W9-CFR-727

The Primary Care and Emergency Medicine Reports® Textbook of

PRIMARY AND ACUTE CARE MEDICINE

Practice • Protocols • Pathways

1st Edition

Editor-in-Chief

GIDEON BOSKER, MD, FACEP

Editor-in-Chief, *Emergency Medicine Reports®*
Editor-in-Chief, *Clinical Consensus Reports®*
Assistant Clinical Professor
Section of Emergency Services
Yale University School of Medicine
Yale-New Haven Hospital
New Haven, Connecticut
Associate Clinical Professor
Oregon Health Sciences University
Portland, Oregon

THOMSON
AMERICAN HEALTH CONSULTANTS

Editor-in-Chief

GIDEON BOSKER, MD, FACEP

Editor-in-Chief, *Emergency Medicine Reports®*
Editor-in-Chief, *Clinical Consensus Reports®*
Assistant Clinical Professor
Section of Emergency Services
Yale University School of Medicine
Yale-New Haven Hospital
New Haven, Connecticut
Associate Clinical Professor
Oregon Health Sciences University
Portland, Oregon

Editor-in-Chief: Gideon Bosker, MD, FACEP
Vice President/Publisher: Milo Falcon
Cover Design: Jeff Dannels
Senior Managing Editor: Suzanne Zunic

NOTE: The indications for and dosages of medications recommended conform to practices at the time of publication of each chapter. References to specific products are incorporated to serve only as guidelines; they are not meant to exclude a practitioner's choice of other, comparable drugs. Every attempt has been made to ensure accuracy and appropriateness.

FIRST EDITION

American Health Consultants
P.O. Box 740056
Atlanta, GA 30374

ISBN# 0-9603332-1-5

Introduction

The fields of primary care and acute care medicine continue to evolve at a rapid rate, especially as they incorporate advances from many different disciplines into their clinical practice spheres. Therapeutic paradigm shifts continue to have an effect on primary and acute care practice in a number of clinical areas, especially those involving acute coronary ischemic syndromes (ACS); prevention of deep venous thrombosis in the non-surgical, medically ill patient; antibiotic selection for infectious diseases; and management of acute and chronic congestive heart failure.

With this challenge in clear focus, the First Edition of the *Primary Care and Emergency Medicine Reports® Textbook of Primary and Acute Care Medicine: Practice, Protocols, and Pathways* has been designed to meet the needs of several clinician subgroups: 1) the hospital-oriented primary care physician, the emergency physician, and the internist seeking clinical excellence in day-to-day, heat-of-battle practice; 2) the teaching center-based academician seeking evidence-based trials, expert analysis, and consensus reports to support specific critical pathways; 3) the primary care, emergency medicine, and internal medicine departmental director interested in identifying outcome-effective treatment protocols and risk-averting management strategies; and 4) the primary and acute care medicine, clinical investigator who wishes to be informed about the latest clinical trials and controversies in primary and acute care.

One of the principal editorial challenges has been to produce a textbook that maintains clinical relevance in an age characterized by databases, protocols, and clinical information that are instantaneously available—and amenable to rapid modification and revision—on electronic platforms. This is a formidable objective, and not surprisingly, textbooks have been perceived by many as "static" resources, whereas electronic, on-line delivery systems have been lauded as "living" resources that are responsive to changes and revisions as supported by evolving clinical data.

This is an over-simplification, especially for the field of primary and acute care medicine. While the rapidity of access and continual updating that characterize on-line information sources are important, there is no substitute for an authoritative, printed resource that combines rigorous analysis, peer review, and evidence-based medicine to generate outcome-effective clinical protocols that will stand the test of time. The First Edition of *The Textbook of Primary and Acute Care Medicine: Practice, Protocols, and Pathways* has been written, edited, and produced with this mission statement in mind.

One of the most important objectives of this volume is to ensure that vital, treatment-oriented information can be accessed rapidly and efficiently. To accomplish this goal, there has been increasing emphasis on "application-oriented" tables, protocols, and pathways that are instantaneously available for use during patient encounters in the primary, acute care, or emergency settings. Specifically, authors have been encouraged to produce detailed, evidence-supported tables, algorithms, and pathways that permit rapid access to treatment-oriented information in the clinical environment.

Whether these primary and acute care medicine protocols involve management of acute myocardial infarction, deep venous thrombosis, migraine headache, community-acquired pneumonia, acute otitis media, unstable angina, or urinary tract infection, as a rule, treatment recommendations included in this resource have been stratified so that "preferred" or "first-line" therapeutic alternatives are clearly identified; these are followed by alternative or second-line options. To support differentiation between a preferred and alternative treatment strategy, rigorous criteria—cost-effectiveness, side effects, risk of drug-drug interactions, consensus statements, and national association recommendations—are used to distinguish among advantages of specific therapeutic positions and drug-based protocols. Whenever possible, these guidelines have been adapted for primary and acute care medicine use and incorporated into rapid access tables or algorithms.

One of the major objectives of the First Edition has been to include recommendations, protocols, and treatment pathways generated by national consensus panels, scientific associations, and expert committees. In chapters on infectious disease, the reader will have access to national guidelines developed by the American Thoracic Society (ATS), the Centers for Disease Control and Prevention (CDC), the American College of Emergency Physicians (ACEP), and the Infectious Disease Society of America (IDSA). In chapters focusing on myocardial infarction and unstable angina, guidelines generated by the American Heart Association (AHA) and the American College of Cardiology (ACC) have been highlighted. If they meet rigorous academic standards and peer review criteria, recommendations issued by other panels also have been included, among them, the ASCAP (Antibiotic Selection for Community-Acquired Pneumonia) and OMBIRT (Outpatient Management of Bacterial Infections of the Respiratory Tract) Panels. When guidelines require adaptation for the primary and acute care medicine environment, such modifications have been made to ensure they are consistent with the intent of the original protocols.

Drawing upon peer-reviewed contributions, expert-endorsed protocols, and clinical perspectives reflecting more than 300 nationally recognized experts in the field of primary and acute care medicine—as well as scholar-physicians from such related fields as pediatrics, infectious diseases, surgery, orthopedics, cardiology, toxicology, and clinical pharmacology—this book has been designed to aid the practicing primary and acute care physician with completing the challenging journey from clinical "information" to hands-on "application." Each chapter includes a detailed discussion of diagnosis, assessment, and management of a specific clinical problem. In the area of pharmacotherapeutics, one of the primary goals of this textbook is to provide primary and acute care physicians with a practical roadmap for both distinguishing among and comparing the myriad treatment options available for a specific condition.

The focus on drug therapy reflects an increasing emphasis within these specialties to make outcome-optimizing choices among agents with similar indications. In addition, many treatment options for heart disease and infectious conditions rely on combination therapies; therefore, the analyses in this resource attempt to clarify these options and identify regimens associated with superior outcomes. The fact is, all medications that belong to a given drug class are rarely created equally. And because the consequences of therapeutic failure and/or drug toxicity can be significant, physicians must be aware of clinically important distinctions among therapeutic alternatives, some which may produce more predictable results than others.

Whenever possible, the contributors to this book have analyzed clinical trials to identify superior agents for conditions under discussion. For example, if two agents have similar indications, but one drug has a more convenient dosing schedule, fewer adverse side effects, a more favorable (i.e., shorter) duration of therapy, a lower risk of drug interactions, and equal or better efficacy, the agent with these advantages will be recommended as a preferred or initial choice. Because noncompliance with medications is a significant problem in primary and acute care practice, medication regimens associated with once-daily therapy, reduced duration of therapy, and better tolerability are highlighted.

Inasmuch as drug-based therapy continues to play an increasingly pivotal role in primary and acute care, there has never been a greater need for a drug selection system that identifies the most outcome-effective agent available for a specific condition. In general, the editorial perspective in this textbook has applied a consistent system—one based on pharmatectural criteria—for making drug comparisons and evaluating the outcome-effectiveness of drug-based therapy. In this regard, the equation for drug selection in this resource incorporates the principles of cost, compliance, side effects, drug-drug and drug-disease interactions, the productivity level of a medication, and its efficacy as supported in evidence-based trials.

This framework for drug selection permits primary and acute care physicians to "upgrade" their prescribing practices from one drug class to another, or from one drug within a class to another drug within a class, as indicated. For example, recent upgrades in the therapeutic arena of primary and acute care medicine have included: 1) increasing use of enoxaparin as a "workhorse" drug for management of acute coronary syndromes and prevention of deep venous thromboembolism (DVT) in non-surgical patients; 2) the increasing importance of specific macrolides and fluoroquinolones as monotherapeutic options for outpatient management of community-acquired pneumonia; 3) the emergence of cyclooxygenase-2 (COX-2) inhibitors for pain management and/or treatment of osteoarthritis; and 4) the evolving role of glycoprotein IIb/IIIa receptor antagonists, such as abciximab, for patients in whom procedural coronary intervention (PCI) is planned. Because application of these pharmacotherapeutic advances is essential for optimizing clinical outcomes, we have provided comprehensive reviews and treatment updates for these rapidly evolving clinical areas.

In the final analysis, optimizing outcomes for patients with acute and/or life-threatening conditions requires superior clinical judgment, a systematic approach to patient assessment, and prompt administration of proven therapies supported by evidence-based medicine. With these challenges in clear focus, the purpose of the First Edition of the *Textbook of Primary and Acute Care Medicine: Practice, Protocols, and Pathways* is to provide an authoritative resource that will guide them from the broad, expansive world of "information" to the targeted, focused arena of clinical "application." If this book can help primary and acute care practitioners, emergency physicians, and other-hospital-based physicians refine their diagnostic skills and upgrade their treatment strategies to enhance patient outcomes in day-to-day practice, it will have served its purpose.

Gideon Bosker, MD, FACEP
Editor-in-Chief, Emergency Medicine Reports®
Editor-in-Chief, Primary Care Medicine Consensus Reports®
Assistant Clinical Professor
Section of Primary and Acute Care Services
Yale University School of Medicine
Associate Clinical Professor
Oregon Health Sciences University

ACKNOWLEDGEMENTS

A work of this scope requires collaboration and support from many colleagues, editors, contributors, peer reviewers, and publishing experts. In this regard, I would like to acknowledge the commitment and support of the academic colleagues; emergency medicine, primary care, and acute care physicians; and clinical scholars who have contributed to this volume. In particular, I am grateful to all the editorial board members, the editors-in-chief, and peer reviewers who, as part of the their association with *Primary Care Reports®, Emergency Medicine Reports®,* and *Pediatric Emergency Medicine Reports®* have committed their time and expertise to ensure that this resource would maintain the highest standards of academic excellence.

First and foremost, I would like to acknowledge the editorial leadership and talents of Dr. Gregory Wise, Editor-in-Chief of *Primary Care Reports®* (American Health Consultants). Many of the chapters on outpatient, primary care topics included in this book have been adapted from or represent revisions and/or updates of reviews published in *Primary Care Reports®.* Dr. Wise's editorial direction and skills—along with the editorial board and peer reviewers of *Primary Care Reports®*—have helped produce definitive analyses and reviews, from which this volume has benefited immensely.

In the area of emergency medicine, among those academicians and teaching scholars who have shown unfaltering commitment and demonstrated academic excellence of the highest caliber, I would especially like to thank Drs. Greg Volturo, Charles Emerman, William Brady, David Howes, Sandra Schneider, Charles Stewart, Kurt Kleinschmidt, David Robinson, and Steve Winograd. In addition, I would like to thank all the members of the academic faculty in the Section of Emergency Medicine at Yale University School of Medicine for their support and ongoing participation in the publishing and educational programs at American Health Consultants. In this regard, the academic excellence, consultation, and peer reviews of Dr. Albert Weihl and Dr. John Schriver deserve special recognition.

The content, analysis, and recommendations for pediatric topics included in this book represent the editorial vision, peer review, and expertise of clinical scholars who have managed the *Pediatric Emergency Medicine Reports®* publishing program. I would especially like to acknowledge Dr. Larry Mellick, Dr. Steven Rothrock, and Dr. Anne Dietrich who, in their capacity as distinguished editors or co-editors of *Pediatric Emergency Medicine Reports,* served as the principal editors for the articles—and corresponding chapters in this edition—on pediatric topics. Their intellectual efforts and professional commitment to publishing excellence are gratefully acknowledged. A complete list of physicians, peer reviewers, and editorial board members who have contributed their time, vision, and talents to this project is included at the beginning of this book.

Even with the support of professional medical colleagues, a project as large and complex in scope as this book requires, above all, a devoted and committed staff of editorial colleagues who, day-to-day, demonstrate the skills, vision, and talent to produce academic publications of the highest standard. I have been fortunate to work on this project with editors, publishers, and production professionals of the highest caliber. I would like to thank David Davenport for his early designs and work on the book during its early stages. The editorial teams responsible for *Primary Care Reports®, Pediatric Emergency Medicine Reports®,* and *Emergency Medicine Reports®,* from which the chapters in this book have been adapted, deserve the highest praise for their commitment to publishing excellence. Among the many participants involved in this award-winning publication, I would like especially to recognize the talents and professionalism of Brenda Mooney, Valerie Loner, and Suzanne Zunic. I would also like to acknowledge Mark Gulledge, whose superb and elegant design schemes for tables and algorithms have made this book a more practical and informative resource. Their efforts have assured that the content and information design features in this book are consistent in quality and that it reflects the highest editorial standards.

A project of this size and vision would not be possible without the vision, consultation, and support of publishers who are willing to commit human and financial resources to advance the state of medical knowledge. In this regard, special praise and appreciation are due to Jeff MacDonald, CEO & President of American Health Consultants, and Tom Kelly, Vice President of Medical Economics Company.

Most important, I would like to recognize those few professional colleagues who made this project part of their day-to-day life for months, and who took made painstaking efforts to ensure this textbook would meet its ambitious editorial and publishing objectives. I am especially grateful to Nancy Saltmarsh, whose exacting editorial standards and design skills were applied with consistency to produce a state-of-the-art textbook. Her devotion to this project and her execution of complicated editorial modifications under time and quality pressures demand the highest praise.

Finally, the lion's share of praise and gratitude for producing and orchestrating this complex, landmark project goes to Milo Falcon, Vice President, Special Projects, American Health Consultants. Mr. Falcon oversaw the day-to-day editorial and publishing requirements for this book, and orchestrated all critical aspects of the project-editorial, design, and production-to ensure this resource would meet the highest standards of publishing excellence. His unflagging commitment to this project, combined with his talents and professionalism, deserve special recognition.

—Gideon Bosker, MD

ACKNOWLEDGEMENTS

To Lena Lencek—scholar, thinker par excellence, and lifelong companion.

Thanks for staying the course. G.B.

Editorial Advisory Boards

Primary Care Reports

Ronald M. Perkin, MD, MA
Professor and Chairman
Department of Pediatrics
The Brody School of Medicine
East Carolina University
Greenville, North Carolina

Steven G. Rothrock, MD, FACEP, FAAP
Department of Emergency Medicine
Orlando Regional Medical Center & Arnold Palmer's Hospital for Women and Children
Orlando, Florida
Clinical Assistant Professor
Division of Emergency Medicine
University of Florida College of Medicine
Gainesville, Florida

Alfred Sacchetti, MD, FACEP
Director of Research
Department of Emergency Medicine
Our Lady of Lourdes Hospital
Camden, New Jersey

John P. Santamaria, MD, FAAP, FACEP
Co-Medical Director
After Hours Pediatrics, Inc.
Medical Director
Wound and Hyperbaric Center
St. Joseph's Hospital
Clinical Associate Professor of Pediatrics
University of South Florida School of Medicine
Tampa, Florida

Robert Schafermeyer, MD
Associate Chairman
Department of Emergency Medicine
Carolinas Medical Center
Charlotte, North Carolina

Jonathan I. Singer, MD
Professor of Emergency Medicine
Pediatrics
Wright State University School of Medicine
Vice Chair and Program Director
Department of Emergency Medicine
Dayton, Ohio

Brian S. Skrainka, MD, FAAP, FACEP
Medical Director, Pediatric Emergency Department
St. Vincent Hospital
Indianapolis, IN

Milton Tenenbein, MD, FRCPC, FAAP, FAACT
Professor of Pediatrics and Pharmacology
University of Manitoba
Winnipeg, Manitoba

Joseph A. Weinberg, MD
Director of Emergency Services
Le Bonheur Children's Medical Center
Memphis, Tennessee

Steven M. Winograd, MD, FACEP
Attending Physician
Department of Emergency Medicine
Jeannette District Memorial Hospital
Jeannette, Pennsylvania
St. Clair Memorial Hospital
University of Pittsburgh Medical Center
Pittsburgh, Pennsylvania

Contributors

Barbara J. Abrams, MD, Assistant Professor, Department of Emergency Medicine, State University of New York at Buffalo School of Medicine and Biomedical Science, Buffalo, NY

Alfred Aleguas, PharmD, College of Pharmacy, University of Rhode Island

Susan H. Allen, MD, PhD, Medical Director, Kettering Osteoporosis Center, Kettering Medical Center, Kettering, OH

Harrison Alter, MS, MD, Chief Resident, Department of Emergency Medicine, Alameda County Medical Center, Highland Campus, Oakland, CA

Michael F. Altieri, MD, FAAP, FACEP, Associate Clinical Professor of Emergency Medicine and Pediatrics, George Washington University; Associate Clinical Professor of Emergency Medicine and Pediatrics, Georgetown University, Washington, DC; Associate Clinical Professor of Pediatrics, University of Virginia, Charlottesville, VA; Chief, Pediatric Emergency Medicine, INOVA Fairfax Hospital, Falls Church, VA; Director, INOVA Fairfax/UVA Pediatric Residency, Falls Church, VA

Sandra Bellantonio, MD, Instructor of Medicine, University of Connecticut School of Medicine Center on Aging

Walter G. Belleza, MD, Department of Emergency Medicine, University of Maryland Medical System, Baltimore, MD

Kevin Berman, MD, Cardiologist, Cardiovascular Diseases and Cholesterol Control Center of Dayton, Inc., Dayton, OH

Richard W. Besdine, MD, FACP, Director, Center on Aging, Professor of Medicine, Travelers Professor of Geriatrics and Gerontology, University of Connecticut Health Center School of Medicine, Farmington, CT

Frank J. Bia, MD, MPH, Professor of Medicine and Laboratory Medicine, Infectious Disease and Tropical Medicine, Yale University School of Medicine, New Haven, CT

David Bienenfeld, MD, Professor and Vice Chair, Department of Psychiatry, Wright State University, Dayton, OH

Bill Billica, MD, FAAFP, Department of Family Practice, Banner Health System, Phoenix, AZ

Tina M.H. Blair, MD, FACEP, Associate Professor, Department of Surgery; Chief, Department of Emergency Services, University of Nebraska Medical Center, Omaha, NE

Glenn H. Bock, MD, Associate Professor of Pediatrics, Uniformed Services of the Health Sciences, Bethesda, MD; Co-Director, Pediatric Kidney Center, INOVA Fairfax Hospital for Children, Falls Church, VA

Phillip Bonanni, MD, Primary Care and Internal Medicine, University of Rochester School of Medicine

Marc Borenstein, MD, FACP, FACEP, Associate Professor, Department of Surgery, Chief, Division of Emergency Medicine, University of Connecticut Health Science Center, Farmington, CT

Gideon Bosker, MD, FACEP, Associate Clinical Professor, Department of Emergency Medicine, Oregon Health Sciences Center, Portland, OR; Assistant Clinical Professor, Section of Emergency Services, Yale University School of Medicine

William J. Brady, Jr., MD, Assistant Professor of Emergency Medicine and Internal Medicine; Medical Director, Chest Pain Center, Department of Emergency Medicine, University of Virginia School of Medicine, Charlottesville, VA

Phillip A. Brewer, MD, Assistant Professor of Surgery (Emergency Medicine), Yale University School of Medicine, New Haven, CT

John A. Brose, DO, FAAFP, Professor of Family Medicine and Assistant Dean, Clinical Research, Ohio University, College of Osteopathic Medicine, Athens, OH

Jane C. Buch, MLS, Medical Library Manager, Kettering Medical Center Network, Kettering, OH

Leslie P. Buchanon, RN, MSN, ENP, Department of Emergency Medicine, University of Virginia Health System, Charlottesville, VA

Blake Bulloch, MD, Fellow, Division of Emergency Medicine, Children's Hospital Medical Center, Cincinnati, OH

Sean P. Bush, MD, Clinical Instructor of Emergency Medicine, Loma Linda University School of Medicine, Loma Linda, CA

Kenneth H. Butler, DO, Chief Resident in Emergency Medicine, Michigan State University Affiliated Emergency Medicine Residency Program, Lansing, MI

Richard Caesar, MD, FACEP, Assistant Clinical Professor, Department of Emergency Medicine, Oregon Health Sciences University; Attending Physician, Legacy Good Samaritan Hospital and Medical Center, Portland, OR

Mary A. Camarca, MD, FAAP, Fellow, Pediatric Emergency Medicine, Department of Emergency Medicine, INOVA Fairfax Hospital, Falls Church, VA

Steven C. Carleton, MD, PhD, Assistant Professor, Department of Emergency Medicine, University of Cincinnati, Cincinnati, OH

James A. Castellone, MD, Senior Resident, University of Connecticut Integrated Residency in Emergency Medicine, Farmington, CT

David Chacko, MD, PhD, Associate Professor, Department of Ophthalmology, University of Nebraska Medical Center, Omaha, NE

Katherine K. Chang, MD, Resident, Osler Housestaff, Department of Medicine, Johns Hopkins Hospital, Baltimore, MD

Judy Cheng, PharmD, BCPS, Long Island University Clinical Pharmacy, Mount Siani Medical Center

Abhinav Chhabra, MD, Department of Orthopedic Surgery, University of Virginia School of Medicine, Charlottesville, VA

William K. Chiang, MD, Assistant Professor of Medicine, Brown University School of Medicine; Attending Physician, Department of Emergency Medicine, Rhode Island Hospital; Consultant, Rhode Island Poison Control Center, Providence, RI

Eric S. Chin, MD, Resident Physician, Loma Linda University Medical Center, Loma Linda, CA

Myron E. Chu, DO, Fellow in Rheumatology, Loma Linda University, Jerry L. Pettis VA Medical Center, Division of Rheumatology, Loma Linda, CA

Robin M. Clemons, MD, MPH, Assistant Professor, Department of Family Medicine, University of Medicine and Dentistry of New Jersey, School of Osteopathic Medicine, Stratford, NJ

Keith K. Colburn, MD, Chief, Rheumatology, Pettis Veterans Medical Center and Loma Linda University Medical Center, Loma Linda, CA

Karim Cole, MD, Assistant Professor of Emergency Medicine, Department of Emergency Medicine, Howard University Hospital Program, Washington, DC

Stephen A. Colucciello, MD, FACEP, Assistant Clinical Professor of Emergency Medicine, University of North Carolina Medical School, Chapel Hill, North Carolina; Director, Clinical Services Trauma Coordinator, Deptartment of Emergency Medicine, Carolinas Medical Center, Charlotte, NC

Kathleen M. Cowling, DO, Department of Emergency Medicine. Michigan State University/Lansing, Lansing, MI

Todd Crump, MD, Resident Physician, Department of Emergency Medicine, Palmetto Richland Memorial Hospital, Columbia, SC

Rita K. Cydulka, MD, FACEP, Residency Director, Emergency Medicine, MetroHealth Medical Center; Assistant Professor, Department of Surgery, Case Western Reserve University, Cleveland, OH

Alan C. Dalkin, MD, Associate Professor of Internal Medicine, Department of Internal Medicine; Program Director, Endocrinology and Metabolism Fellowship Program, Department of Internal Medicine, University of Virginia School of Medicine, Charlottesville, VA

Gregory G. Degnan, MD, Assistant Professor of Orthopedic Surgery, Department of Orthopedic Surgery, University of Virginia School of Medicine, Charlottesville, VA

Sarah Delaney-Rowland, MD, Department of Emergency Medicine, MetroHealth Medical Center, Cleveland, OH

Dawn Demangone, MD, Assistant Professor of Medicine, Division of Emergency Medicine, Temple University School of Medicine, Philadelphia, PA

Paul P. Dobesh, PharmD, BCPS, Division of Pharmacy Practice, St. Louis College of Pharmacy

Gail D'Onofrio, MD, FACEP, Assistant Clinical Professor of Surgery (Emergency Medicine), Yale University School of Medicine, New Haven, CT; and Boston University School of Medicine, Boston, MA

Keith Doram, MD, FACP, MBA, CMD, Chief, Division of General Internal Medicine, Lehigh Valley Hospital, Allentown, PA; Assistant Professor of Medicine, Loma Linda University School of Medicine; Associate Clinical Professor of Medicine, Penn State University School of Medicine

William R. Dubin, MD, Associate General Director of Clinical Services, Belmont Center for Comprehensive Treatment; Professor of Psychiatry, Temple University School of Medicine, Philadelphia, PA

Eileen M. Duffy, MD, FAAP, FACEP, Assistant Professor, Department of Surgery, Division of Emergency Medical Services, Loyola University Medical Center, Maywood, IL

John E. Duldner, Jr., MD, Emergency Physician, Department of Emergency Medicine, MetroHealth Medical Center, Cleveland, OH

Barbara J. Dwyer, RN, MA, HealthCare Communications Associates, Miami Beach, FL

Jonathan A. Edlow, MD, Acting Chief, Division of Emergency Medicine, Beth Israel Deaconess Medical Center, Boston, MA; Instructor, Harvard Medical School

Frank J. Edwards, MD, FACEP, Assistant Professor of Emergency Medicine, Department of Emergency Medicine, University of Rochester School of Medicine, Strong Memorial Hospital, Rochester, NY

Suzanne K. Elliott, MD, Department of Emergency Medicine, Rhode Island Hospital, Providence, RI

Charles L. Emerman, MD, Associate Professor of Emergency Medicine, Case Western Reserve University; Department of Emergency Medicine, MetroHealth Medical Center, Cleveland, OH

Stephen Ernest, PharmD, Clinical Pharmacist, Infectious Diseases

George Eversman, MD, Chief Resident, Department of Emergency Medicine, MetroHealth Medical Center; Emergency Medicine Residency Program, Case Western Reserve University, Cleveland, OH

Susan I. Fesmire, MD, Assistant Professor, Department of Internal Medicine, Aston Ambulatory Care Center, The University of Texas Southwestern Medical Center

Steven F. Fisher, MD, Department of Emergency Medicine, Brown University School of Medicine, Rhode Island Hospital, Providence, RI

Raymond Flores, MD, Fellow of Rheumatology, Loma Linda, CA

Murray Flotre, BSc, MD, CCFP, Clinical Instructor in Family Medicine, Regina General Hospital, Regina, Canada

John P. Foreyt, PhD, Professor, Department of Medicine, Baylor College of Medicine, Houston, TX

Linda P. Fredrickson, MA, RN, CDE, Director, Professional Education and Clinical Services, MiniMed, Sylmar, CA

Alan J. Gelenberg, MD, Professor and Head, Department of Psychiatry, University of Arizona Health Sciences Center, Tucson, AZ

Michael Genco, University of Virginia School of Medicine, Charlottesville, VA

Daren D. Girard, MD, Department of Emergency Medicine, Rhode Island Hospital, Brown University School of Medicine

Claudia R. Gold, MD, FACEP, Chair, Department of Emergency Medicine, Children's Hospital of Orange County, Orange, CA

Steven M. Green, MD, FACEP, Director, Emergency Medicine Residency Program, Associate Professor of Emergency Medicine, Loma Linda University School of Medicine, Loma Linda, CA

Pamela Grim, MD, Department of Emergency Medicine, Mt. Sinai Medical Center, Cleveland, OH

John Gums, PharmD, Professor, Departments of Pharmacology and Medicine, University of Florida, Gainesville

Dayna Lynn Gutsin, MD, Chief, Resident, Department of Emergency Medicine, Emory University School of Medicine

Robert Haddon, MD, Urgency Care Clinics, Cleveland Clinic, Cleveland, OH

Kelley A. Hails, MD, Clinical Instructor, College of Human Medicine, Michigan State University, Michigan State Emergency Medicine Residency, Lansing, MI

Gary Hals, MD, PhD, Department of Emergency Medicine, Palmetto Richland Memorial Hospital, Columbia, SC

Rancie Hannah, MD, Chief Resident, Clinton Memorial Hospital Family Practice Residency Program

Masood Haque, MD, Attending Physician, Newark Beth Israel Medical Center, Newark, NJ

Richard A. Harrigan, MD, Assistant Professor of Medicine, Temple University School of Medicine; Director of Emergency Medicine, Resident Education, Temple University Hospital, Philadelphia, PA

Katherine L. Heilpern, MD, Assistant Professor, Department of Emergency Medicine, Emory University School of Medicine, Atlanta, GA

Clayton F. Holmes, EdD, PT, ATC, Assistant Professor, University of Central Arkansas, Department of Physical Therapy, Little Rock, AK

Dave Howes, MD, FACEP, Program Director and Chairman, Residency Program, Department of Emergency Medicine, University of Chicago Hospitals and Clinics; Associate Professor, Pritzker School of Medicine

F. Allan Hubbell, MD, MSPH, Professor of Medicine and Social Ecology; Chief, Division of Internal Medicine and Primary Care; Director, Center for Health Policy and Research, University of California, Irvine, CA

Jean P. Hubble, MD, Associate Professor, Clinical Neurology, Madden—National Parkinson Foundation of Excellence, Columbus, OH

J. Stephen Huff, MD, Associate Professor of Emergency Medicine and Neurology, Department of Emergency Medicine, University of Virginia Health Sciences Center, Charlottesville

Mark A. Hurst, MD, Clinical Assistant Professor, Department of Psychiatry, Ohio State University, Assistant Medical Director for Addiction Psychiatry, Twin Valley Psychiatric System, Ohio Department of Mental Health, Columbus, OH

Frederic Hustey, MD, Attending Physician, Department of Emergency Medicine, The Cleveland Clinic Foundation; Assistant Clinical Professor, The Ohio State University, Department of Emergency Medicine

William B. Ignatoff, MD, Department of Emergency Medicine, Mt. Sinai Medical Center, Cleveland, OH

David A. Jerrard, MD, FACEP, Associate Professor of Surgery Medicine and Clinical Director, Emergency Care Services, Veterans' Affairs Hospital, Baltimore, MD

Norman M. Kaplan, MD, Professor of Internal Medicine, Department of Internal Medicine, University of Texas Southwestern Medical Center, Dallas, TX

Shivanand S. Karkal, MB, HS, MD, Cornell Medical Center, The New York Hospital, New York, NY

David Karras, MD, Assistant Professor of Medicine, Director of Research, Division of Emergency Medicine, Temple University, Philadelphia, PA

Shira Katz, MD, Second-Year Resident Physician, Clinton Memorial Hospital, Family Practice Residency Program, Wilmington, OH

Jerald Kay, MD, Professor and Chair of Psychiatry, Wright State University School of Medicine, Dayton, OH

Kurt Kleinschmidt, MD, FACEP, Associate Professor, University of Texas Southwestern Medical Center, Dallas, TX; Associate Medical Director, Emergency Services Department, Parkland Memorial Hospital, Dallas, TX

Steven M. Koenig, MD, FCCP, Director, Occupational Lung Disease Program; Director, Outpatient Pulmonary Rehabilitation Program, University of Virginia Health Systems, Charlottesville, VA

Neeraj Kohli, MD, Division of Urogynecology and Reconstructive Pelvic Surgery, University of Cincinnati College of Medicine, Good Samaritan Hospital, Cincinnati, OH

Dick C. Kuo, MD, Assistant Professor, Division of Emergency Medicine, University of Maryland Medical Center, Baltimore, MD

David Lang, DO, Operations Medical Director, Department of Emergency Medicine, Mt. Siani Medical Center, Miami, FL

Robert A. Levine, MD, Professor of Medicine, Department of Medicine, Division of Gastroenterology, State University of New York, Health Science Center at Syracuse

Michael D. Levitt, MD, ACOS for Research, VA Medical Center, Professor of Medicine, University of Minnesota, Minneapolis, MN

Cesar Libanati, MD, Associate Professor of Medicine, Pettis VAMC and Loma Linda University, Loma Linda, CA

Deborah Y. Liggan, MD, Psychiatry Resident, Wright State University School of Medicine, Dayton, OH

Robert Linton, MD, Howard University Hospital, Washington, DC

David R. Little, MD, MS, Wright State University, Department of Family Medicine, Dayton, OH

James J. Londis, PhD, Director of Ethics and Values Integration, Kettering Medical Center, Kettering, OH

Joseph D. Losek, MD, FAAP, FACEP, Director, Emergency Department, Children's Hospitals and Clinics—St. Paul, MN

Stephen R. Luber, MD, FAAP, Rockwood Clinic Faculty, University of Washington Medical School, Spokane, WA

Michael Lynn, MD, Department of Emergency Medicine, Alameda County Medical Center, Highland General Hospital, Oakland, CA

Sharon E. Mace, MD, FACEP, FAAP, Director, Pediatric Education/Quality Assurance, Clinical Director, Observation Unit, Cleveland Clinic Foundation, Associate Professor, Department of Emergency Medicine, Ohio State University

James J. Maciejko, MS, PhD, FACC, Director, Lipid Clinic, Botsford General Hospital, Farmington Hills, MI; and Associate Professor of Medicine, Wayne State University School of Medicine, Detroit, MI

David D. Markoff, MD, FACS, Mountain Eye Associates, Haywood Regional Medical Center, Clyde, NC

Laurence B. McCullough, PhD, Baylor College of Medicine, Center for Medical Ethics and Health Policy, Houston, TX

W. Paul McKinney, MD, Division of General Internal Medicine, University of Louisville, Louisville, KY

Patsy M. McNeil, MD, Resident Physician, Department of Emergency Medicine, University of Cincinnati College of Medicine

Stephen W. Meldon, MD, Assistant Professor, Case Western Reserve University; Department of Emergency Medicine, MetroHealth Medical Center, Cleveland, OH

Santosh G. Menon, MD, Division of Cardiology, University of Kentucky

Gary Merlino, DO, Department of Family Medicine, Mt. Siani Hospital, Miami, FL

Daryl Miller, MD, Fellow, Division of Immunology and Rheumatology, Department of Internal Medicine, The University of Missouri-Columbia, Columbia, MO

Lisa A. Miller, MD, Department of Emergency Medicine, Metro-Health Medical Center, Cleveland, OH

Mary Beth Miller, DO, Assistant Director-Education, Michigan State University Emergency Medicine Residency—Lansing, Michigan Capital Medical Center and Sparrow Hospital, Lansing, MI

Rodanda Miller, MD, Assistant Professor of Medicine, Department of Medicine, Johns Hopkins University School of Medicine, Baltimore, MD

Roger M. Mills, Jr., MD, Division of Cardiology, University of Kentucky

Jean Nappi, PharmD, Department of Pharmacy, Medical University of South Carolina, Columbia, SC

David N. Neubauer, MD, Associate Director, Johns Hopkins Sleep Disorders Center, Assistant Professor, Department of Psychiatry, Johns Hopkins University School of Medicine, Baltimore, MD

Robert L. Norris, MD, FACEP, Associate Director, Division of Emergency Medicine, Stanford Health Services, Stanford, CA

Charles A. Nozicka, DO, FAAP, Assistant Professor of Pediatrics, Medical College of Wisconsin, Children's Hospital of Wisconsin, Milwaukee, WI; Medical Director of Pediatric Services, Columbia Hoffman Estates Medical Center, Hoffman Estates, IL

Edward Onusko, MD, Assistant Professor of Family Medicine, Clinton Memorial Hospital, Family Practice Residency Program, Wilmington, OH

Michael Pallaci, DO, Department of Emergency Medicine, Palmetto Richland Memorial Hospital, Columbia, SC

Arthur M. Pancioli, MD, Assistant Professor, Associate Director of Resident Education, Department of Emergency Medicine, Univeristy of Cincinnati College of Medicine

Kenneth Parsons, MD, MPH, Resident, Emergency Medicine, Department of Emergency Medicine, St. John's Hospital and Medical Center, Detroit, MI

William Franklin Peacock, IV, MD, FACEP, Associate Professor, The Ohio State University, Director of Clinical Operations, Department of Emergency Medicine, The Cleveland Clinic, Cleveland, OH

Margarita E. Pena, MD, FACEP, Clinical Instructor, Emergency Medicine, Department of Emergency Medicine, St. John's Hospital and Medical Center, Detroit, MI

Victor R. Pendleton, PhD, Primary Care Postdoctorate Fellow, Department of Medicine, Baylor College of Medicine, Houston, TX

Ronald Perkin, MD, Director, Pediatric Intensive Care Unit, Loma Linda University Children's Hospital; Professor of Pediatrics, Loma Linda University, Loma Linda, CA

William F. Perry, MA, RN, Clinical Information Specialist, Kettering Medical Center Network, Kettering, OH

Emory Petrack, MD, MPH, FAAP, FACEP, Associate Professor of Pediatrics, Director, Pediatric Emergency Medicine, Rainbow Babies and Children's Hospital, Cleveland, OH

Vincent J. Pflug, DO, Clinical Instructor, Emergency Medicine Residency—Lansing, Michigan State University, East Lansing, MI; Michigan Capital Medical Center and Sparrow Hospital

John Pieper, PharmD, FCCP, BCPS, School of Pharmacy, University of North Carolina

Jessica Pierog, EMT, St. Joseph Hospital, Orange, CA

Madeleine Ponder, MD, DVM, Department of Emergency Medicine, MetroHealth Medical Center, Cleveland, OH

Robert D. Powers, MD, FACP, FACEP, Chief of Emergency Medicine, University of Connecticut School of Medicine, Farmington, CT

Susan B. Promes, MD, Associate Residency Director, Department of Emergency Medicine, Alameda County Medical Center-Highland Campus, Oakland, CA; Assistant Professor of Clinical Medicine, University of California, San Francisco

Jeffrey Proudfoot, DO, FACOEP, Attending Physician, Pediatric Emergency Department, Maricopa Medical Center, Phoenix, AZ

J. Crayton Pruitt, MD, FACS, Founder and Director Emeritus of the Vascular Institute of Florida, St. Petersburg, FL

Tammie Quest, MD, Department of Emergency Medicine, Alameda County Medical Center-Highland Campus, Oakland, CA

Georges Ramalanjaona, MD, DSc, FACEP, Associate Professor of Emergency Medicine, Associate Chairman for Academic Affairs, Department of Emergency Medicine, Seton Hall University School of Graduate Medical Education, South Orange, NJ.

John Rambharose, MD, Assistant Professor of Medicine, Loma Linda, CA

Margaret Rathier, MD, Assistant Professor of Medicine, University of Connecticut School of Medicine Center on Aging, Geriatrics, VA Connecticut Healthcare System

Kevin C. Reed, MD, Department of Emergency Medicine, University of Maryland Medical Center

Samuel R. Reid, MD, Staff Physician, Pediatric Emergency Medicine, Children's Hospitals and Clinics—St. Paul, MN

Earl J. Reisdorff, MD, FACEP, Program Director, Michigan State University Emergency Medicine Residency—Lansing, Michigan Capital Medical Center and Sparrow Hospital, Lansing, MI

Raymond J. Roberge, MD, FACEP, Assistant Director, Medical Emergency Services, Mantefiore University Hospital, University of Pittsburgh Medical Center; Assistant Professor of Medicine, University of Pittsburgh School of Medicine, Pittsburgh, PA

David J. Robinson, MD, MS, Director of Research, Division of Emergency Medicine, The University of Maryland Medical Center, Baltimore, MD

Rob Rogers, MD, Division of Emergency Medicine, The University of Maryland Medical Center, Baltimore, MD

Steven G. Rothrock, MD, FACEP, Research Director, Department of Emergency Medicine, Orlando Regional Medical Center and Arnold Palmer's Hospital for Women and Children, Orlando, FL; Clinical Assistant Professor, Division of Emergency Medicine, University of Florida College of Medicine, Gainesville, FL

Richard M. Ruddy, MD, Professor of Clinical Pediatrics, Director, Division of Emergency Medicine, Children's Hospital Medical Center, Cincinnati, OH

Frank Ruiz, MD, Attending Physician, Emergency Services, San Francisco General Hospital; Assistant Clinical Professor of Surgery, University of California-San Francisco

Elmar P. Sakala, MD, MA, MPH, Professor of Gynecology and Obstetrics, Loma Linda University School of Medicine, Loma Linda, CA

Sam Sandowski, MD, Department of Family Practice, SUNY Medical College

Lori A. Sansone, MD, Family Physician, Kettering Medical Center Physicians, Inc., Dayton, OH

Randy A. Sansone, MD, Associate Professor, Department of Psychiatry, Wright State University School of Medicine, Director Psychiatry Education, Ketterning Medical Center, Kettering, OH

Ian J. Sarembock, MB, ChB, MD, Cardiovascular Division, University of Virginia Health System

Sandra M. Schneider, MD, FACEP, Professor and Chair, Department of Emergency Medicine, University of Rochester School of Medicine, Rochester, NY

Betsy Schrader, MD, Division of Emergency Medicine, Temple University Hospital, Philadelphia, PA

Richard J. Schuster, MD, FACP, Director, Primary Care Education in Internal Medicine, Kettering Medical Center, Associate Clinical Professor, Wright State University School of Medicine, Miamisburg, OH

Robert Schwab, MD, Associate Professor, Department of Emergency Medicine, University of Missouri—Kansas City School of Medicine; Medical Director, Emergency Department, Truman Medical Center, Kansas City, MO

Brian P. Schwartz, MD, Director of Clinical Ethics, Kettering Medical Center, Kettering, OH

Gary Schwartz, MD, FAAP, Assistant Professor of Emergency Medicine and Pediatrics; Assistant Director of the Pediatric Emergency Department, Vanderbilt University Medical Center, Nashville, TN

Susan Schwartz, RN, MSN, ENP, Department of Emergency Medicine, University of Virginia Health System, Charlottesville, VA

Charles Seamens, MD, Assistant Professor of Emergency Medicine, Department of Emergency Medicine, Vanderbilt University Medical Center, Nashville, TN

Les Searls, DO, Assistant Clinical Professor, Michigan State University, Ingham Regional Medical Center, Lansing, MI

Sid M. Shah, MD, FACEP, Assistant Residency Director-Research, Sparrow, Michigan State University Residency Program, Ingham Regional Medical Center, Lansing, MI

Robert M. Sills, DO, FAAP, Director, Pediatric Emergency Medicine, Department of Emergency Medicine, St. John's Hospital and Medical Center, Detroit, MI

Corey M. Slovis, MD, FACP, FACEP, Professor and Chairman, Department of Emergency Medicine, Vanderbilt University School of Medicine, Nashville, TN

Ethel Smith, MD, Department of Family Practice, MetroWest Health Center, Cleveland Clinic, Cleveland, OH

Eric Snoey, MD, Associate Residency Director, Department of Emergency Medicine, Alameda County Medical Center, Highland Campus, Oakland, CA

Michael Sparacino, MD, Professor of Family Medicine, North Iowa Family Practice Residency, Mason City, Iowa

Sarah A. Spinler, PharmD, FCCP, CTAP Scientific Panel Co-Chairperson and Co-Moderator, Philadelphia College of Pharmacy, University of the Sciences in Philadelphia

Stuart J. Spitalnic, MD, Resident, Department of Emergency Medicine, Rhode Island Hospital, Providence, RI

Paul Stander, MD, FACP, Regional Medical Director, Banner Health System, Phoenix, AZ

Andrew C. Steele, MD, Division of Urogynecology and Reconstructive Pelvic Surgery, University of Cincinnati College of Medicine, Good Samaritan Hospital, Cincinnati, OH

Meir Steiner, MD, PhD, FRCPC, Professor of Psychiatry and Biomedical Sciences, McMaster University; Director, Women's Health Concerns Clinic, St. Joseph's Hospital, Hamilton, Ontario, Canada

Charles R. Stephens, MD, Department of Emergency Medicine, Howard University Hospital, Washington, DC

Charles Stewart, MD, FACEP, Emergency Physician, Colorado Springs, CO

Kathleen A. Stringer, PharmD, FCCP, School of Pharmacy, University of Colorado Health Sciences Center

Fabrizis L. Suarez, MD, PhD, Research Associate, University of Minnesota School of Medicine, Minneapolis, MN

Selim Suner, MD, MS, FACEP, Assistant Professor, Department of Emergency Medicine, Brown University School of Medicine, Rhode Island Hospital, Providence, RI

Robert Talbert, PharmD, FCCP, BCPS, Professor and Chair, Clinical Pharmacy Program, University of Texas at Austin

Nicholas J. Talley, MD, Professor of Medicine, Department of Medicine, University of Sydney, Nepean Hospital, Australia

Mark Thanassi, MD, Associate Residency Director, Assistant Professor of Surgery, Yale-New Haven Hospital, Section of Emergency Medicine, Department of Surgery

Wendy T. Thanassi, MA, MD, Yale-New Haven Hospital, Section of Emergency Medicine, Department of Surgery, New Haven, CT

Tamara L. Thomas, MD, FACEP, Assistant Professor of Emergency Medicine, Loma Linda University School of Medicine, Loma Linda, CA

Antoinette Tolbert, MD, Department of Emergency Medicine, Palmetto Richland Memorial Hospital, Columbia, SC

Jeffrey R. Unger, MD, Chino Medical Group, Inc., Chino, CA

Gregory A. Volturo, MD, FACEP, Vice Chairman and Associate Professor, Department of Emergency Medicine, University of Massachusetts Medical School, Worcester, MA

David A. Wald, DO, Assistant Professor of Medicine, Division of Emergency Medicine, Temple University Hospital, Philadelphia, PA

Sara E. Walker, MD, Professor, Division of Immunology and Rheumatology, Department of Internal Medicine, The University of Missouri-Columbia, Columbia, MO

Richard Y. Wang, DO, FACEP, Director of Medical Toxicology, Department of Emergency Medicine, Brown University School of Medicine, Providence, RI

Isak F. Wessels, MMed, FRCSE, FRCOphth, FACS, Department of Ophthalmology, University of Tennessee College of Medicine, Chattanooga Unit

Michael W. Wiederman, PhD, Assistant Professor, Department of Psychological Science, Ball State University, Muncie, IN

Ginger Wilhelm, MD, FACEP, Assistant Professor of Emergency Medicine and Residency Director, University of Texas—Houston Department of Emergency Medicine

Ann Wittkowsky, PharmD, Department of Pharmacy Practice, University of Washington

Robert O. Wright, MD, Massachusetts Poison Control Center, Children's Hospital, Harvard University School of Medicine, Boston, MA

Russell Yang, MD, PhD, Assistant Professor of Medicine, Division of Gastroenterology and Liver Diseases, University of Southern California School of Medicine; Chief, Gastroenterology and Endoscopy, Los Angeles Veterans Administration Outpatient Clinic

Michael J. Zappa, MD, Attending Physician, Department of Emergency Medicine, St. Mary's Hospital, West Palm Beach, FL

Stuart J. Spillane, MD, Resident, Department of Emergency Medicine, Rhode Island Hospital, Providence, RI

Paul Stander, MD, FACP, Regional Medical Director, Banner Health System, Phoenix, AZ

Andrew C. Steele, MD, Division of Laryngology and [illegible], Department of [illegible] Surgery, University of Cincinnati College of Medicine, Good Samaritan Hospital, Cincinnati, OH

Meir Steiner, MD, PhD, FRCPC, Professor of Psychiatry and Biomedical Sciences, McMaster University; Director, Women's Health Concerns Clinic, St. Joseph's Hospital, Hamilton, Ontario, Canada

Charles P. Stephens, MD, Department of Emergency Medicine, Howard University Hospital, Washington, DC

Charles Stevens, MD, FACEP, Emergency Physician, Colorado Springs, CO

Kathleen A. Stringer, PharmD, FCCP, School of Pharmacy, University of Colorado Health Sciences Center, Denver, CO

Rebecca L. Suárez, MD, PhD, Research Associate, University of Minnesota School of Medicine, Minneapolis, MN

Selim Suner, MD, MS, FACEP, Assistant Professor, Department of Emergency Medicine, Brown University School of Medicine, Rhode Island Hospital, Providence, RI

Robert L. Talbert, PharmD, FCCP, BCPS, Professor and Chair, Clinical Pharmacy Program, University of Texas at Austin

Nicholas J. Talley, MD, Professor of Medicine, Department of Medicine, University of Sydney, Nepean Hospital, Australia

[illegible], MD, Associate Residency Director/Assistant Professor of Surgery, Yale–New Haven Hospital, Section of Emergency Medicine, Department of Surgery

Wendy [illegible], MD, Yale–New Haven Hospital, Section of Emergency Medicine, Department of Surgery, New Haven, CT

Tamara E. Thomas, MD, FACEP, Assistant Professor of Emergency Medicine, Loma Linda University School of Medicine, Loma Linda, CA

Antoinette Tolbert, MD, Department of Emergency Medicine, [illegible] Richland Memorial Hospital, Columbia, SC

[illegible], MD, Chief, [illegible] Group, [illegible]

Gregory A. Volturo, MD, FACEP, Vice Chairman and Associate Professor, Department of Emergency Medicine, University of Massachusetts Medical School, Worcester, MA

David C. Wall, MD, Assistant Professor of Medicine, Division of Emergency Medicine, Temple University Hospital, Philadelphia, PA

Sara [illegible] Walker, MD, Professor, Division of Immunology and Rheumatology, Department of Internal Medicine, The University of Missouri School of Medicine, Columbia, MO

Richard Y. Wang, DO, FACEP, Director of Medical Toxicology, Department of Emergency Medicine, Brown University School of Medicine, Providence, RI

[illegible], MD, MPH, FRCOphth, FACS, Department of Ophthalmology, University of Tennessee College of Medicine, Chattanooga, TN

Michael W. Wiederman, PhD, Assistant Professor, Department of Psychological Science, Ball State University, Muncie, IN

Ginger [illegible], MD, FACEP, Assistant Professor of Emergency Medicine and Residency Director, University of Texas—Houston Department of Emergency Medicine, [illegible]

Ann Wittkowsky, PharmD, Department of Pharmacy Practice, University of Washington

Robert O. Wright, MD, [illegible] Children's Hospital, Harvard University School of Medicine, Boston, MA

Russell Yang, MD, PhD, Assistant Professor of Medicine, Division of Gastroenterology and Liver Diseases, University of Southern California School of Medicine; Chief, Gastroenterology, [illegible] Los Angeles Veterans Administration Outpatient Clinic

[illegible], MD, Attending Physician, Department of Emergency Medicine, St. Mary's Hospital, West Palm Beach, FL

Peer Reviewers

Victor J. Aaen, MD, Dph, Clinical Assistant Professor of Family Medicine, University of North Dakota Family Physicians, Minot Air Force Base

Cynthia K. Aaron, MD, Director, Toxicology Service Attending Physician, Department of Emergency Medicine, University of Massachusetts Medical Center, Worcester, MA

Jonathan Abrams, MD, Professor of Medicine, Division of Cardiology, The University of New Mexico, Albuquerque, NM

Nancy Albert, MSN, RN, CCRN, CNA, Clinical Nurse Specialist in Heart Failure, The Cleveland Clinic, Cleveland, OH

Cathy A. Alessi, MD, Director, Geriatric Evaluation Services, Geriatric Research, Education, and Clinical Center, Veterans Administration, Greater Los Angeles Healthcare System

Gwen M. Allen, MD, Associate Professor, Department of OB/GYN, Wake-Forest University, Winston-Salem, NC

H. Gibbs Andrews, MD, Chief, Division of Pediatric Surgery, Associate Professor of Surgery, Pediatrics and Emergency Medicine, Loma Linda University Medical Center, Loma Linda, CA

Jeffrey Arnold, MD, Attending Physician, Department of Emergency Medicine, Cedars-Sinai Medical Center, Los Angeles; Associate Clinical Professor of Emergency Medicine, Kangdong Sacred Heart Hospital, Hallym University School of Medicine, Seoul, Korea

Robert M. Arnold, MD, Director of Clinical Training, Associate Professor of Medicine, University of Pittsburgh Medical Center, Center for Medical Ethics, Pittsburgh, PA

Judith Ashley, PhD, RD, Associate Director, The Nutrition Education and Research Program, University of Nevada School of Medicine

Mickey Ask, MD, FASAM, Medical Director, Addictions Treatment Program, Veterans Hospital, Loma Linda, CA

Grant Bakin, MD, FACEP, Clinical Assistant Professor of Medicine, Mercer University School of Medicine; Attending Physician, DeKalb Medical Center, Decatur, GA

Brien A. Barnewolt, MD, FACEP, Attending Emergency Physician, Department of Emergency Medicine, New England Medical Center, Boston, MA

John W. Becher, DO, Director of Emergency Medicine Residency, Albert Einstein Medical Center, Philadelphia, PA

Anthony J. Billittier IV, MD, FACEP, Clinical Assistant Professor, Department of Emergency Medicine, State University of New York—Buffalo; Director of Prehospital Care, Erie County Medical Center, Buffalo, NY

William M. Blackshear, Jr., MD, Director and Surgeon-in-Chief, Vascular Institute of Florida, St. Petersburg, FL

Howard Blumstein, MD, FAAEM, Assistant Residency Director, Department of Emergency Medicine, Wake Forest University School of Medicine, Winston-Salem, NC

Gideon Bosker, MD, FACEP, Assistant Clinical Professor, Section of Emergency Services, Yale University School of Medicine, New Haven, CT; Associate Clinical Professor, Oregon Health Sciences University, Portland, OR

Jemison Bowers, MD, Associate Professor of Ophthalmology, University of Tennessee College of Medicine, Chattanooga Unit

William J. Brady, MD, FACEP, Assistant Professor, Department of Emergency Medicine, University of Virginia; Clinical Director, Department of Emergency Medicine, University of Virginia Health Sciences Center, Charlottesville, VA

Jeremy Brown, MD, Department of Emergency Medicine, Beth Israel Deaconess Medical Center; Instructor in Medicine, Harvard Medical School, Boston, MA

Raghavan Chari, MD, FACEP, Emergency Medicine Physician, Carolina Hospital System, Florence, SC; Emergency Medicine Physician, Wyoming Valley Health Care System, Wilkes Barre, PA, Chairman, Conquest Health Associates

William K. Chiang, MD, Assistant Professor of Medicine, Brown University School of Medicine; Attending Physician, Department of Emergency Medicine, Rhode Island Hospital, Providence, RI; Consultant, Rhode Island Poison Control Center, Providence, RI

Bonnie I. Chi-Lum, MD, MPH, Editor-in-Chief, American Medical Association web site, Loma Linda, CA

Harold Chin, MD, Clinical Assistant Professor, Department of Medicine, University of Chicago; Attending Physician, Department of Emergency Medicine, Lutheran General Hospital, Park Ridge, IL

Norman C. Christopher, MD, Director, Emergency and Trauma Services, Children's Hospital Medical Center of Akron, Akron, OH

Paul Y. Chung, MD, Assistant Professor of Ophthalmology, Loma Linda University School of Medicine; Chief, Ophthalmology Section at VA Medical Center, Loma Linda, CA

Katherine A. Clark, DO, Assistant Clinical Professor, Wright State University School of Medicine, Department of Family Medicine, Dayton, OH

Melissa E. Clarke, MD, Assistant Professor, Howard University Hospital, Division of Emergency Medicine, Washington, DC

Mark E. Classen, MD, PhD, Associate Professor, Department of Family Medicine, Wright State University School of Medicine, Dayton, OH

Patrick P. Coll, MD, Associate Professor of Family Medicine, Associate Director of Center on Aging, University of Connecticut Health Center, Farmington, CT

Stephen A. Colucciello, MD, FACEP, Assistant Clinical Professor of Emergency Medicine, University of North Carolina Medical School, Chapel Hill, NC; Director, Clinical Services Trauma Coordinator, Department of Emergency Medicine, Carolinas Medical Center, Charlotte, NC

Michael H. Crawford, MD, Robert S. Flinn Professor, Chief of Cardiology, University of New Mexico, Albuquerque

Dawn Demagone, MD, FAAEM, Assistant Program Director, Assistant Professor of Medicine, Division of Emergency Medicine, Temple University Hospital, Philadelphia, PA

Gail D'Onofrio, MD, Research Director, Section of Emergency Medicine, Assistant Professor, Yale University School of Medicine, New Haven, CT

Jonathan Edlow, MD, Acting Chief of Service, Department of Emergency Medicine, Beth Israel Deaconess Medical Center, Boston, MA; Instructor in Medicine, Harvard Medical School, Cambridge, MA

Frank J. Edwards, MD, FACEP, Medical Director, Division of Community and Rural Emergency Medicine, Greater Rochester Health System; Clinical Assistant Professor of Emergency Medicine, University of Rochester, Rochester, NY

Charles L. Emerman, MD, Associate Professor of Emergency Medicine, Case Western Reserve University; Chairman of Emergency Medicine, MetroHealth Medical Center, Cleveland Clinic Foundation, Cleveland, OH

Stephen P. Ernest, PharmD, Clinical Pharmacy Coordinator, Columbia Terre Haute Regional Medical Center, Terre Haute, IN

Carol A. Foster, MD, Fellow, Neurology, UCLA School of Medicine, Departments of Neurology and Head and Neck Surgery, Los Angeles, CA

Theodore G. Ganiats, MD, Associate Professor, Department of Family and Preventive Medicine, University of California-San Diego School of Medicine

Laurence J. Gavin, MD, FACEP, Director, Emergency Department, Presbyterian Medical Center, Philadelphia, PA

Joel Geiderman, MD, FACEP, Associate Director, Emergency Medicine, Cedars Sinai Medical Center; Assistant Clinical Professor, UCLA, Los Angeles, CA

Michael Gerardi, MD, FAAP, FACEP, Director, Pediatric Emergency Medical Services, Saint Barnabas Medical Center, Livingston, NJ

Lowell W. Gerson, PhD, Professor of Epidemiology and Associate Director, Division of Community Health Sciences, Northeastern Ohio Universities College of Medicine, Rootstown, OH

Brian M. Glazer, MD, Associate Clinical Professor of Psychiatry, Harvard Medical School, Massachusetts General Hospital

Deborah T. Gold, PhD, Associate Professor of Medical Sociology, Department of Psychiatry and Behavioral Sciences, Duke University Medical Center, Durham, NC

Lewis Goldfrank, MD, Director of Emergency Medicine, Bellevue Hospital and New York University Medical Center; Associate Professor of Clinical Medicine, New York University, New York, NY

Sydney Goldstein, MD, Division of Head Emeritus, Division of Cardiovascular Medicine, Henry Ford Hospital, Detroit, MI

Steven Green, MD, FACEP, Associate Professor of Emergency Medicine, Loma Linda University School of Medicine, Loma Linda, CA

Jerry M. Greene, MD, Chief, Rheumatology Section, Brockton/West Roxbury VA Medical Center, West Roxbury, MA

Stephen B. Gunther, MD, Assistant Professor of Clinical Orthopaedic Surgery, UCSF, Department of Orthopaedic Surgery, San Francisco, CA

Ralph R. Hall, MD, Prosessor and Associate Dean, University of Missouri at Kansas City School of Medicine, St. Luke's Hospital Division, Kansas City, MO

Brian Hardin, MD, Director of Adolescent Medicine, Adolescent Medicine Section, Arkansas Children's Hospital, Little Rock, AK

Richard A. Harrigan, MD, Assistant Professor of Medicine, Temple University School of Medicine; Attending Physician, Temple University Hospital, Philadelphia, PA

David W. Hawkins, MD, Professor and Chair of Pharmacy Practice, Mercer University, Atlanta, GA

Michael Heller, MD, Clinical Professor of Medicine, Temple University School of Medicine; Program Director, Emergency Medicine Residency of the Lehigh Valley, Philadelphia, PA

Katherine L. Heilpern, MD, Assistant Professor, Division of Emergency Medicine, Emory University School of Medicine, Atlanta, GA

John A. Heit, MD, Associate Professor of Medicine, Director, Thrombophilia Center, Mayo Clinic and Foundation, Rochester, MN

J. Thomas Heywood, MD, Director, Cardiomyopathy Program and Adult Cardiac Transplant, Loma Linda University Medical Center, Loma Linda, CA

Donald M. Hilty, MD, Assistant Professor of Clinical Psychiatry, University of California, Davis, Sacramento, CA

Robert S. Hoffman, MD, Associate Medical Director, Director of Medical Toxicology Fellowship Program, New York City Poison Control Center; Attending Physician, Bellevue Hospital Center, New York, NY

Margaret-Mary Holyst, MD, Research Assistant Professor, Department of Internal Medicine, University of Missouri-Columbia, Columbia, MO

David S. Howes, MD, FACEP, Director, Emergency Medicine Residency Program, Associate Professor of Clinical Medicine, University of Chicago, IL

Mary Ann Howland, PharmD, ABAT, Clinical Professor of Pharmacy, St. John's University College of Pharmacy; Consultant, New York City Poison Control Center and Bellevue Hospital Emergency Department, New York, NY

Joseph C. Howton, MD, FACEP, Assistant Clinical Professor of Medicine, Division of Emergency Medicine, University of Washington Medical Center, Federal Way, WA

Gene G. Hunder, MD, Professor of Medicine, Mayo Medical School, Consultant in Internal Medicine and Rheumatology, Mayo Clinic, Rochester, MN

Thomas Hyers, MD, Clinical Professor of Medicine, St. Louis University School of Medicine, St. Louis, MO

Edward C. Jacobs, MD, Assistant Clinical Professor of Urology, Department of Surgery, Wright State University, Dayton, OH

Edward Jauch, MD, MS, Assistant Professor, Department of Emergency Medicine, University of Cincinnati Medical Center; Member, Greater Cincinnati/Northern Kentucky Stroke Team

Elizabeth B. Jones, MD, Assistant Professor, Department of Emergency Medicine, The University of Texas Health Science Center at Houston

Jeffrey Jones, MD, FACEP, Assistant Professor and Research Director, Department of Emergency Medicine, Butterworth Hospital, Michigan State University College of Medicine, Grand Rapids, MI

Justin Kaplan, MD, Research Co-director, Department of Emergency Medicine, Albert Einstein Medical Center of Philadelphia, Philadelphia, PA

Jerald Kay, MD, Professor and Chair, Department of Psychiatry, Wright State University, Dayton, Ohio.

Donald J. Keller, MD, Clinical Professor, University of Colorado, Boulder

Stephen R. Knazik, DO, FACEP, Assistant Professor, Departments of Pediatric and Emergency Medicine, Wayne State University School of Medicine, Detroit, MI

David Kramer, MD, FACEP, Associate Professor, Program Director, Division of Emergency Medicine, Emory University School of Medicine, Atlanta, GA

Steven Krug, MD, Associated Professor of Pediatrics, Northwestern University Medical School; Head, Division of Pediatric Emergency Medicine, Children's Memorial Hospital, Northwestern University Medical School

Michael J. La Penta, MD, Medical Staff President, Anne Arundel Medical Center, Annapolis, MD

James L. Larson, MD, Assistant Professor of Emergency Medicine, Department of Emergency Medicine, University of North Carolina School of Medicine, Chapel Hill, NC

Roseanna Lechner, MD, Assistant Professor of Surgery, Case Western Reserve University; Department of Neurosurgery, MetroHealth Medical Center, Cleveland, OH

Charles Levenbach, MD, Associate Professor, Department of Gynecologic Oncology, M.D. Anderson Cancer Center, Houston, TX

George S. Levenson, Jr., MD, Editorial Board, *Vascular Ultrasound Today*

Louis J. Ling, MD, Medical Director, Hennepin Regional Poison Center, Minneapolis, MN

Jeffrey Linzer, MD, Assistant Professor of Pediatrics, Emory University School of Medicine; Associate Medical Director, Pediatric Emergency Care Center, Hughs Spalding Children's Hospital, Atlanta, GA

Joseph W. Luria, MD, Assistant Professor of Clinical Pediatrics, Division of Emergency Medicine, Children's Hospital Medical Center, Cincinnati, OH

O. John Ma, MD, Assistant Professor of Emergency Medicine, University of Missouri-Kansas City School of Medicine; Research Director, Department of Emergency Medicine, Truman Medical Center, Kansas City, MO

Gary Maier, MD, Director of Psychiatric Services, Forensics Program, Mendota Mental Health Institute, Madison, WI

David E. Manthey, MD, Research Director, Brooke Army Medical Center, Department of Emergency Medicine, San Antonio Uniformed Services Health Education Consortium, San Antonio, TX

Randall L. McAllister, MD, FACP, FACEP, Medical Director, Quality Initiatives; Attending Physician, Emergency Care Center, Memorial Mission Hospital, Asheville, NC

Maureen McCollough, MD, MPH, FACEP, Assistant Professor of Medicine, UCLA School of Medicine; Director of Pediatric Emergency Medicine, OliveView-UCLA Medical Center, Sylmar, CA

William Michael McCollough, Jr., MD, FACOG, Assistant Clinical Professor, Wright State University School of Medicine, Dayton, OH

Robert C. McKinstry, III, MD, PhD, Assistant Professor, Neuroradiology Section, Mallinckrodt Institute of Radiology, Washington University School of Medicine, St. Louis, MO

Robert M. McNamara, MD, Associate Professor, Department of Emergency Medicine, Medical College of Pennsylvania, Philadelphia, PA

Rajeev Mehta, MD, Assistant Clinical Professor, Wright State University School of Medicine, Dayton, OH

Stephen W. Meldon, MD, Department of Emergency Medicine, MetroHealth Medical Center; Assistant Professor, Case Western Reserve University, Cleveland, OH

Larry B. Mellick, MD, MS, FAAP, FACEP, Chief of Service and Chairman, Director of Pediatric Emergency Medicine, Department of Emergency Medicine, Medical College of Georgia, Augusta, GA

John Miklos, MD, Department of Obstetrics and Gynecology, Division of Urogynecology, Northside Hospital, Atlanta, GA

Felice Milan, MD, Associate Professor of Clinical Medicine, Montefiore Medical Center, Albert Einstein College of Medicine, Irvington, NY

Paul Miller, MD, Medical Director, Colorado Center for Bone Research, Lakewood, CO

Steen Mortensen, MD, Chief of Rheumatology, Wichita Clinic, Wichita, KS

Paula D. Mueller, MD, DABMT, Assistant Clinical Professor, University of Florida School of Medicine; Department of Emergency Medicine, Orlando Regional Medical Center, Orlando, FL

Michael Muszynski, MD, FAAP, Director, Residency in Pediatrics; Chief, Division of Pediatric Infectious Disease, Arnold Palmer Hospital for Women and Children, Orlando, FL

Gary L. Nicholson, MD, Medical Oncologist/Hematologist, Dayton Oncology/Hematology Consultants, Dayton, OH

Robert L. Norris, MD, FACEP, Assistant Professor of Surgery/Emergency Medicine, Stanford University, Stanford, CA

Judith A. Owens, MD, MPH, Director, Pediatric Sleep Disorders Clinic, Rhode Island Hospital, Portsmouth, RI

Edward A. Panacek, MD, Associate Professor and Residency Director, Emergency Medicine, U.C. Davis Medical Center, Sacramento, CA

Andrew D. Perron, MD, Assistant Professor of Emergency Medicine, Department of Emergency Medicine, University of Virginia, Charlottesville, VA

John Peters, MD, Clinical Professor of Ophthalmology, Creighton University, Omaha, NE; Clinical Professor, University of Nebraska Medical Center, Omaha

Norman Peterson, MD, Professor of Surgery and Urology, University of Colorado Health Sciences Center; Associate Director of Surgery and Urology Division Director, Denver Health Medical Center, Denver, CO

Paula M. Podrazik, MD, FACEP, Assistant Professor, Department of Emergency Medicine, Temple University Hospital, Philadelphia, PA

Tammie Quest, MD, Assistant Professor, Department of Emergency Medicine, Emory University, Atlanta, GA

Raymond D. Pitetti, MD, MPH, Assistant Professor of Pediatrics, Division of Pediatric Emergency Medicine, Department of Pediatrics, University of Pittsburgh School of Medicine, Pittsburgh, PA

Walker S. Carlos Poston, MPH, PhD, Assistant Professor, University of Missouri—Kansas City, Mid America Heart Institute

Susan B. Promes, MD, Associate Residency Director, Department of Emergency Medicine, Alameda County Medical Center-Highland Campus, Oakland, CA, Assistant Professor of Clinical Medicine, University of California, San Francisco

Kenneth B. Pugar, MD, Chairman, Section of Neurology, Psychiatry, and Physical Medicine, Grandview/Southview Hospital; Division Head for Neurology, Wallace-Kettering Neuroscience Institute, Kettering Medical Center; Clinical Director, Comprehensive Stroke Management Team, Kettering Medical Center, Kettering, OH

Lucy J. Puryear, MD, Assistant Professor of Psychiatry, Department of Psychiatry; Director, Baylor Psychiatry Clinic; Director, Medical Student Education, Baylor College of Medicine, Houston, TX

Lawrence G. Ratcliff, MD, Assistant Professor of Family Medicine, Wright State University School of Medicine, Dayton, OH

Earl J. Reisdorff, MD, FACEP, Associate Director, Michigan State University, Emergency Medicine Residency—Lansing; Associate Professor, College of Human Medicine, Michigan State University, East Lansing, MI

Kevin J. Roache, MD, FRCP(C), FACG, Associate Medical Director, Internal Medicine and Gastroenterology, Sterling Rock Falls Clinic, Ltd., Sterling, IL

David Robinson, MD, MS, Research Director and Assistant Professor, Department of Emergency Medicine, The University of Texas Houston Medical Center, Director, Diagnostic Observation Center, Memorial Hermann Hospital, Houston, TX

Clifford J. Rosen, MD, Research Professor of Nutrition, University of Maine, Bangor, ME

Steven G. Rothrock, MD, FACEP, Research Director, Department of Emergency Medicine, Orlando Regional Medical Center & Arnold Palmer's Hospital for Women and Children, Orlando, FL; Clinical Assistant Professor, Division of Emergency Medicine, University of Florida College of Medicine, Gainesville, FL

Frank Ruiz, MD, Assistant Professor of Surgery, University of California-San Francisco; Department of Emergency Services, San Francisco General Hospital, San Francisco, CA

Douglas A. Rund, MD. FACEP, Professor and Chairman, Department of Emergency Medicine, The Ohio State University, Columbus, OH

Marshall Salkin, MD, JD, FACEP, FCLM, Attending Physician, Emergency Department of Northwest Community Hospital, Arlington Heights, IL

Richard Salluzzo, MD, FACEP, Associate Professor and Chairman of Emergency Medicine, Albany Medical College, Albany, NY

John P. Santamaria, MD, FAAP, FACEP, Director, Wound and Hyperbaric Center, Attending Physician, Pediatric Emergency Services, St. Joseph's Hospital, Tampa, FL

Jonathan C. Saxe, MD, Associate Professor of Clinical Medicine, Wright State University, Dayton, OH

Robert Schafermeyer, MD, Associate Chairman, Department of Emergency Medicine, Carolinas Medical Center, Charlotte, NC

Robert C. Schenck, Jr., MD, Professor and Division Chief, Sports Medicine Section, University of New Mexico Health Science Center, Albuquerque, NM

Robert E. Schneider, MD, Director of Curriculum, Department of Emergency Medicine, Carolinas Medical Center, Charlotte, NC

Sandra Schneider, MD, FACEP, Professor and Chair, Department of Emergency Medicine, University of Rochester, Rochester, NY

Sabrina Schrager, MD, Assistant Professor, Department of Family Medicine, University of Wisconsin, Madison, WI

Robert A. Schwab, MD, Associate Professor, Department of Emergency Medicine, University of Missouri at Kansas City School of Medicine, Kansas City, MO

Brian Schwartz, MD, FACP, Director of Medical Ethics, Kettering Medical Center, Kettering, OH

Chuck Seamens, MD, FACEP, Assistant Professor of Emergency Medicine, Vanderbilt University Medical Center, Nashville, TN

Warren R. Selman, MD, Associate Professor, Case Western University; Chairman, Subcommittee for GIVE far Non-Neurosurgeons, Department of Neurological Surgery, University Hospitals of Cleveland, OH

Sid M. Shah, MD, FACEP, Assistant Residency Director of Research, Sparrow, Michigan State University Residency Program, Ingham Regional Medical Center, Lansing, MI

Mitchell I. Shiffman, MD, Associate Professor of Medicine; Chief, Hepatology Section; Medical Director, Liver Transplant Program, Medical College of Virginia at Virginia Commonwealth University, Richmond

David Sklar, MD, FACEP, Professor and Chair, Department of Emergency Medicine, University of New Mexico School of Medicine, Albuquerque, NM

David C. Sloan, MD, Pathologist, Pathology Associates of Mason City, Mason City, Iowa

Corey M. Slovis, MD, FACP, FACEP, Professor and Chairman, Department of Emergency Medicine, Vanderbilt University School of Medicine, Nashville, TN

Ramona Slupik, MD, Assistant Professor of Gynecology and Obstetrics, Head of Pediatric and Adolescent Gynecology, Department of Gynecology, Northwestern University Medical School, Chicago, IL

Eric R. Snoey, MD, Residency Director, Department of Emergency Medicine, Highland General Hospital, Oakland, CA; Assistant Professor, University of California, San Francisco Medical Center

Leon Speroff, MD, Professor of Obstetrics and Gynecology, Oregon Health Sciences University, Portland

Perry Stafford, MD, FACS, FAAP, FCCM, Director, Trauma and Surgical Critical Care, Children's Hospital of Philadelphia, PA

J. Stephan Stapczynski, MD, Associate Professor and Chairman, Department of Emergency Medicine, University of Kentucky Medical Center, Lexington, KY

Sidney Starkman, MD, FACEP, UCLA School of Medicine, Departments of Emergency Medicine/Emergency Medicine and Neurology, Director, Comprehensive Emergency Neurology Program, Los Angeles, CA

Joyce M. Stein, DO, Krane and Milicia Obstetrics and Gynecology, City Line Avenue Hospital and Hahnemann University, Hospital of the Tenet System, Philadelphia, PA

Charles Stewart, MD, FACEP, Emergency Physician, Colorado Springs, CO

Jeremy Sugarman, MD, MPH, MA, Associate Professor of Medicine and Philosophy, Duke University, Durham, NC

Paul Suratt, MD, John L. Guerrant Professor of Internal Medicine, Division of Pulmonary and Critical Care Medicine, Director of Sleep Disorders Center, University of Virginia, Charlottesville, VA

Daniel Swagerty, Jr., MD, MPH, Assistant Professor, Departments of Family and Internal Medicine, Associate Director, Center on Aging, University of Kansas Medical Center

Jon M. Sweet, MD, Assistant Professor of Medicine, Wright State University School of Medicine, OH

Ken Tardiff, MD, Professor of Psychiatry and Public Health, Cornell Medical College; Medical Director, Payne Whitney Clinic, New York, NY

Michael E. Thase, MD, Professor of Psychiatry, University of Pittsburgh Medical Center, Pittsburgh, PA

Andrew Ulrick, MD, Assistant Professor, Department of Emergency Medicine, Boston University School of Medicine

Sterling B. Walker, MD, Diplomate ABEM, Emergency Physician, Montrose Memorial Hospital, Montrose, CO

Richard Wang, DO, FACEP, Director of Medical Toxicology, Brown University School of Medicine, Providence, RI

Julia K. Warnick, MD, PhD, Associate Professor of Psychiatry; Director, Clinical Research, University of Oklahoma Health Science Center, Tulsa

Albert C. Weihl, MD, FACEP, Assistant Professor of Medicine and Surgery, Yale University School of Medicine, Section of Emergency Medicine, New Haven, CT

Michael P. Weissberg, MD, Professor of Psychiatry and Director, Emergency Psychiatric Services, University of Colorado Health Sciences Center, Denver, CO

Steven M. Winograd, MD, FACEP, Attending Physician, Department of Emergency Medicine, Sturgis Hospital, Sturgis, MI, and Allegan General Hospital, Allegan, MI

Gerald M. Winslow, PhD, Dean, Division of Religion, Chair, Center for Christian Bioethics, Loma Linda University, Loma Linda, CA

Allan B. Wolfson, MD, FACEP, FACP, Program Director, Affiliated Residency in Emergency Medicine; Professor of Emergency Medicine and Medicine, University of Pittsburgh, Pittsburgh, PA

Keith Wrenn, MD, Associate Professor of Emergency Medicine and Medicine; Residency Director, Department of Emergency Medicine, Vanderbilt University of School of Medicine, Nashville, TN

Martha S. Wright, MD, Associate Professor of Pediatrics, Case Western Reserve University School of Medicine; Associate Director, Pediatric Emergency Medicine, Rainbow Babies and Children's Hospital, Cleveland, OH

Beverly Yamour, MD, FACC, Staff Physician of Ohio Heart Care, Canton, OH

Kimberly A. Yonkers, MD, Assistant Professor, Department of Psychiatry and Department of Obstetrics and Gynecology, The University of Texas Southwestern Medical Center, Dallas, TX

Seymour Zimbler, MD, Clinical Instructor in Orthopedic Surgery, Harvard University, Boston

Michael Zimmerman, MD, FACEP, Assistant Clinical Professor, Department of Emergency Medicine, Oregon Health Sciences University; Attending Emergency Department Physician, St. Vincent's Hospital and Medical Center, Portland, OR

Table of Contents

Part I
Pediatrics

Part II
Infectious Diseases

Part III
Neurological Disorders

Part IV
Pulmonary Disorders

Part V
Cardiovascular and Thrombosis-Related Conditions

Part VI
Gastrointestinal Disease

Part VII
Obstetrics and Gynecology

Part VIII
Eye, Ear, Nose, and Throat

Part IX
Geriatric Medicine

Part XVI
Renal Disease and Urological Conditions

Part XVII
Psychiatric Disorders

Part I

Pediatrics

Initial Approaches for the Febrile Child

Steven G. Rothrock, MD, FACEP
Steven M. Green, MD, FACEP

Typically occurring during the first few years of life, an elevated temperature can be the initial manifestation of benign as well as life-threatening illness. Although "fever" is the most common reason children are brought to the emergency department (ED),[1] "fever phobia," or an irrational fear of a fever and its potential effects, is prevalent among both parents and health care professionals.[2,3] Fortunately, the majority of children with an elevated temperature do not have a serious illness, although a small percentage harbor or may develop a serious bacterial infection. To avoid missing serious conditions associated with fever, the emergency physician must determine which children need further diagnostic evaluation or in-hospital therapy and which patients may be discharged for outpatient treatment and careful follow-up.

Among all pediatric patients with fever, febrile infants 3 months to 3 years old present unique challenges. It should be stressed that children 2 years of age and younger do not invariably manifest signs and symptoms of meningeal irritation when they develop meningitis.[4] Moreover, approximately 3-6% of children in this age group with fever have occult bacteremia.[5,6] This incidence is probably overstated, inasmuch as many previous studies included seriously ill children who were bacteremic from such serious non-occult infections as pneumonia, cellulitis, and meningitis. While most cases of occult bacteremia will resolve without treatment, antibiotic administration may prevent some children from progressing to more serious conditions.[7]

Finally, choice of antibiotics, route of administration, as well as selection of children considered appropriate for empiric therapy are just a few of the controversial issues that have been debated in the pediatric and emergency medicine literature.[8,9] Other related issues that demand a systematic approach to the febrile child include proper route of temperature measurement, treatment modalities for an elevated temperature, whether to treat a fever at all, and finally, whether a response to antipyretics has any diagnostic implications.

Given the wide range conditions and the clinical importance of managing children with temperature elevations, this chapter examines the diagnostic and management approaches to the febrile child in detail.

Temperature Elevation: Interpretation and Pitfalls

Temperature Regulation. Generally speaking, control of body temperature is maintained by the anterior hypothalamus, which attempts to maintain an inherent set point or body temperature near 36°C (98.6°F). Heat loss is controlled by producing alterations in blood flow to various organs (most importantly, the skin), alterations in the metabolic rate, and controlling the exocrine sweat glands (vaporization).[10]

A "true" fever occurs when interleukin-1 or another cytokine or combination of cytokines (e.g., interleukin-6, tumor necrosis factor alpha) is released from monocytes and macrophages in response to any of the following stimuli: infection, tissue injury, drugs, and other inflammatory responses. This increases the body's set point. Important actions of interleukins include attraction of white blood cells, increasing blood flow to the inflammatory site, stimulation of the bone marrow to release white blood cells, and increased muscle breakdown.[10]

By definition, other causes of hyperthermia ("false" fevers) do not directly increase the body's set point and, therefore, are not considered mediators of a "true" fever. Examples include: 1) central nervous system (CNS) disease that directly affects the hypothalamus (e.g., intracranial hemorrhage, infection); 2) diseases that increase the body's production of heat (e.g., hyperthyroidism, malignant hyperthermia, salicylate overdose); 3) excess heat load (e.g., a child left in a car in the heat or placed next to a heater for too long); and 4) defective heat loss mechanisms (e.g., burns, heat stroke, drugs that compromise blood flow and sweating mechanisms).[11]

Normal Temperature vs. Fever. Many controversies exist concerning the exact definition and management of a fever. Until recently, all infants under the age of 2-3 months with a temperature of 38°C (100.4°F) or higher were automatically subjected to a complete septic evaluation, including lumbar puncture, and subsequently were admitted to the hospital. Despite the widespread prevalence of this conservative approach, several recent studies have defined a subset of well-appearing febrile infants in this age group who can be safely managed as outpatients without developing adverse sequelae.[8-10] Nevertheless, several questions still remain regarding management of children younger than 2-3 months of age. These include identifying the exact age cutoff that should trigger concern, the exact temperature at which "fever" is considered pathologically significant, indications for diagnostic testing (e.g., lumbar puncture, urinalysis and culture, chest radiography), and indications for broad-spectrum antibiotic coverage.[12]

This controversy has been fueled by many different concerns. While the body tries to maintain a core temperature of 37 ± 1°C (98.6 ± 1.5°F), there is a normal circadian rhythm in the body's temperature, which is highest (up to 2°C [3°F]) around 6 p.m. and lowest at 6 a.m.[10] This may, in part, account for the increased volume of ED visits that peaks in the evening for children. Of clinical significance is the fact that most true fevers follow this diurnal temperature pattern, whereas false fevers do not.

Normal causes of temperature elevation in children include physical activity, ovulation, and, most importantly, environmental temperature. Excessive clothing (or bundling) and a hot environment can cause up to a 0.8°C (1.5°F) temperature elevation.[10,13] However, a decrease in the environmental temperature generally has less of an effect of the body's overall temperature.

Although the definition of a true fever (one mediated by hypothalamic set point elevation) is generally straightforward, the exact level of temperature elevation that defines a fever—and, more importantly, the level of temperature elevation that should raise suspicion of an infection—is more controversial. A survey of pediatric and emergency medicine residency program directors found that most physicians (30%) defined a fever as 38°C (100.4°F), while 27% used a cut-off of 38.3°C (101°F). About 15% did not formally define a specific temperature cutoff for defining a fever.[14]

However, the majority of studies of febrile infants younger than 3 months old define a fever as a temperature 38°C or more, while a temperature range of 38.0-38.5°C is used as a cutoff for defining fever in those greater than 3 months of age.[14] Regardless of the definition, clinicians should understand that no temperature cutoff is completely reliable for detecting or excluding an infection. In fact, in very young infants and neonates, hypothermia is frequently an important manifestation of serious underlying infection.[15]

Temperature Measurement

Employing a reliable method of temperature measurement is essential for making informed and appropriate decisions in febrile children. Although some methods are better than others, it should be stressed that all temperature measurements are estimates of the body's true core temperature or the temperature of the blood in the central circulation (i.e., in the aorta and pulmonary artery).[16]

Several methods for core temperature assessment are available, including tactile, axillary, esophageal, oral, rectal, and tympanic thermometry. Among these, the rectal temperature, because of its accuracy and lack of variation in response to environmental factors, is considered the gold standard for temperature assessment in the ED. In contrast, both tactile and axillary methods are extremely inaccurate, varying considerably with the environmental temperature.[17,18] Esophageal temperature measurement is accurate, but is highly impractical for routine use, whereas oral thermometry can only be used reliably in appropriately aged children (> 5-6 years) and may vary with respiratory rate and in response to recent ingestions.[19,20]

Recently, tympanic thermometry has been advocated for use in children. Tympanic thermometers are placed in the external auditory canal and use an infrared sensor to measure the temperature of the tympanic membrane, which receives its blood supply from an internal carotid artery source (i.e., from the same blood supply as the anterior hypothalamus).[21] Early examination of this technology showed that measurements correlated well with rectal temperatures.[22] However, several recent studies have shown that tympanic thermometry is less successful for detecting fever in young children, especially those younger than 3 years of age.[18] The five largest studies to date have yielded a sensitivity of 51-79% and specificity of 74-93% for tympanic thermometry in detecting temperatures greater than 38.0-38.5°C in children.[18,23-26] Furthermore, tympanic temperatures varied from rectal temperatures by at least 1°F in 56% of children, at least 2°F in 15%, and at least 3°F in 3% of children in one recent study.[18] Because of its potential for inaccuracy, tympanic thermometry is not recommended for assessment of fever in young children.

Fever Phobia

Background. In the Middle Ages, an elevated temperature was felt to be a marker for either death or divine punishment. Vestiges of this thinking are still held by some parents and health care workers, who are concerned that a true fever will harm their child.[2,3] In fact, parents who bring their children to an ED may be concerned that an elevated temperature will be harmful to their child. In fact, in one survey, one-third of parents thought that a temperature of 38-40°C (100.4-104.0°F) would harm their child, two-thirds thought that a temperature of 40-41°C (104-106°F) would harm their child, and all of them thought that brain damage would occur above 41°C (106°F).[2] Furthermore, 16% felt that if a fever were not treated, it would elevate to 108-120°F—leading to convulsions, death, coma, dehydration, blindness, and stroke.[2,27]

Fortunately, a "true" fever is not harmful to a child if the fever is not due to a serious infection and the temperature elevation is not due to excess heat load, defective heat loss mechanism, CNS damage or disease, or excess heat production.[10]

Physiological Benefits of Temperature Elevation. In normal children, the anterior hypothalamus acts as a thermostat that will not allow the temperature to rise above 41.5°C (107°F).[10] Fever-lowering agents or antipyrogens (e.g., V1 arginine vasopressin, alpha-melanocyte stimulating hormone) are released from the anterior hypothalamus during fever elevations that balance the fever-raising effects of pyrogens.[10] Nevertheless, an elevated temperature can confer many advantages. For example, white blood cells work best and kill the most bacteria at 38-40°C (100.4-104.0°F).[10] There is an increased production of antibacterial substances by neutrophils (e.g., superoxide anion) and increased production and activity of interferon.[10]

In addition, elevated temperatures directly inhibit replication of certain viruses (e.g., Coxsackie and polio viruses).[28] Interestingly, studies have found that children with rubeola and varicella who were treated with acetaminophen had symptoms for a significantly longer duration than those not treated, while children with rubeola who are treated with antipyretics were more likely to develop pneumonia.[28] Finally, there has never been a case of CNS damage from a true fever in a normal child who had no serious underlying infection.[29] Consequently, there is no rational reason to be concerned about a true fever in a normal child who does not have a serious underlying bacterial infection.

Febrile Seizures. While short-term adverse events from true fevers are non-existent, clinicians should be aware that a fever may lower the seizure threshold in patients with underlying seizure disorders, may be a non-specific marker for serious bacterial infection, and may promote insensible water loss and raise the basal metabolic rate (~10% for every 1°C) if the fever persists for a long time. Finally, some authors argue that a rapidly rising temperature or a high temperature may place a child at risk for having a febrile seizure. However, whether the maximum elevation point or the rate of rise in temperature causes febrile seizures is simply not known. However, it has been confirmed that febrile seizures tend to occur early in the course of a febrile illness, usually long before physician intervention can make a difference. Furthermore, simple febrile seizures are benign and occur in up to 5% of the entire pediatric population at some point in their lifetime.[30]

Education and Reassurance. When it comes to the consequences of temperature elevation, a word of caution is required. Physicians may play an important part in perpetuating the myth that a fever is harmful to a child. Sixty-five percent of pediatricians in a recent survey thought that an elevated body temperature alone could be dangerous to a child, whereas 28% did not.[3] Seizures were cited 58% of the time as the most frequent complication of fever, followed by dehydration (23%), brain damage (10%), and obtundation (9%).[3] This study suggests that fever phobia may be due to incorrect messages conveyed by pediatric health providers.

Another misconception fostered by parents as well as some health care workers is that the response of a temperature to acetaminophen is useful for differentiating between serious bacterial infections or bacteremia and more trivial illnesses in the pediatric age group. In fact, following administration of an appropriate dose of acetaminophen (15 mg/kg), most children who have a fever will have a 2-3°F decrease in their temperature over a one- to two-hour period.[31] *(See Figure 1.)* As a rule, their temperature usually will not return to normal. Furthermore, the response or non-response to acetaminophen is virtually useless in distinguishing between viral and bacterial infection.[32,33]

Figure 1. Average Response to a Single Dose of Acetaminophen Over Time

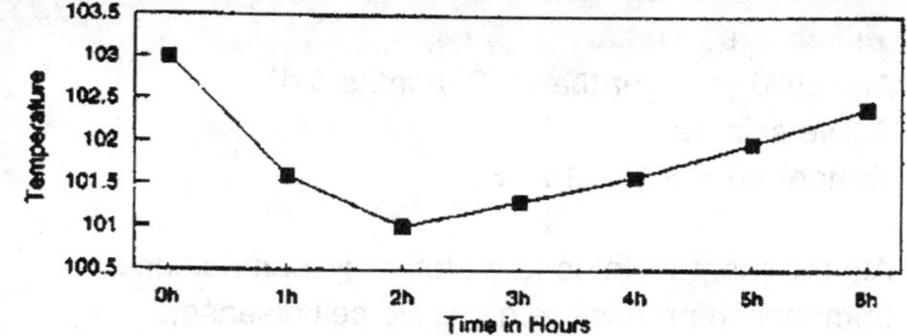

Adapted from: Steele RW. Oral antipyretic therapy. *Am J Dis Child* 1972;123:204.

A lack of parental knowledge concerning fever management is reflected in studies showing that the most common method of temperature measurement used by 86% of parents who brought their child to an ED for evaluation is palpation.[34] Mothers who said their children were febrile were correct only 52% of the time.[34] In fact, in one study, only 10% of parents had measured their child's temperature before bringing him or her to the ED for evaluation of a fever. Furthermore, in one study, up to 90% of suburban parents were unable to correctly read a glass mercury thermometer.[35]

Based on a study in one pediatric clinic, education can play an important part in alleviating parental fears concerning fever. After parents were counseled concerning accurate temperature measurement, appropriate treatment, and the potential beneficial effects of elevated temperatures, the number of inappropriate visits decreased from 40% to 10%, and the number of inappropriate calls regarding fever decreased from 56% to 26%.[27]

Fever Management

Although the presence of fever in a normal child with no underlying infection is of little concern, there are some clinical situations in which febrile children require rapid treatment and evaluation. These patients include children who may not be able to adequately control their own temperature (i.e., those with false fevers) and children who are at risk for serious illness due to temperature elevation. *(See Table 1.)*

Methods of Fever Reduction. There are several approaches—many of them tailored to specific clinical situations—to fever reduction in the pediatric patient. For example, children who are suffering from heat stroke or any other serious disorder that compromises thermoregulation require rapid and aggressive cooling measures (e.g., a fan with continuous cool mist or gastric lavage). In contrast, rapid defervescence and aggressive therapy are almost never required for a normal child with a true fever.

A simple, time-honored technique, sponging with tepid water, is widely used for cooling febrile children. Despite its popularity, however, this method lowers temperature by an average of only 0.5-1.0°F

Table 1. Children Who Need Fever Addressed Promptly

CLINICAL SCENARIO	EXPLANATION
Any child younger than 2-3 months old	Difficult to assess for serious infection
Active seizure	May need temperature control to control seizure
Temperature > 106-107°F	Suggests highest risk for non-interleukin-1 fever (false fever) and bacteremia
Altered mental status (e.g., lethargy, somnolence)	Suggests serious or CNS infection
Immunocompromise (e.g., sickle cell disease, steroids, leukemia)	At risk for serious infection with minimal signs
Hypotension, or extremely fast heart rate or respiratory rate	Suggests sepsis
Suspect non-interleukin-1 fever (e.g., underlying CNS disease or burn or exposed patient)	May not be able to regulate or bring down temperature by normal mechanisms

and, in some children, may actually raise the temperature because it induces increased muscular activity and shivering.[36] In the past, rubbing alcohol (isopropanol) also was used for sponging. However, this technique is mentioned only because it should be condemned; a toxic amount of isopropanol can be absorbed through the skin and respiratory tract, which can potentially lead to seizures and death.

Antipyretics. Treatment with antipyretics generally leads to a temperature decrease of only 1-3°F.[31] This decrease is maximal around two hours after treatment.[31] It should be stressed that, over the short term, the temperature will almost never return to normal. Furthermore, the response or non-response to acetaminophen is virtually useless from a diagnostic perspective. In this regard, the degree of defervescence is similar whether the fever is due to a viral illness, meningitis, or bacteremia.[32,33] And although acetaminophen does not change the mean number of days of subsequent fever or other related symptoms, treated children tend to feel better and are more likely to have an increased level of activity and degree of alertness.

Acetaminophen. Acetaminophen, the most widely used antipyretic in children, blocks the actions of prostaglandins at the hypothalamus in order to bring the set point back to normal. Its effects are primarily antipyretic in nature, and it has no significant anti-inflammatory effects. Although there are no important short-term side effects when appropriately dosed (15 mg/kg q4h), chronic use and acute intoxication can cause renal insufficiency and liver damage. The only absolute contraindication to its use is end-stage liver failure (e.g., liver transplant patients).[37,38]

Ibuprofen. Although the clinical experience with ibuprofen in children is more limited than it is with acetaminophen, ibuprofen should be considered a useful alternate antipyretic that works by decreasing the hypothalamic set point. In contrast to acetaminophen, ibuprofen also has anti-inflammatory effects. The recommended dose is 5-10 mg/kg in a single dose q6h; no more than 30 mg/kg should administered per day. Overdose with ibuprofen elixir is rare and almost uniformly nonfatal as compared to salicylates and acetaminophen. However, on a long-term basis, cases of renal insufficiency, peptic ulcers, and gastritis have been reported. These effects have not been reported during short-term use for fever.

Initial reports indicated that the antipyretic effects of ibupro fen were superior to those of acetaminophen.[37] However, these studies used a substandard dose of acetaminophen and there is no evidence that either drug is superior to the other in terms of antipyretic activity. Contraindications to ibuprofen use include allergy to salicylates or other non-steroidal anti-inflammatory agents, renal disease or insufficiency, bleeding disorders, gastritis, and ulcer disease.[37,38]

Finally, it should be mentioned that because experience with ibuprofen, as compared to acetaminophen, in children is somewhat limited, and because of the link between salicylates and Reye's syndrome, some EDs have opted to maximize dosing of acetaminophen (15-20 mg/kg for short-duration therapy) instead of recommending ibuprofen for home use.

Patient Evaluation in the ED

Significance of Patient Age. The age of the febrile child has a significant effect on guiding diagnostic assessment and therapeutic interventions. Generally speaking, there are three distinct age ranges that have clinical importance regarding the following: 1) etiologic pathogens; 2) the usefulness of clinical examination in detecting serious illness; and 3) differences in the capacity of the immune system to fight certain infections.

Age younger than 3 months. With respect to diagnostic evaluation, children younger than 3 months of age are unique because the physical exam is felt to be unreliable in detecting many serious bacterial infections. Prior to the late 1980s, it was widely recommended that every child in this age group with a temperature 38°C (100.4°F) or more be admitted to hospital and subjected to a complete septic evaluation (lumbar puncture, urine and blood culture, chest radiograph).[39] Recently, this approach has changed. Furthermore, infants younger than 1-2 months of age are at risk for developing infections from such pathogens as *Escherichia coli, Listeria monocytogenes*, and Group B *Streptococcus*. Meningitis from these organisms and other gram-negative rods should always be considered in the newborn or young infant. In addition, their ability to fight infection, as compared to older infants and children, is limited.[39] Historical risk factors that predispose to these infections include maternal fever, maternal HIV infection, and early rupture of membranes.

Age 3-24 months. Children 3-24 months old are at risk for acquiring infections from a different range of infecting organisms, among

Table 2. Yale Observation Scale[40]

OBSERVATION ITEM	1: NORMAL	2: MODERATE IMPAIRMENT	3: SEVERE IMPAIRMENT
Quality of cry	Strong or none	Whimper or sob	Weak **or** moaning, high-pitched, continuous cry or hardly responds
Reaction to parent stimulation	Cries brief or no cry and content	Cries on and off	Persistent cry with little response
State variation	If awake, stays awake **or** if asleep, awakens quickly	Eyes close briefly when awake **or** awakens with prolonged stimulation	No arousal and falls asleep
Color	Pink	Pale extremities or acrocyanosis	Pale **or** cyanotic **or** mottle **or** ashen
Hydration	Skin and eyes normal **and** moist membranes	Skin and eyes normal **and** mouth slightly dry	Skin doughy **or** tented **and** dry mucous membranes **and/or** sunken eyes
Response to social overtures	Smiles or alert (consistently)	Brief smile or alert	No smile, anxious, dull; no alerting to social overtures

A total score of less than 11 signifies a less than 3% probability of serious illness.
A total score of 11-15 signifies a 26% probability of serious illness.
A total score of greater than 15 signifies a greater than 92% probability of serious illness.

them *Streptococcus pneumoniae, Haemophilus influenzae,* and *Neisseria meningitidis.*[7,8] While reliable physical findings of meningitis are present only when children approach 24 months, general observation and physical examination are useful in differentiating ill from well children.[5,40] This age range also reflects the peak incidence for the occurrence of occult bacteremia.[8]

Age greater than 24 months. In children 24 months of age and older, the incidence of occult bacteremia declines, and the physical examination becomes more reliable in differentiating seriously ill from non-ill children; the exam is also more useful for identifying the source of fever. Children also begin to acquire communication skills that permit them to indicate where they hurt and what is bothering them.

Although consideration of a child's age is useful in detailing the risk and site of serious infection, age cutoffs are not absolute in their predictive value. For instance, some experts do not include a 2- to 3-month-old child in the youngest age cutoff, whereas others feel that children 24-36 months or even older should be considered at risk for occult bacteremia.

Differential Diagnosis of Fever

General Principles. Evaluation of febrile children should be directed at detecting three main categories of infectious conditions: 1) meningitis; 2) occult bacteremia; and 3) serious bacterial infections (SBIs), including skin, skeletal, or joint infection, pneumonia, urinary infection, and bacterial diarrhea.

Although meningitis is the most important infection that must be diagnosed in the febrile child, SBIs other than meningitis often can be detected with a thorough physical examination accompanied by specific laboratory and radiological tests. In this regard, extensive guidelines were published in 1993 by the American College of Emergency Physicians concerning appropriate evaluation and management of children with suspected serious infections including cellulitis, omphalitis, sepsis, infectious diarrhea, septic arthritis, pneumonia, and osteomyelitis.[41] According to these guidelines, pneumonia and urinary infections stand out as important common infections that may present with subtle features.

Meningitis. The incidence of meningitis has declined significantly since the introduction of a vaccine that is effective against *Haemophilus influenzae* in the mid-1980s. Overall, the incidence of *H. influenzae*, once the most common organism causing meningitis, has declined by more than 90% in immunized children and more than 70-80% in unimmunized children.[42-44] Nevertheless, cases of pneumococcal and Neisseria meningitis, as well as occasional cases of *H. influenzae* meningitis, still occur. In the neonate, viral pathogens such as herpes simplex virus (HSV) also must be considered. It should be stressed that the diagnosis of meningitis is facilitated if clinicians are aware that classic findings associated with this condition (i.e., nuchal rigidity, Kernig's and Brudzinski's signs) are not consistently present until children reach the age of 2 years.

Signs and symptoms. Signs of meningitis are extremely subtle in infants younger than 3 months of age. In fact, up to 10% of infants with meningitis in this age group may appear clinically well on initial examination; only 15% manifest a bulging fontanelle, and 10-15% have nuchal rigidity. Irritability, altered sleep patterns, vom-

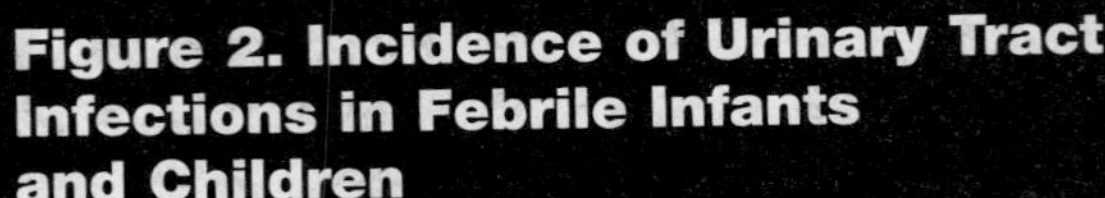

Figure 2. Incidence of Urinary Tract Infections in Febrile Infants and Children

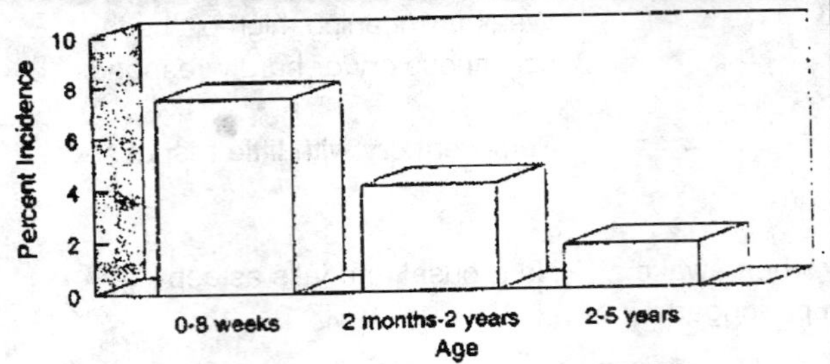

Adapted from: Sclager TA, Lor JA. Urinary tract infection in outpatient febrile infants and children younger than 5 years of age. *Pediatr Ann* 1993;22:505.

iting, a high-pitched cry, or decreased oral intake may be the only symptoms at this age.[45,46] Because up to 1% of all infants with fever greater than 38°C (100.4°F) harbor meningitis,[47] a lumbar puncture is usually recommended for all children in this age group who have a fever, regardless of clinical examination.

Observation variables and CNS-specific symptoms are more useful in identifying meningitis in patients 3-24 months of age.[32] Vomiting, irritability, and lethargy are typical symptoms encountered in meningitis when it occurs in these children. In fact, almost all patients between 3 and 24 months of age with bacterial meningitis will manifest one of the following: meningeal signs, lethargy or coma, or a toxic or moribund state.[5] In infants younger than 12 months of age who have this condition confirmed, lethargy or coma (present in 80%) occur more frequently than meningeal signs (72%).[5]

History. While most children with meningitis manifest meningeal signs or an alteration in mental status, although up to 23% may not have a fever on initial presentation.[48] Furthermore, a large number of children with meningitis at this age have a coexisting upper respiratory infection, with otitis media occurring in 20-30% of individuals and pharyngitis in 5%.[49] These associated conditions may help explain why as many as 30-50% of children younger than 24 months of age with bacterial meningitis have seen a physician in the week prior to their presentation. A significant percentage of these children were initially diagnosed with a trivial illness and many started on oral antibiotics.[49]

Yale Observation Scale. While most signs and symptoms of meningitis are nonspecific and open to subjective interpretation, an objective scale—the Yale Observation Scale—has been evaluated that may assist in determining a whether children between the ages of 3 and 36 months are at high risk of having meningitis or some other serious illness. Although this scale has shown some utility, it is not completely accurate in identifying ill children, and errors will be made if this is the only tool used to identify children with serious illness.[40] *(See Table 2.)*

A total score of less than 11 signifies a less than 3% probability of serious illness. A score of 11-15 signifies a 26% probability of serious illness, and a total score of greater than 15 signifies a greater than 92% probability of serious illness.[43] In one recent study, children with meningitis had a mean Yale Observation Scale of 18, whereas febrile children without serious infection had a mean score of 7-8.[32]

Urinary Tract Infections. Urinary tract infections (UTIs) are a frequent cause of fever in young children, occurring with increased frequency in younger age groups. *(See Figure 2.)* Making the diagnosis is extremely important inasmuch as recurrence rates are 30%, 60%, and 70% following a first, second, and third episode of UTI, respectively.[50,51] Moreover, UTIs can progress to overwhelming sepsis. From 3-25% of children with UTI may have an anatomic obstruction such as posterior urethral valves, ureteropelvic junction obstruction, ureterovesical junction obstruction, or a ureterocele.[51] Vesicoureteral reflux, which occurs in 30-50% of children with UTI, may predispose to renal scarring during years (age 0-5 years) in which renal growth is occurring.[51] Sequelae of renal scarring include renal insufficiency, hypertension, and growth failure. Consequently, it is extremely important to make the diagnosis of UTI in children and to provide follow-up so that the urinary tract can be evaluated for anatomic abnormalities.[50]

Signs and Symptoms. Signs and symptoms of UTIs can be extremely subtle in children. In this regard, a recent series noted the following nonspecific symptoms in children younger than 3 years of age with UTI: irritability (80%), poor feeding (65%), vomiting (40%), diarrhea (30%), cough (< 10-20%), and nasal discharge (< 10-20%). Each of these symptoms occurred with equal frequency in febrile children with and without UTIs. Consequently, these findings are of little help in differentiating between children with and without UTI.[51] Nearly 9% of females with a fever of 39°C or more had a UTI, whereas 7.5% of all patients with fever and no source, 3.5% with fever and otitis media, and 1.5% with fever and an unequivocal source (i.e., pneumonia) had a UTI.[51]

Even above age 2, meningeal signs can be subtle. In this regard, although most patients in this age group have vomiting, headache, photophobia, and stiff neck, about 1-2% do not manifest these classic signs and symptoms of meningitis.[52]

Diagnosis. A urinalysis alone is not reliable in diagnosing a UTI (proven by culture). A positive urine Gram's stain is the most reliable immediate test for UTIs (sensitivity, 94-99%).[53] A urinalysis on unspun specimens with any white blood cells is 77% sensitive, more than five WBCs per high power field (HPF) is 54% sensitive, the presence of any bacteria is 86% sensitive, and positive leukocyte esterase, positive nitrates, or more than five WBC/HPF is 75-85% sensitive in detecting a UTI.[51] Thus, regardless of the initial urinalysis, obtain a urine culture in all children suspected of UTI.

Pneumonia. Generally speaking, pneumonia in children is most often due to viral infection (e.g., respiratory syncytial virus, parainfluenza viruses types 1, 2, or 3, adenoviruses, influenza A, or mycoplasma infection). These agents accounted for 86% of all isolates in one study, although concurrent or subsequent bacterial infection occurs in up to 20% of cases.[54]

The peak incidence of pneumonia in the pediatric age group is during the winter and early spring. This period corresponds with outbreaks of influenza and other viral epidemics, which tend to have their highest prevalence in 2- to 4-year-olds.[55] Other risk factors for childhood pneumonia include ambient cigarette smoke, perinatal infections, immunocompromised state, chronic disease such as cystic fibrosis, children at risk for aspiration (feeding difficulties, neuromuscular weakness, or gastroesophageal reflux), and absence of pertussis immunization.[55]

Table 3. Utility of Tachypnea as a Sign of Pneumonia

AGE GROUP	TACHYPNEA	SENSITIVITY*	NEGATIVE PREDICTIVE VALUE†
0-5 months	≥ 59	85%	99%
6-11 months	≥ 52	67%	98%
11-23 months	≥ 42	71%	96%

* Percent of all pneumonia detected with defined age cutoff for tachypnea.
† Probability that there will be no pneumonia if tachypnea is absent.

Age 0-3 Months. In the first week of life, pneumonia usually is caused by such perinatally acquired organisms as Group B Streptococcus and gram-negative enteric organisms. Unfortunately, newborns with bacterial pneumonia often have few specific signs, among them, mild tachypnea, irritability, lethargy, and poor feeding. Temperature deviation—usually hypothermia rather than fever—bradycardia or tachycardia, and apnea or tachypnea should trigger a search for pneumonia. Of special diagnostic importance is the fact that pleural effusions, skin pustules, rapid progression, and purulent conjunctivitis appearing during the first few weeks suggest staphylococcal pneumonia.[5]

After the first month of life, *Chlamydia trachomatis* is a common cause of afebrile pneumonia, which usually develops between the third and 12th week. Infants with chlamydial pneumonia usually are afebrile and present with progressive nasal congestion, tachypnea, and a staccato cough. The presence of bilateral conjunctivitis in combination with an afebrile pneumonia also should suggest the diagnosis of chlamydia pneumonia. Toxicity or signs of severe illness are rare. The chest radiograph usually reveals hyperinflation and diffuse bilateral infiltrates. Pertussis is another important cause of acute bronchitis in this age group and is occasionally complicated by bacterial pneumonia.[55]

In the past, a chest radiograph was recommended as a routine part of the workup of all infants younger than 3 months of age with fever. However, the clinical examination can be used to determine the necessity for chest radiographs. Generally speaking, a radiograph is not necessary for febrile infants in this age group who have no respiratory signs and symptoms, since the probability of having pneumonia in this subgroup is less than 1%.[56] High-yield findings that indicate a 60% probability of pneumonia at in this age bracket include rales, intercostal retractions, or wheezing.[56] Any of the following also may indicate pneumonia and suggest the need for a chest x-ray: rhonchi, retractions, tachypnea, coryza, grunting, stridor, nasal flaring, or cough.[56] Almost without exception, infants younger than 2 months of age with a pneumonia require admission and IV antibiotics effective against the most common organisms.[55]

Pneumonia in children older than 3 months. Most cases of pneumonia in children between 3 months and 8 years of age are due to viral infection or mycoplasma. *Streptococcus pneumoniae* is the most common bacterial etiology, followed by *H. influenzae*, Bordatella pertussis, and *Staphylococcus aureus*. Nearly half of all cases of *H. influenzae* pneumonia have concurrent otitis media, meningitis, or epiglottitis. In children 8 years of age or older, *Mycoplasma pneumoniae* increasingly becomes an important etiologic agent, followed by *S. pneumoniae*; viral infections and *H. influenzae* are less common.[55]

High-yield findings associated with abnormal radiographs (and pneumonia) in children older than 3 months of age include tachypnea, which is associated with the highest overall sensitivity *(see Table 3)*, rales (33% chance of abnormal chest radiograph), cyanosis, dullness to percussion, decreased breath sounds, and difficulty breathing (suggested by nasal flaring and retractions).[57-59] Low-yield findings include wheezing, prolonged expiration, and rhonchi.[57,58] While these criteria for plain films are not all-inclusive, they should serve as a general guide to ordering chest radiographs.

A major problem with interpreting chest x-rays in children is that the radiographic appearance may not help discriminate between viral and bacterial pneumonia. In fact, 20-40% of children with interstitial infiltrates on chest radiography may have a bacterial rather than viral etiology for their pneumonia.[60] Conversely, a significant number of cases with lobar infiltrates may by due to viral infection.[60] One reason is that lobar or segmental atelectasis, which occurs with pediatric viral pneumonia, is easily mistaken for consolidation. Furthermore, radiographic interpretation is highly subjective, with studies showing poor correlations between interpretations given by radiologists (blinded to the clinical features), non-blinded radiologists, and examining physicians.[61]

Occult Bacteremia

Occult bacteremia (OB) is defined as a positive blood culture in the setting of a well-appearing febrile child in the absence of an apparent focus of infection. Generally speaking, the highest age incidence of OB is observed in children 6-24 months old, although cases do occur outside this range. The most common organisms include *S. pneumoniae* and *H. influenzae*, although with the recent introduction of the *H. influenzae* vaccine, the incidence of *H. influenzae* bacteremia has dropped dramatically.[6] *(See Figure 3 and Figure 4.)*

The incidence of OB has been reported at 3-6% in febrile children 3-36 months of age.[6,7] However, many studies citing a high incidence of bacteremia were simple chart reviews, many of which were limited by the inclusion of children who were ill-appearing or had serious bacterial infections when their blood cultures were obtained, a profile that would have falsely overestimated the incidence of this disorder.[6,7]

Including about 6700 consecutive febrile children, the largest prospective study of OB ever published found that the incidence of OB was about 2.8%.[62] Well-appearing children with upper respiratory infections, otitis media, diarrhea, and wheezing also were included in this study and were found to have a similar incidence of OB com-

Figure 3. Occult Bacteremia Before 1991

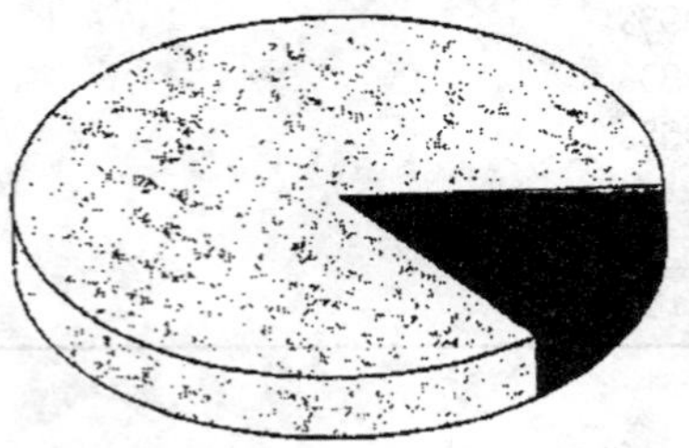

85%: *S. pneumoniae*

< 1: *N. meningitidis*, *Salmonella*, others

< 15%: *H. influenzae*

Adapted from: Harper MB, Fleisher GR. Occult bacteremia in the 3 month old to 3 year old age group. *Pediatr Ann* 1993;22:484-493.

Figure 4. Occult Bacteremia in 1995 (Estimated)

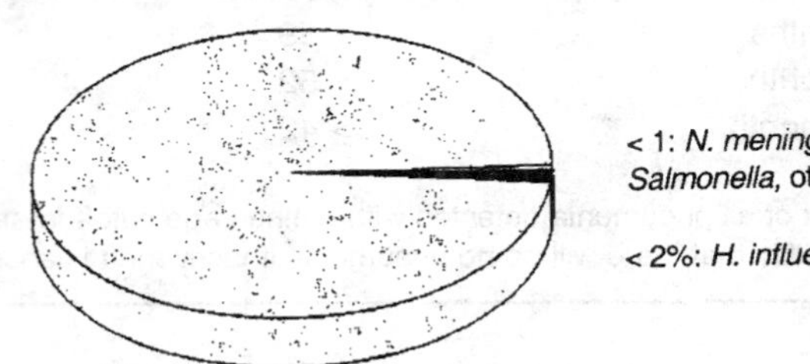

Adapted from: Harper MB, Fleisher GR. Occult bacteremia in the 3 month old to 3 year old age group. *Pediatr Ann* 1993;22:484-493; Adams WG, Deaver KA, Cochi SL et al. Decline of childhood *Haemophilus influenzae* type b (Hib) disease in the Hib vaccine era. *JAMA* 1993;269:221-226; Broadhurst LE, Erickson RL, Kelley PW. Decreases in invasive *Haemophilus influenzae* diseases in US Army children, 1984 through 1991. *JAMA* 1993;269:227-231; Vadheim CM, Greenberg DP, Eriksen E, et al. Eradication of *Haemophilus influenzae* type b disease in Southern California. *Arch Pediatr Adolesc Med* 1994;148:51-56.

pared to those with no apparent source of infection.[62] However, it has been suggested by some authors that children with a minor source (e.g., upper respiratory infections, otitis media) and bacteremia develop serious bacterial infections less frequently than children with no apparent focus of infection.[8,9]

Outcomes in Children with OB. Most cases of OB will clear spontaneously without treatment. However, a subset of bacteremic children will develop serious infections—most importantly, meningitis. A recently published meta-analysis study of patients with OB found that parenteral antibiotics, when administered at the time the blood culture was obtained, were effective in decreasing the risk of meningitis in children with *H. influenzae* OB from 25% to less than 1%.[7] Oral antibiotics were found to be much less effective in preventing sequelae from *H. influenzae* bacteremia.[7] Fortunately, the incidence of *H. influenzae* disease has markedly decreased and is of less concern in fully immunized children.[42-44]

For cases of OB due to *S. pneumoniae*, the risk of progressing to meningitis fell from 6% to less than 1% when either oral or parenteral antibiotics were administered at the time the blood culture was obtained.[7] More recently, this meta-analysis was repeated, excluding studies of ill-appearing children, admitted children, and children who underwent spinal taps (ill-appearing children who underwent a procedure known to seed the CSF) on their initial physician encounter. This repeat meta-analysis found that the risk of *S. pneumoniae* bacteremia progressing to meningitis was less than 3% and that oral antibiotics were not effective in preventing meningitis.[63]

Summary

Fever is a common complaint in infants and children brought to the ED. Although many parents may believe that fever in and of itself can be harmful, there are no adverse consequences from a fever in normal children without serious bacterial infections. Physicians should recognize the limitations of the physical examination for detecting UTIs, pneumonia, and meningitis in febrile infants and children. Although observation variables (e.g., Yale Observation Score) may be useful in identifying those at risk for serious infections such as meningitis and sepsis, they are much more limited in detecting pneumonia and UTIs. An understanding of these factors will improve the emergency physician's ability to diagnose and detect serious infections in infants and children.

References

1. Nelson DS, Walsh K, Fleisher G. Spectrum and frequency of pediatric illness presenting to a general community hospital emergency department. *Pediatrics* 1992;90:1-10.
2. Kramer MS, Naimark L, Leduc DG. Parental fever phobia and its correlates. *Pediatrics* 1984;75:1110-1113.
3. May A, Bauchner H. Fever phobia: The pediatrician's contribution. *Pediatrics* 1992;90:851-854.
4. Kelly-Walsh C, Nelson DB, Smith DS, et al. Clinical predictors of bacterial versus aseptic meningitis in childhood. *Ann Emerg Med* 1992;21:910-914.
5. Baraff LJ. Management of infants and children 3 to 36 months of age with fever without source. *Pediatr Ann* 1993;22:497-504.
6. Harper MB, Fleisher GR. Occult bacteremia in the 3 month old to 3 year old age group. *Pediatr Ann* 1993;22:484-493.
7. Baraff LJ, Oslund S, Prather M. Effect of antibiotic therapy and etiologic microorganisms on the risk of bacterial meningitis in children with occult bacteremia. *Pediatrics* 1993;92: 140-143.
8. Long SS. Antibiotic therapy in febrile children: "Best-laid schemes . . ." *J Pediatr* 1994;124:585-588.
9. Cox RD, Wagner M, Woolard DJ. Infants and children with fever without source. *Ann Emerg Med* 1994;23:598-600.
10. Kluger MJ. Fever revisited. *Pediatrics* 1992;90:846-851.
11. Yarbrough B. Heat Illness. In: Rosen, ed. *Emergency Medicine: Concepts and Clinical Practice*. 3rd ed. St. Louis: Mosby Yearbook, Inc; 1993:946-964.
12. McCarthy PL. The febrile infant. *Pediatrics* 1994;94:

396-397.

13. Cheng TL, Partridge JC. Effect of bundling and high environmental temperature on neonatal body temperature. *Pediatrics* 1993;92:238-240.
14. Baraff LJ. Management of the febrile child: A survey of pediatric and emergency medicine residency directors. *Pediatr Infect Dis J* 1991;10:795-800.
15. Bonadio WA. Defining fever and other aspects of body temperature in infants and children. *Pediatr Ann* 1993;22: 467-473.
16. Milewski A, Ferguson KL, Terndrup TE. Comparison of pulmonary artery, rectal, and tympanic membrane temperatures in adult intensive care unit patients. *Clin Pediatr* 1991;30: Suppl 13-16.
17. Murna BK, Treloar DJ, Wurmlinger K, et al. Comparison of rectal, axillary, and tympanic membrane temperatures in infants and young children. *Ann Emerg Med* 1991;20:41-44.
18. Brennan DF, Falk JL, Rothrock SG, et al. Reliability of infrared tympanic thermometry in the detection of rectal fever in children. *Ann Emerg Med* 1995;25:21-30.
19. Webb GE. Comparison of esophageal and tympanic temperature during cardiopulmonary bypass. *Anesth Analg* 1973;52: 729-733.
20. Tandberg D, Sklar D. Effect of tachypnea on the estimation of body temperature by an oral thermometer. *N Engl J Med* 1983;308:945-946.
21. Beach PS, McCormick P. Clinical applications of ear thermometry. *Clin Pediatr* 1991;30:Suppl 3-5.
22. Terndrup TE. An appraisal of temperature assessment by infrared emission detection tympanic thermometry. *Ann Emerg Med* 1992;21:1483-1492.
23. Terndrup TE, Milewski A. The performance of two tympanic thermometers in a pediatric emergency department. *Clin Pediatr* 1991;30:Suppl 18-23.
24. Kenney RD, Fortenberry JD, Surratt SS, et al. Evaluation of an infrared tympanic membrane thermometer in pediatric patients. *Pediatrics* 1990;85:854-858.
25. Terndrup TE, Wong A. Influence of otitis media on the correlation between rectal and auditory canal temperatures. *Am J Dis Child* 1991;145:75-78.
26. Nypaver M, Ziesserl E, Nachtsheim B, et al. Tympanic membrane thermometers. Caveat emptor. *Am J Dis Child* 1991; 145:403.
27. Schmitt BD. Behavioral aspects of temperature taking. *Clin Pediatr* 1991;Suppl:8-10.
28. Kramer MS. Risks and benefits of paracetamol antipyresis in young children with fever of presumed viral origin. *Lancet* 1991;337:591.
29. Fruthaler GJ. Fever in children: Phobia vs. facts. *Hosp Pract* 1985;20(11A):49-53.
30. Berg AT. Are febrile seizures provoked by a rapid rise in temperature. *Am J Dis Child* 1993;147:1101-1103.
31. Steele RW. Oral antipyretic therapy. *Am J Dis Child* 1972;123:204.
32. Baker RC, Tiller T, Baucher JC, et al. Severity of disease correlated with fever reduction in febrile infants. *Pediatrics* 1989;83:1016-1019.
33. Rothrock SG, Green SM. Fever response to acetaminophen. *Am J Emerg Med* 1995;13:98-100.
34. Banco L, Veltri D. Ability of mothers to subjectively assess the presence of fever in their children. *Am J Dis Child* 1985;138:976-978.
35. Banco L, Jayashekaramurthy S. The ability of mothers to read a thermometer. *Clin Pediatr* 1990;29:343-345.
36. Friedman AD. Efficacy of sponging vs acetaminophen for reduction of fever. *Pediatr Emerg Care* 1990;6:6.
37. Walson PD. Ibuprofen, acetaminophen, and placebo treatment of febrile children. *Clin Pharmacol Ther* 1989;46:9.
38. Amdekar YK. Antipyretic activity of ibuprofen and paracetamol (Tylenol) in children with pyrexia. *Br J Clin* Pract 1985; 39:140-143.
39. Jaskiewicz JA, McCarthy CA. Evaluation and management of the febrile infant 60 days of age or younger. *Pediatr Ann* 1993;22:477-482.
40. McCarthy PL, Sharp MR, Spiesel SZ, et al. Observation scales to identify serious illness in febrile children. *Pediatrics* 1982;70:802-809.
41. American College of Emergency Physicians. Clinical policy for the initial approach to children under the age of 2 years presenting with fever. *Ann Emerg Med* 1993;22:628-637.
42. Adams WG, Deaver KA, Cochi SL et al. Decline of childhood *Haemophilus influenzae* type b (Hib) disease in the Hib vaccine era. *JAMA* 1993;269:221-226.
43. Broadhurst LE, Erickson RL, Kelley PW. Decreases in invasive *Haemophilus influenzae* diseases in US Army children, 1984 through 1991. *JAMA* 1993;269:227-231.
44. Vadheim CM, Greenberg DP, Eriksen E, et al. Eradication of *Haemophilus influenzae* type b disease in Southern California. *Arch Pediatr Adolesc Med* 1994;148:51-56.
45. Lipton JD, Schafermeyer RW. Evolving concepts in pediatric bacterial meningitis—Part I. Pathophysiology and diagnosis. *Ann Emerg Med* 1993;22:1602-1615.
46. Lipton JD, Schafermeyer RW. Evolving concepts in pediatric bacterial meningitis—Part II. Management and therapeutic research. *Ann Emerg Med* 1993;22:1616-1629.
47. Baraff LJ, Oslund SA, Schriger DL, et al. Probability of bacterial infections in febrile infants less than three months of age: A meta-analysis. *Pediatr Infect Dis* J 1992;11:257-265.
48. Bonadio WA. Defining fever and other aspects of body temperature in infants and children. *Pediatr Ann* 1993;22: 467-473.
49. Rothrock SG, Green SM. Pediatric bacterial meningitis: Is preliminary antibiotic therapy associated with an altered clinical presentation. *Ann Emerg Med* 1992;21:146-154.
50. Schlager TA, Lor JA. Urinary tract infection in outpatient febrile infants and children younger than 5 years of age. *Pediatr Ann* 1993;22:505-509.
51. Hoberman A, Chao HP, Keller DM, et al. Prevalence of urinary tract infection in febrile infants. *J Pediatr* 1993;123: 17-23.
52. Callaham M. Fulminant bacterial meningitis without meningeal signs. *Ann Emerg Med* 1989;18:90-93.
53. Lockhart GR, Lewander WJ, Cimini DM, et al. Use of urinary gram stain for detection of urinary tract infection in infants. *Ann Emerg Med* 1995;25:31-35.
54. Murphy TF, Henderson FW, Clyde WA, et al. Pneumonia:

An 11-year study in a pediatric practice. *Am J Epidemiol* 1981;113:12.
55. Barkin R, Dwyer BJ. Managing the unique challenge of pediatric pneumonia. *Emerg Med Rep* 1987;8:89-96.
56. Bramson RT, Meyer TL, Silbiger ML, et al. The futility of the chest radiograph in the febrile infant without respiratory symptoms. *Pediatrics* 1993;92:524-526.
57. Zukin DD, Hoffman JR, Cleveland RH, et al. Correlation of pulmonary signs and symptoms with chest radiographs in the pediatric age group. *Ann Emerg Med* 1986;15:792-796.
58. Grossman LK, Caplan SE. Clinical, laboratory, and radiological information in the diagnosis of pneumonia in children. *Ann Emerg Med* 1988;17:43-46.
59. Taylor JA, Del Beccaro M, Done S, et al. Establishing clinically relevant standards for tachypnea in febrile children younger than 2 years. *Arch Pediatr Adolesc Med* 1995;149: 283-287.
60. Courtoy I. Lande AE, Turner RB. Accuracy of radiographic differentiation of bacterial from nonbacterial pneumonia. *Clin Pediatr* 1989;28:261-265.
61. Kramer MS, Roberts-Bauer R, Williams RL. Bias and overcall in interpreting chest radiographs in young febrile children. *Pediatrics* 1992;90:11-13.
62. Fleisher GR, Rosenberg N, Vinci R, et al. Intramuscular versus oral antibiotic therapy for the prevention of meningitis and other bacterial sequelae in young, febrile children at risk for occult bacteremia. *J Pediatr* 1994;124:504-512.
63. Rothrock SG, Green SM, Clark M, et al. Do oral antibiotics prevent meningitis in children with occult pneumococcal bacteremia? A meta-analysis. *Acad Emerg Med* 1995;2:A.

Current Management Guidelines for the Febrile Child

Steven G. Rothrock, MD, FACEP
Steven M. Green, MD, FACEP

A fever in children is often a cause of great concern for both parents and health care professionals. This chapter on the febrile child reviews specific clinical scenarios, including the management of febrile children younger than 3 months, children with suspected occult bacteremia (OB), and children between the ages of 3 and 36 months with fever but no apparent source. Controversies within these areas, as well as recently published guidelines that attempt to standardize management of febrile children, also are reviewed.[1,2]

Each of these topics is discussed in detail, with an emphasis on current guidelines that have been generated for diagnosis and management of children with OB, febrile infants younger than 3 months of age, and other important disorders that are encountered in febrile children. This chapter presents specific clinical strategies that will improve care, guide diagnostic evaluation, increase cost-effectiveness, and improve patient outcomes.

Management of Specific Clinical Scenarios

The Febrile Young Infant (0-3 months of age). Stratifying the Risk of Serious Bacterial Infection. Prior to the late 1980s, almost all infants less than 3 months of age with a temperature greater than 38°C (100.4°F) were admitted to the hospital and treated with IV antibiotics.[3] Studies show that 7-9% of nontoxic-appearing febrile infants in this age group harbor serious bacterial infections.[3] As might be expected, those patients who are toxic have a much higher risk of serious bacterial infection and should be admitted to the hospital and treated with antibiotics. The choice of antimicrobial agent should be specific to the site of infection and most common infecting organisms; if no source is identified on initial evaluation, a combination of ampicillin and cefotaxime (or ceftriaxone) should be employed. However, if certain criteria are present *(see Table 1)*, and the infant appears non-toxic, the risk of having a serious bacterial infection falls substantially.[3]

Outpatient Management of Well-Appearing Infants. The safety of outpatient treatment of nontoxic febrile infants less than 3 months of age who meet all Rochester criteria has been verified in several prospective studies.[4-6] *(See Table 2.)* Generally, less than 1% of children meeting these criteria will develop a serious bacterial infection.[4-6] Moreover, nearly all serious infections will be detected on follow-up examination, and if a single injection of ceftriaxone (50 mg/kg IM) is administered to infants who are discharged, adverse sequelae will be negligible.[5,6] A single study has demonstrated that management of febrile, nontoxic, low-risk infants without antibiotic therapy also may be safe.[4] Further verification of this approach is necessary before management of all nontoxic febrile infants without antibiotics can be recommended.

Table 1. Appearance of Infants and Incidence of Infectious Disorders[3]

APPEARANCE	BACTEREMIA	SBI*	MENINGITIS
Nontoxic	1%	9%	1%
Nontoxic + low-risk criteria**	1%	< 1%	0.5%
Toxic	10%	17%	4%
Toxic + not meeting criteria**	13%	24%	4%

* SBI = serious bacterial infection
** criteria = Rochester criteria

Table 2. Rochester Criteria

1. Reliable parents and 24-hour follow-up
2. Non-toxic-appearing, born full-term
3. Previously healthy, no current antibiotic use
4. WBC of 5000-15,000 cells/mm^3 with < 1500 bands
5. Stool WBC < 5 per high-power field if diarrhea
6. Normal chest x-ray (may not be necessary in all patients)
7. Normal urinalysis or urine Gram's stain
8. Normal cerebrospinal fluid

Observation Variables in Young Infants

One of the most critical and difficult components on the Rochester criteria is evaluation of a young infant's appearance. As might be expected, many physicians are uncomfortable evaluating children in this age group, inasmuch as distinguishing between the appearance of ill and well children is especially difficult in younger infants. Although the Yale Observation Scale (YOS) is unreliable for evaluating infants less than 8 weeks old,[7] a Young Infant Observation Scale has been described for infants less than 8-12 weeks of age.[8]

In this scale, infants are graded 1 (no compromise), 3 (moderate compromise), and 5 (severe compromise) with respect to three variables: 1) affect; 2) respiratory effort/status; and 3) peripheral perfusion. A single study using this scale found that a total score of less than 7 indicated a 4% probability of having a serious bacterial infection, while a total score greater than 7 indicated a 40% probability of serious infection.[8] Before this scale can be recommended for routine use, it must be verified in larger, more diverse clinical settings.

Does the Degree of Temperature Elevation Matter at this Age? Another important feature in children less than 3 months of age is the degree of temperature elevation. Generally speaking, higher temperature elevations are associated with a greater risk of harboring a serious bacterial infection; therefore, clinicians should have a lower threshold for admission and initiation of empiric antibiotic therapy in this patient subgroup.[9,10]

History of Fever but Fever Not Documented in the ED. A common problem is the infant with a reported fever at home who is afebrile on presentation to the ED. In this situation, an important question to ask the parent is: How was the temperature documented?

For the infant with a documented rectal temperature greater than 38°C (100.4°F), the number who subsequently develop a fever is high (90%), and this subgroup has a high incidence of serious bacterial infections (10-15%).[12,13] Accordingly, all infants in this age group require a complete septic evaluation (lumbar puncture, CBC, urinalysis, blood and urine culture), while all ill-appearing infants and all infants less than 4 weeks old should be admitted to the hospital. Infants in the 4- to 12-week age range should be assessed according to the Rochester criteria.[10,11,13] For infants with a "history" of fever, but no documented temperature elevation at home, the risk of subsequently developing a fever and serious bacterial infection is low (0-4%).[13] Furthermore, virtually all serious bacterial infections will be detected on septic evaluation.[13] Of interest, one study noted that all infants 0-4 weeks of age with a serious bacterial infection had a CBC differential ratio ([% lymphocytes + monocytes] / [% neutrophils + bands]) greater than 1 while all without a serious bacterial infection had a CBC differential ratio less than 1.[13] Since the risk of serious bacterial infection is low, those with a negative work-up who are well-appearing can be safely managed as outpatients with close follow-up and repeat temperature measurement.[12,13]

Infants Younger than 1 Month Old

Many children 1-3 months old with fever can be managed as outpatients, but those less than 1 month of age should still undergo a septic evaluation and admission to the hospital. Although several authors who have examined the Rochester criteria have included children in the 0-1 month age bracket, the data should still be considered is preliminary and incomplete.[6,11] In the future, a subset of febrile infants less than 1 month of age that is appropriate for outpatient therapy may be identified. At present, however, there are no data to support this clinical approach.

Infants 3-24 Months Old

Management of the 3- to 24-month-old child with fever and no major source of infection has generated considerable controversy in the literature. First of all, children in this age range do not consistently manifest nuchal rigidity or other meningeal signs when meningitis is present.[14] Second, they also cannot tell you that they have headaches, earaches, or painful urination. Not surprisingly, this age group is at highest risk for developing occult bacteremia (OB).

Partially Treated Meningitis. One important clinical feature concerning children 3-24 months old is that 30-50% of those patients who are ultimately diagnosed with bacterial meningitis have been seen by a physician within the prior week (usually 1-2 days before) and were diagnosed as having a trivial illness and discharged on oral antibiotics.[15] It follows that these children may have had early meningitis that was missed or OB that progressed to meningitis. The misdiagnosis (or delayed diagnosis) of meningitis is the most common reason that physicians in pediatric EDs are sued, and this condition accounts for the largest percentage of dollars awarded in pediatric malpractice cases.[15]

Misdiagnosed children were generally discharged from EDs and clinics with such diagnoses as upper respiratory infections, otitis media, or gastroenteritis. Furthermore, children with meningitis who had been placed on oral antibiotics were less ill-appearing, more likely to have upper respiratory signs and symptoms, and less likely to manifest fever. Thus, prior treatment with oral antibiotics masks the presentation of meningitis at this age.[15]

Febrile Older Children

Management decisions regarding febrile children older than 24-36 months of age are easier than those for the younger child. First, in this older age range, typical physical findings of meningitis are reliable and children who are bacteremic usually become bacteremic only after developing bacterial infections from a specific site (e.g., cellulitis, pneumonia, urinary tract infections). Obviously, the clinician must search diligently for the source of a fever; however, assessment relies on both objective criteria and findings on physical examination.

Occult Bacteremia

Features Identifying Patients With OB. Because of its potential to progress to meningitis or other serious bacterial infections, OB has received considerable attention in the medical literature.[1,2] This attention is characterized by several published guidelines that attempt to direct care of the potentially bacteremic child.[1,2] In this regard, several clinical parameters have been suggested to help identify patients with a significant risk of having OB. These include: the degree of temperature elevation, immunization status (and overall immune status), the age of the child, the presence or absence of a major or minor source of infection, the white blood cell (WBC) count, other blood tests, blood cultures, and the appearance of the child.

Degree of Temperature Elevation. In the past, the incidence of bacteremia in well-appearing children (3-36 months of age) with a temperature greater than 39°C (102.2°F) has been reported at 3-6%.[2,16] However, this number was actually found to be approximately 2.8% in the largest study of OB.[17] In fact, if children with Haemophilus influenzae are excluded (i.e., if only children who are fully immunized against *H. influenzae* are considered), the incidence of bacteremia falls to less than 2.5%.[17] The risk of a child who is fully immunized against *H. influenzae* developing a serious bacterial infection or meningitis from bacteremia parallels that of OB at different temperatures. *(See Table 3.)*

It is apparent that even at very high temperatures (i.e., > 41°C [105.8°F]), the vast majority (> 90%) of well-appearing children still are not bacteremic and will not develop a serious bacterial infection or meningitis.

Because the risk of bacteremia rises in patients with temperatures greater than 39°C (102.2°F), some authors, including a recent expert panel, recommend obtaining a blood culture (and initiating empiric antibiotic therapy) on all patients with a temperature above this level.[2] However, this approach has been questioned by other investigators.[18,19]

Although the degree of temperature elevation is important, reliance on this parameter alone will not detect all cases of bacteremia. Bacteremia due to *H. influenzae* and *Streptococcus pneumoniae* still occurs at lower temperatures, with up to 13% of children who are bacteremic from these organisms being afebrile on presentation to the ED.[20] On the other hand, a persistent fever after 48 hours of antibiotic therapy is associated with an increased risk of bacteremia and serious bacterial infection.[21]

Table 3. Association of Temperature and Outcome of Bacteremia[17]

TEMPERATURE	RISK OF BACTEREMIA	RISK OF MENINGITIS	RISK OF SBI
39.0-39.4°C	1.6%	0.04%	< 0.2%
39.5-40.0°C	2.8%	0.07%	< 0.3%
40.0-40.4°C	3.7%	0.09%	< 0.4%
40.5-40.9°C	3.8%	0.1%	< 0.4%
≥ 41°C 9	3%	0.25%	< 1%

* Estimation of meningitis and SBI risk based on fully immunized child.

Age of the Child. Prior studies of OB have found that most children who are bacteremic are between the ages of 6 and 18 months.[22] Those who are less than 6 months old retain protective maternal antibodies against common organisms, while those who are more than 18-24 months old are more immune competent and, therefore, are less at risk for developing bacteremia. However, the drop-off in the incidence of bacteremia noted by several authors may be misleading, since clinicians may not look as aggressively for bacteremia in children who are in the 24- to 36- month age bracket.

The White Blood Cell Count. The WBC has been promoted as a useful tool for detecting OB in well-appearing children. Published guidelines recommend a WBC cutoff of greater than 15,000 cells/mm^3 as a threshold for obtaining a blood culture and considering empiric antibiotic therapy.[2] However, this cutoff as a trigger to culture and treat misses up to 35% of bacteremic children.[23] Furthermore, the positive predictive value (PPV; the number of children with a WBC at or above that level [WBC count] who actually have bacteremia) of this cutoff is less than 10% (i.e., > 10 children who are not bacteremic will be treated for every 1 truly bacteremic child).[23] While a lower WBC cutoff of 10,000 cells/mm^3 would detect 92% cases of bacteremia, the PPV falls to less than 3% (i.e., > 30 children who are not bacteremic will be treated as bacteremic for every 1 truly bacteremic child).[2,23] *(See Table 4.)* Finally, the addition of a WBC count to the work-up of every febrile child (whose temperature is > 39°C [102.2°F]) may cause delays in treatment and added expense while contributing little useful information to the evaluation of the well-appearing child.

Other problems with the WBC count exist. For example, in one series, less than 20% of children with *Neisseria meningitides* bacteremia had an elevated WBC count, rendering the test useless in this setting.[24] *H. influenzae* type b bacteremia also does not consistently elevate the WBC count, with only 50-70% showing a WBC greater than 15,000 cells/mm^3.[25,26] In contrast, pneumococcal bacteremia elevates the WBC count to a level greater than 15,000 cells/mm^3 in up to 75% of cases.[27,28]

Other Laboratory Tests. The C-reactive protein and erythrocyte sedimentation rate (ESR) also have been evaluated for utility in detecting OB. An ESR of greater than 30 mm/h or an elevated C-reactive protein (> 0.8 mg/dL) denotes a 10-15% incidence of bacteremia in a febrile child.[29,30] Unfortunately, the high rate of false-positives and false-negatives limits the use of either of these tests for detecting OB. Serum interleukin-6 levels have recently been assessed for utility in detecting bacterial infections. In one small study includ-

Table 4. Utility of WBC for Detecting Occult Bacteremia[16,23]

WBC COUNT	SENSITIVITY	PPV*
10,000 cells/mm^3 or more	92%	5%
15,000 cells/mm^3 or more	67%	8%
20,000 cells/mm^3 or more	40%	13%
25,000 cells/mm^3 or more	23%	19%

*PPV = positive predictive value; the number of children with a WBC count at or above that level (WBC count) who actually have bacteremia

ing only 20 children, the presence of any serum interleukin-6 was 91% sensitive and 98% specific in detecting serious bacterial infections.[31] However, use of this test in detecting OB has not been thoroughly evaluated, and its use is still considered experimental.[31]

Blood Cultures. Blood cultures remain the gold standard for identifying children with bacteremia. Unfortunately, several problems exist with this. First, the average time for cultures to return as positive varies from 24 to 48 hours, which is too late to make initial treatment decisions. Furthermore, more than two-thirds of positive cultures are actually false positives.[32] One recent study found that for true positive blood cultures, 15% of patients were lost to follow-up, 11% returned to a physician prior to the culture turning positive, 31% followed up due to a scheduled appointment, and in only 42% of children did a true positive result potentially affecting therapy prompt a return visit to see a physician.[32]

Several approaches are available for improving the yield and turnaround time for blood cultures. In this vein, increasing blood volume to 3 mL, and doubling the number of cultures obtained will increase the sensitivity for cultures detecting bacteremia and shorten the time that it takes for a culture to turn positive.[33] The culture technique used is also important. Three commonly used techniques include the BACTEC NR660, the BACTEC 9240 (Becton Dickinson Diagnostic Instrument Systems, Sparks, MD), and the BacT/Alert (Organon Teknika Corporation, Durham, NC). With these three techniques, culture bottles are monitored for positivity by instruments that monitor CO2 released from the culture broth during organism growth and metabolism: One technique relies on infrared spectroscopy (BACTEC NR660), one uses fluorescent CO_2 sensors (BACTEC 9240), and one uses a colorimetric method (BacT/Alert).[34,35] The BACTEC NR660 permits reading for positive cultures one or two times per day, while the alternate methods allow continuous monitoring of culture bottles.[34,35] Therefore, laboratories using the BACTEC NR660 method are significantly slower in reporting positive cultures compared to other methods.

A newer blood culture technique (DIFCO ESP) monitors each culture for any increase or decrease in internal atmospheric pressure caused by gas production or use.[35] This technique has a higher total aerobic culture rate and a significantly decreased mean turnaround time for positive cultures.[35] Clinicians should be aware of the specific culture technique used in their laboratory and discuss upgrading to one of the newer techniques with their laboratory pathologist.

There are other problems associated with reliance on blood cultures to make clinical decisions. For example, most cases of occult pneumococcal bacteremia will clear spontaneously without treatment.[36] Moreover, blood cultures may not identify all children who eventually develop serious infections or become ill. In one recent series, 24% of those without bacteremia who were treated with oral antibiotics required a second physician visit during their illness: About 25% developed diarrhea, vomiting, or a rash, and nearly 2% required hospitalization due to antibiotic-related side effects.[17]

Is There a Minor Source of Infection? Debate exists as to whether children with a fever and otitis media, upper respiratory infection, or diarrhea need evaluation for OB. However, bacteremia occurs in a substantial number of children with these minor infectious sources. In a large series of 6700 children with acute fever and no major infectious source, 12.8% of children with otitis media were bacteremic, although only one patient developed a serious bacterial infection.[17] Others have reported a bacteremia rate for children with otitis media of 3-6%, which is similar to the rate for children with fever and no source.[2,37] However, those with focal minor infection (e.g., otitis media, upper respiratory infection) may have lower serum bacterial concentration (< 100 CFU/mL) and thus may be at lower risk for progression to meningitis and other serious bacterial infection.[22,28,39] Consequently, the rate of serious bacterial infections developing following bacteremia may be lower than that of a child with fever and no source.[17,19]

Observation. While observation variables (e.g., the YOS) may be useful in differentiating ill- from non-ill-appearing children, their use in discriminating between bacteremic and non-bacteremic children is less clear. In a study of fever response to acetaminophen, a YOS of greater than 10 was found to be 68% sensitive and 77% specific for detecting bacteremia.[40] This raised the following question: Were these cases of bacteremia truly occult? More recently, another study found that most children with OB had the lowest possible YOS (i.e., 6) although bacteremic children were more likely to have scores of greater than 6 compared to non-bacteremic children.41 Furthermore, 2.5% of children with a YOS of 6 were bacteremic compared to 4.7% with a YOS of 8 or more and 5.7% with a YOS score of 10 or more, although no cutoff had reliable sensitivity or specificity for detecting bacteremia.[41] *(See Table 5.)* This suggests that there is a subtle influence of OB on observation variables, although this influence has limited clinical utility.

Other Factors. Children who are immunocompromised, including those with leukemia or who are HIV-positive, have a higher risk of having bacteremia than normal children when they develop a fever.[42] Furthermore, children not immunized against *H. influenzae* type b run a higher risk of developing serious bacterial infections from this organism, as it is much more invasive and more likely to progress to meningitis compared to *S. pneumoniae*.[36]

An important factor that often is not considered in evaluating and managing children with febrile illness is the preference of the parents. In general, parents prefer to avoid the short-term "risk" of a painful blood draw, urine catheterization, or antibiotic injection while accepting the long-term, possible "risk" of a serious infection developing.[43,44] An informed explanation of the risks and benefits—careful follow-up—may be appropriate for the parent who wishes to avoid a blood culture and empiric antibiotic therapy for OB.

A final factor that must be considered is the reliability of the patient's parents. Compared to all other patient subgroups, children have the poorest compliance with mandatory follow-up (only 16%) to EDs.[45] Furthermore, caretakers who are younger than 21, without

Table 5. Accuracy of Yale Observation Score for Detecting Occult Bacteremia[41]

YOS	# BACTEREMIC	# NOT BACTEREMIC	SENSITIVITY	SPECIFICITY
6	137	5297 (83%)	71%	17%
≥ 8	55	1122 (17%)	29%	83%
≥ 10	32	522	17%	92%
≥ 12	10	210	6%	97%
≥ 14	1	75	0.5%	99%

a car, and who feel that their child is not ill are significantly less likely to comply with mandatory follow-up from the ED.[46] One method to ensure follow-up is employing a visiting nurse. This approach guarantees follow-up and allows for a health care professional to visit the home and evaluate the infant for improvement or progression of their disease at a specified time.[11]

What if the Culture Results Are Known?

Appropriate management of an infant or child with positive blood cultures depends on the infecting organisms and the clinical appearance of the child. All children with true positive blood cultures should be reevaluated by a physician as soon as possible. Those who appear ill on follow-up should receive a lumbar puncture, chest radiograph, repeat blood culture, and be admitted for IV antibiotics. For the child with *S. pneumoniae* bacteremia who is afebrile, without a focus of infection, and appears well on reevaluation, the risk of invasive disease and persistent bacteremia is extremely low (< 1-2%).[47] Appropriate treatment consists of repeat culture and either an injection of a third-generation cephalosporin (e.g., ceftriaxone) or other antibiotics effective against *S. pneumoniae*.

Children with *H. influenzae* bacteremia have a much higher risk of developing invasive disease. Up to 20% who have a serious infection may appear "improved" on follow-up examination.[48] Therefore, appropriate treatment consists of chest radiography, repeat blood culture, lumbar puncture, admission, and administration of a parenteral third-generation cephalosporin effective against *H. influenzae* regardless of clinical appearance. Treatment of bacteremia due to other organisms (i.e., *N. meningitides* and gram-negative enterics) requires admission with IV antibiotics as these organisms are more likely to cause serious infections.

Guidelines for Managing Febrile Children

Two sets of guidelines for managing febrile children have been published. They are intended to standardize and direct the management of febrile children.

ACEP Guidelines. In 1993, the American College of Emergency Physicians (ACEP) published a *Clinical Policy for the Initial Approach to Children Under the Age of 2 Years Presenting with Fever*.[1] This publication outlines both rules (actions reflecting principles of good practice in most cases that should be performed on all children with specific complaints) and guidelines (lists of recommendations that should be considered but may or may not be performed depending on the patient, the circumstances, or other factors). This clinical policy introduces recommendations and defines a standard of care for children with abnormalities of major organ systems, specific infections, and specific complaints (e.g., children of different ages who have fever without a source).

Stated briefly, ACEP recommends that all children 0-8 weeks of age with a history of fever (rectal temperature > 38°C [100.4°F]) receive a complete blood count (CBC), urinalysis, blood culture, urine culture, chest radiograph, lumbar puncture, and admission. These recommendations are only guidelines if there is a history of fever; however, this work-up is a rule for children with documented fever and age of 0-4 weeks.[1]

For children 1-24 months of age and a fever without a source (with a temperature > 38°C [104°F]), ACEP recommends a thorough head-to-toe examination as a rule.[1] Guidelines to consider, depending on the clinical examination, include the following: glucose, CBC, urinalysis, urine culture, blood culture, chest radiography, lumbar puncture, external cooling if temperature is greater than 40.6°C (105°F), antipyretics, antibiotics, and referral for follow-up within 24 hours if not admitted.[1] Although ACEP recommendations were published to set a standard of care, they are broad and leave considerable leeway for interpretation and implementation. In fact, a computer science method known as decision table analysis used to verify ACEP's practice guidelines found more than 23,000 possible options available for managing febrile children.[49] Furthermore, the guidelines were found to be "illogical, incomplete, and inconsistent," with too many "contradictions and undecidable points."[49]

Expert Panel Guidelines. A second expert panel comprised of pediatric emergency physicians, infectious disease specialists, and pediatricians published recommendations primarily for children 0-3 years old.[2] Their recommendations are much more specific, having been written primarily for children with a fever without a source. Admission is recommended for all infants 0-28 days old with a rectal temperature of 38°C (100.4°F). For those who are 28-90 days old and are well-appearing, the authors recommend adherence to the Rochester criteria for deciding which children can be treated as outpatients. The authors also leave a second option of careful observation and a urine culture with close follow-up for this age group. Furthermore, ceftriaxone should only be administered to those infants who receive a lumbar puncture and blood culture to help distinguish partially treated meningitis and bacteremia from a viral syndrome.[2]

The expert panel's recommendations for children 3-36 months old with a fever without a source are also specific.[2] Non-toxic-appearing children (males < 6 months and females < 2 years) with a temperature of 39°C (102.2°F) or more all should receive a urine culture.[2] Blood cultures and empiric antibiotic therapy (parenteral ceftriaxone 50 mg/kg IM or oral amoxicillin 60 mg/kg/d orally for 3 days) are recommended for all children or only those with WBC counts greater than 15,000 cells/mm^3.[2]

Although these guidelines are much more specific and useful from the standpoint of providing a standard or a reference of how to evaluate these children, several problems exist. First of all, WBC cutoffs are either insensitive or nonspecific for detecting bacteremia. Furthermore, these guidelines were written and published based on studies that found a high incidence of *H. influenzae* bacteremia. As mentioned, *H. influenzae* is much more invasive than *S. pneumoniae*. Moreover, a recent meta-analysis found that the incidence of meningitis following streptococcus pneumonia bacteremia is much lower than previously reported (< 3% instead of 5.8%).[50] Furthermore, oral antibiotics were not found to be effective in preventing pneumococcal meningitis.[50] The widespread use of antibiotics for the prevention of bacteremia-related complications in all children with temperatures greater than 39°C may have some negative effects, including: 1) development of partially treated meningitis, making diagnosis more difficult; 2) increased drug resistance; 3) increased delays and costs of ED visits; and 4) side effects requiring a second physician visit in up to 20% of patients (with potential hospital admission in 2%) in those receiving antibiotics.[17]

Finally, obtaining blood cultures and treating all children with temperatures greater than 39°C (102.2°F) will not ensure that all cases of bacteremia will be detected and treated. A single blood culture will miss cases of bacteremia, which does occur in children with a temperature less than 39°C (102.2°F), albeit less frequently.

A Logical Approach

Although there are many opinions regarding management of the febrile child, several consistent recommendations can be made. All infants 0-28 days old with a temperature greater than 38°C (100.4°F) require a complete septic evaluation (spinal tap, urinalysis, blood culture, urine culture), admission, and treatment with IV antibiotics. Toxic-appearing children 28-90 days old should receive the same septic evaluation, IV antibiotics, and admission. Well-appearing infants 28-90 days old with a temperature greater than 38°C (100.4°F) should be evaluated for the presence or absence of Rochester criteria. If Rochester criteria are present, administer ceftriaxone and schedule re-evaluation by a physician in 24 hours.

Several treatment options for managing children 3-36 months old can be considered appropriate. The first option is adherence to the expert panel guidelines recommending obtaining a blood culture and treating all children with a temperature of greater than 39°C (102.2°F) and no source. Emergency physicians should realize that this approach will detect most cases of bacteremia while needlessly treating a large number of children without bacteremia. A second option for clinicians who are extremely comfortable with their ability to assess and manage febrile children is to selectively culture and treat those who are at the highest risk for OB using the following factors: patient age, the degree of temperature elevation, the child's immunization status, the presence or absence of a minor source of infection, parental preference and reliability, and the child's clinical examination (observation).

Blood culture and treatment should be reserved for children with: 1) a high temperature (> 41°C); 2) a YOS greater than 6; 3) less than full H. influenzae type b immunization; 4) no minor source for infection; 5) age of 6-24 months; 6) unreliable parents; or 7) parents who desire treatment (but only if they understand the potential risks and benefits of treatment vs. non-treatment). This approach will potentially miss more cases of bacteremia. Only children at highest risk are cultured and treated, and fewer nonbacteremic children will be subjected to needless evaluation and antibiotic side effects. Regardless of which approach is taken with febrile children 3-36 months old, all males younger than 6 months and females younger than 2 years without a source of fever should receive a urinalysis and culture, as recommended by the expert panel. Most important, all patients should receive a mandatory re-evaluation within 24 hours.

What the Future Holds

Current management of febrile children with a fever and no source is determined by the risk of children with *S. pneumoniae* (and, to a lesser extent, *H. influenzae* type b) bacteremia developing serious infection. In the future, this management approach may change dramatically. First, studies are currently under way to test the effectiveness of childhood vaccines against *S. pneumoniae*.[51] If a vaccine is found to be effective, the incidence of invasive disease due to pneumococcal bacteremia will undoubtedly fall substantially, and OB may become a disease of the past. In the meantime, resistance of *S. pneumoniae* to penicillin is increasing, with a few cases of resistance to third-generation cephalosporins reported.[52-54]

Finally, future tests may be developed that improve our ability to detect bacteremia early in the disease course. Faster turnaround times for blood cultures and immediate tests (e.g., interleukin-6) may be devised that are more sensitive and specific for detecting patients with OB.

Summary

Management of febrile infants and children without an obvious infectious source mandates that clinicians be aware of the limitations of the physical examination in diagnosing serious bacterial infections. All febrile infants younger than 4 weeks old require a septic evaluation, IV antibiotics, and hospital admission. Application of the Rochester criteria to well-appearing infants 1-3 months of age with fever has been proven safe.

Evaluation of the febrile infant and child who is between 3 and 36 months old without a source of fever requires an understanding of the subtle nature of urinary tract infection and meningitis in this age group, as well as the multiple factors that place children within this age range at risk for OB. No single approach will identify and treat all children with bacteremia. Use of the expert panel guidelines will detect most cases of bacteremia, while overtreating a large number of children without bacteremia. Adherence to this approach should be considered by all clinicians who do not evaluate and treat febrile children on a routine basis.

For those clinicians who are experienced and feel comfortable with their ability to assess febrile children and with their knowledge of risk factors for OB, a more selective approach of careful follow-up and selective culturing and treatment only of those at highest risk for OB is acceptable. This approach will detect fewer cases of OB while curtailing the overtreatment of non-bacteremic children. Regardless of which approach is taken, 24-hour follow-up of at-risk children is mandatory, as well as an explanation to the parents of the risks of a febrile illness potentially progressing to more serious illness.

References

1. American College of Emergency Physicians. Clinical policy for the initial approach to children under the age of 2 years presenting with fever. *Ann Emerg Med* 1993;22:628-637.
2. Baraff LJ, Bass JW, Fleisher GR, et al. Practice guidelines for management of infants and children 0-36 months of age with fever without source. *Pediatrics* 1993;92:1-12.
3. Baraff LJ, Oslund SA, Schriger DL, et al. Probability of bacterial infections in febrile infants less than three months of age: A meta-analysis. *Pediatr Infect Dis J* 1992;11:257-265.
4. Baker MD, Bell LM, Avner JR. Outpatient management without antibiotics of fever in selected infants. *N Engl J Med* 1993;329:1437-1441.
5. Baskin MN, O'Rourke EJ, Fleisher GR. Outpatient treatment of febrile infants 28-89 days of age with intramuscular administration of ceftriaxone. *J Pediatr* 1992;120:22-27.
6. Jaskiewicz JA, McCarthy CA, Richardson AC, et al. Febrile infants at low risk for serious bacterial infection—an appraisal of the Rochester Criteria and implications for management. *Pediatrics* 1994;94:390-396.
7. Baker MD, Avner JR, Bell LM. Failure of infant observation scales in detecting serious illness in febrile 4- to 8-week-old infants. *Pediatrics* 1990;85:1040-1043.
8. Bonadio WA, Hennes H, Smith D, et al. Reliability of observation variables in distinguishing infectious outcome of febrile young infants. *Pediatr Infect Dis J* 1993;12:111-114.
9. Bonadio WA, McElroy K, Jacoby PL, et al. Relationship of fever magnitude to rate of serious bacterial infections in infants aged 4-8 weeks. *Clin Pediatr* 1991;30:478-480.
10. Bonadio WA. Defining fever and other aspects of body temperature in infants and children. *Pediatr Ann* 1993;22: 467-473.
11. Hertz AL, Herrod HG, Barrett FF, et al. Outpatient management of selective febrile neonates with ceftriaxone and home nurse visitations. *Acad Emerg Med* 1994;1:A3.
12. Bonadio WA, Hegenbarth M, Zachariason M. Correlating reported fever in young infants with subsequent temperature patterns and rate of serious bacterial infections. *Pediatr Infect Dis J* 1990;9:158-160.
13. Bonadio WA. Incidence of serious infections in afebrile neonates with a history of fever. *Pediatr Infect Dis J* 1987;6:911-914.
14. Kelly-Walsh C, Nelson DB, Smith DS, et al. Clinical predictors of bacterial versus aseptic meningitis in childhood. *Ann Emerg Med* 1992;21:910-914.
15. Rothrock SG, Green SM. Pediatric bacterial meningitis: Is preliminary antibiotic therapy associated with an altered clinical presentation? *Ann Emerg Med* 1992;21:146-154.
16. Harper MB, Fleisher GR. Occult bacteremia in the 3-month-old to 3-year-old age group. *Pediatr Ann* 1993;22:484-493.
17. Fleisher GR, Rosenberg N, Vinci R, et al. Intramuscular versus oral antibiotic therapy for the prevention of meningitis and other bacterial sequelae in young, febrile children at risk for occult bacteremia. *J Pediatr* 1994;124:504-512.
18. Cox RD, Wagner M, Woolard DJ. Infants and children with fever without source. *Ann Emerg Med* 1994;23:598-600.
19. Long SS. Antibiotic therapy in febrile children: "Best-laid schemes . . ." *J Pediatr* 1994;124:585-588.
20. Kline M, Lorin M. Bacteremia in children afebrile at presentation to an emergency department. *Pediatr Infect Dis* J 1987;6:197-201.
21. Jaffe DM, Tanz RR, Todd-Davis A, et al. Antibiotic administration to treat possible occult bacteremia in febrile children. *N Engl J Med* 1987;317:1175-1180.
22. Sinkinson CA, Pichichero ME. Occult bacteremia in children: What are the odds? *Emerg Med Rep* 1991;12:1-10.
23. Jaffe DM, Fleisher GR. Temperature and total white blood cell count as indicators of bacteremia. *Pediatrics* 1991;87: 670-674.
24. Dashefsky R, Teele DW, Klein JO. Unsuspected meningococcemia. *J Pediatr* 1983;102:69-72.
25. Anderson AB, Ambrosino DM, Siber GR. *Haemophilus influenzae* type b unsuspected bacteremia. *Pediatr Emerg Care* 1987;3:82-86.
26. Marshall R, Teele DW, Klein JO. Unsuspected bacteremia due to *Haemophilus influenzae:* Outcome in children not initially admitted to hospital. *J Pediatr* 1979;95:690-695.
27. Bratton L, Teele DW, Klein JO. Outcome of unsuspected pneumococcemia in children not initially admitted to the hospital. *J Pediatr* 1977;90:703-706.
28. Heldrich FJ. Diplococcus pneumonia. *Am J Dis Child* 1970;119:12-17.
29. Bennish M, Beem MO, Orniste V. C-reactive protein and zeta sedimentation ratio as indicators of bacteremia in pediatric patients. *J Pediatr* 1984;104:729-732.
30. McCarthy PL, Jekel JF, Dolan TF. Comparison of acute-phase reactants in pediatric patients with fever. *Pediatrics* 1978;62:716.
31. Saladino R, Erikson M, Levy N, et al. Utility of serum interleukin-6 for diagnosis of invasive bacterial disease in children. *Ann Emerg Med* 1992;1413-1418.
32. Joffe M, Avner JR. Follow-up of patients with occult bacteremia in pediatric emergency departments. *Pediatr Emerg Care* 1992;8:258-261.
33. Karasic RB, Isaacman DJ, Kost SI, et al. Collecting two blood cultures and a larger volume of blood improves detection of bacteremia in children. *Acad Emerg Med* 1994;1:A21.
34. Morello JA, Leitch C, Nitz, et al. Detection of bacteremia by Difco ESP blood culture system. *J Clin Microbiol* 1994;32: 811-818.
35. Zwadyk P, Pierson CL, Young C. Comparison of Difco ESP and Organon Teknika BacT/Alert continuous monitoring blood culture systems. *J Clin Microbiol* 1994;32:1273-1279.
36. Baraff LJ, Oslund S, Prather M. Effect of antibiotic therapy and etiologic microorganisms on the risk of bacterial meningitis in children with occult bacteremia. *Pediatrics* 1993;92: 140-143.
37. Schutzman SA, Petrycki S, Fleisher G. Bacteremia with otitis media. *Pediatrics* 1991;87:48-53.
38. Bell LM, Alpert G, Campos JM, et al. Routine quantitative blood cultures in children with *Haemophilus influenzae* or

Streptococcus pneumoniae bacteremia. *Pediatrics* 1985;76: 901-904.

39. Sullivan TD, LaScolea LJ, Neter E. Relationship between the magnitude of bacteremia in children and the clinical disease. *Pediatrics* 1982;69:699-702.
40. Baker RC, Tiller T, Bauscher JC, et al. Severity of disease correlated with fever reduction in febrile infants. *Pediatrics* 1989;83:1016-1019.
41. Teach SJ, Fleisher GR. Occult Bacteremia Study Group. Efficacy of the Yale Observation Score in detecting occult bacteremia. *Arch Pediatr Adolesc Med* 1994;Suppl 41:148.
42. Pinkert H, Harper MB, Cooper T, et al. HIV-infected children in the pediatric emergency department. *Pediatr Emerg Care* 1993;9:265-269.
43. Kramer MS, Etezadi-Amoli J, Ciampi A, et al. Parents' versus physicians' values for clinical outcomes in young febrile children. *Pediatrics* 1994;93:697-701.
44. Oppenheim PI, Sotiropoulos G, Baraff LJ. Incorporating patient preferences into practice guidelines: Management of children with fever without source. *Ann Emerg Med* 1994; 24:836-841.
45. Vukmir RB. Compliance with ED patient referral. *Am J Emerg Med* 1992;10:413-416.
46. Scarfone RJ, Loiselle JM, Wiley JF. Compliance with scheduled revisits to a pediatric emergency department. *Acad Emerg Med* 1994;1:A41. Abstract.
47. Korones DN, Shapiro ED. Occult pneumoccocal bacteremia: What happens to the child who appears well at reevaluation. *Pediatr Infect Dis J* 1994;13:382-386.
48. Korones DN, Marshall GS, Shapiro ED. Outcome of children with occult bacteremia caused by *Haemophilus influenzae* type b. *Pediatr Infect Dis J* 1992;11:516-520.
49. Wears RL, Stenklyft PH, Luten RC. Using decision tables to verify the logical consistency and completeness of clinical practice guidelines: Fever without a source in children under three. *Acad Emerg Med* 1994;1:A35.
50. Rothrock SG, Green SM, Clark M. Do oral antibiotics prevent meningitis in children with occult pneumococcal bacteremia? A meta-analysis. *Acad Emerg Med* 1995;2:A.
51. Steinhoff MC, Edwards K, Keyeserling H, et al. A randomized comparison of three bivalent *Streptococcus pneumoniae* glycoprotein conjuhate vaccines in young children: Effect of polysaccharide size and linkage characteristics. *Pediatr Infect Dis J* 1994;13:368-372.
52. Mason EO, Kaplan SL, Lamberth LB, et al. Increased isolation of penicillin-resistant *Streptococcus pneumoniae* in a children's hospital and in vitro susceptibilities to antibiotics of potential therapeutic use. *Antimicrob Agents Chemother* 1992;36:1703-1707.
53. Leggiadro RJ, Davis Y, Tenover FC. Outpatient drug-resistant pneumococcal bacteremia. *Pediatr Infect Dis J* 1994;13: 1144-1146.
54. Bradley JS, Connor JD. Ceftriaxone failure in meningitis caused by *Streptococcus pneumoniae* with reduced susceptibility to beta-lactam antibiotics. *Pediatr Infec Dis J* 1991;10:871-873.

Meningitis

Charles A. Nozicka, DO, FAAP

The diagnosis of pediatric meningitis presents the emergency physician with significant clinical challenges and formidable medicolegal risks. Young children and infants with meningitis are notorious for presenting with subtle symptoms and signs, often mimicking other more common illnesses. Although much has been published in the last several years regarding the approach to the febrile infant and child and the treatment of pediatric meningitis, clinicians must continue to approach every febrile child as potentially having bacterial meningitis. There remains the necessity for emergency physicians to continually update their practices and remain current in the diagnosis and treatment of this disease.

Pediatric meningitis continues to be a high-risk diagnosis for clinicians. It often is difficult to diagnose in its early stages and has the potential for serious permanent morbidity and death. Associated lawsuits can take the emergency physician beyond the limits of a malpractice policy, as judgments can be in the millions of dollars. Not only must the diagnosis be suspected and made in a timely matter, but these complicated cases also demand exquisite attention to detail in all aspects of care.

Emergency physicians can improve the outcomes of children by suspecting the disease early and initiating treatment promptly. But which signs and symptoms are most useful for identifying the febrile infant or child that has early meningitis? Is there a point on the continuum from occult bacteremia to meningeal seeding to early meningitis when the diagnosis is impossible to make?

Which child with a febrile seizure needs a lumbar puncture? Is dexamethasone indicated in any child with suspected meningitis? Is there a "gold standard" pertaining to the timing of antibiotics after a child with meningitis presents to the ED?

This chapter addresses these questions and others associated with the latest standards for the diagnosis and treatment of pediatric meningitis. Its recommendations are based on available data; controversies are discussed where they currently exist.

Initiation of Infection

Meningitis is characterized by inflammation of the meninges, connective tissue structures that surround the brain and spinal cord. When pathogens invade the central nervous system, they do so by several potential mechanisms. These include hematogenous dissemination after bacterial colonization and direct spread from a distant focus of infection, such as the mastoid ear cells or paranasal sinuses. In order to invade the nervous system, pathogenic organisms must penetrate the continuous protective cell layer of the blood brain barrier. Any disruption of this normal anatomy by trauma, operative procedures, or congenital deformities may facilitate such penetration. initiating infection.[1]

In cases involving hematogenous dissemination, the child initially has colonization of the nasal pharynx. The organism may then spread into the blood stream via the surrounding mucous membranes and capillaries. If the infecting organism is of sufficient virulence or inoculation, a significant bacteremia ensues which results in eventual meningeal invasion and bacterial replication in the subarachnoid space. The development of a sustained, high-grade bacteremia has been suggested as one important factor in the development of central nervous system invasion. Several investigators have suggested that the treatment of occult bacteremia in the young child or infant with initial empiric intervention during the bacteremic stage may prevent serious bacterial infections such as bacterial meningitis.[2]

Numerous investigators have studied the inflammatory response caused by the penetration of organisms into the central nervous system. Acute inflammatory mediators such as interleukins and cytokines have been implicated in the pathophysiology. This increased inflammatory response after initial antibiotic administration may result in hearing loss and other neurological sequelae; and is the theoretical basis for the use of steroids early in bacterial meningitis.[3] Other various inflammatory mediators, such as superoxides and tissue necrosis factor (TNF), are the subject of numerous recent investigations.[4,5]

Acute Bacterial Meningitis

The bacterial organisms causing acute meningitis in the pediatric age group vary according to the underlying health status and age of the patient. In immunocompetent children, older than 3 months of age, three bacterial species account for the majority of CNS infections: *Haemophilus influenzae, Streptococcus pneumoniae,* and *Neisseria meningitidis*.[6] Over the past five years, the widespread use of *H. influenzae* type B (HiB) conjugate vaccines has decreased the incidents of HiB meningitis in developed countries significantly.[7,8] Between 1987 and 1994, the incidence of HiB meningitis declined 95% in the United States.[8]

Unique organisms such as group B *Streptococcus*, *Escherichia coli,* and *Listeria monocytogenes*, resulting from the infant's contact with the perineum during the birth process, cause infection in the neonatal period (0-1 month).[9] *Table 1* notes the most common organisms causing meningitis in each age group. Nevertheless, it is important to note that these age groups overlap. *Salmonella* meningitis, usually associated with gastroenteritis, is an uncommon cause of acute meningitis in the infant less than 12 months of age.[1] Children with cerebral spinal shunts are susceptible not only to the usual pediatric pathogens, but may also be infected with *Staphylococcus* species.[10] The most commonly cultured organisms in children with these shunts are *Staphylococcus epidermidis* and *S. aureus*.[10] *S. epidermidis* may cause meningitis and sepsis in premature infants.

Clinical Presentation

The clinical presentation of acute bacterial meningitis differs significantly with the age of the child. Older children and adolescents frequently present with headache, fever, altered sensorium, and meningismus. Kernig's or Brudzinski's signs may be absent in up to 50% of adolescents and adults with bacterial meningitis.[1] Their absence does not rule out the diagnosis. Vomiting is seen in more than half the patients presenting in this older age group.[1] Younger pediatric patients may not manifest many of these classic symptoms and signs of bacterial meningitis.[1] Neonates with acute bacterial meningitis often lack meningismus. Clinical clues of meningitis in neonates are temperature instability (hyperthermia or hypothermia), poor feeding, listlessness, lethargy, irritability, vomiting, or respiratory distress. A change in the child's usual feeding pattern or state of alertness may be an important sign of meningitis. However, these findings are nonspecific in the neonate and may be associated with numerous other acute illnesses. A bulging fontanelle may be seen in up to one-third of cases, although it usually appears later in the course of illness.[1]

Suspecting the Diagnosis

Meningitis, especially in children younger than 2 years old, is frequently associated with acute otitis media, pneumonia, and even gastroenteritis. Therefore, the emergency physician must have a low threshold in considering the diagnosis of bacterial meningitis even with these other primary diagnoses. Although febrile children account for approximately 20% of all visits to the ED,[11] it is not necessary to perform a lumbar puncture (LP) in every acutely febrile child with non-specific findings. The most important consideration in suspecting acute bacterial meningitis in the young child or infant is his or her perceived interaction with the surrounding environment. The child who is difficult to console by his or her mother or is paradoxically irritable (increasingly agitated with parental comforting) should be suspect. LP is recommended in the young child or infant who fails to follow your examination, interacts appropriately during a short period of observation, or appears more toxic than usual with an acute febrile illness. Again, the finding of another bacterial focus during the work-up of the young child or infant does not rule out meningitis.

All febrile neonates less than 2 months of age should undergo the full septic work-up, usually with initiation of empiric antibiotic treatment.[12-14] This "work-up" includes bacterial cultures of urine, blood, and CSF.[12-14] The difficulty in assessing the febrile neonate still mandates this aggressive laboratory evaluation.[11-14]

The age group of greatest concern for the practicing emergency physician is the child between the ages of 2 and 24 months. In these younger children, the initial presentation of early meningitis is often non-focal with fever, relative lethargy, irritability, and/or vomiting. Several investigators have studied the frequency of positive meningeal signs in young infants. Samson et al identified 21 infants ages 1-15 months with bacterial meningitis and found only 48% had positive meningeal signs, including nuchal rigidity or Kernig's or Brudzinski's signs.[14] Walsh-Kelly et al found nuchal rigidity in only 27% of infants aged 0-6 months with bacterial meningitis compared to 95% of patients aged 19 months or older.[15] The same investigators found that 28% of infants 12 months of age and younger with bacterial meningitis did not have physical evidence of meningeal irritation.[15] A high index of suspicion for early bacterial meningitis is essential when evaluating the febrile infant 12 months of age or younger.

The "Partially Treated" Child

A child with partially treated meningitis may present atypically.[7] Pretreatment with oral or inadequate parenteral antibiotics may "blunt" the severity of symptoms and signs. Children with partially treated meningitis demonstrate lower average maximum temperatures, more subtle alterations in mental status, and often, a longer duration of symptoms prior to diagnosis.[7] The emergency physician must be cognizant of the often subtle presentations of young children and infants who are partially treated.

The Child with a Cerebrospinal Shunt

The clinician will frequently evaluate a child with a cerebrospinal shunt. The most common of these are ventriculoperitoneal (VP) shunts. These patients are at risk not only for the usual bacterial pathogens, but are also at risk for staphylococcal meningitis. Their presentations are often similar to a "partially treated" child, with more subtle and non-specific symptoms and signs.[16]

The ventricular catheter is attached subcutaneously to a reservoir that may be percutaneously tapped to obtain ventricular fluid for both diagnostic and therapeutic purposes.[17] It is recommended that the emergency physician obtain neurosurgical consultation prior to tapping a shunt reservoir.[17]

The Lumbar Puncture

Analysis of CSF, usually obtained by LP, is the basis for evaluation of the patient with suspected meningitis. In children without evidence of increased intracranial pressure, focal neurological findings, or papilledema, a CT scan is not necessary prior to an LP; it is extremely unlikely that uncal herniation with develop without evidence of increased intracranial pressure on physical examination.[18,19]

With suspected increased intracranial pressure, a blood culture is obtained and empiric antimicrobial therapy initiated while the CT scan is pending.[1,19] This same approach is usually required for patients with HIV, a history of brain tumors or neoplasms, or in whom a brain abscess is suspected from history and physical examination usually require this approach. Although one recent literature search found no evidence of a patient herniating with acute bacterial meningitis as a result of an LP,[19] cerebral herniation occurring after LP in children with a normal CT scan has been reported.[20]

Once obtained, CSF should be sent for cell count, protein, glucose, bacterial culture, and Gram's stain. Opening pressures, helpful in older children and adults, are usually not obtained in the infant age group.

A CSF glucose level of less than 40 mg/dL or a CSF glucose-to-blood glucose ratio of less than 0.3 to 0.5 suggests bacterial meningeal infection, as does a CSF protein of more than 150-170 mg/dL in neonates or 40-50 mg/dL in older infants and children.[17] Children with significant hypoglycorrhachia (CSF glucose < 20 mg/dL) have a poorer prognosis than those with normal CSF glucose. In HIV-positive children, India ink, cryptococcal antigen, acid fast bacillus (AFB) smear and culture, and fungal cultures are included. Children with history of tuberculosis exposure or travel to an area endemic for tuberculosis should have CSF AFB smear and culture. These tests may not be included in the usual CSF panels in many institutions and must be specifically ordered. *Table 2* delineates the usual cerebrospinal fluid characteristics of children. Initial CSF analysis may be unreliable in differentiating aseptic from bacterial meningitis. Finally, infants in the first month of life may have higher baseline WBC counts and protein than older children and adults.

Children with ventriculoperitoneal shunts will have elevated baseline CSF protein and cell counts; however, approximately 90% of those with cell counts greater than 100 cells/mm^3 will be infected.[16]

Table 1. Pediatric Bacterial Meningitis Pathogens

NEONATE TO 1 MONTH

Common:
- Group B streptococci
- *E. coli*
- Other aerobic gram-negative bacilli

Uncommon:
- *Listeria monocytogenes*
- *Enterococcus* sp.

INFANTS 1-3 MONTHS

Common:
- Group B streptococci
- Aerobic gram-negative bacilli
- *H. influenzae* (HiB)
- *S. pneumoniae*
- *N. meningitidis*

Uncommon:
- *Listeria monocytogenes*
- *Salmonella* sp.

3 MONTHS AND OLDER

Common:
- *H. influenzae* (HiB)
- *S. pneumoniae*
- *N. meningitidis*

Uncommon:
- *Salmonella* sp.

CSF (VP) SHUNT

Common:
- Usual organisms for age
- Staphylococcal sp.

Although higher WBC counts (generally > 1000 cell/mm^3) with a predominance of polymorphic neutrophils (PMNs) are associated with bacterial meningitis, a finding of fewer WBCs (or < 50% PMNs) may be seen with early bacterial disease. Several investigators have reported series of patients with essentially normal CSF that were subsequently diagnosed with acute bacterial meningitis.[21,22] Most of the patients in these two studies were less than 2 years of age. These studies indicate that a small number of patients with acute bacterial meningitis may present to a clinician during the early phase of meningeal invasion and have apparently normal CSF indices. Likewise, in early bacterial meningitis, a relatively low WBC cytology, negative Gram's stain and even latex agglutination may mimic a child with aseptic meningitis. A child who clinically appears ill even with normal spinal fluid analysis or the consideration of early sepsis or meningitis mandates immediate empiric antimicrobial therapy and hospital admission. Such is often the case with early meningococcemia without meningitis. In the child admitted as "sepsis" with a "viral-appearing" CSF, repeat LP 12-24 hours later may clarify the situation

Table 2. Typical CSF Characteristics of Normal and Infected Hosts

CASE	COLOR	OPENING PRESSURE	WBC COUNT	GLUCOSE*	PROTEIN**	GRAM'S STAIN	CULTURE	INDIA INK	CRYPTOCOCCAL ANTIGEN
Normal infant	Clear	< 180 mm	< 10/mm³	> 40 mg/dL	90 mg/dL	negative	negative	negative	negative
Normal child or adult	Clear	< 180 mm	0	> 40 mg/dL	< 40 mg/dL	negative	negative	negative	negative
Bacterial meningitis	Cloudy	> 200 mm	200-10000/mm³ (> 80% PMN)	< 40 mg/dL	100-500 mg/dL	usually positive	positive	negative	negative
Viral meningitis	Clear	< 180 mm	25-1000/mm³ (< 50% PMN)	> 40 mg/dL	50-100 mg/dL	negative	negative	negative	negative
Cryptococcal meningitis	Clear	> 200 mm	50-1000/mm³ (< 50% PMN)	< 40 mg/dL	50-300 mg/dL	negative	negative	positive	positive

* Normal CSF glucose is dependent upon serum glucose. A rough guideline is that CSF glucose is normally greater than one-half the serum glucose.

** Each 1000 RBC/mm³ in the CSF typically increases CSF protein by about 1.5 mg/dL.

Adapted from: Lipton JD, Schafermeyer RW. Evolving concepts in pediatric bacterial meningitis—Part 1: Pathophysiology and diagnosis. *Ann Emerg Med* 1993;22:1602-1615.

Clinicians must be very cautious in making a diagnosis of aseptic meningitis based on initial CSF characteristics and electing not to treat with antibiotics.

The Traumatic LP

Traumatic spinal punctures may create a diagnostic challenge. The "traumatic tap" usually will "clear," producing less RBCs in the last sample tube compared to the first, whereas a subarachnoid hemorrhage results in an equal number of RBCs in each sample. The number of WBCs expected in a sample after a traumatic tap may be estimated.[23] This formula estimates:

$$\textbf{\# of WBCs introduced/mm}^3 = \frac{\textbf{(peripheral WBC)} \times \textbf{(CSF RBCs)}}{\textbf{(peripheral RBCs)}}$$

The expected WBC count is compared to the actual CSF WBC result. Another estimate is that for each 1000 RBCs introduced traumatically, 1-2 WBCs will be introduced.[23]

Associated Diagnostic Work-up

Other chemistry and hematological tests are usually obtained in the ED to help facilitate the management of the patient. A CBC is traditionally part of the patients work-up for sepsis, significant bacterial illness, or meningitis in the pediatric patient. A normal WBC count with the absence of a left shift does not exclude a significant bacterial infection and cannot be used to exclude bacterial meningitis. Serum electrolytes and glucose are obtained as a baseline and to exclude the syndrome of inappropriate antidiuretic hormone (SIADH).

Bacterial antigen tests of CSF (latex agglutination and counter immunoelectrophoresis) often routinely ordered, are relatively expensive and are usually of little value in the acute phase of management. An exception is the child on antibiotics for another focus of infection who presents with partially treated meningitis. Although the CSF cytology usually will be abnormal, instances of falsely negative cultures with meningitis previously treated with antibiotics.[1,7,24,25] In these cases, the latex agglutination or other rapid antigen detection test may yield a diagnosis.[26] A clinician must realize, however, that there are many false-positive and false-negative results associated with rapid antigen detection.[26] Use of urine for CIE or latex agglutination has even less specificity when used to identify a bacterial organism in meningitis.[26]

Numerous other laboratory tests have been evaluated to increase the specificity and sensitivity in patients with acute meningitis. CSF limulus lysate, CSF lactate,[27] and CSF leukocyte esterase have been studied to help differentiate between aseptic and bacterial meningitis,[27] but they are rarely indicated over the routine CSF analysis.[17] Blood cultures are obtained, along with CSF, to rule out sepsis or bacteremia and increase the diagnostic yield for a bacterial pathogen.

A Differential Diagnosis

Occult Bacteremia. The pathophysiology of hematogenous dissemination involves the initially asymptomatic child being colonized with a virulent bacterial pathogen. This colonization leads to hematogenous dissemination and an initially "occult" bacteremia. During the early bacteremic phase, the infant or child may have a paucity of non-specific clinical findings. As the pathogens spread from bacteremia to meningeal invasion, a subtle, non-specific presentation including fever, irritability, or vomiting may be the only clinical findings. During the early meningeal phase, the diagnosis may be elusive until more focal signs develop. Clinicians caring for acutely febrile children must be aware that in this early phase, clinical signs and symptoms may be subtle and preclude the diagnosis of bacterial meningitis. Obviously there is a clinical continuum in the development of meningeal irritation in which specific signs of meningitis may be completely absent in the infant with early meningitis—the diagnosis is essentially clinically impossible to make during this period. The clinician evaluating the acutely febrile

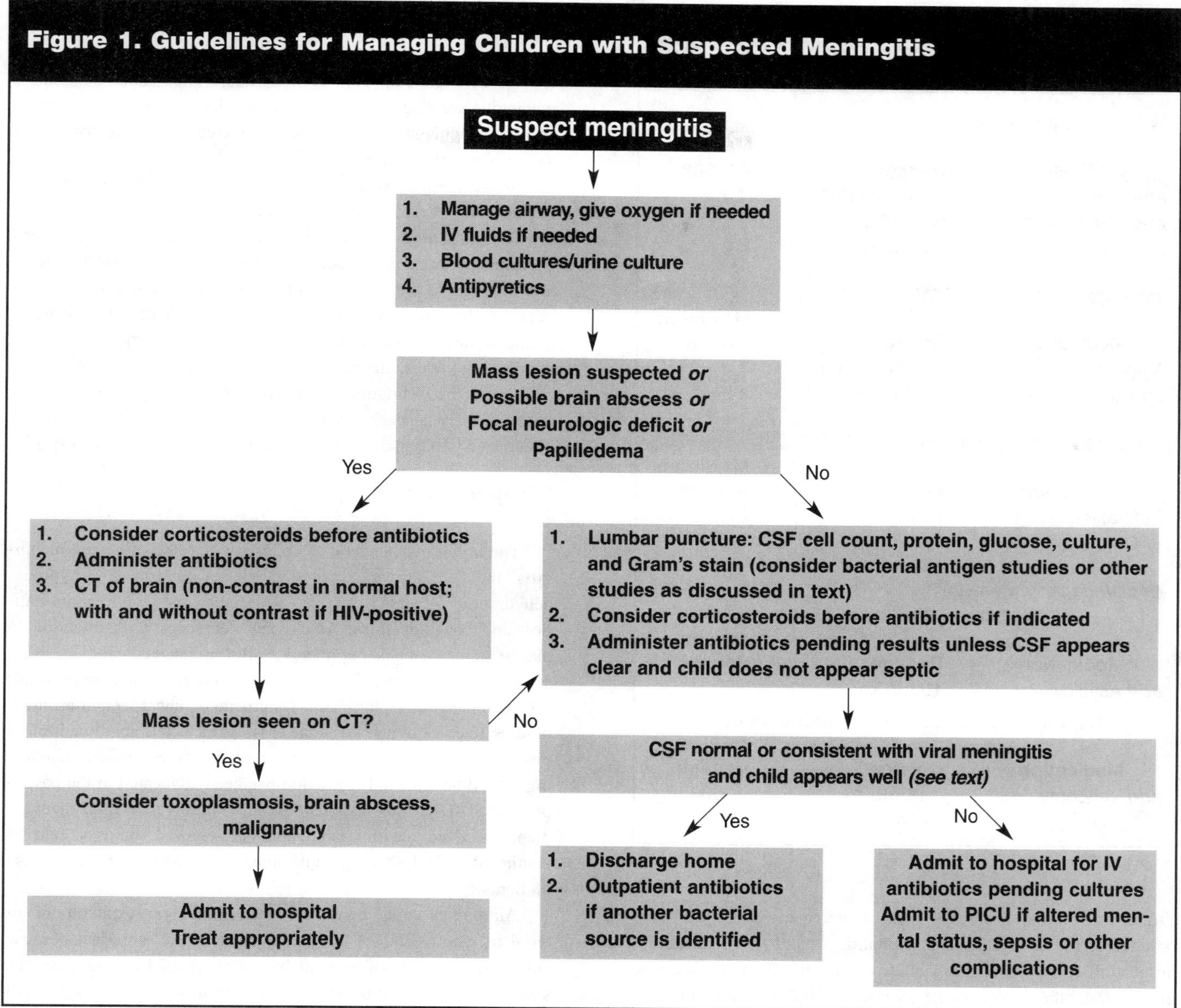

child must explain these issues to parents and provide comprehensive written discharge instructions enabling the parents to follow up quickly if the clinical condition of the child deteriorates.

Sepsis. The same pathophysiology that accounts for the development of meningitis explains the development of sepsis. Colonization leads to occult bacteremia, which, in turn, may lead to dissemination of bacterial infection to distant foci or to overt clinical sepsis.[31] In children with fever, cyanosis, hypothermia, altered mental status, or other non-specific significant clinical presentations, the lack of positive CSF findings does not rule out sepsis. Meningococcemia is an example of a rapidly developing sepsis syndrome that occurs without clinical meningitis, with the child developing sepsis, hypotension, and DIC within a period of only a few hours.[31] The child who presents with significant irritability, altered mental status, or signs of hemodynamic instability mandates stabilization of the ABCs and empiric antibiotic treatment initiated—even in light of a negative spinal tap.

Encephalitis. Encephalitis is an inflammation of the central nervous system, usually of viral etiology, that often mimics meningitis. Encephalitis causes direct inflammation of the brain parenchyma. Patients usually present with profound altered mental status, severe headache, vomiting, autonomic nervous system dysfunction, or ataxia.[32,33] With the exception of HSV, no specific treatment is available for most cases. Herpes simplex virus type 2 (HSV-2) in adolescents, often seen in conjunction with genital HSV, is usually associated with a self-limited form of meningitis, although chronic symptoms and recurrent meningitis does occur.[33] HSV infections in infants are usually caused by HSV-2, a complication of maternal genital infection.[33] Newborn infants usually present within the first week of life with fever or temperature instability and, often, jaundice. Vomiting, lethargy, respiratory distress, cyanosis, and shock may follow shortly. The presence of vesicular lesions (typically on the presenting body part during delivery) is helpful in making the diagnosis. However, skin lesions may be absent in up to 20% of infants.[33] Herpes simplex virus type 1 (HSV-1), may cause a rapidly progressive fatal encephalitis occur-

Table 3. ED (Loading) Antibiotic Dosages in Pediatric Meningitis

NEONATE (< 4 WEEKS)

Medication	Dosage	Maximum dosage
Ampicillin	50-100 mg/kg	2 g
and Cefotaxime	50 mg/kg	
or Gentamicin	2.5 mg/kg	2 g

INFANT (1-2 MONTHS)

Medication	Dosage	Maximum dosage
Ampicillin	50-100 mg/kg	2 g
and Cefotaxime	50-75 mg/kg	2 g

INFANT 3 MONTHS TO ADULT

Medication	Dosage	Maximum dosage
Cefotaxime	75 mg/kg	2 g
or Ceftriaxone	100 mg/kg	2 g

IF CLINICALLY INDICATED:

Herpes Simplex Virus

Medication	Dosage	Maximum dosage
add Acyclovir	10 mg/kg	

Cephalosporin-Resistant Pneumococcus

Medication	Dosage	Maximum dosage
add Vancomycin	15 mg/kg (over 1 hour)	500 mg

ring in approximately three-fourths of untreated cases.[33] Children or adolescents with HSV-1 encephalitis usually have an abrupt onset with fever, chills, headaches, conjunctivitis, myalgias, sore throat, and other non-specific symptoms. Inflammation may be localized to the frontal temporal area with focal findings simulating a mass lesion, or the inflammation may be diffuse, involving both cerebral hemispheres.

LP usually reveals CSF pleocytosis with a predominance of lymphocytes. The diagnosis is suggested by characteristic CSF findings and clinical presentation along with MRI findings suggestive of a characteristic frontal temporal lesion. A brain biopsy may be necessary for confirmation, because HSV is rarely cultured directly from the CSF.[33]

When skin lesions are present, viral antigens can be detected using immunofluorescence, immunoparoxidase, or ELISA techniques. The diagnosis is strongly suggested by characteristic temporal lobe discharges on EEG and by temporal lobe swelling on MRI. Treatment with acyclovir should be initiated early if clinical suspicion for HSV encephalitis is high.[33]

Viral Meningitis. Many other viruses are capable of causing encephalitis[32,33] or meningitis. Enteroviruses and arboviruses are the most common etiologic agents. Measles, mumps, or varicella can cause a post-infectious encephalitis occurring several weeks after the initial illness.[32] These infections, considered diagnoses of exclusion, may mimic bacterial meningitis or HSV encephalitis, diseases which have specific treatments. Likewise, in the immunocompromised or HIV-positive patient, *Cryptococcus neoformans* and tuberculosis meningitis are diagnostic considerations. Lyme disease may present as aseptic meningitis. It should be considered with suggestive historical or physical findings.[34]

Non-Infectious Considerations. Other diagnostic entities that present with altered mental status and fever are toxicological syndromes including salicylates, phencyclidine, and acute lead encephalopathy or rheumatological diseases such as systemic juvenile rheumatoid arthritis, systemic lupus erythematosis (SLE), and, occasionally, Kawasaki's disease. Subarachnoid hemorrhage, although rare in the pediatric population, can produce signs of meningismus with altered mental status. Subarachnoid hemorrhage can usually be distinguished from bacterial meningitis by a sudden onset of severe headache, and lack of prodromal signs in the presence of crenated RBCs in the cerebral spinal fluid with a paucity of WBCs.

Management

The initial management of children suspected of having meningitis includes airway management, evaluation for hypoxia, dehydration, increased intracranial pressure, electrolyte abnormalities, and coagulopathies. Assessment for shock with attention to mental status changes, peripheral profusion, delayed capillary refill, and significant tachycardia with or without hypotension are priorities for the emergency physician. Treatment of shock requires initial boluses 20 cc/kg of normal saline or Ringer's lactate solution. If more than 40 cc/kg is required, consider central venous pressure monitoring.[17,35] Although fluid restriction has been advocated in the past to prevent SIADH, most experts advocate conservative fluid management. Once circulation stabilization is achieved, fluids should be continued at 75-100% of maintenance requirements for the first 24-48 hours.[36]

Antibiotics should be initiated immediately on suspicion of bacterial meningitis. Initial treatment decisions are empirical because culture results will not be available for at least 24 hours. A Gram's stain of the CSF must be examined for organisms, but results should not be the sole basis for initiating empiric therapy. Other considerations in antibiotic selection are age, underlying chronic conditions, and the child's immunologic status. If immediate LP cannot be performed because of cardiovascular instability, technical difficulties, or consideration for increased intracranial pressure, antibiotics should be initiated after obtaining a blood culture with the anticipation that the LP will be completed as early as possible.[35] When bacterial meningitis is suspected and vascular access cannot be achieved quickly, the intramuscular administration of antibiotics in usual parenteral dosages is recommended.[17,31] For the child in shock who needs immediate fluid resuscitation with antibiotics, intraosseous administration is appropriate.[17,31] *Table 3* summarizes appropriate medications for bacterial meningitis.

Treatment Issues

Does Antibiotic Administration Before LP Alter CSF Results? Many physicians are concerned that giving antibiotics before an LP will significantly interfere with CSF analysis and confuse the diagnosis. One study addressing this issue indicates that although the potential for false-negative CSF cultures exist, a combination of using Gram's stains, latex agglutination or counter current immunoelectrophoresis (CIE), and pretreatment blood cultures usually yield the suspected pathogen.[37] The initiation of antibiotics before an LP will rarely alter the CSF enough to interfere with appropriate interpretation. The emergency physician should not wait for LP (or CT) results before starting appropriate antibiotics.

Antibiotics Should Be Initiated Within 30 Minutes of Presentation to the ED. Classic teaching recommends treatment of acute bacterial meningitis with parenteral antibiotics within 30 minutes of patient presentation. Studies have not demonstrated better outcomes with earlier administration of antibiotics,[38,39] and prospective studies designed to address this issue will never be done. Several investigations have demonstrated the average time to administration of antibiotics at 2.1-3.0 hours.[40,41] This is in contrast to the often quoted "gold standard" of 30 minutes.[41] One study attributed the majority of the delay to time after the initial physician encounter, which, thus, is potentially preventable.[40] Theoretical considerations of treating bacterial meningitis mandate appropriate antibiotics without preventable delay; however, the frequently quoted "within 30 minutes" of presentation may be an unreasonable goal and probably does not represent the "gold" standard.[41]

Dexamethasone or Not? That is the Question. Administration of dexamethasone during the treatment of *H. influenzae* (HiB) meningitis reduces the incidence of subsequent sensorineural hearing loss.[42-49] The proposed mechanism of action is inhibition of inflammatory mediators such as cytokine production in the CSF.[47] Dexamethasone has recently been studied with other bacterial pathogens; the benefits and the potential disadvantages are controversial.[42] Several clinical trials have claimed to support the use of dexamethasone in cases of children with pneumococcal meningitis.[42-49] A recent prospective study of 56 children with pneumococcal meningitis demonstrated a significant reduction in neurologic sequelae (most notably hearing loss) in dexamethasone-treated patients.[49] If cephalosporin-resistant pneumococcal meningitis is suspected, vancomycin is indicated in the initial antimicrobial regimen.[34,50] A potential complication using dexamethasone with pneumococcal meningitis has recently been reported: The penetration of vancomycin across the inflamed meninges is maybe decreased with dexamethasone therapy, potentially decreasing drug concentrations in the CSF.[50,51] This is because inflammation of the blood-brain barrier during acute meningitis facilitates vancomycin passage into the subarachnoid space.[42] Since the penetration of rifampin to the CSF is not altered by dexamethasone therapy, some experts have suggested that initial therapy in areas with cephalosporin-resistant organisms consist of cefotaxime or ceftriaxone combined with rifampin. In those patients in whom meningitis may be caused by HSV, concomitant use of dexamethasone could potentially have adverse effects.

The preponderance of data appears to support the use of dexamethasone in children older than 3 months of age with bacterial meningitis.[42-49] Caution is necessary if HSV or cephalosporin-resistant pneumococcal meningitis is a consideration.[17,50] The recommend dosage of dexamethasone is 0.15 mg/kg q6h intravenously for the first four days of therapy.[31,44,47] The therapeutic effect of dexamethasone is maximized if it is administered 10 minutes before the administration of the first dose of antibiotics.[44,47] Recommendations for the use of dexamethasone with tuberculosis meningitis differ and are beyond the scope of this report.[51]

Table 4. Chemoprophylaxis for Pediatric Meningitis

***H. INFLUENZAE* (HiB)**

- Household contacts should receive rifampin only if there is one or more child younger than age 4 living in the household.
- All members of the household, including those previously immunized and the patient, should receive prophylaxis.
- Daycare contacts should consider prophylaxis if two or more cases of invasive HiB disease occur within two months. In smaller daycare settings in which young children (< 2 years) spend more than 24 hours a week together, prophylaxis after a single case may be recommended.
- ***Dosage:*** *20 mg/kg single daily dose (maximum, 600 mg/d) for four days.*

N. MENINGITIDIS

- All household, daycare, and anyone with close contact with oral secretions should receive prophylaxis.
- ***Dosage:*** *20 mg/kg/d (maximum, 600 mg/d) q12h for two days.*

S. PNEUMONIAE

- Chemoprophylaxis not indicated.

Complications

Hypoglycemia. Hypoglycemia may occur as a reaction to stress, poor feeding, or shock. It is most commonly concomitant with meningitis in the first three months of life.[31] Any child with altered mental status should have a bedside blood glucose check. If it is below 50 mg/dL, 25% dextrose should be given at a dosage of 0.25-1.00 g/kg (1-4 cc/kg).[31] In infants less than 1 month of age, using a bolus of 10% dextrose (5 cc/kg) is advisable. This should be followed by IV infusions containing 5% dextrose solutions. Occasionally 10% dextrose-containing solutions may be necessary to maintain acceptable serum glucose levels.

Seizures. Seizures may be seen in up to 25% of children with bacterial meningitis. They are occasionally seen with viral meningitis, and are common with encephalitis, especially HSV infection.

Seizures should be treated with lorazepam 0.05-0.1 mg/kg/dose IV or diazepam 0.1-0.2 mg/kg/dose IV q5-10min (maximum, 10 mg). Rectal diazepam should be considered if venous access cannot be quickly obtained. The intravenous preparation is administered rectally, via a feeding tube or a 1 mL TB syringe, in a dosage of 0.5 mg/kg/dose. If diazepam is used, a longer-acting anticonvulsant such as phenytoin should be initiated. Anatomical abnormalities, such as subdural effusion or cerebral abscesses, and metabolic derangements should be excluded.

Disposition. All pediatric patients with possible bacterial meningitis require hospitalization. Those at risk for associated sepsis with poor profusion, coma, seizures, purpura, or petechia require close monitoring in a pediatric intensive care unit. A patient in whom there is a suspicion for bacterial meningitis despite a CSF analysis appearing normal or consistent with viral meningitis should be admitted for IV antibiotics pending culture results in 48-72 hours. Traditional management is on an inpatient basis; completion of therapy on an outpatient basis may be an option in the near future in uncomplicated patients, thus reducing medical costs.[53]

Chemoprophylaxis. Chemoprophylaxis is indicated in household, day care, and nursery school contacts, as well as anyone with close intimate exposure to oral secretions of patients with meningococcal meningitis.[17,32,55] Household contacts of patients with *H. influenzae* meningitis should receive chemoprophylaxis if there is at least one child 4 years old or younger in the household;[52] then all contacts in the household, including adults, children, and the patients themselves should receive chemoprophylaxis (usually rifampin), including individuals previously immunized.[17,52] Clinicians must be aware that the dosages for rifampin prophylaxis differ between these two pathogens and that prophylaxis does not prevent disease in all cases. Fever in a susceptible contact of a child with bacterial meningitis should be promptly evaluated for possible early invasive disease, even if prophylaxis was given. Pregnant women should not take rifampin.[52] Rifampin causes orange bodily fluids (urine, stool, tears) and may stain soft contact lenses. Chemoprophylaxis and rifampin dosages are summarized in *Table 4*.

Prevention. Immunization with *H. influenzae* conjugate vaccine is now routinely available to children beginning at 2 months of age. Children who are younger than 2 years of age who have recovered from *H. influenzae* meningitis should receive the *H. influenzae* conjugate vaccine, as the disease does not provide consistent long-term protection against reinfection.[17,52] A polyvalent meningococcal vaccine is available but is only recommended for children older than 2 years of age who are at high risk for infection (i.e., those with immunodeficiency syndromes or complement component deficiency). A pneumococcal polyvalent vaccine composed of capsular antigens from 23 serotypes is available. It also is only recommended for children who are older than 2 years of age who are at risk of developing pneumococcal disease (i.e., immunodeficiency syndromes, sickle cell disease, nephrotic syndrome, and recurrent meningitis after head trauma).

Summary

Physicians face many perplexing questions and dilemmas concerning the diagnosis and management of pediatric meningitis. There are a number of important points to bear in mind. First, bacterial meningitis may be difficult to diagnose in the initial stages, especially during the neonatal period; the younger the child, the more subtle the signs and symptoms. Next, children may present with CSF findings indicating a viral infection or within normal limits (rarely) and still have early bacterial meningitis. Importantly, a negative LP never "rules out" sepsis, and empiric antimicrobial therapy should never be delayed to obtain an LP if bacterial meningitis is suspected. In partially treated patients, blood culture and bacterial antigen tests can often identify the causative organism.

Third-generation cephalosporins, cefotaximine, and ceftriaxone are the drugs of choice for pediatric bacterial meningitis. In the neonate, cefotaxime is combined with ampicillin. When cephalosporin-resistant *S. pneumoniae* is suspected, vancomycin is added. Dexamethasone administered with or before initial antibiotics decreases the neurological sequelae of HiB meningitis; its routine use with other bacterial etiologies is controversial.

References

1. Tunkel AR, Scheld WM. Acute meningitis. In: Mandell GL, Bennett JE, Dolin R, eds. *Principles and Practice of Infectious Diseases.* 4th ed. New York: Churchill Livingstone Inc.; 1995:831-865.
2. Singer JI, Vest J, Prints A. Occult bacteremia and septicemia in the febrile child younger than two years. *Emerg Med Clin North Am* 1995;2:381-416.
3. Jafari HS, McCracken GH. Dexamethasone therapy in bacterial meningitis. *Pediatr Ann* 1995;2:82-88.
4. Arditi M, Ables L, Yogev R, et al. Cerebrospinal fluid tumor necrosis factor-M and platelet-activating factor concentrations and seventy of bacterial meningitis in children. *J Infect Dis* 1990;162:139-147.
5. Saez-Horens X, Ramilo O, Mustafa MM, et al. Molecular pathophysiology of bacterial meningitis: Current concepts and therapeutic implications. *J Pediatr* 1990;116:671-684.
6. Bohr V, Hansen B, Jessen O, et al. Eight hundred and seventy-five cases of bacterial meningitis; clinical data, prognosis and the role of specialized hospital departments. *J Infect* 1983;7:21-30.
7. Lipton JD, Schafermeyer RW. Evaluating concepts in pediatric bacterial meningitis: Part I—Pathophysiology and diagnosis. *Ann Emerg Med* 1993;22:1602-1615.
8. Progress toward elimination of *Haemophilus influenzae* type B disease among infants and children. United States 1987-1995. *MMWR Morb Mortal Wkly Rep* 1996;45:901-905.
9. DeLanois J. Acute bacterial meningitis in the newborn. *J Antimicrob Chemother* 1994;34:61-73.
10. Wiedermann BL. Characteristics of pathogenic microbes and infectious syndromes. In: Holbrook PR. *Textbook of Pediatric Critical Care.* Philadelphia: WB Saunders Co.; 1993:898-917.
11. Singer JI. Fever and sepsis. In: Reisdorff EJ, Roberts MR, Wegenstein JG, eds. *Pediatric Emergency Medicine.* Philadelphia: WB Saunders Co.; 1993:556-565.
12. Baraff LJ, Bass JW, Fleisher GR, et al. Practice guidelines for the management of infants and children 0-36 months of age with fever without source. *Pediatrics* 1993;92:1-12.
13. Nozicka CA. Evaluation of the febrile infant less than 3 months of age with no source of infection: new management strategies. *Am J Emerg Med* 1995;13:315-318.
14. Samson JH, Apthorp J, Finely A. Febrile seizures and purulent meningitis. *JAMA* 1969;210:1918-1919.
15. Walsh-Kelly C, Nelson DB, Smith DS, et al. Clinical predictors of bacterial versus aseptic meningitis in childhood. *Ann Emerg Med* 1992;21:910-914.
16. Odio C, McCraken GH, Nelson JD. CSF shunt infections in pediatrics. *Am J Dis Child* 1984;138:249-251.
17. Barkin RM. Bacterial Meningitis. In: Barkin RM, ed. *Pediatric Emergency Medicine: Concepts and Clinical*

Practice. 2nd ed. St. Louis: Mosby-Yearbook, Inc.; 1996

18. Haslem RA. Role of computed tomography in the early management of bacterial meningitis. *J Pediatr* 1991;119:157-159.
19. Archer B. Computed tomography before lumbar puncture in acute meningitis: A review of the risks and benefits. *Can Med Assoc J* 1993;148:961-965.
20 Rennick G, Shann F, de Campo J. Cerebral herniation during bacterial meningitis in children. *BMJ* 1993;306:953-955.
21. Omorato IM, Wormser GP, Nicholas P. "Normal" CSF in bacterial meningitis. *JAMA* 1980;244:1469-1471.
22. Levy DR. Lumbar puncture and the diagnosis of meningitis. *South Med J* 1981;74:28-30.
23. Bonadio WA, Smith DS, Goddard S, et al. Distinguishing cerebrospinal fluid abnormalities in children with bacterial meningitis and traumatic lumbar puncture. *J Infect Dis* 1990;162:251-254.
24. David SD, Hill SR, Feigl P, et al. Partial antibiotic therapy in *Haemophilus influenzae* meningitis: its effect on cerebrospinal fluid abnormalities. *Am J Dis Child* 1975;129:802.
25. Feigin RD, Cherry JD, eds. *Textbook of Pediatric Infectious Diseases*, 3rd ed. Philadelphia: WB SaunderS; 1992.
26. Dougherty JM, Jones J. Cerebrospinal fluid culture and analysis. *Ann Emerg Med* 1986;15:317.
27. Nelson N, Eeg-Olofsson, Larsson L. The diagnostic and predictive value of cerebrospinal fluid lactate in children with meningitis; its relation to current diagnostic methods. *Acta Paediatr Scand* 1986;75:52-57.
28. Lieu TA, Schwartz JS, Jaffe DM, et al. Strategies for diagnosis and treatment of children at risk for occult bacteremia: Clinical effectiveness and cost-effectiveness. *J Pediatr* 1991;118:21-29.
29. Fleisher GR, Rosenberg N, Vinci R, et al. Intramuscular versus oral antibiotic therapy for the prevention of meningitis and other bacterial sequelae in young, febrile children at risk for occult bacteremia. *J Pediatr* 1994;124:504-512.
30. Baker MD, Bell LM, Avner JR. Outpatient management without antibotics Fof fever in selected infants. *N EngL J Med* 1993;329:1437-1441.
31. Fleisher GR. Infectious disease emergencies. In: Fleisher GR, Ludwig S, eds. *Textbook of Pediatric Emergency Medicine.* 3rd ed. Baltimore: Williams and Wilkins; 1993:595-606.
32. Reisdorff EJ. Viral encephalitis. In: Reisdorff EJ, Roberts MR, Weigenstein JG, eds. *Pediatric Emergency Medicine.* Philadelphia: WB Saunders Co.; 1993:1056-1062.
33. Lipton JD, Schafermeyer RW. Central nervous system infections—the usual and the unusual. Pediatric emergencies. *Emerg Med Clin North Am* 1995;13:417-443.
34. Sundel R. Rheumatologic emergencies. In: Fleisher GR, Ludwig S, eds. *Textbook of Pediatric Emergency Medicine.* 3rd ed. Baltimore: Williams and Wilkins; 1993:1074-1078.
35. Bell LM. Shock. In: Fleisher GR, Ludwig S, eds. *Textbook of Pediatric Emergency Medicine.* 3rd ed. Baltimore: Williams and Wilkins; 1993:44-54.
36. Brown LW, Feigin RD. Bacterial meningitis: Fluid balance and therapy. *Pediatr Ann* 1994,23:93-98.
37. Blazer S, Berant M, Alon U. Bacterial meningitis: Effect of antibiotic treatment on cerebrospinal fluid. *Ann J Clin Pathol* 1983;80:386-387.
38. Kallio MJ, Kilpi T, Anttila M, et al. The effect of a previous visit to a physician on outcome after bacterial meningitis. *JAMA* 1994;10:787-791.
39. Radetsky M. Duration of symptoms and outcome in bacterial meningitis: An analysis of causation and the implications of a delay in diagnosis. *Pediatr Inf Dis J* 1992;9:694-701.
40. Talan DA, Gutermann JJ, Overturf GD, et al. Analysis of emergency department management of suspected bacterial meningitis. *Ann Emerg Med* 1989;18:856-862.
41. Meadow WL, Lantos J, Tanz RR, et al. Ought "standard care" be the "standard of care"? A study of the time to administration of antibiotics in children with meningitis. *Am J Dis Child* 1993;147:40-44.
42. Schaad UB, Kaplan SL, McCracken GH. Steroid therapy for bacterial meningitis. *Clin Infect Dis* 1995;20:685-690.
43. Kaplan SL. Dexamethasone for children with bacterial meningitis—should it be routine therapy ? *Am J Dis Child* 1989;143:290-291.
44. American Academy of Pediatrics, Committee on Infectious Diseases. Dexamethasone therapy for bacterial meningitis in infants and children. *Pediatrics* 1990;86:130-133.
45. Odio CM, Faingezicht I, Paris M, et al. The beneficial effects of early dexamethasone administration in infants with bacterial meningitis. *N Engl J Med* 1991;324:1525-1531.
46. Schaad UB, Lips U, Gnehm HE, et al. Dexamethasone therapy for bacterial meningits in children. *Lancet* 1993;342: 457-461.
47. Jafari HS, McCracken GH. Dexamethasone therapy in bacterial meningitis. *Pediatr Ann* 1994;23:82-88.
48. Girgis NI, Farid Z, Kilpatrick ME, et al. Dexamethasone treatment for bacterial meningitis in children and adults. *Pediatr Infect Dis J* 1989;8:848-851.
49. Kanra GY, Ozen H, Secmeer G, et al. Beneficial effects of dexa-methasone in children with pneumococcal meningitis. *Pediatr Infect Dis J* 1995;14:490-494.
50. Chandy JC. Treatment failure with use of a third-generation cephalosporin for penicillin-resistant pneumococcal meningitis: Case report and review. *Clin Infect Dis* 1994;18:188-193.
51. Starke JR. Current chemotherapy for tuberculosis in children. *Infect Dis Clin North Am* 1992;6:215-238.
52. Committee on Infectious Diseases: American Academy of Pediatrics. Report 1994. Elk Grove Village, IL: American Academy of Pediatrics: 1994.
53. Waler J, Rathore MH. Outpatient management of pediatric bacterial meningitis. *Pediatr Infect Dis J* 1995;14:89-92.

Asthma

Blake Bulloch, MD
Richard M. Ruddy, MD

The American Thoracic Society defines asthma as "a disease characterized by an increased responsiveness of the trachea and bronchi to various stimuli and manifested by a widespread narrowing of the airways that changes in severity either spontaneously or as a result of treatment."[1] While this definition was first used in 1962, it remains appropriate today.

In order to establish the diagnosis of asthma, the clinician should determine that 1) the patient has intermittent or recurring symptoms of airflow obstruction; 2) that the obstruction to airflow is reversible; and 3) that the airflow obstruction is not due to other diagnoses.[2] Remember that "all that wheezes is not asthma" and that you must consider other disease entities in acutely wheezing children.[3,4]

To better guide the clinician's assessment of asthma severity and to optimize the management of patients with asthma, guidelines by an expert panel at the National Institutes of Health and the National Heart, Lung, and Blood Institute were published initially in 1991 and updated in 1997.[2] In the 1997 report, the classification of asthma severity has been changed from mild, moderate, and severe to the new classification of mild intermittent, mild persistent, moderate persistent, and severe persistent. This more accurately reflects the clinical and chronic manifestations of asthma. The panel does emphasize that no matter what classification of asthma a patient has, he can have mild, moderate, or severe exacerbations. *(Please see Table 1.)* An asthma exacerbation is a worsening of symptoms, which can be either abrupt in onset or gradual, but which is always associated with a decrease in expiratory airflow. This review will approach the diagnosis, clinical evaluation and management of children presenting with an acute asthma exacerbation.

Epidemiology

Asthma is the most common chronic disease of childhood, with a prevalence of 5-10%.[3,5] Analysis of national data from the CDC during the years 1980 through 1993 indicated that asthma-related mortality and hospitalization rates increased among people younger than 25 years of age.[6] Asthma accounted for approximately 4000 deaths in people younger than 24 years of age during this 14-year interval. During that interval, annual hospitalizations for asthma in this group increased 28%, with a large proportion of this increase in children younger than 4 years of age.[7]

Despite recent advances in treatment, asthma continues to be a substantial economic burden and the leading cause of missed school days. Weiss and associates estimated the direct and indirect costs of asthma in all age groups to be $6.2 billion in 1990.[8] They found that children 17 years of age and younger made up approximately 50% of all visits to the emergency department for asthma-related complaints at a cost of $90.4 million annually. Average inpatient stays for children were five days in length and accounted for greater than $250 million in costs. Asthma resulted in the estimated loss of more than 10 million school days in 1990 in children between 5 and 17 years old, with accompanying loss of workdays for the primary caregiver. Overall, the costs attributed to asthma in this age group amounted to more than $1 billion per year without including medication costs.

Etiology

Episodes of wheezing associated with respiratory infections are common in the first year of life. Many of these infants will have bronchiolitis, an infectious etiology of wheezing, but some have asthma. Martinez and colleagues prospectively studied factors affecting wheezing before the age of 3 years and their relation to wheezing at 6 years of age.[12] They gathered data on four groups of patients: a) patients who never wheezed (51.5%); b) transient wheezers—those with at least one episode of wheezing in the first three years of life associated with a lower respiratory tract infection but no wheezing at 6 years of life (20%); c) late wheezers—children who had wheezing with a lower respiratory tract infection at 6 years of age but none in the first three years of life (15%); and d) persistent wheezers—children who had wheezing in the first three years of life and at 6 years of age (13%). Factors found to be independently associated with persistent wheezing were: maternal asthma, maternal smoking, rhinitis apart from colds, eczema during the first year of life, male sex, and Hispanic background. Among the children with non-recurrent (transient) wheezing, maternal smoking was the only independent factor.

Other studies have revealed that infants with documented viral infections of the lower respiratory tract are at greater risk for wheezing later in life.[13] This includes not only those infants who had severe episodes of bronchiolitis but also those with mild forms of viral lower respiratory tract infections that were managed in the office setting. As well, patients born with impaired lung function at birth may be more susceptible to these infections and, therefore, to wheezing. In contrast, lower respiratory tract infections from bacterial causes do not seem to predispose children to asthma.

Conditions that predispose or that may worsen lower airway disease include rhinitis and sinusitis. With this in mind, patients and parents should be questioned about nasal obstruction, nasal discharge, frequent colds, day and night coughing with post-nasal drip, and sore throat. Treatment of sinusitis will often result in improvement in airway obstruction. Management includes the use of antihistamines, decongestants, and antibiotics for common pathogens.[14] Gastroesophageal reflux may also cause symptoms of dyspnea and wheezing often within a couple of hours of feeding and shortly after being laid supine. These infants often have histories of recurrent vomiting or regurgitation and must be considered as a cause of wheezing in infants.

Pathophysiology

Regardless of the severity, asthma is a chronic inflammatory disorder of the tracheobronchial tree. In general, a variety of physiologic triggers including inhalant allergens, tobacco smoke, pollutants, viral infections, exercise, and emotions enhance the release of the preformed mediators of inflammation from the mucosal mast cells.[15] These mediators include histamine, chemotactic factors, leukotrienes, prostaglandins, and platelet activating factor. These mediators lead to contraction of bronchial smooth muscle and increased vascular permeability leading to edema of the airways and increased mucus production.[16-18] This is the early asthma response, which consists of bronchoconstriction, lasts 1-2 hours, and can be reversed with high-dose beta-agonists.[19]

Up to 80% of patients will go on to develop a late asthma reaction within four hours of exposure to the trigger and lasting up to a week.[4] This late-phase is due to the effect of inflammatory cells attracted to the airways (polymorphonuclear leukocytes, eosinophils, and monocytes) that release proteolytic enzymes leading to mucosal injury and further inflammation.[16-18] It has been shown that cromolyn sodium and corticosteroids may contribute to the alleviation of symptoms in the late phase.

The physiologic consequences of the above include bronchoconstriction and increased mucus production leading to obstruction of both the large and small airways. Due to the airway obstruction, patients experience increased air-trapping that increases dead space ventilation, placing the patient on the compliance/resistance curve at a point where the work of breathing can dramatically increase. This results in ventilation/perfusion mismatching with hypoxia. Lack of effective treatment may lead to patient fatigue, and minute ventilation may decrease leading to CO_2 retention and respiratory failure.

Clinical Evaluation

The clinical evaluation of a patient who presents with an asthma exacerbation should begin with a rapid cardiopulmonary assessment and immediate institution of rescue therapy when required. Focus the assessment on the degree of respiratory distress, which determines the amount of airway obstruction and ventilatory compromise. Ventilation/perfusion changes, spirometry, and patient symptoms have been shown to poorly correlate with each other in a variety of situations. However, in each individual patient, assessing the degree of obstruction is best done by measuring the severity of symptoms and signs displayed on physical exam combined with an objective measure of airway obstruction such as peak expiratory flow rates.

History. The most common presenting symptoms in asthmatics include shortness of breath (SOB), wheezing, cough, and chest tightness. Patients frequently feel SOB although it is not entirely clear why. The chest is hyperinflated due to the air trapping. Because of increased elastic recoil at this distended lung volume, the work of exhalation is lessened but the work of inspiration is greatly increased.[20] Tonic activity of the inspiratory muscles throughout inspiration and expiration has been shown in patients with asthma exacerbations, and this is a major contributor to the sensation of dyspnea. Dyspnea can be clinically assessed by determining the effect on the child's normal speech (i.e., the ability to speak in normal sentences without breaths).

Chest tightness is a manifestation of stimulation of vagal nerve irritant receptors. Subtle airway obstruction may have cough as the only clinical manifestation of an acute exacerbation. In mild cough-variant episodes as described, there may be no wheezing or prolonged expiration on clinical exam. Asthma with acute cough should be enough of a symptom complex to provide the patient with a trial of bronchodilators.

Other important historical data to obtain include the onset and duration of the current exacerbation and possible triggers of the episode. Triggers can be allergic, infectious, or irritant in nature. Viral URI is more common in infants and young children, while environ-

Table 1. Classification of the Severity of Acute Asthma Exacerbation

Signs/Symptoms	Mild	Moderate	Severe
Dyspnea (speed/feeding)	None; talks in sentences	Short of breath with talking; difficulty breathing	Can only speak in 1-2 word sentences; may refuse feeds
Alertness	May be agitated	Usually agitated	Agitated to decreased level of consciousness
Respiratory rate*	Increased	Increased	Increased
Respiratory distress	None	Moderate	Severe
Wheeze	Often only end-expiratory	Loud and throughout expiration	Often both inspiratory and expiratory
Heart rate†	< 100	100-200	> 120
Pulsus paradoxus	Absent	10-20 mmHg	Often 20-40 mmHg
PEFR	> 80% predicted	< 80% predicted	< 50% predicted
Oxygen saturation on R/A	> 95%	91-95%	< 91%
$PaCO_2$	< 42 mmHg	< 42 mmHg	> 42 mmHg

* Guide to rates of breathing in awake children

Age	Normal rate
< 2 months	< 60/min
2-12 months	< 50/min
1-5 years	< 40/min
6-8 years	< 30/min

† Guide to normal pulse rates in children

Age	Normal rate
2-12 months	< 160/min
1-2 years	< 120/min
2-8 years	< 110/min

Modified from: Highlights of the expert panel report 2: Guidelines for the diagnosis and management of asthma. National Institutes of Health, National Heart, Lung and Blood Institute; May 1997. NIH Publication No. 97-4051A. Figure 5-9.

mental allergens/irritants are more common in older children and adolescents. Duration of symptoms for more than 24 hours is likely to suggest a greater component of inflammation. Obtain an inventory of current medications and the dose and frequency of each drug, including the use of systemic corticosteroids over the past several months. Identify patients who have had previous hospital admissions including the need for intensive care to identify the most high-risk patients. Factors that have been identified that increase a patient's risk of a fatal asthma exacerbation include: previous life-threatening exacerbations, hospital admission for asthma in the last 12 months, suboptimal medical management, poor access to medical care, psychological or psychosocial problems, overuse of beta-agonists, black race, and age (with teenagers at increased risk).[9-11] Finally, seek a history of allergies to help identify triggers. Some authors report that up to 90% of children may have allergy/atopy as part of their asthma.[21]

Physical Examination. Initially, the physical exam should be brief and focused. Always begin by assessing the child's general appearance. Work of breathing as evidenced by the presence of chest wall retractions and abdominal excursion, skin color, and level of consciousness can be assessed within seconds and is a good indicator of the severity of respiratory compromise. Assess for an increase in the anterior-posterior diameter of the chest, the "barrel-chest," to estimate the severity of air trapping. Observe the patient's respiratory rate and look for nasal flaring as a sign of distress. Occasionally, patients may grunt if there is significant pneumonia or atelectasis. Evaluate the use of accessory muscles by looking for intercostal, subcostal, and suprasternal retractions. The accessory muscles work to lift the entire rib cage cephalad. This generates high-negative intrapleural pressures in patients whose airways are partially obstructed to assist in ventilation. Use of the accessory muscles of respiration in this fashion places a larger metabolic demand on the child. This leads to more CO_2 production and fatigue that may contribute to respiratory acidosis.

Expiration is impaired in asthma due to intrathoracic small airway obstruction. Prolonged expiration is often subtle in mild asthma but can be pronounced in severe episodes. Most characteristic, but least prognostic, is the degree of wheezing on exam. Wheezing may be auscultated and is caused by rapid, turbulent airflow through the narrowed airways. Wheezing may be heard on both inspiration and expiration and tends to vary in intensity and pitch over time and often changes from place to place. After bronchodilator therapy, it may be louder due to improvement of the obstruction. Be aware of the patient in whom no wheezing is auscultated, as wheezing is not heard when airflow has diminished over severely obstructed airways.

On physical exam, it is useful to calculate a standard score such as a clinical asthma score.[22] *(See Table 2.)* Clinical asthma scores, such as the Wood-Downes' score shown in table 2, were designed to predict patients at high risk for respiratory failure. Many authors have tried to validate updated scores, but only a few have shown reasonable trends. However, these scores are still useful in following the individual patient's response to treatment during an acute exacerbation. The Wood-Downes' clinical system can assist the clinician by showing that a score of greater than 5 is indicative of impending respiratory failure, while a score of greater than 7 indicates existing respiratory failure. Obtain oxygen saturation by pulse oximetry to detect hypoxia and to assist in demonstrating the effect of small airways disease on oxygen shunting.

Table 2. Wood-Downes' Clinical Asthma Score

Parameter	0	1	2
Cyanosis (PaO_2)	None (> 70 mmHg in room air)	Present in room air (< 70 mmHg in room air)	Present in 40% O_2 (< 70 mmHg in 40% O_2)
Inspiratory air entry	Normal	Decreased or asymetric	Decreased or absent
Accessory muscle use	None	Moderate	Severe
Expiratory wheezes	None	Moderate	Severe
Cerebral function	Normal	Agitated or depressed	Comatose

Measurement of pulsus paradoxus is useful in recognizing severe episodes, although it may be difficult to obtain in children. A paradoxical pulse is measured by inflating an appropriate sized blood pressure cuff above the systolic blood pressure, slowly deflating it until you hear the first systolic sounds during expiration. Note this pressure and then continue to lower the pressure until you can hear the systolic sounds throughout the respiratory cycle. The difference is normally less than 4-5 mmHg and is the change in systolic blood pressure between inspiration and expiration. A pulsus paradoxus is present when this value is 10 mmHg or greater and is accurate in identifying patients with a greatly diminished FEV_1.

Laboratory Studies. Bedside pulmonary function tests provide a rapid, objective assessment of the patient and serve as a guide to the effectiveness of therapy. In moderate-to-severe obstruction, these tests may be delayed until after bronchodilators are administered and the patient shows some improvement. The forced expiratory volume in one second from maximal inspiration (FEV_1) and the peak expiratory flow rate (PEFR) can be measured. These studies directly measure the degree of large airway obstruction. Patient cooperation is required for these tests to be reliable. Sequential measurements may be taken to monitor.

Peak expiratory flow (PEF) monitoring has been shown to play a useful role in the ED management of childhood asthma. It is effort dependent and takes practice, so it is not always useful in children under 5 years of age. Appropriate normal values for age, corrected for height, are available. A decrease in PEFR to less than 50% of the patient's personal best indicates a severe exacerbation.[2] Following improvement in PEFR by the titration of rescue medications to response can decrease hospital admissions when performed well.[23]

Pulse oximetry is a useful adjunct in the monitoring of patients with exacerbations, especially in those children younger than 5 years of age who are unable to perform PEFR. It is a noninvasive, painless method of assessing a patient's oxygenation and small airways disease. It is unreliable in cool, underperfused states, and it can be sensitive to movement and lighting. Some literature suggests that patients with initial oxygen saturation less than 91% who respond to treatment well enough to be sent home have a higher incidence of relapse with return visits and often hospitalization. On the other hand, patients with an initial oxygen saturation of 95% or higher rarely relapse acutely.[24] A disadvantage is that pulse oximetry does not reflect a decreased PaO_2 until it has decreased to less than 80 mmHg. It is not reliably consistent when the O_2 saturation is less than 75-80%.

Arterial blood gas (ABG) analysis has not been a good predictor of clinical outcome in patients with acute asthma exacerbations.[25] Hypoxia is a major concern in children with asthma. Pulse oximetry is useful and more convenient for assessing oxygenation, but an ABG is the only way to get an accurate measurement. It is the patient with an acute severe exacerbation in whom we are concerned about respiratory failure (increasing PCO_2 and respiratory acidosis) and who has a significant O_2 requirement in which the ABG may be useful. As such, the ABG can be reserved for those patients who may require intubation and mechanical ventilation or who are clinically difficult to assess. Keep in mind that obtaining an ABG may be difficult, especially in a child younger than 2 years of age, and may further aggravate the patient's respiratory distress.

The use of chest radiographs in patients with wheezing remains controversial. Radiographic findings of hyperinflation, peribronchial thickening, increased central lung markings, and subsegmental atelectasis are frequent findings in asthma exacerbations and usually do not change patient management. Chest radiography has been previously recommended for patients presenting with their first episode of wheezing. However, Gershel and colleagues found 94.3% of radiographs in first-time "wheezers" to be normal.[26] They found that patients with first-time wheezing and a respiratory rate above 60 or a pulse above 160, localized rales or localized decreased breath sounds before treatment, and localized rales and localized wheezing after bronchodilator treatment were more likely to have positive films. Those in support of radiographs argue correctly that all that wheezes is not asthma. However, history and physical examination most often lead the clinician in the right diagnostic direction. It seems wise to follow the patient's response to medical management and, if the clinical picture seems discordant with the history, consider obtaining the radiographs. If a patient fails to respond to medical management or has fever, a radiograph is wise to help exclude pneumonia, pneumomediastinum, or the rare pneumothorax. Sinusitis may be an important co-morbid factor for an asthma exacerbation and, occasionally, it is beneficial to obtain a CT or radiograph of the sinuses.

The need for blood analysis is limited in patients with asthma exacerbations. While a CXR will detect cases of pneumonia, a white blood cell count is a nonspecific indicator of toxicity or of accompanying bacteremia in patients with pneumonia. Keep in mind that the use of corticosteroids or sympathomimetics will result in demargination of white blood cells and possibly cause leukocytosis. As such, the CBC is not a good indicator of infection in asthmatic patients. Beta-agonists have been shown to decrease serum levels of potassium, magnesium, and phosphate, although this is not usually of clinical significance in otherwise healthy children. Beta-agonists stimulate $beta_2$-adrenergic receptors that are linked to membrane-bound sodium-potassium ATPase. In activating this enzyme, there is a direct influx of potassium into cells leading to a decreased serum potassium concentration. Catecholamines have also been shown to cause intracellular shifts of phosphate ions.[27] If a patient is on theophylline at home, it is prudent to check a serum level.

Patients in status asthmaticus may have increased levels of plasma anti-diuretic hormone (ADH). This may occur secondary to hypovolemia, decreased left atrial pressures, or stimulation by adrenergic drugs. If given hypotonic fluids, patients have developed clinically significant hyponatremia. Therefore, hypotonic fluids should be avoided in patients with severe exacerbations, especially if they are not showing a significant response to therapy. ADH levels return to normal once there is relief of the airway obstruction.[28]

On occasion, moderately severe asthma may affect serum electrolytes such as potassium, magnesium, or phosphate. Severe asthmatic patients are hypoxic and may have a respiratory alkalosis from hyperventilating. This, combined with low serum potassium and/or magnesium, may precipitate cardiac dysrrthymias. Hypophosphatemia is reported to cause respiratory muscle fatigue and to cause a decrease in tissue oxygen extraction in patients with asthma exacerbations. Whether the decreases in serum concentrations of potassium, magnesium, or phosphate are clinically significant is unknown, and measurement of these electrolytes on a routine basis is not indicated.

Differential Diagnosis

Wheezing reflects an obstruction to airflow with turbulent flow producing the ausculatory findings. A variety of other conditions may present with wheezing in infants and children as shown in Table 3.[3,29] The wheezing associated with these conditions is rarely rapidly reversible and is often not paroxysmal. For example, the sudden onset of respiratory distress with cough and dyspnea, especially in the child with no prior history of obstructive airway disease, suggests foreign body aspiration. The exam may reveal stridor, unequal air entry, or unilateral chest wall expansion as a means of differentiating it from asthma. A history of possible aspiration should be carefully obtained.

Bronchiolitis is caused by a viral infection, most notably the respiratory syncytial virus (RSV), and presents in a manner clinically similar to asthma. It tends to affect children younger than 2 years and, often, infants who are younger than 6 months. There is often a 1-2 day prodrome of upper respiratory tract infection symptoms, low-grade fever, and similar symptoms in other family members. Recurrent episodes are unusual. The chest radiograph is similar to asthma in that they both may show hyperinflation with focal atelectasis. It is possible to identify the RSV antigen by immunoflorescence of nasopharyngeal aspirates.

Cystic fibrosis (CF) can mimic asthma, especially in the first year of life. Both result in an obstructive respiratory pattern, and chest radiographs may appear similar. Exacerbations are often triggered by infections. Viral infection may exacerbate CF, but bacterial infection ensues from *Staphylococcus* or *Pseudomonas* organisms. Some CF patients have a good response to bronchodilators. Other findings associated with CF include steatorrhea causing failure to thrive, recurrent pneumonia, digital clubbing, rectal prolapse, chronic cough, and nasal polyposis. The definitive diagnosis for CF is the sweat chloride test.

Bronchopulmonary dysplasia is still a common pulmonary problem. It results from prolonged endotracheal intubation, mechanical ventilation, and high-inspired oxygen concentrations in premature infants with respiratory distress syndrome. Some respond well to bronchodilator therapy and corticosteroids. Often, the pulmonary symptoms will resolve by 5 years of age.

Table 3. Differential Diagnoses of Wheezing*

ALLERGIC
Asthma
Anaphylaxis
ACQUIRED
Foreign body aspiration
Bronchopulmonary dysplasia
Gastroesophageal reflux
Aspiration syndrome
CARDIAC
Congestive heart failure
Mitral stenosis, cor triatriatum
CONGENITAL
Laryngotrachomalacia
Tracheoesophageal fistula
Cystic fibrosis
Tracheal or bronchial stenosis
Bronchomalacia
Vascular rings
INFECTIONS
Bronchiolitis
Bacterial, mycoplasma, or viral pneumonia
TB endobronchitis

* Most common conditions encountered in infants and children but not all inclusive.

Gastroesophageal reflux is caused by a laxity in lower esophageal sphincter tone. This may lead to symptoms of dyspnea and wheezing often within a couple of hours of feeding and shortly after being laid supine. These infants often have a history of recurrent vomiting or regurgitation and may develop recurrent pneumonia. Aspiration as a cause of coughing and wheezing in infants must be considered. Tests that may be useful in determining if reflux is present include a 24-hour pH probe or barium swallow.

Other causes of wheezing to consider include fixed obstruction from vascular disease, congenital heart disease, and endobronchial masses such as from bronchogenic cysts or secondary-to-enlarged paratracheal nodes from tuberculosis.

Medications

Asthma medications are now divided into two groups. The first group is the quick-relief or "rescue" medications used to treat acute symptoms and exacerbations.[2] Medications in this group consist of the short-acting beta$_2$-agonists, anticholinergics, and systemic corticosteroids and will be the focus of this section. *(See Table 4.)* The second group is referred to as the long-term control medications and

Table 4. Medications for the Treatment of Asthma Exacerbations

Medication	Dosage	Comments
Oxygen	FiO_2 to maintain saturation > 90%	
Sympathomimetics		
Albuterol		
Nebulizer solution (5 mg/mL)	0.15 mg/kg q 15-20 min for 3 doses (min. dose 2.5 mg, max dose 5 mg/nebulization), then 0.15-0.3 mg/kg up to 10 mg q 1-4 h prn, or 0.5 mg/kg/h by continuous nebulization	Deliver at 6/L min with O_2 to ensure small particle size and optimal delivery
MDI (90 mcg/puff)	4-8 puffs q 20 min up to 4 h, then q 1-4 h prn	Always use with spacing device
Terbutaline (1 mg/mL)	0.01 mL/kg subcutaneously q 15-20 min to a maximum of 0.25 mL	Both terbutaline and epinephrine may be used q 15-20 min for 3 doses subcutaneously. However, there is no proven advantage over inhaled beta-agonists
Epinephrine (1:1000 solution)	0.01 mL/kg subcutaneously q 15-20 min to a maximum dose of 0.3 mL	
Anticholinergics Ipratropium Bromide (0.25 mg/mL)	0.25 mg q 20 min for 3 doses then q 2-4 h prn	May be mixed in same nebulizer as albuterol
Corticosteroids Prednisone Prednisolone Methylprednisolone	2 mg/kg initially then 1 mg/kg q6h for 48 h, then 1-2 mg/kg/d in 2 divided doses with a maximum dose of 60 mg for 3-10 d	No clear advantage in administering IV over po if the patient is able to keep the medication down, is not in severe distress, or has an ileus

are used to achieve and maintain control of persistent asthma.

Quick-relief Medications. Beta-agonists act by increasing levels of cAMP in bronchial smooth muscle and in mast cells by activating the enzyme adenylate cyclase. Increased cAMP leads to increased binding of intracellular calcium to the endoplasmic reticulum, which decreases myoplasmic calcium and causes bronchial smooth muscle relaxation.[16] High-dose, short-acting beta$_2$-agonists, specifically albuterol, remain the treatment of choice for relief of acute symptoms.[19] Bitolterol and pirbuterol are also inhaled short-acting beta$_2$-agonists, but they have not been sufficiently studied. Possible adverse effects from beta-agonist therapy can include a decrease in PaO_2 due to a transient worsening of the ventilation/perfusion ratio, cardiac stimulation (i.e., tachycardia and ectopy), skeletal muscle tremor, and central nervous system stimulation.

Ipratropium bromide (Atrovent) is a quaternary ammonium derivative of atropine that limits its systemic absorption and decreases the side effects that were seen with the use of atropine. As such, it is the only anticholinergic currently used in the treatment of acute asthma exacerbations. It is delivered by aerosolization and inhibits smooth muscle contraction and mast cell mediator release. It has a slower onset of action than beta$_2$-agonists with a peak effect occurring over two hours but lasting up to six hours.[30,31] When compared directly to albuterol, it is not as potent a bronchodilator. Osmond and Klassen reported a meta-analysis of randomized controlled trials using ipratropium bromide with beta$_2$-agonists and found a statistically significant improvement in percentage predicted FEV_1 over beta$_2$-agonists alone.[30] The studies did not find a clinically significant difference, but patients were compared after only one dose of ipratropium bromide and with the use of low-dose beta-agonists. Schuh and colleagues later performed a triple armed, randomized, double-blind placebo controlled trial comparing ipratropium bromide 0.25 mg every 20 minutes for three doses, with a second group receiving one dose of ipratropium bromide during the first hour, and a third group received placebo.[31] All patients received high-dose albuterol (0.15 mg/kg) every 20 minutes for the first hour. Patients showed a statistically significant improvement in FEV_1 with the use of frequently administered ipratropium bromide, and the difference was more marked the more severe the exacerbation.

It is currently recommended that ipratropium bromide be used as a quick relief medication along with beta$_2$-agonists. It may be repeated with the first three beta$_2$-agonist treatments during an acute exacerbation, as it appears there may be a dose response curve. It is available as both a nebulizer solution (0.25 mg/mL) and as an MDI (18 mcg/puff). Only the nebulizer solution is recommended for use in acute asthma exacerbations since the MDI has not been studied under these conditions.

Corticosteroids appear to work by the inhibition of phospholipase A_2 activity, which blocks the release of inflammatory mediators, thereby suppressing the migration of polymorphonuclear leukocytes. They also increase the number and affinity of beta-adrenergic receptors, and reverse the increased capillary permeability seen in exacerbations. A number of studies have verified that systemic corticosteroids improve exacerbations and reduce length of symptoms. They should be routinely prescribed to all asthmatics experiencing an exacerbation.

A meta-analysis by Rowe and colleagues that examined the role of corticosteroids in acute asthma exacerbations came to the following conclusions:[32] Corticosteroid treatment results in a decreased relapse rate in the first week to 10 days. Administration of steroids within 30 minutes in the acute care setting leads to a reduced admission rate.[32,33] Based on their calculations, the number of children you would need to treat early in an emergency department visit in order to prevent one hospital admission would be 6-11 children based on a baseline admission rate of 20%.[32] There is no evidence to suggest that route of administration of the corticosteroid (oral vs intravenous) improves the patient's outcome. Despite this conclusion, clinicians treating severe asthma exacerbations would likely still choose the IV route in specific patients with vomiting, ileus, or evidence of other factors that may delay steroid delivery.

Prednisone, or its active form prednisolone, is the oral corticosteroid of choice while methyprednisolone is the IV steroid of choice. Side effects from the short-term use of corticosteroids are more limited than with chronic use. These include mood changes, hypertension, fluid retention, and an increase in appetite, all of which will resolve with discontinuation of the corticosteroids. Unusual complications of steroid therapy include peptic ulcer disease or aseptic necrosis of the hip.[34] Most children have minimal effect from 3-4 courses of five-day corticosteroid therapy over a year. Children requiring more than four courses of corticosteroids in a year are at greater risk for adrenal suppression and adverse effects on bone calcium. Care needs to be taken to not extend courses to greater than 10 days, nor to fail to initiate corticosteroid therapy because of concern over side effects. Repeated use would be good reason for an allergy or pulmonology referral.

Table 5. Management of Patients with an Acute Asthma Exacerbations

Initial Assessment: History, Physical O_2, Saturation, PEF or FEV_1

FEV_1 or PEF > 50%
- Inhaled beta$_2$-agonist by MDI or nebulizer, up to 3 doses in the first hour
- O_2 to achieve O_2 saturation > 90%
- Oral corticosteroids if no immediate response or if patient recently took oral steroid

FEV_1 or PEF < 50% (severe exacerbation)
- Inhaled high-dose beta$_2$-agonist and anticholinergic by nebulization q 20 min or continuously for 1 h
- O_2 to achieve O_2 saturation > 90%
- Oral systemic corticosteroid

Impending or actual respiratory arrest
- Intubation and mechanical ventilation with 100% O_2
- Nebulized beta$_2$-agonist and anticholinergic
- IV corticosteroid

→ Admit to hospital intensive care setting

Repeat Assessment
Symptoms, physical examination, PEF, O_2 saturation, other tests as needed

Moderate Exacerbation
(FEV_1 or PEF 50-80% predicted/personal best or physical exam revealing moderate symptoms)
- Inhaled short-acting beta$_2$-agonist q 60 min
- Systemic corticosteroids
- Continue treatment 1-3 h, provided there is improvement

Severe Exacerbation
(FEV_1 or PEF < 50% predicted/personal best or physical exam revealing severe symptoms at rest)
- Inhaled short-acting beta$_2$-agonist, hourly or continuous and inhaled anticholinergic
- Oxygen
- Systemic corticosteroids

Good Response
- FEV_1 or PEF > 70%
- Response sustained 60 min after last treatment
- No distress
- Physical exam: normal

Incomplete Response
- FEV_1 or PEF > 50% but < 70%
- Mild to moderate symptoms

Poor Response
- FEV_1 or PEF < 50%
- PCO_2 > 42 mmHg
- Physical exam: symptoms severe, drowsiness, confusion

Individualize decision regarding hospitalization

Discharge Home
- Continue treatment with inhaled beta$_2$-agonist
- Course of oral systemic corticosteroid
- Patient education

Admit to Hospital Ward
- Inhaled beta$_2$-agonist and anticholinergic
- Systemic corticosteroid
- Oxygen
- Monitor FEV_1 or PEF, O_2 saturation, and pulse

Admit to Hospital Intensive Care
- Inhaled beta$_2$-agonist hourly or continuously and inhaled anticholinergic
- Intravenous corticosteroid
- Oxygen
- Possible intubation and mechanical ventilation

Improve

Discharge Home
- Continue treatment with inhaled beta$_2$-agonist
- Course of oral systemic corticosteroid
- Patient education

Management

The approach to the child who presents with an acute asthma exacerbation is outlined by the expert panel report shown in Table 5.[2] As mentioned previously, the initial evaluation begins with a rapid cardiopulmonary assessment with institution of therapy as indicated. A thorough history and physical examination with emphasis on color, ausculatory findings, use of accessory muscles, respiratory rate, and heart rate is performed. Oxygen saturation should be measured, and PEF and FEV_1 should be considered except in children with severe obstruction or in children younger than 5 years of age.

If the patient is in mild-to-moderate distress or has a PEF or FEV_1 50% or greater predicted, then inhaled beta$_2$-agonist by MDI with spacer device or nebulizer is given. Patients should receive up to three treatments in the first hour. Oxygen should be administered as necessary to maintain a saturation of 90% or greater. If the patient does not clear completely with the first dose of beta-agonist, then oral corticosteroid should be given. If there are continued moderate symptoms, then inhaled short acting beta$_2$-agonists should be continued hourly. A good response is indicated by an FEV_1 or PEF 70% or higher that is maintained for at least one hour from the time of the last treatment, no respiratory distress, and a normal physical exam. If the patient demonstrates a good response they may be discharged home.

Patients who present with a severe exacerbation or an FEV_1 or PEF lower than 50% predicted should be treated aggressively. Administer supplemental oxygen to maintain their saturation above 90-95% and initiate high-dose beta$_2$-agonist therapy and anticholinergic continuously for one hour. Corticosteroids should be given parenterally in moderate-to-severe exacerbations and orally in children with mild-to-moderate exacerbation or showing improvement and not vomiting. These patients need to be monitored closely, and, at the end of the first hour of treatment, their response will dictate the extent of continued beta-agonist and anticholinergic frequency.

An incomplete response is indicated by an FEV_1 or PEF 50% or higher but less than 70% after therapy. These patients may benefit from hospitalization or from a short stay admission depending on the facilities available. Hospital admission is also indicated if there is persistent respiratory distress (clinical asthma score greater than 2 or tachypnea) after initial aggressive therapy. Other guidelines include: oxygen saturation less than 93% in room air, previous emergency treatment in the last 24 hours, or an inability to tolerate medications by mouth (i.e., vomiting). Children in high-risk categories should also be considered for admission to the hospital and include those with congenital heart disease, BPD, CF, or neuromuscular disorders.[2,3,15,35]

A poor response is defined as a physical exam that reveals the patient to remain in severe respiratory distress with a high clinical asthma score, a PCO_2 42 mmHg or higher, or an FEV_1 or PEF lower than 50%. These patients should be admitted to an intensive care setting for constant monitoring. Consider intensive care admission if there is 1) impending respiratory failure as evidenced by exhaustion or pulsus paradoxus higher than 25 mmHg, 2) worsening distress despite therapy, 3) requirement for continuous nebulization (beta-agonists less than 1 hour in frequency after the initial 3 treatments), 4) there is evidence of complications from an air leak.[3]

The Child in Respiratory Failure

Most asthma exacerbations do not involve respiratory failure, but almost all exacerbations do involve some degree of reduction in oxygen delivery. A PaO_2 above 50 mmHg affects oxygen saturation much less than a PaO_2 less than 50 mmHg and is part of the definition of type I respiratory failure (i.e., respiratory failure with hypoxia). As an exacerbation evolves, the patient may be unable to maintain minute ventilation due to fatigue, and, eventually, the patient's $PaCO_2$ will begin to rise into the "normal range" and above, signifying type II respiratory failure (i.e., respiratory failure with hypoxia and CO_2 retention).[35,36] Treatment for these patients is limited and may involve the use of intravenous infusions of beta$_2$-agonists and mechanical ventilation. Obviously, these patients need to be monitored closely in an intensive care setting.

At Toronto's Hospital for Sick Children, Bohn and colleagues have used IV infusions of salbutamol (albuterol) in children with imminent respiratory failure and have avoided the need for intubation and mechanical ventilation.[37] It is given as a loading dose of 0.5 mcg/kg, followed by an infusion of 0.2 mcg/kg/min with increases of 0.1 mcg/kg/min every 15 minutes to a maximum of 4 mcg/kg/min monitoring for a decrease in $PaCO_2$ or the development of cardiotoxicity. Since albuterol is not approved by the FDA for use intravenously in the United States, terbutaline can be used in a similar fashion. It is given as a 10 mcg/kg loading dose over 5-10 minutes and then as an infusion of 0.4 mcg/kg/min with increments of 0.2 mcg/kg/min up to a maximum dose of 6 mcg/kg/min.[3]

Intubation and mechanical ventilation is still required in a small number of patients in whom pharmacologic treatment has failed and they are unable to adequately eliminate CO_2. Ketamine (1-2 mg/kg slow IV) is the sedative of choice for intubation in asthmatic patients as it relaxes bronchial smooth muscles, antagonizes the histamine response, and increases the plasma concentration of catecholamines.[38] The concomitant use of benzodiazepines will reduce the risk of emergence phenomena, and the use of an anticholinergic (atropine) will reduce the risk of excessive bronchial secretions associated with the use of ketamine. Exercise caution if rapid sequence intubation with paralytics is performed. Importantly, succinylcholine and pancuronium can cause bronchoconstriction by releasing histamine (potentially worsening hypoxia), while patients with severe bronchoconstriction may be extremely difficult to bag after paralysis due to elevated airway pressures. Histamine release is rare with vecuronium, atracuronium, or rocuronium use.

When volume ventilation is utilized use a low respiratory rate and high inspiratory flow with a long expiratory time and minimal end-expiratory pressure to allow full expiration and enhance venous filling of the heart.[36] You need to allow as full an expiration as possible since air trapping is the underlying problem in asthma. If full expiration is not allowed, the end expiratory pressure continues to increase with subsequent breaths, and this impairs cardiac filling and, subsequently, the patient's blood pressure will fall. By hypoventilating patients, their PCO_2 may increase but they will have a longer expiratory time and be able to decrease their end expiratory pressure. "Even if the $PaCO_2$ doubles from 40 to 80 mmHg, the serum pH will only fall from 7.4 to 7.1. Bicarbonate can be added if needed to raise the pH level to protect the heart from potential adverse effects."[36] This is referred to as permissive hypercapnia and is effective in ventilating asthmatic patients.

Long-term Control Medications

The exact mechanism by which methylxanthines (theophylline and aminophylline) produce bronchodilation is unclear. Though effective bronchodilators, they have a narrow therapeutic window that limits their use. Early appearance of side effects often prevents the goal of optimal smooth muscle relaxation and bronchodilation. Toxic effects include headaches, tremor, nausea, vomiting, dysrrthymias, and seizures. Methylxanthines are no longer recommended for the treatment of acute asthma exacerbations. In several well-designed studies, methylxanthines and steroids have been shown to offer no therapeutic benefit to children with mild-to-severe symptoms but have been associated with more side effects when compared to the use of beta-agonists combined with systemic corticosteroids.[39-41] In the 1997 NIH guidelines, sustained release theophylline is considered a mild-to-moderate bronchodilator and to possibly have some mild anti-inflammatory effects. Its use is primarily as an adjunct to inhaled corticosteroids in the prevention of nocturnal asthma symptoms. For acute exacerbations, unless there is evidence of theophylline toxicity, most authors would continue the long-acting drug.

The leukotriene modifiers are a new class of medications that may play a role in the prevention of symptoms in mild persistent asthma patients. Induction of asthma symptoms, such as bronchospasm, airway edema, mucus secretion, and inflammatory cell migration may be attributed to the leukotrienes. Zafirlukast (Accolate) is a leukotriene antagonist that attenuates the late response to allergens leading to an improvement in pulmonary function and a decrease in asthma symptoms. Zileuton (Zyflo) is a 5-lipoxygenase inhibitor and interferes with the production of leukotrienes. These medications have been shown to partially reverse spontaneous bronchoconstriction and to reduce asthma symptom scores in clinical trials.[42] Their exact role has not yet been defined. They are only recommended for use in children older than 12 years of age.

Salmeterol (Serevent) is a long-acting $beta_2$-adrenoreceptor agonist that is 10 times more potent then albuterol in its bronchodilatory effects. It has a slow onset of action—compared to the short-acting $beta_2$-agonist requiring up to 20 minutes for effect—but has a duration of up to 12 hours. Currently, it is indicated for the long-term prevention of symptoms, especially nocturnal, in combination with an anti-inflammatory agent. It is not recommended as a rescue treatment option for acute asthma exacerbations.[43,44]

Cromolyn Sodium (Intal) and Nedocromil (Tilade) are mast cell membrane stabilizers that are able to suppress both the early and late onset asthma responses. They do not directly produce bronchodilation, but they do decrease bronchial hyper-reactivity and will inhibit the acute phase response from exercise and cold air. These agents require up to two weeks of use to develop therapeutic response and are extremely safe.[45] They are usually initiated for chronic use before inhaled corticosteroids as the first anti-inflammatory medication in the treatment of mild persistent asthma.

Inhaled corticosteroids are useful and effective prophylactic medications that must be differentiated from systemic cortico-steroids. Their clinical effectiveness has been demonstrated in numerous studies, and systemic side effects are extremely low.

Use of Medications

Patients must be educated on how to use their medications and why it is important that they closely follow the instructions. Short-acting $beta_2$-agonists should be prescribed generally as an MDI with spacing device to be administered as 2-6 puffs every 3-4 hours as needed for symptoms of airway obstruction. Prednisone or prednisolone should be prescribed at a dose of 1 mg/kg/dose given once a day or divided twice daily for 3-10 days, up to a maximum dose of 80 mg/day. All patients older than 5 years of age should be given a peak flow meter and taught how to use it correctly. They should also be educated on the use of a diary, to obtain measurements in the morning and evening, and to record the best of three attempts each time. Signs and symptoms of recurrent airflow obstruction should be discussed with the child and family, along with the steps to take if they occur.

Controversial Issues

The use of intravenously administered $beta_2$-angonist has been controversial. In order for beta-agonist to be effective, it must reach the target organ, the small airways, and some investigators believe this initially occurs by systemic absorption of inhaled agents in severe exacerbations. Browne and associates recently performed a double-blind, randomized, placebo-controlled study to determine if a child with severe asthma would have a more rapid initial response to the $beta_2$-agonists if therapeutic salbutamol concentrations could be achieved within 15 minutes of the start of therapy.[46] They found that patients in the intravenous group achieved better pulmonary indices, less distress, a decreased requirement for oxygen, and faster rate of improvement to discharge than inhaled therapy alone.

Except for tremor, there were no other side-effect differences between the two groups, and the tremor was not considered to be clinically significant. Despite small numbers, the results were significant in showing that a 10-minute infusion of IV salbutamol (15 mcg/kg) early in the course of treatment of an acute exacerbation may decrease clinical progression compared to inhaled therapy alone.

The use of oral beta-agonists in children with acute asthma often arises. Louridas and colleagues prospectively compared inhaled salbutamol (albuterol) to oral salbutamol in 10 patients.[47] Pulmonary function tests were performed at 20, 40, 80, and 120 minutes post-medication administration. Within 20 minutes, the FEV_1 in the inhalation group had increased by 7-8% vs. 2-3% in the oral group. This change was even more pronounced at 120 minutes with the FEV_1 increasing by 20% in the inhalation group vs. 5-6% in the oral group. Similar responses were seen in the PEFR. It appears, therefore, that inhaled beta-agonist produces a rapid onset and prolonged upslope in bronchodilatory effects while the oral route has a slower onset and less bronchodilatory effects. The oral form also appears to have more pronounced side effects than the inhaled form. They may be of use in infants with mild asthma, in whom inhaled beta-agonist by MDI may be more difficult to deliver efficiently.

The use of a nebulizer, compared to a MDI, has long been the preferred method of delivery for $beta_2$-agonists in the hospital setting. However, with the addition of spacing devices for use with MDIs, there is increasing evidence that they may be a more reliable method of medication delivery.[48,49] Spacing devices extend the area between the inhaler and the mouth. This allows larger particles that would normally be trapped in the upper airway to be removed in the chamber, thereby reducing systemic absorption and increasing deposition of smaller particles in the airways. The aerosolized particles remain suspended in the spacing device for up to five seconds, which eliminates the need for coordination of MDI activation and inhalation and enhances drug delivery. It has been estimated that an MDI with spacing device delivers up to 20% of the drug to the airways vs. 10% using MDI or nebulizer alone. Current data suggest that between 10-12 inhalations by MDI with spacing device is equivalent to 5 mg of nebulized $beta_2$-agonist.[15]

Amirav and Newhouse recently reviewed 10 articles comparing the use of MDI with spacing devices to nebulizers. Despite administering greater that 2-4 times the dose by nebulizer, the nebulizer never showed any superiority, and, in three of the 10 articles, the MDI with spacing devices was more efficacious.[49] However, the MDI set-up has not been tested in controlled trials using patients with severe obstruction.

It has been proposed that magnesium sulfate stimulates bronchial smooth muscle relaxation by inhibiting calcium flux into smooth muscle cells through the slow calcium channels. The exact mechanism by which decreased magnesium affects bronchospasm is unknown, but there can be a significant decrease in serum magnesium after inhaled bronchodilators. It is unusual for this to be of such significance that it is necessary to measure serum magnesium levels. There have been conflicting studies on its efficacy in the treatment of asthma exacerbations in adults.[50-54] Recently, Ciarallo and colleagues performed a randomized, double-blind, placebo-controlled trial evaluating the efficacy of intravenous magnesium sulfate (IV Mg) in children 6-18 years of age with moderate-to-severe asthma exacerbations.[55] Patients were candidates if, after receiving three $beta_2$-agonist treatments by nebulizer, they continued to have a PEFR less than 60% of their predicted value. Patients in the IV Mg group (25 mg/kg, maximum 2 g in 100-mL normal saline over 20 min) showed improvement by 50 minutes post-treatment. At 110 minutes post-treatment, FEV_1 had improved by 75% in the Mg group vs. 5% in the placebo group. Similar results were seen in PEFR and resulted in fewer hospital admissions. The patients in either group reported no adverse effects, and there were no significant changes in blood pressure. Previously reported side effects were minimal, and these include flushing, mild fatigue, and a burning sensation at the intravenous site. These results revealed more improvement in lung function compared to previous adult studies and are encouraging.

A recent study investigated the use of Heliox (a mixture of 70% helium and 30% oxygen) in children with acute severe asthma exacerbations.[56] The rationale behind its use involved the hypothesis that part of the reason for decreased airflow in asthmatics is turbulent flow. They hypothesized that if you could decrease the density of inspired gas, there should be an improvement in the air exchange. The investigators did not demonstrate a significant effect on pulmonary function.

Antimicrobials were used a great deal in the past in patients with acute asthma exacerbations. While it can be difficult to differentiate a bacterial lower respiratory tract infection from a severe asthma exacerbation, the routine use of antibiotics has not been shown to be beneficial.[57] The diagnosis of pneumonia may be supported by the findings of fever and chills, a left shift in the peripheral white blood cell count, and if the child is old enough to provide a sputum sample, by the finding of a large number of neutrophils in the sputum accompanied by the heavy growth of only 1-2 organisms. Clinically significant infections, such as otitis media or sinusitis, should be treated with amoxicillin, trimethoprim-sulfamethoxazole (Bactrim or Septra), or amoxicillin-clavulanate (Augmentin). If the clinician suspects infection with *Chlamydia pneumoniae* (formerly the TWAR strain), then erythromycin is suggested.

Summary

Asthma is the most common chronic illness of childhood and a leading cause of morbidity. Advances continue to show that inflammation plays a major role in its pathogenesis and severity. The new guidelines by the NHLBI emphasize aggressive anti-inflammatory therapy to control acute exacerbations and chronic symptoms. First-line medications used to control patients with acute asthma exacerbations include $beta_2$-agonists, anticholinergics, and systemic corticosteroids. Further study is needed into therapies such as intravenous magnesium sulfate and salbutamol, which may play an important role in the treatment of patients with moderate-to-severe exacerbations.

References

1. American Thoracic Society: Chronic bronchitis, asthma, and pulmonary emphysema. *Am Rev Respir Dis* 1962;85:762-768.
2. Highlights of the expert panel report 2: Guidelines for the diagnosis and management of asthma. National Institutes of Health, National Heart, Lung and Blood Institute; May 1997. NIH Publication No. 97-4051A.
3. Kulick RM, Ruddy RM. Allergic emergencies. In: Fleisher GR, Ludwig S, eds. *Textbook of Pediatric Emergency Medicine.* 3rd ed. Baltimore, MD: Williams and Wilkens; 1993:858-867.
4. Konig P. Asthma. A pediatric pulmonary disease and a changing concept. *Pediatr Pulmonol* 1987;3:264-275.
5. Nelson DR, Sachs MI, O'Connell EJ. Approaches to acute asthma and status asthmaticus in children. *Mayo Clin Proc* 1989;64: 1392-1402.
6. CDC. Asthma mortality and hospitalization among children and young adults—United States, 1980-1993. *MMWR Morb Mortal Wkly Rep* 1996;45:350-353.
7. Gergen PJ, Weiss KB. Changing patterns of asthma hospitalization among children: 1979 to 1987. *JAMA* 1990;264:1688-1692.
8. Weiss KB, Gergen PJ, Hodgson TA. An economic evaluation of asthma in the United States. *N Engl J Med* 1992;326:862-866.
9. Larsen GL. Asthma in children. *N Engl J Med* 1992;326: 1540-1545.
10. Call RS, Smith TF, Morris E, et al. Risk factors for asthma in inner city children. *J Pediatr* 1992;121:862-866.
11. Newcomb RW, Akhtor J. Respiratory failure from asthma: A marker for children with high morbidity. *AJDC* 1988;142:1041-1044.
12. Martinez FD, Wright AL, Taussig LM, et al. Asthma and wheezing in the first six years of life. *N Engl J Med* 1995;332:133-138.
13. Hall WJ, Hall CB. Bacteria and viruses in etiology and treatment. In: Weiss EB, Stein M, eds. *Bronchial Asthma, Mechanisms and Therapeutics.* 3rd edition. Little, Brown and Company; 1993: 564-576.
14. Senior BA, Kennedy DW. Management of sinusitis in the asthmatic patient. *Ann Allergy Asthma Immunol* 1996;77:6-19.
15. Murphy SJ, Kelly MW. Advances in the management of acute asthma in children. *Pediatr Rev* 1996;17:227-235.
16. McFadden ER. Evolving concepts in the pathogenesis and management of asthma. *Adv Intern Med* 1994;39:357-394.
17. Kaliner MA. How the current understanding of the pathophysiology of asthma influences our approach to therapy. *J Allergy Clin Immunol* 1993;92:144-147.
18. Beasley R, Burgess C, Crane J, et al. Pathology of asthma and its clinical implications. *J Allergy Clin Immunol* 1993;92:148-154.
19. Schuh S, Parker P, Rajan A, et al. High versus low dose frequently administered nebulized albuterol in children with severe acute asthma. *Pediatr* 1989;83:513-518.
20. Williams Jr. MH, Shim C. Clinical evaluation. In: Weiss EB, Stein M, eds. *Bronchial Asthma, Mechanisms and Therapeutics.* 3rd ed. Little, Brown and Company; 1993:447-454.
21. Kaliner M. Goals of asthma therapy. *Ann Allerg Asthma Immunol* 1995;75:169-172.
22. Wood DW, Downes JJ, Lecks MS. A clinical scoring system for the diagnosis of respiratory failure. *AM J Dis Child* 1972;123:227-279.
23. Taylor MRH. Asthma: Audit of peak flow rate guidelines for admission and discharge. *Arch Dis Child* 1994;70:432-434.
24. Geelhoed GC, Landau LI, LeSouef PN. Evaluation of SaO_2 as a predictor of outcome in 280 children presenting with acute asthma. *Ann Emerg Med* 1994;23:1236-1241.
25. Nowak RM, Tomlanovich MC, Sarkar DD, et al. Arterial blood gases and pulmonary function testing in acute bronchial asthma. *JAMA* 1983;249:2043-2046.
26. Gershel JC, Goldman HS, Stein RE. The usefulness of chest radi-

ograph in first asthma attacks. *N Engl J Med* 1983;309:336-339.

27. Bodenhamer J, Bergstrom R, Brown D, Gabow P, et al. Frequently nebulized beta-agonists for asthma: Effects on serum electrolytes. *Ann Emerg Med* 1992;21:1337-1342.
28. Hill NS, Weiss EB. Status asthmaticus. In: Weiss EB, Stein M, eds. *Bronchial Asthma, Mechanisms and Therapeutics.* 3rd ed. Little, Brown and Company; 1993:985-1016.
29. MacDonnell KF, Beauchamp HD. Differential diagnosis. In: Weiss EB, Stein M, eds. *Bronchial Asthma, Mechanisms and Therapeutics.* 3rd ed. Little, Brown and Company; 1993:459-484.
30. Osmond M H, Klassen TP. Efficacy of Ipratropium Bromide in acute childhood asthma: A meta-analysis. *Acad Emer Med* 1995;2: 651-656.
31. Schuh S, Johnson DW, Callahan S, et al. Efficiency of frequent nebulized ipratropium bromide added to frequent high-dose albutrol therapy in severe childhood asthma. *J Pediatr* 1995;126:639-645.
32. Rowe BH, Keller JL, Oxman AD. Effectiveness of steroid therapy in acute exacerbations of asthma: A meta-analysis. *Am J Emerg Med* 1992;10:301-310.
33. Chapman KR, Verbeek PR, White JG, et al. Effect of a short course of prednisone in the prevention of early relapse after the emergency room treatment of acute asthma. *N Engl J Med* 1991;324:788-794.
34. Darr CD. Asthma and bronchiolitis. In: Rosen P, Barkin R, eds. *Emergency Medicine, Concepts and Clinical Practice.* Mosby-Year book, Inc.; 1998:1137-1149.
35. Rubin BK Marcushamer S, Priel I, App EM. Emergency management of the child with asthma. *Pediatr Pulmonol* 1990;8:45-57.
36. Wiener C. Ventilatory management of respiratory failure in asthma. *JAMA* 1993;269:2128-2131.
37. Bohn D, Kalloghlian A, Jenkins J, et al. Intravenous salbutamol in the treatment of status asthmaticus in children. *Crit Care Med* 1984; 12:892.
38. Hemminsen C, Nielson PK, Odorico J. Ketamine in the treatment of bronchospasm during mechanical ventilation. *Am J Emerg Med* 1994;12:417-420.
39. Carter E, Cruz M, Chesrown S, et al. Efficacy of intravenously administered theophylline in children hospitalized with severe asthma. *J Pediatr* 1993;122:470-476.
40. DiGiulio GA, Kercsmar CM, Krug SE, et al. Hospital treatment of asthma: Lack of benefit from theophyline given in addition to nebulized albuterol and intravenously administered corticosteroid. *J Pediatr* 1993;122:464-469.
41. Strauss RE, Wertheim DL, Bonagura VR, et al. Aminophylline therapy does not improve outcome and increases adverse effects in children hospitalized with acute asthma exacerbations. *Pediatrics* 1994;93:205-210.
42. O'Byrne PM, Israel E, Drazen JM. Antileukotrienes in the treatment of asthma. *Ann Intern Med* 1997;127:472-480.
43. Verberne AAPH, Frost C, Roorda RJ, et al. One-year treatment with salmeterol compared with beclomethasone in children with asthma. *Am J Resp Crit Care Med* 1997;156:688-695.
44. Pearlman DS, Chervinsky P, LaForge C, et al. A comparison of salmeterol with albuterol in the treatment of mild-to-moderate asthma. *N Engl J Med* 1992;327:1420-1425.
45. Eigen H, Reid JS, Dahl R, et al. Evaluation of the addition of cromolyn sodium to bronchodilator maintenance therapy in long-term management of asthma. *J Allergy Clin Immunol* 1987;80:612-621.
46. Browne AJ. Penna AS, Phung X, Soo M. Randomized trial of intravenous salbutamol in early management of acute severe asthma in children. *Lancet* 1997;349:301-305.
47. Louridas G, Kakoura M, Galanis N, et al. Bronchodilatory effect of inhaled versus oral salbutamol in bronchial asthma. *Respiration* 1983;44:439-443.
48. Lin YZ, Hsieh KH. Metered dose inhaler and nebulizer in acute asthma. *Arch Dis Child* 1995;72:214-218.
49. Amirav I, Newhouse MT. Metered-dose inhaler accessory devices in acute asthma. Efficacy and comparison with nebulizers: A literature review. *Arch Pediatr Adolesc Med* 1997;151:876-882.
50. Bloch H, Silverman R, Mancherie N, et al. Intravenous magnesium sulfate as an adjunct in the treatment of acute asthma. *Chest* 1995; 107:1576-1581.
51. Skobeloff EN, Spivey WH, McNamara RN, et al. Intravenous magnesium sulfate for the treatment of acute asthma in the emergency department. *JAMA* 1989;262:1210-1213.
52. Noppen M, Vanmaele L, Impers N, et al. Bronchodilation, effect of intravenous magnesium sulfate in acute severe bronchial asthma. *Chest* 1990;97:373-376.
53. Green SM, Rothrock SG. Intravenous magnesium for acute asthma failure to decrease emergency treatment or need for hospitalization. *Ann Emerg Med* 1992;21:260-265.
54. Schiermeyer RP, Finkelstein JA. Rapid infusion of magnesium sulfate obviates need for intubation in status asthmaticus. *Am J Emerg Med* 1994;12:164-166.
55. Ciarallo L, Sauer AH, Shannon MW. Intravenous magnesium therapy for moderate to serve pediatric asthma: Results of a randomized, placebo-controlled trial. *J Pediatr* 1996;129:809-814.
56. Carter ER, Webb CR, Moffitt DR. Evaluation of heliox in children hospitalized with acute severe asthma. A randomized crossover trial. *Chest* 1996;109:1256-1261.
57. Slavin RG. Upper respiratory tract. In: Weiss EB, Stein M, eds. *Bronchial Asthma, Mechanisms and Therapeutics.* 3rd ed. Little, Brown and Company; 1993:533-544.

Immunization Update

Edward Onusko, MD
Shira Katz, MD

Recommendations for routine immunizations has been a dynamic and exciting topic in the field of preventive health services in recent years. This chapter will: present information concerning new vaccines for rotavirus and Lyme disease; update recommendations on established vaccines; highlight opportunities for vaccination at various stages in the life cycle; discuss some useful principles of vaccine administration; and explore various vaccines in development that may be available for clinical use in the near future.

Introduction

The advent of immunizations has greatly reduced the incidence of many infectious diseases. Smallpox has been eradicated worldwide.[1] Poliomyelitis caused by the wild poliovirus has been virtually eliminated in the Western Hemisphere.[2] In the United States, the incidence of many other vaccine-preventable diseases has dropped significantly. (*See Table 1.*) Available vaccines are not always used to their full advantage; however, there are many persons at risk who are not immunized for various reasons. Traditionally, it has been the pediatric population that was regularly immunized. Greater emphasis on adolescent and adult immunization programs has been a more recent development. Even in the pediatric population, there are many problems that contribute to incomplete or undervaccination. There are many studies that show that regular assessment and feedback of vaccination rates to providers result in a significant rise in immunization coverage both in public clinics and the private sector.[3]

It is important that health care providers be aware of the availability of new vaccines and new guidelines for use of older vaccines. This article will present a practical, clinically oriented update on immunizations, with an emphasis on recommendations that are new for 1999.

Immunization of Infants (0-2 years)

Each year, the American Academy of Family Physicians (AAFP), the American Academy of Pediatrics (AAP), and the Advisory Committee on Immunization Practices of the Centers for Disease Control (ACIP) collaborate to provide a recommended childhood immunization schedule (*see Table 2*). This yearly update provides information concerning the addition of newer vaccines and changes in guidelines for older vaccines.

Rotavirus (Rv). For 1999, the rotavirus vaccine (RotaShield—Wyeth Laboratories) has been added to the schedule. Rotavirus is considered to be the most common cause of severe diarrhea among infants and young children in the United States.[4] It has been found to be the major etiology of diarrhea requiring hospitalization. From 1993 to 1995, nearly 500,000 diarrhea-associated hospitalizations were reported in children between the ages of 1 month and 4 years (> 160,000 per year and 13.5% of total hospitalizations in this age group). More than 80,000 of these diarrhea-related hospitalizations (> 26,000 annually) were associated with documented rotavirus infection.[5] (*See Table 3.*) In addition, approximately one of every eight children will seek medical attention due to rotavirus diarrhea in the first five years of life.[4] It has been estimated that a rotavirus immunization program would prevent 39% of cases of rotavirus diarrhea in the first five years of life, with a 55% reduction in physician visits, a 59% reduction in emergency department visits, a 67% reduction in hospitalizations, and a 65% reduction in deaths.[6] (*See Table 4.*)

Rotavirus infections are seasonal, with a peak during the winter months. The virus is highly contagious and most frequently affects children from 6 to 24 months of age. Nearly all children have at least one rotavirus infection before age 5 years. It has been shown that a degree of natural immunity is acquired after exposure to the virus at a young age, but that clinically protective immunity is often acquired only after several infections. It appears that infection can be symptomatic or asymptomatic with the same resulting degree of immunity. The immunity conferred by natural rotavirus infection can range from protection against asymptomatic infection to protection against moderate to severe diarrhea. The highest degree of protection is acquired after at least two infections.[7]

RotaShield is the first rotavirus vaccine to be clinically available. It is an oral, tetravalent vaccine, containing a rhesus rotavirus (serotype 3) and three rhesus-human reassortant viruses (serotypes 1, 2, and 4). These four rotavirus serotypes are responsible for the major portion of rotavirus disease in infants and young children in the United States. The RotaShield vaccine appears to have a good safety profile, with few adverse effects. Fever following administration of the first dose is the main adverse reaction (21% incidence vs 6% with placebo), with occasional excessive irritability or decreased activity. The second and third doses of the vaccine have an incidence of adverse reactions comparable to placebo.[8-10]

The immunity conferred by natural rotavirus infection appears to be most significant in preventing moderate to severe diarrhea.[7] This also appears to be true for the vaccine. In one study in the United States, the efficacy of the vaccine over a single season was 49% for all gastroenteritis; 73% for gastroenteritis needing medical intervention; 80% for severe rotavirus gastroenteritis; and 100% for gastroenteritis with dehydration.[8]

RotaShield is an oral vaccine, scheduled to be given in three doses at 2, 4, and 6 months of age. Other recommendations include: 1) the first dose should not be given before 6 weeks of age; 2) the minimum interval between doses is three weeks; 3) the vaccination series should not be initiated at 7 months of age or older; and 4) all three doses should be completed prior to the first birthday. (Older children seem to have a higher incidence of adverse reactions.) (*See Table 2.*)[6]

The vaccine is contraindicated in infants with a known or suspected immunodeficiency, with an evolving neurological disorder, in acute moderate or severe febrile illnesses, and in infants with persistent vomiting. Precautions in the use of the rotavirus vaccine include prematurity, history of latex sensitivity, chronic gastrointestinal disorders or ongoing diarrhea, and close contact with an immunocompromised individual. The vaccine should not be readministered to a child who vomits, regurgitates, or spits out the dose he or she received (in contrast to oral polio vaccine, which may be readministered).

Due to the newness of the rotavirus vaccine, it may take time to incorporate its use into practice. At the present time, the AAFP is not recommending universal rotavirus immunization, but suggests that the parent or guardian make the decision as to the use of the rotavirus vaccine in consultation with their physician.[11] The U.S. Advisory Committee on Immunization Practices (ACIP) recommends routine use of the vaccine. Cost of the vaccine to the health care provider is about $38 per dose.

Poliovirus—OPV vs. IPV. In 1997, the ACIP revised its recommendations for poliovirus vaccination to allow for three options: 1) sequential—two doses of inactivated poliovirus vaccine (IPV), followed by two doses of oral poliovirus vaccine (OPV); 2) four doses of all IPV; or 3) four doses of all OPV. IPV was first used in the United States in 1955 and was in widespread use until OPV was introduced in 1963. OPV had several advantages over the original IPV: 1) Efficacy—OPV had a more successful immunity profile than IPV (after 3 doses of OPV, 95% of those vaccinated developed long-lasting immunity); 2) Ease of administration—the oral dosing was more readily accepted than injection; 3) In addition to a humoral response, the oral route of administration resulted in the induction of mucosal immunity mediated by secretory IgA, theoretically giving enhanced protection over the IPV; and 4) Excretion of the attenuated poliovirus strain from the gut of the recipient results in secondary transmission and inoculation of susceptible household contacts in 73-96% of cases, depending on the person's age.[12]

Poliovaccine has been effective in preventing wild poliomyelitis. The last naturally occurring case of polio in the United States was in 1979 and the last case in the Western Hemisphere occurred in 1991. Unfortunately, there has been a small incidence of spontaneous reversion of attenuated oral poliovirus to a more virulent form, resulting in vaccine-associated paralytic poliomyelitis (VAPP) at a rate of about one per 2.4 million doses of OPV since 1980. The profile of persons contracting VAPP is: 1) About two-thirds of the cases occur in vaccine recipients. Of these, two-thirds are healthy and one-third have an immunodeficiency (usually a B-cell disorder such as hypogammaglobulinemia, sometimes undiagnosed prior to administration of OPV); 2) About one-third of VAPP occur in contacts of vaccine recipients. Of these, about three-fourths are healthy and one-fourth are immunodeficient; 3) About 80% of VAPP occur after the first dose of OPV vs. subsequent doses. The risk of acquiring VAPP after the first dose of OPV is one case per 750,000. The overall risk of VAPP in healthy recipients (excluding their contacts) is one in 6.2 million doses; and 4) Adult recipients of OPV have a higher rate of VAPP than children. A newer, enhanced-potency IPV was licensed for use in the United States in 1987. It too confers long-lasting immunity in 90-100% of recipients. After several studies were done, the ACIP decided that two IPV followed by two OPV was also an acceptable alternative poliovirus vaccine series, in addition to the four OPV series and the four IPV series.[13]

The reason for using IPV (either exclusively or prior to using OPV) was to reduce the incidence of vaccine-associated paralytic poliomyelitis (VAPP). Two doses of IPV induce protective humoral immunity in more than 90% of recipients, thus preventing VAPP with subsequent doses of OPV. The OPV will then induce mucosal immunity as well, though some virus may be shed from the gut and result in exposure of household or community contacts. The preva-

Table 1. The Maximum Number of Cases of Specified Vaccine-Preventable Diseases Ever Reported for a Calendar Year Compared With the Number of Cases of Disease and Vaccine Adverse Events Reported for 1995—United States

Category	Maximum no. reported cases during prevaccination era	Year(s) maximum no. cases reported	Reported no. cases during 1995*	Percentage change in morbidity
Disease				
Congenital rubella syndrome	20,000†	1964-65	7	(-99.96)
Diphtheria	206,939	1921	0	(-99.99)
Invasive *Haemophilus influenzae*	20,000†	1984	1164	(-99.18)
Measles	894,134	1941	309	(-99.97)
Mumps	152,209	1968	840	(-99.45)
Pertussis	265,269	1934	4315	(-98.37)
Poliomyelitis (wild)	21,269	1952	0	(-99.99)
Rubella	57,686	1969	146	(99.75)
Tetanus	601	1948	34	(97.82)
Vaccine adverse events††	**0**		**10,594**	

*Provisional totals.

†Estimated because national reporting did not exist in the prevaccine era.

††Total number reported to the Vaccine Adverse Events Reporting System (VAERS).

Source: *MMWR Morb Mort Wkly Rep* 45(RR-12):2.

lence of immunity following the sequential series ranged from 96% to 100%.[14]

In 1996, the results of an analysis were published suggesting that using IPV exclusively or in a sequential schedule would not be cost-effective despite the prevention of at least some cases of VAPP. It was eventually decided, however, to incorporate the option of the sequential series in the hopes that it would reduce the anxiety over OPV vaccination and increase public confidence in the safety of vaccination programs.[15] This was also a compromise between "all OPV" advocates and "all IPV" advocates. Since then, the costs of IPV and OPV schedules are similar, so it is now probably cost-effective to use IPV.[12]

The 1999 recommendations now state that either an all-IPV or a sequential 2IPV/2OPV schedule should be used. This would prevent nearly all cases of OPV-associated VAPP in recipients, while ensuring both mucosal and humoral immunity.

OPV is not recommended for use for the first two vaccine doses except in special circumstances: 1) if the parents do not accept the recommended number of injections; 2) if the first dose is being administered late and would require an unacceptable number of injections; or 3) if the infant will be traveling shortly to a country where polio is endemic (therefore increasing the urgency to induce mucosal immunity).[15]

Previously, there had been some questions as to the efficacy and safety of administration of the OPV and the rotavirus vaccine simultaneously. When RRV-TV was used and three doses given, there was no significant suppression of rotavirus or poliovirus antibody response.[16,17] This is less important now since the first two doses of poliovirus vaccine will usually be IPV. Both RotaShield and OPV are effective in inducing immunity in breastfed infants, despite the possible presence of maternal antibodies in the breast milk.

Diphtheria/tetanus/acellular Pertussis (DTaP). Another change in the 1999 recommended immunization schedule is that the combination vaccine diphtheria, tetanus, and acellular pertussis (DTaP), is now the preferred vaccine, rather than the whole cell DTP (DTwP or DTP). The DTaP has one-fourth to one-half of the adverse effects of DTwP. The combination vaccine DTaP-Hib (*H. influenzae* type b) is not recommended for children younger than 1 year of age due to decreased efficacy of the Hib portion of the vaccine.[11]

The recommendations for the use of Hepatitis B vaccine have changed slightly. For infants, the third dose in the series should not be given prior to 6 months of age. (*See Insert.*) Previously, the third dose could be given as early as four months. *H. influenzae* type b (Hib), measles/mumps/rubella (MMR), and varicella vaccine recommendations for infancy are unchanged (*see Table 2*).

Immunization of Preschool Children (ages 4-6 years)

Some school systems and some states are mandating completion of Hepatitis B vaccination by 1 year of age or before entry into

Table 2. Recommended Childhood Immunization Schedule (United States, January-December 1999)

Vaccines[1] are listed under the routinely recommended ages. Bars indicate range of recommended ages for immunization. Any dose not given at the recommended age should be given as a "catch-up" immunization at any subsequent visit when indicated and feasible. Shaded bars indicate vaccines to be given if previously recommended doses were missed or given earlier than the recommended minimum age.

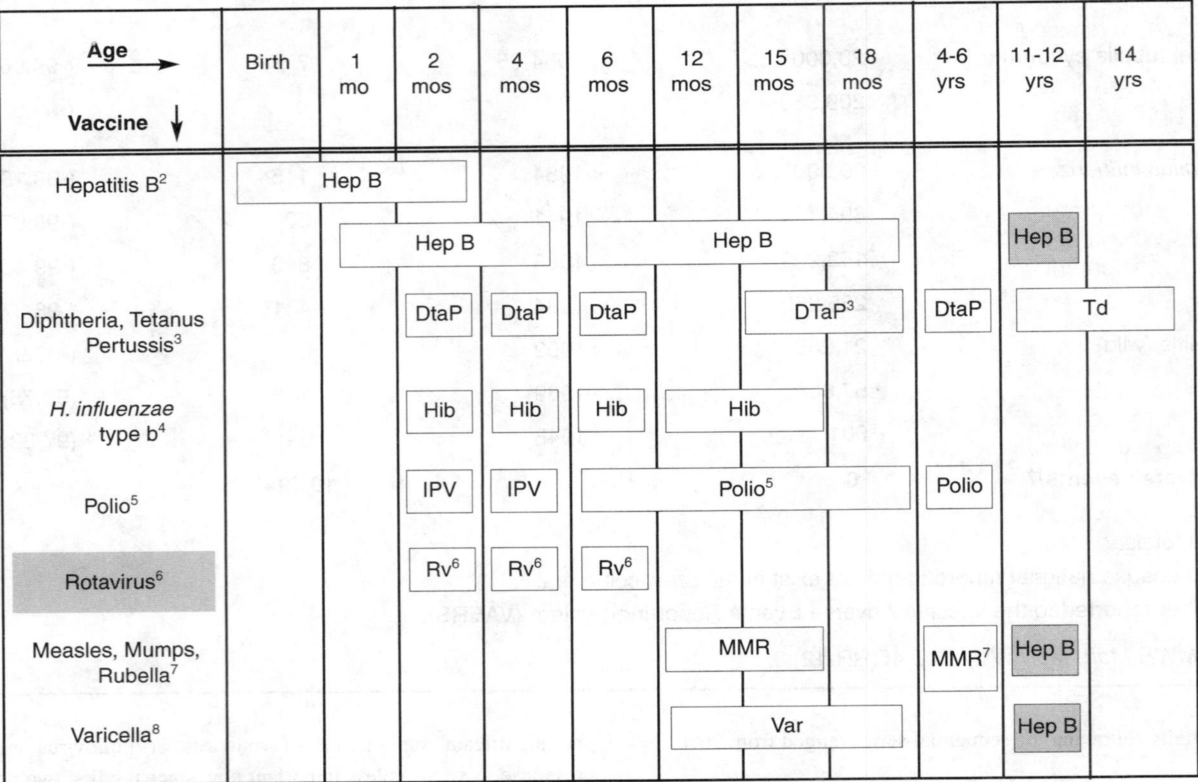

Age → / Vaccine ↓	Birth	1 mo	2 mos	4 mos	6 mos	12 mos	15 mos	18 mos	4-6 yrs	11-12 yrs	14 yrs
Hepatitis B[2]	Hep B										
		Hep B			Hep B					Hep B	
Diphtheria, Tetanus Pertussis[3]			DtaP	DtaP	DtaP		DTaP[3]		DtaP	Td	
H. influenzae type b[4]			Hib	Hib	Hib	Hib					
Polio[5]			IPV	IPV	Polio[5]				Polio		
Rotavirus[6]			Rv[6]	Rv[6]	Rv[6]						
Measles, Mumps, Rubella[7]						MMR			MMR[7]	Hep B	
Varicella[8]						Var				Hep B	

1 This schedule indicated the recommended ages for routine administration of currently licensed childhood vaccines. Combination vaccines may be used whenever any components of the combination are indicated and its other components are not contraindicated. Providers should consult the manufacturers' package inserts for detailed recommendations.

2 Infants born to HBsAg-negative mothers should receive the second dose of hepatitis B vaccine at least one month after the 1st dose. The 3rd dose should be administered at least 4 months after the 1st dose and at least 2 months after the 2nd dose, but not before 6 months of age for infants.
Infants born to HBsAg-positive mothers should receive hepatitis B vaccine and 0.5 mL hepatitis B immune globulin (HBIG) within 12 hours of birth at separate sites. The 2nd dose is recommended at 1-2 months of age and the 3rd dose at 6 months of age.
Infants born to mothers whose HBsAg status is unknown should receive hepatitis B vaccine within 12 hours of birth. Maternal blood should be drawn at the time of delivery to determine the mother's HBsAg status; if the HBsAg test is positive, the infant should receive HBIG as soon as possible (no later than 1 week of age). All children and adolescents (through 18 years of age) who have not been immunized against hepatitis B may begin the series during any visit. Special efforts should be made to immunize children who were born in or whose parents were born in areas of the world with moderate or high endemicity of HBV infection.

3 DTaP (diphtheria and tetanus toxoids and acellular pertussis vaccine) is the preferred vaccine for all doses in the immunization series, including completion of the series in children who have received one or more doses of whole-cell DTP vaccine. Whole-cell DTP is an acceptable alternative to DTaP. The 4th dose (DTP or DTaP) may be administered as early as 12 months of age, provided 6 months have elapsed since the 3rd dose and if the child is unlikely to return at age 15-18 months. Td (tetanus and diphtheria toxoids) is recommended at 11-12 years of age if at least 5 years have elapsed since the last dose of DTP, DTaP, or DT. Subsequent routine Td boosters are recommended every 10 years.

4 Three *H. influenzae* type b (Hib) conjugate vaccines are licensed for infant use. If PRP-OMP (PedvaxHIB) and COMVAX (Merck) are administered at 2 and 4 months of age, a dose at 6 months is not required. Because clinical studies in infants have demonstrated that using some combination products may induce a lower immune response to the Hib vaccine compo-

Table 2. Recommended Childhood Immunization Schedule (United States, January-December 1999) *Continued*

nent, DTaP/Hib combination products should not be used for primary immunization infants at 2, 4, or 6 months of age, unless FDA-approved for these ages.

5 Two poliovirus vaccines are currently licensed in the United States: inactivated poliovirus vaccine (IPV) and oral poliovirus vaccine (OPV). The ACIP, AAP, and AAFP now recommend that the first two doses of poliovirus vaccine should be IPV. The ACIP continues to recommend a sequential schedule of two doses of IPV administered at ages 2 and 4 months, followed by two doses of OPV at 12-18 months and 4-6 years. Use of IPV for all doses also is acceptable and is recommended for immunocompromised persons and their household contacts. OPV is no longer recommended for the first two doses of the schedule and is acceptable only for special circumstances such as: children of parents who do not accept the recommended number of injections, late initiation of immunization which would require an unacceptable number of injections, and imminent travel to polio-endemic areas. OPV remains the vaccine of choice for mass immunization campaigns to control outbreaks due to wild poliovirus.

6 Rotavirus (Rv) vaccine is shaded and italicized to indicate: 1) health care providers may require time and resources to incorporate this new vaccine into practice; and 2) the AAFP feels that the decision to use rotavirus vaccine should be made by the parent or guardian in consultation with their physician or other health care provider. The first dose of Rv vaccine should not be administered before 6 weeks of age, and the minimum interval between doses is 3 weeks. The Rv vaccine series should not be initiated at 7 months of age or older, and all doses should be completed by the first birthday.

7 The 2nd dose of measles, mumps, and rubella (MMR) vaccine is recommended routinely at 4-6 years of age but may be administered during any visit, provided at least 4 weeks have elapsed since receipt of the 1st dose and that both doses are administered beginning at or after 12 months of age. Those who have not previously received the second dose should complete the schedule by the 11-12 year-old visit.

8 Varicella vaccine is recommended at any visit on or after the first birthday for susceptible children (i.e., those who lack a reliable history of chickenpox [as judged by a health care provider] and who have not been immunized. Susceptible persons 13 years of age or older should receive two doses, given at least 4 weeks apart.

Note: This schedule is provided by the American Academy of Family Physicians only as an assistance for physicians making clinical decisions regarding the care of their patients. As such, they cannot substitute for the individual judgment brought to each clinical situation by the patient's family physician. As with all clinical reference resources, they reflect the best understanding of the science of medicine at the time of publication, but they should be used with the clear understanding that continued research may result in new knowledge and recommendations.

Source: *AFP* 1999;59:203-204;206.

primary grades.[18] For example, the Ohio legislature recently approved a law requiring that all kindergarten students show evidence of the Hepatitis B vaccination series beginning with the 1999-2000 school year. Those children in the process of being immunized will be able to enter school but will be monitored to ensure completion of the vaccination series.[19]

It is now recommended that the second dose of MMR be given at age 4-6 years rather than at the preteen years.

It is still recommended that boosters for DTaP and polio be given at age 4-6 years. If the fourth dose of DTaP (or DTwP) is given after the fourth birthday, a fifth dose is not needed. If the third dose of polio is given after the fourth birthday in the all-IPV or all-OPV series, a fourth dose is not needed. If the sequential 2-IPV/2-OPV series is used, all four doses need to be administered.

Immunization of Adolescents/Preteens (ages 11-12 years)

Most vaccination programs focus on infants and children. Many adolescents continue to suffer from vaccine-preventable diseases because they have not been previously vaccinated or have not received indicated booster doses of vaccines. It is now recommended that a routine health care visit be scheduled for age 11-12 years in order to provide preventive health services and to immunize those adolescents who are not up-to-date on their vaccinations.[20] *(See Table 5.)*

Hepatitis B is one of the vaccinations that many adolescents have not received, simply because the vaccine was not in use when they were infants. One of the most common sources of hepatitis B infection in adolescents is sexual activity. Therefore, it is important that those who are not immunized receive the vaccine before becoming sexually active or beginning high-risk behaviors.[20] Many colleges and universities are requiring students to be immunized prior to admission.[18] Universal vaccination with hepatitis B is recommended for all infants and adolescents, regardless of risk factors.

Varicella is another vaccine-preventable disease that most adolescents have not been vaccinated against. It is thought that approximately 20% of adolescents are still susceptible to varicella, despite a high incidence of exposure to natural infection in the community. The varicella vaccine became available in 1995[20] and since 1996 has been a part of the recommended routine immunization schedule.[18] Varicella (chicken pox) can be a debilitating illness in persons 15 years of age or older, with many complications, including death.[20] Therefore, it is recommended to vaccinate those without a convincing history of natural infection. Administering the

Table 3. Age-Specific Proportion of Reported Gastroenteritis (GE) Hospitalizations Associated with Rotavirus (RV) among Children Ages 1-59 Months, 1993-1995

Age group (months)	No. of GE hospitalizations	No. of GE hospitalizations associated with RV (%)	Cumulative no. of RV hospitalizations
1-3	65,943	6761 (10.3)	6761 (8.4)
4-6	47,009	4666 (9.9)	11,427 (14.2)
7-11	88,674	17,245 (19.5)	28,672 (35.7)
12-23	138,234	29,487(21.2)	58,159 (72.3)
24-35	73,164	14,053 (19.20)	72.212 (89.8)
36-47	41,898	6040 (14.4)	78,242 (97.3)
48-59	31,511	2141 (6.8)	80,393 (100)
Total	487,433	80,393 (16.5)	——

Source: Parasher UD. *J Infect Dis* 1998;177:13-17.

vaccine by 12 years of age has the advantage that a single dose of vaccine is sufficient. Older than that age, two doses should be given, with at least four weeks between doses.[18,20,21] Another advantage of the vaccine is that the development of herpes zoster (shingles) later in life seems much less likely in vaccine recipients vs. those who have had natural varicella infection.[22]

Recommendations for mumps, measles, and rubella (MMR) include two doses at 12 months of age or older. Some children have received both doses prior to reaching adolescence. Those who have not could be administered the vaccine at the 11-12 year visit. There are states that now require two doses of MMR before entering elementary school, while others require them prior to entering middle school.[20]

The 11-12 year visit is also a good time to administer a tetanus, diphtheria (Td) booster. If the DTaP was given at age 4-6 years, it is now thought that age 11-12 years is an appropriate time for a Td booster to ensure long-lasting immunity. It has been found that immunity is decreased in persons 9-13 years of age, with up to 36% unprotected. After this booster, doses are recommended at 10-year intervals.

Immunization of Adults

Adults who are not immunized can be at risk for many of the diseases that we consider "childhood diseases." These diseases can be devastating with severe complications, including death. Any adult not immunized against varicella (and without a clinical history of chicken pox) or measles/mumps/rubella should be vaccinated against these diseases. As mentioned with adolescents, a Td booster should be given every 10 years.[18]

The ACIP and AAFP are now recommending that physicians review the immunization status of their adult patients at age 50 in order to determine what routine vaccinations are necessary. In addition, the physician should determine what risk factors might be present, indicating a need for other less routine vaccinations. Among adults 50-65 years old, 30-40% have risk factors that necessitate immunizing with the pneumococcal vaccine and/or the influenza vaccine.[18]

Pneumococcal vaccine. The pneumococcal vaccine has been well documented to provide significant protection against invasive forms of pneumococcal disease, such as bacteremia and meningitis. It is not effective against upper respiratory infections such as otitis media and sinusitis.[22] Likewise, the effectiveness of the vaccine in decreasing the incidence of pneumococccal pneumonia in middle-aged and elderly individuals has been questioned.[24-26] Health care providers often promote this vaccine to their patients as "the pneumonia vaccine." Strictly speaking, it is a vaccine that provides significant protection against pneumococcal bacteremia and meningitis. Adults to be immunized include those 65 years of age or older and those at increased risk of invasive pneumococcal disease. Adults at increased risk are defined later in this article. Although the effectiveness of the vaccine has not been proven in all high-risk groups, vaccination is felt to be justified.[23]

Rates of pneumococcal vaccination (about 30% for individuals with approved indications) have been consistently lower than rates for influenza vaccine.

Influenza vaccine. As with pneumococcal disease, influenza can cause significant morbidity and mortality in individuals older than 65 years of age or in other high-risk groups. Influenza is estimated to cause 10,000-40,000 deaths and 200,000 hospitalizations in the United States annually.[27] There are three strains of influenza virus, but only two cause the seasonal epidemics in the United States. Each year, a new influenza vaccine is prepared with a different antigenic makeup, determined by which virus strains are thought most likely to be circulating the coming winter.[28,29] Influenza vaccination rates in persons aged 65 years or older have improved in recent years to approximately 66%, but rates among at-risk patients younger than 65 years have remained below 30%.[27] The success of the vaccine in attenuating or preventing illness depends on both the extent of a successful match, and by the age and immunocompetence of the vaccine recipient. A recent retrospective cohort study of women aged 15-64 years enrolled in the Tennessee Medicaid program from 1974 to 1993 demonstrated a substantial increase in morbidity and mortality from acute cardiopulmonary events during influenza season, suggesting a possible

Table 4. Rotavirus Health Outcomes and Costs With and Without a Rotavirus Immunization Program*

Variable	No Vaccine Program	With Vaccine Program	Prevented by Vaccine Program	Reduction (%)
Events, No.				
Total rotavirus diarrhea	2,730,000	1,652,000	1,078,000	39
Physician visits	410,000	183,000	227,000	55
Emergency department visits	160,000	65,000	95,000	59
Hospitalizations	50,000	16,400	33,600	67
Deaths	20	7	13	65
Costs, $(thousands)				
Medical costs				
Office visits	51,777	23,144	28,633	55
Emergency department visits	37,264	15,185	22,079	59
Hospital	175,434	43,894	131,540	75
Death (emergency department visits)	15	5	10	67
Vaccine administration	0	192,660	-96,300	. . .†
Cost of vaccine, $20 per dose	0	—	-192,660	. . .†
Total Medical Costs	264,490	371,218	-106,728	-40
Nonmedical costs				
Loss of earnings by caregiver	687,779	311,390	376,389	-55
Other direct nonmedical	28,577	15,654	12,923	45
Lifetime productivity loss of child to death	19,912	6541	13,371	67
Total Nonmedical Costs	732,268	333,585	402,683	55
Total Cost	1,000,758	704,803	295,955	30

*Data are five-year estimates for a birth cohort of 3.9 million.
†Ellipses indicate cost incurred.

Source: Tucker AW. *JAMA* 1998;279(17):1371-1376.

need for routine influenza vaccination in this relatively low-risk population.[27] The majority of persons hospitalized secondary to influenza are not those aged 65 years or older, but are persons younger than 65 years who have chronic underlying conditions—particularly chronic pulmonary disease.[30] At times, the vaccine has been 70-90% effective in preventing disease. Other studies have shown it to be successful in preventing hospital complications and death, especially in nursing home patients.[29]

Immunization of High-Risk Populations

There are many children, adolescents, and adults younger than age 65 who have special needs when it comes to immunizations. These include those with: 1) chronic cardiovascular diseases (such as congestive heart failure or cardiomyopathy); 2) chronic pulmonary diseases (emphysema, chronic bronchitis, asthma); 3) metabolic disorders (including, but not only, diabetes mellitus); 4) chronic renal disorders; 5) chronic liver disorders; 6) sickle cell disease and other hemoglobinopathies; and 7) immunocompromised states, such as asplenia (functional and anatomic), malignancies (leukemia, lymphoma, etc.), patients on chemotherapy or chronic steroid treatment, and patients with HIV infections. (In this last group, the efficacy of immunization has not been proven, but the benefits probably outweigh the risks.) All of these patients need to be immunized with both the pneumococcal and influenza vaccines.[23,28,29] Table 6 shows the recommendations for pneumococcal vaccine and for revaccination. In addition, there are some special indications for influenza vaccine, including children who are on chronic aspirin therapy and would, therefore, be at an increased risk for Reye's syndrome. Also at risk are pregnant women who will be in their second or third trimester during the influenza season and health care workers who could potentially transmit influenza to persons at high risk.[29] A recent randomized trial demonstrated the effectiveness of influenza vaccine in preventing serologically

Table 5. Recommended Vaccination Schedule for Adolescents Ages 11-12 Years

IMMUNOLOGIC	INDICATIONS	NAME	DOSE	FREQUENCY	ROUTE
Hepatitis A vaccine	Adolescents who are at increased risk of hepatitis A infection or its complications	HAVRIX*	720 EL.U†/0.5 mL$^{\delta}$	A total of two doses at 0,¶ 6-12 mos	IM**
		VAQTA*	25 U/0.5 mL	A total of two doses at 0, 6-18 mos	IM
Hepatitis B vaccine	Adolescents not vaccinated previously for hepatitis B	Recombivax HB*	5 mcg/0.5 mL	A total of three doses at 0, 1-2, 4-6 months	IM
		Engerix-B*	10 mcg/0.5 mL	A total of three doses at 0, 1-2, 4-6 mos	IM
Influenza vaccine	Adolescents who are at increased risk for complications caused by influenza or who have contact with persons at increased risk for these complications	Influenza virus vaccine††	0.5 mL	Annually (September-December)	IM
Measles, mumps, and rubella vaccine (MMR)	Adolescents not vaccinated previously with two doses of measles vaccine at ≥ 12 mos of age	MMR II*	0.5 mL	One dose	SC$^{\delta\delta}$
Pneumococcal polysaccharide vaccine	Adolescents who are at increased risk for pneumococcal disease or its complications	Pneumococcal vaccine polyvalent††	0.5 mL	One dose	IM or SC
Tetanus and diphtheria toxoids (Td)	Adolescents not vaccinated within the previous five yrs	Tetanus and diphtheria toxoids, absorbed (for adult use)††	0.5 mL	Every 10 yrs	IM
Varicella virus vaccine	Adolescents not vaccinated previously and who have no reliable history of chickenpox	VARIVAX*	0.5 mL	One dose¶¶	SC

*Manufacturer's product name
†Enzyme-linked immunosorbent assay (ELISA) unit.
$^{\delta}$Alternative dosage and schedule of 360 EL.U/0.5 mL and a total of three doses administered at 0, 1, and 6-12 months.
¶0 months represents timing of the initial dose, and subsequent numbers represent months after the initial dose.
**Intramuscular injection.
††Generic name.
$^{\delta\delta}$Subcutaneous injection.
¶¶Adolescents ≥ 13 years of age should be administered a total of two doses (0.5 mL/dose) subcutaneously at 0 and 4-8 weeks.
Source: *MMWR Morb Mort Wkly Rep* 1996;45(RR-13).

defined influenza A (88% effective) and influenza B (89% effective) in health care professionals.[31]

Those who should be immunized against hepatitis B are health care workers, hemodialysis patients, persons with high-risk sexual behavior, IV drug users, persons receiving clotting factor concentrates and other blood products, adoptees from countries where the disease is endemic, international travelers to those countries, those who are in close personal contact with hepatitis B carriers, and patients with hepatitis C or chronic liver disease.[18,28]

Hepatitis A vaccine is recommended for those with hepatitis C infections, other chronic liver disorders, illegal drug users, homosexual males, travelers to endemic areas, military personnel, and persons with an occupational risk.[18]

General Considerations

The Insert is a table of summaries of the recommended immunizations for children and adults, respectively. These tables include: 1) Indications for the vaccine; 2) The recommended dosing schedule; 3) The minimum dosing intervals. For example, MMR is recommended to be given in two doses at ages 12 months and 4-6 years. However, it is acceptable to give the first dose at 12 months and the second dose as early as 13 months, because the minimum interval between the first and second doses is 28 days (as long as both doses are given after the first birthday); 4) Scheduling guidelines for those who are behind; and 5) Contraindications and precautions.

Live, attenuated-virus vaccines (OPV, MMR, Varicella, and Rv) in general are able to reproduce in the vaccine recipient, thereby increasing the antigenic stimulus and enhancing the body's immune response. What is the risk, however, of these vaccines causing actual clinical infection in the immunized individual or their contacts? All four of the above live virus vaccines can rarely induce clinical infection in the vaccine recipient. (That's why VAPP has occurred with OPV, as discussed previously, and why MMR and Varicella vaccines are contraindicated in pregnancy.) In contacts of vaccine recipients, it is also clear with OPV there is a small risk of contracting VAPP. With MMR administration, however, there is no associated risk of transmission of clinical infection to household or community contacts. Varicella vaccine seems to carry only a very slight risk of transmission—usually only from recipients who develop a herpetic-type rash following vaccine administration. Rotavirus replicates in the intestine of the recipient and is shed in the stool. Although numerous studies have failed to demonstrate transmission of significant infection to contacts of vaccine recipients, caution is still recommended in administering the vaccine if family members or other close contacts are immunocompromised.

Figure. Lyme Disease Distribution

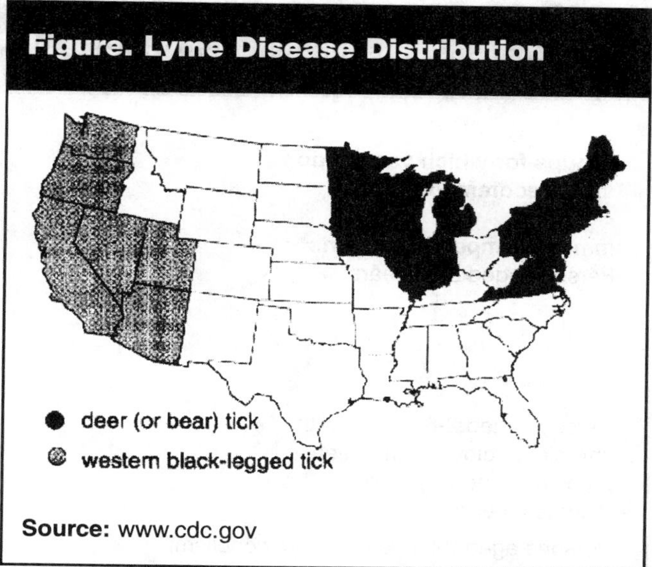

Source: www.cdc.gov

New Vaccines on the Horizon

Lyme Disease. Lyme disease is a tick-borne infection that may result in chronic arthritic, neurologic, cardiac, and other symptoms. It is endemic primarily in the Northeast and Upper Midwest regions of the United States (*see Figure 1*). There is now a vaccine available against Lyme disease. LYMErix (SmithKline Beecham) was approved by the FDA in December 1998 for ages 15-70 years. It has been shown to be efficacious after a three-dose series (initial dose, followed by doses at 1 month and 12 months) of the vaccine.[32-34] Efficacy of immune response was 49-68% after two doses and 76-92% after the third dose. The duration of protection is unknown. Eight months after the third injection, antibody levels had fallen to near the lower limit of protective levels, suggesting that frequent boosters may be necessary.[35] The Lyme disease vaccine caused some adverse effects. These included soreness, redness, and swelling at the site of injection, and some systemic symptoms such as myalgias, fever, and chills. All of these adverse effects were minor and self limited—none lasting longer than several days.[32,33]

The development of this vaccine shows promise in the fight against Lyme disease, but antibiotics alone are generally effective in treating early disease and preventing complications, and the long-term safety and effectiveness of the vaccine are unknown.[35] It should be considered for use in high-risk individuals (adults who live in endemic areas and live, work, or walk in grassy or wooded areas), though its role in this population is still uncertain. Vaccination does not reduce the need for preventive measures such as avoiding tick habitats, wearing protective clothing, promptly removing attached ticks, etc. The vaccine should probably not be used in low-risk populations. The ideal time for the third vaccine may be in March, just prior to the tick season. More studies are needed to test the efficacy and safety of the vaccine in children.

Conjugate Pneumococcal Vaccine. At the present time, research is being done on protein-polysaccharide conjugate vaccines against pneumococcal disease. A vaccine of this type would potentially be more immunogenic and would improve the efficacy of the vaccine. The vaccines being tested at this time include seven serotypes and could potentially protect against bacteremia, meningitis, and otitis media. Preliminary data also suggest that conjugate vaccines may also reduce the incidence of the nasopharyngeal carrier states of the specific serotypes in the vaccine. Although the research at present is focusing on a vaccine for children, it will probably be evaluated for use in adults—especially those who respond poorly to the present vaccine.[23]

Nasal spray influenza vaccine. Also on the horizon is a pediatric nasal spray vaccine for preventing influenza. It is a live, attenuated influenza virus vaccine. Preliminary studies show it to be 95% effective in children ages 1-6 years.[36] It is awaiting FDA approval and may be available for use by the fall of 1999. It appears to have the potential advantage of inducing nasal mucosal immunity because of the route of administration.

Summary

Immunization is an important part of the arsenal in the fight against infectious diseases. It is the responsibility of health care providers to ensure that their patients receive the maximum benefit from available vaccinations. In order to do this, we must keep up-to-date with the development of new vaccines and with changes in the guidelines for established vaccines.

References

1. World Health Organization. The global eradication of smallpox: Final report of the Global Commission for the Certification of Smallpox Eradication. In: *History of International Public Health*. No. 4. Geneva, Switzerland: World Health Organization, 1980.
2. CDC. Certification of poliomyelitis eradication—the Americas, 1994. *MMWR Morb Mort Wkly Rep* 1994;43: 720-722.
3. LeBaron CW, et al. Impact of measurement and feedback on vaccination coverage in public clinics, 1988-1994. *JAMA* 1997;277(8):631-635.
4. Glass RI, et al. The epidemiology of rotavirus diarrhea in the United States: Surveillance and estimates of disease burden. *J Infect Dis* 1996;174(Suppl 1):S5-S11.

Table 6. Recommendations for the Use of Pneumococcal Vaccine

Groups for which vaccination is recommended	Strength of recommendation*	Revaccination†
Immunocompetent persons[δ]		
Persons aged ≥ 65 years	A	Second dose of vaccine if patient received vaccine≥ 5 years previously and were aged < 65 years at the time of vaccination.
Persons aged 2-64 years with chronic cardiovascular disease,¶ chronic pulmonary disease,** or diabetes mellitus	A	Not recommended.
Persons aged 2-64 years with alcoholism, chronic liver disease,†† or cerebrospinal fluid leaks	B	Not recommended.
Persons aged 2-64 years with functional or anatomic asplenia[δδ]	A	If patient is aged > 10 years: single revaccination≥ 5 years after previous dose. If patient is aged≥ 10 years: consider revaccination 3 years after previous dose.
Persons aged 2-64 years living in special environments or social settings.¶¶	C	Not recommended.
Immunocompromised persons[δ]		
Immunocompromised persons aged ≥ 2 years, including those with HIV infection, leukemia, lymphoma, Hodgkin's disease, multiple myeloma, generalized malignancy, chronic renal failure, or nephrotic syndrome; those receiving immuno-suppressive chemotherapy (including corticosteroids); and those who have received an organ or bone marrow transplant.	C	Single revaccination if ≥ 5 years have elapsed since receipt of first dose. If patient is aged ≥ 10 years: consider revaccination 3 years after previous dose.

*The following categories reflect the strength of evidence supporting the recommendations for vaccination:
A = Strong epidemiologic evidence and substantial clinical benefit support the recommendation for vaccine use.
B = Moderate evidence supports the recommendation for vaccine use.
C = Effectiveness of vaccination is not proven, but the high risk for disease and the potential benefits and safety of the vaccine justify vaccination.
†Strength of evidence for all revaccination recommendations is "C"
δIf earlier vaccination status is unknown, patients in this group should be administered pneumococcal vaccine.
¶Including congestive heart failure and cardiomyopathies.
**Including chronic obstructive pulmonary disease and emphysema.
††Including cirrhosis.
δδIncluding sickle cell disease and splenectomy.
¶¶Including Alaskan Natives and certain American Indian populations.

Source: *MMWR Morb Mortal Wkly Rep* 1997;46(RR-8).

5. Parashar UD, et al. Hospitalizations associated with rotavirus diarrhea in the United States, 1993 through 1995: Surveillance based on the new ICD-9-CM rotavirus-specific diagnostic code. *J Infect Dis* 1998;177:13-17.
6. Tucker AW, et al. Cost-effectiveness analysis of a rotavirus immunization program for the United States. *JAMA* 1998; 279(17):1371-1376.
7. Velazquez FR, et al. Rotavirus infection in infants as protection against subsequent infections. *N Engl J Med* 1996;335(14):1022-1028.
8. Rennels MB, et al. Safety and efficacy of high-dose rhesus-human reassortant rotavirus vaccines—Report of the national multicenter trial. *Pediatrics* 1996;97:7-13.
9. *The Medical Letter.* A vaccine for rotavirus. Vol. 41 (Issue 1053):50. May 21, 1999.
10. Joensuu J, et al. Randomised placebo-controlled trial of rhesus-human reassortant rotavirus vaccine for prevention of severe rotavirus gastroenteritis. *Lancet* 1997;350:1205-1209.
11. Zimmerman RK. The 1999 harmonized immunization schedule. *AFP* 1999;59:203-204,206.
12. Zimmerman RK, Spann SJ. Poliovirus vaccine options. *AFP* 1999;59(1):113-118.
13. CDC. Poliomyelitis prevention in the United States: Introduction of a sequential vaccination schedule of inactivated poliovirus vaccine followed by oral poliovirus vaccine; recommendations of the advisory committee on immunization practices (ACIP). *MMWR Morb Mort Wkly Rep* 1997;46(RR-3):1-24.
14. Modlin JF, et al. Humoral and mucosal immunity in infants induced by three sequential inactivated poliovirus vaccine-live attenuated oral poliovirus vaccine immunization schedules. *J Infect Dis* 1997;175(Suppl 1):S228-S234.
15. Miller MA, et al. Cost-effectiveness of incorporating inactivated poliovirus vaccine into the routine childhood immunization schedule. *JAMA* 1996;276(12):967-971.
16. Migasena S, et al. Simultaneous administration of oral rhesus-human reassortant tetravalent (RRV-TV) rotavirus vaccine and oral poliovirus vaccine (OPV) in Thai infants. *Vaccine* 1996;13(2):168-174.
17. Rennels MB, et al. Concurrent oral poliovirus and rhesus-human reassortant rotavirus vaccinations: Effects on immune responses to both vaccines and on efficacy of rotavirus vaccines. *J Infect Dis* 1996;173:306-313.
18. Schaffner W. The bright spot: Immunizations in 1998. *Patient Care* August 15,1998;123-126,135-138,141-142,144,147-148.
19. Smith F. New school entrance law requiring hepatitis B vaccine. Memorandum from the Ohio Department of Health, October 9, 1998.
20. CDC. Immunization of adolescents: Recommendations of the Advisory Committee on Immunization Practices, the American Academy of Pediatrics, the American Academy of Family Physicians, and the American Medical Association. *MMWR Morb Mort Wkly Rep* 1996;45(RR-13).
21. Zimmerman RK. Varicella vaccine: Rationale and indications for use. *AFP* 1996;53(2):647-651,654.
22. CDC. Epidemiology and prevention of vaccine-preventable diseases. 3rd ed. January 1996:197.
23. CDC. Prevention of pneumococcal disease: recommendations of the Advisory Committee on Immunization Practices (ACIP). *MMWR Morb Mort Wkly Rep* 1997;46(RR-8).
24. Ortqvist A, et al. Randomised trial of 23-valent pneumococcal capsular polysaccharide vaccine in prevention of pneumonia in middle-aged and elderly people. Swedish Pneumococcal Vaccination Study Group. *Lancet* 1998;399-403.
25. Fine MJ, et al. Efficacy of pneumococcal vaccination in adults. A meta-analysis of randomized controlled trials. *Arch Intern Med* 1994;154(23):2666-2677.
26. Effectiveness of pneumococcal vaccine. *Lancet* 1998; 351(9111):1283-1285.
27. Neuzil KM, et al. Influenza-associated morbidity and mortality in young and middle-aged women. *JAMA* 1999;281(10):901-907.
28. Adkins SB III. Immunizations: Current recommendations. *AFP* 1997;56(3):865-874.
29. CDC. Prevention and control of influenza: Recommendations of the Advisory Committee on Immunization Practices (ACIP). *MMWR Morb Mort Wkly Rep* 1998;47(RR-6).
30. Glezen WP. Influenza control—unfinished business. *JAMA* 1999;281(10):944-945.
31. Wilde JA, et al. Effectiveness of influenza vaccine in health care professionals. *JAMA* 1999;281(10):908-913.
32. Steere AC, et al. Vaccination against Lyme disease with recombinant *Borrelia burgdorferi* outer-surface lipoprotein A with adjuvant. *N Engl J Med* 1998;339(4):209-215.
33. Sigal LH, et al. A vaccine consisting of recombinant *Borrelia burgdorferi* outer-surface protein A to prevent Lyme disease. *N Engl J Med* 1998;339(4):216-222.
34. Steigbigel RT, Benach JL. Immunization against Lyme disease—an important first step. Editorial. *N Engl J Med* 1998;339(4):263-264.
35. The Medical Letter. Lyme disease vaccine. Vol. 41 (Issue1049):29-30. March 26, 1999.
36. Belshe RB, et al. The efficacy of live attenuated, cold-adapted, trivalent, intranasal influenzavirus vaccine in children. *N Engl J Med* 1998;338:1405-1412.

Pediatric Code and Resuscitation Organization

Larry B. Mellick, MS, MD, FAAP, FACEP

In many settings, pediatric resuscitations are relatively few and far between. In fact, the nursing staff in private offices and many smaller emergency departments (EDs) are typically able to narrate in vivid detail all pediatric resuscitations that have occurred in recent history.

Without doubt, the resuscitation of an infant or young child is an emotionally exacting event that can leave an indelible impression on the mind and emotions of health care providers. Even though the priorities and basic tenets of pediatric advanced life support are, in reality, no different than those for adults, the organizational demands of pediatric resuscitations are complicated by the relative infrequency and unique requirements of these events. Consequently, organization, understanding, and preparation for pediatric resuscitations should be a high priority for EDs and private offices.

The organization of the teams and systems that deliver resuscitative care to emergently ill children and adults clearly needs better definition. Review of the medical literature demonstrates that relatively little has been published concerning pediatric code team organization. While several articles describe the organization of pediatric trauma interventions in algorithmic format,[1,2] there are only a few publications providing insight into the process of code or resuscitation organization.[3-5] This review presents current experience and information on code organization from a pediatric perspective and describes a systems and systematic approach to this topic.

Rationale for Organizing Codes and Resuscitations

Delivering emergency health care foreordains working with health conditions that have clear time limitations for maximal beneficial results. In fact, our rhetoric often reflects these time exigencies with terms such as "time is muscle" and "the golden hour." While team organization cannot unequivocally be associated with improved outcome, it is axiomatic that planning, practice, and organization can result in increased process speed and efficiency. Evidence also exists that the global development and organization of a trauma system can affect patient survival.[6-8] Increased speed and efficiency (i.e., faster transport) has been demonstrated to improve outcomes for trauma patients in EMS settings[9,10] and the Vietnam and Korean war experiences. Finally, there is clear clinical evidence that timely interventions do prevent morbidity and mortality in a host of trauma and medical conditions. In the resuscitation setting, it is this increased speed and efficiency that will most likely benefit the critically ill patient.

Code or Resuscitation Ingredients

The code or resuscitation process is a series of activities that can be generally delineated. The components listed below will vary in degree of application and are patient- and condition-defined.

Table 1. Three Perspectives on Resuscitation Systems: Outline of Component Parts

PATIENT ORGANIZATIONAL VIEW[6]
Prehospital: Historical and observational
Primary survey: ABCDE *(see Table 2)*
Resuscitation: Interventions and checklist
Secondary survey: Complete examination
Definitive care: Appropriate interventions

TEAM ORGANIZATIONAL VIEW[3]
Anticipation phase
Entry phase
Resuscitation phase
Maintenance phase
Family notification phase
Transfer phase
Critique phase

THE GLOBAL OVERVIEW
Prehospital phase
Hospital resuscitative phase
Hospital restorative phase
Rehabilitation phase

- A patient with life or limb at risk or perceived risk
- Time limitations necessitating rapid organization and intervention.
- Personnel response dependent on local resources and prior team organization
- Defined leadership (physician and nursing)
- Protocol or patient needs-driven interventions
- Procedures and interventions exercised on the patient
- Various degrees of medication and equipment delivery and utilization
- Diversity of personnel experience, skills, and expertise potentially required
- Consultants used as indicated

Code Organization Systems and Structures

Resuscitation Systems. The clearest understanding of the resuscitation process comes from a systematic and a systems-oriented analysis. There are three echelons or perspectives from which to view the processes of code and resuscitation organization. These views are the *patient organizational view,* the *team organizational view,* and the encompassing *global overview.* The components of each of these perspectives are listed in *Table 1.*

The Patient Organizational View

The patient organizational view is centered around the structure used in the Advanced Trauma Life Support (ATLS) course.[11] This organization functions well for both trauma and medical resuscitations and includes the following component phases:

Table 2. Primary Survey: Emergency Care Priorities

A:	Airway with cervical spine control
B:	Breathing
C:	Circulation
D:	Disability (neurologic exam)
E:	Expose patient

1. Prehospital: Preparation—historical and observational
2. Primary survey: ABCDE *(See Table 2.)*
3. Resuscitation: Interventions and checklist
4. Secondary survey: Complete examination
5. Definitive care: Appropriate interventions

In addition to being used to provide structure to the resuscitation scenario, those components can be used as section headings during documentation of resuscitation care.

Prehospital. From the hospital setting perspective, there is typically a vague understanding of the prehospital events. Nevertheless, three relevant prehospital components for the hospital-based physician and nurse include preparation, observation, and history acquisition. The preparation component includes prehospital information documentation and distribution, as well as readying the team and resuscitation room for the patient's arrival. The observation component takes place following the patient's arrival and entails making visual note of apparent prehospital interventions and actions. Was the child's cervical spine properly immobilized? Did the patient have an adequate or appropriate airway? Was effective cardiopulmonary resuscitation ongoing and effective? Taking the patient's history is often a juggling act for the emergency physician providing care to a critical patient. The history may be fragmented or acquired in phases. Often, the prehospital personnel must be asked to delay their departure long enough so that a more complete history may be obtained.

There are two primary historical sources, and from each source specific historical elements should be solicited by the health care provider. The sources and elements of the prehospital history are demonstrated in *Table 3.*

Primary Survey. The next component of the patient organization view of resuscitation is the primary survey. The primary survey is an assessment of the patient's physiologic status and is accomplished by evaluating the functional status of the patient's airway, breathing, and circulation. The primary survey may be as short as a 60-second evaluation and usually is accomplished during the patient resuscitation phase.

The patient care interventions occurring during the primary survey are also prioritized, and each of these components must be consecutively managed. The format includes component assessment, correction of documented problems, and reassessment of any resuscitative intervention before the next lower priority is evaluated. The primary survey essentially "leads" the resuscitation phase.

Resuscitation Phase. The resuscitation phase is the third component of the patient-oriented view. Emergency interventions and procedures are accomplished during the resuscitation phase.

A second component of the resuscitation phase is the "checklist

Table 3. Prehospital History Components

PREHOSPITAL HISTORY—PARAMEDIC SOURCE	
V:	Vital signs (at scene and in transport)
I:	Injuries documented (on their examination)
C:	Condition of patient (at scene and in transport) Circumstances (of accident and injury)
T:	Treatments/Therapeutic interventions performed
I:	Intravenous fluids provided (amount/type)
M:	Mental status changes noted
S:	Splints (c-spine protection) Signs and symptoms noted
PREHOSPITAL HISTORY—PATIENT SOURCE	
I:	Identification/Immunization status for tetanus
M:	Medications
P:	Past medical history/pain locations
A:	Allergies
L:	Last meal
E:	Events preceding and precipitating accident
D:	Drug dependencies (HIV, ETOH, etc.)

period." During this segment of time, the primary survey has been accomplished and the majority of the urgent resuscitative interventions have been achieved. This phase is formalized in some medical centers, and specific checklists are displayed (on the wall or clipboard) for the resuscitation team leader. While not typically taught in ATLS or ACLS classes or formally recognized by many caregivers, this aspect of resuscitative care is pivotal to efficient code management and team leadership.

This list includes verification and ordering of appropriate intravenous lines, designating frequency of vital signs, the ordering of specific laboratory test batteries, and oxygen delivery methods. Other components of the checklist phase include ordering x-rays, collection of arterial blood gases, application of splints, tetanus vaccine administration, administration of antibiotics, attachment of monitor leads, chest tube placement, nasogastric tube insertion, Foley catheter placement, requesting old records, and notification of the hospital chaplain.

Secondary Survey. The secondary survey is the fourth component of the patient intervention perspective of code organization. While the primary survey is a physiologic survey, the secondary survey is an anatomic survey. It is a thorough examination from head to toe of the patient's body. The objective of this phase is to discover and document patient injury or discover physical examination clues of a medical illness.

Definitive Care Phase. The fifth phase of the patient intervention scenario is the definitive care phase. During this phase, more definitive emergency care takes place, and may include further investigational studies such as MRI or CT scans, rapid transport to the operating room, or admission for observation. Disposition home or transfer of the patient to another facility may also occur.

Team Organizational View

The team orientation view of a medical or trauma resuscitation involves seven phases.[3] Each phase encompasses temporally important priorities for the resuscitation team.

The Anticipation Phase. The first phase is the anticipation phase. During this phase, the data provided to the hospital by the paramedics is received and analyzed. Subsequently, the team is gathered, leadership is established, duties are delegated, the equipment is prepared and checked, and the team members position themselves in readiness for the arrival of the critically ill patients.

The Entry Phase. Phase two of the team organizational view is the entry phase and involves the exchange of vital signs obtained by the paramedics just prior to their arrival. Additionally, there is the orderly transfer or exchange of the patient to the ED stretcher. Baseline assessments of the patients ABCs are obtained by the hospital resuscitation team members. A concise history is provided by the paramedics and new vital signs are obtained.

The Resuscitation Phase. The third phase is the resuscitation phase. During this phase, the team assesses the patient's ABCs (performs a primary survey) and then carries out any indicated resuscitative interventions. It is especially important during this phase to have strong and unflappable physician and nursing leadership. There should be only one dominant voice, and information is continuously provided to the team leadership. Vital signs are obtained ideally every five minutes, and procedures and medication administration are accomplished. The secondary or anatomical survey is accomplished; when the patient's condition does not improve, the primary or physiologic survey is repeated. Communication between the team members and leadership is extremely important to the effective resuscitation of the patient.

The Maintenance Phase. The next phase is the maintenance phase. During this period of time the major assessment and resuscitative procedures have been accomplished. Continued stabilization of the patient is performed, and intravenous lines and inserted catheters and tubes are stabilized. During this phase, the team's "adrenaline rush" begins to subside as the most critical interventions have been accomplished. This is a most vulnerable time period for the patient. A conscious effort to maintain the team's attention is mandatory.

The Family Notification Phase. The family notification phase is not really a single period in time. In fact, the notification process continues throughout the resuscitation process. It is simply humane for the resuscitation team to designate one member to be a liaison with the family. Frequent, honest status reports and information updates are important to family members and should be carried out with sensitivity.

The Transfer Phase. The transfer phase is another period of time that does not occur specifically at the end of a resuscitation. The transfer process may mean moving the patient to an intensive care unit or to another hospital with tertiary facilities. The resuscitation team must transfer the patient to a team of equal or greater expertise.[4] The potential for delays in necessary emergent care can occur if the transfer process is not managed efficiently. Arranging for transport late into a resuscitation may not be efficient management of the patient's medical or surgical problem.

The Critique Phase. The last period is the critique phase. Every resuscitation is different, and each resuscitation is potentially associated with unique problems. Every team should perform a code critique, no matter how brief.[4] The patient care d`elivered and the team's interdependent performance should be critiqued ideally as soon as possible after every resuscitation. This allows maximal educational benefit from the process and prevents repetition of inefficiencies with future patients.

Finally, due to the nature of the event, all resuscitation team members sustain some degree of emotional trauma. The cumulative process is potentially not unlike a post-traumatic stress syndrome. During the critique phase, defusing processes can also occur that allow team members to begin to manage personal grief or stress reactions.

Team Performance and Organization

Team Performance. While almost everyone has experienced work or play milieus in which they intuitively sensed the benefits and actuality of a "team," the teamwork construct is especially meaningful in the resuscitation process.

The Ideal Team: The Pit-Crew Analogy. The image of an auto racing pit crew best depicts effective resuscitation team performance. Just as with the auto racing pit crew, the ideal resuscitation team shares the characteristics of well-defined leadership, clearly identified responsibilities, specific role or job delineations, emphasis on efficiency and speed, expert accomplishment of individual roles, team performance and dynamics, adequate training and preparation, well-delineated priorities, and appropriate number of team members. The team dynamics of a pit crew also include performance as a unified, concerted, and harmonious effort that is carefully choreographed for flawless timing.

Resuscitation Team Composition. While there are a basic number of roles requiring execution during a code or resuscitation event, several roles may be fulfilled simultaneously or consecutively by one or more team members. Nevertheless, the roles delineated in *Table 4* must typically be achieved as part of the patient resuscitation process.

Resuscitation Team Leadership: Emphasizing the Need for Leadership. It is a non-negotiable fact that someone must take overall responsibility for organizing the care of the critically ill child. Someone must prevent the occurrence of multiple specialists intent on different treatment plans. General team acceptance of strong leadership is mandatory, and designated leaders must not be embarrassed to assume a strong leadership role and take control of the resuscitation process. Effective leadership traits include decisiveness, professionalism, and unflappability.[3]

Central to this premise is the fact that there must be one and only one physician leader at any specific time. This physician functions as the "sinus node" pacemaker for the resuscitation team, and no other "ectopic" loci of team pacing activity is allowed to occur. There should also be well-defined, singular nursing leadership.

Room Positioning of Team Members. Standardization of team member positioning is a relatively important but frequently uncodified component of the code organization planning process. The positioning of specific team members or roles is both dependent on certain local variables as well as being open to more general recommendations. Role identification can be facilitated by team member positioning relative to the patient and the resuscitation room. Certain roles are intuitively assigned to specific room positions because of the particular activities performed by that individual or the location of major equipment (airway physician, therapist, c-spine control, cutdowns, chest tube, chest compression administrator, defibrillator, blood warmers, monitors, etc.). Respiratory therapy, anesthesia, or the emergency physician in charge of airway control would take position at the patient's head. Since physicians traditionally examine patients from the patient's right side, that location will usually be occupied by the team leader, who performs the physical assessment in most settings. During different phases of the resuscitation process and depending on the health condition being treated, the physician leadership location may transition. Concurrently, the lead nurse, who ideally is in continuous communication with the team leader, would be located on the patient's left and directly across from the physician team leader. The location of other team members (right or left) is dependent on the standard location for performing patient procedures and the ease of performing the procedure. The documentation nurse is typically stationed within auditory proximity (which prevents having to request information) at a writing station or table. If a supply cart is located immediately behind and a drug cart in front, the documentation nurse can simultaneously assist with equipment and medication acquisition. Code spectators may or may not be allowed in the resuscitation area, and appropriate room locations may be clearly designated. Signage and markings on the floor or wall will help direct and assign spectators to specific locations. Finally, a wall board can quite effectively delineate and direct the team membership to approximate role locations and associated duties. *(See Figure 1.)*

How To "Run" a Resuscitation

Letting Them Know You Are Boss. In the ED setting as well as the code, a microcosm of the ED, strong physician leadership is recognized as ideal. However, leadership is not always a natural process or event and typically requires certain finite actions to delineate the leadership role. A number of steps or actions that assist in leadership declaration exist. These include physically being located in the resuscitation room prior to the patient's arrival, assembling the team, and leading patient care planning prior to the patient's arrival. Additional

Table 4. Resuscitation Team Roles
Team leadership
Patient disrobing
Room and equipment preparation
Physical assessment
Airway control
Historical intake
Ventilation of lungs
Code process documentation
Chest compressions
Medication administration
Intravenous access
Various physician procedures
Vital sign procurement
Various nursing procedures

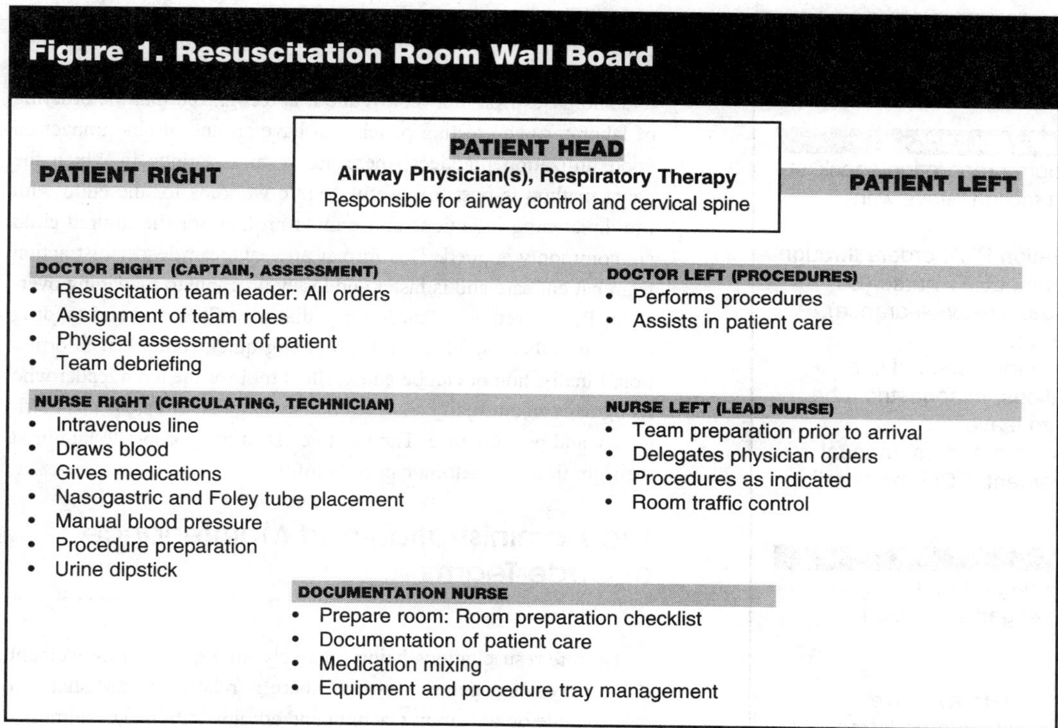

Figure 1. Resuscitation Room Wall Board

steps for leadership declaration include taking responsibility for team member role assignments, positioning oneself in the room at a location typical for the team leader, reception of the paramedic history, and using the local system for team leader identification (colored gown, hat, etc.). Appropriate speaking decibels, behavior, and tone of voice must support the role. Friendly, strong communication that includes eye contact and addressing other team members by name further supports fulfillment of this role. Finally, in some settings the leadership admonition, "take orders only from me," may be necessary and appropriate.

Maintaining Team Ambiance. Resuscitations are emotionally and intellectually demanding settings. Because of these performance demands, there is a natural tendency for mistakes in team ambiance. A tense, excessively serious, or inappropriately flippant demeanor can detract from a team's effective performance. Displays of anger, verbally abusive behavior, or negative, hypercritical, accusatory attitudes are also damaging to the work ambiance.

Pediatric Code Organization Issues. The management of pediatric resuscitations has several unique characteristics. The perennial pediatric problems of intravenous and airway access must be efficiently managed during pediatric resuscitations. Alternative access skills such as intraosseous and rectal administration of medications and fluids or needle cricothyrotomy and bag-valve-mask ventilation must be maintained. Drug calculations are complicated by the need to remember weight-related dosages, have an accurate estimate of the child's weight, and to flawlessly calculate and administrate the medication to the child.[12] A spectrum of equipment sizes to match the entire span of pediatric physical sizes must be available to the resuscitation team and prehospital providers.[13,14] Additionally, the small size of the patient frequently makes team member access for procedures a distinct problem. Complicating the process is the relative infrequency of pediatric resuscitations. Consequently, team member expertise, training, and skill maintenance is more problematic for pediatric resuscitations. Concurrently, there is a distinct (but finite) fund of knowledge and a number of additional assessment and procedural skills necessary for effective management of pediatric resuscitations. Finally, the emotional toll associated with pediatric codes is potentially significant. Effective management of tragedies for family members and the team's own emotional responses or countertransference is mandatory.

Resuscitation Job Aids

Resuscitation Checklists. In most industries and avocations that require a certain level of precision, it is not uncommon to use what are called "job aids." Job aids are essentially checklists containing all the specific task elements for which accuracy and oversight prevention are mandatory. A classic example of a job aid is the checklist used by airline pilots in preparation for flight. Another example is the job aid already widely used in resuscitation settings by those who apply the ABC mnemonic to the primary survey. Potential activities for the application of checklists include resuscitation room preparation *(see Table 5),* secretarial/clerical, and physician resuscitation duties.

Other Job Aids. There are other useful job aids that are not necessarily checklists. Forms, such as well-organized trauma resuscitation records, can greatly increase the efficiency of documentation. Dry erase boards on the resuscitation room wall can assist with documentation of the prehospital history or team role assignments. Wall information charts or posters containing valuable reference information can be strategically placed on resuscitation room walls. Pediatric resuscitation drugs, the Glasgow coma scale, ACLS algorithms, and immunization schedules are examples of information that can be easily posted. A resuscitation team wall chart delineating the roles, duties, and locations of specific team members can be a useful adjunct. *(See Figure 1.)* Such a chart is especially useful in training center settings where team members regularly rotate. Another piece of equipment, the Broselow resuscitation tape, is becoming a standard piece of equipment in most EDs. This tape allows the application of preset drug calculations and equipment sizes using an estimate of the child's weight based on the child's length. This system is a faster and more accurate method of estimating a child's weight, calculating drug doses, and making equipment size selections.

Additionally, well-thought-out systems for equipment organization and display are extremely valuable to code organization. The room location for storage of equipment does affect resuscitation team efficiency. Equipment cupboards with glass doors or open equipment

Table 5. Room Preparation Checklist

IDENTIFICATION OF TEAM MEMBER ROLES

- ❑ Documentation Nurse—Room preparation checklist, documentation, medication mixing, stays with patient.
- ❑ Lead Nurse—Team preparation PTA, orders through RN from resuscitation captain, LEFT nurse (CT placement, peritoneal lavage, airway clearance), traffic control, second to leave.
- ❑ Circulating Nurse—RIGHT nurse (second line, draws blood, gives medications, nasogastric tube placement, urine dip), first to leave.
- ❑ Technician—Places patient on monitors, manual blood pressure, Foley placement, ECG, preparation for procedures.

AIRWAY, BREATHING

- ❑ Appropriate size ventilation bag on bed
- ❑ Oxygen ready (humidified oxygen available for pediatric patients)
- ❑ Suction on and ready
- ❑ Appropriate size suction catheters available
- ❑ Airway kit open at bedside—estimate endotracheal tube size
- ❑ Broselow tape on bed (pediatric patients)
- ❑ Rapid sequence intubation tray at bedside
- ❑ End-tidal CO2 monitoring device (EasyCap)
- ❑ Pulse oximeter on and ready

CIRCULATION

- ❑ Hand and Dynamap cuff at bedside
- ❑ CPR backboard (as needed)
- ❑ Heat lamps on (as needed)
- ❑ IV lines stripped (2)—one line placed on Level I warmer
- ❑ CPR step stool in room
- ❑ Cardiac drugs at bedside
- ❑ Appropriate size infusion catheter available
- ❑ Cardiac monitor on and paper in recorder
- ❑ Defibrillator on with appropriate paddles—external pacer pads if needed
- ❑ Call for blood if needed (give estimated time of arrival of patient as available.)

DISABILITY

- ❑ Otoscope bulb functional
- ❑ Appropriate size soft restraints at bedside

EXPOSURE

- ❑ Trauma scissors available

MISCELLANEOUS

- ❑ Hemocue and Accu-chek at bedside
- ❑ Appropriate size Foley catheter at bedside
- ❑ Appropriate size nasogastric tube at bedside
- ❑ Mayo stands available at bedside
- ❑ Additional personnel paged (as needed)

THINK AHEAD . . .

- ❑ Are the appropriate invasive procedure supplies readily available?

carts allow easy visibility and access of supplies. Interference to flow by mechanical components can be reduced by the delivery of monitors and gases from above.[15] While it is recognized that the ordering of laboratory and testing panels can have an undesirable impact on good utilization practices, there are several settings in which the panel method is possibly useful. Septic workups for the child with life-threatening infections and trauma profiles for the injured child are commonly applied. This format prevents team leader distraction from patient care and is faster and less vulnerable to managing oversight. Pocket reference cards for pediatric, ACLS, and airway drug doses are other useful job aids providing quick sources of information. Finally, humor can be an excellent tool for the team leader who recognizes an unusually tense team or setting that threatens team efficiency and performance. The positive effect of appropriate humor at the right time and setting can be helpful.

The Administration and Maintenance of Code Teams

Despite resuscitations being relatively high quality improvement (QI) or risk management settings, there is relatively little attention paid to code organization teaching and administration. The administrative and maintenance process frequently succumbs to the whims of good intentions. Often, only minimal attention is dedicated to the understanding and definition of the local team process.

Teaching the art of code organization also occurs infrequently. Teaching hospitals are the institutions most frequently interested in code organization, and training using mock codes or other techniques may take place. While the development of skills extrapolated from actual experience is helpful, it is neither fair to the patient nor the young physician for learning to occur in "sink-or-swim" settings. Finally, even though the American Heart Association (AHA) has dedicated several pages in the latest edition of the ACLS textbook to teaching principles of code organization,[4] the *Textbook of Pediatric Advanced Life Support (PALS)* does not yet address code team organization.

Code Organization Committees. There are several formats that allow effective administration of code team organization. Administrative management of code organization can be accomplished in hospital trauma committees' subcommittees. Other settings have both a "code blue" committee, possibly in addition to a trauma committee. Nevertheless, for EDs in which resuscitations are a regular component of its practice, specific code organization administration is necessary. While there are many universal issues, resuscitation organization must be accomplished in the context of each individual hospital. These committees are best organized under a continuous quality improvement (CQI) format; team membership should include nurse educators, staff nurses, charge nurses, and nursing administration. Interested physician representation may include the pediatric emergency medicine attending, the ED medical director, and a member of the surgical service. Departmental clerical staff also should be represented.

The possible scope of activities for such a committee includes definition of team membership and composition, setting criteria for team member credentialing and training, planning specific team roles and assignments, reviewing team performance problems, identification of QI issues, and referring to appropriate QI committee.

Additionally, the committee can plan and orchestrate training activities, oversee new equipment procurement and training, supervise equipment stocking and display, institute training in notification of next of kin, identify areas for resuscitation research, create code organization benchmarks, and participate in prehospital education.

Training and Mock Codes. Mock codes are an ideal tool for resuscitation team training. There are two major areas for training focus. The first approach is the standard "megacode," in which ATLS and ACLS tenets are practiced and reviewed.[11,16] A broad spectrum of resuscitation situations and patient ages and conditions can potentially be incorporated.[17,18] The second training emphasis is the code organization process. Attention to both areas is important. However, while there are formal systems for teaching the megacode aspects of resuscitation (PALS, ACLS, ATLS, BCLS, BTLS), there have been relatively few local systems established for teaching code organization. Finally, other important areas for training include emergency alternatives to intravenous and airway access.[19,20]

Mock codes are most effective as training tools when they are realistic while protecting the self-confidence of those in training. Because of the tendency for attrition of skills and turnover of staff, staging mock codes should be done on a regular basis.

When teaching the process of code organization, the specific ideology and structure for each institution should be reviewed. Common paradigms of team performance and leadership should be reviewed. The importance of team member roles and role interdependence should be emphasized. Practice paradigms for successful team behavior and interface with consultants can also be discussed.

Summary

The process of code team organization for children deserves particular attention, especially since pediatric resuscitations are relatively uncommon and are associated with unique, additional requirements. In this review, a pediatric perspective of current experience and information on code organization and a systems and systematic approach was presented. More specifically, code organization systems, team performance and organization, techniques for running a resuscitation, and the administration and maintenance of code teams were reviewed.

References

1. Eichelberger MR, Randolph JG. Pediatric trauma: An algorithm for diagnosis and therapy. *J Traum* 1983;23:91-97.
2. Eichelberger MR, Zwick HA, Pratsch GL, et al. Pediatric trauma protocol: A team approach. In: Eichelberger MR, Pratsch Gll, eds. *Pediatric Trauma Care.* Rockville, MD: Aspen; 1988:11-31.
3. Burkle FM, Rice M. Code organization. *Am J Emerg Med* 1987;5:235-239.
4. American Heart Association. *Textbook of Advanced Cardiac Life Support: Essentials of ACLS.* Dallas: American Heart Association; 1994:1-69.
5. Harris BH, Latchaw LA, Murphy RE, et al. A protocol for pediatric trauma receiving units. *J Pediatr Surg* 1989;24: 419-422.
6. West JG, Trunkey DD, Lim RC. Systems of trauma care: A study of two counties. *Arch Surg* 1979;114:455.
7. West JG, Cales RH, Cazzaniga AG. Impact of regionalization: The Orange County experience. *Arch Surg* 1983;18:740.
8. Guss DA, Meyer FT, Neuman TS, et al. The impact of a regionalized trauma system on trauma care in San Diego County. *Ann Emerg Med* 1989;18:1141.
9. Gervin AS, Fischer RP. The importance of prompt transport in salvage of patients with penetrating heart wounds. *J Traum* 1982;22:443-448.
10. Baxt WG, Moody P. The impact of a rotorcraft aeromedical emergency care service on trauma mortality. *JAMA* 1983;249:3047-3051.
11. American College of Surgeons, Committee on trauma. *Textbook of Advanced Trauma Life Support.* Chicago: American College of Surgeons; 1993.
12. Koren G, Barzilay Z, Greenwald M. Tenfold errors in administration of drug doses: A neglected iatrogenic disease in pediatrics. *Pediatrics* 1986;77:848-849.
13. Mellick LB, Dierking BH. One size doesn't fit all: Choosing pediatric equipment, Part I. *J Emerg Med Serv* 1991;16:78-82.
14. Mellick LB, Dierking BH. One size doesn't fit all: Choosing pediatric equipment, Part II. *J Emerg Med Serv* 1991;16: 35-46.
15. Yaron M, Ruiz E, Baretich MF. Equipment organization in the emergency department adult resuscitation area. *J Emerg Med* 1994;12:845-848.
16. Emergency Cardiac Committee and Subcommittees, American Heart Association. Guidelines for cardiopulmonary resuscitation and emergency cardiac care. *JAMA* 1992;268: 2172.
17. Baker MD. Current methods of training residents to manage pediatric cardiopulmonary arrests. *Pediatr Emerg Care* 1986;2:82-84.
18. Duncan B, Banner W, Ruggil J. Emergency drills in a pediatric residency training program. *Ann Emerg Med* 1983;12: 164-166.
19. Zimmerman JJ, Strauss RH. History and current application of intravenous therapy in children. *Pediatr Emerg Care* 1989;5:120-127.
20. Orlowski JP. Emergency alternatives to intravenous access: intraosseous, intratracheal, sublingual, and other site drug administration. *Pediatr Clin North Am* 1994;41;1183-1200.

Cervical Spine Injury

Jeffrey Proudfoot, DO, FACOEP

How often do emergency care providers experience the arrival of an immobilized and crying toddler unaccompanied by parents or family members? Typically, the prehospital providers describe a traffic collision or some other significant traumatic event while the frightened, screaming child struggles with the immobilization straps. The child's abraded face is often contorted into pathetic fits of loud crying, and the emergency department (ED) team attempts to soothe or calm the child with distracting activities. Not infrequently, a distraught parent subsequently arrives and pleads repeatedly to pick up and hold the crying child. The countertransference process tempts the emergency care provider to honor the request, but adherence to clinical standards prevails. Efforts at calming either the child or his or her parent are often only partially successful, and the tension mounts when x-ray and cervical spine films are delayed. Without doubt, this scenario occurs on a daily basis in EDs around the country.

Assessment and management of infants and children with possible cervical spine injuries (CSIs) can be a daunting task. While the simple act of cervical spine immobilization may prevent movement and worsening of CSI, this process often causes a frightened child to struggle and cry, further limiting the ability to clinically assess the child for associated injuries or neurologic deficits. Moreover, management decisions are often complex, and the radiographic and clinical assessment of children is underemphasized in many training programs, leaving the clinician with limited training or experience in dealing with possible pediatric CSI. The presence of developmental radiologic variants has the potential to mislead clinicians into overdiagnosing abnormalities or mistakenly judging a true injury to be an anatomic variant. Unfortunately, errors in diagnosis or management of CSI have the potential to lead to catastrophic consequences, including death and permanent disability. Finally, the economic expense associated with evaluation, treatment, and rehabilitation of victims of pediatric CSI is astronomical in a population with a potential for a lifetime of dependency and disability. With these important points in mind, this review provides a detailed discussion of normal and abnormal radiologic variants, pediatric CSI syndromes, as well as a rational approach to dealing with children who may harbor CSI.

Background

Distinct pediatric CSI patterns differ from adults in many important ways when traumatic forces are applied to the growing cervical spine. The immature structural elements, modified biomechanical function, and inherent structural differences of the pediatric vertebral column alter these injury patterns in the pediatric trauma victim. These structural differences include incompletely ossified vertebral elements, ligamentous attachments that are stronger than the bony elements, epiphyseal zones that are highly susceptible to distraction and separation under mechanical stressors, and more horizontally oriented, articular surfaces. Additionally, the pediatric skull repre-

Figure 1. Normal Cervical Vertebrae

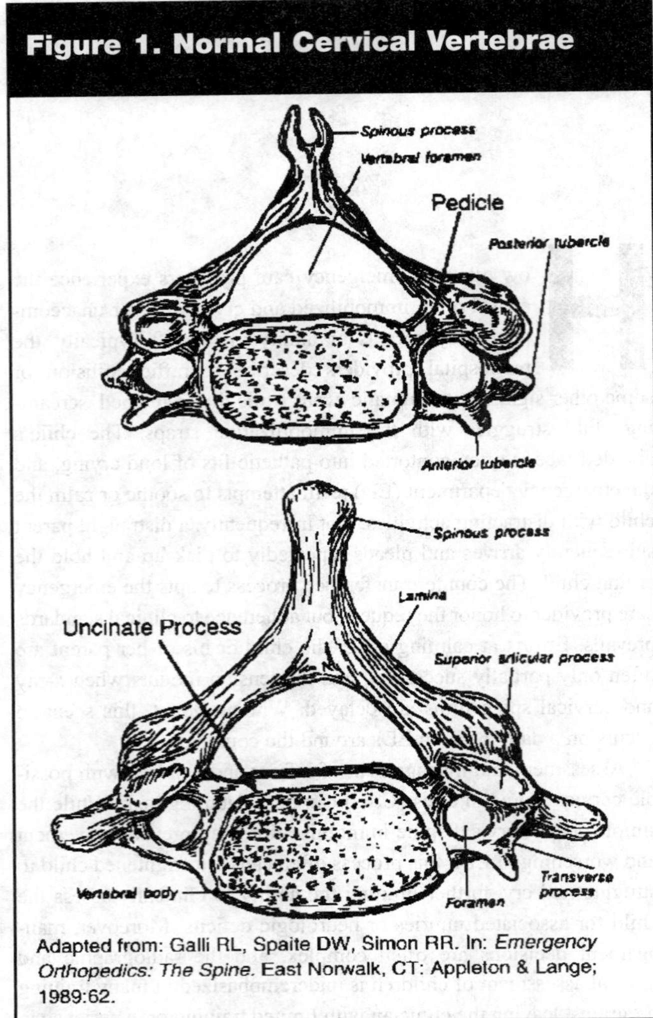

Adapted from: Galli RL, Spaite DW, Simon RR. In: *Emergency Orthopedics: The Spine.* East Norwalk, CT: Appleton & Lange; 1989:62.

sents a relatively larger mass on top of an immature cervical vertebral column with correspondingly poor muscular support. Consequently, the pediatric cervical spine is more susceptible to torsional forces, angular momentum, and an altered fulcrum of motion—effects that are modified as the pediatric spine matures with age and ossification into the adult model.

Epidemiology

Most pediatric victims of trauma have no significant serious injury to the cervical spine. While pediatric CSIs comprise only 1-3% of all pediatric trauma hospital admissions, nearly 1000 children are paralyzed each year.[1-10] Unfortunately, the low incidence can fool the unwary clinician, yet the problem demands that the ED physician maintain a high index of suspicion, particularly with certain mechanisms of injury. Those events most strongly associated with spinal cord injury (SCI) are motor vehicle accidents (MVAs), sports injuries, falls, and concomitant head injury.[11] Although rare, permanent disability, paralysis, or death associated with pediatric SCI is extremely high.[12]

Reviews of pediatric trauma indicate that: 1) low cervical spine injury is uncommon in children less than 8 years old and rare in those under 2-3 years of age; 2) as children reach age 12-13, the injuries are similar in nature to adults; 3) fatality rates, while low, tend to increase with injuries to the higher cervical spine; and 4) probably most disconcerting, some children with CSI have no radiographic evidence of injury.[13]

Pathomechanics

The fact that injury to the developing child's cervical spine manifests in distinct patterns is useful for ED physicians.[1-3,9,12] The recognition of these patterns is assisted by a complete working knowledge of pediatric anatomy, cervical spinal development, and mechanics. Patients with pediatric CSI can be functionally divided into four groups: neonatal, infants and children younger than 8 years old, those 8-12 years old, and those over 12 years old.

Neonatal. Obstetrical trauma during the birth process can cause serious SCIs.[14-19] Most of these relate to abnormal (breech or facial) presentation or use of excessive traction from manipulating the head.[20] These injuries most commonly involve the cervicothoracic junction where the spinal cord has only loose ligamentous attachment. Traction on the head stretches an inelastic spinal cord between anchor points of the brachial plexus superiorly and the cauda equina inferiorly. The bony spine can potentially stretch two inches while the cord will only extend one-quarter inch before disrupting with resultant intramedullary hemorrhage and infarction. The injury is fatal if this occurs superior to the phrenic nuclei. The infant classically presents with hypotonia and apnea.[18]

Infants and Children to Age 8. The anatomic characteristics of a relatively larger head-to-body ratio, underdeveloped cervical musculature, greater laxity of cervical spinal ligaments, incomplete vertebral ossification, and predominately horizontal orientation of articulating facet surfaces make the fulcrum of spinal movement at the C2-C3 level rather than at C5-C6, as in adults. These anatomic distinctions predispose the younger (< 8 years) patient to injury by torsional forces and angular momentum delivered to the high cervical spine. Additionally, young children exhibit low resistance to rotatory and distractive forces applied to their larger and proportionally heavier heads. The vector consequences of applied forces combined with ligamentous attachment to bone, which is often stronger than the bone itself (particularly at physeal growth centers), more commonly results in shearing injury to the atlantoaxial region with its high concentration of synchondroses. As a result, children in this age group are also more likely to suffer subluxation/distraction type injuries rather than the vertebral body or arch fractures more common in older children or adults. The occipito-atlantal junction is tightly bound together via strong ligamentous attachment to allow flexion and extension with almost no rotation. The atlas is tightly connected to the axis by a group of ligaments: the alar, apical dental, the tectorial membrane, and the strong cruciate ligament. Movement at the atlantoaxial joint is limited to approximately 40-50° of axial rotation. Thus, the occipitoatlantoaxial complex is the zone of greatest mobility in the developing pediatric spine, and, consequently, is the area most subject to applied external injury forces. This so-called "juvenile" pattern of pediatric SCI (i.e., a predisposition to injury of C1-C3) has been described as an unrecognized cause of death from apnea and cardiopulmonary arrest with blunt trauma.[21]

In the United States, most trauma leading to CSI in children less than 8 years of age is of the rapid acceleration-deceleration type commonly associated with MVAs (either as passenger or pedestrian) and followed by falls.[11] The high inertial moment exhibited by the young

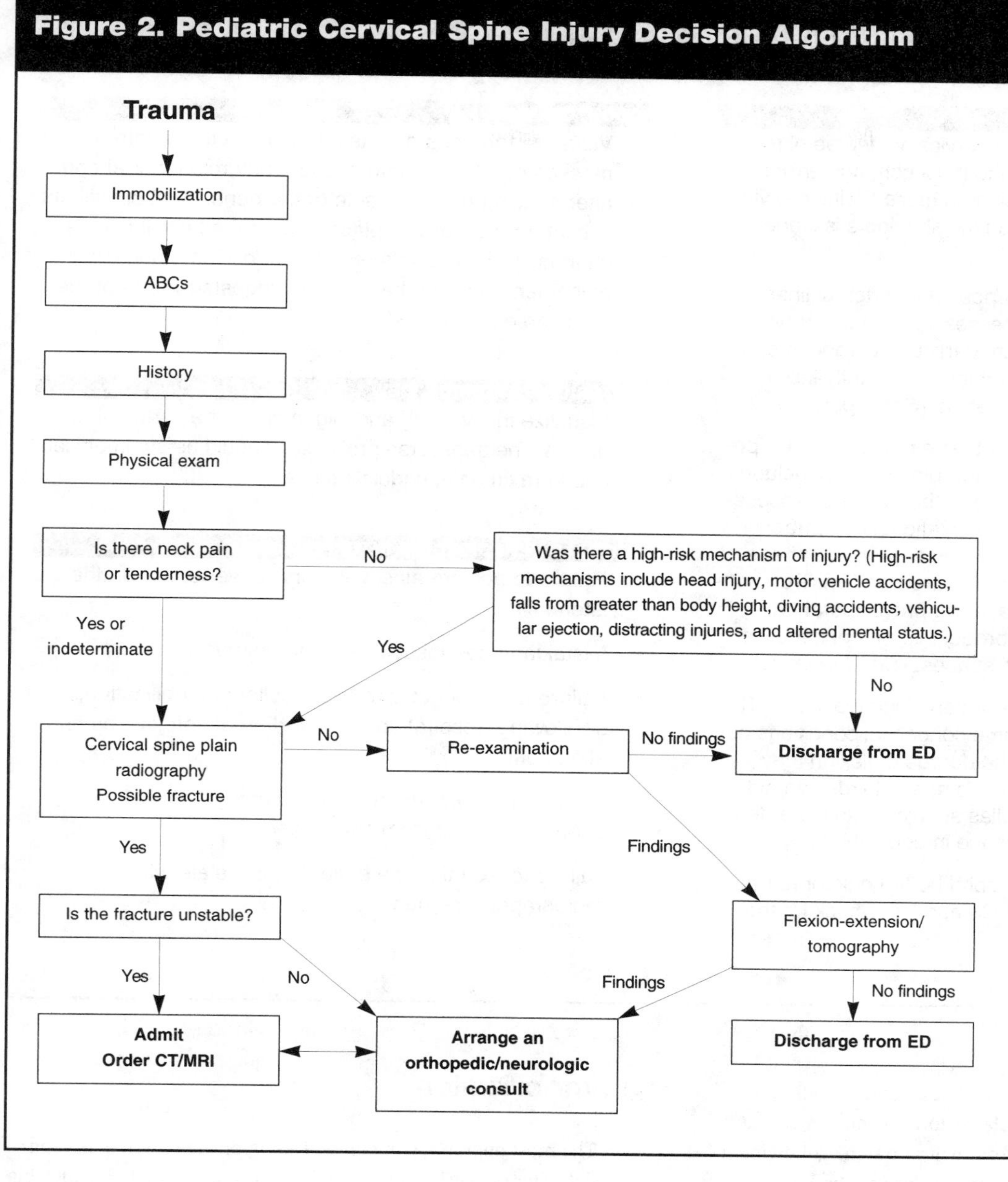

pediatric head to these types of forces results in pronounced sagittal flexion-extension or axial rotation, leading to subluxation at the C1-C3 region. An increased mobility of the C1-C3 segments of the pediatric spine is known to be normal in healthy infants and is magnified by the traumatic forces. Primary injury to the cord most commonly results from impingement on the cord by luxated vertebrae, fragments fractured from the vertebrae itself, or longitudinal traction. While the actual cascade of neurophysiologic/neurochemical events leading to tissue necrosis and functional loss has not been clearly delineated, considerable emphasis has been placed on secondary injury derived from petechial hemorrhage, lipid peroxidation, and tissue ischemia.[22]

External protection that provides support for both head and torso is essential in preventing pediatric CSI and serves as the basis for most car seat restraints and recommendations. Helmets, safety harnesses, and appropriate sports training/ conditioning all help contribute to prevention.

Children Ages 8-12. Children in this group are maturing toward the adult anatomical model. Neck musculature is better developed, ossification of the dens is almost complete, anterior vertebral wedging disappears, facet planes become more vertical, and ligaments tighten. This alters the biomechanics of cervical spine motion to external injury forces by changing the fulcrum of movement to the C3-C5 region. Children older than 8 years old tend to injure the lower cervical spine (although injuries are pancervical) with simple linear and compression or burst fractures of the vertebral bodies associated with radiologically visible abnormalities. There is relatively less worry regarding SCI without radiographic abnormality (SCIWORA), which occurs more frequently in children younger than age 8. Precipitating mechanisms of injury are more likely to be related to sports and recreational accidents (football, water sports, rugby, gymnastics, ice hockey) along with the typical MVAs and falls. This reflects the increased involvement of this age group in organized sports and with hazardous equipment such as boats, jet skis, and trail bikes.[23-25] Fractures associated with dislocation in this group portend a nearly universal lethal outcome.

Children Ages 12 and Older. The preadolescent group of patients manifests the so-called "adult" pattern of CSIs. Typical for this age group are pancervical injuries (with a predominance of low cervical and high thoracic region fractures), radiologic evidence of injury, and a concomitant SCI as evidenced by an immediate neurologic deficit. The fulcrum of cervical spine flexion now rests in the C5-C6 region. SCI tends to result in paraplegia or quadriplegia rather than death if the initial insult is survived.

SCIWORA. SCIWORA accounts for 25-50% of pediatric CSI.[11] This syndrome has been well-documented by Pang and colleagues but has also been described previously by others.[30,69,70] SCIWORA is found primarily in the pediatric population under 8 years of age. An associated history of crush or distraction injury and

Table 1. Standard Radiologic Interpretation

CROSS-TABLE LATERAL

- Visualize and identify all seven cervical vertebrae plus superior aspect of T1. This is the most common error in radiographic interpretation.[34] A swimmer's (Twining's) view may be necessary if traction on the shoulders is inadequate to assess C6, C7, or T1.
- Visualize the general anterior/posterior vertebral lines and the curve of the spinous processes. Loss of the cervical lordosis is common in children, particularly when in cervical collars, which tend to straighten and slightly flex the spine. Check for pseudosubluxation. *(See Figure 4.)*
- Identify and measure the soft-tissue distances (i.e., prevertebral at C3 and inferior to the glottis). This includes examining the distances between the spinous processes that can be indicative of subluxation. Remember pseudothickening can occur depending on the phase of respiration/swallowing that is captured on film. True soft-tissue swelling should displace the prevertebral fat stripe (if present) and be reproducible on consecutive films. Look at individual disc spaces. *(See Figure 4.)*
- Identify and measure the atlantodental interval (ADI). This space may be widened in some congenital conditions but should be less than 5 mm. The degree of flexion may affect the appearance.[11,34] Steel's rule of thirds can aid evaluation: the canal of the atlas should contain the dens, the spinal cord, and empty space in equal thirds.
- Visualize and trace each vertebral body. Look for normal wedging of the upper bodies C3 and C4. Check for the relationship of adjacent bodies.

ODONTOID VIEW

- Visualize the dens and its relationship to the lateral masses of C1. Take into account any rotation that can alter spacing on either side of the dens. Most significant is bilateral outward displacement of the lateral masses characteristic of a Jefferson fracture. Combined displacement of more than 7 mm suggests rupture of the transverse ligament.[37]

ANTERIOR-POSTERIOR VIEW

- Visualize the spacing and alignment of the vertebral bodies. The transverse processes should be symmetrical and form smooth, undulating lines.

PITFALLS IN RADIOLOGIC INTERPRETATION

- Failure to acquire all seven cervical vertebrae on the lateral film
- Mistaking pseudosubluxation for injury
- Failure to account for rotation, collar immobilization, swallowing, respiration for distortion of soft tissues and alignment
- Unfamiliarity with the normal variants of os odontoideum, os terminale
- Failure to examine the patient to correlate with radiographic findings

transient symptoms of paresthesias, weakness, and/or lightning or burning sensation down the spine related to neck movement have been described. This injury results from neural trauma following a self-reducing (but unstable) displacement of the vertebral elements (e.g., vertebral subluxation, disc herniation, ligamentous impingement of the cord with vascular compromise, or stretching traction of the spinal cord itself) without residual, radiographically evident bony damage.

Neurologic deficits may not appear until days (range of 30 minutes to 4 days in one series)[11] after the initial trauma event in patients with SCIWORA. Incidental secondary trauma sometimes precipitates these delayed severe neurologic deficits. Consequently, the clinician should maintain a high index of suspicion in the face of any moderate-to-severe injury with reports of neurologic symptomatology or patients with persistent symptoms or pain. Carefully performed flexion-extensiosn views remain indispensable in detecting ligamentous injury. CT scanning of questionable areas of the cervical region are also helpful. MRI imaging, while useful in delineating spinal cord and soft-tissue injury associated with pediatric CSI, has limited utility in the acute setting. It is the imaging of choice beyond the acute phase for incomplete lesions.

Immobilization

The most appropriate method of immobilization remains controversial. The pediatric "stiff neck" and the traditional Philadelphia collars have found use in older children. However, in the very young, no single collar is available that provides reliable immobilization; therefore, other methods, such as using towels, padding, or sandbags in conjunction with a spine board have been employed. Most children transported on a spine board are not maintained in "radiographically" neutral position (0° of angulation).[26] This is in large part due to the larger occiput of the infant or child relative to the body, which forces some degree of cervical flexion when placed supine on a rigid surface. This is further explained by the finding that 50% of postnatal head circumference is attained by age 18 months while 50% of chest circumference is reached by age 8.[27] Some EMS providers have found use for malleable, soft pediatric immobilization devices that allow for more support and immobilization than the traditional wooden spine board. Some of the pediatric immobilization devices make allowances for the larger occiput with depressions or cutouts in the board itself. Less sophisticated solutions such as raising the back, neck, and shoulders with padding and towels to achieve a more neutral position have been used successfully.[28] A suggested clinical

Figure 3. Normal Spinal Contour Lines

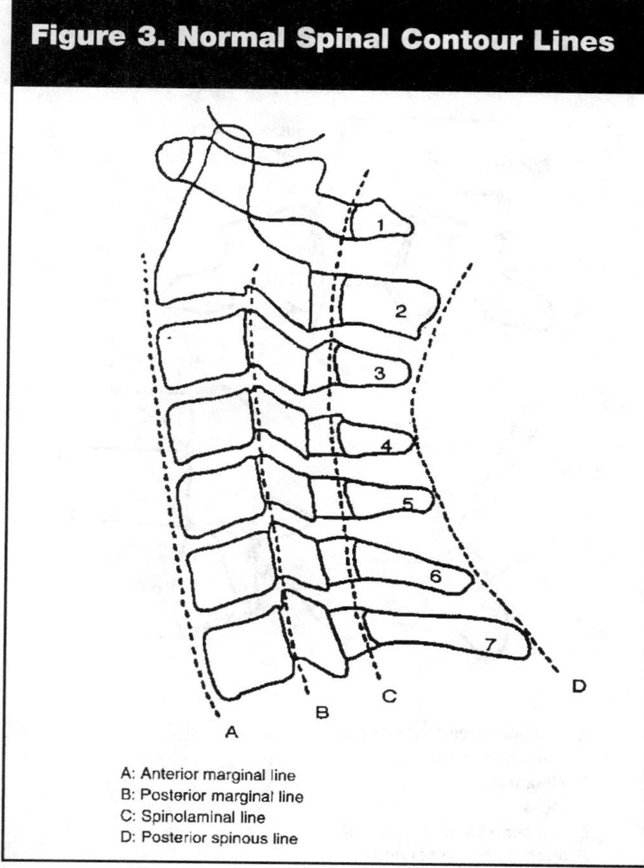

A: Anterior marginal line
B: Posterior marginal line
C: Spinolaminal line
D: Posterior spinous line

Figure 4. Normal Cervical Spine Spaces

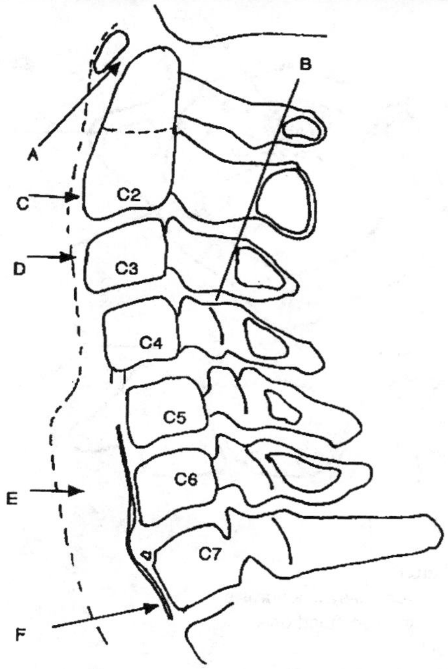

A: Atlantodental interval < 5 mm
B: Posterior cervical line
C: Prevertebral space ≤ 7 mm
D: Limit of normal overriding < 3-5 mm
E: Retrotracheal space < 14 mm
F: Prevertebral fat stripe

guideline recommends aligning the external auditory meatus with the shoulder as a way to avoid anterior displacement and flexion.[29] With small infants, car seats can serve as an immobilization device when appropriate immobilization is accomplished. Finally, unimmobilized patients with anything more than truly minor trauma need to be triaged and adequately immobilized until the physician can examine, interview, and evaluate the patient.

Clinical Evaluation

The injured pediatric patient presents the emergency physician with a perplexing dilemma. Many very young patients are preverbal or unable to communicate symptoms to the examiner, and the classic triad of neck pain, muscle spasm, and limited cervical range of motion is difficult to elicit. Complicating the situation is the fact that the patient has just sustained a traumatic experience, been forcibly restrained in a collar and on a board, separated from family or parents, and thrust into a hectic and unfamiliar environment. The examiner is frequently faced with a crying child or fearful infant who is unwilling or simply unable to cooperate with the examination. Further complicating evaluation is the paucity and delay in appearance of clinical signs and symptoms of pediatric CSI as well as SCIWORA.[30] More often the child is assumed to have pediatric CSI if he or she arrives in the ED with a collar or immobilized spine. By default (rightly or wrongly), as a result of the outliers noted above, a mandatory radiologic examination is performed. Finally, important factors documented to cause a delay in diagnosis include distracting injuries or an obtunded patient, incomplete physical examination, abnormal films interpreted as normal, failure to order radiographs, and patients not brought to medical attention.[31]

History. The most important diagnostic clues will come from a thorough history. This history should include the circumstances of injury, mechanism of trauma, relative magnitude of forces involved, and observations of prehospital personnel, family, or witnesses to the event. Unfortunately, the patient is often too young to give a history, may oversimplify, or may purposefully alter the circumstances fearing punishment. Many injuries are simply unwitnessed or seen only by other young playmates, and it is not unusual to receive pediatric patients in the ED unaccompanied by their parent. An added emphasis on physical examination is usually necessary as a result of these dilemmas in historical acquisition.

Some important considerations in the history and physical examination are:

- Does the patient have a normal level of consciousness? A decreased level of consciousness is an immediate tip-off that CSI is to be presumed.
- Are distracting injuries present? Gross trauma easily catches the examiner's attention and just as easily distorts the child's response to pediatric CSI. The distractibility of children is legendary and often used by clinicians as a treatment tool in the care of injured children.
- Is neck pain present? A common presumption is that a pediatric CSI will cause immediate pain as opposed to the classic

Figure 5. Normal Atlas Anatomy

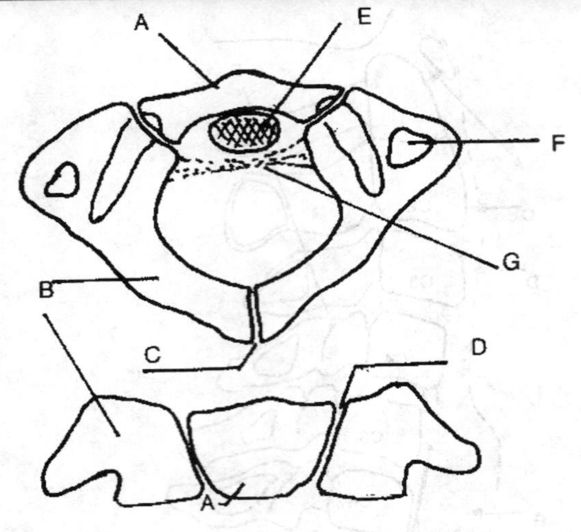

A: Body
B: Neural arch
C: Spinous process synchondrosis
D: Neurocentral synchondrosis
E: Odontoid
F: Foramen transversarium
G: Transverse atlantal ligament

Adapted from: Bailey DK. Normal cervical spine in infants and children. *Radiology* 1952;59:713.

Figure 6. Normal Axis Anatomy

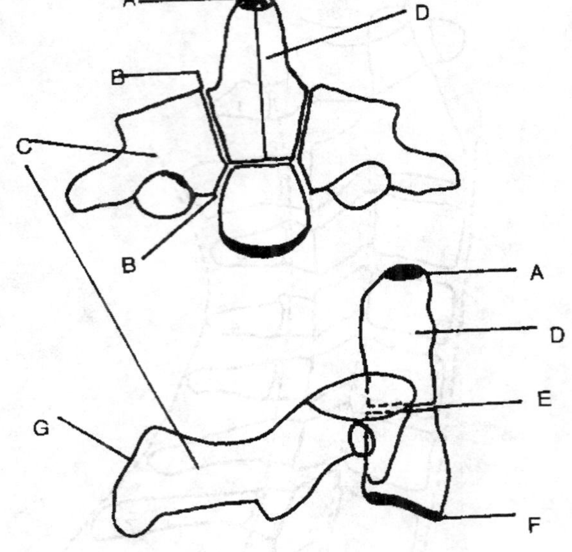

A: Terminal ossification center
B: Neurocentral synchondrosis
C: Neural arch
D: Dens
E: Subchondral synchondrosis
F: Inferior epiphyseal ring
G: Synchondrosis of spinous process

Adapted from: Bailey DK. Normal cervical spine in infants and children. *Radiology* 1952;59:713.

"whiplash" presentation of delayed symptomatology. Remember: Beware of SCIWORA.[30]

- Are (or were) there radicular neurological symptoms present? Again, beware of pediatric CSI and SCIWORA in particular.[30]
- What was the mechanism of injury? Forced hyperextension from striking a fixed object such as a windshield or the bottom of a pool are almost pathognomonic etiologies for unstable pediatric CSI.

The obligatory ABCs must be addressed first for all seriously injured patients. These patients are always presumed to have pediatric CSI until the evaluation can be directed specifically at neurologic and orthopedic systems and correlated with history. All treatments and diagnoses are based on a secured airway, adequate breathing, and stable circulation. This should all be achieved (including intubation) while maintaining cervical spine immobilization either manually with assigned personnel or via the standard immobilization devices until the patient is resuscitated and stable for further evaluation. *(See Figure 2.)*

A carefully executed secondary physical examination and serial neurologic examinations must follow to delineate the extent of injury. Severely injured or neurologically impaired patients are not difficult to diagnose; rather, those with an isolated pediatric CSI without concomitant signs of injury are the most worrisome. Disturbances in breathing patterns and gross motor function relating to spontaneous and purposeful movement of extremities are useful, albeit rare, clues. Unsustained clonus and extensor plantar response can be normal findings before complete myelination of the nerve tracts. Determining a level of sensory impairment can help localize the injury in the spinal cord and can be facilitated by using tickle rather than pinprick and careful repetition. The presence of primitive reflexes may be helpful if the patient is older than age 4. Absence of active movement in a limb indicates injury. Input from parents or family relating to preexisting medical conditions/abnormalities is very helpful in establishing a baseline level of function for each patient (particularly in those with congenital abnormalities such as Down syndrome or cerebral palsy).

Radiologic Clearance

The lack of physical evidence of pediatric CSI tends to push over-reliance on radiographic evaluation to "clear the cervical spine" of injury. Yet, with the almost requisite immobilization for any type injury, pediatric patients may inappropriately undergo obligatory radiologic examination as part of the "clearance" process—a standard operating procedure at many trauma centers. Selective criteria have been applied in using radiography for determination of adult CSI.[32] However, there are few data to suggest that these are useful in children.[33] Radiographic evidence of pediatric CSI should be pursued in patients with injuries known to have high correlation with pediatric CSI (e.g., head injury, multiply traumatized, obtunded patients, and those with demonstrable abnormal neurologic examinations). All mechanisms clearly associated with CSI, such as falls, MVAs, diving injuries, and acceleration/deceleration events involving the head, should also be radiographically evaluated.

Ambulatory or active children with incidental or minor trauma to the head (such as the perennial coffee table laceration) not involving the above criteria can be evaluated without spinal radiography given normal examinations and histories. Children younger than 12-18 months represent a higher risk group due to the prevalence of non-accidental trauma and probably warrant radiographs with anything less than a reliable history and congruent examination or very minor head trauma.

The initial technique of choice is plain film radiography to include cross-table lateral, AP, and odontoid views. *(See Table 1.)* Oblique films add little information to the above films and can be eliminated as an initial screening tool.[34] An appropriate film series is one that: 1) demonstrates all seven cervical vertebrae plus the odontoid and lateral masses; 2) has the patient positioned properly; and 3) provides the correct degree of penetration. Films with the patient overly rotated, flexed, and extended complicate interpretation by presenting nonstandard perspectives and tend to augment shadows and overlapping structures. Repetition of plane films to achieve the correct technique may be very useful given that the standard radiologic technique of brute force positioning and restraint of the pediatric patient may result in unacceptable or nonstandard films. Flexion/extension views are invaluable in the intact/cooperative child. Those who are too young or otherwise do not fit this category are more appropriately evaluated by computerized tomography (CT), particularly in the C1-3 area, which is well-demonstrated with CT scanning.

Evaluation of pediatric CSI with plain radiographs is complicated by variable degrees of ossification and soft-tissue spacing, multiple synchondroses, absence of normal curvatures, normal variants of developing vertebrae, pseudosubluxation, general hypermobility of spinal elements, and finally, the quality of the films themselves. Interpretation of plain films is best performed by a clinician familiar with the injury patterns and knowledgeable about cervical spine development with increasing age.

The concept of "C-spine clearance" is described by many physicians and often delegated to emergency physicians.[35,36] It is the act of the emergency physician "ruling out" the possibility of a cervical spine fracture in the pediatric patient (i.e., clinically and radiographically ascertaining that no pediatric CSI exists) as described in the following three steps: 1) normal initial physical examination; 2) normal radiographic plain film interpretation (with or without flexion/extension/CT as required); 3) subsequent repeat (preferably serial) examination and observation of the patient demonstrating lack of symptomatology and neurologic findings. The concept of SCIWORA may require the patient to remain immobilized until the repeat examination can be performed and is normal. While step two may not be warranted given the individual mechanism, injury, or findings, many clinicians have inaccurately come to interpret clearance as synonymous with only step 2.[35,36] *(See Figure 2.)*

Performance of Flexion/Extension Views. Flexion/extension views are considered indispensable in detecting occult or suspected ligamentous injury to the cervical spine.[1] The standard protocol requires the patient to actively provide the necessary movement to flex or extend the spine under the direct supervision of the emergency physician. This technique is derived from the assumption (unproven) that a patient with a significant injury will not move his or her neck sufficiently (even with verbal encouragement) to worsen an SCI due to the associated pain. This obviously eliminates passive motion initiated by a technician, nurse, or physician since forced flexion is running the risk of precipitating a life-threatening injury. Likewise, no patient with preexisting pain is to undergo flexion/extension studies. While SCIWORA calls into question the validity of the assumption that the patient will have pain with a significant injury, the protocol helps to eliminate further injury caused by forced passive movement.

In the pediatric population, younger patients will exhibit age-proportional decreased ability to participate in flexion/extension maneuvers just because of their lack of ability to understand, and even some older patients cannot or will not cooperate. The evaluation then defaults to tomograms or a CT scan.

Pseudosubluxation

The vertebral bodies of the cervical spine in flexion may show anterior displacement that mimics subluxation but is in reality a normal finding due to the inherent ligamentous laxity and high dynamic fulcrum of the pediatric cervical spine. Anywhere from 25-46% of children younger than age 8 will exhibit as much as 3-5 mm of "pseudosubluxation" of C2 on C3 and a smaller percentage with C3 on C4.[34,38] *(See Figure 4.)* A method of differentiating physiologic pseudosubluxation from true subluxation has been devised by Swischuk.[39,40] This relies on the concept of an imaginary line drawn through the anterior aspect of the spinous processes of C1 to C3. With this reference, the anterior aspect of the spinous process of C2 should fall within 2 mm on either side of this line. A greater than 2 mm deviation is considered evidence of true subluxation; however, a result of less than 2 mm does not absolutely rule out pathology and the rule is only applicable to C2 on C3. In fact, physiologic amounts of flexion subluxation can involve the entire cervical spine in an incremental fashion with each superior vertebral body slightly forward on the adjacent one below it. When this involves multiple vertebrae, the "stair stepping" appearance makes for easy recognition. However, an isolated anterior subluxation of C1, C2, C3 complicates evaluation, but nonetheless can be physiologic given the inherent laxity of the developing cervical spine.[38,41-47]

Soft-Tissue Spacing

Pseudothickening. Soft-tissue swelling/thickening is widely used to suggest occult ligamentous or cervical spine injury. *(See Figure 4.)* However, the soft tissues of the pediatric cervical spine can have a marked variability from what is commonly seen in the adult population. While normal values for prevertebral/anterior vertebral soft tissue widths on lateral radiographs are useful, children can show marked variability in tissue width. Prevertebral soft-tissue depth is affected by phases of respiration, swallowing, and flexion enough to make what appears as a marked increase, physiologic. Normal widths of less than seven mm at C2 and up to 14 mm below the glottis have been proposed.[34,38,48,49] This "pseudothickening" may be a result of adenoidal lymphoid tissue. Deviation of the prevertebral fat stripe found anteriorly to the lower cervical vertebrae in older children may be useful in detecting injury.

ADI Width. The atlantodental interval (ADI) is another area of variability in the pediatric spine. It is common in lateral radiographs of children to find an increase in the distance between the odontoid and the anterior arch of C1 due to laxity of the transverse ligament. While in adults this predental space is considered abnormal if greater than 3 mm, in children it can be up to 5 mm and is commonly 3-4 mm in children younger than age 8. Widening greater than 5 mm is usually attributable to atlantoaxial instability from conditions such as juvenile rheumatoid arthritis (JRA), Down syndrome, or congenital hypoplasia of the dens. Even with dens fractures, the predental space is usually maintained due to the strength of the transverse ligament and the tendency of the C1 and dens to translate as a fixed unit.[34,38,50-56]

Abnormal Curvatures

The loss of cervical lordosis or normal curvature of the cervical spine is another radiographic finding that is often interpreted as suggestive for occult pediatric CSI. In children without injury, the absence of lordosis has been reported as high as 14%.[34] Indeed, children can exhibit absence of normal angulation between adjacent vertebra and absence of flexion curvature between C2 through C7 in flexion.[34]

Variants of Ossification

C3 to C7. Vertebrae C3-C7 all have three primary ossification centers that completely ossify during the first two years of life to form the neural arch. Secondary ossification centers appear during puberty at the tips of the spinous processes and the superior and inferior ring apophyses of the vertebral end plates and fuse by age 25. Both of these areas can mimic fracture sites when seen radiographically. Conversely, these cervical end plates are a weak link in the vertebral complex, and, with severe enough hyperextension trauma (such as MVA or shaken infant), the endplate may become disrupted into the intervertebral space, or typical tear drop fractures may occur from the anterior inferior cortices.

In the very young, the C3-C4 vertebral bodies are often physiologically "wedged," mimicking a compression fracture because of the ossification process. The involvement of several levels with similar appearance helps to describe this as a physiologic variant since compression fractures from a flexion mechanism rarely involve multiple levels. Because fractures and dislocations of the atlas and axis constitute approximately 70% of pediatric CSIs and development differs greatly from the rest of the developing spine, they are considered separately.[57]

Atlas. The atlas has three primary ossification centers, two that form the lateral masses and one that appears as the anterior arch at 1 year of age. Delayed fusion of any of these centers can mimic ring fractures. Widened posterior and irregular anterior synchondroses are developmental variants. Normally, the posterior synchondrosis fuses at age 3 and the anterior body fuses with the neural arches at age 7. Retarded ossification of the posterior synchondrosis can lead to spina bifida occulta and be confused with a fracture but has little clinical significance. At approximately age 4, C1 has reached its adult diameter and will not add much area to the canal occupied by the spinal cord. In younger children, hypermobility of C1 has been noted as a physiologic phenomenon. In extension, C1 remains in close proximity to the occipital condyle and can appear to be riding extraordinarily high on C2, and the same phenomena involving a widened intraspinous distance can be evident in flexion.

Axis. The axis develops from five primary and two secondary ossification centers. At birth, the dens is a fusion of two longitudinal ossification centers that form a synchondrosis with the neural arch and the body of the axis. The tip (ossiculum terminale) forms from a separate ossification center and fuses with the dens at 12 years. The synchondrosis between the dens and the neural arch is the area of weakness that is fractured during an injury to the odontoid, the most common fracture of the upper cervical spine and usually a result of a flexion mechanism. In fact, normally this synchondrosis can be found in all 3-year-olds and is not completely ossified until 4-6 years of age. A remnant of the synchondrosis can be confused with a fracture line on lateral radiographs. Failure of the odontoid to fuse with the body of C2 (os odontoideum) is a well-known congenital anomaly. This is thought to be a result of a flexion-type injury that has subluxated the dens at one time and subsequently failed to fuse.[11,59,60] The vascular supply to the dens is via the apex at the ossiculum terminale and through vessels that enter the body of C2 superior and medial to the synchondrosis. These vessels are spared with the typical juvenile odontoid fracture—a consideration as to why dens fractures usually heal well in pediatric patients.

Failed fusion of the tip of the dens is known as ossiculum terminale. It is a variant that is thought to be benign, although death in a Down syndrome patient has been reported.[61] *(See Figure 6.)*

Specific Pediatric Cervical Spine Injuries

Atlanto-occipital Dislocation (AOD). The pediatric AO joint is susceptible particularly to extension injury because the AO facets lack the angulation that develops with skeletal maturation. The anatomical structures most closely associated with the AO joint are the lower cranial and greater occipital nerves, the medulla, and the proximal SC.

Total dislocation of the AO joint is rarely seen radiographically since the injury involves disruption of the medulla or medullospinal junction of the cord with almost universally lethal results, although survivors have been reported.[63] Clinical consequences of partial disruption have been reported and range from cardiopulmonary arrest to total quadriplegia to minimal neurologic dysfunction of the brainstem, such as cranial nerve palsies or sensory loss that can be transient.[88] Dislocation without fracture also is possible, particularly in those patients with inflammatory conditions known to predispose to this type of injury.[62-66] Survival may depend on maintaining effective immobilization, limiting further displacement, and concomitant respiratory compromise.

Atlas (Jefferson) Fractures. Fractures of the atlas are infrequent and usually result from axial loading of the spine.[67] When this occurs, the occipital condyles may be forced caudally into the lateral masses of the atlas, displacing them laterally though not as much as in adults due to the strength of the transverse ligament. This usually causes a posterior disruption in the ring as well through the neurocentral synchondroses or where the ring is grooved for the vertebral artery. Clinically the patient has occipital or suboccipital pain with or without cord injury.[34] Plain radiography in this region is limited; however, CT scanning is extremely helpful in identifying suspected fractures.

Atlantoaxial Dislocation. This is one of the most common injuries of the pediatric cervical spine, in large part due to the higher fulcrum of flexion and intrinsic ligamentous laxity in the pediatric cervical spine. This ligamentous laxity can be increased by associated inflammatory conditions such as pharyngitis, tonsillitis, JRA, or Down syndrome.[37,51-54] In this injury, the atlas moves forward on the axis either through disruption of the transverse ligament or more commonly from forced rotatory subluxation. Close attention to the atlantodental interval (ADI) (i.e., the distance between the anterior arch of the atlas and the anterior of the dens, normally 3-5 mm in the neutral position) helps to detect the injury, keeping in mind that SCIWORA always is a possibility. Clinically, patients can exhibit torticollis, restricted or painful range of motion, or neck pain with posterior palpation.

Dens Fractures. The dens is anatomically bound to the anterior portion of the atlas via the cruciate ligament. This ligament attaches to the lateral masses forming the atlantotransverse portion, a superior attachment to the foramen magnum and inferior attachment to the body of C2. The atlantotransverse portion is the strongest ligament in the cervical spine and provides the primary stabilization for the atlantoaxial complex. Alar ligaments that attach to the dens from the occipital condyles limit rotation at the atlantoaxial joint.

Dens fractures in children differ significantly from adults. Adults usually exhibit the standard Type I-III fractures involving either the tip of the odontoid, the entire odontoid, or the odontoid and some of the body of C2. In children, because the synchondroses of the axis lie below the lateral facets, the shear forces usually follow the line of the epiphysis. Some investigators have proposed that dens fractures in children are always an epiphyseal distraction. It is suspected that undisplaced dens fractures more commonly occur than actually diagnosed and frequently go undetected.[12]

Children usually exhibit a paucity of findings if they have survived the initial trauma event. This is in part due to the wide diameter of the cervical canal at the level of the axis, which allows for bony injury without impingement on the spinal cord itself. Classically, the patient resists extension on clinical examination. The most common symptom is occipital pain due to injury to the greater occipital nerve. Radiographically the appearance of the dentrocentral synchondrosis can mimic a fracture and complicates diagnosis. An anterior angulated dens is highly indicative of fracture. Soft-tissue swelling in the retropharyngeal area can help in detection; however, with infants and children variability is so common that no definitive measurement is applicable. Typically the subglottic soft tissues are double the width of those above the glottis.[66] In older children and adolescents the synchondrosis is fused to the body, resulting in the more typical adult pattern of fractures. Congenital variations such as absence of the dens, os odontoideum (agenesis of the odontoid) have been reported.[34-68]

Tear Drop Fractures. These fractures are uncommon and involve the lower cervical spine, usually in children older than age 8. Typically these result from compressive forces applied to anterior borders of the vertebral bodies during hyperflexion and buckling of the anterior longitudinal ligament associated with a "diving" type injury. The inferior corner of the vertebral body is then avulsed, forming the triangular or "tear drop" fragment. Conversely, hyperextension injury commonly fractures off the superior corner of the vertebral body as distraction forces are applied to the anterior longitudinal ligament. With the frequent ligamentous disruption, concomitant SCI is common.

Cervical End-Plate Injury. The superior and inferior articulating surfaces of the C3-C7 vertebral bodies contain physeal growth plates, often mistaken on lateral radiographs for fractures. Nevertheless, injury also can occur through these ossification centers. The superior end plate has intrinsic protection from the uncinate processes which articulate with the inferior surface of the vertebrae directly above, thus making the inferior plate more susceptible to fracture. Soft-tissue swelling is a prominent feature of end-plate injury and should suggest apophyseal fracture.[1]

Prevention

Primary Prevention (Injury Prevention). Most pediatric CSIs can be prevented with appropriate attention to restraint of patients traveling in motor vehicles. All 50 states mandate use of seat belts or child car seats for infants and children. Studies have estimated a decrease in mortality of 71% and serious injury by 67% with proper use.[70-76] No benefit is gained when restraints are used incorrectly; this, in fact, may contribute to injury. Some studies have indicated that three-quarters of all car seats are used improperly and as many as a third are installed facing the wrong direction. Current recommendations are use of a size-appropriate rear-facing child restraint seat up to a weight of 9 kg. Recommendations for a change to forward-facing vary but, in general, are age of 1 year and only when the infant can sit unsupported.[77] Proper tethering of the seat with a top anchor when necessary and an integral safety harness to secure the child within the seat are important factors. An intact seat with a restrained child makes for a good immobilization device when towels and tape are added to stabilize the neck. Parents should be encouraged to follow the guidelines for infant and child restraints provided by the American Academy of Pediatrics or those restraint requirements outlined in their specific state's child restraint laws.[78] Some activities, such as transport of children in open pickup truck beds, are to be condemned and are known for their lethality in collisions.

School programs for water safety and sports training are crucial to prepare children for the wide range of potentially hazardous activities they participate in during their younger years. Rule changes in high-impact sports to limit the incidence of cervical spine axial load injuries (e.g., "spearing" in football and "checking" in hockey) have produced a documented decrease in cervical spine fractures and dislocations.[79] Use of spotters has limited injury in trampoline use and gymnastics, other high-risk sports for CSI. Unsupervised diving accidents still remain a major cause of pediatric CSI, with the majority related to diving in shallow water or striking submerged objects.

Secondary Prevention (Prehospital). A well-trained EMS system that can respond to pediatric trauma with the appropriate skill and experience to properly immobilize and transport the pediatric patient is considered of major importance in secondary prevention. Prehospital personnel must be aware that immobilization is as important in pediatric victims as it is in adults.

Tertiary Prevention (Health Care System). Physicians maintaining high indices of suspicion for mechanisms correlative with CSI, typical presentations of SCIWORA, and clinical acumen for subtle signs of CSI will help to maximize outcomes.

Summary

The different patterns of pediatric CSI that occur when traumatic forces are applied to the growing pediatric cervical spine can be explained by the distinct anatomic and developmental differences.

Additionally, patients with pediatric CSI can be functionally divided into four groups according to age. Accordingly, a complete working knowledge of pediatric anatomy, cervical spine development, biomechanics, and pathophysiology is highly useful to the emergency medicine specialist treating injured children.

References

1. Caffey J. *Pediatric X-Ray Diagnosis.* Vol. 1, 7th ed. Chicago: Year Book Medical Publishers Inc; 1978.
2. Anderson JM , Schott AH. Spinal injury in children: A review of 56 cases seen from 1950 through 1978. *Mayo Clin Proc* 1980;55: 499-504.
3. Hadley MN, Zambramski JM, Browner CM, et al. Pediatric spinal trauma: Review of 122 cases of spinal cord and vertebral column injuries. *J Neurosurg* 1988;60:18-24.
4. Hill SA, Miller CA, Kosnick EJ, et al. Pediatric neck injuries. *J Neurosurg* 1984;60:700-706.
5. Melzak J . Paraplegia among children. *Lancet* 1969;2:45-48.
6. Ruge JR, Grant PS, McLone DG, et al. Pediatric spinal injury: The very young. *J Neurosurg* 1988;68:25-30.
7. Nitecki S , Moir CR. Predictive factors of the outcome of traumatic cervical spine fracture in children. *J Pediatr Surg* 1994;29:1409-1411.
8. Bracken MB, Freeman DH, Hellenbrand K. Incidence of acute traumatic hospitalized spinal cord injury in the United States, 1970-1977. *Am J Epidemiol* 1981;113:615-619.
9. Kewalramani LS, Kraus JF, Sterling HM. Acute spinal-cord lesions in a pediatric population: Epidemiological and clinical features. *Paraplegia* 1980;18:206-219.
10. Kewalramani LS, Tori JA. Spinal cord trauma in children; neurologic patterns, radiologic features and pathomechanics of injury. *Spine* 1980;5:11-18.
11. Fesmire FM, Luten RC. The pediatric cervical spine: Developmental anatomy and clinical aspects. *J Emerg Med* 1989;7:133-142.
12. Dietrich Am, Ginn-Pease ME, Bartkowski HM. Pediatric cervical spine fractures: Predominately subtle presentation. *J Pediatr Surg* 1991;26:995-1000.
13. Pang D, Pollack IF. Spinal cord injury without radiographic abnormality in children—the SCIWORA. *J Trauma* 1989;29:654.
14. Bresnan MJ, Abrams IF. Neonatal spinal cord transectionsecondary to intrauterine hyperextension of the neck in breech presentation. *J Pediatr* 1974;84:734-737.
15. Hillman JW, Sprofkin BE, Parrish TF. Birth injury of the cervical spine producing a "cerebral palsy" syndrome. *Am Surg* 1954;20: 900-906.
16. Crothers B. Injury of the spinal cord in breech extraction as an important cause of fetal death and paraplegia in childhood. *Am J Med Sci* 1923;165:94-110.
17. Abrams IF, Bresnan MJ, Zuckerman JE, et al. Cervical cord injuries secondary to hyperextension of the head in breech presentation. *Obstet Gynecol* 1973;41:369-378.
18. Venes JL, DiPietro MA. Spinal cord injury. In: Touloukian RJ, ed. *Pediatric Trauma.* 2nd ed. St. Louis: Mosby Year Book; 1990: 235-244.
19. Leventhal HR. Birth injuries of the spinal cord. *J Pediatr* 1960;56: 447-453.
20. Stauffer ES, Mazur JM. Cervical spine injuries in children. *Pediatr Ann* 1982;11:502-511.
21. Bohn D, Armstrong D, Becker L. Cervical spine injuries in children. *J Trauma* 1990;30:4.
22. Janssen L, Hansebout RR. Pathogenesis of spinal cord injury and newer treatments. A review. *Spine* 1989;14:23-28.
23. Reid DC, Saboe LA, Allan DG. Spine trauma associated with off-road vehicles. *Phys Sports Med* 1988;16:6143-6152.
24. Sneed RC, Stover SL, Fine PR. Spinal cord injury associated with all-terrain vehicle accidents. *Pediatrics* 1986;77:271-274.
25. Haynes CD, Stroud SD, Thompson CE. The three wheeler (adult tricycle): An unstable, dangerous machine. *J Trauma* 1986;26: 643-648.
26. Curran C, Dietrich AM, Bowman MJ, et al. Pediatric cervical-spine immobilization: Achieving neutral position? *J Trauma* 1995;39: 729-732.
27. Snyder RG, Schneider LW, Owings CL, et al. Anthropometry of infants, children and youths to age 18 for product safety design SP-450. Warrendale, PA: Society of Automotive Engineers; 1977.
28. Nypaver M, Treloar D. Neutral cervical spine positioning in children. *Ann Emerg Med* 1994;23:208-211.
29. Herzenberg JE, Hensinger RN, Dedrick DK, et al. Emergency transport and positioning of young children who have an injury of the cervical spine. *J Bone Joint Surg* 1989;71A:15-22.
30. Pang D, Pollack IF. Spinal cord injury without radiographic abnormality in children—the SCIWORA syndrome. *Trauma* 1989;29: 658.
31. Orenstein JB, Klein BL, Ochsenschlager DW. Delayed diagnosis of pediatric cervical spine injury. *Pediatrics* 1992;89:6,1185-1188.
32. Roberge RJ, Wears RC, Kelly M, et al. Selective application of cervical spine radiography in alert victims of trauma. A prospective study. *J Trauma* 1988;28:784-788.
33. Rachesky I, Boyce WT, Duncan B. Clinical prediction of cervical spine injuries in children. *Am J Dis Child* 1987;141:199-201.
34. Swischuk LE. *Emergency Imaging of the Acutely Ill or Injured Child.* 3rd ed. Baltimore; Williams & Wilkins; 1994:653.
35. Ross SE, Schwab CM, David ET, et al. Clearing the cervical spine: Initial radiologic evaluation. *J Trauma* 1987;27:1055-1060.
36. Lally KP, Senac M, Hardin WD. Utility of cervical spine radiograph in pediatric trauma. *Am J Surg* 1989;158:540-542.
37. Galli RL, Spaite DW, Simon RR. Fractures, dislocations, and subluxations. In: *Emergency Orthopedics: The Spine.* East Norwalk, CT: Appleton & Lange; 1989.
38. Cattell HS, Filtzer DL. Pseudosubluxation and other normal variations in the cervical spine in children. *J Bone Surg* 1965;47A: 1295-1309.
39. Swischuk LE. *Radiology of the Newborn and Young Infant.* 2nd ed. Baltimore: Williams & Wilkins; 1980:834-857.
40. Swischuk LE. Anterior displacement of C2 in children—physiologic or pathologic? A helpful differentiating line. *Radiology* 1977;122: 759-763.
41. Harrison RB, Keats TE, Winn HR, et al. Pseudosubluxation in the axis in young adults. *J Can Assoc Radiol* 1980;31:176-177.
42. Jacobson G, Bleecker HH. Pseudosubluxation of the axis in children. *Am J Roentgenol* 1959;82:472-481.
43. Kattarl KR. Backward "displacement" of the spinolaminal line at C2: A normal variation. *Am J Roentgenol* 1977;129:289-290.
44. Pennecot GF, Gouraud D, Hardy Jr, et al. Roentgenographical study

of the stability or the cervical spine in children. *J Pediatr Orthop* 1984;4:346-352.
45. Sullivan CR, Bruwer AJ, Harris LE. Hypermobility of the cervical spine in children: A pitfall in the diagnosis of cervical dislocation. *Am J Surg* 1958;95:636-640.
46. Teng, P, Paptheodorou C. Traumatic subluxation of C2 in young children. *Bull Los Angeles Neurol Soc* 1967;32:197-202.
47. Townsend EH, Rowe ML. Mobility of the upper cervical spine in health and disease. *Pediatrics* 1952;10:567-572.
48. Apple JS, Kirks DR, Merten DF, et al. Cervical spine fractures and dislocations in children. *Pediatr Radiol* 1987;17:45-49.
49. Swischuk LE. *Emergency Radiology of the Acutely Ill or Injured Child.* 2nd ed. Baltimore: Williams & Wilkins; 1986:556-609.
50. Locke GR, Gardner JI, Van Epps EF. Atlas-dens interval (ADI) in children: A survey based on 200 normal cervical spines. *Am J Roentgenol* 1966;97:135-140.
51. Reid GD, Hill RH. Atlantoaxial subluxation in juvenile ankylosing spondylitis. *J Pediatr* 1978;93:531-532.
52. Burkheiser EJ, Seigler F. Non-traumatic dislocations of the atlantoaxial joint. *JAMA* 1931;96:517-519.
53. Burke SW, French HG, Roberts JM et al. Chronic atlanto-axial instability in Down syndrome. *J Bone Joint Surg* 1985:67: 1356-1360.
54. Davidson RG. Atlantoaxial instability in individuals with Down syndrome. A fresh look at the evidence. *Pediatrics* 1988;81: 857-865.
55. Fielding JW, Lochran GVB, Lawsing JP, et al. Tears of the transverse ligament of the atlas. *J Bone Joint Surg* 1974;56A:1683-1691.
56. Kobori M, Takahashi H, Mikawa Y. Atlanto-axial dislocation in Down syndrome. Report of two cases requiring surgical correction. *Spine* 1986;11:195-200.
57. Funk FJ, Wells RE. Injuries to the cervical spine in football. *Clin Orthop* 1975;109:50-58.
58. Sherk HH, Schut L, Lane JM. Fractures and dislocations of the cervical spine in children. *Orthop Clin North Am* 1976;7:593-604.
59. Truex RC, Johnson CH. Congenital anomalies of the upper cervical spine. *Orthop Clin North Am* 1978;9:891-900.
60. Garber JN. Abnormalities of the atlas and axis vertebrae: Congenital and traumatic. *J Bone Joint Surg* 1964;46A:1782-1791.
61. Sherk HH, Nicholson J. Rotatory atlanto-axial dislocation associated with ossiculum terminale and mongolism. *J Bone Joint Surg* 1969;51A:957-960.
62. Bucholz RW, Burkhead WZ. The pathologic anatomy of fatal atlanto-occipital dislocations. *J Bone Joint Surg* 1979; 61A: 248-250.
63. Collalto PM, DeMuth WW, Schwentker EP, et al. Traumatic atlanto-occipital dislocation. *J Bone Joint Surg* 1986;68A: 1106-1109.
64. Gillis FH, Binna J, Sotrel A. Infantile atlanto-occipital instability. *Am J Dis Child* 1979;133:30-37.
65. Davis D, Bohlman H, Walker AE, et al. The pathological findings in fatal cranio-spinal injuries. *J Neurosurg* 1979;34:603-613.
66. Powers B, Milla MD, Kramer RS, et al. Traumatic anterior antlanto-occipital dislocation. *Neurosurgery* 1979;4:12-17.
67. Marlin AE, Williams GR, Lee JF. Jefferson fractures in children. *J Neurosurg* 1983;58:277-279.
68. Fielding JW, Griffin PP. Os odontoideum: An acquired lesion. *J Bone Joint Surg* 1974;56A:187.
69. Yngve DA, Harris WP, Herndon WA. Spinal cord injury without osseous fracture. *J Pediatr Orthop* 1988;8:153-159.
70. Walsh JW, Stevens DB, Young AB. Traumatic paraplegia in children without contiguous spinal fracture or dislocation. *Neurosurgery* 1983;12:439-445.
71. Kahane CJ. An evaluation of child passenger safety: The effectiveness and benefits of safety seats. Washington DC: National Highway Traffic Safety Administration; 1986. U.S. Department of Transportation report DOT HS 806-889.
72. Fuchs S, Barthel MJ, Flannery AM, et al. Cervical spine fractures sustained by young children in forward facing car seats. *Pediatrics* 1989;84:348-354.
73. Torg JS. Epidemiology, pathomechanics, and prevention of athletic injuries to the cervical spine. *Med Sci Sports Exercise* 1985;17:3, 295-303.
74. Nygren A, Tingvall C, Turkell T. Misuse of child restraints in cars and potential hazards from misuse: Road traffic observations and barrier sled tests. *Acta Paediatr Scand* 1987;339(suppl):1-19.
75. Margolis LH, Wagenaar AC, Molnar LJ. Recognizing the common problem of child automobile restraint misuse. *Pediatrics* 1988;81: 717-720.
76. Kahane CJ. An evaluation of child passenger safety: the effectiveness and benefits of safety seats. Washington, D.C. National Highway Traffic Safety Administration, 1986
77. Shellness A, Charles S. Children and car seats. *Pediatrics* 1986;77:256-258.
78. American Academy of Pediatrics. Infant and child restraints: Selecting the appropriate type. Elk Grove Village, IL: American Academy of Pediatrics; 1996.
79. American Academy of Pediatrics Committee on Injury and Poison Prevention. Selecting and using the most appropriate car safety seats for growing children: Guidelines for counseling parents. *Pediatrics* 1996;97:761-763.

Pediatric Burn Injuries

Charles Stewart, MD, FACEP

Thermal burns are perhaps the most devastating injury suffered by an individual. The skin separates us from our environment. It provides the bulk of cooling from the stress of heat, regulates the egress of bodily fluids, and prevents outside agents and bacteria from entering the body. It is the largest organ in the body. When the skin is broached by a burn, we lose some or all of these factors to some degree, depending upon the extent of the burn.

The emergency care provider may find caring for the burned child to be stressful, frightening, and even repugnant.

This chapter reviews current assessment and management strategies for pediatric burns.

Demographics of Burns in Children

Among the environmental injuries sustained by man, by far the most common are thermal burns. The National Consumer Commission has estimated that at least 2 million people in the United States are burned each year. Of these patients, some 100,000 will require hospitalization, and about 12,000 will die.[1] Burns are not only common, they also can be lethal. While a minor burn requires little treatment, a 20% full-thickness burn is an injury equivalent to having both legs crushed.

About 440,000 children will receive treatment each year for burn injuries.[2] Young children and older adults have a higher fatality rate than older children and adults for the same degree and extent of burn, although survival has improved for children younger than age 4.[3,4] The reason for the higher mortality rate in young children is not clear, although it may involve less physiologic reserve, more extensive damage with thinner skin, less margin for error in fluid management, and technical difficulties with vascular access.

Indeed, children younger than age 6 have more burns than any other age group. Burns ranked third as a cause of childhood injury-related mortality in both Canada and the United States.[5,6] Children are most often victims of scald and contact burns, smoke inhalation, and electrical burns.[7,8] Structural fires account for 45% of burn-related deaths, and burns are the leading cause of childhood injury-related death within the home.[9] African American and Native American children are at higher risk of death or injury from burns compared to white children. Both low income and poor quality housing have been blamed for this. Use of alternative heating sources may contribute to the disparity.[10]

Survival of the burn patient is dependent upon the amount and depth of the burn, the age of the patient, and other associated injuries.[11] Determining the degree of injury in a given patient helps when deciding where to transport the patient, the appropriate level of care, and immediate focus of therapy.

Ages 0-2

The young child is at greatest risk to sustain a scald burn. Scald burns fall into two categories: kitchen scalds and bathroom scalds.

With scald burns, the magnitude of injury depends upon the heat transferred from the liquid. This, in turn, depends on the specific heat of the liquid (the amount of heat needed to raise a certain volume of liquid a specific number of degrees). A higher specific heat means that the liquid's capacity to store and release heat is greater. Water has a higher specific heat than most substances found in nature. The heat stored in even small quantities of hot water is sufficient to cause thermal injuries in children. The maximum temperature that liquid water can attain at sea level is 100°C (212°F). Other liquids, such as tar, sulfur, or molten metals, can attain higher temperatures. Sulfur and tar also have higher specific heats than water; thus, the burns from these two substances can be severe.

The length of time a liquid is in contact with the skin also is important. At temperatures greater than 70°C (158°F), water can cause complete necrosis of the epidermis in less than two seconds. It is fortunate that water is not particularly viscous and flows unless impeded by clothing. With immersion scalds, the duration of contact between the hot liquid and skin is considerably longer than when water splashes onto the skin. Consequently, the resulting injury is more severe.

Kitchen scalds are the most dangerous. Grabbing a dangling cord attached to a frying pan, deep fryer, slow cooker, or electric kettle can bring extremely hot water or grease down on a toddler. Pulling a parent's coffee or other hot beverage off the table may scald both child and parent alike.

Bathroom scalds occur from hot tap water. These may occur whenever the water temperature is greater than 128°F. Indeed, when the water temperature is 150°F or greater, a scald burn may occur in less than two seconds. On the other hand, it takes more than five minutes exposure to water of 120°F to cause a scald burn. Simply setting the hot water heater temperature at 120°F can prevent the vast majority of these burns.[12]

Although infrequently reported, aspiration of hot liquid can occur in conjunction with upper-body scald burns, leading to acute compromise of the small pediatric airway.[13] If the early, subtle signs of airway compromise are neglected, the child may develop severe respiratory distress.

Wood- and gas-burning stoves, grills, or fireplaces also can cause burns when the toddler touches the hot metal.[14] Although these burns are common, there are few long-lasting sequelae.[15]

Electrical cords, plugs, and sockets are attractive nuisances to the toddler, and children may suffer electrical injuries when chewing or playing with electrical outlets and cords.

Ages 3-8

Children at this age continue to require both guidance and protection. These children are still developing coordination, and the body is not fully in control, so scald and contact burns persist in this age group.

Fascination with fire, matches, and lighters begins at an early age, before the motor coordination and judgment to handle dangerous items have developed. Experimentation with matches, camp fires, fireplaces, and stoves occurs in solitary or group play situations. This can lead to house fires and clothing ignition. In a Massachusetts study, flame burns ranked second after scalds in the 3- to 8-year-old age group, and the burns requiring hospital treatment often involved a single-ignition, single-victim flame injury.[4]

Fireworks injuries are common in this age group.[16] Many of the injuries will be minor and due to sparklers, firecrackers, bottle rockets, and roman candles. Adult supervision can prevent as many as half of the injuries.

Ages 9-12

Risk-taking behavior and peer pressure become driving forces. There is an increasing wish to be responsible and do adult tasks. This behavior may lead to increased use of flammable liquids such as gasoline for lawn mowers. These youngsters are often unaware of the dangers of these flammable liquids. Many of the hospitalized youngsters in this age group will have flame burns due to careless use of lighter fluids, charcoal lighter, gasoline, or even hair spray. Fireworks injuries also are common in this age group.

Pathophysiology of Thermal Burns

Burns are caused by the transfer of energy to the skin at a faster rate than the body or skin can dissipate it. The depth of a burn depends upon the temperature and duration of the heat applied, and the ability of the tissues to dissipate the transferred energy. The rate of heat transfer is more critical than the total amount of heat transferred.

Vascular Changes in Burned Skin. Almost immediately after the burn, the vessels in the adjacent area are altered. At first, an intense vasoconstriction is caused by the release of numerous vasoactive substances from the injured cells.

After a few hours, the vessels dilate as kinins are released from the damaged mast cells. During the vasodilatation, the capillaries become more permeable, allowing extravasation of plasma into the burned wound.

Ischemia from the initial vasoconstriction and subsequent microthrombus formation may extend the area of the injury. The ischemia may be present to a depth of as much as 3-7 times greater than the area of the cells directly damaged by the heat. Because of this ischemia, final determination of the depth of the burn may be delayed as long as five days.

Many authorities recognize three concentric layers of vascular changes due to the effects of the burn and subsequent ischemia. The center of the burn is often called the zone of coagulation and represents the area of direct cellular destruction by the heat. Within this region, all blood vessels are thrombosed. As the intensity of the heat or the length of the exposure increases, this zone of coagulation will become deeper and wider.

Surrounding the zone of coagulation is a zone of stasis. In this area, there is vasoconstriction and some microvascular thrombosis. Some blood vessels will remain patent, even though blood flow is reduced overall. If circulation is promptly restored, some of the injured cells in this region will survive. However, a delay in treatment can cause more irreversible damage.

Surrounding the area of vascular stasis is an area of minimal damage, the zone of hyperemia. The bright red color that blanches on pressure is noted at the margin of all burn wounds, and, in the most minimal cases, may comprise the entire wound.

Water and Heat Losses. In addition to the direct reactions to a thermal burn, burns that destroy the epidermis will allow increased insensible water losses of up to 15 times normal. As the water evaporates, body heat is lost, which can lead to the development of hypothermia. Caloric requirements increase enormously as the body tries to adjust to this increase in metabolic rate. Major thermal injury also is associated with extreme hypermetabolism and catabolism.

Infection Potential. Following a severe skin burn from any source, the skin undergoes coagulation necrosis and becomes an excellent growth medium for bacteria. Because the local blood supply also is compromised, the local defense mechanisms may be inadequate. The degree and consequences of the resultant bacterial invasion will vary directly with the severity of the wound. Bacterial invasion is one of the most frequent, fatal complications of a serious burn.

Initially, the microflora is gram positive like the normal skin flora. After the fifth day, the wound is colonized with gram-negative organisms. Less severe burns may evolve into deeper burns as tissue is destroyed by infection.

Assessment of the Burn. The assessment of thermal burn injury involves three major factors: the location, depth, and extent of the damage. These three factors help determine the capacity for regeneration and the potential for bacterial invasion. Included in the initial assessment of the burn should be the evaluation of potentially exacerbating factors such as age, prior medical history, allergies, and current medications.

Initial History. Obtain the history of the injury from the patient, parents, relatives, or emergency response crew. Remember that although the burn may ultimately be fatal, if the patient has survived the initial insult, the burn wound itself is not likely to be the *immediate* threat to life. Gas explosions, propane explosions, or other explosive injuries may cause substantial associated injuries. Confinement in an enclosed car or a room may be associated with pulmonary injuries from inhalation of toxic gases. The child may have been involved in an accident that preceded the burn, or may have leapt to escape being more severely burned. These potentially life-threatening injuries may take precedence over the burn wound management and should be dealt with as necessary.

The history should include any associated illnesses such as diabetes, hypertension, metabolic disorders, or cardiac and pulmonary diseases. It is important to find out if there are any allergies and current drug therapies. The patient's age should be noted at this time. Remember that burns occurring to those at the extremes of age will be associated with the highest morbidity and mortality.

The Skin

The epidermis is the outer layer of the skin and is made up of four layers:

1. *Stratum corneum*. This water-retaining layer consists of dead, dried out (keratinized) cells that are constantly being shed.
2. *Stratum lucidum*. This is a clear cell layer in which cells are becoming keratinized.
3. *Stratum granulosum*. In this layer, the epidermal cells gradually die and start to keratinize.
4. *Stratum germinativum*. This is the layer in which new skin cells are produced. Injury to this layer may result in vitiligo, a mottled coloring of the skin. This is the layer that is destroyed in a third-degree burn.

Table 1. Burn Classification Scheme

MAJOR BURN INJURIES
- Second-degree burn greater than 25% TBSA in adults
- Second-degree burn greater than 20% TBSA in children
- Third-degree burns greater than 10% TBSA
- Burns of hands, face, eyes, ears, feet, or perineum
- All inhalation injuries
- Electrical burns
- Burns complicated by fractures or other trauma
- Burns in poor risk patients

MODERATE, UNCOMPLICATED BURN INJURIES
- Second-degree burns greater than 15% TBSA in adults
- Second-degree burns greater than 10% TBSA in children
- Third-degree burns greater than 2% TBSA that do not involve ears, eyes, face, hands, feet, or perineum

MINOR BURN INJURIES
- Second-degree burns less than 15% TBSA in adults
- Second-degree burns less than 10% TBSA in children
- Third-degree burns that are less than 2% and do not involve any of the critical areas

TBSA = Total body surface area

The true skin, dermis, or corium is the inner layer of the skin, and is composed of connective tissues and the pressure sensors, nerves, pain sensors, hair follicles, and sweat glands. This layer also controls heat balance. The germinal layer, stratum germinativum, extends into the dermis where the skin's hair follicles, sweat glands, and other appendages are produced.

Depth of the Burn

The depth of a burn provides the initial clue to the severity of the injury, but it may not be possible to accurately determine the depth of a burn until debridement has been performed. What initially appears to be a second-degree burn may evolve into a third-degree burn by infection or vascular changes from the original burn injuries. Burns may be classified based on depth and percentage of body surface involved. *(See Table 1.)*

First-Degree Burns. A first-degree burn affects only the superficial epidermis. It results in vasodilatation and congestion of the dermal vessels. The resultant erythema will blanch upon pressure. There is no bullae formation, and the wound is painful. Premature cell death often results in desquamation or peeling a few days after the burn.

Healing of the first-degree burn is not normally accompanied by scarring or discoloration, and there is no substantial clinical significance to this injury in the otherwise healthy child. Most first-degree burns take 3-5 days to heal.

Typical etiologies may include thermal and thermal exposure (particularly scalding injuries in children), ultraviolet exposure, and occasionally ionizing radiation exposure.

Second-Degree Burns. A second-degree burn involves a portion of the dermis and produces an epidermolysis. The resultant edema and fluid exudate leads to bullae formation, a hallmark of the second-degree injury. There is a varying depth of destruction, with sparing of dermal appendages such as sweat glands, hair follicles, and sebaceous glands. There is erythema that blanches with pressure. The epidermis is easily separated from the skin.

By definition, the full-thickness dermis is not destroyed in a second-degree burn, and the epidermis can regenerate over a period of time without significant scarring or contracture formation. Since nerve fibers in the skin are often spared, these burns are exquisitely painful. This is the typical scalding injury in children.

The intact blisters provide a sterile water-proof covering for the wound and healing occurs by continued growth of the remaining basal cells. Underlying the blister formation may be an erythematous or waxy base, depending upon the depth of the burn. If the blister is broken, a weeping wound will result. There is then concomitant increase in evaporative water and heat losses, and exposure of naked nerve fibers.

The typical second-degree burn heals in about 14-21 days. There is minimal scar formation with a second-degree burn. Dark-complected children may lose melanin in the burned tissues and develop vitiligo.

Deep second-degree burns occur when the damage is extensive, but the deeper structures retain viable skin elements. This is most often true in deep burns of the back, palms, and soles. At times, the only remaining elements may be very deep in the dermis, such as sweat glands and hair follicles. This burn may develop the same eschar as the third-degree burn. It is important to recognize these deeper second-degree burns in extensively burned patients because the skin may regenerate without skin grafting. This differentiation may become obsolete as more experience is developed with culturing human epithelium from the victim.[17-20]

Although bullae are classically found with second-degree burns, they also may be caused by infection or by superheated steam. Bullae due to second-degree burns develop relatively promptly after the injury. Those bullae noted with infection present later, usually 24 or more hours after the insult. The provider should be suspicious of blisters appearing more than 16 hours after a burn injury. Superheated steam also may cause bullae because the high temperature causes water in the skin to boil and then vaporize, separating the dermis from the epidermis. The burns from superheated steam should be considered third-degree at all times. Note that superheated steam is used only in commercial and marine boilers and is not a common source of injury in children.

When the burn is greater than 10% of the body surface in children, and particularly in infants, the child should generally be admitted to the hospital and therapy started there.

Third-Degree Burns. As the depth of injury increases in more severe burns, all epidermal and supporting structures are destroyed. The surface of a third-degree burn is dry, leathery, and inelastic. The burned skin surface may appear white to gray, waxy, and translucent. Mottling and superficial coagulated vessels may be seen through the surface of the resultant eschar. The leathery eschar permits water losses to an excessive degree and there is no functional barrier to bacterial invasion. These burns are often painless, due to the destruction of the nerve fibers.

By definition, the third-degree burn will not regenerate except from the unburned edges of the skin or from a skin graft. For this reason, surgical intervention usually will be needed. New research with skin cell cloning may help some of these victims.

Only very small third-degree burns in children should be treated in the outpatient setting. Consultation with a plastic surgeon or a surgeon skilled in the treatment of the hand burn is mandatory.

Fourth-Degree Burns. Though not used by all authorities, the classification of fourth-degree burn is applied to burns that extend beyond the depth of the skin to involve underlying fascia, muscle, tendons, nerves, periosteum, and vessels. Occasionally even bone may be involved. This burn classification is most often used with electrical injuries, but severe charring of extremities also may be termed fourth-degree lesions. The natural history of this wound is the same as a third-degree burn, but there is deeper destruction and more dysfunction. There is no difference in the initial treatment of a third-degree burn and a fourth-degree burn.

Fourth-degree burns in children should be treated by hospitalization in all cases. This is beyond the scope of this article.

Extent of the Burn Surface

A variety of methods have been developed to estimate the amount of involved body surface area.

Lund and Browder Chart. Since the proportions of surface areas of the younger patients will vary with age, schemes to approximate the burn surface area will fail unless these variations are taken into account. The most accurate method for determining the extent of the burn is the Lund and Browder Chart, which accounts for changes in the sizes of the body parts that occur during growth.[21] *(See Table 2.)* These calculations can be quite time consuming, and the rule of nines is more frequently used in field emergency services, though it is less accurate for the pediatric population.

Rule of Nines. The rule of nines apportions a 9% segment to each of 11 major body surfaces, and the remaining 1% is apportioned to the groin. This scheme is for the adult human. For children, a greater percentage is assigned to the head and a lesser percentage to the lower extremities.

Rule of Palms. The rule of palms is convenient for measuring small burn surfaces. The patient's hand is roughly 1% of the patient's total body surface area (TBSA). Estimation of the number of hand spans for a small burn will give a rough approximation of the burned surface area. This method is not accurate for large burned surfaces. (Note: Although the Advanced Trauma Life Support course teaches that the patient's palm is 1% of the total surface area, the better approximation is that the patient's hand, including the fingers, is 0.8%.)[22-23]

Location of the Burn

The location of a burn is critical in planning care of the patient's burn. Most facial burns, groin burns, hand burns, and foot burns require inpatient care.

Facial burns should be carefully assessed for associated airway involvement. In general, all but the most superficial facial burns should be admitted. If there is any question of ocular injury, then admission is essential. Burns of the neck can rapidly become macerated and may require in-hospital treatment. Up to 48 hours of

Table 2. Lund and Browder Chart

AGE VS. BODY SURFACE AREA PROPORTIONS (PERCENTAGE)						
Area	**Up to 1 Year**	**1-4 Years**	**5-9 Years**	**10-14 Years**	**15 Years**	**Adult**
Head	19%	17%	13%	11%	9%	7%
Neck	2%	2%	2%	2%	2%	2%
Ant. Trunk	13%	13%	13%	13%	13%	13%
Post. Trunk	13%	13%	13%	13%	13%	13 %
Buttock	2.5%	2.5%	2.5%	2.5%	2.5%	2.5 %
Upper Arm	4%	4%	4%	4%	4%	4%
Lower Arm	3%	3%	3%	3%	3%	3%
Hand	2.5%	2.5%	2.5 %	2.5%	2.5%	2.5%
Thigh	5.5%	6.5%	8%	8.5%	9%	9.5%
Leg	5%	5%	5.5%	6%	6.5%	7%
Foot	3.5%	3.5%	3.5%	3.5%	3.5%	3.5%
Genitalia	1%	1%	1%	1%	1%	1%

Adapted from: Lund CC, Browder NC. The estimation of areas of burns. *Surg Gynecol Obstet* 1944;79:352-358.

observation is wise for any patient with significant facial burns, especially if there is any question of inhalation injury.

Patients with deep or extensive burns of the hands should receive a surgical consultation. These burns are very difficult to manage at home because they often are treated with topical agents, no dressings, and may require debridement. Early evaluation and participation in physical therapy is a major advantage of inpatient care. Deep second-degree, as well as third-degree, burns of the hand may benefit from early excision of the burn eschar.

One of the more trying injuries to treat at home is a foot burn. The necessary elevation and pain on walking make home management very difficult, even in children. If the patient tries to care for himself, severe edema, pain, excessive exudation, and early superficial infection often occur. Burns of the feet are initially best treated in the hospital.

The final critical area is the groin, including both the perineum and the genitalia. Even second-degree burns in this area should be treated with open management. This requires expert nursing care. If these burns macerate, they rapidly develop infection and severe scarring. With good hospital care and treatment, however, these wounds heal extremely well.

The pattern of the burn also should be carefully examined to detect elements of abuse. A child who accidentally pulls a container with hot liquid from a stove will usually have a scalding burn of the anterior head/face, anterior neck, palmar surfaces of the hands and fingers, extended arm or arms, anterior shoulder, axilla, and anterior chest. A scald due to immersion usually involves the lower trunk, buttocks, perineum, and legs. Abusive burns tend to be deeper and larger than accidental burns.

Burns that are seldom accidental include: stocking or glove burns; mirror image burns; burns that spare flexor surfaces; and burns located on the buttocks, perineum, external genitalia, dorsal hands, fingers and feet, and posterior head, neck, shoulders, torso, and extremities. Contact burns are the most common pattern of abuse. Multiple cigarette burns or contact burns, particularly of varying ages, should be considered abuse until proven otherwise.

Finally, very young children or those with pre-existing disease will have more mortality or morbidity as a result of the complications from a burn injury. Those pre-existing diseases that increase the risk of a major burn include (but are not limited to) major cardiovascular or respiratory diseases, hepatic and renal diseases, insulin dependent diabetes, alcoholism, severe psychiatric illness, and head injuries with unconsciousness. Patients with sickle cell disease also should be considered to be in this category because they will frequently develop a sickle cell crisis in response to major burns.

Care of the Burn Patient

Upon arrival at the ED, therapy begins with any chemically contaminated garments being removed and the victim washed with copious amounts of water (with only a few exceptions).

Burns may be inflicted in children as a form of abuse. Contact burns with matches, cigarettes, irons, or hot metal appliances, and scald burns are common forms of this type of child abuse. If the history seems inconsistent with the trauma noted, or if the parent's concern seems inconsistent with the seriousness of the injuries of a child, the physician should be alerted to the possibility of child abuse. Frequent locations of non-accidental burn trauma include burns of the backs of the hands, and legs, buttocks, and feet.

Moist soaks or ice applications are often recommended to relieve the pain of a superficial burn. If the patient has more than a single extremity burned, the patient should not be wrapped in cold compresses or have ice applied.[24] If the burn is third degree, the child also does not need treatment with ice or cold water. With an immersion of this sort in an infant, it is easy to imagine the rapid development of hypothermia. The child with a burn does not need the additional stress of hypothermia and its associated problems.

IV access should not be placed in any burned area, if possible. If IV fluids are not available for any reason, oral fluid replacements may be required. The decision to give oral fluids in this situation should not be made lightly, as about 30% of patients with a burn of 20% or more of the body surface area will develop an adynamic ileus. The complications of an adynamic ileus and administration of oral fluids are obvious. If contraindications to the administration of oral fluids exist, such as abdominal trauma, facial trauma, or unconsciousness are present, oral fluids should not be given.

Care should be taken to keep burned extremities elevated when possible so that excessive edema formation does not occur. Circumferential extremity burns should be treated as outlined below to prevent limb ischemia. Circumferential chest injuries also may necessitate an escharotomy to prevent respiratory embarrassment.

It should be remembered that for the patient with an extensive burn, this is only the beginning of a treatment program that may last for years. The emergency physician's goal is to enhance the maximum chance for survival of both body and burned surfaces for the patient. This may mean that the emergency physician's appropriate role is that of stabilization and referral rather than definitive therapy. Burn care has advanced tremendously during the past 20 years through the joint efforts of cognizant emergency providers and burn researchers in specialized burn units. The average hospital quite simply does not have the resources or training for management of the severely burned patient.

Appraisal of the Burn

Upon arrival of the patient, the physician needs to assess the basics of airway, breathing, and circulation. Airway swelling, respiratory distress, and signs of potential inhalation injury should be sought and corrected immediately.

Although impairment of circulation is not usually a problem in the early management phase of an uncomplicated burned patient, burned patients have frequently sustained additional trauma in the process of exiting the burning area or as a consequence of the burn. The patient should be examined thoroughly for signs of additional trauma. As the formation of local edema in the burn progresses, hypovolemia (burn shock) becomes likely and must be corrected. Locally, circulation to the extremities may be impaired by circumferential burns. This must be promptly treated.

Inhalation Injuries. Postburn lung dysfunction is a major cause of mortality in the burned pediatric patient. Increasing use of plastics and other materials that liberate noxious fumes when ignited has increased the potential for such injuries. Objective criteria for diagnosis of inhalation injuries such as fiberoptic bronchoscopy and Xenon lung scans have demonstrated the presence of pulmonary insult in up to one-third of all burn victims. These problems should not be underestimated. Patients of any age with a burn and inhalation injury have twice the mortality of patients with only a burn.

The presence of a pulmonary or respiratory injury due to the inhalation of products of combustion should be anticipated. Suspect carbon monoxide poisoning in all burned patients and obtain CO levels.

In cases with upper airway damage, rapid intubation may be lifesaving. Stridor is an ominous finding and implies that at least 20% of the airway is occluded in the adult patient. In the young child, small amounts of edema can result in severe occlusions because of the small diameter of a pediatric airway. Ensure that the patient is intubated with an endotracheal tube. Administer 100% humidified oxygen to prevent mucous membrane drying and ensure oxygenation of the patient.

Do not rely on pulse oximeters in burn victims. Because they measure reflectance of bound hemoglobin, they are notoriously inaccurate in the presence of CO-bound and HS-bound hemoglobin.

Burn Shock. Following a severe burn, adult patients may lose up to 10-15 liters of fluid due to increased capillary permeability throughout the body. This isotonic fluid and protein leak from the intravascular compartment to the cellular interstitium has its greatest losses during the first 8-12 hours. If untreated, this transfer of fluid may cause hypovolemic shock.

Fluid resuscitation "budgets" developed over the past two decades have virtually eliminated death due to burn shock. In fact, burn edema due to increased capillary permeability and simultaneous over zealous fluid administration is now the most common complication of a burn.

Fluid resuscitation becomes critical in children who have sustained burns of more than 10% of their body surfaces. The goals of fluid resuscitation are to maintain cardiovascular hemodynamics, prevent renal and pulmonary complications, and to correct acid/base abnormalities.

Calculating Fluid Replacements. In 1952, Evans and associates devised a formula for calculating the fluid and electrolyte requirements of severely burned patients. Our concepts of the fluid and electrolyte replacements called for in the burned patient have been derived from suggestions by many investigators since that time. (*See Table 3.*)

There are several components to the burn budgets listed above. Crystalloid, particularly Ringer's lactate solution, is the most popular resuscitation fluid used today. Proponents of Ringer's lactate feel that other solutions are no better and are substantially more expensive than Ringer's. In major burns, severe hypoproteinemia may result with these crystalloid resuscitation formulas. The hypoproteinemia may result in more edema formation.

These fluid budgets were designed for adult patients with adult burns. In a child with 10-20% burn, the Parkland formula alone would be insufficient for maintenance, much less for burn resuscitation.[25] A child's maintenance fluid requirements can be calculated through a number of different techniques relying on surface area or weight. A useful method of calculating the child's maintenance fluid requirements is:

Maintenance fluid = (100 cc/kg/day for first 10 kg)
+ (50 cc/kg/day for second 10 kg)
+ (20 cc/kg/day for weight in excess of 20 kg)

In the child, burn resuscitation should be the maintenance fluids plus additional fluids to compensate for losses (2-3 cc/kg x % burn surface area). As with the Parkland fluid formula, half should be given during the first eight hours and half during the next 16 hours.

The Caravajal formula uses body surface area instead of weight to estimate the fluid requirements.[26] Although this formula is technically more accurate than adding maintenance fluids to the Parkland formula, it is more difficult in most EDs to calculate the child's body surface area. Caravajal recommends 5000 mL/m^2 per percentage of burned surface area and then adding 2000 mL/m^2 for maintenance fluids. He also recommends giving half of the calculated amount in the first eight hours and half in the ensuing 16 hours.

The physician should administer all fluids to children as normal saline or lactated Ringer's. If the fluid given is hypotonic, there is a distinct risk of iatrogenic hyponatremia with subsequent cerebral edema and seizures. This is particularly true in the patient who is getting large amounts of fluids for extensive burns.

Because the most drastic fluid shifts occur in the first 8-12 hours after the burn, most formulas advocate replacement of half of the cal-

Table 3. Burn Resuscitation Formulas in the First 24 Hours

INVESTIGATOR	ELECTROLYTE	COLLOID	WATER
Evans	1 cc/kg/% burn	1 cc/kg/% burn	D_5W 2000 cc
Brooke Burn Unit	1.5 cc/kg/% burn	0.5 cc/kg/% burn	D_5W 2000 cc
Brooke (Rev. 1979)	2-3 cc/kg/% burn LR	None	None
Baxter (Parkland)	4 cc/kg/% burn LR	None	None
Slater	Lactated Ringer's 2L/24 hours	Fresh frozen plasma 75 cc/kg/24 hours	
Monafo	Hypertonic lactated saline. Fluid contains 250 mEq Na+/L. To maintain urine at 30 cc/hr (About 2 cc/kg/% burn).		
Hypertonic sodium solution (Warden)	Volume to maintain urine output at 30-50 cc/hr. Fluid is lactated Ringer's plus 50 mEq $NaHCO_3$ (180 mEq Na/L), Lactated Ringer's to maintain urine at 30-50 cc/hr beginning 8 hours postburn.		
Dextran formula (Demling)	Lactated Ringer's—volume to maintain urine at 30 cc/hr. Dextran 40 in saline 2 cc/kg/hr for 8 hours. Fresh frozen plasma 0.5 cc/kg/hr for 18 hours, 8 hours after the burn.		

culated fluid requirements for the first 24 hours be given during the first 8-12 hours. When calculating the replacement, be certain to consider the time of the burn, not the time of arrival of the patient in the ED. On the other hand, care must be taken not to overwhelm the patient's cardiovascular system with massive fluid administration rates if the patient arrives late in the course of the burn. Judgment becomes critical when the patient arrives 4-6 hours after a severe burn and has not had adequate fluid resuscitation.

In general, use the formula recommended by the local burn center. Although good results have been obtained with all formulas and "budgets," the local burn team may be more familiar with a different formula. Since they are going to be responsible for the care of this patient for an extended time, it is thoughtful to find out, in advance, the burn center's preferences and make their task easier.

Monitoring the State of Hydration. All of the burn formulas and budgets are merely guidelines, and a rigid application of formulas will ignore the variability of both burn and patient. The burn fluid replacement formulas frequently result in over- or under-hydration at the extremes of weight and burn size. Do not rely on a single parameter to judge the efficacy of fluid replacement. Look for a combination of the following factors:

- Clear sensorium;
- Extremity capillary filling and warmth of extremities;
- Vital signs normal or near normal;
- Decreasing hematocrit; and
- Adequate urine output (30-50 cc/hr in children older than 12 years or 0.5-1 cc/kilogram/hr in younger children).

If more than 1 cc/kg/hr is given, even in a child, there is a risk of iatrogenic pulmonary edema.

Hematocrit, blood pressure, and pulse have significant limitations as indicators of shock in the burned child. As always, obtaining a blood pressure reading in a toddler may be difficult. Even in an older child, it is often quite difficult to obtain an accurate pulse or blood pressure through the thick, tough eschar of a severe burn. Arterial lines may be needed for accurate monitoring of blood pressure. The blood pressure in children and young adults is often stable until late in the clinical picture of shock. Hypertension frequently may be found in severely burned children. With the increased metabolic rates associated with thermal trauma, a pulse in excess of 100 is often found and is compatible with adequate fluid resuscitation.

Hematocrit of 55-60% are common in the first 24 hours after serious burn injuries, even with adequate fluid administration. Decreasing hematocrit is to be expected with adequate fluid resuscitation, but may also be a hallmark of occult bleeding. If the patient apparently requires fluid far in excess of the burn budget, a vigorous search for occult bleeding is indicated.

Circumferential Burns. In severe burns of the extremities, especially those with circumferential or total involvement, it is imperative to establish the adequacy of perfusion. Marked edema from a deep dermal and third-degree burn within the confines of inelastic eschar or the rigid fascial compartments of the extremity can limit the arterial supply and the venous outflow. The resultant tissue hypoxia can cause muscle necrosis that results in further swelling and further decrease in blood supply.

The appropriate preventative measures include early removal of rings and jewelry and elevation of the limbs. If the extremity appears cyanotic distal to the injury, or capillary filling time is increased despite these measures escharotomy should be considered. Doppler flow detectors also may be used to assess small vessel blood flow. If the patient develops weak or absent distal peripheral pulses, progressive neurological signs such as paresthesias, or deep tissue pain, escharotomy is indicated. When in doubt, perform a fasciotomy or escharotomy rather than risk a subsequent amputation. A tissue pressure of greater than 30 mm of mercury, obtained by inserting a needle into the tissues and attempting to infuse saline or by attaching a manometer is indicative of impending vascular compromise.

The escharotomy should be made in both the mid-medial and the mid-lateral line of the limb and carried down to the ends of the fingers or to unburned skin. The incisions should be carried across involved joints and should be incised only to the depth which allows the cut edges of the eschar to separate.

Thoracic escharotomy may be required to prevent respiratory decompensation in the child with a severe chest burn.

Care of the Burn Wound

Care of the burn wound should be directed toward four principles:

- Preventing infection;
- Decreasing of burn fluid losses;

- Relieving of pain; and
- Salvaging of all viable burn tissue.

It should be emphasized that the best coverage for tissue is skin. Although acceptable artificial substitutes are now available, there is still nothing better than the "real thing."[27-29]

Cleansing the Wound. Before cleansing the burn, soak off charred clothing with sterile saline, and clip any hair within about two inches of the burn. Gently cleanse the burn with mild soap and water, debriding it of all foreign particulate matter and charred tissue. The process is easier if the affected area is immersed in warm saline or water. The use of a Hubbard or similar immersion tank is ideal for treatment of larger burns, but washing under running tap water will suffice for smaller burns. Enzymatic debriding preparation may prove useful in the treatment of burns. These agents may help in the removal of necrotic tissue. Debriding also may be less painful.

Once cleansing has taken place, the next step is debridement. Obviously necrotic and partially sloughed epidermis and dermis is removed by using forceps and tissue scissors. This skin is dead, and therefore, insensitive. Local anesthetics are not required.

The question of whether to debride intact bullae has been controversial for more than 20 years.[30-32] Proponents of leaving blisters note that the blister provides a sterile biologic dressing and should be left intact unless it is extremely large or inhibits motion. Adherents to blister removal point out that the fluid within the blister is an ideal culture media for bacteria.

A rational compromise between the two opposing camps is proposed. Intact bullae less than 2 cm in diameter should probably be left intact. Alternately, these may be aspirated using aseptic technique. Intact bullae more than 2 cm in diameter should be debrided because they are easily ruptured and, once violated, the fluid within provides an excellent culture medium for inoculating bacteria. If the blisters are ruptured, hemorrhagic, or purulent, they should be debrided.

Burn Excision

The concept of excising and promptly closing a burn wound is appealing for several reasons. First, when the wound is closed, the risks of fluid losses and infection are markedly decreased. Second, wound closure will allow decrease in pain medications, more effective physical therapy, and potentially faster recovery. There does not appear to be any significant decrease in either hospital stay or mortality.[33]

Obviously, third-degree and some deep second-degree burns are the only candidates for excision of the burn wound. Superficial partial thickness wounds will not require removal of the eschar and will re-epithelialize within three weeks. Following the excision of burned tissue, the wound is covered with either an artificial membrane, autologous donor graft, allograft, or xenografts. Burn excision should be performed by a plastic or general surgeon who will manage the ongoing care of the patient.

Use of Antibiotic Creams, Lotions, and Ointments. There are a number of ways to manage a burn once it has been cleansed. For the early care of a burn, little wound coverage is needed. Dry sheets (sterile if at all possible) will prevent air exposure to the burned tissues and will decrease pain. If something must be applied to the wound, a water-soluble base is mandatory. For long-term therapy, treatment may be open with or without topical agents, or closed with application of a topical agent followed by a dressing. The dressing protects the wound and keeps the topical agent in contact with the wound.

Open Method. The open method with topical creams cannot bc used for a child who must attend school or go to work. In these situations, an occlusive dressing is obviously the only acceptable solution. The purpose of the open method is defeated when clothing is placed over the wound. Burns on the trunk, buttocks, and thighs cannot be treated by the open method.

Facial burns should be treated without dressings or burn creams. No topical agents are usually needed for burns on the face, since the facial vascularity protects against most infections. The face is difficult to dress due to the facial angles and curves. Children may be quite agitated if the eyes are continuously covered. If the face is simply cleansed with mild soap and water twice daily, healing usually proceeds without problems.

Likewise, burns of the perineum are very difficult to dress. In children, frequent soiling is quite common. Open therapy of these burns is essential and hospitalization is usually necessary.

First-degree burns can be dressed with a lubricating lotion. Aloe also has been shown to be of benefit by inhibiting thromboxane A2 and prostaglandins. Pruritus may develop as the first-degree burn heals due to histamine release from mast cells. This can be especially troublesome to small children; diphenhydramine hydrochloride in appropriate doses can be effective in relieving this symptom.

Topical Agents. For smaller burns, treated on an outpatient basis, studies show that any of a variety of medications are appropriate. These medications include povidone-iodine, mafenide, and silver sulfadiazine. There are many opinions, but little concrete data that support one topical agent over another. Likewise, there are few data about using these agents under dressings in closed therapy. Data during development of the agents were obtained from patients with open treatment in burn units, not as outpatient therapy using dressings.

An appropriate first choice for topical therapy is silver sulfadiazine. This drug is readily available in most EDs. It should be avoided in the child who is allergic to sulfa. Silver sulfadiazine is easy to apply and is quite comfortable for the patient. It has been used for years with good effect in both open and closed treatment of burns. Silver sulfadiazine dressings should be changed at least daily. When used in open treatment, silver sulfadiazine should be reapplied at least three times daily. Silver sulfadiazine also softens tissue, thereby maintaining joint movement and facilitating eschar debridement.

Because of its relatively low toxicity and ease of use, silver sulfadiazine is the most widely used topical antimicrobial agent.[34] However, silver sulfadiazine should not be used around the eyes and mouth, in children with hypersensitivity to sulfonamides, or in pregnant women, nursing mothers, and infants younger than 2 months of age (because of the risk of sulfonamide kernicterus). Potential side effects include thrombocytopenia, leukopenia, and a rash.

Mafenide acetate (Sulfamylon) is thought to have better tissue penetration. It may be superior for treatment of electrical and deeply penetrating burns. Mafenide acetate may be appropriate for the patient who is going to have excision of a small third-degree burn followed by grafting or suture repair of the defect. Mafenide penetrates deeply into the eschar and decreases the chance of infection when the wound is subsequently closed.

Unfortunately, it causes pain, dries the wound out, and can cause metabolic acidosis. The metabolic acidosis occurs because of its action as a carbonic anhydrase inhibitor, resulting in excretion of bicarbonate and retention of chloride. Mafenide acetate should never be used under a dressing because it causes severe maceration with tissue breakdown and a contact dermatitis.

Povidone iodine penetrates wounds better than silver sulfadiazine. However, povidone iodine is less well tolerated because it causes pain. Furthermore, iodine toughens and dries the eschar and diminishes joint mobility.

Do not use petroleum-based ointments, unless the burn is caused by sulfur or tar. Polymixin B sulfate and neomycin (Bacitracin and Neosporin) are petroleum based. These agents are hard to clean off and do not penetrate as well as silver sulfadiazine. Bacitracin requires fewer changes than silver sulfadiazine and is a little less expensive, but the difficulty in cleaning it off is not worth the cost benefit.

Gentamycin burn creams should be avoided. Use of gentamycin tends to select for gentamycin resistant *Pseudomonas* species.

Silver nitrate 0.5% is still used in some burn units but is generally unsuitable for outpatient use. It has a very good antimicrobial spectrum against most gram-positive bacteria and many gram-negative bacteria and is cheap to use. It has many disadvantages: It is messy, fails to penetrate eschar well, and can cause hyponatremia, hypochloremia, and methemoglobinemia.

If the child is going to be transferred, please check with the local burn center for their preferences. Some authorities do not wish to have any topical medications applied until they have evaluated the patient themselves.

The Dressing. Since the wound may weep copiously during the exudative phase of the burn, a sufficiently bulky dressing should be used to prevent wicking of bacteria because of a wet dressing. Plain, fine-mesh gauze placed against the burn surface allows the exudate to permeate the bulky dressing. Petrolatum-impregnated gauze often causes maceration of the wound and should not be used. Over the fine-mesh gauze, fluffs of absorbent gauze material should be used. Four or five layers are usually sufficient if the dressing is to be left in place for 24 hours. One or two layers of bias-cut stockinette or Kerlix will provide an external barrier to prevent contamination as well as secure the dressing in place. The dressing should be changed once or twice a day and inspected by a physician every second or third day.

In very young patients, it may be necessary to trim fingernails to prevent scratching of the healing wounds. Occasionally, the child's hands must be wrapped in mitten fashion to prevent digging at the wounds.

Biosynthetic dressings such as DuoDerm, Epigard, Biobrane, Opsite, and others can be used for superficial partial-thickness burns in both children and adults.[35-39] One biosynthetic dressing that has been extensively studied is Biobrane (Woodruff Laboratories, Santa Ana, CA), a knitted nylon fabric bonded to a silicone membrane and coated with covalently bonded collagen peptides. The biosynthetic dressings should be applied directly to the clean burn and will spontaneously separate in 7-14 days. Once adhered to a fresh, partial-thickness wound or donor site, the Biobrane is left in place until epithelialization occurs. The biosynthetic dressings must be applied to a flat surface and can cover only a 1-2% TBSA burn. The biosynthetic dressing should be covered by an absorbent dressing that is changed daily.

As a dressing that remains in place until wound healing occurs, nursing time is minimized, and the cost of multiple dressing changes is saved. These dressings may be better tolerated, are less painful, maintain wound moisture, and reduce the local trauma from frequent dressing changes.

These dressings are costly, and have not been shown to decrease healing time in partial-thickness wounds.[40] Newer dressing materials are constantly being evaluated and may provide good effect for less money.[34] The main disadvantages of these dressings are leakage of wound fluid, premature separation of the dressing, and cost.

Adjunctive Therapies

Nasogastric Suction. Nasogastric suction using a Salem sump or similar tube should be initiated early in the ED. Many patients with a burn of greater than 25% TBSA will develop an ileus in the first 24-48 hours that will often last for several days. If the child has nausea, distention, or vomiting with lesser burns, a nasogastric tube often will make the child more comfortable.

Curling's ulcer (burn stress ulcers) often will be prevented by the use of cimetidine (Tagamet) or other H2 blockers or antacids instilled into the nasogastric tube or given intravenously.

Pain Medication. Patients with extensive, severe burns often experience little pain. More minor burns, paradoxically are much more painful, as the cutaneous nerve endings are damaged but not destroyed. The second-degree burn is perhaps the most painful injury a child can sustain. Deep burns have destroyed the pain fibers, so these burns are not particularly painful.

Burn patients with partial thickness injuries will experience environmental aggravation of the injury and will benefit by simply covering the burn with a sheet.

The emergency physician should routinely ensure that pain and suffering are considered in the child's management. Pain should be controlled with incremental intravenous doses of morphine sulphate or similar agents. There are no contraindications to the intravenous route, and it provides rapid action, assured uptake, and easy control. If using morphine sulphate in the child, a dose of 0.1-0.2 mg/kg intravenously IV every 15-30 minutes may be sufficient: in the older child or adolescent, 3 mg increments are often useful.

Intramuscular and subcutaneous routes are not appropriate for the patient with cardiovascular compromise. Absorption of medications given by these routes are notoriously unpredictable. If the patient becomes hypovolemic for any reason, narcotics injected intramuscularly or subcutaneously will not be absorbed until the circulatory status is restored.

If the burn patient becomes restless or agitated, first check the oxygenation, then check the fluid replacement status. Often, anxiety and agitation are early signs of hypoxia or hypovolemia. Since both conditions are commonly found in association with severe burns, the child must be evaluated for hypoxemia and hypovolemia before each dose of pain medication.

Acetaminophen may be useful for pain control later in the child's course (15 mg/kg/dose). Acetaminophen with codeine is useful before dressing changes (codeine dose is 0.5-1.0 mg/kg) In the pediatric patient with extensive burns, ketamine is commonly used in burn units as a sedation agent for dressing changes, grafts, and similar episodic painful therapies. The child will be completely sedated and will not lose respiratory reflexes.

Blood. Erythrocyte hemolysis may occur after a major burn. The etiology of this hemolysis is not known, but between 3% and 15% of red blood cells may be lost in the first week or two after a patient's burn. A victim of a major burn will very likely need a transfusion for these red cell losses. Ensure that adequate blood is obtained for a cross match in preparation for transfusion.

Antibiotics. In the early post-burn period, antibiotics are rarely indicated. The single exception to this is the patient who has been on antibiotics for an antecedent illness. These patients should be continued on their antibiotics.

During the first week, the wound should be carefully observed for cellulitis. Early stages of infection include the edges of the wound becoming reddened and tender and the patient complaining of increasing pain. The most common causative organism of cellulitis is beta-hemolytic *Streptococcus*. Penicillin, therefore, should be the antibiotic of choice in initial treatment of a mild burn wound cellulitis. If oral antibiotics are not promptly effective, the child should be hospitalized for intravenous antibiotics.

Sunscreen. Healing burn wounds are quite sensitive to sun exposure. An effective sun block (with a sun protection factor of 15 or greater) should be applied to the area of the burn for 6-12 months following treatment. This can help prevent some of the hyperpigmentation seen following burn healing.

Tetanus Immunization. A burn injury is considered a high risk wound for tetanus. If the patient has had a tetanus immunization within five years, no further therapy is needed. If the patient's last tetanus immunization was received more than five years ago, then a tetanus booster of 0.5 cc of age-appropriate toxoid should be given. If the patient has never had a full series of tetanus immunizations, then the patient should receive hyperimmune tetanus anti-toxin and the tetanus immunization series initiated.

Conclusion

Of course, the best way to treat any illness is to prevent it from occurring. In most cases, burns are preventable.

Emergency physicians may have an opportunity to intervene before these tragic accidents occur. When a child is seen in the ED for other illnesses, simply telling the parents about recommended preventive measures may save a child at essentially no cost to the parent, physician, or society. Ideas that should be recommended to parents include: 1) ensuring that electrical cords of appliances are beyond the reach of toddlers; 2) placing cups of hot beverages out of the reach of children; 3) placing pots and pans on the stove so that the handles face away from the child; 4) turning the thermostat on the water heater to about 120°F; 5) discussing the "Stop, Drop, and Roll" protocol with the child; and 6) using smoke detectors and recommending that family members for evacuation in the event of a house fire.

The child who is burned by abuse remains at risk for abuse and neglect after discharge. These children should have a safe environment. The perpetrator, if identified, should be dealt with in a way that ensures the child remains safe.[41]

If the child sustains a severe burn, rapid stabilization and appropriate therapy are mandatory. For minor burns, careful selection of dressings and careful monitoring for infection are usually all that is necessary.

References

1. Accident facts, 1983. Chicago: National Safety Council, 1983.
2. McLoughlin E, McGuire A. The causes, cost, and prevention of childhood burn injuries. *Am J Dis Child* 1990;144:677-683.
3. Chamion HR, Copes WS, Buyer D, et al. Major trauma in geriatric patients. *Am J Public Health* 1989;79:1278-1282.
4. Sheridan RL, Remensnyder JP, Schnitzer JJ, et al. Current expectation for survival in pediatric burns. *Arch Pediatr Adolesc Med* 2000;154:245-249.
5. The health of Canadian children: A CICH Profile. Canadian Institute of Child Health, 1989.
6. A Data Book of Child and Adolescent Injury. Washington, DC, National Center for Education in Maternal and Child Health, 1991.
7. McLoughlin E, McGuire A. The causes, cost, and prevention of childhood burn injuries. *Am J Dis Child* 1990;144:677-683.
8. Mackay A, Halper J, McLoughlin E, et al. A comparison of age specific burn injury in five Massachusetts communities. *Am J Public Health* 1979;69:1146.
9. Injury Control for Children and Youth. American Academy of Pediatrics, 1987.
10. Silverstein P, Wilson R. Prevention of pediatric burn injuries. In: Caravajal H, Parks D, eds. *Burns in Children: Pediatric Burn Management*. St. Louis: Year Book Medical Publishers; 1988.
11. Sheridan RL, Remensnyder JP, Schnitzer JJ, et al. Current expectation for survival in pediatric burns. *Arch Pediatr Adolesc Med* 2000;154:245-249.
12. Erdmann TC, Feldman KW, Rivera FP, et al. Tap water burn prevention: The effect of legislation. *Pediatrics* 1991;88:572-577.
13. Sheridan RL. Recognition and management of hot liquid aspiration in children. *Ann Emerg Med* 1996;27:89-91.
14. Urbancic JM, VanMeter BH, Edlich RF, et al. Gas-fired gravity floor furnace contact burns. *J Emerg Med* 1993;11:539-541.
15. Barret JP, Desai MH, Herndon DN. The isolated burned palm in children: Epidemiology and long term sequelae. *Plast Reconstr Surg* 2000;105:949-52.
16. Smith GA, Knapp JF, Barnet TM, et al. The rocket's red glare, the bombs bursting in air: Fireworks-related injuries to children. *Pediatrics* 1996;98:1-9.
17. Franzi AT, D'Anna F, Zicca A, et al. Histological evaluation of human cultured epithelium before and after grafting. *Burns* 1992; 18:(Suppl 1):S26-S31.
18. DeLuca M, Cancedda R. Culture of human epithelium. *Burns* 1992;18:(Suppl 1):S5-S10.
19. Tomkins RG, Burke JF. Burn wound closure using permanent skin replacement materials. *World J Surg* 1992;16:47-52.
20. Alsbjorn BF. Biologic wound coverings in burn treatment. *World J Surg* 1992;16:43-46.
21. Lund CC, Browder NC. The estimation of areas of burns. *Surg Gynecol Obstet* 1944;79:352-358.
22. Alexander RH, Proctor HJ. Advanced trauma life support course for physicians. 5th ed. Chicago: American College of Surgeons, 1993.
23. Perry RJ, Moore CA, Morgan BDG, et al. Determining the approximate area of a burn: An inconsistency investigated and re-evaluated. *BMJ* 1996;312:1338.
24. Mlcak R, Cortiella J, Desai MH, et al. Emergency management of

pediatric burn victims. *Ped Emerg Car* 1998;14:51-54.

25. Graves TA, Cioffi WG, McManus WF, et al. Fluid resuscitation in infants and children with massive thermal injury. *J Trauma* 1988; 28:1156-1159.
26. Caravajal HF. Fluid resuscitation of pediatric burn victims; A critical appraisal. *Pediatr Nephrol* 1994;8:357-366.
27. Muhart M, McFalls S, Kirsner RS, et al. Behaviour of tissue-engineered skin. *Arch Dermatol* 1999;135:913-918.
28. Bello Y, Phillips TJ. Recent advances in wound healing. *JAMA* 2000;283:716-718.
29. Phillips TJ. Tissue-engineered skin. *Arch Dermatol* 1999;135: 977-978.
30. Swain AH, Azadian BS, Wakeley CL, et al. Management of blisters in minor burns. *Br Med J* [Clin Res] 1987;295:181.
31. Rockwell WB, Ehrlich HP. Should burn blister fluid be evacuated? *J Burn Care Rehab* 1990;11:93-95.
32. Rockwell WB, Erlich HP. Should burn blister fluid be evacuated. *J Burn Care Rehab* 1990;11;93-95.
33. Monafo WW, Bessey PQ. Benefits and limitations of burn wound excision. *World J Surg* 1992;16:37-42.
34. Singer AJ, Mohammad M, Tortora G, et al. Octylcyanoacrylate for the treatment of contaminated partial-thickness burns in swine: A randomized controlled experiment *Acad Emerg Med* 2000;7: 222-227.
35. Waffle GD, Simon RR, Joslin C. Moisture-vapour-permeable film as an outpatient burn dressing. *Bums* 1988;14:66-78.
36. Wyatt D, McGowan DN, Najarian MP, et al. Comparison of a hydrocolloid dressing and silver sulfadiazine cream in the outpatient management of second degree burns. *J Trauma* 1990;30:857-865.
37. Afilalo M, Dankoff J, Guttman, et al. DuoDERM hydroactive dressing versus silver suiphadiazine/Bactigras in the emergency treatment of partial skin thickness burns. *Burns* 1992;18:313-316.
38. Khan U, Rhoer S, Healy C. Use of Biobrane in pediatric scald burns —experience in 106 children by LF Ou, SY Lee, YC Chen, RS Yang, YW Tang. [letter]. *Burns* 1998;24:770.
39. Barret JP, Dziewulski P, Ramzy PI, et al. Biobrane versus 1% silver sulfadiazine in second degree burns. *Plast Reconstr Surg* 2000;105:62-65.
40. Waymack JP, Jenkins M, Warden GD, et al. A prospective study of thymopentin in severely burned patients. *Surg Gynecol Obstet* 1987;164:423-430.
41. Hultman CS, Priolo D, Cairns BA, et al. Return to jeopardy: The fate of pediatric burn patients who are victims of abuse and neglect. *J Burn Care Rehab* 1998;19:367-376.

Cardiac Emergencies

Neda Mulla, MD
Richard Chinnock, MD

Cardiac emergencies are among the most stressful emergency department (ED) presentations in any patient population. In infants and children, the clinical challenges are magnified. Diagnosis and management require a broad understanding of underlying pathophysiologies and therapeutic options, as well as a swift and decisive course of action that often includes consultation with appropriate specialists. Three of the most clinically demanding pediatric cardiac ED presentations are congestive heart failure (CHF), hypercyanotic spells, and heart transplant recipients.

Congenital heart disease (CHD) is one of the most common defects of birth, occurring in 6-10 cases per 1000 live births.[1] Consequently, CHF, a frequent complication of CHD and other cardiac conditions or rhythms, can present at almost any time and in the youngest of infants. Its early recognition and timely management are extremely critical.

While hypercyanotic spells are much less frequent than CHF, their diagnosis and management can be formidable. The pathophysiology of these spells, which present dramatically with a cyanotic and inconsolable child, is still not clear. In fact, these spells actually occur in several types of CHD and have certain pathophysiologic factors in common. The infrequency and complexity of this condition almost guarantee that the ED physician will experience some professional anxiety.

The number of pediatric heart transplant procedures being performed in the United States is rapidly expanding. Consequently, the chance of encountering a pediatric cardiac transplant patient in the community ED is becoming almost a sure bet. Because seemingly simple interventions such as prescribing erythromycin can have disastrous results for the cyclosporine-treated child, a clear understanding of the management of this condition is mandatory.

With these unique considerations in mind, this chapter presents a valuable clinical compendium of these angst-generating conditions in pediatric patients.

Managing CHF in Children

CHF is a broad diagnosis that covers a heterogeneous group of cardiac diagnoses. CHF is a term often attached to a child with a known or suspected cardiac diagnosis who appears ill or distressed. When preparing a management plan for the child, it is important to understand the pathophysiology of the underlying condition. CHF can be divided into four types based on the underlying pathophysiology: 1) pulmonary overflow CHF; 2) CHF due to myocardial impairment; 3) CHF due to obstructive lesions; and 4) tachyarrhythmia-induced CHF.

Pulmonary Overflow CHF. Pulmonary overflow CHF is the most common and presents in children with large left-to-right shunts, such as large ventricular septal defects, large atrioventricular canal, large patent ductus arteriosus (PDA), and arteriovenous malformations. The basic pathophysiology is one of increased pulmonary flow with or without pulmonary hypertension. As the pulmonary vascular resistance drops in the first few weeks of life, there is a progressive increase in the shunt across the intracardiac or extracardiac communication. The increased flow will raise the pulmonary capillary hydrostatic pressure and increase transudation into the lung interstitium, decreasing lung compliance. Frank pulmonary edema may develop in severe cases.[2] Usually, the infant will gradually develop rapid breathing and an active precordium. The parents may notice the infant pausing more often during feeding to catch his or her breath. Additionally, diaphoresis may be noted or increased, especially during feedings. Children with small shunts, however, will not have significant pulmonary overflow and will not have CHF.

Precipitating factors exist that can lead to decompensation and presentation to the ED. The most common precipitating factor is infection.[3] The child with CHF is susceptible to respiratory tract infections. Associated fever also will compromise the child as the increased oxygen consumption will overtax the pulmonary and cardiac reserves. The worst offender is the respiratory syncytial virus (RSV), which has a mortality rate approaching 40% in infants with CHF.[3] In many institutions, therapy with ribavirin is instituted as soon as the diagnosis of RSV infection is suspected. Therapy may be discontinued if the RSV screen is negative. Other precipitating factors are uncommon and include infective endocarditis and tachyarrhythmia.

The physical evaluation will reveal the child to be pink or mildly cyanotic with normal or bounding pulses. The precordium will be active and there may be a right ventricular lift. Although a loud murmur is usually present, infants with large, unrestrictive intracardiac communications may have faint, low-pitched murmurs. The liver is often soft and enlarged. Tachypnea and increased use of accessory muscles are often noted. Breath sounds, however, are usually clear unless there is concomitant pneumonia.[2] Peripheral perfusion is usually normal but can be impaired if there is dehydration or frank pulmonary edema. The documentation of palpable femoral pulses is important since coarctation of the aorta can be an associated diagnosis. The obstruction created by the coarctation will increase resistance to systemic flow and further favor increased flow into the pulmonary circulation.

A chest radiograph is very informative and will show cardiomegaly and increased pulmonary flow. Comparison to a previous chest x-ray is helpful in distinguishing new changes due to pulmonary infection or increased pulmonary overflow.

It is important to understand that certain types of cyanotic congenital heart disease may also have overflow CHF. Examples include transposition of the great vessels, total anomalous pulmonary venous return without obstruction, truncus arteriosus and tetralogy of Fallot with pulmonary atresia, and overflow via aortopulmonary collaterals. Those children will usually have only mild cyanosis.

Initial management consists of diuretic therapy using furosemide 1 mg/kg intravenously or intramuscularly. Control of fever and infection should be initiated. Oxygen therapy should be used with caution since it is a potent pulmonary vasodilator and will increase pulmonary flow. Oxygen therapy should be reserved for infants with significant respiratory discomfort and cases of desaturation due to pulmonary infection. Further management consists of afterload reduction and digoxin therapy, which should be instituted in consultation with a cardiologist. It is extremely important to recognize that fluid balance in children with CHF is very sensitive. While we all realize that fluid overload will worsen CHF, it is also important to remember that infants with overflow CHF actually have decreased systemic flow due to the "steal" into pulmonary circulation. Therefore, dehydration can seriously decrease systemic flow, leading to impaired perfusion and even shock. A diuretic dose instead of a fluid bolus in diuretic-treated children who are volume-depleted due to vomiting or diarrhea can have serious results.

CHF Due to Impaired Myocardium. CHF due to impaired myocardium can be due to myocarditis or cardiomyopathy. It may not be possible to differentiate between myocarditis and cardiomyopathy on initial presentation. The common pathophysiology is low forward output as well as passive venous congestion. In cases of myocarditis, there may be a history of a preceding viral illness with gradual development of CHF symptoms over the course of days or a few weeks. Cardiomyopathy, on the other hand, may be relatively asymptomatic due to adaptation until there is decompensation by a precipitating factor. Precipitating factors include infection, tachy- or bradyarrhythmia, and pulmonary embolism. Symptoms include shortness of breath worsened by activity, ease of fatigue, chest pain, pulmonary edema, abdominal pain, palpitations, and syncope. Abdominal pain is generated by the rapid distention of the liver due to passive congestion. Some patients may also experience post-prandial abdominal pain due to gastrointestinal ischemia. Severely compromised patients will present with a combination of pulmonary edema and shock due to low cardiac output. Physical examination may well show a distressed child with some or all of the following signs: tachypnea, use of accessory muscles, tachycardia, elevated jugular venous pressure, peripheral edema, hepatomegaly, and signs of decreased systemic perfusion. The chest radiograph will show cardiomegaly and pulmonary venous congestion.[2]

Management consists of diuresis, inotropic support, and afterload reduction. Diuretic therapy will relieve pulmonary edema, peripheral edema, and abdominal pain due to liver distention. However, care must be taken not to deplete intravascular volume, causing worsening of systemic perfusion. Inotropic therapy should be instituted either with digoxin or infusion of beta-adrenergic agents such as dobutamine. Afterload reduction is very important and can be instituted with angiotensin-converting enzyme (ACE) inhibitors or intravenous agents such as sodium nitroprusside and nitroglycerin. Afterload reduction will help increase the cardiac output without increasing myocardial oxygen consumption. In cases of cardiomyopathy secondary to acute severe hypertension, afterload reduction is the main form of therapy. Ideally, the patient's cardiologist should be involved in these treatment decisions. Respiratory support and oxygen therapy are indicated for alleviation of symptoms and distress of pulmonary edema. The patient should be evaluated for precipitating factors with an electrocardiogram (ECG) to assess for tachy- or bradyarrhythmia as well as a chest radiograph to evaluate for pulmonary infection.

CHF Due to Obstructive Lesions. CHF due to obstructive lesions is almost always associated with left-sided lesions. Obstructions located in the left ventricular outflow tract, such as aortic stenosis and coarctation, will cause a combination of impaired ventricular function and pulmonary venous congestion. Cardiac output is decreased due to the combination of obstruction and impaired

Table 1. Features of Sinus Tachycardia and Supraventricular Tachycardia

FINDING	SINUS TACHYCARDIA	SUPRAVENTRICULAR TACHYCARDIA
Heart rate	Up to 240 bpm	200-300 bpm
Heart rate variation	Present	Absent
P waves on ECG	Present	Absent
Response to adenosine	No response	Tachycardia stops abruptly

function. Obstructions to left ventricular inflow, such as mitral stenosis and obstructed pulmonary veins, will present with pulmonary edema but without an effect on ventricular function. However, cardiac output also will suffer due to the limited filling of the left ventricle. Often, there is more than one level of left-sided obstruction, hypoplastic left heart syndrome being the extreme form. The most common presentation to the ED is probably the ductal-dependent neonate who has recently closed the patent ductus arteriosus (PDA). Those infants will present in a combination of shock and pulmonary edema. The evaluation of the infant's pulses is the most important part of the physical evaluation. Absence of femoral pulses will alert the physician to the diagnosis. However, the pulse may be weak or of low volume in all extremities, which would point to obstruction at the level of the aortic valve.

In managing these infants, a prostaglandin E_1 infusion at 0.05-0.1 mcg/kg/min should be instituted when there is clinical suspicion of a ductal-dependent lesion. Diuretic therapy is indicated for pulmonary congestion or edema. Inotropic support is needed for the impaired myocardium. Afterload reduction is of no use in the presence of a fixed level of obstruction and is not indicated. If there is inflow obstruction with pulmonary venous obstruction, then diuretic therapy may only offer temporary improvement. Those patients require emergency life-saving surgery.

CHF Due to Tachyarrhythmia. The management of CHF due to tachyarrhythmia is a lengthy subject that is beyond the scope of this article. However, many of the patients with other types of CHF will present in sinus tachycardia as an appropriate physiological response. Often, the ED physician has to determine whether there is sinus tachycardia or supraventricular tachycardia. *(See Table 1.)* Sinus tachycardia is usually below 220 beats per minute (bpm), but in smaller infants it can reach up to 230-240 bpm. With sinus tachycardia, there is fluctuation of the heart rate with anxiety, distress, body temperature, and fluid status. For example, the child's heart rate will decrease when the child is held by the parent and then increase when intravenous access is attempted. Supraventricular tachycardia (SVT), on the other hand, will usually be in the 200-300 bpm range and cause no physiological changes. On the ECG, sinus tachycardia will show the presence of P waves prior to the QRS, although, if the rate is rapid enough, the P wave may begin to merge with the preceding T wave. A 12-lead ECG is often more helpful than a rhythm strip for the detection of P waves. In SVT there is usually absence of the P wave. Some varieties of SVT will have a retrograde P wave. In differentiating sinus tachycardia from SVT, it is helpful to attempt to correct dehydration and alleviate fever, distress, and anxiety. Intravenous adenosine (0.05-0.25 mg/kg) may be used if there is no heart rate variation with the above measures and there is concern that the tachycardia is contributing to the child's compromise. However, it should be noted that sinus tachycardia will also transiently slow with this therapy since adenosine depresses the sinus node. Observing and recording the ECG during the administration of adenosine is very important. The rhythm strip may slow enough to show P waves with sinus tachycardia. Recurrence of tachycardia after adenosine is abrupt in cases of SVT and usually gradual with sinus tachycardia.

Managing Hypercyanotic Spells

"Hypercyanotic spells" is the more appropriate term for what have conventionally been called "tetralogy spells." The reason is simple: These spells are not restricted to tetralogy of Fallot but can occur in other types of congenital heart disease that have certain factors in common. The hemodynamic set-up is one of obstruction or restriction of pulmonary flow and presence of intracardiac communication such as a ventricular septal defect (VSD) or single ventricle. Examples include tetralogy of Fallot, ventricular septal defect with severe valvular pulmonary stenosis, and tricuspid atresia with a restrictive VSD.[2]

Pathophysiology. The pathophysiology of hypercyanotic spells is not entirely clear. However, it is best thought of as an imbalance between pulmonary and systemic vascular resistance favoring decreased pulmonary flow and increased right-to-left shunting into the aorta. In other words, an increasing portion of systemic venous return bypasses the lungs and is directed into the aorta.[2,4] The increasing hypoxemia and developing lactic acidosis will induce further pulmonary vasoconstriction. Hence, a malignant cycle is established: cyanosis, hypoxemia, and acidosis begetting a further reduction of pulmonary flow and hypoxemia. *(See Figure 1.)* Infundibular spasm is no longer considered the etiology of hypercyanotic spells. Spells are known to occur in patients with no element of infundibular subpulmonary stenosis.[2]

Precipitating Factors. There are many precipitating factors that can bring on a hypercyanotic spell. In general, they have the following in common: tachycardia, tachypnea, increased oxygen consumption, and/or decreased systemic vascular resistance. When one considers the clinical features of hypercyanotic spells, tachypnea is always present at the onset of the spell. Tachypnea in and of itself is probably not the cause of the spell but a result of it. One possible explanation is that the augmentation of right-to-left shunt results in an increase in the amount of carbon dioxide that bypasses the lungs, raising the arterial tension of CO_2. This stimulates hyperventilation, which in turn significantly lowers the PCO_2 in pulmonary venous return to help balance the rising arterial PCO_2.

The known precipitating factors include fever, anxiety, exercise, dehydration, tachypnea, tachycardia due to any cause, and drugs that

Figure 1. Pathophysiology and Precipitating Factors of Hypercyanotic Spells

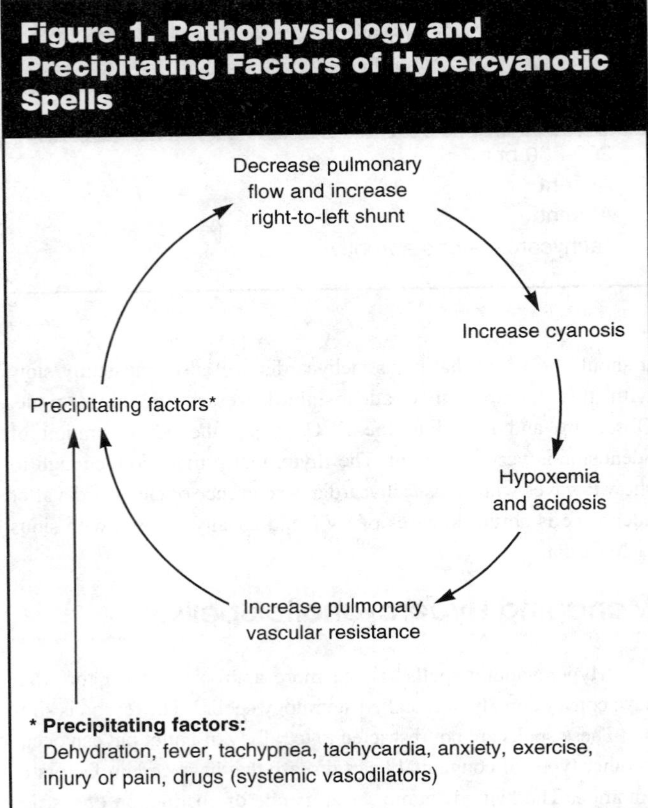

decrease systemic vascular resistance, such as chlorpromazine (Thorazine) and ACE inhibitors. The spells tend to occur in infants with mild-to-moderate cyanosis at rest. They are also more common in the child with cyanosis and iron deficiency.[2]

Clinical Characterization and Physical Examination. Hypercyanotic spells are clinically characterized by sudden onset of labored deep breathing, anxiety, crying, and development of intense cyanosis. Often there is a drop in arterial blood pressure, causing the child's color to become pale, ashen, or gray. The child often looks panicked, distressed, and may be somewhat unresponsive to the parents' attempt to comfort him or her. Spells are often mistaken for other causes that can change an infant's behavior, such as colic, pain, or seizures. Spells can occur at any age, although they become less frequent in older children. Spells can occur at any time of the day, although they occur more frequently early in the morning, after a nap, or after a feeding. Spells do not occur during sleep.

Physical examination during a spell will show a distressed and inconsolable child. The child may be deeply cyanosed or ashen gray. There is tachycardia and tachypnea with a drop in transcutaneous oxygen saturation. As pulmonary blood flow decreases, the intensity of the murmur decreases and may disappear. If the spell is persistent, then the child will lose consciousness and signs of hemodynamic compromise may prevail. Sequelae of hypercyanotic spells include central nervous system damage due to hypoxemia and, if persistent, can lead to death.

Squatting is a behavior noted in older children with tetralogy of Fallot following exercise. Presumably it is a defensive mechanism against spells. Squatting increases systemic vascular resistance acutely, thereby decreasing right-to-left shunt and promoting pulmonary blood flow.

Medical Management. Hypercyanotic spells are a life-threatening emergency that call for medical stabilization followed by surgical intervention to increase pulmonary flow. Medical management *(see Table 2)* starts with comforting the infant. If the parents are present, allow them to hold the child in a knee-chest position so that the knees are flexed and drawn up toward the chest and abdomen. This mimics squatting and will increase systemic vascular resistance. Oxygen therapy should then be established in a non-threatening manner. Do not attempt to use a nasal cannula or mask. Simply hold the oxygen close to the child's face. Most spells will break without further intervention at this point. If the spell is persistent, then proceed to sedate the infant with morphine sulfate 0.1 mg/kg given subcutaneously, intramuscularly, or intravenously. Ketamine is also preferred as a sedative since it will increase systemic vascular resistance. The exact effect of morphine sulfate is unknown and may be related to venodilation, which decreases the amount of systemic venous return, therefore decreasing the right-to-left shunt. A peripheral vagotonic effect has also been postulated.[5] Intravenous access should be established next. Metabolic acidosis will develop rapidly in hypercyanotic patients. Therefore, correction of acidosis with sodium bicarbonate infusion (1 mEq/kg) should be given as soon as a blood gas has been drawn. As the bicarbonate is being drawn up, begin volume infusion with 10 mL/kg. If there are clinical signs of dehydration, then a larger initial bolus can be given. Sodium bicarbonate infusion may be repeated as indicated by the severity of metabolic acidosis on the blood gas. A gradual decrease in heart rate and an increase in oxygen saturation are signals that the spell is breaking. Continue volume and bicarbonate infusion until the child is well-hydrated and acidosis has been corrected.

A severe spell may not be aborted even with the above measures. The next line of therapy involves drugs that can decrease heart rate and contractility, such as phenylephrine and propranolol. Generally, each institution will favor one line of therapy over the other, and in severe cases a combination will be used. Intravenous propranolol is effective in terminating hypercyanotic spells. However, it must be used with caution since it can be profoundly cardioinhibitory. Therefore, prior to giving propranolol, isoproterenol must be available at bedside in case of severe bradycardia. The initial dose of propranolol is 0.05 mg/kg to be diluted in 5-10 mL of fluid and given slowly over 5-10 minutes. A second dose may be given if there is no response. The maximum total dose is 0.1 mg/kg, not to exceed a dose of 1 mg total.[2]

Recently, esmolol, an ultrashort-acting cardioselective beta-blocker, has been successfully used to treat hypercyanotic spells.[6] Esmolol dosage can be titrated with ease and the short half-life will allow reversal of any side effects when the infusion is discontinued. The suggested dosage is an initial bolus of 0.5-1.0 mg/kg followed by an infusion of 100-300 mcg/kg/min.

Phenylephrine, an alpha-agonist, is a peripheral vasoconstrictor and is used to increase systemic vascular resistance, resulting in a decrease in right-to-left shunt and possibly reflex bradycardia. The dose administered is 10 mcg/kg as an initial bolus, aiming for a one-and-a-half increase in systemic blood pressure relative to baseline. The bolus may be repeated with increments of 10 mcg/kg to a maximum of 50 mcg/kg every few minutes until the desired blood pressure response is established. Phenylephrine has a short half-life so that maintenance of the blood pressure effect would require a continuous infusion of 1-10 mcg/kg/min. The cardiologist should be

Table 2. Steps for the Management of Hypercyanotic Spells

MEDICAL MANAGEMENT	COMMENTS
1. Calm the child and establish knee-chest position	The parent is the best person to calm the child.
2. Oxygen	Blow-by O_2
3. Sedation	Morphine: 0.1 mg/kg IV, IM, or SQ Ketamine: 1 mg/kg IV (Administer slowly as bolus infusion can cause respiratory arrest)
4. Establish intravenous access	Draw blood gas (usually capillary or venous). Draw arterial blood gas only if child is well-sedated
5. Correct acidosis	Sodium bicarbonate 1 mEq/kg and repeat as necessary
6. Hydrate	10 cc/kg boluses of crystalloid or colloid
7. Pharmacological therapy:	
a. Propranolol	0.05 mg/kg IV. Maximum dose is 0.1 mg/kg, not to exceed a total of 1 mg. (Be prepared for severe bradycardia)
b. Esmolol infusion	Initial bolus of 0.5-1.0 mg/kg; then continuous infusion of 100-300 mcg/kg/min
c. Phenylephrine	Initial bolus of 10-50 mcg/kg/min; may repeat and double bolus to a maximum of 50 mcg/kg/min; then continuous infusion of 1-10 g/kg/min
8. General anesthesia	
9. Emergency cardiopulmonary bypass or ECMO **or** emergency surgery	Palliative or complete repair

contacted as soon as the diagnosis of hypercyanotic spell is established. The cardiovascular surgeon should also be contacted to perform the necessary emergency shunt, or, in some cases with favorable anatomy, complete repair. General anesthesia, extracorporeal membrane oxygenation (ECMO), and surgery have been used as last resorts to abort hypercyanotic spells when physiologic and pharmacologic therapy have been unsuccessful.[5]

It is important to remember that even if the child's spell self-terminated prior to evaluation in the ED, the child should be admitted and intravenous access established electively. In-hospital observation and emergent surgery are still indicated.

Pediatric Heart Transplant Recipients

Pediatric heart transplantation is an accepted form of therapy for children with end-stage1 cardiac disease. Each year approximately 300 pediatric heart transplantation procedures are performed.[7] Five-year survival rates approach 70%.[7] The increasing numbers of procedures performed and the excellent survival means that there are an increasing number of recipients. Many of these patients are living near their transplant center, but many have moved back to their hometowns. Therefore, there is an increasing likelihood that ED physicians will encounter these patients in their practice. This section explores principles of managing these patients.

There are many aspects to the care of the child who has had a heart transplant. Those aspects of care most relevant to the ED physician, and most likely to engender anxiety on the ED practitioner's part, are the recognition and management of graft rejection, differentiating benign from serious infection, and sorting out the implications of medication side effects.

Evaluation and Management of Graft Rejection. Rejection probably causes the most concern for the treating physician, but it is important to avoid attributing every sign and symptom to rejection. It is tempting to direct the diagnostic evaluation and therapy to the graft. However, non-transplant-related processes are much more common. In one review, cardiac-related diagnoses accounted for only 9% of the ED discharge diagnoses in pediatric heart transplant recipients.[8] A careful history and physical examination, as with all patients, is the best insurance against tunnel vision.

Receiving a new heart begins a lifelong process of accommodation of the host to the graft. Most rejection episodes occur in the first three months after transplantation.[9] Rejection, however, can occur at any time. Factors that predispose a child to a rejection episode, and therefore should be searched for, include medication noncompliance and infections. Infections can cause an upregulation of the recipient's immune system, which initiates a cascade of events leading to rejection. Gastrointestinal infections can cause either an inability to tolerate immunosuppressive medications due to nausea or vomiting or lead to decreased absorption due to diarrhea. Children presenting to the ED following diarrhea of several days' duration may experience very low cyclosporine (CSA) levels, inadequate immunosuppression, and, consequently, rejection of the graft.

The signs and symptoms most likely to be encountered in the ED are more easily understood if one considers the pathophysiologic processes involved. Mild rejection episodes are only rarely accompanied by symptoms. But in the absence of symptoms, the child is unlikely to present to the ED. Hence, this discussion will focus on

Table 3. Findings Consistent with Cardiac Graft Rejection

Clinical signs	Fever, tachycardia, tachypnea, rales, hepatosplenomegaly, new heart murmur, gallop, arrhythmias
Symptoms	Irritability, malaise, poor feeding, nausea, change in sleeping patterns
Echocardiogram	New pericardial effusion, poor ventricular function, thickening of LV posterior wall and septum, new mitral insufficiency, decreasing LV fiber-shortening fraction
Electrocardiogram	25% or greater reduction in QRS voltages, significant change in QRS axis, change in conduction pattern, arrhythmias
Chest x-ray	Advancing global cardiomegaly, pulmonary edema, pleural effusion

moderate-to-severe rejection episodes.

Acute rejection involves focal or diffuse lymphocytic infiltration and/or an antibody-mediated inflammatory process. There is interstitial edema and damage or destruction of the myocardial cells. Poor graft function and altered conduction pathways produce signs and symptoms of CHF and cardiac arrhythmias. Inflammation of the heart, even in the absence of overt CHF, can lead to tachycardia. An ECG may show a decrease in QRS voltage, arrhythmias, ectopy, or conduction defects.[10] The ECG is relatively insensitive, but when findings are present, they should be taken seriously. A chest x-ray will show cardiomegaly and possibly effusions, but only late in the course of acute rejection. A caution in the use of the chest x-ray is that most children get a graft from a donor larger than themselves and therefore will have an apparent cardiomegaly. Careful comparison to prior x-rays, if available, is very helpful in this regard.

Clinical symptoms of rejection vary with age. In the infant recipient, they may have poor feeding, lethargy, or irritability.[11] These symptoms are nonspecific, but their absence is helpful in ruling out rejection. Older children have often presented with complaints of abdominal discomfort, nausea, and vomiting. This is most likely related to poor perfusion to the intestines from a poorly functioning graft. Fever may accompany rejection in any age but is also a very nonspecific sign.

The echocardiograph is a sensitive measure of graft function but is rarely available in the ED. Echocardiographic findings of rejection and a summary of other clinical findings of rejection are found in *Table 3*.

Any child who presents to the ED with signs of significant hemodynamic compromise probably has a serious infection or acute graft rejection. In the absence of fever or history consistent with infection, rejection must be considered and treated aggressively. Along with measures to treat CHF as described previously, the child should be given a large dose of intravenous methylprednisolone. A dose of 20 mg/kg to a maximum of 1000 mg is recommended. The cardiac

Table 4. Changes in Electrolytes Associated with Cyclosporine

↓ Na^+	↑ Cl^-	↑ BUN
↑ K^+	↓ CO_2	↑ Cr

transplant team should be contacted and arrangements made to transfer the child to a facility where an experienced team is available.

Post-Transplant Coronary Artery Disease. Post-transplant coronary artery disease is a rejection-related phenomenon. It involves a diffuse, concentric hyperplasia of the myointima of the coronary vessels. The children rarely, if ever, have anginal symptoms, since the sensory connections are severed when the heart is replaced. Patients present with symptoms of CHF due to poor perfusion of the myocardium. They are also at risk for sudden events such as infarction or arrhythmias.

Evaluation of Infections. Infection is the most common reason a child with a heart transplant will present to the ED.[8] The infant heart transplant recipient has a frequency of usual childhood illnesses similar to the general pediatric population.[12]

The management of febrile illness in transplant recipients requires sound clinical acumen. Fever does not require "automatic" admission for all children. For example, a child with otitis media who looks well and who has a temperature of 38.5°C can be treated similarly to the non-transplanted child. Temperatures greater than 39°C without an obvious source in a relatively well-appearing child should be managed with blood and urine cultures and antibiotic coverage (e.g., ceftriaxone) and close follow-up. Children who have an oral steroid as part of their immunosuppression regimen should be managed more cautiously since fever and other signs of infection may be muted. It should also be noted that some children with complex congenital heart disease are also anatomically or functionally asplenic and at increased risk for bacteremia with encapsulated organisms.[13]

Immunosuppression does increase the risk for more opportunistic infections. The highest risk for serious infection is during the first few months after transplantation and after treatment for rejection. *Pneumocystis carinii* pneumonia (PCP) and cytomegalovirus (CMV) infection are the most common opportunistic infections. Children with PCP present with tachypnea and hypoxia. Diagnosis of PCP requires bronchoalveolar lavage. Infection with CMV may present as sepsis, pneumonia, enteritis, or the CMV syndrome. The CMV syndrome includes persistent fever, low white blood cell count, thrombocytopenia, and often, elevation of liver enzymes. Even though rapid diagnostic tests are not available, obtaining serology for CMV titers and CMV cultures in the ED can facilitate the diagnostic process. Any child suspected of having PCP or serious CMV disease should be admitted for further evaluation and definitive therapy.

Cyclosporine and Changes in Electrolytes, BUN, and Creatinine. Gastrointestinal symptoms are frequently seen in the pediatric heart transplant recipient presenting to the ED. These are most frequently related to infectious disease processes. Examination of electrolytes is frequently performed during the evaluation process. It is important to understand changes in electrolytes that accompany the transplant process. Cyclosporine (CSA) can cause alterations that can be confusing and not necessarily reflective of an

Table 5. Significant Side Effects of Immunosuppressive Medications

MEDICATION	SIDE EFFECT
Cyclosporine	Renal insufficiency
	Gingival hyperplasia
	Hirsutism
	Seizures
	Elevated liver transaminases
Azathioprine	Neutropenia (most common)
	Bone marrow suppression
	Anemia
	Thrombocytopenia
	Elevated liver transaminases
Prednisone	Gastrointestinal bleeding
	Cushingoid appearance
	Adrenal insufficiency
	Osteopenia
	Hyperglycemia
	Myopathy
	Sodium and fluid retention
	Many others

acute process. Changes in electrolytes associated with CSA are illustrated in *Table 4*.

These changes may be confused with acute changes due to dehydration. It is helpful to compare to values obtained during the steady state. Additionally, diarrheal disease can cause a decreased CSA level due to increased GI transit time. An empiric increase of CSA dose from 25-50% (depending on the degree of diarrhea) is often necessary. Obtaining a CSA level in the ED is rarely indicated since few laboratories can provide a rapid turnaround. Also, interpretation of the CSA level is difficult except at "trough." A CSA level obtained when acute rejection is suspected can be helpful to retrospectively assess medication compliance.

Side Effects of Immunosuppressive Medications. Typical "triple" immunosuppression protocols use CSA, azathioprine, and prednisone. All of these medications have side effects beyond their immunosuppressive properties.[14,15] Significant side effects are summarized in *Table 5*.

Drug-Drug Interactions. Cyclosporine has many important drug interactions. One of the most common errors is prescribing erythromycin (especially Pediazole) while a child is on CSA. This causes a two- to threefold increase in CSA level. Erythromycin can be used if absolutely necessary with consultation with the transplant team. Common drug interactions with CSA are summarized in *Table 6*.

Neoplasms in the Transplant Recipient. Neoplasms have been reported in up to 10% of pediatric heart transplant recipients.[16] Most of these will be lymphomas. Presentation can vary from an isolated submandibular mass to CNS mass effects to intra-abdominal symptomatology. Diagnostic vigilance must be maintained. Most of these lymphomas are related to lymphoproliferative effects after Epstein-Barr virus (EBV) infection. If EBV infection is diagnosed or suspected, it is important to relay this information to the transplant team.

Table 6. Common Drug Interactions with Cyclosporine

DRUGS THAT INCREASE CSA LEVELS
Erythromycin
Verapamil
Diltiazem (but not nifedipine)
Metoclopramide
Ketoconazole
Fluconazole
DRUGS THAT DECREASE CSA LEVELS
Rifampin
Carbamazepine
Phenobarbital
Phenytoin
DRUGS WITH A REDUCED CLEARANCE WITH CSA
Prednisone
Lovastatin
Digoxin

Summary

While not an everyday occurrence, pediatric patients with CHF, hypercyanotic spells, and heart transplants will present to the ED for evaluation and treatment. CHF, divided into four types based on underlying pathophysiology, will require pathophysiologic-specific interventions as well as more standard therapies. Hypercyanotic spells, caused by congenital heart diseases besides tetralogy of Fallot, result from an imbalance between pulmonary and systemic vascular resistance that favors decreased pulmonary flow and increased right-to-left shunting into the aorta. Emergency medical care providers for children must know precipitating factors and drugs as well as acute interventions and therapies for hypercyanotic spells. Rejection probably causes the most concern for physicians treating pediatric heart transplant recipients. Nonetheless, it is important to avoid attributing every sign and symptom to rejection. Yet, except in the most trivial of circumstances, the transplant center and the child's primary physician should be contacted.

References

1. Hoffman J. Congenital heart disease incidence and prevalence. *Pediatr Clin North Am* 1990;37:25-43.
2. Garson A, Bricker JT, McNamara DG. *The Science and Practice of Pediatric Cardiology.* 2nd ed. Philadelphia: Lea & Febiger; 1990.
3. Flynn PA, Engle ME, Ehlers KH. Cardiac issues in the pediatric emergency room. *Pediatr Clin North Am* 1992;39: 955-986.
4. Pinsky WW, Arciniegas E. Tetralogy of Fallot. *Pediatr Clin North Am* 1990;37:179-192.
5. Van Roekens CN, Zuckerberg AL. Emergency management

of hypercyanotic crises in tetralogy of Fallot. *Ann Emerg Med* 1995;25:256-258.

6. Nussbaum J, Zane EA, Thys DM. Esmolol for the treatment of hypercyanotic spells in infants with tetralogy of Fallot. *J Cardiothorac Vasc Anesth* 1989;3:200-202.
7. United Network for Organ Sharing and the International Society for Heart and Lung Transplantation; 1996. Personal communication.
8. Chinnock R, Sherwin T, Robie S, et al. Emergency department presentation and management of pediatric heart transplant recipients. *Pediatr Emerg Care* 1995;11:355-360.
9. Chinnock R, Baum M, Larsen R, et al. Rejection management and long-term surveillance of the pediatric heart transplant recipient: The Loma Linda experience. *J Heart Lung Transplant* 1993;12:S255-S264.
10. Johnston JK, Mathis CM. Determination of rejection using noninvasive parameters following cardiac transplantation in very early infancy—The Loma Linda experience. *Prog Cardiovasc Nurs* 1988;3:13-18.
11. Chinnock R, Johnston J, Baum M, et al. Signs and symptoms of graft rejection in the infant heart transplant recipient. *Cardiol Young* 1993;3(Suppl 1):59.
12. Cutler D. Infant infections and immune response. *J Heart Lung Transplant* 1991;10:852-853.
13. Wade JC. Origin of infection in the compromised host. In: Patrick CC, ed. *Infections in Immunocompromised Infants and Children.* New York: Churchill Livingstone; 1992:124.
14. Mason J. Renal side effects of cyclosporine. *Transplant Proc* 1990;22:1280-1283.
15. Min DI, Monaco AP. Complications associated with immunosuppressive therapy and their management. *Pharmacotherapy* 1991;11:119S-125S.
16. Bernstein D, Baum D, Berry G, et al. Neoplastic disorders after pediatric heart transplantation. *Circulation* 1993;88: II230-11237.

Sedation for the Pediatric Patient

Jeffrey Proudfoot, DO, FACOEP
Emory Petrack, MD, MPH, FAAP, FACEP

While pain and suffering are "frequent flyers" as well as long-time customers of emergency department (EDs), sedation and aggresive pain control are relatively new visitors. Contributing to the relatively late arrival of more sophisticated pharmacologic interventions has been the significant controversy that has surrounded the use of sedation agents in the ED. A succession of therapeutic misadventures were documented following the early use of many of these agents. Appropriate concerns about the safety of the varied agents were engendered, and as presented by Green and Wittlake,[1] different organizations have attempted to establish potentially useful guidelines directing the application of these clinically valuable drugs for sedation and analgesia. In this chapter, the authors review six mandatory skills for effective pediatric sedation.

Introduction

Providing sedation and analgesia is an integral part of pediatric medical care in the ED. With pain as one of the most common presenting ED complaints, emergency physicians are in the forefront of the development and implementation of new and effective ways to provide comfort and cooperation for pediatric patients. Long neglected as unnecessary, the rational use of sedative and analgesic agents has been hampered by myths and concerns about dangerous side effects, a paucity of scientific documentation regarding effectiveness, and ignorance of options available to the emergency physician.

Over the last decade, there has been a renewed interest in the effective use of pharmacologic pain control and sedation in the ED. Recent work suggests that the use of analgesia for procedures in the emergency setting increased significantly from 1988 to 1994.[1] Nevertheless, while the increase in analgesic use was seen in all age groups, pediatric patients continue to receive less analgesia for painful procedures than adults.[1a]

With the ready availability of newer, more potent agents for sedation, emergency physicians are becoming increasingly experienced at providing highly effective and safe analgesia and sedation for pediatric patients. This process has been spurred by documentation in the literature of the safety and efficacy of ED use of these agents by experienced emergency physicians. In fact, many subspecialties now rely on the expertise of the emergency physician to provide the requisite level of sedation to manage therapeutic procedures that in the past would have required an expensive operating room charge—a benefit in the managed care environment. Lastly, there is satisfaction of parental expectations that their child will not have to suffer because of lack of experience on the part of the physician.

Pathophysiology

A review of two key pharmacokinetic and pathophysiologic principles can help explain how these medications exert their effect

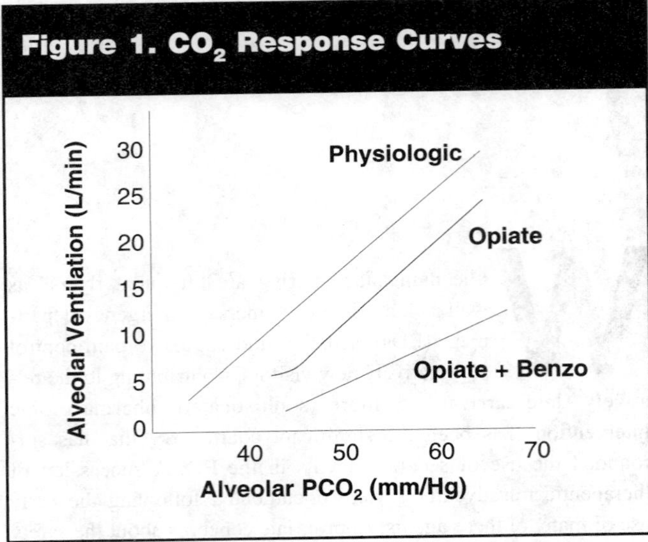

Figure 1. CO_2 Response Curves

and interact with the pediatric metabolism. These mechanisms, which govern the clinical response to and recovery from sedative and analgesic medications, are important principles for effective pediatric sedation and analgesia.

CO_2 Response Curve. Children normally exhibit a linear, concentration dependent increase in minute ventilation with increasing pCO_2. At physiologic pCO_2 levels (e.g., 40), minute ventilation is approximately 5 L/min. *(See Figure 1, curve A.)* Administration of an opiate shifts the curve to the right (i.e., the patient has the same responsive increase in minute ventilation, it simply occurs at a higher pCO_2). *(See Figure 1, curve B.)* Addition of a benzodiazepine to the opiate greatly depresses the response to increasing pCO_2, limiting both the rate of increase in minute ventilation and the threshold of pCO_2 required to stimulate ventilation. This depression in slope is proportional to both the amount and rate of administration of the drug. Children compromised by poor cardiopulmonary reserve such as those with cystic fibrosis, severe asthma, cardiac defects, etc. mimic the curve shift with a combined opiate/sedative. *(See Figure 1, curve C.)*

Drug Redistribution. Most sedative and analgesic medications produce their clinical effect by direct passage into the CNS to occupy specific receptor sites in the brain. Termination of effect is brought about by redistribution of drug down the concentration gradient from lipid-rich brain to other body tissues (i.e., muscle, fat, etc.). The same amount of drug remains in the body until metabolized or excreted but is not physiologically active, having relocated to non-neural tissues.

The Six Skills

1. Keep Your End Point and Goal in Mind

Sedation can relieve anxiety, and analgesics can eliminate or control pain during therapeutic or diagnostic maneuvers, thereby improving patient cooperation and satisfaction of parents. The challenge facing emergency physicians is to select an agent that will achieve the desired end point while minimizing the potential adverse effects that every sedative and analgesic medication possesses. Since the benefits are clear, the goal is knowing the medications in intimate detail, matching the patient and the patient's problem with appropriate technique, controlling the environment, selecting monitoring parameters, and, most importantly, knowing your own limitations. Unfortunately, the ideal medication that is 100% effective, universally safe, with appropriate duration of action, no adverse side effects, and rapid onset and recovery does not yet exist. The medication's selected for a specific patient should be integrated into the physician's knowledge of the relative potency of the drug, its effects on vital organ systems, common side effects, duration of action, and factors that affect elimination. An assessment of patient risk is in essence analysis of vital organ reserve (i.e., cardiovascular, respiratory, and neurological systems). Fortunately, most children have large cardiorespiratory reserves with adequate ventilation and oxygenation to withstand the predictable effects of these medications. On the other hand, some patients are not candidates for ED sedation and are best treated in the operating suite with an empty stomach and a general anesthetic. In summary, the physician using these medications must be intimately familiar with their effects, the specifics and nuances of selection, and be knowledgeable with the techniques used. Remembering the classical admonition, "primum non nocere," first do no harm, physicians must be able to manage any untoward consequences of these drugs.

2. Know How To Get To Where You're Going

After selecting the right patient and drug, a decision must be made on the most appropriate method of administration to get to the planned end point for the task at hand. This may take the form of light (conscious) sedation where the child's anxiety is alleviated and awareness is blunted. Children under light sedation remain responsive to verbal and physical stimuli and maintain their airway, swallowing reflexes, and vital signs independently. The patient receiving transmucosal agents is unlikely to have any deterioration of airway or cardiovascular function, primarily because variable gastrointestinal absorption with delayed onset and hepatic first pass effect creates a ceiling on response and is not effectively titratable. Transmucosal administration is useful for local anesthetic infiltration, IV starts, lumbar punctures, sexual examinations, or painless procedures requiring limited patient cooperation. Many patients require movement along the sedation continuum from simple anxiety reduction to deeper levels of sedation that have the potential to compromise airway reflexes or cardiorespiratory function. This is particularly true for specific end points such as complete immobilization for computerized tomographic (CT) scanning, which can be difficult or impossible to achieve with light sedation. The newer ultrashort agents are especially advantageous at creating deep sedation with minimum time in a compromised state and allowing rapid recovery. Use of these agents allows titration to desired effect in an incremental fashion (i.e., administer drug and observe central nervous system effect and repeating to quiescence or immobilization). Deep sedation mandates continued physician supervision of the patient from beginning to end, and this supervision cannot be performed at a distance.

3. Control the Environment

The venue in which sedation takes place is crucial to success and has been defined by most institutions via institutional sedation poli-

Table 1. Comparison of Sedatives, Analgesics, Hypnotics

Ultrashort	Type	Route	Dose (mg/kg) #	Onset	Duration	Titration	Comment
Midazolam	S†	IV,IM IN po	0.05-0.1 0.2-0.3 0.5	2 min 10-15 min 15-20 min	30 min 45 min 45 min	++++ poor poor	See text, hypotension difficult to titrate
Fentanyl	AΩ	IV, IM	1-4 mcg	1-2 min	20-30 min	++++	Initial dose 1 mcg/kg, then titrate in 1 mcg/kg doses
Alfentanil	AΩ	IV	5 mcg	1-2 min	20-30 min	++++	Does not accumulate, may rebolus
Thiopental	H	IV	3-5	30-60 sec	15 min	++++	Titrate in 1 mg/kg doses
Methohexital	H	IV	0.5-1.0	30-45 sec	10-15 min	++++	Limited experience
Nitrous Oxide	S, A	Inhalation	50:50 mix $N_2O:O_2$	1-2 min		+++	Demand valve mask. Older than 8 years.
Intermediate							
Diazepam	S†	IV	0.05-0.2	2-5 min	1-2 hours	+++	Not recommended IM
Meperidine	AΩ	IV, IM	0.5-1.5	2-5 min	3-4 hours	+	Titrate slowly to 1-1.5 mg/kg
Fentanyl	AΩ	Oralet	5-15 mcg/kg	5-15 min	60-90 min	+	(100, 200, 300, 400 mcg), max 400 mcg
Pentobarbital	H	IV, IM	2-5	2-5 min	30-60 min	++	Titrate in 1 mg/kg doses
Long Acting							
Chloral Hydrate	H	po, pr	20-50 mg/kg	30-60 min	3-4 hrs	poor	Higher doses commonly used. See text.
Morphine	AΩ	IV, IM	0.1	5-10 min	2-4 hrs	++	
Ketorolac	A	IM,IV,po	0.5-1	15-30 min	2-4 hrs	poor	
Butorphanol	A	IN	1 spray	5-10 min	2-3 hrs	poor	
Dissociative							
Ketamine	S, A, H	IM IV	4 1-2	5 min 1-2 min	30-60 min 20-40 min	++ +++	Requires atropinization IV over 1-2 minutes

S - sedative A - analgesics H - hypnotics

† reversible with flumazenil Ω reversible with naloxone # mg/kg unless otherwise indicated

cies. This usually takes the form of limiting procedures and sedation to areas that are adequate to accommodate skilled personnel and all the appropriate monitoring and resuscitation equipment—commonly a critical care area. It is the responsibility of the emergency physician to know his or her facility's capabilities and the expertise level of the personnel assisting in the procedure. The controlled chaos present in most pediatric EDs demands a standardized approach to sedation procedures and is prerequisite for minimizing confusion attendant to sudden deterioration or unexpected problems with either patient or procedure. A room setup that has all necessary medications, reversal agents, airway equipment, and suction immediately available within arm's reach facilitates rapid intervention when necessary.

Monitoring. The American Academy of Pediatrics (AAP) has recommended minimum standards for monitoring of pediatric patients during elective sedation and has defined conscious (light) sedation, deep sedation, and general anesthesia.[2] The optimum monitoring situation is a dedicated, experienced, patient observer performing visual confirmation of respiratory effort and patient color, and surveillance of monitoring instruments in place. This is facilitated with appropriate patient exposure, lighting, and positioning of the head to maintain a patent airway and allow visualization of oral mucosa and chest wall excursions. A second provider, in addition to the physician involved, assumes this responsibility, and thus mandates a minimum of two trained personnel when using deep sedation.

Monitor all patients receiving sedation by parenteral routes with a minimum of continuous pulse oximetry. Pulse oximetry monitors detect hypoxia well in advance of its clinical appearance and sequelae.[3] Using cardiac monitors or combined EKG/oximeter monitors helps sort out inaccurate oximeter readings due to signal loss from sensors or incomplete correlation with high pulse rates common to pediatric patients. End tidal carbon dioxide monitors using nasal cannula sensors are also available, but efficacy as a monitoring adjunct during sedation remains unproven.[3] Children receiving simple or light sedation transmucosally require little in the way of monitoring (pulse oximetry alone should suffice) unless large doses, multiple agents or long-acting agents (e.g., chloral hydrate) are involved. However, infants and children undergoing deep sedation (particularly with multiple agents) require careful monitoring with pulse oximeter, cardiac monitor, and continuous close visual appraisal with interval (usually every 5-10 minutes) documentation of respiratory and pulse rates and blood pressure. The time, route, and dose of medications administered entered on the chart ensure a complete record. Sending a sedated patient to the radiology suite without appropriate monitoring and personnel is a prescription for disaster.

Table 2. Discharge Criteria

INFANTS
- Baseline vital signs and mental status
- Active, able to sit upright or crawl appropriate for age
- Recognizes, interacts with, or is consolable by parent/caregiver
- Responsible parent or guardian present

CHILDREN
- Baseline vital signs and mental status
- Able to follow command and verbalize appropriately
- Demonstrates motor function appropriate for age (e.g., sit or walk unassisted)
- Able to take popsicle or liquids
- Responsible parent or guardian present

4. Select the Right Drug And Route

The most common clinical error is mismatching a patient with the wrong drug and/or route for the right reason. Administering enough of any sedative can alter the response to painful stimuli but should always be coupled with an analgesic if serious discomfort is anticipated. Likewise, analgesics that cause sedation as a side effect are not the best choice for pure sedation or amnesia. Light (transmucosal route) sedation is a uniquely pediatric phenomenon. It is useful for minor or briefly painful indications yet has an efficacy ceiling due to variability in transmucosal absorption, rapid clearance from first pass hepatic metabolism, and unpredictable duration and response from low drug effect.[5] Repeat dosing can increase effectiveness at the cost of delaying the entire procedure. Light (conscious) sedation has the benefit of being minimally invasive, easy to administer, and extremely unlikely to compromise the patient's cardiorespiratory status. Coupled with topical anesthesia, it is effective for minor lacerations, lumbar punctures, and sexual examinations. Intramuscular (IM) administration of sedative or analgesic agents is to be avoided (the exception being ketamine). Depending on the site of the injection, absorption is erratic and carries the risk of oversedation without benefit of vascular access should complications develop. There is little reason to recommend the antiquated "DPT" or "MPC;" a fixed combination of meperidine (Demerol), promethazine (Phenergan), and chlorpromazine (Thorazine) that produces an unpredictable degree of sedation and significant hypotension in many patients with delayed onset (mean, 27 minutes).[5-11]

The gold standard for effective and reliable pediatric sedation to a predictable end point is intravenous (IV) administration. Almost all EDs are accomplished at IV access in pediatric patients. Repeat dosing is easy, painless, and can deliver the medication in a controlled, incremental fashion to peak clinical effect. It is the only route suitable for deep sedation, as it provides access for administration of reversal agents and any necessary resuscitation drugs. Deep sedation is facilitated by the IV use of potent, highly lipophilic, and ultrashort-acting agents such as fentanyl or thiopental. Clinicians can administer a small dose, observe the CNS effect within seconds to minutes, and repeat the process until a desired clinical end point is reached. This "individualizes" the process by allowing a combination of medications to be used such as a sedative and an analgesic. *(See Table 1.)* It also avoids the "hit or miss" phenomenon where a fixed dose of medication is administered and the patient is observed for the window of effect, as is commonly done with chloral hydrate or "DPT." Additionally, it is anticipated that enough drug will have been given to produce the appropriate duration of sedation required to complete the task at hand. Often the patient requiring and receiving repeat doses is committed to a longer recovery.

5. Anticipate Complications

As with all procedures, physicians administering sedation to enough patients will eventually experience a complication. It is paramount that emergency clinicians employing sedation be vigilant for potential complications, be able to recognize adverse effects immediately, and be prepared to intervene rapidly and definitively. The worst case scenario of cardiac or respiratory arrest should be uppermost in the mind of the emergency physician managing the sedation. Correct use of therapeutic sedating agents and close adherence to monitoring policies are essential. Physicians who are uncomfortable with active interventional airway management in children are better off seeking supplemental training and relegating sedation to experienced colleagues.

Avoid "Stacking." One of the most common pitfalls in pediatric sedation is drug "stacking." This process occurs after the physician administers a second or third drug dose before peak clinical effect of the initial administered drug dose. As the first dose is peaking, the subsequent doses that are already delivered literally "stack" up on the initial dose and summate, exaggerating clinical effect and pushing the patient much deeper than was anticipated. Stacking can be prevented by knowing specific pharmacokinetics properties of the medications used. It is much easier to reach a targeted end point with smaller, appropriately timed doses rather than one large dose that has the potential to overshoot the mark. Impatience and an "itchy trigger finger" can lead to an anesthetized and apneic patient.

Beware of the Lost Stimulus. One of the more common times to experience oversedation is at the completion of a painful procedure, particularly orthopedic reductions. With sudden removal of pain and antagonist stimulation, the patient tends to slide deeper into unopposed sedation and can require stimulation to breathe. Keeping close observation at this point can catch apneic episodes before they lead to desaturation. Providing selected, supplemental noxious stimulation is the easiest way to counteract this (e.g., applying pressure to the painful site).

Minimize Crossover Titration. Crossover titration occurs when alternating doses of two different classes of medications are used in a sequential fashion (e.g., midazolam then fentanyl, then midazolam then fentanyl, etc.) This practice is risky because the cumulative effect often is unpredictable and much greater than establishing baseline sedation and titrating to an end point with a single analgesic agent. In addition, repeat doses of drugs with differing times to peak effect make it difficult to estimate subsequent doses. Exactly how much to decrease the standard dose for the second or third administration to prevent the rapid shift of the CO_2 response curve to the right and into apnea territory is at best a guess given the variability in pediatric metabolism. *(See Figure 1, curve C.)* Time to recovery also is prolonged with crossover.

Recognize the Shifting Baseline. Patients who have already received analgesia before their light or deep sedation for procedures such as a fracture reduction represent an increased risk because of their altered baseline. Subsequent administration of sedatives and analgesics must take this into account. Use of the standard doses and techniques can lead to exaggerated effect secondary to interaction with the active drugs already circulating. The same admonition applies to adolescents under the influence of alcohol or drugs of abuse.

Anticipate and Avoid Cumulation. Repeat administration of any of the analgesic agents (the exception is alfentanil) to extend a procedure beyond the normal duration of action of the drug leads to accumulation of that agent in the body. This obligates the physician to use analgesics or sedatives that will be effective for the duration of the procedure contemplated. Most of the ultrashort medications have predictable termination of their clinical effect via redistribution from lipid-rich brain tissue down a concentration gradient into skeletal and other body fat depots. As the level of active drug present in the brain decreases, the patient demonstrates recovery; however, the great majority of the medication is still present in the body. Cumulation is common to a patient who is sedated for fracture reduction and, after x-ray, undergoes repeat sedation to improve the fracture then gets x-rayed again, etc. If body tissue depots become saturated, then redistribution is impeded and the patient will experience prolonged sedation. Recovery time is then dependent on hepatic metabolism or renal excretion of the drug involved and not on redistribution. Alfentanil is a notable exception, as it does not cumulate in the body but is rapidly metabolized to terminate its effect.

6. Recovery And Documentation

Ideal emergence from sedation is characterized by a rapid return to presedation levels of consciousness with minimal distress for the child. This ensures safe discharge home without worries of cardiorespiratory compromise, resedation, aspiration of food (commonly given immediately as a reward), or parental anxiety over ongoing abnormal behavior from the medications used. Discharge criteria that list discrete behavioral, motor, or mental status responses and conditions to be met prior to discharge are the best guidelines for determining readiness for discharge. *(See Table 2.)* Avoid reversal of sedative or analgesic agents with opiate or benzodiazepine antagonists to speed recovery. Sudden reversal of sedation or analgesia, while hastening emergence, also carries with it the return of pain, anxiety, and sympathetic stimulation. Resedation is a possibility, particularly with the longer-acting medications that are metabolized slower than their antagonists. Antagonists are essential adjuncts for the patient who has apnea or respiratory compromise from oversedation. Hopefully, close attention to titration will minimize the duration of apnea or hypotension.

The Ultrashort Agents

Fentanyl. Fentanyl is a synthetic narcotic. It is 100 times as potent as morphine and 7000 times more lipophilic, with rapid uptake by lipid-rich brain within 30-60 seconds of intravenous injection to peak analgesia in 2-3 minutes.[13,14] Because its duration of effect is 20-30 minutes, it is best employed for short, painful procedures.[15]

The drug has been used extensively with good safety and efficacy in the ED for repair of facial lacerations, orthopedic procedures, incision and drainage, and diagnostic procedures including CT sedation.[16,17] The adverse effects of fentanyl relate to either rapid administration or large doses (> 8-10 mcg/kg).[18-21] Large doses or too rapid administration of fentanyl can produce rigidity of the chest wall related to stimulation of the spinal cord inspiratory motor neurons and consequently inspiratory muscles leading to sustained inspiration (i.e., "tight chest syndrome").[20,22,23] A prominent bradycardia occurs from stimulation of the central vagal nucleus and prolongs both atrioventricular node conduction and refractory period; however, fentanyl causes the least hemodynamic changes of any opiate. Additionally, these adverse effects of fentanyl are reportedly reversed by naloxone. Metabolism in infants is prolonged, although children are less likely than adults to suffer respiratory depression,[24,25] and patients will maintain awareness even though appearing to be asleep.[26] While primarily an analgesic, at higher doses it also has sedative effects. It is highly titratable at a dose of 0.5-1.0 mcg/kg slowly, which can be repeated every 2-3 minutes for effect. The usual total dose is 1-4 mcg/kg.

Alfentanil. Alfentanil is an analog of fentanyl that is one-fifth as potent and has one-third the duration of action.[21] As a result of its low pKa, approximately 90% of the drug is non-ionized at physiologic pH, allowing more rapid diffusion across the blood-brain barrier and thus more rapid onset of action than fentanyl.[26,28-30] Termination of action is via rapid redistribution. However, unlike fentanyl, alfentanil does not accumulate with repeat dosing due to its smaller volume of distribution and shorter half-life (elimination half-life 70 minutes as compared with 185 minutes for fentanyl).[31] Alfentanil has the same adverse effect profile as fentanyl and works best for 20- to 30-minute procedures. The usual dose is 5-20 mcg/kg IV administered slowly.[31,32]

Midazolam. As a rapid-acting, water soluble benzodiazepine, midazolam has become the most popular ED agent for sedation. It has 3-4 times the potency of diazepam and rapid onset to a peak effect within 2-3 minutes after intravenous administration.[33,34] The two minutes delay to peak effect makes it more difficult to titrate for deep sedation and an easy drug to "stack" with repeat doses. It is highly water soluble and non-irritating to veins. This is by virtue of a carbon ring structure which closes at a pH greater than four to become water soluble at physiologic pH and therefore does not require a propylene glycol solubilizing agent as necessitated for diazepam. Because midazolam redistributes rapidly, its duration of action is short.

The drug binds GABA receptors in the CNS to inhibit spinal afferent pathways and produces skeletal muscle relaxation, amnesia, and anxiolysis. Midazolam, while altering the response to pain, like all benzodiazepines, does not reduce pain perception and has a propensity to produce apnea by shifting the CO_2 response curve to the right and depressing the slope. *(See Figure 1, curve C.)* At higher doses, midazolam can produce hypotension, particularly in hypovolemic children.[35-37] In low doses, the patient is able to maintain airway reflexes while anxiety is moderated and the patient is calmed. It has the added advantage of providing anterograde and retrograde amnesia.[38,39] When used for painful procedures, addition of an analgesic is recommended. Used intravenously or in conjunction with a narcotic, it is a potent sedative-amnestic and requires extreme vigilance to cardiorespiratory function.[40-43] The effects of midazolam can be reversed with intravenous flumazenil[43] but, as mentioned previously, routine reversal is not recommended. The effectiveness of midazolam in pediatric patients has been well documented.[44-53] The initial IV dosing for children 6 months to five years is 0.05-0.1 mg/kg, then titrated to a maximum of 0.6 mg/kg. For children 6-12 years, the initial IV dose is 0.025-0.05 mg/kg, then titrated to a maximum of 0.4 mg/kg.

Thiopental. Thiopental is an ultrashort-acting, potent barbiturate hypnotic that reaches the brain within 30 seconds of intravenous injection. It produces profound hypnosis and sedation that is highly predictable, lasting 10-15 minutes at subanesthetic doses. Because it is a histamine releaser, it must be used with caution in asthmatics. It can cause significant hypotension through venodilation and a depression of the baroreflex mechanism.[51-54] Thiopental has the advantage of dose dependent depression of cerebral metabolism, cerebral blood flow, and intracranial pressure.[55] It is a highly alkaline solution (pH 10.5) and if extravasated into subcutaneous or dermal sites can cause erythema, edema, and severe tissue necrosis. Sedative dosing is at 1 mg/kg every 1-2 minutes, titrating for effect to a usual total dose of 3-5 mg/kg. Like benzodiazepines, thiopental provides no analgesia and should be combined with an opiate analgesic for painful procedures. Finally, it is active via rectal administration.[56]

Methohexital. Similar to its lipophilic cousin thiopental methohexital is an oxybarbiturate with faster onset, shorter duration of action,[57] and 2-3 times the potency. It has been widely used as an induction agent at doses of 20 mg/kg administered rectally to produce light to deep sedation.[58-62] Methohexital has been used intravenously for sedation during painful pediatric oncologic procedures and as sedation for radiologic studies.[63,64] The intravenous dose is 0.5-1.0 mg/kg. The drug can cause myoclonic jerking of the musculature and has the potential to induce seizures in patients with temporal lobe epilepsy.[65] Respiratory and airway compromise is a concern.[66] Coadministration of an analgesic or use of a local anesthetic is recommended for painful procedures.

Propofol. A unique ultrashort agent in the alkylphenol class unrelated to any of the previous agents, propofol is rapidly becoming a favored agent for ED sedation. Formulated as an aqueous emulsion in intralipid (soybean oil, glycerol, and egg phosphatide), it has the advantage of faster onset than thiopental, twice the potency, rapid emergence, and return to baseline with antiemetic, antipruritic, anticonvulsant, anixiolytic effects.[67-73] Emergence is so rapid that procedures that last longer than 5-10 minutes require a continuous infusion or repeat bolus injection to maintain effect. Propofol produces hypotension, myocardial depression, and apnea that is directly related to dose and rate of injection. It has not been shown to release histamine but does depress the CO_2 response curve by 50%. As many as half of children will experience pain on infusion that can be eliminated by using 0.5 mg/kg lidocaine with the agent, larger veins, or a concomitant analgesic. Unlike thiopental, it is not antianalgesic, yet has no amnestic or analgesic properties and, as such, should be combined with other appropriate agents to maintain amnesia and pain relief. Propofol is administered as intermittent boluses or a continuous infusion at an initial rate of 25-100 mcg/kg/min titrated to effect.[74-79] Patients are exquisitely sensitive to rate of injection of propofol, so much so that "time taken over the injection under most clinical circumstances is of greater importance than volume."[80] Thus, slow gradual infusion of doses yields the fewest adverse effects. Propofol has been most useful as pediatric sedation for CT or MRI where longer periods of immobilization are required and are easily managed by continuous gravity infusions without pumps or other metallic equipment.[81-86] More recently, propofol has been used effectively in the ED setting and the dental suite.[87-89] Apnea and hypotension may be more common than with other agents but are also more transient and self limited. This mandates the usual caveat of use by physicians facile with pediatric airway management. The great benefit of propofol is on-off emergence that limits the time the child is at risk from sedation-related events.

Intermediate-/Medium-Duration Agents

Morphine. Morphine is the classic opiate narcotic to which other analgesics are compared. Morphine provides analgesia, sedation, and diminishes anxiety by its agonist activity at mu and kappa opioid brain receptors. It is more effective for continuous, dull pain than for sudden, sharp, painful stimuli. Because of poor lipid solubility, only small amounts of an administered dose enter the CNS, restricting its usefulness as a titratable sedative.[12,13,26] It does, however, provide effective analgesia for a 3-4 hour duration, low CNS toxicity, and is preferable for painful procedures longer than 30 minutes.[90] Morphine has a relatively slow onset (5 minutes IV, 10-15 minutes IM). It works well when combined with benzodiazepines. Side effects include nausea, hypotension from histamine release, and respiratory depression. Children younger than 2 months of age are particularly susceptible to respiratory depression. The preferred route is intravenously (at 0.1 mg/kg), but it is absorbed intramuscularly, sublingually, and rectally. The drug causes significant histamine release that can lead to hypotension and, like all narcotics, depresses the medullary response to hypercapnia and hypoxia. It has a prolonged half-life and decreased clearance in infants younger than one month of age.[91]

Meperidine. As the most commonly used narcotic in the ED, the synthetic meperidine has a narrow therapeutic margin (i.e., therapeutic dose close to toxic dose). It is not titratable for deep sedation, as it requires 10-20 minutes to peak clinical effect and has a 2-3 hour duration. Accumulation of its principle active metabolite, normeperidine, has the potential to cause CNS stimulation and seizures.[13,26,92,93] Because of this, it is usually administered in conjunction with phenothiazines to potentiate its sedative characteristics. Meperidine is an antiquated favorite of clinicians who shun the newer agents because of its predictable, albeit gradual onset. It offers almost no advantage over morphine and is only one-tenth as potent; it is not recommended routinely for children.

Diazepam. The father of midazolam, diazepam has been the most familiar benzodiazepine to emergency physicians. Solubilized in propylene glycol, diazepam is very irritating to veins on injection and while predictable, has a slower onset to action than midazolam, making it less useful for effective titratation for deep sedation. The side effect profile is similar to midazolam.

Long-Duration Agents

Pentobarbital. Pentobarbital is a long-acting barbiturate that induces sedation within five minutes of IV injection. It has a duration of action of 30-60 minutes and requires monitoring for potential hypoxia. Pentobarbital has found most use in sedation for diagnostic studies that are not painful.[94-97] Dosing is at 2-5 mg/kg.

Chloral Hydrate. Chloral hydrate is a popular hypnotic/sedative for use in infants, particularly among intensivists and pediatric radiologists.[98-101] This agent is active secondary to its hepatic metabolite trichloroethanol and is thus contraindicated in liver failure. Dosages vary from 25-100 mg/kg up to 1000 mg either rectally or orally. In other words, doses higher than recommended by the manufacturer (e.g., 75 mg/kg) are frequently administered. The dose is often repeated if the intended end point is not reached. Chloral hydrate has several disadvantages for the emergency setting. Notably, it has delayed onset up to 60 minutes or more, often resulting in a child who is sedated for several hours with the peak drug effect, minutes to hours beyond the completion of the procedure.[101,102] This possibility mandates extended recovery and observation time. Nausea, vomiting, respiratory depression, and death have been reported.[103] Additionally, some question has been raised regarding possible carcinogenicity of its metabolite.[104]

Meperidine, Promethazine, and Chlorpromazine. Also known as the "lytic cocktail," "DPT," or "MPC," this combination of Demerol (meperidine 25 mg/mL), Phenergan (promethazine 6.5 mg/mL), and Thorazine (chlorpromazine 6.5 mg/mL) has been used widely because of its ease of intramuscular administration and reliable sedating effects. It has also been used inappropriately to chemically immobilize children for non-painful procedures.[105,106] The combination is not titratable and is well known for complications including seizures, dystonic reactions, hypotension, and even death at the standard (0.1 mL/kg) and lower dosage (0.06 mL/kg).[5-11] Combining two phenothiazine class drugs with a long-acting opiate potentiates the respiratory depressant effects of the meperidine and magnifies the toxicity of this combination with duration of action reported as long as 19 hours.[107] Current practice recommends against use of this drug combination in the ED because of these issues. The Agency for Health Care Policy and Research has stated "the efficacy of this mixture is poor when compared with alternative approaches; it has been associated with a high frequency of adverse effects. It is not recommended for general use and should be used only in exceptional circumstances".[108]

Special Agents

Dissociative Sedation. Ketamine is a unique medication that is particularly useful in pediatric sedation. It also has a unique profile of advantages and side effects that must be considered before using it safely. A derivative of phencyclidine that creates the trance-like dissociative state characterized by sedation, amnesia, analgesia, and catalepsy, it has been in use since 1970.[109] The so-called "kiddie-caine" child appears awake with eyes open with a slow nystagmic gaze, intact corneal and light reflexes but unresponsive to painful and visual stimuli—often described as the "lights are on but nobody's home" phenomenon. A functional dissociation is created between the cortical and limbic systems of the brain that interferes with sensory perception of painful stimuli and memory. This occurs by ketamine binding to the NMDA (N-methyl D aspartate) receptors in the brain. The level of sedation is comparable to deep sedation with other agents, yet the patient independently maintains an airway; as a result, ketamine is enjoying increasing use in the ED.[110,111] At low doses ketamine supports cardiovascular function as a positive inotrope that increases blood pressure, heart rate, cardiac output, intracranial pressure (ICP), and shifts the CO_2 response curve to the right.[109,112,113] It also has a bronchodilatory effect on lungs and maintains airway reflexes. Ketamine can also increase airway secretions, salivation, and rarely causes laryngospasm. At high doses, it is a general anesthetic with the usually attendant cardiopulmonary depressive effects. The drug is highly predictable in onset (1-2 minutes IV, 5 minutes IM) and duration (approximately 45 minutes), even via the intramuscular route. Its safety and efficacy in the ED setting have been extensively documented in more than 11,000 cases.[110,111,113,114] Ketamine use mandates several special considerations.

Induction and Administration. Ketamine has been used orally, rectally, and intranasally.[115-121] While active via these routes, it is most efficacious and predictable when given IM or slowly IV. Intramuscular administration is used most commonly and the dose is 4 mg/kg. Intravenous loading of ketamine (1-2 mg/kg) should occur over at least 1-2 minutes. Concerns over increased tracheobronchial secretions and salivation have prompted the recommendation that antisialogogues such as atropine (0.01 mg/kg, maximum 0.5 mg) or glycopyrrollate (0.005 mg/kg, maximum 0.25 mg) be administered prior to or combined with ketamine.[111] Incidence of larygospasm is estimated overall less than 1% to a high of 9% in children with upper respiratory infections.[122] Neonates and infants less than 3 months old have a higher incidence of airway complications including apnea and aspiration.[111]

Emergence. Return from the dissociative process can create an agitated, disoriented, and combative child—a process known as "emergence reaction."[109,111] Risk factors for emergence reactions are age older than 10-15, female gender, a history of vivid dreams, and personality or psychiatric problems. While unusual in children (approx 2%), emergence phenomenon is prevented by coadministration of low-dose midazolam (0.05-0.1 mg/kg) and recovery in a quiet environment. However, use of midazolam may prolong the duration of action. Emesis can occur during recovery but likewise is uncommon (8%). Delayed or long-term effects are almost non-existent.[122]

Patient Selection. Because of its physiologic effects, patient selection is very important. Children with suspected head injury, upper respiratory infections, psychiatric histories, age younger than 3 months or older than 10 years, or those with thyroid or liver diseases are probably not good candidates for dissociative sedation. The nursing staff must be educated to the idiosyncrasies of ketamine. Thorough instructions to the parents regarding persistent nystagmus, ataxia, and behavioral effects of ketamine are necessary to allay parental concerns. Worldwide experience has shown a serious complication rate (apnea, laryngospasm, emergence reaction, aspiration, death) of less than 0.2%.[123] Ketamine appears to be among the safest alternatives for sedation in the pediatric population.

Nitrous Oxide. Nitrous oxide is an inhaled sedative analgesic. It is short-acting, rapid in onset, and is easily administered by demand valve face mask in a 50:50 mixture with oxygen to prevent hypoxia. It seems to be most effective in children older than age 8.[124,126] It is particularly useful in children who are poorly cooperative (developmental delay, mental retardation), as it is non-invasive, requires minimum expertise and monitoring, and produces light sedation. Because it is highly diffusable, it can accumulate in enclosed body cavities such as the middle ear or bowel and potentially cause perforation, but for short use it is very safe.[125-129] When used in conjunction with narcotics or sedatives, it produces deep sedation, and appropriate monitoring is desirable.

Fentanyl "Lollipop." Considerable potential was anticipated with the availability of an oral form of fentanyl (Fentanyl Oralet). Fentanyl citrate is impregnated in the matrix of a sweet lozenge on a holder. The child uses it like a "lollipop" with absorption across oral mucosal surface and into systemic circulation without first-pass effect. There are four oralet dosages (100, 200, 300, 400 mcg). The oralet is contraindicated in children less than 10 kg. Randomized studies have shown it to be effective sedation for painful procedures (bone marrow, lumbar puncture), but with as high as 47% of children manifesting nausea and vomiting and a mean time to discharge of 98 minutes.[130] It has the same risk of respiratory depression as with parenteral fentanyl.[131-137] In addition, some philosophical concern has been raised regarding the use of a medication in "candy" form.

Ketorolac. Ketorolac is the only parenteral nonsteroidal anti-inflammatory analgesic that is currently available for use. Its mechanism of action is inhibition of prostaglandin synthesis.[118] Because it is a non-narcotic medication, it offers analgesia without risk of respiratory depression and nausea commonly associated with use of narcotic agents. It has been widely used intravenously without complications.[138-147] Adverse reactions reported in the adult population include gastrointestinal bleeding, anaphylaxis, renal insufficiency, and platelet dysfunction.[148-155] Pediatric experience is limited due to lack of approval for use in children younger than 12 years of age and has generated some concern over possible prolongation of bleeding times. Clinical trials have shown ketorolac to be an effective analgesic at doses of 0.5-1.0 mg/kg IM without adverse gastrointestinal or renal effects.[156] More commonly, ketorolac has been used post operatively and for renal colic, comparing favorably to morphine or demerol.[157] It also has reduced postoperative opioid requirements in children.[147]

Butorphanol. Recently an intranasal spray of butorphanol tartrate (10 mg/mL) has become available. Butorphanol is an opioid agonist-antagonist analgesic. Its primary agonist activity is at the kappa opioid receptors with some mixed agonist-antagonist function at the mu receptor. While it has the potential of respiratory depression, there is a ceiling on its effects due to the antagonist component. Peak analgesia is within one hour of nasal administration. The recommended dose is one spray in one nostril that delivers approximately 1 mg.[158] It has been used successfully for postoperative pain control in outpatient pediatric surgery settings and for migraine headaches.[159-161] The reader should be cautioned that its use for children has yet to be clearly identified. Contraindications are sensitivity to butorphanol or the preservative benzethonium chloride and the usual precautions attendant to use of narcotics.

Conclusion

It is clear that there has been significant progress in the provision of pediatric analgesia and sedation in the emergency setting. Over the past several years, new agents have been developed with a more desirable profile for use in this setting. In addition, it appears that the actual use of sedation and analgesia for painful procedures is increasing in the pediatric population. The safe use of these agents remain a central concern to practitioners. It is important that clear, written procedures, with appropriate monitoring, be established to ensure patient safety. Physicians using these agents in children must be adept at advanced airway procedures in this special group of patients. The careful selection of the most appropriate agent(s), combined with appropriate skills in drug administration, will lead to decreased distress and enhanced comfort for children requiring relief from pain and anxiety.

References

1. Green S, Wittlake W. Meeting the guidelines and standards for pediatric sedation and analgesia. *Pediatr Emerg Med Rep* 1997;2:67-78.

1a. Petrack EM, Christopher NC, Kriwinsky J. Pain management in the emergency department: Patterns of analgesic utilization. *Pediatrics* 1997;99:711-714

2. American Academy of Pediatrics, Committee on Drugs, Section on Anesthesiology. Guidelines for the elective use of conscious sedation, deep sedation and general anesthesia in pediatric patients. *Pediatrics* 1985;76: 317-321.

3. Wright SW. Conscious sedation in the emergency department: The value of capnography and pulse oximetry. *Ann Emer Med* 1992; 21:551-55

4. American Academy of Pediatrics, Committee on Drugs. Guidelines for monitoring and management of pediatric patients during and after sedation for diagnostic and therapeutic procedures. *Pediatrics* 1992;6:1110-1115.

5. Cohen GH, Casta A, Sapire DW, et al. Decorticate posture following "cardiac cocktail." A transient complication of sedation for catheterization. *Pediatr Cardiol* 1982;2:251-253.

6. Krippaehne JA, Montgomery MT. Morbidity and mortality from pharmacosedation and general anesthesia in the dental office. *J Oral Maxillofac Surg* 1992;50:691-698.

7. Mitchell AA, Louik C, Lacouture P, et al. Risks to children from computed tomographic scan premedication. *JAMA* 1982;247:2385-2388.

8. Nahata MC, Clotz MA, Knogg EA. Adverse effects of meperidine promethazine and chlorpromazine for sedation in pediatric patients. *Clin Pediatr* 1985;24:558.

9. Ros SP. IM MPC in children: Safe and effective or a poor choice? *Ann Emerg Med* 1991;20:1274.

10. Snodgrass WR, Dodge WF. Lytic "DPT" cocktail: Time for rational and safe alternatives. *Pediatr Clin North Am* 1989;36:1285-1291.

11. Sacchetti AD, Schafermeyer RW, Gerardia MJ, et al. Pediatric analgesia and sedation. 1993 Report prepared by the Pediatric Emergency Medicine Committee of the American College of Emergency Physicians, Dallas:1-80.

12. Murphy MR. Opioids. In: Barash PG, Cullen BF, Stoelting KK, eds. *Clinical Anesthesia*. Philadelphia: Lippincott; 1989:255.

13. Murphy MR, Hug CC Jr, McClain DA. Dose-independent

pharmacokinetics of fentanyl. *Anesthesiology* 1983;59: 537-540.

14. Yaster M, Nichols DG, Deshpande JK. Midazolam-fentanyl intravenous sedation in children: Case report of respiratory arrest. *Pediatrics* 1990;86:463.
15. Billmire DA, Neale HW, Gregory RO. Use of IV fentanyl in the outpatient treatment of pediatric facial trauma. *J Trauma* 1985;25:1079.
16. Chudnofsky CR, Wright SW, Dronen SC. The safety of fentanyl use in the emergency department. *Ann Emerg Med* 1989;18:635.
17. Stoeckel H, Hengstmann JH, Schuttler J. Pharmacokinetics of fentanyl as a possible explanation for recurrence of respiratory depression. *Br J Anaesth* 1979;51:741-745.
18. Streisand JB, Bailey PL, LeMaire L, et al. Fentanyl-induced rigidity and unconsciousness in human volunteers. *Anesthesiology* 1993;78:4.
19. Tabatabai M, Kitahata LM, Collins JG. Disruption of the rhythmic activity of the medullary inspiratory neurons and phrenic nerve by fentanyl and reversal with nalbuphine. *Anesthesiology* 1989;70:489.
20. Hubbard AM, Markowitz Rl, Kimmel B, et al. Sedation for pediatric patients undergoing CT and MRI. *J Comp Assist Tomog* 1992;16:3-6.
21. Scamman FL. Fentanyl-O_2-N_2O rigidity and pulmonary compliance. *Anesth Analg* 1983;62:332-334.
22. Koehntop DE, Rodman JH, Brundage DM, et al. Pharmacokinetics of fentanyl in neonates. *Anesth Analg* 1986;65:227-232.
23. Singleton MA, Rosen Jl, Fisher DM. Plasma concentration of fentanyl in infants, children, and adults. *Can J Anesth* 1987;34:152-155.
24. Collins VJ. Intravenous anesthesia: Narcotic and neuroleptic narcotic agents. In: *Principles of Anesthesiology: General and Regional Anesthesia.* 3rd ed. Philadelphia: Lea and Febiger; 1993:712-721.
25. White PF, Coe V, Shafer A, et al. Comparison of alfentanil with fentanyl for outpatient anesthesia. *Anesth Analg* 1986;64:99.
26. Bailey PL, Stanley TH. Narcotic intravenous anesthetics. In: Miller RD, ed. *Anesthesia.* 3rd ed. Churchill Livingstone; 1980:281-365.
27. Goresky GV, Koren G, Sabourin MA. The pharmacokinetics of alfentanil in children. *Anesthesiology* 1987;67:654.
28. Meistelman C, Saint-Maurice C, Lepaul M, et al. A comparison of alfentanil pharmacokinetics in children and adults. *Anesthesiology* 1987;66:13.
29. Murphy MR. Clinical pharmacology of alfentanil and sufentanil. *Anesthesiology Rev* 1984;11:17.
30. Nauata J, deLange S, Koopman D, et al. Anesthetic induction with alfentanil: A new short acting narcotic analgesic. *Anesth Analg* 1982;61:267-72.
31. Fragen RJ, Avram MJ. Non-Opioids. In: Barash PG, Cullen BF, Stoelting KK, eds. *Clinical Anesthesia.* Philadelphia, PA: Lippincott; 1989:227-248.
32. Collins VJ. Barbiturate intravenous anesthetic agents. Thiopental. In: *Principles of Anesthesiology: General and Regional Anesthesia.* 3rd ed. Philadelphia: Lea and Febiger; 1993:665-671.
33. Burnett YL. Midazolam preop. effects on sedation, ventilation, and oxygen saturation in higher risk children. *Anesth Analg* 1993;76:S30.
34. Forster A, Gardaz JP, Suter PM. Respiratory depression by midazolam and diazepam. *Anesthesiology* 1980;53:494-497.
35. Payne K, Mattheyse FJ, Dawes T. The pharmacokinetics of midazolam in pediatric patients. *Eur J Clin Pharmacol* 1989;37:267.
36. Twersky RS, Hartung J, Berger BJ. Midazolam enhances anterograde but not retrograde amnesia in pediatric patients. *Anesthesiology* 1993;78:51.
37. Walters BL. Pain control in the emergency department. In: Reisdorff EJ, Roberts and Weigenstein, eds. *Pediatric Emergency Medicine*. Philadelphia: WB Saunders; 1993:908-915.
38. Bailey PL, Moll JWB, Pace NL. Respiratory effects of midazolam and fentanyl: Potent interaction producing hypoxemia and apnea. *Anesthesiology* 1988;169:A813.
39. Forster A, Gardaz JP, Suter PM. Respiratory depression by midazolam and diazepam. *Anesthesiology* 1980;53:494-497.
40. Wright SW, Chudnofsky CR, Dronen SC, et al. Comparison of midazolam and diazepam for conscious sedation in the emergency department. *Ann Emerg Med* 1993;22:201-205.
41. Votey SR, Bosse GM, Bayer MJ, et al: Flumazenil: A new benzodiazepine antagonist. *Ann Emerg Med* 1991;20:181.
42. Anderson BJ, Exarchos H, Lee K, et al. Oral premedication in children: A comparison of chloral hydrate, diazepam, alprazolam, midazolam and placebo for day surgery. *Anaesth Intens Care* 1990;18:185-193.
43. Diament MJ, Stanley P. The use of midazolam for sedation of infants and children. *Am J Roentgenol* 1988;150:377.
44. Feld LH, Negus JB, White PF. Oral midazolam preanesthetic medication in pediatric outpatients. *Anesthesiology* 1990; 73:831.
45. Karl HW, Keifer AT, Rosenberger JL, et al. Comparison of the safety and efficacy of intranasal midazolam or sufentanil for preinduction of anesthesia in pediatric patients. *Anesthesiology* 1992;76:209-215.
46. Karl HW, Rosenberger JL, Larach MG, et al. Transmucosal administration of midazolam for premedication of pediatric patients. *Anesthesiology* 1993;78:885-891.
47. Lejus C, Renaudin M, Testa S. Midazolam for premediciation in children: Intranasal vs. intrarectal administration. *Anesth Analg* 1993;76:S217.
48. Theroux MC, West DW, Corddry DH, et al. Efficacy of intranasal midazolam in facilitating suturing of lacerations in preschool children in the emergency department. *Pediatrics* 1993;91:624-662.
49. Weldon BC, Watcha MF, White PF. Oral midazolam in children: effect of time and adjunctive therapy. *Anesth Analg* 1992;75:51-55.
50. Wilton NC, Leigh J, Rosen DR, et al. Preanesthetic sedation of preschool children using intranasal midazolam. *Anesthesiology* 1988;69:972-975.
51. Blouin RT, Conard PF, Gross JB. Time course of ventilatory depression following induction doses of propofol and thiopental. *Anesthesiology* 1991;75:940-944.

52. Bready R, Spear R, Fisher B, et al. Propofol infusion: Dose response for CT scans in children. *Anesth Analg* 1992;74:S36.
53. Collins VJ. Barbiturate intrvenous anesthetic agents: Thiopental. In: *Principles of Anesthesiology: General and Regional Anesthesia.* 3rd ed. Philadelphia: Lea and Febiger; 1993:665-671.
54. Fragen RJ, Avram MJ. Barbiturates. In: Miller RD, ed. *Anesthesia.* 3rd ed. Churchill Livingstone; 1980:225-243.
55. Collins VJ. Barbiturate intrvenous anesthetic agents: Thiopental. In: *Principles of Anesthesiology: General and Regional Anesthesia.* 3rd ed. Philadelphia: Lea and Febiger; 1993:665-671.
56. O'Brien JF, Falk JL, Carey BE, et al. Rectal thiopental compared with intramuscular meperidine, promethazine, and chlorpromazine for pediatric sedation. *Ann Emerg Med* 1991;20:644-647.
57. Mitchell AA, Louik C, Lacouture P, et al. Risks to children from computed tomographic scan premedication. *JAMA* 1982;247:2385-2388.
58. Kestin IG, McIlvaine WB,Lockhart CH, et al. Rectal methohexital for induction of anaesthesia in children with and without rectal aspiration after sleep: A pharmaconetic and pharmacodynamic study. *Anesth Analg* 1988;67:1102-1104.
59. Khalil SN, Nuutinen LS, Rawal N, et al. Sigmoidorectal methohexital as an inducing agent for general anesthesia in children. *Anesth Analg* 1988;67:S113.
60. Liu LM, Gaudreault P, Friedman PA, et al. Methohexital plasma concentrations in children following rectal administrations. *Anesthesiology* 1985;62:567-570.
61. Liu LM, Goudsouzian NG, Liu PL. Rectal methohexital premedication in children, a dose comparison study. *Anesthesiology* 1980;53:343-345.
62. Zink BJ, Darfler K, Salluzo RF, et al. The efficacy and safety of methohexital in the emergency department. *Ann Emerg Med* 1991;20:1293-1298.
63. Griswold JD, Liu LMP. Rectal methohexital in children undergoing computerized cranial tomography and magnetic resonance imaging scans. *Anesthesiology* 1987;67:A494.
64. Schwanda AE, Freyer DR, Sanfilippo DJ, et al. Brief unconscious sedation for painful pediatric oncology procedures: Intravenous methohexital with appropriate monitoring is safe and effective. *Amer J Ped Hem Onc* 1993;15:370-376.
65. Rockoff M, Goudsouzian NG. Seizures induced by methohexital. *Anesthesiology* 1981;54:333-335.
66. Daniels AL, Cote CJ, Polaner DM. Continuous oxygen saturation monitoring following rectal methohexitone induction in pediatric patients. *Can J Anaesth* 1992;39:27-30.
67. McNeir DA, Mainous EG, Tieger N. Propofol as an intravenous agent in general anesthesia and conscious sedation. *Anesth Prog* 1988;35:147-151.
68. Mirakhur RK. Induction characteristics of propofol in children: Comparison with thiopentone. *Anesthesiology* 1988;43:593-598.
69. White PF. Propofol: Pharmacokinetics and pharmacodynamics. *Semin Anesthesia* 1988;7:4-20.
70. Borgeat A, Wilder-Smith OHG, Saiah M, et al. Subhypnotic doses of propofol possess direct antiemetic properties. *Anesth Analg* 1992;74:539-541.
71. Fragen RJ, Avram MJ. Non-Opioids. In: Barash PG, Cullen BF, Stoelting KK eds. *Clinical Anesthesia.* Philadelphia: Lippincott; 1989:227-248.
72. Hannallah R, Friedfeld S, Verghese P, et al. Comparison of propofol and thiopental for rapid anesthesia induction in infants. *Anesth Analg* 1992;74:S132.
73. Hannallah RS, Baker SB, Casey W, et al. Propofol. Effective dose and induction characteristics in unpremedicated children. *Anesthesiology* 1991;74:217-219.
74. Aun CT, Sung RT, O'Meara ME, et al. Cardiovascular effects of IV induction in children: Comparison between propofol and thiopentone. *Brit J Anaesthesia* 1993;70:647-653.
75. Collins VJ. Intravenous anesthesia: Nonbarbiturates-Non-narcotics In: *Principles of Anesthesiology: General and Regional Anesthesia.* 3rd. Philadelphia: Lea and Febiger; 1993:768-772.
76. Norreslet J, Wahlgreen C. Propofol infusion for sedation of children. *Crit Care Med* 1990;18:890-892.
77. Westrin P. The induction dose of propofol in infants 1-6 months of age and in children 10-16 years of age. *Anesthesiology* 1991:74:455-458.
78. Valtonen M, Lisalo E, Kanto J, et al. Propofol as an induction agent in children: Pain on injection and pharmacokinetics. *Acta Anaesthesiol Scand* 1989;33:152-155.
79. Patel DK, Keeling PA, Newman GB, et al. Induction dose of propofol in children. *Anaesthesia* 1988;43:949-952.
80. Goodman NW, Black AM. Rate of injection of propofol for induction of anesthesia. (Letter) *Anesth Analg* 1992;74: 938-939.
81. Bloomfield EL, Masaryk TJ, Schubert A. Pediatric sedation for MRI of the brain and spine: A comparative study of pentobarbital vs. propofol. *Anesth Analg* 1993;76:S22.
82. Bready R, Spear R, Fisher B, et al. Propofol infusion: Dose response for CT scans in children. *Anesth Analg* 1992;74:S36.
83. Lefever EB, Potter PS, Seeley NR. Propofol sedation for pediatric MRI. *Anesth Analg* 1993;76:919-920.
84. Frankville DD, Spear RM, Dyck JB. The dose of propofol required to prevent children from moving during magnetic resonance imaging. *Anesthesiology* 1993;79:953-958.
85. Kain ZN, Gaal DJ, Kain TS, et al. A first pass cost analysis of propofol versus barbiturates for children undergoing magnetic resonance imaging. *Anesth Analg* 1994;79:1102-1106.
86. Valtonen M. Anaesthesia for computerised tomography of the brain in children: A comparison of propofol and thiopentone. *Acta Anaesthesiol Scand* 1989;33:170-173.
87 Ewah B, Carr C. Comparison of propofol and methohexitone for dental chair anaesthesia in children. *Anaesthesia* 1993;48:260-262.
88. Swanson ER, Seaberg DC, Mathias S. The use of propofol for sedation in the emergency department. *Acad Emerg Med* 1996;3:234-238.
89. Swanson ER, Seaberg DC, Stypula RW, et al. Propofol for conscious sedation: A case series [letter]. *Acad Emerg Med* 1995.2:661-663.
90. Dahlstrom B, Bolme P, Feychting H, et al. Morphine kinetics in children. *Clin Pharmacol Ther* 1979;26:354-365.
91. Lynn AM, Slattery JT. Morphine pharmacokinetics in early

infancy. *Anesthesiology* 1988;66:136-139.

92. Dahl SG. Active metabolites of neuroleptic drugs. Possible contribution to therapeutic and toxic effects. *Therapeutic Drug Monit* 1982;4:33-40.
93. Mather LE, Tucker GT, Pflug AE, et al. Meperidine kinetics in man: Intravenous injection in surgical patients and volunteers. *Clin Pharmacol Ther* 1975;17:21-30.
94. Cook BA, Bass JW, Nomizu S, et al. Sedation of children for technical procedures current standard of practice. *Clin Pediatr* 1992;31:137-142.
95. Hubbard AM, Markowitz Rl, Kimmel B, et al. Sedation for pediatric patients undergoing CT and MRI. *J Comp Assist Tomog* 1992;16:3-6.
96. Keeter S, Benator RM, Weinberg SM, et al. Sedation in pediatric CT: National survey of current practice. *Radiology* 1990;175:745-752.
97. Strain JD, Campbell JB, Harey LA, et al. IV nembutal: Safe sedation for children undergoing CT. *Am J Rad* 1988;151: 975-979.
98. Binder LS, Leake LA. Chloral Hydrate for emergent pediatric procedural sedation: A new look at an old drug. *Am J Emerg Med* 1991;9:530-534.
99. Moody EH Jr, Mourino AP, Campbell RL. The therapeutic effectiveness of nitrous oxide and chloral hydrate administered orally, rectally, and combined with hydroxyzine for pediatric dentistry. *Assoc J Dent Child* 1986;53:425-429.
100. Greenberg SB,Faerber EN, Aspinall CL, et al. High-dose chloral hydrate sedation for children undergoing CT. *J Comput Assist Tom* 1991;15:467-469.
101. Reimche LD, Sankaran K, Hindmarsh KW, et al. Chloral hydrate sedation in neonates and infants: Clinical and pharmacologic considerations. *Dev Pharmacol Ther* 1989;12:57-64.
102. Rumm PD, Takao TR, Fox DJ, et al. Efficacy of sedation of children with chloral hydrate. *South Med J* 1990;83: 1040-1043.
103. Hunt CE, Hazinski TA, Gora P. Experimental effects of chloral hydrate in ventilatory response to hypoxia and hypercarbia. *Pediatr Res* 1982;16:79-81.
104. Keller DA, Heck HD. Mechanistic studies on chloral toxicity: Relationship to trichloroethylene carcinogenesis. *Toxicol Lett* 1988;42:183-191.
105. Smith C, Rowe RD, Vlad P. Sedation of children for cardiac catheterization with an ataractic mixture. *Can Anaes Soc J* 1958;5:35-40.
106. Terndrup TE, Cantor RM, Madden CM. Intramuscular meperidine, promethazine, and chlorpromazine: Analysis of use and complications in 487 pediatric emergency department patients. *Ann Emerg Med* 1989;18:528.
107. Terndrup TE, Dire DJ, Madden CM, et al. A prospective analysis of intramuscular meperidine, promethazine and chlorpromazine in pediatric emergency department patients. *Ann Emerg Med* 1991;20:31.
108. U.S. Department of Health and Human Services: Agency for Health Care Policy and Research. Acute pain management: Operative of medical procedures and trauma. Februrary 1992
109. White PF, Way WL, Trevor AJ. Ketamine—its pharmacology and therapeutic uses. *Anesthesiology* 1982;56:119-136.
110. Green SM, Nakamura R, Johnson NE. Ketamine sedation for pediatric procedures: Part 1, a prospective series. *Ann Emerg Med* 1990;19:1024-1032.
111. Green SM, Nakamura R, Johnson NE. Ketamine sedation for pediatric procedures: Part 2, review and implications. *Ann Emerg Med* 1990;19:1033-1046.
112. Hazma J, Ecoffey C, Gross JB. Ventilatory response to CO_2 following intravenous ketamine in children. *Anesthesiology* 1989;70:422-425.
113. Morgan M, Loh L, Singer L. Ketamine as the sole anaesthetic agent for minor surgical procedures. *Anaesthesia* 1971;26: 158-165.
114. Bragg CL, Miller BR. Oral ketamine facilitates induction in a combative mentally retarded patlent. *J Can Anesth* 1990;2: 121-122.
115. Gutstein HB, Iohnson KL, Heard MB, et al. Oral ketamine preanesthetic medication in children. *Anesthesiology* 1992;76:28-33.
116. Warner DL, Cabaret J, Velling D. Ketamine plus midazolam—a most effective paediatric oral premedicant. *Paediatric Anaesthesia* 1995;5:293-295.
117. Alderson PJ, Lerman J. Oral premedication for paediatric ambulatory anaesthesia:A comparison of midazolam and ketamine. *Can J Anaesth* 1994;41:3:221-226.
118. Roelofse JA, Joubert JJ, Roelofse PG. A double-blind randomized comparison of midazolam alone and midazolam combined with ketamine for sedation of pediatric dental patients. *J Oral Maxillofac Surg* 1996;54:838-844.
119. Van der Bijl P, Roelofse JA. Rectal ketamine and midazolam for premedication in pediatric dentistry. *J Oral Maxillofac Surg* 1991;49:1050.
120. Louon A, Reddy VG. Nasal midazolam and ketamine for paediatric sedation during computerized tomography. *Acta Anaesthesiologica Scandinavica* 1994;38:259-260.
121. Aldrete JA, Roman de Jesus JC, Russell LJ. Intranasal ketamine as induction adjunct in children: Preliminary report. *Anesthesiology* 1987;67:514.
122 Petrack EM, Marx CM, Wright MS. Intramuscular ketamine is superior to meperidine, promethazine and chlorpromazine for pediatric emergency department sedation. *Arch Pediatri Adolesc Med* 1996;150:676-681.
123. Green SM, CLem KJ, Rothrock SG. Ketamine safety profile in the developing world: Survey of practitioners. *Acad Emerg Med* 1996;3:598-604.
124. Dula DJ. Nitrous oxide analgesia. In: Roberts JR, Hedges JR, eds. *Clinical Procedures in Emergency Medicine.* 2nd ed. Philadelphia: WB Saunders Co.; 1991:508-514.
125. Gamis AS, Knapp JF, Glenski JA. Nitrous oxide analgesia in a pediatric emergency department. *Ann Emerg Med* 1989;8:177-181.
126. McKinnon K. Pre-hospital analgesia with nitrous oxide/oxygen. *Can Med Assoc J* 1982;125:836-840.
127. Muir JJ, Warner M, Offord K. Role of nitrous oxide and other factors in postoperative nausea and vomiting. *Anesthesiology* 1987;66:513-518.
128. Evans JK, Buckley SL, Alexander AH, et al. Analgesia for the reduction of fractures in children: A comparison of nitrous oxide with intramuscular sedation. *J Ped Orthoped* 1995;15:73-77.

129. Hennrikus WL, Shin AY, Klingelberger CE. Self administered nitrous oxide and a hematoma block for analgesia in the outpatient reduction of fractures in children. *J Bone Joint Surg* 1995;77A:335-339.
130. Schutzman SA, Burg J, Liebelt E. Oral transmucosal fentanyl citrate for premedication of children undergoing laceration repair. *Ann Emerg Med* 1994;24:1059-1064.
131. Ashburn MA, Lind GH, Gillie MH, et al. Oral transmucosal fentanyl citrate (OTFC) for the treatment of postoperative pain. *Anesth Analg* 1993;76:377.
132. Feld LH, Champeau MW, van Steennis CA, et al. Preanesthetic medication in children: A comparison of oral transmucosal fentanyl citrate vs. placebo. *Anesthes* 1989;71:374.
133. Friesen RH, Lockhart CH. Oral transmucosal fentanyl citrate for preanesthetic medication of pedatric day surgery patients with and without droperidol as a prophylactic anti-emetic. *Anesthesiology* 1992;76:46-51.
134. Lind GH, Marcus MA, Mears SL. Oral transmucosal fentanyl citrate for analgesia and sedation in the emergency department. *Ann Emerg Med* 1991;20:1117.
135. Neslon PS, Streisand JB, Mulder SM, et al. Comparison of oral transmucosal fentanyl citrate and an oral solution of meperidine, diazepam, and atropine for premedication in children. *Anesthes* 1989;70:616.
136. Streisand JB, Stanley TH, Hague B, et al. Oral transmucosal fentanyl citrate premedi cation in children. *Anesth Analg* 1989;69:28-34.
137. Streisand JB, Varvel JR, Stanski DR, et al. Absorption and bioavailability of oral transmucosal fentanyl citrate. *Anesthesiology* 1991;75:223.
138. Brocks DR, Jamali F. Clinical pharmacokinetics of ketorolac tromethamine. *Clin Pharmacokinet* 1992;23:415-427.
139. Maunuksela EL, Kokki H, Bullingham RE. Comparison of intravenous ketorolac with morphine for postoperative pain in children. *Clin Pharmacol Ther* 1992;52:436-443.
140. Powell H, Smallman JM, Morgan M. Comparison of intramuscular ketorolac and morphine in pain control after laparotomy. *Anaesthesia* 1990;45:538-542.
141. Sevarino FB, Sinatra RS, Paige D, et al. The efficacy of intramuscular ketorolac in combination with intravenous PCA morphine for postoperative pain relief. *J Clin Anesth* 1992; 4:285-288.
142. Watcha MF, Ramirez-Ruiz M, White PF, et al. Perioperative effects of oral ketorolac and acetaminophen in children undergoing bilateral myringotomy. *Can J Anaesth* 1992;39: 641-642.
143. Yee JP, Koshiver JE, Allbon C, et al. Comparison of intramuscular ketorolac tromethamine and morphine sulfate for analgesia of pain after major surgery. *Pharmacotherapy* 1986;6:253-261.
144. Buck ML. Clinical experience with ketorolac in children. *Ann Pharmacother* 1994;28:1009-1013.
145. Sutters KA, Levine JD, Dibble S, et al. Analgesic efficacy and safety of single dose intramuscular ketorolac for postoperative pain management in children following tonsillectomy. *Pain* 1995;61:145-153.
146. Mendel HG, Guarnieri KM, Sundt LM, et al. The effects of ketorolac and fentanyl on postoperative vomiting and analgesic requirements in children undergoing strabismus surgery. *Anesth Analg* 1995;80:1129-1133.
147. Maunuksela E, Kokki H, Bullingham RES. Comparison of intravenous ketorolac with morphine for postoperative pain in children. *Clin Pharmacol Ther* 1992;52;436-443.
148. Horswell JL. Bleeding diathesis after perioperative ketorolac. *Anesth Analg* 1992;74:168-169.
148. Rotenberg FA, Giannini VS. Hyperkalemia associated with ketorolac. *Ann Pharmacother* 1992;26:778-779.
150. Schoch PH, Ranno A, North DS. Acute renal failure in an elderly woman following intramuscular ketorolac administration. *Ann Pharmacother* 1992;26:1233-1236.
151. Steinberg RB, Tessier EG. Gastrointestinal bleeding after administration of ketorolac (letter). *Anesthiology* 1993; 5:1146.
152. Zikowski D, Hord AH, Haddox JD, et al. Ketorolac-induced bronchospasm *Anesth Analg* 1993;76:417-419.
153. Chez MG, Soglin D. Ketorolac tromethamine (Toradol) treatment in children with acute migraine (abstract). *Ann Neurol* 1991;30:494.
154. Watcha F, Ramirez-Ruiz M, White PF, et al. Perioperative effects of oral ketorolac and acetominophen in children undergoing bilateral myringotomy. *Can J Anaesth* 1992;39:649-654.
155. Watcha F, Jones B, Lagueruela RG, et al. Comparison of ketorolac and morphine as adjuvants during pediatric surgery. *Anesthesiology* 1992;76:368-372.
156. Olkkola KT, Maunuksela EL. The pharmacokinetics of postoperative intravenous ketorolac tromethamine in children. *Br J Clin Pharmacol* 1991;31:182-184.
157. Oosterlinck W, Philp NH, Charig C, et al. A double blind single dose comparison of intramuscular ketorolac tromethamine and pethidine in the treatment of renal colic. *J Clin Pharmacol* 1990;30:336-341.
158. Schwesinger WH, Reynolds JC, Harshaw DH, et al. Transnasal butorphanol and intramuscular meperidine in the treatment of postoperative pain. *Adv Therapy* 1992;9: 123-129.
159. Diamond S, Freitag FG, Diamond ML, et al. Transnasal butorphanol in the treatment of migraine headache pain. *Headache Quarterly* 1992;3:164-171.
160. Wetchler BW, Alexander CD, Uhll MA. Transnasal butorphanol tartrate for pain control following ambulatory surgery. *Curr Therap Res* 1992;52:571-580.
161. Tobias JD, Rasmussen GE. Transnasal butorphanol for postoperative analgesia following paediatric surgery in a third world country. *Paediatric Anaesth* 1995;5:63-66.

Acute Respiratory Failure

Sharon E. Mace, MD, FACEP, FAAP

Respiratory diseases are a common problem encountered by physicians who treat pediatric patients.[1] Respiratory disorders account for one out of five pediatric hospital admissions and about 10% of pediatric emergency department p(ED) visits.[2] Respiratory disorders also are a major cause of pediatric mortality.[1,3] About one-half of all deaths in patients younger than age 1 and more than one-third of the deaths in children younger than age 15 are due to pulmonary diseases.[2]

Introduction

Respiratory failure is the inability of the respiratory system to provide adequate oxygen to meet the body's metabolic requirements and/or to excrete the carbon dioxide produced by the body.

There are many disorders, both within the respiratory tract and outside the pulmonary system, that can cause respiratory failure.[4] *(See Table 1.)* Exchange of gases occurs in the pulmonary capillary bed. Failure of the respiratory system to deliver adequate oxygen to the tissues causes hypoxia, and failure to excrete carbon dioxide results in hypercapnia.[5]

Respiratory System: Anatomy

The respiratory system can be conceptualized as a pump consisting of the nervous system (central nervous system [CNS], spinal nerves, peripheral nerves, and the neuromuscular junction); the effector components (the respiratory muscles and chest wall); the conducting airways; and the air exchange system in the alveoli. The pump drives the system, and the respiratory muscles and chest wall do the work of breathing. The conducting airways are the conduit for movement of air from the atmosphere to the alveoli.[6] The alveoli are where actual diffusion of gases occurs. The nervous system regulates respiration. Failure of the respiratory pump leads to hypercapnia, while alveolar disorders primarily cause hypoxemia.[6]

Respiratory Physiology: Process of Oxygenation

Multiple steps are needed to provide sufficient oxygen for the cells to maintain aerobic metabolism and to remove carbon dioxide, which is important in maintaining the body's pH via the bicarbonate buffer system.

The first step in the process is ventilation, which is the movement of gases between the environment and the lungs,[7] followed by intrapulmonary gas exchange.[8] Diffusion of oxygen and carbon dioxide across the pulmonary capillary membrane occurs, allowing mixed venous blood to release carbon dioxide to the lungs and then pick up oxygen. This is followed by gas transport, in which adequate amounts of oxygenated blood are transported to the tissues and cells

Table 1. Causes of Respiratory Failure by Clinical Pathway or Organ System

NEUROLOGIC DISORDERS
- Central nervous system (control abnormalities with a decreased respiratory drive)
- Spinal nerve pathways
- Peripheral nerves
- Neuromuscular junction

RESPIRATORY MUSCLE DISORDERS
- Primary muscle disorders (decreased ability of muscles)
- Respiratory muscle fatigue (resulting from increased work of breathing)

PULMONARY DISORDERS
- Airway disorders (interference with ventilation), airway obstruction
- Alveolar (parenchymal) diseases

CHEST WALL/PLEURA ABNORMALITIES
- Chest wall disorders (decreased chest wall compliance): flail chest
- Ruptured pleural space (limited movement of lungs): pneumothorax, pleural effusion

CARDIOVASCULAR DISORDERS
- Shock (interferes with oxygen/carbon dioxide transports by inadequate blood flow)

HEMATOLOGIC DISORDERS
(Interferes with oxygen transport by red blood cells)
- Severe anemia
- Abnormal hemoglobins

METABOLIC DISORDERS
- Severe metabolic acidosis
- Increased metabolic rate: burns, fever, infection, sepsis
- Abnormal respiratory quotient
- Abnormal cellular oxygen uptake: cyanide poisoning

for aerobic metabolism, and carbon dioxide is transported to the lungs for excretion.[9] Finally, tissue/cellular gas exchange occurs in which oxygen is taken up and used by the tissues, and carbon dioxide is released. These processes are controlled by CNS regulation of respiration in the brainstem.

Thus, respiratory failure may involve a failure of oxygenation, a failure of ventilation, or both.[10] Furthermore, failure of oxygenation can result from non-pulmonary factors, including: cardiogenic shock, severe anemia, abnormal hemoglobins (such as methemoglobinemia), an abnormal oxygen carrying capacity (as with carbon monoxide poisoning), or a failure of cellular oxygen uptake (e.g., cyanide poisoning or septic shock).[10]

Classification

Respiratory failure is classified according to the pCO_2 level. Type I failure, also known as normocapnic or non-ventilatory failure, is

Table 2. Causes of Hypoxemia (Type I) Normocapnic Respiratory Failure*

VENTILATION/PERFUSION (V/Q) ABNORMALITIES
Pulmonary edema, meconium aspiration, pneumonia

SHUNTING
Cyanotic congenital heart disease: right to left shunts (ventricular septal defect, endocardial cushion defect) Intrapulmonary shunts: alveoli are ventilated but not perfused (pneumonia, ARDS)

DIFFUSION ABNORMALITIES
Interstitial fibrosis

INADEQUATE SYSTEMIC BLOOD FLOW
Inadequate cardiac output: shock, cardiomyopathy

INADEQUATE OXYGEN CARRYING CAPACITY
Abnormal hemoglobin (methemoglobinemia, cyanide poisoning), severe anemia

INADEQUATE CELLULAR UPTAKE/UTILIZATION OF OXYGEN
Cyanide poisoning

** This is not an inclusive list. Some disorders are included in each group.*

indicated by hypoxemia (low pO_2) with a normal or low pCO_2. An elevated pCO_2 is the hallmark of Type II failure, also known as ventilatory or hypercapnic failure. A variable degree of hypoxemia also is present with this type.[6]

Type I (normocapnic, non-ventilatory) respiratory failure is commonly due to ventilation/perfusion (V/Q) abnormalities. Other causes of Type I respiratory failure include: impaired diffusion across the alveolar-capillary membrane (as occurs with pulmonary fibrosis) and shunting.[11] *(See Table 2.)*

Type II (hypercapnic) respiratory failure generally is the result of alveolar hypoventilation, increased dead space ventilation, or increased CO_2 production. Factors that impair the central ventilatory drive in the brainstem, restrict ventilation, or increase CO_2 production can cause hypercapnic (Type II) respiratory failure.[11] *(See Table 3.)*

Case No. 1

A 16-year-old male arrives in the ED. No other history is available because the friends who brought him to the ED left.

The vital signs are:
- Temperature (T) = 96°F;
- Pulse (P) = 90 beats/min;
- Respiratory rate (R) = 6 breaths/min;
- Blood pressure (BP) =120/80 mmHg; and
- Pulse oxygen saturation is 76% on room air.

Arterial blood gas (ABG) is: pH = 7.13; pO_2 = 52; pCO_2 = 81; HCO_3 = 26; and oxygen saturation = 75% on room air.

He is unresponsive to painful stimuli, and his pupils are pinpoint. His respirations are shallow. The lungs are clear, and the heart rate is

Table 3. Causes of Hypercapnic (Type II) Respiratory Failure: Hypoxemia (Low PO_2) with Hypercapnia (High PO_2)

ALVEOLAR HYPOVENTILATION

NEUROLOGIC DISORDERS

- Central nervous system inhibition (control abnormalities)
  - Coma
  - Overdose
  - CNS disease
- Spinal/anterior horn cell disorders
  - Cervical spinal cord trauma
  - Myelitis
- Peripheral nerve disease
  - Guillian-Barré
- Neuromuscular junction disorders
  - Myasthenia gravis
  - Paralytic drugs

RESPIRATORY MUSCLE DISORDERS

- Respiratory muscle failure
  - Primary muscle diseases (i.e., muscular dystrophy, poliomyelitis)
- Respiratory muscle fatigue (i.e., excessive work of breathing)

CHEST WALL/PLEURA DISORDERS

- Decreased chest wall compliance
  - Flail chest
  - Diaphragmatic hernia
  - Severe kyphoscoliosis
- Disrupted pleural space
  - Limited movement of lungs: pneumothorax, hemothorax, pleural effusion

AIRWAY DISORDERS

- Upper airway obstruction:
  - Foreign body
  - Edema
  - Infection (croup, laryngotracheobronchitis, epiglottitis, retropharyngeal abscess)
  - Congenital web
  - Subglottic stenosis
  - Tracheomalacia
- Lower airway obstruction (edema, foreign body, tracheobronchomalacia, tumor)

PULMONARY DISEASES

- Increased airway resistance
  - Bronchiolitis, asthma
- Decreased lung compliance
  - Fibrosis, pulmonary edema, vasculardiseases (polyarteritis), interstitial disease (sarcoidosis)
- Ventilation/perfusion (V/Q) abnormalities:
  - Pneumonia
- Increased dead space ventilation
  - Alveoli overdistention
  - Asthma, COPD
- Decreased pulmonary blood flow
  - Severe pulmonic stenosis, pulmonary hypertension

INCREASED CARBON DIOXIDE PRODUCTION

- Increased metabolic rate
  - Infection
  - Sepsis
  - Fever
  - Burns
- Abnormal respiratory exchange quotient

regular. There are needle tract marks on his arms but no signs of trauma. He has a depressed level of consciousness but no focal neurologic findings.

This patient has hypercapnia and hypoxia due to alveolar hypoventilation, resulting in Type II hypercapnic respiratory failure secondary to a control abnormality with a decreased respiratory drive. Of the physiologic events in respiration, diffusion, transport, and the tissue/cellular uptake of oxygen are normal, but ventilation is impaired. His hypoxia and hypercapnia are due to a non-pulmonary mechanism with a narcotic drug (e.g., heroin) overdose depressing his respiratory drive.

He has some signs of respiratory distress, including: abnormal respirations with a decreased tidal volume evidenced by shallow respirations (decreased depth), decreased rate (bradypnea, R = 6 breaths/min), and pattern (apneic at times). He does not have signs of air hunger and increased respiratory effort. He meets the criteria for acute respiratory failure (ARF). *(See Table 4.)* He is given supplemental oxygen, and his ventilations are assisted while other therapy, including naloxone, is given. After observation in the ED, the overdose wears off, and he becomes progressively more alert.

Causes of Respiratory Failure

The etiology of respiratory failure is more diverse than just lung or airway disorders. Respiratory failure can occur from an abnormality in any component of the respiratory system from the CNS to the pulmonary capillary bed where gas exchange occurs,[14] and to the tissues and cells where cellular uptake and utilization of oxygen occur. Nervous system disorders (from the respiratory control center in the medulla and pons via the spinal nerve pathways to the peripheral nerves and the neuromuscular junction), chest wall/pleura disorders, airway disease (e.g., obstruction), pulmonary diseases, and even cellular uptake/utilization disorders all can lead to respiratory failure.

CNS disorders that lead to respiratory failure are control abnormalities that cause Type II (hypercapnic) respiratory failure and usually present without signs and symptoms of respiratory distress (such as dyspnea, retractions, or tachypnea).[15] Common causes of respiratory failure from CNS disorders include: drug overdoses; anesthesia; sedation; seizures; and CNS infections, injuries, and malformations (i.e., meningitis, encephalitis, brain abscesses, congenital malformations, encephalopathy, ischemia, infarcts, tumors, and trauma). These disorders all exert their effect by depressing the respiratory center in the brainstem.

Disorders of the upper motor neurons or spinal nerves also can cause Type II hypercapnic respiratory failure.[16] This may occur with several disorders, including: cervical spinal cord trauma, demyelinating diseases, myelitis (poliomyelitis, transverse myelitis), and Werdnig-Hoffman syndrome. Diseases of the peripheral nerves (i.e., Guillain-Barré syndrome, post-thoracotomy phrenic nerve damage, or a peripheral neuropathy) also can lead to hypercapnic respiratory failure.

Diseases affecting the neuromuscular junction may cause hypercapnic respiratory failure. These diseases include: myasthenia gravis, botulism, tetanus, organophosphate poisoning, and neuromuscular

Table 4. Criteria for Acute Respiratory Failure

CLINICAL FINDINGS OF ACUTE RESPIRATORY DISTRESS (IMPENDING RESPIRATORY FAILURE)

- **Laboratory parameters**
  - Hypoxemia
  - $PaO_2 < 50\text{-}60$ mmHg
  - $SaO_2 < 90\%$
  - PaO_2/FiO_2 ratio < 300
  - $PaO_2 < 60$ mmHg on $FiO_2 > 40$
- **Hypercapnia**
  - $pCO_2 > 55$
  - $pCO_2 > 50$ with acidosis ($pH < 7.25$)
  - $pCO_2 > 40$ with severe distress
- **Pulmonary function parameters**
  - Vital capacity < 15 mL/kg
  - Maximum inspiratory force (pressure) < 20-25 cmH_20
  - VD/VT = Dead space/tidal volume > 0.60

blocking drugs/anesthetics (i.e., pancuronium and succinylcholine). Fatigue of the respiratory muscles also can lead to ARF.[17,18]

Chest wall/pleura disorders lead to respiratory failure by decreasing chest wall compliance, as with flail chest, severe kyphoscoliosis, congenital or genetic deformities of the chest (e.g., severe dwarfism), or by disruption of the pleural space (e.g., pneumothorax or pleural effusion).[19] These disorders cause respiratory failure by mechanical abnormalities and decreased alveolar ventilation, which result in hypercapnia.

Airway obstruction causes increased airway resistance.[3] Airway obstruction can be in the upper airway (e.g., above the vocal cords) or in the lower airway from the larynx distally. The upper airway includes the nose, paranasal sinuses, and the pharynx. The lower airway includes the larynx, bronchi, bronchioles, and the alveoli. Obstruction in children is commonly due to foreign bodies, or infection, and infrequently due to congenital abnormalities such as a laryngeal web or tracheomalacia. Causes of upper airway obstruction include:

- Foreign bodies;
- Infections (epiglottitis, retropharyngeal abscess, or croup);
- Edema (as with anaphylaxis or laryngoedema);
- Congenital defects (web, stenosis, tracheomalacia, etc.);
- Tumors;
- Adenotonsilar hypertrophy; and
- Subglottic stenosis.

Lower airway obstructions include similar etiologies as with upper airway obstruction (e.g. foreign body, edema, congenital defects, and infections), but also reactive airway disease (asthma and bronchiolitis) secondary to bronchospasm.

In children, respiratory failure most often is due to diseases of the lungs.[15] Pulmonary diseases include: pneumonia, near drowning, adult respiratory distress syndrome (ARDS), pneumonitis, vasculitis, pulmonary edema, cystic fibrosis, and tuberculosis. Respiratory failure also may be caused by control abnormalities or by abnormalities in the mechanical function of the lungs. Control abnormalities are the result of decreased respiratory drive and, thus, there are few or no signs of respiratory distress even when there is significant hypercapnia and/or hypoxemia.

Respiratory failure caused by abnormalities in the mechanical function of the lungs and/or chest wall generally raise the ventilatory requirements and increase the work of breathing so the patient has to expend more physical effort to breathe. The patient will have air hunger; complain of dyspnea (secondary to chemoreceptor stimulation); and have an increased respiratory drive with physical signs and symptoms of respiratory distress such as tachypnea, retractions, etc. In children, respiratory failure more commonly is caused by mechanical abnormalities than by control abnormalities.[11]

Case No. 2

An 8-year-old male with muscular dystrophy is seen in his pediatrician's office because of increasing weakness. He is referred by his primary care physician to the ED for evaluation. The parents tell you that everyone in the family, including his sisters, had colds recently.

You observe a boy, who is thin and small for his age, sitting in a wheelchair. The parents tell you he usually walks with assistance but has been too weak to do so for the last day. The child nods appropriately but can speak only one or two syllables at a time, although he usually can talk in full sentences. His speech is slurred.

His vital signs are:

- T = 100.2°F;
- P = 120 beats/min;
- R = 12 breaths/min; and
- BP = 100/70 mmHg; and
- Weight = 20 kg.

A head, ears, eyes, nose, and throat (HEENT) examination reveals rhinorrhea and excessive secretions in the oropharynx. There are scattered rhonchi in the lungs bilaterally. The abdomen is benign. There is no peripheral edema or cyanosis. The neurologic exam is consistent with his diagnosis of muscular dystrophy with muscle weakness.

The respiratory therapist tells you that his maximum inspiratory pressure is 10 cm H_2O, and his vital capacity is 160 cc. Based on these pulmonary function parameters (see Table 4), you diagnose respiratory insufficiency with acute exacerbation of muscle weakness from an upper respiratory infection (URI) in a patient with chronically impaired muscle function secondary to his muscular dystrophy. Other tests confirm your diagnosis. A chest roentgenogram shows areas of plate-like atelectasis.

The ABG is: pH = 7.17; pO_2 = 46; pCO_2 = 78; HCO_3 = 32; and O_2 saturation = 71% on room air. You place him on BiPAP and admit him to the pediatric intensive care unit (PICU) for observation.

This patient has Type II hypercapnic respiratory failure secondary to failure of the respiratory muscles from a primary muscle disorder. He may be able to maintain himself in mild respiratory acidosis with a partially compensated metabolic alkalosis (as noted by the mildly increased bicarbonate) until an acute exacerbation (caused by the URI) weakens his already limited muscle strength and sends him into ARF with a rising pCO_2 and respiratory acidosis.

BiPAP is a reasonable therapy for the patient since he is awake and cooperative. BiPAP has been used in children as young as age 4, although most pediatric patients on BiPAP are older than age 5.

Signs and Symptoms of Respiratory Distress

History. The parents or caregivers of an infant or child who is having respiratory difficulty may report a decreased level of activity (i.e., not playing, not feeding, "not acting right") and a change in mental status (i.e., lethargy, listless, somnolent, restless, agitated, sleepy). Excessive sleepiness or somnolescence may occur with a pCO_2 of more than 45 mmHg and restlessness from hypoxia may occur at a PO_2 of less than 75 mmHg. Older children or adolescents also may report shortness of breath or dyspnea. The older child or adolescent may complain of a headache. Dilatation of the cerebral blood vessels from acute hypoxemia and hypercapnia is responsible for the headache symptoms.

Depending on the etiology of the respiratory failure, there may be a history of a foreign body ingestion, a previous URI, or another infection. The parents may mention noisy breathing or wheezing. They may relate the presence of a fever, cough, sputum, or hemoptysis. The patient may be tired or fatigued due to the increased work of breathing.

Physical Examination

The patient may be confused, combative, restless, irritable, somnolent, lethargic, unresponsive, or comatose. The patient may have assumed a certain posture in an attempt to maintain an open airway or to help decrease the work of breathing. A child who is sitting up and leaning forward in the tripod position is attempting to keep his/her airway open. Drooling, which indicates an inability to swallow one's saliva, can occur with upper airway obstruction or can be caused by a foreign body, or an infection such as epiglottitis or a retropharyngeal abscess.

The vital signs will be abnormal if significant respiratory distress is present. Tachycardia and tachypnea are usual. Bradycardia and bradypnea are ominous signs of impending respiratory failure and/or cardiopulmonary arrest. Hypertension and diaphoresis reflect the body's attempt to compensate by the adrenergic "flight or fight" response. Hypotension suggests significant dehydration or shock. If an infection is the underlying cause of the respiratory failure, then fever may be present, although hypothermia also can occur.

Increased work of breathing is reflected by: intercostal retractions, use of accessory muscles in the neck, flaring of the alae nasi, "see-saw" respirations, paradoxical breathing, abdominal breathing, head bobbing (especially in infants), and pursed lips.[12,13]

Noisy, abnormal respiratory sounds, from audible wheezing to stridor, or crowing or gurgling sounds may be present. Inspiratory stridor indicates obstruction in the upper airway, while prolonged expiration with wheezing is due to lower airway obstruction at the bronchial or bronchiolar level. Stridor may be due to infection (epiglottitis, retropharyngeal abscess, or laryngotracheobronchitis), foreign body aspiration, congenital anomalies (i.e, laryngeal web and vocal cord cyst), or laryngomalacia. Wheezing usually occurs with asthma and bronchiolitis. Expiratory grunting is an attempt to increase airway pressure, thereby maintaining or increasing the functional residual capacity. In early inspiration, premature closure of the glottis, along with active contraction of the chest wall, results in grunting.

The rate (tachypnea, normal, or bradypnea), depth (shallow vs deep), and pattern (irregular, apnea, etc.) of respiration should be noted. Respiratory alternans may be present. Cyanosis is a late sign of respiratory failure. The percentage of desaturated hemoglobin in the blood determines whether cyanosis is present. Weak, thready pulses and delayed capillary fill of the skin suggest decreased peripheral perfusion and shock.

Observation of the chest may reveal an abnormal shape, appearance, or asymmetrical movement. Lung auscultation may detect rales, rhonchi, wheezing, and/or prolonged expiration. Fremitus and dullness to percussion are suggestive of consolidation as with pneumonia. Hyperresonance to percussion with decreased breath sounds is consistent with a pneumothorax.

Physical examination may reveal disorders that increase the risk for respiratory failure (see Table 5) or an underlying etiology for ARF.

Case No. 3

A 4-month-old female who is having trouble breathing is brought into the ED by her mother. She has had a cold for several days. Today she developed a fever, cough, and breathing difficulties.

Neonatal history is significant for prematurity (30 weeks), which was complicated by respiratory distress syndrome requiring a ventilator for two weeks and supplemental oxygen for an additional five weeks. She also had a congenital gastrointestinal problem requiring surgery at 6 weeks of age and has continued to have gastrointestinal problems. She has bronchopulmonary dysplasia and has not received the immunization for respiratory syncytial virus.

Her vital signs are:

- T = 103.5° F;
- P = 190 beats/min;
- R = 64 breaths/min;
- BP = 80/50 mmHg; and
- Pulse oxygen saturation = 82% in room air.

She is small for her age. The infant is in marked respiratory distress with retractions, grunting, flaring, head bobbing, abdominal respirations, and the use of accessory muscles for respiration. Her skin is pale, sweaty, and cyanotic with delayed capillary fill. There are rales in both lung fields. The chest roentgenogram shows diffuse bilateral infiltrates.

The ABG on room air is: pH = 7.61; pO_2 = 56; pCO_2 = 24; HCO_3 = 27; and oxygen saturation is 78%.

This infant has multiple risk factors for ARF: prematurity with bronchopulmonary dysplasia, congenital anomalies, gastrointestinal disorder (with the potential for aspiration), malnutrition with failure to thrive, and her young age (infants have less pulmonary reserve and impaired immunologic capability compared to older children and adults).

She also has all the classic signs of air hunger and is struggling to breathe with increased work of breathing. She has respiratory failure due to pulmonary disease from an alveolar parenchymal disorder. Due to her pneumonia, she has V/Q abnormalities from collapsed alveoli that are perfused but not ventilated (and fail to pick up oxygen), creating an intrapulmonary right to left shunt. She has Type I respiratory failure characterized by hypoxia with low pCO_2. In this case, her CO_2 is low because she is compensating with increased work of breathing and tachypnea.

The cause of her hypoxia by mechanism includes V/Q abnormalities and intrapulmonary shunting. She has numerous criteria for

Table 5. Patients at High Risk for Acute Respiratory Failure

PRE-EXISTING DISORDERS
- Pre-existing pulmonary disease (Cystic fibrosis, bronchopulmonary dysplasia, etc.)
- Congenital cardiovascular disease
- Immunocompromised state (Malignancy, immunosuppression, HIV, etc.)
- Genetic and/or congenital defects

CO-EXISTENT DISEASE STATES
- Coma
- Shock
- Multiple organ system dysfunction (i.e., hypoxic-ischemic encephalopathy)
- Hypermetabolic states (i.e., thyroid storm)

CO-EXISTENT STRESSFUL CONDITIONS
- Multiple trauma
- Central nervous system trauma
- Postoperative (following major surgery)
- Post anesthesia (following general anesthesia)
- Post sedation (following general sedation)

HOST FACTORS
- Malnutrition
- Extremes of age (infants, geriatric patients)

ARF, including acute respiratory distress and laboratory parameters of hypoxemia. She has multiple indications for intubation (see Table 6), including: hypoxia, respiratory distress and need for special therapy; prolonged ventilation (until her pneumonia improves) and need for pulmonary care (suctioning, etc.); and delivery of positive end expiratory pressure (PEEP) to open her collapsed alveoli.

Diagnosis of Respiratory Failure

Respiratory failure can be determined by clinical, laboratory (e.g., ABG), and pulmonary function parameters.

Classically, the hallmark of respiratory failure is hypoxemia and/or hypercapnia.[20] Hypoxia is a decreased amount of oxygen supplied to or utilized by the body's tissues and cells, while hypoxemia refers to a decreased amount of oxygen in the blood or less than the physiologically normal amount of oxygen in the blood.

Normal ABG values are: pO_2 of 80-100 mmHg; pCO_2 of 35-45 mmHg; pH of 7.35-7.45; and SaO_2 of 95-100%. Hypoxemia is any value less than normal for the PO_2 and/or oxygen saturation. The arterial pO_2 in healthy young adults is usually 95-100 mmHg, although some healthy young adults have an arterial pO_2 of 80-90 mmHg. Therefore, the accepted range of normal for arterial pO_2 varies, and some allow a value as low as 80 for a normal pO_2.

Another commonly used method for evaluating oxygenation is the alveolar-arterial oxygen gradient:

$PAO_2 - PaO_2 = P(A\text{-}a)O_2$.

The alveolar-arterial difference (PAO_2-PaO_2) is normally less than 15 mmHg. In a person breathing room air at sea level, the alveolar PO_2 or PAO_2 can be calculated by subtracting the arterial pCO_2 measured in the blood from 150 (PAO_2 = 150-pCO_2) where there is a normal pCO_2 of 40 (the PAO_2 = 150- 40 = 110 mmHg). In patients given supplemental oxygen, a rough approximation of the expected or normal alveolar pO_2 is calculated by multiplying the actual delivered percentage of oxygen by 6. In a patient receiving 100% oxygen, the PAO_2 would equal 600 (100 × 6), while the PAO_2 would equal 360 (60 × 6) in a patient receiving 60% oxygen.

The PaO_2/FiO_2 ratio is yet another method for estimating the oxygenation. The normal PaO_2/FiO_2 ratio is 500-600, which is the arterial pO_2 measured in the blood divided by the fraction of inspired oxygen. This ratio is then used to determine the amount of shunting in the lungs.

The shunt (Qs/QT) represents the fraction of blood that passes through the lung without being oxygenated. The normal amount of physiologic shunting in the lung (also known as venous admixture) is 2-3% and represents the small amount of blood in the bronchial veins that drains into the pulmonary veins and the thebesian veins, which drain into the left atrium.

There are several variables that affect the arterial PO_2 or PaO_2. These are: the concentration or fraction of oxygen in the inspired gases (FiO_2), the amount of alveolar ventilation, the oxyhemoglobin dissociation curve, and the functional capability of the lungs.

The FiO_2 when breathing room air is 21% (or .21), and the addition of supplemental oxygen can increase the FiO_2 up to 100% (or 1.0). At a given FiO_2, the PaO_2 changes with the altitude or height above sea level. The higher the altitude, the lower the PO_2 in the air. For each 10,000-foot increase above sea level, the PaO_2 decreases approximately 3-4 mmHg.

The patient's age also affects pulmonary function. The normal PaO_2 is lower at the extremes of age. A normal, healthy older infant, child, or young adult has an arterial PO_2 of 80-100 mmHg, while a newborn has an arterial PO_2 of 60-90 mmHg. An 80-year-old has an arterial PO_2 of 75-80 mmHg. After age 30, the PaO_2 decreases by approximately 3-4 mmHg in each decade.

The generally accepted values of hypoxemia that define ARF are: PaO_2 less than 50-60 mmHg; SaO_2 less than 90%; PaO_2 less than 60 mmHg on FiO_2 = 40% or PaO_2/ FiO_2 less than 300.

Hypercapnia or hypercarbia is an elevated level of carbon dioxide in the blood. ARF is indicated by the following pCO_2 values: pCO_2 higher than 50 with acidosis (pH < 7.25) or pCO_2 higher than 40 with severe distress, or pCO_2 higher than 55. This assumes that there are no pre-existing pulmonary disorders, such as cystic fibrosis, which cause chronic retention of carbon dioxide. Pulmonary function abnormalities consistent with ARF are: vital capacity less than 15 mL/kg or inspiratory pressure less than 25-30 cmH_20.

ABGs should be interpreted in a clinical setting.[11,20] For example, in a child with an intracardiac right to left shunt, as with a ventricular septal defect and pulmonic stenosis, the arterial PO_2 may be low, yet the patient is not in ARF. In a patient receiving supplemental oxygen, the arterial PO_2 may be in the normal range (pO_2 = 90-100), yet the patient is in respiratory failure. In patients with chronic metabolic alkalosis, the arterial pCO_2 may be elevated although the patient is not in respiratory failure. Patients with a respiratory disease such as asthma may be able to maintain normal blood gas values temporarily by increasing their work of breathing yet be in impending respiratory failure. Furthermore, it takes time to obtain and analyze

Table 6. Causes of Hypoxia by Mechanism

LOW INSPIRED FIO_2

- Deficiency of oxygen in atmosphere (i.e., high altitude)
- Low oxygen content of gas mixture: Suffocation, smoke inhalation, iatrogenic (problem with oxygen inflow during anesthesia, etc.)

HYPOVENTILATION

- Control disorders/central nervous system diseases (i.e.,infection, trauma, infarct, encephalopathy)

NEUROMUSCULAR DISEASES

- Spinal disorders/diseases (i.e., spinal cord injury)
- Peripheral nerve disorders (i.e., Guillain-Barré disease)
- Neuromuscular junction (i.e., botulism, tetanus)

STRUCTURAL DISEASES: CHEST WALL OR PLEURAL DISORDERS

- Flail chest
- Hemothorax
- Pneumothorax

PULMONARY DISORDERS

- Increased airway resistance
  - Airway obstruction (i.e., bronchospasm, mucous plugging foreign body, etc.)
  - Pulmonary edema
- Decreased compliance
  - Decreased chest wall compliance (spinal/chest wall deformities)
  - Decreased lung compliance (i.e., pulmonary edema)
- Impaired alveolar diffusion of oxygen
  - Pulmonary fibrosis
- Ventilation/perfusion abnormalities (V/Q mismatch)
  - Asthma, pneumonia
- Intrapulmonary shunts
  - Blood goes through pulmonary circulation without being oxygenated (i.e., severe pneumonia, pulmonary arteriovenous fistula)

INADEQUATE TRANSPORT/DELIVERY OF OXYGEN

- Hematologic
  - Anemia, abnormal hemoglobins
- Cardiac/circulation
  - Shock, low output states, local circulation abnormality

SHUNTS: CARDIAC

- Ventricular septal defect with pulmonic stenosis

TISSUE/CELL INCAPABLE OF UTILIZING OXYGEN

- Cyanide poisoning, beriberi

an ABG or any other test. Life-saving therapy should not be delayed in order to obtain a blood gas or any other test. Clinical assessment may be the most important parameter in determining respiratory failure, and treatment often should be initiated before the specific laboratory criteria for ARF can be obtained or are fulfilled.

Case No. 4

A 2-month-old is brought to the ED by her mother with a chief complaint of not eating for several days. Vital signs are:

- T = 36.8°C (R);
- P = 180 beats/min;
- R = 58 breaths/min
- BP = 55/30 mmHg; and
- Pulse oxygen saturation is 78% on room air.

Past medical history was unremarkable. She was the full-term product of an uncomplicated pregnancy, labor, and delivery. Her birth weight was 7 lbs, 10 oz, and she had no neonatal problems.

Physical examination reveals a 2-month-old female in respiratory distress with tachypnea, retractions, and cyanosis. The HEENT examination is within normal limits. The neck is supple. The lungs are clear. The heart is tachycardic with no murmurs. The liver edge is down 2 cm. The abdomen is non-tender. There is no edema and no rash.

The chest roentgenogram has no infiltrates and the heart size is enlarged. The WBC is 12,000, with 60% polymorphonuclear leukocytes, 30% lymphocytes, 8% monocytes, 2% eosinophils, and no bands. The urinanalysis is labstick negative, with no WBCs, no RBCs, and no casts.

An ABG reveals: pH = 7.48; pO_2 = 62; pCO_2 = 34; and HCO_3 = 23.

The electrocardiogram shows sinus tachycardia with right ventricular hypertrophy. Because she is afebrile without a marked leukocytosis or a leftward shift, the chest roentgenogram is without infiltrates, and she has a negative urinalysis; your suspicion for sepsis is low. Since there are no pediatric cardiologists or pediatric intensivists at your community hospital, an echocardiogram is not available.

The next test you order will confirm your diagnosis of congenital heart disease. An ABG drawn on 100% FiO_2 shows essentially no change from the room air blood gas: pH = 7.48; pO_2 = 64; pCO_2 = 35; HCO_3 = 23; and O_2 saturation is 79%.

The only disease mechanism that shows essentially no response to supplemental oxygen is a right to left shunt. You already have placed a foley catheter to measure urine output and given furosemide with a good response. On repeat examination: P = 150 beats/min; R = 40 breaths/min; BP = 60/40 mmHg; O_2 saturation is 82%; the liver edge is down 1 cm; and a murmur is heard. After appropriate stabilization, you transfer the patient to a tertiary care hospital. At the tertiary care hospital, after an evaluation by the pediatric cardiologist, the infant is diagnosed with cyanotic congenital heart disease (i.e, pulmonic stenosis and ventricular septal defect with a right to left shunt) and congestive heart failure.

Infants may not have all the classic signs of heart failure, such as peripheral edema or jugular venous distention. Since the cardiac output was poor, no murmur was heard initially. Later, after treatment, she improved clinically and a murmur was heard.

Discussion

Failure to respond to supplemental oxygen is pathognomonic for a right to left shunt of more than 30%. If other tests are not immediately available, ABGs done on room air and 100% oxygen will allow the diagnosis to be made. A shunt can be non-pulmonary, as in this case, with cyanotic congenital heart disease, from a pulmonary arteriovenous fistula, or a shunt can be from a severe pulmonary shunt such as extensive lung disease (although this is uncommon). Whatever the etiology, with a shunt, there is bypass of the pulmonary capillaries bed because of shunting of systemic venous blood to the systemic arterial system. The amount of the shunt can be calculated by the formula for QS/QT.

Respiratory Physiology: Hypoxia

Respiration involves several key physiologic events. Pulmonary ventilation is the movement of air (inflow and outflow) between the environment or atmosphere and the alveoli. Gaseous exchange in the alveoli involves diffusion of oxygen and carbon dioxide across the pulmonary capillary membrane. Oxygen and carbon dioxide are then transported in the blood to and from the cells. The tissues and cells must be able to utilize the oxygen. Finally there is a control process or regulation of the physiologic events involved in respiration.[21,22]

There are numerous causes of hypoxia.[2,23] *(See Table 6.)* The more common causes are: hypoventilation (whether secondary to control abnormalities or pulmonary disorders involving increased airway resistance or decreased compliance), ventilation/perfusion abnormalities, and shunts.[5] Less common etiologies involve: inadequate delivery of oxygen (hematologic or circulation abnormalities), tissue/cellular inability to use oxygen, and oxygen deficiency in the inhaled gases.[5] V/Q abnormalities may be the most common cause of hypoxemia. In the normal lung, ventilation nearly matches perfusion (V/Q = .8), or alveoli that are ventilated also have adequate blood flow. Where there is no alveolar blood flow to a ventilated alveoli, ventilation is wasted and there is increased dead space with increased work of breathing. When there is an alveoli that has normal blood flow but is not ventilated, there is an intrapulmonary shunt whereby some pulmonary blood flow fails to pick up oxygen, which can cause hypoxemia if severe.

Thus, lung units that are perfused but poorly ventilated cause desaturation, while lung units that are well ventilated but poorly perfused (e.g., high V/Q) cause physiologic dead-space, but not hypoxemia. When alveoli that have no blood flow are ventilated, the ventilation of these alveoli is wasted, which adds to the dead space. Dead space refers to areas of the lung that are ventilated but not perfused. Ventilation of the respiratory passageways (conducting airways such as the larynx, trachea, and bronchi) where gas exchange does not occur is anatomic dead space. When there is a large increase in dead space, much of the work of breathing becomes a wasted effort, since most of the ventilated air never reaches the bloodstream. When an area of the lung is perfused but is not ventilated, blood is not oxygenated and an intrapulmonary shunt is present. The shunt fraction (or venous admixture) estimates the amount of pulmonary blood flow that perfuses non-ventilated or underventilated lung.

Alveolar dead space is that part of the inspired air that passes through the anatomic dead space to the alveoli but does not take part in the gas exchange in the pulmonary capillary bed. In the normal lung, alveolar dead space is negligible; however, it is markedly increased in diseases such as ARDS and with pulmonary emboli.

Under normal conditions, there is a small intrapulmonary shunt (2-3%) due to the drainage of bronchial veins into the pulmonary vein and the thebesian veins into the left ventricle. Venous admixture (or pulmonary shunt) of more than 5% is abnormal. Pathologic admixture can be caused by: intracardiac right to left shunts (cyanotic congenital heart disease, such as ventricular septal defect or endocardial cushion defect), or by intrapulmonary shunting from pulmonary diseases such as pneumonia, pulmonary edema, and atelectasis.

Impaired diffusion across the alveolar-capillary membrane can lead to hypoxia. Diseases that impose a barrier to diffusion across the alveolar-capillary membrane include pulmonary fibrosis and pulmonary edema.

Oxygen transport failure results from the inability to deliver adequate amounts of oxygen to the tissues/cells. Oxygen transport failure can occur with hematologic disorders. These include: severe anemia, the presence of abnormal hemoglobins (e.g., methemoglobinemia), and lack of hemoglobin binding to oxygen (e.g., carbon monoxide poisoning). Cardiac diseases with low output (including cardiomyopathies and severe heart failure) and circulatory disorders (e.g., shock) can lead to inadequate oxygen transport to the tissues/cells. Hypoxia secondary to low inspired FiO_2 most often is encountered in cases involving high altitudes, suffocation, or smoke inhalation.

Disorders in which the cells and tissues are presented with oxygen but are unable to use or metabolize oxygen are rare. This does occur with cyanide poisoning and in deficiencies of the oxidative enzymes or tissue oxidation system (e.g., berberi).

Hypoventilation is a common cause of hypoxia and usually also causes hypercapnia (Type II respiratory failure). Hypoventilation can be due to ventilatory pump failure, caused by either control abnormalities (nervous system) or chest wall/pleural mechanical pulmonary abnormalities leading to increased airway resistance or decreased compliance. Airway obstruction and asthma are causes of increased airway resistance.

Case No. 5

A 5-year-old male is seen for a cough of several days duration that is not improving. He developed a cough three days ago after playing outside on a hot, humid day while his father mowed the lawn. Past medical history is unremarkable except for a history of bronchiolitis as an infant, for which he was hospitalized for two days. Family history is positive for asthma in an older sister, two paternal cousins, and the mother. His mother noted that he is usually quite active but hasn't been playing much, and hasn't been eating for the past three days. Tonight he seems worse.

The nursing triage note reads "chief complaint: cough; no fever, emesis, or diarrhea."

Vital signs are:

- T = 96.8°F (O);
- P = 170 beats/min;

Table 7. Indications for Intubation

CATEGORY	CLINICAL EXAMPLE OF DISEASES
Failure of respiratory drive (Control mechanism abnormalities)	CNS disorders (infection, trauma, malformations, infarcts), unresponsiveness, altered mental status, coma
Airway protection	Anesthesia Sedation, alcohol or drug intoxication Loss of gag reflex Severe emesis during procedures (such as gastric lavage)
Cardiac	Cardiac arrest Shock Peripheral vascular collapse
Pulmonary (Clinical signs: tachypnea, retractions, etc.)	Respiratory distress Ineffective ventilation, 2° respiratory muscle injury/disorders (trauma, spinal/peripheral nerve disease, neuromuscular junction disease), etc. Chest wall/pleural disease (flail chest, pneumothorax, etc.) Pulmonary disorders causing hypoxia and/or hypercapnia, ARF
Need for special therapy	Hyperventilation Delivery of PEEP, special need pulmonary care (suctioning, etc.), need for prolonged ventilation

- R = 44 breaths/min; and
- Pulse oximetry is 94% on room air.

On physical examination, there is an alert 5-year-old male sitting up and leaning forward. A lung examination reveals wheezing bilaterally. He is tachypnic with intercostal retractions. Three continuous albuterol aerosols were given by respiratory therapy. An ABG was drawn because of his poor response to aerosol.

An hour after he was triaged, you notice a lethargic 5-year-old male. His lungs are clear, no wheeze or rales, and no retractions. He has dry mucous membranes and pale skin with tenting. You order repeat vital signs and put him on a monitor.

Vital signs are now:

- T = 96.8°F (O);
- P = 102 beats/min;
- R = 16 breaths/min;
- BP = 65/40 mmHg; and
- Pulse oxygen saturation = 86% on room air.

The monitor shows sinus tachycardia with occasional premature ventricular contractions (PVCs). You order an IV, electrolytes, blood urea nitrogen, creatinine, complete blood count, chest x-ray, ABG, repeat aerosol, 100% FiO_2, a bolus of normal saline at 20 cc/kg, and IV steroids. A terbutaline drip also is started.

After the second aerosol, there is bilateral wheezing but poor air entry/exchange and no retractions:

- P = 94 beats/min;
- R = 14 breaths/min;
- BP = 75/45 mmHg; and
- Pulse oximetry is 91% on 100% FiO_2.

He is lethargic, but when aroused by a needle-stick, he is confused and combative. You give a second bolus of normal saline to treat his hypotension.

You decide you need to intubate the patient and perform a rapid sequence induction. You premedicate with atropine and lidocaine, followed by ketamine as the sedating agent and vecuronium as the paralytic agent. He is given an aerosol and 100% FiO_2 via the endotracheal tube. Post intubation, he is difficult to ventilate by bagging. However, the endotracheal tube is checked for tube placement and is documented to be in good position (a chest roentgenogram shows no pneumothorax or infiltrate), and there is some improvement after the aerosol. He is admitted to the PICU.

The laboratory data arrives after the patient is in the PICU. Laboratory results include:

- WBC = 14,600;
- Hematocrit = 52;
- BUN = 60;
- Creatinine = 1.5;
- Sodium = 150; and
- Potassium = 4.0.

The first ABG on room air shows: pH = 7.52; pO_2 = 58; pCO_2 = 24; HCO_3 = 14; and oxygen saturation = 88% on room air.

The second ABG shows: pH = 7.12; pO_2 = 68; pCO_2 = 70; HCO_3 = 14; and oxygen saturation is 90% on 100% FiO_2.

Five days later, he was doing well and was discharged home from the pediatric floor.

Discussion

The patient had hypotension/shock caused by several days of poor oral intake and increased fluid losses from his tachypnea (secondary to the asthmatic attack) and the hot weather. The laboratory data indicate hypernatremic dehydration with an elevated BUN, sodium, and hematocrit (hemoconcentration). The WBC was elevated from the stress of an acute asthmatic attack.

Even without an ABG, the patient had multiple indications for emergent intubation. On initial presentation, he had numerous indications that he might require intubation: signs of severe respiratory distress; wheezing with tachypnea; intercostal retractions; and use of accessory muscles. He was struggling to breathe and had air hunger. Therapy did not improve his air exchange.

A short time later (~ 1 hour), his respiratory rate dropped to the

Table 8. Methods for Administration of Supplemental Oxygen*

METHOD	MAXIMUM POSSIBLE FIO_2
• Isolette (with supplemental oxygen through port)	~ 100%†
• Oxygen hood (head box)α	~ 95%
• Face shield (face tent)	40%
• Oxygen tent	40-50%β
• Nasal cannula (various sizes)	Flow rate (liters/min)
Infant (< 1 year)	
Toddler (1-5 years)	
Pediatric (5-13 years)	
Adolescent (> 13 years)	
Adult	24-25% - 44-45%
• Mouth to mask (with supplemental oxygen)	50-80%
• Face mask	
Venturi face	24, 28, 31, 35, 40, 50%
Simple face mask	40-50%
Reservoir (partial re-breather, no one-way valves)	60-80%
Reservoir bag (non-breather, has two one-way valves)	90-100%
• Bag valve mask ventilation (without reservoir)	40%
• Bag valve mask ventilation (with reservoir)	90-100%
• Anesthesia bag (depending on source gas)	21-100%

FiO_2 depends on the rate, depth, and respiration. A rough guideline is to add ~ 4% to FiO_2 of 21% for room air for each liter per minute.

Legend
* Methods preferred depend on ease of administration, consistency of FiO_2, tolerance by patient, and ability to achieve a specific FiO_2.
† Use with oxygen analyzer
α Difficult to maintain a consistent or stable FiO_2
β Size allows for use in patients up to about 1 year of age

normal range (from 44 to 16). He was so exhausted from the three days of doing excessive work to breathe that he no longer had the energy to struggle to breathe and no longer had retractions or the use of accessory muscles. He no longer had wheezing since he was moving so little air, also indicating a worsening clinical condition. He was no longer alert but now was lethargic, suggesting somnolence due to a rising pCO_2. The confusion and combativeness that occurred when an IV was started was probably due to cerebral hypoxia. He had multiple clinical indicators of respiratory distress. He also had shock secondary to severe dehydration.

In addition to these clinical parameters, he also had laboratory criteria for ARF. The ABG obtained when he was struggling to breathe showed respiratory alkalosis (low pCO_2), and low bicarbonate from his dehydration, shock, and hypoxia ($paO_2 < 60$ mmHg; $SaO_2 < 90\%$; $PaO_2/FiO_2 = 58/0.21 = 276 < 300$). When he was too tired to continue the extra effort of breathing, the second ABG demonstrated hypercapnia with respiratory acidosis and hypoxia.

His underlying pulmonary disorder (asthma) caused increased airway resistance, which resulted in increased work of breathing, which led to impaired movement of air from the atmosphere to the alveoli (ventilation). His respiratory failure was due to respiratory muscle fatigue from increased work of breathing and a cardiovascular disorder (e.g., shock). He had many indications for intubation. *(See Table 7.)* Ketamine is considered the sedative of choice with an acute asthmatic attack because of its bronchodilating effects.

Treatment

The first step is to ensure patency of the airway.[24] If the child has adequate air exchange, then he or she should be allowed to maintain a position of comfort with the head in a neutral sniffing position. Hyperextension of the neck may worsen upper airway obstruction and should be avoided. Similarly, a child may have better ventilation if left in an upright position sitting in his or her parent's lap than if forced to lie down. An upright position on the examining table is usually preferred since the supine position increases the work of breathing by placing the weight of the abdominal organs on the diaphragm.

Suctioning of the airway, clearing the airway of an obstruction, and appropriately positioning the head and neck of the patient may help maintain airway patency.

After a patent airway is obtained, oxygenation and/or ventilation must be assessed and appropriate intervention completed. Respiratory failure may be categorized as a failure of oxygenation, a failure of ventilation, or both. Hypoxia is treated by administering supplemental oxygen by various devices ranging from facemasks or nasal cannulas to hoods. *(See Table 8.)* Administration of supplemental oxygen is indicated in all pediatric patients at risk for respiratory failure, even if there is no obvious hypoxemia or impending ARF. Such aggressive therapy may prevent the at risk patient from proceeding to ARF. Patients with ARF may need assisted ventilation in addition to supplemental oxygen.

Additional therapies also are beneficial in the ARF patient. These include careful attention to fluids and electrolytes; treatment of dehydration; appropriate antibiotics for infection; correcting electrolyte abnormalities; and transfusion if the patient is severely anemic.

Treatment of the underlying cause of the respiratory distress may prevent respiratory failure or reverse/correct the respiratory failure if it is already present. Treatment of an infection such as pneumonia with appropriate antibiotics, relieving an airway obstruction, or initiating bronchodilator therapy in asthma is essential in averting or reversing ARF in specific cases.

In those patients who do develop ARF, various newer therapies, such as high frequency jet ventilation, BiPAP, surfactant, liquid ventilation, nitrous oxide, or extra-corporeal membrane oxygenation, may be beneficial in selected cases.[25-28]

Summary

Pulmonary disease remains a leading cause of mortality in pediatric patients in spite of recent advances in treatment. ARF is a significant cause of morbidity and mortality in infants and children. Careful assessment of pediatric patients can lead to early recognition of respiratory distress, and institution of appropriate therapy may prevent ARF in some patients. The advent of newer therapies also may lead to a decrease in the high morbidity and mortality associated with ARF.

References

1. Thompson AE. Respiratory distress. In: Fleisher GR, Ludwig S, eds. *Textbook of Pediatric Emergency Medicine*. Baltimore, MD: Williams and Wilkins; 1993:450-455.
2. Baker MD, Ruddy RM. Pulmonary emergencies—acute respiratory failure. In: Fleisher GR, Ludwig S, eds. *Textbook of Pediatrics Emergency Medicine*. Baltimore, MD: Williams and Wilkins; 1993:874-877.
3. Airway and ventilation. In: Chameides L, Hazinski MF, eds. *Textbook of Pediatric Advanced Life Support*. Dallas, TX: American Heart Association; 1994:1-22.
4. Durmowicz AG, Stenmark KR. Acute respiratory failure. In: Chernick V, Boat TF, Kendig EL, eds. *Kendig's Disorders of the Respiratory Tract in Children*. 6th ed. Philadelphia: WB Saunders Co; 1998:265-286.
5. Marianai JJ, Wright LA. Acute respiratory failure. In: Baum GL, Celli BR, Crapo JD, et al, eds. *Textbook of Pulmonary Diseases, Vol. 1*. 6th ed. Philadelphia, PA: Lippincott-Raven, 1998:919-940.
6. Grippi MA. Respiratory failure: An overview. In: Fishman AP, Elias JA, Fishman JA, et al, eds. *Fishman's Pulmonary Diseases and Disorders, Vol. 2*. 3rd ed. New York: McGraw-Hill, 1998:2525-2536.
7. Guyton AC. Pulmonary ventilation. In: *Textbook of Medical Physiology*. 8th ed. Philadelphia, PA: WB Saunders Co.; 1991: 402-413.
8. Guyton AC. Physical principles of gaseous exchange: Diffusion of oxygen and carbon dioxide through the respiratory membrane. In: *Textbook of Medical Physiology*, 8th ed. Philadelphia, PA: WB Saunders Co.; 1991:422-432.
9. Guyton AC. Transport of oxygen and carbon dioxide in the blood and body fluids. In: *Textbook of Medical Physiology*, 8th ed. Philadelphia, PA: WB Saunders Co.; 1991:422-432.
10. Greene KE, Peters JL. Pathophysiology of acute respiratory failure. *Clin Chest Med* 1994;15:1-12.
11. Anas NG. Respiratory failure. In: Levin DL, Morriss FC, eds. *Essentials of Pediatric Intensive Care, Vol 1*. 2nd ed. New York: Churchill-Livingstone; 1997:69-82.
12. Seidel JS. Respiratory emergencies and cardiopulmonary arrest. In: Barkin RM, Asch SM, Caputo GL, et al, eds. *Pediatric Emergency Medicine-Concepts and Clinical Practice*. St. Louis: Mosby Year Book; 1992:73-83.
13. Recognition of Respiratory Failure and Shock. In: *Textbook of Pediatric Advanced Life Support*. Dallas, TX: American Heart Association; 1994:1-10.
14. Ludwig S, Kettrick RG. Resuscitation—pediatric basic and advanced life support. In: Fleisher GR, Ludwig S, eds. *Textbook of Pediatric Emergency Medicine*. 3rd ed. Baltimore, MD: Williams and Wilkins; 1993:1-31.
15. Haddad GG, Perez Fontan JI. Respiratory failure. In: Behrman RE, Kliegman RM, Arvin AM, eds. *Nelson Textbook of Pediatrics*. 15th ed. Philadelphia, PA: WB Saunders Co.; 1996:1177-1179.
16. Thompson AE. Respiratory distress. In: Fleisher GR, Ludwig S. eds. *Textbook of Pediatrics Emergency Medicine*. 3rd ed. Baltimore, MD: Williams and Wilkins; 1993:450-455.
17. Kotloff RM. Acute respiratory failure in the surgical patient. In: Fishman AP, Elias JA, Fishman JA, et al, eds. *Fishman's Pulmonary Diseases and Disorders*. New York: McGraw-Hill; 1998:2589-2604.
18. Teba L, Omert LA. Postoperative respiratory insufficiency. *Amer Fam Phys* 1995;51:1473-1480.
19. Kelsen SG, Criner J. Pump failure: The pathogenesis of hypercapnic respiratory failure in patients with lung and chest wall disease. In: Fishman AP, Elias JA, Fishman JA, et al, eds. *Fishman's Pulmonary Diseases and Disorders*. New York: McGraw-Hill; 1998:2605-2626.
20. Recognition of respiratory failure and shock. In: Chameides L, Hazinski MF, eds. *Textbook Pediatric Advanced Life Support*. Dallas, TX: American Heart Association; 1994:1-10.
21. Guyton AC. Regulation of respiration. In: *Textbook of Medical Physiology*. 8th ed. Philadelphia, PA: WB Saunders Co.; 1991: 444-453.
22. Chernick NS, Pack AL. Control of ventilation. In: Fishman AP, Elias JA, Fishman JA, et al, eds. *Fishman's Pulmonary Diseases and Disorders, Vol 1*. 3rd ed. New York: McGraw-Hill; 1998: 163-175.
23. Guyton AC. Regulation of respiration. In: *Textbook of Medical Physiology*. 8th ed. Philadelphia, PA: WB Saunders Co.; 1991: 444-453.
24. Kisson N, Singh N. Airway management and ventilatory support. In: Reisdorff EJ, Roberts MR, Wiegenstein JG, eds. *Pediatric Emergency Medicine*. Philadelphia, PA: WB Saunders Co.; 1993;51-67.
25. Hillberg RE, Johnson DC. Noninvasive ventilation. *N Engl J Med* 1997;337:1746-1752.
26. Clark DR, Lahren KM. Noninvasive positive pressure ventilation. *South Med J* 1997;90:72-74.
27. Arensman RM, Statter MB, Bastawrous AL, et al. Modern treatment modalities for neonatal and pediatric respiratory failure. *Amer J Surg* 1996:172:41-47.
28. Paret G, Dekel B. Vardi A, et al. Heliox in respiratory failure secondary to bronchiolitis: A new therapy. *Pediatr Pulm* 1996;23:322-323.

Summary

Pulmonary disease remains a leading cause of morbidity in pediatric patients. In spite of recent advances in treatment, ARF is a significant cause of mortality and morbidity in infants and children. Careful assessment of pediatric patients can lead to early recognition of respiratory distress and institution of appropriate therapy. [illegible] the advent of newer therapies [illegible] may lead to a decrease in the high morbidity and mortality associated with ARF.

References

1. Thompson AE. Respiratory distress. In: Fleisher GR, Ludwig S, eds. *Textbook of Pediatric Emergency Medicine*. Baltimore, MD: Williams and Wilkins; 1993:[illegible].
2. Baker MD, [illegible]. Pediatric emergencies—acute respiratory failure. In: Fleisher GR, Ludwig S, eds. *Textbook of Pediatric Emergency Medicine*. Baltimore, MD: Williams and Wilkins; 1993:[illegible].
3. Airway and ventilation. In: Chameides L, Hazinski MF, eds. *Textbook of Pediatric Advanced Life Support*. Dallas, TX: American Heart Association; 1994:[illegible]-22.
4. Dunmore AL, [illegible] KR. Acute respiratory failure. In: Chernick V, [illegible] eds. *Kendig's Disorders of the Respiratory Tract in Children*. [illegible] ed. Philadelphia, PA: WB Saunders Co; 1998:[illegible].
5. [illegible] A. Acute respiratory failure. In: Baum GL, Celli BR, [illegible], eds. *Textbook of Pulmonary Diseases*. Vol. [illegible] 6th ed. Philadelphia, PA: Lippincott-Raven; 1998:[illegible].
6. [illegible] MA. Respiratory failure: an overview. In: Fishman AP, Elias JA, Fishman JA, et al, eds. *Fishman's Pulmonary Diseases and Disorders*. Vol. [illegible] 3rd ed. New York: McGraw-Hill; 1998:[illegible].
7. Guyton AC. Pulmonary ventilation. In: *Textbook of Medical Physiology*. [illegible] ed. Philadelphia, PA: WB Saunders Co; 1991:[illegible].
8. Guyton AC. Physical principles of gaseous exchange: Diffusion of oxygen and carbon dioxide through the respiratory membrane. In: *Textbook of Medical Physiology*. [illegible] ed. Philadelphia, PA: WB Saunders Co; 1991:[illegible]-43.
9. Guyton AC. Transport of oxygen and carbon dioxide in the blood and body fluids. In: *Textbook of Medical Physiology*. [illegible] ed. Philadelphia, PA: WB Saunders Co; 1991:[illegible].
10. Greene KE, Peters JI. Pathophysiology of acute respiratory failure. *Clin Chest Med*. 1994;15:1-12.
11. [illegible] Respiratory failure. In: Levin DL, Morriss FC, eds. *Essentials of Pediatric Intensive Care*. [illegible] ed. New York: Churchill Livingstone; 1997:[illegible]-52.
12. Steed [illegible]. Respiratory emergencies and cardiopulmonary arrest. In: [illegible], M. Lampe [illegible], et al, eds. *Respiratory Care: Principles and Clinical Practice*. [illegible]. New York: [illegible].
13. Recognition of respiratory failure and shock. In: *Textbook of Pediatric Advanced Life Support*. Dallas, TX: American Heart Association; 1994:[illegible].
14. Ludwig S, [illegible] KC. Resuscitation—pediatric basic and advanced life support. In: Fleisher GR, Ludwig S, eds. *Textbook of Pediatric Emergency Medicine*. 3rd ed. Baltimore, MD: Williams and Wilkins; 1993:[illegible]-34.
15. Haddad GG, Perez Fontan JJ. Respiratory failure. In: Behrman RE, Kliegman RM, Arvin AM, eds. *Nelson Textbook of Pediatrics*. 15th ed. Philadelphia, PA: WB Saunders Co; 1996:[illegible].
16. Thomas AE. Respiratory distress. In: Fleisher GR, Ludwig S, eds. *Textbook of Pediatric Emergency Medicine*. 3rd ed. Baltimore, MD: Williams and Wilkins; 1993:[illegible]-45.
17. [illegible] Acute respiratory failure in the surgical patient. In: Fishman AP, Elias JA, Fishman JA, et al, eds. *Fishman's Pulmonary Diseases and Disorders*. New York: McGraw-Hill; 1998:[illegible].
18. [illegible] Postoperative respiratory insufficiency. *Amer Rev Dis*. 1995;[illegible].
19. Kelsen SG, [illegible]. Pump failure: The pathogenesis of hypercapnic respiratory failure in patients with lung and chest wall disease. In: Fishman AP, Elias JA, Fishman JA, et al, eds. *Fishman's Pulmonary Diseases and Disorders*. New York: McGraw-Hill; 1998:[illegible].
20. Recognition of respiratory failure and shock. In: Chameides L, Hazinski MF, eds. *Textbook of Pediatric Advanced Life Support*. Dallas, TX: American Heart Association; 1994:1-[illegible].
21. Guyton AC. Regulation of respiration. In: *Textbook of Medical Physiology*. 8th ed. Philadelphia, PA: WB Saunders Co; 1991:[illegible]-455.
22. Cherniack NS, Pack AI. Control of ventilation. In: Fishman AP, Elias JA, Fishman JA, et al, eds. *Fishman's Pulmonary Diseases and Disorders*. Vol. 1. 3rd ed. New York: McGraw-Hill; 1998:[illegible]-175.
23. Guyton AC. Regulation of respiration. In: *Textbook of Medical Physiology*. 8th ed. Philadelphia, PA: WB Saunders Co; 1991:[illegible]-452.
24. [illegible] N, Singh N. Airway management and ventilatory support. In: Reisdorff EJ, Roberts MR, Wiegenstein JG, eds. *Pediatric Emergency Medicine*. Philadelphia, PA: WB Saunders Co; 1993:[illegible].
25. Hillberg RE, Johnson DC. Noninvasive ventilation. *N Engl J Med*. 1997;337:1746-1752.
26. Clark DR, Lauren KA. Noninvasive positive pressure ventilation. *South Med J*. 1997;90:[illegible].
27. [illegible] IM, Soper [illegible], [illegible], et al. Modern treatment modalities for neonatal and pediatric respiratory failure. *Am J Surg*. 1988;[illegible]:[illegible].
28. Pa[illegible] KS, Dodd [illegible], Venti [illegible]. [illegible] respiratory failure secondary to bronchiolitis: [illegible] therapy. *Pediatr Pulmonol*. 1996;23:[illegible].

Pediatric Seizures

Claudia R. Gold, MD, FACEP
Jessica Pierog, EMT

Children with seizures, shaking spells, and other convulsive activity commonly are seen in the emergency department (ED). As many as 10% of all ambulance calls for children are for seizure activity, and approximately 1-2% of total ED visits by children are for seizure-related complaints.[1,2]

Children who experience seizures are a heterogeneous group with a wide range of associated problems. While many children with seizures are otherwise healthy, many also have significant primary and secondary diagnoses, and the initial seizure may be the presenting symptom of serious underlying disease.

Most children who arrive with a complaint of seizure activity can be grouped into one of five categories for emergency evaluation and management: 1) febrile seizure; 2) new-onset nonfebrile seizure; 3) established seizure disorder with recurrence; 4) status epilepticus; or 5) neonatal seizure.

Of these, the management of children with new onset, nonfebrile seizures is the most challenging and controversial. However, the focus in the ED should be the same for patients in all categories: Stabilize the child, identify and manage any life-threatening condition, and arrange appropriate disposition and follow-up. This chapter will provide a rational approach to seizures.

Definitions and Classification

A seizure is defined as a paroxysmal electrical discharge of neurons in the brain resulting in alteration of function or behavior. Seizures may occur in both normal and abnormal brain tissue. The clinical manifestations of a seizure will vary with the number, location, and duration of the electrical discharges involved. Epilepsy is defined as two or more seizures not immediately provoked by a specific event such as fever, trauma, infection, or chemical changes. Neonatal seizures are those that occur during the first 28 days of life (most commonly in the first few days of life), but that do not indicate epilepsy.[3] A febrile seizure is an event in infancy or childhood that usually occurs between 3 months and 5 years of age and is associated with fever but has no evidence of intracranial infection or a definable cause.[4]

Historically, the most widely used terms to describe seizures were grand mal, petit mal, and psychomotor. This language has since been replaced by a classification system introduced by the International League Against Epilepsy. This classification separates seizures into three major categories: partial, generalized, and unclassified.[5] *(See Table 1.)*

While a definitive diagnosis of a particular seizure type often is deferred in the ED, it is important to be familiar with current terminology to accurately describe seizure activity and effectively communicate with consulting physicians.

A generalized seizure implies that the entire cerebral cortex demonstrates simultaneous, synchronous electrical discharges that

Table 1. Seizure Classification

PARTIAL SEIZURES (FOCAL, LOCAL)

Simple Partial Seizures (consciousness not impaired)
- With motor signs
- With somatosensory or special sensory symptoms
- With autonomic signs or symptoms
- With psychic symptoms

Complex Partial Seizures (consciousness impaired)
- Simple partial onset followed by impaired consciousness (with or without automatisms)
- Onset with impaired consciousness (with or without automatisms)

Partial Seizures Evolving into Generalized Seizures
- Simple partial evolving to generalized
- Complex partial evolving to generalized
- Simple partial evolving to complex partial evolving to generalized

GENERALIZED SEIZURES (CONVULSIVE OR NONCONVULSIVE)

Absence Seizures
- Typical absence (brief stare, lapse in awareness, no movement)
- Atypical absence (may have tonic, mild clonic, atonic, automatism, or autonomic features)
- Myoclonic seizures (brief, repetitive, symmetrical contractions)

Clonic Seizures (rhythmic jerking)
Tonic Seizures (sustained muscle contraction)
Tonic-Clonic Seizures (usually begins with tonic phase)
Atonic Seizures (abrupt loss of muscle tone)

UNCLASSIFIED EPILEPTIC SEIZURES

Adapted from: Commission on Classifications and Terminology of the International League Against Epilepsy. Proposal for revised clinical and electroencephalographic classification of epileptic seizures. *Epilepsia* 1981;22:489-501.

result in one of several clinical manifestations: tonic, clonic, tonic-clonic, myoclonic, atonic, or absence seizures. Tonic activity is a continuous muscle contraction resulting in rigidity, whereas clonic seizures are manifested by rhythmic jerking of flexor muscles. Tonic-clonic seizures are a combination of both, usually beginning with the tonic phase. Myoclonic seizures manifest as brief jerks or contractions of a specific muscle or muscle group. Myoclonus is a component of several epilepsy syndromes, and commonly is symmetrical. Atonic seizures result in a sudden loss of postural muscle tone and may result in falling (drop attacks). Absence seizures are characterized by brief staring spells, or loss of awareness, typically lasting less than 10 seconds, and with no post-ictal effects. Patients also may have atypical absence events that differ from simple absence seizures in that the onset occurs at an earlier age, and the electroencephalogram (EEG) findings do not demonstrate the typical absence generalized spike and wave discharges at three per second.[6]

In contrast, partial seizures have a focal onset. A simple partial seizure causes no alteration in consciousness, whereas complex partial seizures are accompanied by a change in consciousness. A partial seizure, both simple and complex, also may secondarily generalize to tonic-clonic activity. It is important to distinguish partial from generalized seizures, as they may respond differently to anticonvulsant medications. In addition, partial seizures more often are associated with a focal area of intracranial pathology that might be amenable to surgical treatment.

Epidemiology

Epilepsy is a common medical condition affecting 0.5-1% of all children. Each year, approximately 150,000 children in the United States will have a newly occurring, single seizure, and one-fifth subsequently will be diagnosed with epilepsy.[7] The incidence of seizures is highest in early childhood, and reaches 4.1 per 1000 in children younger than 11 years of age.[2,8] Febrile seizures occur at least once in approximately 2-5% of children, and account for 30% of all childhood seizures.[8] They are the most common type of seizure in children between 6 months and 5 years of age. In children ages 5-15 years, central nervous system (CNS) infections and head trauma are identified almost equally as the precipitating causes.[9] In the early neonatal period, the most common seizure etiology is hypoxic-ischemic encephalopathy. Other causes include congenital CNS anomalies, pyridoxine deficiency, drug withdrawal, and electrolyte disturbances. In the later neonatal period (after 4 days of age), infections become the most common etiology.[10] *(See Table 2.)*

Clinical Approach to the Child with a Seizure

The emergency evaluation of seizures in children clearly depends on the circumstances of the presentation. During an active seizure, evaluation and treatment must occur simultaneously. In the majority of cases, however, the seizure will have stopped in the prehospital phase, and the evaluation is then guided by whether or not the child has returned to a normal baseline. Frequently, a child will be brought in by his or her parents after a significant amount of time has elapsed since the "event" occurred. The diagnosis then will have to be based primarily on the history, which often is unreliable.

History. It is imperative to determine if a seizure actually occurred. While parents, bystanders, and even medical personnel may report witnessing a seizure, it is important to remember that children manifest a large repertoire of conditions that may be misconstrued as seizure activity. An accurate history may be hampered by the emotional state of the witnesses, and is often subject to interpretation. Bystanders often embellish the motor activity or grossly overestimate the duration of the event. Older pediatric patients may be able to contribute to their own history, especially regarding the circumstances prior to the seizure. However, they frequently have little or no recall of their attacks.

When gathering the history, speak to all available witnesses and attempt to distinguish actual observations from opinions and interpretations of what happened. The patient's personal physician, if available, should be contacted for pertinent medical information.

Important questions should include:

Table 2. Etiology of Seizures in Childhood

INFECTIOUS
- Meningitis
- Encephalitis
- Cerebral abscess
- Shigella
- Roseola

METABOLIC
- Hypoglycemia
- Hyponatremia
- Hypocalcemia
- Hypomagnesemia
- Hypernatremia
- Pyridoxine deficiency
- Hypoxia
- Inborn error of metabolism

TRAUMATIC
- Epidural or subdural hematoma
- Subarachnoid hemorrhage
- Cerebral contusion

TOXIC
- Drug intoxication
- Drug withdrawal

NEOPLASTIC
- Primary CNS tumor
- Metastatic lesions

EPILEPTIC
- Inadequacy of anticonvulsant
- Noncompliance

MISCELLANEOUS
- Idiopathic
- Febrile seizures
- Postimmunization
- Ventriculoperitoneal shunt malfunction
- Neurocutaneous syndromes
- Familial
- Cerebral degenerative disease
- Pregnancy (eclampsia)

- What was the child doing when the attack occurred?
- Did anything seem to precipitate the attack?
- Was there an aura?
- How long did the event last?
- Was there a loss of or change in consciousness?
- What abnormal movements occurred?
- Were there abnormal eye movements or automatisms?
- Was there a change in breathing or color or frothing at the mouth?
- Was there urinary or fecal incontinence?
- Did any injury occur during the event?
- What was the postictal behavior?
- Are there any underlying medical conditions?
- Is there a history of recent fever, head injury, poisoning, or drug use? *(See Table 3.)*
- Is there a possibility of pregnancy?
- Is there a family history of seizures?

Fortunately, many features of true seizures help to distinguish them from other paroxysmal attacks. While some seizures are precipitated by auras or other nonspecific prodromal symptoms, the actual seizure activity begins abruptly. Any attack that develops gradually over many minutes should be considered suspect. The duration of most seizures is brief, usually lasting fewer than two minutes, although prolonged seizures may occur. With the exception of simple partial seizures, all seizures result in some impairment of consciousness. Accordingly, the patient usually has impaired memory of the event. Any attack in which there is significant alteration in consciousness, yet is recalled by the patient in significant detail, is unlikely to be a true seizure. Motor activity during a seizure is usually simple, synchronous, and purposeless (automatisms). Violent thrusting, or movements that change in response to the environment should be considered suspect. True seizures only rarely are provoked by specific stimuli such as sudden emotion or fright. Finally, most seizures, with the exception of simple absence or simple partial types, are followed by a postictal period of lethargy or confusion. Any dramatic convulsive activity followed by a rapid return to normal mental status should prompt a search for an alternative diagnosis.[11]

There are numerous isolated and recurrent events that may be mistaken for seizures. *(See Table 4.)*

Syncope. Syncope is one of the most common events mistaken for seizures. Syncope usually is accompanied by warning signs such as nausea, pallor, lightheadedness, and diaphoresis; however, true sensory auras do not occur. Some convulsive activity as well as incontinence may be seen, however, which adds to the confusion. Recovery is usually immediate with no distinct period of postictal confusion.

Breath-Holding Spells. Breath-holding is common in early childhood, occurring in approximately 5% of children younger than age 2. These attacks follow a precipitating event such as fright, pain, or anger. The child will appear either pale or cyanotic, become limp, and then often stiffen in an apparent tonic seizure. There may be some clonic activity as well. Apnea and severe bradycardia may accompany the spell, though intervention is rarely necessary.[12,13]

Sleep Disorders. Sleep disorders (night terrors, nightmares, nar-

Table 3. Drug-Related Seizures

OVERDOSE
- Cocaine
- Amphetamines
- PCP
- Phenothiazines
- Tricyclic antidepressants
- Hypoglycemics
- Methylxanthines
- Salicylates
- Meperidine
- Propoxyphene
- Antihistamines
- Isoniazid
- Haloperidol
- Beta blockers
- Lead
- Carbon monoxide

WITHDRAWAL
- Alcohol
- Narcotics
- Anticonvulsants

Table 4. Conditions that Mimic Seizures

SYNCOPE
- Vasovagal syncope
- Orthostatic hypotension
- Micturitional syncope
- Cough syncope

BREATH-HOLDING SPELLS
- Pallid spells
- Cyanotic spells

MOVEMENT DISORDERS
- Tics
- Tremors
- Tourette's syndrome
- Shudder attacks
- Spasmus mutans
- Paroxysmal kinesigenic choreoathetosis
- Sandifer's syndrome

SLEEP DISORDERS
- Nightmares
- Night terrors
- Sleepwalking
- Somniloquy
- Narcolepsy

MIGRAINE HEADACHES
- Classic migraine
- Complicated (basilar) migraine

PSYCHOLOGICAL
- Pseudoseizures
- Hyperventilation syndrome
- Hysteria and rages
- Panic attack
- Attention deficit disorder

colepsy, nocturnal enuresis, sleepwalking, and sleeptalking) are common childhood conditions. Night terrors may result in a child suddenly sitting up panic stricken, screaming, sweating, and unresponsive to calming efforts. These episodes are usually followed by a return to sleep, with no memory of the event the next day. Sleep disorders can result in excessive daytime sleepiness due to nighttime disturbances. Narcoleptic behaviors may be misinterpreted as absence seizures. Sleepwalking and nocturnal enuresis are reported in up to 15% of children.[13,14]

Paroxysmal Movement Disorders. Tics and tremors are rapid, brief, and repetitive involuntary movements that occur intermittently, and often in response to stress. There is no change in consciousness with these motor activities. Shudder attacks consist of periods of shivering motion, also with no altered consciousness. Spasms mutans is a disorder seen in children between 4 and 12 months of age that causes head tilt, nodding, and asymmetric nystagmus. Paroxysmal kinesigenic choreoathetosis is a rare movement disorder precipitated by the onset of movement after a period of rest (such as getting out of a chair at the end of a class).[12-14] Sandifers syndrome refers to the infantile tonic posturing, arching of the back, and torticollis, associated with gastroesophageal reflux.[13]

Migraines. Migraines are relatively common in children, and may be associated with only a mild headache. The symptoms may resemble the auras reported by patients with complex partial seizures. Complicated migraines may involve a loss of consciousness, although generally no motor activity occurs. A family history commonly is found.[13]

Psychogenic Seizures. Psychogenic seizures (pseudoseizures) are not rare in children, and may be difficult to distinguish from true seizures. Unfortunately, they often are seen in patients who also have epilepsy. Psychogenic seizures usually are precipitated by stress, and often are more violent in nature, though they rarely lead to injury or incontinence and do not occur during sleep. A test for elevated serum prolactin may be useful if performed within 30 minutes of the event. If positive, it suggests true seizure activity.[11,13,15]

Physical Examination

The physical examination should be directed toward determining any underlying cause of the seizure, as well as any injury resulting from the event. Particular attention should be paid to signs of underlying systemic disease, infection, toxic exposure, or any focal neurological finding. The level of consciousness is most important. Patients found to have impaired consciousness require frequent serial examinations to determine whether a cause other than a simple postictal state is responsible. Vital signs, including pulse oximetry, should be checked initially, and re-evaluated as indicated by clinical condition. The child must be undressed completely to evaluate any dysmorphic features or cutaneous stigmata of underlying systemic disease (café au lait spots, neurofibromas), or infection (rashes). A careful evaluation for trauma is required. Palpation of the head may reveal a skull fracture, hematoma, or bulging fontanelle. Examination of the musculoskeletal system may suggest fractures or dislocations. Oral mucosa lacerations are particularly common. The eye examination should include pupil size, symmetry, and reactivity, as well as assessment of conjugate or disconjugate gaze. A fundal assessment should search for papilledema and retinal hemorrhages. Any signs of meningeal irritation such as photophobia or neck stiffness should be noted. Cardiac assessment should note any significant ectopy or murmurs. Further neurological examination should search for any focal abnormalities and include assessment of motor strength, coordination, sensation, and reflexes. Hyperreflexia and bilateral Babinski signs may occur following a seizure, but should resolve in the postictal period.[9,16] Transient focal findings lasting several hours or more (Todd's paralysis) may be seen after an apparent generalized seizure and suggest a focal etiology.[11] It is helpful to document the patient's mental and physical capacities in descriptive operational terms, rather than vague words such as weak, lethargic, or confused.

Diagnostic Studies

Laboratory. Decisions regarding which laboratory tests to order in patients with seizures should be guided and individualized by the clinical scenario. Although there is little evidence of utility, it is unfortunately still common practice to order routine or baseline lab studies in patients who present with a first, or even a recurrent, seizure.

Known epilepsy patients who present with a typical seizure while on their medications but who have returned to normal, should only require a measurement of their anticonvulsant levels (if the test is available). This assumes, however, there is no comorbidity that would suggest a metabolic derangement.[16-19]

The management of patients presenting to the ED after a first seizure who are alert, oriented, and without clinical findings is controversial. Most authors agree with routinely obtaining a blood glucose, though as a general rule hypoglycemia that is significant enough to result in a seizure will not be associated with a normal clinical exam.[17] The incidence of new onset seizures due to electrolyte abnormalities in neurologically normal patients is extremely low. Therefore, routine measurements should be reserved for those children with an abnormal mental status,with significant underlying medical conditions such as diabetes or renal disease, taking medications such as diuretics, and with significant signs of dehydration or malnourishment. An exception to these guidelines should be made in the case of neonatal seizures, where routine glucose, electrolytes, calcium, and magnesium levels result in a much higher yield.[8]

The complete blood count (CBC) in clinically well patients has shown to be minimally helpful, if at all. Although many studies have demonstrated an abnormal white blood cell (WBC) count in a significant percentage of new onset, as well as recurrent, seizure patients, the values did not affect their management.[8,17]

There are no prospective studies supporting the performance of a lumbar puncture in the diagnostic evaluation of children with a first-time seizure who are alert, oriented, asymptomatic, and immunocompetent. A lumbar puncture should be performed without delay if meningitis or a subarachnoid hemorrhage is suspected. It also should be considered strongly in children with an abnormally prolonged postictal state, fever, a positive HIV history, or those who are otherwise immunocompromised.[16]

In some cases, laboratory studies may be useful in determining if the patient actually had a seizure as opposed to another paroxysmal event. Creatine phosphokinase levels (CPK) may be elevated after a seizure, and metabolic acidemia may be present. Rhabdomyolysis may be detected if the urine tests positive for blood in the absence of red blood cells on microscopic examination. A more specific finding is an elevated blood prolactin level drawn within 30 minutes of the attack; however, a normal prolactin level cannot exclude a true seizure.[11,16] The need for any general or specific toxicology studies should be determined by the history and examination findings.

Neuroimaging. Considerable disagreement exists about the need for neuroimaging in the evaluation of patients presenting with a first seizure. Similarly, controversy exists over the specific study to be done (computed tomography [CT] vs magnetic resonance imaging [MRI]), as well as the urgency with which it should be obtained.

Neuroimaging studies should be considered strongly in the ED in patients with a history of head trauma, persistent alteration in consciousness or other abnormal neurological findings, severe headache, malignancy, immunocompromise, anticoagulation, cerebrospinal fluid (CSF) shunt, or a geographic risk of cystercercosis.[11,13,20] However, in patients who are neurologically normal on exam, the indications for neuroimaging are much less clear.

The most recent clinical policy from the American College of Emergency Physicians (that applies to patients age 6 and older) advises non-contrast CT scanning in the evaluation of all patients with first-time seizures without known cause. It also recommends non-contrast CT scanning as a rule in all previously diagnosed seizure patients with a change in seizure pattern without attributable cause.[17] However, patients who have recovered completely from their seizures, with nonfocal examinations, and have no significant risk factors for intracranial abnormalities may have neuroimaging studies performed electively at a later time, assuming reliable follow-up is planned.[17,20,21]

MRI, though not as readily available, is superior to CT imaging when evaluating children for epileptic lesions. Small tumors in the temporal lobe or close to bony structures may be masked on CT scans.[8,9] Follow-up MRI scans are used to exclude subtle lesions in patients with normal, emergency CT scans, as well as to better characterize lesions previously detected by a CT scan. An argument can be made, then, to defer neuroimaging in low-risk patients until a subsequent MRI can be arranged.[11]

Electroencephalography. An EEG is an extremely important diagnostic tool in the evaluation of seizure patients, though it is rarely available on an emergency basis. An emergent EEG is recommended, however, in patients with persistent altered mental status following the apparent termination of the seizure. This would allow the diagnosis of subtle convulsive, or nonconvulsive status epilepticus (SE). It also may be helpful in making the diagnosis of epilepsy in patients who present with new onset altered level of consciousness of uncertain cause. Another emergent indication for an EEG is monitoring the adequacy of treatment in patients with SE whose convulsions have been suppressed either by muscle paralysis to facilitate intubation, or by barbiturate coma.[22]

Treatment Decisions

The appropriate management of a patient with a first seizure involves controlling any ongoing seizure activity, treatment of any known precipitating cause, and the prevention of seizure recurrence.

A child who has not made a full recovery from the initial seizure, or who has recurrent seizures, requires admission for further observation, evaluation, and treatment. Any underlying disease that may have precipitated the attack must be identified, as it usually will pose a greater risk to the child than the seizure itself. Examples include CNS infections, drug intoxications, severe electrolyte derangements, and mass lesions. Treatment of the underlying disorder may obviate the need for anti-epileptic medication. Moreover, anticonvulsant therapy, if started, may not be effective unless the causative problem is corrected.

The more controversial issue involves the decision to begin anticonvulsant therapy in a child who has fully recovered from an initial seizure and does not require admission to the hospital. It is generally considered reasonable in these patients to allow discharge from the ED, with follow-up neuroimaging and EEG studies as an out-patient. Whether or not to begin antiepileptic medication should be decided by the predicted risk of recurrence. These statistics vary considerably, however, especially if the EEG and neuroimaging results are unknown at the time of discharge.

If the child had an idiopathic seizure, and the EEG is subsequently normal, the risk of recurrence is about 25%. However, if the EEG is abnormal, the risk of recurrence is almost 60%. The majority of seizure recurrences will happen within the first three months, and if there is a second seizure, the likelihood of further seizures rises to

Table 5. Common Seizure Prophylactic Drugs

DRUG	TRADE NAME	MAINTENANCE DOSE (mg/kg/day)	THERAPEUTIC LEVEL	SIDE EFFECTS
Phenytoin	Dilantin	4-8 bid, tid, or qhs	10-20	Gingival hyperplasia, hirsutism, rashes, Stevens-Johnson syndrome, megaloblastic anemia, lymphoma
Phenobarbital	Luminol	2-6 bid	15-40	Sedation, behavioral problems
Carbamazepine	Tegretol	10-40 bid	4-12	Rashes, liver disease, leukopenia, dizziness, rare aplastic anemia
Valproate	Depakene	10-60 tid or qid	50-100	GI upset, weight gain, alopecia, tremor, hepatitis, pancreatitis
Ethosuximide	Zarontin	20-40 bid or qd	40-100	GI upset, headaches, rashes, hiccups, blurred vision, lethargy, SLE
Primidone	Mysoline	10-25 bid or tid	5-12	Behavioral problems, sedation, rashes, ataxia
Clonazepam	Klonopin	0.05-0.2 bid	0.02-0.08	Fatigue, behavioral problems, increased salivation
Gabapentin	Neurontin	20-70 tid	Unknown	Fatigue, dizziness, ataxia, diarrhea
Lamotrigine	Lamictal	3-15, depending on concurrent drugs, qd x 14 d, then bid	1-3	Sedation, dizziness, headaches, nausea

approximately 75%.[13] In children, the sleep state of the first seizure is also predictive, with the risk of recurrence being twice as great if the initial seizure occurred while sleeping.[14]

Treatment decisions also must consider the risks and consequences of beginning antiepileptic medication. *(See Table 5.)* No anticonvulsant drug offers 100% protection against future seizures, and all medications have potential side effects ranging from minor problems (i.e., gastrointestinal upset and sedation) to severe complications (i.e., liver failure, aplastic anemia, agranulocytosis, Lupus-like disease, and Stevens-Johnson syndrome, among others).[6] Additional treatment considerations must include compliance issues, the cost of the medication, and its monitoring requirements.

If medical treatment is initiated in the ED, it should be in consultation with the primary care physician or pediatric neurologist who will be following the child. The drug chosen should be the most appropriate for the seizure type, taking into account the above issues of side effects, cost, and compliance. *(See Table 6.)*

Generalized tonic-clonic seizures may be controlled with phenytoin, phenobarbital, carbamazepine, valproic acid, and primidone. The drugs of choice for partial seizures are phenytoin and carbamazepine. Phenobarbital and primidone also are effective against partial seizures but have a much higher incidence of adverse effects. Absence seizures are typically treated with ethosuximide, but if absence seizures are associated with other seizure types as well, valproic acid is the better choice. Valproic acid also is used in the management of myoclonic and atonic seizure disorders. Clonazepam also has been used to manage myoclonic and atonic epilepsy; however, most patients develop tolerance to its antiepileptic effect.[6]

Over the past decade, several new antiepileptic drugs have been introduced. These include felbamate, gabapentin, lamotrigine, topiramate, tiagabine, and vigabatrine. These newer agents should not be considered as first-line therapy, and they should be used under the direction of a pediatric neurologist.[23-25]

Seizures Unique to Childhood

Febrile Seizures. As defined by the National Institutes of Health (NIH) Consensus Development Conference of Febrile Seizures in 1980, "A febrile seizure is an event in infancy or childhood, usually occurring between 3 months and 5 years of age, associated with fever but without evidence of intracranial infection or defined cause." Seizures associated with fever in children who have suffered a prior nonfebrile seizure are excluded.[26,27] Approximately 2-5% of all children experience at least one febrile seizure before age 5. The peak incidence is from 9-20 months of age.[26,28]

A simple febrile seizure typically occurs early in the course of illness, is brief (fewer than 15 minutes), and does not have focal features. It does not occur more than once in a 24-hour period. Approximately 20% of first febrile seizures are classified as complex. These are defined as being longer than 15 minutes and focal in nature or occurring in a series during a 24-hour period. Febrile epilepticus is defined as any febrile seizure lasting more than 30 minutes, or recurrent seizures lasting a total of more than 30 minutes without regaining consciousness.[26]

Most febrile seizures are associated with viral illnesses such as upper respiratory infections or gastroenteritis, though they also may be associated with bacterial infections. Seizures in children with shigella gastroenteritis are not uncommon, and may occur before the diarrhea stage begins. Classic viral illnesses associated with rashes such as roseola may be the precipitating cause; however, the diagno-

Table 6. Anticonvulsant Therapy in Common Childhood Seizure Disorders

SEIZURE TYPE	PREFERRED DRUG	ALTERNATE(S)
Generalized tonic-clonic	Carbamazepine Phenytoin	Valproate Phenobarbital
Absence	Ethosuximide	Valproate
Atypical Absence	Valproate	Lamotrigine
Myoclonic	Valproate	Clonazepam Lamotrigine
Atonic	Valproate Clonazepam	Lamotrigine Ethosuximide
Partial, simple and complex	Carbamazepine Phenytoin	Valproate Phenobarbital Primidone Gabapentin Lamotrigine Tiagabine Topiramate
Lennox-Gastaut syndrome		Adjunctive treatment with felbamate Lamotrigine
Infantile Spasms	ACTH (corticotropin)	Prednisone Vigabatrin

sis may be missed, as the seizure usually occurs before the rash appears. The height of the fever and the intensity of the illness are thought to affect the seizure threshold, though a direct correlation is unknown. There is a higher risk of febrile seizures in children with a positive family history of this condition.[12,26,29]

As simple febrile seizures are typically very brief, the child usually will not be actively seizing on arrival to the ED, and may have recovered completely from the postictal period. Many parents will not realize their child had a fever until the temperature is taken either by paramedics or in the ED. The evaluation then should focus on finding the cause of the fever by a thorough history and physical examination. Immunization status must be ascertained, and any recent history of antibiotic use is particularly important, as it may lead to the consideration of partially treated meningitis.

There is general agreement that routine laboratory and radiographic studies are not indicated in uncomplicated first or repeat febrile seizures. Appropriate diagnostic studies should be based on the search for the fever source and will vary in individual patients. The greatest controversy arises over the necessity of performing a lumbar puncture. Many protocols advise an age cut-off between 12 and 18 months, based on the general experience that meningeal signs are difficult to appreciate in this age group. However, many also argue that the decision should be based on the clinical characteristics of each case, as well as physician experience and judgment.[26,30,31] Almost all children with meningitis or encephalitis will present with other signs and symptoms in addition to fever and seizures. In one widely cited study of 503 consecutive children with meningitis, none were found to have meningitis manifesting solely as a simple febrile seizure.[30]

Neuroimaging studies are not helpful in the evaluation of febrile seizures unless the history or physical exam suggests intracranial pathology. An EEG is not indicated as it does not reliably predict the risk of recurrence or the future development of epilepsy.[26,27]

The treatment of febrile seizures is based on the underlying cause of the fever, and also is directed toward control of the fever itself. The actual seizure activity rarely requires anticonvulsant medication.

The risk of recurrence is estimated at 25-50%. One-half of the children who have a second febrile seizure also will have a third. Most recurrences happen within 6-12 months of the initial episode, and in approximately 20% the recurrence is within the same febrile illness.[26,29] Routine prophylaxis with antiepileptic medication is not indicated, although both phenobarbital and diazepam historically have been recommended for this purpose in cases of recurrent or complex febrile seizures.

Parents and other caregivers must be counseled regarding the possibility of seizure recurrence. A common fear is that the child has or will suffer brain damage as a result of the seizure. Reassurance should be given that there is no increased risk of neurological damage, learning disorders, or death as a result of a simple febrile seizure alone. Education in the management of an actively seizing child should be provided, as well as instruction on when to seek immediate medical attention.

Neonatal Seizures. Seizures occur more commonly during infancy than at any other time during childhood.[33] Even though the threshold for seizures is high in the neonatal period, the overall incidence is 1 in 200 live births.[10] Neonatal seizures tend to be brief and commonly are quite subtle. Clinical signs may vary from eye blinking and mouth and tongue movements to repetitive "bicycling" motion of the extremities. Autonomic changes in heart rate, blood pressure, and respirations may occur, including apnea, though apnea as a sole manifestation of a seizure is rare in the newborn.[12] Unlike epilepsy in older children, many events thought to be seizure activity do not have concurrent electrical abnormality on the EEG. Likewise, many epileptic discharges in the newborn EEG are not associated with any clinical signs and are thus of questionable significance.[12]

The most common cause of neonatal seizures is hypoxic-ischemic encephalopathy, with an onset usually in the first day of life. Other conditions precipitating early seizures include congenital CNS anomalies, intracranial hemorrhage, electrolyte derangements, infections, drug withdrawal, and pyridoxine deficiency. Hypoglycemia and hypocalcemia commonly are seen in association with infants of diabetic mothers. Infections are the most common cause of neonatal seizures in the second week of life. Intracranial hemorrhage is observed more frequently in premature infants when seizure activity may be particularly difficult to recognize.[10]

Several features of neonatal seizures may help distinguish them from nonseizure events such as "jitters." Nonepileptic spells usually can be both provoked, and inhibited by sensory stimulation, whereas seizures occur independently of such stimuli. Nonepileptic events usually are not associated with the autonomic changes frequently seen in true seizures. Drug withdrawal seizures usually include general tremulousness, tachypnea, vomiting, diarrhea, and sometimes fever.

The management of neonatal seizures must initially focus on maintaining an adequate airway, ventilation, and cardiovascular support. In the presence of acceptable vital signs and oxygenation, aggressive intervention to terminate brief seizure activity is unwarranted as it is not associated with permanent deficits.[10] Blood glucose should be checked immediately and hypoglycemia corrected if found. Other laboratory studies should include electrolytes, calcium, and magnesium. A CBC, blood and urine cultures, and a lumbar puncture for CSF evaluation also should be obtained. TORCH antibody titers will provide information regarding in utero infections with toxoplasmosis, rubella, cytomegalovirus, and herpes. Other appropriate studies will vary with individual cases and may include an arterial blood gas, ammonia level, blood and urine amino acids, liver enzymes, cranial ultrasound, and head CT.[10]

While most neonatal seizures do not require anticonvulsant medication, those that are prolonged or more compromising should be treated with phenobarbital (15 to 30 mg/kg loading dose). Peak concentration is reached within 90 minutes-6 hours. Pyridoxine deficiency should be considered in the case of intractable seizures, as they will not resolve until pyridoxine is replaced.[12]

Lennox-Gastaut Syndrome. This syndrome refers to a mixed seizure disorder, with the usual onset in children younger than 8 years, in which patients have frequent tonic, absence, myoclonic, and atonic seizures.[12,13] These children often are seen in the ED for evaluation of injuries due to falls associated with their seizures. These children almost always are mentally retarded, although they may not be at the disease onset. They also may have severe behavioral disorders. SE occurs frequently in these children, and they also are prone to nonconvulsive status in which they appear to be in a continuous daze. This condition is characterized by its frequent lack of response to usual anti-epileptic medications. Newer drugs, such as felbamate and lamotrigine, have been used with some success. The ketogenic diet also may be used to manage these children, which is especially important to consider in the ED, because the use of glucose-containing solutions can break the induced ketosis state and, subsequently, increase seizure frequency.

Infantile Spasms (West's Syndrome). This syndrome is characterized by the onset of spasms consisting of sudden single jerks of one or more muscle groups resulting in a sudden flexion or extension of the body. Although each spasm is very brief, they usually occur in clusters and may be associated with a short crying sound. They can be misinterpreted as colic.[13] The typical age at onset is between 4 and 12 months. Therapy traditionally involves the use of adrenocorticotropic hormone (ACTH) or corticosteroids, which may help in the early phase, but the overall prognosis is poor. The vast majority of these children become severely disabled, and usually require institutional care.[13]

Benign Rolandic Epilepsy. This is one of the most common childhood epilepsy syndromes, manifesting as simple partial seizures affecting otherwise normal children between 3 and 13 years of age. These seizures almost always occur at night, waking the child, and may secondarily generalize. The child is unable to speak during the episode. This syndrome may be initially difficult to distinguish from other less benign causes of partial seizures, and the definitive diagnosis requires an EEG. The seizures are benign, resolve during the teenage years, and rarely require treatment. However if they are occurring so frequently as to interrupt sleep, they can be managed with carbamazepine.[12,13]

Juvenile Myoclonic Epilepsy. This syndrome generally occurs in normal patients with a peak onset in the early teenage years, and the etiology appears to be genetic. The hallmark of this disorder is myoclonic seizures, typically on awakening, although tonic, tonic-clonic, and absence seizures also may occur. Frequently, the myoclonic events are not recognized, and the syndrome is not discovered until the onset of a tonic-clonic seizure. Often, these seizures are precipitated by stress, lack of sleep, or excessive alcohol consumption. An EEG is required for definitive diagnosis. The treatment of choice is valproic acid, and usually is required indefinitely.

Status Epilepticus

SE is one of the most common life-threatening emergencies in childhood. It is defined as continuous seizure activity lasting more than 30 minutes, or the occurrence of two or more seizures without full recovery of consciousness in between.[34] Of the approximately 150,000 cases of SE reported each year, the greatest proportion occurs in young children and those older than 60 years. As many as 70% of children younger than 1 year with epilepsy experience at least one episode of SE.[35,36]

Significant hemodynamic and metabolic abnormalities may occur with prolonged seizures and can lead to permanent neurological impairment or even death. The repetitive muscle contractions of SE place a great strain on the patient's cardiovascular, respiratory, and renal systems. Tachycardia and other arrhythmias may occur. Acidosis and hyperkalemia develop from the accumulation of lactate, and the development of rhabdomyolysis. Respiratory acidosis and hypoxia also may be seen. Moreover, the medications used to control SE may contribute to these findings. Nevertheless, the mortality rate is determined primarily by the etiology and severity of the underlying disease.[35,36] Although any type of seizure can progress to SE, generalized tonic-clonic seizures are the most common presentation and will be the focus of discussion.

Management of Status Epilepticus. Most seizures in children stop spontaneously in the prehospital phase, without any anticonvulsant medication. Therefore, it is safe to assume that if a child is actively seizing on arrival to the ED, the seizure will continue unless treated. It is important to ascertain if any anti-epileptic medication has been given prior to arrival. It has been shown that the prehospital administration of diazepam can shorten the duration of SE and reduce the risk of recurrence.[37,38]

In an actively seizing child, the initial supportive, therapeutic, and diagnostic measures must occur simultaneously. *(See Table 7.)* Cardiorespiratory support must take precedence over the ultimate goal of ending the convulsions. Several studies have determined that SE is much less dangerous when not associated with hypoxia.[36] Vital signs, pulse oximetry, and cardiac rhythm must be closely monitored. A bedside blood glucose level should be immediately determined, and any hypoglycemia corrected. The initial stabilization phase,

Table 7. Management of Convulsive Status Epilepticus

STABILIZATION

- Protect the patient
- Check airway, breathing, and circulation (ABCs)
- Monitor vital signs with pulse oximetry
- Intubate, if indicated, to secure the airway
- Establish IV or IO access with normal saline
- Draw blood for laboratory tests
- Check for hypoglycemia

INITIAL INTERVENTION

- Give glucose if hypoglycemic
- Give antibiotics if meningitis is suspected
- Cooling measures and antipyretics, if indicated
- First-line IV anticonvulsant medication
  - Lorazepam, 0.1 mg/kg at 2 mg/min, *or*
  - Diazepam, 0.2 mg/kg at 5 mg/min, *or*
  - Midazolam, 0.2 mg/kg
  - Consider the use of rectal diazepam, or IM, IN, *or* buccal Midazolam if there is no IV access
- Add long-acting IV anticonvulsant medication
  - Phenytoin, 20 mg/kg at 1 mg/kg/min, *or*
  - Fosphenytoin, 20 mg PE/kg at 3 mg/kg/min

IF SEIZURES PERSIST

- IV load with second long-acting anticonvulsant
  - Phenobarbital, 20 mg/kg at 100 mg/min
- If seizures continue, add Phenobarbital, 5-10 mg/kg until a maximum of 40 mg/kg or 1 gm

REFRACTORY STATUS EPILEPTICUS

- If not given previously, IV bolus with midazolam 0.2 mg/kg, followed by a drip of 1-10 mcg/kg/min
- Transfer to ICU
- Begin continuous EEG monitoring
- Institute general anesthesia with IV
  - Pentobarbital, 5-15 mg/kg at 25 mg/min, followed by 1-5 mg/kg/hr

which should not delay the administration of anticonvulsants, should be accomplished within the first 10 minutes. This includes establishing either intravenous (IV) or intraosseous (IO) access, obtaining blood for laboratory studies, and a directed history and physical examination. Specific attention should be given to any history or signs of trauma, poisoning or substance abuse, pre-existing epilepsy, and focal neurological findings.

Laboratory tests should be guided by the available history, and may include CBC, chemistry studies, arterial blood gas, toxicology screens, and medication levels as indicated. A lumbar puncture should be performed when the seizures are controlled and the child is hemodynamically stable. However, if meningitis or encephalitis is suspected, antibiotic or antiviral therapy should not be delayed until the lumbar puncture is done. A head CT should be ordered prior to the lumbar puncture whenever intracranial hypertension, hydrocephalus, or a mass lesion is suspected. MRI may be more helpful in a known seizure patient who has had prior CT scans.[34,51]

SE in patients with a tricyclic antidepressant overdose poses a special challenge, as the treatment requires that bicarbonate be given to raise the arterial pH above 7.5.[11] Otherwise, all patients with prolonged convulsions will show a metabolic acidosis, which should not be corrected with bicarbonate as it will resolve once seizure control is achieved.[35] Particular attention also should be paid to preventing hyperthermia, which is another common complication and may contribute to future neurological impairment.[35]

Traditionally, IV benzodiazepines have been the first-line anticonvulsants of choice. Both diazepam (0.1-0.5 mg/kg) and lorazepam (0.05-0.2 mg/kg) administered either IV or IO have proven to be potent, rapidly acting, and effective in terminating seizure activity approximately 75% to 90% of the time.[34,36,39] Lorazepam is currently preferred due to its longer duration of action and its slightly safer profile of adverse effects. Both lorazepam and diazepam have been used rectally with good results, however rectal diazepam has been studied more extensively.[11,34,40] Lorazepam needs to be kept refrigerated, which limits its usefulness outside the hospital.[36] A rectal gel has been formulated containing 5 mg/mL of diazepam packaged in pre-filled syringes.[39] This has been particularly useful in the prehospital phase when no IV or IO access is available. It also has been well received and used extensively by families in many European countries and the United Kingdom. The recommended dosages for rectal diazepam are: ages 2-5 years, 0.5 mg/kg; ages 6-11 years, 0.3 mg/kg; and ages 12 and older, 0.02 mg/kg. Regardless of the method given, both lorazepam and diazepam share the potential for hypotension, respiratory depression, impairment of consciousness, and short-term duration of seizure control.[34,35,39]

Another benzodiazepine, midazolam, rapidly is emerging as an alternative treatment for SE, both as the initial anticonvulsant given and in cases refractory to more traditional therapy.[35,39-46] The water solubility, rapid onset of action, and short elimination half life of midazolam offer clear advantages over other benzodiazepines. The short elimination half life and the relative inactivity of its metabolites allow for a better post seizure neurological evaluation.

Midazolam also offers significant advantages with its versatility of use, including IV, IM, rectal, intranasal, and buccal routes of administration. Recent reports of the successful use of intranasal and buccal midazolam in halting SE may lead to it becoming the treatment of choice, especially in the prehospital phase.[42,43] Midazolam also has been shown to have a good safety profile with low rates of cardiovascular and respiratory depression.[34,35,41]

The majority of seizures will stop following adequate doses of benzodiazepines; however, a longer-acting agent also should be given to prevent recurrence. A second-line drug also will be required in those cases unresponsive to initial therapy. IV phenytoin generally is considered the drug of choice for this purpose. Phenytoin is very effective in both acute and chronic seizure management. When administered as an IV loading dose of 20 mg/kg, peak brain levels are reached in 10-30 minutes.[39] Phenytoin has the advantages of a long duration of action, an easy transition to oral maintenance, and the lack of significant cardiac, respiratory, or CNS depression. The drawbacks of phenytoin use include the necessity of IV use, the association with cardiac arrhythmias requiring continuous cardiac monitoring, and administration at a rate no faster than 50 mg/min. In addition, IV phenytoin must be given in normal saline as any glucose containing IV fluid will cause precipitation. This may require that a second IV line be accessed. Moreover, severe tissue necrosis may result if there is any extravasation.

Fosphenytoin has been approved for use since 1996, and is gaining acceptance as a phenytoin substitute. Fosphenytoin offers significant administration and several safety advantages over phenytoin. It can be given much more quickly by the IV route, and is compatible with glucose-containing solutions. It is much less of a tissue irritant, and the availability of an IM form allows treatment when vascular access is difficult.[39] Fosphenytoin has a peak serum level within 30 minutes after IM use, and at six minutes following IV loading. The dose of fosphenytoin is expressed as phenytoin equivalents (PE) and is 15-20 mgPE/kg. If given IV, the maximum infusion rate is 150 mg /min (3 mg/kg/min).[35,39] The current roadblocks to widespread fosphenytoin acceptance seem mainly related to its high cost and the lack of significant experience in the pediatric population.

Phenobarbital is the next anticonvulsant treatment recommended for those patients who continue to seize even after first- and second-line therapy. The recommended IV dose is 20 mg/kg, given at an infusion rate of 100 mg/min.[34,36] The infusion rate should be slowed if seizures abate prior to completing the dose. Although phenobarbital has a long history of successful use as an antiepileptic agent, it is generally considered second to phenytoin for long-term seizure control due to its marked sedative effects. It is however preferred over phenytoin for the management of SE in neonates.[47] The average time from phenobarbital administration to control of SE is 15-30 minutes. However, due to its long elimination half-life (approximately 100 hours), its effective duration of action is about 48 hours.[34,36] The patient's respiratory status must be closely guarded with phenobarbital use, and intubation may be required. The risk of respiratory depression is significantly increased when phenobarbital is given to a patient who has already received a benzodiazepine. If SE continues after the initial phenobarbital loading, additional doses of 5-10 mg/kg may be given up to a total of 40 mg/kg, or a maximum dose of 1 gm.[47]

SE that persists even after the above treatment is considered refractory, and may require general anesthesia. As previously mentioned, however, recent studies with midazolam have shown promise in terminating SE and would be a good choice in refractory cases prior to consideration of the more traditional barbiturate coma. Several studies report success with midazolam when the prior use of diazepam, lorazepam, phenytoin, and phenobarbital have failed.[41,48-50] The IV dose advised is a bolus of 0.2 mg/kg, followed by a continuous IV drip in a range of 1-10 mcg/kg/min.[51]

Pentobarbital remains the barbiturate of choice for the induction of coma. It penetrates the brain rapidly and is in turn more quickly eliminated than phenobarbital or thiopental. It has no active metabolites, and may also exert a protective effect in cerebral hypoxia, as well as lower intracranial pressure.[34,44,51] Pentobarbital is administered as an IV loading dose of 5-15 mg/kg, followed by a maintenance infusion of 0.5-5.0 mg/kg/hr.[51] All patients with a pentobarbital-induced coma require intubation and ventilatory support. A barbiturate coma suppresses all brainstem function, thus requiring extensive hemodynamic and EEG monitoring. Pentobarbital use is adjusted to produce a burst suppression on continuous EEG monitoring.

Other drugs that have been used in the management of refractory SE include IV lidocaine, IV propofol, IV and rectal valproic acid, rectal paraldehyde, rectal chloral hydrate, and inhalational anesthesia with halothane and isoflurane gases.[36,39,51] However, with the better known pentobarbital coma, and the encouraging use of midazolam, these alternative agents should rarely be required.

Summary

Children with both new onset and established seizure disorders commonly seek care in the ED. The evaluation of each child will vary with the circumstances of presentation. The management of a child with an apparent first seizure is particularly challenging. A patient with active convulsions must be immediately stabilized. In an already stable patient, the approach begins with a careful assessment of the details of the event, with consideration given to various disorders that may mimic seizure activity. The history and physical and diagnostic tests are directed at determining the etiology of the seizure, and guide management. The necessity and appropriateness for both immediate and future anticonvulsant therapy must be determined, and should be coordinated with the child's primary care physician or pediatric neurologist. Disposition must take the child's social situation, compliance issues, and available resources into account. Family education regarding home management is essential, as well as the need for close follow-up.

References

1. Terndrup TE. Clinical issues in acute childhood seizure management in the emergency department. *J Child Neurol* 1998;13(suppl 1):7-10.
2. Smith RA, Martland T, Lowry MF. Children with seizures presenting to accident and emergency. *J Accid Emerg Med* 1996;13:54-58.
3. Freeman JM, Vining EP. Decision making and the child with afebrile seizures. *Pediatr Rev* 1992;13:305-311.
4. Barnett TM, Wasserman GS. Seizures and status epilepticus. In: Reisdorff et al, eds. *Pediatric Emergency Medicine*. Pennsylvania: W.B.Saunders; 1993:1008-1014.
5. Commission on Classification and Terminology of the International League Against Epilepsy. Proposal for revised clinical and electroencephalographic classification of epileptic seizures. *Epilepsia* 1981;22:489-501.
6. Willmore LJ, Wheless JW. Epilepsy. In: Medicine. New York: Scientific American;1999:11(XII).
7. Zupanc ML. Update on Epilepsy in pediatric patients. *Mayo Clin Proc* 1996; 71:899-916.
8. Bradford JC, Kyriakedes CG. Evaluation of the patient with seizures: An evidence based approach. *Emerg Med Clin North Am* 1999;17:203-220.
9. Roth HL, Drislane FW. Seizures. *Neurol Clin North Am* 1998;16: 257-284.
10. Sheth DP. Hypocalcemic seizures in neonates. *Am J Emerg Med* 1997;15:638-641.
11. Pelligrino TR. An emergency department approach to first-time seizures. *Emerg Med Clin North Am* 1994;12:925-939.
12. Murphy JV, Dehkharghani F. Diagnosis of childhood seizure disor-

ders. *Epilepsia* 1994;35(suppl 2):7-17.

13. Vining EP. Pediatric seizures. *Emerg Med Clin North Am* 1994;12:973-987.
14. Rubin DH, Conway EE, et al. Neurologic disorders. In: Rosen, Barkin, eds. *Emergency Medicine: Concepts and Clinical Practice* 4th Ed. St. Louis: Mosby; 1997:1213-1242.
15. Stores G. Practioner review: Recognition of pseudoseizures in children and adolescents. *J Child Psychol Psychiat* 1999;40:851-857.
16. Jagoda A, Richardson L. The evaluation and treatment of seizures in the emergency department. *Mount Sinai J Med* 1997;64:249-257.
17. ACEP Clinical Policies Committee. Clinical policy for the initial approach to patients presenting with a chief complaint of seizure who are not in status epilepticus. *Ann Emerg Med* 1997;29:706-724.
18. Turnbull TL, Vanden Hoek TL, et al. Utility of laboratory studies in the emergency department patient with a new-onset seizure. *Ann Emerg Med* 1990;19:373-377.
19. Baraff LJ, Schriger DL, et al. Compliance with a standard for the emergency department management of epileptics who present after an uncomplicated convulsion. *Ann Emerg Med* 1990;19:367-372.
20. Warden CR, Brownstein DR, Del Becarro MA. Predictors of abnormal findings of computed tomography of the head in pediatric patients presenting with seizures. *Ann Emerg Med* 1997;29: 518-523.
21. American College of Emergency Physicians. Practice Parameter: Neuroimaging in the emergency patient presenting with seizure (summary statement). *Ann Emerg Med* 1996;28:114-118.
22. Privitera MD, Stawsburg RH. Electroencephalographic monitoring in the emergency department. *Emerg Med Clin North Am* 1994;12: 1089-1100.
23. Pellock JM. Managing pediatric epilepsy syndromes with new antileptic drugs. *Pediatrics* 1999;104:1106-1116.
24. Pellock JM, Appleton R. Use of the new antiepileptic drugs in the treatment of childhood epilepsy. *Epilepsia* 1999;40(suppl 6):29-38.
25. Pellock JM, Watemberg N. New antiepileptic drugs in children: Present and future. *Seminars Ped Neurol* 1997;4:9-18.
26. Stenklyft PH, Carmona M. Febrile seizures. *Emerg Med Clin North Am* 1994;12:989-999.
27. Kuturec M, Emoto SE, et al. Febrile seizures: Is the EEG a useful predictor of recurrences? *Clin Pediatr* 1997;36:31-36.
28. Teach SJ, Geil PA. Incidence of bacteremia, urinary tract infections, and unsuspected bacterial meningitis in children with febrile seizures. *Ped Emerg Care* 1999;15:9-12.
29. Freeman JM, Vining EP. Decision making and the child with febrile seizures. *Pediatr Rev* 1992;13:299-304.
30. Green SM, Rothrock SG, et al. Can seizures be the sole manifestation of meningitis in febrile children? *Pediatrics* 1993;91:527-534.
31. Nozica C. Lumbar puncture and the first simple febrile seizure. *Pediatrics* 1997;99:306-307.
32. Baumann RJ, D'angelo SL. Technical report summary: The neurodiagnostic evaluation of the child with a first simple febrile seizure. *Pediatrics* 1996;97:769-771.
33. Nordli DR, Bazil CW, et al. Recognition and classification of seizures in infants. *Epilepsia* 1997;38:553-560.
34. Shepherd SM. Management of status epilepticus. *Emerg Med Clin North Am* 1994;12:941-961.
35. Wheless JW. Treatment of acute seizures and status epilepticus in children. *J Child Neurol* 1999;20(suppl)47-51.
36. Haafiz A, Kissoon N. Status epilepticus: Current concepts. *Pediatr Emerg Care* 1999;15:119-129.
37. Alldredge BK, Wall DB, Ferriero DM. Effect of prehospital treatment on the outcome of status epilepticus in children. *Pediatr Neurol* 1995;12:213-216.
38. Tasker RC. Emergency treatment of acute seizures and status epilepticus. *Arch Dis Child* 1998;79:78-83.
39. Morton LD, Rizkallah E, Pellock JM. New drug therapy for acute seizure management. *Seminars in Pediatr Neurol* 1997;4:51-63.
40. Appleton R, Sweeney A, et al. Lorazepam vs diazepam in the acute treatment of epileptic seizures and status epilepticus. *Dev Med Child Neurol* 1995;37:682-688.
41. Pellock JM. Use of midazolam for refractory status epilepticus in pediatric patients. *J Child Neurol* 1998;13:581-587.
42. Kendall JL, Reynolds M, Goldberg R. Intranasal midazolam in patients with status epilepticus. *Ann Emerg Med* 1997;29:415-417.
43. Scott RC, Besag F, Neville B. Buccal midazolam and rectal diazepam for the treatment of prolonged seizures in childhood and adolescence: A randomized trial. *Lancet* 1999;353:623-626.
44. Holmes GL, Riviello JJ. Midazolam and pentobarbital for refractory status epilepticus. *Pediatr Neurol* 1999;20:259-261.
45. McDonagh TJ, Jelinek GA, Galvin GM. Intramuscular midazolam rapidly terminates seizures in children and adults. *Emerg Med* 1992;4:77-81.
46. Lal Koul R, Raj Aithala G, et al. Continuous midazolam infusion as treatment for status epilepticus. *Arch Dis Child* 1997;76:445-448.
47. Sabo-Graham T, Seay AR. Management of status epilepticus in children. *Pediatr Rev* 1998;19:306-309.
48. Rivera R, Segnini M, et al. Midazolam in the treatment of status epilepticus in children. *Crit Care Med* 1993;21:991.
49. Parent JM, Lowenstein DH. Treatment of refractory generalized status epilepticus with continuous infusion of midazolam. *Neurology* 1994;44:1837-1840.
50. Kumar A, Bleck TP. Intravenous midazolam for the treatment of refractory status epilepticus. *Crit Care Med* 1992;20:483-488.
51. Roberts MR, Eng-Bourquin J. Status epilepticus in children. *Emerg Med Clin North Am* 1995;13:489-507.

Hypoglycemia in Infants and Children

Samuel R. Reid, MD
Joseph D. Losek, MD, FAAP, FACEP

Children with hypoglycemia pose a diagnostic challenge because hypoglycemia is an uncommon pediatric condition and its presenting signs and symptoms may be either nonspecific or suggestive of a pathophysiology other than hypoglycemia. However, prompt recognition is of utmost importance because untreated hypoglycemia may result in permanent neurologic dysfunction.

Hypoglycemia is not a diagnosis in itself but rather a sign suggesting a more specific diagnosis. Although the causes of hypoglycemia in a child are numerous, and many may seem obscure, the clinician must have a working knowledge of the broad diagnostic categories of hypoglycemia so that a timely and appropriate diagnostic investigation can be initiated at the time of recognition and treatment.

This chapter reviews those aspects of pediatric hypoglycemia that are important for emergency department management.

Definition

While it is generally accepted that a plasma glucose concentration of less than 60 mg/dL constitutes hypoglycemia in an older child or adult, the definition of hypoglycemia in the newborn period and during infancy is controversial.[1,2] Attempts to correlate clinical signs with glucose levels have depended on subjective assessments and are inconclusive.[1] A review of 36 pediatric textbooks found cutoff values for hypoglycemia in newborns ranging from 18 to 72 mg/dL.[2] Most authorities, however, would currently accept that a plasma glucose of less than 30 mg/dL in the first 24 hours of life and less than 45 mg/dL thereafter constitutes hypoglycemia in the newborn.[3] Over time, the trend has been to accept higher and higher values of plasma glucose as constituting hypoglycemia in this age group. Some authorities have advocated abandoning a numerical definition of hypoglycemia, arguing that the plasma glucose concentration constituting euglycemia may vary from person to person and from physiologic circumstance to physiologic circumstance.[1,2,4] Until consensus has been reached as to the level of plasma glucose below which neurologic injury occurs, it seems prudent that the emergency medicine physician maintain a low threshold for the diagnosis and treatment of hypoglycemia in newborns and infants.

Measurement

The plasma glucose concentration is felt to closely approximate the amount of glucose available to brain tissue and is therefore considered the "gold standard" for the determination of hypoglycemia.[1,2,5] Whole blood measurements of glucose underestimate the plasma glucose concentration by approximately 10-15% because erythrocytes contain relatively low concentrations of glucose.[1,6] Venous samples are preferred; arterial and capillary samples

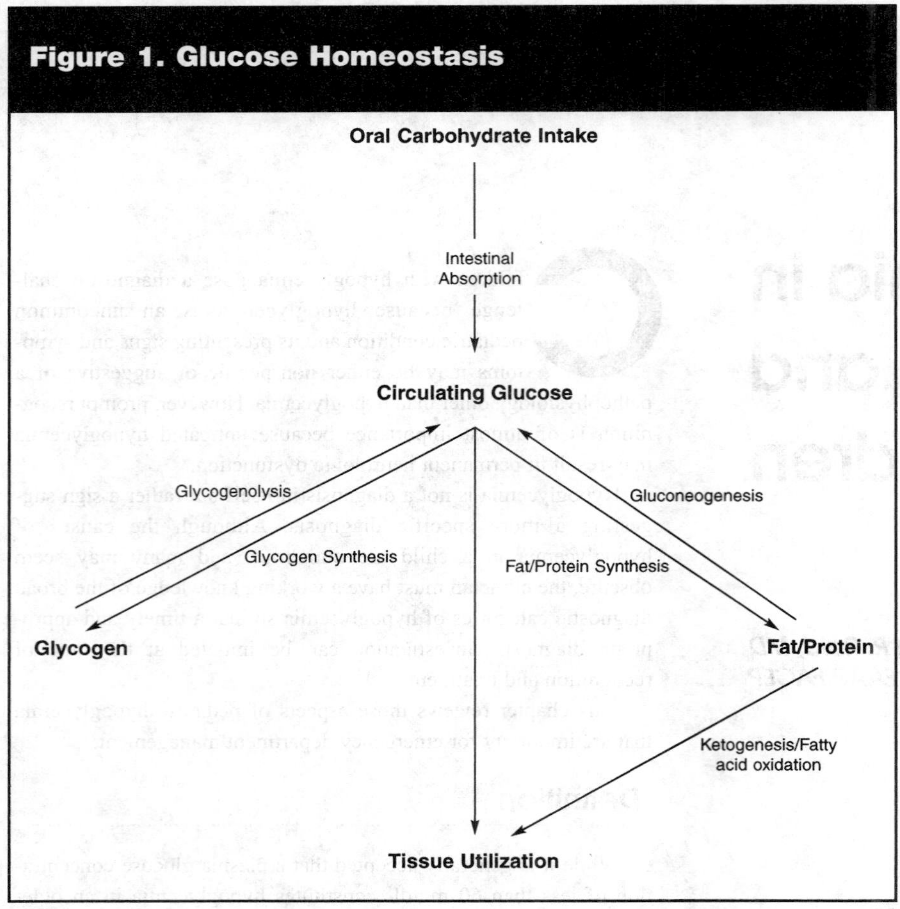

may overestimate the plasma glucose concentration by 10% in nonfasting patients.[1] Specimens should ideally be transported to the laboratory on ice and analyzed promptly to minimize the effect of ongoing glucose consumption by blood cells.[1,7,8]

Bedside glucose determination is a convenient and expeditious method for determining glucose concentration in the emergency department. However, such determinations may not be accurate at low glucose concentrations; both false positives and false negatives occur.[1,7,8] Isopropyl alcohol used for skin preparation may contaminate specimens and cause erroneous results.[1,7,9] A low hematocrit can result in falsely high readings, while a high hematocrit and hyperbilirubinemia can result in falsely low readings.[2,6,7] Some brands of reagent strips are not intended for use in neonates.[7] In a recent study of adult patients, however, bedside glucose determination using a visually interpreted reagent strip was found to be both sensitive and specific for the detection of hypoglycemia.[10] Until these findings have been reproduced for pediatric patients, all children for whom hypoglycemia is a possibility (either on the basis of clinical findings or a suggestive bedside glucose determination) should be treated while awaiting the results of a confirmatory laboratory plasma glucose determination.[3,6,9]

Physiology and Pathophysiology

Glucose homeostasis is an intricate balance between those physiologic mechanisms that reduce circulating glucose (fasting, glucose utilization, and insulin) and those that increase circulating glucose (feeding, gastrointestinal glucose absorption, catecholamines, glucagon, growth hormone, and adrenal corticosteroids).[5,6,11] Figure 1 diagrams glucose homeostasis. The brain is a principal consumer of circulating glucose and for all practical purposes, is dependent on glucose alone for its metabolic needs.[1,5] When the brain is deprived of glucose for prolonged periods or on multiple occasions, injury occurs.[3,5,6,9]

Any disorder that interferes with carbohydrate intake, intestinal absorption, glycogen formation or mobilization, gluconeogenesis, ketogenesis, or fatty acid oxidation places a child at risk for hypoglycemia. Similarly, disorders which result in excessive tissue utilization of glucose (e.g., hyperinsulinism) place a child at risk for hypoglycemia.

In the presence of hypoglycemia, epinephrine and glucagon are released and stimulate glycogenolysis, gluconeogenesis, and ketogenesis. Glycogenolysis acutely increases levels of circulating glucose; gluconeogenesis becomes important when glycogen stores are depleted. After a period of adaptation, the brain can derive a portion of its energy needs by metabolizing the products of ketogenesis and fatty acid oxidation.[12] Concomitantly, increased cardiac output and systemic vascular resistance increase cerebral blood flow and the delivery of glucose to brain tissue. Glucose utilization by muscle tissue is diminished and insulin secretion is suppressed. Growth hormone, adrenal corticosteroids, and non-epinephrine catecholamines also contribute to these physiologic responses.[5,6,11]

A number of factors make the infant and child more vulnerable to hypoglycemia than the adult. Glucose utilization is higher, probably due to the proportionately larger brain.[5] Glycogen stores are smaller and may only be sufficient to provide circulating glucose for a fast of a few hours. Available muscle mass and fat stores from which to generate precursors for gluconeogenesis and ketogenesis are smaller. Most importantly, the developing brain is more prone to hypoglycemic injury.[9]

Electroencephalogram and brain imaging studies in patients who have suffered hypoglycemic events demonstrate characteristic changes.[13-15] Pathologically, neuronal injury primarily affecting the superficial cerebral cortex, dentate gyrus, caudate nucleus, and hippocampus has been described.[3] Clinical outcomes ranging from no detectable sequelae and mild cognitive dysfunction to microcephaly, mental retardation, and epilepsy have been described.[3,16-19] Symptomatic hypoglycemia, particularly that resulting in seizures, seems to be more strongly associated with more adverse neurologic sequelae than asymptomatic hypoglycemia.[3,19] Neonates seem to be most vulnerable to adverse outcomes.[9]

Clinical Features

History. The relationship of a hypoglycemic episode to the most recent meal can be important diagnostically. Hypoglycemia occurring

Table 1. Signs and Symptoms of Hypoglycemia in Infants and Children

	Adrenergic	Neuroglycopenic	Other
INFANTS:	Tachycardia	Poor feeding	Hypothermia
	Tachypnea	Lethargy	
	Pallor	Irritability	
	Cyanosis	Hypotonia	
	Jitteriness	Seizure	
		Coma	
		Apnea	
CHILDREN:	Nausea	Visual disturbance	Hunger
	Anxiety	Parasthesia	Headache
	Weakness	Lethargy	
	Tachycardia	Irritability	
	Pallor	Confusion	
	Diaphoresis	Bizarre behavior	
	Tremor	Incoordination	
		Seizure	
		Coma	

after a short fast (2-3 hours) is suggestive of glycogen storage disease. Hypoglycemia occurring after a long fast (12-14 hours) suggests a disorder of gluconeogenesis. Postprandial hypoglycemia may indicate galactosemia or hereditary fructose intolerance. Hypoglycemia inconsistently related to fasting is seen in patients with hyperinsulinism.[5,20] A family history of sudden infant deaths may be a clue to an unrecognized, inherited metabolic disorder. A history of ingestion of an agent known to cause hypoglycemia (e.g., sulfonylurea) should be sought but may not always be available.

Signs and Symptoms. Signs and symptoms of hypoglycemia are typically divided into two categories: adrenergic and neuroglycopenic. Adrenergic signs and symptoms result from secretion of epinephrine in response to the stress of hypoglycemia. Neuroglycopenic signs and symptoms reflect a circulating supply of glucose which is insufficient for normal brain function. Classic teaching suggests that adrenergic signs and symptoms precede neuroglycopenic signs and symptoms. Recent evidence, however, suggests that not all patients present with such a predictable evolution of symptoms and that some patients will develop no adrenergic phenomena at all. Patients with repeated episodes of hypoglycemia tend to experience similar symptoms with each event; however, their perception of these symptoms may be diminished. Certain symptoms commonly experienced by hypoglycemic patients are not explained by adrenergic stimulation or neuroglycopenia alone.[21]

Infants cannot describe their symptoms and have a limited repertoire of signs with which to manifest illness. Signs of hypoglycemia are therefore particularly nonspecific and may suggest dysfunction in any of several organ systems. Because infants are particularly vulnerable to hypoglycemia, the possibility of hypoglycemia should be considered for all ill patients in this age group. Table 1 summarizes hypoglycemic signs and symptoms for infants and older children. It should be remembered that hypoglycemia may be asymptomatic.

On occasion, hypoglycemia will present with symptoms or signs suggestive of a pathophysiology other than hypoglycemia. Of these, focal neurologic deficits seem to be the most common. Several reports of hemiplegia and hemiparesis affecting pediatric patients can be found in the literature.[22-25] As in adult patients, the pathogenesis is unclear but may reflect a Todd's paralysis following an unrecognized focal seizure, cerebral vasospasm, or selective neuronal susceptibility to hypoglycemia.[23-25]

Other described focal neurologic manifestations of hypoglycemia include cranial nerve palsies, ataxia, cortical blindness, decerebrate posturing, and choreoathetosis.[26-31] Non-neurologic presentations of hypoglycemia suggestive of other disease processes include acute respiratory failure, sinus bradycardia, night terrors, psychosis, and urticaria.[32-36]

Hypoglycemia can also present as a complication of other disease processes such as sepsis, congestive heart failure, alcohol intoxication, dehydration, and trauma.[5,37-40] The clinician should not overlook the possibility of hypoglycemia in any ill-appearing infant or child.[41]

Physical Examination. Certain physical findings are helpful in determining the etiology of hypoglycemia.

Hepatomegally is strong evidence for an inborn error of metabolism or primary hepatic disease. Short stature may reflect growth hormone deficiency. Macrosomia suggests hyperinsulinism. The combination of macrosomia, macroglossia, omphalocele, and organomegally is consistent with Beckwith-Wiedemann syndrome. Hyperpigmentation and ambiguous genitalia are seen with adrenal insufficiency. Cleft palate and micropenis suggest hypopituitarism.

Etiology and Differential Diagnosis

The differential diagnosis of hypoglycemia in infants and children is broad and summarized in Table 2. Selected etiologies are discussed below. Phillip has proposed an algorithm for the diagnostic evaluation of the hypoglycemic child for whom toxin or drug ingestion, malnutrition, liver failure, and extrapancreatic tumors have been excluded.[20]

Neonatal. Neonatal hypoglycemia is not typically encountered in the emergency department. However, earlier postpartum discharges have led to reports of neonatal hypoglycemia presenting as outpatient emergencies.[42] Most cases of neonatal hypoglycemia are transient and result from decreased glucose production (e.g., deficient glycogen stores and impaired gluconeogenesis in small for gestational age infants) or increased utilization (e.g., hyperinsulinism in an infant of a diabetic mother). Hypoglycemia persisting beyond, or occurring after, the third day of life suggests the possibility of an endocrine or metabolic disorder.[43]

Endocrine. Hypoglycemia is a common complication of insulin therapy in children with insulin dependent diabetes mellitus. As efforts to maintain stricter glycemic control in diabetic patients intensify, the risk of hypoglycemia increases.[44,45] If a child does not consume enough glucose-containing foods or beverages following the administration of insulin, hypoglycemia will occur. Diabetic patients who experience multiple episodes of hypoglycemia may develop "hypoglycemia unawareness," a failure to perceive symptoms of hypoglycemia. The mechanism of this phenomenon is unclear but may involve a blunted neurohumoral counterregulatory response to hypoglycemia.[46,47] Such patients are more likely to present with findings of profound neuroglycopenia.[47]

Hyperinsulinism presents as refractory hypoglycemia without ketosis and results from a defect in pancreatic beta cell regulation, pancreatic beta cell hyperplasia, or an islet cell adenoma.[5,8,48]

Table 2. Differential Diagnosis of Hypoglycemia

NEONATAL
- Infant of diabetic mother
- Small for gestational age
- Prematurity
- Asphyxia
- Hypothermia
- Systemic illness (e.g., sepsis, respiratory distress syndrome)
- Adrenal hemorrhage
- Beckwith-Wiedemann syndrome
- Maternal medication (e.g., insulin, beta-blockers)

ENDOCRINE
- Hyperinsulinism (e.g., insulinoma, nesidioblastosis)
- Hypopituitarism
- Growth hormone deficiency
- Adrenocortical deficiency (e.g., congenital adrenal hyperplasia)
- Hypothyroidism
- Glucagon deficiency
- Catecholamine deficiency (e.g., adrenal medullary unresponsiveness)

INBORN ERRORS OF METABOLISM
- Disorders of carbohydrate metabolism (e.g., galactosemia, glycogen storage diseases)
- Disorders of amino acid and organic acid metabolism (e.g., methylmalonic acidemia, biotinidase deficiency)
- Disorders of fat metabolism (e.g., carnitine deficiency)

TOXIC
- Salicylates
- Alcohol
- Oral hypoglycemic agents (e.g., sulfonylureas)
- Insulin (e.g., diabetic therapy, factitious)
- Propranolol
- Antimalarial agents
- Unripe ackee fruit

OTHER
- Fasting
- Intestinal malabsorption
- Idiopathic ketotic hypoglycemia
- Dehydrating gastroenteritis
- Sepsis
- Liver failure (e.g., Reye syndrome, hepatitis)
- Large extrapancreatic tumor (e.g., Wilm's tumor)
- Cyanotic congenital heart disease
- Malnutrition (e.g., anorexia nervosa)
- Trauma

Inappropriately high levels of circulating insulin increase tissue glucose utilization and decrease rates of endogenous glucose production. Intentional misuse of insulin by a diabetic child or an abusive parent will also result in hypoglycemia and can be detected by measuring low serum levels of c-peptide in the setting of high serum levels of insulin.[8] Large, non-pancreatic tumors can occasionally produce an insulin-like substance with resultant hypoglycemia.[49]

Several other endocrine pathways are instrumental to glucose homeostasis. Glucagon, growth hormone, and cortisol play important roles in the physiologic response to hypoglycemia; deficiency of any of them predictably predisposes a child to hypoglycemia. Hypopituitarism results in both ACTH and growth hormone deficiency; therefore, patients with this disorder are especially prone to hypoglycemia. Thyroid hormone may play a role in the production of gluconeogenic substrates and hepatic enzyme function, and its deficiency has occasionally been associated with hypoglycemia. "Adrenal medullary unresponsiveness" is a term applied to children who are found to have low levels of secreted epinephrine in response to hypoglycemia. Some authorities feel these patients constitute a subset of idiopathic ketotic hypoglycemia.[6]

Inborn Errors of Metabolism

Inborn errors of metabolism are rare, but as a group are responsible for a significant portion of childhood hypoglycemia. Most are inherited in an autosomal recessive manner. Presentations vary but hepatomegally, failure to thrive, and metabolic acidosis are common. Burton has recently reviewed the diagnosis of inborn errors of metabolism.[50]

Toxic. Numerous medications and toxins are associated with hypoglycemia. Ethanol causes hepatic enzyme dysfunction and impaired gluconeogenesis.[5] Salicylate toxicity has been associated with hypoglycemia but the mechanism remains unclear.[51] Propranolol inhibits glucagon and epinephrine secretion and the mobilization of glycogen. Beta adrenergic blockade can also mask adrenergic signs and symptoms of hypoglycemia.[6,52] Sulfonylurea oral hypoglycemic agents produce a state of hyperinsulinism.[53] Unripe ackee fruit contains hypoglycin, a substance that inhibits gluconeogenesis.[8]

Other. Idiopathic ketotic hypoglycemia is the most common cause of hypoglycemia in non-diabetic children outside the neonatal period. It characteristically occurs in a child 1-5 years of age after a relatively long fast (more than 12 hours) or when suffering a routine illness. Affected children are typically smaller than their peers and may have been small for gestational age. It is felt that these children have diminished stores of gluconeogenic substrates (low muscle mass) and thus are less tolerant of prolonged fasting. This disorder typically resolves spontaneously by age 10.[5,6]

Fulminant liver disease such as with Reye syndrome or infectious hepatitis may cause hypoglycemia as a result of decreased glycogen stores and impaired gluconeogenesis.[6]

Cyanotic congenital heart disease has been associated with hypoglycemia. Chronic hypoxia may interfere with hepatic glycogen storage and release.[5] Hepatic hypoperfusion leading to impaired gluconeogenesis may be responsible for hypoglycemia in children with acyanotic congenital heart disease and congestive failure.[5] However, poor oral intake and intestinal malabsorption resulting in poor glycogen stores may also contribute.[38]

Reports from underdeveloped nations have associated hypo-

Table 3. Laboratory Studies to Obtain at the Time of Hypoglycemia

BLOOD	URINE
Plasma glucose (confirmatory)	Urinalysis (ketones)
Electrolytes (anion gap)	Reducing substances
Lactate	
Pyruvate	
Beta-hydroxybutyrate	
Acetoacetate	
Insulin	
Glucagon	
Cortisol	
Growth hormone	
Free fatty acids	
Alanine	
Glycerol	

Table 4. Treatment of Hypoglycemia

ORAL	
Juice (orange/apple)	10-20 mL/kg PO/NG/OG
DEXTROSE	
Bolus	
Neonate:	$D_{10}W$ 5-10 mL/kg IV/IO
Child:	$D_{25}W$ 2-4 mL/kg IV/IO
Infusion	
6 mg/kg/min	$D_{10}W$ at (3.6 × weight [kg]) mL/hr
8 mg/kg/min	$D_{10}W$ at (4.8 × weight [kg]) mL/hr
10 mg/kg/min	$D_{10}W$ at (6 × weight [kg]) mL/hr
12 mg/kg/min	$D_{10}W$ at (7.2 × weight [kg]) mL/hr
GLUCAGON	
Neonate:	0.3 mg/kg IV/IM/SQ
Child/Adolescent:	1 mg IV/IM/SQ
DIAZOXIDE	
Neonate:	3-5 mg/kg PO/IV (over 30 minutes)
Child:	1-3 mg/kg PO/IV (over 30 minutes)
Adolescent:	300 mg PO/IV (over 30 minutes)
OCTREOTIDE	
1 mcg/kg SQ	
HYDROCORTISONE	
2.5 mg/kg IV (maximum 100 mg)	

PO = oral; NG = nasogastric tube; OG = orogastric tube; IV = intravenous; IO = intraosseous; SQ = subcutaneous; IM = intramuscular

glycemia with dehydrating gastroenteritis.[39,54,55] Most affected children were young (younger than age 5) and suffered from bacterial gastroenteritis. Malnutrition among these patients was uncommon, suggesting that hypoglycemia was not a result of deficient glycogen stores but rather a result of impaired gluconeogenesis.[39]

Diagnostic Studies

For the infant or child with hypoglycemia not easily explained by history (e.g., a diabetic child who received insulin but failed to eat, or a clear-cut oral hypoglycemic ingestion), the emergency medicine physician plays a vital diagnostic role. While a definitive diagnosis may not be made in the emergency department, collection of appropriate laboratory tests at the time of hypoglycemia can greatly expedite diagnosis and spare the patient an uncomfortable and potentially harmful diagnostic fast. Table 3 lists diagnostic studies indicated at the time of hypoglycemia.[6,8,9,12] Rather than committing this list to memory, it is helpful to develop a "hypoglycemia panel" so that the clinician need only know the quantity of blood and urine to obtain and the appropriate specimen containers in which to put them. Toxicology screening should be considered for patients in whom an unwitnessed ingestion is a possibility. If phlebotomy is unsuccessful after a few minutes, treatment should be administered without obtaining laboratory studies. A first-voided urine following the diagnosis and treatment of hypoglycemia is sufficient for initial urine studies.[12]

Management

When hypoglycemia is suspected, treatment should be started as quickly as possible to reduce the likelihood of permanent neurologic sequelae.[8] For the patient without a clear-cut etiology by history, a few minutes can be spent obtaining the laboratory tests outlined above. Table 4 summarizes the treatment of hypoglycemia and drug dosages.

If a patient is alert and has intact airway protective reflexes, oral liquids containing sugar (e.g., orange juice) can be administered. Case reports of aspiration pneumonitis underscore the risk of treating hypoglycemia orally in patients with depressed consciousness and impaired airway protective reflexes.[56] For the infant or child who will not drink but has intact airway protective reflexes, orogastric or nasogastric administration of oral liquids containing sugar may be performed. Patients with hereditary fructose intolerance will typically vomit beverages containing fructose and may be treated with oral or parenteral dextrose.[5,8]

For patients requiring parenteral therapy, dextrose is administered intravenously or intraosseously. Dextrose in high concentration may cause venous sclerosis and local tissue damage, particularly in newborns.[3,6,11] For this reason, dextrose is administered as $D_{10}W$ in infants and $D_{25}W$ in children. The American Academy of Pediatrics and the American Heart Association recommend administering 0.5-1 g/kg of glucose (5-10 mL/kg of $D_{10}W$ or 2-4 mL/kg of $D_{25}W$) to acutely reverse hypoglycemia.[57] Other authors recommend glucose boluses as small as 0.25 g/kg (2.5 mL/kg of $D_{10}W$ or 1 mL/kg of $D_{25}W$) to acutely reverse hypoglycemia.[3,6,8,9,12] While the administration of concentrated dextrose in adult patients is thought to incur some risk of exacerbating ischemic cerebrovascular disease, no such association has been reported in children.[4]

Following a dextrose bolus, a continuous infusion of $D_{10}W$ to provide glucose at approximately 6-8 mg/kg/minute is recommended.[3,6,8,11,12,33] This infusion is titrated to maintain a plasma glucose concentration above 60 mg/dL.[58] Glucose determinations should be performed serially to assess the adequacy of therapy.

Patients who require more than 10-12 mg/kg/min of glucose and are not ketotic should be suspected to have hyperinsulinism.[3,8,58] Diazoxide inhibits insulin release and may be initiated with close blood pressure monitoring and preferably in consultation with an endocrinologist.[3,5,6,8,9,11] Octreotide is a long-acting somatostatin analog that also inhibits insulin release and has been used successfully in the management of hyperinsulinism.[59]

Glucagon may be used in the emergency management of hypoglycemia.[60] It can be administered intravenously, intraosseously, intramuscularly, and subcutaneously. Intranasal administration of glucagon has been described, but concerns about absorption in the patient with nasal obstruction or rhinitis make it a less attractive option for emergency department care.[61] Glucagon may be useful for patients for whom oral therapy is contraindicated and vascular access is difficult. Effect should be observed within 20 minutes. Administration of glucagon should not, however, end attempts for vascular access and dextrose therapy. Because glucagon requires adequate glycogen stores to be effective, children with poor glycogen stores, children with defects in glycogenolysis, and children with severe liver disease would not be expected to benefit from its administration.[11]

Steroids do not elevate glucose levels quickly enough to be of more than adjunctive value in the acute management of hypoglycemia. Their use in the child with hypoglycemia of unknown etiology may obscure certain endocrine diagnoses.[12] A child with known hypopituitarism or adrenal insufficiency should receive hydrocortisone. Epinephrine is no longer considered appropriate for the management of hypoglycemia.[3,11]

Management of hypoglycemia resulting from sulfonylurea ingestion is similar to that of hyperinsulinism from other etiologies. Active charcoal is administered if the child presents within one hour of ingestion and the plasma glucose concentration is determined. Careful glucose monitoring, not empiric treatment, is recommended for the euglycemic child who may have ingested a sulfonylurea. Dextrose is administered if hypoglycemia evolves. When continuous infusion of relatively high concentrations of dextrose are not effective, an inhibitor of insulin secretion such as diazoxide or octreotide is administered.[51,62]

Disposition

Diabetic patients who experience hypoglycemia as the result of insulin administration, who become asymptomatic after treatment, tolerate oral intake, and have a care giver capable of monitoring their progress may be discharged from the emergency department. In general, all other hypoglycemic patients should be hospitalized for further monitoring, treatment, and diagnostic evaluation.

Summary

The emergency medicine physician should maintain a high index of suspicion for hypoglycemia when evaluating any ill-appearing child. Once suspected, the goals for management are to confirm the diagnosis, initiate an appropriate diagnostic evaluation, and establish euglycemia.

References

1. Halamek LP, Benaron DA, Stevenson DK. Neonatal hypoglycemia, Part I: Background and definition. *Clin Pediatr* 1997;36:675-680.
2. Cornblath M, Schwartz R, Aynsley-Green A, et al. Hypoglycemia in infancy: The need for a rational definition. *Pediatrics* 1990;85:834-837.
3. Halamek LP, Stevenson DK. Neonatal hypoglycemia, Part II: Pathophysiology and therapy. *Clin Pediatr* 1998;37:11-16.
4. Hoffman RS, Goldfrank LR. The poisoned patient with altered consciousness: Controversies in the use of a "coma cocktail." *JAMA* 1995;274:562-569.
5. Haymond MW. Hypoglycemia in infants and children. *Endocrinol Metab Clin North Am* 1989;18:211-252.
6. LaFrenchi S. Hypoglycemia of infancy and childhood. *Pediatr Clin North Am* 1987;34:961-982.
7. Burrin JM, Price CP. Measurement of blood glucose. *Ann Clin Biochem* 1985;22:327-342.
8. Gruppuso PA, Schwartz R. Hypoglycemia in children. *Pediatr Rev* 1989;11:117-124.
9. Goetting MG, Gebara, BM. Hypoglycemia in children. In: Tintinalli JE, et al, eds. *Emergency Medicine: A Comprehensive Study Guide.* 4th ed. New York: McGraw-Hill; 1996:257-259.
10. Scott PA, Wolf LR, Spadafora MP. Accuracy of reagent strips in detecting hypoglycemia in the emergency department. *Ann Emerg Med* 1998;32:305-309.
11. Kohane DS, Tobin JR, Kohane IS. Hypoglycemia. In: Rogers MC, ed. *Textbook of Pediatric Intensive Care.* 3rd ed. Baltimore: Williams and Wilkins; 1996:1272-1275.
12. Hale DE. Hypoglycemia. In: Fleisher GR, Ludwig S, eds. *Textbook of Pediatric Emergency Medicine*. 3rd ed. Baltimore: Williams and Wilkins; 1993:944-946.
13. Bjorgaas M, Sand T, Gimse R. Quantitative EEG in type 1 diabetic children with and without episodes of severe hypoglycemia: A controlled, blind study. *Acta Neurol Scand* 1996;93:398-402.
14. Kinnala A, Rikalainen H, Laoinleimu H, et al. Cerebral magnetic resonance imaging and ultrasonography findings after neonatal hypoglycemia. *Pediatrics* 1999;103:724-729.
15. Murakami Y, Yamashita Y, Matsuishi T, et al. Cranial MRI of neurologically impaired children suffering from neonatal hypoglycemia. *Pediatr Radiol* 1999;29:23-27.
16. Gold AE, Deary IJ, Frier, BM. Recurrent severe hypoglycemia and cognitive function in type 1 diabetes. *Diabetic Med* 1993;10:503-508.
17. Cresto JC, Abdenur JP, Bergada I, et al. Long-term follow up of persistent hyperinsulinaemic hypoglycemia of infancy. *Arch Dis Child* 1998;79:440-444.
18. Duvanel CB, Fawer CL, Cotting J, et al. Long-term effects of neonatal hypoglycemia on brain growth and psychomotor development in small-for-gestational-age preterm infants. *J Pediatr* 1999;134:492-498.
19. Rovet JF, Ehrlich RM. The effect of hypoglycemic seizures on cog-

nitive function in children with diabetes: A 7-year prospective study. *J Pediatr* 1999;134:503-506.

20. Phillip M, Bashan N, Smith CP, et al. An algorithmic approach to diagnosis of hypoglycemia. *J Pediatr* 1987;110:387-390.
21. Service FJ. Hypoglycemic disorders. *N Engl J Med* 1995;332: 1144-1152.
22. Pocecco M, Ronfani L. Transient focal neurologic deficits associated with hypoglycemia in children with insulin dependent diabetes mellitus. *Acta Paediatr* 1998;87:542-544.
23. Spiller HA, Schroeder SL, Ching DS. Hemiparesis and altered mental status in a child after glyburide ingestion. *J Emerg Med* 1998;16:433-435.
24. Wayne EA, Dean HJ, Booth F, et al. Focal neurologic deficits associated with hypoglycemia in children with diabetes. *J Pediatr* 1990;117:575-577.
25. Lala VR, Vedadarayana VV, Ganesh S, et al. Hypoglycemic hemiplegia in an adolescent with insulin-dependent diabetes mellitus: A case report and a review of the literature. *J Emerg Med* 1989;7: 233-236.
26. Rajbhandari SM, Powell T, Davies-Jones GA, et al. Central pontine myelinolysis and ataxia: An unusual manifestation of hypoglycemia. *Diabet Med* 1998;15:259-261.
27. Mukamel M, Weitz R, Nissenkorn I, et al. Acute cortical blindness associated with hypoglycemia. *J Pediatr* 1981;95:583.
28. Garty BZ, Dinari G, Nitzan M. Transient acute cortical blindness associated with hypoglycemia. *Pediatr Neurol* 1987;3:169-170.
29. Gold AE, Marshall SM. Cortical blindness and cerebral infarction associated with severe hypoglycemia. *Diabetes Care* 1996;19: 1001-1003.
30. Siebert DG. Reversible decerebrate posturing secondary to hypoglycemia. *Am J Med* 1985;78:1036-1037.
31. Shaw C, Haas L, Miller D, et al. A case report of paroxysmal dystonic choreoathetosis due to hypoglycemia induced by an insulinoma. *J Neurol Neurosurg Psychiatry* 1996;61:194-195.
32. Luber S, Meldon S, Brady W. Hypoglycemia presenting as acute respiratory failure in an infant. *Am J Emerg Med* 1998;16:281-285.
33. Pollock G, Brady WJ, Hargarten S, et al. Hypoglycemia manifested by sinus bradycardia: A report of three cases. *Acad Emerg Med* 1996;3:700-707.
34. McCabe ER. Disorders of carbohydrate metabolism. In: McMillan JA, et al, eds. *Oski's Pediatrics: Principles and Practice.* 3rd ed. Philadelphia: Lippincott, Williams and Wilkins; 1999:1996-1998.
35. Brady WJ, Duncan CW. Hypoglycemia masquerading as acute psychosis and acute cocaine intoxication. *Am J Emerg Med* 1999;17:318.
36. Sacerdote AS. Hypoglycemic urticaria revisited. *Diabetes Care* 1999;22:861.
37. Miller SI, Wallace RJ, Musher DM, et al. Hypoglycemia as a manifestation of sepsis. *Am J Med* 1980;68:649-654.
38. Benzing G, Schubert W, Hug G. Simultaneous hypoglycemia and acute congestive heart failure. *Circulation* 1969;40:209-216.
39. Bennish ML, Azad AK, Rahman O, et al. Hypoglycemia during diarrhea in childhood. *N Engl J Med* 1990;322:1357-1363.
40. Brady WJ, Butler K, Fines R, et al. Hypoglycemia in multiple trauma victims. *Am J Emerg Med* 1999;17:4-5.
41. Losek JD. Hypoglycemia and ABC'S (sugar) of pediatric resuscitation. *Ann Emerg Med* 1999;34:S95.
42. Moore AM, Perlman M. Symptomatic hypoglycemia in otherwise healthy, breast-fed term newborns. *Pediatrics* 1999;103: 837-839.
43. Haymond MW. Hypoglycemia in infants and children. In: Rudolph AM, et al, eds. *Rudolph's Pediatrics.* 20th ed. Stamford: Appleton and Lange; 1996:1828-1837.
44. Davis EA, Keating B, Byrne GC, et al. Impact of improved glycemic control on rates of hypoglycemia in insulin dependent diabetes mellitus. *Arch Dis Child* 1998;78:111-115.
45. The Diabetes Control and Complications Trial Research Group. Adverse events and their association with treatment regimens in the diabetes control and complications trial. *Diabetes Care* 1995;18:1415-1427.
46. Chiarelli F, Verrotti A, Catino M, et al. Hypoglycemia in children with type 1 diabetes mellitus. *Acta Paediatr Suppl* 1999;427: 31-34.
47. Cydulka R. Diabetes mellitus and disorders of glucose homeostasis. In: Rosen P, Barkin R, eds. *Emergency Medicine: Concepts and Clinical Practice.* 4th ed. St. Louis: Mosby; 1998:2456-2478.
48. de Lonlay-Debeney P, Poggi-Travert F, Fournet JC, et al. Clinical features of 52 neonates with hyperinsulinism. *N Engl J Med* 1999;340:1169-1175.
49. Rose MG, Tallini G, Pollak J, et al. Malignant hypoglycemia associated with a large mesenchymal tumor: Case report and review of the literature. *Cancer J Sci Am* 1999;5:48-51.
50. Burton BK. Inborn errors of metabolism in infancy: A guide to diagnosis. *Pediatrics* 1999;102:E69.
51. Chan JC, Cockram CS, Critchley JA. Drug-induced disorders of glucose metabolism. *Drug Safety* 1996;15:135-157.
52. Chavez H, Ozolins D, Losek JD. Hypoglycemia and propranolol in pediatric behavioral disorders. *Pediatrics* 1999;103: 1290-1292.
53. Spiller HA. Management of sulfonylurea ingestions. *Pediatr Emerg Med* 1999;15:227-230.
54. Daral TS, Singh HP, Sachdev HP, et al. Acute dehydrating diarrhea: Clinical profile in neonates and young infants. *Indian Pediatrics* 1985;22:333-338.
55. Hirschhorn N, Lindenbaum J, Greenough WB, et al. Hypoglycemia in children with acute diarrhea. *Lancet* 1966;2:128-133.
56. Kaneki T, Kubo K, Kawashima A. Acute pulmonary edema caused by accidental aspiration of sweetened water in two cases of diabetes mellitus. *Intern Med* 1998;37:969-972.
57. Chameides L, Hazinski MF, eds. *Pediatric Advanced Life Support.* Dallas: American Heart Association; 1997:6-10.
58. Stanley CA, Baker L. The causes of neonatal hypoglycemia. *N Engl J Med* 1999;340:1200-1201.
59. Barrons RW. Octreotide in hyperinsulinism. *Ann Pharmacother* 1997;31:239-241.
60. Pollack CV. Utility of glucagon in the emergency department. *J Emerg Med* 1993;11:195-205.
61. Stenninger E, Aman J. Intranasal glucagon treatment relieves hypoglycemia in children with type 1 (insulin dependent) diabetes mellitus. *Diabetologia* 1993;36:931-935.
62. Boyle PJ, Justice K, Krentz AJ, et al. Octreotide reverses hyperinsulinemia and prevents hypoglycemia induced by sulfonylurea overdoses. *J Clin Endocrinol Metab* 1993;76:752-756.

Shock

Ronald M. Perkin, MD
Mark S. McConnell, MD

Thankfully, the child presenting in shock to the emergency department (ED) is not an everyday occurrence. Nevertheless, this physiologic state is not uncommon, and even common causes of shock such as dehydration from severe vomiting and diarrhea or hypovolemia from acute blood loss can be a therapeutic challenge.

In children, contrasted to adults, the shock state can occur without obviously contributing or underlying conditions. Furthermore, as with many other conditions, the causes and frequency of shock may vary with age.

Shock is more than simple hypotension. In fact, shock frequently occurs in the presence of a normal blood pressure and a normal or increased cardiac output. Consequently, because of the dramatic responses of the child's systemic vascular resistance, other indicators of shock in children should be astutely and rapidly recognized.

"Shock" is a clinical state characterized by complex circulatory and metabolic derangements, the precise nature of which depends on the inciting etiology, the time course of the disease, and characteristics of the individual patient. Shock is a clinical diagnosis made following a rapid cardiopulmonary assessment by a health care provider. Whatever the underlying cause, a diagnosis of "shock" demands immediate interventions and vigilant, often invasive, monitoring. This chapter presents unusual conditions of pediatric shock that are diagnostic as well as therapeutic challenges to the pediatric emergency health care provider.

Overview

It is currently believed that shock reflects a relative deficiency of oxygen and/or substrate delivery to the tissues. Since shock is perceived as an acute state of oxygen deficiency, we can understand the classification and treatment of shock only by understanding the components of oxygen delivery and how these components interact during severe pathological states.

"Oxygen delivery" is the quantity of oxygen delivered into the systemic circulation and is a function of two components: the oxygen content of blood and the cardiac output. Oxygen content is determined primarily by the concentration of hemoglobin and the extent of oxygen saturation of hemoglobin. Cardiac output is defined as the volume of blood ejected by the ventricle in a given unit of time. Cardiac output is the product of heart rate and stroke volume (the volume of blood ejected by the ventricle per contraction). Stroke volume, in turn, depends on three factors: preload, contractility, and afterload.

Preload is most accurately defined as the left ventricular end-diastolic volume. In a normal heart, an increase in venous return and thus end-diastolic volume will increase cardiac output according to the Frank-Starling relationship. Ventricular end-diastolic volume is not only determined by the fluid volume within the circulation, but it is also dependent on the passive and active diastolic properties of the ventricle. That is, for a stiff, non-compliant ventricle, there will be less ventricular stretch and cardiac output for a given intravascular volume.

Contractility is the capacity of the ventricle to function as a pump, so that for a given preload and afterload, a ventricle with normal contractility will generate a larger stroke volume than a ventricle with poor contractility. Clinical determination of contractility, however, remains an elusive goal, since most commonly used measures (cardiac output, ejection fraction) are dependent on ventricular loading conditions.

Finally, stroke volume also depends on afterload, which is conceptualized as the sum of forces against which the ventricle contracts. Afterload is composed of vascular resistance, arterial stiffness (capacitance), the mass of blood in the arterial column, and the blood viscosity. As afterload increases, stroke volume diminishes and cardiac work increases.

Shock may be classified by the component of oxygen delivery which is primarily compromised. Diseases that result in diminished preload (diarrhea and dehydration, distributive shock) are classified as "hypovolemic shock." Shock which stems from an abnormality in cardiac function is termed "cardiogenic shock." Although "septic shock" has traditionally been listed as "distributive shock," septic shock is instead a combination of hypovolemic, distributive, and cardiogenic shock, in addition to altered metabolism and direct inflammatory injury to the tissues.

The physical signs associated with shock reflect the patient's attempt to compensate for inadequacies in oxygen delivery. For example, a decrease in stroke volume caused by hypovolemia can be compensated by an increase in heart rate, thereby preserving cardiac output and tissue oxygen delivery. Significant decreases in cardiac output may result in peripheral vasoconstriction (poor capillary refill, diminished pulses, and skin temperature) in order to maintain oxygen delivery and perfusion pressure to the heart and brain. The concept of "compensated shock" has been proposed to describe the clinical state in which these physiologic compensatory mechanisms are able to maintain oxygen delivery to vital organs; whereas "uncompensated shock" is a term used to describe the clinical state in which vital tissue oxygen delivery is compromised, anaerobic metabolism dominates, and the patient is at high risk of mortality if interventions are not immediate.

Although the etiologies of shock are distinct, the severe insults that lead to shock are now known to affect common pathogenic pathways, both molecular and cellular, and result in common clinical manifestations. Usual causes of shock are easily recognized and in general respond well to usual therapies. Unusual causes of shock may present differently, may respond less promptly to customary therapies, or may require alternate therapies.

Abnormalities of Heart Rate

Case #1. A 19-day-old female was in her usual state of health until 24 hours prior to admission, when she developed a low-grade fever and vomiting. She was treated symptomatically with acetaminophen and clear liquids. On the morning of admission, the mother found the child to be lethargic, with cool, mottled extremities. The child refused all feeds.

On arrival at the ED, the child had the following vital signs: heart rate, 274; respiratory rate, 60; temperature, 37.4°C (rectal); and her blood pressure was unable to be obtained, even by Doppler. She was lethargic and mottled with cool extremities; capillary refill time was prolonged. Grunting respirations were present; the lung fields were clear on auscultation.

A presumptive diagnosis of supraventricular tachycardia (SVT) was made based on a rhythm strip. Because of the severity of her presentation, the emergency physician elected to intubate the child. With laryngoscopy and intubation of the trachea, the child converted to a sinus rhythm with a rate of 180. This rate change resulted in an improvement of peripheral perfusion, and blood pressure was able to be obtained, with a value of 60/34.

Appropriate blood chemistries and cultures of body fluids were obtained, and the child was started on intravenous antibiotics. A capillary blood gas was obtained after intubation that showed a pH of 7.26 and PCO_2 of 29 mmHg. The child was transported uneventfully to the intensive care unit.

Within one hour of arrival in the ICU, the child again developed SVT with heart rates of 280-300 and signs of cardiovascular collapse. Adenosine was used but required advanced dosing before conversion occurred.

Case Discussion. *Tachydysrhythmias.* Sinus tachycardia occurs in children after exercise, with fever, after volume contraction such as in hemorrhagic shock, with certain drug ingestions, in children with anxiety or hypoxemia, and also usually accompanies heart failure of any cause. Sinus tachycardia is seen quite frequently in children and is not associated with any hemodynamic defect. Indeed, it generally indicates a physiologic response to an underlying pathologic abnormality, which requires an increase in cardiac output. Treatment of sinus tachycardia, which is a normal physiologic compensation for a pathologic state, is not indicated and can be disastrous.

Supraventricular Tachydysrhythmias. SVT can be defined as a sustained, accelerated, non-sinus cardiac rhythm originating above the level of the atrioventricular (AV) junction. The electrophysiologic mechanism is essentially one of two types: 1) an abnormal or enhanced normal automatic rhythm; or 2) a reentrant rhythm.[1-3]

The ECG in SVT shows a narrow QRS complex with regular RR intervals. The P waves may be abnormal in morphology, there may be a prolonged PR interval, and the P wave may be difficult to define. In neonates and infants, heart rates of 200-300 bpm may occur. In older children, heart rates of 150-250 bpm are more common.

Although in neonates and children, the QRS morphology is almost always normal, when aberrant conduction complicates SVT, the ECG may demonstrate wide QRS complexes that most commonly are morphologically similar to the QRS pattern seen with right bundle branch block.

SVT may occur in utero (leading to the birth of an hydropic infant), in the neonatal period, and throughout all age groups. Most commonly, it occurs in children under 6 months of age. Although it frequently reflects underlying Wolff-Parkinson-White (WPW) syndrome, it may be associated with metabolic abnormalities, Ebstein's anomaly, infection, fever, or drugs. Commonly, however, no cause can be identified.

Infants with SVT generally present with congestive heart failure.[2] *(See Table 1.)* Frequently, the picture of supraventricular tachyarrhythmia may be confused with other causes of low-output states associated with tachycardia such as septic shock, fever, sepsis, and even volume contraction secondary to hemorrhagic shock or excessive fluid loss.

Table 1. Symptoms and Signs of SVT

NEWBORN AND INFANT	OLDER CHILD
Tachypnea	Chest discomfort (pain)
Decreased feeding	Heart racing/fluttering
Lethargy	Palpitations
Respiratory distress	Faintness/dizziness
Diminished pulses	Syncope
Vasoconstriction	Cardiac arrest
Hypotension	
Shock	

Treatment Considerations. The first step in evaluation is to check the hemodynamic status. If the child is hypotensive or has poor capillary refill, one must start immediate measures to restore effective perfusion, including securing reliable intravascular access. Cardiopulmonary resuscitation also should be considered, depending on the degree of physiologic decompensation.

Careful assessment of the rhythm is the next priority. No informed action can be taken without first determining the mechanism of the rhythm. A child who has a narrow complex tachycardia greater than 220 bpm, with less than 10 bpm variation is very likely to have SVT.[4] A rapid rhythm with a wide complex may represent SVT with aberrant conduction, but ventricular tachycardia (VT) must be considered until proven otherwise.

The management of SVT is aimed at terminating the abnormal rhythm. If hypotension or poor perfusion is present, synchronized direct current cardioversion (0.5-1.0 J/kg) should be performed without delay. Overdrive pacing through the esophagus is an alternative in some centers. If it is immediately available, administration of adenosine intravenously may be substituted.

In many children, SVT usually is well-tolerated hemodynamically and the approach can be more methodical. Vagal stimulation often can interrupt the reentrant rhythm of SVT by slowing conduction in the atria and AV node. In infants, a useful vagal maneuver involves placing an examination glove filled with ice slurry over the forehead and nose, taking care not to occlude the nose or mouth. Other maneuvers in infants include insertion of a rectal thermometer and gentle abdominal pressure to mimic a Valsava maneuver. In older patients, it may be useful to elicit a gag reflex. Carotid massage is not a favored technique because it can impair cerebral blood flow. Ocular pressure (pressing on the eyeballs) has been associated with retinal detachment and is contraindicated.[4] In this child, vagal stimulation with laryngoscopy resulted in conversion of the SVT.

If vagal stimulation fails to convert SVT, but the patient is hemodynamically uncompromised, one option is to digitalize the hospitalized patient and monitor for conversion over the following 1-2 days. If evidence of congestive heart failure occurs, or if close follow-up is not possible, pharmacologic intervention aimed at immediate conversion is indicated.

Adenosine is a drug with many attractive characteristics. It acts by slowing atrioventricular nodal conduction, thus disrupting a re-entry circuit.[5,6] It has a rapid onset of action and is effective within 10-20 seconds of being given intravenously. It has a short half-life of 10-15 seconds; therefore, side effects, which occur in one-third of the patients treated, are transient and rarely require intervention. Moreover, if adenosine is administered to a child with VT by mistake it will not precipitate ventricular fibrillation. Indeed, a bolus of adenosine can be used in the difficult situation of a wide complex tachycardia as a diagnostic aid to help distinguish VT from SVT. The main disadvantage of using adenosine is that in approximately 30% of cases the tachycardia will reinitiate.

The recommended dose of adenosine is 50 mcg/kg given by rapid IV bolus. This dose can be doubled and repeated every few minutes up to a maximum of 300 mcg/kg. Since adenosine is rapidly taken up and cleared from the plasma, the dosage can be repeated without cumulative effect.

Verapamil is highly effective in terminating SVT in children and has been advocated in the past as the treatment of choice for the acute management of SVT. However, verapamil depresses contractility and suppresses both sinus and atrioventricular node function. Within the last several years, reports have been published of infants responding to verapamil with profound bradycardia and hypotension.[7] In some cases, this vascular collapse has been irreversible despite the use of calcium. Verapamil is contraindicated in children less than 12 months of age and in the presence of congestive heart failure, hypotension, or shock.[4]

Case #2. A previously healthy 3-year-old female presented to the ED with a one-day history of lethargy, pallor, sweating, and tachypnea. There was no history of fever, travel, ingestions, or other ill contacts. Past medical history was insignificant.

On physical examination the temperature was 99°F; pulse, 200 bpm; respirations, 50/min; blood pressure, 75/45 mmHg; and oxyhemoglobin saturation was 94% on room air. In general, she was lethargic but easily arousable, pale, tachypneic with mild grunting, and slightly diaphoretic. Neck exam demonstrated no nuchal rigidity, no lymphadenopathy, and no jugular venous distention. Lungs had fine rales in the bases bilaterally. Heart exam showed tachycardia with regular rate and a II/VI systolic ejection murmur. The liver edge was palpable 3 cm below the costal margin without splenomegaly. The extremities were cool with weak thready pulses that were equal in upper and lower extremities. There was no cyanosis, and capillary refill was delayed at 4 seconds.

Laboratory data were normal. A chest roentgenogram demonstrated mild cardiomegaly with evidence of pulmonary edema. A 12-lead ECG showed a wide complex tachycardia at a rate of 200 bpm, left axis deviation, and an absence of P waves.

A presumptive diagnosis of stable VT was made. The patient was given oxygen by face mask. Adenosine was given with no change in her rhythm. A lidocaine bolus at 1 mg/kg was given followed by a lidocaine infusion without change in the rate or morphology of the tachycardia. The patient was given one bolus of bretylium at 5 mg/kg; again, with no change in the tachycardia. An echocardiogram was done and verified that the patient was in VT. Cardiac anatomy was normal with a slight diminution in contractility. The patient was sedated and DC cardioversion was attempted with only a brief interruption in her tachycardia. The patient was started on a procainamide infusion without change in her cardiac rhythm or rate.

The patient was then transported to a tertiary care children's hospital, where further attempts at DC cardioversion were unsuccessful. The patient was then given a trial of intravenous amiodarone under a compassionate-use protocol, which decreased the heart rate to 120-140 bpm with an underlying rhythm that varied between VT and sinus tachycardia with premature ventricular contractions. The

Table 2. Causes of VT in Children

ELECTROLYTE ABNORMALITIES
Hyperkalemia
Hypokalemia
Hypomagnesemia

ISCHEMIA
Anomalous origin of left coronary artery
Kawasaki's disease
Vasculitis
Systemic lupus erythematosus
Right ventricular overload (pulmonary hypertension)
Myocardial infarction

DRUGS OR TOXINS
Any Class I or III anti-arrhythmic
Sympathomimetic agents (e.g., albuterol, inotropes, isoproterenol)
Cocaine
Amphetamines
Digitalis toxicity
Tricyclic antidepressants
Anesthetic agents (e.g., enflurane, isoflurane, halothane)
Antibiotics (erythromycin, trimethoprim/sulfamethoxazole, pentamidine, ketoconazole)
Antihistamines (terfenadine [Seldane], astemizole [Hismanal])
Cisapride
Phenothiazines
Organophosphates

MYOCARDIAL DISEASE
Cardiomyopathy
Myocarditis
Arrhythmogenic right ventricular dysplasia (ARVD)
Cardiac tumors (hamartomas, purkinje cell tumors, rhabdomyomas)

MISCELLANEOUS
Prolonged QT syndromes
Post-operative cardiac surgery
Hypothermia
Acidosis
Hypoxia
Mitral valve prolapse
Congenital heart disease
Idiopathic

patient remained clinically stable on intravenous amiodarone. An MRI of the chest was done that demonstrated multiple cardiac tumors consistent with hamartomas. The patient was discharged to home on oral amiodarone.

Case Discussion. VT in infants and children is distinctly unusual. Sustained VT is usually secondary to metabolic or electrolyte abnormalities, drug or toxin exposure, or intrinsic myocardial abnormalities. *(See Table 2.)* Children less than 3 years of age who develop VT will often have an incessant rhythm (>10% of the day). These incessant VTs are usually secondary to an underlying myocardial tumor.[8,9]

The clinical manifestations of VT are secondary to the myocardial depression and poor cardiac output that accompanies this rhythm disturbance. With the onset of congestive heart failure, children will demonstrate hepatomegaly, pulmonary edema, and poor peripheral perfusion. Patients may develop central nervous system abnormalities. Infants may tolerate this arrhythmia well and present only with poor oral intake. Older children may present with syncope, chest pain, and palpitations. Exercise-induced syncope in children with structurally normal hearts is most commonly caused by VT.[10]

Treatment of VT begins with accurate diagnosis. Not all wide-complex tachycardias are due to VT. SVTs conducted aberrantly or through an accessory pathway may mimic VT.[11] The ECG diagnosis of VT can be supported by the presence of fusion beats, captured beats, and atrio-ventricular dissociation. The presence of left or right bundle branch blocks is also suggestive of VT. Further confirmation can be obtained through echocardiogram, cardiac catheterization, or electrophysiologic studies.

The medical management of VT in children is similar to adults. In children who are hemodynamically unstable, immediate synchronized cardioversion or defibrillation, if pulses are not present, should be done according Pediatric Advanced Life Support (PALS) guidelines.

Antiarrhythmic drugs for treating VT are listed in *Table 3.* Initial medical therapy should begin with lidocaine. If lidocaine does not successfully convert the rhythm, then procainamide should be used. Procainamide is an excellent drug choice because it will treat both supraventricular and ventricular arrhythmias. Differentiating SVT with aberrancy from VT is difficult and procainamide can be useful in this setting. Patients unresponsive to procainamide or lidocaine may be responsive to bretylium. Other antiarrhythmics include magnesium (useful in treating torsades de pointes), phenytoin, and beta-blocking agents.[12] The use of intravenous amiodarone has become more popular with cardiologists to treat refractory VT in children. Although not currently FDA-approved for use in children, many journal articles support its use in this setting.[13]

Unresponsive Hypovolemia

Case #3. A previously healthy 6-week-old male was brought to the ED with a 24-hour history of vomiting and diarrhea. Six hours prior to admission, the child became lethargic, developed labored respirations with grunting, and his mother felt his color was changing to blue.

In the ED, the child was lethargic, poorly responsive to painful stimuli, and was cyanotic. Vital signs showed a heart rate of 205 bpm; respirations, 42/min with audible grunting; and blood pressure could not be obtained. Peripheral perfusion was poor, capillary refill was prolonged, and the child appeared markedly dehydrated. The abdomen was soft and flat. The rectal exam was normal, and the stool was not tested.

The child was intubated, hand-ventilated, given supplemental oxygen, and vascular access was obtained. Over the next 30 minutes,

Table 3. Antiarrhythmics for Use in Pediatric Patients with Ventricular Tachycardia

DRUG	DOSE	COMMENTS
Lidocaine	Load 1 mg/kg IV q5min up to 3 mg/kg, then continuous infusion 20-50 mcg/kg/min IV	Monitor levels; may cause myocardial depression, seizures, irritability.
Bretylium tosylate	Load 5 mg/kg IV, may repeat load at 10 mg/kg IV	May cause hypotension, nausea and vomiting, myocardial depression.
Procainamide	Load 3-6 mg/kg/dose IV over 5 min (100 mg max dose), then continuous infusion 20-80 mcg/kg/min IV (2 g max in 24 h)	Contraindicated in AV block, torsades de pointes, bundle branch block, or digitalis intoxication. May cause a positive ANA and lupus-like reaction. Monitor serum levels.
Magnesium sulfate	25-50 mg/kg/dose IM or IV. May repeat.	Used primarily for torsades de pointes but may be helpful for other causes of VT. May cause hypotension, paralysis, or respiratory arrest. Monitor serum magnesium levels. Do not administer rapidly.
Phenytoin	Load 5 mg/kg IV over 5-10 min. Repeat if necessary to a total of 15 mg/kg. Begin maintenance dose	May cause hypotension or arrhythmias if given too rapidly. May be helpful for refractory VT or prolonged QT syndrome.
Propranolol	0.01-0.15 mg/kg/dose over 10 min (max 1 mg/dose)	Contraindicated in myocardial depression, asthma. May cause hypotension, nausea, or hypoglycemia.

he received 40 cc/kg of normal saline solution, 30 cc/kg of 5% albumin, and 6 mEq of sodium bicarbonate.

After this fluid resuscitation, the blood pressure was measured at 45/28 and the heart rate was 190. An arterial blood gas showed: pH 6.96, PaO_2 115 mmHg, and $PaCO_2$ 35 mmHg.

A dopamine infusion was started, and arrangements for transfer to the tertiary ICU were made.

Over the next three hours, the patient received 10 cc/kg of blood, and additional 30 cc/kg of 5% albumin, and 7 mEq/kg of sodium bicarbonate. During the course of this massive fluid resuscitation, the infant's abdomen was noted to be enlarging. Vital signs had improved to blood pressure, 70/45 mmHg and heart rate, 180 bpm. Arterial blood gas showed persistent acidosis (pH, 7.22). Plain abdominal films showed air in the stomach and duodenum with no air seen past the duodenum. A barium upper GI series was done that was consistent with malrotation and midgut volvulus.

Case Discussion. Generally, an ill-appearing infant such as the one described above would be immediately considered to have sepsis and reflexively managed as such. While this may be the correct approach, one should remember the other conditions that can produce a similarly ill, septic-appearing infant.[14,15] *(See Table 4.)*

Hypovolemic shock is a clinical state characterized by decreased venous return to the left ventricle (preload), resulting in oxygen delivery insufficient to meet tissue demands. Hypovolemic shock is the type of shock most frequently encountered in the pediatric population, and may be secondary to absolute whole blood loss (internal hemorrhage, external hemorrhage, splenic sequestration), relative whole blood loss secondary to vasodilation and venous pooling (vasodilating drugs, spinal cord injury, anaphylaxis), plasma loss (burns, nephrotic syndrome, intestinal obstruction, hypoproteinemia, Stevens-Johnson syndrome), or fluid and electrolyte losses with inadequate replacement (vomiting, diarrhea, excessive transdermal losses, or urinary losses from renal disease, adrenal insufficiency, or diabetes insipidus).[16]

Physiologic compensatory mechanisms allow otherwise healthy children to tolerate acute volume losses of 10-15%, although they do so at the expense of altered intracardiac and systemic venous pressures and changes in blood flow to various regional circulations.[17] Compensated phases of hypovolemic shock are characterized by decreases in central venous pressure, stroke volume, and urine output with increases in heart rate, systemic vascular resistance, and cardiac contractility. Systemic arterial blood pressure is usually normal, and the mental status is normal or only minimally impaired. The extremities are cool and pale, the volume of peripheral pulses diminished, and capillary refill prolonged. If appropriate resuscitative measures are instituted, compensated hypovolemic shock can be treated with excellent clinical outcome.

When intravascular fluid losses surpass the body's compensatory abilities, decompensated phases appear with pronounced systemic vasoconstriction, ischemia, and stagnant hypoxia. Patients are frequently hypotensive, acidotic, lethargic or comatose, and oliguric. Stroke volume and cardiac output are further decreased. Prolonged severe hypovolemic shock can lead to multiorgan dysfunction, multiorgan failure, and death.

A child with nonhemorrhagic hypovolemic shock should respond to 40 mL/kg of crystalloid solution. If a child remains unresponsive after this amount of fluid resuscitation, the child must be evaluated for complicating factors. Causes of unresponsive shock include unrecognized pneumothorax or pericardial effusion, intestinal ischemia (volvulus, intussusception, necrotizing enterocolitis), sepsis, myocardial dysfunction, adrenocortical insufficiency, and pulmonary hypertension.[18]

Finally, grunting respirations are a sign of serious illness in infants and children.[19,20] Although grunting respirations are usually associated with respiratory diseases, clinicians must be aware that grunting respirations can occur in patients with nonrespiratory conditions.

Cardiogenic Shock—Systolic

Case #4. A previously healthy 12-year-old male was brought to the ED by paramedics following a brief seizure episode associated

Table 4. Differential Diagnosis of Septic-Appearing Infants

INFECTIOUS DISEASES
Sepsis (bacterial, viral)
Meningitis
CARDIAC DISEASE
Congenital heart disease
Supraventricular tachycardias
Myocarditis
Pericarditis
Myocardial infarction or ischemia
ENDOCRINE AND METABOLIC DISORDERS
Congenital adrenal hyperplasia
Inborn errors of metabolism
Hypoglycemia, hypocalcemia
Drug toxicity
GASTROINTESTINAL DISORDERS
Gastroenteritis with dehydration
Pyloric stenosis
Intussusception
Volvulus
Hirschsprung's-associated enterocolitis
NEUROLOGIC DISEASE
Child abuse-intracranial bleed
HEMATOLOGIC DISORDERS
Severe anemia
Methemoglobinemia

with lethargy and shortness of breath. The patient had been previously healthy until one week prior to admission, when he developed symptoms of a viral upper respiratory tract infection that had been improving. Over the past day his parents noted increasing lethargy so that the patient would not respond to verbal commands. Prior to admission the patient experienced a brief tonic-clonic seizure that lasted approximately three minutes and resolved spontaneously.

On admission to the ED, the patient was obtunded, tachypneic, and mottled. Initial vital signs were: temperature, 39°C; pulse, 150; respirations, 30; and blood pressure, 70/40 mmHg. On examination, the patient responded only to painful stimuli. The head was normocephalic with no evidence of trauma, and there was no nuchal rigidity or lymphadenopathy. Jugular venous pulsations were prominent. Lungs demonstrated rales bilaterally. The heart was tachycardic with regular rhythm and normal S1/S2 and a prominent S3. The extremities were cool with diminished pulses and poor capillary refill, and the abdominal exam was significant only for an enlarged liver 3 cm below the costal margin.

The patient was tracheally intubated and placed on mechanical ventilation. An IV line was established, and the patient was given dopamine at 5 mcg/kg/min. The patient received a loading dose of phenytoin and a bolus of furosemide. A chest roentgenogram demonstrated marked cardiomegaly with pulmonary edema and otherwise clear lung fields. An electrocardiogram demonstrated a left bundle branch block pattern with frequent premature ventricular contractions. A creatinine phosphokinase level was elevated with an elevated MB fraction.

An echocardiogram demonstrated normal cardiac anatomy with poor left ventricular function with a shortening fraction of 10%, dilated left ventricle, and an intraventricular thrombus. A right ventricular biopsy specimen was consistent with myocarditis.

The patient became progressively more hypotensive and required increasing inotropic medications, including dopamine, dobutamine, and norepinephrine, in order to maintain blood pressure and cardiac output. The patient was then placed on extracorporeal membrane oxygenation (ECMO) in order to await a cardiac transplantation. While on ECMO, he was weaned from his inotropic medications and his native cardiac function improved.

Case Discussion. Myocarditis has an insidious onset and can present with pulmonary, cardiac, neurologic, or gastrointestinal symptoms.21 The differential diagnosis for an acute dilated cardiomyopathy in infants and children is broad.[22] *(See Table 5.)*

Acute myocarditis may mimic acute myocardial infarction in some children. These patients may present with chest pain, elevated creatinine phosphokinase levels, and ECG findings that are consistent with acute myocardial infarction. A thorough history in a child presenting with chest pain may help to distinguish myocarditis from infarction; however, definitive diagnosis usually requires serial electrocardiograms and right ventricular biopsy.[23,24]

The natural history of myocarditis usually follows a course from a viral upper respiratory tract infection to profound cardiogenic shock over a period of days to weeks. Infection of the myocardium leads to widespread myocyte necrosis from direct viral invasion and from immune-mediated effects.[25,26] Myocyte death leads to severe cardiac dysfunction with ventricular dilatation and diminished ventricular contractile function. This cardiac dysfunction leads to an elevated left-ventricular end-diastolic pressure, pulmonary vascular congestion, right heart failure, and poor systemic perfusion.

Current treatment focuses on modulating the immune response with corticosteroids and improving cardiac function and systemic perfusion. Although inotropic medications have been routinely used to improve cardiac function, inotropes may potentially be harmful in this setting because of their pro-arrhythmic effects.[27] Since there is widespread myocyte death, and since these patients are typically maximally stimulated by endogenous catecholamines with concomitant beta-receptor down-regulation, further stimulation with exogenous catecholamines will likely be futile.[27,28]

Therapy involves good supportive care to maximize oxygen delivery with early tracheal intubation, blood transfusions, fluid restriction, diuresis, afterload reduction with angiotensin-converting enzyme (ACE) inhibitors, and inotropic support with amrinone or milrinone (which increase inotropy through phosphodiesterase activity and not beta-receptor activity). If the patient is hypotensive, then an inotrope/vasoconstrictor may be added (i.e., dopamine, epinephrine, or norepinephrine). Patients with profound shock from myocarditis should be considered for early mechanical cardiac support with either intra-aortic balloon counterpulsation (IABC), left-ventricular assist device (LVAD), or ECMO.

Cardiogenic Shock—Diastolic

Case #5. A 3-year-old male was referred for evaluation with the diagnosis of acute abdominal pain of unknown etiology. A fever was

Table 5. Differential Diagnosis of Dilated Cardiomyopathy in Pediatric Patients

INFECTIOUS (MYOCARDITIS)
Viral
Bacterial
Protozoan
Fungi
Rickettsial
Parasitic
CORONARY ARTERY DISEASE (ISCHEMIA)
Anomalous coronary artery
Kawasaki's disease
Vasculitis
Systemic lupus erythematosus
Rheumatic fever
METABOLIC
Hypoglycemia
Hypothyroid
Thyrotoxicosis
Pheochromocytoma
Defects in fatty acid oxidation
NEUROMUSCULAR DISORDERS
Duchene muscular dystrophy
Myotonic dystrophy
Limb-girdle (Erb)
Friedreich's ataxia
Spinal muscular atrophy
Multiple lentiginosis
MISCELLANEOUS
Chronic tachydysrhythmias
Drugs and toxins
Inborn errors of metabolism
Endocardial fibroelastosis
Genetic/familial
Idiopathic
Congenital heart disease

the child's first evidence of illness two days prior to admission. On the day prior to admission, periumbilical abdominal pain, emesis, and decreased appetite developed along with a persistence of his temperature elevation. The patient had no bowel movements during the two previous days. At the time of his initial evaluation in an outlying ED his vital signs were: temperature, 98.6°F; heart rate, 130 bpm; and respiratory rate, 26. The physical examination was normal except for mild abdominal tenderness and distention. His past medical history obtained was negative.

Laboratory testing during the initial evaluation demonstrated a white blood cell count of 7100/mm^3 with 25% polymorphonuclear cells and 46% bands and a normal urinalysis. Radiographs of the patient's abdomen were interpreted as negative. Following this evaluation, the child was released with a diagnosis of gastroenteritis and supportive care for that diagnosis was advised. During the day the child continued to spike high temperatures, becoming tachypneic and lethargic and seeming to have increasing abdominal pain. He returned to the ED 12 hours later and that time the vital signs were: temperature, 102.5°F; heart rate, 163 bpm; respiratory rate, 45; and blood pressure, 109/87 mmHg. The physical examination showed a lethargic and tachypneic male with abdominal distention and marked abdominal tenderness.

Following admission to an outlying hospital the surgical service was consulted. Laboratory testing was again accomplished. The WBC had fallen to 3500 with 37% PMN cells and 28% band-forms. The urinalysis remained negative except for ketones, serum electrolytes were normal, and a barium enema was interpreted as negative. The child remained tachycardic, tachypneic, lethargic, and febrile. Blood cultures were obtained and the child was started on intravenous fluids and an antibiotic (cefotaxime). Eight hours following admission, the child's temperature spiked to 106°F and he became hypotensive (75 mmHg systolic pressure). Bolus intravenous fluids were administered and arrangements were made for transport to the local pediatric ICU.

On arrival to the ICU, the child appeared ill and was crying because of the pain in his abdomen. Physical examination revealed rhonchi throughout the chest with rales at the right base, liver enlargement, abdominal distention with diffuse tenderness, and absent bowel sounds. Additionally, cool extremities and prolonged capillary refill were noted. No murmur, rub, or gallop was appreciated; however, a pulsus paradoxus of 25-30 mmHg was present.

Aggressive intravenous fluid therapy was given, and a percutaneously placed arterial catheter confirmed the presence of pulsus paradoxus. Chest x-ray showed marked enlargement of the cardiac shadow, perihilar infiltrates, and a right pleural effusion. An electrocardiogram showed diffuse ST-T wave elevation with low voltage in the limb leads. Echocardiography showed a large pericardial effusion that was symmetric around the heart, and there appeared to be some compression of the cardiac structures (i.e., diastolic collapse of the right atrium and the right ventricular outflow tract).

Emergency pericardiocentesis was performed at the bedside. Utilizing the standard sub-xyphoid approach, 145 cc of purulent material was obtained and sent for appropriate laboratory studies and cultures. Removal of this fluid improved the child's blood pressure and heart rate and alleviated the marked pulsus paradoxus. Cultures from pericardial fluid and pleural fluid eventually grew *Haemophilus influenzae* type b that was beta-lactamase negative.

Case Discussion. The pericardium, the fibroserous covering of the heart, is composed of a serous portion that is divided into an outer parietal layer, which lines the surface of the fibrous pericardium, and an inner visceral layer (the epicardium), which is in contact with the surface of the heart. A potential space separates the parietal and visceral layers and may normally contain up to 50 mL of clear fluid in the adult.[29]

Pericardial effusion, an abnormal accumulation of fluid in the pericardial space, may result from a variety of etiologies. *(See Table 6.)* In children, acute pericarditis is much more likely to be of bacterial origin as compared to adults. The majority of cases of bacterial, or acute purulent, pericarditis continue to occur following dissemination from another focus of infection. Pneumonia remains the most commonly associated infection.

Untreated purulent pericarditis is rapidly fatal; therefore, it is important to suspect the disease early and to approach the diagnosis

Table 6. Conditions Associated with Pericardial Effusion

INFECTIOUS
Bacterial (tuberculosis, *Haemophilus influenzae, Meningococcus, Pneumococcus, Staphylococcus aureus)*
Viral (varicella, echovirus, adenovirus, coxsackie virus)
Fungal
Psittacosis
Protozoal
NEOPLASM
CONNECTIVE TISSUE DISEASE
Systemic lupus erythematosus
Rheumatoid arthritis
Rheumatic fever
RENAL
Uremia
ENDOCRINE
Hypothyroidism
TRAUMA
Penetrating
Nonpenetrating
Catheter insertion
POSTOPERATIVE
Pericardiomyotomy
Cardiac transplantation
POST-MYOCARDIAL INFARCTION
Acute/subacute
Chronic (Dressler's syndrome)
DRUGS
Procainamide
Hydralazine
MISCELLANEOUS
Sarcoidosis
Polyarteritis nodosa
Kawasaki's disease

aggressively. The classic signs and symptoms of pericarditis are reported to be precordial pain, pericardial friction rub, evidence of pericardial fluid, and muffled heart sounds.[29-31]

The child presenting with this condition may complain of dyspnea and be febrile. Chest pain, if present, is usually vague and substernal in location, although it may be referred to any portion of the thorax, neck, upper abdomen, or the flank. It is often intensified by deep inspiration, coughing, or trunk rotation. The pain is lessened when the child sits upright or leans forward.

Inflammatory and irritative lesions of the pericardium always produce fluid owing to exudation within the pericardial sac. As pericardial fluid accumulates, intrapericardial pressure rises. The rate of rise is a function of both the speed of accumulation and the compliance of the pericardium. With slow accumulation of fluid, large volumes can be accommodated because of gradual expansion of the parietal pericardium. When the pericardial sac becomes maximally stretched, however, further accumulation of even small volumes of fluid results in an abrupt increase in intrapericardial pressure. If pericardial fluid accumulates at a rapid rate, marked elevation in pericardial pressure may occur with much smaller volumes of fluid (i.e., tamponade may occur with a radiographically normal cardiac shadow). In rapid tamponade caused by hemorrhage, as in trauma, shock dominates the picture. If untreated, it leads to electromechanical dissociation.

The most significant hemodynamic effect of pericardial effusion is restriction of ventricular filling. Cardiac tamponade is the compression of the heart by a tense pericardial sac resulting in a decrease in venous return to the heart and, consequently, a decrease in cardiac output. As was the case in this patient, tachycardia and peripheral vasoconstriction are seen in an attempt to maintain cardiac output.

The definitive treatment of cardiac tamponade is removal of the pericardial fluid by surgical drainage or pericardiocentesis.[30] Removal of even a small volume of fluid can rapidly improve blood pressure and cardiac output. Although bedside needle pericardiocentesis may be lifesaving or necessary for rapid diagnosis, it must be emphasized that it is a blind and potentially very dangerous procedure.

Medical management does not substitute for drainage but may avert a catastrophe until pericardiocentesis or surgical drainage can be performed. The principles of medical management for tamponade include: 1) blood volume expansion to maintain venoatrial gradients; 2) inotropic agents; and 3) afterload reducing drugs in patients with normal systemic arterial blood pressure.[32]

Case #6. A 3-year-old male slipped while running around a swimming pool and struck the back of his head. His parents reported that he acted stunned but did not lose consciousness. During the evening, he became drowsy and began vomiting. He was taken to the ED, where CT of the head showed bilateral occipital epidural hematomas.

Approximately two hours after ED admission, the child became hypoxemic, hypotensive, and bradycardic. He was unresponsive, in marked respiratory distress, and on physical examination had developed an S3 gallop rhythm and rales. He was intubated, hyperventilated, and given a diuretic. Chest x-ray after intubation showed mild cardiomegaly and pulmonary edema.

Echocardiography showed normal ventricular end-diastolic dimension but markedly decreased shortening fraction (13%) and a "still" (poorly moving) left ventricle. Initial ECG showed sinus tachycardia, marked decreased in left ventricular forces, and depressed ST segments with T-wave inversion in leads II, III, and AVF. Placement of a pulmonary arterial catheter demonstrated elevated pulmonary artery pressure and wedge pressure with normal to low central venous pressures.

The child was started on inotropic drugs (dopamine, dobutamine). The hemodynamic variables obtained during the first 72 hours showed a marked disparity between right- and left-sided filling pressures. Creatinine phosphokinase (CPK) levels were also followed and showed a physiologically significant elevation 24 hours post injury.

The child was maintained on the ventilator and received inotropic support , diuretics, and sedation. By the fifth post-operative day, he had improved sufficiently to be extubated. ECG at this time demonstrated reduced ST-segment depression and increased left ventricular forces; echocardiography showed an improved shortening fraction of 30%. A radionuclide (Technetium-pyrophosphate) myocardial scintigram was also done and did not detect myocardial necrosis (no pyrophosphate uptake).

Case Discussion. Since Cushing's original observations of the systemic hypertensive and bradycardic response to elevated intracranial pressure, many reports have described electrocardiographic (ECG) changes and myocardial damage associated with severe brain insults including intracerebral hemorrhage of spontaneous or traumatic origin.[33-40]

Nearly every type of ECG abnormality (rhythm, conformation, and conduction) has been detected in patients with acute neurologic illness or injury.[33,37-39] The ECG changes reported most commonly include prolonged QT intervals, depressed ST segments, flat or inverted T waves, and U waves.[33] Various combinations of these ECG findings have been described in patients with subarachnoid hemorrhage, intracerebral hemorrhages, ischemic cerebrovascular insults, and head trauma. The ST-T wave changes are typical of those seen in myocardial injury of ischemia, and, if present, are associated with greatly increased mortality.[33]

In this patient, the ECG, the echocardiographic changes, and the elevation of creatine phosphokinase and its myocardial isoenzyme all suggested myocardial ischemia as the cause of this child's hemodynamic problems. Evidence of myocardial ischemia and injury have been identified in a variety of intracerebral injury syndromes. The underlying mechanism for the myocardial damage seen after head injury is not clear. A sustained sympathetic hyperactivity, either directly from cardiac sympathetic nerve terminals or indirectly from circulatory catecholamines, is one process that could account for elevations in CPK activity and the observed ECG abnormalities.[34,35,37]

In the patient above, the centrally mediated myocardial ischemia resulted in both systolic and diastolic heart failure. Echocardiography revealed abnormal left ventricular wall motion and decreased shortening fraction suggesting systolic failure but also showed decreased mitral flow velocities suggesting abnormal myocardial relaxation (diastolic failure). Diastolic properties of the left ventricle appear to be the first to become abnormal in patients with myocardial ischemia.[41] Specifically, abnormalities in myocardial relaxation alter left ventricular compliance such that left ventricular pressure is increased at any volume. This is hemodynamically unfavorable, since the increased pulmonary venous pressure can result in pulmonary edema, as it did in this patient. Additionally, increased diastolic stiffness limits cardiac output by reducing filling. Altered left ventricular compliance probably contributed to the marked disparity between central venous pressure and pulmonary capillary wedge pressure. Disparate ventricular function in the pediatric patient appears to be a similar phenomenon to that described in the adult population.[41,42]

This case illustrates that ischemic myocardial injury can occur with head trauma and may jeopardize the hemodynamic stability needed for neurologic recovery. Centrally mediated myocardial injury should be suspected in any patient with a neurologic catastrophe.

Shock: Abnormal Afterload

Case #7. A 2-month-old male infant with Down syndrome presented to the ED with a two-day history of increasing irritability, decreased oral intake, and increasing lethargy. On the day of admission, the patient did not eat and the parents noted rapid, shallow breathing. There was no history of congenital cardiac disease.

On admission to the ED, the patient was noted to be lethargic, poorly responsive to stimuli, and tachypneic. The patient had poor perfusion with mottled lower extremities. Initial vital signs were: temperature, 38.9°C; pulse, 180 bpm; respirations, 60; and blood pressure, 100/45 mmHg. On examination, the fontanelle was flat, pupillary responses were normal, the lungs demonstrated fine rales, the heart demonstrated a tachycardia with a 2/6 systolic ejection murmur at the left sternal border and normal S1/S2, and the abdomen was distended and tense with a liver edge palpable 4 cm below the costal margin. The extremities were cool, and the lower extremities were noted to be mottled with poor pulses and markedly prolonged capillary refill.

The ED team was unable to establish intravenous access, so an intraosseous needle was placed and the patient received a bolus of normal saline. Initial laboratory data showed elevated potassium, BUN, and creatinine. The white blood cell count was elevated, and the platelet count was 90,000/mm^3. Additionally, the PT and PTT were both elevated. A chest x-ray demonstrated mild cardiomegaly with pulmonary edema. An abdominal film demonstrated a large amount of intraluminal air without evidence of obstruction or free intraperitoneal air. An arterial blood gas obtained on 6 L/min of oxygen by face mask was pH 7.20; PCO_2, 30 mmHg; PO_2, 75 mmHg.

The patient was transported to a pediatric intensive care unit. Central venous access was established and the patient received a bolus of sodium bicarbonate, more fluid infusions, antibiotics, intubation, and mechanical ventilation. An abdominal ultrasound showed normal intraperitoneal anatomy with hepatomegaly. In spite of maximal medical therapy, the patient had a progressive metabolic acidosis, which led to cardiovascular collapse requiring cardiopulmonary resuscitation, and ultimately death. On post-mortem examination, the patient was found to have a severe coarctation of the aorta which led to extensive bowel ischemia and infarction.

Case Discussion. The differential diagnosis of shock in the infant and neonate is extensive. Different types of shock may present with similar clinical findings. The age of the patient at presentation may provide an important clinical clue to the etiology of shock.

Since the ductus arteriosus can close within the first few months after birth, one should consider ductal-dependent congenital heart disease syndromes in infants presenting with shock during this time period. Such syndromes include hypoplastic left heart syndrome, tricuspid atresia, transposition of the great vessels, and coarctation of the aorta.

Shock develops in aortic coarctation as the aortic end of the ductus arteriosus closes, which causes a constriction at the juxtaductal aortic narrowing leading to a precipitous increase in left ventricular afterload. The infant myocardium is unable to compensate for this increased afterload, which results in elevated ventricular wall tension and decreased myocardial perfusion.[43]

The key to treating this disease is early diagnosis by astute physicians prior to the development of shock.[44] A majority of patients develop a murmur and upper-extremity hypertension within the first few months of life. However, only 10-30% of infants with physical findings of aortic coarctation are referred to cardiologists with the correct diagnosis.[45,46] Patients with coarctation often are not referred for medical management until they are in shock.

The diagnosis of cardiogenic shock secondary to aortic coarctation may be difficult to distinguish from septic shock in the infant. ED physicians must maintain a high index of suspicion in conjunction with a thorough physical exam that includes four extremity blood pressures. Unfortunately, patients may go on to develop bowel infarction and septic shock as a result of the coarctation in spite of the best efforts by the clinician.

Many cardiologists recommend the early institution of prostaglandin E_1 (PGE_1) in any infant who presents in shock until critical coarctation or other ductal-dependent lesions have been excluded.[43] PGE_1 reverses the cardiogenic shock caused by these lesions due to its vasodilatory effects on the ductus arteriosus. By keeping the ductus open, the shock caused by these cardiac lesions may be reversed or stabilized until more definitive care can be provided. PGE_1 should be started at a dose of 0.05 mcg/kg/min and titrated to a maximum of 0.2-0.4 mcg/kg/min and then reduced to lowest effective dose when the desired results are obtained. PGE_1 is associated with some potentially harmful adverse side effects, including apnea, hypotension, cutaneous vasodilation, rhythm abnormalities, seizures, fever, diarrhea, and, rarely, coagulopathy.

Case #8. The patient is a 2-year-old black female born at 32 weeks' estimated gestational age. Her history included a short neonatal ICU stay for prematurity, without being on the ventilator. She was admitted for severe RSV pneumonia one year earlier, but had otherwise been in good health. One week prior to admission she developed nasal congestion and hoarseness. She suffered from respiratory distress, particularly at night. For two days she had been sleeping restlessly, awakening every 30 minutes and sleeping in an upright position. Her mother denied a history of fever or cough. Further history revealed snoring since birth, which had been progressively worsening.

The patient presented to an outlying ED in mild respiratory distress and was diagnosed with asthma. Subcutaneous epinephrine and nebulized albuterol were administered without evidence of improvement. Because the chest x-ray showed severe cardiomegaly, furosemide and supplemental oxygen were administered. The patient was subsequently transferred to a tertiary center for further evaluation. On arrival, she was noted to be in severe respiratory distress with a markedly decreased mental status. On physical exam the patient was afebrile with a respiratory rate of 18; heart rate, 124 bpm; and blood pressure, 122/67 mmHg. She was barely arousable with marked subcostal retractions and tracheal tugging. Auscultation of the lungs demonstrated minimal air movement and faint expiratory wheezing. There was no apparent stridor. The heart examination demonstrated only a prominent P2 with no other abnormalities. Jugular venous distention and hepatomegaly were present. The extremities had diminished pulses and perfusion with no edema. Chest x-ray showed marked cardiomegaly with no parenchymal opacities. Bilateral atrial enlargement and right axis deviation were noted on the ECG. An arterial blood gas on 85% O_2 mask had a pH of 7.26; PCO_2, 97 mmHg; PO_2, 82 mmHg; and HCO_3, 39 mEq/L.

Following tracheal intubation, the patient was easily ventilated with minimal symptoms of reactive airways disease. An echocardiogram was obtained showing right ventricular enlargement, marked tricuspid regurgitation, and severe pulmonary hypertension with systolic pressures of 75 mmHg. Her pulmonary hypertension and right heart failure were treated with hyperventilation, oxygen, nitroglycerin, dobutamine, and furosemide. Systemic hypertension was also present and was treated with nifedipine. Within 24 hours the patient was noted to have marked improvement of both pulmonary hypertension on echocardiogram and cardiomegaly on chest x-ray. Over the next few days she was weaned off the ventilator and medications. Following extubation she was noted to have radiographic evidence of recurrent cardiomegaly. Additionally, she was also observed to have significant snoring while asleep. Arterial blood gas showed a marked rise in PCO_2 while asleep. While awake, she had a pH of 7.47; PCO_2, 44 mmHg; PO_2, 77 mmHg; and HCO_3, 31 mEq/L. While sleeping, the pH was 7.22; PCO_2, 83 mmHg; PO_2, 168 mmHg; and HCO_3, 32 mEq/L. With supplemental oxygen, her PCO_2 increased to 99 mmHg. Bronchoscopy revealed severely increased compliance of the nasopharynx and hypopharynx with otherwise normal structures.

A multi-channel polysomnogram, including monitoring of EEG channels, eye movements, heart rate, oral-nasal airflow, upper and lower chest wall movement, and oxygen saturation, revealed significant hypoxemia during obstructive apnea events. The O_2 saturation nadir was < 50% (recorded at 8%). Although it is rare to see any obstructive episodes in children, she showed an apnea index (the average number of apnea episodes per hour of total sleep time) of 9/hour. The longest apnea was 20 seconds and occurred during REM sleep. Significant O_2 desaturation was also noted without any apparent apnea event and was thought to be a result of hypoventilation.

Nasal continuous positive airway pressure (CPAP) produced a marked therapeutic change. Once 9.0 cmH_2O pressure was applied, snoring resolved and 100% saturation was maintained throughout sleep. The patient was also noticeably more alert in the daytime.

Case Discussion. Obstructive sleep apnea (OSA) is a common problem in adults and may present as a life-threatening event. It is currently becoming recognized as a significant health concern in children. OSA usually presents more subtly in the child than the adult, yet it can also present in a sudden and severe manner. This case is an example of OSA presenting with pulmonary hypertension and right heart failure, mistaken originally as a severe case of status asthmaticus.

OSA consists of a recurring cycle of events including obstruction of the airway, asphyxia, arousal from sleep (secondary to hypercapnia and hypoxia), and restoration of the airway.[47] OSA occurs in multiple settings, including orofacial anomalies, neuromuscular diseases, tonsillar and adenoidal hypertrophy, deviated nasal septum, mucopolysaccharide storage disorders, obesity, central hypoventilation syndrome, and isolated increased pharyngeal compliance.[48]

Effects of OSA range from daytime hypersomnolence secondary to interruption of sleep continuity, to pulmonary hypertension and right heart failure as a result of hypoxia. Other significant problems noted in children with OSA include learning disabilities, psychological impairment, systemic hypertension, and failure to thrive. Failure to thrive may be the only symptom in some children with serious OSA.[49] Left-sided heart failure has been described and is attributed to a combination of systemic hypertension and increased afterload on the left ventricle resulting from high negative intrathoracic pressures generated during apneic spells.[47]

Treatment of OSA includes weight loss, medication, nasal CPAP, and surgery.[50] Nasal CPAP has been shown to be very effective in adults. While limited data are available to demonstrate its efficacy in children, CPAP also appears effective in children with OSA.[50]

Problems with compliance often arise in the pediatric population. Treatment of OSA with O_2 alone is inadequate as oxygen cannot change airway patency and may reduce the hypoxic drive for ventilation in a patient with chronic CO_2 retention.[51]

This case is an example of life-threatening respiratory and right heart failure resulting from OSA. Although the patient had evidence of chronic CO_2 retention, she showed immediate improvement in pulmonary hypertension, and the CO_2 normalized as soon as the obstructive element was eliminated. Severe pulmonary hypertension and heart failure can occur in patients with OSA. This case emphasizes the importance of clinical evaluation of sleep disorders in children, and the remarkable resolution of OSA symptoms with nasal CPAP.

Summary

Recognition and diagnosis of unusual causes of pediatric shock in the ED require a well-honed diagnostic acumen, a thorough understanding of shock pathophysiology, and a well-endowed differential diagnosis list. In this issue we reviewed the important but uncommon conditions of pediatric shock to assist the emergency healthcare provider in meeting these diagnostic and therapeutic challenges.

References

1. O'Conner BK, Dick M. What every pediatrician should know about supraventricular tachycardia. *Pediatr Ann* 1991;20: 368-376.
2. Ros SP, Fisher EA, Bell TJ. Adenosine in the emergency management of supraventricular tachycardia. *Pediatr Emerg Care* 1991;7:222-223.
3. Ganz LI, Friedman PL. Supraventricular tachycardia. *N Engl J Med* 1995;332:162-173.
4. Erickson LC, Cocalis MW. The acute management of paroxysmal supraventricular tachycardia in children. *Pediatr Rev* 1993;7:273-274.
5. Bertolet BD, Hill JA. Adenosine: Diagnostic and therapeutic uses in cardiovascular medicine. *Chest* 1993;104:1860-1871.
6. Camm AJ, Garratt CJ. Adenosine and supraventricular tachycardia. *N Engl J Med* 1991;325:1621-1629.
7. Garland JS, Berens RJ, Losek JD, et al. An infant fatality following verapamil therapy for supraventricular tachycardia: Cardiovascular collapse following intravenous verapamil. *Pediatr Emerg Care* 1985;1:198-200.
8. Garson A, Smith RT, Moak JP, et al. Incessant ventricular tachycardia in infants: Myocardial hamartomas and surgical cure. *J Am Coll Cardiol* 1987;10:619-626.
9. Gharagozloo F, Porter CJ, Tazelaar HD, et al. Multiple myocardial hamatomas causing ventricular tachycardia in young children: Combined surgical modification and medical treatment. *Mayo Clin Proc* 1994;69:262-267.
10. Noh CI, Fong JY, Kim HS. Ventricular tachycardia and exercise related syncope in children with structurally normal hearts: Emphasis on repolarisation abnormality. *Br Heart J* 1995;73:544-547.
11. Meldon SW, Brady WJ, Berger S, et al. Pediatric ventricular tachycardia: A review of three illustrative cases. *Pediatr Emerg Care* 1994;10:294-300.
12. Tzivoni D, Banai S, Schuger C, et al. Treatment of torsade de pointes with magnesium sulfate. *Circulation* 1988;77: 792-397.
13. Perry JC, et al. Intravenous amiodarone for life-threatening tachyarrhythmias in children and young adults. *J Am Coll Cardiol* 1993;22:95-98.
14. Selbst SM. The septic-appearing infant. *Pediatr Emerg Care* 1985;1:160-167.
15. Marty TL, Matlak ME, Hendrickson M, et al. Unexpected death from enterocolitis after surgery for Hischsprung's Disease. *Pediatrics* 1995;96:118-121.
16. Perkin RM, Levin DL. Shock in the pediatric patient. *J Pediatr* 1982;101:163-168.
17. King DR. Trauma in infancy and childhood: Initial evaluation and management. *Pediatr Clin North Am* 1985;32:1299-1305.
18. Perkin RM. Shock states. In: Fuhrman BP, Zimmerman JJ,eds. *Pediatric Critical Care*. St. Louis: Mosby-Year Book; 1992:287-298.
19. Pook SR, Chetham M, Anderson M. Grunting respirations in infants and children. *Pediatr Emerg Care* 1995;11:158-161.
20. Singer JI, Losek JD. Grunting respirations. Chest or abdominal pathology? *Pediatr Emerg Care* 1992;8:354-358.
21. Bonadio WA, Losek JD. Infants with myocarditis presenting with severe respiratory distress and shock. *Pediatr Emerg Care* 1987;3:110-113.
22. McConnell MS, Perkin RM, Hernandez R. Acute dilated cardiomyopathy as a cluster in children. *West J Med* 1993;158: 522-525.
23. Hoyer MH, Fischer DR. Acute myocarditis simulating myocardial infarction in a child. *Pediatrics* 1991;87:250-253.
24. Narula J, An Khaw B, et al. Brief Report: Recognition of acute myocarditis masquerading as acute myocardial infarction. *N Engl J Med* 1993;328:100-104.
25. Chow LH, Beisel KW, McManus BM. Entervorial infection of mice with severe combined immunodeficiency. *Lab Invest* 1992;66:24-31.
26. Lange LG, Schreiner GF. Immune mechanisms of cardiac disease. *N Engl J Med* 1994;330:1129-1135.
27. McConnell MS, Perkin RM. Inotrope futility in children with myocarditis. [Abstract.] *Sixth Pediatric Critical Care Colloquium* 1993; Philadelphia, PA.
28. Merlet P, et al. Myocardial beta-adrenergic desensitization and neuronal norepinephrine uptake function in idiopathic dilated cardiomyopathy. *Cardiovasc Pharmacol* 1992;19: 10-16.
29. Spodick DH. Pericarditis, pericardial effusion, cardiac tamponade, and constriction. *Crit Care Clin* 1989;5:455-463.
30. Green M, Kaplan EL. Infection of the heart and pericardium. In: Fuhrman BP, Zimmerman JJ, eds. *Pediatric Critical Care*. St. Louis: Mosby-Year Book; 1992:299-304.
31. King DL. Rhabdomyolysis with pericardial tamponade. *Ann Emerg Med* 1994;23:583-585.
32. Perkin RM. Shock states. In: Fuhrman BP, Zimmerman JJ, eds. *Pediatric Critical Care*. St. Louis: Mosby-Year Book; 1992:287-298.
33. Talman WT. Cardiovascular regulation and lesions of the central nervous system. *Ann Neurol* 1985;18:1.
34. Frost EAM. Cardiorespiratory effects of central nervous system derangements. *Anesthesiol Clin North Am* 1987;5:507.
35. McGrath RB, Revtyak G. Secondary myocardial injuries. *Crit Care Med* 1984;12:1024.

36. Hackenberry LE, Miner ME, Rea GL, Woo J, et al. Biochemical evidence of myocardial injury after severe head trauma. *Crit Care Med* 1982;10:641.
37. Drislane FW, Samuels MA. How cardiorespiratoy problems are caused by neurologic disease. *J Respir Dis* 1988;9:31.
38. Hart GK, Humphrey L, Weiss J. Subarachnoid hemorrhage-cardiac complications. *Crit Care Rep* 1989;1:88.
39. Rogers MC, Zakla KG, Nugent SK, et al. Electrocardiographic abnormalities in infants and children with neurological injury. *Crit Care Med* 1980;8:218.
40. Clifton GL, Ziegler MG, Grossman RG. Circulatory catecholamines and sympathetic activity after head injury. *Neurosurgery* 1981;59:447.
41. Katz AM. A physiologic approach to the treatment of heart failure. *Hosp Pract* 1987;22:117.
42. Raper R, Sibbald WJ. Misled by the wedge? *Chest* 1986;89:427.
43. Schwengel DA, Nichols DG, Cameron DE. Coarctation of the aorta and interrupted aortic arch. In: Nichols DG, et al, eds. *Critical Heart Disease in Infants and Children*. St. Louis: Mosby; 1995:669-692.
44. Thoele DG, Muster AJ, Paul MH. Recognition of coarctation of the aorta: A continuing challenge for the primary care physician. *Am J Dis Child* 1987;141:1201-1204.
45. Strafford MA, Griffiths SP, Gersony WM. Coarctation of the aorta: A study in delayed detection. *Pediatrics* 1982;69: 159-163.
46. Ward KE, Pryor RW, et al. Delayed detection of coarctation in infancy: Implications for timing of newborn follow-up. *Pediatrics* 1990;972-976.
47. Strollo PJ, Rogers RM. Obstructive sleep apnea. *N Engl J Med* 1996;334:99-104.
48. Downey R, Perkin RM, Ellis GA, et al. Childhood and infant sleep-disordered breathing. *RT J Respir Care Pract* 1995;8: 39-48.
49. Carroll JL, Loughlin GM. Diagnostic criteria for obstructive sleep apnea syndrome in children. *Pediatr Pulmonol* 1992;14:71-74.
50. Marcus CL, Ward SLD, Mallory GB, et al. Use of nasal continuous positive airway pressure as treatment of childhood obstructive apnea. *J Pediatr* 1995;127:88-94.
51. Brouillette RT, Waters K. Oxygen therapy for pediatric obstructive sleep apnea syndrome. *Am J Respir Crit Care Med* 1996;153:1-2.

Tachyarrhythmias

James C. Perry, MD

The infant presenting with signs of physiologic decompensation and an extremely fast heart rate demands expert management by an emergency health care provider with an in-depth understanding of diagnostic subtleties. While at first glance similarities to adult management may exist, there are potentially dangerous pitfalls that exist if one attempts to indiscriminately apply principles of adult management to pediatric arrhythmias.

Cardiac arrhythmias in the pediatric age group primarily pertain to the diagnosis and management of supraventricular tachycardias (SVTs). These tachycardias differ from those seen in the adult population in terms of modes of presentation, their natural history, prognosis, and overall management schemes. This chapter conveys the pertinent features in the recognition and management of pediatric cardiac tachyarrhythmias, with commentary on the acute therapies, chronic drug therapy, and indications and anticipated success rates for interventional, curative radiofrequency catheter ablative procedures.

Mechanisms of Supraventricular Tachycardia

On the basis of heart rate alone, there can be a fair degree of overlap between sinus tachycardia and abnormal tachyarrhythmia mechanisms. In the face of infection and/or fever, infants can manifest sinus rhythm rates as high as 230-240/minute, young children up to 200/minute, and teenagers up to 180/minute. Heart rates above these parameters should be strongly suspected as representing abnormal mechanisms. Electrocardiographic P waves are generally easy to identify during sinus tachycardia, and the PR interval is shorter than the RP interval.

The diagnosis of SVT is non-specific, as there are at least 16 different types of SVT. *(See Table 1.)* These arrhythmias can be broken down into three distinct physiologic mechanisms: reentry SVTs that utilize an accessory pathway or bypass tract, reentry SVTs that do not utilize an accessory pathway, and automatic tachycardias. Fortunately for the clinician, the majority of these mechanisms are quite rare. The two most overwhelmingly common forms of SVT in pediatrics are accessory pathway-mediated SVTs, such as those that occur in Wolff-Parkinson-White (WPW) syndrome, and typical atrioventricular (AV) node reentry SVT. In children, accessory pathway-mediated SVT is twice as common as AV nodal reentry SVT.

Normal cardiac conduction patterns involve activation from the sinus node complex in the high right atrium through preferential routes of conduction in the right and left atria to the region of the compact AV node above the septal leaflet of the tricuspid valve. There is slow conduction through the AV node, accounting for the bulk of the isoelectric interval seen on the surface electrocardiogram

Table 1. Mechanisms of Supraventricular Tachycardia

REENTRY WITH BYPASS TRACT
Wolff-Parkinson-White
Concealed WPW
More than one accessory pathway
Mahaim (nodoventricular)
Permanent junctional reciprocating tachycardia
Antidromic tachycardia
Atrio-Hisian pathway
REENTRY WITHOUT BYPASS TRACT
Sinus node reentry
Intra-atrial reentry
Typical AV node reentry
Atypical AV node reentry
Atrial flutter
Atrial fibrillation
AUTOMATIC
Atrial ectopic
Chaotic atrial
Junctional ectopic

between the P wave and the QRS complex, and conduction then proceeds to the bundle of His. Rapid activation of the ventricles occurs via the right bundle and the anterior and posterior fascicles of the left bundle system, resulting in a narrow, rapid-frequency QRS complex on the surface ECG. Initial activation of the ventricular septum in a left-to-right direction results in the normal Q wave seen in the lateral (V5-V7) and inferior (II, III, or aVF) ECG leads. This Q wave is important in that its presence verifies that the lateral leads are in fact positioned properly to reflect true left ventricular voltages.

Conduction, repolarization, and depolarization times are typically shorter for the newborn and young child because of decreased overall size and myocardial mass. Normal values for the PR interval vary with heart rate and age. In the newborn, the range of the normal PR interval is 0.07-0.12 seconds. This range increases to 0.12-0.21 seconds by adulthood. Thus, diagnosis of disorders that prolong the PR interval, such as myocarditis, drug-induced AV block, and congenital heart disease (ECD and ASD), becomes more difficult. The QRS interval also has a shorter duration than found in the adult population. The upper limits of a normal QRS interval in an infant is 0.07 seconds, increasing to 0.10 seconds by age 12. Thus, diagnosis of ventricular ectopy, intraventricular blocks, and preexcitation requires a knowledge of age-specific standards. Other important differences between adults include a normal P wave of 0.07 seconds or less in infants, 0.09 seconds or less in children, and 0.11 seconds or less in adults.

Accessory Pathway SVTs. The ECG pattern of what we now call WPW syndrome was first reported in 1930.[1] The classic definition of a WPW pattern on ECG is that of a short PR interval and slurred upstroke of the QRS ("delta wave"). This is due to a microscopic bridge of muscle or accessory connection that "short circuits" the normal ventricular activation and preexcites the ventricles, leading to the early depolarization and appearance of a delta wave. The diagnosis of WPW may be difficult in some children due to higher normal sinus rates and rapid AV node conduction. There are some ECG findings that assist in the diagnosis of "subtle" forms of WPW. The findings of a PR under 100 milliseconds, the lack of a clear septal Q wave in the left precordial leads, and left axis deviation may all suggest "subtle" WPW.[2] A combination of two of these factors is rare in normal patients (2%) but common in those with WPW (> 60%). Not all accessory connections will show the WPW pattern in sinus rhythm. These accessory connections can conduct in the retrograde (ventricle-to-atrium) direction only, allowing SVT to occur. The lack of antegrade (atrium-to-ventricle) conduction precludes the presence of preexcitation during normal sinus beats.

The initiating factors for SVT vary[3] but can include premature atrial or ventricular beats, sinus node acceleration, or sinus pauses with junctional escape beats. During SVT in patients with accessory connections, cardiac electrical activation typically proceeds from the atria to the ventricles via the normal AV node-His-Purkinje system; therefore, a narrow QRS complex may be seen. There is then retrograde activation of the atria via the accessory pathway and back down the AV node, resulting in a reentry form of SVT. The retrograde activation of the atria during SVT of this type can usually be seen by the presence of a P wave buried in the ST segment or the T wave. In children, there is often a beat-to-beat alternation of the amplitude of the QRS complex. This is nearly pathognomonic of an accessory pathway-mediated SVT. Whereas the majority of childhood SVTs have a narrow QRS, there is a notable exception to this rule in patients under 1 year of age. A left bundle branch block pattern, resulting from delayed conduction or functional block in the fascicles of the left bundle system is a common finding in infant SVTs, occurring in more than 25% of cases.[4] This bundle branch block pattern results in a relatively wide QRS tachycardia during SVT with a late, positive deflection in the left chest leads. This phenomenon is one of the many reasons why a full ECG is imperative for accurate techniques in pediatric arrhythmia diagnosis. Fortunately, ventricular tachycardias are rare in young children, so a wide QRS tachycardia (with left bundle branch block), which might be diagnosed as ventricular tachycardia, is essentially SVT with aberrancy until proven otherwise. Nevertheless, the assumption that all wide QRS tachycardias in children are SVT with aberrancy could result in fatal therapeutic mismanagement of ventricular tachycardias.

The other form of arrhythmia of concern in the setting of WPW is that of atrial fibrillation. This chaotic, irregular atrial rhythm disturbance is more common in patients with WPW than those without and is far more common in older patients. Some accessory pathways in WPW can conduct in an antegrade fashion (atria to ventricles) very rapidly. In this setting, rapid conduction during atrial fibrillation may bring about the induction of ventricular tachycardia or ventricular fibrillation. This capability of rapid antegrade conduction of some accessory pathways accounts for the observed phenomenon of sudden death in approximately 1% of patients with WPW. The mean age of induction of atrial fibrillation in children with WPW is around 12 years.[5] The risk of sudden death, therefore, is likely to be near zero before about the age of 10 years. However, chaotic atrial arrhythmias (atrial ectopic tachycardia and chaotic atrial tachycardia) can manifest rates of 300-400 bpm and can occur in children under 18 months of age as well, so a small risk may be present in this age group.

AV Node Reentry. AV node reentry is the second most common form of SVT in children and young adults. AV node reentry is due to an underlying functional division of normal AV conduction into antegrade "fast" and "slow" components. Under the right circumstances, such as properly timed atrial premature beat, conduction may block in the fast pathway and proceed down the slow pathway only. This results in a long PR interval after the premature P wave. In this setting, since the fast pathway has not depolarized (and is therefore not refractory), subsequent retrograde activation of the atria is possible via the fast pathway. Antegrade activation of the ventricles happens at the same time as retrograde atrial activation via the fast pathway, so the QRS complex and P wave occur simultaneously and are superimposed on the surface ECG. This is in contrast to most accessory pathway SVTs, where the retrograde P wave can be seen in the ST segment of T wave.

Atrial Flutter. Atrial flutter tends to occur in postoperative congenital heart disease patients[6] as a rapid and sustained atrial arrhythmia, often conducting to the ventricles with a 2:1 atrioventricular (AV) ratio. Since many postoperative flutters are in the 300/minute range, this results in ventricular rates of 150/minute. Greater degrees of block and variable block also occur, allowing ready detection of classic, saw-tooth flutter waves in some cases. Flutter waves in many postoperative patients (e.g., postoperative Fontan patients) have a smaller amplitude and isoelectric intervals, eliminating the saw-tooth appearance and making diagnosis more difficult.

Atrial flutter can be confused with many other tachyarrhythmias. If 1:1 AV conduction occurs, it can mimic ventricular tachycardia (due to preexisting bundle branch block or rate-related aberrancy) or SVT. Flattened flutter waves with variable AV conduction can resemble atrial fibrillation or atrial ectopic tachycardia, while a fixed 2:1 or 3:1 AV block can fool investigators into believing sinus rhythm is present (as small flutter waves can be hidden in preceding T waves). An elevated or fixed heart rate in any postoperative congenital heart patient must be suspected as indicating an underlying atrial flutter.

Therapy for atrial flutter typically goes beyond the scope of the ED setting, except when rapid AV conduction causes hemodynamic compromise and electrical cardioversion is indicated.

Natural History of SVT in Children

The spectrum of SVT mechanisms varies with age. Essentially, a very small fraction of infant SVT is due to AV nodal reentry. Most cases of SVT use an accessory connection, while rare cases of primary atrial tachycardias occur. Of all infants with an accessory pathway-mediated SVT who experience SVT as newborns (≤ 2 months of age), 93% of them will stop having SVT by the time they are 8-10 months of age, and antiarrhythmic therapy can be discontinued.[5] However, of the SVTs that "go away" in this early part of childhood, nearly one-third will experience a recurrence subsequently at a mean age of 8 years. If SVT due to an accessory pathway is present over the age of 5 years, it will persist into adulthood in 78% of cases.[5] The explanation for these observations is elusive but may be related to the types and frequency of those factors that can initiate SVT, such as premature atrial or ventricular events, sinus pauses with junctional escape beats, and sinus node acceleration.[3] These natural history factors have an important bearing on the type of antiarrhythmic agents used, the duration of antiarrhythmic medical therapy, and the timing for consideration of any interventional therapy.

Presentation of SVT in Children

A number of cardiac evaluations to rule out occult tachyarrhythmias come about when a child has a syncopal episode. The overwhelming majority of these episodes are simple, benign, vasovagal faints, unlikely to recur and never causing any harm. However, the events surrounding the syncopal episode warrant a thorough historical evaluation. Warm days, long duration standing, poor fluid intake, and, interestingly, pulling on hair are common associated findings for benign faints. Syncope is an extremely rare presentation of SVT in children. It needs to be made clear, however, that syncope, especially that which presents during or immediately after exercise, can be due to serious ventricular arrhythmias and warrants a complete investigation.

Most infants can tolerate SVT for many hours. Since they cannot verbally relate their perceptions of tachycardia, subtle signs must be discerned for early diagnosis. These include poor feeding (essentially, a form of exercise for the infant), tachypnea (from pulmonary venous congestion), pallor and diaphoresis (due to a heightened catecholamine state), lethargy, and irritability. These latter signs and symptoms reflect a measure of congestive heart failure and are typically present in infants with SVT lasting several hours. Interestingly, SVT rarely occurs during sleep. The use of heart rate alarms in the home for small children with SVT is generally discouraged.

Older children rarely have symptoms of congestive heart failure due to episodic SVT. Some patients with incessant SVTs, even those that are fairly "slow SVTs" (in the range of 120-150/minute), can develop ventricular enlargement and symptoms of poor exercise tolerance and low cardiac output over time. Older children may complain of a perceived arrhythmia or palpitations. If the tachycardia lasts for half an hour or more, they often feel ill and may have "presyncope" with dizziness and orthostatic hypotension. Perceptions of chest pain and palpitations in children lasting less than one minute generally do not represent a pathologic tachyarrhythmia in young children and teenagers. Tachycardia often occurs at rest in these young patients, while they are sitting, reading, watching television, or in the 5-10 minutes *after* exercise.

Many patients, particularly adolescents, have learned to stop their SVT episodes at home using a number of "home remedies" before coming for evaluation. These maneuvers may include breath-holding (incorporating a Valsalva maneuver), doing a headstand for 30 seconds, putting their face in cold water, or coughing.

Initial Therapy for SVT

Table 2 details the initial therapy for patients with SVT. SVT episodes lasting more than 30 minutes or so in a patient under antiarrhythmic therapy generally should precipitate an ED visit as well as any in which cardiovascular compromise is suspected. Home remedies can be used for the patient with known SVT, but use of the diving reflex with an ice bag to a young infant's face (without obstructing the airway) is recommended only in rare circumstances by sophisticated parents outside the hospital setting. Ocular pressure is *always* contraindicated due to the risk of retinal detachment. Carotid massage is rarely effective in young patients.

Since the advent of adenosine, the ED therapeutic approach for SVTs has been altered forever. Adenosine is an endogenous adenine nucleoside agent with an intravenous half-life measured in seconds.

Table 2. Initial Therapy for Supraventricular Tachycardia

Record ECG before, during, and after conversion attempts!

- Ice bag to face (if infant, approximately 15-20 seconds)
- Vagal maneuvers (Valsalva, headstand)
- Adenosine IV rapid push
- If time and if available, transesophageal (or transvenous) overdrive pacing

Is there hemodynamic compromise?

If Yes: DC cardioversion. Lidocaine first, if on digoxin

If No: Digoxin IV (stop if WPW present)
Verapamil IV or propranolol IV (only if patient is > 1 year old) if no heart failure present
Procainamide IV

It acts to transiently block antegrade AV node conduction (proximal to the bundle of His). Therefore, in tachycardias that utilize the AV node, the SVT can be terminated quite easily. Ventricular ectopy occurs not infrequently after adenosine administration and may actually function to terminate the SVT. Facial flushing and dyspnea are rare. There is a transient hypotension, also lasting seconds, often followed by a mild catecholamine rebound.

Two other intravenous agents, which are commonly employed in adults, are to be avoided in children younger than 1 year of age. Intravenous verapamil and intravenous propranolol both can terminate SVT in these young patients. However, these drugs also result in long-duration adrenergic and calcium-channel blockade, which can lead to cardiovascular collapse, profound bradycardia, and death.[7]

Episodes of SVT in the infant may go unrecognized for many hours and may occasionally extend over 1-2 days. In these cases, the SVT may be either very difficult to terminate at all or may respond to intervention only briefly, with SVT recurring within seconds. In these cases, base deficits on the order of -10 to -15 are not uncommon. Intensive care admission with administration of a long-acting intravenous antiarrhythmic agent is often necessary. Of course, if there is significant cardiovascular compromise at the time of presentation, direct current cardioversion is an appropriate first-line therapy. Repeated use of cardioversion or adenosine for SVTs that recur after initial termination is inappropriate.

Chronic Medical Therapy for SVT

The types of antiarrhythmic agents used in the therapy of pediatric SVT *(see table 3)* has been changed irrevocably due to the success and safety of interventional catheter ablative procedures, which can provide a long-term cure. Many drugs or combinations of drugs can now be avoided. Generally, digoxin is an appropriate initial agent for those patients with SVT who do not have WPW present in sinus rhythm. If WPW is present or if a patient fails initial therapy with digoxin, propranolol or another beta-blocker is typically used next. Other options for problematic arrhythmias include procainamide (although dosing is often difficult in smaller patients due to both large unit dosing and rapid pharmacokinetics), flecainide, sotalol, and amiodarone. Combinations of these agents are rarely necessary and are usually done in conjunction with the advice of pediatric electrophysiologist. Calcium-channel blockers tend to be ineffective in most young patients but may help in some patients with AV node reentry SVTs. Class IC drugs such as flecainide and propafenone are safe in patients with SVT and normal hearts[8] but are contraindicated in those with congenital heart disease or cardiomyopathies.[9] Many forms of drug therapy can have serious adverse effects, worse than the arrhythmias being treated, and no longer need to be considered. Due to the natural history described above, there is often a several-year period wherein patients with newborn SVTs can avoid antiarrhythmic therapy.

Table 3. Chronic Therapy Options for Supraventricular Tachycardia

DRUG	COMMENTS
Digoxin	Most centers do not use if WPW present
Propranolol	Often qid in infants, tid in those older than 6 months
Atenolol	Does not cross the blood-brain barrier, given once or twice daily
Nadolol	Also can be given qd or bid
Flecainide*	Age-dependent kinetics. Do not use if abnormal heart
Propafenone*	Variable metabolism, tid dosing
Procainamide*	Usually q4h dosing in infants. Sustained-release available for older patients
Quinidine*	Many centers avoid its use due to side effects, proarrhythmia (torsades de pointes)
Verapamil	Best for AV node reentry, infrequently effective in children
Sotalol*	Beta-blocker at low dose, class III effects at higher dose
Amiodarone*	Potential side effects require monitoring: thyroid, liver, skin, pulmonary

* Requires in-hospital initiation of drug.

Catheter Ablation of SVTs in Children

The decision to proceed with an interventional procedure to cure SVT is a multifactorial one. First, the natural history must be considered. If the patient is an infant, there is an overwhelming chance that the arrhythmia will disappear, perhaps never to return, and the early use of interventional catheter ablative therapies may be inappropriate. Frequent SVT recurrences, especially on drug therapy, may require multiple ED visits and hospitalizations, adding an ongoing financial burden to the frustration of having a child with SVT. Many adolescents are not compliant with medical intervention and request a curative procedure to remove the need and stigma of drug therapy. Sports activities also come into consideration, particularly in the young teenager participating in interscholastic sports, since most schools will avoid the legal risk of them competing with any chance of having tachycardia by barring them from participation. Increasingly, patient choice is becoming the major determinant in the decision to proceed to the catheterization laboratory.

Catheter intervention for tachyarrhythmias consists of an intracardiac electrophysiology study to determine the mechanism and location of SVT substrates. Four catheters are generally used to induce SVT, determine the mechanism, and pinpoint the location of any accessory connections. Once this has been completed, a catheter ablation procedure is performed at the same time. Radiofrequency catheter ablation employs the delivery of radiofrequency current (about 500 kHz) from the end of the catheter to an indifferent patch on the patient's back. This bipole generates resistive heating of tissue at the tip of the catheter up to a depth of approximately 3-4 mm. If the catheter has been positioned precisely at the location of an accessory pathway, for example, the tissue is heated (essentially desiccated) and the accessory pathway is destroyed. This can result in a non-surgical cure of SVT for the majority of patients. The success rates for radiofrequency catheter ablation depend on the mechanism, accessory pathway location, and experience of the *pediatric* cardiologist performing the procedure.[10] Most centers report a success rate for accessory pathway SVTs on the left side of the heart at close to 95%.[10] Right-sided pathways are more difficult, carrying an approximate success rate of 75-90%, and some have the added risk of proximity to the normal AV conduction system.[10] Inadvertent block of the AV node is a rare but recognized risk of the procedure for pathways adjacent to the AV node and His bundle. It has been determined that the cost of catheter ablation is far less than the previous gold standard, surgical intervention. Additionally, catheter ablation costs for children tend to balance with continued medical therapy after 4-5 years, increasing the appeal for the procedure for most young patients who are otherwise expecting 40-50 years of potential tachycardia episodes.[11]

Ventricular Arrhythmias

Accelerated Ventricular Rhythm. Fortunately, ventricular arrhythmias are extremely rare in children with normal hearts. One benign arrhythmia worthy of mention is called accelerated ventricular rhythm. In this arrhythmia, there is an automatically depolarizing, accelerated ventricular focus, resulting in uniform (monomorphic) ventricular ectopy at a rate just above that of the underlying sinus rate. A heart rate of less than or equal to 15% faster than the sinus rate is generally seen in accelerated ventricular arrhythmias, while ventricular tachycardia generally produces a rate that is greater than 15% faster than the sinus rate. However, the diagnosis cannot be made by ventricular rate alone, since benign accelerated ventricular rates in excess of 150/minute can be seen in the very young patient with more rapid sinus rates. The ECG picture of accelerated ventricular rhythm is one of gradual onset and termination, often with fusion of QRS complexes as the accelerated rate "walks into" the sinus rate.

Ventricular arrhythmias can occur in patients with underlying congenital heart defects.[12] These arrhythmias tend to occur many years after surgical repair of the defect. The cardiac lesions most often cited as presenting with late ventricular arrhythmias are shown in *Table 4*. Once present, these postoperative arrhythmias do not tend to disappear, as seen with many forms of SVT. A search for residual hemodynamic problems (e.g., persistent right ventricular outflow tract obstruction in tetralogy of Fallot) and subsequent surgical revision may eliminate ventricular arrhythmias in many of these patients.[13]

Ventricular Tachycardia. Ventricular tachycardia (VT) is defined as three or more consecutive ventricular beats, generally faster than 120/minute and more than 15% faster than the underlying sinus rate at that time. The QRS morphology must differ from that seen in sinus rhythm. VT can be sustained (> 30 seconds duration), non-sustained and monomorphic (all beats with the same QRS appearance), or polymorphic. In addition to the VT rate, these descriptors often aid in the determination of proper therapeutic options. For example, neither a slow, hemodynamically stable VT nor repeated runs of non-sustained VT should be addressed by direct current cardioversion. Both settings warrant other medical therapies.

The potential causes of VT are shown in *Table 5*. They range from metabolic and electrolyte abnormalities to drug effects to both structural and electrical cardiac disorders.

Therapy for VT depends in large part on whether hemodynamic compromise is present in the face of sustained arrhythmia. *(See Table 6.)* Additionally, more etiology-specific therapies may be indicated, as in the long QT syndrome.

Long QT Syndrome. A significant concern in young patients with ventricular arrhythmia relates to the potential diagnosis of long QT syndrome. Most often, this is manifested as a congenital arrhythmia, rather than an acquired one, in patients with normal hearts.[14] However, many situations can bring about an acquired prolongation of the QT interval on the surface ECG and long QT syndrome. *(See Table 7.)* In the congenital form, the corrected QT is prolonged from birth but may not result in problems until the late toddler or early teen years. The QT is measured as a value corrected for heart rate (the QTc) as in Bazett's formula:

$$QTc = \frac{QT}{\sqrt{RR\ interval}}$$

The QT and RR intervals are measured in seconds. Values in excess of 0.44 may be abnormal, and clearly those greater than 0.46 are abnormal. The abnormality of cardiac repolarization causing the long QT interval can result in spontaneous induction of a form of ventricular tachycardia (VT) called torsades de pointes. This is a potentially lethal arrhythmia resulting in little or no cardiac output. The torsades may be precipitated by emotion, exercise, or any heightened catecholamine state. Syncope is the most common presentation. Nightmares may occur, probably due to episodes of VT and low cardiac output. A thorough investigation of the family history is necessary for seizures, sudden death, and odd accidents, which may actually represent episodes of torsades. Congenital deafness is a rare accompaniment (Jervell and Lang-Nielsen syndrome). There is an annual mortality of close to 5% for this disorder,[14] and the finding of "T waves alternans" in the long QT patient is particularly ominous.

Initial therapy for long QT syndrome usually consists of a beta-blocking agent, especially if the episodes appear to be

Table 4. Cardiac Lesions Associated with Late Ventricular Arrhythmias

Tetralogy of Fallot, double outlet ventricles
Mustard or Senning procedures
Aortic valve operations (including Konno)
Subaortic operations
Cardiomyopathies (resections)
Right ventricular-pulmonary conduits
Anomalous coronary artery reimplantations
Kawasaki's disease

Table 5. Causes of Ventricular Tachycardia

Metabolic: Acidosis, hypoxemia, hypokalemia, hyperkalemia, hypoglycemia, hypercalcemia, hypothermia
Drugs: Digoxin, quinidine, flecainide, propafenone, sotalol, sympathomimetics, tricyclic antidepressants, cocaine, halothane
Cardiac: All defects from Table 4, myocarditis, endocarditis, long QT syndrome (congenital and acquired), arrhythmogenic right ventricular dysplasia, cardiac tumors, muscular/myotonic dystrophies

Table 6. Initial Therapy Options for Ventricular Tachycardia

Is there hemodynamic compromise?*

If Yes: DC cardioversion
Lidocaine IV bolus, then infusion
If available, transvenous ventricular overdrive pacing

If No: Lidocaine IV bolus, then infusion
Propranolol IV (not in patients < 1 year old)
Esmolol IV bolus, then infusion
Procainamide IV bolus, then infusion
Amiodarone IV bolus, then infusion
Phenytoin IV bolus

** In all cases, correct electrolyte abnormalities, acidosis. Treat drug intoxication.*

catecholamine-triggered. However, there are some patients with long QT syndrome who have episodes of torsades after pauses in cardiac rhythm, followed by premature ventricular beats. Many of these "pause-dependent" patients may benefit from cardiac pacing to prevent the inciting pauses. A number of patients eventually require combination therapy of beta-blockers and pacing systems and others may need left stellate ganglionectomy or implantation of an automatic defibrillator to prevent sudden death.[14]

Recent dramatic results from molecular cardiology research have identified two genetic loci for patients with familial long QT syndrome:[15,16] Chromosome 7 has an identified gene defect related to the potassium channel gene and chromosome 3 has a defect in a region

Table 7. Causes of Acquired Prolonged QT on the Electrocardiogram

DRUGS
Class IA IC, III antiarrhythmic agents
Phenothiazines
Tricyclic antidepressants
Lithium

METABOLIC
Hypokalemia, hypocalcemia (long ST segment), hypomagnesemia
Hypothyroidism, anorexia

CENTRAL NERVOUS SYSTEM
Increased intracranial pressure
Subarachnoid hemorrhage

MISCELLANEOUS
Myocardial infarction
Right radical neck dissection
Balloon valvuloplasty
IV erythromycin, organophosphate poisoning

associated with a cardiac sodium channel gene. Future therapy for this life-threatening disease may involve ionic channel-specific agents[17,18] or gene therapy to replace the defective expression of these ion channel genes.

Ventricular Fibrillation. Ventricular fibrillation (VF) is rare in children as a primary rhythm abnormality and more often results as a secondary event due to a preceding VT. All of the causes of VT shown in *Table 5* are potential causes of VF as well. The main goal of VF therapy is to ensure proper diagnosis (e.g., all the ECG leads attached and artifact ruled out) and support for the circulation while preparations are made for defibrillation at 2 J/kg with unsynchronized cardioversion. The myocardium tends to be quite acidotic and resistant to initial defibrillation attempts. When defibrillation succeeds in terminating VF, the result is often a bradycardic rhythm (sinus, escape junctional, or ventricular). Transthoracic pacing (and/or continued CPR) is frequently necessary, and its need should be anticipated.

Summary

In order to effectively diagnose and manage pediatric tachyarrhythmias, there are key points that deserve special emphasis. First, when confronted with a pediatric tachycardia, do not panic. Next, support the circulation while obtaining the data necessary (more than just a monitor strip, most often) to make the diagnosis. Remember that most fast, narrow QRS, regular-rhythm tachycardias are adenosine-responsive, and that they may recur. Furthermore, only a few therapies actually need to be memorized: adenosine (150 mcg/kg IV push, with immediate flush), lidocaine (1 mg/kg, repeated if necessary), and DC cardioversion (0.5-2.0 watt sec/kg). If the patient is very ill with tachycardia, cardioversion is often necessary urgently. If cardioversion is used, all the possible results must be anticipated: sinus rhythm, atrial or ventricular fibrillation, continued tachycardia, bradycardia or asystole.

References

1. Wolff L, Parkinson J, White PD. Bundle branch block with short PR interval in healthy young people prone to paroxysmal tachycardia. *Am Heart J* 1930;5:685-704.
2. Perry JC, Giuffre RM, Garson A Jr. Clues to the electrocardiographic diagnosis of subtle Wolff-Parkinson-White syndrome in children. *J Pediatr* 1990;117:871-875.
3. Dunnigan A, Benditt DG, Benson DW Jr. Modes of onset ("initiating events") for paroxysmal atrial tachycardia in infants and children. *Am J Cardiol* 1986;57:1280-1287.
4. Cecchin F, Fenrich AL, Friedman RA, et al. Wide QRS tachycardia in infancy: Left bundle branch block is common during supraventricular tachycardia. *Pediatr Cardiol* 1994;15: 254. Abstract.
5. Perry JC, Garson A Jr. Supraventricular tachycardia due to Wolff-Parkinson-White syndrome: Early disappearance and late recurrence. *J Am Coll Cardiol* 1990;16:1215-1220.
6. Garson A Jr, Bink-Boelkens M, Hesslein PS, et al. Atrial flutter in the young: A collaborative study of 380 cases. *J Am Coll Cardiol* 1985;6:871-878.
7. Epstein ML, Kiel EA, Victorica BE. Cardiac decompensation following verapamil therapy in infants with supraventricular tachycardia. *Pediatrics* 1985;75:737-740.
8. Perry JC, Garson A Jr. Flecainide acetate for pediatric tachyarrhythmias: Review of world literature on efficacy, safety and dosing. *Am Heart J* 1992;124:1614-1621.
9. Fish FA, Gillette PC, Benson DW Jr. Proarrhythmia, cardiac arrest and death in young patients receiving encainide and flecainide. *J Am Coll Cardiol* 1991;18:356-365.
10. Kugler JD, Danford DA, Deal B, et al. Radiofrequency catheter ablation in children and adolescents: Early results in 572 patients from 24 centers. *N Engl J Med* 1994;330: 1481-1487.
11. Garson A Jr. Children with Wolff-Parkinson-White and supraventricular tachycardia: A model cost effectiveness analysis for pediatric chronic disease. *Am J Cardiol* 1993;72: 502. Abstract.
12. Altman C, Vick GW, Perry JC, et al. Ventricular tachycardia after repair of congenital heart disease. *Prog Pediatr Cardiol* 1995;4:229-236.
13. Deal BJ, Scagliotti D, Miller SM, et al. Electrophysiologic drug testing in symptomatic ventricular arrhythmias after repair of tetralogy of Fallot. *Am J Cardiol* 1987;59: 1380-1385.
14. Garson A Jr, Dick M III, Fournier A, et al. The long QT syndrome in children. An international study of 287 patients. *Circulation* 1993;87:1866-1872.
15. Wang Q, Shen J, Splawski I, et al. SCN5A mutations associated with an inherited cardiac arrhythmia, long QT syndrome. *Cell* 1995;80:805-811.
16. Curran ME, Splawski I, Timothy KW, et al. A molecular basis for cardiac arrhythmia: HERG mutations cause long QT syndrome. *Cell* 1995;80:795-803.
17. Schwartz PJ, Priori SG, Locati EH, et al. Long Qt syndrome patients with mutations of the SCN5A and HERG genes have differential responses to Na+ channel blockade and to increases in heart rate. *Circulation* 1995;92:3381-3386.
18. Sato T, Hata Y, Yamamoto M, et al. Early after depolarizations abolished by a potassium channel activator in a patient with idiopathic long QT syndrome. *J Cardiovasc Electrophysiol* 1995;6:279-282.

Infants and Children with HIV

Steven G. Rothrock, MD, FACEP

Over the past decade, the global pandemic of HIV has spread to every continent, with nearly 13 million cases worldwide.[1] Of these cases, 1 million have occurred in children.[1,2] While the spread of HIV has not abated, medical knowledge concerning the pathophysiology, diagnosis, and management of HIV-infected infants and children has grown exponentially. Early diagnostic and treatment protocols based on data extrapolated from adult studies were the cornerstone of therapy for HIV-infected children. However, research into pediatric-specific aspects of HIV has improved the ability of clinicians to make rational diagnostic and management decisions regarding HIV-infected children.

Several important advances have dramatically changed the approach to children with HIV. Importantly, treatment of infected mothers with AZT has been shown to reduce the rate of vertical transmission of HIV.[3] While diagnosis of HIV infection in adults is relatively straightforward, the presence of maternal anti-HIV IgG, which crosses the placenta, potentially confuses diagnostic efforts in infants younger than 18 months old. However, newer assays allow for accurate identification of most infants as young as 3 months old with HIV. Moreover, age-specific serum markers and other disease-specific tests are important tools for monitoring infants and children with HIV. Thus, choice of laboratory tests used to diagnose and monitor HIV must take into consideration the patient's age, each laboratory's ability, and the sensitivity and specificity of particular lab assays that are currently available.

With an increased ability to diagnose, monitor, and prevent disease progression, it is important that clinicians be able to identify undiagnosed infants and children with HIV. An increased awareness of the varied clinical presentations of HIV in infants and children may serve this goal. An understanding of the normal disease course, common complications of HIV disease, and therapy will improve the ability of clinicians to care for children with HIV who present to the ED. Early intervention, aggressive prophylaxis against common pathogens, and antiretroviral treatment also will likely improve the overall health and survival of HIV-infected infants and children.

Introduction

Since the first childhood cases were reported in 1983, the number of children infected with the HIV virus has grown almost exponentially. As of December 1994, the WHO estimated that over 1 million children had acquired the HIV virus worldwide.[1] By 1993, over 4000 cases of AIDS in children less than 13 years old had been reported to the Centers for Disease Control (CDC), with an estimated 10,000-20,000 children infected with the HIV virus (with most not yet exhibiting severe symptoms).[2] While newer therapies have the potential to decrease vertical transmission (mother to fetus) of HIV, with a resulting decreased rate of new neonatal cases, the number of adolescents (ages 13-19) with HIV is doubling every 2-3 years.[1,3] Furthermore, the median life span of children with perinatally acquired HIV has risen from six years to nine years due to newer therapies and better supportive care.[4] Thus, emergency physicians increasingly will be called upon to care for a larger population of infants and children who are surviving longer with HIV.

HIV and the Immune System

HIV-1 is an RNA virus and is a member of the retroviridae family of viruses—a group of viruses causing disease in goats, sheep, horses, and monkeys in addition to humans.[5] Several unique properties of the HIV virus contribute to its pathogenicity.[5,6]

HIV has an outer envelope docking protein (gp120) that interacts with the CD4 protein lining the outer surface of helper T cells.[6] Another protein (gp41) with other sequences of viral envelope proteins facilitates fusion of the viral envelope with the cellular membrane, allowing viral RNA entry.[6] Once the viral RNA is within the cell, it is transcribed to DNA using the enzyme reverse transcriptase that was originally packaged in the whole viron. Viral replication then occurs with production of new virus particles.[5,6] The life cycle of the virus allows for disruption of the host's immune system and eventual destruction of helper T cells and other cells that carry the CD4 protein on their outer surface (e.g., monocytes, macrophages, astrocytes, oligodendrocytes).[5,6]

Who is at Risk?

To date, 90% of HIV cases in infants and children (<12 years) have been acquired perinatally.[1] Without treatment, the vertical transmission rate of HIV has been reported at approximately 25% (12-52%).[1,7,8] Factors that increase vertical transmission of HIV include mothers with AIDS-defining illness, maternal active sexually transmitted disease, premature rupture of membranes, delivery before 34 weeks' gestation, placental membrane inflammation, maternal p24 antigenemia, maternal CD4 count less than 700 cells/mm^3, maternal HIV-1 RNA levels 190,000 copies/mm^3, and, possibly, vaginal delivery.[1,7-9] In 1994, zidovudine treatment was found to decrease the vertical transmission rate of HIV in neonates from 26% to 8% if initiated in the second trimester, with continuous IV therapy during delivery and oral therapy continued in the newborn infant for six weeks postpartum.[10] Importantly, this therapy has the potential to decrease the number of new neonatal cases of HIV by over 65% per year.[10] Some authors have noted that those who still develop HIV (after mothers were treated with zidovudine) may be more likely to harbor zidovudine-resistant HIV infection.[10,11] This may make treatment of HIV in infants and children more difficult in the future.

Another important route for vertical transmission of HIV is breast feeding. It has been estimated that this route leads to HIV infection in up to 14-20% of infants.[1] For this reason, HIV-infected mothers should not breast feed. The WHO still recommends breast feeding in developing countries with a high rate of death due to malnutrition and diarrheal disease.[1,2]

With today's more accurate testing, the risk of transmitting HIV via transfusion has fallen to 1 in 40,000-60,000.[1,2] New heat treatment techniques for factor VIII concentrates and recombinant factor preparations have virtually eliminated the risk of HIV for hemophiliacs.

For 1% of infants and children 12 years or younger, the route of HIV transmission is unknown.[1] Importantly, clinicians must consider the possibility of sexual abuse in this population. At one pediatric AIDS center, 14 out of 94 cases of pediatric HIV were transmitted through sexual abuse.[12]

The number of AIDS cases occurring in adolescents (13-19 years) is relatively small, with fewer than 1000 cases reported by late 1992.[1] However, underreporting is a problem since a number of states (e.g., Florida) require only that cases of AIDS (severe HIV infection) and not HIV infection be reported. Moreover, the number of new cases of HIV is rising ~77% every two years, making this one of the fastest-growing populations of HIV patients in the country.[1] Unprotected sex and IV drug use are the most common causes within this age group.[1]

HIV is a disease that has spread from several epicenters in the United States, generally areas with large population centers, large homosexual populations, and high rates of IV drug use.[13] Perinatally acquired HIV occurs most frequently in areas with high HIV seroprevalence among childbearing women. National HIV seroprevalence data show the highest incidence of HIV among women of childbearing age in the following locations: New York City (1.25% seroprevalence), Washington DC (0.9%), New Jersey (0.55%), and Florida (0.54%), compared to a national seroprevalence rate of 0.17% (or 1.7 HIV-infected women per 1000 live births).[13]

Classification of HIV

In the past, children and adults were defined as being HIV-positive (a positive blood test without symptoms or with minor symptoms) or as having AIDS (one of a set of serious disorders related to immune dysfunction: currently CDC Clinical Category C).[14] Experts no longer make the distinction between these two definitions for children as all patients are now considered HIV-positive with different levels of symptoms, immunosuppression, and infection.[14]

In 1994, the CDC published a new classification system for children younger than 13 years with HIV.[14] This classification system is simpler than the prior system and is based on the presence of symptoms, the degree of immunosuppression based on CD4 count, and the patient's age.[14] *(See Table 1.)* Importantly, while CD4 counts are used to follow and categorize adults, their variation with age can lead to confusion in children. Infants and young children normally have higher CD4 counts that decline over the first few years of life; therefore, different CD4 counts are used to identify the level of immunosuppression in infants and young children. *(See Table 2.)* Moreover, children may develop opportunistic infections at higher CD4 counts compared to older children and adults.[14,15] With this classification system, children should never be reclassified to a less severe category from a more severe category.[14]

Diagnosis of HIV

Diagnosis of HIV in infants is confounded by the presence of maternal anti-HIV IgG antibodies that cross the placenta, which persists for 12-18 months.[1,15] Therefore, all infants born to HIV-infected mothers are HIV-antibody-positive at birth. For this reason, testing that relies on detection of IgG (e.g., Western blot and ELISA) can give false-positive results until age 18 months and should not be relied upon in patients up to this age.[16] In children older than 18 months, HIV tests consist of an initial ELISA test, which is nearly

Table 1. Pediatric Human Immunodeficiency Virus Classifications

IMMUNOLOGIC CATEGORIES	N: NO SIGNS/ SYMPTOMS	A: MILD SIGNS/ SYMPTOMS	B: MODERATE SIGNS/ SYMPTOMS	C: SEVERE SIGNS/ SYMPTOMS **
No evidence of suppression	N1	A1	B1	C1
Evidence of moderate suppression	N2	A2	B2	C2
Severe suppression	N3	A3	B3	C3

* Children whose HIV status is not confirmed are classified by using the above grid with a letter E (for perinatally exposed) placed before the appropriate classification code (e.g., EN2)

** Both Category C and lymphoid interstitial pneumonitis in Category B are reportable to state and local health departments as acquired immunodeficiency syndrome.

Adapted from: Centers for Disease Control and Prevention. 1994 Revised classification system for human immunodeficiency virus infection in children less than 13 years of age. *MMWR Morb Mortal Wkly Rep* 1994;43(suppl RR-12):1-17.

Table 2. Immune Categories Based on Lymphocyte Profile

IMMUNOLOGIC CATEGORY	AGE < 12 MONTHS mcL	(%)	1- 5 YEARS mcL	(%)	6-12 YEARS mcL	(%)
No evidence of suppression	≥ 1500	≥ 25%	≥ 1000	≥ 25%	≥ 500	≥ 25%
Evidence of moderate suppression	750-1499	15-24%	500-999	15-24%	200-499	15-24%
Severe suppression	< 750	< 15%	< 500	< 15%	< 200	< 15%

Adapted from: Centers for Disease Control and Prevention. 1994 Revised classification system for human immunodeficiency virus infection in children less than 13 years of age. *MMWR Morb Mortal Wkly Rep* 1994;43(suppl RR-12):1-17.

99% sensitive, with positive testing confirmed by the more specific Western blot test.[16]

A diagnosis of HIV infection can now be made with certainty in nearly 50% of neonates and 95% of infants older than 3 months with polymerase chain reaction (PCR), viral culture, or acid-dissociated p24 antigen assays.[17] PCR is an in vitro technique for amplification of specific nucleic acid sequences of HIV to levels that are readily detectable in the laboratory.[16] Sensitivity of PCR has been reported at 27% for neonates 0-4 days old, 55% for those at 0-15 days, and nearly 98% at 16-90 days.[18] It has been postulated that viral levels are much higher in neonates who acquire HIV during pregnancy (intrauterine) compared to those who acquire the disease during delivery (intrapartum).[19] This may explain why PCR detects a subset of cases in neonates (intrauterine infection) but fails to detect most cases of HIV (intrapartum acquisition) within the first few days of delivery.[19] HIV viral blood culture is a technically difficult and expensive test (~$500) with greater than 95% sensitivity for detecting HIV in infants older than 1 month. The p24 antigen tests are performed via an ELISA technique.[20] This technique has less sensitivity (~70% sensitivity at 3 months) compared to other tests, while specificity approaches 95%.[20] In general, demonstration of IgG antibody via ELISA and a confirmatory test (Western blot) establishes the diagnosis of HIV in any child older than 18 months old.[16] Under 18 months, at least two confirmatory assays (any combination of HIV culture, PCR or p24 antigen) for the presence of HIV are required before a definitive diagnosis can be made.[16] *(See Figure 1.)*

Common Clinical Presentations

Early retrospective studies of pediatric HIV painted a bleak picture since they often concentrated on children who were diagnosed early in their disease course and had a rapid clinical deterioration.[21] More recent prospective longitudinal studies have shown that HIV presents in a bimodal pattern, with 20-30% developing severe immune deficiency and AIDS-defining illness (clinical Category C) before age 1 year while most children have a slowly progressive course, with a greater than five-year survival.[1] Those who are very young (< 6-12 months) and those who are greater than 5 years have mortality rates that are 1.5-2.0 times higher than children aged 1-5 years.[22] Currently, it is believed that many infants with early clinical deterioration acquired HIV during pregnancy, allowing the virus to attack an immature immune system and therefore causing a more profound immune deficiency.[19] Increases in mortality after age 5 are primarily associated with a progressive decline in the immune system.[22,23]

Common presentations of HIV in infants include failure to thrive, recurrent bacteremia and bacterial infections, generalized lymphadenopathy, and progressive neurologic decline with failure to attain normal neurologic and developmental milestones.[1] Failure to thrive occurs from chronic infections, malabsorption, chronic diarrhea, increased nutritional requirements, and overall poor nutrition.[24] Encephalopathy is another common presenting feature of HIV, resulting in developmental delay or loss of milestones.[25] HIV directly invades and destroys cells within the central nervous system, while

Figure 1. Diagnostic Testing of Infants Born to HIV-Positive Mothers

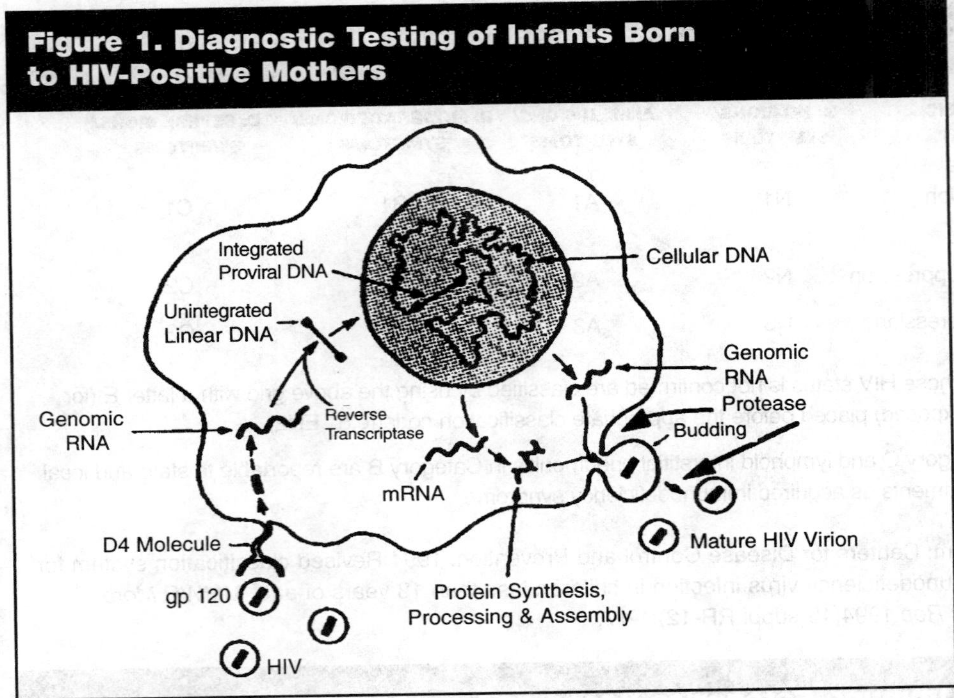

damage also may occur from opportunistic infection, malnutrition, and the effects of toxins.[25]

While HIV causes a progressive decline in T cell lines, immunoglobulin levels are often elevated early in the disease.[26] However, these immunoglobulins are often dysfunctional, and children are unable to mount a prolonged antigen antibody response to bacterial infections.[26] For this reason, recurrent bacterial infections, often with the same agent, are frequently seen in HIV. Recurrent bacteremia, pneumonia, otitis media, and sinusitis due to the usual pathogens seen in normal children are the most common bacterial infections in children with HIV.[1,27] Therefore, initial empiric therapy for simple bacterial infections (e.g., otitis media, sinusitis, cellulitis, and bacterial pneumonia) should parallel treatment used in immunocompetent children. In children with CD4 counts greater than 200 cells/mm^3, IV immunoglobulin has been shown to significantly reduce the incidence of serious bacterial infections, the rate of deterioration of CD4 counts, and total days of hospitalization for infections, although no effect on mortality has been noted.[1,28] A double-blind, placebo-controlled study in symptomatic HIV-infected children found that the benefits of IV immunoglobulin (IVIG) were not greater than standard AZT with PCP prophylaxis with TMP/SMX.[28] Accepted indications for IVIG treatment in pediatric HIV include: 1) recurrent, invasive bacterial disease (especially with encapsulated organisms); 2) HIV related hypogammaglobulinemia; 3) bronchiectasis; 4) documented inability to produce protective antibody to important immunizations (e.g., measles, Hib); and 5) HIV-related ITP.[1,26]

Pinkert et al detailed the presenting features of children with known and unsuspected HIV who presented to one pediatric ED.[29] Fever was the most common presenting complaint (50%), followed by respiratory symptoms (21%), and GI symptoms (8%). Importantly, many children were not receiving appropriate outpatient treatment, as 87% with known HIV had CD4 counts below thresholds for PCP prophylaxis and 52% were not receiving any therapy.[21] The majority of children had an acute infection, with 33% described as serious. Eight of 92 children had positive blood cultures for *S. pneumoniae* (3), *S. faecalis* (2), *E. coli* (1), *Torulopsis glabrata* (1), and *Staphylococcus* species (1—possibly a skin contaminant). Half of the positive blood cultures were in children with temperatures below 38°C, although three-quarters had central lines with a history of a fever. Importantly, a white blood count was useless in discriminating between children with and without bacteremia.[29] Thus, clinicians must diligently search for bacterial infections in all HIV-positive children who present to the ED with a history of fever, regardless of the presenting temperature or white blood cell (WBC) count. Empiric antibiotic therapy should be considered for all of these patients (especially those with central lines). Only children who are well-appearing, with no obvious infection or only minor infection, should be considered for outpatient therapy with closely coordinated follow-up.

For the foreseeable future, many infants and children will be undiagnosed until symptoms related to HIV infection develop. Persaud found that 18% of HIV-infected children cared for at one children's hospital were not diagnosed until they were 4 years old or older.[30] Diagnoses that eventually prompted consideration of HIV in these children included recurrent bacterial infections in 31%, hematological disorders (e.g., ITP, neutropenia, anemia) in 16%, PCP in 9%, followed by developmental delay, recurrent skin conditions, weight loss, malignancy, and nephropathy.[30] This study's findings underscore the need for emergency physicians to consider the diagnosis of HIV in many children who present to the ED with rare or unusual complaints.

While a subset of infants and young children may present with frequent bacterial infections and rapid progression of disease, most children with HIV manifest a more gradual onset of disease, with predominant findings within the reticuloendothelial system (e.g., generalized lymphaden- opathy, parotitis, lymphoid interstitial pneumonia, and hep- atosplenomegaly).[1,2] Children who present with these disorders have a better prognosis and a longer survival compared to infants with onset of disease in the first year of life.[1,2]

Complications and Natural Progression of HIV

While infants and children with HIV are at risk for developing a wide array of bacterial, viral, fungal, and parasitic infections, some diseases are almost ubiquitous in this population. The most common opportunistic infections reported in children with AIDS include *Pneumocystis carinii* pneumonia, recurrent bacterial infections, candidiasis, cytomegalovirus (CMV) disease, and *Mycobacterium avium-intracellulare* complex (MAC).[31] *(See Table 4.)* The absolute CD4 lymphocyte count appears to be an important predictor of the risk of specific infections. HIV-infected children with a CD4 count less than 200 cells/mm^3 are six times more likely than those with a count greater

Table 3. Clinical Categories for Children with HIV Infection

CATEGORY N: NOT SYMPTOMATIC

Children who have no signs or symptoms considered to be the result of HIV infection or who have only one of the conditions listed in Category A.

CATEGORY A: MILDLY SYMPTOMATIC

Children with two or more of the conditions listed below but none of the conditions listed in Categories B and C.

- Lymphadenopathy (≥ 0.5 cm at more than two sites)
- Hepatomegaly, splenomegaly, dermatitis, parotitis, and recurrent or persistent upper respiratory infection, sinusitis, or otitis media

CATEGORY B: MODERATELY SYMPTOMATIC

Children who have symptomatic conditions other than those listed for Category A or C that are attributed to HIV infection. Examples of conditions in clinical Category B include but are not limited to:

- Anemia (< 8 g/dL), neutropenia (< 1000/mm^3), or thrombocytopenia (< 100,000/mm^3) persisting 30 days; bacterial meningitis, pneumonia, or sepsis (single episode); candidiasis, oropharyngeal (thrush), persisting (> 2 months) in children > 6 months of age; cardiomyopathy; CMV infection with onset before 1 month of age; diarrhea that is chronic or recurrent; hepatitis; herpes simplex virus (HSV) stomatitis, recurrent; HSV bronchitis, pneumonitis, or esophagitis with onset before 1 month of age; herpes zoster involving at least two distinct episodes or more than one dermatome; leiomyosarcoma; lymphoid interstitial pneumonia or pulmonary lymphoid hyperplasia complex; nephropathy; nocardiosis; persistent fever (> one month); toxoplasmosis with onset before 1 month of age; varicella that is disseminated.

CATEGORY C: SEVERELY SYMPTOMATIC

Children who have any condition listed in the 1987 surveillance case definition for acquired immunodeficiency syndrome with the exception of LIP.

- Serious bacterial infections; candidiasis (other than oral); coccidiomycoccosis; cryptococcosis; cryptosporidiosis or isosporiasis with diarrhea persisting > one month; encephalopathy; HSV stomatitis persisting > one month or HSV bronchitis, pneumonitis, or esophagitis for any duration affecting a child > 1 month old; histoplasmosis, disseminated; Kaposi's sarcoma; lymphoma; *Mycobacterium* tuberculosis that is disseminated or extrapulmonary; *Mycobacterium* (other species or unidentified disseminated); *Mycobacterium avium*-complex or *Mycobacterium kansasii* that is disseminated; *Pneumocystis carinii* pneumonia; progressive multifocal leukoencephalopathy; nontyphoidal *Salmonella* septicemia; toxoplasmosis of the brain with onset at > 1 month; or wasting syndrome.

than 200 cells/mm^3 to develop opportunistic infections, three times more likely to develop serious bacterial infections, twice as likely to develop viral infections, and slightly more prone to developing minor bacterial infections. The risk of acquiring PCP rises dramatically at CD4 levels less than 200 cells/mm^3, while CMV and MAC infections become more common at CD4 levels less than 50 cells/mm^3.[1,32] Furthermore, after an individual develops an opportunistic infection, they may never be completely cured, and that infection may resurface as immunodeficiency worsens.[33]

Pulmonary Disease. *Pneumocystis carinii* pneumonia (PCP) is the most common opportunistic infection in infants and children who are HIV-positive and may be the first presenting infection.[33,34] Of infants and children with HIV, 43-53% will acquire PCP.[31,34,35] Compared to adults, this is a much more virulent disease, with mortality from a first infection near 50%, rising to nearly 100% for subsequent episodes.[2,31] Early studies found that infants less than 1 year old have a more virulent course (with a 30% one-year survival) after acquiring PCP compared to older infants and children, who have a 48% one-year survival following PCP.[2] While recent improvements in management have decreased mortality, PCP is still an extremely lethal disease. Clinicians must be aware of the typical and atypical presentations of this disorder, key diagnostic features, and appropriate management.

The most common symptoms of PCP are nonproductive cough, fever, and dyspnea, with a gradual or explosive onset.[36] Most cases occur in infants 18 months or younger with rapidly progressive immunosuppression.[34] In contrast to adults, a depressed CD4 count is not required for development of PCP. In fact, 10% of infants with PCP have CD4 counts above 1500 cells/mm^3.[31,37] Typically, fever is present, bilateral rales are heard, and tachypnea is prominent. Infants and children are hypoxic, with a markedly elevated A-a gradient averaging 60-80 mmHg. (A-a gradient at sea level = 150 - [PaO_2 + PCO_2/0.8], with normal A-a gradient < 10-15).[34] Chest radiography may initially appear normal; abnormal blood gas findings can be the only clue to the presence of PCP.[36] As the infection progresses, bilateral perihilar and interstitial infiltrates develop.[38] Advanced disease leads to a ground-glass appearance to the lung fields.[38] PCP may cause subpleural cavities and emphysematous blebs, predisposing patients to recurrent air leaks (e.g., pneumothorax, bronchopulmonary fistulas) that can be extremely difficult to manage.[39] Differentiating PCP from other pulmonary infections (e.g., viral pneumonia and tuberculosis) can be difficult. One clue is an elevated LDH, averaging 780-795 U/L in children with PCP.[34] Children who are old enough to cooperate can have induced sputum sent for PCP prep. However, definitive diagnosis may require bronchoscopy with bronchoalveolar lavage or tracheal aspirate, neither of which is available or practical in the ED setting.[36]

Due to the high rates of respiratory failure, pulmonary complications, and mortality, admission is mandatory for infants and children with PCP.[1,15] Treatment consists of IV TMP/SMX (20 mg/kg/d divided qid), supportive respiratory care, and close monitoring for respiratory failure.[31] TMP/SMX allergy is common problem seen in children with HIV, with rates that surpass those seen in the normal population. Many centers routinely desensitize patients to TMP/SMX if they are allergic. Trimetrexate with leucovorin rescue is often used in patients not responding to TMP/SMX. Pentamidine is an alternative also used for nonresponders.[31] Recently, steroid therapy (either IV methylprednisolone or prednisone 1 mg/kg/d for 5 days

Table 4. Commonly Reported Indicator Infections

Most commonly reported indicator infections in 4249 reported cases of children with AIDS in the United States (1992).

Infection	Cases	%
Pneumocystis carinii pneumonia	1574	(37%)
Recurrent bacterial infection	831	(20%)
Candidiasis	675	(19%)
Esophagus	599	(15%)
Pulmonary	176	(4%)
Cytomegalovirus Disease	394	(10%)
Other than retinitis	339	(8%)
Retinitis	55	(2%)
Mycobacterium avium-intracellulare complex	212	(5%)
Cryptosporidiosis and chronic diarrhea	138	(3%)
Herpes simplex esophagitis/pneumonia/ulcers	142	(3%)
Mycobacterium tuberculosis extrapulmonary	25	(1%)
Other disseminated mycobacterial disease	41	(1%)
Cryptococcosis extrapulmonary	42	(1%)
Toxoplasmosis of brain	34	(1%)
Coccidiomycosis, extrapulmonary	6	(<1%)

Adapted from: Tovo PA, deMartino M, Bagiano C, et al. Prognostic factors and survival in children with perinatal HIV-1 infection. *Lancet* 1992;339:1249-1253.

followed by 0.5 mg/kg/d for 5 days) was shown to reduce the need for mechanical ventilation (from 64% to 24%) and the mortality rate (from 30% to 0%) in children with PCP.[34] Due to its dramatic effects on outcome, steroid therapy should be considered the standard of care for children with PCP.

Prophylaxis for PCP with oral TMP/SMX has been show to decrease the development of PCP by 75% and mortality by 67% in infants and children at risk.[37,40]Alternatives include dapsone and aerosolized pentamidine.[40] The CDC recommends prophylaxis for all HIV-positive infants younger than 12 months since the predictive value of the CD4 count is unreliable at this age.[37,41] Over 12 months, prophylaxis is recommended for severe immunosuppression *(see Table 2),* all children with prior episodes of PCP, most children with rapidly declining CD4 counts or percentage, or severely symptomatic HIV disease (Category C).[33] *(See Table 3.)* While initiation and monitoring prophylaxis for PCP is not necessarily appropriate or feasible in the ED, clinicians can make a significant impact by identifying and rapidly referring children who need prophylaxis.

Lymphoid interstitial pneumonia (LIP) is the most common pulmonary disorder that must be differentiated from PCP. In contrast to PCP, LIP is a chronic disorder that occurs in older children with a less virulent HIV disease course.[1] While the exact cause of LIP is unproven, some evidence links this pneumonia to an atypical pulmonary response to the Epstein-Barr virus.[1] LIP is associated with nodular lymphoid hyperplasia in the bronchi and bronchiolar epithelium that causes alveolar capillary block. A diffuse reticulonodular pattern is seen on chest radiography, often before symptoms are noted.[1] Gradual onset of tachypnea, cough, hypoxia, normal auscultatory findings or minimal rales, digital clubbing, and improvement with oral corticosteroids are typical of this disorder.[1]

Many other causes of pneumonia occur in children with HIV. Bacterial pneumonia due to typical pathogens (e.g., *S. pneumoniae*) is frequent in children, while gram-negative bacteria (e.g., *Pseudomonas aeruginosa)* are often associated with terminal respiratory disease, respiratory failure, and death.[1] Other pathogens causing respiratory disease include MAC, CMV, tuberculosis, *Aspergillus, Cryptococcus, Histoplasma,* RSV, parainfluenza, influenza, adenovirus, and lymphoma.[1]

Radiographic differentiation between various causes of pulmonary disease can be extremely difficult in HIV-infected children. A review of chest x-ray findings in PCP found that diffuse infiltrates were noted in 53%, patchy infiltrates in 32%, focal infiltrates in 10%, while 5% had normal radiographs.[38] A recent study of thin-section low-dose chest CT in children with HIV-associated respiratory disorders found that ground-glass haziness was seen exclusively with PCP, reticulonodular thickening only with LIP, while adenopathy was noted in those with lymphoma, MAC, or *M. tuberculosis*.[42]

In general, all HIV-infected children with new lower-tract respiratory infections require hospital admission, appropriate diagnostic measures, aggressive therapy tailored toward preventing respiratory failure, and antimicrobials effective against the specific organism causing symptoms. Failure to improve with initial therapy should prompt a search for a second infectious agent, as coexisting pathogens exist in 10-20% of HIV-infected children with pneumonia.[38,43]

Cardiac Disease. Nearly 20% of HIV-infected infants and children will develop congestive heart failure or cardiomyopathy.[44] The causes of cardiomyopathy in HIV are varied and include direct toxic effect of HIV, viral infection, malnutrition (especially selenium), pulmonary insufficiency, anemia, and medications.[1] A recent study found that children receiving zidovudine had a 8.4-fold greater risk of developing cardiomyopathy compared to those receiving didanosine.[45] Zidovudine may directly inhibit cardiac mitochondrial DNA chain replication.[45] All children with cardiac or unexplained pulmonary deterioration should be considered for echocardiography. Serial cardiac examination and echocardiography should also be performed on all children receiving zidovudine.[45]

Pericardial effusion, while common in pediatric HIV, is generally non-purulent, nonfibrinous, and usually asymptomatic.

Neurologic Symptoms in HIV. HIV can directly damage several neuronal cell types. Many cells within the central nervous system have CD4 receptors that are recognized by HIV-1. This leads to direct cell infection with eventual damage. Indirect effects from toxins produced by HIV, cytokines, malnutrition, and central nervous system infection also play a role in damaging the developing neurologic system in HIV-infected children.[46]

Developmental delay with an early and persistent delay in motor development and deceleration in mental development in late infancy is typical of HIV infection and may be the initial manifestation of disease.[38] In fact, progressive encephalopathy is the most common neurological finding in HIV, occurring in 50-65% of infected children.[47,48] Impaired postnatal brain growth, cerebral atrophy, secondary microcephaly, and arrest or loss of developmental milestones in infancy are common manifestations.[46,48] Among older

Table 5. Common Opportunistic CNS Infections

Toxoplasma gondii	*Mycobacterium avium-intracellulare*
Candida albicans	Coccidiomycoses
Cytomegalovirus	*Nocardia asteroides*
Cryptococcus neoformans	*Treponema pallidum*
Mycobacterium tuberculosis	Epstein-Barr virus
Papovavirus	Varicella zoster virus
Herpes simplex virus I	

infected children and adolescents, short-term memory loss, hand tremors, slowing in fine motor skills, attention difficulties, apathy, depression, and emotional lability may predominate.[46,47]

Corticospinal deterioration occurs with weakness and initial hypotonia, progressing to spasticity, tremor, ataxia, gait disturbances, and, less commonly, rigidity and extrapyramidal signs.[47] At autopsy, myelin or axonal damage of the corticospinal tracts is found in up to 65% of children.[47]

While gradual developmental decline and corticospinal deterioration are common in HIV, acute neurological decompensation (e.g., seizure or altered mentation) may be a harbinger of a life-threatening disorder. The list of diseases causing neurological decompensation in HIV is extensive. Hypoglycemia and hypoxia should be ruled out immediately in these patients, followed by a search for other serious infectious and metabolic disorders. After initial resuscitation, cranial computerized tomography (with contrast) or magnetic resonance imaging should be performed to rule out mass lesions (e.g., abscesses, lymphoma, or bleeding due to thrombocytopenia). Classic head CT findings in pediatric HIV are cerebral atrophy with or without calcifications of the basal ganglia.[25,46,47] Importantly, chronic progressive disorders, medication-related complications, and many infectious disorders initially will not manifest abnormal CT findings. Lumbar puncture with routine CSF analysis for common bacterial pathogens, in addition to common opportunistic infections *(see Table 5),* should be performed if cranial CT is normal. Finally, cerebrovascular disease must be considered if initial evaluation is negative. Direct damage of the cerebrovascular wall is found in 25% of children with HIV at autopsy.[46] This can lead to acute stroke, occurring in ~1.3% of HIV-infected children per year.[46]

Gastrointestinal Disorders. Gastrointestinal symptoms are prominent in infants and children with HIV. Chronic diarrhea, dysphagia, vomiting, and pharyngitis can lead to malnutrition, inhibit prophylaxis and treatment of infectious disorders, and contribute to new infections. HIV-related disorders can affect any site within the gastrointestinal system. Identification and treatment of such disorders may allow for prolonged symptom-free periods, improved nutrition, and increased ability to fight and treat other serious infections.

The esophagus is commonly involved in HIV infection. Odynophagia and dysphagia occur following infection with *Candida,* herpes simplex virus, and CMV. Mucosal candidiasis is common in advanced disease, occurring in up to 70% of all HIV-positive children.[48] Candidal esophagitis causes discrete linear or irregular filling defects that tend to be longitudinally oriented with a shaggy or cobblestone appearance on barium swallow.[49,50] Thrush is not always present.[49] Treatment with nystatin is ineffective; either fluconazole or ketoconazole is necessary.[49,50] If the patient does not improve, amphotericin B is used. CMV infects the endothelial cells of the capillaries of the enteric mucosa, causing a vasculitis and inflammation that is often limited to the distal esophagus, while HSV-1 causes numerous shallow discrete ulcers at the midesophagus or near the left main bronchus with sparing of the rest of the esophagus.[49] Other disorders that affect the mediastinum (e.g., lymphoma or tuberculosis) can directly compress the esophagus or predispose to fistula or sinus tract formation.[50] Due to the wide array of disorders causing dysphagia and odynophagia, clinicians should consider radiographic evaluation for all children without classic features of candidal disease (e.g., thrush) and all who do not respond to initial therapy.

Table 6. Intestinal Infections in Children with HIV

Protozoa: *Cryptosporidium, Giardia lamblia, Isospora belli, Entamoeba histolytica*

Fungi: *Candida albicans, Histoplasma capsulatum, Coccidiodes imitis, Pneumocystis carinii*

Mycobacteria: *M. avium intracellulare, M. tuberculosis, M. kansasii*

Bacteria: *Salmonella, Shigella, Campylobacter, Vibrio vulnificus, Clostridium difficile,* enteropathic *Escherichia coli, Yersinia, Aeromonas, Plesiomonas*

Viruses: Cytomegalovirus, adenovirus, rotavirus, herpes simplex virus, hepatitis B, Norwalk agent

Source: Lewis JD, Winter HS. Intestinal and hepatobiliary diseases in HIV-infected children. *Gastroenterol Clin North Am* 1995;24:119-132.

The stomach is relatively resistant to opportunistic infection compared to other areas of the GI tract. CMV is the most common organism, with contiguous involvement from a distal esophagus site, GE junction involvement, or involvement of the gastric fundus.[49] CMV may cause clinical and radiographic findings of hypertrophic pyloric stenosis with muscular wall thickening and prepyloric antral narrowing.[49] Biopsy confirms the diagnosis.[49] HIV-related neoplasms (most commonly non-Hodgkin's lymphoma and Kaposi's sarcoma) also affect the stomach.[49]

Recurrent, chronic, and acute diarrhea occurs in 40% of HIV-positive children and is the leading cause of death from HIV in Africa and developing nations.[32,49,50] Causes of diarrhea are varied and include infections, medications, and mucosal injury from malnutrition.[32] *(See Table 6.)* No pathogen or cause can be identified in a significant number of cases.[32]

Common bacterial infections account for a large number of cases of diarrhea. Typical features include fever and bloody or heme-positive stool. Development of bacteremia is common in bacterial diarrhea, with almost half of bacteria isolated from the blood of HIV-infected children identified as enteric pathogens.[32] For this reason, parenteral antibiotic therapy should be considered for most HIV-infected children with fever and presumed bacterial diarrhea. MAC causes infection involving the bone marrow, lungs, liver, mesenteric lymph nodes, and the GI tract.[32] MAC typically occurs late in HIV infection, when CD4 counts fall below 50 cells/mm^3.[32] No effective therapy for MAC infection is available at present, although azithromycin, clarithromycin, ethambutol, ciprofloxacin, amikacin, and rifampin have been used individually with variable success.[32] MAC prophylaxis with rifabutin is recommended for children with CD4 counts less than 75 cells/mcL.[15]

Common parasitic infections include *Giardia* and *Cryptosporidium*. *Giardia* causes a watery diarrhea, bloating, and abdominal pain.[32] Diagnosis is confirmed by stool analysis for ova and parasite or duodenal aspirate.[32] Treatment consists of metronidazole or furazolidone.[32] *Cryptosporidium* causes a chronic secretory diarrhea that can be debilitating and severely compromise a child's nutritional status.[32] *Cryptosporidium* infects the small and large intestines, as well as the mucosa of the gallbladder, bile ducts, and pancreatic duct, resulting in cholangitis and pancreatitis.[32] Typically, serum alkaline phosphatase is elevated when the bile ducts are involved. There is no effective therapy for *Cryptosporidium* infections, although long-term azithromycin has been used with minimal success. Trials with paromycin, petrazuril, atovaquone, and bovine anti-*Cryptosporidium* immunoglobulin are under way in adults.[31]

Rotavirus is the most common cause of viral enteritis in HIV-infected children, although adenovirus, CMV, herpes simplex, astrovirus, picornavirus and calcivirus have been identified. In contrast to immunocompetent children, rotavirus causes a chronic diarrhea that may become disseminated and involve other organs, most notably the liver. Treatment is generally supportive, although enterally administered serum immunoglobulin can be effective. Adenovirus may result in fulminant hepatitis, GI bleeding, and may occur as part of a disseminated adenovirus infection affecting the lungs, bone marrow, heart, and brain. Ribavirin and serum immunoglobulin may be therapeutic. CMV is a common cause of ulcerative lesions anywhere along the GI tract, and treatment consists of ganciclovir or foscarnet.[32]

In general, initial diagnostic evaluation for diarrhea should include stool studies for WBC, blood, and possibly rotavirus. Obtain *C. difficile* toxin if any blood or WBC is found (especially if the patient is on antibiotics). Send stool for ova and parasite and consider colonoscopy with intestinal biopsy if no readily identifiable cause is found. Treatment of dehydration and electrolyte disorders is essential, as are antimicrobials directed against identified pathogens.

Pancreas and liver involvement are common during opportunistic infections. Many organisms (hepatitis B, CMV, HSV, MAC, PCP, fungi, granulomatous disease) and drugs can cause hepatic inflammation and cholestasis.[32] Pancreatitis can occur from direct infection (e.g., CMV) or typically from medications (especially pentamidine and didanosine).[32] Pancreatitis occurs in up to 17% of patients and portends a poor prognosis.[51]

Colitis and proctitis manifest as hematochezia, mucous stools, abdominal pain, and fever in children with HIV. Prominent organisms that cause colitis include *Shigella, Salmonella,* and CMV. CMV has been blamed for the most severe complications in children, including typhilitis, pneumatosis, toxic megacolon, ischemia, and perforation. If these complications are suspected, early surgical consultation should be obtained. CT findings in CMV colitis include bowel wall thickening, distortion and ulceration of the mucosal surface, and pericolic inflammation (especially around the cecum). CMV colitis has been successfully treated with IV ganciclovir.[50]

Malignancy. Malignancies are uncommon in children with HIV. They represent 1.7% of HIV-defining illnesses in children.[52] The most common malignancies include Burkitt's lymphoma, immunoblastic lymphoma, non-Hodgkin's lymphoma, and primary CNS lymphoma.[52] In contrast to adults, Kaposi's sarcoma is rare in children, with only 25 cases reported prior to 1996.[52] However, when Kaposi's sarcoma occurs in children, skin manifestations are rare occurring in only 12%.[53] The primary sites of development include the lymphatic and GI system.[52]

Other Manifestations of HIV. Dental infections and poor oral hygiene are common in HIV. Studies of children referred to ENT specialists and dentists have identified multiple caries in 60%, oral candidiasis in 70%, sialadenitis in 15%, while a significant number of children have parotid gland enlargement, parotitis, gingivostomatitis, aphthous ulcers, herpes labialis, and leukoplakia.[48,54] Severe apthous stomatitis often requires topical steroid (e.g., dexamethasone swish and spit-out or fluoro-steroid in orabase) or even systemic steroids (prednisone). Identification and treatment of oral disorders is essential to keep children from becoming malnourished.

Dermatologic disorders in children with HIV tend to be severe and less responsive to traditional therapy. The occurrence of many skin disorders correlates with CD4 cell counts. Viral diseases are prone to dissemination. Measles is of particular concern, as there have been a significant number of deaths from giant cell pneumonia in these children. The illness may be associated with the characteristic clinical signs and symptoms of generalized rash, coryza, conjunctivitis, cough, and Koplik spots or may frequently occur without the typical rash. Administer gamma globulin to all HIV-positive children exposed to measles whether or not they have been vaccinated.[15] Varicella also can cause severe illness in the immunocompromised host. Therefore, administer varicella immune globulin within 96 hours to all HIV-positive children exposed to varicella; once illness begins, all patients need IV acyclovir.[15] If herpes zoster occurs, oral acyclovir may be used if children are not ill-appearing.[15]

Gram-positive skin infections commonly encountered include ecthyma, cellulitis, erysipelas, furunculosis, folliculitis, and impetigo. The most frequently identified organism is *S. aureus*. Bacillary angiomatosis, a cutaneous vascular disorder caused by rickettsial-like organisms *Bartonella helensii* and *Bartonella quintani,* causes pinpoint papules that grow to become several centimeters in diameter. Although this disorder is less common in children compared to adults, it can be deadly with involvement of viscera.[53]

AIDS nephropathy occurs primarily in older symptomatic children and may result from a direct effect of HIV on renal epithelial cells.[1] Asymptomatic proteinuria and renal salt wasting are common in pediatric HIV. A wide range of renal disorders, including nephrotic syndrome, focal glomerulosclerosis, mesangial hyperplasia, and segmental necrotizing glomerulonephritis, have also been reported in HIV-infected children.[1] Prior to administration of potentially nephrotoxic agents, renal function studies are mandatory.

Ocular disorders and blindness (especially due to CMV) are less common in children with HIV compared to adults.[1] It is expected that as children survive longer with HIV, many uncommon and previously unreported diseases may occur that will necessitate development of new treatment strategies.

Assessing the Environment

Infants and children with perinatally acquired HIV are usually

Table 7. Provisional Public Health Service Recommendations for Chemoprophylaxis after Occupational Exposure to HIV

TYPE OF EXPOSURE	SOURCE MATERIAL	ANTIVIRAL PROPHYLAXIS	ANTIRETROVIRAL REGIMEN
Percutaneous	Blood		
	Highest Risk	*Recommend*	ZDV + 3TC + IDV
	Increased Risk	*Recommend*	ZDV + 3TC ± IDV
	No increased risk	*Offer*	ZDV + 3TC
	Fluid containing visible blood, other potential infectious fluid	*Offer*	ZDV + 3TC
	Other fluid (e.g., urine)	*Do not offer*	
Mucous membrane	Blood	*Offer*	ZDV + 3TC ± IDV
	Fluid containing visible blood, other potential infectious fluid	*Offer*	ZDV ± 3TC
	Other fluid (e.g., urine)	*Do not offer*	
Skin—increased risk*	Blood	*Offer*	ZDV + 3TC ± IDV
	Fluid containing visible blood, other potential infectious fluid	*Offer*	ZDV ± 3TC
	Other fluid (e.g., urine)	*Do not offer*	

ZDV: zidovudine; 3TC: lamivudine; IDV: indinavir

* Increased risk—for skin, risk is increased for exposures involving a high titer of HIV, prolonged contact, an extensive area, or an area in which skin integrity is visibly compromised.

PROTOCOL AND DRUG DOSING FOR HIV EXPOSURE†

- Draw HIV, CBC, liver and renal function, βhCG ± hepatitis exposure workup
- Repeat CBC, liver and renal tests at two weeks, and HIV at six weeks, 12 weeks, and 12 months

zidovudine (ZDV)	200 mg po TID × 4 weeks
lamivudine (3TC)	150 mg po BID × 4 weeks
indinavir (IDV)	800 mg po TID × 4 weeks (may substitute saquinavir 600 mg po TID)

Most common short-term side effects: ZDV: GI, fatigue, headache; 3TC: GI, pancreatitis; IDV: GI, high bilirubin, and kidney stones (may be limited by drinking ≥ 1.5 L of water per day).

† CDC has no recommendations for HIV-exposed pregnant health care workers.

Adapted from: Centers for Disease Control and Prevention. Case control study of HIV seroconversion in healthcare workers after percutaneous exposure to HIV infected blood — France, United Kingdom and United States, January 1988-August 1994. *JAMA* 1996;275:274-275; Centers for Disease Control and Prevention. Update: Provisional public health service recommendations for chemoprophylaxis after occupational exposure to HIV. *MMWR Morb Mortal Wkly Rep* 1995;45:469-472.

cared for by ill parents or caretakers who also harbor the HIV virus. Caretakers often do not have the health, financial ability, or community support to adequately ensure that their child is receiving appropriate ongoing care. In one study, only 48% of HIV-positive children who presented to a large urban pediatric ED were receiving adequate prophylaxis for PCP.[21] Before discharging HIV-positive children with minor or unrelated illness, clinicians can make a significant impact by reviewing the records for recent CD4 counts and medication lists and ensuring that infants and children with HIV are receiving appropriate treatment. Involvement of social service personnel and closely coordinated follow-up will ensure that children receive appropriate nutrition, medication, and social support so that they may lead a longer, healthier life.

Health Care Workers and HIV

Health care workers are at risk for acquiring HIV in the workplace. A recent study of health care workers who acquired HIV at work found that blood from needlesticks accounted for 94% of exposures, while 6% involved other sharp objects. Importantly, only a handful of cases of HIV have ever been reported from urine or feces. Transmission via saliva (which contains < 1 particle/mL) has not been reported. Risk factors for transmission of HIV include: 1) a device visibly contaminated with the patient's blood; 2) a procedure that involved a needle placed directly in a vein or artery; 3) a deep puncture or wound to the health care worker regardless of visible blood; and 4) a terminal illness in the source patient.[55] Treatment with

Table 8. Side Effects of HIV Therapy

MEDICATION	USE/INDICATION	SIDE EFFECTS (NOT ALL-INCLUSIVE)
Acyclovir	HSV, HZV	Nausea, renal insufficiency
Amphotericin B	Fungal infections	Fever, nephritis, anemia, hypocalcemia, phlebitis
Azithromycin	MAC	Nausea, emesis
Clarithromycin	MAC	Nausea, emesis
Dapsone	PCP prophylaxis/treatment	Hemolysis, neuropathy, pancreatitis, GI intolerance
Didanosine (ddI)	Antiretroviral	Pancreatitis, neuropathy, liver dysfunction
Ethambutol	Tuberculosis	Optic neuritis, hepatitis, high uric acid
Fluconazole	Fungal infections	Rash, nausea, hepatitis
Foscarnet	CMV or herpes simplex	Fever, anemia, GI, renal, seizure, low calcium
Ganciclovir	CMV	Bone marrow toxicity, fever, rash, renal, liver dysfunction
Indinavir (Crixivan)	Protease inhibitor	Multiple drug interactions and toxicities
Isoniazid	Tuberculosis	Hepatotoxicity, nausea
Ketoconazole	Fungal infections	Rash, gynecomastia, liver, depressed endocrine function
Lamivudine (3TC)	Antiretroviral	Bone marrow toxicity, liver, GI intolerance
Pentamidine	PCP prophylaxis/treatment	Pancreatitis
Pyrimethamine-sulfadoxine	PCP treatment	Rash, fever, emesis, megaloblastic anemia
Rifabutin	MAC	GI intolerance, yellow skin discoloration
Rifampin	Tuberculosis	Nausea, hepatotoxicity
Saquinavir	Protease inhibitor	Multiple drug interactions and toxicities
Stavudine (d4T)	Antiretroviral	Bone marrow toxicity, hepatitis, GI intolerance
Trimethoprim-sulfamethoxazole	PCP prophylaxis/treatment	Fever, rash, bone marrow toxicity
Zalcitabine (ddC)	Antiretroviral	Neuropathy, mouth sores, rash, pancreatitis
Zidovudine (AZT)	Antiretroviral	Bone marrow toxicity, hepatitis, GI intolerance

Adapted from: Brady MT. Management of children with human immunodeficiency virus infection. *Compr Ther* 1995;21:139-147.

zidovudine reduced the rate of transmission of HIV by 79%.[55] Based on this study, in June 1996, the CDC published recommendations for treating health care workers after occupational exposure to HIV.[55,56] *(See Table 7.)*

Therapy for HIV

The pharmacopoeia of medications used to treat HIV infection is continuously expanding. Importantly, therapies that are intended to prevent or treat disease and prolong life have important side effects that may contribute to clinical deterioration or prompt ED visits in infants and children with HIV. Many therapies adversely affect bone marrow, leading to anemia, neutropenia, or thrombocytopenia. Other common side effects are GI related (vomiting, diarrhea, hepatitis, or pancreatitis). All HIV patients who present to the ED should have their medication lists examined to ensure that symptoms are not related to therapy.[57] *(See Table 8.)*

Summary

As the population of children with HIV expands and improvements in therapy occur, the chance that clinicians who care for children will be confronted with this disease will also grow. The range of complaints and disorders that may prompt an HIV-infected infant or child to visit the ED is broad and can include abnormalities of almost every organ system. With the exception of infectious disease specialists, most clinicians can not be knowledgeable about every complication of HIV infection in children. To ensure the best outcome, however, clinicians must have an understanding of common and life-threatening complications that occur in this population. Prompt diagnosis and treatment of life-threatening complications, a cautious, conservative approach to management, close coordination with each patient's private physician, and attention to details such as nutrition and each child's social situation will ensure the best outcome for HIV-infected children who present to the ED. Finally, every effort should be made to identify HIV infection in pregnant women so that therapies to prevent vertical transmission can be offered.

References

1. Chadwick EG, Yogev R. Pediatric AIDS. *Pediatr Clin North Am* 1995;42:969-992.
2. Annunziato PW, Frenkel LM. The epidemiology of pediatric HIV-1 infection. *Pediatr Ann* 1993;22:L401-405.
3. Connor EM, Sperling RS, Gelber R, et al. Reduction of maternal-infant transmission of human immunodeficiency virus type 1 with zidovudine treatment. *N Engl J Med* 1994; 331:1173-1180.
4. Stein ZA, Tsai RT, Singh T. Changes over time in survival of

children after AIDS diagnosis in New York City. *Am J Prevent Med* 1995;11(3 Suppl):30-33.
5. Kaplan MH. Pathogenesis of HIV. *Infect Disc Clin North Am* 1994;8:279-288.
6. Church JA. Clinical aspects of HIV infection in children. *Pediatr Ann* 1993;22:417-427.
7. Kuhn L, Stein ZA, Thomas PA, et al. Maternal-infant HIV transmission and circumstances of delivery. *Am J Public Health* 1994;84:1110-1115.
8. Lambert JS. Maternal-fetal transmission of HIV-1 infection. *Pediatr Ann* 1993;22:413-416.
9. Husson RN, Lan Y, Kojima E, et al. Vertical transmission of human immunodeficiency virus type 1: Autologous neutralizing antibody, virus load, and virus phenotype. *J Pediatr* 1995;126:865-871.
10. Davis SF, Byers RH, Lindegren ML, et al. Prevalence and incidence of vertically acquired HIV infection in the United States. *JAMA* 1995;274:952-955.
11. Frenkel LM, Wagner LE, Demeter LM, et al. Effects of zidovudine use during pregnancy on resistance and vertical transmission of human immunodeficiency virus type 1. *Clin Infect Dis* 1995;20:1321-1326.
12. Gutman LT, St. Claire KK, Weedy C, et al. Sexual abuse of human immunodeficiency virus-positive children. *Am J Dis Child* 1992;146:1185-1189.
13. Rogers MF, Caldwill MB, Gwinn ML, et al. Epidemiology of pediatric human immunodeficiency virus infection in the United States. *Acta Paediatr Suppl* 1994;400:5-7.
14. CDC. 1994 Revised classification system for human immunodeficiency virus infection in children less than 13 years of age. *MMWR Morb Mortal Wkly Rep* 1994;43(suppl RR-12):1-17.
15. CDC. USPHS/IDSA Guidelines for the prevention of opportunistic infections in persons infected with human immunodeficiency virus: A summary. *MMWR Morb Mortal Wkly Rep* 1995;44(RR-8):1-34.
16. Church JA. The diagnostic challenge of the child born "at risk" for HIV infection. *Pediatr Clin North Am* 1994;41: 715-726.
17. Ammann AJ. Human immunodeficiency virus infection/AIDS in children: The next decade. *Pediatrics* 1994;93:930-935.
18. Cassol S, Butcher A, Kinard S, et al. Rapid screening for early detection of mother-to-child transmission of human immunodeficiency virus type 1. *J Clin Microbiol* 1994;32: 2641-2645.
19. Espanol T, Caragol I, Bertran JM. Evolution of immunological abnormalities in HIV infection by vertical transmission. *Acta Paediatr Suppl* 1994;400:35-38.
20. Miles SA, Balden E, Magpantay L, et al. Rapid serologic testing with immune complex dissociated HIV p24 antigen for early detection of HIV infection in neonates. *N Engl J Med* 1993;328:297.
21. Scott GB, Hutto C, Makuch RW, et al. Survival in children with perinatally acquired human immunodeficiency virus type 1 infection. *N Engl J Med* 1989;321:1791-1796.
22. Turner BJ, Eppes S, McKee LJ, et al. A population-based comparison of the clinical course of children and adults with AIDS. *AIDS* 1995;9:65-72.
23. Tovo PA, deMartino M, Bagiano C, et al. Prognostic factors and survival in children with perinatal HIV-1 infection. *Lancet* 1992;339:1249-1253.
24. Lewis JD, Winter HS. Intestinal and hepatobiliary diseases in HIV-infected children. *Gastroenterol Clin North Am* 1995; 24:119-132.
25. Chase C, Vibbert M, Pelton SI, et al. Early neurodevelopmental growth in children with vertically transmitted human immunodeficiency virus infection. *Arch Pediatr Adolesc Med* 1995;149:850-855.
26. Crow ME. Intravenous immune globulin for prevention of bacterial infections in pediatric AIDS patients. *Am J Health Syst Pharm* 1995;52:803-811.
27. Brady MT. Management of children with human immunodeficiency virus infection. *Compr Ther* 1995;21:139-147.
28. Spector SA, Gelber RD, McGrath N, et al. A controlled trial of intravenous immune globulin for the prevention of serious bacterial infections in children receiving zidovudine for advanced human immunodeficiency virus infection. *N Engl J Med* 1994;331:1181-1187.
29. Pinkert H, Harper MB, Cooper T, et al. HIV-infected children in the pediatric emergency department. *Pediatr Emerg Care* 1993;9:265-269.
30. Persaud D, Chandwani S, Rigaud M, et al. Delayed recognition of human immunodeficiency virus infection in preadolescent children. *Pediatrics* 1992;89:688-691.
31. Nicholas SW. The opportunistic and bacterial infections associated with pediatric human immunodeficiency virus disease. *Acta Paediatr Suppl* 1994;400:43-45.-50.
32. Lewis JD, Winter HS. Intestinal and hepatobiliary diseases in HIV-infected children. *Gastroenterol Clin North Am* 1995; 24:119-132.
33. Glatt AE. The ten commandments of caring for HIV-infected patients. *Infect Dis Clin North Am* 1994;88:275-278.
34. Bye MR, Cairns-Bazarian AM, Ewig JM. Markedly reduced mortality associated with corticosteroid therapy of *Pneumocystis carinii* pneumonia in children with acquired immunodeficiency syndrome. *Arch Pediatr Adolesc Med* 1994;148:638-639.
35. European Collaborative Study. Natural history of vertically acquired human immunodeficiency virus-1 infection. *Pediatrics* 1994;94:815-819.
36. Elvin K. Laboratory diagnosis and occurrence of Pneumocystis carinii. *Scand J Infect Dis* 1993;94 (suppl): 1-34.
37. Thea DM, Lambert G, Weedon J, et al. Benefit of primary prophylaxis before 18 months of age in reducing the incidence of Pneumocystis carinii pneumonia and early death in a cohort of 112 human immunodeficiency virus-infected infants. *Pediatrics* 1996;97:59-64.
38. Sivit CJ, Millre CR, Rakusan TA, et al. Spectrum of chest radiographic abnormalities in children with AIDS and Pneumocystis carinii pneumonia. *Pediatr Radiol* 1995;25: 389-392.
39. Schroeder SA, Beneck D, Dozor AJ. Spontaneous pneumothorax in children with AIDS. *Chest* 1995;108:1173-1176.
40. Hughes WT. Recent advances in the prevention of Pneumocystis carinii pneumonia. *Adv Pediatr Infect Dis*

1996;11:163-186.
41. CDC. 1995 revised guidelines for prophylaxis against PCP for children infected with or perinatally exposed to HIV. *MMWR Morb Mortal Wkly Rep* 1995;(No. RR-4):1-11.
42. Ambrosino MM, Roche KJ, Genieser NB, et al. Application of thin-section low-dose chest CT (TSCT) in the management of pediatric AIDS. *Pediatr Radiol* 1995;25:393-400.
43. Moran CA, Suster S, Pavlova Z, et al. The spectrum of pathological changes in the lung in children with the acquired immunodeficiency syndrome: An autopsy study of 36 cases. *Hum Pathol* 1994;25:877-882.
44. Lipshultz SE, Orav EJ, Sanders SP, et al. Limitations of fractional shortening as an index of contratility in pediatric patients infected with human immunodeficiency virus. *J Pediatr* 1994;125:563-570.
45. Domanski MJ, Sloas MM, Follman DA, et al. Effect of zidovudine and didanosine treatment on heart function in children infected with human immunodeficiency virus. *J Pediatr* 1995;127:137-146.
46. Pavlakis SG, Frank Y, Nocyze M, et al. Acquired immunodeficiency syndrome and the developing nervous system. *Adv Pediatr* 1994;41:427-451.
47. Fowler MG. Pediatric HIV infection: neurologic and neuropsychologic findings. *Acta Paediatr* 1994;400 (Suppl) :59-62.
49. Valdez IH, Pizzo PA, Atkinson JC. Oral health of pediatric AIDS patients: A hospital-based study. *J Dent Child* 1994; 61:114-118.
50. Haller JO, Cohen HL. Gastrointestinal manifestations of AIDS in children. *Am J Radiol* 1994;162:387-393.
51. Stoane JM, Haller JO, Orentlicher RJ. The gastrointestinal manifestations of pediatric AIDS. *Radiol Clin North Am* 1996;34:779-790.
52. Kahn E, Anderson VM, Greco MA, et al. Pancreatic disorders in pediatric acquired immune deficiency syndrome. *Hum Pathhol* 1995;26:765-770.
53. Mueller BU, Pizzo PA. Malignancies in pediatric AIDS. *Curr Opin Pediatr* 1996;8:45-49.
54. Whitworth JM, Janniger CK, Oleske JM, et al. Cutaneous manifestations of childhood acquired immunodeficiency syndrome and human immunodeficiency virus infection. *Cutis* 1995;55:62-72.
55. Principi N. AIDS and the pediatric ENT specialist. *Int J Pediatr Otorhinolaryngol* 1995;32 (suppl):S7-S12.
56. CDC. Case control study of HIV seroconversion in healthcare workers after percutaneous exposure to HIV infected blood—France, United Kingdom and United States, January 1988-August 1994. *JAMA* 1996;275:274-275.
57. CDC. Update: Provisional public health service recommendations for chemoprophylaxis after occupational exposure to HIV. *MMWR Morb Mortal Wkly Rep* 1995;45:469-472.

Sickle Cell Disease

Charles R. Stephens, MD
Robert Linton, MD
Karim Cole, MD

Sickle cell disease (SCD) refers to a group of genetic disorders characterized by the production of hemoglobin S. The spectrum of clinical disease includes sickle cell anemia, hemoglobin SC disease, sickle beta-thalassemia, and sickle O-thalassemia disease. With manifestations that range from mild, discomfort-making symptoms and arthralgia to life- and limb-threatening complications, this well-studied group of disorders is commonly encountered in patients accessing emergency departments (EDs) in large urban centers.

As is well known, SCD afflicts people of African, Mediterranean, Eastern Indian, and Middle Eastern heritage. In the United States, this condition most often affects African-Americans, about 8% of whom carry the sickle cell gene.[1] From a clinical perspective, sickle cell anemia (SCA), or SS disease, occurs in approximately 0.3-1.3% of African-Americans.[1] Other affected populations in the United States include Hispanics from the Caribbean, Central America, and parts of South America.[1,2]

SCD accounts for approximately 75,000 hospitalizations per year in the United States with an estimated average cost of $6,300 per hospitalization.[3] The economic effect is greater than these statistics suggest, inasmuch as these numbers do not reflect extensive (and intensive) ED- and non-hospital-based management efforts, which contribute substantially to the effect of this disease on patients and the health care system.

Given the widespread prevalence of SCD, it is essential that physicians be familiar with current protocols, standards, and critical pathways that, in evidence-based trials, have been shown to improve patient outcomes and reduce hospitalizations. With these issues in clear focus, the purpose of this chapter is to provide an update on state-of-the-art management of acute complications and manifestations of SCD.

Clinical Principles and Overview

SCD is a very serious, debilitating condition and patients who have SCD have a shortened life expectancy. In hard numbers, the median age of death among persons with SS disease is 42 years for males and 48 years for females.[4,5] In those with SCD, the median age of death is 60 years for males and 68 years for females.[4] In the Cooperative Study of Sickle Cell Disease, approximately 85% of children and adolescents with SCA and 95% of patients with sickle cell hemoglobin C disease survived to 20 years of age. Among the patients younger than 20 years of age in that series, mortality peaked between 1 and 3 years of age; the primary cause of death was infection, most often associated with *Streptococcus pneumoniae* sepsis.

Risk factors associated with poor outcomes in SCD have been identified. In particular, low levels of fetal hemoglobin and an elevated, baseline white-cell count were associated with an increased risk of death.[4] In this study, 78% of patients older than 20 years of age died during an acute painful episode or an episode of acute chest syndrome.[4] Interestingly, 33% of these patients were considered relatively healthy (i.e., although they had no chronic organ failure, they died precipitously during a classic episode of painful crisis).[4]

In the same study, 18% of deaths occurred in chronically ill patients with clinically obvious organ-system failure (renal failure, CHF, or chronic debilitating cardiovascular disease (CVA). Acute, hemorrhagic stroke also was an important cause of death in relatively healthy patients. In general, adult patients with SCA, acute chest syndrome, renal failure, seizures, a baseline WBC greater than 15,000 cells per cubic millimeter, and a low level of fetal hemoglobin were associated with an increased risk of early death.[4]

Table 1. Sickle Cell Syndromes

TYPE	GENOTYPE	HCT	RETIC	MCV
HbSS disease	Bs Bsaa/aa	20-22%	15%	85-110 fl
Sickle-a-Thal	Bs Bsa-/a-	26-28%	6-12%	75
Sickle B0	Bs B0aa/aa	20-30%		65
Sickle B+	Bs B+aa/aa	> 30%		65
HbSc disease	Bs Bcaa/aa	20-30%		80
Sickle Trait	Bs Baaa/aa	> 36%		> 82

Terminology and Syndrome Categorization

The hemoglobin molecule contains four heme units and four globulin chains. There are four different types of globin chains: alpha, beta, gamma, and delta. Of the four chains in a hemoglobin molecule, two are always alpha, and the other two are either beta (in hemoglobin A, the normal adult form), delta (in hemoglobin A2, a minor form), or gamma (in hemoglobin F, the fetal form).

SCD arises from a mutation in the beta globulin chain, specifically, a substitution of valine for the normal glutamic acid at position 6. Persons who are homozygous for the mutation (i.e., who inherit the abnormal gene from both parents) are said to have the "SS" genotype and they produce no normal hemoglobin Al. Instead, they produce mostly hemoglobin S and small amounts of hemoglobin F and hemoglobin A2.[6] Hemoglobin C is a structural variant in which the normal glutamic acid at position 6 of the beta chain is replaced by lysine. Combined with the sickle cell gene, it is known as hemoglobin S/C disease. Similarly, the sickle mutation plus hemoglobin O Arab gives rise to hemoglobin S.O Arab.

Thalassemia is a mutation that impairs the synthesis of hemoglobin, but not its structure. Different forms of thalassemia affect alpha and beta globulin chains. As with SCD, persons can be heterozygous or homozygous for thalassemia. The symbol ∃+ indicates that production of the normal beta chain is decreased, whereas "∃O" indicates that the normal beta chain is totally absent.

Of the forms of SCD, SCA is the most common, followed by hemoglobin S/C disease, sickle-∃+ thalassemia, sickle-∃0 thalassemia, and other combinations. In terms of severity, SCD is the most severe, followed by sickle-∃0 thalassemia, hemoglobin S/C disease, and sickle-∃+ thalassemia. However, this scheme does not always apply to the individual patient, and a patient with SCA may have mild disease, whereas an occasional patient with sickle-∃+ thalassemia may have severe disease. *(See Table 1.)*

Sickle Cell Anemia. In sickle cell anemia (SCA), erythrocytes typically have a normal volume and hemoglobin concentration (i.e., they are normocytic and normochromic). The mean corpuscular volume is approximately 90 m^3/cell (normal range, 86 to 98 m^3/cell). The plasma hemoglobin concentration is low, between 7.0 and 8.0 g/dL (normal range, 14 to 18 g/dL for men, 12 to 16 g/dL for women). Both the white blood cell (WBC) count and the platelet count are increased due to increased marrow activity secondary to chronic hemolytic anemia and, in the case of platelets, to "auto-splenectomy," in which platelets are not stored in the spleen. The reticulocyte count is typically elevated.

Thalassemia. In SCA with homozygous alpha-thalassemia, persons have milder anemia, lower reticulocyte counts, low mean corpuscular volume, and high hemoglobin A2 levels. In hemoglobin S/C disease, patients typically have microcytic and hyperchromic red blood cell indices. In SCD with ∃0 thalassemia, patients typically have microcytosis, hypochromia, high hemoglobin A2 levels, and variable hemoglobin F values. In SCD with ∃+ thalassemia, the anemia is mild, usually with microcytosis and a hemoglobin level greater than 10 g/dL. *(See Table 2.)*

Clinical Pathophysiology. SCD results from a single nucleotide change in the sixth position of the beta-globulin chain. The normal glutamic acid at position 6 is replaced by valine-producing hemoglobin S. In persons who are homozygous for the disease, virtually all hemoglobin is hemoglobin S with small amount of hemoglobin F and hemoglobin A2.[6] In person who are heterozygous for the disorder, half of the RBC contain hemoglobin S. In children, hemoglobin F is produced and levels fall to adult levels around 4-5 months. This accounts for the dearth of symptoms seen in this age group.

Vascular occlusion is the hallmark of SCD and is the basis for systemic, clinical manifestations. Hemoglobin S is abnormal in that it polymerizes when in the deoxygenated state. This causes the RBC to assume bizarre shapes, become less deformable, and predispose it to early destruction in the spleen and liver. Due to altered membrane characteristics and less deformability, sickled cells become trapped in the vasculature, causing occlusive symptoms, subsequent ischemia, and acidosis. A cascade that creates a vicious cycle causing more sickling. The presence of other hemoglobins, such as hemoglobin F and C, tend to ameliorate this sickling process and decrease the clinical severity of the disease.[6] Early destruction of sickled red cells causes a chronic hemolytic anemia with elevated reticulocyte count.

Clinical Features

Hyperhemolytic Crisis. Hyperhemolytic crisis, as the name suggests, is a condition characterized by an increased rate of destruction of RBCs in patients with SCD. It is characterized by decreasing hemoglobin levels, increased reticulocyte count, indirect bilirubinemia, and elevated lactate dehydrogenase.[6] The etiology of hyperhemolytic crises is variable, and many precipitants have been identified, including infections (i.e., Mycoplasma), delayed hemolytic transfusion reactions, and co-existent Glucose 6-phosphodisterase

Table 2. Sickle Cell Disease: Clinical Severity and Laboratory Characteristics

DISEASE	CLINICAL SEVERITY	S (%)	F (%)	A2 (%)	A (%)	HB g/dL	RETIC (%)	MCV	RBC MORPHOLOGY
S	Usually marked	> 90	< 10	< 3.5	0	6-11	5-20	80	Sickle cells, normochromia, anisocytosis, target cells, poikilocytosis, Howell-jolly bodies
S∃° Thal	Marked to moderate	> 80	< 20	> 3.5	0	6-10	5-20	< 80	Sickle cells, hypochromia, microcytosis, anisocytosis, poikilocytosis, target cells
S∃⁺ Thal	Mild to moderate	> 60	< 20	> 3.5	10-30	9-12	5-10	< 75	No sickle cells, hypochromia, microcytosis, anisocytosis, poikilocytosis, target cells
SC	Mild/ moderate	50	< 5		0	10-15	5-10	75-95	"Fat" sickle cells, anisocytosis, poikilocytosis, target cells
S HPF-H	Asymptomatic	< 70	> 30	< 2.5	0	12-14	1-2	0	No sickle cell, anisocytosis, poikilocytosis, target cells

(PD) deficiency with oxidant stress. It may also occur during sickle cell painful crisis.

Aplastic Anemia. Aplastic anemia (AA) occurs when erythropoiesis is suppressed, usually in the setting of infection. Although Parvovirus B-19, which replicates exclusively in bone marrow red cell precursors, is the most commonly implicated infectious agent, this condition has also been linked to other infectious organisms, including pneumococci, salmonella, streptococci, and Epstein Barr virus.[7,8] From a clinical perspective, aplastic crisis is characterized by fever, symptomatic anemia, reticulocytopenia (< 2%), serum IgM antibodies to parvovirus B-19, and the presence of B-19 DNA in serum or bone marrow cells.[8]

Aplastic crisis is more common in children than adults; previous exposure may confer subsequent immunity to the virus.[8] Aplastic crisis terminates spontaneously after 5-10 days.[9] Due to leuko-erythoblastosis that is present in the recovery phase, patients who present during the convalescent phase may be mistakenly thought to be in a hyperhemolytic crisis.[9]

Treatment of aplastic crisis is mainly supportive. Patients with hemoglobin SS and S beta 0 Thal disease usually require simple blood transfusion to ameliorate severe, symptomatic anemia.[9] Hematological consultation should be obtained and patients should be placed in respiratory isolation, which is necessary to prevent exposure of pregnant females (i.e., nursing staff), patients with immunodeficiency disorders, and other patients with SCD.[9] It is also important to stress that if the patient has parents or siblings who have SCD, these individuals also are at risk for developing aplastic crisis due to the communicability of the virus.[10]

Megaloblastic Anemia. Megaloblastic crisis in individuals with SCD can result from folate deficiency that is either due to lack of supplementation, poor dietary intake, or both. Folic acid therapy is required in SCD because this vitamin is readily depleted due to enhanced erythropoietic activity. Folate supplementation is extremely important, especially in patients taking dilantin, due to its propensity for causing meagaloblastic anemia. In addition to its therapeutic effects and its usefulness for prevention of megaloblastic anemia in SCD, folic acid also lowers high homocystiene levels, which have been linked to cardiovascular and cerebrovascular disease.[6]

Iron Deficiency Anemia. Iron deficiency anemia also may be encountered in patients with SCD. SCA disease is characterized by normochromic and normcytic morphology. Iron deficiency is heralded by hypochromic and microcytic morphology. Interestingly, iron deficiency has an ameliorating effect on sickling and may improve clinical manifestations of the anemia.[6] However, if oxygen carrying capacity is reduced to a critically low level, these salutary effects are not observed.

Vaso-Occlusive (Painful) Crisis

Vaso-occlusive crisis is the hallmark of SCD and accounts for more than 90% of hospital admissions related to SCA.[6] Vaso-occlusive crisis is believed to be the result of tissue ischemia and/or completed infarction associated with vascular occlusion precipitated by sickled erythrocytes. Current research indicates that vascular endothelium, humoral factors, and even white blood cells may contribute to the genesis of painful crisis.[3,5]

Clinically, conditions which may precipitate vaso-occlusive crisis include dehydration, infection, cold weather, physical and psychological stress, as well as other causes. *(See Table 3.)* Pain in the lower back, chest, abdomen, and extremities, usually without objective signs, is the typical clinical presentation. Most painful episodes can be treated effectively at home.[11] The average length of painful episodes is 4-6 days but symptoms may persist for weeks.[9] Less than 10% of patients with SCD have three or more painful episodes per year that require ED care. In this regard, it is important to note that three or more painful episodes per year has been identified as in indicator of severe disease and early mortality.[12]

Unfortunately, there are no laboratory findings pathognomonic for painful crises. Hemoglobin levels are generally the same as they are at baseline. The WBC count, if elevated above baseline, is strongly suggestive of infection.

Management. ED management of painful crisis should be aggressive and, in nearly all cases, should include administration of parenteral narcotics and a search for precipitating factors. As a rule,

Table 3. Precipitants of Painful Crisis

Hypoxia	Obstructive snoring
Infection	Exposure to cold
Fever	Depression
Dehydration	Anxiety
Menstruation	Physical exhaustion
Sleep apnea	Unknown

patients presenting to the ED have failed home therapy options, among them oral rehydration and oral, non-narcotic and/or narcotic analgesia. Because use of oxygen in non-hypoxic patients with SCD will result in erythroid hypoplasia and suppressed red cell production, oxygen administration, once considered mandatory, should only be used in patients who are documented to be hypoxic.[9]

Hydration. Hydration is a critical component in the treatment of painful crisis, inasmuch as dehydration usually is present due to increased insensible losses, reduced fluid intake, and hyposthenuria.[9] For patients in mild to moderate painful crisis, oral hydration can be attempted as an initial measure, especially if sufficient personnel are available to encourage and monitor oral intake. However, in severe painful crisis, the patient is either unwilling or unable to take oral fluids and IV hydration is mandatory. Regardless of the route, the goal of hydration is to normalize electrolytes and maintain fluid balance. A good rule of thumb is to administer one and one-half times the patient's daily requirements.[9] Due to hyposthenuria, the use of D5, 0.25-0.50 normal saline (NS) is recommended as the initial fluid challenge. Judicious use of IV fluids will prevent overhydration and iatrogenic CHF.[9]

Analgesia. Morphine remains the drug of choice for painful crisis.[9,13] The usual dose is 0.1-0.15 mg/kg every 3-4 hours IV, IM, or SQ with a single-dose maximum of 10 mg.[13] The principal clinical advantages of morphine include a long, established safety record in other chronic pain syndromes, availability in various formulations (immediate release, controlled release, and [investigational] sustained release), and its hydrophilicity, which makes this analgesic suitable for administration by any route (oral, intramuscular, IV, SQ, rectal, intraspinal, etc.).[13] The disadvantages of morphine include a relatively high incidence of pruritus, rash, nausea, and vomiting in patients with SCD.

Morphine 3-glucuronide and morphine-6-glucuronide are the two major metabolites of morphine. Morphine-6-glucuronide has a relatively long half-life (longer than that of morphine) and, therefore, it accumulates with repetitive dosing, especially in the presence of renal failure. In addition, morphine-6-glucuronide is a potent opioid analgesic and because of its long half-life, excessive sedation is possible.[13] In addition, there have been reports of fatal pulmonary edema with the use of morphine in patients with SCA.[13]

Meperidine (Demerol) continues to be the most frequently used narcotic in the treatment of painful crisis of SCD in the United States and Great Britain despite some well-documented disadvantages.[13] The desirable effects of meperidine includes its rapid onset of action, euphoric effect, and the low incidence of severe pruritus, nausea, and vomiting. However, the major disadvantage of meperidine is linked to one of its toxic metabolites, nor-meperidine. Whereas the half-life of meperidine is only three hours, that of nor-meperidine is 18 hours. Also, nor-meperidine is excreted by the kidneys and will accumulate in patients even with normal renal function. Nor-meperidine is a CNS excitotoxin that produces anxiety, tremor, myoclonus, and generalized seizures if it accumulates after repetitive dosing. The incidence of seizures in patients with SCD related to the use of meperidine varies between 1% and 12%. Caution and careful monitoring are required.[13]

Hydromorphone is a hydrogenated ketone of morphine and is a reasonable alternative to morphine and meperidine for treatment of acute painful crisis. The dose of hydromorphone is 0.01-0.02 mg/kg/dose IV or IM every 3-4 hours. Standard doses of 2-4 mg SQ are generally given in the adult patient. Hydrormorphone is metabolized by the liver and excreted renally. Consequently, it may also accumulate after repeated dosing.

Regardless of which analgesic is selected, a consistent approach to treating vaso-occlusive crisis must be employed. The drug should be given at regular intervals in conjunction with oral or IV hydration, and oxygen therapy, if indicated. A CBC with reticulocyte count should be obtained in all patients in which infection is suspected. A chest x-ray is indicated in patients who present with pulmonary symptoms or with a low pulse oximetry reading or abnormal PaO_2 on an arterial blood gas. Evaluation of the effectiveness of analgesia should be objective using visual, analog, verbal, or numerical scales.[13] If pain is not adequately controlled after 3-4 hours, inpatient therapy should be considered.

Acute Chest Syndrome

Acute pulmonary disease is the most common cause of death, and the second most common precipitant of hospitalization in adults with SCD.[8,9] The term "acute chest syndrome" is used to describe acute pulmonary disease observed in SCD, with the understanding that distinguishing between infectious and non-infectious causes is often difficult.

The etiology of acute chest syndrome (ACS) in SCD is multi-factorial. Moreover, the presentation in children and adults is difficult to identify. The incidence of this complication is approximately 24.5 per 100 patient years in children with HbSS disease.[9] A marked, seasonal variation is seen in the pediatric patient, with more cases encountered in winter than in summer.[14] The most common bacterial etiology is *Streptococcus pneumoniae,* followed by *H. influenzae.*[14] In one study, bacteremia was present in 78% of children with ACS associated with pneumococcus.[14] Typically, children present with fever and cough. A fall in hemoglobin of 1-2 gm/dL is accompanied by relative thrombocytopenia and leukocytosis.[14] Upper and/or middle lobe pulmonary infiltrates are the most common radiographic finding.[14]

In adult patients, there is a striking clinical association between ACS and painful crisis; in fact, 30% of patients who develop ACS initially present with extremity crisis.[9,14,15] Etiologic agents in adults may include pneumococcus, streptococcus, mycoplasma, or chlamydia.[15] Other possible causes are rib or sternal infarction, fat or bone marrow embolism, and pulmonary embolism.[8,16,17] Adults usually present with severe chest pain, cough, and dyspnea.[15] Other symptoms include productive cough and hemoptysis. Interestingly, most adult patients are afebrile. Hemoglobin levels are deceased by 1-2gm/dL; leukocytosis and relative thrombocytopenia are common.

Lower lobe disease with pleural effusions is more common in adult patients.[15]

Management of patients with ACS depends on the severity of the disease. Initial management should consist of oxygen therapy to maintain the oxygen saturation ($Pa0_2$) above 92%. IV hydration and narcotics for pain are also mainstays of therapy. Inhaled beta-agonists are a safe and effective adjunct in patients who present with wheezing.[8] Antibiotics should be used empirically to cover *Streptococcus pneumoniae, H. influenzae*, and atypical bacteria. Patients with a PaO_2 greater than 60 mmHg could have a simple blood transfusion to raise the hemoglobin concentration to 10g/dL.[8]

Exchange blood transfusion is recommended for individuals who have severe hypoxia ($Pa0_2 < 60$).[8] Patients who demonstrate pulmonary emboli should be anticoagulated with heparin or enoxaparin. Patients in respiratory failure will require intubation and mechanical ventilation. Hematology consultation should be obtained and exchange transfusions should be performed if indicated. Hydroxyurea and chronic hypertransfusion have been shown to reduce the incidence of recurrence of ACS.[8]

Acute Splenic Sequestration Crisis

Acute sequestration crisis is a well-recognized complication of SCD. It is classically defined as a fall in hemoglobin concentration of at least 2g/dL, an increased reticulocyte count, and an enlarging spleen.[18] It occurs most commonly in children younger than 2 years of age and is unusual in adults with HbSS disease due to autosplenectomy. It is estimated that patients with SS disease have a 30% probability of having an acute splenic sequestration event by 5 years of age, with a potential mortality approaching 15% per event.[18] Splenic sequestration can occur in older patients with HbS/C disease and S beta-Thal whose spleens either remain enlarged or retain the capability to enlarge.[9]

Splenic sequestration is caused by the accumulation of RBCs within the spleen. Clinical findings include sudden weakness, pallor of the lips and mucous membrane, tachycardia, tachypnea, and abdominal fullness. In severe sequestration crisis, the spleen can become so large that it fills the abdomen and pelvis.[9] Laboratory studies reveal a decrease in hemoglobin level of at least 2 gm/dL and marked reticulocytosis. Relative or absolute thrombocytopenia is also a common finding. The fall in hemoglobin can be precipitous and reach 1.5 gm/dL within six hours.[9]

Management. Treatment of acute splenic sequestration crisis requires administration of high flow O_2, restoration of intravascular volume with cystalloids, and/or volume expanders in anticipation of simple blood transfusion. It should be noted that the hemoglobin level rises approximately 3 g/dL more than would be expected from the number of units transfused as the spleen shrinks and expels trapped RBCs.[8] The ultimate goal is to achieve post-transfusion Hgb levels of 6-8 g/dL. Urgent hematological consultation is recommended. All patients with acute splenic sequestration should be admitted to the hospital. Those who are hemodynamically unstable should be admitted to the intensive care unit.

Stroke and CNS Complications

Acute thrombotic or hemorrhagic stroke is a severe complication of SCD that affects both children and adults, occurring in approximately 11% of patients who have SCD by age 20.[19] In the pediatric age group, it is most commonly encountered in the 6- to 10-year-old age group, whereas in adults, it is most common in the 20- to 29-year-old age group.[9,10] In children younger than 10 years of age, cerebral infarction is more common, whereas in adults, hemorrhagic stroke is more common.[19,20] Moreover, recurrent stroke is commonly hemorrhagic due to rupture of fragile, dilated collateral vessels from prior ischemic infarction.

In children, recurrence is higher in the third year post-event and many patients are on chronic exchange transfusion programs to reduce the level of Hb S to less than 30%, a maneuver that has been shown to reduce the incidence of recurrent stroke in well-controlled, prospective studies.[21] Large vessel occlusion, especially affecting the anterior or middle cerebral artery, is found in 80% of cases involving children.[9]

From a diagnostic perspective, hemiplegia is the most common physical finding, but monoparesis, hemianesthesia, visual field deficits, aphonia, cranial nerve palsies, and altered mental status also can be seen as initial presenting signs and symptoms. The diagnosis is confirmed with a non-contrast CT scan. Acute intracerebral bleeding is readily detected with CT, although the scan may be negative in early ischemic stroke. Magnetic resonance imaging (MRI) is also an excellent modality if available on an urgent basis. The use of hyperosmolar contrast agent should only be undertaken with great caution in patients with SCD, since this therapy may promote sickling of RBCs.

Treatment must be aggressive. Increased intracranial pressure must be corrected but hyperventilation should be avoided. Seizures are common and anticonvulsant therapy should be initiated early. Exchange transfusion is indicated in the treatment of ischemic stroke but not for hemorrhagic stroke. Urgent hematologic and neurologic consultations are mandatory.

Gastrointestinal Manifestations

Hepatobiliary System. About two-thirds of people with SCD have hepatomegaly. Cholethiasis, consisting predominantly of calcium bilirubinate stones is present in 75% of patients, and is the result of chronic intravascular hemolysis. Acute hepatic sequestration can also occur and its presence is suggested by an enlarging liver, decreasing hemoglobin levels, and mildly elevated liver function test.[6]

Sickle cell intrahepatic cholestasis is a more severe form of hepatic crises which presents with right upper quadrant pain, increasing bilirubin levels, and elevated PT/PTT and liver function tests. This syndrome can be life threatening. Treatment consists of total blood exchange; whole blood is removed and replaced with packed RBCs and fresh frozen plasma (FFP). The goal of treatment is to reduce the HbS level to less than 30% and normalization of the PT/PTT.

Bone Complications

The bony skeleton is one of the primary organs affected by intravascular sickling. Blockage of the microcirculation causes infarction of bone marrow and adjacent bony structures.[22] The cumulative effect of recurrent episodes of ischemia or infarction within the spongiosa of bone leads to prominent and characteristic radiographic changes of SCD.

Dactylitis (Hand Foot Syndrome). Hand foot syndrome may be the earliest manifestation of SCD.[23,24] This clinical entity is seen primarily in children younger than 6 months of age, but can be encountered in children as old as 4 years old.[24,25] These patients present with fever, pain, and swelling of the hands or feet. There may also be warmth or redness, a presentation that can mimic osteomyelitis.[22] The leukocyte count and erythrocyte sedimentation rate (ESR) may be elevated above baseline, and radiographs may show periosteal elevation, which usually occurs several days after the episode.[23]

Symptoms of dactylitis are usually self-limited, and management of this syndrome is primarily symptomatic. Treatment includes analgesia, hydration, and warm compresses or baths.[26] In light of the similar presentation of osteomyelitis, the clinician must maintain a high suspicion for osteomyelitis. High fever and/or extreme warmth or tenderness over the affected area should alert the clinician to the possibility of bone infection.[27]

Bone Infarction. Bone and bone marrow infarction are well-documented clinical consequences of chronic red cell sickling. During acute vaso-occlusive crisis, multiple marrow infarctions occur which can be demonstrated in bone marrow scintiscan using 99_mT_c sulfur colloid.[28,34] Infarcts most commonly occur in long bones but have been reported in the spine, ribs, sternum, skull, and clavicle.[22,23,26]

The clinical presentation of patients with bone marrow infarction is similar to that described for dactylitis. Patients will complain of pain, tenderness, and, commonly, swelling over the involved area. Once again, any signs of sepsis, unusual sites of pain, persistent fever, or leukocytosis greater than baseline should warrant consideration of osteomyelitis. Bone marrow infarcts usually resolve in 1-2 weeks.[23]

Plain radiographs show a mottled, strand-like increase in density randomly distributed within the medullary region.[35] In the early stages of infarction, plain radiographs are not helpful in distinguishing between bone infarction and osteomyelitis.[23,26] Bone scans, including those using technetium or gallium, are neither highly specific or sensitive in differentiating the two entities.[23,27,31] Blood cultures and culture of material aspirated from beneath the periosteum are essential for establishing a definitive diagnosis of osteomyelitis, in which salmonella remains the most common organism.[22,31,32,37]

ED treatment of bone infarction is similar to that employed in painful crisis. Narcotic analgesics and hydration are required during the acute phase. NSAIDs can be helpful in providing pain relief by reducing the severity of the inflammatory response.[23] No standard treatment is recognized, but the use of NSAIDs and physiotherapy may be of benefit in these patients.

Osteonecrosis (ON). This condition affects patients with all genotypes of SCD, but occurs most often in those with HbSS and alpha thalassemia.[35] ON usually affects the articulating surfaces and heads of long bones. The overall prevalence of ON of the femoral head in SCD patients older than 5 years of age is about 10%. The prevalence of ON of the humeral head is approximately 5%.[35]

Patients typically present with complaints of pain or limitation of motion in the shoulder, hip, or other joints. Some patients describe worsening of their symptoms with movement of the joint (e.g., walking, climbing stairs). Pain also may worsen without movement. Intermittent or persistent groin or buttock pain is also, although less common, a presenting complaint of SCD patients affected by ON.[36]

In the early stages, radiographs appear normal.[26] After several months, however, radiographs may show areas of increased density mixed with areas of increased lucency.[22] Progression of radiographic findings include femoral head molding, segmental collapse, joint space narrowing, and complete joint degeneration.[35]

Presently, initial management of ON consists primarily of avoidance of weight bearing and judicious use of local heat and analgesics for up to six months. Osteotomy with rotation has been used with children with variable results. Core decompression of the femoral head, and also total hip or joint replacement must be considered for individuals beyond adolescence with incapacitating hip pain.[26]

Sickle Cell Nephropathy

Sickle cell nephropathy (SCN) is an important cause of morbidity and mortality in patients with SCD. There are well-characterized manifestations, risk factors, and prognostic features. As SCD patients reach the third and fourth decades of life, the clinical manifestations of SCN become more apparent.[38,39]

Pathophysiology. In addition to its many other effects, chronic sickling serves as the inciting event for renal microvascular damage.[40,41] The arterial bed of the renal micro-vasculature has a low oxygen tension in a low pressure system. This promotes polymerization of HbS and subsequently, microvascular occlusion.[38,42,43] Hemoglobin S polymerization is also facilitated via the low pH and hypertonicity of the renal medulla, which results in increased blood viscosity and interstitial edema. This cascade contributes to renal microvascular ischemia and infarction.[44]

Clinical Presentation. Hyposthenuria, which is defined as the inability to maximally concentrate the urine, is the first clinical manifestation of sickle cell induced renal failure.[38] The initial response of the renal medullary system is increased glomerular filtration rate (GFR) and renal blood flow, which over time results in hyperfiltration-mediated glomerulosclerosis (GS). This leads to decreased GFR, progressive medullary ischemia, and ultimately end-stage renal disease (ESRD).[38,44]

Hematuria. Asymptomatic hematuria is one of the most common presentations of SCN, and one of the few potential manifestations in patients with sickle cell trait.[44] These patients may present to the ED with microscopic-, or less commonly, gross-hematuria. Both microscopic and gross hematuria are usually self-limited, resulting in minimal blood loss. Bed rest and hydration may hasten the resolution of hematuria.[47]

End-Stage Renal Disease (ESRD). The incidence of renal failure in SCD ranges from 5% to 18%.[40,45] ESRD is a poor prognostic indicator in these patients with a mean four-year survival rate after diagnosis in one study.[48] Persistent, increasing proteinuria is the harbinger of glomerular insufficiency and renal failure.[38] It is a frequent finding in patients with SCD and has been shown to be present in up to 30% of patients during long-term follow-up.[41] Nephrotic syndrome is found in 40% of patients with SCN, and may be a clinical marker for ESRD, evolving from the progression of glomerulosclerosis.[41,46,48,49]

In patients with SCN, although renal abnormalities begin at earlier ages, the development of ESRD occurs between the 3rd and 5th decades of life.[39] Hypertension is a major risk factor for renal failure, and adequate management of this risk factor can delay the onset of ESRD in SCD patients.[50] Angiotensin converting enzyme (ACE) inhibitors, such as enalapril, have been shown to achieve blood pressure control and lower urinary protein excretion.[38]

Dietary management with protein restriction is an important part of therapy for SCN. SCN patients who develop ESRD eventually require maintenance dialysis. Complication rates of SCD patients on dialysis are comparable to the dialysis population as a whole.[38]

Priapism. Priapism is characterized by persistent and painful failure of penile detumescence. In SCD, failure of detumescence may be secondary to venous outflow obstruction or to prolonged smooth muscle relaxation, either singly or in combination. During erection, there is a blockade of the alpha adrenergic stimulus resulting in vascular smooth muscle relaxation and increased blood flow. In the flaccid state, alpha-agonist stimulation contracts the corporal smooth muscle and cavernosal arteries resulting in detumescence.[51-53]

Most children with SCD will respond well to noninvasive medical therapy. More than 50% of adults, however, will respond poorly.[54] During the ED evaluation of a SCD patient with priapism, information as to the time of onset and state of recurrence should be obtained. A complete urologic exam is warranted, with particular attention to the penile shaft and glans. A hard shaft, soft glans, and maintenance of the ability to urinate denotes minimal involvement of the corpus spongiosa. Urinary obstruction and glans engorgement are the hallmarks of secondary involvement of the corpus spongiosa which nearly always suggests cavernosa infarction. With repeated episodes, the cavernosa becomes fibrosed, leading to marked reduction in blood flow.[51]

Blood flow measurements should be obtained for SCD patients with priapism. These include technetium scintigraphy, infusion cavernosometry, color doppler cavernosometry, and MRI.[55,56] Inpatient evaluation will require one of these techniques to evaluate blood flow and the degree of spongiosa involvement. Type of technique used will vary depending on the institution.

Standard, initial therapy of priapism in both adults and children begins with the treatment of pain and anxiety using hypotonic IV fluids and analgesics. Heat application increases blood flow and should increase venous return; however, it seems to benefit primarily those patients without infarction-mediated priapism.[51] To date, definitive evidence for or against red cell transfusion is lacking, although this strategy continues to be used in the management of refractory priapism.

Controversy exists over the pharmacologic agent of choice for the treatment of priapism in SCD patients. Alpha agonists and beta agonists are two of the most commonly used agents. Phenylephrine and epinephrine are alpha agonists thought to promote vascular smooth muscle contraction of the helicline arteries of the cavernosa, thus increasing the flow of blood out of the cavernosa into the venous return. Alternately, vasodilators (beta agonists) such as terbutaline, have been used based on the theory that they induce vascular smooth muscle relaxation, favoring the entry of oxygenated arterial blood into the cavernosa, thereby washing out the damaged sickled red blood cells.[57,58] The use of either agent is not supported by studies at the present time. The need for further investigation precludes a definitive pharmacologic therapy at this time.

Aspiration of the corpus cavernosa is a first-line surgical procedure that is used for sickle cell induced priapism. This procedure has not been shown to actually change the course of the episode, but on an acute basis it has the benefit of decreasing cavernous edema and subsequently reducing pain.[51] Some of the other surgical procedures used include the glans-cavernosum (Winter) shunt and the cavernosaphenous shunts. Surgical intervention should be considered if there is no detumescence after 12-24 hours of conservative measures.[38]

Ophthalmologic Manifestations

Ophthalmologic complications of SCD are common and fall into the broad categories of nonproliferative and proliferative retinopathy. Nonproliferative sickle retinopathy includes vascular occlusions, retinal hemorrhages, retinoschisis cavities, iridescent spots, black sunburst, angioid streaks, and macular changes.[9] These changes generally do not affect visual acuity. Proliferative sickle retinopathy is a common cause of visual loss in SCD and is characterized by retinal neovascularization. This is most common in patients with Hb SC disease in the second and third decades.[9,60]

The most important ocular emergency in patients with SCD is blood in the anterior chamber (hyphema), which usually occurs as a result of trauma or surgery. Due to low pH and $P0_2$ in the aqueous humor, red bloods cell containing Hb S tend to sickle and obstruct the flow of aqueous humor. Sharp rises in intraocular pressure may result. Unlike nonproliferative and proliferative retinopathy, hyphema, with its resultant rise in intraocular pressure, can also affect patients with sickle cell trait.[60]

Treatment of hyphema in the patient with SCD and sickle cell trait begins with a test of visual acuity and determination of intraocular pressures. If a globe rupture is suspected, intraocular pressure measurement should not be performed. The patient should be placed in the supine position with his or her head elevated to 30-45 degrees and a fox eye shield placed to prevent further trauma. Increased intraocular pressure (> 24 mmHg in a SCA or sickle cell trait) should be treated with timolol 0.5% ophthalmic bid. Pilocarpine 2% one drop every 15 minutes should also be used. If intraocular pressure (IOP) is still elevated, nepatazane 50mg po q8hr should be given. Acetazolamide should not be used because it further lowers anterior chamber pH and worsens the process. Emergent ophthalmologic consultation and admission to the hospital are warranted for hyphema.

Transfusions in SCD

The role of blood transfusions in SCD is constantly evolving. Indications for transfusions are based on sound clinical research and others on antecdotal reports of efficacy. However, there is little doubt that some complications of SCD require emergent blood transfusion. It is important for the emergency physician to understand the goals, indications, and effects of blood transfusion on the disease process in person with SCD.

In patients without SCD undergoing blood transfusions, oxygen transport increases as blood is transfused until the hematocrit (HCT) reaches 40%. Once the HCT reaches 45%, the viscosity increases dramatically and oxygen transport starts to fall. In patients with SCD, the viscosity of an RBC suspension at full oxygenation is already higher than that of an Hb AA RBC suspension, and the viscosity of the sickle RBC suspension rises progressively with deoxygenation.

When a patient with SCD receives a simple blood transfusion, the increase in HCT with a constant sickle crit (Sct) leads to an increase in viscosity, thus limiting the improvement of oxygen delivery, despite the improved oxygen carrying capacity. It appears that a Sct of greater than 25% causes a disproportionate increase in whole-

Table 4. Indication for Transfusions in Sickle Cell Disease

SIMPLE TRANSFUSION	EXCHANGE TRANSFUSIONS
Symptomatic anemia	Acute chest syndrome
	Acute CVA
Aplastic anemia	Priapism
Splenic sequestration crisis	Hepatic failure
Hepatic sequestration crisis	

blood viscosity related to increasing HCT as compared with Hb AA patients. Thus, in the non-anemic patient with SCD, exchange transfusion instead of simple transfusion results in more efficient delivery of oxygen to tissues.

Simple blood transfusion is indicated in patients with SCD whose hemoglobin levels drops sufficiently to give rise to clinical compromise such as congestive cardiac failure and hypovolemic shock. It is rarely necessary to transfuse an SS patient if the hemoglobin level is greater than 5.0 g/dL, unless there is a reticulocytopenia associated with the falling hemoglobin or clinical evidence that the fall will continue.

In the United States and United Kingdom, the most common cause of an acute fall in hemoglobin is related to the following sequestration syndromes: 1) Splenic sequestration, which most commonly occurs in SS infants; 2) hepatic sequestration, which is more common in adolescents and adults and is associated with septicemia; 3) the acute chest syndrome; and 4) the mesenteric syndrome. Aplastic crisis, generally caused by infection with parvovirus B-19, often occurs within families. In these cases, raising the hemoglobin to between 9 and 10 g/dL by a single transfusion is generally sufficient· In general, a simple transfusion should be used to return the patients hemoglobin to his or her stable state level. The volume to be transfused can be calculated from the following equation:

Volume of RBCs (mLs) = (Hbd - Hbs) × weight (kg) × K*

K* is a constant depending on the hematocrit of blood to be transfused (K = 3 if packed red cells; K = 4 if plasma reduced blood; K = 6 if whole blood).

Hbd is desired hemoglobin in g/dL.

Hbs is starting hemoglobin in g/dL.

Exchange transfusions are more complex procedures and involve the removal of whole blood which is then replaced with RBC and crystalloid. Exchange transfusions are generally not performed in the province of the ED due to the logistics and time needed to prepare for the procedure. Typically, 7-8 units of blood are needed and vascular access with a Quinton catheter is needed for automated systems. However, it is important for the emergency physician to know the indications for this procedure. *(See Table 4.)*

Disposition

Whether to admit a patient with an acute complication of SCD is often a matter of clinical judgment with input from the patient's hematologist. However, in general, patients who have uncontrolled painful crisis, aplastic anemia, splenic sequestration, acute focal neurological deficit, or signs of infection should be admitted to the hospital. *(See Table 5.)*

Table 5. Indications for Admission

Uncontrolled painful crisis	Swollen painful joints
Acute CVA or new neurologic deficit	Acute sickle chest syndrome or pneumonia
Mesenteric sickling and bowel ischemia	Splenic or hepatic sequestration
Cholecystitis	Renal papillary necrosis with severe renal colic or hematuria
Priapism	Hyphema and retinal detachment

Summary

SCD is a group of genetic disorders which can affect every organ system. Emergency physicians who care for these patients must be familiar with the variety of acute crises as well as chronic manifestations of this condition. It is important to remember that the "repeat sickler" who presents to the ED on multiple occasions, who has the most severe disease, and is at increased risk for complications and early death.

In children with SCD, clinical diligence and a low threshold for consultation will serve the emergency physician well. Mortality is greatest in the 1- to 3-year-old age group, and unusual pathology such as stroke and sequestration crisis may be life threatening. It is hoped that new therapies such as bone marrow transplantation and hydroxyurea will ameliorate the effect of this disease on these patients.

References

1. Lawrenz D. Sickle cell disease: A review and update of current therapy. *J Oral Maxillofac Surg* 1999;57:171-178.
2. The sickle cell information center. Atlanta: Emory University School Of Medicine, 1998. (see www.emory.edu/PEDS/SICKLE).
3. Davis H, Moor R, Gergen P. Cost of hospitalization associated with sickle cell disease in the U. S. *Public Health Rep* 1997;54:183-188.
4. Platt O, Brambilla D, Rosse W, et al. Mortality on sickle cell disease: Life expectancy and risk factors for early death. *N Engl J Med* 1994;330:1639-1644.
5. Davis S, Oni L. Management of patients with sickle cell disease. *BMJ* 1997;315:656-660.
6. Ballas S. Complications of sickle cell anemia in adults: Guidelines for effective management. *Cleve Clin J Med* 1999;66;48-58.
7. Kink KE, Ness PM. Sickle cell disease. *Hematol Oncol Clin North Am* 1996;10:1305.
8. Okpala I. The management of crisis in sickle cell disease. *Eur J Hematol* 1998;60:1-6.
9. Division of Blood Diseases and Resources. Management and therapy of sickle cell disease. 3rd. Rev. Bethesda, MD:

National Heart, Lung, and Blood Institute; 1995. (NIH Publication no. 95-2117).

10. McKie V. Sickle cell anemia in children: Practical issues for the pediatrician. *Pediatr Ann* 1998;27:521-524.
11. Westerman M, Aily K, Freels S. Assessment of painful episode frequency in sickle cell disease. *Am J Hematol* 1997;54:183-188.
12. Schnog J, Lard L, Rojer R, et al. New concepts in assessing sickle cell disease severity. *Am J Hematol* 1998;58:61-66.
13. Ballas Sk. Management of sickle pain. *Current Opin Hematol* 1997;4:104-111.
14. Vichinsky E, Styles L, Colangelo L, et al. The Cooperative Study of Sickle Cell Disease. Acute chest syndrome in sickle cell disease: Clinical presentation and course. *Blood* 1997;89: 1787-1792.
15. Vichinsky E, Styles L. Pulmonary Complications. *Hematol Oncol Clin North Am* 1996;10:1275-1285.
16. Vinchinsky E, Williams R, Das M, et al. Pulmonary fat embolism: A distinct cause of severe acute chest syndrome in sickle cell anemia. *Blood* 1994;83:3107-3112.
17. Rucknagel DL, Kalinyak KA, Gelfand M. Rib infarcts and acute chest syndrome in sickle cell disease. *Lancet* 1991;337: 831-833.
18. Mock L, Berman B. Clinical and laboratory profile of acute splenic sequestration in children with sickle cell disease. *Int J Pediatr Hematol/Oncol* 1998. www. Biomednet.com/library /fulltext. 387137c980014.
19. Ohene-Frempong K, Weiner SJ, Sleeper LA,et al. Cerebrovascular accidents in sickle cell disease: Rates and risks factors . *Blood* 1998;91:288-294.
20. NIH Publication No. 95-2117, Revised December 1995 (Third Edition). *Management and Therapy of Sickle Cell Disease.* National Institutes of Health, National Heart, Lung, and Blood Institute. Chapter 9; Stroke.
21. Adams R, Mckie V, Hsu L, et al. Prevention of a first stroke by transfusions in children with sickle cell anemia and abnormal results on transcranial doppler ultrasonography. *N Engl J Med* 1998;339:5-11.
22. Embury SH, et al. *Sickle Cell Disease: Basic Principles and Practice.* Bone & Joint Disease. 1994:645-661.
23. Smith J. Bone disorders in sickle cell disease. *Hematol Oncol Clin North Am* 1996;10:1345-1355.
24. Bainbridge R, et al. Clinical Presentation of sickle cell disease. *J Pediatr* 1985;106:881.
25. Gill FM, et al. Clinical events in the first decade in a cohort of infant with sickle cell disease. Cooperative Study of Sickle Cell Disease. *Blood* 1995;86:776.
26. Management and Therapy of Sickle Cell Disease, 3rd ed. Charache S, et al, eds. US Department of Health and Human Services, Public Health Service, NIH Publ. No.95-2117, revised December 1995.
27. Wethers DL,Grover R. Pitfalls in the diagnosis of osteomyelitis in children with sickle cell disease. *Clin Pediatr* 1983;22:614.
28. Alavi A, et al. Scan detection of bone marrow infarcts in sickle cell disorders. *J Nucl Med* 1974;15:1003-1007.
29. Alavi A, et al. Scintigraphic examination of bone and marrow infarcts in sickle cell disorders. *Semin Roentgenol* 1987;23: 213-224.
30. Milner PF, Brown M. Bone marrow infarction in sickle cell anemia: correlation with hematological profiles. *Blood* 1982;60:1411-1419.
31. Amundsen TR, Siegel MJ, Siegel BA. Osteomyelitis and infarction in sickle cell hemoglobinopathies: Differentiation by combined technetium and gallium scintigraphy. *Radiology* 1984;153:807.
32. Gupta NC, Prezio JA. Radionuclide imaging in osteomyelitis. *Semin Nucl Med* 1988;18:287.
33. Kahn CE Jr, et al. Combined bone marrow and gallium imaging. Differentiation of osteomyelitis and infarction in sickle cell hemoglobinopathy. *Clin Nucl Med* 1988;13:443.
34. Kim HC, Alavi A, Russel MO, et al. Differentiation of bone and bone marrow infarcts from osteomyelitis in sickle cell disorders. *Clin Nucl Med* 1989;14:249.
35. Lee RG, et al. *Wintrobe's Clinical Hematology*. Ch. 51, Sickle cell anemia and other sickling disorders, 10th ed. 1999.
36. Schumacher HR, et al. Arthropathy in sickle cell disease. *Ann Internal Med* 1973;18:203.
37. Burnett MW, Bass JW, Cook BA. Etiology of osteomyelitis complicating sickle cell disease. *Pediatrics* 1998;101:296-297.
38. Smith J. Renal failure in sickle cell anemia. *Hematol Oncol Clin North Am* 1996;10:1321-1329.
39. Cruz IA, Hosten AO, Dillard MG. Advanced renal failure in patients with sickle cell anemia: Clinical course and prognosis. *J National Med Assoc* 1982;74:1103-1109.
40. Saborio P, Scheinman J. Sickle cell nephropathy. *J Am Soc Nephrol* 1999;10:187-192.
41. Van Eps LWS, de Jong PE. Sickle cell disease. In: *Diseases of the Kidney.* 1997:561-590.
42. Briehl RW. Rheology of hemoglobin S gels: Possible correlation with impaired microvascular circulation. *Am J Pediatr Hematol Oncol* 1983;5:390-400.
43. Eaton WA, Hofrichter J. Hemoglobin S gelation in sickle cell disease. *Blood* 1987;70:1245-1266.
44. *Harrisson's Principles of Internal Medicine,* 14th ed. Ch. 277, Vascular injury to the kidney 1998:1561.
45. Scheinman JI. Sickle cell nephropathy. In: *Pediatric Nephrology* 1994: 908-909.
46. Scheinman JI. Sickle cell nephropathy. In: *Primer on Kidney Diseases* 1998:309-313.
47. Lucas WM, Bullock WH. Hematuria in sickle cell disease. *J Urol* 1960;83:733-741.
48. Powars DR, et al. Chronic renal failure in sickle cell disease: Risk factors, clinical course, and mortality. *Ann Internal Med* 1991;115:614-620.
49. Falk RJ, Jenette JC. Sickle cell nephropathy. *Adv Nephrol Necker Hosp* 1994;23:133-147.
50. Falk RJ, et al. Prevalence and pathologic features of sickle cell nephropathy and response to inhibition of angiotensin converting enzyme. *N Engl J Med* 1992;326: 910-915.
51. Smith JP. Sickle cell priapism. *Hematol Oncol Clin North Am* 1996;10:1363-1371.
52. Aboseif SR, Lue TF. Hemodynamics of penile erection. *Urol Clin North Am* 1988;15:1.
53. Broderick GA, Lue TF. Priapism and the physiology of erection. *Am Urol Assoc.* 1988;7:225-232.

54. Sharpsteen JR, Powars D, Johnson C, et al. Multisystem damage associated with tricorporal priapism in sickle disease. *Am J Med* 1994;94:289-294.
55. Bertero EB, et al. Use of perineal color flow doppler sonography in the management of arterial priapism. *J Urol* 1993;149:29a.
56. Hashmat AI, Raju S, Singh I, et al. 99_m T_c penile scan: An investigative modality in priapism. *Urol Radiol* 1989;11:58-60.
57. Molina L, et al. Diluted epinephrine solution for the treatment of priapism. *J Urol* 1989;141:1127-1128.
58. Shantha TR, Finmorthy DP, Rodriguez AP. Treatment of persistent penile erection using terbutaline. *J Urol* 1989;141: 1427-1429.
59. Embury SH, et al. *Sickle Cell Disease: Basic Principles and Practices*. Priapism 1994: 637-644.
60. Charache S. Eye disease in sickling disorders. *Hematol Oncol Clin North Am* 1996;10:1357-1362.

Envenomations in Children

Sean P. Bush, MD
Tamara L. Thomas, MD, FACEP
Eric S. Chin, MD

The bites of venomous snakes, spiders, and scorpions—three of the least appreciated and most avoided creatures on earth—are discussed in this chapter. Though few species can cause significant morbidity or mortality to humans, the threat of envenomation by any of these can interfere with the outdoors enthusiast's peace of mind. While snakes have taken a bum rap throughout history beginning with the Garden of Eden, the snake has also been begrudgingly respected, as demonstrated by the caduceus with its intertwined serpents. For some, including the primary author of this chapter, ophiology, the branch of herpetology dealing with snakes, is a lifelong fascination.

Venomous reptiles encountered in the United States include the pit vipers (rattlesnakes, copperheads, and cottonmouths), coral snakes, venomous lizards, colubrids, and exotic imports. *(See Table 1.)* Arachnids considered dangerous to humans include widow spiders, brown spiders, and bark scorpions.

The science surrounding treatment recommendations for animal envenomations is not yet clear, is often based on speculation and anecdote, and much of the literature is contradictory. Research in humans often involves chart reviews, which may contain region-specific bias. In addition, envenomation is an uncommon occurrence with an extremely variable presentation, ranging from no ill effects to multisystem failure and death. Furthermore, certain envenomations can have very subtle presentations and no visible wound site; a child presenting with unexplained crying, for example, may be the victim of a spider or scorpion envenomation. The clinician must make a quick diagnosis and accurately identify the source of the envenomation to determine the best therapeutic option. Although antivenoms exist for serious envenomations by many species, their use carries considerable risk of serious allergic complications. Although controversy exists, the recommendations in this article represent the majority of current standards of care.

Reptiles

The pediatric population accounts for about 50% of the more than 7000 reptile bites reported to the American Association of Poison Control Centers (AAPCC) in 1995.[1] There have been no pediatric deaths from snakebite reported to the AAPCC since its first annual report in 1983. Although these figures are conservative due to underreporting, they illustrate the relatively low mortality associated with snakebite. While venomous snakes are prevalent, inhabiting every state in the United States except Alaska, Maine, and Hawaii,[2] the highest incidence of envenomations occurs in the southeast and southwest regions of the country during the months of April to October, when snakes are most active.[3]

Pediatric Considerations. Although there are few comparative studies, most authorities agree that children may be affected differently than adults by snakebite.[4-10] Many suggest that children may suffer more morbidity from snakebites than adults because the

Table 1. Envenomations Encountered in the United States

REPTILES
Crotalidae (pit vipers)
Crotalus and *Sistrurus*—rattlesnakes
Agkistrodon—copperheads, cottonmouths
Elapidae—coral snakes
Heloderma—Gila monsters
Colubrids—envenomation rare: e.g., wandering garter snake and Eastern hognose snake
Exotic imports
ARTHROPODS
Latrodectus—widow spiders
Loxosceles—brown spiders
Centruroides—bark scorpion

Table 2. Identification of Pit Vipers

PIT VIPERS	OTHER U.S. SNAKES
Movable fangs	Teeth only
Venom glands	No venom
Heat-sensing pit	No pit
Triangular head	Round or triangular head
Elliptical pupils	Round or elliptical pupils
Undivided, single subcaudal scales	Double row of subcaudal scales
Rattles (rattlesnakes only)	No rattles

venom load is distributed over a smaller body volume.[4,5,8,11] Toxic effects may be dose-related,[4] and children receive a higher dose of venom per kilogram body weight.[8] As a result, children may require more antivenom to neutralize more severe systemic effects.[5,7] Snakebitten children may be at higher risk for certain complications and less prone to others.[4] Finally, assessing envenomation severity in children may be difficult using grading scales designed for adults.[12-14]

Rattlesnakes

Description. The majority of snakebites are caused by pit vipers, with rattlesnakes (*Crotalus* and *Sistrurus*) accounting for two-thirds of all venomous snakebites in the United States. Features that distinguish the pit vipers from other U.S. snakes include moveable fangs, venom glands, a triangular-shaped head with an elliptical pupil and "pits," and a tail with a row of single, undivided scales on the ventral surface (subcaudal) distal to the large anal plate scale.[3] *(See Table 2.)* Rattlesnakes are distinguished in all but one species by a characteristic rattle at the end of the tail.

The "pit," located between each eye and nostril, is a special sensory organ used for the detection of minute quantities of heat. Using this organ, pit vipers have the ability to detect temperature gradients of 0.003°C from about 14 inches away.[3,15,16] The pit is used in conjunction with the snake's keen sense of smell to track warm-blooded prey (such as rodents) before and after envenomation. Snakes lack clarity of vision and are deaf to airborne sounds. In addition, pit vipers estimate how much venom to deliver to subdue prey or deter predators based on an assessment of size using the pit.[2,17] "Dry bites," resulting in no evidence of envenomation, may occur in as many as 25-50% of pit viper bites to humans.[18,19]

Pathophysiology. *Venom and Venom Apparatus.* Pit viper fangs are located in the anterior mouth and fold back when the mouth is closed. When the snake strikes, fangs extend, and venom is injected through the hollow fangs with muscular contraction of the head. Venom is composed of substances adapted to quickly kill and efficiently digest prey as well as deter predators. Venom generally moves through tissue via lymphatics and via direct extension into adjacent tissues; it consists of water, enzymes, nonenzymatic proteins, peptides, and several unidentified substances.[18]

Most U.S. pit viper envenomations cause a predominance of local and hemotoxic effects. Others may lead to more neurologic changes. However, venom cannot be classified as purely "hemotoxic" or "neurotoxic" because of the complexity of its composition, the interactions of its various components, and the physiologic response to venom.[2] Furthermore, the composition of each venom is species-specific and may even vary with geographic range within the same species.[20]

The majority of clinical features seen after envenomation by rattlesnakes are caused by alteration of the vascular endothelium and clotting system. The local reaction is due to altered blood vessel permeability and direct necrosis of the tissue. Altered blood vessel permeability due to injury of vascular endothelial cells causes third spacing, leading to hypovolemic shock, hemoconcentration, and lactic acidosis.

Digestive enzymes cause both local and systemic damage to tissue. Some of the major enzymes include phospholipase A (common to all snake venoms), which damages cell membranes and causes myonecrosis and hemolysis. Hyaluronidase facilitates the spread of venom. Amino acid esterase and thrombin-like enzymes are thought to contribute to defibrination and bleeding. Proteolytic enzymes RNAse, DNAse, and 5' nucleotidase cause myonecrosis and local necrosis.[3,18] Venom A, found in certain populations of Mojave rattlesnakes *(Crotalus scutulatus),* contains neurotoxins that can cause flaccid paralysis and respiratory impairment.

Clinical Presentation. *Local Effects.* Among the initial findings of pit viper envenomation are immediate pain, advancing edema, and ecchymosis of the tissues surrounding the bite site. Edema of the entire extremity can occur as rapidly as one hour or as long as 36 hours post bite.[21] Rapid advancement of edema usually indicates a more severe envenomation. Hemorrhagic blebs and bullae may develop over a six- to 36-hour period.[3]

Compartment syndrome, characterized by pain on passive stretch of muscle, a "rock hard" feel to the muscle, diminished capillary refill, or absence of distal pulses (a late finding), may develop from severe local tissue reaction. True compartment syndrome is rare, even in patients with severe swelling, as most snakebites are subcutaneous.[3,18] Children may be more at risk for compartment syndrome because they have less subcutaneous fat, making compartments more easily accessible to snake fangs.[22,23] In addition, local myonecrosis may develop even in the absence of elevated compartment pressures because of a direct myotoxic effect of venom.[18] Measurement of intracompartmental pressure is the only way to reliably diagnose compartment syndrome. Venom A (from the Mojave rattlesnake) may cause minimal local swelling, leading to underestimation of a severe systemic envenomation.[7,21]

Systemic Effects. In general, systemic response to envenomation is a combination of complex interactions between the varied venom components and human physiology. General systemic effects such as taste changes and fasciculations may occur.[2] Hypotension and shock may be associated with severe envenomation.[3] In children, shock is most often due to third spacing of circulating volume into an extremity.[24] Severe bleeding, which may result from the snakebite, may also cause hypotension. Pit viper envenomation commonly results in coagulopathies associated with defibrination with or without thrombocytopenia, although full-blown disseminated intravascular coagulation (DIC) is rare.[3,25] Hypotension may also be caused by a vasovagal response. Very rarely, venom may cause direct myocardial depression, leading to hypotension. Also rare, venom-induced anaphylaxis with hypotension has been reported.[26]

Severe systemic envenomation may cause hemorrhagic, myotoxic, and/or neurologic effects. In addition, nephrotoxicity and pulmonary injury can result. Rarely, direct cardiotoxicity or allergy to venom may occur. Any organ system(s) may be involved.[3] Autonomic reactions, usually associated with fear and anxiety, may mimic or compound systemic envenomation.[13] Symptoms such as vomiting, tachycardia, or near syncope may be associated with panic or with the envenomation itself. Neurologic symptoms may occur in individuals who are bitten by certain populations of Mojave rattlesnakes *(C. scutulatus)*, resulting in cranial nerve dysfunction, lethargy, and progressive generalized muscle weakness that may lead to respiratory failure.[27] Rhabdomyolysis may occur secondary to direct local or diffuse myotoxicity.[28] Acute renal failure may result from hypotension, hemoglobin or myoglobin deposits in renal tubules, and/or direct nephrotoxicity of venom.[2] Non-cardiogenic pulmonary edema has been reported.[21,24] Infection may occur as a late complication of snakebite, but the incidence is low.[29,30]

Emergency Department Treatment and Disposition. *Prehospital Care.* Individuals who are bitten by venomous snakes should be transported immediately to the nearest facility where antivenom can be given. Airway, breathing, and circulation should be supported as needed. The patient's movements should be restricted as much as possible, as movement may hasten the spread of venom. In cases where an individual is bitten in the wilderness, the risks vs. benefits of hiking out to medical care or waiting until appropriate transportation can be arranged must be weighed considering the conditions of the patient and environment.[2] Jewelry, rings, or constricting items should be removed from the patient in anticipation of swelling, and caffeine, aspirin, and alcohol should be avoided.

A large-bore IV line should be placed in an area unaffected by the snakebite. Mark with ink and time the advancing edge of edema every 15 minutes. As a control, the circumferences of the unaffected extremity may also be measured at corresponding levels. These measurements will provide an indication of venom spread and severity. Rapid progression of edema is an indication of severe envenomation.

The utility of most first aid is limited, and definitive therapy depends on getting to a hospital.[31] Obsolete because of unproven benefit or increased morbidity is field treatment such as cryotherapy, local application of ice, incision across the fang mark with drainage, electric shock, tourniquets (lymphatic constriction bands may benefit, however), elevation of the extremity, mouth suction, alcohol, stimulants, folk therapy, and spending time to capture or kill the snake. An extractor device ("Sawyer's Extractor"), which uses suction without incision, can remove up to 30% of pit viper venom if used within three minutes after bite.[32] Antivenom should not be given in the prehospital setting because of life-threatening complications associated with its use.

History and Exam. Initial ED treatment includes continued support of the patient's airway, breathing, and circulation. A second IV should be started and the patient hydrated with boluses of normal saline. Again, pay close attention to vital signs, including pulse oximetry. Document the time of bite, and continue to mark and time the border of advancing edema and circumference every 15 minutes. Cleanse the bite area and administer pain control as needed. Ask about the size, description, and species of snake, and identify the snake, if possible. If a live or partially killed snake is brought to the ED, make sure the snake is adequately contained. Obtain a history of field therapy and discontinue any potentially harmful first aid. Find out about previous exposure to venom, antivenom, horse serum, allergies, medications, and past history. Perform a complete physical exam, including a neurological exam. Note the location and number of bites, and check for bleeding from the wounds or elsewhere on the body. Check for signs of compartment syndrome, and obtain compartment pressures if indicated. Call Poison Control.

Laboratory. Suggested laboratory studies includes complete blood count with platelets, coagulation profile (including prothrombin time, partial thromboplastin time, fibrin split products, and fibrinogen), monitor for hematologic abnormality, and type and cross match. Electrolytes, blood urea nitrogen, creatinine, and urinalysis may be obtained. If rhabdomyolysis is suspected, creatine phosphokinase, urine myoglobin, calcium, and phosphorus should also be obtained. For respiratory difficulty or neurologic abnormality, an arterial blood gas may be helpful *(See Table 3).*

Grading and Antivenom Administration. The severity of envenomation depends on the size of the snake, the quantity of venom injected, the toxicity of the venom, the size and general health of the victim, the location and depth of the bite, and length of time before definitive therapy begins. Criteria have been developed to estimate the severity of an envenomation and the amount of antivenom to administer.

Grading envenomations in children presents several problems. Various adult guidelines have correlated envenomation severity with centimeters of edema;[12,13] however, this model fails in pediatric patients because proportionally larger areas are involved for any given measurement. Envenomation scales based primarily on local swelling may underestimate a severe envenomation presenting with mild local effects, as in Mojave rattlesnake envenomations. Snake species and size may affect envenomation severity but are frequently unknown in pediatric cases. The possibility of "dry bites" should be considered when evaluating envenomations. The clinical course dictates when antivenom is given. While many grading scales are based predominantly on local effects with some correlation of systemic and laboratory abnormalities,[12] effects of envenomation should more appropriately be divided into three separate parameters: local effects, systemic effects, and laboratory abnormalities. Severity of envenomation may be reflected by a sin-

Table 3. Grade of Envenomation and Treatment Guidelines

Grade of envenomation and treatment guidelines: Determined by most severely affected parameter assessed continuously.

GRADE	LOCAL EFFECTS	SYSTEMIC EFFECTS	LABORATORY	SKIN TEST	INITIAL AV DOSE
"Dry"	None	None	Normal	No	None
Mild	Confined to bite area	None	Normal	No	None
Moderate	Extends beyond immediate bite area, but less than entire part	Mild manifestations (e.g., vomiting, metallic taste, fasciculations)	Mild changes (e.g., thrombocytopenia, hypofibrinogenemia, increased CK)	Physician discretion	5-10, as needed
Severe	Involves entire part	Severe manifestations (e.g., shock, bleeding, neurologic changes, lethargy, respiratory difficulty, renal failure)	Marked changes (e.g., rhabdomyolysis, coagulopathies)	Physician discretion	15, and more as needed

gle parameter without significant changes in the others; therefore, envenomation should be graded according to the most severely affected parameter. Initial antivenom dose is then based on this grade of envenomation.

Swelling should be quantitated in relation to involvement of an extremity, since most bites occur on an extremity. Bites to the head, neck, or trunk may require more aggressive treatment due to potential complications involving vital structures. While only local and systemic effects are immediately apparent for initial grading, additional antivenom should be given as mandated by laboratory data and a changing clinical course until abnormalities in the affected parameter(s) stabilize.

Guidelines for grading pediatric envenomations have been compiled from previous recommendations.[2,7,33] Choice of initial antivenom dose is based on grade of envenomation and should be guided by laboratory data and a changing clinical course. No antivenom should be given for a minimal envenomation, while 5-10 vials of antivenom should be given initially for moderate envenomations. Patients with severe envenomations should be given 15 vials of antivenom with additional doses given as needed for progression of severity or a lack of improvement in signs of envenomation. The importance of serial examinations and laboratory evaluation is emphasized, as envenomation is a dynamic process. Until abnormalities reverse, additional antivenom should be given as necessitated by the changing clinical course. Repeat doses may be given every 30 minutes to two hours as needed.[2] More aggressive antivenom therapy may be initially required for cases of suspected Mojave rattlesnake bite.[3,7] Antivenom is most effective if given as soon as possible after the snakebite, but may reverse coagulation defects even after 72 hours.[3]

Many complications of snakebite can be prevented with the use of aggressive antivenom therapy. Antivenom is the first line of treatment of coagulation defects. Treatment with blood products should be reserved for severe anemia or serious bleeding that persists after antivenom administration.[25] Surgical intervention for compartment syndrome may be avoided with sufficient antivenom therapy.[34] If compartment pressure remains elevated despite antivenom, surgical consult for fasciotomy may be needed.[21,33] However, local wound excision and routine fasciotomy are no longer recommended.

Neurologic effects have been shown to correct with antivenom.[28] Antivenom may also treat myoglobinuric renal failure, along with other measures, such as hydration, diuresis, and possibly alkalinization of urine.

Antivenom and Adverse Reactions. Complications of antivenom administration include anaphylaxis and serum sickness. Anaphylaxis, an immediate, potentially life-threatening allergic reaction, is characterized in its most severe form by urticaria, bronchoconstriction, vomiting, and hypotension. Wyeth Antivenin (*Crotalidae*) Polyvalent is derived from horses immunized to the venoms of two U.S. snakes, Eastern and Western diamondbacks (*C. adamateus* and *C. atrox*, respectively), and two South American snakes, the Tropical rattlesnake (*C. durissus*) and Fer-de-lance (*Bothrops atrox*). Due to the variety of heterologous proteins in hyperimmune equine serum, anaphylaxis may occur in as many as 25% of patients who receive antivenom.[35]

Preparations to treat anaphylaxis should be made prior to administration of antivenom. If anaphylaxis occurs, stop the infusion and treat as needed with airway control, epinephrine, H_1 and H_2 blockers, and steroids. In severe envenomations, antivenom may need to be continued despite anaphylaxis.[28,36] Some authorities recommend pretreatment for anaphylaxis with H_1/H_2 blockers and steroids before antivenom is administered.[2]

Crotalid antivenin is dissolved in 10 mL of any sterile warm diluent and may be diluted 1:2 in normal saline (for example, 5 vials would be dissolved in 50 cc, then diluted into a total volume of 100 cc). Start mixing the antivenom as soon as possible after the decision is made to administer, as it takes about 20 minutes of gentle agitation to go into solution. Start the infusion slowly (at a rate of 1 mL/min) for the first several minutes, with close observation for signs of allergic reaction. If there is no allergic reaction, administer at a rate of 20 mL/kg/h. The initial dose should be administered over 1-4 hours if no allergic reaction occurs after 10 minutes.[2,3,37] Children seem less likely to suffer anaphylaxis than adults.[4]

Serum sickness (manifested as urticaria, arthralgias, and fever) is almost certain to develop 1-4 weeks after treatment when eight or more vials of antivenom are given.[7,35] For this reason, where effects of envenomation are judged to be less severe than potential complications of serum sickness, fewer than eight vials of antivenom should be given. The treatment for serum sickness is antihistamines and steroids given regularly until all signs and symptoms have subsided for 24 hours, followed by gradual tapering.

An experimental affinity purified Fab antivenin derived from sheep serum has recently been produced that may significantly reduce the allergic complications of the existing polyvalent Crotalid antivenin.[38,39] The new antivenom may better neutralize Mojave toxin (Venom A) than the currently available antivenom, but this has not been studied.

Skin Testing. Skin testing is only potentially useful for variably predicting immediate hypersensitivity in moderately envenomated patients in whom there is a question whether the need for antivenom outweighs the risk of anaphylaxis. The test itself is unreliable in its prediction of allergy to antivenom. This may be secondary to the use of pure horse serum for the test followed by administration of antivenom, which contains many different heterologous proteins. The reliability of the test may be improved if antivenom is used for the skin test, but this has not been studied.[2] An option entails slowly infusing the first vial of dilute antivenom while being immediately prepared to treat anaphylaxis.

Skin testing is not indicated for minimal envenomations as it may sensitize individuals to future exposures to antivenom or even precipitate anaphylaxis.[19] It also is not necessary for severe envenomations where antivenom is clearly needed except for medico-legal purposes. Even if the test is positive, antivenom is still indicated for severe envenomations. Since anaphylaxis may occur in up to one-quarter of all patients receiving antivenom, preparative and preventative measures, including possible pre-treatment and airway/epinephrine at bedside, should always be exercised when antivenom is given.[4,35]

Disposition. Patients with mild-to-moderate envenomations may need hospital admission or extended ED observation with close follow-up for delayed progression of envenomation severity, as there are many reports of delayed complications.[40-42] Some authorities recommend admission for all children with envenomations. Patients receiving antivenom should be admitted and monitored in an intensive care setting during infusion of antivenom.[33] Severely envenomated patients and patients suffering anaphylaxis to antivenom should be admitted to an intensive care unit, and admission should be strongly considered for children with confirmed Mojave rattlesnake bites.

Antibiotics. Although infectious microorganisms (such as *Pseudomonas, Proteus, Clostridium,* and *Bacteroides)* are known to inhabit snakes' mouths, there is a low incidence of wound infections.[29] This may be due, in part, to the antibacterial activity of crotalid venom. However, even nonvenomous snakebites without complicating factors (such as a retained tooth) seldom become infected.[30] Although widely prescribed, prophylactic antibiotics are probably not necessary. Local wound care, including irrigation and exploration, may preclude the need for antibiotics. Antibiotics such as ceftriaxone are indicated for infected bites.[43] Up-to-date tetanus prophylaxis is indicated.

Prevention. The pediatric and adolescent population may benefit from education on how to prevent snakebites. Preventative measures, such as wearing protective clothing while in the snakes' environment and not reaching blindly into areas where snakes may hide, may reduce the incidence of snakebites.[18] Children and adolescents should be taught not to harass snakes or keep venomous snakes as pets. Important facts to understand include that a snake can strike up to two-thirds of its body length, a rattlesnake does not always rattle its tail as a warning before striking, and venomous snakes have the capability of envenomating from birth.

Copperheads and Cottonmouths

The copperheads and cottonmouths (*Agkistrodon* sp.) account for 25% and 10% of all venomous bites in the United States, respectively.[18] Small children may be more at risk for severe envenomation requiring antivenom from copperheads and cottonmouths.[18,21] However, most envenomations are mild, requiring only tetanus prophylaxis and pain control,[3,21,44] and there are no deaths reported in the medical literature from copperheads.[14] If an envenomation is more severe, antivenom is indicated, and further treatment is identical to that of rattlesnake envenomations.

Coral Snakes

The coral snakes (*Micrurus* and *Micruroides*) include the eastern (including Texas and South Florida) coral snakes and the Arizona (also known as Sonoran or western) coral snake. Coral snakes make up only 1-6% of all snakebites in the United States per year, and only 13 bites were reported in children and adolescents in 1995.[1,2,45] Although there are no deaths reported in the United States in almost 30 years, eastern coral snakes are capable of delivering a lethal envenomation in adults, with mortality estimated at 10%.[2,46] There has never been a death reported after an Arizona coral snakebite.[2] The eastern coral snakes are indigenous to the southeast and Texas. The Arizona coral snake is found in Arizona and New Mexico.[45] Coral snakes are characterized by an alternating sequence of yellow, red, and black bands, with a black snout. Coral snakes can usually be distinguished from nonvenomous mimics (such as kingsnakes and milksnakes) by their band pattern. Coral snakes in the United States have red bands are adjacent to yellow bands, whereas red bands are adjacent to black bands in mimic snakes. The mnemonic "red touch yellow, kill a fellow" may be helpful in remembering this color scheme. They have round pupils and subcaudal scales in a double row.[18,33] Unlike pit vipers, coral snakes have short, fixed, anterior fangs. When a coral snake bites into a victim's finger, toe, or web space, its venom is inefficiently delivered to the systemic system. Between 40% and 75% of all bites result in significant envenomation.[21,46]

The venom lacks proteolytic enzyme function, which makes local signs of envenomation rare following a bite. There are even reports of envenomation without visible fang marks.[47] Local necrosis does not occur. Coral snake venom does not appear to cause hemolytic coagulation abnormalities or life-threatening arrhythmias.[47] However, rhabdomyolysis has been observed.[46] Systemic symptoms include drowsiness, fasciculations, tremors, nausea and vomiting, slurred speech, paresthesias, miosis, ptosis, diplopia, dysphagia, stridor, excessive salivation, and eventual respiratory paralysis. Signs of systemic envenomation usually present within three hours, but may be delayed greater than 13 hours after the bite.[3,5,33,46] The predominant component of its venom is a neurotoxin that causes a curare-like, postsynaptic, nondepolarizing blockade at the neuromuscular junction by binding competitively to the acetylcholine receptor.[48] Children are prone to seizures, probably because of the cerebral hypoxia secondary to respiratory failure.[47]

Prehospital treatment should include protection of the airway, breathing, and circulation. Venom extraction may be of benefit if immediately available, as above. Constriction bands or pressure immobilization techniques, as described for elapid bites in Australia, may be useful for field first aid for coral snake bites, but their use has not been well-studied.[47,49,50]

In administering Wyeth Antivenin *(Micrurus fulvius)* (equine), physicians must consider precautions for anaphylaxis and serum sickness, as with rattlesnakes. If the patient is bitten by a coral snake, he or she may need to be given antivenom before symptoms appear in order to prevent respiratory failure.[46,47] Patients who develop respiratory paralysis may require ventilatory support for several days to weeks.[3,51] Skin testing is controversial, as above. Recovery has been shown in patients without using antivenom. Some recommend treating patients with possible allergy to antivenom with supportive care only.[47,49] There is no antivenom for bites from the Arizona (Sonoran) coral snake, and treatment is supportive.

Children may require more antivenom than adults. Early treatment with antivenom is indicated for a positively identified coral snake bite with fang marks and a negative skin test[46,47] and may be indicated in other less well-defined situations. Three to 10 vials of antivenom are recommended for pediatric patients diluted in NS and delivered over two hours.[3,33,46] For those presenting late with symptoms, signs of bulbar paralysis may imply impending respiratory failure. Elective intubation should be considered to prevent aspiration.[49] Any child suspected of being bitten by a coral snake should be admitted to the ICU for at least 24 hours.[5,47]

Spiders

Almost 24,000 spider bites were reported to the AAPCC in 1995, one-third of which were in children and adolescents.[1] These data may represent overreporting, since many unexplained lesions are attributed to spiders. No deaths were reported from spiders.

All but two species of spiders in the United States are venomous. However, only about 50 species have fangs large enough to penetrate human skin, and only a few of these deliver a potent enough venom in sufficient quantity to be considered medically significant. Only the widow and brown spiders are considered dangerous to humans.[17,56] Widow spiders are distributed throughout the United States except in Alaska. In the United States, bites occur most often in the southern and western states and are more common in the warm months, when spiders are more active.[56] Brown spiders exist all over the world.

Pediatric Considerations. More aggressive treatment and hospitalization has been recommended by some for children envenomated by widow spiders;[57] however, other sources suggest that children may actually suffer less morbidity than adults.[58] The diagnostic challenge of young children with unexplained crying may represent spider envenomations.

Widow Spider Envenomations

Description. Of the five species of widow spider *(Latrodectus* sp.) found in the United States, only three species are black. The female black widow spider, which is the most common and well-known widow spider, is shiny black in color with a red spot on the ventral surface of the abdomen, often in the shape of an hourglass. Other widow spiders may be brown and have irregular red markings. The male spider is brown, much smaller than the female, and is not capable of envenomating humans.

Widow spiders spin irregular webs in dark, secluded areas such as woodpiles, basements, and garages and may be found in old furniture, shoes, or clothing. The spiders are not aggressive and bite in self-defense when a web is disturbed.

Pathophysiology. *Venom.* Widow spider venom is one of the most potent venoms by volume, even more so than that of pit vipers.[59-61] Venom consists of six active components, with alpha-latrotoxin being the main component producing systemic symptoms.[62] The proposed latrotoxin mechanism of action occurs through glycoprotein and ganglioside binding on neuromuscular presynaptic membranes. This opens cation channels, allowing release of acetylcholine and catecholamines, and inhibits re-uptake of choline. These biochemical changes result in excessive stimulation of the motor end plate.[63-65] The resulting envenomation produces neurotoxic and autonomic symptoms.

Clinical Effects. *Local Effects.* The initial widow spider bite may be painful at the site or go unnoticed.[56] Children, particularly at preverbal ages, may present with unexplained crying as early as 30 minutes post bite, while adults may present as late as 12 hours post bite.[57,61,66] The average time in all patients from envenomation to onset of symptoms is between one and two hours.[57] Within 20 minutes to one hour, a local erythematous reaction or halo-like target lesion with two small puncture wounds (1-2 mm apart) may be seen. The target lesion has been used as a reliable sign of envenomation in certain studies.[63]

Systemic Effects. The earlier the systemic symptoms, the more severe the envenomation. Systemic symptoms can be grouped into muscle pain and general autonomic disturbances. Patients complain of abdominal, thigh, and back pain from increased spasm of the large muscle groups regardless of bite location.[8,66] Pediatric patients may present with refusing to bear weight and difficulty walking.[58] Cholinergic symptoms include local or generalized diaphoresis, vomiting, salivation, lacrimation, and bronchorrhea.[62] Other symptoms include weakness, fasciculations, ptosis, hyperreflexia, and seizures, fever, tachycardia, and hypertension.

The clinical course of widow spider bites in children is reported to be potentially more severe because of the smaller volume for the venom distribution.[67] Status asthmaticus has been described, which may be due to bronchial smooth muscle contraction.[68] Unusual pediatric clinical findings include priapism and hypertension.[69] Widow spider bites are one of the rare occasions in which a child can present in hypertensive crisis. This can result in renal problems, seizures, or cerebral hemorrhage.[67] In a recent review of pediatric spider bites, 92% of cases developed severe hypertension but no complications were reported.[58] Seizures resulting from widow envenomation are thought to be secondary to hypertension. Normotensive seizures have not been described.[56]

A clinically significant effect of the muscle cramping associated

Table 4. Clark's Grading Scale for Widow Spider Envenomations[63]

GRADE	SYMPTOMS
I	Asymptomatic Localized pain Normal vital signs
II	Localized muscular pain Normal vital signs
III	Generalized muscular pain Nausea, vomiting Headache Abnormal vital signs

with widow spider envenomations is muscle fatigue that results in respiratory difficulties. Respiratory failure has been described as one of the main causes of death due to widow spider envenomation. An expiratory grunt thought to be an effort to keep from moving the abdominal wall has been described and was seen more commonly in pediatric patients.[58,66]

An unusual clinical feature described in widow spider envenomation is diaphoresis at the bite site, face, and nose, with the rest of the body being dry. General diaphoresis may be associated with a more severe envenomation.[8,63] There also can be a gradual onset of periorbital edema without other signs of angioedema or anaphylaxis.

Emergency Department Treatment and Disposition. *Prehospital Care.* Maintaining the airway, breathing, and circulation, along with careful observation of respiratory status, is the priority for prehospital care. Seizure precautions may also be indicated.

Grading of Envenomations. A three-class grading system for bites has been developed.[63] *(See Table 4.)* Grade I is relatively asymptomatic with mild local pain. Grade II has progression of pain to localized muscle pain, while Grade III has generalized muscle pain, systemic symptoms, and abnormal vital signs.

Pain Control. Calcium gluconate has traditionally been recommended for pain control of widow spider bites since it has been thought to replenish calcium stores in the sarcoplasmic reticulum of muscles that are depleted by repetitive stimulation. However, calcium gluconate has been reported to be only 4% effective in a more recent study in comparison with a combination of IV opioids and benzodiazepines.[63] Most human experience with calcium is anecdotal, with symptoms often recurring within 20 minutes of calcium infusion. Thus, calcium gluconate is no longer recommended as first-line treatment for widow spider bites.[63]

Dantrolene sodium is controversial therapy for widow spider bites. Plasma concentrations are variable in children, and there is a potential delay in achieving therapeutic levels via the oral route.[67]

Benzodiazepines, such as lorazepam and diazepam, have been used in treatment of widow spider bites with favorable results along with the added benefits of sedation, amnesia, and anxiolytic effects. Muscle relaxants, such as methocarbamol, also have been used, but have been reported to be even less effective than calcium.[70]

Narcotics, such as morphine sulfate and meperidine, are commonly used for widow spider bites. In conjunction with benzodiazepines, this is recommended as the therapy of choice in patients who are not candidates for antivenom.[63]

Antivenom. Latrodectus Antivenin (Merck & Company) has been shown to rapidly and completely relieve symptoms of widow spider envenomation.[58,63] The dose is one vial of antivenom mixed in 50-100 mL of normal saline and infused over 30-60 minutes. This dose may be repeated if needed. Because pediatric patients have been reported to suffer more morbidity from widow spider bites, more aggressive use of antivenom has been recommended.[57] Although effectiveness of the antivenom is supported by the literature, its use is limited by concerns over anaphylaxis, since it is a horse serum derivative.[67] Although there have been no deaths reported from widow spider envenomation in over 30 years,[58] fatality has been reported from anaphylaxis after administration of Latrodectus Antivenin.[63] Skin testing, as previously mentioned, has variable predictability in identifying immediate hypersensitivity. Serum sickness may occur,[64] but because of the relatively small amount of antivenom used, it is less common than with snakebite antivenom.

Widow spider envenomation has been described as a disease of discomfort rather than a deadly one, even in children.[58] Symptoms of widow spider envenomation usually do not require antivenom as most are self-limited, often resolving within a few hours.[64] Occasionally symptoms are prolonged but have been shown to "dramatically" respond to administration of antivenom as late as 30 hours after envenomation.[71] Antivenom should be considered for severe envenomations when symptoms persist despite adequate administration of parenteral narcotics and benzodiazepines, in children without allergic contraindications, or for children with life-threatening complications associated with envenomation.[58,63]

Disposition. Although antivenom may not change outcome after widow spider envenomation,[64] patients receiving antivenom appear to require less hospitalization.[58,63] If high-dose narcotics and benzodiazepines are required to control persistent pain or abnormalities in vital signs persist, hospital admission is recommended.[58] Symptoms from widow spider envenomations may last for several days. Antivenom may resolve pain within the two hours it takes to infuse.[58] Such patients may be discharged home from the ED with good follow-up, preventing hospitalization. Patients suffering anaphylaxis due to antivenom or significant complications to the envenomation itself should be admitted.[63]

Antibiotics. Wound care considerations include cleansing of the wound and tetanus prophylaxis. Prophylactic antibiotic therapy is not routinely indicated.[43]

Brown Spider Envenomations

Description. The brown recluse spider is the most prevalent of the 13 species of brown spiders (*Loxosceles*) distributed throughout the United States. The brown recluse is found in the south central United States, and desert species are distributed in the southwest. All brown spiders cause a similar local reaction, but the brown recluse is thought to cause more severe local and systemic symptoms.[72] Brown spiders are light to dark brown in color and are approximately 1-2 cm long with a 3 cm leg span. Many have an identifying violin or fiddleback marking on the dorsal cephaothorax, although this marking may be faint or even absent on several species.[73] These spiders are reclusive, nocturnal hunters found under woodpiles, rocks, and in garages.[74] Envenomations occur in spring and summer, often when a spider is trapped against the skin. Unlike the black widow spider, both the male and female spider are capable of envenomating humans.[15] Although this discussion focuses on brown spiders, other spiders are capable of causing a necrotic lesion, referred to as necrotic arachnidism.[8,77]

Pathophysiology. *Venom.* Brown spider venom produces a dermonecrotic reaction secondary to proteolytic enzymes designed to initiate digestion of the prey's tissue.[78] The venom is a complex cytotoxin consisting of at least eight separate components (e.g., hyaluronidase, protease, sphingomyelinase D, hemolysins). Several reports identify sphingomyelinase D as the major cytotoxic factor of *Loxosceles* venom.[73,78,79]

Sphingomyelinase D destroys sphingomyelinase in cell-wall membranes and causes release of inflammatory mediators that damage the endothelium of local arterioles and venules. This lyses erythrocytes and activates platelets, which leads to thrombosis, infarction, and necrosis. Further tissue damage may be due to activity of complement and destruction of leukocytes, leading to the release of kinins, enzymes, and histamine.[73,78]

Clinical Effects. *Local Effects.* Local effects from brown spider envenomation are much more common than systemic effects. Initially, the brown recluse spider bite causes little or no pain and may go unnoticed. Fewer than 10% of lesions progress to form large ulcerations.[78,81] In wounds that do progress, a burning sensation occurring 30-60 minutes after the bite has been identified in as many as 90% of bites in one series.[73] The immediate area of bite becomes erythematous. After several hours, a blister forms within a central ischemic ring surrounded by an eccentric ring of erythema, which is sometimes called a "target lesion." Within 3-4 days, a bleb forms with induration and swelling that later ruptures, forming a central necrotic ulcer. The ulcer enlarges and may be covered with an extensive eschar (up to 15 cm). Necrosis may be superficial or involve muscle and fascial layers.[73,82] Fatty areas such as the abdomen, thighs, and buttocks form more extensive necrotic lesions due to the tenuous blood supply to these regions. Ulcerations can require months to heal and may need skin grafting.

Other lesions may resemble the wounds caused by brown spiders, and spiders are probably not responsible for many of the injuries they are thought to have caused. Unless the spider is identified, diagnosis based upon the lesion alone may be inaccurate.[72] In addition, patients may present late because of the insidious progression of the wound, and may not recall being bitten.[79,83]

Systemic Effects A rare systemic reaction has been described associated with brown spider envenomation. Children may experience arthralgias, chills, nausea, vomiting, and rash.[73,79] The combination of high fever and scarlatiniform rash, together with a typical bite lesion, may suggest loxoscelism.[73] Other reported pediatric systemic effects include hemolytic anemia, epiglottis swelling, and disseminated intravascular coagulation.[75,76,80,84] Systemic envenomation may progress to hemolysis, thrombocytopenia, hemorrhage, shock, jaundice, and renal failure. Systemic symptoms are proportional to the amount of venom injected and not necessarily to the size or appearance of the bite.

Emergency Department Treatment and Disposition. Treatment of brown spider envenomation is controversial, and there are no controlled human studies to evaluate different treatment modalities. Tetanus prophylaxis and wound cleansing are recommended to avoid later secondary infection, but no evidence has linked decreased tissue loss with any specific local therapy.[73]

Although some recommend local surgical excision,[85,86] other sources suggest excision of the lesion has not been shown to aid in healing and may even be detrimental.[79] Untreated, many of the envenomations will regress and form a smaller final cosmetic lesion than if excised.[8]

Dapsone has been thought to decrease skin necrosis by inhibiting polymorphonuclear chemotaxis, lessening the inflammatory reaction. It has been anecdotally reported to resolve the ulceration from brown spider bite[73] and eliminate the need for surgical debridement.[83] However, dapsone has recently been shown to have no more effect on lesion size or histopathological response than control in an animal model and is not currently recommended.[81,87] In addition, dapsone is associated with serious side effects, such as hemolytic anemia, methemoglobinemia, and toxic hepatitis. Dapsone is contraindicated in pregnancy, G6PD deficiency, and patients allergic to sulfa.

Hyperbaric oxygen (HBO) therapy is thought to cause neovascularization in necrotic tissues and inactivate enzymes that contain sulfa-hydryl groups, although it has also been shown in animal studies to have no benefit over controls.[81,87]

Antivenom to certain brown spiders has been produced, although there is no commercially available antivenom in the United States.[54] Antivenom may be effective if given early to prevent the activity of sphingomyelinase enzyme but has been reported to be less effective once the inflammatory reaction has developed.[83] This would require earlier and more accurate recognition of brown spider envenomation than currently available.

Systemic steroids have been recommended for systemic envenomations to prevent further hemolysis, although there has been no proof of benefit.[73,81]

Other anecdotal treatments without proven benefit that are possibly dangerous include electric shock, local steroids, heparin, colchicine, cyroheptadine (serotonin antagonist), and vasodilators. Analgesics and antihistamines may provide symptomatic relief. Antibiotics may be needed for secondary infection.[86]

Laboratory tests for evaluation of systemic toxicity include complete blood count with platelets, electrolyte, BUN, creatinine, and baseline clotting parameters. All patients with signs of systemic envenomation should be admitted to the hospital for evaluation for hemolysis, coagulopathies, and renal failure. Patients with local effects from brown spider envenomation should be followed closely as outpatients with wound care instructions and good follow-up. Patients with systemic infections or underlying debilitating disease should be admitted.

Scorpions

Pediatric patients accounted for a little more than one-fourth of the 11,000 scorpion exposures in 1995.[1] No deaths have been reported from scorpion stings since 1968.[88] The bark scorpion (*Centruroides*) is the only U.S. scorpion considered dangerous to humans. All other U.S. scorpions cause local burning pain and swelling but no systemic symptoms.[59,88]

Bark scorpions are nocturnal and dwell in trees. They are distributed mostly in Arizona but may also be found in parts of California, Texas, New Mexico, and Nevada.[59,89] Envenomations have occurred in other areas when scorpions are unknowingly transported in personal belongings.[90,91]

Description. Scorpions have a segmented cephalothorax, abdomen, and tail. They have eight legs and two pincers. Bark scorpions are yellow or brown and about 5 cm in length. They can be distinguished from other scorpions by a small tubercle just below the base of the stinger, slender pincers, a triangular rather than pentagonal central sternal plate, and a rectangular rather than square proximal tail segment.[59,88,92]

Pediatric Considerations. Children suffer greater morbidity and mortality from scorpion envenomation than adults.[33,88,89,92] Prior to modern intensive care units and development of antivenom, death occurred more often in pediatric patients.[88] Young children suffer more from respiratory compromise than adults envenomated by bark scorpions. Although death has not been reported in almost 30 years in the United States from scorpion envenomation, morbidity may be severe; one such case led to quadriparesis.[89] Most authorities agree on more aggressive treatment and admission of children with bark scorpion stings.

Pathophysiology. *Venom Apparatus and Venom.* Scorpions attack humans when threatened, thrusting their tails over their bodies while grasping with pincers and repeatedly stinging.[59] The segmented tail ends in a vesicle containing venom glands, which contract and eject venom during the scorpion sting.[59,90,91] Bark scorpion venom is primarily neurotoxic. Since there are no enzymes to produce tissue destruction, there is minimal inflammatory response.[90,91] The protein neurotoxins activate sodium channels with prolongation of the action potential as well as spontaneous depolarization of the nerves, which enhances repetitive firing of the neurons.[59,90,91] This autonomic stimulation results in catecholamine release.

Clinical Effects. *Local Effects.* Children may have more severe envenomation because the severity of sting symptoms is weight-dependent.[93] After the sting, symptoms of pain and paresthesias begin immediately and progress to maximum severity in about five hours.[88] The area of the sting is very sensitive, and tapping over the site can accentuate the pain, resulting in a positive "tap test."[24,88] Diagnosis in young children may be difficult if the sting is unwitnessed due to the absence of local signs. The only sign of envenomation may be agitation or unexplained crying.[94]

Systemic Effects. Local pain progresses to generalized symptoms that may last up to 30 hours.[88,89] Systemic symptoms are produced by both sympathetic and parasympathetic stimulation. Sympathetic symptoms can be described by the typical sympathetic "overdrive" syndrome—diaphoresis, tachycardia, hypertension, pulmonary edema, and seizures. Parasympathetic symptoms include the "SLUDGE" syndrome (salivation, lacrimation, urination, defecation, gastric emptying), bradycardia, and hypotension.[59] Patients may complain of trouble swallowing.[90,91]

Airway secretions are an important consideration in the treatment of scorpion envenomations. Excessive drooling can be seen, particularly in children, and may be a combination of increased salivation and difficulty in swallowing.[90,91] Fatalities due to scorpion envenomations in infants and children have been attributed to respiratory arrest.[88]

Cranial nerve dysfunction can be described as "roving" eye movements, blurred vision, tongue fasciculations, and difficulties with pharyngeal muscles resulting in stridor and contributing to respiratory arrest.

Excessive somatic muscular activity can be mistaken for seizure activity as the extremities can have uncontrollable jerking. However, unlike seizures, the patient remains awake and alert.[90,91] True seizures are generally not found with bark scorpion envenomation.[88]

Table 5. Grading Scale for Scorpion Envenomations[90,91]

GRADE	SYMPTOMS
I	Local pain
II	Remote pain
III	Either cranial nerve or somatic skeletal neuromuscular dysfunction. **Cranial nerve dysfunction:** Blurred vision, wandering eye movements, hypersalivation, dysphagia, tongue fasciculations, upper airway problems, slurred speech. **Somatic skeletal neuromuscular dysfunction:** Jerking of extremity, restlessness, severe involuntary shaking and jerking that may be mistaken for a seizure.
IV	Both cranial nerve and somatic skeletal neuromuscular dysfunction.

Cardiac dysfunction has been described and is thought to be due to catecholamine effects on myocardial contractility and perfusion causing increasing myocardial oxygen demand in excess of supply.[95]

Emergency Department Treatment and Disposition. *Prehospital.* Extractor devices may be beneficial but are not well-studied for scorpion envenomations. A lymphatic band with elastic wrap may delay venom absorption.

Supportive care with airway control is the number-one priority in treatment of scorpion envenomations. All patients should have intravenous access and continuous monitoring. No laboratory findings are specific for scorpion envenomation. Laboratory studies specific to the patient's supportive care, particularly respiratory status, should be obtained. Creatinine kinase may need to be obtained to evaluate for possible rhabdomyolysis. Treatment of scorpion envenomation is based on correct identification, quantification of poisoning, and comparison of clinical picture with a graded scale of treatment.[59]

Grading and Antivenom Administration. Criteria for estimating the severity of scorpion envenomation have been developed.[90,91] *(See Table 5.)* Grade I includes local pain and paresthesias and grade II envenomations have symptoms progressing to sites remote from the sting site. Grade III envenomations include cranial dysfunction or somatic neuromuscular dysfunction; grade IV includes both.

Grades I and II are subjective and may be combined for young children.[90,91] The majority of grade IV scorpion envenomations occur in children less than 11 years of age. Infants have been reported to reach grade IV envenomations in 15-30 minutes.

Symptomatic relief of local pain and burning can be provided with analgesics and local wound control. Tetanus prophylaxis is indicated. Most grade I and II envenomations have spontaneous resolution of symptoms. Symptoms abate at a rate dependent on the age of victim and grade of envenomation.[88] Pain and paresthesias can persist for as long as two weeks post envenomation.[88,90,91] In grade III envenomations, illness severity can range from mild tongue fasciculations to severe cranial nerve dysfunction. Patients with grade IV envenomations typically appear ill.[90,91]

Analgesics are recommended for pain control. Corticosteroids, antihistamines, calcium, and sympathomimetics have all been administered for symptomatic relief but have no scientific support.[59] Historically, barbiturates have been recommended for neuromuscular activity control in severe envenomations but may be dangerous for patients with airway difficulties. The physician must provide careful respiratory monitoring and support if using them. Barbiturates have been associated with complications and have not been shown to shorten illness duration.[90,91]

USA-APL Scorpion Antivenin for bark scorpion envenomation may be obtained in Arizona but is not approved by the Food and Drug Administration. Developed by Arizona State University, it is a goat serum derivative. Bark scorpion antivenom has not been well-studied but has been reported to have beneficial clinical effects.[90,91,93,95] Antivenom has been shown to benefit patients with grade III and IV envenomations by rapidly resolving symptoms and shortening clinical course. Some physicians prefer hospitalization, sedation, and supportive care.[90,91] Benefits of antivenom, including immediate symptom resolution and avoidance of sedation, paralysis, intubation, and possibly even hospitalization, must be weighed against allergic complications.[89]

Antivenom dose is one vial diluted in 50 cc normal saline intravenously over 15-30 minutes; this may be repeated after one hour. Improvement in severe neurologic symptoms can be seen within minutes, but skeletal symptom resolution can take longer.[88,90,91] Risk of anaphylaxis and serum sickness is present but is less common, probably because antivenom is derived from goat serum and small volumes are given. Some experience with antivenom has suggested that if full symptom resolution occurs rapidly, the patient may be safely discharged home, avoiding a costly hospitalization and an intubation with sedation.[89] Without antivenom, admission or extended critical care observation should be strongly considered, especially for young children with bark scorpion envenomations.

Summary

While the bites and envenomations of snakes, spiders, and scorpions are less common than some presenting pediatric emergencies, they are nevertheless a potential challenge to the clinician. Once the precarious process of recognition and diagnosis is overcome, the clinician is still faced with demanding therapeutic decisions that at times are as risky as the injury itself. This review of the agents of envenomation, the associated pathophysiology, and the available treatments for snake, spider, and scorpion envenomations helps clarify the decision making for the clinician.

References

1. Litovitz TL, Felberg L, White S, et al. 1995 Annual report of the American Association of Poison Control Centers toxic exposure surveillance system. *Am J Emerg Med* 1996;14: 487-537.
2. Norris RL. Snake venom poisoning in the United States: Assessment and management. *Emerg Med Rep* 1995;16: 87-94.
3. Sullivan JB, Wingert WA, Norris Jr. RL. North American venomous reptile bites. In: Auerbach PS, ed. *Wilderness Medicine: Management of Wilderness and Environmental Emergencies.* 3rd ed. St. Louis: Mosby-Year Book, Inc; 1995.
4. Weber RA, White RR. Crotalidae envenomation in children. *Ann Plast Surg* 1993;31:141-145.
5. Erickson T, Herman BE, Bowman MJ. Snake envenomations. In: Strange GR, Ahrens WR, Lelyveld S, et al, eds. *Pediatric Emergency Medicine: A Comprehensive Study Guide.* New York: McGraw-Hill; 1996.
6. Downey DJ, Omer GE, Moneim MS. New Mexico rattlesnake bites: Demographic review and guidelines for treatment. *J Trauma* 1991;31:1380-1386.
7. Wingert WA, Chan L. Rattlesnake bites in southern California and rationale for recommended treatment. *West J Med* 1988; 148:37-44.
8. Banner Jr W. Bites and stings in the pediatric patient. *Curr Probl Pediatr* 1988;1:8-69.
9. Parrish HM, Guldner JC, Silberg SL. Comparison between snakebites in children and adults. *Pediatrics* 1965;36: 251-256.
10. Buntain WL. Successful venomous snakebite neutralization with massive antivenom infusion in a child. *J Trauma* 1983; 23:1012-1013.
11. Cruz NS, Alvarez RG. Rattlesnake bite complications in 19 children. *Pediatr Emerg Care* 1994;10:30-33.
12. Podgorny G. Reptile bites and scorpion stings. In: Tintinalli J, Krome RL, Ruiz E, eds. *Emergency Medicine: A Comprehensive Study Guide.* 3rd ed. New York: Mcgraw-Hill; 1988.
13. Gold BS, Barish RA. Venomous snakebites: Current concepts in diagnosis, treatment, and management. *Emerg Med Clin North Am* 1992;10:249-266.
14. Dart RC, Hurlbut KM, Garcia R, et al. Validation of a severity score for the assessment of crotalid snakebite. *Ann Emerg Med* 1996;27:321-326.
15. Minton SA. Snakebite in the Midwestern region. *Ind Univ Med Ctr Bull* 1952;14:28.
16. Klauber IM. *Rattlesnakes: Their Habitats, Life Histories and Influence on Mankind.* Vol 1, ed 2. Berkeley: University of California Press; 1972.
17. Galli RL, Weber EJ. Vicious venoms and rabid viruses. *Aud Dig Emerg Med* 1994;11(13).
18. Gold BS, Wingert WA. Snake venom poisoning in the United States: A review of therapeutic practice. *So Med J* 1994; 87:579-589.
19. Spaite D, Dart RC, Sullivan JB. Skin testing in cases of possible crotalid envenomation. *Ann Emerg Med* 1988;17:105-106. Letter.
20. Glenn JL, Straight R. Intergradation of two different venom populations of the Mojave rattlesnake (*Crotalus scutulatus scutulatus*) in Arizona. *Toxicon* 1989;27:411-418.
21. Russell FE, Carlson RW, Wainschell J, et al. Snake venom poisoning in the United States. *JAMA* 1975;233:341-344.
22. Henderson BM, Dujon EB. Snake bites in children. *J Pediatr Surg* 1973;8:729-733.
23. Bush SP, Jansen DW. Rattlesnake envenomations in children: Case review of 38 patients. In press.
24. Curry SC. Rattlesnake bites. American College of Emergency Physicians Scientific Assembly. 1996.

25. Burgess JL, Dart RC. Snake venom coagulopathy: Use and abuse of blood products in the treatment of pit viper envenomation. *Ann Emerg Med* 1991;20:795-801.
26. Ryan KC, Caraveti EM. Life-threatening anaphylaxis following envenomation by two different species of Crotalidae. *J Wild Med* 1994:5:263-268.
27. Jansen PW, Perkin RM, van Stralen D. Mojave rattlesnake envenomation: Prolonged neurotoxicity and rhabdomyolysis. *Ann Emerg Med* 1992;21:322-325.
28. Bush SP, Jansen PW. Severe rattlesnake envenomation with anaphylaxis and rhabdomyolysis. *Ann Emerg Med* 1995;25: 845-848.
29. Clark RF, Selden BS, Furbee B. The incidence of wound infection following crotalid envenomation. *J Emerg Med* 1993;11:583-586.
30. Weed HG. Nonvenomous snakebite in Massachusetts: Prophylactic antibiotics are unnecessary. *Ann Emerg Med* 1993;22:220-224.
31. Hultgren HN, Walter FG, Blackman J, et al. Rattlesnake bite. *J Wild Med* 1994;5:216-221.
32. Bronstein AC, Russell FE, Sullivan JB, et al. Negative pressure suction in field treatment of rattlesnake bite. *Vet Hum Toxicol* 1985;28:297. Abstract.
33. Dart RC, Gomez HF. Reptile bites and scorpion stings. In: Tintinalli J, Krome RL, Ruiz E, eds. *Emergency Medicine: A Comprehensive Study Guide.* 4th ed. New York: Mcgraw-Hill; 1996.
34. Christopher DG, Rodning CB. Crotalidae envenomation. *South Med J* 1986;79:159-162.
35. Jurkovich GJ, Luterman A, McCullar K, et al. Complications of Crotalidae antivenin therapy. *J Trauma* 1988;28: 1032-1037.
36. Otten EJ, McKimm D. Venomous snakebite in a patient allergic to horse serum. *Ann Emerg Med* 1983;12:624-627.
37. Wyeth Antivenin (Crotalidae) Polyvalent (equine origin) package insert. 1986.
38. Consroe P, Egen NB, Russell FE, et al. Comparison of a new ovine antigen binding fragment (Fab) antivenin for United States Crotolidae with the commercial antivenin for protection against venom-induced lethality in mice. *Am J Trop Med Hyg* 1995;53:507-510.
39. Decker W, Dart RC. A new antivenom for crotalid snakebite. *Wild Med Lett* 1995;12:8.
40. Bogdan GM, Dart RC. Prolonged and recurrent coagulopathy after North American pit viper envenomation. *Ann Emerg Med* 1996;27:820.
41. Hurlbut KM, Dart RC, Spaite D, et al. Reliability of clinical presentation for predicting significant pit viper envenomation. *Ann Emerg Med* 1988;438-439.
42. Swindle GM, Seaman KG, Arthur DC, et al. The six hour observation rule for grade I crotalid envenomation: Is it sufficient? Case report of delayed envenomation. *J Wild Med* 1992;3:168-172.
43. Sanford JP, Gilbert DN, Sande MA. Guide to Antimicrobial Therapy. 26th ed. Dallas: Gateway Graphics; 1996.
44. Burch JM, Agarwal R, Mattox KL, et al. The treatment of crotalid envenomation without antivenin. *J Trauma* 1988;28: 35-43.
45. Parrish HM, Khan MS. Bites by coral snakes: Report of 11 representative cases. *Am J Med Sci* 1967;253:561-568.
46. Kitchens CS, Van Mierop LHS. Envenomation by the eastern coral snake (*Micrurus fulvius fulvius*): A study of 39 victims. *JAMA* 1987;258:1615-1618.
47. Norris RL, Dart RC. Apparent coral snake envenomation in a patient without visible fang marks. *Am J Emerg Med* 1989;7: 402-405.
48. Kitchens CS, Van Mierop LH. Envenomation by the eastern Coral snake (*Micrurus fulvivus vulvius*). *JAMA* 1987;258: 1615.
49. Dart RC, Sullivan Jr JB. Elapid snake envenomations. In: Harwood-Nuss, et al, eds. *The Clinical Practice of Emergency Medicine.* 2nd ed. Philadelphia: Lippincott-Raven Publishers; 1996.
50. Davidson TM, Eisner J. United States coral snakes. *Wild Env Med* 1996;1:38-45.
51. Pettigrew LC, Glass PJ. Neurologic complications of a coral snake bite. *Neurology* 1985;35:589-592.
52. Hooker KR, Caraveti EM. Gila monster envenomation. *Ann Emerg Med* 1994;24:731-735.
53. Brown DE. Americas Aztec lizard. *Reptiles* 1995;11:8-29.
54. Boyer DM. *Antivenom Index.* The American Zoo and Aquarium Association and The American Association of Poison Control Centers. 1994.
55. Gomez HF, Davis, M, Phillips S, et al. Human envenomation from a wandering garter snake. *Ann Emerg Med* 1994;23: 1119-1122.
56. Hassen LVB, McNally JT. Spider bites. In: Auerbach P, ed. *Wilderness Medicine.* 3rd ed. St Louis: Mosby Year Book; 1995 .
57. Russell F, Gertsch W. For those who treat spider or suspected spider bites. *Toxicon* 1983;21:337.
58. Woestman R, Perkin R, Van Stralen D. The black widow: Is she deadly to children? *Pediatr Emerg Care* 1996;12: 360-364.
59. Allen C. Arachnid envenomations. *Emerg Med Clin North Am* 1992;10:269-298.
60. Kobernick M. Black widow spider bite. *Am Fam Physician* 1984;29:241-245.
61. Curry SC. Spider envenomation. In: Harwood-Nuss, et al, eds. *The Clinical Practice of Emergency Medicine.* Philadelphia: Lippincott-Raven Publishers; 1996:1446-1448.
62. Mack RB. Will the defendant please rise? Black widow spider poisoning. *N Engl J Med* 1994;55:86-88.
63. Clark RF, et al. Clinical presentation and treatment of black widow spider envenomation: A review of 163 cases. *Ann Emerg Med* 1992;21:782-787.
64. Moss HS, Binder LS. A retrospective review of black widow spider envenomation. *Ann Emerg Med* 1987;16:188-192.
65. Lewin NA. Arthropods. In: Goldfrank LJ, et al, eds. *Goldfrank's Toxicologic Emergencies.* 5th ed. Norwalk, CT: Appleton & Lange; 1994.
66. Prince GE. Arachnidism in children. *J Pediatr* 1956;49: 101-108.
67. Reeves JA, Allison EJ, Goodman PE. Black widow spider bite in a child. *Am J Emerg Med* 1996;14:469-471.
68. Bush SP, Naftel J, Farstad D. Injection of a whole black

widow spider. *Ann Emerg Med* 1996;27:532-533.

69. Stiles AD. Priapism following a black widow spider bite. *Clin Pediatr* 1982:174-175.
70. Key GF. A comparison of calcium gluconate and methocarbamol (Robaxin) in the treatment of Latrodectism (black widow spider envenomation). *Am J Trop Med Hyg* 1981;30: 273-277.
71. Suntornthan S, Roberts JR, Nilsen GJ. Dramatic clinical response to the delayed administration of black widow spider antivenin. *Ann Emerg Med* 1994;24:1198-1199.
72. Russell FE, Waldron, WG, Madon MB. Bites by the brown spiders *Loxosceles unicolor* and *Loxosceles arizonica. Toxicon* 1969;7:109-117.
73. Stewart C. Emergency management of arachnid envenomations: Spider bites and scorpion stings. *Emerg Med Rep* 1993;14:9.
74. Herman BE, Erickson T, Bowman MJA. Spider bites. In: Strange GR, Ahrens WR, Lelyveld S, et al, eds. *Pediatric Emergency Medicine: A Comprehensive Study Guide.* New York: McGraw-Hill; 1996.
75. Minton SA, Tolson C. A case of spider bite with severe hemolytic reaction. *Pediatrics* 1964;33:287-294.
76. Vorse H, et al. Disseminated intravascular coagulopathy following fatal brown spider bite. *J Pediatr* 1972;80:1035-1037.
77. Hobbs GD, Harrell RE. Brown recluse spider bites: A common cause of necrotic arachnidism. *Am J Emerg Med* 1989;7: 309-312.
78. Tully SA, Wingert WA. Venomous animal bites and stings. Barkin RM, ed. *Pediatric Emergency Medicine.* 3rd ed. St Louis: Mosby Year Book; 1992.
79. Otten EJ. Venomous animal injuries. In: Rosen PR, ed. *Emergency Medicine.* 3rd ed. St Louis: Mosby Year Book; 1992.
80. Herman TE, McAlister WH. Epiglottic enlargement: Two unusual causes. *Pediatr Radiol* 1991;21:139-140.
81. Hobbs GD, Anderson AR, Greene TJ, et al. Comparison of hyperbaric oxygen and dapsone therapy for *Loxosceles* envenomation. *Acad Emerg Med* 1996;3:758-761.
82. Anderson JE. Recognizing the recluse spider bite in children: Necrotic arachnidism. *Louisiana St Med Soc J* 1987;139: 33-36.
83. Rees R, Campbell D, Rieger E, et al. The diagnosis and treatment of brown recluse spider bites. *Ann Emerg Med* 1987;16: 945-949.
84. Madrigal GC, Ercolani RL, Wenzl JE. Toxicity from a bite of brown spider *(Loxosceles reclusus). Clin Pediatr* 1972;11: 641-644.
85. Hollabaugh RS, Fernandes ET. Management of the brown recluse spider bites. *J Pediatr Surg* 1989;24:126-127.
86. Salluzo RF. Insect and spider bites. In: Tintinalli J, Krome RL, Ruiz E, eds. *Emergency Medicine: A Comprehensive Study Guide.* 4th ed. New York: Mcgraw-Hill; 1996.
87. Phillips S, et al. Therapy of brown spider envenomation: A controlled trial of hyperbaric oxygen, dapsone, and cyroheptadine. *Ann Emerg Med* 1995;25:363-368.
88. Connor DA, Seldon BS. Scorpion envenomations. In: Auerbach PS, ed. *Wilderness Medicine.* 3rd ed. St Louis: Mosby; 1995:831-842.
89. Bond GR. Antivenin administration for *Centruroides* scorpion sting: Risks and benefits. *Ann Emerg Med* 1992;21:788-791.
90. Curry SC. Scorpion envenomations. *Clin Pract Emerg Med* 1996;378:1465-1467.
91. Curry SC, Vance MV, Ryron PJ, et al. Envenomation by the scorpion *Centruroides sculpturatus. J Toxicol Clin* 1984;21: 417-449.
92. Ellenhorn MJ, Barceloux DG. *Medical Toxicology: Diagnosis and Treatment of Human Poisonings.* Baltimore: Elsevier; 1985.
93. Amitai Y, et al. Scorpion stings in children. *Clin Pediatr* 1985;24:136-140.
94. Rimza ME, Zimmerman DR, Bergenson PJ. Scorpion envenomation. *Pediatrics* 1980;66:298-302.
95. Sofer S, Shahak E, Gueron M. Scorpion envenomation and antivenom therapy. *J Pediatr* 1994;124:973-978.

Electrical Injuries

Charles Stewart, MD, FACEP

There are about 2000 burn unit admissions and about 1000 deaths per year due to electrical injuries in adults and children.[1] Much of the literature about electrical injuries focuses on the serious complications associated with severe injuries due to high voltage or long-duration exposure. Fortunately, few of these serious injuries occur in children. Articles about low voltage injuries focus on the life-threatening complications of apnea and ventricular fibrillation. Less serious complications and injuries receive scant attention. This is unfortunate, since low-voltage electricity is the leading cause of electrical burn injury in children and adults.

With the emphasis in the literature clearly focused on major complications of high-voltage injuries, the recommendation for admission of the patient with a minor electrical injury for 24-48 hours is widespread.[2-7] Many emergency department (ED) practitioners clearly have noted that most injuries to children are minor and require no monitoring or invasive procedures.[3,4,8,9] Research needs to be conducted to determine the spectrum of electrical injuries and guidelines for care.

This chapter puts these issues into proper perspective and gives the emergency physician counsel about both the common, minor injuries and the much rarer life-threats.

Epidemiology

The people who are most commonly injured by electricity are, of course, those who work with it, such as electricians and construction workers. About 93% of electrical injury victims are male and the bulk of these are in their 20s.[10-11] Electrical injury is the fifth leading cause of occupational deaths.

Most electrical injuries in children are due to faulty electrical equipment or to children playing with extension cords and outlets.[12-13] Although we have created multiple safeguards for electrical outlets, most injuries occur with extension cords. The most common ages of injury are between 1 and 5 with the peak occurring in 2-year-olds. Most injuries occur between 10 a.m. and noon and between 4 and 6 p.m. Of the objects inserted into wall sockets, the most common are pins, keys, and fingers.

Pediatric emergency physicians also will see youths who are bent on exploration, often in dangerous places such as high-voltage transformer enclosures or near high tension lines. Other youths who are commonly involved in an electrical accident are hobbyists who are working with radios, computers, and similar electrical appliances and devices.

Physics of Electrical Injuries

The effect of the passage of electricity on various inorganic substances may be one of the most widely studied phenomenon in science. There is a huge body of literature that describes these studies and predicts effects of the passage of electricity through a substance. These effects are unchanged in the organic human model, but since humans are not uniform in composition, the descriptions become more complex.

In the inorganic model, the most important determinants of the extent of changes induced by electrical current are the intensity of the current and the duration of the contact.

Direct current (DC) is a constant current in a single direction. Sources of direct current include electronic power supplies, battery chargers, arc welders, and third rails for some transportation devices such as subways and trams. DC current injuries are not common, as few DC sources deliver much more than 30 volts. The exception to this is the subway third rail.

Alternating current (AC) is current that switches polarity on a regular basis. It is defined by the number of cycles per second as it switches from positive to negative. 60-cycle AC will have 60 negative half cycles and 60 positive half cycles per second. Common frequencies for AC include 60 cycles (U.S. household current), 50 cycles (European household current), and 400 cycles per second, used in some aircraft and military applications. When the frequency of alternating current is greater than 10,000 cycles per second, it is often referred to as high frequency current. Greater than about 30,000 cycles per second is considered radio frequency.

A transformer only works with AC, so most commercial high tension power lines are AC to allow for more efficient change of voltage. Some long distance, very high tension lines may be DC to increase the efficiency of transmission over long distance, but this is infrequent. Virtually all electrical injuries due to commercial current at any voltage are due to AC supplies.

A volt is the unit of electromotive force or "tension" on the line. Multiple descriptions from high school texts to college physics tomes use a familiar example of the water-filled pipe or hose to describe the passage of electrons through a conductor. Voltage is the pressure that forces the electrons through the line.

Voltage can be measured between the terminals on a battery or between the black wire and either the green ground or the white wire. Common voltages encountered in United States and Canadian households are 120 and 240 volts. Business users may encounter 440 volt lines, while the transformer on the street corner will be supplied by a 1200- or 2400-volt line. Europeans often will use 220 volts as household current.

High voltage is arbitrarily defined as a driving force of greater than 1000 volts.

An ampere is the unit of current flow. In the plumbing illustration mentioned previously, an ampere would represent the filling of a bucket at the end of the hose. If the bucket fills rapidly, then there is higher current flow. An ampere represents the passage of approximately 1023 electrons per second through a wire.

The resistance of a substance to the passage of electricity is measured in ohms. Dry skin has a resistance of about 100,000 ohms. In the plumbing simile, the size of the hose or pipe would represent the resistance to flow. A smaller hose would mean more resistance to the flow of current.

Intensity of current flow is governed by Ohm's law, which states that the electrical current is directly proportional to the voltage difference between two points and inversely proportional to the resistance between these two points.

Ohm's Law: $E_{(voltage)} = I_{(current)} \times R_{(resistance)}$

This equation is accurate and applicable for a copper wire of uniform composition. In the organic model, this law still is applicable, but the resistance may not be constant. Resistance in human skin is dependent on perspiration, contact area, variability of skin and underlying tissue, grounding, and the pathway of the current.

The production of heat by the passage of electrical current is significant. This heat is generated by the passage of electrical current through a resistance and is expressed by Joule's law. A watt is one ampere of current flow for one second. One watt of power for one second produces 0.24 calories of heat. One watt-second also is called a joule.

Joule's Law: $Heat_{(power)} = 0.24\ I^2 \times R \times T_{(time)}$

In this equation, the voltage can be substituted for I × R in the $I^2 \times R$ component, so heat produced is directly proportional to the driving voltage:

$Heat_{(power)} = 0.24\ I \times E \times T$

If all other factors are constant, dangerous current passage is more likely as the voltage increases and the time of exposure increases. Of these factors, time may be more important in human electrical burns than voltage.

The amount of current passing through a conductor also varies as the size of the conductor increases. When the current flows through a smaller area, the intensity of the current increases. This leads to the familiar contact burn on a finger touching the current source, while a foot immersed in water may have no burn at all.

An equal number of deaths from high- and low-voltage electrocutions occurred in a study of 220 fatalities.[14] This study did not discuss the duration of exposure.

Four separate tissue effects due to the passage of the current can be found in the electrical burn: 1) direct tissue heating (Joule heating); 2) contact burns (entry and exit point burns); 3) arc burns; and 4) thermal burns from ignition of clothing.

In addition to these tissue effects, distant effects on the body from the effects of the electrical passage are found in the cardiac and respiratory center effects, the nervous system effects, and the late effects. Additionally, mechanical trauma may result from the contractions induced by the current or from a fall caused by loss of consciousness.

Tissue Heating Effects

As noted, passage of current through the tissues will cause heating of the tissues. This heating can cause vascular spasm and thrombosis, peripheral and central neurologic injury, and muscle necrosis. As the current continues to heat the tissues, it literally cooks the tissues from within. This thermal injury is similar to a crush injury.

Different tissues have varying resistance to electric current. *(See Table 1.)* The least resistance is, of course, encountered in the nervous system, which is designed to carry electric current. Blood vessels and muscles carry electricity well because of their high electrolyte composition. Skin, tendon, fat, and bone are rather resistant to the flow of electricity. Unfortunately, if the voltage is high enough, the current will flow through all resistant structures, and the heating becomes greatest in the most resistant tissues. When the contact is prolonged, fat and tendons will melt. Bone heats, and this may cause periosteal damage.

Muscle necrosis, or rhabdomyolysis, second to electrical injury has potentially serious systemic consequences.

Table 1. Tissue Resistance to Electricity

LISTED IN ORDER OF LEAST RESISTANT (MOST CONDUCTIVE) TO MOST RESISTANT (LEAST CONDUCTIVE)
• Nerves
• Blood vessels
• Muscles
• Wet skin
• Dry skin
• Tendon
• Fat
• Bone

Classically, the diagnosis of rhabdomyolysis is made by the finding of dark urine that is strongly positive for hemoglobin but without red cells or red cell fragments. Such urine should be quantitatively assayed for myoglobin. The finding of creatinine phosphokinase (CPK) levels in excess of 5000 units clinches the diagnosis. In most cases, the CPK is greater than 20,000 units.

Contact Lesions

The contact lesions (entry and exit) consist of three characteristic areas: a charred, blackened center; a middle zone of grayish white coagulation necrosis; and a periphery of partial tissue damage. *(See Figure 1.)*

As noted earlier, these contact lesions are due to the current density and local tissue heating at the points of entry and exit. If the patient has contact with the current source over a wide area, either an exit or entry point may be absent. Current traveling through a dry finger can create an impressive burn, whereas the patient sitting in a tub of water may have no exit or entrance burns. Extensive electrothermal damage at the entry and exit points indicates that there has been significant current flow and the child has an increased risk of deep tissue damage.

Lip Burns. Specific mention must be made of lip burns. These injuries occur most frequently in 1- and 2-year-olds, and generally (60%) in boys. These burns can damage the mouth and lips, leaving a permanent scar. They almost uniformly occur in toddlers who bite on an electric cord (29.9%) or suck on an extension cord socket (53.7%). *(See Figure 2.)* Sucking an electric outlet accounts for only 1.8% of these burns. Worn insulation on cords may contribute to the incidence of such injuries.

Lip burns most commonly occur when an arc is formed between two wires and the child's electrolytic saliva conducts the electricity. The saliva rapidly is heated by the current source and a burn occurs. These injuries are local in nature and have no systemic involvement. Such injuries are characterized by local tissue destruction and hemorrhage that may occur 5-10 days following the accident. They may be associated with lip contractures bony injury, dental injury, and delayed bleeding from the labial artery. An electric burn of the lip should be managed by a surgeon familiar with this injury. The family of any child who is discharged should be counseled about the possibility of and care for hemorrhage within 5-10 days of discharge. Discharged children should have a scheduled follow-up.

Flexor Crease. Flexor crease burns may occur across any joint whenever the current produces tetanic contractions of the adjacent muscles. The contractions put the joint in extreme flexion, and this forces the skin from either side of the joint into close proximity. The close apposition allows current to travel from one skin surface to the other, burning both. Flexor crease burns commonly are seen when the hand becomes stuck to an electrical source and tetanic muscle contractions cause the elbow to flex, forming electric current arcs from the forearm to the biceps.

Figure 1. Electrical Entry/Exit Burn

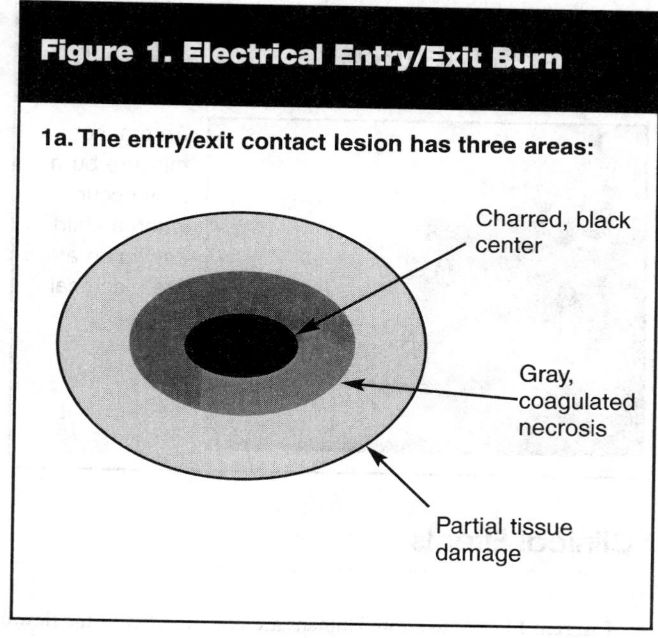

Arc Burns

The second potential effect from an electrical injury is the arc burn, which results from the external passage of high voltage current. This spark consists of ionized, heated plasma with temperatures from 5000-20,000°C and arcs about one inch for each 10,000 volts. It is the arc burn that causes the charred, central portion of the electrical injury with high voltages. The severity of the surface burns will depend upon the proximity of the skin to the arc. Arc burns may be seen at both entry and exit points if very high voltage is involved.

Arc burns usually do not result from household voltage (even with 220 volts) because the arc formed is so small.[15] Arc burns are, therefore, not a significant component of household burns.

Faraday Effect. Very high-frequency, alternating current tends to flow on the outside of a conductor rather than through the conductor. This phenomenon was first described by Michael Faraday and is now called the Faraday effect. This effect means that little deep tissue effects are found with radio frequency electrical currents. Indeed, instructors demonstrate the Faraday effect using very high-frequency, high-voltage current in science museums and physics classes on a daily basis.

Thermal Burns

The exceedingly hot plasma arc also can ignite flammable materials such as clothing. This creates the third type of local burn effect, the thermal burn. Thermal burns should be treated in conjunction with the local burn unit or burn surgeon.

Figure 2. Lip Burn

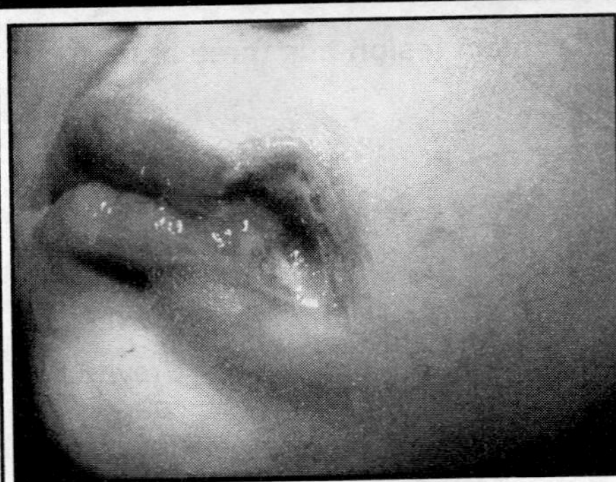

An oral commissure burn may occur when a child chews on a live electrical cord.

Clinical Effects

Current Flow Sensation. Humans are very sensitive to the flow of electric current. The most sensitive organ is the tongue, where the first sensations are detected at only 45 microamperes. When 60-cycle current is passed through the body, an unpleasant tingling sensation is felt at about 1.1 milliamperes current flow. Direct current requires substantially more current to be detected and is felt as increasing warmth.

Muscular Contraction. With increasing flow of alternating current, the unpleasant tingling sensation soon is replaced by muscular contractions. As a sufficiently high level of alternating current is reached, the subject is no longer able to release a grasp on the conductor (the "let go current").

This tetanizing effect on muscles is most pronounced in frequencies from 15-150 cycles per second. The strong muscle contractions cause frequent and well-documented fractures and dislocations, particularly bilateral scapular fractures and shoulder dislocations. As the frequency increases above 150 cycles per second, the tetanizing effects fall off and are not noted above 500,000 cycles per second.[16]

Since direct current does not change polarity, there is no tetany. Direct current does not have a "let-go" threshold, it produces continuous muscle contractions and heat sensations. The abrupt exposure to direct current may cause a muscle contraction that may throw the victim back some distance.

Cardiovascular and Respiratory Effects. Most of the mortality involved in electrical injuries, whether from high- or low-tension lines, is due to cardiovascular and respiratory effects. When the current path crosses either the respiratory center or the heart, then either respiration or the heart may be affected. The path the current takes through the body is a major determinant of morbidity and mortality but it is very difficult to predict. When high voltages travel hand-to-hand, traversing the chest, mortality may be as high as 60%. The mortality associated with high voltages passing hand-to-foot and foot-to-foot is approximately 20% and 5%, respectively.

Many mechanisms have been proposed to account for the myocardial and conducting tissue damage seen in electrical injury. These include the induction of coronary artery spasm, direct thermal injury, ischemia secondary to arrhythmia-induced hypotension, chemoreceptor stimulation producing acute hypertension, catecholamine-mediated injuries, and coronary artery ischemia as part of a generalized vascular injury.[17]

As many as one-third of patients with significant electrical injury may have some significant cardiac component. The shock produces ventricular fibrillation with alternating current and asystole with direct current. If the respiratory center is involved, a respiratory arrest may be produced. Indeed, early research on cardiopulmonary resuscitation was motivated by the effects of electrical current on the heart and respiratory system and funded by the electrical utility companies.

Ventricular fibrillation is the most common cause of death in both high and low voltage electrical injuries.[18]

Multiple experimental studies show AC to be more dangerous to the heart than DC.[19] These animal studies consistently showed that DC injury is less hazardous and produces fewer arrhythmias, myocardial infarctions, and lethalities. One researcher felt that the type of irregularity is related to the current density to which the heart is exposed.[20] At current density up to 25 mA, the cardiac rhythm is unchanged. At about 25-75 mA, the heart stops momentarily and resumes an irregular heart beat. At around 75-100 mA, ventricular fibrillation develops and persists unless stopped by defibrillation. Beyond 4 A, the heart locks in spasm, but resumes a normal beat provided the current is discontinued before ischemic damage. *(Please see Table 2.)*

Additional studies on the effects of frequency on the ventricular fibrillation threshold in animals show that the greatest hazard occurs at about 50-60 cycles—the frequency of power lines.[21]

It should be emphasized that these currents are surface currents. With a low-resistance conductor in the heart, alternating current "leakage" into the system would be dangerous in an amount that is a hundred times less than that required to produce fibrillation via surface electrodes. The increased danger of electrodes directly on the heart has been recognized for many years.[22]

The respiratory arrest often persists after the patient's ventricular fibrillation has been corrected. Ventilation must be continued until the patient has spontaneous respirations.

Electrocardiogram (ECG) findings are usually that of a diffuse coronary ischemia. The electrical injury often does not correlate well with standard patterns of ischemia, since the injury may not follow the coronary vessels. Posterior myocardial injury is a frequent ECG finding of ischemia, however.

Electrical injury may lead to long-term disease of conducting tissue or myocardial damage.[23] Subtle abnormalities, particularly of sinus node function, may pose diagnostic difficulties and may not present for many years. Long-term follow-up of patients with serious electrical burns may help to define the clinical spectrum of cardiac presentations of electrical injury.

Central Nervous System Effects. Central nervous system (CNS) dysfunction is a prominent feature of high-tension electrical injuries. Both acute and delayed central and peripheral neurologic effects have been described.

Acute CNS complications include respiratory arrest, seizures, mental status changes, coma, amnesia, quadriplegia, and localized paresis. Motor deficits appear to occur more frequently than sensory losses. If the current passes through the skull, coagulation of the brain parenchyma, epidural and subdural hematomas, and intraventricular hemorrhages may occur.

Peripheral nerve injury may result from the direct heating effects of the passage of current through the nerves or vascular damage from the current. Compartment syndromes, as discussed below, frequently compress nerves and cause subsequent peripheral neuropathy.

Unusual manifestations of electrical injury are delayed neurologic complications. These delayed complications include ascending paralysis, transverse myelitis, and amyotrophic lateral sclerosis. Mechanisms of these late manifestations are unclear and the prognosis for recovery after development of late complications is not good.[15]

Renal Injuries. The renal manifestations found in electrical injuries are similar to those found in crush injuries. Electrical injuries are associated with a higher incidence of renal failure than burns. Myoglobinuria occurs frequently and is proportional to the amount of muscle damaged by the electric current. As a direct toxin to the kidney, myoglobin causes acute renal failure.

Vascular Injuries. Vascular injuries fall into two broad categories: those due to the passage of the current and those due to the damage to the surrounding tissue.

Compartment Syndrome. The loss of intravascular fluid into an extremity damaged by high current flow results in marked swelling of the contents of the relatively inelastic fascial compartments. The fascial investments limit the amount of swelling with a resultant rising of the interstitial pressure and a consequent reduction of capillary perfusion pressure. The consequences of the decrease in capillary perfusion are tissue hypoxia, resultant increased capillary permeability, and extravasation of further fluid. This vicious cycle results in increased interstitial pressure of the compartment.

Since this is primarily an ischemic phenomenon due to damage to the surrounding tissues, it is potentially a reversible injury. After six hours of this cycle, however, the muscle damage is usually irreversible.[16] The compartment syndrome can be recognized by the classic symptoms of peripheral vascular disease: pain, pallor, paresis, and pulselessness. The most consistent finding is deep diffuse pain that is out of proportion to the purported injury. This may be difficult to assess in child with an electrical injury. Passive movement of the extremity frequently intensifies the pain and may be an early indication. Absent pulses, capillary refill, and pallor are late signs of a compartment syndrome.

In a flame burn or an electrical burn with a component of thermal injury, these diagnostic signs may be difficult to apply because the leathery eschar may render the skin insensitive. The treatment of both flame burns and electrical injuries with potential compartment syndromes is identical. Escharotomy and possibly fasciotomy is indicated early to ensure salvage of the ischemic limb. Any conservation of tissue in the burned upper extremity is of great significance in reconstruction. Hand and digital escharotomy, in particular, reduces the frequency of phalangeal losses.[17,24]

Another complication of the compartment syndrome is a consequence of the necrosis of muscle by ischemia. The resulting breakdown of muscle releases CPK and myoglobin. The results are indistinguishable from the muscle injury due to primary electrical burn of the muscle.

Myoglobinuria can be treated with an initial bolus of 25 gm of mannitol in the adult or 0.5-1 g/kg in the child. This bolus should be followed with a drip of 0.5 g/kg/h. Fluid resuscitation *must* be assured when using this drug. Acidosis should be corrected with bicarbonate and is best guided with arterial blood gases.

Direct Vascular Trauma. Because blood vessels are basically pipes carrying electrolytes, they carry electricity efficiently. Electrical energy tends to flow along blood vessels and may cause severe injury. The veins tend to thrombose first because they are low flow and do not dissipate heat as well as the higher flow arterial pathways. The resulting flow into an extremity without outflow provides rapid swelling, capillary damage, and subsequent compartment syndrome.

Table 2. Effects of Various Current Densities

CURRENT DENSITY	EFFECTS
1 mA	Threshold of perception
5 mA	Accepted as maximum harmless current
10-20 mA	"Let go current"
50 mA	Pain, fainting, exhaustion, and mechanical injury. Heart and respiratory function are normal
100-300 mA	Ventricular fibrillation threshold
300 mA-4 A	Sustained myocardial contraction followed by a normal cardiac rhythm or ventricular fibrillation. Ventricular fibrillation is common. Respiratory paralysis occurs and is temporary. Burns may result if current density is high.

Other Complications. *Cataracts.* In electrical injuries involving the head and neck, the delayed development of cataracts is not uncommon. Cataracts caused by electric injury often occur 4-6 months after the accident and usually are associated with a point of contact near the affected eye. Those at highest risk are patients who have been exposed to greater than 1000 volts and those with injuries about the head or neck.[25] The incidence in these patients is between 5% and 20%. Ophthalmologic referral and long-term follow-up is indicated in all high-voltage injuries of the upper chest, neck, and head.

Abdominal Injury. A wide spectrum of intra-abdominal complications have been reported following high-voltage electrical injury. These injuries may result from either the passage of electrical current through the abdominal viscera or vessels supplying it or through direct injury to the intra-abdominal structures from an entry or exit point. Nausea, vomiting, and adynamic ileus are seen in up to 25% of electrical injuries. Stress ulcer (Curling's burn ulcer) is frequently reported in conjunction with severe electrical injuries. Injuries to the pancreas, gallbladder, and intestines all have been reported in association with major electrical burns.[26] Bowel injuries are particularly troublesome, because ascertaining viability of tissue is often difficult. Both wound and bowel anastomoses have a high frequency of dehiscence after electrical injuries.[27]

Fractures and Bone Complications. Patients with an electrical injury must be inspected for fractures and dislocations caused by severe muscle contractions. Falls after the shock also may be associated with fractures.

The high resistance of bone to the passage of the electrical current may result in local bone destruction that is difficult to diagnose at the time of initial debridement of the wound. Long-term complications of bony areas are common and should be suspected.

Infection. Infection secondary to tissue necrosis is a common complication of the electrical injury and may be the most common cause of death in those who survive the initial resuscitation period. With the large amounts of necrotic tissue found with major electrical injury, patients are at increased risk for clostridial infections to include both gas gangrene and tetanus. Topical antibiotics rarely penetrate sufficiently and debridement is preferable. A burn surgeon should be consulted prior to administration of any antibiotics for prophylaxis. Tetanus prophylaxis should not be overlooked.

Pregnancy and Electrical Shock. Management of the pregnant woman following an accidental electric shock should address the well-being of both the mother and the fetus. Multiple prior case reports have noted that electrical shock to the mother is likely to be fatal to the fetus in as many as 76% of shocks.[28] These were case reports and, thus, biased to more severe injury. Interestingly, the only prospective cohort study of electric shock injury in pregnancy noted that low-voltage injuries are unlikely to damage the fetus.[29] In their study of 31 patients, there were only two miscarriages following electric shock, well within the expected number for that many pregnancies. The authors hypothesize that prior studies suffered from substantial reporting bias.

A potential concern for the pregnant woman in what looks like a trivial electric shock is the remote possibility of late cardiac arrhythmia. An electrocardiogram should be done in any woman who has had an electric shock of greater than 220 volts and probably any time if she was wet or had tetany or if a current pathway that crossed the heart. Cardiac monitoring for 24 hours should be done in any woman with an abnormal initial electrocardiogram or with a history of loss of consciousness or any cardiovascular symptoms. To detect fetal movement and assure that the fetus is still alive, fetal heart Doppler monitoring should be done after the electric shock.

Prehospital Management

The most important factor in the prehospital management of the electrical injury is the safety of the rescuer. If the injury occurs because a child is playing with a power socket, there is usually no danger to the rescuer. Likewise, when an electrical appliance has contacted water, it only needs to be unplugged. The dangerous situation for the rescuer occurs when high-voltage power lines are involved in the accident. If the power line is intact, this is not usually a problem. If the power line is down, there has been an accident, or the current source is still active, then the rescuer needs special equipment and training. If circuit breakers are readily available, these should be shut down.

Numerous items have been advocated for removal of downed power lines including brooms, ropes, sticks, and tree branches. All of these techniques are hazardous. Special-purpose electrical gloves, if tested and kept in good condition, will allow handling of the downed power line. Unfortunately, gloves that are not inspected and sealed prior to use may have unacceptably dangerous current leaks. "Hot sticks" and polypropylene throw lines are somewhat safer when dry but also conduct well when wet. None of these techniques is safe when dealing with the very high-tension line. The safest technique is to allow the electric utility company to remove the downed power line. This may mean leaving a victim until the utility company can respond.

Victims in cars, trains, and buses pose a special circumstance. They are actually safe and should be advised to stay where they are, unless there is another reason, such as fire, which forces an evacuation.

As soon as the patient has been removed from the current source, the ABCs assume priority. Oxygenation, cardiopulmonary resuscitation, and intubation remain the mainstays of care. Arrhythmias will respond to the same medications as for any medical emergency. Cervical spine immobilization is indicated if there is any suspicion of cervical injury by either mechanism of injury or findings. The EMS provider should always presume cervical injury in the unconscious patient with an electrical injury.

Since cardiac and vascular injuries are so common in the major electrical burn, these patients should be carefully monitored in the field. Pulses and capillary refill should be checked in all extremities, documented, and repeated at frequent intervals. Cardiac monitoring is essential for all patients with major electrical injuries.

Fluid requirements in the major electrical burn are often far greater than the surface burns would indicate. Large-bore intravenous lines should be started in at least two locations. Access should be avoided in extremities which have entrance or exit points, if possible. Slowly developing vascular thrombosis will render intravenous lines in involved extremities worthless. Either Ringer's lactate or normal saline is appropriate for an intravenous solution.

The major electrical burn victim should be transported by the most expeditious means available to the closest facility able to handle the special problems of the electrical injury. Any patient with a serious electrical injury should be sent to a burn center that is equipped to handle the major, multiple systems injuries involved. These centers also usually have integral physical and occupational therapy and can manage the patient who may require amputations and subsequent therapy and counseling.

Minor electrical injuries can be safely transported to the closest medical facility that is equipped to deal with the child. These patients should have electrocardiographic monitoring during transport. An intravenous line is discretionary. Cervical immobilization is not usually necessary unless there has been a loss of consciousness.

Emergency Management

Hopefully, the diagnosis of an electrical injury will be obvious. In suspected cases, with unconscious patients, a careful examination of the patient's body may show characteristic burns of exit and entry wounds. Kissing burns of the flexor creases at the wrist, elbow, or axilla may help affirm the diagnosis. The palmar surface of the hands and fingers and the mouth are the most likely site for entrance wounds in toddlers. In older children, scalp wounds may be involved. In rare cases, a history of finding the patient in a tub or shower with an electric appliance with the patient may give the diagnosis.

High-Voltage Injuries. The high-voltage injury is an infrequent event with substantial morbidity and mortality. Upon arrival at the ED, the patient's cardiac and respiratory status should be reassessed and corrected as needed. *(See Table 3.)* The estimated voltages involved, contact times, and prior medical illnesses, history, and allergies should all be ascertained. The patient should be carefully examined for other actual and potential injuries.

Because many patients will be persistently apneic, the patient should be ventilated with high-flow oxygen and intubation strongly considered. The cervical spine should be immobilized prior to intubation.

An abnormal neurologic status may result from intracerebral hemorrhage, blunt injury, vascular spasm, hemorrhage, electrical effects, or thermal injury to the brain. Deterioration of the level of consciousness should prompt evaluation for an intracranial injury and rapid cranial computed tomography scanning.

Radiography of the cervical spine and skull should be considered in those patients who have sustained falls or cranial burns. A chest x-ray is useful as a baseline. Other specific x-rays are indicated in those with complaints or findings of fracture or dislocation.

If not already in place, two large-bore intravenous lines should be started in uninvolved extremities. Blood should be drawn for arterial blood gases, complete blood count, electrolytes, blood sugar, creatinine, blood urea nitrogen, CPK, prothrombin time, partial thromboplastin time, calcium, uric acid, and phosphates at a minimum.[30-32] A type and crossmatch of blood should be considered in all high voltage electrical injuries. A Foley catheter should be inserted and urine sent for analysis and myoglobin determination.

After the ABCs are assured, a complete physical survey to evaluate the extent of injuries should be done. The wounds and associated fractures and dislocations should be managed with usual techniques. Neurologic deficits should be recorded and peripheral pulses confirmed with Doppler flow techniques.

Fluid Replacement. Fluid replacement is essential and adequate rates are far more difficult to estimate than with the thermal injury. A crystalloid challenge of 20- 40 mL/kg is an appropriate starting point for fluid replacement. Fluid losses are greatest in the first 24 hours, and urine output and vascular pressure monitoring should be used as a guide for fluid replacements in all major electrical injuries. Urine output should be maintained at about 0.5 to 1.5 mL/kg/hr. Serial measurements of the hematocrit and electrolytes may aid in estimation of the fluid requirements.

As previously noted, hypovolemia, combined with myoglobinuria, will lead quickly to an acute tubular necrosis. Hypovolemia may be quite pronounced in these patients due to the large masses of tissue damaged. Intravenous bicarbonate to alkalinize the urine may be used based upon appropriate urine and blood pH measurements. A blood pH below 7.2 should mandate sodium bicarbonate administration to correct the pH in the electrically injured patient.

Debridement. Debridement is best done by the burn surgeon who is going to manage the patient on a long-term basis. Muscle debridement is particularly difficult because the current flow is often not uniform and leaves spotty areas of necrosis within muscles. Amputation and repair of damage should be left to the burn specialist.

Remember that the compartment syndrome is far advanced when the examiner waits for signs of pulselessness. Measurement of compartment pressures and prompt fasciotomy for decompression are the mainstays of therapy in this common complication of electrical injuries. Fasciotomy and escharotomy should, however, be performed whenever there is vascular or respiratory compromise; do not wait for a burn surgeon or transfer to a burn unit.

Low-Voltage Injuries. Unlike the extensive coverage in modern medical literature about major injuries, minor electrical injuries have limited coverage in the usual medical text or review article. In one recent exhaustive review totaling some 44 pages, scant attention was paid to the low voltage minor injury. Indeed, when talking about low-voltage injuries the author pointed out that 400-600 volt transportation accidents were defined as low voltage injuries.[33] When injuries with this voltage range are reviewed by other authors, there is indeed substantial morbidity and mortality, enough that the article proposes an intermediate voltage category or redefining high voltage to include 500+ volts.[34]

This emphasis on high-voltage injury is truly referral bias, since the vast bulk of household electrical injuries are neither admitted nor require any surgery. In one series of 145 electrical burns, there were 128 low-voltage injuries admitted.[35] Of these patients, only the patients with high-voltage injuries had any complications beyond 24 hours. All patients with complications had those complications on arrival in the ED. The authors suggest that if there are no cardiac complications on arrival to the ED with a low-voltage injury, then the patient is unlikely to develop any cardiac problems. Other authors echo this feeling that these patients are unlikely to develop other systemic problems.[2,4,5,36-38]

Typical findings are local burns which are limited to points of contact where the current entered or exited the body, and involve mainly distal parts of the limbs or the skull.

An ECG and observation for a few hours should be all that is needed for most minor electrical injuries.[2-5,8] Referral to a burn unit appears to be unnecessary. Obviously, the local injury should dictate the need for consultation and more extensive therapy and evaluation. Lip injuries should be referred to a plastic surgeon, orofacial surgeon, or surgeon familiar with management of this injury.

Tetanus. The burn is a tetanus prone wound and electrical injuries are no exception to this. Tetanus immunization should be ascertained and corrected if needed. Standard tetanus prophylaxis is appropriate.

Laboratory Determinations. The laboratory investigations that are most frequently recommended for evaluation of the electrical injury include CPK, CPK isoenzymes, and urinalysis with measurement of urinary myoglobin

Table 3. Treatment Algorithm for Major Electrical Injuries

PERFORM PRIMARY ASSESSMENT

- Check ABCs
- Establish airway if necessary
- Oxygen
- Ventilate if necessary
- Establish intravenous access
- Give CPR if necessary
- Immobilize cervical spine
- Give fluid resuscitation as needed
- Monitor cardiac function

PERFORM SECONDARY ASSESSMENT

- Order lab tests, x-ray films, and CT scans as indicated by the secondary assessment
- Monitor urine output
- Give tetanus prophylaxis if needed
- Treat specific injuries
- Treat entry/exit wounds and burns

ADMIT PATIENTS WHO HAVE THE FOLLOWING:

- Cardiac arrest
- Major bums or trauma
- ECG abnormalities
- Lip commissure burn
- Loss of consciousness
- Hypoxia
- Myoglobinuria or markedly elevated CPK
- Transthoracic current path
- Exposure to high voltage (> 1000 volts)

Creatinine phosphokinase. Breakdown of the muscle leads to elevated CPK and myoglobin in both serum and urine. Mild elevation of the CPK is quite common in even minor electrical injuries. Markedly elevated CPK reflects the deep muscle damage found with high tension electrical injuries.

In low-voltage burns of children, CPK may be modestly elevated, but this does not usually correlate with any negative outcome or complication.[3] In one study, 16 of 88 (18.1%) had abnormal CPK determinations.[8] Therefore, it could be inferred that a modest elevation in total CPK level is not a diagnostic indicator of muscle injury in the low-voltage electrical burn patient with small surface area burns.

Urinalysis. Urinalysis with determination of the urinary myoglobin is recommended, but multiple studies have shown few abnormalities and none that required therapy in patients with minor electrical injury.[3,8] This is not true for the patient with a high-tension electrical injury or when the patient has been partially immersed in water during the electrical injury.

Local Therapy. Many authorities advocate mafenide acetate (Sulfamylon) as a topical agent in the electrically injured patient due to its greater penetration through the skin.[30,39] If this is not readily available, silver sulfadiazine may be substituted. Metabolic acidosis and pain at the site of application are frequent complications of mafenide acetate. Lip and oral cavity burns should be cleansed and dressed. Splints and tube feedings may be prescribed for some oral electrical burn patients.

The patient's family should be cautioned about the incidence of labial artery bleeding associated with oral electrical burns. The family can be taught the technique of direct pressure for bleeding control. These careful discharge instructions change the whole character of the repeat visit if the child does suffer a delayed bleed.

Admission or Transportation Decisions

The major electrical burn injury is difficult to treat and carries abundant complications and pitfalls. It is, perhaps, the one injury for which the emergency physician should consider rapid stabilization and transport to a specialized burn center to be the most appropriate therapy. Any patient with significant electrical injuries should receive the care offered by trained burn specialists with equally trained supporting staffs.

During transport of these patients, they should be monitored for both cardiac arrhythmias and hemodynamic stability. Unlike the thermal injury, these patients are quite likely to become hypovolemic early in transport. Although airway edema is not potentially as dangerous in the electrical burn, cardiac dysrhythmias and late apnea are more common.

Relatively benign appearing wounds can be associated with life-threatening cardiac arrhythmias, limb-threatening vascular compromise, and acute renal failure secondary to myoglobinuria. These concerns have led to the widespread practice and recommendations for admission of all electrical bums for 24-48 hours of observation, cardiac monitoring, and laboratory evaluation, with no distinction between patients injured by low-voltage vs. high-voltage injury.

Where there is little argument about management of the severe high-tension electrical injury, care of the minor electrical injury is more controversial. There is a growing body of evidence that healthy children with household voltage injuries with a small partial-thickness burn, a normal electrocardiogram, and who have no evidence (over the first few hours) of cardiac or neurovascular injury, do not appear to need hospital admission.[2-5,37]

Other associated injuries may require admission but should be assessed independently. Certainly, the oral low-voltage electrical burn may be successfully managed by many plastic or oral surgeons. Low-voltage injuries rarely cause deep tissue destruction. The smaller, lower voltage isolated wound of an extremity also may be successfully managed by orthopedic, general, or plastic surgeons. Guidelines for these minor burns should be arranged in advance to expedite the care and decisions.

Prevention

There are two dominant themes in pediatric electrical injuries.[40] Household electrical cords are the major hazard for electrical injuries in children younger than 12 years of age. Oral contact was by far the most common etiology in this younger age group. Interestingly enough, most injuries were caused by electrical extension cords. Although many campaigns have focused on wall socket safety, and blank plugs are commonly recommended by pediatricians, wall sockets caused less than half of the injuries that extension cords caused.

Extension cords are found in many households and the digital age has increased the number in use. Emergency physicians could help by encouraging parents to discard old, frayed, and damaged extension cords.

In children older than 12 years of age, greater than 90% are high tension electrical injuries. Most of these were associated with the well-known, risk-taking behaviors of teenagers. Children who climb trees, poles, transformer towers, and high tension line towers can also sustain fractures during falls from these high places, when electrical injuries occur.

Summary

Since the vast majority of electrical injuries are preventable, injury prevention should be paramount. A careful history and physical examination should characterize the injury as high-voltage or low-votage. High-voltage injuries require aggressive resuscitation. The majority of low-voltage injuries require a comprehensive assessment and appropriate care of any tissue injuries.

References

1. Cooper MA. Electrical and lightning injuries. *Emerg Med Clin North Am* 1984;2:489-501.
2. Wilson CM, Fatovich DM. Do children need to be monitored after electric shocks? *J Paediatr Child Health* 1998;34:474-476.
3. Wallace BH, Cone JB, Vanderpool RD, et al. Retrospective evaluation of admission criteria for paediatric electrical injuries. *Burns* 1995;21:590-593.
4. Fatovich DM, Lee KY. Household electric shocks: Who should be monitored? *Med J Aust* 1991;155:301-303.
5. Goodwin CW, Finkelstein JL, Madden MR. Burns. In: Schwartz SI,

Shires GT, Spencer FC, et al, eds. *Principles of Surgery*, 6th ed. New York: McGraw-Hill; 1994:227.

6. Rakel RE, ed. *Textbook of Family Practice*, 4th ed. Philadelphia: Saunders; 1990:978.
7. Hathaway WE, Hay WW, Groothius JR, et al, eds. *Current Pediatric Diagnosis and Treatment*, 11th ed. Norwalk: Appleton and Lange; 1993:270.
8. Zubair M, Besner GE. Pediatric electrical burns: Management strategies. *Burns* 1997;23:413-420.
9. Bailey B, Gaudreault P, Thivierge RL, et al. Cardiac monitoring of children with household electrical injuries. *Ann Emerg Med* 1995; 25:612-617.
10. Robinson M, Seward PN. Electrical and lightning injuries in children. *Pediatr Emerg Care* 1986;2:186.
11. Celikoz B, Sengezer M, Selmanpakoglu N. Four limb amputations due to electrical burn caused by TV antenna contact with overhead electric cables. *Burns* 1997;23:81-84.
12. Garcia CT, Smith GA, Cohen DM, et al. Electrical injuries in a pediatric emergency department. *Ann Emerg Med* 1995;26: 604-608.
13. Baker MD, Chiaviello C. Household electrical injuries in children: Epidemiology and identification of avoidable hazards. *Am J Dis Child* 1989;1:59.
14. Wright RK, Davis JH. The investigation of electrical deaths: A report of 220 fatalities. *J Forensic Sci* 1980;25:514-521.
15. Levine NS, Atkins A, McKeel DW. Spinal cord injury following electrical accidents: Case reports. *J Trauma* 1975;15:549.
16. Stewart CE. Crush Injuries. *Emergency Medicine Reports* 1993;26: 227-236.
17. Salisbury RE, Taylor JW, Levine NS. Evaluation of digital escharotomy in burned hands. *Plast Reconstr Surg* 1976;58:440-443.
18. Sances A, Larson SJ, Myklebust J, et al. Electrical injuries. *Surg Gynecol Obstet* 1979;149:97.
19. Arya KR, Taori GK, Khanna SS. Electrocardiographic manifestations following electrical injury. *Int J Cardiol* 1996;57:100-101.
20. Hughes JBW. Electrical shock and associated injuries. *Br Med J* 1957;1:852-856.
21. Geddes LA, Baker LE. Response to passage of electric current through the body. *J Assoc Advancement Med Instr* 1971;5:13-18.
22. Zoll PM, Linenthal AJ. Long term electric pacemakers for Stokes-Adams disease. *Circulation* 1960;22:341-345.
23. Robinson NMK, Chamberlain DA. Electrical injury to the heart may cause long-term damage to conducting tissue: A hypothesis and review of the literature. *Int J Cardiol* 1996;53:273-277.
24. Salisbury RE, Hunt JL, Warden GD, et al. Management of electrical burns of the upper extremity. *Plast Reconstr Surg* 1973;51:648-652.
25. Portello M, Orlin SE, Kozart DM. Electric cataracts. *Arch Ophthal* 1996;114:1022-1023.
26. Baxter CR. Present concepts in the management of major electrical injury. *Surg Clinic North Am* 1970;50:1401-1418.
27. Goodwin CW, McManus WB, Mason AD Jr, et al. Management of abdominal wounds in thermally injured patients. *J Trauma* 1982;22:92-97.
28. Fish R. Electric shock, Part II, nature and mechanism of injury. *J Emerg Med* 1993;11:457-462.
29. Einarson A, Bailey B, Inocencion G, et al. Accidental electric shock in pregnancy: A prospective cohort study. *Am J Obstet Gynecol* 1997;176:678-681.
30. Yakuboff KP, Kurtzman LC, Stern PJ. Acute management of thermal and electrical burns of the upper extremity. *Orth Clinic NA* 1992;23:161-169.
31. Pawel B. Electrical and lightning injuries. In: Strange GR, Ahrens W, Lelyveld S, et al, eds. *Pediatric Emergency Medicine: A Comprehensive Study Guide*. New York: McGraw-Hill; 1996:609.
32. Dubinsky I. Electrical Injury. In: Rosen P, Barkin RM, Hayden SR, et al, eds. *The 5 Minute Emergency Medicine Consult*. Philadelphia: Lippincott Williams & Wilkins; 1999:358-359.
33. Lee RC. Injury by electrical forces: Pathophysiology, manifestations, and therapy. *Curr Prob Surg* 1997;34:677-764.
34. Rabban J, Adler J, Rosen C, et al. Electrical injury from subway third rails: Serious injury associated with intermediate voltage contact. *Burns* 1997;23:515-518.
35. Arrowsmith J, Usaocar RP, Dickson WA. Electrical injury and the frequency of cardiac complications. *Burns* 1997;23:576-578.
36. Wilson CM, Fatovich DM. Do children need to be monitored after electric shocks. *J Pediatric Child Health* 1998;34:474.
37. Purdue G, Hunt J. Electrocardiographic monitoring after electrical injury: Necessity or luxury. *J. Trauma* 1986;26:166-167.
38. Wallace BH, Cone JB, Vanderpool RD, et al. Retrospective evaluation of admission criteria for paediatric electrical injuries. *Burns* 1995;21:590-593.
39. Rouse RG, Dimick AR. The treatment of electrical injury compared to burn injury: A review of the pathophysiology and comparison of patient management protocols. *J Trauma* 1978;18:43.
40. Rabban JT, Blair JA, Rosen C, et al. Mechanisms of pediatric electrical injury. *Arch Pediatr Adolesc Med* 1997;151:696-700.

Pediatric Submersion Injuries

Charles Stewart, MD, FACEP

Death from submersion incidents is the second leading cause of accidental death in children, with one-third of all survivors sustaining significant neurological damage.[1-3] The exact percentage of the vast number of minor submersion incidents that result in a lethal outcome is controversial. A 1977 study in South Carolina reported that at least 15% of school children had at least one submersion incident during the prior year.[4] With a reported drowning rate of 7.4 per 100,000 in that state, the authors calculated that at least one-half million incidents per year occurred that presented a serious risk of drowning in South Carolina alone. This chapter presents a review of the types of submersion injuries, management strategies, and ways to prevent these occurrences.

Introduction

Every year, drowning claims between 6000 and 8000 people in the United States.[5] Most of these victims are young, under the age of 24.[6] *(See Table 1.)* Drowning is the second largest cause of injury-related death in people of this age group, and it is the third leading cause of death for 1- to 15-year-olds. At all ages, boys will drown three times more often than girls. Most drownings occur within 10 feet of safety, and two-thirds of the victims cannot swim.[7] Boating accidents and floods are other well-known scenarios of drowning.

Adolescents (or parents) using alcohol and drugs not only are at increased risk of drowning themselves, they also increase the risk of those around them.[8] Whether impaired judgment or loss of self-protective reflexes is at fault is moot. The use of other, more illicit drugs is thought to play a relatively major role in drownings, but again, the true incidence is not known.

Since all water-related activities increase with warm weather, the incidence of drownings will naturally increase in warmer climates and weather. Drowning is a problem in all states, including the arid desert states.[9] The most common sites of drownings include home swimming pools, bathtubs, and open bodies of water.

About 6% of drownings may represent child abuse or neglect.[10-12] In one study, as many as 67% of bathtub submersion incidents were found to have a history consistent with abuse or neglect.[13] Bathtubs are the usual site of drowning in children younger than 1 year of age.[14]

Definitions

In order to discuss the circumstances of submersion injuries, a uniform terminology is needed. The following terms are frequently used and have been adapted from Modell and others.[15]

Drowning. Drowning is suffocation by submersion in a fluid, whether or not the fluid is aspirated into the lungs. This is considered the cause of death if the death occurs within 24 hours of the insult.[16]

Near Drowning. Near drowning is survival beyond 24 hours after suffocation by submersion and implies that recovery has

Table 1. Statistical Risk Factors

- Age (40% of victims are younger than 4 years)
- Location (home swimming pools or bathtubs)
- Sex (Boys drown three times more often than girls)
- Drugs (particularly alcohol)
- Trauma (diving or falls)
- Predisposing illnesses (particularly epilepsy)[21-23]
- Warm weather (50% occur between May and August)

occurred after the insult. This may be termed a submersion injury or submersion incident in some of the literature. Note that this definition has been challenged and some feel that near drowning should be redefined as "survival, at least temporarily, after aspiration of fluid into the lungs." These authors feel that aspiration of fluid may lead to complications even without a history of loss of consciousness.[17]

Secondary Drowning. Secondary drowning implies that the victim is initially resuscitated but death occurs minutes to days after the initial resuscitation. The definition of secondary drowning is controversial, and the term probably is inappropriate. This condition also is termed delayed death subsequent to near drowning. Death may result from either the respiratory insult or any other cause. Since the cause of death does not matter in this definition, many of these patients die from severe neurologic dysfunction related to the initial insult. Patients with respiratory causes for secondary drowning usually have clear symptoms of respiratory compromise immediately after submersion.[18]

Immersion Syndrome. The immersion syndrome is a form of drowning caused by sudden exposure to very cold water (< 20°C or 68°F). This may be due to a vagally induced dysrhythmia. The two most commonly proposed arrhythmias are asystole and ventricular fibrillation.[19,20] Ingestion of alcohol and other intoxicants is thought to be a predisposition to this syndrome.

Immersion Hypothermia. Drowning can also result from hypothermia due to prolonged immersion. When the core body temperature reaches about 32-33°C (89.6-91.4°F), the victim will lose purposeful activity. At that point, swimming and other self-protective action ceases, and drowning may occur. If the patient becomes sufficiently hypothermic (e.g., in arctic waters), death may occur from hypothermia alone.

Problems with Definitions. The definitions of near drowning and drowning are, of course, retrospective. There is no prognostic import to any of the definitions. The emergency physician should treat *all* patients as near-drowning casualties, unless there is an obvious injury that is incompatible with life. Only after documented submersion times are greater than 1 hour should the emergency department (ED) consider that the patient is non-resuscitatable. These times may be shortened considerably if the water is warm.

Pathophysiology: Mechanism of Drowning

The sequence of events that follows submersion has been abundantly described in animal studies, providing us with a model of drowning.

Stage I: Panic and Struggle. In most drownings, a period of panic and struggle followed by exhaustion are the initial events.[24] During the 1890s, Brouardel described this as the "stage of surprise" and described it as lasting about 5-10 seconds.[25] Another researcher noted that this stage lasts 20-60 seconds in humans. During this stage, the victim will attempt to reach or remain at the water's surface. Frantic hyperventilation occurs as long as the head can be held above water. Other clues that identify potential drowning victims are an open but not vocalizing mouth and a rolled back (far hyperextended) head. Modell noted that some victims are swimming and calmly become motionless or quietly disappear below the water after diving.[26]

Stage II: Breath Holding. Breath-holding apnea begins with submersion and lasts about 60 seconds. The mouth is shut and respirations voluntarily are stopped.

Stage IIIA: Aspiration. Brouardel also described a stage where agitation ceases, and the victim may swallow water and begin to vomit. Approximately 90% of drowning victims aspirate the water and vomitus, cough violently, and then gasp involuntarily, flooding the lungs and air passages with water.

Stage IIIB: Laryngospasm. The other 10% die of asphyxia thought to be secondary to laryngospasm. No evidence of aspiration is found in these victims. This entity is also called "dry drowning" or "drowning without aspiration." Fluid in the larynx in humans can result in severe and prolonged laryngospasm. This suggests that in humans, breath holding may be followed by laryngospasm of variable duration. Ultimately, of course, asphyxia relaxes the glottis, and the lungs will flood with water. Although only about 15% of victims fit into this category, 90% of the successfully resuscitated patients come from this subset.

Stage IV: Respiratory Arrest. Brouardel then described the "second stage of respiratory arrest" where no thoracic movements occurred and the animals became unconscious.

Stage V: Agonal Movements and Death. Agonal respiratory movements, cardiac arrest, and death then ensue in both types of drowning.

Mitigating Circumstances

There are several exceptions to this sequence of events:

Hypothermia. In very cold water, as noted previously, hypothermia may rapidly disable a victim, and little or no exhaustion, panic, or struggle may occur before the victim ceases to swim and aspirates water.

Unconsciousness. Events that render the victim unconscious, such as use of drugs or alcohol, seizures, or head trauma will also prevent a struggle and exhaustion prior to aspiration.[27-30] Divers who sustain neck injuries may be conscious but unable to resurface. Children with seizure disorders have a far greater risk of drowning, particularly in a bathtub, when compared with children without seizure disorders.[31]

Voluntary Hyperventilation. Another cause is hyperventilation prior to swimming underwater. By hyperventilation, swimmers can rapidly lower their $PaCO_2$ to 20 mmHg, but the PaO_2 will be only modestly increased. As the victim exercises, his $PaCO_2$ will return to between 40 and 47 mmHg, which is not sufficient to trigger the urge to breathe. Simultaneously, the PaO_2 will fall to 30-40 mmHg, causing unconsciousness, with subsequent drowning.[32,33]

Rapidly Moving Water. It is unknown whether the same struggles take place in rapidly moving water. It is conceivable that the force of the moving water and objects struck underwater may cause rapid loss of consciousness due to trauma. In surf and in mountain streams, both drowning and near drowning often are associated with physical evidence of multiple trauma.

Type of Aspirated Fluid

Aspiration of even small quantities of fluid can lead to a drastic change in PO_2. The differentiation between aspiration of salt or fresh water is often emphasized in some medical texts, but the presence of contaminants (i.e., silt, mud, sewage, bacteria, and diatoms) is probably of more consequence in actual practice. Aspiration of acidic stomach contents and other debris (i.e., sewage, sand, mud, diatoms, or algae) profoundly contribute to the pulmonary injury and the development of aspiration chemical pneumonitis.

Theoretically, there should be electrolyte and blood volume differences between fresh and salt-water submersion victims if a significant amount of fluid has been aspirated. Few survivors of submersion incidents aspirate enough water to cause any significant changes in either blood volume or serum electrolytes. Experimental studies show that if less than 20 mL/kg of body weight is aspirated, no life-threatening electrolyte abnormalities occur, and at least 11 mL/kg is necessary to cause changes in blood volume. This means that a 20 kg child must aspirate 400 mL of solution in order to have significant electrolyte disturbances. Although the lungs can hold far more than that, most adults have somewhat less than 150 mL of solution in the lungs at the time of death by drowning. The main reason for the lower volume of aspiration in human vs. animal studies appears to be the previously described laryngospasm that is induced in humans by fluid in the posterior pharynx.

Clinical information on submersion patients indicates that there is no significant difference in serum electrolytes and hematocrit values among fresh, salt, and brackish water aspiration. Following fresh and salt-water submersion in experimental models, the ultrastructure and light microscopy findings of the lungs are remarkably similar.

Profound electrolyte changes can be found in Dead Sea submersion victims, even with aspiration of only modest amounts of fluid.[34] One might expect similar results for submersion victims from the Great Salt Lake, but no cases have been reported in the literature. Hypernatremia from seawater ingestion is thought to be due to swallowed water rather than aspiration.[35]

There are important differences in aspiration of fresh and seawater that do not involve electrolyte imbalance, however. Aspiration of seawater is twice as lethal as fresh water per unit volume because of the impurities and bacteria it contains. Seawater contains more than 20 known pathogenic bacteria, including *Pseudomonas putrefaciens*, *Staphylococcus aureus*, and *Vibrio parahaemolyticus*.[36]

Salt water also appears to produce a larger direct insult to the lung than fresh water.[37] When a significant amount of seawater is aspirated, the salt diffuses into the blood, with rapid elevation of the plasma sodium. Osmotic forces pull protein-rich fluid from the circulation into the pulmonary interstitium. The result is a fulminant pulmonary edema with direct parenchymal damage. With salt-water aspiration, hypovolemia may develop, especially if a large volume of water has been swallowed.

Immediate Sequelae of Aspiration

The most important abnormality from a submersion incident is a profound hypoxemia resulting from asphyxia. The immediate effect of asphyxia is a rapidly decreasing arterial PO_2 with a concomitant increase in the pCO_2 that leads to a combined respiratory and metabolic acidosis. The sequelae of this hypoxia may affect the brain, heart, and kidneys.

As previously noted, about 15% of patients have asphyxia from the laryngospasm without significant aspiration at the time of resuscitation. These patients rapidly recover from asphyxia if they are successfully resuscitated before cardiac arrest or irreversible brain damage occurs.

Aspiration of as little as 1-3 mL of fluid per kg of body weight results in persistently abnormal pulmonary functions from a combination of several mechanisms. *(See Table 2.)* Immediate vagal reflexes cause pulmonary vasoconstriction and a pulmonary hypertension after the aspiration of the fluid. Passage of water through the alveolar epithelium, the basement membrane, and the endothelial capillary lining causes a rapid disruption of the pulmonary ultrastructure.[38,39] Loss or inactivation of pulmonary surfactant causes an alveolar collapse, with a subsequent decrease in pulmonary compliance.

This combination of mechanisms results in increased membrane permeability, exudation of proteinaceous material into the alveoli, and pulmonary edema. The other result of these mechanisms is a profound ventilation/perfusion mismatch and subsequent hypoxemia. These abnormalities cause a rapid elevation of the $PaCO_2$ and a fall of the PaO_2.

Hypothermia

Hypothermia is a more frequent cause of death in the water than formerly realized. When the Titanic sank in 1°C water, 1500 people died within 90 minutes, yet there were ample life preservers to go around.[40] Unconsciousness occurs when the core body temperature reaches about 32-33°C (89.6-91.4°F); in the water, swimming efforts cease, and the unprotected person will drown.

In cold water, hypothermia will develop in a short time in unprotected adults.[41] If the water is not only cold, but also moving quickly, hypothermia may develop at an incredibly rapid rate. A child's temperature drops even more quickly because of the relatively large surface-area-to-mass ratio and the lack of subcutaneous fatty insulation.

Studies on human subjects in cold water (as low as 4.5°C or 40.1°F) show that the maximum heat loss occurs from the head, the neck, the sides of the chest, and the groin.[42] Swimming and other motion enhances this loss, increasing the risk of hypothermia.

Since movement enhances the cooling process, the better swimmers often die first because they are more likely to try to tread water or swim rather than just float. Likewise "drown proofing," a technique of bobbing in the water, will markedly increase the heat loss as water circulates about the head. Based upon these studies, a heat escape lessening posture (the HELP position) was devised in which the victim draws the knees up close to the chest, presses the arms to the sides, and remains as quiet as possible. For three or more persons, huddling quietly and closely together will decrease the heat loss from the groin and front areas of the body.

Detrimental Effects. Hypothermia presents a therapeutic dilemma in the management of the near-drowning victim. On one hand, the

Table 2. Potential Consequences of Aspiration of Fluids

- Pulmonary edema
- Increasing shunt
- Direct toxicity of aspirated fluid
- Washout of surfactant
- Inactivation of surfactant
- Direct alveolar membrane injury

cardiovascular complications of hypothermia include hypotension, bradycardia, conduction deficits, and ventricular fibrillation. Electrical defibrillation of the heart is difficult at low core body temperatures. Drugs, such as antiarrhythmics and insulin, may be ineffective and accumulate, reaching toxic levels due to the slowed metabolism and excretion.

Protective Effects. On the other hand, it should be emphasized that the development of hypothermia prior to the final anoxic insult protects the brain for a considerable period following a cardiopulmonary arrest. The combination of hypothermia (no matter what means of induction) and the diving reflex probably plays a major role in salvage after prolonged submersion.

The development of hypothermia protects the brain by decreasing metabolic demands and slowing the development of cerebral hypoxia. This process has been confirmed by extensive clinical experience in cardiovascular surgery. Since the late 1950s, physicians have been extending cerebral hypoxic survival times for neurosurgical and cardiovascular procedures by profound hypothermia. Of course, the submersion victim is not a well-controlled, well-oxygenated operative patient.

To protect the brain from hypoxic damage, it is necessary to cool the brain very rapidly, at least 7°C in 10 minutes. This rate of cooling will double survival times during cerebral hypoxia.[43] Unfortunately, surface cooling rates associated with immersion are too slow to cool the brain sufficiently to protect it from anoxia caused by drowning, even in children. If cerebral hypoxia is the mechanism for survival in protracted submersion, then an alternative metabolic method of rapid brain cooling must be evoked.

The Diving Reflex

The diving reflex is found in all mammals and consists of bradycardia, profound systemic vasoconstriction, and suppression of respiratory activity.

The diving reflex is evoked by the presence of cold water on the victim's face or nose. Anxiety and very cold water enhance the response. A "dry" suit that prevents rapid cooling of the cutaneous thermal receptors but leaves the face exposed to the environment also enhances it.[44-46]

The diving reflex plays a powerful role in oxygen conservation in diving animals and allows some to remain submerged for as long as 30 minutes. The inhibition of respirations apparently continues until the brain shuts down due to hypoxia. The reflex is strongest in young animals and with colder water. It is present but not particularly strong in adult humans. The diving reflex, which is most active in infants and small children, may drop a child's heart rate to about 8-10 beats per minute, while core body temperature rapidly falls to about 28-30°C (82.4-86°F).

Aspiration of Water. Recent canine studies suggest that swallowing and aspiration of icy water will enhance the cooling rate.[47,48] Indeed, this aspiration of cold water and rapid induction of hypothermia may play a role in cases where preservation of neurologic function occurs despite prolonged anoxia.

It should be emphasized that the simultaneous onset of anoxia with hypothermia carries a less favorable prognosis than when the hypothermia precedes the anoxia. When cardiac arrest finally occurs, there may be only an additional 10- to 15-minute period before the brain is irreversibly damaged in the anoxic hypothermic patient. Even with this understanding, the prolonged periods of submersion that have a subsequent good outcome and total recovery are not quite so miraculous as they appear.

Studies of submersion victims in warmer climates show lower survival and higher morbidity. This is probably due to the loss of protective reflexes and protective hypothermia. The difference is so marked that practitioners who see warm-water submersion patients from the Southern states have an entirely different outlook on this disease than Northerners who deal with cold-water submersion victims. Indeed, the worst outcome appears to be in victims of hot tub submersion incidents.

Emergency Management: Rescue and Initial Resuscitation

Submersion Times. Time is crucial in the management of the submersion victim. Full neurologic recovery is not likely if the victim has been submerged for longer than 30 minutes in cold, fresh water or longer than 15 minutes in warm, fresh water. In hot springs and hot tubs, successful resuscitations are unlikely after even shorter times.[49] In very cold water, victims of submersion have had documented survival times of up to 66 minutes with little or no neurologic deficit.[50]

Submersion time is often inaccurate and should serve only as a rough estimate. The emotional excitement at the time of submersion is so intense that few observers are able to reliably document the duration of submersion. Unless the immersion time exceeds 1 hour in cold water and is unquestionably documented, it is best to attempt resuscitation on all victims. The times at which rescuers were called and help arrived are often known, and in extreme cases, may be used to approximate the submersion time.

Rescue. The attempt to rescue a drowning child has claimed many a rescuer's life. Although a poor swimmer or untrained rescuer should not attempt an in-water rescue, most victims are well within reach of a moderately trained rescuer. The American Red Cross and the YMCA provide abundant courses in proper water rescue techniques for simple water rescue. This material is easily available, and thus, will not be repeated here. Complex water rescue, such as at the foot of dams and in floodwaters, is well beyond the scope of this article.

Mechanisms of Injury

All patients who are involved in boating accidents; fall into rapidly moving water, rapids, or surf; fall from a height greater than 10 feet; or are involved in head-first diving accidents should be considered to have multiple trauma and potential cervical spine injuries.[51] The easiest and quickest splint that can be used for these critical submersion victims is the long backboard. No time should be wasted in meticulous splinting techniques for the patient who is not breathing or who is in respiratory distress from a submersion injury. Likewise, the patient should not be subjected to any movement without appropriate cervical splinting precautions. Once on shore, the long backboard will provide a surface suitable for CPR if needed.

Injuries are likely in rapidly moving water, falls from heights into the water, and ice rescues. Fractures to the lower extremities are more likely in ice accidents and falls from a height, but spinal injuries are common with any head-first entrance into water. Falls into fast-moving water may have any combination of injuries, as the victim may tumble and smash into rocks and other debris. Cervical spine precautions should be taken for all of these patients.

Airway Maneuvers. Since the primary mechanism of injury for this disease is hypoxia, maneuvers to restore ventilation are of paramount importance. If the victim is apneic, mouth-to-mouth breathing should be initiated as soon as possible. It can be started as soon as the patient can be placed on a flotation device or the rescuer can stand. If neck injury is suspected, the head-tilt method should not be used, as it markedly flexes the neck. Use of the jaw-thrust method of airway management will give better protection for the cervical spine and should open the airway sufficiently.

Except for placing the victim in a relatively head down position, most clinicians do not recommend maneuvers designed to expel water from the chest.[52,53] Because of the higher rate of complications from seawater aspiration, some authors advocate postural maneuvers for draining seawater out of the lungs but never at the expense of expeditious CPR.

There are no data to support the use of a Heimlich maneuver in a submersion victim who does not have a particulate matter foreign body obstruction.[54,55] Care must be taken to prevent aspiration of gastric contents since vomiting is very common with this maneuver.

It is imperative that no time be wasted with this or other maneuvers. Since animal studies and human post-mortem studies show that most victims do not aspirate significant amounts of liquid, the overall clinical significance of this or any other maneuver designed to "clear the water out of the lungs" is open to many questions.

Suction. Suction equipment must be available since many of these patients will vomit, which may result in aspiration. If vomiting occurs or seems imminent, the lateral decubitus position is recommended. Early intubation of the patient will protect the patient from further aspiration and allow both suctioning and administration of high-flow oxygen.

Supplemental Oxygen. Supplemental oxygen is a mainstay in the prehospital care of the near-drowning victim. Early efforts should include 100% oxygen, which should be administered immediately by bag-valve-mask, and followed by rapid intubation in the unconscious patient. Field intubation techniques should be modified to protect the spine if trauma is suspected.

Cardiopulmonary Resuscitation. Immediate and adequate resuscitation is of paramount importance and is the single most important factor influencing survival. The immediate actions of the primary responder have the potential to significantly affect the outcome for the near-drowning victim.

If the patient has no pulse or is not breathing, CPR should be initiated. It is difficult to provide effective chest compressions while the patient is still in the water, but ventilations can be instituted immediately. The patient may be extricated from the water on a backboard or a Stokes' basket litter. Chest compression may be started as soon as the backboard can be supported. Initial advanced cardiac life support (ACLS) measures do not otherwise differ from those used in other patients.

Post-Resuscitation Management. If the patient responds to initial management, oxygen must be started at high flow with a non-rebreathing facemask. An intravenous line should be started if available and within the rescuer's ability and training. Wet clothing should be removed, if possible, and the patient covered with blankets. Constant attention should be paid to vital signs, the potential of vomiting, and the possibility of deterioration of the patient during transport. Potential problems include pulmonary edema and shock from associated trauma. The potential for cervical spine trauma in diving accidents cannot be overemphasized.

Emergency Department Management

Initial management of the victim in the ED involves three priorities: 1) assessment of the ABCs; 2) treatment of the hypoxia; and 3) protection of the cervical spine.

Assessment of the ABCs. Airway management and restoration of ventilation and circulation are the first priority tasks. These tasks should not be delayed in an ED to drain the lungs of fluid. As noted above, most patients aspirate only small quantities of fluid. Better survival is found with rapid restoration of ventilation and circulation.

If the patient is not receiving 100% oxygen, this should be instituted immediately, followed by rapid intubation of the unconscious victim. If the child is combative, then rapid sequence intubation should be used. If the child is completely alert, awake, and appropriately mentating on arrival to the ED, then observation with 100% oxygen by facemask is appropriate. If there is any question, the error should be on aggressive management of the airway.

Cardiac monitoring is needed for all patients, as both the acidosis and the hypoxia will decrease the fibrillation threshold. An intravenous line for medications should be started at this time if it is not already present. Core body temperature should be measured, and measures to dry off the patient and conserve the patient's body temperature should be undertaken. Warming lights or warming blankets are always appropriate for unclothed, wet children.

Defibrillation of the patient in ventricular fibrillation should be accomplished in the field if possible. If hypothermia is found, successful defibrillation may be possible only after core rewarming is accomplished. A cold heart is always difficult to restart, so it is important to not give up too soon. There have been reports of complete recovery after CPR times of up to two hours following a cold-water submersion, particularly in small children. Resuscitation efforts should be continued until circulation and respiration are re-established or cerebral death has occurred.[56] The rescuers and clinicians should be reminded that a dry environment is safer during attempts at defibrillation.

Treatment of Hypoxia. Management of the pulmonary system abnormalities of near drowning begins with airway management and continues until final disposition of the patient.

Oxygen should be administered at the highest FiO_2 available. Immediate arterial blood gas (ABG) determinations and an initial chest x-ray are necessary. The goal of routine respiratory management is to achieve a PaO_2 of 70-100 mmHg. Although some patients will be able to maintain this PaO_2 with supplemental oxygen alone, more than 70% of patients will require more aggressive therapy. The initial ABG should be correlated with pulse oximetry and end title CO_2 if the child is intubated.

Rapid intubation allows both protection of the airway and administration of higher oxygen concentrations. Positive end expiratory pressure (PEEP) or continuous positive airway pressure (CPAP) with intermittent mandatory ventilation (IMV) can be used easily on the intubated patient. Ideally, PEEP should be started in the ED and the patient's oxygenation monitored by blood gases as the patient's course progresses. Nasal CPAP also may be used in the conscious and unintubated patient with respiratory distress.[57]

In experimental near drowning in pigs, 5 cm of PEEP increased arterial oxygen tension, even when instituted 20 minutes after the insult.[58] The addition of PEEP will decrease the degree of intrapulmonary shunting, decrease the V/Q mismatch, and increase the functional residual capacity. The increased PaO_2 from the use of PEEP and CPAP will occur regardless of whether the patient has suffered fresh water or seawater submersion. Fresh water submersion victims may require the use of either PEEP or CPAP to maintain the patency of the surfactant-deficient small airways.

Bronchospasm may be treated with a variety of bronchodilators that are administered by nebulizer. The standard dosages of these agents should be used.

Fiberoptic or rigid bronchoscopy may be indicated in patients who have aspirated particulate matter or contaminated fluids. It is particularly noteworthy that a high percentage of patients have had silt or sand in the trachea and lungs after falling in rapidly moving streams or in surfing accidents. These densities may be seen as "sand bronchograms" on plain films of the chest. Chest CT may be indicated for patients who have possible aspiration of sand or other particulate matter. Imaging of the sinuses also is indicated to assess possible nasal inhalation of foreign material.

Protection of the Cervical Spine. The cervical spine should be evaluated rapidly in all submersion victims. This is particularly important if there are signs of trauma or if the patient is unconscious. The cervical spine should be protected by a cervical collar and long spine board, and cervical spine x-rays should be obtained as soon as possible. An appropriate exception to this would be if the incident had been witnessed and there was obviously no trauma involved.

Adjunctive Immediate Therapy. Victims of submersion exhibit a combined respiratory and metabolic acidosis. The respiratory component should be corrected with prompt airway control and ventilation. Severe metabolic acidosis is common and may require correction with sodium bicarbonate. ABG results can be used to guide therapy.

Rewarming Methods. The evaluation and treatment of hypothermia, whether wet or dry, on land or in the water, is essentially the same.[59] The most basic method of prevention of heat loss should be used from the very start of the resuscitation; the patient should be dried. Evaporation causes rapid heat losses, and wet clothes rarely protect sufficiently from heat losses. Wet clothing should be removed as soon as possible in the resuscitation, and the patient should be covered with warmed, dry blankets.

The rewarming method of choice in the hypothermic non-breathing, cold-water submersion victim is probably cardiopulmonary bypass with in-line heat exchanger. This method has the very practical advantage of rewarming the core and oxygenating the brain at the same time.

Water baths for rewarming are dangerous for both patient and staff if cardiovascular monitoring is employed. Other methods (i.e., peritoneal dialysis and hemodialysis) may be used for rapid rewarming. For the conscious patient without significant respiratory embarrassment, active external heating may suffice. Although heated, moistened oxygen and warmed intravenous fluids do not contribute significant heat calories to the resuscitation, this form of adjunctive warming will often balance heat losses.

History. After all of the immediate resuscitative efforts are underway, it is appropriate to obtain as much medical history as is available, paying particular attention to those factors that will influence the prognosis and possible complications. The physician should attempt to document what kind of fluid the patient was submerged in, the temperature of the solution, a rough approximation of duration of submersion, what resuscitative efforts were made at the scene, and the response to these efforts. The patient's age should be estimated, if not readily available, and any pre-existing diseases that are known should be identified. In many cases, these data will be readily available from friends or family, but some victims are never identified. If possible, obtain details of the accident while questioning the patient or those accompanying him. The details may provide clues to other injuries, such as fractures or intra-abdominal injuries, which may go unrecognized temporarily during the excitement of the resuscitation.

If the victim is an infant or a child, the possibility of child abuse must be considered. Children may be forcibly submerged under water as a form of punishment. If other evidence of trauma or child abuse is noted, or the examination is not consistent with the given story, this should be carefully documented.

In the majority of child submersion incidents, at least one parent is near the scene of the accident.[60] Most parents are emotionally distressed, devastated, and remorseful. The parents often relate that the child was playing, and they momentarily lost sight of the child, only to find him floating face down or submerged in the backyard pool. Another classic story is that the child was left playing in the bathtub for a few moments and the caretaker returned to find the child face down in the tub. If the parents are not reacting appropriately or give an overly detailed or unusual story, the examiner's suspicions should be heightened.

Cessation of Resuscitation. After rescue, the victim may appear to be clinically dead, either because a true cardiac arrest has occurred or because the bradycardic weak pulse is not palpable. The development of immersion hypothermia prior to the anoxic insult may be protective for the brain. All cold-water submersion victims should have a trial of resuscitation with immediate ventilation and closed chest massage. Brain death is difficult to determine at lower body temperatures, so rewarming the patient to at least 30°C. is required before abandoning CPR. CPR exceeding two hours has been successful, and victims have survived submersion times as long as 40 minutes.

Adjuvant Hospital Therapy

Antibiotics. The mortality of pneumonia associated with near drowning is 60%.[61] There is little evidence for, and substantial logic against, the use of prophylactic antibiotics. In one study where 21 patients were given prophylactic antibiotics, 16 developed pneumo-

Table 3. Factors Affecting Prognosis*

- Duration of the submersion
- Duration and degree of hypothermia (water temperature)
- Age of the patient
- Water contaminants
- Duration of respiratory arrest
- Duration of cardiac arrest
- Rapidity and effectiveness of resuscitation
- The diving reflex

*Without controlled studies, it is difficult to determine which factors have the greatest effect on the outcome of the patient after a submersion incident.

nia from an organism resistant to the antibiotic used.[62] No reduction in pneumonia or mortality was noted when prophylactic antibiotics have been used.

Less controversy exists over the use of prophylactic antibiotics when the patient aspirates grossly contaminated water such as from sewers or septic tanks. With such contamination of the lungs, most authorities recommend antibiotics.

Glucose. Hypothermia and alcohol, alone or in combination, may cause hypoglycemia, and all drowning victims should have their glucose checked and hypoglycemia corrected.

Steroids. Corticosteroid therapy for pulmonary injury of drowning has not been demonstrated to be helpful in either canine or human studies.[63,64] They should probably not be used for treatment of the pulmonary injury.

Surfactant. Surfactant is washed out or destroyed by both salt water and fresh water aspiration. Addition of artificial surfactant will theoretically improve the gas exchange in submersion survivors. Artificial surfactant has been used in the treatment of submersion victims with some success.[65,66] Animal studies have conflicting results, and this treatment will need additional study before it can be routinely recommended.

Cardiopulmonary Bypass. Cardiopulmonary bypass provides fast rewarming, maintains tissue perfusion and oxygenation, and assists the cold and inefficient heart during the resuscitation. It may have a significant adjuvant role beyond rewarming in the treatment of the cold-water submersion victim in cardiac arrest.

Central Nervous System Protection. Early studies advocated the use of hypothermia, intracranial perfusion monitoring, and barbiturates to improve outcome.[67,68] There is now a general consensus that early barbiturate loading, mild hypothermia, and control of intracranial pressure (ICP) does not improve the overall outcome. Currently, ICP monitoring is not recommended, but if it is done, an elevated ICP bodes a poor prognosis for the patient.

Prognosis

The prognosis of a submersion patient may be difficult to estimate. *(See Tables 3 and 4.)* If the patient has made a first respiratory effort within 30 minutes of rescue, the prognosis is good.[69] The adult patient who arrives at the hospital with a beating heart has a good chance of recovering all neurologic function. Survival after the submersion event appears to depend upon a number of interrelated factors.

Table 4. Good Prognostic Factors Following a Submersion Incident

- Alert and awake on arrival to ED
- Cold, fresh water
- Short submersion
- Older child or young adults
- On-scene advanced cardiac life support or basic life support
- Healthy

In warm water submersion, a clinical picture that includes one or more of the following features will imply a severe neurologic impairment or mortality, even in children:[70-72]

- Submersion for greater than 5 minutes;
- Absence of pupillary light reflex (in the ED);
- Pulseless on arrival to the ED;
- No CPR for 10 minutes or more;
- Rural location of incident;
- CPR longer than 25 minutes;
- pH less than 7.1 on arrival at the hospital;
- Need for in-hospital resuscitation or ventilation;
- High initial blood glucose concentration;
- Male sex;
- Abnormal chest radiograph findings; and/or
- History of epinephrine administration in field or ED.

Many investigators have proposed predictive rules incorporating one or more of these variables. Most of these predictive rules are more appropriately applied in the ICU after initial resuscitation than in the ED. An interesting exception is a tool designed for the ICU — the Pediatric Risk of Mortality Score (PRISM).[73] This tool appeared to be more effective when used in the ED than in the ICU.[74]

In the absence of any unusual circumstance, such as cold water immersion or barbiturate use, a reasonable guideline is to continue resuscitation for 30-40 minutes. After that time, consider stopping all efforts if no effective cardiac activity has been restored.

The same prognostic factors cannot be applied to submersion in cold water. As has been noted before, there is a profound protective effect of hypothermia on cerebral survival.

There is some controversy about what to do when the victim arrives in the ED awake, alert, and without significant signs of aspiration. As noted earlier, pulmonary edema can have a delayed onset (secondary drowning). Observation of the patient with a history of submersion is commonly recommended. Any child with tachypnea, oxygen requirements, or an abnormal chest radiograph should be admitted. Children who have no pulmonary symptoms may be observed for a period of time. At least one study suggests that these patients may be safely sent home.[75,76] An observation period of several hours is a reasonable compromise in low-risk patients with good parental supervision and close medical follow-up.

Prevention

Like all diseases, it is much easier to prevent a submersion incident than it is to treat one. Many of the major factors that contribute to a submersion incident are preventable, such as an inability to swim, failure to wear proper protective gear, consumption of drugs or alcohol, and stunts. Because the greatest proportion of drownings occur in non-swimmers, the protection afforded by swimming lessons is easy to support and has been known for ages.

Children require special preventative measures.[77] A child with "water wings" or in a floating support, without adequate supervision immediately available, is a fatality waiting for a place to happen. Overestimation of swimming skills and trauma associated with horseplay may contribute to a child's demise.

Fences around pools markedly reduce the incidence of submersion injuries in those areas where they are required.[78-80] Because fencing requires no training or action on the part of the child or the parent, it deserves a very high priority in prevention efforts. The fencing should be at least 4 feet high and include self-locking gates. Immersion alarm systems for unattended pools will further decrease deaths but should not be used as a primary means of drowning prevention.

The adult who is intoxicated not only cannot supervise a child, he or she also cannot supervise personal actions. To reach the "legally drunk" 100 mg/dL level, the average 70 kg person needs to consume only four beers or two mixed drinks in the space of an hour. Any steps that reduce intoxication among swimmers will reduce the frequency of injury and death.

Patients with seizure disorders or other handicaps must be properly supervised, as their risk is higher.[81] For these patients, buddy swimming and proper supervision is mandatory. For these parents, cardiopulmonary resuscitation training should be strongly advocated.[82]

For those who are exposed to the elements, particularly at sea in the higher latitudes, instructions in methods of conserving the body heat during immersion should be mandatory. Proper protective gear should be worn at all times in these areas, including both survival suit and approved flotation devices.

Conclusion

Between 6000 and 8000 drownings occur each year in the United States, and there is a similar number of near-drownings that are reported.

The single most important factor in recovery of the patient is the time from submersion until definitive airway management.

Younger victims in cold water have the best prognosis for long-term survival. Those who are submersed in hot tubs have the worst prognosis. All patients deserve a full and aggressive resuscitation. Unfortunately, there is no proven way to predict which person will survive intact, which will die, or which will survive with neurologic damage.

Finally, the best treatment for this disease is prevention. Age-specific swimming lessons, water safety, and adequate supervision should be stressed for children. Liquor and other intoxicants should be banned from swimming areas.

References

1. Zuckerman GB, Gregory PM, Santos-Damiani SM. Predictors of death and neurologic impairment in pediatric submersion injuries. *Arch Ped Adolesc Med* 1998;152:134-140.
2. Orlowski JP. Drowning, near-drowning, and ice-water drowning. *JAMA* 1988;260:390-391.
3. Quan L, Kinder D. Pediatric submersions: Prehospital predictors of outcome. *Pediatrics*. 1992;90:909-913.
4. Schuman SH, Rowe JR, Glaxer HM, et al. Risk of drowning: An iceberg phenomenon. *J Am Coll Emerg Physicians* 1977;6:139-143.
5. Metropolitan Life Insurance Co. Statistical bulletin. May 1977;2-3.
6. Joseph MM, King WD. Epidemiology of hospitalization for near-drowning. *Southern Med J* 1998;91:253-255.
7. Smith DS. Sudden drowning syndrome. *Physician Sportsmed* 1980;8:76-83.
8. Neal JM. Near-Drowning. *J Emerg Med* 1985;3:41-51.
9. Davis S, Ledman J, Kilgore J. Drownings of children and youths in a desert state. *West J Med* 1985;143:196-201.
10. Orlowski JP. Prognostic factors in pediatric cases of drowning and near-drowning. *J Am Coll Emerg Physicians* 1979;8:176-179.
11. Gillenwater JM, Quan L, Feldman KW. Inflicted submersion in childhood. *Arch Pediatr Adolesc Med* 1996;150:298-303.
12. Schmidt P, Madea B. Death in the bathtub involving children. *Forensic Sci Int* 1995;72:147-155.
13. Lavelle JM, Shaw KN, Seidl T, et al. Ten-year review of pediatric bathtub near-drownings: Evaluation for child abuse and neglect. *Ann Emerg Med* 1995;25:344-348.
14. Gastiglia PT. Drowning. *J Ped Health Care* 1995;9:185-186.
15. Modell JH. Drown vs near-drown: A discussion of definitions. *Crit Care Med* 1989;9:351-352.
16. Modell JH. Drowning. *N Engl J Med* 1993;328:253-256.
17. Golden FS, Tipton MJ, Scott RC. Immersion, near-drowning and drowning. *Brit J Anaesthesia* 1997;79:214-225.
18. Pratt FD, Haynes BE. Incidence of secondary drowning after salt-water submersion. *Ann Emerg Med* 1986;15:1084-1087.
19. Goode RC, Duffin J, Miller R. Sudden cold water immersion. *Respir Physiol* 1975;23:301.
20. Keating WR, Hayward MG. Sudden death in cold water and ventricular arrhythmia. *J Forensic Sci* 1981;26:459.
21. Wirrel EC, Camfield PR, Camfield CS, et al. Accidental injury is a serious risk in children with typical absence epilepsy. *Arch Neurol* 1996;53:929-932.
22. Strauss D, Shavelle R, Anderson TW, et al. External causes of death among persons with developmental disability: The effect of residential placement. *Am J Epidemiol* 1998;147:855-862
23. Spitz MC. Injuries and death as a consequence of seizures in people with epilepsy. *Epilepsia* 1998;39:904-907.
24. Suzuki T. Suffocation and related problems. *Forensic Sci Int* 1996;80:71-78.
25. Hermann LK. Drowning, a common tragedy. *Rocky Mountain Medical J* 1979;76:169-173.
26. Modell JH. Drowning. *N Engl J Med* 1993;328:253-256.
27. Franks CM, Golden FS, Hamptom IFG, et al. The effect of blood alcohol on the initial responses to cold water immersion in humans. *Eur J Appl Physiol* 1997;75: 279-281.

28. Spitz MC. Injuries and death as a consequence of seizures in people with epilepsy. *Epilepsia* 1998;39:904-907.
29. Osamura T, Fushiki S, Yoshioka H, et al. An autopsy case of bathtub drowning in epilepsy. *Brain & Development*, 1997;19:499-501.
30. Orlowski JP, Rothner AD, Leuders H. Submersion accidents in children with epilepsy. *Am J Dis Child* 1982;136:777-780.
31. Diekema DS, Quan L, Holt VL. Epilepsy as a risk factor for submersion injury in children. *Pediatrics* 1993;91:612-616.
32. Craig AB Jr. Causes of loss of consciousness during underwater swimming. *J Appl Physiol* 1961;16583-586.
33. Craig AB Jr. Summary of 58 cases of loss of consciousness during underwater swimming and diving. *Med Sci Sports* 1976;8:171.
34. Yagil Y, Stalkikowicz R, Michaeli J, Mogle P. Near drowning in the Dead Sea: Electrolyte imbalances and therapeutic implications. *Arch Int Med* 1985;145:50-53.
35. Ellis RJ. Severe hypernatremia from sea water ingestion during near-drowning in a hurricane. *West J Med* 1997;167:430-433.
36. Sims JK, Enomoto PI, Frankel RI, et al. Marine bacteria complicating seawater near-drowning and marine wounds: A hypothesis. *Ann Emerg Med* 1983;12:212-216.
37. Karch SB. Pathology of the lung in near-drowning. *Am J Emerg Med* 1986;4:4-9.
38. Pearn J. Pathophysiology of drowning. *Med J Aust* 1985;142: 586-588.
39. Nopanitanya W, Gambill TG, Brankhous KM. Fresh water drowning: Pulmonary ultrastructure and systemic fibrinolysis. *Arch Pathol* 1974;98:361-366.
40. Redding JS. Drowning and near-drowning. *Postgrad Med* 1983;74:85-97.
41. Steinman AM. Immersion hypothermia. *Emerg Med Serv* 1977;6:22-25.
42. Collis ML. Survival behavior in cold water immersion. In: *Proceedings of the Cold Water Symposium*. Toronto: Royal Life Saving Society of Canada: 1976.
43. Hunter AR. *Neurosurgical Anesthesia*. 2nd ed. Oxford: Blackwell Scientific Publications, 1975.
44. Tipton MJ, Kelleher PC, Golden FS. Supraventricular arrythmias following breath-hold submersions in cold water. *Undersea and Hyperbaric Medicine* 1994;21:305-313.
45. Tipton MJ. The initial responses to cold water immersion in man. *Clinical Sci* 1989;77:581-588.
46. Tipton MJ. The effect of clothing on "diving bradycardia" in man during submersion in cold water. *Eur J App Physiol* 1989;59: 360-364.
47. Conn AL, Miyasaka K, Katayama M, et al. A canine study of cold water drowning in fresh versus salt water. *Crit Care Med* 1995;23:2029-2037.
48. Golden F. Mechanisms of body cooling in submersed victims. *Resuscitation* 1997;35:107-109.
49. Tron VA, Baldwin VJ, Pirie GE. Hot tub drownings. *Pediatrics* 1985;75:789-790.
50. Chochinov AH, Baydock BMS, Bristow GK, et al. Recovery of a 62-year-old man from prolonged cold water submersion. *Ann Emerg Med* 1998;31:127-131.
51. Lukas GM, Hutton JE Jr, Lim RC, et al. Injuries sustained from high velocity impact with water: An experience from the Golden Gate Bridge. *J Trauma* 1981;21:612-618.
52. Orlowski JP. Heimlich maneuver for near-drowning questioned. (letter). *Ann Emerg Med* 1982;11:111.
53. Wilder RJ, Wedro BC. Heimlich maneuver for near-drowning questioned.(letter). *Ann Emerg Med* 1982;11:111.
54. Heimlich HJ. Subdiaphragmatic pressure to expel water from the lungs of drowning persons. *Ann Emerg Med* 1981;10:476-480.
55. Ornato JP. The resuscitation of near-drowning victims. *JAMA* 1986;256:75-77.
56. Orlowski JP. Drowning, near-drowning, and ice-water submersions. *Ped Clin North Am* 1987;34:75-92.
57. Dottorini M, Eslami A, Baglioni S. Nasal-continuous positive airway pressure in the treatment of near-drowning in freshwater. *Chest* 1996;110:1122-1124.
58. Lindner KH, Dick W, Lotz P. The delayed use of positive end expiratory pressure during respiratory resuscitation following near drowning with fresh or salt water. *Resuscitation* 1983;10:197-211.
59. Samuelson T, Doolittle W, Hayward J, et al. Hypothermia and cold water near drowning treatment guidelines. *Alaska Med* 1982;24:106-111.
60. Fandel I, Bancalari E. Near-drowning in children: Clinical aspects. *Pediatrics* 1976;58:573-579.
61. Ender PT, Dolan MJ. Pneumonia associated with near-drowning. *CID* 1997;25:896-907.
62. Oakes DD, Sherck JP, Maloney JR, et al. Prognosis and treatment of victims of near-drowning. *J Trauma* 1982;22:544-549.
63. Calderwood HW, Modell JH, Ruiz BC. The ineffectiveness of steroid therapy for treatment of fresh-water near-drowning. *Anesthesiol* 1975;43:642-650.
64. Orlowski JP. Drowning, near-drowning and ice-water submersions. *Pediatr Clin North Am* 1987;34:75-92.
65. McBrien M, Katumba JJ, Mukhtar AI. Artificial surfactant in the treatment of near-drowning. *Lancet* 1993;342:1485-1486.
66. Staudinger T, Bankier A, Strohmaier W. Exogenous surfactant therapy in a patient with adult respiratory distress syndrome after near drowning. *Resuscitation* 1997;35:179-182.
67. Nussbaum E, Galant SP. Intracranial pressure monitoring as a guide to prognosis in the nearly drowned, severely comatose child. *J Pediatr* 1983;102:215-218.
68. Dean JM, McComb JG. Intracranial pressure monitoring in severe pediatric near drowning. *Neurosurgery* 1981;9:627-630.
69. Pearn J. The management of near drowning. *Br Med J* 1985;291:1447-1452.
70. Danzl D. Pediatric near-drowning: Aggressive CPR is best. *Patient Care* 1987;August 15:14-16.
71. Robinson MD, Seward PN. Submersion injury in children. *Ped Emerg Care* 1987;3:44-49.
72. Graf WD, Cummings P, Quan L, Brucatao D. Predicting outcome in pediatric submersion victims. *Ann Emerg Med* 1995;26: 312-319.
73. Pollack MM, Ruttimann UE, Getson PR. Pediatric Risk of Mortality (PRISM) Score. *Crit Care Med* 1988:16:1110-1116.
74. Zuckerman GB, Gregory PM, Santos-Damiani SM. Predictors of death and neurologic impairment in pediatric submersion injuries. *Arch Ped Adolesc Med* 1998;152:134-140.
75. Van Berkel M, Bierens JJLM, Lie RLK, et al. Pulmonary oedema, pneumonia and mortality in submersion victims; a retrospective study in 125 patients. *Intensive Care Med* 1996;22:101-107.
76. Noonan L, Howrey R, Ginsburg CM. Freshwater submersion injuries in children: A retrospective review of seventy-five hospi-

talized patients. *Pediatrics* 1996;98:368-371.

77. Spyker DA. Submersion injury: Epidemiology, prevention, and management. *Ped Clin North Am* 1985;32:113-125.
78. Pearn J III, Hsia EY. Swimming pool drownings and near-drownings involving children. A total population study from Hawaii. *Milit Med* 1980;190:15-18.
79. DeNicola LK, Falk JL, Swanson ME, et al. Submersion injuries in children and adults. *Critical Care Clin* 1997;13:477-502.
80. Rivara FP, Grossman DC, Cummings P. Injury prevention (Second of two parts.) *N Engl J Med* 1997;337:613-618.
81. Rivara FP. Pediatric injury control in 1999: Where do we go from here? *Pediatrics* 1999;103:883-888.
82. O'Flaherty JE, Pirie PL. Prevention of pediatric drowning and near-drowning: A survey of members of the American Academy of Pediatrics. *Pediatrics* 1997;99:169-174.

Medical Hardware

Gary Schwartz, MD, FAAP
Charles Seamens, MD

Without question, technological advances in modern medicine have afforded critically ill children increased survival and improved outcomes from conditions that until recently had only dismal chances for any reasonable life expectancy or quality of life. Thousands of children every day are implanted with medical hardware such as cerebral spinal fluid shunts, central venous lines, and gastrostomy feeding devices. Unquestionably, these devices have prolonged and improved the quality of life for thousands of children. Unfortunately, accompanying the profound benefits of these new technologies are myriad complications and new risks to the "high-tech" child. For these reasons, emergency medical healthcare providers should be knowledgeable about the various medical hardware devices and their complications. These treatment modalities and the management of the most commonly associated complications are reviewed in this chapter.

Cerebral Spinal Fluid Shunts

Hydrocephalus is not an uncommon pediatric disease, occurring in one of every 2000 births.[1] Each year neurosurgeons insert approximately 18,000 cerebral spinal fluid (CSF) shunts, making this the most common pediatric neurosurgical procedure.[2-4] Unfortunately, shunt placement also has a very high complication rate; consequently, patients with CSF shunts are frequently brought to the ED with a wide spectrum of complaints. Because shunt problems are potentially life-threatening, any complaints consistent with a shunt malfunction should prompt emergent neurosurgical consultation.

The central nervous system is enclosed in a bony non-compliant structure and is composed of parenchyma, fluid, and vascular structures. Due to the noncompliance of the skull, any change in one of these components will require a compensatory change in the other components. Hydrocephalus occurs when the increased component is cerebral spinal fluid (CSF). CSF is produced in the choroid plexus at a rate of 0.35 cc/min and flows through the ventricles into the spinal canal and subarachnoid space, where it is absorbed by the extensive venous plexus.[5] Any disruption to this process results in hydrocephalus. Disruptions in CSF flow can be divided into three categories: increased production (e.g., choroid plexus tumor), obstruction of flow (e.g., congenital malformation or acquired process such as mass lesion or post infectious), or decreased absorption.

Shunt Function. Most patients with hydrocephalus need a CSF shunt.[3] Medical modalities have had limited success in treating this condition regardless of the etiology. There are several types of CSF shunts, all of which are named according to where the CSF is drained. The most common type of shunt is the ventriculoperitoneal shunt, which drains into the peritoneal cavity. Much less commonly used is the ventriculoatrial shunt, which drains directly into the right atrium.[6] This type of shunt used to be the most popular but is now infrequently used because of significant complications, such as endocarditis, thrombosis, and cardiac arrhythmias.[7] Shunts that drain into the pleural space, ureter, or gallbladder are very rarely used.[2]

Regardless of the type of shunt used, the same basic design principles apply. The proximal tubing is inserted though a Burr hole in the occipital or frontal bones, and preferentially ends up in the anterior part of the lateral ventricle. This procedure is frequently performed using external landmarks, rather than direct visualization.[3] Therefore, misplacement of the catheter tip is possible. The distal end of the tubing may have a preset 90° bend for insertion through the cranium to prevent kinking.[8]

The proximal tubing is usually attached to a valve system, which has both inlet and outlet valves separated by a chamber. There are several types of valves in use, each with unique features.[8,9] Each valve system functions by releasing fluid after the preset pressure differential between the valves is reached. Unfortunately, pressure differences between the valves can be influenced by body position. When standing, the pressure difference can increase dramatically due to the low intra-abdominal pressure compared to the CNS pressure. This pressure differential can lead to overdrainage unless an antisiphon valve is installed.[8,9]

Some patients, especially those undergoing intraventricular chemotherapy, have a reservoir attached to the proximal catheter. The reservoir does not have a proximal valve. Therefore, medications injected into the reservoir can flow into the ventricle.

The distal tubing is connected to the outlet valve and tunneled under the skin to its final destination. The valve and tubing may be one piece or connected pieces.[3,7] Since shunts are frequently placed in the newborn period, a large amount of extra distal tubing is inserted in order to allow for patient growth. Generally, the extra tubing does not appear to increase complications.[3]

Complications. *Obstruction.* Although CSF shunts are actually quite simple devices, complications do occur. The most common complication, which accounts for half of all shunt complications, is obstruction.[3,10,11] Obstruction occurs most often in the proximal portion of the tubing (50%) during the first two years following shunt placement.[11] In fact, obstruction in this area is most common immediately after insertion. Postoperative obstruction is usually due to debris, clots (from postoperative bleeding), or misplacement. Later on, obstruction is usually due to choroid plexus entrapment around the tubing, ependymal reaction, or immune reaction.[3]

The second place for obstruction to occur is at a valve. Malfunction due to manufacturing problems is very infrequent. More commonly, malfunction is due to cellular debris or infection. Again, immune complex-mediated malfunction may also play a role.[3]

Finally, malfunction may occur in the distal catheter, from pseudocyst formation at the tip, kinking, thrombosis, or occlusion of the tip with omentum.[12] Distal obstruction is most common for shunts that have been in place for more than two years.[11]

Infection. Shunt infection is another frequent concern for patients with CSF shunts. Infections have an occurrence rate of approximately 5%.[13,14] Half of the infections occur in the first two weeks and 75% in the first two months after shunt placement.[6,15] Children less than 1 year of age are at highest risk.[14]

Infections are categorized as either wound or shunt infections. Wound infections are usually located over the site of the reservoir or in the abdominal wall in patients with VP shunts. These infections occur at the time of placement and manifest as a cellulitis with redness, warmth, and possible purulent discharge at the affected surgical site. Staphylococcal species are the most frequently cultured etiologic bacteria.[6]

The second type of infection involves the shunt itself. Infection at this site is also frequently acquired at the time of insertion. These infections are usually caused by a less virulent organism and significant signs of inflammation are often not present. The most commonly cultured organisms are *Staphylococcus epidermidis* (40-63%) and *Staphylococcus aureus* (20-27%).[6,14,15] Gram-negative organisms are less commonly cultured and occur most frequently in patients with VP shunts (6-20%).[15] Patients with gram-negative infections are usually more ill-appearing.[16] It also is not uncommon to find mixed flora (10-15%).[6,15] Mixed flora infections are often felt to be related to bowel perforation.[6] Additionally, a higher risk of meningitis with traditional pathogens such as *Pneumococcus, Haemophilus influenzae*, and meningococcemia may exist for patients with shunts.[6] Finally, infection rates are the same for VP and VA shunts, although infections in the latter may lead to other more serious complications. Some of these serious complications include sepsis, nephritis, endocarditis, and thromboembolic events.[17,18]

Overdrainage. Another complication that may be encountered is overdrainage of the CSF. This can cause the slit ventricle syndrome, which involves chronic overdrainage with collapse of the ventricles and transient obstruction of CSF flow.[19] Symptoms may include headache, nausea, vomiting, lethargy, diplopia, and paresis of upward gaze.[20] Symptoms are often alleviated when the patient lies down or lowers his or her head.[20]

Computerized tomography of the head will demonstrate small ventricles in 53-65% of patients with a shunt.[21,22] Only a small fraction (11%) of patients with small ventricles will actually have the slit ventricle syndrome, and only a small number (6%) of these patients will need surgical treatment.[21] Slit ventricle syndrome is less frequently seen now with the use of more sophisticated valves and antisiphon devices.

Other complications of shunts include migration of the distal tip of the peritoneal catheter, hernias, abdominal adhesions, volvulus, and bowel obstruction.[12,23]

Clinical Presentation. Headache, vomiting, and lethargy are classic symptoms of increased intracranial pressure. Any of these symptoms should prompt evaluation of the shunt because headache is present in only 13%, vomiting in only 26%, and lethargy in 40% of patients with shunt obstruction.[24]

Headache, lethargy, fever, and meningismus are classic symptoms of shunt infection. Unfortunately, these classic presentations are also infrequently seen. In studies of children with shunt infection diagnosed by CSF analysis, meningismus was only present in 20-29% of the cases. Other classic symptoms are also not common, with headache occurring in 5-14% and lethargy in 12% of patients.[13,17] Fever is found most commonly and occurs in 73-95% of the patients.[13,17,25]

Patients may also present with complaints of both an obstructive and infectious process since one-third of obstructed patients also have a shunt infection.[13] More common are nonspecific presentations such as fever without a source, poor feeding, and not acting right.[15] This makes it difficult to tell which children have shunt malfunction. One study, which evaluated referral patterns of children with a shunt malfunction, found parents to be as good as general practitioners in identifying shunt malfunction.[26] For this reason, a high level of suspicion for shunt malfunction should be maintained in children whose complaints cannot be explained by another process. This is especially true if the child is very young or the shunt has been recently revised or replaced. Due to the nonspecific complaints, the average delay from the onset of symptoms until shunt revision is 11.5 days.[24]

Patients with peritoneal shunts can present with shunt-related abdominal problems without neurologic complaints. These usually present with abdominal pain. Possible causes include peritonitis due to infection of the distal tubing, intestinal perforation, or volvulus.[27,28]

Diagnosis. Any child presenting with complaints that are suspicious for a shunt problem should be evaluated with a thorough history and physical examination. If shunt malfunction remains in the differential diagnosis afterward, further evaluation is required. Since other laboratory tests are of limited value, analysis of the CSF is necessary. It may be tempting to decide on whether to tap a shunt based on an abnormal peripheral white blood cell count, but in 25% of patients with documented shunt infection, the white blood cell count is normal.[15]

Evaluation of a shunt involves at least two sequential components: radiographic imaging and CSF evaluation.

Radiograph imaging starts with evaluation of ventricular size with cranial computed tomography (CT). Frequently these children do not have normal baseline ventricular size even with a normally functioning shunt. Therefore, comparison with a previous study is essential. Even with a CT scan unchanged from baseline, there is a chance early obstruction may be present (3-35%).[26,29] Therefore, plain radiographs of the shunt valve and tubing are also needed to assess the continuity of the system and to rule out kinking of the tube.

After imaging studies, CSF analysis is necessary. A shunt tap is preferred to a lumbar puncture since the latter procedure will occasionally miss infections.[30] Moreover, an LP is useless in the diagnosis of concurrent shunt obstruction, and both procedures have an exceptionally low risk of introducing an infection into the CSF.[15]

To perform a shunt tap, sterilely prepare the shunt site with betadine followed by alcohol. Insert a 23 gauge butterfly needle attached to a manometer into the valve chamber while occluding the outlet valve. By occluding the outlet, the manometer will reflect the ventricular pressure (opening pressure). Inability to obtain fluid will signify an occlusion proximal to the valve. After the pressure is recorded, the outlet is released and fluid drains into the distal catheter. Distal obstruction is present if the fluid will not drain from the manometer. Normal opening pressure is less than 5-10 cm (less than the valve's preset opening pressure). All patients with a pressure over 20 cm have shunt obstruction and require urgent shunt revision. An opening pressure of 10-20 cm is indeterminate and may benefit from a radionuclide clearance study.[31] Some neurosurgeons also recommend checking a drip interval, the time between drops of CSF as fluid is collected, and closing pressure.[32]

The CSF should be analyzed for cell count, culture, Gram's stain, glucose, and protein. Organisms on Gram's stain confirm the diagnosis of infection. Unfortunately, there is variability in the literature on the acceptable number of WBCs in the CSF obtained from a shunt. In one study, in non-infected shunt patients with shunt dysfunction, the median number of CSF WBCs was 18 cells/mm^3, while in infected patients, it was 79 cells/mm^3.[6] There was a large overlap in each group since 47% of infected patients with a positive CSF culture had less than 20 WBCs.[15] Interestingly, eosinophilia in the CSF has also been associated with shunt infection.[33] CSF also should be analyzed for protein and glucose even though the glucose is normal in 80% of infected patients.[25] If the CSF glucose is low, gram-negative organisms are more likely to be cultured.[16] Even with normal CSF analysis, 17% of patients may have a positive culture.[13] Tapping the shunt should be performed by the neurosurgeon since there is a small risk of infecting the hardware. More importantly, there can be difficulty in interpreting the CSF cell count and opening pressure.

Another test that is sometimes performed is pumping the shunt to check for obstruction. If the shunt cannot be pumped, a distal obstruction is presumed; the absence of filling following pumping indicates a proximal obstruction. Unfortunately, this test is of limited value, with only 20% sensitivity for identifying an obstruction.[34]

Treatment. Treatment of an obstructed shunt involves revision or replacement of the obstructed part. The timing of this will depend on the severity of the presenting symptoms. Children who are minimally symptomatic may have the procedure delayed for several hours. Children who have symptoms of increased pressure will need emergent relief with shunt revision.

If no neurosurgeon is available and emergent action is necessary, the physician can try several maneuvers to relieve the obstruction. For a distal obstruction, manually withdraw fluid from the reservoir by serial aspirations. The emergency healthcare provider should remove fluid slowly to prevent intracranial bleeding resulting from rapid fluid shifts. Cerebral spinal fluid should be removed until the manometer reading is less than 20 cm.[35]

A second method for relief of obstruction is to flush a small amount of saline through the distal tubing. Occlude the proximal valve prior to injection to unclog the distal end. The method for a proximal obstruction is similar, except as the fluid is flushed, the distal catheter is occluded, forcing proximal fluid flow.

If this does not relieve the obstruction and the patient is deteriorating emergently, intubate and hyperventilate while administering an osmotic diuretic such as mannitol.[2] If these maneuvers do not help, an emergent ventricular puncture may be necessary. If time allows, consultation with a neurosurgeon should be obtained before the procedure is attempted. Restrain the child in a supine position. Shave the child's hair and sterilely prep over the sagittal and coronal sutures. If the anterior fontanelle is open, a spinal needle is inserted 1 cm lateral to the sagittal suture along the coronal suture. If the suture is closed, the spinal needle is inserted 2-3 cm lateral to midline and just anterior to the coronal suture. If the skull cannot be penetrated by the spinal needle, use a bone marrow needle to make a hole in the skull. Insert and direct the spinal needle toward the inner canthus of the ipsilateral eye. The ventricle should be encountered by a depth of 5.5 cm or less. Remove fluid slowly until the pressure is less than 20 cm.[36,37]

Treatment for an infected shunt most often involves removal of the infected part, antibiotics, and externalization of the shunt. This is the most successful means to eradicate infection (96%).[17,38] The antibiotic frequently chosen is vancomycin due to its excellent staphylococcal coverage. A third-generation cephalosporin or an aminoglycoside also can be administered to cover gram-negative organisms until CSF or blood cultures are available. The antibiotics should be administered intravenously or intraventricularly if CNS penetration of the chosen antibiotics is not sufficient. When the CSF is sterile, a new shunt is inserted.[16,40] If the infected shunt is not removed and antibiotics alone are used, there is a higher risk of infection recurrence (23-50%).[6,33] However, when the infectious agents are the more common meningitis pathogens such as *Haemophilus influenzae*, *Pneumococcus*, or *Neiserria meningitidis*, antibiotics alone may adequately clear the infection.[39-41]

Complications of Indwelling Venous Devices

More than 500,000 indwelling venous devices are inserted annually.[42] Chronically ill children are surviving longer, and these lines often provide long-term access for any patient needing blood sampling, prolonged infusions (chemotherapy, crystalloids, and blood products), or hyperalimentation.[42,43] More and more patients and their families care for these devices at home. These indwelling lines are available to ED staff to draw blood and administer medications, blood products, and IV fluids.[44] While ED physicians are not usually responsible for placing these lines, they often are confronted with complications of these devices. Consequently, they should be familiar with the recognition and treatment of these complications.

Originally introduced by Broviac et al in 1979, these lines are now known by a variety of names such as Hickman, Broviac, and Groshong catheters. Each has slight differences in construction. As a group, they consist of a silastic catheter with one, two, or three lumens that is tunneled subcutaneously and inserted into the right atrium via subclavian approach.[42,45] The subcutaneous portion of the catheter includes a Dacron cuff that becomes adherent to scar tissue (which may take 2-3 weeks), forming an internal anchor for the catheter and a barrier against ascending infection along the catheter from the skin surface.[43,45-47] The external end separates into individual catheters for each lumen, each of which contains a reinforced sleeve with clamp and terminates in a disposable luer lock.[42] A common exit point is the anterior chest wall.[45] Broviac catheters are most often used in children and Hickman catheters in adults.[48]

There are a few important differences in construction of these devices. Hickman and Broviac catheters are open-ended and blood may back up into the catheter, causing clotting and obstruction. Therefore, a clamp is necessary when the catheter is not in use, and frequent heparin flushing is necessary to prevent clotting.[43] Groshong catheters are similar to Hickman-type catheters with a few exceptions. First, the distal tip (residing in the superior vena cava) of the catheter is solid and blunt. Second, the lateral wall of the distal end has a pressure-sensitive two-way valve that eliminates the need for catheter clamping and frequent heparin flushes. Normal venous pressure results in the valve remaining closed with no backflow of blood into the catheter. External pressure exerted by the infusion of fluids opens the valve. Continued aspiration at the injection port also results in the valve opening and the ability to aspirate blood through the catheter. While this unique design precludes the use of heparin, Groshong catheters have to be flushed with saline every seven days.[43,46] On the other hand, because of the design of the distal valve, Groshong catheter malfunction rates are 3-7 times higher than Hickman-type catheter rates.[45] Finally, the proximal end of the catheter (external to the body) is removable for easier insertion and replacement without splicing.[45]

The Portacath is different in that it has a subcutaneous port with a silastic tube inserted into the right atrium via subclavian approach. The proximal end is a short segment tunneled subcutaneously that terminates in a titanium housing with a hard rubber dome. This infusion port will generally be found subcutaneously on the anterior chest wall. A recent variation on this theme is the forearm subcutaneous port. In these patients, the catheter enters a larger arm vein, either axillary or brachial.

Percutaneously inserted central catheters (PICC lines) are smaller silastic catheters inserted into the right atrium via an antecubital vein.[44] These catheters are like the Hickman catheters in structure, and the proximal end is also outside the skin.

When accessing these catheters, rigorous sterile technique is mandatory.[44] Hickman-like catheters and PICC lines can be accessed easily enough by removing the luer lock adapter on the end and by attaching a syringe or IV tubing directly to the catheter. Subcutaneous ports (Portacaths) need to be punctured with a noncoring needle (Huber needle, 19-22 gauge) for access. This needle has a deflected point and side opening to prevent coring or creating holes in the rubber dome.[43] If standard (coring or hollow) needles are used to repeatedly access a subcutaneous port, there is the risk of creating a permanent, nonsealing hole in the rubber dome of the port, which might allow air embolization to occur. However, in a critical situation, any 18 or 21 gauge needle can be used. The dome of most ports is made of a hard rubber that is similar in consistency to a hockey puck. Therefore, the amount of force that is necessary to insert the needle through the dome is significant.[44] The needle cannot be inserted too far, since it will contact the metal base of the port on deep insertion and a familiar "tick" will occur.[42,44]

Place an ice pack or a topical anesthetic such as EMLA cream to the area over the subcutaneous port prior to painful needle insertion attempts.[43] An approximate 30-minute delay is necessary for EMLA cream to produce topical anesthesia. The needle can then be attached to either a syringe or IV tubing. This technique should allow approximately 2000 punctures.[42] Hickman-like catheters and PICC lines can be used immediately after placement and confirmation of location by x-ray.[49] Subcutaneous ports are usually not accessed for one or more days after placement.[44] Showering and bathing are permitted for patients with healed incisions and no other complications.[43]

After access is achieved, one may phlebotomize by withdrawing 2-4 cc of the heparinized blood from the catheter, reclamping, and then using a separate syringe to remove the desired amount of blood. Coagulation tests are notoriously inaccurate when drawn through indwelling access devices, even when large amounts of blood are initially discarded.[44]

After blood is drawn, intravenous tubing may be connected directly to the external end of the catheter of the Huber needle. Since the internal diameter of the indwelling catheter will limit the rate of fluid administration, a larger-bore needle will not be advantageous.[42] Flow rates without a positive pressure infusion pump can be achieved at 200-250 mL/h with smaller central venous catheters and up to 500 mL/h with larger catheters.[45]

To ensure patency, inject 1-5 mL of heparin (100 U/mL), clamp the line, and reposition the cap upon completion.[44] An "antibiotic lock," a solution of antibiotics (vancomycin, amikacin, and minocycline) and heparin, may decrease the incidence of infectious complications, according to one study.[50]

Subcutaneous ports should be flushed as the needle is being withdrawn from the port. The portacath requires a heparinization flush after each infusion, and at least monthly, if not used more frequently.[45]

Table 1. Complications of Indwelling Venous Catheters

OCCLUSION
INFECTION
Exit site, Tunnel, Line sepsis, Endocarditis
THROMBOSIS
Subclavian/Axillary vein, Superior vena cava syndrome, Thrombophlebitis
FRACTURE
Intravenous, Subcutaneous, External
OTHERS
Extravasation, Air embolism, Migration, Hemorrhage, Cardiac dysrhythmias

Hickman-type catheters and PICC lines should be flushed at least twice weekly with 5 mL heparinized saline. Daily flushing of these designs is not necessary and leads to an increased rate of infection. Groshong catheters need only be flushed once a week to insure patency.[44] All of the currently used ports and catheters are safe for use in CT and MRI scanners provided they do not have a metal needle in place for access.[44,51]

Complications of indwelling vascular devices are common. They include occlusion, infection, thrombosis, and mechanical fracture of the catheter. *(See Table 1.)*

Occlusion. Indwelling venous catheters may become either partially or totally occluded during the course of use. Partial occlusion usually allows fluids to be readily infused into the device but without blood return.[44] It has been estimated that 20% of long-term catheters will eventually fail to yield blood samples.[51,52] Difficulty in drawing blood from a central venous catheter may be due to decreased vascular volume, catheter position or malfunction, and fibrin clot formation at the catheter tip.[44] Several maneuvers can be helpful in obtaining a blood return from these devices when decreased vascular volume is suspected. First, place the patient in the Trendelenberg position to engorge the subclavian system. Patients who are markedly dehydrated may require IV fluid administration before blood return from the access can be demonstrated. Extending the arm on the side of the device above the head will sometimes permit blood return.[44] Other maneuvers may be helpful, including turning the patient's head, coughing, changing position, taking a deep breath, or performing a Valsalva maneuver.[43,51] If occlusion occurs with a subcutaneous port, make certain that the Huber needle has fully penetrated the septum and is not occluded by the silicone dome. The port should be reaccessed to ensure correct placement of the needle.[51] It is possible for the needle to be positioned in a subcutaneous pocket around the port. In this case, no blood will be able to be withdrawn, but flushing will be easy because the fluid is infusing into the pocket. To see if this is the case, infuse a small amount of fluid and watch for any swelling around the port or along the track of the catheter.[43]

Positioning of the catheter's distal tip against a vessel wall or overzealous withdrawal on the syringe (excessive negative pressure) may be other causes of partial occlusion. Rapid infusion of fluid may help to reposition a catheter tip that is against a vessel wall.[42,51] If not successful, a clot or precipitate should be suspected of occluding the catheter.[47]

Probably the most common cause of partial or total occlusion is formation of a fibrin clot at the tip of the catheter, which acts as a one-way valve. When aspiration occurs, the intimal surface of the vein or fibrin sheath is drawn into the tip, preventing blood from entering. The incidence of fibrin clot formation varies from weekly to yearly depending on the frequency of use and flushing of the device.[43,44] An attempt may be made to aspirate a clot into a 10 mL syringe half filled with saline using a gentle push-pull motion. Since clots are unlikely to be aspirated through a needle, the syringe should be connected directly to the luer lock. If the catheter is still occluded after several attempts, a radiographic dye study should be performed to locate the site of the occlusion.[47]

Lack of blood return from one of these devices, however, is not an absolute contraindication to use. If the device has a long-term history of satisfactory use and a chest x-ray confirms the proper placement of the catheter tip in the superior vena cava, the device can be used for the infusion of fluids and medications even if no blood can be aspirated.[42] When there is no blood return and resistance is felt to infusion of fluids, do not force the flush.[43,46]

If it is important that blood withdrawal is an integral part of the catheter's function or the catheter is totally occluded, then thrombolytic infusion should be considered. The thrombolytics, urokinase and streptokinase, have been used successfully to reestablish catheter patency. Most practitioners prefer to use urokinase because it is associated with fewer anaphylactic reactions that seem to plague the use of streptokinase. These reactions are manifest by pruritis, fever, nausea, headache, and shock.[53]

The standard treatment for partial occlusion is a bolus of 0.5-1.0 mL of urokinase (5000 mcg/mL). The amount of time that the urokinase dwells in the access device is variable. The urokinase may be flushed out within 10 minutes or may be allowed to dwell for an hour or even overnight.[42,44] In the systemic circulation, urokinase has a half-life of approximately 20 minutes.[52] A urokinase flush successfully declots the line in up to 95% of cases.[42] This process may usually be repeated once. Patients with central venous access systems that fail to respond to two trials of a urokinase bolus may be admitted for a continuous infusion of urokinase (100-200 units per kg of body weight per hour)[47] until the catheter becomes patent.[44,46,54] Alteplase (tPA) has been used when urokinase was not successful.[52,53]

Chemical precipitates may accumulate within the device, causing occlusion.[55] The inner diameter of the catheter also influences the rate of occlusion, as particulate material is prone to deposit in catheters with smaller diameters.[51] Precipitates are formed by poorly soluble intravenous fluid components or the interaction of incompatible solutions. Medications that are incompatible through multiple lumen catheters should not be infused because turbulence at the catheter tip permits mixture.[42] Drugs that commonly result in a precipitate when infused incorrectly include calcium, diazepam, phenytoin, heparin, and TPN.[52] Patency can be restored by improving the solubility of the precipitate; however, the decision of whether increasing or decreasing pH will improve the solubility of a precipitate is often difficult. In practice, if altering the pH one way

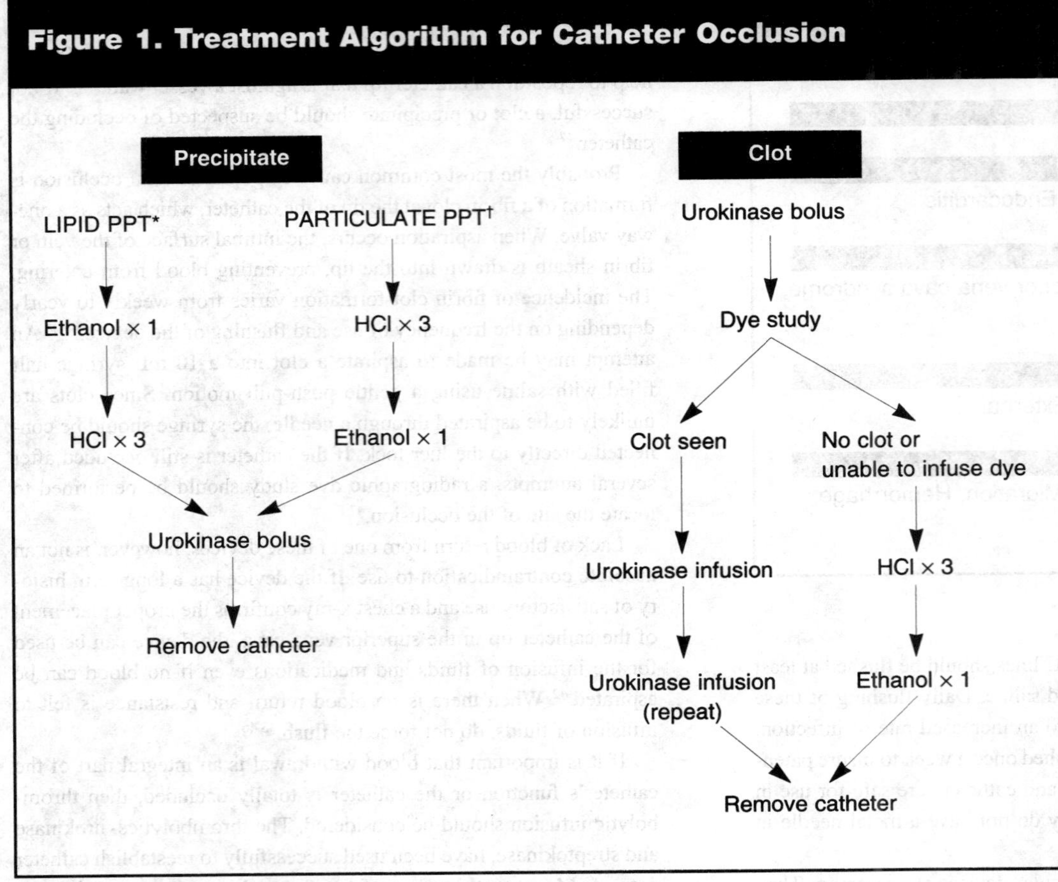

does not result in restoring patency, it is reasonable to try to alter the pH in the opposite direction.[53]

Hydrochloric acid has been used to restore patency successfully to catheters obstructed by drug precipitates. To lower the pH of the precipitate, the catheter is instilled with 0.2-1.0 mL of 0.1% HCl using a tuberculin syringe over one hour.[51] This small amount of HCl should not cause a metabolic acidosis.[53] On the other hand, a common side effect of this technique is a febrile reaction, occurring in up to 42% of patients.[46,52]

Phenytoin precipitates are most difficult to resolve but have been cleared using sodium bicarbonate. Ethanol solutions have been used to clear lipid occlusions with success (take 3.5 mL of 98% dehydrated alcohol for injection and add 1.5 mL of sterile water to make 5 mL 70% ethyl alcohol).[52,53] *(See Figure 1.)*

An uncommon condition, the "pinch-off" syndrome, may cause intermittent flush resistance and catheter compression and malfunction. It is recognized on chest x-ray as a narrowing of the catheter between the clavicle and first rib.[56] When the patient is upright, the weight of the shoulder narrows the area and pinches off the catheter. Changing the shoulder position will temporarily relieve the obstruction of the catheter so that fluids can easily be infused.[43] Compressed catheters are subject to shearing that can lead to catheter fracture and embolization of the tip.[55] Since there is a risk of transection and embolization of the catheter, this condition is an indication for catheter removal.[43] The time course of this process is variable but usually occurs within 3-6 months.[55] Other causes of total occlusion include kinking and coiling of the catheter, which should be detected by x-ray.[51]

Infection

The incidence of catheter-related infection is reported to range from 4% to 60%. The wide variability is related to such factors as insertion techniques, routine maintenance, and the physical condition of the individual patient and the definition of infection.[52] The presence of bacteria may be related to differing clinical scenarios from contamination to colonization to true infection.[57]

Risk Factors. Risk factors include age (< 1 year, > 60 years), altered host defense mechanisms, severity of underlying disease, remote infections, catheter type, catheter material, type of placement, and duration of use.[57] Patients between 1 and 4 years of age have a greater risk of multiple septic complications.[42] Infusate contamination has also been implicated in the pathogenesis of catheter-related septicemia.[46,57]

Catheter sepsis rates are very similar for single- and triple-lumen catheters, although there may be a trend to higher infection rates with triple lumen catheters.[57] Antimicrobial agents can be chemically bonded to catheter surfaces and may decrease the incidence of catheter-related bacteremia.[57,58]

The insertion site may be dressed with sterile gauze or transparent film. Transparent dressings increase the risk of developing catheter-related infection.[57,58] Chlorhexidine, rather than povidone-iodine and alcohol, is the preferred substance for skin disinfection with dressing changes. Topical antimicrobial agents confer only a modest benefit in protecting against catheter-related infection. If an ointment is to be used, the recommended agent is polymyxin/neomycin/bacitracin.[57]

Infections in vascular access devices take two forms, either local or systemic. Local infections occur at the site where the device exits the body and may be classified as exit-site infection or tunnel infection.

Exit-Site Infections. Exit-site infections are diagnosed by the appearance of erythema, tenderness, induration, and purulence at the exit site of the catheter.[42] The exudate should be cultured when present. These local infections can be treated with stringent site care and either oral or intravenous antibiotics for 10-14 days. Since catheter removal is seldom necessary to clear these infections, it is reasonable to attempt a cure by treating with antibiotics without removing the catheter.[46,52]

Empiric therapy may be started with vancomycin since the majority of exit-site infections are due to coagulase-negative

Staphylococcus. If the infection does not respond in a few days, the catheter should be removed.[48] If the infection is due to *Candida,* the catheter should be removed before antifungal therapy is initiated.[48] Unfortunately, this class of infection is unlikely to clear without removal.

Tunnel Infections. Catheter tunnel infections are more extensive than exit-site infections. These are diagnosed in the patient with fever and redness and tenderness along the subcutaneous tract. Pus is rarely expressed from the catheter and blood cultures are usually negative. These tunnel infections are most commonly caused by gram-positive organisms, which also routinely respond to vancomycin or amikacin/cefoxitin combination. However, there is a high rate of recurrence when antibiotics are stopped, and many physicians commonly remove devices with a tunnel infection without waiting for a clinical response to antibiotics.[44,48,52]

Line Sepsis. The other form of infection is device-related bacteremia or line sepsis. In the ED, this diagnosis is suspected after excluding other sources of fever. In device-related bacteremia, the vascular access device itself appears clinically normal. The diagnosis is often indirectly evaluated by quantitative blood cultures, drawn simultaneously via the device and via a peripheral site. If the blood from the catheter contains 5-15 times or more of the colonies than the peripheral blood, the presence of infection is confirmed.[52,57] These infections most commonly involve gram-positive skin flora.[42] A probable catheter-related septicemia is diagnosed when an organism is isolated from blood cultures and no other apparent source except the catheter. More confidence can be made in the diagnosis of catheter-related septicemia when the same organism is isolated from the exit site and blood or when the same organism is isolated from the catheter and a peripheral site. It may also be present when septicemia is refractory to antibiotic therapy but resolves when the catheter is removed.[48,52]

A more definitive method of diagnosis is to culture a segment of the catheter's distal tip. However, this requires removal of the device and may represent only colonization of the catheter and not true infection.[52,59] Culture of the tip is performed by rolling a 5 cm catheter segment across a blood agar plate in a defined reproducible manner.[57] Staphylococci, streptococci, and diphtheroid organisms as well as *Candida* species are cultured most frequently from infected indwelling catheters. *Staphylococcus epidermidis*, a common skin organism, is the most frequently cultured organism.[51,55,59] Gram-negative bacteria occur less frequently and may be associated with neutropenia.[42,45] Fungal infections occur less frequently but are virulent. Children are common victims of fungal infections, and they often present with low-grade fever, bradycardia, thrombocytopenia, apnea, and a predominance of immature PMNs.[42]

Most often, the source of bacteremia is never established in the patient with a long-term catheter. Therapy of bacteremia is usually attempted with the catheter in place after at least the two sets of blood cultures have been obtained. Empiric therapy should be initiated with vancomycin and gentamycin. For patients with neutropenia, start a third-generation cephalosporin with antipseudomonal activity or an antipseudomonal penicillin.[48]

If the infection responds to antibiotic therapy, treatment should continued for 2-3 weeks. If no response is seen in 48-72 hours after initiation of antimicrobial coverage, the line should be pulled. The catheter should be removed immediately if either *Pseudomonas* or fungal species are isolated.[48,53]

The success rate of clinical response may be increased with the addition of a urokinase infusion to standard antibiotic regimens.[44] A fibrin sheath can act as a nidus for reinfection by sequestering the organism to continually seed the circulation with each routine use.[51] The rate of catheter-related septicemia leading to systemic sepsis is relatively low, occurring in less than 1% of individuals.[57]

Port Pocket Infections. Port pocket infections usually exhibit erythema, tenderness, and induration at the edge of the portal body.[51] The port should not be accessed unless already in use. In this case, leave the needle in place for blood drawing and antibiotic infusion.[46,52]

If there is no evidence of skin necrosis over the reservoir, port pocket infections may initially be treated with two weeks of intravenous antibiotics without removal of the port. Purulent exudate in the subcutaneous space should be aspirated or drained.[48] If there is skin necrosis present, the reservoir should be removed. Empiric antibiotic therapy may be started with vancomycin and an aminoglycoside or a third-generation cephalosporin.[48]

Other infectious complications include septic thrombophlebitis and endocarditis. Clinical manifestations of septic thrombophlebitis combine those of infection (fever and rigors) and those of thrombosis (an elevated jugular venous pulse, swelling of the arm, shoulder, neck and face) as well as an obstructed catheter. Reported causative organisms include *S. viridans*, *S. epidermidis*, *S. aureus*, *K. pneumoniae*, and *E. coli*. Diagnosis may be made by venography but is best made by a contrasted CT scan, which has the advantage of excluding other conditions that can compress blood vessels in the area.[48]

Catheter-related endocarditis presents in a fashion similar to endocarditis from other causes. However, the appearance of a new or changing cardiac murmur and peripheral stigmata of endocarditis are frequently absent. Chest x-ray may show multiple nodular densities in the pulmonary parenchyma suggestive of septic pulmonary embolization due to endocarditis on the tricuspid valve.[48] Like other causes of endocarditis, diagnosis is usually made by echocardiography in addition to positive blood cultures. The catheter should be removed if either septic thrombophlebitis or endocarditis are suspected.[48]

PICC Line Complications. The most common complication of PICC lines is a sterile mechanical phlebitis, which is manifested by pain at the insertion site and up the arm, presence of a palpable venous cord, and reddening and swelling along the vein.[43] Unfortunately, these physical findings are difficult to distinguish from a tunnel infection. This phlebitis is caused by a nonspecific inflammatory reaction to the catheter.[55] The catheter can remain in place, and the patient is encouraged to use conservative measures such as warm compresses for 20 minutes throughout the day and to elevate the arm. If this condition does not resolve within 72 hours, the catheter should be removed.[43]

Another complication of PICC lines is bleeding that occurs at the insertion sites. Bleeding occurs most often the day after insertion. After this period, excessive bleeding is usually due to an underlying coagulopathy or excessive use of the arm.[43]

Only about 1 inch of catheter should be visible external to the insertion site.[43] Extreme care must be taken when the dressing for a PICC line is removed since only tape holds the catheter in place. Consequently, it is very easy to inadvertently pull out several inches of the catheter.

On the other hand, PICC lines may also become "stuck" within the arm vein as a result of venospasm, which impedes withdrawal.[55]

If resistance is encountered as the catheter is withdrawn, do not apply excessive traction because the catheter could fracture. Instead, apply heat to the vein of the upper arm and flush the catheter with normal saline and try again. Other reasons for resistance include phlebitis, valve inflammation, and thrombosis.[60]

During removal of a PICC line, it may appear that only part of the catheter is removed. It is possible that the most internal part of the catheter has fractured and remained in the body. During insertion, the catheter is measured and cut to the appropriate length so that the tip lies either in the superior vena cava, subclavian, or axillary vein. This measurement should be recorded on insertion to allow verification that the catheter is intact when removed. The catheter length should be removed and compared with the length on insertion.[43]

Thrombosis. Factors that may predispose to subclavian vein thrombosis include catheter material composition, accelerated coagulation system, reduced flow in the venous system secondary to intrapulmonary or mediastinal disease, and possibly catheter size.[61] Specific tumors such as adenocarcinoma of the lung seem to increase the risk for thrombus formation. Intrapulmonary disease, mediastinal disease, or hypercoagulability associated with malignancy also have been associated with increased risk for thrombus formation, catheter or not. Placement of the catheter tip deep into the right atrium can cause arrhythmias, and increase the chance for thrombosis.[50] Left subclavian catheter placements have been associated with a significantly higher incidence of thrombus.[51]

The clinical presentation of thrombosis is generally insidious in evolution and is characterized by nonspecific pain on the chest wall, neck, or in the scapular area.[61]

Subclavian/axillary vein thrombosis may present with arm swelling while superior vena cava syndrome presents as face or neck swelling.[61] In either case, these are not consistent findings.[61] Since many patients will probably be aware of problems accessing their vascular devices, thrombosis is usually diagnosed before progression to the superior vena cava syndrome. However, thrombosis of the central vasculature may remain unrecognized until total venous obstruction occurs. Signs of venous obstruction include collateral circulation across the chest wall, distended neck veins, and edema in the supraclavicular areas.[51] Clinical examination is usually satisfactory to consider the diagnosis; however, duplex sonography is the preferred method to confirm clinical findings. Venography will not only document clot in symptomatic patients but will show clot in 25% of asymptomatic patients.[44]

Pulmonary embolism is a most worrisome complication but a relatively unlikely event only associated with approximately 12% of the thromboses.[44,61] Pulmonary embolism immediately following catheter flushing is unlikely.[42]

Patients with newly diagnosed thrombosis should be admitted. Venous thrombosis is treated with full anticoagulation.[55] If no contraindications exist and chronic access is required, the catheter is left in place and a trial of thrombolytic therapy may be warranted. Streptokinase is often used but is more effective in the setting of acute occlusions, while line thrombosis is more subacute in progression.[61] If lytic therapy fails or is contraindicated, long-term anticoagulation and/or device removal is required.[43,44] The device should be removed if it is nonfunctional or if the thrombotic symptoms progress despite appropriate anticoagulation therapy.[55,61]

Vigilant flushing between drugs, routine flushing with urokinase, and the avoidance of incompatible infusions are the cornerstones to thrombosis prevention. Chronic oral warfarin has been helpful in preventing thrombosis.[51]

Fracture. Damage to the cannula in the form of small holes or tears can occur when the pressure inside the lumen becomes too high. Excessive pressures can occur when small syringes are used; larger syringes create lower pressures.[62] Fractures of indwelling venous catheters are divided into fractures that occur intravenously, subcutaneously, and those that occur at the external end of Hickman-type catheters.

Pieces of catheter that break off in the venous system need to be retrieved emergently before they embolize to the arterial system. Fracture and embolism of the intravascular catheter tip is a rare but potentially lethal complication of indwelling access devices. Symptoms include the abrupt onset of dyspnea, palpitations, or atypical chest pain. Signs include hypoxia and atrial fibrillation. All of the catheter tips are radiopaque and can be visualized on routine chest x-ray.[49] Many of these emboli can be removed nonsurgically depending on the exact location and size of the catheter fragment.[44]

Fractures that occur subcutaneously become manifest when the patient attempts to flush the catheter. Swelling and/or pain develops at some point in the subcutaneous tunnel when injection into the catheter is attempted. Almost invariably, these catheters must be removed. Repair cannot usually be accomplished.

Fractures of the external end of Hickman-type catheters are usually traumatic but may occur spontaneously. They are diagnosed by observing an obvious break in the catheter or leakage of fluid from a pinhole in the catheter when it is flushed.[45] External fractures more than two inches from the exit may often be repaired in the ED with manufacturer-specific repair kits available for some but not all catheters.[44,47,55]

Other Complications. Additional complications of indwelling lines include mediastinitis, cardiac dysrhythmias, subcutaneous tunnel hematoma, and septic atrial thrombus.[42] Local trauma to the intima may result in erosion of a catheter through the vessel wall with resultant hemorrhage. Gross mishandling of the external portion of the catheter can result in hemorrhage at the venous insertion site, the location of the Dacron cuff, or the skin exit point. Mishandling also increases the potential for air embolus.[45] Although not common, retrograde perfusion into the cerebral circulation of parenteral solutions administered through indwelling catheters has been reported to cause neurologic complications such as stroke-like syndromes.

Port reservoirs may separate from the attached catheter and lead to extravasation of infused fluids manifest by a stinging or burning sensation at the infusion site.[55] This usually results when the needle dislodges from the port. Other mechanisms of extravasation include catheter fracture resulting from compression, fibrin sheath formation, and slippage of port access needles from the reservoir.[55] The degree of damage to the skin and subcutaneous tissues depends upon the type of drug extravasated, the duration of exposure, and site of extravasation.[51]

Air embolism may occur during catheter insertion, during infusions, or during catheter removal. Patients with low central venous pressures and those with compromised pulmonary function are at highest risk for this occasionally fatal complication.[55]

If the catheter has been placed into the right atrium, complications may include arrhythmias, endocardial damage, and risk of perforation and pericardial tamponade.[63,64]

Catheter migration into the jugular system may simply be monitored and is not a cause for catheter removal, although interventional radiographic techniques may be used to reposition the catheter.[61]

Physicians charged with caring for patients with central indwelling venous catheters should be aware of the common complications of these devices as well as their initial treatment.

Complications of Gastrostomy Tubes

Gastrostomy tubes, which are inserted into the stomach through the abdominal wall, allow the chronically ill, neurologically devastated patients with dysphagia to have their nutritional needs met. However, few studies have evaluated long-term complications of these tubes. The most common complications appear to be tube dislodgement or occlusion of the tube.[65]

If a tube comes out and needs replacement, it may simply be reinserted into the tract, provided firm adhesions are formed between the gastric and abdominal walls. When the tract has matured, it is usually safe to replace the tube. There is disagreement as to when the gastrocutaneous fistula tract has matured, ranging from seven days to three months.[66,67] If the tube is inserted when adequate adhesions have not had a chance to form, there is a risk of inserting the tube into the peritoneal space as well as allowing leakage of gastric contents into the peritoneum, causing peritonitis. Air may leak through this tract as well, presenting as pneumoperitoneum, which is usually of no consequence. This must, however, be differentiated from a perforated viscous.[68] Viscous lidocaine lubricant may decrease the discomfort of reinsertion of a tube.[68] The common practice of replacing the tube and insufflating air while listening over the gastric area to confirm placement has resulted in a fatal air embolus in at least one case.[74] Once a tube has been removed, the stoma will often close within 24-48 hours, but this may take up to 10-12 days.[66]

In the event that a regular PEG tube or button is not available, a Foley catheter may be inserted to keep the stoma open and allow tube feedings to continue.

Temporary short-term use of Foley catheters has minimal complications. There are two complications, however, to keep in mind with this technique: 1) rupture of the balloon, allowing the catheter to slip out; and 2) migration of the balloon, causing obstruction. The thin-walled balloon can tolerate the acid medium of the stomach for about three weeks. Gastrostomy tubes with balloons have been reported to cause gastric outlet obstruction or duodenal obstruction, usually presenting with abdominal pain and vomiting.[70-72] Abdominal radiographs are diagnostic. The obstruction may be relieved by simply releasing the balloon.[73] It is important to properly fix the tube to the abdominal wall (with sutures, if need be), so that the balloon is adherent to the gastric and abdominal wall and migration of the balloon is prevented.

To prevent clogged or occluded tubes, it is necessary to flush them with water after intermittent feedings or administration of medications. Crushed pills should be avoided (especially if they are sustained-release medications that depend on the pill matrix for their time-release characteristics) because they are a common cause of malocclusion.[76]

Leakage of gastric contents around the tube may be a manifestation of distal obstruction of the gastrostomy tube or simply of a stoma that is too large.[70,71] If the former has been excluded, simply inserting a larger tube exacerbates the problem by enlarging the stoma even more. Sutures should be placed to tighten the orifice by physicians familiar with revision of stomal orifices.

Infections, such as superficial wound infections and cellulitis, may present as erythema and induration in the peristomal area or may progress to necrotizing fasciitis. This condition manifests as tender red streaks of the abdominal skin often associated with creptitus. Fever is invariably present, as well as systemic toxicity. It is usually caused by a mixture of aerobic and anaerobic bacteria. Necrotizing fasciitis requires emergent management with surgical debridement and intravenous antibiotics.[66,71]

Since complications may have subtle presentations, a water contrast radiologic study should be considered and used liberally to evaluate for extraluminal placement of gastrostomy tubes and such conditions as gastric obstruction, gastric ulcers, gastric perforations, fractured catheters, gastric torsions, intraperitoneal leak, tube migration, intussusception, intestinal obstruction, gastric fistulas, and obstruction of the catheter itself.[75]

Summary

Even though CSF shunts, indwelling venous catheters, and gastrostomy tubes are life-saving devices for children with complex medical conditions, they are associated with significant risks to the pediatric patient. As more of these medical devices are used to facilitate treatment in children, it is incumbent upon physicians to be familiar with the various devices, their functional mechanics, their indications, and the commonly associated complications as well as the treatment.

References

1. Wiswell TE, Tuttle DJ, Northam RS, et al. Major congenital neurologic malformations. *Am J Dis Child* 1990;144:6167.
2. Bondurant CP, Jimenex DF. Epidemiology of cerebrospinal fluid shunting. *Pediatr Neurosurg* 1995;23:254-259.
3. Sainte-Rose C. Hydrocephalus in childhood. In: Youmans JL. *Neurological Surgery.* 4th ed. Philadelphia: WB Saunders; 1996;890-926.
4. Peacock WJ. Prevention and manage of cerebrospinal fluid shunt complication. *Prog Neurol Surg* 1990;13:114.
5. Cutler RW, Page L, Galicich J. Formation and absorption of cerebrospinal fluid in man. *Brain* 1968;9:707-720.
6. Odio C, McCracken G, Nelson JD. CSF shunt infections in pediatrics—seven year experience. *Am J Dis Child* 1984;138: 1103-1108.
7. McLauren RL. Ventricular shunts: Complications and results. In: McLauren RL, Shute L, Venes JL, et al. *Pediatric Neurosurgery: Surgery of the Developing Nervous System.* Philadelphia: WB Saunders; 1989.
8. Turner MS. The treatment of hydrocephalus: A brief guide to shunt selection. *Surg Neurol* 1995;43:314-323.
9. Post EM. Currently available shunt systems: A review. *Neurosurgery* 1985;16:257-260.
10. Keucher TR, Mealey J. Long term results after ventriculoatrial and ventriculoperitoneal shunting for infantile hydrocephalus. *J Neurosurg* 1979;50:179-186.
11. Kast J, Duong D, Nowzari F, et al. Time-related patterns of ventricular shunt failure. *Child Nerv Syst* 1994;10:524-528.
12. Grosfeld J, Cooney D, Smith J, et al. Intra-abdominal compli-

cations following ventriculoperitoneal shunt procedures. *Pediatrics* 1974;54:791-796.

13. Ronan A, Hogg GG, Klug GL. Cerebrospinal fluid shunt infections in children. *Pediatr Infect Dis J* 1995;14:782-786.
14. Walters BC, Hoffman HJ, Hendrick EB, et al. Cerebrospinal fluid shunt infection. Influences on initial management and subsequent outcomes. *J Neurosurg* 1984;60:1014-1021.
15. Schoenbaum SC, Gardner P, Shillito J. Infections of cerebrospinal fluid shunts: epidemiology, clinical manifestations and therapy. *J Infect Dis* 1975;131:543-552.
16. Yogev R. Cerebrospinal fluid shunt infections: A personal view. *Pediatr Infect Dis* 1985;85:113-118.
17. Kontny U, Hofling B, Gutjahr P, et al. CSF shunt infections in children. *Infection* 1993;21:89-92.
18. Forrest DM, Cooper DG. Complications of ventriculo-atrial shunts a review of 455 cases. *J Neurosurg* 1968;29:506-512.
19. Coker SB. Cyclic vomiting and the slit ventricle syndrome. *Pediatr Neurol* 1987;3:297-299.
20. Foltz EL, Blanks JP. Symptomatic low intracranial pressure in shunted hydrocephalus. *J Neurosurg* 1988;68:401-408.
21. Walker ML, Fried A, Petronio J. Diagnosis and treatment of the slit ventricle syndrome. *Neuorsurg Clin North Am* 1993; 4:707-714.
22. Serlo W, Saukkonen AL, Heikkinen E, et al. The incidence and management of the slit ventricle syndrome. *Acta Neurochir* 1989;99:113-116.
23. Engelhard HH, Miller FB. Abdominal pain resulting from cerebrospinal fluid pseudocyst and cholithiasis. *South Med J* 1992;85:851-852.
24. Sekhar LN, Moossy J, Guthkelch N. Malfunctioning ventriculoperitoneal shunts clinical and pathological features. *J Neurosurg* 1982;56:411-416.
25. Forward KR, Fewer D, Stiver HG. Cerebrospinal fluid shunt infections a review of 35 infections in 32 patients. *J Neurosurg* 1983;59:389-394.
26. Watkins L, Hayward R, Andar U, et al. The diagnosis of blocked cerebrospinal fluid shunts: A prospective study of referral to a paediatric neurosurgical unit. *Child Nerv Syst* 1994;10:87-90.
27. Sakoda TH, Maxwell JA, Brackett CE. Intestinal volvulus secondary to a ventriculoperitoneal shunt. *J Neurosurg* 1971;35:95-96.
28. Hubschmann OR, Countee RW. Acute abdomen in children with infected ventriculoperitoneal shunts. *Arch Surg* 1980; 115:305-307.
29. Cantrell P, Fraser F, Carty P. The value of baseline ct head scans in the assessment of shunt complications in hydrocephalus. *Pediatr Radiol* 1993;23:485-486.
30. Myers MG, Schoenbaum SC. Shunt fluid aspiration. *Am J Dis Child* 1975;129:220-222.
31. Uvebrant P, Sixt R, Roos A. Evaluation of cerebrospinal fluid shunt function in hydrocephalic children using 99Tc-DTPA. *Child Nerv Syst* 1992;8:76-80.
32. Sood S, Kim S, Canady AI, et al. Useful components of the shunt tap test for evaluation of shunt malfunction. *Child Nerv Syst* 1993;9:157-162.
33. Vinchon M,Vallee L, Prin L, et al. Cerebro-spinal fluid eosinophilia in shunt infections. *Neuropediatrics* 1992;23:235-240.
34. Piatt J. Physical examination of patients with cerebrospinal fluid shunts: Is there useful information in pumping the shunt? *Pediatrics* 1992;89:470-473.
35. Guertin SR. Cerebrospinal fluid shunts evaluation, complications and crisis management. *Pediatr Clin North Am* 1987;34:203-217.
36. Lang RG. Neurologic procedures. In: Roberts, Hedges, eds. *Clinical Procudures in Emergency Medicine.* Philadelphia: WB Saunders; 1991.
37. Madsen MA. Emergency department management of ventriculoperitoneal cerebrospinal fluid shunts. *Ann Emerg Med* 1986;15:1330-1343.
38. Morissette I, Gourdeau M, Francoeur J. CSF shunt infections: A fifteen-year experience with emphasis on management and outcome. *Can J Neurol Sci* 1993;20: 118-122.
39. Hellbusch LC, Penn RG. Treatment of haemophilus influenzae type b cerebrospinal fluid shunt infection with ceftriaxone and rifampin: Case report. *Nebr Med J* 1995;80: 27-29.
40. Bayston R. Hydrocephalus shunt infections. *J Antimicrob Chemother* 1994;34:75-84.
41. Leggiadro RJ, Atluru VL, Katz SP. Meningococcal meningitis associated with cerebrospinal fluid shunts. *Pediatr Infect Dis* 1984;4:489-496.
42. Howell JM. Obtaining access in patients with indwelling vascular access devices. *Emerg Med Clin North Am* 1994; 12:679-689.
43. Hogle ME, McDonagh JM, Rapp CJ, et al. Patients with long-term vascular access devices: Care and complications. *Orth Nurs* 1994;13:41-52.
44. Gryn J, Sacchetti A. Emergencies of indwelling venous catheters. *J Emerg Med* 1992;10:254-257.
45. Johnson JC. Complications of vascular access devices. *Emerg Med Clin North Am* 1994;12:691-705.
46. Wickham RS. Advances in venous access devices and nursing management strategy. *Nurs Clin North Am* 1990;25: 345-364.
47. Dyer BJ, Weiman MG, Ludwig S, et al. Central venous catheters if the emergency department: Access, utilization, and problem solving. *Pediatr Emerg Care* 1995;11:112-117.
48. Mayhall CG. Diagnosis and management of infections of implantable devices used for prolonged venous access. *Curr Clin Top Infect Dis* 1992;12:83-110.
49. Fisher KL, Leung AN. Radiographic appearance of central venous catheters. *AJR Am J Roentgenol* 1996;166:329 337.
50. Messing B, Peitra-Cohen S, Debure A, et al. Antibiotic lock technique: A new approach to optimal therapy for catheter-related sepsis in home parenteral nutrition patients. *J Parenter Enterol Nutr* 1988;12:185-189.
51. Camp-Sorrell D. Implantable parts: Everything you always wanted to know. *J Intravenous Nurs* 1992;15:262-273.
52. Rumsey KA, Richardson DK, et al. Management of infection and occlusion associated with vascular access devices. *Semin Oncol Nurs* 1995;11:174-183.
53. Holcombs BJ, Forloines-Lynn S, Garmhausen LW, et al. Restoring patency of long term central venous access

devices. *J Intraven* 1992;15:36-41.

54. Tshirhart JM, Rao MK. Mechanism and management of persistent withdrawal occlusion. *Am Surg* 1988;54:326-328.
55. Whitman ED. Complications associated with the use of central access devices. *Curr Probl Surg* 1996;33:309-378.
56. Aitken DR, Minton JP. The "pinch-off sign." A warning of impending problems with permanent subclavian catheters. *Am J Surg* 1984;148:633-639.
57. Norwood S, Ruby A, Civetta J. Catheter-related infections and associated septicemia. *Chest* 1991;99:968-975.
58. Reed CR, Sessler CN, Glauser FL. Central venous catheter infections: Concepts and controversies. *Intensive Care Med* 1995;21:177-183.
59. Whitman ED, Boatman AM. Comparison of diagnostic specimens and methods to evaluate infected venous access ports. *Am J Surg* 1995;170:665-669.
60. Hadaway LC. Comparison of vascular access devices. *Sem Oncol Nurs* 1995;111:154-166.
61. Lokich JJ, Bothe A, Benetti P, et al. Complications and management of implanted venous access catheters. *J Clin Onc* 1985;3:710-717.
62. Hadaway LC. An overview of vascular access device inserted via the antecubital area. *J Intraven Nurs* 1990;13: 297-306.
63. Zarshenas Z, Sparschu RA. Catheter placement and misplacement. *Crit Care Clin* 1994;10:417-436.
64. Keeney SE, Richardson CJ. Extravasation of fluid as a complication of central venous lines in the neonate. *J Perinatol* 1994;15:284-288.
65. Ganga UR, Ryan JJ, Schafer LW, et al. Indications, complications, and long term results of percutaneous endoscopic gastrostomy: A retrospective study. *SD Med J* 1994;47: 149-152.
66. Broscious SK. Preventing complications of PEG tubes dimensions. *Crit Care Nurs* 1995;14:37-41.
67. Foutch PG, Talbert GA, Gaines JA, et al. The gastrostomy button: A prospective assessment of safety, success, and spectrum of use. *Gastrointest Endosc* 1989;35:41-44.
68. Larson DE, Burton DD, Schroeder KW, et al. Percutaneous endoscopic gastrostomy: Indications, success, complications, and mortality in 314 consecutive patients. *Gastroenterol* 1986;93:48-52.
69. Gauderer MWL, Olsen MM, Stellato TA, et al. Feeding gastrostomy button: Experience and recommendations. *J Pediatr Surg* 1988;23:24-28.
70. Wolfsen HC, Kozarte RA, Ball TJ, et al. Tube dysfunction following percutaneous endoscopic gastrostomy and jejunostomy. *Gastrointest Endosc* 1990;36:261-263.
71. Moran BJ, Taylor MB, Johnson CD, et al. Percutaneous endoscopic gastrostomy. *Br J Surg* 1990;77:858-862.
72. McGovern R, Baskin JS, Goldberg RI. Duodenal obstruction: A complication of percutaneous endoscopic gastrostomy tube migration. *Am J Gastroenterol* 1990;85: 1037-1038.
73. Gowen GF. The management of complications of Foley feeding gastrostomies. *Am Surg* 1988;9:582-585.
74. McQuaid KR, Little TE. Two fatal complications related to gastrostomy "button" placement. *Gastrointest Endosc* 1992;38:601-603.
75. DiLorenzo J, Dalton B, Miskoritz P. Percutaneous endoscopic gastrostomy. *Postgrad Med* 1992; 91:277-281.
76. O'Keefe KP. Complications of percutaneous feeding tubes. *Emerg Med Med Clin North Am* 1994;12:815-826.

Urinary Tract Infections

Michael F. Altieri, MD
Mary A. Camarca, MD, FAAP

If one were to personify pediatric urinary tract infections, two words come to mind, "sneaky and sly." Doesn't it always seem to be the urinary tract infection (UTI) that catches us by surprise when evaluating febrile infants and children? At one time or another, all of us have breathed a sigh of relief that we followed our clinical conscience while evaluating that febrile child with an equivocal presentation. Our diagnostic dilemmas are understandable when one considers that in patients younger than age 3, symptoms of UTI include irritability (80%), poor feeding (65%), vomiting (40%), diarrhea (30%), and upper respiratory symptoms in up to 15% of children.[1] Furthermore, Hoberman found that symptoms were not very helpful for differentiating between children with fever who did and did not have a UTI.[1]

As if its commonly subtle clinical presentation is not vexing enough, the management and follow-up of pediatric UTI can be equally demanding. Additionally, there is always the threat of permanent damage to the child's renal parenchyma hanging over the head of the clinician. In this chapter, the authors provide an in-depth and cutting-edge review of the evaluation and management of pediatric UTIs.

Introduction

The diagnosis of a UTI should be considered in all febrile infants and children presenting to the ED. To date, however, there is no consensus on the optimal approach to evaluating a child for a UTI, the proper interpretation of laboratory data, and the most efficient and effective treatment and follow up.

The significance of UTIs as an important cause of acute febrile illness has been recently reaffirmed.[1] In this study, febrile infants ages 1 year and younger underwent bladder catheterization and urine culture. Of all febrile infants evaluated, 5.3% were suffering from a UTI. Among white female infants in this study, 16.9% had a UTI. Of particular interest, approximately one out of three infected infants had an initial diagnosis other than UTI. These results suggest that UTIs may be under-diagnosed in febrile infants and suggests difficulty in the clinical diagnosis of UTIs in young children. Thus, when the source of fever is equivocal, UTI always should be included in the differential diagnosis, particularly in infants during the first two years of life. The information that follows can be used to formulate a rational basis for the selection of children for UTI evaluation and treatment.

Epidemiology and Infection Etiology

Age and gender are major determinants of prevalence rates of UTI in children. UTIs will occur in up to 1% of full-term infants and in as many as 3% of premature infants. During infancy, males and females have comparable risks for UTI. Thereafter, females comprise the major risk group. Symptomatic UTIs will develop in about 2% of

Table 1. Children at Risk for UTI

- Premature infants
- Children with immunologic or systemic disease
- Children with anatomic urinary tract abnormalities
    - Ureterpelvic junction obstruction
    - Congenital megaureter
    - Ectopic ureters
    - Ureterocele
    - Ureteral polyps
    - Extrinsic ureteral compression
        - Neoplasms
        - Inflammatory diseases (Crohn's disease)
        - Hematomas
    - Bladder outlet and ureteral obstructions
        - Posterior urethral valves
        - Bladder diverticula
        - Urethral strictures
        - Urethral atresia
        - Meatal stenosis
        - Renal calculi
        - Urethral foreign bodies
        - Phimosis
- Sexual activity
- Neurogenic bladder
- Voiding dysfunction
- Constipation
- Family history of UTI
- Lack of circumcision
- Voluntary retention

children ranging in age from 1 to 5 years, and in 2.5% of school aged females.[2] Accurate diagnosis is complicated by the fact that 1.2-1.8% of school-aged girls may have asymptomatic bacteriuria.[3]

The importance of UTI as a cause of infectious illness in infants and young children goes beyond the risks of severe local or systemic bacterial infection. Many of these children also suffer permanent injury to renal parenchyma. Those at particularly high risk for kidney injury include children with systemic or immunologic disease and those with a variety of structural urinary tract abnormalities. *(See Table 1.)* For instance, kidney stones or urolithiasis is a relatively uncommon condition in the pediatric patient, but it does occur. In a study by Gearhart et al, 47% of 54 children (birth to 17 years) with urolithiasis had concomitant UTIs.[4] Several of these patients, however, had prior urinary tract surgery and had other risk factors for UTI. The most common infecting organisms were *E. coli, Pseudomonas aeruginosa, Proteus mirabilis, Klebsiella,* and *Proteus vulgaris*.

Additional risk factors include, urethral foreign bodies, phimosis, sexual activity, neurogenic bladders, voiding dysfunction, a family history of UTI, and constipation. Blethyn et al showed an association between fecal loading (on x-ray) and a significant increase in UTI, mainly in females.[5] Vesicoureteral reflux (VUR) may be found in 30-50% of children with UTIs, but is rarely found in normal children.[6] Additionally, a number of studies have demonstrated the significantly increased risk of UTI among uncircumcised male children when compared to those who were circumcised.[7,8] Despite this observation, there remains a degree of controversy over whether the increased risk of UTIs in uncircumcised males is sufficient alone to justify circumcision.

Host susceptibility and virulence factors of the invading pathogen are important variables in the pathogenesis of UTIs. Recently improved understanding of factors enhancing bacterial virulence in UTI show promise for the prevention of UTI in the future. However, at the present time, host immunity and structural/functional aspects of the urinary tract remain the factors of greatest importance.

During the neonatal period, UTIs are presumed to originate via hematogenous spread. In most cases beyond the neonatal period, bacteria are presumed to ascend the urinary tract following perineal colonization. In the female, the short urethra and its proximity to the anal opening explains at least in part the predominance of UTIs in females. Commonly occurring functional and behavioral factors also increase the risk of UTI in females. These include wiping forward after bowel movements, voluntary deferral of micturition, incomplete bladder emptying, and the failure of voiding promptly after coitus. The presence of foreign bodies in the introitus, frequent masturbation, and pinworm infection also are factors that promote UTIs.[13]

Gram-negative enteric bacteria are the most common organisms that cause UTIs.[3,14] *(See Table 2.) E. coli* accounts for the vast majority (80%) of cases of UTI, particularly first infections. Other organisms that must be considered include *Proteus mirabilis, Klebsiella pneumonia, Pseudomonas aeruginosa, Enterobacteraciae, Streptococcus viridans,* and *Candida albicans*. Coagulase-negative staphylococcus UTI occurs in teens and young adults. Acute cystitis may also be caused by adenovirus, occurring more commonly in young male children. These patients often have fever, intense dysuria, and gross hematuria.

Isolated urethritis can also cause symptoms of a UTI such as dysuria. In clinical urethritis, colony counts in urine culture may be as low as 10^2 CFU/mL of a single organism, which is considerably lower than the conventional threshold of 5×10^4 to 1×10^5 CFU/mL for cystitis. Other etiologies of urethritis that must be considered, particularly in adolescents, are *Chlamydia trachomatous, Neisseria gonorrhoeae, Ureaplasm urealyticum,* and Herpes simplex viruses.

Types of Urinary Tract Infections

It is useful to consider UTI in two categories: uncomplicated lower tract infections and upper tract infections. From a practical standpoint, upper tract infections are distinguished as those in which kidney parenchymal injury can be demonstrated. Lower UTIs include cystitis and urethritis. While symptoms of lower UTI among older children are more specific, clinical findings in younger children are often vague. After infancy, cystitis occurs 3-5 times more

Table 2. Organisms Responsible for Pediatric UTI

E. coli
Proteus mirabilis
Klebsiella pneumoniae
Pseudomonas aeruginosa
Enterobacter species
Streptococcus viridans
Coagulase-negative staphylococci
Candida albicans
Chlamydia trachomatous
Neisseria gonorrhoeae

frequently in females than in males and is the most common primary infection in healthy individuals. Among females, the incidence of first time cystitis gradually diminishes during the first decade of life and then increases during the second decade, correlating with the onset of sexual activity. Recurrent lower tract infections occur in nearly 30% of affected females but are rare in males.

Upper UTIs involve infection of the renal parenchyma (pyelonephritis). Pyelonephritis in children is often associated with VUR voiding dysfunction, or other of the risk factors listed above. In most cases the renal parenchyma is infected by bacterial pathogens ascending the urinary tract rather than dissemination via the hematogenous route. Several anatomic factors associated with the growing kidneys places the younger child at particularly high risk for penetration of bacterial pathogens into renal parenchyma, thereby increasing the risk of renal injury. As with lower UTI, pediatric patients experiencing an episode of pyelonephritis are at increased risk for subsequent episodes, particularly during the ensuing two years.

Asymptomatic bacteriuria may confound an evaluation for possible UTI. Although asymptomatic bacteriuria during infancy and in males beyond infancy is associated with a high incidence of urinary tract abnormalities and necessitates prompt diagnosis and treatment,[9] asymptomatic bacteriuria occurs in nearly all age groups and is found predominately in females. The prevalence of asymptomatic bacteriuria in children differs with age. In premature infants, the prevalence is approximately 3%, while in full-term infants it is less than 1%. In preschool females, the incidence is 0.08%, while nearly negligible in males. School-age females have a prevalence of 2%, and approximately 5% of females will have asymptomatic bacteriuria prior to finishing high school. While these patients generally have no abnormalities on urinalysis, many have associated voiding behavioral disturbances. There is often no history of preceding UTI, and usually there is no evidence of anatomic abnormalities or renal parenchymal scarring by radiographic studies. This condition will resolve in approximately half of all patients without treatment. Nevertheless, identification of prepubertal children with asymptomatic bacteriuria is of importance since some may have VUR and an increased risk of recurrent symptomatic infections.[10,11] Although controversial, the routine treatment of asymptomatic bacteriuria in non-pregnant females appears to be of little benefit. Most prospective studies of girls older than 5 with asymptomatic bacteriuria have failed to demonstrate decreased glomerular filtration rates, impaired renal growth, or progressive parenchymal damage in kidneys that are normal at the time of initial evaluation.[12]

Clinical Aspects of UTI

The diagnosis of a UTI often presents a challenge to ED physicians, especially in infants and children. Accompanying this challenge is the urgency that a delay in diagnosis and treatment increases the risk of parenchymal damage.[16,17] Few symptoms, other than fever, are consistently found in infants and young children who are ultimately diagnosed with UTI.[15] Instead, they present with nonspecific signs and symptoms that often refer to other organ systems. Neonates with UTIs commonly present with jaundice, poor feeding, irritability, and lethargy. Infants and young children may demonstrate gastrointestinal signs and symptoms such as abdominal pain, vomiting, change in appetite, and behavioral changes such as unexplained bouts of crying or new onset bed wetting. The diagnosis, on the other hand, is frequently more obvious in older children and adolescents with uncomplicated UTIs who present with the classic signs of dysuria, urinary frequency, urgency, and/or hesitancy. Nevertheless, because of clear vulnerability, particular attention should be given to neonates with a history of prematurity, infants and children with functional or anatomic urinary tract abnormalities, those with previous UTIs, and children with a history of immunologic deficiencies.

Even more challenging is differentiation between lower (uncomplicated) and upper tract (complicated) infections, especially in the younger age groups. The distinction is specifically relevant when considering treatment options, long-term sequelae, and recommendations for follow up. Both lower and upper tract infections are more easily understood as clinical syndromes which, in general, encompass a constellation of signs and symptoms.

Unfortunately, the symptoms of infection anywhere along the urinary tract may be nonspecific or overlapping. Thus, symptoms of cystitis (dysuria, frequency, hesitancy, and urgency) also occur in other lower tract syndromes. For example, urethritis and vulvovaginitis are relatively common conditions in younger children. A history of trauma, masturbation, poor hygiene, foreign bodies, bubble bath, or other perineal irritants is helpful in differentiating the diagnosis. A careful history should include queries about behavioral and voiding disturbances including infrequent voiding, daytime enuresis, squirming, and urinary frequency. Close physical examination of the perineum and external genitalia may reveal irritation or vaginal discharge. Urethral discharges are rare in children. When they are observed, sexual abuse should be considered, and various sexually transmitted diseases should be considered as the possible idealogy. In these cases, cultures for gonorrhea, chlamydia, and other sexually transmitted organisms should be obtained. Urethral discharge in the adolescent should also prompt the consideration of a sexually transmitted disease. Bladder irritation due to cystitis will usually produce more intense symptoms of urethral irritation as well as symptoms of bladder spasm such as urgency and frequency. Other signs and symptoms of cystitis may include abdominal pain, low back pain, and fever. Parenthetically, viral hemorrhagic cystitis may present with symptoms indistinguishable from bacterial lower UTI.

Table 3. Interpretation of Positive Urine Culture

Method of Collection	Quantitative Culture: UTI Present
Suprapubic aspiration	Growth of urinary pathogens in any number (exception of up to 2-3 × 10^3 coagulase-negative staphylococci)
Catheterization	Febrile infants or children with ≥ 5 × 10^4 CFU/mL of single pathogen*
Midstream clean-void	Symptomatic patients with ≥ 10^5 CFU/mL of a single urinary pathogen
Midstream clean-void	Asymptomatic patients with two specimens on different days with ≥ 10^5 CFU/mL of the same organism

* Infection may be present with counts as low as 10-50 × 10^3 CFU/mL

Adapted from: Hellerstein S. Urinary tract infections: Old and new concepts. *Ped Clin North Am* 1995;42:1433-1459.

Upper urinary tract syndromes (complicated UTI, pyelonephritis) imply some degree of renal parenchymal involvement and may or may not demonstrate symptoms of cystitis. The clinical syndrome of upper tract disease often includes more systemic symptoms that may or may not be proceeded by lower tract symptoms. Upper tract infections may consist of fever, chills, nausea, vomiting, and a toxic appearance. The inherent difficulty in distinguishing between upper and lower UTIs is the subjectivity of interpreting clinical indicators of severity. Consequently, it is important to pay close attention to history and clinical symptoms, as well as maintaining a high index of suspicion.

Laboratory Evaluation

The most important reason, obviously, for accurate and timely identification of a UTI in the ED is to allow for immediate implementation of appropriate treatment. Concurrently, accurate diagnosis is necessary for other reasons. For patients without primary care physicians, appropriate counseling and referral can be initiated. Additionally, proper confirmation supports the subsequent work-up by primary care providers and specialists looking for underlying structural and functional abnormalities that may lead to renal scarring, hypertension, and possible end-stage renal disease.[18,19]

While urine culture is the gold standard in the diagnosis of UTIs, culture results are rarely, if ever, available to the physicians in the ED. Therefore, the emergency physician must rely on clinical data and other laboratory tests while obtaining a urine culture to subsequently confirm the diagnosis. On occasion for the very young infant, a leukocyte response is limited, and the microscopic examination of the urine is not diagnostic. In this setting, only the urine culture establishes the diagnosis.

A specimen for urinalysis and culture should be obtained through direct bladder sampling (catheterization, suprapubic sampling) or through a cleanly voided specimen in males and older female patients. Bagged urine specimens are not acceptable. Besides being difficult to obtain because of the time waiting for the child to void, bag specimens have an unacceptably high rate of contamination. If treatment with antibiotics is to commence prior to the availability of culture results, diagnostic uncertainty exists when contaminated specimens produce growth of multiple organisms on culture.[14] In general, children who do not yet have voiding control (< 2 years) should undergo sterile in-and-out catheterization or, when necessary, suprapubic aspiration. Urine specimens from older children with voiding control should be obtained from a cleanly voided mid-stream clean catch. Parents should be instructed on proper technique to avoid contaminated specimens. Periurethral contamination of specimens can be avoided by having the female child sit backwards (facing the rear) on the toilet. This position favors labial retraction and better exposure of the urethral meatus.

Unfortunately, bacterial contaminates grow rapidly at room temperature. When urine samples cannot be cultured immediately, spurious culture results are diminished considerably by maintaining the specimen on ice or at 4°C.

The urinalysis (UA) is by far the most frequently used adjunctive diagnostic test for possible UTI. While the UA frequently identifies urinary abnormalities, an understanding of the proper interpretation of these abnormalities is essential to avoid under- or over-diagnosis of UTI. Urine chemical test strips are a quick means of initial urine screening for the detection of leukocyte esterase and urinary nitrites. Esterases are released into the urine after the breakdown of white blood cells. Nitrates are converted to nitrites by gram-negative urinary pathogens. Both tests provide indirect evidence of pyuria and bacteriuria, respectively. Hematuria, proteinuria, and pyuria are commonly associated with UTI but are nonspecific and occur in the absence of infection. The presence of bacteria in catheterized urinary sediment has also been used as laboratory support for the presence of a UTI. In reality, all of these UA findings have limitations in the diagnosis of a UTI. In most studies, the sensitivities of a positive test for urinary leukocyte esterase or nitrate for a positive urine culture are less than 50%. The combined presence of pyuria (> 5 WBC/HPF) and bacteriuria on urine microanalysis improves the sensitivity to approximately 65%, and other approaches to urinary microscopic interpretation have been reported to yield better results. Nonetheless, the relatively poor sensitivity and positive-predictive value of the UA make it difficult to use alone as a presumptive test for UTI. By contrast, however, the specificity and negative-predictive values of the UA for both the dipstick indices and microscopic findings are consistently in the greater than 95% range. Hoberman et al has described the use of an "enhanced" urinalysis that uses a hemocytometer in the evaluation of uncentrifuged urine.[20] This method reduces the variability of results caused by centrifugation and resuspension, it enables evaluation of a fixed volume of urine, and it facilitates accurate counting by providing a marked visual field with uniform illumination. The centrifuged specimen is also Gram-stained under conditions that standardize the number of drops in urine. A positive-enhanced urinalysis is defined as 10 or more white blood cells per

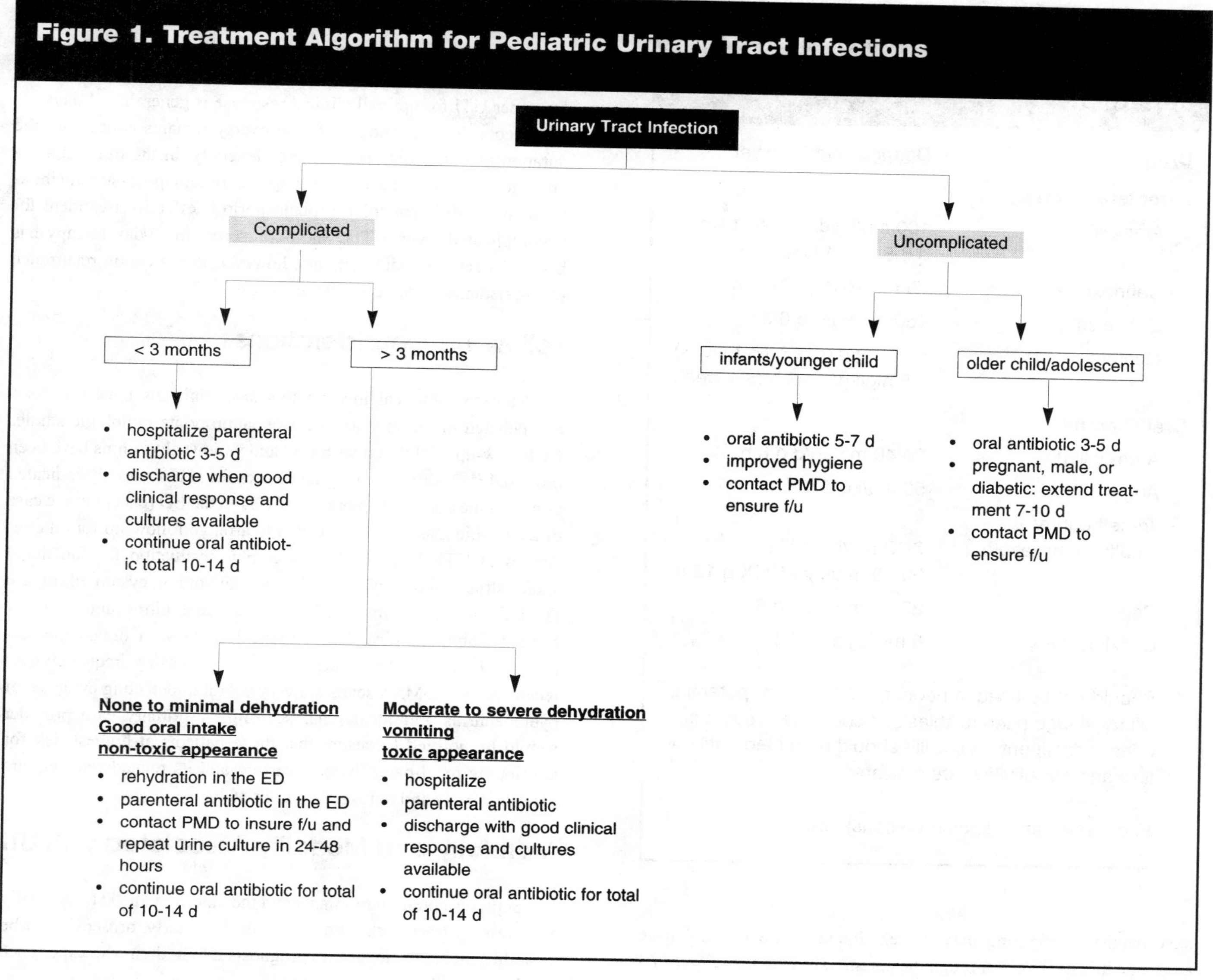

cubic millimeter and bacteriuria is defined as the presence of any bacteria per 10 oil immersion fields on the Gram-stained smear. The sensitivity of the enhanced urinalysis to predict a positive urine culture was 84.5%, compared to 65.6% with the standard urinalysis. The positive-predicted value of enhanced urinalysis was 93.1%, compared with only 80.8% in the standard urinalysis. Although one can reasonably conclude that febrile infants older than 3-6 months of age and older children without symptoms referable to the urinary system with a normal urinalysis are likely to have UTIs, routinely obtaining a urine culture can arguably be cost-effective in nearly all cases. Hoberman describes three scenarios in which urine cultures should be obtained regardless of the results of urinalysis.[20] The scenarios are: children with previous UTIs, children with abnormal urinary tracts, and those who will be treated empirically with antibiotics. The reality of pediatric emergency practice, however, with its inherit difficulties in patient compliance and patient follow up, seems to dictate a more universal approach to culturing the urine in the workup of the febrile child.

A positive urine culture obtained by mid-stream clean catch is defined by greater than 1×10^5 CFU/mL of a single organism. *(See Table 3.)* Catheterized specimens yielding greater than 5×10^4 CFU/mL should also be considered significant. Additionally, growth of a single gram-negative organism in any amount from a suprapubic aspiration should also be considered diagnostic of UTI. While these values are useful, it should be remembered that the urine bacterial concentration may be altered by urine volume, the duration of urine storage in the bladder, and the site of infection. Peripheral white blood cell counts and erythrocyte sedimentation rates are nonspecific tests that should only be interpreted in conjunction with the urinalysis and urine culture.

Treatment Options

As mentioned, early treatment of UTIs especially in infants and young children decrease the risk of kidney damage. Inpatient management should be instituted for any child younger than 3 months of age with a febrile UTI, for those children who have significant dehydration or appear toxic, or when outpatient compliance and follow-up is questionable. In general, children older than 3 months with febrile UTIs who appear only mildly dehydrated and do not

Table 4. Common Antimicrobial Drugs Used in Pediatric Urinary Tract Infections

Drug	Dosage and Interval
Parenteral Therapy	
Ampicillin	100 mg/kg/d 12 h (< 1 week) q 6-8 h (> 1 week)
Ceftriaxone*	75 mg/kg/d q 12-24 h
Cefotaxime	150 mg/kg/d q 6-8 h
Gentamicin	5 mg/kg/d q 12 h (< 1 week) 7.5 mg/kg/d q 8 h (> 1 week)
Oral Therapy	
Amoxicillin†	20-40 mg/kg/d q 8 h
Augmentin	50 mg/kg/d q 8 h
Trimethoprim/ Sulfamethoxazole	6-12 mg/kg/d TMP, 30-60 mg/kg/d SMX q 12 h
Cephalexin	25-50 mg/kg/d q 6 h
Cefixime	8 mg/kg/d q 12 h

* Should not be used in neonates because of potential biliary sludge pseudolithiasis. If cocci are present in urinary sediment, ampicillin should be added until culture and sensitivities are available.

† *E. coli* resistance should be considered

have persistent vomiting may be rehydrated in the ED and have antibiotic therapy begun through the parenteral route. *(See Figure 1.)* Prior to discharge, however, patients should demonstrate adequate oral intake with arrangement for appropriate follow-up. Contact with a primary care physician should be obtained and documented to assure follow-up of urine culture and sensitivities and further treatment and evaluation. Long acting, broad spectrum antibiotic coverage with a third-generation cephalosporin, such as ceftriaxone 50-75 mg/kg IV or IM, is an appropriate choice for most patients clinically considered to have upper tract infection who can be managed as outpatients. However, recent preliminary data suggest satisfactory outcomes in non-toxic infants older than 2 months of age treated with oral cefixime alone.[21] Ampicillin 100 mg/kg should be added if gram-positive cocci are noted in urinary sediment or gram stain. Nitrofurantoin therapy is inadequate if parenchymal infection is considered. Children allergic to cephalosporins should receive a single dose of gentamicin 2.5 mg/kg IV or IM prior to discharge while ensuring that oral therapy is initiated with an appropriate antibiotic such as TMP/SMX or a third-generation cephalosporin. *(See Table 4.)* For patients requiring inpatient management, parenteral antibiotic therapy should be initiated in the ED. Older children should receive broad-spectrum antibiotic coverage with a third-generation cephalosporin, while neonates should receive gentamicin and ampicillin to cover the usual neonatal pathogens and other *Enterobacteraciae.* Ceftriaxone should be avoided in this age group due to the displacement of bilirubin from albumin and biliary pseudolithiasis.[22] The total duration of therapy for upper UTI for optimal clinical response is generally 14 days.

A considerable amount of controversy remains concerning the duration of outpatient oral therapy. Generally, in the older child, a three- to five-day course of trimethoprim, trimethoprim-sulfamethoxazole, or a third-generation cephalosporin is effective treatment for uncomplicated lower UTIs. Short-course or single-day therapy has been advocated in adult patients; however, the infection recurrence rate in pediatric patients precludes its use.[23]

Follow-Up Considerations

Numerous clinical investigators and clinicians have discussed and debated in recent years the most appropriate radiologic studies for follow-up of children with UTI and various algorithms have been proposed.[24-26] Although imaging studies for UTI are rarely indicated as part of the diagnostic work-up of UTI in the ED (except in the case of a palpable mass), it is important to arrange follow-up for all children with UTI. In general, radiographic evaluation for functional and/or structural causes of UTI begin with voiding cystourethrogram (VCUG) to demonstrate reflux and a renal ultrasound to show anatomic abnormalities. Renal cortical scans with dimercaptosuccinic acid (DMSA) have been used with increasing frequency over recent years.[27] DMSA scans are very useful in detecting evidence of pyelonephritis and focal renal scarring. A primary care provider should be notified to ensure that those patients at highest risk for developing renal parenchymal scarring and its related sequelae are identified early and managed appropriately.

Morbidity and Mortality Associated with UTI

Sepsis is common in infants and the elderly with UTI, especially with urinary tract obstruction; as with the elderly, urosepsis can be fatal. In general, the long-term prognosis for children who experience a UTI is excellent provided there is prompt and adequate treatment instituted at the time of diagnosis. Prompt treatment has been shown to minimize the risk of renal scarring. Renal scarring is also the consequence of recurrent UTI and some at-risk children may require antibiotic prophylaxis for extended periods of time.

The main clinical consequences of recurring renal damage caused by pyelonephritis are arterial hypertension and renal insufficiency. Reflux nephropathy, renal injury attributed to the combination of VUR, and recurring infection, is responsible for up to 15% of the cases of end stage renal failure in children in the United States. Because of these potentially serious consequences, it is imperative for the emergency physician to consider the UTI as a cause of fever in the young child, to perform the appropriate diagnostic studies, and to render adequate therapy.

Summary

The diagnosis of a urinary tract infection should be considered in all febrile children, especially when the diagnosis is unclear. The spectrum of infection signs and symptoms is broad because potential sites of infection span the entire urinary tract. Additionally, the differentiation between upper vs. lower urinary tract locations is a recognized challenge; and treatment decisions are dependent on the child's condition and presenting signs and symptoms. The decision to admit or to treat as an outpatient requires careful consideration of the child's overall appearance, oral intake and adequacy of hydration. Urinalysis and culture results must be evaluated carefully as potential errors in collection and sample management can result in spurious results. Finally, because of the potential sequelae of pediatric urinary tract infections appropriate and timely patient follow-up by a primary care provider is a necessity.

References

1. Hoberman A, Chao H-P, et al. Prevalence of urinary tract infections in febrile infants. *J Pediatr* 1993;123:17.
2. Gonzalez R. Urinary Tract infections. In: Behrman R, Klieman R, et al, eds. *Nelsons Textbook of Pediatrics.* 15th ed. New York: W B Saunders; 1996:1528-1532.
3. Orga PL, Faden HS. Urinary tract infections in childhood: An update. *J Pediatr* 1985;106:1023.
4. Blethyn AJ, Jenkins HR, et al. Radiological evidence of constipation in urinary tract infection. *Am J Disease Child* 1995;73:534.
5. Zelikovic I, Adelman RD. Urinary tract infections in children: An update. *West J Med* 1992;157:554.
6. Craig JC, Knight JF, et al. Effect of circumcision on incidence of urinary tract infection in preschool boys. *J Pediatr* 1996;128:21.
7. Wiswell TE, Hachey, WE. Urinary tract infections and the uncircumcised state: An Update. *Clin Pediatr* 1993;32: 130-134.
8. Zahanel GG, Harding GK, et al. Asymptomatic bacteriuria: Which patients should be treated? *Arch Intern Med* 1990; 150:1389-1396.
9. Smellie JM, Normand IC. Urinary tract infections in children. *Post Graduate Med* 1985;61:895.
10. Minninberg DT. Preventing complications of vesicoureteral reflux. *Infect Surg* 1986;5:203-214.
11. Verrier Jones K, Asscher W, et al. Renal functional changes in schoolgirls with covert asymptomatic bacteriuria. *Contrib Nephrology* 1984;39:152.
12. Bock GH. Urinary Tract Infections. In: Hockerman R, ed. *Primary Pediatric Care.* 3rd ed. St. Louis: Mosby-Year Book Inc; 1997:1640-1644.
13. Naylor GR. A 16-month analysis of urinary tract infections in children. *J Med Microbiology* 1984;17:31.
14. Gearhart P, Herzberg G, et al. Childhood urolithiasis: Experiences and advances. *Pediatrics* 1991;87:445-450.
15. Smellie JM, Hodsom, CJ et al. Clinical and radiological features of UTI. *BMJ* 1964;2:1222-1226.
16. Miller T, Phillips S. Pyelonephritis: The relationship between infection, renal scarring, and antimicrobial therapy. *Kidney Int* 1981;19:654-662.
17. Winberg J, Bollgren I, et al. Clinical pyelonephritis and focal renal scarring. *Pediatr Clin North Am* 1982;29: 801-814.
18. Rance CP, Arbus GS, et al. Persistent systemic hypertension in infants and children. *Pediatr Clin North Am* 1974;2: 801-824.
19. Arant BS. Vesicoureteral reflux and renal injury. *Amer J Kidney Disease* 1991;17:491-511.
20. Hoberman A, Wald E. Urinary tract infections in young febrile children. *Pediatr Infect Dis J* 1997;16:11-17.
21. Hoberman A, Wald ER, et al. Oral vs. intravenous therapy for acute pyelonephritis in children 2-24 months (abstract). *Peditr Res* 1996;39:134.
22. Hellerstein S. Urinary tract infection Old and new concepts. *Pediatr Clin North Am* 1995;42:1433-1459.
23. Moffatt M, Embree J, et al. Short-course antibiotic therapy for urinary tract infections in children. *Amer J Dis Child* 1988;142:57-61.
24. Dick PT, Feldman W. Routine diagnostic imaging for childhood urinary tract infection: A systematic overview. *J Pediatr* 1996;128:15-22.
25. Conway J, Cohn R. Evolving role of nuclear medicine for diagnosis and management of urinary tract infections. *J Pediatr* 1994;124:87-90.
26. Andrich MP, Majd M. Diagnostic imaging in the evaluation of the first urinary tract infection in infants and young children. *Pediatrics* 1992;90:436-441.
27. Goldraich N, Goldraich I. Update on dimercaptosuccinic acid renal scanning in children with urinary tract infection. *Pediatr Nephr* 1995;9:221-226.

Chronic Renal Failure

Walter G. Belleza, MD

The patient with end-stage renal disease (ESRD) is a diagnostic and therapeutic challenge for the primary care physician. Clinical presentations range from the nearly asymptomatic patient with laboratory evidence of mild hyperkalemia to the patient with fulminate pulmonary edema or cardiac arrest. Within a narrow window of time, the physician must initiate potentially treacherous therapeutic maneuvers for a patient functioning within narrow metabolic boundaries.

By definition, ESRD occurs when a patient's kidneys can no longer sustain life without the aid of dialysis therapy or a renal transplant. It is at the end point of chronic renal failure where the majority of clinical complications occur. Chronic renal failure (CRF) implies that an irreversible reduction in renal function exists, and recovery of that function is unlikely.

Nearly every organ system suffers in ESRD. If profound enough and not treated accordingly, ESRD results in the uremic syndrome. The uremic syndrome is a constellation of multisystemic complications that result from the accumulation of nitrogenous wastes and metabolic by-products. Symptoms may range from fluid overload and congestive heart failure to encephalopathy and coma. To prevent this and other systemic derangements, patients are started on either peritoneal dialysis or hemodialysis. Dialysis therapy can be life-saving but also can cause its own complications. This chapter reviews the complex constellation of problems associated with ESRD.

Demographics

An estimation of the number of patients suffering from ESRD is provided by the United States Renal Data Systems (USRDS). Current worldwide estimates indicate a gradual increase in the number of patients entering dialysis therapy, with the United States having the highest rate.[1] As of 1993, statistics from USRDS demonstrate that more than 220,000 patients suffer from ESRD, with an annual growth rate of 8-9%.[2] Some projections indicate that the number of dialysis enrollees will exceed 250,000 by the year 2000.[4] The increase in numbers also may be due to more diabetic and elderly patients being accepted for dialysis therapy. In addition, there is a growing population of patients with predialysis renal insufficiency who may require treatment. As of 1990, this group was estimated to number between 648,000 and 708,000 patients.[5]

In the United States, the most common causes of chronic renal failure, in decreasing incidence, are: diabetes, hypertension, glomerulonephritis, cystic renal disease, and interstitial nephritis.[6] A disproportionate number of patients with ESRD

Table 1. Differential Diagnosis of Altered Mental Status in Patients with ERSD

STRUCTURAL LESIONS	METABOLIC
Subdural hematoma	Elemental intoxication (copper, nickel)
Normal pressure hydrocephalus	Drug intoxication
Cerebrovascular accident (hemorrhagic, embolic)	Meningitis/encephalitis
Cerebral abscess	Seizures
Post traumatic	Hypermagnesemia
CARDIOVASCULAR	Hypernatremia/hyponatremia
Arrhythmia	Hypoxia
Myocardial infarction	Hypercalcemia
Hypertension/hypotension	Hyperglycemia/hypoglycemia
OTHER	Hyperparathyroidism
Excessive ultrafiltration	Nonketotic hyperosmolar coma
Wernicke encephalopathy	Hypophosphatemia
Dialysis/dementia	

are young, urban-dwelling blacks who suffer from severe, untreated hypertension.[1,4]

Pathophysiology

After receiving a pathogenic insult, the kidney can either recover and continue to function normally, develop chronic renal insufficiency, or progress to ESRD. Factors that influence disease progression include the severity and type of the primary insult, presence of other chronic diseases (hypertension, diabetes, HIV), age, and continuing insult (infection, obstruction). Once chronic renal insufficiency is established, and plasma creatinine exceeds 1.5-2.0 mg/dL, progression to ESRD occurs with an almost linear decline in the glomerular filtration rate (GFR).[7] Although the aforementioned exogenous factors can serve to accelerate functional decline, disease progression still occurs in their absence. This is due to many intrinsic processes that are poorly understood.

If the original insult results in irreversible injury, the remaining functional glomerular units become hyperperfused. This results in increases in glomerular capillary pressure that become injurious by inducing histological changes that cause glomerular hypertrophy, fusion of epithelial foot processes, and mesangial expansion.[7-9] The mesangial expansion causes the eventual collapse of the capillary lumens and the eventual appearance of patchy glomerulosclerosis.

In addition to causing cellular changes, this hyperfunction induces an "injury response" that involves cellular elements, chemical mediators, and biologically active compounds and results in glomerular and tubulointerstitial damage. Implicated cellular elements include macrophages, monocytes, leukocytes, and platelets.[8,9] Once attracted to the damaged area, these elements help initiate an inflammatory cascade involving chemical mediators such as interleukin-1, platelet activating factor, thromboxane A2, and heparinase.[8,9] The chemical mediator interleukin-1 promotes attachment of inflammatory cells such as neutrophils and monocytes and stimulates the release of thromboxane A2. Thromboxane A2 serves as a vasoconstrictor that decreases glomerular perfusion and promotes platelet aggregation. Platelets, in turn, release platelet-derived growth factor that promotes growth of fibroblasts and proliferation of smooth muscle cells and the release of prostaglandins and leukotrienes that perpetuate the inflammatory cascade.

Clinical Effects

Cardiovascular Complications. Cardiovascular and cerebrovascular complications account for 15-30% of deaths in patients suffering from chronic renal failure.[19-22] Although not considered an independent risk factor for heart disease, chronic renal failure may coexist with other proven cardiac risk factors, such as diabetes, hypertension, and hypercholesterolemia. In addition, ESRD makes control of these conditions more difficult. Cardiovascular conditions that are likely to require emergent evaluation and treatment are hypertension, congestive heart failure (CHF) or pulmonary edema, myocardial ischemia, pericardial disease, and dysrhythmias.

Hypertension. Hypertension in the patient with chronic renal failure is a multifactorial problem. Secondary complications of renal failure, such as volume overload, sodium imbalance, elevated catecholamine levels, and derangements in the renin-angiotensin system, can be superimposed on a pre-existing hypertensive condition.[23,24] A hypertensive emergency exists when signs of severe progressive end-organ damage (e.g., encephalopathy, CHF, cardiac ischemia) occur in the presence of elevated blood pressure. Although a hypertensive emergency does not usually occur until the diastolic blood pressure exceeds 130 mmHg, it can occur at levels as low as 110 mmHg.

Congestive Heart Failure/Pulmonary Edema. As with other complications in renal failure, CHF involves multiple pathophysiologic mechanisms. In addition to primary cardiac dysfunction, volume overload, positive sodium balance, high output failure from anemia, and arteriovenous fistulas are major contributing factors. Cardiac dysfunction can result from hypertension, left ventricular hypertrophy, cardiac ischemia, cardiomyopathy, electrolyte abnormalities, dysrhythmias, and hyperparathyroidism.[21,23,24,26-28] Although the most common cause of CHF and pulmonary edema in patients with ESRD is volume overload, all of the previously mentioned factors can cause heart failure and should be considered in the differential diagnosis. Volume overload may range between 5-10 L and can result from a seemingly innocuous ingestion of food or fluid.

Pericardial Disease. Prior to widespread dialysis therapy, pericarditis occurred in more than 50% of ESRD patients and was a harbinger of early demise. However, the current incidence is between 2%-19% and can occur in patients not

Table 2. Cannulation of Dialysis Vascular Grafts

- Avoid improper placement by documenting function (bruit, thrill) and avoid cannulation of possible aneurysms and pseudoaneurysms
- Adhere to strict sterile technique and firmly, but not occlusively, compress access site for 5-10 min after use
- Avoid use of tourniquets (use finger compression) and multiple punctures
- If IV infusions are to be performed:
  —safely secure all catheters with tape
  —use infusion pump or "pressure bag" apparatus if high-pressure access is cannulated
  —standard intravenous infusion devices may be used if low pressure access is cannulated, or if a precise infusion rate is not required

Adapted from: Wolfson AB, Levy M. The patient with chronic renal insufficiency following renal transplantation. In: *Emergency Care of the Compromised Host.* Philadelphia: J.B. Lippincott Co.; 1994:413-432.

Figure 1. Suspected Pericardial Effusion

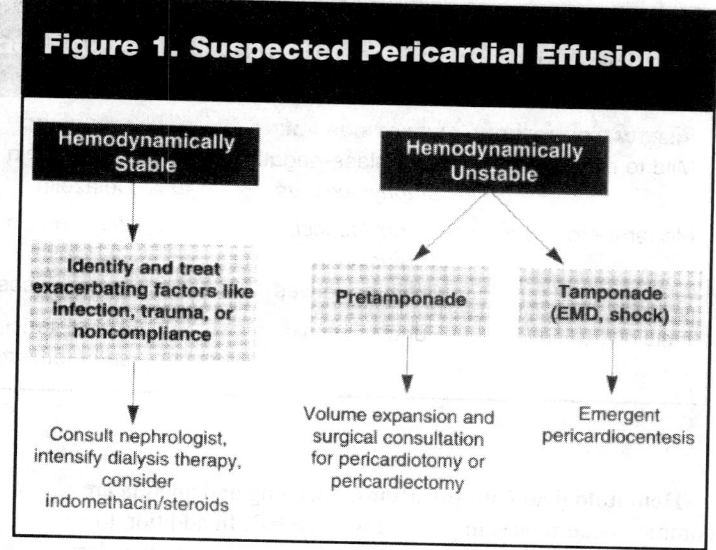

receiving dialysis as well as those undergoing dialysis.[35] In patients not receiving dialysis, its presence indicates the need to initiate therapy. In patients currently on dialysis, pericarditis indicates the presence of stresses such as trauma and infection or the need for a more aggressive dialysis regimen. The exact pathophysiologic process in under-dialyzed patients is unknown but is thought to be secondary to retained metabolic by-products.

The most common chief complaint is substernal, nonexertional, sharp pleuritic chest pain. The pain can increase by moving, yawning, and lying supine. It is relieved by sitting upright and can predate diagnostic evidence by 1-2 weeks. Other complaints include shortness of breath, cough, weight loss, fever, and malaise. Clues that indicate significant effusion are new dysrhythmias, frequent episodes of hypotension during dialysis, or a decreasing need to medically control hypertension in a previously hypertensive patient.[23]

Dysrhythmia. Coronary artery disease (CAD), cardiac dysfunction, electrolyte disorders, and the use of potentially proarrhythmic medication are common occurrences in patients with ESRD.[14,39,40] These factors, along with pericardial disease, decreased oxygen delivery from chronic anemia, and dialysis-induced hypotension, can predispose patients to dysrhythmias. Common dysrhythmias include atrial fibrillation and flutter, PVCs, and non-sustained ventricular tachycardia.[41-44] Dysrhythmias may be precipitated by any condition that impairs cardiac oxygen delivery, and electrolyte disorders such as hyperkalemia, hypercalcemia, and hypermagnesemia.

Coronary Artery Disease. CAD and myocardial ischemia commonly occur in patients with ESRD.[19-22,43] The presence of left ventricular hypertrophy, an AV fistula, and fluid overload may increase cardiac oxygen demand, while chronic anemia can decrease oxygen availability. It was previously thought that the incidence of myocardial ischemia was more prevalent among patients with renal failure and ESRD. Recent studies have shown that, when adjustments are made for age and coexisting disease, there is no significant difference between this population and others. The differential diagnosis of chest pain should include pericarditis, pleural effusion, aortic dissection, pneumothorax, infection, and pulmonary embolism.

Acute Neurologic Complications. Neurologic dysfunction is a well-known consequence of ESRD and can involve the central and peripheral nervous systems.[65,66] Complications range from neuropathies and the restless leg syndrome to lethargy and coma. The challenge for the physician is to distinguish between acute, chronic, and potentially life-threatening disorders. Two significant problems that may be seen are the dialysis disequilibrium syndrome and mental status changes.

Dialysis Disequilibrium Syndrome. This well-known complication usually occurs during or shortly after dialysis. Neurologic symptoms include headache, weakness, restlessness, confusion, seizures, and coma. The syndrome results when the removal of solutes from the blood is too rapid to allow an equilibration between the central nervous system and the rest of the body.[24,48] It occurs more frequently in patients who have more severe metabolic derangements prior to dialysis and in those undergoing a more aggressive dialysis regimen. The syndrome is a diagnosis of exclusion, and other etiologies, such as infection, CVA, uremic encephalopathy, hypoxia, subdural hematoma, and drug intoxication, should be considered.

Altered Mental Status. The list of problems that can cause mental-status change in patients with ESRD is extensive. *(Please see Table 1.)* In addition to common conditions such as stroke, medication effects, and hypoglycemia, complications from the dialysis process must be considered. These include hypotension, the disequilibrium syndrome, dysrhythmia, and spontaneous CNS hemorrhage.[63] Acute onset may indicate cerebrovascular accidents, dysrhythmias, or trauma. A history of slow onset and dialysis noncompliance may indicate uremic encephalopathy.

Table 3. Antibiotic Treatment for CAPD-Associated Peritonitis

CLINICAL CONDITION	INFECTIOUS AGENT	ANTIBIOTIC	IV DOSE	IP DOSE	DURATION
Mild to moderate	Coagulase-negative *Staphylococcus*	Vancomycin	1.0-1.5 mg	30 mg/kg/2 L	7-10 d
		Cefazolin	1.0 g	250 mg/2 L	
Moderate to severe	*Staphylococcus aureus*	Vancomycin	1.5 g	30 mg/kg/2 L	10-14 d
		Cefazolin	1.0 g	250 mg/2 L	
	Gram negatives	Aminoglycoside	1.7 mg/kg	10 mg/2 L	10-14 d
Insidious to severe	Fungi	Amphotericin+ catheter removal	0.5-1.0 mg	2-6 mg/6 L	7-10 d

Hematological Complications. Bleeding and anemia are common occurrences in patients with ESRD. In addition to an underlying platelet dysfunction, bleeding can occur secondary to concurrent heparin administration during dialysis. Anemia can be a consequence of ESRD but can result from an acute hemorrhagic episode. The challenge for the physician is to identify the acuity of these conditions and initiate appropriate therapy.

Common sites of bleeding include vascular access sites and the gastrointestinal tract.[72] Spontaneous hemorrhage into the subdural, retropharyngeal, and retroperitoneal spaces can also occur.[12,61-63] Any area of progressive swelling and pain may harbor occult hemorrhage.

Infectious Complications. Infection is the second most common cause of mortality and morbidity in patients with ESRD and accounts for 15-40% of deaths in this population.[26,46] In addition to compromised humoral and cellular immune responses, patients often have indwelling peritoneal or vascular access devices that serve as ports of entry for infectious agents.[47,48] Conditions that may act as immunosuppressants are chronic uremia, malnutrition, iron overload from transfusion, and electrolyte disorders. Areas such as the urinary tract and lungs have diminished local defenses, making them more susceptible to infection. Other contributing factors to urinary infection include bladder stasis, dysmotility, and underlying structural disease. Complaints of dysuria and frequency may be absent because of decreased urinary flow.

The patient with ESRD should be viewed as an immunocompromised host. Because of this, the presence of fever should prompt an extensive evaluation. Patients may present with fever, chills, hypothermia, joint pain, constitutional complaints, and symptoms referable to the site of infection. Common sites of infection include the lung, urinary tract, vascular access sites, and the peritoneum. Vascular access sites and peritoneal catheters are the most common sources of infection in patients undergoing hemodialysis and peritoneal dialysis, respectively.[50-52]

Electrolyte Complications. Electrolyte abnormalities are the hallmark of chronic renal failure. While many of these complications are not life-threatening and respond to hemodialysis, hyperkalemia, hypercalcemia, and hypermagnesemia can result in clinical decompensation if not treated. These conditions are rare in the compliant and adequately dialyzed patient but can occur due to dietary indiscretion and dialysis noncompliance.

Hyperkalemia. Causes of hyperkalemia include pharmacological agents, dietary and dialysis noncompliance, rhabdomyolysis, metabolic acidosis, and catabolic states. Medications that produce hyperkalemia include: nonselective beta blockers, calcium channel blockers, succinylcholine, and digoxin if taken in toxic doses.[54,55] Tissue breakdown from rhabdomyolysis results in release of intracellular potassium. Extracellular potassium shifts occur with metabolic acidosis.

There are no specific clinical or physical manifestations that can aid in early diagnosis of hyperkalemia. Because clinical presentation can range from cardiac arrest to mild constitutional symptoms, a high index of suspicion for this problem should be maintained in any patient with ESRD. Although most patients are asymptomatic, the most common complaint is weakness.[34] Because the most important consequence of hyperkalemia is increased cardiac irritability, an ECG should be obtained early.

Hypercalcemia and Hypermagnesemia. Hypercalcemia and hypermagnesemia by themselves, or in conjunction with hyperkalemia, can increase cardiac irritability and potentiate cardiac dysrhythmias. Though not a common consequence of renal failure, hypercalcemia and hypermagnesemia can occur due to the inadvertent use of common medications—phosphate binders, vitamin D analogues, and calcium supplements in hypercalcemia, and magnesium-containing antacids and lithium therapy in hypermagnesemia. As in hyperkalemia, patients often present with a variety of clinical complaints that range from weakness and malaise to cardiopulmonary instability and coma.

Patients with mild hypercalcemia are often asymptomatic but generally have clinical signs once the level exceeds 11.5 mg/dL. Presentation may include nausea, vomiting, fatigue, muscle weakness, and abdominal pain. Mental status changes, such as lack of concentration, confusion, and coma also may occur.[24] Although most physical findings are nonspecific, signs of long-standing hypercalcemia such as band keratopathy may be present.

Hypermagnesemia inhibits the presynaptic release of acetylcholine and norepinephrine. Although most side effects involve neural tissue, magnesium also affects vascular smooth muscle and cardiac tissue. Nausea and vomiting can occur at levels of 4-5 mEq/L (2.0-2.5 mmol/L), loss of deep tendon reflexes and mental status changes occur at levels of 4-7 mEq/L (2.0-3.5 mmol/L), and respiratory paralysis occurs at levels of 10-15 mEq/L (5.0-7.5 mmol/L). Other signs include hypotension, lethargy, and paralysis.

Emergent Complications of Dialysis Therapy

The objective of dialysis therapy is the removal of toxins, metabolic waste products, and excess volume from the vascular space. Through the processes of ultrafiltration and diffusion, solutes and material pass from the vascular space to a dialysate solution by crossing semipermeable membranes located either intraperitoneally (peritoneal dialysis) or externally (hemodialysis). By adjusting the duration of therapy and the nature of the dialysate material, specific changes can be made in the constitution of a patient's plasma. Although many complications can occur from dialysis therapy, those likely to require emergent evaluation involve instability during the dialysis process, mechanical defects, and infection. Because unique problems occur in peritoneal dialysis and hemodialysis, they will be discussed separately.

Peritoneal Dialysis. Peritoneal dialysis involves the sterile introduction of dialysate fluid into the peritoneum through a surgically implanted catheter. The dialysate fluid is then allowed to equilibrate with the patient's plasma for a specific amount of time (dwell time). By adjusting the dialysate material and the length of dwell time, the consistency of a patient's plasma can be adjusted. The fluid is later withdrawn under sterile conditions. Although multiple modalities of peritoneal dialysis are available, the one most commonly used is continuous ambulatory peritoneal dialysis (CAPD). In this modality, the dwell time lasts from 4-6 hours and treatment is performed by the patient four times daily. Because of its ease of use, avoidance of hemodynamic instability from rapid volume shifts, and freedom from use of a dialysis center, CAPD is favored by younger patients, the elderly, and those with severe cardiovascular problems. Because CAPD is relatively stable, conditions such as hypotension, chest pain, and neurological deficits should not be attributed to the dialysis process.

Mechanical Complications. Mechanical complications include obstruction and leakage from the catheter site. Patients will notice either an inability to infuse or properly remove dialysate fluid. This can be due to kinking of the catheter tubing, intraperitoneal migration, or obstruction from overlying omentum or peritoneal debris.[59]

Infection. Infection is the most common complication that afflicts the patient receiving peritoneal dialysis, and it occurs an average of once every nine months.[30] In addition to diffuse abdominal pain and dialysate fluid that becomes cloudy, infected peritoneal dialysis patients may experience nausea, vomiting, fevers, and chills. The most common infectious agents are skin-inhabiting *Staphylococcus epidermidis* and *Staphylococcus aureus*.[46,50,67] Infection is usually due to a break in aseptic technique during dialysis exchange. Other organisms include gram-negative organisms such as *Escherichia coli, Pseudomonas, Enterobacter,* and fungal species such as *Candida*.[46,50,67]

In addition to microbial infection, peritonitis can occur secondary to allergic reactions to the dialysis catheters (eosinophilic peritonitis) or dialysate fluid (sclerosing peritonitis). While eosinophilic peritonitis is a self-limited condition, sclerosing peritonitis may result in abdominal adhesions that require discontinuation of peritoneal dialysis. If adhesions are severe, surgical lysis may be required.

Hemodialysis. Hemodialysis involves exchanges between a patient's plasma and a dialysate bath through semipermeable membranes. Vascular access is achieved either through a temporary large intravenous double lumen catheter or repeated cannulation of a permanent, surgically constructed, arteriovenous fistula. Fistula construction uses either native or animal vasculature or synthetic material. The fistula usually connects the patient's radial artery to a large vein in the patient's nondominant arm in an end-to-side or side-to-side fashion. Complications involve mechanical obstruction, infection, hemorrhage, and hemodynamic instability during or after dialysis therapy.

Mechanical Complications. The most common mechanical problem with vascular access devices is obstruction from thrombosis, which is usually caused by venous hyperplasia at the venous end of the graft's anastomotic site. Thrombosis can also result from trauma, inadvertent compression while sleeping, or during compression of a graft hemorrhage. Mechanical obstruction may result from inadvertent kinking of the graft site. The likelihood of obstruction is increased following dialysis from a combination of a low-flow state and hypercoaguable condition.[30,68] Obstruction can also occur in temporary double lumen devices.

History may reveal a loss of the bruit or thrill at the fistula site. If obstruction of a double lumen occurs, severe extremity edema can result. Temporary devices may be inadvertently or intentionally removed with resultant hemorrhage.

Infection. The most common source of infection in patients undergoing hemodialysis treatment is the access site. In addition to symptoms of a localized process, infection of access sites can cause metastatic infection involving the vertebrae, joints, and cardiac valves.[34] Joints commonly infected include the wrist, knee, and shoulder. The aortic valve is most frequently infected from metastatic infections. As in peritoneal dialysis, gram-positive skin flora such as *S. aureus* and *S. epidermidis* are the usual causative agents. Infection usually results from frequent handling and cannulation as well as breaks in aseptic technique.

Although localized warmth, tenderness, and erythema may indicate infection, their absence does not exclude the possibility of infection. In fact, as many as one-third of patients will have no localizing signs and may only complain of constitutional symptoms such as malaise, fever, chills, nausea, and vomiting.[23,30]

Hemorrhage. Bleeding is a common problem with vascular access sites. This is due to frequent cannulation, platelet dysfunction, and use of heparin during dialysis. Unlike "natural grafts," the walls of synthetic devices cannot collapse and are more prone to hemorrhage and formation of pseudoaneurysm. A pseudo-aneurysm is a pulsatile hematoma with a pseudocapsule, while an aneurysm is a true expansion of the vessel wall. Both can produce hemorrhagic complications. An additional cause of bleeding is the AV fistula or graft that is used prematurely prior to adequate maturation after implantation.

Hemodynamic Instability. Hypotension commonly occurs during dialysis and is usually due to a combination of underlying autonomic dysfunction and decreased cardiac output from acute depletion in intravascular volume. The decrease in vascular volume occurs from fluid removal in patients who enter dialysis either euvolemic or relatively hypovolemic. Other possibilities include: cardiac dysfunction from ischemia, arrhythmia, or pericardial effusion, infection, sepsis, antihypertensive use, pulmonary embolism, air embolism, and anaphylaxis. Anaphylaxis can occur at the initiation of dialysis treatment and may be a reaction to the dialyzer membrane, the sterilizer used in cleaning the dialysis machine, or bacterial endotoxins.[63] Dialysis personnel should provide records that document the time of occurrence, any coexisting symptoms, and any diagnostic or therapeutic measures.

Air Embolism. Air embolism is a rare but potentially lethal complication of dialysis therapy that results from passage of air from either an external mechanical malfunction in the circuit or from the dialyzer itself. The dialyzer may be a source of air if refrigerated dialysate containing dissolved air is used.

Clinical presentation depends on the amount of air introduced and the position that the patient is in at the time. Although complications can result from as little as 5 mL of air, larger amounts are required to produce cardiovascular collapse. If the patient is upright, a rushing sensation to the head may soon be followed by neurological dysfunction. Patients lying supine may complain of chest pain or shortness of breath. Those in the Trendelenburg position are fortunate because air will pass into the lower extremities, sparing the heart but demonstrating patchy cyanosis on the lower extremities.

Prehospital Care

Initial prehospital support emphasizes the ABCs with initiation of any required resuscitative measures per pre-established ACLS protocols and rapid transport to an appropriate institution. If an airway is required, EMS personnel should be aware that patients with ESRD can have clotting dysfunction and that tracheal intubation may result in inadvertent hemorrhage.[10-12] If the patient can breathe spontaneously, the sitting position may be helpful. Oxygen should be administered via high-flow delivery systems. Efforts to obtain peripheral IV access should be made but should not delay transport. Field attempts at cannulation of vascular grafts should be avoided. Although pharmacologic therapy is limited in the field, early measures include the use of furosemide (Lasix) and nitroglycerin if congestive heart failure is suspected. Nitroglycerin also addresses cardiac ischemia.

Pre-hospital caregivers should attempt to obtain historical information from the patient and family members. Aside from the past medical history, helpful information includes length, frequency, compliance, and duration of any dialysis and medical treatments, previous renal complications, prescription and non-prescription drug use, and any illicit drug use.

Emergency Care

General Resuscitative Measures. Patient status must be assessed quickly and stabilized prior to initiating any diagnostic evaluation. As with any medical emergency, the ABCs (airway, breathing, circulation) consistently take precedence. In addition to stabilization measures, patients should be placed on a cardiac monitor and continuous pulse oximeter, receive an ECG, and have appropriate laboratory studies obtained shortly after arrival. If hemorrhage is suspected, blood should be sent for type and crossmatch.

Airway. The patient with ESRD can develop respiratory distress from conditions that afflict the general population (pneumonia, myocardial infarction, pulmonary embolism) and those that occur with increasing frequency among dialysis patients (volume overload, cardiac/pleural effusion).

The airway can be secured by a variety of measures, including nasotracheal or oral intubation. If mechanical ventilation is chosen, extreme care should be taken to avoid traumatic intubation. Patients with ESRD may have a severe bleeding diathesis and may bleed spontaneously into the retropharyngeal space.[10-12] Although succinylcholine can cause hyperkalemia, its use is not contraindicated in patients with ESRD unless severe hyperkalemia is suspected as the cause of compromise.[13,14] Vecuronium (Norcuron) may also be used, but pancuronium should be avoided in patients with glomerular filtration rate (GFR) less than 10 mL/min because of possible recurarization after initial recovery.

Breathing. Once the airway has been secured, adequate oxygenation should be administered via high-flow oxygen or by mechanical means. A possible option is the use of continuous positive airway pressure (CPAP) techniques. CPAP's efficacy in avoiding intubation in patients with pulmonary edema secondary to cardiac dysfunction and fluid overload from ESRD has been shown in several studies.[14-18]

Circulation. To avoid any complications with vascular graft cannulation, peripheral access is ideal. If this is not possible, or if intravascular monitoring is required, central venous access should be obtained. If neither of these can be done and IV access is needed quickly, the vascular graft can be cannulated as a last resort. *(Please see Table 2.)*

Diagnostic Evaluation. *History/Physical.* As with any other medical problem, treatment begins with a thorough history and physical examination. Information should be obtained from the patient, family members, other physicians, and dialysis center personnel. The history should ideally seek to establish the patient's baseline functional and medical status; the duration, etiology, and any complications from ESRD; and the level of compliance with dialysis, medical, and dietary therapy.

Evaluation of cardiovascular complications such as myocardial ischemia, dysrhythmias, and hypertensive crisis should be approached in the same manner as in those patients with normal renal function. The physical exam must include a thorough cardiopulmonary, cerebrovascular, and neurological evaluation. Signs of volume overload must be sought in patients with congestive heart failure. Complaints of chest pain should prompt consideration of aortic dissection and pericarditis as well as cardiac ischemia. Signs of aortic dissection may include a new diastolic murmur and pulse/pressure differentials in the extremities.

The evaluation of pericarditis can be difficult because physical findings such as the pericardial friction rub may not be audible until well after the onset of symptoms.[35] The rub is best auscultated along the left sternal border at the third and fourth intercostal spaces using the diaphragm of the stethoscope. It can have a one-, two-, or three-component character, and its presence along with pain is highly suggestive of pericarditis.[36] The presence of pulsus paradoxus, a decrease in systolic blood pressure greater than 10 mmHg during inspiration, should raise suspicion of significant pericardial effusion.

The patient with ESRD should be viewed as an immunocompromised host, and nonspecific complaints as well as fever should prompt consideration of infection. Significant information includes the duration of symptoms, focal complaints, previous infectious complications, HIV status, recent hospitalizations, vaccination status, any recent dental or medical instrumentation, and any illicit drug use. If the patient is sexually active, a social history with an emphasis on high-risk behavior is important. If the patient is receiving dialysis, the time and occurrence of any fever should be sought. Fever that occurs early in dialysis or shortly after cessation is usually secondary to infection. If fever occurs during dialysis, a "pyrogen" reaction may be causative.

The physical exam must include close inspection of the likely infectious sites, such as the lung, urinary tract, peritoneum, and catheter access sites. If the patient is diabetic, the oropharynx, integument, and extremities should be carefully inspected. A cardiopulmonary exam should focus on any new murmurs, signs of pulmonary consolidation, and manifestations of embolic disease. If the patient has fever and abdominal pain signs of other intra-abdominal processes, such as pancreatitis, appendicitis, cholecystitis, or mesenteric ischemia, an abscess must be sought before the diagnosis of CAPD peritonitis is made. Sexually active patients should receive a thorough pelvic and rectal exam. Joints should be checked for metastatic infection if a vascular graft is infected.

If patients are receiving peritoneal dialysis or hemodialysis, catheter and vascular access sites should be closely examined for erythema, fluctuance, discharge, and tenderness. As mentioned previously, an alarming one-third of patients with vascular access infections will manifest no symptoms.[23,30,50] If a vascular shunt is used, its functional integrity should be established. Loss of the bruit or thrill may indicate occlusion. Signs of aneurysm or pseudoaneurysm may include pain, thinning of the overlying skin, exposure of graft material, or impingement of adjacent structures. Aneurysms are a common nidus of infection and may "seed" distant sites, such as the joints, vertebrae, and cardiac valves.

Diagnostic Studies. Because nonspecific complaints may indicate a serious condition, initial diagnostic studies should include at least a 12-lead ECG, electrolytes, and cardiac monitoring. If clinically indicated, a CBC, coagulation studies, ABG, chest x-ray, blood cultures, urinalysis, lumbar puncture, therapeutic drug levels, and toxicology screen should be obtained. It should be noted that patients undergoing hemodialysis can demonstrate low leukocyte counts following dialysis, and, because of impaired cellular response, may not show the expected "left shift" of immature forms in the setting of infection.

The 12-lead ECG is an important tool because it may detect subtle changes secondary to pericardial disease, electrolyte disorders, and ischemia. Early ECG changes in pericarditis include diffuse ST segment elevations with a concave upward contour as well as PR segment depression. Later, the ST segments may return to baseline. The T wave amplitude may decrease and eventually invert in those leads that had ST segment elevation.[73] However, ECG diagnosis can be complicated by the presence of baseline ST-T wave changes often present in this population. ECG evidence of tamponade includes widespread decreases in QRS voltage and electrical alternans. Electrical alternans refers to changing levels of QRS voltage heights in an ECG that occurs when the heart changes position because of its suspension in a fluid-filled pericardium.

Electrolyte disorders such as hyperkalemia, hypercalcemia, and hypermagnesemia may produce characteristic ECG changes. The ECG changes found in hyperkalemia may not correlate with the level of elevation.

In hypercalcemia, a decreased QT interval is the most reliable ECG change and usually occurs at levels greater than 13 mg/dL.[7] Additional changes include prolongation of the PR interval and QRS complex, increased QRS voltage, and T-wave flattening.[7] At higher levels, atrioventricular block can progress to complete heart block. Hypermagnesemia may demonstrate bradycardia, heart block, and asystole. Morphologic changes include prolongation of the PR, QRS, and QT intervals.

Interpretation of chest radiographs may be difficult. Chronic volume overload may make radiographic diagnosis of pneumonia difficult if prior films are not available for comparison.

If peritonitis is suspected in patients receiving CAPD, at least 150 cc of peritoneal fluid should be obtained. Peritoneal fluid should be grossly examined for color and character and sent for Gram's stain, cell count, and culture. Peritonitis is diagnosed by the presence of a white cell count greater than 100 cells/mm^3 with a predominance of polymorphonuclear cells.[67] If a predominance of eosinophils or mononuclear cells is found, diagnoses of eosinophilic peritonitis or tubercles peritonitis, respectively, should be considered. Although a Gram's stain exam has a low predictive value, it may help in the early diagnosis of fungal peritonitis. Blood cultures are usually negative in peritonitis.

Additional studies may include a CT scan for suspected intracranial processes or an echocardiogram for suspected pericardial effusion or tamponade.

Specific Treatment Modalities

Hypertensive Complications. Hypertensive complications in patients with ESRD are usually due to volume overload or medical noncompliance. The ideal treatment for hypertensive emergencies caused by volume overload is dialysis. If emergent dialysis is unavailable, parenteral therapy should be started.

The treatment goal in a hypertensive emergency is to reduce the blood pressure in a rapid and controlled fashion. Reasonable goals are to reduce the blood pressure by 20-30% or to a level of 160/100 mmHg in the first 24 hours.[7,23] If a cerebrovascular accident is suspected, drastic reduction should be avoided and a mean arterial pressure (MAP) maintained at a level of 120-160 mmHg to insure adequate cerebral perfusion.[7,25]

If signs of hypertensive crisis exist, parenteral therapy using nitroprusside at an initial dose of 0.3 mcg/kg/min is the drug of choice. It acts as both an alpha- and beta-adrenergic blocker and can reduce both cardiac preload and afterload. Potential thiocynate toxicity can be avoided by limiting infusion to less than 48 hours, initiating early dialysis, and maintaining levels between 5 and 10 mg/dL.

If nitroprusside is unavailable, nitroglycerin may be used and is a safe and effective venodilator. If immediate intravenous access is unavailable, nitroglycerin can be given sublingually every five minutes x 3 with blood pressure checked frequently. Subsequently, nitroglycerin can be infused intravenously at an initial rate of 5 mcg/min.

Other potentially useful agents include combination alpha- and beta-blockers (IV labetalol), diuretics, IV ACE inhibitors, and calcium-channel blockers. 100 mL of 30% sorbitol given orally or rectally may be used if the hypertensive condition exists in the presence of pulmonary edema. It acts by creating an osmotic gradient between the gastrointestinal tract and the vascular space.

Congestive Heart Failure/Pulmonary Edema. The most common exacerbating factor causing congestive heart failure in patients with ESRD is volume overload, but other factors to consider are cardiac ischemia, dysrhythmia, hypertensive emergency, and medication/dialysis noncompliance. The first goal of treatment is to ensure hemodynamic stability. Presence of cardiogenic shock may require infusion of vasopressor agents such as dopamine or inotropes such as dobutamine. If anemia is suspected of causing high-output failure or contributing to myocardial ischemia, infusion of packed red cells should be considered. Central venous pressure monitoring may be required with these modalities to avoid volume overload.

Hemodialysis or peritoneal dialysis are the preferred methods of removing excess volume. Because lack of immediate availability may limit their use in some centers, pharmacotherapy should be used as a temporizing measure.

Safe and effective agents immediately available include nitroglycerin, morphine sulfate, and furosemide.[30-33] These agents act by reducing cardiac preload through venodilation. Nitroglycerin 0.4 mg SL q 5 can be given initially and followed by an IV drip started at 5 mcg/min titrated to effect while avoiding hypotension. Morphine 2-5 mg IV decreases preload and decreases patient anxiety. Frequent dosing should be avoided to prevent respiratory depression. Though ineffective in initiating diuresis in an anuric patient, furosemide 80-120 mg IV can cause venodilation with consequent decreases in left ventricular filling pressures and pulmonary capillary wedge pressures.[33]

Additional agents include nitroprusside and sorbitol. Nitroprusside started at 0.3 mcg/kg/min acts as both a preload and afterload reducer, thereby decreasing left ventricular pressure and cardiac oxygen demand; 100 mL of 30% sorbitol given orally or rectally promotes an osmotic shift between the vascular space and the gut.[7,34] Its late onset of action (1-6 hours) and copious diarrhea may make management difficult. Phlebotomy should be avoided.

Pericardial Disease. The patient's hemodynamic status will dictate the therapeutic approach to pericarditis or pericardial tamponade. *(Please see Figure 1.)* If the patient is hemodynamically stable, exacerbating factors such as trauma, infection, dialysis non-compliance, and medications should be identified and corrected. The patient's nephrologist should be informed, and arrangements should be made to either initiate dialysis or intensify the patient's current regimen. If the patient is complaining of pain or fever, indomethacin or steroids may be used for relief once other sources of fever and chest pain have been ruled out.

If the patient is hemodynamically unstable, the patient should be prepared for pericardiocentesis. Because of potential complications such as myocardial laceration, dysrhythmia, iatrogenic tamponade and hepatic laceration, pericardiocentesis should be deferred for those patients in shock.[38] If the patient is mildly unstable but responds to volume expansion with saline or mannitol, immediate surgical consultation should be made and the patient prepared for either pericardiotomy or pericardiectomy.

Dysrhythmias. Treatment of specific dysrhythmias should follow currently recommended guidelines, with specific dose adjustment. If cardiac arrest exists, hyperkalemia should be suspected and 10-20 mL of 10% calcium chloride or 15-20 mL of 10% calcium gluconate should be given over 10-15 minutes. Calcium should be avoided if digitalis toxicity is suspected, as it may worsen the dysrhythmia. The only ACLS protocol drug to avoid is bretylium. If ischemia is suspected, treatment should include aspirin, nitrates, heparin, and possible thrombolytics.

Cardiac Ischemia. There is no significant alteration in the management of myocardial infarction and ischemia in patients suffering from chronic renal failure and ESRD.

Aspirin, nitrates, heparin, and thrombolytics should be used according to currently established guidelines. Because underlying anemia impairs oxygen delivery, transfusion with packed red blood cells should be considered. Hemodialysis should be avoided during this period.

Infections

General Considerations. Specific treatment regimens are based on likely foci of infection and the patient's underlying renal function. In the unstable septic patient, cultures should be obtained and vancomycin 1g IV and gentamycin 1.7 mg/kg started empirically. This regimen provides coverage for the likely gram-positive and gram-negative organisms that commonly infect this population. Diabetics, patients with HIV, and those suspected of nosocomial pathogens require therapy tailored to likely pathogens, local resistance patterns, and any previous culture results.

Pneumonia is a common source of infection, and the most likely agent is streptococcal pneumonia. If recent hospitalization has occurred, infection with gram-negative and nosocomial pathogens should be suspected, and antibiotics should be chosen accordingly. If the patient is extremely ill, infection with gram-negative organisms, *Staphylococcus,* and *Legionella* should be suspected. Tuberculosis also should be considered, especially among groups at higher risk, such as the institutionalized, the poor, and those with HIV.[53]

If a urinary source is suspected, the physician should consider whether the patient suffers from polycystic kidney disease. These patients require lipid-soluble antibiotics (clindamycin, chloramphenicol, trimethoprim/sulfamethoxazole) and surgical consultation if intra-renal or perinephric abscesses are suspected.

Peritonitis. Care of peritoneal dialysis patients with peritonitis should include quick dialysate exchange (which helps alleviate pain and remove peritoneal debris) and intravenous and intraperitoneal antibiotics. The initial antibiotics chosen should have anti-staphylococcal coverage. Additional considerations should be made for gram-negative organisms and methicillin-resistant strains of *Staphylococcus.*

Other therapeutic agents include heparin and rifampin. Heparin given intraperitoneally at a dose of 500 units/lL of dialysate for 3-5 days helps prevent obstruction of the catheter and prevents formation of fibrin that acts as a haven for microbial growth. Rifampin is usually administered for relapsing peritonitis. It acts by penetrating the bacterial protective sanctuaries of peritoneal cellular debris and the biofilm located in and around dialysate catheters. Fortunately, the majority of patients with peritonitis can be treated as outpatients if they are clinically stable, reliable, and able to maintain adequate nutrition. *(Please see Table 3.)*

Hospital admission is mandatory for patients who cannot maintain nutritional balance, who show signs of clinical instability, and are suspected of having either fungal or sclerosing peritonitis. Fungal peritonitis requires removal of the dialysis catheter, systemic antifungal therapy, and nutritional support. Sclerosing peritonitis requires removal of the catheter, discontinuation of peritoneal dialysis, and surgery for complications secondary to abdominal adhesions.

Vascular Access Infection. If access site infection is suspected, the patient's nephrologist should be informed. Concerns of vascular access site aneurysms or thrombosis should lead to vascular surgery consultation as well. Initial treatment should be vancomycin 1g IV × 1, and gentamycin 1.7 mg/kg × 1 if gram-negative infection is suspected. The long half-life (5-7 days) and antimicrobial spectrum of these agents make them ideal agents for outpatient treatment. Patients with hemodynamic instability, graft compromise, or inability to maintain adequate nutrition require admission.

Electrolyte Disorders

Hyperkalemia. Treatment goals in hyperkalemia are to insure cardiac stability, facilitate translocation of extracellular potassium, and enhance excretion. The immediate goal in hyperkalemia is to stabilize the myocardium by administering 10% calcium chloride or 10% calcium gluconate. These agents should be given immediately to patients in cardiac arrest or to patients exhibiting signs of rhythm instability.

Following initial stabilization, agents that help translocate extracellular potassium should be administered. These include beta-agonists, IV insulin, and sodium bicarbonate.

Beta-agonists and insulin act by stimulating the cellular Na+K+ ATPase pump to translocate extracellular potassium.[54,55,56] Albuterol, 20 mg in 4 mL NS given by nebulizer can lower potassium by 1.0 mmol/L and has few side effects. Ten to 20 units of regular insulin IV along with 50 cc of D50 can lower potassium levels by 0.6-1.0 mmol/L over one hour. Because hypoglycemia is a potential side effect, initial therapy should be followed by IV D5W.

The role of sodium bicarbonate is controversial. Some studies have not proven its efficacy, but current emergency medicine sources advocate its use. The dose is 50 mEq IV over 5-10 minute.[7,57-60,71]

The ideal means of potassium removal is dialysis, but its rapid availability limits its use. Sodium polystyrene sulfate (Kaexylate) can be given either orally or rectally and exchanges potassium for sodium using the gastrointestinal tract. Kaexylate 25 g/25 cc of 70% sorbitol orally, or 50 g/50 cc of 70% sorbitol rectally, removes 0.5-1.0 mmol of potassium for every gram of kaexylate. Sodium overload can result from Kaexylate treatment, so close monitoring is required.

Disposition. Patients who are symptomatic require admission to a monitored setting. Those having cardiovascular instability need an intensive care unit. Patients with mild elevations (5.5-6.0) who demonstrate no ECG manifestations and who are asymptomatic may receive conservative therapy (albuterol, insulin/glucose, and Kaexylate) and be discharged, if the patient's nephrologist is notified and agrees. Such patients must be reliable, and hemodialysis must be arranged in a timely fashion. If compliance is in question, the patient should be admitted to ensure that dialysis takes place.

Hypercalcemia. Unlike patients with normal renal function, fluids and diuretics are ineffective in the treatment of hypercalcemic patients with ESRD. Those with levels between 12 mg/dL and 15 mg/dL can often await timely dialysis. Those with levels greater than 15 mg/dL require emergent treatment regardless of symptoms. This involves IV fluids if the patient's volume is depleted, salmon calcitonin intravenously at 5 MRC U/kg q6hr, and prompt dialysis. Although the effects of steroids are delayed, their use should be considered.

Hypermagnesemia. Treatment goals are to ensure respiratory stabilization, cardiac stability, and magnesium elimination.

Mechanical ventilation may be required if respiratory depression is significant. Ten mL of 10% calcium chloride or calcium gluconate IV should be given for cardiac instability and may be repeated twice every 5-20 minutes. Elimination is best achieved through hemodialysis.

Hematologic Complications

Spontaneous Hemorrhage. Treatment involves ensuring hemodynamic stability and preventing further hemorrhage. Resuscitative measures include direct pressure, establishing large-bore IV access, and infusion of crystalloid and/or packed red blood cells as appropriate. If compression is required at the dialysis catheter site, excessive pressure should be avoided to prevent occlusion of the catheter. Persistent bleeding may indicate the presence of an aneurysm or pseudoaneurysm. Tourniquet use above the vascular catheter should be avoided unless fulminate hemorrhage is present

Correction of suspected coagulopathy may require specific pharmacological therapy. If heparin is a suspected factor in major bleeding, protamine 0.5 mg/100 units of heparin used can be given. It is best given within 30 minutes of the last heparin dose. To correct platelet dysfunction, DDAVP, 0.3 mcg/kg in 50 cc of NS IV or 3 mcg/kg nasally can be administered.[64] A subcutaneous dose of 0.4 mcg/kg can also be used, but absorption may be erratic. Ten bags of Cryoprecipitate can also be administered.[11] Dialysis can help correct the bleeding diathesis, but its emergent use may be limited by lack of immediate availability.

Traumatic Hemorrhage. The patient with ESRD who is injured should be approached in the same fashion as other trauma victims. Resuscitation should follow standard ATLS protocols.

Volume resuscitation should use both crystalloid solutions and blood products as indicated. Because lactated Ringer's solution contains 4 mEq/L of potassium, it should be avoided because of its potential to cause hyperkalemia. Anemia is a common occurrence among patients with ESRD, and even minor blood loss may impair oxygen delivery; transfusion with packed red blood cells should be considered early. Crossmatching patients may be difficult due to the presence of red cell antibodies from previous transfusion.

Neurologic Complications

Altered Mental Status. In general, the evaluation and management of altered mental status in the patient with ESRD is the same as for other patients. A higher index of suspicion, however, should be maintained for spontaneous subdural hemorrhage. In addition, the dialysis disequilibrium syndrome should be kept as a diagnosis of exclusion. Treatment involves infusion of osmotically active fluid such as mannitol or hypertonic saline. The patient's nephrologist should be consulted prior to initiating therapy.

If a seizure occurs or is suspected, there is no contraindication to using phenytoin, phenobarbital, or diazepam. Because of decreased protein binding, phenytoin should be loaded to achieve a level between 5-10 mcg/mL.

Dialysis-Associated Complications

Peritoneal Catheter Obstruction. Treatment should include manipulating the patient's position in an attempt to relieve the obstruction. Definitive treatment using a trochar device and thrombolytic agents necessitates a surgical consultant.

Vascular Catheter Obstruction. Since it is difficult to differentiate between a mechanical and thrombotic obstruction, angiography must be performed promptly. Urokinase 2500-5000 IU can be given if the obstruction is acute, and the vascular surgeon has been consulted. This should be done as soon as possible to preserve function.

If a double-lumen catheter device is obstructed, gentle aspiration may be corrective. Urokinase or streptokinase also may be given. Forceful irrigation must be avoided to prevent distal embolization.

Vascular Access Hemorrhage. Treatment of hemorrhage includes firm, nonocclusive pressure for 5-10 minutes and identification of any correctable bleeding disorder. Observation should continue for 1-2 hours to assure homeostasis. A vascular surgeon should be consulted if functional compromise, rapid expansion, or if imminent rupture is suspected. If rupture occurs, a tourniquet should be applied proximal to the site and resuscitative measures begun.

Air Embolism. If air embolism is suspected, all venous lines should be clamped immediately; the patient should be placed in the left lateral decubitus position and given 100% oxygen. This allows the air to be trapped at the apex of the right ventricle. If the patient develops air embolism while in Trendelenburg, he or she should be left in that position. If the patient is in arrest, percutaneous aspiration of air with an intracardiac needle is required. Additional treatments include IV corticosteroids for cerebral edema and heparin or low molecular weight dextran to improve microcirculation.

Dialysis-Induced Hypotension. Treatment should be tailored to the underlying condition. Most episodes of hypotension respond to volume infusion administered in the dialysis unit. If a patient presents with continuing instability despite early resuscitative measures, etiologies other than modest volume deficits must be investigated. To treat the hypotension, small aliquots of volume in 100-200 mL increments should be given with close monitoring. If a patient is mildly symptomatic and all underlying factors, such as arrhythmia, cardiac dysfunction, and infection, can be ruled out, the hypotension may be treated with food and fluids containing sodium.

Summary

The incidence of ESRD has been progressively increasing over the past two decades. Because of an increasing geriatric population and acceptance of patients with conditions such as severe hypertension, diabetes, and HIV into dialysis therapy, this trend will most likely continue. As a result, the primary care physician is increasingly likely to encounter the many potential complications of ESRD.

ESRD and its complications are difficult entities to manage in both the chronic and acute care settings. The problems that cause rapid decompensation of the ESRD patient involve cardiovascular conditions, infections, metabolic disorders, and complications secondary to dialysis therapy. Thorough knowledge is required if the primary care physician is to successfully evaluate and treat this complicated patient population.

References

1. Port FK. Worldwide demographics and international trends in end stage renal disease. *Kidney Int* 1993;43:S4-S7.
2. United States Renal Disease System. 1993 Annual Data Report. National Institute of Diabetes and Digestion and Kidney Diseases. Bethesda, MD; 1993:1-100.
3. Eggers PW. Projections of the end stage renal disease population to the year 2000. In: Challenges for Public Health Statistics in the 1990s: Proceedings of the 1989 Public Health Conference on Records and Statistics. Hyatsville, MD: U.S. Dept of Health and Human Services, Centers for Disease Control, National Center for Health Statistics; 1989:121-126.
4. Moore MA, Blythe WB, and the National High Blood Pressure Education Program. National High Blood Pressure Education Program Working Group report on hypertension and chronic renal failure. *Arch Intern Med* 1991;151:1280-1287.
5. Strauss MJ, Port FK. An estimate of the size of the U.S. predialysis population with anemia. *Am J Kidney Dis* 1993;21:264-269.
6. Ismail N, Becker BN. Treatment options and strategies in uremia: Current trends and future directions. *Semin Nephrol* 1994;14: 282-299.
7. Wolfson AB. Chronic renal failure and dialysis. In: Rosen P, Barkin RM. *Emergency Medicine Concepts and Clinical Practice.* 3rd ed. St. Louis: Mosby-Year Book; 1992:1928-1943.
8. Klahr S, Schreiner G, Ichikawa I. The progression of renal disease. *N Engl J Med* 1988;318:1657-1666.
9. Jacobson HR. Chronic renal failure: pathophysiology. *Lancet* 1991;338:419-425.
10. Minno GD, Martinez J. Platelet dysfunction in uremia. *Am J Med* 1985;79:552-559.
11. Janson PA, Jubelirer SJ. Treatment of the bleeding tendency in uremia with crypoprecipitate. *N Engl J Med* 1980;303:1318-1322.
12. Handa SP, Colwell B. Spontaneous retropharyngeal bleeding in a patient on chronic hemodialysis. *Nephron* 1993;64:485-486.
13. Nancarrow C, Mather LE. Pharmacokinetics in renal failure. *Anaes Intensive Care* 1983;11:350-358.
14. Huff SJ, Whelan TV. CPAP as adjunctive treatment of severe pulmonary edema in patients with ESRD. *Am J Emerg Med* 1994;12: 388.
15. Vainasen IT, Rasanen J. Continous positive airway pressure and supplemental oxygen in the treatment of cardiogenic pulmonary edema. *Chest* 1994;92:481-485.
16. Fitzpatrick M, Nelson J. Continous positive airway pressure as an adjunct in treatment of cardiogenic pulmonary edema. *Ann Emerg Med* 1990;21:1045.
17. Bersten AD, Holt AE., et al. Treatment of severe cardiogenic pulmonary edema with continous positive airway pressure delivered by face mask. *N Engl J Med* 1991;325:1825-1836.
18. Ansari A, Kaupke CJ. Cardiac pathology in patients with end stage renal disease maintained on hemodialysis. *Int J Artif Organs* 1993;16:31-36.
19. Ma KW, Greene EL, Raij L. Cardiovascular risk factors in chronic renal failure and hemodialysis populations. *Am J Kidney Dis* 1992;19:505-513.
20. Rostand SG, Brunzell JD, et al. Cardiovascular complications in renal failure. *J Am Soc Nephrol* 1991;2:1053-1061.
21. Greaves SC, Sharpe DN: Cardiovascular disease in patients with end-stage renal failure. *Aust N Z J Med* 1991;22:152-159.
22. Kreastinos D, Paraskevaidis I, et al. Painless myocardial ischemia in chronic hemodialyzed patients: A real event? *Nephron* 1992;60: 164-170.
23. Zarconi J, Phinney, B. Special considerations in the patient with chronic renal failure in the ICU. In: *The High Risk Patient: Management of the Critically Ill.* Baltimore: Williams & Wilkins; 1995.
24. Kim KE, Swartz C. Cardiovascular complications in end-stage renal disease. In: Schrier RW, Gottschalk CW. Diseases of the Kidney, 5th ed. Boston: Little, Brown, and Co; 1993:2817-2844.
25. Calhou DA, Oparil S. Treatment of hypertensive crisis. *N Engl J Med* 1990;323:1177-1183.
26. Harney JD, Parfrey PS. Cardiac disease in uremia. *Semin Nephrol* 1994;14:245-252.
27. Parferey PS, Harnett JD. Congestive heart failure in dialysis patients. *Arch Intern Med* 1988;148:1519-1526.
28. Gehm L, Propp DA. Pulmonary edema in the renal failure patient. *Am J Emerg Med* 1989;7:336-338.
29. Kohen, JA, Opsahl JA. Deceptive patterns of uremic pulmonary edema. *Am J Kidney Dis* 1986;8:456-460.
30. Hodde LA, Sandroni S. Emergency department evaluation and management of dialysis patient complications. *J Emerg Med* 1992;10:317-334.
31. Sacchetti A, McCabe H. ED management of acute congestive heart failure in renal dialysis patients. *Am J Emerg Med* 1993;11: 644-647.
32. Wolfson AB, Singer I. Hemodialysis-related emergencies—part II. *J Emerg Med* 1987;5:533-543.
33. Kraus PA, Lipman J, Becker PJ. Acute preload effect of furosemide. *Chest* 1990;98:124-128.
34. Cloonan CC, Gatrell CB, Cushner HM. Emergencies in continous dialysis patients: Diagnosis and management. *Am J Emerg Med* 1990;134-148.
35. Rostand SC, Rutsky EA. Pericarditis in end-stage renal disease. *Cardiol Clin* 1990;8: 701-707.
36. Shabetai R. Diseases of the pericardium: Pericardial disease. In: Hurst JW, Schlant RC. *The Heart,* 7th ed. New York: Mcgraw Hill; 1992;1348-1374.
37. Kim KE, Swartz C. Cardiovascular complications of end-stage renal disease. In: Schrier RW, Gottschalk CW. *Diseases of the Kidney.* 5th ed. Boston: Little, Brown, and Co.; 1993:2817-2844.
38. Hammerman H, Kloner RA. Pericardial diseases. In: Kloner RA. *The Guide to Cardiology.* 2nd ed. New York: Le Jacq

Communications; 1990:383-394.

39. Parfrey PS. Cardiac and cerebrovascular disease in chronic uremia. *Am J Kidney Dis* 1993;21:77-80.
40. Parfrey PS, et al.: Congestive heart failure in dialysis patients. *Arch Intern Med* 1988;148:1519-1523.
41. Shapira OM, Bar-Khayim Y. ECG changes and cardiac arrhythmias in chronic renal failure patients on hemodialysis. *J Electrocardiog* 1992;25;273-279.
42. Blumberg A, Hausermann M, et al. Cardiac arrhythmias in patients on maintenance hemodialysis. *Nephron* 1983;33:91-95.
43. Morrison G, Michelson EL, et al. Mechanisms and prevention of cardiac arrhythmias in chronic hemodialysis patients. *Kidney Int* 1980;17:811-819.
44. Kimura K, Tabei K. Cardiac arrhythmias in hemodialysis patients. *Nephron* 1989;53:201-207.
45. Singhal PC, Barth RH, Ginsberg NS, et al. Determinants of creatinine kinase activity in dialysis patients. *Am J Nephrol* 1988;8: 220-224.
46. Goldman M, Vanherwheghen JL. Bacterial infections in chronic hemodialysis patients: Epidemiologic and pathophysiologic aspects. *Adv Nephrol* 1990;19:315-332.
47. Zibaria GB, Rohr MS, et al. Complications from permanent hemodialysis vascular access. *Surgery* 1988; 681-686.
48. Jameson MD, Wiegamann TB. Principles, uses, and complications of hemodialysis. *Med Clin North Am* 1990;74:945-960.
49. Goldblum SE, Reed WP. Host defenses and immunologic alterations associated with chronic hemodialysis. *Ann Intern Med* 1980;93:597-613.
50. Dobkin JF, Miller MH, et al. Septicemia in patients on chronic hemodialysis. *Ann Intern Med* 1978;88:28-33.
51. Andrew OT, Shoenfield PY, et al. Tuberculosis in patients with end-stage renal disease. *Am J Med* 1980;68:59-67.
52. Rimmer JM, Horn JF, Gennari J. Hyperkalemia as a complication of drug therapy. *Ann Intern Med* 1987;147:867-869.
53. Papadakis MA, Wexman MP, Fraser C, et al. Hyperkalemia complicating digoxin toxicity in a patient with renal failure. *Am J Kidney Dis* 1985;5:64-66.
54. Allon M. Treatment and prevention of hyperkalemia in end-stage renal disease. *Kidney Int* 1993;43:1197-1209.
55. Liou HH, Chiang SS. Hypokalemic effects of IV infusion on nebulization of salbutamol in patients with chronic renal failure: Comparative study. *Am J Kidney Dis* 1994;23:266-271.
56. Allon M, Copkney C. Albuterol and insulin for treatment of hyperkalemia in hemodialysis patients. *Kidney Int* 1990;38:869-972.
57. Blumberg A, Weidmann P, Shaw S, et al. Effect of various therapeutic approaches on plasma potassium and major regulating factors in terminal renal failure. *Am J Med* 1988;85:507-512.
58. Blumber A, Weidmann P, Ferrari P. Effects on prolonged bicarbonate administration on plasma potassium in terminal renal failure. *Kidney Int* 1992;41:369-374.
59. Wolfson AB, Levy M. The patient with chronic renal insufficiency following renal transplantation. In: Herr RD, Cydulka RK. *Emergency Care of the Compromised Patient.* 1st ed. Philadehphia: JP Lippincott Co.; 1994:416-432.
60. Walter FG, Lowe RA. Disorders of potassium metabolism. In: Harwood-Nuss A, Linden C, et al. *The Clinical Practice of Emergency Medicine,* 1st ed. Philadelphia: JP Lippincott Co.; 1991:999-1001.
61. Ellison R, Corroa W, Fox M, et al. Spontaneous mediastinal hemorrhage in patients on chronic hemodialysis. *Ann Intern Med* 1988;95: 704-706.
62. Bora S, Kleinfled M. Subcapsular liver hematoma in a patient on chronic hemodialysis. *Ann Intern Med* 1980;93:574.
63. Blagg CR. Acute complications associated with hemodialysis. In: Maher JF. *Replacement of Renal Function by Dialysis.* 3rd ed. Dordecht: Kluwer Academic Publishers; 1989:750-771.
64. Carvalho ACA. Bleeding in uremia: A clinical challenge. *N Engl J Med* 1983;308:38-39.
65. Nielsen VK. The peripheral nerve function in chronic renal failure. *Acta Med Scand* 1971;190:105-111.
66. Fraser CL, Arieff AI. Nervous system complications in uremia. *Ann Intern Med* 1988;109:143-153.
67. Saklayen MG. CAPD peritonitis: Incidence, pathogens, diagnosis, and management. *Med Clin North Am* 1990;74:997-1010.
68. Wolfson AB, Singer I. Hemodialysis-related emergencies—Part 1. *J Emerg Med* 1987;5:533-543.
69. Bernstein JM, Erk SD. Choice of antibiotics, pharmacokinetics, and dose adjustments in acute and chronic renal failure. *Med Clin North Am* 1990;74:1059-1076.
70. Bennett WM, Aronoff GR, et al. Drug prescribing in renal failure: Dosing guidelines for adults. *Am J Kidney Dis* 1993;3:155-180.
71. Wilson RF. Fluid and electrolyte problems. In: Tintinalli JE, Krome RL, Ruiz E. *Emergency Medicine: A Comprehensive Study Guide.* 3rd ed. New York: McGraw-Hill; 1992:72-74.
72. Nichols, A. Atherosclerosis in chronic renal failure: A historical perspective. *Scott Med J* 1983:28:270.
73. Pratt DF, Bissen HA. Acute pericarditis and cardiac tamponade. In: *The Clinical Practice of Emergency Medicine.* 2nd ed. Philadelphia: Lippincott-Raven; 1996:617-619.

Sexually Transmitted Diseases

Eileen M. Duffy, MD, FAAP, FACEP

Sexually transmitted diseases (STDs) are occurring in epidemic proportions in sexually active adolescents. This age group accounts for approximately 25% of the 12 million cases of STDs occurring annually in the United States.[1] The prevalence of *Neisseria gonorrheae, Chlamydia trachomatis*, and possibly even human papilloma virus (HPV) infections are highest among the adolescent age group. In 1996, of the 325,000 people infected with gonorrhea in the United States, about 60% of cases occured in young adults between the ages of 15 and 24.[2] Approximately 4 million cases of chlamydia occur each year in the United States. Although age-specific rates are not available for chlamydial infections, a study from family planning clinics showed the prevalence to be three times higher in females younger than 18 years of age than in those older than 29 years of age.[3] The rate of HPV infection also is reported to be 2-3 times higher in young women.[4] This article comprehensively reviews a variety of STD syndromes, their clinical presentations, diagnostic evaluation, and management.

Introduction

In the 1997 Youth Risk Behavior Surveillance Survey, almost 50% of high school students polled had been sexually active.[5] Several factors place these adolescents at increased risk of acquiring STDs. First, this age group is more likely to practice unprotected intercourse. According to the risk behavior survey, only 57% of respondents reported that either they or their partner had used a condom the last time they had intercourse. Adolescents also are biologically more susceptible to infection than adults. In addition, health care services are less readily accessible to adolescents.

Long-term sequelae may occur in up to 25% of patients with certain STDs,[6] and management in an emergency department (ED) setting is frequently based on a presumptive diagnosis as results of definitive tests are not immediately available—making follow-up a critical aspect of ED care. The vulnerability of this age group mandates a careful, thorough ED evaluation and scheduled follow-up.

History and Physical Examination

Clinicians must appreciate the value adolescent patients place on confidentiality. In most states, they can consent to the diagnosis and treatment of STDs without parental knowledge. Likewise, adolescents can consent to HIV counselling and testing in many states. Familarity with state laws governing STDs and adolescents is essential to the ED physician's ability to provide care.

Eliciting accurate information from adolescents can be challenging. The medical history should be obtained privately, without parents present. If the patient's presentation may be consistant with an STD, information obtained should include date of last menstrual period, sexual activity, number of partners and their health, contraceptive use, history of STDs, and symptoms suggestive of STDs.

Since STDs may present with a wide variety of findings, the examination must include inspection of the skin, oropharynx, lymph nodes, abdomen, genitalia, and anorectal region. Cultures and serologic testing should be obtained as indicated, and all females should have a pregnancy test. Screening for syphilis and HIV should be considered in all patients with STDs.

Urethritis

Urethritis. *N. gonorrheae.* Urethritis is divided into gonococcal and non-gonococcal etiologies. *N. gonorrheae* is a gram-negative diplococcus that accounts for 15-32% of urethritis in symptomatic adolescent males. The incubation period is 3-7 days after exposure. Gonorrheal infections of the urethra are symptomatic in 85-90% of cases.[8] Patients who practice oral or receptive ano-rectal sex also may develop gonorrheal pharyngitis or proctitis. As many as 20% of males with gonococcal urethritis are coinfected with chlamydia.[9]

Chlamydia trachomatis. *Chlamydia trachomatis* is an obligate intracellular parasite that accounts for 23-55% of non-gonococcal urethritis (NGU) in adult men.[10] Chlamydia may be more prevalent in adolescents. Studies have isolated the organism in 83-89% of patients with urinalysis evidence of NGU.[11] The incubation period to symptomatic disease is 7-14 days. Of note, approximately 5-10% of sexually active males are infected with chlamydia but remain asymptomatic.[12]

Other sexually transmitted organisms causing NGU include *Ureaplasma urealyticum, Mycoplasma genitalium*, and *Trichomonas vaginalis.*[10] Herpes simplex virus (HSV) also may cause urethritis; however, this is usually accompanied by typical skin lesions. In approximately 20% of cases, the cause of urethritis is unknown.[13]

The microbiology of sexually transmitted urethritis in females has not been extensively studied. It is thought to be similar to that seen in males.

Clinical Presentation. Urethritis in males most commonly presents as dysuria and/or urethral discharge. Other symptoms may include urinary urgency or frequency, scrotal pain, and meatal irritation. The differential includes other causes of urethral irritation such as foreign bodies, ulcers, or other lesions.

Urethritis also may occur in females, with symptoms simulating a urinary tract infection (UTI). Typically, concurrent signs and symptoms of a cervical infection are present when the etiology is due to a sexually transmitted organism.

It is difficult to differentiate gonococcal vs. non-gonococcal urethritis on exam alone. Classically, gonorrhea is associated with expression of a purulent urethral discharge, while a serous or mucoid discharge is usually associated with NGU.

Diagnosis. Urethritis may be diagnosed when any of the following is present:

1. Mucopurulent or purulent urethral discharge;
2. Gram stain of discharge with five or more white blood cells (WBCs) per oil immersion field. A presumptive diagnosis of gonorrhea can be made if intracellular gram-negative diplococci are present; or
3. Positive leukocyte esterase test or demonstration of more than 10 WBCs per high powered field on a first-void urine.[10]

Identifying the organism is important for infection control. The gold standard of using culture techniques to isolate gonorrhea and chlamydia are largely being replaced by non-culture tests. DNA amplification techniques using polymerase chain reaction (PCR) or ligase chain reaction (LCR) and nucleic acid hybridization (NAH) techniques have been shown to be more sensitive and nearly as specific in identifying these agents. NAH and LCR offer the advantage of requiring one swab to test for both gonorrhea and chlamydia. Specifically, studies have shown that PCR and LCR detect these agents in urine with more sensitivity than culture techniques, thus eliminating the need for urethral swabbing.[7,14] Direct fluorescent antibody (DFA) staining and enzyme immunoassay (EIA) tests are also available to detect chlamydia.

Urethral cultures are still indicated in cases of abuse and rape as non-culture methods have a small potential for false-positive results. Swabs with cotton tips and wooden shafts should be avoided, as they may interfere with the culture. Specimens for gonorrhea are plated on chocolate agar and modified Thayer-Martin media and transported in CO_2 containing systems. Culture of chlamydia is more difficult and requires a laboratory staff experienced in the technique and handling of specimens. Even in an experienced laboratory setting, the sensitivity is only about 70-90%.[15]

Treatment. Since it is difficult to distinguish gonococcal from non-gonococcal causes of urethritis on physical exam, treatment should include coverage for both gonorrhea and chlamydia in symptomatic patients.[10] *(See Table 1.)* Single-dose regimens are strongly recommended given the high rate of compliance when administered under direct observation. Patients with HIV should be treated with the same regimen as those who are HIV negative. Quinolones are not approved for the treatment of patients younger than 18 years of age. Fluoroquinolone-resistant strains of gonorrhea are widespread in Asia but have only been reported sporadically in the United States and, therefore, have not altered current treatment recommendations.[10] Patients should be advised to abstain from sexual intercourse until treatment is completed and clinical symptoms have resolved.

Complications. Left untreated, the symptoms of urethritis usually resolve spontaneously, although infectivity persists. Symptomatic complications of urethritis include epididymitis, Reiter's syndrome, and disseminated gonococcal infection. Reiter's syndrome consists of the triad of a reactive arthritis, NGU, and conjunctivitis. Although typically occuring after an enteric infection, Reiter's syndrome has also been associated with chlamydial urethritis. The majority of patients are HLA-B27 positive and therefore genetically predisposed.[16]

Epididymitis

Etiology. Gonorrhea and chlamydia are responsible for 67% of cases of epididymitis in sexually active adolescents and young men. Gram-negative enteric organsims are a more common cause of epididymitis in men older than 35 years and in younger males who practice anal intercourse.[17]

Clinical Presentation. Scrotal pain and swelling are the most common symptoms associated with epididymitis. Onset may be acute or gradual, with the scrotum eventually becoming warm and erythematous. Symptoms of urethritis are usually present. Occasionally the patient will be febrile.

On examination, the scrotum is typically swollen, erythematous, and warm. Differentiating epididymitis from testicular torsion can be difficult. With epididymitis, palpation revels exquisite tenderness over the epididymus. Scrotal swelling may make it difficult to discern this structure. A urethral discharge may be present. The cremasteric reflex is usually preserved in epididymitis and absent in testicular torsion. However, 30% of normal males do not have an elicitable reflex.[7]

Diagnosis. As with urethritis, gonorrhea and chlamydia may be diagnosed by culture or non-culture methods. A mid-stream, clean-catch urine culture can identify infections caused by gram-negative enteric organisms. If testicular torsion cannot be ruled out on clinical exam, a testicular scan or Doppler ultrasound should be performed. A urologist should be notified as soon as the diagnosis of torsion has been made or if there is going to be any delay in getting a testicular scan or ultrasound.

Treatment. When the etiology is gonorrhea or chlamydia, treat-

Table 1. Treatment of Urethritis, Epididymitis, and Cervicitis

RECOMMENDED REGIMENS FOR THE TREATMENT OF GONOCOCCAL INFECTIONS
Cefixime 400 mg po (single dose)
or
Ceftriaxone 125 mg IM (single dose)
or
Ciprofloxacin 500 mg po (single dose)
or
Ofloxacin 400 mg po (single dose)
Plus
RECOMMENDED REGIMENS FOR THE TREATMENT OF CHLAMYDIA
Azithromycin 1 gm po (single dose)
or
Doxycycline 100 mg po bid for 7 days

ment is the same as for urethritis.[10] *(See Table 1.)* Partners should be notified and treated and patients should abstain from sexual intercourse until fully treated and asymptomatic.

Disseminated Gonococcal Infection

Left untreated, gonorrheal mucosal infection can spread hematologically, causing a disseminated disease in 0.5-3% of cases.[18] The incubation period ranges from 7 to 30 days, and symptoms include a migratory asymmetric tenosynovitis of multiple joints, fevers, and skin lesions. The rash occurs in about 75% of cases and is characterized by papular lesions that may progress to pustular or purpuric lesions.[9] In the early phase of disseminated gonococcal infection (DGI), blood cultures may be positive, however, joint aspirates are typically negative. As DGI progresses, septic arthritis will develop in one or more joints, most commonly the knee, followed by the elbow, ankle, wrist, foot, and hand. In patients younger than 45 years, gonorrhea is the most common etiology of septic arthritis.[19] In this phase, blood cultures will be negative, whereas joint aspirates will reveal gonococcus. Cultures should also be obtained from the genital tract. Endocarditis and meningitis may complicate DGI. Patients with DGI are hospitalized for IV therapy.[10] *(See Table 2.)* These patients also should be treated presumptively for chlamydial infection. Therapy is generally switched to an oral regimen 24-48 hours after clinical improvement is noted.

Cervicitis

Etiology. Gonorrhea and chlamydia are the most common infectious agents causing cervicitis. Symptomatic gonococcal cervicitis typically presents within 10 days of contact with an infected person. Approximately 25% of women infected with gonorrhea will be asymptomatic.[20] As many as 50% of patients with gonococcal cervicits are coinfected with chlamydia.[21] Chlamydia has an incubation period of 7-14 days to symptomatic disease. Approximately 30-80% cases of cervicitis due to chlamydia are asymptomatic.[20]

Clinical Presentation. Females with cervicitis typically present with vaginal discharge. Dysuria may be a predominent symptom if there is a concomittant urethritis. Presenting complaints also may include abnormal vaginal bleeding, post-coital vaginal bleeding, and dyspareunia.

Table 2. Treatment of Disseminated Gonococcal Infection

RECOMMENDED INITIAL REGIMEN
Ceftriaxone 1 g IV every 24 hours
ALTERNATIVE INITIAL REGIMEN
Cefotaxime 1 g IV every 8 hours
or
Ceftizoxime 1 g IV every 8 hours
FOR PERSONS ALLERGIC TO BETA-LACTAM DRUGS
Ciprofloxacin 500 mg IV every 12 hours
or
Ofloxacin 400 mg IV every 12 hours
or
Spectinomycin 2 g IM every 12 hours

On pelvic exam, a cervical discharge usually is noted. Traditionally, the discharge associated with gonorrhea is purulent while the discharge seen with chlamydia cervicitis is mucoid. In reality, it is usually difficult to distinguish the etiology based on physical examination alone. A positive Q-tip sign occurs when a sample of the discharge changes the color of the white cotton tip. Cervical edema, erythema, and friability may be present. It is not unusual to see vaginal spotting during culture collection.

The oropharynx and anorectal areas should be inspected as well. Gonorrhea may cause pharyngitis or proctitis with minimal symptomatology in patients who practice oral or anorectal receptive sex.

Diagnosis. Screening for both gonorrhea and chlamydia should be performed on any female suspected of having cervicitis. Culture specimens must be taken from the endocervical canal and plated as described in the section on urethritis. The specifity of culture techniques is 100%; however, the sensitivity for gonorrhea and chlamydia is less (80-95% and 70-80%, respectively).[21] Although culture techniques remain the gold standard for diagnosis, they are more commonly reserved for cases where legal issues arise (i.e., rape and abuse). DFA, EIA, and NAH are both sensitive and specific for identifying gonorrhea and chlamydia from endocervical samples. Recent studies have demonstrated DNA amplification tests (LCR, PCR) on first-void urines to be as sensitive and specific as endocervical cultures.[1,21]

Treatment. Empiric treatment of cervicitis must cover both gonorrhea and chlamydia.[10] *(See Table 1.)* In order to ensure compliance, single-dose regimens are recommended; however, quinolones are not recommended in patients younger than 18 years. Doxycycline and quinolones are contraindicated during pregnancy.[10] *(See Table 3.)* HIV-infected patients are treated the same as HIV-negative patients. Sexual partners should be evaluated and tested as well.

Complications. Disseminated gonococcal infection (see prior section) and pelvic inflammatory disease (PID) are potential significant complications of untreated cervical infections.

Pelvic Inflammatory Disease

PID is a bacterial infection of the upper genital reproductive tract in

Table 3. Treatment of Cervicitis in Pregnant Women

RECOMMENDED REGIMENS FOR THE TREATMENT OF GONORRHEA
Cefixime 400 mg po (single dose)
or
Ceftriaxone 125 mg IM (single dose)
or (if unable to tolerate cephalosporins)
Spectinomycin 2 g IM (single dose)
Plus
RECOMMENDED REGIMENS FOR THE TREATMENT OF CHLAMYDIA
Erythromycin base* 500 mg po qid for 7 days
or
Amoxicillin 500 mg po tid for 7 days
* erythromycin estolate is contraindicated in pregnancy

Table 4. CDC Guidelines for the Diagnosis of PID

MINIMUM CRITERIA
Lower abdominal tenderness,
Adnexal tenderness, *and*
Cervical motion tenderness
ADDITIONAL CRITERIA SUPPORTING A DIAGNOSIS OF PID
Oral temperature > 101°F (38.3°C)
Abnormal cervical or vaginal discharge
Elevated erythrocyte sedimentation rate
Elevated C-reactive protein
Laboratory documentation of cervical infection with *N. gonorrhoeae* or *C. trachomatis*

females. Each year, more than 1 million cases occur in the United States, with adolescents comprising about 20% of the total.[22] Significant, long-term sequelae occur in 25% of women with a history of PID.[23] Adolescents are at particular risk for sequelae due to a delay in seeking treatment and non-compliance with therapy.

Etiology. Studies of direct cultures from the upper genital tract have shown PID to be polymicrobial in nature.[24,25] The most important causative agents remain chlamydia and gonorrhea, which account for more than 50% of the cases.[6] Other pathogens isolated represent microflora from the vagina and bowel, including *Escherichia coli, Bacteroides* species, anaerobic cocci, *Mycoplasma hominis,* and *Ureaplasma urelyticum.*[6]

Clinical Presentation. Lower abdominal pain is the most common presenting symptom. Typically, the pain is bilateral and sharp. Local peritoneal symptoms may cause patients to walk stooped over with a shuffling gait. An abnormal vaginal discharge is reported in up to 50% of patients. Other symptoms include dysfunctional uterine bleeding, dysuria, dyspareunia, nausea, vomiting, and fever. Women may have asymptomatic PID, which is not recognized until evaluation for infertility reveals tubal scarring and serum antibodies to chlamydia and gonorrhea.[22]

Pelvic examination typically shows signs of cervicitis, including a mucopurulent discharge. Uterine and/or adnexal tenderness may be present. Cervical motion tenderness is a hallmark of acute PID, although it is not reliably present in all cases. Peritoneal signs may be elicited on abdominal exam.

Diagnosis. Laparoscopy is considered the gold standard for diagnosing PID, but because of the expense and invasiveness of this procedure, it is not routinely used in the emergency diagnosis of PID. The Centers for Disease Control and Prevention (CDC) recommended criteria for diagnosing PID rely on clinical findings through a direct physical examination and selected lab tests.[10] *(See Table 4.)* Endocervical cultures for gonorrhea and chlamydia should be obtained, although most cases of PID also involve other aerobic and anaerobic organisms. It is also important to obtain a pregnancy test, as this will affect treatment. An ultrasound study can aid in differentiating PID from other conditions with similar presentations, including appendicitis, ovarian torsion, and ovarian cysts. Ultrasound is mandatory in the symptomatic pregnant patient to exclude the diagnosis of ectopic pregnancy.

Treatment. Empiric treatment for PID should be administered if the minimal CDC criteria are present without another identifiable etiology. Current CDC criteria for hospitalization no longer include mandatory admission of adolescent females; however, the clinician must have a low threshold for admitting adolescents if compliance or follow-up is in question.[10] *(See Table 5.)* Due to the polymicrobial etiology of PID, treatment must include broad-spectrum antibiotics. Current guidelines for in-patient treatment are listed in Table 6.[10] Patients admitted for parenteral therapy may be discharged 24 hours after showing clinical improvement on a regimen of doxycycline or clindamycin to complete a total of 14 days of treatment. Patients initally managed with an out-patient oral regimen should be reevaluated within 72 hours and admitted if no improvement is noted. *(See Table 7.)*[10]

Complications. Acute complications of PID include tubo-ovarian abscess (TOA) formation, peritonitis, and peri-hepatitis (Fitz-Hugh-Curtis syndrome). Patients with a TOA usually appear ill and typically present with fever and severe lower abdominal pain. Exam reveals localized tenderness over an adnexal mass. Ultrasound can be used to confirm the presence of an abscess. A ruptured TOA represents a surgical emergency. Treatment of an unruptured TOA is more controversial but generally involves conservative management with IV antibiotics in a regimen similar to that used for PID.

Peritonitis results when microorganisms exit the fallopian tubes and enter the peritoneal cavity. Infection that tracks up the paracolic gutter causing inflammation of the liver capsule is known as the Fitz-Hugh-Curtis syndrome. Patients typically present with sudden onset of severe right upper quadrant pain that may refer to the right shoulder. Pain in the right upper quadrant may overshadow pelvic pain, making the diagnosis more elusive. In a few cases, ultrasound was helpful in demonstrating peritoneal fluid around the liver and spleen and ruling out cholelithiasis.[26]

Significant long-term complications from PID result from tubal and intra-abdominal scarring and include chronic pelvic pain, infertility, and increased risk of ectopic pregnancies. The risk of infertility following the first episode of PID is 12% and increases following each subsequent episode.[27] The risk for ectopic pregnancy is 7- to 10-fold greater in women with a history of PID.[27]

Vaginitis

Patients with vaginitis typically present with vaginal discharge

Table 5. CDC Criteria for Hospitalization to Treat PID

- ❑ Diagnosis is in question
- ❑ Pregnancy
- ❑ Patient fails outpatient treatment
- ❑ Patient is unable to follow or tolerate an outpatient oral regimen
- ❑ Patient has nausea, vomiting, or high fever
- ❑ Patient has a tubo-ovarian abscess
- ❑ Patient is immunodeficient (i.e., HIV with low CD4 counts)

accompanied by irritation, itching, burning, and/or dyspareunia. Candidiasis, trichomonas infection, and bacterial vaginosis are the most common causes of an abnormal vaginal discharge. Candidal infection will not be discussed here as it is not usually transmitted sexually.

Trichomonas Infection. Women infected with the protozoa *T. vaginalis* will usually complain of a malodorous discharge that is frequently accompanied by pruritus, dyspareunia, and post-coital bleeding. As many as 25-50% of infected women will be asymptomatic.[28] On examination, the discharge is typically purulent; however, the classic "frothy" discharge is only seen in 12% of cases.[28] Punctate hemorrhage of the cervix (strawberry cervix) is seen in only 2% of patients.[28]

Testing for the presence of amines by mixing a sample of secretions with a drop of 10% KOH will produce the characteristic fishy odor (Whiff test). Diagnosis is made by identifying motile, flagellated trichomonads by saline microscopy. The sensitivity for this test ranges around 60%.[28] Culture techniques are available when a more definitive diagnosis is required. PCR tests may be available in the near future to further aid in the diagnosis.

Metronidazole is the only effective treatment for trichomonas vaginitis. The recommended regimen is 2 gm orally in a single dose. The alternative regimen is 500 mg twice a day for seven days.[10] Patients who are allergic to metronidazole should be desensitized. HIV-infected patients should receive the same treatment protocol. Sexual partners also should be treated.

Bacterial Vaginosis. Bacterial vaginosis, formerly known as non-specific or *Gardnerella vaginitis*, is a polymicrobial infection of the vagina. Fifty percent of women will be asymptomatic.[28] Symptoms that may be present include a thick, malodorous vaginal discharge that is associated with pruritus or irritation in up to 67% of cases.[28] Meeting three of Amsel's criteria is sufficient to make the diagnosis:

1. Homogeneous gray or white discharge on exam;
2. Vaginal pH greater than 4.5;
3. Positive whiff test; and/or
4. Clue cells on saline microscopy.[29]

Treatment regimens for bacterial vaginosis are listed in Table 8.[10] HIV-positive patients are treated similarly. Routine treatment of sexual partners is not recommended.

STDs Associated with Lesions

In the United States, herpes simplex virus (HSV) accounts for the majority of genital ulcers. Other disease processes that may be associated with lesions include syphilis and chancroid. In developing nations, chancroid and granuloma inguinale predominate. More than one infectious agent is found in 3-10% of cases.[30] Of note, these infectious diseases are associated with an increased risk of HIV infection.

Table 6. Parenteral Treatment of PID

REGIMEN A

Cefotetan 2 g IV every 12 hours
or
Cefoxitin 2 g IV every 6 hours
Plus
Doxycycline 100 mg IV or po every 12 hours

REGIMEN B

Clindamycin 900 mg IV every 8 hours
Plus
Gentamicin loading dose 2 mg/kg IV *or* IM followed by a maintenance of 1.5 mg/kg every 8 hours (single daily dosing may be substituted)

Herpes Simplex Virus. It is estimated that 20% of the United States population older than 12 years is infected with HSV.[31] HSV1 is associated with oral or facial lesions, while HSV2 typically affects the genital area (however cross-over does occur). The organism is highly contagious, with an 80% transmission rate after a single sexual exposure to an individual actively shedding the virus.[32]

Primary infection with HSV follows an incubation period of 2-10 days after sexual contact. Manifestations include mucosal and/or cutaneous lesions as well as systemic symptoms. It is not uncommon for patients to experience a 1- to 2-day prodrome of localized tingling, burning, and irritation before lesions appear. Painful, itchy, vesicular, or ulcerated lesions with an erythematous base develop. Lesions may coalesce and cause significant swelling and pain. As a result, patients may present with urinary retention as a chief complaint.[33] Extra-genital lesions due to self-innoculation may be seen on the buttocks, fingers, hands, or legs in 20% of cases.[34] The sores and pain may last up to six weeks. Mucopurulent discharge occurs with urethral or cervical involvement. Dysuria occurs in males and females with HSV urethritis. As many as 50% of patients also will experience fever, myalgias, arthralgias, nausea, vomiting, and headache. Aseptic meningitis occurs in up to 8%.[34] Often, tender, non-fluctuant lymphadenopathy is present. Pharyngitis is seen in 10-15% of cases.[33] Herpes proctitis is associated with severe rectal pain, tenesmus, and rectal discharge. Immunosuppressed patients are at risk for more disseminated infection.

Following the primary infection, HSV travels to the dorsal root ganglia where it remains latent until reactivation occurs.[35] Secondary outbreaks occur in up to 90% of patients with initial genital involvement.[36] Reactivation also may be heralded by a prodrome of burning or paresthesias. These episodes tend to be less painful and of shorter duration than the primary infection. Lesions occur in the same nerve distribution as the primary infection but are fewer in number and last for only 5-10 days. Constitutional symptoms are uncommon with reactivation. Patients may have reactivation without a clear history of primary infection. Up to 25% of recurrent episodes are asymptomatic; however, viral shedding still occurs.[34]

The characteristic ulcerated lesion usually makes HSV an easy diagnosis on clinical grounds alone. A Tzanck test, whereby a vesicle is unroofed and material from the base is stained with Giemsa or

Table 7. Oral Treatment of PID

REGIMEN A
Ofloxacin 400 mg po twice a day for 14 days
Plus
Medtronidazole 500 mg po twice a day for 14 days
REGIMEN B
Ceftriaxone 250 mg IM (single dose)
or
Cefoxitin 2 g IM *plus* Probenecid 1 g po (single dose)
Plus
Doxycycline 100 mg po twice a day for 14 days

Table 8. Treatment of Bacterial Vaginosis

RECOMMENDED REGIMEN
Metronidazole 500 mg po twice a day for 7 days
or
Clindamycin cream 2%, one applicator full intravaginally for 7 days
or
Metronidazole gel 0.75%, one applicator full intravaginally twice a day for 5 days

Wright's stain, can confirm the diagnosis by demonstrating multinucleated giant cells. This test is very specific for HSV but is only 30-50% sensitive.[37] EIA and DFA tests also are available, as well as viral cultures.

Some antivirals have been shown to reduce the duration of viral shedding and symptoms with primary infection when started within five days of symptom onset.[35] If taken during the prodrome period or within one day after onset of lesions in a reactivation infection, the duration of symptoms may shorten by 1-2 days.[38] Treatment does not prevent latency of the virus or reactivation of disease.[38] Patients should be advised to avoid intercourse when an active herpetic infection is present.

Oral acyclovir, famciclovir, and valacyclovir are approved for the treatment of primary and reactivation herpes. *(See Table 9.)*[10] The topical form of acyclovir is far less effective and therefore not recommended. Intravenous therapy is recommended for patients with more severe, systemic infection, including patients with disseminated infections, pneumonitis, hepatitis, or meningitis.

Initial episodes of herpes proctitis and oral infections may require higher dosages of acyclovir (400 mg 5 times daily).[10] Valacyclovir and famciclovir have not been adequately studied for these particular infections. HIV patients may require higher doses of antivirals as well.

Syphilis

Syphilis is caused by the spirochete *Treponema pallidum,* which is spread after contact with infectious lesions. The majority of cases are acquired by sexual exposure; however, syphilis also can be transmitted by kissing, transfusion of fresh blood from an infected person, and congenitally.[39]

Between 1985 and 1990 there was a 75% increase in the incidence of syphilis in the United States.[39] An increase in the prevalence of HIV in the 1980s may have played a role. Approximately 15% of persons with syphilis are also HIV positive.[40] Since 1990, rates of syphilis have declined.

Syphilis is divided into clinical stages (primary, secondary, latent, and late), although there is considerable overlap of symptoms between stages.

Primary syphilis occurs following an incubation period of 9-90 days, with an average of three weeks, following exposure.[41] This stage manifests as one or more painless papules originating at the site of innoculation. The lesion(s) erode and develop into the classic chancre with a well-defined raised border and a hard, ulcerative base. Chancres are most commonly located on the external genitalia but, dependent on site of innocuation, also may occur on the cervix, the perianal area, or the oropharynx. These lesions are teeming with spriochetes. Chancres are accompanied by painless regional lymphadenopathy (LAN) in about 50% of patients.[40] It is not uncommon for chancres to go unnoticed. They resolve spontaneously in 3-6 weeks without treatment.

Hematogenous and lymphatic spread of *T. pallidum* will cause more disseminated disease in untreated individuals. Secondary syphilis develops in 9-90 days, with an average of three weeks following the onset of the chancre.[41] Rash, LAN, and flu-like symptoms characterize this stage. A painless, non-pruritc, generalized eruption is a prominent feature of secondary syphilis. This rash may mimic other dermatologic conditions, however, there are several characteristics that implicate syphilis as the cause. The rash may be macular, papular, pustular, or a combination of these but is not vesicular. The lesions tend to be pink or red in color, symmetric, discrete, and well demarcated. In addition, the rash is more prominent on the upper extremities and has a predilection for palms and soles. When hair follicles are involved, patients may develop patchy alopecia including loss of the lateral third of eyebrows. The rash may last a few weeks to several months.

Some patients with secondary syphilis may develop mucus patches. These shallow, painless ulcerations with slightly raised borders can develop on any mucosal surface. Mucus patches are packed with spirochetes.

Condyloma lata are raised, flat, grayish papular lesions which are found in moist areas of the body including the anus, vulva, and scrotum. These lesions also are teeming with *T. pallidum.*

Generalized LAN is a common finding in secondary syphilis. This painless lymph node enlargement usually precedes skin manifestations.

Constitutional symptoms including headaches, fever, malaise, nasal discharge, sore throat, and arthralgias are common. Aseptic meningitis occurs in 1-2% of infected patients.[39] Cranial nerve involvement is occasionally seen.

Without treatment, the symptoms of secondary syphilis resolve spontaneously in 1-2 months and patients enter the latent phase. The latent phase is divided into early (less than 1 year duration) and late periods. Typically, patients are asymptomatic during this phase, however, relapses of secondary syphilis may occur, particularly in the first two years.

Late syphilis is rarely seen in the United States. Manifestations often occur 10-20 years following the primary infection and involve the CNS, cardiovascular system, skin, and/or bone.

Testing for syphilis should be considered in any patient with another STD as there is a 6% incidence of coinfection.[42] In addition, patients with multiple partners, groin adenopathy, an unexplained

Table 9. Genital Herpes: Recommended Regimens for Treatment

RECOMMENDED REGIMEN
Acyclovir 400 mg po three times a day for 7-10 days
or
Acyclovir 200 mg po five times a day for 7-10 days
or
Famciclovir 250 mg po three times a day for 7-10 days
or
Valacyclovir 1 g po twice a day for 7-10 days
RECOMMENDED REGIMEN FOR RECURRENT INFECTION
Acyclovir 400 mg po three times a day for 5 days
or
Acyclovir 200 mg po five times a day for 5 days
or
Acyclovir 800 mg po twice a day for 5 days
or
Famciclovir 125 mg po twice a day for 5 days
or
Valacyclovir 500 mg po twice a day for 5 days
SEVERE DISEASE
Acyclovir 5-10 mg/kg IV every 8 hours for 5-7 days or until clinical resolution is noted

generalized rash, or history of cocaine abuse in exchange for sex should undergo screening.

Scrapings of lesions seen in primary and secondary disease will reveal moving, corkscrew-like spriochetes under dark field microscopy. The non-specific serologic tests (VDRL, RPR) use reaginic, cardiolipin-lechithin-cholesterol antigens to detect antibodies to *T. pallidum.* These quantitative levels correlate with disease activity. They become detectable shortly after patients enter the primary stage and remain elevated through the early latent stage if left untreated. During the late latent period, levels will decrease even without treatment. In the absence of reinfection, properly treated patients with primary syphilis will become seronegative within one year. Patients treated with secondary syphilis will become seronegative within two years. Those with late syphilis should convert in five years following successful treatment. False-positive results may occur with collagen vascular disorders, pregnancy, other spirochete infections, and some viral illnesses.

The treponemal specific tests (FTA-ABS, MHA-TP, and TPI) are more expensive and technically demanding. They are generally reserved to confirm positive non-treponemal tests. Once a patient becomes positive, they are generally positive for life despite adequate treatment.

Parenteral penicillin G is the first-line therapy for all stages of syphilis.[10] *(SeeTable 10.)* Patients who are allergic to penicillin may be tried on doxycycline or tetracycline with close follow-up for treatment failure. For patients with neurosyphilis or syphilis during pregnancy, parenteral penicillin G is the only proven treatment. If these patients are penicillin allergic, they should be desensitized and then treated with penicillin. The Jarisch-Herxheimer reaction, characterized by acute onset of fever, rigors, and possibly hypotension may occur within 24 hours of initiating treatment for syphilis. There is no natural

Table 10. Primary and Secondary Syphilis

RECOMMENDED REGIMEN
Benzathine penicillin G 2.4 million units IM (single dose)
REGIMEN FOR PENICILLIN ALLERGIC PATIENTS
Doxycycline 100 mg po twice a day for 2 weeks
or
Tetracycline 500 mg po four times a day for 2 weeks

immunity to syphilis so reinfection is possible despite appropriate treatment. Sexual partners should be identified and evaluated serologically for syphilis.

Chancroid

Chancroid, which is caused by the bacteria *Haemophilus ducreyi,* is endemic in tropical and semi-tropical regions but is uncommon in the United States. Symptoms of infection appear 1-21 days following exposure and present as a papule or pustule at the site of innoculation that eventually erodes into one or more deep, soft, painful ulcers with ragged edges. A yellow-gray exudate usually covers the base of the ulcer. Lesions are usually located on the penis in males and vaginally in females. Painful unilateral or bilateral inguinal lymphadenopathy is present in about 50% of patients.[30] These nodes may suppurate and form large bubos in up to 25%.[30]

Generally, the diagnosis of chancroid is based on a clinical presentation and exclusion of HSV and syphilis. Gram stain of an aspirated bubo or swab of an ulcer may reveal gram-negative coccobacilli in clusters or chains. Culture of *H. ducreyi* is difficult and requires special media not available in all laboratories. Sensitivity for cultures is less than 80%.[10] Recent studies have shown PCR to be sensitive and specific for detecting *H. ducreyi.*

Treatment is usually based on clinical presentation after considering the more common causes of genital ulcers, including syphilis and HSV. *(See Table 11.)*[10] Resistance to ceftriaxone has been reported in Africa but not in the United States.[43] HIV-positive patients can receive the same treatment as HIV-negative patients. All sexual contacts should be treated regardless of symptomatology. Successful treatment results in clinical improvement within three days. Ulcers and lymphadenopathy may take more than two weeks to completely resolve. Fluctuant nodes should be drained by aspiration.

Lymphogranuloma Venereum

Lymphogranuloma venereum (LGV) is caused by *Chlamydia trachomatis* serotypes L_{1-3}. It is rare in the United States. Following an incubation period of 3-30 days, infection is manifested by small, painless papules, vesicles, or ulcers that heal spontaneously in 2-3 days. Occasionally the primary lesion goes unnoticed. This is followed in 2-3 weeks by painful, typically unilateral, inguinal LAN. Systemic symptoms, including fever, malaise, and headache, may occur with the LAN. The nodes enlarge, coalesce, and eventually ulcerate. Open lesions may drain a purulent discharge. Diagnosis may be made by aspirating lymph nodes and testing for chlamydia by EIA or DFA techniques. Treatment involves a prolonged course of antibiotics due to poor penetration into the lymph nodes. *(See Table 12.)*[10] Fluctuant

Table 11. Treatment of Chancroid

RECOMMENDED REGIMEN
Azithromycin 1 g po (single dose)
or
Ceftriaxone 250 mg IM (single dose)
or
Ciprofloxacin 500 mg po twice a day for 3 days
or
Erythromycin base 500 mg po four times a day for 7 days

nodes may be aspirated. All partners having sexual contact with the patient within 30 days of symptom onset must also be treated. HIV-infected patients are treated as outlined in Table 12.

Granuloma Inguinale

Granuloma Inguinale (GI), another rare sexually transmitted disease in the United States, is caused by *Calymmatobacterium granulomatis.* Following an incubation period ranging from eight days to 12 weeks, the clinical symptoms of GI take on one of four possible forms. The most common presentation, the ulcerovegetative form, manifests as large, friable, painless ulcerations with a rolled border and beefy red base. There is usually no lymph node involvement. If left untreated, the infection may spread to surrounding tissue, causing extensive destruction of the genitalia. *C. granulomatis* cannot be readily cultured. Diagnosis depends on identifying the organism within cytoplasmic vacuoles of macrophages (Donovan bodies) in biopsy specimens taken from the advancing edge of the ulceration.

Prolonged antibiotic therapy is required and relapses are not uncommon. *(See Table 13.)*[10] Persons having sexual contact with the patient within 60 days of the onset of symptoms must be treated as well. HIV patients are treated the same as HIV-negative patients.

Human Immunodeficiency Virus (HIV)

AIDS was the seventh leading cause of death among persons 15-24 years of age in 1997.[44] Although AIDS is a reportable disease in the United States and has reliable prevalence and incidence data, HIV infection is not. Given that the incubation period between HIV infection and manifestations of AIDS has a mean of 10 years, the true magnitude of HIV in adolescents may not be recognized until they are adults. Early diagnosis of HIV is important for several reasons. Therapy, which is available to delay the decline in immune function, is most effective early in the course of the disease. Prophylactic medications may be initiated, which can prevent the development of certain opportunistic infections. In addition, patients can be counselled on methods to prevent the transmission of infection to others.

Recent reports suggest that one in four new infections are occurring in persons younger than 21 years of age.[45] HIV infection in adolescents is acquired primarily through heterosexual or homosexual encounters or through intravenous drug use. It is important to identify this group at risk for HIV infection, particularly patients presenting with other sexually transmitted diseases, in order to counsel them about high-risk activities and offer a means for testing for early identification of disease.

Table 12. Treatment of Lymphogranuloma Venereum

RECOMMENDED REGIMEN
Doxycycline 100 mg po twice a day for 21 days
ALTERNATIVE REGIMEN
Erythromycin base 500 mg po four times a day for 21 days

Table 13. Recommended Treatment of Granuloma Inguinale

RECOMMENDED REGIMEN
Trimethoprim-Sulfamethoxazole double-strength tablet po twice a day for 3 weeks
or
Doxycycline 100 mg po twice a day for 3 weeks
ALTERNATIVE REGIMEN
Ciprofloxacin 750 mg po twice a day for 3 weeks
or
Erythromycin base 500 mg po four times a day for 3 weeks

Informed consent must be obtained before HIV testing is performed. HIV is tested for using HIV-1 antibody tests. A positive screening test, such as the EIA, must be confirmed by a supplemental test such as the Western blot or immunofluorescence assay. Ninety-five percent of affected persons will have positive tests within six months of infection.[45]

HIV testing should only be offered in the setting where appropriate pretest and post-test counseling can be given.

Summary

Due to the prevalence of STDs in the adolescent age group, physicians caring for these patients must consider this in the differential diagnosis of patients who present with abdominal pain, dysuria, vaginal or penile discharge, arthralgias, pharyngitis, or a rash. Obtaining an accurate history may be difficult especially if parents are allowed to stay in the room. A thorough physical is essential as STDs can present with a wide variety of signs.

Chlamydia and gonorrhea are more prevalent in adolescents than adults. Symptomatic disease includes cervicitis, urethritis, and PID. However, a significant number may actually be asymptomatic and present with long-term complications such as infertility or after a partner has been diagnosed.

Herpes is the most common STD presenting with lesions and is diagnosed clinically by the characteristic vesicular or ulcerative lesion with an erythematous base. Although the prevalence of syphilis has declined recently, it must be considered in any patient with a diffuse rash, particularly those involving the hands and feet. Screening for syphilis is recommended for patients presenting with other STDs. Chancroid, lymphogranuloma venereum, and granuloma inguinale are rare in the United States.

Finally, any patient who is sexually active should be offered testing for HIV, particularly those presenting with other STDs. Since the emergency department is typically not a suitable setting for a formal discussion on HIV infections, adolescents at risk should be referred to the appropriate clinic.

References

1. Shafer MB, Pantell RH, Schachter J. Is the routine pelvic examination needed with the advent of urine-based screening for sexually transmitted diseases? *Arch Pediatr Adolesc Med* 1999;153:119-125.
2. Centers for Disease Control and Prevention (CDC). Summary of Notifiable Diseases, US 1996. *Morb Mortal Wkly Rep MMWR* 1997;45(S3).
3. Centers for Disease Control and Prevention (CDC). Sexually Transmitted Disease Surveillance, 1995. Atlanta, GA; 1996.
4. Rosenfeld W, Vermund SH, Wentz SJ, et al. High Prevalence rate of human papillomavirus infection and association with abnormal papanicolaou smears in sexually active adolescents. *Am J Dis Child* 1989;143:1443-1447.
5. Centers for Disease Control and Prevention (CDC). Youth risk behavior surveillance, 1995. *Morb Mortal Wkly Rep MMWR* 1997;46(SS-6):1-56.
6. McCormack WM. Pelvic inflammatory disease. *N Engl J Med* 1994;330:115-119.
7. Lappa S, Moscicki A. The pediatrician and the sexually active adolescent. *Pediatr Clin North Am* 1997;44:1405-1445.
8. Stewart C, Bosker G. Common sexually transmitted diseases (STDs): Diagnosis and treatment of uncomplicated gonococcal and chlamydial infections. *Emerg Med Reports* 1999;20:173-182.
9. Sung L, MacDonald NE. Gonorrhea: A pediatric perspective. *Pediatr Rev* 1998;19:13-16.
10. Centers for Disease Control and Prevention (CDC). 1998 Guidelines for treatment of sexually transmitted diseases. *Morb Mortal Wkly Rep MMWR* 1998;47(RR-1).
11. Chambers CV, Shafer MA, Adger H, et al. Microflora of the urethra in adolescent boys: Relationships to sexual activity and non-gonococcal urethritis. *J Pediatr* 1987;110:314-321.
12. Shafer MA, Prager V, Shalwitz J, et al. Prevalence of urethral *Chlamydia trachomatis* and *Neisseria gonorrhoeae* among asymptomatic, sexually active adolescent boys. *J Infect Dis* 1987;156:223-224.
13. Janier M, Lassau F, Casin I, et al. Male urethritis with and without discharge: A clinical and microbiological study. *Sex Transm Dis* 1995;22:244.
14. Koumans EH, Johnson RE, Knapp JS, et al. Laboratory testing for *Neisseria gonorrhoeae* by recently introduced nonculture tests: A performance review with clinical and public health considerations. *Clin Infect Dis* 1998;27:1171-1180.
15. Darville T. Chlamydia. *Pediatr Rev* 1998;19:85-91.
16. Keat A. Reiter's syndrome and reactive arthritis in perspective. *N Engl J Med* 1983;309:1606-1614.
17. Berger RE, Alexander ER, Harnisch JR, et al. Etiology, manifestations and therapy of acute epididymitis: Prospective study of 50 cases. *J Urol* 1979;121:7500-754.
18. Zenilman JM. Update on bacterial sexually transmitted diseases. *Urol Clin North Am* 1992;19:25-34.
19. Cucurull E, Espinoza LR. Gonococcal arthritis. *Rheum Dis Clin North Am* 1998;24:305-322.
20. Golden NH. Vaginitis and cervicitis in adolescents. *Emerg Office Pediatr* 1997;10:44-48.
21. Gevelber MA, Biro FM. Adolescents and sexually transmitted diseases. *Pediatr Clin North Am* 1999;46: 747-766.
22. Pletcher JR, Slap GB. Pelvic inflammatory disease. *Pediatr Rev* 1998;19:363-367.
23. Peterson HB, Galaid EI, Cates W Jr. Pelvic inflammatory disease. *Med Clin North Am* 1990;74:1603-1615.
24. Eschenbach DA, Buchanan TM, Pollock HM, et al. Polymicrobial etiology of acute pelvic inflammatory disease. *N Engl J Med* 1975;293:166-171.
25. Sweet RL, Mills J, Hadley KW, et al. Use of laparoscopy to determine the microbiologic etiology of acute salpingitis. *Am J Obstet Gynecol* 1979;134:68-74.
26. Dinerman LM, Elfenbein DS, Cumming WA, et al. Clinical Fitz-Hugh-Curtis syndrome in an adolescent. *Clin Pediatr* 1990;29:532-535.
27. Labadie LL, Rhule RL. Management of genital infections. *Emerg Med Clin North Am* 1987;5:443.
28. Nyirjesy P. Vaginitis in the adolescent patient. *Pediatr Clin North Am* 1999;46:733-746.
29. Amsel R, Totten PA, Spiegel CA, et al. Nonspecific vaginitis: Diagnostic criteria and microbial and epidemiologic associations. *Am J Med* 1983;74:14.
30. Rosen T, Brown TJ. Genital ulcers. *Dermat Clin* 1998;16: 673-685.
31. Brown HP. Recognizing STDs in adolescents. *Contemp Pediatr* 1989;6:17-36.
32. Fleming DT, McQuillan GM, Johnson RE, et al. Herpes simplex virus Type 2 in the United States, 1976 to 1994. *N Engl J Med* 1997;337:1105-1111.
33. Maccato ML, Kaufman RH. Herpes genitalis: Clinical and laboratory features and relationship to cancer. *Res Staff Phys* 1991;37:34-40.
34. Corey L, Adams HG, Brown ZA, et al. Genital herpes simplex virus infections: Clinical manifestations, course and complications. *Ann Int Med* 1983;98:958-972.
35. Stewart C, Bosker G. The diverse and challenging spectrum of sexually transmitted diseases: Current diagnostic modalities and treatment recommendations; Part II, STDs with skin manifestations: Herpes, syphilis, lymphogranuloma venereum, chancroid, and human papillomavirus. *Emerg Med Reports* 1995;16:1-12.
36. Guinan MF, Wolinsky SM, Reichman RC. Epidemiology of genital herpes simplex virus infection. *Epidemiol Review* 1985;7:127-146.
37. Emans SJH, Goldstein DP. *Pediatric and Adolescent Gynecology.* Boston, MA: Little, Brown and Co., Inc.; 1990.
38. Bryson YJ, Dillon M, Lovett M, et al. Treatment of first episodes of genital herpes simplex virus infection with oral acyclovir. *N Engl J Med* 1983;308:916-921.
39. Darville T. Syphilis. *Pediatr Rev* 1999;20:160-164.
40. Sung L, MacDonald NE. Syphilis: A pediatric perspective. *Pediatr Rev* 1998;19:17-22.
41. Fiumara NJ. Infectious syphilis. *Dermatol Clin* 1983;1:3-21.

42. Augenbraun MH, McCormack WM. Sexually transmitted diseases in HIV-infected persons. *Infect Dis Clin North Am* 1994;8:439-448.
43. Tyndall M, Malisa M, Plummer FA. Ceftriaxone no longer predictably cures chancroid in Kenya. *J Infect Dis* 1993;167:469-471.
44. Centers for Disease Control and Prevention (CDC). Trends in HIV-related sexual risk behaviors among high school students—Selected U.S. cities, 1991-1997. *Morb Mortal Wkly Rep MMWR* 1999;48:440-443.
45. Gourevitch MN. The epidemiology of HIV and AIDS. *Med Clin North Am* 1996;80:1223.

Chronic Renal Failure

Georges Ramalanjaona, MD, DSc, FACEP

Emergencies in children with chronic renal failure (CRF), although uncommon, represent a special clinical entity that requires rapid recognition and appropriate management by the emergency physician. The challenge with these children is to identify both reversible causes of chronic renal failure which— if left untreated—will further compromise their renal function, and potentially life-threatening conditions that require immediate interventions.

Current practices and recommendations regarding management have changed significantly during the past few years. For example, intravenous or inhaled albuterol has been shown to be an effective, rapid, and safe treatment for moderate hyperkalemia in children.

Appropriate management of these emergencies requires a knowledge of the basic pathophysiology and treatment regimens currently being used for children with CRF, since many of these emergencies may be treatment-related.

Emergency department (ED) physicians must be familiar with advances in dialysis techniques and indications as well as complications that may be associated with the use of this technology. In addition, the increasing use and success of renal transplantation has created a subgroup of pediatric patients with special needs that must be identified and met in the ED.

Each child with chronic renal failure presenting to the ED should be carefully evaluated and final disposition made in conjunction with the nephrologist.

Introduction

Chronic renal failure (CRF) is defined as an irreversible and progressive reduction in the glomerulofiltration rate (GFR) to below 25% of normal level (decline of 30 mL/min/1.73 m^2) for at least three months.[1] Creatinine clearance (CCr) is a good indicator of GFR and is helpful in monitoring renal function of children in various age groups. *(See Table 1.)*

The estimated incidence of CRF ranges from one to three children per million in a population younger than 16 years of age. Complications of CRF vary with the degree of renal insufficiency and the nature of primary renal disease. In children younger than 5 years, congenital renal diseases, such as renal hypoplasia, renal dysplasia, and obstructive uropathy, are the most common cause of CRF.[2] In older children, hereditary diseases, metabolic diseases and acquired etiologies occur more frequently. Hereditary diseases include juvenile nephritis, cystic kidney, and Alport syndrome. The most frequent metabolic causes are cystinosis and oxalosis, and the principal acquired etiology is chronic glomerulonephritis.[3,4]

Pathophysiology

Emergencies in CRF constitute a special entity in the pediatric population. To understand its development, the emergency physician (EP) must understand the basic pathophysiology leading to this disease.

The kidney plays an essential role in maintaining homeostasis. Thus, renal dysfunction affects electrolytes and water balance, acid-

Table 1. Mean CCr Values

NORMAL VALUES
Newborn: 38 mL/min/1.73 m^2
At 1 year of age: 77 mL/min/1.73 m^2
Between 4 and 10 years: 109 for female, 124 for male
Adult values (for reference): 117 for female, 131 for male.

base balance, blood pressure control, calcium and phosphate metabolism, hemoglobin level, and the clearance of endogenous toxins, known as azotemia. The classic signs of CRF occur as each of these systems is affected. *(See Table 2.)*

The precise mechanisms resulting in progressive, irreversible functional deterioration of the nephron remains unclear; however, several factors may play critical roles, including immunologic injury, dietary protein and phosphorus intake, hemodynamically mediated hyper-filtration in the remaining glomeruli, and systemic hypertension with persisting proteinuria.[5]

Deposition of immune complex or anti-glomerular basement membrane antibodies in the glomerulus may result in persistent glomerular inflammation leading to sclerosis.

Experimental and human studies of chronic renal insufficiency have shown that a high-protein diet accelerates the development of renal failure.[6] Conversely, a diet low in protein and phosphorus reduces the functional deterioration of nephrons. Although the exact mechanism is still unclear, once renal function starts to decline, compensatory mechanisms develop in the remaining nephrons to maintain a normal homeostasis (internal environment). However, when the GFR drops below 25% of normal values, complex clinical, biochemical, and metabolic abnormalities occur that constitute the uremic state.

Hyperfiltration injury in the surviving glomeruli may represent an important, final, common pathway of glomerular destruction, regardless of the initial mechanism of renal injury. When nephrons are lost, the surviving ones undergo a structural and functional hypertrophy mediated by an increase in glomerular blood flow. This high hydrostatic pressure is associated with dilatation of afferent arterioles and vasoconstriction of efferent arterioles and will result in changes in the integrity of capillary wall, leading to an increase in passage of proteins across the wall. This will result in changes in mesangium and epithelial cells, with the development of glomerular sclerosis. As sclerosis progresses, the surviving nephrons show an increase in a number of fuctions. Their excretory functions result in a vicious cycle of increasing glomerular blood flow and hyperfiltration.

Finally, systemic hypertension from any etiology or persistent proteinuria directly may affect the glomerular capillary wall, leading to sclerosis and more hyperfiteration injury.

Dialysis

Dialysis remains one of the standard treatments of CRF. However, when it is delayed or improperly applied, complications may ensue; thus, the EP should know the different modalities of dialysis in children and its common indications and complications.

A GFR of less than 5% of normal is usually an indication for dialysis treatment in children with CRF. It is used to regulate solutes and fluid abnormalities. Common indications for emergent dialysis in this subset of the population include fluid overload (pulmonary edema/congestive heart failure [CHF]), hyperkalemia, severe hyponatremia, metabolic acidosis, malignant hypertension, bleeding diathesis, and uremic encephalopathy. Less frequent indications are drug overdose, severe hypocalcemia or hypermagnesemia, cardiac tamponade, and pericarditis.

There are two major dialysis modalities: peritoneal dialysis (PD) and hemodialysis. Each is based on the principle of filtering the patient's blood through a semi-permeable membrane bathed in a balanced physiologic solution. Because of osmotic gradients between these two fluids, water and solutes will diffuse across the membrane, thus normalizing the patient's blood composition.

Peritoneal Dialysis. PD requires the insertion of a catheter into the peritoneal cavity for the instillation of a dialysis solution for 4-8 hours, 4-5 times a day. The retained body solute will diffuse from the blood to dialysate via the peritoneum.

Two types of PD are available for children with CRF: continuous ambulatory peritoneal dialysis (CAPD) and continuous cyclic peritoneal dialysis (CCPD).[7-10]

CAPD is the standard technique for the majority of the pediatric population. It is a continuous procedure that has the advantage of allowing the maintenance of satisfactory levels of blood urea nitrogen (BUN) and creatinine, smoother control of fluid and hypertension, and avoidance of the use of anti-coagulants.

In CAPD, dialysis across the peritoneal membrane removes excess body water through an osmotic gradient created by the glucose concentration in the dialysate. Resulting wastes are removed by diffusion from the capillaries into the dialysate. The peritoneal cavity is accessed by the insertion of a Tenckoff catheter via a midline infra-umbilical incision. Then, the catheter is brought out through the skin by a subcutaneous tunnel and connected to an extension tube with a spike for insertion into the dialysis bag. Family members are taught this technique of spiking the bags of dialysate, allowing the dialysate to run and remain in the peritoneal cavity for the allotted period, and then draining the dialysate into the bag. Such exchanges are performed on a regular basis (usually 3-5 times a day) over a 24-hour period. Since the benefits of CAPD far outweigh the risks (see Table 3), it still remains the optimal form of chronic dialysis for the majority of children.

CCPD is an acceptable and equally effective alternative to CAPD, and it uses the same principle as CAPD. However, this procedure reverses the schedule of CAPD by allowing automatic exchanges at night only, using a simple cycler machine. The use of this device permits an uninterrupted day of activities, a decrease in the number of connections and disconnections, less time spent to perform dialysis, and a reduction in parental burnout.[11]

Hemodialysis (HD). In this modality, the patient's heparinized blood is pumped through an extra-corporal circuit where it comes into contact with an artificial membrane across which fluid and solute movement occurs. The amount of fluid transferred can be controlled by adjusting the pressure under which blood is pumped through the dialyzer. This technique requires special vascular access to the patient's circulation through a surgically created arterio-venous fistula or an implanted artificial graft. This vascular access should be treated with caution, since careless manipulation can result in bleeding, infection, or thrombosis and lead to a loss of the access. HD is usually performed three times a week for 3-5 hours per session, either at home or at a specially staffed dialysis unit.[12,13]

Emergencies in Children with CRF

In the ED, clinical manifestations of CRF in children present serious challenges for the EP's diagnostic skills due to a variety of reasons, including:

1. A child with a new diagnosis of CRF, especially one who has not yet started dialysis, often presents to the ED with non-specific complaints of insidious onset (i.e., weakness, poor appetite, and altered mental status), thus masking the etiology and severity of the condition.

2. Although CRF is typically irreversible and progressive, the EP must exclude potentially reversible factors and identify treatable causes of CRF (see Table 4), which if properly managed, may allow for some return of renal function. Furthermore, with an early diagnosis and aggressive management, the EP may be in the unique position of making a significant difference in the patient's outcome.

3. Also, in the context of a pediatric patient with CRF presenting to the ED with an acute problem, the EP should promptly identify and manage intercurrent illness that results in clinical decompensation of CRF, and restore the patient to a stable compensated state. Therefore, these conditions need to be treated vigorously and in a timely manner. These reversible factors include:

- Volume depletion, which will lead to decreased renal perfusion in the already impaired kidney's ability to concentrate fluid and solute.
- Increased protein catabolism secondary to stressful events such as intercurrent infection, trauma, surgery, or gastro-intestinal bleeding, which are responsible for worsening azotemia.
- Cardiac insufficiency of any etiology may decrease renal perfusion and further deteriorate renal function.
- Accelerated hypertension (HTN) with severe vasoconstriction may rapidly impair renal function, as in patients with scleroderma, that can be readily reversed with angiotension-converting enzyme (ACE) inhibiting drugs.

Side effects of the drugs themselves constitute an important group of reversible factors.

Diuretics may exacerbate renal insufficiency by causing volume depletion. Anti-hypertensive agents (i.e., ACE inhibitors) may decrease renal function in patients with bilateral renal stenosis. Non-steroidal anti-inflammatory drugs (NSAIDs) may produce acute interstitial nephritis. Radiocontrast agents can cause acute tubular necrosis.

Post-renal reversible causes are important because of their frequency. They include reflux nephropathy and papillary necrosis in children with diabetes mellitus, sickle cell disease, or a history of long-term use of analgesics.

4. Finally, clinical presentations of CRF in children may manifest as potentially life-threatening conditions even in the dialyzed patient. They include: volume overload; metabolic disturbances (i.e., hyperkalemia, hyponatremia, and metabolic acidosis); hypertensive crisis; infection; complications related to treatment; peritonitis; PD catheter malfunction; graft emergencies; post-dialysis problems (i.e., hypotension); and fever and rejection in post-transplant patients.

The following sections review the clinical manifestation of these true emergencies and outline their ED management.

Table 2. Classic Manifestations of CRF

- Azotemia
- Metabolic acidosis
- Anemia
- Bleeding diathesis
- Infection
- CNS changes
  - Altered mental status
  - Peripheral neuropathy
- Hypertension
- Pericarditis
- Hyperkalemia
- Growth retardation
- Renal osteodystrophy
- Sodium retention/wasting

Volume Overload

The most common emergency complaint in children with CRF is fluid overload, and it may manifest with a variety of complaints, including pulmonary edema or CHF. Frequently, the etiology is extra fluid or salt in excess of the patient's greatly diminished excretory capacity. A decrease in the kidney's filtering capacity usually does not result in volume overload unless the GFR is less than 10% of normal for age.[14]

Typically, the child presents to the ED with dyspnea on exertion or paroxysmal nocturnal dyspnea. Further history reveals recent weight gain (more than 5 lbs) and weakness, and physical examination may show the expected signs of pulmonary edema or CHF, which may be confirmed by chest radiograph.

However, presenting signs may be subtle (except for weight gain and increasing dyspnea), and in the absence of other etiology of dyspnea in CRF, the EP should assume the diagnosis of volume overload and treat the patient accordingly.

Temporizing measures which may be instituted include:

- Placement of the child in a sitting position, with administration of high flow oxygen and fluid restriction;
- IV or sublingual nitroglycerin (NTG) to decrease both preload and afterload;
- IV nitroprusside as an alternative to NTG. It may be more effective in producing arteriolar dilatation than NTG; and
- IV morphine to decrease preload. Its routine use as a first-line drug in pulmonary edema has become less frequent;
- IV diuretics (i.e., furosemide at a dose of 1 mg/kg/dose). Although less effective in patients with advanced CRF, it is still a powerful pulmonary venodilator, and its use may result in relief of dyspnea. In addition, patients with residual renal function may respond to a large IV dose of furosemide.

The approach to treatment of volume overload in patients with CRF is different from that for children with normal kidney function, in that the main priority is to arrange for an emergent dialysis, which is currently the most effective means of reducing intravascular load in the absence of renal function.

In summary, temporary measures may be utilized, in consultation with the child's nephrologist, to treat volume overload while awaiting dialysis or to delay dialysis in a patient with residual renal function. The EP and the pediatric nephrologist should discuss definite treatment and appropriate disposition.

Metabolic Disturbances

Major metabolic crisises that may be encountered include hyperkalemia, hyponatremia, and metabolic acidosis.

Hyperkalemia. This is potentially the most rapidly lethal complication of CRF, especially since it is usually clinically silent until it presents with life-threatening manifestations. Therefore, the EP must

Table 3. Benefits and Risks of CAPD

BENEFITS	RISKS
• Technical simplicity • Cheaper than hemodialysis • Fewer blood transfusions than hemodialysis • Minimal dietary restrictions • Better/steady control of solutes • Greater flexibility	• Catheter malfunction • Infection • Parental burnout • Hyperlipidemia

Table 4. Treatable Causes of CRF

- Malignant hypertension
- Renal artery stenosis
- Acute interstitial nephritis
- Hypercalcemic nephropathy
- Multiple myeloma
- Vasculitis
  - Lupus erythematosis
  - Polyarteritis

look for hyperkalemia in any child with CRF, especially when GFR falls below 5% of normal for age.

Hyperkalemia can be exacerbated even by modest exogenous and endogenous loads. The use of drugs such as ACE inhibitors and beta-adrenergic blockers, which usually have only minimal effects on serum K^+ in normal subjects, may have devastating consequences in a child with deteriorating renal function.

When hyperkalemia is suspected, an electrocardiogram (ECG) should be rapidly obtained to look for electrical signs of hyperkalemia (peaked T waves, widened QRS complexes, flattened P waves, ectopic rhythms, and intra-ventricular block). If electrical changes are present, then appropriate treatment should be initiated before laboratory confirmation of hyperkalemia. Also, ECG changes may be absent when hyperkalemia is severe; therefore, a normal ECG does not make laboratory confirmation of serum K^+ level unnecessary.[15,16]

A serum K^+ greater than 6 mEq/L should be evaluated for its accuracy and signs of cardiac toxicity, since false increases of 1-2 mEq/L in serum K^+ may be due to hemolysis of the specimen or to local muscle release of K^+ from prolonged tourniquet application. However, when in doubt, it is appropriate to treat hyperkalemia while awaiting the results of a repeat potassium test since reducing a normal potassium level rarely causes any adverse events, whereas delaying treatment for hyperkalemia can be potentially harmful, even fatal. In the case of a patient with known CRF who presents to the ED in cardiac arrest, hyperkalemia should be assumed and treated accordingly.

The most rapidly effective treatment is IV administration of 10% calcium gluconate 0.2-0.5 mL/kg slowly over 2-5 minutes for the presence of electrical signs of hyperkalemia. Calcium transiently reverses the ECG signs of hyperkalemia without changing the serum K^+ level or total body K^+.

The next temporizing measure consists of administering IV sodium bicarbonate 1-2 mEq/kg and/or IV glucose D50W 0.5-1 gm/kg followed by infusion of D25W with IV insulin 1 unit per 4 gm of glucose infused to maintain blood sugar between 120 and 300 mg/dL. Use D10W in a child weighing less than 10 kg, and D25W in a child weighing 10-30 kg. Intravenous glucose and insulin drive potassium into cells, thus reducing the serum potassium level. This combination is effective, but requires more time to achieve the desired effects than intravenous sodium bicarbonate. However, repeated doses of bicarbonate should be avoided, since it may precipitate fluid overload in a CRF patient with limited ability to tolerate volume and solute.[17]

The use of inhaled or intravenous albuterol recently has been advocated to shift potassium into cells and lower the serum potassium by 1-1.5 mEq/L. The authors of several clinical trials concluded that this drug administered via nebulizer or intravenously is an effective, rapid, and safe treatment for hyperkalemia in children and advocated its use as a first-line emergency treatment for this disorder in their centers.[18-22]

All of these temporary measures are helpful in altering the distribution of potassium or decreasing the cardiac sensitivity to hyperkalemia, but they do not diminish the total body's potassium content. The total body potassium can be decreased by administration of the exchange resin sodium polystyrene sulfonate (Kayexlate), which is a resin that exchanges sodium for potassium in colonic mucosa. Each gram of resin/kg of body weight will decrease the serum potassium level by 1 mEq/L. Kayexlate may be administered orally or rectally. It is usually given with sorbitol (20% solution) to decrease the associated constipation, which affects its efficacy. The rectal administration acts more rapidly to decrease potassium levels, and should be given as an enema to ensure prolonged contact between the colonic mucosa and drug. Since administration of this medication results in potassium being exchanged for sodium, the process may result in a significant sodium burden, which may lead to hypertension (HTN) or volume overload in CRF children.

While these temporizing maneuvers are necessary, more definite measures to decrease potassium load, such as dialysis, should be discussed with the pediatric nephrologist.

Hyponatremia. Hyponatremia may cause malaise, altered mental status, or seizures in a child with CRF. It is almost never due to sodium depletion, but rather purely dilutional since total body sodium is usually normal. Treatment consists of water restriction, hypertonic saline, and urgent dialysis.[23,24]

Metabolic Acidosis. Acidosis will frequently occur in children with CRF and should not be corrected unless the serum bicarbonate falls below 20 mEq/L.[25]

Treatment consists of intravenous infusion of sodium bicarbonate to achieve a pH greater than 7.2 and a serum bicarbonate level above 20 mEq/L. The amount of bicarbonate required may be calculated by this formula:

Base deficit = 0.6 × body weight in kg × (mEq/L desired HCO_3 Level - observed level), divided by 2.

The EP should give half of the replacement in the first 2-3 hours and then infuse the remaining amount over 22 hours. As previously noted, children with CRF may not tolerate the administration of this quantity of sodium. For these situations an acceptable alternative is the use of thromethamine (Tham) in 0.3 m solution.

The correction of significant metabolic acidosis will necessitate the admission of the child to the appropriate inpatient unit for close monitoring.

Hypertensive Crisis

The prevalence of HTN in childhood is between 0.5% and 5%,

and renal disease is the most common cause.[26] Although the true definition of HTN in the pediatric population remains controversial, the accepted definition of blood pressure (BP) norms comes from the 1987 report on the second task force on BP control in children from the National Heart, Lung, and Blood Institute.[27] The resulting figures, correlated with height-weight, are based on experiences, and consensus and may be used in the ED.

Definition. Normal blood pressure is defined as a systolic and diastolic less than the 90th percentile for age- and sex-specific norms, high normal as between 90th and 95th percentile, and HTN as systolic and diastolic equal and greater than 95th percentile. The task force further defines two classes of HTN in children: Significant hypertension is between the 95th and 99th percentile, and severe hypertension is at or above the 99th percentile. In order to establish HTN, measurements should be obtained on at least three readings, and the correct BP cuff size must be used.

Physiology and Etiology. The physiologic basis of HTN depends on the underlying cause, and it is estimated that in 79-98% of cases, pediatric HTN is usually secondary to a specific etiology, the most frequent being renal (80%).

Renal HTN is caused by vasoconstriction to the afferent arteriole of the glomerulus, resulting in the secretion of renin from the juxtaglomerular complex. This leads to aldosterone secretion, which results in sodium retention and potassium loss in the kidneys. Sodium retention produces hypervolemia and increased cardiac output, which leads the renin-angiotensin system to increase peripheral vascular resistance, which increases the HTN.

HTN may be the presenting sign or complication of significant renal diseases, including chronic infection, post-streptococcal glomerulonephritis, reflux nephropathy, hemolytic-uremic syndrome, and anaphylactic purpura.

Following renal disease, the second leading cause of secondary HTN in children is coarctation of aorta (2%). Even after surgical correction, HTN may persist secondary to the hyperdynamic state, persistent pressure gradient, and increased sympathetic tone, based on how long the condition went unimpaired.

Endocrine causes (i.e., pheochromocytoma) represent an important but a small percentage of children with HTN.

HTN can also be secondary to acute stress situations such as major trauma, burns, central nervous system (CNS) infections, and autonomic dysfunction.

Drug ingestion should always be considered in any unexplained HTN in children.

Essential or idiopathic HTN is also a possibility in the pediatric population, and is probably the result of interaction of genetic, environmental, and constitutional factors.

Treatment. The decision to treat HTN in children with CRF is based on a combination of BP readings and symptomatology.[14,28,29]

In a child with chronic HTN, higher blood pressures may be necessary to maintain end-organ perfusion. Thus, a rapid decrease in BP may compromise perfusion of vital organs (i.e., brain, heart, and kidneys). The goal of treatment is to limit cardiovascular sequelae as well as diminish the rate of progression of CRF with a reduction of BP to the 50th percentile for age or 15-25% in mean arterial pressure.

In severe HTN, appropriate treatment is indicated to prevent hypertensive encephalopathy, stroke, or CHF. Since HTN in children with CRF is due to expanded vascular volume because of salt and water retention, and activation of renin-angiotensin system, any treatment of HTN in those children should include salt and water restriction and/or diuretics, and other anti-hypertensive drugs targeted at these two mechanisms.

Most children will require anti-hypertensive drugs as a single agent or in combination with others to effectively control HTN in the ED. As a rule of thumb, a single agent should be initiated at less than maximal dose, then increased to its maximum before adding a second drug. Careful and regular monitoring of BP is necessary to avoid rapid decreases in BP that may further compromise the GFR. A wide variety of agents can be used in the ED to effectively control HTN.

ACE Inhibitor Agents. This class of agents is useful for the treatment of renin-mediated HTN, which is frequent in children with CRF. Captopril is particularly useful in children who develop hypertension following the use of an umbilical artery catheter. Disadvantages of this medication include slow incremental dosing, which limits its use in the ED, and its potential to precipitate acute renal failure (ARF) in patients with renal arterial stenosis. The initial dose is 0.3 mg/kg orally, doubled every two hours to a maximum of 2-6 mg/kg or until the desired effect is achieved.

Enalapril is an acceptable alternative, since it has fewer side-effects and its dose is one-tenth that of captopril. However, serum potassium should be monitored with administration of this medication because it may result in hyperkalemia.

Diuretics. A trial of diuretics to stimulate remaining renal function may be useful in the hypertensive child with volume overload. Furosemide can be used at a dose of 1 mg/kg every two hours with the maximum effect usually within 30 minutes.

Beta-Adrenergic Blocking Agents. The most frequently used drug of this class is labetalol, a combined alpha- and beta-blocker, that is effective for the treatment of significant/severe HTN. An initial loading dose of 0.2-1 mg/kg is administered intravenously and followed by escalating doses of 0.5-1 mg/kg, followed by a constant infusion of 1-3 mg/kg/hour. It is contraindicated in patients with bradycardia, bronchospasm, or CHF.

Calcium Channel Blockers. In general, as these agents decrease BP, vascular volume increases, thus requiring the use of diuretics. Furthermore, vasodilatation results in tachycardia, which necessitates the concommitant use of beta-blockers.

The choice of an agent depends on severity of HTN and size of the child.

The short-acting nifedipine acts within 30 minutes when given orally or rectally, but results in wide variation of BP. The dose is the same as the long-acting preparation.

Other Agents. Minoxidil is a very potent agent, usually effective in children with refractory HTN, at dose of 0.1-2 mg/kg. The most significant side-effects are hypotension and hirsutism.

Intravenous nitroprusside is both an arterial and venous dilator and is reserved for severe or refractory HTN. Patients usually require continuous BP monitoring via an arterial line, and admission to an ICU. The drug is given at a continuous infusion rate of 0.1-10 mcg/kg/min, and BP should be titrated against infusion rate as the onset of action is within a few seconds. If hypotension occurs, the infusion should be slowed or stopped. Cyanide toxicity is one side effect that is increased in CRF, and can cause metabolic acidosis.

Infection

Infection is a leading cause of morbidity and mortality in children with CRF. These children have an increased susceptibility to infection most likely secondary to defects in both cellular and humoral immunity. Thus, the potential for serious infection should always be entertained even when the classic signs are not evident. For instance, the presence of fever alone may be due to occult bacteremia or sepsis, and pneumonia may present as atypical dyspnea, which must be differentiated from volume overload. In the setting of a child with fever or dyspnea, all diagnoses should be considered, ancillary tests performed, and children placed on empiric broad-spectrum antibiotics (dose corrected for CRF) until the proper etiology has been established.

Emergencies Related to Treatment

Peritonitis. Peritonitis remains the primary complication of long-term peritoneal dialysis in children. The incidence of peritonitis in CCPD is one episode per year, with a slightly higher rate in CAPD.

The potential routes for peritoneal contamination include the lumen of the peritoneal catheter, the sinus tract around the catheter, the blood stream or peritoneal lymphatics, and across the walls of an intraperitoneal hollow viscus.[30] Important factors that influence the development of peritonitis include skin infections of the hand, infection of sites in proximity to the catheter exit site, or catheter exit site infection.

The signs and symptoms of peritonitis include fever, vomiting, diarrhea, and abdominal pain or tenderness. The peritoneal fluid is usually cloudy. A peritoneal fluid sample is obtained prior to initiation of antibiotics, and sent for Gram's stain, cell count, and cell culture. A WBC of more than 100 cells/cm with more than 50% neutrophils is suggestive of peritonitis.

The majority of infections (60-70%) are caused by gram-positive cocci (*Staphylococcus epidermidis and Streptococcus viridans*) which frequently occur at the exit site. The most serious form of peritonitis is fungal peritonitis and is commonly associated with an episode of bacterial peritonitis and use of antibiotic therapy in the preceding month.[31,32] Microscopic examination of peritoneal fluid using gram stain-identified yeast infections with budding yeast or pseudohyphae in up to 30% of cases. Fungal peritonitis is significantly associated with morbidity and mortality, and commonly results in abdominal adhesions that ultimately destroy the functional ability of the peritoneal membrane to dialyze.[33]

In a patient with CRF and abdominal pain it is important to remember that peritoneal dialysis patients are still at risk for serious intra-abdominal events such as appendicitis, pancreatitis, and cholecystitis, which are especially important to consider when the peritoneal culture reveals multiple organisms.

The goals in treatment of peritonitis include elimination of peritoneal infection, preserving the integrity of the peritoneal membrane, and not aggravating the child's underlying condition.

The accepted therapeutic regimen consists of peritoneal lavage and antibiotic administration. When peritonitis is identified, the care giver should perform three rapid flushes with peritoneal dialysate and heparin (500 U/L.)

Most peritonitis episodes can be treated with intra-peritoneal antibiotics (IP) or with intravenous antibiotics in moderate to severe cases. Antibiotics which are useful in the treatment of peritonitis include penicillin G, gentamycin, vancomycin, clindamycin, and tobromycin. Practically, the choice of an initial antibiotic is guided by the gram stains of the peritoneal fluid, which are positive in 30-50% of cases. Antibiotic therapy is then modified according to the findings of the peritoneal dialysis fluid culture. Most antibiotics (with the exception of Penicillin G) retain at least 75% of their bioactivity when used in dialysate solute.

When patients develop antibiotic resistant peritonitis, or fungal peritonitis, hospitalization is indicated. The Tenckoff catheter should be removed (even if functioning), surgical consult obtained, and hemodialysis initiated.

Peritoneal Dialysis Catheter Malfunction. These technical difficulties are commonly encountered and may be simple or complex. The two most frequent complications are leakage and obstruction.

Leakage. The incidence of leakage varies from 5% to 25%. Risk factors include previous abdominal surgery (i.e., previous catheter insertion) debilitated or obese patients, and children treated with corticosteroids.

Early leakage leads to infection at the exit site and in the subcutaneous tissue. Late leakage may result in peritoneal tears that lead to fluid dissecting into the abdominal wall, scrotum or vagina, or chest wall.

Minimal leakage usually does not necessitate catheter removal as it usually spontaneously resolves. Late or significant leakages may require discontinuation of dialysis to allow the peritoneal tear to heal (about 8-10 days). During this time patients will benefit from short-term hemodialysis. Patients who develop a hydrothorax (incidence 2%) are managed by cessation of the peritoneal dialysis and temporary use of hemodialysis. In some instances, thoracotomy may be required to repair the defect.

Overflow Obstruction. One of the main mechanical complications of peritoneal dialysis is failure of the dialysate to drain. Major causes include catheter migration and fibrin clots. Catheter migration usually leads to removal of the catheter in 90% of cases. Fibrin clots may occur as a result of bleeding after catheter implantation or after an episode of peritonitis.[34,35]

Large amounts of heparin (i.e., 5000 U) or thrombolytic drugs in a small volume of dialysis can be used to dissolve the fibrin clots during an irrigation of the catheter. If successful, subsequent exchanges are done with 1000 units of heparin added to each liter of dialysate. Catheter replacement is necessary when the above attempts have failed.

Graft Emergencies

Graft emergencies constitute special emergencies necessitating both technical knowledge of hemodialysis and timely diagnosis and management of its potential complications.

Hemodialysis requires the ability to access the vascular space and to provide significant extracorporeal blood flow. The most commonly used access to the pediatric patient weighing more than 20 kg is an arterio-venous (AV) fistula. There are two types of AV fistulas which are used: an autogeneous fistula or a synthetic graft. Autogeneous fistulas surgically anastomose the cephalic vein and radial artery using a side-to-side vein to artery connection in the non-dominant arm, called a brachio-cephalic fistula. A synthetic graft can also be utilized in the arm with either a straight or loop configuration. These synthetic grafts include polytetrafluroethylenl, PTFE Gore-Tex, or Impra. In general, autogenous fistulas last longer than synthetic grafts and are less prone to thrombosis, stenosis, and infection. Young children and infants have smaller size vessels for AV fistulas and require vascular access in the subclavian or internal jugular vein for hemodialysis.[36-38]

Common emergencies that occur with hemodialysis include bleeding, thrombosis, and infection. The occurrence of these complications mandate vascular surgery and pediatric nephrology consultations.

Persistent Bleeding. Surgical trauma or technical errors may result in persistent bleeding in 30% of patients. In most cases, the bleeding spontaneously subsides. Instances that fail to resolve may require transfusion and surgical repair.

The necessity of infusing anticoagulants (i.e., heparin) in hemodialysis patients predisposed to bleeding may also lead to persistent bleeding. Clinical manifestations include petechial skin hemorrhage, sub-capsular liver hematoma, retroperitoneal hematoma, and gastro-intestinal bleeding. Treatment consists of supportive therapy, transfusion, and altering the patient's heparinization prescription (i.e., low dose, intermittent, or regional heparin) or starting on peritoneal dialysis. Studies have reported the successful use of hemodialysis without anticoagulant during the perioperative period in adults, but data are not yet available for the pediatric population.[37]

External blood loss may be due to breaks in the dialyzing membrane, manufacturing defects, or separation of blood lines. Most membrane leaks are due to rupture of a dialysis membrane and require clamping of arterial and venous blood connections and discontinuation of dialysis. The EP's decision to transfuse blood will depend on the amount of blood loss, clinical severity of symptoms, and the pre-dialysis hemoglobin level.

When separation of the blood line is a cause of blood loss, reconnection and continuation of dialysis treatment is feasible.

Thrombosis. Thrombosis is a common cause of loss of vascular access and should be rapidly recognized with every effort made to salvage the access. Many factors have been implicated in the genesis of thrombosis.

Hypercoagulable states (i.e., clotting factor abnormalities) are similar to those seen in children with nephrotic syndrome, including low serum protein, high levels of fibrinogen and factor VII, and reduced half life for fibrinogen may exist. If the clotting defect is diagnosed prior to dialysis, correction of the abnormal factor may be achieved prior to initiation of dialysis.

Technical factors during surgical anastomosis may result in thrombosis and should be corrected as soon as possible to prevent loss of the vascular access. The diagnosis is established clinically by the loss of the thrill or bruit over the anastomosis. Surgical repair is the usual treatment.

Insufficient or inadequate heparinization prior to or during dialysis may result in thrombosis. This condition is easily corrected through adjusting to the optimal dose during each dialysate.

Late-graft thrombosis (after 48 hours) is usually caused by anastomotic failure or infection. Late anastomotic failure is produced by intimal hyperplasia on the distal graft which in turn facilitates the formation of clots. Treatment consists of intravenous thrombolytic therapy to dissolve the clots or surgical thrombectomy.

Graft Infection. Graft infection will result in a non-functional anastomosis with thrombosis, which is commonly managed by intravenous antibiotics and graft removal.

Bacterial contamination, usually gram-positive cocci, may occur during surgery. A culture and sensitivity from the site should be obtained, and the patient should receive intravenous antibiotics. Consultation with the surgeon who operated on the patient should be obtained.

Post-Dialysis Problems

Hypotension, muscle cramps, and dialysis dysequilibirum are all potential post-dialysis complications.

Hypotension. Hypotension is the most frequently encountered complication of hemodialysis in children. It varies in severity, ranging from transient to severe. The incidence ranges from 20% to 30%, and patients often manifest with the sudden onset of nausea, vomiting, abdominal cramping, and tachycardia.

Hypotension may result from excessive blood loss (internal or external), rapid ultrafiltration, autonomic nervous system dysfunction, or acetate use.

Hypotension can be prevented by limiting intradialytic weight loss to less than 5% of body weight and slowing the rate of fluid exchange during dialysis.

Muscle Cramps. Muscle cramps are another frequent complication of hemodialysis. Although the pathogenesis of this condition remains unclear, three predisposing factors have been implicated:

- Hemodialysis induced hypotension;
- Rapid and excessive ultrafiltration below the child's dry weight; and
- Use of sodium poor dialysate (muscle cramps appear twice as frequently in patients dialyzed against a solution with a sodium concentration of 132 vs 145 mEq/L).

Treatment consists of volume expansion with hypertonic saline (17.5% or 3 mol/liter), 50% glucose (25% glucose in children under 30 kg), or sequential ultrafiltration. Oral quinine sulfate has been shown to reduce both the frequency and severity of muscle cramps in a double-blind study, and is effective in patients who have persistent cramping post-dialysis.

Dialysis Dysequilibrium Syndrome (DDS). DDS is a spectrum of systemic and neurologic symptoms that can occur during or post-dialysis. Initial symptoms include restlessness, headache, nausea, and vomiting. Subsequently, muscle twitching, hypertension, disorientation, and myoclonic seizures may occur and lead to life-threatening complications such as seizures, coma, and cardiac arrhythmias if left untreated.[39]

EEG features include loss of alpha wave, bursts of delta waves, and slow wave activities.

Although the pathophysiology is still unclear, the most plausible explanation is that the rapid correction of uremia leads to the development of acute cerebral edema. Patients prone to develop DDS are patients receiving their first dialysis sessions with newly diagnosed CRF in whom aggressive dialysis clearances are used. Other suggested mechanisms include rapid lowering of serum sodium, acute changes in the pH of the cerebral spinal fluid, dialysis with a low glucose dialysate, and a high rate of removal of blood urea vs. brain urea.

Prevention of DDS is preferable to the actual treatment of DDS, and is easily achieved by simple technical maneuvers.

When severe symptoms develop, dialysis should be discontinued and diagnostic evaluation (i.e., EEG) should be performed to rule out another etiology. The patient should be admitted, and pediatric nephrologist consultation is advisable.

Renal Transplant Patients

Specific emergencies that may occur following renal transplant include fever and transplant rejection. The transplanted kidney may originate from a related living donor (or identical twin 18 years or older), an unrelated living donor, or a cadaveric donor. Among these options, live-related donation among immediate family members appears to achieve better long-term renal function than the others, with minimal long-term risks to the donor.

Rejection. Renal transplantation is the preferred treatment for children with chronic renal failure over dialysis for several reasons:[40]

1. It allows an unrestricted lifestyle and more normal quality of life, including growth and development, and maximum cognitive and physical development.

2. It improves patient survival. Current five-year graft survival is 70% in the first year and continues to increase with the advent of new and less toxic immune suppressive drugs.

3. It is cost effective.

There are three types of rejection: acute, sub-acute, and chronic rejection.

Pre-operative evaluation for both living or cadeveric donors include a donor-recipient cross-match of the donor's lymphocytes against the recipient to identify preformed cytotoxic antibodies.

An acute rejection occurs when preformed cytotoxic antibodies against ABO or HLA antigens, due to a typing cross-mismatching. Rejection may be immediate or late, occurring as long as 3-4 years post-transplantation. Clinical signs include fever, malaise, anorexia, hypertension, abdominal pain, or steady increase in BUN and creatinine, and renal biopsy will show evidence of rejection. In this setting, the EP should admit the patient and obtain a nephrology consult.

Immunosuppressive drugs are usually prescribed for the life of the transplanted graft to prevent rejections and include a combination of Prednisone, Azathioprine, and Cyclosporine given in doses based on the child's weight.

Acute rejection itself can often be halted with a higher dose of intravenous methylprednisone and OKT3, which can lead to preservation of renal function.

Repeated acute rejection episodes can produce sub-acute or chronic rejection, which also may be caused by a chronic humoral rejection. This later condition is usually refractory to anti-rejection therapy and eventually leads to graft failure.

Other transplant-related complications include renal arterial and venous stenosis, thromboembolism, osteonecrosis, medication side effects (i.e., hypertension from cyclosporine), and recurrence of original disease in the grafted kidney.

In summary, prevention of long-term and late complications of renal transplant are essential and begin during the planning phase of medical management of children with CRF.

The five-year success rate of kidney transplants in children approaches that for adults, and shorter duration and less toxic drugs should improve the ability to prevent acute and chronic rejection.[41]

Fever. Fever is not an uncommon event after and during renal transplants. Known causes of febrile episodes are multiple: [42]

- Defective granulocytic function seen in CRF;
- Impaired cellular immune function;
- Drugs used before, during, or after transplant (i.e. Bleomycin);
- Serious-illness such as sepsis, rejection, pneumonia, meningitis; and
- Minor, incidental illness.

Regardless of the causes, the final pathway is the genesis of endogenous pyrogen which alter the hypothalamus heat regulatory set-point and result in heat generation and conservation. Fever is also a part of inflammatory response produced by cytokin-mediated host defense mechanisms.

True fever is accompanied by tachycardia and sweating. Ancillary tests are useful in establishing the etiology of the fever and include CBC, blood cultures, radiographs of the chest, and in appropriate situations, renal biopsy.

The EP should act promptly to hospitalize toxic-appearing children for diagnostic evaluation, antibiotic administration, and close observation. Antipyretics, such as acetaminophen, are indicated to control fever after a complete evaluation is done. Ibuprofen is to be avoided. Parenteral antibiotics should be given early to high-risk children ages 2-24 months who display signs of bacterial infection. Continuation of antibiotic therapy will be guided by results of appropriate cultures.

Conclusion

In summary, emergencies in children with CRF, although an infrequent event, represent a special entity requiring comprehensive diagnostic and decision-making skills.

The unique presentations of these true emergencies may be due to reversible causes which should be identified and treated. Life-threatening conditions should be recognized and aggressively managed. Consultation with the pediatric nephrologist is advised before final disposition of the patient in the ED.

References

1. Foreman JW, Chan JCM. Chronic renal failure in infants and children. *J Pediatr* 1988;113:793-799.
2. Kaplan BS, Kaplan P, Ruchelli E. Inherited and congenital malformations of the kidneys in neonatal period. *Clin Perinatol* 1992;19:197-211.
3. Moxey-Mims M. Renal tubular disoders in the Neonate. *Clin Perinatol* 1992;19:159-178.
4. Kashtan CE. Alport syndrome, basement membrane and collagen. *Pediatr Nephrol* 1990;4:523-527.
5. Ritz E, Bundschu HD, Massry SG. Chronic Renal Insufficiency. In: Massry SG, Glassock RJ, eds. *Textbook of Nephrology, Volume II* (3rd Ed.). Baltimore: Williams and Wilkins; 1995:1474-1481.
6. Knight F, Gorynski L, Bentson M, et al. Hemodialysis of the infant or small child with chronic renal failure. ANNA Journal 1993;20:315-323.
7. Leichter HE, Kher KK. Management of End-Stage Renal Failure. Dialysis Therapy. In: Kher KK and Makkur SP, eds. *Clinical Pediatric Nephrology.* New York: McGraw-Hill; 1992:559-593.
8. Evans ED, Greenbaum, LA, Ettenger, RB. Principles of renal replacement therapy in children. *Pediatr Nephrol* 1995;42:1579-1596.
9. Maher JF. Physiology of the peritoneum: Implication for peritoneal dialysis. *Med Clin North Am* 1990;74:985-996.
10. Alexander SR. Peritoneal Dialysis. In: Holliday M, Barratt MT, Avner ED, eds. *Pediatric Nephrology, Ed. 3*, Baltimore: Williams and Wilkins; 1994:1339-1353.
11. Bishop NA, Welch TR, Strife CF. Continuous hemofiltration in children. *Pediatrics* 1990;85:819-824.
12. Bunchman TE. Continuous arterio-venous hemofiltration in infants and children. *Pediatr Nephrol* 1994;8:96-100.
13. Harmon WE, Jabs K. Hemodialysis in Children. In: Holliday M, Barratt MT, Avner ED, eds. *Pediatric Nephrology.* 1994:1354-1372.
14. Port FK. Mortality and causes of death in patients with end-state renal failure. *Am J Kidney Dis* 1990;15:215-225.
15. Brem AS. Disorders of K^+ homeostasis. *Pediatr Clin North Am* 1990;37:419-440.
16. Morris KP, Skinner JR. Cardiac abnormalities in chronic renal failure. *Arch Dis Child* 1993;68:637-643.
17. Blumberg A, Wiedmann P, Ferrari P. Effect of prolonged bicarbonate administration on plasma K in terminal renal failure. *Kidney Int* 1992;41:369-374.
18. Kemper MJ, Harps E, Muller-Wiefel DE. Hyperkalemia: Therapeutic options in acute and chronic renal failure. *Clin Nephrol* 1996; 46:67-69.
19. McClure RJ, Prasad VK, Brocklebank JT. Treatment of hyperkalemia using IV and nebulized salbutamol. *Arch Dis Child* 1994;70: 126-128.
20. Allon M, Copkney C. Albuterol and insulin for the treatment of hyperkalemia in hemodialysis patients. *Kidney Int* 1990;38:869-872.
21. Murdoch IA. Treatment of hyperkalemia with IV salbutamol. *Arch Dis Child* 1991:66:527-528.
22. Chang LH, Wu SC, Huang TP. Hypokalemic effects of IV or nebulization of salbutamol in patients with CRF. *Am J Kidney Dis* 1994;23:266-271.
23. Berry PL, Belsha CW. Hyponatremia. *Pediatr Clin North Am* 1990; 37: 351-358.
24. Conley SB. Hypernatremia. *Pediatr Clin North Am* 1990;37:257-260.
25. Brewer ED. Disorders of Acid-Base. *Pediatr Clin North Am*

1990;37:429-440.

26. Hanna HD, Chan JCM, Gill JR Jr. Hypertension and the kidney. *J Pediatr* 1991;118; 327-341.
27. From Task Force on BP Control in Children: Report of the Second Task Force on Blood. *Pediatrics* 1987;79:1-25.
28. Calhoun DA, Oparil S. Treatment of Hypertensive Crisis. *N Engl J Med* 1990;323:1177-1183.
29. Cetta F. Malignant hypertension. *J Pediatr* 1991;118:981-986.
30. Leehey DJ. Peritonitis and Exit-Site Infection. In: Daugirdas JT, Ing TS, eds. *Handbook of Dialysis*. Boston: Little Brown; 1994:338-362.
31. Levy M, Balfe JW. Optimal approach to the prevention and treatment of peritonitis in children undergoing CAPD and CCPD. *Seminars in Dialysis* 1994;7:442-449.
32. Port FK. Risk of peritonitis and technique failure by CAPD connection technique: A national study. *Kidney Int* 1992;42: 967-974.
33. Michael G. Fungal peritonitis in patients on peritoneal dialysis. *Am J Nephrol* 1994;14:113-20.
34. Hakim RM, Depner TA. Adequacy of dialysis. *Am J Kidney Dis* 1992;20:107-123.
35. Fine RN. Dialysis in Infants and Children. In: Daugirdas JT, Ing TS, eds. *Handbook of Dialysis*. Boston: Little Brown; 1994:553-568.
36. Fan PY, Schuab SJ. Vascular access: Concepts for the 1990s. *J Am Soc Nephrol* 1992; 3:1-10.
37. Bregman H, Daugirdas JT, Ing TS. Complications During Hemodialysis. In: Daugirdas JT, Ing TS, eds. *Handbook of Dialysis,* 2nd ed. Boston: Little Brown; 1994:149-168.
38. Jameson MD, Wiegmann TB. Principles, uses and complications of hemodialysis. *Med Clin North Am* 1990;74:945-959.
39. Warady BA. The use of the peritoneal equilibration test to modify peritoneal dialysis modality in children. *Seminars in Dialysis* 1994;7: 403-408.
40. Meyer KE, Weiland H, Thomson PD. Pediatric renal transplant non-compliance. *Pediatr Nephrol* 1995;9:189-192.
41. Welch TR. Treatment options for end-stage renal disease in children. *Clin Trans* 1990;5:146-149.
42. McKay DB, Milford EL, Seyegh MH. Clinical Aspects of Renal Transplant. In: Brenner BM, ed. *The Kidney,* 5th Ed., Vol. 2. Philadelphia: W.B. Saunders; 1996:553-568.

Occult Bacteremia

Steven G. Rothrock, MD, FACEP

Occult bacteremia in children: treacherous, confusing, and controversial. How treacherous? How confusing? Put simply, identifying and treating occult bacteremia (OB) in the pediatric age group is a risk management and risk stratification nightmare. In fact, few life-threatening conditions present such difficult—and, sometimes, ambiguous—triage and treatment decisions.

The scenario is familiar to seasoned practitioners of emergency medicine. Typically, an infant or young child arrives in the emergency department (ED) with a temperature greater than 39°C, appears to be ill, but no source of minor or major infections is readily identified. The clinical dilemma quickly thickens and the physician must arrive at answers to a number of critical questions. What is the likelihood this patient has OB? How extensive should the laboratory evaluation be? What clinical features can help distinguish between "low-risk" and "high-risk" patients? Is empiric antibiotic treatment justified? Will an oral agent suffice? Is hospitalization necessary?

Although definitive guidelines for managing these patients are still a matter for debate, recent studies help point the emergency physician toward outcome-effective assessment and treatment strategies.[1-4] For example, whereas *Haemophilus influenzae* Type b once was the most common cause of OB, today the most common etiologic agent causing OB in children who have been immunized against *H. influenzae* is *Streptococcus pneumoniae*.[5,6] Complicating the development of strict guidelines for antibiotic use is the fact that most recommendations for antimicrobial intervention were made prior to the dramatic decline in *H. influenzae* disease, which can be extremely invasive and produce such sequelae as meningitis and pneumonia.[7,8]

Despite the emergence of expert guidelines and recommendations, many issues surrounding this important clinical syndrome remain unanswered. With these uncertainties and gaps in knowledge in mind, this review presents a systematic, evidentiary-based analysis of OB. By emphasizing possible causes, risk factors, and predictive clinical signs, this issue will permit ED practitioners to make informed and logical decisions that will help optimize care in children suspected of having OB.

Definitions and Risk Management Issues

OB occurs when a well-appearing child, with no major focus of infection, is bacteremic. The highest age incidence of OB is 6-24 months, although cases occur outside this range.[9] The most common organisms implicated in OB include *S. pneumoniae* and *H. influenzae* type B, accounting for approximately 99% of all cases. With the recent introduction of the *H. influenzae* vaccine, however, the incidence of *H. influenzae* bacteremia has decreased dramatically.[1-3,5,6]

The incidence of OB has been reported to be as high as 2.8-11.1% in febrile children 3-36 months old.[5,10-13] Many prior

Figure 1. Temperature and Outcome of Bacteremia

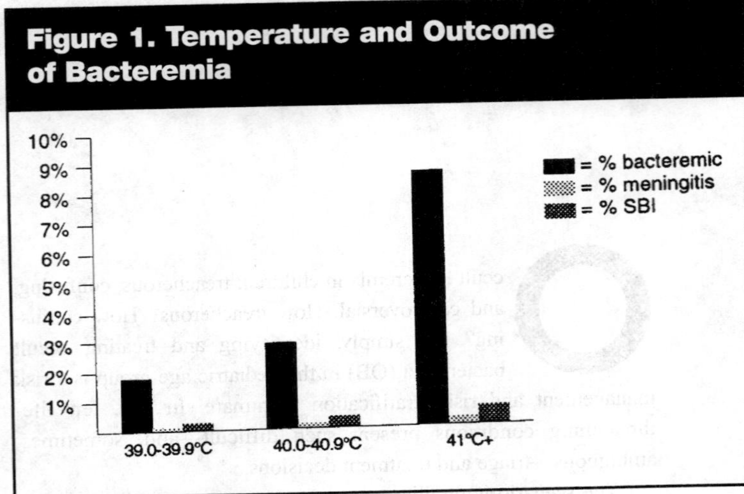

studies citing a high incidence of bacteremia were simple chart reviews limited by the inclusion of children who were ill-appearing or had serious bacterial infections when their blood cultures were obtained; consequently, they falsely overestimated the incidence of this disorder.[5,10-13] Recently, the largest prospective study of OB ever published (including ~ 6700 consecutive febrile children) found that the incidence of OB was 2.8% in well-appearing children 3-36 months old with temperatures of 39°C or higher.[5] This single study was larger than all other OB studies combined, had rigorous criteria for patient inclusion (defined age, temperature, and criteria for well-appearance), and thorough follow-up; as a result, it conveys a more accurate estimate of the prevalence of OB. Well-appearing children with upper respiratory infections, otitis media, diarrhea, and wheezing were included in this study and were found to have a similar incidence of OB compared to those with no apparent source of infection.[5]

Natural History of Occult Bacteremia?

Fortunately, most cases of OB will clear spontaneously. However, a subset of bacteremic children will develop serious infections—most importantly meningitis.[4] A recently published meta-analysis of OB studies found that parenteral antibiotics administered at the time the blood culture was obtained were effective in decreasing the risk of meningitis in children with *H. influenzae* OB from 25% to less than 1%.[4] Oral antibiotics, however, were found to be ineffective in preventing sequelae from *H. influenzae* bacteremia.[4] Fortunately, the incidence of *H. influenzae* disease has markedly decreased and is of less concern in fully immunized children.[1-3] For cases of OB due to *S. pneumoniae,* the risk of progression to meningitis fell from 6% to less than 1% when either oral or parenteral antibiotics were administered.[4] More recently, this meta-analysis was repeated, excluding studies of ill-appearing children, admitted children, and children who underwent spinal taps (ill-appearing children who underwent a procedure known to seed the CSF) on their initial physician encounter. This repeat meta-analysis found that the risk of *S. pneumoniae* bacteremia progressing to meningitis was less than 3% and that oral antibiotics were not effective in preventing meningitis.[8]

Risk Stratification and Predictive Value of Clinical Findings

Several findings may be useful for identifying the presence of OB and its progression to more serious disease. These include:

- The degree of the temperature elevation;
- The age of the child;
- The white blood cell count;
- Other blood tests;
- Blood cultures;
- The presence of a minor or major source of infection;
- Immune status; and
- The appearance of the child.

Height of the Temperature. While the incidence of OB in well-appearing children (3-36 months of age) with a temperature of 39°C (102.2°F) or higher has been reported at 2.8-11.1%,[5,10-13] this number was actually found to be about 2.8% in the largest study of OB.[5] In fact, if children with *H. influenzae* are excluded (i.e., if only children who are fully immunized against *H. influenzae* are considered), the incidence of bacteremia falls to less than 2.5%.[5] The risk of harboring OB rises with the height of a child's temperature, although even at temperatures of 41°C or higher, most well-appearing children are not bacteremic.[6] Moreover, the risk of a child who is fully immunized against *H. influenzae* developing a serious bacterial infection or meningitis increases as the temperature rises. *(See Figure 1.)*

It is apparent that even at very high temperatures (41°C [105.8°F] or higher), the vast majority of well-appearing children (well over 90%) are not bacteremic and will not develop a serious bacterial infection.

Because the risk of bacteremia rises with temperatures higher than 39°C (102.2°F), some authors, including a recent expert panel, recommend obtaining a blood culture (and initiating empiric antibiotic therapy) on all patients with a temperature above this level or obtaining a blood culture and initiating treatment only on those with an elevated temperature (above 39°C) and a white blood cell count greater than 15,000 cells/mm^3.[7] However, this approach has been questioned.[14,15]

While the height of the temperature has a positive correlation, reliance on this parameter alone will not detect all cases of bacteremia. In fact, bacteremia (due to *H. influenzae* and *S. pneumoniae*) still occurs at lower temperatures, with up to 13% of bacteremic children afebrile on presentation to an ED.[16] On the other hand, the persistence of a fever after 48 hours of antibiotic therapy is associated with an increased risk of bacteremia and infectious complications.[12]

The Child's Age. Prior studies of OB have found that most children who are bacteremic are between the ages of 6 and 18 months.[9] *(See Figure 2.)* Those who are younger than 6 months old retain protective maternal antibodies against common organisms, whereas those older than 18-24 months are more immunocompetent and at lower risk for developing bacteremia. However, the drop-off in the incidence of bacteremia noted by several authors may be misleading since clinicians may not look for bacteremia in children older than 24 months or younger than 3-6 months.

The White Blood Cell Count. The white blood cell (WBC) count has been promoted as a useful tool for evaluation of well-appearing children suspected of having OB. Published guide-

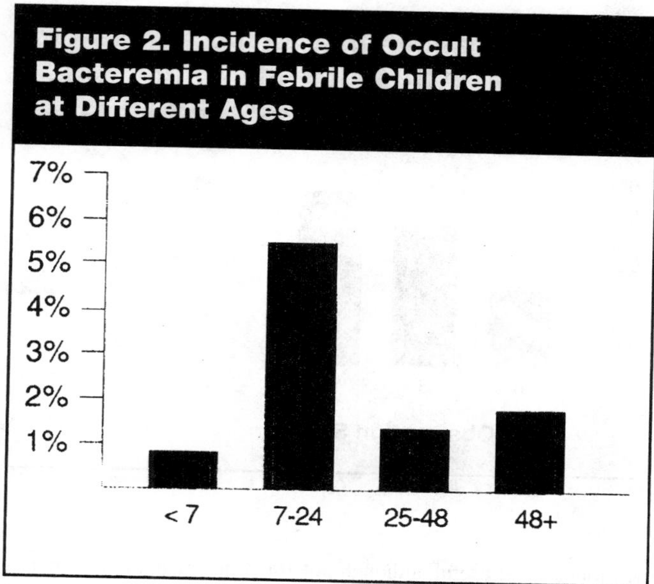

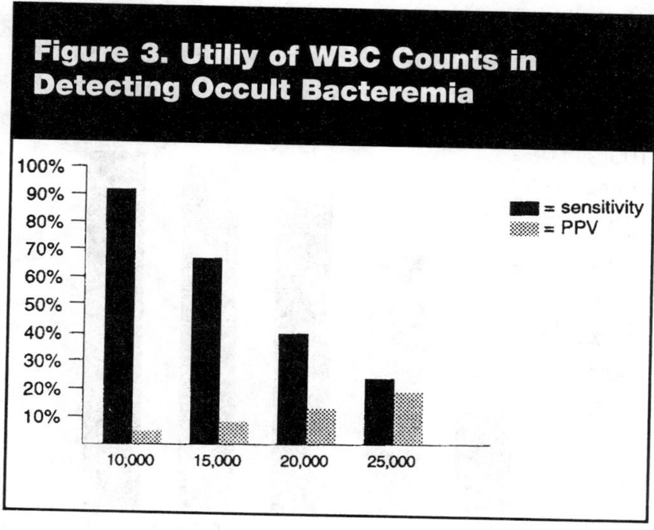

lines recommend a WBC cut-off of 15,000 cells/mm³ or greater as a trigger for obtaining a blood culture and consideration of empiric antibiotic therapy.[7] However, using this cut-off as a trigger for culture and treatment misses up to 35% of bacteremic children.[13] Furthermore, the positive predictive value of this cut-off is less than 10% (i.e., < 1 in 10 children with a WBC count of ≥ 15,000 cells/mm³ will be bacteremic). While a lower WBC cut-off of 10,000 cells/mm³ would detect 92% of bacteremia cases, the positive predictive value falls to less than 3% (i.e., < 3 in 100 children with a WBC count ≥ 10,000 cells/mm³ will be bacteremic).[7,13] *(See Figure 3.)* Finally, the addition of a WBC count to the work-up of every febrile child with a temperature of 39°C (102.2°F) or greater may cause delays in treatment and added expense while contributing little useful information to the evaluation of the well-appearing child.

Other Laboratory Tests. The C-reactive protein and erythrocyte sedimentation rate have been evaluated for detecting OB. A sedimentation rate of greater than 30 mm/h or an elevated C-reactive protein denotes a 10-15% incidence of bacteremia in a febrile child.[17,18] Unfortunately, the high rate of false positives and false negatives limits the use of these tests for detecting OB.

Blood Cultures—An Unreliable Gold Standard. Blood cultures are considered the gold standard for identifying children with bacteremia. Unfortunately, several problems exist with this test that diminish its clinical usefulness. The average time for cultures to return as positive varies from 24 to 48 hours—too late to make initial treatment decisions. Furthermore, more than two-thirds of positive cultures are actually false positives.[19,20] One recent study found that 58% of all children with true positive blood cultures were either lost to follow-up, returned to a physician prior to the culture turning positive, or followed up due to a scheduled appointment prior to the culture returning positive.[21] In the remainder, the blood cultures prompted an unscheduled return visit.

Recent evidence suggests that increasing volume to 3 mL may increase the sensitivity for cultures detecting bacteremia and shorten the time that it takes for a culture to turn positive.[22]

The culture technique used also is important. Three common systems include the BACTEC NR660, the BACTEC 9240 (Becton Dickinson Diagnostic Instrument Systems, Sparks, MD) and the BacT/Alert (Organon Teknika Corporation, Durham NC). With these three techniques, culture bottles are monitored for positivity by instruments that detect the CO_2 released from the culture broth during organism growth and metabolism using infrared spectroscopy (BACTEC NR 660), fluorescent CO_2 sensors (BACTEC 9240), or a colorimetric method (BacT/Alert).[23,24] The BACTEC NR 660 permits reading for positive cultures one or two times per day, while the alternate methods allow continuous monitoring of culture bottles.[23,24] Thus, laboratories using the BACTEC NR 660 method are significantly slower in reporting positive cultures compared to other methods. A newer blood culture technique (DIFCO ESP) monitors each culture for any increase or decrease in internal atmospheric pressure due to gas production or use.[24] This technique has a higher total aerobic culture rate, and a significantly decreased mean turnaround time for positive cultures compared to BacT/Alert.[24] Clinicians should be aware of the specific culture technique used in their laboratory and, if necessary, consider advocating an upgrade to one of the newer techniques.

Other problems exist with reliance on blood cultures to make decisions. Most cases of *S. pneumoniae* OB will spontaneously clear.[4] Moreover, blood cultures may not identify all children who eventually develop serious infections or become ill. Additionally, in one recent series, 24% of those without bacteremia who were treated with oral antibiotics required a second physician visit during their illness. In this same series, about 25% developed diarrhea, vomiting, or a rash, and a significant number required hospitalizations due to antibiotic-related side effects.[5]

Minor Infections: Implications. Debate exists as to whether children with a fever and otitis media, upper respiratory infection, or diarrhea require evaluation for OB. It should be stressed that bacteremia can occur in a substantial number of children with these minor infectious sources. In the large series of 6700 children with acute fever and no major infectious source, 12.8% of children with otitis media were bacteremic, although only one patient developed a serious bacterial infection.[5] Others have reported a bacteremia rate for children with otitis media of 3-6%, which is similar to the child with fever and no source.[7,25] However, those with focal minor infection (e.g., otitis media, upper respiratory infections) may have lower serum bacterial concentration (< 100 CFU/mL) and thus may be at lower risk for progression to meningitis and other serious bacterial

Figure 4. Age and Reliability of Meningeal Signs

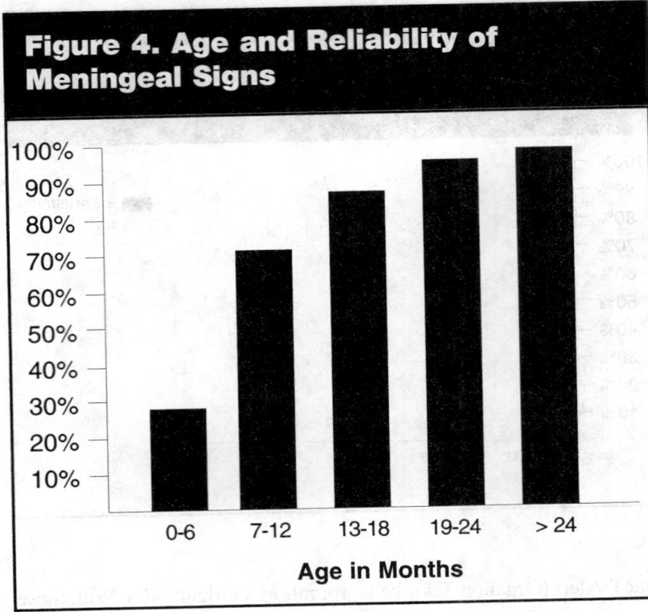

Figure 5. Association of Occult Bacteremia with Yale Observation Score

6%
5%
4%
3%
2%
1%
■ = % bacteremia
6
8
10
Yale Observation Score

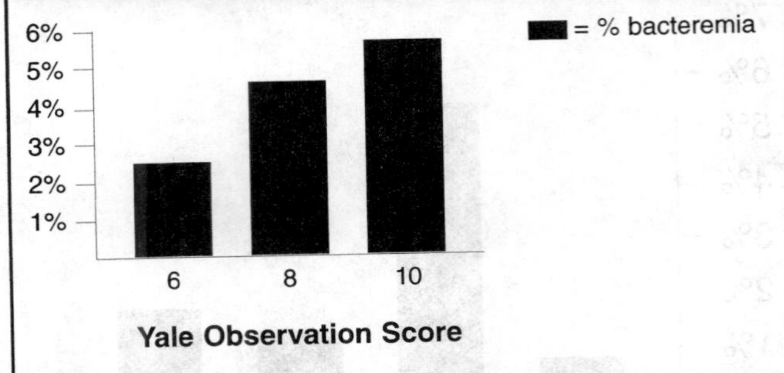

infection.[9,26,27] Thus, the rate of serious bacterial infections developing following bacteremia may be lower in these patients than that of a child with fever and no source.[5,15]

Missing Major Infection. Prior to considering the diagnosis of OB in febrile children with no obvious infectious source, clinicians must consider whether a major focus of infection is present with only minimal clinical signs. Most importantly, clinicians must consider and exclude the diagnosis of meningitis either by history and physical examination or by performing a lumbar puncture. While most children older than 24 months manifest nuchal rigidity and other meningeal signs when they develop meningitis, those who are under the age of 18-24 months and those who have been pretreated with antibiotics may not uniformly manifest meningeal signs or an altered mental status.[28] *(See Figure 4.)* Furthermore, as many as 30% with meningitis may concurrently display signs and symptoms of upper respiratory infections including, but not limited to, otitis media and pharyngitis—thus, potentially leading to diagnostic delays.[29]

Urinary tract infections (UTIs) are another important class of infections that may present with few or no localizing signs and symptoms. In one series of children younger than age 3, 80% with UTIs manifested irritability; 65%, poor feeding; 40%, vomiting; 30%, diarrhea; and a smaller percentage had a cough or nasal discharge.[30] Each of these symptoms occurred with equal frequency in febrile children with and without UTIs and, thus, were useless diagnostically.[30] Moreover, nearly 9% of females with fever 39°C or higher, 7.5% of all children with fever and no source, 3.5% with fever and otitis media, and 1.5% with fever and an unequivocal source (e.g., pneumonia) had a UTI.[30] Thus, UTIs must be considered and excluded in most children at risk for OB.

Finally, minimal localizing signs and symptoms may occur in infants and children with osteomyelitis, septic arthritis, bacterial diarrhea, pneumonia, and other serious bacterial infections. To exclude these disorders, a thorough evaluation must be performed before determining that no source for a child's fever is present.

Clinical Support Tools. When the Yale Observation Scale (YOS) was first described by McCarthy and colleagues in 1982, it was found to be useful, although not 100% accurate, in discriminating ill- from non-ill-appearing children.[31] This scale allowed clinicians to apply an objective description to their clinical assessment of febrile children. *(See Table 1.)* Two separate reports have examined the utility of the YOS in detecting bacteremia. In an earlier study of the fever response to acetaminophen, a YOS score of greater than 10 was found to be 68% sensitive and 77% specific in detecting bacteremia.[31] A larger prospective study by Teach and associates found that 71% of febrile children with OB had the lowest possible YOS, 6.[32] Importantly, this score was only 17% specific for diagnosing OB.[32] As the YOS increased to 8 or greater, specificity for diagnosing OB increased to 83%, while sensitivity dropped to 29%.[32] *(See Figure 5.)* Thus, no YOS cut-off had reliable sensitivity or specificity for detecting bacteremia, limiting the utility of this single feature in accurately diagnosing or excluding OB.

Immune Status and Other Risk Factors. Children who are immunocompromised, including those with leukemia or HIV, are more likely to harbor bacteremia than normal children when they develop a fever. A recent study found a 9% prevalence of bacteremia in HIV-positive children who presented to one pediatric ED.[33] Organisms responsible for bacteremia were frequently atypical: for example, *Streptococcus faecalis, Escherichia coli, Torulopsis glabrata,* and non-*aureus Staphylococcus* species. Importantly, one-half of all HIV-positive children with positive blood cultures had temperatures below 38°C, although most had central lines and a history of a fever.[33]

Immunization status is another important consideration in children at risk for bacteremia. Children not immunized against *H. influenzae* Type b run a higher risk of developing serious bacterial infections from this organism, as it is much more invasive and more likely to progress to meningitis compared to *S. pneumoniae*.[4]

Important risk factors for invasive *S. pneumoniae* disease include institutional day care center attendance (36-fold increased risk), family day care center attendance (4.4-fold increase), and frequent otitis media (8.8-fold increase).[34] The presence of any of these risk factors should heighten the suspicion that *S. pneumoniae* OB is present.

The Role of Parents. An important factor that often is not considered in evaluating and managing children with febrile illness is the preference of the parents. In general, parents prefer to forego the short-term definite risk of a painful blood draw, urine catheterization, or antibiotic injection while accepting the long-term possible risk of a

Table 1. Yale Observation Scale

OBSERVATION ITEM	NORMAL = 1	MODERATE IMPAIRMENT = 3	SEVERE IMPAIRMENT = 5
Quality of cry	Strong or none	Whimper or sob	Weak **or** moaning, high-pitched, continuous cry or hardly responds
Reaction to parent stimulation	Cries brief **or** no cry and content	Cries on and off	Persistent cry with little response
State variation	If awake, stays awake **or** if asleep, awakens quickly	Eyes close briefly when awake **or** awakens with prolonged stimulation	No arousal and falls asleep
Color	Pink	Pale extremities **or** acrocyanosis	Pale **or** cyanotic **or** mottled **or** ashen
Hydration	Skin and eyes normal **and** moist membranes	Skin and eyes normal **and** mouth slightly dry	Skin doughy **or** tented **and** dry mucous emmbranes **and/or** sunken eyes
Response to social overtures	Smiles or alert (consistently)	Brief smile or alert	No smile, anxious, dull; no alerting to social overtures

A total score of less than 11 signifies a less than 3% probability of serious illness.
A total score of 11-15 signifies a 26% probability of serious illness.
A total score of greater than 15 signifies a greater than 92% probability of serious illness.

serious infection developing.[35,36] An informed explanation of the risks and benefits with careful follow-up may be appropriate for parents who wish to avoid a blood culture and empiric antibiotic therapy for OB.

A final factor to be considered is the reliability of parents. Children have the poorest compliance with mandatory follow-up (only 16% in one series) of all types of patients who present to EDs.[37] Furthermore, caretakers who are younger than 21 years old, without a car, and who feel that their child is not ill are significantly less likely to comply with mandatory follow-up from the ED.[38] One method to ensure follow-up is employment of a visiting nurse. This approach virtually guarantees follow-up and allows for a health care professional to visit the home and evaluate the infant for improvement or progression of their disease at a specified time while also saving money.[39]

Guidelines for Managing Occult Bacteremia

Two sets of guidelines for managing febrile children with possible OB have recently been published. In 1993, the American College of Emergency Physicians published a *Clinical Policy for the Initial Approach to Children Under the Age of 2 Years Presenting with Fever*.[40] This publication details Rules (actions reflecting principles of good practice in most cases that should be performed on all children with specific complaints) and Guidelines (lists of recommendations that should be considered, but may or may not be performed, depending on the patient, the circumstances, or other factors.) This clinical policy details recommendations for the care of children with abnormalities of major organ systems, specific infections, and specific complaints (e.g., children of different ages who have fever without a source). Deviations from rules are acceptable if a detailed explanation or reason is documented in writing.

For children 1-24 months of age and a fever without a source (with a temperature > 40°C [104°F]), ACEP recommends a thorough head-to-toe examination as a rule.[40] Guidelines to consider depending upon the clinical examination include the following: glucose, CBC, urinalysis, urine culture, blood culture, chest radiography, lumbar puncture, external cooling if the temperature is greater than 40.6°C (105°F), antipyretics, antibiotics, and referral for follow-up within 24 hours if not admitted.[40] No specific recommendations were made regarding management of children with suspected OB. Importantly, a temperature cut-off for considering blood cultures was listed as 104°F. Moreover, the route and choice of antibiotic was left to the discretion of the treating clinician in children with fever and no source. While ACEP recommendations were published to set a standard of care, they are broad, attempt to cover a wide variety of pediatric infectious diseases, and leave considerable leeway for interpretation and implementation. In fact, a computer science method known as decision table analysis used to verify ACEP's practice guidelines found more than 23,000 possible options available for managing febrile children.[41] Furthermore, according to the authors of this abstract, the guidelines were found to be "inconsistent," with too many "contradictions and undecidable points."[41]

A second expert panel comprised of pediatric emergency physicians, infectious disease specialists, and pediatricians published recommendations primarily for children 0-3 years old.[7] The expert panel's recommendation for children 3-36 months old with a fever without a source are more specific than those devised by ACEP. Non-toxic children (males < 6 months and females < 2 years) with a temperature of 39°C (102.2°F) or higher all should receive a urine culture.[7] Blood cultures and empiric antibiotic therapy (parenteral ceftriaxone 50 mg/kg IM or oral amoxicillin 60 mg/kg/d for 3 days) are recommended for all children or only those with WBC counts of 15,000 cells/mm^3 or higher.[7] While these guidelines are much more specific and useful from the standpoint of giving a standard or a reference of how to evaluate these children, several problems exist. Importantly, WBC cutoffs are either insensitive or nonspecific for detecting bacteremia. Furthermore, these guidelines were written and published based on studies that found a high incidence of *H. influenzae* bacteremia. *H. influenzae* is much more invasive than *S. pneumoniae,* and its dramatic decline in incidence means that most future cases of bacteremia will clear spontaneously.

Moreover, a recent meta-analysis published as an abstract found that the incidence of meningitis following *S. pneumoniae* bacteremia may be much lower than previously reported (< 3% instead of 5.8%).[8] Furthermore, oral antibiotics were not found to be effective in preventing pneumococcal meningitis.[8] The widespread use of antibiotics for the prevention of bacteremia complications in all children with temperatures of 39°C or higher may have some negative effects, including: 1) development of partially treated meningitis, making diagnosis more difficult; 2) increased drug resistance; 3) increased delays and costs of ED visits; and 4) side effects requiring a second physician visit in up to 20% (with potential hospital admission)[5] in those receiving antibiotics.

Finally, obtaining blood cultures and treating all children with temperatures of 39°C or higher will not ensure that all cases of bacteremia will be detected and treated. Obtaining only one blood culture does not provide the sensitivity or reliability to detect bacteremia consistently. In addition, arbitrary use of 39°C as a temperature cut-off for empiric antibiotic treatment is based on an erroneous assumption that bacteremia does not exist when the temperature is less than 39°C.

A Systematic Approach

Several treatment options for managing children with possible OB exist. The first option is adherence to the expert panel guidelines of obtaining a blood culture and treating all children with a temperature of 39°C or higher and fever without a source. Clinicians should realize that this approach will detect most cases of bacteremia while needlessly treating a large number of children without bacteremia.

A second option for emergency physicians who are extremely comfortable with their ability to assess and manage febrile children is to selectively culture and treat those who are at the highest risk for OB using the following factors: patient age, the height of the temperature, the child's immune status, the presence or absence of a minor source of infection, parental preference and reliability, and the child's clinical examination (observation). Blood culture and treatment should be considered in children with temperatures of 40°C or higher or temperatures of 39°C or higher with: 1) YOS score > 6; 2) less than full *H. influenzae* Type B immunization; 3) no minor source for infection; 4) age of 6-24 months; 5) unreliable parents; or 6) parents who desire treatment—if they understand an explanation of the potential risks and benefits of treatment vs. non-treatment. This approach will potentially miss more cases of bacteremia, while only children at highest risk are cultured and treated and fewer non-bacteremic children will be subjected to needless evaluation and antibiotic side effects. Most importantly, all patients should receive a mandatory re-evaluation within 24 hours regardless of which approach is taken.

Summary

Evaluation of infants and children who have fever without a source requires understanding the subtle nature and presentations of UTIs and meningitis at this age as well as the multiple factors that place children within this age range at risk for OB. No single approach will identify and treat all children with bacteremia. Use of the expert panel guidelines will detect the most cases of bacteremia while overtreating a large number of children without bacteremia. Adherence to this approach should be considered by all clinicians who do not treat and evaluate febrile children on a routine basis. For those clinicians who are experienced and feel comfortable with their ability to assess febrile children and with their knowledge of risk factors for OB, a more selective approach of careful follow-up and selective culturing and treatment of only those at highest risk for OB is acceptable. This approach will detect fewer cases of OB while curtailing the over-treatment of non-bacteremic children. Regardless of which approach is taken, 24-hour follow-up of at-risk children, as well as an explanation to the parents or caretaker of the risks of a febrile illness potentially progressing to more serious illness, are mandatory. Re-evaluation by a physician may be the best way to ensure that no serious bacterial infection has developed in those at risk for OB.

References

1. Adams WG, Deaver KA, Cochi SL, et al. Decline of childhood *Haemophilus influenzae* Type b (HIB) disease in the HIB vaccine era. *JAMA* 1993;269:221-226.
2. Broadhurst LE, Erickson RL, Kelley PW. Decreases in invasive *Haemophilus influenzae* diseases in U.S. Army children, 1984 through 1991. *JAMA* 1993;269:227-231.
3. Vadheim CM, Greenberg DP, Eriksen E, et al. Eradication of *Haemophilus influenzae* Type b disease in Southern California. *Arch Pediatr Adolesc Med* 1994;148:51-56.
4. Baraff LJ, Oslund S, Prather M. Effect of antibiotic therapy and etiologic microorganisms on the risk of bacterial meningitis in children with occult bacteremia. *Pediatrics* 1993; 92:140-143.
5. Fleisher GR, Rosenberg N, Vinci R, et al. Intramuscular versus oral antibiotic therapy for the prevention of meningitis and other bacterial sequelae in young, febrile children at risk for occult bacteremia. *J Pediatr* 1994;124:504-512.
6. Harper MB, Fleisher GR. Occult bacteremia in the 3-month-old to 3-year-old age group. *Pediatr Ann* 1993;22:484-493.
7. Baraff LJ, Bass JW, Fleisher GR, et al. Practice guidelines for management of infants and children 0-36 months of age with fever without source. *Pediatrics* 1993;92:1-12.
8. Rothrock SG, Green SM, Clark M. Do oral antibiotics prevent meningitis in children with occult pneumococcal bacteremia? A meta-analysis. *Acad Emerg Med* 1995;2:A.
9. Sinkinson CA, Pichichero ME. Occult bacteremia in children: What are the odds? *Emerg Med Rep* 1991;12:1-10.
10. Teele DW, Pelton SI, Grant MJA, et al. Bacteremia in febrile

children under 2 years of age: Results of cultures of 600 consecutive febrile children seen in a walk-in clinic. *J Pediatr* 1975;87:227-230.

11. Schwartz, RH, Wientzen RL. Occult bacteremia in toxic appearing febrile infants. a prospective clinical study in an office setting. *Clin Pediatr* 1982;21:1175-1180.
12. Jaffe DM, Tanz RR, Todd-Davis A, et al. Antibiotic administration to treat possible occult bacteremia in febrile children. *N Engl J Med* 1987;317:1175-1180.
13. Jaffe DM, Fleisher GR. Temperature and total white blood cell count as indicators of bacteremia. *Pediatrics* 1991;87: 670-674.
14. Cox RD, Wagner M, Woolard DJ. Infants and children with fever without source. *Ann Emerg Med* 1994;23:598-600.
15. Long SS. Antibiotic therapy in febrile children: "Best-laid schemes . . . " *J Pediatr* 1994;124:585-588.
16. Kline M, Lorin M. Bacteremia in children afebrile at presentation to an emergency department. *Pediatr Infect Dis J* 1987;6:197-201.
17. Bennish M, Beem MO, Orniste V. C reactive protein and zeta sedimentation ratio as indicators of bacteremia in pediatric patients. *J Pediatr* 1984;104:729-732.
18. McCarthy PL, Jekel JF, Dolan TF. Comparison of acute-phase reactants in pediatric patients with fever. *Pediatrics* 1978;62: 716.
19. Lyman JL. Use of blood cultures in the emergency department. *Ann Emerg Med* 1986;15:308-331.
20. Stair TO, Linheart M. Outpatient blood cultures: Retrospective and prospective audits in one ED. *Ann Emerg Med* 1984;13: 986-987.
21. Joffe M, Avner JR. Follow-up of patients with occult bacteremia in pediatric emergency departments. *Pediatr Emerg Care* 1992;8:258-261.
22. Karasic RB, Isaacman DJ, Reynolds EA, et al. Effect of number of blood cultures and volume of blood on detection of bacteremia in children. *J Pediatr* 1996;128:190-195.
23. Morello JA, Leitch C, Nitz, et al. Detection of bacteremia by Difco ESP blood culture system. *J Clin Microbiol* 1994;32: 811-818.
24. Zwadyk P, Pierson CL, Young C. Comparison of Difco ESP and Organon Teknika BacT/Alert continuous monitoring blood culture systems. *J Clin Microbiol* 1994;32:1273-1279.
25. Schutzman SA, Petrycki S, Fleisher G. Bacteremia with otitis media. *Pediatrics* 1991;87:48-53.
26. Bell LM, Alpert G, Campos JM, et al. Routine quantitative blood cultures in children with *Haemophilus influenzae* or *Streptococcus pneumoniae* bacteremia. *Pediatrics* 1985;76: 901-904.
27. Sullivan TD, LaScolea LJ, Neter E. Relationship between the magnitude of bacteremia in children and the clinical disease. *Pediatrics* 1982;69:699-702.
28. Kelly-Walsh C. Nelson DB, Smith DS, et al. Clinical predictors of bacterial versus aseptic meningitis in childhood. *Ann Emerg Med* 1992;21:910-914.
29. Rothrock SG, Green SM. Pediatric bacterial meningitis: Is preliminary antibiotic therapy associated with an altered clinical presentation? *Ann Emerg Med* 1992;21:146-154.
30. Hoberman A, Chao HP, Keller DM, et al. Prevalence of urinary tract infection in febrile infants. *J Pediatr* 1993;123: 17-23.
31. McCarthy PL, Sharp MR, Spiesel SZ, et al. Observation scales to identify serious illness in febrile children. *Pediatrics* 1982;70:802-809.
32. Teach SJ, Fleisher GR. Efficacy of an observation scale in detecting bacteremia in febrile children three to thirty-six months of age, treated as outpatients. *J Pediatr* 1995;126: 877-881.
33. Pinkert H, Harper MB, Cooper T, et al. HIV-infected children in the pediatric emergency department. *Pediatr Emerg Care* 1993;9:265-269.
34. Takala AK, Jero J, Kela E, et al. Risk factors for primary invasive pneumococcal disease among children in Finland. *JAMA* 1995;273:859-864.
35. Kramer MS, Etezadi-Amoli J, Ciampi A, et al. Parents' versus physician's values for clinical outcomes in young febrile children. *Pediatrics* 1994;93:697-701.
36. Oppenheim PI, Sotiropoulos G, Baraff LJ. Incorporating patient preferences into practice guidelines: management of children with fever without source. *Ann Emerg Med* 1994;24: 836-841.
37. Vukmir RB. Compliance with ED patient referral. *Am J Emerg Med* 1992;10:413-416.
38. Scarfone RJ, Loiselle JM, Wiley JF. Compliance with scheduled revisits to a pediatric emergency department. *Acad Emerg Med* 1994;1:A41. Abstract.
39. Hertz AL, Herrod HG, Barrett FF, et al. Outpatient management of selective febrile neonates with ceftriaxone and home nurse visitations. *Acad Emerg Med* 1994;1:A3.
40. American College of Emergency Physicians. Clinical policy for the initial approach to children under the age of 2 years presenting with fever. *Ann Emerg Med* 1993;22:628-637.
41. Wears RL, Stenklyft PH, Luten RC. Using decision tables to verify the logical consistency and completeness of clinical practice guidelines: Fever without a source in children under three. *Acad Emerg Med* 1994;1:A35.

Pneumonia

Sharon E. Mace, MD, FACEP, FAA

The clinical challenge of diagnosing and treating viral and bacterial pneumonia in children is familiar to every practitioner of emergency medicine. Unlike adults, in whom the diagnosis of pneumonia is usually straightforward and for whom quantitative triage criteria have been established, in children the clinical picture is frequently less than straightforward. For example, in infants and toddlers, the auscultatory findings may not be helpful in making the diagnosis, and the x-rays frequently are equivocal. Even when an infiltrate is present, the distinction between viral, atypical, and bacterial pneumonia can be difficult, thereby undermining the approach to pharmacotherapy.

Outcome-effective management of pneumonia in infants and children requires a meticulous understanding of etiologic organisms responsible for producing pneumonia in the pediatric age groups. For example, whereas neonates with lower respiratory tract infections are likely to be infected with Group B streptococci or gram-negative enteric bacteria, the toddler or preschooler is more likely to be affected by *Streptococcus pneumoniae*, *Haemophilus influenzae*, or atypical organisms. Not surprisingly, these etiologic patterns govern initial selection of empiric antibiotic therapy, both in the hospital and in the outpatient setting.

With these clinical issues in mind, the purpose of this review is to outline a systematic, diagnostic approach to children suspected of having pneumonia. In addition, the authors provide an age group-by-age group analysis of etiologic agents repsonsible for pneumonia in the pediatric population, and highlight antitibiotics of choice for these infections, reviewing the role of newer macrolide agents—such as azithromycin and clarithromycin—in patient management.

Introduction

Acute respiratory tract infections are the most common illnesses in pediatrics[1] and account for the majority of pediatric emergency department (ED) visits.[2] It is estimated that children may have as many as 10 or more respiratory infections yearly in early childhood.[2] Pneumonia accounts for approximately 15% of all respiratory tract infections.[1] Worldwide, about 3 million children die each year from pneumonia, with the majority of these deaths occurring in developing countries.[1]

In spite of antibiotics and other treatment modalities, pneumonia remains a significant cause of morbidity.[3]

The highest incidence of pneumonia is in the youngest patients with the incidence decreasing gradually with increasing age. The attack rates for pneumonia are: infants (< 1 year), 1 per 100; preschool age, 4 per 100; school age (5-9 years), 2 per 100; and ages 9-15 years, 1 per 100.[4] In infants (age < 2 years) with a fever without source, pneumonia, as diagnosed by positive chest roentgenogram, was found in 13%.[5]

Pneumonia is an inflammation of the lung parenchyma. Although pneumonia is almost always caused by a microorganism, there are a

Table 1. Noninfectious Causes of Pneumonia

- Hypersensitivity reactions
- Drug-induced pneumonitis
- Radiation-induced pneumonitis
- Hydrocarbons/lipoid substance
- Aspiration of food and/or gastric acid
- Foreign bodies

few noninfectious etiologies.[6,7] *(See Table 1.)* Since the infectious etiology and antibiotic treatments may differ, pneumonia is often divided into categories: pneumonia in the immunocompromised patient (such as the patient with HIV) and in the immunocompetent patient (the otherwise normal infant and child). Community-acquired pneumonia is pneumonia not acquired in a hospital or an extended care facility.[8,9] Our focus will be on community-acquired pneumonia in the nonimmunocompromised pediatric patient.

Pathogenesis: Normal Pulmonary Defense Mechanisms

The lungs are protected by various mechanisms.[10-13] *(See Table 2.)* Inspired air is filtered by the nares. Warming, humidification, and filtration occurs in the upper airway. The trachea and bronchi are lined with ciliated epithelial cells and goblet cells. The goblet cells and the mucous glands of the airway secrete a mucous layer. The action of the cilia moves the mucous layer toward the pharynx so the mucous layer with entrapped particles can then be expectorated or swallowed.

Particles larger than 10-15 mcg are filtered by the coarse nasal hairs. Particles 5-10 mcg land on the nasal surface and are removed by mechanisms including the ciliary action of the epithelium and by sneezing. Particles 1-5 mcg land on the tracheobronchial mucosal blanket and are removed by ciliary action. Particles smaller than 1 mcg may reach the respiratory bronchioles and air spaces, where some may be exhaled. Particles in the alveoli may be removed by the mucociliary system, phagocytosis by alveolar macrophages, or via the lymphatics or bloodstream.

Opsonins and small lymphocytes act to enhance the phagocytosis and killing of living particles. Secretory immunoglobins, especially secretory IgA, can neutralize some viruses and toxins and assist in the lysis of bacteria. IgG and IgM are secreted when lung inflammation occurs. Other substances including interferon, lactoferrin, and lysozymes may also be a part of the defensive mechanisms of the lung.

Pathogenesis: Impaired Pulmonary Defense Mechanisms

Any process that adversely affects any of the pulmonary defense mechanisms predisposes to pneumonia.[14,15] *(See Table 3.)* Factors that impair host defenses can be congenital (ranging from anatomic abnormalities to impaired immunity) or acquired (generalized disorders such as human immunodeficiency virus [HIV] or pulmonary diseases such as pulmonary fibrosis) or even iatrogenic (drugs, anesthetics, intubation, and tracheostomy). *(See Table 4.)*

Table 2. Defense Mechanisms of the Lung

SPECIFIC PULMONARY MECHANISMS

Filtration of inhaled particles

Humidification, warming of inspired air

Absorption of noxious fumes/gases by the vascular upper airway

PULMONARY REFLEXES

Reflex mechanisms to expel foreign particles: reflexly shallow breathing, temporary cessation of respiration, laryngospasm, bronchospasm

Closure of epiglottis (prevents aspiration of food, secretions, foreign bodies)

MUCOCILIARY SYSTEM

CELLULAR MECHANISMS

Phagoycytosis of particles by alveolar macrophages

Phagocytosis of particles by lymphocytes then transport into regional lymph nodes or bloodstream

Enhancement of phagocytosis-killing process by: opsonins, small lymphocytes

HUMORAL MECHANISMS

Secretory immunoglobulins (IgA, IgG, IgM)

Other substances: interferon, lactoferin, lysozymes

There also are environmental factors that are associated with an increased incidence and severity of respiratory infections. These include cigarette smoke, crowded living conditions, poverty, malnutrition, daycare attendance, and inhalation of pollutants from wood-burning stoves.[16-18] *(See Table 5.)*

In children, probably the most common factor that renders the lung susceptible to pneumonia is a preceding viral infection. At least 50% of the time, a viral upper respiratory infection (URI) precedes the onset of pneumonia.[19] Such a viral URI impairs host defenses by disrupting the normal epithelium of the respiratory tract that impairs the mucociliary system, altering normal secretions, modifying the native bacterial flora, and even inhibiting phagocytosis.

Organisms can gain access to the lungs by several routes. Most often, organisms colonizing the upper respiratory tract are aspirated into the lungs.[20] Less commonly, organisms access the lung via the bloodstream during a primary bacteremia or from a distant focus of infection.[20] Once the microorganism invades the lung, an inflammatory response occurs. This results in the migration of polymorphonuclear leukocytes, the release of oxidative enzymes and mediators of inflammation, the loss of surfactant, and the leakage of plasma. These pathophysiologic changes inter-

Table 3. Impaired Pulmonary Defense Mechanisms Predisposing to Pneumonia*

LOSS OF/DEPRESSED REFLEXES
- Neurologic diseases
- Muscle weakness
- Drugs that impair cough reflex
- Anesthesia, sedation
- Chemical/physical agents (smoke, ethanol ingestion, steroids, hypoxemia, starvation, narcotics, some anesthetics)
- Cystic fibrosis
- Bronchitis
- Ciliary dyskinesia
- Alpha 1 antitrypsin disease

BYPASS OF UPPER AIRWAY
- Intubation
- Tracheostomy

CONGENITAL ANATOMIC ABNORMALITIES
- Cleft palate
- Tracheoesophageal fistula
- Sequestration

ALTERATIONS IN PULMONARY PARENCHYMA
- Noninfectious inflammatory conditions: aspiration
- Changes in pulmonary blood flow
- Damage to respiratory epithelium (certain lung diseases: pulmonary fibrosis, etc.)
- Fluid in the lungs (congestive heart failure, pulmonary edema)
- Anatomic abnormalities: pulmonary sequestration

IMPAIRMENT OF MUCOCILIARY SYSTEM
- Viral infection(s)
- Bronchial obstruction (foreign body, etc.)

IMMUNOSUPPRESSION
- Malignancies
- Drugs: steroids, others
- Chemotherapeutic agents
- Radiation therapy
- HIV

IMMUNODEFICIENCY DISORDERS/DISEASE
- Cellular
- Alveolar macrophage: steroids, chemotherapy, chronic granulomatous disease
- Leukocytes: decreased numbers: chemotherapy, congenital neutropenia; Decreased mobility-WBC motility disease; Lymphocytes: decreased number/fiction

* *Impaired defense mechanism with some examples of disorders that predispose to pneumonia are listed.*

Table 4. Clinical Conditions that Predispose to Pneumonia

DISORDERS OF IMMUNE SYSTEM
Congenital/Acquired defects/deficiencies in cellular immunity; Congenital/Acquired defects/deficiencies in humoral immunity

IMMUNOSUPPRESSED PATIENTS
Malignancies; Patients on chemotherapeutic agents; Patients on radiation therapy; Patients on steroids, other drugs; Transplant patients; HIV

PULMONARY DISEASES
Bronchopulmonary dysplasia; Cystic fibrosis; Asthma

CERTAIN NEUROLOGIC OR NEUROMUSCULAR DISEASES

GASTROINTESTINAL DISEASES
Tracheosophageal fistula; Severe reflux; Aspiration

SICKLE CELL DISEASE

CERTAIN CONGENITAL HEART DISEASES

fere with respiration and lead to the clinical signs and symptoms of pneumonia.

Clinical Presentation by Age

The clinical signs and symptoms depend primarily on the age of the patient, the causative organism, and the severity of the disease.

Neonates. Neonates generally present with nonspecific signs and symptoms including lethargy, irritability, poor feeding, isolated fever or hypothermia, vomiting, and poor muscle tone.[21] Neonates often do not have the usual signs and symptoms such as a cough or rales as found in older children, adolescents, and adults.[21]

Neonates do not have fully developed immunologic capabilities and, thus, are highly susceptible to any infection.[22] A diagnosis of pneumonia in a neonate mandates an appropriate diagnostic evaluation including initiation of antibiotics and hospital admission. A septic workup in a neonate includes a chest roentgenogram even if pulmonary findings, such as tachypnea and rales, are not present.[23]

Infants. Classic findings of pneumonia that occur in adults and older children, such as cough and rales, are often absent in infants and toddlers.[24] Infants may also have the same nonspecific signs and symptoms that can occur in the neonates.[25-27] Pneumonia in infants, including neonates, may also present as sepsis or as a "fever without a source."[28-30]

Infants with chlamydia pneumonia often are afebrile with only a cough and a surprising lack of physical examination findings, while those with a bacterial pneumonia may have a fever and signs of respiratory distress, such as tachypnea and retractions.

Toddler or Young Child. The young child with pneumonia usually has a fever and a cough.[31] However, gastrointestinal symptoms are common and may be the presenting complaint. Vomiting and anorexia are common as is abdominal pain, especially with lower lobe infiltrates. Occasionally, the abdominal pain may be mistaken for appendicitis or an acute abdomen.[2]

Older Children and Adolescents. In older children and adolescents with pneumonia, the presentation is similar to that of adults with pneumonia.[31] Cough is often, but not always, present.[32] Chest pain may occur and is usually pleuritic.

Clinical Presentation Based on Etiology

The typical presentation of a pediatric patient with bacterial pneumonia is the sudden onset of high fever with lower respiratory

Table 5. Environmental Factors Associated with Increased Incidence and Severity of Pulmonary Infections

- Cigarette smoking in household
- Crowded living conditions
- Daycare attendance
- Poverty
- Malnutrition
- Inhaled pollutants from wood burning stoves

symptoms (e.g., cough) with rales on the lung examination indicative of pulmonary consolidation.[31,32] The usual history in a child with a viral pneumonia is a gradual onset of respiratory symptoms, which may include wheezing, along with a low-grade fever. Unfortunately, children with pneumonia (viral or bacterial) may have a varied presentation.[31,32] Therefore, one cannot always predict whether the pneumonia is bacterial or viral.[33] However, given the clinical signs and symptoms, laboratory findings, the chest radiograph, epidemiologic factors (the time of year or seasonal variation and an outbreak of the pathogen in the community or within a family), and patient factors (e.g., age, comorbidity, past medical history), a reasonable prediction of the etiology *(see Table 6)* or pneumonia syndrome usually can be made. *(See Table 7.)*

History

The history is important since it may determine the patient management. Are there any underlying diseases or conditions that make the infant or child more susceptible to a severe and/or more frequent pneumonia? This includes bronchopulmonary dysplasia, cystic fibrosis, asthma, sickle cell disease, congenital heart disease, malignancies, immunosuppressed patients (such as those with HIV and congenital disorders of the immune system), some neurologic diseases, certain gastrointestinal disorders, (e.g., tracheoesphageal fistula, significant reflux, aspiration, etc). *(See Table 4.)* If the patient has had a recent infection with measles or varicella, the pneumonia may represent a serious complication of the initial infection. Infants (younger than 3-6 months of age) with pneumonia may have apnea, so admission is recommended in these patients.

Has the child been able to take oral fluids and/or medicines? Is the child having symptoms of dehydration or respiratory distress? Has the child been on treatment as an outpatient and failed to respond? Are there psychosocial issues complicating the child's care, whether it be concerns about compliance with therapy or follow-up? Such issues or concerns may affect the decision for hospital admission. *(See Table 8.)* History should also recognize any exposures, travel, or other risk factors for pneumonia caused by unusual organisms *(see Table 9)* or even for the possibility of tuberculosis.

Physical Examination

The first step in the physical examination is an assessment of the general appearance and level of activity or behavior of the child. This is to determine if the child has any complications of pneumonia such as sepsis, shock, or respiratory failure, and if emergent resuscitation is needed. Is the child toxic and ill appearing or nontoxic, smiling, playful, and behaving appropriately?

The vital signs should be assessed. Pediatric patients with bacterial pneumonia generally have a fever except for the septic infant who may be hypothermic or the infant with the afebrile pneumonia syndrome. The blood pressure and pulse may reflect the child's hydration status and rarely shock.

Tachypnea may be the only sign of pneumonia in an infant or young child and is reported to be the best single parameter for pneumonia, but it is not always present.[34-37] Since fever can cause tachypnea, the respiratory rate should be rechecked after the patient has defervesced. Is the respiratory rate elevated to an extent that cannot be explained just by the fever or persists after the fever has dissipated?

Signs of respiratory distress may or may not be present depending on the severity of the disease. Indeed, no one sign or symptom or group of signs and symptoms can always predict pneumonia.

Findings typical of pneumonia in an adult including rales, wheezing, decreased breath sounds, dullness to percussion, and decreased fremitus may sometimes be found in the older child or adolescent but are often absent in the young child or infant. Rales may not be heard in the infant or young child. This is because the transmission of sounds throughout the chest prevents localization, or there may be a poor inspiration, or noisy upper airway sounds may be present.

The abdomen may appear distended due to gastric dilatation from swallowed air or to an ileus. Downward displacement of the right diaphragm may give the false impression of hepatomegaly. Children with pneumonia in the upper lobes may have meningismus without meningeal infections.

A thorough physical examination should be done in order to find clues to the possible source of the pneumonia or to the etiologic agent. Other infections, such as otitis media, sinusitis, meningitis, pericarditis, and bone, soft tissue, or skin infections, may be implicated in the hematogenous spread of a microorganism to the lungs. Extrapulmonary findings may suggest a specific infectious agent. Various skin exanthems are associated with viral and bacterial pathogens. Pharyngitis may indicate a mycoplasma or streptococcal infection. Conjunctivitis is present in about half of the infants with *Chlamydia pneumonia*.[38] Rhinorrhea and other findings may implicate a previous or coexistent URI.

Laboratory Data

With a viral pneumonia, the white blood cell count may be normal or mildly elevated, often with a lymphocytosis. In bacterial pneumonia, there is generally a leukocytosis in the range of 15,000-40,000 cells/mm^3, with an increased percentage of polymorphonuclear leukocytes and band forms. Leukopenia (WBC < 5000/mm^3) may indicate a poor prognosis. A markedly elevated WBC count (> 30,000 mm^3) almost always denotes a bacterial pneumonia, often with bacteremia and a higher risk of complication.[7] Eosinophilia may be present with *C. pneumonia*[38] or a parasitic infection. Leukocytosis, with severe lymphocytosis, occurs with pertussis,[7] although this may not be present in infants younger than 6 months old.[39] A normal WBC count is typical of mycoplasma, or *C. pneumonia*. The erythrocyte sedimentation rate and C-reactive pro-

Table 6. Likely Etiologic Organisms for Various Pediatric Age Groups

Age	Most Common Etiologic Group	Most Common Specific Organisms in the Given Age Group		
		Bacterial	**Viruses**	**Atypical**
Neonate (< 1 month)	1. Bacterial 2. Viruses	Group B streptococci Gram-negative enteric bacteria *(E. coli, Klebsiella)* *Listeria monocytogens* Other gram-positive cocci Staphylococci	Cytomegalovirus Herpes simplex Measles	
Infant (1-4 months)	1. Atypical (Chlamydia) 2. Viruses 3. Bacteria	Same as for neonates plus *Streptococcus pneumoniae* *Haemophilus influenzae* *Staphylococcus aureus*	Respiratory Syncytial virus (RSV)	Chlamydia
Toddler/ Preschooler	1. Virus 2. Bacteria 3. Atypical (Mycoplasma)	*S. pneumoniae* *H. influenzae* *S. aureus*	RSV Parainfluenza Adenovirus Influenza Other (enterovirus, rhinovirus)	Mycoplasma
School-age children and adolescents	1. Atypical (Mycoplasma) 2. Viruses 3. Bacteria	*S. pneumoniae*	Parainfluenza Adenovirus Influenza Others	Mycoplasma

tein are usually elevated but are so non-specific that they are not helpful in management.[7]

The use of sputum cultures is limited since children (especially younger than 10 years of age) rarely produce sputum, and it is difficult to get a good quality sputum sample that is not contaminated by the indigenous flora of the mouth and pharynx.[40] High-quality sputum samples should have more than 25 polymorphonuclear cells per field, 40 squamous cells per field, and the presence of mucous.[41] Sputum samples and morning gastric aspirate samples are helpful to confirm tuberculosis. Nasopharyngeal and throat cultures are not usually helpful and are often misleading in establishing an etiologic agent for bacterial pneumonia because of a high rate of false-positive tests.[2,20]

Overall, blood cultures are positive in about 10-30% of patients with bacterial pneumonia.[19,40] However, a much higher yield occurs with certain bacterial pneumonias such as pneumococcal (25%)[41,42] or *Haemophilus influenza* type B (up to 95%),[41] or *Staphylococcus aureus* (33% and up to 89% if disseminated disease is present).[42] There are differences in opinions concerning whether or not blood cultures should be obtained. Those in favor feel that blood cultures will provide a specific bacteriologic diagnosis; those against state that blood cultures almost never alter the treatment or outcome for previously healthy children presenting with pneumonia.[43]

Rapid screening tests to detect bacterial antigens in serum or urine using latex particle agglutination or countercurrent immunoelectrophoresis (CIE) generally have had a low sensitivity and specificity,[40,41,45,46] but some studies have found better results.[47,48] With improved techniques, bacterial antigen testing of the urine may become useful in the future.[44,48] Generally, serologic testing has also not been useful since paired acute and convalescent serum are needed.[40]

However, in selected cases, such as mycoplasma, cytomegalovirus, or measles, a rise in the immunoglobulin M antibody may confirm the diagnosis.[44] Pneumonia caused by group A streptococci can be diagnosed by detecting an elevated level of streptococcal antibodies (e.g., Antistreptolysin O, streptozyme, or anti Dnase B titers), although an elevated titer may reflect a previous infection.[43] Rapid antigen detection tests, using the immunofluorescent antibody test (IFA) or the enzyme-linked immunosorbent assay (ELISA) on nasopharyngeal secretions has been helpful with the diagnosis of RSV.[20]

Mycoplasma infection results in a positive cold agglutinin titer (> 1:32) in about half (from 1/3 to 3/4) of infected patients. However, elevated titers can occur with other diseases; such as adenovirus, Epstein-Barr virus, measles, lymphoma, and some tropical diseases.[49,50] A "bedside" test for cold agglutinins is done by putting 0.3-0.4 cc of blood in a lavender hematology tube with ethylenediaminetetracetic acid (EDTA) or in a blue prothrombin tube with sodium citrate. The tube is put in ice water for 15-30 seconds then tilted on its side and examined. A positive test is indicated by the presence of coarse floccular agglutination that disappears when the tube is rewarmed. A positive test corresponds to a cold agglutinin titer of more than 1:64. No agglutination or fine granularity is a negative test.[49,50]

Table 7. Differential Diagnosis of Pneumonia by Etiologic Category/ Pneumonia Syndromes*

Signs and Symptoms	Bacterial	Viral	Chlamydia	Mycoplasma	Tuberculosis
History			Afebrile pneumonia of infancy		
Age	Any, especially neonates	Any, especially toddlers/preschoolers	1-4 months (3-16 weeks)	School age adolescent	Any age > 4 months
Onset	Sudden (> 50% occur after URI)	Gradual	Gradual	Gradual	Usually gradual, may be acute
Cough	Often productive	Dry cough	Dry cough can be only symptom	Usually dry cough	Cough often productive, sometimes hemoptysis
Other signs	Sometimes pleuritic chest pain	Sometimes coryza sore throat, rash	Conjunctivitis in ~ 50% (may precede or occur with pneumonia)	Sometimes sore throat, rash, bullous otitis media, headache	Weight loss, night sweats
Physical Examination					
Appearance of Fever	May be toxic usually high (> 39°C)	Nontoxic usually low grade	Nontoxic usually afebrile	Nontoxic usually low grade	Usually nontoxic variable
Lung Auscultation	Rales, decreased breath sounds	Rales, wheezing rhonchi	Rales wheezing	Sometimes rales	Variable
Laboratory	**Bacterial**	**Viral**	**Chlamydia**	**Mycoplasma**	**Tuberculosis**
White Blood Cell**	Increased WBC	Normal or slightly increased	Normal or slight increase WBC up to 15,000 range; May have eosinophia	May have atypical lymphocytes, lymphocytosis	Variable
Other laboratory tests	Obtain blood culture	Nasal washing for RSV may be helpful	Nasal washings may be helpful	Cold agglutinins often positive, bedside test	Sputum, gastric aspirates for skin testing (ppd)
Chest Roentgenogram	Consolidation Pleural effusion Think *S. aureus* if Pneumatoceles pleural effusions, lung abscess	Hyperinflation Interstitial infiltrates	Hyperinflation Interstitial infiltrates	Variable patchy Interstitial infiltrates are most common	Variable, often adenopathy, Other: infiltrates cavitation, effusions

* *These are the generally observed characteristics for a given category of pneumonia. Any given patient may have all, some, or none of the given characteristics even when proven to have a specific infection. This is a general guide, not an absolute for every patient.*

** *Pertussis characteristically has an elevated WBC usually 15,000-40,000/mm^3 with a marked lymphocytosis, although this may not be present in infants.*

Table 8. Indications for Hospital Admission with Pneumonia

Neonate	Hypoxemia
Young infant ≤ 3-6 months	Complications of pneumonia (lung abscess, emphysema, fistula, etc.)
Inability to tolerate fluids or medications	Bacteremia
Lack of response to outpatient therapy	Sepsis
Psychosocial issues (compliance with therapy, follow-up)	Dehydration
Comorbidity (bronchopulmonary dysplasia, sickle cell disease, etc.)	Suspicion of specific virulent pathogens (e.g., *P. carinii, S. aureus)*
Respiratory distress	

If tuberculosis is suspected, a mantoux tuberculin test with 5 units of purified protein derivative (PPD) should be done. Skin tests for candida and histoplasmosis can also be done in selected cases, although these skin tests can be positive with past exposure as well as with active infection.

Currently, the laboratory detection of the etiologic agent causing pneumonia is limited. However, the use of polymerase chain reaction (PCR) testing along with other technological improvements looks promising and may lead to more widespread use of serologic type tests for the diagnosis of pneumonia in the future.

Invasive diagnostic techniques are generally done only in patients who lack a definitive diagnosis (e.g., noninvasive tests have not yielded a diagnosis) and who are deteriorating clinically, especially if they are immunocompromised.

If there is a significant pleural effusion, then thoracentesis, with removal of pleural fluid, may be diagnostic and therapeutic. Pleural fluid should be sent for analysis including appropriate cultures. Flexible bronchoscopy with bronchoalveolar lavage has mostly been used in HIV-infected children who have pulmonary disease. It has been a fairly safe and effective procedure (27-75% diagnostic yield).[52] Transbronchial biopsy has not been widely used in pediatrics except in lung transplant patients because of the bronchoscope size. Open lung biopsy has been done in critically ill patients in whom noninvasive procedures have failed to yield a diagnosis.[53]

Radiograph Evaluation

Although the diagnosis of bacterial vs. viral pneumonia can not be made solely on the basis of a chest roentgenogram, the radiographic appearance can be helpful.[54] The accuracy of the chest radiograph in predicting the etiologic agent causing the pneumonia varies widely from 42-73% to more than 90%.[44,56]

Pulmonary infiltrates can be classified into three categories: interstitial, alveolar, or bronchopneumonia.[54] An interstitial pattern has increased bronchovascular markings, peribronchial cuffing, and hyperaeration. Occasionally, there may be patchy consolidation due to atelectasis. Viral and mycoplasmal pneumonia generally have this radiographic appearance.

Table 9. Risk Factors/Association with Unusual Causes of Pneumonia

Pneumonia	Risk Factor Association
Coccidiomycosis	Location/recent travel to Southwestern U.S. (San Joaquin Valley, S. California, New Mexico, S. Arizona, SW Texas)
Histoplasmosis	Mississippi/River Valley
Hantavirus	SW U.S. (4 corner area of Arizona, New Mexico, Australia, SE Asia, Guam)
Meliodosis	South/Central America, W. Indies, Australia, SE Asia, Guam
Animal Exposure	
Psittaci	Exotic birds (parrots, cockatoos, etc.), turkeys, pigeons
Anthrax	Cattle, horses, swine, animal hides
Brucellosis	Unpasteurized dairy products, cattle, goats, pigs
Bubonic Plague	Lagomorphs (squirrels, rabbits, chipmunks, etc.), rats
Hantavirus	Rodent excretions, urine, saliva, droppings
Histoplasmosis	Soil with bird or bat droppings
Leptospirosis	Water contaminated with animal urine, wild dogs, cats, rodents, cattle, horses, pigs
Pasteurella multocida	Infected dogs, cats
Q Fever	Secretions of infected animals or contact with the animals (cattle, sheep, goats, other domestic animals)
Tularemia	Hunting, trapping, skinning of infected animals
Other Risk Factors	
Legionnaires' disease	Contaminated aerosols (hospital water supply, air coolers, etc.)
Tuberculosis	Exposure to someone with tuberculosis

Consolidation with air bronchograms is the radiographic pattern found with alveolar or air space disease. Bacterial infections, such as pneumococcal pneumonia, generally exhibit this radiographic appearance. The third radiographic pattern is bronchopneumonia. This is characterized by a diffuse bilateral pattern, increased peribronchial markings, and small fluffy infiltrates that extend into the periphery of the lung. Bacterial infections, including *S. aureus*, tend to have a bronchopneumonic pattern on the chest roentgenogram.

A nonlobar patchy infiltrate(s) or an interstitial pattern is the usual radiographic appearance with the atypical pneumonias. Thus, the chest roentgenogram with mycoplasma can be consistent with a viral or a bacterial infection. Bilateral diffuse interstitial infiltrates with hyperaeration can be seen with *C. pneumonia*.

Table 10. Disorders that can Present as Pneumonia

CHRONIC INFECTIONS
- Tuberculosis
- Fungal diseases
- Parasitic diseases

PRIMARY PULMONARY DISEASES
- Alpha 1-antirysin deficiency
- Acute respiratory distress syndrome
- Atelectasis
- Asthma
- Bronchopulmonary dysplasia
- Cystic fibrosis
- Pleural effusions
- Pulmonary infarction
- Sickle cell vasoocclusive crisis
- Pulmonary emboli

AUTOIMMUNE DISORDERS (COLLAGEN VASCULAR DISEASES)
- Systemic lupus erythematous, etc.
- Others

MALIGNANCIES/GROWTHS

CONGENITAL PULMONARY MALFORMATIONS
- Bronchogenic cysts
- Pulmonary sequestrations
- Cystic adenomatoid malformations

OTHER
- Pulmonary hemosiderosis

RADIOLOGIC TECHNIQUES/FACTORS THAT MAY APPEAR AS PNEUMONIA ON CHEST ROENTGENOGRAM
- Underpenetration
- Uneven grid on the film
- Poor inspiration
- Thymus shadow
- Breast shadow

Occasionally, the chest roentgenogram may reveal a "round" pneumonia. This is a consolidative pneumonia usually caused by a bacteria. It has a spherical shape, indistinct borders, can be large, and is a solitary lesion. Initially, it may suggest a tumor.

Occasionally, there are other factors that may give the appearance of pneumonia on the chest radiograph. These include radiologic technique and noninfectious causes. *(See Table 10.)* Radiologic techniques that may simulate a pneumonia are an underpenetrated film, an uneven grid on the film, poor inspiration, breast shadow, and thymus shadow.[57-59]

Atelectasis also can be confused as pneumonia.[57-59] Atelectasis has many causes. These include extrinsic compression of a bronchi (from a congenital malformation, lymphadenopathy, tumor, cardiovascular disease, web or ring), and intrinsic bronchial obstruction (foreign body, edema, inflammation, bronchomalacia or stenosis, tumor, and mucous plug secondary to cystic fibrosis or asthma). Noninfectious pulmonary diseases can also cause atelectasis from hyaline membrane disease to adult respiratory distress syndrome or pulmonary edema. External pulmonary compression for whatever reason from a growth or tumor to a pleural effusion also can result in atelectasis.

A chest roentgenogram can assist in the detection of complications of pneumonia, including a large pleural effusion, pneumatocoles, or a lung abscess. Such complications suggest a bacterial infection, particularly, *S. aureus* and, less commonly, *H. influenza*.

Although a positive chest radiograph is the gold standard for the diagnosis of pneumonia, an occasional patient with clinical symptoms and signs of pneumonia may have a normal chest roentgenogram.[20] The radiographic finding is said to "lag behind" the clinical picture.[7] If a child is dehydrated, especially early in the course of illness, an initial chest x-ray may be negative while a repeat film after therapy may then become positive.[20]

Likewise, the patient may have clinically recovered from the pneumonia, yet still have findings of pneumonia on the chest roentgenogram.[7] Thus, most clinicians will wait 6-8 weeks before repeating the chest roentgenogram in patients with lobar consolidation in order to confirm resolution of the pneumonia and to rule out an underlying anatomic abnormality of the lung.

Some physicians feel that a chest radiograph is not essential in a nontoxic well-appearing infant or child with no risk factors who appears to have a mild pneumonia and who has close follow-up, especially it if is during a viral outbreak or other family members have evidence of a viral infection.[32,36] However, other physicians disagree and feel that a chest roentgenogram is indicated in any infant or child seen in the ED in whom the diagnosis of pneumonia is suspected.[14,20]

Nevertheless, the practice of ordering radiographs on all febrile infants as part of a standard work-up deserves reflection. Febrile infants subsequently diagnosed with pneumonia generally will have evidence of pulmonary disease. Several studies based on both meta-analysis prospective, and retrospective reviews of x-rays and patient records demonstrated that most infants less than 2-3 months with pneumonia had respiratory signs and symptoms such as tachypnea, rales, ronchi, retractions, wheeze, cough, or rhinorrhea.[60-62]

Pneumonia in Infants and Children: Etiologic Agents

Nonbacterial (e.g., viral) pneumonias account for about 60-80% of all pneumonias in pediatric patients. The most common viruses are respiratory syncytial virus (especially in infants), parainfluenza virus, adenovirus, and influenza virus. The atypical pneumonias are the most common pneumoniae in school age children and adolescents (age > 5 years). *Mycoplasma pneumoniae* is the most common atypical pneumoniae followed by *C. pneumoniae*, previously called the TWAR strain of *Chlamydia trachomatis*. The most common bacterial pneumonias are *Streptococcus pneumoniae*, *Staphylococcus aureus*, and *H. influenzae* type B. *(See Table 6.)*

Table 11. Organisms Causing Pneumonia and Empiric Therapy in Pediatrics

Age Group	Bacterial	Viral	Empiric Therapy
Neonate (0-28 days)	Group B streptococcus, gram-negative enteric *(E. coli, Klebsiella, Listeria* monocytogenes, *S. aureus,* other gram-positive)	Cytomegalovirus Herpes simplex	Ampicillin and aminoglycoside (gentamicin or tobramycin or amikacin, or third-generation cephalosporin). *Note: Avoid ceftriaxone 2° to bilirubin*
Infants 3-16 weeks; afebrile pneumonia infancy		*Chlamydia trachomatis* *Ureaplasma urealyticum* Cytomegalovirus *Pneumocystis carinii*	Erythromycin Sulfonamide
Infants febrile or ill appearing age 1-3 months	Same organisms as for neonate plus *S. pneumoniae, H. influenzae, S. aureus*	Not applicable	Antibiotic (nafcillin, oxacillin, or methacillin) Broad-spectrum cephalosporin *(e.g., cefotaxime)*
Toddler or preschool age	*S. pneumoniae,* *H. influenzae* *M. pneumoniae,* *Chlamydia*	RSV Parainfluenza Adenovirus Influenza	Azithromycin Amoxacillin-clavulanate: not active against atypical organisms (Mycoplasma, Chlamydia)

The pathogens are listed in order of frequency, with the most common pathogen occurring first.

Whenever S. aureus is a pathogen, penicillinase-resistant penicillin is recommended. Depending on resistance patterns, methicillin may be used (if no resistance in community or vancomycin MRSA-methicillin-resistant S. aureus).

Pneumonia in Various Pediatric Age Groups: Etiology and Therapy

Neonate. Pneumonia in neonates is usually due to an organism acquired during passage through the birth canal. The most common pathogens causing pneumonia in the first month of life are group B streptococci followed by enteric gram-negative bacteria, usually *Escherichia coli* and *Klebsiella pneumonia*. Other pathogens include *Listeria monocytogenes*, other gram-positive cocci, viruses (most commonly, cytomegalovirus and herpes simplex virus), and *S. aureus*.

Thus, antibiotic coverage should include group B streptococci, enteric gram-negative bacteria, and listeria. Generally, penicillin-type antimicrobials are the drug of choice for the gram-positive pathogens, with ampicillin being preferred because of better in-vitro activity against enterococcus, listeria, and some gram-negative bacilli.

If *S. aureus* is a possibility, then a penicillinase-resistant penicillin is indicated. Methicillin is the usual choice although methicillin-resistant *S. aureus* has been found in some neonatal nurseries. Antibiotic coverage for the gram-negative bacilli depends on recent antimicrobial susceptibility patterns for newborns in that community and hospital; an aminoglycoside is usually chosen. This could be gentamicin, tobramycin, or amikacin.

Another acceptable alternative to ampicillin plus an aminoglycoside is the third-generation cephalosporin, cefotaxime. Ceftriaxone is not recommended in the neonate because the drug may cause displacement of bilirubin.

Regardless of their clinical appearance, all neonates with pneumonia, fever without a source, or sepsis should have an evaluation (including a CBC, chest roentgenogram, and appropriate cultures of blood, urine, and cerebrospinal fluid) followed by an initial dose of antibiotics and hospital admission. The empiric therapy would be ampicillin plus an aminoglycoside or ampicillin plus a cephalosporin.

Infants. Pneumonia in infants (older than 1 month but younger than 1 year) can be categorized into two groups: afebrile well-appearing infant vs. the febrile and/or ill-appearing infant.

"Afebrile pneumonia of infancy" generally occurs at the age of 3-4 weeks up to 16 weeks or from 1-4 months of age. It is due to organisms that colonized the infant at birth. It is also referred to as "chlamydia pneumonitis" since the most common pathogen is *Chlamydia trichomatis*, followed by (in order of decreasing frequency) ureaplasma urealyticum, cytomegalovirus, and *Pneumocystis carinii*. Classically, the infant has a gradual onset of symptoms with nasal congestion followed by a dry cough. Conjunctivitis usually precedes or occurs with the respiratory symptoms and is present in about half the patients. The infant is usually afebrile. Rarely is a low-grade fever present. The cough is probably the most prominent feature of "afebrile pneumonia of infancy." Often, the infant is alert and active and looks well, with the only symptom being a cough and the only physical examination finding being conjunctivitis. The cough may or may not interfere with the infant's usual activities such as feeding or sleeping. The cough may be paroxysmal like pertussis. Respiratory distress with tachypnea and retractions may occur. Rales are often but not always present. Wheezing may be present. This is usually a mild disorder, but respiratory distress, hypoxia, and/or apnea may occur.

Ancillary studies usually reveal a normal WBC count with eosinophilia and an interstitial pneumonia on chest radiograph. A culture or fluorescent antibody stain of nasopharyngeal secretions is positive for *Chlamydia*. The drug of choice, erythromycin (or sulfonamide), decreases the symptom duration. Outpatient therapy is the

Table 12. Antimicrobial Therapy for Specific Pathogens

Organism	Antimicrobial
BACTERIA	
S. pneumoniae	Penicillin (if not resistant). Vancomycin (if resistant to penicillin)
H. influenzae	Azithromycin or Amoxicillin (if not resistant)
Beta lactamase	Cefuroxime or third-generation cephalosporin (if beta lactamase + and resistant)
S. aureus	Methicillin (if not resistant) Vancomycin (if MRSA-methicillin resistant *S. aureus*) if penicillin allergy: vancomycin, clindamycin
ATYPICAL	
Chlamydia	Azithromycin (other macrolides); alternative, sulfa drugs
Mycoplasma	Azithromycin (other macrolides); alternative, tetracycline (if older than 8 years)
VIRUSES	
RSV	Ribavirin (optional)
Influenza	Amantadine (if severe)

Table 13. Factors Influencing Antibiotic Choice

INDIVIDUAL (PATIENT) FACTORS

- Patient's condition (co-morbid factors, respiratory/overall status)
- Recent antibiotic use
- Allergies
- Age (drug metabolism, age-related side effects)

DRUG FACTORS

- Efficacy/side effect profile of particular antibiotic
- Drug resistance patterns in the community
- Frequency of administration
- Duration of administration
- Cost

rule except if there are complications such as hypoxia, respiratory distress, dehydration, or apnea.

Infants (Febrile or Ill-Appearing). Infants (1-4 months) who are febrile and/or ill-appearing are presumed to have a bacterial pneumonia. Empiric antibiotic therapy for the febrile infant in this age group should include coverage for the usual neonatal pathogens as well as for the three pathogens most common in the toddler age group (*S. pneumoniae*, *H. influenza*, and *S. aureus*). A broad spectrum cephalosporin, such as cefotaxime, would cover the common neonatal pathogens as well as *S. pneumoniae* and *H. influenza*. A penicillinase-resistant penicillin, such as nafcillin, methicillin, or oxacillin, is added to provide antistaphylococcal coverage. One choice for empiric therapy would be cefotaxime and an antistaphylococcal antibiotic (nafcillin, oxacillin, or methacillin).

There have been reports of resistance of *S. pneumoniae* to penicillin (up to 20%), macrolides (about 10% combined for erythromycin, azithromycin, and clarithromycin), trimethoprim-sulfamethoxazole (18%), and various cephalosporins (from 3-12%).[63] However, there has not yet been documented penicillin failures in pneumococcal pneumonia. If there is penicillin resistance, then other antibiotics such as vancomycin can be used.[64]

Toddler/Preschooler. In this age group, the majority of the pneumoniae are due to viral infections.[65] The usual pathogens are respiratory syncytial virus (RSV), parainfluenza, adenovirus, influenza, other viruses (enterovirus and rhinovirus), and mycoplasma.

There is a seasonal variation with the various organisms. RSV tends to occur in the winter months, parainfluenza in the late summer and autumn, and influenza in the winter during influenza epidemics.

Given an appropriate scenario (e.g., toddler with no risk factors who looks well, with an outbreak of a given virus in the community so there is an appropriate epidemiologic setting) and reliable follow-up, then some feel a chest radiograph is optional and the patient may be observed as an outpatient without instituting antibiotic therapy. However, daily outpatient follow-up is mandatory since an occasional bacterial pneumonia may initially have a benign presentation like that of a virus, and a more severe secondary bacterial pneumonia may occur following a viral pneumonia.

If the toddler or preschooler is febrile or appears ill, then a bacterial pneumonia is likely. *S. pneumoniae* is the most common bacterial pathogen followed by *H. influenza*. Other less common bacterial organisms causing pneumonia are *Neisseria meningitides* and *S. aureus*. When *N. meningitides* pneumonia is present, generally it is in the content of meningococcemia and sepsis, so other signs and symptoms (such as petechiae) are present.

In the hospitalized toddler or preschooler, a broad-spectrum parenteral cephalosporin is a reasonable choice. If the patient looks well, has no risk factors or co-morbid conditions, or complications and close follow-up is assured, then possible antibiotic choices are a macrolide (azithromycin, clarithromycin, or erythromycin), amoxicillin/clavulanate, a broad-spectrum cephalosporin, or amoxicillin.[66] Although there is a 20-30% incidence of beta lactamase-positive resistance in most communities, amoxicillin remains an acceptable choice in those with mild disease because it is inexpensive as well as other factors.[66] *(See Table 12.)*

School Age Children and Adolescents. Once children enter school (ages 5-18 years), the atypical organisms are the most common cause of pneumonia followed by viral then bacterial pathogens. Mycoplasma is responsible for about one-fifth of all cases of pneumonia in the general population. The incidence of *M. pneumonia* increases during childhood, about 9-16% in school-age children (ages 5-12 years), 16-21% in adolescents (ages 12-18 years), and up to 30-50% in college students and military recruits.

The greatest incidence of pneumococcal pneumonia is in infants younger than 2 years. The macrolides (erythromycin, clarithromycin, and azithromycin) are the drugs of choice.[67] Those with severe disease should be hospitalized and also receive antibiotic coverage for other organisms including nontypeable *H. influenzae*. A third-generation cephalosporin plus a macrolide would be a good choice in these patients.

From the perspective of pediatric emergency medicine practice—with its primary emphasis on providing definitive, cost-effective, compliance-promoting, and drug-drug-interaction-minimizing therapy—the newer macrolide antibiotics, which include both azithromycin and clarithromycin, have recently emerged—along with amoxicillin-clavulanate—as drugs of choice for outpatient management of community-acquired pneumonia, as well as otitis media in children.[72] When used as oral agents, they play a central role in ED-based management of pneumonia in otherwise healthy children who do not require hospitalization. Unlike penicillins, cephalosporins, and sulfa-based agents, these drugs have the advantage of showing in vitro activity against both atypical and bacterial offenders implicated in pneumonia. The most common side effects include gastrointestinal upset and a metallic taste in the mouth, which are more common in clarithromycin.

These agents also have the advantage of a simplified dosing schedule, especially azithromycin, which is given once daily for five days. Clarithromycin requires a longer course of therapy and is slightly more expensive. In general, the decision to use a macrolide is based on weighing the cost of a course of therapy with azithromycin against its real-world advantages, which include a more convenient dosing schedule, its broader spectrum of coverage, its favorable drug interaction profile, and its decreased incidence of gastrointestinal side effects, which occur in 3-5% of patients taking a five-day, multiple-dose regimen.[73]

Azithromycin is approved in a palatable suspension formulation for the treatment of acute otitis media and pneumonia in children. The cost for a course of therapy is usually less than $30, and the once-daily, five-day course introduces compliance-enhancing features that, to a great degree, permit parental, day care, and grade school drug administration problems to be circumvented.[74] A well-accepted palatability profile, combined with an overall discontinuation rate of about 0.9%, are favorable as far as patient resistance is concerned.[75-77] When the five-day course of the suspension is used for treatment of otitis media, the reported incidences of side effects includes diarrhea/loose stools (2%), abdominal pain (2%), vomiting (1%), and nausea (1%).

From the perspective of drug resistance, the oral suspension of azithromycin is characterized by acceptable in vitro coverage of beta-lactamase-producing *H. influenzae* and *M. catarrhalis*, as well as in vitro coverage of *S. pneumoniae*, for which the overall resistance rate is estimated to be about 5-12%.[75-77]

The antimicrobial role of azithromycin and other macrolides in the ED, pediatric, and primary care setting is supported by rigorous otitis media studies that have been published comparing the safety and efficacy of azithromycin to amoxicillin-clavulanate for the treatment of acute otitis media in children.[75,78,79] In these large trials, clinical cure rates of up to 87.5% are reported, and azithromycin was as effective as, but better tolerated than, amoxicillin-clavulanate for the treatment of acute otitis media in the pediatric age group.[74,78-80] Although azithromycin does not affect a single IV dose of theophylline, caution is advised if multiple doses of theophylline are used. Accordingly, prudent clinical monitoring of theophylline levels is recommended in these patients.

The most common viral causes of pneumonia in this age group (5-18 years) are influenza, parainfluenza, and adenovirus. The most common cause of bacterial pneumonia in this age group remains *S. pneumoniae*.

Specific Pathogens

Streptococcus pneumoniae. *S. pneumoniae* is the most common cause of bacterial pneumonia in all pediatric age groups after the newborn period. The classic case of pneumococcal pneumonia is abrupt onset with fever, chills, cough, and dyspnea. Adolescents and adults with pneumococcal pneumonia may have hemoptysis or a blood tinged sputum. Asymptomatic carriage of *S. pneumoniae* in the nasopharynx occurs in up to 60% of individuals. The highest rates of carriage are in infants followed by families with children.

The greatest incidence of *S. pneumoniae* is in infants younger than 2 years old with the peak attack rate occurring at 3-5 months and peak hospitalization at 13-18 months. It is more frequent in the winter and spring months. Pneumonia from *S. pneumoniae* is greater in African-Americans and in males. There is a marked predilection for pneumococcal pneumonia in sickle cell disease, asplenia (whether congenital, surgical, or functional), and in immunosuppressed patients.

There is a 23 valent pneumococcal vaccine available, but it is poorly antigenic in young children (< 2 years of age), so it is currently used only in "at-risk" children older than 2 years of age, such as those with sickle cell disease or asplenia.[64] There are newer pneumococcal vaccines currently being evaluated that are promising.

Haemophilus influenzae. *H. influenzae* is still a cause of pneumonia, although there has been a marked decrease in disease secondary to *H. influenzae* since the advent of the hemophilus B conjugate (HIB) vaccine.[69,70] *H. influenzae* pneumonia is most prevalent in young children, with more than 80% of pneumonia occurring in children younger than 4 years of age. Like *S. pneumoniae*, *H. influenzae* may also colonize the nasopharynx and is more common in the winter and springs. Like the other bacterial pneumoniae, *H. influenzae* pneumonia usually begins with the abrupt onset of fever and cough. Extrapulmonary infections are more frequent with *H. influenzae* than with *S. pneumoniae* pneumonia. Infections ranging from otitis media, meningitis, pericarditis, and epiglottitis have been found in almost half of the patients with *H. influenzae* pneumonia. Positive blood cultures occur in 75-90% of children with *H. influenzae* pneumonia.

If the *H. influenzae* is beta-lactamase negative, then ampicillin can be used. Since there is increasing resistance to ampicillin from B-lactamase producing strains (up to 36%),[71,72] chloramphenicol or a broad spectrum cephalosporin, such as, cefotaxime, ceftriaxone, cefuroxime, can be used.

There can be secondary transmission of invasive *H. influenzae* type B so rifampin prophylaxis is recommended. Rifampin prophylaxis is indicated for close (household) contacts, of all ages (including adults) if there is an immunocompromised child in the household (regardless of vaccination status); if there is an incompletely vaccinated or unvaccinated child younger than 4 years of age in the household; if there is an incompletely vaccinated or unvaccinated child younger than 2 years in a day-care setting; and if there is an incompletely or unvaccinated child (children) in a day-care setting where more than two cases of invasive disease has occurred within two months.[73]

Staphylococcus aureus. *S. aureus* is an uncommon but important cause of pneumonia that can occur in any age group. *S. aureus* is a rapidly progressive fulminant illness so patients with this disease should be hospitalized. *S. aureus* is found on the skin, nasal mucosa, and other mucous membranes. *S. aureus* pneumonia may be primary or secondary. Primary disease is defined as pneumonia with no extra-pulmonary site of infection. Secondary pneumonia indicates the presence of one or more nonpulmonary sites of infection. Blood cultures are positive in 20-30% of patients with primary *S. aureus* pneumonia. The pleural effusions should be drained by thoracentesis or, if large, by a chest tube. Pneumatoceles are also common and are found in 45-60% of patients of patients with *S. aureus* pneumonia.

Antistaphylococcal penicillin (methicillin, oxacillin, or nafcillin) are the drugs of choice. In community-acquired pneumonia, methicillin-resistant *S. aureus* (MSRA) is rare. In hospitalized patients or patients in a long-term care facility, MSRA is more frequent, making vancomycin a better choice. If the patient has a penicillin allergy, then alternative antibiotics include vancomycin, clindamycin, or cefazolin.

Mycoplasma. *Mycoplasma* infections occur all year round with sporadic outbreaks in the fall and early winter. *M. pneumonia* generally has a gradual onset of symptoms that include a low-grade fever and a nonproductive cough. Headaches, myalgias, abdominal pain, and vomiting are other symptoms that can occur. Examination of the lungs may reveal rales or decreased breath sounds or a normal auscultation. The WBC count is usually normal. The cold agglutinins are positive, and the liver transaminase enzymes are often elevated. A small percentage of patients with mycoplasma pneumonia develop neurologic complications (about 7%) that range from meningoencephalitis to transverse myelitis, Guillan-Barré syndrome, to cerebellar ataxia. The preferred antibiotic for mycoplasma infection is the macrolides (erythromycin, clarithromycin, and azithromycin).[62,63]

Pertussis. Pertussis (whooping cough) usually occurs in infants younger than 6 months of age. It occurs in three clinical stages: catarrhal, paroxysmal, and convalescent stage.

The catarrhal stage lasts approximately 1-2 weeks. It begins with mild upper respiratory tract symptoms (coryza) and a cough. The paroxysmal stage, lasting 2-4 weeks, is characterized by a severe paroxysmal cough that may end with the classic inspiratory "whoop." Pertussis emesis often occurs. The characteristic whoop is frequently absent in infants. Generally, the patient is afebrile. The physical examination is fairly unremarkable between the paroxysms, which may be precipitated by gagging the patient. During the convalescent stage, the patient improves with the symptoms gradually disappearing.

The chest roentgenogram may be normal with clear lung fields or have a "shaggy" right heart border. Leukocytosis is generally present with a WBC count higher than 15,000/mm^3 up to 40,000/mm^3 and a marked lymphocytoses. The *Bordella pertussis* organism can be detected by culture or by fluorescent antibody staining of nasopharyngeal secretions during the catarrhal or early paroxysmal stages.

The antibiotic of choice for pertussis is erythromycin. In infants, pertussis is especially severe with frequent complications, therefore, all pediatric patients younger than 1 year of age should be hospitalized for monitoring and supportive care. Complications can include secondary bacterial pneumonia, apnea, seizures, encephalopathy, and death.

Respiratory Syncytial Virus. Respiratory syncytial virus (RSV) is the most common pediatric viral pneumonia, especially in infancy. RSV is most prevalent during the winter months, although epidemics may occur throughout the year. The hallmark of RSV infection is bronchiolitis. However, many infants with bronchiolitis (about one-third) will have pneumonia. Indeed, it is difficult to differentiate the two diseases (RSV bronchiolitis vs RSV pneumonia). Generally, if bronchospasm (e.g., wheezing) is present, the disease is classified as bronchiolitis, irrespective of whether or not pneumonia is also present.

The usual clinical signs of RSV infection include low-grade fever and signs of an upper respiratory infection. Generally, the temperature is less than that seen with bacterial pneumonia. A cough may be present. Wheezing and rales may be present simultaneously or may alternate during the 5-7 day course of the illness with wheezing present on one examination and rales on the next examination or vice versa. A normal or minimally elevated white blood cell count with a lymphocytosis is typical. The radiographic findings with RSV pneumonia are variable, but atelectasis is common.

Treatment is somewhat controversial. Some clinicians use bronchodilators if wheezing is present. There have been conflicting results from clinical trials on ribavirin, prompting the Committee on Infectious Diseases of the American Academy of Pediatrics to revise its recommendations.[74,75] Ribavirin should be considered "based on the clinical circumstances and physicians' preferences."[76] Studies on the use of intravenous RSV immunoglobulin (RSV-IGIV) and intramuscular RSV monoclonal antibodies are in progress. Preliminary results suggest that RSV-IGIV is effective in preventing RSV infection in preterm infants but not effective in treating RSV infections.[76]

Unusual Causes of Pneumonia

Other unusual causes of pneumonia can be related to certain exposures, travel, or hobbies. *(See Table 9.)* Tuberculosis has a variable clinical presentation and radiologic findings and is in the differential diagnosis of pneumonia. Histoplasmosis is endemic to the Mississippi river valley region. Coccidiomycosis is endemic to the Southwestern United States as is Hantavirus, which is especially associated with the "four corner" region of Arizona, New Mexico, Utah, and Colorado. *Chlamydia psittaci* pneumonia is transmitted via exotic birds. *Francisella tularensis* pneumonia could occur in a teenager or child who has been hunting with his/her parent.

Clinical Course of Pneumonia

Bacterial pneumonias generally resolve quickly once treatment including appropriate antibiotics is started unless complications occur. *(See Table 13.)* Generally, the patient will defervesce and feel significantly better within 24-48 hours of instituting therapy. Viral and atypical pneumonia have a more gradual onset and a slower resolution of symptoms.

Clearing of the abnormalities on the chest radiograph takes longer than resolution of the clinical symptoms and may not clear for weeks (up to about 6 weeks). In patients with an acute pneumonia discharged from the ED, follow-up especially in infants and young children may be in two stages: initial (24 hours) to check for deterioration or complications and delayed (about 6 weeks) in order to document radiographic resolution.

In the pediatric patient with nonresolving or recurrent pneumonia, other conditions need to be considered. These include: chronic infections, (tuberculosis is a major consideration, but fungal and parasitic infections may be present), primary pulmonary diseases (ranging from asthma to cystic fibrosis), aspiration (whether due to foreign body, chemicals, toxins, or anatomic/physiologic factors), malignancy, pulmonary infarction (pulmonary emboli or sickle cell vasoocclusion), congenital disorders (sequestration, cysts), autoimmune disease (lupus pneumonitis), and immunologic diseases. *(See Table 10.)*

When encountering such a patient with recurrent or nonresolving "pneumonia," treat for an acute infectious pneumonia with appropriate antibiotics until an infectious cause can be ruled out. Depending on the clinical situation, other studies (skin tests, laboratory tests, fungal or tuberculosis cultures, etc.) can be done.

Management. Management of pneumonia includes supportive care, the appropriate use of antimicrobials, *(see Tables 11 and 13)* and hospitalization in selected cases. The patient's age, the likely pathogen, *(see Tables 6 and 7)* and the severity of the illness direct the management. Hospital admission is mandatory in any patient with hypoxemia, respiratory distress, a neonate, or underlying disease (including: sickle cell disease, malignancy, immunosuppression, etc.). *(See Table 8.)* Hospitalization is warranted if complications of the pneumonia are present, such as empyema, lung abscess, a moderate to large pleural effusion, bacteremia, or sepsis. Other indications for hospital admission include: dehydration, inability to take oral fluids or medications, and/or failure to respond to outpatient therapy. Presumed or proven pneumonia due to certain highly virulent organisms, such as *S. aureus* or meningococcus warrants inpatient therapy. *(See Table 8.)*

If bacterial pneumonia is suspected (or proven), selection of an appropriate antibiotic is based on factors including: the patient's age, clinical presentation (signs and symptoms including their overall appearance, respiratory status, and vital signs), laboratory and radiographic findings, epidemiologic considerations, etc. Empiric antibiotic therapy may need to be chosen *(see Table 11)* and therapy modified when culture and ancillary laboratory results are available.

A determination of whether the pneumonia is bacterial, viral, or an atypical (e.g., mycoplasma or chlamydia) pneumonia is also based on the above factors since there is no one definitive test (or sign or symptom) that is pathognomonic (except perhaps for a positive blood culture that is not available when the patient is initially seen). Unfortunately, since a definitive diagnosis is not often available when the patient first presents to the physician, treatment is based on a presumptive etiology. *(See Tables 6 and 7.)*

Supportive care includes: hydration (sometimes intravenous), control of fever, management of complications, and respiratory support. Respiratory care may range from oxygenation, bronchodilators for wheezing, humidification or mist, suctioning, and postural drainage, intubation and mechanical ventilation.

An empyema and some pleural effusions (especially if interfering with respiration) of moderate to large size may need to be drained either by thoracentesis or a chest tube. Empyema usually requires a chest tube. Thoracentesis of a pleural effusion may also need to be done for diagnostic purposes.

Pneumonia secondary to a foreign body may require removal of the foreign body before the pneumonia will resolve. Apnea and respiratory failure may occur precipitously in infants with bacterial pneumonia (ages 3-6 months) consequently monitoring and hospitalization is appropriate.

Antiviral agents may be indicated in certain high-risk patients: former premature infants with bronchopulmonary dysplasia, chronic lung diseases (such as cystic fibrosis), certain congenital heart diseases, and immunodeficiencies. The two common antiviral agents are ribavirin (for respiratory syncytial virus) and amantadine for influenza. *(See Table 12.)*

Summary

Pneumonia in pediatric patients encompasses a wide spectrum of etiologies and illness from mild to severe and life threatening. Fortunately, most pediatric patients with pneumonia have mild disease and can be treated as an outpatient.

Outpatient therapy should include an antibiotic if a bacteria or atypical bacteria (chlamydia or mycoplasma) is suspected. No antibiotics are necessary for viral pneumonia. Outpatient supportive therapy also includes fever control and maintenance of hydration. Close follow-up is necessary in order to detect any secondary bacterial infection or the development of complications. Pediatric patients, especially infants and young children, diagnosed with pneumonia in the ED should have follow-up within 24 hours. Use of parenteral antibiotics (e.g., intramuscular ceftriaxone) may expand our ability to treat pediatric patients with pneumonia as outpatients.

References

1. Campbell PW, Stokes DC. Pneumonia. In: Loughlin GM, Eigen H, ed. *Respiratory Disease in Children. Diagnosis and Management.* Baltimore: Williams and Wilkins; 1994: 351-372.
2. Chase PS, Hilton NS. Pneumonia. In: Reisdorff EJ, Roberts MR, Wiegenstein JG. eds. *Pediatric Emergency Medicine.* Philadelphia: WB Saunders Co.; 1993:280-289.
3. Letourneau MA, Schuh S, Gauschem. Respiratory Disorders-Pneumonia. In: Barkin RM, Asch SM, Caputo GL, et al, eds. *Pediatric Emergency Medicine.* St. Louis: Mosby Yearbook; 1992:1011-1016.
4. Murphy TF, Henderson FW, Clyde WA Jr., et al. Pneumonia: An eleven-year study in a pediatric practice. *Am J Epidemiol* 1981;113:12-21.
5. Fosarelli PD, DeAngelis C, Winkelstein J, et al. Infectious diseases in the first two years of life. *Pediatr Inf Dis* 1985;4: 153-159.
6. Baker MB, Scanlin TF. Pulmonary emergencies. In: Fleischer GR, Ludwig S, Silverman BK, eds. *Synopsis of Pediatric Emergency Medicine.* Baltimore: Williams and Wilkins; 1996:489-501.
7. Prober CG. Pneumonia. In: Nelson WE, Behrman RE, Kliegman RM, et al, eds. *Nelsons Textbook of Pediatrics,* 15th ed. Philadelphia: WB Saunders Co.; 1996:716-721.
8. Meeker DP, Longworth DL. Community-acquired pneumonia: An update. *Cleveland Clin J Med* 1996;63:16-30.
9. Musher DM, Spindel SJ. Community-acquired pneumonia. *Curr Clin Topics Infect Dis* 1996;16:102-124.
10. O'Brodovich HM, Haddad GG. The functional basis of respi-

ratory pathology and disease. In: Chernick V, Boat TF, Kendig EL, eds. *Kendig's Disorders of the Respiratory Tract in Children.* 6th ed. Philadelphia: WB Saunders Co.; 1998: 27-73.

11. Mercer RR, Crapo JD. Normal anatomy and defense mechanisms of the lung. In: Baum GL, Celli BR, Crapo JD, et al, eds. *Textbook of Pulmonary Diseases* Vol 1. 6th ed. Philadelphia: Lippincott-Raven Publishers; 1998:23-45.
12. Said S. Metabolic and endocrine functions of the lung. In: Chernick V, Boat TF, Kendig EL, eds. *Kendig's Disorders of the Respiratory Tract in Children.* 6th ed. Philadelphia: WB Saunders Co.; 1998:74-84.
13. Reynolds HY, Elias JA. Pulmonary defense mechanisms against infections. In: Fishman AP, Elias JA, Fishman JA, et al, eds. *Fishman's Pulmonary Diseases and Disorders.* Vol 1. 3rd ed. New York: McGraw Hill; 1998:265-274.
14. Ashbourne JF, Downey PM. Pneumonia. In Rosen P, Barken RM, Braen CR, et al, eds. *Emergency Medicine—Concepts and Clinical Practice.* Vol 2. 3rd ed. St. Louis Mosby Year Book; 1992:1162-1177.
15. Blinkhorn RJ Jr. Community-acquired pneumonia. In: Baum GL, Celli BR, Crapo JD, et al, eds. Vol 1. 6th ed. Philadelphia: Lippincott-Raven Publishers; 1998:503-542.
16. Committee on Environmental Hazards. Involuntary smoking—a hazard to children. *Pediatrics* 1986;77:755-757.
17. Denny FW, Collier AM, Henderson FW. Acute respiratory infections in daycare. *Rev Infect Dis* 1986;8:527-532.
18. Morris K, Morganlander M, Coulehan JL, et al. Woodburning stoves and lower respiratory tract infections in American Indian Children. *Am J Dis Child* 1990;1;4:490.
19. Connors K, Terndrup TE. Viral and bacterial pneumonia in children. In: Tintinalli JE, Ruiz E, Kroma RL, eds. *Emergency Medicine—A Comprehensive Study Guide.* New York; McGraw-Hill, 1996:622-625.
20. Schutzman SA, Caputo GL. Pneumonia. In: Rosen P, Barkin RM, Braen GR, et al, eds. *Emergency Medicine-Concepts and Clinical Practice.* Vol 3. 3rd ed. St. Louis: Mosby Year Book; 1992:2761-2769.
21. Miller MJ, Fanaroff AA, Martin PJ. The respiratory system-pneumonia. In: Fanaroff AA, Martin RJ, eds. *Neonatal-Perinatal Medicine.* Vol 2. 5th ed. St. Louis: Mosby Year Book; 1992:838-839.
22. Feigin RD, Adcock LM, Edwards MS. The immune system. In: Fanaroff AA, Martin RJ, eds. Vol 2. 5th ed. St. Louis: Mosby Year Book; 1992:587-690.
23. Baraff LJ, Bass JW, Fleisher GR, et al. Practice guidelines for the management of infants and children 0-36 months of age with fever without source. *Pediatrics* 1993;92:1-12.
24. Baraff LT, Bass JW, Fleisher GR, et al. Health Care Policy and Research. Practice guidelines for the management of infants 0-36 months of age with fever without source. *Ann Emerg Med* 1993;22:1198-1210.
25. Mace SE, Le Nga. Controversies in the evaluation and management of a febrile infant or young child. *J Clin Outcomes Man* 1997;4:52-63.
26. Gotoff SP. Infections of the newborn-neonatal sepsis. In: Behrman RE, Kliegman RM, Nelson WE, et al, eds. *Nelson Textbook of Pediatrics.* 14th ed. Philadelphia: WB Saunders Co.; 1992:501-504.
27. Modlin JF. Bacterial pneumonia. In: Oski FA, DeAngelis CD, Feigin RD, et al, eds. *Principles and Practice of Pediatrics.* 2nd ed. Philadelphia: JB Lippincott Co.; 1994:1472-1474.
28. Prober CG. Pneumonia in the neonate. In: Behrman RE, Kliegman RM, Arvin AM, eds. *Nelson Textbook of Pediatrics.* 15th ed. Philadelphia: WB Saunders Co; 1996:537-539.
29. Singhi S, Dharvan A, Kataria S, et al. Clinical signs of pneumonia in infants under 2 months. *Arch Dis Child* 1994;70: 413-417.
30. Margolis PA, Ferkal TW, Marsocci S, et al. Accuracy of the clinical examination in detecting hyperoxemia in infants with respiratory illness. *J Pediatr* 1994;24:552-560.
31. Connors K. Pneumonia. In: Strange GR, Ahrens WR, Lelyveld S, et al, eds. *Pediatric Emergency Medicine—A Comprehensive Study Guide.* New York: McGraw-Hill; 1996:176-180.
32. Schidlow DV, Callahan CW. Pneumonia. *Pediatr Review* 1996;17:300-310.
33. McCarthy PL, Klig JE, Shapiro EL, et al. Fever without apparent source on clinical examination, lower respiratory tract infections in children, other infectious diseases and acute gastroenteritis, and diarrhea of infancy and early childhood. *Curr Opin Pediatr* 1996;8:75-93.
34. Paternack MS. Pneumonia in childhood. In: Fishman AP, Elias JA, Fishman JA, et al, eds. *Fishman's Pulmonary Diseases and Disorders.* New York: McGraw-Hill; 1998: 1997-2010.
35. Peter G. In: Burg FD, Ingelfinger JR, Wald ER, eds. *Gellis and Kgan's Current Pediatric Therapy.* Philadelphia: WB Saunders Co.; 1993:563-567.
36. Korppi M. Physical signs in childhood pneumonia. *Pediatric Infect Dis J* 1995;14:405-406.
37. Harari M, Shann F, Spooner V, et al. Clinical sign of pneumonia in children. *Lancet* 1991;338:928-930.
38. Fleicher GR. Infectious Disease Emergencies-Chlamydial Pneumonia In: Fleisher GR, Ludwig S, Henretig FM, et al, eds. *Textbook of Pediatric Emergency Medicine.* 3rd ed. Baltimore: Williams and Wilkins; 1993:624-625.
39. Law BJ. Pertussis. In: Chernick V, Boat TF, Kendig EL, eds. *Kendig's Disorders of the Respiratory Tract in Children.* Philadelphia: WB Saunders Co.; 1998:1018-1025.
40. Donowitz GR, Mandell GL. Acute pneumonia. In: Mandell GL, Bennett JE, Dolin R, eds. *Mandell, Douglas and Bennet's Principles and Practice of Infectious Diseases.* Vol 1. 4th ed. New York: Churchill Livingstone;1995:619-637.
41. Correa AG, Starke JR. Bacterial pneumonia. In: Chernick V, Boat TF, Kendig EL, eds. *Kendig's Disorders of the Respiratory Tract in Children.* 6th ed. Philadelphia. WB Saunders Co; 1998:485-503.
42. Chartrand SA, McCracken GH. *Staphylococcal pneumonia* in infants and children. *Pediatr Infect Dis J* 1982;1:19-23.
43. Hickey RW, Bowman MJ, Smith GA. Utility of blood cultures in prediatric patients found to have pneumonia in the emergency department. *Ann Emerg Med* 1996;27:721-725.
44. Correa AG. Diagnostic approach to pneumonia in children. *Semin Resp In* 1996;11:131-138.
45. Rusconi F, Rancilio L. Assael BM, et al. Counterimmuno-

electrophoresis and latex particle agglutination in the etiologic diagnosis of presumed bacterial pneumonia in pediatric patients. *Pediatr Infect Dis J* 1988;7:781-785.
46. Isaacs D. Problems in determining the etiology of community acquired childhood pneumonia. *Pediatr Infect Dis* 1989;8: 143-148.
47. Ramsey BW, Marcuse EK, Foy HM, et al. Use of bacterial antigen detection in the diagnosis of pediatric lower respiratory tract infections. *Pediatrics* 1986;78:1-9.
48. Turner RB, Hayden FG, Hendley JD. Counterimmunoelectrophoresis of urine for the diagnosis of bacterial pneumonia in pediatric patients. *Pediatric* 1983;71:780-783.
49. Fernald GW. Infections of the respiratory tract due to mycoplasma pneumoniae. In: Chernick V, Boat TF, Kendig EL, eds. *Kendig's Disorders of the Respiratory Tract in Children.* 6th ed. Philadelphia: WB Saunders Co., 1998: 526-532.
50. Baum SG. *Mycoplasma pneumoniae* and atypical pneumonia. In: Mandell GL, Bennett JE, Dolin R, eds. *Mandell, Doughlas and Bennett's Principles and Practice of Infectious Diseases.* Vol 2, 4th ed. New York: Churchill Livingstone; 1995:1704-1713.
51. deBlic J, McKelvie P, leBourgeois M, Blanche S, Benoist MR, Scheinmann P. Value of bronchoalveolar lavage in the management of severe acute pneumonia and interstitial pneumonias in the immunocompromised child. *Thorax* 1987;42: 759-765.
52. Wood RE. The diagnostic effectiveness of the flexible bronchoscope in children. *Pediatric Pulmonol* 1985;1:188-192.
53. Pianosi P. Diagnostic and therapeutic procedures. In Chernick V, Boat TF, Kendig EL, eds. *Kendig's Disorders of the Respiratory Tract in Children.* 6th ed. Philadelphia; 1998: 106-129.
54. Swischuk LE. Respiratory system-postnatal pulmonary infections. In: *Imaging of the Newborn Infant and Young Child.* Baltimore: Williams and Wilkins; 1997:108-125.
55. McCarthy PL, Spiesel SZ, Stashwick CA, et al. Radiographic findings and etiologic diagnosis in ambulatory childhood pneumonias. *Clin Pediatr* 1981;20(11):686-691.
56. Davies HD, Wang EE-L, Manson D, et al. Reliability of the chest radiogrpah in the diagnosis of lower respiratory tract infections in young children. *Pediatr Inf Dis* 1996;15: 600-604.
57. Oermann CM, Moore RH. Foolers: Things that look like pneumonia in children. *Semin Resp Infect* 1996;11:204-213.
58. Swischuk LE. Respiratory System-other pulmonary abnormalities. In: *Imaging of the Newborn Infant and Young Child.* Baltimore: Williams and Wilkins; 1997:126-142.
59. Harris JH, Harris WH, Novelline RA. The Chest. In: *The Radiology of Emergency Medicine.* Baltimore: Williams and Wilkins; 1993:469-622.
60. Bramson RT, Meyer TL, Blickman JG, et al. The futility of the chest radiograph in the febrile infant without respiratory symptoms. *Pediatrics* 1993;92:524-526.
61. Heulitt MJ, Ablow RC, Santos CC, et al. Febrile infants less than 3 months old: Value of chest radiography. *Radiology* 1988;167:135-137.
62. Crain EF, Bulas D, Bijur PE, et al. Is a chest radiograph necessary in the evaluation of every febrile infant less than 8 weeks of age? *Pediatrics* 1991;88:821-824.
63. Doern GV, Brueggemann A, Holley HP J, Rauch AM. Antimicrobial resistance of *Streptococcus pneumoniae* recovered from outpatients in the United States during the winter months of 1994 to 1995: Results of a 30-center national surveillance study. *Antimicrob Agents Chemother* 1996;40: 1208-1213.
64. Bartlett JG, Procter RA eds. Etiology/Causative Agents-Resistance and Emergency Patterns. Respiratory Infection in the Year 2000. Managing Community-Acquired Pneumonia and Acute Exacerbations of Chronic Bronchitis-Consensus Conference Proceedings—1998. University of Wisconsin 1998;1-24.
65. Glezen WP. Viral Pneumonia. In: Chernick V, Boat TF, Kendig EL, eds. *Kendig's Disorders of the Respiratory Tract in Children.* 6th ed. Philadelphia: WB Saunders Co; 1998: 518-525.
66. Harris JS. Antimicrobial therapy of pneumonia in infants and children. *Semin Resp Inf* 1996;11:139-147.
67. Bosker G. Antibiotic update 1998: outcome effetive treatment guidelines for bacterial infections managed in the primary care and emergency department settings. *Emerg Med Reports* 1997;18:1-24.
68. Committee on Infectious Diseases of the American Academy of Pediatrics "Pneumococcal Infection, Active immunization 1997 Red Book." *Report of the Committee on Infectious Diseases.* 24th ed. Elk Grove, Illinois: American Academy of Pediatrics; 1997:416-418.
69. Mulholland K, Hilton S, Adegbola R, et al. Randomized trial of *Haemophilus influenza* type-b tetanus protein conjugate vaccine [corrected] for prevention of pneumonia and meningitis in Gambian infants. *Lancet* 1997;249:1191-1197.
70. Liptak GS, McConnochie KM, Roghmann KJ, et al. Decline of pediatric admissions with *Haemohpilus influenzae* type-b in New York State, 1982 through 1983: Relation to immunizations. *J Pediatr* 1997;130:923-930.
71. Barry AL, Pfaller MA, Fuchs PC, Packer RR. In vitro activities of 12 orally administered antimicrobial agents against four species of bacterial respiratory pathogens from U.S. medical centers in 1992 and 1993. *Antimicrob Agents Chemother* 1994;38:2419-2425.
72. Doern GV. Trends in antimicrobial susceptibility of bacterial pathogens of the respiratory tract. *Am J Med* 1995;99(suppl 6B):3S-7S.
73 Committee on Infectious Diseases of the American Academy of Pediatrics. *Haemophilus influenzae* infections—rifampin chemoprophylaxis. 1997 Red Book. Report of the Committee on Infectious Diseases. 24th ed. American Academy of Pediatrics; Elk Grove, Illinois; 1997:222-226.
74. Committee on Infectious Diseases of the American Academy of Pediatrics. Reassessment of indications for ribavirin therapy. *Pediatrics* 1996;97:137-140.
75. Committee on Infectious Diseases of the American Academy of Pediatrics. Use of ribavirin in the treatment of respiratory syncytial virus infection. *Pediatrics* 1993;92:501-504.
76. Committee on Infectious Diseases of the American Academy of Pediatrics. Respiratory syncytial virus-treatment. *1997 Red*

Book. Report of the Committee on Infectious Diseases. 24th ed. American Academy of Pediatrics. Elk Grove, Illinois; 1997:445-447.

Stridor in Children

Steven G. Rothrock, MD, FACEP
Ronald Perkin, MD

The clinical presentation has life or death written all over it. And for good reason. An acutely ill child who presents to the emergency department (ED) with stridor invariably triggers consideration of an extensive differential diagnosis that includes both mild and life-threatening conditions. Because complete airway obstruction, respiratory collapse, and operative intervention are potential elements of the clinical scenario, swift action is mandatory. The best clinical outcome is achieved through implementation of a systematic, proven protocol for managing patients with stridor.

From a diagnostic perspective, several issues will challenge the emergency practitioner: First, what is the etiology of the stridor? Croup? Epiglottitis? Retropharyngeal abscess? Next, are diagnostic studies necessary to confirm the diagnosis? Or will they delay definitive intervention and precipitate clinical deterioration? Is immediate control of the airway required? If so, should a team experienced in pediatric airway control be assembled to provide support? Finally, what pharmacotherapeutic measures can provide rapid improvement without delaying targeted management of the airway?

Fortunately, the management of children with stridor has become increasingly focused and systematic. For one thing, the infectious agents producing clinical syndromes associated with stridor have changed dramatically since the introduction of vaccines directed against *Haemophilus influenzae* type B, which is fading from the scene as the principal offender in epiglottitis. More and more, the ED physician must have a high index of suspicion for atypical offenders, among them *Candida* species, herpes simplex, and Staphylococcal organisms.[1]

Changes in the causative organisms for stridor syndromes have been accompanied by significant departures from the accepted management catechism for diseases such as epiglottitis and croup. For example, whereas the use of racemic epinephrine once mandated admission to the hospital, recent studies have questioned this dogma.[2] Moreover, the strict admonition against direct examination of the hypopharynx also has been questioned, with current recommendations permitting such evaluation providing specific clinical criteria are satisfied. Finally, newer treatment regimens, including nebulized epinephrine (L isomer) and intramuscular steroids, have proven effective in clinical management.[3]

With these evolving issues in clear focus, the purpose of this review is to provide a systematic, targeted approach that examines diagnostic options and management pathways that will improve outcomes for this common—yet anxiety-provoking—clinical problem.

What is Stridor?

Stridor is a musical, high-pitched sound of respiration that is a sign of partial obstruction of the upper airway, which begins with the pharynx and includes the trachea and the main bronchi. The Venturi effect explains the sounds that are heard.[6] The pressure exerted on a partially closed tube by a gas is equal in all directions except during linear movement. Linear flow creates additional pressure in a forward direction in the tube with a corresponding fall in lateral wall pressure. In other words, during inspiration, areas of the airway that are easily collapsible (e.g., posterior pharynx and above the glottis) are "suctioned" closed; during expiration, these areas are forced open. Thus, sounds are created due to the changing shape and size of the airway.

The fact that different parts of the airway are more collapsible than others accounts for differences in presentation of airway disease. For example, above the glottis (vocal cords), there is only soft tissue and no cartilage; therefore, this area collapses more easily during inspiration compared to airway at the vocal cords and the glottis. The trachea, on the other hand, is less collapsible. Therefore, obstructive lesions at this level lead to stridor that changes little during inspiration and expiration.

Clinical and Anatomical Correlations

Anatomically, the upper airway can be divided into three main areas: 1) the supraglottic airway (above the vocal cords); 2) the glottic and subglottic airway; and 3) the intrathoracic airway. Depending on the location of obstruction, disorders that cause stridor have a variable propensity to develop complete obstruction, and they have different clinical features. *(See Figure 1.)*

Supraglottic Airway. The supraglottic airway comprises the section of the airway from the nose to just above the vocal cords. Importantly, this part of the airway is easily distensible and easily collapsible because there is no cartilaginous support. Due to the presence of multiple tissue planes, localized infections can spread easily and form abscesses. In young children (especially < 2 years old), the retropharyngeal space contains lymph nodes that may serve as a nidus for formation of abscesses. Eventually, these retropharyngeal lymph nodes atrophy, and the risk of abscess formation decreases as children age.

Classic important diseases that cause obstruction or stridor at this level include supraglottitis (epiglottitis), retropharyngeal abscess(es), and diphtheria, although many other supraglottic conditions also produce this finding. Stridor from supraglottic obstruction generally produces a sound that is heard primarily on inspiration, since the airway easily collapses from the negative pressure exerted with inspiration. With exhalation, the airway is reinflated and the obstruction improves. Drooling can be a prominent feature, since the obstruction is above the level of the esophagus and patients may be unable to swallow. A muffled or "hot-potato" voice also may be prominent. This is caused by an obstruction between the listener and the vocal cords, as the vocal cords are generally uninvolved. Therefore, the sound produced by the vocal cords is normal while the obstruction muffles what the examiner is hearing.

It should be stressed that disorders causing supraglottic obstruction have the potential to rapidly obstruct the airway. Obstruction may be swift and lethal since this part of the airway collapses the most easily.

Glottic and Subglottic Airway. The glottic and subglottic airway extends from the vocal cords to the trachea before entering the thoracic cavity. This part of the airway is not as collapsible as the supraglottic airway because cartilage (cricoid cartilage and incomplete tracheal cartilaginous rings) surrounds the majority of its length.

The most common disorder causing obstruction at this level is laryngotracheobronchitis (croup). Many congenital disorders can also cause stridor or partial obstruction at this level, including laryngomalacia, tracheomalacia, and vocal cord paralysis. The ED physician should appreciate that inflammation or obstruction at the glottis (vocal cords) leads to a hoarse-sounding voice and not muffling, as seen with supraglottic disease. Stridor may occur during inspiration *(see Figure 1)* or during inspiration and expiration since the shape and size of this part of the airway changes little during respiration. Although drooling implies obstruction above or at the esophagus and not at the level of the glottis or trachea, a large obstructing tracheal lesion or foreign body can compress the posterior wall of the trachea, leading to esophageal obstruction and drooling. Therefore, the presence of drooling should not be considered concrete evidence that a lesion is not at the level of the glottis or trachea.

Intrathoracic Airway. The intrathoracic airway is comprised of the trachea that lies within the thoracic cavity and the mainstem bronchi. Intrathoracic airway obstruction causes stridor that is loudest on expiration since intrathoracic pressure rises on expiration and tends to cause airway collapse. During inspiration, intrathoracic pressures fall, and the thoracic airway (and any existing obstruction) tends to expand, leading to a quieter sound. Congenital disorders are also a prominent cause of obstruction at this level (e.g., vascular slings and webs). Furthermore, although foreign bodies frequently lodge at this level, they can lodge at any site within the upper or lower airway.

Systematic Assessment of Stridor

The Seven Airway A's. Seven important clues can be used to help identify the cause of a child's upper airway obstruction or stridor. These include:

- Age;
- Acuity of onset;
- Associated symptoms;
- Appearance;
- Acoustics (the quality of sound);
- Air-shadow interface (radiographs); and
- Airway examination.

Age is an important factor that can help identify the etiology of a child's stridor. While generalizations can be made about the age at which certain disorders present, most non-congenital disorders can produce stridor at any age. Generally, congenital disorders (e.g., vocal cord paralysis, laryngomalacia, and tracheomalacia) present during the first few weeks of life. At about 6 months of age, infants begin to explore their environment and place objects in their mouth, which can lead to foreign body aspiration. Developmentally, the pediatric patient's ability to grasp small, potentially aspirated objects progresses from a raking motion at 7 months to a distinct pincer grasp at 1 year of age. The incidence of foreign body aspiration peaks at around 2-3 years of age and tapers off by age 5. Croup also occurs primarily in infants younger than 3 years old. Importantly, retropharyngeal abscesses are most common in those youner than age 4, since retropharyngeal lymph nodes generally atrophy after this age.

In the past, epiglottitis was described as a disease that usually occurred in children 2-7 years of age. However, epiglottitis can occur at *any* age, from neonate to adult. In fact, since the introduction of the *H. influenzae* type B vaccine, the overall incidence of epiglottitis has

Figure 1. Critical Pathway in Emergency Medicine: Stridor CPEM

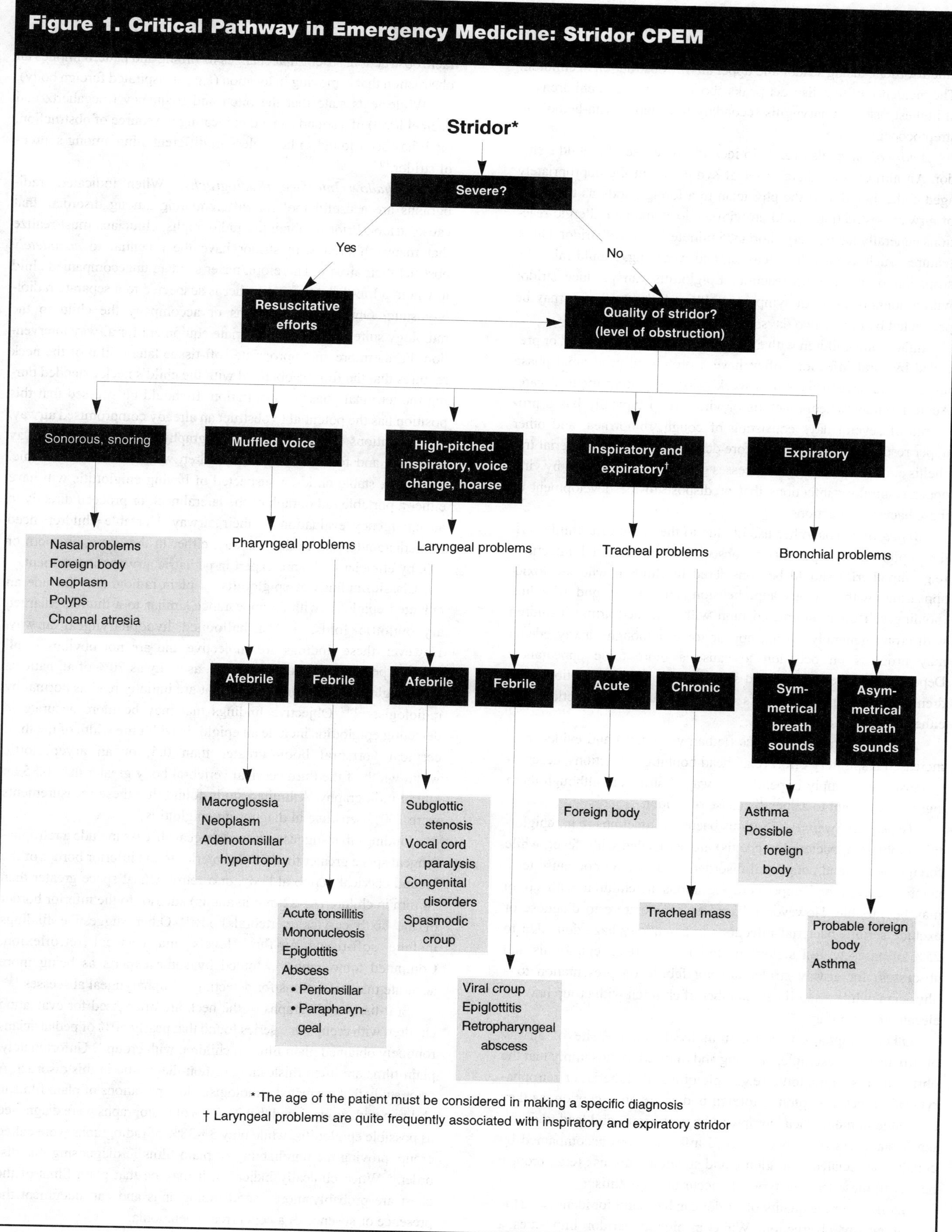

* The age of the patient must be considered in making a specific diagnosis

† Laryngeal problems are quite frequently associated with inspiratory and expiratory stridor

dropped dramatically, and the peak age incidence for epiglottitis is now greater than 7 years.[1] Peritonsillar abscesses are another important disorder causing stridor and upper airway obstruction in children. The incidence of this disorder peaks above age 10, when children are at highest risk for pharyngitis secondary to group A beta-hemolytic streptococci.[7]

Acuity of onset also can help identify the cause of a child's stridor. An almost immediate onset of symptoms in the appropriately aged child should alert the physician to a foreign body as the cause of airway obstruction. Children with angioedema and allergic reactions generally have a very short (< 5 minutes) onset of stridor. Other features, such as rash, hypotension, and wheezing, should raise the suspicion of an allergic reaction. Epiglottitis can produce stridor within hours of onset of symptoms, although the prodrome may be protracted by one or two days.

Infants and children with airway disorders that are caused or preceded by viral infections often have a protracted prodromal phase lasting from several days to a week prior to seeking medical care. Acute laryngotracheobronchitis or viral croup typically has a prodrome of several days consisting of cough, rhinorrhea, and other upper respiratory symptoms before developing stridor. Bacterial tracheitis and retropharyngeal abscesses generally are preceded by viral upper respiratory infections that predispose to the development of these bacterial infections.

Appearance is another useful clue to the cause of a child's stridor. Epiglottitis, upper airway abscesses, and bacterial infections (e.g., diphtheria) should be considered in children who are toxic-appearing, with obvious apprehension, air hunger, and tripoding (holding self up in sitting position with extended arms). Children with croup generally do not appear toxic, although airway edema may progress on occasion to cause a more toxic appearance. Depending on the location and severity of airway obstruction, children with congenital disorders and foreign body obstruction may either appear toxic or nontoxic.

Alterations in mental status (lethargy, anxiety) and evidence of increased respiratory effort (e.g., head bobbing, retractions, accessory muscle use) imply impending airway obstruction, although these signs do not point to a specific cause of stridor.

Associated Symptoms. Serious bacterial infections (e.g., epiglottitis, diphtheria, bacterial tracheitis) are associated with fever, while foreign bodies and congenital disorders as a rule do not cause temperature elevation. Temperature elevations in children with croup may be variable. However, reliance on temperature to diagnose or exclude serious bacterial infections is potentially hazardous. Up to 25% of cases with a serious bacterial cause (e.g., epiglottitis and abscesses) for airway stridor are *not* febrile on presentation to a physician, while a significant number of children with croup have an elevated temperature.[8,9]

Other symptoms may assist in localizing the site of airway obstruction. For example, drooling and muffled sounds imply that the obstruction is supraglottic (e.g., epiglottitis, diphtheria, or retropharyngeal abscess). Aspirated foreign bodies are an exception, as they can lodge in the trachea, compress the esophagus, and lead to drooling. Hoarseness (due to vocal cord inflammation) accompanied by cough is associated with glottic and subglottic disease (e.g., croup), neither of these features typically occur in epiglottitis.

Acoustics or the quality of stridor can be useful for identifying the site of airway obstruction. While inspiratory stridor implicates a supraglottic obstruction, biphasic stridor implicates glottic or subglottic obstruction, and expiratory stridor is indicative of intrathoracic obstruction, stridor that changes its timing and pattern implies an obstruction that is moving in location (e.g., an aspirated foreign body).

While texts state that the pitch and frequency (megahertz and decibel level) of a sound can aid in locating the source of obstruction, pitch has been found to be useless in differentiating among sources of stridor.[10]

Air-Shadow Interface (Radiographs). When indicated, radiographs are a useful tool for differentiating among disorders that cause stridor. Prior to obtaining radiographs, clinicians must realize that many children with stridor have the potential to *completely* obstruct their airway. Therefore, never send an unaccompanied child in whom a life-threatening disorder is suspected to a separate radiology suite. Obtain portable films or accompany the child to the radiology suite and bring appropriate equipment for airway intervention. Furthermore, an appropriate soft-tissue lateral film of the neck requires that the film be obtained with the child's neck extended during the terminal phase of inspiration. It should be stressed that this position has the potential to obstruct an already compromised airway.

Indications for plain film radiography include upper airway abscesses and foreign bodies in children who are clinically stable. Generally, stable children suspected of having epiglottitis will have either a portable radiograph of the lateral neck or proceed directly to an emergency evaluation of their airway. Unstable children need immediate attention to their airway, either in the operating room or ED, by clinicians who are expert in pediatric airway management.

Classic findings of epiglottitis on plain radiography include an enlarged epiglottis with an appearance similar to a thumb, enlarged aryepiglottic folds, and a ballooned hypopharyngeal airway. However, these findings are subjective and are not obvious in all cases of pediatric epiglottitis. In fact, as many as 70% of all patients with epiglottitis have radiographs that are initially read as normal by radiologists.[11,12] Objective findings that may be more accurate in detecting epiglottitis include an epiglottis width/the width of the third cervical vertebral body greater than 0.5, or an aryepiglottic width/width of the third cervical vertebral body greater than 0.35 on lateral radiography. A limited study found that these measurements were 100% sensitive in diagnosing epiglottitis.[12]

Findings that suggest retropharyngeal abscess include a retropharyngeal space greater than 7 mm anterior to the inferior border of the second cervical vertebral body, or a retrotracheal space greater than 14 mm in children (> 22 mm in adults) anterior to the inferior border of the sixth cervical vertebral body.[13] Other suggestive findings include soft-tissue air-fluid levels and cervical retroflexion. Computed tomography is touted by some experts as being more accurate than plain films for detecting retropharyngeal abscesses.[14]

Soft-tissue radiographs of the neck are often used for evaluating children with croup. One series found that nearly 50% of pediatricians routinely obtained plain films in children with croup.[15] Unfortunately, plain films are often misleading or non-diagnostic in this disorder. A prior study that evaluated radiologists' interpretations of plain films in children with croup found that 24-28% of radiographs were diagnosed as possible epiglottitis, while only 33-38% of radiographs were called croup, proving the unreliability of plain films in diagnosing this disorder.[16] When clinically indicated, it may be that plain films of the chest are probably more useful radiographs and can document the presence or absence of a concurrent pneumonia.

Airway foreign bodies are also a final important cause of stridor that can be detected with plain films. Unfortunately, less than 10% of aspirated foreign bodies are radiopaque.[17] Furthermore, even more sensitive radiographic indicators of a bronchial foreign body, such as mediastinal shift, unilateral atelectasis or hyperexpansion, and persistent expansion with expiration, may not completely rule out a foreign body. Therefore, never rely on plain films to exclude an airway foreign body when there is a strong clinical suspicion. In these cases, other airway visualization techniques (e.g., direct laryngoscopy or bronchoscopy) should be considered.

Airway Examination. Direct visualization is an important tool to consider for diagnosing the cause of a child's stridor. In the past, it was commonly taught that direct visualization of the hypopharynx and use of a tongue blade or mirror (indirect laryngoscopy) was a hazardous technique that should be avoided at all costs in children with stridor and possible epiglottitis. However, several bodies of evidence suggest that this risk is overstated. A literature review dating back to 1964 reveals no recorded cases of tongue blade laryngospasm in children with epiglottitis.[18] Furthermore, there has never been a case of laryngospasm in the more than 1000 adult cases of epiglottitis reported.[19]

Finally, several studies have evaluated the safety of direct visualization in children with suspected epiglottitis. At one pediatric ED, a policy of sequential visualization of the epiglottis in 155 consecutive stridorous children was safely performed by first having the child open his or her mouth.[2] If the epiglottis was not visualized, a tongue blade was applied to the anterior tongue while the child was sitting up, then a laryngoscope was used while the child was sitting up; and, finally, direct laryngoscopy was performed while the child was lying down. Using these sequential techniques, the epiglottis was correctly identified in 148 of 149 children with croup and six of six children with epiglottitis. No complications occurred during direct visualization.

Two other series totaling 126 children with epiglottitis found that direct laryngoscopic visualization with care not to touch the epiglottis and hypopharynx was uniformly safe.[11,20] While these reviews suggest that stable children will usually tolerate careful laryngoscopy or application of a tongue blade to the mid or anterior tongue, only clinicians who are comfortable with all aspects of pediatric airway management should perform these techniques. Furthermore, equipment should be available to intervene if stridor worsens or laryngospasm occurs. In general, it is best to use these techniques only in children with a moderate or low suspicion of epiglottitis who are deemed clinically stable. Finally, each institution should develop protocols that outline clinical pathways for children who present with severe, acute, upper airway obstruction.

Specific Upper Airway Disorders. The list of disorders that can precipitate stridor is extensive. *(See Table 1.)* However, ED physicians must be aware of those disorders that are common (e.g., croup) and potentially life-threatening (e.g., bacterial infection, foreign bodies).

Epiglottitis

Prior to the late 1980s, *Haemophilus influenzae* type B (HIB) was the most common etiology of epiglottitis. With the introduction of an effective vaccine against this organism, the incidence of all diseases due to HIB dropped dramatically. In 1980, *H. influenzae* meningitis occurred in 19.3 of every 100,000 children under the age of 5.[22] By 1991, only 3.7 of every 100,000 children at this age developed meningitis—a greater than fivefold decrease.[22] Furthermore, the average annual incidence of epiglottitis dropped from 11 cases per 10,000 hospital admissions prior to 1990 to fewer than two cases per 10,000 admissions.[1]

Finally, the changing pattern of epiglottitis is reflected by a newer age spectrum for this disease. Prior to 1990, the median age for children with epiglottitis was approximately 3 years, with a typical range of 2-5 years.[1] Additionally, up to 24% of children with epiglottitis were less than 2 years of age.[23] However, since 1990, the median age has risen to 7 years, with adolescents, teenagers, and even adults more frequently affected.[1]

Prior to 1990, HIB accounted for 85-90% of all childhood cases of epiglottitis.[1] With the introduction of an effective HIB vaccine over the past decade, HIB currently accounts for only 25% of all cases.[1] Due to a decrease in HIB cases and an increase in the number of immunocompromised patients (due to rising HIV rates, more children living with cancer, etc.), atypical organisms are more frequently recognized as a cause of epiglottitis, including *Candida,* herpes simplex, *Staphylococcus aureus,* and *Streptococci.*[1,24] Acute supraglottitis secondary to varicella has also recently been reported.[25]

Presentation. Classically, children with epiglottitis present with high fever, toxicity, acute onset of stridor, drooling, the absence of a cough, and a preference for sitting up. Importantly, the triad of drooling, agitation, and the absence of a cough have been found to be useful in differentiating epiglottitis from croup.[2] Although the median age for epiglottitis has risen from 3 years to 7 years, epiglottitis can occur at any age.

While early studies indicate that those younger than age 2 with epiglottitis generally present with subtle clinical features easily confused with croup,[23] more recent comparisons indicate that features probably do not differ dramatically between those over and under the age of 2.[8] However, adolescents, teenagers, and adults often present with atypical features.[19] Older children may simply complain of a sore throat, without evidence of stridor or other features of airway obstruction and with few or no findings of inflammation on examination of the pharynx.[19] Importantly, hyoid tenderness is present in almost all older patients.[19] Furthermore, while initial clinical features may be subtle, the propensity to develop airway obstruction is still present.

Diagnosis. The method chosen to diagnose this disorder depends on the clinical stability of the patient, as well as the physician's airway expertise and comfort level.

If a child with severe stridor, toxicity, or other features strongly suggestive of epiglottitis presents to the ED, assessment and management must be swift and directed. Although a portable radiograph of the lateral neck soft tissues can be obtained, generally it is recommended to avoid radiography, as this wastes valuable time. If the child has an airway that is patent and maintained, do not disturb or manipulate the airway. A team consisting of an anesthesiologist and surgeon skilled in invasive airway surgical techniques should be assembled immediately in the operating room. Preferably, the composition of this team should be predetermined by protocol. If time allows, anesthetic induction with an inhalational agent should take place in the operating room under controlled circumstances by the physician most skilled in airway management. In children who are clinically stable, nasotracheal intubation is preferred, although oral endotracheal intubation is often necessary in unstable patients.

Table 1. Differential Considerations of Stridor

ALLERGIC
Anaphylaxis
Hereditary angioneurotic edema

CONGENITAL ANATOMIC
Laryngomalacia
Tracheomalacia/tracheal stenosis
Vascular abnormality
Vocal cord cysts/paralysis
Webs (bronchial or laryngeal)
Tracheoesophageal fistulas

INFECTIONS
Bacterial tracheitis
Epiglottitis
Peritonsillar abscess
Retropharyngeal abscess
Viral croup (acute laryngotracheobronchitis)

NEOPLASMS
Cystic hygroma
Hemangioma
Lymphoma/lymphangioma
Neuroblastoma
Rhabdomyosarcoma
Teratoma
Papillomas

NEUROLOGIC
CNS malformation
Hypoxic encephalopathy

TRAUMA
Facial
Ingestion (especially caustic)
Inhalation injury
Postintubation edema, granuloma, stenosis
Retropharyngeal hematoma
Laryngeal/tracheal swelling or fracture

OTHER
Foreign bodies (airway/esophageal)
Juvenile rheumatoid arthritis (cricoarytenoid arthritis)
Kartagener's syndrome (bronchiectasis, sinusitis, situs inversus)
Hysterical stridor
Exercise

Adapted from: Santamaria JP, Schafermeyer R. Stridor: A review. *Pediatr Emerg Care* 1992;8:229-234.

If airway compromise occurs prior to assembling an operating team, proceed with bag-mask ventilation. Mask ventilation can be easily accomplished in most patients with epiglottitis, since airway compromise is usually due to diaphragmatic fatigue rather than complete airway obstruction from a floppy, heavy epiglottis.[11] Higher airway pressures than normal may be necessary to sufficiently balloon the hypopharynx and help mechanically lift the epiglottis to open the airway. If mask ventilation is unsuccessful, proceed with endotracheal intubation. It can generally be stated that with epiglottitis, unsuccessful mask ventilation means improper head position, and, consequently, a closed airway. Use a MacIntosh (curved) laryngoscope blade to avoid direct manipulation of the epiglottis. Prepare several endotracheal tubes that are 0.5 and 1.0 mm smaller than expected for that age with stylets. If vocal cords and the airway are not visualized, have an assistant apply gentle pressure to the sternum. Frequently, this maneuver will produce an air bubble between the vocal cords, allowing for airway visualization. Surgical airway techniques (cricothyrotomy vs tracheostomy), depending on the child's age, are final options in children with complete airway obstruction. Finally, transtracheal jet ventilation is relatively contraindicated in children with complete airway obstruction due to the high risk from barotrauma in this group of patients.[26]

For patients who are stable, nontoxic, and have only minimal-to-moderate stridor, several evaluation and management options should be considered. First, assemble airway intervention equipment in case clinical deterioration occurs. Do not allow the patient to be unattended or to leave the department (e.g., to obtain radiographs). Plain film radiography may reveal an enlarged epiglottis, confirming the diagnosis of epiglottitis. However, false-negative (or falsely normal) radiographs have been reported in up to 70% of all cases.[12] Alternately, clinicians who are comfortable with their airway skills may consider direct visualization of the epiglottis in children who are clinically stable and have a low-to-moderate suspicion of epiglottitis.

Management. To prevent sudden airway obstruction, all children with epiglottitis require intubation under controlled circumstances. In the past, children who were expectantly managed without intubation in intensive care units had a mortality rate greater than 5%.[19] In contrast, mortality in intubated children is less than 1%.[19] Consequently, all children with epiglottitis should be intubated until airway swelling resolves. Diligently search for concurrent infections (e.g., pneumonia, upper respiratory infections, meningitis, septic arthritis) in all children with epiglottitis, as 20-25% of children have a second infectious source.[1,11] Administer antibiotics that are effective against HIB and other common organisms that cause epiglottitis (e.g., a third-generation cephalosporin). Steroids have not been proven effective in epiglottitis and are not recommended.[27] No controlled studies have addressed the utility of racemic epinephrine; theoretically, use of this treatment modality might induce laryngospasm.

Retropharyngeal Abscesses

Retropharyngeal abscess is a rare but serious cause of supraglottic airway obstruction. This infection generally occurs in very young children prior to atrophy of retropharyngeal lymph nodes. The infection is often polymicrobial, and common oral pathogens are the most frequent causative organisms (e.g., *Bacteroides, Peptostreptococci, Fusobacteria,* Group A streptococci, *Streptococcus viridans,* and *Staphylococcus aureus*).[13]

Most children with retropharyngeal abscesses are younger than 4 years old.[13] There is often a preceding viral upper respiratory infection with eventual seeding of the retropharyngeal lymph nodes by bacteria. With spread of the bacterial infection, an abscess forms, and children develop fever, drooling, stridor, and toxicity. Because of the abscess site adjacent to the cervical spine, the head is often hyperextended. Direct visualization carries the same theoretic risk of airway obstruction as epiglottitis. If the pharynx can be visualized without worsening the symptoms, unilateral or bilateral swelling of the posterior pharyngeal wall may be evident. However, this finding may not be obvious on clinical examination, especially if swelling is bilateral. In addition to airway obstruction, complications of mediastinitis, aspiration, and sudden death can occur with rupture of the abscess into adjacent tissue planes, airway, or vascular structures (e.g., jugular vein or carotid artery).[13]

Diagnosis. Rapid diagnosis and management are required to avoid complete airway obstruction. As in patients with suspected epiglottitis, children who are toxic with severe stridor, drooling, or other evidence of impending airway obstruction must be taken directly to the operating room. Gentle airway management and induction with a general anesthetic is necessary before the abscess ruptures, with leakage of contents into the lungs.

Although plain film radiography may reveal air-fluid levels or soft-tissue swelling anterior to the vertebral bodies (> 7 mm anterior to C2 or > 14 mm anterior to C6), computed tomography (CT) is more accurate at identifying retropharyngeal abscesses.[14] Only children who are clinically stable should be allowed to proceed to CT. Furthermore, always ensure that airway equipment and personnel who are capable of managing airway compromise accompany the patient.

Management. If immediate airway intervention is required in a child with a retropharyngeal abscess, consider positioning the head in a downward and hyperextended position to avoid aspiration should the abscess rupture. Following airway management, surgical drainage of the abscess will be required. Antibiotics effective against oral pathogens including anaerobes should be administered. Penicillin is the recommended drug of choice. Clindamycin is an acceptable alternative. Additional coverage with a third-generation cephalosporin or an antistaphylococcal penicillin should be strongly considered.

Bacterial Tracheitis

Bacterial tracheitis is a rare disorder in children that causes features similar to those of epiglottitis and upper airway abscesses. Only 100 cases had been reported in the literature prior to 1989.[28]

Typically, patients with bacterial tracheitis develop a viral upper respiratory infection. Symptoms are initially mild and mimic those of croup. They consist of a cough, rhinorrhea, and low-grade fever. Over an ensuing three- to seven-day period, a bacterial superinfection of the trachea occurs with *S. aureus*. A purulent exudate of the trachea leads to severe stridor, and systemic toxicity occurs. Fifty percent of patients have an associated pneumonia.[28] Intubation is generally required to secure the airway and prevent obstruction. Following intubation, frequent suctioning may be required in addition to bronchoscopy in order to unplug the airway and prevent total airway occlusion. Anti-staphylococcal antibiotics also are required.

Foreign Body Aspiration

Foreign body aspiration is an important and potentially fatal cause of acute stridor. Aspiration most commonly occurs in children younger than age 6, with 80% of cases occurring in those younger than age 3.[29] This is the leading cause of home-related deaths in the United States for children younger than age 6, with 2000 deaths occurring each year.[29] Fortunately, with the passage of the Consumer Products Safety Act of 1979, home safety has improved and the incidence is decreasing. Infants and children older than 6 months are particularly at risk because they lack dentition, are inherently curious, are still crawling, do not have a completely coordinated swallowing mechanism, and are increasingly adept at picking up small objects.[29,30,31]

Identifying children who have aspirated foreign bodies can be extremely difficult. Only 20-46% present within 24 hours of the initial aspiration while 17% wait more than 30 days from aspiration before seeking medical care.[30] Generally, those with upper respiratory foreign bodies present more acutely than those with foreign bodies that have lodged in the lower respiratory tract. Furthermore, 24% of children with aspirated foreign bodies have previously been misdiagnosed, usually as having a respiratory illness such as pneumonia or bronchitis.[30] In 25-50% of children, no history of foreign body ingestion can be elicited. Fewer than 10% of aspirated foreign bodies are radiopaque, which underscores the ease with which they can be missed on radiologic examination.[32]

Most foreign bodies (80-85%) lodge in the bronchial tree. Although the mainstem bronchi of a child branch at equal angles from the trachea, the right side is the most common position for a bronchial foreign body to lodge. Only 2-12% of foreign bodies lodge within or above the larynx, while 3% lodge within the trachea.[30] Esophageal foreign bodies can also cause airway compromise through compression on the trachea.

Children with bronchial foreign bodies usually present subacutely, with recurrent cough, wheezing, or other respiratory symptoms. In contrast, children with laryngotracheal foreign bodies more frequently present with acute stridor or cardiopulmonary arrest. However, there is considerable overlap in the symptoms manifested by children with upper and lower airway foreign bodies. *(See Figure 2.)*

Diagnosis. The most difficult assignment in identifying a lodged foreign body is considering the diagnosis in a child with upper or lower respiratory symptoms. This diagnosis should be considered in any child with acute stridor or cardiopulmonary arrest. Never rely on plain films to exclude the diagnosis of an upper or lower respiratory foreign body. It should be stressed that most foreign bodies (> 90%) will not be visible on plain radiographs.[32] Furthermore, inspiratory/expiratory films and decubitus films to detect air trapping have only a 67% sensitivity in detecting bronchial foreign bodies.[32] Typical features of a lower respiratory foreign body include recurrent wheezing, pneumonia, or bronchitis, or a persistent cough. When the clinical suspicion is high for an airway foreign body, consider laryngoscopy or bronchoscopy regardless of radiographic findings.

Management. Immediate treatment of a child with an upper airway foreign body and respiratory failure consists of a series of five back blows and chest thrusts in those under 1 year of age. For children older than 1 year, substernal abdominal thrusts are recommended with the child in the upright or supine position.

Table 2. Clinical Scoring System for Assessing Children with Stridor

SIGN	0	1	2	3
Stridor	None	With agitation	Mild at rest	Severe at rest
Retraction	None	Mild	Moderate	Severe
Air entry	Normal	Mild	Moderate	Severe
Color	Normal		Cyanotic	
Level of consciousness	Normal	Restless if disturbed	Restless if undisturbed	Lethargic

Suggested management if total score adds up to:

< 5: Mild severity
Treat as outpatient with mist only.

5-6: Mild severity
Treat as outpatient only if patient improves after mist in ED, is older than 6 months, and has a reliable family. Racemic epinephrine may be used.

7-8: Moderate severity
Admit and use racemic epinephrine.

> 8: Severe
Treat as above; admit to ICU.

Adapted from: Tausig LM, Castro O, Biandry PA, et al. Treatment of laryngotracheitis (croup): Use of intermittent positive pressure breathing and racemic epinephrine. *Am J Dis Child* 1975;129:790-795.

Directly inspect the oropharynx between thrusts and do *not* perform blind finger sweeps. If these maneuvers are unsuccessful, directly inspect the hypopharynx, and inspect the larynx via laryngoscopy. Remove the foreign body with Magill forceps if it is accessible. If this procedure is unsuccessful, consider endotracheal intubation or needle cricothyrotomy.

Laryngotracheobronchitis (Croup)

Laryngotracheobronchitis or viral croup is the most common infectious cause of acute upper airway obstruction in children, accounting for greater than 90% of all cases of stridor and 20,000 hospital admissions per year.[7] Most cases occur in the late fall and early spring. Viruses, including parainfluenza, respiratory syncytial virus (especially in patients < 12 months), rhinoviruses, and influenzae A and B, are responsible for croup.[7]

Stridor in children with croup occurs from mucosal and submucosal edema of the subglottic portion of the airway. The mucosa in this region is loosely adherent, permitting significant edema formation and potential airway compromise. In infants, 1 mm of subglottic edema will cause a 50% decrease in the cross-sectional area of the trachea.[33] The subglottic portion of the airway is the narrowest portion of a child's airway, which further increases the propensity for obstruction. In addition to the upper airway, inflammation often spreads to the trachea and bronchi, causing signs and symptoms of lower respiratory tract disease.

Clinical features include inspiratory and expiratory stridor, a cough (similar to the bark of a seal), hoarseness from vocal cord inflammation, fever, and, occasionally, lower tract symptoms such as wheezing. In contrast to viral croup, a non-seasonal allergic variant known as spasmodic croup may occur. This disorder typically has an abrupt onset, with no preceding upper respiratory infection and no fever.[7]

Diagnosis. Diagnosis of croup is primarily based on clinical features. The typical age is 2 years. Most children have a few days of prodromal upper respiratory tract symptoms, including nasal congestion, a mild cough, and fever, before stridor develops. Stridor is usually biphasic, although it is often louder on inspiration. Importantly, clinicians must rule out other more immediately life-threatening diseases, including epiglottitis, abscesses, and foreign bodies. Plain radiography has been promoted for the diagnosis of this disorder; however, the main use for this modality is to exclude other serious disorders.

Assessment of Severity. While most children with croup have mild symptoms that will not progress, a small subset of children may develop airway obstruction. Several clinical scoring systems have been proposed for assessing children with stridor. *(See Table 2.)* Features suggestive of impending airway obstruction have been identified, including age less than six months, rest stridor, cyanosis, decreased level of consciousness, hypoxia, and hypercarbia.[7,33] Importantly, an experienced clinician's evaluation may be more accurate than any scoring system for evaluating the degree of stridor.

Pulse oximetry and capnometry have been evaluated as tools for assessing the severity of a child's stridor. Pulse oximetry should be routinely obtained on all children with stridor. One recent study

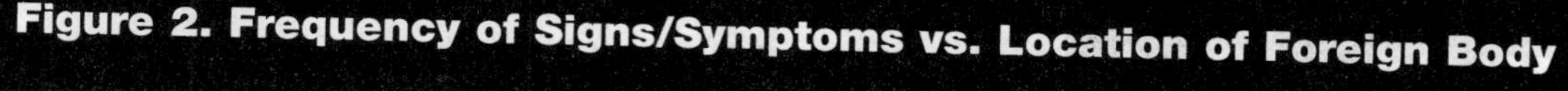

Figure 2. Frequency of Signs/Symptoms vs. Location of Foreign Body

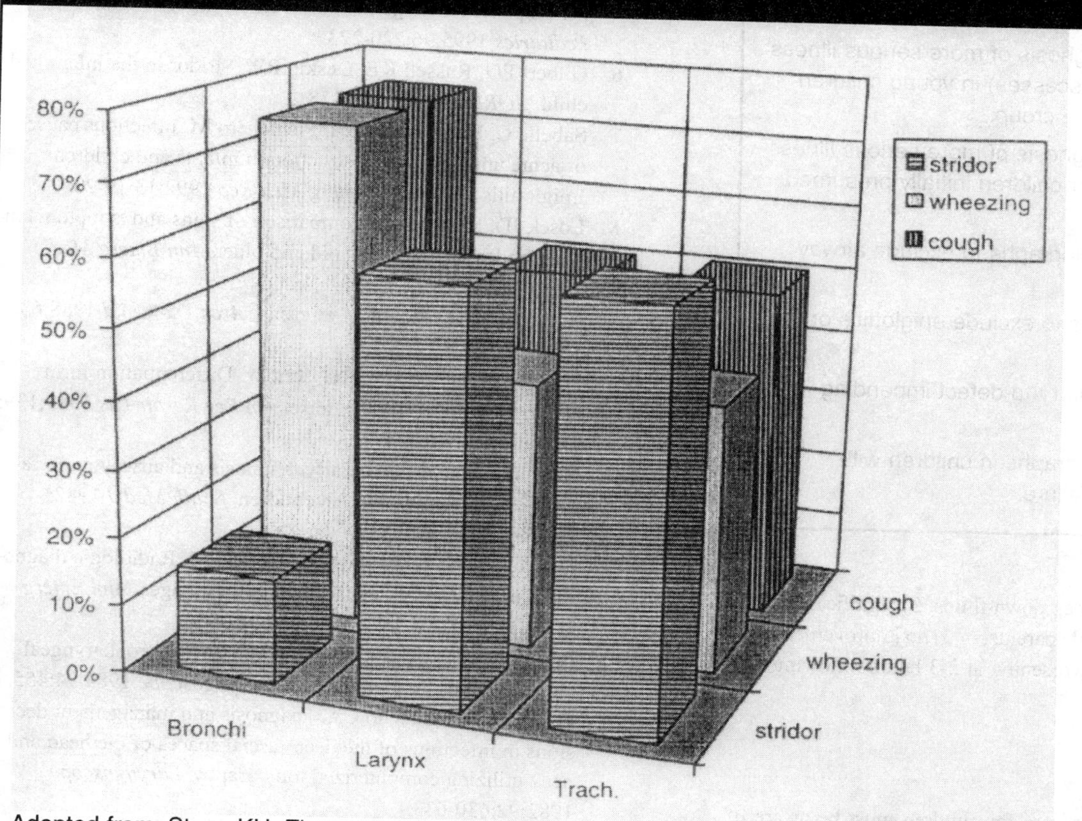

Adapted from: Steen KH, Zimmerman T. Tracheobronchial aspiration of foreign bodies in children: A study of 94 cases. *Laryngoscope* 1990;100:525; Wiseman NE. The diagnosis of foreign body aspiration in childhood. *J Pediatr Surg* 1984;19:531-535.

found that clinicians were only 33% sensitive in identifying hypoxemia in children with acute respiratory disease.[35] Importantly, a normal oxygen saturation also may serve to falsely reassure clinicians. Hypoxia generally indicates advanced disease and impending respiratory failure. While hypoxia signifies fatigue and impending airway obstruction, hypercarbia (detected by capnography or capnometry) has been found to be a much better (and earlier) predictor of clinical deterioration and the need for intubation in children admitted to an intensive care unit.[36]

Treatment. Humidified mist is usually recommended as first-line treatment for children with croup, although no controlled studies have proven its efficacy. The mist may directly decrease inflammation or reflexly slow respiration through an undefined mechanism.[37] Oxygen administration may also benefit a subset of children.

Racemic epinephrine has been promoted as an effective treatment for croup. Racemic epinephrine is composed of 50% D and 50% L isomers of epinephrine. It was first used because the D isomer has 1/30 of the alpha effects of the pure L isomer (e.g., hypertension, tachycardia). However, racemic epinephrine is much more expensive than the L isomer (the form used for all other purposes—asthma, allergy, anaphylaxis, and cardiac arrest). Moreover, direct comparisons of racemic epinephrine to an equal amount of the L isomer have shown no differences in outcome for the treatment of croup, including croup scores, side effects, heart rate, blood pressure and respiratory rate.[3] Given the apparent rapid efficacy and significant cost differences, the L isomer is the recommended form of epinephrine for the treatment of acute laryngotracheobronchitis.[3] The administered dose of the L isomer is 5 cc of the 1:1000 concentration.[3]

In the past, administration of epinephrine to children with croup mandated admission to observe for potential rebound or further closing of the airway after the medication wore off. This approach has been challenged for several reasons. First, the half-life of epinephrine is only 1-2 hours. Four studies of racemic epinephrine use in children with rest stridor have shown that the effects of epinephrine will wear off within two hours.[38,39,40,41] Outpatient management was deemed safe in all children with mild symptoms who had been observed in the ED for two or three hours after epinephrine administration without a worsening of their stridor. In addition, a large number of children received intramuscular steroids in addition to epinephrine in these studies.[38,39,40,41] Therefore, observe all children for at least 2-3 hours and administer steroids to all who receive epinephrine.

Steroids are an accepted adjunctive treatment for children with croup. Nebulized budesonide (2 mg) has been shown to decrease croup scores by 50% at two hours in admitted children with moderate-to-severe croup.[4,42,43] A meta-analysis that included more than 1200 children with croup from 10 studies found that intramuscular dexamethasone (0.6 mg/kg) decreased croup scores at 12 and 24 hours and intubation rates in admitted children with croup.[44] A single study also found that children treated as outpatients with moderately severe croup who received 0.6 mg/kg of dexamethasone IM were improved significantly at the 24-hour follow-up.[5] Although clinical studies on outpatient experience with steroids in children with croup are limited, their use for this purpose is widespread in the pediatric community.[45]

Finally, the decision to admit or discharge a child with croup can be difficult. Generally, admit all children with: 1) a toxic appearance;

Table 3. Pitfalls in the Diagnosis and Management of Stridor

1. Not considering the diagnosis of more serious illness (e.g., foreign bodies, abscesses) in young children initially presumed to have croup.
2. Not considering the diagnosis of more serious illness (e.g., epiglottitis) in older children initially presumed to have pharyngitis.
3. Reliance on normal radiographs to exclude airway foreign bodies.
4. Reliance on radiographs to exclude epiglottitis or to diagnose croup.
5. Reliance on pulse oximetry to detect impending respiratory failure.
6. Wasting time with radiographs in children with impending respiratory failure.

2) dehydration or inability to keep down fluids; 3) significant stridor or retractions at rest; 4) unreliable parents; or 5) no improvement with epinephrine administration or worsening at 2-3 hours following epinephrine administration.

Conclusion

Emergency physicians who care for children must be aware of both common and life-threatening causes of stridor. While most children with stridor do not have a serious illness, an important subset will harbor a serious illness that may progress to complete airway obstruction. Clues from the history and physical examination can be used to guide the assessment and management of most children with stridor. *(See Table 3.)* Importantly, clinicians must be aware of the limitations of plain film radiography in diagnosing the cause of a child's stridor. In the past, direct visualization of the airway was felt to be uniformly contraindicated in children with stridor. However, this simple technique may provide useful information for clinicians who are trained and equipped to manage a child's airway. Finally, clinicians must be aware of the different treatments available, as well as indications for emergent and urgent airway intervention in children with stridor.

References

1. Gorelick MH, Baker MD. Epiglottitis in children, 1979 through 1992: Effects of *Haemophilus influenzae* type B immunization. *Arch Pediatr Adolesc Med* 1994;148:47-50.
2. Mauro RD, Poole SR, Lockhart CH. Differentiation of epiglottitis from laryngotracheitis in the child with stridor. *Am J Dis Child* 1988;142:679.
3. Waisman Y, Klein BL, Boenning DA, et al. Prospective randomized double-blind study comparing L-epinephrine and racemic epinephrine aerosols in the treatment of laryngotracheitis (croup). *Pediatrics* 1992;89:302-306.
4. Husby S, Agertoft L, Mortensen S, et al. Treatment of croup with nebulised steroid (budesonide): A double-blind, placebo-controlled study. *Arch Dis Child* 1993;68:352-355.
5. Cruz MN, Stewart G, Rosenberg N. Use of dexamethasone in the outpatient management of acute laryngotracheitis. *Pediatrics* 1995;96:220-223.
6. Gilbert EG, Russell KE, Deskin RW. Stridor in the infant and child. *AORN J* 1993;58:23-38.
7. Sabella C, Fontanarosa PM, Pichichero M. Infectious causes of acute upper airway obstruction in infants and children: Epiglottitis and croup. *Emerg Med Rep* 1992;13:19-28.
8. Losek JD. Epiglottitis: Comparison of signs and symptoms in children less than 2 years old and older. *Ann Emerg Med* 1990;19:55.
9. Couriel JM. Management of croup. *Arch Dis Child* 1988;63: 1305-1309.
10. Baughman RP, Loudon RG. Stridor: Differentiation form asthma and upper airway noise. *Am Rev Respir Dis* 1989;139: 1407-1410.
11. Diaz JH, Lockhart CH. Early diagnosis and airway management of acute epiglottitis in children. *South Med J* 1982; 75:399.
12. Rothrock SG, Pigniatello G, Howard RM. Radiologic diagnosis of epiglottitis: objective criteria for all ages. *Ann Emerg Med* 1990;19:978.
13. Barratt GE, Koopman CF, Coulthard SW. Retropharyngeal abscess—a ten year experience. *Laryngoscope* 1984;94:455.
14. Endicott JN, Saraceno CA. Diagnosis and management decisions in infections of the deep fascial spaces of the head and neck utilizing computerized tomography. *Laryngoscope* 1982;92:630-633.
15. Mills JL, Spackman TJ, Borns P, et al. The usefulness of lateral neck roentgenorgrams in laryngotracheobronchitis. *Am J Dis Child* 1979;133:1140.
16. Stankiewicz JA, Bowes AK. Croup and epiglottitis: A radiologic study. *Laryngoscope* 1985;95:1159.
17. Steen KH, Zimmerman T. Tracheobronchial aspiration of foreign bodies in children: A study of 94 cases. *Laryngoscope* 1990;100:525.
18. Rothrock SG. Recognition and management of pediatric upper airway disorders. *Critical Care for the Acutely Ill and Injured*. Orlando, FL; 1994. Lecture.
19. Mayosmith MF, Hirsch PJ, Wodzinski SF, et al. Acute epiglottitis in adults. An eight-year experience in the state of Rhode Island. *N Engl J Med* 1986;314:1133.
20. Greenberg LW, Schiagall R. Acute epiglottis in a community hospital. *Am Fam Physician* 1979;19:123-127.
21. Santamaria JP, Schafermeyer R. Stridor: a review. *Pediatr Emerg Care* 1992;8:229-234.
22. Adams WG, Deaver KA, Cochi SL, et al. Decline of childhood *Haemophilus influenzae* type B (HIB) disease in the HIB vaccine era. *JAMA* 1993;269:221-226.
23. Brilli RS, Benzing G, Cotcamp DH. Epiglottitis in infants less than two years of age. *Pediatr Emerg Care* 1989;5:16-21.
24. Balsam O, Sorrano D, Barax C. Candida epiglottitis presenting as stridor in a child with HIV infection. *Pediatr Radiol* 1992;22:235-236.
25. Narasimhan N, van Stralen DW, Perkin RM. Acute supraglottitis caused by varicella. *Pediatr Infect Dis J* 1993;12: 619-620.

26. Mace SE. Cricothyrotomy. In: Roberts JR, Hedges JR, eds. *Clinical Procedures in Emergency Medicine.* Philadelphia: WB Saunders; 1991:40-59.
27. Fleisher GR. Infectious disease emergencies. In: Fleisher GR, Ludwig S, eds. *Textbook of Pediatric Emergency Medicine.* Baltimore: Williams & Wilkins; 1993:596-652.
28. Rabie I. Bacterial tracheitis. *J Laryngol Otol* 1989;103: 1059-1062.
29. Cantrill SV. Aspirated foreign bodies. In: Reisdorff EJ, ed. *Pediatric Emergency Medicine.* Philadelphia: WB Saunders; 1993:298-301.
30. Steen KH, Zimmerman T. Tracheobronchial aspiration of foreign bodies in children: A study of 94 cases. *Laryngoscope* 1990;100:525.
31. Wiseman NE. The diagnosis of foreign body aspiration in childhood. *J Pediatr Surg* 1984;19:531-535.
32. Losek JD. Diagnostic difficulties of foreign body aspiration in children. *Am J Emerg Med* 1990;8:348.
33. Bank DE, Krug SE. New approaches to upper airway disease. *Emerg Med Clin North Am* 1995;13:473-487.
34. Tausig LM, Castro O, Biandry PA, et al. Treatment of laryngotracheitis (croup): Use of intermittent positive pressure breathing and racemic epinephrine. *Am J Dis Child* 1975;129: 790-795.
35. Mancker AJ, Petrack EM, Krug SE. Contribution of routine pulse oximetry to evaluation and management of patients with respiratory illness in a pediatric emergency department. *Ann Emerg Med* 1995;25:36-40.
36. Fanconi S, Burger R, Maurer H, et al. Transcutaneous carbon dioxide pressure for monitoring patients with severe croup. *J Pediatr* 1990;117: 701-705.
37. Sasake CT. The respiratory mechanism of aerosol inhalation in the treatment of partial airway obstruction. *Pediatrics* 1977;59:689-694.
38. Kelley PB, Simon JE. Racemic epinephrine use in croup and disposition. *Am J Emerg Med* 1992;181-183.
39. Pendergast M, Jones JS, Hartman D. Racemic epinephrine in the treatment of laryngotracheitis: Can we identify children for outpatient therapy? *Am J Emerg Med* 1994;12:613-616.
40. Ledwith C, Shea L, Mauro RD. Safety and efficacy of nebulized racemic epinephrine in conjunction with oral dexamethasone and mist in the outpatient treatment of croup. *Ann Emerg Med* 1995;25:331-337.
41. Wussow K, Krug S, Yamashita T. Duration of clinical response to racemic epinephrine in children with croup. *Pediatr Emerg Care* 1992;8:306. Abstract.
42. Klassen TP, et al. Nebulized budesonide for children with mild-to-moderate croup. *N Engl J Med* 1994;331:285-289.
43. Landau LI, Geelboed GC. Aerosolized steroids for croup. *N Engl J Med* 1994;331:322-323.
44. Kairys SW, Olmstead EM, O'Conner GT. Steroid treatment of laryngotracheitis: A meta-analysis of the evidence from randomized trials. *Pediatrics* 1989;83:683-693.
45. Connors K, Gavula D, Terndrup T. The use of corticosteroids in croup: A survey. *Pediatr Emerg Care* 1994;10:197-199.
46. Handler SD. Stridor. In: Fleisher GR, Ludwig S, eds. *Textbook of Pediatric Emergency Medicine.* Baltimore: Williams & Wilkins; 1993:477.

Treatment of Acute Otitis Media

Gideon Bosker, MD, FACEP

Acute otitis media: common, unpredictable, challenging, and now more than ever, fiercely debated at the front lines of clinical practice and in the ivory towers of medicine. In fact, the continuing controversy surrounding outcome-effective treatment strategies has attracted the interest of nationally recognized clinicians, epidemiologists, and clinical scholars from the disciplines of emergency medicine, pediatrics, and infectious diseases. As might be expected, each expert or consensus panel brings its own set of biases to the challenge of establishing critical pathways for this common condition. One group may emphasize *Streptococcus pneumoniae* resistance patterns (PRSP), while another will put a priority on dosing schedule, side effects, and compliance-enhancement.

In response to PRSP species and emerging resistance among some antibiotics, the Centers for Disease Control and Prevention (CDC) was prompted to convene experts in the management of otitis media to form the Drug-Resistant *Streptococcus pneumoniae* Therapeutic Working Group. The objective was to provide consensus recommendations for the management of acute otitis media (AOM) and strategies for surveillance of drug-resistant *Streptococcus pneumoniae.*

In this concluding part of our two-part series, we closely examine the CDC recommendations. They are carefully evaluated against the backdrop of evidence-based trials, practical considerations, resistance surveillance studies, and national expert opinion that may offer other treatment strategies and that diverge in some aspects from these published pathways. Moreover, this review discusses, in detail, the prescription, parent, patient, and drug resistance (PPPD) approach to antibiotic selection for AOM—a drug selection framework that includes a number of disease management factors, including cost, compliance, patient toleration, taste, side effects, dosing schedules, and convenience factors, all of which can affect the journey from prescription pad to clinical cure.

Finally, this review of AOM also will examine the implications of recent evidence-based trials that have investigated the role of bacteriologic eradication in producing clinical cure in patients with AOM and effective approaches to AOM treatment failures.

Predictors of Patient Outcomes

Regardless of the specific antibiotic selected for AOM, there appears to be a relationship between early bacterial eradication of the organism from the middle ear and cure rates in children with AOM.[1] To determine the relation between early bacteriologic eradication and clinical outcome of AOM in infants and young children treated with various antibiotics, an Israeli group studied patients ages 3 to 24 months seen in a pediatric emergency department.

Patients enrolled in this trial presented with symptoms and physical findings consistent with AOM of 7 days or less duration. Moreover, the following criteria were met: 1) there was no spontaneous perforation or tympanostomy tubes; 2) there was a positive initial middle ear fluid culture; and 3) a follow-up culture on at least Day 10 ± of the study, with a second culture performed 72-96 h after initiation of antibiotic treatment. Any patient with a positive middle ear fluid culture 72-96 h after initiation of antibiotic treatment was considered to have bacteriologic failure.[1]

Otologic evaluation was done by an otolaryngologist unaware of the culture results and of the study drug allocation. A clinical score based on body temperature, report of irritability and ear tugging observed by the parents, and the appearance and redness of the ear drum as observed by the otolaryngologist was also used for clinical evaluation.

Of the 123 patients evaluated in the study, 57 (46%) had positive middle ear fluid 72-96 h after initiation of antibiotic treatment. Clinical failure was observed in 21 of 57 (37%) patients in whom bacteriologic eradication did not occur vs. only two of 66 (3%) patients with bacteriologic eradication after 3-4 days of treatment ($P < 0.001$). Clinical score for both moderate and severe disease decreased significantly faster in those with bacteriologic eradication than in those in whom middle ear fluid was still culture-positive 72-96 h after initiation of treatment.[1]

The investigators concluded that clinical failures in their population were associated with inability to eradicate the causative organisms of AOM from the middle ear fluid within 3-4 days after initiation of antibiotic therapy. Most patients (including those without bacteriologic eradication) improved after 3-4 days of treatment, but patients with sterile middle ear fluid felt better after 3-4 days of treatment than patients in whom middle ear fluid was still culture-positive.[1]

Short Course Therapies for AOM. One of the important, practical questions when selecting an antibiotic for AOM is how long a course of therapy should be in order to maximize clinical outcomes. Some practitioners have advocated 7- to 10-day treatment courses, even though studies show that medication noncompliance rates with 10-day regimens can be as high as 92% by the last day of drug therapy.[2-6]

Unfortunately, a recent working group statement from the CDC did not address the issue of short courses for AOM in a systematic manner.[7] Evaluating the efficacy of short duration therapy for AOM, however, must be addressed in a drug-specific manner, inasmuch as all short courses do not have the same pharmacokinetic properties. For example, some short half-life antibiotics are given for a short duration and, as predicted, provide only short duration "bug-drug" contact at the locus of infection (i.e., the middle ear). In contrast, other agents such as azithromycin, offer the potential convenience and compliance advantages of a short five-day course, while maintaining longer duration, MIC-effective bug-drug contact at the tissue level for an additional 5-7 days after the last dose.[8]

To shed light on this aspect of the AOM treatment controversy, one group of investigators conducted a meta-analysis of randomized, controlled trials of antibiotic treatment of AOM in children to determine whether outcomes were comparable in children treated with antibiotics for less than seven days or at least seven days or more.[8] Current Contents and Science Citation Index searches were conducted to identify randomized controlled trials of the treatment of AOM in children with antibiotics of different durations. Studies were included if they met the following criteria: subjects were between the ages of 4 weeks and 18 years; they had a clinical diagnosis of AOM; there was no antimicrobial therapy at time of diagnosis; and patients were randomized to less than seven days of antibiotic treatment vs. seven days or more of antibiotic treatment.[8]

Trial methodological quality was assessed independently by seven reviewers; outcomes were extracted as the number of treatment failures, relapses, or reinfections. Trials evaluated in this meta-analysis were grouped by antibiotic used in the short course. There were: 1) 15 short-acting oral antibiotic trials (penicillin V potassium, amoxicillin, amoxicillin/clavulanate, cefaclor, cefixime, cefuroxime, cefpodoxime proxetil, and cefprozil); 2) four intramuscular ceftriaxone sodium trials; and 3) 11 oral azithromycin trials.

The summary odds ratio for treatment outcomes at 8-19 days in children treated with short-acting antibiotics for five days vs. 8-10 days was 1.52 (95% confidence interval [CI], 1.17-1.98), but by 20-30 days outcomes between treatment groups were comparable (odds ratio, 1.22; 95% CI, 0.98 to 1.54). The risk difference (2.3%; 95% CI, -0.2% to 4.9%) at 20-30 days suggests that 44 children would need to be treated with the long course of short-acting antibiotics to avoid one treatment failure. This similarity in later outcomes was observed for up to three months following therapy (odds ratio, 1.16; 95% CI, 0.90-1.50). Comparable outcomes were shown between treatment with ceftriaxone or azithromycin, and at least seven days of other antibiotics. The authors of this meta-analysis concluded that five days of short-acting antibiotic use is effective treatment for uncomplicated AOM in children.[8]

In a European trial, a comparison was made of the clinical effectiveness of azithromycin (once daily for 3 days at a dose of 10 mg/kg in children or 500 mg/d in adults) and amoxicillin/clavulanic acid and cefaclor (standard doses for 7-14 days) in acute ear, nose, and throat infections in an open, randomized study.[9] The group with azithromycin included 37 patients with otitis media, 24 with pharyngotonsillitis, and six with maxillary sinusitis ($n = 67$). The amoxicillin/clavulanic acid group included 22 patients with otitis media, 19 with pharyngotonsillitis, and six with maxillary sinusitis ($n = 47$). The cefaclor group had 15 patients with otitis media, 12 with pharyngotonsillitis, and four with maxillary sinusitis ($n = 31$).[9]

Fifteen days after beginning treatment, 97% (65 of 67) of the patients who received azithromycin had improved or cured, compared with 85% (40 of 47) of those who received amoxicillin/clavulanic acid, and 84% (26 of 31) of those treated with cefaclor ($P < 0.02$).[9] Pathogens were not eradicated in 3% (2 of 58) of the patients who received azithromycin, compared with 13% (4 of 28) who received amoxicillin/clavulanic acid and 15% (4 of 28) who received cefaclor.[9]

Patients with azithromycin showed an earlier clinical improvement and more rapid normalization of the leukocyte count, erythrocyte sedimentation rate (ESR), and acute phase proteins. No patient with azithromycin had adverse effects vs. 15% (7 of 47) of patients with amoxicillin/clavulanic acid and 16% (5 of 31) with cefaclor-treated patients. Treatment compliance was 100%, 83% (39 of 47) and 84% (26 of 31), respectively ($P < 0.01$).[9] It should be pointed out that three-day courses of azithromycin for AOM are not currently approved in the United States, nor is azithromycin indicated for maxillary sinusitis.

Another open, randomized, multicenter study compared the clinical efficacy of a short 5-day course of cefuroxime axetil (CAE) suspension with that of amoxicillin/clavulanate (A/CA) suspension for 8 or 10 days.[10] Children ages 6 to 36 months with AOM with effusion, diagnosed by tympanocentesis and microbiologic culture, were randomized to receive CAE (30 mg/kg/d in two divided doses for 5 days) or A/CA 40 mg/kg/d in three divided doses for 10 days (A/CA-10). In French centers, A/CA was given at 80 mg/kg/d in three divided doses for 8 days (A/CA-8). Patients were assessed 1-4 days after completing the course (post-treatment) and followed-up 21-28 days after completing the course.[10]

Of the 716 patients randomized, 252 were treated with CAE, 255 with A/CA-10, and 209 with A/CA-8. In the clinically evaluable population, the proportions of patients with clinical cure at post-treatment were 175 of 203 (86%), 181 of 205 (88%), and 145 of 164

(88%) in the CAE, A/CA-10, and A/CA-8 groups, respectively, demonstrating equivalence among the three treatments. For patients older than 18 months, clinical cures occurred in 111 of 134 (83%), 116 of 131 (89%), and 83 of 99 (84%) in the CAE, A/CA-10, and A/CA-8 groups, respectively; equivalence was also demonstrated. At follow-up, 130 of 175 (74%) CAE patients, 121 of 172 (70%) A/CA-10, and 112 of 142 (79%) A/CA-8 had maintained cure.

A total of 837 pretreatment pathogens were isolated from middle ear fluid in 73% (522 of 716) of patients, the majority of isolates were *S. pneumoniae* (30%) and *H. influenzae* (27%). The most common adverse events were gastrointestinal, the incidence of drug-related diarrhea being higher in the A/CA-10 group (18%) than in either the CAE or A/CA-8 groups (10%). The investigators concluded that a 5-day course of CAE, given twice daily, was shown to be equivalent to the two regimens of A/CA for treatment of AOM with effusion in children.[10]

Treatment Failures. The value of intramuscular ceftriaxone for use in those children who have failed initial oral therapy for AOM deserves careful consideration by pediatricians, emergency physicians, and pediatric emergency medicine specialists. The most compelling data, perhaps, has been generated by a multicenter, non-comparative, nonrandomized study evaluating the clinical efficacy and safety of ceftriaxone for treating AOM in children following clinical failure of oral antibiotic therapy. Middle-ear fluid samples were collected on day 0 and on day 3, 4, or 5 (day 3 to 5) and were used to test whether ceftriaxone therapy can eradicate *Streptococcus pneumoniae* isolates with increased resistance to penicillin (MIC ≥ 1 mg/L). At the first visit, on day 0, middle-ear fluid was sampled for bacteriological testing by tympanocentesis or otorrhea pus suction.[11]

Patients were administered 50 mg of ceftriaxone/kg of body weight/day, injected intramuscularly once daily, for 3 days. A second sample was collected by tympanocentesis if a pneumococcus isolate for which the MIC of penicillin was 1 mg/L or greater was detected in the day-0 sample and if the middle-ear effusion persisted on days 3 to 5. This second sample was tested for bacterial eradication. One hundred eighty-six children ages 5 months to 5 years, 10 months, with AOM clinical failure were enrolled and treated in this trial. On day 10-12, 145 (83.8%) of the 173 patients evaluable for clinical efficacy were clinically cured. Of the 59 patients infected by pneumococci, 36 had isolates for which the MICs of penicillin were 1 mg/L or higher. Of those patients, on day 10-12, 32 (88.9%) were clinically cured.[11]

Middle-ear fluid samples collected by day 3-5 following the onset of treatment with ceftriaxone were sterile for 24 of the 27 (88.9%) patients who were infected as of day 0 by pneumococci for which the MICs of penicillin were 1 mg/L or higher and who were evaluable for bacteriological eradication. On day 10-12, 81.4% of *S. pneumoniae*-infected children and 87.5% of *Haemophilus influenzae*-infected children were clinically cured. No discontinuation of treatment due to adverse events, particularly due to local reactions at the injection site, were reported.[11]

Only 11 adverse events which had doubtful, probable, or possible links with the study treatment were recorded. Both the bacteriologically assessed eradication of pneumococci for which the MICs of penicillin were 1 mg/L or higher and the clinical cure rates demonstrate that ceftriaxone is of value in the management of AOM unresponsive to previous oral antibiotic therapy. The role of ceftriaxone as an initial agent for treatment of AOM is potentially compromised by the "semi-invasive" nature of an intramuscular injection, cost, parental and patient acceptance, necessity for a brief observation period, and necessity for three injections in the outpatient office setting.[11]

Centers for Disease Control and Prevention Guidelines: Drug-Resistant *Streptococcus pneumoniae* Therapeutic Working Group

The concern about evolving resistance to *S. pneumoniae* prompted the CDC to convene experts in the management of otitis media to form the Drug-Resistant *Streptococcus pneumoniae* Therapeutic Working Group. The objective was to provide consensus recommendations for the management of AOM and strategies for surveillance of drug-resistant *Streptococcus pneumoniae* (DRSP).

The Group addressed five principal questions: 1) Can amoxicillin remain the best initial antimicrobial agent for treating AOM, especially in the current period of increasing prevalence of DRSP? 2) What are suitable alternative agents for use if amoxicillin fails? 3) Should empiric treatment of AOM vary by geographic region? 4) Where can clinicians learn about resistance patterns in their patient populations? And, 5) What modifications to laboratory surveillance would improve the utility of the information for clinicians treating AOM?

The recommendations were made on the basis of both published and unpublished data summarized from the scientific literature and experience from the experts present. After group presentations and review of background materials, subgroup chairs prepared draft responses to the five questions, discussed the responses as a group, and edited those responses.[7]

Although the precise universe of studies included or excluded and the process by which data were used for making specific antibiotic recommendations was not discussed in detail, the Group did issue recommendations. And even though the consensus group was limited to a relatively small number of experts, they issued rather rigid recommendations limited to four agents, among them, that oral amoxicillin should remain the first line antimicrobial agent for treating AOM. They proposed that in view of the increasing prevalence of DRSP, the safety of amoxicillin at higher than standard dosages, and evidence that higher dosages of amoxicillin can achieve effective middle ear fluid concentrations, an increase in the dosage used for empiric treatment from 40 to 45 mg/kg/d to 80 to 90 mg/kg/d was recommended.[7]

For patients with clinically defined treatment failure after three days of therapy, the group presented a limited number of useful alternative agents that included oral amoxicillin/clavulanate, cefuroxime axetil, and intramuscular ceftriaxone. They noted that many of the 13 other FDA-approved otitis media drugs lack good evidence for efficacy against DRSP, but did not specify which drugs did and which ones did not.

They also concluded that, currently, local surveillance data for pneumococcal resistance that are relevant for the clinical management of AOM are not available for most areas in the United States. Their recommendations to improve surveillance include establishing criteria for setting susceptibility breakpoints for clinically appropriate antimicrobials to ensure relevance for treating AOM, testing middle ear fluid or nasal swab isolates in addition to sterile site isolates, and the testing of drugs that are useful in treating AOM.

Challenging the Guidelines, Resistance Surveys, and Implications For Clinical Practice. For a number of reasons, the Working Group recommendations have fueled controversy and well-reasoned, evidence-based counter-responses from a number of experts and investigative groups. For example, one Cleveland Clinic group conducted an exhaustive study of the susceptibilities of *Streptococcus pneumoniae* (1476 strains) and untypeable *Haemophilus influenzae* (1676 strains) to various oral beta-lactam, macrolide-azalide, and fluoroquinolone antimicrobial agents. Resistance patterns were

Table 1. Organisms Isolated by Tympanocentesis in Acute Otitis Media

COMMON
Streptococcus pneumoniae
Haemophilus influenzae
Moraxella catarrhalis
LESS COMMON
Streptococcus pyogenes
*Staphylococcus aureus**
Gram-negative enteric bacteria*
Anaerobic bacteria
Viral pathogens:
• respiratory syncytial virus
• rhinovirus
• adenovirus
• influenza
• parainfluenza
* relatively common in neonates (< 1 month of age)

determined by broth microdilution. Organisms were isolated from specimens obtained from outpatients in six geographic regions of the United States. MIC data were interpreted according to pharmacodynamically derived breakpoints applicable to the oral agents tested.[12]

Overall, 94% of *S. pneumoniae* isolates were susceptible to amoxicillin and amoxicillin/clavulanate, 69% were susceptible to azithromycin and clarithromycin, 63% were susceptible to cefprozil and cefuroxime, 52% were susceptible to cefixime, 22% were susceptible to cefaclor, and 11% were susceptible to loracarbef. Based on these susceptibility data, it may be difficult to decipher why the CDC recommended cefuroxime as a second line alternative to amoxicillin but did not not include a short-course macrolide option such as azithromycin, even though in this surveillance study, as well as others cited below, it had marginally superior activity against *S. pneumoniae* as compared to the cephaloporin.[12-15]

In this regard, the activity of macrolides against *S. pneumoniae* and other etiologic agents has been confirmed in other surveillance data as well.[13] For example, the susceptibility of Canadian isolates of three respiratory tract pathogens (*Haemophilus influenzae, Moraxella catarrhalis,* and *Streptococcus pneumoniae*) to several antimicrobial agents were tested by two different methods. Beta-lactamase was produced by 68 of 211 (32.2%) *H. influenzae* isolates and 64 of 75 (85.3%) *M. catarrhalis* isolates. For *S. pneumoniae,* 19 of 156 (12.2%) isolates were resistant to penicillin (MIC ≥ 0.12 mg/L) and two isolates had MICs of 1.5 mg/L. For some combinations of agents and organisms, different methods gave different values for the proportion of isolates susceptible.[13]

Regardless of methodology, for *H. influenzae* the most active antimicrobials based on proportion of strains susceptible were ciprofloxacin (100%) and cefpodoxime (98.5-100%). For *M. catarrhalis*, the most active agents were azithromycin, cefaclor, cefixime, cefpodoxime, cefuroxime, ciprofloxacin, clarithromycin, and loracarbef (100% each); the least active was ampicillin.

Against penicillin-sensitive and -resistant pneumococci, the activity was not significantly different for azithromycin and clarithromycin (93.4-100%) and ciprofloxacin (MIC_{90} 2.0 and 1.5 mg/L, respectively), but was different for cefuroxime (99.3% and 31.6%, respectively), cefaclor (MIC_{90} 0.75 and ≥ 256 mg/L, respectively), cefpodoxime (MIC_{90} 0.047 and 1.5 mg/L, respectively), and loracarbef (MIC_{90} 0.75 and ≥ 256 mg/L, respectively). This study indicates the increasing incidence, in Canada, of beta-lactamase resistance in *H. influenzae* and *M. catarrhalis* and penicillin resistance in *S. pneumoniae*. The authors concluded that macrolides provide excellent in vitro activity against the three most common bacterial offenders—*H. influenzae, M. catarrhalis,* and *S. pneumoniae*—encountered in AOM.[13] *(See Table 1.)*

As part of the ongoing multinational SENTRY antimicrobial resistance surveillance program, a total of 1047 respiratory tract isolates of *Streptococcus pneumoniae*, 845 from 27 United States medical centers and 202 from seven Canadian institutions, were collected between February and June 1997 and characterized in a central laboratory. In the United States, the overall percentages of penicillin-intermediate strains and strains with high-level resistance to penicillin were 27.8% and 16.0%, respectively. In Canada, these values were 21.8% and 8.4%, respectively. Among the 31 centers in the United States and Canada that contributed at least 19 isolates, the combined rate of intermediate plus resistant strains varied between 24.0% and 67.8%.[14]

The in vitro activity of 19 other antimicrobials was assessed against all study isolates. Overall rates of resistance among selected agents in the United States and Canada, respectively, were as follows: amoxicillin, 18.1% and 10.5%; cefaclor, 38.3% and 26.2%; cefuroxime, 19.5% and 12.9%; cefpodoxime, 18.6% and 11.4%; cefepime, 8.2% and 4.5%; cefotaxime, 4.0% and 3.0%; macrolides (i.e., erythromycin, azithromycin, and clarithromycin), 11.7-14.3% and 5.0-7.4%; clindamycin, 3.5% and 3.5%; chloramphenicol, 3.9% and 4.0%; tetracycline, 10.2% and 10.9%; and trimethoprim-sulfamethoxazole, 19.8% and 15.8%.[14]

Divergence in Expert Opinion. Because of the ample body of literature supporting macrolide activity against common etiologic agents in AOM, and the growing number of published studies demonstrating effectiveness of short-course therapy with azithromycin and some cephalosporins, pediatric, emergency medicine, and infectious disease experts have expressed well-reasoned reservations about strict adherence to a dogmatic, guidelines-directed treatment strategy in AOM.[16]

Some experts prefer to consider a more multi-factorial view of organisms implicated in AOM, middle ear drug levels, and the possible emergence of atypical organisms as causes of infection.[17] The Kentucky Research Group notes that *S. pneumoniae, H. influenzae,* and *M. catarrhalis* are the most frequently isolated pathogens in patients with AOM. Other potential causative pathogens include *Streptococcus pyogenes* in older children and *Chlamydia pneumoniae* in younger children. The recent emergence of penicillin-resistant *S. pneumoniae* and the increasing frequency of beta-lactamase-producing strains of *M. catarrhalis* and *H. influenzae* are creating concerns regarding the use of amoxicillin as traditional first-line empiric therapy for AOM in younger children.[17]

The omission of specific antibiotics has elicited counterpoint positions by a significant number of pediatric experts, pharmacologists, and clinical scholars. Both the in vitro antibiotic activity against these more resistant causative pathogens and the antibiotic concentrations achieved in middle ear fluid must be considered when selecting antibiotics for treatment of refractory AOM. The newer macrolides, azithromycin and clarithromycin, provide reasonable in vitro coverage against penicillin-resistant *S. pneumoniae* and beta-lactamase-producing *H. influenzae,* although azithromycin is more active against the latter. Both drugs also achieve notably higher, sustained concentrations in middle ear fluid than do beta-lactam antibiotics. Thus, according to this evaluation based on in vitro data and epidemiological trends, the newer macrolides represent important new, rational alternatives for the management of AOM.[17]

In a roundtable session discussing the potential pitfalls in the

Table 2. Factors Considered in Determining Total Outcome Costs for Otitis Media in Children

- Cost of *initial* physician (or extended provider) visit
- Cost of the first antibiotic prescription
- Cost of subsequent human resource time (telephone consultations, re-evaluations, etc.) expended by nurses, physicians, and other providers to service queries about the drug, its side effects, dosing schedule, and other questions
- Cost of practitioner re-evaluation time to assess cause of treatment failures
- Cost of subsequent antibiotic prescriptions (i.e., additional courses of therapy) in response to treatment failures
- Economic opportunity costs sustained by parents or guardians because of time lost from work to care for child or in order to administer medication
- Cost of medications or other measures (diapers) to service gastrointestinal side effects (diarrhea) of antibiotics
- Cost of managing sequelae related to treatment failure: recurrent infections, tympanostomy, mastoiditis, hearing loss, learning disability, otitis media with effusion, etc.

CDC working group recommendations, several key points were emphasized.[16] At least two members felt the guidelines were limiting. Dr. Jeffrey Blumer, Chief of Pediatric Pharmacology at the University Hospitals of Cleveland, suggested that the antibiotic choices in the published guidelines "are, in some ways, problematic." Specifically, he expresses concern that the guidelines may have "left out a number of useful agents that may perform as well as other agents," adding that he is not sure he is in "full concurrence [with the CDC guidelines]." Appropriately, Blumer emphasizes that there are about "17 agents [labeled by the FDA] for use in acute otitis media," and "none of them is labeled as second-line agents." He summarizes his position this way: " I think the consensus statement and guidelines fall short by not encompassing anything that really points out the similarities and differences [among available antibiotics]."[16]

The fact is, studies and surveillance data are inconsistent in identifying specific outcome data confirming the efficacy of one antibiotic vs. another in AOM.[10,12-16,18] Although Dr. Scott F. Dowell, medical epidemiologist at the CDC, stressed that the working group recommendations focused specifically on antibiotic issues as they relate to *S. pneumoniae* resistance, other roundtable participants concurred with Dr. Blumer and emphasized the shortcomings of the published guidelines. Dr. Itzhak Brook, Professor of Pediatrics at Georgetown University, expressed concern "that the guidelines are limiting us to only three options, and each of the three options have their own problems." Potential limitations cited by the pediatrician included the diarrhea associated with amoxicillin/clavulanate, the poor taste toleration of cefuroxime in liquid form, and the potential discomfort of three intramuscular injections of ceftriaxone. Brook concluded with an opinion that clinicians "should also consider other agents that would be able to achieve similar goals," and then added that it might be difficult "following these less-than-practical guidelines, which will only result in frustration."

Table 3. PPPD Factors Influencing Antibiotic Selection for Acute Otitis Media in Children

PRESCRIPTION AND PHARMACY RESISTANCE BARRIERS

Cost of course of therapy
Prescription coverage by health plan
Formulary status/availability
Previous experience with medication
Physician and pharmacist-based patient education
Written instructions for parent/guardian regarding medication intake
Emphasizing importance of medication compliance

PARENT RESISTANCE BARRIERS

Number of days required to complete a course of therapy
Daily dose frequency of the medication (once-daily dosing is optimal)
Day care considerations: Can all doses of the antibiotic be given by the parent without reliance on day care personnel or other caretakers to ensure administration?
Can medication be taken with or without food, or are special timing considerations required?
Do side effects (diarrhea, GI discomfort, etc.) deter parents from completing a full course of therapy?
Does the drug require refrigeration?

PATIENT RESISTANCE BARRIERS

Taste of medication: Does the suspension have a pleasant and appealing flavor, and a palatable consistency? Or, is the taste excessively bitter and the consistency granular and unappealing to the child?
Gastrointestinal tolerance profile: GI distress? Diarrhea? Nausea? Rash?
Discontinuation rate of antibiotic
Does child feel "forced" to take antibiotic?

DRUG RESISTANCE BARRIERS

What are clinical cure rates in well-designed clinical trials?
Does antibiotic show increasing in vitro resistance to *S. pneumoniae* species?
Does antibiotic show increasing in vitro resistance to beta-lactamase-positive middle ear pathogens, *H. influenzae,* and *M. catarrhalis?*
What are regional or local antibiotic resistance patterns?

The PPPD Approach to Selecting Antimicrobial Suspensions in Children

Given the diversity of opinion, variability in study designs for AOM, and conflicting results of surveillance trials, as well as the continuing controversies surrounding antibiotic selection in AOM, another approach to antibiotic may be considered. Specifically, this framework for antibiotic selection attempts to account not only for *S. pneumoniae*

Table 4. PPPD Approach to Selection of Oral Antibiotic Suspensions for Treatment of Acute Otitis Media in Children[4-6,10,19-25,31,32,34,50]

ORAL ANTIBIOTIC SUSPENSION (Generic name)	PRESCRIPTION RESISTANCE (Cost for course of therapy < $40)	PARENTAL RESISTANCE (Once-daily dosing)	PATIENT RESISTANCE (Palatability and GI effect profile considered extremely favorable)	DRUG RESISTANCE (Less than 30% of *S. pneumoniae* isolates from middle ear show in vitro resistance and drug shows adequate coverage of beta-lactamase-producing *H. influenzae* and *M. catarrhalis)*
Amoxicillin	++ ($7.49)	± (BID)	+	–
Amoxicillin-clavulanate	+ ($39.40)	± (BID)	– (diarrhea)	+
Azithromycin	+ ($30.35)	+ (QD)	+	+
Cefaclor	+ ($39.40)	– (BID/TID)	+	±
Cefixime	– ($47.20)	+ (QD)	+	±
Cefpodoxime	– ($56.00)	+ (QD)	– (poor taste)	+
Cefprozil	– ($47.35)	± (BID)	– (poor taste)	+
Cefuroxime	– ($64.84)	± (BID)	+	+
Clarithromycin	– ($44.60)	± (BID)	– (poor taste)	+
Erythromycin-sulfisoxazole	+ ($23.60)	– (TID or QID)	– (poor taste, GI intolerance)	±
Loracarbef	– ($57.20)	± (BID)	+	+
Trimethoprim-sulfamethoxazole	++ ($6.63)	± (BID)	– (allergic reactions)	±
Ceftriaxone	± ($24-72)	± QD (1-3 days)	– (intramuscular injection)	+

(+) Satisfies specific PPPD category criterion; (-) Does not usually satisfy specific PPPD category criterion; (±) Possibly satisfies PPPD category criterion

resistance, but also such other factors as: pharmacokinetic parameters, beta-lactamase producing species of *H. influenzae* and *M. catarrhalis*, regional variations, and real world barriers (cost, compliance, patient toleration, taste, side effects, dosing schedules, convenience factors, etc.) that can affect the journey form prescription pad to clinical cure. It can be argued that this is a more comprehensive, outcomes-oriented approach—one that is also evidence-based—because it attempts to account for all potential barriers that may obstruct or compromise optimal clinical outcomes in the real world.[1,4-6,10,15,17,19,30-33,35-37,51]

PPPD Resistance Barriers for Oral Antibiotic Therapy. In the best and most cost-effective of all worlds, the antibiotic selection process for AOM would be based on an outcome-oriented assessment of the total cost of cure for this common, and sometimes recurrent and distressing, infection in the pediatric age group. *(See Tables 1 and 2.)* Close examination of Table 2 underscores the importance of identifying therapeutic agents that, because of favorable cost, compliance, and coverage features, are able to reduce barriers to achieving clinical cure.

Antimicrobial agents that satisfy these criteria (acceptable spectrum of coverage, reasonable cost, excellent toleration, acceptable taste, and streamlined dosing schedule) will likely improve "first time around" cure rates and thereby reduce overall outcome costs. Among the factors that would be included in such an outcome analysis (i.e., the total costs associated with diagnosis, management, and cure of otitis media) are the following: cost of the medication used for the initial course of therapy, cost of the initial physician visit, human resource time (telephone time, revisits, etc.) required to service queries regarding the drug and/or its side effects, the cost of practitioner re-evaluations for treatment failures, the cost of additional courses of therapy for therapeutic failures, the economic opportunity cost sustained by parents because of time lost from work to care for their child, the cost of medications or other devices (diapers, etc.) to service the gastrointestinal side effects (diarrhea) of the medication, and the short- and long-term sequelae of treatment failure or repeated episodes of infection (hearing loss, linguistic difficulties, tympanostomy tubes, mastoiditis, otitis media with effusion, etc.).

Although comprehensive, outcome-directed studies addressing all of these variables for AOM are not currently available, other outcome-sensitive drug therapy assessment tools can be pressed into service for the purpose of drug selection. In this regard, the prescription, parent, patient, and drug resistance (PPPD) approach to drug selection permits pediatricians, family practitioners, and pediatric emergency physicians to evaluate and compare the clinical success profiles (CSPs) of one antibiotic vs. another. *(See Table 3.)* These comparisons are based on a synthetic approach constructed according to established specifications and parameters such as price, daily dosing frequency, duration of therapy, in vitro resistance data from numerous studies, palatability, side-effect profile, and spectrum of coverage.[1,2,10,15,17,20,21,26-29,31-39,51]

From the perspective of prescribing antibiotics in the outpatient setting, it must be emphasized that each of these four resistance barriers is important, and that if one or more of these barriers (cost, side-effect profile, lack of convenience, inadequate coverage) is of sufficient magnitude, it may influence the overall real-world cure rate.[2,15,21,28]

Optimal PPPD Profiles.[6] Optimal PPPD profiles are characterized by antibiotics with low prescription, parent, patient, and drug resistance barriers. In this regard, the most desirable agent—in other words, the antibiotic producing the greatest likelihood of clinical success in the real-world patient encounter—will satisfy the following criteria: 1) It will be priced attractively enough to encourage prescription filling and/or its cost is sufficiently competitive to ensure formulary acceptance at cost-sensitive, managed care health plans and HMOs; 2) it is easy enough to store, prepare, and give to encourage parental administration; 3) it is sufficiently well-tolerated by the patient to promote ingestion of the drug without undue patient resistance; and 4) the agent demonstrates in vitro activity against all the anticipated bacterial pathogens in AOM (*S. pneumoniae, H. influenzae* [including beta-lactamase producing species], and *M. catarrhalis*) so that its empiric use will provide appro-

Table 5. Antibiotics of Choice for Pediatric Otitis Media[4-6,10,19-25,31,32,34,50]

First-Line Antibiotic Suspensions for Acute Otitis Media in Children (cost for course of therapy usually < $10)

GENERIC NAME	TRADE NAME	DOSAGE	DURATION	COST	COMMENTS
Amoxicillin	Amoxil	80-90 mg/kg/d in two or three divided doses	10 days	$6.02-$8.13	Significant resistance to beta-lactamase-producing *H. influenzae* and *M. catarrhalis.* Up to 25% of *S. pneumoniae* resistant at lower doses. Widely used as first-line agent.

Second-Line Antibiotic Suspension for AOM (cost < $10)

GENERIC NAME	TRADE NAME	DOSAGE	DURATION	COST	COMMENTS
Trimethoprim-Sulfamethoxazole	Septra or Bactrim	8/40 mg/kg/d	10 days	$5.36-$7.70	Increasing resistance (up to 30%) to *S. pneumoniae* species Allergic reactions: Stevens-Johnson (rare)

First-Line Antibiotic Suspensions for Acute Otitis Media in Children (cost for course of therapy usually < $45)

GENERIC NAME	TRADE NAME	DOSAGE	DURATION	COST	COMMENTS
Amoxicillin-clavulanate	Augmentin	80/20 mg/kg/d	10 days	$38.10-$44.30	Diarrhea common (16% of patients)
Azithromycin	Zithromax	10 mg/kg day 1, 5 mg/kg days 2-5	5 days	$28.40-$32.20	Compliance-enhancing. Good in vitro coverage of beta-lactamase-producing *H. influenzae* and *M. catarrhalis.* Clinical cure rates in pediatric otitis media comparable to those seen with amoxicillin/clavulanate.

First-Line Antibiotic Suspensions for Acute Otitis Media in Children (cost for course of therapy usually > $40)

GENERIC NAME	TRADE NAME	DOSAGE	DURATION	COST	COMMENTS
Cefuroxime	Ceftin	30 mg/kg/d	10 days	$62.84	
Ceftriaxone	Rocephin	50 mg/kg/d IM	1-3 days	$24-$72	Intramuscular dosing may be inconvenient

Second-Line Antibiotic Suspensions for Acute Otitis Media in Children (cost for course of therapy usually > $40)

GENERIC NAME	TRADE NAME	DOSAGE	DURATION	COST	COMMENTS
Clarithromycin	Biaxin	15 mg/kg/d	10 days	$42.40-$44.10	Palatability may be consideration
Cefpodoxime	Vantin	10 mg/kg/d	10 days	$54.00-$57.20	Palatability may be consideration

priate coverage with initial therapy, thereby reducing the necessity for pharmacologic reservicing due to treatment failures. A drug with an acceptable drug resistance profile will also have demonstrated in clinical studies that it is effective in treating AOM.

Based on the parameters outlined above, it is possible to categorize and compare antibiotic suspensions according to whether and how consistently they satisfy specific PPPD criteria. The antibiotic with the most favorable overall PPPD profiles is azithromycin, followed by amoxicillin/clavulanate and ceftriaxone. *(See Table 4.)*

Antibiotics of Choice

The outcome-sensitive, cost-effective oriented criteria considered in the PPPD system can be used to guide initial selection of antibiotics for otitis media. *(See Table 4.)* Because price is an important issue, especially in managed care environments, Table 4 presents therapeutic recommendations that have been broken down according to price categories (i.e., suspensions costing < $40 for an entire course vs those costing > $40). As discussed, many authorities still consider amoxicillin to be the drug of first choice for AOM because of its efficacy, low cost, and tolerability.[38] A more critical look at changing resistance patterns to PRSP species has induced the CDC group to recommend a dosing schedule of amoxicillin 80-90 mg/kg/d.

Introduction of new antimicrobial options with shorter courses and more convenient dosing schedules has forced a re-evaluation of this agent's time-honored position among many pediatric and infectious disease experts.[15-17,29,34-37,39] Nevertheless, because amoxicillin has been an "institution" in the therapeutic arsenal for otitis media, it justifies inclusion among first-line options costing less than $10 per course of therapy, albeit with some reservations. In this regard, amoxicillin may be a less-than-optimal initial agent in patient subgroups at higher risk for treatment failure due to poor medication compliance and in communities where a high percentage of penicillin-resistant *S. pneumoniae* isolates and beta-lactamase producing species have been documented.[3,5,29,40]

Among agents that cost more than $20 but less than $40, three agents with acceptable PPPD profiles merit inclusion in the first-tier group: azithromycin, amoxicillin/clavulanate, and ceftriaxone (when administered as a single dose). Based on azithromycin's PPPD profile, which reflects a reasonable acquisition cost ($29.40-$31.60 per course of therapy), its once-daily, five-day therapeutic course, low discontinuation rate (< 1% due to side effects) efficacy studies confirming cure rates comparable to amoxicillin/clavulanate, and acceptable in vitro activity against implicated bacterial species, azithromycin justifiably can be positioned as a first-line-or alternate to amoxicillin-agent for AOM in children.[19,41-45] Amoxicillin/clavulanate, which also merits inclusion in this "first-line" group, has the advantages of appropriate spectrum of coverage and evidence-based trial support for its efficacy. Ceftriaxone, another first-line PPPD recommendation, has the advantage of established efficacy in treatment failures, and an acceptable level of activity against the three most common organisms implicated in AOM, including PRSP species. It must be administered by the intramuscular route, and in one study three days of once-daily IM injections were required, which may adversely affect patient and parental acceptance. *(See Table 5.)*

Antibiotics such as trimethoprim-sulfamethoxazole can be very useful when cost issues predominate in drug selection and in patients with penicillin allergies.[46] However, evolving *S. pneumoniae* resistance makes trimethoprim-sulfamethoxazole a less-than-ideal choice as compared to high dose amoxicillin (90 mg/kg), which also has cost advantages. Among medications usually costing in excess of $40 for a course of therapy, first-line agents would include cefuroxime, a CDC working group alternative to amoxicillin. Second-line agents in this category would include clarithromycin and cefpodoxime, both of which may pose palatability problems. Cefpodoxime has the advantage of once-daily dosing and a short course of therapy.

Disposition and Follow-up

The majority of children with AOM can be treated successfully as outpatients. Indications for hospitalization include toxic appearance, refractory vomiting, severe volume depletion, and intracranial or intratemporal extension, including acute mastoiditis and meningitis. Febrile neonates in the first month of life with otitis media should be managed as inpatients because of their relatively immunocompromised state and because of the risk of sepsis from gram-negative organisms and *S. aureus*.

Afebrile neonates younger than 1 month of age with otitis media can be treated as outpatients if they are well-appearing and have close follow-up.[47] Selected febrile infants between 4 and 12 weeks of age can be treated for AOM as outpatients, provided they are non-toxic in appearance, have a white blood cell count of less than 15,000 cells/mm^3, and have been carefully evaluated to exclude other sources of infection (including examination of cerebrospinal fluid, if indicated).[48] It is imperative that discharged neonates have a reliable caretaker with a telephone and that prompt follow-up is assured.

Older infants and children with AOM who are well-appearing, have no underlying disease, and an otherwise normal examination do not require further laboratory evaluation in the ED. Well-appearing febrile children with otitis media have the same rate of occult bacteremia as well-appearing febrile children with no obvious source for their infection. Complete blood counts, which generally show a mild leukocytosis, and blood cultures are not routinely indicated, and results do not correlate with severity of illness or risk of complications.

Follow-Up. Upon discharge, parents and caretakers of children treated for AOM should receive careful discharge instructions highlighting potential problems related to treatment failure. In order to identify patients with infections refractory to initial antibiotic therapy, parents should be instructed to return for re-evaluation if fever, ear pain, or other signs and symptoms of acute infection are persisting 48 hours after initiation of antibiotic therapy.

Parents should also be instructed to return for re-evaluation immediately if the child exhibits evidence of worsening illness, including rising temperature, increasing irritability, anorexia, vomiting, or the development of lethargy. Signs and symptoms of infection will resolve within two days in most children treated for AOM. Assuming that the child recovers as expected, a follow-up examination in 2-3 weeks is generally recommended. The purpose of the re-evaluation is to document resolution of infection and to detect chronic effusion or other sequelae of AOM.

The necessity for routine follow-up in all cases of AOM has recently been questioned. In healthy children older than 15 months of age, parental impression of infection resolution and absence of symptoms appear to be accurate predictors of otitis resolution. Therefore, routine follow-up visits at 2-3 weeks may only be required of children 15 months of age or younger, those who have persistent symptoms of otitis media, or whose parents believe that the infection has not resolved.[49] Children not meeting these high-risk criteria would still require follow-up at a later date to assess for persistent effusion, but this visit can be delayed for up to three months.

References

1. Dagan R, Leibovitz E, Greenberg D, et al. Early eradication of pathogens from middle ear fluid during antibiotic treatment of acute otitis media is associated with improved clinical outcome. *Pediatr Infect Dis J* 1998;17:776-782.
2. Finney JW, Friman PC, Rapoff MA, et al. Improving compliance with antibiotic regimens for otitis media: Randomized clinical trial in a pediatric clinic. *Am J Dis Child* 1985;139:89-95.
3. Nelson JD. Clinical importance of compliance and patient intolerance. *Infect Dis Clin Pract* 1994;3:158-160.
4. Cockburn J, Gibberd RW, Reid AL, et al. Determinants of non-compliance with short-term antibiotic regimens. *BMJ Clin Res* 1987;295:814-818.
5. Greenbery RN. Overview of patient compliance with medication dosing: A literature review. *Clin Ther* 1984;6: 592-599.
6. Bosker G. *Pharmatecture: Minimizing Medications to Maximize Results.* St. Louis: Facts and Comparisons; 1996.
7. Dowell SF, Butler JC, Giebink GS, et al. Acute otitis media: Management and surveillance in an era of pneumococcal resistance-A report from the Drug-resistant *Streptococcus pneumoniae* Therapeutic Working Group. *Pediatr Infect Dis J* 1999;18:1-9.
8. Kozyrskyj AL, Hildes-Ripstein GE, Longstaffe SE, et al. Treatment of acute otitis media with a shortened course of antibiotics: A meta-analysis. *JAMA* 1998;279:1736-1742
9. Garcia Callejo FJ, Velert Vila MM, Orts Alborch MH, et al. Comparison of azithromycin, amoxicillin/clavulanic acid and cefaclor in the treatment of acute ENT infections. *Acta Otorrinolaringol Esp* 1998;49:306-312.
10. Pessey JJ, Gehanno P, Thoroddsen E, et al. Short course therapy with cefuroxime axetil for acute otitis media: Results of a randomized multicenter comparison with amoxicillin/clavulanate. *Pediatr Infect Dis J* 1999;18:854-859.
11. Gehanno P, Nguyen L, Barry B, et al. Eradication by ceftriaxone of *Streptococcus pneumoniae* isolates with increased resistance to penicillin in cases of acute otitis media.

Antimicrob Agents Chemother 1999;43:1532.

12. Jacobs MR, Bajaksouzian S, Zilles A, et al. Susceptibilities of *Streptococcus pneumoniae* and *Haemophilus influenzae* to 10 oral antimicrobial agents based on pharmacodynamic parameters: 1997 U.S. Surveillance study. *Antimicrob Agents Chemother* 1999;43:1901-1908.
13. Blondeau JM, Suter M, Borsos SJ. Canadian Antimicrobial Study Group. Determination of the antimicrobial susceptibilities of Canadian isolates of *Haemophilus influenzae, Streptococcus pneumoniae* and *Moraxella catarrhalis. Antimicrob Agents Chemother* 1999;43(Suppl A):25-30.
14. Doern GV, Pfaller MA, Kugler K, et al. Prevalence of antimicrobial resistance among respiratory tract isolates of *Streptococcus pneumoniae* in North America: 1997 results from the SENTRY antimicrobial surveillance program. *Clin Infect Dis* 1998;27:764-770.
15. McLinn S, Williams D. Incidence of antibiotic-resistant *Streptococcus pneumoniae* and beta-lactamase-positive *Haemophilus influenzae* in clinical isolates from patients with otitis media. *Pediatr Infect Dis J* 1996;15(9 Suppl):S3-S9.
16. Dowell SF, (Moderator) Blumer JL, Brook I, Culpepper L, et al. (Panel Members). Acute Otitis Media: Challenging the Guidelines and Course of Antibiotic Therapy. *Medical Crossfire*. 1999;1: June 15, 1999.
17. Block SL. Causative pathogens, antibiotic resistance and therapeutic considerations in acute otitis media. *Pediatr Infect Dis J* 1997;4:449-456.
18. Haddad J JR, Saiman L, Chin NX, et al. Penicillin-nonsusceptible pneumococcus in acute otitis media in New York City. *Otolaryngol Clin North Am* 1994;27:431-441.
19. McLinn S. Double blind and open label studies of azithromycin in the management of acute otitis media in children: A clinical review. *Pediatr Infect Dis J* 1995;14: S62-S66.
20. Demers DM, Scotik Chan D, Bass JW. Antimicrobial drug suspensions: A blinded comparison of taste of twelve pediatric drugs including cefixime, cefpodoxime, cefprozil, and loracarbef. *Pediatr Infect Dis J* 1994:13:87-89.
21. Chinburapa V, Larson LN. The importance of side effects and outcomes in differentiating between prescription drug products. *J Clin Pharm Ther* 1992;17:333-342.
22. Beardon PH, McGilchrist MM, McKendrick AD, et al. Primary noncompliance with prescribed medications in primary care. *BMJ* 1993;307:846-848.
23. Berg JS, Dischler J, Wagner DJ, et al. Medication compliance: A healthcare problem. *Ann Pharmacother* 1993;27:S1-24.
24. Litchman HM. Medication noncompliance: A significant problem and possible strategies. *R I Med* 1993;76:608-610.
25. McNally DL, Wertheimer D. Strategies to reduce the high cost of patient noncompliance. *Md Med J* 1992;41:223-225.
26. Anonymous. Writing prescription instructions. *Can Med Assoc J* 1991;44:647-648.
27. Coleman TJ. Non-redemption of prescriptions. *BMJ* 1994; 308:135.
28. Roth HP, Caron HS. Accuracy of doctor's estimates and patient's statements on adherence to a drug regimen. *Clin Pharm Ther* 1978;23:361-370.
29. Eisen SA, Miller DK, Woodward RS, et al. The effect of prescribed daily dose frequency on patient medication compliance. *Arch Intern Med* 1990;150:1881-1884.
30. Amsden GW. Pneumococcal macrolide resistance—Myth or reality? *J Antimicrob Chemother* 1999;44:1-6.
31. Dagan R, Leibovitz E, Fliss DM, et al. Bacteriologic efficacies of oral azithromycin and oral cefaclor in treatment of acute otitis media in infants and young children. *Antimicrob Agents Chemother* 2000;44:43-50.
32. Scaglione F, Demartini G, Dugnani S, et al. Interpretation of middle ear fluid concentrations of antibiotics: Comparison between ceftibuten, cefixime and azithromycin. *Br J Clin Pharmacol* 1999;47:267-271.
33. Brook I, Gober AE. Microbiologic characteristics of persistent otitis media. *Arch Otolaryngol Head Neck Surg* 1998;124: 1350-1352.
34. Cohen R, Navel M, Grunberg J, et al. One dose ceftriaxone vs. ten days of amoxicillin/clavulanate therapy for acute otitis media: Clinical efficacy and change in nasopharyngeal flora. *Pediatr Infect Dis J* 1999;18:403-409.
35. Thompson D, Oster G, McGarry LJ, et al. Management of otitis media among children in a large health insurance plan. *Pediatr Infect Dis J* 1999;18:239-244.
36. Thornsberry C, Jones ME, Hickey ML, et al. Resistance surveillance of *Streptococcus pneumoniae, Haemophilus influenzae* and *Moraxella catarrhalis* isolated in the United States, 1997-1998. *J Antimicrob Chemother* 1999;44:749-759.
37. Howie VM. Eradication of bacterial pathogens from middle ear infections. *Clin Infect Dis* 1992;14(Supp 2):209-210.
38. Anonymous. Drugs for treatment of acute otitis media in children. *Med Lett Drugs Ther* 1994;36:19-21.
39. McCarty JM. Bacterial susceptibility and tympanocentesis in acute otitis media. *Pediatr Infect Dis J* 1995;14:S45-50.
40. Friedland IR, McCracken GH. Management of infections caused by antibiotic-resistant Streptococcus pneumoniae. *N Engl J Med* 1994;331:377-382.
41. Neu HC. Otitis media: Antibiotic resistance of causative pathogens and treatment alternatives. *Pediatr Infect Dis J* 1995;14:S51-56.
42. Barry AL, et al. In vitro activity of 12 orally administered antibiotics against four species of respiratory pathogens from U.S. medical centers in 1992 and 1993. *Antimicrob Agents Chemother* 1994;38:2419-2425.
43. Hopkins SJ, Williams D. Clinical tolerability and safety of azithromycin in children. *Pediatr Infect Dis J* 1995;14:S87-91.
44. Khurana C, McLinn S, Block S, et al. Trial of Azithromycin (AZ) vs Augmentin (AUG) for treatment of acute otitis media (AOM) [Abstract M61-64] Presented at the 34th Interscience Conference on Antimicrobial Agents and Chemotherapy, Orlando, FL, Oct. 4-7, 1994.
45. Brown SD, Burton P, Rich T, et al. Susceptibility surveillance of U.S. respiratory pathogen isolates to newer macrolide and azalide antibiotics. Presented at the 94th General Meeting of The American Society for Microbiology, Las Vegas, NV, May 23-27, 1994.
46. Berman S. Otitis media in children. *N Engl J Med* 1995;332: 560-1565.
47. Fleisher GR. Infectious disease emergencies. In: Fleisher GR,

Ludwig S, eds. *Textbook of Pediatric Emergency Medicine*. 3rd ed. Baltimore: Williams & Wilkins; 1993.

48. Baker MD, Bell LM, Avner JR. Outpatient management without antibiotics of fever in selected infants. *N Engl J Med* 1993;329;1437-1441.
49. Hathaway TJ, Katz HP, Dershewitz RA, et al. Acute otitis media: Who needs post-treatment follow-up? *Pediatrics* 1994; 94:143-147.
50. McLinn S, Williams D. Incidence of antibiotic-resistant *Streptococcus pneumoniae* and beta-lactamase-positive *Haemophilus influenzae* in clinical isolates from patients with otitis media. *Pediatr Infect Dis J* 1996;15(9 Supp):S3-S9.
51. Chater RW. Dosing tips for tots. *Am Pharm* 1993;NS33:55-56.

Antibiotic Selection for Acute Otitis Media

Gideon Bosker, MD, FACEP

Outcome-effective management of patients with acute otitis media (AOM) remains one of the most debated, investigated, and controversial areas in outpatient medicine. A number of factors account for the wide spectrum of recommendations and approaches used in this patient population. Among the most important issues is the emergence of resistant organisms causing AOM, a trend that has complicated its treatment, and more specifically, identification of first-line antimicrobials for initial management of children with AOM.

The clinical burden of AOM in pediatric and emergency practice has been well-documented. It is estimated that the number of physician visits for AOM has increased from 9 million in 1975 to more than 25 million by the 1990s.[1] In one large study, investigators identified and retrospectively followed 22,000 children younger than 10 years of age who had one or more episodes of AOM.[2] Study subjects averaged 2.9 physician office visits for management of otitis media; among children younger than 2 years of age, one-fourth had six or more such visits. Amoxicillin was prescribed as initial therapy in more than one-half (56.6%) of all episodes of acute otitis media, followed by cephalosporins (18.3%), trimethoprim-sulfamethoxazole (12.3%), macrolides (6.4%), and amoxicillin-clavulanate (6.0%). Over multiple episodes, however, use of amoxicillin declined by about 50%.[2]

Organisms commonly responsible for causing AOM include *Streptococcus pneumoniae, Haemophilus influenzae*, and *Moraxella catarrhalis*. The evolution of pneumococcal resistance to penicillins, trimethoprim-sulfamethoxazole, and oral cephalosporins may require use of other agents as initial therapy. Moreover, beta-lactamase-producing *H. influenzae* and *M. catarrhalis* are becoming increasingly resistant to penicillins, trimethoprim-sulfamethoxazole, oral cephalosporins, and erythromycin.

Mechanisms of resistance include changes in penicillin-binding proteins, production of beta-lactamase, alterations in target enzymes, and inhibition of drug access to the site of action. Regional variations also are present. One study reported that the prevalence of penicillin-nonsusceptible (intermediate and resistant) pneumococci was highest in the South Atlantic (44%) and East South Central (43%) regions and lowest in the Mid-Atlantic (28%) and New England (28%) regions.[3] Because of changing resistance patterns and the increasingly limited spectra of activity of many currently available antimicrobials, new agents have been developed in the hope of improving therapeutic outcomes.

Selecting an antibiotic for initial treatment of AOM—as well as for treatment failures—has become the subject of intensive analysis by pediatricians, emergency physicians, and infectious disease specialists. While amoxicillin and trimethoprim-sulfamethoxazole are still considered appropriate first-line agents by some experts and panels, children at risk for resistant infections—as well as those risk-stratified into a more serious subgroup—may be treated initially with cefuroxime axetil, azithromycin, or amoxicillin-clavulanate.

Additional debate has focused on the necessity—or lack thereof—of treating mild or initial cases of AOM. Although some experts point out antibiotics may not be routinely indicated in all cases—especially mild or first episodes—of AOM, it remains the position of

Table 1. Risk Factors for Otitis Media

- Day care attendance
- Siblings at home
- Second-hand cigarette smoke
- Lack of exclusive breast feeding for the first four months
- Male sex
- White race
- Native American race
- Craniofacial abnormalities, including cleft palate
- Family history of otitis media
- Family history of atopy
- History of otitis media

the CDC and most U.S. experts that antibiotics should be used to treat documented cases of AOM. Certainly, this is the accepted standard for children with risk factors for poor outcome. Finally, there has been substantial investigation into the value, effectiveness, and potential compliance-enhancement associated with short-course (5 days or less) therapy for AOM.

With these issues in clear focus, the purpose of this review is to present a rational and evidence-based approach to an analysis of current treatment strategies, published recommendations, and clinical support tools designed to maximize clinical outcomes in children with AOM.

Etiology

The primary reason for colonization of the middle ear with pathogenic bacteria is eustachian tube dysfunction. It occurs in infants and children mainly because of the abnormal tubal compliance, leading to collapse of the eustachian tube and delayed innervation of the tensor veli palatini muscle, which serves to open the tube. The three most common bacteria involved in AOM are *Streptococcus pneumoniae, Haemophilus influenzae*, and *Moraxella catarrhalis*. Anaerobic organisms, as well as viruses, also can contribute to the infection. One study recently determined the prevalence of various respiratory viruses in the middle ear fluid of children (ages 2 months to 7 years) with AOM.[4] In 168 of 456 children, the etiology for their respiratory tract infection was viral. Respiratory syncitial virus was the most common virus found in middle ear fluid during AOM, followed by parainfluenza virus, influenza A or B virus, enteroviruses, and adenoviruses. The risk factors that lead to AOM are shown in Table 1.[5] The factors that most increase the occurrence of AOM are child care outside the home and parental smoking.[6]

Clinical Features

Most commonly, a viral upper respiratory infection precedes AOM. Sudden development of ear pain and fever in one-third to one-half of patients can signal the onset of AOM. In infants, the symptoms can be less localized and can include irritability, vomiting, diarrhea, and fever.

Middle ear effusion (MEE) is the hallmark of otitis media. If MEE is associated with symptoms such as pain or fever, the condition is called AOM. When MEE is asymptomatic, the condition is called otitis media with effusion (OME). Erythema of the tympanic membrane without associated MEE is myringitis or tympanitis.[7]

Table 2. Common Signs and Symptoms of Inflammation and Fluid in the Middle Ear[5]

- Otalgia
- Ear pulling
- Diminished hearing
- Fever
- Loss of appetite
- Irritability
- Vomiting
- Vertigo
- Tinnitus
- Otorrhea

Examination of the tympanic membrane is best accomplished with pneumatic otoscopy to determine movement. A normal tympanic membrane is flaccid, and lack of motion when the ear is insufflated implies middle ear fluid. Tympanometry also can be used to assess MEE. Table 2 lists the signs and symptoms seen most commonly when there is inflammation and fluid in the middle ear.[5]

Differential Diagnosis

Although otalgia is the number one symptom of patients presenting with AOM, a substantial number of patients presenting with this symptom will have normal-appearing ear canals and tympanic membranes.[8] When the ear appears normal, the physician must consider the possibility of referred pain to the ear.

The sensory innervation is supplied through a combination of cranial nerves five, seven, nine, 10, and a number of cervical nerves. The convergence of these cranial and upper cervical somatic afferents into a common synaptic region can explain the occurrence of referred pain in the head and neck region. Common sources of referred otalgia include abscessed teeth, malocclusion, temporomandibular joint disorders, myofascial pain syndromes (especially in the masseter muscles), nasopharyngeal carcinoma, infections in the paranasal sinuses, pharynx and salivary glands, carotodynia, temporal arteritis, cervical arteritis, and neuralgias.[9] The age of the patient can allow exclusion of many of the above possible causes.

In most developed countries (except the Netherlands), the standard treatment for AOM is antibiotic therapy. However, in 1992, the U.S. Institute of Medicine warned of the growing threat posed by resistant bacteria, and in 1996, the Centers for Disease Control and Prevention convened the Drug-resistant *Streptococcus Pneumoniae* Therapeutic Working Group made up of pediatricians, family physicians, internists, and public health practitioners to determine how best to use antimicrobial resistance data to make informed decisions for treatment of AOM.[10] Penicillin resistance has been found everywhere that surveillance data are available. The proportion of invasive disease caused by penicillin nonsusceptible *S. pneumoniae* (minimum inhibitory concentration [MIC] 0.1 mcg/mL) ranges from 8% to 34%, with the higher rates in children rather than adults, especially if the children are in day care or have received antibiotic therapy within the preceding three months.[11] One study found the rate of ampicillin resistance of bacteria in effusions to be three times higher during recurrent AOM as compared to an initial untreated episode of AOM.[12]

General Principles, Issues, and Controversies

From a practical, clinical perspective, it is well accepted that antibiotic prescribing for AOM is almost always empiric in nature and rarely benefits from microbiological identification or susceptibility results. Some clinicians note that mild cases—especially those with low-grade fever and no risk factors for poor outcomes—may either have viral etiologies and/or not benefit greatly from antibiotic therapy. However, experts point out that distinguishing among patients who, on the basis of clinical grounds alone, do and do not require antimicrobial intervention can be a formidable challenge for the front-line practitioner.

In addition, there are other "real world" issues that enter the equation, even after antibiotic therapy is chosen. Even if an antibiotic with an appropriate spectrum of coverage is identified, there is always the "give" and "take" issue associated with antibiotic administration (i.e., parents have to "give" the antibiotic, and in turn, children must be willing to "take" the drug). This give-and-take interaction is fundamental to maximizing cure rates in the real-world environment.

Making matters worse is the difficulty of identifying an appropriate, cost-effective antibiotic that is "smart" enough to provide coverage against the most likely offending organisms in any individual patient. For example, in children with otitis media, a so-called "high-performing" or "correct spectrum" antibiotic must have a sufficiently targeted spectrum to cover appropriate—and increasingly, penicillin-resistant—species of *Streptococcus pneumoniae* (PRSP), *Haemophilus influenzae,* and *Moraxella catarrhalis.*

Moreover, because time-honored agents such as amoxicillin, especially at previously recommended, so-called low doses of 40 mg/kg/d, have demonstrated inconsistent in vitro activity against beta-lactamase-producing bacterial isolates as well as against PRSP species, many experts have recommended alternative agents or new dosing protocols for established agents, among them, ceftriaxone, cefuroxime, amoxicillin-clavulanate, advanced macrolides (azithromycin) and amoxicillin (80-90 mg/kg).[2,13-20]

Finally, the road from the prescription pad to clinical cure depends on many factors beyond spectrum of coverage, including prescription, parent, patient, and drug resistance (PPPD factors). The PPPD approach to antimicrobial selection in otitis media attempts to account for all the factors and potential "barriers" that go into the equation for clinical cure, such as cost of the medication, compliance profile, palatability issues, duration of therapy, gastrointestinal side-effect profile, convenience of dosing, spectrum of coverage, resistance patterns, and day care administration concerns. Overcoming all these barriers to clinical cure is essential for enhancing clinical outcomes and reducing the costs of therapy and complications of the disease.

Antibiotic Selection in Acute Otitis Media: The Case for and Against Routine Antibiotic Therapy

Who should be treated? When are antibiotics indicated, and when is watchful waiting with close follow-up the most appropriate course? The majority of pediatricians, family practitioners, and emergency physicians—and, in fact, many parents of children with otitis media—are aware that the necessity to routinely treat otitis media with antibiotics has been the subject of heated debate over the past decade.

In this regard, a number of factors are widely cited as evidence that current indications for antibiotic treatment should be re-evaluated. Four placebo-controlled trials examining the effect of withholding antibiotic therapy in acute otitis media found that 76% of untreated children demonstrated "spontaneous cure" or significant improvement without treatment.[21] A recent meta-analysis of 30 studies evaluating 5400 cases of acute otitis media found an 81% rate of spontaneous symptom resolution and improvement in the appearance of the tympanic membrane.[22] While some of these spontaneously resolving cases may represent patients with ear infections of viral etiology, the high percentage of recovery without treatment suggests that a significant percentage of bacterial infections will also clear without antibiotic therapy.

These data have led some practitioners to view AOM as a self-limited disease that does not generally require medical (i.e., antimicrobial) intervention. In Europe, particularly in Scandinavia and the Netherlands, watchful waiting is an accepted standard of care for AOM. Most physicians in these countries will initiate antibiotic therapy only when fever and symptoms persist for more than 24-72 hours or when complications develop.[22-24] By withholding antibiotics for the majority of patients, it has been argued, unnecessary antibiotic treatment with its attendant costs and side effects is minimized, and the rise of multidrug-resistant bacterial organisms may be curtailed.

These studies, however, should be interpreted with great caution, since the majority of the trials included in the meta-analysis did not follow children over the long term and, therefore, could not evaluate the risk of recurrent infections, hearing loss, development of otitis media with effusion, and other complications. Moreover, the rate of spontaneous recovery appears to be bacterial species-specific, with some organisms associated with better non-treatment recovery rates than others. In this regard, one study reported that in about 50% of patients with *H. influenzae*, 80% of those with *M. catarrhalis*, and in only 20% of those with *S. pneumoniae*, was there a spontaneous recovery.[25] Unfortunately, because confirmation of a specific etiologic diagnosis is the exception rather than the rule in AOM, it is almost impossible to predict which patients will and will not benefit from antibiotic therapy. Accordingly, most experts in the United States do not favor withholding antibiotic therapy in AOM.

Moreover, European studies, it has been noted, do not have sufficient power to detect low complication rates and represent only children not prone to recurrent infections.[21,26] It is argued that complications such as intratemporal or intracranial infections, which are now rare, occurred in up to 20% of patients with AOM in the pre-antibiotic era.[21] In particular, antimicrobial therapy was largely responsible for reducing the incidence of mastoiditis as a sequela of otitis media from 17% to less than 1%.[27] Furthermore, a recent rise in the number of cases of acute mastoiditis in German infants and children has been attributed to inadequate or absent antibiotic treatment of AOM.[28]

In addition to the limitations of the aforementioned studies, recent investigations and meta-analyses demonstrate antibiotic therapy to be significantly more effective than a strategy of watchful waiting.[22,29] Despite the high spontaneous cure rate, treatment with antimicrobial agents improves the incidence of symptom resolution in AOM by about 15% and reduces treatment failure eightfold compared to observation alone.[22,30] In light of these studies, and given the dramatic reduction in complications since the introduction of antibiotics, most pediatric and emergency medicine authorities—as well as the CDC—in the United States recommend routine antibiotic treatment for acute otitis media suspected to be of bacterial origin.[1,31]

The Pediatric Antimicrobial Armamentarium: The Challenge of Making Sound Therapeutic Choices

Although one of the principal concerns when choosing antibiotic therapy is the drug's in vitro efficacy against the most likely infective organisms—including potentially resistant species—many studies have found that a number of available antimicrobial agents are virtually equally effective in treating otitis media.[32] In this regard, it also should be noted that a drug's efficacy in a clinical trial setting and its therapeutic worthiness in the "real-world environment"—which is characterized by well-recognized impediments to clinical cure such as day care-mediated administration of the drug, palatability of the medication, cost considerations, and discontinuation due to side effects—often diverge depending on the clinical environment and patient population. Development of agents permitting more convenient administration but which also maintain in vitro coverage against the appropriate bacterial species represents an attempt to mitigate these potential barriers.

The most commonly isolated bacterial pathogens in both acute and recurrent otitis media are *Streptococcus pneumoniae*, *Haemophilus influenzae* (nontypable), and *Moraxella catarrhalis*.[33,34] Consequently, first-line agents should demonstrate adequate in vitro coverage against this spectrum of organisms. In children between 1 month and 10 years of age, *S. pneumoniae* and *H. influenzae* each account for about 40% of infections; *M. catarrhalis* accounts for about 20%.[35] It should be stressed that neonates may also develop infections with gram-negative enteric bacilli and *Staphylococcus aureus*, together accounting for 15-20% of otitis media cases in this age group.[26] Other pathogenic bacteria include *Streptococcus pyogenes* and anaerobic organisms.[36] Children younger than 6 years of age with patent tympanostomy tubes and acute symptoms have pathogens similar to other children, while *Pseudomonas aeruginosa* and *Staphylococcus aureus* are occasionally isolated from older children with tubes.[37]

Drug resistance among bacteria involved in otitis media is rapidly emerging.[13,34] In this regard, beta-lactamase production is common among isolates of *H. influenzae* and *M. catarrhalis*, rendering about 30-50% of *H. influenzae* and up to 80% of *M. catarrhalis* isolates resistant to ampicillin.[38] The emergence of PRSP has dominated current concerns about antimicrobial therapy.[19,20] Although variable from patient to patient and region to region, these emerging resistance patterns may explain the failure rates associated with such traditional therapeutic approaches—and older dosing recommendations—as amoxicillin.[13,34]

Accordingly, the evolution of antibiotic-resistant bacterial strains implicated in otitis media has fueled interest in alternatives and backup therapy to amoxicillin, which, primarily because of its cost, has been the traditional first-line agent for this infection, despite showing increasing resistance. This problem can be circumvented by adding a beta-lactamase inhibitor such as clavulanic acid to amoxicillin (i.e., amoxicillin-clavulanate), increasing the dose of amoxicillin, or by choosing alternative antibiotics, among them, azithromycin, cefuroxime, or ceftriaxone.

A far more disturbing trend is the emergence of penicillin-resistant *S. pneumoniae*. Although the incidence of resistant strains demonstrates regional variations, the continued prevalence of *S. pneumoniae* as the principal etiologic agent in otitis media has important therapeutic implications. In addition to the older, so-called "standard antibiotics," most notable among them the penicillins such as amoxicillin and TMP/SMX, there are many newer oral agents, particularly cephalosporins and macrolides, that play an important role in treating bacterial infections commonly encountered in children.

Typically, antibiotics have been evaluated by comparing spectrum of activity, clinical efficacy, toxicity (adverse drug reactions and interactions), pharmacokinetics, convenience, compliance with dosing, and cost. When antibiotics are indicated, however, the choice is often more complicated than it may seem to be on the surface. Addressing resistance issues is important, but other aspects of the treatment plan also require evaluation.

The newer antibiotic suspensions, although possessing variable increases in the spectrum of activity and convenience factors over older agents, have uniformly been shown in clinical trials to be equally, but rarely more, efficacious than standard therapy. It should be stressed, however, that within the context of clinical trials, patients are frequently counseled and followed with pill counts to ensure compliance with their regimens. As a result, outcomes in these studies may deviate (i.e., they may be better than) from those observed in the "real world," where noncompliance with antibiotics is a major barrier impeding the pathway from the prescription pad to clinical cure.[39-42] Consequently, it may be difficult to extrapolate from cure rates published in idealized clinical trials to observed results at the front lines of clinical practice.

Special Therapeutic Considerations in AOM: Evidence-Based Analysis of Treatment Options

The clinical debate surrounding outcome-effective therapy for AOM has been fueled by the need to consider a multiplicity of issues that go into the equation for drug selection. For example, while adequate in vitro activity against increasingly resistant *S. pneumoniae* may be the focus of one panel evaluating therapeutic options, another group may focus its attention on β-lactamase-producing organisms, i.e., *H. influenzae* or *M. catarrhalis* species. And while in vitro activity against organisms implicated in AOM is certainly an important parameter to follow, other experts have generated their recommendations based on the antibiotic levels achieved in the middle ear, as well as intracellular drug concentrations and the effect on bacterial infection.

Although identification of emerging resistance patterns is an essential component of developing treatment pathways (see Figure), it is acknowledged that the precise relationship between antimicrobial resistance (as measured by in vitro studies) and real-world clinical results in children with AOM is far from conclusive. Some observers have challenged surveillance studies reporting resistance to certain antibiotics, pointing out the "disconnect" between in vitro results, tissue levels of the antibiotic, and clinical outcomes.[1,18,43-46] These experts also emphasize the inconsistency in findings reported by such surveys, which are conducted according to different study designs. Still other trials have focused on the efficacy of short treatment courses, and stress that many consensus panels have failed to account for the usefulness of this approach in AOM treatment protocols.[1-3,25,47-49] Finally, there is the issue of treatment failures and identifying second-line agents that predictably produce acceptable cure rates in patients who have failed their first course of therapy.

What is clear is that any treatment recommendation for AOM must account for as many of the potential variables, resistance patterns, pharmacokinetic parameters, regional variations, and real world barriers—cost, compliance, patient toleration, taste, side effects, dosing schedules, and convenience factors—that can affect the journey from prescription pad to clinical cure. The PPPD approach to antibiotic selection for AOM (see next section) attempts to account for all these factors, including the CDC working group recommendations. In the sections that follow, an evidence-based approach to evaluating critical issues in AOM management is presented.

Antibiotics For Beta-Lactamase-Producing Organisms: Treatment Implications. From Nov. 1, 1997, to April 30, 1998, 726 *Moraxella catarrhalis* isolates and 1529 *Haemophilus influenzae* isolates were obtained from 34 medical centers throughout the United

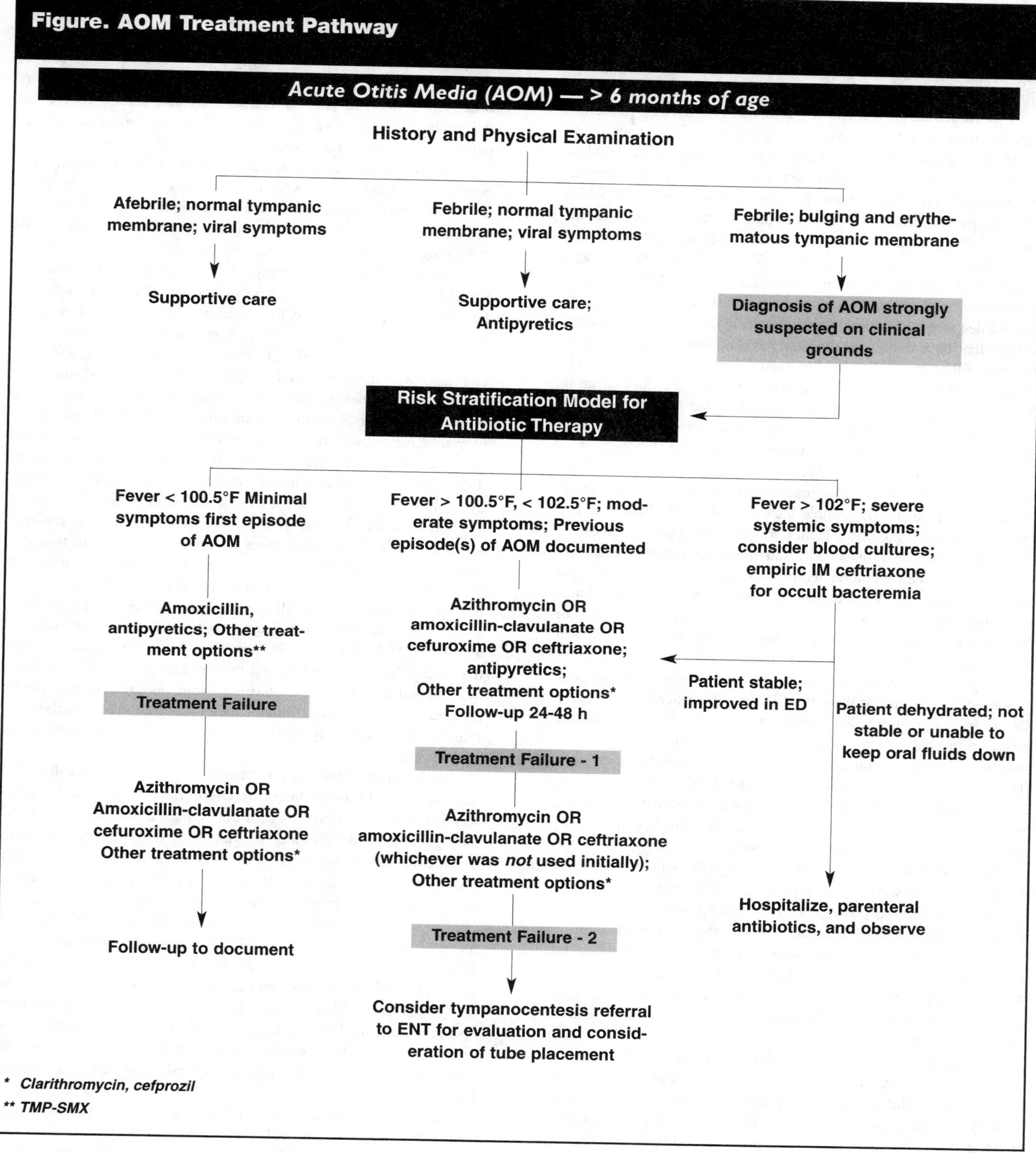

States. Rates of beta-lactamase production were 94.6% among *M. catarrhalis* and 31.1% among *H. influenzae* strains. Susceptibility rates of *M. catarrhalis* isolates to selected antimicrobial agents were greater than 99% for amoxicillin-clavulanate, cefixime, cefpodoxime, cefuroxime, cefaclor, loracarbef, clarithromycin, azithromycin, chloramphenicol, and tetracycline, 97.8% for cefprozil, 50.4% for trimethoprim-sulphamethoxazole, and 28.1% for ampicillin.[50]

Of the antimicrobials tested against *H. influenzae*, the only agents with susceptibility rates below 96% were loracarbef (87.6%), cefprozil (83.4%), cefaclor (82.7%), trimethoprim-sulphamethoxazole (67.3%) and ampicillin (64.7%). The clarithromycin susceptibility rate was 67.4% but this agent was not tested in the presence of its 14-OH metabolite. This survey supports the susceptibility of beta-lactamase-producing strains of both *H. influenzae* and *M.*

catarrhalis to such agents as azithromycin, amoxicillin-clavulanate, and cefpodoxime. Conversely, its suggests potentially less-than-optimal susceptibility rates to these species for such agents as ampicillin and trimethoprim-sulfamethoxazole. The precise implications on clinical cure and failure rates cannot be assessed from the study.[50]

Pneumococcal Macrolide Resistance: Drug Selection Implications. At least one consensus panel report has attempted to justify downgrading the use of macrolides for treatment for AOM on the basis of in vitro resistance patterns reported with *Streptococcus pneumoniae*. This has created a formidable debate about which agents—amoxicillin, amoxicillin-clavulanate, azithromycin, or the cephalosporins—represent the best initial choice for AOM.

According to some experts—as well as clinicians who have had excellent clinical results using macrolides for AOM in their own practice—justification for this cautious assessment of some macrolides is questionable, especially in light of rigorous clinical studies that have compared the safety and efficacy of azithromycin to amoxicillin-clavulanate for the treatment of acute otitis media in children.[13,15,20,51,52] In these large trials, clinical cure rates of up to 87.5% were reported, and the authors concluded that azithromycin was as effective as, but better tolerated than, amoxicillin-clavulanate for the treatment of AOM in the pediatric age group.[14-16,18,51]

How, then, does one reconcile expert recommendations with antimicrobial sensitivity data, practitioner experience, and in vivo clinical trial results? The simple answer: only with difficulty. The controversy over antibiotic selection for AOM has been fueled by the observation that use of macrolides and amoxicillin over the past several years has been accompanied by increases in resistance. Despite this trend—which, to some degree or another applies to all antibiotics including cephalosporin—some investigators propose that use of macrolides, in particular, for such conditions as AOM be evaluated according to parameters other than in vitro results exclusively.

To provide a balanced approach to this dilemma, it has been proposed by one author from the Clinical Pharmacology Research Center in Cooperstown, NY, that microbiology laboratories should return to the habit of providing the clinician with MIC values for pathogenic isolates rather than generic susceptibility reports ([S]usceptible, [I]ntermediate, [R]esistant) that are based on standard disc diffusion testing. Although agar dilution MIC testing is a bulky and labor-intensive practice, it provides the best data when conducted in the appropriate environment.

Secondly, and more importantly, these MIC values need to be compared with in vivo antibiotic pharmacokinetics and pharmacodynamics. Although it is possible to compare MIC values directly with serum concentrations of beta-lactams and aminoglycosides, this is not a valid practice, it has been suggested by Amsden, for azithromycin or the macrolides. Rather, MICs of azithromycin and the macrolides must be compared with the infection site and phagocytic cell concentrations to determine the utility, or lack thereof, of one of these agents.[18]

In this regard, the author appropriately emphasizes that there are differences among the macrolides. For example, whereas azithromycin cellular penetration potentially allows maximal pharmacodynamics, perhaps even against moderately or highly resistant pneumococci, other macrolides may do so less optimally. Although there are no reports of widespread clinical failures resulting from macrolide/azalide resistance in pneumococci, it is expected that such reports will appear if and when these isolates become consistently highly resistant. This is likely to affect the macrolides, erythromycin and clarithromycin, before the azalide, azithromycin owing to the differences in pharmacokinetics of these drugs.[18]

Until then, it will be important to determine the MICs of not just one macrolide, but of all the specific macrolides and azalides for the isolates evaluated. This approach will permit clinicians to make pharmacokinetically and pharmacodynamically sound choices and distinctions. The author of this analysis proposes that by choosing clinical MIC breakpoints of 4-8 mg/L for oral macrolides and 32 mg/L or less for oral azithromycin, rather than the present standard breakpoints, the clinician can make a macrolide/azalide choice that will optimize the pharmacodynamics of the drug against the isolated pathogen and result in the best possible clinical outcome.[18]

The aforementioned theoretical advantages of azithromycin have been supported by other in vitro investigations as well as clinical trials.[18,46,52] As emphasized, the prevalence of PRSP and beta-lactamase-producing *Haemophilus influenzae* in otitis media infections is increasing; emergence of these pathogens has complicated treatment. This study attempted to evaluate the incidence of penicillin resistance and the in vitro activity of amoxicillin/clavulanate, cefaclor, loracarbef, cefixime, trimethoprim-sulfamethoxazole, azithromycin, and clarithromycin in *S. pneumoniae* isolates.[47]

The in vitro activity of azithromycin, clarithromycin, and cefaclor also was evaluated in beta-lactamase-positive and -negative isolates of *H. influenzae*. Bacterial isolates of *S. pneumoniae* and *H. influenzae* were obtained by tympanocentesis and subsequent culture of middle ear effusion from children with acute otitis media enrolled in a multicenter trial. Susceptibility to test agents was assessed by disk diffusion and broth dilution techniques with criteria established by the National Committee for Clinical Laboratory Standards.

Nineteen (31%) of the 61 *S. pneumoniae* isolates were resistant to penicillin. A significantly lower percentage of the *S. pneumoniae* isolates were resistant to azithromycin (16%) and clarithromycin (11%) than to penicillin, amoxicillin-clavulanate, cefaclor, loracarbef, or cefixime (31% in all cases). Azithromycin also was more active than cefaclor and significantly more active than clarithromycin against the 55 *H. influenzae* isolates. The investigators concluded that the susceptibility of resistant and nonresistant strains of *S. pneumoniae* to azithromycin and clarithromycin and of isolates of *H. influenzae* to azithromycin, coupled with penetration of azithromycin into the middle ear, may provide a significant advantage in the treatment of otitis media.

Antimicrobial Resistance Patterns and Clinical Results: The Test Tube-Real World Outcomes Disconnect Syndrome. One reason that clinicians disagree about the optimal initial agent for AOM management is the diversity in trial designs evaluating antibiotic treatment for AOM, the diversity of opinion regarding MIC levels and their relationship to in vivo patient outcomes, and the variable clinical end points used to evaluate antimicrobial efficacy.

For example, one study evaluated the susceptibilities of *Streptococcus pneumoniae* (1,476 strains) and untypable *Haemophilus influenzae* (1,676 strains) to various oral beta-lactam, macrolide-azalides, and fluoroquinolone antimicrobial agents using broth microdilution techniques. Organisms were isolated from specimens obtained from outpatients in six geographic regions of the United States. MIC data were interpreted according to pharmacodynamically derived breakpoints applicable to the oral agents tested.[43]

In this study, overall, 94% of *S. pneumoniae* isolates were susceptible to amoxicillin and amoxicillin-clavulanate, 69% were susceptible to azithromycin and clarithromycin, 63% were susceptible to cefprozil and cefuroxime, 52% were susceptible to cefixime, 22% were susceptible to cefaclor, and 11% were susceptible to loracarbef.[43]

However, another study looking exclusively at AOM isolates reported different (i.e., more advantageous) resistance patterns for the macrolides—patterns, in fact, suggesting the clinical usefulness of such agents as azithromycin for this condition. In light of the prevalence of penicillin-resistant *Streptococcus pneumoniae* and beta-lactamase-producing *Haemophilus influenzae* in otitis media infections, a group of investigators set out to evaluate the incidence of penicillin resistance and the in vitro activity of amoxicillin-clavulanate, cefaclor, loracarbef, cefixime, trimethoprim-sulfamethoxazole, azithromycin, and clarithromycin in *S. pneumoniae* isolates. The in vitro activity of azithromycin, clarithromycin, and cefaclor was also evaluated in beta-lactamase-positive and -negative isolates of *H. influenzae.*[44]

In this straightforward and well-designed study, bacterial isolates of *S. pneumoniae* and *H. influenzae* were obtained by tympanocentesis and subsequent culture of middle ear effusion from children with AOM enrolled in a multicenter trial. Susceptibility to test agents was assessed by disk diffusion and broth dilution techniques with criteria established by the National Committee for Clinical Laboratory Standards.[44]

These investigators found that 19 (31%) of the 61 *S. pneumoniae* isolates were resistant to penicillin. A significantly lower percentage of the *S. pneumoniae* isolates were resistant to azithromycin (16%) and clarithromycin (11%) than to penicillin, amoxicillin-clavulanate, cefaclor, loracarbef, or cefixime (31% in all cases). As might be expected, azithromycin also was more active than cefaclor and significantly more active than clarithromycin against the 55 *H. influenzae* isolates. Based on these results, this pediatric investigative group concluded that the susceptibility of resistant and nonresistant strains of *S. pneumoniae* to azithromycin and clarithromycin and of isolates of *H. influenzae* to azithromycin, coupled with penetration of azithromycin into the middle ear, may provide a significant advantage for this agent in the treatment of otitis media.[44]

Other studies have supported the activity of macrolides in penicillin-resistant *S. pneumoniae*. For example, in one urban study, a pediatric team tried to determine the proportion of children with AOM presenting in New York City who were infected with nonsusceptible *Streptococcus pneumoniae*, and to determine the susceptibility of these organisms to penicillins and other antibiotics commonly used to treat AOM.[53]

The children were seen in ambulatory clinics and the emergency department of a tertiary care, inner-city medical center. During a two-year period from 1993 to 1995, 115 children (ages 6 months to 12 years) with AOM underwent tympanocentesis. Patients did not receive antibiotics for at least one week before tympanocentesis.[53]

Investigators found that 31 children were infected with *S. pneumoniae*, and 83.9% of isolates were susceptible to penicillin. Of the 16.1% strains that were nonsusceptible, most (4 of 5 strains) were intermediately resistant, and only one exhibited high-level resistance to penicillin. Of all the cephalosporins tested, only cefotaxime had consistent activity against the intermediately resistant strains. Notably, all nonsusceptible pneumococci were inhibited by macrolides.[53] In contrast to the conclusions of the aforementioned U.S. studies[44] demonstrating clinically useful activity of advanced generation macrolides such as azithro-mycin, an Israeli group reported bacteriologic failure rates suggesting that the susceptibility breakpoints for *H. influenzae* should be considerably lower than the current ones for both cefaclor and azithromycin for AOM caused by *H. influenzae.*[45]

What is clear from these and other investigations, consensus reports, and reviews, is that there is a tremendous variability—and not uncommonly, contradiction and inconsistencies—in both the design of trials and in results of antibiotic efficacy and resistance patterns for organisms causing AOM.

Middle Ear and Tissue Antibiotic Levels. Clearly, variables other than MIC tube dilutions and serum blood levels play an integral role in determining clinical outcomes. In one study designed to determine the potential influence of variables such as the cell content in the fluid and serum levels on the concentrations of ceftibuten, cefixime, and azithromycin in the middle ear fluid of patients suffering from AOM, the authors found that the penetration of antibiotics into the middle ear fluid is influenced by its serum concentrations as well as by the cell content in the fluid. In particular, while ceftibuten and cefixime concentrations are negatively influenced by the cell content in the middle ear fluid, in contrast, the concentration of azithromycin in the middle ear fluid is positively influenced by the cell content in the fluid.[46]

Moreover, studies suggest that among patients who failed to respond to antimicrobial therapy—and have persistent otitis media—certain microbiological characteristics are associated with specific agents used for treatment. In an attempt to identify the pathogens isolated from children with AOM who did not respond to antimicrobial drug therapy, one Georgetown group performed a retrospective analysis of cultures obtained by tympanocentesis from 46 children.[54]

Organisms were recovered from 34 children (74%), and 43 isolates were recovered from these individuals. The organisms included *Streptococcus pneumoniae* (16 isolates), *Haemophilus influenzae* non-type B (12 isolates), *Moraxella catarrhalis* (5 isolates), *Streptococcus pyogenes* (5 isolates), *Staphylococcus aureus* (3 isolates), and *Peptostreptococcus* species (2 isolates).[54]

Resistance to the antimicrobial agent used was found in 27 (63%) of 43 isolates found in 22 patients (48%). Of patients who did not respond to amoxicillin therapy, infection with *H. influenzae* predominated. *Streptococcus pneumoniae* was recovered from five (56%) of nine of those who did not respond to trimethoprim and sulfamethoxazole therapy, four (44%) of nine patients after azithromycin therapy, three (25%) of 12 patients after amoxicillin therapy, and two (40%) of five patients after cefixime therapy. *Streptococcus pyogenes* was recovered from two (40%) of five patients after trimethoprim and sulfamethoxazole therapy and from two (40%) of five patients after cefixime therapy. The authors emphasize the relationship between resistance to antimicrobial drug therapy and failure of patients with otitis media to improve.[54]

References

1. Dowell SF (moderator), Blumer JL, Brook I, Culpepper L, Phillips WR (panel members). Acute otitis media: Challenging the guidelines and course of antibiotic therapy. *Medical Crossfire* 1999;1:5.
2. Thompson D, Oster G, McGarry LJ, et al. Management of otitis media among children in a large health insurance plan. *Pediatr Infect Dis J* 1999;18:239-244.
3. Thornsberry C, Jones ME, Hickey ML, et al. Resistance surveillance of *Streptococcus pneumoniae, Haemophilus influenzae* and *Moraxella catarrhalis* isolated in the United States, 1997-1998. MRL Pharmaceutical Services, Brentwood, TN. Utrecht, The Netherlands. 13665 Dulles Technology Drive, Suite 200, Herndon, VA. Ortho-McNeil Pharmaceutical, Raritan, NJ.
4. Heikkinen T, et al. Prevalence of various respiratory viruses in the middle ear during acute otitis media. *N Engl J Med* 1999;340:260-264.
5. O'Handley JG. Acute otitis media. In: Rakel RE (ed.) *Manual of Medical Practice*. 2nd ed. Philadelphia:WB Saunders; 1996:78-79.
6. Uhari M, et al. A meta-analytic review of the risk factors for acute otitis media. *Clin Infect Dis* 1996;22:1079-1083.
7. Rosenfeld RM. An evidence-based approach to treating otitis media. *Pediatr Clin N Am* 1966;43:1165-1181.

8. Kriesberg MK, Turner J. Dental causes of referred otalgia. *Ear Nose Throat J* 1987;66:30-48.
9. Thaller SR, DeSilva A. Otalgia with a normal ear. *Am Fam Phys* 1987;36:129-136.
10. Dowell SF, et al. Acute otitis media: Management and surveillance in an era of pneumococcal resistance—A report from the Drug-resistant *Streptococcus Pneumoniae* Therapeutic Working Group. *Pediatr Infect Dis J* 1999;18:1-9.
11. Dowell SF, Schwartz B. Resistant pneumococci: Protecting patients through judicious use of antibiotics. *Am Fam Phys* 1997;55:1647-1654.
12. Harrison CV, Marks MI, Welch DF. Microbiology of recently treated acute otitis media compared with previously untreated acute otitis media. *Pediatr Infect Dis J* 1985;4:641-646.
13. Neu HC. Otitis media: Antibiotic resistance of causative pathogens and treatment alternatives. *Pediatr Infect Dis J* 1995;14:S51-56.
14. McLinn S. Double blind and open label studies of azithromycin in the management of acute otitis media in children: A clinical review. *Pediatr Infect Dis J* 1995;14: S62-66.
15. Hopkins SJ, Williams D. Clinical tolerability and safety of azithromycin in children. *Pediatr Infect Dis J* 1995;14:S87-91.
16. Khurana CM. Issues concerning antibiotic use in child care settings. *Pediatr Infect Dis J* 1995;14:S34-38.
17. Aspin MM, Hoberman A, McCarty J, et al. Comparative study of the safety and efficacy of clarithromycin and amoxicillin-clavulanate in the treatment of acute otitis media in children. *J Pediatr* 1994;125:136-141.
18. Amsden GW. Pneumococcal macrolide resistance—Myth or reality? *J Antimicrob Chemother* 1999;44:1-6.
19. Kozyrskyj AL, Hildes-Ripstein GE, Longstaffe SE, et al. Treatment of acute otitis media with a shortened course of antibiotics: A meta-analysis. *JAMA* 1998;279:1736-1742.
20. Garcia Callejo FJ, Velert Vila MM, Orts Alborch MH, et al. Comparison of azithromycin, amoxicillin/clavulanic acid and cefaclor in the treatment of acute ENT infections. *Acta Otorrinolaringol Esp* 1998;49:306-312.
21. Giebink GS, Canafax DM, Kempthorne J. Antimicrobial treatment of acute otitis media. *J Pediatr* 1991;119:495-500.
22. Rosenfeld RM, Vertrees JE, Carr J, et al. Clinical efficacy of antimicrobial drugs for acute otitis media: Meta-analysis of 5400 children from 33 randomized trials. *J Pediatr* 1994;154: 355-367.
23. Van Buchem FL, Dunk JHM, van't Hof MA. Therapy of acute otitis media: Myringotomy, antibiotics, or neither. *Lancet* 1981;883-887.
24. Van Buchem FL, Peters MF, van't Hof MA. Acute otitis media: A new treatment strategy. *BMJ* 1981;290:1033-1037.
25. Howie VM. Eradication of bacterial pathogens from middle ear infections. *Clin Infect Dis* 1992;14 (Suppl 2):209-210.
26. Giebink GS, Le CT. Risk of mastoiditis in typical otitis media not managed by antibiotics. *Lancet* 1982;111.
27. Rudberg RD. Acute otitis media: Comparative therapeutic results of sulfonamide and penicillin administered in various forms. *Acta Otolaryngol* 1954;113(Suppl):9-79.
28. Hoppe JE, Köster S, Bootz F, et al. Acute mastoiditis—Relevant once again. *Infection* 1994;22:178-182.
29. Ruuskanen O, Arola M, Heikkinen T, et al. Viruses in acute otitis media: Increasing evidence for clinical significance. *Pediatr Infect Dis J* 1991;10:427.
30. Burke P, Bain J, Robinson D, et al. Acute red ear in children: Controlled trial of non-antibiotic treatment in general practice. *BMJ* 1991;303:558-562.
31. Paradise JL. Managing otitis media: A time for change. *Pediatrics* 1995;96:712-715.
32. Anonymous. Drugs for treatment of acute otitis media in children. *Med Lett Drugs Ther* 1994;36:19-21.
33. Bluestone, et al. Ten-year review of otitis media pathogens. *Pediatr Infect Dis J* 1992;11:S7-11.
34. Barry AL, et al. In vitro activity of 12 orally administered antibiotics against four species of respiratory pathogens from US medical centers in 1992 and 1993. *Antimicrob Agents Chemother* 1994;38:2419-2425.
35. Stair TO. Otolaryngologic disorders. In: Rosen P, Barkin RM, eds. *Emergency Medicine*. 3rd ed. St. Louis: Mosby-Year Book; 1992:2460-2466.
36. Berman S. Otitis media in children. *N Engl J Med* 1995;332: 1560-1565.
37. Mandel EM, Casselbrant ML, Kurs-Lasky M. Acute otorrhea: Bacteriology of a common complication of tympanostomy tubes. *Ann Otol Rhinol Laryngol* 1994;103:713-718.
38. Cockburn J, Gibberd RW, Reid AL, et al. Determinants of non-compliance with short-term antibiotic regimens. *BMJ Clin Res* 1987;295:814-818.
39. Chater RW. Dosing tips for tots. *Am Pharm* 1993;NS33:55-56.
40. Finney JW, Friman PC, Rapoff MA, et al. Improving compliance with antibiotic regimens for otitis media: Randomized clinical trial in a pediatric clinic. *Am J Dis Child* 1985;139:89-95.
41. Nelson, JD. Clinical importance of compliance and patient intolerance. *Infect Dis Clin Pract* 1994;3:158-160.
42. Osterholm MT, Reves RR, Murph JR, et al. Infectious diseases and child care. *Pediatr Infect Dis J* 1992;11:S31-41.
43. Jacobs MR, Bajaksouzian S, Zilles A, et al. Susceptibilities of *Streptococcus pneumoniae* and *Haemophilus influenzae* to 10 oral antimicrobial agents based on pharmacodynamic parameters: 1997 U.S. Surveillance study. *Antimicrob Agents Chemother* 1999; 43:1901-1908
44. McLinn S, Williams D. Incidence of antibiotic-resistant *Streptococcus pneumoniae* and beta-lactamase-positive *Haemophilus influenzae* in clinical isolates from patients with otitis media. Scottsdale Pediatric Center.
45. Dagan R, Leibovitz E, Fliss DM, et al. Bacteriologic efficacies of oral azithromycin and oral cefaclor in treatment of acute otitis media in infants and young children. *Antimicrob Agents Chemother* 2000;44:43-50.
46. Scaglione F, Demartini G, Dugnani S, et al. Interpretation of middle ear fluid concentrations of antibiotics: Comparison between ceftibuten, cefixime and azithromycin. *Br J Clin Pharmacol* 1999;47:267-271.
47. McLinn S, Williams D. Incidence of antibiotic-resistant *Streptococcus pneumoniae* and beta-lactamase-positive *Haemophilus influenzae* in clinical isolates from patients with otitis media. *Pediatr Infect Dis J* 1996;15(9 Suppl):S3-9.
48. Cohen R, Navel M, Grunberg J, et al. One dose ceftriaxone vs.

ten days of amoxicillin/clavulanate therapy for acute otitis media: Clinical efficacy and change in nasopharyngeal flora. *Pediatr Infect Dis J* 1999;18:403-409.

49. Block SL. Causative pathogens, antibiotic resistance and therapeutic considerations in acute otitis media. *Pediatr Infect Dis J* 1997;16:449-456.
50. Richter SS, Brueggemann AB, Huynh HK, et al. 1997-1998 national surveillance study: *Moraxella catarrhalis* and *Haemophilus influenzae* antimicrobial resistance in 34 U.S. institutions. Department of Pathology, University of Iowa College of Medicine, Iowa City 52242, USA.
51. Khurana C, McLinn S, Block S, et al. Trial of azithromycin (AZ) vs augmentin (AUG) for treatment of acute otitis media [Abstract M61-64] Presented at the 34th Interscience Conference on Antimicrobial Agents and Chemotherapy, Orlando, FL, Oct. 4-7, 1994.
52. Doern GV, Pfaller MA, Kugler K, et al. Prevalence of antimicrobial resistance among respiratory tract isolates of *Streptococcus pneumoniae* in North America: 1997 results from the SENTRY antimicrobial surveillance program. *Clin Infect Dis* 1998;7:764-70.
53. Haddad J JR, Saiman L, Chin NX, et al. Penicillin-nonsusceptible pneumococcus in acute otitis media in New York City. *Otol Head Neck Surg* 1999;121:27-30.
54. Brook I, Gober AE. Microbiologic characteristics of persistent otitis media. *Arch Otolaryngol Head Neck Surg* 1998;124:1350-1352.

The Battered Child

Robert M. Sills, DO, FAAP
Margarita E. Pena, MD, FACEP
Kenneth Parsons, MD, MPH

Acute musculoskeletal injury accounts for a large percentage of all visits to the emergency department (ED). Although fairly straightforward in adults, managing these injuries in children presents special challenges. The clinician must keep in mind that fracture patterns can often be different in children, various growth centers in the bones can simulate fractures, the history is often given by a caretaker and not the injured child, and the physical exam often is more difficult to perform on a child. In addition, it is important to keep in mind that any injury presenting to the ED may be the result of child abuse. The reported frequency of fractures associated with child abuse varies from 11-55%.[1] To effectively manage these injuries, one must develop a systematic approach to evaluating the injured child. This approach must include a thorough history and physical, an understanding of the types of injuries children can sustain, a basic knowledge of pediatric radiographs, and most importantly, an understanding of how to diagnose and manage the intentionally injured (or abused) child. A discussion of the definitive treatment of pediatric fractures can be found in most pediatric, emergency, and orthopedic textbooks and will not be emphasized here. The authors will review skeletal injuries in children with an emphasis on the evaluation and initial treatment of the abused child.

It is well known that commonly occurring childhood fractures (e.g., femur fractures) can be the result of abuse, and that fractures that raise the suspicion of abuse (e.g., spiral fractures) can be accidental.[2,3,4] Therein lies the rift. This article will review the pathophysiology and types of common childhood fractures, and will aid the clinician in deciding which injuries are abusive and which are not. Keep in mind that there is a vast gray area in which the determination is difficult to make. In these cases, experts in this area (i.e., child maltreatment specialists, social service personnel, and pediatric orthopedic surgeons) can assist in making the determination.

Child Abuse

There are many ways to define child abuse. A practical definition of physical abuse for the clinician is: "An injury to a child caused by a caretaker for any reason . . . Injury includes tissue damage beyond erythema or redness from a slap to any area other than the hand or buttocks. Physical discipline should not be used on children who are younger than 12 months of age. The child should be normal developmentally, emotionally, and physically. Tissue damage includes bruises, burns, tears, punctures, fractures, rupture of organs, and disruption of functions. The use of an instrument on any part of the body is abuse. The injury may be caused by impact, penetration, heat, a caustic, a chemical, or a drug."[5] This is not only a thorough definition, but it can aid the clinician in defining which injuries are considered beyond accepted disciplinary measures.

The prevalence of child maltreatment, in all forms, continues to rise. Compared to younger children, children older than 3 years of age

Figure 1. Anatomy of a Growing Long Bone

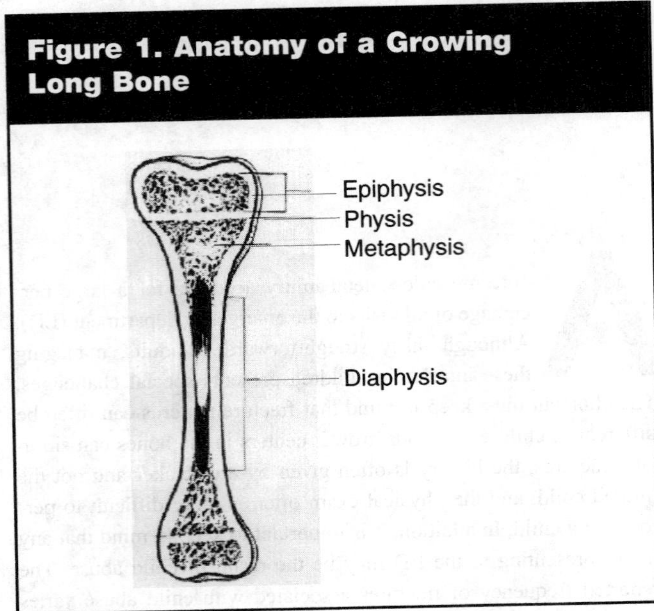

Figure 2. Common Fractures in Childhood

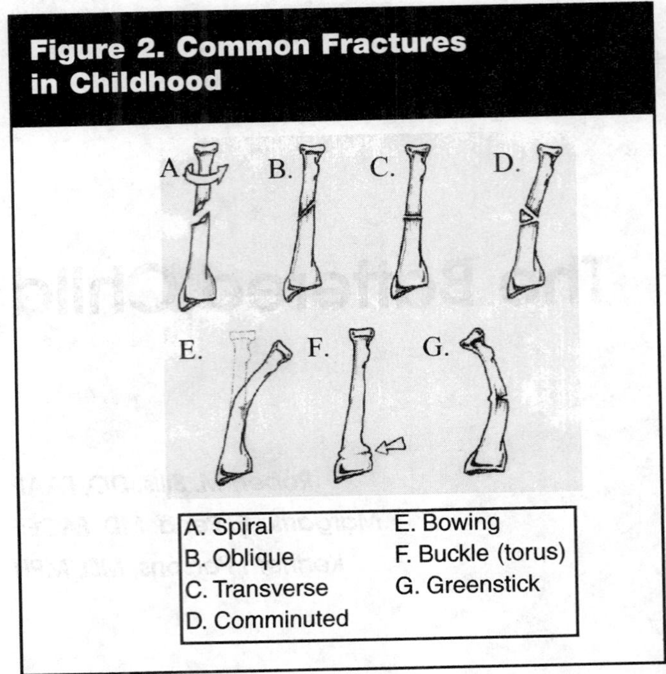

are much more likely to suffer physical and sexual abuse.[6] However, life-threatening injuries and fractures secondary to abuse are much more common in children younger than 5 years of age, with 80% of abuse fractures occurring in this age group.[1,8] In fact, age is the single most important risk factor in the increase of abuse-related skeletal injuries.[1] These are, unfortunately, the patients whose history is most difficult to obtain, and a physical exam harder to perform.

It is important to remember that physical abuse occurs throughout all strata of society and not just in the indigent population.[6] Many of the pitfalls that occur in diagnosing abuse deal with health care professionals' personal beliefs and experiences. Physicians tend to believe that abuse does not occur in pleasant, well-spoken, and well-dressed families. Don't be fooled—all patients should be treated and evaluated with the same systematic approach to avoid missing the diagnosis of child abuse.

Multiple social and cultural factors and family stresses contribute to a child's risk for abuse. Some of the more important risk factors include: the child who is perceived as different (i.e., such as the child with mental or physical handicaps, or behavioral problems); social stressors, such as poverty, unemployment, poor family support, or poor parental relationship; and/or parent produced stresses, such as low self-esteem, being a product of an abusive parent, depression, substance abuse, or ignorance of child rearing. Child abuse can occur when a triggering event, such as a family conflict or substance abuse, is associated with any or all of the above risk factors.[7]

The Growing Bones

The bones of a child need to be able to grow with the child. There are special features of the young bone that allow this to happen. *(See Figure 1.)* A typical long bone allows growth by having growth centers that consist of four distinct anatomic regions. The first region, the metaphysis, is a flared out area between the shaft and the physis. The second region, the physis, is a cartilaginous growth area consisting of several zones. In the physis, a matrix upon which new bone is formed is produced. When the bone stops growing, this cartilaginous area becomes filled with bone. The third region is the epiphysis, which is the bony plate atop the physis that serves as a support for the articular cartilage of that bone. If the end of the bone does not form a joint but attaches to muscles or tendons, it is called an apophysis. Finally, the diaphysis is the shaft of a long bone. Any injury to the growth plate can arrest growth and, subsequently, result in limb deformities. The physis is relatively weak compared to the strong ligamentous attachments between the bones and, when injured, usually will result in a fracture rather than a sprain. Therefore, as a general rule, younger children are more likely to break their bones than have sprains.[9]

A growing child's bones are less dense and have more cartilaginous features than the bones of an adult. The periosteum of a young bone is thicker and has more bone-forming potential than its adult counterpart. These characteristics of the periosteum allow far less displacement of the fracture fragment and quicker healing. Another important feature of the young bone is its ability to remodel. Because of its rapid active growth, the young bone can overcome many imperfections in alignment depending on the location and type of fracture.[9,11] Because of the unique features of the young bone, there are specific fractures that occur in children that do not exist in adults. *(See Figure 2.)* A Buckle or Torus fracture occurs when a compressive force results in failure of the bone, usually at the metaphyseal-diaphyseal junction of the radius or tibia. These fractures can be very subtle both clinically and radiographically. This type of injury occurs in the long bones, which is uncommon in abuse situations. A plastic deformity or bowing fracture occurs when the bone is bent beyond its ability to recoil and remains in a bowed or curved position. Presentation of plastic deformity on x-rays are often subtle. In this situation, comparison films with the normal extremity are beneficial. Greenstick fractures also occur because of the decreased density of the younger bone, resulting in an incomplete fracture involving only one cortex. They are often associated with a bowing deformity. Growth plate fractures involve the physis and/or the metaphysis and epiphysis. They occur in growing bones and can

Figure 3. Salter-Harris Classification of Growth Plate Injuries

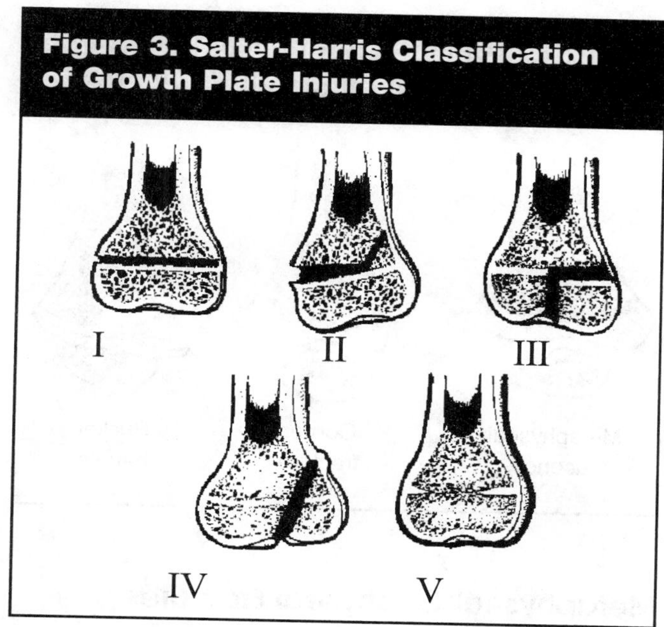

Table 1. Developmental Milestones

AGE	MOTOR SKILLS	FINE MOTOR SKILLS
4-5 months	Rolls front to back	Hands come together
7 months	Sits without support; rolls back to front	Transfers object from hand to hand
9 months	Crawls; pulls to stand	Mature grasp
12 months	Walks with hand	Pat-a-cake; objects in and out of box
15 months	Runs	Use of cup and spoon
2 years	Walks up and down steps	Tower of 6-7 cubes
3 years	Rides a tricycle	Tower of 10 cubes

affect subsequent growth. The Salter-Harris classification system is used to describe the five most common injuries to the growth plate. The higher the number type, the greater likelihood of long-term effect on bone growth. *(See Figure 3.)*[9,10,11]

Other common fracture patterns in childhood, include longitudinal, transverse, oblique, spiral, and comminuted fractures.[9,10,11] All of the previously mentioned fractures can occur in child abuse. However, some are more common than others.

History

In all injuries to children, a thorough history and physical must be obtained to avoid missing the diagnosis of abuse. When evaluating the injured child, it is important to have a complete understanding of the events surrounding the injury. The history can be supplied by the child (if verbal), the parent, or other witnesses. When possible, it should be substantiated by as many witnesses as possible. It is important to ask open-ended questions. Asking the patient, "Why are you here today?" or "What happened to you?" may give a more complete representation of the events rather than a yes or no question, such as "Did your brother push you?" Let the historian supply as much information as possible without leading them. The information should be detailed and include such questions as, what happened, when, where, who was present, and how did it happen? The history also should include previous injuries, fractures, lacerations, burns, hospitalizations, and any significant past or present history of disease processes (i.e., hemophilia, cerebral palsy, failure to thrive, and osteogenesis imperfecta). Injuries not consistent with the history should raise the suspicion of abuse. Injury should be considered in the context of normal developmental milestones. *(See Table 1.)* A pre-ambulatory 7-month-old child, for instance, should not sustain a femur fracture by walking and then falling, nor should a fall from a crib produce multiple fractures or serious injury. The history of the event should be precise and any inconsistencies should be documented. Suspicious histories are usually vague and in two studies were more likely to involve a change in behavior (i.e., child is irritable or not moving an extremity) or a noted abnormality (i.e., swelling of the skull) rather than a history of actual trauma.[3,4] In fact, 63% of abused children in one study and 52% in another who had fractures related to abuse had no history of trauma.

A common type of history given in both abusive and unintentional injuries is a fall. A history of a fracture in a minor fall should be investigated, but single unintentional fractures can occur from falls of less than two feet, and falls from less than four feet can result in injury to more than one bone.[3] Changing stories with repeated histories should also raise suspicion. It is usually best to question the child and the caregiver separately about the events. The child may feel safe in the company of a compassionate health care worker and may be more likely to supply pertinent information than in the presence of a threatening caregiver. Remember, the purpose of the interview in the ED is not to place blame on a specific person but to discover the details of the event. The detective work needed to find the culprit should be left to police investigators. The physician should be a family advocate, as well as a patient advocate. It is best to remain as neutral and objective as possible and assure the family that your ultimate goal is to ensure the safety of the child and not break up the family unit.

Physical Examination

To obtain an informative and complete physical exam on an injured child, it should be performed in a gentle and nonthreatening manner. To gain the child's trust, examine the obviously injured area last and inform the child of each step of the exam. Distractions, such as toys, may help the examiner pinpoint the painful area. Observe first, then palpate. If a child is extremely anxious, he or she may let the parent do the exam. This may help in deciding which films to order. Remember that all injuries can be the result of abuse, and it is important that a complete head-to-toe exam be performed. Undress all areas at some point during the exam. Attention should be paid to the child's modesty. Look for multiple injuries in different stages of healing (pathognomonic for child abuse).[1] Areas often missed on physical exam that are frequently injured in the abused child include the buttocks, genital region, behind the ears, the scalp, the hands, and the feet. Perform the exam in a well lit area to detect subtle bruises and texture changes that may be difficult to discern in darker skinned patients.[15] When examining the injured part of the body, perform a thorough exam including evaluation of neurovascular and motor function as well as inspection, palpitation, color, and temperature assessment.

Physical signs of neglect, which may add evidence to your suspicion of abuse, are easily missed. These signs include, but are not limited to, a dirty, unkempt appearance, severe diaper rash (from infrequent diaper changes), bald spots to the scalp, a withdrawn or shy child, and failure to thrive.

Radiographic Evaluation

Plain films are an important part of the investigation of an injured child. Most fractures can be picked up with two views of the bone at 90° to each other. Insist on perfect postero-anterior (PA) and lateral films. Oblique views are rarely indicated in long bone injuries except in cases where a clinically obvious fracture is not seen on the PA and lateral view.[12] Oblique films are routinely indicated when the hand or foot are injured to avoid missing fractures. Multiple growth areas that change in appearance with age can be confused with fractures, and having a book of normal x-ray variants nearby is helpful. Although comparison views of the unaffected extremity may help in certain cases, routine comparison films are costly and may not be required.

When child abuse is strongly suspected in young children, an additional series of plain films can be helpful in the abuse work-up. Finding multiple fractures in different stages of healing is a classic finding in child abuse.[1] A skeletal survey may pick up these older fractures. The skeletal survey includes two views of the skull, spine, and chest, and one view of the rest of the skeleton and has been shown to aid in the diagnosis of abuse in up to 31% of selected patients.[3] A routine skeletal survey is indicated in all infants younger than 2 years of age who have clinical evidence of physical abuse, and in infants younger than 1 year of age who show evidence of significant neglect and deprivation. A selective approach to complete skeletal examination is suggested for older infants and children to age 5 years. Thereafter, a skeletal survey is rarely indicated.[13] Follow-up skeletal surveys are suggested if abuse is strongly suspected. These follow-up surveys yielded additional fracture information in 61% of cases. Most were previously undetected metaphyseal-epiphyseal lesions.[14] Follow-up skeletal surveys done approximately two weeks after the initial survey are suggested if abuse is strongly suspected.

Although classic x-ray findings exist that are diagnostic for abuse, these findings are often absent and the diagnosis must be made on history and physical alone. Multiple fractures in different stages of healing, fractures not consistent with the patient's developmental level, metaphyseal-epiphyseal fractures, and posterior rib fractures in an infant, are all consistent, if not diagnostic, for child abuse.[1]

Fractures of the long bones in children are common. Distinguishing between intentional and unintentional injuries to the long bones can be a challenge. Abuse fractures are typically divided into diaphyseal and metaphyseal-epiphyseal fractures. Abused infants are more likely to have metaphyseal-epiphyseal injuries than are older children. Abused children older than 1 year of age are more likely to have diaphyseal fractures.[19]

Figure 4. Classic Metaphyseal-Epiphyseal Injuries of Child Abuse

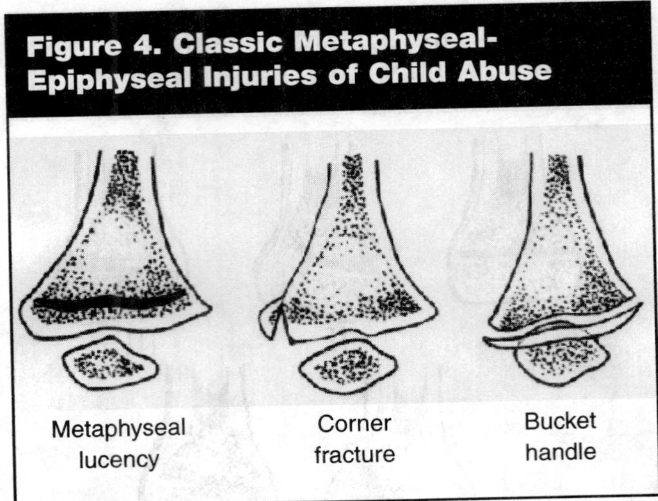

Metaphyseal-Epiphyseal Fractures

Metaphyseal-epiphyseal injuries are classic fractures of child abuse and can occur in any long bone adjacent to a growth plate.[15,18] The intensity and direction of force needed to cause this injury do not occur in typical "accidents." Although previously thought to be due to an avulsion of a metaphyseal fragment at the site of fixed periosteal attachment, it is now known that a different mechanism is involved.[19] Shaking and jerking associated with large accelerating-decelerating forces cause a shearing effect that results in a fracture through the weak spongiosum bone layer. Depending on the size of the injury, the degree of involvement of the periphery of the bone, and the radiographic projection, the following lesions may result: the bucket handle fracture, the corner fracture, or the metaphyseal lucency.[19] *(See Figure 4.)* In contrast, spurring and cupping of the metaphysis of the long bones are common, normal variants in infants under 8 months of age.[11]

Diaphyseal Fractures

Although much more common in abuse than metaphyseal-epiphyseal fractures, diaphyseal injuries are much less specific for abuse.[2] Isolated diaphyseal fractures can present the most difficulty in making the diagnosis of abuse. Since no diaphyseal fracture in and of itself is pathognomonic for abuse, the clinician must take into account the history and physical, developmental age of the child, skeletal survey, social service report (if indicated), and the appearance of fracture. Even with all of this information, it can be difficult to determine how the fracture occurred.

Diaphyseal fractures including transverse, greenstick, spiral, oblique, and comminuted can occur in both intentional and unintentional injuries.[2,4,20] However, the injury should be considered abusive when occurring in conjunction with other skeletal or extraskeletal injuries as well as in cases without adequate history. Long-bone fractures from abuse are more likely to occur in the middle and distal third of the bone.[2,4] Spiral fractures of the femur, although classically considered abusive, can occur in a child who is running then trips and falls.[4] However diaphyseal fractures in nonambulatory children should be considered highly suspicious.[2,4]

Dating a Fracture

Although not an exact science, the physician should have an idea of how fractures appear in different stages of healing on plain films. Immediately after the injury, soft-tissue swelling and inflammation are apparent up until about four days following the injury.[15] Periosteal reaction usually takes approximately 7-10 days to become apparent.[1,16] Hard callus formation usually occurs 14-21 days after the injury.[1] In infants and children, the fracture site can appear normal in as early as six months.[15] Periosteal reaction can be physiologic in infants between 1 and 6 months because of the active growth occurring at this time and should not be mistaken as a fracture. It is more likely to be bilateral and involve the diaphysis of long bones.[16]

Regional Injuries

Skull. Skull fractures are the second most common bony injury seen in child abuse.[13,15,21] The mechanism of injury is a forceful direct impact against a flat surface or from an object or fist. Of intentional skull fractures, 80% occur in infants younger than 1 year of age.[1] The prevalence of skull fractures in abused infants is almost 50%. Infants have a six-fold greater risk of sustaining a skull fracture than an older child.[17,2,21]

The majority of abusive skull fractures are linear, nondepressed parietal fractures. Interestingly, linear parietal fractures are most common whether unintentional or secondary to abuse. Linear skull fractures can be seen in accidental falls less than two feet, and falls from less than four feet can result in complicated fractures. However, fractures that are multiple, depressed, diastatic more than 3 mm, bilateral, or cross suture lines are more suggestive of intentional injury, especially coupled with a suspicious history.[3,22,28,29]

Plain radiographs of the frontal and lateral views of the skull are the best initial screening modality for the skull, except for basilar skull fractures, which usually require computed tomography (CT) for detection. Cranial CT with bony windows are helpful in visualizing the extent of injury of depressed and complicated fractures as well as associated intracranial injuries. Radionuclide skeletal scintigraphy has a low sensitivity for detecting skull fractures.[13]

Humerus. The humerus is the most commonly fractured bone in battered children.[2,20] Several authors have reports that the majority (46-81% in 5 different studies) of humerus fractures in children younger than 3 years of age are intentional, and in infants younger than 15 months, 67-100% of humerus fractures are thought to be secondary to abuse.[4,3,22,25,26] Strait et al studied 164 humeral fractures, more than in any other series, in children younger than 3 years of age and used strict abuse criteria and excluded children with known abuse prior to discovery of the humeral fracture.[20] In this study, only 8% of fractures under age 3 and 36% under 15 months were due to abuse. These significantly lower percentages may have resulted from excluding known abuse cases, thereby underestimating the percent due to abuse.

The most common fracture types associated with abuse are spiral/oblique and transverse.[20,2] The most common fracture locations are midshaft or metaphyseal. Rotational or twisting injuries result in spiral/oblique fractures, while metaphyseal-epiphyseal injuries occur with tractional forces or when the child is grabbed by the arms or shaken.[3,4]

Classic metaphyseal lesions (CML) have been used to describe the metaphyseal-epiphyseal injuries seen in abuse. CML of the humerus are seen radiographically as lateral corner fractures, metaphyseal radiolucencies and irregularities, a discrete fracture line, or flame-shaped metaphyseal extensions.[27] Subperiosteal new bone formation also may be seen. These radiographic changes are most evident in healing or chronic injuries. Acute injuries may have no radiographic signs of injury. Therefore, repeat and/or high-detail radiographs should be performed if abuse is suspected. These lesions are most evident with the humerus in external rotation, as is seen in a standard antero-posterior chest view.

Salter-Harris type fractures (i.e., distal physeal fractures) are less commonly seen than CML injuries and are the result of violent traction or twisting of the arm associated with a greater magnitude of force than seen with CML injuries.[13,12] Abuse should be strongly considered when these injuries are present. Although plain radiographs are not very sensitive in detecting these injuries because of the nonossified epiphysis, there are some characteristic findings of these distal physeal fractures. The radius and ulna are displaced posteromedially relative to the distal humerus, there is displacement of the medial epicondyle or capitellar ossification center, and a distal humeral metaphyseal fragment may also be present.[13] Without a history of birth trauma, distal physeal fractures are almost always secondary to abuse.[29] Distal physeal injuries can easily be confused with supracondylar fractures or elbow dislocations on plain radiographs, both of which are not commonly associated with abuse. Ultrasound, magnetic resonance imaging, and arthrography can be useful in identifying these injuries as well as guiding orthopedic management by determining Salter type and therefore management type in order to prevent complications of inadequate reduction such as cubitus valgus and varus.

Supracondylar fractures, a common childhood fracture, are almost always accidental and are consistent with a history of an ambulatory child falling on an outstretched dorsiflexed hand with the elbow hyperextended or directly on a flexed elbow.[29] Although, previously, these fractures had always been thought not to be associated with abuse, Strait et al found that supracondylar fractures were secondary to abuse in 20% of children less than 15 months of age. In this age group, greater consideration of the reported mechanism of injury and time of presentation may be warranted. Accidental proximal humeral fractures may be the result of birth trauma, direct impact to the posterolateral aspect of the shoulder, or a fall backward onto an outstretched dorsiflexed hand with the elbow extended. Accidental humeral shaft fractures are rare and seen as a result of a direct impact or falling on an outstretched arm.

Radius and Ulna. Fractures of the radius and ulna represent 10-20% of all bony injuries from child abuse. Diaphyseal fractures can be seen in abuse and are usually transverse due to the same mechanism as "nightstick" fractures (i.e., blocking injuries of direct impact to the forearm). Most metaphyseal-epiphyseal injuries are distal and present as corner fractures or metaphyseal lucencies.[15]

The distal radius, overall, is the most commonly fractured long bone in children. Most accidental fractures are greenstick or torus fractures and result from a fall on an outstretched hand. Physeal fractures of the distal radius and ulna are most commonly Salter-Harris type I or II. Torus fractures are not commonly abusive. Physeal fractures, therefore, can be seen both in accidental and nonaccidental trauma. A compatible history in an ambulatory child would reflect an accidental injury whereas physeal injuries in nonambulatory infants would be much more suggestive of abuse.

Ribs. Rib fractures are seen in 5-26% of abused children with 90% of abuse-related fractures occurring in children under 2 years of age.[11,21] In infants, rib fractures represent the most frequent fracture of abuse.[22,31] In general, rib fractures in children are much less common than in adults owing to their more compliant chest walls. Therefore, rib fractures, especially multiple fractures or fracture of the first rib, are almost pathognomonic for abuse in children younger than 2 years of age in the absence of major blunt trauma or prior bone pathology.[15,32]

Fractures occur when the infant is manually grabbed around the thoracic cage and violently squeezed and shaken. *(See Figure 5.)* This anteroposterior compressive force results most frequently in multiple, symmetrical, posterior rib fractures where mechanical stress is at its greatest. With increasing force, lateral then anterior fractures occur.[13] This mechanism of injury usually does not present with overlying bruising. Rib fractures resulting from direct blows to the chest, seen most often in children older than 2 years of age, are often associated with an overlying bruise.[15] Of importance, rib fractures from cardiopulmonary resuscitation are rare in infants and young children.[33]

Figure 5. Rib Fractures in Child Abuse

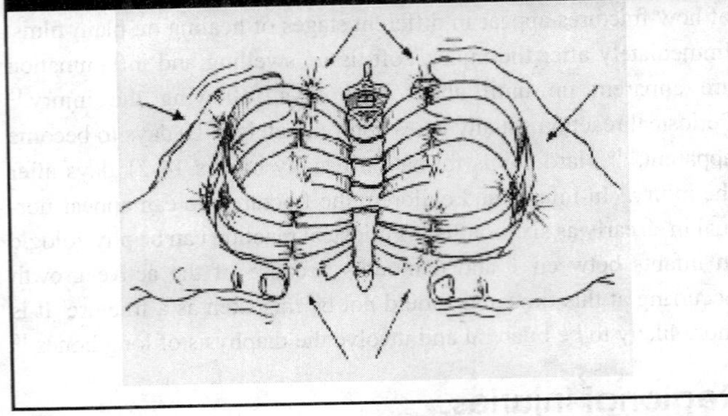

Acute rib fractures are very difficult to detect radiographically because of location, age, and orientation of the fracture line or fragment. A postmortem study of 31 abused infants showed that only 36% (30/84) of rib fractures were seen on skeletal survey even though most were healed fractures.[17] A subtle radiographic sign of an early healing fracture is an extrapleural opacity corresponding histologically to organizing hematoma and cartilaginous callus. Signs of further healing include bony callus formation seen after two weeks, new subperiosteal bone formation, and a "hole in the rib" appearance resulting from bone resorption at the fracture line with surrounding new bone formation. Costochondral junction fractures involve the osteochondral junction, and as in CML seen in long bones, a radiolucency extending into primary spongiosa can be seen. Radiographs with high detail and oblique views are best for detection of rib fractures. Highly sensitive bone scans are useful for hard to see costovertebral rib fractures as well as other acute, nondisplaced fractures.

Pelvis. Mention of pelvic fractures due to non accidental trauma in child abuse literature is rare. Since non accidental femoral fractures are much more frequently seen in abuse, it has been suggested that careful evaluation of the adjacent pelvis for fractures would be prudent.[15]

Femur. Femur fractures are very commonly seen in battered children. In infants younger than 1 year of age, 60% are intentional.[2,4] Oblique/spiral femur fractures in nonambulatory children should arouse a high suspicion of abuse. A history of a fall from less than three feet should also arouse suspicion, as midshaft fractures are unlikely to result from this height.[35] The amount of force required to cause a midshaft femur fracture in an infant is substantial and requires a major acceleration-deceleration injury. Accidental fractures of the femoral shaft can be the result of a running fall with twisting injury in young ambulatory children.[29]

According to several studies, there is no one fracture type that is characteristic of abuse,[4,36] although shaft fractures are more common than metaphyseal-epiphyseal fractures in abused children.[2,15] In the study by Kleinman et al of 31 postmortem infants younger than 1 year of age, they found that the vast majority of femoral fractures (15/17) are metaphyseal-epiphyseal fractures, and all of these fractures involved the distal growth plate. This propensity for distal involvement is seen in abused children of all ages with bilateral involvement often associated with violent shaking.[34] Proximal metaphyseal-epiphyseal injuries are difficult to visualize radiographically because of the multiple growth plates in this region that are initially nonossified. Subtle radiographic findings include soft tissue injury or abnormal alignment of the shaft relative to the pelvis. Although less common, it is important to identify them early since they can result in greater long-term sequelae such as avascular necrosis, nonunion, or growth disturbances. Bone scans, MRI, or arthrography are very useful modalities for detecting these subtle injuries.[11,15]

Tibia and Fibula. The tibia is a very common site for the CML[17,2] with proximal growth plate involvement more common than distal.[23] In a study using specimen radiology and histology of tibial fractures in abused children, Kleinman and Marks, describing CML, found that the medial margin of all proximal tibial fractures were involved.[23] They hypothesized that anatomically the subperiosteal bone collar is not continuous with cortex at the medial metaphyseal margin of the proximal tibia as this is where remodeling occurs. This exposes medullary trabeculae, and therefore the bone is less dense than the lateral margin where subperiosteal bone is continuous with cortex. It is thought that this medial margin is more susceptible to the various mechanical forces involved in abuse. Involvement of the lateral metaphysis is seen in more significant injury but always concurrently with medial metaphyseal involvement.

The proximal tibial CML may have several appearances radiologically. The fracture line first undercuts a thick posteromedial metaphyseal bony fragment, then the classic corner fracture is seen on the AP view. The bucket handle appearance, better seen using a beam with caudal angulation, is just an extension of this fracture line anterolaterally and may involve the tibial tubercle region. The most subtle finding of an acute fracture is a radiolucent line extending laterally from the medial metaphyseal margin and is referred to as a metaphyseal lucency. Similar radiographic findings are seen with distal growth plate fractures.

Non accidental injury should be strongly suspected in infants younger than 9 months with diaphyseal tibial fractures. Direct impact injury or violent grabbing and twisting can produce transverse and spiral/oblique fractures, respectively. Fracture lines are not always seen, but periosteal reaction with healing can commonly be seen.

Unintentional oblique/spiral fractures of the tibia (toddler's fracture), however, can be seen in novice walkers younger than 3-4 years of age.[11,34]

Fibular fractures secondary to abuse are rare, but, when they occur, they are from direct blows to the shaft seen concurrently with tibial shaft fractures.

Spine. Skeletal injury to the spine is not commonly seen in battered children. However, in infants without a history of trauma, any vertebral fracture should raise suspicion for abuse, as half of intentional spine injuries are seen in infants younger than 1 year of age.[15] Most of these injuries are asymptomatic but commonly result in persistent vertebral body deformities and may present years later with a severe kyphosis or growth disturbance.[37]

Most intentional fractures involve the vertebral bodies of the thoracolumbar spine and are caused by severe hyperflexion-hyperextension associated with violent shaking or direct blows. Violent shaking of an infant also results in spinous process avulsion and interspinous ligament disruption. *(See Figure 6.)* Initial radiographs are usually negative because of the cartilaginous nature of the spinous processes in early infancy. Subsequent radiographs may prove useful in demonstrating signs of healing. Irregularly shaped spinous processes with adjacent ossification corresponding to ossification of the avulsed cartilaginous part of the spinous process and/or adjacent soft tissues may be seen.[13,15]

Anterior compression fractures from the hyperflexion aspect of shaking are most common in the lower thoracic and upper lumbar regions. These present radiographically as loss of bone or sclerosis of the fracture line on the anterosuperior or less commonly anteroinferior margin of the vertebral body.[13,15] Spinous processes avulsions (clay-shoveler fractures) of the lower cervical or upper thoracic region can also be seen with intentional hyperflexion injury and are most commonly found in older children.[38] Anterior or posterior and, less commonly, lateral subluxation may also be seen in child abuse and is best seen on lateral spine radiographs. Fracture dislocations of the cervical or lumbar spine from abuse have been reported but are rare.[39]

Accidental spine fractures in older children are rare and predominantly caused by falls, motor vehicle accidents (MVA), or sports/recreational activities in older children. Most cervical spine injuries in children involve the upper cervical region above C3. Odontoid fractures are among the most common types and can result from trivial head trauma.[9] Children with Down's syndrome are at risk for chronic atlantoaxial and atlantooccipital instability. Significant displacement with neurologic compromise can occur with relatively minor trauma from activities involving significant neck flexion such as somersaults or contact sports. Chronic atlantoaxial instability is also seen in children with juvenile rheumatoid arthritis, Reiter's syndrome, Larsen's syndrome, and bone dysplasias.[9] Pseudosubluxation of C2-C3 is common in children and should not be confused with an acute injury. Pseudosubluxation of C3-C4 can also occur, but less frequently, and is seen mostly in younger children. Spinal fractures secondary to forward flexion over a lap-belt during an MVA can result in Chance Fractures usually involving L1-L4.[9] These fractures consist of anterior compression fractures with distraction of the posterior vertebral elements.

Plain radiographs remain the best modality for detection of spine injuries due to abuse. Bone scintigraphy is useful in detecting subtle fractures of the transverse and spinous processes. However, it has poor sensitivity for detection of vertebral body fractures.

Figure 6. Spinous Process Avulsion and Interspinous Ligament Disruption Associated with Severe Hyperflexion-Hyperextension Injury

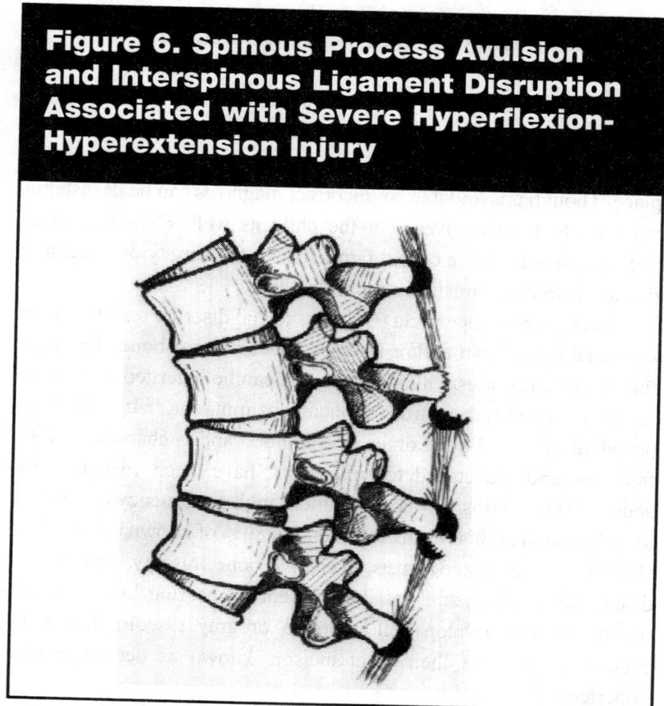

Shoulder Girdle. The clavicle is the most commonly fractured bone in children.[11] Midshaft fractures of the clavicle are typically accidental and consistent with a history of an ambulatory child falling on his or her shoulder or outstretched arm or a newborn child with a history of a traumatic birth.[1,15] Fractures seen two weeks after birth, with no callous formations, suggest the fracture did not occur at delivery.[40] A suspicious history or a delay in seeking care may be the only clues to a non accidental midshaft clavicular fracture. Intentional clavicular fractures are uncommon. One large series found that clavicular fractures represent only 7% of all skeletal injuries in child abuse.[21] Lateral or medial avulsion fractures of the clavicle result from violent shaking or arm traction and are much more specific for abuse.[13] Associated proximal humeral injury may be seen with clavicular avulsion fractures.[5]

Accidental scapular fractures in children are rare and result from severe direct trauma such as an MVA or fall from a great height. Without this type of history, any scapular fracture should raise high suspicion for abuse. Non accidental avulsion fractures of the acromion process or, less commonly, fractures of the coracoid process are due to violent arm traction or shaking. Glenoid fractures and fractures to the body of the scapula from direct blows are rare fractures of abuse.[15,21]

Plain radiographs are best for evaluating fractures of the shoulder girdle. Bone scans may be helpful for the more subtle scapular fracture.[15]

Hands And Feet. Hand or foot fractures are not common fractures of abuse, but when they occur they are usually seen in older children. Both metaphyseal-epiphyseal and shaft fractures can be seen in abuse. Injuries are usually seen in the metacarpal or metatarsal areas and frequently involve multiple digits as the result of direct blows with an object or deliberate stomping.[15]

Accidental fractures of the distal metacarpals, especially the fifth (boxer's fracture), are usually seen in adolescent males as a result of striking a person or object with a closed fist.[29]

Diseases Mistaken for Child Abuse

Making the diagnosis of child abuse is challenging and requires that the history, clinical, radiographic, and laboratory findings are all taken into account to responsibly suspect such an action has taken place. Though unavoidable, an incorrect diagnosis can be devastating not only to the caregivers but the child as well. Physicians must become astutely aware of and familiar with the variety of conditions that are commonly mistaken for child abuse.

Osteogenesis imperfecta (OI) is a skeletal disorder resulting from increased breakdown and/or reduced production of bone. There are four major categories with subtypes that can be inherited as an autosomal dominant trait or from spontaneous mutation.[42] It is the most prevalent of the OI syndromes in childhood and is characterized by fractures and skeletal deformities that have been mistaken for abuse.[43] Type I OI is the most common, with a frequency of approximately one in 30,000 births representing 80% of known cases.[42] It is characterized by osteoporosis, excessive bone fragility, joint laxity, distinct blue sclera, and possible subsequent hearing loss.[42] Nearly two-thirds will develop yellow-brown or gray discoloration with enamel fractures of their front incisors known as dentinogenesis imperfecta.[44]

Type II OI affect 1 in 60,000 live births and is the lethal form of OI. Their skull is soft with multiple palpable bony islands and long bones are crumpled. Type III OI is manifested in the newborn or infant with severe bone fragility and multiple fractures. The sclera is blue at birth but fades with age. Their birth weight and length tend to be normal but are reduced by subsequent fractures and bowing deformities of long bones. Few reach adult life. Type IV OI is rare but more difficult to diagnose. The sclera is normal, family history may not be present, and radiographs can be normal. The diagnosis may not be made until teeth have formed and dentinogenesis imperfecta is seen.[45]

Other skeletal abnormalities are seen with copper deficiency or Menke's syndrome, which is an X-linked recessive disorder that involves inadequate copper absorption.[46] These children have profound mental and physical retardation, alopecia, osteoporosis of the long bones, rib fractures, wormian bones, and metaphyseal fractures similar to those seen in child abuse.[47,48]

Rickets and scurvy also produce radiologic bone abnormalities resembling child abuse. Rickets results in cupping and fraying of the metaphysis and increased distance between the metaphysis secondary to deposition of uncalcified bone as well as demineralization and thinning of the cortex and epiphysis.[49,50] With scurvy, the epiphysis is outlined by an increased density of the zone of provisional calcification where fractures traverse into the metaphysis. With healing, the elevated periosteum may become calcified giving a radiologic finding similar to fractures seen in child abuse.[48] Congenital syphilis, congenital insensitivity to pain and certain drugs including vitamin A, methotrexate, and prostaglandins also may have bony abnormalities associated with them that may be suggestive of child abuse.[51,52]

The misdiagnosis of child abuse also is made with several diseases that manifest their presence with cutaneous lesions mistaken for bruising. Mongolian spots are grayish-blue, present from birth in dark-skinned-children, located usually over the buttocks and/or lower back, and are non-tender. Coagulopathies such as hemophilia and Von Willebrand disease, ingestion of anticoagulants (salicylates, rat poison), leukemia, and neuroblastoma may produce purpura suggesting abuse.[53,54]

Folk Remedies or Child Abuse?

Many folk remedies have been mistaken for child abuse. "Cupping" is practiced by Mexican and Eastern European immigrants to restore appetite, relieve vertigo, and reduce inflammation. Alcohol is placed in a cup and ignited then placed on the skin creating a vacuum which results in a circular echymotic ring.[55] Cao Gio ("coining") and Quat Sha ("spooning"), practiced by Southeast Asians for fever and headache, is performed by rubbing a coin or spoon heated in hot oil on an ill child's neck, spine, and ribs until echymotic lesions appear.[56,57,58] Caida de Mollera or sunken fontanelle is believed by Hispanics to be the cause of vomiting, diarrhea, and lethargy. An attempt is made to elevate the fontanelle by holding the child upside down and vigorously shaking, thus resulting in retinal hemorrhages[53,59] Moxibustion and Maquas are two additional forms of folk medicine where induced burns are believed to draw out illnesses.[60]

Reporting Suspected Child Abuse

Every state has a statute for discovering and reporting child abuse with the reporter being immune from both civil and criminal liability, but penalized if he or she does not report.[61] Mandated reporters include physicians, dentists, podiatrists, nurses, psychologists, speech pathologists, coroners, medical examiners, child day care center employees, childrens' service workers, social workers, and school teachers.[15] Reportable conditions include non accidental physical injury, neglect, sexual abuse, and emotional abuse. However, each state defines them differently.[15] For child protective service agencies, the primary purpose is to protect and ensure the safety of children who have been or are at risk of maltreatment, and to provide services to alter the conditions that create risk of maltreatment in the future.[62] Child abuse reporting statutes dictate when a report must be made. Most statutes require reporters to make an immediate oral report by telephone to one of four traditional agencies: social service agencies, police department, health department, or juvenile court.[15]

Documentation is critical, and the interview and physical examination should be performed by the most experienced individual. The aid of social workers should not be delayed. After the work-up and reporting has been completed, and if it is believed the that the child is not safe, he or she should be hospitalized pending further evaluation.

Summary

While accidents happen, the incidence of child maltreatment has reached epidemic proportions. In order to distinguish between intentional and unintentional injury, the physician needs to be familiar with the common unintentional pediatric fractures and their mechanism of injury as well as fractures that are commonly abusive. *(See Table 2.)* They must also have an understanding of the normal developmental stages of childhood. While there are fractures that are classic for the diagnosis of child abuse, most fractures that are abusive are not in this category. Almost any type of fracture can occur in the abused child and it is imperative to perform a thorough history

Table 2. Summary of Regional Injuries and the Likelihood of Abuse

FRACTURES MORE LIKELY TO BE ABUSIVE

- Metaphyseal-epiphyseal fractures (i.e., corner, bucket handle, and metaphyseal lucency)
- Rib fractures—especially posterior
- Fractures in different stages of healing
- Fractures inconsistent with history or developmental age of the child
- Avulsion fractures of the clavicle or acromion process
- Skull—multiple, depressed, bilateral, or across suture lines
- Pelvic and spinal fractures without a history of significant force
- Femur fractures in a child younger than 1 year of age
- Fractures with delayed onset of seeking care

FRACTURES LESS LIKELY TO BE ABUSIVE

- Clavicle fractures
- Toddler's fracture of the tibia
- Supracondylar fractures of the humerus
- Fractures of the hands and feet
- Torus fractures of the long bones
- Pelvic or spinal fractures with a history of significant force

and physical on every injured patient to help determine the origin of each injury. It is the responsibility of all clinicians to become familiar with the signs of child abuse and consider every pediatric fracture as a possible fracture of abuse.

References

1. Reece DM. *Child Abuse: Medical Diagnosis and Management.* Philadelphia: Lea and Febiger; 1994:23-50.
2. King J, Diefendorf D, Apthorp J, et al. Analysis of 429 fractures in 189 battered children. *J Ped Ortho* 1988;8: 585-589.
3. Leventhal JM, et al. Fractures in young children—distinguishing child abuse from unintentional injuries. *Am J Dis Children* 1993;147:87-92.
4. Thomas SA, Rosenfield NS, Levanathal JM, et al. Long-bone fractures in young children: Distinguishing accidental injuries form child abuse. *Pediatrics* 1991;88:471-476.
5. Johnson CF. Inflicted injury vs. accidental injury. *Peds Clin North Am* 1990;37:791-811.
6. Cappelleri JC, Eckenrode J. The epidemiology of child abuse: Findings from the second national incidence and prevalence study of child abuse and neglect. *Am J Public Health* 1993;83:1622-1624.
7. Newberger E. Child physical abuse. *Ped Clin North Am* 1993;20:317-327.
8. McClain PW, Sacks JJ, et al. Estimates of fatal child abuse and neglect, United States, 1979 through 1988. *Pediatrics* 1993;91:338-343.
9. Rockwood CA, Wilkins KC, King RE. *Fractures in Children.* 3rd ed. Philadelphia, PA: Lippincott Co; 1991:1-6.
10. Rang, Mercer. *Children's Fractures.* 2nd ed. Philadelphia, PA: Lippincott Co; 1983:1-15.
11. England SP, Sundberg S. Management of common pediatric fractures. *Ped Clin North Am* 1996;43:991-1013.
12. Swischuk LE. *Emergency Imaging of Acutely Ill or Injured Child.* 3rd ed. Baltimore: Williams and Wilkins; 1994: 361-363.
13. Merten DF, Carpenter BC. Radiologic imaging of inflicted injury in the child abuse syndrome. *Ped Clin North Am* 1990;37:815-837.
14. Kleinman PK, Nimkin K, et al. Follow-up skeletal surveys in suspected child abuse. *Am J Radiology* 1996;167:893-896.
15. Broduer AE, Monteleone JA. *Child Maltreatment. A Clinical Guide and Reference.* St. Louis: GW Medial Publishing, Inc; 1994:32.
16. Pergolizzi R, Oestrich AE. Child abuse fracture through physiologic reaction. *Pediatr Radiol* 1995;25:566-567.
17. Kleinmen PK, Marks SC, Richmond JM, et al. Inflicted skeletal injury: A postmortem-radiologic-histopathologic study in 31 infants. *Am J Radiol* 1995;165:647-650.
18. Silverman FN, Kuhn JP, eds. *Caffey's Pediatric X-Ray Diagnosis: An Integrated Imaging Approach.* St. Louis: The CV Mosby Co.; 1992:1814-1816.
19. Kleinman PK, Marks SC, Blackbourne B. The metaphyseal lesion in abused infants: A radiographic histologic study. *Am J Radiol* 1986;146:895-905.
20. Strait RT, Siegel RM, Shapiro RA. Humeral fractures without obvious etiologies in children younger than 3 years of age: When is it abuse? *Pediatrics* 1995;96:667-671.
21. Merten DF, Radkowski MA, Leonidar JC. The abused child: A radiologic reappraisal. *Radiology* 1983;146:377-381.
22. Worlock P, Stower M, Barbor P. Patterns of fractures in accidental and nonaccidental injury in children: A comparative study. *BMJ* 1986;293:100-102.
23. Kleinman PK, Marks SC. A regional approach to the classic metaphyseal lesion in abused infants: The proximal tibia. *Am J Radioliogy* 1996;166:421-426.
24. Hobbs CJ. Skull fracture and the diagnosis of abuse. *Arch Dis Child* 1984;59:246-252.
25. Kowal-Vern A, Paxton TP, Ross SP, et al. Fractures in the under 3-year-old cohort. *Clin Pediatr* 1992;31:653-659.
26. Rosenberg N, Bettenfield G. Fractures in infants: A sign of child abuse. *Ann Emerg Med* 1982;11:178-218.
27. Kleinman PK, Marks SC. A regional approach to the classic metaphyseal lesion in abused infants: The proximal humerus. *Am J Radiol* 1996;167:1399-1403.
28. Meservy CJ, Towbin R, McLaurin RL, et al. Radiographic characteristics of skull fractures resulting from child abuse. *Am J Radiol* 1987;149:173-174.
29. Reisdorff EJ, Roberts MR Wiegenstein JG, eds. *Pediatric Emergency Medicine.* Philedelphia: W.B. Saunders Co.;1993.
30. O'Neill JA. Patterns of injury in the battered child syndrome. *J Trauma* 1973;13:332-339.
31. Kleinman PK, Marks SC, Mimkin K, et al. Rib fractures in 31 abused infants: Postmortem radiologic-histopathologic study. *Radiology* 1996;200:807-810.
32. Strouse PJ, Owings CL. Fractures of the first rib in child

abuse. *Radiology* 1995;197:763-765.
33. Feldman KW, Brewer DK. Child abuse, cardiopulmonary resuscitation, and rib fractures. *Pediatrics* 1984;73:339.
34. Kleinman PK. *Diagnostic Imaging of Child Abuse.* Baltimore: Williams and Wilkins; 1987.
35. Helfer RE, Slouis TL, Black M. Injuries resulting when small children fall out of bed. *Pediatrics* 1977;60:533.
36. Anderson WA. The significance of femoral fractures in children. *Ann Emerg Med* 1982;11:174-177.
37. Dickson RA, Leatherman KD. Spinal injuries in child abuse: Case report. *J Trauma* 1978;18:811-812.
38. Kleinman PK, Zito JL. Avulsion of the spinous processes caused by infant abuse. *Radiology* 1984;151:389-937.
39. McGrory BE, Fenichel GM. Hangmans fracture subsequent to shaking an infant. *Ann Neurol* 1977;2:82.
40. Kogutt MS, Swishuck LE, Feagan CJ. Pattern of injury and significance of uncommon fractures in the battered child syndrome. *Am J Radiol* 1974;121:143.
41. Cummings WA. Neonatal skeletal fractures: Birth trauma or child abuse. *J Can Assoc Radiol* 1979;30:30-33.
42. Gahagan S, Rimsza ME. Child abuse or osteogenesis imperfecta: How can we tell? *Pediatrics* 1191;88:987-992.
43. Ojima K, Matsumoto H, Hayase T, et al. An autopsy case of osteogenesis imperfecta initially suspected as child abuse. *Forensic Sci Int* 1994;65:97-104.
44. Wright JT, Thornton JB. Osteogenesis imperfecta with dentinogenesis imperfecta: A mistaken case of child abuse. *Pediatric Dentistry* 1983;5:207-209.
45. Augarten A, Laufer J, et al. Child abuse, osteogenesis imperfecta and the grey zone between them. *J Med* 1993;24:171-175.
46. Danks DM, et al. Menke's kinky hair syndrome. *Pediatrics* 1972;50:188-201.
47. Martin LA, McNemar A, O'Brien E. Menke's kinky hair disease. *MCN* 1994;19162-164.
48. Brill PW, Winchester P. Differential diagnosis of child abuse. In: Kleinman PK, ed. *Diagnostic Imaging of Child Abuse.* Baltimore: Williams & Wilkins; 1987:221-241.
49. Kaplan S. *Clinical Pediatric Endocrinology.* Philadelphia: Saunders; 1990:442-443.
50. Zeiss J, Wycliffe ND. Radiological case of the month. *Am J Dis Child* 1988;142:1367-1368.
51. Stewart GM, Rosenberg NM. Conditions mistaken for child abuse. *Pediatr Emerg Care* 1996;12:116-121.
52. Lim HK, Smith WL, et al. Congenital syphilis mimicking child abuse. *Pediatr Radiol* 1995;25:560-561.
53. Bays J. Conditions mistaken for child abuse. In: Reece R., ed. *Child Abuse: Medical Diagnosis and Management.* Philadelphia: Lea & Febiger; 1994:358-385.
54. Haddad LM, Winchester Jf, eds. *Clinical Management of Poisoning and Drug Overdose.* Philadelphia: WB Saunders; 1990;914-915.
55. Sandler AP, Haynes V. Nonaccidental trauma and medical folk belief: A case report of cupping. *Pediatrics* 1978;61: 921-922.
56. Yeatman FW, Shaw C, Barlow Mj, et al. Pseudo-battering in Vietnamese children. *Pediatrics* 1976;58:616-618.
57. Leung AKC. Ecchymosis from spoon scratching simulating child abuse. *Clin Pediatr* 1986;25:98.
58. Gellis S, Feingold M. Cao Gio: Pseudobattering in Vietnamese Children. *Am J Dis Child* 1976;130:857-858.
59. Guarnaschelli J, Lee J, Pitts FW. Fallen fontanelle (Caida de Mollera): A variant of the battered child syndrome. *JAMA* 1972;222:1545.
60. Stewart GM, Rosenberg NM. Conditions mistaken for child abuse. *Pediatr Emerg Care* 1996;12:116-121.
61. Landers J. Flood: 17 California, 3d 399, 551, p. 2d; 389, 131 Cal Rpt. 1976; 69.
62. Cunningham C, Horowitz R. *Child abuse and Neglect: Cases, Text, and Problems.* American Bar Association, National Legal Resource Center for Child Advocacy and Protection, Washington, DC 1989.

Part II

Infectious Diseases

Meningitis

Dayna Lynn Gutsin, MD
Katherine L. Heilpern, MD

Meningitis, or inflammation involving the meninges and cerebral spinal fluid (CSF), is a life-threatening emergency that may be associated with devastating neurologic sequelae or death if not promptly recognized and treated. Its causative organisms have been changing over the years and so has the treatment for this disease. Because of its myriad presentations, it is crucial that the emergency physician be able to diagnose acute bacterial meningitis (ABM) and differentiate this condition from other disease processes that may cause or mimic meningitis.

The incidence of bacterial meningitis is approximately 4-10 cases per 100,000 people in the United States, and this infection is responsible for more than 2000 deaths per year.[1] However, a 1997 study reported a 55% reduction in all cases of bacterial meningitis between 1986 and 1995. Specifically, there was an 87% reduction in meningitis in children between ages 2 months and five years, a group that accounted for two-thirds of all cases reported in 1986.[2] The introduction of the *Haemophilus influenzae* Type b (Hib) vaccine has dramatically reduced the incidence of what was once the most prevalent organism responsible for bacterial meningitis. Currently, the age group at greatest risk for ABM includes children between 1 and 24 months of age, followed by a gradual increase in risk of infection from age 22 years until old age.[3] Adults older than age 60 account for 1000-3000 cases of ABM per year in the United States and for more than 50% of all deaths related to meningitis.[4]

Understanding age groups at risk and characterization of likely pathogens aids the emergency physician in confirming the diagnosis and implementing life-saving treatment. With these clinical challenges in mind, the purpose of this chapter is to review critical decisions involved in the diagnosis and management of adult meningitis.

Overview and General Principles

The pathogens responsible for bacterial meningitis are thought to originate in the nasopharyngeal mucosa. From this location, pathogens invade the intravascular space, cross the blood brain barrier (BBB), and eventually enter the CSF. Viruses (enterovirus) are more likely to spread via the fecal-oral route. In this scenario, viral replication occurs in the gastrointestinal (GI) tract, which leads to viremia and subsequent invasion of the BBB.[5] Generally speaking, host defenses in the subarachnoid space are inadequate and inefficient; therefore, once organisms gain entry in to the CSF, bactericidal activity is lacking[6] and pathogens may propagate.

The deleterious consequences of ABM are, to a great extent, caused by the inflammatory response generated by the host. Inflammation involves many cascades and cellular responses, including activated polymorphonuclear leukocytes (PMNs) and inflammatory mediators such as interleukin-1 (IL-1), tumor necrosis factor (TNF), and platelet activating factor (PAF).[7] The consequences of this inflammatory response include cerebral edema, vasculitis, increased intracranial pressure (ICP), decreased cerebral blood flow, loss of autoregulation, and cortical hypoxia.[1] Similar pathophysiologic consequences occur with non-bacterial (aseptic) meningitis; however, recruitment of leukocytes and activation of inflammatory mediators are not as intense as they are in ABM.

Patients at Risk

A number of underlying medical illnesses and epidemiologic risk factors are associated with an increased risk of bacterial meningitis. Extremes of age, anatomic or functional asplenia (e.g., sickle cell disease), alcoholism, cirrhosis, malnutrition, chronic liver or renal disease, immunoglobulin or complement deficiencies, HIV, malignancy, and diabetes mellitus increase the risk for acquiring meningitis. In addition, patients with recent head injury or neurosurgery, cerebroventricular shunt or CSF leak, or who attend day care or live in close living quarters (i.e., military barracks or college dorms) are at increased risk. Finally, local extension or bacteremia leads to an increased risk of meningitis in persons with such concomitant conditions as otitis media, sinusitis, mastoiditis, brain abscess, or pneumonia.[1,6,8,9]

Patients in whom the diagnosis of ABM is being considered should be isolated in a respiratory isolation room. This is required to prevent potential transmission of *Neisseria meningitidis* and *Haemophilus influenzae*, both of which are spread via respiratory droplets.

Clinical Presentation

It should be stressed that only 10-20% of patients eventually diagnosed with ABM present with fulminant symptoms over a 24-hour period; the remaining 80-90% of individuals develop symptoms over 1-7 days. Eighty-five percent of patients with bacterial meningitis eventually present with fever, headache, meningismus or nuchal rigidity, and altered mental status.[8] Other common signs and symptoms include photophobia, vomiting, back pain, myalgias, diaphoresis, and malaise. Generalized seizures can occur in up to 40% of patients with ABM.[1] Kernig's sign (resistance to extension of the leg while the hip is flexed) and Brudzinski's sign (involuntary flexion of the hip and knee when the patient's neck is abruptly flexed while laying supine) are observed in up to 50% of patients and are suggestive of meningitis. However their presence or absence does not rule in or rule out meningitis.[1,5,8]

Papilledema is present in fewer than 1% of patients on initial exam; in fact, its presence may suggest an alternative diagnosis, such as venous sinus thrombosis, brain abscess, subdural empyema, or syphilis.[8,9] Cranial nerve palsies, especially those involving CN III, IV, VI, and VII can occur in up to 20% of patients; visual field defects, dysphasia, and hemiparesis are encountered less frequently. Coma, hypertension, and signs of impending herniation are late findings.[1] Importantly, about 50% of patients with *N. meningitidis* may present with a rash that begins as an erythematous macular rash, and then eventually progresses to petechiae and purpura.[1,3,4]

From a clinical perspective, it is important to note that viral meningitis shares several clinical features of bacterial meningitis including fever, headache, nausea and vomiting, and back pain. These signs and symptoms may be preceded by several days of a nonspecific acute febrile illness characterized by malaise and anorexia.[10] The symptoms can develop abruptly or they can evolve over several weeks. Although seizures occur less often in viral meningitis, certain viruses such as Arbovirus, mumps, and Varicella-Zoster virus are associated with seizures and encephalitis.[10] An erythematous macular rash may be present as well. Although many physicians feel that viral meningitis presents with a more indolent, or less "toxic," course, this is not always the case, and, therefore, CSF evaluation is mandatory in all suspected cases.

It should be emphasized that certain groups of patients present with atypical signs and symptoms that may be confused with aseptic meningitis or other illnesses. In particular, elderly patients may present only with lethargy or obtundation, with or without fever or signs of meningeal irritation. In fact, fever may be absent in up to 40% of elderly patients with ABM; instead, some cases may present with hypothermia.[8,9] Confusion occurs in more than half of elderly patients, while headaches occur in 20-80% of all cases. Nuchal rigidity, which is present in about 60-90% of cases, is neither sensitive nor specific in the geriatric patient. One review suggests that approximately 35% of elderly patients have had nuchal rigidity without meningitis. In these cases, nuchal rigidity is due to such other diseases as cervical spondylosis or Parkinson's disease.[4] Accordingly, the emergency physician should maintain a high index of suspicion for meningitis in all elderly patients with altered level of consciousness, whether or not they have fever, headache, or meningismus.

Although this article focuses on bacterial meningitis in adults, it should be pointed out that neonates comprise an important group of patients with atypical presentations; these include poor feeding, listlessness, and altered respiratory pattern. Patients with head trauma (in particular, penetrating wounds) are at increased risk for developing meningitis; however, the emergency physician may erroneously believe the symptoms are secondary to the trauma and may forego performing an LP. Neutropenic or immunosuppressed patients, which include patients with HIV, chronic steroid therapy, or metastatic disease, may not be able to mount the characteristic CSF inflammatory response. Therefore, typical signs of meningeal irritation may be absent. In patients with a cerebroventricular shunt, malfunction may result in shunt infection and, conversely, shunt infection may result in malfunction. These patients often present with headache, nausea, lethargy, with or without fever, and alterations in level of consciousness.[9]

Fungal meningitis usually presents in an indolent fashion with focal neurologic signs and altered mental status. Tuberculous meningitis, like fungal meningitis, may be characterized by a slowly evolving course and absence of frank meningeal signs. Cranial nerve deficits, ophthalmoplegia, facial droop, seizures, and altered mental status are common findings.[4] In patients with AIDS, cryptococcal meningitis may present with a paucity of signs and symptoms (mild headache, constitutional symptoms); therefore, emergency physicians should maintain a high suspicion for fungal or tuberculous meningitis in patients with HIV, even if patients present with minimal symptoms. Partially treated bacterial meningitis may be clinically indistinguishable from aseptic meningitis, consequently, a thorough history of recent antibiotic use is important in all patients who are being evaluated for meningitis.

Finally, there are many infectious and noninfectious causes of meningeal irritation. In patients who have an indeterminate CSF, the ED physician should consider unusual pathogens, multisystem disease, or drug reactions. *(See Table 1.)*

Table 1. Differential Diagnosis of Acute Bacterial Meningitis (ABM)

INFECTIOUS	NON-INFECTIOUS
• Parameningeal focus	• Systemic disease
Brain abscess	Sarcoidosis
Subdural empyema	Kawasaki disease
Epidural abscess	SLE
Pansinusitis	Multiple sclerosis
• Bacterial infection	Migraine headache
Partially treated ABM	Guillain-Barre
Lyme disease	Behcet's disease
Syphilis	Malignancy
Leptospirosis	Leukemia
Neurobrucellosis	Lymphoma
• Fungal infection	• Vaccine reaction
• Mycobacterial infection	Mumps
• Parasitic infection	MMR
• Viral Infection	Polio
Adenovirus	Poison
Arbovirus	Lead
CMV	Mercury
Coronavirus	• Trauma
Enterovirus	Subarachnoid hemorrhage
EBV	s/p Neurosurgery
HSV	Traumatic LP
HIV	• Drugs
Influenza virus	Azathioprine
Parainfluenza virus	Ibuprofen
Rabies virus	IVIG
LCV	Isoniazid
Rhinovirus	OKT3
Rotavirus	Sulfamethizole
VZV	Trimethoprim-sulfamethoxazole

Adapted from: Maxson S, Jacobs RF. Viral meningitis. *Postgrad Med* 1993;93:153-166; Nelsen S, Sealy DP, Schneider EF. The aseptic meningitis syndrome. *Am Fam Phys* 1993;48:809-815.

Patient Evaluation: Timing and Critical Decisions

Computerized Tomography (CT). One of the most important factors contributing to delayed diagnosis and treatment of bacterial meningitis is the decision to perform cranial CT imaging prior to lumar puncture.[11] Historically, a subset of practitioners has been concerned about the remote risk of herniation that may occur during lumbar puncture (LP). Systematic guidelines help risk stratify these patients. When evaluating patients for meningitis, patients who require CT prior to LP include those with focal neurologic findings, papilledema, focal seizures, or abnormalities on exam that suggest increased intracranial pressure.[1,4] Such findings can also suggest alternative diagnoses such as brain abscess, venous sinus thrombosis, mass lesion, subdural empyema, obstructive hydrocephalus, or tuberculous or fungal meningitis. Any expert would agree that it is usually safe to perform an LP on patients who have a reliable history of generalized tonic-clonic seizures, but who present without neurologic deficits. One other group of patients who should have CT evaluation done prior to LP are those in whom atypical presentations are common. For example, patients with immunosuppression (i.e., HIV, multiple myeloma or metastatic cancer, or patients receiving chronic steroids or chemotherapy) are at risk for mass lesions with or without clinical evidence of elevated ICP. Frequently, elderly patients present atypically (without fever or meningismus) and may have comorbid illnesses that cause altered mentation (stroke, hemorrhage). Alcoholics comprise another high-risk group; not only are they immunosuppressed, but they are at increased risk for subdural hematoma.

The most compelling argument for obtaining a CT prior to performing an LP is that a mass lesion may not be clinically evident, and that empiric treatment can be instituted before the scan. Moreover, some authorities suggest that the delay in time to LP does not affect its accuracy or outcome of the results.[11] Opponents feel that CT is usually a waste of time and valued resources, and, that CSF culture results may be affected by empiric therapy. If bacterial meningitis is a strong consideration, and the decision is made to perform a CT prior to LP, two sets of blood cultures should be obtained and antibiotics should be administered promptly before sending the patient for neuroimaging. Urine cultures may be helpful in the very young and very old.

Antibiotic Administration Timing

Delaying administration of antibiotics in patients suspected of having bacterial meningitis is a frequent precipitant of malpractice litigation. Typical arguments take the position that a delay in antibiotic therapy may result in increased morbidity and mortality.[11,12,13] Although there is still some controversy concerning clinical outcomes and their relationship to the timing of antibiotic administration, most physicians would agree that meeting the following standard of care is advisable. Antibiotics should be administered within 30 minutes of clinical suspicion/presentation of ABM. Often, patients who appear "sick" or have symptoms such as hypotension, abnormal mental status, or a temperature greater than 40°C will receive antibiotics more quickly, as will children in the age group of 2-10 years, and infants with a bulging fontanelle. Interestingly, the presence of headache is associated with delayed use of antibiotics, probably because alternative diagnoses for headache are sought.[13] It is essential to initiate antibiotics quickly in high-risk patients with atypical presentations. Blood cultures followed by antibiotic administration within 30 minutes of presentation is mandatory in all patients suspected of having bacterial meningitis and in whom CT precedes LP.

Although prompt administration of antibiotics is the rule rather than the exception, there are two groups of patients in whom it may be reasonable to withhold antibiotics pending LP results. In this regard, patients who are young, healthy and "nontoxic" in appearance, and in whom the physician is strongly suspicious of aseptic meningitis or an alternate diagnoses (i.e., there is a very low suspicion for bacterial meningitis), comprise one group. The second group consists of patients who are nontoxic, do not require CT, but in whom the diagnosis of ABM is likely and in whom LP results can be obtained within a reasonable time limit, (i.e., 30-60 minutes).

It should be stressed that, despite immediate initiation of antibiotic therapy, there is a minimal alteration in CSF parameters (cellular and metabolic composition) for 12-24 hours; consequently, there is a sufficient diagnostic window within which to perform LP and still make an accurate diagnosis.[8] However, it must be stressed that the diagnostic yield of CSF Gram's stain and culture decreases by approximately 20% and 30%, respectively, if antibiotics are initiated prior to LP.[22] Although Gram's stain and cultures may be negative shortly after initiation of antibiotics, as a rule, cell counts, percentage of cell morphologies, and protein and glucose levels remain unaltered for about 24 hours after initiation of IV antibiotics.[10]

Table 2. Cerebrospinal Fluid Parameters in Meningitis

	NORMAL	BACTERIAL	VIRAL	FUNGAL	TB	PARAMENINGEAL FOCUS OR ABSCESS
WBC count (WBC/uL)	0-5	> 1000	100-1000	100-500	100-500	10-1000
% PMN % lymph	0-15	90 > 50	< 50 > 50	< 50 > 80	< 50	< 50
Glucose (mg/dL)	45-65	< 40	45-65	30-45	30-45	45-65
CSF:blood glucose ratio	0.6	< 0.4	0.6	< 0.4	< 0.4	0.6
Protein (mg/dL)	20-45	> 150	50-100	100-500	100-500	> 50
Opening pressure (cm H_2O)	6-20	++	NL or +	++	++	N/A

Adapted from: Segreti J, Harris A. Acute bacterial meningitis. *Inf Dis Clin North Am* 1996;10:797-809.

Interpretation of Lumbar Puncture

Examination of the CSF is mandatory for diagnosis evaluation of meningitis. *(See Table 2.)* The typical CSF findings for ABM can be found in Table 3. Fortunately, prediction rules have been generated to help characterize and confirm the diagnosis of bacterial meningitis. These predictors have been tested in many situations and have performed reliably as individual predictors of bacterial meningitis.[15] The following prediction rules developed by Spanos and others have demonstrated certainty of higher than 99% for the diagnosis of ABM:[1,3,8,9,15]

1. CSF glucose < 34 mg/dL
2. CSF:blood glucose ratio < 0.23
3. CSF protein > 220 mg/dL
4. Total CSF leukocyte count > 2 x 10^6 /L
5. Total CSF neutrophil count > 1180 x 10^6 /L.

In addition, this author has produced an excellent nomogram for estimating the probability of bacterial vs. viral meningitis.[3]

In many patients, the LP results will fall in an indeterminate category (i.e., an elevated CSF leukocyte count higher than 500/mcL with near normal CSF glucose and protein). In 25% of patients with bacterial meningitis, no organisms are seen on Gram's stain, and in 30-40% of these patients, the CSF parameters will be nondiagnostic.[3,15] In other words, 10% of patients with subsequent confirmation of ABM will have an LP that yields a negative Gram's stain—as well as a total CSF WBC lower than 1000/mcL—and only mild abnormalities in the CSF glucose and protein.

If antibiotics are not given prior to the LP, the accuracy of the Gram's stain is between 60-90%. Overall, the Gram's stain performs poorly as a screening test, with a sensitivity of only 40-60%; however, specificity is greater than 90%.[1,8] Furthermore, the sensitivity decreases by 20% if the patient has been pretreated with antibiotics.[14] CSF cultures are positive in about 70-85% of cases without prior antibiotic administration and decrease to less than 50% with prior therapy.[1,8] Given the relative insensitivity of the Gram's stain and culture, obtaining two sets of blood cultures prior to antibiotic administration is imperative and may help compensate for the decrease in positive CSF culture results.

Preadministration of oral antibiotics prior to presentation does not appear to decrease the total CSF white blood cell count, the glucose, the glucose serum ratio, or the percentage of patients with a positive Latex agglutination (LA). There is, however, a decrease in percentage of neutrophils, a decrease in CSF protein, and a decrease in the percentage of positive Gram's stains. Intravenous antibiotics given 1-2 days prior to LP may not significantly alter the CSF cell count, protein, or glucose concentration, but will substantially decreases the positivity of the Gram's stain and culture.[16]

Ancillary CSF tests can be employed to help confirm the diagnosis. For example, if the CSF parameters are nondiagnostic, or the patient has been treated with prior oral antibiotics, and, therefore, the Gram's stain and/or culture are likely to be negative, then LA may be helpful. This test requires a small amount of bacterial antigen to produce a positive test.[1] It has a variable sensitivity rate, ranging between 50-100%, and high specificity. Latex agglutination tests are available for Hib, *Streptococcus pneumoniae*, *N. meningitidis*, *Escherichia coli* K1, and *S. agalactiae* (Group B strep).[8] Up to 25% of patients pretreated with antibiotics have a positive LA, so it may be helpful in a small subgroup of patients who have received antibiotics prior to ED

Table 3. Typical CSF Findings in Patients with Bacterial Meningitis

CSF PARAMETER	TYPICAL FINDINGS
Opening pressure	> 180 mm H_2O[a]
White blood cell count	1000-5000/mcL (range, < 100 to >10,000)[b]
Percentage of neutrophils	> 80% [c]
Protein	100-500 mg/dL
Glucose	< 40 mg/dL[d]
Lactate	> 35 mg/dL
Gram's stain	Positive in 60-90%[e]
Culture	Positive in 70-85%[f]
Bacterial antigen detection	Positive in 50-100%

[a] Values over 600 mm H_2O suggest the presence of cerebral edema, intracranial suppurative foci, or communicating hydrocephalus.

[b] Patients with very low CSF white blood cell counts (0 to 20/uL) tend to have a poor prognosis.

[c] About 30% of patients with *Listeria monocytogenes* meningitis have an initial lymphocyte predominance in CSF.

[d] The CSF-serum glucose ratio is < 0.31 in ~70% of patients.

[e] The likelihood of detecting the organism by Gram's stain correlates with the concentration of bacteria in the CSF; concentrations of < 103 cfu/mL is associated with positive Gram's stain ~25% of the time and concentrations > 105 cfu/mL leads to positive microscopy in up to 97% of cases.

[f] Yield of CSF cultures may decrease in patients who have received prior antimicrobial therapy.

Adapted from: Tunkel AR, Scheld WM. Acute bacterial meningitis in adults. In: Remington JS, Swartz MN, eds. *Current Clinical Topics in Infectious Diseases.* Boston: Blackwell Science, 1995:220.

presentation.[9] Given the cost of antigen testing (approximately $100) and its limited clinical utility, most experts do not recommend bacterial antigen testing of CSF, except in patients who have received prior antibiotics or who have a negative Gram's stain.[4] CSF C-reactive protein (CRP) has been found to be significantly elevated in children with ABM compared to those individuals with aseptic meningitis; however, there are no established recommendations for adults.[10] In children, a CRP greater than 20mg/L corresponds to bacterial meningitis with 100% sensitivity and 96% specificity.[5] CSF lactate and pH are also under investigation for their clinical utility in predicting ABM.[10]

CSF Cryptococcal antigen and India ink stain should be considered in all patients who have known HIV disease or HIV risk factors, including those who live in an area with a high incidence of HIV. Cryptococcal antigen is positive in 95% of confirmed cases, and India ink is positive in 50-75% of cases.[4]

In the nontoxic patient with a nondiagnostic lumbar puncture, the LP should be repeated in 8-12 hours to help differentiate between bacterial and viral (aseptic) meningitis, regardless of whether the ED physician has administered antibiotics.[10] Early in the course of viral meningitis, there may be a predominance of neutrophils in the CSF initially; this will shift toward a lymphocytic cell line after a few hours.[3,8,10] This also holds true for bacterial meningitis that may initially present with a lymphocytic predominance in the CSF. A repeat LP can be performed in EDs with observation units, or as an outpatient in patients with reliable caretakers and guaranteed follow up. Outpatient LP is not appropriate for patients who have already received antibiotics within the week prior to presentation or in children younger than 1 year of age.[10]

A traumatic tap will raise both red and white blood cell counts. To interpret the actual number of CSF white blood cells, a quick rule of thumb is as follows :

True WBC CSF = (WBC actual CSF - WBC blood) × RBC CSF - RBC blood

In addition, 1000 RBCs in the CSF artificially increase the CSF protein by 1mg/dL.[16]

Acute Viral Meningitis (AVM)

The typical presentation of acute viral meningitis (AVM) is characterized by acute onset of fever, headache, nausea and vomiting, with or without meningismus. AVM occurs most commonly in children between 1 and 10 years of age and has a peak incidence in summer and early fall. Patients with AVM are generally easily arousable and have a nonfocal physical exam.[17] Approximately one-half of patients with AVM will present with nuchal rigidity. Myalgias and photophobia are other commonly encountered complaints. Seizures are rare in AVM, except in young children with high fever or in those with a preexisting seizure disorder.[18] Most cases (85%) are secondary to enteroviral infection, and, consequently, other evidence of enteroviral illness may accompany the clinical symptoms of meningitis, including pharyngitis, conjunctivitis, rash (macular, maculopapular, petechial or vesicular), pleurodynia, pericarditis, or myocarditis.[19] AVM may be preceded by a nonspecific acute febrile illness with malaise and anorexia suggesting viral disease.[18] Typically, the headache of AVM improves significantly after the LP is performed.[20] The absence of other sites of bacterial infection such as pneumonia or otitis media supports the diagnosis of AVM. Finally, disease in the community or in a close contact supports the diagnosis of AVM.[20] The spread of enterovirus is via the fecal-oral route and has an incubation period of 4-6 days. The illness usually lasts between 1-2 weeks.[19]

The annual incidence of AVM is between 11 and 27 cases per 100,000 population. Over 7000 cases are reported annually in the United States.[17] AVM is well known to result in community-wide outbreaks often leading to infection in greater than 1000 patients during an epidemic.[21] Many studies have been done to evaluate the effectiveness of the ED in evaluating patients with acute meningitis during an epidemic in order to develop a protocol that minimizes the overuse of valuable resources, while still maintaining the safety of the population at large.

Evaluating AVM

In every patient evaluated for acute meningitis, the ED physician must form a pretest probability of whether the patient has AVM or

Table 4. Antibiotic Choice Based on Age and Comorbid Medical Illness

AGE	ORGANISM	ANTIBIOTIC
Neonate	*E. coli*, Group B strep, *Listeria monocytogenes*	Ampicillin and third-generation cephalosporin
1-3 months	*S. pneumoniae, N. meningitidis, H. influenzae, S. agalactiae, Listeria, E. coli*	Ampicillin and third-generation cephalosporin
3 months to 18 years	*N. meningitidis, S. pneumoniae, H. influenzae*	Third-generation cephalosporin
18-50 years	*S. pneumoniae, N. meningitidis*	Third-generation cephalosporin
Older than 50 years	*N. meningitidis, S. pneumoniae,* Gram-negative bacilli, *Listeria,* Group B strep	Ampicillin and third-generation cephalosporin

MEDICAL ILLNESS	ORGANISM	ANTIBIOTIC
Neurosurgery/ head injury	*S. aureus, S. epidermidis,* Diphtheroids, Gram-negative bacilli	Vancomycin and Ceftazidime
Immunosuppression	*Listeria,* Gram-negative bacilli *S. pneumoniae, N. meningitidis* (consider adding Vancomycin)	Ampicillin and Ceftazidime
CSF shunt	*S. aureus,* Gram-negative bacilli	Vancomycin and Ceftazidime

Third generation cephalopsorin = ceftriaxone or cefotaxime

ABM. This is based on the clinical appearance and exam, the characteristics of the patient (age and comorbidities), and epidemiological factors (ill contacts, local epidemics and the time of year). Once the pretest probability for AVM has been established, the ED physician should proceed to the LP to help confirm the diagnosis and rule out other life-threatening illnesses such as ABM or subarachnoid hemorrhage. The typical CSF findings of AVM are outlined in Table 2.

AVM Lumbar Puncture

As many as two-thirds of all patients ultimately diagnosed with AVM demonstrate an initial neutrophilic predominance in the CSF.[22] As a result, many patients receive several days of IV antibiotics and hospitalization, even though 48 hours later, blood and CSF cultures are negative. Several studies have evaluated the utility of a second LP to differentiate patients with AVM vs. ABM. Feigin and Shackelford recognized the concept of leukocyte shifting during a retrospective study as early as 1973.[23] They found that 85 of 230 patients with a discharge diagnosis of aseptic meningitis demonstrated an initial LP with neutrophilic predominance (37 of these patients received antibiotics after the initial LP and were removed from the study). The remaining 48 patients comprised the study group. These patients were not toxic and all had a total CSF WBC count less than 1000/mcL with a neutrophilic predominance, a near normal CSF glucose concentration, and a negative Gram's stain. None of these patients received IV antibiotics. These 48 patients had a second LP performed 6-72 hours after the initial LP (31 of 48 had it repeated within 6 to 8 hours). In this study, 87% of patients had a clear shift from a polymorphonuclear cell line in the CSF to a mononuclear line between the initial LP and one performed 6-8 hours later ($p < 0.001$). Ninety-four percent shifted to a mononuclear cell line 12-72 hours after the initial LP. No significant change occurred in CSF total cell count, glucose, and protein. They concluded that, in most cases, if the patient has not received prior antibiotics, a brief period of observation followed by a repeat LP in 6-12 hours helps the ED physician distinguish between AVM and ABM.

A similar study was conducted by another group prospectively in 1979.[22] It included 16 patients with a history and physical exam consistent with AVM, who received supportive care only (i.e., no antibiotics). The LP was repeated 18-48 hours later in the 10 patients who failed to show significant clinical improvement. Additionally, 11 of 16 patients had an LP performed prior to discharge (5-12 days after the initial LP), although all were asymptomatic at discharge. All patients in this study had a total CSF WBC count less than 500/mcL on the initial LP with a mean percent of PMNs of 41.75 ± 29.00. The percent of PMNs in the CSF fell significantly to a mean percent of 8.0 ± 8.8 ($P < 0.001$) in all 10 patients who had repeat LP performed; the neutrophil percent remained low at 5-12 days. Total leukocyte count, glucose, and protein content in the CSF showed no significant change throughout the acute phase of the illness. In this study of patients with AVM, all patients undergoing serial LP demonstrated a

Table 5. Antibiotic Choice Based on Gram's Stain

STAIN RESULTS	ORGANISM	ANTIBIOTIC
Gram's (+) cocci	*S. pneumoniae, S. aureus, S. agalactiae (Group B)*	Vancomycin and third-generation cephalosporin
Gram's (-) cocci	*N. meningitidis*	Penicillin G
Gram's (-) coccobacilli	*H. influenzae*	Third-generation cephalosporin
Gram's (+) bacilli	*Listeria monocytogenes*	Ampicillin, Penicillin G + Gentamycin
Gram's (-) bacilli	*E.coli, Klebsiella, Serratia, Pseudomonas*	Ceftazidime +/- aminoglycoside

shift in the cell line from neutrophils to mononuclear cells; none of these patients received antibiotics, and all had good outcomes.

Another study in 1989 confirmed that the season and the patient's age are also important predictors because patients at the extreme of age are more likely to have ABM and young adults are more likely to have AVM. In this study, neutrophils predominated in the initial spinal tap in 40% of cases eventually diagnosed with AVM. Conversely, 15% of patients with a discharge diagnoses of ABM had lymphocytosis in the CSF on initial LP. In 70% of the patients diagnosed with AVM, the fall in proportion of PMNs in the CSF was seen during the first two days of hospitalization, reaffirming the shift from polymorphic to monomorphic cell lines on repeat LP.

In 1991, a study suggested that the shift from polymorphic to monomorphic cells in the CSF occurs approximately 24 hours after the initial symptoms.[24] This prospective study was performed during an outbreak of enteroviral meningitis in Israel. Special attention was paid to the time of onset of symptoms. A second LP was performed 6-14 hours after the initial LP on all patients who did not improve clinically and had a CSF analysis suggestive of AVM, but with a neutrophilic predominance. The patients were divided into four groups according to the interval between onset of symptoms and time of the first LP (LP performed within 12 hours of symptom onset; 12-24 hours of symptom onset; 24-36 hours after symptom onset; and more than 36 hours). The percentage of PMNs in the CSF of the patients who had the initial LP in the first 24 hours of onset of the illness fell significantly more than the patients in the latter group ($P < 0.01$). In all samples obtained more than 24 hours after the onset of symptoms, fewer than 50% of the cells were PMNs. This study affirmed that a second LP is helpful in distinguishing between AVM and ABM, but that the time interval between the onset of symptoms and the LP may influence the trend toward monomorphic cells. Previous studies have recommended repeating the tap in 6-12 hours after the initial tap, whereas this trial suggests deferring the second tap until 24 hours have elapsed after the onset of symptoms (assuming that the patient has presented within the first few hours of his or her illness) in order to provide more conclusive information. A predominance of neutrophils 2-3 days after the initial onset of the symptoms would be unusual in AVM.

Early Bacterial Meningitis vs. AVM

In 1984, Powers reported a CSF lymphocytic predominance in 14 of 103 cases of bacteriologically proven acute bacterial meningitis.[15] Classically, ABM presents with CSF leukocyte counts greater than 1000/ mm^3. In this study however, 41 patients with ABM had CSF leukocyte counts less than 1000/mm^3 and 13 of the 41 patients had CSF lymphocytosis as well. Five of the 14 patients in this study were younger than 2 months old. Many of the patients had other CSF parameters that suggested ABM including low glucose (7 of 14), elevated protein (6 of 14) or a positive Gram's stain (7 of 14). There was no difference between the groups in terms of bacterial type or pretreatment with antibiotics. There is not adequate data regarding the shift of monomorphs to polymorphs in the CSF of patients infected with early ABM. However, the study by Powers suggests that up to 10% of patients with ABM may present with a total CSF WBC count less than 1000/mcL and a lymphocytic predominance. In most cases, other CSF parameters will be abnormal and suggestive of ABM.

The majority of the evidence seems to support the use of serial lumbar puncture to aid the ED physician in differentiating between AVM and ABM in patients with a total CSF WBC count less than 500/mcL. The patient who appears toxic or has other CSF parameters consistent with ABM is admitted and given IV antibiotics. The patient who is nontoxic and has clear evidence of AVM by LP (CSF WBC count less than 500/mcL with a lymphocytic predominance, normal CSF glucose, normal or slightly elevated CSF protein, and a negative Gram's stain) may be discharged home with supportive care (for pain, fever, and dehydration). The patients in whom the history and clinical exam suggest a viral etiology, but the LP results are ambiguous (i.e. a CSF WBC count less than 500/mcL, a neutrophil predominance, a normal glucose, and a slightly elevated protein with a negative Gram's stain), warrant a period of observation and, if symptoms persist, a repeat LP 6-12 hours later.

The patient can be discharged from the ED if he has guaranteed follow-up and a family member or friend to closely observe him in the interim. This is not appropriate for the extremes of age, patients with immunocompromising comorbidities (cancer, HIV, steroid therapy, diabetes, chronic alcoholism), or in patients whose mental status cannot be followed. These patients require admission and close observation. In most of the studies mentioned in this article, the majority of patients had a total CSF WBC count less than 500/mcL. There is no available data on whether a repeat LP is valuable in patients with a CSF WBC between 500 and 1000 with a neutrophil predominance, normal glucose, normal protein, and a negative Gram's stain.

The repeat lumbar puncture is most valuable in the group of patients suspected to have AVM who have a neutrophil predominant CSF and persistent CNS symptoms. Patients with persistent headache or meningismus should undergo repeat LP to differentiate AVM from early bacterial meningitis.

Table 6. Recommended Dosages of Antibiotics

ANTIBIOTIC	DOSAGE
May need to adjust for renal or hepatic disease	
Ampicillin	2 g IV q 4 h
Cefotaxime	2 g IV q 4-6 h
Ceftazidime	2 g IV q 8 h
Ceftriaxone	2 g IV q 12 h
Gentamycin	Load 1.5 mg/kg IV then 1-2 mg/kg q 8 h
Nafcillin/Oxacillin	1.5-2 g IV q 4 h
Penicillin G	4 million units IV q 4 h
Rifampin	600 mg po q 12-24 h
Trimethoprim-sulfamethoxazole	10 mg/kg IV q 12 h
Vancomycin	1.5-2 g IV q 12 h

Adapted from: Segreti J, Harris A. Acute bacterial meningitis. *Inf Dis Clin North Am* 1996;10:797-809; Martin JB, Tyler KL, Scheld WM. Bacterial meningitis. In: Tyler KL, Martin JB, eds. *Infectious Diseases of the Central Nervous System (Contemporary Neurology Series).* Philadelphia: FA Davis, 1993:176-178; Ashwal S. Neurologic evaluation of the patient with acute bacterial meningitis. *Neurol Crit Care* 1995;13:549-577.

Antimicrobial and Corticosteroid Therapy

The initial choice of antibiotic depends upon the patient's age, comorbid medical illnesses, and trends in the community for antimicrobial resistance. *(See Table 4.)* Clearly, the antibiotic should have a high degree of CSF penetration, achieve a high concentration in the CSF, and have intrinsic activity in infected fluid.[11]

Knowledge of the patient's underlying medical condition will help in antibiotic selection. For example, *Listeria monocytogenes* is seen in patients older than 60 years of age, in patients with renal or liver failure, in individuals with connective tissue disease, cancer, diabetes, chronic steroid therapy, and in alcoholics.[8,9] *Listeria monocytogenes* can account for up to 25% of cases of ABM in patients older than 60 years.[4] *S. aureus* is a common pathogen in patients who have undergone neurosurgery, in those who have a CNS shunt, and in patients with a head injury and CSF leak. Enteric Gram-negative bacilli (Klebsiella, *E. coli*, *Pseudomonas,* and *Serratia*) are implicated in neurosurgery patients, in elderly and immunosuppressed patients, and in patients with Gram negative sepsis. *S. agalactiae* (Group B strep) is also found in the elderly and in parturient women, as well as in patients with liver and kidney failure.[9] HIV patients are at increased risk for toxoplasmosis, and for cryptococcal tuberculous and CMV meningitis.[6]

Knowledge of resistance patterns in your community is important when deciding upon empiric therapy. For example, a 1994 CDC study of Atlanta demonstrated that 25% of cases of invasive pneumococcal infection were resistant to penicillin, and 7% were highly resistant and resistant to third generation cephalosporins.[8,11] In some areas, *H. influenzae* shows a 15-30% resistance to ampicillin for type B and non-type B strains.[8] In addition to local epidemiology, awareness of the habitat of the patient is helpful; *N. meningitidis* in more commonly seen in outbreaks in populations living in close confines such as military barracks, dormitories, or day care.[9] In most circumstances, the emergency physician will administer empiric therapy based on age and underlying disease. If he or she is able to obtain Gram's stain results quickly, therapy may be stain-directed.

S. pneumoniae once was adequately covered by use of penicillin G or ampicillin, but with emerging and increasing resistance across the United States, a third-generation cephalosporin is a more prudent initial choice. In areas characterized by high resistance to penicillin, vancomycin plus a third-generation cephalosporin ought to be the first line therapy in the ED.[9,11,16] This can be tailored after resistance patterns are obtained from cultures. *H. influenzae* is usually adequately covered by a third-generation cephalosporin. The drug of choice for *N. meningitidis* is penicillin or ampicillin, because little resistance has emerged to this organism. In patients who are at risk for *Listeria meningitis*, ampicillin must be added to the regimen. *S. agalactiae* (Group B) is covered by ampicillin as well, and adding an aminoglycoside provides synergy. *Pseudomonas* and other Gram-negative bacilli should be treated with a broad spectrum third-generation cephalosporin (ceftazidime) plus an aminoglycoside. *S. aureus* may be covered by nafcillin or oxacillin; vancomycin may be needed if the patient is at risk for methicillin-resistant *S. aureus*.[9,11,16] *(See Table 5.)(See Table 6 for recommended antibiotic dosages.)*

If it is possible to obtain a Gram's stain within 30 minutes of the patient's presentation, it may be possible to tailor therapy to the organisms seen by microscopy. These results should be interpreted in conjunction with the patient's underlying risk factors (i.e., a 25-year-old with no medical problems with Gram-positive cocci is more likely to have *S. pneumoniae* than *S. aureus meningitis).*

Corticosteroids

Dexamethasone reduces the inflammatory response that, to a great degree, is responsible for the morbidity associated with meningitis. In particular, the literature demonstrates that audiologic and neurological sequelae in infants older than two months of age are markedly reduced by early administration of dexamethasone in patients with *H. influenzae* (Hib) meningitis. There is also some evidence that dexamethasone also may be beneficial in children with pneumococcal meningitis. However, there is no clear evidence of any beneficial effect of dexamethasone in adult meningitis, although the issue has not been adequately studied.[7,26]

For optimal effect, dexamethasone should be given at a dose of

Figure 1. Algorithm for the Evaluation of Patients with Probable Viral Meningitis

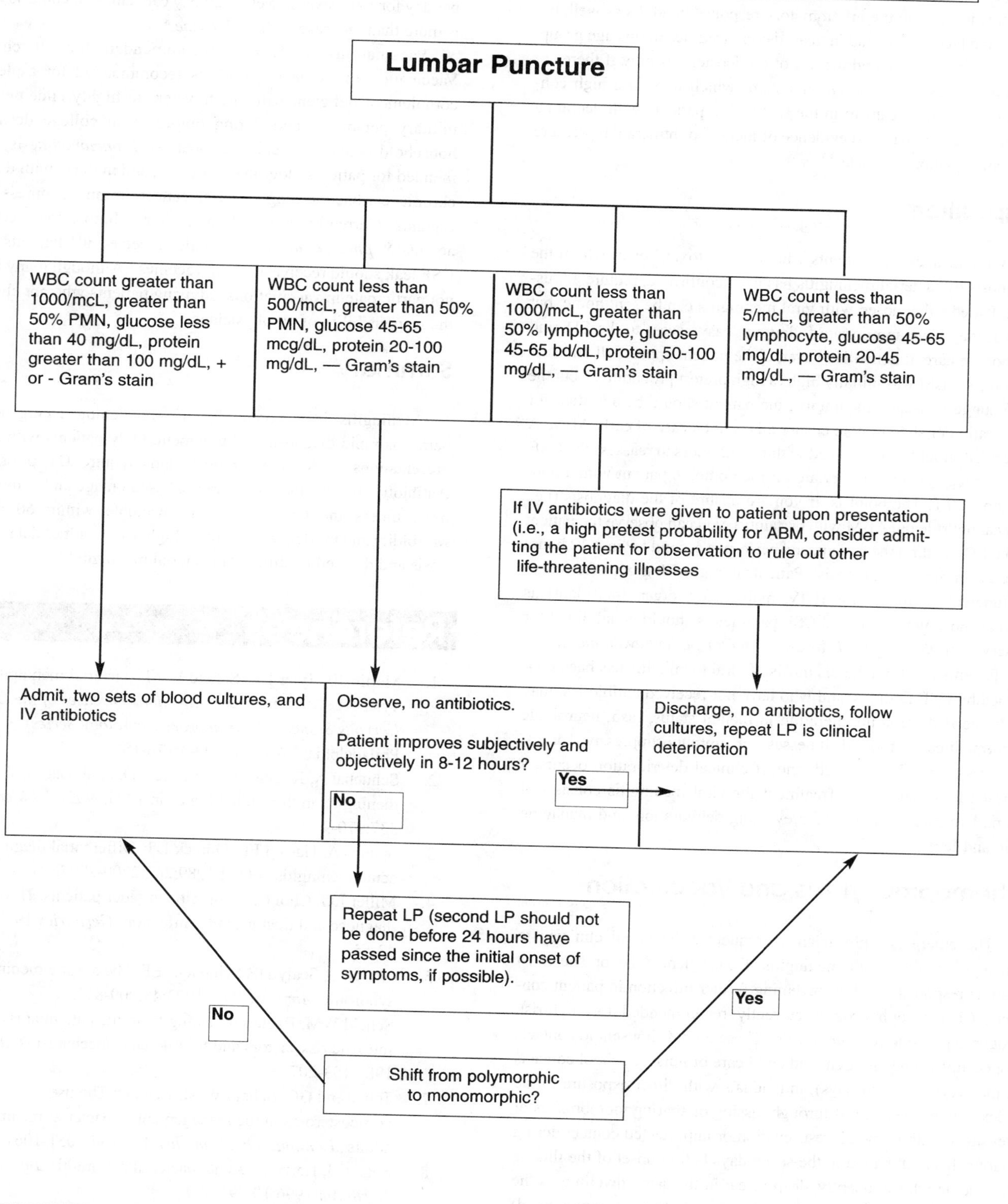

0.15mg/kg every six hours IV for 2-4 days to children with suspected Hib or pneumococcal meningitis. The dose should be given just prior to or with the initiation of antibiotics.[7,11] Increasing *S. pneumoniae* resistance to penicillin has created concern with regard to interactions between vancomycin and dexamethasone. Animal studies suggest that dexamethasone may decrease vancomycin penetration into the CSF, but a recent study in children did not bear this out.[27] It is reasonable to believe that dexamethasone should be effective in diluting the inflammatory response in adults as well, but due to the lack of data and increased comorbidities in this age group, some experts recommend the use of corticosteroids only if there are organisms present on the Gram's stain (which implies a high concentration of the organism in the CSF) or in patients with declining mental status (coma), and evidence of increased intracranial pressure by exam or laboratory data.[9,7]

Disposition

Without question, patients who appear "toxic," or in whom the diagnosis of bacterial meningitis has been confirmed, require admission. Patients diagnosed with viral meningitis can be sent home, but only if they have appropriate follow up, easy access to the ED, and supportive care at home. However, if the patient appears ill and suspicion for ABM was initially high (a high pretest probability), but the CSF suggests aseptic meningitis, the patient should be admitted for observation or short-stay to ensure this is not a case of early ABM. A repeat LP should be performed within 8-12 hours to reassess the CSF. This strategy also is appropriate for the nontoxic patient with a nondiagnostic LP. The point is, if you are unsure of the diagnosis (i.e., you cannot rule out ABM with certainty), you can observe the patient in the ED or admit the patient, and perform a second LP in 8-12 hours later to confirm the diagnosis. Patients in high-risk groups for fungal or tuberculous meningitis (HIV, malignancy, organ transplant) as well as those with abnormal CSF parameters should be admitted for observation. *(See Figure 1 for algorithm for patient evaluation.)*

Patients in whom the diagnosis of viral meningitis has been confirmed by CSF findings, and who have not received antibiotics, may go home if there is no alteration in mental status, rash, neurologic abnormalities, comorbid illnesses, or immunosuppressive drugs. Cultures should be followed, and, if clinical deterioration occurs, a repeat LP is mandatory. Treatment for viral meningitis consists of supportive care: treating and preventing dehydration, and managing pain and fever.

Chemoprophylaxis and Vaccination

The emergency physician is frequently the initial clinician to manage a patient with meningitis. Consequently, he or she must assume responsibility for preventing further infection in patient contacts. Chemoprophylaxis is currently recommended for high-risk groups exposed to *N. meningitidis*. These include household contacts (especially young children, and child care or nursery school contacts in the previous seven days), individuals with direct exposure to the index patient's secretions through kissing or sharing toothbrushes or utensils, mouth to mouth resuscitation or unprotected contact during endotracheal intubation in the seven days before onset of the illness, and people who frequently sleep or eat in the same dwelling as the index patient. Low-risk groups (no prophylaxis recommended) include casual contacts or indirect contact, and medical personnel not directly exposed to the index patient's oral secretions. Rifampin 10mg/kg every 12 hours for four doses (max 600 mg) is the current drug of choice. Ceftriaxone, ciprofloxacin, and sulfasoxazole are alternatives.[28] Chemoprophylaxis is also recommended for *H. influenzae* if there is another child younger than 4 years old in the same household as the index case. In this case, all members of the household should be treated with rifampin 20 mg/kg (max 600 mg) per day for four days, as well as all day care children contacts if there is more than one case of *H. influenzae*.[8]

Vaccination for Hib is recommended for all children. Vaccination for *N. meningitidis* is recommended for asplenic or complement deficient patients, travelers to highly endemic areas, military personnel, and during outbreaks in college dorms and household contacts. Vaccination against *S. pneumoniae* is recommended for patients older than 65 years, and in those with diabetes, chronic cardiac or lung disease, cancer immunosuppression, or asplenia. Currently, only 10% of patients eligible for vaccination against *S. pneumoniae* have actually received it.[4] Patients with a CSF leak should receive all three vaccines.[8] Although many EDs do not participate in vaccinations, advising patients who are eligible is the responsibility of all physicians.

Summary

Meningitis is a potentially life-threatening emergency that demands rapid diagnosis and treatment. Only patients with atypical presentations or focal neurologic signs require CT prior to LP. Antibiotic choice should be empiric, based on age and comorbid illness, unless the Gram's stain is available within 60 minutes. Morbidity and mortality still remain high, as a result of delayed diagnosis and delayed treatment of bacterial meningitis.

References

1. Martin JB, Tyler KL, Scheld W M. Bacterial meningitis. In: Tyler KL, Martin JB, eds. *Infectious Diseases of the Central Nervous System (Contemporary Neurology Series)*. Philadelphia: FA Davis; 1993:176-187.
2. Schuchat A, Robinson K, Wenger JD, et al. Bacterial meningitis in the United States in 1995. *N Engl J Med* 1997; 337:970-976.
3. Spanos A, Harrell FE, Durack DT. Differential diagnosis of acute meningitis. *JAMA* 1989;262:2700-2707.
4. Miller LG, Choi C. Meningitis in older patients: How to diagnose and treat a deadly infection. *Geriatrics* 1997;52: 43-55.
5. Nelsen S, Sealy DP, Schneider EF. The aseptic meningitis syndrome. *Am Fam Phys* 1993;48:809-815.
6. Scheld WM. Bacterial meningitis in the patient at risk: Intrinsic risk factors and host defense mechanisms. *Am J Med* 1984;193-207.
7. Townsend GC, Scheld W M. Review: The use of corticosteroids in the management of bacterial meningitis in adults. *J Antimicrob Chemother* 1996;37:1051-1061.
8. Segreti J, Harris A. Acute bacterial meningitis. *Infect Dis Clin North Am* 1996;10:797-809.

9. Tunkel AR, Scheld WM. Acute bacterial meningitis in adults. In: Remington JS, Swart MN, eds. *Current Clinical Topics in Infectious Diseases.* Boston: Blackwell Science; 1995: 215-239.
10. Maxson S, Jacobs RF. Viral meningitis. *Postgrad Med* 1993; 93:153-166.
11. Quagliarello VJ, Scheld WM. Treatment of bacterial meningitis. *N Engl J Med* 1997;336:708-716.
12. Radetsky M. Duration of symptoms and outcome in bacterial meningitis: An analysis of causation and the implications of a delay in diagnosis. *Pediatr Infect Dis J* 1992;11:694-698.
13. Talan DA, Zibulewsky J. Relationship of clinical presentation to time to antibiotics for the emergency department management of suspected bacterial meningitis. *Ann Emerg Med* 1993;22:1733-1738.
14. Greenlee JE. Approach to diagnosis of meningitis. *Infect Dis Clin North Am* 1990;4:583-598.
15. McKinney W, Heudebert GR, Harper SA, et al. Validation of a clinical prediction rule for the differential diagnosis of acute meningitis. *J Geriatr Intern Med* 1994;9:8-12.
16. Ashwal S. Neurologic evaluation of the patient with acute bacterial meningitis. *Neurol Crit Care* 1995;13:549-577.
17. Anderson M. Management of cerebral infection. *J Neurol Neurosurg Psychiatry* 1993;56:1243-1258.
18. Maxson S, Jacobs RF. Viral meningitis. *Postgrad Med* 1993;93:153-166.
19. Lipton JD, Schafermeyer RW. Central nervous system infections. *Emerg Med Clin North Am* 1995;13:417-443.
20. Overall JC. Is it bacterial or viral? Laboratory differentiation. *Pediatr Rev* 1993;14:255-257.
21. Rice SK, Heinl RE, Thornton LL, et al. Clinical characteristics, management strategies, and cost implications of a statewide outbreak of enterovirus meningitis. *Clin Infect Dis* 1995;20:931-937.
22. Varki AP, Puthuran P. Value of second lumbar puncture in confirming a diagnosis of aseptic meningitis. A prospective study. *Arch Neurol* 1979;36:581-582.
23. Feigin RD, Shackelford PG. Value of repeat lumbar puncture in the differential diagnosis of meningitis. *N Engl J Med* 1973;289:571-573.
24. Amir J, Harel L, Frydman M, et al. Shift of cerebrospinal polymorphonuclear cell percentage in the early stage of aseptic meningitis. *J Pediatr* 1991;119:938-941.
25. Powers WJ. Cerebrospinal fluid lymphocytosis in acute bacterial meningitis. *Am J Med* 1985;79:216-219.
26. McIntyre PB, Berkey CS, King SM, et al. Dexamethasone as adjunctive therapy in bacterial meningitis. *JAMA* 1997;278: 925-931.
27. Klugman KP. Bactericidal activity against cephalosporin-resistant *S. pneumoniae* in CSF of children with acute bacterial meningitis. *Antimicrob Agents Chemother* 1995;39:1988-1992.
28. American Academy of Pediatrics (Section 3). In: Peter G, ed. *1997 Red Book: Report of the Committee on Infectious Diseases.* 24th ed.1997:222-3;359-360.

Evaluation of Fever

Sid M. Shah, MD, FACEP
Les Searls, DO

Fever is a nonspecific body response to a variety of environmental and internal factors. It is among the most frequent reasons for patients to present to the ED, accounting for 6% of adult and 20-40% of pediatric visits.

Unlike the pediatric patient, in whom fever most frequently reflects an infectious etiology, fever in an adult can be due to noninfectious conditions such as collagen vascular diseases, malignancy, embolic disease, and other conditions. Fever at the extremes of age or in an immunocompromised patient remains a diagnostic challenge. An ill-appearing elderly or immunocompromised patient suspected of harboring an infection who presents without fever can be difficult to assess, since the "septic elderly" may not mount the expected febrile response. Symptoms of infection may be masked in adults with chronic diseases or altered sensorium. Moreover, recent expansion in the use of "medical hardware" increases the risk of "occult" infection in the elderly.

This chapter reviews definitions of fever, clinical evaluation, and differential diagnosis of the febrile adult patient.

Fever: Clinical Considerations

Normal body temperature is controlled within a narrow "physiologic" range through a variety of behavioral and physiologic mechanisms. The preoptic area of the hypothalamus is the body's thermoregulatory center. It consists of thermosensitive neurons whose rate of discharge is affected by the temperature of the local blood supply, and has neural connections with temperature sensors distributed in skin and muscle. These neurons also are affected by a variety of hormones, cytokines, and neurotransmitters. In response to these signals, the hypothalamus directs efferent nerve pathways, resulting in actions that lead to heat generation or loss; for example, peripheral vasoconstriction and shivering cause heat generation, and peripheral vasodilatation causes heat loss.

Generally, fever represents a controlled elevation of "normal" body temperature and is associated with a reset of the hypothalamic set point. In humans, the normal set point ranges between 36°C and 37.8°C. The daily variation of body temperature of approximately 1°C is referred to as the circadian rhythm. Typical body temperatures are lowest in the early morning and highest in the late afternoon.

Hyperthermia is defined as an elevation of normal body temperature that occurs when peripheral heat-dissipating mechanisms become overwhelmed, as with vigorous exercise, environmental exposure, hyperthyroidism, or the use of anticholinergic or phenothiazine medications. In almost all cases, a temperature higher than 41.5°C reflects "hyperthermia" rather than true fever. Behavioral mechanisms also are important, as is exemplified by the use of blankets or warmer clothing during a chill in the early phase of infection.[1] *(See Table 1.)*

Whether temperature elevation represents a significant defense mechanism in humans has been debated. Temperature elevation

Table 1. Ranges of Fever and Associated Neurological Symptoms

- Normal: between 36°C and 37.8°C
- Circadian rhythm: daily variation of approximately 1°C
- Hyperthermia: > 41°5 C
- Alteration of mental status: > 41°C
- Loss of consciousness: > 42°C (neurological damage may occur if these temperatures are sustained for a prolonged period of time)

results in increased oxygen and caloric demands, and poses potential damage to neural tissue. Fever also is associated with excessive protein breakdown and with increased gluconeogenesis,[2] perhaps, in part, mediated by interleukin-1.[3] A patient's basal metabolic rate may be increased as much as 15% for each degree Celsius rise in temperature. This "response" to temperature elevation can drain metabolic reserves in a critically ill or an elderly patient.

Neurological damage is the most important complication of significant elevations in temperature. This complication is most often encountered with hyperthermia. Alteration of mental status is common at temperatures above 41°C. Temperatures greater than 42°C may produce loss of consciousness, and neurological damage may occur if these temperatures are sustained for a prolonged period of time.

Moderate elevations in temperatures are usually well tolerated by the patient and may aid to some degree in "host defense." In this regard, increases in body temperature directly inhibit replication of such viruses as coxsackie and polio. The only infections in which fever has clearly been shown to inhibit microbial growth, however, are neurosyphilis and a disseminated gonococcemia.[1]

The genesis and maintenance of fever represents a complex interaction between various biochemical predicters that elevate the hypothalamic set point. Pyrogens, which are capable of inducing fever, can either be endogenous or exogenous. Endogenous pyrogens are produced within the body, whereas exogenous pyrogens are introduced by infecting microrganisms. Exogenous pyrogens may be either the microorganisms themselves, or they may represent metabolic products or toxins produced by the offending agent. They generally cause fever by inducing the host to produce endogenous pyrogens.

Endogenous pyrogens are a heterogeneous collection of cytokines that include interleukin-1 (IL-1), interleukin-6 (IL-6), tumor necrosis factor (TNF), interferon-a and -b, and others. In response to infectious, inflammatory, or immunological stimuli, monocytes and macrophages produce endogenous pyrogens, which travel via the blood to the thermoregulatory center of the hypothalamus. There, arachidonic acid is released, which is associated with production of prostaglandin E2 (PGE2). When the hypothalamic set point is raised, efferent signals lead to peripheral vasoconstriction, increased internal heat production, and behavioral changes that conserve heat. Ultimately, the new thermostatic set point is reached, and a new equilibrium for body temperature prevails. Fever is maintained as long as the levels of endogenous pyrogen remain steady and the effects of pyrogens are not inhibited. If the levels of endogenous pyrogen fall, the thermostat is reset at a lower level. Cyclo-oxygenase inhibitors, such as aspirin, decrease temperature by blocking production of PGE2.

Clinical Evaluation of the Febrile Adult

A detailed history, when available, can generate a useful differential diagnosis in most febrile patients presenting to the emergency department (ED). The history will suggest specific aspects of the physical examination. The majority of febrile illnesses are infectious, and, therefore, clinical findings indicating involvement of a specific organ system may suggest a diagnosis. Overall, the diagnosis of 70-85% of adult febrile illnesses can be made on the basis of a history and a physical examination.[4,5]

The origin and duration of the current illness should be considered, including an inquiry into the time and the magnitude of fever. A history of associated symptoms, if any, should be elicited. Consider infectious (e.g., amoebiasis, malaria) and non-infectious conditions (e.g., pulmonary embolus) in patients with a recent history of travel. A history of chronic illness, recent and past surgeries, presence of "medical hardware," and medication use (prescription and nonprescription) is important; immunization status also should be considered. A recent hospitalization should prompt consideration of a nosocomial infection, whereas a history of exposure to animals, toxic fumes, raw or poorly cooked meats, or unpasturized dairy products can provide important clues to fever in an adult without an obvious source of infection. The patient should be questioned about sexual activity and the use of protective measures.

Vital Signs. Blood pressure, temperature, heart rate, and respiratory rate are noted. Pulse oximetry is useful in selected patients who are severely ill. Temperature is measured either orally or rectally. Axillary and tympanic temperatures are unreliable, as are oral temperatures measured after recent intake of hot or cold beverages, smoking, or hyperventilation.[6] Rectal temperatures are approximately 17.2°C higher than the oral temperature.[6] Serial temperatures measured via the same route provide additional information. The heart rate can be expected to increase by approximately ten beats per minute per 17.2°C of temperature elevation. Relative bradycardia or temperature-pulse dissociation is seen in such conditions as typhoid fever, brucellosis, leptospirosis, drug-associated fevers, and factitious fever.[6] The physician should consider rheumatic fever, Lyme disease, viral myocarditis, bacterial endocarditis, presence of underlying cardiac conduction disease, or concurrent use of medications such as beta-blockers in a febrile patient with frank bradycardia. Tachypnea, a sign of dyspnea, suggests pulmonary disease. In the absence of dyspnea, tachypnea can be a nonspecific sign of sepsis.[7]

Sensorium. Mental status changes, especially in the elderly and the chronically ill patient, require evaluation for infection. Altered mental status can present as decreased level of consciousness, confusion, lethargy, agitation, anorexia, weakness, lightheadedness, vertigo, falls, incontinence, or memory loss. Severe agitation or coma in a febrile patient on neuroleptic medications raises the possibility of neuroleptic malignant syndrome. Rigors, which generally suggest bacteremia, can occur in noninfectious diseases such as lymphoma. Rigors are absent in more than half of bacteremic patients.[8]

Physical Examination

Skin. The skin should be examined for exanthema. Viral exanthema is frequently maculopapular. Purpuric lesions are characteristic of meningococcemia, and petechial lesions are characteristic of vasculitis or thrombocytopenia. Decubitus ulcers can be a portal of entry for systemic infection. The characteristic hot red lesions of cellulitis can be missed if not specifically sought. Specific rashes associated with fever are reviewed later.

Head and Neck. Palpebral conjunctivitis is characteristic of several viral infections, while bulbar conjunctivitis can be associated with leptospirosis. Scleral icterus may suggest hepatitis, biliary tract obstruction, or hemolysis. Funduscopic abnormalities associated with fever include fluffy, white exudates associated with disseminated candidiasis; retinal hemorrhage associated with leukemia; emboli associated with endocarditis; or yellow nodules associated with miliary tuberculosis.[9] Erythema of the tympanic membrane or air fluid levels on otoscopic examination suggest otitis media. Bullae on the tympanic membrane are characteristic of *Mycoplasma* infection. The presence of erythema, epithelial debris, and exudate along with pain on auricular manipulation are characteristic of otitis externa, whereas tenderness on palpation of the mastoid process may indicate mastoiditis.

Stridor is a late finding associated with supraglottitis or epiglottitis in adults.[10,11] The presence of an enlarged erythematous uvula is seen in uvulitis, which has been associated with epiglottitis. Poor dentition and oral hygiene is associated with gingival infection, periodontal abscess, and aspiration pneumonia. Tonsils and peritonsillar tissues should be examined for swelling, erythema, injection, soft palate petechiae, and exudates. Severe tonsillitis can present with stridor. Unilateral tonsillar swelling with unilateral soft palate edema and erythema and uvular deviation suggest peritonsillar abscess. Tonsillar exudates are seen with a number of infectious agents and are not pathognomonic of Group A beta hemolytic strep infection.

The neck should be examined for lymphadenopathy, masses, and thyroid enlargement. Nuchal rigidity is suggestive of meningitis, but this sign is frequently absent in the elderly or chronically debilitated individual. Soft tissue infections in the neck, such as parapharyngeal or retropharyngeal abscess can present with sore throat with or without stridor, drooling, and muffled or "hot potato" speech.

The differential diagnosis of fever associated with lymphadenopathy includes autoimmune disorders, malignancy, drug-related side effects and a variety of infections. Lymphadenopathy caused by infections is usually tender, whereas malignant lymphadenopathy is usually painless, rubbery, hard, and firm. Infectious agents usually cause bilateral cervical lymphadenopathy. Unilateral cervical lymphadenopathy is more often malignant. Supraclavicular nodes can be felt in association with fungal infections such as cocciodomycosis and histoplasmosis, but are more common with malignancies of lung, abdominal, or pelvic organs.

Epitrochlear nodes may be encountered in hand infections as well as in non-Hodgkin's lymphoma and secondary syphilis. Axillary and inguinal lymphadenopathies are commonly associated with infection, although malignancies (specifically breast and melanoma) also can present in this manner. Infections that cause generalized lymphadenopathy include acute viral infections, brucellosis, leptospirosis, and AIDS. Non-infectious etiologies of generalized lymphadenopathy associated with fever include: lymphoma, sarcoidosis, collagen vascular disorders, immune globulin disorders, myeloproliferative and lymphoproliferative diseases, and side effects of such drugs as phenytoin, methyldopa, and procainamide.

Chest. Auscultation of the chest may yield findings associated with pneumonia or congestive heart failure; ronchi and wheezes may reflect bronchospasm caused by bronchitis, reactive airway disease, or exacerbation of chronic obstructive pulmonary disease.The presence of a pericardial rub on auscultation can indicate pericarditis. A new murmur in an IV drug user or elderly patient should suggest the possibility of endocarditis. New onset of congestive heart failure can be seen with myocarditis.

Abdomen. The abdomen should be examined for distention, the presence of atypical "tinkles and rushes" associated with evolving obstruction, areas of tenderness, signs of peritoneal irritation, intraperitoneal fluid, and organ enlargement. Rectal examination may demonstrate perianal or perirectal abscesses. Prostatic tenderness indicates prostatitis, which can be a source of recurrent infections. Intra-abdominal infections such as cholecysitis, diverticulitis, appendicitis, and abscesses of the liver, spleen, or pancreas are a common cause of fever that may be difficult to diagnose.

Noninfectious causes of fever with abdominal pain include inflammatory bowel disease and pancreatitis. Elderly patients, as well as patients with diabetes or those on chronic corticoidsteroid therapy, may lack typical physical findings. The clinician should note the low sensitivity and specificity of "classic" predictors (temperature > 37°C, white blood cell count > 14,000, rebound, and vomiting) of appendicitis in patients 60 years and older.[12]

Genitourinary. External genitalia should be examined for ulcerations, swelling, discharge, and nodules. The foreskin, if present, should be examined and retracted. Urethral discharge suggests urethritis that is caused by a sexually transmissible disease. An enlarged, tender testicle requires evaluation for orchitis or torsion. The epididymis is palpated for enlargement and tenderness, findings that suggest epididymitis.

Suprapubic tenderness associated with dysuria and/or urinary frequency should prompt a urinalysis to evaluate for urinary tract infection, a common cause of fever in the elderly and debilitated patient. A pelvic examination is performed routinely to evaluate for the cervical motion tenderness and cervical discharge of pelvic inflammatory disease, as well as adenexal tenderness or mass associated with tubo-ovarian abscess or ovarian cyst.

Musculoskeletal and Extremities. Examination of the extremities and axial skeleton is often overlooked in the evaluation of the febrile patient. Palpation of the spine may reveal tenderness that can indicate spinal osteomyelitis, discitis, or epidural abscess. The latter is common in intravenous drug abusers and alcoholics. Palpation and inspection of the extremities can reveal osteomyelitis, cellulitis, deep venous thrombosis, ruptured Baker's cyst, diabetic ulcers, or acute septic arthritis.

Differential Diagnosis of Fever

The differential diagnosis in patients presenting to the ED with fever is broad. Age and underlying medical conditions are the most important considerations in generating a list of differential diagnosis in an adult febrile patient. For example, a young, healthy patient is more likely to have a benign viral illness, whereas an elderly diabetic is more likely to have a serious bacterial infection. Since infections are responsible for most fever-related visits to the ED, an initial evaluation directed toward infectious etiologies is most likely to be rewarding.

In general, the goal of ED evaluation of a febrile adult is to detect either a "treatable infection" (which in most cases is a bacterial ill-

Table 2. Laboratory and Radiological Studies in the Febrile Patient

- Leukocyte counts
- Acute phase reactants
- Strep screen and throat culture
- Sputum gram stain
- Urine analysis and culture
- Blood cultures
- Cerebrospinal fluid examination
- Stool evaluation

ness) or a serious, life-threatening noninfectious cause of fever (such as pulmonary embolus). The ED investigation is a time-restricted process that includes a history, physical examination, and limited ancillary tests. In the majority of cases, safe discharge from the ED or the decision to hospitalize an adult febrile patient is made on the basis of clinical information and physical examination rather than on ancillary tests.

Laboratory and Radiological Studies

Judicious use of laboratory and radiologic tests guided by a careful history and physical examination—and a well developed differential diagnosis—can provide high quality, yet cost efficient, patient care. *(See Table 2.)*

Leukocyte Counts. The leukocyte (WBC) count frequently is used to evaluate the febrile patient in order to distinguish bacterial from viral etiologies of fever, and to gauge the severity of infection. Although a leukocytosis suggests a higher likelihood of occult bacterial infection, even with a left shift, viral illness is still possible. As a result, the usefulness of the absolute leukocyte count, with or without an increase in immature cell forms, is limited.[13-18] Leukocyte count is neither sensitive nor specific for the type or severity of infection. Demargination of neutrophils in response to strenuous exercise can account for a leukocytosis as high as 35,000/mm.[6,17] Neutrophilia with a "left shift" can be a nonspecific reaction to acute emotional stress, acute or chronic inflammation, benign or malignant tumors, other non infectious states, or medications such as steroids, lithium, and epinephrine.[17] Although relatively inexpensive to perform, the true cost of a leukocyte count includes the cost of over treatment in response to abnormal, but clinically irrelevant, leukocytosis.[18] In one study, only two out of 860 leukocyte counts with differentials had a clearly beneficial effect on patient care.[16]

However, the leukocyte count is useful in the assessment in *selected* febrile patients. It should be interpreted and correlated with the entire clinical picture and used as one of several tools to aid in the decision making process. The leukocyte count can be used to increase the suspicion of a bacterial illness in the following selective clinical conditions: 1) febrile elderly patients, 2) febrile adults without a definite source of infection, and 3) immunocompromised febrile adults.

Acute Phase Reactants. In the febrile patient, the erythrocyte sedimentation rate (ESR) and C-reactive protein (CRP) are sometimes used to screen for an inflammatory or infectious processes. As with the leukocyte count, these tests can be misleading if they are not interpreted cautiously.

ESR, a simple and an inexpensive test, is an index of the suspension stability of red blood cells in citrated blood. ESR measures the distance in millimeters that erythrocytes fall in one hour. In clinical practice, the ESR is used to monitor progression or improvement of a documented disease and response to therapy. In the ED, ESR is primarily used to identify the presence or absence of a disease such as temporal arteritis in an older patient with headache and fever. Numerous studies have reported the inconsistent sensitivity and poor specificity of the ESR. However, the ESR does not help discriminate between those patients who have serious bacterial infection and those who do not.[19-26]

Although less than ideal, CRP is both more sensitive and more specific than ESR.[23,24] With serial measurements, CRP is more useful in monitoring response to therapy.[26] CRP rises faster in infectious states than does ESR,[24,25] which enhances its usefulness in emergency medicine. In a cohort study of elderly patients, neither ESR nor CRP satisfactorily discriminated between patients with and without ongoing active or chronic disease.[27] In addition, the same study reported elevation of ESR and CRP with infection, although neither had an advantage over the other.[27] In some chronic illnesses, such as diabetes and chronic renal failure, a rise in CRP is considered to be more specific for infection.[20,28]

Strep Screen and Throat Culture. Viral and bacterial pharyngitis are self-limited illnesses in most immunocompetent patients. However, a variety of symptoms accompanying bacterial-mediated "sore throat" resolve more quickly with prompt (early) initiation of antibiotic therapy. In addition, the association of Group A beta hemolytic strep (GAS) with rheumatic heart disease is well documented.

Throat cultures have been the "gold standard" for diagnosis of bacterial, and, specifically, streptococcal pharyngitis. However, throat cultures can be falsely positive and indicate a carrier state or they may be falsely negative. Multiple commercial rapid strep screens are available, with sensitivities ranging from 55% to 96% and specificities ranging from 50% to 98%.[29-33] A newer technique, optical immunoassay, has a reported sensitivity of 97.4-98.9% and a specificity of 95.6-98.0%, which is more sensitive than bacterial culture.[33]

These screening tests only detect GAS, while other organisms commonly implicated in pharyngitis, such as *Chlamydia trachomatis, Mycoplasma pneumonia,* and gonococcus, are not detected by a screening test.

The most outcome-effective treatment protocol for acute pharyngitis is controversial. Some experts recommend antibiotic treatment on the basis of a history and physical examination, while others advocate treating only those with positive cultures or rapid assays.[32] As a rule, a strep screen is not indicated when the clinical suspicion for GAS is high and antibiotics will be prescribed based on clinical presentation alone. The prudent use of antibiotics in the treatment of acute pharyngitis is based on the results of a strep screen in patients with sore throat and recent exposure to GAS; those with a history of rheumatic fever, diabetes, or fever higher than 38.8°C; and those with the presence of a scarlatiniform rash or sore throat that persists for longer than six days.[34]

Sputum Gram Stain. In the febrile patient with a productive cough, a sputum gram stain is sometimes helpful. An appropriate sample of sputum has more than 25 neutrophils and less than 10 epithelial cells/HPF on gram stain. Sputum cultures are often not as helpful due to the presence of fastidious anaerobes that fail to grow or to the overgrowth of oral flora. In cases of pneumococcal pneumonia, bacteria fail to grow in approximately one-half of cases in which it was demonstrated on gram stain.[35,36]

Urine Analysis and Culture. Dysuria, urgency, and frequency of urination accompanied by suprapubic tenderness and a urinalysis demonstrating pyuria and bacteruria confirm the diagnosis of urinary tract infection. As a rule, young adult females with no prior episodes of cystitis do not require further microbiological evaluation other than consideration of a curvical culture to rule out *Chlamydia* infection. Males with urinary infection require urine *culture* and sensitivity, as well as rectal examination to evaluate prostatic pathology. Examination of the urine after prostatic massage may reveal increased leukocytes suggesting prostatitis.

Despite a few studies challenging the usefulness of its ability to screen for infection, dipstick urine analysis is widely used and relatively accurate.[37] A positive leukocyte esterase test, in conjunction with positive urine tests for nitrite and blood on dipstick test, suggest the presence of urinary infection. The dipstick test has been reported to have a sensitivity and specificity of greater than 88%.[37] The sensitivity is lower when there are less than 10 WBC/HPF. However, a positive dipstick test does not always indicate a urinary infection. Non-infectious causes such as interstitial nephritis, nephrolithiasis, or vaginal discharge also can produce pyuria. As false-negative tests for infection are common with dipstick urine testing, a microscopic urinalysis is recommended when urine dip stick testing is negative in a patient with a strong clinical suspicion of urinary infection.

The presence or absence of a "true" urinary tract infection is difficult to confirm in light of controversy regarding the precise criteria indicating urinary infection. Colony forming unit (CFU) count or "colony count" higher than 100,000 CFUs/mL of urine has been traditionally used as a marker for urinary tract infection. However, infections can be documented with much lower CFUs. Bacteremia, too, can occur with lower concentrations of bacteria in the urine.[37] Not suprisingly, in the literature, the presence of urine infection has been characterized according to many different criteria: 10,000-100,000 CFUs/mL of a *single* urinary pathogen; 1000 CFUs/mL of a single urinary pathogen from a catheterized specimen; or 100 CFUs/mL of a single urinary pathogen in a "symptomatic" female patient.

In the absence of any risk factors, a urine culture usually is *not* necessary in most cases of uncomplicated urinary tract infection when symptoms suggest only "lower urinary tract" infection. However, in the presence of normal microscopic and dipstick urine tests and a *high* clinical suspicion of urinary tract infection, urine culture is recommended. Urine culture also is indicated in the patient with recurrent urinary tract infections or when urinary symptoms persist for more than seven days, and in those patients with a history of recent hospitalization, catheterization, pregnancy, or diabetes.[38] Urine culture is mandatory in the febrile, toxic-appearing adult and in the chronically debilitated patient with a fever who has an indwelling urinary catheter or surgically altered urinary tract.

In the absence of a uniform definition of a urine culture that indicates a urine infection, the results of urine analysis and urine culture must be interpreted in association with clinical findings. This is particularly relevant when evaluating a female with acute dysuria. Since the results of a urine analysis can be misleading, the cause of acute dysuria in women (cystitis, urethritis and vaginitis) should be made clinically.

Table 3. Patient Subgroup and/or Clinical Conditions Benefitting from Blood Culture Studies

- Signs of sepsis, which may include fever, chills, tachycardia, and/or hypertension
- Acute alteration of mental status, especially in the elderly
- Identifying the causative organism in established cases of pneumonia, meningitis, osteomyelitis
- Unexplained leukocytosis in an ill-appearing patient
- Ill-appearing, immunocompromised patient
- New onset of organ failure such as renal failure, liver failure, etc.

Blood Cultures. Blood cultures are performed to recover organisms that may be responsible for infection. Blood cultures are expensive, with a cost ranging from $25-$60 per set. False positive and false-negative results are common. Studies have reported that of *all* blood cultures drawn, true-positive results are obtained in less than 5% of samples.[39-41] Interestingly, the incidence of contamination is also approximately 5%.[39,41]

Although spiking fever and chills are typical signs of a bacteremic episode, well-defined clinical criteria that predictabaly identify bacteremia are lacking. When a bacteremic episode is suspected, two or three sets of blood cultures should be drawn by separate venipuncture for each set of blood cultures. Femoral vessels and vessels underlying skin the with dermatological disease should be avoided. The site is prepared with 70% isopropyl alcohol in a concentric fashion starting at the center. After allowing time for drying, the site is then prepared a second time with providine-iodine 10% solution in the same fashion and allowed to dry. Improvement in blood culture accuracy by using "a dedicated blood culture team" of phlebotomists has been reported.[39] A minimum of 10 mL and a maximum of 30 mL of blood is required for appropriate blood culture.[41]

Selected patient subgroups and/or clinical conditions that can benefit from blood culture studies *(see Table 3)* include:

- Signs of sepsis, which may include fever, chills, tachycardia, and/or hypotension;
- Acute alteration of mental status, especially in the elderly;
- Identifying the causative organism in established cases of pneumonia, meningitis, osteomyelitis, etc.;
- Unexplained leukocytosis in an ill-appearing patient;
- Ill-appearing immunocompromised patient; and
- New onset of organ failure such as renal failure, liver failure, etc.

Cerebrospinal Fluid Examination. Lumbar puncture for collection of cerebrospinal fluid (CSF) is indicated whenever the diagnosis of central nervous system (CNS) infection, a CNS inflammatory process such as lupus cerebritis or a CNS neoplastic process, is suspected. Cardinal signs and symptoms of adult meningitis include fever, headache, and signs of meningeal irritation such as nuchal rigidity, Kernig's sign, and Brudzinski's sign.

The diagnosis of CNS infection in the elderly and the chronically ill can be difficult inasmuch as the classic signs of meningeal irritation are frequently absent. Accordingly, a low threshold for the examination of CSF in these patients is prudent.

Table 4. Liver Enzyme Elevation in the Febrile Patient

MEASUREMENT OF HEPATIC ENZYMES CAN BE HELPFUL IN THE EVALUATION OF:

- Suspected infectious or inflammatory hepatitis
- Sepsis
- Lower lobe pneumonia
- Legionnaire's disease

Cerebrospinal fluid is analyzed for cell count and differential, gram stain, culture and sensitivity testing, glucose, protein, and testing for bacterial antigens. The opening pressure is elevated in most cases of meningitis. The CSF may be clear, cloudy, or frankly purulent. The leukocyte count is frequently elevated with neutrophilic predominance. Low cell counts in *bacterial* meningitis are associated with poor prognosis. CSF pleocytosis with predominant polymorphonuclear leukocytes does not always indicate a "bacterial" infection. The CSF may or may not show pleocytosis in viral infections. Protein levels are elevated in bacterial meningitis. CSF glucose falls to less than 40 mm/dL in approximately 60% of cases, and a CSF-to-serum glucose ratio of less than 0.31 is seen in 70% of cases.[42] Reports of xanthochromia or even frank blood in CSF in cases of meningitis have been reported.[42]

The CSF gram stain demonstrates the offending bacteria with an overall sensitivity of 75%. The CSF culture is positive in 70-85% of patients with cofirmed bacterial meningitis.[42] Prior antibiotic therapy decreases the sensitivity of the CSF gram stain and the culture. A variety of immunologic tests are available for identifying bacterial antigens in the CSF; some have a sensitivity and specificity in the 95% range.[42] However, a negative antigen test *does not* rule out bacterial meningitis.

Stool Evaluation. Most cases of diarrheal illness are mild and self-limited and, therefore, stool evaluation is not helpful. Laboratory evaluation of the stool is helpful in the following conditions: chronic or subacute diarrhea; a cluster of diarrheal illness; severe diarrhea; or a diarrhea accompanied by abdominal pain, tenesmus, or hematochezia.

A Wright's (or leukocyte) stain is used to evaluate leukocytosis in the stool. Stool examination for the presence of fecal leukocytes is the most useful diagnostic study in patients with acute diarrhea. When correlated with stool cultures, the fecal leukocyte test is 82% sensitive and 83% specific for detecting a bacterial pathogen.[43] Diarrhea caused by invasive pathogens, such as enteroinvasive *E. coli, Salmonella* sp., *Shigella* sp., *Campylobacter* sp., *Yersinia* sp., *Vibrio* sp., *E. histolytica,* and *C. difficile,* are associated with presence of fecal leukocytes. Diarrheal illness caused by *Vibrio cholera*, enteropathic, enterotoxic *E. coli*, rotavirus, Norwalk agent, adenovirus, Giardia, Cryptosporidium, Strongyloides, and *Staphylococcus aureus, Bacillus cereus,* and *Clostridium* sp., are not associated with fecal leukocytes in the absence of mixed infection. It should be stressed that routine stool culture does not provide much help in detecting the offending pathogen in the absence of fecal leukocytes on stool gram stain. The false-negative incidence of a fecal leukocyte test is approximately 15%.[44]

C. difficile-induced diarrhea should be considered when a diarrheal illness occurs following a recent course of antibiotic therapy. Diagnosis is made by detecting *C. difficile* toxin in the stool.

Parasite-induced diarrheal illness is diagnosed by identification of parasites in the stool or, occasionally, in the small bowel aspirates.

Other Laboratory Tests. Measurement of hepatic enzymes can be helpful in evaluation of suspected infectious or inflammatory hepatitis. Hepatic enzymes also may be elevated in sepsis, lower lobe pneumonia, and Legionnaires disease. *(See Table 4.)* Serum glucose determination can reveal occult diabetes and should be considered in patients with infected leg ulcers and soft tissue infections such as lower extremity cellulitis. Genital cultures are useful for diagnosis of gonorrhea and chlamydial infections; however, nuclear acid hybridization (DNA probe) technology is rapidly replacing genital and urethral cultures due to its high specificity, rapidity, and ease of performance. Routine cultures of eye, ear, nose, and sinus drainage are discouraged since these are almost universally contaminated by normal flora. Cultures of skin, soft tissue wounds, and decubitus ulcers also are likely to be contaminated with skin flora. The offending agents are more reliably found with culture of surgically obtained biopsy material. Aspiration of infected intact vesicles or bullae following meticulous skin preparation can isolate causative organisms. Fluid accumulation may occur in a variety of body organs, cavities, or spaces in response to infection or inflammation that may be amenable to aspiration (arthrocentesis, paracentesis, thoracentesis, etc.) and subsequent culture.

Microscopic detection of infective organisms with stains other than Gram's stain, such as acid fast stain, methylene blue stain, KOH prep, and malaria smears should be performed as indicated. Specialized immune microscopy techniques include fluorescent antibody tests—either direct (DFA) or indirect (IFA)—that detect antigens or antibodies for such organisms as *S. pyogenes, B. pertussis, C. parvum, Brucella* Spp., *Francisella tularensis, Y. pestis, Legionella, C. trachomatis, P. carinii,* and selected viruses (herpes, rabies, influenza, parainfluenza, and RSV). Enzyme-linked immunosorbant assay (ELISA or EIA) is used for detection of antibodies to HIV, hepatitis A, B, or C, parasitic agents, fungi, *C. difficile* toxin, and Group A strep, among others. Latex agglutination is useful for determining streptococcal groups.

Radiologic Studies. Selected diagnostic imaging studies can help determine the etiology of fever. The chest radiograph, which is the the most frequently performed diagnostic radiological study, provides a wealth of information at relatively low cost. In a febrile patient, chest radiography should be performed as a "diagnostic test" rather than a "screening test." Numerous studies have reported the difficulty of using clinical findings for predicting bacterial pneumonia. In this regard, lack of auscultatory findings are reported in 6-25% patients with proven radiological presence of lung infiltrates.[45,46] In contrast, in patients with "normal" chest radiographs, abnormal auscultatory findings are reported to be present in 20-62% of patients in some studies.[47-49]

One study attempted to validate low-yield criteria for chest radiography, but was unable to derive or validate parameters that were any more useful than a "seasoned clinician's probability estimate of pneumonia."[47] Clinical findings associated with a positive finding on a chest radiograph include: fever, cough, chills/rigors, tachypnea, abnormal breath sounds, tachycardia, chest pain, dyspnea, wheezing, occupational exposure of toxins, weight loss, old age, alteration of mental status, a history of tobacco use, substance abuse (particularly intravenous drug use), stroke, COPD, or AIDS. *(See Table 5.)*

Abdominal radiographs rarely provide additional information beyond that available from a clinical examination of an adult febrile

Table 5. Clinical Findings Associated with Abnornal Chest X-ray in the Febrile Patient

- Fever
- Cough
- Chills/rigors
- Tachypnea
- Abnormal breath sounds
- Tachycardia
- Chest pain
- Dyspnea
- Wheezing
- Occupational exposure of toxins
- Weight loss
- Old age
- Alteration of mental status
- History of tobacco use
- Substance abuse (particularly intravenous drug use)
- Stroke
- COPD
- AIDS

patient. Selected findings on plain abdominal radiographs that may suggest an intra-abdominal pathology include: obstructive pattern, air fluid levels and ileus (bowel obstruction), local ileus (appendicitis), free air (bowel perforation), appendicolith (appendicitis), psoas shadow obliteration and haziness over the sacroiliac joint (appendicitis), "thumbprinting" or gas in the bowel wall and portal system (mesenteric ischemia), and gall stones and kidney stones. *(See Table 6.)* Although plain radiography is rarely useful in the diagnosis of acute cholecystitis, ultrasonographic examination *is* useful. Helical (or spiral) CT imaging can help in high-risk cases of suspected appendicitis. Helical CT imaging is now the imaging modality of choice in many cases of suspected pulmonary embolus. Pelvic ultrasound is helpful in evaluation of tubo-ovarian abscess or free fluid secondary to pelvic inflammatory disease. Intra-abdominal abscesses are frequently occult, presenting with spiking fever and vague abdominal complaints; they are best assessed with CT imaging.

Plain radiographs of the extremities may show gas formation in soft tissue infections, suggesting infection with gas forming, anaerobic organisms. Advanced osteomyelitis can be apparent on plain radiographs, although triple phase bone scan is more sensitive and becomes positive much earlier.

Sinus radiography is not recommended for the routine diagnosis of community-acquired sinusitis because of a lack of specificity.[50] Viral rhinosinusitis associated with the common cold is the most common form of sinusitis. Bacterial conversion is reported to be estimated at 0.5% to 2% of cases. Complete unilateral opacification of the adult sinus represents disease in approximately 75% of cases; an air fluid level also correlates with bacterial infection in 75% of cases. Mucosal thickening, in contrast, correlates with sinus pathology in fewer than 50% of cases.[50] Mastoid films can establish the diagnosis of mastoiditis, which is quite rare, however CT is more sensitive and specific.

Table 6. Intra-abdominal Findings Suggesting Pathology in the Febrile Patient

- Obstructive pattern
- Air fluid levels and ileus (bowel obstruction)
- Local ileus (appendicitis)
- Free air (bowel perforation)
- Appendicolith (appendicitis)
- Psoas shadow obliteration and haziness over the sacroiliac joint (appendicitis)
- "Thumbprinting" or gas in the bowel wall and portal system (mesenteric ischemia)
- Gall stones and kidney stones

References

1. Kluger MJ, Ringler DH, Anvar MR. Fever and survival. *Science* 1980;166:166.
2. Beisel WR. Magnitude of the host nutritional responses to infection. *Am J Clin Nutr* 1977;30:1236.
3. Dimarelle CA. Interleukin-1 and the pathogenesis of the acute phase response. *N Engl J Med* 1984;311:1413.
4. Stapczynski JS. Evaluation of the febrile adult in the emergency department. *Ann Emerg Med* 1990;19:481.
5. Keating HJ, Klimek JJ, Levine DS, et al. Effects of aging on the clinical significance of fever in ambulatory adult patients. *J Am Geriatr Soc* 1984;32:282-287.
6. Gelfand JA, Dinarello CA. Alterations in body temperature. In: Fauci AS, Martin JB, Braunwald E, et al. (eds). *Harrison's Principles of Internal Medicine*. New York: McGraw-Hill; 1998:84-90.
7. Stollerman GH. Infectious diseases. In: Cassel CK, Meier DE, Resnick NM, et.al, eds. *Geriatric Medicine*. New York: Spring-Verlag; 1997:599-626.
8. Fontanarosa PB, Kaeverlein SJ, Gerson LW, et al. Difficulty in predicting bacteremia in elderly emergency patients. *Ann Emerg Med* 1992;21:842-848.
9. Saunders MD, Graham EM. Ocular disorders associated with systemic diseases. In: Vaughn D, Ashbury T, eds. *General ophthalmology.* Norwalk: Lange; 1986:262-301.
10. Deeb ZE. Acute supraglottitis in adults: Early indicators of airway obstruction. *Am J Otolar* 1997;18:112-115.
11. McNamare R, Koobatian T. Simultaneous uvulitis and epiglottitis in adults. *Am J Emerg Med* 1997;15:161-163.
12. Elangovan S. Clinical and laboratory findings in acute appendicitis in the elderly. *JABFP* 1996;9:75-78.
13. Pfitzenmeyher P, Decry H, Auckenthaler R, et al. Predicting bacteremia in older patients. *JAGS* 1995;43:230-235.
14. Wenz B, Gennis P, Canova C, et al. The clinical utility of the leukocyte differential in emergency medicine. *LAJCP* 1986;86:298-303.
15. Badgett RG, Hansen CJ, Rogers CS. Clinical usage of the leukocyte count in emergency room decision making. *J Gen Intern Med* 1990;5:198-200.

16. Calaham M. Inaccuracy and expense of the leukocyte count in making urgent clinical decisions. *Ann Emerg Med* 1986;15: 774-781.
17. Young GP. CBC or not CBC? That is the question. *Ann Emerg Med* 1986;15:367-371.
18. Leibovici L, Greenshtain S, Cohen O, et al. Bacteremia in febrile patients. A clinical model for diagnosis. *Arch Intern Med* 1991;151:1801-1806.
19. Sox HC Jr, Liang MH. The erythrocyte sedimentation rate. Guidelines for rational use. *Ann Intern Med* 1986;104: 515-523.
20. VanEden SF, Strachan AF, Hough SF. Circulating acute phase reactive proteins as indicators of infection in poorly controlled diabetes mellitus. *Diabetes Res Clin Pract* 1988;5:99-105.
21. Lindback S, Hellgren U. Julander I, et al. The value of C-reactive protein as a marker of bacterial infection in patients with septicaemia/endocarditis in influenza. *Scand J Infect Dis* 1989;21:543-549.
22. Groulie M, Hjortdahl P. The erythrocyte sedimentation rate; its use and usefulness in primary health care. *Scand J Prim Health Care* 1991;9:97-102.
23. Hjortdahl P, Landaas S, Urdal P, et al. C-reactive protein: A new rapid assay for managing infectious disease in primary health care. *Scand J Prim Health Care* 1991;9:3-10.
24. Buess T, Ludwig C. Diagnostic value of C-reactive protein in comparison with erythrocyte sedimentation as routine sdmission diagnostic test. *Schweiz Med Wochenschr* 1995;125:120-124.
25. Melbye H, Magnus AK. Relation between erythrocyte sedimentation and C-reactive protein in serum of adults with lower respiratory tract infections. Significance of microbiological agents. *Tidsskr Nor Laegeforen* 1995;115:1607-1609.
26. Olaison L, Hogevik H, Alestig K. Fever, C-reactive protein, and other acute phase reactants during treatment of infective endocarditis. *Arch Int Med* 1997;157:885-892.
27. Katz PR, Gutman SI, Richman G, et al. Erythrocyte sedimentation rate and C-reactive protein compared in the elderly. *Clin Chem* 1989;35:466-468.
28. Isak R, Hassan K. The erythrocyte sedimentation rate, C-reactive protein, plasma fibrinogen and viscosity in chronic renal disease patients with infection. *Malays J Pathol* 1989;Aug 11:22-31.
29. Hoffman S. Detection of group A streptococcal antigen from throat swabs with five diagnostic kits in general practice. *Diag Microbiol Infect Dis* 1990;13:209-215.
30. Chu JM, Chen JM, Wu MH, et al. Rapid diagnosis of streptococcal pharyngitis with enzyme immunoassay. *Acta Paediatr Sin* 1990;31:151-157.
31. Hasin M, Furst A. Sore throat in family practice: Comparison of blood agar throat culture with a repid enzyme immunoassay test for diagnostic purposes. *J R Coll Gen Pract* 1989;39:332-334.
32. Centor RM, Dalton HP, Campbell MS, et al. Rapid diagnosis of streptococcal pharyngitis in adult emergency room patients. *J Gen Intern Med* 1986;1:248-251.
33. Hurbeck RJ, Teague J, Crossen GR, et al. Novel, rapid optical innumoassay technique for detection of group A streptococci from pharyngeal specimens: Comparison with standard culture methods. *J Clin Microbiol* 1993;31:839-844.
34. Karas SJ, Cantrill SV, Josephson G, et al. Guidelines for cost containment in emergency medicine. *Am Coll Emerg Phys Dallas* 1983;93-96.
35. Barrett-Connor E. The nonvalue of sputum culture in the diagnosis of pneumococcal pneumonia. *Am Rev Resp Dis* 1971;103:845.
36. Lepow ML, Balassanian N, Emmili I, et al. Interrelationships of viral, mycoplasmal, and bacterial agents in uncomplicated pneumonia. *Am Rev Resp Dis* 1968;97:533.
37. Roberts FJ. Quatitative urine culture in patients with urinary tract infection and bacteremia. *Am J Clin Pathol* 1986;85: 616-618.
38. Stamm WE. Protocol for diagnosis of urinary tract infection: Reconsidering the criterion for significant bacteruria. *Urology* 1988;32:6-12.
39. Weinbaum FI, Lavie S, Danek M, et al. Doing it right the first time: Quality improvement and the contaminant blood culture. *J Clin Microbiol* 1997:35:563-565.
40. Spitalnic SJ, Woolard RH. The significance of changing needles when innoculating blood cultures: A meta-analysis. *Clin Infect Dis* 1995;21:1103-1106.
41. Smith-Elekes S, Weinstein MP. Blood cultures. In: Washington JA, ed. *Laboratory Diagnosis of Infectious Disease. Infect Disease Clinics of North America.* Philadelphia: Saunders; 1993:221-234.
42. Scheld MW. Bacterial meningitis, brain abscess, and other suppurative intracranial infections. In: Fauci AS, Martin JB, Braunqald E, et al, eds. *Harrison's Principles of Internal Medicine.* New York: Mc Graw-Hill; 1998:2419-2426.
43. DuBois D, Binder L, Nelson B. Usefulness of the stool Wright's stain in the emergency department. *J Emerg Med* 1998;7:263-268.
44. Siegel D, Cohen PT, Neighbor M, et al. Predictive value of stool examination in acute diarrhea. *Arch Pathol Lab Med* 1987;111:715-718.
45. Mellors JW, Horowitz, RI,Harvey MR, et al. A simple index to identify occult bacterial infection in adults with acute unexplained fever. *Arch Intern Med* 1987;147:666-671.
46. Osmer JC, Cole BK. The stethoscope and roentenogram in acute pneumonia. *Soth Med J* 1966,59:75-77.
47. Singai BM, Hedges JF, Radack KL. Decision rules and clinical prediction of pneumonia: evaluation of low-yield criteria. *Ann Emerg Med* 1989;18:37-44.
48. Gennis P, Gallagher J, Falvo C, et al. Clinical criteria for detection of pneumonia in adults: Guidelines for ordering chest roetenograms in the emergency department. *J Emerg Med.* 1989;7:263-68.
49. Heckerling PS, Tape TG, Wigton RS, et al. Clinical prediction rule for pulmonary infiltrates. *Ann Intern Med* 1990;113: 664-670.
50. Gwaltney JM Jr. Acute community acquired sinusitis. *Clinical Infec Dis* 1996;23:1209-1223.

Causes of Fever

Sid M. Shah, MD, FACEP

Les Searls, DO

Frequently, the diagnosis of fever is obvious—the elderly patient with urinary tract infection, the alcoholic with aspiration pneumonia, the acute bacterial exacerbation of COPD—but in many cases, the etiology of fever is not immediately apparent, especially when the underlying cause is non-infectious or when the patient is elderly, immunocompromised, or has a history of multiple medication usage. Not only is the treatment course unclear in these cases, but the triage decision can be especially difficult.

To a great degree, these ambiguous cases require the physician to, first, generate a comprehensive, targeted differential diagnosis, and second, to perform a systematic exclusion or inclusion of these diagnostic possibilities based on historical, laboratory, and radiographic data. Once a likely cause for fever is ascertained, appropriate treatment measures are implemented. In the case of infectious etiologies (pneumonia, urinary tract infection, abdominal infection, prostatitis, skin and soft tissue infections, etc.), authoritative, empirical treatment protocols are available. For such non-infectious causes of fever as arthritis, vasculitis, and other inflammatory disorders, the management often is less straightforward, and frequently requires subspecialty consultation. *(See Table 1.)*

With these issues in mind, this chapter on the febrile adult highlights issues in the differential diagnosis of the adult febrile patient. Both infectious and non-infectious etiologies are discussed in detail, and fever in specific patient subgroups—post-partum, the diabetic, the elderly, the alcoholic individual—is analyzed.

Non-infectious Causes of Fever

Drug-Related Fever. Drug fever is defined as a temperature-elevation fever that coincides temporally with the administration of a drug and resolves after the drug is discontinued in a patient in whom other causes of fever have been excluded. Since there are no definitive diagnostic tests for drug fever, this entity remains a diagnosis of exclusion. *(See Table 2.)*

A large number of drugs are capable of producing fever through myriad mechanisms. These include: 1) febrile responses caused by impurities in the drug, 2) disorders in thermo-regulation, 3) induction of pyrogen release, and 4) hypersensitivity reactions.

Certain antibiotics, clot-dissolving medications such as streptokinase, and certain chemotherapeutic agents contain microbial products that are not completely removed during the drug manufacturing process. Vancomycin used to be a problem in this regard, but newer and cleaner preparations have essentially eliminated this issue. Other drugs may induce fever by either increasing internal heat production or interfering with external heat dissipation. Thyroxine, amphetamines, and dinitrophenol are capable of elevating body temperature by causing an increase in heat production. Epinephrine induces vasoconstriction, and atropine impairs perspiration, both of which can lead to decreased heat dissipation. Antiparkinsonian drugs, as well as other

Table 1. Causes of Fever

NON INFECTIOUS	INFECTIOUS
Drug fever	Viral
Thrombo-embolic disease	Bacterial
Tumor fever	Fungal
Rheumatic illness or collagen	Opportunistic
Granulomatous diseases (sarcoidosis)	Pathogens
Idiosyncratic reactions (Malignant hyperthermia, transfusion reaction, etc.)	
Neuroleptic malignant syndrome	
Miscellaneous (familial Mediterranean fever, profound type V hyperlipidemia, etc.)	

Table 2. Pharmacologic Agents Causing Hyperthermia

INCREASED MUSCULAR ACTIVITY
Amphetamines
PCP
Monoamine oxidase inhibitors
Cocaine
Tricyclic antidepressants
Halothane, succinylcholine ("malignant hyperthermia")
Antipsychotics, lithium ("neuroleptic malignant syndrome")
INCREASED METABOLIC RATE
Salicylates
Thyroid hormone
IMPAIRED THERMOREGULATION
Phenothiazines
Ethanol
IMPAIRED HEAT DISSIPATION
Anticholinergics
Antihistamines
Tricyclic antidepressants
Phenothiazines

drugs with anticholinergic effects, have similar results. In addition to their atropine-like effects, phenothiazines and butyrophenones depress hypothalamic function, which can result in hyperthermia. However, the majority of drug-induced febrile episodes are caused by drug-induced hypersensitivity reactions. These are associated with antibody production in response to the offending agents, development of drug-antibody immune complexes, and subsequent release of endogenous pyrogens. Although these reactions may be accompanied by eosinophilia, oftentimes the eosinophil count is normal.

Unfortunately, no single pattern of drug-induced fever is sufficiently specific to permit differentiation from other causes of fever. Although low-grade fevers are characteristic, patients may present with shaking rigors suggestive of bacteremia with sepsis. In fact, dramatic temperature elevations can be seen with reports of temperatures as high as 43°C.[1] In most cases, however, the degree of temperature elevation is more moderate; drug fever rarely is associated with hypotensive events.

Although a relative bradycardia may be associated with drug fever, it is an unusual finding. A minority of patients complain of headaches and myalgias. In one large study of drug-induced fever, leukocytosis was present in 22% of cases and eosinophilia in another 22%.[1] Rashes were observed in 18% of patients. In this study, although death was a rare event, in a small percentage of cases, the drug reaction appeared to contribute to the patient's demise.[1]

It should be stressed that drug fever may occur at any time during therapy with a particular agent. However, certain therapeutic classes have characteristic lag times prior to the onset of fever. For instance, antineoplastic agents tend to cause drug fever during the first day of therapy and then again at the point of neutrophil nadir. Antimicrobial agents frequently induce fever about one week after onset of therapy. Cardiac and antiepileptic medications have been reported to cause fever both early and after several months of therapy. It must be emphasized that, because of the marked degree of variability, timing of onset of fever cannot be reliably used to implicate any particular agent.

Malignant hyperthermia is a syndrome characterized by profound temperature elevation that occasionally follows anesthesia induction with succinylcholine and potent inhalational anesthetics, such as halothane.[2] It typically is associated with muscular rigidity, tachypnea, metabolic acidosis, ventricular ectopy, and circulatory instability. It may be complicated by severe rhabdomyolysis and acute renal failure. The mortality rate of malignant hyperthermia ranges from 28% to 70%.[1] Although the precise mechanism is unclear, it appears that, in genetically predisposed individuals, skeletal muscle inappropriately releases calcium when exposed to certain anesthetic agents. *(See Table 3.)*

Neuroleptic malignant syndrome (NMS) is a rare, potentially lethal disorder that occurs after use of major tranquilizers.[3] The most common causative agent is haloperidol, but phenothiazines and thioxanthenes also have been implicated. NMS is characterized by profound hyperthermia, muscle rigidity, autonomic dysfunction, and altered mentation. Clinicians should be aware that NMS is an idiosyncratic reaction, and is not related to the dosage or duration of the inciting agent. It appears to be caused by central dopaminergic blockade, leading to sustained muscle contraction, internal heat production, and inappropriate peripheral vasoconstriction. This cascade results in profound hyperthermia, dehydration, and physical exhaustion. Although therapy is somewhat controversial, most authorities recommend a peripheral muscle relaxant, such as dantrolene, in association with physical cooling measures.[3]

Pulmonary Thromboembolism. Approximately two-thirds of patients with angiographically proven pulmonary thromboemboli will exhibit fever.[4] Although the precise pathophysiology is not clearly understood, suspected contributing factors include infarction with tissue necrosis, hemorrhage with extravasation of blood, atelectasis, vascular inflammation, and occult infection. Moreover, as many as 20% of patients with pulmonary emboli have fever in the absence of pulmonary infarction.[5]

Table 3. Medical Conditions Causing Fever/Hyperthermia

Infectious disorders	Neoplastic disease
Mechanical trauma	Vascular accidents
Crash injury	Immune disorders
	Collagen vascular disease

The fever associated with pulmonary emboli can be relatively high. In this regard, 10% of patients in one study were found to have temperatures greater than 39.5°C .[6] The duration of fever may last as long as a week or even longer, but a rectal temperature higher than 38.5°C persisting for more than four days or a temperature greater than 38°C lasting more than six days is unusual. Accordingly, persistent fevers beyond this time should provoke an evaluation for recurrent emboli or intercurrent infection.

Tumor Fever. Various malignancies are capable of generating a febrile response either as a result of the primary disease process, drug-induced temperature elevation, or infection. As with drug fever, however, this is a diagnosis of exclusion. Patients with malignancy, especially if they have undergone chemotherapy or radiation therapy, are prone to a wide variety of infections. The most common malignancies associated with fever are Hodgkin's and non-Hodgkin's lymphomas, leukemia, hypernephroma, hepatoma, and atrial myxoma. Other malignancies associated with fever include metastatic tumors to the liver, neuroblastoma, central nervous system tumors, and adenocarcinoma of the gastrointestinal tract, breast, and lung.

The cause of fever from malignancy is not completely understood. In some instances, endogenous pyrogens are produced by the tumor, leukocytes, or other cells. This mechanism has been demonstrated in Hodgkin's disease and hypernephroma. In other tumors that undergo rapid growth with subsequent necrosis, fever may be produced as a result of monocyte/macrophage recruitment, with subsequent release of endogenous pyrogens.

As a rule, evaluation of a febrile patient with a malignancy in the emergency department (ED) will require pursuit of an infectious process as the likely cause of fever.

Rheumatic Illnesses and Connective Tissue Disorders. Some rheumatic illnesses present with fever as their sole, initial manifestation. In particular, juvenile rheumatoid arthritis, systemic lupus erythematosus (SLE), and a variety of vasculitic disorders present in this fashion. Adult-onset Still's disease is a disorder characterized by arthritis, pharyngitis, splenomegaly, lymphadenopathy, and leukocytosis. Daily temperature spikes often reach 39.6-40.0°C, and may be the only manifestation of the disease for several months. Rheumatoid factor is not present in these patients, and the diagnosis is frequently delayed until symptoms other than fever are apparent.

Fever is the only initial symptom of SLE in approximately 5% of patients. Serologic studies may help clarify the diagnosis. Temporal arteritis (TA) should be considered in the elderly patient who presents with prolonged, recurrent fevers in the absence of "localizing" findings. Symptoms such as headache, jaw claudication, temporal artery tenderness, and visual disturbances may help confirm the diagnosis, but these findings can be absent. Although a high sedimentation rate is typical of temporal arteritis, a normal sedimentation rate does not rule out TA. In an elderly patient at risk, with prolonged fever, temporal artery biopsy should be considered.

Factitious and Self-Induced Fever. Factitious fever and self-induced illness are more common than generally recognized. The patient will typically present with an "unusual" systemic illness, but appears to be clinically well. As a rule, there is no evidence of illness other than fever. The majority of patients with factitious or self-induced fever are women, many of whom have a medical background.[7,8] Oftentimes there is an underlying, severe personality disorder, conversion reaction, or psychosis. In some instances, there is some degree of perceived secondary gain; for example, prisoners may find hospitalization preferable to incarceration.

Recognition of self-induced fever may require checking multiple, simultaneous temperatures at different body sites (i.e., axilla, mouth, and rectum), while observing the patient. Another technique is to check the temperature of freshly voided urine.

Patients with self-induced temperature elevations use a number of methods. Fever may be generated by injecting themselves with feces, urine, dirty water, or other noxious or infectious substances. The presence of polymicrobial bacteremia in an immunocompetent patient without underlying malignancy or GI, GU, or biliary tract pathology should alert the clinician to this possibility. Occasionally, a patient may ingest a medication to which he or she has a known hypersensitivity. This has been reported with phenolphthalein.

Miscellaneous Disorders. Various noninfectious disorders not previously discussed also may present with fever. *(See Table 4.)* For example, disorders such as granulomatous hepatitis, sarcoidosis, and inflammatory bowel disease can present with fever. Inherited disorders such as familial Mediterranean fever and profound type V hyperlipidemia, with or without pancreatitis, can also present with isolated fever. Moreover, the central nervous system can generate a febrile response in the absence of active infection. This is observed in patients who have pathologic processes such as tumors, hemorrhage, vascular abnormalities, or degenerative disease occurring in or near the hypothalamic thermoregulatory center. Laennec's cirrhosis is commonly associated with fever, especially when laboratory and pathologic evidence of active hepatic disease is present. Although it may not be possible to confirm diagnosis of these disorders in the emergency setting, clinicians should maintain a high index of suspicion.

Treatment of Fever

The definitive therapy for fever generally requires treatment of the underlying cause. Infections, endocrinopathies, neoplasms, connective tissue diseases, and other causes of fever should be diagnosed and treated expeditiously. Availability of safe and effective pharmacological agents directed at fever reduction also has facilitated patient management. Although, in most cases, antipyretics do not affect the underlying illness, the patient frequently feels subjectively improved.

In patients with an asymptomatic, low-grade temperature, it is not necessary to prescribe antipyretic agents routinely. In the symptomatic patient, however, it is reasonable to prescribe fever-lowering drugs. Patients frequently feel most ill when the temperature is rising or falling. After the fever has reached a plateau, patients are frequently asymptomatic.

Agents most frequently used in adults for treatment of fever include aspirin, acetaminophen, and non-steroidal anti-inflammatory

Table 4. Chronology and Manifestations of Post-operative Fever

Cause and etiology	Post-operative time frame
Physiological	**24 h**
Tranfusion and drug reaction hours	Generally within 24 h
Malignant Hyperthermia	**Generally within 30 min. of anesthesia**
Metabolic derangements (prolonged hypotension with poor tissue perfusion)	Within 6 h
Endocrine derangements (unmasking thyroid storm or pheochromocytoma)	**within 6 h**
Pulmonary causes	24 h
Urinary tract infection	**2nd/3rd d**
Wound infection	3rd/4th d
Thromboembolic disease	**Beyond 3-5 d**
Post-operative pancreatitis	3 d
Post-operative suppurative parotisis	**Within 2 weeks**
Post-operative maxillary sinusitis	Within 2 weeks

Table 5. Factors Associated with Bacteriuria in Elderly Patients

- Incontinence
- Instrumentation
- Immobility
- Indwelling catheter
- Residual urine in the bladder
- Condom catheter

agents (NSAIDs). These agents lower the hypothalamic set point in febrile patients, while having no significant effect on the temperature of afebrile individuals. It should be stressed that these agents have little or no effect on patients suffering from hyperthermia because the elevated temperatures are not caused by an elevation of their hypothalamic set points, but by altered heat production or dissipation mechanisms.

Extremely high temperatures associated with hyperthermia require emergent application of local cooling measures. Lukewarm baths or sponge baths are effective and augment the body's ability to dissipate heat through evaporation. Cooling blankets and fans are also helpful. These measures, however, may be deleterious in the patient with "true fever" if used without central hypothalamic set point lowering agents because the body will simply expend more energy to produce more heat in order to achieve its hypothalamic goal.

Special Patient Subgroups

Fever and Rash. Patients with fever and a rash frequently are encountered in the ED. The etiology can be infectious or noninfectious, and treatment should be specific or symptomatic depending on the etiology. A thorough history should be undertaken, including a search for the site of onset of the rash, direction of spread, symptoms (pruritus, dyspnea, etc.), documentation of medications taken within the past month, possible exposure to animals, plants or other toxins, travel, immunization state, risk factors for arthropod bites, and recent exposures to ill persons, individuals with sexually transmitted disease, or known allergens. Physical examination should focus on the rash morphology as well as a search for associated signs.

Fever in the Elderly and Nursing Home Patient. Elderly and debilitated patients frequently present to the ED with fever, but with minimal or no localizing signs and symptoms. Urinary tract infection is the most common cause of bacteremia and sepsis in the elderly, especially in those with indwelling urinary catheters or recent urethral manipulation (e.g., post TURP).[9,10] *(See Table 5.)* Pneumonia, which is the leading cause of death due to infection in the elderly,[9,10] may present with vague symptoms of malaise, weakness, anorexia, or behavioral changes; cough or sputum production may or may not be present, even if there is significant hypoxia. *(See Tables 6 and 7.)* Intra-abdominal infections may present without the typical localizing tenderness or signs of peritoneal irritation. The incidence of gangrene of the gallbladder and appendix is high in this age group,[9,10] as is diverticulitis.

Febrile patients on peritoneal dialysis with abdominal pain should have dialysate gram stain and, if indicated, culture and sensitivity should be performed. Significant peritonitis in theses patients can develop without the usual rebound, guarding, and rigidity.

Soft tissue infections (e.g., pressure ulcers, wound infections, and cellulitis) are common sources of seemingly occult infections in the elderly. The possibility of tetanus must also be considered, as many of these patients are inadequately immunized. Meningitis is easily missed in the elderly, as is endocarditis, tuberculosis, and septic arthritis. Patients with recent travel history should be evaluated for infections endemic to the area in which they traveled.

The elderly demonstrate a blunted fever response to infection, as well as diminished leukocytosis. Bandemia (especially greater than 6%), even with normal leukocyte count, is suggestive of sepsis in the elderly. A low threshold for performing ancillary tests such as peripheral smear and blood count, blood culture, chest radiograph, UA, and CSF examination is prudent in this vulnerable group of patients.

Fever of Unclear Etiology. Patients of any age may present to the ED with fever without localizing signs or symptoms. Certain infections are well known for their paucity of localizing symptoms. These include infections of the genitourinary and biliary tracts, intra-abdominal abscess, and endocarditis. Rocky Mountain spotted fever, Lyme disease, Q-fever, malaria, and typhoid fever should be considered in travellers or those who live in endemic areas.

Immunocompromised patients on chemotherapy who have neutropenia should be aggressively evaluated for common infections, as well as less common entities such as coagulase-negative staphylococcal sepsis or fungemia. Special attention is paid to those with

Table 6. Factors Associated with Pneumonia in Elderly Patients

- Pharyngeal colonization with gram-negative bacilli
- Aspiration
- Poor clearance of aspirated material
- Poor systemic response to sepsis

indwelling intravascular access devices. One study reported a rise from 7% to 16% between January 1993 and April 1995 in the frequency of primary bloodstream infections related to intravascular devices.[11] Unless there are obvious local signs of infections at the site, the diagnosis may require removal and culture of the device.

Post Partum Fever. Post partum fever occurs in about 2-4% of vaginal deliveries and in 5-35% of cesarean deliveries, depending on whether the C-section was planned or performed after prolonged labor and ruptured membranes. These rates almost double in indigent populations.[12]

In the first few hours after delivery, thyroid storm may present as a rare, non-infectious etiology of fever. In this early period, infectious etiologies include early group B streptococcal infection or chorioamnionitis. Over the next few days, pulmonary atelectasis, pneumonia, UTI, and wound infection begin to emerge as important causes of fever. Breast engorgement may produce fever in some women. By the end of the first post partum week, mastitis and septic pelvic vein thrombophlebitis should be considered as possible etiologies of fever. Wound abscess, pulmonary embolism, or mastitis are late causes of puerperal fever.

Endometritis is a polymicrobial uterine infection caused by normal vaginal flora that gain access to the upper genital tract or beyond as a result of vaginal examinations during labor or surgical manipulation. The onset of fever associated with the entity typically occurs within 36 hours of delivery, and is accompanied by malaise, lower abdominal pain, uterine tenderness, and foul smelling lochia. Common pathogens include group B strep, anaerobic strep, aerobic gram-negative bacilli (*E. coli, K. pneumoniae,* and *Proteus* sp.), and *Bacteroides* spp. *Chlamydia* must be considered in late-presenting endometritis (after the first post partum week).

Fever from breast engorgement rarely exceeds 30°C and does not require antibiotic therapy. It begins within 2-3 days of delivery and usually lasts for less than one day. Mastitis is associated with higher fever, erythema of the breast, and usually occurs two weeks or more post partum.

Septic pelvic vein thrombophlebitis occurs in 1:2,000 pregnancies and can be associated with endometritis (approximately 1% of patients with endometritis develop septic pelvic vein thrombophlebitis).[12] Onset is usually within 48-96 hours of delivery and is signaled by fever, pain, and tenderness in the lower abdomen, which is usually unilateral. Nausea, vomiting, and bloating may be present. Physical examination reveals localized tenderness, guarding, and in 50-70% of patients, a rope-like mass is palpable in the area of the cornua extending laterally and cephalad. Other considerations include: ovarian torsion, pelvic abscess, broad ligament hematoma, appendicitis, ureterolithiasis, and upper urinary tract infection. The diagnosis of septic pelvic vein thrombosis can be confirmed by CT imaging or magnetic resonance angiography. Treatment is intravenous heparin for 7-10 days in addition to appropriate antibiotic therapy.[12]

Table 7. Clinical Features of Pneumonia in Elderly Patients

- Insidious onset
- Chest pain uncommon
- Fever may be absent
- Cough weak or absent
- Delirium common
- Sputum minimal or absent

Fever in the Neutropenic Cancer Patient. Patients with cancer are at increased risk for fever both as a result of their underlying disease state and as a consequence of their cancer treatment. Infection is of greatest concern, especially in the neutropenic patient, but other causes such as drug fever (most commonly in response to antibiotics such as the penicillins, cephalosporins, and amphotericin B, cardiovascular drugs, phenytoin, and other CNS drugs, cytotoxics, and immunotherapy), tumor fever, transfusion-related fever, or fever due to thromboembolism also must be considered.

Fever in the neutropenic cancer patient represents medical emergency. Specifically, fever in neutropenia is defined as a single oral temperature greater than 38.3°C or persistent temperature greater than 38°C on at least two occasions greater than four hours apart within a 24-hour period in a patient with an absolute neutrophil count of less than 500 cells/mm.[13] The degree and duration of neutropenia are independent risk factors for infection.[13] As these patients are at risk for rapidly aggressive infections with high morbidity and mortality, it is imperative that evaluation and empiric treatment be assigned high priority. A thorough history includes information about type of the cancer, details of chemotherapy, and any potential exposures to infection. Ancillary studies include at least two sets of blood cultures, urine culture, as well as cultures of any other suspected sites of infection. A leukocyte count with differential and a chest radiograph are helpful in this subset of febrile adults.

Based on knowledge of the most likely organisms involved and guided by specific risks for the individual patient, the choice of initial therapy is a broad spectrum antibiotic. Historically, gram-negative organisms were the leading cause of infection in neutropenic cancer patients, but in the last 10 years, gram-positive organisms have predominated and currently account for more than two-thirds of infections.[14] Fungal infections caused by such organisms as *Candida* and *Aspergillus* also must be considered.

Treatment options for neutropenic febrile patients continue to evolve in response to the changes in types of infective organisms, antibiotic development, and emerging antibiotic resistance. Treatment with single antibiotic therapy continues to be evaluated and shows promise,[15,16] although most experts recommend two or more agents providing broad spectrum coverage. Outpatient treatment has been shown to be acceptable in low-risk neutropenic patients.[17] Vancomycin, widely used in this setting, must be used judiciously because of increasing incidence of vancomycin-resistant pathogens.

Fever in the Diabetic Patient. Patients with diabetes are at risk for a variety of infections secondary to compromised immune func-

Table 8. Life-Threatening Infections Associated with Diabetes

Infection	Characteristics
Malignant otitis externa	Pseudomonal infection with risk of craniofacial osteomyelitis, meningitis, subdural empyema
Rhinocerebral mucormycosis	Fungal infection of upper respiratory tract with risk of CNS and vascular thromboses
Emphysematous cholecystitis	Symptoms of cholecystitis but gas forms in and around the gall bladder. 50% are acalculus
Emphysematous pyelonephritis	Gas forming renal infection, usually *E. coli*. CT is diagnostic; IVP contraindicated
Necrotizing fasciitis	Polymicrobial infection of decubitus ulcers, perineum, and lower extremities

tion apparently related to impaired leukocyte function. Microangiopathy and neuropathy contribute to the increased risk of infection.

Certain life threatening infections unique to the diabetic patient include: necrotizing fasciitis, malignant (necrotizing) otitis externa, rhinocerebral mucormycosis, and emphysematous cholecystitis.[18] *(See Table 8.)* Malignant otitis externa, also known as invasive or necrotizing, primarily affects the elderly diabetic patient. As is the case with common otitis externa, this infection is frequently caused by *Pseudomonas* sp., and presents with otalgia, otorrhea, and periauricular tenderness. Otoscopy may reveal a mass of granulation tissue in the external auditory canal. While these patients may not appear to be "toxic," they are at risk for cranial and facial bone osteomyelitis; contiguous infection, including involvement of the temporomandibular joint can lead to cranial nerve palsies, meningitis, lateral and sigmoid sinus thrombosis, and subdural empyema. CT imaging can establish the degree of bony involvement, while MRI will demonstrate soft tissue and central nervous system involvement. Traditional treatment has required dual antibiotic therapy (beta-lactam plus aminoglycoside) and surgical debridement.

Rhinocerebral mucormycosis is a rare fungal infection seen in poorly controlled diabetic patients. Common soil and food fungi can infect the upper respiratory passages and invade local vasculature, causing hemorrhage, thrombosis, and tissue infarction. Infections can spread in to the brain. Rhinocerebral mucormycosis presents with abrupt onset of lethargy and headache along with fever. Facial pain and swelling occurs early, and is followed by necrosis of the palate and/or nasal turbinates. Visual impairment and proptosis are common. Black, necrotic pus may drain from the eyes. Known complications include cavernous sinus thrombosis, carotid artery thrombosis, and cranial nerve palsies (CN V and VII). Brain involvement is signaled by seizures or coma. Diagnosis is established by biopsy of any necrotic eschars that are present. CT and MR imaging are useful ancillary tests. Treatment involves normalization of blood sugars, parenteral amphotericin B, and surgical debridement.

Emphysematous cholecystitis presents with signs and symptoms typical of "infective cholecystitis," but gas develops in or around the gallbladder within 48 hours of onset of infection. Demonstration of gas by plain radiography, CT, or ultrasound establishes the diagnosis. This entity should be suspected in all diabetics with acute cholecystitis. The gallbladder is acalculus in nearly one-half of cases. Treatment is open cholecystectomy plus antibiotic coverage for clostridia and anaerobic gram-negative bacilli, usually with a penicillin, clindamycin, and an aminoglycoside.

Emphysematous pyelonephritis is a gas-forming infection in the renal collecting system most commonly caused by *E. coli,* although *K. pneumoniae, E. aerogenes, P. mirables,* and *P. aeruginosa* are the other offending pathogens. Rarely, fungal infections also have been implicated in emphysematous pyelonephritis. Emphysematous pyelonephritis, which can be confirmed by CT imaging, should be suspected when a diabetic with UTI fails to respond to the usual antimicrobial regimen. Failure of intensive antibiotic therapy may require nephrectomy.

Diabetics also are at risk for necrotizing fasciitis and cellulitis, which are usually polymicrobial infections involving the perineum, decubitus ulcers, or the lower extremities. These patients appear toxic with high, unremitting fevers. Lesions are typically anesthetic, draining ulcers, or bullae, with varying amounts of necrosis, although in some cases the skin may appear normal. Diagnosis is based on clinical presentation confirmed by cultures of excised tissue. Treatment is surgical debridement or amputation and antibiotics, which may include imipenem. Hyperbaric oxygen therapy has been shown to be helpful in selected cases.[19]

Febrile illnesses, especially respiratory or gastrointestinal illnesses, may precipitate diabetic ketoacidosis. Any evidence of infection should be sought in any patient presenting with diabetic ketoacidosis or hyperosmolar, hyperglycemic, nonketotic diabetic states.

The Alcoholic Patient. Alcoholics are at risk for febrile illness due to a variety of infectious and noninfectious processes. The most common cause of noninfectious fever in the alcoholic patient are alcohol withdrawal, delirium tremens, prolonged postictal state, hepatitis, pancreatitis, and, infrequently, unrecognized subarachnoid hemorrhage.[19] Pneumonia has been identified as the most common cause of an infection in the alcoholic patient.[19] *Streptococcus pneumoniae* and *Hemophilus influenza* are the most common pathogens, although tuberculosis and other atypical infections are also precipitants in the alcoholic population. These patients are also at risk for aspiration pneumonia (polymicrobial infections are common) that is often indolent and can present with minimal symptoms.

Spontaneous bacterial peritonitis should be considered in alcoholic patients with cirrhosis or ascites. These infections, which usually spread to the ascitic fluid hematogenously, are most commonly caused by pneumococci or gram-negative enteric bacteria. The diagnosis is established by paracentesis demonstrating ascitic fluid with greater than 300 leukocytes/mm^3, a pH less than 7.35, and a lactate greater than 25 mg/dL. A gram stain and culture of the ascitic fluid may yield an etiologic diagnosis.

Alcoholics with liver disease are also at risk for spontaneous bacteremia, most commonly secondary to *E. coli* due to hepatic reticuloendothelial system dysfunction. A rare but aggressive cause of sepsis associated with bullae, cutaneous ecchymosis, and subcutaneous necrosis is seen in alcoholics infected with *Vibrio vulnificus* from ingestion of infected shellfish.

Intravenous Drug Users. Intravenous drug users (IVDUs) frequently present to the ED with fever. While the fever may be due to common or minor infections, IVDUs are at risk for specific life-threatening infections. The increased incidence of HIV and viral hepatitis among IVDUs is well established. Patients with history of IVDU who present with fever without a clear cause should be evaluated for HIV infection.

Infective endocarditis is a major cause of hospitalization of IVDUs. *Staphylococcus aureus* is the most common offending agent, although a number of other bacteria or fungi can be responsible for infective endocarditis. The diagnosis may be difficult and the course of the illness indolent.

Fever resulting from other infectious processes in an alcoholic patient include pneumonia (*S. pneumoniae* and *H. influenza*), cellulitis at injection sites, tetanus, septic pulmonary emboli, or tuberculosis. Common non infectious causes of fever in the IVDU are due to opioid withdrawal or pyogenic reactions secondary to drug adulterants.[20]

HIV Infected Patients. The differential diagnosis of a febrile, HIV-infected patient is extensive. Primary HIV infection usually presents with fever associated with lymphadenopathy, pharyngitis, rash, and myalgias. The natural history of HIV infection is an "acute retroviral syndrome" occurring 2-4 weeks after infection during which seroconversion has not occurred. During this stage, the diagnosis can be established by HIV viremia and high levels of p24 antigen. During the latent period (months to years), there is a gradual decrease in CD4 count. When the CD4 count is below 500/mm^3, the patient is increasingly prone to infections with relatively virulent, community-acquired pathogens. If the CD4 counts drop below 200/mm^3, infection with opportunistic organisms is more common.

Infections in HIV-infected patients with CD4 counts greater than 500/mm^3 include pneumonia due to *S. pneumoniae, S. aureus,* and *H. influenzae,* bronchitis, sinusitis, PID, pyelonephritis, cellulitis, viral respiratory infections, and tuberculosis (pulmonary and/or extra-pulmonary).

Febrile, HIV-infected patients with CD4 counts less than 200 must be evaluated for infections with opportunistic pathogens and for neoplasms such as non-Hodgkin's lymphoma and visceral Kaposi's sarcoma. Opportunistic infections include *Pneumocystis carinii* pneumonia (PCP), disseminated *Mycobacterium avium* complex (MAC), *Histoplasma capsulatum*, cryptococcal meningitis, and others. Disseminated cytomegalovirus (CMV) infection does not typically present with persistent fever although, on rare occasions, fever may be the only manifestation.[21]

PCP classically presents with fever, cough, dyspnea, chest discomfort, and general malaise that develops over days to weeks. The incidence of PCP has decreased significantly over the past several years.[22] The chest radiograph may fail to show an infiltrate in 20% or more of cases. Resting or exercise-induced oxygen desaturation and elevated serum lactate dehydrogenase support the diagnosis of PCP. Diagnosis is confirmed by presence of cysts in sputum or lavage specimens.

MAC, a complex infection associated with advanced immunosuppression, presents with indolent fever with weight loss, anorexia, night sweats, weakness, and diarrhea. The diagnosis is usually established by isolation of the organism from blood, however, the process typically takes several weeks.

Disseminated CMV is an opportunistic infection that occurs late in HIV, typically in patients with CD4 counts less than 25/mm^3. The most common form is retinitis, but it may cause other problems such as colitis, enteritis, gastritis, esophagitis, or, less commonly, encephalitis, hepatitis, or pancreatitis. The diagnosis is made by tissue stain or culture from infected organs or by identification of the characteristic fundoscopic changes.

Noninfectious causes of fever in a HIV-infected patient are common when CD 4 counts are below 200/mm^3. Neoplasms such as Kaposi's sarcoma, non-Hodgkin's lymphoma, and primary CNS lymphomas can induce febrile episodes. Late stage HIV patients are unusually susceptible to drug fever, and this may be seen with drugs such as TMP-SMZ, clindamycin, dapsone, amphotericin B, antivirals, antimycobacterial agents, erythropoietin, granulocyte colony stimulating factor, and several antineoplastic agents.[21]

Evaluation is guided by the stage of the disease as well as the history and physical of the current illness. Laboratory evaluation includes CBC, blood culture, urinalysis, and chest radiograph. When indicated, appropriate body specimen fluids should be sent for acid fast stain and mycobacterial culture. Abdominal CT imaging can help identify intra-abdominal infections (especially involving the liver) in patients with abdominal pain and hepatosplenomegaly.

References

1. Mackowiak PA, LeMaistre CF. Drug fever: A critical appraisal of conventional concepts through an analysis of 51 episodes diagnosed in two Dallas hospitals and 97 episodes reported in the English literature. *Ann Intern Med* 1987; 106:728.
2. Gronert GA. Malignant hyperthermia. *Anesthesiol* 1980; 53:395.
3. Szabadi E. Neuroleptic malignant syndrome. *BMJ* 1984; 288:313.
4. Murray HW, Ellis GC, Blumenthal DS, et al. Fever and pulmonary thromboembolism. *Am J Med* 1979;67:232.
5. Israel HL, Goldstein F. The varied clinical manifestations of pulmonary embolism. *Ann Intern Med* 1957;47:202.
6. Fred HL. Bacterial pneumonia or pulmonary infection. *Chest* 1969;55:422.
7. Reich P, Gottfried LA. Factitious disorders in a teaching hospital. *Ann Intern Med* 1983;99:240.
8. Aduan RP, Fauci AS, Dale DC, et al. Factitious fever and self-induced infection. A report of 32 cases and review of the literature. *Ann Intern Med* 1974;90:230.
9. Stollerman GH. Infectious diseases. In: Cassel CK, Meier DE, Resick NM, et al, eds. *Geriatric Medicine.* New York; Spring-Verlag, 1997:599-626.
10. Yoshikawa TT. Approach to the diagnosis and treatment of the infected older adult. In: Hazzard WR, Birman EL, Blass JT, et al, eds. *Principles of Geriatric Medicine.* New York; McGraw-Hill, 1994:1157-1163.
11. Zaleznik DF. Hospital-acquired and intravascular device related infections. In: Fauci AS, Martin JB, Braunwald E, et al, eds. *Harrison's Principles of Internal Medicine.* New York; McGraw-Hill, 1998:846-849.
12. Duff P. Maternal and prinatal infection. In: Gabbe SG, Niebyl JR, Simpson JL. *Obstetrics: Normal and Problem*

Pregnancies. New York; Churchill Livingstone, 1996:1193-1246.

13. Hathorn JW, Lyke K. Empirical treatment of febrile neutropenia: evolution of current therapeutic approaches. *Clin Infect Dis* 1997;(2 supp)S256-265.
14. Cleary JF. Fever and sweats: Including the immunocompromised hosts. In: Berger A, Portenoy RK, Weissman DE. *Principles and Practice of Supportive Oncology*. Philadelphia; Lippincott-Raven, 1998:119-131.
15. Cometta A, Glauser MP. Emperic antibiotic monotherapy with carbapenems in febrile neutropenia: A review. *J Chemother* 1996;8:357-381.
16. Aparicio J, Oltra A, Llorca C, et al. Randomized comparison of ceftazidine and imipenem as monotherapy for febrile episodes in neutropenic cancer patients. *Eur J Cancer* 1996;32A:1739-1743.
17. Escalante CP, Rubenstein EB, Rolston KU. Outpatient antibiotic treatment in low-risk febrile neutropenic cancer patients. *Support Care Cancer* 1996;4:358-363.
18. Smitherman KO, Peacock JE. Infectious emergencies in patients with diabetes mellitus. In: Ober KP. *Endocrine Emergencies.The Medical Clinics of North America*. Philadelphia: WB Saunders; 1995:53-77.
19. Wrenn KD, Larson S. The febrile alcoholic in the emergency department. *Am J Emerg Med* 1991;9:57-60.
20. O'Connor PG, Samer JH, Stein MD. Management of hospitalized intravenous drug users: Role of the internist. *Am J Med* 1994;96:551-558.
21. Gleckman R, Czachor JS. Assessment of fever in HIV-infected patients. *Postgrad Med* 1996:99;78-102.
22. Sullivan M, Feinberg J, Bartlett J. Fever in patients with HIV infection. In: Cunha BA. *Fever. Infectious Disease Clinics of North America*. Philadelphia: Saunders; 1996:149-165.

Fever in the Returning Traveler

Mark Thanassi, MD
Wendy T. Thanassi, MA, MD

In the current environment, emergency medicine physicians are more likely than ever before to be asked to carry out the difficult task of evaluating and treating returned travelers presenting with febrile illness. As globalization of the world economy accelerates, people have more time and financial support for international business trips and more disposable income for pleasure travel. Worldwide "adventure" travel also is a rapidly expanding pastime.

These travelers are faced with immunization decisions that are becoming increasingly complex, and many are departing with inadequate immunoprophylaxis. The emergency department (ED) often is the first stop for evaluation. The goal of this chapter is to assist physicians in the management of the returned traveler with a febrile illness by increasing the understanding of pathogens involved, their geographic distributions, and the presenting clinical signs.

Introduction

The number of travelers at risk for febrile illness is significant. More than 500 million people cross international borders each year. [1] More than 45 million of these travelers are U.S. citizens, one-half of whom visit tropical or developing countries.[16] It is reported that up to 5% of all international travelers, or 2.25 million Americans, will consult a physician upon their return.

In a Swiss study, 4% of travelers who visited developing countries for approximately three weeks developed either chills or a high fever over several days, and 61-71% of them remained febrile upon returning home.[2]

Moreover, public awareness of problems associated with travel-related medical illness is poor. Of each 100 unimmunized travelers who visit a developing country for a month or more, 1-2 will contract hepatitis A (HAV).[3,4] A recent survey of 353 North American passengers boarding an international flight found that 72% had not obtained any pre-travel immunizations, despite their impending departure to regions highly endemic for hepatitis A.[5] Surveys given to these same passengers revealed that 78% incorrectly reported the mode of transmission of hepatitis A and 95% were unable to identify fever, abdominal pain, and jaundice as symptoms of hepatitis infection.[6] Furthermore, 88% of the flight crew members surveyed were not immunized, thus posing an additional potential threat to the traveling public.[17]

Historical Evaluation of the Returning Traveler with Fever

The evaluation of the febrile patient begins with a thorough travel history. This history is used to determine the risks of exposure to pathogens and should include a general medical history, a pre-travel history, and a travel history. *(See Table 1.)*

Table 1. Key Aspects of the History in the Febrile Returned Traveler[14]

MEDICAL HISTORY

Is the patient immunocompromised?
Does the patient have decreased gastric acidity?
Is there a history of chronic respiratory disease?

PRE-TRAVEL HISTORY

Did the patient seek a pre-travel consult?
To what extent did the patient comply with the recommendations?
What current, documented immunizations does the patient have?
Did the patient receive chemoprophylaxis against disease?

TRAVEL HISTORY

What was the exact itinerary?
What precautions, if any, did the patient take against disease while traveling?
Did any activities increase the risk of disease exposure?

Medical History. Underlying risk factors for contracting diseases are elicited. Immunocompromised patients are at risk for severe bacterial and viral infections. Medications that decrease gastric acidity, such as H2 blockers, place the traveler at increased risk for intestinal illnesses, such as cholera and typhoid fever. Patients with chronic respiratory disease are at higher risk for pneumococcal infection and influenza; patients with functional asplenia are more likely to contract diseases caused by encapsulated organisms. Sickle cell trait and G6PD deficiency, on the other hand, confer some protection against *Plasmodium falciparum* malaria.[7,8]

Pre-travel History. Establish the vaccination status of the patient. Generally speaking, the likelihood of a patient contracting a disease is inversely related to the individual's degree of protection against that illness. Immunizations for polio and tetanus should be boostered prior to international travel in most cases. Persons born between 1957 and 1980 should have received an adult measles booster, with either measles antigen alone or the measles-mumps-rubella trivalent vaccine.

Between 250,000 and 300,000 new cases of hepatitis B are diagnosed in Americans each year;[9] since it has only recently been added to the childhood vaccination schedule, the vast majority of U.S. adults remain unprotected against this serious illness. Remember, foreign-born individuals may have never had their primary childhood immunizations.

It should be stressed that the most common causes of fever in travelers are the same as those encountered in non-travelers. Accordingly, inquire as to whether the patient received an influenza or (in the elderly or those with pulmonary disease) pneumococcus immunization. The flu season occurs year-round in most of the Southern hemisphere and very few travelers receive the appropriate vaccination.

Knowledge of the relative efficacies of vaccines helps narrow the list of possible pathogens. *(See Table 2.)* For instance, immunizations for yellow fever, polio, and hepatitis B are nearly 100% effective, whereas the vaccine for cholera is only 50% efficacious and, for typhoid fever, only 50-80% protective.[9-11]

It is essential to ask the patient about pre-travel medical consults, medications prescribed, and follow-through with recommendations. Most travelers fail to seek pre-travel medical advice and, of those who do, many fail to act on the recommendations received. Rather than asking if the patient was placed on malaria chemoprophylaxis, determine which antimalarial was prescribed, the dosing schedule, and patient compliance. Antimalarial compliance is notoriously poor because of the side-effects of gastrointestinal upset, sleep disturbances, and severe mood alterations.[21]

Travel History. This is one of the most important elements of the history. The physician should determine the dates of travel, the countries of travel, the type (business/urban vs. pleasure/rural) of travel, and what precautions were taken (i.e., insect repellents).

Because different diseases have different incubation periods, defining the dates of travel and date of return will help narrow the list the possible pathogens. For example, diseases with short incubation periods (less than one week) include bacterial gastrointestinal pathogens, dengue fever, yellow fever, and plague. *P. falciparum* malaria, typhoid fever, trypanosomiasis, and brucellosis have incubations of 1-2 weeks, whereas clinical signs of *P. ovale* and *P. malariae* malaria, rabies, tuberculosis, schistosomiasis, and viral hepatitis may appear more than three weeks after infection. *(See Table 3.)*

In addition, knowledge of the traveler's exact itinerary aids in estimating the traveler's risk of having encountered certain diseases. For example, yellow fever does not exist in Southeast Asia, while Japanese encephalitis only occurs in that region. Southeast Asia also has the greatest typhoid fever risk, whereas dengue fever is most often imported from the Caribbean.[12,13]

However in 1998, Vietnam's Ministry of Health is reporting record numbers of dengue fever, with 70,000 cases and 166 deaths in just the first six months of the year. Malaria resides in tropical regions worldwide. Eighty to ninety percent of all cases of imported *P. falciparum* malaria are in travelers returning from Sub-saharan Africa.[14,15] The first documented importation of yellow fever in the United States since 1924 occurred in 1996 in an unimmunized traveler upon return from Brazil. The patient died on the sixth day of hospitalization.[16]

Inquire if the patient resided in an urban or rural setting. This is an important distinction because water and food-borne illnesses are more common in household settings where the water source may be the local stream, than in urban hotels where bottled water is readily available. Diseases transmitted via insect or animal vectors are most often encountered in rural settings such as beaches, villages, farms, or mountainsides. Schistosomiasis is contracted through contact with any fresh water that harbors the snail host, which is endemic to sub-Saharan Africa.

The physician should determine if the traveler took precautions against disease exposure. Beverages should be bottled or carbonated; unclean water carries hepatitis A, typhoid fever, and gastrointestinal pathogens. Foods that are boiled, cooked, or peeled are generally safe. Lettuce, tomatoes, and carrots are among the foods that may have been grown in fields with human manure, washed with dirty water, or handled by unclean hands. Dairy products in developing countries are often unpasteurized and can harbor salmonella, brucellosis, and tuberculosis.

Table 2. Relative Efficacies of Vaccines[6]

VACCINE	EFFICACY	DURATION
Cholera	50%	3-6 months
Typhoid fever (all)	50-80%	3-5 years
Immune globulin	70-80%	3-5 months*
Japanese encephalitis	85%	3 years
Meningococcus	85-95%	3 years
Hepatitis B	> 90%	> 7 years
Hepatitis A vaccine	> 90%	> 10 years
Polio booster	90-100%	Life
Yellow fever	~ 100%	10 years

* Dose-dependent (0.02 cc/kg for 3 months, 0.06 cc/kg for 5 months)

Inquire about the use of insect repellents and bednets. Mosquitoes that spread dengue fever bite from dawn to dusk, while those that transmit malaria feed from dusk to dawn. Japanese encephalitis is spread by rice-field breeding mosquitoes that bite at night, so the average tourists' exposure is minimal. As with any thorough history, questions regarding sexual contacts and drug use can point out exposure to HIV and hepatitis B.

Clinical Presentation of Diseases Commonly Acquired During Foreign Travel

The number of possible pathogens that cause fever in the returned traveler can seem overwhelming to the clinician. However, a careful approach to these patients, as described below, will permit the emergency physician to gather information that can lead to the diagnosis. Most diseases have certain characteristic clinical features that distinguish them from other illnesses. Although physicians often look for specific physical exam findings to suggest a certain disease, the characteristics and pattern of the fever can be equally important.

Fever. Fever often is the symptom that prompts patients to seek medical care. A thorough fever history includes information about the date of onset, the fever pattern, and temperature range.

A continuous fever has little variation over time and is seen in typhoid fever and typhus. Remittant fevers have daily fluctuations of greater than 4° F, with a low point near normal body temperature. Trypanosomiasis and pulmonary tuberculosis produce a remittant fever. A fever that seems to resolve for periods during the day but then returns is characteristic of intermittant fever and is seen with malaria and pyogenic abscesses. Relapsing fevers also come and go but the period between fever and normal temperature is measured in days to weeks. The classic pathogen causing relapsing fever is *Borrelia*, but dengue, malaria, and leptospirosis also can produce this fever pattern.[17] Fevers of greater than 104°F are highly suspicious for malaria, meningitis, measles, and severe bacterial infections.[18]

The date of the fever's onset provides clues to the incubation period and, therefore, may suggest specific pathogens. The mode of onset is another important clinical feature: A high fever that has

Table 3. Incubation Periods of Tropical Pathogens

INCUBATION		
Short (< 1 week)	Medium (1-2 weeks)	Long (> 3 weeks)
GI bacterial pathogens	Malaria (falciparum)*	Viral hepatitis
Dengue fever	Typhoid fever	Schistosomiasis
Yellow fever	Brucellosis	Malaria (vivax, ovale, malariae†)
Plague	Trypanosomiasis	Tuberculosis
		Amoebic liver abscess
		Rabies
		Visceral leishmaniasis (kala azar)

* Minimum incubation, 8 days; 75-88% present in < 4 weeks.

† 25% will present > 6 months after exposure[13]

an abrupt onset and is accompanied by rigors suggests malaria or pyogenic infections, whereas a fever of gradual onset is more typical of subacute or chronic infections such as viral hepatitis or tuberculosis.[10]

Symptoms. There are several key symptoms in the ill traveler that will help the emergency physician generate a differential diagnosis. Severe myalgias and retro-orbital pain are frequently seen in dengue fever. Chills can be indicative of many febrile illnesses, but are particularly prominent in malaria, dengue, and bacterial infections. Spontaneous bleeding or bruising may suggest a hemorrhagic viral infection such as ebola, yellow fever, dengue hemorrhagic fever, or Lassa fever.

Fever and Diarrhea. Diarrhea, in combination with fever, is typically caused by bacterial pathogens such as *Escheria, Campylobacter, Salmonella,* and *Shigella* species. These organisms may even cause septicemia and produce fevers as high as 104° F, both before and during the onset of diarrhea. About 15% of individuals with traveler's diarrhea (*E. coli*) also will be febrile.[27] Diarrhea is a complaint in 30-50% of patients with typhoid fever. Viral causes of diarrhea (Norwalk, rotavirus) will usually produce a fever of less than 102°F. Viral, protozoal, and helminth infections, such as *Entamoeba histolytica* and even malaria, also can produce an enteritis as a component of their presentation.

Respiratory Complaints With Fever. The list of pathogens that can cause respiratory symptoms with fever is extensive. Influenza, *Mycoplasma*, *Streptococcus*, and *Staphylococcus* are still the most likely agents, but there are a few highly toxic, travel-acquired pathogens that deserve consideration. Hantavirus pulmonary syndrome is a pan-American viral zoonosis that has been identified in Canada, Argentina, Brazil, Chile, Paraguay, Uraguay, and the United States; it has a case-fatality rate of 47.5%. Twenty-two cases were confirmed in the United States in 1996, while 138 cases were reported in just the first four months of 1997.[16]

Pulmonary tuberculosis is common among immigrants arriving from other countries,[19] though it is uncommon among short-term travelers. Patients with *P. falciparum* malaria may have an adult respiratory distress syndrome that is often fatal. Schistosomiasis can cause bronchospasm. Extraintestinal amebiasis may present as cough, pneumonitis, or pleural effusion. However, the usually related liver abscess should be apparent.

Physical Examination. The physical exam begins with a review of the vital signs. Pulse-temperature irregularities can be a clue to the diagnosis of typhoid and yellow fevers, which can produce a fever with relative bradycardia. As one proceeds with a "head-to-toe" exam, look for signs consistent with tropical diseases.

The ears, nose, and throat exam may reveal conjunctivitis, which is classic for measles and typhus, and for scleral icterus, which is seen in acute hepatitis and yellow fever. A cranial neurologic screen to assess for meningitis is particularly prudent in travelers returning from Saudi Arabia and sub-Saharan Africa.

Careful examination of the skin may reveal the petechial rash of meningococcemia or dengue hemorrhagic fever. A positive "tourniquet test," in which a tourniquet applied to the biceps produces a petechial rash, may indicate capillary fragility seen in classic dengue fever. "Rose spots" are transient crops of 2-3 mm pink macules on the chest or abdomen that blanche with pressure and signify possible typhoid infection. Measles cause a maculopapular rash, and the rash of schistosomiasis is urticarial. A chancre is classic for African trypanosomiasis, and eschar is classic for typhus (rickettsial). Jaundiced skin may be seen with hepatitis, yellow fever, and malaria, although in the latter it is usually mild.

Examination of the lymph nodes may reveal localized, inguinal node swelling indicative of sexually transmitted diseases, or generalized swelling that may be seen in viral syndromes such as dengue, hepatitis B, and HIV. Bilateral posterior cervical adenitis ("Winterbottom's sign") is seen with African trypanosomiasis. Locally swollen glands, or "buboes," occur in bubonic plague (*Yersinia pestis*). Approximately 13 cases of plague are reported each year in the United States, but, thus far, all have been domestically acquired.[16]

Auscultation of the heart and lungs for rales, ronchi, or cardiac murmurs should be performed, as pneumonias are common in any febrile person, and subacute bacterial endocarditis is a consideration in all occult fevers.

A tender liver on abdominal exam can be a clue to hepatitis, malaria, or typhoid fever. Splenomegaly is a nonspecific but notable finding, arguing strongly for the diagnosis of a tropical disease such as chronic malaria or Kala-Azar, and reducing the likelihood of common North American illnesses. Acute schistosomiasis manifests with hepato- or splenomegaly.

The secondary exam should be guided by the findings of the primary exam, with special attention paid to specifics of the patient's history (i.e., if the traveler was sexually active, a thorough genital examination is in order).[18]

Diagnostic Studies

The history and physical exam direct the laboratory workup of the febrile returned traveler. Initial focus should be on diagnosing those diseases that have a high morbidity and mortality such as falciparum malaria and typhoid fever. Thick and thin smears and blood cultures, therefore, are essential initial diagnostic studies. False-negative smears for malaria can occur. Sensitivity is increased by repeating the smears every 12 hours, independent of fever, until the diagnosis can be ruled out. Bone marrow smears can be obtained if the suspicion of malaria is high. Blood smears also should be obtained 24 hours after treatment is initiated to document decreasing parasitemia. In addition to blood and urine cultures, stool cultures for *Salmonella typhi* are helpful in diagnosing typhoid fever.

The initial laboratory workup of the febrile patient also should include a complete blood count (CBC) with platelets and differential, stool examination for ova and parasites, and liver enzymes. It can be helpful to draw an extra acute-phase serum sample for future confirmatory tests at a reference laboratory such as the Centers for Disease Control and Prevention (CDC).

The CBC may be especially useful in this patient population. Bacterial infections generally produce a leukocytosis with a left shift, whereas leukopenia is seen in viral infections such as dengue fever. An acutely (< 2 weeks) increased white blood cell count (WBC) can indicate pyogenic infection, *Borrelia* species, or leptospirosis, while typhus, dengue, and typhoid fever do not elevate the WBC. A chronically depressed WBC (> 2 weeks) is seen in disseminated TB, malaria, visceral leishmaniasis, and brucellosis. Eosinophilia represents invasive helminthic infection, schistosomiasis, visceral larva migrans, or lymphatic filariasis. Thrombocytopenia points to dengue fever or malaria.

An elevation of liver enzymes is nonspecific and is seen in many viral and bacterial infections; however, a significant increase can point to viral hepatitis. Travelers overseas for a prolonged period of time or exposed to TB should receive a purified protein derivative test and, if respiratory symptoms are present, a chest x-ray. The passage of Schistosomal eggs through the bladder wall can result in microscopic or gross hematuria. Granulomatous lesions from Schistosomal infection can cause ureteral obstruction, hydroureter, and bacterial pyelonephritis. Urinalysis should reveal schistosome eggs.

Management and Targeted Therapy

Once the pathogen-causing illness has been determined, specific therapy is started. Current guidelines from sources such as the CDC can help the clinician begin appropriate treatment. *(See Recommended Reading.)* There are several principles of management of the febrile returned traveler that are important to review.

The majority of fevers in travelers represent benign, self-limiting viral illnesses that will resolve spontaneously. Returned travelers who are acutely ill or toxic may have life-threatening bacterial or malarial infections. Early treatment with broad spectrum antimicrobials and antimalarials can reduce morbidity and mortality in these patients. Consider hospitalization for patients with signs of infections that might progress rapidly such as high fevers (> 104°F), petechial rash, or mental status changes. Clinically stable patients in whom the diagnosis is uncertain should keep fever logs and return for re-evaluation and culture results in 48 hours.

Commonly Encountered Tropical Febrile Illnesses

Although estimates vary, it is generally agreed that malaria, hepatitis A, dengue fever, and typhoid fever are the most common tropical causes of febrile illness in travelers, together comprising more than 80% of identified tropical diseases in returned traveler with fever. Additional information on these important illnesses follows.

Malaria. Physicians must always consider malaria in the return traveler.[20] In fact, malaria is probably the most important diagnosis to contemplate in the traveler returning from malarious areas. Malaria is spread by the female Anopheles mosquito, which bites between dusk and dawn. No prophylactic regimen is perfectly effective, and falciparum malaria has become mefloquine-resistant in areas of Southeast Asia (particularly Thailand) and West Africa. Of the four malarial species (*Plasmodium falciparum, malariae, ovale,* and *vivax*), *P. falciparum* is the most prevalent worldwide (200-250 million cases/year) and is also the most deadly, accounting for 95% of all deaths from malaria.[21]

Approximately 8 million Americans visit areas with active risk of malaria annually. Ninety percent of the approximately 1,000 U.S. travelers who acquire malaria will not develop symptoms until they return home.[19,22] Malaria's "classic" periodic or intermittent fever does not usually occur until the illness has persisted for more than a week. Only *P. falciparum* malaria causes fevers higher than 104°F, though a low-grade fever does not rule out this pathogen. The concurrent gastrointestinal complaints may mislead physicians to pursue enteric illnesses rather than malaria.

All four species induce similar early clinical features of fever (~100%), chills (~65-80%), vomiting (~40-60%), and headache (74%).[32] Yet, if the diagnosis of falciparum malaria is missed, the patient can become rapidly worse over the next 1-2 days as the parasitemia rises in circulating red blood cells. These cells then tend to sludge in the capillaries, impeding microcirculation and leading to symptoms of end-organ damage including renal failure, cerebral edema, septic shock, adult respiratory distress syndrome, and even death.

Each year, several hundred cases of falciparum malaria are reported to the CDC, with a case fatality rate of approximately 4%. More than 75% of these fatal *P. falciparum* infections and 90% of all *P. falciparum* cases in Americans are contracted in sub-Saharan Africa.[23,11] When falciparum malaria is suspected, it should be considered a medical emergency.

The incubation period is 8-30 days for *P. falciparum*, with 75-88% of cases presenting within 30 days and 95% of cases presenting within 60 days. *P. ovale* and *P. vivax* have a longer incubation, with only 50% becoming clinically evident in these first two months and fully 25% initially presenting more than six months after exposure. Note that the shorter incubation period in *P. falciparum* may be misleadingly extended by the use of only partially effective chemotherapeutic agents.

Laboratory tests will reveal thrombocytopenia in 50-80% of patients with malaria. When malaria is suspected, thick blood films (more sensitive for light infections) and thin smears (better for determining the species) should be obtained once or twice daily, even in the absence of fever, until the diagnosis is made. New products such as Para Sight F assay based on antigen detection and the quantitative buffy coat QBC method, both by Becton-Dickinson Inc., may prove useful adjuncts when skilled microscopists are unavailable.

Therapy for malaria varies depending on the suspected species and drug sensitivities. If a patient is severely ill and malaria is suspected, it is prudent to treat the patient for both systemic bacterial illness and malaria, with a combination of tetracycline and quinine sulfate orally, or doxycycline and quinidine gluconate parenterally,[25] with admission and cardiac monitoring for quinidine toxicity. Patients with malaria who cannot be discharged home should return the following day for a repeat smear to document decrease in parasitemia.

Table 4. Approximate Number of Cases Reported Annually to the CDC[28]

Disease	Cases
Hepatitis B	25,000*
Hepatitis A	27,000~ (1994)
Tuberculosis	21,000
Malaria	1,000 (1985-96)
Typhoid fever	400 (as of 1990)
Dengue fever	91† (1994)

* the first hepatitis B vaccine was introduced in 1982

~ The CDC estimates the actual number of HAV infections at 143,000 per year (# from foreign travel 1,350-7,150)[31]

† Includes only those cases submitted with specimens

Hepatitis A. Hepatitis A (HAV) is the most common vaccine-preventable disease in travelers. Two inactivated live viral hepatitis A vaccines, Havrix and Vaqta, were recently licensed by the FDA. Protection against hepatitis A is 90% effective 10 days after receipt of the initial dose, and, after four weeks, persons are considered nearly 100% protected for the next 6-12 months. Unfortunately, the vast majority of patients are still not receiving this vaccine. A minority of travelers still receive a gamma globulin (IgG) injection, which is only 60-70% effective and lasts only for 3-5 months.

Hepatitis A is endemic in virtually every country except Canada, Australia, New Zealand, Japan, and nations in Scandinavia and western Europe. Spread by fecally contaminated food and water, the risk of unprotected travelers contracting hepatitis A is as high as two cases per 100 persons per four week stay in a developing country.[3,4] Hepatitis A infection is 10-100 times more frequent than typhoid fever (2 per 1,000-10,000) and 1,000 times more common than cholera infection (2 per 100,000) in the unimmunized traveler.[4] *(See Table 4.)*

Hepatitis A virus is one of several hepatitis viruses that cause a systemic infection with pathology in the liver. HAV is usually a benign self-limited disease. In adults, fever is common in the preicteric period, while patients who present with jaundice, dark urine, and anorexia may be afebrile or have only a low grade fever. In children, HAV tends to be mild or asymptomatic. HAV does not cause chronic hepatitis or the carrier state and only rarely causes fulminant hepatitis. Symptoms occur weeks to months after exposure and last 2-6 weeks. Treatment is supportive. The overall fatality rate for HAV infection is approximately 1 per 1,000 cases.

Dengue Fever. While the etiologies of dengue fever and dengue hemorrhagic fevers are the same, dengue fever is a benign, self-limited illness and dengue hemorrhagic fever is fatal in 2-10% of cases.[13] In 1990, 102 cases of imported dengue were reported to the CDC, no doubt representing only a small fraction of actual dengue morbidity.[25] Dengue was most often imported from the Caribbean. For a variety of reasons—principally, increased frequency of travel and decreased mosquito control programs—the incidence of dengue fever is on the rise.

This viral illness is distributed worldwide, with more than one-half the population of the world at risk for infection. In 1907, dengue fever was the second human disease found to be of viral origin (yellow fever was the first).[26] Dr. Albert Sabin, the famed polio researcher, was the first to isolate the four different strains of the virus, DE-1, DE-2, DE-3, and DE-4.

Dengue fever, known as "breakbone fever" for its predilection to cause severe bony pains, is an acute febrile illness transmitted by the *Aedes* mosquito species. Note that in contrast to the malaria carrying Anopheline, Aedes mosquitoes are urban dwellers that bite during the day. The only prophylaxes against disease are long clothes and insect repellents.

Symptoms usually begin within a week of exposure, and the duration of acute illness is generally 3-5 days. A viral prodrome of nausea and vomiting is common, followed by the sudden onset of high fever (103-106°F), severe headache, and bony pains. Retrobulbar pain accentuated by eye movement is "classic." Chills and malaise may precede the fever by a few hours. Similarly, facial flushing, eyelid puffiness, and suffused conjunctival capillaries, known as "dengue facies," may occur. Diarrhea is rare. A fine, blanching macular rash may appear in the first 24-48 hours and a secondary morbilliform rash that spares the palms and soles may be coincident with or follow defervescence. This second rash can last 1-5 days and may be accompanied by pruritis and scaling. At this point, the fever may rise again, producing the characteristic "saddleback" or biphasic fever present in 60% of dengue infections.

Dengue hemorrhagic fever causes vascular permeability and abnormal hemostasis. Patients with the hemorrhagic form are severely ill with bleeding, hypotension, obtundation, and a paradoxically increased hematocrit secondary to capillary leakage and hemoconcentration. As overt bleeding is not always present, petechiae, pupura, or mucosal bleeds should raise suspicion. All infants are at risk for the hemorrhagic form, as are adults with their second dengue infection.

It is because of this dangerous clinical quality that no vaccine is available yet. That is, a person who is sensitized to one strain of dengue via infection or immunization is at greater risk for hemorrhagic fever if they become infected with a different strain. Therefore, the immunized person could suffer greater morbidity than the unimmunized person unless the vaccine afforded protection against all four viral serotypes. Efforts toward tetravalent vaccine development are underway.

Laboratory examination may reveal neutropenia alone or neutropenia with thrombocytopenia to as low as 80,000/cc platelets. Viral isolation can be made from a serum sample taken during the first five days of illness and sent on dry ice to a public health laboratory. Dengue serologies are also available. Dengue hemorrhagic fever is a clinical diagnosis, though laboratory values consistent with DIC are found in the late stages.

Treatment of dengue fever is supportive. Because of the thrombocytopenia, aspirin and NSAIDs should be avoided. Additionally, some risk of Guillan-Barré and Reye's syndrome may exist with the concurrent use of aspirin.

Typhoid/Enteric Fever. Enteric fever is caused by *Salmonella typhi* and is acquired by fecal contamination of food or water. Current vaccines are only 60-70% effective. The United States has between 400 and 500 cases per year reported to the CDC,[22] with a case-fatality rate of 1.3-8.4%.[27] While Nepal has the highest incidence of typhoid fever in the world, most imported cases come to the United States from Mexico.

Fever is the most characteristic sign of the disease, and incubation periods vary from approximately 10-21 days depending on the inoculum size and host factors. The fever is usually low-grade at onset, coincident with the period of active invasion, and is generally followed by nonspecific constitutional symptoms such as headache and cough, which mimic the course of an influenza-type illness. Approximately 2-4 weeks after ingestion of the organisms, the fever increases to 102-103°F and gastointestinal symptoms arise. Many patients present with only a persistent fever of 2-3 weeks duration. When malaria has been ruled out, enteric fever is the most common tropical cause of fever lasting 10 or more days.[11]

Commonly cited, but rarely seen clinical clues, include relative bradycardia, rose spots (10-20% of cases), and hepatosplenomegaly. Typical laboratory results include a normal-low leukocyte count and anemia. The organism itself can be cultured from the blood in more than 80% of cases in the first week of illness.

Multi-drug resistance to antimicrobials has now been reported in the United States, with fully 33% of *S.typhi* (termed DT104) isolates in 1996 resistant to trimethoprim/sulfamethoxazole, ampicillin, and chloramphenicol.[22]

Summary

A systematic review of the patient's itinerary, vaccination status, and clincal symptoms will usually point to a specific diagnosis in the returned traveler with a febrile illness. CBC finding and a peripheral smear also will aid in the diagnosis. Currently, such conditions as malaria, hepatitis, dengue fever, typhoid fever, and common pathogens must be considered in the differential diagnosis.

References

1. Wilson M. Travel and the emergence of infectious diseases. *Emerg Infec Dis* 1995;1:39-46.
2. Steffen R, Rickenbach M, Wilhelm U, et al. Health problems after travel to developing countries. *J Infect Dis* 1987;156: 84-91.
3. Rose S. Hepatitis. 1995.
4. Steffen R. Risk of hepatitis A in travelers: The European experience. *J Infec Dis* 1995;171:S24-28.
5. Thanassi W, Abhyankar S, Weiss E. Travelers neglecting to seek pretravel medical advice. American Public Health Association (1998) session #2125.
6. Thanassi W, Abhyankar S, Weiss E. Ignorance of hepatitis A among travelers to Southeast Asia. American Public Health Association (1998) session #2027.
7. Marin S, et al. Severe malaria and glucose-6-phosphate dehydrogenase deficiency: A reappraisal of the malaria/G6PD hypothesis. *Lancet* 1979;1:524.
8. Nagel R, Roth, Jr. E. Malaria and red cell genetic defects. *Blood* 1989;74:1213-1221.
9. Thompson R. Special immunizations. 1998.
10. Saxe S, Gardner P. The returning traveler with fever. *Infec Dis Clin North Am* 1992;6:427-439.

11. Humar A, Keystone J. Evaluating fever in travellers returning from tropical countries. *BMJ* 1996;312:953-956.
12. Mathieu J, Henning K, Bell E, et al. Typhoid fever in New York City, 1980-1990. *Arch Intern Med* 1994;154:1713-1718.
13. Lange W, Beall B, Denny S. Dengue fever: A resurgent risk for the international traveler. *Am Fam Physician* 1992;45: 1161-1168.
14. Svenson J, MacLean J, Gyorkos T, et al. Imported malaria: Clinical presentation and examination of symptomatic travellers. *Arch Intern Med* 1995;155:861-68.
15. Centers for Disease Control and Prevention. Recommendations for the prevention of malaria among travelers. *MMWR Morb Mortal Wkly Rep* 1990;39:1.
16. Centers for Disease Control and Prevention. Summary of notifiable diseases, United States, 1996. *MMWR Morb Mortal Wkly Rep* 1996;45.
17. Liles C, Van Voorhis W. Travel-acquired illnesses associated with fever. 1995.
18. Hill D. Evaluation of the returned traveler. *Yale J Biol Med* 1992;65:343-356.
19. Molyneux M, Fox R. Diagnosis and treatment of malaria in Britain. *BMJ* 1993;306:1175-1180.
20. Jong E, McMullen R. Travel medicine problems encountered in emergency departments. *Emerg Med Clin N Am* 1997;15:261-81.
21. Stanley J. Malaria. *Emerg Med Clin N Am* 1997;15:113-155.
22. Centers for Disease Control and Prevention. Summary of notifiable diseases, United States, 1996—Graphs. *MMWR Morb Mortal Wkly Rep* 1996;45:
23. Strickland T. Fever in the returned traveler. *Med Clin North Am* 1992;76:1375-1392.
24. White N, Nosten F. Advances in chemotherapy and prophylaxis of malaria. *Curr Opin Infect Dis* 1993;6:323-330.
25. Centers for Disease Control and Prevention. Imported dengue—United States, 1991. *MMWR Morb Mortal Wkly Rep* 1992;41:725, 731-732.
26. Ashburn P, Craig C. Experimental investigations regarding the etiology of dengue fever. *J Infect Dis* 1997;4:440-75.
27. Christie A. Infectious diseases: Epidemiologic and clinical practice. 1987.

Recommended Reading

Issue on Returning Travelers. *Infectious Disease Clinics of North America*, June 1998.

Centers for Disease Control and Prevention. Health Information for International Travel, 1996-1997. Includes up-to-date malaria resistence information for every country as well as general vaccine information. Available bi-annually from the Superintendent of Documents, U.S. Government Printing Office, Washington, DC, 20402. (202) 512-1800.

Travel-Related Emergencies. in: Shoff W, Shepherd S, eds. *Emergency Medicine Clinics of North America*, 2nd ed. Chapter specific to issues of emergency medicine. Philadelphia: WB Saunders and Co.; 1997. 800-654-2425.

Jong E, McMullen R. *The Travel and Tropical Medicine Manual*, 2nd ed. Philadelphia: WB Saunders and Co.; 1995.

Auerbach P, ed. Wilderness Medicine: Management of Wilderness and Environmental Emergencies, 3rd ed. Includes travel medicine chapters. St. Louis: Mosby-Yearbook; 1995.

Bia F, ed. *Travel Medicine Advisor.* Loosefleaf library with bi-monthly updates. Atlanta: American Health Consultant; 1998. 800-688-2421.

Thanassi W, Weiss E. Immunizations and travel. *Emerg Med Clin N Am* 1997;15:43-70.

Thanassi W, Weiss E. Evaluation of febrile illness in the returned tropical traveler. *Hos Med* 1997;9-19.

Jong E, McMullen R. The travel and tropical medicine manual. 1995.

Thanassi W, Abhyankar S, Weiss E. Flight attendants and hepatitis A. American Public Health Association (1998) session #2058.

Community-Acquired Pneumonia

ASCAP Panel

A common cause for admission to the hospital, community-acquired pneumonia (CAP) is a serious, growing health problem in the United States. It has an incidence estimated at 5.6 million cases annually.[1,2] Approximately 1.7 million hospitalizations for CAP are reported each year at an annual cost of about $23 billion.[1,3] The elderly consume the majority of these expenses, account for the majority of CAP-related hospitalizations, and have longer lengths of stay. Mortality rates among the most seriously affected patients with CAP (the majority of whom are in the geriatric age group) approaches 40%, and causative pathogens are identified in fewer than 50% of patients.[4] Accordingly, empiric antibiotic regimens frequently are chosen in hospitalized patients with CAP on the basis of results of clinical trials and expert panel recommendations.

Despite a general consensus that empiric treatment of CAP requires, at the least, mandatory coverage of such organisms as *Streptococcus pneumoniae, Haemophilus influenzae,* and *Moraxella catarrhalis,* as well as atypical organisms (*Mycoplasma pneumoniae, Chlamydia pneumoniae,* and *Legionella pneumophila*), antibiotic selection strategies for achieving this spectrum of coverage vary widely. To provide physicians and pharmacists current, evidence-supported standards for antimicrobial therapy in CAP, new treatment guidelines have been issued by a number of national panels and/or associations, including the American Thoracic Society Guidelines (2001); Infectious Disease Society of America (IDSA); the ASCAP Panel (Antibiotic Selection for Community-Acquired Pneumonia); and the Centers for Disease Control and Prevention, Drug-Resistant *Streptococcus pneumoniae* Therapeutic Working Group (CDC-DRSPWG).

As might be expected, although there are consistencies among expert-endorsed recommendations, there also are variations, with some panels prioritizing one treatment strategy over another. In some cases, panel recommendations lag behind the emergence of new data that would force a reevaluation of current practices. For example, beginning in January 2002, the National Committee on Clinical Laboratory Standards (NCCLS) officially adopted new breakpoint minimum inhibitory concentrations (MIC) for two third generation cephalosporins for non-meningeal sources of *Streptococcus pneumoniae.* Stemming from discrepancies between microbiologic failure and clinical cure, the NCCLS reviewed and accepted revised breakpoint MICs for ceftriaxone and cefotaxime. Based on the new microbiologic standards, a drug-resistant *Streptococcus pneumoniae* (DRSP) of non-meningeal sources is defined with a breakpoint MIC of ≥ 4 mcg/mL to cefotaxime or ceftriaxone. Since the only treatment guidelines that recognized the new NCCLS breakpoints for cefotaxime and ceftriaxone are those published by the CDC-DRSPWG, the clinical implications of the revised breakpoints will be widespread as the remaining treatment guidelines reevaluate the role of third generation cephalosporins for initial therapy of all in-patients with CAP.

Deciphering the strengths, subtleties, and weaknesses of recommendations issued by different authoritative sources can be problematic and confusing. Because patient disposition practices and treatment pathways vary among institutions and from region to region, management guidelines for CAP in the geriatric patient must be "customized" for the local practice environment. Unfortunately, no single set of guidelines is applicable to every patient or practice environment; therefore, clinical judgment must prevail. This means taking into account local antibiotic resistance patterns, epidemiological and infection incidence data, and patient demographic features.

It also is becoming clear that outcomes in patients with CAP can be maximized by using risk-stratification criteria that predict mortality in various patient subgroups with CAP. Associated clinical findings such as hypotension, tachypnea, impaired oxygen saturation, multi-lobar involvement, elevated blood urea nitrogen, and altered level of consciousness are predictive of more serious disease, as are age and acquisition of CAP in a nursing home environment. These factors may assist clinicians in initial selection of intravenous antibiotic therapy for hospitalized patients.

Because of important advances, changes, and refinements that have occurred in the area of CAP treatment over the past year, this landmark review presents a comprehensive, state-of-the-art assessment of antimicrobial guidelines for management of the geriatric patient with CAP. Special emphasis has been given to both epidemiological data demonstrating the importance of correct spectrum coverage with specific cephalosporins (ceftriaxone, Rocephin®) in combination with a macrolide (azithromycin, Zithromax®) or monotherapy with a fluoroquinolone, as well as the selection of initial intravenous antibiotics for in-hospital management of CAP. In addition to antibiotic therapy, comprehensive management of the patient with CAP includes not only supportive respiratory and hemodynamic measures, but also risk-stratifying patients according to the Fine Pneumonia Severity Index (PSI) to evaluate their risk for deep venous thrombosis (DVT) and its associated, life-threatening complications. Accordingly, the ASCAP Consensus Panel has addressed the need to provide prophylaxis against venous thromboembolic disease (VTED) in immobilized patients with pneumonia, congestive heart failure (CHF), and/or respiratory failure.

In addition, a detailed analysis and comparison of two-drug (ceftriaxone plus a macrolide) approaches vs. monotherapeutic options (azithromycin or advanced generation fluoroquinolones [moxifloxacin, levofloxacin, gatifloxacin]) are provided. In this regard, although one national association (2001 American Thoracic Society Guidelines) has proposed the option of intravenous monotherapy with a macrolide for inpatient management of CAP in selected, younger patients without co-morbidity, most experts and national panels agree that hospitalized patients are at sufficiently high risk for CAP-related morbidity, complications, and mortality to require combination therapy that includes a cephalosporin (i.e., ceftriaxone, cefotaxime, etc.) with significant activity against *S. pneumoniae, H. influenzae,* and *M. catarrhalis,* along with a macrolide to provide activity against atypical organisms. Moreover, one recent study suggests that CAP patient outcomes in those with bacteremic, pneumococcal pneumonia may be improved with two-drug, combination regimens as compared to monotherapeutic approaches using fluoroquinolones or other agents.[5] Detailed discussions of this important controversy and practical, antibiotic selection implications of the year 2002 NCCLS breakpoints are presented to provide evidence-based guidance in the area of empiric drug selection for CAP.

Finally, to ensure that clinicians are current with and can apply the latest evidence-based strategies for CAP treatment to their patient populations, detailed antibiotic selection guidelines (please see Table 1, ASCAP 2002 Consensus Panel Guidelines) issued by the ASCAP (Antibiotic Selection for Community-Acquired Pneumonia) Consensus Panel are provided. Drawing upon consensus panels and association guidelines, these antimicrobial protocols are linked to risk-stratification criteria and specific clinical profiles of patients presenting to the hospital or acute ambulatory setting with CAP.

Introduction: The ASCAP (Antibiotic Selection for CAP) 2002 Consensus Report® Panel and Scientific Roundtable

To address the complex issues surrounding antibiotic selection and care of the hospitalized patient with pneumonia, the ASCAP Year 2002 Consensus Panel and Scientific Roundtable was convened. Its mission statement was to review, analyze, and interpret published, evidence-based trials assessing the safety and efficacy of antibiotic therapy for CAP. In addition, the ASCAP Consensus Panel was charged with developing strategies that would ensure appropriate use of antibiotics in this patient population, and making recommendations for how patients with respiratory infections should be evaluated and managed in the inpatient setting.

Treatment guidelines generated by the ASCAP 2002 Consensus Panel, and reported in this consensus statement, were based on evidence presented from well-designed clinical trials, and focused on hospital management by the emergency physician, hospitalist, internist, critical care specialist, and/or infectious disease specialist. Detailed review and analyses of national consensus guidelines issued by the American Thoracic Society (ATS), Infectious Disease Society of America (IDSA), CDC Drug-Resistant *Streptococcus pneumoniae* Working Group (CDC-DRSPWG), and the Year 2001 Antibiotic Selection in Community-Acquired Pneumonia (ASCAP) Panel also were evaluated and included in the decision-making process. *(Please see Tables 2 and 3.)*

Table 1. ASCAP 2002 Guidelines — Empiric Antimicrobial Therapy of Choice for Outpatient‡ and In-Hospital Management of Patients with CAP

PATIENT PROFILE/ETIOLOGIC AGENTS	FIRST-LINE ANTIBIOTIC THERAPY†	ALTERNATIVE FIRST-LINE ANTIBIOTIC THERAPY
Otherwise Healthy **< 60 years of age** (Patients deemed to be suitable for outpatient/oral therapy, i.e., no systemic toxicity, high likelihood of compliance, and supportive home environment)*	Azithromycin PO	Moxifloxacin PO (preferred) *OR* Levofloxacin PO *OR* Clarithromycin *OR* Gatifloxacin PO
Otherwise Healthy **> 60 years of age** (Patients deemed to be suitable for outpatient/oral therapy, i.e., no systemic toxicity, high likelihood of compliance, and supportive home environment)*	Azithromycin PO	Moxifloxacin PO (preferred) *OR* Levofloxacin PO *OR* Clarithromycin *OR* Gatifloxacin PO
In-Hospital (not in intensive care unit) underlying risk factors or comorbid conditions: In-Hospital management (COPD, history of pneumonia, diabetes, etc.)	Ceftriaxone IV plus azithromycin IV†††	Moxifloxacin *OR* Levofloxacin IV *OR* Gatifloxacin IV
CAP acquired in the nursing home environment (increased likelihood of gram-negative, *E. coli, Klebsiella pneumoniae*)	Ceftriaxone IV plus azithromycin IV	Moxifloxacin *OR* Levofloxacin IV *OR* Gatifloxacin IV
CAP in the elderly individual with chronic alcoholism (Increased likelihood of *Klebsiella pneumoniae* infection)	Ceftriaxone IV plus azithromycin IV	Cefotaxime†† plus erythromycin IV *OR* Levofloxacin IV *OR* Cefepime IV plus azithromycin IV
Severe bacteremic CAP with documented *S. pneumoniae* species showing high-level resistance to macrolides and/or penicillin, but maintaining high sensitivity to extended spectrum quinolones and cephalosporins	Ceftriaxone IV plus moxifloxacin *OR* Ceftriaxone IV plus levofloxacin IV	Vancomycin¶ plus azithromycin IV
Severe CAP complicated by structural disease of the lung (bronchiectasis): Increased likelihood of *Pseudomonas* and polymicrobial infection	Cefepime IV plus levofloxacin IV plus/minus aminoglycoside *OR* Ciprofloxacin IV plus aminoglycoside IV plus azithromycin IV	Ciprofloxacin IV plus cefepime IV plus azithromycin IV *OR* Carbapenem IV plus azithromycin IV plus aminoglycoside
CAP in a patient with suspected aspiration (increases the likelihood of gram-negative and anaerobic infection**)	Ceftriaxone IV plus azithromycin IV plus clindamycin IV	Levofloxacin IV plus clindamycin IV *OR* Levofloxacin IV plus metronidazole IV *OR* Gatifloxacin IV plus clindamycin IV
Severe CAP in a compromised host with a previous hospitalization for, or who resides in a community or facility with a high reported incidence of methicillin-resistant *S. aureus* (MRSA)***	Moxifloxicin IV plus vancomycin IV *OR* Levofloxacin IV plus vancomycin IV	Gatifloxacin IV plus vancomycin IV
CAP patient with severe pneumonia requiring ICU hospitalization***	Ceftriaxone IV plus levofloxacin IV plus/minus aminoglycoside (*Pseudomonas* strongly suspected) *OR* Ceftriaxone IV plus azithromycin IV plus/minus anti-pseudomonal agent	Cefepime IV plus aminoglycoside IV plus azithromycin IV *OR* Carbepenem IV plus aminoglycoside IV plus azithromycin IV

* Oral therapy/outpatient treatment recommendations are appropriate only for those otherwise healthy patients with CAP of mild enough severity that they are judged to be suitable candidates for outpatient management with oral antibiotics.
§ Quinolones are restricted for use in patients > 18 years of age.
¶ If *S. pneumoniae* demonstrates complete resistance to extended spectrum quinolones (very rare), third-generation cephalosporins, and macrolides, then vancomycin may be required as part of initial therapy, although this would be necessary only in rare circumstances.
† First-line therapy recommendations take into consideration cost of the drug (which may vary from one institution to another), convenience of dosing, daily dose frequency, spectrum of coverage, side effects, and risk of drug-drug interactions.
†† Cefotaxime IV should be dosed on a q 8° basis when used for treatment of CAP.
††† Some institutions may use oral macrolide therapy for patients with mild-to-moderate CAP.
** When anaerobic organisms are suspected as one of the possible etiologic pathogens in a patient with CAP, clindamycin or a β-lactam/β-lactamase inhibitor (ampicillin/sulbactam, tricarcillin/clavulanate, or ticarcillin/tazobacatam) is recommended.
*** High community prevalence of, previous history of hospitalization, or increasing local incidence of methicillin-resistant *S. aureus* (MRSA) in a patient with a clinical presentation consistent with *S. aureus* pneumonia; vancomycin should be considered as component for initial therapy.
‡ Adapted from references 2, 3, 9, 12, 20-31
§§ Cefotaxime may be substituted for ceftriaxone, although ceftriaxone is preferred because of its once-daily dosing.

With these objectives in clear focus, the purpose of this comprehensive review, which includes the ASCAP 2002 Consensus Panel report on assessment strategies and treatment recommendations, is to provide an evidence-based, state-of-the-art clinical resource outlining, in precise and practical detail, clinical protocols for the acute management of CAP. To achieve this goal, all of the critical aspects entering into the equation for maximizing patient outcomes, while minimizing costs, including systematic patient evaluation, disposition decision trees, and outcome-effective antibiotic therapy, will be discussed in detail. In addition, because appropriate disposition of patients with CAP has become essential for cost-effective patient management, this review includes critical pathways and treatment tables which incorporate risk stratification tools that can be used to identify and distinguish those patient subgroups that are appropriately managed in the outpatient setting from those more appropriately admitted to the hospital for more intensive care.

Community-Acquired Pneumonia: Epidemiology, Diagnosis, and Evaluation

CAP affects 5.6 million adults annually in the United States, with 1.7 million patients requiring hospitalization.[6] It is the sixth leading cause of death overall and the most common cause of death from infection,[6,7] with an overall case-fatality rate of about 5%. Mortality is substantially greater (about 13.6%) among hospitalized patients.[8] Expert committees have published treatment guidelines intended to improve the care of pneumonia patients, but the guidelines have not been prospectively validated.[9,10] Prior studies of pneumonia guidelines have reported decreased lengths of stay, admission rates, and costs, but no change in clinical outcomes.[11-13] Expert guidelines are difficult to implement, and traditional continuing medical education has little effect on physician practice.[14-19]

The introduction of antibiotic agents dramatically reduced mortality from pneumococcal pneumonia. However, the mortality rate from bacteremic pneumococcal CAP has shown little improvement in the past three decades, remaining between 19% and 28% depending on the population and institution studied. The aging population, increased prevalence of comorbid illnesses, human immunodeficiency virus, and increasing microbial resistance all have probably contributed to maintaining the high mortality rate despite advances in medical care. However, even allowing that some patients are seen too late to benefit from the antibiotic therapy, the continued high mortality rate, despite apparently appropriate antibiotic therapy, is a cause for concern.

The annual incidence of pneumonia in patients older than age 65 is about 1%.[20] The typical presentation of pneumococcal pneumonia with fever, rigors, shortness of breath, chest pain, sputum production, and abnormal lung sounds is easy to recognize. Unfortunately, the changing epidemiology of pneumonia presents a greater diagnostic challenge, especially in the aging patient. Atypical agents or opportunistic infections in

Table 2. IDSA — Year 2000 Guidelines. Empirical Selection of Antimicrobial Agents for Treating Patients with CAP

OUTPATIENTS

- Generally preferred are (not in any particular order): doxycycline, a macrolide, or a fluoroquinolone
- Selection considerations (see text, *Management of Patients Who Do Not Require Hospitalization*)
- These agents have activity against the most likely pathogens in this setting, which include *Streptococcus pneumoniae, Mycoplasma pneumoniae,* and *Chlamydia pneumoniae*
- Selection should be influenced by regional antibiotic susceptibility patterns for *S. pneumoniae* and the presence of other risk factors for drug-resistant *S. pneumoniae*
- Penicillin-resistant pneumococci may be resistant to macrolides and/or doxycycline
- For older patients or those with underlying disease, a fluoroquinolone may be a preferred choice; some authorities prefer to reserve fluoroquinolones for such patients

HOSPITALIZED PATIENTS

- General medical ward
- Generally preferred are: an extended-spectrum cephalosporin combined with a macrolide or a β-lactam/β-lactamase inhibitor combined with a macrolide or a fluoroquinolone (alone)

INTENSIVE CARE UNIT

- Generally preferred are: an extended-spectrum cephalosporin or β-lactam/β-lactamase inhibitor plus either a fluoroquinolone or macrolide
- Alternatives or modifying factors (see text, *Management of Patients Who Are Hospitalized, Special considerations)*
- Structural lung disease: antipseudomonal agents (piperacillin, piperacillin-tazobactam, carbapenem, or cefepime) plus a fluoroquinolone (including high-dose ciprofloxacin)
- β-lactam allergy: fluoroquinolone ± clindamycin
- Suspected aspiration: fluoroquinolone with or without clindamycin, metronidazole, or a β-lactam/β-lactamase inhibitor

Note: β-lactam/β-lactamase inhibitor: ampicillin-sulbactam or piperacillin-tazobactam. Extended-spectrum cephalosporin: cefotaxime or ceftriaxone. Fluoroquinolone: gatifloxacin, levofloxacin, moxifloxacin, or other fluoroquinolone with enhanced activity against *S. pneumoniae* (for aspiration pneumonia, some fluoroquinolones show in vitro activity against anaerobic pulmonary pathogens, although there are no clinical studies to verify in vivo). Macrolide: azithromycin, clarithromycin, or erythromycin ± with or without.

Table 3. Recommended Year 2000 CDC DRSP-WG Empiric Regimens for Treating Community-Acquired Pneumonia*

Empiric treatment**	Penicillin MIC ug/mL ≤ 0.06	0.12-1	2	4	≥ 8	Comments
Outpatients						
Macrolide (erythromycin, clarithromycin, or azithromycin)	+++	+	±	-	-	Covers atypical pathogens (*Mycoplasma* species *Chlamydia* species, and *Legionella* species)
Doxycycline (or tetracycline)	+++	++	+	-	-	Covers atypical pathogens; not FDA-approved for children younger than 8 y
Oral β-lactam (cefuroxime axetil, amoxicillin, or amoxicillin-clavulanate potassium)	+++	++	+	-	-	Does not cover atypical pathogens, alternatively cefpodoxime or cefprozil may be used
Fluoroquinolones (levofloxacin, moxifloxacin, or gatifloxacin)†	+++	+++	+++	++	++	Not first-line treatment because of concerns about emerging resistance; not FDA approved for use in children; covers atypical pathogens
Hospitalized (Nonintensive Care Unit) Patients						
Parenteral β-lactam (cefuroxime, cefotaxime sodium, ceftriaxone sodium, or ampicillin sodium-sulbactam sodium) plus macrolide (erythromycin, clarithromycin, or azithromycin)	+++	+++	++	±	-	Ceftriaxone and cefotaxime have superior activity against resistant pneumococci in comparison with ampicillin-sulbactam and with cefuroxime
Fluoroquinolones (e.g., moxifloxacin, levofloxacin, gatifloxacin, or trovafloxacin)†	+++	+++	+++	++	++	See previous comments about fluoroquinolones
Intubated or Intensive Care Unit Patients‡						
Intravenous β-lactam (ceftriaxone or cefotaxime sodium) plus intravenous macrolide (erythromycin or azithromycin)	+++	+++	++	±	-	Ceftriaxone or cefotaxime are preferred over other β-lactams because of their superior activity against resistant pneumococci; clarithromycin has no intravenous formulation
Intravenous β-lactam (ceftriaxone or cefotaxime) plus fluoroquinolone (e.g., gatifloxacin, levofloxacin, moxifloxacin, or trovafloxacin)†	+++	+++	++	++	++	Ceftriaxone or cefotaxime are preferred over other β-lactams; see previous comments about fluoroquinolones
Fluoroquinolones (e.g., moxifloxacin, levofloxacin, gatifloxacin, or trovafloxacin)†	++	++	++	++	++	See previous comments about fluoroquinolones; efficacy of monotherapy for critically ill persons with pneumococcal pneumonia has not been established

* FDA indicates Food and Drug Administration. Ratings estimate clinical efficacy and in vitro susceptibility among persons with pneumococcal pneumonia. In-depth information on empiric treatment of pneumonia is given by the Infectious Disease Society of America and the American Thoracic Society guidelines.

† The relative antipneumococcal activity of these agents differs slightly, with that of trovafloxacin equal or superior to that of grepafloxacin, which equals that of sparfloxacin, which is superior to that of levofloxacin. Because of new data showing an association with serious liver damage, the FDA issued a public health advisory recommending that trovafloxacin be used only for patients with serious and life- or limb-threatening infections who receive initial treatment in an inpatient health care facility and for whom physicians believe that the benefit of the agent outweighs its potential risk.

‡ Vancomycin hydrochloride may be indicated for the treatment of selected critically ill children with community-acquired pneumonia for whom coverage of drug-resistant *Streptococcus pneumoniae* must be ensured.

** Adaptations made to reflect introduction of new agents since report was published.

immunocompromised individuals have a much more subtle presentation. In particular, pneumonia in older patients frequently has an insidious presentation and fewer characteristic features of pneumonia, which may be confused with CHF or respiratory compromise associated with chronic lung disease.

The definitive, etiologic diagnosis of pneumonia is verified by the recovery of a pathogenic organism(s) from either the blood, sputum, or pleural fluid in the setting of a patient with a radiographic abnormality suggestive of pneumonia. In the case of atypical organisms, the diagnosis usually is made by the comparison of acute and convalescent sera demonstrating a rise in appropriate titers, or by other sophisticated techniques such as direct florescent antibody testing. The gram stain is occasionally helpful with establishing the diagnosis, but requires practitioners or technicians who are highly skilled in this diagnostic methodology. An adequate Gram's stain must have fewer than 25 epithelial cells per low-powered field. The finding of more than 10 gram-positive, lancet-shaped diplococci in a high-powered field is a sensitive and specific predictor of pneumococcal pneumonia. Unfortunately, the Gram's stain rarely will be helpful in determining other causes of pneumonia. The IDSA Guidelines recommend Gram's stain, whereas the ATS considers gram stain optional.

Transtracheal aspiration or bronchial washings are a more accurate means of obtaining specimens for gram stain and culture, although this procedure rarely is indicated in the outpatient setting. Overall, fewer than 50% of patients with CAP will be able to produce sputum. Of these, one-half of the sputum specimens obtained will be inadequate. When an adequate gram stain is obtained, however, it has a negative predictive value of 80% when compared to a sputum culture. The blood culture is helpful in about 15% of patients, while serology will establish the diagnosis in 25% of patients.[9,20] About 40% of sputum cultures will identify a pathologic organism. Bronchoscopy and thoracentesis may occasionally be necessary, but these procedures generally are reserved for seriously ill patients, particularly those who require management in the intensive care unit (ICU) setting.[3,9,21]

Signs and Symptoms. Especially in the elderly patient, the signs and symptoms of pneumonia may be mimicked by many disorders, including pulmonary embolism (PE), CHF, lung cancer, hypersensitivity pneumonitis, tuberculosis, chronic obstructive pulmonary disease (COPD), granulomatosis disease, and fungal infections. A variety of drugs also can induce pulmonary disease. Cytotoxic agents; non-steroidal anti-inflammatory drugs (NSAIDs); and some antibiotics, including sulfonamides and certain antiarrhythmics (e.g., as amiodarone or tocainide), can mimic pulmonary infection. In addition, common analgesics, including salicylates, propoxyphene, and methadone, also may precipitate acute respiratory symptoms. Such collagen vascular diseases as systemic lupus erythematosus, polymyositis, and polyarteritis nodosa may cause fever, cough, dyspnea, and pulmonary infiltrates, thereby mimicking symptoms of pneumonia. Rheumatoid arthritis can cause an interstitial lung disease, although it does not usually cause fever or alveolar infiltrates.

Initial Stabilization and Adjunctive Measures. Prompt, aggressive, and adequate supportive care must be provided to geriatric patients who present to the hospital with pneumonia. As is the case with other serious conditions, supportive care frequently must be performed in conjunction with the history, physical examination, and diagnostic testing. Among initial stabilization measures, managing the airway and ensuring adequate breathing, oxygenation, ventilation, and perfusion are of paramount importance.

Upon arrival to the hospital, oxygenation status should be assessed immediately using pulse-oximetry. Patients with an arterial oxygen saturation of less than 90% should receive supplemental oxygen, and should be considered candidates for admission, prompt evaluation, and treatment if the diagnosis is confirmed. Arterial blood gases are especially helpful in patients suspected of hypercarbia and respiratory failure. This laboratory modality may be useful in patients with COPD, decreased mental status, and fatigue. Patients with hypoxia who do not respond to supplemental oxygen, as well as those with hypercarbia accompanied by respiratory acidosis, may be candidates for mechanical ventilation. This patient population also has a poorer prognosis. Support may be accomplished with either intubation and mechanical ventilation or non-invasive ventilation (bilevel positive pressure ventilation [BiPAP]). Recent studies have shown BiPAP to be successful for treatment of patients with respiratory failure due to pneumonia.[10] When this technique is available, it may avert the need for endotracheal intubation and its potential complications. Finally, patients with evidence of bronchospasm on physical exam, as well as those with a history of obstructive airway disease (asthma or COPD), may benefit from inhaled bronchodilator therapy.

Evidence of inadequate perfusion may range from mild dehydration with tachycardia to life-threatening hypotension due to septic shock. Patients with septic shock usually will show evidence of decreased tissue perfusion, such as confusion and oliguria in association with a hyperdynamic circulation. In either case, initial therapy consists of intravenous fluids (normal saline or lactated Ringer's solution) administered through a large bore IV. In elderly patients, fluid overload is a potential complication, and it is prudent to administer IV fluids with frequent assessment of clinical response.

Risk Stratification and Patient Disposition: Outpatient Vs. Inpatient Management

Determining whether to admit or discharge patients suspected of having CAP, is one of the most important decisions an emergency physician, pulmonologist, or internist can make. For this reason, there have been increasing efforts to identify patients with CAP who can appropriately be treated as outpatients.[11-13,32] The disposition decision for geriatric patients with pneumonia should take into account the severity of the pneumonia, as well as other medical and psychosocial factors that may affect the treatment plan and clinical outcome.[33-35]

Patient Disposition. In the absence of respiratory distress or other complicating factors, many young adults can be adequately treated with appropriate oral antibiotic therapy. In fact, guidelines issued by the IDSA and ATS support oral antibiotic therapy in patients deemed to be at low risk for complications and/or mortality associated with CAP. This option is utilized less frequently in the case of elderly patients with CAP because comorbid conditions and other risk factors that may complicate the course of the illness frequently are present. Even following appropriate treatment and disposition, patients may have symptoms, including cough, fatigue, dyspnea, sputum production, and chest pain that can last for several months. To address the issue of patient disposition and treatment setting, a variety of investigators have proposed risk-stratification criteria to identify patients requiring hospitalization.

Among the factors most physicians use to make admission decisions for pneumonia are the presence of hypoxemia, overall clinical status, the ability to maintain oral intake, hemodynamic status, and the patient's home environment. Such factors as hypotension, tachypnea, multi-lobar involvement, elevated BUN, and confusion have been linked to inferior outcomes in patient with CAP. Using clinical judgment, however, physicians tend to overestimate the likelihood of death from pneumonia.[33] These findings have led some investigators to employ more stringent prediction rules. For example, the chest radiograph may help identify patients who are at high risk for mortality. The presence of bilateral effusions, moderate-size pleural effusions, multi-lobar involvement, and bilateral infiltrates are associated with poorer outcomes.

A landmark study outlined below presented a prediction rule (Pneumonia Severity Index [PSI]) to identify low-risk patients with CAP.[12] Using such objective criteria as patient age, coexistent medical conditions, and vital signs, patients are assigned either to a low-risk class, which has a mortality rate of about 0.1% in outpatients, or to higher risk categories. Patients with any risk factors are then evaluated with a second scoring system that assigns individuals to one of three higher risk categories, which have mortality rates ranging from 0.7% to 31%.[33] In addition to the factors noted in this prediction rule, patients who are immunocompromised as a result of AIDS or chronic alcohol use frequently require hospitalization.

Once the clinician has determined hospitalization is required, the need for ICU admission also must be evaluated. A variety of factors are associated with an increased risk for mortality, including increasing age (> 65 years), alcoholism, chronic lung disease, immunodeficiency, and specific laboratory abnormalities, including azotemia and hypoxemia. These patients may require admission to the ICU.

Prognostic Scoring. There have been many efforts to assess severity and risk of death in patients with pneumonia.[34,36,37] The study by Fine and colleagues has received considerable attention and is used as a benchmark by many clinicians.[33] This study developed a prediction rule, the PSI (Pneumonia Severity Index), to assess 30-day mortality in patients with CAP. The rule was derived and validated with data from more than 52,000 inpatients, and then validated with a second cohort of 2287 inpatients and outpatients as part of the Pneumonia PORT (Pneumonia Patient Outcomes Research Team Cohort) study. Subsequent evaluation and validation has been performed with other cohorts, including geriatric patients and nursing home residents.[38,39]

In this risk-stratification model, patients are assigned to one of five risk classes (1 is lowest risk, 5 is highest risk) based upon a point system that considers age, co-existing disease, abnormal physical findings, and abnormal laboratory findings. Elderly patients cannot be assigned to Class 1, as a requirement is age younger than 50 years. In older patients, age contributes the most points to the overall score. For example, it should be noted that males ages older than 70 years and females ages older than 80 years would be assigned to Class 3 on the basis of age alone, without any other risk factor. In the Fine study, patients assigned to Classes 1 and 2 were typically younger patients (median age, 35-59 years) and patients in Classes 3-5 were older (median age, 72-75 years).

Outpatient management is recommended for Classes 1 and 2, brief inpatient observation for Class 3, and traditional hospitalization for Classes 4 and 5.[34] For a geriatric patient to qualify for outpatient treatment based on these recommendations, he or she would have to be younger than age 70 if male or younger than age 80 if female, and have no additional risk factors. Inpatient observation or traditional hospitalization would be recommended for all other patients based on this rule. Other studies have suggested outpatient management for Class 3 patients, but most authorities consider Class 3 patients to be appropriate candidates for hospital admission or for management in an observation unit.[12,40]

As a rule, patients considered eligible for management as outpatients must be able to take oral fluids and antibiotics, comply with outpatient care, and be able to carry out activities of daily living (ADLs) or have adequate home support to assist with ADLs. Other factors cited in previous studies but not included in the PSI also have been found to increase the risk of morbidity or mortality from pneumonia. These include: other comorbid illnesses (diabetes mellitus, COPD, post-splenectomy state), altered mental status, suspicion of aspiration, chronic alcohol abuse or malnutrition, and evidence of extrapulmonary disease.[9] Additional laboratory studies that may suggest increased severity of illness include white blood cell count less than 4000 or greater than 30,000; absolute neutrophil count less than 1000; elevated protime or partial thromboplastin time; decreased platelet count; or radiographic evidence of multilobar involve- ment, cavitation, and rapid spreading.[9]

Severe pneumonia may require ICU admission. In the Fine study, 6% of patients in Class 3, 11% of patients in Class 4, and 17% of patients in Class 5 required ICU admission.[33] The ATS guidelines define severe pneumonia as the presence of at least one of the following: respiratory rate greater than 30, severe respiratory failure ($PaO_2/FIO_2 < 250$), mechanical ventilation, bilateral infiltrates or multilobar infiltrates, shock, vasopressor requirement, or oliguria (urine output < 20 cc per hour). The presence of at least one of these is highly sensitive (98%) but only 32% specific for the need for ICU management.[41] It is emphasized that the above guidelines for admission should not supercede clinical judgment when assessing the need to hospitalize patients.[9,33,34,42]

Antibiotic Selection for Hospitalized CAP Patients: An Overview of Current Controversies, Issues, and Guidelines

Introduction. Antibiotic therapy is the mainstay of management for patients with CAP. It should be stated at the outset that antibiotic therapy should be initiated promptly, as soon as the diagnosis is strongly suspected or confirmed, and after appropriate microbiological studies or samples have been obtained. More and more, institutional guidelines are mandating administration of antibiotics within 4 to 8 hours of patient presentation to the hospital, since mortality rates rise when antibiotic administration is delayed beyond eight hours.[43] Because the elderly are at high risk for acquiring pneumonia, many of the guidelines issued by consensus panels, clinical experts, and scientific associations, including those of the IDSA, the ATS, ASCAP Consensus Panel, and the CDCDRSP-WG, apply directly to this patient population. Therefore, these recommendations should be studied in detail to arrive at sensible, empiric pharmacotherapeutic interventions for the elderly patient with pneumonia. Although the CDC group makes no specific recommendations for geriatric patients, their guidelines apply to all adult patients; hence, their conclusions are applicable to the geriatric patient with CAP.

Consensus Panels. It should be stressed that there is no absolute or consistent consensus about precisely which drug, or combination of drugs, constitutes the most outcome-effective choice for pneumonia in patients with CAP, although a recent study suggests improved mortality rates with regimens using two-drug combinations rather than monotherapy in patients with bacteremic pneumococcal pneumonia.[5] Most panels and guideline documents agree that antimicrobial coverage must include sufficient activity against the principal bacterial pathogens *S. pneumoniae, H. influenzae,* and *M. catarrhalis,* as well as against the atypical pathogens *Mycoplasma, Legionella,* and *C. pneumoniae.* Therefore, such regimens as ceftriaxone/cefotaxime plus azithromycin, or monotherapy with advanced generation fluoroquinolones—given some qualifications regarding outcomes and resistance issues to be discussed later—have emerged as preferred options for treatment of inpatients with CAP.

Beyond this non-negotiable caveat mandating coverage for the six aforementioned pathogens, there are important differences among recommendations and expert panels for empiric treatment of pneumonia. Variations among the guidelines usually depend upon: 1) their emphasis or focus on the need to empirically cover drug-resistant *Streptococcus pneumoniae* (DRSP) species as part of the initial antimicrobial regimen; 2) their concern about using antimicrobials (fluoroquinolones) with an over-extended (too broad) spectrum of coverage; 3) their concern about the potential of growing resistance to a class (fluoroquinolones) which has agents that currently are active against DRSP species; 4) their preference for monotherapeutic vs. combination therapy; 5) when the guidelines were released (recent vs several years old); and 6) their emphasis on drug costs (please see Table 4), patient convenience, and options for step-down (IV to oral) therapeutic approaches. Clearly, these factors and the relative emphasis placed on each of them will influence antimicrobial selection for the geriatric patient with pneumonia.

Table 4. Daily Drug Cost (WAC)*

DRUG AND DOSAGE	COST/DAY
Azithromycin IV 500 mg	$18.96
Ceftriaxone 1 gm IV qd	36.06
Levofloxacin 500 mg IV qd	33.00
Erythromycin 500 mg IV qid	5.20
Ciprofloxacin 400 mg IV bid	48.00
Cefotaxime 1 g IV tid	25.00
Tricarcillin-clavulanate 3.1 g qid	48.32

* WAC = Wholesale acquisition cost.
Hospital formulary pricing guide, August 1999. WAC may not necessarily reflect actual pharmacy costs or costs associated with drug administration cost comparisons.

With these issues and drug selection factors in mind, the most recent guidelines issued by the CDC Drug-Resistant *Streptococcus pneumoniae* Therapeutic Working Group and American Thoracic Society attempt to both risk-stratify and "drug-stratify" patients according to their eligibility for receiving agents as initial empiric therapy that have activity against DRSP (drug-resistant *Streptococcus pneumoniae*). Before presenting a detailed discussion of the current treatment landscape for CAP, the following points from the ASCAP expert's panel should be emphasized. First, the relative importance of *S. pneumoniae* as a cause of outpatient CAP is difficult to determine. Nevertheless, a review of the literature suggests that *S. pneumoniae* accounts for 2-27% of all cases of CAP treated on an outpatient basis.[20,44] In addition, surveillance studies have suggested that about 7% of invasive *S. pneumoniae* species in the United States show a significant degree of penicillin resistance.[45] Hence, this group estimates that only 0.14% (7% of 2%) to 1.9% (7% of 27%) of outpatients with bacterial pneumonia have pneumococcal infections with levels of resistance high enough to warrant consideration of alternative treatment.

This analysis has prompted the CDC panel to conclude that because CAP in patients who are appropriately triaged and risk-stratified is generally not immediately life-threatening and because *S. pneumoniae* isolates with penicillin MICs of no less than 4 mcg/mL are uncommon, antibiotics with predictable activity against highly penicillin-resistance pneumococci are not necessary as part of the initial regimen. From a practical, drug-selection perspective, the working group, therefore, suggests that oral fluoroquinolones are not first-line treatment in outpatients with CAP because of concerns about emerging resistance. Consequently, oral macrolide or beta-lactam monotherapy is recommended by the CDC-DRSPWG as initial therapy in patients with pneumonia considered to be amenable to outpatient management. Because atypical pathogens are an important cause of outpatient CAP, the ASCAP Consensus Panel recommends macrolides over beta-lactam monotherapy for outpatients.

It should be noted, however, that even for hospitalized (non-ICU) patients, this panel, while noting the effectiveness of monotherapy with selected fluoroquinolones, recommends the combination of a parenteral beta-lactam (ceftriaxone, cefotaxime, etc.) plus a macrolide (azithromycin, erythromycin, etc.) for initial therapy.[2] Regardless of the panel or critical pathway, one of the important consistent changes among recent recommendations for initial, empiric management of patients with CAP is mandatory inclusion of a macrolide (which covers atypical pathogens) when a cephalosporin (which has poor activity against atypical pathogens) is selected as part of the regimen. For critically ill patients, first-line therapy should include an intravenous beta-lactam, such as ceftriaxone or cefotaxime, and an intravenous macrolide, such as azithromycin (please see discussion below).

The option of using a combination of a parenteral beta-lactam (ceftriaxone, etc.) plus a fluoroquinolone with improved activity against DRSP also is presented. Once again, however, the committee issues clarifying, and sometimes cautionary, statements about the role of fluoroquinolone monotherapy in the critically ill patient, stating that caution should be exercised because the efficacy of the new fluoroquinolones as monotherapy for critically ill patients has not been determined.[2] Based on this cautionary statement, it is recommended that a parenteral beta-lactam such as ceftriaxone be used in combination with a fluoroquinolone in ICU patients with serious CAP.

Clearly, however, fluoroquinolones are an important part of the antimicrobial arsenal in the elderly, and CDC-DRSPWG has issued specific guidelines governing their use in the setting of outpatient and inpatient CAP. In general, this panel has recommended that fluoroquinolones be reserved for selected patients with CAP, and these experts have identified specific patient subgroups that are eligible for initial treatment with extended-spectrum fluoroquinolones. For hospitalized patients, these include adults for whom one of the first-line regimens (e.g., ceftriaxone plus a macrolide) has failed, those who are allergic to the first-line agents, or those who have a documented infection with highly drug-resistant pneumococci (i.e., penicillin MIC = 4 mcg/mL).[2] The rationale for this approach is discussed in subsequent sections.

Emergence of Fluoroquinolone Resistance in *Streptococcus pneumoniae*

Ironically, the only treatment guideline that recognizes the potential impact of widespread fluoroquinolone resistance also is the only treatment guideline that recommends that fluoroquinolones be reserved for selected patients with CAP (CDC-DRSPWG). With revised breakpoint MICs for cefotaxime and ceftriaxone, the percent of resistant *Streptococcus pneumoniae* to these third generation cephalosporins is expected to drop below 3-5% nationally. This will require clinicians to re-examine the published treatment guidelines that recommend fluoroquinolones as initial therapy for CAP.

Moreover, widespread, indiscriminate use of fluoroquinolones may be associated with rising resistance rates to selected gram-positive and gram-negative organisms. Previous assumptions that fluoroquinolones will be more clinically effective vs. DRSP than ceftriaxone or cefotaxime must be reevaluated. Based on the 2002 NCCLS guidelines, both ceftriaxone and cefotaxime are expected to provide comparable microbiologic end points and clinical cures in patients with non-meningeal *Streptococcus pneumoniae* as compared to the anti-pneumococcal fluoroquinolones. The clinician will be asked to incorporate geographic specific resistance rates and the ecology of micro-organisms into his/her decision about how to empirically treat the patient with CAP.

When first introduced in 1987, ciprofloxacin was promoted for the treatment of respiratory tract infections, including those due to *S. pneumoniae.* Early trials demonstrated clinical success for patients with respiratory infections.[46,47] However, subsequent studies found that the use of ciprofloxacin against *S. pneumoniae* was associated with poor eradication rates both in acute exacerbations of chronic bronchitis (AECB) and pneumonia.[48-50] Reports of the development of resistance soon appeared.[51-55] Knowing the pharmacodynamics parameters of ciprofloxacin and *S. pneumoniae,* this is not unexpected. The AUC24/MIC generally accepted to be most predictive of bacterial eradication and clinical success is > 35.[56-59] The C_{max}/MIC ratio generally accepted to be most predictive for prevention of resistance selection is > 4.[60,61] Following a 750 mg oral dose of ciprofloxacin the C_{max} is only 3 mg/L and the AUC24 is 31 mg·h/L.[62] The MIC_{90} of *S. pneumoniae* is 1 mg/L giving a C_{max}/MIC of 3 and an AUC/MIC of 31.[63]

Although ciprofloxacin was not promoted or widely used for the treatment of CAP, it was used for the treatment of AECB at a dose of 500 mg twice daily. Eradication rates of *S. pneumoniae* in AECB varied from 63% to 90%.[64,65] This failure to eradicate was associated with the development of resistance during therapy in some patients.[64,65] This may, in part, explain the emergence of pneumococci with reduced susceptibility to the fluoroquinolones and, in particular, to ciprofloxacin.

Emergence of resistance in *S. pneumoniae* to the fluoroquinolones has been described in Canada, Spain, Hong Kong, and Northern Ireland. In Canada, Chen et al found that the prevalence of ciprofloxacin-resistant pneumococci (MIC ≥ 4 mcg/mL) increased from 0% in 1993 to 1.7% in 1997-1998 (P = 0.01).[66] In adults, the prevalence increased from 0% in 1993 to 3.7% in 1998. This was associated with an increase in the consumption of fluoroquinolones. Overall, the number of fluoroquinolone prescriptions increased from 0.8 to 5.5 per 100 persons per year between 1988 and 1997.[66] In addition to the increase in prevalence of pneumococci with reduced susceptibility to fluoroquinolones, the degree of resistance also increased. From 1994 to 1998, there was a statistically significant increase in the proportion of isolates with a MIC for ciprofloxacin of ≥ 32 mcg/mL (P = 0.04).

Linares et al found an increase of ciprofloxacin-resistant pneumococci in Spain from 0.9% in 1991-1992 to 3% in 1997-1998.[67] Ho and colleagues documented a marked increase in the overall prevalence of non-susceptibility to the fluoroquinolones when comparing results of surveillance carried out in Hong Kong in 1998 and 2000.[68,69] Over a two-year period, the prevalence of levofloxacin non-susceptibility increased from 5.5% to 13.3% among all isolates and from 9.2% to 28.4% among the penicillin-resistant strains. In Northern Ireland ciprofloxacin resistance was linked to penicillin resistance. Eighteen (42.9%) of 42 penicillin-resistant pneumococci were resistant to ciprofloxacin.[70] Current rates of resistance in the United States are low.[71-74] Doern et al[72] reported ciprofloxacin resistance rates of 1.4%. The Centers for Disease Control and Preventions Active Bacterial Core Surveillance (ABCs) program carried out during 1995-1999 reported levofloxacin resistance rates of 0.2%.[71] They have not included ciprofloxacin as one of the agents they test.

One study group reviewed 181 *Streptococcus pneumoniae* isolated in Hong Kong in 1998. Hong Kong is an area with high rates of resistance, which gives us a picture of what high levels of *Streptococcus pneumoniae* resistance can look like.[68] Within three years, the resistance of *Streptococcus pneumoniae* to fluoroquinolones has increased from less than 0.5% to ofloxacin, to 5.5% for levofloxacin. Also, 4% of penicillin resistance isolates also were resistant to trovafloxacin, an agent that was only approved for use in October 1998, demonstrating the cross resistance to newer quinolones. Resistance to levofloxacin and trovafloxacin was found only in isolates that also were penicillin resistant.

One abstract detailed changes in *Streptococcus pneumoniae* resistance among different drug classes. Unfortunately, although no MICs or breakpoints are given, *Streptococcus pneumoniae* resistance grew from 0.1% to 0.6%, a growth rate over the period of about 600%. While *Streptococcus pneumoniae* grew in several antibiotic classes and among various agents, including macrolides, TMP/SMX, and cefuroxime, the greatest growth in resistance was seen with levofloxacin.[75] In another study evaluating emergent resistance[76] it was found, that compared to cephalosporins and combination therapy, fluoroquinolones were associated with the greatest risk for acquiring emergent resistance during therapy, had the highest treatment failure due to emergent resistance, the largest increase in treatment duration due to resistance, and the largest decrease in clinical response due to emergent resistance.[76]

Clinical Implications. Although treatment failures due to beta-lactams, macrolides, and TMP-SMX resistance in pneumococci have been reported with meningitis and otitis media, the relationship between drug resistance and treatment failures among patients with pneumococcal pneumonia is less clear.[77,78] However, fluoroquinolone resistance in pneumococci causing pneumonia in association with clinical failures, although anecdotal, has been well described.[48-51,79,80]

Reports of the development of resistance and clinical failures appeared shortly after the introduction of the ciprofloxacin in 1987.[51-55] Weiss and colleagues described a nosocomial outbreak of fluoroquinolone-resistant pneumococci.[80] Over the course of a 20-month period, in a hospital respiratory ward where ciprofloxacin was often used as empirical antimicrobial therapy for lower respiratory tract infections, 16 patients with chronic bronchitis developed lower respiratory tract infections caused by a strain of penicillin- and ciprofloxacin-resistant *S. pneumoniae* (serotype 23 F). The MIC of ciprofloxacin for all isolates was ≥ 4 mcg/mL. All five patients with AECB due to the resistant strain who were treated with ciprofloxacin, failed therapy. Davidson et al report four cases of pneumococcal pneumonia, treated empirically with oral levofloxacin, that failed therapy.[79] All cases were associated with the isolation of an organism that was either resistant to levofloxacin prior to therapy or which had acquired resistance during therapy. Two of the four patients had been or were on fluoroquinolones prior to initiating levofloxacin.

From these and other studies, a number of risk factors may identify the patients who are likely to be colonized or infected with a fluoroquinolone-resistant pneumococci: patients who are older than age 64, have a history of chronic obstructive lung disease, and/or a prior fluoroquinolone exposure.[66,69,71,74,81] None of the CAP position papers published since the introduction of the fluoroquinolones for the treatment of pneumococcal pneumonia has suggested that a history of previous fluoroquinolone use should be a reason for caution when using one of these antimicrobials.

Year 2002 NCCLS Breakpoints: Evidence-Based Support for Adoption of New Standards

Prior to revising the NCCLS MIC breakpoints for *S. pneumoniae,* the clinical significance of the original S, I, R breakpoints (originally published in NCCLS document M100-S9) of the parenteral aminothiazolyl cephalosporins ceftriaxone/cefotaxime in systemic non-meningeal pneumococcal infections (N-MPI) was not full elucidated.

To evaluate clinical outcomes in patients managed with ceftriaxone/cefotaxime, one group, during the period January, 1994 through October, 2000, studied 522 episodes (in 499 adult patients) of N-MPI (448 of severe pneumonia—clinical and x-ray findings together with positive blood or invasive lower respiratory tract cultures—and 74 of bacteremia from other origin). Of the 522, 74% had serious underlying diseases, 14% nosocomial, and 7% polymicrobial infections.[82] The 30-day mortality rate was 21%. Ceftriaxone/cefotaxime minimum inhibitory concentrations (MICs) according to NCCLS were determined by microdilution methods and Mueller-Hinton broth with lysed horse blood. The frequency distribution in terms of ceftriaxone/cefotaxime MICs of strains was S <= 0.5 mcg/mL 413 (79%), I = 1 mcg/mL 79 (15%), R = 2 mcg/mL 30 (6%); no strain with a ceftriaxone/cefotaxime MIC > 2 mcg/mL was found.

In ceftriaxone/cefotaxime-resistant strains the most commonly encountered serotypes were 14, 9, 23, and 6. In the 429 episodes of community-acquired pneumococcal infection (polymicrobial and nosocomial cases were excluded), we correlated the ceftriaxone/cefotaxime MICs and antibiotic therapy (prescribed according to the attending physician's criteria) with the 30-day mortality rate. In 185 episodes treated with 1 g/d of ceftriaxone (n = 171) or 1.5-2 g/8 h of cefotaxime (n = 14), the mortality rates for patients with S, I, and R strains were 18% (26/148), 13% (3/24), and 15% (2/13), respectively (P = 0.81). In the 244 patients treated with other antibiotics, the mortality rates for patients with S, I, and R strains were 18% (36/200), 12% (4/33), and 9% (1/11), respectively (P = 0.55).[82]

Hence, patients infected with pneumococci with ceftriaxone/cefotaxime MIC of 1 or 2 mcg/mL categorized as I or R by NCCLS did not show an increased mortality rate compared to S strains in N-MPI when treated with ceftriaxone (1 g/d) or cefotaxime (1.5-2 g/8h). These data support the higher breakpoints for ceftriaxone/cefotaxime by the NCCLS that went into effect in January 2002 for non-meningeal pneumococcal infections. This study demonstrates that parenteral aminothiazolyl cephalosporins such as ceftriaxone (1 g/day) or cefotaxime (1.5-2 g/8 h) work well in adult patients with systemic non-meningeal pneumococcal infections caused by strains with ceftriaxone/cefotaxime MIC up to 1 mcg/mL. Based on their limited experience, they concluded it also is probable that this observation is true for strains with ceftriaxone/cefotaxime MICs of 2 mcg/mL.

Moreover, the available data in children[83] and adults suggest the NCCLS interpretive breakpoints were appropriately modified for systemic non-meningeal pneumococcal infections, and considered susceptible up to a ceftriaxone/cefotaxime MIC of 1 mcg/mL (NCCLS publication M100-S12 which went into effect January 2002). Until further experience with isolates with ceftriaxone/cefotaxime MIC = 2 mcg/mL accumulates, the investigators strongly recommend continued monitoring of the MIC of aminothiazolyl cephalosporins in all invasive pneumococcal isolates, and assessment of clinical and bacteriological outcomes.[83]

Antimicrobial Therapy

With these considerations in focus, the purpose of this antimicrobial treatment section is to review the various recommendations, consensus panel statements, clinical trials, and published guidelines. A rational analysis of this information also will be performed, to generate a set of guidelines and protocols for specific populations as these issues relate to the geriatric patient.

Antibiotic Overview. A brief overview of agents that have been used for treatment of CAP will help set the stage for outcome-effective drug selection. *(Please see Table 1.)* The first generation cephalosporins have significant coverage against gram-positive organisms. By comparison, third generation cephalosporins have less gram-positive coverage and increased coverage against aerobic gram-negative rods.[84] Ceftazidime has coverage against *Pseudomonas*, while cefoperazone has a somewhat higher MIC. Some of the second generation cephalosporins, such as cefoxitin, cefotetan, and cefmetazole, provide coverage against *Bacteroides* species. Imipenem has broad coverage against aerobic and anaerobic organisms. Aztreonam provides significant coverage for gram-negative bacilli such as *Pseudomonas*.

Among the beta-lactams, the CDC-DRSPWG identifies cefuroxime axetil, cefotaxime sodium, ceftriaxone sodium, or ampicillin-sulbactam as recommended empiric agents. The group notes, however, that among these agents, ceftriaxone and cefotaxime have superior activity against resistant pneumococci when compared with cefuroxime and ampicillin-sulbactam.[2] Because it is recommended that cefotaxime be administered on a q8h basis for treatment of CAP,[2,85] and because the efficacy and safety of once-daily ceftriaxone for inpatient CAP is well established, ceftriaxone is recommended by most experts and the ASCAP Consensus Panel as the cephalosporin of choice for management of CAP.[85]

The aminoglycosides are active against gram-negative aerobic organisms. These agents are generally used for elderly patients with severe CAP, particularly when *Pseudomonas* infection is suspected. As a rule, the aminoglycosides are combined with a third generation cephalosporin or an extended spectrum quinolone antibiotic, monobactam, or an extended spectrum penicillin when used in these circumstances.[86]

The tetracyclines are active against *Streptococcus pneumoniae, H. influenza, Mycoplasma, Chlamydia,* and *Legionella.* There is, however, a growing incidence of *S. pneumoniae* resistance to tetracyclines.[89] These agents are alternatives to the macrolide antibiotics for empiric therapy for CAP in young, healthy adults.[88] Convenience and coverage advantages of the new macrolides, however, have thrust the tetracyclines into a secondary role for managing CAP. Clindamycin has activity against anaerobes, such as *B. fragilis.*[89,90] Its anaerobic coverage makes it a consideration for the treatment of pneumonia in nursing home patients suspected of aspiration. Metronidazole also has activity against anaerobic bacteria such as *B. fragilis.* It is used in combination with other antibiotics for the treatment of lung abscesses, aspiration pneumonia, or anaerobic infections.

Appropriate and Adequate Intensity of Antimicrobial Coverage. Because macrolides and extended spectrum quinolones have indications for monotherapeutic treatment of CAP, they frequently get equal billing as initial choice agents for management of CAP. However, the macrolides and extended spectrum quinolones have clinically significant differences that should be considered in the antibiotic treatment equation for CAP. Accordingly, a careful analysis of the benefits and potential pitfalls of these agents should include a full accounting of the relevant similarities and differences. It will help emergency physicians, hospitalists, infectious disease specialists, and intensivists develop criteria that suggest the appropriateness and suitability that each of these classes may have in specific patient subgroups.

Although the previously cited six organisms (*S. pneumoniae, H. influenzae,* and *M. catarrhalis,* and atypical pathogens *Mycoplasma, Legionella,* and *C. pneumoniae)* are the most commonly implicated pathogens in elderly patients with CAP, this patient population also is susceptible to infection with gram-negative enteric organisms such as *Klebsiella, Escherichia coli,* and *Pseudomonas.* In other cases, the likelihood of infection with DRSP is high. When infection with these pathogens is likely, intensification of empiric coverage should include antibiotics with activity against these gram-negative species.[3,20,21] From a practical, antibiotic selection perspective, this requires that macrolides be used in combination with a cephalosporin such as ceftriaxone as initial, empiric therapy, or alternatively, an advanced generation fluoroquinolone.

Clinical features or risk factors that may suggest the need for intensification and expansion of bacterial and/or atypical pathogen coverage include the following: 1) increasing fragility (> 85 years of age, comorbid conditions, previous infection, etc.) of the patient; 2) acquisition of the pneumonia in a skilled nursing facility; 3) the presence of an aspiration pneumonia, suggesting involvement with gram-negative or anaerobic organisms; 4) chronic alcoholism, increasing the likelihood of infection with *Klebsiella pneumoniae;* 5) pneumococcal pneumonia in an underlying disease-compromised individual who has not been vaccinated with pneumococcal polysaccharide antigen (Pneumovax); 6) history of infection with gram-negative, anaerobic, or resistant species of *S. pneumoniae;* 7) history of treatment failure; 8) previous hospitalizations for pneumonia; 9) patient requires or has had previous ICU hospitalization for pneumonia; 10) acquisition of pneumonia in a community with high and increasing resistance among *S. pneumoniae* species; and 11) immunodeficiency and/or severe underlying disease. Many of the aforementioned risk groups also can be treated with the combination of a third-generation cephalosporin plus a macrolide, in combination with an aminoglycoside when indicated.

As emphasized earlier in this report, most consensus panels, infectious disease experts, textbooks, and peer-reviewed antimicrobial prescribing guides recommend, as the initial or preferred choice, those antibiotics that, within the framework of monotherapy or combination therapy, address current etiologic and mortality trends in CAP. As a general rule, for empiric initial therapy in patients without modifying host factors that predispose to enteric gram-negative or pseudomonal infection, they recommend those antibiotics that provide coverage against the bacterial pathogens *S. pneumoniae, H. influenzae,* and *M. catarrhalis,* as well as against atypical pathogens *Mycoplasma, Legionella,* and *C. pneumoniae*.[36]

Treatment Guidelines for CAP: Outcomes, Value, and Institutional Implementation

Based on a review of the available literature and personal communications among the panel members, the ASCAP Consensus Panel recommends implementation of institution-wide guidelines for patients with CAP. A strong case can be made for adopting such a strategy, especially when educational, process of care, and quality review/improvement measures are put into place.

In one study reviewed,[91] a pneumonia guideline developed at Intermountain Health Care included admission decision support and recommendations for antibiotic timing and selection, based on the 1993 ATS guideline.[91] The study included all immunocompetent patients older than age 65 with CAP from 1993 through 1997 in Utah; nursing home patients were excluded. The investigators compared 30-day mortality rates among patients before and after the guideline was implemented, as well as among patients treated by physicians who did not participate in the guideline program.

Overall, the research group observed 28,661 cases of pneumonia, including 7719 (27%) that resulted in hospital admission. Thirty-day mortality was 13.4% (1037 of 7719) among admitted patients and 6.3% (1801 of 28,661) overall. Mortality rates (both overall and among admitted patients) were similar among patients of physicians affiliated and not affiliated with Intermountain Health Care before the guideline was implemented. For episodes that resulted in hospital admission after guideline implementation, 30-day mortality was 11.0% among patients treated by Intermountain Health Care-affiliated physicians compared with 14.2% for other Utah physicians. The guideline used ceftriaxone without or without a macrolide such as azithromycin or clarithromycin.

An analysis that adjusted by logistic regression for age, sex, rural vs. urban residences, and year confirmed that 30-day mortality was lower among admitted patients who were treated by Intermountain Health Care-affiliated physicians (odds ratio [OR]: 0.69; 95% confidence interval [CI]: 0.49 to 0.97; P = 0.04) and was somewhat lower among all pneumonia patients (OR: 0.81; 95% CI: 0.63 to 1.03; P = 0.08). The investigators concluded that implementation of a pneumonia practice guideline in the Intermountain Health Care system was associated with a reduction in 30-day mortality among elderly patients with pneumonia.

Explanations offered by the investigators for the decreased mortality after guideline implementation include selection of more appropriate antibiotics, timing of initial antibiotic administration, and use of heparin prophylaxis against thromboembolic disease. For example, one study[92] reported that mortality was about 25% lower among inpatients when the initial, empiric antibiotic regimen combined a third-generation cephalosporin with a macrolide compared with cephalosporins alone, whereas another investigation[41] showed a 15% reduction in mortality when antibiotics were administered within eight hours of hospitalization. The guideline that was evaluated by Intermountain Health Care recommended that antibiotics should be administered before a patient with pneumonia leaves the outpatient site of diagnosis. In addition, admission orders included prophylactic heparin.

Another group conducted a comprehensive review of the medical literature to determine whether guideline implementation for CAP reduces mortality and resource costs.[93] These investigators noted that studies have shown significant changes in the processes of care after implementation of guideline recommendations for treatment of patients with CAP.[94-96] The most extensive of these studies consisted of a randomized trial that was conducted in 19 hospitals and which included 1743 patients.[12] This study design provided reasonable internal validity (i.e., it is likely that the differences in the process of care between the nine intervention hospitals and the 10 control hospitals were due to the implementation of the critical pathway). The trial's motivation was a desire to find means of cost-containment, inasmuch as the primary hypothesis was that the critical pathway would reduce the use of institutional resources without compromising the safety and efficacy of therapy.[12]

Two other studies have demonstrated an improvement in outcome after implementation of guidelines: improvement of patient response to antibacterial treatment in one[97] and lower mortality rates in the other.[98] Both studies used an uncontrolled, before-and-after design, but in one of the studies, the changes in the mortality rate in the intervention hospital were compared with data from 23 other hospitals.[98] In both of these studies, the improvement in outcome was accompanied by a reduction in the cost of care. A third study used an uncontrolled, before-and-after design to show that a quality improvement program reduced time to initiation of antibacterial treatment of patients with CAP, which is likely to improve patient outcome. However, there was no direct measurement of outcome. The reviewers conclude that the best-quality evidence about the effects of guideline implementation shows that they can be used to reduce unnecessary use of resources without compromising the quality of care or patient outcomes.[40,97]

Correct Spectrum Coverage: Outcome-Optimizing Regimens for CAP

Because beta-lactams, advanced generation macrolides, and extended spectrum quinolones constitute the principal oral and intravenous treatment options for CAP, the following sections will discuss indications, clinical trials, side effects, and strategies for their use in CAP. The discussion will focus on antibiotics that: 1) provide, as combination therapy or monotherapy, appropriate coverage of bacterial and atypical organisms causing CAP; 2) are available for both outpatient (oral) and in-hospital (IV) management; and 3) are supported by national consensus panels or association guidelines.

Beta-Lactams: Ceftriaxone for Combination Therapy in CAP. The safety and efficacy of ceftriaxone for managing hospitalized patients with CAP has been well-established in numerous clinical trials, including recent investigations confirming its equal efficacy as compared to new generation fluoroquinolones. In this regard, one recent study attempted to determine the comparative efficacy and total resource costs of sequential IV to oral gatifloxacin therapy vs. IV ceftriaxone with or without IV erythromycin to oral clarithromycin therapy for treatment of CAP patients requiring hospitalization.[99]

Two hundred eighty-three patients were enrolled in a randomized, double-blind, clinical trial, data collected included patient demographics, clinical and microbiological outcomes, length of stay (LOS), and antibiotic-related LOS (LOSAR). Overall, 203 patients were clinically and economically evaluable (98 receiving gatifloxacin and 105 receiving ceftriaxone). It should be noted that IV erythromycin was administered to only 35 patients in the ceftriaxone-treated group, thereby putting a significant percentage (about 62%) of the ceftriaxone cohort at a "spectrum of coverage" disadvantage because of the failure to include an agent with coverage against atypical organisms. Despite this, oral conversion was achieved in 98% of patients in each group, and the investigators concluded that clinical cure and microbiological eradication rates did not differ statistically between ceftriaxone (92% and 92%) and gatifloxacin (98% and 97%).[99]

Given the concern about DRSP in hospitalized CAP patients, there has been robust debate about the effectiveness of ceftriaxone in pulmonary infections caused by DRSP. Attempting to shed light on this issue, an important study evaluating actual clinical outcomes in patients treated with beta-lactams for systemic infection outside of the central nervous system (CNS) which was caused by isolates of *Streptococcus pneumoniae* considered nonsusceptible to ceftriaxone (MIC ≥ 1.0 mcg/mL) by pre-2002 NCCLS breakpoints has recently been published by the Pediatric Infectious Diseases Section, Baylor College of Medicine.[100]

The objective of the study was to determine the actual clinical outcomes of patients treated primarily with beta-lactam antibiotics for a systemic infection outside of the CNS caused by isolates of *Streptococcus pneumoniae* nonsusceptible to ceftriaxone (MIC ≥ 1.0 mcg/mL). A retrospective review was performed of the medical records of children identified prospectively with invasive infections outside of the CNS caused by isolates of *S. pneumoniae* that were not susceptible to ceftriaxone between September 1993 and August 1999. A subset of this group treated primarily with beta-lactam antibiotics was analyzed for outcome. Among 2100 patients with invasive infections outside the CNS that were caused by *S. pneumoniae,* 166 had isolates not susceptible to ceftriaxone.

One hundred patients treated primarily with beta-lactam antibiotics were identified. From this group, 71 and 14 children had bacteremia alone or with pneumonia, respectively, caused by strains with an MIC of 1.0 mcg/mL. Bacteremia or pneumonia caused by isolates with a ceftriaxone MIC ≥ 2.0 mcg/mL occurred in six and five children, respectively. Three children with septic arthritis and one with cellulitis had infections caused by strains with an MIC to ceftriaxone of 1.0 mcg/mL. Most were treated with parenteral ceftriaxone, cefotaxime, or cefuroxime for one or more doses followed by an oral antibiotic. All but one child were successfully treated. The failure occurred in a child with severe combined immune deficiency and bacteremia (MIC = 1.0 mcg/mL) who remained febrile after a single dose of ceftriaxone followed by 12 days of cefprozil. The investigators concluded that ceftriaxone, cefotaxime, or cefuroxime are adequate to treat invasive infections outside the CNS caused by pneumococcal isolates with MICs up to 2.0 mcg/mL. Accordingly, the NCCLS breakpoints, as of January 2002, for the beta-lactam ceftriaxone and cefotaxime were modified and up-calibrated so that currently about 95% of all *S. pneumoniae* species are considered sensitive to ceftriaxone, as well as cefotaxime.[10]

Observational Trends from The ARM Database: Ceftriaxone Vs. Cefotaxime for *Streptococcus pneumoniae*

The Antimicrobial Resistance Management (ARM) program was established to help individual institutions define their antimicrobial resistance problems and establish cause-effect relationships that could lead to strategic interventions. To date, the ARM program has entered more than 100 community and teaching hospitals into a web-centered database. This observational database currently has susceptability data on up to 19 different organisms and up to 46 different antibiotics. As of January 2002, the ARM program had collected data on more than 10 million total isolates, and sensitivity data on more than 60,000 separate isolates of *Streptococcus pneumoniae*.[101]

Evaluation of national *Streptococcus pneumoniae* sensitivity data for ceftriaxone and cefotaxime revealed differences between the third-generation cephalosporins. Using the pre-2002 NCCLS breakpoint MICs for ceftriaxone and cefotaxime, the ARM database demonstrated *Streptococcus pneumoniae* sensitivities to ceftriaxone and cefotaxime of 80.4% and 69.2%, respectively. Since the 2002 NCCLS breakpoint MICs were adjusted equally for ceftriaxone and cefotaxime, the observed sensitivity differences are not expected to change once the new breakpoints are superimposed from the new data.

The sensitivity differences between ceftriaxone and cefotaxime observed nationally also were seen in select geographic sections of the country. Discrepancies in *Streptococcus pneumoniae* sensitivities between ceftriaxone and cefotaxime were demonstrated in the Southeast region of the United States. However, the Northeast cohort of the ARM database showed no differences in sensitivity percentages between ceftriaxone and cefotaxime.[101]

Since the ARM program was originally designed as an observational database to use antibiogram trending to identify resistance patterns for individual hospitals, it is not capable of isolating the specific reason why national sensitivity differences exist between ceftriaxone and cefotaxime. Additionally, for similar reasons, the ARM program is not designed to identify why certain geographic sections of the United States demonstrate the discrepancies in sensitivities and others do not. However, subanalysis of the data suggests that the discrepancy between the third-generation cephalosporins did not exist through the whole database. The difference in sensitivity percentages appeared to emerge during the last half of the 1990-2000 decade. This coincides with the push to use cefotaxime on a twice a day basis vs. a more traditional three times daily dosing regimen.[101]

Since cefotaxime exerts its antimicrobial activity as a function of its time above the MIC of *Streptococcus pneumoniae,* a drop in dosing frequency from TID to BID will increase the percent of time that the organism is exposed to subinhibitory concentrations.[102] Without any significant post-antibiotic effect, the sensitivities of cefotaxime to *Streptococcus pneumoniae* may fall. Further and more specific MIC analysis is required to determine if the reduced dosing frequency is causally related to the emergence of a sensitivity discrepancy between cefotaxime and ceftriaxone.

Advanced Generation Macrolides. The established new generation macrolide antibiotics include the erythromycin analogues azithromycin and clarithromycin.[103,104] Compared to erythromycin, which is the least expensive macrolide, the major advantages of these newer antibiotics are significantly decreased gastrointestinal side effects, which produce enhanced tolerance, improved bioavailability, higher tissue levels, and pharmacokinetic features that permit less frequent dosing and better compliance, as well as enhanced activity against *H. influenzae*.[105,106] In particular, the long tissue half-life of azithromycin allows this antibiotic to be prescribed for a shorter duration (5 days) than comparable antibiotics given for the same indications. Given the cost differences between azithromycin and clarithromycin, as well as the improved compliance patterns associated with short-duration therapy, any rational approach to distinguishing between these agents must consider prescription, patient, and drug resistance barriers.

From the outset, it is fair to say that these macrolides—especially azithromycin—to a great degree, have supplanted the use of erythromycin in community-acquired infections of the lower respiratory tract.

From the perspective of providing definitive, cost-effective, and compliance-promoting therapy, the newer macrolide antibiotics, which include intravenous azithromycin for hospital-based management, have recently emerged as some of the drugs of choice—along with the new, extended spectrum quinolones—for outpatient management of CAP.[107] When used as oral agents, they play a central role in management of pneumonia in otherwise healthy elderly individuals who do not require hospitalization.

From an emergency medicine and in-hospital management perspective, the value and desirability of macrolide therapy has been significantly enhanced by availability of the intravenous formulation of azithromycin, which has been approved for hospitalized patients with CAP. Unlike penicillins, cephalosporins, and sulfa-based agents, azithromycin has the advantage of showing in vitro activity against both atypical and bacterial offenders implicated in CAP.[25,26]

The macrolides also have the advantage of a simplified dosing schedule, especially azithromycin, which is given once daily for only five days (500 mg po on day 1 and 250 mg po qd on days 2-5). Clarithromycin requires a longer course of therapy and is more expensive. Clarithromycin costs approximately $68-72 for a complete, 10-day course of therapy vs. $42-44 for a complete course of therapy with azithromycin.

Clarithromycin, however, is another alternative among macrolides for outpatient treatment of CAP. It is now available in once-daily formulation (1000 mg/d for 10 days) for oral use, but an intravenous preparation is not currently available. In general, the decision to use a macrolide such as azithromycin rather than erythromycin is based on weighing the increased cost of a course of therapy with azithromycin against its real-world advantages, which include a more convenient dosing schedule; its broader spectrum of coverage; its favorable drug interaction profile; and its decreased incidence of gastrointestinal side effects, which occur in 3-5% of patients taking a five-day, multiple-dose regimen.[108] The introduction of a tablet formulation permits consumption of the antibiotic without regard to food ingestion.

Azithromycin-Coagent (i.e., with Ceftriaxone) For Combination Therapy in Hospitalized CAP. Intravenous azithromycin can be used for the management of hospitalized patients with moderate or severe CAP.[27,28,109] Currently, azithromycin is the only advanced generation macrolide indicated for parenteral therapy in hospitalized patients with CAP due to *C. pneumoniae, H. influenzae L. pneumophila, M. catarrhalis, M. pneumoniae, S. pneumoniae,* or *Staphylococcus aureus.*[25,26,109,110] This coverage would be considered correct spectrum coverage for empiric therapy of CAP in most patients. However, for hospitalized patients, who tend to have co-morbid conditions, including underlying cardiorespiratory disease, the addition of a beta-lactam (ceftriaxone/cefotaxime) is considered mandatory by the ASCAP Consensus Panel.

Azithromycin dosing and administration schedules for hospitalized patients are different than for the five-day course used exclusively for outpatient management, and these differences should be noted. When this advanced generation macrolide is used for hospitalized patients with CAP, 2-5 days of therapy with azithromycin IV (500 mg once daily) followed by oral azithromycin (500 mg once daily to complete a total of 7-10 days of therapy) is clinically and bacteriologically effective. For patients requiring hospitalization, the initial 500 mg intravenous dose of azithromycin should be given in the ED.

Like the oral formulation, IV azithromycin appears to be well-tolerated, with a low incidence of gastrointestinal adverse events (4.3% diarrhea, 3.9% nausea, 2.7% abdominal pain, 1.4% vomiting), minimal injection-site reactions (less than 12% combined injection-site pain and/or inflammation or infection), and a low incidence of discontinuation (1.2% discontinuation of IV therapy) due to drug-related adverse patient events or laboratory abnormalities.[111]

Community-Acquired Pneumonia (CAP): ASCAP Consensus Panel Recommendations for Outpatient Management

Despite a general consensus that empiric, outpatient treatment of CAP requires, at the least, mandatory coverage of such organisms as *S. pneumoniae, H. influenzae,* and *M. catarrhalis,* as well as atypical organisms (*Mycoplasma pneumoniae, Chlamydia pneumoniae,* and *Legionella pneumophila*), antibiotic selection strategies for achieving this spectrum of coverage vary widely. New treatment guidelines for CAP have been issued by such national associations as the IDSA (2000), the ATS (2001), and the CDC (CDCDRSP-WG, 2000).

Deciphering the strengths, subtleties, and differences among recommendations issued by different authoritative sources can be problematic and confusing. Because patient disposition practices and treatment pathways vary among institutions and from region to region, management guidelines for CAP in the geriatric patient must be "customized" for the local practice environment. Unfortunately, no single set of guidelines is applicable to every patient or practice environment; therefore, clinical judgment must prevail. This means taking into account local antibiotic resistance patterns, epidemiological and infection incidence data, and patient demographic features.

Patient Management Recommendations. The ASCAP 2002 Consensus Panel concurred that appropriate use of antibiotics requires radiographic confirmation of the diagnosis of CAP. In this regard, physicians should use clinical judgement when ordering chest x-rays, with the understanding that the diagnostic yield of this radiographic modality in CAP is increased in patients with fever greater than 38.5°C; presence of new cough; and abnormal pulmonary findings suggestive of consolidation, localized bronchoconstriction, or pleural effusion.

Accordingly, a chest x-ray is recommended and encouraged by the ASCAP Consensus Panel, as well as by such national associations as the IDSA, ATS, and American College of Emergency Physicians (ACEP), to confirm the diagnosis of outpatient CAP; however, the panel acknowledges that, on occasion, logistical issues may prevent radiographic confirmation at the time of diagnosis and treatment.

The approach to antibiotic therapy usually will be empiric, and must account for a number of clinical, epidemiological, and unpredictable factors related to antibiotic resistance patterns and respiratory tract pathogens. As a general rule, appropriate antibiotic choice for the patient with CAP requires consideration of strategies that will yield clinical cure in the patient "today," combined with antibiotic selection strategies that prevent accelerated emergence of drug-resistant organisms that will infect the community "tomorrow."

Based on the most current clinical studies, the principal six respiratory tract pathogens that must be covered on an empiric basis in individuals with outpatient CAP include: *S. pneumoniae, H. influenzae, M. catarrhalis, Chlamydia pneumoniae, M. pneumoniae,* and *Legionella pneumophila.* In addition, the ASCAP Consensus Panel emphasized that there may be a "disconnect," (i.e., an incompletely understood and not entirely predictable relationship between an antibiotic's MIC level and its association with positive clinical outcomes in CAP). This "disconnect" may be explained by the unique qualities of an antimicrobial, such as tissue penetration and/or pharmacokinetics, patient medication compliance, and other factors.

Double-blinded, prospective clinical trials comparing new generation macrolides vs. new generation fluoroquinolones demonstrate similar outcomes in terms of clinical cure and bacteriologic eradication rates in outpatients with CAP.[100] However, emergence of resistance among *S. pneumoniae* species to new generation fluoroquinolones has been reported in a number of geographic regions, including the United States, Hong Kong, and Canada, and this may have implications for treatment.

The frequency of DRSP causing outpatient CAP, as estimated by the CDC, is very low (i.e., in the range of 0.14-1.9%). The CDC-DRSPWG cautions against overuse of new generation fluoroquinolones in outpatient CAP, and recommends their use as alternative agents when: 1) first-line therapy with advanced generation macrolides such as azithromycin fails; 2) patients are allergic to first-line agents; or 3) the case is a documented infection with DRSP.[112]

Given concerns about antibiotic overuse, the potential for emerging resistance among DRSP to fluoroquinolones, and the increasing recognition of atypical pathogens as causative agents in patients with outpatient CAP, the panel concurs with the CDCDRSP-WG recommendation advocating macrolides as initial agents of choice in outpatient CAP. The ASCAP Consensus Panel also noted that the Canadian Consensus Guidelines for CAP Management and the 2001 ATS Consensus Guideline Recommendations also include advanced generation macrolides as initial therapy for outpatient CAP.

In this regard, two safe and effective advanced generation macrolides, azithromycin and clarithromycin, currently are available for outpatient, oral-based treatment of CAP (IV azithromycin also is indicated for in-hospital management of patients who are risk-stratified as having more serious disease). Based on outcome-sensitive criteria such as cost, daily dose frequency, duration of therapy, side effects, and drug interactions, the ASCAP Consensus Panel recommends as first-line, preferred initial therapy in CAP, azithromycin, with clarithromycin or doxycycline as an alternative agents; and as second-line therapy, moxifloxacin, gatifloxacin, or levofloxacin when appropriate, according to CDC guidelines and other association-based protocols. Among the advanced generation fluoroquinolones, moxifloxacin is preferred by the ASCAP Consensus Panel because it has the most favorable MICs against *S. pneumoniae,* and a more focused spectrum of coverage against gram-positive organisms than levofloxacin or gatifloxacin.

Physicians are urged to prescribe antibiotics in CAP at the time of diagnosis and to encourage patients to fill and begin taking their prescriptions for CAP on the day of diagnosis. Ideally, patients should initiate their first course of oral therapy within eight hours of diagnosis, a time frame that appears reasonable based on studies in hospitalized patients indicating improved survival in patients who received their first IV dose within eight hours of diagnosis. Primary care practitioners also are urged to instruct patients in medication compliance, and in the case of short (5-day) courses of therapy, educate their patients that although they are only consuming medications for a five-day period, the antibiotic remains at the tissue site of infection for about 7-10 days and continues to deliver therapeutic effects during that period.

Either verbal or on-site, reevaluation of patients is recommended within a three-day period following diagnosis and initiation of antibiotic therapy. Follow-up in the office or clinic within three days is recommended in certain risk-stratified patients, especially the elderly, those with co-morbid illness, and those in whom medication compliance may be compromised. More urgent follow-up may be required in patients with increasing symptoms, including dyspnea, fever, and other systemic signs or symptoms. Follow-up chest x-rays generally are not recommended in patients with outpatient CAP, except in certain high-risk groups, such as those with right middle lobe syndrome, and in individuals in whom the diagnosis may have been uncertain.

In-Hospital Management of CAP: Monotherapy Vs. Combination Therapy. Outcomes Analysis and ASCAP Treatment Guidelines

As emphasized earlier, prompt administration of intravenous antibiotics in the ED can improve clinical outcomes in patients with CAP. Consequently, once diagnostic tests, including cultures and radiographs (when appropriate), have been performed, initial antibiotic therapy for hospitalized patients should be administered in the ED, especially if delays in getting the patient admitted are anticipated.

Although antibiotic recommendations based on risk-stratification criteria, historical features, sites where the infection was acquired, and other modifying factors play a role, institutional protocols, hospital-based critical pathways, resistance features, and other factors also will influence antibiotic selection. Despite variations in hospital or departmental protocols, certain requirements regarding drug selection for CAP are relatively consistent. For example, from an empiric antibiotic selection perspective, what appears to be non-negotiable for managing the majority of patients with CAP, is providing mandatory antimicrobial coverage against *S. pneumoniae, H. influenzae, M. catarrhalis, Legionella, M. pneumoniae,* and *C. pneumoniae.* As mentioned earlier, consensus reports and national guidelines support this strategy (please see section on Consensus Guidelines for Antibiotic Therapy, below).

When combination cephalosporin/macrolide therapy is the accepted hospital protocol, among the beta-lactams available, IV ceftriaxone is recommended by the ASCAP 2002 Consensus Panel because of its evidence-based efficacy in moderate-to severe CAP, once-daily administration, spectrum of coverage, and because it is supported by all major guideline panels. One study evaluated antibiotic resistance data using data derived from community-based medical practices. Data was gathered from July 1999 to April 2000. Four of the most common isolates were: *Moraxella catarrhalis* (27%), *Haemophilus influenzae* (25%), *Staphylococcus aureus* (14%), and *Streptococcus pneumoniae* (12%); atypical organisms were not assessed.

Among *Streptococcus pneumoniae* isolates, levofloxacin exhibited a 4.8% level of resistance; for ceftriaxone, the resistance rate was only 5.8% (based on pre-2002 NCCLS MIC breakpoint). For *Staphylococcus aureus,* both ceftriaxone and levofloxacin inhibited all isolates. And for *M. catarrhalis* and *H. influenzae,* no resistance was observed for either levofloxacin or ceftriaxone. The investigators concluded that levofloxacin and ceftriaxone exhibited equivalent susceptibility/resistance patterns to organisms encountered in CAP.[113]

Although ceftriaxone was introduced to the market in 1985, and despite 18 years of use, its susceptibility to multiple gram-positive and gram-negative isolates has not changed significantly. In this regard, ceftriaxone has retained potent activity against the most commonly encountered enteric species (i.e., *E. coli, K. pneumoniae, K. oxytocia,* and *P. mirabilis*), at a level of 93-99%.[113]

Azithromycin is recommended as the co-therapeutic macrolide agent (i.e., in combination with ceftriaxone) in patients with CAP for the following reasons: 1) it can be administered on a once-daily basis, thereby minimizing human resource costs associated with drug administration; 2) it is the only macrolide indicated for in-hospital, intravenous-to-oral stepdown, monotherapeutic management of CAP caused by *S. pneumoniae, H. influenzae, M. catarrhalis, Legionella pneu-*

mophila, M. pneumoniae, C. pneumoniae, or *S. aureus*—an important efficacy and spectrum of coverage benchmark; 3) at $19-22 per day for the intravenous dose of 500 mg azithromycin, its cost is reasonable; 4) the intravenous-to-oral step-down dose of 500 mg has been established as effective in clinical trials evaluating hospitalized patients with CAP; and 5) azithromycin has excellent activity against *Legionella pneumophila,* a pathogen commonly implicated in the geriatric patient with CAP. The decision to use azithromycin as a monotherapeutic agent, or in combination with a cephalosporin for initial therapy of CAP, will be determined by intrainstitutional pathways and protocols, based on consensus recommendations and association guidelines as presented in this article.

Critical Pathways and Protocols. When patients with CAP are hospitalized in the ICU or there is a significant likelihood of gram-negative infection (i.e., *Klebsiella, E. coli,* or *P. aeruginosa*), monotherapy with a macrolide is not appropriate, and CDC group's recent consensus report stresses the importance of using an IV macrolide in combination with other agents, in particular, third-generation cephalosporins such as ceftriaxone.[2] In these patients, a macrolide should be used in combination with a cephalosporin (i.e., ceftriaxone), and when anti-pseudomonal coverage is necessary, an anti-pseudomonal cephalosporin and/or an aminoglycoside also may be required. Or alternatively, an extended spectrum fluoroquinolone such as levofloxacin should be considered, although combination therapy that includes a cephalosporin such as ceftriaxone also has been advocated with this agent in severely ill patients.[2] When anaerobic organisms are suspected, clindamycin or a beta-lactam/beta-lactamase inhibitor is appropriate.

Accordingly, a number of critical pathways for pneumonia therapy recommend use of two-drug therapy for CAP. The therapy typically is the combination of an IV cephalosporin such as ceftriaxone plus a macrolide, which usually is administered, initially, by the intravenous route when the patient's condition so warrants. Perhaps the important change in CAP treatment since publication of the ATS guidelines in 1993 is the current general consensus, including guidelines presented at the 2001 ATS Scientific Conference, that atypical organisms such as *L. pneumophila, C. pneumoniae,* and *M. pneumoniae* must be covered empirically as part of the initial antibiotic regimen. Whereas previous consensus guidelines indicated that macrolides could be added to a cephalosporin on a "plus or minus" basis for initial CAP treatment, it is now felt that coverage of the atypical spectrum, along with coverage of *S. pneumoniae, H. influenzae,* and *M. catarrhalis,* is mandatory.[2] New guidelines from the IDSA, ATS, ASCAP, and CDC now reflect this strategy.

Although virtually all protocols using combination cephalosporin/macrolide therapy specify intravenous administration of the cephalosporin, guidelines specifying whether initial macrolide therapy should occur via the intravenous or oral route are less concrete. Recent CDC-DRSPWG guidelines recommend an intravenous macrolide therapy for patients hospitalized in the ICU, while oral therapy is permissible in conjunction with an IV cephalosporin in the medical ward patient.[2] Because atypical infections such as *L. pneumophila* are associated with high mortality rates, especially in the elderly, and because hospitalized patients with CAP, by definition, represent a sicker cohort, it is prudent and, therefore, advisable that initial macrolide therapy in the hospital be administered by the intravenous route. The ASCAP Consensus Panel, therefore, recommends IV azithromycin therapy as the preferred initial, empiric agent in combination with ceftriaxone. The Panel acknowledges, however, that some institutions will use intravenous ceftriaxone in combination with an oral macrolide in non-ICU patients, an approach supported by a number of national panels. In patients on combination cephalosporin/macrolide therapy, step-down to oral therapy with azithromycin can be accomplished when the patient's clinical status so dictates, or when culture results suggest this is appropriate.

Monotherapy Vs. Combination Therapy. It should be pointed out that while some consensus panels (ATS Guidelines, 2001) support the use of IV azithromycin in very carefully selected hospitalized CAP patients (mild disease) as monotherapy or as the macrolide component of combination therapy, other panels, such as CDC-DRSPWG and the IDSA 2000 Guidelines, support its use specifically as the macrolide component of combination therapy (i.e., to be used in combination with such agents as ceftriaxone).

As emphasized, advanced generation fluoroquinolones also provide a monotherapeutic option for management of CAP, and advocates of this approach argue that these agents, on an empiric basis, provide an adequate spectrum of coverage against expected respiratory pathogens at lower drug acquisition costs. Other experts make the case that although monotherapy for pneumococcal pneumonia is standard practice in many institutions, and is identified as a treatment option in many national association guidelines, there may be a survival benefit from using a combination beta-lactam and macrolide therapy.[5] To address this issue, a group of investigators evaluated a patient data base to determine whether initial empirical therapy with a combination of effective antibiotic agents would have a better outcome than a single effective antibiotic agent in patients with bacteremic pneumococcal pneumonia.

The investigators conducted a review of adult bacteremic pneumococcal pneumonia managed in the Methodist Healthcare System, Memphis, Tennessee, between Jan. 1, 1996 and July 31, 2000. Empirical therapy was defined as all antibiotic agents received in the first 24 hours after presentation. On the basis of culture results, empirical therapy was classified as single effective therapy (SET), dual effective therapy (DET), or more than DET (MET). Acute Physiology and Chronic Health Evaluation II (APACHE II)-based predicted mortality, and PSI scores were calculated.[5]

Two hundred twenty-five subjects met the inclusion criteria for analysis. An additional seven cases of CAP with pneumococcal bacteremia were identified but were excluded from the study because the isolate was resistant to the empirical therapy the patient received. Investigators noted that the subjects who received MET were significantly sicker than the subjects who received SET or DET, as measured by the PSI ($P = 0.04$) and APACHE II-based PM ($P = 0.03$). Of special significance was the fact that there was no statistically significant difference between the prevalence of chronic disease states between the SET and DET groups.

Levofloxacin was the most commonly chosen fluoroquinolone (70.4%), with only four subjects treated with ciprofloxacin (1 in the SET group, 2 in the DET group, and 1 in the MET group, all with no fatalities). Eight subjects who received more than one antibiotic agent as empirical therapy were classified as SET on the basis of the isolate being resistant to azithromycin (5 subjects), cefotaxime (2 subjects), or combined ticarcillin-clavulanate potassium (1 subject). Twenty-nine subjects (12.9%) died. A Kaplan-Meier plot of mortality over time for each antibiotic therapy group demonstrated that mortality with the SET group was significantly higher than with the DET group (P = 0.02; OR, 3.0 [95% CI, 1.2-7.6]). Even when the DET and MET groups are combined, the mortality was still significantly higher in the SET group (P = 0.04; OR, 2.3 [95% CI, 1.0-5.2]). Because only a few subjects received MET and the subjects who received MET were significantly sicker than the other subjects, subsequent analysis is confined to the SET and DET groups.

Because subjects who received SET had a lower PM than those who received DET, a logistic regression model was used to calculate the OR for death of SET vs. DET adjusted for PM, which was 6.4 (95% CI, 1.9-21.7). All deaths occurred in patients with a PSI score higher than 90 (PSI classes IV and V). In subjects with PSI class IV or V CAP who were given SET, the PM-adjusted OR for death was 5.5 (95% CI, 1.7-17.5). Because antibiotic therapy would be expected to have little influence on early deaths, the investigators reanalyzed SET vs. DET groups after excluding all deaths that occurred within 48 hours of presentation (n = 4, 3 in the SET group and 1 in the DET group). Univariate analysis of this subgroup showed a trend to better outcome with DET compared with SET (94% survival vs 85%, respectively; P = 0.06). Multivariate analysis again confirmed that SET was an independent predictor of worse outcome (P = 0.01), with the PM-adjusted odds ratio for death in subjects given SET being 4.9 (95% CI, 1.6-18.3). Subgroup analysis did not show any significant trends to suggest any advantage or disadvantage of any specific antibiotic agents or combinations of antibiotic agents within the SET or DET groups.

Of the 225 patients with CAP who were identified, 99 were classified as receiving SET, 102 as receiving DET, and 24 as receiving MET. Compared with the other groups, patients who received MET statistically had significantly more severe pneumonia as measured by the PSI score (P = 0.04) and predicted mortality (P = 0.03). Mortality within the SET group was significantly higher than within the DET group (P = 0.02; OR, 3.0 [95% confidence intervals, 1.2-7.6]), even when the DET and MET groups (P = 0.04) were combined. In a logistic regression model including antibiotic therapy and clinical risk factors for mortality, SET remained an independent predictor of mortality with a predicted mortality-adjusted odds ratio of death of 6.4 (95% CI, 1.9-21.7). All deaths occurred in patients with a PSI score higher than 90, and the predicted mortality-adjusted odds ratio for death with SET in this subgroup was 5.5 (95% CI, 1.7-17.5).

In comparably matched patients, this group found that SET is associated with a significantly greater risk of death than DET. On the basis of these results, they concluded that monotherapy may be suboptimal for patients with severe bacteremic pneumococcal pneumonia who have PSI scores of greater than 90.[5]

While acknowledging its limitations, the results of this retrospective study strongly suggest that bacteremic patients with pneumococcal CAP who receive at least two effective antibiotic agents within the first 24 hours after presentation to a hospital have a significantly lower mortality than patients who receive only one effective antibiotic agent. In fact, among high-risk patients (PSI classes IV or V), receiving only one effective antibiotic agent increases mortality by more than five-fold as compared with patients receiving two effective antibiotic agents. Although these findings need to be confirmed by a prospective study, the authors suggest that current approaches to the empirical therapy of severe CAP may need to be reevaluated.[5] Accordingly, the ASCAP 2002 Consensus Panel evaluated this study and found its results and conclusions—as well as its clinical implications—to be sufficiently compelling to recommend combination therapy with ceftriaxone plus a macrolide as the initial approach-of-choice in managing moderately-to-severely ill patients suspected of having bacteremia associated with pneumococcal pneumonia.

Extended Spectrum Fluoroquinolones: Intensification of Coverage and Patient Selection

The extended spectrum quinolones, moxifloxacin, levofloxacin, and gatifloxacin, are indicated for treatment of CAP. Each of these agents is available as an oral and intravenous preparation. Quinolones have been associated with cartilage damage in animal studies; therefore, they are not recommended for use in children, adolescents, and pregnant and nursing women.

Moxifloxacin. Among the new fluoroquinolones, moxifloxacin has the lowest MICs against *S. pneumoniae* and more specific gram-positive coverage; therefore, it is recommended by the ASCAP Consensus Panel as the fluoroquinolone of choice—when a fluoroquinolone is indicated—for managing patients suspected of CAP caused by *S. pneumoniae.* Moxifloxacin is generally well tolerated. In clinical trials, the most common adverse events were nausea (8%), diarrhea (6%), dizziness (3%), headache (2%), abdominal pain (2%), and vomiting (2%). The agent is contraindicated in persons with a history of hypersensitivity to moxifloxacin or any quinolone antibiotic. The safety and effectiveness of moxifloxacin in pediatric patients, adolescents (> age 18), pregnant women, and lactating women have not been established.

Although clinical reports of clinical problems are rare, moxifloxacin has been shown to prolong the QT interval of the electrocardiogram in some patients. The drug should be avoided in patients with known prolongation of the QT interval, patients with uncorrected hypokalemia, and patients receiving Class lA (e.g., quinidine, procainamide) or Class III (e.g., amiodarone, sotalol) antiarrhythmic agents due to the lack of clinical experience with the drug in these patient populations. Pharmacokinetic studies between moxifloxacin and other drugs that prolong the QT interval such as cisapride, erythromycin, antipsychotics, and tricyclic antidepressants have not been performed. An additive effect of moxifloxacin and these drugs cannot be excluded; therefore, moxifloxacin should be used with caution when given concurrently with these drugs.

The effect of moxifloxacin on patients with congenital prolongation of the QT interval has not been studied; however, it is expected that these individuals may be more susceptible to drug-induced QT prolongation. Because of limited clinical experience, moxifloxacin should be used with caution in patients with ongoing proarrhythmic conditions, such as clinically significant bradycardia or acute myocardial ischemia. As with all quinolones, moxifloxacin should be used with caution in patients with known or suspected CNS disorders or in the presence of other risk factors that may predispose to seizures or lower the seizure threshold.

Gatifloxacin. Gatifloxacin, a broad-spectrum 8-methoxy fluoroquinolone antibiotic, has been approved for the safe and effective treatment of approved indications, including community-acquired respiratory tract infections, such as bacterial exacerbation of chronic bronchitis (ABE/COPD); acute sinusitis; and CAP caused by indicated, susceptible strains of gram-positive and gram-negative bacteria. The recommended dose for gatifloxacin is 400 mg once daily, for all individuals with normal renal function. Dosage adjustment is required in patients with impaired renal function (creatinine clearance, < 40 mL/min).

Gatifloxacin is primarily excreted through the kidneys and less than 1% is metabolized by the liver. In clinical trials, gatifloxacin has been found to be a well-tolerated treatment in 15 international clinical trials at 500 study sites. Gatifloxacin may have the potential to prolong the QTc interval of the electrocardiogram in some patients, and due to limited clinical experience, gatifloxacin should be avoided in patients with known prolongation of the QTc interval, in patients with uncorrected hypokalemia, and in patients receiving Class IA (e.g., quinidine, procainamide) or Class III (e.g., amiodarone, sotalol) antiarrhythmic agents. Gatifloxacin should be used with caution when given together with drugs that may prolong the QTc interval (e.g., cisapride, erythromycin, antipsychotics, tricyclic antidepressants), and in patients with ongoing proarrhythmic conditions (e.g., clinically significant bradycardia or acute myocardial ischemia).

Gatifloxacin should be used with caution in patients with known or suspected CNS disorders or patients who have a predisposition to seizures. The most common side effects associated with gatifloxacin in clinical trials were gastrointestinal. Adverse reactions considered to be drug related and occurring in greater than 3% of patients were: nausea (8%), vaginitis (6%), diarrhea (4%), headache (3%), and dizziness (3%).

Oral doses of gatifloxacin should be administered at least four hours before the administration of ferrous sulfate; dietary supplements containing zinc, magnesium, or iron (such as multivitamins); aluminum/magnesium-containing antacids; or Videx (didanosine, or ddI). Concomitant administration of gatifloxacin and probencid significantly increases systemic exposure to gatifloxacin. Concomitant administration of gatifloxacin and digoxin did not produce significant alteration of the pharmacokinetics of gatifloxacin; however, patients taking digoxin should be monitored for signs and/or symptoms of digoxin toxicity.

Levofloxacin. Levofloxacin, the S-enantiomer of ofloxacin, is a fluoroquinolone antibiotic that, when compared with older quinolones, also has improved activity against gram-positive organisms, including *Streptococcus pneumoniae.* This has important drug selection implications for the management of patients with CAP and exacerbations of COPD. The active stereoisomer of ofloxacin, levofloxacin is available in a parenteral preparation or as a once daily oral preparation that is given for 7-14 days. Levofloxacin is well-tolerated, with the most common side effects including nausea, diarrhea, headache, and constipation. Food does not affect the absorption of the drug, but it should be taken at least two hours before or two hours after antacids containing magnesium or aluminum, as well as sucralfate, metal cations such as iron, and multivitamin preparations with zinc. Dosage adjustment for levofloxacin is recommended in patients with impaired renal function (clearance < 50 mL/min).

Although no significant effect of levofloxacin on plasma concentration of theophylline was detected in 14 health volunteers studied, because other quinolones have produced increases in patients taking concomitant theophylline, theophylline levels should be closely monitored in patients on levofloxacin and dosage adjustments made as necessary. Monitoring patients on warfarin also is recommended in patients on quinolones.

When given orally, levofloxacin is dosed once daily, is well absorbed orally, and penetrates well into lung tissue.[114] It is active against a wide range of respiratory pathogens, including atypical pathogens and many species of *S. pneumoniae* resistant to penicillin.[115,116] In general, levofloxacin has greater activity against gram-positive organisms than ofloxacin and is slightly less active than ciprofloxacin against gram-negative organisms.[117,118]

Levofloxacin is available in both oral and parenteral forms, and the oral and IV routes are interchangeable (i.e., same dose). Levofloxacin is generally well tolerated (incidence of adverse reactions, < 7%). Levofloxacin is supplied in a parenteral form for IV use and in 250 mg and 500 mg tablets. The recommended dose is 500 mg IV or orally qd for 7-14 days for lower respiratory tract infections. All quinolones have been associated with cartilage damage in animal studies, and therefore, they are not recommended for use in children, adolescents, and pregnant and nursing women.

Levofloxacin is indicated for the treatment of adults (> 18 years) with mild, moderate, and severe pulmonary infections, including acute bacterial exacerbation of chronic bronchitis and CAP.[119] It is active against many gram-positive organisms that may infect the lower respiratory tract, including *S. pneumoniae* and *Staphylococcus aureus,* and it also covers atypical pathogens, including *Chlamydia pneumoniae, Legionella pneumophila,* and *Mycoplasma pneumoniae.* It also is active against gram-negative organisms, including *E. coli, H. influenzae, H. parainfluenzae, Klebsiella pneumoniae,* and *Moraxella catarrhalis.* Although it is active against *Pseudomonas aeruginosa* in vitro and carries an indication for treatment of complicated UTI caused by *Pseudomonas aeruginosa,* levofloxacin does not have an official indication for CAP caused by this gram-negative organism.

Several studies and surveillance data suggest that some newly available, expanded spectrum fluoroquinolones, including levofloxacin (which is approved for PRSP), are efficacious for the treatment of *S. pneumoniae,* including penicillin-resistant strains.[2,29,120] In one study, microbiologic eradication from sputum was reported among all 300 patients with pneumococcal pneumonia treated with oral levofloxacin.[29] In a study of in vitro susceptibility of *S. pneumoniae* clinical isolates to levofloxacin, none of the 180 isolates (including 60 isolates with intermediate susceptibility to penicillin and 60 penicillin-resistant isolates) was resistant to this agent.[120] In addition, a surveillance study of antimicrobial resistance in respiratory tract pathogens found levofloxacin was active against 97% of 9190 pneumococcal isolates and found no cross-resistance with penicillin, amoxicillin-clavulanate, ceftriaxone, cefuroxime, or clarithromycin.

Fluoroquinolones: Resistance Concerns and Over-Extended Spectrum of Coverage. Despite high level activity against pneumococcal isolates and a formal indication for levofloxacin use in suspected DRSP lower respiratory tract infection, the CDC-DRSPWG recent guidelines do not advocate the use of expanded spectrum fluoroquinolones (among them, levofloxacin) for first-line, empiric treatment of pneumonia.

This is because of the following: 1) their broad, perhaps, over-extended spectrum of coverage that includes a wide range of gram-negative organisms; 2) concern that resistance among pneumococci will emerge if there is widespread use of this class of antibiotics; 3) their activity against pneumococci with high penicillin resistance (MIC = 4 mcg/mL) makes it important that they be reserved for selected patients with CAP; 4) use of fluoroquinolones has been shown to result in increased resistance to *S. pneumoniae* in vitro; and 5) population-based surveillance in the United States has shown a statistically significant increase in ofloxacin resistance among pneumococcal isolates between Jan. 1, 1995, and Dec. 31, 1997 (unpublished data, Active Bacterial Core Surveillance, CDC).[2]

The CDC-DRSPWG concerns about inducing fluoroquinolone resistance not only to *S. pneumoniae,* but also to other pathogenic organisms has support in the medical literature.[121-123] Individual fluoroquinolone use in U.S. hospitals, as measured by inpatient dispensing, is changing over time. Selective pressure exerted by fluoroquinolone use may be causally related to the prevalence of ciprofloxacin resistant *P. aeruginosa.* In fact, databases support growing concern about emerging fluoroquinolone resistance. In this regard, recent NNIS surveillance data indicates that resistance for *P. aeruginosa* to fluoroquinolones is increasing, possibly as a result of increasing use of this drug class.[121-123] To shed light in this possible associate, the SCOPE-MMIT network of 35 hospitals tracked inpatient fluoroquinolones dispensing since 1999, and obtained hospital antibiograms to assess for associations between use and resistance rates.

MediMedia Information Technology (MMIT, North Wales, PA) collected data of inpatient-dispensed drugs from each participating hospital information system. Grams of individual fluoroquinolones are converted each quarter to defined daily dose/1000 patient days (DDD/1000PD). Antibiograms (1999) testing susceptibility of *P. aeruginosa* to ciprofloxacin were available from 22 hospitals. The relationship between total fluoroquinolone use and percentage resistance for *P. aeruginosa* to ciprofloxacin was assessed by linear regression. Results indicated that total fluoroquinolone use between 1999 and 2001 remained at ~ 140DDD/1000PD, although mean levofloxacin increased significantly and ciprofloxacin use declined slightly. There was a significant positive relationship between total fluoroquinolone use and resistance to *P. aeruginosa* ($r = 0.54$, $P = 0.01$).

Investigators concluded that mean total fluoroquinolone dispensing in the 35 hospitals studied was stable, although there were significant differences in use between individual fluoroquinolones. There was a positive relationship between total fluoroquinolone use and resistance to ciprofloxacin for *P. aeruginosa,* but it was not yet possible to determine if the relationship was causal or which fluoroquinolones are most likely responsible. The SCOPE-MMIT network will continue to evaluate the quantitative relationships between antibiotic use and resistance as antibiotic use changes over time, and as resistance rates respond to these changes in selective pressure.[121-123]

Fluoroquinolones and MRSA. Methicillin-resistant *Staphylococcus aureus* (MRSA) is a substantial problem in antibiotic therapy, and its origin is now recognized to be both from the hospital and the community.[1] There are a variety of well-known risk factors for the development of MRSA in the hospital, including extensive prior broad-spectrum antibiotic use, admission to an ICU, prolonged hospitalization, presence of an indwelling catheter, severe comorbid diseases, surgery, and exposure to MRSA-colonized patients. However, there has arisen a substantial amount of new data that fluoroquinolones are a risk factor for the increase in MRSA. Given the widespread use of oral fluoroquinolones in the community over the last several years, and the increase in community-acquired MRSA, it is prudent to consider the possibility that fluoroquinolone overuse may be associated with increasing emergence of MRSA.[124]

To address this question, one study evaluated prior antibiotic exposure and the development of nosocomial MRSA bacteremia in patients admitted to a 750-bed tertiary care hospital.[124] All patients with nosocomial bacteremias from Jan. 1, 1996, to June 30, 1999, were evaluated. For each patient, investigators documented all antibiotics administered prior to the development of the bacteremia. They performed a case-controlled evaluation comparing fluoroquinolone-exposed patients to non-fluoroquinolone-exposed patients in relation to the development of MRSA bacteremia. A chi-squared analysis and relative risk (RR) were calculated.

A total of 514 nosocomial bacteremias occurred over the study period with 78 (15%) MRSA. The percentage of MRSA bacteremias/nosocomial bacteremias increased from 10% in 1996 to 22% in 1999 (P < 0.05). MRSA as a percent of all *S. aureus* clinical isolates increased from 29% to 40%. Prior fluoroquinolone exposure and MRSA bacteremia rose significantly from 25% of cases in 1986 to 65% of cases in 1999 (40% fluoroquinolone alone and 25% fluoroquinolone and other antibiotics) (P < 0.05). Cephalosporin exposure alone and the development of MRSA bacteremia dropped significantly from 50% of cases in 1996 to 0% of cases in 1999 (P < 0.01). Overall, 52% of fluoroquinolone-exposed patients developed MRSA bacteremia vs. 8% methicillin-sensitive *S. aureus* (MSSA) bacteremia (P < 0.05). In 1996 the RR of fluoroquinolone exposure and the development of MRSA bacteremia was 2.27 (ns), whereas during 1997-99 the RR of fluoroquinolone exposure was significant, ranging from 3.25 to 4.68 (P < 0.05). Fluoroquinolone usage increased hospital-wide over the study period.[124]

The study group noted a significant increase in nosocomial MRSA bacteremias in fluoroquinolone-exposed patients and a significant decrease in patients with cephalosporin exposure over the study period. fluoroquinolone-exposed patients had a 3-4 times greater risk of developing nosocomial MRSA bacteremia than non-fluoroquinolone-exposed patients. Because increasing fluoroquinolone usage may have contributed to the increased selection and development of MRSA bacteremias, the study group implemented policies to limit fluoroquinolone utilization to attempt to control the selection and development of nosocomial MRSA bacteremias in the future.[124]

Selective Fluoroquinolone Use. Based on observational, surveillance, and other published data and emerging trends, from a practical, drug selection perspective, the CDC-DRSP-WG has recommended that fluoroquinolones be reserved for selected patients with CAP, and these experts have identified specific patient subgroups that are eligible for initial treatment with extended-spectrum fluoroquinolones such as levofloxacin. For hospitalized patients, these include adults and elderly patients for whom one of the first-line regimens (cephalosporin plus a macrolide) has failed, those who are allergic to the first-line agents, or those who have a documented infection with highly drug-resistant pneumococci (i.e., penicillin MIC = 4 mcg/mL).[84]

Whereas, until recently, fluoroquinolone resistance to *Streptococcus pneumoniae* was not considered an urgent clinical issue, the *Morbidity and Mortality Weekly Report* recently reported the appearance of, and increasing levels of, fluoroquinolone resistance to what was once a susceptible organism. Ofloxacin-resistance of 3.1% in 1995 had increased to 4.5% in 1997 (P = 0.02), whereas levofloxacin-resistance of 0.2% in 1998 was reported to be 0.3% in 1999 (P value not significant).[125]

In support of the CDC-DRSPWG's position on restricting fluoroquinolone use, the editors of *Morbidity and Mortality Weekly Report* also report that while prescriptions in the United States for all antibiotics decreased between 1993 and 1998, the prescriptions for fluoroquinolones increased from 3.1 to 4.6 prescriptions per 100 persons per year, respectively, thus greatly increasing the exposure to these broad spectrum agents.[125]

For this reason, the *Morbidity and Mortality Weekly Report* concluded that, "appropriate use of antibiotics is crucial for slowing the emergence of fluoroquinolone resistance." It is for these reasons, plus concerns for increased gram-negative resistance to fluoroquinolones, that specific recommendations were issued from the CDC-DRSPWG. This recommendation, in essence, reserved fluoroquinolone use to patients who were allergic to first-line therapy, who had failed first-line therapy, or who had proven high level (MIC ≥ 4 mcg/mL) penicillin resistance. This report also does not recommend fluoroquinolone monotherapy for critically ill persons with pneumococcal pneumonia, because its efficacy in such patients has not been established.[125]

Empiric Antibiotic Coverage for CAP: Matching Drugs with Patient Profiles

A variety of antibiotics are available for outpatient management of pneumonia. Although the selection process can be daunting, as mentioned, a sensible approach to antibiotic selection for patients with pneumonia is provided by treatment categories for pneumonia generated by the Medical Section of the American Lung Association and published under the auspices of the ATS.[30] This classification scheme helps make clinical assessments useful for guiding therapy, but it also is predictive of ultimate prognosis and mortality outcome.

The most common pathogens responsible for causing CAP include the typical bacteria: *S. pneumoniae, H. influenzae,* and *M. catarrhalis,* as well as the atypical pathogens: *Mycoplasma, Legionella,* and *Chlamydia pneumoniae*.[126] *H. influenzae* and *M. catarrhalis* are both found more commonly in patients with COPD. Clinically and radiologically, it is difficult to differentiate between the typical and atypical pathogens; therefore, coverage against all these organisms may be necessary. In patients producing sputum containing polymorphonuclear leukocytes, the sputum Gram's stain may contain a predominant organism to aid in the choice of empiric therapy. For most patients, therapy must be entirely empiric and based on the expected pathogens.[31,127]

Therefore, for the vast majority of otherwise healthy patients who have CAP, but who do not have comorbid conditions and who are deemed well enough to be managed as outpatients, therapy directed toward *S. pneumoniae, H. influenzae, M. pneumoniae, Chlamydia pneumoniae, Legionella pneumophila,* and *M. catarrhalis* is appropriate. From an intensity and spectrum of coverage perspective, coverage of both the aforementioned bacterial and atypical species has become mandatory.

In these cases, one of the newer macrolides should be considered one of the initial agents of choice. The other monotherapeutic agents available consist of the extended spectrum quinolones, which provide similar coverage and carry an indication for initial therapy in this patient subgroup.

For the older patient with CAP who is considered stable enough to be managed as an outpatient, but in whom the bacterial pathogen list also may include gram-negative aerobic organisms, the combined use of a second- or third-generation cephalosporin or amoxicillin-clavulanate plus a macrolide has been recommended. Another option may consist of an advanced generation quinolone.

Some experts emphasize that in non-smoking adults without COPD (i.e., patients at a low risk for having *H. influenzae),* therapy with erythromycin should be strongly considered.[31] This is a matter of clinical judgment, but in any event, the newer macrolides, azithromycin and clarithromycin, are recommended in cases of erythromycin intolerance. In patients with COPD, either TMP-SMX or doxycycline usually provides adequate coverage against *S. pneumoniae* and *H. influenzae,* but TMP-SMX will not cover atypical pathogens.

Use of the older quinolones is not recommended for empiric treatment of community-acquired respiratory infections, primarily because of their variable activity against *S. pneumoniae* and atypical organisms. Although the older quinolones (i.e., ciprofloxacin) generally should not be used for the empiric treatment of CAP, they may provide an important option for treatment of bronchiectasis, particularly when gram-negative organisms such as *Pseudomonas* are cultured from respiratory secretions.[128] In these cases, ciprofloxacin should be used in combination with another anti-pseudomonal agent when indicated.

The most important issue for the emergency physician or pulmonary intensivist is to ensure that the appropriate intensity and spectrum of coverage are provided, according to patient and community/epidemiological risk factors. In many cases, especially when infection with gram-negative organisms is suspected or there is structural lung disease, this will require shifting to and intensifying therapy with an extended spectrum quinolone. However, in most cases of non-ICU patients admitted to the hospital, IV ceftriaxone plus azithromycin IV is recommended, depending on institutional protocols.

In this regard, determining which of these antibiotics (macrolides vs extended spectrum quinolones) should be considered "workhorse" drugs in the ED or hospital setting, for initial CAP treatment requires thoughtful analysis that takes into account cost, convenience, spectrum of coverage, host risk factors, and patient risk stratification.

In the case of azithromycin, its five-day duration of therapy; $39-$42 cost per course of treatment; and targeted coverage of *S. pneumoniae, H. influenzae, M. catarrhalis, Chlamydia,* and *M. pneumoniae* must be weighed against the longer duration and slightly greater cost per treatment course for the quinolones and the fact that their spectrum of coverage includes not only the appropriately targeted, aforementioned organisms commonly implicated in CAP, but also extensive activity against gram-negative organisms, which may not always be required, especially in otherwise healthy individuals. This over-extended spectrum of coverage may exert resistance pressure on gram-negative organisms frequently encountered in a hospital setting; therefore, quinolone use should be risk-stratified to an appropriate subset.

Finally, there is an increasing problem in the United States concerning the emergence of *S. pneumoniae* among hospitalized pneumonia patients that is relatively resistant to penicillin and, less commonly, to extended-spectrum cephalosporins. These isolates also may be resistant to sulfonamides and tetracyclines.[30,129,130] Except for vancomycin, the most favorable in vitro response rates to *S. pneumoniae* are seen with extended spectrum quinolones. Please see Table 1 for a summary of current recommendations for initial management of outpatient and in-hospital management of patients with CAP.

Antimicrobial Therapy and Medical Outcomes. A recent study has helped assess the relationship between initial antimicrobial therapy and medical outcomes for elderly patients hospitalized with pneumonia.[92] In this retrospective analysis, hospital records for 12,945 Medicare inpatients (65 years of age) with pneumonia were reviewed. Associations were identified between the choice of the initial antimicrobial regimen and three-day mortality, adjusting for baseline differences in patient profiles, illness severity, and process of care. Comparisons were made between the antimicrobial regimens and a reference group consisting of patients treated with a non-pseudomonal third-generation cephalosporin alone.

Of the 12,945 patients, 9751 (75.3%) were community-dwelling and 3194 (24.7%) were admitted from a long-term care facility (LCF). Study patients had a mean age of 79.4 years ± 8.1 years, 84.4% were white, and 50.7% were female. As would be expected, the majority (58.1%) of patients had at least one comorbid illness; and 68.3% were in the two highest severity risk classes (IV and V) at initial examination. The most frequently coded bacteriologic pathogens were *S. pneumoniae* (6.6%) and *H. influenzae* (4.1%); 10.1% of patients were coded as having aspiration pneumonia, and in 60.5% the etiologic agent for the pneumonia was unknown.

The three most commonly used initial, empiric antimicrobial regimen in the elderly patient with pneumonia consisted of the following: 1) a non-pseudomonal third-generation cephalosporin only (ceftriaxone, cefotaxime, ceftizoxime) in 26.5%; 2) a second-generation cephalosporin only (cefuroxime) in 12.3%; and 3) a non-pseudomonal third-generation cephalosporin (as above) plus a macrolide in 8.8%. The 30-day mortality was 15.3% (95% CI, 14.6%-15.9%) in the entire study population, ranging from 11.2% (95% CI, 10.6%-11.9%) in community-dwelling elderly patients to 27.5% (95% CI, 26%-29.1%) among patients admitted from a long-term care facility.[92]

As might be predicted, this study of elderly patients with hospitalization for pneumonia demonstrated significant differences in patient survival depending upon the choice of the initial antibiotic regimen. In particular, this national study demonstrated that, compared to a reference group receiving a non-pseudomonal third-generation cephalosporin alone, initial therapy with a non-pseudomonal plus a macrolide, a second generation cephalosporin plus a macrolide, or a fluoroquinolone alone was associated with 26%, 29%, and 36% lower 30-day mortality, respectively. Despite that these regimens are compatible with those recommended by the IDSA and CDC, only 15% of patients received one of the three aforementioned regimens associated with reduced mortality rates.

For reasons that are not entirely clear, patients treated with a beta-lactam/beta-lactamase inhibitor plus a macrolide or an aminoglycoside plus another agent had mortality rates that were 77% and 21% higher than the reference group, respectively.

Role of Specific Pathogens in CAP. Prospective studies evaluating the causes of CAP in elderly adults have failed to identify the cause of 40-60% of cases of CAP, and two or more etiologies have been identified in 2-5% of cases. The most common etiologic agent identified in virtually all studies of CAP in the elderly is *Streptococcus pneumoniae,* and this agent accounts for approximately two-thirds of all cases of bacteremic pneumonia.

Other pathogens implicated less frequently include *H. influenzae* (most isolates of which are other than type B), *Mycoplasma pneumoniae, C. pneumoniae, S. aureus, Streptococcus pyogenes, Neisseria meningitidis, M. catarrhalis, Klebsiella pneumoniae,* and other gram-negative rods, *Legionella* species, influenza virus (depending on the time of year), respiratory syncytial virus, adenovirus, parainfluenza virus, and other microbes. The frequency of other etiologies, (e.g., *Chlamydia psittaci* [psittacosis], *Coxiella burnetii* [Q fever], *Francisella tularensis* [tularemia], and endemic fungi [histoplasmosis, blastomycosis, and coccidioidomycosis]), is dependent on specific epidemiological factors.

The selection of antibiotics, in the absence of an etiologic diagnosis (gram stains and culture results are not diagnostic), is based on multiple variables, including severity of the illness, patient age, antimicrobial intolerance or side effects, clinical features, comorbidities, concomitant medications, exposures, and the epidemiological setting.

Consensus Guidelines for Antibiotic Therapy

Consensus Report Guidelines: Infectious Disease Society of America. The IDSA, through its Practice Guidelines Committee, provides assistance to clinicians in the diagnosis and treatment of CAP. The targeted providers are internists and family practitioners, and the targeted patient groups are immunocompetent adult patients. Criteria are specified for determining whether the inpatient or outpatient setting is appropriate for treatment. Differences from other guidelines written on this topic include use of laboratory criteria for diagnosis and approach to antimicrobial therapy. Panel members and consultants were experts in adult infectious diseases.

The guidelines are evidence-based where possible. A standard ranking system is used for the strength of recommendations and the quality of the evidence cited in the literature reviewed. The document has been subjected to external review by peer reviewers as well as by the Practice Guidelines Committee, and was approved by the IDSA Council in September 2000. *(Please see Table 2.)*

Centers for Disease Control Drug-Resistant *Streptococcus pneumoniae* Therapeutic Working Group (CDC-DRSPWG) Guidelines. One of the important issues in selecting antibiotic therapy for the elderly patient is the emerging problem of DRSP. To address this problem and provide practitioners with specific guidelines for initial antimicrobial selection in these patients, the CDC-DRSPWG convened and published its recommendations in May 2000.[2] Some of the important clinical issues they addressed included the following: 1) what empirical antibiotic combinations (or monotherapeutic options) constituted reasonable initial therapy in outpatients, in hospitalized (non-ICU) patients, and in hospitalized intubated or ICU patients; 2) what clinical criteria, patient risk factors, or regional, epidemiological features constituted sufficient trigger points to include agents with improved activity against DRSP as initial agents of choice; and 3) what antibiotic selection strategies were most appropriate for limiting the emergence of fluoroquinolone-resistant strains.

Their conclusions with respect to antibiotic recommendations overlap significantly with the IDSA recommendations and the existing ATS guidelines. The specific differences contained in the CDC-DRSPWG primarily involve the sequence in which antibiotics should be chosen to limit the emergence of fluoroquinolone-resistant strains, a preference for using combination drug therapy, cautionary notes about using fluoroquinolones as monotherapy in critically ill patients, reserving use of fluoroquinolones for specific patient populations, and detailed guidance regarding the comparative advantages among agents in each class. *(Please see Table 3.)*

Oral macrolide (azithromycin, clarithromycin, or erythromycin) or beta-lactam monotherapy is recommended by the CDC working group as initial therapy in patients with pneumonia who are considered to be amenable to outpatient management. For inpatients not in an ICU (i.e., medical ward disposition), this group recommends for initial therapy the combination of a parenteral beta-lactam (ceftriaxone or cefotaxime) plus a macrolide (azithromycin, erythromycin, etc.).[2] Hence, one of the most important, consistent changes among recent recommendations for initial, empiric management of patients with CAP is mandatory inclusion of a macrolide (which covers atypical pathogens) when a cephalosporin (which has poor activity against atypical pathogens) is selected as part of the initial combination regimen.

For critically ill patients, first-line therapy should include an intravenous beta-lactam, such as ceftriaxone, and an intravenous macrolide such as azithromycin. The option of using a combination of a parenteral beta-lactam (ceftriaxone, etc.) plus a fluoroquinolone with improved activity against DRSP also is presented. Once again, however, this committee issues clarifying, and sometimes cautionary, statements about the role of fluoroquinolone monotherapy in the critically ill patient, stating that caution should be exercised because the efficacy of the new fluoroquinolones as monotherapy for critically ill patients has not been determined.[2]

Clearly, fluoroquinolones are an important part of the

antimicrobial arsenal in the elderly, and the CDC-DRSPWG has issued specific guidelines governing their use in the setting of outpatient and inpatient CAP. It recommends fluoroquinolones be reserved for selected patients with CAP, among them: 1) adults, including elderly patients, for whom one of the first-line regimens (cephalosporin plus a macrolide) has failed; 2) those who are allergic to the first-line agents; or 3) those patients who have a documented infection with highly drug resistant pneumococci (i.e., penicillin MIC > 4 mcg/mL).

Prevention of Deep Venous Thromboembolism (DVT)

Background. Although antibiotic therapy, oxygenation, and maintenance of hemodynamic status are the primary triad of emergency interventions in elderly patients with pneumonia, there has been an increasing recognition of the risk for venous thromboembolic disease (VTED) incurred by immobilized elderly patients with infections such as pneumonia, especially when accompanied by CHF and/or respiratory failure. Emergency physicians, as well as attending physicians admitting such patients to the hospital, should be aware that the risk of VTED is significant enough to require prophylaxis in elderly patients with CAP who are likely to be immobilized for a period of three days or more (i.e., can ambulate less than 10 meters per day), and who have such risk factors as obesity, previous history of VTED, cancer, varicose veins, hormone therapy, chronic heart failure (NYHA Class III-IV), or chronic respiratory failure.[131]

From a practical perspective, this subset of patients should be strongly considered for prophylaxis to reduce the risk of VTED. Based on recent studies, the presence of pneumonia in a patient age 75 or older is, in itself, a criterion for prophylaxis against VTED; when these factors are accompanied by CHF (Class III-IV) or respiratory failure, prophylaxis should be considered mandatory if there are no significant contraindications.[131] It should be added that The American College of Chest Physicians (ACCP) guidelines[132] and International Consensus Statement[133] also cite risk factors for VTED and emphasize their importance when assessing prophylaxis requirements for medical patients.

Evidence for Prophylaxis. The data to support a prophylactic approach to VTED for serious infections in the elderly is growing. The studies with subcutaneous unfractionated heparin (UFH) are inconclusive, although this agent is used for medical prophylaxis. Despite the recognition of risk factors and the availability of effective means for prophylaxis, DVT and PE remain common causes of morbidity and mortality. It is estimated that approximately 600,000 patients per year are hospitalized for DVT in North America.[134] In the United States, symptomatic PE occurs in more than 600,000 patients and causes or contributes to death in up to 200,000 patients annually.[135]

With respect to the risk of VTED in older patients with infection, one study group randomized infectious disease patients ages older than 55 years to UFH 5000 IU bid or placebo for three weeks. Autopsy was available in 60% of patients who died. Deaths from PE were significantly delayed in the UFH group, but the six-week mortality rate was similar in both groups. Non-fatal VTE was reduced by UFH. The findings of previous trials of prophylaxis in medical patients have been controversial, as the patient populations and methods used to detect thromboembolism and the dose regimens vary, undermining the value of the findings. Comparative studies with clearly defined populations and reliable end points were therefore required to determine appropriate patient subgroups for antithrombotic therapy.[136]

The MEDENOX Trial. In response to the need for evidence to clarify the role of prophylaxis in specific non-surgical patient sub groups, the MEDENOX (prophylaxis in MEDical patients with ENOXaparin) trial was conducted using the low molecular weight heparin (LMWH) enoxaparin in a clearly identified risk groups.[131] In contrast to previous investigations, the MEDENOX trial included a clearly defined patient population (patients immobilized with severe chest [cardiopulmonary] disease), and was designed to answer questions about the need for prophylaxis in this group of medical patients and to determine the optimal dose of LMWH.[131]

Patients in the MEDENOX trial were randomized to receive enoxaparin, 20 or 40 mg subcutaneously, or placebo once daily, beginning within 24 hours of randomization. They were treated for 10 (4 days in hospital and followed up in person or by telephone contact on day 90 [range, day 83-110]). During follow-up, patients were instructed to report any symptoms or signs of VTE or any other clinical events. The primary and secondary efficacy end points for MEDENOX were chosen to allow an objective assessment of the risk of VTE in the study population and the extent of any benefit of prophylaxis. The primary end point was any venous thromboembolic event between day 1 and day 14. All patients underwent systematic bilateral venography at day 10 or earlier if clinical signs of DVT were observed. Venous ultrasonography was performed if venography was not possible. Suspected PE was confirmed by high probability lung scan, pulmonary angiography, helical computerized tomography, or at autopsy.[131] The primary safety end points were hemorrhagic events, death, thrombocytopenia, or other adverse event or laboratory abnormalities.[131]

A total of 1102 patients were included in the MEDENOX trial, in 60 centers and nine countries. The study excluded patients who were intubated or in septic shock. Overall, the mean age was 73.4, the gender distribution was 50:50 male/female, and the mean body mass index was 25.0. The mean patient ages, gender distribution, and body mass index were similar in all three treatment groups; there were slightly more males than females in the placebo and enoxaparin 20 mg groups, and more females than males in the enoxaparin 40 mg group, but this difference was not significant. The reasons for hospitalization of randomized patients varied.

The majority of patients were hospitalized for acute cardiac failure, respiratory failure, or infectious disease, with pneumonia being the most common infection in those older than age 70. For the study population as a whole, the most prevalent risk factor in addition to the underlying illness was advanced age (50.4%). By day 14, the incidence of VTE was 14.9% in the placebo group and 5.5% in the enoxaparin 40 mg group, representing a significant 63% relative risk reduction (97% CI: 37-78%; P = 0.0002) in VTE.

The primary conclusions of the MEDENOX trial can be applied directly to clinical practice. First, acutely ill elderly medical patients with cardiopulmonary or infectious disease are at significant risk of VTE. Second, enoxaparin, given once daily at a dose of 40 mg for 6-14 days reduces the risk of VTE by 63%; and third, the reduction in thromboembolic risk is achieved without increasing the frequency of hemorrhage, thrombocytopenia, or any other adverse event compared with placebo. This study strongly suggests that elderly, immobilized patients admitted to the hospital with severe pneumonia, especially if accompanied by respiratory failure or Class III-IV CHF, should, if there are no contraindications to the use of anticoagulants, be considered candidates for prophylaxis with enoxaparin, 40 mg SC qd upon admission to the hospital to prevent VTED.

—Acknowledgement: The ASCAP 2002 Panel Members sincerely thank Dr. Donald Low, Mount Sinai Hospital and Toronto Medical Laboratories, Department of Microbiology, for his analysis, research, and contributions to the sections on emerging fluoroquinolone resistance and its clinical implications.

The ASCAP Panel*

Panel Members: **Gideon Bosker, MD, FACEP,** Section of Emergency Medicine, Yale University School of Medicine and Oregon Health Sciences University, ASCAP Panel Moderator and Chairman, Editor-in-Chief, *Emergency Medicine Reports;* **Charles Emerman, MD, FACEP,** ASCAP Panel Associate Chairman, Chairman, Department of Emergency Medicine, Cleveland Clinic Hospitals and Metro Health Center, Cleveland, Ohio; **Stephen Ernest, PharmD,** Clinical Pharmacist, Infectious Diseases; **John Gums, PharmD,** Professor, Departments of Pharmacology and Medicine, University of Florida, Gainesville; **Dave Howes, MD, FACEP,** Program Director and Chairman, Residency Program, Department of Emergency Medicine, University of Chicago Hospitals and Clinics, Associate Professor, Pritzker School of Medicine; **Kurt Kleinschmidt, MD, FACEP,** Associate Professor, Department of Emergency Medicine, University of Texas Southwestern Medical School, Parkland Memorial Medical Center, Dallas, Texas; **David Lang, DO,** Operations Medical Director, Department of Emergency Medicine, Mt. Sinai Medical Center, Miami, Florida; **Sandra Schneider, MD, FACEP,** Professor and Chairman, Department of Emergency Medicine, University of Rochester/Strong Memorial Hospital, Rochester, New York; and **Gregory A. Volturo, MD, FACEP,** Vice Chairman and Associate Professor, Department of Emergency Medicine, University of Massachusetts Medical School, Worcester, Massachusetts.

*** ASCAP—Antibiotic Selection for Community-Acquired Pneumonia**

References

1. Sue DY. Community-acquired pneumonia in adults. *West J Med* 1994;161:383-389.
2. Heffelfinger JD, Dowell SF, et al. A report from the Drug-resistant *Streptococcus pneumoniae* Therapeutic Working Group. Management of community-acquired pneumonia in the era of pneumococcal resistance. *Arch Int Med* 2000;160:1399.
3. Bartlett JG, Mundy M. Community-acquired pneuominia. *N Engl J Med* 1995;333:1618-1624.
4. Fine MD, Smith MA, et al. Prognosis and outcomes of patients with community acquired pneumonia. A meta-analysis. *JAMA* 1996;275:134-141.
5. Waterer GW, Somes GW, Wunderink RG. Monotherapy may be suboptimal for severe bacteremic pneumococcal pneumonia. *Arch Intern Med* 2001;161:1837-1842.
6. Niederman MS, McCombs JS, Unger AN, et al. The cost of treating community-acquired pneumonia. *Clin Therapeut* 1998;20: 820-837.
7. Medicare and Medicaid statistical supplement, 1995. *Health Care Financ Rev* 1995:16.
8. Fine MJ, Smith MA, Carson CA, et al. Prognosis and outcomes of patients with community-acquired pneumonia. *JAMA* 1995;274: 134-141.
9. American Thoracic Society: Guidelines for the Initial Management of Adults with Community-Acquired Pneumonia: Diagnosis, assessment of severity, and initial antimicrobial therapy. *Am Rev Respir Dis* 1993;148:1418-1426.
10. Confalonieri M, Potena A, Carbone G, et al. Acute respiratory failure in patients with severe community-acquired pneumonia. A prospective randomized evaluation of noninvasive ventilation. *Am J Respir Crit Care Med* 1999;160:1585-1591.
11. Hoe LK, Keang LT. Hospitalized low-risk community-acquired pneumonia: Outcome and potential for cost-savings. *Respirology* 1999;4:307-309.
12. Marrie TJ, Lau CY, Wheeler SL, et al. A controlled trial of a critical pathway for treatment of community-acquired pneumonia. *JAMA* 2000;283:749-755.
13. Dean NC, Suchyta MR, Bateman KA. Implementation of admission decision support for community-acquired pneumonia. A pilot study. *Chest* 2000;117:1368-1377.
14. Davis DA, Thomason MA, Oxman AD, et al. Evidence for the effectiveness of CME. A review of 50 randomized controlled trials. *JAMA* 1992;268:111-1117.
15. Lomas J, Anderson GM, Domnick-Pierre KD, et al. Do practice guidelines guide practice? The effect of a consensus statement on the practice of physicians. *N Engl J Med* 1989;321:1306-1311.
16. Gleicher N. Cesarean section rates in the United States: The short-term failure of the national consensus development conference in 1980. *JAMA* 1984;252:3273-3276.
17. Greco PJ, Eisenberg JM. Changing physician's practices. *N Engl J Med* 1993;329:1271-1273.
18. Mittman BS, Tonesk X, Jacobson PD. Implementing clinical practice guidelines. *Qual Rev Bull* 1992;18:413-422.
19. Tunis SR, Hayward RSA, Wilson MC, et al. Internists' attitudes about clinical practice guidelines. *Ann Intern Med* 1994;120: 956-963.

20. Marrie TJ. Community-acquired pneumonia: Epidemiology, etiology, treatment. *Infect Dis Clinic North Am* 1998;12:723-740.
21. Bates JH, Campbell AL, et al. Microbial etiology of acute pneumonia in hospitalized patients. *Chest* 1992;101:1005-1012.
22. Fang GD, Fine M, Orloff, et al. New and emerging etiologies for community-acquired pneumonia with implications for therapy-prospective multicenter study of 359 cases. *Medicine* 1990;69: 307-316.
23. Antibiotic Update 1998: Outcome-effective treatment for bacterial infections managed in the primary care and emergency department setting. *Emerg Med Rep* 1997;18:1-24.
24. Fang GD, Fine M, Orloff J, et al. New and emerging etiologies for community-acquired pneumonia with implications for therapy. *Medicine* 1990;69:307-316.
25. Plouffe J, Schwartz DB, Kolokathis A, et al. Clinical efficacy of intravenous followed by oral azithromycin monotherapy in hospitalized patients with community-acquired pneumonia. *Antimicrob Agents Chemother* 2000;44:1796-1802.
26. Vergis EN, Indorf A, et al. Azithromycin vs cefuroxime plus erythromycin for empirical treatment of community-acquired pneumonia in hospitalized patients. A prospective, randomized, multicenter trial. *Arch Int Med* 2000;160:1294-1300.
27. The choice of antibacterial drugs. *Med Lett Drugs Ther* 1996;38: 25-34.
28. Clarithromycin and azithromycin. *Med Lett Drugs Ther* 1992;34: 45-47.
29. File TM, Dunbar L, et al. A multicenter, randomized study comparing the efficacy and safety of intravenous and/or oral levofloxacin versus ceftriaxone and/or cefuroxime in treatment of adults with community-acquired pneumonia. *Antimicrob Agents Chemother* 1997;41:1965-1972.
30. American Thoracic Society, Medical Section of the American Lung Association. *Am Rev Respir Dis* 1993;148:1418-1426.
31. American Thoracic Society. Guidelines for the initial management of adults with community-acquired pneumonia: Diagnosis, assessment of severity, and initial antimicrobial therapy. *Am Rev Respir Dis* 1993;148:1418-1426.
32. Flanders WD, Tucker G, Krishnadasan A, et al. Validation of the pneumonia severity index: Importance of study-specific recalibration. *J Gen Intern Med* 1999;14:333-340.
33. Fine MJ, Auble TE, Yealy DM, et al. A prediction rule to identify low-risk patients with community-acquired pneumonia. *N Engl J Med* 1997;336:243-250.
34. Auble TE, Yealy DM, Fine MJ. Assessing prognosis and selecting an initial site of care for adults with community-acquired pneumonia. *Infect Dis Clin North Am* 1998;2:741-759.
35. Dean NC. Use of prognostic scoring and outcome assessment tools in the admission decision for community-acquired pneumonia. *Clin Chest Med* 1999;20:521-529.
36. Farr BM, Sloman AJ, Fisch MJ. Predicting death in patients hospitalized for community-acquired pneumonia. *Ann Intern Med* 1991;
115:428-436.
37. Conte HA, Chen YT, Mehal W, et al. A prognostic rule for elderly patients admitted with community-acquired pneumonia. *Am J Med* 1999;106:20-28.
38. Ewig S, Kleinfeld T, Bauer T, et al. Comparative validation of prognostic rules for community-acquired pneumonia in an elderly population. *Eur Respir J* 1999;14:370-375.
39. Mylotte JM, Naughton B, Saludades C, et al. Validation and application of the pneumonia prognosis index to nursing home residents with pneumonia. *JAGS* 1998;46:1538-1544.
40. Atlas SJ, Benzer TI, Borowsky LH, et al. Safely increasing the proportion of patients with community-acquired pneumonia treated as outpatients. An interventional trial. *Arch Intern Med* 1998; 158:1350-1356.
41. Ewig S, Ruiz M, Mensa J, et al. Severe community-acquired pneumonia. Assessment of severity criteria. *Am J Respir Crit Care Med* 1998;158:1102-1108.
42. Marston BJ, Plouffe JF, et al. Incidence of community-acquired pneumonia requiring hospitalization. Results of a population-based active surveillance study in Ohio. The Community-Based Pneumonia Incidence Study Group. *Arch Int Med* 1997;157: 1709-1718.
43. Marsten. *JAMA* 1997;2780-2080.
44. Brentsson E, Lagergard T. Etiology of community-acquired pneumonia in outpatients. *Eur J Clin Microbiol* 1986;5:446-447.
45. Whitney CG, Barrett N, et al. Increasing prevalence of drug-resistant *Streptococcus pneumoniae* (DRSP): Implications for therapy for pneumonia. In: Programs and Abstracts of the 36th Annual Meeting of the Infectious Disease Society of America, Nov. 12-15, 1998. IDSA, Abstract 51.
46. Ball AP. Overview of clinical experience with ciprofloxacin. *Eur J Clin Microbiol* 1986;5:214-219.
47. Fass RJ. Efficacy and safety of oral ciprofloxacin in the treatment of serious respiratory infections. *Am J Med* 1986;82:202-207.
48. Davies BI, Maesen FP, Baur C. Ciprofloxacin in the treatment of acute exacerbations of chronic bronchitis. *Eur J Clin Microbiol* 1986;5:226-231.
49. Hoogkamp-Korstanje JA, Klein SJ. Ciprofloxacin in acute exacerbations of chronic bronchitis. *J Antimicrob Chemother* 1986;18: 407-413.
50. Maesen FP, Davies BI, Geraedts WH, et al. The use of quinolones in respiratory tract infections. *Drugs* 1987;34(Suppl 1):74-79.
51. Thys JP. Quinolones in the treatment of bronchopulmonary infections. *Rev Infect Dis* 1988;10(Suppl 1):S212-S217.
52. Cooper B, Lawlor M. Pneumococcal bacteremia during ciprofloxacin therapy for pneumococcal pneumonia [see comments]. *Am J Med* 1989;87:475.
53. Gordon JJ, Kauffman CA. Superinfection with *Streptococcus pneumoniae* during therapy with ciprofloxacin. *Am J Med* 1990; 89:383-384.
54. Lee BL, Kimbrough RC, Jones SR, et al. Infectious complications with respiratory pathogens despite ciprofloxacin therapy. *N Engl J Med* 1991;325:520-521.
55. Perez-Trallero E, Garcia-Arenzana JM, Jimenez JA, et al. Therapeutic failure and selection of resistance to quinolones in a case of pneumococcal pneumonia treated with ciprofloxacin. *Eur J Clin Microbiol Infect Dis* 1990;9:905-906.
56. Ambrose PG, Grasela DM, Grasela TH, et al. Pharmacodynamics of fluoroquinolones against *Streptococcus pneumoniae* in patients with community-acquired respiratory tract infections. *Antimicrob Agents Chemother* 2001;45:2793-2797.
57. Craig WA. Pharmacokinetic/pharmacodynamic parameters: Rationale for antibacterial dosing of mice and men. *Clin Inf Dis* 1998; 26:1-12.

58. MacGowan AC, Rogers, K. Bowker. The use of in vitro pharmacodynamic models of infection to optimize fluoroquinolone dosing regimens. *J Antimicrob Chemother* 2000;46:163-170.
59. Wright DH, Brown GH, Peterson ML, et al. Application of fluoroquinolone pharmacodynamics. *J Antimicrob Chemother* 2000;46: 669-683.
60. Madaras-Kelly KJ, Demasters TA. In vitro characterization of fluoroquinolone concentration/MIC antimicrobial activity and resistance while simulating clinical pharmacokinetics of levofloxacin, ofloxacin, or ciprofloxacin against *Streptococcus pneumoniae. Diagn Microbiol Infect Dis* 2000;37:253-260.
61. Thorburn CE, Edwards DI. The effect of pharmacokinetics on the bactericidal activity of ciprofloxacin and sparfloxacin against *Streptococcus pneumoniae* and the emergence of resistance. *J Antimicrob Chemother* 2001;48:15-22.
62. Gonzalez MA, Uribe F, Moisen SD, et al. Multiple-dose pharmacokinetics and safety of ciprofloxacin in normal volunteers. *Antimicrob Agents Chemother* 1984;26:741-744.
63. Mazzulli TA, Simor E, Jaeger R, et al. Comparative in vitro activities of several new fluoroquinolones and β-lactam antimicrobial agents against community isolates of *Streptococcus pneumoniae. Antimicrob Agents Chemother* 1990;34:467-469.
64. Anzueto A, Niederman MS, Tillotson GS. Etiology, susceptibility, and treatment of acute bacterial exacerbations of complicated chronic bronchitis in the primary care setting: Ciprofloxacin 750 mg b.i.d. versus clarithromycin 500 mg b.i.d. Bronchitis Study Group. *Clin Ther* 1998;20:885-900.
65. Chodosh S, Schreurs A, Siami G, et al and the Bronchitis Study Group. Efficacy of oral ciprofloxacin vs. clarithromycin for treatment of acute bacterial exacerbations of chronic bronchitis. *Clin Infect Dis* 1998;27:730-738.
66. Chen D, McGeer A, de Azavedo JC, et al and The Canadian Bacterial Surveillance Network. Decreased susceptibility of *Streptococcus pneumoniae* to fluoroquinolones in Canada. *N Engl J Med* 1999;341:233-239.
67. Linares J, De La Campa AG, Pallares R. Fluoroquinolone resistance in *Streptococcus pneumoniae* [letter]. *N Engl J Med* 1999;341:1546-1547.
68. Ho PL, Que TL, Tsang DN, et al. Emergence of fluoroquinolone resistance among multiply resistant strains of *Streptococcus pneumoniae* in Hong Kong. *Antimicrob Agents Chemother* 1999;43: 1310-1313.
69. Ho PL, Yung RW, Tsang DN, et al. Increasing resistance of Streptococcus pneumoniae to fluoroquinolones: Results of a Hong Kong multicentre study in 2000. *J Antimicrob Chemother* 2001; 48:659-665.
70. Goldsmith CE, Moore JE, Murphy PG, et al. Increased incidence of ciprofloxacin resistance in penicillin-resistant pneumococci in Northern Ireland [letter; comment]. *J Antimicrob Chemother* 1998; 41:420-421.
71. Centers for Disease Control. Resistance of *Streptococcus pneumoniae* to fluoroquinolones-United States, 1995-1999. *Morbid Mortal Weekly Rep MMWR* 2001;50:800-804.
72. Doern GV, Heilmann KP, Huynh HK, et al. Antimicrobial resistance among clinical isolates of Streptococcus pneumoniae in the United States during 1999-2000, including a comparison of resistance rates since 1994-1995. *Antimicrob Agents Chemother* 2001; 45:1721-1729.
73. Sahm DF, Karlowsky JA, Kelly LJ, et al. Need for annual surveillance of antimicrobial resistance in *Streptococcus pneumoniae* in the United States: 2-year longitudinal analysis. *Antimicrob Agents Chemother* 2001;45:1037-1042.
74. Sahm DF, Peterson DE, Critchley IA, et al. Analysis of ciprofloxacin activity against *Streptococcus pneumoniae* after 10 years of use in the United States. *Antimicrob Agents Chemother* 2000;44:2521-2524.
75. Thornsberry C, et al. Longitudinal analysis of resistance among *Streptococcus pneumoniae* (SP) isolated from 100 geographically distributed institutions in the United States during the 1997-1998 and 1998-1999 respiratory seasons. Abstract of the 39th Interscience Conference on Antimicrobial Agents and Chemotherapy, San Francisco, Sept. 26-29, 1999.
76. Fish DN, Piscitelli SC, Danziger LH. Development of resistance during antimicrobial therapy: A review of antibiotic classes and patient characteristics in 173 studies. *Pharmacotherapy* 1995;15:279-291.
77. Deeks SL, Palacio R, Ruvinsky P, et al. Risk factors and course of illness among children with invasive penicillin-resistant *Streptococcus pneumoniae*. The Streptococcus pneumoniae Working Group. *Pediatrics* 1999;103:409-413.
78. Straus WL, Qazi SA, Kundi Z, et al. Antimicrobial resistance and clinical effectiveness of co-trimoxazole versus amoxycillin for pneumonia among children in Pakistan: Randomised controlled trial. Pakistan Co-trimoxazole Study Group. *Lancet* 1998;352: 270-274.
79. Davidson RJ, Cavalcanti R, Brunton JL, et al Resistance to levofloxacin and failure of treatment of pneumococcal pneumonia. *N Engl J Med* 2002;346:747-750.
80. Weiss K, Restieri C, Laverdiere M, et al. A nosocomial outbreak of fluoroquinolone-resistant *Streptococcus pneumoniae. Clin Inf Dis* 2001;33:517-522.
81. Ho PL, Tse W, Tsang KW, et al. Risk factors for acquisition of levofloxacin-resistant *Streptococcus pneumoniae:* A case-control study. *Clin Infect Dis* 2001;32:701-707.
82. Pallares R, Capdevila O, Liñares J, et al. Hospital Bellvitge, University of Barcelona, Spain; Clinical Relevance of Current NCCLS Ceftriaxone/Cefotaxime Resistance Breakpoints in non-Meningeal Pneumococcal Infections. Abstract Poster, 2001.
83. Kaplan SL, Mason EO, Barson WJ, et al. Outcome of invasive infections outside the central nervous system caused by *Streptococcus pneumoniae* isolates nonsusceptible to ceftriaxone in children treated with beta-lactam antibiotics. *Pediatr Infect Dis J* 2001;20:392-396.
84. Cleeland R, Squires E. Antimicrobial activity of ceftriaxone: A review. *Am J Med* 1984;77:3.
85. ASCAP Panel (Antibiotic Selection for Community-Acquired Pneumonia). Jackson, Wyoming, Dec. 6, 2000. A Panel of emergency physicians, internal medicine specialists, and pharmacists assessing treatment guidelines for community-acquired pneumonia.
86. Mandell LA. Antibiotics for pneumonia therapy. *Med Clin N Am* 1994;78:997-1014.
87. Gopalakrishna K, Lerner P. Tetracycline-resistant pneumococci: Increasing incidence and cross resistance to newer tetracyclines. *Am Rev Respir Dis* 1973;108:1007.
88. Mandell L. Community-acquired pneumonia: Etiology, epidemi-

ology and treatment. *Chest* 1995;108(supp):35S-42S.
89. Edelstein P. Legionnaires' disease. *Clin Infect Dis* 1993;16:741.
90. Garrison D, DeHaan R, Lawson J. Comparison of in vitro antibacterial activities of 7-chloro-7-deoxylincomycin, lincomycin, and erythromycin. *Antimicrob Agents Chemother* 1968;1967:397.
91. Dean NC, Silver MP, Bateman KA, et al. Decreased mortality after implementation of a treatment guideline for community-acquired pneumonia. *Am J Med* 2001;110:451-457.
92. Gleason PP, Meehan TP, Fine JM, et al. Associations between initial antimicrobial therapy and medical outcomes for hospitalized elderly patients with pneumonia. *Arch Intern* Med 1999;159: 2562-2572.
93. Nathwani D, Rubinstein E, Barlow G, et al. Do guidelines for community-acquired pneumonia improve the cost-effectiveness of hospital care? *CID* 2001;32:728 (1 March, 2000).
94. People G, Kapoor WN, Stone RA, et al. Medical outcomes and antimicrobial cost with the use of the American Thoracic Society guidelines for outpatients with community-acquired pneumonia. *JAMA* 1997;278:32-9.
95. Dowell SF. The best treatment for pneumonia: New clues, but no definitive answers. *Arch Intern Med* 1999;159:2511-2512.
96. Canadian Coordinating Office for Health Technology Assessment. Clinical and economic considerations in the use of fluoroquinolones: technology overview. Pharmaceuticals. Ottawa: Canadian Coordinating Office for Health Technology Assessment (CCOHTA), 1997;10:1-13.
97. Al-Eidan FA, McElnay JC, Scott MG, et al. Use of a treatment protocol in the management of community-acquired lower respiratory infection. *J Antimicrob Chemother* 2000;45:387-397.
98. McGarvey RN, Harper IJ. Pneumonia mortality reduction and quality improvement in a community hospital. *QRB Qual Rev Bull* 1993;19:124-130.
99. Dresser LD, Niederman MS, Paladino JA. Cost-effectiveness of gatifloxacin vs ceftriaxone with a macrolide for the treatment of community-acquired pneumonia. *Chest* 2001;119:1439-1448.
100. Kaplan SL, Mason EO Jr, Barson WJ, et al. Outcome of invasive infections outside the central nervous system caused by *Streptococcus pneumoniae* isolates nonsusceptible to ceftriazone in children treated with beta-lactam antibiotics. *Pediatr Infect Dis J* 2001;20:392-396.
101. Gums JG. Abstract/poster presentation; American College of Chest Physicians (ACCP), 2001. Antimicrobial susceptibility trends from 1990-2000: Preliminary results of the antimicrobial resistance management (ARM) program. *Pharmacotherapy* 2001;21:1300-1301.
102. Fraschini F, Scaglione F. Study on the relationship between pharmacokinetics and antibacterial activity: Comparison between ceftriaxone and cefotaxime within the respiratory tract. *Chemotherapy* 1989;45:77-82
103. Enoxacin-A new fluoroquinolone. *Med Lett Drugs Ther* 1992;34: 103-105.
104. Cooper B, Lawer M. Pneumococcal bacteremia during ciprofloxacin therapy for pneumococcal pneumonia. *Am J Med* 1989;87:475.
105. Flynn CM, et al. In vitro efficacy of levofloxacin alone or in combination tested against multi-resistant *Pseudomonas aeruginosa* strains. *J Chemother* 1996;8:411-415.
106. Dholakia N, et al. Susceptibilities of bacterial isolates from patients with cancer to levofloxacin and other quinolones. *Antimicrob Agents Chemother* 1994;38:848-852.
107. Habib MP, et al. Intersci Conf Antimicrob Agents Chemother 1996;36. Abstract L002. 36th Interscience Conference on Antimicrobial Agents and Chemotherapy. New Orleans, LA. Sept. 15-18, 1996.
108. File TM, et al. Abstr Intersci Conf Antimicrob Agents Chemother 1996;36. Abstract L001 (LM1). 36th Interscience Conference on Antimicrobial Agents and Chemotherapy. New Orleans, LA. Sept. 15-18, 1996.
109. Pfizer, Inc. Azithromycin package insert.
110. Pfizer product monograph. Azithromycin for IV injection.
111. Data on file, Pfizer, Inc. New York, NY.
112. de Klerk GJ, van Steijn JH, Lobatto S, et al. A randomised, multicentre study of ceftriaxone versus standard therapy in the treatment of lower respiratory tract infections. *Int J Antimicrob Agents* 1999;12:121-127.
113. Mayfield DC, et al. TSN Database, USA, 1996-2000, on file at Roche Laboratories In Vitro Evaluation of Ceftriaxone activity against recent gram negative clinical isolates: results from the TSN Database.
114. Levaquin Product Information. Ortho-McNeil Pharmaceuticals. January 1997.
115. Vincent J, et al. Pharmacokinetics and safety of trovafloxacin in healthy male volunteers following administration of single intravenous doses of the prodrug, alatrofloxacin. *J Antimicrob Chemother* 1997;39(supp B):75-80.
116. Spangler SK, et al. Activity of CP 99,219 compared with those of ciprofloxacin, grepafloxacin, metronidazole, cefoxitin, piperacillin, and piperacillin-tazobactam against 489 anaerobes. *Antimicrob Agents Chemother* 1994;38:2471-2476.
117. Child J, et al. The in-vitro activity of CP 99,219, a new naphthyridone antimicrobial agent: A comparison with fluoroquinolone agents. *J Antimicrob Chemother* 1995;35:869-876.
118. Brighty KE, et al. The chemistry and biological profile of trovafloxacin. *J Antimicrob Chemother* 1997;39(supp B):1-14.
119. Mundy LM, et al. Community-acquired pneumonia: Impact of immune status. *Am J Respir Crit Care Med* 1995;152:1309-1315.
120. Kulgman KP, Capper T, et al. In vitro susceptibility of penicillin-resistant *S. pneumoniae* to levofloxacin, selection of resistant mutants, and time-kill synergy studies of levofloxacin combined with vancomycin, telcoplanin, fusidic acid, and rifampin. *Antimicrob Agents Chemother* 1996;40:2802-2804.
121. Polk R, Johnson C, Clarke J, et al. Virginia Commonwealth University, Richmond, Va; Trends in Fluoroquinolone (FQ) Prescribing in 35 U.S. Hospitals and Resistance for *P. aeruginosa:* A SCOPE-MMIT Report. MultiMedia Info. Technologies Abstract.
122. Fridkin S, Steward CD, Edwards JR, et al. Surveillance of antimicrobial use and antimicrobial resistance in United States hospitals: project ICARE phase.
123. Project Intensive Care Antimicrobial Resistance Epidemiology (ICARE) hospitals. *Clin Infect Dis* 1999:29:245-252.
124. Graham KK, Hufcut RM, Copeland CM, et al. Flurorquinolone exposure and the development of nosocomial MRSA bacteremia. *Infect Cont Hosp Epidemiol* 2000;21:90.
125. Resistance of *Streptococcus pneumoniae* to fluoroquinolones—United States, 1995-1999. *MMWR Morbid Mortal Wkly Rep* 2001;50:800-804.

126. Fine MJ, et al. The hospital discharge decision for patients with community-acquired pneumonia. Results from the Pneumonia Patient Outcomes Research Team cohort study. *Arch Intern Med* 1997;157:47-56.
127. Zimmerman T, Reidel KD, Laufen H, et al. Intravenous toleration of azithromycin in comparison to clarithromycin and erythromycin. In: Abstracts of the 36th Interscience Conference on Antimicrobial Agents and Chemotherapy. Washington, DC: American Society Microbiology; 1996:16 Abstract A82.
128. Thys JP, Jacobs F, Byl B. Role of quinolones in the treatment of bronchopulmonary infections, particularly pneumococcal and community-acquired pneumonia. *Eur J Clin Microbiol Infect Dis* 1991;10:304-315.
129. Piscitelli SC, Danziger LH, Rodwold KA. Clarithromycin and azithromycin: New macrolide antibiotics. *Clin Pharm* 1992;11: 137-152.
130. Ortquist A, et al. Oral empiric treatment of community-acquired pneumonia. *Chest* 1996;110:1499-1506.
131. Samama MM, Cohen AT, Darmon JY, et al. A comparison of enoxaparin with placebo for the prevention of thromboembolism in acutely ill medical patients. Prophylaxis in Medical Patients with Enoxaparin Study Group. *N Engl J Med* 1999;341:793-800.
132. Clagett GP, Andersen FA, Heit JA, et al. Prevention of venous thromboembolism. *Chest* 1998;114(5 suppl):531S-560S.
133. Nicolaides AN, Bergquist D, Hull R, et al. Consensus statement. Prevention of venous thromboembolism. *Int Angiol* 1997:16:3-38.
134. Anderson FA, Wheeler HB, Goldberg RJ, et al. A population-based perspective of the hospital incidence and case-fatality rates of deep vein thrombosis and pulmonary embolism. The Worcester DVT study. *Arch Intern Med* 1991;151:933-938.
135. Sandler DA, Martin JF. Autopsy proven pulmonary embolism in hospital patients: Are we detecting enough deep vein thrombosis? *J Royal Soc Med* 1989;82:203-205.
136. Gardund B for the Heparin Prophylaxis Study Group. Randomized, controlled trial of low-dose heparin for prevention of fatal pulmonary embolism in patients with infectious diseases. *Lancet* 1996;347:1357-1361.

Outpatient Management of Bacterial Infections in the Lower Respiratory Tract

*The OMBIRT Panel**

Antibiotic guidelines for treatment of community-acquired pneumonia (CAP) and acute bacterial exacerbations of chronic obstructive pulmonary diease (ABE/COPD) vary from institution to institution, and depending upon antimicrobial resistance patterns, such protocols also may vary from region to region. The variability among antimicrobial strategies is exemplified by the somewhat different approaches advocated by national associations, infectious disease experts, and published reviews in the medical literature. As a general rule, however, outcome-effective antibiotic selection, which is the subject of this consensus review, means taking into account local antibiotic resistance patterns, epidemiological and infection incidence data, and patient demographic features; then, against the background of clinical judgment, it also means determining the most appropriate agent for an individual patient.

To address these complex issues, the OMBIRT (Outpatient Management of Bacterial Infections in the Respiratory Tract) Consensus Panel and Scientific Roundtable met in August 2001 to review, analyze, and interpret published, evidence-based trials assessing the safety and efficacy of antibiotic therapy for managing ABE/COPD and community-acquired pneumonia (CAP). In addition, the OMBIRT Panel was charged with developing strategies that would ensure appropriate use of antibiotics in this patient population, and making recommendations for how patients with respiratory infections should be evaluated in the outpatient setting.

Treatment guidelines generated by the OMBIRT Panel were based on evidence presented from well-designed clinical trials, and focused on out-of-hospital management by the primary care practitioner. Detailed analysis of national consensus guidelines issued by the American Thoracic Society (ATS), Infectious Disease Society of America (IDSA), CDC Drug-Resistant Streptocococcus pneumonaie Working Group, and the Antibiotic Selection in Community-Acquired Pneumonia (ASCAP) Panel also were evaluated and included in the decision-making process.

With these objectives in clear focus, the purpose of this comprehensive review, which includes the OMBIRT Panel guidelines, assessment strategies, and treatment recommendations, is to provide a state-of-the-art clinical resource outlining, in precise and practical detail, clinical protocols for acute management of CAP and ABE/COPD. To achieve this goal, all of the critical aspects entering into the equation for maximizing outcomes, while minimizing costs, including systematic patient evaluation, disposition decision trees, and outcome-effective antibiotic therapy, will be discussed in detail. In addition, because appropriate disposition of patients with CAP and ABE/COPD has become essential for cost-effective patient management, this review includes critical pathways and treatment tables that incorporate risk stratification protocols and intensification-of-treatment trigger (IOTT) criteria that can be used to identify those patient subgroups that are suitably managed in the outpatient setting and those more appropriately admitted to the hospital for more intensive care.

Introduction

Evaluating advantages and disadvantages among recommendations and protocols issued by different authoritative sources can be problematic and confusing, to say the least. And although management guidelines for CAP must be "customized" for the local practice environment and for the individual patient, there appears to be a consensus regarding one aspect of CAP management: the outpatient with CAP generally requires treatment with an antibiotic that provides adequate coverage against *S. pneumoniae, H. influenzae, M. catarrhalis, M. pneumoniae, C. pneumoniae,* and *L. pneumophila.* In contrast, the uncomplicated outpatient with ABE/COPD typically requires coverage against *S. pneumoniae, H. influenzae,* and *M. catarrhalis.* In both conditions, antibiotics that provide activity against these organisms may be considered "correct spectrum" coverage. Accordingly, those agents—most important among them, advanced generation macrolides and advanced generation fluoroquinolones—that provide this range of coverage within the framework of monotherapy, represent appropriate, initial choices for these conditions

Unfortunately, no single set of guidelines or critical pathways is applicable to every patient or practice environment; therefore, clinical judgment must take in account other factors that suggest the need for "intensifying" therapy with antibiotics whose spectrum extends beyond the six aforementioned organisms and includes other gram-negative species. In this regard, when patients with CAP present with risk factors or historical features that strongly suggest the likelihood of infection with such gram-negative organisms as *Klebsiella pneumoniae* (chronic alcoholism) or *E. coli* (infection acquired in a nursing home), it is appropriate to use an agent (an advanced generation fluoroquinolone) providing this spectrum of coverage. However, a cautionary note is in order. When, in the setting of CAP, the probability of gram-negative infection with *E. coli, Pseudomonas* sp., or other enterobacteria is relatively low, using an extended spectrum quinolone as initial therapy may represent "over-extended" coverage, in the sense that resistance pressure may be exerted against organisms not typically implicated in such infections, among them *E. coli, Pseudomonas*, and other enterobacteria.

Identifying treatment trigger points and historical features that support amplifying spectrum of coverage from a "correct spectrum" macrolide to an "extended spectrum" fluoroquinolone are essential for outcome-effective antibiotic use. As a rule, clinical results in ABE/COPD and CAP can be optimized by using risk-stratification criteria. Such clinical findings as hypotension, tachypnea, impaired oxygen saturation, multi-lobar involvement, elevated blood urea nitrogen, and altered level of consciousness are predictive of more serious disease in CAP, as is acquisition of CAP in a nursing home environment. These patients generally will need to be treated as inpatients.

With these antibiotic selection issues in clear focus, the OMBIRT Panel will review current strategies for evaluating and managing oupatients with bacterial infection of the respiratory tract and present a set of consensus guidelines outlining antibiotic selection for these patients.

Acute Bacterial Exacerbations of Chronic Onstructive Pulmonary Disease (ABE/COPD) — General Principles

ABE/COPD are common, costly, and above all, complex to manage. In fact, few conditions produce such a broad range of outcomes, require such customized approaches, or present so many options for treatment.[1,2]

Although there have been important advances in patient assessment techniques and therapeutics, including pulmonary function testing, capnometry, pulse oximetry, disposition support tools, and antimicrobial therapy, ABE/COPD continues to be a leading cause of morbidity and mortality in the United States.[2] From patient disposition to antimicrobial selection, optimizing management of these patients requires the clinician to integrate a number of clinical, laboratory, radiologic, and etiologic factors, and then initiate a course of action that accounts for all the risks, costs, and benefits of an individualized treatment plan.

Despite a number of guidelines and the availability of new, targeted spectrum antibiotics, the management of ABE/COPD in the outpatient setting remains extremely challenging. More than ever, it requires a multifactorial analysis of myriad clinical, historical, and laboratory parameters that predict success or possible failure for each individual case. In this regard, clinical decision-making in ABE/COPD can be problematic for the primary care physician.

Achieving optimal patient outcomes for this common and debilitating condition requires the primary care physician to consider several features of each individual case. Factors that must be considered include the patient's age, response to medical therapy, overall pulmonary function, character and severity of previous exacerbations, bacterial colonization status of the patient, previous requirements for mechanical ventilation, and local antimicrobial resistance patterns. With this in mind, a Severity-of-Exacerbation and Risk Factor (SERF) pathway can be employed to help guide patient disposition, empiric antibiotic selection, and necessity for additional diagnostic investigation.

The antibiotic selection process for ABE/COPD in the office-based setting offers multiple options. Currently, the pathogens most often responsible for causing "uncomplicated and typical" cases of ABE/COPD that can be treated in the outpatient environment include the bacterial organisms, *S. pneumoniae, H. influenzae*, and *M. catarrhalis*. Because it may be difficult, if not impossible, to identify a specific pathogen at the time of initial patient assessment, empiric antimicrobial coverage against all expected pathogens usually is necessary to minimize treatment failures. Patients with advanced disease and multiple risk factors may have exacerbations caused by *Klebsiella spp., Pseudomonas aeruginosa,* and other gram-negative species. As will be discussed below, these patients may require intensification of therapy with agents that are active against gram-negative organisms.

In this vein, the development of advanced generation macrolides (e.g., azithromycin), as well as extended spectrum quinolones, has made it possible to treat most patients using monotherapy. Finally, because there is a growing incidence of resistance among common bacterial agents that cause CAP (in some areas of the United States, intermediate-to-complete resistance to penicillin among *Streptococcus pneumoniae* is reported to be greater than 25%), antibiotic selection must be guided by local and/or regional resistance patterns.

Acute Bacterial Exacerbations of COPD — OMBIRT Panel Overview and Recommendations

Although certain recommendations can be made regarding management of patients with ABE/COPD, the OMBIRT Panel noted that the number, quality, and design of studies evaluating and comparing effectiveness of and indications for antibiotic therapy are less than optimal, and in general, inferior to those available for CAP. In addition, upon review of multiple studies comparing advanced generation macrolides (azithromycin or clarithromycin) and advanced generation fluoroquinolones, no significant differences in clinical outcomes could be observed in outpatients managed with these antibiotic regimens.

The tendency to overuse antibiotics in patients with ABE/COPD should be recognized by primary care practitioners, and only patients meeting clinical criteria for antibiotic therapy should receive antibiotics for their exacerbations. The OMBIRT Panel recommendations for outpatient management of ABE/COPD are summarized in this section, and supportive evidence, analysis of clinical trials, and adjunctive approaches to managing ABE/COPD are discussed in subequent sections.

Appropriate Use of Antibiotics. As a rule, the clinical criteria for initiating antibiotic therapy in patients with a documented history of COPD, and who are suspected of having ABE/COPD, include the presence of at least two of the following three symptoms: increasing purulence of sputum, increasing volume of sputum production, and increasing cough and/or dyspnea. In contrast, patients with symptoms of acute tracheobronchitis who have no previous history of COPD initially should not be treated with antibiotics, since antibiotics have not been shown to improve outcomes in this patient population.

However, it was recognized by the panel that in real world practice a significant percentage of patients fall into a clinical gray zone. In particular, those outpatients with persistent (i.e., > 10-14 days) symptoms of acute tracheobronchitis, and who have no previous history of COPD may be considered appropriate candidates for antibiotic therapy, especially if clinical assessment suggests that persistent symptoms may be due to infection with such atypical organisms as *Chlamydia pneumoniae* or *Mycoplasma pneumoniae.*

Appropriate use of antibiotics in ABE/COPD requires clinical confirmation of the diagnosis, which is usually made on the basis of symptom exacerbation and clinical history. As a rule, chest x-ray is not recommended or encouraged for typical cases of ABE/COPD, but should be considered in patients who present with an atypical presentation and in whom CAP is suspected.

Appropriate antibiotic use and selection is designed to accomplish the following: 1) return patient's respiratory status (FEV_1, oxygenation, respiratory rate, symptoms, etc.) back to baseline; 2) reduce the number and frequency of exacerbations; and 3) prevent hospitalization. The principal respiratory tract pathogens that must be covered on an empiric basis in individuals with moderate-to-severe ABE/COPD in the outpatient setting include *S. pneumoniae, H. influenzae, M. catarrhalis, H. parainfluenzae,* and *Staphylococcus aureus.* Some patients, especially those with severe disease, a recent history of mechanical ventilation and hospitalization, and/or high-dose chronic steroid therapy are more susceptible to infection with *Pseudomonas* species.

Treatment. The majority of double-blinded, prospective clinical trials comparing new generation macrolides (azithromycin and clarithromycin) vs. new generation fluoroquinolones (moxifloxacin, gatifloxacin, and levofloxacin) demonstrate comparable outcomes in terms of clinical cure and bacteriologic eradication rates at days 7, 14, and 28 days in outpatients with either moderate or severe ABE/COPD. Emergence of resistance among *S. pneumoniae* to new generation fluoroquinolones has been reported in a number of geographic regions, including the United States, Hong Kong, and Canada. Given the emergence of such strains and the presence of numerous studies demonstrating comparable effectiveness between macrolides and advanced generation fluoroquinolones the OMBIRT Panel supports cautious, restrictive use of fluoroquinolones for appropriately selected patients with ABE/COPD, and recommends the advanced generation macrolide, azithromyzin, as the initial agent of choice for managing appropriately risk-stratified outpatients with ABE/COPD. *(Please see Table 1.)*

Table 1. Factors Influencing Patient Disposition in AECOPD

- Age of patient
- Overall respiratory status
- Respiratory rate
- O_2 saturation
- Degree of hypercarbia
- Patient's status compared to baseline
- Mental status
- Home environment
- Likelihood of acceptable medication compliance
- Nighttime emergency department visit
- Previous pattern of frequent relapse
- Pulmonary function tests
- FEV_1 less than 40% of predicted normal
- Multiple ED courses of aerosolized β-agonists

The frequency of drug-resistant *Streptococcus pneumoniae* (DRSP) causing ABE/COPD is not known, but is presumed to be less than or equal to the incidence of DRSP causing outpatient CAP. There is currently no evidence to support initial outpatient therapy directed at DRSP for patients with ABE/COPD. As it does in the management of CAP, the panel cautions against overuse of new generation fluoroquinolones as initial agents in outpatients with ABE/COPD, and recommends their use as alternative agents when: 1) first-line therapy with advanced generation macrolides such as azithromycin fails; 2) patients are allergic to first-line agents; or 3) patients have documented or suspected infection with gram-negative organisms.

Given concerns about antibiotic overuse, the potential for emerging resistance among DRSP to fluoroquinolones, the panel concurs with other guideline panels specifying advanced generation macrolides as initial therapy for outpatient ABE/COPD and use of fluoroquinolones as alternative agents in patients who fail therapy or who have risk factors predictive of gram-negative infection. Patients who do not respond to oral therapy with one class of antibiotics (relapse) may be treated with a course of antibiotics with different gaps in coverage. Reinfections should be treated with antibiotics that have been shown to be effective in previous exacerbations.

Unfortunately, limited data exist to guide physicians in the cost-effective treatment of acute exacerbation of chronic bronchitis (ABE/COPD). One important study, however, attempted to determine the antimicrobial efficacy of various agents and compared total outcome costs for patients with ABE/COPD. For the purpose of this analysis, a retrospective review was performed of 60 outpatient medical records of individuals with a diagnosis of COPD associated with acute episodes seen in the pulmonary clinic of a teaching institution. Empirical antibiotic choices were divided into first-line (amoxicillin, co-trimoxazole, tetracyclines, erythromycin); second-line (cephradine, cefuroxime, cefaclor, cefprozil); and third-line (azithromycin, amoxicillin-clavulanate, ciprofloxacin) agents.

Table 2. OMBIRT (Outpatient Management of Bacterial Infections of the Respiratory Tract) Consensus Panel Antibiotic Treatment*† Recommendations for Acute Bacterial Exacerbations of Chronic Obstructive Pulmonary Disease (ABE/COPD)

SERF CATEGORY A**

CONDITION • SEVERITY • SUSPECTED PATHOGENS

Acute Bacterial Exacerbation of COPD (ABE/COPD)
Mild severity based on SERF (severity of exacerbation and risk factors) pathway and IOTT (intensity of treatment triggers) criteria
— Suspected pathogens: *Streptococcus pneumoniae, Haemophilus influenzae, Moraxella catarrhalis*

Initial (preferred agent, any class) first-line therapy: Azithromycin 500 mg on day 1, followed by 250 mg qd for 4 days
Alternative first-line agents (macrolides): Clarithromycin 500 mg PO qd x 7 days
Alternative first-line agents (fluoroquinolones): Moxifloxacin (preferred) 400 mg PO qd x 5 days; Gatifloxacin 400 mg PO qd x 7 days; Levofloxacin 500 mg PO qd x 7 days
Alternative first-line agents (other classes, including generic formulations): Amoxicillin-clavulanate 875 mg PO q 12 hours x 10 days; Doxycycline 100 mg PO bid x 7-14 days; Trimethoprim-sulfamethoxazole 1 DS tablet PO bid x 7-14 days

SERF CATEGORY B

CONDITION • SEVERITY • SUSPECTED PATHOGENS

Moderate-to-severe bacterial exacerbation of COPD (ABE/COPD)
Severity based on SERF (severity of exacerbation and risk factors) pathway and IOTT (intensity of treatment triggers) criteria
— Suspected pathogens: *Streptococcus pneumoniae, Haemophilus influenzae, Moraxella catarrhalis*

Initial (preferred agent, any class) first-line therapy: Azithromycin 500 mg on day 1, followed by 250 mg qd for 4 days
Alternative first-line agents (macrolides): Clarithromycin 500mg PO qd x 7 days
Alternative first-line agents (fluoroquinolones): Moxifloxacin (preferred) 400 mg PO qd x 5 days; Gatifloxacin 400 mg PO qd x 7 days; Levofloxacin 500 mg PO qd x 7 days
Alternative first-line agents (other classes): Amoxicillin-clavulanate 875 mg PO q 12 hours x 10 days

SERF CATEGORY C

CONDITION • SEVERITY • SUSPECTED PATHOGENS

Severe and/or frequently recurrent bacterial exacerbation of COPD (ABE/COPD)
Severity based on SERF (severity of exacerbation and risk factors) pathway and IOTT (intensity of treatment triggers) criteria
— Associated risk factors and/historical features: Recent hospitalization for ABE/COPD and documented infection with gram-negative organisms such as: *Klebsiella, Pseudomonas,* and other enterobacteria; patients with structural lung disease (bronchiectasis); or patients who have failed first-line macrolide therapy.
— Suspected pathogens: *Streptococcus pneumoniae, Haemophilus influenzae, and Moraxella catarrhalis,* in addition to possible infection with gram-negative organisms known to cause exacerbations in patients who are risk-stratified to a more severe category (see above)

Initial (preferred agent, any class) first-line therapy: Moxifloxacin (preferred) 400 mg PO qd x 5 days; Gatifloxacin 400 mg PO qd x 7 days; Levofloxacin 500 mg PO qd x 7 days
Alternative first-line agents (fluoroquinolones): Ciprofloxacin 500 mg PO bid x 10 days (Although effective in clinical trials and recommended for acute, documented gram-negative exacerbations of COPD, ciprofloxacin is not the agent of choice when ABE/COPD is thought to be secondary to *S. pneumoniae* infection)
Alternative agents (other classes): Amoxicillin-clavulanate 875 mg PO q 12 hours x 10 days

* Approved Indications for recommended antimicrobial agents:
Azithromycin: Indicated for acute bacterial exacerbations of COPD caused by susceptible species of *Streptococcus pneumoniae, Moraxella catarrhalis,* and *Haemophilus influenzae.*
Clarithromycin: Indicated for acute bacterial exacerbations of COPD caused by susceptible species of *Streptococcus pneumoniae, Moraxella catarrhalis, Haemophilus influenzae,* and *Haemophilus parainfluenzae*
Moxifloxacin: Indicated for acute bacterial exacerbations of COPD caused by susceptible species of *Streptococcus pneumoniae, Moraxella catarrhalis, Haemophilus influenzae, Staphylococcus aureus, Klebsiella pneumoniae,* and *Haemophilus parainfluenzae*
Gatifloxacin: Indicated for acute bacterial exacerbations of COPD caused by susceptible species of *Streptococcus pneumoniae, Moraxella catarrhalis, Haemophilus influenzae, Staphylococcus aureus,* and *Haemophilus parainfluenzae*
Levofloxacin: Indicated for acute bacterial exacerbations of COPD caused by susceptible species of *Streptococcus pneumoniae, Moraxella catarrhalis, Haemophilus influenzae, Staphylococcus aureus,* and *Haemophilus parainfluenzae*

† OMBIRT Panel recommendations and preferences are based on a critical analysis and evaluation of published clinical trials, FDA indications, association guidelines, and pharmatectural criteria including cost, spectrum of coverage, compliance parameters (daily dose frequency, duration of therapy, and side effects), pregnancy category, and risk of drug-drug and/or drug-disease interactions.

** SERF - Severity of Exacerbation and Risk Factor clinical assessment strategy.

In this study, patients receiving first-line agents (amoxicillin, co-trimoxazole, tetracyclines, erythromycin) failed significantly more frequently (19% vs 7%; $P < 0.05$) than those treated with third-line agents (azithromycin, amoxicillin-clavulanate, ciprofloxacin). Moreover, patients prescribed first-line agents were hospitalized significantly more often for ABE/COPD within two weeks of outpatient treatment as compared with patients prescribed third-line agents (18.0% vs 5.3% for third-line agents; $P < 0.02$). Time between subsequent ABE/COPD episodes requiring treatment was significantly longer for patients receiving third-line agents compared with first-line and second-line agents ($P < 0.005$).

Two advanced generation macrolides—azithromycin and clarithromycin—are available for treating ABE/COPD. Based on outcome-sensitive criteria and pharmatectural considerations such as cost, daily dose frequency, duration of therapy, side effects, and drug interactions, the panel recommends azithromycin as first-line, preferred initial therapy in moderate-to-severe, non-hospitalized patients, with clarithromycin or doxycycline as an alternative agent; and, as second line therapy, moxifloxacin, gatifloxacin, or levofloxacin. Amoxillin-clavulanate is another alternative agent. When historical or clinical factors in the SERF (Severity of Exacerbation and Risk Factor) pathway suggest the presence of gram-negative infection, a new generation fluoroquinolone would be considered the agent of choice. Physicians are urged to prescribe antibiotics in ABE/COPD at the time of diagnosis and to encourage patients to fill and begin taking their prescriptions on the day of diagnosis.

Primary care physicians are discouraged from using antibiotics for "chronic prophylaxis" against ABE/COPD, since studies do not support the efficacy of this strategy for preventing acute exacerbations. Patients should be instructed about issues related to the importance of medication compliance, and in the case of short (5-day) courses of therapy, they should be educated that although they are only consuming medications for a five-day period, such antibiotics as azithromycin remains at the tissue site of infection for about nine days and continue to deliver therapeutic effects during that period.

Either verbal or on-site, re-evaluation of patients is recommended within a three-day period following diagnosis and initiation of antibiotic therapy. Follow-up in the office or clinic within three days is recommended in certain risk-stratified patients, especially the elderly, those with co-morbid illness, signifcantly impaired FEV_1, and those in whom medication compliance may be compromised.[3] More urgent follow-up may be required in patients with increasing symptoms, including dyspnea, fever, and other systemic signs or symptoms. Follow-up chest x-rays generally are not recommended in patients with outpatient ABE/COPD, except in certain high-risk groups.

Antibiotic Therapy for ABE/COPD: The SERF Pathway for Ouctome-Effective Drug Selection

Patients in whom exacerbation of COPD is associated with acute respiratory infection are at high risk for relapse unless treated.[3] Patients with acute bronchitis that is unrelated to COPD probably do not benefit from antibiotic therapy. It should be noted, however, that for patients with COPD, antibiotics appear to have a role in the treatment of exacerbations caused by bacterial bronchitis (i.e., ABE/COPD). The outpatient with an increase in sputum quantity and/or a change in character or color, especially if accompanied by increasing cough and dyspnea, should be treated with a course of outpatient antibiotics.

It should be stressed that many patients with COPD have colonization of their tracheal tract with *Streptococcus pneumoniae, Haemophilus influenzae,* or *Moraxella catarrhalis.*[4] Other organisms, such as *Klebsiella* species, *Mycoplasma pneumoniae, Pseudomonas, Staphylococcus aureus, Proteus* species, or *Chlamydia TWAR* also may be seen. Unfortunately, making an etiologic bacteria-specific diagnosis in ABE/COPD is usually not possible. Consequently, most patients will require empiric therapy directed at the most likely etiologic organisms.

Although a number of clinical decision support tools, consensus guidelines, and recommendations have been issued, none has universal support. In large part, this is because the etiologic agents responsible for ABE/COPD, the outcome-effectiveness of various antibiotics, and risk-stratification parameters are not as thoroughly elaborated as they are for community-acquired pneumonia (CAP). Consequently, several authors have argued that there is an immediate need for guidelines on antibiotic use in COPD. The OMBIRT Panel has reviewed published trials and generated a set of guidelines based on evidence-based trials. Several attempts to formulate such protocols have resulted in broadly similar recommendations. Although the guidelines inevitably have been hampered by the lack of well-designed prospective studies, they have taken a practical approach that seems to be logical and can be used in the primary care setting. It must be emphasized, however, that the concepts on which the guidelines are based have not yet been verified by prospective clinical trials.[5-7]

Antibiotics. A number of relatively inexpensive, well-tolerated antibiotics are available, including amoxicillin, trimethoprim-sulfamethoxazole, doxycycline, and tetracycline. Antimicrobial resistance, particularly involving *H. influenzae, M. catarrhalis,* and *S. pneumoniae,* has become an increasing problem with many of these agents, specifically with older members of each of these drug classes. There is an increase in amoxicillin-resistant, beta-lactamase-producing *H. influenzae.* New agents are providing solutions to these difficulties. The azalide antibiotic azithromycin has the advantage of an appropriate spectrum of coverage, an acceptable safety profile, reasonable cost, and a patient-dosing schedule that improves patient compliance.

The newer fluoroquinolones, moxifloxacin, gatifloxacin, and levofloxacin, are advantageous when gram-negative bacteria predominate; ciprofloxacin is an excellent choice in this subgroup, especially for those with structural lung disease such as bronchiectasis and documented infection with gram-negative species (e.g., *Pseudomonas species).* Amoxicillin-clavulanate also has in vitro activity against beta-lactamase-producing *H. influenzae* and *M. catarrhalis,* as well as *S. peumoniae;* moreover, the agent's clinical efficacy in lower respiratory tract infection attributable to enzyme-producing strains has been demonstrated.

Severity of Exacerbation and Risk Factors Pathway. The Severity of Exacerbation and Risk Factors (SERF) pathway for antibiotic selection in outpatients with ABE/COPD is a clinical decision, consensus-driven support tool based on epidemiology, efficacy, and prognostic data generated by many published clinical trials.[5,23] In general, the need for intensification and amplification of antimicrobial coverage in patients with acute exacerbations of chronic obstructive lung disease (ABE/COPD) depends on the likelihood of infection with gram-negative enterobacteria, colonization status, the patient's history of exacerbations and antimicrobial treatment response record, the patient's ability to tolerate a treatment failure given his or her respiratory status, and other factors.

The SERF Pathway (*please see Table 2*), which is based on evi-

Table 2. The SERF Risk-Stratification Pathway for Antibiotic Selection in ABE/COPD

SEVERITY OF EXACERBATION AND RISK FACTOR (SERF) SUPPORT TOOL

RATIONALE

The need for intensification and amplification of antimicrobial coverage in patients with acute exacerbations of chronic obstructive lung disease (ABE/COPD) depends on:

- Likelihood of infection with gram-negative enterobacteria
- Colonization status
- Patient's history of exacerbations and antimicrobial treatment response record
- Ability of patient to tolerate a treatment failure given his or her respiratory status
- Other factors requiring sound clinical judgment.

THE SERF PATHWAY

- Based on evidence-based trials and consensus opinion
- Designed as a clinical decision support tool to help guide empiric antibiotic therapy for outpatients with ABE/COPD.

Final decisions regarding drug selection should be made by the clinician on a patient-by-patient basis using on a comprehensive database including history, physical examination, and other diagnostic information.

Table 3. SERF Pathway: Intensification of Treatment Trigger (IOTT) Criteria for Risk-Stratification in ABE/COPD

INTENSIFICATION-OF-TREATMENT TRIGGER (IOTT) CRITERIA SHOULD BE CONSIDERED WHEN SELECTING AN ANTIBIOTIC FOR EMPIRIC OUTPATIENT TREATMENT OF ABE/COPD.

WHEN IOTT CRITERIA ARE PRESENT, CLINICIANS SHOULD CONSIDER NEWER AGENTS WITH EVIDENCE-BASED SUPPORT AS INDICATED AND RECOGNIZE POSSIBLE LIMITATIONS OF OLDER AGENTS SUCH AS SULFONAMIDES, PENICILLINS, AND TETRACYCLINES

IOTT criteria include the following:

- History of multiple bacterial exacerbations of COPD within a short time period (more than 3 exacerbations in < 4 months)
- Multiple antimicrobial treatment exposures
- Documentation of gram-negative (enterobacteria, pseudomonas, Klebsiella, etc.) respiratory tract colonization
- History of requiring mechanical ventilation after ABE/COPD treatment failure
- History of gram-negative nosocomial lower respiratory tract infection
- Chronic, systemic corticosteroid use
- Multiple emergency department visits with relapse within a 10-day period
- Supplemental home oxygen
- Smoking
- High prevalence (documented) *S. pneumoniae* resistance to penicillin
- Chronic alcoholism associated with history of gram-negative (Klebsiella) lower respiratory tract infection
- Serious co-morbidity (immunosuppression, HIV, underlying malignancy, etc.)

dence-based trials and consensus opinion, is designed as a clinical support tool to help guide empiric antibiotic therapy for outpatients with ABE/COPD. Final decisions regarding drug selection should be made by the clinician on a patient-by-patient basis using a comprehensive database including history, physical examination, and other diagnostic information. Specifically, the SERF pathway identifies a number of IOTT criteria that have been generated from consensus reports, reviews, and prospective trials in ABE/COPD. These factors should be considered when selecting an antibiotic for empiric outpatient treatment of ABE/COPD. The OMBIRT Panel notes there is ample support in the medical literature for using clinical parameters identified in the SERF pathway and using IOTT criteria. *(Please see Tables 2 and 3.)*

Approximately one-half of all exacerbations of COPD can be attributed to bacterial infection, and antibiotic therapy has been demonstrated to improve clinical outcomes and accelerate clinical and physiologic recovery. The major pathogen continues to be *H. influenzae*, and resistance to beta-lactam antibiotics such as ampicillin can be expected in 20-40% of isolated strains.[24] Certain high-risk patients, in whom the cost of clinical treatment failure is high, can be identified by simple clinical criteria.

Studies suggest, for example, that patients with significant cardiopulmonary comorbidity, frequent purulent exacerbations of COPD, advanced age, generalized debility, malnutrition, chronic corticosteroid administration, long duration of COPD, and severe underlying lung function may be more likely to fail therapy with older drugs, such as ampicillin, and that early relapse can be expected.[24] Treatment directed toward resistant pathogens using appropriate agents may be expected to lead to improved clinical outcomes and overall lower costs, particularly if hospital admissions and respiratory failure can be prevented. Future studies examining the role of antibiotics should enroll these high-risk patients to determine if new therapies have significant clinical, quality-of-life, and economic advantages over older agents.[24]

Other authors have proposed different classification schemes. There is general agreement that acute exacerbations of chronic bronchitis (AECB) can be defined as the presence of increases in cough/sputum, sputum purulence, and dyspnea. However, recent investigations suggest that the severity of AECB also may be divided into three stages based on the history of the patient: 1) previously healthy individuals; 2) patients with chronic cough and sputum and infrequent exacerbations; and 3) persons with frequent exacerbations or more severe chronic airflow limitation.

Comparative Trials of Antibiotic Efficacy in Acute Bacterial Exacerbations of COPD. The goals of therapy for ABE/COPD are to resolve the infection expeditiously, maintain an infection-free interval for as long as possible, and select an antibiotic with the fewest adverse effects and most favorable compliance profile. Because patients with COPD frequently are on complicated, multi-modal drug therapy (consumption of many medications with a complicated dosing schedule is not uncommon), identifying effective, compliance-enhancing regimens for ABE/COPD is an important clinical objective. (*Please see Table 4.*)

Moreover, because the key meta-analysis study supporting the efficacy of antibiotics in ABE/COPD was based on older trials with "older" agents, it is important that practitioners are aware of more recent studies evaluating effectiveness of newer antibiotics for this condition.

One randomized, multicenter, investigator-blinded, parallel-group study compared a five-day, once-daily course of azithromycin (two 250 mg capsules on day 1, followed by one 250 mg capsule on days 2-5) with a 10-day, three-times-daily course of amoxicillin-clavulanate (one 500 mg tablet tid) in 70 patients with ABE/COPD.[23] At the end of therapy, all 29 (100%) efficacy-assessable patients treated with azithromycin were cured or improved, compared with 25 (93%) of 27 assessable patients given amoxicillin-clavulanate (P = NS). Bacteriologic eradication rates were 86% (25 of 29 isolates) with azithromycin and 87% (20 of 23 isolates) with the comparative agent. Azithromycin was well tolerated; adverse events considered related or possibly related to treatment were reported in 28% of azithromycin recipients, compared with 39% of amoxicillin-clavulanate recipients (P = NS). The authors concluded that the five-day, once-daily regimen of azithromycin is comparable to a standard agent in the treatment of patients with ABE/COPD.[23]

The results of this study indicated that the administration of azithromycin once daily for five days is comparable to amoxicillin-clavulanate in the treatment of patients with ABE/COPD. The dosing schedule of azithromycin described in this trial is among the the shortest and simplest regimens among commonly prescribed oral antibiotics for ABE/COPD.[23] Because reduced frequency of dosing and shorter therapy duration may improve patient compliance, and potentially outcomes, practitioners should be aware of differences among effective agents as they relate to these compliance-sensitive parameters.

The safety and efficacy of macrolides vs. fluoroquinolones have been compared in clinical trials, all of them demonstrating, in a rather consistent manner, comparable clinical outcomes in patients with ABE/COPD.[49,50] In one study, 986 patients were randomized to receive either moxifloxacin 400 mg PO qd for either 5 or 10 days, or clarithromycin, 500 mg PO bid for 10 days.[49] The main outcome measures were bacteriologic response rate at the end of therapy (post-therapy, days 0-6) and at follow-up (post-therapy, days 7-17), as well as overall clinical response. Two patient populations were analyzed: efficacy-valid (i.e., those with a pretherapy pathogen) and intent-to-treat (all subjects who took a drug).

In 420 efficacy valid patients, overall clinical resolution was 89% for five days of moxifloxacin vs. 91% for 10 days moxifloxacin, vs. 91% for 10 days clarithromycin. Bacteriologic eradication rates at the end of therapy were 94% and 95% for five-day moxifloxacin and 10-day moxiflloxacin, respectively, and 91% for the clarithromycin group. Overall, moxifloxacin 400 mg once daily was found to be clinically and bacteriologically equivalent to a 10-day course of clarithromycin for treatment of ABE/COPD.[49]

A safety and efficacy study comparing moxifloxacin, an oral advanced generation fluorooqunolone, with azithromycin was conducted between October 1998 and April 1999. In all, 576 patients with ABE/COPD were enrolled in 37 centers across the United States and Canada; 280 (49%) of those enrolled had acute bacterial exacerbations of chronic bronchitis (i.e., pretherapy pathogen). Patients were randomized to receive either moxifloxacin 400 mg administered once daily for five days or azithromycin for 500 days (500 mg qd x 1, then 250 qd x 4). For the purposes of study blinding, all patients received encapsulated tablets.[25]

The main outcome measure was clinical response at the test-of-cure visit (14-21 days post-therapy). Three patient populations were analyzed for efficacy: clinically-valid, microbiologically-valid (i.e., those with a pretherapy pathogen), and intent-to-treat (i.e., received at least 1 dose of the study drug).

Table 4. Multi-Modal Pharmacotherapy for ABE/COPD: Checklist of Agents Requiring Consideration

- Beta-agonists (selective agents preferred)
- Anticholinergic drug
- Home oxygen
- Systemic corticosteroids
- Inhaled corticosteroids
- Antibiotics (advanced generation macrolides and quinolones preferred)
- Theophylline (efficacy is controversial)

For the efficacy-valid group, clinical response at the test-of-cure was 88% for patients in each treatment group. In 237 microbiologically-valid patients, corresponding clinical resolution rates were 88% for five-day moxifloxacin vs. 86% for five-day azithromycin. Bacteriological eradication rates at the end of therapy were 95% for five-day moxifloxacin and 94% for the azithromycin. Corresponding eradication rates at the test-of-cure visit were 89% and 86%, respectively. Among the 567 intent-to-treat patients (283 moxifloxacin and 284 azithromycin), drug-related events were reported for 22% and 17% respectively. Diarrhea and nausea were the most common drug-related events reported in each group.

The investigators concluded that a five-day course of azithromycin was clinically and bacteriologically equivalent to moxifloxacin 400 mg once daily for five days for treatment of patients with ABE/COPD of proven bacterial etiology.[25] Similar results and conclusions were reached in a prospective, multicenter, phase IIIb clinical trial evaluating patients with signs and symptoms of ABE/COPD. Patients randomly received either a five-day oral course of azithromycin (500 mg qd x 1, then 250 qd x 4) or moxifloxacin (400 mg once-daily), and rates of clinical success were assessed at follow-up 14-21 days after completion of therapy. Clinical resolution at 14-21 days was 85% for moxifloxacin- and 81% for azithromycin-treated patients (95% CI, -6.0% to 14%).[26]

In another prospective, multicenter, double-blind study, the efficacy of ciprofloxacin was compared with that of clarithromycin as therapy for patients with ABE/COPD from whom a pretherapy pathogen was isolated; the efficacy was measured by the infection-free interval. Patients randomly received either ciprofloxacin or clarithromycin (500 mg twice a day for 14 days). Three hundred seventy-six patients with acute exacerbations of chronic bronchitis were enrolled in the study, 234 of whom had an ABE/COPD. Clinical resolution was observed in 90% (89 of 99) of ciprofloxacin recipients and 82% (75 of 91) of clarithromycin recipients for whom efficacy could be evaluated. The median infection-free interval was 142 days for ciprofloxacin recipients and 51 days for clarithromycin recipients (P = 0.15). Bacteriologic eradication rates were 91% (86 of 95) for ciprofloxacin recipients and 77% (67 of 87) for clarithromycin recipients (P = 0.01). The investigators concluded that compared with clarithromycin, treatment of ABE/COPD with ciprofloxacin was associated with a trend toward a longer infection-free interval and a statistically significantly higher bacteriologic eradication rate.[32]

Infectious Precipitants of ABE/COPD. The role of bacterial and viral-mediated infection as precipitants of acute respiratory decompensation in the setting of COPD has been controversial. Certainly, numerous studies have confirmed the role of viral infection in acute exacerbations of COPD.[33-35] In one study, 32% of patients with an acute exacerbation had evidence of viral infection.[34] In these and other investigations evaluating the role of viral infection, the most common agents identified include influenza virus, parainfluenzae, and respiratory syncytial (RSV) virus.[33-37]

Interestingly, although many treatment guidelines for ABE/COPD do not mandate empirical antimicrobial coverage of atypical organisms (e.g., *Mycoplasma pneumoniae, Chlamydia pneumoniae,* and *Legionella)* for patients with ABE/COPD, studies show that atypical organisms such as mycoplasma or chlamydia occasionally may be associated with decompensation in patients with COPD. In fact, many patients with COPD have serologic evidence of previous *Chlamydia* infection. On the other hand, recent studies suggest that acute *Chlamydia pneumoniae* infection occurs in only about 5% of acute exacerbations of COPD.[35,36]

Epidemiology. The precise role of bacterial infection is more difficult to ascertain, and equally problematic to confirm in the individual patient. Nevertheless, it is clear that bacterial precipitants play an important etiologic role in ABE/COPD. In one Canadian study enrolling 1687 patients (80% of which had ABE/COPD), sputum cultures were obtained in 125 patients (7.4%). Normal flora was found in 76 of 125 sputum specimens (61%), and a pathogen was found in 49 (39%). Of all the patients having sputum cultures, *H. influenzae* was the most common pathogen, occurring in 24 cases (19%), followed by *Streptococcus pneumoniae* in 15 (12%) and *Moraxella catarrhalis* in 10 (8%).[4] Complicating confirmation of a linkage between acute bacterial infection and clinical deterioration in COPD is the fact that patients with COPD have chronic colonization of the respiratory tree with such organisms as *Streptococcus pneumoniae, Hemophilus influenzae,* and *Hemophilus parainfluenzae.*[37] In addition, *Moraxella catarrhalis* is being recognized with increasing frequency.

Role of Antibiotics. It should be noted that many studies were performed prior to the availability of more potent, compliance-enhancing agents, many of which, such as azithromycin and the new-generation fluoroquinolones, are not only active against atypical organisms, but also against beta-lactamase-producing *H. influenzae* and *M. catarrhalis.* Furthermore, the failure rate of older antibiotics may be as high as 25%.[39,40]

One approach to delineating the precise role of bacterial infection in ABE/COPD is to evaluate the efficacy of antibiotics in producing symptomatic and functional improvement in patients during an acute exacerbation of COPD. A number of trials have been performed to assess the relationships between antibiotic treatment and resolution of symptoms, many of them using tetracycline as the therapeutic agent.[33] Some of these studies demonstrated a role for antibiotics during the acute exacerbation, while others did not find a significant advantage.

However, a landmark meta-analysis of nine studies performed between 1957 and 1992 confirms that there is a small, but statistically significant benefit when antibiotics are used for acute exacerbations of COPD.[38] The benefits are relatively greater for those patients with ABE/COPD who require hospitalization.

Clinical studies of acute exacerbations of COPD are difficult to interpret because of the heterogeneous nature of COPD, diffuse symptoms that can vary spontaneously, and difficulties in defining clinical response both in the short and long term. Although the role of bacterial infection—and as a result, empiric use of antibiotics—in COPD is somewhat controversial, the most currently available evidence shows that bacterial infection has a significant role in acute exacerbations, but its role in disease progression is less certain. Moreover, based on the preponderance of published evidence, antibiotic therapy is recommended in all patients with ABE/COPD who present with infectious symptoms (i.e., increased sputum production, change in character of the sputum, increased coughing and shortness of breath) suggesting that antimicrobial therapy will produce a better outcome.[4,41-44]

Upper respiratory tract commensals, such as nontypable *Haemophilus influenzae,* cause most bronchial infections by exploiting deficiencies in the host defenses.[41] Some COPD patients are chronically colonized by bacteria between exacerbations, which represents an equilibrium in which the numbers of bacteria are contained by the host defenses but not eliminated. When an exacerbation occurs, this equilibrium is upset and bacterial numbers increase, which incites an inflammatory response. Neutrophil products can further impair the mucosal defenses, favoring the bacteria, but if the infection is managed, symptoms resolve. However, if the infection persists, chronic inflammation may cause lung damage. About 50% of exacerbations involve bacterial infection, but these patients are not easy to differentiate from those who are uninfected, which means that antibiotics should be given empirically to the majority of patients who present with ABE/COPD. Further research is needed to characterize those patients in whom bacterial infection may play a more important role and in whom more intensive antibiotic coverage is required.

Old vs. New Agents. The antibiotic arsenal available for treatment of ABE/COPD includes a wide range of older and newer agents representing several drug classes. Although many of the studies confirming efficacy of antibiotics in ABE/COPD were performed with such older agents as amoxicillin and tetracycline, usage patterns are changing in favor of newer agents such as macrolides and advanced generation fluoroquinolones with a broader spectrum of coverage and which also have compliance-enhancing features.

There is evidence-based justification for this evolution in prescribing practices.[4,41-43] In the past, antibiotics such as amoxicillin, ampicillin, tetracycline, erythromycin, and co-trimoxazole were widely employed. Many of the meta-analysis trials demonstrating the usefulness of antibiotics drew upon studies using these agents. But resistance patterns have changed.[41-46] In particular, during the last 10 years, there has been a steady rise in the frequency of beta-lactamase production by *H. influenzae* and *M. catarrhalis,* and more recently, strains of penicillin-resistant pneumococci have emerged.[41-47]

Fortunately, these older antibiotics have been joined by newer agents with either a wider spectrum of activity in vitro, better pharmacokinetics, lower incidence of side effects, more convenient dosing, and/or a shorter duration of therapy. Among the antibiotics approved for ABE/COPD, and which also have evidence-based support for their effectiveness in this condition, the azalide azithromycin, the macrolide clarithromycin, and quinolones such as moxifloxacin, gatifloxacin, and evofloxacin are playing an increasingly important role.[43-48] In addition, beta-lactamase inhibitors, including second and third generation cephalosporins, also are available.[41] A more detailed discussion of antibiotic therapy and the selection process are presented in subsequent sections of this review.

Antibiotic Outcome-Effectiveness and Total Cost of Therapy. Unfortunately, limited data exist to guide physicians in the cost-effective treatment of acute exacerbation of chronic bronchitis

(ABE/COPD). One important study, however, attempted to determine the antimicrobial efficacy of various agents and compared total outcome costs for patients with ABE/COPD.[51] For the purpose of this analysis, a retrospective review was performed of 60 outpatient medical records of individuals with a diagnosis of COPD associated with acute episodes seen in the pulmonary clinic of a teaching institution.

The participating patients had a total of 224 episodes of ABE/COPD requiring antibiotic treatment. Before review, empirical antibiotic choices were divided into first-line (amoxicillin, co-trimoxazole, tetracyclines, erythromycin); second-line (cephradine, cefuroxime, cefaclor, cefprozil); and third-line (azithromycin, amoxicillin-clavulanate, ciprofloxacin) agents. The designations "first-line," "second-line," and "third-line" were based on a consensus of resident pulmonologists, and was not intended to indicate superiority of one group of drugs vs. another. The residents were asked, "What antibiotic would you choose to treat a patient with ABE/COPD on their initial presentation, on their second presentation, and on a subsequent presentation, if each episode was separated by 2-4 weeks?"[52]

The results have potentially interesting implications for antibiotic selection in the outpatient environment. In this study, patients receiving first-line agents (amoxicillin, co-trimoxazole, tetracyclines, erythromycin) failed significantly more frequently (19% vs 7%; $P < 0.05$) than those treated with third-line agents (azithromycin, amoxicillin-clavulanate, ciprofloxacin). Moreover, patients prescribed first-line agents were hospitalized significantly more often for ABE/COPD within two weeks of outpatient treatment as compared with patients prescribed third-line agents (18.0% vs 5.3% for third-line agents; $P < 0.02$). Time between subsequent ABE/COPD episodes requiring treatment was significantly longer for patients receiving third-line agents compared with first-line and second-line agents ($P < 0.005$).[51] The high failure rate with such older agents as amoxicillin, tetracycline, and erythromycin correlates well with recent reports of increasing antibiotic resistance.[52-54]

As might be expected, initial pharmacy acquisition costs were lowest with first-line agents (first-line U.S. \$10.30 ± 8.76; second-line U.S. \$24.45 ± 25.65; third-line U.S. \$45.40 ± 11.11; $P < 0.0001$), but third-line agents showed a trend toward lower mean total costs of ABE/COPD treatment (first-line U.S. \$942 ± 2173; second-line, U.S. \$563 ± 2296; third-line, U.S. \$542 ± 1946). The use of so-called third-line antimicrobials, azithromycin, amoxicillin-clavulanate, or ciprofloxacin, significantly reduced the failure rate and need for hospitalization, prolonged the time between ABE/COPD episodes, and were associated with a lower total cost of management for ABE/COPD. Well-designed, prospective studies are needed to confirm these findings and determine how critical pathways should be constructed to maximize outcome-effectiveness of antibiotics used for ABE/COPD.

Based on these results, the authors of this retrospective analysis suggest that these trends should be of interest to the following groups: 1) managed care decision-makers involved in the formulary selection process; 2) physicians whose objective is to optimize outcome-effectiveness of antibiotic therapy; and 3) to patients with ABE/COPD, since definitive treatment of the initial presentation is necessary to minimize work disability, permit continuance of normal activities, reduce hospitalizations requiring more intensive therapy, and prevent further clinical deterioration from bronchitis to pneumonia.[52]

In addition, the reduction in hospitalization rate observed with second-line and third-line agents, when compared with first-line agents, may have potential impact on the mortality of patients with COPD. In a recent study of 458 patients with COPD who required admission to hospital for AECB, mortality was 13% after a median length of stay of 10 days; mortality at 180 days was 35%.[55] The severity of ventilator-related impairment of lung function in patients with COPD is strongly related to death both from obstructive lung disease and from all causes.[55,56] Moreover, patients who experience frequent episodes of ABE/COPD are at risk for accelerated loss of lung function and effective antibiotic therapy may slow this decline. The use of third-line antibiotics in the outpatient setting could decrease the number of hospitalizations and the degenerative disease process, and thus prolong the survival of patients with COPD. Further evaluation of this hypothesis is required.[252,54-57]

Based on data collected in this study, the use of azithromycin, amoxicillin-clavulanate, or ciprofloxacin for the treatment of ABE/COPD resulted in significantly fewer physician office visits and appeared to prevent hospitalizations when compared with first- or second-line antimicrobial therapy.[52] Whether there is any difference among these agents remains to be evaluated longitudinally. Additionally, the repetitive nature of return visits to the emergency department or outpatient clinic for ABE/COPD may assist in identifying patients who require initial treatment with more effective agents in order to prevent ABE/COPD-related hospital admissions and progression of the disease.

Pharmacotherapy for Patient Stabilization: A Multi-Modal Approach for Optimizing Clinical Outcomes

Optimizing outcomes in patients with ABE/COPD requires prudent but prompt administration of pharmacological agents directed at relieving bronchoconstriction and improving oxygenation. A multi-modal approach to initial stabilization is the rule rather than the exception. As might be expected, pharmacological approaches for chronic maintenance therapy differ somewhat from those used for acute management. In both cases, it should be stressed that the response to various pharmacotherapeutic modalities may vary from one patient to another; hence, sequencing and combining therapy (using such agents as oxygen, beta-agonists, anticholinergics, and/or corticosteroids) according to previously documented patterns of clinical response may represent the most logical approach in the majority of patients. The role of antibiotic therapy is discussed in a separate section.

Home-Based Treatment Plans for Primary Care Practice

After evaluation and initial treatment in the office or clinic setting, several adjustments to the patient's outpatient medical regimen may be considered.

Oxygen. First, patients with severe COPD may be eligible for home oxygen therapy. Although this is generally not initiated as part of the emergency department treatment, patients may benefit from a referral for subsequent consideration for home oxygen therapy. Patients with a PaO_2 of less than 55 mmHg at rest or a PaO_2 between 55-60 mmHg with evidence of cor pulmonale may meet Medicare criteria for reimbursable oxygen supplementation. It has been shown that home oxygen therapy prolongs survival, reduces polycythemia, decreases the risk of pulmonary hypertension, and reduces the risk of right ventricu-

Table 5. Characteristics of Bronchodilators Delivered by Metered-Dose Inhalers

Medication	Dose (mg)/Puff	Beta-1-Agonist*	Beta-2-Agonist*	Anticholinergic*	Onset (Min)	Peak (Min)	Duration (Min)
Isoproterenol	0.08	+ + +	+ + +	-	3-5	5-10	60-90
Isoetharine	0.34	+ +	+ +	-	3-5	5-20	60-150
Metaproterenol	0.65	+	+ + +	-	5-15	10-60	60-180
Terbutaline	0.20	+	+ + + +	-	5-30	60-120	180-360
Albuterol	0.09	+	+ + + +	-	5-15	60-90	240-360
Bitolterol	0.37	+	+ + + +	-	5-10	60-90	300-480
Pirbuterol	0.20	+	+ + +	-	5-10	30-60	180-240
Salmeterol	0.04	+	+ + + +	-	10-20	180	720
Ipratropium	0.18	-	-	+ + + +	5-15	60-120	240-480

* The number of plus signs denotes the relative level of activity.

lar failure. Accordingly, patients who meet these criteria should be referred to appropriate providers who can arrange for home oxygen supplementation.

Bronchodilators. Long-term management of the patient with COPD almost always requires use of various bronchodilating agents. Studies have shown that most patients with COPD respond to bronchodilators.[58,59] (*Please see Table 5.*) Significant improvements in pulmonary function may occur in response to inhaled beta-agonists, inhaled anticholinergic agents, and oral methylxanthines. Accordingly, appropriate patients should be discharged on bronchodilators, beginning with either inhaled beta-agonists or inhaled anticholinergics. Although the older, non-selective beta-agonists are effective in COPD, when used for long-term therapy, patients should be on one of the newer, longer acting, beta-2 selective agonists such as metaproterenol, albuterol, terbutaline, or bitolterol. For long-term maintenance, these agents are typically used in a dose of two puffs up to four times a day by metered dose inhaler. (*Please see Table 6.*) Some patients, however, may require larger doses, and studies in patients with chronic disease have found dose-related improvements up to 1600 mcg.[60]

In large studies, albuterol has been found to improve pulmonary function for stable patients with COPD.[60] The effectiveness, however, decreases over time. Albuterol is safe for the long-term management of COPD, as the incidence of drug-related adverse events are low. Patients with COPD tend to be older, and as such, have decreased sensitivity to adrenergic compounds. Some authors have found that the response to anticholinergic compounds in chronic therapy may be superior to beta-agonists for routine use.

Anticholinergic Agents. Anticholinergics should probably be used for routine maintenance in most patients with COPD. Inhaled quaternary ammonium anticholinergic agents have been found in some studies to lead to greater bronchodilation than beta-agonists or theophylline. Since older patients have a decrease in responsiveness to the adrenergic receptors, the cholinergic receptors become even more important in the older patients with COPD. Ipratropium is the primary agent used by metered-dose inhaler in this country. It is relatively safe, with side effects generally limited to dry mouth or the sensation of a "metallic" taste in the mouth. Again, this agent leads to increasing bronchodilation as the dose increases up to 600 mcg. Ipratropium is available in 500 mcg doses by metered-dose inhaler.

A meta-analysis of seven long-term studies comparing ipratropium with beta-agonists demonstrated that ipratropium leads to greater improvement in FEV_1 and even greater improvements in force vital capacity over the course of 90 days. Ipratropium leads to greater improvements in quality-of-life measurements. The improvements in pulmonary function are greatest in patients who have stopped smoking compared to current smokers. Furthermore, patients using ipratropium are less likely than patients using beta-agonists to develop a decreased response over time.[61] Ipratropium has minimal side effects that primarily are related to dry mouth or leaving a bad taste in the mouth.

Inhalers. Prior to discharge from the primary care clinic or office, patients should be instructed in the proper means of using meter-dose inhalers. Many patients will benefit from the use of a spacer device. A typical discharge regimen will include albuterol by meter dose inhaler either on an as needed basis for rescue therapy or for chronic maintenance therapy.[62,63] In addition, most patients with COPD should be using ipratropium by meter-dose inhaler for chronic maintenance therapy. These drugs are available as combination therapy in meter-dose inhalers. Patients who have prominent nighttime symptoms may benefit from a long-acting beta-agonist such as salmeterol. Patients should be counseled, however, that salmeterol should not be used for rescue therapy.

Theophylline. Theophylline does have dose-related effects on pulmonary function in patients with stable COPD. This drug may be used for patients who cannot or will not use meter-dose inhalers, patients who are not responding to otherwise maximal therapy, or patients who have prominent nighttime symptoms. Therapy is usually initiated at a dose of 300 mg twice a day with monitoring of the theophylline level. Therapeutic theophylline levels are considered to be between 10 and 20 micrograms per cc, although the FDA has changed labeling requirements for these drugs to suggest that consideration be given to maintain the level between 10 and 15 micrograms per cc. Theophylline metabolism is affected by a number of factors and patients should be cautioned not to increase their dose without seeking medical advice.

Corticosteroids. About 25% of patients with COPD will respond to oral steroids. Patients with a significant degree of reversibility of pulmonary function on baseline testing are most likely to respond to steroids.[64] It seems reasonable to initiate a two-week trial of oral steroids for patients with COPD. Studies indicate that there may be a role for inhaled corticosteroids in patients with COPD. In this regard, one study found that the addition of inhaled corticosteroids over the

Table 6. Beta-Agonist Dosages

Albuterol (Proventil, Ventolin)	2-4 puffs q4h	0.5 cc (2.5 mg) in 2.5 cc NS
Bitolterol (Tornalate)	2 puffs q8h	0.5 cc (0.2% [1mg]) in 2 cc NS
Isoetharine (Bronkosol)	4 puffs q4h	0.5 cc (0.25%) in 3 cc NS
Isoproterenol (Isuprel)	5-15 puffs (1:200) q4h	0.5 cc (0.5%) in 3 cc NS
Metaproterenol (Alupent, Metaprel)	2-3 puffs q3-4h	0.3 cc (1.5 mg) in 2.5 cc NS
Pirbuterol (Maxair)	2 puffs q4-6h	
Terbutaline (Brethine)	2 puffs q4-6h	
Salmeterol (Serevent)	2 puffs q12h	

course of two years decreased morbidity and improved airway obstruction when used in conjunction with an inhaled beta-2 agonist.[65] A more recent study found a short-term improvement in lung function in smokers with COPD treated with inhaled steroids, but this then was followed by continued deterioration in lung function.[66]

Antibiotics: Summary

While many episodes of acute exacerbation of COPD are caused by viral infection, the weight of evidence seems to indicated that patients respond to oral antibiotics—especially when the exacerbation is associated with signs and symptoms of acute, bacterial bronchitis that is superimposed on COPD with a presentation characterized by fever, dyspnea, increase in sputum production, or change in the color of sputum.[61] Available antibiotics with evidence-based support for their efficacy and which have indications for ABE/COPD have been discussed in detail.

Patients with ABE/COPD who are deemed suitable for oral, outpatient therapy and who do not have signficant IOTT criteria in the SERF pathway (*please see Table 3*) that suggest the specific need for more extensive gram-negative coverage, should be discharged with a compliance-sensitive antibiotic that provides adequate coverage of *S. pneumoniae, H. influenzae,* and *M. catarrhalis.*

Macrolides/Azithromycin. Based on evidence-based trials and pharmatectural criteria (duration of therapy, reduced dosing frequency, drug interaction profile, cost, and spectrum of coverage), macrolides such as azithromycin should be considered a first-line agent in patients with ABE/COPD who, on the basis of clinical judgement, are likely to be infected with *S. pneumoniae, H. influenzae,* or *M. catarrhalis.*[6,7,15-18,68-70]

It should be stressed that one of the advanced macrolides, azithromycin, has the advantage of a simplified dosing schedule; it is given once daily for only five days (500 mg PO on day 1 and 250 mg PO qd on days 2-5). Azithromycin (500 mg on day 1 and 250 mg on days 2-5) did not affect the plasma levels or pharmacokinetics of theophylline administered as a single intravenous dose. However, because the effect of azithromycin on plasma levels or pharmacokinetics of theophylline is not known, until further data are available, prudent medical practice dictates careful monitoring of plasma levels of theophylline in COPD patients receiving azithromycin and theophylline concomitantly. The same precaution should be applied to patients receiving warfarin and azithromycin concomitantly. Other macrolides generally require a similar monitoring strategy.

Clarithromycin, another advanced generation macrolide, requires a longer course of therapy and, as a 7-day course, is more expensive ($58-$68 for a 7-day course) than a five-day course of azithromycin ($43-$46). In general, the decision to use a macrolide such as azithromycin is based on consideration of its generally acceptable cost ($43-$46 for a five-day treatment regimen), as well as its real-world advantages, which include convenient, once-daily dosing; a correct spectrum of coverage; favorable drug interaction profile; and toleration data (gastrointestinal side effects occur in about 3-5% of patients taking a five-day, multiple-dose regimen). The oral tablet formulation permits consumption of the antibiotic without regard to food ingestion.

Fluoroquinolones. Patients who are macrolide treatment failures, are suspected of gram-negative infection with enterobacteria, and/or present with multiple IOTT points on the SERF pathway may be effectively served by a fluoroquinolone such as levofloxacin, moxifloxacin, gatifloxacin, or ciprofloxacin, the latter of which is not recommended when *S. pneumoniae* is the presumed causative agent. Levofloxacin is well-tolerated, with the most common side effects, including nausea, diarrhea, headache, and constipation. Food does not affect the absorption of the drug, but it should be taken at least two hours before or two hours after antacids containing magnesium or aluminum, as well as sucralfate, metal cations such as iron, and multivitamin preparations with zinc. Dosage adjustment for levofloxacin is recommended in patients with impaired renal function (clearance < 50 mL/min).

Although no significant effect of levofloxacin on plasma concentration of theophylline was detected in 14 health volunteers studied, because other quinolones have produced increases in patients taking concomitant theophylline, theophylline levels should be closely monitored in patients on levofloxacin and dosage adjustments made as necessary. Monitoring patients on warfarin also is recommended in patients on quinolones. All quinolones have been associated with cartilage damage in animal studies, and therefore, they are not recommended for use in children, adolescents, and pregnant and nursing women. Cephalosporins are also available and effective for treatment of ABE/COPD.

Moxifloxacin is the only fluoroquinolone antibiotic indicated in the United States for a five-day treatment of ABE/COPD. Other fluoroquinolones are indicated for seven, 7-10, or 7-14 days for the treatment of ABE/COPD. Moxifloxacin is generally well tolerated. In clinical trials, the most common adverse events were nausea (8%), diarrhea (6%), dizziness (3%), headache (2%), abdominal pain (2%), and vomiting (2%). The agent is contraindicated in persons with a history of hypersensitivity to moxifloxacin or any quinolone antibiotic. The safety and effectiveness of moxifloxacin in pediatric patients, adolescents (> age 18), pregnant women, and lactating women have not been established.

Moxifloxacin has been shown to prolong the QT interval of the electrocardiogram in some patients. The drug should be avoided in patients with known prolongation of the QT interval, patients with uncorrected hypokalemia, and patients receiving Class lA (e.g., quinidine, procainamide) or Class lll (e.g., amiodarone, sotalol) antiarrhythmic agents, due to the lack of clinical experience with the drug in these patient populations. Pharmacokinetic studies between moxifloxacin and other drugs that prolong the QT interval such as cisapride, erythromycin, antipsychotics, and tricyclic antidepressants have not been performed. An additive effect of moxifloxacin and these drugs cannot be excluded; therefore, moxifloxacin should be used with caution when given concurrently with these drugs.

The effect of moxifloxacin on patients with congenital prolongation of the QT interval has not been studied; however, it is expected that these individuals may be more susceptible to drug-induced QT prolongation. Because of limited clinical experience, moxifloxacin should be used with caution in patients with ongoing proarrhythmic conditions, such as clinically significant bradycardia or acute myocardial ischemia. As with all quinolones, moxifloxacin should be used with caution in patients with known or suspected central nervous system (CNS) disorders or in the presence of other risk factors that may predispose to seizures or lower the seizure threshold.

Gatifloxacin, a broad-spectrum 8-methoxy fluoroquinolone antibiotic, has been approved for the safe and effective treatment of approved indications, including community-acquired respiratory tract infections, such as bacterial exacerbation of chronic bronchitis (ABE/COPD); acute sinusitis; and CAP caused by indicated, susceptible strains of gram-positive and gram-negative bacteria. The recommended dose for gatifloxacin is 400 mg once daily, for all individuals with normal renal function. Dosage adjustment is required in patients with impaired renal function (creatinine clearance, < 40 mL/min).

Gatifloxacin is primarily excreted through the kidneys and less than 1% is metabolized by the liver. In clinical trials, gatifloxacin has been found to be a well-tolerated treatment in 15 international clinical trials at 500 study sites. Gatifloxacin may have the potential to prolong the QTc interval of the electrocardiogram in some patients, and due to limited clinical experience, gatifloxacin should be avoided in patients with known prolongation of the QTc interval, in patients with uncorrected hypokalemia, and in patients receiving Class IA (e.g., quinidine, procainamide) or Class III (e.g., amiodarone, sotalol) antiarrhythmic agents. Gatifloxacin should be used with caution when given together with drugs that may prolong the QTc interval (e.g., cisapride, erythromycin, antipsychotics, tricyclic antidepressants), and in patients with ongoing proarrhythmic conditions (e.g., clinically significant bradycardia or acute myocardial ischemia).

Gatifloxacin should be used with caution in patients with known or suspected CNS disorders or patients who have a predisposition to seizures. The most common side effects associated with gatifloxacin in clinical trials were gastrointestinal. Adverse reactions considered to be drug related and occurring in greater than 3% of patients were: nausea (8%), vaginitis (6%), diarrhea (4%), headache (3%), and dizziness (3%).

Oral doses of gatifloxacin should be administered at least four hours before the administration of ferrous sulfate; dietary supplements containing zinc, magnesium, or iron (such as multivitamins); aluminum/magnesium-containing antacids; or Videx (didanosine, or ddI). Concomitant administration of gatifloxacin and probencid significantly increases systemic exposure to gatifloxacin. Concomitant administration of gatifloxacin and digoxin did not produce significant alteration of the pharmacokinetics of gatifloxacin; however, patients taking digoxin should be monitored for signs and/or symptoms of digoxin toxicity.

Patients with a greater risk of respiratory failure are more likely to benefit from antibiotic therapy. This would include patients of advanced age and patients with significant lung impairment, impairment due to other comorbid conditions, frequent exacerbations, or steroid use. Accordingly, a small percentage of these patients may require intensification and amplification of antibiotic therapy (i.e., the movement from azithromycin to a fluoroquinolone) to cover gram-negative organisms in addition to the three common offenders cited above.

Less expensive and still widely used in certain institutions and health plans, many of the older agents (sulfa-derivatives, tetracyclines, and amoxicillin) are becoming resistant to *S. pneumoniae* or do not cover beta-lactamase-producing organisms and, as a result, may no longer represent the best choice for empiric therapy of ABE/COPD.[71-77] The finding in one retrospective study that such antimicrobials as azithromycin, amoxicillin-clavulanate, or ciprofloxacin significantly reduced the failure rate and need for hospitalization, prolonged the time between ABE/COPD episodes, and were associated a lower total cost of management for ABE/COPD compared to the older agents is extremely provocative and requires further investigation.[76]

Even until clarification of outcome-effectiveness is forthcoming, clinicians should be aware that a number of newer antibiotic agents are available, including advanced generation macrolides and quinolones, which have the advantage of a broader spectrum of activity, simplified dosing regimens, and lower resistance rates.[78]

Pneumonia in Patients with COPD. The development of pneumonia in a patient with COPD frequently will provide an indication for admission. However, there are younger patients with very mild COPD who have good ventilatory status and who do not have other concomitant medical diseases who, on the basis of clinical judgement, may be given a trial of outpatient antibiotic therapy. Protocols for treatment of CAP are widely published. *(Please see Table 7.)* However, most patients with COPD complicated by pneumonia will require admission. The small percentage of patients who are discharged, and therefore judged appropriate for outpatient treatment, should be treated for the most common causative agents, which include *S. pneumoniae, H. influenzae, M. catarrhalis, M. pneumoniae,* and *C. pneumoniae.* Given the spectrum of organisms encountered, it is probably preferable to initiate therapy with either a macrolide/azalide such as azithromycin or, as an alternative, an advanced generation fluorquinolone.

Community-Acquired Pneumonia (CAP)—OMBIRT Panel Overview and Recommendations for Outpatient Management

Despite a general consensus that empiric, outpatient treatment of CAP requires, at the least, mandatory coverage of such organisms as *S. pneumoniae, H. influenzae,* and *M. catarrhalis,* as well as atypical organisms (*Mycoplasma pneumoniae, Chlamydia pneumoniae,* and *Legionella pneumophila*), antibiotic selection strategies for achieving this spectrum of coverage vary widely. New treatment guidelines for CAP have been issued by such national associations as the Infectious Disease Society of America (IDSA, 2000), the American Thoracic Society (ATS, 2001) and the Centers for Disease Control and Prevention (CDC) Drug-Resistant Streptococcus pneumoniae Therapeutic Working Group (CDCDRSP-WG, 2000).

Deciphering the strengths, subtleties, and differences among recommendations issued by different authoritative sources can be problematic and confusing. Because patient disposition practices and

Table 7. OMBIRT Panel Guidelines—Empiric Antimicrobial Therapy of Choice for Outpatient‡ and In-Hospital Management of Patients with Community-Acquired Pneumonia (CAP)

PATIENT PROFILE/ETIOLOGIC AGENTS	FIRST-LINE ANTIBIOTIC THERAPY†	ALTERNATIVE FIRST-LINE ANTIBIOTIC THERAPY
Outpatients Patients deemed to be suitable for outpatient/oral therapy, i.e., no systemic toxicity, high likelihood of compliance, and supportive home environment*	Azithromycin PO	Moxifloxacin PO (preferred) *OR* Levofloxacin PO *OR* Gatifloxacin PO *OR* Clarithromycin PO
In-Hospital management of mild severity CAP (excludes nursing home patients, immunosuppressed patients; patients with sepsis, renal failure, aspiration; the elderly; and patients with other serious, co-morbid conditions)	Azithromycin IV plus ceftriaxone IV	Azithromycin IV††
In-Hospital CAP (not in intensive care unit) with underlying risk factors or comorbid conditions: In-Hospital management (COPD, history of pneumonia, diabetes, etc.)	Azithromycin IV plus ceftriaxone IV	Levofloxacin IV *OR* Gatifloxacin IV *OR* Cefotaxime** plus azithromycin IV
CAP acquired in the nursing home environment (increased likelihood of gram-negative, *E. coli, Klebsiella pneumoniae* infection)	Azithromycin IV plus ceftriaxone IV	Levofloxacin IV *OR* Gatifloxacin IV *OR* Cefotaxime plus azithromycin IV
CAP in the elderly individual with chronic alcoholism (Increased likelihood of *Klebsiella pneumoniae* infection)	Azithromycin IV plus ceftriaxone IV	Cefepime IV plus azithromycin IV *OR* Levofloxacin IV *OR* Gatifloxacin IV

* Oral therapy/outpatient treatment recommendations are appropriate only for those otherwise healthy patients with CAP of mild enough severity that they are judged to be suitable candidates for outpatient management with oral antibiotics.

§ Quinolones are restricted for use in patients > 18 years of age.

¶ If *S. pneumoniae* demonstrates complete resistance to extended spectrum quinolones (very rare), third-generation cephalosporins, and macrolides, then vancomycin may be required as part of initial therapy, although this would be necessary only in rare circumstances.

† First-line therapy recommendations take into consideration cost of the drug (which may vary from one institution to another), convenience of dosing, daily dose frequency, spectrum of coverage, side effects, and risk of drug-drug interactions.

†† Identifying hospitalized patients with CAP that is mild enough to warrant azithromycin monotherapy is difficult; therefore combination therapy with ceftriaxone is preferred in almost all hospitalized patients.

** Cefotaxime requires q 8 hour dosing for treatment of CAP.

treatment pathways vary among institutions and from region to region, management guidelines for CAP in the geriatric patient must be "customized" for the local practice environment. Unfortunately, no single set of guidelines is applicable to every patient or practice environment; therefore, clinical judgment must prevail. This means taking into account local antibiotic resistance patterns, epidemiological and infection incidence data, and patient demographic features.

Patient Management Recommendations. The OMBIRT Panel concurs that appropriate use of antibiotics requires radiographic confirmation of the diagnosis of CAP. In this regard, physicians should use clinical judgement when ordering chest x-rays, with the understanding that the diagnostic yield of this radiographic modality in CAP is increased in patients with fever greater than 38.5°C; presence of new cough; and abnormal pulmonary findings suggestive of consolidation, localized bronchoconstriction, or pleural effusion.

Accordingly, a chest x-ray is recommended and encouraged by the OMBIRT Panel, as well as by such national associations as the IDSA, ATS, and American College of Emergency Physicians (ACEP), to confirm the diagnosis of outpatient CAP, however, the panel acknowledges that, on occasion, logistical issues may prevent radiographic confirmation at the time of diagnosis and treatment.

The approach to antibiotic therapy usually will be empiric, and must account for a number of clinical, epidemiological, and unpredictable factors related to antibiotic resistance patterns and respiratory tract pathogens. As a general rule, appropriate antibiotic choice for the patient with CAP requires consideration of strategies that will yield clinical cure in the patient "today," combined with antibiotic selection strategies that prevent accelerated emergence of drug-resistant organisms that will infect the community "tomorrow."

Based on the most current clinical studies, the principal six respiratory tract pathogens that must be covered on an empiric basis in individuals with outpatient CAP include: *S. pneumoniae, H. influenzae, M. catarrhalis, Chlamydia pneumoniae, M. pneumoniae,* and *Legionella pneumophilia.* In addition, the OMBIRT Panel emphasized that there may be a "disconnect," i.e. an incompletely understood and not entirely predictable relationship between an antibiotic's MIC level and its association with positive clinical outcomes in CAP. This disconnect may be explained by the unique qualities of an antimicrobial, such as tissue penetration and/or pharmacokinetics, patient medication compliance, and other factors.

Double-blinded, prospective clinical trials comparing new generation macrolides vs. new generation fluoroquinolones demonstrate similar outcomes in terms of clinical cure and bacteriologic eradication rates in outpatients with CAP.[79] However, emergence of resistance among *S. pneumoniae* species to new generation fluoroquinolones has been reported in a number of geographic regions, including the United States, Hong Kong, and Canada, and this may have implications for treatment.

The frequency of DRSP causing outpatient CAP, as estimated by the CDC, is very low (i.e., in the range of 0.14-1.9%). The CDC working group panel on drug-resistant Streptococcus pneumoniae (CDCDRSP-WG) cautions against overuse of new generation fluoroquinolones in outpatient CAP, and recommends their use as alternative agents when: 1) first-line therapy with advanced generation macrolides such as azithromycin fails; 2) patients are allergic to first-line agents; or 3) the case is a documented infection with DRSP.[80]

Given concerns about antibiotic overuse, the potential for emerging resistance among DRSP to fluoroquinolones, and the increasing recognition of atypical pathogens as causative agents in patients with outpatient CAP, the panel concurs with the CDCDRSP-WG recommendation advocating macrolides as initial agents of choice in outpatient CAP. The OMBIRT Panel also noted that the Canadian Consensus Guidelines for CAP Management, and the 2001 ATS (American Thoracic Society) Consensus Guideline Recommendations also include advanced generation macrolides as initial therapy for outpatient CAP.

In this regard, two safe and effective advanced generation macrolides, azithromycin and clarithromycin, currently are available for outpatient, oral-based treatment of CAP (IV azithromycin also is indicated for in-hospital management of patients who are risk-stratified as having more serious disease). Based on outcome-sensitive criteria and pharmatectural considerations such as cost, daily dose frequency, duration of therapy, side effects, and drug interactions, the OMBIRT Panel recommends as first-line, preferred initial therapy in CAP, azithromycin, with clarithromycin or doxycycline as an alternative agents; and as second-line therapy, moxifloxacin, gatifloxacin, or levofloxacin when appropriate, according to CDC guidelines and other association-based protocols.

Physicians are urged to prescribe antibiotics in CAP at the time of diagnosis and to encourage patients to fill and begin taking their prescriptions for CAP on the day of diagnosis. Ideally, patients should initiate their first course of oral therapy within eight hours of diagnosis, a time frame that appears reasonable based on studies in hospitalized patients indicating improved survival in patients who received their first IV dose within eight hours of diagnosis. Primary care practitioners also are urged to instruct patients in medication compliance, and in the case of short (5-day) courses of therapy, educate their patients that although they are only consuming medications for a five-day period, the antibiotic remains at the tissue site of infection for about 7-10 days and continues to deliver therapeutic effects during that period.

Either verbal or on-site, re-evaluation of patients is recommended within a three-day period following diagnosis and initiation of antibiotic therapy. Follow-up in the office or clinic within three days is recommended in certain risk-stratified patients, especially the elderly, those with co-morbid illness, and those in whom medication compliance may be compromised. More urgent follow-up may be required in patients with increasing symptoms, including dyspnea, fever, and other systemic signs or symptoms. Follow-up chest x-rays generally are not recommended in patients with outpatient CAP, except in certain high-risk groups, such as those with right middle lobe syndrome, and in individuals in whom the diagnosis may have been uncertain.

Risk Stratification and Patient Disposition: Outpatient vs. Inpatient Management

Overview. The OMBIRT Panel concurred that determining whether to admit or discharge a patient with pneumonia is one of the most important decisions made by a primary care physician when managing patients suspected of having CAP. For this reason, there have been increasing efforts to identify patients with CAP who can appropriately be treated as outpatients.[73-75,81] The disposition decision for patients with pneumonia should take into account the severity of the pneumonia, as well as other medical and psychosocial factors that may affect the treatment plan and clinical outcome.[82-84]

In the absence of respiratory distress or other complicating factors, many young adults can be adequately treated with appropriate oral antibiotic therapy. This is less often the case for the elderly patient with CAP, because comorbid conditions and other risk factors may complicate the course of the illness. Even when following appropriate treatment and dispositon, patients may have symptoms, including cough, fatigue, dyspnea, sputum production, and chest pain that can last for several months. To address this issue of patient disposition and treatment setting, a variety of investigators have proposed criteria to identify patients requiring hospitalization. Patients felt to be at low risk have a median length of stay of seven days, while those at medium risk have a median length of stay of 12-13 days.

Among the factors most physicians use to make admission decisions for pneumonia are the presence of hypoxemia, overall clinical status, the ability to maintain oral intake, hemodynamic status, and the patient's home environment. Using clinical judgment, however, physicians tend to overestimate the likelihood of death from pneumonia.[82] These findings have led some investigators to employ more stringent prediction rules. For example, the chest radiograph may help identify patients who are at high risk for mortality. The presence of bilateral effusions, moderate-size pleural effusions, multi-lobar involvement, and bilateral infiltrates are associated with a higher risk of mortality.

A landmark study presented a prediction rule (Pneumonia Severity Index [PSI]) to identify low-risk patients with CAP.[73] Using such objective criteria as patient age, coexistent medical conditions, and vital signs, patients are assigned either to a low-risk class, which has a mortality rate of about 0.1% in outpatients, or to higher risk categories. Patients with any risk factors are then evaluated with a second scoring system that assigns individuals to one of three higher risk categories, which have mortality rates ranging from 0.7% to 31%.[82] In addition to the factors noted in this prediction rule, patients who are immunocompromised as a result of AIDS or chronic alcohol use frequently require hospitalization.

Once the clinician has determined hospitalization is required, the need for intensive care unit (ICU) admission also must be evaluated. A variety of factors are associated with an increased risk for mortality, including increasing age (> age 65), alcoholism, chronic lung disease, immunodeficiency, and specific laboratory abnormalities, including azotemia and hypoxemia. These patients may require admission to the ICU.

Prognostic Scoring. There have been many efforts to assess severity and risk of death in patients with pneumonia.[83,85-88] The study by Fine and colleagues has received considerable attention and is used as a benchmark by many clinicians.[82] This study developed a prediction rule, the PSI, to assess 30-day mortality in patients with CAP. The rule was derived and validated with data from more than 52,000 inpatients, and then validated with a second cohort of 2287 inpatients and outpatients as part of the Pneumonia PORT study. Subsequent evaluation and validation has been performed with other cohorts, including geriatric patients and nursing home residents.[89,90]

In this risk-stratification scheme, patients are assigned to one of five risk classes (1 is lowest risk, 5 is highest risk) based upon a point system that considers age, co-existing disease, abnormal physical findings, and abnormal laboratory findings. Elderly patients cannot be assigned to Class 1, as a requirement is age younger than 50 years.[82]

In older patients, age contributes the most points to the overall score. For example, it should be noted that males older than age 70 and females older than age 80 would be assigned to Class 3 on the basis of age alone, without any other risk factor. In the Fine study, patients assigned to Class 1 and 2 were typically younger patients (median age, 35-59 years) and patients in Class 3-5 were older (median age, 72-75 years).[82]

Outpatient management is recommended for Classes 1 and 2, brief inpatient observation for Class 3, and traditional hospitalization for Classes 4 and 5.[83,91] For a geriatric patient to qualify for outpatient treatment based on these recommendations, he or she would have to be younger than 70 years of age if male or younger than 80 years of age if female, and have no additional risk factors. Inpatient observation or traditional hospitalization would be recommended for all other patients based on this rule. Other studies have suggested outpatient management for Class 3 patients.[73,92]

Patients considered eligible for management as outpatients must be able to take oral fluids and antibiotics, comply with outpatient care, and be able to carry out activities of daily living (ADLs) or have adequate home support to assist with ADLs.[82-84] Other factors cited in previous studies but not included in the PSI also have been found to increase the risk of morbidity or mortality from pneumonia. These include: other comorbid illnesses (diabetes mellitus, COPD, post-splenectomy state), altered mental status, suspicion of aspiration, chronic alcohol abuse or malnutrition, and evidence of extrapulmonary disease.[93] Additional laboratory studies that may suggest increased severity of illness include white blood cell count less than 4 or greater than 30, absolute neutrophil count less than 1, elevated protime or partial thromboplastin time, decreased platelet count, or radiographic evidence of multilobar involvement, cavitation, and rapid speeding.[93]

Severe pneumonia may require ICU admission. In the Fine study, 6% of patients in Class 3, 11% of patients in Class 4, and 17% of patients in Class 5 required ICU admission.[82] The ATS guidelines define severe pneumonia as the presence of at least one of the following: respiratory rate greater than 30, severe respiratory failure ($PaO_2/FIO_2 < 250$), mechanical ventilation, bilateral infiltrates or multilobar infiltrates, shock, vasopressor requirement, or oliguria (urine output < 20 cc per hour). The presence of at least one of these is highly sensitive (98%) but only 32% specific for the need for ICU management.[94] It is emphasized that the above guidelines for admission should not supercede clinical judgment when assessing the need to hospitalize patients.[82,83,91,93]

Antibiotic Selection in the Patient with Pneumonia

Introduction. Antibiotic therapy is the mainstay of management for outpatients with CAP. As previously emphaszied, antibiotic therapy should be initiated promptly, as soon as the diagnosis is strongly suspected or confirmed, and after appropriate microbiological studies or samples have been obtained. Chest x-rays should be performed to confirm the diagnosis.

It should be stressed that there is no absolute or consistent consensus on precisely which drug, or combination of drugs, constitutes the most outcome-effective choice for managing CAP in outpatients. However, virtually all panels and guideline documents, including the OMBIRT Panel, agree that antimicrobial coverage, as a baseline spectrum of coverage, must include sufficient activity against the following bacterial pathogens: *S. pneumoniae, H. influenzae,* and *M. catarrhalis,* as well as against the atypical pathogens *Mycoplasma, Legionella,* and *C. pneumoniae.* Therefore, such macrolides as azithromycin and advance generation fluoroquinolones which, because of their activity against both bacterial and atypical pathogens commonly encountered in CAP, have supplanted cephalosporins and amoxicillin-clavulanate as preferred monotherapeutic options for treatment of outpatients with CAP.

Beyond this non-negotiable caveat mandating coverage for the six aforementioned pathogens, there are important differences among recommendations and expert panels for empiric treatment of pneumonia. Variations among the guidelines usually depend upon: 1) their emphasis or focus on the need to empirically cover drug-resistant Streptococcus pneumoniae (DRSP) species as part of the initial antimicrobial regimen; 2) their concern about using antimicrobials (fluoroquinolones) with an over-extended (too broad) spectrum of coverage; 3) their concern about the potential of growing resistance to a class (fluoroquinolones) which has agents that currently are active against DRSP species; 4) their preference for monotherapeutic vs. combination therapy; 5) the date when the guidelines were released (recent vs several years old); and 6) their emphasis on drug costs, patient convenience, and options for step-down (IV to oral) therapeutic approaches. Clearly, these factors and the relative emphasis placed on each of them will influence antimicrobial selection for the patient with pneumonia.

With these issues and drug selection factors in mind, the most recent guidelines issued by the IDSA, CDCDRSP-WG, and ATS attempt to both risk-stratify and "drug-stratify" patients according to their eligibility for receiving agents as initial empiric therapy that have activity against DRSP. Before presenting the OMBIRT Panel's detailed analysis of the current treatment landscape for CAP, a number of points should be emphasized. First, the relative importance of *S. pneumoniae* as a cause of outpatient CAP is difficult to determine. Nevertheless, a review of the literature by the CDCDRSP-WG suggests that *S. pneumoniae* accounts for about 2-27% of all cases of CAP treated on an outpatient basis.[95-97] In addition, surveillance studies have suggested that about 7% of invasive *S. pneumoniae* species in the United States showed a significant degree of penicillin resistance.[98] Hence, this group estimates that only 0.14% (7% of 2%) to 1.9% (7% Of 27%) of outpatients with bacterial pneumonia have pneumococcal infections with levels of resistance high enough to warrant consideration of alternative treatment.

This analysis has made the CDC panel conclude that because CAP in outpatients who are appropriately triaged and risk-stratified is generally not immediately life-threatening and because *S. pneumoniae* isolates with penicillin MICs of no less than 4 mcg/mL are uncommon, antibiotics with predictable activity against highly penicillin-resistance pneumococci are not necessary as part of the initial regimen. From a practical, drug-selection perspective, the working group, therefore, suggests that oral fluoroquinolones are not first-line treatment in outpatients with CAP because of concerns about emerging resistance. Consequently, oral macrolide or beta-lactam monotherapy is recommended by the CDC working group as initial therapy in patients with pneumonia considered to be amenable to outpatient management.

Community-Acquired Pneumonia (CAP) Outpatient Management

Appropriate and Adequate Intensity of Antimicrobial Coverage. Because macrolides and extended spectrum quinolones are effective, appropriate agents for treatment of CAP, they frequently get equal billing as initial choice agents for management of CAP. Despite their excellent track record and proven efficacy, however, the macrolides and extended spectrum quinolones have clinically significant differences that should be considered in the antibiotic treatment equation for CAP. Accordingly, a careful analysis of the benefits and potential pitfalls of these agents should include a full accounting of the relevant similarities and differences. It will help emergency physicians and intensivists develop criteria that suggest the appropriateness and suitability that each of these classes may have in specific patient subgroups.

Although the previously cited six organisms (*S. pneumoniae, H. influenzae,* and *M. catarrhalis,* and atypical pathogens *Mycoplasma, Legionella,* and *C. pneumoniae)* are the most commonly implicated pathogens in patients with CAP, there are patients who are susceptible to infection with gram-negative enteric organisms such as *Klebsiella, E. coli,* and *Pseudomonas.* In other cases, the likelihood of infection with DRSP is high. When infection with these pathogens is likely, intensification of empiric coverage should include antibiotics with activity against these gram-negative species and/or DRSP. However, it should be noted that patients with infections caused by the aforementioned respiratory pathogens usually are managed on an *inpatient* basis.

Clinical features or risk factors that may suggest the need for intensification and expansion of bacterial and/or gram-negative pathogen coverage include the following: 1) increasing fragility (> age 85, comorbid conditions, previous infection, etc.) of the patient; 2) acquisition of the pneumonia in a skilled nursing facility; 3) the presence of an aspiration pneumonia, suggesting involvement with gram-negative or anaerobic organisms; 4) chronic alcoholism, increasing the likelihood of infection with *Klebsiella pneumoniae;* 5) pneumococcal pneumonia in underlying disease-compromised individual who has not been vaccinated with pneumococcal polysaccharide antigen (Pneumovax); 6) history of infection with gram-negative, anaerobic, or resistant species of *S. pneumoniae;* 7) history of treatment failure; 8) previous hospitalizations for pneumonia; 9) patient requires or has had previous ICU hospitalization for pneumonia; 10) acquisition of pneumonia in a community with high and increasing resistance among *S. pneumoniae* species; and 11) immunodeficiency and/or severe underlying disease.

As emphasized earlier in this review, most consensus panels, infectious disease experts, textbooks, and peer-reviewed antimicrobial prescribing guides recommend, as the initial or preferred choice, those antibiotics that, within the framework of monotherapy or combination therapy, address current etiologic and mortality trends in CAP. As a general rule, for empiric initial therapy in patients without modifying host factors that predispose to enteric gram-negative or pseudomonal infection they recommend those antibiotics that provide coverage against the bacterial pathogens *S. pneumoniae, H. influenzae,* and *M. catarrhalis,* as well as against atypical pathogens *Mycoplasma, Legionella,* and *C. pneumoniae.*[99]

Correct Spectrum Coverage. When antimicrobial monotherapy is desirable, cost-effective, and/or clinically indicated, extended spectrum quinolones and advanced generation macrolides best satisfy the empiric coverage requirements for patients with CAP. These antimicrobial agents are among the therapeutic classes of choice for management of CAP in the outpatient setting. *(Please see Table 7.)*

Although third generation cephalosporins, beta-lactam antibiotics, and TMP/SMX (trimethoprim-sulfamethoxazole) are still deemed valuable by many authorities and practitioners (in particular, in combination with other agents for in-hospital management of CAP), these agents, for the most part, have been allocated to alternative status for oral therapy. This is because they are not, as a rule, clinically indicated for treatment of atypical organisms, including *Mycoplasma, Legionella,* and *C. pneumoniae,* whose increasing importance now mandates initial empiric coverage of atypical organisms.

Because advanced generation macrolides and extended spectrum quinolones constitute the principal oral treatment options for CAP, the following sections will discuss indications, clinical trials, side effects, and strategies for their use in CAP. The focus of the discussion will be on newer antibiotics that: 1) provide coverage of bacterial and atypical organisms causing CAP; and that, 2) are able, when indicated, to provide compliance-enhancing and cost-effective treatment within the context of antimicrobial monotherapy. It should be stressed that these agents also may be used as part of combination therapy for CAP.

Advanced Generation Macrolides: Correct Spectrum Coverage in Outpatient CAP

The established new generation macrolide antibiotics include the erythromycin analogues azithromycin and clarithromycin.[100,101] Compared to erythromycin, which is the least expensive macrolide, the major advantages of these newer antibiotics are significantly decreased gastrointestinal side effects, which produce enhanced tolerance, improved bioavailability, higher tissue levels, and pharmacokinetic features that permit less frequent dosing and better compliance, as well as enhanced activity against *H. influenzae.*[102,103] In particular, the long tissue half-life of azithromycin allows this antibiotic to be prescribed for a shorter duration (5 days) than comparable antibiotics given for the same indications.

Macrolides in CAP Therapy: An Overview. Given the cost differences between azithromycin and clarithromycin, as well as the improved compliance patterns associated with short-duration therapy, any rational approach to distinguishing between these agents must consider prescription, patient, and drug resistance barriers. From the outset, it is fair to say that these macrolides, to a great degree, have supplanted the use of erythromycin (as well as cephalosporins and tetrayclines) in community-acquired infections of the lower respiratory tract.

In some institutions, this is not the case. Although erythromycin, in particular, has been considered by some to be the antibiotic of choice for CAP, its lack of efficacy against *H. influenzae,* as well as its adverse gastrointestinal side effects, potential for drug-drug interactions, and poor compliance profile, are now recognized as clinically important liabilities in emergency practice.[104,105] It is, however, effective against pneumococcal pneumonia, Mycoplasma pneumonia, and many atypical infections, including Legionella. Food decreases the absorption of erythromycin, which interferes with drug metabolism; therefore, many experts caution this drug should not be considered for use in elderly patients on theophylline or warfarin.[90,99]

From the perspective of providing definitive, cost-effective, and compliance-promoting therapy, the newer macrolide antibiotics, which include both azithromycin and clarithromycin, have recently emerged as some of the drugs of choice-along with the new, extended spectrum quinolones-for outpatient management of CAP.[106] When used as oral agents, they play a central role in management of pneumonia in otherwise healthy elderly individuals who do not require hospitalization.

Macrolides have the advantage of a simplified dosing schedule, especially azithromycin (Zithromax®), which is given once daily for only five days (500 mg PO on day 1 and 250 mg PO qd on days 2-5). Clarithromycin (Biaxin® XL) requires a longer (1000 mg/d for 7-days) course of therapy and costs more. In general, the decision to use a macrolide such as azithromycin rather than erythromycin is based on weighing the increased cost of a course of therapy with azithromycin against its real-world advantages, which include a more convenient dosing schedule, its broader spectrum of coverage, its favorable drug interaction profile, and its decreased incidence of gastrointestinal side effects, which occur in 3-5% of patients taking a five-day, multiple-dose regimen.[107] The introduction of a tablet formulation permits consumption of the antibiotic without regard to food ingestion.

Comparative Studies. Although advanced generation fluoroquinolones have enhanced coverage against DRSP as compared to macrolides, most studies suggest comparable outcomes. One prospective, double-blind, multicenter trial reviewed the safety and efficacy of moxifloxacin and clarithromycin in adult patients with radiographically documented CAP.[79] Patients were treated for 10 days with either oral moxifloxacin 400 mg qd, or clarithromycin 500 mg bid. Among 382 patients, both drugs were highly effective, with 95% clinical resolution rate and 96% bacterial resolution. Drug-related adverse events occurred at comparabel rates with the two antibiotics, although nausea and/or vomiting was a more frequent cause of premature discontinuation in the clarithromycin group than in the moxifloxacin group. Taste perversion was almost twice as common in those given clarithromycin (7%) as in those given moxifloxacin (4%).[79]

Extended Spectrum Fluoroquinolones, Indication for Initial Empiric Use: Intensification of Coverage and Patient Selection

The extended spectrum quinolones-moxifloxacin, levofloxacin, and gatifloxacin-are indicated for treatment of CAP because they are active against many gram-positive organisms that may infect the lower respiratory tract, including *S. pneumoniae* and *Staphylococcus aureus,* as well as covering atypical pathogens, including *Chlamydia pneumoniae, Legionella pneumophila,* and *Mycoplasma pneumoniae.* Levofloxacin also is active against gram-negative organisms, including *E. coli, H. influenzae, H. parainfluenzae, Klebsiella pneumoniae,* and *Moraxella catarrhalis.*

Several studies and surveillance data suggest that some of newly available, expanded spectrum fluoroquinolones, including levofloxacin (which is approved for PRSP), are efficacious for the treatment of *S. pneumoniae,* including penicillin-resistant strains.[76,80,108] In one study, microbiologic eradication from sputum was reported among all 300 patients with pneumococcal pneumonia treated with oral levofloxacin.[108] In a study of in vitro susceptibility of *S. pneumoniae* clinical isolates to levofloxacin, none of the 180 isolates (including 60 isolates with intermediate susceptibility to penicillin and 60 penicillin-resistant isolates) was resistant to this agent.[76] In addition, a surveillance study of antimicrobial resistance in respiratory tract pathogens found levofloxacin was active against 97% of 9190 pneumococcal isolates and found no cross-resistance with penicillin, amoxicillin-clavulanate, ceftriaxone, cefuroxime, or clarithromycin.

Despite high level activity against pneumococcal isolates and a formal FDA approval/indication for levofloxacin use in suspected DRSP lower respiratory tract infection, the CDCDRSP-WG recent guidelines do not advocate the use of expanded spectrum fluoroquinolones for first-line, empiric treatment of pneumonia. This is because: 1) of their broad, perhaps, over-extended spectrum of coverage that includes a wide range of gram-negative organisms; 2) of concern that resistance among pneumococci will emerge if there is widespread use of this class of antibiotics; 3) their activity against pneumococci with high penicillin resistance (MIC = 4 mcg/mL) makes it important that they be reserved for selected patients with CAP; 4) use of fluoroquinolones has been shown to result in increased resistance to *S. pneumoniae* in vitro; and 5) population-based surveillance in the United States has shown a statistically significant increase in ofloxacin resistance among pneumococcal isolates between Jan. 1, 1995, and Dec. 31, 1997 (unpublished data, Active Bacterial Core Surveillance, CDC).[80]

From a practical, drug selection perspective, the CDCDRSP-WG has recommended that fluoroquinolones be reserved for selected patients with CAP, and these experts have identified specific patient subgroups that are eligible for initial treatment with extended-spectrum fluoroquinolones. However, outpatients with CAP, according to the CDCDRSP-WG and OMBIRT Panel recommendations, are managed preferentially with an oral macrolide (or doxycycline).

For hospitalized patients, advanced generation fluoroquinolones are recommended for adults and elderly patients in whom one of the first-line regimens (cephalosporin plus a macrolide) has failed, those who are allergic to the first-line agents, or those who have a documented infection with highly drug-resistant pneumococci (i.e., penicillin MIC = 4 mcg/mL).[109] Other guideline panels and recommendations, such as those issued by the IDSA (2000) and the ATS (2001), do not prioritize between two-drug, combination (cephalosporin plus macrolide) vs. advanced generation fluoroquinolone monotherapy.

OMBIRT Summary for Empiric Antibiotic Selection in Outpatients with ABE/COPD and CAP—Matching Bugs with Drugs

A variety of antibiotics are available for outpatient management of pulmonary infections. Although the selection process can be daunting, as mentioned, a sensible approach, accompanied by specific recommendations for antibiotic selection in patients with outpatient bacterial infections of the respiratory tract has been generated by the OMBIRT Panel. Regardless of the specific antimicrobial selected, one of the most important issues for the primary care practitioner is to ensure that the appropriate intensity and spectrum of coverage are provided, according to patient and community/epidemiological risk factors and patterns. The significant majority of cases of both ABE/COPD and CAP are appropriately managed with a macrolide. In the minority of cases (i.e, those in which infection with gram-negative organisms is suspected or if there is structural lung disease), the practitioner, based on clinical judegement, may consider shifting to and intensifying therapy with an extended spectrum quinolone.

ABE/COPD. As a rule, the clinical criteria for initiating antibiotic therapy in patients with a documented history of chronic obstructive pulmonary disease (COPD), and who are suspected of having ABE/COPD, include the presence of at least two of the following three symptoms: increasing purulence of sputum, increasing volume of sputum production, and increasing cough and/or dyspnea. In contrast, patients with symptoms of acute tracheobronchitis who have no previous history of COPD initially should not be treated with antibiotics, since antibiotics have not been shown to improve outcomes in this patient population.

Given concerns about antibiotic overuse, the potential for emerging resistance among DRSP to fluoroquinolones, the panel concurs with other national guidelines specifying advanced generation macrolides such as azithromycin (or clarithromycin) as initial therapy for outpatient ABE/COPD and use of fluoroquinolones or amoxicillin-clavulanate as alternative agents in patients who fail therapy or who have risk factors predictive of gram-negative infection. Patients who do not respond to oral therapy with one class of antibiotics (relapse) may be treated with a course of antibiotics with different gaps in coverage. Reinfections should be treated with antibiotics that have been shown to be effective in previous exacerbations.

A number of relatively inexpensive, well-tolerated antibiotics also are available, including amoxicillin, trimethoprim-sulfamethoxazole, doxycycline, and tetracycline. Antimicrobial resistance, particularly involving *H. influenzae, M. catarrhalis,* and *S. pneumoniae,* has become an increasing problem with many of these agents, specifically with older members of each of these drug classes. There is an increase in amoxicillin-resistant, beta-lactamase-producing *H. influenzae.* New agents are providing solutions to these difficulties. The azalide antibiotic azithromycin has the advantage of an appropriate spectrum of coverage, an acceptable safety profile, reasonable cost, and a patient-dosing schedule that improves patient compliance.

The newer fluoroquinolones, moxifloxacin, gatifloxacin, and levofloxacin are advantageous when gram-negative bacteria predominate; ciprofloxacin is another appropriate choice in this subgroup, especially those with structural lung disease such bronchiectasis and documented infection with gram-negative species such as *Pseudomonas* species. When there is documented infection with DRSP, levofloxacin or moxifloxacin are prudent choices. Amoxicillin-clavulanate also has in vitro activity against beta-lactamase-producing *H. influenzae* and *M. catarrhalis,* as well as *S. peumoniae;* moreover, the agent's clinical efficacy in lower respiratory tract infection attributable to enzyme-producing strains has been demonstrated.

CAP. The overwhelming majority of well-designed, double-blinded, prospective clinical trials comparing new generation macrolides (azithromycin and clarithromycin) vs. new generation fluoroquinolones (moxifloxacin, gatifloxacin, and levofloxacin) demonstrate comparable outcomes in terms of clinical cure and bacteriologic eradication rates in outpatients with CAP. However, emergence of resistance among *S. pneumoniae* species to new generation fluoroquinolones has been reported in a number of geographic regions, including the United States, Hong Kong, and Canada, and this may have implications for treatment.

Although not precisely known, the frequency of DRSP causing outpatient CAP, as estimated by the CDC, is very low (i.e., in the range of 0.14-1.9%). Accordingly, the CDCWG-DRSP cautions against overuse of new generation fluoroquinolones in outpatient CAP, and recommends their use as alternative agents when: 1) first-line therapy with advanced generation macrolides such as azithromycin fails; 2) patients are allergic to first-line agents; or 3) the casess are documented infection with DRSP.

Given concerns about antibiotic overuse, the potential for emerging resistance among DRSP to fluoroquinolones, and the increasing recognition of atypical pathogens as causative agents in patients with outpatient CAP, the OMBIRT Panel concurs with the CDCDRSP-WG recommendation advocating macrolides as initial agents of choice in outpatient CAP. The OMBIRT Panel also noted that the Canadian Consensus Guidelines for CAP Management and the 2001 ATS (American Thoracic Society) Consensus Guideline Recommendations also specify advanced generation macrolides as initial therapy for outpatient CAP.

In this regard, two safe and effective advanced generation macrolides, azithromycin and clarithromycin, currently are available for outpatient, oral-based treatment of CAP (IV azithromycin also is indicated for in-hospital management of patients who are risk-stratified as having more serious disease). Based on outcome-sensitive criteria and pharmatectural considerations such as cost, daily dose frequency, duration of therapy, side effects, and drug interactions, the OMBIRT Panel recommends as first-line, preferred initial therapy in CAP, azithromycin, with clarithromycin or doxycycline as alternative agents; and, as second-line therapy, moxifloxacin, gatifloxacin, or levofloxacin when appropriate, according to CDCDRSP-WG guidelines, epidemiological patterns in the local community, and other association-based protocols issued by the IDSA and ATS.

The OMBIRT Panel*

The OMBIRT Consensus Panel and Scientific Roundtable†: **Gideon Bosker, MD, FACEP**, Panel Chairman and Moderator, Yale University School of Medicine; **Bill Billica, MD FAAFP**, Department of Family Practice, Banner Health System, Phoenix, AZ; **Phillip Bonanni, MD**, Primary Care and Internal Medicine, University of Rochester School of Medicine; **Susan I. Fesmire, MD,** Assistant Professor, Department of Internal Medicine, Aston Ambulatory Care Center, The University of Texas Southwestern Medical Center; **Robert Haddon, MD**, Urgency Care Clinics, Cleveland Clinic, Cleveland, OH; **Gary Merlino, DO**, Department of Family Medicine, Mt. Sinai Hospital, Miami, FL; **Sam Sandowski, MD**, Department of Family Practice, SUNY Medical College; **Ethel Smith, MD**, Department of Family Practice, MetroWest Health Center, Cleveland Clinic, Cleveland, OH; **Paul Stander, MD, FACP,** Regional Medical Director, Banner Health System, Phoenix, AZ; **Gregory Volturo, MD, FACEP,** University of Massachusetts Medical School.

* OMBIRT - Outpatient Management of Bacterial Infections in the Respiratory Tract. *The OMBIRT Consensus Panel & Scientific Roundtable assembled in San Juan, Puerto Rico, August 10-13, 2001.*

References

1. Statistics VaH. Current Estimates from the National Health Interview Survey. NHS Publication. 1990:1643.
2. Cydulka R, McFadden E, Emerman C, et al. Patterns of hospitalization in elderly patients with asthma and chronic obstructive pulmonary disease. *Am J Respir Crit Care Med* 1997;156: 1807-1812.
3. Kanner RE, Renzetti AD, Jr, Stanish WM, et al. Predictors of survival in subjects with chronic airflow limitation. *Am J Med* 1983;74:249-255.
4. Salit IE, Mederski B, Morisset R, et al. Azithromycin for the treatment of acute LRTIs: A multicenter, open-label study of infections in medicine. *Infect Med* 1998;15:773-777.
5. Wilson R. The Role of Infection in COPD. *Chest* 1998;113: 242S-248S.
6. Shu D, et al. A Controlled Randomized Multicenter Trial Comparing 5 Days Of Azithromycin to 10-14 Days of Clarithromycin for the Treatment of Acute Bacterial Exacerbations of Chronic Bronchitis. In: American Society for Microbiology, ed. 37th Interscience Conference on Antimicrobial Agents and Chemotherapy; Sept. 28-Oct. 1, 1997; Toronto, Ont. Washington, D.C.; pg. 372
7. Rosen MJ. Treatment of exacerbations of COPD. *Am Fam Phys* 1992;45:693-697.
8. Cydulka R, McFadden E, Emerman C, et al. Patterns of hospitalization in elderly patients with asthma and chronic obstructive pulmonary disease. *Am J Respir Crit Care Med* 1997;156:1807-1812.
9. Celli BR, Snider GL, Heffner J. Standards for the diagnosis and care of patients with chronic obstructive pulmonary disease. *Am J Respir Crit Care Med* 1995;152:S77-S120.
10. Kanner RE, Renzetti AD, Jr, Stanish WM, et al. Predictors of survival in subjects with chronic airflow limitation. *Am J Med* 1983;74:249-255.
11. Gump DW, Philips CA, Forsyth BR. Role of infection in chronic bronchitis. *Am Rev Respir Dis* 1976;113:465-474.
12. Blasi F, Legnani D, Lombardo VM, et al. *Chlamydia pneumoniae* infection in acute exacerbations of COPD. *Eur Respir J* 1993;6: 19-22.
13. Beaty CD, Grayston JT, Wang SPP, et al. *Chlamydia pneumoniae,* strain TWAR, infection in patients with chronic obstructive pulmonary disease. *Am Rev Respir Dis* 1991;144:1408-1410.
14. Rodnick JE, Gude JK. The use of antibiotics in acute bronchitis and acute exacerbations of chronic bronchitis. *West J Med* 1988;149:347-351.
15. Wallace RJ Jr. Newer oral antimicrobials and newer etiologic agents of acute bronchitis and acute exacerbations of chronic bronchitis. *Semin Respir Infect* 1988;3:49-54.
16. Wallace RF Jr, Steele LC, Brooks DL, et al. Amoxicillin/clavulanic acid in the treatment of lower respiratory tract infections caused by β-lactamase-positive *Haemophilus influenzae* and *Branhamella catarrhalis*. *Antimicrob Agents Chemother* 1985;27:912-915.
17. Hopkins SJ. Clinical toleration and safety of azithromycin in adults and children. *Rev Contemp Pharmacother* 1994;5:383-389.
18. Nightingale CH, Belliveau PP, Quintiliani R. Cost issues and considerations when choosing antimicrobial agents. *Infect Dis Clin Pract* 1994;3:8-11.
19. Eller J, Ede A, Schaberg T, et al. Infective exacerbations of chronic bronchitis: Relation between bacteriologic etiology and lung function. *Chest* 1998;113:1542-1548.
20. Knaus WA, Harrell FEJ, Lynn J, et al. The SUPPORT Program prognostic model. Objective estimates of survival for seriously ill hospitalized adults. Study to understand prognosis and preferences for outcomes and risks of treatments. *Ann Intern Med* 1995:122:191-203.
21. Lange P, Nyboe J, Appleyard M, et al. Relationship of ventilatory impairment and of chronic mucous secretion to mortality from chronic obstructive lung disease and from all causes. *Thorax* 1990:45:579-585.
22. Sherman CB, Zu X, et al. Longitudinal lung function decline in subjects with respiratory symptoms. *Am Rev of Resp Dis* 1992:146:855-859.
23. Warren Whitlock on behalf of the Multicenter Chronic Obstructive Pulmonary Disease Study Group. Multicenter comparison of azithromycin and amoxicillin/clavulanate in the treatment of patients with chronic obstructive pulmonary disease. *Curr Therapeutic Res* 1995;56:10.
24. Grossman RF. The value of antibiotics and the outcomes of antibiotic therapy in exacerbations of COPD. *Chest* 1998;113:249S-255S.
25. DebAbate CA, Mathew CP, Warner JH, et al. The safety and efficacy of a short course (5-day) moxifloxacin vs. azithromycin in the treatment of patients with acute exacerbation of chronic bronchitis. *Respir Med* 2000;94:1029-1037.
26. Kreis S, Herrera N, Golzar N, et al. A comparison of moxifloxacin and azithromycin in the treatment of acute exacerbations of chronic bronchitis. *JCOM* 2000;7:33-37.
27. Bauernfreind A., Jungwirth R., Eberlein E. Comparative pharmacodynamics of clarithromycin and azithromycin against respiratory pathogens. *Infection* 1995;23:316-321.
28. Guggenbichler JP, Kastner H. The influence of macrolide antibiotics on the fecal and oral flora. *Infect Medicate* 1998;15(Suppl D):17-25.
29. Adam D, Grimm H, Lode H, et al. Comparative pharmacodynamics of clarithromycin and azithromycin against respiratory pathogens. *Infection* 1996;24:270.
30. Retsema JA. Susceptibility and resistance emergence studies with macrolides. *Int J Antimicrob Agents* 1999;11:S15-S21.
31. Girard AE, Cimochowski CR, Faiella JA. Correlation of increased azithromycin concentrations with phagocyte infiltration into sites of localized infection. *J Antimicrob Chemother* 1996;37(Suppl C): 9-19.
32. Chodosh S, Schreurs A, Siami G, et al. Efficacy of oral ciprofloxacin vs. clarithromycin for treatment of acute bacterial exacerbations of chronic bronchitis. The Bronchitis Study Group. *Clin Infect Dis* 1998;27:730-738.
33 Fagon JY, Chastre J. Severe exacerbations of COPD patients: The role of pulmonary infections. *Semin Respir Infect* 1996;11:109-118.
34. Gump DW, Philips CA, Forsyth BR. Role of infection in chronic bronchitis. *Am Rev Respir Dis* 1976;113:465-474.
35. Blasi F, Legnani D, Lombardo VM, et al. *Chlamydia pneumoniae* infection in acute exacerbations of COPD. *Eur Respir J* 1993;6: 19-22.
36. Beaty CD, Grayston JT, Wang SP, et al. *Chlamydia pneumoniae,* strain TWAR, infection in patients with chronic obstructive pulmonary disease. *Am Rev Respir Dis* 1991;144:1408-1410.
37. Eller J, Ede A, Schaberg T, et al. Infective exacerbations of chronic

bronchitis: Relation between bacteriologic etiology and lung function. *Chest* 1998;113:1542-1548.

38. Saint S, Bent S, Vittinghoff E, et al. Antibiotics in chronic obstructive pulmonary disease exacerbations. A meta-analysis [see comments]. *JAMA* 1995;273:957-960.
39. Ball P, Harris JM, Lowson D, et al. Acute infective exacerbations of chronic bronchitis. *QJM* 1995;88:61-68.
40. Macfarlane JT, Colville A, Guion A, et al. Prospective study of etiology and outcome of adult lower-respiratory-tract infections in the community. *Lancet* 1993;341:511-514.
41. Wilson R. The role of infection in COPD. *Chest* 1998;113:242S-248S.
42. Shu D, et al. A controlled randomized multicenter trial comparing 5 days of azithromycin to 10-14 days of clarithromycin for the treatment of acute bacterial exacerbations of chronic bronchitis. In: American Society for Microbiology, ed. *37th Interscience Conference on Antimicrobial Agents and Chemotherapy*; 1997 Sept.-Oct. 28-1; Toronto, Ont. Washington, D.C.; 1997:372
43. Rosen MJ. Treatment of exacerbations of COPD. *Am Fam Phys* 1992;45:693-697.
44. Rodnick JE, Gude JK. The use of antibiotics in acute bronchitis and acute exacerbations of chronic bronchitis. *West J Med* 1988;149:347-351.
45. Wallace RJ, Jr. Newer oral antimicrobials and newer etiologic agents of acute bronchitis and acute exacerbations of chronic bronchitis. *Semin Respir Infect* 1988;3:49-54.
46. Wallace RF Jr, Steele LC, Brooks DL, et al. Amoxicillin/clavulanic acid in the treatment of lower respiratory tract infections caused by β-lactamase-positive *Haemophilus influenzae* and *Branhamella catarrhalis*. *Antimicrob Agents Chemother* 1985;27:912-915.
47. Hopkins SJ. Clinical toleration and safety of azithromycin in adults and children. *Rev Contemp Pharmacother* 1994;5:383-389.
48. Nightingale CH, Belliveau PP, Quintiliani R. Cost issues and considerations when choosing antimicrobial agents. *Infect Dis Clin Pract* 1994;3:8-11.
49. Chodosh S, DeAbate CA, et al. Short-course moxifloxacin therapy for treatment of acute bacterial excaerbations of chronic bronchitis. *Respir Med* 2000;94:18-27.
50. Wilson R, Kubin R, et al. Five-day moxifloxacin comparedd with 7 day clarithromycin for the treatment of acute exacerbations of chronic bronchitis. *J Anitimicrob Ther* 1999;44:501-513.
51. Destache CJ, Dewan N, O'Donohue WJ. et al Clinical and economic considerations in the treatment of acute exacerbations of chronic bronchitis. *J Antimicrob Chemother* 1999;43:A107-A113.
52. Davies. J. Inactivation of antibiotics and the dissemination of resistance genes. *Science* 1994;264:375-382.
53. Jorgensen JH, Doern GV, Maher LA, et al. Antimicrobial resistance among respiratory isolates of *Haemophilus influenzae, Moraxella catarrhalis,* and *Streptococcus pneumoniae* in the United States. *Antimicrob Agents Chemother* 1990;34:2075-2080.
54. Doern GV. Trends in antimicrobial susceptibility of bacterial pathogens of the respiratory tract. *Am J Med* 1995;99:3S-7S.
55. Knaus WA, Harrell FEJ, Lynn J, et al. The SUPPORT Program prognostic model. Objective estimates of survival for seriously ill hospitalized adults. Study to understand prognosis and preferences for outcomes and risks of treatments. *Ann Intern Med* 1995:122:191-203.
56. Lange P, Nyboe J, Appleyard M, et al. Relationship of ventilatory impairment and of chronic mucous secretion to mortality from chronic obstructive lung disease and from all causes. *Thorax* 1990;45:579-585.
57. Sherman CB, Zu X, et al. Longitudinal lung function decline in subjects with respiratory symptoms. *Am Rev of Resp Dis* 1992:146;855-859.
58. Tashkin DP, Bleecker E, Braun S, et al. Results of a multicenter study of nebulized inhalant bronchodilator solutions. *Am J Med* 1996;100:62S-69S.
59. Cazzola M, Di Perna F, Noschese P, et al. Effects of formoterol, salmeterol or oxitropium bromide on airway responses to salbutamol in COPD. *Eur Respir J* 1998;11:1337-1341.
60. Corris PA, Neville E, Nariman S, et al. Dose-response study of inhaled salbutamol powder in chronic airflow obstruction. *Thorax* 1983;38:292-296.
61. Colice GL. Nebulized bronchodilators for outpatient management of stable chronic obstructive pulmonary disease. *Am J Med* 1996;100:11S-18S.
62. Rennard Sa, Serby Ca, Ghafouri Ma, et al. Extended therapy with ipratropium is associated with improved lung function in patients with COPD. *Chest* 1996;110:62-70.
63. Friedman M. A multicenter study of nebulized bronchodilator solutions in chronic obstructive pulmonary disease. *Am J Med* 1996;100:30S-39S.
64. Chanez P, Vignola AM, O'Shaugnessy T, et al. Corticosteroid reversibility in COPD is related to features of asthma. *Am J Respir Crit Care Med* 1997;155:1529-1534.
65. Kerstjens Ha, Brand Pa, Hughes Ma, et al. A comparison of bronchodilator therapy with or without inhaled corticosteroid therapy for obstructive airways disease. *N Engl J Med* 1992;327:1413-1419.
66. Pauwels R, Claes-Goran L, Laitinen L, et al. Long-term treatment with inhaled budesonide in persons with mild chronic obstructive pulmonary disease who continue smoking. *N Engl J Med* 1999;340:1948-1953.
67. Saint S, Bent S, Vittinghoff E, et al. Antibiotics in chronic obstructive pulmonary disease exacerbations. A meta-analysis [see comments]. *JAMA* 1995;273:957-960.
68. Bosker G. *Pharmatecture: Minimizing Medications To Maximize Results*. St. Louis: Facts and Comparisons; 1999.
69. Salit IE, Mederski B, Morisset R, et al. Azithromycin for the treatment of acute LRTIs: A multicenter, open-label study. *Infect Med* 1998;15:773-777.
70. Destache CJ, Dewan N, O'Donohue OJ, et al. Clinical and economic considerations in the treatment of acute exacerbations of chronic bronchitis. *J Antimicrob Chemother* 1999;43:107-113.
71. Bartlett JG, Mundy M. Community-acquired pneuominia. *N Engl J Med* 1995;333:1618-1624.
72. Fine MD, Smith MA, et al. Prognosis and outcomes of patients with community acquired pneumonia. A meta-analysis. *JAMA* 1996;275:134-141.
73. Marrie TJ, Lau CY, Wheeler SL, et al. A controlled trial of a critical pathway for treatment of community-acquired pneumonia. *JAMA* 2000;283:749-755.
74. Dean NC, Suchyta MR, Bateman KA. Implementation of admission decision support for community-acquired pneumonia. A pilot study. *Chest* 2000;117:1368-1377.
75. Flanders WD, Tucker G, Krishnadasan A, et al. Validation of the pneumonia severity index: Importance of study-specific recalibra-

tion. *J Gen Intern Med* 1999;14:333-340.

76. Kulgman KP, Capper T, et al In vitro susceptibility of penicillin-resistant *S. pneumoniae* to levofloxacin, selection of resistant mutants, and time-kill synergy studies of levofloxacin combined with vancomycin, telcoplanin, fusidic acid, and rifampin. *Antimicrob Agents Chemother* 1996;40:2802-2804.
77. Levaquin Product Information. Ortho-McNeil Pharmaceuticals. January 1997.
78. Vincent J, et al. Pharmacokinetics and safety of trovafloxacin in healthy male volunteers following administration of single intravenous doses of the prodrug, alatrofloxacin. *J Antimicrob Chemother* 1997;39(supp B):75-80.
79. Fogarty C, Grossman C, et al. Efficacy and safety of moxifloxacin vs clarithromycin in community-acquired pneumonia. *Infect Med* 1999;16:11.
80. Heffelfinger JD, Dowell SF, et al. A report from the Drug-resistant Streptococcus pneumoniae Therapeutic Working Group. Management of community-acquired pneumonia in the era of pneumococcal resistance. *Arch Int Med* 2000;160:1399.
81. Hoe LK, Keang LT. Hospitalized low-risk community-acquired pneumonia: Outcome and potential for cost-savings. *Respirology* 1999;4:307-309.
82. Fine MJ, Auble TE, Yealy DM, et al. A prediction rule to identify low-risk patients with community-acquired pneumonia. *N Engl J Med* 1997;336:243-250.
83. Auble TE, Yealy DM, Fine MJ. Assessing prognosis and selecting an initial site of care for adults with community-acquired pneumonia. *Infect Dis Clin North Am* 1998;2:741-759.
84. Dean NC. Use of prognostic scoring and outcome assessment tools in the admission decision for community-acquired pneumonia. *Clin Chest Med* 1999;20:521-529.
85. Farr BM, Sloman AJ, Fisch MJ. Predicting death in patients hospitalized for community-acquired pneumonia. *Ann Intern Med* 1991;115:428-436.
86. Fine JM, Smith MA, Carson CA, et al. Prognosis and outcomes of patients with community-acquired pneumonia. *JAMA* 1996;275:134-141.
87. Houston MS, Silverstein MD, Suman VJ. Risk factors for 30-Day mortality in elderly patients with lower respiratory tract infection. *Arch Intern Med* 1997;157:2190-2195.
88. Conte HA, Chen YT, Mehal W, et al. A prognostic rule for elderly patients admitted with community-acquired pneumonia. *Am J Med* 1999;106:20-28.
89. Ewig S, Kleinfeld T, Bauer T, et al. Comparative validation of prognostic rules for community-acquired pneumonia in an elderly population. *Eur Respir J* 1999;14:370-375.
90. Mylotte JM, Naughton B, Saludades C, et al. Validation and application of the pneumonia prognosis index to nursing home residents with pneumonia. *JAGS* 1998;46:1538-1544.
91. Marston BJ, Plouffe JF, et al. Incidence of community-acquired pneumonia requiring hospitalization. Results of a population-based active surveillance study in Ohio. The Community-Based Pneumonia Incidence Study Group. *Arch Int Med* 1997;157: 1709-1718.
92. Atlas SJ, Benzer TI, Borowsky LH, et al. Safely increasing the proportion of patients with community-acquired pneumonia treated as outpatients. An interventional trial. *Arch Intern Med* 1998;158: 1350-1356.
93. American Thoracic Society: Guidelines for the Initial Management of adults with Community-Acquired Pneumonia: Diagnosis, Assessment of Severity, and Initial Antimicrobial Therapy. *Am Rev Respir Dis* 1993;148:1418-1426.
94. Ewig S, Ruiz M, Mensa J, et al. Severe community-acquired pneumonia. Assessment of severity criteria. *Am J Respir Crit Care Med* 1998;158:1102-1108.
95. Marrie TJ. Community-acquired pneumonia: Epidemiology, etiology, treatment. *Infect Dis Clinic North Am* 1998;12:723-740.
96. Brentsson E, Lagergard T. Etiology of community-acquired pneumonia in outpatients. *Eur J Clin Microbiol* 1986;5:446-447.
97. Langille DB, Yates L, Marrie TJ. Serological investigation of pneumonia as it presents to the physician's office. *Can J Infect Dis* 1993;4:328.
98. Whitney CG, Barrett N, et al. Increasing prevalence of drug-resistant Streptococcus pneumoniae (DRSP): Implications for therapy for pneumonia. In: *Programs and Abstracts of the 36th Annual Meeting of the Infectious Disease Society of America*, November 12-15, 1998. IDSA, Abstract 51.
99. Antibiotic Update 1998: Outcome-effective treatment for bacterial infections managed in the primary care and emergency department setting. *Emerg Med Rep* 1997;18:1-24.
100. Enoxacin-A new fluoroquinolone. *Med Lett Drugs Ther* 1992;4: 103-105.
101. Cooper B, Lawer M. Pneumococcal bacteremia during ciprofloxacin therapy for pneumococcal pneumonia. *Am J Med* 1989;87:475.
102. Flynn CM, et al. In vitro efficacy of levofloxacin alone or in combination tested against multi-resistant *Pseudomonas aeruginosa* strains. *J Chemother* 1996;8:411-415.
103. Dholakia N, et al. Susceptibilities of bacterial isolates from patients with cancer to levofloxacin and other quinolones. *Antimicrob Agents Chemother* 1994;38:848-852.
104. Garibaldi RA. Epidemiology of community-acquired respiratory tract infections in adults. Incidence, etiology, and impact. *Am J Med* 1985;78:32-37.
105. Fang GD, Fine M, Orloff J, et al. New and emerging etiologies for community-acquired pneumonia with implications for therapy. *Medicine* 1990;69:307-316.
106. Habib MP, et al. Intersci Conf Antimicrob Agents Chemother 1996;36. Abstract L002. 36th Interscience Conference on Antimicrobial Agents and Chemotherapy. New Orleans, LA. Sept. 15-18, 1996.
107. File TM, et al. Abstr Intersci Conf Antimicrob Agents Chemother 1996;36. Abstract L001 (LM1). 36th Interscience Conference on Antimicrobial Agents and Chemotherapy. New Orleans, LA. Sept. 15-18, 1996.
108. File TM, Dunbar L, et al. A multicenter, randomized study comparing the efficacy and safety of intravenous and/or oral levofloxacin versus ceftriaxone and/or cefuroxime in treatment of adults with community-acquired pneumonia. *Antimicrob Agents Chemother* 1997:41:1965-1972.
109. Cleeland R, Squires E. Antimicrobial activity of ceftriaxone: A review. *Am J Med* 1984;77:3.

Key, Selected References

1. Sethi S. Infectious exacerbations of chronic bronchitis: Diagnosis

and management. *J Antimicrob Chemother* 1999;43(Suppl A): 97-105. Review.

2. Sachs FL. Chronic bronchitis. *Clin Chest Med* 1981;2:79-89. Review.
3. Ball P, Tillotson G, Wilson R. Chemotherapy for chronic bronchitis. Controversies. *Presse Med* 1995;24:189-194. Review.
4. Grossman RF. Acute exacerbations of chronic bronchitis. *Hosp Pract* 1997;32:85-89, 92-94.
5. Sethi S. Infectious etiology of acute exacerbations of chronic bronchitis. *Chest* 2000;117(5 Suppl 2):380S-3855S. Review.
6. Zuck P, Rio Y. [Antibiotic therapy in exacerbations of chronic bronchitis]. *Presse Med* 1997;26:1492-1494. French.
7. Read RC. Infection in acute exacerbations of chronic bronchitis: A clinical perspective. *Respir Med* 1999;93:845-850. Review.
8. Niederman MS. [Clinical contribution of the newer fluoroquinolones in acute bacterial exacerbation of chronic bronchitis]. *Medicina* (B Aires). 1999;59(Suppl 1):23-30. Spanish.
9. Nicotra MB, Kronenberg RS. Con: antibiotic use in exacerbations of chronic bronchitis. *Semin Respir Infect* 1993;8:254-258. Review.
10. Verghese A, Ismail HM. Acute exacerbations of chronic bronchitis. Preventing treatment failures and early reinfection. *Postgrad Med* 1994;96:75-76, 79-82, 87-89. Review.
11. Isada CM. Pro: Antibiotics for chronic bronchitis with exacerbations. *Semin Respir Infect* 1993;8:243-253. Review.
12. Adams SG, Anzueto A. Antibiotic therapy in acute exacerbations of chronic bronchitis. *Semin Respir Infect* 2000;15:234-247. Review.
13. Carbon C. Acute and chronic bronchitis. *Microb Drug Resist* 1995;1:159-162. Review.
14. Buchenroth M. [Antibiotic therapy in bronchial infections. 1: Acute and chronic bronchitis]. *MMW Fortschr Med* 1999;141: 49-50. German.
15. Grossman RF. Management of acute exacerbation of chronic bronchitis. *Can Respir J* 1999;6(Suppl A):40A-45A. Review.
16. Wilson R. Ten years of ciprofloxacin: the past, present and future. Acute exacerbations of chronic bronchitis. Introduction. *J Antimicrob Chemother* 1999;43(Suppl A):95-6.
17. Wilson R, Wilson CB. Defining subsets of patients with chronic bronchitis. *Chest* 1997;112(6 Suppl):303S-309S. Review.
18. McHardy VU, Inglis JM, Calder MA, et al. A study of infective and other factors in exacerbations of chronic bronchitis. *Br J Dis Chest* 1980;74:228-238.
19. Grossman RF. How do we achieve cost-effective options in lower respiratory tract infection therapy? *Chest* 1998;113(3 Suppl): 205S-210S.
20. Wilson R, Grossman R. Introduction: The role of bacterial infection in chronic bronchitis. *Semin Respir Infect* 2000;15:1-6. Review.
21. Niroumand M, Grossman RF. Airway infection. *Infect Dis Clin North Am* 1998;12:671-688. Review.
22. Adams SG, Anzueto A. Treating acute exacerbations of chronic bronchitis in the face of antibiotic resistance. *Cleve Clin J Med* 2000;67:625-628, 631-633. Review.
23. Ayoub A, Rekik WK. [Chronic bronchitis exacerbations: justifications and indications of antibiotic therapy]. *Tunis Med* 1996;74: 271-276. Review. French.
24. Ball P, Make B. Acute exacerbations of chronic bronchitis: An international comparison. *Chest* 1998;113(3 Suppl):199S-204S.
25. Riise GC, Larsson S, Larsson P, et al. The intrabronchial microbial flora in chronic bronchitis patients: A target for N-acetylcysteine therapy? *Eur Respir J* 1994;7:94-101.
26. Donner CF. Infectious exacerbations of chronic bronchitis. ORI-ONE Board. *Monaldi Arch Chest Dis* 1999;54:43-48. Review.
27. Allegra L, Catena E, Pozzi E, et al. [Effectiveness of and tolerance to ceftibuten in the treatment of chronic bacterial bronchitis exacerbations in an elderly population]. *Minerva Med* 1996;87: 479-485. Italian.
28. Niederman MS. Antibiotic therapy of exacerbations of chronic bronchitis. *Semin Respir Infect* 2000;15:59-70. Review.
29. Ball P, Harris JM, Lowson D, et al. Acute infective exacerbations of chronic bronchitis. *QJM* 1995;88:61-68.
30. Ball P. Infective pathogenesis and outcomes in chronic bronchitis. *Curr Opin Pulm Med* 1996;2:181-185. Review.
31. Paster RZ, McAdoo MA, Keyserling CH, et al. A comparison of a five-day regimen of cefdinir with a seven-day regimen of loracarbef for the treatment of acute exacerbations of chronic bronchitis. *Int J Clin Pract* 2000;54:293-299.
32. San Pedro G, George R. Treating acute exacerbations of chronic bronchitis. *Hosp Pract* (Off Ed). 2000;35:43-50. Review.
33. Grossman RF. Guidelines for the treatment of acute exacerbations of chronic bronchitis. *Chest* 1997;112(6 Suppl):310S-313S. Review.
34. Finch RG. A review of worldwide experience with sparfloxacin in the treatment of community-acquired pneumonia and acute bacterial exacerbations of chronic bronchitis. *Int J Antimicrob Agents* 1999;12:5-17. Review.
35. Shteingardt IN, Bukreeva EB, Khristoliubova EI, et al. [Etiologic structure of exacerbations in chronic bronchitis]. *Ter Arkh* 1988;60:93-95. Russian.
36. Gonzales R, Sande MA. Acute bronchitis in the healthy adult. *Curr Clin Top Infect Dis* 2000;20:158-173. Review.
37. Melbye H, Berdal BP. [Acute bronchitis in adults. Clinical findings, microorganisms and use of antibiotics]. *Tidsskr Nor Laegeforen* 1994;114:814-817. Norwegian.
38. Robertson CE, Ford MJ, Munro JF, et al. The efficacy of a new formulation of trimethoprim and sulphadiazine in acute exacerbations of chronic bronchitis. *Methods Find Exp Clin Pharmacol* 1983;5:127-129.
39. Staley H, McDade HB, Paes D. Is an objective assessment of antibiotic therapy in exacerbations of chronic bronchitis possible? *J Antimicrob Chemother* 1993;31:193-197. Review.
40. Hamacher J, Vogel F, Lichey J, et al. Treatment of acute bacterial exacerbations of chronic obstructive pulmonary disease in hospitalised patients—a comparison of meropenem and imipenem/cilastatin. COPD Study Group. *J Antimicrob Chemother* 1995;36(Suppl A):121-133.

Urinary Tract Infection: Diagnosis and Evaluation

Kenneth H. Butler, DO, FACEP
Kevin C. Reed, MD
Gideon Bosker, MD, FACEP

In the constantly shifting landscape of drug resistance, antibiotic options, and pharmacoeconomic considerations, urinary tract infection (UTI) continues to be one of the most frequently diagnosed conditions in patients presenting to emergency department and hospital-based settings.

It is estimated that practitioners manage seven million new cases of cystitis in the United States each year and that, overall, UTIs now account for approximately 1 million hospitalizations annually.[1,2] Moreover, UTIs are the leading cause of gram-negative bacteremia in patients of all ages, and are associated with a high risk of morbidity and mortality, especially in the elderly.[3] The total annual cost of treatment is in the billions of dollars.[4]

Among common infections managed in the emergency department and acute hospital setting, few conditions have treatment guidelines, antibiotic selection strategies, or diagnostic protocols that have changed or evolved as rapidly as those used for UTI. Despite a general consensus that empiric treatment of UTI in adult women requires, at the very least, mandatory coverage of *Escherichia coli* and other gram-negative organisms, antibiotic selection strategies—including initial choice of therapy and duration of treatment—vary widely among practitioners and institutions.

There are many reasons for inconsistencies in the current approach to UTI management among hospital-based physicians. Unfortunately, deciphering the strengths and weaknesses of recommendations issued by different authoritative sources can be problematic and confusing, especially since resistance patterns of infecting uropathogens may vary among geographic regions, and because outcome-effectiveness, failure rates, total-resource costs to achieve clinical cure, the risk of recurrent infection, and evolving bacterial resistance issues are not always entered into the drug selection equation.

Because no single set of guidelines is applicable to every patient or hospital practice environment, management guidelines for UTI must be "customized" for the local practice setting and, as always, clinical judgment must prevail. This means taking into account local antibiotic resistance patterns, epidemiological and infection incidence data, and patient demographic features.

Even when these factors are considered, a number of important questions about drug selection issues for UTI still remain: 1) What is the appropriate initial, empiric choice for uncomplicated UTI? Ciprofloxacin or trimethoprim/sulfamethoxazole (TMP/SMX)? 2) What are the specific "intensification and treatment trigger" criteria that support amplifying initial spectrum of coverage from TMP/SMX to a fluoroquinolone such as ciprofloxacin? 3) How should evolving resistance of *E. coli* to TMP/SMX affect initial antimicrobial therapy in hospitalized patients with UTI? 4) What is the role of risk-stratification guidelines for initial antibiotic selection in elderly patients with UTI? 5) What is the optimal duration of therapy for uncomplicated UTI? Complicated UTI? 6) What type of therapy and its duration can be characterized as "optimal"?

and 7) Which antibiotic currently provides "correct spectrum" coverage, safety, and reliability for outpatient and inpatient treatment of UTI?

Although optimizing cure rates with so-called convenient, dose- and duration-friendly branded agents that provide appropriate and predictable coverage with a low risk of antimicrobial resistance may be perceived as costly on a drug-acquisition basis, it is important to stress the following point: Antimicrobial agents with more predictable coverage against pathogens implicated in UTI can help avoid the unnecessary costs of treatment failures, disease progression, patient re-evaluations, return visits, patient dissatisfaction, and the pharmacological reservicing costs associated with initiating a second course of antibiotics.[5]

In this sense, antibiotics that lower barriers to clinical cure and provide a predictable spectrum of coverage can be seen as "productivity tools" that improve efficiency of clinical care, and potentially reduce the overall costs associated with inpatient and acute outpatient management of UTI. These benefits are especially important in the older patient in whom repeated hospitalizations increase the risk of nosocomial infections and drug-related complications.

In light of the important advances, changes, and refinements that have occurred in the area of UTI treatment recently, this comprehensive, state-of-the-art review presents a revised and updated set of guidelines outlining UTI epidemiology and management in the emergency department and hospital-based setting. Special emphasis has been given to both epidemiological data demonstrating the importance of "correct spectrum" coverage with specific fluoroquinolones, such as ciprofloxacin, and to the selection of initial antibiotics for patients deemed suitable for discharge.

In addition, detailed evidence-based analyses comparing ciprofloxacin and TMP/SMX are presented to guide antibiotic selection in patients with uncomplicated UTI and pyelonephritis.[5] Cautionary notes about the overuse of extended-spectrum fluoroquinolones are outlined, and evidence-based studies confirming ciprofloxacin's workhorse role in hospital-based treatment of UTI is discussed. Drawing upon consensus panels, expert opinion, and clinical trials, this clinical consensus report presents antimicrobial protocols and treatment guidelines linked to, and driven by, risk-stratification criteria, evidence-based trials, and specific clinical profiles of patients presenting to the hospital with symptoms and signs suggestive of UTI.

Introduction

The prevalence of UTIs varies greatly with age, race, and gender. Between 4.1% and 7.5% of serious bacterial infections in febrile pediatric patients are attributed to UTIs, with the prevalence highest (17%) in white females.[6,7] The majority of patients with UTIs are female, with close to a 50% lifetime occurrence rate.[3,4] As both sexes age, the incidence of bacteriuria increases from less than 5% in young adult women and less than 0.1% in young adult males to at least 20% of women and 10% of men older than age 65.[8]

Because younger patients are at low risk for occult genitourinary tract abnormalities and are less likely to have comorbid conditions, they respond predictably to empiric antibiotic therapy. Certain patient subgroups, however, have complicating conditions that increase the risk for acquiring invasive, systemic infection or for failing therapy. Complicated UTI may occur in men, children, and pregnant women, but it is especially common in the elderly as well as in immunocompromised patients and in individuals with neurologic disorders.

Severity of infection in these patient subgroups ranges from mild cystitis to life-threatening urosepsis, which may be more difficult to treat because of: 1) associated structural or functional genitourinary tract abnormalities; 2) resistant organisms, and/or; 3) inadequate host defenses. Accordingly, special consideration to antibiotic selection must be given to elderly patients, who require prompt, appropriate therapy and thorough evaluation of their UTIs to avoid prolonged infection or serious renal sequelae.

Diagnosis—Screening, Culture, and Radiographic Studies

Confirming the clinical diagnosis of UTI may present challenges in both the younger and older patient populations. Detection of UTI is especially important in these patient subgroups because inadequate or delayed therapy may lead to renal deterioration and life-threatening systemic toxicity.

The Elderly. Urinary tract infection in the elderly may present in a manner that is different from its typical presentation in younger adults. For example, the classic lower tract symptoms of frequency, urgency, and dysuria, accompanied by upper tract findings of chills, flank pain, and tenderness, may be altered or absent in the geriatric patient. Moreover, the fever may be absent and some patients are hypothermic.[9] Although acute pyelonephritis in the elderly typically exhibits a septic syndrome manifested as fever, tachycardia, and altered mental status, UTIs in the elderly may present with a wide range chief complaints, which may include mental status deterioration, nausea, vomiting, abdominal pain, or respiratory distress.[10,11]

In a study of community-dwelling adults older than 50 years of age, bacteremic UTI most commonly presented as confusion, cough, and dyspnea. New urinary symptoms were the chief complaint in only 20% of cases.[11] In another study, only one-half of older bacteremic UTI patients were febrile. However, older patients were no more likely to be afebrile than were younger bacteremic patients (40% of whom had normal temperatures).[12] Because of the wide range of presenting symptoms, the misdiagnosis of UTI in the geriatric patient ranges from approximately 20% to 40%.[5,10,13]

The high misdiagnosis rate can be attributed to patients presenting with non-urinary complaints. In light of the difficulties identifying elderly patients with UTI—and the significant mortality rate associated with inadequate or delayed therapy—clinicians must maintain a high index of suspicion for this condition. In addition, certain laboratory and microbiological procedures, in combination with uncharacteristic clinical findings will optimize detection of UTI in this geriatric patient.

It may be clinically impossible to ascertain whether fever in the bacteriuric elderly patient lacking urinary symptoms is an invasive urinary infection. The majority of febrile episodes in the bacteriuric, non-catheterized elderly are unlikely to be due to invasive infection.[14,15] Foul-smelling urine is sometimes considered a symptom in the elderly adult, especially in the institutionalized patient. Urinary bacteria produce polyamines, which account for the odor, and although antibiotic therapy may ameliorate the odor, use of antibiotics for this exclusive purpose is not advocated.[14] Management of incontinence and improved hygiene, especially in the institutionalized patient, will usually solve this problem.

Pediatric Age Group. Extensive research has been conducted over the past few years to evaluate the diagnostic approach to the diagnosis of UTI in children > 5 years of age—and especially, in those younger than 2 years of age. The difficulty in making this diagnosis is evident from studies showing that fever and irritability are the most common complaints in children in this age group.[17,18] In fact, up to 80% of infants with culture-proven UTIs present with only fever or failure to thrive as their chief symptom.[17-19] Furthermore, the presence of nonspecific symptoms in children with UTIs also are common to other childhood infections, including viral syndromes, gastroenteritis, otitis media, and upper respiratory infections.[17,18]

In one study of 200 febrile infants with UTI diagnosed by urine culture, 64% initially were felt by the examining physician to have another diagnosis as a source of their fever.[20] Pediatric investigators have identified risk factors associated with an increased risk of UTI in children younger than 2 years of age. They include: temperature higher than 39°C, fever for longer than two days, white race, age less than one year, and no other obvious source of fever.[20] The presence of two or more of the above risk factors yielded a sensitivity of greater than 99% and specificity of 71% for detection of UTI in children in this age group.[20]

Screening and Culture. The most common screening tests for UTI include urine dipstick and microscopic urinalysis, with a combination of leukocyte esterase (LE) and nitrate testing achieving sensitivities of 78% to 92% and specificities of 65% to 98%.[21,22] Enhanced microscopic analysis of centrifuged urine from pediatric patients has been found to have a sensitivity of 94% and a specificity of 84-92%.[21] The authors of a recent study using enhanced urinalysis (coupling a white blood cell [WBC] count by hemocytometer and a gram stain on uncentrifuged urine) recommend a urine dipstick as a reliable and economic screening test. In their view, enhanced urinalysis should reserved for use in neonates (infants < 8 weeks of age) and in patients with comorbid conditions, including underlying anatomic renal abnormalities.[21]

Urine culture remains the definitive test for confirming the diagnosis of UTI.[17,19] Recommendations for culture differ depending upon the risk group. Adult patients who require hospitalization for presumptive UTI should be cultured to confirm an etiologic diagnosis. In children, the approach is more complicated. The updated American Academy of Pediatric recommendations[19] for diagnosis of UTI in children age 2 months to 2 years with an unexplained fever offer the following guidelines regarding urine culture: 1) Culture a specimen obtained by suprapubic aspiration (SPA) or bladder catheterization or; 2) Obtain a urine specimen by the most convenient method and analyze it by urine dipstick or urinalysis; if it is positive for LE or nitrite, obtain a culture by SPA or bladder catheterization. The importance of accurate diagnosis in infants and young children, in part, is related to the concern over renal scarring, subsequent hypertension, and end stage renal disease, which may manifest years later in approximately 10-15% of patients who have had pyelonephritis.[18,23]

Urine cultures are rarely indicated to diagnose simple cystitis in otherwise healthy adults. However, they should be obtained from pregnant women for detection of both asymptomatic and symptomatic bacteriuria. They are also required if the patient has: 1) continued symptoms of UTI while on treatment; 2) suspected pyelonephritis; 3) a history of recurrent UTI; 4) history of recent antibiotic use; or 5) any comorbid neurologic or anatomic abnormalities.[24] Blood cultures can be obtained in children younger than 6 months of age with presumed pyelonephritis, although bacteremia is rare in this age group.[25]

A recent study of 391 pregnant women with pyelonephritis found that initially prescribed antibiotics were changed in only 1% of cases after confirmation of bacteremia (positive blood cultures).[26] In addition, these patients had a similar clinical course as those without bacteremia. Based on this work and previous studies, the authors suggest eliminating blood cultures in the routine management of pyelonephritis in pregnant women, citing possible significant cost savings (approximately $15 million annually) and no significant compromise in patient care.

Radiographic Advances—Imaging and Ultrasound. The goal of radiologic evaluation is: 1) to identify renal scarring or parenchymal damage at the time of diagnosis; 2) to identify the presence of underlying functional or anatomic abnormalities that predispose the patient to UTIs or renal damage; and 3) to provide a baseline for further comparisons.[27,28] As a rule, a renal ultrasound is the first step for identifying parenchymal disease or signs of obstructive uropathy such as a hydroureter or hydronephrosis in infants, children with suspected pyelonephritis, and children with a known immunodeficiency or suspected anatomic abnormality.[17,19,28] Renal ultrasound can be performed at any time during the course of treatment. A voiding cystourethrogram (VCUG) is excellent for identifying vesico-ureteral reflux, the most common abnormality associated with UTI in infants; this condition is present in more than 50% of infants younger than 1 year of age.[3]

A recent advance in imaging is the development of a fluoroscopic VCUG, which allows continued monitoring of the urinary system for intermittent reflux, which may be missed with conventional modalities.[3] A VCUG is generally performed when there is evidence of urine sterilization. Some experts wait for four weeks after treatment initiation due to concerns that bladder spasms will interfere with the quality of the study.[28] A 99mTc-DMSA (technetium99-labeled dimercaptosuccinic acid) nuclear cortical scan is generally considered the gold standard for identifying previous renal parenchymal damage. It is recommended in patients with abnormalities noted on renal ultrasound or VCUG and for toxic patients unresponsive to parenteral antibiotic treatment.[29] These tests have generally replaced intravenous pyelography (IVP) as the studies of choice, although in certain cases IVP is still performed.

Recently introduced, power Doppler ultrasonography was developed as an alternative to standard B-mode ultrasound. This technique has demonstrated great promise, as it displays an image analogous to a perfusion map that is sensitive to low-flow states seen in acute pyelonephritis.[30] Preliminary reports reveal an 89% sensitivity relative to CT and a 75% sensitivity relative to nuclear renal scans. This test is noninvasive, avoids radiation, intravenous injection, and sedation for the majority of patients. In the future, it may replace CT or nuclear scans for suspected pyelonephritis.[30] Limitations of this modality are that is operator and reader dependent, as well being motion sensitive and difficult to perform on an uncooperative child.

Imaging studies are rarely indicated in adult patients with UTI. Patients with fever for longer than 48 to 72 hours despite antibiotic treatment and with signs of systemic toxicity or bacteremia should be suspected of having a complicated infection with renal or perirenal abscess, anatomic obstruction, or nephrolithiasis.[31] Ultrasound has become more available in the emergency department (ED) and has been recommended by the American College of Emergency Physicians as a valuable tool for the emergency department evaluation of selected medical and traumatic conditions.[32]

One group of investigators retrospectively studied the use of ultrasound by emergency physicians for the diagnosis of renal abscess in the emergency department setting.[33] The physicians were trained at least three months in the use of abdominal ultrasonography by the radiology department, and senior radiologists verified that the emergency physicians were able to recognize the imaging of renal abscess. Although a high rate of success was achieved for diagnosis of renal abscesses, the study was limited by the small numbers of enrolled patients and lack of control patients.

Clearly, a prospective study of ultrasonographic evaluation of emergency physicians for screening high-risk patients suspected of having renal abscesses is needed to obtain sensitivity and specificity rates.[33] Currently, this study group recommends that emergency physicians focus on patients with diabetes, renal stones, history of renal transplant, immunosuppression, longer duration of symptoms of UTI, and renal failure. Ultrasound should be used promptly in the ED to aid in the early diagnosis of renal abscess. This procedure also is useful for establishing adequate vascular perfusion in renal transplant recipients.

Bacteriologic Resistance Patterns

The emergence of resistance to antibiotics, especially to TMP/SMX is changing initial selection patterns in patients with uncomplicated and complicated UTI. To appreciate the scope of the problem, a brief review of the common uropathogens is warranted. The most common uropathogens identified in adult patients with UTI include enteric gram-negative bacteria, with *E. coli* being the most common (in 60-80% of UTIs). *(Please See Table 1.)* The remainder of infections are caused by coagulase-negative *Staphylococcus saprophyticus* (10-20%), while *Proteus mirabilis, Klebsiella*, and *Enterococcus* account for less than 5%.[3,8,34] Other aerobic gram-negative bacteria of the *Enterobacteriacea* family include *Citrobacter, Enterobacter, Serratia*, and *Salmonella*.[7,19,23] Non-enteric aerobic gram-negative rods such as *Pseudomonas* and aerobic gram-positive cocci such as *Enterococcus* are less prevalent in immunocompetent hosts. *(Please See Table 1)*. Group B streptococci infection is observed in neonates secondary to inoculation from a colonized mother during delivery through the vaginal canal.

Anaerobic bacteria are rarely pathogenic despite their prevalence in fecal flora. The *Lactobacillus* species, coagulase-negative staphylococci, and *Corynebacterium* are not considered clinically significant isolates in the urine of healthy children between 2 months and 2 years of age.[18,19] *Corynebacterium, Lactobacillus*, and *Streptococcus* species are identified only rarely; when they are present, they nearly always represent contamination of the specimen rather than a true pathogen. In complicated UTI, in addition to *E. coli* there is a higher prevalence of *Pseudomonas, Enterobacter* species, *Serratia, Acinetobacter, Klebsiella*, and enterococci.[31] There are anecdotal reports of treatment for *Gardnerella vaginalis, Lactobacilli, Chlamydia trachomatis*, and *Ureaplasma urealyticum* in pregnant women, but it is unclear whether these organisms represent true pathogens in this population.[35,36] Candidal species are now emerging in greater numbers, especially catheterized patients and those who received previous treatment for enterococcal UTIs.[31]

The high incidence of UTIs, the potential for complications, and the associated costs of treatment emphasize the importance of appropriate antibiotic therapy. Microbial resistance to nearly all classes of antimicrobials continues to rise despite increasing awareness and concerns worldwide. European studies have shown *E. coli* resistance rates to multiple antibiotics, specifically TMP/SMX, in as many as one-third of patients.[37,38] Similar trends in the United States have prompted a shift to fluoroquinolones such as ciprofloxacin as preferred initial agents for empiric intravenous and/or oral therapy of UTI in the hospital and emergency department setting.[39]

In a cross-sectional survey of emergency department urine cultures from an urban tertiary care center in the United States, microbial resistance was as high as 48% to ampicillin, 25% to tetracycline, 14-28% to TMP/SMX, and 13% to nitrofurantoin.[40] Similar studies have shown that the resistance to ciprofloxacin among common uropathogens, including *E. coli*, frequently encountered in hospital-managed UTI is as low as 1-2%.[41-45] These epidemiological data have important treatment implications, since recent studies are already also demonstrating outcome differences in clinical efficacy and patient cure rates between UTI patients managed on TMP/SMX and those managed on ciprofloxacin.[46] As would be expected, maintenance of predictable antimicrobial activity by ciprofloxacin against the anticipated spectrum of uropathogens has solidified the role of this antibiotic in treatment pathways for UTI among all institutional settings.

Hospitals affiliated with managed care organizations also have been prompted to re-evaluate their initial approach to antibiotic selection for UTI. A cross-sectional survey of 4,000 urine cultures obtained from women ages 18 to 50 years in an HMO setting between 1992 and 1996 showed *E. coli* prevalence to be 86%, with the resistance rate to TMP/SMX increasing over this period from 9% to 18%. Recent data suggest that in some regions of the country, especially the West and Southwest, and in most major urban centers, the resistance rate to TMP/SMX has risen to as high as 35%.[5,37,38,47-50] The overall resistance to multiple groups of antimicrobials, including the penicillins, cephalosporins, and sulfa drugs, doubled from 8% to 16%.[51] In pregnant patients, *E. coli* resistance to ampicillin which, at one time was a drug of choice for UTI in this population, is now about 20% to 30%.[36]

Fortunately, one class of antimicrobials to which sensitivity rates have remained consistently high is the fluoroquinolone group, of which ciprofloxacin, is the most frequently used as the agent in the adult population. A two-tiered study from 1989 to 1991 and 1996 to 1997 at an urban sexually transmitted disease clinic evaluated young, sexually active females diagnosed with a UTI and found *E. coli* resistance rates to ampicillin, cephalosporins, or tetracycline in as many as 25% of patients. There was very little change in the low prevalence of organisms resistant to fluoroquinolones.[52]

Additional studies at student health clinics in California over a five-year period demonstrated significant increases in the resistance of *E. coli* to ampicillin (30%-45%), tetracycline (29%-40%), and TMP/SMX (15%-32%), with resistance to fluoroquinolones in $< 5\%$ of organisms.[34] In a recent analysis of young women with uncomplicated pyelonephritis, *E. coli* was isolated in more than 90% of cultures and was resistant to TMP/SMX in 18%, compared with a 0.4% resistance to ciprofloxacin. A significant variance in resistance patterns existed in different geographic regions, with resistance to

Table 1. Pathogens Responsible for Uncomplicated and Complicated Urinary Tract Infections§

1) *Escherichia coli*
2) *Staphylococcus saprophyticus*
3) *Klebsiella pneumoniae*
4) *Proteus mirabilis*
5) *Enterococcus* faecalis*
6) *Pseudomonas aeruginosa*
7) *Enterobacter cloacae*
8) *Citrobacter*

§ = Listed in order of decreasing frequency
* = Gram-positive organisms

TMP/SMX as high as 35% on the West Coast of the United States as opposed to 14% in the Midwest and 7% on the East Coast.[46] One caveat regarding bacterial resistance is that in vitro sensitivity results may not correlate with clinical cure rates and in vivo sensitivity. Eradication of a uropathogen depends on the concentration of antibiotics in the urine as opposed to serum, which may be higher than the levels used in in vitro studies.[31]

Antibiotic Selection for UTI—General Principles and Overview of Therapeutic Options

The optimal antibiotic for in-hospital management of UTI requires evidence-based trials demonstrating high clinical and bacteriocidal cure rates and a low potential for resistance. It also should be associated with a reasonable acquisition cost, a convenient dosing schedule conducive to patient compliance, minimal side effects, and be easily available to prescribing practitioners and their patients. *(Please See Table 2.)*

Fluoroquinolones—Agents of Choice. With rapidly changing resistance patterns among the common uropathogens, standard first-line treatments are being replaced in many instances by one of the newest classes of antimicrobials, the fluoroquinolones. The mechanism of action, side effects, drug interactions, and contraindications of the fluoroquinolones are reviewed in Table 3.

Derivatives of nalidixic acid, fluoroquinolones were discovered accidentally in the early 1960s during the synthesis of the anti-malarial agent, chloroquine.[39] To date, more than 10,000 analogues of nalidixic acid have undergone initial screening, and the first flouroquinolone antibiotic was approved for clinical use in the late 1980s.[39] These highly effective antimicrobials act on bacterial topoisomerases, a class of enzymes that is essential for maintaining the physicochemical stability and biological activity of bacterial DNA.[39] In general, the newer quinolones have longer serum half-lives with proven post-antibiotic effects from one to six hours, allowing patient-friendly single- or twice-daily dosing and higher peak levels for maximum bactericidal activity.[39]

In addition, fluoroquinolones are well-absorbed from the gastrointestinal tract, and in the case of ciprofloxacin, equivalent clinical outcomes in selected patient populations with moderate to severe UTI have been established between patient groups who received this drug intravenously and those who received oral therapy.[41,43,53] The fluoroquinolones have excellent penetration into various tissues; they are well-distributed intracellularly, and they have the added benefit of eliminating perineal, vaginal, and perirectal reservoirs of uropathogens without altering normal bowel or vaginal flora.[39,54]

As mentioned, the high oral bioavailability of fluoroquinolones allows switching from intravenous to oral therapy without dosage adjustments.[55] Excretion is primarily renal, although some of the compounds have exclusive hepatic metabolism or a combination of the two.[39] They have an extended spectrum of bactericidal activity against gram-negative rods, including *Pseudomonas*, gram-positive cocci, and intracellular pathogens.[54,55] Fluoroquinolones remain classified as category C drugs, requiring practitioners to rule out pregnancy before prescribing them to potentially pregnant patients.[39]

The armamentarium of commonly used fluoroquinolones is expanding at a rapid rate. Ciprofloxacin (Cipro®), which has been a clinically proven gold standard for oral and intravenous-based therapy of UTI has been joined by other agents, many of which also are indicated for community-acquired pneumonia (CAP). Newer members of this class include enoxacin (Penetrex®), gatifloxacin (Tequin®), levofloxacin (Levaquin®), lomefloxacin (Maxaquin®), and ofloxacin (Floxin®). Low levels of resistance to fluoroquinolones are beginning to appear through two mechanisms: chromosomal mutations or alterations affecting the ability of fluoroquinolones to permeate the bacterial cell well.[39] Fortunately, separate isomerases are required to produce this form of resistance; therefore, the emergence of a predictably resistant organism would require a rare double mutation.[39]

An extensive body of clinical research confirms that fluoroquinolones are extremely effective for the treatment of UTIs ranging in severity from uncomplicated cystitis to urosepsis.[56] As would be expected, many studies evaluating newly introduced quinolones compare clinical trial outcomes to the established track record of ciprofloxacin, which has become a standard choice for initial, empiric therapy for most UTIs. In a clinically controlled trial comparing three days of oral ciprofloxacin with seven days of TMP/SMX or nitrofurantoin, bacteriologic cure rates for uncomplicated UTI after four to six weeks were 91%, 79%, and 82%, respectively.[57] Clinical cure rates after four to 10 days were similar among the three groups, as was the overall incidence of adverse events. The superior efficacy of ciprofloxacin as compared to TMP/SMX also has been confirmed in patients with acute pyelonephritis.[46]

In certain studies of acute uncomplicated cystitis, levofloxacin has shown preliminarily to have equal efficacy in single doses as in the standard longer dosing regimens.[59,62] Ciprofloxacin and norfloxacin are effective in either single daily or double dosing regimens in uncomplicated UTI.[63,64] For complicated UTIs, including pyelonephritis, levofloxacin and lomefloxacin have equivalent bacteriologic and clinical cure rates as ciprofloxacin. Of the newer fluoroquinolones, only levofloxacin is approved for both upper and lower UTIs.

Overuse of the extended-spectrum fluoroquinolones—levofloxacin, and gatifloxacin—for hospital-based management of UTI must be considered in light of recommendations made by the Centers for Disease Control and Prevention (CDC), and concerns about emerging resistance to pathogens implicated in CAP. The fluoro-

Table 2. Recommended Oral Antibiotics for Uncomplicated UTI and Intravenous Agents for Hospital-Based Management of Pyelonephritis[19,25,34,39,56-58,63,64,66,82,84,86,91,98,104]

Agent	Dosage
ACUTE UNCOMPLICATED UTI IN ADULTS, CYSTITIS (3-DAY REGIMEN)	
First-line agents:	
Fluoroquinolone (initial agent of choice)	
Ciprofloxacin (preferred)	250 mg po BID x 3 days
Fluoroquinolone (alternative)	
Enoxacin	200 mg po BID x 3 days
Gatifloxacin	200-400 mg po QD x 3 days
Levofloxacin	250 mg po QD x 3 days
Ofloxacin	200 mg po BID x 3 days
Lomefloxacin	400 mg po QD x 3 days
Norfloxacin	400 mg po BID x 3 days
Secondary Alternatives:	
Trimethoprim/sulfamethoxazole*	160/800 mg po bid x 3 days

*Only if *E. coli* resistance is < 10%-15% in patient population (based on regional resistance surveillance data).
**Alternatives: Oral cephalosporin, nitrofurantoin, doxycycline, trimethoprim, or amoxicillin/clavulonic acid.

Agent	Dosage
ACUTE UNCOMPLICATED PYELONEPHRITIS, OUTPATIENT TREATMENT: A FLUOROQUINOLONE FOR 7 DAYS*	
Preferred:	
Ciprofloxacin	500 mg po BID x 7 days
Alternative:	
Enoxacin	400 mg po QD x 7 days
Levofloxacin	250-500 mg po QD x 7 days
Ofloxacin	200-400 mg po BID x 7 days
Lomefloxacin	400 mg po QD x 7 days
Norfloxacin	400 mg po BID x 7 days

*Recommendations for other (alternative) fluoroquinolones based on limited studies and generalization of efficacy of ciprofloxacin, which has greatest body of evidence-based trials in UTI.
**Secondary Alternatives: amoxicillin/clavulonic acid, cephalosporin, TMP/SMX-DS for 14 days.

Agent	Dosage
ACUTE UNCOMPLICATED PYELONEPHRITIS, INPATIENT TREATMENT FLUOROQUINOLONE IV	
Initial Empiric Agent of Choice:	
Ciprofloxaxin (preferred)	400 mg IV BID
Alternative:	
Gatifloxacin	400 mg IV QD
Levofloxacin	250-500 mg IV QD
Ofloxacin	400 mg IV BID
Ampicillin plus gentamicin	150-200 mg/kg/day divided Q4H° 5-7 mg/kg QD
Cefotaxime	1-2 g Q4-12°
Ceftriaxone	1-2 g IV QD
Piperacillin	3 g IV Q6°
COMPLICATED PYELONEPHRITIS, UROSEPSIS, OR INDWELLING CATHETER	
Ciprofloxacin plus (tobramycin)* (+ 5-7 mg/kg/day)	400 mg IV Q8H
Ampicillin (+ tobramycin)* (+ 5-7 mg/kg/day)	150-200 mg/kg/day IV divided Q4°
Piperacillin/tazobactam	3.375 g IV Q6 or 4.5 g Q8
Ticarcillin/clavulinic acid	3.1 g IV Q4-6H
Imipenim	0.5 g IV Q6

* amikacin or gentamicin (alternatives)
Note: Any patients receiving advanced generation penicillins and aminoglycosides or fluoroquinolones may need adjustments of their dosing and or intervals if they have renal impairment.

quinolone ciprofloxacin is a preferred oral agent for the treatment of *Pseudomonas aeruginosa* urinary infections.[46] It should be emphasized that although other quinolones may demonstrate activity against, and may be indicated for treatment of gram-negative organisms implicated in UTI, some of these antibiotics, especially the extended-spectrum fluoroquinolones used for initial, empiric treatment of CAP, also are approved for or active against drug-resistant *Streptococcus pneumoniae* (DRSP). Consequently, the use of such quinolones as an initial, first-line agent for UTI should be considered with reservation, because of concerns about emerging resistance among DRSP implicated in CAP. This cautionary approach is supported by a recent guidelines document issued by the Centers for Disease Control (CDC) Drug-Resistant Streptococcus pneumoniae Therapeutic Working Group.

In this regard, because of significant concerns about emerging resistance, the CDC panel has recommended that extended-spectrum fluoroquinolones (i.e., levofloxacin, gatifloxacin, etc.) with activity against DRSP be "reserved" for selected patients with CAP. In light of this position, it appears prudent to limit the potential for inducing resistance in these pathogens, and reserve such antibiotics as alternative agents in patients with UTI, especially because effective and safe fluoroquinolones such as ciprofloxacin are available that do not have significant activity against DRSP. Accordingly, ciprofloxacin is recommended as the initial fluoroquinolone of choice for managing patients with UTI.

Fluoroquinolones are not approved by the Food and Drug Administration (FDA) for patients younger than age 18 in the United States. This status is based on studies in young animals showing damage to articular cartilage in weight-bearing joints.[17,39,65,66] The association and true incidence of quinolone-induced arthropathy in children is still uncertain. It should be emphasized that fluoroquinolones have been used in more than 8 million children and infants worldwide, most commonly for the treatment of *Pseudomonas* infections in patients with cystic fibrosis, with a 1.3% incidence of reversible arthralgias.[65,67] There have been no reported cases of unequivocal quinolone-induced arthropathy. However, there have been three cases of suspected quinolone-induced arthropathy in children without underlying medical disorders such as cystic fibrosis or salmonellosis (baseline rates of arthropathy in these specific populations are approximately 10% and 7%).[65] All three cases involved the use of the fluoroquinolone perfloxacin. One patient required surgical intervention and arthroplasty, and the remaining two showed complete resolution of pain one to eight weeks after perfloxacin was discontinued.[65] The safety and side effect profiles of fluoroquinolones in children are otherwise similar to those in adults.[65] Until clinically controlled trials determine the true efficacy, safety, and optimal dosing regimens of fluoroquinolones in the pediatric population, these drugs should be used only as a last alternative in a multidisciplinary approach to treatment.

Side effects that may be observed in the quinolone anti-infective class are outlined in Table 3. The most common side effects are neurologic (headache, dizziness), gastrointestinal (nausea, diarrhea), and dermatologic (photosensitivity).[58] Patients taking fluoroquinolones that have a greater propensity to cause photosensitivity reactions should be advised to avoid exposure to the sun, bright natural light, and ultraviolet rays throughout the duration of treatment and for five days after completion of treatment.

More than 300 cases of fluoroquinolone-induced tendonitis, arthralgias, and tendon rupture in adult patients have been documented in the literature.[65] Those identified to be at risk included patients older than age 60 and patients on long-term steroid therapy.[65,67] The pathophysiology of fluoroquinolone-induced tendon disorders is unclear, and the onset of symptoms can occur within one or two days after starting therapy. Patients affected typically develop joint pain and swelling (arthralgia), followed by difficulty with movement; some progress to tendon rupture, with accompanying nodules and ecchymoses.[65,67] Diagnosis is usually made clinically, although ultrasound is helpful as an adjunct evaluation. Tendon rupture may require surgical intervention and has caused prolonged disability.[65] In response to these reports, the FDA has asked clinicians to alert their patients to this potential side effect and has requested that manufacturers revise the package inserts to include similar warnings.[65]

Drug Interactions. The potential for drug interactions between fluoroquinolones and other medications has been well-documented. Serious, but rare, adverse events include cardiotoxicity (QT prolongation, torsade de pointes, cardiac arrest).[58] In this regard, sparfloxacin, grepafloxicin, gatifloxacin, and moxifloxacin are generally contraindicated in patients taking other medications (such as cisapride, Class Ia and III antiarrhythmics, and phenothiazines) that prolong the QT interval.[39,58,68] Quinolones have been reported to enhance the effects of warfarin anticoagulation when administered concomitantly. No specific dosage adjustments are needed with either medication, but prothrombin time (PTT) and the internationalized ratio (INR) should be monitored closely to prevent bleeding complications.[68] The mechanism of this interaction is unclear.

Patients receiving digoxin and quinolones may have an increased risk of digoxin toxicity and should be monitored for clinical signs of this interaction, including nausea, vomiting, and cardiac arrhythmias.[68] Selected fluoroquinolones inhibit the cytochrome p450 1 A2 isoenzyme, an enzyme responsible for metabolization of methylxanthine derivatives, including theophylline.[39] Increases in serum theophylline levels secondary to decreases in total body clearance can be as high as 30% to 84% (ciprofloxacin vs. enoxacin).[69] These levels have been associated with theophylline toxicity manifesting as nausea, vomiting, and, in rare cases, seizures. Gatifloxacin, levofloxacin, and moxifloxacin do not alter theophylline metabolism. Grepafloxacin, levofloxacin, and ofloxacin, in rare cases, have been shown to have a synergistic interaction with nonsteroidal anti-inflammatory agents, resulting in an altered seizure threshold. The mechanism involves inhibition of gamma-aminobutyric acid (GABA), resulting in central nervous system (CNS) excitation; therefore, caution should be used in patients with baseline seizure disorder or those with increased risk of seizure activity.[39,68] Theoretically, this risk extends to the entire class of fluoroquinolones.

Ciprofloxacin has been noted in rare cases to cause fluctuations in phenytoin levels, but this appears to have little clinical significance.[68] Case reports have documented that interactions between ciprofloxacin and glyburide resulted in resistant hypoglycemia in patients receiving glyburide therapy.[68,70] It is unclear if this hypoglycemia was secondary to ciprofloxacin inhibition of the cytochrome P-450 hepatic enzyme that metabolizes glyburide. Ciprofloxacin, enoxacin, and ofloxacin also have been shown to increase caffeine levels, resulting in increased CNS stimulation. Patients should be cautioned to decrease or avoid caffeine while on

Table 3. Adverse Effects of Fluoroquinolones[16,34,36,38-45,49-54]

	Ciprofloxacin	Levofloxacin	Lomefloxacin	Ofloxacin	Gatifloxacin*
Skin/ Mucocutaneous					
Photosensitivity[a,b]	✓	✓	✓	✓	
Rash	✓	✓			
Pruritus	✓	✓			
Gastrointestinal					
Dyspepsia	✓	✓			
Gastrointestinal upset	✓	✓			
Diarrhea	✓	✓	✓	✓	
Vomiting					
LFT abnormalities[c]	✓				✓
Taste perversion					✓
Adbominal pain		✓			✓
Nausea		✓		✓	✓
Neurologic					
Headache	✓	✓			✓
Insomnia					✓
Somnolence	✓				
Dizziness	✓	✓			✓
Seizure[d]	✓	✓	✓	✓	✓
Cardiovascular					
Prolongation of QT interval[e,f]					✓
Theophylline toxicity	✓			✓	
Digoxin toxicity[f]	✓	✓	✓	✓	✓
Warfarin potentiation[g]	✓	✓	✓	✓	✓
Musculoskeletal					
Arthritis	✓	✓		✓	
Tendonitis	✓	✓		✓	
Tendon rupture[h]	✓	✓		✓	
Genitourinary					
Vaginitis	✓	✓			✓

LFT, liver function test

[a]Photosensitivity is rare in association with ciprofloxacin and levofloxacin (< 1.0%) and high with sparfloxacin (8%).

[b]Caveat to Note a: up to 50% photosensitivity in patients with cystic fibrosis.

[c]LFT abnormalities are mild and of unclear significance. No clear evidence of hepatitis or hepatoxicity except in association with trovafloxacin.

[d]Seizures are rare. Concomitant use of NSAIDs may lower seizure threshold.

[e]Gatifloxacin is contraindicated in patients taking medications that prolong the QT interval.

[f]Flouroquinolones may elevate digoxin levels. Watch for signs of toxicity (nausea, vomiting, CNS disturbances, arrythmias).

[g]Closely monitor PPT and INR to prevent bleeding complications.

[h]Rare

*Other very infrequent side effects include drug fever, serum-sickness-like reaction, angiodema, anaphylaxis, vasculitis.

these quinolones. Sucralfate and antacid products containing aluminum, magnesium, iron, calcium, and zinc can significantly decrease the bioavailability of the fluoroquinolones.[39] Administration of these medications should be staggered, giving the fluoroquinolones two hours before or four hours after the other agent.

Antibiotic Treatment Guidelines: A Disease- and Syndrome-Specific Stratification Model for Antimicrobial Therapy

Asymptomatic Bacteriuria. Asymptomatic bacteriuria (ASB) is generally not treated in most patients, since multiple studies have shown treatment to have little long-term significance in an otherwise healthy adult population.[71] A recent prospective study of asymptomatic bacteriuria in sexually active young women found prevalence rates of approximately 5%, with 8% of those women developing symptomatic UTI within one week.[72] Specific groups benefiting from antibiotic treatment include pregnant women, neutropenic patients, patients with abnormal renal function, renal transplant recipients in the early post-transplantation period, and men and women planning to undergo urologic procedures.[3,72]

Infants with ASB represent a low-risk population for the development of UTIs, with a tendency toward spontaneous abacteriuria within a few months, and do not generally require antibiotic treatment.[73] School-age children are usually left untreated; however, patients with underlying voiding disorders should be referred appropriately for further evaluation and treatment.

Pregnant women with ASB should be treated with a three- to seven-day course of antibiotics, followed by a subsequent culture to ensure sterilization of urine. Despite increasing resistance rates to ampicillin, amoxicillin and cephalosporins remain a first-line choice in these patients. Nitrofurantoin is becoming a first-line drug, because it is efficacious, inexpensive, and well-tolerated. The only contraindication to using this drug is in patients with G6PD deficiency, in whom hemolysis can occur. TMP/SMX remains a first-line agent in areas of low resistance but should be avoided in the first and third trimesters secondary to possible teratogenic effects and the risk of kernicterus from competitive binding of TMP/SMX to bilirubin binding sites. At this time there is no clear evidence to support a single-dose regimen over a typical three- to seven-day course.[35,74,75] A properly sized randomly controlled trial is recommended for comparison of these regimens, as a single dose has lower cost, fewer adverse effects, and increased compliance compared with longer treatment regimens.[74]

Initial evidence in the elderly population has suggested an increased risk of morbidity and mortality in patients with ASB. More recent studies have challenged these reports, however, failing to identify a connection between ASB and an increase in long-term sequelae such as hypertension or end-stage renal disease. Up to 40% of the elderly will have ASB at some time. Aggressive screening and treatment have little effect on decreasing symptomatic or clinically significant infection and associated complications.[3] Catheterized patients, including those with neurologic disorders or spinal cord injuries, rarely require aggressive work-up and treatment, unless symptoms intervene.[76] Interestingly, a recent study of catheterized patients found that catheter-associated UTIs are rarely symptomatic and infrequently cause bacteremia (< 1%). No significant differences were noted between symptomatic and asymptomatic bacteriuria groups with regard to signs and symptoms commonly associated with infection (fever, dysuria, urgency, or flank pain) or leukocytosis.[77] Investigations have noted that both groups are a major reservoir for antibiotic resistant organisms in the hospital setting.

Symptomatic UTI in Children. Pediatric patients with UTI require early antibiotic treatment and proper referral with follow-up to prevent renal scarring and the subsequent, severe complications of hypertension and end-stage renal disease. Simple cystitis in the pediatric population can be treated with a three- to seven-day course of antibiotics.[73] *(Please See Table 4.)* Some studies recommend that prepubertal children should not be treated for less than five to 10 days unless clear documentation exists that the patient has no underlying urinary tract abnormalities.[18,78] Based on a meta-analyses of 14 controlled trials, there is insufficient evidence to recommend single-dose treatment in this population, with a tendency toward a higher failure rate and reinfection in single-dose groups.[73]

Oral antibiotic choices in the pediatric age group include the penicillins, cephalosporins, sulfonamides, TMP/SMX, and nitrofurantoin. Because of increasing resistance against amoxicillin and ampicillin, other antibiotics should be considered.[79] Amoxicillin/clavulinic acid (Augmentin) is an alternative penicillinase-resistant drug with a wide spectrum of coverage, but it is not recommended as first-line therapy, because of concerns about emerging resistance, higher cost, and greater number of side effects. There is a negligible difference in clinical outcomes with amoxicillin-clavulanate as compared with other common regimens.[17,66,73] TMP/SMX is an acceptable alternative due to its minimal levels of resistance in most pediatric populations and its low cost.[79] Tetracyclines are contraindicated in children because of the drug's effects on teeth.

Cephalosporins are used widely in the management of pediatric UTIs. Cefaclor, an oral second-generation cephalosporin, has been associated with serum sickness in as many as 0.5% of patients, thus limiting its use in children.[54] Cefprozil and Loracarbef, also second generation agents, are approved for patients ages 6 months and older. They have been found to be effective and have a lower rate of gastrointestinal side effects than Augmentin. Cefixime (Suprax®), an oral third-generation cephalosporin, is an attractive alternative, as it maintains a high urinary excretion level and bactericidal action, it can be dosed once daily, has a relatively pleasant taste, and can be stored at room temperature for up to two weeks.[54,79] Mild gastrointestinal effects occur in as many as 25% of patients after an oral dose.

The third-generation agent, cefpodoxime (Vantin®) also is effective in the treatment of urinary infection, including pyelonephritis in infants older than 1 month.[35] Side effects are similar to those of other cephalosporins, with diarrhea occurring in 4-17% of patients (higher percentage in infants); vomiting is uncommon. Cephalosporins should be avoided in patients with known severe reactions to penicillins, as a 5-10% cross-reactivity has been cited.[66] If there is a history of only mild skin rash, a small test dose can be administered and the patient observed for 30-45 minutes prior to continuing use.

Adult Females. Young, sexually active females with symptomatic uncomplicated UTI typically can be treated for three days, with effective elimination of infection in a majority of patients. Three-day regimens are as effective as 5-, 7-, and 10-day regimens and have the

Table 4. Treatment of Pediatric Patients with UTI[17,19,23,73,108]

ACUTE, UNCOMPLICATED UTI (3-5 DAYS)	
Amoxicillin	30-50 mg/kg/day po divided TID[a]
Amoxicillin/clavulanic acid	45 mg/kg/day po divided BID[b]
Trimethoprim/sulfamethoxazole	8-10 mg/kg/day of TMP po divided BID
Nitrofurantoin	5-7 mg/kg/day po divided QID[c,d]
Cefixime	8 mg/kg/day po divided BID
Cephalexin	25-50 mg/kg/day po divided QID
Cefuroxime	10-15 mg/kg/day po BID (max 1 g/d)[e]
Cefaclor	20-40 mg/kg/day po divided TID[e,f]
Cefprozil	15-30 mg/kg/day po divided BID (max 1 g/)[e,f]
Loracarbef	15-30 mg/kg/day po divided BID (max 0.8 g/d)[e,f]
COMPLICATED UTI OR UTI REQUIRING ADMISSION (14 DAYS)	
Ampicillin +	100 mg/kg/day IV divided QID
gentamicin	5-7 mg/kg/day IV divided TID[g,h]
Ceftriaxone	50-100 mg/kg/day IV/IM[i]
Ceftazidime	30-50 mg/kg IV TID[i]
Cefotaxime	150 mg/kg/day IV divided TID[i]

[a]Increasing resistance rates limiting efficacy; trimethoprim/sulfamethoxazole is superior in recent studies.
[b]Reserved for patients with amoxicillin-resistant organism.
[c]Not used in patients younger than 6 weeks of age.
[d]Avoid in patients with G6PD deficiency.
[e]Not as effective in patients with *Enteroccocus* infection.
[f]Only in patients older than 28 days old.
[g]Associated with ototoxicity and nephrotoxicity; adjust according to renal function and follow serum levels.
[h]Intramuscular form may be used in outpatient setting for patients with a history of allergy to cephalosporins.
[i]Significant concern about resistant enterococci; not recommended as first-line drug for recurrent infections.

advantage of fewer side effects, lower cost, and higher levels of patient compliance.[34,80] Single-dose regimens appear to have lower effectiveness than other regimens.[81,82] Recently updated and published guidelines from the Infectious Disease Society of America recommend that TMP/SMX remain the standard first-line drug in uncomplicated cystitis in young adult women in areas of *E. coli* resistance less than 10-20%.[57] However, the resistance landscape and preferences for initial empiric therapy are changing as a result of evidence-based trials.

For acutely symptomatic young women with cystitis, the preferred treatment is a three-day course with ciprofloxacin or TMP/SMX. TMP/SMX may be considered a first-line agent in women who can tolerate this agent and in areas in which resistance is infrequent. Its status, however, is changing, as resistance to TMP/SMX has emerged as a common clinical problem. Accordingly, with increasing resistance by *E. coli* to TMP/SMX, ciprofloxacin is becoming the initial antibiotic of choice, even in uncomplicated UTI. Ciprofloxacin should be considered first-line in patients with allergies to other drugs or in areas where trimethoprim/sulfamethoxazole resistance is high (> 10%).

Total-cost outome studies comparing antibiotics (i.e, TMP/SMX vs quinolones) used for cystitis suggest that the high cure rates, excellent compliance, and predictable and sustained antimicrobial activity against *E. coli* (resistance rates among *E. coli* < 1%), as well as the low relapse rates associated with ciprofloxacin, make this antibiotic a cost-effective first choice in patients with uncomplicated UTI. Even in cost-conscious environments—among them, managed care settings, HMOs, military hospitals, and emergency departments—ciprofloxacin (250 mg po BID X three days) represents an outcome-effective antibiotic for initial therapy of uncomplicated UTIs. In certain regions, and especially in urban areas, resistance to TMP/SMX has risen to 24%. Over the past four years, a pattern that has relegated TMP/SMX to a secondary or alternative agent for management on cystitis and uncomplicated UTI.[83,84]

When resistance is not an issue, trimethoprim is effective in clearing the pathogenic organism, has minimal adverse effects on the vaginal and fecal flora, and is generally well-tolerated.[34,57,86] As already stressed, fluoroquinolones are a better choice in areas of higher TMP/SMX resistance (> 10-20%), for patients with allergies to sulfa or other drugs, and in patients returning for failed antibiotic treatment of recently diagnosed UTI.[57] Due to the increased costs and the concern for promoting resistance in this class of antibiotics, the panel does not recommend that they be used in all patients with uncomplicated UTI. However, other sources, including an updated antimicrobial therapy guide, now recommend fluoroquinolones such as ciprofloxacin as first-line agents and TMP/SMX as a second-line agent for all acute uncomplicated UTI infections, citing resistance to TMP/SMX in more than 18% of *E. coli* infections.[83,84] *(Please See Table 2.)* Physicians should be aware of local resistance patterns when devising antibiotic selection strategies.

In a recent study, nitrofurantoin was found to have equal efficacy as other antibiotics with sustained concentration in the urine and appears to have a superior level of efficacy in vitro against multiresistant *Enterobacteriaceae*, including *E. coli*.[85] The authors suggest that nitrofurantoin be reconsidered as a first-line agent in the treatment of uncomplicated UTI. However, nitrofurantoin is much less effective against *Staphylococcus saprophyticus* and is not effective against *Pseudomonas* and *Proteus* species. It has minimal effects on the resident fecal and vaginal flora and leads to a low incidence of bacterial resistance.[86] Nitrofurantoin should be dosed in a seven-day regimen to ensure efficacy.[87]

An alternative for acute cystitis treatment may be fosfomycin tromethamine, which is administered as a 3-gm oral single dose.[35,88,89] This antibiotic is active against common uropathogens, including organisms resistant to other antibiotics.[88] The single dose is well-absorbed, produces therapeutic concentrations in urine for 2-4 days, and has been shown in clinical trials to be as effective as 7- to 10-day regimens of nitrofurantoin, norfloxacin, and TMP/SMX. Ampicillin should no longer be used because of high resistance rates.[36] The suprapubic discomfort or dysuria common to UTI can be treated with oral analgesics (Tylenol, Motrin) or phenazopyridine (Pyridium) with a TID dose of 100-200 mg for no more than 48 hours.[18] Elderly females with lower UTI symptoms and no systemic complications may be treated for three days with similar regimens as prescribed for younger women.[90]

In patients suspected of having a complicated UTI, including patients with symptoms lasting longer than one week, diabetic patients, immunocompromised individuals, and nontoxic febrile patients without evidence of acute pyelonephritis, the treatment duration should be between five and seven days.[31] Because these patients are less able to tolerate treatment failures, and are more susceptible to recurrent infection, ciprofloxacin is recommended as the initial agent of choice. Moreover, in these patients, a urine culture is recommended prior to administration of antibiotics to ensure proper management and identification of the uropathogen in the event of treatment failure or recurrence.[31]

Urethritis is common in males younger than age 50 and should be treated as such based on history and physical examination. Urinalysis, urine culture, and/or urethral cultures are recommended. Therapy for acute cystitis in men typically lasts one or two weeks, four weeks for acute bacterial prostatitis, and six to 12 weeks for chronic bacterial prostatitis.[91] Ciprofloxacin is recommended, because these fluoroquinolones penetrate prostatic tissue and secretions. Candidal infections are usually treated with oral fluconazole or, in catheterized patients, by continuous bladder irrigation with amphotericin B for two to five days.[31]

Pyelonephritis

Adults. Adult patients with pyelonephritis can be managed on an inpatient or outpatient basis, depending upon clinical severity *(Please See Table 2.)* A retrospective comparison of inpatient and outpatient management of pyeloenphritis suggested that general guidelines for admission should include the following: 1) underlying anatomical urinary tract abnormality; 2) an immunocompromised host (diabetes mellitus, cancer, sickle cell disease, transplant patients); 3) urinary tract obstruction; 4) failed outpatient management of pyelonephritis; 5) progression of uncomplicated UTI; 6) persistent vomiting; 7) renal failure; 8) suspected urosepsis; 9) age older than 60 years; 10) poor social situation; and, 11) inadequate access to follow-up.[92] If these criteria are used for making in-hospital dispositions, it is estimated that 70% of all patients who are treated for pyelonephritis can be managed as outpatients.[82]

The general consensus for emergency department management of pyelonephritis is to begin parenteral therapy with a fluoroquinolone (ciprofloxacin) intravenously in patients who meet admission criteria.[80] Non-toxic patients with uncomplicated pyelonephritis suitable for outpatient management may receive oral ciprofloxacin for a total of 7-14 days, depending on clinical judgment and hospital protocols.[80] Other parenteral therapies include a combination of ampicillin or a third-generation cephalosporin plus an aminoglycoside in extended-interval dosing (i.e., every 24-48 hours).[36,93-95] The extended-spectrum cephalosporins, such as ceftriaxone, should be considered for serious urinary infections because of the high urinary concentrations that are achieved.[96]

If gram-positive cocci are the causative organism, ampicillin/ sulbactam with or without an aminoglycoside is recommended.[97] Admitted patients with suspected enterococci may require extended-spectrum penicillins (Timentin® or Zosyn®) or alternative therapies, including nitrofurantoin to treat isolated vancomycin-resistant enterococci (VRE). Because multi-drug resistance is common in VRE isolates, susceptibility testing is recommended for ampicillin, aminoglycosides, chloramphenicol, fluoroquinolones, minocycline (a tetracycline), and rifampin.[96] UTI caused by *Pseudomonas* will often require double antimicrobial coverage. *(Please see Table 2.)*

As with children, admitted patients who remain afebrile for 24 to 48 hours and tolerate oral intake can be switched safely to an oral medication to complete a 14-day course. A multidisciplinary approach to complicated patients is encouraged to provide adequate empiric treatment, with subsequent adjustments based on identification and sensitivities, while preventing the development of further resistance.

To evaluate the efficacy and cost of antibiotics used in pyelonephritis, a recent randomized, double-blind multicenter trial analyzed 255 women with acute uncomplicated pyelonephritis. These patients received either ciprofloxacin, 500 mg BID for seven days, or TMP/SMX, 160/180 mg BID for 14 days.[46] More than 90% of UTI culture isolates from both groups were *E. coli*. Bacteriologic and clinical cure rates were greater at four to 11 days in the ciprofloxacin group (99% and 96%) than the TMP/SMX group (89% and 83%). At 22 to 28 days, bacteriologic and clinical cure rates were 84% vs. 74% and 82% and 74%, respectively. Bacterial and clinical cure rates with TMP/SMX in patients found to be infected with resistant *E. coli* were only 50% and 35%, respectively. Adverse effects were similar among groups occurring in 24% with ciprofloxacin and 33% with TMP/SMX. Health care resource use and estimated total treatment costs were calculated, from initial evaluation to "prescription pad" to "cure," including needed hospitalization, lab testing, office visits, and other procedures. Mean total cost per patient was 29% higher for TMP/SMX-treated patients than for ciprofloxacin-treated patients.[46]

Because of additional interventions and antibiotic prescriptions required in the TMP/SMX group to achieve a cure, the mean cost per cure also was 25% higher in the TMP/SMX group than in the ciprofloxacin-treated patients. These studies help confirm that knowledge of local resistance rates is imperative in deciding which antibiotics should be used in the treatment of UTI. They support the use of ciprofloxacin as a first-line agent in the management of uncomplicated pyelonephritis. With the current outcome- and cost-sensitive environment of managed care, clinicians must make informed choices in the management of their patients.[46,97] A related randomized trial found that oral and intravenous ciprofloxacin were equally effective in the empiric treatment of severe pyelonephritis or complicated UTIs, provided that severe sepsis, obstruction, and focal renal suppuration are not present.[98] Since all patients in this study were hospitalized, a direct comparison between inpatient and outpatient treatment with ciprofloxacin is still needed.

Pregnancy. In pregnant women, pyelonephritis tends to occur more commonly during the second half of pregnancy.[2] In general, outpatient treatment is not the standard of care for pregnant women. Inpatient treatment with intravenous antibiotics and close monitoring are usually required to maximize outcomes. Treatment options are similar to other adult regimens, including ampicillin with gentamicin, cephalosporins, and extended-spectrum penicillins or aztreonam.[2] Patients may be discharged safely and parenteral therapy stopped after defervescence within 48 to 72 hours of admission.[86] Persistent fever or symptoms require further evaluation and consultation.

A study of more than 100 women with uncomplicated pyelonephritis at less than 24 weeks' gestation found that almost 10% of those treated initially as outpatients eventually required hospitalization.[99] Two additional studies suggest that, in very carefully selected patients, outpatient treatment may be a safe option.[100,101] However, without concise, evidence-based protocols or guidelines to guide this decision, the acceptable and prudent choice in pregnant women is to admit them for initial parenteral antibiotics and supportive care. In both nonpregnant adults and pregnant patients, failure to respond to appropriate antibiotics requires emergent radiologic studies, including ultrasound and possible CT scan, to evaluate for obstruction, masses, and renal and perirenal abscess. All patients should have follow-up urine cultures 1-2 weeks after completion of therapy to ensure eradication of infection.

Children. Traditionally, infants younger than 1 year of age with a fever and UTI (nearly pathognomonic for pyelonephritis) were hospitalized and treated with intravenous antibiotics and hydration.[102] *(Please see Table 4.)* More recently, admission recommendations have been modified to focus on certain high-risk groups, including febrile infants younger than 3 months of age, infants and children with dehydration who are unable to tolerate oral hydration or medication, immunocompromised children, and patients with a high risk of noncompliance with medication and early follow-up.[17,103] Neonates should have continued parenteral therapy for 7-14 days. Parenteral antibiotics should be continued in admitted infants and children until the patient has been afebrile for 24-48 hours and tolerating oral intake well. The switch to oral antibiotics can be made safely based on original identification and sensitivities of the identified uropathogen.

The total treatment duration should be from 10 to 14 days.[17,19,23,65,72] Parenteral regimens include ampicillin plus an aminoglycoside or a third-generation cephalosporin until culture identification and sensitivities return.[17,23] The greatest concern with using aminoglycosides is the possibility of developing nephrotoxicity or ototoxicity. Available data do not support the generally accepted belief that ototoxicity is directly related to elevated serum levels; rather, it appears instead that it is related to duration of therapy, repeat courses of aminoglycosides, or high cumulative doses.[104] Daily dosing regimens currently being studied in children and neonates, including very-low-birth-weight infants (< 1500 g), appear to yield enhanced antibacterial efficacy and decreased toxicity.[39,105] If *Enterococcus* is the expected organism, vancomycin is recommended because of high levels of penicillin resistance and lack of resistance to a cephalosporin.

Ticarcillin/clavulinate (Timentin®) and pipercillin/tazobactam (Zosyn®), both extended-spectrum penicillins, are not approved for use in children younger than 12 years of age.[39] In a European randomized controlled trial of 300 children with pyelonephritis (ages 1 month to 12 years), both cefepime and ceftazidime given intravenously (50 mg/kg every eight hours) for at least 48 hours after defervescence, followed by TMP/SMX for 12-14 days, were equally effective and well-tolerated.[106] Clinical cure rates after 4-6 weeks were 98% and 96%, with bacteriologic cure rates of 86% and 83%, respectively.

A recent multicenter, randomized, clinical trial evaluated the efficacy of initial oral cefixime vs. initial intravenous cefotaxime in children ages 1 to 24 months with febrile UTIs.[103] All patients had positive urine cultures, had negative sonograms for urinary tract abnormalities upon enrollment, and received a total of 14 days of antibiotics (the IV group changed over to oral cefixime after three days or after the child was afebrile for 24 hours).[103] In the outpatient arm, the initial oral cefixime dose was 16 mg/kg given in the ED, followed by 8 mg/kg once daily. Both groups of patients were placed on oral cefixime prophylaxis for two weeks following treatment (4 mg/kg QD) until a VCUG was performed. There were no statistically significant differences in cure rates, reinfection rates, or higher grades of renal scarring based on DMSA scan.[103]

Mean costs for children treated intravenously were at least twofold higher, including outpatient re-evaluation, follow-up cultures, and radiologic imaging after appropriate referral. The authors concluded that non-toxic, young children with fever and UTI may be treated safely with oral cefixime on an outpatient basis, with the additional benefit of a significant decrease in cost compared with hospitalization. Other authors have recommended that children over the age of 3 months who are non-toxic in appearance receive initial parenteral treatment with a long-acting third-generation cephalosporin such as ceftriaxone and then have close follow-up on continued oral antibiotics for 14 days, with subsequent prophylaxis.[73]

Transplant Recipients

While infection-related mortality rates in transplant recipients have dropped from 70% in the first decades of renal transplantation to less than 5% today, persistent prevention and effective treatment of infectious complications remain major concerns.[107] Immunosuppression secondary to transplant-related treatments, exposure to infectious agents in the community and hospital (especially immunomodulating viruses such as cytomegalovirus, Epstein-Barr virus, and hepatitis B and C), leukopenia, and metabolic abnormalities in patients with end stage renal disease awaiting transplant all determine a patient's risk for infection.[107] In the first month after transplantation, urinary infections are a major complication, occurring in 35% to 79% of patients. Uropathogens include enteric gram-negative isolates, including *Pseudomonas aeurginosa*, enteroccocci, and staphylococcal and fungal species. Most bacterial infections can be treated with a 10- to 14-day course of antibiotics, which may be followed by continued prophylaxis with low-dose ciprofloxacin.

Recurrent infections require further radiologic imaging, including ultrasound, CT scan, and/or nuclear imaging studies.[107]

Fungal urinary infections are common, often presenting as a relatively asymptomatic candiduria or cystitis. Severe infections caused by obstructing fungal balls result in ascending infection, overt candidial pyelonephritis, and significant fungemia.[107] Patients on large doses of corticosteroids; those with a history of multiple episodes of allograft rejection or poor allograft function; or those with baseline hyperglycemia, leukopenia, prolonged antibiotic use, or older age have an increased risk of developing fungal infections.

Aggressive treatment of suspected fungal pyelonephritis is warranted. This includes fungal stains and culture of the urine or blood, possible fine-needle aspiration of the kidney, and prompt administration of antifungal therapy. Oral fluconazole is acceptable for mild to moderate infections caused by *Candida albicans*, but amphotericin is the drug of choice in *C. krusei* and *C. glabrata* infections and in disseminated disease. Patients with evidence of nephrotoxicity can be treated with the liposomal formulation of intravenous fluconazole.[107] Patients receiving antimycobacterial therapy may develop hepatic dysfunction, hyperuricemia, and potential drug interactions with cyclosporine, which may lead to nephrotoxicity.

Bacteremia and Urosepsis

UTIs associated with obstruction caused by calculi, congenital abnormalities, an enlarged prostate gland, or any underlying neurologic condition leading to incomplete bladder emptying predispose to urosepsis.[51] Bacteremic patients usually present with classic signs and symptoms of UTI. Additional manifestations of a septic process seen in bacteremic patients include shaking chills, fever or hypothermia (associated with worse prognosis), tachycardia, tachypnea, respiratory alkalosis and hyperventilation, changes in mental status (lethargy or possible agitation), and skin lesions (e.g., petechial rashes seen in *P. aeruginosa* bacteremia).[108]

These symptoms usually develop within the first 24 hours of infection, except in bacteremia caused by *S. marcescens*, in which symptoms typically develop several days later. Patients who progress to septic shock will manifest severe hypotension; metabolic acidosis; and hemocoagulative disorders, including thrombocytopenia and disseminated intravascular coagulation. Immunocompromised or neutropenic patients may have a more insidious onset secondary to an altered inflammatory response to infection. Fever, dysuria, and pyuria may be absent, with compensatory hyperventilation and changing mental status serving as important clues.[107] Overall mortality rates for septic shock in critical care unit patients range from 20% to 80%.[108]

The diagnosis of urosepsis is usually made clinically, with blood and urine cultures obtained to guide management. Additional laboratory studies that follow cytokine plasma levels (correlation to endotoxin) and procalcitonin (closely related to plasma levels of TNF-alpha and IL-6) have been utilized in certain hospitals in selected cases for the management and follow-up of patients with sepsis.[108] Treatment requires aggressive monitoring of airway patency, breathing, and circulation. Initial interventions include obtaining intravenous access, preferably central access, to allow invasive monitoring of the hemodynamic clinical status and to guide fluid and electrolyte management. Fluid resuscitation with either crystalloids or colloids is a top priority, along with the use of inotropes or pressors to treat hypotension. Dopamine is recommended as the initial drug because of its inotropic and vasopressor action, with alternative drugs including dobutamine and norepinephrine.

Broad-spectrum empiric antimicrobial therapy should be started immediately. The combination of a fluoroquinolone with antipseudomonal activity (ciprofloxacin) or a beta-lactam (a semisynthetic penicillin associated with a beta-lactamase inhibitor or fourth-generation cephalosporin) plus an aminoglycoside is recommended as the first-line regimen.[108] Pipercillin/tazobactam or ticarcillin/clavulanate should be considered for two reasons: the increasing prevalence of enterococci (especially in nosocomial patients) and the decreased risk of expanded-spectrum, beta-lactamase-producing, gram-negative pathogens.[108]

Amakacin is more active than gentamicin or tobramycin against both *Enterobacteriaceae* and *P. aeruginosa*.[93] Amphotericin B or fluconazole is the preferred treatment option for UTI caused by *Candida*.[108] Once uropathogen identification and sensitivities from urine and blood cultures are available, a single agent with a narrow spectrum is recommended to decrease drug toxicity, cost, and the emergence of resistant strains.[93] Adjunctive therapies previously studied, including high-dose corticosteroids and monoclonal antibodies against endotoxins released by aerobic gram-negative bacteria, are no longer recommended.[108] Imaging to evaluate for obstruction, renal abscess, or perinephric abscess is recommended in patients with persistent fever or clinical sepsis.

Catheterized Patients

Bacteremia associated with urinary catheterization is usually asymptomatic, occurring in up to 10% of patients, with fewer than 1% of patients developing symptomatic bacteremia.[108] However, with symptomatic urinary catheter-related bacteremia mortality is as high as 30% and therefore the symptomatic patient requires aggressive diagnosis and therapeutic interventions. Over the past decade there has been a shift from more susceptible pathogens (*E. coli, Proteus mirabilis, Klebsiella pneuominiae*) to more resistant pathogens (staphylococci, enterococci, *Enterobacter sp., Pseudomonas aeruginosa,* and *Candida albicans*).[51,108] However, *E. coli* remains the most prominent organism isolated. In most cases, bacteriuria in patients with short-term catheterization is caused by a single organism, while polymicrobial infections are more common in subjects with chronic indwelling catheters.[108] Recurrent instrumentation of the urinary tract is associated with infection caused by *P. aeruginosa* and other resistant uropathogen infections.[51] A fluoroquinolone such as ciprofloxacin, with good antipseudomonal coverage, often in combination with an aminoglycoside or a beta-lactam, is appropriate as initial therapy.

References

1. Lifshitz E, Kramer L. Outpatient urine culture: Does collection technique matter? *Arch Intern Med* 2000;160:2537-2540.
2. Roberts JA. Management of pyelonephritis and upper urinary tract infections. *Urol Clin North Am* 1999;26:753-763.
3. Orenstein R, Wong ES. Urinary tract infections in adults. *Am Family Phys* 1999;59:1225-1234.
4. Saint S, Scholes D, Fihn SD, et al. The effectiveness of a clinical practice guideline for the management of presumed uncomplicated urinary tract infection in women. *Am J Med* 1999;106:636-641.
5. Talan DA, Stamm WE, Hooton TM, et al. Comparison of ciprofloxacin (7 days) and trimethoprim-sulfamethoxazole (14 days) for acute uncomplicated pyelonephritis in women. *JAMA* 2000;283:12.
6. Rushton HG. Urinary tract infections in children: Epidemiology, evaluation and management. *Pediatr Clin North Am* 1997;44:1133-1169.
7. Steele RW. The epidemiology and clinical presentation of urinary tract infections in children 2 years of age through adolescence. *Pediatr Ann* 1999;28:653-658.
8. Lutters M, Vogt N. Antibiotics duration for treating uncomplicated, symptomatic lower urinary tract infections in elderly women. *Cochrane Database of Systematic Rev* 2000;2.
9. Kunin C. *Urinary tract infections: detection, prevention, and management,* 5th ed. Baltimore, MD: Williams & Wilkins; 1997:150-154.
10. Nickel JC, Pidutti R. A rational approach to urinary tract infections in older patients. *Geriatrics* 1992;47:49-55.

11. Barkham TMS, Martin FC, Eykyn SJ. Delay in the diagnosis of bacteremic urinary tract infection in elderly patients. *Age Ageing* 1996;25:130-132.
12. Richardson JP. Bacteremia in the elderly. *J Gen Intern Med* 1993;8:89-92.
13. Ackerman RJ, Monroe PW. Bacteremic urinary tract infection in older people. JAGS 1996;44:927-933.
14. Nicolle LE. Urinary tract infection in the elderly. *J Antimicrob Chemother* 1994;33(Supp A):99-109.
15. Nicolle LE, McIntyre M, Zacharias H, et al. Twelve-month surveillance of infections in institutionalized elderly men. *J Am Geri Soc* 1984;32:513-519.
16. Le Saux N, Pham B, Moher D. Evaluating the benefits of antimicrobial prophylaxis to prevent urinary tract infections in children: A systematic review. *Can Med Assoc J* 2000;163:523-529.
17. Kelly LA, Shortliffe LMD. Evaluation and management of pediatric urinary tract infections. *Urol Clin North Am* 1999;26:719-728.
18. Shaw KN, Gorelick MH. Urinary tract infection in the pediatric patient. *Pediatr Clin North Am* 1999;46:1111-1124.
19. American Academy of Pediatrics. Practice parameter: The diagnosis, treatment, and evaluation of the initial urinary tract infection in febrile infants and young children. *Pediatrics* 1999;103:843-852.
20. Gorelick MH, Shaw KN. Screening tests for UTI in children: A meta analysis. *Pediatrics* 1999;104:e54.
21. Shaw KN, McGowan KL, Gorelick MH, et al. Screening for urinary tract infection in infants in the emergency department: Which test is best? *Pediatrics* 1998; 101:E1.
22. Winberg J. Commentary: Progressive renal damage from infection with or without reflux. *J Urol* 1992;148:1733-1734.
23. Jacobson SH, Eklof O, Eriksson CG, et al. Development of hypertension and uremia after pyelonephritis in childhood: 27 year follow up. *BMJ* 1989;299:703-706.
24. Andriole VT. When to do culture in urinary tract infections. *Int J Antimicrob Agents* 1999;11:253-255.
25. Berry V, Page R, Satterfield J, et al. Comparative efficacy of gemifloxacin in experimental models of pyelonephritis and wound infection. *J Antimicrob Chemother* 2000;45(suppl S1):87-93.
26. Wing DA, Park AS, Debuque L, et al. Limited clinical utility of blood and urine cultures in the treatment of acute pyelonephritis during pregnancy. *Am J Obstet Gynecol* 2000;182:1437-1440.
27. Pennington DJ, Zerin JM. Imaging of the urinary tract in children. *Pediatr Ann* 1999;28:678-685.
28. Andrich MP, Majd M. Diagnostic imaging in the evaluation of the first urinary tract infection in infants and young children. *Pediatrics* 1992;90:436-441.
29. Alon US, Ganapathy S. Should renal ultrasonography be done routinely in children with first urinary tract infection. *Clin Pediatr* 1999;38:21-25.
30. Auringer ST. Pediatric uroradiology update. *Urol Clin North Am* 1997;24:673-681.
31. Wood CA, Abrutyn E. Urinary tract infection in older adults. *Clin Geriatr Med* 1998;14:267-283.
32. American College of Emergency Physicians. Use of ultrasound imaging by emergency physicians (policy number 400121, approved June 1997). http://www.acep.org/library/index.cfm/id./684.htm, November 2000.
33. Yen DHT, Hu SC, Tsai J, et al. Renal abscess: Early diagnosis and treatment. *Am J Emerg Med* 1999;17:192-197.
34. Anderson R. Management of lower urinary tract infections and cystitis. *Urol Clin North Am* 1999;26:729-735.
35. Connoly AM, Thorp JM. Urinary tract infections in pregnancy. *Urol Clin North Am* 1999;26:779-787.
36. Delzell JE, Lefevre ML. Urinary tract infection in pregnancy. *Am Fam Phys* 2000;61:713-721.
37 Newell A, Riley P, Rogers M. Resistance patterns of urinary tract infections diagnosed in a genitourinary medicine clinic. *Int J STD AIDS* 2000;11:499-500.
38. Baerheiy A, Digranes A, Hunskar S. Are resistance patterns published by microbiological laboratories valid for general practice? *APMIS* 1999;107:676-680.
39. O'Donnell JA, Gelone SP. Antibacterial therapy: Fluoroquinolones. *Infect Dis Clin North Am* 2000;14:489-513,xi.
40. Marco CA, Parker K. Antimicrobial resistance among organisms causing urinary tract infections [letter]. *Acad Emerg Med* 1997;4:159-160.
41. Mombelli G, Pezzoli R, Pinoja-Lutz G, et al. Oral vs. intravenous ciprofloxacin in the initial empirical management of severe pyelonephritis or complicated urinary tract infections. A prospective randomized clinical trial. *Arch Intern Med* 1999;159:53-8.
42. Flanagan PG, Davies EA, Stout RW. A comparison of single-dose vs. conventional-dose antibiotic treatment of bacteriuria in elderly women. *Age Aging* 1991;20:206-211.
43. Wiseman LR, Balfour JA. Ciprofloxacin, a review of its pharmacological profile and therapeutic use in the elderly. *Drugs & Aging* 1994;2:145-173.
44. Li-McLeod J, Cislo P, Gomolin IH. Cost analysis of ciprofloxacin oral suspension vs. trimethorim/sulfamethoxazole oral suspension for treatment of acute urinary tract infections in elderly women. Presented at the American Society of Consultant Pharmacists Annual Meeting, Nov. 1-4, 2000, Boston, MA. Abstract #3.
45. Stapleton A, Stamm WE. Prevention of urinary tract infection. *Infect Dis Clin North Am* 1997;11:719-733.
46. Talan DA, Stamm WE, Hooton TM, et al. Comparison of ciprofloxacin (7 days) and trimethoprim-sulfamethoxazole (14 days) for acute uncomplicated pyelonephritis in women. *JAMA* 2000;283:1583-1590.
47. Blaine WB, Yu W, Summe JP. Epidemiology of hospitalization of elderly Medicare patients for urinary tract infections, 1991-1996, Abstract L-87, Presented at the 38th Interscience Conference on Antimicrobial Agents and Chemotherapy; Sept. 15-18, 1996. San Diego, Ca.
48. Patton JP, Nash DB, Abrutyn E. Urinary Tract Infection: Economic considerations. *Med Clin North Am* 1991;75:495-513.
49. Haley RW, Culver DH, White JW. The nationwide nosocomial infection rate: A new need for vital statistics. *Am J Epidemiol* 1985;121:159-167.
50. Boscia JA, Kobasa WD, Knight RA, et al. Epidemiology of bacteriuria in an elderly population. *Am J Med* 1986;80:208-214.
51. Simon D, Trenholme G. Antibiotic selection for patients with septic shock. *Crit Care Clin* 2000;16:215-231.
52. Gupta K, Hooton TM, Wobbe CL, Stamm WE. The prevalence of antimicrobial resistance among uropathogens causing acute uncomplicated cystitis in young women. *Int J Antimicrob Agents* 1999;11:305-308.
53. Gomolin IH, Siami P, Haverstock D, et al. Efficacy and safety of oral ciprofloxacin suspension vs. TMP/SMX for treatment of communi-

ty- and nursing home-residing elderly women with acute urinary tract infection. Presented at the 6th International Symposium on New Quinolones; November 15-17, 1998; Denver, Colorado.

54. San Joaquin VH, Stull TL. Antibacterial agents in pediatrics. *Infect Dis Clin North Am* 2000;14:341-355,viii.
55. Langtry HD, Lamb HM. Levofloxacin: Its use in infections of the respiratory tract, skin, soft tissues and urinary tract. *Drugs* 1998;56:487-415.
56. Ronald A. The quinolones and renal infection. *Drugs* 1999;58(suppl 2):96-98.
57. Iravani A, Klimberg I, Briefer C, et al. A trial comparing low-dose, short-course ciprofloxacin and standard 7 day therapy with co-trimoxazole or nitrofurantoin in the treatment of uncomplicated urinary tract infection. *J Antimicrob Chemother* 1999;43(suppl A):67-75.
58. Henry DC, Nenad RC, Iravani A, et al. Comparison of sparfloxacin and ciprofloxacin in the treatment of community-acquired acute uncomplicated urinary tract infection in women. Sparfloxacin Multicenter Uncomplicated Urinary Tract Infection Study Group. *Clin Ther* 1999;21:966-981.
59. Koyama Y, Mikami O, Matsuda T, et al. [Efficacy of single-dose therapy with levofloxacin for acute cystitis: Comparison to three day therapy.] [Japanese] *Hinyokika Kiyo* 2000;46:49-52.
60. Henry D, Ellison W, Sullivan J, et al. Treatment of community-acquired uncomplicated urinary tract infection with sparfloxacin vs. ofloxacin: The Sparfloxacin Multi Center UUTI Study Group. *Antimicrob Agents Chemother* 1998;42:2262-2266.
61. Dowzicky M, Nadler H, Dorr MB, et al. Comparison of the in vitro activity of and pathogen responses to sparfloxacin with those of other agents in treatment of respiratory tract, urinary tract, and skin and skin-structure infections. *Clin Ther* 1999;21:790-805.
62. Perry CM, Barman-Balfour JA, Lamb HM. Gatifloxacin. *Drugs* 1999;58:683-696.
63. Krcmery S, Naber KG. Ciprofloxacin once vs. twice daily in the treatment of complicated urinary tract infections. German Ciprofloxacin UTI Study Group. *Int J Antimicrob Agents* 1999;11:133-138.
64. Pimentel FL, Dolgner A, Guimaraes J, et al. Efficacy and safety of norfloxacin 800 mg once-daily vs. norfloxacin 400 mg twice-daily in the treatment of uncomplicated urinary tract infections in women: A double blind, randomized clinical trial. *J Chemother* 1998;10:122-127.
65. Alghasham AA, Nahata MC. Clinical use of fluoroquinolones in children. *Ann Pharmacother* 2000;34:347-358.
66. Henry NK, Hoecker JL, Rhodes KH. Antimicrobial therapy for infants and children: Guidelines for the inpatient and outpatient practice of pediatric infectious diseases. *Mayo Clin Proceedings* 2000;75:86-97.
67. Zabraniecki L, Negrier I, Vergne P, et al. Fluoroquinolone induced tendinopathy: Report of 6 cases. *J Rheumatol* 1996;23:516-520.
68. Fluoroquinolones. Micromedex Healthcare Series. Micromedex, Inc. 2000;Vol. 6.
69. Lowe MN, Lamb HM. Gemifloxacin. *Drugs* 2000;59:1137-1147.
70. Roberge RJ, Kaplan R, Frank R, et al. Glyburide-ciprofloxacin interaction with resistant hypoglycemia. *Ann Emerg Med* 2000;36:160-163.
71. Nicolle LE. Asymptomatic bacteriuria-important or not? *N Engl J Med* 2000;14:1037-1039.
72. Hooton TM, Scholes D, Stapleton AE, et al. A prospective study of asymptomatic bacteriuria in sexually active young women. *N Engl J Med* 2000;343:992-997.
73. Rushton HG. Urinary tract infections in children: Epidemiology, evaluation and management. *Pediatr Urol* 1997;44:1133-1167.
74. Villar J, Lydon-Rochelle MT, Gülmezoglu AM, et al. Duration of treatment for asymptomatic bacteriuria during pregnancy (Cochrane Review). In: The Cochrane Library, Issue 3, 200. Oxford: Update Software.
75. Vazques JC, Villar J. Treatments for asymptomatic urinary tract infections during pregnancy (Cochrane Review). In: The Cochrane Library, Issue 3, 2000. Oxford: Update Software.
76. Alrajhi AA. Urinary tract infection in spinal cord injury patients. *Saudi Med J* 1999;20:24-28.
77. Tambyah PA, Maki DG. Catheter-associated urinary tract infection is rarely symptomatic: A prospective study of 1497 catheterized patients. *Arch Intern Med* 2000;160:678-682.
78. Johnson CE. New advances in childhood urinary tract infections. *Pediatr Rev* 1999;20:335-343.
79. Bennett J, St. Geme III JW. Bacterial resistance and antibiotic use in the emergency department. *Pediatr Clin North Am* 1999;46: 1125-1143.
80. Klimberg IW, Cox CE II, Fowler CL, et al. A controlled trial of levofloxacin and lomefloxacin in the treatment of complicated urinary tract infections. *Urology* 1998;51:610-615.
81. Anonymous. Single-dose antibiotic treatment for symptomatic urinary tract infections in women: a meta-analysis of randomized trials. In: Database of Abstracts of Reviews of Effectiveness, Volume 1, 2000. NHS Center for Reviews and Dissemination.
82. Lutters M, Herrmann F, Dayer P, et al. [Antibiotic utilization in a university geriatric hospital and drug formularies]. [French] *Schweiz Med Wochenschr* 1998;128:268-271.
83. Gilbert DN, Moellering RC, Sande MA. The Sanford Guide to Antimicrobial Therapy. 30th edition. Hyde Park, VT: Antimicrobial Therapy, Inc.;2000:24-25, 120.
84. Tice AD. Short-course therapy of acute cystitis: A brief review of therapeutic strategies. *J Antimicrob Chemother* 199;43(suppl A): 85-93.
85. Cahen P, Honderlick P. [Nitrofurans: A modern treatment for uncomplicated urinary infection?] [French] *Pathol Biol* (Paris) 2000;48:470-471.
86. Engel JD, Schaeffer AJ. Office management of urologic problems: Evaluation of and antimicrobial therapy for recurrent urinary tract infections in women. *Urol Clin North Am* 1998;25:685-701.
87. Hooton TM, Stamm WE. Diagnosis and treatment of uncomplicated urinary tract infection. *Infect Dis Clin North Am* 1997;11: 551-581.
88. Stein GE. Single-dose treatment of acute cystitis with fosfomycin tromethamime. *Ann Pharmacother* 1998;32:215-219.
89. Stein GE. Fosfomycin tromethamime: Single-dose treatment of acute cystitis. *Int J Fertil Womens Med* 1999;44:104-109.
90. Satlan M, Kaye D. Antibacterial therapy: Antibiotic agents in the elderly. *Infect Dis Clin North Am* 2000;14(2):
91. Lipsky BA. Prostatitis and urinary tract infection in men: What's new: What's true? *Am J Med* 1999;106:327-334.
92. Safrin S, Siegel D, Black D. Pyelonephritis in adult women: Inpatient vs. outpatient therapy. *Am J Med* 1988;85:793-798.
93. Anonymous. A meta-analysis of studies on the safety and efficacy of aminoglycosides given either once daily or as divided doses. In:

Database of Abstracts of Reviews of Effectiveness, Volume 1, 2000. NHS Center for Reviews and Dissemination.

94. Anonymous. A meta-analysis of extended-interval dosing vs. multiple daily dosing of aminoglycosides. In: *Database of Abstracts of Reviews of Effectiveness,* Volume 1, 2000. NHS Center for Reviews and Dissemination.
95. Anonymous. A meta-analysis of the relative efficacy and toxicity of single daily dosing vs. multiple daily dosing of aminoglycosides. In: *Database of Abstracts of Reviews of Effectiveness*, Volume 1, 2000. NHS Center for Reviews and Dissemination.
96. Virk A, Steckelberg JM. Clinical aspects of antimicrobial resistance [symposium on antimicrobial agents-part XVII]. *Mayo Clin Proc* 2000;75:200-214.
97. Bosker GB. *Pharmatecture: Minimizing medications to maximize results: A systematic approach to outcome-effective drug selection.* St. Louis, Missouri: Facts and Comparisons; 1999.
98. Mombelli G, Pezzoli R, Pinoja-Lutz G, et al. Oral vs intravenous ciprofloxacin in the initial empirical treatment of severe pyelonephritis or complicated urinary tract infections: A prospective randomized clinical trial. *Arch Intern Med* 1999;159:53-58.
99. Millar LK, Wing DA, Paul RH, et al. Outpatient treatment of pyelonephritis in pregnancy: A randomized controlled trial. *Obstet Gynecol* 1995;86:560-564.
100. Wing DA, Hendershott CM, Debuque L, et al. A randomized trial of three antibiotic regimens for the treatment of pyelonephritis in pregnancy. *Obstet Gynecol* 1998;92:249-253.
101. Wing DA, Hendershott CM, Debuque L, et al. Outpatient treatment of acute pyelonephritis in pregnancy after 24 weeks. *Obstet Gynecol* 1999;94:633-638.
102. Hoberman A, Wald ER. Treatment of urinary tract infections. *Pediatr Infect Dis J* 1999;18:1020-1021.
103. Hoberman A, Wald ER, Hickey RW, et al. Oral vs. initial intravenous therapy for urinary tract infections in young febrile children. *Pediatrics* 1999;104:79-96.
104. Santucci RA, Krieger JN. Gentamicin for the practicing urologist: Review of efficacy, single daily dosing and "switch" therapy. *J Urol* 2000;163:1076-1084.
105. Lundergan FS, Glasscock GF, Kim EH, et al. Once-daily gentamicin dosing in newborn infants. *Pediatrics* 1999;103(6 Pt 1):1228-1234.
106. Schaad UB, Eskola J, Kafetzis D, et al. Cefepime vs. ceftazidime treatment of pyelonephritis: A European, randomized, controlled study of 300 pediatric cases. European Society for Paediatric Infectious Diseases (ESPID) Pyelonephritis Study Group. *Pediatr Infect J* 1998;17:639-644.
107. Sia IG, Paya CV. Infectious complications following renal transplantation. *Surg Clin North Am* 1998;78:95-112.
108. Paradisi F, Corti G, Mangani V. Urosepsis in the critical care unit. *Crit Care Clin* 1998;14:165-180.

Antibiotic Therapy for Urinary Tract Infection

Kenneth H. Butler, DO, FACEP
Kevin C. Reed, MD
Gideon Bosker, MD, FACEP

For the first time in the United States, adults older than 60 years of age outnumber children ages 14 years and younger. This population is expected to double to nearly 80 million by the year 2050.[1] Hence, there are compelling reasons for developing consistent, outcome-effective treatment guidelines for managing urinary tract infection (UTI) in the elderly. Analysis of 1991-1996 Medicare claims demonstrates that urinary tract infection was the most common diagnosis in women older than the age of 65.

The scope of this problem in the elderly makes a major impact on the this population. More than 50% of bacteremic episodes in the institutionalized elderly are caused by UTIs, many of which are associated with long-term catheterization. Even in the independent, community-dwelling elderly population, about 6% of men and 16%-18% of women have significant bacteriuria. In the long-term care facility (LCF) environment, the prevalence of significant bacteriuria increases to 17%-55% in women and to 15%-31% in men without catheters; when chronic, indwellling catheters are present the risk of bacteriuria is almost 100%. Finally, fatal outcomes for hospitalization among the elderly were 4.3%, emphasizing the importance of early detection and prompt, definitive antimicrobial therapy.[2]

The elderly population is very sensitive to the incorrect use, selection, or dosage of antibiotics because of pharmacokinetic alterations associated with age, reduced homeostatic functional reserve, multiple underlying diseases (e.g., renal failure), and polypharmacy (leading to drug interactions and side effects).[3] Moreover, the elderly have multiple risk factors for developing UTI. (*Please see Table 1.*) Physicians must be aware of these unique factors in the elderly population when managing their illnesses and selecting antimicrobial therapy.

It is becoming clear that using risk-stratification criteria for predicting treatment failure and/or progression to complications and more serious disease can maximize clinical outcomes for UTI in the geriatric patient. In this regard, associated clinical findings or risk factors such as flank pain, hypotension, age over 65, diabetes, neurological disease, immunosuppression, and recurrent infection are predictive of more serious disease, as are urinary tract manipulation, catheterization, and acquisition of UTI in a nursing home or nosocomial environment. Presence of these factors may assist clinicians in initial selection of intravenous antibiotic therapy for hospitalized patients. Moreover, because indwelling catheters and bacteriuria are common in chronically ill elderly patients residing in LCFs, it is important to identify precise indications for initiating antibiotic therapy in this subgroup of patients.

With these issues in focus, the purpose of this second part of a two-part series on UTI management is to present a disease-stratification model for patient evaluation and antibiotic selection. Pharmacoeconomic considerations are highlighted and specific guidelines for antimicrobial selection are presented.

Table 1. Risk Factors in the Elderly for Developing Urinary Tract Infection

- Previous urinary tract infection
- Prolonged hospitalization in LCF
- Immobilization
- Less frequent urination
- Incomplete bladder emptying
- Prostate disease (men)
- Neuropathic diseases
- Immune response deterioration
- Increased incidence of renal/bladder/prostatic calculi
- Iatrogenic genitourinary instrumentation

Antimicrobial Therapy—Treatment Guidelines Based on Disease Stratification Model

Antibiotic treatment should be considered for patients of any age with symptomatic UTIs. Strategies differ in the healthy, community-dwelling elderly patient seen in the office as compared to the frail, institutionalized patient. Choice and intensity of antimicrobial treatment should be determined by several factors, including susceptibility of the infecting organism, patient tolerance, severity of the illness, and cost. In both the institutionalized elderly patient and the outpatient, there may be local patterns of infecting organisms or antimicrobial resistance that will direct antimicrobial choices.[4]

Cystitis. For the acutely symptomatic, elderly woman with cystitis, the preferred treatment is a three-day course with ciprofloxacin or trimethoprim-sulfamethoxazole (TMP-SMX). For drug cost acquisition reasons, TMP-SMX may be considered by some clinicians a first-line agent in women who can tolerate this agent, and who do not have underlying risk factors (the elderly, diabetics, previous history of UTI) and in areas in which resistance is infrequent. Its status as the initial agent of choice, however, is changing as fluoroquinolones have become increasingly favored as agents of first choice in the majority of patients. In particular, with increasing resistance of *E. coli* to TMP-SMX, ciprofloxacin is becoming the initial antibiotic of choice, even in uncomplicated UTI.[5,6] Ciprofloxacin should be considered the first-line antimicrobial in patients with UTI who have allergies to other drugs, in the elderly, in patients with recurrent infections, in diabetics, in patients with underlying diseases that predispose to serious infection, and in geographic areas where *E. coli* resistance to TMP-SMX is high (> 10-20%).

Total-cost outcome studies comparing antibiotics (i.e., TMP-SMX vs quinolones) used for acute pyelonephritis suggest that the high cure rates, excellent compliance, and predictable and sustained antimicrobial activity against *E. coli* (resistance rates among *E. coli* < 1%), as well as the low relapse rates associated with ciprofloxacin make this antibiotic a cost-effective first choice in patients with uncomplicated and complicated UTI.[7-9] Even in cost-conscious environments, ciprofloxacin (250 mg po BID x three days) represents an outcome-effective antibiotic for initial therapy of uncomplicated UTIs. In certain regions, and especially in urban areas, resistance among *E. coli* to TMP-SMX has risen to 24% over the past four years, a pattern that has relegated TMP-SMX to a secondary or alternative agent for management of cystitis and uncomplicated UTI.[5,6]

Single-dose therapy has lost favor because of fewer cures and increased recurrence rates, while the seven-day course of some drug classes exhibits greater potential for side effects, is more expensive, and has not been shown to improve the therapeutic effect. Some sources would suggest that patients with UTI symptoms for greater than five days, the elderly, diabetics, immunocompromised patients, males, those with flank pain but no fever, and those with fever but no other constitutional findings, require longer than three days of therapy.[10,11] For patients with severe dysuria, one to two days of analgesics, such as phenazopyridine 200 mg TID, may be helpful.[12]

Pyelonephritis. Patients suspected of having acute pyelonephritis should be treated with oral or intravenous agents that predictably cover the spectrum of implicated organisms, and therefore are likely to lead to clinical cure during the initial course of therapy. This is particularly important in the elderly, diabetic patients, immunocompromised individuals, men, and patients with chronic bacteriuria with signs of infection after GU procedures. In these high-risk subgroups, serious morbidity may be prevented by rapid administration of effective therapy.[13]

The optimal duration of treatment for women with acute, uncomplicated pyelonephritis is less clearly defined than for acute uncomplicated cystitis. Generally, a 10- to 14-day course of a quinolone such as ciprofloxacin is recommended. Ciprofloxacin is the antibiotic of choice in this subgroup because of its predictable coverage of gram-negative organisms—among them, *E. coli, Proteus sp., Pseudomonas sp.,* and others—known to cause invasive infection among hospitalized patients. Patients must be stratified into those who can be managed as outpatients with oral antibiotic therapy, and those who are ill enough to warrant inpatient, parenteral ciprofloxacin therapy.

No study has specifically compared oral vs. parenteral therapy in febrile, elderly patients with UTI in order to determine which route of administration produces better clinical outcomes. However, studies examining the use of oral therapy in patients of all ages with acute febrile pyelonephritis suggest that parenteral administration offers few benefits over oral therapy. In this regard, studies comparing IV and oral fluoroquinolone regimens for management of acute pyelonephritis suggest that the two routes yield comparable outcomes. A study comparing oral and IV ciprofloxacin in 141 patients (ages 18 to 96) with acute pyelonephritis showed no significant difference in outcomes for the regimens.[14,15]

Among the fluoroquinolones, the depth of clinical experience for treating UTI in the elderly has been greater with ciprofloxacin than with other agents, including other expanded-spectrum fluoroquinolones. Furthermore, studies evaluating ciprofloxacin in the elderly population confirm that safety and efficacy profiles in this subgroup are similar to those seen in a younger population; recent product labeling changes reflect these findings.[16,17]

It should be emphasized that although other quinolones may demonstrate activity against, and may be indicated for treatment of gram-negative organisms implicated in UTI, some of these antibiotics, especially the extended spectrum fluoroquinolones used for initial, empiric treatment of community-acquired pneumonia also are approved for or active against drug-resistant *Streptococcus pneumoniae* (DRSP). Consequently, the use of such quinolones as an initial, first-line agent for UTI in the elderly should be considered with reservation, because of concerns about emerging resistance among DRSP implicated in community-acquired pneumonia (CAP). This cautionary approach is supported by a recent guidelines document issued by the Centers for Disease Control (CDC) Drug-Resistant Streptococcus pneumoniae Therapeutic Working Group.

In this regard, because of significant concerns about emerging resistance, the CDC panel has recommended that extended-spectrum fluoroquinolones (i.e., levofloxacin and gatifloxacin) with activity against DRSP be "reserved" for selected patients with CAP. In light of this position, it appears prudent to limit the potential for inducing resistance in these pathogens, and reserve such antibiotics as alternative agents in patients with UTI, especially because effective and safe fluoroquinolones such as ciprofloxacin are available which do not have significant activity against DRSP. Accordingly, ciprofloxacin is recommended as the initial fluoroquinolone of choice for managing patients with UTI.

Finally, recent evaluations of antimicrobial resistance patterns confirm that ciprofloxacin has maintained an excellent level of susceptibility among commonly occurring uropathogens. A recent in vitro study in 1999 showed ciprofloxacin to be the most potent agent tested, with 96.8% of *E. coli*, 86.9% of *P. mirabilis*, 95.8% of *K. pneumoniae*, and 99.7% of *S. saprophyticus* susceptible to ciprofloxacin.[5]

The decision to use the oral vs. parenteral route of administration for initial therapy should be made by the physician based on the patient's condition. More specifically, the need for parenteral therapy should be dictated by the clinical condition of the patient (i.e., the likelihood of septicemia, metabolic abnormalities, fluid status, inability to take oral medication, and cardiovascular signs) rather than the patient's temperature. If these therapeutic limitations are not present, empiric treatment with oral fluoroquinolones is safe and effective for most patients with pyelonephritis.[14,15,18,19]

Cost-effectiveness of UTI treatment may be enhanced by using oral antimicrobials to manage elderly patients in the LCF or outpatient setting, if outpatient management is deemed safe and appropriate in an individual patient. Increasing attention is being given to cost-containment strategies—in the office, hospital, and managed care settings—and the issue of whether a specific subgroup of elderly patients with UTI can be managed with oral medications in the LCF or outpatient setting, rather than in the hospital, has important implications for clinical practice and antibiotic selection. In fact, from an efficacy and cost-effectiveness perspective, there is considerable evidence-based support for the use of oral ciprofloxacin in the management of severe urinary tract infections.[15]

In one multicenter, prospective, randomized trial oral ciprofloxacin (500 mg twice daily) was compared with intravenous ciprofloxacin (200 mg twice daily) in the initial empiric management of elderly, hospitalized patients (mean age, 66 years) with serious forms of UTI. The study population included 66 women with pyelonephritis, 43 patients with community-acquired UTIs, and 32 patients with hospital-acquired UTIs. The frequency of bacteremia was 42% in patients with pyelonephritis and 33% of those with complicated UTIs. Patients with severe sepsis were excluded from the study.[14,15]

Overall, there were no infection-related deaths and no patients required an early change of antibiotics because of worsening clinical status during the initial phase of treatment. The mean duration of fever was 1.7 days in patients treated by the oral route, compared to 1.9 days in patients treated by the intravenous route ($P = 0.15$). The rates of microbiological failure (3% in the oral vs. 2% in the intravenous treatment group) and of unsatisfactory clinical response (4% in the oral group vs 3% in the intravenous group) were low. A treatment alteration was eventually required in 14% of the patients assigned to the oral ciprofloxacin group and 7% of those to the intravenous group, primarily because of the isolation of enterococci or ciprofloxacin-resistant organisms during pre-therapy urine specimens.[14,15] Investigators concluded that in the hospital setting, oral ciprofloxacin is as effective as an intravenous regimen in the initial empirical management of serious UTIs, including bacteremic forms, in patients without severe sepsis, obstruction, or renal foci of suppuration.

Patients with severe pain, nausea, vomiting, dehydration, inability to take oral fluids or medications, or concerns about compliance or complicating factors should be admitted for parenteral antibiotics.[2,20] When the patient has been afebrile for 24-48 hours, the antibiotic can be changed to oral form to complete 14 days of therapy. Ciprofloxacin is first-line therapy for mild to moderate illness because its spectrum of activity is broad and high renal parenchymal levels are achieved following oral administration. If the two-week regimen fails, a longer course of four to six weeks should be considered because renal parenchymal disease is more difficult to eradicate than bladder mucosal infections.

Infections with *Enterococcus* and *Pseudomonas* are difficult to treat and may need longer therapy. Inpatient therapy, with intravenous antibiotics (ciprofloxacin, ampicillin and gentamicin, ceftriaxone, or some combination) initially, may be required if the patient's clinical condition suggests a toxic picture or inability to tolerate oral antibiotics. If fever has not resolved by 72 hours, radiologic imaging studies such as ultrasonography or intravenous pyelography should be performed to rule out obstruction.

Antibiotic Choices In The Elderly: Evidence-Based Support for Outcome-Effective Therapy. Diagnosis of UTI in the elderly may be difficult. *(Please see Table 2.)* Although a number of antibiotics are approved for managing UTIs in the geriatric patient, this consensus report has identified ciprofloxacin as a "workhorse" antibiotic with unique advantages and evidence-based support in this patient population. *(Please see Table 3.)* First, the availability of effective antimicrobial therapy in oral suspension can facilitate UTI management in the LCF or acute hospital setting. Convenience of administration may improve medication compliance which, in turn, may enhance therapeutic outcomes.[21] Please note that ciprofloxacin oral suspension should not be administered via feeding tubes due to physical characteristics of the formulation.

In this regard, bioequivalence of the oral suspension of ciprofloxacin (500 mg/10 mL) with ciprofloxacin 500 mg tablets has been documented in comparative studies evaluating the efficacy and safety of ciprofloxacin oral suspension vs. TMP-SMX oral suspension in community- and nursing home elderly women with UTI.[22] In one investigation of 261 patients, resistance rates of pretreatment bacteria was 4% to ciprofloxacin and 13% to TMP-SMX. Clinical resolution was observed in 96% of patients on ciprofloxacin and 87% of those on TMP-SMX. In addition, adverse events were lower following ciprofloxacin (17%) vs. TMP-SMX (27%) treatment regimen including premature discontinuation (2% ciprofloxacin vs 11% TMP-SMX; $P < 0.01$). Based on these results, the authors of the study concluded that ciprofloxacin oral suspension was more effective and better tolerated than TMP-SMX and can be considered a drug of choice among elderly women with UTI.

Table 2. Diagnostic Approaches for Identifying Elderly Patients With UTI: Assessment Strategies in the Acute Hospital Environment

RISK FACTORS/INCREASED SUSPICION FOR UTI
Frail elderly
Previous history of UTI
Indwelling catheter
Recent GU manipulation
Anticholinergic medications
Bacteriuria
ATYPICAL FINDINGS
Fatigue
Lethargy
Confusion
Cough
Weakness
Dyspnea
Afebrile
Abdominal pain
CLASSICAL FINDINGS
Dysuria
Urgency
Frequency
Flank pain
Back pain
Shaking chills/rigors
Fever
Tachycardia
Hypotension (urosepsis)
LABORATORY AND MICROBIOLOGICAL EVALUATION
Urine collection
Midstream clean catch or catherization
Leukocyte esterase
Microscopic bacteriuria
Pyuria
Urine culture
Blood culture
FINDINGS SUGGESTIVE OF BACTEREMIC UTI
Elevated serum creatinine
Increased leukocyte count
Fever
Presence of diabetes mellitus
Low serum albumin

The use of ciprofloxacin as a foundation antibiotic in a number of settings has been confirmed by a review of 127 articles in the medical literature on drug therapy in the elderly. The authors of the review conclude that: 1) ciprofloxacin is an effective agent for infections that commonly occur in the elderly population, including the full range of infections involving the urinary tract; 2) oral ciprofloxacin manifests potent antimicrobial activity that is sufficient to permit cost-effective therapy for serious infections in and out of the acute hospital setting; and 3) ciprofloxacin offers correct spectrum coverage of multiple pathogens known to cause UTI in this population.[17,23]

As mentioned previously, elderly patients can be placed on prophylaxis for as long as one to three months (low-dose TMP-SMX, nitrofurantoin, flouroquinolone, two or three times weekly) following recurrences.[24] Female patients may benefit from topical vaginal cream or oral estrogen replacement to counteract hormonal changes in the vaginal mucosa that increase the risk for reinfection.[24,25] recent randomized trial evaluated the efficacy of prevention with an estradiol-releasing silicone ring (Estring) compared with no estrogen treatment in postmenopausal women.[26] The cumulative likelihood of remaining free of UTIs during treatment was 45% in women with the vaginal ring compared with 20% in the control group after 36 weeks, and no significant adverse effects were found. High levels of intravaginal estrogens appear to promote the growth of commensurate bacteria such as lactobacilli, which suppress the growth of uropathogenic bacteria.[25] With regard to a preventive measure more commonly used by both younger females and older women, definitive evidence is lacking to support the use of cranberry juice for the prevention of bacteriuria.[27]

Catheterized patients require a scrupulous technique for the placement and replacement of indwelling catheters, as well as for collection of urine specimens. The best way to prevent infection is to remove the catheter as soon as possible. For patients requiring long-term catheterization, the use of clean intermittent catheterization four times daily is an alternative effective strategy. In males, the use of condom catheters also lowers the risk of infection, and several studies have suggested a lower risk of bacteriuria.[15] Catheters coated with silver oxide may delay bacteriuria during short-term use, but silver alloy catheters seem more effective.[15] Long-term antibiotic prophylaxis can lead to increased resistance and thus is not recommended.[28]

A study evaluating nitrofurantoin prophylaxis in an attempt to eradicate bacteriuria in patients with chronic neurogenic bladder receiving clean intermittent catheterization also showed persistently high levels of bacteriuria despite treatment (65% vs 74% in placebo).[28] Of greater concern was the finding that the most common pathogen found in the placebo group, *E. coli*, was replaced in the treatment group with resistant *Klebsiella sp.* and *Pseudomonas sp.* In a similar study using ciprofloxacin, the common organisms were eradicated in all cases; new organisms emerged as uropathogens, including methicillin-resistant *Staphylococcus aureus* (MRSA), enterococci, and *Acinetobacter sp.*[18] It is important to note, however, that this altered pattern of colonization did not translate into increased urinary tract infections or associated morbidity.[28]

Pharmacoeconomic Considerations—Cost of Resistance Vs. Resistance to Drug Cost

Pharmacoeconomic Considerations: Antibiotic Selection Process. Whether at the formulary level or in the practice setting, the selection process for antibiotics is never easy, even for well-educated practitioners and pharmacists at the front lines of hospital practice. Experienced hospital-based clinicians are particularly aware of the current debate: to choose a newer, conveniently dosed, shorter-dura-

Table 3. Antibiotic Treatment Guidelines* for Urinary Tract Syndromes in the Elderly

ASYMPTOMATIC BACTERIURIA
Evaluation and monitoring for symptoms, renal function, continuing bacteriuria
URINARY INCONTINENCE PLUS OTHERWISE ASYMPTOMATIC BACTERIURIA
Evaluate and treat underlying cause of incontinence
ACUTE SYMPTOMATIC CYSTITIS
Ciprofloxacin 250mg PO BID x 3 days (preferred) TMP-SMX DS One tab DS PO BID x 3 days (alternative, avoid in areas where *E. coli* resistance to TMP-SMX is > 10%)
CATHETERIZED PATIENT: LOWER ABDOMINAL PAIN OR NEW SYMPTOMS SUGGESTIVE OF UTI/WITHOUT FEVER OR SYSTEMIC SIGNS
Ciprofloxacin 250-500 mg PO BID x 7 days (preferred)
CATHETERIZED PATIENT: LOWER ABDOMINAL PAIN WITH FEVER OR SIGNS OF BACTEREMIA
Ciprofloxacin 500 mg PO BID x 7-10 days (preferred) Norfloxacin/ofloxacin/levofloxacin (alternative)
ACUTE PYELONEPHRITIS: MILD
Ciprofloxacin 500 mg PO BID x 7-10 days (preferred) Norfloxacin/ofloxacin/levofloxacin (alternative) Amoxicillin/clavulanate 500 PO BID x 7-10 days
ACUTE PYELONEPHRITIS: SYSTEMIC TOXICITY AND SIGNS OF BACTEREMIA
Ciprofloxacin 500 mg IV x 7-10 days (preferred) Cefotaxime IV (alternative) Levofloxacin (alternative)

*Empiric therapy

tion, and usually, more costly medication with documented track record of antimicrobial activity, patient friendliness, and more predictable antibacterial coverage; or, to choose a less expensive, vintage, workhorse drug-one that is "report card" and formulary-friendly—but one that requires a longer duration of therapy, is compromised by evolving resistance, and that has less predictable clinical cure rates. It should be stressed that especially in elderly patients who are frail and have comorbid conditions there are powerful incentives, from a cost, practice perception, and patient satisfaction perspective to identify agents that will cure infections the first time around (i.e., within the framework of the first prescription or antibiotic order).

Although optimizing cure rates with so-called convenient, dose- and duration-friendly branded agents that provide appropriate coverage with a low risk of antimicrobial resistance may be perceived as costly on a drug acquisition basis, it is important to stress the following points: antimicrobials with these properties also can help avoid the unnecessary costs of treatment failures, patient re-evaluations, return visits, patient dissatisfaction, and the pharmacological retreatment costs associated with initiating a second course of antibiotics. In this sense, antibiotics that lower barriers to clinical cure can be seen as "productivity tools" that approve efficiency of clinical care, and potentially, reduce the overall costs associated with both outpatient and hospital-based treatment of infections.

Antibiotic Choices In UTI: Evidence-Based Support for Outcome-Effective Therapy. Although a number of antibiotics are approved for managing UTIs, this review has identified ciprofloxacin as a "workhorse" antibiotic with unique advantages and evidence-based support in a number of adult populations. *(Please see Table 4.)* First, the availability of effective antimicrobial therapy in oral suspension can facilitate UTI management in the elderly in hospital setting. Convenience of administration may improve medication compliance which, in turn, may enhance therapeutic outcomes.[29] Please note that ciprofloxacin oral suspension should not be administered via feeding tubes due to physical characteristics of the formulation.

In this regard, bioequivalence of the oral suspension of ciprofloxacin (500 mg/10 mL) with ciprofloxacin 500 mg tablets has been documented in comparative studies evaluating the efficacy and safety of ciprofloxacin oral suspension vs. TMP-SMX oral suspension in community-dwelling and nursing home elderly women with UTI.[30] In one investigation of 261 patients, resistance rates of pretreatment bacteria was 4% to ciprofloxacin and 13% to TMP-SMX. Clinical resolution was observed in 96% of patients on ciprofloxacin and 87% of those on TMP-SMX. In addition, adverse events were lower following ciprofloxacin (17%) vs. TMP-SMX (27%) treatment regimen including premature discontinuation (2% ciprofloxacin vs. 11% TMP-SMX; $P < 0.01$). Based on these results, the authors of the study concluded that ciprofloxacin oral suspension was more effective and better tolerated than TMP-SMX and can be considered a drug of choice among elderly women with UTI.[30]

The safe and effective use of ciprofloxacin as a foundation antibiotic in the hospital and emergency department settings has been confirmed by a review of 127 articles in the medical literature on drug therapy in the elderly. The authors of the review conclude that: 1) ciprofloxacin is an effective agent for infections that commonly occur in the elderly population, including the full range of infections involving the urinary tract; 2) oral ciprofloxacin manifests potent antimicrobial activity that is sufficient to permit cost-effective therapy for serious infections in and out of the acute hospital setting; and 3) ciprofloxacin offers correct spectrum coverage of multiple pathogens known to cause UTI in this population.[16]

Cost of Resistance. With respect to barriers that can compromise clinical cure, in vitro activity and in vivo effectiveness against implicated pathogens are critical for cost-effective care. This is especially true for management of urinary tract infections such as cystitis and pyelonephritis. Fortunately, recent studies now are available that have compared bacteriologic and clinical cure rates of ciprofloxacin with older agents increasingly compromised by emerging resistance.[8]

It is important to stress that the road from the clinician's prescription pad to clinical cure, in the setting of urinary tract infection, depends on many factors including prescription resistance (the cost of the medication to the patient or health plan); patient resistance (tolerability, side effects, daily dose frequency, duration of therapy, quality of patient's life, and other patient-oriented factors that affect medication compliance); and drug resistance (the likelihood that the selected antibiotic will provide predictable coverage against organisms implicated in the infection, i.e., *E. coli* in patients with UTI).[31]

The prescription, patient, and drug resistance (PPD) approach to antibiotic selection permits pharmacists and physicians to evaluate and compare the clinical success profiles of one antibiotic vs. another. These comparisons are a synthetic approach based on multiple drug-related factors, including price, total resource cost, daily dose frequency, duration of drug therapy, side effect profile, and spectrum of coverage (bacteriologic cure rates).

With these cost and cure efficacy issues in clear focus, a well-designed, randomized, double blind comparative study—the lead author of which is an emergency department physician—was conducted to compare the efficacy and safety of a seven-day ciprofloxacin regimen and a 14-day TMP-SMX regimen for the treatment of acute pyelonephritis in women.[8] A total of 255 patients (all ages) were included in the analysis. Patients were randomized to oral ciprofloxacin, 500 mg twice per day for seven days (with or without an initial 400 mg intravenous dose) followed by placebo for seven days (n = 128 included in analysis) vs. TMP-SMX, 160/800 mg twice per day for 14 days (with or without intravenous ceftriaxone, 1 g) (n = 127 included in the analysis). The main outcome measure was continued bacteriologic and clinical cure, such that alternative antimicrobial drugs were not required, among evaluable patients through the four- to 11-day post-therapy visit, compared by treatment group.

Clinical Cure Rates: Ciprofloxacin Superiority Established. This was an important study because trial results indicate superior efficacy for the ciprofloxacin group. At 4-11 days post-therapy, bacteriologic cure rates were 99% (112 of 113) for the ciprofloxacin regimen and 89% (90 of 101) for the TMP-SMX regimen (95% confidence interval [CI] for difference 0.04-0.16; P = .004). Clinical cure rates were 96% (109 of 113) for the ciprofloxacin regimen and 83% (92 of 111) for the TMP-SMX regimen (95% CI, 0.06-0.22; P = 0.002).

Adverse drug events occurred in 24% of 191 ciprofloxacin-treated patients and in 33% of 187 TMP-SMX-treated patients, respectively (95% CI, -0.001 to 0.2). Gastrointestinal events, headache, and rash tended to occur more frequently in the TMP-SMX group. Adverse events causing study drug discontinuation occurred in 11 (6%) of the ciprofloxacin-treated patients and 21 (11%) TMP-SMX-treated patients.

E. coli, which caused more than 90% of infections, was more frequently resistant to TMP-SMX (18%) than to ciprofloxacin (0%; P < 0.001). Among TMP-SMX-treated patients, drug resistance was associated with greater bacteriologic and clinical failure rates (P < 0.001 for both). Drug-related adverse events occurred in 24% of 191 ciprofloxacin-treated patients and in 33% of 187 TMP-SMX-treated patients, respectively (95% CI, -0.001 to 0.2). To summarize, in this study of outpatient treatment of acute uncomplicated pyelonephritis in women, a seven-day ciprofloxacin regimen was associated with greater bacteriologic and clinical cure rates than a 14-day TMP-SMX regimen, especially in patients infected with TMP-SMX-resistant strains.

Total Outcome Costs. The current shift to outpatient management and treatment of elderly patients in the LCF has placed an emphasis on cost-saving strategies; clinicians and pharmacists must now critically evaluate total treatment costs-beyond those associated with drug acquisition costs alone-associated with regimens used to manage acute, uncomplicated pyelonephritis. Physicians practicing in cost-conscious settings, including LCFs, need evidence-based trials to determine whether higher cure rates linked to drugs with a more predictable spectrum of coverage can reduce overall treatment costs for conditions such as pyelonephritis. The improved bacteriologic and cure rates observed with ciprofloxacin in this study suggests this may be the case. In another study, ciprofloxacin suspension showed higher clinical success and bacteriologic eradication rates compared to TMP-SMX for both community- and nursing home-residing elderly women with acute urinary tract infections.[30] In addition, ciprofloxacin was associated with significantly lower rates of adverse events and premature discontinuations compared to TMP-SMX.[30]

To assess the possible advantages conferred by regimens that produce more predictable cure rates, the investigators of the pyelonephritis study conducted a health resource use and cost analysis for both ciprofloxacin and TMP-SMX treatment regimens. All health care resources used were prospectively collected. Additional resources required for achieving clinical cure were defined as those associated with managing clinical or bacteriologic failure, or adverse drug events. The perspective of the cost analysis was that of the third-party payer. Direct medical costs were assigned retrospectively and were reported in 1997 dollars.

All significant real-world costs associated with completing the journey from "prescription pad" to "clinical cure" were considered and included the following resource cost components: 1) the cost of the initial physician visit, including site of care (i.e., office or emergency department); 2) antimicrobial cultures, urinalysis, and urine culture; 3) a single follow-up visit (if there was at least one follow-up visit) with urinalysis and urine culture; and 4) additional resources used associated with failures and adverse drug events including subsequent nonstudy-required medical visits, laboratory and radiology tests, hospitalizations, therapeutic adjuncts, and other antimicrobials, through the patient's last visit.

Costs of hospitalizations, office visits, laboratory tests, and other procedures were estimated by multiplying relative value units by an estimate of the average cost per relative value unit. Cost per cure was calculated based on the total costs for all patients divided by the number of cured patients in each treatment group. Safety, health resource use, and costs were evaluated for all 378 enrolled patients.

Cost Comparisons. Of special clinical importance was the finding that the total treatment costs for the seven-day course of ciprofloxacin was less than it was for those individuals treated with TMP-SMX. Additional health resource use (i.e., excluding resources required for initial management, and post-therapy follow-up visits for patients without earlier treatment failure) was higher in all categories for patients treated with TMP-SMX than ciprofloxacin, with the exception of radiological procedures. Since more TMP-SMX-treated

Table 4. Recommended Oral Antibiotics for Uncomplicated UTI and Intravenous Agents for Hospital-Based Management of Pyelonephritis[19,25,34,39,56-58,63,64,66,82,84,86,91,98,104]

Agent	Dosage
ACUTE UNCOMPLICATED UTI IN ADULTS, CYSTITIS (3-DAY REGIMEN)	
First-line agents:	
Fluoroquinolone (initial agent of choice)	
Ciprofloxacin (preferred)	250 mg po BID x 3 days
Fluoroquinolone (alternative)	
Enoxacin	200 mg po BID x 3 days
Gatifloxacin	200-400 mg po QD x 3 days
Levofloxacin	250 mg po QD x 3 days
Ofloxacin	200 mg po BID x 3 days
Lomefloxacin	400 mg po QD x 3 days
Norfloxacin	400 mg po BID x 3 days
Secondary Alternatives:	
Trimethoprim/sulfamethoxazole*	160/800 mg po BID x 3 days

*Only if *E. coli* resistance is < 10%-15% in patient population (based on regional resistance surveillance data).
**Alternatives: Oral cephalosporin, nitrofurantoin, doxycycline, trimethoprim, or amoxicillin/clavulonic acid.

Agent	Dosage
ACUTE UNCOMPLICATED PYELONEPHRITIS, OUTPATIENT TREATMENT: A FLUOROQUINOLONE FOR 7 DAYS*	
Preferred:	
Ciprofloxacin	500 mg po BID x 7 days
Alternative:	
Enoxacin	400 mg po QD x 7 days
Levofloxacin	250-500 mg po QD x 7 days
Ofloxacin	200-400 mg po BID x 7 days
Lomefloxacin	400 mg po QD x 7 days
Norfloxacin	400 mg po BID x 7 days

*Recommendations for other (alternative) fluoroquinolones based on limited studies and generalization of efficacy of ciprofloxacin, which has greatest body of evidence-based trials in UTI.
**Secondary alternatives: Amoxicillin/clavulonic acid, cephalosporin, TMP/SMX-DS for 14 days.

Agent	Dosage
ACUTE UNCOMPLICATED PYELONEPHRITIS, INPATIENT TREATMENT FLUOROQUINOLONE IV	
Initial Empiric Agent of Choice:	
Ciprofloxaxin (preferred)	400 mg IV BID
Alternative:	
Gatifloxacin	400 mg IV QD
Levofloxacin	250-500 mg IV QD
Ofloxacin	400 mg IV BID
Ampicillin plus	150-200 mg/kg/d divided Q4H°
gentamicin	5-7 mg/kg QD
Cefotaxime	1-2 g Q4-12°
Ceftriaxone	1-2 g IV QD
Piperacillin	3 g IV Q6°
COMPLICATED PYELONEPHRITIS, UROSEPSIS, OR INDWELLING CATHETER	
Ciprofloxacin plus (tobramycin)* (+ 5-7 mg/kg/d)	400 mg IV q 8 hr
Ampicillin (+ tobramycin)* (+ 5-7 mg/kg/d)	150-200 mg/kg/d IV divided Q4°
Piperacillin/Tazobactam	3.375 g IV Q6 or 4.5 gm Q8
Ticarcillin/clavulinic acid	3.1 g IV Q4-6H
Imipenim	0.5 g IV Q6

* Amikacin or gentamicin (alternatives)
Note: Any patient receiving advanced generation penicillins and aminoglycosides or fluoroquinolones may need dosing adjustments and/or interval adjustment if they have renal impairment.

patients had clinical failures, it is not surprising these patients accrued high total service costs. In this regard, the mean total cost per patient was greater for TMP-SMX-treated patients ($687) than for ciprofloxacin-treated patients ($531) by 29% or $156 (95% CI, -$118 to $443).

Since TMP-SMX-treated patients ultimately required more interventions and additional antimicrobial prescriptions to achieve cure, the mean cost per cure was higher for TMP-SMX ($770) than for ciprofloxacin-treated patients ($615) by 25% or $155 (range of difference based on upper and lower bounds of the 95% CI in cure rates, $102-$207).

Implications for Hospital Clinical Practice. The data from this landmark study suggest that excessive total treatment costs and inferior clinical cure rates associated with TMP-SMX therapy may be the consequence of an unexpectedly high prevalence of in vitro resistance to TMP-SMX among *E. coli* strains causing acute uncomplicated pyelonephritis. In fact, the evolving resistance is a phenomenon that appears to be significant enough to alter clinical practice patterns related to antibiotic selection. As the authors point out, in 1994, prior to beginning the study, resistance rates to TMP-SMX among uropathogens associated with acute uncomplicated pyelonephritis were generally less than 10% at investigative sites.

They emphasize, however, that increasing rates of TMP-SMX resistance—reported to be as high as 25%, especially in Western states—have been observed among urinary *E. coli* isolates and that in this study, in vitro resistance to TMP-SMX was strongly associated with bacteriologic and clinical failure. They conclude that, based on their data, TMP-SMX may no longer be appropriate as empiric therapy in certain geographic areas where a fluoroquinolone should be strongly considered as the initial agent of choice.[8,30]

Although the trial was not powered to show statistical significance in the economic differences between treatment groups for health care resource use, there was a discernible trend for more intensive resource use in all categories among TMP-SMX-treated patients, with the exception of radiological procedures. Of special importance is that despite the fact the prescription cost of the ciprofloxacin regimen was greater than that of the TMP-SMX regimen, patients treated with the TMP-SMX regimen tended to have greater overall costs, particularly those related to subsequent hospitalizations, office visits, and laboratory tests.

In addition, from a pharmatectural perspective, the findings of this study—in particular, the superior bacteriologic and clinical cure rates seen with a seven-day course of ciprofloxacin as well as reduced overall treatment costs—support ciprofloxacin's favorable PPD profile and suggest it should considered the agent of choice in female patients with outpatient pyelonephritis. Finally, the results, conclusions, and comparative analyses from this well-designed clinical trial suggest that in the current outcome- and cost-sensitive environment of hospital practice, ciprofloxacin represents a more outcome-effective agent—as this relates to cost, bacteriologic eradication, and clinical cure rate parameters—than does TMP-SMX for management of acute uncomplicated pyelonephritis.

Future Treatments and Directions for Research

Clinical Trials and Literature Review. No clinical randomized controlled trials have conclusively shown a benefit of silver alloy catheters for prevention of UTI. However, a recent analysis using silver-coated catheters in a hypothetical cohort of hospitalized patients requiring short-term catheterization (two to 10 days) theoretically reduced the incidence of UTI and bacteremia, along with saving an estimated $4 per patient despite the $5 higher initial cost of the special catheter.[32] A large randomized, controlled trial is warranted to evaluate this type of catheter, as more than 80% of nosocomial UTIs are related to indwelling catheters. In vitro studies of catheters impregnated with quinolones or chlorhexidine gluconate have shown promising early results in the prevention of UTI. A very interesting avenue of research in in vitro and animal models involves the application of electric current to catheter surfaces, with relatively good efficacy at reducing UTIs; a practical clinical application of this technology awaits further study.[15]

In one novel study, clinicians administered an immunostimulating bacterial extract by mouth to patients with persistent recurrent UTI, with subsequent beneficial curative action and decreased frequency and severity of recurrent infections long term.[25] Similar success was found in a study using Uro-Vaxom, an oral drug prepared from immunogenic fractions extracted from *E. coli*.[25] Phase II trials have been completed for a multi-strain vaccine administered as a vaginal suppository in women susceptible to recurrent UTI. Intervals to reinfection while off antibiotics were longer in those taking the vaccine than in the placebo group: 13 weeks vs. 8.7 weeks.[25] No serious side effects were noted.

The same research group found that this vaccine had greater efficacy in patients with a specific human leukocyte antigen phenotype (HLA-DR).[35] In patients with spinal cord injuries and a mean of 3.1 symptomatic UTIs per year, a small trial using intravesical inoculation with *E. coli* 83972, a benign pathogen, showed that successfully colonized patients had no symptomatic infection over a mean duration of 12.3 months.[34] Colonized subjects also reported subjective improvement in quality of life with respect to this improved prevention of UTIs. Authors suggest that colonization with *E. coli* 83972 may be used safely to reduce the rate of UTI in spinal-cord patients with a neurogenic bladder.

Laboratory Models. In an animal model, adjunctive oral prednisolone appeared to be effective in diminishing renal scarring in severely affected kidneys.[35] Based on these results, clinical prospective trials are planned to further evaluate the possibility of oral steroids as an adjunct to the present treatment of pyelonephritis in children.[35] Additional research trials in rats found that the addition of ibuprofen to antibiotic therapy decreases renal scarring due to acute pyelonephritis, even when treatment is delayed 72 hours.[36] Further study to understand the mechanisms responsible for this finding may lead to additional treatment options for patients with pyelonephritis.

In the future, research will focus on understanding factors that lead to infection in order to develop nonantimicrobial strategies for preventing symptomatic infections. These areas of investigation include possible vaccination, colonization of patients with a virulent organism that prevents uropathogen inoculation, and selective interference with bacterial adhesion proteins or cell surface receptors.[19] One such study that is being conducted in animal models and in humans has focused on the development of a vaccine against pyelonephritis. This approach is based on current knowledge of virulence factors such as adhesive molecules on the tip of pili in some *E. coli* strains that allow binding to human uroepithelial calls.[37]

Experimental research also is ongoing being evaluating administration of nitric oxide synthase inhibitors involved in the pathogeneisis of sepsis.[38] Other investigational studies of inflammatory cytokines (IL-10), soluble TNF-alpha or IFN-gamma receptors, anti-IFN gamma monoclonal antibody, platelet-activating factor receptor antagonists, and antibodies directed against endotoxin-binding proteins also may provide insight and lead to new treatments for severe urinary tract infections.[38]

Antimicrobials. The management of severe multidrug resistant infections continues to become more challenging. Newer alternatives to standard therapies that may be used for UTIs include 1) Synercid (Quinupristin/dalfopristin), the first injectable streptogramin antibiotic with substantial efficacy against VRE, and 2) Colistin, a polymyxin, that, in a small trial, showed improved outcomes in patients with severe infections with multidrug-resistant *Pseudomonas aeruginosa* and *Acinetobacter baumanni*.[39,40]

Summary

Outcome-effective management of urinary tract infections equires a detailed clinical history, careful physical examination, and limited initial laboratory testing. This approach is essential for appropriate triaging of patients and initial management. Populations at risk for increased morbidity and mortality include neonates, patients of any age with signs of systemic toxicity, pregnant women, immunocompromised patients (those with the human immunodeficiency virus and transplant recipients), and any adult or elderly patient with significant co-morbid illnesses.

Rapid assessment and resuscitation are mandatory for hemodynamic instability or shock, accompanied by prompt antimicrobial treatment. Initial empirical choice of antibiotics and duration of treatment have been influenced by the rapid emergence of significant resistance to nearly all classes of antibiotics used in the management of urinary tract infections. In this regard, previous first-line agents, including amoxicillin and TMP-SMX, can no longer be recommended in the setting of *E. coli* resistance higher than 10%-20%. In this increasingly common situation, ciprofloxacin has emerged as the preferred agent. A thorough understanding of the common side effects, drug interactions, and contraindications is essential for preventing any untoward consequences in patients with UTI.

Recent trials have shown that appropriately selected patients that once required admission for parenteral treatment may be discharged safely and treated with oral regimens. The greatest experience and trial data have been reported with ciprofloxacin, although other fluoroquinolones also may provide advantages of outpatient management. Close follow-up and appropriate referral are key to successful management of these patient populations.

Advances in biotechnology and molecular science are enhancing our understanding of the establishment of urinary tract infection as well as the cascade of events leading to renal damage. This expanded knowledge base may lead eventually to newer, more effective prevention strategies and treatment regimens and, in the process, decrease morbidity and mortality associated with UTI.

References

1. Stalam M, Kaye D. Antibacterial therapy-antibiotic agents in the elderly. *Infect Dis Clin North Am* 2000;14:357-369.
2. Kunin C. *Urinary tract infections: detection, prevention, and management*, 5th edition. Baltimore, MD; Williams & Wilkins: 1997:150-154.
3. Lutters M, Herrmann F, Dayer P, Vogt N. [Antibiotic utilization in a university geriatric hospital and drug formularies]. [French] *Schweiz Med Wochenschr* 1998;128:268-271.
4. Shaw KN, Gorelick MH. Urinary tract infection in the pediatric patient. *Pediatr Clin North Am* 1999;46:1111-1124.
5. Gupta K, Scholes D, Stamm WE. Increasing prevalence of antimicrobial resistance among uropathogens causing acute uncomplicated cystitis in woman. *JAMA* 1999;281:736-738.
6. Wright SW, Wrenn KD, Haynes ML. Trimethoprim-sulfamethoxazola resistance among urinary coliform isolates. *J General Intern Medical* 1999:14:606.
7. Orenstein R, Wong ES. Urinary tract infections in adults. *Am Family Phys* 1999;59:1225-1234.
8. Talan DA, Stamm WE, Hooton TM, et al. Comparison of ciprofloxacin (7 days) and trimethoprim-sulfamethoxazole (14 days) for acute uncomplicated pyelonephritis in women. *JAMA* 2000;283:12.
9. Patton JP, Nash DB, Abrutyn E. Urinary tract infection: Economic considerations. *Med Clin North Am* 1991;75:495-513.
10. Nordenstam GR, Brandberg CA, Oden AS, et al. Bacteriuria and mortality in an elderly population. *N Engl J Med* 1986;314: 1152-1156.
11. Wolfson SA, Kalmanson GM, Rubini ME, et al. Epidemiology of bacteriuria in a predominantly geriatric male population. *Am J Med Sci* 1965;89:168-173.
12. Winberg J. Commentary: progressive renal damage from infection with or without reflux. *J Urol* 1992;148:1733-1734.
13. Newell A, Riley P, Rogers M. Resistance patterns of urinary tract infections diagnosed in a genitourinary medicine clinic. *Int J STD AIDS* 2000;11:499-500.
14. Mombelli G, Pezzoli R, Pinoja-Lutz G, et al. Oral vs. intravenous ciprofloxacin in the initial empirical management of severe pyelonephritis or complicated urinary tract infections. A prospective randomized clinical trial. *Arch Intern Med* 1999;159:53-58.
15. Sedor J, Mulholland SG. Infections in urology: Hospital acquired urinary tract infections associated with the indwelling catheter. *Urol Clin North Am* 1999;26:821-828.
16. Wiseman, LR, Balfour, JA. Ciprofloxacin, a review of its pharmacological profile and therapeutic use in the elderly. *Drugs Aging* 1994:145-173.
17. Nicolle LE. Asymptomatic bacteriuria-important or not? *N Engl J Med* 2000;14:1037-1039.
18. Waites KB, Canupp KC, Brookings ES, et al. Effect of ciprofloxacin on bacterial flora of perineum, urethra, lower urinary tract in men with spinal cord injury. *J Spinal Cord Med* 1999;22:192-198.
19. O'Donnell JA, Gelone SP. Antibacterial therapy: Fluoroquinolones. *Infect Dis Clin North Am* 2000;14:489-513,xi.
20. Barnett BJ, Stephens DS. Urinary tract infection: An overview. *Am J Med Sci* 1997;314:245-249.
21. Rushton HG. Urinary tract infections in children: epidemiology, evaluation and management. *Pediatr Clin North Am* 1997;44:1133-1169.
22. Roberge RJ, Kaplan R, Frank R, et al. Glyburide-ciprofloxacin interaction with resistant hypoglycemia. *Ann Emerg Med*

2000;36:160-163.

23. Lutters M, Vogt N. Antibiotics duration for treating uncomplicated, symptomatic lower urinary tract infections in elderly women. *Cochrane Database of Systematic Rev* 2000;2.
24. Wood CA, Abrutyn E. Urinary tract infection in older adults. *Clin Geriatr Med* 1998;14:267-283.
25. Engel JD, Schaeffer AJ. Office management of urologic problems: Evaluation of and antimicrobial therapy for recurrent urinary tract infections in women. *Urol Clin North Am* 1998;25:685-701.
26. Erikson B. A randomized, open, parallel-group study on the preventative effect of an estradiol releasing vaginal ring (ESTRING) on recurrent urinary tract infections in postmenopausal women. *Am J Obstet Gynecol* 1999;180:1072-1079.
27. Jepson RG, Mihaljevic L, Craig J. Cranberries for preventing urinary tract infections. *Cochrane Database Sys Rev* 2000;2.
28. Schlager TA, Anderson S, Trudell J, Hendley JO. Nitrofurantoin prophylaxis for bacteriuria and urinary tract infection in children with neurogenic bladder on intermittent catheterization. *J Pediatr* 1998;123:704-708.
29. Haley RW, Culver DH, White JW. The nationwide nosocomial infection rate: A new need for vital statistics. *Am J Epidemiol* 1985;121:159-167.
30. Gomolin, IH, Siami, P Haverstock, D. Heyd, A; Efficacy and safety of oral ciprofloxacin suspension vs. TMP-SMX for treatment of community- and nursing home-residing elderly women with acute urinary tract infection. Presented at the 6th International Symposium on New Quinolones; Nov. 15-17, 1998; Denver, Colorado.
31. Bosker GB. PharmatectureÆ: *Minimizing Medications To Maximize Results—A Systematic Approach to Outcome-Effective Drug Selection.* St. Louis, MO: Facts and Comparisons; 1999
32. Saint S, Veenstra D, Sullivan S. The potential clinical and economical benefits of silver alloy urinary catheters in preventing urinary tract infections. *Arch Intern Med* 2000;160:2670-2675.
33. Hopkins WJ, Heisey DM, Uehling DT. Association of human leukocyte antigen phenotype with vaccine efficacy in patients receiving vaginal mucosal immunization for recurrent urinary tract infection. *Vaccine* 1999;17:169-171.
34. Hull R, Rudy D, Donovan W, et al. Urinary tract infection prophylaxis using *Escherichia coli* 83972 in spinal cord injured patients. *J Urol* 2000;163:872-877.
35. Pohl HG, Rushton HG, Park JS, et al. Adjunctive oral corticosteroids reduce renal scarring: The piglet model of reflux and acute experimental pyelonephritis. *J Urol* 1999;12:815-820.
36. Huang A, Palmer L, Hom D, et al. Ibuprofen combined with antibiotics suppresses renal scarring due to ascending pyelonephritis in rats. *J Urol* 1999;162:1396-1398.
37. Johnson CE. New advances in childhood urinary tract infections. *Pediatr Rev* 1999;20:335-343.
38. Paradisi F, Corti G, Mangani V. Urosepsis in the critical care unit. *Crit Care Clin* 1998;14:165-180.
39. Levin AS, Barone AA, Penco J, et al. Intravenous colistin as therapy for nosocomial infections caused by multidrug-resistant *Pseudomonas aeruginosa* and *Acinetobacter baumannii. Clin Infect Dis* 1999;28:1008-1011.
40. Moellering RC, Linden PK, Reinhardt J, et al. The efficacy and safety of quinupristin/dalfopristin for the treatment of infections caused by vancomycin-resistant *Enterococcus faecium:* Synercid Emergency-Use Study Group. *J Antimicrob Chemother* 1999;44:251-261.

Tuberculosis

Dawn Demangone, MD
David Karras, MD

Since 1985, the number of new tuberculosis cases in the United States has risen about 18% annually.[1] Many consider the resurgence of this disease to be a failure of the American health care system or a symptom of government cuts in health care spending and social programs. Probably, the most important factor in the rise of tuberculosis, however, is the rapid increase in the number of immunocompromised hosts.[2] The present epidemic of tuberculosis is largely a by-product of AIDS, whose victims frequently live in crowded conditions and can easily transmit the disease to immunocompetent individuals.

Coincident with the rise in the number of tuberculosis cases is a striking increase in multidrug-resistant strains of the organism. Poor compliance with antibiotic therapy has led to a crisis of drug-resistant tuberculosis, long a common problem in developing countries but uncommon in the United States prior to the 1990s.[3] Nationally, more than 14% of new tuberculosis cases are resistant to at least one drug, and fully one-third of isolates in New York City are isoniazid-resistant.[3] Multidrug-resistant strains pose a serious threat not only to the control of the disease in the population but also to health care workers.

With these issues in focus, this article reviews the epidemiology and pathogenesis of tuberculosis, focusing on the features of the disease salient to emergency physicians. The authors discuss diagnostic options and unusual clinical presentations of this protean disease, as well as specific manifestations in high-risk subgroups. In addition, the most current tuberculosis treatment recommendations of the Centers for Disease Control and Prevention (CDC) are described. Finally, this review provides detailed discussions about tuberculosis (TB)-related issues that are relevant to emergency medicine, including prophylaxis of exposed health-care workers and infection control professionals in the emergency department (ED).

Epidemiology

Infection with *Mycobacterium tuberculosis* continues to be a worldwide problem. Approximately one-third of the world's population is currently infected.[4] Ten million newly infected individuals are diagnosed each year, resulting in 30 million cases of active tuberculosis and 3 million deaths annually. Infection with *M. tuberculosis* is responsible for 6% of deaths worldwide.[5]

The recent resurgence in tuberculosis in the United States has been attributed to immigration from endemic areas, homelessness, intravenous drug use, and perhaps most importantly, the HIV epidemic.[1,6,7] Infection with tuberculosis is frequent among the elderly, institutionalized individuals (such as those in nursing homes and prisons), the urban poor, minority groups, and those infected with HIV. Non-whites have twice the risk of infection, with the highest rates in African-Americans and immigrants from regions with high tuberculosis prevalence, including Asia, Africa, Latin America, and the Caribbean.[8,9] Children of immigrants have a four-fold increased infection rate over children with U.S.-born parents.[7] The largest concentration of cases is in those between the ages of 25 and 44 years, and males are infected 2.5 times more frequently than females.[5,7] In 1992, African-American men between 35 and 44 years of age had a rate of tuberculosis infection 53 times the national average.[5]

Transmission

Mycobacteria are slow-growing aerobic rods with characteristic cell-wall lipids that account for their acid-fast staining properties. Four subspecies of mycobacteria make up the "tuberculosis complex," each of these organisms can cause tubercular disease: *M. tuberculosis, M. microti, M. africanum,* and *M. bovis. M. tuberculosis* accounts for the majority of human disease.[1,6,10]

Transmission occurs primarily through inhalation of aerosolized bacilli. While as few as 1-10 bacilli entering the alveoli can cause infection, only about one-fifth of exposed individuals become infected.[2,11] After a sneeze or cough by an infectious individual, aerosolized microdroplets are expelled into the environment. Large droplets are usually trapped in the upper airway, which contain multiple mechanical barriers resistant to infection.[12] However, the droplets may partially evaporate into droplet nuclei and remain suspended in air for extended periods of time, where they are easily carried by air currents. These droplet nuclei are very small particles of the right size (1-5 mm), contain 1-3 tubercle bacilli, and have about a 50% chance of reaching the alveoli after inhalation. Micrometer-sized particles evade the mucociliary apparatus. Because they are too small to be entrapped, they can reach alveoli and produce infection. In addition, it should be stressed that droplet nuclei can remain suspended in a room, even if the patient is no longer present, an important factor when it comes to infection control measures.

Establishment of infection is influenced by many factors, including the intensity of exposure, the number of bacilli to reach the alveoli, viability of the bacilli, and the microbicidal activity of host alveolar macrophages.[13] Specific infectious sites are associated with higher rates of transmission: patients with laryngeal tuberculosis, endobronchial disease, or extensive cavitary pulmonary disease are considered highly infectious, while extra-pulmonary tuberculosis is typically not considered transmissible.[9] Tuberculosis is more effectively transmitted when acid-fast bacilli are present in the infected individual's sputum, when exposure occurs in a small, enclosed space, or occurs in rooms that do not have adequate ventilation and there is recirculation of contaminated air.[9] Nosocomial transmission is more common when the prevalence of tuberculosis is high in the community, there exists close contact with infectious individuals, and with the performance of certain procedures, notably endotracheal intubation, bronchoscopy, respiratory secretion suctioning, open abscess irrigation, and autopsy.[9] The most important host factor bearing on an exposed individual's susceptibility to infection is previous mycobacterial infection, which protects against re-infection. Genetic predisposition and the presence of underlying disease may also affect the risk of infection.[2] Among factors predisposing to tuberculosis infection, the most important are HIV infection, end-stage renal disease, cancer, diabetes, malnutrition, corticosteroid use, intravenous drug use.[15]

Primary Infection

Once present in the alveoli, the bacilli may replicate extracellularly or, more typically, are ingested by alveolar macrophages where they are either killed or replicated intracellularly. If infection is established, localized granulomas, or tubercles, develop within 2-6 weeks and are characterized by caseation necrosis and calcification. The bacilli also are transported to regional lymph nodes, where the infection may also be contained. Evidence of this primary infection is the "Ghon complex," defined as a peripheral lung lesion (the tubercle) and calcified hilar lymph nodes.[2,15,16,17]

Some individuals develop clinically apparent primary tuberculosis with fever, cough, and infiltrates on chest radiograph. Others will develop symptoms of pleurisy with an effusion, representing a local hypersensitivity reaction to the tubercle bacilli. Usually, however, the immune system limits replication and spread of the bacilli during this primary infection. Patients are typically asymptomatic, although the organisms may remain viable and dormant for many years. In these individuals, the only indication of primary infection is conversion to a positive reaction to the tuberculin purified protein derivative (PPD) skin test. Acid-fast bacilli are not present in the sputum.[2]

Tubercle bacilli also may enter the bloodstream via the thoracic duct, resulting in widespread dissemination. However, the majority of bacilli do not survive hematogenous dissemination. Tuberculosis requires high amounts of oxygen and blood flow to maintain viability and the ability to grow. These environmental requirements are readily available in the apical or posterior segments of the upper lobes of the lungs, superior segment of the lower lobes of the lungs, and, less commonly, the renal cortex, meninges, long bone epiphyses, and vertebrae.

Reactivation Disease

Reactivation of tuberculosis is the most common form of clinically apparent disease. Immunocompetent individuals with tuberculosis infection will have a 10% chance of developing reactivation disease during their lifetimes.[13] The risk appears to be greatest during the initial two years following exposure, and is highest in young adults. In immunocompromised individuals and the pediatric population, transition to active disease may occur rapidly.[13,14] Overall, in HIV positive patients, the risk of acquiring active TB is approximately 10% per year.[15]

Reactivation tubercular disease occurs after a variable latent period when the immune system can no longer contain foci of dormant bacilli. Typical triggers for reactivation are advancing age, malignancy, AIDS, corticosteroid therapy, viral illness, malnutrition, and even emotional stress.[2] Disease is accompanied by the signs and symptoms of a chronic wasting illness in the majority of patients. Individuals may experience generalized, nonspecific symptoms such as malaise, night sweats, low grade fever, weight loss, as well as symptoms specific to the site where reactivation occurs.[4,8,15,11,19]

Pulmonary Disease

Eighty percent of individuals with reactivation tuberculosis exhibit pulmonary disease. Most commonly, the apical and posterior segments of the upper lobes or the superior segments of the lower lobes are involved. Disease may range from virtually no symptoms to severe, destructive disease. Without effective therapy, active pulmonary tuberculosis pursues a progressive and chronic course. The overall death rate of untreated pulmonary disease may be as high as 60%, with a median time to death of 2.5 years after onset. With proper treatment, diseased areas may heal with very little permanent damage.[4,8,15]

Chronic cough with scant sputum production and hemoptysis are the principal respiratory symptoms. Hemoptysis is typically limited to blood streaking of sputum. As the pulmonary lesions progress, they undergo central caseation necrosis. Pulmonary architecture may be lost and there may be pulmonary fibrosis, volume loss, and upward retraction of the lungs. The lesions can erode into bronchi, with resultant spread throughout the airways and bleeding. Bronchopulmonary fistulas may cause severe respiratory compromise and require operative management. Cavitary lesions also can rupture into the pleural space causing empyemas, which require surgical drainage. The lesions also may erode into pulmonary blood vessels. "Rasmussen's aneurysm," or rupture of a terminal pulmonary artery into a cavitary site, is a catastrophic complication.[4,8,15,11,19]

Table 1. Historical and Symptomatic Clues to Infection with Tuberculosis

Consider the diagnosis of tuberculosis in any patient presenting to the ED with the following symptoms:
- Cough > 3 weeks duration
- Night sweats
- Bloody sputum/hemoptysis
- Weight loss
- Fever
- Anorexia

Or with a history of:
- Exposure to tuberculosis
- Institutionalization
- HIV infection
- Positive PPD

Extrapulmonary Disease

Tubercle bacilli may reach a number of extrapulmonary sites through hematogenous or lymphatic dissemination. Extrapulmonary tuberculosis may develop during the primary tuberculosis infection or with reactivation disease. It may present with localized symptoms, reflecting focal infection, or with dramatic systemic symptoms, most notably in the case of miliary tuberculosis.[2,11] Extrapulmonary disease, regardless of site, tends to respond well to systemic antituberculosis medical therapy.

Miliary tuberculosis results from hematogenous spread of tubercle bacilli, with tuberculous lesions developing synchronously throughout the body. Patients typically experience generalized symptoms of fever, chills, and weight loss. Although a cough may be present, acid-fast organisms will rarely be seen in the sputum. When occurring during reactivation disease, miliary tuberculosis progresses in a much more destructive and fulminant pattern.[8] On physical exam, hepatomegaly, splenomegaly, and adenopathy may be apparent. Patients generally become ill-appearing prior to the development of the characteristic radiographic findings. Diagnosis can be made via bronchoscopy, bronchial alveolar lavage, or bone marrow biopsy.[11]

Pleural disease typically has an abrupt onset and is characterized by significant pleuritic pain. Young individuals without evidence of pulmonary tuberculosis infection are most likely to develop pleurisy. If left untreated, the symptoms resolve spontaneously; however, two-thirds of these patients progress to active pulmonary disease within five years.[8] Asymptomatic pleural effusions commonly occur with reactivation disease as a peripheral lesion erodes into the pleural space.

Pericarditis may present with fever, pericardial pain, and possibly a pericardial friction rub. As with pericarditis of other etiologies, complications can include pericardial tamponade and chronic constrictive cardiac dysfunction.[11]

Peritonitis presents with ascites and is frequently erroneously attributed to cirrhosis. The course is insidious in onset and indolent in nature. Acid-fast stains as well as cultures of the ascitic fluid are rarely positive, making diagnosis difficult.

Laryngeal tuberculosis is of special concern as it is highly infectious. It develops in association with advanced pulmonary disease. The laryngeal mucosa is seeded with infectious bacilli that are expelled with expectoration. The infection may be a superficial ulceration or granuloma, but other structures including the epiglottis or hypopharynx may also be affected. The chief complaint, in addition to pulmonary symptoms, is typically hoarseness.[2,8,11,17,20]

Lymph node infection (adenitis) secondary to tuberculosis may occur anywhere but is most common in the cervical chain. Scrofula is a chronic lymphadenitis of the cervical nodes, usually located just inferior to the mandible. The nodes are non-tender and initially have a rubbery consistency but harden as infection progresses. Chronic infection may lead to draining cutaneous fistulas.[11,17,20]

Skeletal System. Tuberculosis may infect any bone but is frequently found in the long bone epiphyses, particularly those of large weight-bearing bones, and in the vertebral bodies. Pott's disease, infection of the vertebral bodies, most commonly affects the mid-thoracic region and may present as spontaneous compression fractures and associated spinal cord injury.[2,4,8,15,17,20]

Genitourinary System. Renal tuberculosis presents with hematuria or microscopic sterile pyuria. If untreated, patients can develop cavitation and permanent destruction of the renal parenchyma, in addition to scarring and strictures of the ureters and bladder. The prostate, seminal vesicles, and epididymis may all be infected, becoming edematous and indurated but remaining non-tender. Tuberculosis salpingitis can result in sterility.

Central nervous system (CNS) infection is more likely to be acute in children and chronic in adults. Acute infection is characterized by typical signs and symptoms of meningitis: fever, headache, neck stiffness. Chronic infection manifests with similar signs and symptoms; however, the course may be more indolent. Interestingly, approximately 30% of patients with chronic meningitis exhibit cranial nerve deficits. Cranial nerve deficits are caused by spread of infection to the meninges, where a basilar meningitis can develop. Focal tuberculomas can produce focal neurologic deficits that can include cranial nerve palsies ranging from hoarseness to diplopia and visual disturbances.[2,4,8,11,17,20]

Diagnosis

Infection with *M. tuberculosis* is sometimes difficult to diagnose due to the variety of presentations and the time required for cultures to develop. However, it is an important consideration in the ED, as proper isolation procedures and diagnostic measures should be undertaken as quickly as possible. Pulmonary tuberculosis should be considered in any patient demonstrating the characteristics described in *Table 1*.[9] Immediate steps, including facial masks and isolation procedures, should be implemented to limit the spread of infection when tuberculosis is suspected.

Laboratory Diagnosis. Samples of sputum or other body fluids suspected of infection should be sent for both acid-fast stain and tuberculosis culture. While up to 80% of patients with active pulmonary infection will demonstrate acid-fast organisms on the initial sputum smear, a negative acid-fast-stain does not eliminate the possibility of infection.[8] Sputum culture is the "gold standard" for diagnosing tuberculosis infection, but it can require 3-6 weeks to obtain final results.[11] Blood cultures for mycobacteria may be obtained; while cultures are positive in the minority of patients, they may yield a diagnosis faster than sputum cultures.[21] Newer, commercially available DNA probes that use polymerase chain reactions (PCR) are available for more rapid identification of tuberculosis in sputum, tissue specimen, and blood samples.[22-24] Their use is limited by cost and the time required to obtain results.

To ensure identification, smears and cultures should be performed on three different days in patients with high risk of infection.[9] If sputum is not available, samples may be obtained via nasotracheal aspiration, bronchoscopy, bronchoalveolar lavage or early morning gastric aspiration. Positive acid fast-stains are unusual with tuberculosis-related pleural effusions. Occasionally surgical biopsy of an infected site is indicated (particularly with tuberculous adenitis) and a microbiologic diagnosis is made from the biopsy specimen. All cultures should have susceptibility testing performed as well.

Other laboratory studies generally yield nonspecific results. The CBC may show a minor anemia and monocytosis of between 8-12%. The sedimentation rate is typically elevated. Patients with miliary tuberculosis may also develop hyponatremia, thrombocytopenia, and leukopenia. Cerebrospinal fluid (CSF) analysis must be performed if tuberculous meningitis is suspected. Infected CSF shows low glucose and high protein levels, while cell counts reveal granulocytosis in acute disease and lymphocytosis with chronic disease.[11] It should be stressed that the diagnosis of tuberculous meningitis is difficult to make, and that additional quantities of CSF may be required to enhance culture results and improve yield of AFB positive smears. Analysis of tuberculous pleural effusions shows exudative properties with low pH, low glucose, and high protein. Again, granulocytes predominate in acute effusions, lymphocytes in chronic effusions.

Chest radiographs are critical to the diagnosis of pulmonary tuberculosis. While serial films are generally necessary to distinguish active from non-active infection, a single chest x-ray can be invaluable in identifying potentially infectious individuals. The classic finding in symptomatic primary infection is a small, parenchymal infiltrate in any region of the lung associated with unilateral hilar adenopathy. As the primary infection resolves, this lesion calcifies into a nodule. Other patients with primary infection may exhibit unilateral pleural effusions or no radiologic abnormalities at all.

The chest x-ray in patients with reactivation pulmonary tuberculosis classically demonstrates infiltrates in the apical and posterior segments of the upper lobes or in the superior segments of the lower lobes. Cavitation is frequently present in regions of substantial infiltration. Lordotic views, taken in an anterior-posterior fashion with the patient leaning backward against the x-ray plate, allow better visualization of the lung apices and may be helpful in identifying infiltrate in regions that may be obscured by the upper ribs or the clavicles.[25] The typical finding in miliary tuberculosis are soft, fine, uniformly distributed nodules throughout both lung fields.

As the tubercular lesions heal, fibrotic scarring with loss of pulmonary volume is apparent. The lungs and hilar regions may be retracted upward and medially, the trachea may be deviated and atelectasis may be present. Atypical chest x-ray findings may manifest more frequently in certain patient populations, particularly the immunocompromised, and are discussed in the section on special considerations.

Skin Testing. The Mantoux skin test is used to measure delayed-type hypersensitivity to the tubercle bacillus. It is commonly referred to as the "PPD," as tuberculosis purified protein derivative is introduced beneath the skin of the volar or dorsal aspect of the forearm. The test is a reliable method of recognizing prior infection, however, it is neither perfectly sensitive nor specific.[9] The test should be interpreted by trained individuals 48-72 hours following placement. The diameter of the region of induration, not erythema, should be measured. *Table 2* describes criteria for positive reactions.[9]

False-positive reactions are possible as a result of exposure to non-pathological mycobacterial disease (e.g., *M. avium* complex), but not as a result of allergy to PPD components or previous testing. False-negative reactions are seen with advancing age, in individuals who have received BCG, have had recent tuberculosis infection, and are immunosuppressed.[8] In fact, as many as 25% of all individuals with active tuberculosis may have a negative skin test at the time of initial presentation due to transient immunosuppression, and the majority of patients with miliary tuberculosis will have negative tests.[2] Such individuals may be responsive to skin testing performed a few weeks later. This is called the "booster phenomenon." An anergy panel (skin testing with antigens to which most individuals will be hypersensitive) should be performed when a PPD test is negative in a patient suspected of having tuberculosis.

Treatment

Post-Exposure Prophylaxis. Because tuberculosis is a disease of relatively low communicability, post-exposure prophylaxis is generally not indicated unless the PPD skin test is positive. The exception to this is in children younger than 5 years of age, in whom empiric therapy with isoniazid (10 mg/kg/d) is indicated after tuberculosis exposure. Therapy may be discontinued if the PPD is negative at three months. Immunocompetent adults who remain PPD negative do not require empiric therapy.

Positive PPD Test. Prophylactic therapy should be considered for individuals with positive PPD reactions and negative chest x-rays. Criteria for initiating preventative treatment are listed in *Table 3*.[9] The potential risks and benefits of prophylactic therapy should be analyzed and may differ between patients. The likelihood of a positive PPD secondary to tuberculosis, and not other mycobacterial infection, should be assessed. The risk of progression to active disease should be weighed against the very small risk of hepatitis or other adverse reaction to drug therapy. Because health care workers are at higher risk for contracting tuberculosis and have the potential to transmit infection to large numbers of ill individuals, special considerations are made when determining whether or not to offer preventative treatment to this group.

Table 2. Interpretation of PPD Results

1. **Induration greater than or equal to 5 mm considered positive in:**
   - HIV positive individuals
   - persons with recent close contact to individual with active tuberculosis
   - persons with chest x-ray consistent with healed tuberculosis
2. **Induration greater than or equal to 10 mm considered positive in:**
   High-Risk Groups
   - intravenous drug users who are HIV negative
   - patients with chronic illness at risk for reactivation (silicosis, chronic renal failure, diabetes mellitus, chronic steroid use, hematologic disorders, malignancy)
   - children younger than 4 years of age

   High-Prevalence Groups
   - immigrants from endemic regions (Asia, Africa, Latin America, Caribbean)
   - residents of long-term care facilities (nursing homes, prisons, etc.)
   - persons from medically underserved, low-income populations
3. **Induration greater than or equal to 15 mm considered positive in all persons.**
4. **Recent conversion criteria:**
   - increase greater than or equal to 10 mm within two years in individuals younger than 35 years of age
   - increase greater than or equal to 15 mm within two years in individuals 35 years of age or older
5. **Interpretation of PPD testing in health care workers:**
   - follow guidelines 1-3
   - facilities with a high prevalence of tuberculosis patients may consider induration 10 mm in individ uals without other risk factors as a positive reaction
   - recent conversion is increase in induration 10 mm in two-year period in high-prevalence facilities, 15 mm in low-prevalence facilities

Table 3. Preventive Therapy Considerations

GENERAL POPULATION
- Individuals < 35 years of age with positive reaction to PPD (including children)
- HIV-positive patients with positive PPD reactions
- Anergic Individuals with recent, known contact to person(s) with active tuberculosis
- Children with known TB exposure, even if PPD negative

HEALTH CARE WORKERS
(in addition to above recommendations)
- Recent PPD conversion
- Close contact of individual with active tuberculosis
- HIV positive, regardless of PPD reaction
- Intravenous drug users
- Medical condition that increases risk of progression to active disease

Table 4. Preventive Therapy Recommendations

ISONIAZID
300 mg po daily in adults
10 mg/kg po daily in children

DURATION
6-12 months in otherwise healthy adults
9 months in children
12 months in HIV positive individuals

Specific recommendations for medical prophylaxis are described in *Table 4*.[9] If the risk of primary infection with multi-drug resistant tuberculosis is high, multi-drug preventative therapy should be considered.[9] In individuals with positive reactions to PPD and chest radiographs demonstrating either silicosis or fibrotic disease, but who are without evidence of active infection, preventative therapy with isoniazid and rifampin for four months, or isoniazid alone for 12 months is acceptable.[9]

Treatment of Active Disease. Single-drug therapy is no longer recommended because of the prevalence of drug-resistant tuberculosis. Currently, four-drug initial therapy is recommended until specific susceptibilities of isolates are known. *Table 5* and *Table 6* outline specific therapeutic regimens.[9,16] Adherence to these guidelines will effectively treat at least 95% of patients.[16] Additionally, sputum culture conversion to negative will occur more rapidly using a four- rather than three-drug regimen.[16] Approximately 85% of patients will become culture negative within two months of starting therapy.[4,15] Administration of drugs in a directly observed therapy program increases the effectiveness of therapy and may benefit individuals in whom compliance is questionable. Practitioners should consult other sources for information regarding medicolegal considerations pertaining to quarantine, mandatory hospitalization, and noncompliance with treatment.

Special Considerations

Tuberculosis in HIV Infection. Infection with HIV has played an important role in the recent resurgence of tuberculosis. Infection with tuberculosis is 500 times more common in AIDS patients than the general population. The demographic groups with the highest increase in prevalence of HIV infection, that is African-American and Hispanic males between 25-44 years of age, have also demonstrated the largest increase in tuberculosis infection. Additionally, cities and states with large numbers of HIV-infected persons have the largest increase in tuberculosis infection.[6] In the United States, co-infection

Table 5. Dosage Recommendations for Treatment of Tuberculosis in Children and Adults

DRUG	DAILY		TWO TIMES/WEEK		THREE TIMES/WEEK	
	Children	Adults	Children	Adults	Children	Adults
Isoniazid (INH)	10-20 mg/kg Max. 300 mg	5 mg/kg Max. 300 mg	20-40 mg/kg Max. 900 mg	15 mg/kg Max. 900 mg	20-40 mg/kg Max. 900 mg	15 mg/kg Max. 900 mg
Rifampin (RIF)	10-20 mg/kg Max. 600 mg	10 mg/kg Max. 600 mg	10-20 mg/kg Max. 600 mg	10 mg/kg Max. 600 mg	10-20 mg/kg Max. 600 mg	10 mg/kg Max. 600 mg
Pyrazinamide (PZA)	15-30 mg/kg Max. 2 g	15-30 mg/kg Max. 2 g	50-70 mg/kg Max. 4 g	50-70 mg/kg Max. 4 g	50-70 mg/kg Max. 3 g	50-70 mg/kg Max. 3 g
Ethambutol (EMB)	15-25 mg/kg Max. 2.5 g	5-25 mg/kg Max. 2.5 g	50 mg/kg Max. 2.5 g	50 mg/kg Max. 2.5 g	25-30 mg/kg Max. 2.5 g	25-30 mg/kg Max. 2.5 g
Streptomycin (SM)	20-30 mg/kg Max. 1 g	15 mg/kg Max. 1 g	25-30 mg/kg Max. 1.5 g	25-30 mg/kg Max. 1.5 g	25-30 mg/kg Max. 1 g	25-30 mg/kg Max. 1 g

is most frequent in those patients who acquired HIV via intravenous drug use, or in immigrants from Haiti or Central Africa.[12] The risk of development of active disease is 10% per year in these groups, compared to a 10% lifetime risk in immunocompetent individuals.[13]

Active tuberculosis infection develops in more than half of AIDS patients previously infected with tuberculosis. Tuberculosis typically presents sooner than other AIDS-defining illnesses, thus making it an AIDS-defining illness in HIV-positive individuals.[6,8,11] Patients with co-infection progress faster to active tuberculous disease following primary exposure than do HIV-negative patients.[6] Mortality rates of co-infection can be as high as 14-44%.[11]

Impaired host immunity is the most likely cause of the high morbidity and mortality of co-infection. Macrophage microbicidal activity is abnormal in AIDS patients, due to a lack of activation factors supplied by CD4+ cells.[1] It has also been suggested that tuberculosis may increase the active expression of HIV, thereby further weakening an already impaired immune system.[4] Interpretation of the PPD skin test can certainly be confused by this immunodeficient state. Of patients with culture proven infection and CD4+ counts greater than 100, only 64% displayed positive reactions to PPD. That percentage dropped to 0% in patients with CD4+ count less than 100.[13] Thus, a negative reaction to PPD does not rule out infection. HIV-positive patients suspected of tuberculosis infection should receive anergy panel testing to assess the effectiveness of their immune response when their PPD is negative.

The vast majority of AIDS patients with tuberculosis will develop pulmonary manifestations of disease. However, tuberculosis may be difficult to distinguish from other HIV-related pulmonary infections.[5] Other considerations include Kaposi's sarcoma, lymphoma, fungal infections, and *Pneumocystis carinii*. Approximately half of patients display atypical patterns on chest x-ray, but in the majority, the pattern is suggestive of tuberculosis.[8,13,26] The most frequent findings are hilar adenopathy, pleural effusion, predominate upper lobe infiltrate, miliary pattern, or cavitation.[13] Patterns consistent with miliary disease are more common after the CD4+ count falls below 100, whereas cavitation and pleural effusion are more common when CD4+ counts are higher than 200. The presence of HIV infection does not affect the frequency with which sputum cultures are positive for acid-fact bacilli.[27] Mycobacterial bacteremia, however, may be more common in HIV-infected patients, adding to the diagnostic yield of blood cultures in these individuals.[21]

The rate of extrapulmonary tuberculosis is very high in HIV-infected individuals: 70% of AIDS patients with TB exhibit extrapulmonary manifestations of primary infection or reactivation.[8,26] There appears to be an inverse relationship between the frequency of extrapulmonary disease and CD4+ counts: 64% of patients with CD4+ counts less than 100 experience extrapulmonary disease, compared to 37% in those with counts greater than 200. Most frequently, extrapulmonary disease is manifested by lymphadenitis and bacteremia. It should be stressed that fever is often absent in HIV-infected patients, and that the presentation may be limited to headache in a non-toxic appearing patient. Thus, blood cultures should be performed in addition to other studies in all patients with suspicion of tuberculosis infection.[13] Patients commonly present with tender adenopathy, fever, and weight loss. Overall, blood cultures are positive in 26-42% of AIDS patients with active tuberculosis, but again this rate varies inversely with CD4+ count. Meningitis is not uncommon, with a five-fold higher rate than in patients without associated HIV infection. CNS mass lesions and intraparenchymal disease are also more common.[13]

Treatment. Response to tuberculosis therapy in HIV-infected patients is similar to that in immunocompetent individuals.[28,29] Treatment of active disease is therefore the same as that outlined for the general population in *Table 6*. The American Thoracic Society/CDC guidelines stipulate that a slow or suboptimal response—clinically or microbiologically—may necessitate prolonging the treatment course. AIDS patients experience an increased incidence of adverse drug reactions, which may lead to alteration of treatment regimens.[26,29] Malabsorptive states can certainly impair the absorption of antituberculosis medications in HIV-infected individuals, although dosage adjustment is not recommended at this time.[30] Treatment failure rates vary between 0-16%, and of those patients with an adequate response, 0-15% will relapse.[11] There is a significant potential for interaction with anti-HIV medications and thus regimens often require adjustment. Protease inhibitor therapy should be stopped during tuberculosis treatment.[28] Long-term anti-tuberculous maintenance therapy is not recommended.[29]

Multidrug-Resistant Tuberculosis

Perhaps the most concerning aspect of the recent resurgence of tuberculosis is the increasing occurrence of drug resistant strains. Multidrug-resistant tuberculosis (MDR-TB) is defined as resistance to both isoniazid and rifampin, and possibly other drugs.[31] Incomplete, sporadic, or erratic treatment of tuberculosis creates selective influences favoring growth of drug resistant bacilli over those that are susceptible.[1,31] Other factors contributing to the rise in drug resistance are inappropriate therapy, the change from in-patient to poorly supervised out-patient management, delay in diagnosis, ineffective infection control, and transmission in institutionalized settings.[1,3,6]

The strongest predictor of the presence of MDR-TB is previous treatment with anti-tuberculous medications.[6,31] Yet, at least 15% of newly diagnosed cases of tuberculosis are due to infection with MDR strains. A study conducted in New York City demonstrated that 79% of MDR-TB infections represented primary disease.[32] In a 1991 CDC survey, 14.2% of tuberculosis cases were resistant to at least one drug.[3] Of the resistant strains, more than half were resistant to one drug, one-quarter were resistant to two drugs, and 4% were resistant to five or more drugs. Drug-resistant strains are concentrated in large, urban regions: New York City had 54 times the rate of MDR-TB as the rest of the country. Minorities have a dramatically higher rate of MDR-TB. Transmission of MDR-TB to health care workers has been described, as has nosocomial transmission of MDR-TB via contaminated bronchoscopes.[1,3,6,33]

Pulmonary disease develops in more than 90% of patients with active MDR-TB.[3] These patients are more likely than drug-susceptible patients to have positive acid fast smears and are more likely to transmit infection to other individuals.[3] In some outbreaks of MDR-TB, up to 96% of patients with active disease also are HIV infected.[13,34] Immunocompromised patients develop disease much more rapidly, with a median time to death of 4-16 weeks, and have a mortality as high as 89%.[3,6] Other predictors of MDR-TB disease include persistent fever lasting more than two weeks and presence of hilar or mediastinal lymphadenopathy.[6]

Treatment should be based on the local rates of drug resistance. In regions with rates of MDR-TB higher than 4%, all patients with newly diagnosed tuberculosis should be treated with at least four drugs until susceptibility results are available. In regions with rates lower than 4%, treatment with three drugs is appropriate.[6,31] Treatment strategies are outlined in *Table 6*.[1,16]

Table 6. Initial Treatment Options for Tuberculosis in Adults and Children

HIV NEGATIVE

Option 1
INH + RIF + PZA + (EMB or SM) daily for eight weeks followed by INH + RIF daily or 2-3 times weekly for 16 weeks
Regimen may be tailored following results of susceptibility testing.

Option 2
INH + RIF + PZA + (EMB or SM) daily for two weeks followed by same drugs two times/week for six weeks followed by:
INH + RIF two times/week for 16 weeks.

Option 3
INH + RIF + PZA + (EMB or SM) 3 times/week for six months

HIV POSITIVE

Option 4
Options 1, 2, or 3 for a total of nine months and at least six months following culture conversion to negative.

Tuberculosis in Children

The rise in tuberculosis in the pediatric population reflects the increase in adult transmission.[35] Tuberculosis is present primarily in minority children living in large urban regions. While the majority are born in the United States, they may have parents who immigrated from endemic regions. There appears to be no gender predilection.[18] Approximately 60% of infected children are younger than age 5—those who are at highest risk to develop active disease.[18]

Diagnosing tuberculosis in children can be difficult, and similar studies should be obtained on children as in the adult population. Skin testing with PPD should be interpreted in the same manner as adults, but 5% of children with culture-proven tuberculosis have negative reactions to PPD.[10] Chest x-ray findings mimic those of adults, with presence of a Ghon complex indicating healed primary infection.[35] Sputum or other appropriate cultures should be obtained, including early morning gastric aspiration in children unable to produce adequate sputum cultures. All cultures should have susceptibility testing performed.

The primary infection is commonly asymptomatic, manifesting only as a positive PPD reaction with normal chest x-ray.[17] Progression to active disease is more frequent in infants and immunocompromised children, possibly due to their less developed or impaired immune systems. Active pulmonary disease develops in 40% of untreated children younger than 1 year old, 24% of children 1-5 years old, and 15% of children 11-15 years old.[14]

Progressive primary pulmonary infection occurs when the primary peripheral infectious focus forms a large caseous lesion, which may drain into a bronchus, forming a cavitary lesion and leading to disseminated disease.[17] These children appear ill, with fever, weight loss, malaise, and chronic cough.[17] Chest x-ray findings are similar to those of adults. Uncommonly, children develop chronic pulmonary tuberculosis which is analagous to reactivation pulmonary tuberculosis in adults.

The pediatric population demonstrates a higher rate of extrapulmonary tuberculosis than adults, with 30% of children with active tuberculosis developing extrapulmonary disease.[18] Lymphadenitis is the most common, followed by meningeal, pleural, miliary, musculoskeletal, and other infection manifestations.[17] The hilar and mediastinal nodes are most commonly affected and can become significantly enlarged, leading to bronchial obstruction.[18]

Tuberculous meningitis is the most common cause of pediatric death due to tuberculosis.[17] It is most frequent in children younger than age 6, and develops within 3-6 months from the time of primary infection.[18] Disease is characterized by an insidious onset over 1-3 weeks and consists of three stages. Stage 1 typically occurs over 1-2 weeks and demonstrates non-specific signs and symptoms of fever, anorexia, emesis, personality changes, apathy, and loss of play interest. During this stage, no neurologic deficits are evident. Stage 2 begins as intracranial pressure increases, with signs of meningeal irritation and cerebral dysfunction such as drowsiness, emesis, stiff neck, seizures, tremors, and slurred speech. Focal neurological deficits, such as asymmetric pupils and cranial nerve palsies, may be present. Stage 3 is characterized by obtundation, decerebrate or decorticate posturing, irregular respirations, and coma.[17]

Another serious complication of disseminated disease in children is miliary tuberculosis. Infants appear to be at highest risk. Disease is characterized by acute onset of fever, lethargy, anorexia, and generalized weakness. Respiratory signs and symptoms are usually absent. Physical exam may reveal hepatomegaly, splenomegaly, and lymphadenopathy. One-third to one-half of patients with miliary disease also will develop meningitis.

Transmission Prevention

Minimizing the risk of exposure to and transmission of tuberculosis is a concern to all health care workers. PPD conversion in health care workers is not infrequent, and occurs with both drug-susceptible and drug-resistant strains of tuberculosis. As emergency physicians, the likelihood of caring for patients with active, and potentially transmittable disease is high. Thus, proactive measures must be taken to prevent exposure and transmission.

Effective tuberculosis control policies should exist in all facilities. Three levels of preventative measures should be used to minimize the risk of transmission.

Level I: Administrative Measures. This first level of transmission prevention attempts to reduce risk through education of health care workers and implementation of policies to identify and isolate potentially infectious individuals.[9] Education and training regarding effective preventative measures (e.g., respiratory protection and proper use of isolation rooms) should be provided to all health care workers.[9] Policies outlining identification and isolation of high-risk patients should be developed, implemented, and emphasized. Additionally, annual PPD screening of all health care workers should be performed, except in areas with high risk of exposure. These areas require PPD screening on a bi-annual basis.

Level II: Environmental/Engineering Controls. Effective environmental controls can significantly reduce risk of transmission but do not completely eliminate risk. These interventions help contain the spread and reduce the number of infectious droplet nuclei present in the air.

Source control is important in reducing transmission. Once high-risk patients are identified, they should be instructed to cover their mouth and nose when coughing and sneezing; a surgical mask may be placed on the patient for the same purpose. These interventions are not entirely effective in preventing dissemination of droplet nuclei.

High-risk patients should be placed in an adequate, single-patient, isolation room. Negative pressure rooms prevent flow of droplet nuclei into adjacent areas of the facility. The door should remain closed and, if possible, an anteroom with relatively positive pressure should separate the isolation room from the common corridor. Adequate ventilation is perhaps the most important intervention, and at least six complete room air exchanges per hour are necessary.[9] The exhaust from the rooms should be filtered via high-efficiency particulate filters and directed outside the hospital. The exhaust should never be recirculated into the general facility ventilatory system.

Mycobacteria were first hypothesized to be susceptible to ultraviolet (UV) germicidal irradiation after the observation that tuberculosis was rarely transmitted outdoors during daylight. While research has demonstrated the ability of UV light to destroy bacilli, no clinical trials have proven its efficacy in the clinical setting.[12] Despite this, UV light is widely used as an adjunct to air exchange. The source light should be placed above eye level (to prevent keratitis) and in a location where room air has maximal exposure.

Level III: Personal Respiratory Equipment. Use of personalized, fitted masks with efficient filters by health care workers is required by OSHA to further discourage transmission. However, their use remains controversial as their safety and efficacy has yet to be proven.[16]

Summary

Tuberculosis presents many different faces and requires customized treatment and diagnostic strategies depending upon the patient subgroup in which the disease is encountered. Although long-term treatment and definitive diagnosis of TB occur beyond the province of the ED, the ED physician must be able to recognize the wide spectrum of possible clinical presentations and measures for disease prevention. Finally, the ED physician must be aware of indications for treatment and prophylaxis, and the problems posed by multi-drug resistant TB.

References

1. Kent JH. The epidemiology of multidrug-resistant tuberculosis in the United States. *Med Clin North Am* 1993;77:1391-1409.
2. Ellner JJ. Tuberculosis. In: Kelley WN, ed. *Textbook of Internal Medicine.* New York: Lippincott; 1989:1569-1577.
3. Bloch AB, Cauthen GM, Onorato IM, et al. Nationwide survey of drug-resistant tuberculosis in the United States. *JAMA* 1994;271:665-671.
4. Bloom, BR, Murray CJL. Tuberculosis: Commentary on a reemergent killer. *Science* 1992,257:1055-1064.
5. Rom WN, Zhang Y. The rising tide of tuberculosis and the human host response to *Mycobacterium tuberculosis. J Lab Clin Med* 1993;121:737-741.
6. Segal-Maurer S, Urban C, Rahal JJ, et al. Current perspectives on multidrug-resistant bacteria. *Infect Dis Clin N Am* 1996;10:

939-957.

7. Cantwell MF, Snider DE, Cauthen GM, et al. Epidemiology of tuberculosis in the United States, 1985 through 1992. *JAMA* 1994;272:535-539.
8. Daniel TM. Tuberculosis. In: Wilson JD, et al, eds. *Harrison's Principles of Internal Medicine.* 12th ed. New York: McGraw Hill; 1991:637-645.
9. Centers for Disease Control and Prevention. Guidelines for preventing the transmission of *Mycobacterium tuberculosis* in health care facilities, 1994. *MMWR Morb Mortal Wkly Rep* 1994;43:1-111.
10. Abernathy RS. Tuberculosis: An update. *Pediatr Rev* 1997;18: 50-58.
11. Welch RD. Tuberculosis. In: Tintinalli JE, et al, eds. *Emergency Medicine—A Comprehensive Study Guide.* 4th ed. New York: McGraw Hill; 1996:422-425.
12. Nardell EA. Environmental control of tuberculosis. *Med Clin North Am* 1993;77:1315-1334.
13. Barnes PF, Le HQ, Davidson PT. Tuberculosis in patients with HIV infection. *Med Clin North Am* 1993;77:1369-1389.
14. Starke JR. Childhood tuberculosis in the 1990's. *Pediatr Ann* 1993;22:550-560.
15. ATS/CDC. Treatment of TB and tuberculosis infection in adults and children. *Am J Crit Care Med* 1994;149:1359-1374.
16. Centers for Disease Control and Prevention. Initial therapy for tuberculosis in the era of multidrug resistance. *MMWR Morb Mortal Wkly Rep* 1993;42:1-7.
17. Waagner DC. The clinical presentation of tuberculous disease in children. *Pediatr Ann* 1993;22:622.
18. Starke JR. Childhood tuberculosis in the 1990's. *Pediatr Ann* 1993;22:550-560.
19. Schutze GE, Jacobs RF. Treatment of tuberculosis infection and disease. *Pediatr Ann* 1993;22:631-39.
20. Vallejo JG, Ong LT, Starke JR. Clinical features, diagnosis and treatment of tuberculosis in infants. *Pediatrics* 1994;94:1-7.
21. Bouza E, Diaz-Lopez MD, Moreno S, et al. *Mycobacterium tuberculosis* bacteremia in patients with and without HIV. *Arch Intern Med* 1993;153:496-500.
22. Condos R, McClune A, Rom WN. Periperal blood-based PCR assay to identify patients with active pulmonary tuberculosis. *Lancet* 1996;347:1082-1085.
23. Bradley SP, Reed SL, Catanzaro A. Clinical efficacy of the amplified *M. tuberculosis* direct test for diagnosis of pulmonary tuberculosis. *Am J Resp Crit Care Med* 1996;153:1606-1610.
24. Rish JA, Eisenach KD, Cave MD, et al. Polymerase chain reaction detection of *M tuberculosis* in formalin-fixed tissue. *Am J Resp Crit Care Med* 1996;153:1419-1423.
25. Squire LF, Novelline RA. *Fundamentals of Radiology,* 4th ed. Cambridge: Harvard University Press, 1998:16.
26. Perlman DC, el-Sadr WM, Nelson ET, et al. Variation of chest x-ray pattern in pulmonary TB by degree of HIV-related immune suppression. *Clin Infect Dis* 1997,25: 242-246.
27. Smith RL, Yew K, Berkowitz KA. Factors affecting the yield of acid-fast sputum smears in patients with HIV and tuberculosis. *Chest* 1994;106:684-686.
28. Sanford JP, Gilbert DN, Moellering RC, et al. *Guide to Antimicrobial Therapy,* 27th ed. Vienna, VA: Antimicrobial Therapy, Inc; 1997:74-76.
29. Small PM, Schecter GF, Goodman PC, et al. Treatment of tuberculosis in patients with advanced HIV infection. *N Engl J Med* 1991;342:289-294.
30. Sahai J, Gallicano K, Swick L, et al. Reduced plasma concentrations of antituberculosis drugs in patients with HIV infection. *Ann Intern Med* 1997;127:289-293.
31. Iseman MD. Treatment of multidrug-resistant tuberculosis. *N Engl J Med* 1993;329:784-791.
32. Friedman CR, Stoeckle MY, Krieswirth BN, et al. Transmission of multidrug-resistant tuberculosis in a large urban setting. *Am J Resp Crit Care Med* 1995;152:355-359.
33. Jereb JA, Klevens RM, Privett TD, et al. Tuberculosis in health care workers at a hospital with an outbreak of MDR-TB. *Arch Intern Med* 1995;155:854-859.
34. Frieden TR, Sherman LF, Maw KL, et al. A multi-institutional outbreak of highly drug-resistant tuberculosis. *JAMA* 1996;276: 1229-1235.

Lyme Disease

Jonathan A. Edlow, MD

With the thaws and blossoms of spring arrive other, less-welcome offerings of nature: ticks and their propensity for producing an eclectic range of serious and sometimes life-threatening disorders. Human tick-borne diseases (TBD), which can cause significant morbidity and mortality in all age ranges, represent an important diagnostic challenge for emergency physicians, especially during the summer months.

Not surprisingly, clinical presentations for tick-related infections are highly variable. Signs, symptoms, and target organ damage can result from myriad mechanisms, including non-infectious inflammatory responses (hypersensitivity and toxin-mediated reactions), secondary bacterial infection associated with skin trauma, and primary inoculation into the skin of infectious agents that produce conditions ranging from babesiosis to Lyme disease (LD).

The most common vector-borne disease in the United States, LD was first described as a unified clinical entity in 1977 following an outbreak of statistically improbable childhood arthritis associated with a distinctive rash called erythema migrans (EM).[1] The description and geographical spread of LD, the recognition of two forms of human ehrlichiosis, and a growing appreciation of domestic babesiosis have sparked a renewed interest in TBD over the last 20 years. These three diseases, caused by different classes of microorganisms, share a common tick vector, and their increased prevalence is at least in part related to changes in our environment and the way we relate to it. Expansion of the deer herd in the Northeast, the incursion of people into more rural habitats, and increased recognition of TBD all play a role.[2,3]

Patients with TBD frequently develop acute illness and seek care in the ED. Thus, clinicians must know when antimicrobial therapy is indicated, indications for serological testing, and clinical findings that require lumbar puncture or hospitalization. This report will focus primarily on the early manifestations of LD but also will describe clinical manifestations of Rocky Mountain spotted fever (RMSF), babesiosis, and ehrlichiosis. Diagnostic tests will be highlighted and vaccines will be mentioned.

Epidemiology and Infectious Patterns

LD is by far the most common TBD in the United States and has been reported in nearly every state. Over the past several years, about 10,000 annual cases have been reported to the CDC,[4-6] though it is likely that 10 times that number occur.[7] In 1995, LD was reported in 43 states, but its frequency is highly patchy, with eight states (Connecticut, New York, Rhode Island, New Jersey, Delaware, Maryland, Pennsylvania, and Wisconsin), accounting for more than 80% of cases.[6] The seven states in which LD was not seen were Alaska, Hawaii, Colorado, Idaho, Montana, and North and South Dakota.

The incidence varies widely, from nine cases per 100,000 people in Maryland to 839 per 100,000 on Nantucket island off the

Massachusetts coast. Even within a given state, incidence varies widely by county. The overall incidence in the United States is 4.4 per 100,000.[6]

As would be expected, people whose jobs or recreational activities expose them to ticks have an increased risk of acquiring TBD. There appears to be no sex or age predilection. Nevertheless, CDC data show a bimodal peak, with 24% of cases occurring in children younger than 15 and another 24% of cases in adults between 35 and 49 years of age.[6] It should be emphasized that, in endemic areas, infected ticks can survive in well-maintained lawns.[8,9] Infection with LD and other tick-borne diseases also can occur in urban areas.[10]

Clinical Manifestations: Three Phases

The likelihood of acquiring infection following a single tick bite is low.[11,12] Following inoculation with *Borrelia burgdorferi*, the infecting organism of LD, three outcomes are possible with respect to the spirochete. First, the organisms can be completely eliminated by host defense mechanisms. Second, *Borrelia* can remain localized but viable in the skin.[13,14] Last, they can disseminate to other organs via bloodstream or lymphatics. Dissemination can occur quite rapidly.[15-17] With respect to clinical findings, *B. burgdorferi* appears to have a tropism for cutaneous, cardiac, nervous, and musculoskeletal tissues.[18]

From a practical, clinical perspective, LD has been divided into three stages: early localized disease (EM), early disseminated disease, and late disseminated disease. *(Please see Table 1.)* Typical late manifestations—including joint, skin, and nervous manifestations—occur many months to years after infection and are not discussed in this review. Asymptomatic patients presenting after tick bite will be discussed first.

Table 1. Lyme Disease: Clinical Stages

TICK BITE
EARLY, LOCALIZED DISEASE
Erythema migrans, solitary lesion
EARLY, DISSEMINATED DISEASE
Cutaneous—multiple erythema migrans
Neurologic—lymphocytic meningitis, cranial nerve palsies, meningoradiculitis
Cardiac—fluctuating degrees of AV block, myopericarditis, LV dysfunction
Musculoskeletal—migratory pain in joints and peri-articular soft tissues
Lymphatic—lymphadenopathy, splenomegaly
GI—abnormal hepatic transaminases
Ocular—conjunctivitis, keratitis, iritis
LATE, DISSEMINATED DISEASE
Cutaneous, neurologic, rheumatologic

Tick Bites: To Treat or Not to Treat

Tick-bite studies suggest that 24-48 hours of tick attachment is usually required for infection to occur.[19-21] The time delay is explained by the fact that in most unfed ticks, the spirochetes are localized to the midgut. After the tick attaches to the host for a blood meal, the organisms migrate to the salivary glands, a journey that requires hours to days.[22-24]

Although many authors state categorically that more than 24 hours of attachment is required for transmission, clinical and experimental data suggest that transmission is clearly possible within a shorter duration, although the frequency of this occurrence in North America is unknown. In one European study of 231 culture-confirmed cases of EM, data were reported on those 34 patients who specifically recalled not only the tick bite but also the duration of attachment. In nine of the 34, the duration of attachment was less than six hours, and in an additional 16 of the 34, it was less than 24 hours.[25] Moreover, clinical LD also has been documented after as little as six hours of attachment in North America.[26] This probably occurs because some ticks are infected systemically, and these ticks could transmit the disease faster.

Endemic Areas. Several studies have examined the likelihood of developing clinical infection with *B. burgdorferi* in individuals who have had a tick bite in areas endemic for LD.[11,12] Showing fairly consistent results, these studies demonstrate that 1-3% of patients develop the marker rash for EM after placebo treatment for a tick bite, even when the affected ticks had an infection rate of between 15-30%. Late symptoms or seroconversion were not seen in the placebo group. One possible methodological flaw in a larger study of more than 300 patients was that serologic follow-up was only done at six weeks and three months.[11,12] Only 75% of LD patients develop the marker rash of EM.[27] While serologic conversion likely would have occurred within the three-month window, it is possible that some patients who never developed EM could have seroconverted after the three months and developed late disease after one year of clinical follow-up.

Treatment Considerations. Based on these investigations, the official recommendation is not to treat tick bites with prophylactic antibiotics. As a general rule, this represents a prudent, outcome-effective approach to clinical management. However, each case should be considered individually, and the clinical decision in the emergency-medicine setting should be based on a number of relevant risk factors, historical features, and physical findings.

Without question, duration of tick attachment is a critical parameter influencing the likelihood of acquiring clinical infection. Generally speaking, the longer the duration of attachment, the greater the likelihood of disease transmission. The species of biting tick is also important because, as a rule, only *Ixodes* ticks are capable of transmitting the disease. Characterizing the species of tick in the ED, however, may be difficult. The morphological stage of the tick should also be documented, since adult ticks are twice as likely to be infected as nymphs, and larvae are very rarely infected.[3] Geography can play a decisive role in determining the need for emergency treatment. For example, in hyper-endemic areas, up to 50% of the *Ixodes scapularis* ticks can be infected, while in other areas, the rate is much lower.[26,28]

From a frontline, practical perspective, patient preference must enter into the management equation. Some patients, particularly those who live in endemic areas, are so anxious about acquiring LD that even after a thorough, reassuring explanation of the risks and options, a significant percentage will insist on antimicrobial prophylaxis and threaten go elsewhere if antibiotics are not prescribed. While there is no standard of "prophylactic" therapy for these situations, tick-bite studies that used a 10-day antibiotic course (amoxicillin in children, doxycycline in adults) have found no disease in the treatment groups.[11,12]

Early States of Lyme Disease: Localized Disease

Early localized LD refers to solitary EM, which is found in about 75% of infected patients.[27] Classic EM starts as a red macule or papule that characteristically appears 1-33 days (average, 7-10) after the tick bite and expands centrifugally while clearing centrally.[29] EM is generally flat, although the borders may be slightly raised. A central punctum resulting from the bite also may be present in some cases.[30] Median size of the rash is 15-16 cm, but EM can attain a sizes up to 73 cm. [25,27,29]

As a rule, the location of the rash reflects areas of the body where ticks frequently stop and feed, including the popliteal fossa, gluteal folds, groin, axilla, as well as areas where an elastic band of clothing presses against the skin. Despite a predilection for these sites, EM lesions can occur anywhere, though the hands and feet are distinctly unusual locations.[25,27,29]

The size of EM tends to be a function of the duration of infection. Typically, EM enlarges day by day, rather than over hours, and it does not remain stable over months. EM is associated with mild systemic symptoms such as fatigue, arthralgia, myalgia, headache, fever, chills, and stiff neck in about 40% of patients. Mild pruritis or pain sometimes accompanies the skin lesions.[29]

The emergency physician must be aware that atypical manifestations of EM are not uncommon and can include vesicular scaling and necrotic lesions.[31] In addition, EM can occur in unusual shapes, and both linear and triangular configurations have been reported. EM can also be characterized by either central darkening or have a uniform color.[25,27,29,32] EM can be mistaken for cellulitis, urticaria, contact dermatitis, tinea corporis, granuloma annulare, fixed drug eruption, and localized toxic or hypersensitivity reactions to arthropod bites.[25,27,29,32-34] Finally, because few patients with LD recall their tick bite, a history of this event is not required for the diagnosis.

When EM findings are classical, the ED physician can confirm the diagnosis by performing a careful physical examination. In equivocal cases, the practitioner may elect to measure the lesion and then re-examine the patient in 2-3 days. The diagnosis of EM is suggested by a lesion that has expanded a few centimeters over this period, though it should be stressed that the features of evolving lesions can be extremely variable.[31] Moreover, since EM can be evanescent—in fact, it will disappear after a few weeks even without antibiotic treatment—the clinician must be cautious when trying to draw definitive conclusions using this approach.

Although a culture of the advancing rim of the lesion will be positive in about 50-66% of cases, this microbiological test is not routinely available in most hospitals, and is not usually indicated.[25,30,35] Complicating the diagnosis of LD is the fact that only 30-40% of patients are seropositive at this early stage of the illness. As a result, blood testing is not necessary in most cases.[36] There are exceptions to this rule. In atypical or ambiguous cases, because most patients seroconvert by enzyme-linked immunosorbent assay (ELISA) test or IgM immunoblot even when treated promptly and appropriately, acute and convalescent testing can be of value in establishing the diagnosis.[36]

Early Disseminated Disease: Cutaneous and Systemic Manifestations

Disseminated hematogenously, multiple EM lesions are observed in about 20-50% of patients.[25,27,29,32] The secondary lesions are generally smaller than the original lesion and lack a central punctum.[30] Of special clinical, differential, and diagnostic significance is the fact that disseminated lesions tend to be found everywhere, except for palms, soles, and mucous membranes.[31] Accordingly, accurate evaluation of these findings requires that the patient be fully unclothed.

A flu-like illness without a rash also occurs at this stage, though the incidence of this is unknown.[37] This "spring or summer flu syndrome" can challenge the ED physician to distinguish among a number of conditions, ranging from trivial viral infections to several other tick-borne entities, including ehrlichiosis, babesiosis, and spotless Rocky Mountain spotted fever (RMSF), which can be fatal.

Because most patients with TBD are unaware of their tick bite, it is mandatory that the emergency physician not just ascertain whether a tick bite has occurred but whether one is likely to have occurred. Clues that suggest a tick bite include the season and participation in outdoor activities. Remember, however, that nothing more exotic than mowing the lawn or playing in the backyard is required.

Neurologic Manifestations. To reduce morbidity and improve patient outcomes, the ED physician must be able to recognize neurological signs and symptoms associated with LD. In this regard, it should be stressed that about 15-40% of untreated patients eventually develop neurologic sequelae that involve both the peripheral (PNS) and the central nervous system (CNS).[18,38] The three common early neurologic syndromes that ED physicians must recognize present relatively early in the course of the disease (i.e., within weeks to months of the tick bite). These include lymphocytic meningitis, cranial neuropathy, and radiculoneuritis. Other reported neurological syndromes include acute myelitis, encephalitis, ataxia, and myositis.[39] A pseudotumor cerebri-like syndrome also has been described in North American children.[40] Timing of presentations is variable. Neurologic symptoms can precede the onset of EM, can occur without a prior history of EM, and can occur concurrently with the rash.[41]

Meningitis. Lyme meningitis results from direct invasion of the CNS by borrelial organisms.[42] Symptoms, which are usually described as mild, are similar to those associated with other causes of meningeal irritation and include headache, stiff neck, and fatigue. Occasionally, patients have an element of mild encephalopathy and may present with such symptoms as forgetfulness and irritability.[42] One clue to a borrelial etiology is symptoms that wax and wane over hours or days. Fever and severe meningismus are mild or absent.[42] Otherwise, physical examination is unremarkable, unless a concurrent EM or seventh nerve palsy (7-NP) is present. Lumbar puncture shows lymphocytic pleocytosis and elevated protein. Collecting and saving extra CSF may be of subsequent value to the primary care physician, who may wish to perform other tests such as PCR and/or anti-*B. burgdorferi* antibodies at a later point in the clinical course.

As in all LD syndromes, a high index of suspicion and a careful history are the ED physician's most powerful allies. Diagnosis is confirmed by culture in only about 5% of patients.[42] Although most Lyme meningitis patients are seropositive, an occasional patient may be negative.[42] There are many other etiologies for these symptoms. One Connecticut-based study of patients presenting with acute meningitis with a negative Gram's stain of CSF found that only four patients of 168 had Lyme meningitis.[43] In 71% of cases, a specific etiology was never established.

Cranial Neuropathy. Paralysis of the seventh cranial nerve is found in approximately 11% of patients with LD and is bilateral in 25% of cases.[44] Paralysis of the second side generally occurs sequentially, days to weeks after the first. Bilateral 7-NP is an important clue to the diagnosis of LD, inasmuch as the other causes of bilateral 7-NP palsy (e.g., Guillain-Barré syndrome, neurosarcoidosis, and basilar meningitides like tuberculosis) are distinctly uncommon. In pediatric patients with 7-NP, LD needs to be excluded, as the idiopathic variety is less common in patients of this age group.[45] One investigator reported that facial erythema and swelling is a clue that a 7-NP is borrelial in etiology and suggested that the 7-NP was frequently ipsilateral to the tick bite.[46]

The incidence of idiopathic Bell's palsy is about 20 cases per 100,000 of population.[47] In an endemic state like Connecticut, the incidence of LD is 46 per 100,000.[6] If 11% of patients with LD get 7-NP, then the expected number of cases of 7-NP secondary to LD would be about 5 per 100,000 (or 20% of the total). Several studies have found incidence figures in this range, but others have not.[47-51] Since idiopathic Bell's palsy has no seasonal variance, 7-NP occurring during the summer months should be suspected of being borrelial in origin.

Although the majority of LD patients with 7-NP are seropositive, some patients are sero-negative. Hence, an initially negative serology does not rule out borrelial infection.[47] Many clinicians advocate doing a lumbar puncture on these patients. The rationale is that patients with a pleocytosis should be treated with parenteral antibiotics, whereas those with normal CSF can be treated orally.[18] Although this hypothesis does have some common-sense appeal, there are no controlled trials evaluating efficacy or clinical outcomes. Finally, the outcome of 7-NP in LD is excellent. In one early study of over 100 patients, not all of whom received antibiotics, the recovery rate was 99%.[44]

Radiculoneuritis. Radiculoneuritis appears to be more common in Europe (where it is known as Bennwarth's syndrome) than in North America.[38] This syndrome generally presents as a painful limb and may mimic the presentation of an acute herniated disc.[39,52] The distribution of pain, however, is more characteristic of a plexitis, multiple radiculitis, or a mononeuritis multiplex.[39,52] Like the other Lyme syndromes, these symptoms generally resolve without antibiotics after 5-6 months, but improve more quickly with antibiotic therapy.[39]

Cardiac Involvement. Fewer than 10% of untreated patients will develop cardiac manifestations of LD.[18,53] On occasion, cardiac disease can even be the presenting feature. When it occurs, cardiac involvement generally presents weeks to months after the tick bite and is typically short-lived (days to weeks).[53,54] Like most manifestations of LD, symptoms usually resolve spontaneously, even in the untreated patient. Symptoms include palpitations, light-headedness, syncope, dyspnea, and chest pain.[53,55] Cardiac involvement is more common in men.[53-55]

Conduction abnormalities, especially varying degrees of atrioventricular (AV) block, are the most common cardiac manifestations, with complete, transient heart block occurring in about 50% of patients with cardiac involvement.[53,55] Myocarditis, pericarditis, and myopericarditis also occur, and there is a single case report of pericarditis with tamponade.[53-57]

Despite the tendency for spontaneous improvement, anti-borrelial chemotherapy is indicated at this stage of disease, both to hasten resolution and to prevent progression of symptoms. Because patients with complete heart block from LD almost never require a permanent pacemaker, establishing the diagnosis is particularly important. Serologies are almost always, but not universally, positive at this stage of the illness.

Early Disseminated Syndromes

Ocular Syndromes. Ocular involvement occurs in the early and late stages of LD.[58-60] Non-specific follicular conjunctivitis occurs in up to 10% of patients with early disease. Episcleritis and keratitis can be seen early in the disease, and blindness has been reported from panophthalmitis.[57-61] The spirochete has been cultured from iris biopsy.[62] Later stages of the disease include retinal vasculitis, inflammation of the retina, optic atrophy, and disc edema.[58] Patients with ocular disease can be seronegative.[59]

Arthritis. Although classic Lyme arthritis is a late phenomenon, there are musculoskeletal manifestations that occur early in the natural history of the disease. Patients may experience migratory pains in muscles, tendons, joints, and bursae that may wax and wane over hours or days.[63] Some patients will develop arthritis within weeks to months, which is usually is characterized by mono- or oligo-articular inflammation of large joints, typically the knee.

Hepatic. Liver involvement, suggested by abnormalities in the hepatic transaminases, is common.[64] However, symptomatic hepatitis does not occur; splenomegaly develops occasionally.[65,66]

Other Tick-Borne Diseases: Differential Diagnosis

Ehrlichiosis. Caused by a rickettsial organism, two forms of human ehrlichiosis have been described: human granulocytic ehrlichiosis (HGE) and human monocytic ehrlichiosis (HME). HGE is common in geographical areas populated with *I. scapularis* ticks, while HME is transmitted by the lone-star tick (*Amblyomma americanum*), which predominates in the Southern and Midwestern states.[67-69] Both entities present as a nonspecific febrile illness, with fever, chills, fatigue, headache, myalgias, and arthralgias. The accompanying rash can be macular, papular, or petechial.[67-70] Adult respiratory distress syndrome has been reported with both HGE and HME.[71,72]

The diagnosis can be confirmed by the presence of berry-like inclusions called morulae in white blood cells on the peripheral smear. Morulae are found commonly in HGE, and rarely in HME. Associated diagnostic clues include leukopenia, thrombocytopenia (occasionally, pancytopenia), and elevated hepatic transaminases.[67-69]

From an emergency medicine perspective, the diagnosis is made on clinical grounds and requires a high index of suspicion. Making the diagnosis is important, inasmuch as ehrlichiosis is fatal in about 5% of cases, but can be treated with doxycycline.[68,69,73]

Babesiosis. Babesiosis is a protozoan disease that is carried by *I. scapularis*. It causes a non-specific febrile illness. Seroprevalence studies show that in endemic areas such as Block Island, up to 10% of individuals tested positive.[74] One species of *Babesia, B. microti,* leads to a milder disease than that in Europe, where *B. divergens* frequently attacks asplenic patients and often leads to massive hemolysis, renal failure, and death.[75] Domestic babesiosis is fatal in about 5% of patients.[76]

Symptoms of babesiosis are similar to those described above for ehrlichiosis.[75,76] However, anemia is more likely to be encountered in babesiosis, which also may be accompanied by proteinuria and hemaglobinuria.[75] The diagnosis can be made by examining a Giemsa-stained blood smear for intra-erythrocytic protozoa.[75] Severe cases of babesiosis in asplenic patients, the immunocompromised, and the elderly are treated using a combination of clindamycin and quinine. Finally, studies indicate that co-infection of ehrlichiosis, babesiosis, or both can occur in combination with LD.[77-82]

Rocky Mountain Spotted Fever. RMSF also presents as a summer flu for the first three days and remains "spotless" in 10% of cases.[83,84] Most patients, however, will exhibit a petechial rash on the third or fourth day of illness.[84,85] Increased fatalities occur in RMSF patients who present during the first three days of symptoms, out of season, (October through April), and/or without a rash.[86] Even with the much larger Dermacentor tick vector, 40% of RMSF victims do not recall the tick bite.[85] Treatment with chloramphenicol or tetracycline has dramatically reduced the fatality rate from about 70% to roughly 5%.[87]

Confirming the Diagnosis of LD

The Centers for Disease Control and Prevention (CDC) case definition for confirming the diagnosis of LD can be summarized as physician-diagnosed EM of more than 5 cm diameter, or any late manifestations of the disease—neurological, cardiac, arthritis, etc.—associated with a positive Lyme serology. It is important to note that this CDC definition is tailored for epidemiologic surveillance purposes and should not dictate management for any individual patient.[88]

History and Physical Examination. Emergency physicians—especially those practicing in the northeastern United States—must maintain a high index of suspicion for LD between May and October. In many cases, the diagnosis of LD is no more complicated than taking a history and performing a detailed physical exam that reveals characteristic EM or other signs of early disseminated LD. In this regard, asking a patient, "Have you been bitten by any ticks?" is not sufficient, and can be misleading, since most patients who eventually develop LD simply do not recall being bitten by a tick. Instead, the inquiry should be directed toward uncovering the possibility that the individual has been the victim of a tick bite.

A fruitful line of questioning would entail asking the patient with a rash where he or she has been during the month prior to presentation. Remember, a patient with 7-NP who lives in Arizona, where the prevalence of LD is low, may have been vacationing in Rhode Island, which is endemic for the disease. In addition, patients should be asked about specific recreational activities—gardening, hiking, camping or fishing—that might have placed them at higher risk for being bitten by a tick. Furthermore, the season of onset for these early syndromes can be suggestive. However, patients can present with TBD in all months and, in fact, the mortality rate is higher in patients with RMSF who present "out of season."[86] Finally, while affirmative responses to these questions point toward TBD, negative responses do not rule out tick-mediated pathology.

In the appropriate geographical setting and within the targeted temporal window, the presence of classic EM is diagnostic of LD and no additional testing is indicated. However, because EM can be associated with atypical presentations, the emergency physician must become familiar with these clinical variants. Another example in which diagnostic testing may not be necessary is the presence of lymphocytic meningitis in combination with facial nerve palsy in the characteristic setting. This combination overwhelmingly suggests LD. In most other cases, laboratory testing for antibodies to borrelial proteins will be required to corroborate the diagnosis.

Serological Testing. To confirm the diagnosis of LD, the CDC currently recommends a two-step procedure similar to that used for HIV testing (i.e., a screening ELISA followed by a confirmatory Western blot in positive or borderline ELISA).[89] This approach is supported by recent studies that suggest that a standardized ELISA test followed up by Western blot for all positive or borderline tests yields fairly specific results.[90] As with most tests in medicine, higher specificity generally comes at the price of lower sensitivity.[91] Despite widespread use of these serological methods, there is no universally agreed upon standard for what constitutes a positive Western blot.[92-94]

Current testing, while vastly improved, is still imperfect, and misinterpretation of either false-negative and false-positive results can have serious clinical consequences. Therefore, ED physicians who order these tests must understand their intrinsic limitations. Measurable host antibodies to borrelial proteins frequently take several weeks to develop.[36-95] Early seronegativity does not exclude the diagnosis of LD.

False-positive tests by ELISA occur with many different infectious conditions, including Epstein-Barr viral infection, varicella, endocarditis, ehrlichiosis, gingivitis from non-pathogenic spirochetes normally present in the mouth, other spirochetal infections, immunologic conditions (systemic lupus erythematosus [SLE], rheumatoid arthritis [RA]), and malignancies.[95,96-99] Another potential source of error is encountered in the patient who has a previous history of LD. In this regard, it should be emphasized that antibodies can persist for many years.[92-94,100] Finally, routine lab tests such as CBC and ESR are generally normal, although 40% of patients will have one or more abnormalities on liver function testing.[64,100]

In the ED setting, treatment decisions will be based upon clinical and epidemiologic parameters. While early treatment may cause later seronegativity, most patients with culture-proven EM will seroconvert even with treatment.[18,36,95,101] Specific diagnostic tests (culture and PCR) are not routinely available to the emergency physician.

Management Guidelines and Disposition

Asymptomatic Tick Bites. In most cases, no treatment is recommended in patients who present with an asymptomatic tick bite. However, if after considering all the relevant historical and epidemiological factors, the ED physician, in collaboration with the patient, decides that antimicrobial treatment is the most prudent clinical approach, the following recommendations can be made. A 10-day course of amoxicillin (250-500 mg po tid) for children and 10-day course of doxycycline (100 mg po bid) in adults is appropriate. *(Please see Table 2.)*

Tick Removal. Removal of ticks is best accomplished by grasping the tick as close as possible to the skin with very fine tweezers and pulling slowly, but firmly, and perpendicularly away from the

Table 2. Guidelines for Treatment of Tick-Borne Diseases

SYNDROME	EXAM FINDINGS	LAB AIDS	THERAPY (SEE BELOW)	COMMENTS
Tick bite	None, tick may be present, may have minor erythema at the site	None (Lyme serology only reflects prior exposure)	If treat at all, use 10-14 days of doxycycline or amoxicillin—same dose as for EM	This can be a complicated decision; many authorities recommend no treatment.
Solitary EM	Delayed rash at the site of tick bite that may take on various morphologies	Serologies often negative at this point; may see an IgM response	2-4 weeks of: amoxicillin (500 mg tid) doxycycline (100 mg bid-tid), cefuroxime (500 mg tid), or erythromycin (250 mg tid)	Azithromycin not as effective. Doxycycline also covers ehrlichiosis and RMSF. Examine the patient head-to-toe for evidence of secondary EM lesions
Lymphocytic meningitis and radiculoneuritis	Findings of meningeal irritation, other signs of LD	Lyme serology, CSF shows pleocytosis, elevated protein, may show antibody production in CSF	IV ceftriaxone, 2 g/d for 2-4 weeks, penicillin G 20 million U/d in divided doses	Studies have shown po doxycycline 200-300 mg/d for 30 days treats Lyme meningitis, but most authorities recommend parenteral treatment
7th nerve palsy	Peripheral-type facial nerve lesion; other signs of LD	Lyme serology, spinal tap?	If CSF is negative: same as for EM; if CSF is positive: same as for meningitis	Some authorities recommend spinal tap in all patients with 7th nerve palsy possibly due to LD
Lyme carditis	Arrhythmia, signs of CHF; other signs of LD	ECG, Lyme serology	Same as for meningitis, but 2 weeks' duration is generally recommended	Need for permanent pacemaker rare. Tamponade has been reported. 1° AVB can be treated with oral regimens
Babesiosis	Flu-like syndrome, occasionally splenomegaly	CBC, serology examination of blood smear for intra-erythrocytic inclusions	Clindamycin 1.2 g bid IV or 600 mg tid po and quinine 650 mg tid po	Patients with splenectomy do worse. Treatment indicated in immunocompromised, elderly, splenectomized, and severely symptomatic patients
Human ehrlichiosis monocytic and granulocytic	Flu-like syndrome, occasionally non-specific rash	CBC, examination of blood smear for morulae, LFTs, PCR	Doxycycline 100 mg bid PO or IV depending on clinical situation. Possibly chloramphenicol	May be worse in young and old patients. Chloramphenicol not active in vitro but shows some activity in vivo
Rocky Mountain spotted fever	Flu-like syndrome; 90% with acral red maculo-papular rash	CBC, serum sodium, serology, skin biopsy	Doxycycline 100 mg bid, or chloramphenicol 1 g q6h IV	Increased mortality for patients diagnosed after day 3, without rash, or "out of season"

Notes: 1. Avoid doxycycline in children younger than 9 and pregnant or lactating women. 2. **Pediatric doses of medications** (duration same as for adults): amoxicillin, 25-50 mg/kg/d po bid; cefuroxime, 125 mg po bid; erythromycin, 30 mg/kg/d po tid; ceftriaxone, 75-100 mg/kg/d IV once daily; penicillin G, 300,000 U/kg/d IV in divided doses q4h; clindamycin 20-40 mg/kg/d in divided doses; quinine, 25 mg/kg/d in three doses; chloramphenicol, 100 mg/kg IV for first day (to total of 3 g) then 50 mg/kg/d po. 3. **Pregnant women:** no treatment recommended for *asymptomatic* seropositivity; for EM, amoxicillin 500 mg po tid for 3-4 weeks; for any disseminated disease, penicillin G 20 million U/d/IV in divided doses. 4. Erythromycin probably not as effective and should be last choice. 5. Remember the phototoxicity of doxycycline; advise use of strong sun block.

skin.[102] Retained tick parts may predispose to secondary bacterial infection but will not increase the risk of LD.[103] Some physicians advocate injecting a small wheal of lidocaine with epinephrine using a fine-gauge needle directly beneath the tick.[104]

Gloves should be worn and the skin should be thoroughly disinfected after tick removal. The tick's body should not be squeezed, since there is a theoretical possibility that this might "inject" infectious material into the patient's skin. It should be re-emphasized that most manifestations of LD will go away without treatment with antibiotics, but treatment will shorten the duration of symptoms and prevent development of subsequent manifestations.

Conclusive data regarding the effect of LD on the fetus in pregnant women are lacking.[105,106] In general, however, the threshold for treating pregnant patients and for using parenteral medications should be lower. Tetracyclines are contraindicated in pregnant women and in children less than 9 years of age. *(Please see Table 2.)*

Solitary Erythema Migrans. Solitary EM requires antibiotic therapy—the only question being the choice and duration. Oral doxycycline or amoxicillin are considered by most experts to be the drugs of choice.[18,107] Alternatives include phenoxymethyl penicillin, tetracycline, and cefuroxime, the only drug approved by the FDA for this use.[18] Erythromycin and azithromycin have been used as alternatives but a recent study comparing amoxicillin and azithromycin, showed amoxicillin to be superior.[108] Varying durations of therapy have been recommended in the literature, ranging between 10 and 30 days.[18] Most physicians recommend 14-21 days of therapy. [107] A three-week course seems prudent, until controlled trials dictate otherwise. Patients with systemic symptoms and those with a longer duration of disease should be treated with four weeks of therapy.

Summer Flu Syndrome. When the geographical and historical circumstances so dictate, the "summer flu" syndrome can probably be treated as EM. Doxycycline has the advantage of activity against RMSF and ehrlichiosis.

Early Disseminated Disease. Early disseminated disease usually is treated with parenteral antibiotics.[107] Patients in whom parenteral therapy is mandatory include those with meningitis, radiculoneuritis, and high-degree heart block. Some physicians treat isolated 7-NP with oral antibiotics, but for a longer duration (21-30 days).[107] Some experts advocate doing a spinal tap on all patients with Lyme-associated 7-NP. Their reasoning is that those with pleocytosis require parenteral therapy, whereas those without cells can be treated orally. As is the case for many treatment decisions regarding LD syndromes, there are insufficient scientific data to resolve this issue.

Meningitis and radiculoneuritis are treated intravenously for 2-3 weeks. Ceftriaxone has excellent activity against *B. burgdoferi* and has the pharmacologic advantage of a long half-life. Intravenous penicillin G also can be used.[18] Symptoms usually resolve over days, although resolution of motor signs and symptoms can take longer. Treatment of chronic LD syndromes is outside the purview of the emergency physician.

Prevention

Preventing TBD requires implementation of specific environmental, personal, and vaccine-related strategies. Proven environmental techniques include insecticide application and wildlife management (i.e., fencing to exclude deer from a given area).[3]

Personal measures, including the use of insect repellants and prompt tick removal also can be helpful. Wearing light-colored clothing to make ticks more visible, long pants and sleeves, and tucking pant legs into the socks are all recommended, although difficult to comply with in hot summer weather. Staying to the center of trails when hiking may reduce tick exposure. Daily tick inspections with removal of any that are found may help to identify ticks before they can transmit disease. Finally, application of permethrin to clothing and DEET to skin are effective tick repellants. Caution is necessary in children, who can develop neurotoxicity from DEET if used in high concentrations.

Phase 3 human vaccine trials are currently ongoing in endemic areas. Phase 1 and 2 trials of a vaccine to Osp A, a borrelial surface protein, were shown to be safe and immunogenic. Vaccine is presently available on a protocol basis only.

Summary

Patients with TBD frequently present to the ED with signs and symptoms that can be confused with many common disorders, including allergic conditions, viral infections, and non-specific "summer flu" syndromes. Because LD can progress from a benign condition to a serious, disseminated condition with serious neurological, cardiac, and rheumatological sequelae, the emergency physician must maintain a high index of suspicion for tick-related conditions and be familiar with indications for treatment, especially in the appropriate epidemiologic setting.

References

1. Steere AC, Malawista SE, Snydman DR, et al. Lyme arthritis: An epidemic of oligoarticular arthritis in children and adults in three Connecticut communities. *Arthritis Rheum* 1977;20: 7-17.
2. Barbour AG, Fish D. The biological and social phenomenon of Lyme disease. *Science* 1993;260:1610-1616.
3. Fish D. Environmental risk and prevention of Lyme disease. *Am J Med* 1995;98:2S-8S; discussion 8S-9S.
4. Lyme Disease—United States, 1991-1992. *MMWR Morb Mortal Wkly Rep* 1993;42:345-348.
5. Lyme Disease—United States, 1994. *MMWR Morb Mortal Wkly Rep* 1995;44:459-462.
6. Lyme Disease—United States, 1995. *MMWR Morb Mortal Wkly Rep* 1996;45:481-484.
7. Coyle BS, Strickland, GT, Liang, YL. The public health impact of Lyme disease in Maryland. *J Infect Dis* 1996;173: 1260-1262.
8. Falco RC, Fish D. Prevalence of *Ixodes dammini* near the homes of Lyme disease patients in Westchester County, New York. *Am J Epidemiol* 1988;127:826-830.
9. Maupin GO, Fish D, Zultowsky J, et al. Landscape ecology of Lyme disease in a residential area of Westchester County, New York. *Am J Epidemiol* 1991;133:1105-1113.
10. Salgo MP, Telzak EE, Currie B, et al. A focus of Rocky Mountain spotted fever within New York City. *N Engl J Med* 1988;318:1345-1348.
11. Costello CM, Steere AC, Pinkerton RE, et al. A prospective

study of tick bites in an endemic area for Lyme disease. *J Infect Dis* 1989;159:136-139.

12. Shapiro ED, Gerber MA, Holabird NB, et al. A controlled trial of antimicrobial prophylaxis for Lyme disease after deer-tick bites [see comments]. *N Engl J Med* 1992;327:1769-1773.
13. Strle F, Cheng Y, Cimperman J, et al. Persistence of *Borrelia burgdorferi* sensu lato in resolved erythema migrans lesions. *Clin Infect Dis* 1995;21:380-389.
14. Asbrink E, Hovmark A. Successful cultivation of spirochetes from skin lesions of patients with erythema chronica migrans afzelius and acrodermatitis chronica atrophicans. *Acta Pathol Microbiol Immunol Scand* 1985;93:161-163.
15. Goodman JL, Bradley JF, Ross AE, et al. Bloodstream invasion in early Lyme disease: Results from a prospective, controlled, blinded study using the polymerase chain reaction. *Am J Med* 1995;99:6-12.
16. Luft BJ, Steinman CR, Neimark HC, et al. Invasion of the central nervous system by *Borrelia burgdorferi* in acute disseminated infection. [Published erratum appears in *JAMA* 1992;268:872.] [see comments]. *JAMA* 1992;267:1364-1367.
17. Nadelman RB, Pavia CS, Magnarelli LA, et al. Isolation of *Borrelia burgdorferi* from the blood of seven patients with Lyme disease. *Am J Med* 1990;88:21-26.
18. Nocton JJ, Steere AC. Lyme disease. *Adv Intern Med* 1995;40:69-117.
19. Piesman J, Mather TN, Sinsky RJ, et al. Duration of tick attachment and *Borrelia burgdorferi* transmission. *J Clin Microbiol* 1987;25:557-558.
20. Piesman J, Maupin GO, Campos EG, et al. Duration of adult female *Ixodes dammini* attachment and transmission of *Borrelia burgdorferi,* with description of a needle aspiration isolation method. *J Infect Dis* 1991;163:895-897.
21. Piesman J. Dynamics of *Borrelia burgdorferi* transmission by nymphal *Ixodes dammini* ticks. *J Infect Dis* 1993;167: 1082-1085.
22. Ribiero J. Role of saliva in blood-feeding by arthropods. *Ann Rev Entomol* 1987;32:463-478.
23. Zung JL, Lewengrub S, Rudzinska MA, et al. Fine structural evidence for the penetration of the Lyme disease spirochete, *Borrelia burgdorferi* through the gut and salivary tissues of *Ixodes dammini. Can J Zoo* 1989;67:1737-1748.
24. Benach JL, Coleman JL, Skinner RA, et al. Adult *Ixodes dammini* on rabbits: A hypothesis for the development and transmission of *Borrelia burgdorferi. J Infect Dis* 1987;155: 1300-1306.
25. Strle F, Nelson J, Ruzic-Sabljic E, et al. European Lyme borreliosis: 231 culture-confirmed cases involving patients with erythema migrans. *Clin Infect Dis* 1996;23:61-65.
26. Patmas MA, Remorca C. Disseminated Lyme disease after short-duration tick bite. *J Spirochet Tick-Borne Dis* 1994;1: 77-78.
27. Malane MS, Grant-Kels JM, Feder HM, et al. Diagnosis of Lyme disease based on dermatologic manifestations. *Ann Intern Med* 1991;114:490-498.
28. Bosler EM, Ormiston BG, Coleman JL, et al. Prevalence of the Lyme disease spirochete in populations of white-tailed deer and white-footed mice. *Yale J Biol Med* 1984;57: 651-659.
29. Nadelman RB, Nowakowski J, Forseter G, et al. The clinical spectrum of early Lyme borreliosis in patients with culture-confirmed erythema migrans. *Am J Med* 1996;100:502-508.
30. Melski JW, Reed KD, Mitchell PD, et al. Primary and secondary erythema migrans in Central Wisconsin. *Arch Dermatol* 1993;129:709-716.
31. Berger BW. Dermatologic manifestations of Lyme disease. *Rev Infect Dis* 1989;11:S1475-S1481.
32. Nadelman RB, Wormser GP. Erythema migrans and early Lyme disease. *Am J Med* 1995;98:15S-23S; discussion 23S-24S.
33. Feder HM, Jr., Hunt MS. Pitfalls in the diagnosis and treatment of Lyme disease in children. *JAMA* 1995;274:66-68.
34. Feder HM, Jr., Whitaker DL. Misdiagnosis of erythema migrans. *Am J Med* 1995;99:412-419.
35. Mitchell PD, Reed KD, Vandermause MF, et al. Isolation of *Borrelia burgforferi* from skin biopsy specimens of patients with erythma migrans. *Clin Microbiol Infect Dis* 1992;99: 104-107.
36. Aguero-Rosenfeld ME, Nowakowski J, Bittker S, et al. Evolution of the serologic response to *Borrelia burgdorferi* in treated patients with culture-confirmed erythema migrans. *J Clin Microbiol* 1996;34:1-9.
37. Feder HM, Jr., Gerber MA, Krause PJ. Early Lyme disease: A flu-like illness without erythema migrans. *Pediatrics* 1993;91: 456-459.
38. Coyle PK. Neurologic complications of Lyme disease. *Rheum Dis Clin North Am* 1993;19:993-1009.
39. Garcia-Monco JC, Benach JL. Lyme neuroborreliosis. *Ann Neurol* 1995;37:691-702.
40. Belman AL, Iyer M, Coyle PK, et al. Neurologic manifestations in children with North American Lyme disease. *Neurology* 1993;43:2609-2614.
41. Reik L, Jr., Burgdorfer W, Donaldson JO. Neurologic abnormalities in Lyme disease without erythema chronicum migrans. *Am J Med* 1986;81:73-78.
42. Pachner AR. Early disseminated Lyme disease: Lyme meningitis. *Am J Med* 1995;98:30S-37S; discussion 37S-43S.
43. Elmore JG, Horwitz RI, Quagliarello VJ. Acute meningitis with a negative Gram's stain: Clinical and management outcomes in 171 episodes. *Am J Med* 1996;100:78-84.
44. Clarke JR, Carlson RD, Pachner AR, et al. Facial paralysis in Lyme disease. *Laryngoscope* 1985;95:1341-1345.
45. Christen H, Bartlau N, Hanefield F, et al. Peripheral facial palsy in childhood: Lyme borreliosis to be suspected unless proven otherwise. *Acta Pediatr Scand* 1990;79:1219-1224.
46. Markby DP. Lyme disease facial palsy: Differentiation from Bell's palsy. [See comments]. *BMJ* 1989;299:605-606.
47. Halperin JJ, Golightly M. Lyme borreliosis in Bell's palsy. Long Island Neuroborreliosis Collaborative Study Group. [see comments]. *Neurology* 1992;42:1268-1270.
48. Olsson I, Engervall KA, Hovmark A. Tick-borne borreliosis and facial palsy. *Acta Otolaryngol* (Stockholm) 1988;105: 100-107.
49. Roberg M, Ernerudh J, Forsberg P, et al. Acute peripheral facial palsy: CSF findings and etiology. *Acta Neurol Scand* 1991;83:55-60.
50. Puhakka HJ, Laurikainen E, Viljanen M, et al. Peripheral

facial palsy caused by *Borrelia burgdorferi* and viruses in south-western Finland. *Acta Otolaryngol* [supplement] 1992;492:103-106.

51. Kuiper H, Devriese PP, de Jongh BM, et al. Absence of Lyme borreliosis among patients with presumed Bell's palsy. *Arch Neurol* 1992;49:940-943.
52. Halperin JJ. Neuroborreliosis. *Am J Med* 1995;98:4A-52S-59S.
53. Sigal LH. Early disseminated Lyme disease: Cardiac manifestations. *Am J Med* 1995;98:25S-28S; discussion 28S-29S.
54. Steere AC, Batsford WP, Weinberg M, et al. Lyme carditis: Cardiac abnormalities of Lyme disease. *Ann Intern Med* 1980;93:8-16.
55. van der Linde MR. Lyme carditis: Clinical characteristics of 105 cases. *Scand J Infect Dis* [supplement] 1991;77:81-84.
56. Horowitz HW, Belkin RN. Acute myopericarditis resulting from Lyme disease. *Am Heart J* 1995;130:176-178.
57. Bruyn GA, De Koning J, Reijsoo FJ, et al. Lyme pericarditis leading to tamponade. *Br J Rheumatol* 1994;33:862-866.
58. Lesser RL. Ocular manifestations of Lyme disease. *Am J Med* 1995;98:60S-62S.
59. Karma A, Seppala I, Mikkila H, et al. Diagnosis and clinical characteristics of ocular Lyme borreliosis. *Am J Ophthalmol* 1995;119:127-135.
60. Aaberg TM. The expanding ophthalmologic spectrum of Lyme disease. *Am J Ophthalmol* 1989;107:77-80.
61. Steere AC, Duray PH, Kauffmann DJH, et al. Unilateral blindness caused by infection with the Lyme disease spirochete, *Borrelia burgdorferi. Ann Intern Med* 1985;103:382-384.
62. Preac-Mursic V, Pfister HW, Spiegel H, et al. First isolation of *Borrelia burgdorferi* from an iris biopsy. *J Clin Neuroophthalmol* 1993;13:155-161; discussion 162.
63. Steere AC. Musculoskeletal manifestations of Lyme disease. *Am J Med* 1995;98:44S-48S; discussion 48S-51S.
64. Horowitz HW, Dworkin B, Forseter G, et al. Liver function in early Lyme disease. *Hepatology* 1996;23:1412-1417.
65. Steere AC, Malawista SE, Hardin JA, et al. Erythema chronicum migrans and Lyme arthritis: The enlarging clinical spectrum. *Ann Intern Med* 1977;86:685-698.
66. Ilowite NT. Muscle, reticuloendothelial, and late skin manifestations of Lyme disease. *Am J Med* 1995;98:63S-68S.
67. Dumler JS, Bakken JS. Ehrlichial diseases of humans: Emerging tick-borne infections. *Clin Infect Dis* 1995;20:1102-1110.
68. Fishbein DB, Dawson JE, Robinson LE. Human ehrlichiosis in the United States, 1985 to 1990. *Ann Intern Med* 1994;120:736-743.
69. Walker DH. Human ehrlichiosis: More trouble from ticks. *Hosp Pract* 1996;31:47-57.
70. Ratnasamy N, Everett ED, Roland WE, et al. Central nervous system manifestations of human ehrlichiosis. *Clin Infect Dis* 1996;23:314-319.
71. Wong S, Grady LJ. Ehrlichia infection as a cause of severe respiratory distress (letter). *N Engl J Med* 1996;334:273.
72. Vugia DJ, Holmberg E, Steffe EM, et al. A human case of monocytic ehrlichiosis with adult respiratory distress syndrome in northern California. *West J Med* 1996;164:525-528.
73. Bakken JS, Krueth J, Wilson-Nordskog C, et al. Clinical and laboratory characteristics of human granulocytic ehrlichiosis. *JAMA* 1996;275:199-205.
74. Krause PJ, Telford SR, Pollack RJ, et al. Babesiosis: An underdiagnosed disease of children. *Pediatrics* 1992;89:1045-1048.
75. Boustani M, Gelfand J. Babesiosis. *Clin Infect Dis* 1996;22:611-615.
76. Meldrum SC, Birkhead GS, White DJ, et al. Human babesiosis in New York State: An epidemiological description of 136 cases. *Clin Infect Dis* 1992;15:1019-1023.
77. Mitchell PD, Reed KD, Hofkes JM. Immunoserologic evidence of coinfection with *Borrelia burgdorferi, Babesia microti,* and human granulocytic *Ehrhichia* species in residents of Wisconsin and Minnesota. *J Clin Microbiol* 1996;34:724-727.
78. Paparone PW, Glenn WB. Lyme disease with concurrent ehrlichiosis. *J Am Osteopath Assoc* 1994;94:568-570, 573, 577.
79. Benach JL, Coleman JL, Habicht GS, et al. Serological evidence for simultaneous occurrences of Lyme disease and babesiosis. *J Infect Dis* 1985;152:473-477.
80. Grunwaldt E, Barbour AG, Benach JL. Simultaneous occurrence of babesiosis and Lyme disease [letter]. *N Engl J Med* 1983;308:1166.
81. Krause P, Telford S, Spielman A, et al. Concurrent Lyme disease and babesiosis—evidence for increased severity and duration of illness. *JAMA* 1996;275:1657-1660.
82. Marcus LC, Steere AC, Duray PH, et al. Fatal pancarditis in a patient with coexistent Lyme disease and babesiosis: Demonstration of spirochetes in the myocardium. *Ann Intern Med* 1985;103:374-376.
83. Westerman EL. Rocky Mountain spotless fever: A dilemma for the clinician. *Arch Intern Med* 1982;142:1106-1107.
84. Weber DJ, Walker DH. Rocky Mountain spotted fever. *Infect Dis Clin North Am* 1991;5:19-35.
85. Helmick CG, Bernard KW, D'Angelo LJ. Rocky Mountain spotted fever: Clinical, laboratory, and epidemiological features of 262 cases. *J Infect Dis* 1984;150:480-488.
86. Kirkland KB, Wilkinson WE, Sexton DJ. Therapeutic delay and mortality in cases of Rocky Mountain spotted fever. *Clin Infect Dis* 1995;20:1118-1121.
87. Woodward TE. Rocky Mountain spotted fever: Epidemiological and early clinical signs are keys to treatment and reduced mortality. *J Infect Dis* 1984;150:465-468.
88. Case definitions for public health surveillance. *MMWR Morb Mortal Wkly Rep* 1990;39:19-21.
89. Recommendations for test performance and interpretation from the Second National Conference on Serologic Diagnosis of Lyme Disease. *MMWR Morb Mortal Wkly Rep* 1995;44:590-591.
90. Johnson BJ, Robbins KE, Bailey RE, et al. Serodiagnosis of Lyme disease: Accuracy of a two-step approach using a flagella-based ELISA and immunoblotting. *J Infect Dis* 1996;174:346-353.
91. LeWitt MH. Biostatistics for the clinical physician. *Hosp Phys* 1996:41-44.
92. Dressler F, Whalen JA, Reinhardt BN, et al. Western blotting in the serodiagnosis of Lyme disease [see comments]. *J Infect*

Dis 1993;167:392-400.

93. Engstrom SM, Shoop E, Johnson RC. Immunoblot interpretation criteria for serodiagnosis of early Lyme disease. *J Clin Microbiol* 1995;33:419-427.

94. Zoller L, Burkard S, Schafer H. Validity of western immunoblot band patterns in the serodiagnosis of Lyme borreliosis. *J Clin Microbiol* 1991;29:174-182.

95. Magnarelli LA. Current status of laboratory diagnosis for Lyme disease. *Am J Med* 1995;98:10S-12S; discussion 12S-14S.

96. Feder HM, Jr., Gerber MA, Luger SW, et al. False-positive serologic tests for Lyme disease after varicella infection [letter]. *N Engl J Med* 1991;325:1886-1887.

97. Kaell AT, Volkman DJ, Gorevic PD, et al. Positive Lyme serology in subacute bacterial endocarditis: A study of four patients. *JAMA* 1990;264:2916-2918.

98. Magnarelli LA, Miller JN, Anderson JF, et al. Cross-reactivity of nonspecific treponemal antibody in serologic tests for Lyme disease. *J Clin Microbiol* 1990;28:1276-1279.

99. Magnarelli LA, Anderson JF, Johnson RC. Cross-reactivity in serological tests for Lyme disease and other spirochetal infections. *J Infect Dis* 1987;156:183-188.

101. Dattwyler RJ, Volkman DJ, Luft BJ, et al. Seronegative Lyme disease. Dissociation of specific T- and B-lymphocyte responses to *Borrelia burgdorferi.* [see comments] *N Engl J Med* 1988;319:1441-1446.

100. Feder HM, Jr., Gerber MA, Luger SW, et al. Persistence of serum antibodies to *Borrelia burgdorferi* in patients treated for Lyme disease. *Clin Infect Dis* 1992;15:788-793.

102. Needham GR. Evaluation of five popular methods of tick removal. *Pediatrics* 1985;75:997-1002.

103. Rossignol P, Feinsod FM. Arthropods directly causing human injury. In: Warren KS, Mahmoud AAF, eds. *Tropical and Geographic Medicine.* 2nd ed. New York: McGraw-Hill Information Sevices Company; 1990:519-532.

104. Murakami E. Lyme disease case in the Lower Mainland and a new wood-tick removal technique. In: Ziska M, ed. *VIIIth Annual LDF International Scientific Conference on Lyme Borreliosis and Other Spirochetal and Tick-borne Diseases.* Vancouver, Canada; 1995.

105. MacDonald AB. Gestational Lyme borreliosis. Rheumatic diseases. *Clin North Am* 1989;15:657-677.

106. Markowitz LE, Steere AC, Benach JL, et al. Lyme disease during pregnancy. *JAMA* 1986;255:3394-3396.

107. Rahn DW, Malawista SE. Lyme disease: Recommendations for diagnosis and treatment [see comments]. *Ann Intern Med* 1991;114:472-481.

108. Luft BJ, Dattwyler RJ, Johnson RC, et al. Azithromycin compared with amoxicillin in the treatment of erythema migrans. A double-blind, randomized, controlled trial. *Ann Intern Med* 1996;124:785-791.

Influenza

Stephen R. Luber, MD, FAAP
Charles L. Emerman, MD

Misery, suffering, and prostration: a distinctly unpleasant triad of sensations that say, "influenza." Every experienced clinician can recognize the classical symptoms of this common viral infection that every year, almost like clockwork, rears its unpredictable antigenic heads, in which neuraminidase and hemagglutinin surface proteins play musical chairs, thereby defying enduring host immunity.

The incentives for ameliorating the signs and symptoms of influenza are well known. The abrupt onset of fever, myalgias, malaise, sore throat, and cough that characterize influenza turn even the most robust individual into a compromised creature who begs for symptomatic relief. The bad news is the influenza season is here. The good news is we finally have a potent, well-tolerated arsenal of antiviral agents that can positively affect clinical outcomes.

From all apparent signs, the influenza season of 2000-2001 has been problematic. Vaccine manufacturers have experienced lower than expected yields for a component strain—the A/H3N2/Panama component has been especially difficult to grow—required for the year 2000-2001 vaccine.[1] Currently, the Centers for Disease Control and Prevention (CDC) predicts that 40-70 million doses will be available this year. Last year, more 80 million vaccine doses were available.[1]

Add to this looming problem that approximately 10,000-40,000 Americans die from influenza each season and that the economic and productivity costs linked to this viral infection are staggering. Even when mortality is not the outcome of influenza infection, the disease produces significant morbidity that ranges from transient, disabling symptoms to secondary bacterial infections (e,g., sinusitis, bronchitis, and pneumonia). Although symptomatic relief using supportive measures and over-the-counter pain relievers were once the accepted approach for managing flu-mediated discomfort and misery, recent evidence-based studies have clarified the outcome-effectiveness and clinical value of neuraminidase inhibitors such as oseltamivir and zanamivir in this patient population.

Put simply, currently approved neuraminidase inhibitors—oseltamivir, which is available in an orally administered preparation, and zanamivir, which requires inhalation—are active against their intended targets, produce minimal side effects, and are associated with low level of induction of drug resistance. To maximize the therapeutic benefits for patients, however, prompt recognition of flu symptoms and early diagnosis are required. Moreover, it should be stressed that neither drug should be considered a substitute for proper vaccination of target populations; vaccination remains the bulwark of defense against infection, spread, and secondary complications.

With these issues in mind, the author of this evidence-based review evaluates the current clinical approach to the patient with influenza. A detailed discussion of epidemiological patterns and diagnostic strategies is complemented by a thorough assessment of

Figure 1. Influenza Surface Proteins

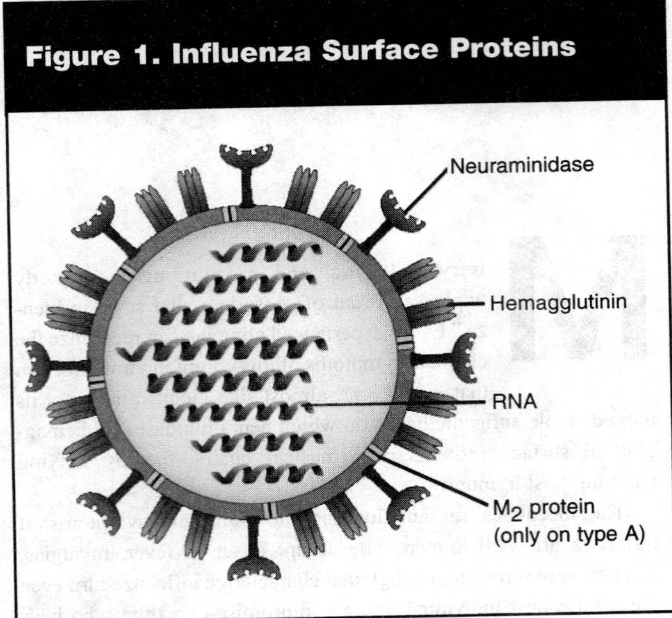

therapeutic benefits offered by neuraminidase inhibitors, which range from reduction of symptom severity and duration to potential prophylactic use and reduction of intra-household viral transmission.

Influenza Viruses: Architecture and Action

Influenza viruses are small RNA viruses belonging to the Orthomyxoviridae family. There are three major types of influenza virus, two of which have been documented to cause infection in the human population. Influenza Type A is the most common and is responsible for major worldwide pandemics. It may infect pigs, horses, seals, whales, and birds as well as humans. Different strains of Influenza A infect some but not all hosts. Influenza Type B, a derivative strain, infects only humans. This strain is simpler and more stable, although it may cause regional epidemics. Its impact is not as global as Type A, but this virus can cause a significant public health problem. Type C belongs to an entirely different genus and does not appear to cause human disease.

Viral Architecture. The architecture of the influenza virus helps explain its unique capacity for infecting the human host and its pathogenic durability over time. Simply speaking, the influenza virus may be visualized as a ball studded with "spikes." These spikes or protuberances represent surface proteins (hemagglutinin and neuraminidase). *(Please see Figure 1.)* Hemagglutinin binds the virus to the target epithelial cell receptor, while neuraminidase degrades the receptor, permitting the virus to enter the cell. Neuraminidase then facilitates release of newly formed viral particles, or virions, which promote spread of the infection within the organism.

These proteins also are the antigens that initiate immune system surveillance. As would be expected, host recognition of these specific proteins by the immune system confers long-lasting immunity against the specific virus. They also reveal the specific identity of the virus and allow epidemiologists to track various strains of influenza that are infecting a population over time or from region to region. Currently, 15 hemagglutinin and nine neuraminidase subtypes have been identified. Interestingly, only three hemagglutinin and two neuraminidase subtypes are commonly associated with human infection. Individual subtypes show minor sequence differences that characterize the various strains, each of which is named according to type, geographic origin, strain sequence number, and year of isolation.[2] *(Please see Figure 2.)*

Antigenic Drift. The RNA core genome of the virus is composed of multiple, segmented single strands of nucleic acids. Lacking the quality control of complementary strand DNA replication, translation errors are frequent. Most mutations are lethal to the virus but some variations (e.g., hemagglutinin is particularly labile) survive and propagate new antigenic variants. These variations are recognized as new strains; they have diminished immunological recognition in the community, thereby permitting the virus to spread infection. From a temporal perspective, this antigenic drift is of clinical significance from the perspective of changes in annual infection patterns and is responsible for periodic, winter epidemics of influenza. In the case of antigenic drift, major subtypes of the hemagglutinin and neuraminidase antigens remain the same.[3]

Antigenic Shift. Antigenic shifts are characterized by major changes in surface antigens on influenza A and are associated with severe illness and worldwide pandemics. Such antigenic shifts originate from the genetic recombination of two strains within a single infected cell and subsequent propagation of the progeny virus manifesting a new configuration of surface antigens. Antigenic shift is facilitated by the segmented nature of the RNA genome. From a clinical perspective, shift is significant for its association with diminished, or complete lack of, contemporary human immunity and, as a result, sets the stage for widespread disease in the susceptible population.

The major subtype(s) of hemagglutinin and/or neuraminidase will change with antigenic shift. For example, the Asian flu pandemic of 1957 was characterized by a shift from a H1N1 to a H2N2 influenza strain. Seventy thousand deaths were reported in the United States alone. The recombination of avian and human viral subtypes within infected hogs appears to be the primary crucible for development of new strains with pandemic potential. Modern pandemics have had a propensity for originating in China, where pigs, birds, and people live in close proximity. Figure 3 illustrates the cycles of epidemics and pandemics that derive from antigenic drifts and shifts, respectively.[2,3]

The influenza B virus is more stable and does not demonstrate the antigenic shifts characteristic of influenza A. It is implicated primarily in regional epidemics rather than worldwide pandemics and, accordingly, this virus typically receives less attention from the professional and lay press. This pathogen, however, can produce widespread disease and accounted for 80% of influenza infections in the winter of 1991-1992. Military installations and schools appear especially susceptible, and specific complications, such as Reye's syndrome and myositis, are encountered more commonly with influenza B infection.

Pandemic Potential. In 1997, six people in Hong Kong died from a particularly lethal strain of influenza, which had a reported mortality rate of 30%.[4] Prior to these reported cases, the H5N1 strain isolated from these patients had been known to infect only birds.[5] Public health officials rapidly isolated the source as commercial poultry, a significant percentage of which were infected with the responsible strain. After transmission from bird to human was documented, an unprecedented public health decision was made to slaughter 2 million birds.[6]

Although person-to-person transmission was documented in some cases, the virus had not yet developed the ability to transmit readily from person to person. If the virus had acquired that capability, the consequences could have been catastrophic. Computer models estimated that up to one-third of the world's population could have died.[2] Development, manufacture, and distribution of a vaccine to contain the virus would have taken six months.[4] Unfortunately, modern transportation networks would have carried the virus around the world in epidemic proportions within four months. The case for effective therapeutic agents was made.

Figure 2. Naming Influenza Viruses

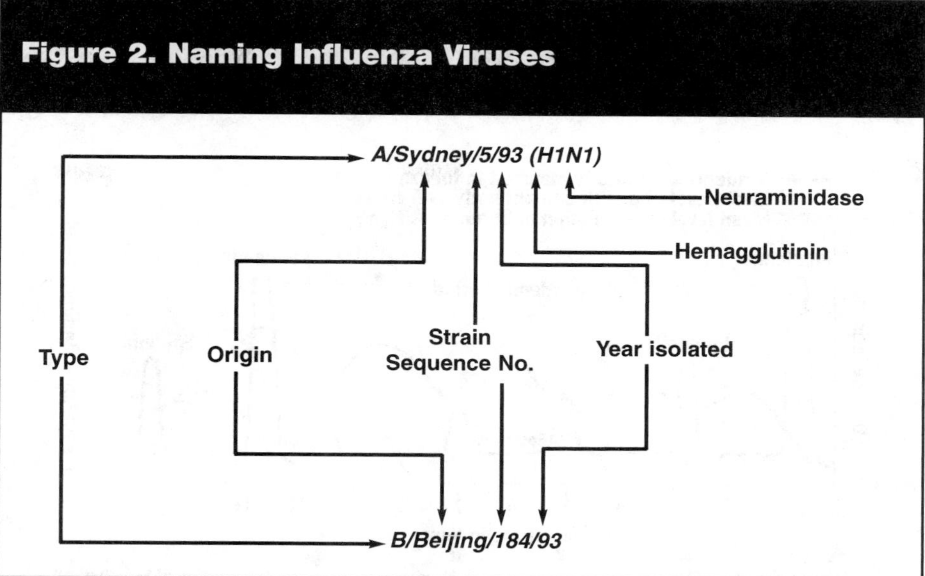

Epidemiology and Infectious Patterns in the Community

Community influenza epidemics typically are short, widespread, and infect a substantial segment of populations. In addition, the onset of a community epidemic is abrupt and peaks within several weeks, with the entire flu "season" lasting 1-2 months during the winter in temperate climates. The first sign of community involvement is an increased incidence of respiratory infection in children that is associated with widespread school absenteeism. As a rule, up to 30% of local children will be involved.

Transmission. Characteristic transmission patterns for influenza have been documented in both the adult and pediatric populations. In this regard, transmission is highest in families with school children.[7] Adults typically acquire the disease from children, a transmission pattern that is accompanied by an increase in physician and emergency room visits for "flu." Interestingly, hospitalization rates are higher at the end of the season. Up to 20% of adults in the community may be infected, with even greater penetration in closed, at-risk communities such as nursing homes, schools, and military installations.[7] While it has been customary to focus on the increased risk and complication rate among the elderly, children younger than age 1 also are susceptible to infection and have an increased mortality rate.

Respiratory secretions generated by coughing and sneezing transmit individual infections. Hand-to-hand contact also has been implicated. Infection is limited to the respiratory epithelium, and ciliated columnar cells initially are involved. Viral replication proceeds over 4-6 hours, is followed by rapid, local invasion of all cell types, and culminates with cell death and necrosis. The infection spreads by local extension throughout the respiratory tract, with clinical symptoms appearing as early as 18 hours after inoculation. The patient remains infectious for 2-5 days following the appearance of symptoms. Although extensive systemic signs, such as fever, generalized malaise, myalgias, and headache, are the hallmark of influenza, the virus rarely is found outside the respiratory tract, and viremia is not a characteristic of most infections.[7]

Host Response. The host reaction to viral invasion is rapid and complex. Humoral immunity, which is mediated by IgG and secretory IgA antibodies directed against the hemagglutinin antigen, appears early and plays an important role in immunity.[8] The antibody levels against hemagglutinin antigens are used as markers for disease activity and for confirming immunity. The cell-mediated response is intense; increased concentrations of tumor necrosis factor (TNF), interferon gamma, and interleukin 6 parallel disease severity in clinical studies.[9] Immunity to a specific strain is clinically protective and long lasting. Immunological durability was confirmed by reemergence of the H1N1 "Russian" flu strain in 1977, which was identical to a strain responsible for epidemics between 1947 and 1950. The pandemic primarily affected those younger than age 25. Individuals exposed to the virus prior to 1950 had developed and maintained effective immunity.[2]

Presentation and Natural History

Overview. The clinical spectrum of influenza illness is well documented and, more often than not, is recognized by the astute clinician. The classic constellation of signs and symptoms includes sudden onset of elevated temperature, generalized malaise, headache, and fever. The initial temperature rise can be precipitous, with fever and associated systemic symptoms remitting over 2-3 days. These signs and symptoms are associated with such respiratory complaints as sore throat, cough, and sputum production, which develop several days after the initial systemic complaints. The respiratory symptoms become more prominent as the illness matures, with the cough lasting up to two weeks.

Because of fatigue, weakness, and other lingering symptoms of the respiratory tract, full recovery from influenza often takes several weeks.[10] Patients may miss an entire week of employment or school. During the 1994 influenza season, 90 million Americans contracted the disease; they spent 170 million days in bed and missed 69 million days of work.[2] Complications of influenza are not uncommon and often are the major source of morbidity and mortality. Primary influenza viral pneumonia is the most common, and also one of the most serious, complications. It occurs early and is characterized by rapid progression of fever, dyspnea, and cyanosis. Chest x-ray (CXR)

Figure 3. Occurrence of Influenza Pandemics and Epidemics

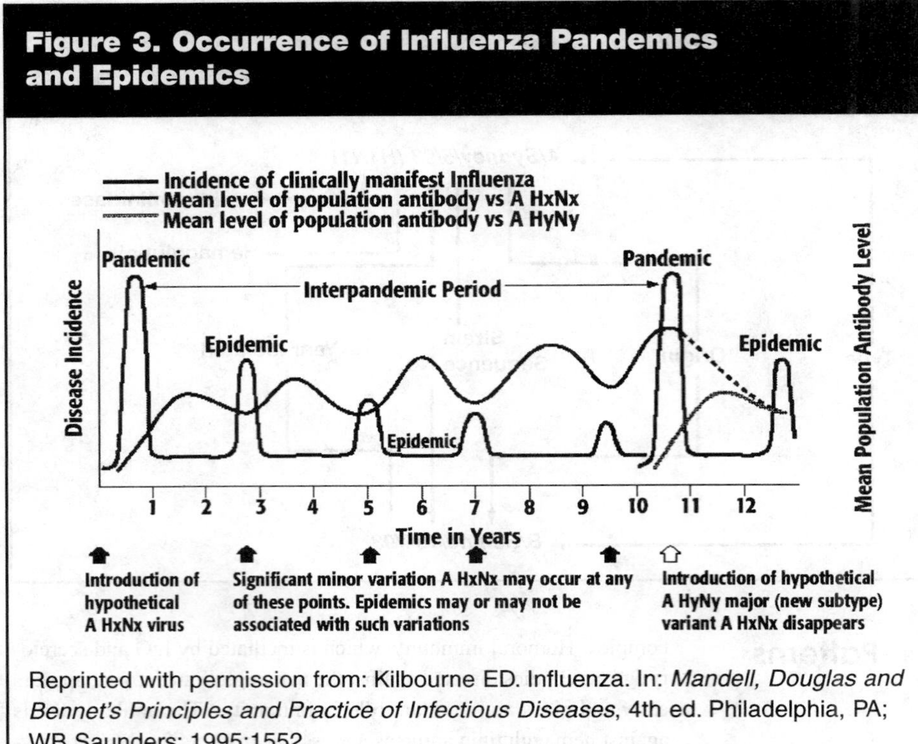

Reprinted with permission from: Kilbourne ED. Influenza. In: *Mandell, Douglas and Bennet's Principles and Practice of Infectious Diseases*, 4th ed. Philadelphia, PA; WB Saunders: 1995;1552.

demonstrates diffuse, non-focal findings and the clinical course is rapid, with findings and a clinical course similar to that seen with adult respiratory distress syndrome. Secondary bacterial pneumonia also may occur, especially in the very young and very old. *Staphylococcus aureus* and *Streptococcus pneumoniae* are common bacterial pathogens, and when suspected, require antimicrobial therapy.

Diagnosis. It may be difficult to differentiate influenza from a number of common respiratory illnesses on clinical grounds alone. Other viral illnesses or bacterial or atypical respiratory infections (e.g., *Mycoplasma pneumoniae, Chlamydia pneumoniae*, and early bacterial pneumonia) can be difficult to rule out. Even streptococcal throat infections can present in a manner that may make it difficult, especially during the early stages, to distinguish from the flu. In the very young and elderly, differentiation from respiratory syncytial virus (RSV) infection is difficult on clinical grounds and may require laboratory confirmation.[11,12] When influenza is widespread and documented serologically and/or clinically within a community, however, the signs and symptoms of this infection usually are specific enough to permit timely diagnosis.

From a practical clinical perspective, a detailed, thorough history and physical examination usually are sufficient to make the diagnosis. Clearly, the positive predictive value of a test, laboratory measurement, or diagnostic strategy for any specific infection increases significantly as the incidence of the disease rises within the population being evaluated. This finding also applies to the predictive value of signs and symptoms elicited in the course of a history and physical examination. For example, when the influenza virus is confirmed by local authorities, state health departments, or the CDC to be present in a region or a community, persons with fever, muscle aches, and cough most likely will have influenza.[13] Several studies have shown a clinical accuracy of as high as 85% during confirmed outbreaks. During clinical trials with zanamivir, it was found that experienced physicians using key factors in the history demonstrated a diagnostic accuracy rate as high as that reported in recently marketed rapid immunoassay kits.[14]

The importance of epidemiological surveillance cannot be overemphasized. The Influenza Diagnosis Working Party (IDWP), an international expert panel, determined that epidemiological support is essential for accurate clinical diagnosis.[15] Although many studies have attempted to differentiate influenza by symptoms alone, the protean nature of this viral illness (as well as most others) hampers diagnostic distinction in the absence of supportive epidemiological data and support.[16] Knowledge of a local outbreak or known contact with a patient with influenza is key to the effectiveness of clinical diagnosis. Accordingly, local health departments and the CDC have long monitored influenza activity. Commercial monitoring by pharmaceutical companies has been initiated during the past two years and increasingly detailed information is now available to the practitioner. Detailed maps of influenza activity are available to the lay public via cable TV and on the Internet. Surveillance sites are noted in Table 1.

From a diagnostic perspective, the most important factors in the patient history are the presence of systemic symptoms: headache, fever, myalgias, malaise, and chills accompanied by cough and sore throat. The onset of these signs and symptoms typically is abrupt, and patients often can tell the physician exactly when they fell ill.[11] Young, otherwise healthy patients are often surprised by how poorly they feel. In the setting of known disease, these historical features will point to the correct diagnosis. Typically, physical findings are nonspecific and often minimal.[13] The patient may look ill, but specific signs of influenza are remarkable for being unremarkable. An elevated temperature of 39°C or 40°C is present for the first 2-3 days. The skin may appear moist and flushed. The chest exam is often normal. Indeed, the presence of chest findings suggest the possibility of complications or underlying medical problems.[13]

Laboratory Examination. Typical, rapidly available laboratory findings are nonspecific in patients suspected of having influenza. For example, white blood cell (WBC) counts are variable and, not infrequently, are normal. While a low WBC with a left shift has been associated with influenza, the absolute count and differential are not diagnostic and offer little help in differential diagnosis. The virus is readily recovered from nasopharyngeal washes, but 48-72 hours are required for culture confirmation of infection. Serologic documentation requires 14 days. The CXR is normal in uncomplicated cases. As a result, obtaining a "routine" CBC and CXR in uncomplicated cases adds little to the diagnostic accuracy,[11,13] and is responsible for overloading ancillary support services better utilized for other patients.

It should be stressed that a CXR is indicated when physical findings or clinical course point to pneumonia. The presence of such underlying medical conditions as chronic obstructive pulmonary disease (COPD), asthma, or cardiac disease also may dictate the need for CXR. Rapid assay kits are now being marketed for the detection of influenza A and B; they will be useful for confirmation of clinical diagnosis. Results may be available in as little as 15 minutes, and these tests have few hands-on steps. They are regulated by the Clinical Laboratories Improvement Act and carry a rating of intermediate complexity, which limits their use in many private practice settings. These tests will be of great benefit to local community practitioners for determining local infection rates. It can be expected that rapid assay tests will subjectively enhance patient confidence in the diagnosis and will provide evidence-based support for increasing the prescription rate of antiviral therapy.

It is well appreciated that many patients with symptoms of the "flu" have come to "expect" antibiotic treatment for their illness. Positive results from on-site immunoassay tests that support a viral diagnosis may help discourage these patients from seeking inappropriate antibiotics and bolster the practitioner's resolve to withhold these medications if not indicated. Use of diagnostic kits in a children's hospital emergency department has led to a significant decrease in antibiotic use while increasing the use of appropriate antiviral therapy.[17] Table 2 outlines diagnostic kits that are currently available.

Age Considerations. Compared to the young and middle-age adult population, the elderly individual and the very young child are more likely to suffer from influenza infection and its complications. In addition, the diagnosis may be more problematic at the extremes of age. While most adults present with a classical picture, the presentation in young children is often more subtle, with signs and symptoms mimicking other common childhood diseases. In particular, the distinctive clinical picture of adult influenza often is muddied by the subjective nature of the pediatric history and its interpretation by concerned parents.

First, the child's ability to describe the myalgias, headache, and malaise of influenza is limited. Gastrointestinal symptoms of vomiting and diarrhea, which are rare in adults with influenza, are not uncommon in children. Alternatively, the infection may present to the clinician as acute laryngotracheitis/croup or classic bronchiolitis. Infants may present with severe bronchiolitis progressing to respiratory failure. Differentiation from parainfluenza or RSV infections frequently require culture or immunoassay. The very young infant/neonate may appear moribund and require a septic workup.

Table 1. Influenza Surveillance Networks, 2000-2001

CENTERS FOR DISEASE CONTROL AND PREVENTION (CDC)
www.cdc.gov/ncidod/diseases/flu/fluvirus.htm
Weekly culture and mortality reports collated with state health department reports and sentinel physician surveys.

NATIONAL FLU SURVEILLANCE NETWORK (NFSN)
www.fluwatch.com
Network of practicing physicians using ZstatFlu diagnostic kits. Uses CDC reports for specific typing of virus.

FLUTRACK
www.flutrack.com
Community level surveillance service provided by Glaxo-Wellcome. Updated weekly.

FLUSTAR
www.FluSTAR.com
Roche provides local epidemiological information as well as generalized public educational information about influenza.

Finally, febrile seizures are not uncommon in the infant.[18]

The elderly patient also may represent a diagnostic dilemma, because in this population, the findings of influenza may be understated. In the geriatric patient, neurological symptoms of confusion, lassitude, and decreased mental acuity with high fever may predominate. Nasal stuffiness is common. The classic abrupt onset often is missed, and the malaise, myalgias, and cough, although present, may be dominated by the more pronounced mental symptoms.[15] The elderly patient with underlying health problems is more likely to develop complications of influenza. They also may suffer a prolonged convalescence with pronounced lassitude. Termed post-influenza asthenia, this post-acute phase can affect the patient's ability to manage his or her own affairs.[13] There may be a need to assess the living situation, with a possible need for placement, as the elderly are at risk for a progressive, gradual deterioration of multiple organ system function leading to a persistent generalized decreased level of health or death.[13]

Table 2. Rapid Diagnostic Tests

CLIA Certified Office-Based Tests*				Detect Viral Antigen		
NAME	COST (DOLLARS)	TIME (MIN.)	STEPS	SENSITIVITY‡	SPECIFICITY‡	COMMENT
Directigen Flu A+B	19.00	15	11	88%	92%	Flu A + B
Flu OIA	16.50	15	5	95%	64%	
QuickVue	20.00	10	3	73%	95%	
ZstatFlu	18.00	20	4	62%	98%	Pharyngeal swab
Influenza Rapid Test	NA	10	4	85%	81%	

* = Average reimbursement $35.00

‡ = Nasopharyngeal swab

Complications. A number of pulmonary, cardiac, and hepatic complications have been reported in patients with influenza. Viral pneumonia is a serious, potentially life-threatening complication. Mortality is high and patients do not respond to antibiotics. Bacterial pneumonia is seen in about 1-3% of patients as a secondary infection, often in the recovery phase of the illness. The findings and clinical course are that of classic lobar pneumonia in a host weakened by a prior viral infection. Typical pathogens isolated are *Streptococcus*

Table 3. Candidates for Influenza Vaccine

INDICATED FOR:

- Health care workers
- Homeless persons
- Persons at high risk of severe consequences of contracting influenza
- Patients ≥ 50 years of age
- Presence of a chronic health condition, including: asplenia, asthma, chronic pulmonary disease, diabetes, heart disease, hemoglobinopathy, HIV infection, immuno-suppression, metabolic disease, renal disease
- Patients maintained on long-term aspirin therapy
- Pregnant women in the second or third trimester
- Public safety workers
- Staff and residents of nursing homes and residential facilities such as dormitories and prisons
- Travelers to foreign countries where influenza activity is reported

CONTRAINDICATED FOR:

- Persons with a history of anaphylactic reactions to eggs
- Persons with hypersensitivity to vaccine components
- Persons with acute febrile illnesses

Sourcees: Recommendations of the Advisory Committee on Immunization Practices. *MMWR Morb Mortal Wkly Rep* 1999;48(RR-4); Update: Influenza activity-United States and worldwide, 1998-99 season and composition of the 1999-2000 influenza vaccine. *MMWR Morb Mortal Wkly Rep* 1999;48:374-378.

pneumoniae, Staphylococcus aureus, and *Haemophilus influenzae*. The response to appropriate antibiotic therapy in patients suffering from bacterial infection is rewarding. It should be stressed that a "mixed" pattern of pneumonia—one showing characteristics and a time course incorporating features of both primary viral and secondary bacterial pneumonia—has been recognized with increased frequency. Therapy, which has included antibiotics and supportive care, has produced good outcomes.[10,13]

Virtually all healthy patients will suffer some transient deterioration of pulmonary function during an episode of influenza. Those with underlying problems are at higher risk. Adults with COPD frequently experience exacerbation of chronic bronchitis and are at increased risk for developing either viral or bacterial pneumonia. Patients with asthma may develop status asthmaticus. Children with cystic fibrosis (CF) may suffer severe compromise. Respiratory failure is the leading source of mortality.[13] Myositis with exquisite pain in the legs may occur. The calf muscle is most commonly involved and creatine phosphokinase (CPK) is elevated. It is most common in children with influenza B.[18]

Reye's syndrome is characterized by acute fatty deterioration of the liver with accompanying liver failure and encephalopathy. It occurs after many viral infections, especially with the use of aspirin, which is a precipitating epidemiologic cofactor. It has occurred after both influenza A and B infections but is more commonly seen after infection with influenza B. It is typically recognized as the patient recovers from the antecedent viral infection. The patient begins to vomit and may go on to have an altered mental status. Frank encephalopathy may progress to coma, decorticate posturing, brain stem abnormalities, and death.

Liver abnormalities may be encountered. Laboratory examination in these patients reflects hepatic insult and encephalopathy with elevated transaminases, serum ammonia, and prothrombin time. According to some experts, the liver biopsy is characteristic and is essential for confirming the diagnosis. Treatment is supportive and aimed at correcting biochemical abnormalities while reducing intracranial pressure. Fortunately, there has been a sharp decline in incidence as the use of aspirin had decreased, which should not be prescribed for symptoms of influenza because of the risk of Reye's syndrome in children.[18]

Other complications encountered less frequently include central nervous disease with encephalitis, Guillain-Barré syndrome, and transverse myelitis.

Cardiac complications are becoming less common. Although myocarditis and pericarditis were reported early in the 20th century, these complications have become less common in recent epidemics. ECG changes with influenza most often represent deterioration of underlying cardiac problems rather than direct invasion of the myocardium.[13]

Prevention

Immunization with inactivated flu virus vaccines remains the cornerstone of public health efforts to reduce the effect of influenza.[19] Such vaccines are typically trivalent and active against the two strains of influenza A and one strain of influenza B that are predicted to be epidemic in the coming flu session. The inactivated vaccine stimulates specific humoral immunity against the selected strain. As explained earlier, antigenic drift requires new viral preparations each year and annual vaccination. The CDC publishes recommendations for annual vaccination. *(Please see Table 3.)* Prevention of disease is possible in nearly 80% of patients younger than 65 years and declines with age. Although vaccines are less effective in preventing illness in the frail elderly, vaccinations maintain effectiveness in the prevention of complications, hospitalizations, and death in nursing home populations.[19]

It should be stressed that manufacturers experienced lower than expected yields for a component strain required for the year 2000-2001 vaccine.[1] In particular, the A/H3N2/Panama component was especially difficult to grow. Currently, the CDC predicts that only 40-70 million doses will be available this season. Last year, more than 80 million doses were available.[1] Moreover, initiation of vaccination programs was delayed one month and was restricted to high-risk individuals. The level of concern about vaccine shortfalls is demonstrated by a pilot project to determine efficacy of half-dose immunization. Volunteers at St. Louis University School of Medicine have been entered into a blinded study using a full or half-dose of vaccine. Serum antibody titers three weeks after inoculation will be used to determine immunogenicity.[20]

A live attenuated, cold-adapted, trivalent intranasal virus vaccine has undergone successful trials and has demonstrated efficacy that is as good or greater than traditional inactivated vaccines. No adverse events were reported.[21] Developed by Aviron, the live virus vaccine stimulates cellular immunity in addition to humoral immunity. The T-lymphocytes are able to respond to closely related strains of the specific selected components. The robustness of this broadened immunity has been demonstrated with induced antibody and endurable resistance to new strains in a second flu season after vaccination. Recipients developed antibody to the circulating A/Sydney strain without inclusion of this strain in the vaccine.[22] The vaccine was 86% effective in preventing infection.[22]

The intranasal delivery system is particularly attractive for the pediatric population. Acceptance of this vaccine with increased childhood immunizations may have significant effect on propagation of annual epidemics. FDA approval has been sought for the coming 2000-2001 flu season. Development of intranasal vaccines to specific immunogenic components (HA) of influenza virus also is underway. These vaccines would not be dependent on the unpredictable process of harvesting virus using fertilized eggs. The recombinant technology could produce vaccines with 2- to 3-month lead times, thereby increasing their usefulness for controlling pandemic infection.[2]

The CDC appropriately emphasizes the importance of vaccination. Prophylaxis with effective antiviral agents is not considered a substitute for effective prevention.[19] Unfortunately, this year's decreased vaccine inventories will likely lead to a less effective disease prevention program and an increased demand for treatment with neuraminidase inhibitors.

Treatment Strategies for Influenza: The Mandate for Neuraminidase Inhibitor Therapy

Overview. Until effective, well-tolerated, and convenient antiviral therapy became available, the treatment of influenza and "flu-like" illnesses was primarily symptomatic. In this model, the emphasis has been on bed rest, increased fluid consumption, and fever control. Supportive therapy also extended to treatment of complications. Unfortunately, many influenza patients who do not have bacterial infections as a secondary component of their flu—and who, therefore, would more likely be eligible for antiviral therapy—inappropriately are prescribed antibiotics. In one study that surveyed outpatient treatment for flu-like symptoms, investigators found that more than 50% of patients received antibiotics. The most commonly prescribed antimicrobial class was the macrolides. Only 21% received antiviral therapy.[23]

The temporal window for successful antiviral intervention in patients with influenza is relatively small. Because the illness is usually self-limited and significant resolution can be expected without therapy in most patients within 5-7 days of symptom onset, treatment must be initiated early in the course of illness if clinicians intend to limit the significant morbidity associated with influenza. The first antiviral agents, amantadine and rimantadine, were marketed for influenza with recommendations that they be prescribed early in the course of the illness. Recently introduced neuraminidase inhibitors have indications for use within the first two days of symptoms.

Amantadine (Symmetrel). Specific antiviral therapy for influenza began about 30 years ago with the introduction of amantadine. This drug targets the M2 membrane protein of influenza A and is effective in reducing the duration of symptoms of established illness. Timely use reduces fever and other symptoms of influenza by 1-2 days.[24] It also is an effective prophylactic agent during epidemics affecting both adults and children.[24] Rapid emergence of resistance and lack of activity against influenza type B compromise its usefulness. Resistance has been documented within single households, in which treated index cases transmitted resistant virus to other family members.[25] Significant neurologic side effects associated with amantadine, including lightheadedness, nervousness, confusion, and insomnia, occur most frequently in the elderly.[26]

Rimantadine (Flumadine). This anti-influenza agent produces fewer neurologic side effects but, like amantadine, is subject to rapid emergence of resistance, lacks efficacy against type B, and is not indicated for acute therapy in children. If rimantadine is started during the first 48 hours of illness, it has been found to reduce symptoms of influenza by 1-2 days as compared to placebo in young adults.[27] Trials in elderly patients have produced similar results. Controlled trials have shown that this antiviral agent is 70-90% effective in preventing disease in populations ranging from school children to elderly nursing home residents.[28] Neither amantadine nor rimantadine has been shown to decrease mortality or complications of influenza.

Neuraminidase Inhibitors: Zanamivir and Oseltamivir. The two prominent surface proteins of the influenza virus, hemagglutinin and neuraminidase, have been investigated extensively as part of the ongoing effort to develop more effective antiviral agents. In particular, neuraminidase has proven to be a suitable target for antiviral therapy, inasmuch as inhibition of neuraminidase activity prevents spread of virus within the host and aborts the infection.[29,30] Although recognition sites for human antibodies to neuraminidase vary across strains of influenza, the active binding site for sialic acid, and hence for biologic activity, is fixed. Molecular modeling of the neuraminidase protein indicated there is conservation of the active sialic acid binding site across known types and subtypes of influenza viruses. As a result, successful inactivation of the binding site via neuraminidase inhibition will hinder virtually all strains and limit development of resistance.[29,30]

Zanamivir (Relenza). The first active neuraminidase developed was zanamivir which, because it has minimal activity against mammalian neuraminidase, limits toxicity and side effects. Clinical studies with experimental and natural infection demonstrated decreased length of viral shedding, decreased symptoms, and reduced severity in both Type A and B influenza infections.[29,31] The critical measure in clinical trials of time to relief of all symptoms was 1.5-2.0 days in several Phase III studies of patients with naturally occurring influenza. Symptom relief was 2.5 days earlier in high-risk patients and this was accompanied by a decrease in complications.[29,30,32] Specific studies also showed efficacy with influenza B infections.[33] In vaccinated elderly patients with active influenza infection, zanamivir was effective in reducing symptom duration vs. placebo suggesting synergistic benefit with vaccination in high-risk elderly patients.[34]

Zanamivir's ionic nature mandated direct delivery of the drug to the respiratory mucosa by inhalation. Side effect profiles in trials reported such patient complaints as nasal and throat discomfort, headache, and cough; these symptoms were similar in frequency to control groups. Questions were raised about possible deterioration of respiratory function in patients with existing COPD and asthma. In this regard, bronchospasm has occurred in patients with asthma.[31,32]

Table 4. Antiviral Agents for Influenza

Generic Name	Trade Name	Indications	Dosage	Whilesale Cost - Treatment	Comments
M2 INHIBITORS — INFLUENZA A					
Amantadine	Symmetrel	Treatment > age 1 Prophylaxis > age 1	100 mg bid × 7 days 100 mg qd	\$6.45 (generic) \$14.38 (branded)	CNS side effects > age 65 — dose decreased to 100 mg qd If CrCl < 80 mL/min — decrease dose
Rimantadine	Flumadine	Treatment > age 14 Prophylaxis > age 1	100 mg bid × 7 days 100 mg qd	\$32.60	If CrCl < 20 mL/min — decrease dose
NEURAMINIDASE INHIBITORS — INFLUENZA A AND B					
Zanamivir	Relenza®	Treatment ≥ age 7	2 blisters bid × 5 days	\$46.18	Disk inhalation device Caution with history of bronchospasm
Oseltamivir phosphate	Tamiflu™	Treatment ≥ age 1 Prophylaxis ≥ age 13 (see Table 5 for pediatric dosing)	75 mg bid × 5 days 75 mg qd × at least 7 days	\$59.54	Mild GI side effects

Moreover, the package insert contains important precautionary information regarding the use of zanamivir in patients with underlying airways disease. Drug interactions have not been reported, and no adjustment in dosage for patients with renal disease is recommended.[35] *(Please see Table 4.)* The drug is taken as a five-day course using a proven dischaler design. It is indicated for patients 7 years of age and older with fewer than 48 hours of signs and symptoms of influenza A or B.

Oseltamivir Phosphate (Tamiflu™). The need for an orally active drug led to the development of oseltamivir. The original compound GS 4071 proved as effective as zanamivir in early trials. Conversion of a prodrug, GS 4104 (oseltamivir), permitted oral absorption. Double blind studies in experimentally induced influenza with A/Texas/36/91 (H1N1) demonstrated this agent was effective both for prophylaxis and as an early treatment modality.[9,14,36] Phase III clinical trials evaluating naturally occurring influenza in a total of 1384 patients worldwide confirmed clinical efficacy of oseltamivir.[31]

Reducing the time required for relief of all major, acute influenza symptoms was the critical measure of therapeutic success demanded by regulatory agencies for clinical trial design and drug approval. With these end points and parameters in mind, oseltamivir reduced duration of disease by 30% (1.3 days) in the U.S. trial. In addition, measures of disease severity declined by 40% and time to resumption of usual activities declined by more than two days. Of special importance was the observation that such complications as otitis media, sinusitis, bronchitis, and pneumonia were reduced by about 50%.[31,37] Specific efficacy also was demonstrated against influenza B infection, with a decrease in symptom duration by 25%.[32,38]

Taken orally as a 75 mg dose twice daily for five days, oseltamivir was well tolerated in clinical trials and the drug's safety profile was excellent. The original trials reported nausea in 17-19% of patients and vomiting in 13-15% of patients in the treatment group. These gastrointestinal symptoms were described as transient and mild by the recipients and led only one patient to withdraw from the study.[39,40] Subsequent studies demonstrated a significant reduction of gastrointestinal symptoms with concomitant consumption of food.[39] Moreover, resistant strains were uncommon and, when present, represented viruses with limited infectivity in humans. Drug interactions were minimal with no dosage adjustments required for concurrent medications; elderly patients also required no dosage adjustment. However, patients with renal disease should have their dosage decreased to once a day if they have a CrCl less than 30 mL/min. Oseltamivir has not been studied in patients with CrCl less than 10 mL/min.[39] Oseltamivir is indicated for patients older than age 18 with a presumptive diagnosis of influenza who present with symptoms of fewer than two days duration.

Although Phase III trials report similar efficacy with oseltamivir and zanamivir, there are no reported studies comparing these neuraminidase inhibitors in a head-to-head trial. Neither are there comparative data with respect to the established drugs, amantadine and rimantadine. Physician and patient preference will be determined by side effect profiles and mode of delivery. There are no published data evaluating the use of neuraminidase inhibitors in pregnant women.

Prophylaxis. The neuraminidase inhibitors also have been shown to be effective for prevention of influenza infection. In pivotal clinical trials, neuraminidase inhibitors showed efficacy with 1- to 2-day decreases in time to alleviation of all significant symptoms of influenza. Zanamivir once a day was 79% effective in prevention of influenza transmission within families with a confirmed index case.[41] A double blind, placebo-controlled study with 1107 patients tested the effectiveness of zanamivir for prevention of influenza over a 28-day period during a local epidemic. Laboratory examination confirmed that influenza occurred in 2% of treated patients vs. 6% of placebo recipients. Inhaled zanamivir was proven effective for reducing transmission of influenza A and B in a nursing home during an influenza outbreak.[42]

Orally administered oseltamivir, 75 mg once daily, was 92% effective in protecting close family contacts against influenza and reduced

Table 5. Oseltamivir Pediatric Dosing

BODY WEIGHT IN KG	BODY WEIGHT IN LBS	RECOMMENDED DOSE
≤ 15 kg	≤ 33 lbs	30 mg twice daily
> 15 kg to 23 kg	> 33 lbs to 51 lbs	45 mg twice daily
> 23 kg to 40 kg	> 51 lbs to 88 lbs	60 mg twice daily
> 40 kg	> 88 lbs	75 mg twice daily

transmission within households by 89%.[40,43] Long-term studies of frail elderly patients taking oseltamivir 75 mg qd in a residential home care setting provided 92% protection against influenza.[43] Mean age of the recipients was 81 years. Application for a prophylaxis indication in adolescents and adults 13 years of age and older with oseltamivir was approved in November 2000.

Ongoing studies of the neuraminidase inhibitors also have shown efficacy in childhood. A double blind, placebo-controlled study of zanamivir in the 1998-1999 Northern hemisphere flu season recruited 471 children with flu-like symptoms. Among these, 346 had culture-proven influenza; dischaler therapy significantly shortened time to alleviation of symptoms and time to resumption of normal activity, and the treatment group used less relief medication. Complications and associated antibiotic use were deceased by 16% and 12%, respectively.[44]

Oseltamivir also has been studied in pediatric populations. A study of 695 patients 1-12 years of age showed a statistically significant 37% reduction in duration of influenza symptoms and allowed patients to return to normal activity 40% faster than placebo-controlled patients. The incidence of acute otitis media was reduced by 43%, and use of antibiotics to treat secondary complications was reduced by 40%.[45] Oseltamivir was well tolerated, with an incidence of gastrointestinal side effects similar to adult studies.

The FDA approved the pediatric indication of the neuraminidase inhibitor oseltamivir marketed as Tamiflu in December 2000. Oseltamivir is approved for treatment of influenza in children from one to twelve years of age. It is delivered as a tutti-frutti flavored suspension with concentration of 60 mg per 5 cc. Dosing is on a per kilogram basis. *(Please see Table 5.)* A graduated measuring device is included with the 100cc bottles to facilitate accurate delivery of the medication.

Oseltamivir is not currently indicated for prophylaxis in children younger than 13 or treatment in children younger than age 1 year. Zanamivir, an inhaled neuraminidase inhibitor is currently indicated for adults and children ages 7 or older. There are no immediate plans to seek indication for younger children. All neuraminidase inhibitors are indicated for patients with less than 48 hours of symptoms and must be administered early in the course of illness to be maximally effective.

Knowledge of local influenza infection is often key to the clinical diagnosis and prompt management of the disease. To this end, surveillance programs have been set up and active websites are available to provide the public and physicians with timely information. Roche pharmaceutical has established the FluSTAR system at www.FluSTAR.com to provide local epidemiological information as well as generalized public educational information about influenza. Professional information is available at www.Tamiflu.com.

Pharmacoeconomic Considerations. Some health maintenance organizations and other third-party payers have questioned the outcome-effectiveness of neuraminidase inhibitors, and as a result, these drugs frequently have been excluded from such panels. The perception by some evaluators that there is only marginal efficacy with these antiviral medications stands in stark contrast to the clinical observations of patients, physicians, and investigators who have prescribed or consumed these medications and evaluated their efficacy first hand.

In an effort to reconcile clinical impressions in real world practice with trial data, investigators followed 1408 patients who were prescribed zanamivir in Australia during the 1999 flu season. Symptom relief was reported by more than 50% of patients within 24 hours and by 77% of patients within 48 hours of drug administration.[46] Of the 400 elderly patients included, 78% were satisfied with their treatment, with 59% reporting symptom relief within 24 hours.[46] The survey concluded that zanamivir was associated with early return to normal activities. They also noted the prolonged nature of residual cough in treated influenza after systemic symptoms of fever, headache, myalgia, and malaise had resolved. Investigators speculated that residual cough prolonged the temporal end point in the clinical studies and, thus, the true clinical effects of treatment may have been underestimated.

Resistance to zanamivir and oseltamivir has been induced in influenza A and B both in vitro and in vivo. In the laboratory, multiple passages through cell culture are required.[47] Resistance during clinical trials has been detected but is infrequent.[48] It appears that alterations of neuraminidase sialic acid binding site that confer resistance also diminishes the virus' ability to propagate. Post-marketing studies to detect significant resistance are under way.

Timely Therapeutic Intervention and New Standards for Influenza Treatment. Neuraminidase inhibitors represent a significant step forward in antiviral drug development. Pending new drug applications promise extension of indications for children and prophylaxis. Ongoing clinical trials are examining efficacy in high-risk patients, especially in individuals residing in long-term, skilled care facilities. Reduction of complications continues to be examined.

Emerging data, however, are very positive and suggest that this class of agents has the capacity to accomplish one or more of the following clinical, prophylactic, or epidemiological objectives:

- Reduce duration and severity of flu symptoms;
- Reduce incidence of secondary bacterial infections;
- Reduce spread of disease by making vectors less infectious;
- Possibly reduce mortality, especially in the elderly;
- Achieve pharmacoeconomic benefits including decreased use of antibiotics;
- Reduce patient load in acute care facilities; and/or
- Prevent development of flu epidemics (by reducing transmission rates).

Clearly, outcome-effective use of these medications demands prompt diagnosis of influenza and timely response by the medical care provider. The classic advice that adheres to the principles of "go home, go to bed, take a couple of aspirin, and call in the morning if you are not better," does not take advantage of the symptom- and complication-ameliorating benefits offered by neuraminidase.[18,19,30] The historical option of offering a patient an appointment with his or her personal physician or clinic in a couple of days if they do not feel better misses the window of opportunity to treat influenza with neuraminidase inhibitors, which are safe and well-tolerated agents that can positively affect the natural history of the disease. In this regard, providing relief of symptoms using only traditional over-the-counter analgesics and decongestants or even more problematic, inappropriately prescribing antibiotics, ignores the opportunity to minimize duration of symptoms afforded by neuraminidase inhibitor therapy.

Moreover, it can be expected that a reasonable standard of care for patients early in their course of influenza will consist of effective antiviral therapy that shortens illness, decreases symptoms, and reduces the risk of complications. In an age characterized by empowered health care consumers, informed patients will want, and predictably will even request, medications that permit them to return to work promptly while reducing complications, decreasing viral transmission within their household, and potentially returning children to school without prolonged absenteeism.

Inevitably, medical professionals, public health personnel, and pharmaceutical manufacturers, working cooperatively, will educate the public about new therapies that have become available for influenza. To this end, prospective patients eligible for antiviral therapy should be prepared to seek medical attention if they develop symptoms of a febrile respiratory illness in the setting of a local influenza outbreak. Recognizing the abrupt onset of flu symptoms is essential so therapy can be initiated promptly.

Summary

Those working in outpatient clinics, emergency departments, and urgent care centers, as well as office based primary care physicians should meet the prevention and therapeutic challenges presented by yearly influenza epidemics. Telephone triage systems should be established to screen for those individuals with classic symptoms of influenza and promptly direct them where they can be evaluated and treated with minimal delay.[18,19,30] The opportunity to reduce viral transmission within households should not be underestimated. Accordingly, specific time slots dedicated to prompt evaluation and treatment of afflicted patients should be established during anticipated flu seasons. Treatment protocols emphasizing clinical diagnosis, recognition of complications, and use of effective antiviral medications need to be prepared and distributed to the health care team.

References

1. Reuters Health Information: U.S warns of possible flu vaccine shortage. Aug. 23, 2000.
2. Laver W, Bischofberge N, Webster RG. Disarming flu viruses. *Sci Am* 1999:280:78-87.
3. Webster RG. Evolution of influenza viruses. Poster, ICAAC 1999.
4. Keavey S. Preparing for the next influenza outbreak—or (inevitably) pandemic. *JAAPA* 1999;11:28-40.
5. Class EC, Osterhaus AD, van Beek R, et al. Human influenza A/H5N1 virus related to a highly pathogenic avian influenza virus. *Lancet* 1998;351:472-477.
6. Tangley L. Detecting secrets of a potential killer. *US News and World Report* 1998;26:60-61.
7. National Institute of Allergy and Infectious Diseases. Fact Sheet: Flu. December 1997.
8. *Mandell, Douglas and Bennet's Principles and Practice of Infectious Diseases*, 4th ed. Philadelphia, PA: WB Saunders; 1995: 1554-1567.
9. Hayden FG, Treanor JJ, Betts RF, et al. Safety and efficacy of the neuraminidase inhibitor GG167 in experimental human influenza. *JAMA* 1996;275:195-199.
10. Nicholson KG. Clinical features of influenza. *Semin Resp Inect* 1992;7:26-37.
11. Cate TR. Clinical manifestations and consequences of influenza. *Am J Med* 1987;82(supp 6A):15-19.
12. Flamaing J, Engelman M, van Ranst M, et al. Influenza and respiratory syncytial virus inflection in the elderly: A prospective study. Poster Session, ICAAC; 1999.
13. Dolin R. Influenza. In: Fauci A, Braunwald E, Isselbacher K, et al. *Harrison's Principles of Internal Medicine.* 14th ed. New York: McGraw Hill; 1998.
14. Aoki F, Osterhaus A, Rimmelzwan G, et al. Oral GS4104 successfully reduces duration and severity of naturally acquired influenza [abstract]. 38th Interscience Conference of Antimicrobial Agents and Chemotherapy. Sept. 24-27, 1998. San Diego, USA.
15. Govaert TH, Dinant GJ, Aretz K, et al. The predictive value of influenza symptomology in elderly people. *Fam Prac* 1998;15:16-22.
16. Snacken R, Osterhaus A, Hayden FG, et al. Managing influenza in primary care: A practical guide to clinical diagnosis: The Influenza Diagnosis Working Party.
17. Noyola D, Demmler GJ. Effect of rapid diagnosis on management of Influenza A infections. *Ped Infect Dis J* 2000;19:303-307.
18. Henderson F. Viral Respiratory Infection. In: Rudolph A, Hoffman J, Rudolph C. *Rudolph's Pediatrics,* 20th ed. Stamford, CT: Appleton & Lange; 1996.
19. Center for Disease Control and Prevention. Prevention and control of influenza: Recommendations of the Advisory Committee on Immunization Practices. (ACIP). *MMWR Morb Mortal Wkly Rep* 1999:48(RR-04):1-28.
20. Reuters Health Information: Flu vaccine shortage prompts US to test half-doses. Aug. 3, 2000.
21. Belshe RB, Mendelman PM, Treanor J, et al. The efficacy of live attenuated cold adapted trivalent intranasal virus vaccine in children. *N Engl J Med* 1998;338:1465-1472.
22. Belshe RB, Gruber WC, Mendelman PM, et al. Efficacy of vaccination with live attenuated, cold adapted, trivalent intranasal influenza virus vaccine against a variant (A/Sydney) not contained in the vaccine. *J Pediatr* 2000;136:168-175.
23. Schweinle J, Mathews D, Petriello K, et al. Flu attitudes for the new millennium: Opportunities to optimize effectiveness of neuraminidase inhibitors to treat influenza. Poster Session, ICAAC 1999.
24. Amantadine: Does It Have a Role in the Prevention and Treatment of Influenza? *NIH Consens Statement* 1979;2:51-56.
25. Hayden FG, Belshe RB, Clover RD, et al. Emergence and apparent transmission of rimantadine-resistant influenza A virus in families. *N Eng J Med* 1989;321:1696-1702.
26. Hayden FG, Gwaltney JM Jr., van de Castle RL, et al. Comparative toxicity of amantadine hydrochloride and rimantadine hydrochloride in healthy adults. *Antimicrob Agents Chemother* 1981;19:226-233.
27. Hayden FG, Monto AS. Oral rimantadine hydrochloride therapy of

influenza A virus H3N2 subtype infection in adults. *Antimicrob Agents Chemother* 1986;29:339.

28. Crawford SA Clover RD, Abell TD, et al. Rimantadine prophylaxis in children: A follow-up study. *Pediatr Infect Dis J* 1988;7: 379-383.
29. Boivin G, Goyette N Aoki F, et al. Clinical and virological efficacy of zanamivir in the treatment of influenza A virus infections during the 1997-1998 flu season. Poster Session, ICAAC 1999.
30. Centers for Disease Control and Prevention. Neuraminidase inhibitors for treatment of influenza A and B infections. *MMWR Morb Mortal Wkly Rep* 1999:48(RR-14)1-9.
31. Hayden FG, Osterhaus AD, Treanor JJ, et al. Efficacy and safety of the neuraminidase inhibitor zanamivir in the treatment of influenza virus infections. *N Engl J Med* 1997;337:874-880.
32. Monto A, Fleming D, Henry D, et al. Efficacy and safety of the neuraminidase inhibitor zanamivir in the treatment of influenza A and B virus infections. *J Infect Dis* 1999;180:254-261.
33. Osterhaus AD, Makela MJ, Webster A, et al. The efficacy of inhaled zanamivir in the treatment of influenza B. Poster Session, ICAAC 1999.
34. Gravenstein S, Freund B, McElhaney J, et al. Greater effectiveness from zanamivir treatment of influenza with antecedent influenza vaccination in older adults. Poster Session, ICAAC; 1999.
35. Lumpkin M. Safe and appropriate use of influenza drugs. Food and Drug Administration Public Health Advisory. Jan. 12, 2000.
36. Hayden FG, Treanor JT, Fritz RS, et al. Use of the oral neuraminidase inhibitor oseltamivir in experimental human influenza: Randomized controlled trials for prevention and treatment. *JAMA* 1999;282:1240-1246.
37. Nicholson KG, Ward P, Kinnersley N, et al. Oral GS4104 in the treatment of influenza in adults is effective and reduces influenza complications and need for antibiotic treatment [abstract/poster]. 21st International Congress of Chemotherapy; July 4-7, 1999. Birmingham, England.
38. Hayden F, Robson R, Jennings L, et al. Efficacy of oseltamivir in experimental human influenza B virus infection. Poster 670, ICAAC 2000.
39. Bardsley-Ellit A, Noble S. Oseltamivir. *Drugs* 1999;58:851-860.
40. Hayden FG, Atmar RL, Schilling M, et al. Use of the selective oral neuraminidase inhibitor oseltamivir to prevent influenza. *N Engl J Med* 1999;341:1336-1343.
41. Monto A, Robinson D, Herlocher M, et al. Zanamivir in the prevention of influenza among healthy adults: A randomized controlled trial. *JAMA* 1999;282:31-35.
42. Schilling M, et al. Efficacy of zanamivir for chemoprophylaxis of nursing home influenza outbreaks. *Vaccine* 1998;16:1771-1774.
43. Peters PH, Norwood P, De Bock V, et al. Oseltamivir is effective in the long term prophylaxis of influenza in vaccinated frail elderly. Leon Valley Diagnostic Clinic, San Antonio, TX.
44. Hedrick J, Barzilai A, Behre U. Zanamivir for treatment of symptomatic influenza A and B infection in children five to 12 years of age: A randomized controlled trial. *Pediatr Infect Dis J* 2000;19: 410-417.
45. Whitley RJ, Hayden FG, Reisinger KS, et al. Oral oseltamivir treatment of influenza in children; submitted for publication, June 2000.
46. Silagy C, Watts R. Zanamivir, a new targeted therapy in the treatment of influenza: A patient perspective assessed by questionnaire. *Clin Drug Invest* 2000; 19:2:111-121.
47. Gubavera L, Bethell R, Hart GJ, et al. Characterization of mutants of influenza A virus selected with the neuraminidase inhibitor 4-guanidino-Neu5Ac2en. *J Virol* 1996;70:1818-1827.
48. Barnett J, Dempsey M, Tisdale M, et al. Susceptibility monitoring of influenza virus clinical isolates to the neuraminidase inhibitor zanamivir (GG167) during Phase II clinical efficacy trials. Abstracts: ICAAC 1997:230.

Skin and Soft Tissue Infections

Charles Stewart, MD, FACEP

Bacterial infections of the skin and underlying soft tissues are among the most common complaints encountered in emergency medicine and in acute ambulatory care settings, including urgent care facilities and office-based practices. Although most skin infections—among them, cellulitis, folliculitis, furunculosis, and trauma- and wound-related infections—can be managed expeditiously, some variants, especially when associated with comorbid conditions and/or bacteremia, may lead to hospital admission and, in selected patients, can produce substantial morbidity.

Fortunately, the majority of uncomplicated skin and soft tissue infections respond to oral antibiotic therapy with a cephalosporin (cephalexin), with a macrolide such as azithromycin or penicillin (dicloxacillin), although a significant minority will pose diagnostic and therapeutic problems. Moreover, it should be emphasized that there is variation among antimicrobial agents with respect to daily dose frequency, duration of therapy, side effects, and patient convenience, all of which may enter in the equation for drug selection.

Although most uncomplicated infections respond predictably to local measures or antibiotics, the course of complicated, serious skin infections can be fulminant, and the mortality rate can be as high as 75%.[1] To produce optimal outcomes in these patients, the emergency physician must have a thorough understanding of the various etiologies, syndromes, and presentation patterns associated with a wide range of skin infections.

As might be expected, changes in the etiologic agents causing skin infections—whether it be cellulitis, infections associated with mammalian bites, or diabetic foot ulcers, as well as changes in sensitivity to antimicrobials, have heightened interest in these infections and options for outcome-effective management.

Worldwide re-emergence of streptococcal strains responsible for streptococcal group A sepsis and streptococcal septic shock syndrome have kindled renewed interest in these diseases. Add changes in the patient population to these microbial and resistance factors, and the stage has been set for an increase in atypical and unusual infections. Recent increases in transplant surgery, cancer chemotherapy, and changing demographic patterns in HIV-infected patients have resulted in more immunocompromised patients seen in emergency departments for skin-related infections. Many of these individuals, along with diabetics, are at increased risk for complications related to these conditions.

With these clinical issues in clear focus, the purpose of this review is to outline diagnostic strategies, detailed management approaches, and antimicrobial selection strategies for common skin infections encountered in the emergency department, with a special emphasis on differential diagnosis and outcome-effective antibiotic selection.

Table 1. Signs, Symptoms, and Microbiology of Folliculitis

- Reddened papules or pustules, 2-5 mm in diameter
- Near hair follicles
- Common locations: beard, upper back, buttocks, chest, forearms
- Pruritic or painful, especially when pustular
- Most common organisms: *S. aureus* or *S. pyogenes*
- "Hot tub" folliculitis: *P. aeruginosa*

Uncomplicated Skin and Soft Tissue Infections

Pyodermas Impetigo. Impetigo is an indolent, superficial pyoderma that can be caused by either *S. aureus* or by *S. pyogenes* (with or without co-infection), with *S. aureus*.[1] Although the literature implicates *Streptococcus* as the most common cause of pyoderma, *S. aureus* increasingly has been identified as the sole pathogen.[2]

It should be emphasized that impetigo is probably the most common skin infection in the pediatric population. Typically, the infection originates with small pinpoint papules that gradually enlarge to form pustules and vesicles. The vesicles rupture and leave a characteristic honey-colored scaling over an inflammatory base. Impetigo usually presents on the face, and will typically manifest as erythematous lesions near the mouth and nose. Impetigo also may occur at the site of minor trauma, especially near abrasions or insect bites. The common, epidemic variety appears most frequently during the late summer and early fall, when warm, humid weather predisposes to the disease.

A variant of impetigo is bullous impetigo, which is usually caused by *S. aureus*.[3] Clinically, bullous impetigo is characterized by large, flaccid bullae with yellow fluid. These bullae frequently rupture to leave a "scalded skin" appearance that is accompanied by superficial erosion of the skin surface. The same bacterial toxin that causes these bullae also causes the systemic staphylococcal scalded skin syndrome.[4-6] A gram stain of the vesicular fluid or exudates will demonstrate characteristic gram-positive cocci.

For many patients, topical treatment and good hygiene may be sufficient. Mupirocin 2% ointment (Bactroban®) is applied three times daily. Bacitracin is less effective but less expensive. If topical therapy fails, an oral anti-staphylococcal agent is appropriate. Recurrent infections are often the result of nasal colonization with *S. aureus*. Mupirocin 2% ointment in a calcium base (Bactroban® Nasal Ointment) applied twice daily for five days will usually cure this problem. For recurrent infections, some clinicians recommend that topical and oral agents be used simultaneously.

Ecthyma. *S. aureus* and *S. pyogenes* are the most common causes of impetigo. Ecthyma resembles impetigo clinically, but the process is more extensive and also includes the subcutaneous tissue. The typical lesion of ecthyma is a "punched-out" ulceration with adherent, necrotic crusts and raised, inflammatory borders. Vesicles or pustules are occasionally seen. The most commonly affected anatomic area is the legs, especially the dorsum of the feet and the anterior shin.

Table 2. Local and Antimicrobial Management of Folliculitis

INITIAL THERAPY:

- Warm compresses and topical treatment.
- Area should be cleaned with a topical benzoyl peroxide soap, cleansing lotion, or an antibacterial soap.
- After thorough cleansing, a topical antibiotic (1% clindamycin) may be applied.

IF TOPICAL THERAPY FAILS:

- Systemic, oral anti-staphylococcal therapy (to methicillin-susceptiple *S. aureus*) may be necessary if local, skin-directed measures fail.
- Cephalexin 500 mg PO BID x 10 days continues to remain a standard and effective therapeutic option. Another initial, first-line option would be azithromycin (500 mg PO on day one, 250 mg PO days 2-5), which permits a relatively shorter course of therapy (5 days) and decreased daily dose frequency (once-daily) as compared to cephalexin or other cephalosporins (cefuroxime, cefadroxil).

Metastatic seeding of the skin from *Pseudomonas* septicemia may cause a syndrome with a similar appearance called ecthyma gangrenosum.[7] These patients are often gravely ill, unlike those seen with streptococcal ecthyma. Crowded living conditions, poor hygiene, heat, humidity, and compromised nutrition contribute to this disease. Ecthyma often follows insect bites and excoriations associated with other minor trauma, including lacerations or wound closures, involving the skin. Varicella lesions also may provide a portal of bacterial entrance to the skin.

Treatment of choice is an oral anti-staphylococcal agent. Necrotic areas should be gently debrided and crusts removed. Fluctuant vesicles or pustules should be drained and the area washed with an anti-staphylococcal soap. Ecthyma is slow to heal and, unlike impetigo, often causes scarring at the site of the infection.

Folliculitis, Furuncles, and Carbuncles. Folliculitis is a superficial infection characterized by reddened papules or pustules about the hair follicles which are 2-5 mm in diameter. Common sites for folliculitis include the beard, upper back, chest, buttocks, and forearms. Folliculitis may be pruritic or painful, especially when it is pustular. Most cases of folliculitis are caused by *S. aureus*, although *Pseudomonas aeruginosa* also is implicated in hot tub or swimming pool folliculitis. "Hot tub folliculitis" usually will be most prominent on parts of the body covered by a bathing suit. Gram stain of the pustular fluid may identify the causative organism. *(Please see Tables 1 and 2.)*

Extension of the follicular infection into the subcutaneous tissue will result in a furuncle. Furuncles or boils are deep-seated, painful nodules adjacent to the hair follicle. Confluence of several furuncles and further extension can create a carbuncle with interconnecting sinus tracts and fibrosis. Furuncles can occur in any hair-bearing area including the face and auditory canal, but the lesions usually occur on the posterior portion of the neck, the back, or the thighs. *(Please see Table 3.)*

Furuncles can enlarge rapidly and, not infrequently, these lesions are associated with severe pain and erythema. Fluctuance also may

Table 3. Signs, Symptoms, and Microbiology of Furunculosis and Carbunculosis

- Furuncles (or boils) are deep-seated, painful nodules adjacent to hair follicles
- Confluence of several furuncles may create a carbuncle with confluent tracks
- Fluctuance and erythema are common
- Carbuncles may be associated with systemic signs (fever, malaise)
- When fluctuance develops, surgical drainage is advised
- Most common organisms: *S. aureus* or *S. pyogenes*

develop. Carbuncles are often associated with more systemic symptoms than observed with furuncles, including fever, malaise, and lymphadenopathy, which are the most common findings. Recurrent furunclulosis can be a challenging problem in diabetic patients, in alcoholics, in those who are malnourished or obese, and in individuals with atopic dermatitis. Immunosuppressed patients and those with immunoglobulin deficiencies or defects in neutrophil function are also at increased risk of recurrence of furuncles. Occlusive clothing and poor hygiene contribute to the problem.

Some patients will develop recurrent furuncles due to skin or nasal colonization with *S. aureus*.[8] Bacteremia can occur when a furuncle is manipulated (i.e., squeezing the lesion). As a rule, the bacteremia is transient although bacterial metastases to heart, bones, joints, meninges, and deep tissues have been reported.

Antimicrobial Therapy. Carbuncles and furuncles associated with cellulitis and fever should be treated with an anti-staphylococcal drug. *(Please See Table 4.)* Surgical incision and drainage are indicated for all fluctuant masses. A cruciate incision and undermining may be needed for large furuncles and carbuncles. Patients with staphylococcal carrier states will benefit from an oral anti-staphylococcal antibiotic and nasal mupirocin cream for eradication of the *Staphylococcus*. These patients also can be treated with rifampin for a 10-day course.[9] Topical use of nasal mupirocin has also been reported to decrease carrier states.

For many patients with isolated furuncles, appropriate treatment consists of warm compresses and topical treatment. The area should be cleaned with a topical benzoyl peroxide soap, cleansing lotion, or an antibacterial soap. After thorough cleansing, the patient should apply a topical antibiotic such as mupirocin 2% or clindamycin 1%. For more extensive disease or when topical antibiotics fail, an oral anti-staphylococcal agent indicated for uncomplicated, *S. aureus* skin and soft tissue infections, such as azithromycin (a macrolide) or cephalexin (a cephalosporin), should be added. Among those agents that have been shown to be effective for uncomplicated skin and soft tissue infections are azithromycin, cephalexin, cefadroxil, cefuroxime, ciprofloxacin, clindamycin, dicloxacillin, levofloxacin, and loracarbef. *(Please see Table 5.)*

Although there are several effective, excellent options for treatment of furuncles, cellulitis, and folliculitis, because compliance can be an important determinant of treatment outcome, when possible, antimicrobial agents selected for skin infections should be conveniently dosed and they should be well-tolerated.[10-20] Cephalexin continues to be a commonly used, drug of initial choice in the emergency and office-based management of folliculitis, furuncles, and other uncomplicated skin and soft tissue infections. Although it remains a reasonable choice, alternative agents, among them, the macrolide azithromycin, has also demonstrated efficacy in these conditions, and as a result, it should be considered an excellent alternative to cephalexin, especially when compliance, pharmacokinetics, and convenience are entered into the drug selection equation. For example, intracellular accumulation of the antibiotic within macrophages and skin fibroblasts, accompanied by adequate tissue levels of the antimicrobial, may help to account for the excellent clinical results demonstrated when azithromycin is used for uncomplicated skin and soft tissue infections. Studies have also demonstrated that medications dosed less frequently are associated with better compliance profiles.[62, 64, 71] Specifically, as a result of its long tissue half-life, azithromycin, can be prescribed for a shorter duration (5 days) than comparable antibiotics, among them, cephalosporins. Azithromycin also has the advantage of a simplified dosing schedule, which is given once daily for only five days (500 mg po on day 1 and 250 mg po qd on days 2-5) for treatment of uncomplicated skin and soft tissue infections caused by *Staphylococcus aureus*, *Streptococcus pyogenes*, or *Streptococcus agalactiae*.

In addition, its well-tolerated gastrointestinal side effect profile may also be conducive to maintaining compliance and reducing discontinuation of the regimen, which occurred in about 0.7% of patients in clinical trials taking the multiple-dose regimen of azithromycin.[21] Overall, the most common side effects in adults taking the 5-day treatment course were related to the gastrointestinal system with diarrhea/loose stools (5%), nausea (3%), and abdominal pain (3%) being the most frequently reported.[21] The introduction of a tablet formulation permits consumption of the antibiotic without regard to food ingestion. Azithromycin is contraindicated in patients with know hypersensitivity to azithromycin, erythromycin, or any macrolide antibiotic.

Table 4. Management of Furunculosis

INITIAL THERAPY:
- Initial topical measures are usually ineffective once furunculosis or carbunculosis has developed.
- Systemic, oral anti-staphylococcal therapy (for methicillin-susceptiple *S. aureus*) may be necessary if local, skin-directed measures fail.
- Cephalexin 500 mg PO BID x 10 days continues to remain a standard and effective therapeutic option. Another initial, first-line option would be azithromycin (500 mg PO on day one, 250 mg PO days 2-5), which permits a relatively shorter course of therapy (5 days) and decreased daily dose frequency (once-daily) as compared to cephalexin or other cephalosporins (cefuroxime, cefadroxil).
- Large carbuncles with extensive sinus tracts and fluctuance will require surgical drainage.

Table 5. Antibiotic Options for Uncomplicated Skin and Soft Tissue Infections in Adults

PREFERRED INITIAL AGENTS (WHEN COMPLIANCE AND/OR COST FACTORS PREDOMINATE)

- Cephalexin
- Azithromycin

ALTERNATIVE AGENTS

- Cefadroxil
- Cefuroxime
- Ciprofloxacin
- Clindamycin
- Dicloxacillin
- Levofloxacin
- Loracarbef

From a practical, clinical perspective, azithromycin is indicated for uncomplicated skin and skin-structure infections due to *S. aureus*, *S. pyogenes*, or *S. agalactiae*, with one clinical trial confirming its comparable efficacy to cephalexin in treating this condition. In a randomized, third-party-blinded study, patients with uncomplicated skin and skin-structure infections received either 500 mg of azithromycin on day 1, followed by 250 mg/day on days 2 through 5, or 500 mg of cephalexin bid for 10 days.

Clinical responses were assessed on day 11, and were defined at the end of therapy as: 1) Cured (based on complete resolution of signs and symptoms); 2) improved (based on improvement, but incomplete resolution of signs or symptoms); or 3) failed (based on no improvement in signs or symptoms). In this study, which evaluated 102 patients in the azithromycin group and 36 patients in the cephalexin group, 67% were cured and 37% improved among the azithromycin patients, and 59% were cured and 37% improved among the cephalexin subjects, an overall cure/improvement rate that was comparable and differences that were not statistically significant between the two treatment arms.[22]

Bacteriologic eradication also was evaluated and compared. Bacteriologic response at the end of therapy was classified as eradication, if the susceptible pathogen present at baseline was eradicated; or persistent, if the susceptible pathogen was still present. In this study azithromycin produced comparable eradication rates (99%; 135/137 isolates) compared to cephalexin (98%, 58/59 isolates).[22]

Cellulitis. Cellulitis is a deep infection of the skin that extends to the subcutis. It begins as a painful, tender, erythematous, warm area that spreads rapidly and produces indistinct borders. Fever, chills, rigors, and sweats are frequent. The infection most often begins at the site of antecedent trauma, which may be minor or major. It also may occur as a result of infection associated with closure of non-sterile wounds and at the site of sutures. Cellulitis frequently extends via the lymphatic system and can produce lymphangitis, lymphadenopathy, abscesses, and bacteremia.

Prior to the age of antibiotics, lymphatic spread of cellulitis was a surgical emergency mandating immediate amputation to prevent septicemia and death.[23] Etiologic agents include *S. aureus*, *S. pyogenes*, Group A beta-hemolytic streptococci, and *Haemophilus influenzae* (primarily in children). Group B *Streptococcus* species is seen in newborns. With the advent of *H. influenzae* vaccine, *H. influenzae* has become an uncommon etiology for this type of infection.

Diagnostic yield of cultures, aspirates, and blood cultures in most cases is low.[24] Cultures from aspirates of the leading edge of the cellulitis may be useful for diagnosis.[3,25] In the typical patient, cellulitis should be presumed to be of staphylococcal or streptococcal origin. For severely ill and immunocompromised patients, cultures should be obtained, despite the poor yield, to identify unusual causative organisms. Cellulitis can extend to deeper underlying tissues and has been associated with osteomyelitis and septic arthritis. Septicemia can complicate the picture, with metastatic arthritis, meningitis, and seeding of cardiac valves.

Antimicrobial Treatment. Initial treatment of cellulitis that is suspected of being caused by *S. aureus* or *S. pyogenes* should include administration of an oral antibiotic such as a cephalosporin or azithromycin. If the patient does not respond rapidly to oral therapy, has systemic toxicity, or has extensive disease, then parenteral antibiotics are indicated.

Wound infections are common in the emergency medicine and urgenct care settings. In these patients, uncomplicated, localized cellulitis associated with traumatic, non-bite-related injuries to the skin, post-skin closure wound infections, and/or suture-related infections is most often due to *S. aureus* or *S. pyogenes*. Multiple treatment options are available. Historically, the standard treatment regimen in emergency and urgent care practice has been cephalexin, which continues to be an acceptable and effective approach for managing patients with cellulitis. Other agents, including amoxicillin-clavulanate, dicloxacillin, and more recently, fluoroquinolones also have been used. However, when medication compliance, clinical efficacy, acceptable side effect profile, and reduced duration of treatment (i.e., < 7-10 days of therapy) are deemed desirable—as they frequently are in the emergency department setting—azithromycin should be considered. As discussed, azithromycin has the advantage of a simplified dosing schedule, which is given once daily for only five days (500 mg po on day 1 and 250 mg po qd on days 2-5) for treatment of uncomplicated skin and soft tissue infections, including cellutlits, caused by *S. aureus*, *S. pyogenes*, or *S. agalactiae*.

Immunocompromised patients should always be admitted and treated with parenteral antibiotics. Warm compresses, elevation of affected limbs, and drainage of any fluctuant area are important adjuvant therapy. When cellulitis is associated with diabetic or decubitus ulcers, initial treatment will consist of a broad-spectrum antibiotic such as an advanced-generation cephalosporin, or an aminoglycoside plus clindamycin as discussed below.

Erysipelas. Known in the Middle Ages as St. Anthony's fire or ignis sacer, erysipelas is characterized by a rapidly progressing, erythematous, indurated, painful, and sharply demarcated area of superficial skin infection caused by *S. pyogenes*.[26] On rare occasions, erysipelas can be cased by non-group A streptococci (B, C, or G), *H. influenzae*, *S. aureus*, and *Streptococcus pneumoniae*.[27] An advancing border can be identified with sequential observation. There is no central clearing of the lesions.

The initial site of entry is often trivial or not apparent. It is more common in the very young and elderly patient. Systemic symptoms such as chills, fever, rigors, and sweats are frequent. About 5% of patients with erysipelas will have bacteremia. Erysipelas may rapidly progress to cellulitis, abscess formation, or even fasciitis.[28] Regional lymphadenopathy is common.

Predisposing factors include venous stasis, diabetes mellitus, alcoholism, and chronic lymphatic obstruction. About one-third of cases are recurrent, mostly in patients who have either lymphatic or venous stasis. Erysipelas is relatively common in individuals with lymphedema following radical mastectomy and chest wall irradiation. Neonates may develop erysipelas in the umbilical stump and the infection may spread over the abdomen.

The differential diagnosis includes cellulitis, herpes zoster, and contact dermatitis. Rapid spreading across dermatomes tends to rule out both contact dermatitis and herpes zoster. Because cultures of the skin rarely yield organisms, the diagnosis should be made on the basis of clinical findings.

Treatment. Treatment consists of penicillin 250-500 mg orally four times daily, although the emergence of beta-lactam-resistant *S. pyogenes* may soon make this therapy obsolete, and require administration of cephalosporins. Three or four days of antibiotic therapy are usually necessary before the signs and symptoms resolve. Resolution of systemic symptoms should be evident within the first 48 hours. The skin changes may resolve more slowly.

Bite Wounds and Associated Infections

Bites from dogs, cats, and humans are common problems encountered in emergency and urgency care practice. It is estimated that dogs bite 1-1.5 million people each year in the United States.[29] In locations where animal bites are a reportable condition, dogs account for 90% of all bites, cats for about 5%, and humans and rodents for about 2-3% each; all other animal species produce less than 1% of all bites.[30] It is estimated that animal and human bite wounds account for about 1-2% of all emergency department visits annually.

Although many bites appear to be minor shortly after they have been inflicted, these injuries can produce serious local tissue effects as well as systemic complications. *(Please see Table 6.)* The most common complication is infection, which may lead to sepsis, joint injury, tendon injury, and in serious cases, even amputation of the limb. Assessment of these wounds may be difficult. *(Please see Table 7.)*

Bacteriology. Whether a bite is caused by a dog, cat, human, or another animal, when a tooth penetrates human skin, it has the potential to inoculate tissues with high concentrations of bacteria. In this regard, the mammalian mouth is a "microbial incubator" that supports growth of more than 200 species of bacteria. In particular, mammalian gingival material contains large quantities of anaerobic streptococci, spirochetes, and *Bacteroides* species.[31] Other organisms commonly recovered from mammals include *Streptococcus viridens, S. aureus*, and *Pasturella multocida.*

As might be expected, infections caused by animal bites may be associated with a wide variety of organisms, and mixed bacterial infections often predominate. Although any of the plethora of organisms that abound in the oral flora of the animal may cause the infection, some infections are species-specific (see below).

Anatomic Location. In many cases, the anatomic location of bites can help determine the risk of serious infection and guide antimicrobial therapy. Generally, wounds that involve deep structures—bones, joints, tendons, vessels, nerves, or viscera—are at high risk of infection and associated systemic complications. Moreover, puncture wounds usually are considered high-risk wounds because they are difficult to irrigate and decontaminate. Cat and human bites of the hand also place patients at high risk for subsequent infection. Initially, human bites may be ignored by the patient because of the influence of alcohol and because of social embarrassment. In infants and small children, scalp and facial wounds are at risk of penetration through the thin membranous bones of the skull. In adults, these same areas are low risk for infection because of the good vascular flow.

Table 6. Complications of Animal Bites

- Localized cellulitis
- Abscess formation
- Septic arthritis
- Tenosynovitis
- Osteomyelitis
- Sepsis
- Endocarditis
- Meningitis

Dog Bites. Dog bites are the most common mammalian bites inflicted on human beings. One author estimates that more than 1000 patients per day seek emergency care for dog bites and that there may be a much greater number who do not.[32] Despite this vast amount of clinical material encountered in the ED on a daily basis, only a few controlled studies have been conducted, most of which involve a relatively small number of patients.

The majority of studies and reviews suggest that a disproportionate number of dog bites are inflicted by German shepherds, Rottweilers, Doberman pinschers, pit bulls, and Alaskan/malamutes.[33] Most dogs that produce human bites are managed in a household rather than being strays, and more than half of the victims are children.[34,35] It is estimated that dog bites account for about 80% of all animal bite injuries in the United States. In one study, about 5% of dog bites returned to the emergency department with a complication.[35] About 1% of dog bite victims will require hospitalization.[30]

Many dog bites produce more than a trivial contusion or laceration. It should be stressed that these bites may be delivered with a force of 150-450 pounds per square inch, which is enough to create a crush injury, in addition to puncture and tear wounds.[23] Severe injuries, including penetrating wounds of the skull, facial avulsions, arterial lacerations, and avulsions of lip or ear have been reported.[37-40] Trauma accompanied by significant blood loss, rib fracture, airway compromise, pneumothorax, and even death, may result from dog bites produced by the larger breeds.[41]

About 75% of all dog bites involve the extremities, with upper and lower extremities affected almost equally.[37-39] Most dog bites in children are relatively minor, usually involve an extremity, and tend to be seen promptly in an emergency department. Severe facial lacerations caused by dog bites occur almost exclusively in children younger than age 10, and most of these involve the cheeks and lips.[35,42] The short stature of children places them at higher risk for facial bites. In addition, children are more likely to place their faces in close proximity to the dog in an effort to inspect or "kiss" the dog.

The microbiology of dog bite wounds is complex. *(Please see Table 8.)* Many authors have reported that the results of initial cultures of non-infected dog bite wounds do not correlate with subsequent cultures of infected wounds.[43-46] Bacteria that are fre-

Table 7. Assessment of Low- Vs. High-Risk Wounds

LOWER RISK
- Larger lacerations
- Wounds on face or scalp

HIGH RISK
- Punctures
- Cat bites
- Most human bites
- Bites or wounds on hand, wrist, or foot
- Immunocompromised patients
- Diabetic patients
- Patients with vascular disease

quently cultured from newly infected wounds include the following: *P. multocida* (wound infections within 24 hours); enterobacteria; *Pseudomonas*; *S. aureus*; *Bacillus subtilus*; and streptococci species, most notably, *S. viridens*.[46,47] Moreover, there appears to be an increased incidence of *Pasteurella* infection in patients younger than 4 years and older than 55 years of age.[44]

Capnocytophaga canimorsus (formerly called CDC group DF-2) has been documented to cause sepsis, gangrene, purpura, and disseminated intravascular coagulopathy about 7-14 days after dog bites in some patients.[48-52] If the patient is immunosuppressed or has no spleen, DF-2 infection after a dog bite may be more common. The organism responsible for this infection is a gram-negative aerobic bacillus found in normal oral flora in dogs. Local signs of infection may not be present with DF-2 infections.[53] The organism responds to penicillin G.

The majority of published studies note that infected dog bite wounds frequently involve multiple bacterial species.[48-52] As might be expected, infection with variable, multiple flora limits the clinical usefulness of the gram stain, and when antibiotic therapy is indicated, it must be empiric in nature. Similarly, routine culturing of the wound may yield minimal information regarding the appropriateness of specific antibiotic therapy. Because culture and sensitivity results typically take 48-72 hours to return, close clinical observation of the wound may yield more information regarding necessity for antimicrobial treatment.

These same studies have concluded that antibiotic administration does not predictably reduce the likelihood of subsequent wound infection in all recent dog bites, but they stress that exceptions to this policy include high-risk wounds as discussed above (i.e., bites to hand and face; deep soft tissue penetration; involvement of tendons, bone, and similar structures; and bites in immunocompromised individuals). In addition to previously cited risk factors, the incidence of wound infection following a dog bite does appear to be markedly increased if the patient is older than 50, has a puncture or hand wound, or if the wound is sutured.[54] As might be predicted, there is an increase in the incidence of wound infections if the patient has waited more than 24 hours to seek medical care or if there was inadequate wound care at the time of the first visit.

Although drugs of choice frequently cited in the literature include penicillin, penicillinase-resistant penicillin, or a cephalosporin,

Table 8. Microbiology of Bite Wounds—Most Common Pathogens

DOG AND CAT BITES	HUMAN BITES
P. multocida	*Streptococcus* species
S. aureus	*S. aureus*
Streptococcus	*E. corrodens*
Corynebacterium	*Bacteroides*
Fusobacterium	*Fusobacterium*
Bacteroides	*Peptostreptococcus*
Porphyromonas	
Prevotella	

amoxicillin-clavulanate probably has the most appropriate spectrum of antimicrobial activity for dog bites and is a generally accepted as a standard of care. Cephalosporins are an acceptable alternative choice. Quinolones also may be effective, with better activity against gram-negative than gram-positive organisms.

Cat Bites and Scratches. Although not as common as dog bites, cat bites are associated with a higher incidence of wound infection than dog bites.[55] Overall, about 29% of cat scratch and bite injuries will develop infectious complications.[35,55,56] In particular, the potential for involvement of tendons and tendon sheaths with *Pasteurella* infections in cat bites is high. The sharp-pointed feline teeth seem to act as hypodermic injectors of *Pasteurella* into the tendon. These puncture wounds are virtually impossible to debride.

Interestingly, cat bites and scratches are more common in women than in men, and about 25% of these injuries occur while playing with the animal.[35,56] In one large study, the peak incidence of bites occured in children younger than 6 years old.[43] The most common organisms recovered from cat bites include *P. multocida* and *Streptococcus viridens,* as well as other strains of *Streptococcus*, *S. aureus*, and strains of *Bacteroides*. Cat scratches are thought to be bacteriologically similar to cat bites, perhaps because of the manner in which cats groom themselves. Accordingly, wounds due to cat scratches have been considered equivalent to cat bites in severity, although at least one study did not find this supposition to be true.[56] As a result, uninfected cat scratches probably do not require empiric antibiotic therapy. When treatment is indicated, amoxicillin-clavulanate is considered the agent of choice.

Cat-Scratch Disease. Cat-scratch disease is caused by an unclassified gram-negative bacterium, inoculated by the scratch of a cat or other animal. The inoculation may be caused by a scratch, lick, or bite. Although the name "cat-scratch disease" implies that cats are the primary vector, dogs also may cause this condition. It is most often seen in young patients who have been scratched by a kitten. The incidence is estimated to be about 3.3 per 100,000 patients. Eighty percent are younger than 21 years of age. There is a slight male predilection, despite the fact that most cat bites occur in females.[35,56]

Patients with cat-scratch disease usually are not ill-appearing. Typically, however, after a 3- to 10-day incubation period, a tender papule develops at the site of the scratch. Impressive regional lymphadenopathy, fever, malaise, and a headache follow in about two weeks. This usually is followed by spontaneous resolution after a few weeks to months. Uncommon presentations of cat scratch disease include encephalitis, oculoglandular syndrome with conjunctivitis, lytic bone lesions, or fever of unknown etiology.[57,58] The conjunctiva may be inoculated in some cases, but the mechanism for inoculation is unknown.

The literature is conflicting about the use of antibiotics in this disease. Much of the literature states that there is no effective antibiotic or that no antibiotic is needed, whereas some sources note that the patient may be treated with doxycycline and rifampin, ciprofloxacin, or erythromycin.[59] Quinolones cannot be used in children and pregnant women due to the effects on developing cartilage.

Culture of the organism is quite difficult, but pus from the lymph nodes may be stained with Warthin-Starry silver stains. Diagnosis is usually made with the assistance of the following findings or observations: history of cat contact and presence of scratch; positive cat-scratch disease skin test; negative studies of other causes of lymphadenopathy; and characteristic histopathology on biopsy of nodes.[60]

Evaluation, Disposition, and Antibiotic Therapy for Animal Bites. All patients with mammalian bites should be examined carefully and all life-threatening problems should be addressed in the usual manner. The priorities of airway, breathing, and circulation (ABCs) should be managed as necessary. Life-threatening hemorrhage should be controlled, and wounds that penetrate body cavities are cared for in customary fashion. The emotional care of the child who has just been attacked by an animal is a top priority and the child should be comforted.

History. Historical data required to properly evaluate and treat dog bites include the following:

- General information about the patient
- Patient's general state of health
- Age of the patient
- Current and past medical history
- History of immunocompromising disease or treatment
- Status of tetanus prophylaxis
- Time elapsed since the bite occurred
- Status of rabies prophylaxis for both animal and human
- Animal status (i.e., rabies prophylaxis in domesticated animals)
- Status of human prophylaxis if patient is an animal handler
- General information about the dog
- Health of the animal
- Species of the animal inflicting the bite
- Whether it is a domestic, wild, or stray animal
- Whether the bite was provoked or unprovoked
- History of prior attacks
- Current location of the animal
- Ownership

Physical Examination. Multiple bite sites are common and, therefore, the patient should be examined carefully to ensure that no lesions are missed. The wounds should be inspected for depth and extent of injury, and the integrity of neurovascular and motor systems should be ascertained. Remember that in a frightened child, it may be difficult to properly evaluate the neuromuscular and vascular systems. Verbal "sedation" of the child by parents and friends may help the examination.

Wound Care. Without question, one of the most important factors in managing an animal bite is proper care of the wound. *(Please see Table 9.)* In this regard, adequate wound management should include mechanical cleansing to remove contaminated material, such as broken teeth and fragments of clothing. The physician should ensure that tetanus prophylaxis is current. Following mechanical cleansing, the wound should be irrigated with a minimum of 250 cc of saline. It should be stressed that irrigation of the wound and wound debridement have been shown to decrease the rate of infection by a factor of almost thirty-fold.[61]

Addition of antiseptics to the irrigation solution is controversial, and there is no conclusive evidence that this increases the efficacy of irrigation alone. It should be noted that puncture wounds are very difficult to irrigate, and some clinicians recommend excising a small plug of tissue around the puncture wound or enlarging the puncture wound with scalpel or needle to facilitate the irrigation. These procedures have not been studied, information is anecdotal only, and their effectiveness is not known.

In cases complicated by a high risk of rabies transmission, the wound should be irrigated with a 1% benzalkonium chloride solution. This solution has been shown to be effective in killing the rabies virus.[62] Decisions regarding wound closure and use of antibiotics are made independently of decisions about rabies prophylaxis. Debridement of the bite wound should include removal of embedded soil, clots, and organisms that may not have been removed by irrigation alone. Tissue that has potential vascular compromise also may be removed at this time. A limited debridement is appropriate for wounds of the face, fingers, and for those areas where neurovascular or motor function may be impaired by extensive debridement. Sharp debridement in other areas will remove the crushed tissue and help clean up lacerations.

If the injury has the potential to involve a body cavity, head, face, joint or boney structures, x-ray films are appropriate. When swelling is present, regardless of the cause, elevation of the area is essential. Immobilization also may be required in the case of hand and lower extremity wounds. Hyperbaric oxygenation has been advocated in human bite infections and the clenched fist injury from human teeth.[63] This therapy remains controversial.

Wound Closure. Primary closure of animal bites is controversial. As a general principle, wound therapy should be individualized for the patient, type of injury, and other risk factors. Nevertheless, certain principles should be applied to the management of these injuries. Fortunately, most wounds are minor, and only 10% will require suturing or surgical care.[30] Wounds that may be sutured relatively safely after they are appropriately cleansed include those involving the face, scalp, trunk, or proximal extremities. Facial wounds are almost always closed primarily, but only after appropriate cleansing, irrigation, and debridement.

Wounds associated with risk factors for infection usually are not sutured immediately. When possible, in the case of human bites, the wound is preferably left open with a delayed primary closure at 48 to 72 hours after first care of the wound. In the case of cat bites or scratches to the hand, a similar policy should apply. As emphasized, high-risk wounds, or wounds in high-risk patients, should not be sutured immediately. Rather, these wounds should be cleansed and debrided, then loosely packed with fine mesh gauze soaked in saline solution. If the wound remains uninfected for 48 to 72 hours, it can be re-irrigated and closed on a return visit, usually on or around the fourth post-bite day. This delayed primary closure has produced excellent results in heavily contaminated wounds.[64]

Loosely suturing the wound, using surgical staples, or applying Steristrips are functionally equivalent to suturing the wound. Wounds

Table 9. General Bite Wound Management Techniques

1. Cleanse the wound. Povidone-iodine solution is recommended for periphery cleansing. The standard solution is diluted 10:1 with saline and can serve as both the cleansing agent and irrigant.
2. After thoroughly scrubbing the wound periphery, irri gate copiously with high pressure using a 19-gauge needle, catheter, or splash shield attached to a 20 mL or 35 mL syringe. Deliver diluted povidone-iodine solution directly into the wound.
3. Debride all devitalized tissue and wound edges. This is essential to reduce the possibility of wound infection.
4. Irrigate after debridement to provide greater exposure of the wound.
5. To facilitate effective irrigation of fang wounds, par ticularly slender cat teeth wounds, the entry site can be widened with a simple 1-1.5 cm incision across the puncture with a #15 knife blade. Retract the new wound with a hemostat or forceps to permit irrigation. Leave these incisions to close without sutures. If the edges are devitalized, trim back to viable skin.
6. Culture purulence or suspected infection. If antibiotics appear advisable, a beta-lactam with lactamase inhibitor or second-generation cephalosporin is recommended. Consult Table 5 for alternatives.
7. Ensure proper tetanus immunization.
8. Assess and treat for rabies exposure if necessary.

Source: Trott A. *Wounds and Lacerations: Emergency Care and Closure.* 2nd ed. St. Louis: Mosby; 1997.

that are not amenable to closure by customary suturing techniques probably should not be closed by these techniques as an alternative. If the wound becomes infected, it should be opened if it was closed, sutures should be removed, and the wound irrigated with copious amounts of saline. The wound should then be debrided and packed open. Consideration should be given to admitting the patient to the hospital for treatment with intravenous antibiotics.

Extensive complex facial lacerations or multiple animal bite wounds are often better managed in an operating room under appropriate anesthesia. Particularly in children with facial wounds or extensive wounds, general anesthesia may be the most appropriate choice.

Antibiotic Therapy. There have been few, if any, controlled, prospective, large-scale studies of the role of antibiotics in the treatment of animal bites, according to anatomic location, patient type, and nature of injury. The studies currently available to guide therapy have been small in scale, confined to one institution, or retrospective.[47,64-66] Most emergency department-based studies have very poor follow-up and the patient who does not have an infection has little incentive to return. Accordingly, there is not a definitive database upon which to make concrete recommendations for antibiotic therapy for the management of animal bites.

No single antibiotic agent is consistently active against all of the numerous potential bite wound pathogens. *(Please see Table 8.)* The recommendations outlined in this review are based upon current information and are designed as a rational approach to management.

For abrasions, contusions, and other injuries that do not require sutures, antibiotics probably are not indicated in the majority of patients. The major exception to this policy is the puncture wound, from either a tooth or claw. Other low-risk wounds will also have little benefit from antibiotics. In the remainder of cases, although the term "prophylactic" antibiotics is used universally, this is not strictly correct. Antibiotics are often given empirically, before a clinical infection has become manifest; a so-called "prophylactic antibiotic" would actually have to be given before the injury occurred.

The choice of an empiric antibiotic is the same, since cultures of the wound at the time of first care inadequately reflect pathologic organisms cultured from infections. Studies with dicloxacillin, penicillin, or cephalexin have failed to show any strong advantages of one drug over the others.[47,65] The combination drug, amoxicillin-clavulanate potassium, ampicillin-sulbactam, and other beta-lactams, have also been reported to be efficacious for initial empiric therapy.[66]

Between 18% and 50% of *Pasteurella multocida* species are resistant to the first-generation cephalosporins and the semisynthetic penicillins.[58] Given the unusual spectrum of sensitivity of *P. multocida,* penicillin G or amoxicillin-clavulanate is the most appropriate antibiotic for the infection that develops rapidly (within 12 to 24 hours after the bite). Considering the frequency and severity of *P. multocida* infections, the poor in-vitro activity of erythromycin, and reports of sepsis in patients who are treated with erythromycin, this macrolide should not be used for animal bite infections.[68]

In the case of a human bite, *Eikenella corrodens* is often found and this organism may be resistant to the semisynthetic penicillins, such as methicillin. However, it is sensitive to penicillin, ampicillin, and some of the cephalosporins. A logical choice for human bites is probably combination of amoxicillin and clavulanic acid.[69] The addition of the latter improves the drug's action against staphylococcal species.

In all cases, tetanus prophylaxis should be current. Hyperimmune serum should be used in the standard dosages for those who have never been immunized. These wounds should be treated as having high tetanus potential, and tetanus immunization should be renewed if more than five years have elapsed since the last immunization.

Human Bites. Human bites are similar to dog and cat bites with two notable exceptions: the location of the bite and the presence of *E. corrodens* in the wound. Like dog bites, the most common pathogens in human bites include *Streptococcus* and *S. aureus*. As the interval from injury to treatment increases, anaerobes become more frequent, particularly *E. corrodens*.

E. corrodens is a slow-growing gram-negative rod that is commonly isolated from human bite infections (10-30%).[70] *Eikenella* exhibits synergism with *Streptococcus*, *S. aureus*, *Bacteroides* species, and gram-negative organisms.[71] This organism has an unusual antibiotic sensitivity pattern. It is resistant to oxacillin, methicillin, nafcillin, and clindamycin. However, it appears to be sensitive to ampicillin, penicillin, and the cephalosporins. Other diseases, such as hepatitis B, however, have occasionally been transmitted by the bite of a human. Abrasions and contusions that do not penetrate the full thickness of the skin are unlikely to become infected. Wounds of the extremities other than the hand or trunk produce less risk for infection.

One important issue that is specific to the human bite is the "human" factor. The victim may not be forthcoming about the mechanism of injury, which confuses matters. The victim may be embarrassed and delay in seeking therapy. The most common reason for delay in hand bites may be recovery time from a binge during which the fight took place. As the patient delays, the flora changes to ivolve more "malignant" anaerobic bacteria. Patients who present within 24 hours often have a benign clinical course and have excellent function after healing, whereas delays in treatment are associated with a more complicated course.[71]

One unique problem that should be emphasized is the "clenched fist syndrome." When a person strikes an opponent's mouth, an irregular laceration occurs over the dorsum of the metacarpophalangeal joint. Dorsal expansion hoods do not cover the joint, and teeth may easily penetrate the joint space or tendon sheath. When the victim extends his fingers, movement of the tendon carries the saliva further into the joint and tendon sheath. The small entrance wound into the metacarpophalangeal joint is frequently overlooked, and may conceal a multilayer violation of skin, subcutaneous tissues, joint capsule, and extensor tendons.

These bites are most likely to occur during the summer months in men ages 20-35 and are on the dominant hand.[72] Unfortunately, the usual picture is that of a small draining wound over the third or fourth metacarpal in a patient who has delayed seeking medical care. Underlying the draining wound is often an infected joint space or tendon sheath that progresses to osteomyelitis or joint involvement.

Deep or full-thickness human bites of the hand have a high incidence of infectious complications, even when treated early. These infections are difficult to treat. Some teaching services recommend that the patient be admitted and intravenous antibiotics started in all cases of suspected human bites to the hand that involve either the joint space or tendon.[73]

Human bite wounds more than 24 hours old require exploration and drainage. This is best accomplished under anesthesia. Many will also need arthrotomy or drainage of the tendon sheath or both, if the joint space or tendon sheath has been violated. Intravenous antibiotics should be initiated as soon as possible.

Diabetic Foot Infection

Potentially serious and usually difficult to treat, infections of the lower extremity frequently are encountered in diabetic patients and are among the most common causes for hospital admission of the older diabetic patient. Most of these individuals will be admitted for both diagnostic studies and parenteral antibiotic therapy. A wide range of aerobic and anaerobic bacterial species are responsible for these infections, and it is estimated that up to 20% of these patients have involvement of underlying bone.

General Principles. The diabetic foot is susceptible to soft tissue infections because of three principal factors: 1) sensory neuropathy; 2) chronic ischemia; and 3) alteration of host defenses. The mere presence of a foot ulcer does not necessarily mean that it is infected. The peripheral neuropathy associated with diabetes permits repeated painless trauma to pressure points on the foot. Over time, these mechanical factors contribute to ulceration. The prevalence of diabetic neuropathy increases with duration of the disease and is exacerbated by poor metabolic control of diabetes. Multiple studies show that those patients with neuropathy and loss of protective sensation of the foot are at greatest risk of amputation, serious infection, or delayed healing of ulcers.[74]

In addition, decreased circulation to the soft tissue plays a major role in the impairment of host defenses in the diabetic. Arterial insufficiency occurs in up to 60% of patients with non-healing ulcers, and about 50% of those who require amputation.[2] The presence of peripheral vascular disease predisposes to infection and slows ulcer healing. Patients with poorly controlled diabetes (i.e., elevated blood glucose and glycosylated hemoglobin levels) also may have impairment of polymorphonuclear leukocyte function. Chemotaxis, adherence, phagocytosis, and intracellular bactericidal activity are found to be depressed in this patient subgroup.[75] Subsequent ulceration provides a pathway for secondary infection that is typically polymicrobial.

Presentation and Diagnosis. Diagnostic confirmation of soft tissue infection in the diabetic foot requires data gleaned from both the history and physical examination. Erythema and purulent drainage are characteristic findings of an infected diabetic foot ulcer. Since many of these patients have neuropathy, pain may not be present. Erythema, increased drainage, crepitance, and/or pain in the leg or ankle may be the signs of limb-threatening infections. It should be stressed that fever is frequently absent. However, unexplained hyperglycemia may offer an early clue to the presence of a serious soft tissue infection.

Minor foot infections are characterized by less than 2 cm of erythema surrounding the ulcer, they are superficial, and systemic signs are typically absent. If the patient has systemic signs, if there is extension of the cellulitis beyond the wound margins, or if there is full thickness ulceration, then the infection is serious. Other findings that suggest a poor prognosis are rapid progression, gangrene of the overlying tissues, or gas in the ulcer or wound, all of which are associated with life- or limb-threatening infection. Moreover, such comorbid conditions as renal failure, malignancy, malnutrition, obesity, cardiac disease, or immunosuppression should prompt placing the patient in a more serious category.

Most infections are polymicrobial, with an average of 2-6 aerobic and/or anaerobic organisms cultured from most diabetic wounds.[76] Secondary infection is common. Culture of the base of the ulcer after the wound has been surgically debrided offers the best opportunity for identifying causative organisms. From a diagnostic perspective, radiographs of the foot and soft tissues are important. Soft tissue films may demonstrate gas or spread of the infections along fascial planes, whereas bone abnormalities may suggest osteomyelitis, a diagnosis that is difficult to make in the diabetic patient.[76, 77] Nuclear scans are occasionally helpful.

Treatment. The two principal objectives of treatment include preventing spread of the infection and avoiding amputation. Control of diabetes, drainage of abscesses, and debridement of necrotic tissue are important components of therapy. Elevation of the limb can help decrease edema. The patient should always be counseled to avoid weight bearing.

Optimal antimicrobial therapy for diabetic foot infections is still a matter of clinical controversy. Because a wide variety of both anaerobic and aerobic bacteria have been implicated in these infections, broad-spectrum antibiotic therapy is appropriate. As rule, minor infections will require coverage for the aerobic gram-positive cocci. Clindamycin, cephalexin, or dicloxacillin are effective when aerobic gram-positive organisms predominate.

However, for infections that are potentially limb-threatening, multiple agents that provide coverage for gram-positive cocci, gram-negative aerobes, and anaerobic organisms are usually necessary. Intravenous therapy is preferred for initial treatment. Tricarcillin-clavulanate, piperacillin combined with tazobactam, ampicillin-sulbactam, other beta-lactams, and cefoxitin are reasonable single agents. Ciprofloxacin is an excellent choice for diabetic foot infections, especially when gram-negative organisms predominate; when empiric coverage is started with ciprofloxacin, it is recommended that anaerobic coverage be added with clindamycin. Adding anaerobic coverage with such agents as ceftazidime or ofloxacin is another effective alternative. After the patient's wound has shown significant improvement, step-down therapy to oral antibiotics may be used.

As emphasized, most patients with diabetic foot infections usually are hospitalized for intravenous antibiotics. However, there is a recent trend to use intravenous antibiotics on an outpatient basis. When this approach is selected, the patient must return for therapy once or twice daily. In selected patients, this method can both reduce costs and be more comfortable to the patient. It requires a responsible and compliant individual to whom detailed follow-up instructions are provided.

Noninflamed ulcers of the foot usually can be considered uninfected, and therefore they may be treated successfully without antibiotics. This clinical distinction, however, may be difficult. Nevertheless, careful wound care and attempts to relieve mechanical pressures at the site of the ulcer are important therapeutic measures. Before discharging the patient, the emergency physician must ensure that the patient has adequate follow-up.

Finally, surgery can play an integral role in the treatment of diabetic foot ulcers. All necrotic and infected soft tissue must be debrided both to control infection and to promote subsequent healing. Diabetic patients with osteomyelitis may require complete resection of the affected bone—or intensive debridement of the affected bone—usually in combination with a prolonged course of antibiotics. Limb-sparing procedures are preferred for surgical therapy of this disease. Unfortunately, despite the best therapy, amputation may be necessary to control the infection. Of the approximately 125,000 lower extremity amputations performed each year, about 50% are directly attributable to diabetes.[5]

References

1. Davison AJ, Rotsein OD. The diagnosis and management of common soft tissue infections. *Can J Surg* 1998;31:333-336.
2. Blumer JL, Lemon E, O'Horo J, Snodgrass DJ. Changing therapy for skin and soft tissue infections in children: Have we come full circle? *Pediatr Infect Dis J* 1987;6:117-122.
3. Carson SC, Prose NS, Berg D. Infectious disorders of the skin. *Clin Plast Surg* 1993;20:67-76.
4. Prose NS, Mayer Fe. Bacterial skin infections in adolescents. *Adolescent Medicine: State of the Art Reviews*. 1990;1:325-332.
5. Schachner L, Taplin D, Scott GB, et al. A therapeutic update of superficial skin infections. *Pediatr Clin North Am* 1983;30:397-403.
6. Scott MA. Bacterial skin infections. *Prim Care* 1989;16:591-602.
7. Ben-Amitai D, Ashkenazi S. Common bacterial skin infections in childhood. *Pediatr Ann* 1993;22:225-233.
8. Hedstrom SA. Treatment and prevention of recurrent staphylococcal furunculosis: Clinical and bacteriological follow-up. *Scand J Infect Dis* 1985;17:55-58.
9. Wheat LG, Kohler RB, Luft FC, et al. Long-term studies of the effect of rifampin on nasal carriage of coagulase-positive staphylococci. *Rev Infect Dis* 1983; 5(Suppl 3):S459-S462.
10. Nelson JD. Clinical importance of compliance and patient intolerance. *Infect Dis Clin Pract* 1994;3:158-160.
11. Cockburn J, Gibberd RW, Reid AL, et al. Determinants of non-compliance with short-term antibiotic regimens. *BMJ Clin Res* 1987;295:814-818.
12. Greenbery RN. Overview of patient compliance with medication dosing: A literature review. *Clin Ther* 1984; 6:592-599.
13. Bosker G. Pharmatecture: *Minimizing Medications to Maximize Results*. St. Louis: Facts and Comparisons; 1999.
14. Chinburapa V, Larson LN. The importance of side effects and outcomes in differentiating between prescription drug products. *J Clin Pharm Ther* 1992;17:333-342.
15. Beardon PH, McGilchrist MM, McKendrick AD, et al. Primary noncompliance with prescribed medications in primary care. *BMJ* 1993;307:846-848.
16. Berg JS, Dischler J, Wagner DJ, et al. Medication compliance: A healthcare problem. *Ann Pharmacother* 1993;27:S1-S24.
17. Litchman HM. Medication noncompliance: A significant problem and possible strategies. *R I Med* 1993;76:608-610.
18. McNally DL, Wertheimer D. Strategies to reduce the high cost of patient noncompliance. *Md Med J* 1992; 41:223-225.
19. Roth HP, Caron HS. Accuracy of doctor,s estimates and patients, statements on adherence to a drug regimen. *Clin Pharm Ther* 1978;23:361-370.
20. Eisen SA, Miller DK, Woodward RS, et al. The effect of prescribed daily dose frequency on patient medication compliance. *Arch Intern Med* 1990;150:1881-1884.
21. Azithromycin package insert (Azithromycin tablets and capsules). Pfizer Labs, A Division of Pfizer, Inc. September, 1999.
22. Mallory SB. Azithromycin compared with cephalexin in the treatment of skin and soft tissue infections. *Am J Med* 1991;91(suppl 3a):36S-39S.
23. Ahrenholz DH. Necrotizing soft-tissue infections. *Surg Clin North Am* 1988;68:199-214.
24. Aly AA, Roberts NM, Seipo KS, MacLellan DG. Case survey of management of cellulitis in a tertiary teaching hospital. *Med J* Aust 1996;165:553-556.
25. Fleishcer G, Ludwig S, Campos J. Cellulitis, bacterial etiology, clinical features and laboratory findings. *J Pediatr* 1980;97:591-593.
26. Feingold DS, Hirschmann JV, Leyden JJ. Bacterial infections of the skin. *J Am Acad Derm* 1989;20:469-475.
27. Finch R. Skin and soft tissue infections. *Lancet* 1988;1:164-168.
28. Ramage L, green K, Pyskir D, Simor AE. An outbreak of fatal nosocomial infections due to group A streptococcus on a medical ward. *Infect Cont Hosp Epidemiol* 1996;17:429-431.
29. Moore RM Jr, Zehmer RB, Moulthrop JI, et al. Surveillance of animal bite cases in the United States, 1971-1972. *Arch Environ Health* 1977;32:267-270.
30. Callaham ML. Human and animal bites. *Top Emerg Med* 1982;4: 1-15.
31. Edlich RF, Morgan RF, Mayer NE, Rodeheaver GT. Mammalian

bites. *Cur Concepts Wound Care* 1986; Summer;15-22.

32. Heller MB. Management of bites: Dog, cat, human, and snake. *Res Staff Physician* 1982;Feb:75-84.
33. Avner JR, Baker MD. Dog bites in urban children. *Pediatrics* 1991;88:55-57.
34. Karlson TA. The incidence of facial injuries from dog bites. *JAMA* 1984;251:3265-3267.
35. Kizer KW. Epidemiologic and clinical aspects of animal bite injuries. *JACEP* 1979;8:134-141.
36. Goldstein EJC, Richwald GA. Human and animal bite wounds. *Amer Fam Phys* 1987;36:101-109.
37. Miller SJ, Copass M, Johansen K, et al. Stroke following Rottweiler attack. *Ann Emerg Med* 1993;22:262-264.
38. Ruskin JD, Laney TJ, Wendt SV, et al. Treatment of mammalian bite wounds of the maxillofacial region. *J Oral Maxillofac Surg* 1993;51:174-176.
39 Snyder KB, Pentecost MJ. Clinical and angiographic findings in extremity arterial injuries secondary to dog bites. *Ann Emerg Med* 1990;19:983-986.
40. Baack BR, Kucan JO, Demarest G, et al. Mauling by pit bull terriers: Case report. *J Trauma* 1989;29:517-520.
41. Sacks JJ, Sattin RW. Dog bite-related fatalities from 1979 through 1988. *JAMA* 1989;262:1489-1492.
42. Lackmann GM, Tollner U. More on dog-bite injuries [letter] *Pediatrics* 1991;122:356.
43. Boenning DA, Fleisher GR, Campos JM. Dog bites in children: Epidemiology, microbiology, and penicillin prophylactic therapy. *Am J Emerg Med* 1983;1:17-21.
44. Callaham ML. Treatment of common dog bites: Infection risk factors. *JACEP* 1978;7:83-87.
45. Spencer RC, Matta H, Ferguson DG, et al. Routine culture of dog bites [letter]. *Ann Emerg Med* 1987;16:730.
46. Ordog GJ. The bacteriology of dog bite wounds on initial presentation. *Ann Emerg Med* 1986;15:1324-1329.
47. Rosen RA. The use of antibiotics in the initial management of recent dog-bite wounds. *Am J Emerg Med* 1985;3:19-23.
48. Anderson CR. Animal bites. *Postgrad Med* 1992;92:134-149.
49. Malnick H, Adhami ZN, Galloway A. Isolation and identification of Capnocytophaga canimorsus (DF-2) from blood culture.[letter]. *Lancet* 1991;338:384.
50. Hantson P, Gautier PE, Vekemans MC, et al. Fatal Capnocytophaga canimorsus septicemia in a previously healthy woman. *Ann Emerg Med* 1991;20:93-94.
51. Peek RM, Truss C. Secretary diarrhea following a dog bite. *Diges Dis Sci* 1991;36:1151-1153.
52. Kullberg BJ, Westendorp RGJ, Vant Wout JW, et al. Purpura fulminans and symmetrical peripheral gangrene caused by *Capnocytophaga canimorsus* (formerly DF-2) septicemia—A complication of dog bite. *Medicine* 1991;70:287-292.
53. Chretien JH, Garagusi VF. Infections associated with pets. *Amer Fam Phys* 1990;41:831-845.
54. Brown CG, Ashton JJ. Dog bites: The controversy continues [editorial]. *Am J Emerg Med* 1985;3:83-84.
55. Aghababian RV, Conte JE. Mammalian bite wounds. *Ann Emerg Med* 1980;9(s):79-83.
56. Dire DJ. Cat bite wounds: Risk factors for infection. *Ann Emerg Med* 1991;20:973-979.
57. Harvey RA, Misselbeck WJA, Uphold RE. Cat-scratch disease: An unusual cause of combative behavior. *Am J Emerg Med* 1991;9:52-53.
58. Tobin EH, McDaniel H. Oculoglandular syndrome: Cat-scratch disease without the cat scratch. *Postgrad Med* 1992;91:207-210.
59. Holley HP, Jr. Successful treatment of cat-scratch disease with ciproflaxin. *JAMA* 1991;265-1563.
60. Margileth AM. Update on cat-scratch disease. *Hosp Med* 1989;Dec:61-81.
61. Newcomer VD, Young EM. Unique wounds and wound emergencies. *Derm Clinics* 1993;11:715-727.
62. Hopman L, Stewart CE. Rabies. *Emerg Med Serv* 1986;May:22G-22J.
63. Lehman WL Jr, Jones WW, Allo MD, et al. Human bite infections of the hand: Adjunct treatment with hyperbaric oxygen. *Infect Surg* 1985;4:460.
64. Wounds and injuries of the soft tissues. In: *Emergency War Surgery First Unites States Revision of Emergency War Surgery NATO Handbook.* Washington, DC: US Government Printing Office; 1975.
65. Elenbaas RM, McNabney WK, Robinson WA. Prophylactic oxacillin in dog bite wounds. *Ann Emerg Med* 1982;248-51.
66. Goldstein EJ, Reinhardt JF, Murray PM, et al. Outpatient therapy of bite wounds: Demographic data, bacteriology and a prospective randomized trial of amoxicillin/clavulanic acid versus penicillin +/- dicloxacillin. *Int J Dermatol* 1987;26:123-127.
67. Stevens DL, Higbee JW, Oberhofer TR, et al. Antibiotic susceptibilities of human isolates of *Pasteurella multocida. Antimicrob Agents Chemother* 1979;16:322-324.
68. Levin JM, Talan DA. Erythromycin failure with subsequent Pasturella multocida meningitis and septic arthritis in a cat-bite victim. *Ann Emerg Med* 1990;19:1458-1461.
69. File TM, Tan JS. Treatment of skin and soft tissue infections. *Am J Surg* 1995;169(5A Suppl):26S-33S.
70. Bilos ZJ, Kuchararchuk A, Metzger W. *E. corrodens* in human bites. *Clin Orthop* 1978;134:320-324.
71. Basadre JO, Parry SW. Indications for surgical debridement in 125 human bites to the hand. *Arch Surg* 1991;126:65-67.
72. Rest JG, Goldstein EJC. Management of human and animal bite wounds. *Emerg Med Clin North Am* 1985;3:117-126.
73. Taylor GA. Management of human bite injuries of the hand. *Can Med Assoc J* 1985;133:191-192.
74. The Diabetes Control and Complications Trial Research Group. The effect of intensive treatment of diabetes on the development and progression of long-term complications in insulin-dependent diabetes mellitus. *N Engl J Med* 1993;329:977-986.
75. Caputo GM, Joshi N, Weitekamp MR. Foot infections in patients with diabetes. *AFP* 1997;56:195-202.
76. Lipsky BA, Baker PD, Landon GC, et al. Antibiotic therapy for diabetic foot infections: Comparison of two parenteral-to-oral regimens. *Clin Infect Dis* 1997;24:643-648.
77. Lipsky BA, Pecoraro RE, Wheat LJ. The diabetic foot: Soft tissue and bone infection. *Infect Dis Clin North Am* 1990;4:409-432.
78. Armstrong DG, Lavery LA, Quebedeaux Tl, et al. Surgical morbidity and the risk of amputation due to infected puncture wounds in diabetic vs non-diabetic adults. *South Med J* 1997;90:321-389.

HIV Infection: Diagnosis and Treatment

Dawn Demangone, MD, FAAEM
Betsy Schrader, MD

The AIDS epidemic in the United States has changed in ways that affect the practice of medicine. With newer antiretroviral regimens, the length of time for progression from human immunodeficiency virus (HIV) infection to acquired immunodeficiency syndrome (AIDS), and from AIDS to death, has increased.[1] Individuals infected with HIV are living longer, healthier lives. Both the number of AIDS cases and deaths from AIDS decreased in the United States in 1996 for the first time. Yet, the incidence of new HIV infections continues to grow, but at a slower rate than was seen in earlier years.[1]

Consequently, as the prevalence of persons living with HIV continues to increase in the United States, it is likely that an increased number of patients with HIV will seek emergency department (ED) care at some point during their illness. Accordingly, it is imperative that emergency physicians remain abreast of variable presentations of this illness, side effects of polypharmacy drug regimens, and drug interactions characteristic of current treatment protocols.

In addition, emergency physicians may be involved in counseling and evaluation of health care workers at risk for acquiring HIV and other blood-borne disease transmission following exposure to potentially contaminated fluids. At times, prompt initiation of antiretroviral therapy may be required. As the public becomes more informed regarding post-exposure prophylaxis, patients may present to the ED requesting evaluation and treatment following non-occupational exposure. These post-exposure prophylaxis assessments present an opportunity for emergency physicians to have a significant affect on disease progression in those with recently acquired HIV infection.

Given the evolving changes in transmission and treatment recommendations in HIV infection, this review will first outline the epidemiology of HIV infection. The pathophysiology of HIV infection will be described, with an emphasis on disease manifestations, prognostic factors, and treatment objectives. The acute retroviral syndrome associated with recent HIV acquisition and its potential effect on emergency medicine practice will be explored. Current treatment medications, side effects, and drug interactions will be presented. Finally, the current recommendations for post-exposure evaluation and prophylaxis (both occupational and non-occupational) will be discussed in detail.

Epidemiology

Worldwide, as of December 1999, it has been estimated that 33.6 million people are living with HIV. The majority of these individuals live in the developing world, with almost 70% living in sub-Saharan Africa. Most of these individuals are expected to die within the next 10 years, adding to the 16.3 million who have already died as a result of AIDS.[2] The worldwide prevalence rate in 1998 was estimated at 1.1%, that is, 1.1 out of every 100 people in the world were infected with HIV. Sub-Saharan Africa had a prevalence rate of 8% during this period.[2]

Table 1. Source Factors that Increase Risk of HIV Transmission[9,10]

- High viral titer
  - Primary HIV infection
  - Advanced or pre-terminal AIDS
- Menstruation
- Other vaginal bleeding
- Presence of inflammatory or ulcerative genital lesions

Table 2. Risk of Transmission Per Episode of Contact[9-16]

BLOOD TRANSFUSION	
Recipient of 1 unit	95%
NON-SEXUAL, NON-OCCUPATIONAL	
IV drug abuse/needle sharing/ other percutaneous	0.67%
OCCUPATIONAL	
Percutaneous	< 0.5%
SEXUAL	
Penile—anal contact (receptive partner)	0.1-3%
Penile—anal contact (insertive partner)	0.03%
Penile—vaginal contact (receptive partner)	0.1-0.2%
Penile—vaginal contact (insertive partner)	0.03-0.09%

In the United States, approximately 900,000 Americans were living with HIV in 1998, giving North America a prevalence rate of 0.56%.[1-3] Approximately 417,000 Americans had died as result of AIDS by this time.[3] The number of AIDS cases and deaths due to AIDS steadily increased in the United States until a decline was first noted in 1996.[1] However, the number of Americans infected with HIV continues to rise, with approximately 40,000 new infections reported every year.[1] The groups with the highest rates of new HIV diagnoses include African-Americans, women, Hispanics, and individuals between the ages of 13 and 24.[1] Prevention efforts should be aimed at these high-risk subgroups.

Pathophysiology

As would be expected, understanding the pathophysiology of HIV infection is critical for identifying the natural history of this condition and the distinct phases of the illness that are amenable to intervention. HIV is classified as a retrovirus (more specifically a lentivirus), which contains its genetic information in a single strand of RNA. The virus is contained within a lipid bilayer, and a protein "core" structure encloses the genetic information and other enzymes essential to its life cycle.

As is characteristic of retroviruses, HIV shows a propensity for mutation. Two main types, HIV-1 and HIV-2, have been identified, with several groups and subgroups also identified within viral types. HIV-1 infection predominates worldwide, and is the type generally referred to as "HIV." HIV has a predilection for cells that express the CD4 molecule on their surface, but it also may infect other mononuclear or glial cells.[4]

Infection begins with binding of the viral envelope (env) protein to the CD4 molecule, followed by fusion of the virus and host cell membranes. The viral contents then enter the host cell cytoplasm, and eventually its nucleus. Viral reverse transcriptase is activated and a DNA copy of the viral RNA information is produced. The new, viral-derived DNA is incorporated into the host cell genome. The infection of the host cell is now complete, and permanent. Targeting the virus for elimination without injury to the host cell now becomes much more difficult. All progeny cells will carry the viral genes.[4]

After insertion into the host cell genome, the viral DNA information may remain quiescent for future activation, or it may be reproduced immediately. When activated, the viral DNA information is translated into novel, viral-derived proteins using host resources. The viral proteins are packaged into virions, which are released into the extracellular space to infect more susceptible cells. This active replication is highly toxic to the host cell, and eventually leads to its death.[4] It has been estimated that each infected host cell will result in the infection of 19 more host cells through its viral progeny.[5]

Following exposure, epidermal dendritic cells acquire the virus and "present" it to cells of the immune system so that systemic dissemination can begin. This does not occur immediately; it has been estimated that dissemination requires several hours to days.[6,7] During early HIV infection, the viral burden is concentrated in the hematopoietic and lymphatic systems, where uninfected immune system cells frequently migrate and gain exposure to the virus. The immune cells respond to the virus with the production of cytokines, which can contribute to the damage of the immediate surrounding host tissues.[4,8] HIV infection eventually destroys the microstructure of the lymph nodes, further compromising immune functions and the immune system as a whole.[4]

Transmission

Transmission: Blood and Body Fluid Source Factors. The likelihood of HIV transmission has been linked with specific, "source patient" characteristics. *(See Table 1.)* Individuals with high HIV viral titers (i.e., those with primary HIV infection, advanced HIV disease, or pre-terminal AIDS) are more likely to transmit the virus than those with lower levels of circulating HIV.[9] One occupational exposure study demonstrated that HIV transmission is more likely if the source patient dies within two years following the exposure incident.[10] Menstruation, other sources of vaginal bleeding, and the presence of inflammatory or ulcerative genital lesions also have been associated with an increased likelihood of transmission.[9]

HIV can be transmitted through several mechanisms: transfusions, sexual contact, perinatal transmission, occupational, and non-sexual/non-occupational vectors. Currently, the most frequent transmission route worldwide is sexual activity. The risks of transmission based on exposure type are listed in Table 2.[9-16]

Transfusions. Blood and/or blood product transfusion remains the most efficient manner of HIV transmission. Individuals receiving a single unit of infected blood have approximately a 95% chance of acquiring the virus.[11] All blood donated in the American Red Cross system is screened for HIV via donor self-disclosure questionnaires and antibody testing.[17] However, the possibility does exist of an indi-

Table 3. Factors that Increase HIV Transmission Risk after Occupational Percutaneous Exposure[10]

- ❑ Deep injury
- ❑ Percutaneous exposure to a visibly bloody device
- ❑ Percutaneous exposure to a needle previously inserted into an artery or vein
- ❑ Terminal illness or AIDS in the source patient

Table 4. Factors that Increase Risk of HIV Acquisition Through Sexual Activity[9]

- ❑ Presence of ulcerative genital lesions
- ❑ Presence of inflammatory genital lesions
- ❑ Cervical ectopy
- ❑ Absence of circumcision

vidual who has been infected but is not yet antibody positive donating blood. One group has estimated the risk of blood donation during the antibody negative period of HIV infection as being one in 493,000. They concluded that adding viral nucleic acid testing to routine blood bank testing for antibody to virus potentially would identify only up to 19 more HIV-infected donations per 12 million units collected annually.[17]

Occupational Exposure. The overall risk of acquiring HIV through percutaneous occupational exposure has been identified as less than 0.5% per exposure episode.[10,15] However, certain circumstances associated with percutaneous exposure increase the risk of disease acquisition. *(See Table 3.)* They include: deep injury; exposure to a visibly bloody device; exposure to a needle previously inserted in the source patient's vein or artery; and terminal illness or AIDS in the source patient.[10] One study reviewed 94 reported cases of occupationally acquired HIV infection. Eighty-two (or 91%) of these cases followed a single percutaneous exposure, eight cases (8.5%) followed mucocutaneous exposure alone, two cases (2%) followed simultaneous percutaneous and mucocutaneous exposure, and one case (1%) occurred after two separate percutaneous exposures.[10] Additional, detailed information regarding occupational HIV exposure and transmission will be presented in a section covering occupational post-exposure evaluation and prophylaxis in the second part of this two-part series.

Sexual Transmission. The most common mechanism of HIV transmission is through sexual contact.[18] A number of source and recipient factors increase the likelihood of transmission and influence the risk of acquiring the virus through sexual activity.[9] *(See Table 4.)* Individuals with ulcerative/inflammatory genital lesions, cervical ectopy, or those who are not circumcised have a higher risk of acquiring HIV.[9,19] Risks for transmission have been estimated based on participative sexual activity and are listed in Table 2.[9-16]

Although probably less efficient as a transmission mechanism than other forms of sexual activity in HIV transmission, oral-genital contact should be considered a potentially important vector.[20] One study found that patients with primary HIV infection had participated in oral-genital contact 10 times more frequently than in anal-genital contact. In addition, participants used condoms during only 3-4% of their oral-genital contacts, compared with 42% of their anal-genital contacts.[20] It appears that the public perceives this behavior as less "risk-linked" than other sexual activities. Even though the risk has not yet been estimated, oral-genital contact appears to carry a substantial risk for HIV transmission based on the high frequency of unprotected encounters.[20]

Non-Sexual/Non-Occupational Exposure. Non-sexual/non-occupational exposures occur in many situations. Potentially significant percutaneous exposures can occur via needle sharing in intravenous drug use, body piercing or tattooing, or other cuts with sharp objects or inadvertent needlesticks with discarded needles. Skin or mucous membrane contact with blood or other body fluids is especially concerning when exposed areas are chapped, abraded, affected by dermatitis, or cover large regions of the skin.[21] Oral mucous membrane contact with contaminated blood has been associated with occupationally acquired infection, and this has been suggested as the source of transmission in one reported case of infection of a woman by her HIV-infected husband.[10,22]

Transmission through human bites is rare, but has been reported. One such case involved a man who came to the aid of his neighbor, an end-stage AIDS patient. The victim was not aware of his neighbor's HIV status and attempted to maintain an open airway during a grand mal seizure. The man was unintentionally bitten, producing a small wound near his fingernail. Later, he noticed blood in the mouth of the seizing man. Despite starting post-exposure prophylaxis with zidovudine (AZT) 10 hours after the bite, the victim developed symptoms consistent with a mild acute retroviral syndrome 33 days following the incident, and seroconverted to HIV antibody positive two weeks later.[23] Although this case demonstrates transmission via oral secretions, it was more likely that the viral source was the blood contamination of the saliva, and not the saliva itself.[23] One investigator cited findings suggesting that saliva is actually a poor vector for transmission, as it inhibits the infectivity of HIV, and the virus only infrequently has been identified in saliva.[23]

HIV Testing in the Emergency Department

Even when the emergency physician is not called upon to perform HIV testing, it is important to understand the testing protocol to counsel the patient and to recommend testing to those with occupational or other potential exposures. Standard HIV laboratory protocols are used when testing for HIV-specific antibodies. Most commonly, an enzyme-linked immunoassay (ELISA) is performed first, and if this is negative, further testing is not pursued on a routine basis since this patient is considered HIV negative. Of course, false-negative tests can occur, especially in primary HIV infection, during a period in which antibodies have not yet developed. If the ELISA test is positive for HIV antibodies, a confirmatory Western Blot is performed. The patient is considered HIV positive only if both the ELISA and Western Blot are positive for antibodies to HIV.[24]

Regardless of the time elapsed between acquisition of the virus and presence of clinical symptoms, a high index of suspicion for primary HIV infection should prompt further testing. Evaluation for the presence of viral components should be pursued. Testing for specific viral proteins, such as the p24 core antigen, may be indicated, or poly-

Table 5. Most Commonly Reported Symptoms in Patients with ARS

REFERENCE NUMBER§	1	2	3	4	5	6
Fever	95%	100%	77%	87%	92%	96%
Fatigue	90%	51%	66%	26%	*	61%
Sore throat	70%	43%	16%	48%	75%	*
Weight loss	68%	20%	*	13%	*	*
Myalgias	60%	*	18%	42%	92%	*
Headache	58%	*	51%	39%	58%	61%
Nausea	58%	*	*	26%	67%	*
Cervical adenopathy	55%	80%	16%	*	75%	*
Night sweats	50%	33%	*	*	92%	*
Diarrhea	50%	7%	*	32%	33%	*
Vomit	40%	*	*	23%	67%	*
Rash	35%	20%	56%	67%	50%	67%
Abdominal pain	*	*	*	32%	*	*
Arthralgia	*	*	*	29%	*	*
Cough	*	*	*	26%	*	*
Oral ulcers	*	*	*	13%	*	*

* = Symptom/sign not reported
§ = References

1. Schacker T, Collier A, Hughes J, et al. Clinical and epidemiologic features of primary HIV infection. *Ann Int Med* 1996;125:257-264.
2. Dorrucci M, Rezza G, Vlahov D, et al. Clinical characteristics and prognostic value of acute retroviral syndrome among injecting drug users. *AIDS* 1995;9:597-604.
3. Vanhems P, Allard R, Cooper DA, et al. Acute human immunodeficiency virus type 1 disease as a mononucleosis-like illness: Is the diagnosis too restrictive? *Clin Infect Dis* 1997;24:965-970.
4. Kinloch-de Loes S. Symptomatic primary infection due to human immunodeficiency virus type 1: Review of 31 cases. *Clin Infect Dis* 1993;17:59-65.
5. Cooper DA. Acute AIDS retrovirus infection. Definition of a clinical illness associated with seroconversion. *Lancet* 1985;1:537-540.
6. Perrin LU, Balavoine JF, Schockmell GA, et al. Post-exposure prophylaxis and sexual HIV transmission between husband and wife. Int Conf AIDS 1998;12: 630 (abstract no. 33189).

merase chain reaction for viral RNA and/or DNA may be helpful in identifying patients who have not yet produced antibodies to HIV. Rapid screening tests are available, but are limited by their sensitivities and specificities.[24]

Performance of HIV testing requires time, confidentiality, patient consent, and both pre- and post-test counseling. This is a formidable commitment for an already busy ED staff. However, one group of investigators has suggested that ED-based HIV screening is feasible, and can play a significant role in the early identification of HIV infection, particularly in regions with high HIV prevalence rates.[25,26] In these studies, rather than adding another task to the responsibilities of the ED physicians and nurses, trained counselors performed HIV pre-test counseling in parallel with the patient's ED course.[25,26]

Post-test counseling appointments were made at the time of the initial ED visits. A rapid screening test, conventional ELISA, and confirmatory Western Blot studies for HIV were coordinated through the ED program, as were post-test counseling, delivery of results, and arrangement of follow-up care. They demonstrated the effectiveness of an ED-coordinated HIV screening program for diagnosing a large number of new HIV-positive individuals in a high-risk population.[25,26] Whether more hospitals caring for populations with a high HIV prevalence will begin offering HIV testing services to the public has yet to be determined. However, one group has found that HIV testing is already performed routinely in some academic EDs in cases of occupational exposures, rape, disease consistent with AIDS, and even in patients treated for sexually transmitted diseases.[27]

Primary HIV Infection

Primary HIV infection is defined as the period between initial HIV acquisition and the time of HIV specific antibody production.[28] Primary infection symptoms can range from none to a severe acute retroviral syndrome (ARS) requiring hospitalization.

Pathophysiology of Primary HIV Infection. Massive viremia quickly follows initial infection with HIV because of rapid viral replication, with an estimated doubling time of 10 hours.[5,28-30] However, absolute viral levels are variable among individuals throughout primary infection.[5,29] Typically, viremia appears to peak somewhere between 21 days and one month after viral acquisition.[5,29] Following this early peak, viral levels begin a rapid decline, and may even fall to undetectable levels, presumably in response to an activated immune system.[19] This decline continues until about post-exposure days 54-120, at which time viral levels again begin to climb.[5,29] Viral levels at this inflection point appear to be significant in predicting the subsequent disease course.[29]

Without therapy, the CD4+ T cell counts fall at a rapid rate shortly after infection until post exposure day 160, when the decline continues but at a slower rate.[5,28,29] Like viral levels, CD4+ T cell counts vary greatly among individuals throughout primary infection.[5] The immune system responds to HIV infection by producing large numbers of CD8 T cells and various cytokines.[8,28] This initial immune response appears to be another important factor predicting the ultimate disease course.[31]

Eventually, the immune system stabilizes and a "set point" or equilibrium is achieved between the virus and the host, typically at 4-12 months following infection.[29] This "set point"—and more specifically, the viral load—is an important predictor of the rate and severity of the subsequent disease course. Although there is no correlation between early viral loads and rate of CD4+ T cell count declines, higher viral levels at 120-365 days after infection are associated with a significantly faster fall in CD4+ T cell counts throughout disease.[29] But prior to the "set point" (approximately postexposure day 120), disease progression or CD4+ T cell depletion cannot be estimated.[29,31]

Table 6. Physical Examination Findings in ARS[20,28,34,38]

- Fever
- Rash
- Lymphadenopathy
- Oral manifestations
- Postural hypotension
- Hepatomegaly
- Neurological disorders such as meningitis, radiculopathy

Table 7. Differential Diagnosis of ARS[18,19]

- Epstein-Barr viral mononucleosis
- Cytomegalovirus infection
- Toxoplasmosis
- Secondary syphilis
- Viral hepatitis
- Enteroviral infection
- Primary herpes simplex virus infection
- Drug reaction[36]

Primary HIV infection ends with the appearance of HIV specific antibodies, which have been first detected in as little as eight days after infection and as long as one year after infection.[8,28] About 95% of patients with primary infection will test positive for antibodies within six months following infection.[32] It should be stressed that the overall disease course already may have been established 4-6 months following viral acquisition, and therefore, early recognition represents an opportunity for appropriate treatment and establishing follow-up care.[19,20,29,31]

Acute Retroviral Syndrome. A syndrome of clinical symptoms associated with primary HIV infection was first described in 1984, in association with an occupationally acquired infection.[33] In 1985, several cases were reviewed by a group that described a mononucleosis-like illness in 11 of 12 patients with acute seroconversion.[34] One group has defined ARS as the "development of high-level viremia accompanied by immunological activation in the presence of clinical manifestations" of HIV infection.[28] In 1997, another group of investigators suggested that because only 20% of their patients with ARS experienced a mononucleosis-like illness, the term ARS should be applied to a more generalized acute febrile illness rather than limited to the earlier mononucleosis-like definition.[35] In this regard, fever appears to be the most common symptom reported by several authors, while sore throat is much more variable.[20,34-38]

It is essential to recognize ARS because symptomatic seroconverters have been reported to progress to AIDS and death from AIDS more rapidly than asymptomatic seroconverters. One study reported that 27% of symptomatic converters progressed to AIDS and 26% to death within 48 months, compared to only 6.5% progressing to AIDS and 2.8% to death in asymptomatic seroconverters.[37] Symptomatic patients also have faster rates of CD4+ T cell decline.[37] While some studies found that patients whose ARS symptoms lasted longer have progressed to AIDS faster than those with a shorter duration of symptoms, others have not.[29,37] Therefore, early recognition is imperative to identify patients who are likely to experience a more rapid disease course.

Why some individuals develop symptoms with acute infection and others do not is not understood. One study reported no demographic differences between symptomatic and asymptomatic converters.[20] It has been theorized that ARS may represent greater disease dissemination or an inadequate immune response to recent HIV acquisition.[29] Publications have reported that symptomatic seroconversion occurs in between 10% and 90% of acutely HIV-infected individuals.[20,28,34-38]

Symptoms can range from mild to a degree of severity warranting hospitalization. Indeed, ARS may even present as an AIDS-defining illness, or with a CD4+ T cell count less than 400.[20,28,34-38] Typically, the onset of ARS symptoms has been reported between five and 30 days following exposure to the virus.[19,20,28,35] Symptoms can persist from seven to more than 28 days, and then this phase may be followed by a prolonged asymptomatic period.[2,5,7,28,34-37,67] There is no difference in CD4+ T cell counts during acute infection between symptomatic and asymptomatic seroconverters.[37]

The most common symptoms reported during ARS in six different studies are listed in Table 5. The more common complaints include: fever, fatigue, sore throat, lymphadenopathy, weight loss, myalgias, headache, nausea, vomiting, diarrhea, and rash.[20,34-35,37-38] Two studies reported that symptoms were severe enough to require hospitalization in 17% and 42% of the symptomatic subjects, respectively.[20,38] Obviously, these complaints commonly are evaluated in the ED and, therefore, present an opportunity for early recognition in high-risk patients.

Findings on physical exam can include fever, rash, lymphadenopathy, oral manifestations, and postural hypotension.[20,28,34,38] *(See Table 6.)* The average temperatures reported were 38.6°C and 38.9°C.[20,38] The rash most commonly has been described as a maculopapular erythematous truncal rash (with or without an urticarial component), but also may present on the face and extremities or as ulcers involving the mouth or genitalia or urticaria.[34,38] Adenopathy is most often observed in the cervical distribution, but also may be found in axillae, inguinal, and epitrochlear regions.[38] Oral manifestations can include exudative pharyngitis, oral ulcers, and thrush.[20,28,34] The differential diagnoses of ARS should be considered based on the presenting complaints and physical findings.[18,19] Some diseases to consider in the differential diagnosis are listed in Table 7 and include several infectious diseases.[18,19]

Clinical Implications of ARS Recognition. As stressed earlier, individuals with ARS more quickly progress to AIDS and death due to AIDS than asymptomatic converters. Moreover, failure to recognize acute HIV infection may mean missing an opportunity for early treatment, which may substantially improve the course of the illness and prevent further transmission to others. Therefore, prompt recognition of ARS by health care professionals is crucial; unfortunately, this phase of the illness frequently is not recognized. One study demonstrated that a significant majority (88%) of patients sought medical evaluation during onset of ARS symptoms. One-half went to their primary care physician; the other half sought care in an ED or walk-in clinic. Importantly, among patients undergoing medical evaluation for their symptoms, ARS was considered in only 26%, despite

Table 8. Medications Used for Treatment of HIV Infection[21,46]

GENERIC	BRAND
NUCLEOSIDE REVERSE TRANSCRIPTASE INHIBITORS (NRTI)	
Zidovudine (AZT)	(Retrovir)
Stavudine (d4T)	(Zerit)
Didanosine (ddI)	(Videx)
Lamivudine (3TC)	(Epivir)
Zalcitabine (ddC)	(Hivid)
Zidovudine plus lamivudine	(Combivir)
Abacavir (ABC)	(Ziagen)
NON-NUCLEOSIDE REVERSE TRANSCRIPTASE INHIBITORS (NNRTI)	
Nevirapine	(Viramune)
Delavirdine	(Rescriptor)
Efavirenz	(Sustiva)
PROTEASE INHIBITORS (PI)	
Saquinavir	(Invirase, Fortovase)
Ritonavir	(Norvir)
Indinavir	(Crixivan)
Nelfinavir	(Viracept)
Amprenavir	(Agenerase)

Table 9. Web Sites of Interest

- **Centers for Disease Control and Prevention:** www.cdc.gov
- **HIV/AIDS Treatment Information Service:** www.hivatis.org
- **HIV InSite (University of California at San Francisco):** hivinsite.ucsf.edu
- **Pediatric AIDS Clinical Trials Group:** pactg.s-3.com
- **AIDS Education and Research Trust:** www.avert.org
- **Joint United Nations Programme on HIV/AIDS:** www.unaids.org

awareness on the part of health care professionals of high-risk activities among these individuals.[20]

Another study reported that 32% of symptomatic patients presented to an ED for evaluation.[38] These studies suggest a large number of patients with ARS seek medical evaluation during their symptoms, but that their diagnosis is frequently overlooked during the initial encounter. Seeking medical attention for symptoms of ARS may be another factor associated with faster disease progression, in addition to experiencing symptomatic seroconversion. One group reported that patients with ARS who sought medical attention had lower CD4+ T cell counts at six months and progressed to AIDS faster than those whose symptoms did not prompt them to seek care.[20,29] Based on the significant number of patients presenting to the ED with ARS, an opportunity exists for emergency physicians to identify and have an effect on the symptomatic, acutely HIV-infected patient.

While the emergency physician may not perform the HIV testing, or even begin antiretroviral treatment, alerting the patient to the possibility of acute HIV infection and advising appropriate follow-up testing and care may ultimately lead to an improvement in the patient's quality and length of life. Without question, earlier identification ARS or primary HIV infection will permit earlier initiation of antiretroviral therapy. In this regard, some experts believe that early, aggressive treatment will inhibit viral replication during the critical stages of early infection.[21] In addition, during initial stages of infection, the viral load is relatively homogenous, since the virus has had limited time to mutate; therefore, it is less likely to have developed antiretroviral resistance and may be more susceptible to treatment.[21,39,40]

One trial reported that using AZT alone during primary infection led to patients with higher CD4+ T cell counts and a delay in HIV-associated infections (zoster, thrush, oral hairy leukoplakia) compared to placebo-treated patients.[41] In fact, AZT-treated patients displayed monthly gains in their CD4+ T cell counts, while the placebo group demonstrated a decline.[41] However, no significant differences in viral loads existed between treated and placebo patients throughout the study.[41] It is hoped that early treatment favorably will alter the initial "set point" following acute HIV acquisition, leading to lower viral loads and, potentially, to improvement in the course of the disease. Lower HIV viral titers 4-6 months after infection potentially could slow and make the disease course more indolent for those patients at risk for a rapid disease progression.[21,28,40]

More recent studies have used triple drug regimens (AZT, lamivudine, and either indinavir or didanosine) for treatment of primary HIV and found continually decreasing viral levels throughout treatment.[39,42] One study reported that triple antiretroviral therapy successfully suppressed viral replication in all treated subjects to undetectable levels at 24 weeks.[42] Subjects in that study also demonstrated CD4 T cell counts at levels close to normal during treatment.[42] However, these studies followed patients a maximum of 36-44 weeks or eight months, and therefore, long-term benefits are unclear at present.[39,42] Despite these encouraging reports, it should be noted that discontinuing therapy started during primary HIV infection might result in a rapid rebound of the virus and its effects, although at a slower rate of viral replication than the rate in primary infection.[5]

In addition to improving the health of patients infected with HIV, counseling them with regard to high-risk activities may prevent further transmission. It has been estimated that HIV transmission is 4-12 times more frequent during primary HIV infection than during the later seropositive stages.[43-45] Both high viral loads typical of primary HIV infection and the patient's lack of awareness of newly acquired HIV infection are likely to contribute to the increased frequency of transmission.[43-45] Moreover, because symptomatic converters have higher viral titers than asymptomatic seroconverters, these patients present a greater risk for transmission—again reinforcing the need for early identification.[20]

Current Treatment Options. Three medication classes are currently approved for treatment of HIV. Table 8 contains the current classifications and names of medications recommended for the treatment of HIV.[21,46] Monotherapy is contraindicated with any medication because of the development of resistance. The one exception is AZT, when used during pregnancy for patients with high CD4+ T cell counts and low viral load to prevent HIV transmission to the fetus.[21] The most recent information regarding specific combination therapy recommendations are available as a living document on the Internet. *(See Table 9.)*

Treatment regimens frequently require adjustment throughout the disease course due to failure, development of resistance, and/or clinical intolerance.[21] Present thinking suggests that no regimen completely eliminates the virus from all locations, although strategic combinations can postpone AIDS-related complications and extend length of life by diminishing viral replication and promoting immune system function.[21] Accordingly, the primary goal of therapy is to suppress viral replication for as long as possible. Current recommendations support offering treatment to all symptomatic and asymptomatic patients with: CD4+ T cell counts less than 500; viral loads (HIV RNA) greater than 10,000 (6DIUA) or more than 20,000 copies (RT-PCR); ARS; recent, documented seroconversion (within 6 months); and symptoms of illness related to HIV infection.[21]

References

1. Center for Disease Control and Prevention. Trends in the HIV and AIDS Epidemic 1998. http://www.cdc.gov/nchstp/hivaids/stats/trends98.pdf (accessed 1/9/2000).
2. Joint United Nations Programme of HIV/AIDS. AIDS epidemic update: December 1999. http://www.unaids.org/publications/documents/epidemiology/surveillance/wad1999/Una99c53.doc (accessed 1/9/2000).
3. Centers for Disease Control and Prevention. United States HIV and AIDS Statistics. http://www.avert.org/usastaty.htm (accessed 1/9/2000).
4. Terwilliger, FF. Biology of HIV-1 and treatment strategies. *Emerg Med Clin North Am* 1995;13:27-41.
5. Little S, McLean A, Spina CA, et al. Viral dynamics of acute HIV-1 infection. *J Exp Med* 1999;190:841-850.
6. Jochimsen EM. Failures of zidovudine postexposure prophylaxis. *Am J Med* 1997;102:52-55.
7. Centers for Disease Control and Prevention. Guidelines for treatment of sexually transmitted diseases. *MMWR Morb Mortal Wkly Rep* 1998;47:109-111.
8. Daar ES. Virology and immunology of acute HIV Type 1 infection. *AIDS Res Hum Retroviruses* 1998;14:S229-S234.
9. Dong B. Prophylaxis after nonoccupational exposure to HIV. *Am J Health Syst Pharm* 1999;56:1011-1016.
10 Ippolito G, Puro V, Heptonstall J, et al. Occupational human immunodeficiency virus infection in health care workers: Worldwide cases through September 1997. *Clin Infect Dis* 1999;28:365-383.
11. Center for Disease Control and Prevention. Management of possible sexual, injecting drug use, or other nonoccupational exposure to HIV, including considerations related to antiretroviral therapy: Public Health Service statement. *MMWR Morb Mortal Wkly Rep* 1998;47(RR-17):1-14.
12. Katz MH, Gerberding JL. The care of persons with recent sexual exposure to HIV. *Ann Int Med* 1998;128:306-312.
13. Katz MH, Gerberding JL. Postexposure treatment of people exposed to human immunodeficiency virus through sexual contact or injection drug use. *N Engl J Med* 1997;336:1097-1100.
14. Mastro TD, deVincenzi I. Probabilities of sexual HIV-1 transmission. *AIDS* 1996;10(Suppl A):S75-80.
15. Cardo DM, Culver DH, Cieselski CA, et al. A case control study of HIV seroconversion in health care workers after percutaneous exposure. *N Engl J Med* 1997;337:1485-1490.
16. Kaplan EH, Heimer R. A model-based estimate of HIV infectivity via needle sharing. *J Acquir Immun Defic* 1992;5:1116-1118.
17. Schreiber GB, Busch MP, et al. Compliance with universal precautions among emergency department personnel: Implications for prevention programs. *N Engl J Med* 1996;334:1685-1690.
18. Katsufrakis PJ, Daar ES. HIV/AIDS management in office practice. *Prim Care* 1997;24:479-496.
19. Schacker T. Primary HIV infection. *Postgrad Med* 1997;102:143-151.
20. Schacker T, Collier A, Hughes J, et al. Clinical and epidemiologic features of primary HIV infection. *Ann Int Med* 1996;125:257-264.
21. Department of Health and Human Services, Henry J. Kaiser Family Foundation. Guidelines for the use of antiretroviral agents in HIV infected adults and adolescents. *MMWR Morb Mortal Wkly Rep* 1998;47(RR5):43-82.
22. Center for Disease Control and Prevention. Transmission of HIV possible associated with exposure of mucous membrane to contaminated blood. *MMWR Morb Mortal Wkly Rep* 1997;46:620-624.
23. Vidmar L. A human bite: Possible mode of HIV-1 transmission. Int Conf AIDS July 7-12, 1996;11:362 (abstract no. Tu.C.2563).
24. Hansen K. HIV testing. *Emerg Med Clinic North Am* 1995;13:43-59.
25. Kelen GD, JB Shahan, Quinn TC, et al. Emergency department-based HIV screening and counseling: Experience with rapid and standard serologic testing. *Ann Emerg Med* 1999;33:147-155.
26. Kelen GD, Hexter DA, Hansen KN, et al. Feasibility of an emergency department-based, risk-targeted voluntary HIV screening program. *Ann Emerg Med* 1996;27:687-692.
27. Wilson SR, Mitchell C, Bradbury DR, et al. Testing for HIV: Current practices in the academic ED. *Am J Emerg Med* 1999;17:354-356.
28. Rosenberg E, Cotton D. Primary HIV infection and the acute retroviral syndrome. *AIDS Clin Care* 1997;9:21-25.
29. Schacker T, Hughes J, Shea T, et al. Biological and virologic characteristics of primary HIV infection. *Ann Int Med* 1998;128:613-620.
30. Jolles S. Primary HIV-1 infection: A new medical emergency? (editorial). *BMJ* 1996;312:1243-1244.
31. Pantaleo G, Demarest J, Schacker T, et al. The qualitative nature of the primary immune response to HIV infection is a prognosticator of disease progression independent of the initial level of plasma viremia. *Proc Natl Acad Sci U S A* 1997;94:254-258.
32. Ciesielski C, Metler R. Duration of time between exposure and seroconversion in healthcare workers with occupationally acquired infection with human immunodeficiency virus. *Am J Med* 1997;102(5B):115-116.
33. Anonymous. Needlestick transmission of HTLV-III from a patient infected in Africa (editorial). *Lancet* 1984;2:1376-1377.
34. Cooper DA. Acute AIDS retrovirus infection. Definition of a clinical illness associated with seroconversion. *Lancet* 1985;1:537-540.
35. Vanhems P, Allard R, Cooper DA, et al. Acute human immunodeficiency virus type 1 disease as a mononucleosis-like illness: Is the diagnosis too restrictive? *Clin Infect Dis* 1997;24:965-970.
36. Kopko P, Calhoun L, Petz L, et al. Distinguishing immunosilent AIDS from the acute retroviral syndrome in a frequent blood donor. *Transfusion* 1999;39:383-386.
37. Dorrucci M, Rezza G, et al. Clinical characteristics and prognostic value of acute retroviral syndrome among injecting drug users. *AIDS* 1995;9:597-604.
38. Kinloch-de Loes S. Symptomatic primary infection due to human immunodeficiency virus type 1: Review of 31 cases. *Clin Infect Dis* 1993;17:59-65.
39. Perrin L, Markowitz M, Calandra G, et al. An open treatment study of acute HIV infection with zidovudine, lamivudine and indinavir

sulfate. 4th Conf Retro and Opportun Infect Jan. 22-26, 1997;108 (abstract no. 238).

40. Raines CP. Antiretroviral treatment in HIV infection. *Prim Care Pract* 2000;4:83-100.
41. Perrin LU, Balavoine JF, Schockmell GA, et al. Post-exposure prophylaxis and sexual HIV transmission between husband and wife. Int Conf AIDS 1998;12:630(abstract no. 33189).
42. Carcelain G, Blanc C, Leibowitch J, et al. T cell changes after combined nucleoside analogue therapy in HIV primary infection. *AIDS* 1999;13:1077-1081.
43. Jacquez JA. Role of the primary infection in epidemics of HIV infection in gay cohorts. *J Acquir Immun Defic* 1994;7:1169-1184.
44. Koopman JS. The Role of Primary Infection in Epidemic HIV Transmission. Int Conf AIDS June, 6-11, 1993;9:100 (abstract no. WS-C19-5).
45. Koopman JS. The role of early HIV infection in the spread of HIV through populations. *J Acquir Immune Defic Syndr Hum Retrovirol* 1997;14:249-258.
46. Hovanessian H. New developments in the treatment of HIV disease: An overview. *Ann Emerg Med* 1999;33:546-555.

HIV Infection: Drug Therapy and Prophylaxis

Dawn Demangone, MD, FAAEM
Betsy Schrader, MD

The risk of occupational exposure to human immunodeficiency virus (HIV) remains a concern among health care workers. Despite the risks, a significant percentage of health care workers fail to comply with universal precautions. To minimize transmission of HIV in occupational settings, evaluation and treatment protocols have been established according to size of inoculum and titers. A careful consideration of these and other factors will determine the potential usefulness of antiretroviral therapy. Non-occupational exposures may be more difficult to evaluate, and there is less consensus about the effectiveness of post-exposure prophylaxis.

This second part of a two-part chapter (see Chapter 44) will present a systematic approach for evaluating exposures to HIV and risk-stratifying patients according to their need for pharmaco-propylaxis. In this chapter, specific regimens are discussed and potential complications, drug toxicities, and interactions are highlighted.

Pharmacotherapy for HIV: Protocols, Side Effects, and Adverse Events

Nucleoside Reverse Transcriptase Inhibitors (NRTIs). Medications in this drug class inhibit viral reverse transcriptase, thus preventing or interfering with the production of a DNA copy of the viral RNA, therefore, preventing its replication and/or ultimate insertion into the host cell genome following infection.[4] Intracellular activation is required for nucleoside reverse transcriptase inhibitor (NRTI) effectiveness. Medications in this class primarily are metabolized through renal mechanisms.[2,5] Current regimens frequently include one or two medications from this class; however, stavudine and zidovudine (ZDV) should not be used concurrently because of antagonistic activities.[6] Some side effects are common to all medications in this group, and drug-specific side effects can occur. *(Please see Table 1.)*[1-4]

Peripheral neuropathy can occur with some of the NRTIs. Interestingly, there is a correlation with disease stage and development of peripheral neuropathy (i.e., those with more advanced disease have a greater likelihood of developing this side effect).[6] Symptoms begin as distal extremity numbness or burning, which can progress to a constant, severe burning sensation, or intermittent, sharp shooting pains.[6] Hepatic steatosis and lactic acidosis also can occur with this group of medications.[2]

Of special note is that abacavir has been associated with a drug-specific side effect that must be recognized by the emergency physician. Two percent of patients treated with abacavir develop a potentially fatal hypersensitivity reaction.[7] Misdiagnosis or delaying diagnosis can allow continuation or re-introduction of this medication in the patient's treatment regimen, which can have life-threatening implications. Patients can develop more severe symptoms within hours that may include life-threatening hypoten-

Table 1. Side Effects of NRTIs[1-4]

MEDICATION	SIDE EFFECTS
ZIDOVUDINE (AZT, ZDV, RETROVIR)	
	Headache
	Insomnia
	Asthenia
	Bone marrow suppression (anemia +/- neutropenia)
	Lactic acidosis with hepatic steatosis
	Myopathy
DIDANOSINE (DDI, VIDEX)	
	Peripheral neuropathy
	Pancreatitis
	Nausea
	Diarrhea
	Lactic acidosis with hepatic steatosis
	Retinal depigmentation
ZALCITABINE (DDC, HIVID)	
	Peripheral neuropathy
	Pancreatitis
	Stomatitis
	Rash
	Lactic acidosis with hepatic steatosis
	Esophageal ulceration
	Fever
STAVUDINE (D4T, ZERIT)	
	Peripheral neuropathy
	Pancreatitis
	Transaminitis
	Agitation
LAMIVUDINE (3TC, EPIVIR)	
	Peripheral neuropathy
	Pancreatitis
	Nausea
ABACAVIR (ZIAGEN)	
	Nausea
	Headache
	Hypersensitivity syndrome

sion and death.[2,7] Presentations can vary, but any patient on abacavir with fever, rash, fatigue, respiratory symptoms, or gastrointestinal (GI) symptoms (nausea, vomiting, diarrhea, abdominal pain) should discontinue the drug as soon as hypersensitivity reaction is considered. Such cases should be reported to the ABC Hypersensitivity Registry at 1-800-270-0425.[2,3,6,7]

Respiratory symptoms recently have been recognized as a presentation of hypersensitivity reaction. Approximately 20% of patients with a hypersensitivity reaction to abacavir experience cough, dyspnea, or pharyngitis.[7] It should be noted that patients have died after being initially diagnosed with an acute respiratory illness, such as bronchitis, pneumonia, or flu-like illness, rather than hypersensitivity reaction to abacavir.[7] *(Please see Table 2.)*[4,7-9]

Table 2. Symptoms Associated with Abacavir Hypersensitivity Reaction

- Fever
- Skin rash
- Fatigue
- Gastrointestinal symptoms
  - Nausea
  - Vomiting
  - Diarrhea
  - Abdominal pain
- Respiratory symptoms
  - Pharyngitis
  - Dyspnea
  - Cough

Non-Nucleoside Reverse Transcriptase Inhibitors (NNRTIs). Medications in this class directly bind viral reverse transcriptase, preventing transcription of viral RNA into DNA copies.[6] Metabolism of NNRTIs is largely via the cytochrome p450 system, which must be considered when prescribing other medications metabolized in the same manner. Resistance quickly develops to the NNRTIs through viral mutations; consequently, they are only recommended as part of combination therapy, and never in combination with each other.[3,6] The most common side effect of the NNRTIs is a maculopapular rash that typically is self-limited.[3] Between 1.7% and 7% of patients taking NNRTIs discontinue the medication due to the rash. Stevens-Johnson syndrome has been associated with NNRTI use on rare occasions.[2] *(Please see Table 3.)*

Protease Inhibitors. Protease inhibitors (PIs) appear to be the most potent anti-retroviral medications.[3] These drugs prevent precursors of viral proteins from being activated into mature, potentially infective viral proteins.[4,6] Metabolism is via the cytochrome p450 system, and again, care must be taken when prescribing other medications metabolized by this mechanism. Carefully following dosing schedules for these medications is especially important, as resistant mutations have been associated with low trough levels.[3]

Fat redistribution and abnormal metabolism of lipids and glucose are side effects common to all PIs.[2,6] Fat may accumulate at the base of the neck, or in the abdomen or mesentery. Terms such as "protease paunch" or "crix belly" have been coined to describe this side effect. Women may experience an increase in breast size. Losses of fat occur in the arms, legs, and face. It is unclear whether these effects are reversible with discontinuation.[3] Additionally, all PIs can increase bleeding in hemophiliacs.[2]

Indinavir is associated with nephrolithiasis in 3-5% of patients. Typically, the symptoms develop after taking indinavir for approximately 18 weeks. Patients may present with dysuria and urgency or with symptoms suggestive of renal colic, although they may or may not have evidence of stones. Drinking 1.5-2.0 liters of water daily is encouraged to prevent crystallization of indinavir in the urine.[3]

Drug Interactions. Drug interactions frequently occur with the anti-retroviral medications. Although absolute contraindications for drug interactions are listed in Table 4, many other interactions also exist. Before adding any medications to the regimen of patients on

Table 3. Side Effects and Contraindicated Drug Interactions of NNRTIs[2,3]

SIDE EFFECTS	DRUG INTERACTIONS
NEVIRAPINE (VIRAMUNE)	
Rash	Protease inhibitors
Nausea	Rifampin, rifabutin
Transaminitis	Oral contraceptives
Hepatitis	Triazolam, midazolam
DELAVIRDINE (RESCRIPTOR)	
Rash	Terfenadine, astemizole
Nausea	Alprazolam, midazolam, triazolam
Transaminitis	Rifampin, rifabutin
	Ergot derivatives
	Amphetamines
	Nifedipine
	Anticonvulsants
	Cisapride
EFAVIRENZ (SUSTIVA)	
Altered dreams	Astemizole, cisapride
Dizziness	Midazolam, triazolam
Somnolence	Ergot derivatives
Insomnia	
Transaminitis	
Impaired concentration	
Confusion	
Hallucinations	
Amnesia	

anti-retroviral therapies, consultation with their primary care physician or a pharmacist is prudent.

Evaluating and Managing Exposures to HIV

Occupational Exposure. Health care workers are at risk for exposure to HIV. Standard (universal) precautions for all health care workers are strongly encouraged to prevent acquisition of HIV and other blood-borne pathogens. However, not all health care workers may be fully aware of or regularly comply with standard precautions. One Level-1 trauma center presented a questionnaire to its emergency department (ED) staff (physicians, nurses, and technicians) and found personnel were not knowledgeable of risks for blood-borne pathogen infection, did not report all exposures, and were not compliant with universal precautions.[11] Other studies have shown similar findings, with rates of physician compliance with universal precautions ranging between 54% and 94%, with 44% of physicians reporting that they do recap needles contaminated with blood.[9]

Among surveyed emergency medicine residents, only 36.6% always followed standard precautions, 54% frequently followed them, and 9.4% sometimes, rarely, or never followed them.[12] One group has suggested barrier precautions for all but the most uncomplicated procedures performed in the ED. Face protection should be considered during invasive procedures, such as lumbar puncture or examination of the bleeding patient, since face splashes are not uncommon.[13]

Risk Factors for Occupational Transmission. Needle stick injuries can occur any time a needle is used or exposed, and in fact, needle stick injuries account for 80% of reported occupational exposures.[14] One group studied the effect of time into shift on exposure rate and found higher exposure rates during the first hour and last two hours of a shift among the workers in their hospital.[15] Following standard precautions and infection control recommendations could prevent a significant number of exposures.

Some activities that appear to be particularly dangerous for injury include recapping needles, improper disposal of used needles, and transferring body fluids between different containers.[16] Of 326 needle stick injuries in one study, 17% occurred during device use and 13% during disposal or after disposal. The great majority (70%) occurred after use, but before disposal. Recapping needles accounted for 17.8% of injuries. Contact of a used needle that had penetrated through the cap accounted for another 12.3% of injuries. Exposed needles left on working surfaces were contacted after use for 10.7% of injuries, and 8.9% contacts occurred with used needles protruding from trash.[17] In addition, one group found that the risk of injury was further influenced by the type of device being used. Particularly, devices that required disassembly had increased risks. It appears that special care should be taken when disassembling and disposing of equipment.[17]

Institution of needles with safety devices has been shown to lower the number of percutaneous injuries.[17-20] One group reported that 83% of needle sticks from hollow bore needles could be prevented by using protective devices.[21] Safer needle devices have been created in an attempt to minimize potential health care worker contact with the needle. These devices should provide a permanent barrier between the health care worker and the needle, keep workers hands behind the needle at all times, remain in effect after disposal, and be simple to use. Other devices, such as blunt needles and pre-penetrated intravenous catheter tips, also are useful for diminishing risk of injury.[22]

Compliance with these measures, in addition to following standard precautions, can reduce the health care worker's risk of injury, but cannot eliminate risk completely. Other factors that are not always the health care worker's control can contribute to exposures to blood and body fluids. One study found that latex gloves can leak, exposing health care workers' skin to blood or other body fluids. They also found increased glove perforations when gloves were worn for longer periods, used during critical care procedures, or worn during more than one procedure.[23]

After an exposure, health care workers should report the contact to the employee health service. Studies have found frequent underreporting. One study found that 70% of surgeons never or rarely reported their needle stick injuries, despite an average of 11 needle sticks every three years.[24] Among surveyed emergency medicine residents, 56.1% had at least one significant exposure during their training, and only 46.7% of the most recent exposures had been reported.[12]

According to the Centers for Disease Control and Prevention (CDC) HIV/AIDS surveillance report that was published in 1997, there were 52 documented cases of HIV seroconversion after occupational exposure to the virus, with an additional 114 cases of seroconversion possibly due to an occupational exposure.[25] Again, the most effective way to prevent transmission of HIV is by primary pre-

Table 4. Side Effects and Contraindicated Drug Interactions of Protease Inhibitors[2-4,32]

	SIDE EFFECTS	USE CONTRAINDICATED WITH
SAQUINAVIR (FORTOVASE)	Headache Transaminitis Hyperglycemia Fat redistribution Lipid abnormalities Diarrhea Abdominal pain Dyspepsia Nausea	Rifampin, rifabutin Terfenadine, astemizole Cisapride Ergot alkaloids Triazolam, midazolam
RITONAVIR (NORVIR)	Nausea, vomiting Diarrhea Peri-oral paresthesias Extremity paresthesias Hypertriglyceridemia Taste changes Fat redistribution Transaminitis Hepatitis Hyperglycemia Asthenia	Amiodarone, encainide, flecainide Propafenone, quinidine Astemizole, terfenadine Bepridil Bupropion Cisapride Clozapine, clorazepate Diazepam, estazolam, midazolam Triazolam, flurazepam, zolpidem Meperidine, piroxicam Propoxyphene
INDINAVIR (CRIXIVAN)	Nausea Hyperbilirubinemia Nephrolithiasis Fat redistribution Hyperglycemia Headache Dizziness Rash Metallic taste Thrombocytopenia Blurred vision	Astemizole, terfenadine Cisapride Triazolam, midazolam Ergot alkaloids
NELFINAVIR (VIRACEPT)	Nausea Diarrhea Hyperglycemia Ergot alkaloids	Astemizole, terfenadine Cisapride Triazolam, midazolam
AMPRENAVIR (AGENERASE)	Nausea	Astemizole, terfenadine Cisapride Triazolam, midazolam Ergot alkaloids

vention or avoiding percutaneous, mucous membranes, or non-intact skin exposure by using standard precautions.[26]

It has been estimated that the average risk of HIV seroconversion after a percutaneous exposure is 0.3%, and average risk after a mucous membrane exposure is 0.09%.[21,27] The actual risk of seroconversion after an exposure, however, is dependent on many factors. An increased risk of transmission was noted with exposures that involve deep injuries, injuries with a device contaminated with visible blood, or injuries involving a procedure in which a device is placed directly into an artery or vein of the source patient.[28] It also has been shown that exposures involving blood from a patient with terminal AIDS carries an increased risk of transmission.[29]

Post-Exposure Management. After an exposure has occurred, the use of medications for post-exposure prophylaxis (PEP) may reduce the risk of seroconversion. Although there have been no prospective, randomized studies proving the effectiveness of PEP in reducing the rate of seroconversion, use is based on animal and human studies. Some animal studies have shown the use of ZDV as PEP was successful in preventing infection.[29] In addition, a prospective trial has proven that the use of ZDV during pregnancy, labor, and delivery decreases the risk of maternal-fetal transmission by 67%.[30] A retrospective case-control study reviewing seroconversion in health care workers after an exposure showed an 81% reduction in the odds of HIV infection by those who took ZDV as PEP.[28]

In 1996, the Public Health Service (PHS) interagency, comprised of representatives from the CDC, FDA, and National Institutes of Health, published recommendations for PEP for health care workers with occupational exposures to HIV.[31] In 1998, the PHS revised the recommendations in light of emerging data and new medications.[26] The following is a summary of the recommendations.

Step 1. The first step is evaluating the exposure incident for risk of transmission. There is a risk of transmission if the health care worker is exposed to blood, body fluids containing visible blood, semen, vaginal secretions, cerebrospinal fluid, synovial fluid, pleural fluid, peritoneal fluid, pericardial fluid, or amniotic fluid.[26] If the exposure occurred to intact skin, no PEP may be required. Exposures that occur to mucous membranes or non-intact skin that involve a small amount of body fluid or a short duration of exposure are considered small inoculums exposures. Those involving a large amount of body fluid or a long duration of exposure to mucous membranes or non-intact skin are considered moderate inoculums exposures. Percutaneous injuries with solid needles or those resulting in superficial scratches are moderate inoculums exposures, and those involving hollow-bore needles and deep injuries are large inoculums exposures.[29] *(See Figure 1.)*

Step 2. The second step in evaluating an occupational exposure to HIV is determining the status of the source patient. If the source patient is known, laboratory data, medical records, clinical symptoms, or history may determine HIV status. If consent can be obtained, the patient can be tested for HIV, but if consent cannot be obtained, further HIV testing depends upon state and local laws. If the source patient is unknown, risk of transmission should be determined by the prevalence of HIV among the population.[29] If the source patient is HIV negative with no signs or symptoms of the disease, no further testing is required and PEP is not necessary. It has not yet been determined whether further testing should be performed on source patients with recent potential exposures to HIV. If the source patient is HIV positive, patients with high CD4 + T cell counts who are asymptomatic are considered low titer exposures. Exposures to patients with end-stage AIDS, low CD4+ T cell counts, and high viral loads are considered high titer exposures.[29] *(Please see Figure 2.)*

Figure 1. Evaluate the Exposure

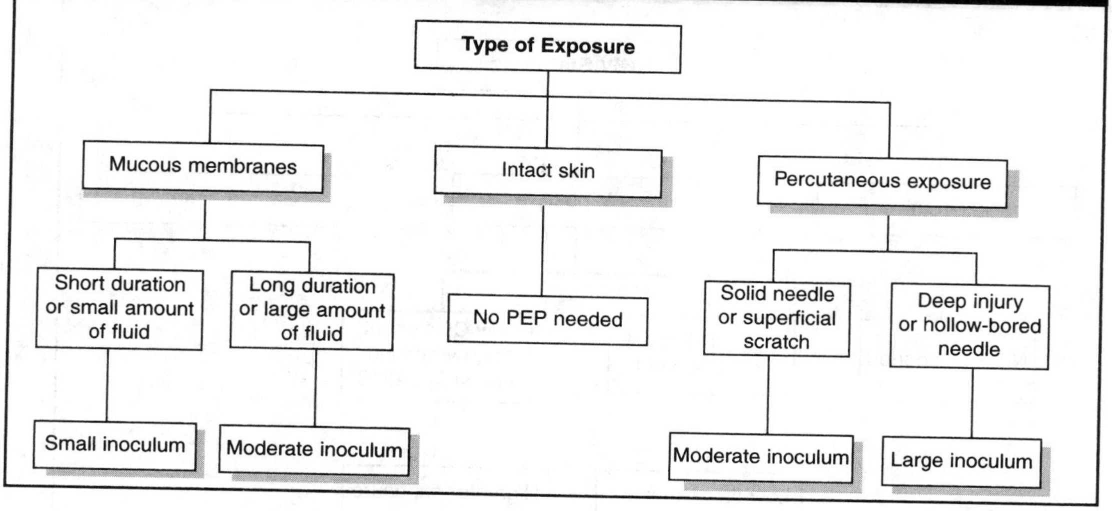

Step 3. The third step in determining an appropriate PEP regimen involves comparing the exposure risk with the HIV status of the source patient. Exposures that are considered small inoculums, low-titer exposures are not associated with a risk of transmission and may not require PEP. Small inoculums, high-titer exposures are associated with a relatively low risk of transmission.In these cases, a basic PEP regimen should be considered. The basic regimen for adults consists of four weeks of ZDV 600 mg daily in divided doses and lamivudine 150 mg twice a day. Most commonly, health care workers experience moderate inoculums, low-titer exposure. This type of exposure requires the basic PEP regimen. Injuries associated with a higher risk of transmission, which include moderate inoculums, high-titer exposures, and large inoculums with either low- or high-titer exposures require an expanded PEP regimen. The expanded regimen consists of the basic regimen plus either indinavir 800 mg every eight hours or nelfinavir 750 mg three times a day. Indinavir should be taken on an empty stomach with increased fluid intake, and nelfinavir should be taken with meals.[29]

Initiation of Therapy: Timing and Special Considerations. PEP medications should be started immediately after an exposure. This recommendation is based on information suggesting that there is a short period between exposure to the virus and replication within its target cells. Animal studies have shown a decrease in transmission of HIV when PEP was given within 24 hours of exposure, but no difference was seen when given after 72 hours. Since no data are available on humans, PEP should still be given even up to two weeks following an exposure with a high risk of transmission.[29] *(Please see Table 5.)*

Certain situations require special consideration when choosing a PEP regimen. Exposure to drug-resistant HIV may effect which medications are chosen. Avoid medications to which the virus may have developed resistance. If the virus is resistant to one class of medications, the use of a medication in another class may be warranted. Also, consider using a third or fourth drug until expert consultation can be obtained.[67]

Another group requiring special consideration is the pregnant health care worker. The pregnant health care worker should make an informed decision about PEP based on information about what is known and not known about the risks and benefits of PEP, the potential risks to the fetus, and the risk of transmission of HIV. Information on the medications and their usage in pregnancy should be relayed to the health care worker. ZDV has been used in pregnancy, and data suggest that there are no short-term risks associated with its use.

Data on long-term risk, as well as short- and long-term risks of lamivudine are limited. The dosages for ZDV and 3TC are the same in pregnancy. The use of protease inhibitors in pregnancy has not yet been studied, but many HIV-positive pregnant women on aggressive antiretroviral therapy continue on these drugs or resume them during pregnancy, so data should be forthcoming.[29]

HIV testing for all health care workers with an exposure should occur at the time of exposure and at six weeks, 12 weeks, and six months post exposure. There is no clear recommendation as to whether 12-month follow-up is beneficial, but it may considered in health care worker's who receive highly potent PEP regimens or who also were exposed to Hepatitis C. If the health care worker experiences symptoms consistent with acute retroviral syndrome (ARS), repeat testing should be performed. Although no prospective, randomized trials have proven the effectiveness of PEP, its benefits often outweigh the risks when used after an occupational exposure to HIV. If the clinician is unsure which PEP medications to give, it is recommended to start ZDV and 3TC immediately rather than to delay treatment. For questions regarding medications or special situations, consultation may be obtained through the National Clinicians Post-Exposure Prophylaxis Hotline at 1-888-448-4911.[29]

Non-Occupational Exposure

Emergency physicians are likely to encounter patients inquiring about PEP following non-occupational exposures, particularly as the public becomes more aware of its existence. Probably the most effective manner to prevent acquisition of HIV is to abstain from the behaviors at risk for transmission. Obviously, this message must continue to be emphasized as the primary means to prevent acquisition, and should never be replaced by post-exposure antiretroviral therapy.

Occupational exposures actually account for very few HIV infections; the majority of infections occur through needle sharing and

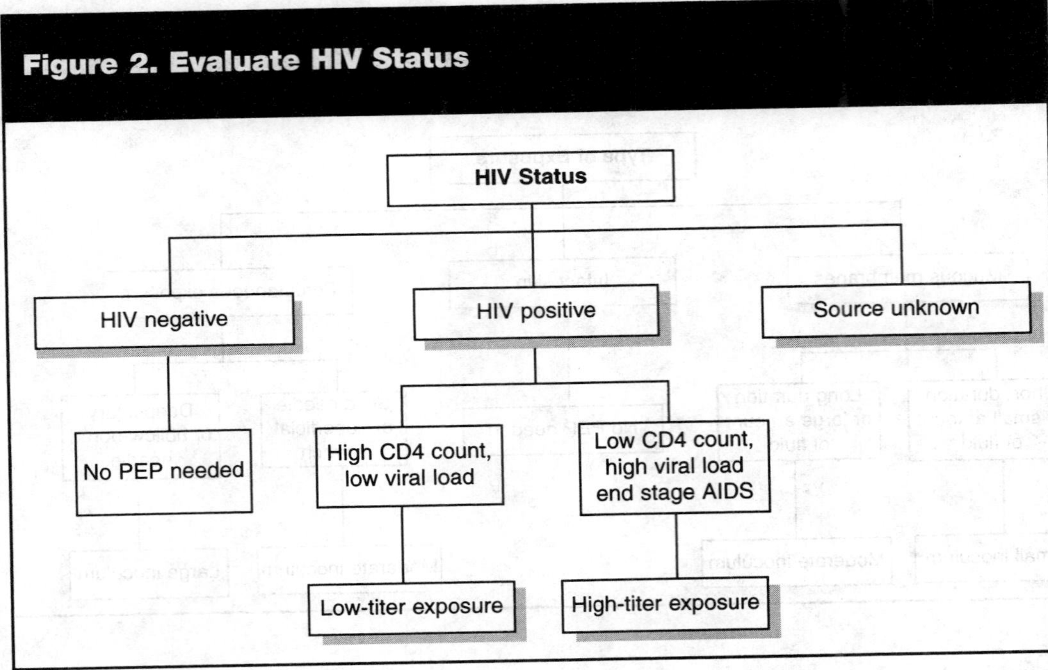

sexual activity. Certain high-risk behaviors, such as sharing needles and receptive anal or vaginal intercourse, carry similar or higher risks of transmission to that of occupational exposures. Many believe that since PEP has been found to be effective in preventing infection in occupational contacts,[29,30,33] it also should be offered to other potential victims of similar transmission risk.[34-36] Indeed, physicians do prescribe PEP for non-occupational exposures, even though no data exist on its efficacy.[37] Some recommend PEP after unprotected receptive and insertive anal and vaginal intercourse with HIV+ or high-risk partners, or after receptive fellatio with ejaculation.[34,35,38] However, the CDC recommends only considering therapy, not necessarily providing therapy, after unprotected receptive anal and vaginal intercourse with an HIV+ partner.[37]

Most advocates of PEP for non-occupational exposures support using the same medication combinations as those recommended for occupational exposures by the CDC.[35,36,38,39] However, the potential risks of medication toxicity, lowered compliance with protective behaviors, and resistance development must be considered prior to beginning therapy.[37,38] In addition, the same behaviors that put patients at risk for acquiring HIV also include risk for other transmissible diseases. Evaluation for hepatitis B and C (as well as other sexually transmissible diseases) and pregnancy also should be pursued.[37,38,40] Behavioral modification also should be considered part of non-occupational PEP.[41]

The prescribing physician must carefully consider several issues, which make the decision to provide PEP for non-occupational exposures more complex than for occupational exposures. As stated above, the efficacy of PEP for non-occupational exposures has not yet been proven. Failures are known to occur with occupational exposures, and have now been reported with non-occupational exposures.[8,42] It is unlikely that PEP for non-occupational exposures will ever be investigated through clinical trials because an extremely large number of participants would be required, and some argue that it is not ethical to use a placebo when treatments are known to be effective.[34,35] Patients must be made aware of the unknown efficacy, and the possible risks and benefits of PEP prior to beginning treatment.[38]

Several questions must be considered before beginning PEP treatment. As with the health care worker with occupational exposures, perhaps the first item to address is evaluation for the risk of the exposure. The specific activity and circumstances of the contact must be elicited from the patient. Some activities actually have higher estimated risks of HIV transmission than occupational exposures. Beside the specific activity, characteristics of both the source and exposed individuals can influence the risk for transmission and should be examined.

The HIV status of the exposure source should be estimated. This information frequently is available or can be obtained in the occupational environment. Some patients with non-occupational exposures may know the status of the source, such as couples who may have experienced an isolated exposure event, but most probably will not. The local seroprevalence rates can be helpful in estimating the likelihood of a HIV-positive source.

The time from exposure also should be determined. Current occupational exposure recommendations support starting PEP for occupational exposures up to two weeks after contact but are believed to be most effective within 72 hours based on PEP efficacy animal studies.[29] Several physicians currently prescribing non-occupational PEP recommend limiting the time limit to 72 hours.[34,37,43] The likelihood of repeated or continued exposures should be evaluated. Occupational exposure usually is not repeated willingly, however, needle sharing and high-risk sexual contacts frequently are. Most agree that PEP has no role in the treatment of individuals likely to continue in their high-risk behaviors.[34,36] Perhaps these patients would be better served by participating in educational programs that discourage high-risk exposures. Individuals with episodic exposures, such as condom slippage, sexual assault, or relapsing intravenous drug use, can be considered for PEP according to non-occupational PEP advocates.[34-36]

Patient compliance should be estimated. In a study of occupational exposures, 31% of individuals receiving PEP discontinued therapy due to side effects of AZT alone.[44] One group reported that 75% of health care workers receiving PEP with combination therapy experienced one or more side effects. Of those health care workers with sources of unknown or HIV+ status, 47% discontinued medications due to side effects.[45] The benefits of taking the medications in an otherwise healthy population may not justify the risks of the potential toxicities.[36,37] Additionally, poor or sporadic compliance could lead to the development of resistance to current standard therapies. Even if taken properly, therapy can be ineffective and may select out resistant strains.[37] Based on the aforementioned criteria, one study found that only one of 42 patients (or 2%) with non-occu-

Table 5. Determining Appropriate PEP Regimen

Small inoculum	➔➔	Low titer	➔➔	PEP may not be necessary
Small inoculum	➔➔	High titer	➔➔	Consider basic PEP regimen
Moderate inoculum	➔➔	Low titer	➔➔	Basic PEP regimen recommended
Moderate inoculum	➔➔	High titer	➔➔	Expanded PEP regimen recommended
Large inoculum	➔➔	Low or high titer	➔➔	Expanded PEP regimen recommended

pationally acquired primary HIV infection would have qualified for receiving PEP, and in that one case, only if the patient had presented in a timely manner.[43] The majority of these participants were not aware of the HIV exposure, and did not seek medical care until symptomatic. Of those infected through sexual contact, only one knew of his partner's HIV positive status. Whether the patients were aware of the existence of PEP was not reported, but may not have made much of a difference, as few identified the specific event that allowed for disease transmission.

These authors concluded that PEP probably would not prevent significant numbers of new, non-occupationally acquired infections.[43] However, as public awareness of PEP increases, more patients are likely to present for evaluation. A legitimate concern of making PEP available for non-occupational exposures is a potential increase in high-risk activities. More people may increase their high-risk activities if they are already receiving PEP, or if it is easily available and they perceive it as a "cure."[35] And, since PEP is not 100% effective in preventing infection, the number of infections could actually increase.[35] One study found that the recent successes in the treatment of HIV infections negatively have influenced compliance with protection during high-risk activities. Of 54 studied men who had sex with men, 15% reported they had "taken a chance of getting infected when having sex" because of the effectiveness of new treatments. Whether their attitudes were influenced by availability of PEP or the recent improvement in HIV treatment is unclear.[46]

Despite these findings, some believe that this is not an adequate reason to withhold therapy.[36] In summary, before offering PEP, several issues must be considered. Risks and benefits of treatment must be considered. The probability that the source is HIV positive, the time from exposure, the risk of transmission via the particular exposure, and patient compliance must all be estimated.[37] Additionally, baseline HIV testing, evaluation for other transmissible diseases, pregnancy evaluation, prevention counseling, and arranging follow-up care are crucial.

Rape. Offering PEP following sexual assault has been recommended by the CDC; however, no specific protocols were offered.[47] Treating the victim of sexual assault poses multiple complexities. Frequently, the HIV status of the aggressor is not known. The victim may present within 72 hours of exposure, and rape typically is not a repeated behavior by the victim.[40] In addition to attending to other needs of the sexual assault patient, circumstances that influence HIV transmission should be addressed. The emergency physician must assess the amount of trauma to the patient, the probability of blood and body fluid exposure, and the presence of any sexually transmitted diseases or other ulcerations. Guidelines for occupational and non-occupational exposures should be followed when evaluating and treating the victim of sexual assault for HIV transmission.[40]

Summary

As current anti-retroviral therapies are proving effective in prolonging lives of those infected with HIV, and as the number of HIV cases continues to increase, the likelihood of encountering HIV-positive patients in the ED is high. Recognizing the signs and symptoms associated with primary HIV infection (i.e., ARS) is important for improving patient disease course and to prevent further disease transmission. Emergency physicians must be aware of the contraindications and side effects of the currently recommended medications when evaluating patients on antiretroviral regimens. Familiarity with transmission risks is imperative for evaluating both health care workers and the general public, for potential exposure to HIV, and for potentially prescribing PEP.

References

1. Schacker T, Collier A, Hughes J, et al. Clinical and epidemiologic features of primary HIV infection. *Ann Int Med* 1996;125: 257-264.
2. Department of Health and Human Services, Henry J. Kaiser Family Foundation. Guidelines for the use of antiretroviral agents in HIV infected adults and adolescents. *MMWR Morb Mortal Wkly Rep* 1998;47(RR5):43-82.
3. Shaker I, Bartlett J. Strategies of antiretroviral therapy in adults. *Urol Clinic North Am* 1999;26:809-820.
4. Abramowicz M. Drugs for HIV infection. *Med Lett* 1997;39: 111-116.
5. Raines CP. Antiretroviral Treatment in HIV infection. *Prim Care Pract* 2000;4:83-100.
6. Hovanessian H. New Developments in the Treatment of HIV Disease: An Overview. *Ann Emerg Med* 1999;33: 546-555.
7. GlaxoWellcome. Important drug warning Re: Fatal hypersensitivity reactions, respiratory symptoms, and Ziagen (abacavir sulfate). Letter, February 2000.
8. Perrin LU, Balavoine JF, Schockmell GA, et al. Post-exposure prophylaxis and sexual HIV transmission between husband and wife. *Int Conf AIDS* 1998;12:630(abstract no. 33189).
9. Michalsen A, Delclos G, Felknor SA, et al. Compliance with universal precautions among physicians. *J Occup Env Med* 1997;39: 130-137.
10. Kinloch-de Loes S. Symptomatic primary infection due to human immunodeficiency virus type 1: Review of 31 cases. *Clin Infect Dis* 1993;17:59-65.
11. Kim LE, Evanoff BA, Parks RL, et al. Compliance with universal precautions among emergency department personnel: Implications for prevention programs. *Am J Infect Control* 1999;27:453-455.

12. Lee CH, Carter WA, Chiang WK, et al. Occupational exposures to blood among emergency medicine residents. *Acad Emerg Med* 1999;6:1036-1043.
13. Kelen GD, Hansen KN, Green GB, et al. Determinants of emergency department procedure and condition-specific universal (barrier) precaution requirements for optimal provider protection. *Ann Emerg Med* 1995;25:743-750.
14. Jagger J, Hunt EH, Brand-Elnagger J, et al. Rates of needlestick injury caused by various devices in a university hospital. *N Engl J Med* 1988;319:284-288.
15. Macias DJ, Hafner J, Brillman JC, et al. Effect of time of day and duration into shift on hazardous exposures to biological fluids. *Acad Emerg Med* 1996;3:605-610.
16. Department of Health and Human Services. Preventing needlestick injuries in health care settings. DHHS (NIOSH) Publication 1999. www.cdc.gov; (accessed 1/31/00).
17. Jagger J. Reducing occupational exposure to bloodborne pathogens: Where do we stand a decade later? *Infect Control Hosp Epidemiol* 1996;17:573-575.
18. Lawrence LW, Delclos GL, Felknor SA, et al. The effectiveness of a needless intravenous connections system: An assessment by injury rate and user satisfaction. *Infect Control Hosp Epidemiol* 1997;18:175-182.
19. Gartner K. Impact of a needleless intravenous system in a university hospital. *Am J Infect Control* 1992;20:75-79.
20. Yassi A, McGill ML, Khokhar JB. Efficacy and cost-effectiveness of a needless intravenous access system. *Am J Infect Control* 1995; 23:57-64.
21. Ippolito G, Puro V, Heptonstall J, et al. Occupational human immuodeficiency virus infection in health care workers: Worldwide cases through September 1997. *Clin Infect Dis* 1999;28:365-383.
22. Office of Occupational Health Nursing. Safer Needle Devices: Protecting the Health Care Workers. *OSHA* 1997:www.osha-slc.gov. (accessed 1/26/00).
23. Hansen KN, Korniewicz DM, Hexter DA, et al. Loss of glove integrity during emergency department procedures. *Ann Emerg Med* 1998;31:65-72.
24. Patterson J, Novak C, Mackinnon SE, et al. Surgeons' concern and practices of protection against bloodborne pathogens. *Ann Surg* 1998;228:266-272.
25. Centers for Disease Control and Prevention. HIV/AIDS surveillance report 1997;9:15.
26. Centers for Disease Control and Prevention. Update: Universal precautions for prevention of transmission of human immunodeficiency virus, hepatitis B virus, and other bloodborne pathogens in health-care settings. *MMWR Morb Mortal Wkly Rep* 1988;37:377-82, 387-388.
27. Bell DM. Occupational risk of immunodeficiency virus infection in healthcare workers: an overview. *Am J Med* 1997;102(supp 5B):9-15.
28. Cardo DM, Culver DH, Cieselski CA, et al. A case control study of HIV seroconversion in health care workers after percutaneous exposure. *N Engl J Med* 1997;337:1485-1490.
29. Centers for Disease Control and Prevention. Public Health Service guidelines for the management of health-care worker exposures to HIV and recommendations for postexposure prophylaxis. *MMWR Morb Mortal Wkly Rep* 1998;47(RR-7):1-33.
30. Connor EM, Sperling RS, Gelber R, et al. Reduction of maternal-infant transmission of human immunodeficiency virus type 1 with zidovudine treatment. *N Engl J Med* 1994;331: 1173-1180.
31. Public Health Service. Update: Provisional Public Health Service recommendations for chemoprophylaxis after occupational exposure to HIV. *MMWR Morb Mortal Wkly Rep* 1996;45:468-480.
32. Dorrucci M, Rezza G, Vlahov D, et al. Clinical characteristics and prognostic value of acute retroviral syndrome among injecting drug users. *AIDS* 1995;9:597-604.
33. Little S, McLean A, Spina CA, et al. Viral dynamics of acute HIV-1 infection. *J Exp Med* 1999;190:841-850.
34. Katz MH, Gerberding JL. The care of persons with recent sexual exposure to HIV. *Ann Int Med* 1998;128:306-312.
35. Katz MH, Gerberding JL. Postexposure treatment of people exposed to human immunodeficiency virus through sexual contact or injection drug use. *N Engl J Med* 1997;336:1097-1100.
36. Lurie P, Miller S, Hecht F, et al. Postexposure prophylaxis after nonoccupational HIV exposure: Clinical, ethical and policy considerations. *JAMA* 1998;280:1769-1733.
37. Centers for Disease Control and Prevention. Management of possible sexual, injecting drug use, or other nonoccupational exposure to HIV, including considerations related to antiretroviral therapy: Public Health Service statement. *MMWR Morb Mortal Wkly Rep* 1998;47(RR-17):1-14.
38. Dong B. Prophylaxis after nonoccupational exposure to HIV. *Am J Health Syst Pharm* 1999;56:1011-1016.
39. Schacker T. Primary HIV infection. *Postgrad Med* 1997;102: 143-151.
40. Bamberger J, Waldo C, Gerberding JL, et al. Postexposure prophylaxis for human immunodeficiency virus (HIV) infection following sexual assault. *Am J Med* 1999;106:323-326.
41. Kegebein VR, Bamberger JD, Katz MH, et al. Post-exposure prophylaxis: Community controversies in San Francisco. Int Conf AIDS. 1988;12:628 (abstract no. 251/33179).
42. Jochimsen EM. Failures of zidovudine postexposure prophylaxis. *Am J Med* 1997;102:52-55.
43. Sudre P, Schmockel G, Fagard C, et al. Post HIV exposure prophylaxis: Who may benefit? Int Conf AIDS. 1998;12:630 (abstract no. 33188).
44. Postexposure treatment not easy to swallow. *AIDS Alert* 1998;13:107.
45. Swotinsky R, Steger K, Sulis C, et al. Occupational exposure to HIV: Experience at a tertiary care center. *J Occup Env Med* 1998; 40:1102-1109.
46. Dilly JW, Woods WJ, McFarland W. Are advances in treatment changing views about high-risk sex? (Letter). *N Engl J Med* 1997; 337:501-502.
47. Centers for Disease Control and Prevention. Guidelines for treatment of sexually transmitted diseases. *MMWR Morb Mortal Wkly Rep* 1998;47:109-111.

Part III

Neurological Disorders

Diplopia

Izak F. Wessels, MMed, FRCSE, FRCOphth, FACS

When patients complain about double vision, primary care physicians often tune out and simply refer these patients to an ophthalmologist. This chapter outlines how to develop a differential diagnosis, distinguish an emergency or urgent condition from the more mundane, and know when to refer to the specialist. Internuclear ophthalmoplegia is also a not uncommon presentation of patients, and this chapter provides an algorithm for helping the practitioner sort out a differential diagnosis and management plan.

Normal binocular vision requires that all the ocular structures involved with movement and alignment (muscular and neurologic), as well as the intricate processes controlling conjugate gaze and cortical fusion, be intact. The not-so-uncommon complaint of double vision can simply be normal physiology or a serious omen with catastrophic significance.[1,2] A good history and specific examination can greatly help resolve the problem.[3-5] While the primary care provider should be able to refine the diagnostic possibilities, gatekeepers very poorly manage this symptom, overinvestigating as many as one in four patients, with an overcharge rate of more than 700%.[6]

Introduction

Diplopia occurs when one object appears double; it is often the first manifestation of many systemic (muscular or neurologic) disorders.[7,8] The primary care provider can greatly facilitate triage; a correct evaluation correlates well with appropriateness of urgent referral to neurology clinics.[2]

A systematic history and examination can help to delineate the specific anatomical (and often) pathophysiologic processes causing diplopia.[3,4] This article presents some typical case histories in the context of a series of 10 questions.

Does the Diplopia Persist When Covering Either Eye?

Case 1. *Mr. T, a very tall college senior, comes to see you for chest pains whenever he plays basketball. He reports seeing two blurry objects despite covering the left eye, but not when covering the right eye, which he blames on his contact lenses being dirty. Examination reveals a loud diastolic murmur over the precordium, and the blood pressure is 60/20 in the right arm and 140/85 in the left.*

Diagnosis. *Marfan's syndrome, with a dissecting aneurysm of the ascending aorta, and partially dislocated crystalline lens.*

Figure 1. The Extraocular Muscles

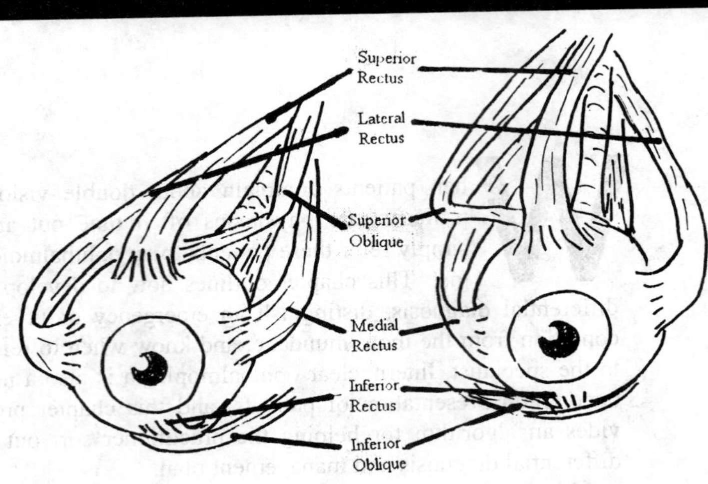

The six muscles controlling the position of each eye can be divided into the following groups: Two with horizontal action (medial and lateral rectus); two with primarily vertical action (superior and inferior rectus); and two with primarily torsional action (superior and inferior rectus). Because the superior and inferior recti insert at an angle to the sagittal plane, they also will have some torsional effect. Likewise, the oblique muscles will have a slight vertical effect. The superior oblique and lateral rectus each have their own nerve supply (IV and VI) while all the other muscles (including the pupil and lid elevator) are innervated by III.

Monocular diplopia is comparatively rare. Possible causes include:

- Severe astigmatism (e.g., keratoconus);[8]
- Additional openings in the iris that function as pupils;
- Cataracts or media opacities;[9]
- Dislocated or subluxated lens (e.g., Marfan's syndrome, intraocular lens);[10] and
- Retinal abnormalities (e.g., macular scarring)

Obviously, closing the affected eye will make the diplopia go away, but it will persist if the unaffected (other) eye is closed. Three, four, or more images may be seen, depending on the cause of the problem.[11]

Binocular diplopia (double vision only if both eyes are open) indicates mal-alignment of the eyes and inability to suppress the image from the deviating eye. A child with crossed eyes will *not* have double vision, since the developing brain can suppress the "wrong" image. If untreated, the vision in the deviating eye may be irreversibly damaged, called amblyopia.

Is the Diplopia Physiologic?

Case 2. *Miss J, a 56-year-old spinster, complains of frequent diplopia and headaches. Her double vision is only for nearby objects, which she demonstrates by holding up one finger close to her face and explaining that it appears double when she looks across the room. When she then looks directly at her finger, she only sees one. Her new glasses also make everything double when she looks to either side.*

Diagnosis. *Physiologic diplopia.*

Physiologic diplopia is a normal phenomenon because the visual axes cannot possibly intersect at all distances at the same time.[11] Suddenly noticing the diplopia represents a disturbance of higher cerebral function, especially of attention.[12] Other causes of "normal diplopia" include the edge effect of a bifocal lens, as well as a thick spectacle lens inducing a prismatic effect that convergence disparities notice more readily.[13]

Are the Eye Movements Normal?

Three cranial nerves dynamically balance the six extraocular muscles. *(Please see Figure 1.)* Four of the muscles are the recti—the medial recti adduct move the eyes inward horizontally, while the lateral recti abduct move the eyes outward horizontally and remain in dynamic balance.

The superior recti elevate and the inferior recti primarily depress the globe. However, because the superior and inferior recti both insert at 23° to the sagittal plane, they also intort and extort the eye (rotate the 12 o'clock position inward or outward). By slightly abducting the eye, the cornea will align with the superior and inferior recti and pure elevation or depression results.

The two remaining muscles (superior and inferior obliques) insert at 51° and counterbalance the torsional effects of the vertical recti. The superior oblique intorts and depresses, while the inferior oblique extorts and elevates. Therefore, in upgaze, the superior rectus and inferior oblique act in concert, and in downgaze, the inferior rectus and superior oblique act in concert. Neuronal reflexes achieve a remarkably stable interrelationship and dynamic balance between the different muscles in the various directions of gaze.

Inability of the eye to move in a certain direction will result in double vision when attempting to look in that direction. The cause may be neurologic or muscular.

Three cranial nerves control eye movements, III, IV, and VI. The Oculomotor (III) nerve supplies the lid elevator, pupil constrictor, and all but two of the six extraocular muscles. Therefore, classic III nerve lesions result in inability to elevate, adduct, or depress, and ptosis, as well as a dilated nonreactive pupil. Since the ptosis is usually total, the diplopia is often masked by the lid covering the pupil.

The abducens nerve (VI) only supplies the lateral rectus. Lesions of VI result in inability to abduct (lateral movements) with horizontal diplopia. The trochlear nerve (IV) supplies only the superior oblique. Lesions of IV result in vertical and torsional deviations and vertical diplopia.

Figure 2. The Field of Action of the Extraocular Muscles

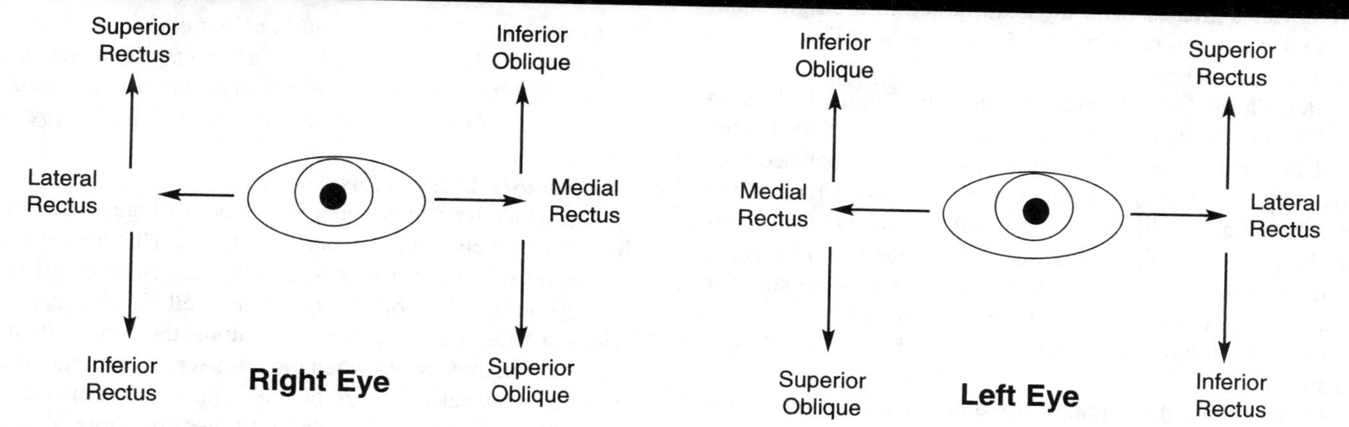

By moving the eye along a path describing a capital letter "H," the individual muscles can be isolated. The vertically acting muscles all have a torsional component as well, which the "bowlegged" diagram emphasizes. Note that the superior oblique moves the eye down, seemingly counterintuitive when the superior rectus moves the eye upward.

Observe the range of movements of each eye separately as well as both together as the patient's eyes fixate on the six cardinal positions, first, left and right, and then up and down in left or right gaze, like the lines of a capital letter "H." By observing up and down movements only when the eye is turned outward or inward, the superior and inferior recti as well as the inferior and superior obliques can respectively be isolated. *(Please see Figure 2.)* Note that the vertical muscles also have a torsional effect.

Is the Diplopia Worse in any Particular Direction of Gaze?

This evaluation is more sensitive than observing a decreased range of movement, since it relies on the dynamic balance between the muscles of both eyes. Attempting to move a weak muscle requires a greater neurologic stimulus that results in the opposite eye "overshooting" as the complementary muscle responds to a greater degree. For example, when looking toward the left, the left lateral rectus and right medial rectus contract equally due to equal innervation. If the left lateral rectus is weak, it requires greater stimuli but will contract less than it should. The right medial rectus receives the same excessive stimulation and will contract more. Thus, the patient may have normal vision when looking to the right, but intolerable diplopia to the left. The patient can usually tell in which direction the two objects are farthest apart. An oblique or vertical muscle weakness is more complex, as is described next.

Is There an Abnormal Head Posture?

Case 3. *Mr. J, a 60-year-old male, complains of a worsening neckache due to a "slipped disk." There is no limitation or pain on neck movement, but he believes he has a "pinched nerve," causing him to see objects double or on top of one another.*

He has a pronounced head tilt to the left. With the head held normally, the right eye is higher than the left and the deviation worsens when he tilts or turns the head to the right, or when both eyes look to the left.

Diagnosis. *Right superior oblique weakness, trochlear (IV) nerve palsy.*

A compensatory head, face, or chin posture minimizes the diplopia arising from a weak muscle. As discussed above, turning the eyes to the opposite side of the field of action of a weak muscle minimizes the need for that muscle to act. The head posture allows the patient to see straight ahead without moving the eyes from this "neutral position."[14] The Parks three-step test may help elucidate which of the four muscles with a vertical effect (total of 8 in both eyes) is weak and, therefore, responsible for the vertical diplopia and compensatory head tilt.[15] Although the test may appear impossibly complex at first, it follows a logical procession.

Note which eye is higher: first with the head normally positioned, second with the head turned left or right, and, finally, with the head tilted to the left or right.

Step One. Which eye is higher in primary gaze? This reduces the possibilities from eight to four. A subtle deviation can be confirmed by covering one eye and watching whether the other moves up or down to take up fixation. By alternating the cover, the same effect will be evident in the eye just uncovered. Alternatively, ask the patient in which eye the image appears lower to identify the eye deviating upward.

If the right eye is higher, the weakness resides in the depressors on the right (right inferior rectus and right superior oblique) or in the elevators on the left (left superior rectus and left inferior oblique).

Step Two. Is the deviation greater with left or right head turn? This halves the possibilities from four to two. If the right eye deviates greatest with the head turned to the right (both eyes are gazing to the left), the right superior obliques or the left superior rectus remain.

Step Three. Is the deviation greater when tilting the head to the left or to the right? This is the Bielschowski head tilt and the final elimination step. It relies on the torsional balance provoked by tilting the head. The higher eye extorts (due to the inferior oblique), while the lower eye intorts (due to the superior oblique). If the diplopia is worse with head tilt to the right, then the weak muscle in the lower (right) eye is the superior oblique and in the higher (left) eye is the inferior oblique. Combining all three steps identifies the right superior oblique as affected.

Occasionally, the findings are subtle, which confuses the casual observer, more so if other nerves (e.g., III) are also partially affected. Vestibular diplopia can also cause confusion, since a head tilt may occasionally stabilize the dysfunction.[16] However, typically these patients have symptoms of vertigo, hearing loss, and tinnitus.[17]

The astute clinician can "short cut" the process by realizing that of all the muscles, the superior oblique is most likely involved. A head tilt to the same side will exacerbate the diplopia, also the eye highest in adduction points at the affected muscle.

The IV cranial nerve emerges dorsally and has the longest brainstem course. Congenital weakness is often overlooked, and the patient may be unaware of a long-standing head tilt until old photographs (or the driver's license) reveal the long-standing head tilt.

Is the Diplopia Variable or Does it Fatigue?

Case 4. Mr. P, a retired 68-year-old colonel with arthritis complains of excessive fatigue and weakness for the past few months. The labs are all normal except for a widened mediastinum on chest x-ray. He wants a "tonic" to relieve his fatigue that is causing droopy eyelids and double vision.

***Diagnosis.** Myasthenia gravis.*

Ocular deviations that do not fit a clear-cut neurologic pattern are usually myogenic. Myasthenia is easily overlooked and can involve any eye muscle, including the lids (ptosis) but *not* the pupil. The symptoms are variable but usually worse in the evening, and a thymoma may be associated.[18] To confirm the diagnosis, give a short-acting cholinesterase inhibitor ("Tensilon" edrophonium chloride 10 mg/mL) intravenously. First, inject 1 mg as a test dose and observe for possible hypersensitivity. If there has been no effect, inject the remaining 9 mg. A cholinergic response includes salivation, lacrimation, flushing, and a dramatic brief reversal of the weakness. Because the generalized cholinergic response includes an increased vagal tone, the patient may experience fainting or severe bradyarrhythmias. Atropine must be available as an antidote.[19] Other myopathies (e.g., progressive external ophthalmoplegia, myotonia) may present similarly but will not respond to Tensilon.

Has There Recently Been Trauma to the Eye?

Case 5. Mr. T, a 21-year-old college quarterback, has a very bruised and swollen right eye after a fistfight. His cheek is allegedly totally numb, and when he lifts the lid, he has vertical double vision and the eye elevates and depresses very poorly.

***Diagnosis.** Classic blow-out fracture.*

Diplopia after blunt trauma to the cheek suggests an orbital floor fracture entrapping orbital soft tissue. This prevents up- or downward eye movement, and the parasthesia suggests damage to the infraorbital nerve as well. Urgent surgical release of the muscle and reconstituting the orbital floor is probably only necessary when there is severe enophthalmos.[20] Waiting two weeks or more for the hematoma, tissue edema, and inflammation to subside will identify those patients absolutely needing surgery.[21] The clear-cut history and typical findings rule out more serious intracranial pathology.[22] The entrapped inferior rectus (a restrictive myopathy) resists upward eye movement, which can be confirmed by a forced duction test: Instill topical anesthetic, grasp the globe at the limbus (between the cornea and sclera) with forceps, and evaluate the ease of movement in all directions except upward. Although pushing the anesthetized eye in different directions with a moistened cotton-tip applicator applies much less force, similar information can be gained.[23]

Closed head injury also can be associated with nonspecific VI weakness.[24] However, despite the eyes being misaligned, only about one-third of patients will experience diplopia after head trauma.[25] Other "traumatic" causes include a misdirected dental local anesthetic injection or hematomas after a peribulbar block for cataract surgery.[26,27]

Is There Any Proptosis or Orbital Mass?

Case 6. Miss M, a 50-year-old nervous white widow, successfully received radioactive iodine for acute hyperthyroidism 18 months ago and is well maintained on replacement therapy. She suffers from increasingly gritty, red, and watery eyes that see double whenever she looks up or down. The only positive findings are reduced upgaze, and the left eye appears proptosed.

***Diagnosis.** Early thyroid ophthalmopathy.*

Although any orbital space-occupying lesion can cause ocular displacement and diplopia, the most common cause remains thyroid eye disease with enlarged muscles. Imaging studies can identify the pathological cause, including congenital defects (encephalocele); inflammation (orbital cellulitis and abscess, pseudotumor, thyroid eye disease); benign or malignant neoplasms (e.g., secondary metastases from breast, primary rhabdomyosarcoma, neurofibromatosis, optic nerve gliomata, etc.); and vascular abnormalities (arteriovenous fistulae, hemangiomata). Lesions also may arise from the paraocular sinuses.[28] Diplopia and orbital pain may be the earliest signs of posterior communicating or basilar arterial aneurysm or a carotid-cavernous sinus fistula.[29,30]

Although laboratory tests can confirm an abnormal thyroid function, the diagnosis of thyroid eye disease is made clinically. The findings include ocular discomfort, lid retraction, and lag, diplopia, exophthalmos, and optic nerve dysfunction.[31] Specific and classic signs include:

Lid Lag. The upper lid follows the eye downward at the same rate. Lid lag shows as a delay in lid movement, making the sclera temporarily visible as the eye moves down.

Lid Retraction. The upper lid margin overlaps the cornea by 2 mm (1/6 of the vertical diameter), while the lower lid margin lies at the lower limbus. Lid retraction causes both the upper and lower lids to pull away, creating a staring, "bug-eyed" appearance.

Proptosis. Evaluate protrusion of one eye by standing behind the seated patient with his or her head extended backward as far as possible and look along the face from the top of the head across the forehead toward the chin. Lift both lids up and note if one or both eyes stands out forward with respect to the eyebrows. Precise measurements require a Hertel exophthalmometer to quantitate the degree of proptosis and permit careful follow-up.[32]

Diplopia from thyroid disease usually follows inflammation and secondary fibrosis of the inferior recti, which forced duction tests will confirm.

A useful classification of the severity of thyroid ophthalmopathy has seven components (the mnemonic NO SPECS) that progressively indicate more serious disease.[33]

N. No signs or symptoms (the patient is dysthyroid, but the eyes are not yet involved).

O. Only signs (the patient shows some mild changes, without experiencing ocular irritation, redness, etc.).

S. Soft tissues: At this stage, there is lid lag and lid retraction. Although the eye may not be proptosed, there is a staring appearance.

P. Proptosis: The swelling of the orbital contents (lymphocytic infiltration of the muscles and fat of the orbit) results in a forward displacement of the eye. Tarsorrhaphy (suturing the lateral half of the eyelids together) and/or decompressing the orbital pressure into the ethmoid or maxillary sinus can help reduce the proptosis.

E. Extraocular muscles: The increasing chronic inflammatory process has resulted in muscle thickening (evident on MRI or CT scan) with restriction of globe movement. The inferior rectus, inferior oblique, and medial rectus muscles are affected in order of frequency. Treatment includes prisms in the glasses, radiation therapy, and, eventually, muscle surgery to remedy the fibrosed and contracted muscles. Carefully following the range of extraocular motion and diplopia fields is a relevant measure to determine the choice of therapy in clinical trials.[34] The enlarged muscles may also be seen with idiopathic orbital myositis.[35]

C. Cornea: The proptosis, lid problems, and inability to roll the eyes upward during sleep (Bell's phenomenon) all result in corneal exposure, drying, and ulcers. Lubricants (especially ointments at night) and possibly tarsorrhaphy and orbital decompression are urgently indicated.

S. Scotoma or sight: The increasing proptosis may damage the optic nerve that develops focal blind spots (scotomata) and decreased vision. Urgent orbital decompression may be required to save vision and is best managed by maxillofacial or ophthalmic plastic surgeons.[36]

Smoking worsens ocular symptoms, proptosis, and diplopia up to three-fold.[37]

Is the Diplopia Part of a Classic Neurologic Syndrome?

The classic pattern of neurological abnormalities allow recognition in most cases; establishing an etiology is not always simple.[38] Causes for neurologic diplopia include interruptions of the blood supply (diabetes); inflammation and demyelination (multiple sclerosis and herpes zoster); tumors and aneurysms; or trauma. Lesions at or surgery to the skull base may result in diplopia, as well as oscillopsia.[39] Intracranial hypertension can present with diplopia and papilledema, visual obscurations, tinnitus, etc.[40]

Possibly III Nerve?

Case 7. *Mrs. S, a 48-year-old frail white female, has been confined to a wheelchair due to multiple sclerosis. She has been wearing an eye patch for a few weeks due to double vision whenever looking to the left. The only finding is an inability of the right eye to adduct, but there are no other signs of a III palsy since the pupil and eyelid move normally.*

Diagnosis. *Internuclear ophthalmoplegia.*

This case demonstrates interruption of the connection between the brain stem nuclei.

The yoke muscles responsible for left gaze (left lateral rectus and right medial rectus) receive stimulation from the abducens (VI) and oculomotor (III) nuclei, respectively. The initial stimulus reaches VI first, which is then relayed to the opposite III via the medial longitudinal fasciculus (MLF), the internuclear connection (there is simply no direct connection to III for horizontal gaze). Damage to the MLF on the right (ischemia, MS, etc.) effectively denervates the right medial rectus only.[41]

Case 8. *Mrs. M, a 55-year-old black female, has maturity onset diabetes that is poorly controlled by oral agents due to obesity. She recently developed a persistent headache, followed by diplopia and then a droopy left eyelid. The pupil responses are normal, but the eye can only abduct and intort.*

Diagnosis. *Pupil-sparing III palsy: Diabetic mononeuritis multiplex.*

Diabetics especially may develop acute neuropathies of any nerve, including those supplying the eye. These almost invariably resolve completely over a six-week period. A diabetic III nerve neuritis spares the pupil because the pupillomotor fibers run on the surface of the nerve and are less affected by a microangiopathic ischemia. The headache is presumably vasculitic ischemia. Therapy includes patching the eye until spontaneous recovery has taken place.[42]

Pupil-sparing III nerve palsies are considered "medical." Usually, the ptosis causes more concern than the diplopia—simply because the lid covering the eye prevents them from

Table 1. Diplopia Algorithm[60]

1. **Is it monocular?**
   Check for corneal or lenticular opacities and for extra openings in the iris by the red reflex using a direct ophthalmoscope. A dislocated lens will be evident in the pupil.
2. **Is it physiologic?**
3. **Are the eye movements normal?**
   Isolate the weak muscle by tracing an H pattern.
4. **Is it worse in any direction of gaze?**
5. **Is there an abnormal head posture?**
   Possible oblique muscle (IV) dysfunction. Which eye is higher in:
   Step one: In primary gaze?
   Step two: With the head turned left or right?
   Step three: With the head tilted left or right?
6. **Does it vary during the day?**
   Possible myasthenia gravis. 10 mg IV Tensilon test.
7. **Has there recently been trauma to the eye?**
   Is there loss of sensation over the cheek?
   Probably blow out fracture: X-ray the floor of the orbit and the maxillary sinus.
8. **Is there any proptosis or signs of an orbital mass?**
   Use Werner classification: NOSPECS to determine severity
   Probably thyroid ophthalmopathy. Confirm muscle enlargement by CT scan of orbit.
9. **Is it part of a classic neurologic syndrome?**
   Possible III nerve: Pupil sparing: medical third nerve lesion: observe
   Pupil involved: Surgical third nerve. Tumor, aneurysm likely.
   Possible IV: Evaluate head posture
   Possible VI
10. **Are any other factors present?**
    Infections, metabolic diseases.

seeing double. Management includes reassurance and control of blood pressure and blood glucose because, as a rule, they fully recover.

On the other hand, III nerve palsies involving the pupil are considered "surgical" because a compressive lesion (aneurysm of the posterior communicating artery of the circle of Willis, brain tumor, other space occupying lesion, etc.) is often associated. Other physical signs (loss of consciousness, meningismus, etc.) may make the presentation more serious and dramatic, such as the familiar "Hutchison's" dilated pupil on the side of an expanding intracranial mass.[43]

Diplopia also can be associated with ischemia from giant cell arteritis, but the optic neuropathy and visual loss usually dominate.[44] An atypical "migraine" episode may show the same signs, and only by very careful specific history and subtle examination (as well as neuroimaging) can a more sinister cause be excluded.[45]

Possibly IV Nerve (Trochlear)?

This has been discussed above. The Bielschowski head tilt test identifies the affected superior oblique muscle and nerve.[46] The head turn and tilt frequently decompensate in middle age, when degenerative joint disease restricts neck mobility, or after head injury, fever, or intoxication.

Possibly VI Nerve (Abducens)?

The abducens (VI) nerve supplies only the lateral rectus. Weakness causes the eye to be adducted and unable to abduct. The head is usually turned toward the side of weakness (i.e., with a left VI weakness the head will be turned to the left). (Note that a IV weakness tilts the head to the opposite side.) The forced duction test shows easy and full lateral movements, proving the medial rectus is not tight. Only 16% of nontraumatic IV palsies failed to recover, and, of these, 40% had serious underlying pathology.[47]

The localizing value of an abducens palsy is limited, since it is a nonspecific sign of other problems, including increased intracranial pressure and pineal tumors.[48,49]

Are Any Other Factors Present?

Infrequently, other diseases, including epilepsy, can adversely affect eye movements.[50]

Case 9. *A 9-year-old white patient on total parenteral nutrition fell out of bed but did not suffer a head injury. The patient now has an ataxic gait, diplopia, and nystagmus.*

Diagnosis. *Classic Wernicke's encephalopathy.*

Diplopia was the first indication of a nutritional deficiency in a series of patients on total parenteral nutrition when there was a temporary shortage of appropriate multivitamin infusions.[51] It may also develop during pregnancy as a result of increased metabolic demand.[52] Other rare metabolic diseases include Wilson's disease, malabsorption, and vitamin B1 deficiency.[53,54]

Infections also can cause diplopia: Black tar heroin injections may result in wound botulism, causing diplopia, dysphagia, dysponia, and descending paralysis.[55] Opportunistic infections in HIV-positive patients can result in diplopia, a sign of severe disease.[56]

Conclusion

This particular outline can guide evaluation and management of most cases of diplopia. *(Please see Table 1.)* If the cause (e.g., IV palsy, thyroid disease, etc.) results in permanently abnormal ocular alignment, then surgical intervention may be successful to reduce symptoms.[57,58] In other cases, an opaque contact lens is less cosmetically significant than wearing a patch.[59]

References

1 Richardson LD, Joyce DM. Diplopia in the emergency department. *Emerg Med Clin North Am* 1997;15:649-664.

2 Robertson NP, et al. Urgent neurology out-patient referrals from primary health care providers. *Quart J Med* 1998;91:309-313.

3. Kutschke PJ. Taking a history of the patient with diplopia. *Insight* 1996;21:92-95.

4. Fraser H. Diagnosis of double vision in adults. *Aust Fam Physician* 1995;24:1014-1015.

5. Yardley CJ, Hedges TR. Diplopia: The role of the ophthalmic medical assistant. *J Ophthalmic Nurs Technol* 1995;14: 259-263.

6. Dillon EC, et al. Diagnostic management by gate keepers is not cost effective for neuro-ophthalmology. *Ophthalmology* 1994;101:1627-1630.

7. Campbell C. Corneal aberrations, monocular diplopia, and ghost images: Analysis using corneal topographic data. *Optom Vis Sci* 1998;75:197-207.

8. Tan AK, Yeow YK. Warning symptoms of sinister headache. *Singapore Med J* 1994;35:294-297.

9. Miedziak A, Carty J. Chromatic visual phenomenon caused by subluxed intraocular lens. *J Cataract Refract Surg* 1996;22: 637-638.

10. Hapert M, BenEzra D. Surgery of the hereditary subluxated lens in children. *Ophthalmology* 1996;103:681-686.

11. Woods RL, et al. Monocular diplopia caused by ocular aberrations and hyperopic defocus. *Vision Res* 1996;36:3597-3606.

12. Stangler-Zuschrott E. Disturbing physiologic diplopia. *Klin Monatsbl Augenheilkk* 1979;174:370-373.

13. Lasley DJ, et al. Stereo discrimination between diplopic images in clinically normal observers. *Invest Ophthalmol Vis Sci* 1984;25:1316-1320.

14. Dengis CA, et al. Learning to look with one eye: The use of head turn by normals and strabismics. *Vision Res* 1996;36: 3237-3342.

15. Brazis PW, Lee AG. Binocular vertical diplopia. *Mayo Clin Proc* 1998;73:55-66.

16. Safran AB. Vestibular neuritis: A frequently unrecognized cause of diplopia. *Klin Monatsblat Augenheilkd* 1995;206:413-415.

17. Baloh RW. Approach to the dizzy patient. *Baillieres Clin Neurol* 1994;3:453-465.

18. Marzo ME, et al. Ocular myasthenia: Clinical course and strategies for treatment. *Rev Neurol* 1998;26:398-400.

19. Pourmand R. Myasthenia gravis. *Dis Mon* 1997;43:65-109.

20. Shumrick KA, et al. Criteria for selective management of the orbital rim and floor in zygomatic complex and midface fractures. *Arch Otolaryngol Head Neck Surg* 1997;123:378-384.

21. Bhattacharya J, et al. The role of plain radiography in the management of suspected orbital blow-out fractures. *Br J Radiol* 1997;70:29-33.

22. Wojno TH. The incidene of extraocular muscle and cranial nerve palsies in orbital floor blow out fractures. *Ophthalmology* 1987;94:682-685.

23. Fingeret M, et al. Forced duction test. *Atlas of Primary Eyecare Procedures*. Norwalk, CT: Appleton & Lange; 1990:138-144.

24. Hollis GJ. Sixth cranial nerve palsy following closed head injury in a child. *J Accid Emerg Med* 1997;14:172-175.

25. Fowler MS, et al. Squints and diplopia seen after brain damage. *J Neurol* 1996;243:86-90.

26. Goldenberg AS. Transient diplopia as a result of block injections. Mandibular and posterior superior alveolar. *N Y Stage Dent J* 1997;63:29-31.

27. Capo H, et al. Vertical strabismus after cataract surgery. *Ophthalmology* 1996;103:918-921.

28. Palmer-Hall AM, Anderson SF. Paraocular sinus mucoceles. *J Am Optom Assoc* 1997;68:725-733.

29. Kasner SE, et al. Neuro-ophthalmic aspects of aneurysms. *Neuroimaging Clin N Am* 1997;7:679-692.

30. Day JD, Fukushima T. Direct microsurgery of dural arteriovenous malformation type carotid-cavernous sinus fistula: Indications, technique, and results. *Neurosurgery* 1997;41: 1119-1124.

31. Gladstone GJ. Ophthalmologic aspects of thryoid-related orbitopathy. *Endocrinol Metab Clin North Am* 1998;27:91-100.

32. Fledelius HC. Exopthalmometry and thyroid disease. The value of Hertel measurements evaluated by a group of patients with thyroid disease and a control group. *Ugeskr Laeger* 1994;156:6528-6531.

33. Werner SC. Modification of the classification of the eye changes of Graves' disease: Recommendations of the Ad Hoc Committee of the American Thyroid Association. *J Clin Endocrinol Metab* 1977;44:203-204.

34. Gorman CA. The measurements of change in Graves' ophthalmopathy. *Thyroid* 1998;8:539-543.

35. Scott IU, Siatkowski RM. Idiopathic orbital myositis. *Curr Opin Rheumatol* 1997;9:504-512.

36. Tallsted L. Surgical treatment of thyroid eye disease. *Thyroid* 1998;8:447-452.

37. Pfeilschifter J, Ziegler R. Smoking and endocrine ophthalmopathy; impact of smoking severity and current vs lifetime cigarette consumption. *Clin Endocrinol (Oxf)* 1996;45:477-481.

38. Batocchi AP, et al. Ocular palsies in the absence of other neurological or ocular symptoms: Analysis of 105 cases. *J Neurol* 1997;244:639-645.

39. Ing E, Kennerdell JS. The evaluation and treatment of extraocular motility deficits. *Otolaryngol Clin North Am* 1997;30: 877-892.

40. Kabat AG. Intracranial hypertension. *Optom Clin* 1996;5: 153-179.

41. Miller NR. *Walsh and Hoyt's Clinical Neuro-Ophthalmology. Lesions of the supranuclear ocular motor pathways*. 4th ed. Baltimore, MD: Williams & Wilkins; 1985:707-715.

42. Polak BC, Heine RJ. Eye symptoms and latent diabetes. *Ned Tijdschr Geneeskd* 1997;141:73-75.

43. Hart AJ, et al. Malignant meningioma of the oculomotor nerve without dural attachment. Case report and review of the literature. *J Neurosurg* 1998;88:1104-1106.

44. Hayreh SS, et al. Occult giant cell arteritis: Ocular manifestations. *Am J Ophthalmol* 1998;125:521-526.

45. Krishna R, et al. Pseudotumor cerebri sine papilledema with unilateral sixth nerve palsy. *J Neuroophthalmol* 1998;18:53-55.

46. Bielschowski A. Disturbance of vertical motor muscles of the eyes. *Arch Ophthalmol* 1938;20:175-200.

47. King AJ, et al. Spontaneous recovery rates for unilateral sixth

nerve palsies. *Eye* 1995;9(Pt 4):476-478.

48. Galimberti CA, et al. Epileptic skew deviation. *Neurology* 1998;50:1469-1472.
49. Cho BK, et al. Pineal tumors: Experience with 48 cases over 10 years. *Childs Nerv Syst* 1998;14:53-58.
50. Adams RJ. Nursing assessment of visual function in children with neurologic diagnosis. *ABNF J* 1996;7:85-87.
51. Hahn JS, et al. Wernicke Encephalopathy and Beriberi during total parenteral nutrition attributable to multivitamin infusion shortage. *Pediatrics* 1998;101:E10.
52. Rees JH, et al. Two pregnant women with vomiting and fits. *Am J Obstet Gynecol* 1997;177:1539-1540.
53. Berman EL. Clues in the eye: Ocular signs of metabolic and nutritional disorders. *Geriatrics* 1995;50:34-36.
54. Kolling GH. Reflections on expert assesment of double vision and forced head position. *Klin Monatsbl Augenheilkd* 1996;208:63-65.
55. Anderson MW, et al. Wound botulism associated with black tar heroin. *Acad Emerg Med* 1997;4:805-809.
56. Seminari E, et al. Clinical significance of diplopia in HIV infection. Assesment of a personal caseload and review of the literature. *Minerva Med* 1996;87:515-523.
57. Gill MK, Drummond GT. Indications and outcomes of strabismus repair in visually mature patients. *Can J Ophthalmol* 1997;32:436-440.
58. Buckley SA, Elston JS. Surgical treatment of supranuclear and internuclear ocular motility disorders. *Eye* 1997;11(pt 3): 377-380.
59. Astin CL. The use of occluding tinted contact lenses. *CLAO J* 1998;24:125-127.
60. Schachat AP, et al. Diplopia. In: *Diagnostic Diagrams: Ophthalmology.* Williams & Wilkins: Baltimore, Md.; 1984: 101-107.

Alzheimer's Disease: Diagnosis and Management

Margaret Rathier, MD
Sandra Bellantonio, MD
Richard W. Besdine, MD, FACP

The incidence and prevalence of Alzheimer's disease (AD) increases dramatically with age, and a four-fold increase in the prevalence of AD is expected in the next millennium. Primary care providers play an important role for AD patients by assuring that an accurate diagnosis is made and an appropriate treatment plan is instituted.

Ongoing research into the etiology of AD has greatly enhanced our knowledge of the disease. Control of hypertension and treatment of atherosclerosis are known to reduce mortality from myocardial infarction. An added benefit of these therapies may be a decreased likelihood of being diagnosed with AD. Three genes have been identified that cause AD, but these account for a small proportion of known cases. Variations in the course or symptoms of patients diagnosed with AD might be explained by the coexistence of two separate pathologic processes.

Treatment of AD is a three-step process involving treatment of disease symptoms, treatment of the underlying pathology, and treatment of the caregiver. The goal of therapy in AD is to prevent excess disability, since it is not yet possible to reverse the process that triggers the death of neurons. Appropriate management of co-existing disease, treatment of depression when present in early dementia, and prompt treatment of delirium in AD will markedly improve cognitive function in the patient with AD.

Current drug therapy slows the progression of AD in some patients. Tacrine and donepezil, cholinesterase inhibitors, replace depleted acetylcholine stores and result in preserved cognitive as well as physical function. Anti-oxidant therapy is thought to inhibit the inflammatory process surrounding dying neurons. Trials using selegiline, vitamin E, and gingko biloba have slowed the progression of AD by preserving physical function.

The act of caring for a patient with AD can impair the physical and emotional health of the caregiver. Caregivers need education about the course and symptoms of AD and referral to community agencies that can assist with information and appropriate services. Caring for the caregiver will allow the AD patient to remain well cared for at home for as long as possible.

Ongoing research will identify the trigger responsible for AD. AD research has shifted to treatment, looking for agents that will delay time to symptom onset. Several case-control studies have shown that AD is diagnosed less frequently in subjects who have taken estrogen and nonsteroidal antiinflammatory drugs (NSAIDs). The ability to delay the onset of AD symptoms by five to 10 years will substantially reduce the resources devoted to the care of patients with AD.

In 1907, Alois Alzheimer described a 50-year-old woman with a rapidly progressive dementia, who had what we now call plaques and tangles on microscopic examination of her brain. The more typical presentation of AD is one of progressive decline in cognitive function over 8-10 years in an adult older than the age of 65. More than 4 million Americans have AD, and this number is expected to increase to 14 million by 2050 as a result of increased numbers of aging baby boomers, increased disease detection, and increased longevity.

Diagnostic Criteria for AD

AD most commonly presents as a deficit in short- and, eventually, long-term memory, but the diagnosis requires documentation of deficits in additional areas of cortical function. (Please *see Table 1.*) Deficits of cortical function most often seen in AD include aphasia, apraxia, agnosia, and disturbances in executive functioning. The disease usually has a gradual onset with a continuous decline.

In addition, cognitive deficits in AD must represent a significant decline from the patient's baseline and must impair the patient's activities of daily living. The deficits cannot result from other medical or psychiatric diseases. The accuracy of a clinical diagnosis in experienced hands is more than 90%.

Table 1. DSM-IV Criteria for AD

- Development of cognitive deficits manifested by memory impairment and one or more of the following:
  - — aphasia
  - — apraxia
  - — agnosia
  - — disturbance in executive functioning
- The cognitive deficits represent a significant decline from previous baseline
- The deficits cause significant impairment in functioning
- The deficits are not caused by other medical or psychiatric diseases

Clinical Evaluation

Patients are brought in for dementia evaluation when their cognitive deficits have progressed enough to impair their ability to function independently in the community or when their deficits are identified on mental status screening.[1,2] A history of cognitive loss should be obtained from the patient and caregivers with attention to the duration of loss and rate of change. Does the patient keep appointments, pay the bills, take medications, shop, and keep up his or her home? The patient's history can be approached as a life review, and this can identify the extent of long-term memory deficits. Depressive symptoms and a history of substance abuse should be probed. The family should be asked if a personality change has occurred. The extent and duration of comorbid illnesses should be identified, in particular hypertension, cardiovascular disease, cerebrovascular disease, and depression. The presence of hallucinations, paranoia, or delusions should be ascertained. A review of all prescribed and over-the-counter medications is necessary to identify agents with the potential to adversely affect cognition. The ability of the patient to function safely in the community should be determined by asking questions about cooking, driving, wandering, and falls. *(Please see Figure 1.)*

The objective of the physical examination is to identify remediable abnormalities that influence cortical functioning. The physical examination should determine the presence of hearing and vision deficits. Focal abnormalities on neurologic exam may aid in the differential diagnosis of dementia. An assessment of the patient's physical function also should be done to document any difficulty getting out of a chair, walking, or going to the bathroom.

The role of laboratory data in the work-up of a patient with cognitive impairment is to exclude reversible or treatable conditions that affect cognitive performance. Blood tests to be obtained include complete blood count, electrolytes, glucose, blood urea nitrogen, creatinine, calcium, thyroid-stimulating hormone, vitamin B_{12}, and syphilis serology. HIV testing should be obtained if the patient has a history of unprotected sexual intercourse, IV drug use, or transfusions of multiple blood products. There is no single diagnostic test with high enough sensitivity and specificity to make the diagnosis of AD.

Routine brain imaging is not necessary in the work-up of the patient with dementia, but a CT scan without contrast should be obtained if there is a history of head trauma, if focal neurologic deficits are found on physical examination, or if the clinical picture is not typical of AD. Brain imaging may be useful in determining the etiology of dementia; clinically silent cerebrovascular disease can be found on CT scan in the presence of a normal neurologic exam.

A formal mental status examination is the best way to document the areas of cognitive impairment and to gauge its severity. The Mini-Mental State Examination, a screening test for cognitive impairment developed by Folstein, is widely used, easy to administer, and has been translated into several languages *(please see Figure 2)*.[3] A score of 24 or higher is considered normal, but higher cut-off values have been established for patients with advanced education.[4] Likewise, subjects with less than an eighth grade education may have scores less than 24 and no evidence of dementia.

Referral for further neuropsychological testing should be pursued if questions remain regarding the differential diagnosis of dementia, especially in the presence of established psychiatric or neurologic disease.

Differential Diagnosis

It is important to determine the etiology of a patient's dementia, given the long clinical course of AD and the availability of treatments specific to AD.[5] Once cognitive impairment is confirmed, the first step is to confirm that dementia, rather than depression or delirium, is the cause. Patients with depression exhibit impaired concentration and impaired memory. Depression is commonly present early in the course of AD. Delirium has an acute onset with a fluctuating course; impaired attention and fluctuating level of consciousness are universally present.

AD is the most common dementia in those older than the age of 65, presenting gradually with progressive decline. Numerous diseases can cause dementia *(please see Table 2)*. AD is slightly more common in women. AD involves the parietal and temporal lobes of the brain. Presence of language deficits, word finding difficulty, or difficulty naming objects is very helpful in distinguishing AD from other dementias. The speech of patients with AD often is described as a fluent aphasia, void of detail.

Figure 1. Recognition and Initial Assessment of Alzheimer's Dementia and Related Dementias

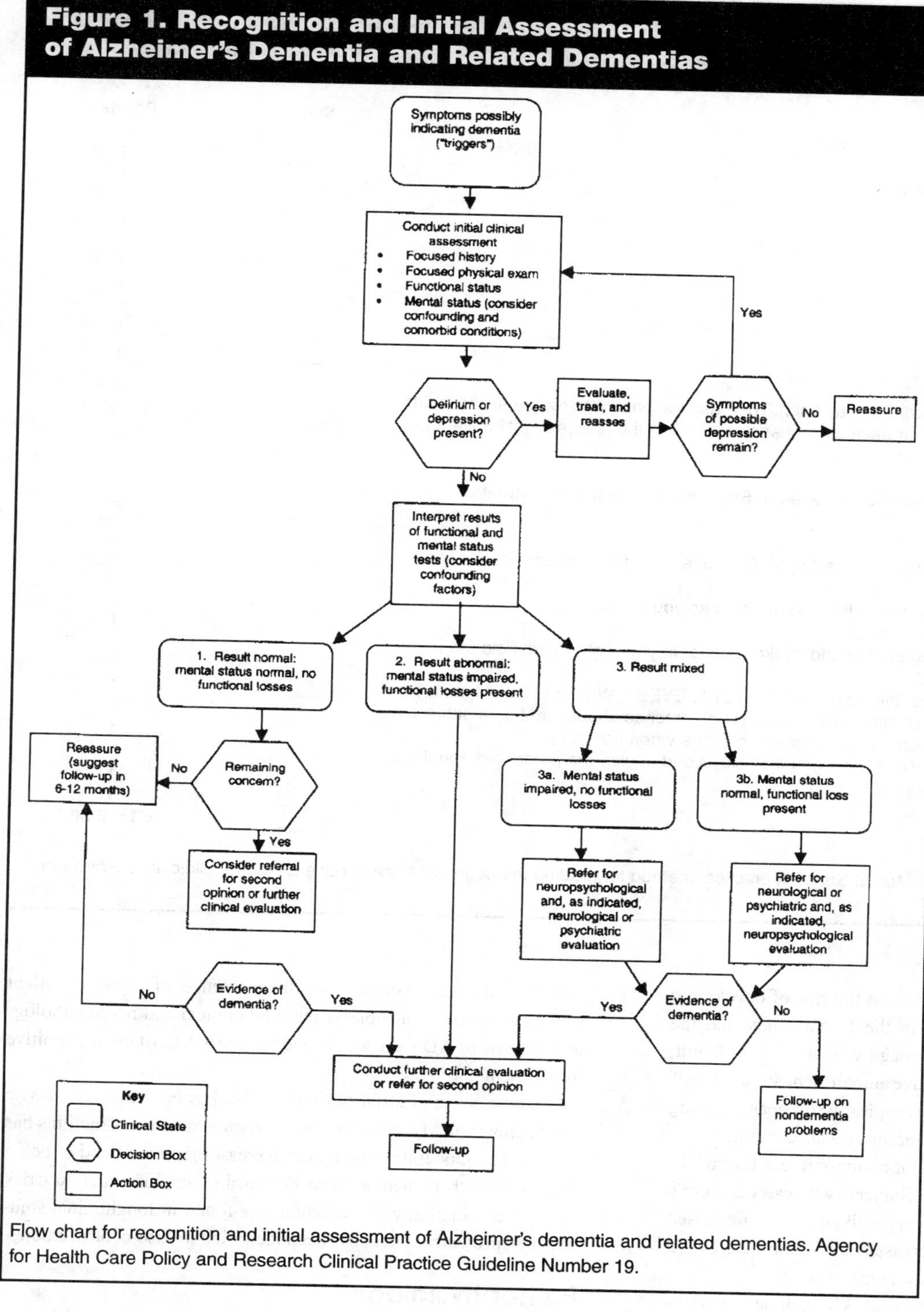

Flow chart for recognition and initial assessment of Alzheimer's dementia and related dementias. Agency for Health Care Policy and Research Clinical Practice Guideline Number 19.

Vascular dementia is defined as the onset of cognitive deficits following a stroke.[6] Focal neurologic signs and symptoms and evidence of cerebrovascular disease on brain imaging confirm the diagnosis. The presentation of dementia due to multiple infarcts is abrupt in onset with a step-wise deterioration, but the spectrum of vascular dementia includes several different subtypes with varied presentation *(please see Table 3)*.

Approximately 30% of patients with established Parkinson's disease develop dementia. In Parkinson's disease, Lewy bodies, (intracytoplasmic eosinophilic inclusion bodies) are found in subcortical nuclei. Cases of dementia have been identified with diffuse Lewy bodies in the cortex as well as subcortical regions, whose clinical presentation is not consistent with Parkinson's disease. Diffuse Lewy body dementia (LBD) is more prevalent in males by a 2:1 ratio, and 80% of patients present with neuropsychiatric symptoms, including prominent visual hallucinations, delusions, and psychosis.[7] The clinical course fluctuates daily, as does the patient's attention level. Neurologic examination is remarkable for rigidity and a gait disorder, but little tremor. Dementia occurs late in the disorder. Overlap between diffuse LBD and AD exists; 50% of patients with diffuse Lewy bodies also meet neuropathologic criteria for AD.

Epidemiology

The incidence and prevalence of AD varies by the age of the population studied; studies of all subjects older than the age of 65 yield prevalence rates ranging from three to 11.[8] The prevalence increases to 20-50% if the age of the population studied is limited to those 85 years of age and older *(please see Figure 3)*.

Risk Factors. Established risk factors are listed in Table 4. Advanced age is the primary risk factor for developing AD; the incidence and prevalence increase exponentially after the age of 65. More than 90% of cases of dementia occur in those older than age 70. A family history of dementia in a first-degree relative confers a four-fold increase in the risk for developing dementia. A history of loss of consciousness associated with head injury also has been associated with a two-fold increased risk of developing AD.

As patients with Down's syndrome (Trisomy 21) enter middle age, they can sustain a deterioration in cognitive function, and brains with Down's syndrome have neuropathology identical to AD. These facts led to a search for an AD gene on chromosome 21.

Education reduces the risk of developing AD; having less than an eighth-grade education or being employed in a non-managerial

Figure 2. Mini-Mental State Examination (MMSE)

Add points for each correct response.		Score	Points
Orientation			
1. What is the:	Year?	____	1
	Season?	____	1
	Date?	____	1
	Day?	____	1
	Month?	____	1
2. Where are we?	State?	____	1
	Country?	____	1
	Town or city?	____	1
	Hospital?	____	1
	Floor?	____	1
Registration			
3. Name three objects, taking one second to say each. Then ask the patient to repeat all three after you have said them. Give one point for each correct answer. Repeat the answers until patient learns all three.		____	3
Attention and calculation			
4. Serial sevens. Give one point for each correct answer. Stop after five answers. Alternate: Spell WORLD backward.		____	5
Recall			
5. Ask for names of three objects learned in question 3. Give one point for each correct answer.		____	3
Language			
6. Point to a pencil and a watch. Have the patient name them as you point.		____	2
7. Have the patient repeat "No ifs, ands, or buts."		____	1
8. Have the patient follow a three-stage command: "Take a paper in your right hand. Fold the paper in half. Put the paper on the floor."		____	3
9. Have the patient read and obey the following: "CLOSE YOUR EYES." (Write it in large letters.)		____	1
10. Have the patient write a sentence of his or her choice. (The sentence should contain a subject and an object and should make sense. Ignore spelling errors when scoring.)		____	1
11. Have the patient copy the design. (Give one point if all sides and angles are preserved and if the intersecting sides form a quadrangle.)		____	1
		____	1
		____	= Total 30

Adapted from: Folstein MF, et al. "Mini-Mental State." A practical method for grading the cognitive state of patients for the clinician. *J Phychiatr Res* 1975;12:189-198.

job is associated with a two-fold increase in the risk of developing AD.[9] Snowden and associates found in the Nun's Study that the more complex a subject's written language was as a young adult, the less likely she was to have cognitive impairment in late life.[10] Fewer grammatical details and less complex writing as a young adult increased the likelihood of developing AD as an adult.

A gene on chromosome 19 codes for apolipoprotein E (Apo-E) and is associated with late-onset AD.[11] Subjects who carry one copy of the Apo-E (4 allele are 2-4 times more likely to be diagnosed with AD, and homozygosity for (4 increases risk 5-18 times. The (2 allele is associated with a reduced prevalence of AD.

New vascular risk factors identified for AD include hypertension and atherosclerosis, disorders more commonly associated with vascular dementias. A longitudinal population-based study from Sweden showed that diastolic blood pressure elevation at age 70 independently predicts the diagnosis of AD at age 80.[12] This association between hypertension and AD has also been confirmed in the Framingham, Honolulu Heart, and Systolic Hypertension in Europe studies.[13] The presence of atherosclerosis, determined by the presence of carotid artery plaque and decreased ankle-brachial blood pressure ratio, has also been found to independently predict the diagnosis of AD; this risk was increased four-fold if the subject carried a copy of the Apo-E (4 allele).[14] Additional data from the Nun's Study demonstrated that the presence of clinically silent strokes on autopsy in subjects with the clinical and neuropathologic diagnosis of AD were associated with more substantial cognitive impairment.[15]

The presence of atrial fibrillation also has been associated with the diagnosis of AD, but noninsulin-dependent diabetes mellitus has not. Mild-to-moderate wine intake decreases the likelihood of being diagnosed with dementia. Data concerning smoking and AD risk vary; no association with dementia was found in longitudinal studies, but a protective effect has been identified in case-control studies.

Pathophysiology

The neuropathologic diagnosis of AD requires the presence of neuritic plaques, neurofibrillary tangles (NFTs), and cerebral amyloid angiopathy. The neuritic plaque is an extracellular structure containing a core of (-amyloid protein ((-AP) surrounded by degenerating neurons, activated microglia, and reactive astrocytes. (-AP is a 42 amino acid protein that is cleaved from a much larger precursor protein. Plaques are found in high numbers in the associative cortex and limbic system, and are most dense in the hippocampus. Neurons in these regions predominantly use acetylcholine as a neurotransmitter, and the first attempts to treat AD tried to replace acetylcholine.

Table 2. Diseases Associated with Dementia

Degenerative
- Alzheimer's disease
- Frontotemporal atrophy without Pick bodies
- Huntington's disease (chorea)
- Lewy body disease (paralysis agitans)
- Parkinson's disease
- Pick's disease
- Progressive supranuclear palsy
- Spinocerebellar degeneration

Vascular
- Binswanger's disease
- Cardiac disorders
- Vasculitis of central nervous system
- Delayed effects of irradiation
- Hemorrhage (subdural hematoma, subarachnoid hemorrhage, cerebral hemotama, vascular malformations)
- Hypoperfusion (cardiac arrest, profound hypotension, watershed ischemia)
- Multiple infarcts (amyloid angiopathy, large complete infarcts, lacunae of the basal ganglia and pons, frontal white matter lacunae)
- Strategic single infarct (thalamic, posterior cerebral artery, bilateral carotid occlusion, parietal infarct)
- Senile leukoencephalopathy (also related to amyloid angiopathy)

Mixed-vascular and Alzheimer's

Infectious
- Bacterial meningitis (chronic or partially treated)
- Whipple's disease of central nervous system
- Creutzfeldt-Jakob disease
- Fungal or tuberculous meningitis
- Neurosyphilis
- Viral encephalitis (herpes, human immunodeficiency virus [HIV])

Inflammatory
- Demyelinating disease (for example, multiple sclerosis)
- Limbic encephalitis
- Lupus erythematosus
- Sarcoidosis
- Sjögren's syndrome

Neoplastic
- Meningeal carcinomatosis
- Primary tumors (frontal globe or corpus callosum gliomas)
- Metastatic lesions

Traumatic
- Hypoxemic anoxia (respiratory failure, pure asphyxia)
- Subdural hematoma
- Traumatic brain injury

Toxic
- Alcohol
- Heavy metals (arsenic, lead, mercury)
- Histotoxic anoxia (carbon monoxide, cyanide)
- Medications (e.g., anticholinergic, antihistaminic, polypharmacy)

Metabolic
- Vitamin B_{12} or folate deficiency
- Cushing's disease
- Hypopituitarism
- Parathyroid disease
- Porphyria
- Thyroid disease (hyperthyroidism, hypothyroidism)
- Uremia
- Wilson's disease

Psychiatric
- Depression

Hydrocephalus
- Nonobstructive vs. obstructive
- Normal pressure

Reprinted with permission from: Fleming KC, et al. Dementia: Diagnosis and evaluation. *Mayo Clin Proc* 1995;70:1093-1107.

Table 3. Categories of Vascular Dementia

Category	Clinical Presentation
Multiple infarctions	Step-wise appearance
Single strategic infarction	Sudden onset, deficits dependent on location
Lacunar infarction	Progressive dementia, history of stroke may be absent
White matter infarctions (small vessel disease)	Dementia with gait disorder
Mixed AD-vascular dementia	Progressive dementia with history of stroke

Reprinted with permission from: Knopman D. The differential diagnosis of dementia in the elderly. *Mediguide to Geriatric Neurology* 1997;1(1):1-7. Copyright ©1997, Lawrence DellaCorte Publications, Inc. All rights reserved.

Plaques are also found in the brains of 80% of older adults without dementia, but the plaques are present in a diffuse fashion and in much smaller numbers. Apo-E has also been found in neuritic plaques.

NFTs are intracellular dense bundles of paired helical filaments derived from altered forms of tau, a microtubule-associated protein. NFTs are found in the hippocampus and temporal lobe cortex of brains with AD but can also be found in other neurodegenerative diseases. The gene that codes for tau is found on chromosome 17, which is not known to be associated with AD.

Amyloid is deposited in small- and medium-sized blood vessel walls in the cortex and leptomeninges of brains with AD. This cerebral amyloid angiopathy is more severe in the brains of AD patients who are Apo-E (4 positive. Current research is examining the effect of amyloid deposition on the aggregation of platelets and fibrin, which might result in small vessel disease, helping to explain the association between AD and vascular disease.

Variations in the clinical course of AD may reflect the co-existence of several pathologies. A more rapid decline in cognitive function than typical for AD may be the result of silent small vessel strokes. If plaques and tangles are present with diffuse Lewy bodies, the patient with AD may have a gait disorder and rigidity on neurologic exam.

Genetics

Currently there are four genes that have an association with AD; three genes are associated with familial autosomal dominant AD (FAD), which starts prior to the age of 60 (*see Table 5*).[17] FAD accounts for 5% of patients with AD. The gene on chromosome 21 codes for the (-amyloid precursor protein and results in increased production of (-AP. Mutations in this gene account for 2-3% of cases of FAD. Mutations in the presenilin-1 gene on chromosome 14 account for 80% of FAD cases. The genes on chromosomes 14 and 1 code for proteins or presenilins, which also result in the increased production of (-AP.

A potential role for mutations in mitochondrial genes exists in AD. Alterations in cellular metabolism have been detected in patients with AD, and different forms of cytochrome oxidase have been identified.

At this time, a gene that is directly associated with typical, late-onset AD has not been identified. It is likely that one exists, since twin studies show increased concordance in monozygotic as compared to dizygotic twins (67% vs 22%).[18] However, the late age of onset of usual AD, in association with the presence of fatal comorbid disease before AD is detected, makes the study of genetics in typical AD difficult.

The association between Apo-E and AD was first described in 1993.[19] Apo-E is a major component of circulating lipoproteins and is made by astrocytes. It can be found in neurons and the extracellular space. The gene that codes for Apo-E has been identified on chromosome 19. There are three common alleles; one or two copies of (4 is associated with an increased risk of AD. It is thought that Apo-E may interact with tau to form NFTs and precipitate cell death.

Patients with AD who are homozygous for (4 will develop AD at an earlier age (70 vs 90). The association between Apo-E (4 and AD in African-Americans or Hispanics is less strong.[20] Having one or two copies of (4 is associated with increased amounts of (-AP in the neuritic plaques.[21] However, Apo-E (4 is neither necessary nor sufficient for the diagnosis of AD. Data from the Framingham study show that the sensitivity of Apo-E (4 as a predictor of AD is 49% and the specificity is 81%. The positive predictive value for (4 homozygotes is 30%.[22] Most major medical societies agree that there is no role for Apo-E genotyping in the diagnostic work-up for AD.[23] Apo-E genotype testing might help confirm a clinical diagnosis of AD.

Management

The goals of therapy are to maximize independence for the person with AD, to enhance quality of life for the patient and for his/her caregiver(s), and to maintain the patient's cognition as long as possible. Primary care physicians (PCPs) have a pivotal role in the management of AD. PCPs must understand the different needs of patients with AD and of their caregivers at various stages of the illness, including the unique needs of the person with end-stage AD. Knowledge of medications commonly used in the treatment of AD, of the available supportive services, and of options for living location as the disease progresses is crucial for the PCP caring for persons with AD. Caring for persons with AD is complex; thus, PCPs should be aware of consultants, such as geriatricians, geriatric psychiatrists, and neurologists, available to assist with the management of persons with AD.

Treatment of Cognitive Symptoms

Reality orientation and memory retraining should be avoided, since they are potentially frustrating for persons with AD and are only transiently effective.[5] Persons with AD should be encouraged to engage in mentally stimulating activities, such as puzzles, reading, and playing cards, since there is evidence that persons with more years of education have a lower prevalence of AD compared to those with fewer years of education.[9]

Pharmacological Treatment

Cholinesterase Inhibitors. Cholinesterase inhibitors diminish the breakdown of acetylcholine, thus, increasing the supply of acetylcholine in the brain. Cholinesterase inhibitors do not alter the underlying course of AD, but in one-third of persons with AD,

Figure 3. Incidence Rates of Dementia and Alzheimer's Disease in Rochester, MN

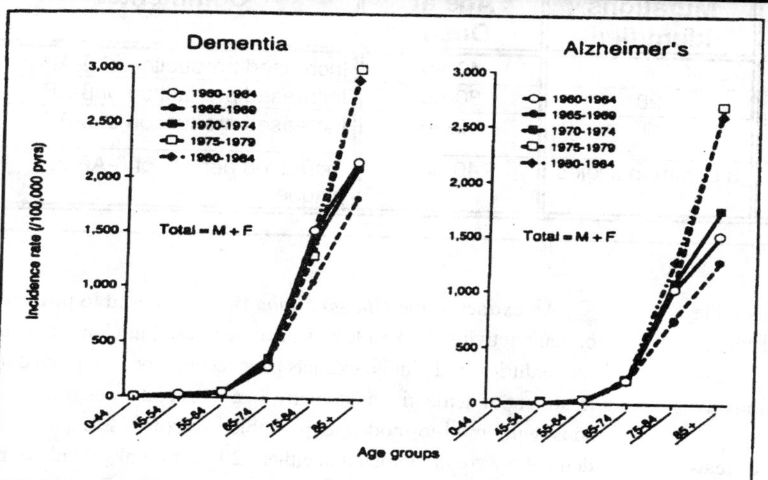

Incidence rates of dementia and Alzheimer's disease in Rochester, Minnesota, stratified by age for five quinquennial periods (1960-1984). Pyrs = person-years. Reprinted with permission from: Kokmen E, et al. Epidemiology of dementia in Rochester, MN. *Mayo Clin Proc* 1996;71:275-282.

cholinesterase inhibitors attenuate disease progression by 6-12 months.[24] Two cholinesterase inhibitors have been approved for use in the treatment of AD in the United States: tacrine and donepezil.

Tacrine hydrochloride, the first FDA-approved treatment for mild-to-moderate AD, became available for use in the United States in September of 1993. Although more than 600 persons with AD were enrolled in a randomized, controlled trial designed to evaluate the efficacy and safety of tacrine, approximately two-thirds of the participants at the most effective dose did not complete the 30-week study.[25] Withdrawal from the study was primarily attributed to adverse effects. More than half of those enrolled developed abnormalities of liver function tests; other commonly reported side effects included nausea and/or vomiting (35%), diarrhea (18%), and anorexia (12%). Participants who completed the study demonstrated mild-to-modest improvement in cognitive function compared to those treated with placebo; however, the clinical use of tacrine is limited by the high incidence of adverse events associated with its use and the need for frequent measurement of liver function.

In 1995, the FDA approved the use of donepezil hydrochloride for the treatment of mild-to-moderate AD. Donepezil is highly selective for acetylcholinesterase in the central nervous system; thus, its use is associated with a relatively low incidence of peripheral cholinergic events. Nearly 90% of persons with mild-to-moderate AD completed a 12-week trial designed to evaluate the efficacy and safety of donepezil (5 mg/d) vs. placebo.[26] In this study, donepezil (5 mg/d) was associated with mild-to-modest enhancement of cognitive function compared to placebo. Donepezil use was not associated with hepatotoxicity, although 10% of the participants experienced nausea/vomiting or diarrhea. In a 24-week randomized trial of nearly 500 persons with mild-to-moderate AD, donepezil (10mg/d) was more effective than either donepezil (5 mg/d) or placebo in enhancing cognitive function.[27] However, 68% of the persons randomized to donepezil (10 mg/d) vs. 85% of those randomized to donepezil (5 mg/d) completed the trial. Those randomized to the higher dose of donepezil had a higher incidence of nausea/vomiting, diarrhea, fatigue, and muscle cramps compared to those randomized to donepezil 5 mg/d or to placebo. The investigators reported that the higher percentage of cholinergic side effects experienced by the donepezil 10 mg/d group was related to a rapid titration protocol used during the study. Thus, the recommended starting dose of donepezil is 5 mg/d; if a patient tolerates donepezil 5 mg/d, then the dose should be increased to 10 mg/d in 4-6 weeks. The improvement in cognition disappeared during the six-week washout period.

Cholinesterase inhibitors have not been studied in persons with severe AD or in persons who live in nursing facilities (NF). Thus, the efficacy of cholinesterase inhibitors for the treatment of severe AD or for the treatment of NF residents is unknown. Moreover, studies guiding the timing of cessation of therapy with a cholinesterase inhibitor are lacking.

Anti-oxidants. The accumulation of free radicals may play a role in the pathogenesis of AD by leading to neuronal degeneration in the brain.[28] Three agents with anti-oxidant properties have been shown to slow the progression of AD: selegiline, an agent that delays the onset of disability in persons with AD,[29] alpha-tocopherol or vitamin E, and *Ginkgo biloba*, a plant extract.

In a two-year trial of 341 community-living persons with moderately severe probable AD, patients randomized to selegiline 5 mg twice daily, alpha-tocopherol 1000 IU twice daily, or both combined, demonstrated delayed progression of AD by an average of 6.5 months compared to patients receiving placebo.[30] AD progression was defined as the time to reach any one of four end points (death, institutionalization, loss of activities of daily living [ADL] independence, or severe dementia). When the four outcomes were analyzed separately, alpha-tocopherol use was associated with delayed institutionalization and delayed loss of ADL independence. Neither selegiline nor alpha-tocopherol use was found to have a

Table 4. Risk Factors for AD

INCREASED RISK ASSOCIATED WITH AD	DECREASED RISK ASSOCIATED WITH AD
Age	Advanced education
Family history	Estrogen use
Head injury with loss of consciousness	NSAID use
Down's syndrome	Apolipoprotein-E ε2
Hypertension	
Atherosclerosis	
Apolipoprotein-E ε4	

Table 5. Genes Associated with AD

Gene Name	Location	Mutations Identified	Age at Onset	Comments
Amyloid Precursor Protein	Chromosome 21	4	40-65	Increased production of β-AP
Presenilin-1	Chromosome 14	28	30-55	Increased production of β-AP
Presenilin-2	Chromosome 1	3	40-90	Increased production of β-AP
Apolipoprotein-E	Chromosome 19	3 common alleles	40-90	Increased density of β-AP in plaque

measurable effect on cognitive status. There was no demonstrable additive effect of combined treatment with selegiline and alpha-tocopherol. In fact, the combined treatment group had worse outcomes compared to the group receiving either selegiline or alpha-tocopherol.

Falls and syncope were more frequently reported in the treatment groups—especially in the group receiving combined therapy compared to placebo (16% vs 4%). Selegiline may have other side effects (nausea, headache). Although high doses of alpha-tocopherol E may increase bleeding tendency in persons who are vitamin K-deficient or who are receiving warfarin, none of the 88 healthy older persons receiving 800 IU of vitamin E for four months experienced bleeding complications.[31] A trial is underway to determine the effectiveness of vitamin E in delaying the onset of AD.

Table 6. Commonly Used Medications in the Treatment of Behavior/ Psychiatric Symptoms

MEDICATION	DOSE RANGE	SIDE EFFECTS	COMMENTS
DEPRESSION			
Tricyclic antidepressants (TCA)		Sedation, anticholinergic effects, orthostatic hypotension, Intraventricular conduction delay	
Nortriptyline	10-100 mg/d	Least orthostatic hypotension	Safest TCA for use in older patients
Desipramine	10-100 mg/d	Least anticholinergic effects	
Amitryptyline			Avoid using due to excessive anticholinergic effects
Selective serotonin reuptake inhibitors (SSRIs)		Insomnia, anxiety, nausea, diarrhea, headache; impotence	Less anticholinergic and hypotensive effects compared to TCAs
Sertraline	25-200 mg/d		
Paroxetine	10-40 mg/d		Higher incidence of mild anticholinergic side effects compared to other SSRIs
Fluoxetine			Avoid using due to agitation and anorexia
Serotonin/norepeinephrine reuptake inhibitors			
Venlafaxine	50-150 mg/d	Diastolic hypertension, nausea, somnolence	
Heterocyclic antidepressants			
Bupropion	50-300 mg/d	Insomnia, nausea, restlessness	No anticholinergic or hypotensive effects
Trazodone	25-100 mg/d	Excessive postural hypotension	Avoid using due to sedation

An extract of the *Ginkgo biloba* tree is believed to possess antioxidant activity. Ginkgo leaves have been used in Chinese medicine for centuries, and ginkgo extracts have recently been approved for the treatment of dementia in Germany. In a recent 52-week trial, 327 persons with mild-to-moderate probable AD (n = 251) or vascular dementia were randomized to either 120 mg of ginkgo daily or placebo.[32] Ginkgo was found to have a modest positive effect on cognition compared to placebo. However, fewer than half the participants completed the trial; the most commonly reported reasons for withdrawal from the study were caregiver request (15% of the treatment group vs 19% of the placebo group) and noncompliance with the protocol (8% of the treatment group vs 9% of the placebo group). Only 4% of the treatment group and 3% of the placebo group withdrew secondary to adverse events; the most commonly reported side effects were gastrointestinal. The National Institute on Aging (NIA) is sponsoring additional investigations of ginkgo in the treatment of AD.

Estrogen Replacement Therapy (ERT). In case-control and epidemiological studies,[33-36] women who used estrogen were less likely to develop AD. Prospective data from the Baltimore Longitudinal Study of Aging demonstrated a 54% reduction in the incidence of AD in estrogen users among nearly 500 women.[37] Clinicians must interpret these results with caution since the relative value of epidemiological studies is considerably weaker when compared to randomized, controlled trials. Although several small, nonrandomized trials have demonstrated a beneficial effect of estrogen on cognitive function,[38-40] data conclusively demonstrating that estrogen has a role in preventing or treating AD are lacking. The Women's Health Initiative Memory Study, a randomized, controlled trial of women older than age 65, should provide conclusive information regarding the benefits of ERT on cognitive function. The study will end in 2005 and data should be available by 2007.

Estrogen is believed to enhance cognition through several direct and indirect mechanisms. In vitro studies have demonstrated that estrogen functions as a neurotropic factor that prolongs neuronal survival and enhances neuronal growth. Estrogen indirectly affects brain cells by stimulating the production of other neurotropic factors and by improving cerebral blood flow.[41] Finally, estrogen exhibits antioxidant activity.[42]

Potential side effects of estrogen use include breast tenderness, vaginal bleeding, thromboembolic disease, and uterine and breast cancer. Given the lack of conclusive data demonstrating estrogen's role in the prevention of AD, estrogen should not be recommended to prevent cognitive loss. The FDA has approved estrogen for the prevention and treatment of osteoporosis; the majority of evidence suggests that estrogen use has benefits in preventing heart disease. Thus, women should be counseled about estrogen use based on its proven benefits to bone and cardiovascular health.

Anti-inflammatory Agents. Numerous case control and cross-sectional studies have demonstrated an association between NSAID use and a decreased risk of developing AD.[43,44] Prospective data from the Baltimore Longitudinal study of Aging demonstrate a 60% reduction in the incidence of AD among persons who have used NSAIDs for at least two years.[45] Although these data are promising, they do not conclusively demonstrate that NSAID use prevents AD, only that NSAID use is associated with a lower risk of developing AD. The mechanism by which NSAID use could potentially prevent AD is unclear. Inflammation is clearly part of the neuropathology of AD, but whether the inflammation is a cause or an effect of AD is unknown.

NSAID use is associated with potentially serious side effects such as peptic ulcer disease, fatal gastrointestinal hemorrhage, heart failure, and renal failure. Given the lack of conclusive evidence demonstrating the role of NSAIDs in preventing AD, they should not be considered in the prevention of AD until additional data are available.

A selective COX-II inhibitor, celecoxib, has recently become available for use in the symptomatic treatment of osteoarthritis and rheumatoid arthritis. COX II inhibitors may be useful in studying the effects of NSAIDs and AD, and because they potentially have fewer side effects than other available NSAIDs, there has been some recent concern about the safety of celecoxib. The NIA is currently sponsoring a clinical trial designed to establish the safety and efficacy of prednisone in preventing AD.

Table 7. Other Commonly Used Medications in the Treatment of Behavior/Psychiatric Symptoms

MEDICATION	DOSE RANGE	ADVERSE EFFECTS	COMMENTS
ANTIPSYCHOTICS			
Olanzapine	2.5-7.5 mg/d	Weight gain	Lowest incidence of extrapyrimidal side effects and orthostatic hypotension
Risperidone	0.5-2 mg/d	Weight gain, Orthostatic hypotension	Decrease dosage in patients with renal failure
Haloperidol	0.25-2 mg/d	Extrapyrimidal effects	
Thioridazine	10-100 mg/d	Most likely to cause sedation, orthostatic hypotension and anticholinergic effects	Use only when sedation desired
ANXIOLYTICS			
Alprazolam	0.125-0.75 mg/d	Sedation, delirium, falls	
Lorazepam	0.25-2 mg/d	Sedation, delirium, falls	
Buspirone	10-60 mg/d	Headache, dizziness, nausea	Nonsedating, therapeutic effect in 1-3 weeks
ANTICONVULSANTS			
Carbamazepine	200 mg bid	Sedation, gait disturbance, diplopia	Induces metabolism of other drugs (warfarin, haldol)
Valproic acid	250 mg bid	Nausea, vomiting, weight gain, sedation	Enteric coated divalproex can reduce nausea and vomiting

Treatment of Behavioral/Psychiatric Symptoms

Prior to considering therapeutic intervention in the management of behavioral or psychiatric symptoms associated with AD, a comprehensive evaluation must be conducted to assure that medical reasons for the decline do not exist. In particular, new or worsened behavioral or psychiatric symptoms may be due to delirium. Many potentially serious conditions can lead to delirium in the patient with dementia, particularly infections (such as pneumonia and urinary tract infection) and medications (such as psychotropics and agents with anticholinergic effects).

Nonpharmacological Treatment

Agitation (aggression, combativeness, shouting, disinhibition) is common among persons with AD. In one study, up to half of persons with middle-to-late stage AD experienced agitation in one form or another.[5] Agitation and other behavior disorders common in AD, such as wandering, reversal of the sleep-wake cycle, and resistance to care, usually respond poorly to pharmacological interventions. Recreational activities, reminiscence therapy, and support groups may diminish behavioral and psychiatric symptoms associated with AD.[46-49] Keeping the environment simple, structured, and as constant as possible minimizes confusion and may alleviate difficult-to-control symptoms. Often, keeping the patient safe is the only intervention required, as in the case of wandering. If nonpharmacological therapy is ineffective in controlling behaviors that are potentially harmful to the patient or to others, pharmacotherapy may be necessary.

Pharmacological Treatment

Among behaviors that respond relatively well to pharmacological intervention are depression, psychosis, and anxiety. Depressive symptoms, such as loss of sleep, loss of appetite, or irritability, are common among persons with AD and should be treated aggressively, even if the patient fails to meet criteria for depression.[5] The choice of drug therapy should be guided by the medication side effects profile and by the patient's comorbid conditions (*see Tables 6 and 7*).

Psychotic symptoms are less common than depressive symptoms among persons with AD. Psychotic features are more common in the middle-to-later stages of the illness, and include paranoia, delusions, and hallucinations. Psychotic symptoms can be very distressing to persons with AD and may lead to self-harm or danger to others. In such cases, it is appropriate to initiate therapy with an antipsychotic medication. Some of the newer agents, such as olanzapine, are less sedating and have fewer anticholinergic side effects than older antipsychotic medications; however, they are significantly more costly. Older antipsychotic medications that are relatively inexpensive, such as haloperidol, are appropriate for use during acute episodes of

Table 8. Additional Resources

RESOURCES	PHONE NUMBERS	WEB SITES
Organizations		
National Association of Professional Geriatric Care Managers	520-881-8008	www.caremanager.org
National Association for Home Care	202-547-7424	www.nahc.org
National Association for Area Agencies on Aging	202-296-8130	www.n4a.org
Assisted Living Federation of America	703-691-8100	www.alfa.org
National Academy of Elder Law Attorneys	520-881-4005	www.naela.org
Services		
Meals-on-Wheels		
Local senior citizens centers		
Local church/community groups		
Adult day centers		
Hospice care services		
Respite care services		
Skilled nursing facility care		
Information/Education about AD		
Alzheimer's Association	800-272-3900	www.alz.org
American Geriatrics Society	212-308-1414	www.americangeriatrics.org
American Disease Education and Referral Centers	800-438-4380	www.alzheimers.org

psychosis or for chronic use at a low dose (0.25-2 mg/d).

Severe anxiety, which manifests with phobias and panic attacks, responds well to benzodiazepines. Benzodiazepines with a shorter half-life are preferred (oxazepam and lorazepam) to longer acting agents (diazepam and chlordiazepoxide), which tend to be more sedating due to the accumulation of active metabolites. However, all benzodiazepines have been associated with increased risk of falls, and their use should be minimized.

Agitation, as described above, often does not respond to pharmacotherapy. Agitated behavior that has not responded to nonpharmacological measures and that is potentially harmful to the patient or to others, may warrant a trial of pharmacotherapy. If behavior does not respond to antipsychotic medications, other ("second-line") agents such as carbamazepine, valproate, or buspirone may be helpful. Although trazodone should be avoided for use as an antidepressant due to its excessively sedating properties, it may be helpful in treating agitated behaviors, especially at night when sleep is a desired side effect.

Involvement of Specialty Consultations

Although the PCP is often able to manage persons with AD, especially in the early stages of the disease, situations often arise when consultation with other professionals is helpful. Geriatricians or geriatric psychiatrists may be helpful in managing difficult behaviors or severe psychiatric problems. Geropsychologists skilled at individual or family therapy may help persons with AD and their caregivers gain skills in coping with the disease. Neurologists may be helpful in evaluating a patient with a rapidly progressing clinical course. Social workers, especially case managers, can help patients and caregivers access community resources. Attorneys specializing in eldercare are able to provide legal advice surrounding long-term financial planning.

Maximizing General Health

It is imperative to maximize the general health of persons with AD by detecting and treating underlying medical conditions, such as hypertension, cerebrovascular disease, thyroid disease, and B_{12} deficiency, which if left untreated, could potentially further impair cognitive and functional status. Preventive measures, such as screening mammography and fecal occult blood testing, should be undertaken only if the patient and/or caregiver are prepared to treat a detected breast or colorectal cancer. Influenza and pneumococcal vaccinations are appropriate for persons with early as well as advanced AD, both as a preventive measure for an individual patient and to diminish risk of disease transmission. As AD advances, managing conditions such as continence and malnutrition may become important.

Caregiver Education/Support

More than 70% of persons with AD are living at home and receiving care by families and friends.[50] Family caregivers, most often middle-aged spouses or daughters, provide an average of 17.6 h/week of care, and more than half are employed.[51] It is not surprising that caregivers frequently report depressive and physical health symptoms.[52] Thus, caregiver support is crucial in the management of persons with AD. In a longitudinal study of 206 persons with AD, participation in counseling sessions and support groups by spouse caregivers and families delayed NF placement by 329 days compared to the control group.[53] Despite the proven benefits of caregiver support and education, studies have demonstrated that many physicians are unaware of available community services for patients with dementia.[54,55] It is encouraging that more than half of physicians who participated in a project designed to improve caregiver education and support stated they had learned more about available community resources by referring patients with AD and their caregivers to a local chapter of the Alzheimer's Association.[56] Thus, encouraging caregiver support benefits the caregiver by alleviating stress, the patient by delaying NF placement, and the PCP by increasing awareness of community services available to persons with AD *(please see Table 8)*.

Management of End-Stage AD

The primary goal of caring for a person with advanced AD is to maintain comfort and to avoid suffering. Restricting interventions to those therapies that enhance or maintain quality of life is central to good care for persons with end-stage AD. Decisions regarding the appropriateness of tube feeding, antibiotics, transfusions, and hospitalization are facilitated by discussions between the physician, the patient, and the caregivers early in the course of the disease when the patient is still able to express his or her wishes regarding care at the end of life. Providing care to persons with advanced AD that is consistent with his or her values and beliefs requires that physicians initiate discussions regarding advanced directives, such as a living will and durable power of attorney soon after they begin caring for the person with early AD.

References

1. Fleming KC, et al. Dementia: Diagnosis and evaluation. *Mayo Clin Proc* 1995;70:1093-1107.
2. Geldmacher DS, Whitehouse PJ. Evaluation of dementia. *N Engl J Med* 1996;335:330-336.
3. Folstein MF, et al. "Mini-Mental State." A practical method for grading the cognitive state of patients for the clinician. *J Psychiat Res* 1975;12:189-198.
4. Tombaugh TN, McIntyre NJ. The mini-mental state examination: A comprehensive review. *J Am Geriatr Soc* 1992;40:925-935.
5. Small GW, et al. Diagnosis and treatment of Alzheimer's disease and related disorders. *JAMA* 1997;278:1363-1371.
6. Nyenhuis DL, Gorelick PB. Vascular dementia: A contemporary review of epidemiology, diagnosis, prevention and treatment. *J Am Geriatr Soc* 1998;46:1437-1448.
7. Gomez-Tortosa E, et al. Dementia with Lewy bodies. *J Am Geriatr Soc* 1998;46:1449-1458.
8. Kokmen E, et al. Epidemiology of dementia in Rochester, Minnesota. *Mayo Clin Proc* 1996;71:275-282.
9. Stern Y, et al. Influence of education and occupation on the incidence of Alzheimer's disease. *JAMA* 1994;271: 1004-1010.
10. Snowdon DA, et al. Linguistic ability in early life and cognitive function and Alzheimer's disease in late life. Findings from the Nun Study. *JAMA* 1996;275:528-532.
11. Roses AD. Apolipoprotein E alleles as risk factors in Alzheimer's disease. *Annu Rev Med* 1996;47:387-400.
12. Skoog I, et al. 15-year longitudinal study of blood pressure and dementia. *Lancet* 1996;347:1141-1145.
13. Forette F, et al. Prevention of dementia in randomised double-blind placebo-controlled systolic hypertension in Europe (Syst-Eur) trial. *Lancet* 1998;352:1347-1351.
14. Hofman A, et al. Atherosclerosis, apolipoprotein E, and prevalence of dementia and Alzheimer's disease in the Rotterdam Study. *Lancet* 1997;349:151-154.
15. Snowdon DA, et al. Brain infarction and the clinical expression of Alzheimer disease. The Nun Study. *JAMA* 1997;277:813-817.
16. Ott A, et al. Atrial fibrillation and dementia in a population-based study. The Rotterdam Study. *Stroke* 1997;28:316-321.
17. Selkoe DJ. Alzheimer's disease: Genotypes, phenotype, and treatments. *Science* 1997;275:630-631.
18. Gatz M, et al. Heritability for Alzheimer's disease: The study of dementia in Swedish twins. *J Gerontol A Biol Sci Med Sci* 1997;52:M117-M125.
19. Roses AD. Alzheimer's disease: The genetics of risk. *Hosp Pract* 1997;51-69.
20. Farrer LA, et al. Effects of age, sex and ethnicity on the association between apolipoprotein E genotype and Alzheimer disease. A meta-analysis. *JAMA* 1997;278: 1349-1356.
21. Polvikoski T, et al. Apolipoprotein E, dementia, and cortical deposition of beta-amyloid protein. *N Engl J Med* 1995; 333:1241-1247.
22. Myers RH, et al. Apolipoprotein E E4 association with dementia in a population-based study: The Framingham Study. *Neurology* 1996;46:673-677.
23. NIA/Alzheimer's Association Working Group. Apolipoprotein E genotyping in Alzheimer's disease. A consensus statement. *Lancet* 1996;347:1091-1095.
24. Aging Research & Training News. Scientists Outline Current Thinking on Alzheimer's Disease Treatments. 1998; 127.
25. Knapp MJ, et al. A 30-week randomized controlled trial of high-dose tacrine in patients with Alzheimer's disease. *JAMA* 1994;271:985-991.
26. Rogers SL, Friedhoff LT, and the Donepezil Study Group. The efficacy and safety of donepezil in patients with Alzheimer's disease: Results of a U.S. multicentre, randomized, double-blind, placebo-controlled trial. *Dementia* 1996;7:293-303.
27. Rogers SL, et al. A 24-week, double-blind, placebo-controlled trial of donepezil in patients with Alzheimer's disease. *Neurology* 1998;50:136-145.
28. Smith MA, et al. Oxidative damage in Alzheimer's. *Nature* 1996;382:120-121.
29. The Parkinson Study Group. Effects of tocopherol and deprenyl on the progression of disability in early parkinson's disease. *N Engl J Med* 1993;328:176-183.
30. Sano M, et al. A controlled trial of selegiline alpha-tocopherol, or both as treatment for Alzheimer's disease. *N Engl J Med* 1997;336:1216-1222.
31. Meydani SN, et al. Assessment of the safety of supplementation with different amounts of vitamin E in healthy older adults. *Am J Clin Nutr* 1998;68:311-318.
32. LeBars PL, et al. A placebo-controlled, double-blind, randomized trial of an extract of *Gingko biloba* for dementia. *JAMA* 1997;278:1327-1332.
33. Henderson VW, et al. Estrogen replacement therapy in older women: Comparisons between Alzheimer's disease cases and non-demented control subjects. *Arch Neurol* 1994;51: 896-900.
34. Mortel KF, Meyer JS. Lack of postmenopausal estrogen replacement therapy and the risk of dementia. *J Neuropsychiatry Clin Neurosci* 1995;7:334-337.
35. Tang M-X, et al. Effect of estrogen during menopause on risk and age at onset of Alzheimer's disease. *Lancet* 1996; 348:429-432.

36. Paganini-Hill A, Henderson VW. Estrogen deficiency and risk of Alzheimer's disease in women. *Am J Epidemiol* 1994;140:256-261.
37. Kawas C, et al. A prospective study of estrogen replacement therapy and the risk of developing Alzheimer's disease. The Baltimore Longitudinal Study of Aging. *Neurology* 1997; 48:1517-1521.
38. Fillit H, et al. Observations in a preliminary open trial of estradiol therapy for senile dementia—Alzheimer's type. *Psychoneuroendocrinology* 1986;11:337-345.
39. Honjo H, et al. Senile dementia-Alzheimer's type and estrogen. *Horm Metab Res* 1995;27:204-207.
40. Ohkura T, et al. Long-term estrogen replacement therapy in female patients with dementia of the Alzheimer's type: 7 case reports. *Dementia* 1995;6:99-107.
41. Birge SJ. Is there a role for estrogen replacement therapy in the prevention and treatment of dementia? *J Am Geriatr Soc* 1996;44:865-870.
42. Niki E, Nakano M. Estrogens as antioxidants. *Methods Enzymol* 1990;186:330-333.
43. McGeer PL, et al. Arthritis and anti-inflammatory agents as possible protective factors for Alzheimer's disease: A review of 17 epidemiologic studies. *Neurology* 1996;47:425-432.
44. Rozzini R, et al. Protective effect of chronic NSAID use on cognitive decline in older persons. *J Am Geriatr Soc* 1996; 44:1025-1029.
45. Stewart WF, et al. Risk of Alzheimer's disease and duration of NSAID use. *Neurology* 1997;48:626-632.
46. Mintzer JE, et al. Behavioral intensive care unit (BICU): A new concept in the management of acute agitated behavior in elderly demented patients. *Gerontologist* 1993;33: 801-806.
47. Teri L, Uomoto J. Reducing excess disability in dementia patients: Training caregivers to manage patient depression. *Clin Gerontol* 1991;10:49-63.
48. Teri L, et al. Treatment of depression in dementia patients: A controlled clinical trial. *J Gerontol B Psychol Sci Soc Sci* 1997;52:159-166.
49. Patterson MB, Bolger JP. Assessment of behavioral symptoms in Alzheimer disease. *Alzheimer Dis Assoc Disord* 1994;8(suppl 3):4-20.
50. *Alzheimer's Disease: Statistics*. Chicago, IL: Alzheimer's Disease and Related Disorders Assoc. Inc.; September 1996; IRS 230Z.
51. *Who Cares? Families Caring for Persons with Alzheimer's Disease*. Washington, DC: Alzheimer's Association and the National Alliance for Caregiving; February 1999.
52. Geroge LK, Gwyther LP. Caregiver well-being: A multidimensional examination of family caregivers of demented adults. *Gerontologist* 1986;26:253-259.
53. Mittleman MS, et al. A family intervention to delay nursing home placement of patients with Alzheimer disease. *JAMA* 1996;276:1725-1731.
54. Glosser G, et al. Physicians' and families' perspectives on the medical management of dementia. *J Am Geriatr Soc* 1985;33:383-391.
55. Fortinsky RH, et al. Primary care physicians' diagnostic, management, and referral practices for older persons and families affected by dementia. *Research on Aging* 1995; 17:124-148.
56. Fortinsky RH. How linked are physicians to community support services for their patients with dementia? *J App Gerontol* 1998;17:480-498.

Update on Parkinson's Disease

Jean P. Hubble, MD

There is growing awareness and interest in Parkinson's disease in the medical community and general public. This stems from remarkable achievements in our understanding of this illness and its treatments. Also playing a role is the media attention directed to Parkinson's disease because of public figures who have disclosed their diagnosis. Finally, there is the growing realization that this and other age-related noncurable ailments will constitute a large socioeconomic burden for the foreseeable future.

Clinical Presentation and Diagnosis: Diagnosis

The term "parkinsonism" refers to a symptom complex consisting of two or more of the following: resting tremor, rigidity, or bradykinesia (slowed movement). *(Please see Table 1.)* Whereas parkinsonism can occur as part of various disorders of the central nervous system (CNS), it most commonly takes the form of idiopathic Parkinson's disease. Parkinson's disease is a progressive, disabling condition affecting approximately 1% of the U.S. population older than 60 years of age.

Many conditions can mimic Parkinson's disease. *(Please see Table 2.)* A careful history and thorough neurological examination usually establish the diagnosis. Testing, including blood work and brain imaging, may be warranted in those instances when unusual signs or symptoms exist.

Symptoms of Parkinson's disease usually begin during the sixth decade of life or later. Motor signs and symptoms usually begin on one side of the body and progress to involve the opposite side. Although resting tremor is frequently considered the most obvious feature of Parkinson's disease, its presence does not appear to be essential to the diagnosis. Thus, stiffness and discomfort in a single limb may be the initial presentation. Other early features of the disease may include small shaky handwriting (micrographia); voice changes (loss of volume, stuttering); decrease in facial expression; stooped posture; and slowed, shuffling gait.

Nonmotor Features

Psychological disturbances are common in Parkinson's disease and may include alteration in effect, personality, and cognition. Significant cognitive impairment (dementia) can occur, particularly in aged patients or in patients with advanced disease. Depression also is common. Other nonmotor features may include sensory disturbances, loss of the sense of smell, skin changes, and autonomic dysfunction (constipation, sweat abnormalities, and orthostatic hypotension).

Table 1. Clinical Features of Parkinsonism

- Resting (or postural) tremor
- Rigidity
- Bradykinesia (slowed movement)

Pharmacotherapy: Levodopa

Levodopa often is called the "gold standard" of the treatment of Parkinson's disease because it typically produces a prompt and dramatic alleviation of motor signs and symptoms. A total absence of response to levodopa at high doses (e.g., 1000-2000 mg of levodopa per day given in conjunction with carbidopa) argues against the diagnosis of Parkinson's disease. Not all the signs and symptoms of Parkinson's disease respond equally to levodopa. Rigidity and bradykinesia tend to respond best. Tremor is variably affected. It is usually suggested that levodopa therapy be started when the illness is clearly resulting in disability or limitations in the individual's day-to-day functioning. Most of the symptoms of Parkinson's disease are due to the dopamine depletion within the striatum of the brain. Dopamine is not an effective oral remedy for Parkinson's disease as it is not well absorbed in the gut and it does not readily enter the brain from the bloodstream. Levodopa is a precursor to dopamine. The therapeutic effect of levodopa depends upon its passage from the bloodstream into the brain, where it is decarboxylated into dopamine and exerts its symptomatic benefit in Parkinson's disease.

Acute side effects from levodopa constituted a major problem when the drug was first introduced in the late 1960s. *(Please see Table 3.)* Large amounts of levodopa (6-8 g/d) were required to achieve a good response (i.e., improved mobility). These high doses were needed because more than 90% of orally administered levodopa is systemically metabolized before it can reach the brain. Metabolized levodopa is wasted and has no therapeutic benefit in Parkinson's disease. The aromatic amino acid decarboxylase pathway is the major peripheral levodopa metabolic pathway, resulting in accumulation of systemically circulating dopamine. The systemic side effects of dopamine can include incapacitating nausea and vomiting and orthostatic hypotension. Decarboxylase inhibiting drugs are coadministered with levodopa in order to limit systemic metabolism and peripheral dopaminergic side effects. Carbidopa is the decarboxylase inhibitor available in the United States. The addition of carbidopa to each dose of levodopa permits more levodopa to enter the brain and usually prevents side effects such as nausea. Virtually all levodopa prescribed in the United States is given in a tablet form that contains levodopa and carbidopa. Various doses of carbidopa/levodopa are available in both brand name and generic products. Two common brand names for carbidopa/levodopa are Sinemet and Atamet.

Other potential side effects of levodopa include hallucinations and psychosis. These reactions are more common in patients of advanced age and those with underlying cognitive impairment. Visual hallucinations are the most common form of levodopa-induced hallucinations. These hallucinations frequently consist of nonthreatening people or animals; insight initially may be retained.

Table 2. Differential Diagnosis of Parkinsonism and Tremor

Idiopathic, Typical Parkinson's Disease

- Rest tremor is common
- Begins with asymmetric limb involvement
- Responds to levodopa (and related) drugs

Atypical Parkinsonism

- Example: progressive supranuclear palsy
- Advances more quickly
- Truncal rigidity, falling, and other neurological symptoms are common
- Fails to respond to levodopa (and related) drugs

Secondary Parkinsonism

- Symptoms are attributable to a specific cause
- A common cause is chronic exposure to dopamine-blocking drugs (e.g., haloperidol)
- Symptoms will usually resolve if the precipitating cause can be remedied (e.g., discontinuation of the offending drug)

Essential Tremor

- Most common form of tremor
- Muscle rigidity and bradykinesia are absent
- Family history is often positive
- Often responds to ethanol
- Tremor is usually accentuated with sustained posture (e.g., outstretched arms)

Such hallucinations may signal incipient psychosis. Lowering the dosage of levodopa can be tried but is often a problem because it results in a decline in motor function. Another approach to the treatment of levodopa-induced hallucinations is the use of antipsychotic medications. Because these antipsychotic agents block dopamine receptors in the brain, some will cause worsening of the motor features of Parkinson's disease. More recently, the antipsychotic compound clozapine has been successfully used for levodopa-induced psychosis.[1] This drug does not worsen Parkinson's disease symptoms, but frequent blood counts are needed because of a rare blood disorder (agranulocytosis) associated with its use. Newer antipsychotic drugs (e.g., quetiapine) may also be used to safely control drug-induced psychosis in Parkinson's disease.

The most frequent and troublesome problem associated with levodopa use is motor fluctuations. Response to levodopa is usually stable for the first several years. Thereafter, the length of benefit from a single dose tends to decline ("wearing off"), peak-dose dyskinesia (involuntary wiggly movements) may occur, and overall predictable efficacy lessens. Patients' motor status may wax and wane throughout the day in relation to their levodopa dosing. Some patients may have random, abrupt motor fluctuations termed *on-off phenomena*. Levodopa can be given in multiple small doses in an attempt to alleviate fluctuations. However, smaller doses may not control symptoms, and larger total daily levodopa dose may result in side effects. Alternative strategies include switching to controlled-release carbidopa/levodopa or adding adjunctive drugs, as described below.

Carbidopa/Levodopa Preparations

To minimize peripheral side effects and enhance penetration into the brain, levodopa is usually administered with carbidopa, an enzyme decarboxylase inhibitor. Available formulations of carbidopa/levodopa denote the amount of carbidopa (mg) in the numerator and the amount of levodopa (mg) in the denominator as follows: standard formulation 10/100, 25/100, 25/250, and controlled release 25/100, 50/200. A reasonable starting dosage of standard formulation carbidopa/levodopa is one 25/100 tablet taken three times per day. The medicine is usually best given during the daytime, and it should be taken without food when possible (30 minutes before or 1 hour after meals). The drug dosage and timing of administration can be adjusted based on efficacy and side effects. Additional carbidopa (Lodosyn) can be given in conjunction with carbidopa/ levodopa if nausea is a dose-limiting side effect.

Controlled-Release Carbidopa/Levodopa

Controlled-release carbidopa/levodopa can be used to attempt to control motor fluctuations.[2] This formulation provides longer duration levodopa blood levels and may reduce motor fluctuations. Less frequent dosing of the controlled-release levodopa is needed, as compared with the conventional standard formulation (reduction in the number of doses by one-third to one-half). Because of altered bioavailability, a greater total amount of daily levodopa may need to be given in the form of controlled-release carbidopa/levodopa.

The slower onset of clinical effect of controlled-release carbidopa/levodopa may actually be experienced as disadvantageous by some individuals (i.e., patients may prefer the brisk and more pronounced effects of the standard formulation particularly when first arising in the morning). In these instances, additional standard formulation carbidopa/levodopa can be given along with the controlled-release tablets to provide a more rapid onset of therapeutic effect.

In addition to its role in treatment of advancing Parkinson's disease, controlled-release carbidopa/levodopa can be used when levodopa therapy is first instituted—1-2 tablets daily may be sufficient. Early initiation of controlled-release carbidopa/levodopa does not seem to delay onset of motor fluctuations.[3] As with all antiparkinsonian drugs, successful use of the controlled release carbidopa/ levodopa requires careful adjustment of dose depending on the patient's clinical status and levodopa tolerance.

Table 3. Possible Side Effects of Levodopa

- Nausea/vomiting
- Sedation
- Hallucinations, psychosis
- Dyskinesia (involuntary wiggly movements)
- Nonsustained or unpredictable response (motor fluctuations)

Dopamine Receptor Agonists

Dopamine agonists can provide symptomatic relief in Parkinson's disease. *(Please see Table 4.)* The drugs act independently of levodopa by directly activating dopamine receptors.[4] Bromocriptine (Parlodel) and pergolide (Permax) are ergoline compounds that have been available for use in Parkinson's disease for several years.[5] These two compounds have been most widely tested and used as adjunctive therapies along with levodopa in patients with more advanced disease and motor fluctuations.

Two newer dopamine agonists are now available in the United States.[6-9] These compounds, pramipexole (Mirapex) and ropinirole (Requip), received approval from the Food & Drug Administration in the United States for use in both early and advanced Parkinson's disease. In clinical trials, approximately 30-40% of patients with mild to moderate disease have received sufficient benefit from pramipexole or ropinirole so as to be able to postpone levodopa therapy for up to three or more years. The dopamine agonist ropinirole has been compared to carbidopa/levodopa in a five-year, double-blind study.[10] By the end of the study, about two-thirds of the subjects assigned to the ropinirole group also were receiving open-label supplemental carbidopa/levodopa because of progression of motor symptoms. Dyskinesias (a form of motor fluctuations) developed in nearly one-half of those assigned to start with carbidopa/levodopa therapy but in only 20% of those initially assigned to the ropinirole group. Thus, the relative early use of dopamine agonists can postpone initiation of levodopa therapy and therefore may delay the onset of levodopa complications.

All the dopamine agonists currently available in the United States have been approved for use in more advanced Parkinson's disease as adjunctive therapy used along with levodopa. Large-scale, controlled comparison studies of the dopamine agonists are lacking. There is no clear evidence to suggest that one drug is more effective or safer than the other drug. Potential side effects of dopamine agonists include: nausea, vomiting, hallucinations, sedation, insomnia, worsening of dyskinesia, and low blood pressure. Rarely has this class of drugs been associated with fibrosis or scarring of the membranous lining of internal organs or body cavities (e.g., pleural fibrosis).

Successful use of these drugs depends upon the introduction of a small dose, with incremental dose escalation every 4-7 days. Dose escalation schedules are provided by the drugs' manufacturers. Based on clinical experience, target dosing ranges are provided:

Table 4. Dopamine Agonists Used to Treat Parkinson's Disease

- Bromocriptine (Parlodel)
- Pergolide (Permax)
- Pramipexole (Mirapex)
- Ropinirole (Requip)

bromocriptine: 2.5-5.0 mg t.i.d. (or more frequently); pergolide 0.25-1.0 mg t.i.d.; pramipexole: 0.5-1.5 mg t.i.d.; ropinirole: 3-8 mg t.i.d. There is growing use of this class of drug as monotherapy in relatively early Parkinson's disease in an effort to postpone the introduction of levodopa with the hope of postponing levodopa complications such as motor fluctuations.[11]

Selegiline

Selegiline blocks a brain chemical called monoamine oxidase type B. Selegiline, when used at the recommended dose (10 mg daily), does not react with red wine and smoked meats and cheeses. No dietary restrictions are required with selegiline, which is in contrast to the older types of monoamine oxidase inhibitors used to treat depression. Selegiline's effects in the brain are complex; thus, its potential effects in Parkinson's disease may be multiple. Selegiline provides modest symptomatic relief and is approved as an adjunctive therapy with levodopa in patients with moderate to advanced disease.[12] In addition, clinical trials with selegiline in early untreated Parkinson's disease indicate that its use permits postponement of levodopa therapy; thus, it can be considered as monotherapy for early disease.[13]

For patients who are untreated or who are taking small doses of levodopa, selegiline therapy can usually begin at 5 mg twice daily at breakfast and lunch. Dosing late in the day is best avoided because it can produce or worsen insomnia. Other potential adverse effects include headache, confusion, hallucinations, dizziness, exacerbation of peptic ulcer disease, dyskinesia, nausea, and postural hypotension. Some of these side effects may be more common when given in conjunction with other antiparkinsonian medications. Similar to other monoamine oxidase inhibitors, selegiline can produce serious adverse reactions when taken with the pain reliever meperidine (Demerol). Selegiline should be used cautiously, if at all, with antidepressant drugs because of the potential for drug-drug interactions.

Other Therapies

Amantadine and anticholinergic drugs also can provide relief of symptoms for some patients with Parkinson's disease.[14] The efficacy of these drugs is usually modest compared with that of levodopa. The drugs typically may be given as adjunctive therapy with levodopa or as monotherapy to patients who are intolerant of other drugs or who have mild early disease. Anticholinergic drugs are reputed to be especially useful in reducing tremor while amantadine has recently been demonstrated to have antidyskinetic effects.[15]

Table 5. COMT Inhibition as an Augment to Levodopa Therapy

- Extends the duration of action of each dose of levodopa
- May cause levodopa-related side effects
- May cause harmless urine discoloration
- Entacapone (Comtan): 200 mg with levodopa dose (maximum of 8 tablets per day)
- Tolcapone (Tasmar): see revised manufacturer's labeling due to potential hepatotoxicity

Not all of the clinical problems associated with Parkinson's disease can be remedied with antiparkinsonian medications. Urinary difficulties, constipation, hypotension, skin disorders, anxiety, and depression are examples of nonmotor manifestations that may occur. Medications directly targeting these symptoms can be used (e.g., antidepressants can be prescribed). No specific antidepressant has been demonstrated to be uniquely safe and effective for depression in Parkinson's disease.[16] Other nonpharmacologic therapies can often be of help, especially for more advanced cases. These include physical, occupational, and speech therapy. The home can be outfitted with safety equipment (e.g., handrails, elevated toilet seat) as needed.

The nonambulatory patient with advanced Parkinson's disease is susceptible to all of the medical complications associated with immobility, including pneumonia, urosepsis, and venous thrombosis with pulmonary embolization. The ongoing care of such patients is complex and usually requires the assistance of a general medical practitioner. Availing the patient and family of social assistance may also be valuable in advanced cases. Lay support groups can serve as a remarkable resource throughout all stages of the illness. Such organizations are able to provide educational materials, plan social meetings, offer caregiver support and respite, develop exercise programs, and sponsor research activities.

COMT Inhibition

The catechol-*O*-methyl transferase (COMT) inhibitors comprise a novel class of drugs recently introduced for the treatment of Parkinson's disease. *(Please see Table 5.)* These drugs reduce the systematic metabolism of levodopa, thereby extending the duration of benefit of orally administered carbidopa/levodopa. The COMT inhibitors are adjunctive drugs exerting no clinical effect when used alone. COMT inhibitor drugs can precipitate or worsen levodopa-related side effects such as dyskinesia or hallucinations. Such side effects can usually be managed by reducing the dose of levodopa. These compounds can cause a harmless reddish-brown urine discoloration.

Entacapone (Comtan) has recently been approved for use in the United States. Entacapone is indicated for the treatment of "wearing off" experienced at the end of carbidopa/levodopa dosing.[17-18] Patients with "wearing off" may find that the therapeutic effects of a dose of carbidopa/levodopa lasts only 1-3 hours and then tremor, slowness, and poor mobility re-emerge. Studies have shown that the addition of entacapone can provide 1-1½ hours of improved mobility per day in such patients. Suggested dosing for entacapone is 200 mg tablets: one tablet with each dose of carbidopa/levodopa for a maximum of eight tablets per day.

Tolcapone (Tasmar) is also a COMT inhibitor.[19] It has a longer half-life compared to entacapone. Tolcapone has been associated with diarrhea, elevated liver function tests, and potential hepatotoxicity (liver damage). Frequent liver function blood test monitoring is recommended with the use of tolcapone. Because of the risk of hepatotoxicity, tolcapone is now recommended only for patients with motor fluctuations who are not candidates for other therapies. Prescribing physicians need to be fully aware of these safety issues. Patients need to be informed of potential risks and a written consent document is recommended. Suggested dosing of tolcapone is 100 or 200 mg three times daily at approximate six-hour intervals.

Surgeries for Parkinson's Disease

There are both conventional and investigational surgical treatment options for Parkinson's disease. Pallidotomy is an established stereotactic neurosurgical procedure that involves selective destruction of a part of the globus pallidus of the brain.[20-21] Although the surgery is not considered experimental, some issues regarding its use remain uncertain. Results published to date suggest that the procedure is most helpful in reducing levodopa-induced dyskinesia but its beneficial effects on other features of Parkinson's disease may be less dramatic. Experience regarding the long-term effects of pallidotomy is limited. Proper patient selection appears important. Some patients, including the aged or those with dementia, may be at higher risk for poor outcome and complications.

Deep brain stimulation (DBS) is a novel therapy for the treatment of Parkinson's disease. DBS involves the stereotactic implantation of an electrical lead within the brain; high-frequency stimulation is then delivered to the targeted brain region with the use of an implanted pulse generator analogous to a cardiac pacer device. The ventral intermediate nucleus of the thalamus is targeted to provide tremor control in Parkinson's disease and other tremor disorders.[22-23] Alternatively, the stimulator lead tip can be implanted in the globus pallidus or subthalamic nucleus to alleviate other features of Parkinson's disease, including rigidity, bradykinesia, tremor, and drug-induced dyskinesia.[24-25] Thus, thalamic DBS is analogous in its effect to the older lesion thalamotomy, whereas pallidal or subthalamic DBS is analogous to pallidotomy. The putative advantages of DBS over lesion surgery include its nondestructive nature and the capability to adjust stimulation parameters, thereby improving symptomatic benefit or lessening side effects postoperatively. Thalamic DBS for disabling parkinsonian tremor has been approved for use in the United States under the brand name Activa Tremor Control Therapy. Other uses of DBS are being developed.

Investigational Therapies

Other investigational therapies for Parkinson's disease that require surgical intervention include brain cell transplantation and direct instillation of neurotrophic factor in the brain.[26-27] Also under study are antiparkinsonian compounds that can be administered by skin patch, injection, or via rapidly dissolving tablets on or under the tongue. New types of drugs that differ from the mechanism of action of levodopa and related dopaminergic compounds are being tested. It is hoped that these new strategies may offer the means to halt or delay this degenerative disease.

References

1. Friedman JH, Lannon MC. Clozapine in the treatment of psychosis in Parkinson's disease. *Neurology* 1989;39: 1219-1221.
2. Cedarbaum JM, Hoey M, McDowell FH. A double-blind crossover comparison of Sinemet CR4 and standard Sinemet 25/100 in patients with Parkinson's disease and fluctuating motor performance. *J Neurol Neurosurg Psychiatry* 1989; 52:207-212.
3. Block G, Liss C, Reines S, Irr J, Nibbelink D. The CR First Study Group. Comparison of immediate-release and controlled release carbidopa/levodopa in Parkinson's disease. A multicenter 5-year study. *Eur Neurol* 1997;37:23-27.
4. Jenner P. The rationale for the use of dopamine agonists in Parkinson's disease. *Neurology* 1995;45(suppl):S6-S12.
5. Goetz CG, Shannon KM, Tanner CM, et al. Agonist substitution in advanced Parkinson's disease. *Neurology* 1989;39:1121-1122.
6. Adler CH, Sethi KD, Hauser RA, et al. Ropinirole for the treatment of early Parkinson's disease. *Neurology* 1997; 49:393-399.
7. Brooks DJ, Torjanski N, Burn DJ. Ropinirole in the symptomatic treatment of Parkinson's disease. *J Neural Transm Suppl* 1995;45:231-238.
8. Hubble JP, Koller WC, Cutler NR, et al. Pramipexole in patients with early Parkinson's disease. *Clin Neuropharmacol* 1995;18:338-347.
9. Shannon KM, Bennett JP Jr, Freidman JH. The Pramipexole Study Group. Efficacy of pramipexole, a novel dopamine agonist, as monotherapy in mild to moderate Parkinson's disease. *Neurology* 1997;49:724-728.
10. Rascol O, Brooks DJ, Korczyn AD, et al. A five-year study of the incidence of dyskinesia in patients with early Parkinson's disease who were treated with ropinirole or levodopa. *N Engl J Med* 2000;342:1484-1491.
11. Olanow CW, Koller WC. An algorithm (decision tree) for the management of Parkinson's disease: Treatment guidelines. *Neurology* 1998;50(suppl 3):S1-S57.
12. Gollbe LI. Long-term efficacy and safety of deprenyl (selegiline) in advanced Parkinson's disease. *Neurology* 1989;39:1109-1111.
13. The Parkinson Study Group. Effects of tocopherol and deprenyl on the progression of disability in early Parkinson's disease. *N Engl J Med* 1993;328:176-183.
14. Jabbari B, Scherokman B, Gunderson CH, et al. Treatment of movement disorders with trihexyphenidyl. *Mov Disord* 1989;4:202-212.
15. Verhagen Metman L, Del Dotto P, van den Munckhof P, et al. Amantadine as treatment for dyskinesias and motor

fluctations in Parkinson's disease. *Neurology* 1998;50: 1323-1326.

16. Tom T, Cummings JL. Depression in Parkinson's disease: Pharmacological characteristics and treatment. *Drugs Aging* 1998;12:55-74.
17. The Parkinson's Study Group. Entacapone improves motor fluctuations in levodopa-treated Parkinson's disease patients. *Ann Neurol* 1997;42:747-755.
18. Rinne UK, Larsen JP, Siden A, et al. Entacapone enhances the response to levodopa in parkinsonian patients with motor fluctuations. *Neurology* 1998;51:1309-1314.
19. Adler CH, Singer C, O'Brien C, et al. Randomized, placebo-controlled study of tolcapone in patients with fluctuating Parkinson disease treated with levodopa-carbidopa. Tolcapone Fluctuator Study Group III. *Arch Neurol* 1998; 55:1089-1095.
20. Baron MS, Vitek JL, Bakay RA, et al. Treatment of advanced Parkinson's disease by posterior GPi pallidotomy: 1-year results of a pilot study. *Ann Neurol* 1996;40:355-366.
21. Laitinen LV, Bergenheim AT, Hariz MI. Leksell's posteroventral pallidotomy in the treatment of Parkinson's disease. *J Neurosurg* 1992;76:53-61.
22. Hubble JP, Busenbark KL, Wilkinson S, et al. Effects of thalamic deep brain stimulation based on tremor type and diagnosis. *Mov Disord* 1997; 12:337-341.
23. Koller W, Pahwa R, Busenbark K, et al. High-frequency unilateral thalamic stimulation-treatment of essential and parkinsonian tremor. *Ann Neurol* 1997;42:292-299.
24. Pahwa R, Wilkinson S, Smith D, et al. High-frequency stimulation of the globus pallidus for the treatment of Parkinson's disease. *Neurology* 1997;49:249-253.
25. Limousin P, Pollak P, Benazzouz A, et al. Effect of parkinsonian signs and symptoms of bilateral subthalamic nucleus stimulation. *Lancet* 1995;345:91-95.
26. Fahn S. Fetal-tissue transplants in Parkinson's disease. *N Engl J Med* 1992;327:1589-1590.
27. Lindvall O. Neural transplantation: A hope for patients with Parkinson's disease. *Neuroreport* 1997;8:iii-x.

Obstructive Sleep Apnea Syndrome

Steven M. Koenig, MD, FCCP

The classic example of a disorder due to abnormal breathing during sleep is the obstructive sleep apnea (OSA) syndrome. Classically, the OSA syndrome is characterized by repetitive episodes of complete or partial upper airway obstruction during sleep, which results in significant physiologic consequences such as sleep disruption and oxyhemoglobin desaturation. Once thought to be an uncommon disorder, a recent community-based study estimated that 2-4% of randomly chosen middle-age working adults have this condition.[1] Evidence indicates OSA syndrome is associated with an increased rate of automobile and work-related accidents. OSA syndrome also has been associated with an increased prevalence of hypertension, coronary artery disease (CAD), cerebrovascular accidents, and increased mortality.

The purpose of this chapter is to outline the clinically relevant underlying pathophysiology, presenting symptoms, and signs, diagnosis, and treatment of OSA syndrome. Because OSA is clearly a major public health problem, and because many cases are often unsuspected, it is essential that primary care physicians as well as the public at large become more aware of the clinical presentation of this common disorder.

Pathogenesis

Narrowing of the human pharynx or upper airway and the resultant elevated upper airway resistance are responsible for all the consequences associated with OSA syndrome. Therefore, individuals with this condition must have some abnormality or abnormalities of the determinants of the caliber of their upper airway. These determinants include the baseline pharyngeal area, which is determined by both craniofacial (bony) and soft tissue structures (i.e., fat around the airway), the collapsibility of the airway, the pressures inside the airway and in the tissues surrounding the pharyngeal wall, the outward pressure exerted by pharyngeal dilating muscles, the shape of the upper airway, and lung volume. Disorders that predispose to the development of OSA do so by influencing one or more of these determinants of upper airway size. Such predisposing conditions include anatomic abnormalities such as retrognathia; obesity; hypothyroidism; acromegaly; neuromuscular disorders; alcohol; sedative-hypnotics; nasal congestion; the supine position; and sleep deprivation. Such predisposing factors should be looked for in all patients suspected of having OSA syndrome.[2]

Physiologic Consequences

The physiologic consequences of OSA syndrome can be divided into two categories—those due to arousal from sleep, and that secondary to oxyhemoglobin desaturation and hypercapnia. *(Please see Tables 1 and 2.)* Daytime sleepiness and visual motor incoordination are the presumed cause of the increased rate of automobile and work-related accidents in patients with OSA compared with the

Table 1. Consequences of Arousal from Sleep

- Sleep fragmentation
  - — Excessive daytime sleepiness
  - — Personality changes
  - — Intellectual deterioration
  - — Visual-motor incoordination
  - — Impotence
- Insomnia
- Restlessness
- Choking, gagging, gasping, resuscitative snorting

Table 2. Consequences of Nocturnal Hypoxia/Hypercapnia

- Polycythemia
- Pulmonary hypertension
- Cor pulmonale
- Chronic hypercapnia
- Morning and nocturnal headache
- Left-sided congestive heart failure
- Cardiac dysrhythmias
- Nocturnal angina
- Diurnal systemic hypertension

general population.[3] Unrecognized sleep apnea occurs in approximately 20-30% of hypertensive patients in the United States.[4] OSA syndrome is also associated with increased prevalence of CAD and cerebral vascular accidents as well as excess mortality.[5-7] Because current morbidity and mortality data are based on retrospective studies, the true effect of sleep disordered breathing on society remains unknown. A randomized trial is clearly required and, in fact, is presently ongoing.

Definitions

An apnea is defined as the complete or near complete cessation of airflow that lasts for at least 10 seconds.[8] A hypopnea is defined as a 50% or higher decrease in airflow or less than a 50% decrease with either an oxyhemoglobin desaturation of 3% or more or an arousal from sleep lasting at least 10 seconds.[8] Both abnormal breathing events are associated with similar sequelae and are treated in the same manner. They often occur together in the same patient.

Apneas and hypopneas are further divided into obstructive, central, and mixed. They are considered obstructive if there is continued or increasing respiratory efforts despite absent or diminished airflow, and central if there is absent respiratory effort. An event is labeled mixed if it begins as a central apnea or hypopnea and is terminated by an obstructive event. *(Please see Figure 1.)*

The upper airway resistance syndrome (UARS) is a newly described syndrome in which upper airway narrowing alone, without an associated apnea, hypopnea, or oxyhemoglobin desaturation, causes arousal from sleep.[9] These repetitive episodes of upper airway narrowing and consequent arousals lead to excessive daytime sleepiness (EDS) or tiredness. Since both obstructive hypopneas and increased upper airway resistance alone can have profound physiological consequences, the term OSA is not, strictly speaking, applicable to the entire spectrum of sleep-disordered breathing. It is best reserved for those individuals with the most severe form of the disease. The term obstructive sleep-disordered breathing (OSDB) syndrome better describes the entire spectrum of obstructive breathing abnormalities during sleep. On one end of the continuum of upper airway narrowing and consequent increased upper airway resistance is primary, asymptomatic snoring. This is followed by the UARS, then the obstructive sleep hypopnea syndrome, and finally by the OSA syndrome *(Please see Figure 2.)*

Indicators of the severity of OSDB syndrome include the apnea index, which is the number of apneas per hour of sleep, the hypopnea index, which is the number of hypopneas per hour of sleep, the respiratory disturbance index (RDI), which is the number of apneas plus hypopneas per hour of sleep and the oxyhemoglobin desaturation index, which is the number of oxyhemoglobin desaturation episodes 3-4% or more per hour.

Diagnosis

The possibility of sleep disordered breathing should be *considered* in any patient with *any* of the predisposing factors, signs, or symptoms mentioned above. *(Please see Tables 1 and 2.)* Talking with the bed partner, family members, friends, or fellow employees can be helpful, as they will often notice signs such as apneas or falling asleep unintentionally that the patient may be unaware of or deny. The next step is to estimate a clinical likelihood or pretest probability of sleep disordered breathing based on a focused history and physical examination. This evaluation should include searching for alternative explanations for symptoms such as insufficient sleep or shift work causing EDS. *(Please see Table 3.)* Although commonly reported, the following symptoms of EDS do not distinguish sleep apnea from other nonpulmonary sleep disorders: unrefreshing or nonrestorative sleep, morning headaches, cognitive impairment, depression, nocturnal esophageal reflux, nocturia or enuresis, hearing loss, automatic behavior, sleep drunkenness (disorientation, confusion upon awakening), hypnagogic hallucinations and night sweats.

In any patient presenting with a complaint of daytime sleepiness, the degree of sleepiness should be quantitated. The sleepier the individual, the more likely he has sleep disordered breathing or some other significant disorder, and the more severe the condition, the latter influencing treatment. A reasonable approach is to divide sleepiness into mild, moderate, and severe, based on the frequency of sleep episodes, the degree of impairment of social and occupational function, and in what situations sleep episodes occur. With *mild* sleepiness, sleep episodes are infrequent, may not occur every day, and occur at times of rest or when little attention is required, such as while watching TV, reading, or traveling as a passenger.

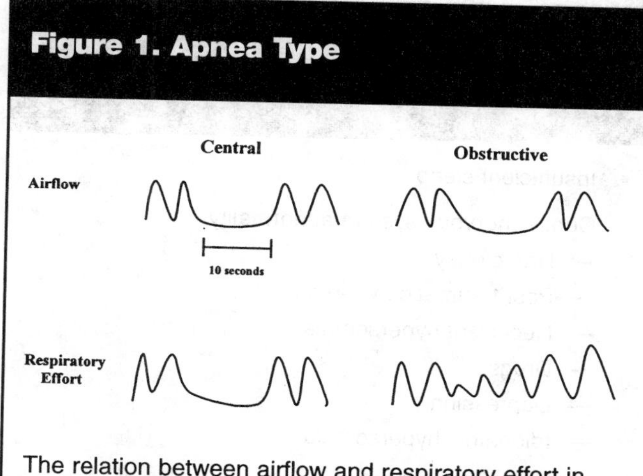

The relation between airflow and respiratory effort in central and obstructive apnea. During a central apnea there is cessation of airflow for at least 10 seconds with no associated respiratory effort. An obstructive apnea is defined as a similar cessation of airflow but with continued respiratory effort.

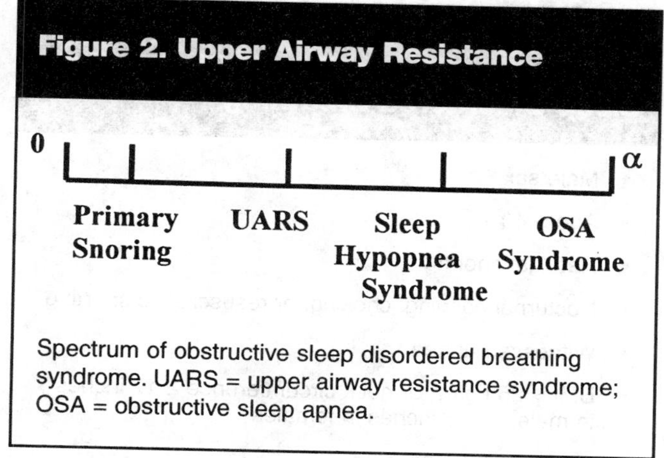

Spectrum of obstructive sleep disordered breathing syndrome. UARS = upper airway resistance syndrome; OSA = obstructive sleep apnea.

Sleepiness is considered *severe* when it is present daily, and when sleep episodes occur even during activities requiring sustained attention such as eating, conversation, walking, and driving. *Moderate* sleepiness lies somewhere in between these extremes. It is important to remember that daytime sleepiness is underreported.[10,11] Fatigue may be the only symptom. Thus, the absence of sleepiness cannot be used to reliably exclude OSA. In addition, sleep disordered breathing is not the only cause of EDS. *(Please see Table 4.)* That is, EDS is not specific for sleep disordered breathing either.

Those physical examination findings that significantly increase the likelihood of sleep disordered breathing are listed in Table 3. Other features that should be searched for include craniofacial and upper airway abnormalities, such as retrognathia, tonsillar hypertrophy (especially in children), and an enlarged soft palate. The size and consistency of the tongue; presence of pharyngeal edema or abnormal reddish coloring of the pharynx; appearance of the soft palate; size, length, and position of the uvula; and evidence of trauma. Nares, including whether they collapse with inspiration, particularly while the patient is supine, should also be noted.

Unfortunately, subjective impression alone, based on history and physical examination, lacks both sensitivity (52-78%) as well as specificity (50-79%).[12-15] Although plugging clinical variables into regression formulas improves these operating characteristics somewhat (sensitivity [79-92%], specificity [50-51%]), many involve complicated mathematical formulas, which limits their usefulness.[13,15,16] Moreover, even if the clinical likelihood is low, the post-test probability for OSA, defined as a respiratory disturbance index (RDI) greater than 10, still varies between 16% and 21%.[13,16,17] In addition, patients with symptoms secondary to UARS would have been missed in these studies, decreasing the sensitivity of clinical assessment even further. Whether a post-test probability for OSA of 16-21% is low enough will depend on the threshold at which a physician is willing to accept diagnostic uncertainty. The threshold for pursuing further diagnostic testing should be lower in patients with severe daytime sleepiness, comorbid illnesses such as CAD, a driving accident record, and certain occupations (i.e., school bus driver).

If further diagnostic testing is deemed necessary, options include a formal sleep study or polysomnogram (PSG) and a variety of portable monitoring systems. The gold standard for diagnosing OSA syndrome is a PSG. Variables typically recorded include the following: electroencephalogram (EEG), electrooculogram (EOG), and submental electromyogram (EMG) to stage sleep; airflow and respiratory effort to detect and diagnose hypoventilation or the type of apnea or hypopnea; oxygen saturation; electrocardiogram (ECG); and tibialis anterior EMG to detect periodic leg movements, a cause of excessive daytime sleepiness. To decrease the cost of PSG and facilitate treatment, a split night study can be performed. With a split night study, the initial portion of the evening is spent determining whether sleep disordered breathing is present. If sleep disordered breathing is documented, the remainder of the night is spent finding and titrating the most effective treatment.

Because of the cost and frequent unavailability of PSG, investigators have sought less expensive alternatives to formal sleep studies performed in sleep laboratories. These portable recording devices differ in the number and types of parameters measured, varying from pulse oximetry alone to all those variables measured in the sleep laboratory. Each is associated with its own advantages as well as disadvantages. Advantages of these portable systems include lower cost, greater availability, and ability to perform in the patient's home. Of those devices that have been studied and the results published in peer reviewed journals, their sensitivities vary from 78% to 100%, and their specificity varies from 67% to 100%, depending on the particular system, the number of variables monitored, and the definition of sleep apnea.[18]

The major disadvantage of portable systems and pulse oximetry is the possibility of false-negative results. The likelihood of a false-negative study depends on the number of variables monitored and is due to not staging sleep, observing body position, or detecting UARS. In addition, these systems cannot diagnose other etiologies of excessive sleepiness such as periodic leg movements and narcolepsy. Finally, even if these portable systems were 100% specific, a formal PSG is still required if significant sleep disordered breathing is documented. The optimum nasal continuous positive airway pressure (CPAP) must be determined and, at least at the present time, this is done primarily in a sleep laboratory. However, with the advent of self-titrating or Auto-CPAP devices, some of which have the capability to diagnose sleep disordered breathing as well as ini-

Table 3. Features Most Useful for Determining Probability of Obstructive Sleep-Disordered Breathing

- Male sex
- Age > 40
- Habitual snoring
- Nocturnal gasping, choking, or resuscitative snorting
- Witnessed apnea
- BMI > 25 kg/m^2 or neck circumference ≥ 17 inches in males, ≥ 16 inches in females
- Systemic hypertension

tiate treatment, this situation may soon change. A recent study comparing the cost-utility of treating OSA syndrome based on polysomnography, home testing, and bedside diagnosis concluded that polysomnography was superior.[19]

At the present time, the following is the approach the author of this piece uses to determine the presence of OSDB *(please see Figure 3)*: 1) Consider the diagnosis of sleep disordered breathing in anyone with any predisposing factor, sign, or symptom consistent with the diagnosis; 2) Estimate a clinical likelihood or pretest probability based on the number and predictive value of the patient's signs and symptoms and predisposing factors, as well as the presence of alternative explanations (i.e., insufficient sleep or shift work as the cause of their daytime sleepiness); 3) Take into account the potential consequences of missing the diagnosis. That is, have a lower threshold for pursuing the diagnosis in a school bus driver, someone who has already had an auto accident, or someone with underlying CAD. A Multiple Sleep Latency Test (MSLT) consists of a series of four or five opportunities to sleep administered at two-hour intervals using standard procedures. Sleepiness is measured as the speed of falling asleep (sleep latency); the presence of rapid eye movement (REM) sleep is also noted. An average sleep latency for all naps of less than five minutes is considered severely sleepy; 5-8 minutes moderately sleepy; 8-10 minutes mildly sleepy; and 10 minutes or more normal. The appearance of REM sleep in two or more naps is suggestive of narcolepsy. A positive oximetry study is defined as one with a *pattern* of repetitive, short duration oxyhemoglobin desaturation.[20] No absolute (i.e., ≤ 90%) or relative (i.e., ≥ 3-4%) decrease in oxyhemoglobin saturation is used. With this criteria, the negative predictive value of nocturnal pulse oximetry is good (96.9%), but the positive predictive value is not (61.4%). Consequently, every abnormal oximetry requires follow-up. Finally, for any other constellation of signs or symptoms, perform a split night PSG.

Treatment

The author of this piece uses the following definitions of OSDB syndrome: AI > 20 or RDI ≥ 30 regardless of symptoms; RDI ≥ 5 or number of arousals due to respiratory effort-related arousal > 10 *plus*

Table 4. Differential Diagnosis of Excessive Daytime Sleepiness

- Insufficient sleep
- Central nervous system abnormality
  - — Narcolepsy
  - — Post-traumatic hypersomnia
  - — Recurrent hypersomnia
  - — Drugs
  - — Depression
  - — Idiopathic hypersomnia
- Circadian rhythm disorder
- Sleep fragmentation
  - — Periodic limb movement disorder
  - — Sleep disordered breathing
  - — Medical disorders (i.e., arthritis)
  - — Neurological disorders (i.e., Parkinson's disease)

some physiologic consequence, such as excessive daytime sleepiness, impaired cognition, mood disorder, insomnia, or documented cardiovascular disease such as hypertension, ischemic heart disease, or stroke.[8] Since the optimum therapy for OSDB depends on the severity of disease, the first task is to estimate this severity. *(Please see Table 5.)*

The goals of treatment are the elimination, in all sleep positions and sleep stages, of all evidence of increased upper airway resistance, which includes hypopneas and apneas; an oxyhemoglobin saturation 88-90% or above; no sleep disruption from respiratory effort-related arousals, hypopneas, or apneas; and no snoring. Therapeutic options for sleep disordered breathing can be divided into conservative, medical, and surgical.

Conservative Treatment

Although the importance of avoiding factors that can increase the severity of sleep disordered breathing should be discussed with all patients, if the patient has mild disease and a clear predisposing factor, conservative therapy may be all that is required. Patients should avoid factors that can increase the severity of upper airway resistance such as sleep deprivation, alcohol, and sedative-hypnotic agents. In some individuals, sleep disordered breathing occurs only in the supine position. Training individuals to sleep primarily in the supine position may completely alleviate their sleep disordered breathing, though the long-term effectiveness of this intervention is unclear. One technique is to place one or more tennis balls (or a similar object) in a pocket sewn in the back of a nightshirt or in a sock that is then pinned to the garment. Hopefully in time, the person will be "trained" to sleep in the lateral recumbent position and, therefore, no longer require the tennis ball(s). Some patients may benefit from elevating the head of the bed at a 30-60° angle. The head-up or lateral recumbent position also may benefit the patient who is

Figure 3. Obesity and Sleep-Disordered Breathing

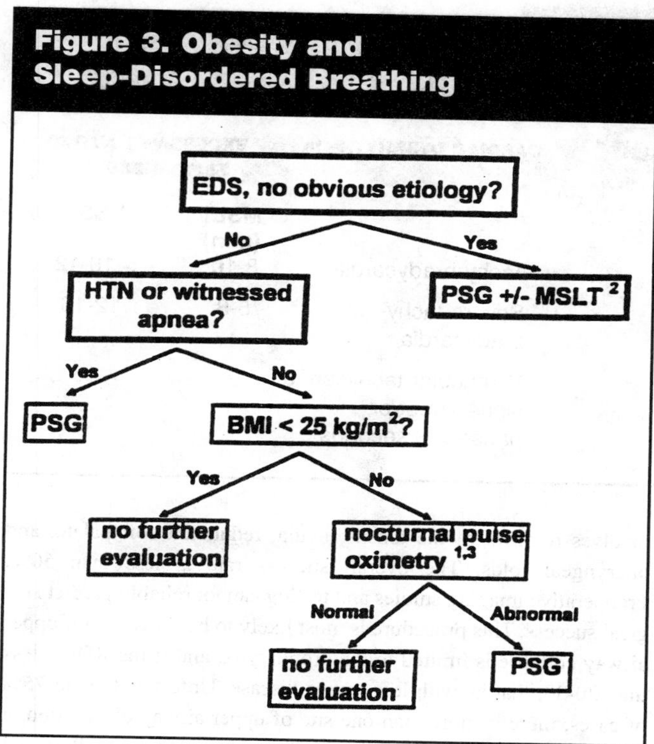

suboptimally treated on maximally tolerable positive-pressure therapy such as CPAP. If present, treatment of increased nasal resistance with a combination of nasal steroids, decongestants, and/or antihistamines should be undertaken. Likewise, hypothyroidism and acromegaly should be appropriately treated. Since treatment of hypothyroidism without concomitant treatment of OSA may result in more severe oxyhemoglobin desaturation due to increased oxygen consumption, both should be treated concurrently (i.e., with nasal CPAP). Nasal CPAP treatment may be discontinued after treatment of the endocrine abnormality, if a follow-up PSG no longer demonstrates significant sleep disordered breathing. In obese individuals, dietary weight loss can significantly improve OSA.

Medical Treatment

Nasal Continuous Positive Airway Pressure (CPAP).[21] For patients with moderate-to-severe disease, conservative treatment alone is rarely adequate, and treatment with nasal CPAP becomes the next therapeutic option. With this device, CPAP is applied to the upper airway with a nasal mask, nasal prongs, or an oronasal mask. Although there are numerous proposed mechanisms, CPAP acts predominantly by providing a "positive pressure or pneumatic splint" to the upper airway, preventing the airway narrowing that occurs when dilator muscle activity decreases at sleep onset. *(Please see Figure 4.)*

If tolerated, nasal CPAP is effective in the majority of cases of OSDB. Thus, the major limiting factor is compliance, with subjective estimates by the patient being much higher than objective measurements. In one study, only 46% of patients complied with treatment.[22] Compliance appears more closely linked to relief of daytime symptoms such as decreased alertness than to the severity of the RDI.[23] It can be improved with simple interventions such as weekly phone calls and written information about sleep apnea and the importance of regular CPAP use.[24]

At least part of the reason for the poor compliance with nasal CPAP is side effects, which can be divided into nasopharyngeal (congestion, dry nose/mouth, sinus discomfort, headache, ear discomfort/infection, epistaxis) and pressure-related (chest wall discomfort, ear discomfort, smothering sensation, and barotrauma [pneumothorax, pneumomediastinum, pneumoencephalos] symptoms). Mouth opening, claustrophobia, conjunctivitis, bridge of nose bruise/ulceration, allergic reaction, and the inconvenience of being attached to a machine may also be problematic. Although the precise cause of the nasopharyngeal symptoms is unknown, they likely result from the machine's cool, dry air injuring the lining epithelium and/or stimulating nerves in the nasopharynx. *(Please see Table 6.)* The function of the ramp option found on most CPAP machines is to allow the CPAP pressure to gradually increase to the prescribed level over a period of 5-45 minutes.

Devices that automatically adjust or self titrate the nasal CPAP based on the pressure required to maintain upper airway patency have recently been developed. Some of these "Auto-CPAP" devices are effective in determining the optimal CPAP setting for most OSA patients.[25] They allow reduction in the average nasal CPAP required and titration of CPAP without the immediate involvement of a technologist. Treatment with auto-titrating nasal CPAP systems have shown slight increases in adherence when compared to fixed-pressure nasal CPAP.[26,27] Additional studies, particularly in the home setting, are needed to determine the optimal role of "autotitrating" CPAP devices in the treatment of OSDB. At the present time, it would be reasonable to use one of these devices in patients having difficulty tolerating "fixed" CPAP due to pressure-related symptoms.

Nasal Bilevel Positive Airway Pressure. Bilevel positive airway pressure systems differ from nasal CPAP in that the former allows the independent adjustment of inspiratory positive airway pressure (IPAP) and expiratory positive airway pressure (EPAP). With nasal CPAP, the IPAP and EPAP must be the same. Depending on the particular machine, bilevel systems also allow the operator to set a back-up respiratory rate, change the IPAP percentage, and adjust the flow sensitivity. Thus, unlike nasal CPAP, bilevel systems permit ventilation of the patient. However, ventilation is typically not required with OSDB, unless hypoventilation coexists.

Since a higher pressure is required to maintain adequate upper airway patency during inspiration than expiration, if a bilevel system is used, the EPAP can usually be decreased. This lower EPAP may diminish problems with exhaling or a "smothering" sensation, the risk of barotrauma (due to a lower mean alveolar pressure), the risk of hypercapnia (since ventilation can be instituted), and significant mask air leakage. However, although patient acceptance may be better with bilevel systems, compliance is similar to that with CPAP.[28] BiPAP is the bilevel system manufactured by Respironics, Inc., in Murrysville, PA.

Oral Appliances. Currently, oral or dental appliances are considered useful for primary snoring but are considered second-line therapy for OSDB. These devices are most effective for patients with mild OSA who do not respond to conservative measures. Since some patients with moderate-to-severe disease may respond as well, I consider an oral appliance in such individuals if they are intolerant of, refuse, or are not candidates for nasal CPAP, a bilevel system, or surgery. Nonobese individuals and those with OSDB predominantly in the supine position are more likely to improve with an oral appliance. Those devices that work appear to do so by increasing the

Table 5. Severity Scale for Sleep-Disordered Breathing

SEVERITY	RESPIRATORY DISTURBANCE INDEX (RDI)	MINIMUM OXYGEN SATURATION	CARDIAC DYSRHYTHMIA	EXCESSIVE DAYTIME SLEEPINESS	
				MSLT (min)	ESS
Mild	> 5-20	≥ 85%	Tachy-bradycardia	8-10	> 10-12
Moderate	21-50	65-84%	Severe tachy-bradycardia	5-8	12-16
Severe	> 50	< 65%	Ventricular tachycardia; sinus arrest or pause > 3 seconds		> 16

posterior airway space by providing a stable anterior position of the mandible, by advancing the tongue or soft palate, and possibly by changing genioglossus muscle activity. Close cooperation between physician and dentist is necessary to ensure optimal patient selection and follow-up and to avoid potential side effects. Problems include tongue, gum, or temporomandibular joint (TMJ) soreness and orthodontic problems. Compliance ranges from 50% to 100% and, in a recent study, was preferred over nasal CPAP. As for surgical procedures for OSA, it is difficult to predict success, and treatment may improve OSA somewhat, but the patient is still left with significant residual disease. Consequently, a follow-up sleep study is required for moderate-to-severe disease, but not primary snoring or mild OSA.[29-33]

Medications. Overall, medications are not effective in the treatment of OSDB or OHS. With the exception, perhaps, of fluoxetine and tricyclic antidepressants in patients with mild OSDB, oxygen for central apnea and hypoventilation, and anorexiant drugs for weight loss, medications for the treatment of OSDB should be limited to patients who refuse, cannot tolerate, or have contraindications to weight loss, nasal positive airway pressure, oral appliances, and surgery. When used, follow-up PSG in patients who appear to have responded to treatment is mandatory. Fluoxetine and tricyclic antidepressants work by suppressing REM sleep and increasing upper airway dilator muscle tone. These agents may also allow a decrease in high nasal CPAP. The role of anorexiant drugs in the treatment of OSA remains unclear.[34]

Moreover, the association of fenfluramine and phentermine with cardiac valvulopathies and primary pulmonary hypertension has resulted in their being removed from the market.

Surgical Treatment

The goal of surgery is to improve one or more of the determinants of upper airway caliber.[35]

Nasal Surgery. Nasal surgery alone is rarely curative but is often used in conjunction with other surgical procedures (i.e., as part of Phase 1 surgery for OSA).

Adenotonsillectomy. Although this procedure can be curative in children and adolescents with OSA, it is not usually helpful in adults.[36] However, in carefully selected adults, it may be the only treatment required.[37]

Uvulopalatopharyngoplasty (UPPP).[38-41] The most commonly performed surgical procedure for OSDB is UPPP. The procedure involves removal of the tonsils, uvula, redundant soft palate, and pharyngeal folds. The overall success rate is less than 50%. Preoperative imaging studies and testing cannot reliably predict surgical success. This procedure is most likely to be successful if upper airway collapse is limited to the oropharynx, and if the RDI is less than 20-30, that is, with less severe disease. Unfortunately, in 75% of cases, there is more than one site of upper airway obstruction, a fact that is the likely explanation for the poor success rate. Potential complications include nasal reflux and speech problems. Post-operative pain is significant.

Laser-assisted Uvulopalatoplasty (LAUP).[38,42-45] LAUP has recently been introduced as an outpatient treatment for snoring and potentially for OSDB. It involves removing part of the uvula and associated soft palate with a CO_2 laser in 1-7 sessions. Unlike the surgical UPPP, neither the tonsils nor the lateral pharyngeal tissues are removed or altered. Compared to UPPP, LAUP is less expensive, bloodless, requires less time off from work, does not require general anesthesia and hospitalization, and is not associated with velopharyngeal insufficiency or stenosis. Although less painful than UPPP, 60-75% of patients report severe postoperative pain from one to eight and, up to, 21 days. Snoring is *subjectively* cured or softer in 76-90% of cases, with best results occurring when a long uvula or a draping soft palate is present. Considering the advantages over UPPP, it may be the most appropriate surgical treatment for snoring. Although not previously recommended for the treatment of OSDB, recent evidence indicates that in carefully selected patients with mild, moderate, or severe disease, LAUP may be considered a surgical option. However, some patients may have worse OSDB postoperatively and LAUP may decrease nasal mask tolerance. Thus, if performed for OSDB, a postoperative PSG to document efficacy is essential. One potential problem with LAUP is that the elimination of snoring removes one of the signs of OSDB and may provide a false sense of security.

Maxillofacial Surgery. Because of the poor and unpredictable results with UPPP, a variety of other procedures have been developed to further increase the size of the upper airway. Such surgeries ideally have both an otorhinolaryngologist and oral surgeon involved. Inferior sagittal mandibular osteotomy plus genioglossal advancement, with or without a hyoid myotomy and suspension, enlarges the retrolingual (behind the tongue) airway. These procedures may be performed in conjunction with a UPPP and nasal surgery. With success being defined as an RDI less than 20 and a

Figure 4. Schematic Representation of the Effect of CPAP on the Upper Airway in Obstructive Sleep Apnea

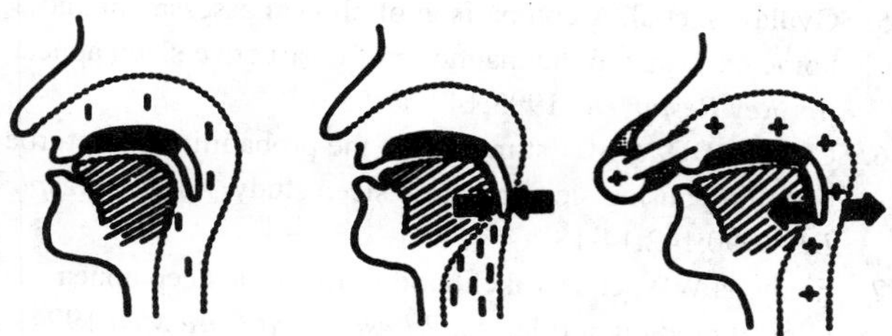

The top panel demonstrates that negative airway pressure is generated during inspiration and that muscle tone is needed to prevent airway collapse. The middle panel represents airway occlusion resulting from negative intra-airway pressure exceeding muscle forces tending to maintain airway patency. The lower panel shows the theoretical effect of reversing the negative airway pressure with continuous positive pressure.

Reprinted with permission from: Sullivan CE, Berthon-Jones M, Issa FG, et al. Medical Treatment for the sleep apnea syndrome. *Lancet* 1981;1:862-865.

50% or more decrease, there is a 66-67% response rate to this Phase 1 surgery. Complications include need for a root canal, numbness, dysesthesia of the chin for 3-6 months, and facial contour changes.[42,46,47]

If the patient has significant craniofacial abnormalities and/or has not responded to "Phase 1" surgery, maxillomandibular osteotomy and advancement is an option. This procedure further advances the tongue and enlarges the retropalatal airway as well. In the right hands, results have been good, with more than a 90% success rate being reported.[46] Average hospital stay is two days, the major complications being dysesthesia or paresthesia of the face that lasts six weeks to six months.

Tongue Reduction Surgery. Laser midline glossectomy also is an option for those who fail the above mentioned surgical procedures. However, this procedure is associated with a long difficult recovery, speech problems, and some persistent sensory loss. The substantial associated edema requires placement of a temporary tracheostomy.

Tracheostomy. With the many surgical options and, in particular, the advent of nasal CPAP and BiPAP, tracheostomy is infrequently used as treatment for OSA. This procedure should be required in less than 5% of cases. Nonetheless, there is a small subgroup of patients with severe OSDB who cannot tolerate or do not respond to other therapeutic options. In these individuals, tracheostomy, which completely bypasses the upper airway obstruction, can provide dramatic improvement and can be lifesaving. However, the potential for additional medical as well as psychological morbidity needs to be taken into account.[48,49]

Radiofrequency Volumetric Tissue Reduction.[50] Performed in the office under local anesthesia, radiofrequency volumetric tissue reduction has recently been FDA approved for the treatment of snoring but not OSDB. Its role in the surgical management of OSDB remains to be defined.

Table 6. Treatment of Adverse Effects of Nasal CPAP

- Nasopharyngeal symptoms
  - — Humidification
    - Nasal salt solution/spray
    - Add humidifier to machine
  - — Nasal steroids
  - — Other
    - For nasal congestion:
      - Infrequent: alpha-adrenergic spray
      - Frequent: alpha-adrenergic pill
      - Intractable: oronasal mask
    - For rhinorrhea:
      - Anticholinergic spray
    - Nasal nedocromil
    - Nasal cromolyn sodium
- Pressure-related symptoms
  - — Ramp
  - — BiPAP
  - — Auto-CPAP
  - — Relaxation techniques
- Mouth opening
  - — Chin strap
  - — Form fitting mouth guard
  - — Oronasal mask
- Claustrophobia
  - — Different mask
  - — Relaxation techniques
  - — Desensitization
- Conjunctivitis
  - — Adjust mask fit
  - — Different mask
- Bridge of nose bruise/ulceration
  - — Reinforce area
  - — Different mask
- Allergic reaction
  - — Different mask

Bariatric Surgery.[51] For significantly obese individuals with either OSDB, surgical weight loss procedures are another option. Weight-loss surgical procedures that have been studied include gastric bypass, jejuno-ileal bypass, and gastroplasty. Results have been impressive and include a weight change of 31-72.5%, an increase in RDI of 89% to 98%, improved nocturnal oxyhemoglobin saturation, decreased cardiac dysrhythmias, improved subjective daytime somnolence, and improved sleep continuity and architecture (increased total sleep time, % slow wave sleep, % REM sleep). Unfortunately, all studies of the effect of weight loss on sleep disordered breathing thus far are poorly designed, and are little more than a series of case reports. Moreover, good data on the risks and benefits of surgery, the effects of bariatric surgery on waking performance, and long-term follow-up on either the weight loss or improvements in sleep and sleep-disordered breathing are lacking. Clearly more and better-controlled studies are needed.

Summary

OSA syndrome is a common disorder and a clinically significant disease affecting 6% of the middle-age adult working population. It is associated with significant adverse health effects, can present subtlely, and is frequently overlooked. If undiagnosed, OSA syndrome may be associated with significant morbidity and even mortality. Moreover, it is readily and noninvasively diagnosed, and typically easily treated. Consequently, it would behoove all primary care physicians to at least consider obstructive sleep disordered breathing in any patient who has any predisposing factor, sign, or symptom associated with this disease.

References

1. Young T, et al. The occurrence of sleep-disordered breathing among middle-aged adults. *N Engl J Med* 1993;328: 1230-1235.
2. Isono S, Remmers JE. Anatomy and physiology of upper airway obstruction. Krieger MH, Roth T, Dement WC, eds. In: *Principles and Practice of Sleep Medicine*. Philadelphia, Pa: W.B. Saunders Company; 1994:642-656.
3. Teran-Santos J, et al. The association between sleep apnea and the risk of traffic accidents. *N Engl J Med* 1999;340: 847-851.
4. Bonsignore MR, et al. The cardiovascular effects of obstructive sleep apnoeas: Analysis of pathogenic mechanisms. *Eur Respir J* 1994;7:786-805.
5. Hung J, et al. Association of sleep apnoea with myocardial infarction in men. *Lancet* 1990;336:261-264.
6. Partinen M, Guilleminault C. Daytime sleepiness and vascular morbidity at seven-year follow-up in obstructive sleep apnea patients. *Chest* 1990;97:27-32.
7. He J, et al. Mortality and apnea index in obstructive sleep apnea. Experience in 385 male patients. *Chest* 1988;94:9-14.
8. Loube DI, et al. Indications for positive airway pressure treatment of adult obstructive sleep apnea patients: A consensus statement. *Chest* 1999;115:863-866.
9. Guilleminault C, et al. A cause of excessive daytime sleepiness: The upper airway resistance syndrome. *Chest* 1993;104:781-787.
10. Kribbs NB, Getsy JE, Dinges DF. Investigation and management of daytime sleepiness in sleep apnea. Saunders NA, Sullivan CE, eds. In: *Sleeping and Breathing*. New York, NY: Marcel Dekker; 1993:575-604.
11. Walsleben JA. The measurement of daytime wakefulness. *Chest* 1992;101:890-891.
12. Hoffstein V, Szalai JP. Predictive value of clinical features in diagnosing obstructive sleep apnea. *Sleep* 1993;16:118-122.
13. Viner S, et al. Are history and physical examination a good screening test for sleep apnea? *Ann Intern Med* 1991;115: 356-359.
14. Kapuniai LE, et al. Identifying sleep apnea from self-reports. *Sleep* 1988;11:430-436.
15. Gyulay S, et al. A comparison of clinical assessment and home oximetry in the diagnosis of obstructive sleep apnea. *Am Rev Respir Dis* 1993;147:50-53.
16. Crocker BD, et al. Estimation of the probability of disturbed breathing during sleep before a sleep study. *Am Rev Respir Dis* 1990;142:14-18.
17. Flemons WW, et al. Likelihood ratios for a sleep apnea clinical prediction rule. *Am J Respir Crit Care Med* 1994; 150:1279-1285.
18. Practice parameters for the use of portable recording in the assessment of obstructive sleep apnea. *Sleep* 1994;17: 372-377.
19. Chervin RD, et al. Cost-utility of three approaches to the diagnosis of sleep apnea: polysomnography, home testing, and empirical therapy. *Ann Intern Med* 1999;130:496-505.
20. Series F, et al. Utility of nocturnal home oximetry for case finding in patients with suspected sleep apnea hypopnea syndrome. *Ann Intern Med* 1993;119:449-453.
21. Strollo PJ, et al. Sleep disorders: Positive pressure therapy. *Clin Chest Med* 1998;19:55-68.
22. Kribbs NB, et al. Objective measurement of patterns of nasal CPAP use by patients with obstructive sleep apnea. *Am Rev Respir Dis* 1993;147:887-895.
23. Indications and standards for use of nasal continuous positive airway pressure (CPAP) in sleep apnea syndromes. *Am J Respir Crit Care Med* 1994;150:1738-1785.
24. Chervin RD, et al. Compliance with nasal CPAP can be improved by simple interventions. *Sleep* 1997;20:284-289.
25. Lloberes P, et al. Comparison of manual and automatic CPAP titration in patients with sleep apnea/hypopnea syndrome. *Am J Respir Crit Care Med* 1996;154: 1755-1758.
26. Series F, Marc I. Efficacy of automatic continuous positive airway pressure therapy that uses an estimated required pressure in the treatment of obstructive sleep apnea syndrome. *Ann Intern Med* 1997;127:588-595.
27. Konermann M, et al. Use of conventional and self-adjusting nasal continuous positive airway pressure for treatment of severe obstructive sleep apnea syndrome. *Chest* 1998;113: 714-718.
28. Reeves-Hoche MK, et al. Continuous versus bilevel positive airway pressure for obstructive sleep apnea. *Am J Respir Crit Care Med* 1995;151:443-449.
29. Ferguson KA, et al. A randomized crossover study of an oral appliance vs nasal-continuous positive airway pressure in the treatment of mild-moderate obstructive sleep apnea. *Chest* 1996;109:1269-1275.
30. Schmidt-Nowara W, et al. Oral appliances for the treatment of snoring and obstructive sleep apnea: A review. *Sleep* 1995;18:501-510.
31. Practice parameters for the treatment of snoring and obstructive sleep apnea with oral appliances. *Sleep* 1995; 18:511-513.

32. Marklund M, et al. The effect of a mandibular advancement device on apneas and sleep in patients with obstructive sleep apnea. *Chest* 1998;113:707-713.
33. Millman RP, et al. Oral appliances in the treatment of snoring and sleep apnea. *Clin Chest Med* 1998;19:69-75.
34. Hudgel DW, Thanakitcharu S. Pharmacologic treatment of sleep-disordered breathing. *Am J Respir Crit Care Med* 1998;158:691-699.
35. Powell NB, et al. Surgical management of obstructive sleep apnea syndrome. *Clin Chest Med* 1998;19:77-86.
36. Aubert-Tulkens G, et al. Failure of tonsil and nose surgery in adults with long-standing severe sleep apnea syndrome. *Arch Intern Med* 1989;149:2118-2121.
37. Miyazaki S, et al. Effectiveness of tonsillectomy in adult sleep apnea syndrome. *Psychiatry Clin Neurosci* 1999;52: 222-223.
38. Barthel SW, Strome M. Snoring, obstructive sleep apnea, and surgery. *Med Clin North Am* 1999;83:85-96.
39. Sher AE, et al. The efficacy of surgical modifications of the upper airway in adults with obstructive sleep apnea syndrome. *Sleep* 1996;19:156-177.
40. Shepard JWJ, et al. Evaluation of the upper airway in patients with obstructive sleep apnea. *Sleep* 1991;14: 361-371.
41. Powell NB, et al. *Principles and Practice of Sleep Medicine.* Philadelphia, Pa: W.B. Saunders Company; 1994:706-721.
42. Practice parameters for the use of laser-assisted uvulopalatoplasty. Standards of practice committee of the american sleep disorders association. *Sleep* 1994;17: 744-748.
43. Walker RP, et al. Laser-assisted uvulopalatoplasty for the treatment of mild, moderate, and severe obstructive sleep apnea. *Laryngoscope* 1999;109:79-85.
44. Pribitkin EA, et al. Efficacy of laser-assisted uvulopalatoplasty in obstructive sleep apnea. *Otolaryngol Head Neck Surg* 1998;119:643-647.
45. Coleman JAJ. Laser-assisted uvulopalatoplasty: Long-term results with a treatment for snoring. *Ear Nose Throat J* 1998;77:22-34.
46. Riley RW, et al. Obstructive sleep apnea syndrome: A review of 306 consecutively treated surgical patients. *Otolaryngol Head Neck Surg* 1993;108:117-125.
47. Johnson NT, Chinn J. Uvulopalatopharyngoplasty and inferior sagittal mandibular osteotomy with genioglossus advancement for treatment of obstructive sleep apnea. *Chest* 1994;105:278-283.
48. Guilleminault C, et al. Obstructive sleep apnea syndrome and tracheostomy. Long-term follow-up experience. *Arch Intern Med* 1981;141:985-988.
49. Conway WA, et al. Adverse effects of tracheostomy for sleep apnea. *JAMA* 1981;246:347-350.
50. Powell NB, et al. Radiofrequency volumetric tissue reduction of the palate in subjects with sleep-disordered breathing. *Chest* 1998;113:1163-1174.
51. Strobel RJ, Rosen RC. Obesity and weight loss in obstructive sleep apnea: A critical review. *Sleep* 1996;19: 104-115.

Recognition and Management of Sleep Disorders

David N. Neubauer, MD

Sleep problems are widespread in our society, and primary care medicine is at the front lines of sleep disorder recognition and management. National Sleep Foundation surveys show that about one-half of U.S. adults have some problem with their sleep. It is clear that sleep disorders not only have major consequences for individuals, they also cause significant public health problems and a considerable societal economic burden. The challenge in primary care includes the identification of sleep-disordered patients, as well as the appropriate management of those patients presenting with sleep complaints.[1] Identifying sleep problems is especially important since many patients either are not aware that they have a sleep disorder or they raise it as a problem to their physician. Sleep apnea, for example, is relatively common and may have significant consequences, but may not be evident to the affected individual.

The symptoms of sleep disorders are quite varied, ranging from the inability to sleep at desired times (insomnia) to the inability to stay awake at appropriate times (excessive daytime sleepiness), and even to assorted behaviors and physiological events that emanate from sleep (parasomnias). These symptom-based categories, while overlapping in some patients, nevertheless are useful in organizing the common sleep disorders and helpful in leading to appropriate evaluation and treatment.

Three major nosologies attempt to define and organize sleep disorders.[2-4] Each has strengths and weaknesses. The DSM-IV and ICD-10 use rather broad categories, while the International Classification of Sleep Disorders (ICSD) lists scores of common and esoteric disturbances of sleep. Diagnostic coding requirements most commonly determine which nosology is used.

This sleep disorders review initially will consider the characteristics and regulation of normal sleep. Following this will be three sections reviewing the symptoms, causes, and treatment of disorders related to insomnia, excessive daytime sleepiness, and the parasomnias. These will emphasize the more common and important disturbances encountered in primary care practice. Finally, there will be a review of guidelines in the evaluation of sleep complaints and the potential value of sleep center consultation and testing.

Normal Sleep

An understanding of general sleep characteristics is necessary to appreciate the context of subjective patient complaints and the physiological processes that may undermine sleep and wakefulness. The regulation of the sleep-wake cycle involves two processes that usually operate in concert, but which can be dissociated under naturalistic (e.g., shift work) and experimental circumstances.[5] The homeostatic process represents the overall balance of sleep and wakefulness with an approximate 1:2 ratio—eight hours of sleep and 16 hours of wakefulness. Sleep deprivation, acute or chronic, builds up homeostatic pressure resulting in sleepiness.[6] Sleep discharges the pressure. Brain energy storage and metabolism may be important in this process.

A circadian process is responsible for the typical nighttime sleepiness and daytime alertness cycle driven by the suprachiasmatic nucleus (SCN), the brain's timekeeper. This rhythm influences the typical nighttime pattern of melatonin production and secretion. Generally, circadian sleepiness peaks toward the end of the normal sleep period (about 4:00 a.m. - 5:00 a.m.), while circadian alertness peaks toward the end of the waking period (about 7:00 p.m. - 8:00 p.m.). In addition to the late night sleepiness peak, inherent in the normal daily rhythm is the familiar afternoon increase in sleepiness. Often sleep-wake problems occurring in the context of schedule changes (e.g., shift work and jet lag) can be understood in terms of the interaction of the homeostatic and circadian influences.

Under normal circumstances the homeostatic and circadian processes operate together to allow eight hours of sleep and 16 hours of wakefulness. The entire system is strongly influenced by the photoperiod, and for most people the timing of the clock is reset daily with dawn light. The circadian oscillator has a period of slightly more than 24 hours, producing a progressive phase delay tendency.[7] The biological influence of light has significant therapeutic implications for selected patients.

Although many people sleep from about 11:00 p.m. until about 7:00 a.m., others have sleep-wake cycle phases with considerably earlier (early bird) or later (night owl) patterns. There is a general developmental tendency for adolescents to be phase delayed, with a later sleep onset and arising in the morning. With aging the phase advances, culminating in the common elderly pattern of early evening sleepiness and early morning awakening.

Sleep varies considerably during the night, with dramatic EEG pattern changes and periods of rapid eye movements and decreased muscle tone. Rapid eye movement (REM) sleep, typically accounting for 15-25% of total sleep, is quite distinct from the remainder of sleep, termed non-REM (NREM). By convention, NREM is divided into four stages of increasing depth defined by EEG characteristics, with the deeper stages associated with marked high-amplitude EEG slowing in the delta (0.5-3.0 Hz) range. A typical night's sleep follows a general pattern of REM beginning about 90 minutes following sleep onset and repeating about every 90 minutes for a total of four to five episodes during the night. The REM episodes tend to increase in duration throughout the night, so the greater amount of REM sleep usually is during the latter part of the night. In contrast, most deep sleep (NREM, stages 3 and 4) occurs during the first few hours of a night's sleep. These patterns are useful in diagnosing certain parasomnias.

With aging, the REM sleep duration and pattern are preserved; however, deep sleep diminishes considerably.[8,9] There also are increased arousals and awakenings, as well as the above noted phase advance. Elderly individuals may have greater difficulty maintaining sustained nighttime sleep; however, it is not clear that the need for sleep decreases with aging.[10]

Insomnia

Insomnia, the most common sleep complaint, is the report of inadequate and unrefreshing sleep. The description may be difficulty initiating or maintaining sleep, and the presentation may include early morning awakening and inadequate total sleep time. Usually there is an integral daytime component, such as fatigue and exhaustion.[11] The episode may be transient or chronic, single or recurrent, and of varying degrees of severity. The potential causes of insomnia are plentiful.[12] *(Please see Table 1.)* It is important to consider long-term vulnerabilities and more acute precipitants in evaluating patients with insomnia complaints, as treatment may need to be multifaceted.

Table 1. Causes of Insomnia

- Situational disturbances
- Psychiatric disorders
- Medical disorders
- Medication effects
- Stimulants (e.g., caffeine, nicotine)
- Primary sleep disorders
- Psychological conditioning
- Environmental factors (e.g., light, noise)
- Sleep-wake habits

Everyone is vulnerable to situational disturbances that can interfere with sleep, at least transiently. Stressful episodes with insomnia mostly relate to life problems; however, excitement also can impair sleep. Psychiatric disorders account for a large percentage of insomnia.[13] Major depression predictably promotes insomnia with sleep disturbance throughout the night, not just the classic early morning awakening. Most other psychiatric disorders, especially anxiety disorders, during acute phases readily can cause insomnia. A multitude of medical conditions associated with pain, discomfort, and fear can undermine the ability to sleep soundly. Examples include arthritis, chronic back pain, gastroesophageal reflux, hyperthyroidism, chronic lung disease, renal insufficiency, and fibromyalgia. Insomnia is a potential side effect of many medications, including some antidepressants and antihypertensives, corticosteroids, and decongestants.[14] Nicotine is stimulating, and caffeine can continue to exert its alerting effects for eight hours or more. Bedtime alcohol, while initially sedating, after a few hours then promotes hyperarousal and increased awakenings during the night. Patients with primary sleep disorders, including circadian rhythm disorders, sleep-disordered breathing, restless leg syndrome, and periodic limb movement disorder, may present with insomnia as the chief complaint. Psychological conditioning of mental hyperarousal associated with attempts to sleep and the fear of not sleeping can perpetuate insomnia symptoms indefinitely. Finally, the fundamental processes promoting normal sleep can be undermined by assorted behaviors, routines, and habits. These may include irregular and changing schedules, inadequate evening relaxation, and strenuous exercise within a few hours of bedtime.

Surveys demonstrate that more than one-third of adult populations complain of at least occasional insomnia, and about 10-15% experience severe or persistent symptoms. Although insomnia occurs in all population subgroups, increased risk is recognized for the elderly and for women, especially with menopause and thereafter.[10] Lower socioeconomic status, divorced and single status, and living alone additionally represent increased risk.

The consequences of insomnia include not only the immediate distress of sleeplessness, but also significant decrements in concentration, performance, mood, and other quality-of-life measures.[15] Several studies have established the increased risk of new onset major depression in the context of persistent insomnia.[13,16-18] The total direct costs of insomnia in the United States are estimated in the billions of dollars.[19] Such values include office visits and medications (prescription and OTC), but not the huge indirect costs, such as those related to mistakes, accidents, and absenteeism.[20] Sleep-wake cycle disruption may also contribute to the nursing home placement of individuals who otherwise might be managed by family members at home.

The multitude of potential insomnia causes demonstrate the need for a broad-based evaluation of patients complaining of sleep disturbance. Insomnia treatment first should address underlying disorders (medical, psychiatric, and other sleep disorders) and potential undesired stimulating or sedating medication effects. Specific questions for the patient and bed partner should address snoring and the breathing pattern, as well as body movements during sleep. Patient education about normal sleep will promote realistic expectations and create the foundation for any necessary schedule and behavior changes. Good sleep habits should be reviewed. *(Please see Table 2.)* The physician and patient may work in partnership in trying to isolate key factors that seem particularly influential on that person's sleep. The use of a daily sleep log detailing times in and out of bed, estimated sleep onset and awakenings, daytime functioning, as well as behavior changes and medication trials can be quite useful for diagnostic and treatment efficacy purposes. For selected patients, more directive behavioral strategies can be therapeutic. One approach, termed stimulus control, is to have the patient with excessive mental arousal (e.g., "mind racing") while in bed spend more time out of bed when he or she is unable to sleep. The patient is instructed to go to bed only when sleepy, and to leave the bed if unable to fall asleep quickly or during extended nighttime awakenings. This can help decondition the association between being in bed and the experience of persistent frustration and agitation. A technique called sleep restriction involves limiting the time in bed available for sleep. A normal morning wakeup time remains constant and the bedtime, initially rather late, is gradually scheduled earlier as the percentage of sleep time increases. Psychotherapeutic techniques can address personal conflicts and distressing life situations, as well as help reframe cognitive distortions about sleep.[21-23] These behavioral and psychotherapeutic strategies often are combined successfully with the use of short-acting hypnotics.

Table 2. Sleep Habit Issues

- Wakeup time
- Bedtime
- Napping
- Evening routines
- Sleep environment
- Exercise
- Caffeine
- Alcohol

Circadian rhythm influences are present in many insomnia cases. These are obvious in the context of jet lag and shift work, but also are important with the severe early birds (advanced sleep phase syndrome) suffering with chronic early morning awakening, and the severe night owls (delayed sleep phase syndrome) with chronic initial insomnia and a desire to sleep well into the daylight hours. In these situations treatment should include attention to the patient's exposure to light and darkness. One approach to the advanced sleep phase problem is maximizing bright light exposure in the evening and minimizing light exposure around dawn. Therapeutic light boxes may be used in the evening. Dark curtains or an eye mask can help decrease the morning light. Generally, the individual with a delayed pattern may benefit from minimizing evening bright light and maximizing morning light.

Medications may play a valuable role in the treatment of acute and chronic insomnia for selected patients. Clearly, antidepressants are important when a depressive disorder is present. Antidepressant selection is complicated by potential side effects, including worsened insomnia due to stimulating action or daytime somnolence from the relatively long half-lives of many medications. The combination of an antidepressant and a hypnotic may be beneficial.

OTC antihistamines (diphenhydramine, hydroxyzine, doxylamine, and pyrilamine) are used widely because of the availability and perceived safety. Possible problems with these include morning grogginess after bedtime use because of the long duration of action, and also potential anticholinergic side effects. Theses may include dry mouth, constipation, urinary retention, and confusion. The anticholinergic effects may be especially detrimental for elderly individuals.

Most prescription hypnotics in current usage are positive allosteric modulators of the GABAA receptor complex and function as benzodiazepine receptor agonists.[24] These include the traditional benzodiazepines and newer nonbenzodiazepine agonists, zolpidem and zaleplon. These newer agents are short half-life preparations, minimizing daytime sedation. Nightly use of long half-life agents increases the pharmacokinetic risk of accumulation and subsequent daytime sedation. The newer short-acting hypnotics generally are safe, efficacious, and well tolerated. These medications are appropriate for a variety of short-term uses (days to weeks). Selected patients appear to benefit from longer-term usage; however, further research regarding such extended hypnotic use is necessary to establish appropriate indications and guidelines.[25] Intermittent dosing with general directions of the maximum number of pills per week or month can offer the patient a sense of control in dealing with the sleep disturbance. This strategy can be therapeutic even on those nights the medication is not taken since the fear of unending sleeplessness may be reduced. Dosing should follow the prescribing guidelines for each medication. Typically this involves a reduced dose for the elderly and those with hepatic impairment. Considering the current selection of available hypnotics *(please see Table 3)*, there is no reason to consider the barbiturates and rarely an indication for the long-acting benzodiazepines in the management of insomnia. Certainly, hypnotics

Table 3. Hypnotic Medications

GENERIC NAME	BRAND NAME	DOSAGE RANGE (MG)
Long-acting		
Flurazepam	Dalmane	15-30
Quazepam	Doral	7.5-15
Intermediate-acting		
Temazepam	Restoril	7.5-15
Estazolam	ProSom	1-2
Short-acting		
Triazolam	Halcion	0.125-0.25
Zolpidem	Ambien	5-10
Zaleplon	Sonata	5-10

should be used in the greater context of attention to the assortment of factors that may be stimulating and perpetuating the insomnia.

Excessive Daytime Sleepiness

Excessive sleepiness during desired times of wakefulness is a major societal problem. The U.S. Department of Transportation estimates there are 100,000 fatigue-related driving accidents annually. Workplace accidents due to sleepiness are common, particularly in shift work situations. Chronic sleepiness and fatigue plague millions of people in our society, representing about 5% of the population. By far, the most common cause of excessive sleepiness is simply sleep deprivation resulting from inadequate time allotted for sleep; however, several sleep disorders may be primary causes. Due to the safety and health implications, complaints of excessive daytime sleepiness always warrant clinical evaluation.

Sleep-Disordered Breathing

Sleep-disordered breathing (SDB), which includes sleep apnea, involves repeated interruptions in airflow exclusively during sleep.[26] Complete airflow cessation for at least 10 seconds is termed an apnea, while a partial (50% or greater) reduction is a hypopnea. The events typically are associated with a transient decrease in blood oxygen saturation. There also may be EEG-defined arousals, of which the sleeper generally is unaware. The frequency of the combined apneas and hypopneas is reported as the respiratory disturbance index (RDI) or apnea hypopnea index (AHI), which is the same value derived from polysomnographic studies. These may be listed separately for NREM and REM sleep. The former is more significant, since NREM sleep constitutes the majority of the night, although the rate during REM sleep may be greater due to the normal decrease in muscle tone associated with that sleep state. A minimum of five events per hour of sleep defines SDB, although a greater frequency is necessary for clinical significance. A general guideline is five to 29 events per hour being mild, 30-59 events being moderate, and 60 and above being severe. The degree of oxygen desaturation also will contribute to the assessment of severity. Apneic and hypopneic events may recur hundreds of times during a night's sleep. The airflow reduction causes the oxygen decrease and an increase in carbon dioxide, which, in turn, triggers an arousal and normal breaths until the cycle repeats. Profound fragmentation of sleep can result. SDB has been reported to be present in a healthy community sample in 4% of women and 9% of men.[27] The typical natural course is chronic and progressive.

Obstruction of the airway is by far the most common cause of SDB. Individuals may be anatomically predisposed for airway collapse during sleep, and severe cases may be seen in childhood. Enlarged tonsils and adenoids may contribute to the obstruction, especially in children. Obesity is a major risk factor, as is a large neck, particularly a collar size of 17 and greater. It is most common among males; however, the risk for women increases following menopause. Loud and interrupted snoring is common. Gasping and choking episodes may occur. The cessation of breathing may be evident and frightening for a bed partner, who feels the need to nudge him or her repeatedly throughout the night to maintain breathing. The patient may be completely unaware of the breathing disruption and arousals, and only report a sense of unrefreshing sleep and subsequent daytime sleepiness.

The daytime sleepiness resulting from SDB can be quite profound and dangerous, resulting in workplace and driving accidents. There are likely cumulative health detriments. There is a strong association with hypertension.[28] Further, untreated sleep-disordered breathing increases the risk for other cardiovascular diseases (e.g., stroke, myocardial infarction, and arrhythmias).

The treatment of obstructive SDB depends upon the severity. For those who are overweight, weight reduction can be beneficial. In mild cases, weight loss alone may be sufficient to normalize breathing. Continuous positive airway pressure (CPAP), which supplies a prescribed amount of air pressure through a nasal mask, is the most common approach for clinically significant cases. CPAP can maintain airway patency and eliminate the repeated obstructive events. Selected patients may benefit from surgical approaches or oral appliances. Experimental methods are exploring alternate techniques to increase the upper airway muscle tone. In rare cases, hypothyroidism may be identified as an underlying cause. Treatment of the thyroid condition subsequently can improve the SDB.

Central apneas and hypopneas result from a decreased respiratory drive, which may be cardiovascular or neurological in origin. With congestive heart failure there may be an increased blood circulation time causing a cyclic pattern of increased and decreased respiration (Cheyne-Stokes). Cerebral, brainstem, and spinal cord lesions may impair the functioning of the respiratory center, thus affecting the breathing pattern. Treatment of the underlying disorder is necessary; however, the administration of oxygen and/or CPAP also may be helpful in some of these cases.

Suspected SDB is evaluated with a polysomnographic study to document the frequency of apneas and hypopneas, degree of oxygen desaturations, percentage of associated arousals, and the type of events: obstructive, central, or mixed. A sleep study also will be performed for proper titration of CPAP. A daytime multiple sleep latency test (MSLT) also may be performed to objectively document the degree of daytime sleepiness. This evidence can further direct treatment.

Restless Leg Syndrome/Periodic Limb Movement Disorder

Restless leg syndrome (RLS) is characterized by an uncomfortable and disconcerting motor restlessness and desire to move the limbs (especially the legs) in the evening when the person is at rest.[29] With increasing severity, the restlessness is more intense and may begin earlier in the evening or afternoon. Sleep onset commonly is delayed, and once the person does sleep, usually it is interrupted. Most RLS patients experience episodes of repeated brief involuntary periodic limb movements (PLM) during sleep, and sometimes during waking. These most commonly are expressed as leg kicks and may be associated with arousals. The clinical course of RLS tends to be chronic, and often there is a positive family history. RLS is most prevalent among the elderly. It is exacerbated with caffeine use and may occur transiently during pregnancy. The risk is increased with anemia or simply low iron stores as indicated by a low ferritin level (< 50 mcg/L). Iron supplementation often is beneficial for these patients, so the ferritin level always should be checked in patients presenting with RLS symptoms. More generally, dopaminergic precursors (carbidopa/levodopa) and agonists (e.g., pergolide) have the greatest efficacy for the RLS and PLM symptoms. Secondary pharmacologic approaches include opioids and benzodiazepines. Caffeine elimination and either increases or decreases in evening exercise may benefit some RLS cases.

The PLMs noted above also may occur independent of RLS, and may be recorded in up to 10% of the adult population. These involuntary contractions range from 0.5 to 5 seconds in duration, and from 4 to 120 seconds in periodicity. The contractions involve one or both legs (hip and knee flexion, foot/great toe dorsiflexion), but may generalize to the arms to entire body. These "jerks" may awaken the individual, and may be quite evident to bed partners. The severity of the PLM disorder is represented by the frequency of the contractions and the percentage causing EEG-defined arousals. People with the vulnerability for PLM disorder often experience an increased severity while taking most antidepressants. While RLS is a clinical diagnosis based on the history, PLM disorder is documented with a sleep laboratory study.

Narcolepsy

Narcolepsy is a genetically influenced disorder with a prevalence in less than 0.1% of the population. Symptoms usually emerge by the late teens or early 20s; however, the onset often is insidious, and diagnosis and treatment may await many years. The primary symptom in narcolepsy is persistent excessive sleepiness with superimposed episodes of irresistible sleep. These symptoms may be debilitating, with effects in all aspects of one's life: relationships, education, and occupation. Cataplexy, hypnogogic hallucinations, and sleep paralysis also may be seen as part of the narcolepsy symptom complex. Unlike hypnogogic hallucinations and sleep paralysis, cataplexy occurs almost exclusively with narcolepsy and its presence greatly strengthens the narcolepsy diagnosis. It is a sudden and transient (lasting several minutes) muscle weakness during wakefulness in response to an emotional stimulus (e.g., fear, laughter, competition, sexual excitement). It can be rather debilitating for those with frequent and severe episodes. The muscle weakness may be felt in the face and neck, trunk, and/or limbs, and may result in the individual being unable to speak or remain upright. Similarly, sleep paralysis, which may occur idiopathically, is a transient muscular paralysis; however, it occurs at sleep onset or with an awakening. Hypnogogic hallucinations are dreamlike sensory experiences associated with sleep onset. Narcolepsy is diagnosed by the history and polysomnographic and multiple sleep latency testing revealing rapid sleep onset during repeated daytime naps.

Both behavioral and pharmacologic measures may be useful in the treatment of patients with narcolepsy. Planned periods of activity and scheduled brief naps may reduce intrusive sleepiness. Maximizing nighttime sleep opportunities may be beneficial in reducing further daytime sleepiness. Strategic use of caffeinated beverages may temporarily promote alertness. Prescribed stimulants (pemoline, methylphenidate, modafinil, and dextroamphetamine) play a valuable role in combating sleepiness. Although pemoline (Cylert) has been used successfully for many years in the treatment of narcolepsy, the recent recognition of an increased risk of serious hepatic effects has resulted in the recommendation of biweekly liver function monitoring. Stimulants should be used relatively early in the day to avoid insomnia. The medications need not be used daily. Specific times to promote alertness may be scheduled on different days. REM-suppressant medications (most antidepressants) are useful in treating cataplexy. The newer generation antidepressants (e.g., SSRIs, venlafaxine) are desirable in not adding further sedation and minimizing anticholinergic and other side effects.

Parasomnias

An assortment of behaviors and other symptoms can emerge from and possibly interrupt sleep with subtle to dramatic results. While often benign, some of these events can be quite distressing for the patient and other household members, and there may even be dangerous consequences. Among the parasomnias are symptoms of medical and neurological disorders that for some individuals are

Table 4. Sleep Web Resources

Web Site	Web Address
The Sleep Well	www.stanford.edu/~dement/
The Sleep Medicine Home Page	www.users.cloud9.net/~thorpy/
Sleep Home Pages	www.sleephomepages.org
The American Academy of Sleep Medicine	www.aasmnet.org/
National Sleep Foundation	www.sleepfoundation.org
The National Center on Sleep Disorders Research	rover.nhlbi.nih.gov/about/ncsdr/
The Restless Legs Syndrome Foundation	www.rls.org
The Narcolepsy Network	www.websciences.org/narnet/
The American Sleep Apnea Association	www.sleepapnea.org

more likely to be manifest in sleep. Examples of these include sleep-related seizures and asthmatic episodes. Discomfort from gastroesophageal reflux may occur with muscle relaxation and the recumbent position during sleep. As REM and NREM sleep are markedly different physiological states, certain parasomnias are more likely to be related to specific sleep stages.

Normal characteristics of REM sleep include the rapid eye movements, skeletal muscle atonia, intense mental activity experienced as dreaming, and relative to NREM sleep, greater lability and irregularity of the heart rhythm, blood pressure, and breathing pattern. Especially intense and frightening dreaming can awaken the individual with a nightmare, which may be associated with considerable anxiety. Generally the person awakens fully with a recollection of the dream, usually a complex, emotion-laden narrative that may be bizarre and illogical. As greater REM occurs during the later part of the night, so do nightmares. Factors that lighten sleep and therefore decrease the arousal threshold, such as the stimulating effects of some medications, may temporarily increase the frequency of nightmares.

During REM sleep the brain is as active as when awake. With dreaming the motor areas are activated; however, in the brainstem a mechanism prevents the motor impulses from being transmitted, thus the normal atonia. REM behavior disorder results from faulty disinhibition of this mechanism with subsequent physical activity during dreaming. Examples include simple behaviors, such as repeatedly swinging an arm while dreaming about playing tennis, to physically aggressive behaviors during combat dreams. Thrashing during sleep may be observed. Injuries to patients and bed partners have been reported. This disorder is more common among the elderly, and in some cases may be associated with other neurological disorders.

The parasomnias specific to NREM sleep are more likely related to the difficulty in awakening fully from the deeper sleep with intense slow wave activity, and correspondingly these events are more likely to occur during the first few hours of the night. Most of the NREM parasomnias are more common in children, but may be seen in adults as well. Typically there is incomplete or delayed awakening, resulting in an apparent confusional state. Sleepwalking is one example. Confusional arousals are extended periods when one does not fully awaken. Sleep terrors occur suddenly with the individual sitting up or even bolting from bed, possibly screaming. The person appears intensely frightened, but usually unaware of his surroundings and is unresponsive to others who may be attempting to calm him. He may return to sleep with no memory of an event that might be quite memorable to others sleeping nearby. If the person does awaken fully during the event, generally he can describe a very concentrated fear, perhaps from being chased, but usually there is not the lengthy and complex narrative typical of a dream. Sleep-related eating occurs primarily in adults and may combine sleep walking with eating behavior. After initially sleeping, the individual arises, seeks food, and eats. It is more common among women. She may or may not have a clear memory of the event, and may be aware of the eating only because of crumbs, missing food, and empty wrappers. It tends to occur nightly for many years.

Decisions regarding the treatment of the parasomnias depend upon the frequency, severity, and dangerousness of the events. Of course, treatment of underlying medical, neurological, and psychiatric disorders should be optimized. Some REM and NREM parasomnias occur during stressful periods, so treatment efforts may be intensified at these times. Sleep deprivation with subsequent increased deep sleep may increase the frequency of the NREM events, so regular sleep schedule habits may be therapeutic. In significantly disruptive and/or dangerous situations, REM behavior disorder and sleep terrors in adults may be treated successfully with clonazepam 0.5-1.0 mg at bedtime. Safety precautions to minimize injury during partial arousals also should be considered.

Sleep Evaluation

The first and most important step in the recognition of potential sleep disorders is asking patients about their sleep and wakefulness. Questions regarding sleep should be included in the routine history and review of systems (ROS). A sleep category should be added to chart ROS forms and sleep questions should be incorporated into patient-completed history questionnaires. A few screening items about nighttime sleep and daytime alertness may be satisfactory to determine whether a significant clinical problem exists. At that point, more detailed questioning about specific symptoms may be pursued. With insomnia complaints, the duration and pattern will be important in developing a differential diagnosis. The sleep disturbance must be considered in the context of the 24-hour sleep-wake cycle. Daytime sleepiness should be reviewed in terms of actual situations during which inadvertent sleep would be likely. This may range from mild (reading) to severe (driving). A bed partner may be an invaluable informant, especially regarding snoring, breathing patterns, and physical movements during sleep. Having the patient maintain a sleep log can be helpful in identifying patterns, such as obviously inadequate time in bed and the advanced and delayed sleep phase syndromes. A routine physical examination also is an essential component of the evaluation of a sleep disturbance.

Consultation with a sleep specialist may be valuable in challenging clinical situations in patients with insomnia, excessive daytime sleepiness, and parasomnias. Excessive daytime sleepiness can be especially dangerous and cause marked impairment in daytime functioning; therefore, the threshold for sleep laboratory testing should be very low in theses cases. Accordingly, suspected SDB and narcolepsy should be referred for sleep testing. The sleep specialist may be helpful with further evaluation and treatment of patients with intractable insomnia symptoms.

Sleep and the Worldwide Web

A wide variety of sleep medicine resources are available for physicians, patients, and the general public on the Internet. Table 4 lists the Web addresses of several consumer information, professional society, governmental, and sleep disorder-oriented organizations.

References

1. National Commission on Sleep Disorders Research. Report of the National Commission on Sleep Disorders Research. DHHS Publication. Washington DC: U.S. Government Printing Office, 1992.
2. American Psychiatric Association. *Diagnostic and Statistical Manual of Mental Disorders*. 4th ed. Washington, DC: American Psychiatric Association, 1994.
3. Diagnostic Classification Steering Committee, Thorpy MJ, Chairman. *International Classification of Sleep Disorders: Diagnostic and Coding Manual*. Rochester, Minn: American Sleep Disorders Association, 1990.
4. Buysse DJ, et al. Diagnostic concordance for sleep disorders using proposed DSM-IV categories: A report from APA/NIMH DSM-IV field trial. *Am J Psychiatry* 1994;151:1351-1360.
5. Dijk D-J, Edgar DM. Circadian and homeostatic control of wakefulness and sleep. In: Turek FW, Zee PC, eds. *Regulation of Sleep and Circadian Rhythms*. New York, NY: Marcel Dekker; 1999:111-147.
6. Borbely AA, Achermann P. Sleep homeostasis and models of sleep regulation. *J Biol Rhythms* 1999;14:557-568.
7. Czeisler CA, et al. Stability, precision, and near-24-hour period of the human circadian pacemaker. *Science* 1999;284(5423):2177-2181.
8. Bliwise DL. Sleep in normal aging and dementia. *Sleep* 1993;16:40-81.
9. Neubauer DN. Sleep problems in the elderly. *Am Fam Physician* 1999;59:2551-2558.
10. Foley DJ, et al. Sleep complaints among elderly persons: an epidemiologic study of three communities. *Sleep* 1995;18:425-432.
11. Bonnet MH, Arand DL. Hyperarousal and insomnia. *Sleep Med Rev* 1997;1:97-108.
12. Neubauer DN, et al. Sleep disorders. In: Barker LR, et al, eds. *Principles of Ambulatory Medicine*. 5th ed. Baltimore, Md: Williams & Wilkins; 1999:1314-1328.
13. Ford DE, Kamerow DB. Epidemiologic study of sleep disturbances and psychiatric disorders: An opportunity for prevention? *JAMA* 1989;262:1479-1484.
14. Obermeyer WH, Benca RM. Effects of drugs on sleep. *Neurol Clin* 1996;14:827-840.
15. Zammit GK, et al. Quality of life in people with insomnia. *Sleep* 1999;22(suppl 2):S379-S385.
16. Breslau N, et al. Sleep disturbance and psychiatric disorders: A longitudinal epidemiological study of young adults. *Biol Psychiatry* 1996;39:411-418.
17. Weisman MM, et al. The morbidity of insomnia uncomplicated by psychiatric disorders. *Gen Hosp Psychiatry* 1997;19:245-250.
18. Roberts RE, et al. Sleep complaints and depression in an aging cohort: A prospective perspective. *Am J Psychiatry* 2000;157:81-88.
19. Walsh JK, Engelhardt CL. The direct economic costs of insomnia in the United States for 1995. *Sleep* 1999;22(suppl 2):S386-S393.
20. Simon GE, VonKorff M. Prevalence, burden, and treatment of insomnia in primary care. *Am J Psychiatry* 1997;154:1417-1423.
21. Kupfer DJ, Reynolds CF 3d. Management of insomnia. *N Engl J Med* 1997;336:247-253.
22. Morin CM, et al. Nonpharmacologic treatment of chronic insomnia. *Sleep* 1999;8:1134-1156.
23. Chesson Jr. AL, et al. Practice parameters for the nonpharmacologic treatment of chronic insomnia. *Sleep* 1999;8:1128-1133.
24. Nowell PD, et al. Benzodiazepines and zolpidem for chronic insomnia: a meta-analysis of treatment efficacy. *JAMA* 1997;278:2170-2177.
25. Bunney WE Jr, et al. Report of the Institute of Medicine Committee on the efficacy and safety of halcion. *Arch Gen Psychiatry* 1999;56:349-352.
26. Strollo PJ Jr, Rogers RM. Current concepts: Obstructive sleep apnea. *N Engl J Med* 1996;334:99-104.
27. Young T, et al. The occurrence of sleep-disordered breathing among middle-aged adults. *N Engl J Med* 1993;328:1230-1235.
28. Fletcher EC. The relationship between systemic hypertension and obstructive sleep apnea: Facts and theory. *Am J Med* 1995;98:118-128.
29. Walters AS. Toward a better definition of restless legs syndrome. *Mov Disord* 1995;10:634-642.

Suggested Reading

1. Kryger MH, et al, eds. *Principles and Practice of Sleep Medicine*, 2nd ed. Philadelphia, Pa: W.B. Saunders; 1994.
2. World Health Organization. Insomnia: Report of an international consensus conference. *Sleep* 1999;(suppl 3):S415-S450.
3. Sateia MJ, et al. Evaluation of chronic insomnia. *Sleep* 2000;23:243-308.

Neuromuscular Transmission Failure

Masood Haque, MD

Muscle weakness, double vision, and respiratory failure of acute onset: the classical triad of neuromuscular transmission failure, these symptoms frequently are the only indication of a life-threatening illness that requires aggressive supportive care and pharmacologic intervention. So often, unfortunately, such conditions as myasthenia gravis, paraneoplastic syndromes causing muscle weakness, medication-induced disorders of the neuromuscular junction, and botulism are not recognized by the physician, which leads to delays in intervention and suboptimal clinical outcomes.

Although disease states associated with neuromuscular malfunction only occasionally initially present in the emergency department (ED), these conditions are potentially fatal ailments; therefore, they must be considered in all patients who present with isolated or generalized muscle weakness of unknown etiology. Ranging from immune-mediated disorders such as myasthenia gravis to toxin-based poisonings such as botulism, these conditions have the ability to impair neuromuscular transmission at presynaptic or postsynaptic sites. Pharmacologic stimulation tests (Tensilon®), electrophysiologic testing, historical features, and the physical examination usually can pinpoint a specific diagnosis and guide therapy.

With these issues in mind, the purpose of this chapter is to provide a practical review of disease states characterized by neuromuscular transmission failure and a systematic approach to initial diagnosis and management in the ED.

Overview

The neuromuscular junction is the critical link between the central nervous system and the musculoskeletal system. From an electrochemical perspective, a wave of depolarization along the neuronal sheath induces release of neurotransmitters at the nerve terminal. Upon release, the neurotransmitter, acetylcholine, binds to the muscle fiber and initiates another wave of depolarization, which culminates in muscular contraction. Maintaining integrity of neuromuscular transmission is essential for effective communication between nerve and muscle and is required for maintaining skeletal muscle function, including the mechanism of breathing. Moreover, a failure or deterioration of neuromuscular transmission must be considered in the differential diagnosis of rapidly progressive muscular weakness, especially when bulbar musculature or the respiratory apparatus is involved. *(Please see Figure 1.)* Although disorders of neuromuscular transmission are rare, these conditions may be fatal, due to compromise of the respiratory system. Fortunately, the majority of these disorders initially present with more benign symptoms, permitting life-saving intervention early in the course of the illness. In milder forms of transmission failure, subtle bulbar manifestations will predominate, among them double or blurry vision, drooping eyelids, difficulty chewing or swallowing, or changes in speech. In their more fulminant form, disorders of neuromuscular transmission present as a

Figure 1. Differential Diagnosis of Muscular Weakness

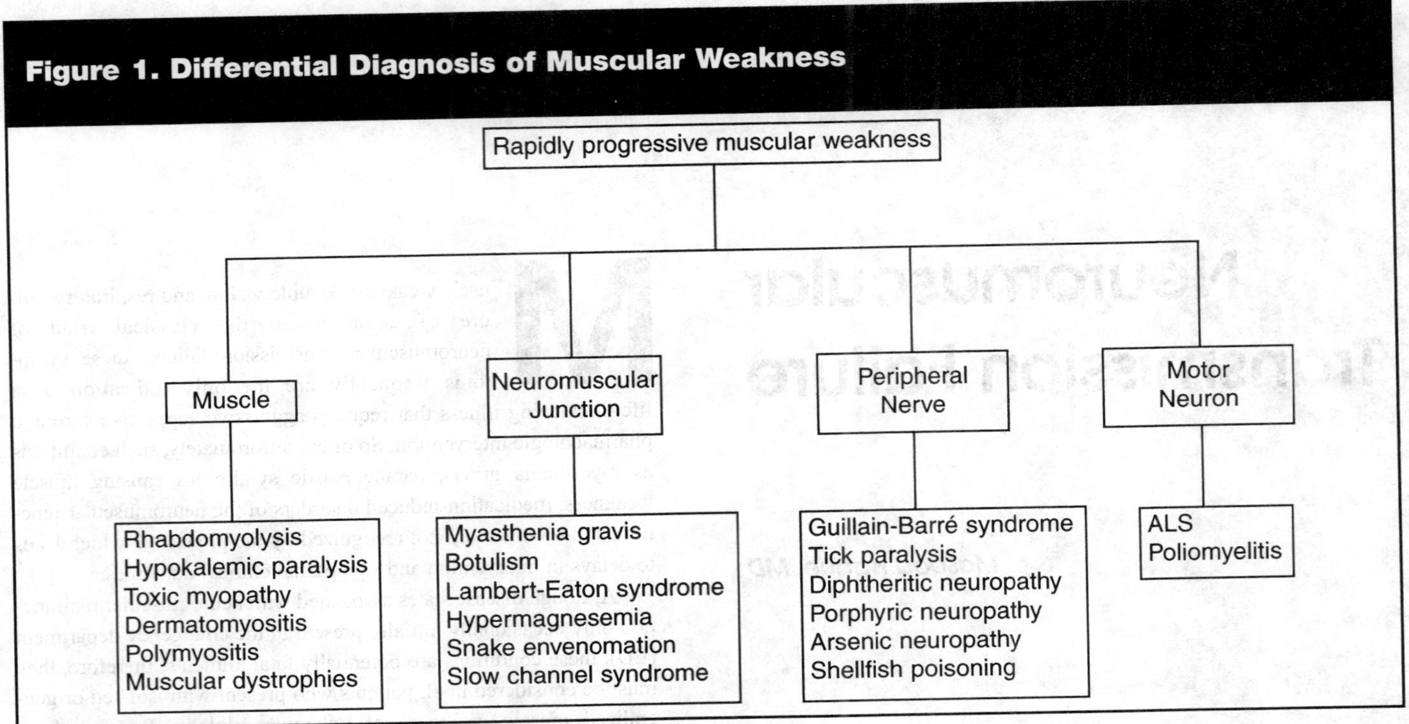

failure to maintain structural integrity of the airway or mechanism of breathing, each of which can result in respiratory failure.

An understanding of normal neuromuscular anatomy and electrophysiology is essential for optimizing clinical management of patients suffering from disorders of neuromuscular transmission.

The Neuromuscular Junction

The neuromuscular junction consists of the presynaptic membrane, the postsynaptic membrane, and the synaptic cleft. The heavily myelinated motor axon of the anterior horn cell branches into many nerve terminals, each of which terminates at a single muscle fiber. The nerve terminal is comprised of a presynaptic membrane, which is separated from the muscular postsynaptic membrane by the synaptic cleft. The portion of the muscle fiber that directly surrounds the nerve terminal is the motor end plate; it is located approximately half way along the length of the muscle fiber. The neuromuscular junction is a nicotinic synapse, which distinguishes it from muscurinic synapses that interface between the CNS and the autonomic system. Transmission failure at the nicotinic synapse produces a predictable type of muscular weakness, whereas impaired transmission at the muscurinic synapse results in systemic anticholinergic symptoms. Generally speaking, disorders limited to the postsynaptic membrane involve limited nicotinic receptors, whereas synaptic and presynaptic derangements may involve both nicotinic and muscurinic receptors. A critical neurochemical feature of the the presynaptic membrane is inclusion of an active zone—voltage gated calcium channels (VGCC)—that facilitates rapid influx of calcium as the depolarization wave reaches the nerve terminal. Increased calcium concentration is required for release of acetylcholine (ACh). Through interactions with the membrane proteins, vesicles containing ACh fuse with the presynaptic nerve terminal and the transmitter is released into the synaptic cleft. Each vesicle contains about 5000-20,000 ACh molecules and represents a quanta of the neurotransmitter. Vesicles containing ACh are segregated into two pools in the nerve terminal, one that is available immediately and another reserve pool that is mobilized during sustained muscular activity.[1,2]

The acetylcholine receptors (ACh-Rs) located on the postsynaptic membrane, are transmembrane allosteric glycoproteins with a molecular weight of 250 kd. Each receptor is comprised of five subunits arranged around a central channel; each of the two alpha subunits has an ACh-binding site located extracellularly, which is localized in the vicinity of amino acids 192 and 193.[3] Sequencing and cloning of genes that script for all receptor subunits in human ACh-Rs have been accomplished over the past several years. Genetic engineering technology has made it possible to produce fusion proteins consisting of large stretches of entire subunits of ACh-Rs. These structurally and functionally intact ACh-Rs have been produced by inserting subunits of messenger RNA into cells such as frog oocytes; clearly, receptors generated using these techniques may have important therapeutic implications in the future.[4]

Finally, ACh-Rs are continually turning over at the neuromuscular junction. Among other factors, motor innervation and stimulation appear to be important regulators of ACh-R synthesis, sub-unit composition, as well as distribution and degradation of postsynaptic receptors. In fact, impaired transmission has been shown to increase transcription of the ACh-R genes, a response that facilitates complete recovery or neuromuscular transmission in patients whose postsynaptic receptors have been destroyed by autoimmune mechanisms.[5]

Neuromuscular Transmission. In the resting muscle, small fluctuations in membrane potential occur at the end-plate region. These fluctuations, also called miniature end-plate potentials (MEPPs), are produced by spontaneous release of packets or quanta of ACh from the motor nerve terminal. As the nerve action potential arrives, it transiently depolarizes the nerve terminal, which opens up the VGCC. The rapid influx of calcium into the nerve terminal stimulates the fusion of

Table 1. Etiologies of Neuromuscular Transmission Failure

• Congenital	Congenital myasthenia gravis, acetylcholinesterase deficiency
• Infectious	*C. botulinum*
• Autoimmune	Myasthenia gravis, Lambert-Eaton syndrome
• Toxins	Snake/Scorpion envenomation, organophosphate poisoning
• Drugs	Magnesium, D-penicillamine, aminoglycosides, chloroquine, fluoroquinolones

Table 2. Division of Neurotransmission Derangements by Categories

Presynaptic	Synaptic	Postsynaptic
Lambert-Eaton syndrome	Organophosphate poisoning	Myasthenia gravis
Botulism	Acetylcholinesterase deficiency	Congenital myasthenia
Hypermagnesemia		Snake venom
Scorpion toxin		

ACh-containing vesicles with the axonal terminal and the subsequent release of hundreds of quanta of ACh into the synaptic cleft.[6,7]

After diffusing across the synaptic cleft, ACh binds to receptors located on the postsynaptic membrane. The ion channel of the ACh-R is closed during the resting state; binding of ACh to the postsynaptic receptor sites alters the receptor configuration, thereby opening the central ion channel and permitting sodium (Na) influx. This produces a local electrical current within the end-plate region known as the end-plate potential (EPP), which then activates the peri-junctional Na channels and initiates propagation of an action potential that activates the muscle fiber and generates a compound muscle action potential (CMAP). The action potential then propagates across the muscle fiber bidirectionally. The depolarization of muscle fiber results in the release of calcium from the sarcoplasmic reticulum, which, in turn, produces muscle contraction. The ACh molecules that are bound to the receptors are hydrolyzed by the enzyme, acetylcholinesterase, into its component. The choline entity then undergoes re-uptake by the nerve terminal and is recycled.[8]

A critical EPP amplitude is required to trigger a CMAP. Attaining the threshold EPP depends upon two factors: 1) a sufficient quantity of neurotransmitters; and 2) an adequate number of receptors on the postsynaptic membrane. If either of these features is quantitatively or qualitatively impaired, the electrical current at the EPP will not reach the critical amplitude required to trigger an action potential. Pathophysiologically, the result is suboptimal recruitment of enough muscle fibers to sustain muscular activity. Symptomatically, this failure of transmission clinically manifests as weakness. Fortunately, the EPP generated is almost five times greater than required to trigger an action potential, representing a comfortable "safety margin." In particular, susceptibility of the bulbar musculature to neuromuscular transmission disorders, in part, can be explained by its low safety margin, which makes this group more sensitive to depletion of either transmitter or receptor.

Disorders of Neuromuscular Transmission: A Classification Scheme

As outlined, neuromuscular transmission is a complex process that requires multiple components and biochemical pathways to support normal muscular function. The transmission is sensitive to failure at several levels. Neurotransmission disorders can be broadly divided into two major categories, those characterized by inadequate transmitter release and those in which there is an inadequate number of receptors. Failure may occur at the level of transmitter release or may result from compromised interaction between ACh and the receptor. Although transmission failure may be congenital, it usually is related to autoimmune disorders or toxins. In addition, there are several drugs that can compromise neuromuscular transmission, and their introduction may unmask a vulnerability to neuromuscular transmission failure or exacerbate failure of an existing neuromuscular transmission deficiency state.

For clinical and diagnostic purposes, it is convenient to divide derangements of neurotransmission into three different categories, according to location and nature of dysfunction. *(Please see Tables 1 and 2.)*

Postsynaptic Disorders. This is the most common etiology of clinical disorders characterized by neuromuscular transmission dysfunction. Failure is usually due to loss of ACh-R, either because of autoimmune-mediated destruction (myasthenia gravis) or congenital deficiency of ACh-Rs. Although autoimmune-mediated destruction usually is idiopathic, several medications also have been implicated, most notably D-penicillamine. Moreover, postsynaptic receptors also are vulnerable to such toxins as snake venom, which produces a slowly evolving, non-depolarizing block of neuromuscular transmission. Clinical impairment of neuromuscular function results from occupation and blockade by alpha-bungarotoxin and cobra neurotoxins of ACh-Rs on the post synaptic membrane of the muscle fiber.

Presynaptic Disorders. Failure at the presynaptic terminal almost always represents insufficient transmitter (ACh) release. In its congenital form, this is characterized by inadequate synthesis and/or packaging of neurotransmitter vesicles. In its acquired form, this disorder results from an interruption of transmitter release. This malfunction may be a consequence of impaired calcium influx (magnesium intoxication, Eaton-Lambert syndrome) or inhibition of transmitter exocytosis (botulinum toxin). ACh release may also be inhibited by exposure to black widow spider venom (alpha-latroxin) or scorpion toxin, both of which cause depletions of the neurotransmitter from the nerve terminal. Failure at the presynaptic level leads to compromised synaptic transmission in both nicotinic and muscurinic receptors; as a result, muscular weakness may be accompanied by anticholinergic symptoms.

Synaptic Transmission Disorders. This group of disorders is characterized by persistent acetylcholine in the synapse. The consequence is depolarization block of the neuromuscular junction. Synaptic disorders result from the inability to clear the neurotransmitter from the synaptic cleft. The disorder is caused by toxins that

Table 3. Clinical Features of Neuromuscular Transmission Failure

- Cranial and proximity muscle weakness
- Respiratory muscle involvement
- Postsynaptic: Improvement in strength after rest
- Presynaptic: Improvement after initiation of activity
- Presynaptic: Autonomic involvement

disable acetylcholinesterase or from a congenital lack of acetylcholinesterase.

Neuromuscular Transmission Failure: Clinical Presentation

The hallmark of weakness associated with failure in neuromuscular transmission is fatigability. The patient may present to the ED with complaints of gradual weakness followed by the precipitous onset of muscular exhaustion. Typically, muscle weakness resolves briefly after a short rest and then worsens again. Frequently, the patients can be specific about the muscle weakness, narrowing the involvement to a single muscle group. Typically, symptoms will be directed at the bulbar musculature or respiratory function, although some patients have predominant extremity weakness. The key is to consider neuromuscular transmission in the clinical context of bulbar symptoms (blurry or double vision, difficulty speaking or swallowing, or alteration in taste). There are specific questions the ED physician should ask to determine whether failure of neuromuscular transmission is responsible for the symptoms related to muscle dysfunction. For example, it is helpful to determine if the patient's vision becomes blurry after prolonged reading, or is it more difficult to swallow at the *end* of a meal? Does the tonality of speech change with talking? Neuromuscular transmission failure should also be considered in patients who report complaints of more generalized symptoms such as chronic fatigue and shortness of breath, especially when there is no other obvious explanation for the clinical presentation.[9]

It is essential to inquire about associated autonomic symptoms, such as constipation, erectile dysfunction, dry mucosal surfaces, or loss of sweating. All of the presynaptic neuromuscular disorders are accompanied by autonomic symptomatology, and, therefore, complaints of autonomic dysfunction can help localize the precise area of transmission failure and may even help delineate a specific etiology. Consideration should also be given to medications that might interfere with neuromuscular transmission, most notable among them, D-pencilliamine, fluoroquinolones, magnesium, and aminoglycosides. An inquiry should made into the patient's dietary habits and any dietary profile should be asked about, as well as any exposure to toxins, including those associated with animal and insect bites. If the patient is unable to provide any history, the clinician should, nevertheless, maintain a high index of suspicion for neuromuscular transmission failure in individuals with etiology of any rapidly progressive weakness. *(Please see Table 3.)*

Physical examination of patients with a suspected neuromuscular transmission disorder should incorporate provocative testing as a diagnostic maneuver to elicit muscle weakness. For example, if a patient complains of weakness in a set of muscles, repeated activity of this group should induce profound muscular fatigue soon after the onset of exertion. In this regard, if a patient complains of droopiness in an eyelid, the ED physician should have the patient stare at the ceiling for few minutes and then re-examine the patient to see if the ptosis worsens. In individuals who present with unexplained shortness of breath (SOB), especially when accompanied by unexplained fatigue of the respiratory musculature, it is important to measure the vital capacity in order to rule out muscular weakness. Clinical features of neuromuscular respiratory failure include confusion and headache, respiratory muscle weakness without evidence of parenchymal disease (i.e., no rales or wheezes can be appreciated), prominent use of accessory muscles of respiration, and paradoxical abdominal movement due to diaphragmatic weakness.[10]

Diagnostic Evaluation. Routine hematological studies and blood chemistry may help rule out underlying systemic illness or sepsis. Respiratory function assessment is an essential component of the initial ED database, and measurement of vital capacity should be performed in every patient presenting with respiratory symptoms that may be related to neuromuscular failure. Patients who present with vital capacity of 2 L or less should have additional tests and elective intubation should be given strong consideration.[11,12]

Although usually not performed in the ED setting, electrodiagnostic testing provides vital information that can help establish the diagnosis and, more specifically, localize the disorder to the neuromuscular junction. The electrodiagnostic procedures most often used to evaluate the integrity of neurotransmission are repetitive nerve stimulation and analysis of "Jitter" with single-fiber electromyography (SFEMG).[4] *(See SFEMG section below.)*

Repetitive Nerve Stimulation (RNS). RNS is the most frequently used electrodiagnostic test for assessment of neuromuscular transmission. Abnormal results usually are not diagnostic of a specific clinical disorder, but they can localize the disorder to the neuromuscular junction and help distinguish between pre- and postsynaptic disorders.

In presynaptic disorders of the neuromuscular junction, such as botulism or Lambert-Eaton syndrome (LES), nerve conduction studies are normal except for the finding of a low motor evoked response that can be demonstrated to increase after 10-15 seconds of isometric contraction of the muscle that is stimulated. This post activation facilitation is a hallmark of presynaptic disorders.

In postsynaptic conditions such as myasthenia gravis (MG), initial motor amplitudes are generally normal, but there is a decremental motor response exceeding 10% with nerve stimulation at low rates of 2-3 Hz.[13]

Single Fiber Electromyography (SFEMG). This test is performed by placing a fine needle electrode between two muscle fibers innervated by a single nerve. The variation in the action potential of the two muscle fibers is recorded and is referred to as a "Jitter." It detects delayed or failed neuromuscular transmission in pairs of muscle fibers supplied by branches of a single nerve fiber. Although a sensitive test, it is not very specific for a failure of neuromuscular transmission.[13]

Prognosis. Prognosis of patients with neuromuscular transmission depends upon the severity of the underlying condition. If the condition is autoimmune in nature, a number of treatment options are available, including immunosuppression. If a toxin is involved in neuromuscular transmission failure, the treatment will include supportive care and administration of a specific antitoxin. Finally, it is important to consider the role that drugs may play in compromising neuromuscular transmission. Implicated medications should be discontinued in patients in whom the diagnosis of neuromuscular transmission failure has been established.

Myasthenia Gravis

MG is the most common disorder producing clinical symptoms caused by failure at the postsynaptic membrane of the neuromuscular junction. Autoimmune-mediated destruction of ACh-Rs is the key pathophysiologic event producing a fluctuating, fatigable weakness of voluntary muscles. The literal meaning of MG is "grave muscle weakness." Although this condition has been described in medical literature for more than 300 years, it is only over the last three decades that the underlying pathophysiology has been elucidated. Currently, it is the best understood of all the autoimmune diseases and has become a prototype for evaluating other autoimmune derangements.

The incidence of myasthenia is estimated to be about 14 per 100,000 in the general population; total cases of myasthenia in the United States are estimated to be 36,000.[14] The incidence is age- and sex-related with two distinct peaks. The first peak is observed in the second and third decades and a later peak is reported in the sixth and seventh decades, when the disease is more likely to afflict men; in contrast, women predominate in the early peak.[15] Later onset MG does not differ in its clinical presentation, although the disease may be more severe. There is an increased incidence of associated thymoma and serologic positivity when the disease presents later in life.[16]

Clinical Pathophysiology. MG is a well established, prototypical autoimmune disease. Antibodies directed against the ACh-R destroy postsynaptic receptors, reducing the number of available binding sites at the neuromuscular junction. Antibody mediated loss of ACh-R is mediated by three mechanism: 1) accelerated endocytosis and degradation of the receptors; 2) complement-mediated damage; and 3) functional blockade of ACh-R (probably only a minor effect).[17] Morphologic changes at the postsynaptic membrane of patients with MG demonstrate a simplified membrane with loss of receptor sites, synaptic folds, and an increased gap between the nerve terminal and the postsynaptic membrane. This reduction of postsynaptic ACh-R results in EPPs of diminished amplitude; consequently, there is a failure to trigger action potentials in some muscle fibers, a characteristic feature of MG.

There is a substantial body of evidence confirming the autoimmune nature of MG, including its association with other autoimmune diseases; a chronic, fluctuating course; and demonstration of anti-ACh-R antibodies. Other evidence suggesting an autoimmune process includes the presence of complement at the receptor; the reduction of ACh-R on the postsynaptic membrane; and the favorable, clinical response to immunosuppression (perhaps the most convincing evidence for autoimmunity transferability of MG to mice using IgG from patients with MG).

Although the role of antibody-mediated destruction of the ACh-R is well-established, the triggering factor for this autoimmune attack remains elusive. However, there is compelling evidence that the thymus gland plays a central pathophysiological role. In this regard, thymic hyperplasia has been reported in 70% of MG patients, and a thymoma is identified in up to 15%.[18,19] The beneficial effects of thymectomy and the fact that the disease is more aggressive clinically in those with thymic hyperplasia and thymic malignancies substantiate the role of thymic abnormalities.[18-21]

Table 4. Signs and Symptoms of Myasthenia Gravis

• Ptosis, diplopia, blurred vision	53%
• Leg weakness	10%
• Generalized fatigue	10%
• Dysphagia	5%
• Slurred or nasal speech	5%
• Difficulty chewing	5%

Clinical Features. MG is a symmetrical descending paralysis with a prominent bulbar component. Almost 75% of patients have bulbar palsy at the time of initial presentation. Intermittent diplopia and ptosis are the most common manifestations and most patients develop these signs within two years of onset of MG. Drooping of the eyelid with a persistent upward gaze and double vision while reading indicate fatigability at the myasthenic, neuromuscular junction.[1,2,8,22] *(Please see Table 4.)* Other prominent, bulbar manifestations include weakness of the tongue and soft palate, which may lead to a change in voice; patients may complain of nasal or slurred speech, especially with continued talking. During a meal, persistent chewing may make the jaw muscles so weak that the patients may have to manually support masticatory functions. Weakness of muscles involved in coughing and swallowing may lead to dysphonia and/or choking on food and secretions, while diminished strength in neck muscles may cause fatigue and require manual assistance for holding up the head. Hearing may be impaired. Weakness of the tensor tympani may cause muffling of low tones, and stapedius weakness may cause hyperacusis.[23]

Limb weakness is the initial symptom in fewer than 10% of the patients.[11,16,24] Although any limb or truncate muscle may be weak, upper extremity weakness is more prominent than lower extremity weakness, and this weakness tends to be symmetrical and proximal when present. Dyspnea is an uncommon initial presentation, although when present, tends to be exertional.[9]

On physical examination, findings usually are limited to the motor system; generally, there is no loss of reflexes and no alteration of sensation or coordination. Ptosis tends to be asymmetrical and worsens with upward gaze after 30 seconds; extraocular muscle weakness is symmetrical and fluctuating. Pupillary responses are normal. A combination of ocular palsy with ptosis in the presence of a normal pupillary response strongly suggests a disorder of neuromuscular transmission, including muscular dystrophy. Other maneuvers that may be used to unmask underlying neuromuscular fatigability include having the patient count up to 100 or chew for 30 seconds and observing signs of functional deterioration.

Onset of the aforementioned symptoms usually is insidious and can take place over weeks or months. Occasionally, symptoms are initiated by emotional upset or infection (usually respiratory), or symptoms may appear during pregnancy or in response to drugs used during anesthesia. Once symptoms become manifest, progression inevitably follows.

In one landmark study evaluating clinical course of MG with 1487 patients, investigators characterized the pattern of weakness, outcomes, and severity of symptoms during the first three years after onset of illness. In 15% of patients, weakness remained localized to the extraocular muscles, whereas in 85%, the disease became generalized, usually within the first year. Maximum severity of the illness was observed in about 50% of patients within the first year and in 85% within the first five years. Moreover, the course of the illness is extremely variable. Rapid spread from one muscle group to another occurs in some individuals, but in others the disease remains unchanged for months before progression ensues. Remissions may take place without explanation, but this happens in less than 50% of cases. If the disease remits for a year or longer and then recurs, it tends to be progressive.[18]

The risk of death from MG is greatest in the first year after the onset of the disease. A second phase characterized by life-threatening progression occurs 4-7 years after onset. After this time, the disease tends to stabilize and risk of severe relapse diminishes.[18]

Diagnostic Evaluation. In addition to the distinct clinical features of MG, there are several other modalities that aid in establishing the diagnosis of MG.

Tensilon Test. (Please see Figure 2.) Intravenous edrophonium (Tensilon) is an anticholinesterase inhibitor with rapid a onset of action (i.e., about 30 seconds) and a short duration of action (i.e., about 5 minutes). Administration produces rapid improvement of ocular symptoms in patients with MG. Theoretically, although any muscle group can be tested, this provocative test is most useful and is most sensitive when improvement of ptosis and double vision are used as diagnostic end points.[25] Despite its advantages, edrophonium should be used with caution, especially in cardiac patients, because of its potential for causing bradycardia. Accordingly, the patient should be placed on a monitor when this test is performed and atropine should be available at the bedside. A "test dose" of 0.1 or 0.2 mg of edrophonium should always be given, due to extreme sensitivity in certain patients. Interpretation of this test may be difficult due to a possible placebo effect or the subjective nature of improvement in muscular strength. The key is to identify precisely which muscle or muscles are being tested. Objective improvement in strength is more important than the patient's perception of improvement, which may be due to the placebo effect.

Immunologic Testing. Measurement of ACh-R antibodies is a highly specific test for MG. Ach-R antibodies are present in 90-95% of patients with MG, but the percentage is lower (70%) in patients with the purely ocular form of the disease. In the right clinical context, the test is specific enough to obviate the need for further diagnostic testing. Generally, there is no correlation between the level of antibody titers and disease activity. Overall, up to 19% of the patients with MG do not have ACh-R antibody detectable by radioimmunoassay. Nevertheless, the clinical presentation and natural history of the disease in these patients are similar to those patients who are seropositive. It is interesting to note that almost all patients with thymoma have elevated ACh-R antibody levels.

Electrophysiologic Studies. Repetitive nerve stimulation shows a decremental response in MG; a 15% decrease in successive action potential is considered a positive response. SFEMG shows increased "Jitter" in up to 95% of the patients with MG.

Management. Currently, there are five, major therapeutic options in managing patients with MG. These modalities have significantly improved the prognosis and quality of life of patients with this condition.

Anticholinesterase Agents. Anticholinesterases are considered first-line agents for treatment of MG. Their primary action is to increase the concentration of ACh at the synapse; pyridostigmine is the most frequently used agent in this class. The exact dosage and dosing schedule of this medication can be tailored to the needs and clinical response of the patient. The starting dose is 15-60 mg q4h. Despite an initial improvement in symptoms, however, many patients find that muscle weakness does resolve and that anticholinesterase agents lose their efficacy over time. Consequently, additional treatment modalities are almost always required.

Immunosuppression. Immunosuppressive therapy has been used to treat patients with MG since the 1950s. It usually is added to the medication regimen of patients whose symptoms are inadequately controlled by anticholinesterase drugs. Among immunosuppressive agents, corticosteroids represent initial agents of choice; however, other agents such as azathioprine, cyclosporine, or cyclophosphamide also can be introduced, if steroids are contraindicated or ineffective.

Corticosteroids reduce the levels of ACh-R antibodies. Initiation of steroid therapy may require hospitalization because of risk of inducing transient exacerbation of MG. This risk is the greatest during the first few weeks following initiation of therapy and may be seen in up to one-half of patients started on corticosteroids. Gradually increasing the steroid dose, with close clinical follow-up, tends to diminish these risks. Recently, a double-blind study using single IV methylprednisolone pulse therapy has shown promise and may be useful in selected patients.[26]

Thymectomy. Thymectomy is indicated in selected patients younger than 60 years of age who have the generalized form of MG, as well as in those individuals who have thymoma. The improvement may be dramatic after the thymectomy, but the course remains unpredictable. If weakness persists one year after the surgical procedure, the disease is unlikely to remit. Overall, about 59% of patients with MG have sustained improvement after thymectomy.[18-20]

Short-term Treatment. Plasmapheresis and IV immunoglobulin are two short-term therapeutic options that are particularly useful when rapid clearance of antibody is required either to improve symptoms in myasthenic crisis or in patients in whom immunosuppressive treatment has been initiated. It is also useful in patients who are being prepared for surgery.

Plasmapheresis removes circulating anti-ACh-R antibodies from the plasma. This therapeutic option is indicated when a rapid, significant reduction of circulating antibodies is required. Despite several open, uncontrolled clinical trials suggesting plasmapheresis induces short-term improvement in patients with MG, as well as numerous anecdotal reports, a controlled trial has never been performed.[27,28] A newer modality, which uses protein A immunoadsorption, can remove IgG, with high efficacy, from plasma, without significant modification of other plasma proteins.[27] A majority of patients with MG show temporary improvement after plasma exchange; maximum improvement may be achieved as early as the first exchange or it may be delayed for several weeks. Clinical improvement can be maintained for weeks to months following plasmapheresis.[29,30]

Intravenous Immune Globulin (IVIG). Several studies have shown a favorable response to IVIG. Although several attractive hypotheses

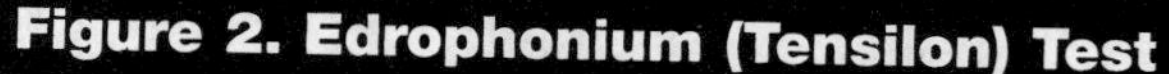

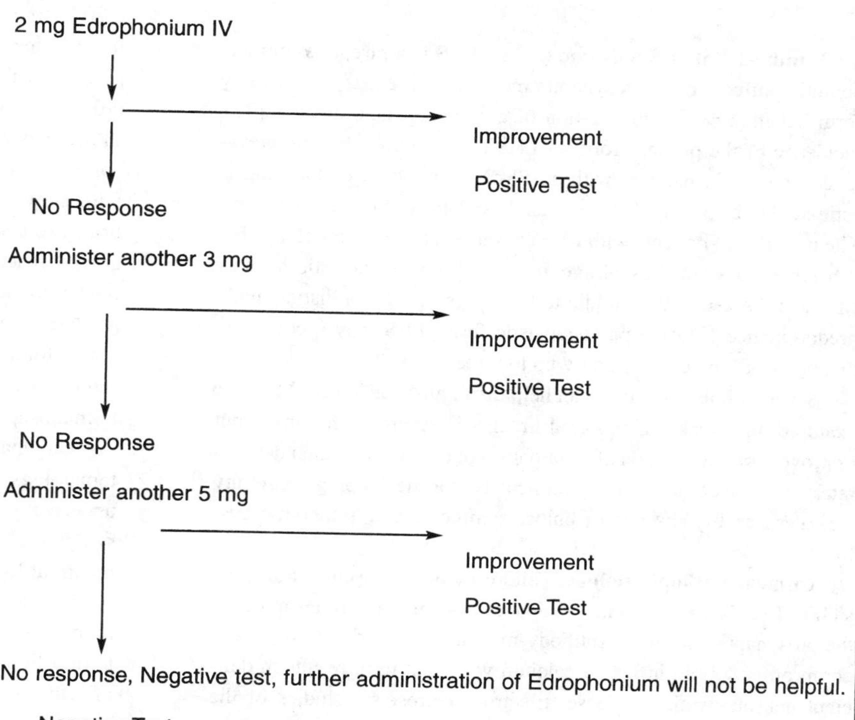

have been proposed for its benefits, including down regulation of antibody production, the mechanism of IVIG in MG remains unknown. The usual dose is 400 mg/kg/d for five days, and the improvement begins within 4-5 days following administration.[27,30]

Myasthenic Crisis. Involving respiratory muscles (including those maintaining the upper airway, intercostal muscles, or the diaphragm), myasthenic crisis is a true emergency and usually requires respiratory support. Up to 20% of myasthenic patients will experience at least one episode of myasthenic crisis.[31] Patients who survive one episode of myasthenic crisis are at risk for a recurrent attack; as many as one-third of these patients will experience another episode. About 75% of myasthenic crises occur within the first two years after the onset of disease, with a median of eight months following onset of initial symptoms. Patients with an associated thymoma are at a much higher risk of experiencing myasthenic crisis.[31]

In the majority of patients with myasthenic crisis, an underlying precipitating event can be identified. Infection is the most common risk factor, followed by aspiration pneumonitis and changes in medication (especially initiation or withdrawal of corticosteroid). In up to one-third of the patients with myasthenic crisis, no precipitating factor can be identified.

Patients in whom the diagnosis of MG has been established and who are taking anticholinesterase agents present a management dilemma, especially in the setting of suspected crisis. Often, these patients will increase their medication dosage as the weakness progresses. This can lead to progressive weakness as a result of depolarizing blockade of the postsynaptic membrane (cholinergic crisis). This makes it difficult to distinguish between a true deterioration associated with underlying MG and an iatrogenic complication of therapy. As a rule, in cholinergic crisis, worsening muscle weakness should be accompanied by symptoms of cholinergic excess, including salivation, lacrimation, urination, diarrhea, gastric distress (cramps), emesis, miosis, and bradycardia. Edrophonium can be a useful tool; this agent should make myasthenic weakness better and should exacerbate the cholinergic crisis. Unfortunately, edrophonium has limited use in an acutely decompensating, apprehensive patient. Therefore, it is recommended that all anticholinesterase medications be stopped in myasthenic crisis.[11,31]

Management of the patient with myasthenic crisis requires general supportive measures and rapid reduction in anti-ACh-R antibody load. Patients suffering from myasthenic crisis will require admission to the ICU, where vigilant monitoring of respiratory status is mandatory. The decision to intubate the patient will depend on the patient's clinical status and respiratory parameters. These values suggest respiratory failure requiring intubation. Plasmapheresis is beneficial in myasthenic crisis, and improvement in the patient's clinical status can be seen within a few days. Intravenous immunoglobulin (IG) should also be considered. In a critically ill patient with a secured airway, high-dose steroid therapy should be initiated immediately. All medications that may impair neuromuscular transmission should be discontinued.

Despite a significant reduction in mortality in myasthenic crisis, this emergency continues to carry a mortality rate as high as 10%. This high mortality is the result of associated complications, including sepsis and cardiac or respiratory arrest.[31]

The ED physician's approach to patients with MG depends upon the severity of the patient's symptoms. Bella and Chad's classification of myasthenia severity is particularly helpful in the ED setting.[11] They classify MG as mild, moderate, and/or severe based upon neurologic function and respiratory compromise. Early neurologic consultation is important. If the patient has limited, mild bulbar symptoms and a disorder of neuromuscular transmission is suspected, close follow-up with the neurologist is mandatory.

Presynaptic Disorders of Neuromuscular Transmission

Lambert-Eaton Syndrome (LES). LES is a rare, autoimmune condition affecting the presynaptic membrane. It exists in a primary form but may be a manifestation of a paraneoplastic disorder. The incidence of the primary form of LES is not known, but the prevalence of LES in patients with small-cell carcinoma of the lung is estimated to be 3%. It also has been described with other neoplasms. The majority of patients with LES are older than 60 years of age, but it has been described in all age groups. The paraneoplastic form of LES is a disease of the middle to late years; there is a distinct male predominance.[32] In the paraneoplastic form, LES may precede the diagnosis of lung carcinoma by up to three years.

Several clinical features can help distinguish LES from MG. For example, the weakness reported in LES is severe at the onset, but improves somewhat soon after initiation of activity, and then deteriorates. Moreover, there is a propensity for developing extremity weakness, in the absence of bulbar symptoms and autonomic dysfunction.

Clinical Pathophysiology. Failure of neuromuscular transmission in LES is due to the insufficient release of a neurotransmitter at the presynaptic terminal. Antibody-mediated blockade of the VGCC compromises rapid influx of calcium which, in turn, results in deficient neurotransmitter release. Electron microscope studies of the presynaptic membranes of patients with LES show depletion of the active zone, which represents the VGCC; depletion of the active zone is secondary to autoimmune destruction.[33] The evidence for an autoimmune etiology comes from several observations: LES is associated with other organ-specific autoimmune diseases,[34] the disease responds to immunosuppressive therapy,[32] and it can be passively transferred to mice with purified IgG from LES patients.[33] Also, immunocolonization of the motor end plate provides direct evidence for the autoimmune nature of this disorder.[33] More recently, calcium channel autoantibodies have been detected in up to 60% of the patients with LES.[35] In paraneoplastic cases, the antigenic stimulus for antibody production is believed to be present in the membranes of small-cell carcinoma cells.[36]

Clinical Features. Primary and paraneoplastic forms of LES generally present with similar clinical manifestations.[36] Due to the vague nature of initial symptoms and the insidious onset of this condition, the diagnosis of LES is often delayed. However, the classic triad of muscle weakness, hyporeflexia, and autonomic dysfunction in an elderly patient should lead to the consideration of LES

Muscle weakness in LES tends to be symmetrical and is most pronounced in the lower extremities. Altered gait after prolonged walking usually is the initial symptom. This may progress to inability to rise from a chair or walk up stairs. Ocular and bulbar symptoms are not common and are mild in nature when present. Autonomic symptoms are common and occur in more than half of the patients. Prominent among anticholinergic symptoms are dry mouth and erectile dysfunction.[34] On physical examination, proximal muscle weakness is the most prominent clinical finding. The peculiar weakness in LES patients may be demonstrated during hand grip. The initial grip may be weak but gets stronger only to weaken again. Autonomic findings, especially pupillary abnormalities and dryness of the oral mucosa may also be appreciated. Hyporeflexia is usually most prominent in the weakest muscles. The diagnosis can be confirmed by the presence of VGCC antibodies and electrophysiologic studies.

Calcium channel antibodies are found in both the primary and the paraneoplastic forms of LES. They are detected in 50-60% of patients with LES.[35] Electrophysiologic studies, although not specific for LES, will localize the problem to the presynaptic terminal. In muscles with weakness due to presynaptic disorders, the resting compound muscle action potential is low and a decrement is noted with slow, repetitive stimulation. With rapid stimulation or after brief exercise, the compound muscle action potential facilitates to at least twice its baseline amplitude. This post-tetanic facilitation is the hallmark of presynaptic disorders.

Management. Management of patients with LES includes a search for and treatment of an underlying tumor, potentiation of neuromuscular transmission through anticholinesterase medication, and immunosuppression.

Malignancy is a more common cause of rapidly evolving symptomatology in patients with LES. Successful treatment of the underlying malignancy often results in remission of neuromuscular symptoms.[8] Occasionally, tumor recurrence may be heralded by recurrent LES.

Like MG, enhancement of neuromuscular transmission is the primary objective of therapy. Anticholinesterase agents, such as pyridostigmine, provide some relief, but in many cases may not to be effective. Other neurotransmitter enhancers, such as aminopyridines, have shown more promise in LES. Aminopyridines are potassium channel blockers that enhance the release of neurotransmitters. Blocking of the potassium channels prolongs the action potential that keeps the calcium channels open for a longer period of time. The resulting increase in calcium influx facilitates neurotransmitter release. Two common agents in this class, 4-aminopyridine (4-AP) and 3,4-diaminopyridine (3,4-DAP), are currently in favor.[28,37] Immunosuppressive regimens are also used but tend not to be as effective as they are in MG and have a slower onset of action.[32] The prognosis of the paraneoplastic form of LES depends on the status of the underlying malignancy.

Botulism

Clostridium botulinum is a spore-forming, anaerobic, gram-positive bacillus that is the source of one of the most lethal neurotoxins known to man. The toxin's actions are linked to its effect on neuromuscular transmission, which can lead to respiratory failure. *C. botulinum* toxin irreversibly binds to the presynaptic membrane and prevents release of ACh. A rapidly progressive descending paralysis follows and is accompanied by prominent, autonomic symptoms and respiratory involvement.

Botulinum Neurotoxins. Seven strains of *C. botulinum* (designated type A through G) have been identified. Only some of these have been implicated in human disease, and they have a geographical distribution. Type A causes disease primarily west of Mississippi and type B east Mississippi. Type E is found in the Pacific Northwest; it usually is restricted to fish and seafood and is capable of growing and producing toxin in near-freezing temperatures. Neurotoxins from A, B, E, and F are well-established causes of human botulism, while C and D primarily cause illness in other animals.[38]

C. Botulinum spores proliferate in an anaerobic environment and can survive under the most adverse conditions. They can withstand boiling (100°C) for hours and produce a neurotoxin that is lethal at a concentration of 0.05-0.1 mcg. *C. Botulinum* can cause human disease when either the spores or the toxin are ingested (classical, food-borne), when spores colonize the GI tract (infant botulism and its closely related, poorly defined adult form), or when the spores germinate and produce the toxin in a traumatic wound (wound botulism). In the United States, infant botulism is the most common form and wound botulism is the rarest form of botulism, although wound botulism has been reported in intravenous drug abusers.

The seven strains of *C. Botulinum* produce related, heat labile neurotoxins. The human neuromuscular junction seems to be sensitive primarily to strains A, B, and E, although toxin C has shown toxicity in vitro.[39] The neurotoxin consists of a light (50 kd) and a heavy chain (100 kd) linked together by a disulfide bond. Due to the high molecular weight of these neurotoxins, they are rapidly inactivated by heat, but not by the acid or proteolytic activity of the stomach. In its natural form, it exists in complex with several other proteins from which it disassociates in the alkaline environment of the intestines.[40,41] The neurotoxin exerts its inhibitory effects against the excretory apparatus that facilitates neurotransmitter release. The neurotoxin binds to the presynaptic membrane (the exact binding site varies with toxin type but is confined to the presynaptic membrane), and after endocytosis it interacts with three crucial SNARE proteins that are responsible for synaptic vesicle fusion; SNARE proteins include synaptobrevin, syntaxin, and SNAP-25. Zinc-dependent catalytic action prevents the synaptic vesicle from fusing with the membrane, thereby inhibiting neurotransmitter release. The exact molecular target for various toxin types may be different, but all produce the same end result.[42,43]

Clinical Presentation. Cranial nerve findings in the presence of GI symptoms should alert the ED physician to the diagnosis of botulism. The history should confirm the initial impression. Although the neurologic signs of botulism may be delayed for weeks, more typically the onset is within 12-36 hours after ingestion of the toxin. The most prominent symptoms relate to the bulbar musculature. Patients most commonly will complain of blurry or double vision, dysarthria, and dysphagia. Skeletal muscle paralysis follows, with a symmetrical, descending, and progressive weakness that may abruptly culminate in respiratory failure. Progression from onset of symptoms to respiratory failure can occur in as little as 24 hours, making this the most fulminant of all the neuromuscular transmission disorders. The presence of anticholinergic symptoms aids in the diagnosis.[44-46]

On physical examination, the patient remains alert, oriented, and without fever. Postural hypotension may be noted, along with dry mucous membranes. Eyelid ptosis and pupillary abnormalities are important early bulbar signs; pupils tend to be dilated and, at times, fixed. Patients may have a compromised gag reflex. The extent of extremity weakness varies depending upon the degree of progression. Deep tendon reflexes range from normal to absent and correlate with the extent of muscular weakness.

The presentation of wound botulism is similar, with prominent bulbar findings associated with a history of a traumatic wound. It should be appreciated that the current target population for wound botulism appears to be IV drug abusers. In any active IV drug abuser presenting with bulbar findings, botulism should be the initial diagnostic consideration. Symptoms present within 3-4 days, although a lag of up to three weeks has been described. The median age for all the cases is 19 years with a range of 6 to 44 years. Symptoms and signs are identical to those in other forms of botulism.[47-49]

Infant botulism should be considered in a listless baby with a weak cry, poor suck, and constipation. This may evolve into generalized weakness in an acute or subacute manner. The pattern remains symmetrical and evolves into a descending paralysis. On physical exam, the child is hypotonic and, therefore, frequently described as "floppy." Cranial nerve findings include sluggish pupillary response to light, ptosis, ophthalmoplegia, and diminished gag reflex. Bowel sounds are hypoactive and there is poor anal sphincter tone. Severity can range from mild infection to a fulminant, fatal course including respiratory failure with respiratory arrest.[50]

Diagnosis requires isolation of *C. botulinum* toxin from a suspected food source, stool, or wound. Isolation of *C. botulinum* from the stool is helpful, but not always present in those with clinical botulism. Up to 40% of the patients may not have *C. botulinum* in their stool and only 36% may be positive after three days. If there is a delay in securing serum sample, two days after a toxin ingestion the chances of obtaining a positive test is less than 30%. Electrophysiologic studies aid when lab data is pending or non-confirmatory. Electrophysiologic studies show classic pattern of presynaptic neuromuscular defect with decreased amplitude of muscle action potential, an incremental response of the muscle action potential (MAP) to slow rates of nerve stimulation, and post-tetanic facilitation.

Management. Treatment of all forms of botulism consists of meticulous supportive care with special attention to respiratory status. Infant botulism does not require antitoxin administration and antibiotic treatment is not required (antibiotics can lead to bacterial cell death and toxin release).[50] Antitoxin administration in other forms of botulism also is controversial because of lack of efficacy in many cases and the risk of allergic reactions. Beneficial effects are more likely with type A and E botulism. To be of benefit, antitoxin must be given early while the toxin is still in the blood and before it is internalized and bound to the nerve terminal. Serious side effects related to antitoxin therapy occur in as many as 20% of the patients. In a series of 268 patients, there was a 3% rate of anaphylaxis.[51] Most commercially available botulinum antitoxins are of equine origin, and allergic reactions are attributed to antibody products of non-human origin. Currently, administration of antitoxin is recommended by most experts regardless of delay in diagnosis.[52]

Guanidine and 4-aminopyridine have been studied and seem to be helpful in patients with bulbar symptoms, although these agents have no effect on respiratory paralysis. Both of these drugs have serious side effects that limit their use.

The prognosis of patients with botulism has improved significantly with advances in critical care. Respiratory management and good supportive care are key to improved survival. Despite a protracted course, complete recovery follows, which requires regeneration of terminal motor neurons and formation of new motor nerve end plates.

Medications that Interfere with Neuromuscular Transmission

The neuromuscular junction is vulnerable to the effects of several medications. Drugs can act presynaptically, postsynaptically, or in combination to produce neuromuscular transmission disturbances. Administration of these drugs can unmask venerability of the neuromuscular junction to transmission failure. It is important to avoid such medications in those with an established diagnosis of neuromuscular transmission failure and recognize that these medications can produce worsening of symptoms in patients with underlying neuromuscular transmission failure.

The best studied medication producing neuromuscular transmission failure of is D-penicillamine, a medication used in Wilson's disease and in several other rheumatologic disorders. D-penicillamine is known to be an iatrogenic cause of MG, with MG occurring in up to 7% of patients on this medication. Serologically and electrophysiologically, drug-induced inhibition of neuromuscular transmission is indistinguishable from idiopathic forms of MG, although its clinical course tends to be milder.[53]

Among drugs causing presynaptic inhibition, magnesium is of particular interest. Despite its increasing popularity, it should be stressed that hypermagnesemia can lead to impaired neuromuscular transmission and respiratory paralysis. At the presynaptic membrane, magnesium regulates calcium influx through VGCC; specifically, hypermagnesemia interferes with neuromuscular transmission by competitively blocking calcium influx at the motor nerve terminal, thereby preventing calcium-mediated exocytosis of the neurotransmitter.[54-56] This presynaptic action produces autonomic cholinergic blockade. Use of magnesium potentiates the action of neuromuscular blocking agents and is responsible for prolonged respiratory muscle weakness. This has been effectively demonstrated in women who had C-section after treatment with magnesium for eclampsia.[55]

Several antibiotics also are known to compromise neuromuscular transmission and exacerbate symptoms in patients with MG. Chief among them are aminoglycosides, chloroquine, and fluoroquinolones.[37,51] All of these agents have pre- and postsynaptic effects.[57,58]

Summary

Disorders of neuromuscular transmission represent a category of life-threatening conditions of which the ED physician should be aware. These potentially fatal disorders should be considered in patients with muscle weakness of unknown etiology. Supportive management, including intubation and pharmacologic intervention should be initiated in a systemic approach to patient care.

References

1. Gutman L. Disorders of Neuromuscular Transmission. *Clin Neurol* 1994;4:1-20.
2. Graus Y, DeBates M. Myasthenia gravis: An Autoimmune response against the acetylcholine receptor. *Immunol Res* 1993;12:78-100.
3. Kachalsky SG, Aladjem M, Barchan D, et al. The ligand binding domain of the nicotinic acetylcholine receptor: Immunological analysis. *FEBS Lett* 1993;318:264-268.
4. Witzeman V, Barg B, Nishikawa Y, et al. Differential regulation of muscle acetylcholine receptor mRNAs. *FEBS Lett* 1987;223:104-112.
5. Ramsay DA, Drachman DB, Drachman RJ, et al. Stabilization of acetylcholine receptors at the neuromuscular synapse: The role of the nerve. *Brain Res* 1992;581:198-207.
6. Maselli R. Pathophysiology of myasthenia gravis and Lambert-Eaton syndrome. *Neurol Clin N Am* 1994;12: 285-303.
7. Kaminski HJ, Suarez JI, Ruff RL. Neuromuscular physiology in myasthenia gravis: Isoforms of the acetylcholine receptors in extraocular muscle and the contribution of the sodium channel to safety factor. *Neurology* 1997;48(supp 5):8-17.
8. Drachman D. Myasthenia gravis. *N Engl J Med* 1994;330: 1797-1809.
9. Dushay KM, Zibrak JD, Jensen WA. Myasthenia gravis presenting as isolated respiratory failure. *Chest* 1990;97: 232-234.
10. Huges R. Management of acute neuromuscular paralysis. *J R Coll Physicians Lond* 1998;32:254-259.
11. Bella I, Chad D. Neuromuscular disorders and acute respiratory failure. *Neurol Clin N Am* 1998;16:391-417.
12. Keesey J. A treatment algorithm for autoimmune myasthenia in adults. *Ann N Y Acad Sci* 1998;841:753-768.
13. Maselli R. Electrodiagnosis of disorders of neuromuscular transmission. *Ann N Y Acad Sci* 1998;841:696-711.
14. Phillips LH. The epidemiology of myasthenia gravis. *Neurol Clin N Am* 1994;12:264-271.
15. Donaldson DH, Ansher M, Horan S. The relationship of age to outcome in myasthenia gravis. *Neurology* 1990;90:56-66.
16. Aarli J. Late-onset myasthenia gravis: A changing scene. *Arch Neurol* 1999;56:25-27.
17. Pumplin DW, Drachman DB. Myasthenic patients' IgG causes redistribution of acetylcholine receptors: Freeze-fracture studies. *J Neurosci* 1983;3:576-584.
18. Grob D, Arsura EL, Brunner NG. The course of myasthenia gravis and therapies affecting outcome. *Ann N Y Acad Sci* 1987;505:472-499.
19. Levy Y, Afet A, Yaniv S, et al. Malignant thymoma associated with autoimmune diseases: A retrospective study and review of the literature. *Semin Arthritis Rheum* 1998;28:73-79.
20. Grip S, Hilgers K, Wurm R, et al. Thymoma: Prognostic factors and treatment outcomes. *Cancer* 1998;83:1495-1450.
21. Lubke E, et al. Strational autoantibodies in myasthenia gravis patients recognize I-band titin epitopes. *J Neuroimmunol* 1998;81:98-108.
22. Osserman KE. *Myasthenia gravis*. New York: Grune & Stratton; 1958:80.
23. Massey JM. Acquired myasthenia gravis. *Neurol Clin* 1997; 15:577-595.
24. Heitmiller RF. Myasthenia gravis: Clinical features, pathogenesis, evaluation, and medical management. *Semin Thorac Cardiovasc Surg* 1999;11:41-46.
25. Seybold ME. The office Tensilon test for ocular myasthenia gravis. *Arch Neurol* 1986;43:842-843.
26. Lindberg C, Andersen O, Lefvert AK. Treatment of

myasthenia gravis with methylprednisolone pulse: A double blind study. *Acta Neurol Scand* 1998;97:370-373.
27. Seybold ME. Plasmapheresis in myasthenia gravis. *Ann N Y Acad Sci* 1987;505:584-587.
28. Corneli F, Antozzi C, Confalonieri P. Plasma treatment in diseases of neuromuscular junction. *Ann N Y Acad Sci* 1998;841:803-810.
29. Intravenous immunoglobulin for the treatment of acquired myasthenia gravis. *Neurology* 1998;51(Supp 5):S30-36.
30. Thornton, CC, R Griggs. Plasma exchange and intravenous immunoglobulin treatment in neuromuscular disease. *Ann Nerurol* 1994;35:260-268.
31. Thomas CE, Mayer SA, Gungor BS. Myasthenic crisis, clinical features, mortality, complications, and risk factors for prolonged intubation. *Neurology* 1997;48:1253.
32. Newsom-Davis J, Murray NMF. Plasma exchange and immunosuppressive drug treatment in the Lambert-Eaton myasthenic syndrome. *Neurology* 1984;34:480.
33. Bednarik J, Bourgeois P, Carton H, et al. Myasthenic syndrome caused by the direct effect of chloroquine on neuromuscular junction. *Arch Neurol* 1989;46:464-468.
34. O'Neil JH, Murray NMF, Newsom-Davis J. The Lambert-Eaton myasthenic syndrome. A review of 50 cases. *Brain* 1988;111:577.
35. Leys K, Lang B, Johnston I, et al. Calcium channel autoantibodies in the Lambert-Eaton myasthenic syndrome. *Ann Neurol* 1991;29:307-314.
36. Harrington GM, Murray NM, Spiro SG, et al. Neurologic paraneoplastic syndromes in patients with small-cell lung cancer. A prospective study of 150 patients. *J Neurol Neurosurg Psychi* 1991;54:746.
37. Sanders DB, Howard JF, Massey JM. 3,4 Diaminopyridine in Lambert-Eaton myasthenic syndrome and myasthenia gravis. *Ann NY Acad Sci* 1993;681:588.
38. Maselli R. Pathogenesis of human botulism. *Ann N Y Acad Sci* 1998;13:122-139.
39. Coffield JA, Bakry N, Zang J, et al. In vitro characterization of botulinum toxin types A, C, and D. Action on human Tissue: Combined electrophysiologic, pharmacologic, and molecular biologic approaches. *J Pharmacol Exp Ther* 1997;280:1489-1498.
40. Simpson, L. The origin, structure, and pharmacological activity of botulinum toxin. *Pharmacol Rev* 1981;33:155-188.
41. Hatheway CL. Toxigenic clostridia. *Clin Microbiol Rev* 1990;3:66-98.
42. Lacy BD, Tepp W, Cohen CA, et al. Crystal structure of botulinum neurotoxin type A and implications for toxicity. *Nat Struct Biol* 1998;5:898-902.
43. Montecucco C, Schiavo G. Structure and function of tetanus and botulinum neurotoxins. *Quarterly Rev Biophys* 1995; 28:423-472.
44. Cherington M. The clinical spectrum of botulism. *Muscle Nerve* 1998;21:701-710.
45. Chia JK, Clark JB, Ryan CA, et al. Botulism in the adult associated with food-borne intestinal infection with *C. botulinum*. *N Engl J Med* 1986;315:4:239-241.
46. Lecour H, Ramos H, Almeida B, et al. Food-borne botulism: A review of 13 outbreaks. *Arch Intern Med* 1988;148: 578-580.
47. Burningham M, Walter F, Mecem C, et al. Wound botulism. *Ann Emerg Med* 1994;24:1184-1187.
48. Maselli R, Mandler R, Knox S, et al Cluster of wound botulism in California. Clinical, electrophysiologic, and pathologic study. *Muscle Nerve* 1997;20:761-770.
49. MacDonald KL, Rutherford GW, Friedman SM, et al. Botulism and botulism-like illness in chronic drug abusers. *Ann Intern Med* 1985;102:616-618.
50. Midura TF. Update: Infant botulism. *Clin Microbiol Rev* 1996;9:119-125.
51. Black RE, Gunn RA. Hypersensitivity reactions associated with botulinal antitoxin. *Am J Med* 1980;69:567-570.
52. Tacket C, Wayne S, Mann J, et al. Equine antitoxin use and other factors that predict outcome in type A food-borne botulism. *Am J Med* 1984;76:794-798.
53. Drosos AA, Christou L, Falanopoulou B, et al. D-Penicillamine induced myasthenia gravis: Clinical, serological, and genetic findings. *Clin Exp Rheumatol* 1993;11:387-391.
54. Altura, B Altura B. Role of magnesium in patho-physiological processes and the clinical utility of magnesium ion selective electrode. *Scand J Clin Lab Invest* 1996;56: 211-234.
55. Fuchs-buder T, Tassonyi E. Magnesium sulphate enhances residual neuromuscular block included by vecuronium. *Br J of Anaesth* 1996;76:565-566.
56. Krendal DA. Hypermagnesemia and neuromuscular transmission. *Semin Neurol* 1990;10:42-45.
57. Feldman S, Karalliedde L. Drug interaction with neuromuscular blockers. *Drug Saf* 1996:15:261-273.
58. Pascuzzi RM. Drugs and toxins associated with myopathies. *Curr Opin Rheum* 1998;10:511-520.

Recommended Reading

- Engel AG, Tsujihata M, Lindstrom JM, et al. The motor end plate in myasthenia gravis and in experimental autoimmune myasthenia gravis: A quantitative ultrastructural study. *Ann N Y Acad Sci* 1976;274:60-79.
- Changeux JP, Devillers-Thiery A, Chemouili P. Acetylcholine receptor: An allorsteric protein. *Science* 1984;225:1335-1345.
- Draschman DB, Adams RN, Josifet LF, et al. Functional activities of autoantibodies to acetylcholine receptors and the clinical severity of myasthenia gravis. *N Engl J Med* 1982; 307:769-775.
- Sanders DB. Clinical neurophysiology of disorders of neuromuscular junction. *J Clin Neurophysiol* 1993;10: 167-180.
- Huang D, et al. No evidence for interleukin-4 gene conferring susceptibility to myasthenia gravis. *J Neuroimmunol* 1998;92: 208-211.
- Bril V, Kojic J, Canani A. The long-term clinical outcome of myasthenia gravis in patients with thymoma. *Neurology* 1998;51:1198-2000.
- Chisakuta A, Tasker R. Respiratory failure in myasthenia gravis and negative pressure support. *Pediatr Neurol* 1998;19:225-226.

- Bach JF, Koutouzov S, Van Endert PM. Are there unique autoantigens triggering autoimmune diseases? *Immunol Rev* 1998;164:139-155.
- Maselli R. Electrophysiology of postsynaptic activation. *Ann N Y Acad Sci* 1998;841:857.
- Gajdos P, Chevret S, Clair B, et al. Plasma exchange and intravenous immunoglobulin in autoimmune myasthenia gravis. *Ann N Y Acad of Sci* 1998;841:720-726.
- Vincent A, Willcox N, Hill M. Determinant spreading and immune response to acetylcholine receptors in myasthenia gravis. *Immunol Rev* 1998;164:157-168.
- Katz JS, Wolfe GI, Burns DK, et al. Isolated neck extensor myopathy: A common cause of dropped head syndrome. *Neurology* 1996;46:917-921.
- Dushay KM, Zibrak JD, Jensen WA. Myasthenia gravis presenting as isolated respiratory failure. *Chest* 1990;97: 232-234.
- Sieb JP. Fluoroquinolone antibiotics block neuromuscular transmission. *Neurology* 1998;50:804-807.
- MacDonald, KL, Cohen ML, Blake BA. The changing epidemiology of adult botulism in the United States. *Am J Epidemiol* 1986;124:794-799.
- Sanders D. 3,4-Diaminopyridine (DAP) in the treatment of Lambert-Eaton myasthenic syndrome (LEMS). *Ann N Y Acad Sci* 1998;13:811-813.

Subarachnoid Hemorrhage

Jonathan A. Edlow, MD

One of the primary goals of emergency medicine is prompt diagnosis and treatment of treatable, life-threatening conditions. Although emergency physicians are constantly on the alert for these so-called "cannot miss diagnoses," clinical vigilance may be hindered by a variety of factors, among them, time constraints of a busy emergency department (ED), the financial pressures of managed care, the relative infrequency of these conditions, and variations in clinical presentation.

Severe headache is among the most worrisome of symptoms suggesting catastrophic intracranial pathology. As far as headache,[1] subarachnoid hemorrhage (SAH) is not the only "cannot miss diagnosis," and the physician is well-served to keep in mind the entire list of conditions that present with this chief complaint. *(Please see Table 1.)* In fact, studies show that about 3-5% of patients presenting to an ED with headache will harbor serious neurologic pathology, and about 1% will have SAH.[2,3] Differentiating these patients from those whose headache is associated with more benign etiology is critical, but difficult. Unfortunately, patients who are misdiagnosed often present with mild symptoms and are the most likely to benefit from current therapies.[4,5] In this regard, two recent studies suggest that patients who are initially misdiagnosed are more likely to clinically deteriorate than those in whom the diagnosis is established at the time of presentation.[5,6]

Early diagnosis is essential to improve morbidity and mortality in SAH. Overall, 40-50% of patients with SAH die within one month of their hemorrhage, and one-third of survivors develop major neurologic disability.[7] Although the incidence of other causes of stroke have declined over the last few decades, the incidence of SAH has remained constant.[8] Moreover, there is evidence that new treatments and more aggressive surgical intervention have led to a decline in the mortality rate over this period.[8,9]

Given the importance of prompt and precise diagnosis, it is essential that physicians understand the myriad, atypical presentations of SAH, as well as the limitations of diagnostic tests, to avoid misdiagnosis and improve patient outcomes. Although this chapter will discuss many clinical issues related to SAH, it will focus on the diagnostic strategies, clinical presentations, and implications for outcome-effective management.

Clinical Anatomy and Epidemiology

SAH is defined as extravasation of blood into the subarachnoid space of the central nervous system (CNS). Excluding head trauma, which is the most common cause of SAH, ruptured intracerebral aneurysm accounts for about 80% of cases of SAH. Other causes include mycotic aneurysms,[10,11] arteriovenous malformations (AMV),[12-14] dissection of intracranial arteries,[15,16] Moyamoya disease,[17] and idiopathic cases.[12,14] Aneurysms also can occur but as rare, late complication of head injury.[18,19]

Table 1. Cannot Miss Diagnosis* Presenting as a Headache

- Bacterial meningitis
- Subarachnoid hemorrhage
- Space-occupying lesion
  - Brain tumor
  - Brain abscess
  - Subdural and epidural hematoma
  - Others including other parameningeal infections
- Pseudotumor cerebri
- Hypertensive encephalopathy
- Acute narrow-angle glaucoma
- Temporal arteritis
- Cerebral venous and dural sinus thrombosis (including cavernous sinus)
- Carbon monoxide poisoning
- Stroke
- Bacterial sinusitis (can lead to complications on the list)

** Defined as medical conditions that are simultaneously life, limb, or vision threatening and treatable.*

Unless otherwise specified, the term SAH, as it is used in this review, refers only to those cases caused by intracerebral aneurysm. Most of these aneurysms arise from arteries at the base of the brain, located in the circle of Willis and its branches. Eighty-five percent of aneurysms are derived from the anterior circulation,[7] most often at its sites of vessel bifurcation. The most common sites are the junction of the internal carotid artery (ICA) and posterior communicating artery (PCoA), the anterior cerebral-anterior communicating artery (ACoA) complex, and the bifurcation of the middle cerebral artery (MCA).

Aneurysms arising from the posterior circulation are most likely to occur at the bifurcation of the basilar artery and at the junctions of the basilar artery with the vertebral and the posterior inferior cerebellar vessels. At the time of initial presentation, about 25% of patients will have multiple aneurysms (usually 2-3), although as many as 13 aneurysms in the same patient have been reported.[7] Generally, cerebral aneurysms form in areas that are deficient in medial layers and where the internal elastic lamina is thin or absent.[7] Hemodynamic stress is thought to play a primary role in the formation of aneurysms.[20,21]

Once an aneurysm develops, the rules of physics govern its subsequent behavior. LaPlace's law[14,22] states that the tension on the wall of a chamber is a function of the radius of that chamber and the pressure gradient across the wall. Thrombus forms in the aneurysm, usually in the dome,[14] and, as the aneurysm enlarges, the medial layer becomes even more tenuous and the adventitia and intima are separated only by variable amounts of connective tissue.[7,8]

The reported incidence of saccular, intracranial aneurysms varies according to the epidemiological techniques used to identify this condition. For example, in autopsy series, they are found in up to 6% of the population, although many of these aneurysms are quite small.[7] Based on cerebral angiographic studies, it is estimated that 0.5-1.0% of individuals have aneurysms.[7] A recent expert panel sponsored by the American Heart Association estimated that approximately 2 million Americans harbor unruptured aneurysms.[13]

In the United States, the annual incidence of SAH is about 30,000, or roughly 10 cases per 100,000 population.[7,13,14] In Japan, the rate is about three times that number.[23] The variable natural history of cerebral aneurysms accounts for the difference between the estimated 2 million Americans who harbor aneurysms and the 30,000 of those who rupture. Overall, the risk of rupture is about 0.5-2.0% per year[7] and, as LaPlace's law would predict, small aneurysms are less likely to rupture than large ones.

SAH can occur at any age, but it is rare in children[24] and the mean age at the time of presentation is about 50 years. Overall, there is a female:male ratio of 3:2; however, in patients younger than age 40, men are more often afflicted than women.[7] All ethnic groups are affected. However, first degree relatives (especially siblings) of patients who have had SAH have a four-fold increased risk compared to the general population of developing SAH.[7] Patients with a prior SAH are six times more likely to have a second hemorrhage later in life.[7]

A number of underlying conditions are associated with an increased risk of aneurysm formation, including autosomal dominant polycystic kidney disease, Ehlers-Danlos syndrome (type 4), neurofibromatosis type 1,[25] Marfan's syndrome,[26] pseudoxanthoma elasticum, fibromuscular dysplasia, and coarctation of the aorta.[14] Other situations associated with SAH include patients with CNS angitis[27] and users of cocaine[28] and methamphetamine.[29] Well-documented risk factors for aneurysm rupture include smoking, alcohol use (especially binge drinking), and hypertension.[7,30] Although aneurysms may become symptomatic during pregnancy,[31] there is no documented association.[32]

Natural History of Intracerebral Aneurysms

Prior to discussion of *ruptured* intracranial aneurysm, it is essential for the ED physician to understand the clinical manifestations and natural history of individuals who have intact cerebral aneurysms.

In one landmark study of 111 patients who had 132 *unruptured* aneurysms,[33] patients were divided into three groups: Group 1 presented with acute symptoms; Group 2 presented with chronic (> 2 weeks in duration) symptoms; and Group 3 were asymptomatic and had been diagnosed either incidentally or during the course of being treated for an aneurysm that had ruptured. Typically, Group 1 patients presented with symptoms related to cerebral ischemia (TIA or stroke),[34,35] which was usually the result of an aneurysmal clot that embolizes distally into the territory of the affected vessel. Other symptoms in Group 1 were acute headache, seizures, and cranial neuropathy.

Patients in Group 2 had headache, visual symptoms, long-tract dysfunction, and facial pain. The three patients with facial pain all had anterior circulation aneurysms, two of which were located within the cavernous sinus, through which the first two divisions of the trigeminal nerve traverse. Not surprisingly, the investigators also noted that the patients in Groups 1 and 2 had larger aneurysms (mean diameter, 2.1 cm) than did the asymptomatic patients in Group 3 (mean diameter, 1.1 cm). The clinical importance of aneurysmal size has been noted by other authors.[36-38] As a rule, aneurysms that pre-

Table 2. Classification Systems for Subarachnoid Hemorrhage

HUNT AND HESS

Grade 0	Unruptured aneurysm
Grade 1	Asymptomatic or mild headache
Grade 2	Moderate-severe headache, nuchal rigidity, ± cranial nerve deficits
Grade 3	Confusion, lethargy, or mild focal symptoms
Grade 4	Stupor, ± hemiparesis
Grade 5	Comatose, ± extensor posturing

WORLD FEDERATION OF NEUROLOGIC SURGEONS

Grade	Glasgow coma scale	Motor deficits
1	15	absent
2	13-14	absent
3	13-14	absent
4	7-12	present or absent
5	3-6	present or absent

sent with findings suggestive of a mass effect are generally larger and, therefore, carry a higher risk of rupture (estimated at 6% per year). Because surgical therapy has become relatively safe, some experts advocate more aggressive surgical treatment of unruptured aneurysms,[39,40] especially those that are greater than 2.5 cm in diameter.[41] It should be stressed that even very small aneurysms can bleed, which suggests that clinical vigilance is required for all individuals with unruptured aneurysm.[42]

The neuro-opthalmic symptoms of unruptured aneurysms fall into two broad categories: visual loss and diplopia.[43] Visual loss can result from intraocular bleeding or *compression* of the visual pathways. Hemorrhage in the retina, sub-hyaloid space, or vitreous occurs in 25-40% of patients[44,45] and may be the only clue to SAH in a comatose patient. In the setting of anterior communicating artery aneurysm, ocular bleeding is referred to as Terson's syndrome; vitreous bleeding in this setting may require a vitrectomy to restore vision.[45] Bleeding is thought to occur as a result of the acute rise in intrcranial pressure (ICP), which leads to venous outflow obstruction.[43]

Because of their proximity to the circle of Willis and the anterior visual pathways, cerebral aneurysms can produce visual field cuts or impairments in ocular function. Symptoms often develop over months to years, but acute increases or even fluctuations in symptoms can occur secondary to periodic dilation of the aneurysms, thrombosis, or changes in ICP.[43] A number of visual deficits can occur depending on the location of the aneurysm and the segment of the visual pathway involved; the most common is 3rd cranial nerve (CN) palsy. About, 30% of 3rd nerve palsies are aneurysmal, and most occur at the junction of the PCoA and the ICA.[46] However, patients may not complain of diplopia because of a coexistent ptosis caused by involvement of the levator palpebrae muscle. This lesion is usually associated with a dilated pupil. Early operation is advised.[46]

Although many entities can produce a 3rd cranial nerve palsy (cavernous sinus syndrome, lesions of the midbrain and orbit, basilar meningitides, neuromuscular disease, and uncal herniation), the most important entity in the differential diagnosis is microvascular infarct resulting from diabetes. Typically a diabetic 3rd cranial nerve palsy spares the pupil, whereas aneurysmal 3rd cranial nerve lesions do not; however, exceptions to this rule occur in a significant percentage of cases.[43,47,48]

Ruptured Aneurysm. Once an aneurysm ruptures, patients may present with a wide range of signs and symptoms; they may be ambulatory and fully conscious or comatose. Several clinical grading systems are used for patients with SAH. The two most widely improved are the Hunt and Hess (H&H)[49] and the World Federation of Neurologic Surgeons classifications, the latter of which is based on the Glasgow coma scale. *(Please see Table 2.)*

The classical textbook history for patients with a ruptured aneurysm includes: abrupt onset of the worst headache of life associated with exertion, transient loss of consciousness with or without nausea, vomiting, and new neurologic deficits. Physical examination may yield a number of associated findings, such as acute hypertension and low-grade fever. Level of consciousness (LOC) may be diminished. The presence of ocular hemorrhage, especially subhyaloid bleeding, is an important clue. Other neuro-ophthalmic findings due to a mass effect have been described above and should be actively sought since they may provide useful clues to both the diagnosis and localization. Meningismus may also be present. The presence of any focal neurologic findings mandates a detailed neurologic examination.

Diagnostic Pitfalls

Despite clues to the diagnosis of SAH, there are numerous pitfalls that can compromise prompt evaluation and subsequentmanagement. These pitfalls fall into three major categories. *(Please see Table 3.)*

1. Failure to consider the *diagnosis* of SAH.
2. Failure to understand the *limitations* of a computerized tomographic (CT) scan.
3. Failure to understand the *limitations* of the lumbar puncture (LP).

Failure to Consider Diagnosis. From a diagnostic perspective, it is important to discuss the warning bleed, a concept introduced in the medical literature in 1958 by a Scottish neurosurgeon, F. John Gillingham,[50] who wrote: "It would appear from the fresh appraisal of many case histories, that a patient's first episode of SAH is commonly of minor severity; a mere leak of blood from the sac." He is also given credit for coining the term "warning leak" nine years later.[51] Since then, there have been numerous references in the literature about warning bleed, warning leak, sentinel bleed, and sentinel leak.[52-61] This symptom usually is also associated with a thunderclap headache, described as an abrupt (develops in seconds), very intense (like a thunderclap, reaching maximal intensity in minutes) headache that is *new* for the patient and lasts for hours to days. Typically, it is focal (bifrontal, bioccipital, vertex, or unilateral),[55,62] and differs from the very brief "jabs and jolts" headache whose intensity, but not duration (seconds), rivals that of the thunderclap headache.[63]

Retrospective reviews of hospitalized patients with SAH estimate that "warning bleeds" occur in 20-60% of patients with SAH a mean

Table 3. Pitfalls in the Diagnosis of Subarachnoid Hemorrhage (SAH)

FAILURE TO CONSIDER THE DIAGNOSIS OF SAH

- Over-reliance on the classic presentation
- Lack of appreciation of the warning bleed
- Atypical presentation—neck pain, flu-like illness, meningitis, coma, mild symptoms
- Focus on head trauma resulting from the SAH
- Focus on the ECG abnormalities or the hypertension
- Failure to realize that the headache of SAH can improve spontaneously or with OTC analgesics
- Lack of knowledge of exception to the rule of the pupil regarding 3rd nerve palsy

FAILURE TO UNDERSTAND THE LIMITATIONS OF A COMPUTERIZED TOMOGRAPHIC (CT) SCAN

- The issue of timing—sensitivity drops off rapidly with time
- Density of the blood (if Hct < 30, CT may be negative)
- Volume of blood—CT may be negative with small bleed (warning bleeds)—spectrum bias
- Technical factors—may be false negative if too thick cuts (10 mm) are made at base of brain

FAILURE TO UNDERSTAND THE LIMITATIONS OF THE LUMBAR PUNCTURE (LP)

- Failure to do an LP (if CT is negative) in patients with high pretest likelihood
- Failure to recognize that LP is often negative in first 12 hours
- Failure to realize that visual inspection for xanthochromia is insensitive
- Failure to distinguish a traumatic tap from truly bloody CSF

of 14 days before the major bleed (range, 1 day to 4 months). A neurologic examination performed at the time is usually normal. Since the mechanism of warning headaches is thought to be a very small leak in the aneurysm, an LP will almost always demonstrate abnormal cerebrospinal fluid (CSF). There is one fatal case on record where this mechanism was documented pathologically.[64] An alternative hypothesis is that the warning headache represents bleeding into the wall of the aneurysm; however, this would not account for the bloody CSF.

If the latter hypothesis were true, then one would expect some patients presenting with thunderclap headache to have a negative CT and LP and go on to develop a SAH within the next several weeks. Indeed, one such patient has been reported,[65] arguing the notion that patients presenting with thunderclap headache and negative CT and LP should undergo cerebral angiography. Subsequent retrospective[66] and prospective[62,67-69] studies have investigated this problem and concluded that a more tempered approach is both safe and effective. The largest of these studies[66] evaluated 71 patients with thunderclap headache for an average of 3.3 years. All patients had negative CT and CSF. Four patients had six angiograms (2 for recurrences) that also were negative. They concluded that cerebral angiography is *not* necessary for patients presenting with thunderclap headache who have a negative CT and normal CSF. It is important to stress, however, that both the CT and LP are necessary to exclude a SAH, inasmuch as these patients are clinically indistinguishable from those with SAH on presentation.[62,67]

From an emergency diagnostic perspective, the thunderclap headache has a differential diagnosis. Upon evaluation with CT and LP, a substantial proportion of patients will have documented SAH. For patients in whom CT *and* LP are *negative*, the diagnosis of aneurysm is essentially excluded. There may be an occasional patient with a very high, pre-test likelihood of SAH (e.g., strong family history or polycystic kidney disease with a good story) for whom additional neurologic or neurosurgical consultation is appropriate. Other explanations for this symptom include migraine,[67] benign exertional cephalgia,[70] and benign sexual headache,[70] but these diagnoses should be considered only if the CT and LP are negative.[22,71] Also in the differential is cortical vein thrombosis.[72] Identifying this condition is one reason to always measure the CSF pressure when performing an LP; the pressure is often high in this "cannot miss" condition.[73]

The natural history of the warning bleed is unpredictable. A recent publication of a prospective, community-based study investigated whether general practitioners could accurately identify these warning bleeds and whether early identification would alter patient outcomes.[74] Investigators followed 148 patients with "thunderclap headache" seen by 252 general practitioners in the Netherlands over a five-year period. One quarter of these patients had SAH and another 12% had other serious neurologic problems. The remainder of patients, who were followed for at least a year, had either a negative angiogram or a benign outcome.

Despite this study, there is no doubt that early diagnosis leads to better outcomes. This hypothesis was recently tested by Mayer and colleagues, who retrospectively examined 217 patients with symptomatic cerebral aneurysms.[5] Their principle conclusions were: 1) 25% of patients were initially misdiagnosed by a physician; 2) misdiagnosed patients were more likely to be of lower grade (38% of patients with a modified H & H grade 1 or 2 were misdiagnosed); and 3) those who were correctly diagnosed on initial presentation had better clinical outcomes. These investigators also found that patients presenting with a seizure or mass effect were more likely to be misdiagnosed.

Conditions most likely to be confused with SAH included viral meningitis, migraine, headache of unknown etiology, stroke, sinus headache, hypertension, tension headache, and depression. These results are similar to those of another study examining pitfalls in the diagnosis of SAH.[4] In this trial, 41 of 181 (23%) patients were misdiagnosed with conditions nearly identical to that in Mayer's study.[5] Still another study showed a remarkable 51% (69 of 131 patients) rate of delayed diagnosis; two-thirds of the patients suffered recurrent bleeding leading to worse outcomes prior to correct diagnosis.[6] Other investigators have examined the rate of late diagnosis in the same geographical area over time and found no change in the rate of delayed referral over the last 15 years.[75]

Why is This Diagnosis Missed? One reason the diagnosis of SAH is missed is over-reliance on the classic teaching. For example, the classic teaching that the leak occurs at time of stress or Valsalva was supported in only 43% of patients in one series of 500 consecutive patients.[22] In 12% of patients, the hemorrhage occurred during rest or sleep. Moreover, some patients did not have abrupt onset of symptoms.[4,69] New-onset headache or a distinct change in a patient's prior headache pattern requires diagnostic evaluation. At the very least, this should include a very detailed history and physical examination, with the goal being to exclude "cannot miss" possibilities. Furthermore, the headache of SAH can be relieved with non-narcotic analgesics[76] and may improve spontaneously during observation in the ED.[69]

It should be stressed that there is a wide range of atypical symptoms, or symptom complexes, that may confuse the clinician. One common presentation is primary neck pain and/or stiffness. The erroneous diagnosis of neck arthritis or musculoskeletal neck pain (in the absence of trauma) is identified with some regularity in studies on misdiagnosis.[4,9,77] Similarly, viral meningitis, which can be mimicked by chemical irritation from blood, is another common misdiagnosis.[4-6] Hypertension, which frequently accompanies SAH, also can confuse physicians. Headache caused by hypertensive encephalopathy should resolve promptly after lowering the blood pressure.

Another potential source of confusion is head injury that results from a fall or injury secondary to the transient syncopal episode sometimes associated with SAH.[29] Sakas reported on four patients in whom mild to moderate head injury followed a fall that resulted from a spontaneous SAH.[78] On initial presentation, there was confusion as to cause and effect between the subarachnoid blood and the trauma. Some unusual presentations include shock,[79] cardio-respiratory arrest,[80] and psychosis from a frontal aneurysm.[81]

ECG abnormalities also can lead to diagnostic confusion.[82,83] The ECG changes in SAH range from T-wave flattening and inversions to prolonged QTc intervals, to life-threatening brady-and-tachyarrhythmias. An ECG pattern simulating acute myocardial infarction has also been reported. These changes may be related to subendocardial ischemia.[84] One prospective study identified arrhythmia in 91% of patients and a potentially dangerous arrhythmia in 41%.[85] The vast majority of patients with SAH have headache, a symptom that is uncommon in acute MI, unless it is accompanied by administration of nitrates. Reversible pump dysfunction may also occur.[86]

Limitations of CT. Once the diagnosis of SAH is considered, a systematic diagnostic strategy is mandatory. The non-contrast CT scan is the first step in evaluation.[87, 88] The advantage of CT is that it is non-invasive, relatively inexpensive, readily available, and has high sensitivity in the first 24 hours.[87-89] Another advantage is that it can yield other important information and identify other diagnostics such as intraventricular or intracerebral hemorrhage[87,88] and subdural hematoma, which can occur secondary to SAH.[87,88,90,91]

Moreover, the pattern of blood identified on CT can sometimes predict the bleeding site. For example, interhemispheric blood between the frontal lobes suggests aneurysm of the ACA or ACoA, whereas blood localized to the Sylvian fissure suggests a lesion in the MCA. This can be useful information if the angiogram shows multiple aneurysms. Furthermore, there is a syndrome characterized by isolated perimesencephalic blood which, if no aneurysm is found on initial angiography, carries an extremely benign prognosis and obviates the need for repeat angiography (assuming the first test is negative).[92,93] Using a protocol of very thin cuts (3 mm) through the region of the circle of Willis helps pick up small bleeds.[88]

Sensitivity with CT is high during the first hours of SAH.[87-89,94,95] In two studies that specifically evaluated CT scans performed within the first 12 hours using a *third generation* scanner, one demonstrated 98% sensitivity (2 of 119 false negatives) 94 and the other 100% sensitivity (0 of 80 false negatives).[95] Therefore, although the CT is an excellent test, especially during the first 12 hours, it is not infallible. If one extends the time window to the first 24 hours, however, sensitivity drops to 93-95%.[87,89] Overall, SAH is detected in about 90% of patients after one day, 58-80% after five days, and roughly 50% after seven days.[87,88]

In addition to timing, other important factors affecting sensitivity of CT for detection of SAH are density and quantity of blood.[88] Blood with a hemoglobin count of less than 10 g/dL may not show up on CT scanning; likewise, small amounts of blood can be missed. False positives can also occur from calcification of dural and vascular structures at the base of the brain, as well as from artifact caused by patient movement and partial volume averaging.

Accordingly, the majority of patients with suspected SAH whose CT scans are *negative* should undergo LP.[87-89,94,95] In making this decision, the clinician should consider the pre-test likelihood of the disease before deciding whether or not to proceed with an LP after a negative CT. There are two major factors to be considered. The first is the likelihood of the disease based on purely clinical parameters, and the second is the timing of the CT, since the sensitivity is highly dependent upon temporal factors. Generally, if the pre-test probability is low, and the CT has been done during the *first 12 hours* on a third generation scanner, and it is negative, then the likelihood of SAH approaches zero.[96] Magnetic resonance imaging (MRI) is not as sensitive in diagnosis of acute SAH, although MR angiography may play some role in defining the aneurysms.

Limitations of the Lumbar Puncture (LP). There are several pitfalls in diagnosis of SAH related to the LP. The first is failure to recognize that it may take up to 12 hours post-ictus for the CSF sampled from the lumbar theca to reflect the pressure bleed,[94,97,98] which can take the form of frank blood or xanthochromia. Xanthochromia is a yellow-golden discoloration of CSF caused by the enzyme-dependent breakdown of hemoglobin into oxyhemoglobin and bilirubin; this may account for the delay.[99] There are two ways of detecting xanthochromia: 1) visual inspection of the CSF with the naked eye; and 2) examination of the fluid by spectrophotometry. Depending on the quantity of breakdown products, xanthochromia may or may not be visible to the naked eye. Only about 50% of specimens that are positive by spectrophotometry are also positive visually.[100] Although it is well established that it may take up to 12 hours for xanthochromia to be visible, some investigators have reported it to be visible with the naked eye as early as four hours after symptoms.[101]

This had led to some controversy about the significance of bloody CSF without xanthochromia in a patient suspected of having SAH. If an LP yields bloody fluid, it should immediately be centrifuged and the supernatant should be examined for xanthochromia. It should be compared to water, and both specimens should be examined against a white background. If xanthochromia is present visually, SAH is strongly suggested. If it is negative to the naked eye, the specimen should be examined for optical density by spectrophotometry. If it is *negative* by spectrophotometry and the fluid was obtained between 12 hours and two weeks after the onset of headache, this suggests *a traumatic* LP rather than SAH.

Although there are several methods that can help to distinguish a traumatic tap from blood associated with SAH, none is error-free. Two time-honored methods include: 1) looking for diminishing redness (and RBC counts) in sequential tubes of CSF; and 2) examining the fluid for xanthochromia. The former approach is useful, but is not foolproof,[102] and absence of xanthochromia (as measured by spectrophotometry) strongly suggests a traumatic tap.

In one study of 12 patients with sudden onset of headache, normal CT, bloody CSF, and no xanthochromia by spectrophotometry, none had subsequent SAH diagnosed during a mean follow-up of four years. This suggests that absence of xanthochromia is strong evidence in favor of a SAH. Another technique is to re-tap one interspace higher, which should yield non-bloody or less bloody fluid if the first tap was traumatic. One other method to distinguish traumatic tap from acute bleed that has proved to be without value is looking for crenated red cells in the CSF.[101] These data always should be interpreted in the clinical context.

The best strategy is to avoid a traumatic tap. Proper attention to procedural detail is imperative. The most important factor is patient preparation—both physical and mental. The plane of the patient's back must be perpendicular to the floor, with hips and shoulders directly on top of their counterparts. Sometimes having the patient push his back out toward the operator "like a cat arching its back" will help spread the spinous processes. Taking time to feel the landmarks and identify the midline are keys for success. Advancing the needle so that one's finger (or thumb) tip is applying the pressure to the hub of the needle assists the operator to feel the decrease in resistance on dural entry.

It is important to avoid post-LP headache in patients being evaluated for SAH for two reasons. First, minimizing pain and discomfort will be in the patient's best interest. Second, to the extent that the mechanism of post-LP headache involves persistent leakage of CSF through the dural rent, this would also decrease the pressure gradient across the aneurysm wall (see LaPlace's law, above). Proven factors that reduce the likelihood of this event are needle size (smaller is better), design (pencil point, non-cutting needle may be better), and orientation (bevel should split rather than transect dural fibers).[103] Reinsertion of the stylet on needle removal may also help.[104]

In some patients who are being evaluated for SAH, bacterial meningitis will be in the differential diagnosis. One should not delay LP in order to perform a CT[105] in these patients, except in those with abnormal level of consciousness, focal neurologic findings, or papilledema. If these findings are present in a patient in whom meningitis is a serious consideration, the appropriate sequence is to treat with antibiotics, scan, and then tap (if there is no contraindication by CT).[106]

There is a small potential for deterioration following LP in patients with SAH.[107,108] In one study of 283 patients, there was a documented complication rate of 2.2%. These four cases were all initially alert prior to the LP. Others have investigated the same phenomenon and found no patients who deteriorated post-LP.[109] While this is another reason that CT has been proposed as the diagnostic method of choice for patients suspected of having SAH, it should be stressed that in patients in whom meningitis is a strong possibility, one must proceed with either treatment or LP prior to CT.

Complications and Management: General Principles

Once the diagnosis is secure, prompt consultation with a neurologist and/or neurosurgeon is mandatory to arrange for angiography and definitive treatment. While this has a high priority, there are a number of urgent or emergent issues that will require prompt attention in the ED.

Attention to the ABCs is paramount. Patients with loss of protective airway reflexes should be intubated with attention to blunting reflex elevations in intracranial and systemic blood pressure. Lidocaine and short-acting barbiturates have been used. A short-acting paralytic such as succinylcholine would lead to rapid resumption of the baseline neurologic status. Succinylcholine's lack of producing hyperkalemia has been specifically studied in this setting.[110]

In general, ED care of the patient with SAH should be focused on prevention or treatment of major complications, among them: rebleeding, vasospasm, seizures, and obstructive hydrocephalus. Prevention of other, longer term sequelae, such as thromboembolic disease, peptic ulcer, and long-term control of hypertension, will not be discussed, but the reader is referred to excellent references.[13,14]

Severe, systemic hypertension should be treated with drugs such as labetalol or possibly hydralazine, but one must factor in the patient's pre-morbid pressure and not aim for any pre-set value.[14]

Seizures occur in 10-25% of cases.[14] In these patients, phenytoin, 17 mg/kg, should be administered intravenously to prevent additional seizures, which can provoke re-bleeding.[13,14] Patients undergoing painful procedures should be treated with short-acting analgesics such as fentanyl.[7] Anxiety in the awake, alert patients can be treated with small doses of short-acting benzodiazepines such as midazolam to minimize the catecholamine release that pain and anxiety may provoke.[14]

Acute obstructive hydrocephalus can be seen within the first 24 hours and is manifested by diminished level of consciousness, stupor, and coma.[13,111] In one series of 473 patients admitted within 72 hours of SAH, 91 (19%) had hydrocephalus on the initial scan.[112] Diagnosis is by CT, and emergency ventriculostomy is indicated for drainage.[14] Patients will often have a dramatic response to this procedure. Care should be taken not to reduce the ICP too rapidly as this will increase the pressure gradient across the wall of the aneurysm and increase the likelihood of rebleeding.[14]

Nimodipine, 60 mg, administered either by mouth or nasogastric tube within the first 12 hours is important for prevention of vasospasm.[13,14] This can be administered in the ED. Vasospasm is a serious and common complication of SAH, and is seen by angiography in as many as 75% of patients.[14] Symptoms will depend on which vessel(s) is in spasm—in the same way that stroke symptoms reflect the vascular territory supplied by the thrombosed vessel. There is a wide range of treatments for vasospasm, including calcium channel blockers, hemodynamic therapy to increase blood pressure and intravascular volume, percutaneous transluminal angioplasty and intrathecal papaverine and tissue plasminogen activator.[14] These therapies fall within the province of the neurointensivist.

The risk of early rebleeding is high—approximately 4% during the first day and 1-2% per day for the next two weeks,[14,113] and rebleeding carries a high mortality. Once a clot is formed around an aneurysm, fibrinolysis begins to occur in the CSF. For many years, antifibrinolytics were administered to reduce clot dissolution. However, they produced no improvements in mortality because what is gained by reduction of rebleeding is lost due to cerebral ischemia and thromboembolic complications.[13,14]

Patients with SAH should not be "run dry" (i.e., dehydrated), although data to support this approach are lacking. There is a tendency for these patients to become volume contracted and hyponatremic, possibly from SIADH. These patients should not be fluid restricted but should be given isotonic or slightly hypertonic saline.[1] Ensuring that patients stay well- or even overhydrated has led some to recommend so-called triple-H therapy (hypertension-hypervolemia-hemodilution) to increase diminished cerebral blood flow seen after SAH.[13,114]

After the patient is stabilized, four-vessel angiography is performed by the neuroradiologist to ascertain the cause of the bleed and the location of the aneurysm. Visualization of all four cerebral arteries is important, even in those cases where the CT shows the likely source of bleeding, because of the frequency of multiple aneurysms. In 15-20% of cases, no aneurysm is demonstrated.[113,115] This group of patients is heterogeneous: some have aneurysms that are not visualized because the feeder vessel is in spasm; about two-thirds have the previously described perimesencephalic pattern of bleeding that is thought to be venous in origin; some have occult aneurysm and others have an other diagnosis, such as dissection, AVM, or a bleeding disorder. Angiography is remarkably safe when carried out by qualified individuals;[116] it has a mortality rate of less than 0.1%.[113] Although conventional angiography is still the gold standard, magnetic resonance angiography is playing an increasingly important role.[117]

Timing of Surgery. Definitive therapy requires isolating the aneurysm from the general circulation. The time-honored method is surgical clipping of the aneurysm. For many years, there was controversy regarding the timing of surgery. Some felt early surgery was better because the risk of rebleeding was reduced; others thought that delaying surgery until after the acute inflammation had receded was a better method. In 1990, the results of an international cooperative trial of 3521 patients partly resolved this controversy.[118,119] While there was no difference in mortality outcomes for patients with H & H grades 1-3, patients operated on early (0-3 days) did better than those operated on late (11-14 days). The international study found that predictors of mortality were decreased level of consciousness, increased age, thickness of clot on CT, elevated blood pressure, co-morbid conditions and basilar aneurysms.

As a result, the general recommendation currently is that H&H grades 1-3 undergo early surgery.[29] The benefits of early surgery are reduced risk of rebleeding, opportunity to clear blood from the subarachnoid cisterns, and ability to aggressively treat vasospasm with triple-H and other therapies.[29]

The timing of surgery for H & H grades 4 and 5 is less clear and the results in these patients are not very encouraging. Some advocate using the endovascularly placed coil to obliterate the aneurysm at the time of initial angiography and then to consider surgical therapy if the patient improves.[29] Others advocate a more aggressive approach in these high-grade patients.[120] There also may be a place for surgery immediately following CT scan in the rare patient who has an aneurysm that ruptures directly into the brain parenchyma, leading to an acute mass effect.[29]

The most recent advance in treatment of intracranial aneurysms is endovascular placement of a variety of balloons or coils that either obliterate the fundus of the aneurysm or decrease flow to the parent vessel. This field is undergoing constant revision as technology changes, and it would seem that these non-surgical techniques will be used more rather than less in the future.[111] Nevertheless, more long-term data are needed to establish the precise indications for this novel method.[29] One recently published study of more than 400 patients treated with the Guglielmi detachable coil showed promising results.[121] Some experts argue that endovascular treatment is indicated for aneurysms which are technically difficult to operate on and in patients with H & H grades 4 and 5 who would normally not be operated on immediately.[111]

These innovative treatments are more useful in patients diagnosed earlier rather than later. Therefore, emergency physicians must strive to identify patients with SAH early in the natural history of their disease.

References

1. Anonymous. Clinical policy for the initial approach to adolescents and adults presenting to the emergency department with a chief complaint of headache. *Ann of Emerg Med* 1996;27:821-844.
2. Dhopesh V, Anwar R, Herring C. A retrospective assessment of emergency department patients with complaints of headache. *Headache* 1979;19:37-42.
3. Leicht M. Non-traumatic headache in the emergency department. *Ann of Emerg Med* 1980;9:404-409.
4. Adams HP, et al. Pitfalls in the recognition of subarachnoid hemorrhage. *JAMA* 1980;244:794-796.
5. Mayer PL, et al. Misdiagnosis of symptomatic cerebral aneurysm: Prevalence and correlation with outcome at four institutions. *Stroke* 1996;27:1558-1563.
6. Neil-Dwyer G, Lang D. 'Brain attack'-aneurysmal subarachnoid hemorrhage: Death due to delayed diagnosis (see comments). *J Royal Coll of Physicians of London* 1997;31:49-52.
7. Schievink WI. Intracranial aneurysms (see comments). *N Engl J Med* 1997;336:28-40.
8. Ingall TJ, et al. Has there been a decline in subarachnoid hemorrhage mortality? *Stroke* 1989;20:718-724.
9. Hop JW, et al. Case-fatality rates and functional outcome after subarachnoid hemorrhage: A systematic review. *Stroke* 1997;28:660-664.
10. Barrow DL, Prats AR. Infectious intracranial aneurysms: comparison of groups with and without endocarditis. *Neurosurgery* 1990;27:562-72; discussion 572-573.
11. Clare CE, Barrow DL. Infectious intracranial aneurysms. *Neurosurgery Clin N Am* 1992;3:551-566.
12. Lasner TM, Raps EC. Clinical evaluation and management of aneurysmal subarachnoid hemorrhage. *Neuroimaging clin N Am* 1997;7:669-678.
13. Mayberg MR, Batjer HH, Dacey R. Guidelines for the management of aneurysmal subarachnoid hemorrhage. *Stroke* 1994;25:2315-2328.
14. Miller J, Diringer M. Management of aneurysmal subarachnoid hemorrhage. *Neurologic Clinics* 1995;13:451-478.
15. Lanzino G, et al. Intracranial dissecting aneurysm causing subarachnoid hemorrhage: The role of computerized tomographic angiography and magnetic resonance angiography. *Surg Neur* 1997;48:477-481.
16. Massoud TF, Anslow P, Molyneux AJ. Subarachnoid hemorrhage following spontaneous intracranial carotid artery

dissection. *Neuroradiology* 1992;34:33-35.
17. Fukui M. Current state of study of Moyamoya disease in Japan. *Surg Neur* 1997;47:138-143.
18. O'Brien D, J, OD, MW, Eversol A. Delayed traumatic cerebral aneurysm after brain injury. *Arch Phys Med & Rehabil* 1997;78:883-885.
19. Quattrocchi KB, et al. Traumatic aneurysm of the superior cerebellar artery: Case report and review of the literature. *Neurosurgery* 1990;27:476-479.
20. Stehbens WE. Pathology and pathogenesis of intracranial berry aneurysms. *Neur Res* 1990;12:29-34.
21. Stehbens WE. Etiology of intracranial berry aneurysms. *J Neurosurg* 1989;70:823-831.
22. Schievink WI, et al. Circumstances surrounding aneurysmal subarachnoid hemorrhage. *Surg Neur* 1989;32:266-272.
23. Inagawa T. What are the actual incidence and mortality rates of subarachnoid hemorrhage. *Surg Neur* 1997;47:47-53.
24. Ostergaard JR. Aetiology of intracranial saccular aneurysms in childhood. *British J Neurosurg* 1991;5:575-580.
25. Muhonen MG, Godersky JC, VanGilder JC. Cerebral aneurysms associated with neurofibromatosis. *Surg Neur* 1991;36:470-475.
26. Schievink WI, et al. Intracranial aneurysms in Marfan's syndrome: An autopsy study. *Neurosurg* 1997;41:866-870; discussion 871.
27. Kumar R, et al. Isolated angiitis of the CNS presenting as subarachnoid hemorrhage. *J Neurol Neursurg Psychiatry* 1997;62:649-651.
28. Fessler RD, et al. The neurovascular complications of cocaine. *Surg Neur* 1997;47:339-345.
29. Zager EL. Surgical treatment of intracranial aneurysms. *Neuroimaging Clin N Am* 1997;7:763-782.
30. Teunissen LL, et al. Risk factors for subarachnoid hemorrhage: A systematic review. *Stroke* 1996;27(3):544-549.
31. Reichman OH, Karlman RL. Berry aneurysm. *Surg Clinics N Am* 1995;75:115-121.
32. Ortiz O, Voelker J, Eneorji F. Transient enlargement of an intracranial aneurysm during pregnancy: Case report. *Surg Neurol* 1997;47:527-531.
33. Raps ED, et al. The clinical spectrum of unruptured intracranial aneurysm. *Arch Neur* 1993;50:265-268.
34. Ohno K, et al. Unruptured aneurysms in patients with transient ischemic attack or reversible ischemic neurological deficit. Report of eight cases. *Clin Neurol Neurosurg* 1989;91:229-233.
35. Parenti G, Fiori L, Marconi F. Intracranial aneurysm and cerebral embolism. *European Neurol* 1992;32:212-215.
36. Wiebers DO, et al. The significance of unruptured intracranial saccular aneurysms. *J Neurosurg* 1987;66:23-29.
37. Wiebers DO, Whisnant JP, O'Fallon WM. The natural history of unruptured intracranial aneurysms. *N Engl J Med* 1981; 304:696-698.
38. Juvela S, Porras M, Heiskanen O. Natural history of unruptured intracranial aneurysms: A long-term follow-up study. *J Neurosurg* 1993;79:174-182.
39. Yoshimoto T, Mizoi K. Importance of management of unruptured aneurysms. *Surgical Neurol* 1997;47:522-526.
40. Yasui N, et al. Long-term follow-up study of unruptured intracranial aneurysms. *Neurosurg* 1997;40:1155-1159; discussion 1159-1160.
41. Hamburger C, Schonberger J, Lange M. Management and prognosis of intracranial giant aneurysms. A report on 58 cases. *Neurosurgical Rev* 1992;15:97-103.
42. Schievink WI, Piepgras DG, Wirth FP. Rupture of previously documented small asymptomatic saccular intracranial aneurysms. Report of three cases. *J Neurosurg* 1992;76: 1019-1024.
43. Kasner SE, Liu GT, Galetta SL. Neuro-ophthalmic aspects of aneurysms. *Neuroimaging Clinics N Am* 1997;7:679-692.
44. Garfinkle AM, et al. Terson's syndrome: A reversible cause of blindness following subarachnoid hemorrhage. *J Neurosurg* 1992;76:766-771.
45. Frizzell RT, et al. Screening for ocular hemorrhages in patients with ruptured cerebral aneurysms: a prospective study of 99 patients. *Neurosurg* 1997;41:529-533; discussion 533-534.
46. Fujiwara S, et al. Oculomotor nerve palsy in patients with cerebral aneurysms. *Neurosurgical Rev* 1989;12:123-132.
47. Kissel JT, et al. Pupil-sparing oculomotor palsies with internal carotid-posterior communicating artery aneurysms. *Ann Neurol* 1982;13:149-154.
48. Trobe JD. Third nerve palsy and the pupil. *Arch Ophthal* 1988;106:601-602.
49. Hunt WE, Hess RM. Surgical risk as related to time of intervention in the repair of intracranial aneurysms. *J Neurosurg* 1968;28:14-20.
50. Gillingham FJ. The management of ruptured intracranial aneurysm. *Ann Royal Coll Surgeons, English* 1958;23: 89-117.
51. Gillingham FJ. The management of ruptured intracranial aneurysm. *Scottish Med J* 1967;12:377-383.
52. Okawara SH. Warning signs prior to rupture of an intracranial aneurysm. *J Neurosurg* 1973;38:575-580.
53. Duff GP. The warning leak in spontaneous subarachnoid hemorrhage. *Med J Australia* 1983;1:514-516.
54. LeBlanc R. The minor leak preceding subarachnoid hemorrhage. *J Neurosurg* 1987;66:35-39.
55. Verweij RD, Wijdicks EF, van Gijn J. Warning headache in aneurysmal subarachnoid hemorrhage. A case-control study (see comments). *Arch Neurol* 1988;45:1019-1020.
56. Bassi P, et al. Warning signs in subarachnoid hemorrhage: A cooperative study. *Acta Neurologica Scandinavica* 1991; 84:277-281.
57. Hauerberg J, et al. Importance of the recognition of a warning leak as a sign of a ruptured intracranial aneurysm. *Acta Neurologica Scandinavica* 1991;83:61-64.
58. Juvela S. Minor leak before rupture of an intracranial aneurysm and subarachnoid hemorrhage of unknown etiology. *Neurosurg* 1992;30:7-11.
59. Jakobsson KE, et al. Warning leak and management outcome in aneurysmal subarachnoid hemorrhage. *J Neurosurg* 1996;85:995-999.
60. Edner G, Ronne-Engstrom E. Can early admission reduce aneurysmal rebleeds? A prospective study on aneurysmal incidence, aneurysmal rebleeds, admission and treatment delays in a defined region. *Brit J Neurosurg* 1991;5:601-608.

61. Ostergaard JR. Headache as a warning symptom of impending aneurysmal subarachnoid hemorrhage. *Cephalalgia* 1991;11:53-55.
62. Markus HS. A prospective follow-up of thunderclap headache mimicking subarachnoid hemorrhage. *J Neurol Neurosurg Psychiatry* 1991;54:1117-1125.
63. Pareja JA, et al. Idiopathic stabbing headache (jabs and jolts syndrome). *Cephalgia* 1996;16:93-96.
64. Ball MJ. Pathogenesis of the "sentinel" headache preceding berry aneurysm rupture. *Canadian Med Assoc J* 1975;112: 78-79.
65. Day JW, Raskin NH. Thunderclap headache: Symptom of unruptured cerebral aneurysm. *Lancet* 1986;ii:1247-1248.
66. Wijdicks EFM, Kerkhoff H, van Gijn J. Long-term follow-up of 71 patients with thunderclap headache mimicking subarachnoid hemorrhage. *Lancet* 1988;ii:68-69.
67. Harling DW, et al. Thunderclap headache: Is it migraine? *Cephalgia* 1989;9:87-90.
68. Abbot RJ, van Hille P. Thunderclap headache and unruptured aneurysm. *Lancet* 1986;ii:1459.
69. Liedo A, et al. Acute headache of recent onset and subarachnoid hemorrhage: A prospective study. *Headache* 1994;34: 172-174.
70. Pascual J, et al. Cough, exertional, and sexual headaches: An analysis of 72 benign and symptomatic cases. *Neurol* 1996; 46:1520-1524.
71. Haykowsky MJ, Findlay JM, Ignaszewski AP. Aneurysmal subarachnoid hemorrhage associated with weight training: Three case reports. *Clin J Sport Med* 1996;6:52-55.
72. De Bruijn SF, Stam J, Kappelle LJ. Thunderclap headache as first symptom of cerebral venous sinus thrombosis. CVST Study Group. *Lancet* 1996:348:1623-1625.
73. Ameri A, Bousser MG. Cerebral venous thrombosis. *Neurologic Clin* 1992;10:87-111.
74. Linn FH, et al. Prospective study of sentinel headache in aneurysmal subarachnoid hemorrhage. *Lancet* 1994;344: 590-593.
75. Sved PD, Morgan MK, Weber NC. Delayed referral of patients with aneurysmal subarachnoid hemorrhage. *Med J Australia* 1995;162:310-311.
76. Seymour JJ, Moscati RM, Jehle D. Response of headache to nonnarcotic analgesics resulting in missed intracranial hemorrhage. *Am J Emerg Med* 1995;13:43-45.
77. Schattner A. Pain in the neck (letter). *Lancet* 1996;348: 411-412.
78. Sakas DE. Dias LS, Beale D. Subarachnoid hemorrhage presenting as head injury (see comments). *BMJ* 1995;310: 1186-1187.
79. Gipe B, McFarland D. Subarachnoid hemorrhage: An unusual presentation of shock. *Ann Emerg Med* 1995;26:85-89.
80. Tabbaa MA, Ramirez-Lassepas M, Snyder BD. Aneurysmal subarachnoid hemorrhage presenting as cardiorespiratory arrest. *Arch Int Med* 1987;147:1661-1662.
81. Hall DP, Young SA. Frontal lobe cerebral aneurysm rupture presenting as psychosis. *J Neurol Neurosurg Psychiatry* 1992;55:1207-1208.
82. Pine DS, Tierney Jr. L. Clinical problem-solving. A stressful interaction (see comments). *N Engl J Med* 1996;334: 1530-1534.
83. Raymer K, Choi P. Concurrent subarachnoid hemorrhage and myocardial injury. *Can J Anaesth* 1997;44(5 pt 1):515-519.
84. Mayer S, LiMandri G, Sherman D. Electrocardiographic markers of abnormal left ventricular wall motion in acute subarachnoid hemorrhage. *J Neurosurg* 1995;83:889-896.
85. Andreoli A, et al. Subarachnoid hemorrhage: Frequency and severity of cardiac arrhythmias; A survey of 70 cases studied in the acute phase. *Stroke* 1986;18:558-564.
86. Wells C, et al. Reversibility of severe left ventricular dysfunction in patients with subarachnoid hemorrhage. *Am Heart J* 1995;129:409-412.
87. Vermeulen M, van Gijn J. The diagnosis of subarachnoid hemorrhage. *J Neurol Neurosurg Psychiatry* 1990;53: 365-372.
88. Latchaw RE, Silva P, Falcone SF. The role of CT following aneurysmal rupture. *Neuroimaging Clinics N Am* 1997;7: 693-708.
89. Sames TA, et al. Sensitivity of new-generation computed tomography in subarachnoid hemorrhage. *Academic Emerg Med* 1996;3:16-20.
90. Ishibashi A, Yokokura Y, Sakamoto M. Acute subdural hematoma without subarachnoid hemorrhage due to ruptured intracranial aneurysm-case report. *Neurologia Medico-Chirurgica* 1997;37:533-537.
91. Kamiya K, et al. Subdural hematoma due to ruptured intracranial aneurysm. *Neurologia Medico Chirurgica* 1991;31:82-86.
92. Schwartz TH, Solomon RA. Perimesencephalic nonaneurysmal subarachnoid hemorrhage: Review of the literature (see comments). *Neurosurg* 1996;39:433-440; discussion 440.
93. Rinkel GJ, et al. Nonaneurysmal perimesencephalic subarachnoid hemorrhage: CT and MR patterns that differ from aneurysmal rupture. *Am J Neuroradiology* 1991;12:829-834.
94. van der Wee N, et al. Detection of subarachnoid hemorrhage on early CT: Is lumbar puncture still needed after a negative scan? *J Neurol Neurosurg Psychiatry* 1995;58:357-359.
95. Sidman R, Connolly E, Lemke T. Subarachnoid hemorrhage diagnosis: lumbar puncture is still needed when the computed tomography scan is normal (see comments). *Academic Emerg Med* 1996;3:827-831.
96. Singal BM. A tap in time? (editorial; comment). *Academic Emerg Med* 1996;3:823.
97. Anonymous. Xanthochromia. *Lancet* 1989;ii:658-659.
98. Vermeulen M, et al. Xanthochromia after subarachnoid hemorrhage needs no visitation. *J Neurol Neurosurg Psychiatry* 1989;52:826-828.
99. Roost KT, et al. The formation of cerebrospinal fluid xanthochromia after subarachnoid hemorrhage. *Neurol* 1972;22: 973-977.
100. Soderstrom CE. Diagnostic significance of CSF spectrophotometry and computerized tomography in cerebrovascular disease: A comparative study in 231 cases. *Stroke* 1977;8: 606-612.
101. Matthews WF and Frommeyer WB. The in vitro behavior of erythrocytes in human cerebrospinal fluid. *J Lab Clin Med* 1955;45:508-515.
102. Buruma OJS, et al. Blood-stained cerebrospinal fluid:

Traumatic puncture or hemorrhage. *J Neurol Neurosurg Psychiatry* 1981;44:144-147.

103. Liebold RA, et al. Post-dural puncture headache: Characteristics, management and prevention. *Ann Emerg Med* 1993;22:1863-1870.
104. Strupp M, Brandt T. Should one reinsert the stylet during lumbar puncture. *N Engl J Med* 1997;336:1190.
105. Archer BD. Computed tomography before lumbar puncture in acute meningitis: A review of the risks and benefits. *Can Med Assoc J* 1993;148:961-965.
106. Talan DA, et al. Role of empiric parenteral antibiotics prior to lumbar puncture in suspected bacterial meningitis: State of the art. *Rev Inf Dis* 1998;10:365-376.
107. Duffy GP. Lumbar puncture in spontaneous subarachnoid hemorrhage. *BMJ* 1982;285:1163-1166.
108. Hillman J. Should computered tomography scanning replace lumbar puncture in the diagnostic process in suspected subarachnoid hemorrhage? *Surg Neurol* 1986;26:547-550.
109. Patel MK, Clarke MA. Lumbar puncture and subarachnoid hemorrhage. *Postgrad Med* 1986;62:1021-1024.
110. Manninen PH, et al. Succinylcholine does not increase serum potassium levels in patients with acutely ruptured cerebral aneurysms. *Anesthesia Analgesia* 1990;70:172-175.
111. Nelson PK, et al. Neuroendovascular management of intracranial aneurysms. *Neuroimag Clin N Am* 1997;7:739-762.
112. Hasan D, et al. Management problems in acute hydrocephalus after subarachnoid hemorrhage. *Stroke* 1989;20:747-753.
113. Bagley LJ, Hurst RW. Angiographic evaluation of aneurysms affecting the central nervous system. *Neuroimaging Clin N Am* 1997;7:721-737.
114. Guterman LR, et al. Hypertensive, hypervolemic, hemodilutional therapy for aneurysmal subarachnoid hemorrhage: If is efficacious? Yes. *Arkh Patol* 1971;33:47-53.
115. Rinkel GJ, van Gijn J, Wijdicks EF. Subarachnoid hemorrhage without detectable aneurysm. A review of the causes. *Stroke* 1993;24:1403-1409.
116. Dion JE, et al. Clinical events following neuroangiography: A prospective study. *Stroke* 1987;18:997-1005.
117. Atlas SW. Magnetic resonance imaging of intracranial aneurysms. *Neuroimaging Clin N Am* 1997;7:709-720.
118. Kassell NF, et al. The International Cooperative Study on the Timing of Aneurysm Surgery. Part 1: Overall management results. *J Neurosurg* 1990;73:18-36.
119. Kassell NF, et al. The International Cooperative Study on the Timing of Aneurysm Surgery. Part 2: Surgical results. *J Neurosurg* 1990;73:37-47.
120. Gumprecht H, et al. Therapeutic management of grade IV aneurysm patients. *Surg Neurol* 1997;47:54-59.
121. Vinuela F, Duckwiler G, Mawad G. Guglielmi detachable coil embolization of acute intracranial aneurysm: Perioperative anatomic and clinical outcome in 403 patients. *J Neurosurg* 1997;86:475-482.

Stroke: Clinical Presentations

John E. Duldner, Jr., MD
Charles L. Emerman, MD

Thrombotic and embolic infarction of the brain is a major cause of morbidity and mortality in the United States, with the estimated annual medical costs of stroke care reaching approximately $30 billion per year. About 20% of these expenditures occur in the first 90 days after an acute event.[1] Cerebral vascular disease is a leading cause of death, second only to cardiovascular disease and cancer.[2] Overall, approximately 500,000 strokes of all types occur each year, and they are responsible for about 150,000 deaths. Seventy-five percent of all strokes occur in patients older than age 65.

The emergency department (ED) frequently is the first point of contact for stroke victims. Although many patients currently present after a substantial delay following onset of symptoms, the role of the physician in the acute management of stroke is likely to expand as newer therapies are shown to improve morbidity and mortality.[3] Though patients may present to the ED with a devastating neurological picture, substantial improvement may occur over time, even in the absence of specific therapy. About 20% of patients who survive the initial event eventually have full or partial resolution of hemiparesis. Hemineglect, a common finding in early stroke, resolves in most patients.[4] Although the risk of repeated stroke is highest within the first 30 days, 25-40% of patients will have a repeat stroke within five years.[5] Early recurrence is associated with a significant increase in morbidity and mortality.

Eighty-five percent of strokes are ischemic in origin, whereas hemorrhagic strokes occur in about 15% of patients.[1] The one-month mortality rate for stroke varies according to etiology. It is approximately 15% for ischemic stroke, 50% for subarachnoid hemorrhage, and may be as high as 80% for intracerebral hemorrhage.[4,6,7] Cardiovascular complications account for 35% of stroke deaths, recurrent stroke for 25%, and pulmonary complications—either pneumonia or embolism—for another 25%.[8]

With these clinical challenges in focus, this chapter will provide a systematic review of clinical presentations and stroke syndromes.

Prehospital Considerations

The goals for prehospital management of stroke patients include priority dispatch, early recognition, brief evaluation, appropriate intervention, and rapid transport. In fact, stroke is considered a medical emergency and the prehospital response should be commensurate with this urgency. Prehospital care for stroke begins with EMS dispatch, for which the priority should be high. Although the majority of prehospital providers will recognize symptoms of a large hemispheric stroke, prehospital personnel should be taught basic neurological assessment skills to detect subtle presentations. A brief neurological examination including assessment of level of consciousness, Glasgow Coma Scale, pupil size and reactivity, and gross motor function may suffice, but a more specific neurological exam may improve diagnostic sensitivity. Several cities have implemented prehospital stroke scales to improve detection, and their sensitivity is being tested. A stroke-specific prehospital protocol may improve clinical outcomes in the field.

The field evaluation should be focused. In addition to evaluating the patient for evidence of cardiovascular or traumatic illness, EMS personnel should evaluate the patient for conditions that mimic stroke and can be readily reversed. These conditions include hypoglycemia, drug overdose, and seizures. In addition to evaluating the ABCs, patients should receive at least the following: cardiac monitor, placement of intravenous catheter, supplemental oxygen, and a rapid blood sugar screen. Providers should avoid administration of excess intravenous (IV) fluids or inappropriate use of dextrose (D50). Scene time should not be delayed with field interventions, and patients should be transported rapidly to an appropriate facility with the capability to manage acute stroke. Prehospital personnel should be instructed to notify the receiving hospital to facilitate prompt mobilization of resources, particularly specialized stroke teams where available.

Table 1. Risk Factors for Stroke

RISK FACTORS	COMMENTS
Hypertension	Primary risk factor
Increased age	Older than age 65
Male gender	Patients younger than age 60
Atrial fibrillation	Particularly with CHF or valvular disease
Cigarette use	
Diabetes	Particularly with women
Family history	Both paternal and maternal
Alcohol use	Heavy
Prior TIA	Highest risk in first year
Hyperlipidemia	Possible role

Definitions

According to the World Health Organization (WHO) definition, stroke is characterized by a neurological deficit of sudden onset accompanied by focal dysfunction and symptoms lasting more than 24 hours that are presumed to be of a non-traumatic vascular origin.[9] A transient ischemic attack (TIA) is diagnosed on the basis of neurological events that have a duration shorter than 24 hours, followed by complete return to baseline. An additional sub-category of stroke includes reversible ischemic neurological deficit (RIND), a category that is used when the deficit resolves completely, usually within three days, but always within three weeks.

It should be stressed that a variety of disorders may mimic strokes. In general, the diagnosis of stroke is correctly made on the basis of the initial clinical examination by non-neurologists in more than 95% of the cases. A few trials have found higher misdiagnosis rates, although these studies were performed at tertiary referral centers, which tend to see more complicated patients. Misdiagnosis occurs more commonly in younger patients and those with complex or atypical symptomatology.[10] The differential diagnosis includes complex migraine headache with hemiparesis, post-ictal paresis (Todd's paralysis), hypoglycemia, cerebral tumor, cerebral infection, subdural hematoma, drug intoxication, and malignant hypertension.

Risk Factors

The risk of stroke increases with age, particularly in patients older than age 65. In patients younger than 60, there is a male predominance to stroke in a 3:2 ratio. There is a familial association with stroke including both a paternal and maternal history of cerebral vascular and cardiovascular disease.[11]

It is estimated that almost 50% of strokes can be prevented by control of treatable risk factors.[12] *(Please see Table 1.)* Hypertension is the primary risk factor for stroke. Patients with hypertension have 4-5 times the risk of stroke than that of nonhypertensive patients. Even in patients with normal blood pressures, the risk of stroke diminishes as the diastolic blood pressure falls. In addition, isolated systolic hypertension also has been recognized as a risk factor for stroke. Cardiovascular and cerebrovascular disease coexist in more than 80% of stroke patients.[13] Atrial fibrillation occurring in the setting of mitral stenosis, congestive heart failure, or cardiomyopathy, as well as in patients with mechanical cardiac valves, carries a risk of stroke on the order of 6% per year.[14,15] The annual risk of atrial fibrillation-associated stroke increases with age and is as high as 36% in the very old.

Cigarette use and diabetes also increase the risk of stroke, particularly in women. Diabetics have a four-fold increase in stroke risk. The incidence and mortality of stroke is higher in African-Americans.[16] This may be attributable to differences in access to health care, although there may be a higher incidence of hypertension, glucose intolerance, and hyperlipidemia in this population.[16] The association between hypercholesterolemia and stroke is less clear, and reduction of cholesterol has recently been shown to reduce stroke risk.[17] Heavy alcohol use increases the risk of stroke, especially subarachnoid hemorrhage.[18] TIAs are strong predictors of stroke with an annual risk that is around 8%, although most strokes are not preceded by a TIA.

Clinical Features

Stroke usually involves the development of a focal neurological deficit, the nature of which can help localize the involved vascular territory. Although transient loss of consciousness may occur from global cerebral hypoperfusion, it is not generally a symptom of stroke unless accompanied by other vertebrobasilar symptoms that localize the vascular insult. Seizures may accompany stroke, although again, in the absence of focal neurological deficits, this finding alone does not confirm the diagnosis of stroke. Headache occurs in a substantial minority of patients with stroke and is most common in patients younger than age 70, in non-smokers, and in patients with cerebellar infarcts.[19] Headache that occurs with stroke is frequently, though not always, diffuse in nature. Vomiting, seizures, headache, or coma occur more commonly with hemorrhagic stroke but may be seen on occasion with ischemic infarction.

Careful clinical evaluation can identify the site of infarction in about 90% of the cases. *(Please see Table 2.)* The variety of neurological deficits seen in stroke relate to the area of the brain involved and the vascular territory perfused by cerebral vessels. Among patients undergoing angiography for atherosclerotic stroke, 62% have stenosis or occlusion of the internal carotid artery (ICA), 10% have

Table 2. Typical Stroke Syndromes

VASCULAR TERRITORY	CLINICAL PICTURE
Internal carotid artery	Variable but may involve hemiparesis and aphasia in dominant hemisphere
Anterior watershed	Hemiparesis greatest in leg with sensory loss
Posterior watershed	Hemianopia
MCA watershed	Hemiparesis, hemisensory loss, aphasia in dominant hemisphere
Superficial ACA	Contralateral leg weakness, sensory loss
Deep ACA	Movement disorders
Superficial ACA	Hemianopia
Deep ACA	Dysesthesia
Lacunar	Pure motor or sensory loss
Vertebral Artery	Impaired contralateral pain and thermal sense, ipsilateral Horner syndrome, nystagmus, vertigo, ipsilateral limb ataxia
MCA, Superior division	Contralateral face, arm, leg sensory and motor deficit, ipsilateral head and eye deviation, Broca aphasia
MCA, Inferior division	Homonymous hemianopia, Wernicke aphasia
Basilar artery	Coma, quadriplegia, "locked-in" syndrome

Key: ACA = anterior cerebral artery
ICA = internal carotid artery
MCA = middle cerebral artery

occlusion or stenosis of the middle cerebral artery (MCA), whereas 15% have blockage of the vertebrobasilar (VB) arteries.[23]

Conditions Causing Focal Neurologic Lesions

Overview. The most common cause of focal neurologic deficits is thrombotic cerebral infarction.[20-28] Because most thrombotic strokes cause abrupt neurologic deficits, that is an important differential point for establishing the diagnosis. Metabolic disorders, however, may also have an abrupt onset, so it is necessary first to distinguish stroke from other conditions, such as brain tumors, brain abscess, and intracranial lesions—in which neurologic dysfunction usually progresses gradually but may initially manifest as seizures or postictal focal paralysis.

Once conditions mimicking primary neurologic disorders have been eliminated, the emergency physician should attempt to identify which of the three categories of cerebro-occlusive disease has occurred—thrombosis, embolism, or hemorrhage—because initial therapy will depend upon the underlying cause.

Physical Examination. A rapid but comprehensive neurologic exam includes assessment of the following nine major neurologic functions: mental status, station and gait, skull and spine, meninges, motor function, sensation, proprioception, cranial nerves, and cerebellar function. Nonspecific, initial vital signs may also give important information. For example, reflex sinus bradycardia and elevated systemic blood pressure frequently occur with catastrophic intracranial events, such as subarachnoid intracerebral hemorrhage. And blood pressure discrepancy between the arms may herald a dissecting aortic aneurysm. The carotid pulses may reveal bruits, and the cardiac exam may suggest embolic causes for focal neurologic deficits: atrial fibrillation, paradoxical movement of the left ventricle (aneurysm with possibility of mural thrombus), and murmurs suggesting valvular disease associated with bacterial or marasmic endocarditis.

Thrombotic Infarction. Cerebral occlusions result in well-described, sudden, focal neurologic deficits. They occur without or with less severe headache and vomiting than intracerebral hemorrhages. Significant obtundation or depression of consciousness is unusual unless the occlusion involves a massive amount of brain, the brainstem, or a previously diseased brain. A full-blown deficit usually develops in seconds with emboli, and from minutes to hours with cerebral thrombotic infarction.

Cerebral artery thrombosis usually develops at night during sleep, with symptoms perceived by the patient or family upon awakening in the morning.[23-25] As a rule, the patient falls asleep without a deficit and awakens with a hemiparesis or speech disturbance.

Usually, thrombotic cerebral infarction does not present with severe depression of consciousness unless the basilar artery system is involved or unless there has been massive internal carotid thromboembolism resulting in acute cerebral edema and secondary compression of the brainstem structures.[26] Moreover, thrombotic infarction rarely causes seizures in the acute phase of the illness, although focal seizures do occur as sequelae in regions that have been scarred as a result of the previous cerebral infarction.

Suspect a diagnosis of thrombotic cerebral infarction in patients with extensive arteriosclerosis and in those with hypercoagulable states due to malignancy, thrombocytosis associated with collagen vascular disorders, and hyperosmolar states, which can lead to venous thrombosis.

Embolic Infarction. Embolic infarction is the next most common cause of focal neurologic deficits.[28-32] In contrast to thrombotic infarction, cerebral embolism is apt to occur at any time of the day or night and frequently occurs during periods of vigorous physical activity.[25]

When evaluating the possibility of cerebral embolic infarction, identifying a source, if possible, is essential. Common sources include atrial thrombi in elderly patients with long-standing chronic atrial or paroxysmal atrial fibrillation, valvular vegetations caused by bacterial endocarditis, thromboembolism in myocardial infarction, and, in patients with extracranial vascular disease, ulcerated plaques in the carotid system. It is, at present, a neurologic axiom that when atrial fibrillation and focal neurologic deficits coexist, cerebral embolization has occurred.[27,29]

As mentioned, embolic infarction usually occurs when the patient is awake, and does not present with severely impaired mental status unless there has been a complette occlusion of the carotid artery, leading to massive cerebral edema, or unless the vasuclar insult involves the ascending reticular activating system (ARAS). The acute phase of embolic infarction may be accompanied by seizures, which can be either focal of diffuse, in up to 20% of cases.[27] At present, it is recommended that patients who have had cerebral embolism due to an intracardiac thrombosis associated with atrial fibrillation be anticoagulated immediately with heparin therapy.[25,28] Anticoagulation should be preceded by CT scanning to exclude the possibility of hemorrhagic infaction.

Transient Ischemic Attacks. TIAs manifest as stereotyped, short-lived, focal neurologic deficits lasting, by definition, less than 24 hours. The time from onset to the maximal deficit is usually only a few minutes, and TIAs rarely last more than eight hours. Most resolve within 15-60 minutes.[30]

Although the definition of TIA is straightforward, management is complex and controversial. In one study, 30% of patients originally diagnosed as having TIAs were subsequently considered misdiagnosed on review of their medical records by a stroke specialist.[29,31,32] Physicians, including neurologists, perceive the management of TIAs as difficult, and many are frequently uncertain about how to best evaluate and manage such patients.

From the viewpoint of emergency practice, the greatest clinical significance of TIAs is that they are harbingers of ischemic cerebral infarction, with its potentially devastating consequences. Estimates of the incidence of infarction following TIA vary, but in the absence of systematic treatment, approximately 5-10% of patients will have a stroke within a month and 12% within a year. At the end of two years, stroke will have occurred in an estimated 20-40% of TIA patients.[31,32] Therefore, emergency physicians must recognize the occurence or increasing frequency of TIAs and institute appropriate measures to reduce the patient's risk of stroke.

Transient focal deficits may be caused by neurologic disorders other than focal ischemia. Features in the history and physical examination may provide clues to underlying disorders. For example, a throbbing unilateral headache (often occurring after disappearance or improvement of a focal deficit) and scintillating scotomas and accompanying nausea suggest migraine, especially in younger patients. Clonic motor activity and abrupt loss of consciousness followed by confusion, or a history of epilepsy or traumatic brain surgery suggest a seizure disorder. A recent history of headache, a clouded sensorium, or depressed level of consciousness with a focal neurologic deficit following a head injury may indicate a subdural hematoma. Remember, they also may occur without any preceding head injury, especially in the elderly.

Although systemic hypotension rarely produces focal symptoms, hemodynamic obstruction of a cerebral artery may decrease regional blood flow enough to cause dysfunction. In addition, cardiogenic emboli are well-known causes of TIA and stroke. Emboli arising from the heart may occur in association with valvular or nonvalvular atrial infarction, cardiomyopathy, mitral stenosis or prosthetic heart valves. Mitral valve prolapse, especially in younger patients, may also be associated with cerebral embolism. Occasionally, septic emboli will originate from a diseased endocardium. So-called paradox emboli originating in the lung or venous system and traveling through a patent foramen ovale may also occur.

Intracranial Hemorrhage. Hemorrhagic strokes, subarachnoid and intracranial hemorrhage, typically occur during stress or exertion. Precipitating events include sexual intercourse, Valsalva's maneuver, and labor and delivery. Recent evidence also suggests that alcohol consumption contributes to hemorrhagic stroke, especially subarachnoid.[33,34] In most cases, focal deficits rapidly evolve and many are associated with confusion, coma, or immediate death.

Excruciating headache is the cardinal symptom of intracranial hemorrhage and is classically described as "the worst" in the patient's life. It may be accompanied by nuchal rigidity on physical exam. Arteriovenous malformations (AVM) may bleed into the subarachnoid space, but when they involve the cerebral parenchyma, lateralizing signs will be present. Lack of focal findings and young age at presentation help distinguish subarachnoid from intracerebral hemorrhage. Except for the occasional field cut, oculomotor palsy of aneurysmatic compession, or focal seizure, lateralizing focal neurologic lesions are notably absent with subarachnoid hemorrhage. On the other hand, intracranial hemorrhage is characterized by prominent focal findings because of its intraparenchymal location.

There are two main types of intracranial hemorrhage: intracerebral and extracerebral. In the elderly population, intracerebral hemorrhage is most common as a complication of long-standing hypertension or anticoagulation therapy. Hypertensive intracerebral hemorrhage has a predilection for certain sites and usually occurs, in order of frequency, in the thalmus, putamen, cerebellum, or brainstem. It most often develops when the patient is awake and active. Detecting cerebellar hemorrhage or hematoma is especially important, as intracranial bleeding in that location is amenable to neurosurgical intervention.[35]

Spontaneous subarachnoid hemorrhage usually results from a ruptured intracranial aneurysm. Onset usually consists of a sudden severe headache during vigorous activity, which is sometimes likened by patients to an abrupt blow on the head. Hemorrhagic infarction, which is the third most common cause of focal deficits in patients with cerebrovascular disease, should be considered in patients with hypertension or those who are taking anticoagulants, who have had previous craniocerebral trauma, or who have a history of unexplained headaches. Unlike thrombotic and embolic cerebral infarction, hemorrhagic infarction frequently presents with severely impaired consciousness and/or seizures and may be accompanied by severe headache and nuchal rigidity.

Noncerebrovascular Causes of Focal Neurological Deficits

Hyperosmolar states (hypernatremia, hyperglycemia), hypoxia, hypotension, carbon monoxide poisoning, hyponatremia, hypoglycemia, hypocalcemia, and hypophosphatemia can cause focal neurologic deficits.[27,28,36-38] CNS findings in patients with metabolic disorders may be diffuse or focal, with diffuse involvement produc-

Figure 1. Anterior View of the Cerebral Arteries

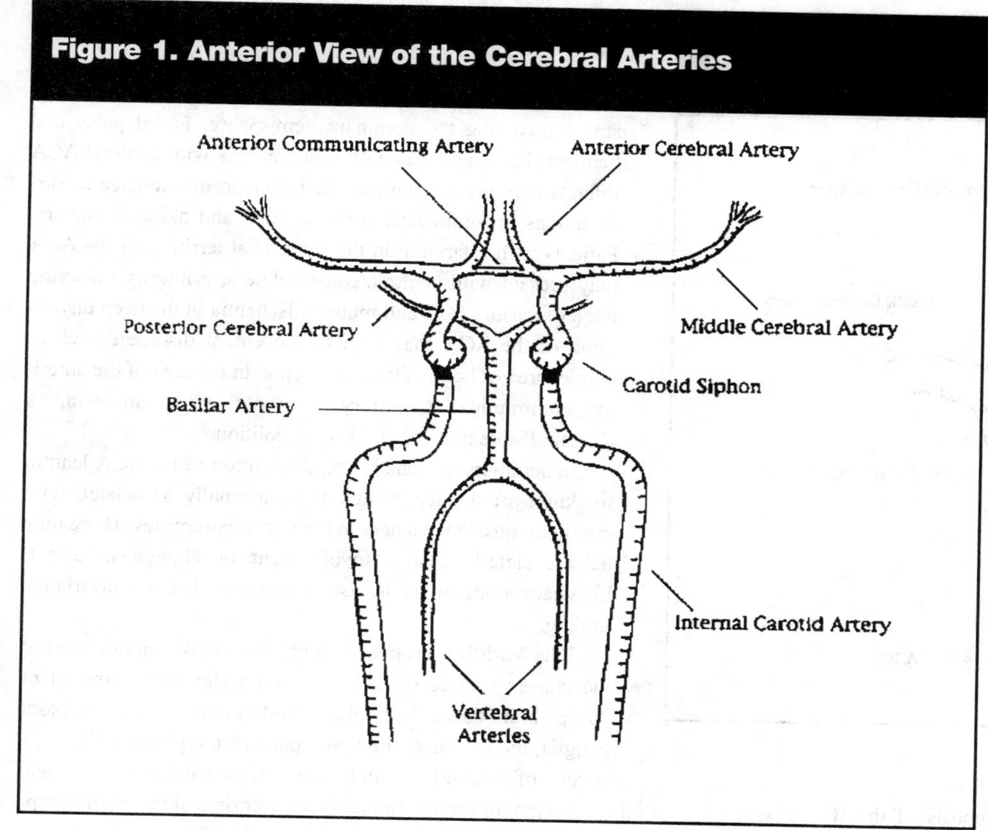

ing alterations in consciousness that range from drowsiness to psychosis to coma. In general, those changes progress in severity as the metabolic derangement worsens, but they may, at times, develop rapidly. The vast majority of diffuse and focal CNS abnormalities caused by metabolic derangements clear completely and promptly once the derangement is corrected.

Symptoms and signs of focal brain dysfunction resulting from metabolic derangement are especially common in the elderly. Those abnormalities probably represent the unmasking of preexisting subclinical structural brain damage by profound metabolic changes within the brain—changes induced by electrolyte or osmolar derangements.[39] The biochemical basis for focal neurologic deficits in metabolic disorders is unclear. However, alterations in brain cell volume seem to play a major role. In hyperosmolar states, intracellular water moves into the extracellular space across the semipermeable cell membrane to maintain equality in tonicity between the two compartments. The resulting shrinkage in intracellular volume then leads to cerebral dysfunction. Conversely, hypo-osmolarity results in fluid movement into the cellular compartment and leads to cerebral edema and CNS symptoms.

Syndromes of Ischemia and Infarction in the Acute Stroke

Cerebral Arterial Anatomy. The anterior portion of the brain involving the frontal, temporal, and parietal lobes, is usually supplied by the carotid arteries, whereas the posterior portion including the occipital lobe, cerebellum, and brainstem is perfused by the VB system. *(Please see Figure 1.)* The carotid artery arises from the innominate artery on the right and directly from the aortic arch on the left. It divides into the internal and external carotid arteries at its extracranial bifurcation. The ICA courses through the skull in segments termed the carotid siphon. The first two branches of the ICA are the ophthalmic and anterior choroidal arteries. The MCA is the largest of the two terminal branches of the carotid artery and divides into two or three main trunks. The MCA perfuses the cortex, parietal lobe, temporal lobe, internal capsule, and portions of the basal ganglia along its course. The anterior cerebral artery (ACA) is the second of the terminal branches of the ICA. It forms the anterior portion of the circle of Willis and supplies portions of the frontal lobe. The posterior cerebral artery (PCA) occasionally arises from the carotid system, although typically it is the terminal portion of the basilar artery, supplying the occipital lobe and selected areas of the thalamus. There may be collateral flow provided to these vascular territories by the circle of Willis.

The vertebral arteries (VA) arise from the subclavian arteries and give off branches supplying the medulla and portions of the cerebellum. The basilar artery (BA) is formed by the junction of the two vertebral arteries and gives off a variety of penetrating arteries supplying the brainstem and portions of the basal ganglia before dividing into the posterior cerebral arteries. *(Please see Figure 2.)*

The Carotid Artery. Obstructing lesions of the carotid artery frequently occur at bifurcation points. In asymptomatic patients, ICA disease may be diagnosed on the basis of a carotid bruit. Approximately half of patients with moderate stenosis (greater than 50% occlusion) will have a carotid bruit, and about 90% of patients with a carotid bruit have at least moderate stenosis.[40,41] Recent studies have demonstrated that treatment of patients with asymptomatic, high-grade carotid stenosis (more than 70% stenosis) can reduce the risk of stroke.[42,43] Patients with carotid artery stenosis may also present with TIA. TIAs occurring in the distribution of the ICA usually have focal symptoms that are rapid in onset and last 2-15 minutes. In general, episodes that last only seconds are not due to TIAs. Attacks in the ICA distribution that involve the dominant hemisphere may present with myriad symptoms such as motor dysfunction, amaurosis fugax, numbness, and/or aphasia. TIAs in the distribution of the ICA of the non-dominant hemisphere have similar symptomatology but without aphasia.

Clinical symptoms of ICA occlusion vary greatly due to variation in collateral flow. Major deficits at initial presentation may resolve partially as emboli migrate to smaller branch vessels. Most symptoms of ICA occlusion reflect ischemia in the middle cerebral artery territory and present with hemiparesis and, in the case of dominant hemispheric lesions, aphasia. Other patterns may occur including hemiparesis with hemianopia or a variety of aphasic patterns without hemiparesis.

Figure 2. The Circle of Willis

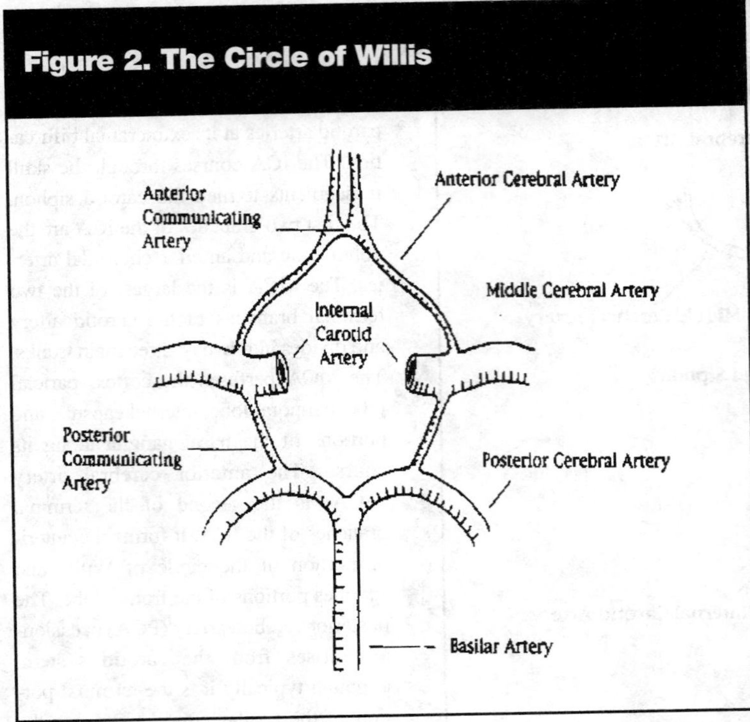

Watershed Infarctions. High-grade stenosis of the ICA also may render the brain susceptible to infarction during periods of relative hypotension. These so called "watershed" infarcts occur in vulnerable areas supplied by distal distribution of the anterior and middle cerebral arteries, the distal distribution served by the middle and posterior cerebral arteries, and the superficial and deep branches of the middle cerebral artery.[44] Patients with watershed infarction between the anterior and middle cerebral arteries present with hemiparesis, predominantly in the leg.[45] There is usually an associated decrease in sensation in the same distribution. In dominant hemisphere infarctions, there is a decrease in verbal ability with preserved comprehension. Infarction involving the posterior watershed area presents with homonymous hemianopia. There may be hypoesthesia in the face and legs. Motor weakness is rare in this type of infarction. Finally, watershed infarction may also occur in the area between the deep and superficial branches of the MCA and nearly all of these patients present with hemiparesis. Hemisensory deficit and language disorder are common in dominant hemisphere infarctions.

The Anterior Cerebral Artery. The ACA forms the anterior portion of the circle of Willis and supplies portions of the frontal lobe and medial portions of the parietal lobe. *(Please see Figure 3.)* Infarction in the distribution of the ACA leads primarily to symptoms involving the distal leg, such as weakness or clumsiness. There may be speech disturbances. The anterior limb of the internal capsule may be affected leading to face and arm weakness. Lesions of the anterior choroidal artery can cause hemiplegia and sensory loss, along with homonymous hemianopia. Frontal lobe infarctions are estimated to occur in about 20% of initial cerebral vascular accidents.[46] About 15% of patients with symptomatic strokes involving other areas of the brain also have frontal lobe infarctions on computed tomography.[47]

A variety of frontal lobe syndromes may occur with anterior cerebral artery infarction. The superior medial syndrome is associated with higher cortical dysfunction: difficulty in task preparation, apraxia, agraphia, volitional movement, loss of bi-manual coordination, and grasp reflex. Aphasia may occur in ACA stroke involving the dominant hemisphere. Facial palsy and hemi-neglect may also be present. Patients with bilateral ACA infarcts may present with docile behavior, indifference to surroundings, incontinence, confabulation, and akinetic mutism. Patients with infarction in the superficial territory of the ACA may present with contralateral weakness, primarily involving the leg, sensory loss, and mutism. Ischemia in the deep distribution of the ACA may lead to movement disorders such as hemichorea or hemiballism. Infarction in the area of the anterior communicating artery presents with amnesia, a Korsakoff-like picture, and loss of volition.

In summary, lesions in the distribution of the ACA lead to weakness of the leg, which is occasionally associated with proximal muscle weakness in the upper extremities. There may be associated sensory involvement or change in affect. Language impairment is also a common, but not invariable, finding.

The Middle Cerebral Artery. The MCA supplies most of the convex surface of the brain and a significant amount of "deep" brain tissue. It supplies blood to almost the entire basal ganglia, the putamen, the upper parts of the globus pallidus, a portion of the head, and all the body of the caudate nucleus, and a substantial part of the anterior and posterior rims of the internal capsule. Not surprisingly, occlusion of the MCA is responsible for the majority of stroke syndromes, with embolism from either the ICA or the heart to the MCA being the most common cause of cerebral infarction. Thrombosis of the MCA accounts for only 2% of ischemic events in the MCA territory.[45] Usually, occlusion of the MCA results in a large infarct that affects both superficial and deep areas supplied by this vessel. However, in some cases, adequate collateralization can minimize the degree of tissue loss.

Occlusion of the trunk or upper division of the MCA produces a large infarct characterized by contralateral hemiplegia, deviation of the head and eyes toward the side of the infarct, global aphasia (in the dominant hemisphere), hemianopia, hemianesthesia, and hemineglect. Hemiparesis affects the leg less than the arm and face. While dominant hemisphere infarction results in aphasia of the Broca-type, occlusion of the lower division of the MCA results in a Wernicke-type aphasia when occlusion involves the dominant hemisphere and hemianopia. Interruption of blood flow in the small penetrating arteries results in lacunar infarction and manifests clinically as pure hemiparesis without sensory, language, or behavioral manifestations.[48,49]

Common findings in MCA infarction include loss of consciousness, hemiplegia and hemiparesis, eye and head deviation, sensory disturbances, visual field disturbances, neglect, and movement disorders. These findings are typical for infarction occurring in either the dominant or nondominant hemisphere.[45,48,49] Immediate loss of consciousness at the onset of the ischemic insult is uncommon. However, delayed loss of consciousness occurring at a point 36 hours to several days after the ischemic insult is more consistent and is usually caused by increased peri-infarct edema, elevated intracranial pressure, and cerebral herniation.

Hemiplegia and hemiparesis can result from infarction of the deeper arterial distribution as well as the superficial distribution.

Figure 3. Lateral View of the Cerebral Arteries

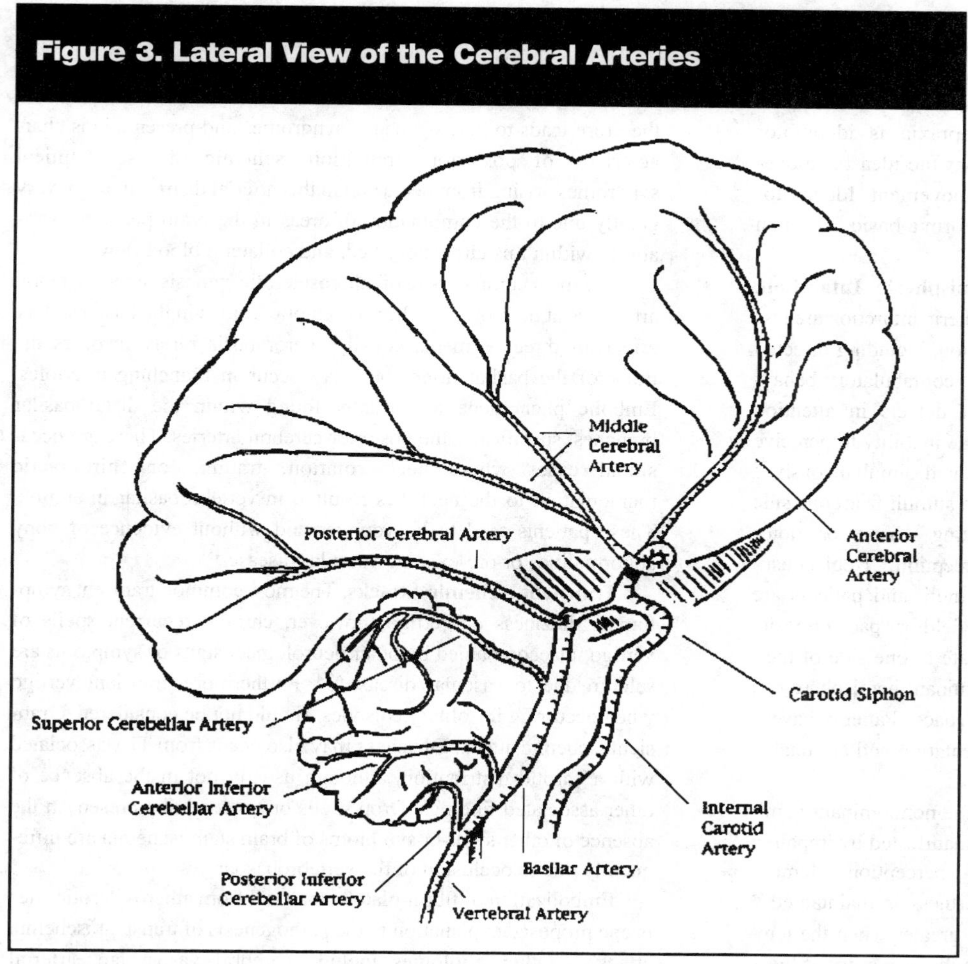

Only when infarction of the lower division of the MCA occurs is a motor deficit unlikely. Head and eye deviation are well-described in middle cerebral artery occlusion and should be expected after massive infarction of the entire middle cerebral artery territory.[44] Eye deviation tends to be more common in right hemispheric infarction, and it may be accompanied by a neglect syndrome of the contralateral side, which, in most cases, resolves after 1-2 weeks. Although sensory deficits are frequently overshadowed in MCA infarctions, profound loss of sensory modalities are common with MCA infarction, particularly if there is involvement of the anterior parietal cortex.[50] Visual field disturbances are common in large infarcts of the middle cerebral artery. Hemianopia is the most common visual field disturbance, however, parietal infarction can result in a quadrantanopia due to involvement of parietal radiations of visual fibers.[48]

As mentioned previously, patients suffering a stroke in the territory of the MCA may develop neglect syndromes. These may involve motor, verbal, or visual neglect. Neglect is manifested clinically by a patient's partial or complete inability to respond or recognize stimuli from one side of the patient's body. Frequently, a patient will fail to respond to a stimulus presented on the right side, for example, in response to motor or auditory stimulus on that side, or a deficiency in naming objects that lie or are positioned on the right side of the patient. Movement disorders including hemichorea, athetosis, or dystonia are infrequently observed after MCA occlusion.[48-52]

Dominant vs. Nondominant Hemisphere Infarction

Characteristics of Dominant Hemispheric Infarction. Because the two middle cerebral arteries supply opposite hemispheres, infarction of the dominant hemisphere will demonstrate clinical findings different from that of infarction of the nondominant hemisphere. Although the contralateral hemiplegic syndromes and other associated abnormalities described earlier still occur, hemisphere-specific symptoms and signs permit more accurate determination of right- or left-hemispheric involvement.

Speech Disorders. It is important to note the patient's hand dominance to infer hemisperhic dominance. The majority of right-handed, and most left-handed patients, have dominance for speech and language located in the left hemisphere. Left hemispheric infarction is characterized by aphasia, both motor and sensory, and apraxia. Speech and language dominance located in the right hemisphere is found infrequently.[49] Global or total aphasia usually results from occlusion of the trunk of the middle cerebral artery or its upper division. Motor aphasia, also known as Broca's aphasia, results from infarction of the insular cortex and fronto-parietal operculum. During the period of acute infarction, total aphasia is more likely, with a true motor aphasia evolving over time. Broca's speech disturbance manifests as hesitant and broken responses. This is especially true when a patient attempts to speak polysyllabic words and is due to the dyspraxia between the oropharynx and the respiratory elements that permit smooth vocalization.[49,53] This speech pattern is nonfluent and displays agrammatism, characterized by simple utterings, usually single words or nouns that are spoken in short and disjunctive phrases.

Wernicke's aphasia, also known as sensory aphasia, occurs with occlusion of the lower division of the middle cerebral artery and generally results from a large infarct encompassing the posterior temporal, inferior parietal, and lateral temporo-occipital regions.[49,53] These patients show no deficit in the ability to vocalize, speak in phrases, make smooth transitions, or properly pronounce their words. However, in the acute phase, attempts at speech contain few understandable words. This condition, known as jargon paraphasia, results in distorted phonetic structure, involves consonants, substituted words, and perseveration.[33] In some cases, the extent of the language disturbance is not evident in simple conversation and requires more extensive evaluation. Generally, there is a deficit in writing that parallels the spoken element. In cases where hemiparesis is not involved, the writing is legible with abnormal content.

Apraxia represents an abnormality in the execution of a task. It is generally an acquired problem in that it results in an inability to perform a previous task that cannot be explained by loss of coordination, weakness, dementia, or aphasia. Apraxia results from a loss of motor programs stored in left hemisphere dominant individuals.[51,52] The most common type of apraxia is ideomotor apraxia where the affected brain area contains the idea for movement and the motor areas that lead to this movement. Ideomotor apraxia is tested by asking the patient to perform a basic task such as combing hair.

Characteristics of Nondominant Hemispheric Infarction. Syndromes produced by nondominant hemispheric infarction are less predictable and may include defects of attention, including directed and focused attention, spacial operations, and confabulatory behaviors. Two common, characteristic forms of defects in attention include extinction and neglect. Extinction is the inability to perceive a stimulus when a second stimulus is presented simultaneously.[54] Neglect is manifested by a lack of response to stimuli from one side of the body in the absence of any pre-existing sensory or motor deficit severe enough to account for this imperception.[49] Neglect usually involves auditory, visual, and tactile stimuli, and patients are frequently found to act to stimuli only in the field or space opposite the affected side. These patients can only relate to one side of their body or surroundings. Damage to the nondominant hemisphere can also affect the ability to localize objects in space. Patients have a diminished capacity to determine spacial orientation and are unable to localize sounds in space.

Behavioral changes due to infarction of the nondominant hemisphere include acute confusion and delirium manifested by impaired orientation, diminished attention, and altered perception. Memory and thought processes are impaired, but alertness is maintained.[48] The incidence of behavioral abnormalities is greater when the temporal lobe is affected, and this is likely due to the proximity of these lesions to the limbic system. Constructional apraxia may occur and results in the inability to arrange, draw, or build objects due to the inability to manipulate objects in space.

The Posterior Cerebral Artery. The posterior cerebral artery generally arises from the VB system. Among the clinically significant areas supplied are the occipital lobe and thalamus.[55]

Thalamic Lesions. Posterior communicating artery infarction may lead to a number of thalamic syndromes. These patients usually have sensory symptoms involving loss of tactile, temperature, and pain sensation. Patients typically complain of numbness and tingling on one side of the body, occasionally associated with dysesthesia. Proprioception is frequently spared. There may be some motor weakness or ataxia, which may indicate involvement of the adjacent internal capsule. Infarction in the paramedian area may involve transient loss of consciousness followed by confusion, amnesia, and confabulation. Hypoesthesia is common and movement disorders may also be associated with this lesion.

Occipital Lesions. The superficial portion of the PCA supplies the occipital area.[56] Typically, lesions in this area lead to a homonymous visual field defect which may be a hemianopia or a quadrantanopia. Macular vision tends to be spared in PCA infarction due to collateral supply from the MCA. Dominant hemisphere lesions may lead to alexia. Bilateral lesions can cause cortical blindness or tunnel vision. Lesions of the PCA may cause midbrain disturbances including oculomotor palsy or internuclear ophthalmoplegia. There may be associated dyslexia, memory loss, and confusion.

The Vertebrobasilar Circulation

Vascular anatomy of the vertebrobasilar system is complex and therefore leads to heterogeneous syndromes and presentations characteristic of posterior circulation ischemic disease. Clinical syndromes arising from occlusion in this arterial distribution can vary greatly due to the combination of areas in the brain perfused, variability within this circulatory bed, and collateral blood flow.

The most common site of atherosclerotic stenosis in the vertebral arteries is at their origin, whereas stenotic lesions in the basilar artery affect all three segments equally. Thrombosis rarely involves the trunk of the basilar artery but may occur in branching arterioles. Embolic phenomena are usually found within the distal basilar branches, specifically the posterior cerebral arteries. There are occasional cases where neck rotation, trauma, or chiropractic manipulation to the neck has resulted in vertebrobasilar infarction. These patients tend to be younger and without evidence of bony abnormalities or pre-existing vascular disease.[45]

Transient Ischemic Attacks. The most common transient symptom is dizziness or vertigo; however, chronic recurrent spells of vertigo unaccompanied by other neurological signs or symptoms are seldom due to vascular disease.[45,48] Furthermore, transient vertigo when occurring in solitary episodes, should not be considered a transient ischemic attack. Dizziness may also occur from TIA associated with a carotid distribution, although usually not in the absence of other associated findings. Drop spells or syncope that present in the absence of other signs or symptoms of brain stem ischemia are infrequently due to occlusion of the vertebrobasilar system.

Embolization of fibrin-platelet material from atherosclerotic sites is one proposed explanation in the pathogenesis of transient ischemia attacks.[57] Other etiologies include cerebral vasospasm, arterial hypotension with fixed stenotic lesions, and, more rarely, TIAs induced by exercise, emotional outbursts, and polycythemia.[58,59] Multiple episodes of transient neurologic dysfunction consisting of different patterns suggest an embolic phenomenon, whereas a fixed patterns of signs and symptoms suggests atherosclerotic or thrombotic lesions.

The classic findings of vertebrobasilar TIA include perioral numbness, dizziness or vertigo, horizontal or vertical diplopia, dysarthria, paresis of either one complete side or both sides of the body, or numbness of all of one or both sides of the body. Other manifestations may include headache; ataxia; decreased vision, including darkening, blurring and tunnel vision, partial or complete blindness, and pupillary and gaze abnormalities; vomiting; hiccups; and impaired hearing.[45]

Weakness or numbness may involve the fingers and face in some TIA episodes but only the fingers in others. Dizziness and ataxia may occur in some attacks, while in others diplopia may be part of the picture. TIAs due to basilar artery disease may affect each side of the body alternately, and affected parts may be involved simultaneously or spread from one region to another. The attacks may cease abruptly or fade gradually.[57,58]

Infarction Syndromes of the Vertebrobasilar System. Subclavian steal presents with symptoms referable to the posterior circulation. Classically, stenosis of the subclavian artery proximal to the origin of the vertebral artery results in augmented flow through the opposite vertebral artery and reversal of flow through the vertebral artery on the same side as a subclavian stenosis. In this case, activity in the upper extremities results in flow reversal and blood being "stolen" from the intended cerebral bed. Patients with subclavian steal present with headache, intermittent episodes of cerebral ischemia, or claudication pain in the ischemic arm. Subclavian steal is more common in the left subclavian artery.[45] The cerebral manifestations of subclavian steal are worse when patients have coexistent carotid artery disease. Diagnosis is based on physical examination that reveals a diminished pulse and blood pressure in the affected extremity; clinical suspicion is required, and Doppler ultrasonography can confirm the diagnosis.

The vertebral arteries are the main source of blood flow to the medulla. Consequently, occlusion can lead to several clinical syndromes, including the lateral medullary syndrome and the medial medullary syndrome. In 80% of cases, the lateral medullary syndrome, also known as Wallenberg syndrome, is usually caused by lesions in the vertebral artery near the take-off of the PICA.[48] This lesion produces infarction in a lateral wedge of the medulla and results in vertigo, headache, facial pain, feelings of disequilibrium, nausea and vomiting, ataxia, and hiccups; diminished sensation in the ipsilateral face, diminished pain and temperature sensation of the contralateral body, Horner's syndrome, ataxia of gait and limb, nystagmus, slight weakness of the ipsilateral face, paralysis of the ipsilateral vocal cord, and weakness of the ipsilateral palate also may occur.[45,48] Contralateral hemiparesis or a positive Babinski's sign are not components of the lateral medullary syndrome. The medial medullary syndrome results in contralateral hemiparesis sparing the face, loss of tactile, proprioceptive, and vibratory sense. There is preservation of pain and temperature sensation, and ipsilateral tongue paralysis.[47,48,60-63]

PICA Syndrome. Occlusion of the posterior inferior cerebellar artery (PICA) is the most common cerebellar artery syndrome and may lead to the lateral medullary syndrome described above. PICA infarcts are associated with greater involvement of the cerebellum and have a worse prognosis. Involvement of the anterior inferior cerebellar artery (AICA) generally results in pontine and cerebellar infarction. Extensive cerebellar infarction is uncommon with AICA occlusion, and it tends to have a more benign prognosis. Patients with AICA infarction have ipsilateral facial weakness and hypesthesia, deafness, Horner's syndrome, ataxia, vertigo, nystagmus, and contralateral limb and trunk hypesthesia.[45,48] Occasionally, infarction of the AICA or the PICA results in a pure vestibular syndrome and patients may be misdiagnosed as having labyrinthitis.[45,48] Isolated superior cerebellar artery (SCA) occlusion is unusual. The SCA infarction syndrome includes ipsilateral limb ataxia, a Horner's syndrome, contralateral thermoanalgesia involving the face, arm, trunk and leg, and a fourth cranial nerve palsy.[48,64]

Vertebrobasilar infarction usually is due to occlusion of a branch of the basilar artery rather than complete infarction of the trunk (basilar branch disease). The basilar artery supplies portions of the midbrain, the pons, and regions of the cerebellum. Three branches are involved: small paramedian penetrators, short circumferential branches, and long circumferential branches (AICA and SCA). Occlusion of the basilar artery trunk results in bilateral infarction of the basis pontis and cerebellar tegmentum. Clinical manifestations include coma, abnormal breathing patterns, quadriplegia with decerebrate posturing ,and bilateral sensory loss. Cranial nerve abnormalities include bilateral reactive pupillary miosis, horizontal ophthalmoplegia (not overcome by oculocephlic maneuvers) and ocular bobbing.[45,48,58] The "locked-in" syndrome results from sparing of the tegmentum with infarction of the basis pontis. Patients are conscious, however they are quadriplegic, anarthric, and have complete sensory impairment but may communicate using eye movements. Occlusion of the distal end of the basilar artery results in the "top of the basilar" syndrome. Patients with bilateral infarction present with motor, sensory, visual, oculomotor, and behavioral findings, absent vertical gaze palsy, nystagmus, third nerve palsy, bilateral ptosis, internuclear ophthalmoplegia, unreactive pupils, homonymous hemianopia, cortical blindness, and hemianesthesia or hemihypesthesia.[45,48,65,66] Pontine lesions due to occlusion of small perforating arteries results in several minor syndromes, indistinguishable from those seen in cerebral lacunar infarction.[45,60]

Lacunar Infarction

While large vessel occlusions have stereotypical symptomatology, there is a separate set of symptoms associated with lesions of the small penetrating branch arteries, commonly termed lacunar infarctions. Lacunar strokes are characterized by the lack of impairment of consciousness, aphasia, or visual disturbances.[67-69] Lacunar infarctions are very common and involve the deep central regions of the brain, particularly the basal ganglia, basis pontis, and thalamus, leading to characteristic syndromes. Pure motor hemiparesis is a frequent result of lacunar infarction. These rarely involve monoplegia, and usually result in hemiparesis of the face, arm, and leg. Pure sensory stroke is the most common lacunar infarction in some series again involving the face, arm, and leg. A third variety of lacunar infarction involves ataxia and leg hemiparesis. Finally, the clumsy hand-dysarthria syndrome, is caused by a lesion in the basis pontis or in the anterior limb of the internal capsule. Lacunar infarctions tend to have a good prognosis. The mortality rate in patients with lacunar infarction is markedly lower than in patients with middle cerebral artery infarction and tend to be due to non-neurologic causes such as pneumonia or cardiovascular events. Patients with lacunar infarction are more likely to recover fully than are patients with large artery occlusions. Approximately 60% of patients with lacunar infarctions will be independent at one year following the stroke.

References

1. Dobkin B. The economic impact of stroke. *Neurology.* 1995; 45(suppl):S6-S9.
2. Whisnant J. Changing incidence and mortality rates for stroke. *J Stroke Cerebrovasc Dis* 1992;2:42.
3. Feldman E, Gordon N, Brooks J, et al. Factors associated with early presentation of acute stroke. *Stroke* 1993;24: 1805-1810.
4. Broderick J, Phillips S, Whisnant J. Incidence rates of stroke in the eighties: The end of the decline in stroke? *Stroke* 1989; 20:577-582.
5. Sacco R, Wolfe P, Kannel W, et al. Survival and recurrence following stroke: The Framingham Study. *Stroke* 1982;13: 290-295.
6. Garraway W, Whisnant J, Drury I, et al. The changing pattern of survival following stroke. *Stroke* 1983;14:699-703.
7. Sacco R, Wolf P, Kannel W, et al. Survival and recurrence fol-

lowing stroke: The Framingham Study. *Stroke* 1982;13: 290-295.

8. Vitanen M, Winblad B, Asplund K, et al. Autopsy-verified causes of death in hemiplegia. *Acta Med Scan* 1987;222: 401-405.
9. WHO Task Force on Stroke and Other Cerebrovascular Disorders. *Stroke* 1989;20:1407.
10. Sacco R. Risk factors and outcomes for ischemic stroke. *Neurology* 1995;45:S10-S14.
11. DeGraba T, Penix L. Genetics of ischemic stroke. *Curr Opin Neurol* 1995;8:24-29.
12. Gorelick P. Stroke prevention: an opportunity for efficient utilization of health care resources during the coming decade. *Stroke* 1994;15:220-224.
13. Wolf P, Cobb J, D'Agostino R, et al. Epidemiology of stroke. In: Barnett JGM, Hohr JP, Stein BM, et al, eds. *Stroke: Pathophysiology, Diagnosis, and Management.* 2nd ed. New York: McGraw-Hill; 1992:3-27.
14. The Boston Area Anticoagulation Trial for Atrial Fibrillation Investigators. The effect of low-dose warfarin on the risk of stroke in patients with nonrheumatic atrial fibrillation. *N Engl J Med* 1990;323:1505-1511.
15. Stroke Prevention in Atrial Fibrillation Investigators. Stroke prevention in atrial fibrillation study: final results. *Circulation* 1991;84:527-539.
16. Gaines K, Burke G. Ethnic differences in stroke: Black-white differences in the United States population. *Neuroepidemiology* 1995;14:209-239.
17. Atkins D, Psaty B, Koepsell T, et al. Cholesterol reduction and the risk for stroke in men: A meta-analysis of randomized, controlled trials. *Ann Intern Med* 1993;119:136-145.
18. Gorelick P. The status of alcohol as a risk factor for stroke. *Stroke* 1989;12:1607-1610.
19. Ferro J, Melo T, Oliveira V, et al. A multivariate study of headache associated with ischemic stroke. *Headache* 1995:315-319.
20. Calandre L, Gomara S, Bermujo F, et al. Clinical CT correlations in TIA, RIND, and strokes with minimum residum. *Stroke* 1986;17:699.
21. Khaw KT, Barrett-Connor E, Suarez L, et al. Prediction of stroke-associated mortality in the elderly. *Stroke* 1984;15:244.
22. Andrews BT, Pitts LH, Lovely MP, et al. Is computed tomographic scanning necessary inpatients with tentorial herniation? Results of immediate surgical exploration without comptued tomography in 100 patients. *Neurosurgery* 1986; 19:409.
23. Schmidley JW, Messing RO. Agitated confusional states inpatients with right hemispheric infarctions. *Stroke* 1984;15:883.
24. Lehman LB. Coma in the elderly: Evlauation and treatment. *Hosp Pract* 1987;22:136.
25. Harrison MJH, Marshall J. Atrial fibrillations, TIAs, and completed strokes. *Stroke* 1984;15:441.
26. Toole JF. Vascular diseases—Etiology and pathogenisis. In: Rowland LP, ed. *Merritt's Textbook of Neurology* Philadelphia: Lea & Febringer; 1984.
27. Ernest MP. Emergency diagnosis and management of brain infarctions and hemorrhages. In: Ernest MP, ed. *Neurologic Emergencies* New York: Churchill Livingstone; 1983.
28. Rosen P, et al. *Emergency Medicine* St. Louis; CV Mosby Company; 1988.
29. Bucknall CA, Morris GK, Mitchell JR. Physicians' attitudes to four common problems: Hypertension, atrial fibrillation, transient ischemic attacks, and angina pectoris. *Brit Med J* 1986;293:739.
30. Furlan AJ. Transient ischemic attacks: Strategies for minimizing stroke risk. *Postgrad Med* 1984;75:183.
31. Tuhrim S, Reggia JA. Management of transient ischemic attacks. *Am Fam Phys* 1986;315:1041.
32. Morris PJ, et al. *Transient Ischemic Attacks* New York: Marcel, Dekker, 1982.
33. Gill JS, Zezulka AV, Shipley MJ, et al. Stroke and alcohol consumption. *N Engl J Med* 1986;315:1041.
34. Donahue R, et al. Alcohol and hemorrhagic stroke. *JAMA* 1986;255:2311.
35. Melamed N, Satya-Murti S. Cerebellar hemorrhage: A review and reappraisal of benign cases. *Arch Neurol* 1984;41:425.
36. Bosker G, Schwartz G. *Principles and Practice of Acute Geriatric Medicine* 2nd ed. St. Louis: CV Mosby Company; 1988.
37. Lowenstein SR, Crecenzi CA, Kern DC, et al. Care of the elderly in the emergency department. *Ann Emerg Med* 1986;5:15.
38. Braaten JR. Hyperosmolar nonketotic diabetic coma: Diagnosis and management. *Geriatrics* 1987;42:83.
39. Miller M. Fluid and electrolyte balance in the elderly. *Geriatrics* 1987;42:65.
40. Wiebers D, Whisnant J, Sanok B, et al. Prospective comparison of a cohort with asymptomatic carotid bruit and a population-based cohort without carotid bruit. *Stroke* 1990; 21:984-988.
41. Ingall T, Homer D, Whisnant J, et al. Predictive value of carotid bruit for carotid atherosclerosis. *Arch Neurol.* 1989; 46:418-422.
42. North American Symptomatic Carotid Endarterectomy Trial Collaborators. Beneficial effect of carotid endarterectomy in symptomatic patients with high-grade carotid stenosis. *N Engl J Med* 1991;325:445-453.
43. European Carotid Surgery Trialists' Collaborative Group. MRC European Carotid Surgery Trial: interim results for symptomatic patients with severe (70-99%) or with mild (0-20%) carotid stenosis. *Lancet* 1991;337:1235-1243.
44. Bogousslavsky J, Regli F. Borderzone infarctions distal to internal carotid artery occlusion: prognostic implications. *Ann Neurol* 1986;20:247-350.
45. Caplan L, Pessin M, Mohr J. Vertebrobasilar occlusive disease. In: Barnett HJM, et al. eds. *Stroke Pathophysiology, Diagnosis and Management.* 2nd ed. New York: McGraw-Hill; 1992:443-515.
46. Bogousslavsky J, FanMelle G, Regli F, et al. for the Lausanne Stroke Registry Group. The Lausanne Stroke Registry. Analysis of 1000 consecutive patients with first stroke. *Stroke* 1988;19:1083-1092.
47. Vingerhoets F, Bogousslavsky J. L'ischemie cerebrale silencieuse. In: Rancural G, ed. *La prevention des accidents ischemiques cerebraux.* Paris; Phase 5: 1994:185-192.
48. Gavrilescu T, Kase C. Clinical stroke syndromes: Clinical-

anatomic correlation. *Cerebrovasc Brain Metabolism Reviews* 1995;7:218-239.
49. Mohr J, Gautier J, Hier D, et al. Middle cerebral artery disease. In: Barnett HJM, et al., eds. *Stroke: Pathophysiology, Diagnosis and Management.* 2nd ed. New York: McGraw-Hill; 1992:361-441.
50. Kim J, Lee M. Stroke and restricted sensory syndromes. *Neuroradiology* 1994;36:258-263.
51. Derouesne C, Cambon H, Yelnik A, et al. Infarcts in the middle cerebral artery territory: Pathological study of mechanisms of death. *Acta Neurol Scand* 1993;87:361-366.
52. Tei H, Uchiyama S, Maruyama S, et al. Capsular infarcts: Location, size and etiology of pure motor hemiparesis, sensorimotor stroke and ataxic hemiparesis. *Acta Neurol Scan* 1993;88:264-268.
53. Kim J. Pure dysarthria, isolated facial paresis, or dysarthria-facial paresis syndrome. *Stroke* 1994;26:1994-1998.
54. Schwartz A, Marchok P, Kreinick C, et al. The asymmetric lateralization of tactile extinction in patients with unilateral cerebral dysfunction. *Brain* 1979;102:669-674.
55. Bogousslavsky J, Reglie F, Uske A, et al. Thalamic infarcts: Clinical syndromes, etiology, and prognosis. *Neurology* 1988;38:837-848.
56. Pessin M, Lathi E, Cohen M, et al. Clinical features and mechanism of occipital infarction. *Ann Neurol* 1987;21: 290-298.
57. Barnett H, Eliaszie M, Meldrum H, et al. Drugs and surgery in the prevention of ischemic stroke. *N Engl J Med* 1995;332: 238-248.
58. Victor M, Adams R. Cerebrovascular diseases. In: *Principles of Neurology*. 5th ed. New York: McGraw-Hill; 1993: 669-748.
59. Ueda F, Toole J, McHenry L, et al. Carotid and vertebral transient ischemic attacks: Clinical and angiographic correlation. *Neurology* 1978;29:1094-1099.
60. Kim J, Kim H, Chung C, et al. Medial medullary syndrome. *Stroke* 1995;26:1548-1522.
61. Ricci S, Celani M, Righetti E, et al. Clinical methods for diagnostic confirmation of stroke subtypes. *Neuroepidemiology* 1994;13:290-295.
62. Schneider R, Gautier J. Leg weakness due to stroke: Site of lesions, weakness patterns and causes. *Brain* 1994;117: 347-354.
63. Bogousslavsky J, Maeder P, Regli F, et al. Pure midbrain infarction: Clinical syndromes, MRI, and etiologic patterns. *Neurology* 1994;44:2032-2040.
64. Barth A, Bogousslavsky J, Regli F, et al. The clinical and topographic spectrum of cerebellar infarcts: A clinical-magnetic resonance imaging correlation study. *Ann Neurol* 1993;33:451-456.
65. Steinke W, Sacco R, Mohr J, et al. Thalamic stroke: Presentation and prognosis of infarcts and hemorrhages. *Arch Neurol* 1992;49:703-710.
66. Nicolai A, Lazzarino L. Acute confusional states secondary to infarctions in the territory of the posterior cerebral artery in elderly patients. *Ital J Neurol Sci* 1994;15:91-96.
67. Nelson R, Pullicino P, Kendall B, et al. Computed tomography in patients presenting with lacunar syndromes. *Stroke* 1980;11:256-261.
68. Ghika J, Bogousslavsky J, Regli F, et al. Infarcts in the territory of the deep perforators from the carotid system. *Neurology* 1989;39:507-512.
69. Chimowitz M, Furlan A, Sila C, et al. Etiology of motor or sensory stroke: a prospective study of the predictive values of clinical and radiological features. *Ann Neurol* 1991;30: 519-525.

Stroke: Evaluation and Managment

John E. Duldner, Jr., MD
Charles L. Emerman, MD

Put simply, acute stroke care is a treacherous, unpredictable enterprise that is just now coming out of its infancy. And, if anything is certain, we know this treatment arena will witness growing pains. In fact, few life-threatening conditions are linked to interventions that require the emergency physician to balance on a tightrope between pharmacotherapies that have the potential to produce, on the upside, so much good, but on the downside, so much potential irreversible damage to vital neurological structures.

Not surprisingly, the management of acute ischemic stroke has become a team effort that combines the skills of prehospital personnel, emergency physicians, and neurological specialists. This intensive multi-disciplinary effort is required because stroke management is no longer a primarily "passive" exercise simply requiring an appropriate triage decision, but now demands a careful assessment of treatment options, including aspirin therapy, blood pressure-lowering medications, anticoagulation, and, in a very small percentage of eligible patients, treatment with thrombolytic drugs.

Because pharmacotherapy directed against the clotting system has the potential of producing undesirable, life- and neurological function-compromising complications—specifically, the conversion of bland, thrombotic cerebral infarctions into hemorrhagic stroke—the most challenging aspect of stroke management is identifying patient subgroups who will benefit from anticoagulation or thrombolytic therapy without incurring the substantial complications associated with their use.

The patient selection process frequently falls within the province of the emergency physician, who must make rapid, time-pegged decisions in collaboration with the consulting neurologist, radiologist, primary care physician, as well as the patient and his or her family. This process requires precise documentation of onset of symptoms, a careful review of exclusionary and inclusionary criteria for thrombolytic protocols, and a determination of the likely risks of therapy based on patient factors, location of the stroke, early radiographic findings, and presentation.

This chapter presents an up-to-date approach for managing patients presenting with stroke syndromes, with a special emphasis on indications for CT scanning, strategies and target parameters for blood pressure reduction, and a discussion of the current status of thrombolytic therapy in this patient population.

Management of Acute Ischemic Syndromes

General Comments. Until recently, emergency physicians managing patients who were suffering an acute stroke had little to offer other than supportive measures. Over the past decade, however, we have seen significant advances in the management and treatment of stroke, as well as a new focus on this devastating disease.[1] Since the

Figure 1. Algorithm for the ED Evaluation of Acute Stroke

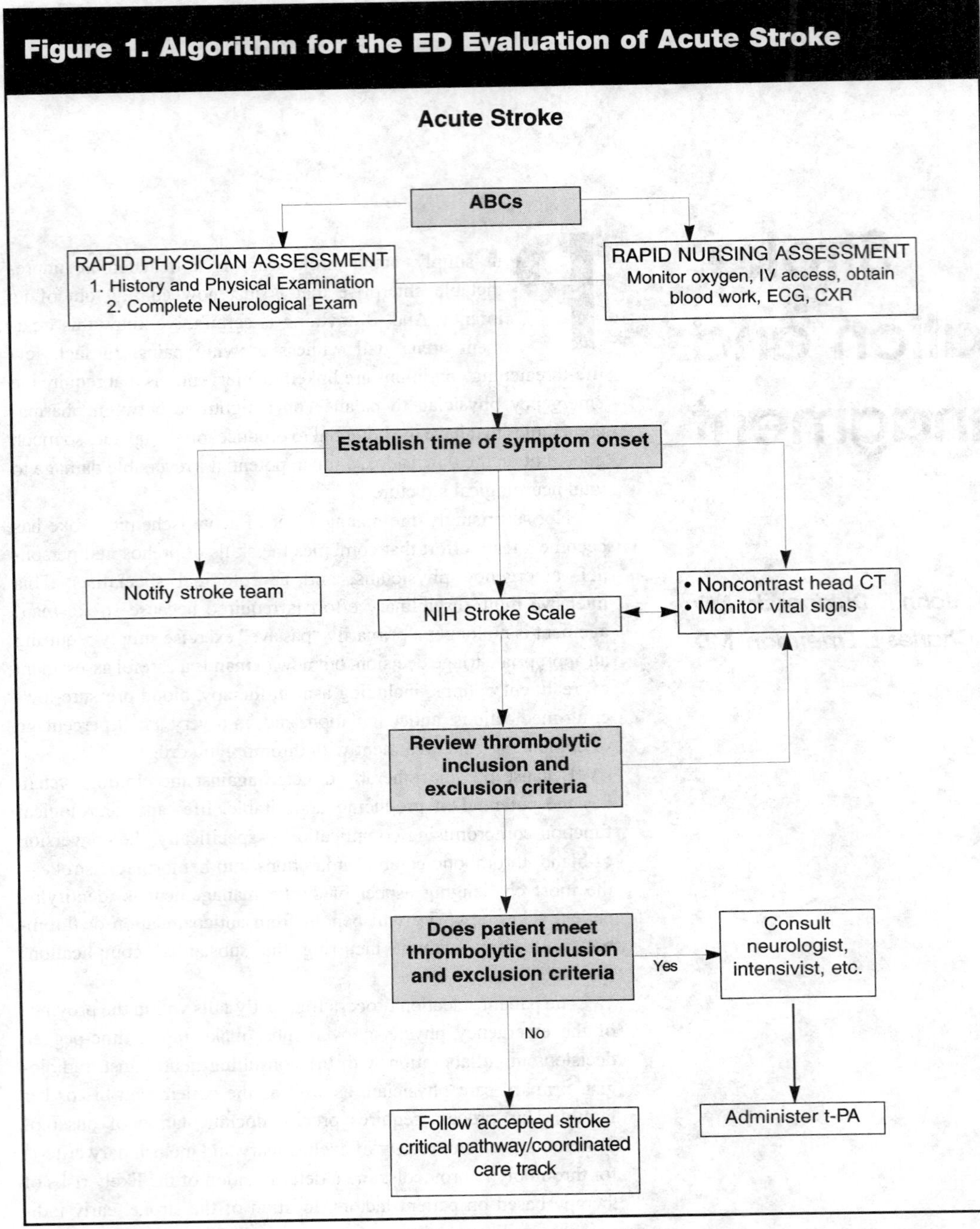

approval of tissue plasminogen activator (t-PA) for use in treating acute ischemic stroke, there has been an increasing awareness of new stroke therapies by both the public and the medical community. Emergency physicians are the first medical contact for a large percentage of stroke victims, and they can play an important role in initiating therapy.

A Systems Approach. The management of the acute stroke patient involves a multidisciplinary approach requiring participation of prehospital personnel, emergency nurses, emergency physicians, primary care providers, neurologists, and, in some cases, intensive care and rehabilitation specialists. The National Institutes of Neurological Disorders and Stroke (NINDS)/t-PA Stroke Study group recently outlined a "systems approach" for evaluation and management of stroke.[2] In outlining a methodology to improve clinical outcomes in acute stroke patients, this group of investigators stated that, "It is critical to develop efficient hospital-based methods for hyperacute stroke patient screening, evaluation, and intervention at both community-based and tertiary care academic centers."[2] Ideally, this stroke awareness and quality improvement program would include community education and public awareness campaigns, education of prehospital providers, systematic protocols for rapid ED evaluation—including a noncontrast head CT, accurate establishment of time of symptom onset, review of thrombolytic inclusion and exclusion criteria, and prompt treatment. In the eight centers included in this report, each had well-developed plans and protocols with defined goals. Each of the leading enrollment centers in the NINDS stroke trial incorporated the use of a "stroke team." Several other stroke programs have demonstrated success using stroke protocols and specialized systems for the care of the stroke patient.[3-7]

Stroke Teams. The number and the training background of personnel participating in a hospital-based stroke team depend on the availability of human and financial resources. At some institutions, the stroke team may consist of an emergency physician, who serves as the primary coordinator of care and uses phone consultation to communicate issues to a number of other team members (research coordinators, cerebrovascular nurse clinicians, neurologists, and intensive care specialists). Regardless of the size of a stroke team, the emergency physician should be able to lead the group, initiate a systematic diagnostic assessment plan, and manage the patient with appropriate medications or resuscitative interventions.

ED Evaluation. The ED evaluation of the acute stroke patient should adhere to a systematic treatment algorithm. *(Please see Figure 1.)* In this regard, it should be stressed that, although the FDA has approved the use of t-PA in selected patients with acute ischemic stroke, it has been postulated that *fewer* than 10% of patients with an

Table 1. Modified Version of the National Institutes of Health Stroke Scale Summary

Item	Name	Response
1A	Level of Consciousness	0=Alert 2=Not alert 3=Unresponsive
1B	Level of Questions	0=Answers both correctly 1=Answers one correctly 2=Answers neither correctly
1C	Level of Commands	0=Performs both tasks correctly 1=Performs one task correctly 2=Performs neither task
2	Best Gaze	0=Normal 1=Partial gaze palsy 2=Total gaze palsy
3	Visual Fields	0=No visual loss 1=Partial hemianopsia 2=Complete hemianopsia 3=Bilateral hemianopsia
4	Facial Palsy	0=Normal 1=Minor paralysis 2=Partial paralysis 3=Complete paralysis
5	Motor Arm a. Left b. Right	0=No drift 1=Drift before 10 seconds 2=Falls before 10 seconds 3=No effort against gravity 4=No movement
6	Motor leg a. Left b. Right	0=No drift 1=Drift before 5 seconds 2=Falls before 5 seconds 3=No effort against gravity 4=No movement
7	Ataxia	0=Absent 1=One limb 2=Two limbs
8	Sensory	0=Normal 1=Mild loss 2=Severe loss
9	Language	0=Normal 1=Mild aphasia 2=Severe aphasia 3=Mute or global aphasia
10	Dysarthria	0=Normal 1=Mild 2=Severe
11	Extinction/inattention	0=Normal 1=Mild 2=Severe
12	Distal Motor a. Left arm b. Right arm	0=Normal 1=Some extension after 5 seconds 2=No extension after 5 seconds

acute ischemic neurological event will qualify for thrombolytic treatment. However, the presence of stroke critical pathways or protocols will improve care for all stroke patients.

Initial Evaluation. Although there is a tendency to focus on neurologic disability, the clinician should focus on airway and circulatory stabilization. It is important to rule out other diseases that may mimic an acute stroke, including seizure disorder, hypoglycemia, complex migraine, dysrhythmia, or syncope. The assessment should include a thorough history and physical examination and an appropriate neurological exam. The time of symptom onset also needs to be accurately determined for consideration of thrombolytic therapy. In patients whose symptoms were present upon awakening, their time of symptom onset is estimated from the last time that the patient's neurological status was known to be normal, or the time just prior to going to sleep. Vital signs should be monitored at least every 10-15 minutes, and a noncontrast cranial computed tomography (CCT) scan should be obtained quickly if thrombolytics are considered.

Moreover, an NIH Stroke Scale (NIHSS) should be included as part of the physician evaluation. *(Please see Table 1.)* A clinical examination scale that was developed to assess neurological function,[8] the NIHSS score is linked to severity of neurological deficit; the higher the score, the worse the neurological deficit, with scores ranging from 0-42. The NIHSS is frequently used in acute stroke trials and may be used to supplement the neurological exam. The NIHSS is available as a training video that requires less than two hours to complete.

The NIHSS, like the Glasgow Coma Scale, standardizes the assessment of stroke severity and allows treating physicians to document and communicate the severity of neurological insult according to a standardized "severity of illness" scale. Moreover, it permits clini-

Table 2. Inclusion and Exclusion Criteria for Administration of t-PA

INCLUSION CRITERIA

- Ischemic stroke
- t-PA can be administered within 3 hours of symptom onset
- Neurological deficit measured by NIH Stroke Scale
- Clearly defined time of symptom onset

EXCLUSION CRITERIA

- Evidence of acute intracerebral or intracranial hemorrhage on non-contrast CT of the head
- Early CT evidence of acute infarction
- Other stroke, serious head trauma, or intracranial surgery in past 3 months
- Intracranial neoplasm, arteriovenous malformation, or aneurysm
- Uncontrolled hypertension, i.e. not reduced to 185/110 or lower within 30 minutes by oral agents, nitroglycerine paste, labetalol, or esmolol
- Rapidly improving or minor neurological symptoms
- Symptoms suggesting subarachnoid hemorrhage
- History of intracranial hemorrhage
- Major surgery in past 14 days
- Known bleeding diathesis
- Gastrointestinal or genitourinary tract bleeding in the past 3 weeks
- Arterial puncture at a noncompressible site in the past 7 days
- Seizure at the onset of stroke
- Patients with a prothrombin (PT) time greater than 15 seconds
- Patients on warfarin (coumadin) with a PT time greater than 15 seconds
- Heparin within the past 48 hours and elevated activated partial thromboplastin time (aPTT)
- Platelet count less than 100,000
- Serum glucose less than 50 mg/dL or greater than 400 mg/dL

cians to compare the status of the patient by performing repeat evaluations to measure either the improvement or worsening of a patient's clinical condition. A comprehensive form for recording patient information includes more detailed instructions for scoring the patient examination. The complete scale with instructions can be obtained from the NINDS.

Thrombolytic therapy inclusion and exclusion criteria should be reviewed. *(Please see Table 2.)* Vital signs, particularly blood pressure should be monitored frequently and treated when appropriate. For all acute stroke patients, therapy to minimize cerebral injury should be administered according to hospital-based critical pathways.

Transient Ischemic Attacks

Evaluation. The primary objective when evaluating a patient with a transient ischemic attach (TIA) is to determine whether the ischemic insult has occurred in the anterior or posterior circulation and whether the patient falls into a high-risk category. The first point to stress is that most TIAs are, in fact, very transient. Almost 25% of patients will have resolution of their symptoms within five minutes, and 50% of patients will have resolution within 30 minutes of noticing symptoms.[9] If the patient's deficit still persists after one hour, there is only a 15% chance that the neurological symptoms will abate over the next 24 hours. Since the patient may be neurologically normal by the time they arrive in the ED, a careful history is essential in establishing the diagnosis. Not infrequently, the emergency physician will have to seek information from EMS personnel, family members, or observers who may have observed the deficit.

Distinguishing between TIAs that involve the anterior circulation from those involving the posterior circulation has important diagnostic and treatment implications. Symptoms associated with anterior circulation ischemia usually include motor or sensory deficits of the extremities or face, amaurosis fugax, aphasia, and/or homonymous hemianopia. In contrast, patients with symptoms involving the posterior circulation ischemia may complain of motor or sensory dysfunction, but commonly such symptoms will occur in association with diplopia, dysphasia, dysarthria, ataxia, and/or vertigo.

The patient should be questioned about co-existing vascular or cardiac disease. For example, a careful inquiry may reveal that the patient may have experienced neurological symptoms but did not seek medical attention. The patient may have symptoms suggesting vasculopathies, connective tissue disorders, or intracranial mass lesions. Patients younger than age 40 should be questioned about family history of early stroke, drug use, or symptoms suggestive of a hypercoagulable state.

The physical examination should be directed at uncovering subtle signs of neurological deficit. Attention should also be focused on determining whether the patient has evidence of cardiovascular disease. In this regard, a carotid bruit is not specific for high-grade stenosis, although, in the setting of a TIA, a carotid bruit is 85% specific for at least moderate stenosis.

Almost all patients should undergo a non-contrast enhanced CT. About 20% of patients who have a TIA will have abnormalities on CT scanning.[10,11] Additionally, the CT may be helpful in ruling out mass lesions or intracranial hemorrhage. An MRI is generally not be part of the ED evaluation. Patients who suffer a TIA are at increased risk for a stroke. After the first year, the risk of subsequent stroke decreases to around 8% per year. There is no difference in stroke rate between patients with an anterior or posterior circulation TIA, but the combination of TIAs in both vascular territories does carry a higher risk.

Patients should be considered to be at high-risk for subsequent stroke if they have had multiple TIAs within the two weeks prior to arrival in the ED, if the deficit associated with the TIA was very severe, or if the patient had crescendo symptoms. In addition, patients should be considered to be at high risk if the TIA was caused by cardioembolic events. Patients who have had a history of recurrent TIAs should be questioned to determine whether symptoms experienced during the attack occurred within the same arterial distribution, indicating a vascular source, or whether symptoms reflect variable circulatory territories suggesting a cardioembolic source.

Risk factors for cardioembolism include atrial fibrillation, mitral stenosis, bioprosthetic and mechanical heart valves, myocardial infarction within the previous six months, documented left ventricular thrombus, known atrial myxoma, and dilated cardiomyopathy.[12] Other cardiac abnormalities that may be minor risk factors for transient ischemic attack include sick sinus syndrome, foramen ovale, aortic stenosis, and atrial septal aneurysm.[12,13]

Patients in the high-risk group should be hospitalized as should those individuals with TIA who cannot undergo a rapid outpatient assessment. If cardioembolism is the suspected etiology for TIA, consideration should be given to heparinization, starting with a loading dose of 5000-10,000 IU followed by 1000-1200 units per hour guided by the PTT. Anticoagulation should be withheld until the CT scan is available in order to rule out a hemorrhagic stroke. In addition, consultation with a neurologist or the patient's primary care physician is strongly advised since the evidence in favor of heparinization in TIA is not definitively established.

Patients in the low-risk group may be discharged to home as long as adequate follow-up is available and an expeditious outpatient work-up can be completed within one week.[14] Patients with symptoms of anterior circulation ischemia should undergo either duplex carotid ultrasound or oculoplethysmography. Duplex Doppler ultrasound is very accurate for detection of carotid stenosis. Ocular plethysmography will detect lesions of at least 50% stenosis with about 90% sensitivity.[15,16] Magnetic resonance angiography (MRA) is a non-invasive means of assessing both the extra- and intracranial circulation. MRA is limited by difficulty in distinguishing between very high grade stenosis and complete occlusion. Patients considered for surgery will generally require conventional angiography. Patients with symptoms consistent with posterior circulation ischemia may be evaluated using a transcranial Doppler ultrasonography. This test is about 75% sensitive for detecting significant stenosis.[17] Alternatively, MRA again can be used to assess the posterior circulation.

Patients who are going to be discharged to home should be started on aspirin therapy, which has been shown to decrease the risk of stroke by about 23%.[18] There is considerable controversy about the appropriate doses of aspirin with recommendations ranging from 75-1300 mg/d. At the present time, 75 mg/d of aspirin appears to be an adequate dose.[19] Patients who cannot tolerate aspirin or who have had a TIA while already on aspirin therapy for another purpose may be started on ticlopidine. Ticlopidine is generally initiated at 250 mg bid. The use of ticlopidine is limited by such side effects as diarrhea and occasional neutropenia, which occur in the first three months of use. Some patients may require anticoagulation with warfarin; however, these patients usually will be admitted, rather than discharged from the emergency department on oral anticoagulants.[20] Patients with symptoms of posterior circulation TIA also may be started on either aspirin or ticlopidine.

Acute Stroke: Management Considerations

ED evaluation of a stroke patient includes a complete blood count (CBC) including platelets, prothrombin time (PT), activated partial thromboplastin time (aPTT), and serum electrolytes. A rapid blood glucose should also be obtained. A noncontrast cranial computed tomography scan, ECG, and chest x-ray should be ordered. If the patient is a candidate for thrombolytic therapy, then the patient should be typed and cross-matched. Arterial blood gas and lumbar puncture should be obtained when indicated.[21,22]

Computed Tomography in Acute Stroke. CT scan is the diagnostic image of choice for acute neurological disease under evaluation in the ED. Previously, it was thought that infarction is not visible on CT scan until 24 hours after the onset of symptoms. However, subtle CT signs of early infarction may be seen within the first six hours after symptom onset with attenuation of brain tissue secondary to cytotoxic edema. Early CT manifestations of acute stroke have prognostic significance in that patients with early infarct changes on CT scan are more likely to have cerebral hemorrhage after t-PA.[23,24] The major signs of early infarction include peri-infarct edema, mass effect, sulcal effacement, or hemorrhage. Patients with *early* infarct signs on CT should not receive thrombolysis.

Blood Pressure. Acute stroke produces an increase in blood pressure in approximately 80% of patients.[8] Regardless of the treatment for stroke, blood pressure should be monitored frequently. Control of blood pressure is especially important in the setting of thrombolytic therapy for several reasons. First, significant elevation in blood pressure is an exclusion criteria for t-PA. In addition, management of blood pressure after administration of t-PA is important because elevated BP is associated with an increased risk of intracerebral hemorrhage.[2,25]

Minimal or moderate elevations in blood pressure do not require urgent pharmacological treatment, since there generally is a spontaneous decline in blood pressure over time.[8,26] As a guideline, antihypertensive intervention is not required unless the calculated *mean* arterial blood pressure is greater than 130 mmHg or the systolic blood pressure is greater than 230 mmHg. Systolic blood pressures between 180-230 mmHg or diastolic pressures 105-120 mmHg may be treated with labetalol hydrochloride. This dose may be repeated or doubled every 10-20 minutes up to a dose of 150 mg. If adequate reductions in blood pressure are not achieved, intravenous sodium nitroprusside may be infused at a starting dose of 0.5 mcg/kg/min. Remember that a *rapid* reduction in the blood pressure is unnecessary and may be harmful.[25] Although there is no definitive data to support an "ideal" blood pressure, a reduction to systolic blood pressures of 200-230 mmHg and to diastolic pressures of 100-120 mmHg is probably adequate. Other agents that may be effective for reduction of blood pressure include intravenous nitroglycerin, sodium nitroprusside, esmolol, and intravenous ACE inhibitors.[26,27] The use of sublingual nifedipine should be avoided because of its rapid and unpredictable hypotensive effect. Hypotension is a rare phenomenon in acute ischemic stroke. If present, the etiology (e.g., volume depletion) should be sought.[25]

Anticoagulation. Although studies are ongoing, the efficacy of heparin in acute ischemic stroke is not well-established. Despite this, heparin is used commonly in the setting of acute stroke. The role of antithrombotic agents in acute stroke also now includes the use of low molecular weight heparins (LMWH) and heparinoids. Initial studies suggest that LMW heparins reduce disability and death even six months after stroke.[28] Two other trials, the International Stroke Trial (IST) [29] and the TOAST trial (Trial of Org 10172 in Acute Stroke Treatment) may lend additional information to support the use of these agents. The use of intravenous heparin should be considered only in consultation with a neurologist or other physicians experienced in stroke management.

A noncontrast CT should be obtained prior to the initiation of heparin therapy. Specifically, heparin has been recommended in: 1) patients who have suffered minor strokes; 2) patients who do not have hemorrhages with their strokes but have evolving signs and symptoms; 3) patients whose stroke is caused by large vessel atherothrombosis; and, 4) patients with cardioembolic stroke.[30] A history of bleeding disorders, recent surgery or trauma, and gastrointestinal bleeding disorders are usually contraindications to the use of heparin. A rectal exam including stool guaiac should be performed prior to heparin administration.

The use of antiplatelet agents in the acute setting of stroke is not well studied. There are two trials that have investigated the role of aspirin in acute stroke. In the IST, patients received 300 mg of aspirin vs. no-aspirin.[29] The mortality reduction was .3% and the reduction in recurrent stroke was .7% in the aspirin group. In the Chinese Aspirin Stroke Trial (CAST), the use of aspirin vs. placebo resulted in decreased mortality, but the overall disability rate was not improved. These studies suggest a role for aspirin or other antiplatelet agents, but the data must be interpreted carefully because patients were enrolled as late as 24 hours after stroke onset.

Hyperglycemia. There has been considerable discussion regarding the effect of elevated serum glucose in the setting of acute stroke. Animal data suggest that hyperglycemia enlarges infarct size; however, clinical studies have not supported this finding.[25,27] Nevertheless, it is important to recognize and treat hyperglycemia and hypoglycemia, as these disorders may present with focal neurological findings.

Antipyretics. Although there is experimental data to support the protective effects of hypothermia in reducing infarct size, clinical data are lacking.[31] Hyperthermia is likely to indicate co-morbid disease, with one study indicating that acute infection may constitute a risk factor for ischemic stroke.[32]

Seizures. The frequency of seizures during an acute stroke approaches 43% and are more likely to occur in the setting of hemorrhagic infarction.[33-35] If seizure occurs, it is more likely to manifest within the first 24 hours and usually presents as a partial seizure.[33,36] In a recent study, patients who had more severe strokes were more likely to have a seizure during the early phase of a stroke. Even when other variables were considered, including atrial fibrillation, diabetes, and admission blood glucose, initial stroke severity was the most important variable predictive of seizure activity. Other factors including age, gender, history of ischemic heart disease, or hypertension did not influence likelihood of seizure.[37] From a practical perspective, early seizures were more likely to occur in younger patients, in individuals with acute confusional states, in those with involvement of the cortex, and in patients who had suffered large stroke. Patients with lacunar infarction are less likely to experience early seizures.[37]

The efficacy of prophylactic anticonvulsant therapy in patients with acute stroke has not been established. However, if seizures are present, they may be controlled with benzodiazepines—either lorazepam or diazepam. Phenytoin is recommended in patients with recurrent seizures.[21]

Corticosteroids. There is currently no role for the use of corticosteroids in the management of acute stroke. Several clinical trials have investigated the use of corticosteroids; however, no improvement in outcome after stroke was demonstrated. Furthermore, the incidence of infection was greater in patients treated with steroids.[21,25,38-40]

Cerebral Edema. The use of hypoosmolar fluids should be avoided. Instead, restrict IV fluids as a means of minimizing cerebral edema. Identify and treat factors that may worsen intracranial pressure such as hypoxia, hypercarbia, and hyperthermia. Elevating the head to 20-30° may also be helpful. Osmotic diuresis using mannitol or furosemide is not recommended.[21] Decompression or evacuation of large cerebellar infarctions that compress the brain stem may be helpful in selected cases.[25]

Special Considerations: Thrombolytic Therapy

The recent approval of tissue plasminogen activator (t-PA) for use in acute ischemic stroke now provides the emergency physician with an additional therapeutic option in stroke management. Despite the controversy surrounding the administration of intravenous thrombolysis, the NINDS study demonstrated a benefit for patients with ischemic stroke in the carotid or vertebrobasilar circulation.[2] The clinical improvement with thrombolysis was found to be beneficial irrespective of gender.[2] It should be stressed that age is not an exclusion criterion for administration of thrombolytic therapy, and, in the NINDS trial, the benefit of therapy was seen in all age groups.[25] The incidence of spontaneous intracerebral hemorrhage, however, does increase significantly with age.[41] Treatment was beneficial for patients regardless of the etiology of the stroke, including small vessel occlusive disease, large vessel occlusive disease, and cardioembolic stroke. Patients with extensive, severe neurological deficit, or proximal middle cerebral artery occlusion may respond only to intravenous thrombolytic therapy. If followed with precision and prudence, the management guidelines recommended by the trial investigators provide an acceptable degree of benefit vs. risk for the patient. In institutions where thrombolysis for stroke is an accepted arm of the stroke management pathway, a primary focus should be to streamline evaluation of stroke patients to determine their stability for t-PA administration.

Informed Consent. A good faith effort to obtain informed consent should be undertaken. Though it is an accepted treatment, there are risks to the patient and it is important that patients and families are made aware of these risks and are able to make an informed decision.

NIH Stroke Scale Score. The NIH Stroke Scale (NIHSS) can be an important part of the diagnostic evaluation of the stroke patient. The scale can guide the decision analysis for thrombolysis because it is linked to severity of neurological deficit. Though not a formal exclusion criteria, patients with NIHSS scores higher than 22 will likely have extensive deficits and may have an increased risk of intracerebral hemorrhage (ICH).[25]

Issues in Thrombolysis. *Dosage and Administrations.* The exclusionary and inclusionary criteria should be reviewed prior to administration of t-PA. *(Please see Table 2.)* The dose of t-PA administered for acute ischemic stroke is 0.9 mg/kg with a maximum dose of 90 mg. Ten percent of the dose is given as a bolus dose, and the remainder is given over 60 minutes. The drug should be administered through a dedicated intravenous catheter site.

Temporal Issues. The present guidelines permit the administration of intravenous thrombolytics *only within three hours of symptom onset.* Accordingly, it is critical to accurately establish time of symptom onset and question the patient, family, or other witnesses to confirm the time of onset accurately. This three-hour window has been chosen to reduce the risk of hemorrhage and to maximize the potential for recovery. In the ECASS trial, which treated patients up to six hours after time of symptom onset, the higher 30-day mortality in the treated cohort outweighed any demonstrated benefit on functional, neurological, and economic outcomes.[24]

In contrast, the NINDS trial focused on evaluation and treatment only in patients with onset of symptoms that occurred within three hours of presentation to the physician. In this select population, the study demonstrated improved outcome in the thrombolytic-treated group.[2] The ATLANTIS trial is presently underway; it is designed to evaluate the administration of t-PA after three hours but within five hours of symptom onset. Results of this study may show that the temporal window can be safely extended. Presently, however, thrombolysis *cannot* be recommended for individuals with symptoms with onset occurring more than three hours prior to ED presentation.

Blood Pressure Management in Thrombolytic Therapy. Meticulous attention to blood pressure management in the setting of thrombolysis is mandatory in order to minimize the risk of ICH. In this view, blood pressure should be monitored at least every 15 minutes for the first two hours after infusion has started, every 30 minutes thereafter for the next six hours, and then every hour, for a total of 24 hours. The presence of hypertension with systolic blood pressures (SBP) exceeding 185 mmHg or diastolic blood pressures (DBP) exceeding 110 mmHg on two or more readings separated by 10-15 minutes is an exclusion criteria. If thrombolytic therapy is administered, blood pressure must be maintained at a systolic value less than 185 mmHg and a diastolic reading of less than 110 mmHg. If the blood pressure on two consecutive readings 5-10 minutes apart shows a SBP greater than 180 mmHg or DBP 110 mmHg, labetalol hydrochloride should be administered at an initial dose of 10 mg IV over 1-2 minutes. The dose may be repeated or doubled every 10-20 minutes up to a dose of 150 mg. If the response is unsatisfactory, then an infusion of sodium nitroprusside starting at a dose of 0.5 mcg/kg/min is recommended. If the DBP is greater than 140 mmHg, then begin with an infusion of sodium nitroprusside, starting at 0.5 mcg/kg/minute.

Other agents that may be effective for reducing of blood pressure include intravenous nitroglycerin, esmolol, and or ACE inhibitors (such as enalapril 0.625-2.5 mg). These medications may be particularly helpful if labetalol is contraindicated.[25]

Concomitant Therapy. The administration of intravenous, subcutaneous, or oral anticoagulants for the first 24 hours of thrombolytic therapy is not recommended. Patients taking oral anticoagulants at the time of stroke should be excluded from the thrombolytic therapy if their INR is increased.

In addition, anti-platelet agents should not be used during the first 24 hours. It is important to note that patients who are taking antiplatelet agents at the time of their stroke are not excluded from the administration of t-PA; however antiplatelet agents should be discontinued for 24 hours.[25]

Complications of Thrombolytic Therapy. The administration of intravenous thrombolysis is not without risk; among possible complications, intracranial hemorrhage is the most worrisome and, potentially, the most devastating. Though more likely to occur within the first few hours of infusion, ICH after t-PA may occur up to 36 hours after administration of therapy.[2]

Vascular access should be performed only as necessary. Central venous or arterial punctures should be restricted during the first 24 hours. In the event IV sodium nitroprusside is required, the risk must be weighted with respect to bleeding complications and the need for intra-arterial blood pressure measurements. Placement of an indwelling bladder catheter should be avoided during the infusion and for 30 minutes thereafter. Insertion of a nasogastric tube should be avoided for 24 hours after treatment.[25]

Bleeding complications are generally classified into those involving the central nervous system (CNS) and those involving other organs.[25] Hemorrhage, superficial or deep, is the most serious complication, and the treatment of bleeding due to thrombolytic therapy is guided by the location and size of the hematoma, likelihood that bleeding can be controlled with direct pressure the interval between the administration of the drug and onset of the hemorrhage, and the risk of neurological worsening or death.

CNS Hemorrhage. ICH should be suspected if there is a significant change in patient's neurological status or if vomiting or increasing headache occurs. Patients with acute ICH generally have an elevated blood pressure as part of their clinical course. If ICH is suspected, the patient should have a hematocrit, PT, PTT, platelet count, and fibrinogen levels drawn. Patients should have blood typed and cross-matched including four units of packed red blood cells, 4-6 units of cryoprecipitate or fresh frozen plasma, and 1-2 units of platelets. Immediate neurosurgical consultation should be obtained following the demonstration of ICH on the CT scan.[25]

Non-CNS Hemorrhage. Direct pressure should be applied for bleeding at compressible sites, including arterial or venous puncture sites. If the bleeding is not stemmed by mechanical compression, the ongoing infusion of drug should be halted. Occult bleeding may occur at noncompressible sites. Subtle signs and symptoms may be present for patients with retroperitoneal or gastrointestinal bleeding. Frequent exams and monitoring of vital signs may provide clues. Unlike CNS hemorrhage, patients with retroperitoneal or GI hemorrhage are more likely to present with hypotension. Fluid resuscitation should be instituted, and appropriate diagnostic studies should be obtained before initiating medical or surgical therapy.

Neurosurgical Consultation. Neurosurgical consultation or support must be available for all patients undergoing thrombolytic therapy.[25] However, it should be noted that there has been some controversy whether neurosurgical support must be immediately available at the treating institution. This issue is of considerable importance to the community physicians since neurosurgical consultation may not be as readily available as in the academic setting. In the community or rural setting, patients should not be eliminated from consideration for t-PA for lack of "in-house" neurosurgical backup. Efforts should be made with the regional tertiary centers to accept patients in the event of complications. Rapid transport via aeromedical means or ground ambulance are acceptable strategies.

Thrombolytic Therapy in the Rural or Community ED. At smaller hospitals, local physicians or hospital administrators may be unable to commit the substantial resources required to support a thrombolytic protocol for ischemic stroke. In these situations, the emergency physician should contact a regional tertiary referral center to establish an acute stroke coordinated care track (CCT) for patient transfer.

An aeromedical coordinated care track to transfer patients from surrounding rural hospitals to a referral center facility using a helicopter transport service may be established at the outlying ED. In this case, t-PA can be administered in the evaluating ED, and the infusion is continued while en route assuming that entry criteria can be adequately evaluated.

Emerging Stroke Therapies

Unfortunately, the overwhelming percentage of stroke patients do *not* meet selection criteria for thrombolytic therapy. The primary focus for new acute stroke therapies is in the area of "neuro-protective" or "cyto-protective" agents. These drugs target the ischemic penumbra, the area where blood supplies are inadequate to main clinical and electrophysiological functions but that represent areas of tissue that may be viable for several hours after the occlusive event. The peri-infarct cellular milieu resulting in tissue death involves depletion of energy stores, ion pump failure, membrane destabilization, and free radical formation.

Free Radical Scavengers. Free radicals are formed in the ischemic penumbra and are believed to be directly toxic to nerve cells.[25] One agent, a steroid lipid peroxidation inhibitor, tirilazad mesylate, has been studied; however, it did not improve overall functional outcome at three months in two separate trials.

Membrane-Stabilizing Compounds. The plasma membrane is a barrier to neurotransmitters and ions. In the ischemic setting, the plasma membrane loses its protective capacity. Membrane stabilizing agents, such as a monoganglioside, are believed to enter the plasma membrane and block harmful excitotoxic effects. Three clinical studies, however, failed to show improved outcome three months after stroke; however, subanalysis did suggest that early treatment within 4-6 hours may offer benefit, but this requires further investigation.[42]

Ion Channel Blockers. Sodium channel blockers are involved with glutamate release. Fosphenytoin, a pro-drug of phenytoin, blocks the sodium receptor and decreases release of glutamate, resulting in diminished excitotoxic side effects. Nimodipine, a calcium channel blocker already recommended for use in subarachnoid hemorrhage, is being investigated for the use of stroke. One study did not show benefit; however, study medication was administered up to 48 hours after the onset of stroke. An ongoing study, the Very Early Nimodipine Use in Acute Stroke (VENUS) trial, is evaluating the effect of oral nimodipine started within six hours after onset of ischemic symptoms.[43]

Glutamate Receptor Antagonists. Glutamate is considered an excitotoxic amino acid because stimulation of glutamate receptors leads to uncontrolled entry of calcium into the neuron resulting in cell death. The NMDA receptor is located on the cell surface and has a glutamate binding site. NMDA receptor antagonists may be protective to cells reducing glutamate release due to the ischemic insult. Eliprodil was an NMDA antagonist that showed promise, however, a Phase III trial did not demonstrate efficacy. Another compound, Cerestat (aptiganel hydrochloride) is presently under evaluation.

Enhanced Activity of GABA. GABA is the main inhibitory neurotransmitter in the brain. The pharmacological strategy for its use involves counteracting excito-toxicity by enhancing the inhibitory activity of GABA. One compound, chlormethiazole, increases the effect of GABA by working directly at the GABA receptor. The efficacy results are pending from the recent completion of a trial.[42]

Monoclonal Antibody Therapy. White blood cells are present after ischemic insult and may be destructive to the microcirculation and may release cytokines that enhance neuronal tissue damage. Enlimomab is a murine monoclonal antibody that binds to intercellular adhesion molecule-1 (ICAM-1). ICAM-1 is increased in the setting of focal ischemia and results in an influx of white blood cells. By administering the monoclonal antibody, it is believed to reduce the destructive effects of the white blood cells.

Though there are several neuroprotective strategies under investigation, additional agents are under development that involve opioid receptor antagonists, protein synthesis inhibitors, and growth factor compounds.

Intra-Arterial Thrombolysis. The use of micro-angiographic techniques for the visualization of clot in the cerebral circulation followed by the administration of thrombolytic agents is possible. One ongoing study, PROACT, uses pro-urokinase administered angiographically within six hours of symptom onset. Patient recruitment efforts are still underway, and the efficacy results are pending. Except for the investigational studies, intra-arterial administration of thrombolysis is not indicated or FDA-approved for the treatment of stroke. Until trials are completed, intra-arterial administration of thrombolytic therapy should be considered strictly investigational.

Summary

Maximizing clinical outcomes in stroke patients requires a systematic approach to diagnosis and management. Prompt CT scanning will be required to guide therapy in most cases, and a careful history documenting symptom onset is mandatory for determining which patients will be eligible for thrombolytic intervention. Although thrombolysis is becoming established as primary modality in some major centers, the precise inclusionary and exclusionary criteria for patient selection are still being refined. In patients who are poor candidates for thrombolytic protocols, or who are managed in centers which do not yet include this therapy in their treatment pathways, eligibility for other interventions, including aspirin and anticoagulation with heparin, should be considered.

References

1. Camarata P, Heros R, Latchaw R, et al. Brain attack: The rationale for treating stroke as a medical emergency. *Neurosurgery* 1994;34:144-158.
2. The National Institutes of Neurological Disorders and Stroke rt-PA Stroke Study Group. Tissue plasminogen activator for acute ischemic stroke. *N Engl J Med* 1995;333:1581-1587.
3. Bowen J, Yaste C. Effect of a stroke protocol on hospital costs of stroke patients. *Neurology* 1994;44:1961-1964.
4. Gomez C, Malkoff M, Sauer C, et al. An attempt to shorten in-hospital therapeutic delays. *Stroke* 1994;25:1920-1923.
5. Webb D, Fayad P, Wilbur C, et al. Effects of a specialized team on stroke care: The first two years of the Yale Stroke Program. *Stroke* 1995;26:1353-1357.
6. Brass L. Stroke teams. In: De Keyser J, et al, eds. *Acute Stroke: Current Approaches to Management* Washington:

Elsevier; 1996;2:3-6.

7. Mitchell J, Ballard D, Whisnant J, et al. What role do neurologists play in determining the costs and outcomes of stroke patients? *Stroke* 1996;27:1937-1943.
8. Broderick J, Brott T, Barsan W, et al. Blood pressure during the first minutes of focal cerebral ischemia. *Ann Emerg Med* 1993;22:1438-1443.
9. Levy DE. How transient are transient ischemic attacks? *Neurology* 1988;38:674-677.
10. Davalos A, Matias-Guiu J, Torrent O, et al. Computed tomography in reversible ischemic attacks: clinical and prognostic correlations in a prospective study. *J Neurol* 1988;235: 155-158.
11. Evans G, Howard G, Murros K, et al. Cerebral infarction verified by cranial computed tomography and prognosis for survival following transient ischemic attack. *Stoke* 1991;22: 431-436.
12. Brickner ME. Cardioembolic stroke. *Am J Med* 1996;100: 465-474.
13. Feinberg WM, Albers GW, Barnett HJM, et al. Guidelines for the management of transient ischemic attacks. *Stroke* 1994; 25:1320-1335.
14. Brown RD, Evans BA, Wiebers DO, et al. Transient ischemic attack and minor ischemic stroke: An algorithm for evaluation and treatment. *Mayo Clin Proc* 1994;69:1027-1039.
15. Steinke W, Hennerici M, Rautenberg W, et al. Symptomatic and asymptomatic high-grade carotid stenoses in Doppler color-flow imaging. *Neurology* 1992;42:131-138.
16. Riles TS, Eidelman EM, Litt AW, et al. Comparison of magnetic resonance angiography, conventional angiography, and duplex scanning. *Stroke* 1992;23:341-346.
17. Caplan LR, Brass LM, DeWitt LD, et al. Transcranial Doppler sonographic findings in middle cerebral artery disease. *Neurology* 1990;40:696-700.
18. Shivkumar K, Jafri SM, Gheorghiade M. Antithrombotic therapy in atrial fibrillation: A review of randomized trials with special reference to the Stroke Prevention in Atrial Fibrillation II (SPAF II) trial. *Prog Cardiovasc Dis* 1996;38: 337-344.
19. Patrono C, Roth GJ. Aspirin in ischemic cerebrovascular disease. *Stroke* 1996;27:756-760.
20. Morely J, Marinchak R, Rials SJ, et al. Atrial fibrillation, anticoagulation, and stroke. *Am J Cardiol* 1996;77:38A-44A.
21. Adams HP Jr, Brott TG, Crowell RM, et al. Guidelines for the management of patients with acute ischemic stroke. *Circulation* 1994;90:1588-1601.
22. Adams R. Management issues for patients with ischemic stroke. *Neurology* 1995;45(suppl 1):S15-S18.
23. VonKummer R, Bozzao L, Manelfe C. *Early CT Diagnosis of Hemispheric Brain Infarction* Strpinger: Berlin: 1995.
24. Hacke W, Kaste M, Fieschi C, et al. Intravenous thrombolysis with recombinant tissue plasminogen activator for acute hemispheric stroke. *JAMA* 1995;274:1017-1025.
25. Adams H, Chair Special Writing Group of the Stroke Council. Guidelines for thrombolytic therapy for acute stroke: A supplement to the guidelines for the management of patients with acute ischemic stroke. *Circulation* 1996;94: 1167-1174.
26. Alberts M. Management of hypertension in acute ischemic stroke. In: De Keyser J, et al., ed. *Acute Stroke: Current Approaches to Management* Washington: Elsevier; 1996;2: 12-14.
27. Hacke W, Stingele R, Steiner T, et al. Critical care of acute ischemic stroke. *Intensive Care Med* 1995;21:856-862.
28. Kay R, Wong K, Yu Y, et al. Low-molecular-weight heparin for the treatment of acute stroke. *N Engl J Med* 1995;333: 1588-1593.
29. International Stroke Trial Pilot Study Collaborative Group. Study Design of the International Stroke Trial (IST), baseline data and outcome in 984 randomized patients in the pilot study. *J Neurol Neurosurg Psychiatry* 1996;60:371-376.
30. Furlan A. Stroke: Prevention still the best treatment. *Cleveland Clin J Med* 1995;62:6-8.
31. Maher J, Hachinski V. Hypothermia as a potential treatment for cerebral ischemia. *Cerebrovasc Brain Metabolism Reviews* 1993;5:277-300.
32. Bova I, Bornstein N, Korczyn A, et al. Acute infection as a risk factor for ischemic stroke. *Stroke* 1996;27:2204-2206.
33. Gupta S, Naheedy M, Elias D, et al. Postinfarction seizures. *Stroke* 1988;19:1477-1481.
34. Horning C, Butner T, Hufnagel A, et al. Epileptic seizures following ischemic cerebral infarction. Clinical picture, CT findings, and prognosis. *Eur Arch Psychiatry Neurol Sci* 1990;239:379-383.
35. Kilpatrick C, Davis S, Tress B, et al. Epileptic seizures in acute stroke. *Arch Neurol* 1990;47:157-160.
36. Reith J, Jorgensen H, Nakayama H, et al. Seizures in Acute Stroke: Predictors and Prognostic Significance. *Stroke* 1997; 28:1585-1589.
37. Arboix A, Garcia-Eroles L, Massons JB, et al. Predictive factors of early seizures after acute cerebrovascular disease.
38. Norris J, Hachinski V. High-dose steroid treatment in cerebral infarction. *BMJ*1986;292:21-23.
39. Mulley G, Wilcox R, Mitchell J, et al. Dexamethasone in acute stroke. *BMJ* 1978;2:994-996.
40. Bauer R, Tellez H. Dexamethasone as treatment in cerebrovascular disease. A controlled study of acute cerebral infarction. *Stroke* 1973;4:547-555.
41. Brott T, Thalinger K, Hertzberg V. Hypertension as a risk factor for spontaneous intracerebral hemorrhage. *Stroke* 1986;17: 1078-1083.
42. De Keyser J. Opportunities for neuroprotection. In: *Current Approaches to Stroke Acute Stroke Management.* Washington: Elsevier; 1996;2:6-12.
43. Mohr JP, Orogozo JM, Harrison MJH, et al. Meta-analysis of oral nimodipine trials in acute ischemic stroke. *Cerebrovasc Dis* 1994;4:197-203.

Spinal Cord Injuries

David A. Wald, DO

It is estimated that approximately 10,000 new cases of spinal cord injury occur annually in the United States.[1-4] Acute traumatic spinal cord injury predominantly is a disease affecting young males. According to statistics from the National Spinal Cord Injury Database, 81% of these victims are male, with an average age of 31.5 years. Since 1991, motor vehicle accidents have accounted for 36% of all reported cases, followed by acts of violence, falls, recreational/ sporting activities, and other non-traumatic conditions. The most commonly injured area is the lower cervical spine (C_5-C_6), followed by the thoracolumbar junction,[3,5] although the elderly may be more likely to sustain injuries to the upper cervical spine.[6] At the present time, there roughly is an equal distribution between patients sustaining an injury resulting in quadraplegia (cervical) and an injury resulting in paraplegia (thoracic or lumbar), and there is a trend toward incomplete rather than complete injuries.[7]

The financial burden of spinal cord injuries is overwhelming. For example, it has been estimated that, for patients with a complete spinal cord injury, the cost of life-long medical expenses and lost wages exceeds $2,000,000.[2] In the first year post injury alone, it is estimated that health care and living expenses for a patient with a high cervical cord injury are in excess of $400,000.[1] With an estimated prevalence of 200,000 spinal cord injured patients in the United States requiring some form of medical care,[8,9] the yearly cost for these patients easily translates into billions of dollars.

The purpose of this review is to provide a categorization scheme for acute spinal cord injuries, and an outcome-effective evaluation and treatment protocol for emergency medicine practice.

Spinal Cord Injury: Clinical Pathophysiology and Anatomy

Spinal cord injury most often results from functional impairment of the cord, rather than from an actual anatomic transection.[2,4,10,11] The initial or primary insult usually occurs as a consequence of various physical forces that cause direct injury to the spinal cord. Forces responsible for producing impairment of function include compression, shear, laceration, and distraction.[2,12] As a result of primary injury, a cascade of secondary cellular changes occurs that can play a significant role in spinal cord injury. For example, after the primary event, there is a decrease in regional blood flow to the injured spinal tissue. This will lead to post-traumatic tissue ischemia and the initiation of a complex cascade of events causing an accumulation of free radicals, increased lipid peroxidation, increased intracellular calcium, and loss of cellular integrity.[2,4,8,10,13] The deficit in neuronal transmission responsible for the neurologic deficit can be caused by local spinal cord hypoxia, which may lead to ischemia, and eventually, tissue infarction.[11]

The vertebral column consists of 33 vertabrae: seven cervical vertebrae, 12 thoracic vertebrae, five lumbar vertebrae, five fused sacral vertebrae, and a variable number (3-5) of coccygeal vertebrae. Within the confines of the vertebral column lies the spinal cord, which originates at the cervico-medullary junction just caudal to the foramen magnum and, in adults, terminates at the level of the 2nd lumber vertebrae. The inferior portion of the spinal cord lies below the lumbosacral enlargement and is known as the conus medullaris, below which there is a continuation of nerve roots known as the cauda equina.

Blood supply to the spinal cord originates from the anterior spinal artery and the two, paired posterior spinal arteries, each of which originate as branches from the vertebral arteries. The anterior spinal artery extends for the entire length of the spinal cord and supplies the anterior two-thirds of the spinal cord. The two posterior spinal arteries supply the remaining, posterior one-third of the spinal cord. The spinal cord receives additional blood supply from radicular arteries of the aorta, including the radicular artery of Adamkiewicz, which enters the spinal canal in the lower thoracic region but sends branches as far cephalad as T_4.

When viewed in cross section, the spinal cord is composed of central gray matter containing cell bodies of neurons and surrounding white matter carrying ascending and descending motor and sensory tracts. The white matter can be divided into three major motor and sensory tracts: 1) the dorsal (posterior) column; 2) the lateral corticospinal (pyrimidal) tract; and 3) the anterior spinothalamic tract. Each of these motor and sensory tracts can be clinically evaluated. The dorsal column carries nerve fibers for the transmission of proprioception, vibration, and touch. Ascending fibers will decussate at the cervico-medullary junction. The lateral corticospinal tract carries nerve fibers for the transmission of voluntary motor function. Ascending fibers for the upper extremities are medially located, while fibers for the lower extremities are positioned to more lateral locations at the periphery of the spinal cord. These ascending fibers also decussate at the cervico-medullary junction. The anterior spinothalamic tract carries fibers for transmission of pain, temperature, and light touch. These fibers will decussate in the anterior white commisure about one level above the point at which they enter the spinal cord. Understanding the topographic relationship and function of the spinal cord tracts will enhance accuracy of diagnosis of incomplete spinal cord injury syndromes.

Initial Assessment and Evaluation

Bystanders and prehospital personnel often are the first people to encounter individuals who may have sustained a spinal cord or spinal column injury. The initial care that is provided may determine whether a patient will ultimately regain normal neurologic function or suffer permanent injury. As in all trauma patients, an initial survey focusing on respiratory and cardiovascular stabilization is essential.[14] It is imperative that proper, spinal immobilization is implemented early if this type of injury is suspected. The head should be maintained in a neutral position and all attempts should be made to limit flexion or axial loading of the cervical spine.[15] Many iatrogenic spinal injuries that occur following trauma result from a combination of flexion and axial loading.[15] A properly sized rigid cervical collar should be applied to all patients suspected of having a spine injury. Lateral stabilization of the head should be maintained with either sand bags or application of towel rolls and taping of the head. Although helpful, these maneuvers do not completely immobilize the cervical spine, since some flexion may still occur. It is recommended that all patients with suspected spine injuries be transported on a spine board.[15] Prolonged exposure of any bony prominence (i.e., the occiput, scapula, sacrum, and calcaneus) may lead to the development of pressure sores. Hence, if a patient will be immobilized for an extended period of time, consider padding these areas. In helmeted patients, a two-person technique can be employed to remove the helmet to gain better access to the airway and to permit further inspection of the head.[16] One author recommends transporting spinal cord injured patients in the Trendelenberg position in order to minimize the risks of aspiration and shock, two major causes of death in the prehospital phase of treatment.[14,17] In the quadriplegic patient, vital capacity may be diminished by Trendelenberg positioning because the mass of the abdominal compartment can displace the diaphragm rostrally. Appropriate management of the airway may be required.

Prehospital personnel should have a low threshold for determining which patients should be immobilized to avoid missing a potential spine injury. In this regard, it also is important to consider spinal immobilization in high-risk patient groups, including individuals who are post-ictal or intoxicated, and patients with an altered mental status who may be victims of occult trauma. Because spinal cord injuries are not always evident, it is preferable to be conservative when the decision is made to immobilize the spine. As a general rule, the following patients usually require spinal immobilization: any potential victim of trauma with neurologic deficits, and/or head, neck, or back pain; or any trauma victim with an altered mental status. In the field, a brief neurologic examination should be performed on all patients and should include an assessment of the level of consciousness, pupillary function, and evaluation of gross motor and sensory function of the upper and lower extremities.

Airway. It is critical that cervical spine control be maintained if, at any time, it is determined that the patient requires intubation. If the front of the cervical collar needs to be removed for inspection of the neck, application of Sellick's maneuver, or airway management, an assistant will be required to maintain manual, in-line cervical stabilization. The assistant's primary goal is to maintain the neck in a neutral position. The airway must be evaluated for patency and adequacy of ventilation and oxygenation. Any patient who has a vital capacity less than 15 mL/kg, a PaO_2 of less than 60-70 mmHg, or a $PaCO_2$ above 45 mmHg will likely require urgent intubation.[2,18] Hypoxia and hypercarbia also may cause an excessive increase in blood flow to the spinal cord leading to tissue edema.[18]

Intubation Techniques

A number of intubation techniques have been used to secure an airway in patients suspected of having spinal cord injuries. These include orotracheal intubation; nasotracheal intubation; light wand assisted, retrograde, fiberoptic intubation; and cricothyroidotomy.[5,17-19] The optimal technique used will vary according to specific circumstances and the comfort level of the operator. If succinylcholine is used for rapid sequence intubation, it should be stressed that this agent may cause an increase in the serum potassium in patients who have spinal cord injuries. This can result from the hypersensitization of denervated muscle below the level of injury.[18] Typically, because this reaction does not occur prior to 48 hours, succinylcholine is safe to use in acute spinal cord injuries.

Cardiovascular System. All patients with suspected spine injuries should have large bore intravenous access, supplemental oxygen, and cardiac monitoring (i.e., the "ED safety net"). Vital signs should be closely monitored. In patients with a high thoracic or cervical cord injury, neurogenic shock may occur as a result of impaired sympathetic innervation to the heart.[2] These patients may present with hypotension, absolute or relative bradycardia, and warm peripheral extremities. Hypotension may occur in patients who are normovolemic as a result of increased venous capacitance. Cardiovascular stabilization should be directed at reversing hypoxia and hypotension to help prevent further secondary tissue injury.[14] Autoregulation is usually lost in the acutely injured spinal cord, and as a guideline the mean arterial pressure should be kept above 70 mmHg to prevent further ischemia.[2] Initially, these patients may be resuscitated with crystalloids, but vasopressor support eventually may be needed. Atropine can be used to treat symptomatic bradycardia.[18] An acute spinal cord injury also may leave the patient poikilothermic. This mandates the need for close monitoring of body temperature.

A careful evaluation should be sought for associated injuries that may be masked by the spinal cord injury. In any patient with sensory abnormalities, it may be necessary to perform a bedside diagnostic peritoneal lavage or an abdominal/pelvic CAT scan to rule out an associated intra-abdominal injury.[17] All patients should have an indwelling foley catheter placed to monitor urine output and prevent urinary retention. A nasogastric tube may need to be placed to decrease the likelihood of aspiration.

Radiographic Studies. After all life threatening conditions are identified and treated, radiographic evaluation may begin. Never delay initial management and stabilization to obtain radiographic studies. The cross-table lateral radiograph, which has long been considered the gold standard for evaluating the cervical spine, is not sensitive enough to radiographically clear the cervical spine.[20-24] Moreover, no single radiographic view can completely exclude an injury to the cervical spine.[17,20-24] In fact, various studies have shown that a single lateral cervical spine view is only 70-80% sensitive for identifying cervical spine fractures.[20-22,25] An initial cervical spine trauma series often consists of a cross-table lateral cervical spine radiograph followed by an anteroposterior and odontoid view. The sensitivity of this series has been noted in two studies to be as high as 93%.[21,23] One author recommends adding bilateral supine trauma oblique radiographs to the cervical spine series.[24]

A CAT scan may be indicated in patients with normal films but a high index of clinical suspicion, in patients with inadequate or equivocal plain films, to delineate fractures noted on plain film, or in patients with neurologic deficits. Magnetic resonance imaging (MRI) may be helpful in determining the extent of acute spinal cord compression, disc herniation, soft tissue changes, or ligamentous injury.[2] Flexion-extension views may be indicated in patients who are alert, non-intoxicated, and cooperative, but who have persistent neck pain, negative radiographs, and who are neurologically intact. If these views are performed, a physician should accompany the patient into the x-ray suite and assist with active range of motion. Under no circumstance should the patient's head be passively moved.[24] If a patient has a cervical spine fracture identified radiographically, there is approximately a 10% incidence of a second, non-contiguous vertebral fracture.[2,16] Therefore, it is important to obtain full spine radiographs if a fracture is identified, or if the patient is intoxicated, has a neurologic deficit, or an alteration in consciousness that precludes a complete physical examination.[26]

It is not uncommon to have an associated head and spine injury. In fact, it has been reported that 5-10% of head injured patients have an associated spinal injury, and that 25-50% of patients with a spine injury have an associated head injury.[16,28] Alcohol use often is associated with spinal cord injury. In one series, 87% of patients with spinal cord injuries were intoxicated upon arrival to the trauma center.[5] This also may present a diagnostic challenge when trying to identify major associated injuries.

After completion of the primary survey and initiation of resuscitative efforts, a detailed and systematic secondary survey should to be performed. While conducting the secondary survey, it is important to continue proper spinal immobilization. It has been reported that up to 10% of spinal cord injuries can occur when patients with unstable fractures are moved.[3,4,13,16] In patients with a suspected spinal cord injury, an understanding of the mechanism of injury may help reveal injury patterns. It is important to question the patient about complaints of neck pain, paresthesias, paralysis, weakness, or loss of consciousness at the time of the injury. The presence of any of these findings may suggest spinal cord involvement. Any patient with an altered mental status or who is intoxicated should heighten the physician's index of suspicion for spinal injury. A complete head to toe secondary survey should be performed in accordance with ATLS guidelines, including a careful examination of the head, neck, and axial skeleton.[16]

Neurological Examination. A thorough and detailed neurologic examination should attempt to determine the presence, severity, and level of neurologic dysfunction—these findings will be used as a basis for future comparison. The neurologic examination can begin with simple patient observation. How is the patient positioned? How does the patient hold his or her extremities? Abnormal extremity positioning in a conscious and alert patient may be a clue to a cervical cord injury The patient's breathing pattern also will need close observation. In lower cervical and upper thoracic cord injuries, there may be loss of innervation to the intercostal muscles resulting in a paradoxic (diaphragmatic) respiratory pattern. With a high cervical cord injury at or above the level of C_4, hypercapneic respiratory failure may ensue because of impaired phrenic nerve innervation to the diaphragm.

A detailed motor and sensory examination (pinprick and light touch) should also be performed as outlined in the American Spinal Cord Injury Association (ASIA) standard neurologic classification form. *(Please see Figure 1 and Table 1.)* Additional dorsal column functions (vibration and joint position) can be tested using a 128 Hz tuning fork or by evaluating proprioception of the great toe or index finger. Cord-mediated deep tendon reflexes, cranial nerve testing, and an evaluation of sacral sparing and islands of sparing should be noted. Sacral sparing is the presence of voluntary anal sphincter contraction or sensory function in the perianal region (S_{3-5}) or slight flexor toe movement of the great toe (S_1).[16] If present, this indicates that the lesion is incomplete and improves the prognosis for functional recovery. The presence of "islands of sparing" of sensation within an affected dermatome or below the level of apparent total dysfunction, even in the presence of complete motor paralysis, indicates a chance of functional motor recovery. The preservation of pinprick sensation between the level of injury and the sacral dermatomes may be the best prognostic indicator for useful motor recovery.[29]

Figure 1. Standard Neurological Classification of Spinal Cord Injury

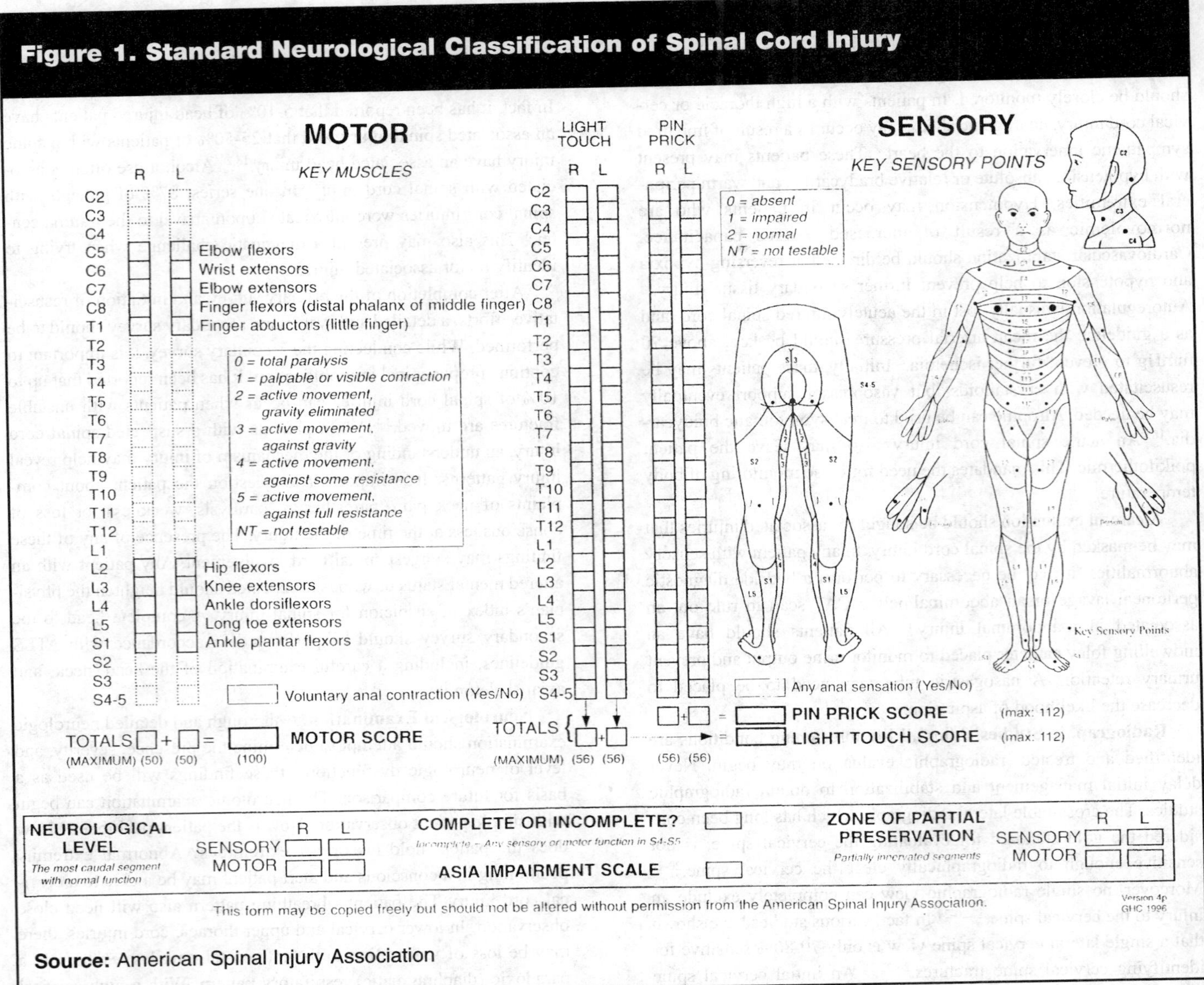

MOTOR

KEY MUSCLES

	R	L	
C2			
C3			
C4			
C5			Elbow flexors
C6			Wrist extensors
C7			Elbow extensors
C8			Finger flexors (distal phalanx of middle finger)
T1			Finger abductors (little finger)
T2–T12, L1			
L2			Hip flexors
L3			Knee extensors
L4			Ankle dorsiflexors
L5			Long toe extensors
S1			Ankle plantar flexors
S2			
S3			
S4-5			Voluntary anal contraction (Yes/No)

0 = total paralysis
1 = palpable or visible contraction
2 = active movement, gravity eliminated
3 = active movement, against gravity
4 = active movement, against some resistance
5 = active movement, against full resistance
NT = not testable

TOTALS ☐ + ☐ = ☐ MOTOR SCORE
(MAXIMUM) (50) (50) (100)

SENSORY

KEY SENSORY POINTS

LIGHT TOUCH R L — PIN PRICK R L (C2 through S4-5)

0 = absent
1 = impaired
2 = normal
NT = not testable

S4-5: Any anal sensation (Yes/No)

TOTALS ☐ + ☐ = ☐ PIN PRICK SCORE (max: 112)
☐ + ☐ = ☐ LIGHT TOUCH SCORE (max: 112)
(MAXIMUM) (56) (56) (56) (56)

Key Sensory Points

NEUROLOGICAL LEVEL — The most caudal segment with normal function — R L — SENSORY ☐ ☐ MOTOR ☐ ☐

COMPLETE OR INCOMPLETE? ☐ — Incomplete = Any sensory or motor function in S4-S5

ASIA IMPAIRMENT SCALE ☐

ZONE OF PARTIAL PRESERVATION — Partially innervated segments — R L — SENSORY ☐ ☐ MOTOR ☐ ☐

This form may be copied freely but should not be altered without permission from the American Spinal Injury Association.

Version 4p GHC 1996

Source: American Spinal Injury Association

Early neurosurgical consultation should be obtained in patients with spine injuries. Carefully screened patients with minor, stable vertebral column injuries such as thoraco-lumbar compression fractures, who are neurologically intact, can be discharged from the emergency department (ED). Bedside neuro/surgical consultation should be obtained for all patients with an unstable vertebral column or an acute spinal cord injury. Early stabilization and transfer of these patients to a regional spinal cord injury treatment center is advocated. These centers are able to provide the specialty care that is required, which consists of a team of specially trained physicians, nurses, and other allied health professionals.

Additional Complications of Spinal Cord Injuries. It is not uncommon for a patient with a prior spinal cord injury to present to the ED seeking medical attention. These patients are at higher risk than the general population for a variety of medical illnesses and conditions. In patients with high thoracic and cervical cord injuries, an impaired ability to clear respiratory secretions increases the incidence of pneumonia. Venous stasis secondary to paralysis also increases the incidence of deep venous thrombosis leading to pulmonary embolism. Pressure on insensate skin often leads to the development of decubitus ulcers. Heterotopic ossification occurs in some spinal cord injury patients, leading to ossification of muscle tissue and a decreased range of motion of the affected joint. Joint contractures and muscle spasticity also are common in this patient population. All patients with chronic indwelling foley catheters are at risk for urinary tract infections. Autonomic hyperreflexia or "mass reflex" is a unique condition affecting spinal cord injury patients. Patients may present with severe hypertension, diaphoresis, or pallor that can lead to seizures. This can occur as a result of hollow organ over distention (bladder or rectum)—initial treatment is directed at relieving the underlying problem (urinary retention or fecal impaction).

Spinal Cord Injury Syndromes

A complete spinal cord injury is one in which there is a complete loss of motor and sensory function below the level of the lesion. If any evidence of sacral sparing or islands of sparing is present, then the lesion is incomplete and there is some chance of functional recovery. In addition, a condition known as spinal shock may mimic a complete cord injury. Spinal shock, which usually occurs in conjunction with a severe spinal cord injury, is a concussive injury to the spinal cord producing total neurologic dysfunction distal to the site of the injury. Clinically, a patient may present with flaccid paralysis, areflexia, and complete anesthesia distal to the injury. Spinal shock also can result in autonomic dysfunction because of interruption of sympathetic innervation and can lead to hypotension, relative bradycardia from unopposed vagal stimulation, and warm peripheral extremities. Cessation of spinal shock is usually heralded by return of the bulbocavernosus reflex. To test this reflex, one has to perform a digital rectal examination and then gently tug on a properly placed foley catheter or squeeze the glans of the penis. A positive reflex is elicited if one feels contraction of the anal sphincter. The symptoms of spinal shock are often variable, but it can be assumed that motor and sensory deficits last only about one hour, although the reflex and autonomic nervous system deficits may persist for days to months.[27]

Incomplete spinal cord lesions can often be classified into one of three clinical syndromes: 1) anterior cord syndrome; 2) central cord syndrome; or 3) the Brown-Sequard syndrome.[13] The anterior cord syndrome often occurs as a result of forced hyperflexion. These patients typically present with a loss of motor function and loss of pain and temperature sensation below the injury; dorsal column functions (joint position, touch, and vibration) are preserved. Prognosis for this type of injury remains poor. The central cord syndrome usually occurs as a result of forced hyperextension. This injury may be associated with buckling of the ligamentum flavum or underlying degenerative arthritis. Patients will present with a neurologic deficit that is more pronounced in the upper extremities than in the lower extremities because of the central location of the ascending and descending motor fibers of the upper extremities. The classic finding is loss of distal upper extremity pain, temperature, and strength, with relative preservation of lower extremity strength and sensation. The Brown-Sequard syndrome can be thought of as a functional hemisection of the spinal cord. The mechanism is often secondary to penetrating trauma, and these patients classically present with loss of ipsilateral motor strength, vibratory and joint position sense, and loss of contralateral pain and temperature sensation below the level of the injury. Usually, some bowel and bladder function is retained, and the prognosis is good.

Other less common, incomplete cord syndromes also have been noted. The cervico-medullary syndrome may mimic a central cord lesion, and can present with sensory loss over the face conforming to the onion skin or Dejerine pattern. The conus medullaris syndrome can present with bilateral lower extremity motor and sensory deficits, in addition to bowel and bladder deficits. This type of injury may appear similar to the cauda equina syndrome, but the former usually is associated with little or no radicular pain, while the latter often has radicular pain as a major complaint.

Another syndrome that is somewhat unique to children is the syndrome of spinal cord injury without radiographic abnormality (SCIWORA). The cause of injuries in this patient population seems to be similar to their adult counterparts.[30] Although often less commonly reported, one series of pediatric spinal cord injuries reported a 67% incidence of SCIWORA.[30] Young children also appear to be more likely to suffer a severe, upper cervical spinal injury.[30] Interestingly, in this group of patients, 27% had delayed onset of neurologic deficits, and some children were noted to have recurrent neurologic injury days to weeks after the initial trauma. These findings raise the concern of prolonged spinal instability. The majority of the cases associated with delayed deficits had transient but definite neurologic symptoms immediately following trauma. The transient symptoms included subjective paralysis, distal parathesias, and the Lhermitte phenomenon. The increased incidence of SCIWORA, as compared to adults, may be related to the relative elasticity of the spinal supporting ligaments and the immature osseous structure of the pediatric spinal column.[4,30]

Table 1. ASIA Impairment Scale

- ❑ **A = Complete:** No motor or sensory function is preserved in the sacral segments S4-S5.
- ❑ **B = Incomplete:** Sensory but not motor function is preserved below the neurological level and includes the sacral segments S4-S5.
- ❑ **C = Imcomplete:** Motor function is preserved below the neurological level, and more than half of key muscles below the neurological level have a muscle grade less than 3.
- ❑ **D = Incomplete:** Motor function is preserved below the neurological level, and at least half of key muscles below the neurological level have a muscle grade of 3 or more.
- ❑ **E = Normal:** Motor and sensory function is normal.

CLINICAL SYNDROMES

- ❑ Central Cord
- ❑ Brown-Séquard
- ❑ Anterior Cord
- ❑ Conus Medullaris
- ❑ Cauda Equina

Spinal Cord Injuries in Athletes

Sports and recreational activities account for 5-15% of all spinal cord injuries.[7,9,31-33] Two-thirds of these injuries occur as a result of diving accidents and an overwhelming majority occur in the lower cervical spine, leading to complete spinal cord injury.[7,9,34] In organized sports, football accounts for the greatest number of spine injuries.[32,35] Generally speaking, spinal injuries in athletes can be divided into three types.[35-37] Type 1 injuries consist of athletes who suffer permanent spinal cord injury. This group of patients can have either a complete or incomplete injury, or any of the previously mentioned spinal cord injury syndromes. It is safe to assume that either the clinical or radiographic evidence of a spinal cord injury will preclude return to contact sports.[33,36,37] A type 2 injury is one in which a transient neurologic deficit occurs without an identifiable bony injury. The presence of transient quadriplegia or the presence of bilateral neurologic symptoms should raise the suspicion of spinal cord compromise. This injury may occur as a result of an underlying spinal canal stenosis. The burning hands syndrome, as described by Maroon, is an example of this type of injury.[38] It can be considered analogous to the central cord syndrome seen in older adults. The mechanism of this injury usually is hyperextension. A key point is that painful dysesthesias or burning hands may be the only complaint of patients with spinal cord injuries. One author recommends that if an athlete has spinal cord symptoms from a sports-related injury and is shown to have functional spinal canal stenosis on MRI, he or she should not be allowed to return to contact sports.[39]

In addition, there is a commonly encountered football-related injury called a stinger or burner. This type of injury is not a true spinal cord injury. The mechanism of injury is usually related to traction on the brachial plexus or nerve root impingement.[36,37,40] In most situations, symptoms last seconds to minutes and involve pain, burning, or tingling down an arm; this may be accompanied by localized weakness. These symptoms are most commonly noted in the C_5-C_6 nerve root distribution,[34,35] are always unilateral, and never involve the lower extremities. When evaluating an athlete who has suffered a suspected stinger injury, a careful distinction must be made between this type of injury and a true spinal cord injury. A type 3 injury includes an injury to the vertebral column without neurologic deficits. Also included in this category are ligamentous injuries and herniated intervertebral discs.

Another entity called spear tackler's spine also has been identified. Permanent neurologic injury has occurred in athletes with the following abnormalities noted on cervical spine films: 1) Developmental narrowing of the cervical spinal canal; 2) straightening or reversal of the normal cervical lordotic curve; and 3) pre-existing minor post-traumatic radiographic evidence of bony or ligamentous injury. In addition, the athletes were documented as using spear tacking techniques.[33,36,37] The decision as to whether to allow an athlete to return to contact sports after he or she has experienced a type 2 or 3 injury is often complex and will need to be made on an case-by-case basis.

Pharmacologic Therapy of Acute Spinal Cord Injury

Initial animal studies simulating spinal cord injury models performed in the 1970s served as the basis for future clinical trials. Glucocorticoids have long been known for their anti-inflammatory properties. Initially, it was thought that glucocorticoids could help prevent secondary spinal cord edema.[41] In 1979, the National Acute Spinal Cord Injury Study Group (NASCIS) performed the first multicenter, randomized, clinical trial evaluating the use of methylprednisolone (MPS) in the treatment of acute spinal cord injury.[42] The study, NASCIS I, compared the efficacy of a 1 gm bolus dose of MPS followed by 1 gm daily for 10 days with a similar dosing regimen of 0.1 gm of MPS. There was no significant difference between the two dosing regimens observed in neurologic recovery of motor or sensory function (pinprick and touch) one year after injury. At the time that the study was conducted, it was felt that steroids were beneficial and that withholding them would be unethical; as a result, there was no placebo control.

NASCIS II was based on extensive studies of MPS in an experimental model of spinal cord injury.[41] The mechanism by which steroids work is still somewhat unclear, but a leading theory is that steroids limit post-traumatic lipid peroxidation.[43] NASCIS II, published in 1990, was the first randomized, double-blind, placebo-controlled trial that unequivocally demonstrated that steroids could modify recovery from a severe, non-penetrating spinal cord injury.[44,45] This study compared three treatment arms: MPS 30 mg/kg bolus, followed by 5.4 mg/kg/hr for 23 hours, naloxone hydrochloride, and a third placebo arm. Initial data analysis did not reveal a difference between the three treatment groups. Subgroup stratification showed that increased recovery rates of neurologic function at six weeks, six months, and one year occurred in patients treated with MPS within eight hours of injury, as compared to those treated with either naloxone or placebo.

In 1991, a study was published that reported the results of a randomized, double-blind, placebo-controlled study evaluating the use of GM-1 gangliocide in acute spinal cord injury.[11] Experimental evidence suggests that these agents augment neurite growth in vitro, and may induce regeneration of neurons and restore neuronal function after injury in vivo.[4] The study consisted of two treatment arms: GM-1 gangliocide 100 mg administered intravenously daily for 18-32 days, and a second placebo arm. In addition, both groups received MPS 250 mg intravenously followed by 125 mg every six hours for 72 hours. Data analysis showed a statistically significant improvement in neurologic function at one year in patients treated with GM-1 gangliocide as compared to placebo. Improvement in patient scores resulted from greater recovery for the lower extremities as compared to the upper extremities, and it appeared that a pattern of recovery was noted in patients who initially had complete paralysis as compared to weak muscles.

In 1997, the results of NASCIS III were published.[46] This study was a randomized, double-blind trial evaluating the use of a 24- or 48-hour protocol of MPS or tirilazad mesylate, a potent lipid peroxidase inhibitor. All three treatment arms received a 30 mg/kg intravenous bolus of MPS prior to randomization. One arm then continued a MPS infusion of 5.4 mg/kg/hr for 23 hours, the second arm continued the infusion for 48 hours, and the third arm received tirilazad as a 2.5 mg/kg bolus every six hours for 48 hours. The 48-hour MPS regimen showed statistically significant improvement in motor recovery at six weeks and six months among patients whose therapy was initiated 3-8 hours after injury. Patients treated with tirilazad for 48 hours showed motor recovery rates equivalent to patients who received MPS for 24 hours.

At the present time, administration of high-dose glucocorticoids has become standard of care in patients with acute, non-penetrating spinal cord injury. All patients should receive an initial intravenous bolus of 30 mg/kg of MPS within eight hours of injury, followed by 5.4 mg/kg/hr for 23 hours.[2,12,17] Steroid administration should be initiated as soon as the neurologic deficit is recognized. Recently published studies, including NASCIS III and other investigational agents, will require further validation before these recommendations are changed.

Summary

In a previously healthy person, an acute spinal cord injury can be devastating. Continued prevention strategies aimed at young adults who are most likely to suffer a spinal cord injury may help reduce the incidence of these injuries occurring. Federal and state legislation addressing the use of seat belts, motorcycle helmets, and drunk driving are playing a role in the reduction of spinal cord injuries.[9] As emergency medicine specialists we must continue to be systematic in our approach to these patients; prompt, efficient, and expert care can play a significant role in improving outcomes.

References

1. Spinal Cord Injury Facts and Figures at a Glance. National Spinal Cord Injury Statistical Center, 1998.
2. Fehlings MG, Louw D. Initial stabilization and medical management of acute spinal cord injury. *Am Fam Prac* 1996;54:1.
3. Meyer PR, Cybulski GR, Rusin JJ, et al. Spinal cord injury. *Neurologic Clinics* 1991;9:3.
4. Highland T, Salciccioli G, Wilson RF. Spinal Cord Injuries. In: Wilson RF, Walt AJ (eds). *Management of Trauma, Pitfalls and Practice*, 2nd ed. Williams & Wilkins; 1996.
5. Shatney CH, Brunner RD, Nguyen TQ. The safety of orotracheal intubation in patients with unstable cervical spine fracture or high spinal cord injury. *Am J Surg* 1995;170:676-679.
6. Daffner RH, Goldberg AL, Evans TC, et al. Cervical vertebral injuries in the elderly: A 10 year study. *Em Rad* 1998.
7. Spinal Cord Injury Statistical Information. National Spinal Cord Injury Statistical Center, 1996.
8. Marion D, Clifton. Injury to the Vertebrae and Spinal Cord. In: Moore EE, Mattox KL, Feliciano DV. (eds) *Trauma*. Appleton & Lange; 1991.
9. Lobosky JM. The Epidemiology of Spinal Cord Injury. In: Narayan RK, Wilberger J, Povlishock JT (eds). *Neurotrauma*. McGraw Hill; 1996.
10. Young W. Spinal Cord Injury Pathophysiology and Therapy. In: Narayan RK, Wilberger J, Povlishock JT (eds). *Neurotrauma*. McGraw Hill; 1996.
11. Geisler FH, Dorsey FC, Coleman WP. Recovery of motor function after spinal cord injury—A randomized, placebo controlled trial with GM-1 ganglioside. *N Engl J Med* 1991;324:26.
12. Mahoney BD. Spinal Cord Injuries. In: Harwood-Nuss A, Linden C, Luten RC, et al (eds). *The Clinical Practice of Emergency Medicine*. 2nd ed. Lipponcott-Raven Publishers; 1996.
13. Hockberger RS, Kirshenbaum K, Doris P. Spinal Trauma. In: Rosen P, Barkin RM, et al (eds). *Emergency Medicine concepts and Clinical Practice.* 3rd ed. Mosby Year Book; 1992.
14. Green BA, Klose KJ, Eismont FJ, et al. Immediate Management of the Spinal Cord Injured Patient. In: Lee BY, et al (eds). *The Spinal Cord Injured Patient Comprehensive Management.* W.B. Saunders; 1991.
15. Benzel EC, Doezema D. Prehospital Management of the Spinally Injured Patient. In: Narayan RK, Wilberger JE, Povlishock JT (eds). *Neurotrauma.* McGraw Hill; 1996.
16. Advance Trauma Life Support Student Course Manual. 6th ed, 1997.
17. Chestnut RM. Emergency Management of Spinal Cord Injury. In: Narayan RK, Wilberger JE, Povlishock JT (eds). *Neurotrauma.* McGraw Hill; 1996.
18. Teeple E, Heres EK. Anesthesia Management of Spinal Trauma. In: Narayan RK, WilbergerJE, Povlishock JT (eds). *Neurotrauma*, McGraw Hill; 1996.
19. Wood PR, Lawler PGP. Managing the airway in cervical spine trauma. *Anaesthesia* 1992;47:792-797.
20. Blahd W, Iserson KV, Bjelland JC. Efficacy of the post-traumatic cross table lateral view of the cervical spine. *J Emerg Med* 1985;2:243-249.
21. Ross SE, Schwab CW, David ET, et al. Clearing the cervical spine: Initial radiologic evaluation. *J Trauma.* 1987;27:9.
22. Mace S. Emergency evaluation of cervical spine injuries: CT versus plain radiographs. *Ann Emerg Med* 1985;14:10.
23. Streitwiesser DR, Knopp R, Wales LR, et al. Accuracy of standard radiographic views in detecting cervical spine fractures. *Ann Emerg Med* 1983;12:9.
24. Daffner RH. Evaluation of cervical vertebral injuries. *Semin Roent* 1992;27:4.
25. Rizzolo SJ, Cotler JM. Unstable cervical spine injuries: Specific treatment approaches. *J Am Acad Orthop Surg.* 1993;1:11.
26. Terregino CA, Ross SE, Lipinski MF, et al. Selective indications for thoracic and lumbar radiography in blunt trauma. *Ann Emerg Med* 1995;26:2.
27. Tator CH. Classification of Spinal Cord Injury Based on Neurological Presentation. In: Narayan RK, Wilberger JE, Povlishock JT. (eds). *Neurotrauma*. McGraw Hill; 1996.
28. Tator CH. Management of Associated Spine Injuries in Head Injured Patients. In: Narayan RK, Wilberger JE, Povlishock JT. (eds). *Neurotrauma.* Mcgraw Hill; 1996.
29. Katoh S, Masry WS. Motor recovery of patients presenting with motor paralysis and sparing following cervical spinal cord injuries. *Paraplegia* 1995;33:9.
30. Pang D, Pollack IF. Spinal cord injury without radiographic abnormality in children—The SCIWORA syndrome. *J Trauma* 1989;29:5.
31. McSwain NE, Martinez JA, Timberlake GA. Cervical Spine Trauma, Evaluation and Acute Management. Thieme Medical Publishers Inc., 1989.
32. Yashon D. Spinal Injury. Appleton-Century-Crofts; 1986.
33. Wilberger JE. Athletic spinal cord and spine injuries. *Clin Sport Med* 1998;17:1.
34. Clarke KS. Epidemiology of athletic neck injury. *Clin Sport Med 1998;*17:1.
35. Bailes JE, Hadley MN, Quigley MR, et al. Management of athletic injuries of the cervical spine and spinal cord. *Neurosurgery* 1991;29:4.
36. Warren WL, Bailes JE. On the field evaluation of athletic neck injury. *Clin Sport Med* 1998;17:1.
37. Cantu RC, Bailes JE, Wilberger JE. Guidelines for return to contact sport after a cervical spine injury. *Clin Sport Med* 1998;17:1.
38. Maroon JC. Burning hand's in football spinal cord injuries. *JAMA* 1977;238:19.
39. Cantu RC. The cervical spinal stenosis controversy. *Clin Sport Med* 1998;17:1.
40. Weinstein SM. Assessment and rehabliitation of the athlete with a "Stinger." *Clin Sport Med* 1998;17:1.
41. Ducker TB, Zeidman SM. Spinal Cord Injury: Role of Steroid Therapy. *Spine* 1994;19:20.
42. Bracken MB, Shepard MJ, Hellenbrand KG, et al. Methylprednisolone and neurologic function 1 year after spinal cord injury. *J Neurosurgery* 1985;63:704-713.

43. Savitsky E. Role of glucocortucoids in treatment of acute spinal cord injury. *WJM* 1996;164:1.

44. Bracken MB, Shepard MJ, Collins WF, et al. A randomized, controlled trial of methylprednisolone or naloxone in the treatment of acute spinal cord injury. *N Engl J Med* 1990;322:20.

45. Bracken MB, Shepard MJ, Collins WF, et al. Methylprednisolone or naloxone treatment after acute spinal cord injury: 1 year follow up data. *J Neurosurgery* 1992;76:23-31.

46. Bracken MB, Shepard MJ, Holford TR, et al. Administration of methylprednisolone for 24 or 48 hours or tirilazad mesylate for 48 hours in the treatment of acute spinal cord injury. *JAMA* 1997;277:20.

Spinal Epidural Abscess

Kenneth H. Butler, DO, FACEP

Back pain is one of the most common complaints among individuals who come to emergency departments (EDs). As for most ED presentations, the physician will initially consider life-threatening conditions (e.g., ruptured abdominal aortic aneurysm) as well as nonurgent conditions (e.g., musculoskeletal strain); unfortunately, spinal epidural abscess (SEA) is rarely included in the differential. Many patients in whom SEA should be considered have a history of narcotic abuse and are written off as coming to the ED to refill their narcotic prescriptions. Others are "bounce-back" patients, who were seen recently in an ED or an outpatient clinic for assessment of back pain and discharged with analgesics but who continued to have pain and thus have returned for medical help.

The clinician must have a high index of suspicion for SEA to make an early and accurate diagnosis and to prevent the development of permanent neurologic dysfunction. Depending on the level of spinal involvement, root pain may mimic a variety of other conditions, including classic sciatica, and therefore, the patient might be discharged home inappropriately. About half of patients with SEA are febrile during the course of the disease; in addition, patients may exhibit mild leukocytosis as well as an elevation in the erythrocyte sedimentation rate (ESR). The classic clinical presentation of SEA consists of four sequential phases: 1) spinal pain; 2) radicular pain; 3) muscular weakness, sensory loss, and sphincter dysfunction; and, finally, 4) complete paralysis. The point at which neurologic dysfunction begins is critical because, once initiated, the time from onset of weakness to complete paralysis is often less than 24 hours and may be as short as 30 minutes. This feature of SEA emphasizes the need for rapid diagnosis and emergency surgical intervention.

The cornerstone of the diagnosis of SEA lies in contemporary neuroimaging studies. Magnetic resonance imaging (MRI) with gadolinium is currently the diagnostic procedure of choice. Prompt neurosurgical consultation should be initiated as early as possible. Traditionally, the management of SEA has consisted of immediate surgery followed by antibiotic therapy. Surgical management has advantages, most importantly the ability to decompress compromised neural tissues, thereby preventing further neurologic deterioration. In certain patients who are neurologically intact and for whom the surgical morbidity rate is unacceptably high, conservative medical management may be appropriate. An acute epidural abscess should be suspected in patients with back pain and fever, particularly in those who have abused drugs intravenously.

Introduction

Epidural abscess of the spinal column is a rare but potentially devastating disease. When it is recognized early and treated appropriately, the outcome can be excellent. However, because this disease process and its associated illnesses frequently advance rapidly, the mortality rate is as high as 20%, even in modern series.[1-3] MRI aids greatly in the diagnostic process and should be obtained, if available, as soon as epidural abscess is suspected. Surgical therapy is preferable in the majority of cases, and as newer surgical techniques and approaches are developed, the indications for medical therapy have become narrower.[4-9]

Abscesses in the spinal subdural space or in the spinal cord proper are even more unusual but also can lead to complete and irreversible loss of neurologic function if not diagnosed and treated rapidly.

An acute epidural abscess should be suspected in patients with back pain and fever, particularly in those with underlying risk factors.[8,10]

Figure 1. Branches of a Typical Spinal Nerve

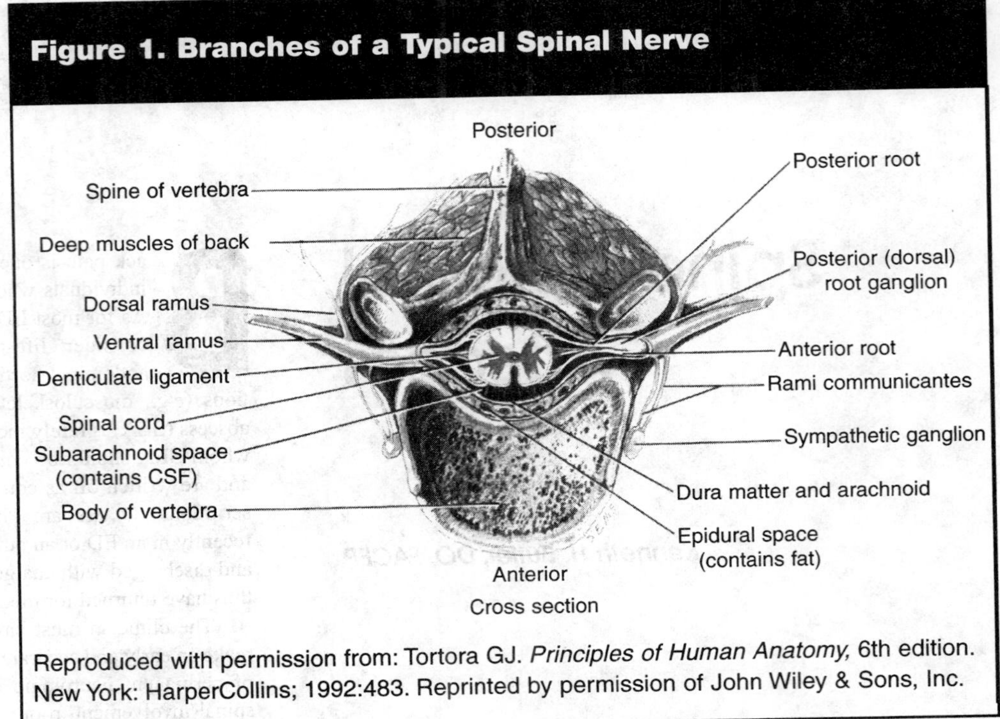

Reproduced with permission from: Tortora GJ. *Principles of Human Anatomy,* 6th edition. New York: HarperCollins; 1992:483. Reprinted by permission of John Wiley & Sons, Inc.

Epidemiology

A bacterial infection in the epidural space can lead to the formation of a pyogenic SEA, resulting in the accumulation of purulent fluid or infected granulation tissue. Although now well recognized as a distinct clinical entity of growing neurosurgical significance, not so long ago SEA was regarded as a relatively rare condition. The incidence of SEA has been estimated at 0.2 to 1.2 cases per 10,000 hospital admissions per year, but more recent series have documented an increasing incidence during the past 10 years.[9,11-13] A number of reasons for this increase can be cited, including an aging population, increased intravenous drug abuse, and an increase in the use of spinal instrumentation and epidural anesthesia. Finally, one cannot exclude the possibility that contemporary imaging procedures have enhanced our ability to detect this disorder.

Blunt trauma contributes to the formation of SEA in 17-30% of cases. The thoracic spine is reportedly involved in 31-63% of cases, the lumbar spine in 21-44%, and the cervical spine in 14-26%. Older studies found that the male-to-female ratio for this disease was about 1; more recent data indicate that men are more likely to be affected.[11,13,14]

Pathophysiology

The mechanism by which neurologic deficit occurs in patients with SEA has been attributed to a variety of factors, including mechanical compression of the neural elements; thrombosis of major arteries and/or veins supplying and draining the cord, respectively; impairment of the intrinsic microcirculation of the cord; and infectious vasculitis. Since SEA is a space-occupying lesion, mechanical compression usually contributes to the observed deficit.

The spinal epidural space is the area surrounding the thecal sac and separating the dura from its bony encasement. *(Please see Figure 1.)* It is not a uniform space.[12] Instead, it is a metameric segmented structure in which some areas contain loose, areolar tissue, fat, and numerous veins (please see Figure 2) and, in others, the dura is in direct contact with bone or ligament (thus creating only a "potential space"). In addition, individual metamers are separated, preventing free communication between the anterior and posterior epidural space. This anatomic arrangement may explain why the majority of epidural abscesses are caused by hematogenous spread and are located posteriorly. In general, the infection does not involve the anterior epidural space or circumferentially surround the thecal sac. In contrast, cases associated with discitis or vertebral osteomyelitis typically involve the anterior epidural space and, possibly because these cases commonly occur after surgery, the abscess may be circumferential because of the disruption of the normal anatomic septations. The metameric segmentation of the epidural space may also limit the longitudinal spread of the pyogenic process. In most cases, the extent of the abscess is usually limited to an average of three to four vertebral segments.[2,6,9]

The spinal epidural space is limited to the dorsal aspect of the spinal canal; ventrally, the dura is tightly adherent to the posterior aspect of the vertebral bodies and their ligaments from the first cervical through the second sacral vertebra. It is only caudal to S2 that the epidural space becomes circumferential, surrounding the dura on all sides.

An important anatomic feature that affects the distribution of SEA is the regional variation in the size of the epidural space. In the cervical spine, the epidural space is more a potential than an actual space. The epidural compartment becomes more apparent at the cervicothoracic junction and becomes wider in a rostral-to-caudal direction. The space then tapers between approximately T11 and L2, caudal to which the epidural space attains its greatest depth. These factors account for the rostral-caudal distribution of SEA, as well as its preference for the dorsal epidural space.[15] *(Please see Figure 3.)*

The precise pathophysiologic cause of the neurologic impairment is not known. Many patients suffer rapid and irreversible deterioration, which has prompted several authors to postulate an ischemic mechanism from either arterial occlusion or venous stasis.[15,16] Other studies using an experimental rabbit model of SEA demonstrated that the progressive neurologic deficits were secondary to compression.[17-20] It seems likely that the cause of the neurologic deficit is multifactorial, with compression being the major component, and ischemia induced by this compression adding to spinal cord damage.

Risk Factors and Underlying Disease

Various risk factors and underlining illnesses are often identified in patients with SEA. *(Please see Table 1.)* Studies have identified factors associated with altered immune status in more than 50% of these patients, notably those with diabetes mellitus, chronic alcoholism, chronic renal failure, and underlying malignancy.[9,21,22] Intravenous drug abuse, HIV infection, and acquired immunodeficiency syndrome (AIDS) have become increasingly important factors that predispose individuals to the development of SEA.[3,11,23,24]

Suppurative processes within the epidural space can develop in three ways: 1) by direct extension from a contiguous site of infection, such as in vertebral osteomyelitis; 2) by hematogenous seeding from a remote source of infection (intravenous drug abuse, skin infections, urinary tract infections, respiratory infections, pharyngeal or dental abscess, subacute bacterial endocarditis, long bone osteomyelitis, pulmonary abscesses); or 3) by direct contamination during invasive procedures, such as spinal surgery, administration of an epidural anesthetic, CT-guided biopsy, or lumbar puncture.[2,6,25]

Figure 2. The Vertebral Venous Plexuses

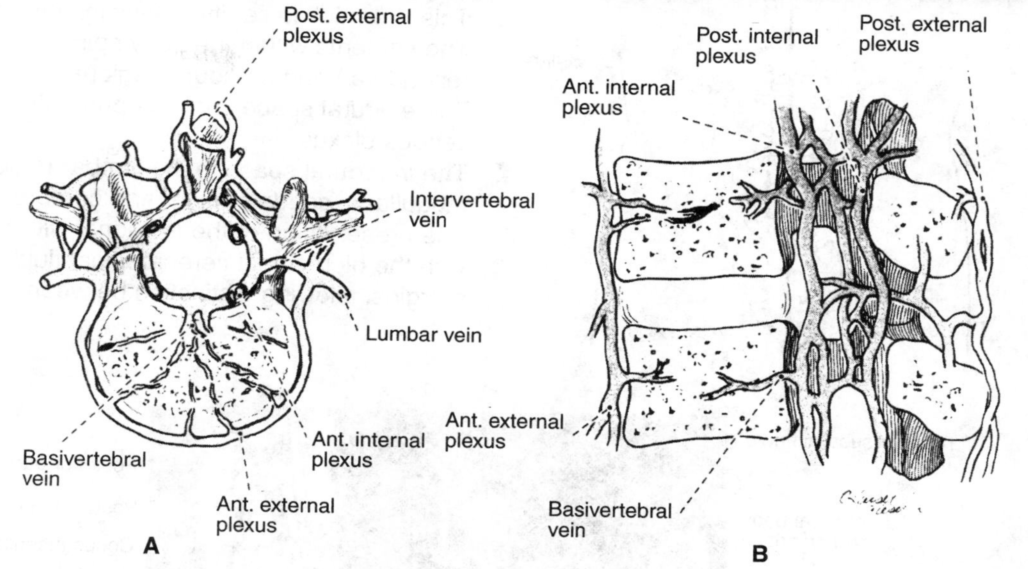

Post. external plexus
Intervertebral vein
Lumbar vein
Ant. internal plexus
Basivertebral vein
Ant. external plexus
A
Post. internal plexus
Post. external plexus
Ant. internal plexus
Ant. external plexus
Basivertebral vein
B

A. Transverse section. **B.** Sagittal section.

Reprinted with permission from Rosse C, Gaddum-Rosse P. *Hollinshead's Textbook of Anatomy*, 5th edition. Philadelphia: Lippincott-Raven; 1997:164.

If carefully sought, a definitive etiology for SEA can be found in more than 50% of patients. SEA most often results from hematogenous seeding of the epidural space from a metastatic source of infection, most commonly skin or soft tissue.[2,9,26,27] Other relatively common sources of infection include urinary or respiratory tract infections, intra-abdominal abscesses, subacute bacterial endocarditis, and septic arthritis. SEA frequently occurs as a complication of vertebral body osteomyelitis.[28] In some cases where an infectious source cannot be found, patients may have only a history of minor spinal trauma.[28-30]

Clinical Presentation

Back pain and fever are the most common symptoms and signs of spinal epidural abscesses. SEA has been described as a "painful, febrile, spinal syndrome," which remains the best summation of the clinical presentation of this disease.[10]

A high index of suspicion remains necessary to diagnose SEA and to prevent the development of permanent neurologic dysfunction. In patients with chronic back pain or narcotic-seeking behavior, this is most difficult.[30] Caution is warranted when evaluating a patient who previously visited an ED or an outpatient clinic complaining of back pain and was discharged on analgesics, only to return with persistent or worsening symptoms (the "bounce-back" patient).[8]

One of the most important aspects of SEA is the variable clinical presentation. Early findings can be subtle, and underlying illness may dominate the clinical picture. The variability in the clinical presentation of SEA is related to a number of factors, including the region of the spine involved, whether the infection is due to hematogenous seeding or to extension of a local process, the immune status of the patient, and the virulence of the infectious agent. From a diagnostic perspective, the triad of pain, fever, and progressive neurological deficits is seen in a minority of patients; consequently, the diagnosis may be delayed in a large percentage of patients. Finally, about 10% of patients with SEA present with encephalopathy.

The classic presentation of SEA consists of four phases that evolve in the following sequence: 1) spinal pain; 2) radicular pain; 3) muscular weakness, sensory loss, and sphincter dysfunction; and finally, 4) complete paralysis.[26,31] *(Please see Table 2.)* The rapidity of progression from one stage to another depends on the factors outlined above. With spontaneous abscess resulting from hematogenous seeding, progression from spinal to radicular pain and neurologic dysfunction tends to occur more rapidly, and systemic manifestations are often a prominent part of the clinical picture. In cases of SEA that result from local extension of adjacent vertebral osteomyelitis, the evolution tends to be slower, at times progressing over weeks or even months until the infection becomes clinically apparent.

Spinal pain is almost universally present with SEA and in most patients is associated with localized spinal tenderness to palpation or percussion. Once spinal pain occurs, it becomes progressively more severe and intractable.[6,8] Most patients also develop radicular pain, which usually follows the onset of spinal pain.[32] Depending on the level of spinal involvement, root pain may mimic a variety of other conditions, including classic sciatica, an acute abdominal process, or herpes zoster.[9] Two-thirds to three-fourths of patients will be febrile, with temperature in excess of 38°C at some point during the course of the illness. Headache and nucal rigidity may occur, reflecting a parameningeal reaction or, in some cases, frank meningitis.[33-35]

Unfortunately, SEA is all too frequently diagnosed after the onset of neurologic dysfunction, which occurs in as many as 90% of

Figure 3. Sectional Anatomy by MRI

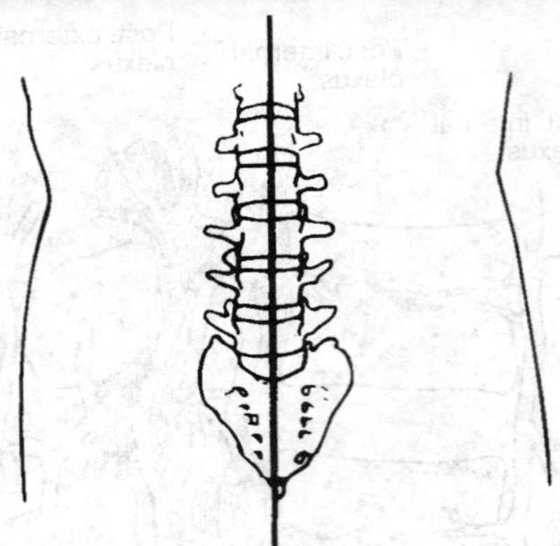

1. This is a midline sagittal T2-weighted fast spin-echo image.
2. The contents within the bony spinal canal are divided into epidural (extradural) and intradural regions.
3. The epidural space contains primarily fat and the internal vertebral venous plexus.
4. The intradural space in the lumbar region contains the conus medullaris, cauda equina, and cerebrospinal fluid.
5. The preservation of the fat signal with this technique, combined with the high-signal cerebrospinal fluid, delineates the dural margins, allowing distinction between the epidural and intradural spaces.

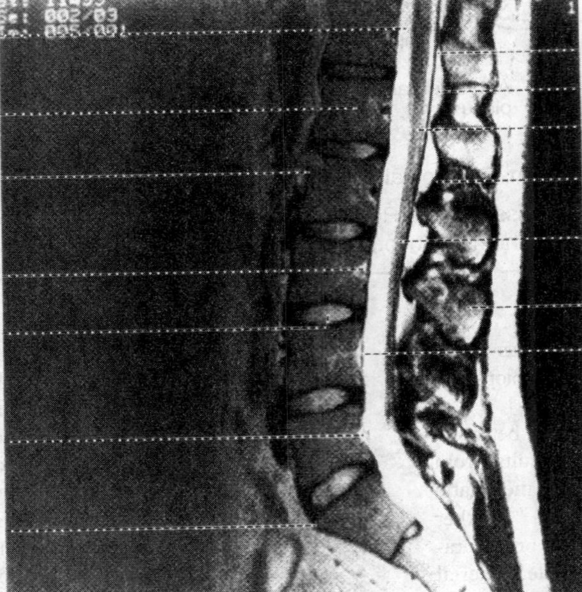

Reproduced with permission from: El-Khoury GY, Bergman RA, Montgomery WJ. *Sectional Anatomy by MRI*, 2nd edition. New York: Churchill Livingstone; 1995:88.

patients.[2,3] Most patients with SEA have some degree of motor weakness, which may be unilateral or bilateral or involve a single extremity. Sensory loss is usually incomplete and may occur in a radicular pattern or present at a discrete sensory level. The point at which neurologic dysfunction begins is especially critical because, once initiated, the time from onset of weakness to complete paralysis is often less than 24 hours and can occur in as little as 30 minutes. This deterioration is a feature of SEA that emphasizes the need for rapid diagnosis and emergency surgical intervention.[36] Continued and timely neurologic examinations should performed in the ED and the results documented, because the neurologic status of these patients can change quickly.

Pediatric Considerations

The characteristic features of SEA may not be prominent in children. The clinical picture may be dominated by nonspecific findings such as fever, malaise, irritability, headache, and vomiting. Reluctance of the child to lie prone, irritability with movement, and rigidity of the spine may be the only clues to the diagnosis prior to the onset of neurologic deficit. The classic four-stage sequence described in Table 2 may not occur. Back pain may be absent.[26]

Differential Diagnosis

The differential diagnosis in a patient with suspected SEA includes common conditions that share the clinical features of epidural infection. Acute transverse myelitis, which is more common than SEA, should be part of the differential diagnosis in patients with back pain, fever, and progressive neurologic deficit. The two can be differentiated on myelography, which is often normal in transverse myelitis but classically shows a subtotal to complete block in SEA. The routine use of MRI may obviate the

Table 1. Risk Factors for Spinal Epidural Abscess

- Altered immune status
- Diabetes mellitus
- Alcoholism
- Chronic renal failure
- Malignancy
- AIDS
- Intravenous drug abuse
- Skin or soft tissue infection
- Steroid dependency
- Antecedent trauma
- Acupuncture
- Tattooing

need for invasive studies. Metastatic neoplasms of the spine (lymphoma in particular), as well as spontaneous intraspinal hematomas, may mimic the presentation of SEA.[23,37-43]

Diagnostic Studies

Laboratory Findings. Routine laboratory studies in patients with SEA are nonspecific; in fact, no one laboratory study is pathognomonic of this condition. Most patients have a mild leukocytosis (10,000 to 13,000/mm^3) and an elevated ESR, usually in excess of 30 mm/hr.[44] Blood cultures may isolate an organism in more than half of patients and should be obtained routinely.[8] Lumbar puncture is generally discouraged in patients with SEA, especially those with dorsal lumbar abscesses, because of the risk of introducing infection into the cerebrospinal fluid (CSF). Moreover, unless there are clinical features suggesting concomitant meningitis, CSF analysis yields little information. If a lumbar puncture is performed, the CSF usually shows evidence of a parameningeal process manifested by pleocytosis, elevated protein levels, and normal glucose concentration. The CSF also can be entirely normal or reveal frank pus, consistent with accompanying bacterial meningitis.

Plain Films. Bony changes on plain film may be evident in only 33-65% of all patients.[21,22] Up to 70% of patients with chronic epidural abscess may be expected to show such changes, but only about 10% of acute cases have positive findings on plain films. It takes time for bone erosion, sclerosis, vertebral collapse, disc space changes, and paravertebral infection to become radiologically evident.[8]

The findings are usually nonspecific, showing degenerative changes or signs of discitis or osteomyelitis, such as disc-space narrowing or vertebral end-plate destruction. *(Please see Figure 4.)* If osteomyelitis is not yet apparent on plain film, nuclear bone scans may confirm the diagnosis.

Myelography. Myelography is a highly reliable method for diagnosing SEA. Myelography can diagnose or confirm infection in virtually all cases, but unless contrast is injected above the collection, the rostral extent of involvement may not be delineated. In performing myelography for suspected SEA, one should enter the epidural space with great caution to avoid introducing bacteria into the subarachnoid space.

Myelography was the diagnostic study of choice before MRI, but now, with the almost universal availability of MRI and the inherent risk of inserting a needle in the thecal sac in the face of infection, myelography is rarely indicated.[45,46] Myelography should be performed if SEA is suspected but not found by newer imaging techniques.

Table 2. Signs and Symptoms of Spinal Epidural Abscess

STAGE I
- Fever
- Back pain
- Malaise

STAGE II
- Radiculopathy
- Paresthesias

STAGE III
- Motor deficits
- Sensory deficits
- Bladder dysfunction
- Bowel dysfunction

STAGE IV
- Paralysis

Computer-Assisted Tomography. Computed tomography (CT) alone has about an even chance of diagnosing SEA. If it is combined with intravenous contrast, the rate of successful diagnosis approaches 100%. CT reveals an extra-axial mass compressing adjacent structures. It may better define destructive bony changes and may be more sensitive in detecting subtle osseous changes not apparent on plain film.[47]

Magnetic Resonance Imaging. Recently, MRI has become an increasingly important modality in the evaluation of patients with suspected SEA. In many EDs, it has supplemented myelography as the procedure of choice.[45,48,49] MRI has a sensitivity equivalent to that of CT-myelography. Additionally, MRI can exclude many entities included in the differential diagnosis, such as herniated disc, neoplasm, spinal hematoma, and transverse myelitis.[50] MRI also provides greater anatomic detail in demonstrating the rostral-caudal extent of the lesion, spinal cord compression, and the status of the spinal cord. The degree of thecal sac compression seen on MRI examination tends to correlate well with the severity of neurologic deficit detected on physical examination. *(Please see Figure 5.)* Patients who use drugs intravenously tend to have abscesses in locations that correlate with their sites of injection.

MRI may not allow diagnosis of SEA in the presence of meningitis or encephalopathy if excessive motion artifact is present.[50]

Bacteriology

Staphylococcus aureus is the most common organism isolated from patients harboring SEA and may account for more than 90% of cases.[2,6,9] *S. aureus* is implicated, in most cases, secondary to skin and soft tissue infections, in cases related to intravenous drug abuse, and in patients with infections following spinal surgery. It also is the most common organism encountered in children. Other gram-positive cocci such as *Staphylococcus epidermidis, Streptococcus pneumoniae*, and *Streptococcus viridans* account for an additional 10% of cases. In recent years, gram-negative aerobes (*Escherichia*

Figure 4. Discitis Secondary to Osteomyelitis

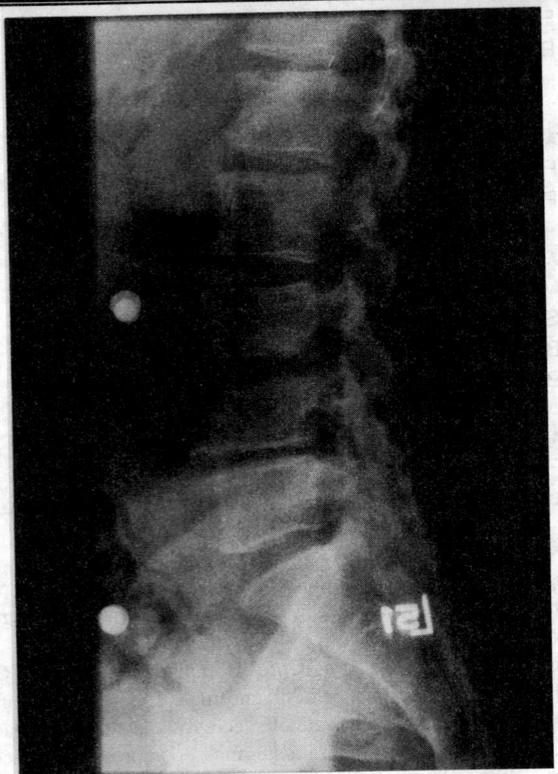

Destruction of the inferior end plate of L5 anteriorly as well as irregularity of the L3 inferior end plate. Consistent with L3-L4 discitis associated with osteomyelitis.

Figure 5. MRI Findings Consistent with L3-L4 Discitis with Associated Adjacent Osteomyelitis

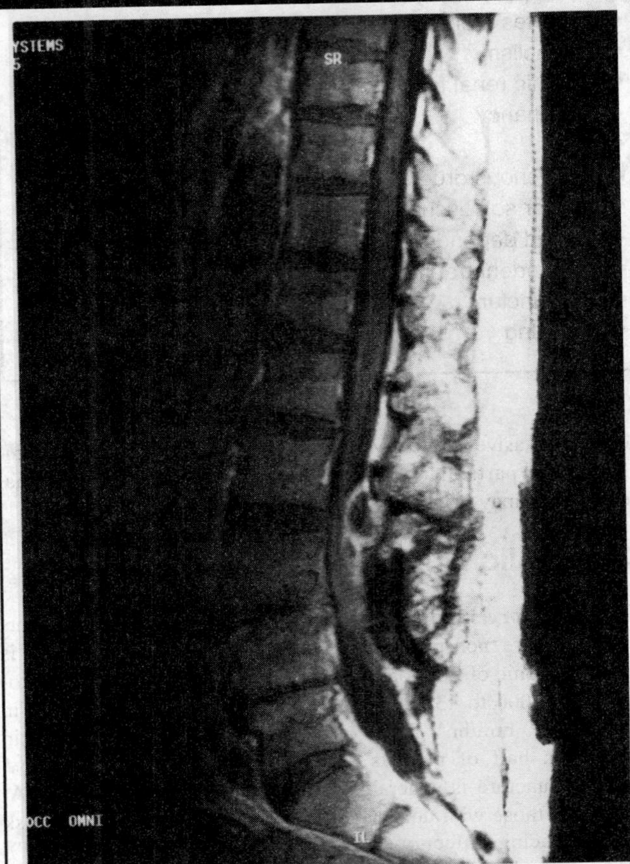

Abnormally enhanced epidural soft tissue at the L3-L4 level. The cord is encased and compressed at this level. Fluid collection extends from the mid portion of L2 through the top of L5, causing posterior compression on the thecal sac.

coli, Pseudomonas aeruginosa, Citrobacter, and *Klebsiella pneumoniae*) have been responsible for a larger percentage of cases. Mycobacterium tuberculosis continues to play an important role in this disease, particularly in economically depressed countries and large urban areas, where tuberculosis accounts for nearly one-fourth of cases.[51] Fungal infections caused by *Echinococcus, Cryptococcus, Brucella, Blastomyces,* and *Aspergillus* organisms also have been reported.

Management

Once the diagnosis of SEA is made, management depends on the condition of the patient. Surgical decompression with specific antibiotic therapy remains the mainstay of treatment. Patients who present in good clinical condition with no neurological compromise or findings, as well as those who are too ill for surgical intervention, may be considered candidates for medical therapy alone. This decision should be made in consultation with a spinal surgeon.

Emergency Department Management. Patients who present with a high clinical probability of SEA require emergent neurosurgical consultation and should not be subjected to any unnecessary delays in the ED before surgery. Intravenous fluid resuscitation, if required, should be performed. Patients should be made NPO and have appropriate OR laboratory tests (complete blood count, electrolytes, and coagulation factors), electrocardiogram, and chest film. Specimens for blood cultures should be drawn prior to administration of any intravenous antibiotic. Cultures should be done for aerobic, anaerobic, and fungal organisms and tuberculosis.

Antibiotics should be initiated in the ED in patients who appear septic or show neurologic deterioration. If presurgical antibiotic administration is deemed prudent, broad-spectrum antibiotics, including those for methicillin-resistant organisms, should be used. Antibiotic agents chosen must be active against *Staphylococcus aureus* because this is the most common organism isolated. If surgery is scheduled within a few hours and the patient with suspected SEA has not been started on antibiotics, is not septic, and has good neurologic status, many neurosurgeons prefer not to start antibiotics until cultures have been taken at surgery. This approach maximizes the probability of obtaining organism growth so the most specific antimicrobial therapy can be given. Steroids may adversely affect outcome and are not indicated.

Surgery

Decompressive laminectomy and drainage of purulent material

Table 3. Proposed Criteria for Exclusive Medical Treatment in Spinal Epidural Abscess

- Poor surgical candidates because of severe, concomitant medical problems
- Patients in which the abscess involves a considerable length of the spinal canal and who have an epiduritis from the cervical to the lumbar level
- Patients not suffering from severe loss of spinal cord or cauda equina function
- Patients with complete paralysis for more than three days

Reproduced with permission from: Leys D, Lesion F, Viaud C, et al. Decreased morbidity from acute bacterial spinal epidural abscesses using computed tomography and nonsurgical treatment in selected patients. *Ann Neurol* 1985;17:350-355.

or debridement of granulation tissue is the best method of preventing neurologic deficits and, if performed quickly after the onset of deficits, may allow full recovery. This is followed by antibiotic therapy of variable duration, usually a four-week course of intravenous antibiotics, which may be extended to eight weeks if vertebral osteomyelitis is present.

Pyogenic epidural abscesses should be considered a neurosurgical emergency because patients, even those receiving appropriate antibiotics, may deteriorate neurologically, rapidly, and unpredictably. The effects of cord compression, especially in the cervical region, can be devastating. If the infection is in the cervical or thoracic area, decompression should be undertaken expeditiously. If the epidural infection involves the lumbar region adjacent to the cauda equina, the surgeon has a little more leeway regarding surgical timing.

Medical Management

Although SEA has traditionally been considered a surgical disease, some authors have advocated conservative treatment, particularly in patients who are neurologically intact and in selected patients in whom the surgical morbidity is unacceptably high.[47,52-54] *(Please see Table 3.)* This approach is predicated on early identification of the organism so that specific antibiotic therapy can be initiated. In selected patients who are neurologically intact, this has been a reasonable approach, particularly applicable in patients with abscesses in the lumbar region, where the epidural space is relatively large and the spinal cord terminates. However, these patients require vigilant monitoring, as neurologic deterioration is not uncommon despite appropriate antibiotic therapy.

Morbidity and Mortality

The functional outcome of the SEA depends greatly on timely diagnosis and rapid institution of therapy. It is therefore imperative that the diagnosis is confirmed quickly and that appropriate consultations be obtained by the emergency physician.

The ability to diagnose SEA in a timely fashion, coupled with improvements in antibiotics and surgical technique, has resulted in a steady decline in mortality rates. Despite these advances, the mortality rate among patients with SEA remains unacceptably high. Additionally, 20-30% of patients who survive will be left with significant neurologic impairment resulting in long-term disability.[55] The outcome in patients who survive primarily depends on the degree and duration of neurologic impairment at the time of diagnosis. Not surprisingly, patients with severe neurologic deficit have a much poorer prognosis than do patients who are neurologically intact. The single most important factor in reducing morbidity is early diagnosis and institution of treatment prior to the onset or progression of neurologic deficit.

Summary

Once thought of as a rare disease entity, and usually a postoperative or surgical complication, epidural abscesses have been increasing in occurrence during the past decade. This increase is related to several factors: widespread intravenous drug abuse (even among adolescents); routine use of epidural anesthesia; and the use of the ED as the primary care provider by uninsured, debilitated, alcoholic, and/or immunosuppressed individuals, particularly those with HIV infection or AIDS. Routine use and increasing availability of MRI has also brought this neurosurgical emergency to light. Infections may reach the spinal epidural space by direct extension from an inflammatory process in adjacent tissues, by metastasis, or by perforating wounds. Skin and soft tissue infections (e.g., "skin-popping ulcers" from substance abuse or abscesses), urinary tract infections, dental infections, chronic pulmonary disease, decubitus ulcers, acupuncture, and tattooing have all been associated with SEA.[56,57] The usual focus is an adjacent vertebral osteomyelitis with direct extension into the epidural space. Surgical wounds, retroperitoneal abscesses, and lumbar punctures represent other potential causes. As these risk factors echo so many of our ED patients, a high index of suspicion for SEA must be maintained when treating patients with back pain and fever.

Staphylococcus aureus remains the most common etiologic agent in adults as well as children and is usually related to an underlying skin or soft tissue infection. Fungal organisms as well as *Mycobacterium tuberculosis* are common in urban areas.

The differential diagnosis of back pain presents a clinical challenge and may be difficult and exhausting in a patient with drug-seeking behavior. The emergency physician should be weary of "red flags" in the patient's history as well as in the physical examination, such as repeated visits for the same complaint, risky social behaviors and associated risk factors, underlying fever in the course of their disease, or a change in neurologic examination results from previous encounters. Since we so often associate a delay in time as a critical factor for an organ system's salvageability in a surgical emergency (e.g., testicular torsion), patients with SEA must be thought of in the same context. The time between emergence of neurologic dysfunction and complete paralysis may be less than one hour.

References

1. Youmans JR, ed. *Neurological Surgery*, Part XI, Infection. 4th ed. Philadelphia: WB Saunders; 1996:3275-3304.
2. Hlavin ML, Kaminski HJ, Ross JS, et al. Spinal epidural abscess: A ten-year perspective. *Neurosurgery* 1990;27: 177-184.
3. Kaufman DM, Kaplan JG, Litman N. Infectious agents in spinal epidural abscesses. *Neurology* 1980;30:844-850.
4. Angtuaco EJL, McConnell JR, Chadduck WM, et al. MR

imaging of spinal epidural sepsis. *AJR Am J Roentgenol* 1987;149:1249-1253.

5. Bertino RE, Porter BA, Stimac GK, et al. Imaging spinal osteomyelitis and epidural abscess with short TI inversion recovery (STIR). *AJNR Am J Neuroradiol* 1988;9:563-564.
6. Del Curling O Jr, Gower DJ, McWhorter JM. Changing concepts in spinal epidural abscess: A report of 29 cases. *Neurosurgery* 1990;27:185-192.
7. Erntell M, Holtas S, Norlin K, et al. Magnetic resonance imaging in the diagnosis of spinal epidural abscess. *Scand J Infect Dis* 1988;20:323-327.
8. Nussbaum ES, Rigamonti D, Standiford H, et al. Spinal epidural abscess: A report of 40 cases and review. *Surg Neurol* 1992;38:225-231.
9. Danner RL, Hartman BJ. Update on spinal epidural abscess: 35 cases and review of the literature. *Rev Infect Dis* 1987;9: 265-274.
10. Hancock DO. A study of 49 patients with acute spinal extradural abscess. *Paraplegia* 1973;10:285-288.
11. Baker AS, Ojemann RG, Swartz MN, et al. Spinal epidural abscess. *N Engl J Med* 1975;293:463-468.
12. Martin RJ, Yuan HA. Neurosurgical care of spinal epidural, subdural, and intramedullary abscess and arachnoiditis. *Orthop Clin North Am* 1996;27:125-136.
13. Rigamonti D, Liem L, Sampath P, et al. Spinal epidural abscess: Contemporary trends in etiology, evaluation, and management. *Surg Neurol* 1999;52:189-197.
14. Wheeler D, Keiser P, Rigamonti D, et al. Medical management of spinal epidural abscess: Case report and review. *Clin Infect Dis* 1992;15:22-27.
15. Spinal Infections. In: Grossman RG, Loftus CM, eds. *Principles of Neurosurgery*. 2nd ed. Philadelphia: Lippincott-Raven; 1999:619-626.
16. Russell NA, Vaughan R, Morley TP. Spinal epidural infection. *Can J Neurol Sci* 1979;6:325-328.
17. Feldenzer JA, McKeeven PE, Schaberg DR, et al. Experimental spinal epidural abscess: A pathophysiological model in the rabbit. *Neurosurgery* 1987;20:859-867.
18. Feldenzen JA, McKeever PE, Schaberg DR, et al. The pathogenesis of spinal epidural abscess: microangiographic studies in an experimental model. *J Neurosurg* 1988;69: 110-114.
19. Heusner AP. Nontuberculosis spinal epidural infection. *N Engl J Med* 1948;239:845.
20. DeGirocami U, Zivin JA. Neuropathology of experimental cord ischemia in the rabbit. *J Neuropathol Exp Neurol* 1982; 41:129-149.
21. Rea GL, McGregor JM, Miller CA, et al. Surgical treatment of the spontaneous spinal epidural abscess. *Surg Neurol* 1992;37: 274-279.
22. Redekop GJ, Del Maestro RF. Diagnosis and management of spinal epidural abscess. *Can J Neurol Sci* 1992;19:180-187.
23. Sapico FL. Pyogenic hematogenous spinal infections. *Infect Dis Clin Pract* 1999;8:267-269.
24. Prendergast H, Jerrard D, O'Conner J. Atypical presentations of epidural abscesses in intravenous drug abusers. *Am J Emerg Med* 1997;15:158-160.
25. Osenbach RK, Hitchon PW, Menezes AH. Diagnosis and management of pyogenic vertebral osteomyelitis in adults. *Surg Neurol* 1990;33:266-275.
26. Fischer EG, Greene CS Jr, Winston KR. Spinal epidural abscess in children. *Neurosurgery* 1981;9:257-260.
27. Ravicovitch MA, Spaccone A. Spinal epidural abscess: Surgical and parasurgical management. *Eur Neurol* 1982;21: 347-357.
28. Ericsson M, Algers G, Schliamser SE. Spinal epidural abscesses in adults: Review and report of iatrogenic cases. *Scand J Infect Dis* 1990;22:249-257.
29. Maslen DR, Jones SR, Crislip MA, et al. Spinal epidural abscess: Optimizing patient care. *Arch Intern Med* 1993;153: 1713-1721.
30. Lange M, Tiecks F, Schielke E, et al. Diagnosis and results of different treatment regimens in patients with spinal abscesses. *Acta Neurochir (Wien)* 1993;125:105-114.
31. McGee-Collett M, Johnston IH. Spinal epidural abscess: presentation and treatment: a report of 21 cases. *Med J Aust* 1991;155:14-17.
32. Liveson JA, Zimmer AE. A localizing symptom in thoracic myelopathy: A variation of Lhermitte's sign. *Ann Intern Med* 1972;76:769-771.
33. Verner EF, Musher DM. Spinal epidural abscess. *Med Clin North Am* 1985;69:375-384.
34. Jeffrey RB, Callen PW, Federle MP. Computed tomography of psoas abscess. *J Comput Assist Tomogr* 1980;4:639-641.
35. Peterson JA, Paris P, Williams AC. Acute epidural abscess. *Am J Emerg Med* 1987;5:287-290.
36. Schlossberg D, Shulman JA. Spinal epidural abscess. *South Med J* 1977;70:669-673.
37. Flynn MW, Felson B. The roentgen manifestations of thoracic actinomycosis. Am J Roentgenol Radium *Ther Nucl Med* 1970;110:707-716.
38. Fraser RA, Ratzan K, Wolpert SM, et al. Spinal subdural empyema. *Arch Neurol* 1973;28:235-238.
39. Altrochhi PH. Acute transverse myelopathy. *Arch Neurol* 1963;9:111-119.
40. Lipton HL, Teasdall RD. Acute transverse myelopathy in adults: A follow-up study. *Arch Neurol* 1973;28:252-257.
41. Markham JW, Lynge HN, Stahlman GEB. The syndrome of spontaneous spinal epidural hematoma: Report of three cases. *J Neurosurg* 1967;26:334-342.
42. Herrick MK, Mills PE Jr. Infarction of spinal cord: Two cases of selective gray matter involvement secondary to asymptomatic aortic disease. *Arch Neurol* 1971;24:228-241.
43. Mullins GM, Flynn TPG, el-Mahdi AM, et al. Malignant lymphoma of the spinal epidural space. *Ann Intern Med* 1971;74:416-423.
44. Mahendru V, Bacon DR, Lema MJ. Multiple epidural abscesses and spinal anesthesia in a diabetic patient: Case report. *Reg Anesth* 1994;19:66-68.
45. Kokes F, Iplikcioglu AC, Camurdanoglu M, et al. Epidural spinal abscess containing gas: MRI demonstration. *Neuroradiol* 1993;35:497-498.
46. Angtuaco EJ, McConnell JR, Chadduck WM, et al. MR imaging of spinal epidural sepsis. AJR *Am J Roentgenol* 1987;149:1249-1253.
47. Leys D, Lesoin F, Viaud C, et al. Decreased morbidity from

acute bacterial spinal epidural abscesses using computed tomography and nonsurgical treatment in selected patients. *Ann Neurol* 1985;17:350-355.

48. Smith AS, Blaser SI. Infectious and inflammatory processes of the spine. *Radiology Clin North Am* 1991;29:809-827.
49. Erntell M, Holtas S, Norlin K, et al. Magnetic resonance imaging in the diagnosis of spinal epidural abscess. *Scand J Infect Dis* 1988;20:323-327.
50. Post MJ, Quencer RM, Montalvo BM, et al. Spinal infection: Evaluation with MR imaging and intraoperative US. *Radiology* 1988;169:765-771.
51. Lobosky JM, Hitchon PW, McDonnell DE. Transthoracic anterolateral decompression for thoracic spinal lesions. *Neurosurgery* 1984;14:26-30.
52. Bouchez B, Arnott G, Delfosse JM. Acute spinal epidural abscess. *J Neurol* 1985;231:343-344.
53. Messer HD, Lenchner GS, Brust JCM, Resor S. Lumbar spinal abscess managed conservatively: case report. *J Neurosurg* 1977;46:825-829.
54. Wheeler D, Keiser P, Rigamonti D, Keay S. Medical management of spinal epidural abscesses: Case report and review. *Clin Infect Dis* 1992;15:22-27.
55. Krauss WE, McCormick PC. Infections of the dural spaces. *Neurosurg Clin North Am* 1992;3:421-433.
56. Yazawa S, Ohi T, Sugimoto S, et al. Cervical spinal epidural abscess following acupuncture: successful treatment with antibiotics. *Intern Med* 1998;37:161-165.
57. Chowfin A, Pitti A, Paul A, et al. Spinal epidural abscess after tattooing. *Clin Infect Dis* 1999;29:225-226.

Seizures: Classification and Diagnosis

Charles M. Seamens, MD
Carey M. Slovis, MD, FACP, FACEP

Seizures: So many diagnostic and therapeutic opportunities to seize, and yet so little time to seize them. When it comes to patients with acute convulsive disorders, experienced physicians appreciate that the risks are formidable, misdiagnosis is common, there is little margin for error, and pharmacotherapeutic intervention can be either life-saving or life-threatening: put simply, a formula for disaster. In fact, few life-compromising encounters challenge the talents and skills of emergency physicians more than patients with generalized, tonic-clonic seizures.

With its vast, complex, and pitfall-peppered clinical spectrum, this potentially devastating condition puts emergency physicians on notice. Unfortunately, seizures have the potential to wreak havoc on every organ system—respiratory arrest, orthopedic injuries, rhabdomyolysis, and reversible metabolic acidosis are just a few of the well-known complications—and, consequently, a broad range of anatomic, pharmacologic, and metabolic investigations must be performed simultaneously.

From the perspective of emergency medicine, the approach to individuals with new-onset seizures, status epilepticus, drug-induced convulsions, and/or febrile seizures requires a unique mix of street-smarts, team coordination, and clinical sophistication. And the clock is always ticking. More often than not, managing patients with acute status seizures requires stabilization techniques that must be performed within parsimonious, heat-of-battle response times, targeted laboratory and radiographic evaluations, and pharmacotherapeutic virtuosity. Moreover, because etiologies for both focal and generalized tonic-clonic seizures range in spectrum from long-festering malignancies and idiopathic causes to drug-related toxicity and hemorrhagic intracranial catastrophes, diagnostic evaluation must be swift, systematic, and appropriately sequenced.

With these concerns in clear focus, this chapter presents a comprehensive, clinically useful review of seizure categories, strategies, and indications for diagnostic evaluations.

Classification

Accurate classification of acute seizures is a prerequisite to appropriate management in the emergency department (ED). As a rule, seizures are classified into two broad categories: generalized and partial (focal) seizures. Generalized seizures are further subclassified according to the presence or absence of various patterns of convulsive movements (e.g., tonic, tonic-clonic, atonic, myoclonic).[1] Partial seizures are subclassified according to whether consciousness is maintained (simple partial seizures) or impaired (complex partial seizures, formerly imprecisely labeled temporal lobe or psychomotor seizures). Most adults with generalized tonic-clonic ("grand mal") seizures have partial seizures that have secondarily generalized. In addition, some patients may experience

Table 1. Determining the Cause of Status Seizures

Test	Causes
VITAL SIGN ABNORMALITIES	
Test	**Causes**
Blood pressure	Shock, hypertensive encephalopathy
Pulse, ECG	Bradycardia, tachycardia
Respiration	Hypoventilation-induced hypoxia
Temperature	Febrile seizure, meningitis
TOXIC-METABOLIC ABNORMALITIES	
Test	**Causes**
SMA-18	
Glucose	Hypoglycemia, hyperglycemia
Sodium	Hyponatremia
Bicarbonate	Profound acidosis
BUN/Creatinine	Renal failure
Calcium	Hypocalcemia
Arterial blood gases	Hypoxia
	Profound acidosis
	Carbon monoxide
Medical history	Aspirin
Drug history	Cocaine
Toxicologic testing	Cyclic antidepressants
	INH
	Lidocaine
	Theophylline
	Strychnine
ETOH level	Alcohol withdrawal
STRUCTURAL ABNORMALITIES	
Test	**Causes**
CT scan	Tumor, trauma, intracranial hemorrhage
EEG	Focal lesion
Lumbar puncture	CNS hemorrhage, abscess
INFECTION	
Test	**Causes**
CBC	Sepsis
Urinalysis	Sepsis
Lumbar puncture	Meningitis
Blood cultures	Sepsis, endocarditis
IDIOPATHIC EPILEPSY	
Test	**Causes**
Medical history	Medical noncompliance
Antiseizure medication levels	Medical noncompliance
EEG	Seizure focus

more than one type of seizure. Generally speaking, choice of antiepileptic drug (AED) therapy will depend on seizure type.

Etiologies

Potential causes of seizures may be grouped into five categories: 1) seizures associated with vital sign abnormalities; 2) toxic or metabolic causes; 3) structural cerebral disease; 4) infectious etiologies; and 5) idiopathic epilepsy. *(Please see Table 1.)* Febrile seizures are the most common variety of convulsions caused by vital sign abnormalities, while alcohol withdrawal, cocaine and other illicit drug intoxication, hypoglycemia, hypoxia, and hyponatremia are the most common causes of seizures associated with toxic or metabolic insults.[2-6]

Structural etiologies of seizures include primary and metastatic tumor and cerebrovascular disease, with studies demonstrating that brain tumors are present in 1-5% of patients who present with their first seizure.[7] Seizures, although rare during the acute phase of thrombotic cerebral infarction, are most likely to develop in the setting of embolic infarction with hemorrhage.[8] Seizures due to intracranial infection also are unusual, although meningitis, brain abscess, and encephalitis have been reported to produce convulsions.[8]

New-Onset Seizures: Clinical Acumen Required

Because any transient alteration in consciousness may be mistaken for an epileptic seizure, obtaining a clear history from witnesses is perhaps the most critical step in confirming the diagnosis of a seizure disorder. Disorders that may mimic seizures include hyperventilation, breath-holding spells in children, migraines, transient global amnesia, cerebral vascular disease (such as transient ischemic attacks and vertebrobasilar insufficiency), narcolepsy, some movement disorders (e.g., parosysmal choreoathetosis, tic disorders), and psychogenic seizures.[6]

Syncope vs. Seizure. A syncopal event caused by reversible cerebral anoxia may be difficult to distinguish from a seizure disorder. Of 946 patients referred because of episodic attacks of unconsciousness, epilepsy was diagnosed in 377 and syncope in 417: In both seizures and syncope, there is transient neurologic alteration, but syncope also involves a loss of muscle tone. In addition, vasovagal syncope may be associated with distinct symptoms prior to the event, including nausea, malaise, light-headedness, diaphoresis, and palpitations. Recovery is usually quick and complete in a vaso-vagal syncopal episode, there is usually no postictal period, and injury is uncommon.[9]

Unfortunately, even after interviewing witnesses, it may still be difficult to distinguish syncope from seizures. Postictal serum creatinine kinase (CK) has been used as a nonspecific indicator of recent generalized tonic-clonic seizure.[10] Practically speaking, elevated CK levels have only moderate sensitivity, but this may be improved if measured more than three hours after the event.[11]

Mild tonic-clonic and partial absence, or psychogenic seizures, can produce minor elevations in total CK. Importantly, false-positive elevations of this enzyme (i.e., false-positive for seizures) also may occur in the setting of unrecognized myocardial infarctions and unrelated trauma.[10]

Pseudoseizures. Psychogenic or pseudoseizures are probably more prevalent than once thought, and distinguishing between this clinical entity and neurogenic seizures may be problematic. Often confounding the diagnosis is the occurrence of psychogenic and true seizures in the same patient.[12] The incidence of psychogenic seizures appears to decrease after the age of 35 years and is rare after age 50.[13] From a differential diagnosis perspective, patients with true neurogenic seizures tend to have a single seizure pattern, whereas psychogenic seizure patients frequently have multiple patterns.[13] Moreover, psychogenic seizures usually are not followed by a postictal period; the event is often recollected by the patient. In contrast, individuals who have a neurogenic generalized seizure usually have a postictal period and cannot recall the ictal event.

Some experts have suggested that out-of-phase limb movements, forward pelvic thrusting, and side-to-side head movements are more common with psychogenic seizures,[14] although others have not been able to confirm these patterns.[15] Whereas most tonic-clonic seizures are less than 60 seconds in duration, psychogenic seizures may last considerably longer.[13] Finally, it should be stressed that urinary incontinence and injury have been described in as many as 20% of patients with pseudoseizures.[13]

Provocative Maneuvers and Evaluation. Several maneuvers can be used to help distinguish between psychogenic and neurogenic seizures. Non-noxious stimuli, such as tickling the nose, passive eye opening, geotropic eye testing, dropping the patient's arm over his or her face, or corneal stimulation, may elicit a response from those suffering a psychogenic seizure.[13] In addition, noxious stimuli, such as applying an ammonia capsule under the nose, have also been effective. Patients with psychogenic seizures are particularly susceptible to verbal suggestion, which may be used to both induce and terminate these episodes.[13]

Arterial blood gas (ABG) analysis, serum prolactin levels, and video EEG monitoring help distinguish true seizures from psychogenic seizures. Blood gas analysis has been shown to be useful in identifying patients with true neurogenic, tonic-clonic seizures, since this patient subgroup usually has some degree of reversible metabolic acidosis following the ictal event.[13,16,17] Although serum prolactin levels are increased consistently in generalized tonic-clonic seizures, these elevations are not observed in complex partial, absent, or pseudoseizures.[13]

Breath-holding Spells. Breath-holding spells occur in children 6-18 months of age, resolve with age, and, in some cases, can be confused with seizures.[9] These episodes begin with crying. usually in response to pain, anger, or frustration. The child then holds his or her breath in expiration and becomes pale or cyanotic. If the breath-holding is prolonged, the child may lose consciousness, stiffen, and, in unusual cases, exhibit clonic movements and experience urinary incontinence. Breath-holding spells overlap clinically with reflexic anoxic seizures.[9]

Seizures in Patients with an Established History of Epilepsy

Assessment of patients with an established seizure disorder differs only slightly from evaluation of the patient with new-onset seizures. Initially, all vital sign abnormalities should be investigated and addressed promptly. For stable patients, the history should focus on any provoking factors, such as medication usage, noncompliance with anti-epileptic medication, recreational drug use, and alcohol ingestion. Signs or symptoms of recent head trauma, symptoms of CNS infection, fever, or recent sleep deprivation should be sought. The type of seizure the patient has experienced in the past and seizure frequency should be noted.

For instance, the patient who has been seizure-free for three years but who now presents with several seizures over the past week is more worrisome and requires a more extensive evaluation than the patient who normally has a seizure every few months. The emergency physician should also inquire about the patient's past and current AED regimen, dosages, compliance patterns, recent AED serum levels, and whether or not there have been any recent additions, substitutions, or alterations in the therapeutic program.

Physical Examination. Physical examination should consist of a brief, but focused, neurologic exam and an evaluation to exclude seizure-related orthopedic injuries. It should be stressed that any deviation from the patient's *baseline* neurologic exam should prompt further evaluation with imaging studies.

Routine measurement of electrolytes in patients with a known seizure disorder is not generally required unless there is a specific clinical indication. Anticonvulsant drug levels, however, should routinely be performed.[3] In one study in which seizure patients had electrolytes and AED levels measured, 96 patients had subtherapeutic AED levels, two had hypoglycemia, and one was found to be hyperglycemic.[18] Sub-therapeutic levels of AED may be the consequence of poor patient compliance or may reflect increased clearance of AED associated with concurrent medication intake, producing accelerated drug metabolism.

Status Epilepticus

Status epilepticus is defined as more than 30 minutes of continuous seizure activity or two or more sequential seizures without full recovery of consciousness between seizures. It may take several forms, including: 1) repeated generalized convulsive seizures with persistent postictal depression of neurological function between seizures; 2) nonconvulsive seizures that produce a continuous fluctuating "epileptic twilight" state characterized by non-responsiveness; and 3) repeated partial seizures.[19]

One thing is clear: *Status epilepticus requires prompt recognition and treatment.* A landmark article on this condition recommends that seizures be terminated within 60 minutes of onset in order to prevent permanent sequelae and death.[20] These guidelines were based on a review of a study in which the median seizure duration was 13 hours in patients who died, 10 hours in those who developed permanent sequelae, and 1.5 hours in those who escaped both. Similarly, many animal studies confirm that permanent brain damage and death may be expected after 1-2 hours of contInuous seizure activity.[21-24]

Febrile Seizures

Febrile seizures (FSs) are the most common type of seizure in childhood, occur in 2-4% of all children, and account for 30% of all childhood seizures.[25-30] As a rule, they occur in children between the ages of 6 months and 5 years.[31] About 85% of FSs are generalized, and the remainder are focal.[32] Most FSs are brief, and only 8% last longer than 15 minutes.[25] Approximately 4% of FSs progress to status epilepticus.[26]

Clinical Features. FSs usually occur during the initial 24 hours of fever activity, and most investigations have concluded there is a correlation between the degree of temperature elevation and the incidence of FS.[33] This makes antipyretic prophylaxis difficult, because by the time a febrile illness has been identified, seizures may have already occurred. Most children have a temperature of 39°C (102.2°F) or greater at the time of their FS[27] although some children may seize at lower temperatures, ranging from 37.7-38.3°C (100-101°F). Children who seize at lower temperatures seem to have higher rates of recurrence.[34] It is interesting to note that, although firmly entrenched in pediatric teaching, there is still no good evidence that FSs are caused by a precipitous rise in body temperature.[33]

Only 25-30% of children who have a single FS will have another, whereas about half of those who have two FSs will have a third occurrence,[28] with most recurrences taking place within 6-12 months of the initial seizure.[28]

Classification. It is important to distinguish simple FS from complex FS, as it will affect the initial evaluation and helps to predict recurrence. Complex FS is defined as a seizure longer than 15 minutes, more than one FS within a 24-hour period, or seizures with focal features.[25,26] Certain historical features may help to predict recurrences of FSs. The younger the child during the first temperature-related-convulsion, the more likely that further FSs will be encountered. A family history of seizures also increases the likelihood of recurrent FSs,[35] whereas the presence of complex FS or abnormal psychomotor development has yielded conflicting results regarding recurrence.[30,34] Of interest, attendance in day-care increased the risk of initial FS.[29] Finally, a FS itself increases the risk of subsequent FSs.[26]

Evaluation of FS. When caring for a child with a FS, the emergency physician must squarely address the following two issues: 1) What is the cause of fever?; and 2) Does the child have meningitis? To address these issues, many experts have debated the need to perform a lumbar puncture (LP). Unfortunately, there is no consensus on clinical indications for performing this procedure in children with a first-time seizure associated with a febrile illness.[35-37] Some authors advocate an LP after all initial FSs, whereas others qualify this approach for children under the age of 18 months.[35,36] Without question, an LP is indicated in any child with petechiae, nuchal rigidity, coma, persistent drowsiness, continued seizures, paresis, or paralysis.[36] Moreover, it is unusual for a child with bacterial meningitis to present with only a seizure and no other associated symptomatology.

Clearly, children who are postictal, lethargic, or irritable are difficult to assess clinically. On the other hand, wasting precious time in order to permit a child to "wake up" for the purpose of additional assessment can potentially delay diagnosis and antibiotic therapy. Consequently, an immediate LP is mandatory in this situation.[35] In contrast, a child who has had a seizure prior to ED presentation and is smiling, happy, playful, and without other signs or symptoms of meningitis probably does not require an LP. This general rule, however, does not apply to a child with a FS who has been taking antibiotics. These patients should undergo an LP to exclude partially treated meningitis. Finally, there is also no universal consensus on initiating antiseizure prophylaxis after a FS.[28,30]

Prophylaxis. The child who has had a single complex FS or recurrent FS has an increased risk of developing epilepsy, but there is no evidence that prophylaxis against FSs prevents subsequent development of a convulsive disorder later in life. In addition, continuous anticonvulsant prophylaxis with phenobarbital should not be routinely recommended as it may affect higher cortical functions on a long-term basis.[37] Sodium valproate also has been used as prophylaxis and is generally a safe medication, although it has been reported to cause fatal liver failure. Intermittent prophylaxis with diazepam is probably just as effective as continuous prophylaxis with phenobarbital or valproate.[38,39] The best treatment is probably reassuring the child's parents that consequences of another FS are minimal.

For patients with recurrent FS, episodic therapy is probably better than continued use of an AED. A rectal diazepam solution at a dose of 0.5 mg/kg may be prescribed in cases in which the parents strongly desire the ability to treat their child's condition, for patients who tend to have prolonged seizures, or for those children who live a considerable distance from medical facilities. Parents should be counseled on the side effects of diazepam and the appearance of generalized seizures vs. paroxysmal non-epileptic events, such as chills associated fever, breath-holding spells, or myoclonic jerks during sleep.

Post-Traumatic Seizures

Within the first year after head trauma, the probability of experiencing post-traumatic seizures is more than 12 times the general population's risk for developing a seizure disorder.[40] The latency period between head injury and the development of epilepsy varies, although one study demonstrates that 57% of patients will have onset within one year of injury.[40] Post-traumatic epilepsy may present as immediate seizures, early post-traumatic seizure, and late post-traumatic seizures. Immediate seizures occur within the first 24 hours after trauma. They may cause hypoxia, acidosis, hypertension, and increased intracranial pressure in an acutely injured patient.[41] Immediate seizures, which make up 50-80% of early post-traumatic seizures, are particularly frequent among children with severe: head injuries.

Early post-traumatic seizures refer to those that occur within the first week after head injury. The incidence of early seizures is approximately 5% among patients with a closed head injury and is higher in young children.[42] They are occasionally observed in children with mild head injury but are rare among adults with mild head injury.[42] Late post-traumatic seizures occur beyond the first week following a traumatic episode. The overall incidence of late post-traumatic seizures in hospitalized patients following closed head injury is approximately 4-7%.[41] Late seizures are observed less frequently in children.[41] Long-term prophylaxis of late post-traumatic seizures with phenytoin is generally ineffective. There is, however, convincing evidence for the effectiveness of phenytoin in preventing immediate and early post-traumatic seizures during the first week after a serious head injury.[42]

Alcohol Withdrawal Seizures

Alcohol withdrawal seizures (AWSs), which usually occur 24-48 hours after discontinuation of alcohol in patients who abuse alcohol,[43,44] are one of the most common causes of seizures in adults. The classic syndrome of AWSs most often occurs in men during their fifth

Table 2. The Alcoholic 'Cocktail'

1. 5% dextrose in normal saline (D_5NSS)
2. Multivitamin solution
3. Folate 1-5 mg
4. $MgSO_4$ 5 g
5. KCl 40 meq, if indicated

Administer thiamine 100 mg IV to all alcoholics with seizures or those receiving glucose.

or sixth decade. Patients typically have a long history of alcohol abuse and have recently stopped their alcohol intake.[43] AWS is more common in binge drinkers, and the average duration of the binge prior to seizure activity is approximately two weeks. The majority of patients experience either one or two tonic-clonic seizures, and a small percentage have more than six.[45,46] The entire seizure period usually lasts six hours or less, although, infrequently, seizures may continue for up to 12 hours.[47] A single episode of AWS is associated with an increased risk of future episodes of AWS.[47]

General Principles. Initially, patients with new-onset AWSs are treated as any other patient with a first-time seizure. Care must be taken not to allow a belligerent intoxicated person to obstruct a thorough evaluation. History is essential in the initial work-up, and attempts should be made to ascertain whether the patient has a prior history of AWS, idiopathic, or post-traumatic epilepsy. Specific questions on use and compliance with anticonvulsant drugs as well as speaking with witnesses to the events surrounding the seizure is essential. Finally, it should be noted that AWS rarely progresses to status epilepticus, although status seizures occur in approximately 3% of cases of AWS.[48] Accordingly, status seizures mandate a complete evaluation for other potential causes.

Initial Assessment. The patient with an AWS should have an immediate bedside glucose determination, and blood should be sent for electrolytes and AED levels.[5] Alcohol inhibits gluconeogenesis and can lead to hypoglycemia by depletion of liver glycogen. In addition, alcoholism is a common cause of hypo-magnesemia, which increases the likelihood of tremor, confusion, hallucinations, and seizures.[5,47] An elevated anion or "wide-gap" metabolic acidosis may occur secondary to seizure-induced lactic acidosis, alcoholic ketoacidosis, or another toxic ingestion.[5] Toxicologic screening is required if there is a suspicion of concomitant illicit drug use.

Laboratory Evaluation. Although there is some controversy regarding the need to perform a head CT scan in alcoholics with a first-time AWS and a normal neurologic examination,[49,50] a head CT scan appears to be an appropriate, prudent procedure in these high-risk patients because heavy alcohol abusers have an increased incidence of brain infarction, hemorrhagic stroke, and subarachnoid hemorrhage, as well as head trauma.[47] In one study of 268 patients with presumed AWS and no suspicion of a traumatic. structural, or toxic metabolic cause, 6.2% of patients had a mass lesion.[46] An EEG may be scheduled as an outpatient but is not essential as the majority of AWS patients will have nondiagnostic EEGs.[51,52]

Alcoholics with new-onset seizures should be evaluated with CBC, electrolytes, blood urea nitrogen (BUN), creatinine, and head CT scan. Because a single magnesium level is unreliable in malnourished and dehydrated patients. we do not routinely recommend serum magnesium levels in all alcoholics with first-time seizures. However. when specific signs or symptoms suggest the possibility of magnesium insufficiency, a level should be obtained. Patients should be observed in the ED for six hours following the seizure. Stable patients may be discharged to a detoxification unit or into the care of individuals who can assist the patient during detoxification.

If the patient has new-onset partial or focal seizures, an urgent head CT scan is indicated to rule out structural lesions. If partial seizures have been documented in the past and the patient has returned to his or her neurological baseline, the patient may also be observed and discharged to a detoxification center if possible.

Management. Treatment of the stable alcoholic patient should include: I) IV fluids containing 50/c dextrose; 2) thiamine 100 mg IV; 3) multivitamins; 4) magnesium and potassium; and 5) a benzodiazepine. *(Please see Table 2.)*

The goals of treatment are to relieve symptoms and to prevent progression to later stages of alcohol withdrawal. This is generally accomplished by replacing alcohol with a pharmacologically similar medication that is then slowly withdrawn over time. Benzodiazepines are presently the mainstay of treatment because they are cross-tolerant with alcohol and reduce symptoms of alcohol withdrawal. They have minimal respiratory depressive effects and have excellent anticonvulsant properties. Numerous benzodiazepines have been studied. and no one is clearly superior.[53] Triazolam, however, should never be used because of its short half-life and capacity for inducing coma.[53]

An initial test dose of lorazepam (1-2 mg), diazepam (5-10 mg), chlordiazepoxide (50-100 mg) can be given orally in the ED. The patient may be discharged with a tapering dosage over 3-6 days if any of these oral benzodiazepines is effective in abating the patient's symptoms over a few hours. If the test dose is insufficient, additional doses should be administered and the tapering regimen started at a higher dose.[46] Highly agitated patients should receive their initial doses intravenously until they are calm.

Selected Drug-Induced Seizures

Cocaine. It is now estimated that 5-10 million Americans use cocaine regularly and that approximately 15% will suffer at least one seizure.[54,55] The development of status seizures is one of the major determinants of mortality in cocaine intoxication.[54-56]

Seizures caused by cocaine are due in part to a hypersympathetic state and are often associated with hyperthermia and high lactate levels.[56,57] They are usually self-limiting, but in cases of status epilepticus, they should be treated with high doses of a benzodiazepine in conjunction with a beta-blocker.[58] These seizures may require extremely high doses of diazepam or lorazepam (e.g., in excess of the usual maximum doses of 20 mg and 8 mg, respectively). Thiopental should be used in refractory cases.

Cyclic Antidepressants. Seizures from cyclic antidepressant overdose result from the drug's central anticholinergic effects and are especially likely to occur with the newer agents amoxapine and maprotiline.[58-63]

Seizure management in cyclic antidepressant overdose begins with securing the patient's ABCs and alkalinizing the patient to a pH of 7.5-7.55 to counteract the drug's sodium-blocking toxic effects.[59,60] Alkalinization with 2-3 ampules of sodium bicarbonate increases the drug's protein binding and probably decreases the free (or active) form of the drug available in the CNS. During the bicarbonate infusion, aggressively administer up to 20 mg of diazepam and follow with thiopental if the diazepam is ineffective. Phenytoin's efficacy in seizure control or prophylaxis for cyclic antidepressant overdose is unproven,[60,63] and the drug should not be used in unstable patients. Physostigmine has no role in seizure management.[63]

Isoniazid (INH). INH-induced seizures are associated with a high mortality rate.[64] Seizures typically occur within 30-120 minutes of an acute overdose[65] and are due to the INH's inability to form a complex with vitamin B6 (pyridoxine), resulting in the brain's depletion of the CNS inhibitory neurotransmitter GABA.[14,63,64] When seizures develop, they are usually refractory to standard antiseizure medications.[64,65]

Treat these patients with IV pyridoxine on a mg by mg basis according to the amount of INH ingested. If that amount is unknown, administer 5 g of pyridoxine in a 50 cc solution over three minutes[66] and give diazepam or lorazepam concurrently. Do not use phenytoin. If not enough pyridoxine is available, deep thiopental coma is an alternative.

Theophylline. Theophylline-induced seizures are often intractable and are associated with a mortality rate of 20-50%.[67,68] The mechanism by which theophylline causes seizures remains unclear but appears to be related to a hyper-sympathetic state in association with high CNS levels of cyclic AMP and cyclic GMP.[68,69] Chronic theophylline intoxication carries a greater risk of seizures than acute intoxication. Thus, acute overdoses rarely lead to seizures unless theophylline levels exceed 100 mg/L (550 mmol/L). In contrast. chronically intoxicated patients may seize with levels below 60 mg/L (330 mmol/L).[68]

No established treatment protocol exists for status seizures in theophylline overdose.[67-70] Most series have reported using multiple drugs in an attempt to control the seizures.[65-68] Diazepam, in conjunction with other drugs, is generally considered effective, whereas phenytoin, especially when used alone, is not.[67-70]

Because theophylline-induced seizures are associated with such a high mortality and usually occur in patients with underlying pulmonary disease, they mandate aggressive treatment and early airway control. Begin with rapid benzodiazepine titration and proceed with thiopental loading and IV infusion. Once the seizure is controlled, consider the use of charcoal hemoperfusion to eliminate the toxic levels of theophylline.[71-73]

Summary

It is not surprising that seizures are commonly encountered in the emergency setting, inasmuch as one out of every 11 Americans who lives to be 80 years old will have at least one seizure during their lifetime. As expected, the most likely cause of acute status seizures varies according to patient age. For example, febrile seizures represent the most common etiology for convulsive disorders in young children between 6 months and 5 years of age. On the other hand, idiopathic epilepsy, as well as illicit drug use, are likely etiologies in adolescence and young adulthood, whereas alcohol withdrawal seizures and sequelae associated with cerebrovascular disease are the most precipitating factors in adults greater than 60 years of age. Finally, malignancy should always be considered a cause of seizures, especially in the elderly.

References

1. Locharemkul C, Primrose D, Pilcher WH, et al. Update in epilepsy. *NYS J Med* 1992;92:14-17.
2. Earnest MP. Seizures. *Neural Clin* 1993;11:563-572.
3. Eisner RF, Tumbull TN, Howes DS, et al. Efficacy of a "standard" seizure workup in the emergency department. *Ann Emerg Med* 1986;15:33-39.
4. Tumbull TL, Vanden Hook TN, Howes DS, et al. Utility of laboratory studies in the emergency department patient with a new-onset seizure. *Ann Emerg Med* 1990;19:373-376.
5. Powers RD. Serum chemistry abnormalities in adult patients with seizures. *Ann Emerg Med* 1985;14:416-420.
6. Alldredge BK. Seizures associated with recreational drug abuse. *Neurology* 1989;39:1037-1039.
7. Rosenthal RH, Heim ML, Waeckerle JF. First-time major motor seizures in an emergency department. *Ann Emerg Med* 1980;9:242-245.
8. Slovis C. ED management of unstable patients with status seizure. *Emerg Med Rep* 1989;10:65-72.
9. Morrell MJ. Differential diagnosis of seizures. *Neurol Clin* 1993;11:737-753.
10. Libman MD, Potvin L, Coupal L, et al. Seizure vs. syncope: Measuring serum creatinine kinase in the emergency department. *J Gen Intern Med* 1991;6:408-412.
11. Wyllie E, Lueders H, Pippenger C, et al. Postictal serum creatinine kinase in the diagnosis of seizure disorders. *Arch Neurol* 1985;42:123-126.
12. Primrose D, Locharemkul C, Pilcher WH, et al. Part II: Special considerations in the treatment of epilepsy. *NYS J Med* 1992:53-56.
13. Jagoda A, Riggio S. Psychogenic convulsive seizures. *Am J Emerg Med* 1993;11:626-631.
14. Gates J, Ramani V, Whalen S, et al. Ictal characteristics of pseudoseizures. *Arch Neurol* 1985;42:1183-1187.
15. Leis AA, Ross MA, Summers AK. Psychogenic seizures: Ictal characteristics and diagnostic pitfalls. *Neurology* 1992;42:95-99.
16. Orringer C, Eustace J, Christian D, et al. Natural history of lactic acidosis after grand mal seizures. *N Engl J Med* 1977;297:796-799.
17. Simon R. Physiologic consequences of status epilepticus. *Epilepsia* 1985;26:S66-S85.
18. Rothstein E. Prevention of alcohol withdrawal seizures. The roles of phenytoin and chlordiazepoxide. *Am J Psych* 1973; 1301:381-382.
19. Working Group on Status Epilepticus. Treatment of convulsive status epilepticus. *JAMA* 1993;270:854-859.
20. Delgado-Escueta AV, Wasterlain C, Treiman OM, et al. Current concepts in neurology-Management of status epilepticus. *N Engl J Med* 1982;306:1337-1340.
21. Wasterlain CG. Mortality and morbidity from serial seizures. *Epilepsia* 1974;15:155.
22. Meldrum BS. Horton RW. Physiology of status epileptic us in primates. *Arch Neurol* 1973;28:1.
23. Meldrum BS, Brierley JB. Prolonged epileptic seizures in primates. *Arch Neurol* 1973;28:10.

24. Meldrum BS, Vigouroux RA. Brierley JB. Systemic factors and epileptic brain damage. *Arch Neurol* 1973;29:82.
25. Rosman NP. Febrile seizure. *Emerg Med Clin North Am* 1987;5:719-737.
26. Monsen RF, Graham WM, Snell GF, et al. Febrile seizure. *Postgrad Med* 1991;90:217-226.
27. Freeman JM. What have we learned from febrile seizures? *Pediatr Ann* 1992;21:355-361.
28. Bethune P, Gordon K, Dooley J, et al. What child will have a febrile seizure? *Am J Dis Child* 1993;147:35-39.
29. Freeman JM, Vining EPG. Decision making and the child with febrile seizures. *Pediatr Rev* 1992;13:298-304.
30. Leung, AK, Robson WLM. Febrile convulsions. *Postgrad Med* 1991;89:217-224.
31. Berg AT. Are febrile seizures provoked by a rapid rise in temperature? *Am Dis Child* 1993;147:1101-1103.
32. Pellock J. Seizures and epilepsy in infancy and childhood. *Neurol Clin* 1993;11:755-768.
33. Berg AT, Shinnar S, Hauser W A, et al. A prospective study of recurrent febrile seizures. *N Engl J Med* 1992;327: 1122-1127.
34. Berg AT, Shinnar S, Hauser W A, et al. Predictors of recurrent febrile seizures: A meta analytic review. *J Pediatr* 1990;116:329.
35. Offringa M, Derksen-Lubsen G, Beishuizen A, et al. Seizures and fever: Can we rule out meningitis on clinical grounds alone? *Clin Pediatr* 1992:514-522.
36. Green SM, Rothrock SG. Lumbar puncture for febrile seizures: Do we need a "maxim"? *Am J Emerg Med* 1991;9:624.
37. Farwell JR. Phenobarbital for febrile seizures-Effects on intelligence and on seizure recurrence. *N Engl J Med* 1990;322:364.
38. Knudsen FU. Intermittent diazepam prophylaxis in febrile convulsions. *Acta Neurol Scand* 1991;135:1-24.
39. Sopo SM, Pesaresi MA, Celestini E, et al. Short-term prophylaxis of febrile convulsions. *Acta Pediatr Scand* 1991;80:248-249.
40. Willmore LJ. Post-traumatic seizures. *Neurol Clin* 1993;11: 823-831.
41. Yablon SA. Post-traumatic seizures. *Arch Phys Med Rehab* 1993;74:983-997.
42. Temkin NR, Dikmen SS, Wilensky AJ, et al. A randomized, double blind study of phenytoin for the prevention of post-traumatic seizures. *N Engl J Med* 1990;323:497-502.
43. Victor M, Brausch C. The role of abstinence in the genesis of alcoholic epilepsy. *Epilepsia* 1967;8:1-20.
44. Ng S, Hauser WA. Alcohol consumption and withdrawal in new onset seizures. *N Engl J Med* 1988;319:666-673.
45. Sellers EM, Kalant H. Alcohol intoxication and withdrawal. *N Engl J Med* 1976;294:757- 762.
46. Freedland ES, McMicken DB. Alcohol related seizures. Part II: Clinical presentation and management. *J Emerg Med* 1993;11:605-618.
47. Freedland ES, McMicken DB. Alcohol related seizures. Part I: Pathophysiology, differential diagnosis, and evaluation. *J Emerg Med* 1993;11:463-473.
48. Lechtenberg R, Worner TM. Seizure risk with recurrent alcohol detoxification. *Arch Neurol* 1990;47:535-538.
49. Feussner JR, Linfors EW, Blessing CL, et al. Computed tomography brain scanning in alcohol withdrawal seizures valve of the neurologic examination. *Ann Intern Med* 1981; 94:519-522.
50. Earnest MP, et al. Intracranial lesions shown by CT in 159 cases of first alcohol-related seizures. *Neurology* 1988;1561-1565.
51. Romach MK, Sellers EM. Management of the alcohol withdrawal syndrome. *Ann Rev Med* 1991;42:323-340.
52. Thompson WL. Management of alcohol withdrawal syndromes. *Arch Intern Med* 1978;138:278-283.
53. Browne M, Anton RF, Malcolm R, et al. Alcohol detoxification and withdrawal seizures: Clinical support for a kindling hypothesis. *Biol Psychiatry* 1988;23:507-514.
54. Brody SL. Cocaine—Actions, abuse, and emergencies. *Emory Univ J Med* 1988;2:257.
55. Myers JA, Earnest MP. Generalized seizures and cocaine abuse. *Neurology* 1984;34:675.
56. Catravas JD, Waters JW. Acute cocaine intoxication in the conscious dog: Studies on the mechanism of lethality. *J Pharmacol Exp Ther* 1981;217:350.
57. Jonsson S, O'Meara M, Young JB. Acute cocaine poisoning. *Am J Med* 1983;75:1061.
58. Brody S, Slovis CM. Recognition and management of complications related to cocaine abuse. *Emerg Med Rep* 1988;9:41.
59. Callaham M. Tricyclic antidepressant overdose *JACEP* 1979;8:413.
60 Slovis CM. Cyclic antidepressant OD: Five classic patient types. *Emerg Med Rep* 1987;8:113
61. Kulig K, Romack BH, Sullivan JB, et al. Amoxapine overdose—Coma and seizures without cardiotoxic effects. *JAMA* 1982;248:1092.
62. Bernad PG, Levine MS. Maprotiline-induced seizures. *South Med J* 1986;79:1179.
63. Kulig K. Management of poisoning associated with "newer" antidepressant agents. *Ann Emerg Med* 1986;15:1039.
64. Orlowski JP, Paganini EP, Pippenger CE. Treatment of a potentially lethal dose isoniazid ingestion. *Ann Emerg Med* 1988;17:73.
65 Yarbrough BE. Wood JP. Isoniazid overdose treated with high-dose pyridoxine. *Ann Emerg Med* 1983:12:303.
66. Parish RA, Brownstein D. Emergency department management of children with acute isoniazid poisoning *Pediatr Emerg Care* 1986:2;88.
67. Singer EP, Kolischenko A. Seizures due to theophylline overdose. *Chest* 1985;87:755.
68. Paloucek FP, Rodvo!d KA. Evaluation of theophyllic overdose and toxicities. *Ann Emerg Med* 1988;17:135.
69. Nakada T, Kwee IL, Lerner AM, et al. Theophylline-induced seizures: Clinical and pathophysiologic aspects. *West J Med* 1983;371.
70. Olson KR, Benowitz NL, Woo OF, et al. Theophylline overdose: Acute single ingestion versus chronic repeated overmedication. *Am J Emerg Med* 1985;3:386.
71. Greenberg A, Paraino BH, Kroboth PD, et al. Severe theophylline toxicity-Role of conservative measures,

antiarrhythmic agents, and charcoal hemoperfusion. *Am J Med* 1984;76:854.

72. Klein-Schwartz W. Theophylline poisoning. *Am J Emerg Med* 1985;3:475.
73. Jefferys DB, Raper SM, Belliwell M, et al. Haemoperfusion for theophylline overdose. *BMJ* 1980:280:1167.

Seizures: Patient Stabilization and Pharmacologic Interventions

Charles M. Seamens, MD
Carey M. Slovis, MD, FACP, FACEP

The pharmacologic approach for acute seizure management is based on prudent and sequential administration of medications that not only increase seizure threshold, but also have the capacity for producing serious side effects. With patient stabilization and treatment as its primary focus, this chapter presents a comprehensive discussion of anti-epileptic drugs—including route of administration, dosage, monitoring needs, and adverse effects—used to manage acute convulsive episodes, including status epilepticus.

Although drug therapy for acute seizure management once relied almost exclusively on the workhorse benzodiazepine, diazepam, in recent years, another drug in this class, lorazepam, with its longer duration of action and shorter half-life, has emerged as the drug of choice in most patients with generalized seizures. And while many patients are still appropriate candidates for IV phenytoin administration, oral loading with phenytoin has simplified the departmental management of patients who can be safely discharged and who require establishment of therapeutic serum phenytoin levels within several hours following their seizure. In addition, it should be stressed that the pharmacotherapeutic approach to status epilepticus often requires careful titration of three or more classes of antiseizure medications in combination with vigilant support of the respiratory and cardiovascular system.

Finally, comprehensive management of the patient with status seizures requires precise delineation of the underlying pathology responsible for the convulsive episode. To guide physicians toward additional treatment modalities that may be required—for example, antimicrobials for infection, surgery for mass lesions, or metabolic interventions for electrolyte disorders—a framework for radiographic and laboratory evaluation of seizure patients in the emergency setting is fleshed out in detail.

Approach to the Patient

Initial Stabilization. Patients who appear to be having a generalized seizure require prompt intervention, including establishment of an airway, breathing maintenance, and circulation support, if necessary. *(Please see Table 1.)* Once these are secured, a fingerstick glucose analysis should be performed while an IV line is being started. Cachectic, malnourished, and alcoholic patients, as well as patients who are hypoglycemic, should receive 50 cc of $D_{50}W$, if indicated, followed by 100 mg of IV thiamine. Initial stabilization maneuvers should be followed promptly by a thorough neurologic exam, which, unfortunately, is sometimes omitted as a result of the clinician's anxiety, preoccupation, and concern with seizure cessation. If a psychogenic seizure is suspected, provocative avoidance maneuvers described below may be attempted at this time. It should be stressed that delays in distinguishing between these two entities can either result in the inappropriate use of anticonvulsant drugs, or delay psychiatric treatment that may be required for patients with psychogenic seizures.

Table 1. Initial Evaluation of First-Time Seizure Patients

1. Secure ABGs
2. Bedside glucose analysis
3. Oximetry and ECG monitoring
4. Head CT scan*
5. Additional studies (e.g., laboratory studies, EEG) as indicated by physical examination, as well as neurologist or primary care consultants

* Some may prefer MRI based on availability, patient age, history, or other factors.

Laboratory Examination. More often than not, an accurate history will point to an etiologic diagnosis. However, if a thorough history and physical examination fail to reveal a cause for the convulsion, a broad-based laboratory evaluation—which generally includes a CBC, serum electrolytes, a urinalysis, an electrocardiogram, and, when indicated by clinical findings, an arterial blood gas analysis and serum anti-epileptic drug levels—should be considered an integral part of the initial evaluation. Calcium and magnesium measurements are not routinely recommended. They should be considered, however, in profoundly malnourished patients, those on continuous IV feedings, and cancer patients receiving chemotherapeutic agents that are known to cause hypomagnesemia. One retrospective study accurately identified the need for hospital admission in 90 of 91 patients using the database outlined above.[1]

In contrast, other authors have found seizures caused by electrolyte abnormalities to be quite rare.[2-6] Moreover, among seizures associated with electrolyte disturbances, the majority were due to hypoglycemia or hyperglycemia, both of which are easily detected by simple bedside analysis.[3,4] Of 136 patients with new-onset seizures, 11 (8%) had a correctable laboratory abnormality as the cause of the seizure, including four patients with hypoglycemia, four with hyperglycemia, two with hypocalcemia. and one with hypomagnesemia.[3]

Radiographic Modalities. From the standpoint of cost-effective clinical guidelines and outcome analysis, virtually all ED physicians now agree that skull radiographs have no use in the evaluation of patients who present with their first seizure.[7,8] Of 61 patients receiving skull films for evaluation of seizures in one study, only two had an abnormality, neither of which changed management. In contrast, a head CT scan is much more likely to provide useful information and is now considered the imaging study of choice due to its ease, accuracy, and availability.[9,10]

Generally, all new-onset seizure patients, as well as patients with established convulsive disorders with new abnormalities in their neurologic exam, should undergo an imaging study (i.e., a head CT scan). As expected, the incidence of abnormal CT scans increases with age.[9] In patients with normal neurologic exams after a first-time seizure, 15-24% of head CT scans were abnormal. Most abnormalities reflected cerebral atrophy and acute or chronic infarctions.[9,10] As magnetic resonance imaging (MRI) becomes more widely available, it may supplant CT scanning because of its superiority in identifying abnormalities in cortical architecture. In particular, MRI can detect subtle changes, especially in the temporal lobes, which is an important advantage, since abnormalities in this region cause a significant percentage of seizures.[11]

Electroencephalography (EEG). Although some experts support the use of EEG in the ED to evaluate new-onset seizures,[12] most clinicians advocate emergent EEG evaluation only to confirm the diagnosis of nonconvulsive status epilepticus or to establish the presence of status epilepticus in a patient who has been given long-acting paralytic agents to facilitate intubation.[13]

Pharmacotherapeutic Strategies for Acute Seizure Management

No one drug fulfills the role of an ideal anti-status seizure medication. *Table 2* lists medications that are effective in status, along with their major advantages and disadvantages. These drugs fit into three families: phenytoin, the benzodiazepines, and the barbiturates.

Phenytoin. Phenytoin is the most commonly prescribed anticonvulsant, and its blood levels are easily measured. Levels reflect only total serum concentration of the drug.[14] This may be an important distinction as a large portion of phenytoin is protein-bound, and bound phenytoin does not cross into the brain to exert an anticonvulsant effect.[15]

Loading. When confronted with a patient with a subtherapeutic phenytoin level, the question is how best to achieve therapeutic levels. If the goal is to achieve a therapeutic level by the time the patient leaves the ED, the only practical method is to load the patient intravenously .

In the past, undiluted phenytoin has been injected manually into a vein or IV line. Phenytoin tends to crystallize in dextrose-containing solutions,[16] and the addition of phenytoin to lactated Ringer's solution produces variable phenytoin concentrations.[14] At present, most intravenously administered phenytoin is diluted with saline and delivered at a rate of 25-50 mg/min (see below).[16,17]

If the patient has very low or absent phenytoin serum levels, the amount of the loading dose should be 15-20 mg/kg. Although phenytoin may be given at rate up to 50 mg/min, many emergency physicians prefer to standard-load patients, at a rate of approximately 25 mg/min in order to minimize the chance of cardiovascular complications. When patients are loaded at the dose of 18 mg/kg, serum phenytoin levels greater than 10 mcg/mL will be achieved for at least 24 hours in most patients.[18,19]

One group of investigators has developed a method to achieve a desired plasma concentration in patients with a subtherapeutic phenytoin level, using the equation:

$$\textbf{Loading dose} = [0.75\ \text{L/kg}][\text{body weight (kg)}][C_{desired} - C_{observed}] / 0.92$$

where 0.75 L/kg is the volume of distribution, $C_{desired}$ is the desired concentration, $C_{observed}$ is the observed concentration of phenytoin, and 0.92 is the fraction of phenytoin sodium present as phenytoin.[20] Therefore, to raise the serum concentration of a 70 kg man from 5 mcg/mL to 15 mcg/mL, one would need to administer approximately 570 mg intravenously .

Oral loading of the drug has been advocated, since administering phenytoin intravenously has been associated with various complications, including cardiac arrest[21] Assuming typical daily doses of 300 mg/d, it would take 3-4 days to achieve therapeutic blood levels (10-

Table 2. Acute Seizure Management: Drug Therapy

Generic	Brand	Most Common Dose	Effectiveness	Advantages	Disadvantages
BENZODIAZEPINES					
Lorazepam	Ativan	2-8 mg (IV)	2-8 hours	Rapid acting Longer duration of action than diazepam	May depress CNS for hours
Diazepam	Valium	5-20 mg (IV)	5-15 minutes	Rapid acting	Short effective half-life
PHENYTOIN					
Phenytoin	Dilantin	500-1000 mg (IV) (18 mg/kg)	24 hours	No CNS depression No respiratory depression	May be ineffective in status from nonidiopathic causes Hypotension and arrhythmias at high infusion rates Takes 20-40 minutes to administer
BARBITURATES					
Phenobarbital	Luminal	500-1000 mg (IV, IM)	1-3 days	Long-lasting	Long-lasting CNS depression
Thiopental	Pentothal	250-500 mg (IV)	Minutes	Immediate onset	Short effective half-life Respiratory depression Respiratory arrest Hypotension Myocardial depression
Pentobarbital	Nembutal	250-500 mg (IV)	Minutes	Immediate onset	Short effective half-life Respiratory depression Respiratory arrest Hypotension Myocardial depression

20 mg/mL) required for seizure prophylaxis. Consequently, oral loading with larger doses is required.

One study using stat oral doses of 18 mg/kg phenytoin obtained therapeutic blood levels in 64% of patients at eight hours.[22] Few patients in this study achieved therapeutic levels if they were given less than a 1.2 g dose.[22] This study and others have demonstrated the safety of oral loading doses.[23,24] Few patients developed cardiovascular, gastrointestinal, or neurological symptoms. Most symptomology is mild and transient, although some patients may become drowsy or ataxic, delaying immediate ED discharge.

Adverse Effects. The most common adverse cardiovascular effect of phenytoin infusion is hypotension, which can usually be reversed by decreasing the rate of infusion or temporarily suspending phenytoin administration.[16,25,26] Hypotension is not related to the total dose of the drug given, so the full loading dose may be administered after the patient's vital signs have normalized.[27,28] Other cardiovascular complications of IV phenytoin administration include development of dysrhythmias, especially bradycardia.[26] Phenytoin infusions should never be given faster than 50 mg/min, as higher rates significantly increase the likelihood of adverse cardiac effects. A 1000 mg loading dose of phenytoin usually requires more than 20 minutes in order to minimize toxicity .

In addition to the cardiovascular complications of phenytoin, adverse neurological side effects may also occur.[27,28] A cerebellar syndrome consisting of nystagmus and ataxia is the most common neurological side effect.[27] although a 1-2 g infusion of phenytoin rarely causes significant neurologic symptomology, CNS depression, confusion, dizziness, and drowsiness have been noted. Nausea and vomiting also have been described, especially with higher total phenytoin doses.[18] Neither drug concentration nor rate of administration seems to correlate with these symptoms.[8] Slowing the rate of phenytoin infusion decreases such local complications as pain and bumming at the infusion.[20]

Serum Levels. It should be noted that published therapeutic levels should only be used for guidance and do not represent standards. AED levels should be increased to levels that are high enough to stop seizures but less than levels that cause toxicity. Some patients may experience toxic effects at low serum levels, while others may not show signs of toxicity despite having higher AED levels than those in the therapeutic range. Levels should be remeasured routinely if the patient is begun on additional AEDs, becomes pregnant, or develops renal or hepatic dysfunction.[18,27,28]

Generic vs. Brand Name. Although, in general, generic medications have the same bioavailability as their brand-name counterparts, most generic antiepileptic drugs are not recommended because of their varied and unpredictable bioavailability.[29] Dilantin Kapseals, the Parke-Davis brand, are the only phenytoin capsules approved by the FDA for once-daily dosage. Generic phenytoin is more reliably absorbed than Dilantin Kapseals. However, generics generally have a shorter and more erratic half-life. If a patient is switched to generic phenytoin, it is imperative to monitor serum levels.[30]

Benzodiazepines. In general, two benzodiazeepines, lorazepam and diazepam are most often used intravenously to control status seizures. Both are highly lipophilic and cross rapidly into the CNS, where their antiseizure activity related to their gamma-amino butyric acid (GABA)-agonist properties.

It should be emphasized that anticonvulsant management with benzodiazepines may result in respiratory depression and may mandate the need for temporary respiratory support or endotracheal intubation. Intubation is necessary more often with diazepam as compared to phenobarbital, phenytoin,[31] or lorazepam.[32] The principles of management of status epilepticus in adults apply to status epilepticus in children. Lorazepam is the preferred benzodiazepine for acute treatment of status epilepticus.[33-37] It has a rapid onset of action (2-3 minutes), which is similar to that of diazepam, but has a longer duration of action. The duration of action of diazepam is only 5-15 minutes as compared to lorazepam, which has a duration of action that can last for several hours. The initial dose of lorazepam is 0.05-0.10 mg/kg, and a dose of 1-2 mg may be repeated every 10-15 minutes. Most authorities recommend administration of a longer-acting anticonvulsant such as phenytoin while control is initiated with a benzodiazepine.[35-39]

Diazepam. Diazepam is the best-studied and widely used medication for status. Its onset is generally within 30 seconds to two minutes and, in approximately 80-90% of cases, takes effect within five minutes of IV administration.[40] Diazepam has a long pharmacologic half-life—30 hours or more—but a short duration of action.[41] Seizures often recur within 5-15 minutes of administration.[42-44] Because of this short duration, a second drug is usually required for long-term seizure control.[45-47] Diazepam has been reported to be ineffective in up to 8-12% of cases of status seizures.[44,48]

The most commonly recommended dosage of diazepam is 5-20 mg IV over several minutes.[42,43,45,46,49-52] It is safest to give 2-5 mg over the first 1-2 minutes and 2 mg per minute thereafter. Diazepam may be given by continuous infusion at 2-8 mg/h and also per rectum.[43] The intramuscular route should not be used because of erratic absorption.

High doses of the drug may cause hypotension, hypoventilation, and apnea. These complications are especially common when diazepam is combined with barbiturate administration.[43,47,48] Physicians should be prepared for any abrupt changes in a patient's airway status and be ready for a controlled intubation. Hypotension is best treated with volume expansion and Trendelenburg positioning.

Lorazepam. Lorazepam is another benzodiazepine with very potent antiseizure activity when given intravenously.[44,52,53] Like diazepam, its onset of action is within minutes, but its effects last considerably longer.[41] The dose of lorazepam is 2-8 mg IV, and its serum half-life is approximately 13-15 hours.[41,44,53] The drug may also be given IM, although the effectiveness of this route has not been well studied. Based on our experience and that reported by others, lorazepam's antiseizure effects generally last for approximately 2-8 hours.[41-44,54]

Whether lorazepam is truly superior to diazepam is debated by some. In the only double-blind study comparing the two drugs, researchers noted few significant differences.[44] Both drugs controlled 92-93% of the patients with tonic-clonic generalized seizures, and both drugs caused respiratory depression and respiratory arrests in four patients.[44] At present, the choice of diazepam or lorazepam depends on the physician's preference. Diazepam allows the patient to arouse sooner, but it also allows the patient to reseize sooner. Its use requires administering a second drug when more than short-term seizure control is required. In contrast, lorazepam may obviate the need for repeated dosing or continuous infusion and the administration of a second anticonvulsant. Keep in mind, however, that respiratory depression may occur up to an hour after seizures have initially been controlled with lorazepam.

Midazolam. Midazolam is a short-acting water-soluble IV-administered benzodiazepine that has been used to control seizures via the IM route as well.[55] It is not yet approved by the FDA for seizure control but appears to be an excellent choice for actively seizing patients in whom an IV line cannot be secured. In one of the few reports of its IM use in seizure control, a single 10 mg dose stopped convulsions within five minutes of administration.[55] Midazolam has also been effective in cases of diazepam-resistant status.[55] Because of its very short effective half-life, most patients would require a continuous infusion, Although this might be considered a disadvantage, the drug might prove useful in patients with a rapidly reversible cause of seizures.

Barbiturates. Barbiturates most commonly used in controlling status seizures are phenobarbital, thiopental (pentothal), and pentobarbital. Until recently, they were considered third- or fourth-line drugs.[40-43,45,47,49-51] These agents exert their antiseizure effects via their global CNS depressant effects on almost all areas of the brain. Such depression occurs via a GABA-receptor-agonistic activity similar to that of the benzodiazepines.[40]

Phenobarbital. Phenobarbital is a long-acting barbiturate with a variable half-life of 60-150 hours.[41] Due to its lower lipid solubility, the drug may not take effect as rapidly as some of the other barbiturates[41,54] and may take 20 or more minutes to obtain maximum effectiveness.[41,45,47,56] The loading dose is 10-20 mg/kg, and may be given IV or IM.[41-43]

One study demonstrated phenobarbital's efficacy in acute seizure control.[57] In a randomized, nonblinded study, patients treated with 100 mg/min of phenobarbital stopped seizing within a median time of five minutes vs. nine minutes for a matched group treated with concurrent 2 mg/min of diazepam and 40 mg/min of phenytoin.[57] Interestingly, the side effects of hypotension, arrhythmias, and respiratory depression were equal in both groups.

Thiopental and Pentobarbital. Thiopental and pentobarbital are short-acting barbiturates that work very rapidly to stop seizure activity. Only a few studies, though, have evaluated these drugs in status seizures.[57-64] Thiopental may be administered as bolus doses of 50-100 mg/min until the seizure is controlled.[57,59-64] However, one early study in a general hospital ward reported that a dose of just 2 mg/min successfully controlled seizures.[61] The larger the dose, the more likely hypotension and respiratory arrests are to ensue.[60]

Pentobarbital's effects are very similar to those of thiopental.[57,59] It usually may be given as boluses of 50-100 mg/min, or, for immediate seizure cessation, as an IV load of up to 5 mg/kg.[57,59] At this higher dose, respiratory arrest" are common, occurring within 30-60 seconds of administration.

Lidocaine. Widely used as a cardiac antiarrhythmic, IV lidocaine has also been reported to be an effective anticonvulsant.[65-69]

Lidocaine may be an appropriate pharmacologic adjunct in patients with status epilepticus, especially in those patients with limited pulmonary reserve. Lidocaine has few sedative properties, making it useful in those who have already received IV benzodiazepines. The dose of lidocaine that is generally used is 1.5-2.0 mg/kg given intravenously over 1-2 minutes. An IV drip of 3 mg/min may be instituted if the bolus is successful.64 The IV infusion in children is 6 mg/kg/h.[70]

Alternate Routes of AED Administration. Intraosseous (IO) infusion of benzodiazepines, phenobarbital, or phenytoin is another option for managing status seizures in children. The same doses recommended for IV administration are used for IO administration and produce the same pharmacokinetics and toxic side effects.[70] Rectal administration of anti-seizure medications offers an excellent alternative to the challenging proposition of starting an IV or IO line in an actively seizing child or neonate.

Rectal diazepam has successfully terminated seizures within five minutes after administration.[71] I with adequate serum levels achieved within about 10 minutes of administration.[72-74] The initial dose recommended is 0.5 mg/kg of diazepam for injection into the rectum. A second dose of 0.25 mg/kg of diazepam may be given in 10 minutes if seizure activity continues.[75] Some may choose to begin with 5 mg administered via a Foley catheter inserted into the rectum or via a retention enema. Adequate serum concentrations are achieved within approximately 10 minutes.[72-74] Better absorption may be achieved by keeping the child on his or her side or prone with buttocks compressed to prevent leakage of the drug.

A Systematic Approach to Managing Unstable Status Seizures

Successful management of status seizures demands clear thinking with meticulous attention to detail. Our treatment protocol consists of five steps. *(Please see Table 3.)*

Table 3. Five-Step Treatment Protocol

1. **Attempt stabilization**
   Secure ABCs (0_2, IV, ECG)
   Assess need for Narcan, glucose, thiamine
2. **Titrate benzodiazepine**
   Diazepam 5-20 mg over 5-10 minutes
   or Lorazepam 2-8 mg over 5-20 minutes
3. **Assess for reversible causes**
4. **Begin phenytoin loading (if indicated)**
   25-40 mg/min
   Total dose 18-20 mg/kg
5. **Induce barbiturate coma**
   Phenobarbital 50-100 mg/min up to 1 000 mg
   or Thiopental 50-100 mg/min*
   or Pentobarbital 50-100 mg/min*

*Usually also requires continuous infusion; start at 2 mg/kg/h

Step 1: Attempt Stabilization. During this step, undertake standard ED life-support measures. Follow airway control and oxygen administration by hooking up an ECG monitor and starting at least one (preferably 2) large-bore IVs. Because the patient may later be turned left side down to decrease the risk of aspiration from the vomiting that may complicate seizures, start the IV in the right arm.

All patients with altered mental status (including seizures) are candidates for naloxone, glucose, and thiamine administration. Although narcotics do not cause seizures, give 2 mg of naloxone to eliminate any confounding CNS depressant effects in unstable patients. A bedside glucose determination will ascertain the need for hypertonic glucose. If a bedside analysis cannot be readily obtained, administer at least 50 cc of 50% dextrose in water (D50) to adult patients. Any patient who receives hypertonic glucose should also receive 100 mg of IV thiamine. To avoid missing Wemicke's encephalopathy, administer thiamine to any alcoholic, AIDS, or malnourished seizing patient regardless of whether hypertonic glucose has been given.

Step 2: Titrate Benzodiazepine. Either diazepam or lorazepam can be used in doses of up to 20 mg or 8 mg, respectively.[41-43,47,48,54,76] Administer diazepam in 2-5 mg boluses or lorazepam in 1-2 mg boluses every 1-2 minutes. Once the maximum dosage has been reached, quickly move to another agent. But if the patient has known idiopathic epilepsy, start a phenytoin infusion in another IV at 25-40 mg/min to run concurrently with the diazepam.

Step 3: Assess for Reversible Causes. As previously noted, almost all patients with idiopathic epilepsy are readily controlled within 5-15 minutes of initiation of benzodiazepine and phenytoin therapy.[40,45,46,51] In patients who are not well controlled, physicians should seek a secondary cause.

Step 4: Begin Phenytoin Loading, Consider Lidocaine. In stable patients who have an underlying seizure focus and whose seizures do not have a toxic or metabolic cause, phenytoin is the drug of choice.[41-4. 45,46] Unstable patients, however, should receive phenytoin only as an adjunct; irreversible brain damage may occur in the 20-30 minutes it takes for phenytoin to work, and the drug is often ineffective in seizures caused by drug overdose. We recommend that clinicians also consider administering lidocaine to patients who have continued to seize after receiving a benzodiazepine. Lidocaine should be administered at a dose of 1.5-2.0 mg/kg over approximately 30-60 seconds. An additional advantage to administering lidocaine is that if the patient requires intubation during the inducement of barbiturate coma (see below), lidocaine also is an excellent pre-intubation medication.

Step 5: Induce Barbiturate Coma. For patients who are still seizing at this point, administer phenobarbital at 100 mg/min or thiopental at 50-100 mg/min. Do not spend time trying to decide whether general anesthesia can be given in the ED. Unless immediate seizure cessation is required, phenobarbital appears to be very safe and effective.[47] For truly unstable patients with life-threatening cardiorespiratory abnormalities, toxic-metabolic-induced seizures, or those who are already compromised by underlying medical illness, rapid-acting thiopental is our agent of choice.

Thiopental Loading. Table 4 depicts the stepwise management protocol for thiopental administration. The patient should be maximally preoxygenated, and BP, pulse, ECG leads, and IV lines should be checked and secured. Keep high-flow 100% O_2 by mask over the patient's mouth and nose. All intubation equipment should be checked and available at the bedside, including a Yankauer suction catheter and an endotracheal tube pre loaded with a stylet.

Table 4. Thiopental Therapy for Status Seizures

1. **Maximize ABCs**
   a. Preoxygenate
   b. Secure two large-bore IVs
   c. Recheck blood pressure
   d. Monitor ECG

2. **Confirm presence and function of intubation equipment**
   a. Check operation of all airway equipment
   b. Prepare one stylet-loaded ET tube
   c. Verify presence of strong-wall suction and large-bore Yankauer suction catheter

3. **Titrate thiopental**
   a. 50-100 mg every 30-60 seconds as IV boluses
   b. Monitor airway, breathing, pulse, and blood pressure
   c. Provide cricoid pressure

4. **Intubate as respiratory rate falls or ceases**
   a. Provide cricoid pressure

5. **Provide long-term control**
   a. Rebolus with thiopental; begin thiopental drip at 2 mg/kg/h, or
   b. Load with phenobarbital; give 50-100 mg/min until 20 mg/kg administered starting at 2 mg/kg/h and titrating upward.

Administer thiopental in bolus doses of 50-100 mg every 30-60 seconds until the seizure is controlled. Maintain cricoid pressure during drug administration to minimize the risk of aspiration. Blood pressure may fall dramatically during this phase, mandating frequent monitoring.

As the patient's respiratory rate falls or ceases, perform a careful orotracheal intubation. Slowly give additional thiopental until the seizure is completely controlled. The patient may then be loaded with phenobarbital or maintained on a thiopental drip starting at 2 mg/kg/h and titrating upward.

Note that this form of therapy should be performed only by a physician who is an expert at airway management. If the treating physician feels uncomfortable doing this type of crash intubation, an anesthetist or anesthesiologist should be summoned to the ED before administering any thiopental. If hypotension develops, push fluids and place the patient in the Trendelenburg position. For persistent hypotension, administer dopamine or other pressor agents.

Disposition

Stable, compliant patients with a new-onset, non-status seizure in whom a metabolic, toxic, structural (i.e., CT scan), and infectious work-up fails to demonstrate an etiology can usually be discharged from the ED. It should be stressed that appropriate anti-epileptic therapy and acute neurologic consultation, including follow-up for possible EEG evaluation and measurement of AED serum levels, are mandatory. Patients with non-status exacerbations of a pre-existing seizure disorder can be discharged so long as the most recent seizure does not reflect an escalating or variant pattern of seizure activity and attempts to restore therapeutic serum levels of anti-epileptic drugs have been initiated (if indicated).

Before discharging any patient, follow-up must be arranged with the patient's primary care physician or neurologist. The patient must be warned of the risks of driving and engaging in high-risk activities. Even in states without mandatory reporting, physicians are legally obligated to report people with seizures who could constitute substantial foreseeable public risk or danger (e.g., a bus driver or pilot).

Summary

In general, successful management of this condition is guided by practicing within a systematic framework for assessment, laboratory/radiological evaluation, and targeted pharmacotherapeutic intervention according to the following patient subgroups: 1) new-onset (i.e., first-time) seizures; 2) recurrent seizures in patients with confirmed epilepsy; 3) febrile seizures; 4) post-traumatic seizures; and 5) alcohol- and drug-related convulsions. Distinguishing between psychogenic and neurogenic epilepsy is essential, and a step-by-step approach to managing status epilepticus will minimize morbidity and maximize outcomes.

From the perspective of cost-effectiveness, sound clinical management includes the following: Patients with new-onset seizures who are neurologically normal should undergo a head CT scan after fingerstick glucose measurement. Additional laboratory evaluation may be performed, but it is not required. However, for those with abnormal mental status or neurological exam, the extended workup also should include a CBC, electrolytes, BUN, creatinine, calcium, toxicology screen, and urinalysis. All patients with a first-time seizure who are cleared by radiographic and laboratory evaluation should have their long-term care discussed with a neurologist or primary care physician prior to discharge from the ED.

References

1. Rosenthal RH, Heim ML, Waeckerle JF. First-time major motor seizures in an emergency department. *Ann Emerg Med* 1980;9:242-245.
2. Eisner RF, Tumbull TN, Howes DS, et al. Efficacy of a "standard" seizure workup in the emergency department. *Ann Emerg Med* 1986;15:33-39.
3. Tumbull TL, Vanden Hook TN, Howes DS, et al. Utility of laboratory studies in the emergency department patient with a new-onset seizure. *Ann Emerg Med* 1990;19:373-376.
4. Powers RD. Serum chemistry abnormalities in adult patients with seizures. *Ann Emerg Med* 1985;14:416-420.
5. Nypaver MM, Reynolds SL, Tanz RR, et al. Emergency department laboratory evaluation of children with seizures: Dogma or dilemma. *Pediatr Emerg Care* 1992;8:13-16.
6. Kenney RD. Absence of serum chemistry abnormalities in pediatric patients presenting with seizures. *Pediatr Emerg Care* 1992;65.
7. Bessen HA, Rothstein R. Futility of skull radiogrdphy for

nontraumatic conditions. *Ann Emerg Med* 1982;11:605-609.

8. Tress B. Skull radiography in epilepsy; Dementia and nonspecific neurological symptoms. *BMJ* 1989;289:160.
9. Ramirez-Lassapas, McIpolle RJ, Morillo LR, et al. Value of computed tomographic scan in the evaluation of adult patients after their first seizure. *Ann Neurol* 1984;15: 536-543.
10. Russo LS, Goldstein KH. The diagnostic assessment of single seizures is cranial computed tomography necessary? *Arch Neurol* 1983;40:744-746.
11. Dodson WE, Leppik lE, Pedley TA. Are you up-to-date on seizures? *Patient Care* 1991;162-190.
12. Hooshmand H, Maloney M. The role of EEG in the emergency room. *Clin Electroenceph* 1980;11:163-168.
13. Jagoda A, Riggio S. Refractory status epilepticus in adults. *Emerg Med* 1993;22:1337-1348.
14. Levine M, Chang T. Therapeutic drug monitoring of phenytoin. *Clin Pharmacokinet* 1990;19:341-358.
15. Ramsay RE, Hammond EJ, Perchalski RJ, et al. Brain uptake of phenytoin, phenobarbitol and diazepam. *Arch Neurol* 1979;36:535-539.
16. Carducci B, Hedges JR, Beal JC, et al. Emergency phenytoin loading by constant intravenous infusion. *Ann Emerg Med* 1984;1027-1031.
17. Donovan PJ, Cline D. Phenytoin administration by constant intravenous infusion: Selective rates of administration. *Ann Emerg Med* 1991;30:139-142.
18. Cranford RE, Leppik IE, Patrick B, et al. Intravenous phenytoin clinical and pharmacokinetic aspects. *Neurology* 1978;28:874-880.
19. Cranford RE, Leppik lE, Patrick B, et al. Intravenous phenytoin in acute treatment of seizures. *Neurology* 1979;29: 1474-1479.
20. Dela Cruz FG, Kanter MZ, Fischer JH, et al. Efficacy of individualized phenytoin sodium loading doses administered by intravenous infusion. *Clin Pharmacol* 1988;7:219-223.
21. York RC, Coleridge ST. Cardiopulmonary arrest following intravenous phenytoin loading. *Am J Emerg Med* 1988;6: 255-259.
22. Osburn H, Zisfein J, Sparano R. Single-dose oral phenytoin loading. *Ann Emerg Med* 1987;16:407-412.
23. Evens RP, Fraser DG, Ludden TM, et al. Phenytoin toxicity and blood levels after a large oral dose. *Am J Hosp Pharm* 1980;37:232-235.
24. Record KE, Rapp RP , Young AB, et al. Oral phenytoin loading in adults: Rapid achievement of therapeutic plasma levels. *Ann Neurol* 1979;268-270.
25. Salem RB, Wilder BJ, Yost RL, et al. Rapid infusion of phenytoin sodium looding doses. *Am J Hosp Pharm* 1981; 38:354-357.
26. Earnest MP, Marx JR, Drury LR. Complications of intravenous phenytoin for acute treatment of seizures. *JAMA* 1983;249:762-765.
27. Murphy JM, Motiwala R, Devinsky O. Phenytoin intoxication. *South Med J* 1991;84:1023-1199.
28. Pienge KL. The toxicity of the major anticonvulsants. *Ariz Med* 1978;177-179.
29. Morrell MJ. Differential diagnosis of seizures. *Neurol Clin* 1993;11:737-753.
30. Dilantin vs. generic phenytoin sodium. *Med Lett* 1980;22:49.
31. Orr RA, Dimand RJ, Venkatararnan ST, et al. Diazepam and intubation in emergency treatment of seizures in children. *Ann Emerg Med* 1991;20:1009-1013.
32. Chiulli DA, Temdrup TE, Kanter RK, et al. The influence of diazepam or lorazepam on the frequency of endotracheal intubation in childhood status epilepticus. *J Emerg Med* 1919;9:13-17.
33. Carnfield PR. Treatment of status epilepticus in children. *Can Med Assoc J* 1983;128:671.
34. Lacey DJ, Singer WD, Horwitz SJ, et al. Lorazepam therapy of status epilepticus in children and adolescents. *J Pediatr* 1986;108:771-774.
35. Browne TR. Drug therapy reviews: Drug therapy of status epilepticus. *Am J Hosp Pharm* 1978;35:915-922.
36. Treiman DM. The role of benzodiazepines in the management of status epilepticus. *Neurology* 1990;40:32.
37. Levy RJ, Krall RL, et al. Treatment of status epilepticus with lorazepam. *Arch Neurol* 1984;41:605-611.
38. Mitchell WG, Crawford TO, et al. Lorazepam is the treatment of choice for status epilepticus. *J Epilepsy* 1990; 3:7-10.
39. Gabor AJ. Lorazepam versus phenobarbital: Candidates for drug of choice for treatment of status epilepticus. *J Epilepsy* 1990;3:3-36.
40. Delgado-Escueta AV, Wasterlain CG, Treiman DM, et al. Status epilepticus: Summary. In: Delgado-Escueta AV, Wasterlain CG, Treiman DM, et al, eds. *Advances in Neurology*. New York: Raven Press; 1983.
41. Van der Kleijn E, Baars AM, Vree TM, et al. Clinical pharmacokinetics of drugs used in the treatment of status epilepticus. In: Delgado-Escueta AV, Wasterlain CG, Treiman DM, et al, eds. *Advances in Neurology*. New York: Raven Press; 1983.
42. Browne TR, Mikati M. Status epilepticus. In: Ropper AH, Kennedy SF, eds. *Neurological and Neurosurgical Intensive Care*. Rockville, MD: Aspen Publishers; 1988.
43. Miller JA, Hallenbeck JM. Pharmacological approach to acute seizures. In: Chemow B, ed. *The Pharmacologic Approach to the Critically Ill Patient*. Baltimore: Williams & Wilkins; 1988.
44. Leppik lE. Derivan AT, Homan RW, et al. Double-blind study of lorazepam and diazepam in status epilepticus. *JAMA* 1983;249:1452.
45. Delgado-Escueta AV, Wasterlain C, Treiman DM, et al. Current concepts in neurology—management of status epilepticus. *N Engl J Med* 1982;306:1337.
46. Celesia CG. Modem concepts of status epilepticus. *JAMA* 1976; 235:1571.
47. Shaner DM, McCurdy SA, Herring MO, et al. Treatment of status epilepticus: A prospective comparison of diazepam and phenytoin versus phenobarbital and optional phenytoin. *Neurology* 1988;38:202.
48. Tassinari CA, Daniele O, Michelussi R, et al. Benzodiazepines: Efficacy in status epilepticus. In: Delgado-Escueta AV, Wasterlain CG, Treiman DM, et al, eds. *Advances in Neurology*. New York: Raven Press; 1983.

49. Leppik lE. Status epilepticus. *Neurol Clin* 1986;4:633.
50. Hall S. Status epilepticus. *Am Fam Physician* 1983;28:117.
51. Fisher RS. Emergency treatment for status epilepticus. *J Crit Illness* 1987;2:27.
52. Meldrum BS, Vigouroux RA, Brierley JB. Systemic factors and epileptic brain damage. *Arch Neurol* 1973;29:82.
53. Gillman AG, Goodman LS, et al, eds. *The Pharmacological Basis of Therapeutics*. 7th ed. New York: MacMillan Publishing Co; 1985.
54. Walker JE, Homan RW, Vasko MR, et al. Lorazepam in status epilepticus. *Ann Neurol* 1979;6:207.
55. Mayhue FE. IM midazolam for status epilepticus in the emergency department. *Ann Emerg Med* 1988;17:643.
56. Treiman DM. General principles of treatment: Responsive and intractable status epilepticus in adults. In: Delgado-Escueta AV, Wasterlain CG, Treiman DM, et al, eds. *Advances in Neurology*. New York: Raven Press; 1983.
57. Lowenstein DH, Aminoff MJ, Somon RP. Barbiturate anesthesia in the treatment of status epileptieus: Clinical experience with 14 patients. *Neurology* 1988;38:395.
58. Lemmen LJ, Klassen M, Duiser B. Intravenous lidocaine in the treatment of convulsions. *JAMA* 1978;239:2025.
59. Rashkin MC, Youngs C, Penovich P. Pentobarbital treatment of refractory status epilepticus. *Neurology* 1987;37:500.
60. Goldberg MA, Mclntryre HB. Barbituratcs in the treatment of status epilepticus. In: Delgado-Escueta AV, Wasterlain CG, Treiman DM, et al, eds. *Advances in Neurology*. New York: Raven Press; 1983.
61. Brown AS, Horton JM. Status epilepticus treated by intrdvenous infusions of thiopensone sodium. *BMJ* 1967;1:27.
62. Cloyd JC, Wright BD, Perrier D. Pharmacokinetic properties of thiopental in two patients treated for uncontrollable seisures. *Epileptic* 1979;20:313.
63. Onowski JP, Erenberg G, Lueders H, et al. Hypothermia and barbituric coma for refractory status epilepticus. *Crit Care Med* 1984;12:367.
64. Partimen M, Kovanca J, Nilsson E. Status epilepticus treated by barbiturate anesthesia with continuous monitoring of cerebrdl function. *BMJ* 1981;282:520.
65. Aggerwal P, et al. Lidocaine in refractory status epilepticus: A forgotten drug in the emergency department. *Am J Emerg Med* 1993;11:243-244.
66. Morris HH. Lidocaine: A neglected anticonvulsant? *So Med J* 1979;72:1564-1566.
67. Pascual J, Ciudad J, Berciano J, et al. Role of lidocaine in managing status epilepticus. *J Neuro Neurosurg Psych* 1992;55:49-51.
68. Pascual J, Sedano MI, Polo JM, et al. Intravenous lidocaine for status epilepticus. *Epilepsia* 1988;29:584-590.
69. Bernard CG, Bohm E, Hojeberg S, et al. A new treatment of status epilepticus. *Arch Neurol Psych* 1955;74:208-214.
70. Tunik MG, Young GM. Status epilepticus in children. *Pediatr Clin North Am* 1992;39:1007-1030.
71. Knudsen FU. Rectal administration of diazepam in solution in the acute treatment of convulsions in infants and children. *Arch Dis Child* 1979;54:855-857.
72. Hoppu K, Santaruori P, et al. Diazepam rectal solution for home treatment of acute seizures in children. *Acta Paediatr Scand* 1981;70:369-372.
73. Soander H, Arnold E, Nilsson K, et al. Effects of the rectal administration of diazepam. *Br J Anaesth* 1985;57:578-580.
74. Dhillon S, Ngwane E, Richens A, et al. Rectal absorption of diazepam in epileptic children. *Arch Dis Childhood* 1982;57:264-267.
75. Albano A, Reisdorff EJ, Wiegenstein JG, et al. Rectal diazepam in status epilepticus. *Am J Emerg Med* 1989;T:6-72.

Dizziness, Vertigo, and Syncope

Frank J. Edwards, MD, FACEP

On virtually every shift in the emergency department (ED), at least one patient presents with dizziness, vertigo, near-syncope, syncope, or some variation or combination thereof. Behind these disparate symptoms lurks a large list of possible diagnoses, making the patient history crucial to the diagnosis. Yet, as if to confound the clinician, patients possess a vast array of vague and misleading vernacular terminology to describe the signs and symptoms of these conditions. It's no surprise, as one author put it, that physicians sometimes experience a "slight decline in spirits" when confronted with a similar case.[1]

Fortunately, careful history taking and a directed approach to physical examination and laboratory testing will rapidly uncover the most likely underlying diagnosis. If a patient has the abrupt onset of positional vertigo, the odds favor a peripheral etiology, which is usually benign and self-limited. A focused neurologic examination can exclude the more serious central causes. Certain vertigo patients benefit from immediate CT or MRI, or referral to an otolaryngologist, for audiological and vestibular evaluation testing. The most common cause of syncope is a neurologically mediated decrease in vascular tone and cardiac output. Other etiologies include cardiac arrhythmias, postural hypotension, and psychiatric disorders.

This chapter addresses the difficult clinical problem of the evaluation of the emergency patient with dizziness, vertigo, or syncope. The author reviews the current literature on the classification of these perplexing disorders, presents useful strategies for their acute assessment and treatment, and discusses the issue of which patients demand more extensive evaluation.

The Diagnostic Dilemma of Dizziness

Dizziness is a common problem in the ED as well as in other outpatient health care settings. According to the National Ambulatory Medical Care Survey, dizziness was the chief complaint of 1% of all patients presenting to primary care physicians, and the incidence increased steadily among older age groups.[2] In a study that examined all presenting complaints—chief and otherwise—in 1000 medical outpatients, dizziness was the third most frequent symptom.[3] In another evaluation of l06 "dizzy" patients, the investigators reported that physicians ended up making 46 different diagnoses.[4] A study of 125 dizzy ED patients revealed that 43% were related to peripheral vestibular disorders; 27% to cardiovascular etiologies (including vasovagal reactions, postural hypotension, and dysrhythmias); 10% remained "unknown;" and 6% were psychogenic in natures.[5] *(Please see Table 1.)*

Clinical Approach. The major initial challenge in dealing with dizzy patients is the English language. The word "dizziness" has become synonymous in the minds of many people with just about any imaginable alteration of consciousness or balance, including lightheadedness, wooziness, a sense of strangeness, faintness, fogginess, swaying, positional instability, swirling, feeling intoxicated,

Table 1. Etiology of Dizziness in 125 ED Patients

Peripheral vestibular disorder	43%
Cardiovascular	21%
Unknown	10%
Medication-induced	7%
Post-traumatic	6%
Other	6%
Psychogenic	6%
Hyperventilation	5%
Endocrine	4%
Infectious	3%
Seizure	2%
Anemia	2%
Meniere's syndrome	1%
Multiple sensory deficit	1%

Adapted from: Herr R, Zun L, Mathews I. A directed approach to the dizzy patient. *Ann Emerg Med* 1989;18:664-672.

giddy, imbalanced, or "out-of-it."[6] With the use of a helpful classification scheme, most dizzy patients can be placed into one of four symptom categories:[7] 1) patients with vertigo, (i.e., a sense of movement); 2) patients with the "graying out" feeling of pre-syncope; 3) patients with a feeling of imbalance or dysequilibrium not associated with a sense of movement and in whom the symptom becomes prominent while standing or walking but tends to resolve when sitting or lying; and 4) patients who describe a vague sense of lightheadedness or non-specific wooziness. *(Please see Table 2.)* When confronted by a patient complaining of dizziness, the clinician's first task is to determine the precise sequence and quality of sensations. Two adages apply: l) banish the word dizzy from the history-taking session; and 2) sit down at the bedside and allow the patient sufficient time to paint a complete picture of the symptomatology. Obtain a thorough medication history, especially for antidepressants, beta-adrenergic blocking agents, and calcium channel antagonists.[8] Inquire about exacerbating or ameliorating maneuvers, lingering symptoms, previous similar episodes, and other illnesses, such as cardiovascular disease, diabetes, migraine,[9] or psychiatric disorders. It may be helpful to ask about current stressors in the patients life.

Understanding Vertigo: Definitions and Pathophysiology

Compared with dizziness, the term vertigo has greater precision. Vertigo is described as either an "illusion" or an "hallucination" of movement.[6,10] Both vertigo and dysequilibrium imply a loss of balance, but vertigo also connotes a sense of motion. Vertigo is a range of sensations centered around a visceral awareness of change in one's relationship to gravity and the earth. Mild vertigo is a feeling that the earth is shifting slightly or tilting and would be difficult to distinguish from "pure" dysequilibrium. Severe vertigo is a profoundly unpleasant sense of whirling. The patient usually describes the room spinning, but may perceive themselves as spinning and the room staying still.[11] This distinction, and that of the spin direction, are primarily of academic interest. Vertigo also includes sensations of linear movement, acceleration, and propulsion (i.e., being thrust to the ground).

Oscillopsia is related to vertigo and consists of the visual illusion of environmental movement, not necessarily accompanied by the sensation of motion. Oscillopsia can be produced by a bilateral decrease in vestibular function. For instance, aminoglycoside toxicity results in impairment of the vestibulo-ocular reflex, which provides compensatory eye movements during head turning. For example, the patient with oscillopsia has difficulty reading street signs unless he holds his head extremely steady.[12]

Maintaining Equilibrium. Normal equilibrium is maintained by the synchronous effort of three sensory systems: the vestibular apparatus of the inner ear; vision; and proprioception.

Vestibular Apparatus. The inner ear (membranous labyrinth) sits in a bony chamber (osseous labyrinth) and consists of: 1) the three semicircular canals, the utricle, and the saccule (collectively

Table 2. Classification of Dizziness

TYPE I: VERTIGO

Indicates an illusion of motion, which is frequently rotary (whirling), but may be rocking, swaying, or a sense of linear propulsion, and can be of varying degrees of intensity and persistence. For example, vertigo may be severe, acute, and related to changes in head position, or it may be mild, continuous, and chronic.

TYPE II: PRE-SYNCOPAL SYMPTOMS

Pre-syncope involves a transient sensation that a faint is about to occur. During the episode, the patient often senses vision growing dark or dim, and may feel some degree of nausea, weakness, or shortness of breath, possibly accompanied by a sense of anxiety. The hallmark of these symptoms is their transient nature, with resolution occurring more or less rapidly.

TYPE III: DYSEQUILIBRIUM

This is a feeling of unsteadiness or imbalance, without an actual illusion of movement or without a "sense of faintness," and usually is more noticeable when the patient walks or stands unassisted.

TYPE IV: NON-SPECIFIC, VAGUE LIGHTHEADEDNESS, WOOZINESS, GIDDINESS

This category holds the remainder of symptoms under dizziness that do not reasonably fit into the first three, more specific, categories. A higher percentage of patients displaying this type of dizziness will, once other causes have been excluded, be classified as having psychological dizziness.

known as the vestibular organ); and 2) the organ of hearing called the cochlea. This entire interconnected structure floats in "perilymph" and contains "endolymph." Only the cochlea is not involved in equilibrium. Otoliths (tiny hair-like structures with a denser deposit at their tips) in the saccule and utricle give orientation to gravity, whereas tiny hair-like projections in the trio of semicircular canals sense motion in their respective dimensions. Afferent cholinergic fibers from the utricle, the saccule, and the canals merge to form the vestibular portion of the acoustic nerve (cranial nerve [CN] VIII). Blood supply is from the labyrinthine artery, a branch of the vertebrobasilar system.[13]

Visual Input. For maintenance of equilibrium, sensory input from both inner ears must be in synchrony with the input from the visual and position-sensing systems. The central processor and relay station for this system is the brainstem vestibular nuclei complex that integrates the tonic input and relays information to other brainstem nuclei and higher brain structures. The false sense of movement that occurs with vertigo arises when discordant stimuli affect the vestibular nuclei. Reading in the back seat of a moving car is a good example. The vestibular organ senses movement, the eyes do not. The resulting tonic imbalance creates a "hallucination" of motion. Standing at the edge of a cliff causes vertigo by a similar imbalance because standard visual clues have suddenly been erased.

The importance of vision to our sense of equilibrium is illustrated by the elderly person whose balance system is marginal due to the effects of aging, but whose balance is reasonably normal during the day. However, in a fashion similar to standing on the cliff edge, when darkness falls and visual clues diminish, the elderly patient may become extremely unsteady.[14] Glaucoma, refraction problems, and eye muscle problems, therefore, can also be sources of dysequilibrium and gait-unsteadiness in elderly people.

Proprioception. Any disorder of proprioception secondary to various peripheral neuropathies or myelopathies (e.g., diabetic, pellagra, tabes dorsalis, etc.) likewise can disturb equilibrium. The Romberg test—staying in balance while closing the eyes—tests the proprioceptive aspect of the balance triad.

The term "multi-sensory dizziness syndrome" is used to describe the elderly person with age-related sensory deficits. This syndrome has been found in as many as one-third of elderly patients with non-specific complaints of dizziness or unsteadiness, particularly when diabetes is present.[7] The association of dizziness with falls in the elderly is a well-recognized and serious complication of aging.[15]

Clinical Evaluation of the Patient with Vertigo

Vertigo is not a common feature with isolated disturbances of vision or position sense. For all practical purposes, vertigo itself arises from a lesion of some sort involving either the labyrinth, the vestibular portion of CN VIII, the vestibular nuclei, or the brainstem structures close to the vestibular nuclei. Although 80 separate conditions ranging from the benign to the devastating have been noted to present with vertigo,[1] the acute assessment and management is straightforward. The clinician must decide whether the vertigo is caused by a disturbance at or near the end organ or whether it arises from a more central process. This distinction is normally unambiguous. *(Please see Table 3.)*

Table 3. Characteristics of Peripheral and Central Vertigo

	PERIPHERAL	CENTRAL
Intensity	Moderate to intense	Mild to moderate
Temporal pattern	Brief, episodic	Chronic, continuous
Onset	Abrupt	Gradual
Nystagmus	Rotatory/ horizontal	Any kind, including bizarre/vertical
Nausea/ vomiting	Common	Uncommon
Hearing loss	Possible	Unlikely
Neurological deficits	Otherwise none	Often present

Peripheral Vertigo. Approximately 85% of ED patients with vertigo have a peripheral etiology,[16] with dysfunction of one of the vestibular organs. The resulting asymmetry of input to the vestibular nuclei causes a sensation of rotation identical to motion sickness. Autonomic symptoms of nausea, pallor, diaphoresis frequently occur. The vestibular nuclei adjust to the asymmetric input. The vertigo, nystagmus, and autonomic symptoms may diminish or cease. However, the next time the patient moves his or her head, the process reoccurs.[17] Positional vertigo lasts seconds. Acute vestibulopathy lasts hours to days. Vertigo due to a severed vestibular nerve "adapts" in 1-3 months.

Peripheral vertigo is intense, episodic, worsened by head motion, and often accompanied by nausea, vomiting, and diaphoresis. Some degree of nystagmus may be found. Nystagmus is rotatory or horizontal (but not purely vertical) with peripheral vertigo, and the slow phase often points toward the dysfunctional vestibular organ (as would be the case if cold water were instilled into a healthy ear).[11] Positional nystagmus tends to "fatigue" and disappear rapidly, and most nystagmus due to peripheral causes also diminishes if the patient visually fixates on an object. In patients with peripheral vertigo, except for nystagmus, the remainder of the neurologic examination should be perfectly normal.

Central Vertigo. In many ways, patients with central vertigo display the opposite of these findings. Central vertigo generally is not episodic, is not abrupt in onset, and is less often associated with autonomic symptoms. Central vertigo tends to have a gradual onset and may remain continuous for days, weeks, or months and is less likely to produce severe whirling sensations. Central vertigo usually is not worsened by changes in head position, and when nystagmus is present, it commonly remains continuous and is not diminished by visual fixation. The presence of asymmetric or pure vertical nystagmus also points to a central process.

Central vertigo is frequently accompanied by neurologic abnormalities. Look especially for signs indicating compromise of other structures near the vestibular nuclei and CN-VIII, such as decreased corneal reflex (CNV), facial weakness (CN-VII), and problems with the gag reflex and swallowing (CN-IX and CN X). Also, because the cerebellum is close to sites of potential pathology causing central ver-

Table 4. Causes of Peripheral Vertigo

- Benign positional vertigo
- Labyrinthitis or vestibular neuronitis
- Meniere's disease
- Middle ear effusions
- Physiologic motion sickness
- Perilymphatic fistula
- Otosclerosis
- Mastoiditis
- Local trauma
- Toxic chemicals
  - Alcohol
  - Aminoglycosides
  - Chloramphenicol
  - Minocycline
  - Quinine
  - Qunidine
  - Cisplatin
  - Aspirin
  - Phenytoin
  - Furosemide
  - Ethacrynic acid

tigo, the clinician should be alert for accompanying signs of cerebellar dysfunction such as truncal ataxia (patient weaves when trying to sit unsupported), limb ataxia (finger-to-nose), and gait ataxia.[6]

Peripheral Vertigo: Diagnosis and Management

Benign Positional Vertigo. Benign positional vertigo (BPV) is by far the most common overall cause of peripheral vertigo, and the incidence increases markedly after age 50.[7,18] BPV is followed in frequency by labyrinthitis or vestibular neuronitis, Meniere's disease, and a number of other less common causes. *(Please see Table 4.)*[19] In children, vertigo is often associated with otitis media and chronic middle ear effusions. BPV is thought to be due to the presence of free-floating "coproliths" in the endolymph which stimulate fibers of the posterior semicircular canal.[20,21] BPV generally follows an episodic course and has a good prognosis. In one series, approximately one-third of patients with BPV experienced spontaneous resolution of symptoms after one month.[22] BPV is characterized by abrupt, transient spells of whirling sensations instigated by changes in head position, and is frequently accompanied by nystagmus. Nausea may or may not be present. A common scenario is for the episode to begin after the patient rolls over in bed. A history of recent head injury is sometimes associated with BPV.[23]

The Hallpike (Nylen-Barany) maneuver is diagnostic for BPV. The full maneuver involves rapidly laying the patient supine from a sitting position until the patient's head is extended 30-45° past horizontal and beyond the edge of the stretcher. This maneuver is repeated with the head turned to the left and the head turned to the right. The test is positive when vertigo and nystagmus begin after a latent period of 2-20 seconds. The vertigo and nystagmus then disappear within one minute, and the nystagmus diminishes ("fatigues") with repeated testing. The ear down when vertigo occurs is the one containing the "coproliths," which enter the posterior semicircular canal with the head in that position.[6]

Labyrinthitis. Labyrinthitis and vestibular neuronitis are terms often used interchangeably to describe self-limited, benign episodes of peripheral vertigo that occur in otherwise healthy young to middle-aged adults. There will usually be only a single episode that lasts one to several days, is characterized by intense paroxysms of whirling vertigo. Symptoms are worsened by head movement and usually are accompanied by typical peripheral-type spontaneous undirectional nystagmus. The remainder of the neurological examination is normal.

This syndrome has often been noted to occur after respiratory infections and may appear in epidemics.[17] The distinction between the terms labyrinthitis and vestibular neuronitis appears to have no clinical or prognostic importance. If tinnitus or other auditory symptoms are present, involvement of the entire labyrinth (including the cochlea) is likely and the term labyrinthitis is appropriate. If only vertigo is present, inflammation of the vestibule or the vestibular portion of CN-VIII is presumed, and the episode is termed vestibular neuronitis. Because of the self-limited nature of this condition, the exact site of pathology is seldom located.

Peripheral vertigo symptoms arising suddenly after a forceful cough or sneeze suggest the creation of traumatic "perilymphatic fistula" at the round or oval window. The vertigo often recurs when the patient coughs, strains, or sneezes again. Hennebert's sign, which is recurrence of vertigo with pneumo-otoscopy, confirms the diagnosis of this generally self-resolving condition.[6]

Meniere's Disease is characterized by the triad of vertigo, tinnitus, and sensorineural hearing loss. The hearing loss tends to be transient at first, but may become fixed.[17] Meniere's disease is a chronic relapsing illness,[24] possibly with a familial component, and pathologically characterized by a build-up of endolymphatic pressure in the labyrinth, hence the name "endolymphatic hydrops." Patients with Meniere's disease have recurrent episodes of severe whirling vertigo and nystagmus, usually accompanied by tinnitus and loss of auditory acuity. The attack can begin so abruptly that the patient appears to have been thrown to the ground and the condition may be confused with a "drop attack." Otherwise, the neurologic examination is normal.

In most cases, to make a working diagnosis of either BPV, labyrinthitis or vestibular neuronitis, or Meniere's disease, the history and physical examination are sufficient. When presented with a patient displaying the classic clinical findings of these entities, with whirling positional vertigo, and having no associated neurological deficits, routine laboratory studies are not likely to yield any important new information, and the need for further studies can be guided by the general clinical situation.[5]

Types II (pre-syncope), III (dysequilibrium), and IV (illdefined) dizziness have very broad differential diagnoses, and these patients usually require basic laboratory work-up in the ED. For example, if anemia is suspected to be a complicating factor for the patient's symptoms, a hemoglobin and hematocrit would be indicated. Common electrolyte abnormalities, such as hypokalemia, would be worth seeking in patients with histories of nonspecific dizziness and weakness, especially in patients who are taking diuretics or are poorly nourished, elderly, or who have multiple major medical illnesses.[6]

Dehydration is certainly in the differential diagnosis of Type II dizziness (presyncope), especially when the symptoms are induced when the patient stands. Laboratory confirmation of this through serum electrolytes, BUN, and creatinine, urinespecific gravity and hemoconcentration would be useful if clinical suspicion is high, (e.g, if there are predisposing factors to dehydration and the examination reveals decreased skin turgor, dry membranes, and orthostatic vital sign changes.)[5,10]

Although it is a common observation that dizziness of any sort seems to mandate among nurses and paraprofessionals that consideration of hypoglycemia is a causal factor, there is no mention in the current literature of hypoglycemia being directly related to true paroxysmal Type I vertigo. With other types of dizziness, however, (including dysequilibrium,) pre-syncope, and Type IV (vague, non-specific dizziness), hypoglycemia or hyperglycemia may be involved in the production of symptoms, and the work-up of these patients should include a glucose determination, especially when diabetes mellitus coexists.[6,10]

The clinician should consider obtaining an electrocardiogram in patients having Type II (pre-syncopal) dizziness. This type of dizziness can arise from compromised cardiac output secondary to ischemic heart disease or arrhythmia. Patients with rapid new onset atrial fibrillation may have primary complaints of "dizziness," lightheadedness, or dysequilibrium.[10]

Vertebrobasilar TIAs belong in the differential diagnosis of all four types of dizziness. These episodes of vascular insufficiency in the posterior circulation can produce many brainstem signs and symptoms, including diplopia, ataxia, dysarthria, facial weakness, syncope, pre-syncope, lightheadedness, and vertigo.[12,19] But vertigo as the sole event precipitated by a vertebrobasilar TIA is uncommon. A series of 40 patients with well-defined events of vertebrobasilar insufficiency did not identify vertigo as the only symptom.[15]

Although some vercebrobasilar TIAs may be due to ischemia of a labyrinthine organ, the anatomy of the vertebrobasilar system is such that ischemia is more likely to occur at the level of the brainstem.[12] Most authors suggest that vertebrobasilar TIAs usually are accompanied by other brainstem symptoms, such as ataxia or diplopia or facial weakness, and that simple, transient isolated episodes of vertigo alone are seldom the result of vertebrobasilar TIAs.[6,12,15,19,25]

Acute Management of Peripheral Vertigo. Some patients with peripheral vertigo will benefit from etiology-specific treatment; those patients with otitis media, for example, will need antibiotic therapy (amoxicillin, sulfamethoxazole-trimethoprim, etc.), and if the vertigo is secondary to a cerumen impaction, then cerumen removal by irrigation would be curative and provide symptomatic relief. But more often, the cause of peripheral vertigo is beyond immediate reach and the clinician must focus on relieving the intensely discomforting symptoms by using various pharmacological agents. *(Please see Table 5.)*

Many commonly used medications for the relief of peripheral vertigo symptoms, such as meclizine and atropine have anticholinergic properties. The afferent neurons traveling from labyrinth to the brainstem are cholinergic. Because peripheral vertigo occurs when an imbalance of stimuli from the labyrinthine organs—one operating normally, its counterpart dysfunctional—affects the vestibular processing center in the brainstem, it stands to reason that anticholinergic agents may work by muting this imbalance.

Table 5. Medications for Acute Peripheral Vertigo

MEDICATION	DOSAGE (ADULT)	ROUTE
Meclizine (Antivert)	25-50 mg	PO
Lorazepam	1-2 mg	IV/PO
Diazepam	5 mg	IV/PO
Atropine	0.5 mg	IV
	0.4 mg	Sublingual
Dimenhydrinate (Dramamine)	50 mg	IV/PO
Promethazine (Phenergan)	25 mg	PO/IM
	12.5 mg	IV
Prochlorperzine (Compazine)	10 mg	IV/IM

There is anecdotal literature support, however, for a wide variety of other medications for the treatment of peripheral vertigo symptoms, include benzodiazepines, dimenhydrinate (Dramamine), trimethobenzamide (Tigan), procholorperazine (Compazine), promethazine (Phenergan), and chlorpromazine (Thorazine). A recent study from Germany suggests that the calcium channel antagonist, flunarizine, also may be an effective drug for the suppression of vertigo.[27]

The most commonly used agent to treat vertigo is oral meclizine, with benzodiazepines and phenothiazines being the next most common agents, especially when the parenteral route is necessary due to protracted vomiting. There is a lack of clinical trials comparing the effectiveness of these commonly used antivertigo agents.

If, upon clinical grounds, the patient is found to have true peripheral vertigo, characterized by episodic whirling sensations brought on by changes in head position and often accompanied by nausea and nystagmus, and if there are no neurological deficits, and if the patient is in good underlying health and has an appropriate degree of help at home-discharge from the ED can be accomplished once the symptoms are controlled and the patient can ambulate. The majority of episodes of peripheral vertigo are self-limited (e.g., labyrinthitis, BPV, Meniere's) and most patients do well at home with symptomatic treatment including vestibular exercise therapy.[2,20]

But if two hours of treatment and observation in the ED fail to bring remarkable relief, the patient should be admitted for bed rest, nursing care, parenteral medication, and possible consideration of further evaluation, including neurologic consultation, CT scan, or MRI.

When patients with peripheral vertigo are discharged, the question of follow-up must be adequately addressed. Otolaryngologists and neurotologists can use a number of specialized testing modalities (such as pure tone audiometry, typanometry, stapedius reflex testing, electronystagmography, etc.) to localize the anatomic site of a peripheral vertigo process. But to automatically refer each patient with peripheral vertigo to an otolaryngologist is unnecessary.

The ideal follow-up situation includes re-evaluation by the primary care physician, who can keep track of the patient's condition and arrange further evaluation if the patient does not improve.

Table 6. Causes of Central Vertigo
Cerebellopontine angle tumors (majority are acoustic neuromas)
Vertebral-basilar circulation vascular events
Vestibular nuclei area TIA or stroke
Cerebellar infarction or hemorrhage
Lateral medullary infarct (Wallenberg's syndrome)
Multiple sclerosis
Complex partial seizures (temporal lobe epilepsy)
Migraine with vertiginous symptoms
Post raumatic brainstem injury (postconcussive syndrome)
Infections (meningitis, encephalitis)

Accurate Identification of Patients with Central Vertigo

Central vertigo is a more serious condition and when suspected, warrants the initiation of a work-up. This work-up can be performed either on an inpatient or outpatient basis, depending upon the severity of illness and the adequacy of the patient's ability to follow-up with the necessary arrangements. It would be preferable to admit a patient with central vertigo of a suspicious nature who is not acutely ill, than to lose them to follow-up. The causes are numerous and include acoustic neuromas (schwannomas), multiple sclerosis, and brainstem and cerebellar infarcts or hemorrhages. *(Please see Table 6.)* The classic clinical presentation of an acoustic neuroma is a gradual onset of hearing changes followed by chronic vertigo and additional cranial nerve deficits.[17]

Although clinicians usually can differentiate between central and peripheral vertigo, infarcts or hemorrhages in certain areas in and near the brainstemespecially the cerebellummay cause an abrupt onset of intense, positional whirling vertigo with nystagmus and produce a clinical picture that closely resembles peripheral vertigo. However, there invariably will be neurological deficits when this occurs.[28-30] The physician should check carefully for truncal and limb (finger-to-nose) ataxia, or the presence of other cranial nerve deficits. If cerebellar involvement is suspected, an urgent CT scan with thin slices of the posterior fossa or MRI (the better choice if available) is indicated.

If a cerebellar infarct is misdiagnosed as peripheral vertigo and the patient is discharged home, serious deterioration can occur secondary to delayed cerebellar edema in the posterior fossa;[10] hence the importance of a good neurological examination.

TIAs of the labyrinth should be suspected in older patients with acute onset of non-positional vertigo lasting minutes. These episodes should be considered peripheral veriebro-basilar TIAs, just as amaurosis fugax episodes are for the anterior circulation.

If a TIA affecting the vestibular system is suspected in any given patient based upon the clinical criteria described above, the patient should be considered a candidate for admission, neurological consultation, and probably should receive a CT or MRI to rule out other posterior fossa processes such as a small brainstem hemorrhage or infarct, particularly if symptoms persist or increase.

All patients with a suspected central etiology for their dizziness will require further work-up. Because the hallmarks of the classic presentation of central vertigo include a chronic indolent course with symptoms evolving slowly over months (with the exception of acute brainstem vascular events), many patients with central vertigo can receive outpatient work-ups, assuming they are completely stable and reliable follow-up can be arranged before their discharge from the ED. But, if there is any question that a patient might be lost to follow-up, admission may be needed and the work-up should probably begin in the ED with a CT scan including thin cuts of the posterior fossa, or an MRI if feasible, and ideally a neurological consultation.

When central vertigo arises from a brainstem vascular event such as a hemorrhage or infarct, these imaging studies and admission become mandatory.

Central vertigo is seldom the presenting symptom of a patient with a central nervous system infection (meningitis or encephalitis), but such a scenario is possible. If fever is present and imaging studies are negative, a lumbar puncture is indicated. Nuchal rigidity is not present with encephalitis.[10]

Approach to the Patient with Syncope

The word syncope is synonymous with fainting, and denotes a transient loss or near-loss (pre-syncope) of consciousness. Unlike vertigo, syncope is an objective sign as well as a symptom. Both syncope and pre-syncope share the same list of causes, and have an etiologic profile distinct from that of vertigo. However, patients with syncope and vertigo may present with a similar chief complaints—"dizziness."[31]

One study suggests that as many as 3% of all ED visits may be related to syncope and pre-syncope, and that no definite cause ultimately can be discovered in at least half of these cases.[32] Nonetheless, the initial task for the emergency physician is to determine if the underlying cause of the episode represents an acute life-threatening process. *(Please see Table 7.)*

The most important issue for the emergency physician is to identify patients who might have cardiac disease or hypovolemia as a cause of syncope. Patients with cardiac syncope have been convincingly demonstrated to be at increased risk for mortality during the year following the syncopal event.[33] Rhythm disturbances—sinoatrial disease, high-grade AV blocks, ventricular and supraventricular tachycardias—are among the most frequent reasons for cardiac syncope.[32] Half of all pacemakers in the United States are implanted in patients with sinoatrial disease, initially manifested as "dizziness" or syncope.[34]

The majority of syncopal patients will have fainted from a neurovascular etiology, most commonly the "vasovagal reflex" (neurally mediated hypotension and bradycardia).[35] A history of the event often reveals predisposing circumstances and prodromal symptoms including nausea, a sense of "graying-out," becoming diaphoretic.[32]

Another important consideration in the ED evaluation is to distinguish a syncopal episode from a seizure. Because the mechanism of syncope is for the brain to become relatively hypoxic, 2-3 beats of tonic-clonic activity occasionally is observed. A syncopal episode is usually briefer and the seizurelike activity much slighter than with a tonic-clonic epileptic seizure. Additionally, the patient should not have a post-ictal phase after syncope, but rather should become alert as soon as the fainting spell resolves.

Table 7. Causes of Syncope and Pre-Syncope

Neurovascular
Vasovagal
Postural hypotension
Post-micturation
Post-tussive
Post-prostate exam
Deglutitional syncope
Breath-holding syncope
Carotid body hypersensitivity
Stroke and transient ischemic attack
Cardiovascular
Dysrhythmias
Myocardial infarction
Valvular heart disease
Atrial myxoma
Structural (e.g., IHSS)
Miscellaneous
Hyperventilation
Panic disorder
Hypoglycemia

Clinical Evaluation. There is no single best method for evaluating patients with syncope. At best, only 25% will receive a definitive diagnosis during ED evaluation and observation.[36] Of those patients ultimately referred to a syncope clinic for in-depth evaluation, 24% in one series received psychiatric diagnoses, usually "panic attack." Compared with patients with cardiac syncope, these patients tended to be younger, had a higher frequency of prodromal symptoms, and had more frequent syncopal episodes.

For young and otherwise healthy patients who have a brief syncopal episode with rapid return to full consciousness and who had a clearly identifiable precipitating stressor and experienced the usual prodrome of nausea, lightheadedness, and diaphoresis—and especially if this patient has a history of similar episodes under similar conditions—then laboratory testing is probably not necessary. The patient can be discharged after a brief observation period including cardiac monitoring, orthostatic vital signs, and a pregnancy test for childbearing-age females.

Most syncopal patients, however, do not present with such classic stories; a high percentage of syncopal patients will be elderly, have major underlying medical problems, or will have atypical features (no prodrome, for example) that mandate further work-up. A full syncopal work-up, which is beyond the scope of ED care, may include continuous cardiac monitoring, CT scan, complete blood work, toxicologic screens, echocardiography, carotid doppler studies and an EEG. Some guidelines to help the clinician decide what degree of work-up will be needed for any given patient and in what setting it should be conducted are:

• Elderly patients generally should be considered for admission for their syncope work-up. They are at high epidemiologic risk for syncope due to dysrhythmias and for injuries related to falling.

• Patients with pre-existing cardiac disease and a new syncopal episode should be admitted for observation and monitoring. This would include patients with a history of major arrhythmias. The minimal ED work-up of these patients includes an ECG and cardiac monitoring while in the ED. An external pacemaker should be applied when such patients display bradycardic rhythms or high-degree heart blocks in the ED.

• Patients who do not fall into the preceding categories (i.e., are relatively young and do not have major cardiac problems) and who do not have obvious signs of having experienced a cerebrovascular event, but who cannot be readily placed into the category of a vasovagal-type syncope, clearly need further work-up, perhaps even the full diagnostic regimen described above. These patients will occasionally turn out to have unusual causes for their syncope, such as brain masses or atrial myxoma. If definite follow-up can be arranged by the emergency physician and the patient is reliable, most of the work-up can be conducted on an outpatient basis after the patient has received routine laboratory studies and an ECG in the ED. But if the patient may be lost to follow-up, prudence would dictate consideration for admission in order to complete the work-up in a definite and time-efficient manner.

References

1. Oosterveld W. Current diagnostic techniques in vestibular disorders. *Acta Otolargyngol* (Stockh) 1991;479:29-34. Supplement.
2. Sloane P. Dizziness in primary care: Results from the National Ambulatory Medical Care Survey. *J Fam Prac* 1989;29:33-38.
3. Kroenke K, Mangelsdorff A. Common symptoms in ambulatory care: Incidence, evaluation, therapy, and outcome. *Am J Med* 1989;86:262-266.
4. Skiendzielewski H, Martyak G. The weak and dizzy patient. *Ann Emerg Med* 1980;9:353-56.
5. Herr R, Zun L, Mathews J. A Directed approach to the dizzy patient. *Ann Emerg Med* 1989;18:664-672.
6. Little N. Vertigo and Dizziness. In: Tintinalli J, Krome R, Ruiz E, eds. *Emergency Medicine: A Comprehensive Study Guide*, 3rd ed. New York:McGraw-Hill Inc.;1992:799-803.
7. Drachman D, Hart C. An approach to the dizzy patient. *Neurol* 1972;22:323-334.
8. Jeunne C, Hugues F, Munera Y, et al. Dizziness in the elderly and calcium channel antagonists. *Biomed & Pharmacother* 1991;45:33-36.
9. Cutter F, Balch R. Migraine-associated dizziness. *Headache* 1992;32:300-304.
10. Daroff R. Dizziness and Vertigo. In: Wilson J, Braunwald E, Isselbacher K, et al, eds. *Harrison's Principle of Internal Medicine*, 12th ed. New York: McGraw-Hill, Inc.; 1991: 140-142.
11. Cohen N. The dizzy patient: Update on vestibular disorders. *Med Clin North Am* 1991;75:1251-1260.
12. Baloh R. Dizziness in older people. *JAGS* 1992;40:713-721.
13. Williams P, Warwick R, Dyson M, et al. *Gray's Anatomy*, 37th ed. Edinburgh: Churchill Livingstone; 1989:1229-1243.
14. Ura W, Pfaltz C, Allum J. The effect of age on the visuo- and vestibulo-ocular reflexes of elderly patients with vertigo. *Acta Otolaryngol* (Stockh) 1991;481:399-402. Supplement.

15. Luxon L. Disturbances of balance in the elderly. *Br J Hosp Med* 1991;41:22-26.
16. Paparella M, Alleva M, Bequer N. Dizziness. *Prim Care* 1990;17:299-308.
17. Adams R, Victor M. *Principles of Neurology*, 5th ed. New York: McGraw-Hill Inc.;1993:247-269.
18. Sloane P, Baloh R. Persistent dizziness in geriatric patients. *JAGS* 1989;37:1031-1038.
19. Warner E, Wallach P, Adelman H, et al. Dizziness in primary care patients. *J Gen Int Med* 1992;7:454-463.
20. Froehling D, Silverstein M, Mohr D, et al. Benign positional vertigo: Incidence and prognosis in a population-based study in Olmsted County, Minnesota. *Mayo Clin Proc* 1991;66: 596-601.
21. Shutty M, Dawdy L, McMahon M, et al. Behavioral treatment of dizziness secondary to benign positional vertigo following head trauma. *Arch Phys Med Rehab* 1991;72:473-476.
22. Epley J. The canalith repositioning procedure for treatment of benign paroxysmal positional vertigo. *Otol H N Surg* 1992;107:399-403.
23. Parties L, McClure J. Posterior semicircular canal occlusion in the normal hearing ear. *Otol H N Surg* 1991;104:52-57.
24. Stable J, Friberg U, Svedberg A. Long-term progression of Meniere's disease. *Acta Otolaryngol* (Stockh) 1991;485:78-83. Supplement.
25. Adams R, Victor M. *Principles of Neurology*, 5th ed. New York: McGraw-Hill; 1993:704.
26. Aantaa E: Treatment of acute vestibular vertigo. *Acta Otolaryngol* (Stockh) 1991;479:44-47. Supplement.
27. Schmidt R, Oestreich W. Flunarizine in the treatment of vestibular vertigo: Experimental and clinical data. *J Cardiovasc Pharmacol* 1991;18(Suppl 8):S27-S30.
28. Mazagri R, Shuaib A, Denath F. Medullary hemorrhage causing vertigo and gaze nystagmus. *ENT J* 1992;71: 402-403.
29. Millikan C, Futrell N. Vertigo of vascular origin. *Arch Neurol* 1990;47:12-13.
30. Grad A, Balch R. Vertigo of vascular origin: Clinical and electronystagmographic features in 84 Cases. *Arch Neurol* 1989;46:28184.
31. Sloane P, Linzer M, Pontinen M, et al. Clinical significance of a dizziness history in medical patients with syncope. *Arch Intern Med* 1991;151:1625-1628.
32. Benditt D, Remole S, Milstein S, et al. Syncope: Causes, clinical evaluation, and current therapy. *Anna Rev Med* 1992;43:283-300.
33. Brignole M, Menozzi C, Gianfranchi L, et al. Carotid sinus massage, eyeball compression, and head-up tilt test in patients with syncope of uncertain origin and in healthy control subjects. *Am Heart J* 1991;122:1644-1651.
34. Bass E, Elson J, Fogoros R, et al. Long-term prognosis of patients undergoing electrophysiologic studies for syncope of unknown origin. *Am J Cardiol* 1988;62:1186-1191.
35. Parsonnet V, Berstein A, Galasso D. Cardiac pacing practices in the US in 1985. *Am J Cardiol* 1988;62:71-77.
36. Wilson A. Syncope. In: Tintinalli J, Krome R, Ruiz E, eds. *Emergency Medicine: A Comprehensive Study Guide*, 3rd ed. New York: McGraw-Hill Inc.; 1992:141-143.

Headache

Richard Caesar, MD, FACEP

The pearls and pitfalls of acute headache management are legendary in emergency medicine. Few clinical problems, in fact, are so agonizing for both patient and physician. After all, the presentation of acute headache can be either subtle or dramatic, the consequences life-threatening or benign. And the pressures to provide cost-effective care—especially as it relates to appropriate use of neuroimaging procedures and drug therapy—have mounted with the growth of managed care.

This is not an easy group of patients. Perhaps more than any other subset of clinical encounters, individuals who present to the emergency department (ED) with severe headache are given to vivid, anxiety-provoking imagery: "It was as if someone jammed a white-hot poker through my eyebrow," and "My temples feel like they are being squeezed in a vise," are typical accounts. In particular, patients with headache caused by migraine, subarachnoid hemorrhage (SAH), and other intracranial catastrophes frequently describe their symptoms as "the worst pain of my life." There is a sense of no possible escape. Add to this scenario a symptom complex consisting of nausea accompanied by the sudden appearance of unexplainable neurologic symptoms, and the formula for abject misery is complete.

From the emergency physician's perspective, the clinical challenge of assessment, treatment, and disposition frequently is no less painful. The differential diagnosis is complex, ranging from migraine, tension, and cluster headaches to drug-induced causes, intracranial hemorrhage, and toxic exposures.

Although patient histories and etiologies are variable, management of these patients often comes down to this: "To CAT scan or not to CAT scan—that is the question." The fact is, a chronic migraine sufferer can develop an SAH, and a previously healthy teenager can present with a meningioma. Which patients, then, should be scanned and tapped? Which can be reassured and treated? And who should be referred for drug counseling and pain management programs?

This chapter characterizes the etiologies of acute headache to provide a framework for assessment and management of these patients in the ED. A detailed approach to differential diagnosis and therapeutic strategies for cost-effective management of headaches are presented.

Epidemiology

Approximately three out of four Americans experience a non-traumatic headache each year, although only 5% of these individuals seek medical attention for this condition.[1] Combined causes of headache produce 18 million patient visits yearly in this country and are responsible for 30 million days of lost productivity costing 12 billion dollars annually.[2] Not surprisingly, migraine remains the most common reason for seeking headache care in the emergency setting, although tension headaches are five times more common in the general population.[3]

The prevalence and etiology of headache vary considerably with

Figure 1. Assessing and Managing Patients With Traumatic vs. Non-Traumatic Headaches

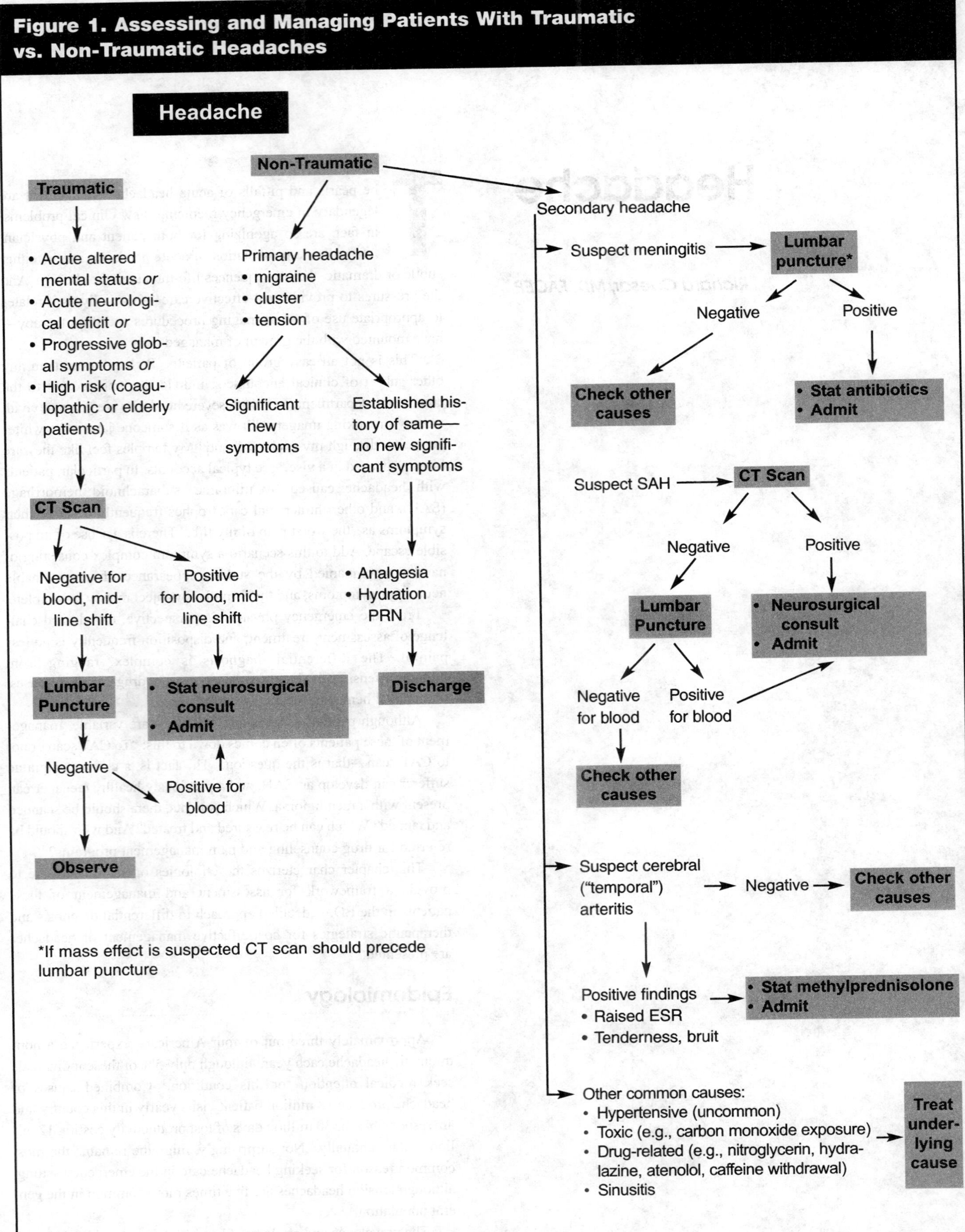

age and gender. For example, primary headaches (e.g., migraine, cluster, tension) decline with age, while headaches secondary to other conditions (e.g., temporal arteritis or lesions with mass effect) increase with age.[3] With respect to gender, female migraineurs outnumber males 2.5 to 1, while in the case of cluster headache, males outnumber females 10 to 1.[4]

Clinical Categorization

From a practical perspective, the emergency physician should categorize patients by distinguishing traumatic from non-traumatic headaches. *(Please see Figure 1.)*

Post-Traumatic Headache. For the patient with post-traumatic—as well as non-traumatic—headache, the development of any new neurologic deficit, including altered mental status and progressive global symptoms (agitation, fatigue, disorientation, dizziness), requires prompt computed tomography (CT) scanning. The indications for CT scanning in patients with vague neurological symptoms and soft findings is controversial. Since 10-20% of SAHs in this setting can be missed on CT, a lumbar puncture (LP) checking for red blood cells (RBCs) in the cerebrospinal fluid (CSF)—or, for xanthochromia in less recent injuries—is frequently recommended for patients with negative CT findings.[5-7] Patients with either positive CT findings or abnormal LP require prompt neurosurgical consultation and admission.

Non-Traumatic Headache. Non-traumatic headaches are conceptually divided into primary and secondary etiologies. As a rule, patients with primary headaches (those with established histories of migraine, cluster, or tension headache) in whom presenting complaints are not significantly different from previous attacks may be treated symptomatically and released.

In contrast, non-traumatic secondary headaches can result from a wide variety of etiologies, many of which require immediate evaluation and therapy. For example, the patient with fever, chills, neck stiffness, and leukocytosis will require an LP to rule out meningitis. In contrast, the appearance of a sudden, excruciating headache, noted as the patient's "first or worst headache ever," is suspicious for SAH. Immediate CT scanning is mandatory; however, if the scan is negative and the index of suspicion for SAH is still high, most experts recommend an LP to rule out the diagnosis.[5-7]

Patients 30 years of age or older who present with a new and unexplained persistent headache, with or without neurologic deficits, should be considered for urgent CT to rule out tumor, unruptured arteriovenous malformation (AVM), pseudotumor cerebri, or abscess. Temporal arteritis usually presents as a new- or recent-onset localized headache in a patient older than 50 (particularly women). Clinical findings include temporal artery tenderness, bruit or diminished pulse, and an elevated erythrocyte sedimentation rate (ESR). These patients require admission for high-dose corticosteroids and observation to prevent such grave complications as unilateral blindness.

The History

An accurate, detailed history is the most important part of evaluating the acute headache patient. The five principal areas to be covered in the headache history are: 1) medication and recreational drug use; 2) duration; 3) location; 4) character; and 5) precipitating factors. Characteristic findings associated with each of these historical areas can guide the clinician toward a specific diagnosis that can be confirmed with noninvasive radiographic, toxicological, or laboratory studies.

Medication History. A careful and detailed medication history, including both prescribed and recreational agents that have been used or recently terminated, should be obtained, since headache is among the most common side effects associated with drug therapy. Otherwise normal individuals with the history of recent cessation of daily caffeine ingestion (as little as 2 cups of coffee a day), may develop severe migraine-like pain after 24-48 hours of abstinence. Administration of Cafergot, or even a double espresso, is diagnostic and therapeutic.

A number of prescribed medications may elicit headache as a side effect. Common offenders include nitroglycerin, hydralazine, calcium-channel blockers, digitalis, and estrogen. Recreational drugs such as nicotine, alcohol, marijuana, and amphetamines can also induce headache. Finally, patients with prolonged exposure to automobile exhaust, fire, faulty heating equipment, and certain paint removers will complain of headache as the earliest symptom of carbon monoxide poisoning. Treatment includes 100% O_2 via mask—or, when indicated, endotracheal intubation—and hyper baric oxygen in severe cases.

Duration. With respect to duration, symptoms that have persisted for many weeks or even months should suggest muscle-contraction/ tension headache, while intense, episodic pain with symptom-free intervals suggests a vascular (migraine or cluster) etiology. The story of a new headache worsening over a four- to six-week period is suspicious for raised intracranial pressure (ICP), which is most commonly due to mass effect (e.g., tumor). In contrast, a patient with a headache characterized by sudden, severe, unprecedented pain of short duration, with or without neurologic deficit, should be investigated for ruptured aneurysm or SAH. The patient who awakens with a headache should be evaluated for hypertensive, cluster, or neoplastic headache, whereas the headache that begins later and worsens as the day progresses is more likely to be tension in origin. Headache that occurs in the setting of diastolic blood pressure greater than 130 mmHg should be considered a manifestation of hypertensive encephalopathy and treated accordingly with pharmacotherapeutic maneuvers aimed at immediate reduction of blood pressure.

Location. Location of the headache is occasionally useful for making an etiologic diagnosis. Unilateral headache suggests a migraine, whereas a headache that progresses from a unilateral to bilateral location (usually bitemporal) may be due to raised ICP.[5] Lesions on the falx or other midline structures tend to cause unilateral eye pain, and cerebellopontine angle tumors produce pain behind the ear. A reasonably valid generalization states that headache due to a mass causes ipsilateral pain, while pain due to a vascular lesion is contralateral to the lesion.[5] Pain that is localized to the back of the neck, with radiation up the occiput, should suggest tension headache.

Character. Characterization with respect to intensity may vary from patient to patient, but a description of the quality of the pain can be useful. "Bursting" or "exploding" pain, especially when associated with bending forward, coughing, or Valsalva maneuver, is suspicious for raised ICP. A pulsatile headache that correlates with the pulse usually indicates a vascular etiology, while a pulsatile or throbbing cephalgia not correlated with the pulse is non-specific.

Table 1. Drug Treatment of Migraine

TYPE OF DRUG	RECOMMENDED DOSAGE	TIME TO PEAK PLASMA CONCENTRATION	IMPORTANT SIDE EFFECTS
Analgesic			
Aspirin	500-650 mg	1 hour	Dyspepsia, gastrointestinal hemorrhage
Acetaminophen	500 mg	1 hour	Dyspepsia
Propoxyphene	65 mg	1 hour	Addiction
Codeine	60 mg	1 hour	Addiction, constipation
NSAID			
Naproxen sodium	750-825 mg	1-2 hours	NSAIDs can cause dyspepsia, gastric erosions and ulcerations, renal insufficiency, and asthma in susceptible individuals.
Tolfenamic acid	200-400 mg	1-2 hours	
Flufenamic acid	250-400 mg	1-2 hours	
Mefanamic acid	500 mg	1-2 hours	
Flurbiprofen	300 mg	1-2 hours	
Diclofenac sodium	50-100 mg	1-2 hours	
Ibuprofen	200 mg	1-2 hours	
Ketorolac (IM)	30-60 mg	0.5-1.0 hour	
Serotonin receptor agonist			
Ergotamine			
Oral	2-4 mg	1-2 hours	Nausea, vomiting, abdominal pain, diarrhea, muscle cramps, limb paresthesia, vasoconstriction
Suppository	2 mg	0.5-2.0 hours	Same as above
Sublingual	2-4 mg	—	Same as above
Dihydroergotamine (SQ)	0.75-1.0 mg	0.25-0.5	Same as for ergotamine, but less severe
Sumatriptan			
Subcutaneous	6 mg	0.25 hours	Flushing, heat, tingling, neck pain, chest heaviness, pressure, pain
Oral	100 mg	1.5 hours	Same as above
Dopamine antagonist			
Metoclopramide (IV)	10 mg	< 0.25 hours	Dystonia
Chlorpromazine (IV)	0.1 mg/kg	< 0.25 hours	Tardive dyskinesia
Prochlorperazine (IV)	10 mg	< 0.25 hours	Tardive dyskinesia

Adapted from: Hoffert MJ. Treatment of migraine: A new era. *Am Fam Physician* 1994;49:1951.

Steady, constant, diffuse pain is unlikely to be vascular. Sharp, lancinating pain across the face may represent trigeminal neuralgia (e.g., tic doloreaux). When behind the eye, it may be a manifestation of cluster headache. A dull, constant, constricting, band-like occipitofrontal pain is characteristic of a tension headache. Any change in headache pattern, or the presence of a unilateral headache that never changes sides ("side-locked headache"), or the occurrence of neurologic symptoms during the headache rather than preceding its onset (as would be typical of migraine aura) demands neuroimaging.[6]

Precipitating Factors. When a correlation is noted between headache and turning the head, coughing, or bending forward, mass effect should be considered. Headache associated with stress, sleep deprivation, menstrual cycle, hunger, specific types of food ingestion, or contraceptive (or other estrogen) usage suggests migraine.

Finally, any history of head trauma (recent or remote) warrants careful evaluation. The relationship between a traumatic event and neurological symptoms and complaints may be obvious in many cases. However, elderly patients in particular may present with little more than a mild headache, confusion, lethargy, or personality change as the only manifestations of subacute or chronic subdural hematoma resulting from a fall several days or weeks earlier. Consequently, only aggressive pursuit of the history and a high index of suspicion will avert misdiagnosis in such cases.

Physical Examination

General Features. Physical assessment of the headache patient includes palpation and percussion of the sinuses, teeth, temporomandibular joints (TMJs), pericranial, and paracervical muscles. Nuchal rigidity suggests meningeal irritation, which may reflect either infectious or hemorrhagic etiologies. In older patients, the superficial temporal arteries should be palpated for tenderness in order to rule out temporal arteritis. An exquisitely tender, erythematous, papulovesicular rash of the scalp, face, or neck that does not cross the midline is likely herpes zoster. (Not uncommonly, the pain and tenderness will precede the rash by several days.) Severe headache, vomiting, visual changes, and an injected sclera are the hallmarks of acute glaucoma, and may closely mimic migraine, unless this diagnosis is considered and the eyes are evaluated for signs of elevated intraocular pressure.

Neurologic Examination. Thorough mental status, cranial nerve, sensorimotor, skull, spine, and cerebellar examinations are mandatory for evaluation of the patient who presents with acute headache. The presence of new focal neurologic deficits, seizures (focal or generalized), or cognitive impairments should suggest the need for immediate imaging studies. Fundoscopic assessment may reveal papilledema and supply the only finding suggestive of increased ICP and its associated conditions. Similarly, acute ischemic or hemorrhagic cerebrovascular disease may present with little more than a headache and visual field defects (as do migraine headaches). The patient's age, history, risk factors, and the timing of the field defects in relation to the pain become critical in distinguishing the two etiologies (i.e., visual auras in migraine generally precede the headache and subside with its onset, whereas the headache of an ischemic event has no predictable pattern in relation to visual symptoms). Ophthalmoplegia is a rare symptom of migraine. The ophthalmoplegia of peripheral unilateral third- or bilateral sixth-nerve palsy, which can occur with intracranial mass lesions and with which it may be confused, is a manifestation of increased ICP, tonsillar herniation, or cerebral aneurysm.[8]

Migraine

General Features. Depending on the institution surveyed, approximately 2-6% of all patients seeking care at EDs have headache as their primary complaint, and 22% of these cases will have migraine.[9] The primary clinical manifestations include headache, photophobia, and nausea with or without vomiting. Generally speaking, migraine headache is an affliction of young and middle-aged individuals, with 80% of patients having had their first attack before age 30.[3] A significant majority of patients reflect a familial predisposition. About 75% of migraine headaches occur without auras (common migraine), while 20% occur with an aura (classic migraine).[3] Less than 5% are so-called migraine variants, which include hemiplegic and ophthalmoplegic varieties, as well as the painless migraine sine cephalgia, a group that usually requires a neurologist and brain imaging to confirm the diagnosis.[10]

Aura. The aura of a classic migraine usually is characterized by sensory—most often visual—symptoms. These range from haziness to shimmering heat waves, to bright or dark holes in the visual field, to frank hemianopia. Apparent distortion of body size or other visual illusions (metamorphopsia) also may occur. Sensory symptoms consist of tingling paresthesias of the face or upper extremity. Legs and trunks are seldom involved.[11] In the majority of cases, the aura is replaced by the full-blown migraine headache, usually within 30 minutes, but sometimes after as long as several hours. In almost all cases, the neurologic deficit is fully reversible, but in rare cases of ophthalmoplegic or retinal migraine, repeated episodes of vasospasm-induced ischemia will produce infarction, accompanied by a permanent neurological deficit.

Pain Characteristics. The headache itself is paroxysmal, often unilateral at onset, and often associated with nausea and vomiting. Along with the cephalgia of cluster and SAH, migraine pain is the most severe of headache pain syndromes. Because migraine headaches almost always begin in childhood or adolescence, the onset of a "new" or "different" headache with migrainous features beginning in a patient more than 35 years of age strongly suggests an alternative diagnosis. The pain of migraine may occur anywhere in the head or face, but is most common over one or both temples. Like the headache of malignant arterial hypertension and that of SAH, migraine pain is throbbing and pulsatile, as opposed to the steady ache of meningitis and brain tumor or the "constricting band" of the tension headache.[1]

Whereas the headache of brain tumor and those caused by post-lumbar "spinal headaches" are exacerbated by sitting or standing, the reverse is true for migraine. In addition, migraine headache is typically precipitated by stress, fatigue, under- or oversleeping, seasonal patterns, fasting, and exercise (e.g., "footballer's migraine" and "coital cephalgia"). A wide variety of foods have been implicated as triggers, particularly high-tyramine-content red wines and certain cheeses. Interestingly, the pre-menstrual state is a common trigger, while pregnancy often results in remission. Those suffering from migraines tend to be irritable and withdrawn, avoiding company and responsibility. Thus it is said that while the tension headache patient will accept attention and care, the migraineur just wants to be left alone.[1]

Migraine Variants. Although hemiplegic migraine is uncommon, knowledge of this clinical subtype may help avoid lengthy, superfluous consultations and unnecessary diagnostic workups. When observed in the setting of migraine, hemiplegia is actually a type of aura and may include motor, sensory, or speech disturbances. By definition, these symptoms last more than one hour and less than one week; neuroimaging is always normal. There is an autosomal dominant inherited form of this syndrome, but unless a family history can be established or the history of previous similar attacks in the patient can be elicited, the presentation of acute headache and hemiparesis will mandate immediate CT evaluation.[12] In the younger patient with a family history of hemiplegic or other migraine with aura, expectant observation coupled with standard migraine therapy is appropriate and full recovery can be expected.

Ophthalmoplegic migraine, a syndrome most commonly seen in children and adolescents, is characterized by transitory paresis of one or more of the extraocular motor cranial nerves (III, IV, VI), which typically occurs at the height of the cephalgia but can persist for days or weeks after the headache ceases. The paresis is unilateral, and the pain is periorbital and ipsilateral to the paresis. Prognosis for recovery is excellent following initial attacks; with recurrent attacks, progressive limitation of extraocular muscle function, probably due to vasospastic microinfarcts of the involved nerves, may occur.[13]

Treatment. *(Please see Table 1.)* Most patients seeking emergency care for migraine have not responded to first- or second-line home treatment: dark, quiet room; nonsteroidal anti-inflammatory drugs (NSAIDs) with or without caffeine; oral ergotamines; oral opiates; and oral or rectal phenothiazines. Although some departments have standardized, critical pathways for management of patients with migraine headaches, most practitioners currently use agents with which they are most familiar and that have been shown to be cost-effective. The principal objective of therapy is to provide prompt, definitive pain relief. Whether this can be accomplished with a narcotic (meperidine plus antiemetics) or non-narcotic agent, the patient should be placed in a quiet, dark room and exposed to minimal stimulation. Antiemetics may or may not be required. The advantages and disadvantages of newer and older agents are discussed below.

Figure 2. DHE-45 Protocol for the Acute Treatment of Migraine

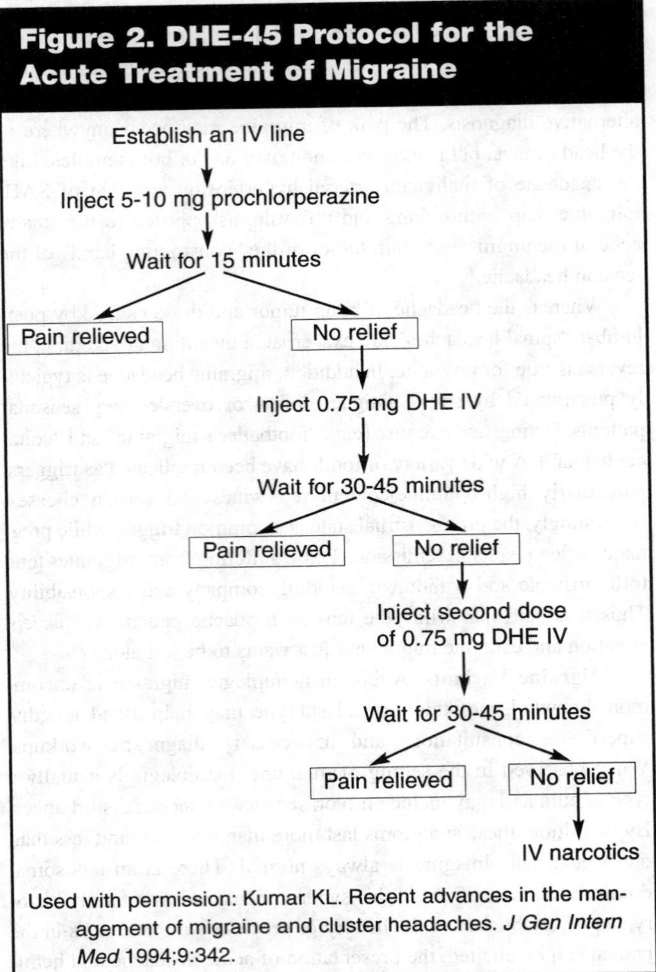

Used with permission: Kumar KL. Recent advances in the management of migraine and cluster headaches. *J Gen Intern Med* 1994;9:342.

Sumatriptan. Sumatriptan is a specific, selective agonist of serotonin receptors on cranial blood vessels. This agent alleviates pain by constricting distended, edematous arteries and by decreasing release of vasoactive peptides which, in turn, minimizes sterile inflammation within involved cerebral vessels.[14] Sumatriptan has no central nervous system (CNS) effects and does not even cross the blood-brain barrier. The standard 6 mg subcutaneous (SQ) dose relieves pain in 77% of patients within one hour of administration and 83% of patients within two hours of administration.[15] Nausea, photophobia, and phonophobia are relieved as well, usually obviating the need for concomitant antiemetics. Its selectivity of receptor site activity explains the relative absence of side effects such as the nausea and peripheral vasoconstriction associated with ergot alkaloids.

Although sumatriptan therapy has played an increasingly important role in the emergency management of migraine headache, its limitations should be recognized. Although its onset of action is more rapid than that of dihydroergotamine (DHE), recurrence of headache within 24 hours is more frequent with sumatriptan, occurring in about 40% of patients treated.[15] While these recurrences are usually milder and respond to a repeat dose of sumatriptan, it has been found that if the initial attack does not respond to sumatriptan treatment, repeat dosing during the initial visit is unlikely to be successful.

The maximum dose consists of two 6 mg injections within 24 hours, with each administration separated by at least an hour. Ergotamines and sumatriptan should not be used within 24 hours of each other in order to prevent prolonged vasospastic episodes resulting from the additive effect of the two drugs.[14] In addition, cautious use in patients with documented cerebrovascular disease is probably warranted. Finally, pharmacy costs are about $30 per injection, which makes this agent among the more expensive options used to treat migraine. Oral sumatriptan (100 mg tablets) will soon be marketed in the United States, and an intranasal spray is currently being investigated.

Sumatriptan kits for patient self-administration are recommended for patients who respond to this pharmacologic agent. Use of these kits may prevent unnecessary ED visits.

DHE-45. As emergency treatment for migraine has moved away from narcotic therapy, there has been renewed interest DHE-45, another serotonin receptor agonist and cranial vasoconstrictor. It has fewer and milder side effects compared with related ergotamine preparations (e.g., Cafergot), although nausea, vomiting, diarrhea, and ischemic symptoms can still be problematic. Overall, it has a 75% success rate and is generally given along with an antiemetic (prochlorperazine or metaclopramide).[16]

One controlled, double-blinded study confirmed that the combination of IV DHE-45 plus IV metaclopramide was consistently more effective than the combination of IV meperidine plus hydroxyzine.[17] *(Please see Figure 2.)* DHE can be administered by the IV, IM, or SQ route. An intranasal form is being used in Europe, although it is less effective than the other routes. As with the other ergotamines, it is contraindicated in patients with coronary disease, peripheral vascular disease, or uncontrolled hypertension. Unlike ergotamine, dependency and rebound phenomena are not seen with DHE-45. The cost of a single dose is $7-10.

Metaclopramide. This is a non-phenothiazine central dopamine antagonist that traditionally has been used as an antiemetic but more recently has been used for migraine therapy. One study demonstrated that 67% of patients had significant relief from one 10 mg IV dose compared with 19% given placebo.[18] The success rate climbs to more than 80% when used in combination with DHE-45. While providing its own analgesic effect, the anti-gastric stasis effect of metaclopramide will enhance the absorption of any concomitantly administered oral medication. There is no rebound or abuse potential, few significant side effects are reported, and the cost is about $4 per therapeutic dose.[14]

Butorphanol Titrate. This is a synthetic, mixed agonist-antagonist analgesic (like nadolol and nalbuphine), with significantly less tolerance and abuse risk compared with standard opiates. Like other mixed agonist-antagonists, it can be given IV, IM, and via metered nasal spray. The standard 2 mg IM dose is equivalent to meperidine 100 mg IM. The cost is approximately $5 per dose of nasal spray.[14]

Phenothiazines. This class of compounds is effective for treatment of both nausea and pain associated with migraine headache. Consequently, phenothiazines can be administered alone or in combination with other drugs. They exert their powerful antiemetic effect via central dopamine blockade of the chemoreceptor trigger zone. These drugs also affect serotonergic, adrenergic, and cholinergic neurotransmitter systems, so their precise mechanism(s) of action on pain and other symptoms remains speculative.[19]

In a meta-analysis of five studies encompassing 336 patients treated for migraine in the emergency setting, both IV chlorpromazine and IV prochlorperazine were more effective than IV meperidine and resulted in fewer side effects.[20] (The chlorpromazine groups were pretreated with normal saline 500 cc IV to prevent postural hypotension.) These agents also were more effective alone than DHE-45 alone, but they were not compared with the DHE-plus-metaclopramide regimen. Consistently better results were seen with IV as opposed to IM administration.[20]

With a success rate of 80-90% (as defined by relief of pain requiring no additional medication), many experts currently recommend chlorpromazine 10 mg IV after pretreatment with 0.5 L of normal saline. The dose can be repeated in 30-60 minutes if needed. As an alternative, prochlorperazine 10 mg IV may be given without saline pretreatment and repeated once after 30 minutes if needed. Extrapyramidal side effects such as akathisia are effectively treated with diphenhydramine 50 mg IV. While phenothiazines are safe, effective, and inexpensive, the necessity for IV access (and, in some cases, saline infusion) may offset their cost savings as compared to sumatriptan.

Most acute, severe migraine patients seeking emergency care will have significant nausea and/or vomiting over the preceding hours or days. Those patients who are volume-depleted should be treated with at least one liter of D_5 LR or D_5 NS. Hydration will potentiate the effectiveness of other agents.

Cluster Headache

Distinct from migraine sufferers, 90% of patients with cluster headaches are male, and there is no familial predisposition.[14] This headache profile is characterized by discrete, daily episodes of excruciating unilateral pain, generally lasting from 30 minutes to 2 hours (average, 45 minutes). The pain usually centers around one orbit and radiates to the ipsilateral frontal, temporal, or mandibular region. Compared with migraine, these headaches are briefer, more focal, more intense, and never associated with aura.

Typically, cluster headaches strike at night, usually commencing an hour or two after sleep. In addition, they often recur at the same time(s) each night ("alarm-clock headache") and there may be tearing and injection of the ipsilateral eye; a transient Horner's syndrome is seen in 25% of cases.[4] The daily clusters generally last from 1-4 months and may recur at the same time annually. In contrast to the withdrawn, subdued migraineur, these patients pace the floor, cry, even bang their heads. Vasodilators, particularly alcohol, can precipitate attacks, and sublingual nitroglycerin administered during the cluster period is a reliable provocative test, although it is rarely performed in the ED. When the ED physician is confident of the diagnosis of cluster headache, treatment should focus on rapid pain relief. All medications shown to be effective in migraine are useful in patients with cluster headache. Although cluster headaches are frequently more painful than migraine, their shorter duration and lack of nausea and vomiting make treatment more straightforward. Sumatriptan or DHE with metaclopramide is an appropriate first-line choice.[14] If these agents fail to provide adequate pain relief, parenteral opiates should be used when appropriate.

Tension Headache

Tension headaches are the most frequent type of headache reported, occurring in up to 78% of the general population.[21] Because it is the least distinct of all headache etiologies, tension headache is often a diagnosis of exclusion. The lack of clinical distinction is reflected

Table 2. Findings on Day of Subarachnoid Hemorrhage from Aneurysmal Rupture

NEUROLOGICAL (1721 CASES)	
Consciousness	
alert	41%
drowsy	32%
stuporous	13%
comatose	14%
Speech	
normal	67%
dysphasic	10%
no verbal response	24%
Orientation	
normal	52%
impaired	48%
Response to commands	
appropriate	66%
inappropriate	34%
Motor response deficit	
normal	69%
mild focal	13%
severe focal	7%
abnormal flexor	3%
abnormal extensor	5%
no response	3%
Meningeal signs	
none	13%
headache	66%
stiff neck	74%
Cranial nerve deficit	
none	87%
third	9%
other	4%

RADIOLOGICAL (1553 CASES)	
Subarachnoid hemorrhage	
diffuse	56%
thin	16%
thick	33%
Intraventricular hemorrhage	20%
Intracerebral hematoma	19%
Hydrocephalus	16%
Mass effect	8%
Aneurysm	5%
Subdural hematoma	2%
Decreased density	1%
Normal	3%

Used with permission: Weir BK. Headaches from aneurysms. *Cephalagia* 1994;14:80.

in the multiplicity of names used to characterize this entity: muscle-contraction headache, psychomyogenic headache, stress headache, ordinary headache, essential headache, idiopathic headache, and psychogenic headache.

Tension headaches are episodic, produce pain that is mild-to-moderate in intensity, and last from minutes to days. The pain is typically "constricting" in character, bilateral in location, and rarely is accompanied by nausea or exacerbated by physical activity. In decreasing order of frequency, the location is frontal, temporal, parietal, and occipital.[22] Anorexia is often present, but nausea is uncommon. On physical examination, manual palpation of pericranial, paracervical, and masticatory muscles may identify trigger points and tender muscle groups,[22] findings that may help rule in the diagnosis.

Finally, it should be stressed that clinical features of tension headache overlap those of most other headache etiologies. In this regard, many experts view tension headache as occupying one pole of a continuum, with classical migraine at the other end.[23,24] However, one investigator goes so far as to state that in patients with either tension headache or migraine, "nausea, throbbing pain, a unilateral distribution, and scalp muscle tenderness all occur at rates predicted only by chance in patients described as having either type of headache. Quantitation of these factors fails to suggest distinct pathophysiologies."[7]

Table 3. Causes of Delay in Referral of 163 Cases to Neurosurgeon After Subarachnoid Hemorrhage from Aneurysmal Rupture

Physician misdiagnosis	**34%**	Hypertensive encephalopathy	6%
Migraine	13%	Cervical myositis	5%
Meningitis	10%	Labyrinthitis	4%
Ischemic stroke	8%	Other*	26%
Myocardial infarction	8%	**Delayed referral policy**	**17%**
Tension headache	7%	**Logistics**	**23%**
Sinusitis	7%	**Patient misdiagnosis**	**12%**
Flu	6%	**Unstable condition**	**7%**
		Other	**6%**

*Other includes brain tumor, eyestrain, alcoholic intoxication, food poisoning, cardiac arrhythmia, syncope, psychiatric illness, epilepsy, morning sickness, hypokalemia, strep throat, low back syndrome, temporal arteritis, and glaucoma.

Used with permission: Weir BK. Aneurysms Affecting the Nervous System. Baltimore: Williams & Wilkins; 1987:82.

Table 4. Headache and Other Patient Chacteristics Predictive of Stroke Subtype

STROKE SUBTYPE	PREDICTOR VARIABLES
Subarachnoid hemorrhage	Onset headache Vomiting Younger age
Intraparenchymal hemorrhage	Onset headache Higher systolic and diastolic blood pressures
Ischemic stroke	Absence of onset headache Absence of vomiting Lower systolic blood pressures Older age

* Determined by stepwise logistic regression analysis

Used with permission: Gorelick P. Headaches in strokes. In: Olsen J, et al, eds. *The Headaches*. New York: Raven Press; 1993:643.

Treatment. The patient who presents to the ED with tension headache is likely to need education and reassurance. If a patient meets the criteria for having tension headache and has no history of trauma, fever, evidence of systemic/metabolic disorder, drug or toxin exposure, and has a normal neurologic exam, the mere act of attention, sympathy, reassurance, and patient education on the part of the physician will often be helpful.[25] When drug therapy is needed, NSAIDs (including aspirin), acetaminophen, and muscle relaxants (in selected patients) will be useful, as may application of moist heat and massage. Sumatriptan, ergotamine, neuroleptics, and barbiturates are contraindicated, and the use of opiates should be avoided.

Subarachnoid Hemorrhage

The pain of SAH is sometimes distinguished from the pain of other cephalgias by its suddenness of onset and severity, which classically results in a scream of pain and, occasionally, an abrupt loss of consciousness. Unfortunately, as with most classical paradigms, the majority of patients will deviate from this profile. SAH is one of the most common causes of sudden death in apparently healthy younger people. The average age of occurrence is 50, with fewer than 10% of cases occurring before age 30.[26] Interestingly, in the first decade of life, males with aneurysms outnumber females 4 to 1.[26] By age 40 the ratio equalizes, and by age 70, females outnumber males 10 to 1.[26] While a majority of cases are due to rupture of an intracranial aneurysm, this condition can also result from trauma, venous thrombosis, blood dyscrasias, and a variety of metabolic conditions.

About one-third of patients with SAH give a history of previous, unusual headache in the past weeks or months ("premonitory leaks").[27] At the time of rupture, two-thirds of patients have some depression of consciousness, one-third have impaired speech, and about half of all cases will have impaired orientation.[27] *(Please see Table 2.)* Commonly, these patients demonstrate confusion, irritability, and even combativeness. Autonomic hyperactivity can include diaphoresis, hypertension, shivering, and episodic hyperventilation. About 75% of patients will have neck stiffness upon presentation, about 15% will present with new-onset seizures, and more than half will develop electrocardiogram changes (prolonged QT, ST elevation or depression, prominent U-waves).[27] The variety of associated signs and symptoms is reflected in documented misdiagnoses on initial presentation observed in one large study of 163 cases.[27] *(Please see Table 3.)*

Approximately 10-20% of SAHs secondary to rupture will be missed on CT scan,[27,28] a false-negative rate that is affected by the location of the bleed and timing of the scan. Because of the risk of tentorial or tonsillar herniation, a CT scan is mandatory prior to LP and CSF examination. In cases where no blood is seen on CT, the absence of shifting or any other mass effect on the scan will make the chances of an LP-induced herniation almost negligible. CSF exam will reveal erythrocytes in acute bleeds, and xanthochromia (from metabolized hemoglobin) will be present for up to one month post-bleed in most cases.[28] For the patient with a suggestive history and physical who demonstrates SAH on CT or LP, four-vessel cerebral angiography is the gold standard for the diagnosis and localization of hemorrhage in preparation for surgical repair (when feasible). In the future, magnetic resonance angiography (MRA) will likely become the procedure of choice.

Headache in Stroke

Headache is frequently an important presenting feature of both ischemic and hemorrhagic stroke, although it is often overshadowed by the presence of sensorimotor and/or cognitive impairment. Headache may precede, accompany, or follow a hemorrhagic or thromboembolic stroke and, on occasion, may be a harbinger of an imminent vascular event.[29] Conversely, the headache may dominate the clinical picture, and a permanent neurologic deficit may be noted only later. Consequently, the frequency of headache in the setting of stroke and any consistent correlation between pain and stroke subtype have been difficult to establish.

Generally speaking, however, the presence of headache is most highly correlated with a large artery, occlusive (thrombotic) stroke. It is reported with intermediate frequency in cerebral embolism and is least common in lacunar infarct.[30] Patients with cortical lesions (on CT) have been found to have headache more often than individuals with deeper infarcts; headache is more common with posterior circulation infarcts as compared with anterior circulation lesions.[31] And while there appears to be no correlation between the location of the pain and the site of the lesion, certain predictive correlations between signs, symptoms, and stroke subtype have been identified. *(Please see Table 4.)*

Post-Lumbar Puncture Headache

Post-LP headache is typically frontal or occipital in location and occurs following 10-30% of all LPs.[32] Usually beginning within 48 hours of the LP, this headache may be associated with nausea, vomiting, dizziness or tinnitus. Invariably, the symptoms improve or disappear upon lying down. The etiology of the pain is persistent leakage of CSF from the dura and consequent traction upon intracranial pain-sensitive structures (e.g., venous sinuses).

Studies have shown that the larger-bore (and smaller-gauge) spinal needles cause larger dural perforations and a higher incidence of headache—a 36% incidence of headache using a 22-gauge needle and a 12% incidence using a 26-gauge needle was observed in one study.[33] Surprisingly, there is no correlation between the volume of CSF withdrawn and the incidence of headache, as long as it is less than 10% of the total CSF volume.[33] The body produces 500 cc of CSF per day, and so the pain is thought to be more related to ongoing hydrostatic shifts from persistent leakage than to the absolute initial volume deficit.

Treatment of post-LP headaches centers around the stabilizing effects of hydration and bedrest. A single 300 mg oral dose of caffeine can also produce symptomatic relief.[34] When conservative measures fail, an epidural blood patch is 90-100% effective.[35] In this procedure, autologous blood is injected epidurally at or around the site of the previous LP, effectively tamponading the dural leak. Since the blood spreads both circumferentially and longitudinally over as many as nine spinal segments, the precision of the second puncture is not critical, so long as the epidural space is injected.

Non-Traumatic Headaches: Miscellaneous Causes

Sinus Headache. The mucosa of all the sinuses and the nose is considered by many rhinologists to be one and the same organ, which reacts as a whole to allergic or inflammatory diseases.[36] In acute sinus headache, the patient presents with purulent nasal discharge, which frequently is associated with fever and leukocytosis. The pain itself is often described as a deep, dull, heavy fullness that is sometimes pulsatile. The pain of maxillary sinusitis pain is localized below the eye, in the gums and teeth of the upper jaw, and occasionally in the temporal region.

Frontal sinusitis is localized across the forehead, sphenoid sinusitis is felt at the vertex and behind the eye, and ethmoid sinusitis results in tenderness of the eyeball(s) and exacerbation of pain with eye movements. Sinus headache is seldom associated with nausea and, while intense, does not reach the degree of pain observed with cluster headache or migraine. Shaking or flexion of the head, coughing, and sneezing exacerbate the pain.[37]

Benign Exertional Headache. Benign exertional headache occurs more frequently in men than women (at a ratio of 4:1) and in individuals more than 40 years of age (at a ratio of 2:1).[38] It may be precipitated by activities such as weightlifting, sneezing, bending, laughing, or swimming, and may even occur during defecation. As a rule, benign exertional headaches are bilateral (but may be unilateral in up to 35% of cases), are prompt in onset, intensely painful, and usually last for a few seconds or minutes.[38] In some patients, the headache may produce a dull, aching pain lasting for a few hours, which may make it difficult to distinguish from potentially serious causes.

The physiological mechanism responsible for these headaches is not entirely clear, but they are believed to result from transient increases in intracranial venous pressure and dilation of venous sinuses with stretching of pain-sensitive intracranial structures. In most cases, reassurance is all that is required. Analgesic use prior to activities that predictably precipitate the headache may also be beneficial.

Benign Cough Headache. This headache is usually bilateral in location and occurs suddenly after a paroxysm of intense coughing. Generally, cough headache is of very brief duration, lasting only a few seconds to minutes (maximum, 10 minutes) with no pain between attacks. There is no associated nausea, vomiting, lacrimation, nasal congestion, or neurological symptoms. The majority of patients with cough headache have a benign course that warrants reassurance, treatment with analgesics, or measures to prevent the cough in order to avert headache.

Headache Associated with Sexual Activity. This headache, which can be precipitated by coitus or masturbation, begins as a dull, bilateral ache as sexual excitement increases and suddenly becomes intense at orgasm in the absence of intracranial pathology. These headaches are believed to be uncommon, although the exact incidence is uncertain because patients may be reluctant to provide detailed sexual histories. They are four times more common in men than women, occur erratically, and are associated with other risk factors such as obesity, hypertension, fatigue, lack of exercise, history of migraine, and peripheral vascular disease. The presence of neurological signs or symptoms in association with these headaches should prompt evaluation for organic causes.

Cold Stimulus Headache. This headache results from either external exposure to cold or ingestion of a cold substance ("ice-cream headache"). The pain is non-pulsatile and reaches a peak intensity about 25-60 seconds after exposure. The great majority of patients with migraine also experience ice-cream headache. No treatment is necessary, and in the case of ice-cream headache, the headache can usually be avoided by stirring the ice cream to a semi-solid consistency.

Toxic Headache

Headaches that are secondary to drugs or environmental exposure are extremely common and often go undiagnosed. Such exposures may generate migraine, tension, hypertensive, or some unspecified variety of headache. Generally speaking, these headaches tend to be generalized, persistent, throbbing, and increase in intensity with increased exposure (or ingestion). With severe exposures, encephalopathy causes consciousness to deteriorate, and these findings may dominate the clinical picture.[39] The drugs most frequently implicated in side-effect headache are vasoactive and do not cross the blood-brain barrier. These are often described as migraine-like in character and include atenolol, nifedipine, cimetidine, ranitidine, and various estrogens.[40] Other commonly implicated substances are discussed in the following sections.

Nitrates/Nitrites. This type of headache correlates with peak vasodilator effect at about three minutes after absorption and disappears roughly 30 minutes later.[41] The pain of nitrate-induced headache is throbbing, bilateral, and sometimes is accompanied by facial flushing. Chemically related medications with similar side effects include dipyridamole, nimodipine, papaverine, and tolazoline.[42] In addition to medications, nitrites in cured meats may bring on the same symptoms (e.g., "hot-dog headache").

Monosodium Glutamate. The monosodium glutamate (MSG)-induced headache associated with the "Chinese-restaurant syndrome" is also throbbing, bifrontal or bitemporal, and begins roughly 20 minutes after ingestion. It is associated with pressure and tightness across the face and chest, dizziness, flushing, nausea, and abdominal discomfort. About one-third of the population is susceptible to the syndrome, which is felt to be secondary to the vasoconstrictor effect of high concentrations of glutamate.[43]

Carbon Monoxide. Chronic mild intoxication in heavy smokers or certain vulnerable individuals in regions of high air pollution is well-established. It results from the inhalation of the byproducts of combustion (especially wood, gasoline, and certain plastics) and is implicated in the morbidity and mortality of fire victims, "closed-garage suicides," and those exposed to faulty heating equipment and certain solvents. The headache is pulsatile and diffuse; nausea, vomiting, and blurred vision accompany the increasingly severe cephalgia until roughly a 30-40% blood CO concentration is reached, at which point obtundation intercedes. Once suspected, the diagnosis is confirmed by measuring venous or arterial CO saturation levels.

Alcohol. Both ingestion of and withdrawal from alcohol can result in headaches, although the latter is more common. After ingestion, the so-called "cocktail headache" is felt to be secondary to interference with cerebral autoregulation and depressed serotonin turnover.[44] The alcohol withdrawal or "hangover" headache usually begins several hours after ingestion, at which point alcohol levels have fallen to near zero. The pain is throbbing, diffuse, and is aggravated by movement of the head and coughing. There is associated nausea, pallor, and irritability; the fact that pilots often find that they get relief from hangovers by inhaling oxygen is consistent with the hypothesis that the syndrome is due to a delay in the metabolic recovery of the redox state modified by alcohol ingestion.[45]

Post-Traumatic Headache

Epidural Hematoma. Classically, the patient with an epidural hematoma has a history of head trauma followed by a brief period of unconsciousness and then a return to normal mental status. Then, after a period of minutes to hours, the hematoma, a result of arterial bleeding, expands and pushes the dura inward. Signs of rising ICP manifest as severe, diffuse, constant headache, pupillary dilatation, hemiplegia, and eventually obtundation as herniation approaches. Unfortunately this "lucid interval" feature is neither sensitive nor specific. Both subdural and intracerebral hemorrhage may generate similar patterns, and up to 20% of patients with epidural hematoma will remain unconscious from the original injury. The condition carries a 25-50% mortality rate largely because of delay in diagnosis.[46]

Subdural Hematoma. This post-traumatic entity is much more common than epidural hematoma and is caused by venous as opposed to arterial bleeding.[46] Since the bleeding is inside the dura, the blood spreads out beneath the dura, giving a broader, convex-outward appearance on CT, as opposed to the more focal, convex-inward bulge of the epidural. Subdural hematoma generally evolves more slowly and, therefore, is less acute in its mass effect than is the epidural. A similar progression of symptoms leading to eventual brainstem herniation may occur, but this process may require as long as two weeks in the case of the subacute form and 2-4 weeks in the chronic variety.

Subarachnoid Hemorrhage (Post-Traumatic). It should be emphasized that post-traumatic SAH is the most common location for bleeding following acute head trauma. The presentation is similar to the spontaneous variety, with stiff neck and other signs of meningeal irritation, but the condition is not usually amenable to surgery.

The headache patient with severe trauma, altered mental status, or a prolonged period of unconsciousness or other neurologic deficit poses little diagnostic dilemma for the emergency clinician. Emergency CT scanning and appropriate neurosurgical consultation are always mandatory. Less dramatic presentations are more problematic, particularly without objective findings. In addition to headache, these patients may complain of forgetfulness, irritability, poor concentration, fatigue, dizziness (usually not vertigo), somnolence, insomnia, anxiety, and other global symptoms.

Unless such complaints are clearly progressive, some authors feel there is little support for the emergent scanning of the neurologically and cognitively intact post-traumatic headache patient.[4] Nonetheless, several warnings need to be emphasized: Intoxicated patients with head injuries must either be scanned immediately or closely observed until their altered status clearly improves. A much lower threshold for scanning patients with hypocoagulable states (e.g., hemophilia, warfarin therapy) must be maintained. The chronic alcoholic must be presumed to be coagulopathic in these circumstances. Finally, an especially low threshold for scanning should be maintained for the elderly patient, in whom the history of head injury may be remote or unclear, the complaints poorly articulated, and the possibility of chronic subdural hematoma more likely.

Summary

A systematic approach to headache assessment can help prevent pitfalls of both "overdiagnosis," with its inappropriate and expensive work-ups, and "underdiagnosis," which can have life-threatening consequences. From a careful history, the basic critical distinctions of traumatic vs. spontaneous, acute vs. chronic, and episodic vs. continuous are established, along with qualitative description of the pain, precipitating factors, and concurrent symptoms. From physical examination a differential diagnosis is generated, and decisions regarding further testing, consultation, and treatment are prioritized.

As a general rule, post-traumatic headache in the absence of both neurologic findings and specific risk factors may be treated symptomatically. Any new neurologic deficit warrants immediate CT evaluation. Nontraumatic headache may be divided into primary etiologies, such as migraine, cluster, or tension, and headaches secondary to other causes (e.g., infectious, toxic, hypertensive). Primary headaches typical of previous episodes may be treated symptomatically, while those with significant new findings (e.g., ptosis, nuchal rigidity) demand immediate investigation.

Secondary headaches demand an aggressive search for underlying causes, including such entities as cerebral arteritis, SAH, or meningitis. Unfortunately, patients with nonspecific, overlapping signs and symptoms, as well as those who are poor historians, frequently do not fall into neat categories. In such cases, the presence of any of the following features should prompt urgent diagnostic evaluation: 1) first or worst headache; 2) a headache associated with fever, nausea, and vomiting that is not explained by systemic (non-CNS) illness; 3) a subacute headache that worsens progressively over days or weeks; 4) a headache associated with new neurologic findings, including sensorimotor deficit, cerebellar signs, or changes in consciousness or cognition. Finally, neurological or neurosurgical consultation is recommended for patients with severe headaches in whom a definitive diagnosis cannot be established.

References

1. Dalessio DJ. Diagnosing the severe headache. *Neurology* 1994;44(suppl 3):S6-S12.
2. Rapoport AM. Update on severe headache. *Neurology* 1994; (suppl 3):S5.
3. Pearce JMS. Cluster headache and its variants. *Postgrad Med J* 1992;68:517.
4. Pearce JMS. Headache. *J Neurol Neurosurg Psychiatry* 1994;57:134-143.
5. Welch KMA. Headache in the emergency room. In: Olesen J, et al, eds. *The Headaches.* New York: Raven Press; 1993: 855-863.
6. Frishberg B. Utility of neuroimagery in headache patients with normal neurologic examinations. *Neurology* 1994;44: 1191-1197.
7. Dalessio DJ, Kudrow L. Treatment of idiopathic headache. In: Bosker G, et al, eds. *Emergency Medicine Desk Reference.* Atlanta: American Health Consultants; 1994:8.59-8.82.
8. Round R, Keane J. The minor symptoms of raised ICP. *Neurology* 1988;38:1461-1464.
9. Baumel B. Migraine: A pharmacologic review. *Neurology* 1994;44 (suppl):13.
10. Stewart WF, Shechter A, Lipton RB. Migraine heterogeneity. *Neurology* 1994;44(6 Suppl 4):S17-S23.
11. Cutler RP. Headache. In: Runenstein E, Federman DD, eds. *Scientific American Medicine*. New York: Scientific American; 1993;11(XI):2.
12. Whitty CW. Familial hemiplegic migraine. In: Rose FC, ed. *Handbook of Clinical Neurology*. Amsterdam: Elsevier; 1986:141-153.
13. Coppetto JR, Lessell S, Sciarra R, et al. Vascular retinopathy in migraine. *Neurology* 1986;36:267-270.
14. Kumar KL. Recent advances in management of migraine and cluster headaches. *J Gen Intern Med* 1994;9:339-348.
15. Plosker GL, McTavish D. Sumatriptan: A reappraisal of its pharmacology and efficacy. *Drugs* 1994;47:622-651.
16. Saddah HA. Abortive headache therapy with IM DHE. *Headache* 1992;32:18-20.
17. Belgrade L, Ling I, Schleevogt MB. Comparison of single dose meperidine, butorphanol, and DHE in treatment of vascular headache. *Neurology* 1989;39:590-592.
18. Tek DS, McClellan D, Olshaker JS. Metaclopramide for the control of migraine in the emergency department. *Ann Emerg Med* 1990;19:1083-1087.
19. Zagami AS. Pathophysiology of migraine and tension headache. *Curr Opin Neurol* 1994;7:272-277.
20. Lipton R. Neuroleptics. In: Olesen J, et al, eds. *The Headaches*. New York: Raven Press; 1993:350.
21. Russwell M, Rasmussen BK. The diagnostic headache diary. *Cephalalgia* 1992;12:369-374.
22. Iversen HK, Langemark M, Andersson PG. et al. Clinical characteristics of migraine and tension-type headaches. *Headache* 1990;30:514-519.
23. Ziegler DK. The headache symptom. How many entities? *Arch Neurol* 1985;23:27-33.
24. Kunkel RS. Tension-type headache: Evaluation and treatment. *Mod Med* 1989;57:60-63.
25. Blanchard EB, Kirsch CA, Applebaum KA, et al. *Management of Chronic Headaches: A Psychological Approach*. New York: Pergamon Press; 1985.
26. Weir BK. *Aneurysms Affecting the Nervous System*. Baltimore: Williams & Wilkins; 1987:74-82.
27. Weir BK. Headaches from aneurysms. *Cephalalgia* 1994;14: 79-87.
28. Leblanc R. The minor leak preceding subarachnoid hemorrhage. *J Neurosurg* 1987;66:35-39.
29. Gorelick PB. Headache in acute cerebrovascular disease. *Neurology* 1986;36:1445-1450.
30. Koudstaal PJ. Headache in transient or permanent cerebral ischemia. *Stroke* 1991;22:754-759.
31. Gorelick PB. Ischemic stroke and intracranial hematoma. In: Olesen J, et al, eds. *The Headaches*. New York: Raven Press; 1993:642.
32. Raskin NH. Lumbar puncture headache: A review. *Headache* 1990;30:197-200.
33. Morgenlander JC. Lumbar puncture and CSF examination. *Postgrad Med* 1994;95:125-131.
34. Camann WR, Murray RS, Mushlin PS. Effects of oral caffeine on postdural puncture headache : A double-blind, placebo-controlled trial. *Anaesth Analg* 1990;70:181-184.
35. Olsen KS. Epidural blood patch in the treatment of post lumbar puncture headache. *Pain* 1987;30:293-301.

36. Ryan RE. Headache of nasal origin. *Headache* 1979;19: 173-176.
37. Saunte C, Soyka D. Headache related to ear, nose and sinus disorders. In: Olesen J, et al, eds. *The Headaches*. New York: Raven Press; 1993:754-755.
38. Indo T, Takahashi A. Swimmer's migraine. *Headache* 1990; 30:485-487.
39. Askmark H, Lundberg P. Drug-related headache. *Headache* 1989;29:441.
40. Atkins FM. A critical evaluation of clinical trials in adverse reactions to foods in adults. *J Allerg Clin Immunol* 1986;78: 174-182.
41. Horowitz LD, Herman MV. Clinical response to nitroglycerine as a diagnostic test for coronary disease. *Am J Cardiol* 1972;29:149-153.
42. Lance JW. Mechanism and Management of Headache. London: Butterworth; 1982:146.
43. Merrit JE, Williams PB. Vasospasm contributes to MSG-induced headache. *Headache* 1990;30:575-580.
44. Altura BM. Alcohol-induced spasm of cerebral blood vessels. *Science* 1983;220:331-333.
45. Ogata S, Hosoi T, Saji H. Studies on acute alcohol intoxication. In: Olesen J, et al, eds. *The Headaches*. New York: Raven Press; 1993:717.
46. Pons P. Head trauma. In: Rosen P, Baker F, et al, eds. *Emergency Medicine*. St. Louis: CV Mosby; 1983:264-280.

Migraine

William B. Ignatoff, MD
Pamela Grim, MD

Migraine headaches were first described more than 4,000 years ago.[15] Aretaeus of Cappadocia gave them the name "hemicrania"[15] (or "heterocrania") in 100 AD, and the current term "migraine" was introduced by Galen 50 years thereafter.[19] They have been described as "a familial disorder characterized by recurrent attacks of headache widely variable in intensity, frequency, and duration. Attacks typically are unilateral and frequently are associated with anorexia, nausea, and/or vomiting. In some cases they are preceded by or associated with neurologic or mood disturbances."[15]

While an "unified theory" of the pathophysiology of migraine has not yet been fully elucidated, some recent findings have produced a new model for the development of migraine headaches. Recent modalities for the acute management of migraines have, therefore, also changed to some extent. While many of the medications currently used for emergency treatment of migraine have been available for many years, there has been a shift in recommendations regarding use of these abortive medications. Moreover, several new agents have been developed in the last decade for acute migraine therapy. Finally, narcotics are not considered agents of choice for management of severe headaches, due to the risks associated with tolerance and dependence.[19] With these clinical issues in focus, this review will discuss recent theories of migraine pathophysiology and diagnosis, and will outline currently available therapeutic options for emergency department (ED) management of migraine headache.

Epidemiology

Headache is the ninth most common chief complaint for which patients visit a physician in the United States;[19] about 40% of Americans suffer from "severe" headaches,[19,20] while 64% suffer "bothersome" headaches at least occasionally.[19] Ten percent of Americans see a doctor episodically for headache relief.[19,20] It is estimated that migraine headaches alone affect approximately 23 million Americans, or about 12% of the population.[20] These estimates vary, with some sources estimating the incidence of migraine at between 5-10%[19] and 15-20%[15] of the population. Up to 90% of the headaches evaluated in emergency and outpatient departments and by primary care physicians are thought to be due to muscle contraction or migraine.[19] There is a significant female predominance among migraine sufferers, with about a 4:1 female to male ratio. There often is a definite relationship between migraine headache frequency and menses; this frequency sometimes decreases (or increases) during pregnancy and after menopause. Migraine headaches often begin in childhood, but they also may be noted first during or after puberty. It is unusual for migraine headaches to start after age 40.[19]

Classification

The once accepted definition of "vascular headaches of the

Table 1. IHS Criteria (1988)

MIGRAINE WITHOUT AURA (COMMON MIGRAINE)

A. Duration 4-72 hours
B. Two or more of the following:
   1. Unilateral location
   2. Pulsating quality
   3. Moderate to severe intensity
   4. Aggravated by routine physical activity
C. At least one of the following:
   1. Nausea and/or vomiting
   2. Photophobia and phonophobia
D. Five or more attacks fitting the above criteria
E. Exclusion of secondary cause of headache

MIGRAINE WITH AURA (CLASSIC MIGRAINE)

A. At least three of the following:
   1. One or more fully reversible aura symptoms indicating brain dysfunction
   2. One aura symptom developing in at least 4 minutes, or two or more symptoms in succession
   3. No aura symptom lasting more than one hour
   4. Headache follows aura within one hour
B. At least two attacks fitting the above criteria
C. Exclusion of secondary cause of headache

AURAS[10,19]

- Positive scotomas (arc of scintillating lights in a herring-bone-like pattern)
- Negative scotomas (blind spots)
- Teichopsia/fortification spectra (luminous appearance before the eyes)
- Photopsia (flashing lights)
- Homonymous visual disturbance
- Unilateral paresthesias/numbness
- Unilateral weakness
- Aphasia/unclassifiable speech difficulty
- Visual or auditory hallucinations
- Diplopia
- Ataxia
- Vertigo
- Syncope
- Hyperosmia

migraine type" was generated by the Ad Hoc Committee on Classification of Headache of the National Institute of Neurologic Disease and Blindness in 1962.[19] It was supplanted in 1988 by the International Headache Society (IHS) criteria, which are more specific and, therefore, ensure consistency in the diagnosis of migraine headaches.[20]

The IHS criteria for diagnosis and classification of migraine headaches are presented in *Table 1*. Common migraines, which account for 80% of all migraine headaches, may have vague prodromes of varying duration; visual changes generally are not associated with common migraines. Photophobia, sonophobia, anorexia, nausea, vomiting, and malaise are frequent findings. Classic migraine, which accounts for 12% of migraine headaches, has a sharply defined prodromal phase, lasting up to one hour prior to the onset of the headache. The most common auras are characterized by temporary, scintillating scotomas or homonymous hemianopsia progressing from the central visual fields to the periphery. Other aura symptoms are listed in Table 1 in the section on IHS criteria for migraine with aura. As with common migraines, classic migraine also is associated with nausea, vomiting, photophobia, and/or sonophobia.[19,20]

Several other migraine variants have been described in the medical literature, although specific inclusion criteria and classification scales have not been developed for their diagnosis. Hemiplegic migraine is manifested by hemiparesis ranging from mild weakness to full hemiplegia. This may persist for some time after resolution of the headache pain. Unless the patient has a history of similar migraines, this is strictly a diagnosis of exclusion, and CT scanning may be necessary to rule out an intracranial process.[10,19]

Ophthalmoplegic migraine is a rare variant usually seen in young adults. The headache pain, which tends to be less intense than a classic migraine, is associated with ipsilateral ophthalmoplegia including extraocular paralysis (usually involving CN III), ptosis, ocular muscle weakness, and occasionally pupillary changes. The Tolosa-Hunt syndrome is a periarteritis of the carotid siphon, which may simulate an ophthalmoplegic migraine. Steady retroorbital pain, oculomotor paralysis, and variable involvement of visual function are suggestive symptoms, which may persist for days to weeks. As with hemiplegic migraine, this is a diagnosis of exclusion, as the differential diagnosis includes carotid artery aneurysm.[10,19]

Basilar artery migraine (or vertebrobasilar migraine) may include severe headache and paroxysmal neurologic deficits, as well as associated symptoms such as vertigo, dysarthria, ataxia, paresthesias, and visual changes. These symptoms should precede the headache and persist only for the duration of the headache, usually from six to eight hours. Basilar artery migraine is most common among females in their teens and 20s. Neuroradiologic scanning may be necessary to exclude posterior fossa tumors, thrombosis of the vertebral/basilar system, and cerebellar hemorrhage or infarct.[10,19]

Status migrainosus refers to any migraine headache persisting for longer than 24 hours. This classification has clinical importance in that headache management may be more difficult in this population, and sequelae such as dehydration are more likely to be present.

Migraine equivalent refers to a condition in which a migraine sufferer experiences autonomic nervous system effects resulting in tachycardia, edema, vertigo, chest pain, thoracic, and abdominal pain, or pelvic pain with little or no headache. Only about 10% of migraineurs suffer this type of migraine variant.[19]

Cluster headaches are sometimes classified as migraine variants, since they are considered to be vascular in origin. They account for between 2% and 9% of migraine headaches. Cluster headaches are characterized by unilateral, excruciating facial pain that rarely lasts for more than two hours. Sufferers also may experience ipsilateral nasal congestion, lacrimation, and conjunctival injection. Attacks occur several times a day for weeks to months with pain-free intervals. They often follow ingestion of alcohol, nitroglycerin, or histamine-containing compounds, or they may be related to stress, climate changes, or allergies. This migraine variant predominates in the male population, usually beginning in mid-adult life.[19]

Clinical Pathophysiology

Multiple physiologic mechanisms for migraine headache have been postulated, some of which may play a role in the clinical pain syndrome of this condition. While all *extracranial* structures are pain-sensitive, the majority of the *intracranial* compartment is insensate. However, the venous sinuses and major arteries at the base of the brain do sense pain, while smaller, intraparenchymal arteries lack pain sensation. The dura mater covering the base of the brain and the dural arteries are somewhat pain-sensitive. The remainder of the intracranial cavity is insensate.

Headache may be produced due to traction, distention, or inflammation of the pain-sensate areas of the head and neck. For example, muscular tension headaches are due to contraction of the extracranial muscles of the neck and scalp. Traction headaches are the result of stress applied on intracranial structures due to mass effect (tumor, intracranial bleed, etc.). In contrast, vascular headaches are secondary to dilatation and distention of the pain-sensitive, intracranial vascular structures. The resulting pain is usually throbbing in nature, fluctuating with the patient's heartbeat. Migraine falls into this category, as do hypertensive headaches and vasodilator headaches (as seen with certain toxins and drugs, such as nitroglycerin). Inflammatory headaches result from inflammation of the peripheral nerves of the head and neck and/or of the basal meninges.

While migraine is primarily a vascular dilatory problem, it also may have a significant inflammatory component.[19] Accordingly, migraine syndromes have long been thought to result from dysfunction of the central autonomic nervous system. This theory (Wolff's vascular theory) postulates that migraines begin with a phase of intracranial arterial vasoconstriction, which is followed by ischemic changes in the corresponding vascular distribution in the brain, which leads to prodromal symptoms. This is followed by a vasodilatation phase, involving primarily those of the extracranial arteries, which causes the characteristic headache of migraine. A "steal syndrome," in which blood is shunted away from cortical areas and into vasodilated extracranial arteries, produces some of the signs and symptoms of migraine. Neuroactive substances released as the migraine develops may produce some of the other symptoms of the headache.[19]

A more current theory of migraine pathogenesis focuses on central serotonergic transmission abnormalities, trigeminovascular neuronal transmission dysfunction, vascular structures, and neurogenic inflammation. Platelet aggregation precipitated by release of vasoactive substances and prostaglandin synthesis also may be involved in the genesis of migraine headache. In this model, activation of the trigeminovascular system induces vasodilatation and neurogenic inflammation.[20] Several recent therapies (i.e., the "triptans") have been developed based on the concept of modulating this system through stimulation of serotonin receptors. A recent review suggests that, in addition to serotonin and neuropeptides, dopamine plays a significant role in the pathophysiology of migraine headaches.[29]

Dopaminergic stimulation (with apomorphine) can induce migraine symptoms and does so more in migraineurs than in a control group (86% of migraineurs developed headache, 0% of controls did). This strongly suggests dopaminergic hypersensitivity as a possible etiology of migraine. The presence of nausea and vomiting as concomitant symptoms in migraine also suggest a dopamine-related etiology, inasmuch as dopamine receptors modulate central emetic centers in the chemotrigger receptor zone. Neuroendocrinologic studies have also demonstrated dopaminergic receptor supersensitivity in migraineurs. Finally, dopamine antagonists (prochlorperazine, haloperidol, chlorpromazine, and metoclopramide) that have long been used empirically for treatment of migraine headaches and their associated symptoms have been successful even as single-agent therapies.

Dopamine activity appears to be a key component of migraine. Some experts consider it to be the "endogenous protagonist in the pathophysiology of the disorder." Serotonin, on the other hand, is viewed as an "endogenous antagonist," since drugs that stimulate serotonin receptors can relieve symptoms of migraine.[29] A unified theory of migraine headache pathophysiology has yet to be developed. Multitudinous therapeutic options available for this disorder, suggesting that at least some of the theories play a significant role in migraine pathogenesis.

Clinical Features

The diagnosis of migraine headache is based on 1) a history consistent with the IHS criteria definition of migraine; and 2) ruling out other organic causes of severe headache. For all practical purposes, then, it is a diagnosis of exclusion. Unfortunately, there are no consistent physical, laboratory, or radiographic findings associated with migraine headache that confirm this diagnosis, although ancillary testing may be indicated to rule out other possible causes of head pain.

History. A history in the headache patient should identify the quality, location, temporal factors (speed of onset, timing of maximal intensity, duration, frequency), mitigating factors, prodromal symptoms, and associated symptoms, as well as other historical features (medical history, family history, occupational history) that may have diagnostic implications. Although a complete analysis of the differential diagnostic implications of various headache syndromes is beyond the scope of this chapter, it should be emphasized that the typical migraine headache can be described as: unilateral (location); throbbing/pulsatile (quality); gradually progressive in onset, and variably associated with prodromal symptoms; usually accompanied by nausea, vomiting, photophobia, and/or phonophobia; and most commonly encountered in patients with a prior history and/or family history of similar headaches. The intensity of headache is not as important as is the entire constellation and evolution of symptoms for distinguishing migraine from more serious causes of head pain.[19]

Certain features of headache should prompt a search for more serious non-migraine etiologies. These include: 1) first-time headache, or worst headache ever (especially if acute in onset with noted neurological deficit); 2) change in character or quality of usual headache; 3) progressively worsening pain over days to weeks with subacute onset; 4) fever, nausea, and vomiting without signs of systemic illness; 5) neck stiffness; 6) or no evident etiology after careful history-taking.[20]

A complete history also should address the patient's prior response to migraine therapies. Most migraine patients presenting to the ED are quite knowledgeable about their condition. They usually are familiar with their symptoms and can identify medications that have helped them obtain relief in the past.[33] Because there is currently no "optimal" therapy for migraine headaches—patient response can be variable—the clinician should determine which classes of therapeutic agents have worked for a patient in the past to guide current therapy.

Physical Examination. As emphasized, physical examination of the migraine patient is aimed at ruling out more dangerous etiologies of headache. As a general rule, most life-threatening causes of headache have demonstrable physical findings,[19] although this is not always the case, and vital signs should be noted in any patient complaining of headache; fever may suggest meningitis, encephalitis, brain abscess, or sinus infection. Severe hypertension may cause head pain, and may predispose to stroke or intracerebral hemorrhage. Respiratory rate may be elevated in patients with hypoxia, hypercarbia, CO or CN poisoning, or anemia as the cause of headache.

Palpation of the scalp, sinuses, neck muscles, oral cavity (teeth and gums), temporomandibular joints, and temporal arteries may reveal other sources of pain. Trigeminal neuralgia may be discovered by tapping over the root of cranial nerve V. The ocular examination may reveal iritis or glaucoma; papilledema should prompt a search for causes of increased intracranial pressure. Retinal hemorrhages may be seen in subarachnoid hemorrhage or hypertensive crisis. Pupillary changes may indicate an intracranial process. Ear examination for otitis media or otitis externa also is important. Meningismus, especially flexion rigidity, suggests meningeal irritation, possibly due to meningitis.

The importance of the neurological examination cannot be overstated. Any patient presenting for headache should undergo careful motor and sensory exams, cranial nerve testing, mental status assessment, and some cerebellar evaluation (gait, tandem walk, finger-to-nose). Abnormalities in any of these evaluations should prompt an intensive search for organic intracranial lesions.

Laboratory Examination. Laboratory and other ancillary studies are reserved for confirming suspected causes of headache other than those caused by migraine. CT scanning is useful for excluding vascular or space-occupying lesions. It is recommended for patients who present with a recent change in headache pattern, seizures, or focal neurological symptoms or signs.[30] Lumbar puncture may be necessary if subarachnoid hemorrhage or an infectious source of headache (meningitis, encephalitis) is suspected. Other tests may include ESR (for temporal arteritis), hemoglobin (for anemia), ABG (for hypoxia/hypercarbia), glucose, WBC, and CO level (or other toxins). If no significant historical or physical exam findings suggest other possible etiologies of headache, and if the headache description is typical of migraine, no laboratory or other testing is required.

It also is important to note that response to therapy is *not* diagnostic of migraine. There are several case reports in the literature of patients with secondary headaches that responded transiently to symptomatic therapies such as DHE and sumatriptan.[42]

Differential Diagnosis. The differential diagnosis of migraine headaches is broad.[19] *(Please see Table 2.)* The key to migraine diagnosis lies in ruling out these other possible causes of head pain (in a patient with an otherwise consistent history and description of current headache quality and associated symptoms).

Table 2. Differential Diagnosis of Migraine Headache

NONMIGRAINOUS VASCULAR HEADACHE
Fever
Hypoxia/hypercarbia
Carbon monoxide poisoning
Hypertensive headache
Anemia
Altitude headache
Stroke
Effort/coital headache
Hypoglycemia
Hypothyroidism/hyperthyroidism
Hypoadrenalism
Menopausal hormone cessation
TRACTION HEADACHE
Tumor
Arteriovenous malformation
Cerebral aneurysm/subarachnoid hemorrhage
Pseudotumor cerebri
Brain abscess
Subdural hematoma/epidural hematoma
Postspinal puncture headache
INFLAMMATORY HEADACHE
Temporal arteritis
INFECTIOUS CAUSES
Meningitis
Encephalitis
Abscess (brain, dental)
Sinus headache
MISCELLANEOUS
Trigeminal neuralgia
Glaucoma
Temporomandibular joint (TMJ) syndrome
Post-traumatic (post-concussive) headache
Ventricular shunt headache
Cervical headache (rheumatoid arthritis, spondylosis, trauma)
Postictal headache
Muscle contraction headache

Management

There is no ideal, universally consistent and successful therapy for all migraine sufferers. The wide variety of therapeutic agents used for treatment of migraine headaches supports this contention. *(Please*

Table 3. Emergency Department Therapy for Migraine

	Medication Name: Generic (Trade)	Dosage/Route of Administration	Comments/Side Effects/ Precautions
FIRST LINE	Prochlorperazine (Compazine)	5-10 mg IV	10 mg IM or 25 mg PR not as effective; Extrapyramidal side effects (dystonia/akathisia), sedation, orthostasis
	Metoclopramide (Reglan)	10 mg IV	IM route not effective as single agent; Less effective than prochlorperazine; Same side effects, but less common
	Ketorolac (Toradol)	30-60 mg IM	Good choice if no IV access; Risk of GI upset, renal impairment; GI upset worse with PO administration; Avoid use in elderly, known renal disease, hypertension, or GI bleeding problems
	Chlorpromazine (Thorazine)	25 mg IM	High risk of orthostatic hypotension; Always pre-treat with 5 cc/kg IV normal saline bolus; Extrapyramidal side effects and sedation are more common than with other antiemetics
	Sumatriptan (Imitrex)	6 mg SQ 25 mg PO	Not to be used within 24 hours of ergots; Contraindications: hypertension, coronary artery disease, other vascular insufficiency; Side effects: injection site discomfort, pressure or tightness in chest or throat, dizziness, vertigo; High rate of headache recurrence
SECOND LINE	Dihydroergotamine (DHE)	1 mg IV/IM	Tends to worsen GI symptoms; use only with concomitant antiemetic; Cannot be used if sumatriptan has already been taken during current attack; Contraindications: coronary artery disease, uncontrolled hypertension, pregnancy; Side effects: transient worsening of headache, chest tightness, hypertension, claudication
	Isometheptene (Midrin)	2 capsules PO	Consider for refractory headache if DHE and sumatriptan are contraindicated
THIRD LINE	Meperidine (Demerol) Stadol (Butorphanol)	50-100 mg IV/IM 2 mg IM	Opioids less efficacious than other treatment modalities; Higher relapse rate; Risk of addiction; Side effects: sedation, dysphoria, psychomimetic effects, respiratory depression; Last resort rather than withholding therapy
	Steroids	Multiple regimens	Only for status migrainosus, severe refractory headaches; Risks: GI bleeding, infection, cataracts, aseptic necrosis, memory disturbances; Consider antacids, H2-blockers for GI protection

see Table 3.) Nevertheless, there are a number of agents available for migraine treatment which have a high rate of success in a large percentage of patients; some of these medications have significant adverse side effects and should not be used in certain populations. Some therapies (particularly opioids) have the potential to induce dependence, and should not be prescribed casually. Other agents have a safer treatment profile, but may be less than ideally effective in eliminating migraine headaches. One way to determine the agent of choice for a particular migraine sufferer is to ask what has worked for them in the past. For those patients who do not know what therapies have been effective or have not received prior medical therapy for migraine, there are several options, all of which have a large number of proponents as well as detractors.

Analgesics. First-line therapy for migraine patients who experience a mild headache or prodrome is an analgesic such as aspirin, acetaminophen, or a NSAID (e.g., naproxen sodium, ibuprofen). These medications are more likely to be effective early in the attack[17] and, therefore, are unlikely to relieve head pain serious enough to bring a patient to the ED. In one study, only 44% of patients reported that they obtained relief from aspirin or acetaminophen, while 25% occasionally reported relief with these agents.[24] Intestinal absorption of drugs may be impaired in patients experiencing migraine, and these agents may not be adequately absorbed to be efficacious. Concomitant administration of an antiemetic improves absorption and makes other agents more effective.

This is not meant to suggest that aspirin and NSAIDs do not play a role in migraine treatment. Aspirin, ibuprofen, and naproxen have all proven more effective than placebo in alleviating mild attacks in randomized, controlled trials.[30] One review suggests that, in combination with metoclopramide (10 mg), 900 mg aspirin is as effective as oral sumatriptan, and causes fewer side effects. Acetaminophen has not been demonstrated to be effective as single-agent migraine therapy,[30] although it can be helpful in combinations such as Excedrin Migraine (with aspirin and caffeine) or acetaminophen/codeine preparations. Other combination therapies will be discussed in subsequent sections of this review.

The most common side effects of aspirin and NSAIDs are gastrointestinal upset and renal impairment,[17,30] and their use should be avoided in the elderly and those with known renal disease or GI bleeding problems. Patients who overuse analgesics are more likely to develop rebound headaches and chronic daily headache, and should be warned against frequent use of symptomatic treatments.[30]

One NSAID that has received unique attention in migraine treatment research is ketorolac (Toradol). Intramuscular (IM) ketorolac (60 mg) provides acceptable or complete pain relief in about 60% of migraine patients.[17] The IM route produces less GI upset than oral administration, and more rapid absorption.[27] It should be stressed that studies have produced mixed results regarding the efficacy of ketorolac. One randomized, double-blind, prospective trial compared the effectiveness of 60 mg of ketorolac to that of 100 mg of meperidine plus 50 mg of hydroxyzine, both given intramuscularly. In this study, 60% of the ketorolac group and 56% of the meperidine/hydroxyzine group had complete or significant relief of their headache pain at 60 minutes, and the ketorolac group experienced fewer side effects.[11] Another trial compared ketorolac 60 mg IM to meperidine 75 mg and promethazine 25 mg IM, and found no statistically significant difference between the two groups with regard to headache or nausea reduction.[9] Another study suggested that ketorolac is less effective than meperidine in the treatment of severe migraine, but only 30 mg of IM ketorolac was used (compared to 75 mg of meperidine). Clearly, the lack of efficacy may have been due to subtherapeutic ketorolac dosing.[26] Comparisons of ketorolac to the phenothiazines also have resulted in mixed results. Ketorolac 60 mg IM compared favorably with chlorpromazine 25 mg IV.[35] Ketorolac 30 mg IV, however, was less effective than prochlorperazine 10 mg IV in another prospective double-blind comparison.[34] Once again, the dosing of ketorolac may have been an issue in this study. Overall, the clinical studies supporting the efficacy of ketorolac are substantial.

Interestingly, it has been suggested that migraine patients "either respond to ketorolac or they do not." In one trial, 74% of patients treated with ketorolac 60 mg IM had a significant reduction in their headache pain within 30-60 minutes, and this effect lasted at least six hours. Ketorolac reaches peak blood levels 45 minutes after IM administration, and its half-life is about six hours. In those individuals whose headache responds to ketorolac, nausea and photophobia are also reduced or eliminated. Those patients with no response after one hour are unlikely to have any additional relief of their head pain.[8] Home administration of IM ketorolac has been studied in an attempt to reduce ED usage; of note is that 87% of patients reported sufficient relief to avoid an ED visit; in this study, rectal antinauseants were offered to patients whose symptoms necessitated such therapy.[39]

Phenothiazines/Antiemetics. Significant attention has been directed toward evaluating the role of phenothiazines in migraine treatment. While prochlorperazine, chlorpromazine, metoclopramide, and other phenothiazine derivatives have long been used for managing the nausea that accompanies many migraine attacks, only recently have these agents been recognized as single-agent therapeutic modalities for migraine headache. At present, the efficacy of the phenothiazines is thought to be due to their modulation of dopaminergic transmission.[29] The phenothiazines should be considered for migraineurs with known or suspected coronary artery disease, since other agents known to be effective in migraine may be associated with serious side effects in the setting of coronary heart disease.

Prochlorperazine can be considered a first-line agent for management of migraine headaches. Because most patients who access the ED with a migraine headache have already tried NSAIDs or mild narcotics without adequate relief, an intravenous antiemetic may be an effective initial ED therapy.[27] Prochlorperazine is a potent dopamine receptor antagonist and has been proven as an effective, single-agent treatment for migraine. In one prospective, randomized, double-blind trial, prochlorperazine 10 mg IV provided complete relief in 74% and partial relief in 14% of patients within 60 minutes of administration (mean of 21 minutes).[24,29] No significant side effects were noted, and no patient returned to the ED within 48 hours.[24] Another study reported that prochlorperazine 10 mg IV was effective in 82% of patients within 30 minutes; there were no recurrences of headache within 24 hours and two dystonic reactions among the 22 patients studied.[29] It should be noted that when prochlorperazine is administered by a route other than the intravenous route, it is not as consistently efficacious. However, one placebo-controlled study of rectal (25 mg) prochlorperazine demonstrated efficacy (at least 50% reduction in pain intensity) at 120 minutes in all patients. It is important to note that 50% of the control patients in this study had relief from placebo, and that no significant difference between study and control patients was seen at 30 or 60 minutes.[21]

Two studies have compared prochlorperazine with another phenothiazine-related compound, metoclopramide. The first trial compared 10 mg of IV prochlorperazine, 10 mg of IV metoclopramide, and placebo. Prochlorperazine achieved patient satisfaction and at least 50% reduction in headache in 82% of patients, in contrast to 48% of metoclopramide patients and 29% of placebo patients. Nausea reduction was also more pronounced with prochlorperazine, and headache recurrence was less common in the prochlorperazine group.[7] The second study compared 10 mg of IM prochlorperazine, 10 mg of IM metoclopramide, and placebo. Prochlorperazine produced significant headache reduction in 67% of patients, metoclopramide in 34%, and placebo in 16%. Thirty-two percent of patients who received prochlorperazine had complete headache relief vs. 14% of the metoclopramide group and 7% of the placebo group. Nausea was completely relieved in 74% of subjects with prochlorperazine, 52% with metoclopramide, and 13% with placebo.[22] No significant difference was found between the two agents in terms of adverse effects. In summary, current studies suggest prochlorperazine is significantly more effective than metoclopramide; however, prochlorperazine administered by intramuscular route did not achieve complete headache relief in a sufficient percentage of patients to justify IM prochlorperazine as an appropriate choice for single-agent therapy.[22]

Single-agent therapy with metoclopramide has met with mixed reviews.[15,24,29] This agent is commonly used in Europe as an adjunctive agent to improve oral absorption of other analgesics. It has been shown to have a beneficial effect as a *prophylactic* agent for migraine patients. It is only moderately effective for acute migraine therapy as a single agent, however, because it has less affinity for dopamine receptors than other phenothiazines.[29] *Intramuscular* metoclopramide, in fact, is no more effective than placebo for pain reduction, although IV metoclopramide has provided adequate relief for ED discharge in 67% of patients (vs 19% with placebo).[24] Other studies have found IV metoclopramide efficacious in treatment of both the pain and nausea of migraine, independent of the concomitant use of other medications.[15] One comparative study evaluating IV metoclopramide and IV chlorpromazine found the two to be equally efficacious for migraine treatment.[4]

Intravenous chlorpromazine is reportedly 89-94% effective for ED treatment of migraine.[24-29,38] Intramuscular chlorpromazine has also relieved both headache and nausea in 96% of patients in the ED setting. However, 18% of patients treated with IM chlorpromazine developed orthostatic hypotension.[24,29,38] Consequently, some authorities recommend that patients who receive chlorpromazine should be *pretreated* with a bolus of normal saline (5 mL/kg).[30] Several other studies have shown chlorpromazine to be effective for treatment of migraine headache, but this agent does not appear to produce relief in as high a percentage of patients as prochlorperazine, and it is more commonly associated with side effects.[24] In one study, about 32% of patients indicated they would not be willing to take chlorpromazine again for future treatment of migraine.[38]

Other phenothiazines and related compounds have been evaluated in Canadian migraine headache studies. For example, methotrimeprazine was found to be comparable to meperidine with dimenhydrinate for treating severe migraines.[36] Granisetron, a selective serotonin antagonist with potent antiemetic properties, was not significantly different from placebo in relieving migraine headaches.[32] Neither of these medications is currently available in the United States.

Although haloperidol is a butyrophenone, as opposed to a phenothiazine, its mode of action is the same as the phenothiazines, and it is therefore discussed in this section. Haloperidol is a potent dopamine receptor antagonist with antiemetic activity. One case series has studied relief of migraine headache with intravenous haloperidol (5 mg). All six patients achieved complete or substantial headache relief within 65 minutes, with minimal or nonexistent side effects.[16] Haldol may be of use in the treatment of migraine headaches, though this small study is insufficient to allow its recommendation as a first-line therapeutic agent.

Side effects of the phenothiazines (and butyrophenones) include extrapyramidal reactions such as dystonia and akathisia.[17] Sedation and orthostasis are also significant risks, and may limit the use of these agents in patients with poor cardiac function and in the elderly.[27]

Ergots. Ergotamine compounds have been used for decades as an *abortive* agent for migraine attacks. Once a migraine headache has ensued, there is no role for ergotamine. Its mechanism of action is vasoconstriction, which counteracts the dilatation of extracranial arteries and arterioles. In order to prevent rebound headaches, ergotamine should not be used more often than every five days. It also *cannot* be used concomitantly with sumatriptan, so ergotamine should not be administered if the patient has already taken sumatriptan during the current attack. Due to severe side effects, parenteral ergotamine is no longer available in the United States. However, sublingual ergotamine (Ergostat) and oral or rectal ergotamine/caffeine combinations (Cafergot, Wigraine) are still available.[10] Rectal administration results in higher blood levels than oral administration. A high rate of side effects and rebound headaches makes this a less than optimal therapy for most patients.[24]

For parenteral therapy, dihydroergotamine (DHE) can be given by the IV or IM route, and it is often given concomitantly with an antiemetic to manage the nausea of migraine as well as the GI upset induced by DHE.[10] DHE has less vasoconstrictive action than ergotamine and produces fewer rebound headaches and fewer side effects.[24,38] In a prospective, double-blind trial, patients received either 1 mg of DHE or 1.5 mg/kg of meperidine intramuscularly. Both agents were given concomitantly with hydroxyzine as an antiemetic. DHE compared favorably with meperidine (no statistically significant difference in outcomes) and it produced fewer CNS side effects, such as dizziness. Another trial compared DHE 1 mg IV plus metoclopramide 10 mg IV with both butorphanol and meperidine plus hydroxyzine. More than 90% reduction in headache was achieved for 38% of patients treated with DHE/metoclopramide compared with 16% treated with butorphanol.[24] Another study found IV DHE superior to IM meperidine, but it must be interpreted with caution because the two medications were given by different routes.[25] DHE has also been tried by both the intranasal and the subcutaneous routes, but with poor efficacy.[24,38] Home administration of DHE by the intramuscular and subcutaneous routes has also been studied as a way of avoiding an ED visit. Results have been promising, but application may be limited by patients' reluctance to inject themselves and by the high rate of side effects.[43]

Contraindications to the use of ergotamine/DHE include uncontrolled hypertension and coronary artery disease (due to risk of vasoconstriction)[27] and pregnancy (due to oxytocic effects).[10] Severe side effects, such as peripheral vascular insufficiency requiring prostaglandin infusion for limb salvage, have been reported after ergotamine use.[13] Other side effects include transient worsening of headache, chest tightness, hypertension, and claudication.[17] Gastrointestinal distress tends to worsen, rather than improve with DHE use. In fact, more than 25% of patients given DHE in one study said they would refuse the drug in the future, mostly due to the GI side effects that affected 58% of the study patients.[38] The decision to use ergots for migraine therapy should be made with caution, especially in patients at risk for vascular insufficiency.

Sumatriptan. The "triptans" represent the newest class of migraine therapeutic agents. Sumatriptan (Imitrex) was first introduced to the market in 1993 in injectable form, and later as a tablet and nasal spray. Three congeners have been subsequently introduced: zolmitriptan (Zomig), naratriptan (Amerge), and rizatriptan (Maxalt). From a practical, clinical perspective, none of these has supplanted sumatriptan. Moreover, none has proven as potent as parenteral sumatriptan, although some patients may have a particular preference among the "triptans." For the purposes of this review, only sumatriptan will be considered.

Sumatriptan's mechanism of action is vasoconstriction, which is mediated through serotonin, dopamine, and adrenergic receptor sites.[24] As mentioned above, it cannot be given concomitantly with (or within 24 hours of) ergots, due to a theoretical additive effect. At least one report has documented severe side effects from the combination of these two medications; renal papillary necrosis developed from renal ischemia after coadministration of sumatriptan, DHE, and ketorolac (all three of these agents probably contributed).[45] Like the ergots, sumatriptan is contraindicated in patients with known hypertension, coronary artery disease, or other vascular insufficiency. It does not worsen GI distress as do ergots. In fact, it tends to relieve headache and nausea,[27] as well as other associated symptoms of migraine.[10] Residual nausea, however, may necessitate addition of antiemetics for up to 25% of patients receiving sumatriptan.[38]

Rare, but potential life-threatening effects of sumatriptan include cardiac arrhythmia, including cardiac arrest and myocardial infarction, and stroke in the setting of occult coronary disease or atherosclerotic vascular disease. Relative contraindications to the use of sumatriptan include poorly controlled hypertension, history of diabetes mellitus, angina, or asthma.[46]

Side effects of administration of sumatriptan include local injection site symptoms (warmth, redness, tingling) and pressure or tightness in the throat or chest.[17] Dizziness and vertigo have also been reported.[1] Sumatriptan is associated with a 40% headache recurrence rate at 24 hours following administration.[17,24,27] One study found that of patients successfully treated with sumatriptan, 42% required rescue medication by eight hours after discharge, 61% by 24 hours postdischarge; only one-third of patients were pain free at the 24-hour follow-up.[38] Sumatriptan costs about $12 for a 25-mg tablet and about $40 for a single injection. Due to these limitations, sumatriptan has been recommended by some authorities as a second-line therapy for migraine patients who have failed to obtain relief after IV antiemetic administration.[27] Other experts, however, are sufficiently impressed with the drug's clinical efficacy, as well as evidence-based trials confirming its value in migraine treatment to position it as a first-line agent in appropriate patient subgroups.

Sumatriptan is effective if taken at any time during a migraine attack, but it should not be taken during the aura phase of a classical migraine, since at least one study has found it ineffective at this stage.[30] Sumatriptan administered by the intravenous route has been effective in 90% of cases in one study.[24] Orally, it provided significant relief for 70-80% of subjects within two hours of administration. Subcutaneous injection improved headache severity in 86-92% of patients at two hours, compared to 37% of placebo controls.[24] Another study of subcutaneous sumatriptan found that 6 mg resulted in complete or almost complete resolution of pain in 70-77% of patients within 60 minutes and 81-87% within two hours. Giving more than 6 mg initially, or repeat dosing later, did not provide any additional benefit.[17] Other authors have recommended repeat dosing at one hour if no relief has been obtained (up to 12 mg in 24 hours).[10] One clinical trial of subcutaneous sumatriptan in the ED found that 75% of patients obtained meaningful relief after 6 mg, vs. 35% with placebo. At discharge, a 100-mg tablet of oral sumatriptan was offered in case of headache return. Sixty-two percent of patients with mild or no pain at discharge took the oral form within 24 hours, and 65% of these patients obtained relief within two hours.[1]

The starting oral dose of sumatriptan is 25 mg, repeated in two hours if needed. This can be increased in 25 mg increments with subsequent dosing, up to a total of 200 mg in 24 hours. As is the case with ergots, a five-day hiatus is recommended between treatment days.[10]

Isometheptene. Isometheptene is a mild vasoconstrictor, and it is available in combination with acetaminophen and dichloralphenazone (a sedative metabolized to chloral hydrate) known as Midrin.[42] This is generally not considered a first-line agent, but it may be considered in patients with contraindications to ergots or sumatriptan, or if medication is still needed on the second or third day of an attack.[10] Patients should take two tablets initially for optimal effect.[42]

Caffeine. Caffeine, a vasoconstrictor, is not a single-agent therapy for migraine, but it has been found helpful as an adjunct in combination medications. Preparations containing caffeine may have greater efficacy because caffeine acts as an analgesic, as well as promoting absorption across mucous membranes.[42] Fioricet and Fiorinal contain acetaminophen and aspirin, respectively, plus caffeine and butalbital. Excedrin contains aspirin, acetaminophen, and caffeine. Wigraine and Cafergot are comprised of ergotamine and caffeine.

Opioids. One of the factors fueling development of new treatment modalities and protocols for migraine is the concern that traditional therapy with opioid medications has the capacity to produce narcotic dependence in migraine sufferers if they require frequent treatment. A cross-sectional survey in 1993 determined that narcotics continue to be a common medication class used for migraine therapy; in fact, they were the most common choice in the study.[2] Many other studies cite the potential for abuse and addiction,[10,27,30] as well as lower efficacy and higher headache relapse rates[38] as reasons to avoid narcotic use for migraines, except as a last resort.[27,30]

As noted in previous sections of this review, many agents have been compared to meperidine to rate their efficacy, and most of them have proven superior. In a study of meperidine for migraine, 1.5 mg/kg of meperidine was given and repeat dosing was required in 43% of participants. Even after two injections, 63% of patients required further rescue medications before discharge, and 28% of patients had headache relapse within 24 hours.[5] Several other studies have confirmed poor results with narcotic injections.[11,36]

Some patients obtain relief from narcotic agents and fail with other therapies. If this is the case, the emergency physician should be willing to use narcotics rather than withholding treatment.[38] Nevertheless, narcotic agents remain a second-line therapy for use in treatment failures.[6]

Oral and transnasal opioids have been recommended for patients requiring narcotic medication for migraine treatment. A 1996 review introduced an oral narcotic protocol using oral meperidine or hydromorphone in combination with pretreatment phenothiazine and metoclopramide, as well as a sedative.[41] This approach was safe and cost-effective protocol, in that it reduced subsequent emergency visits. This approach is unlikely to be used in the ED setting.

Butorphanol (Stadol) is a mixed agonist-antagonist opioid analgesic available for parenteral administration as well as in a transnasal preparation for migraine.[10] One puff in one nostril is equipotent with 5 mg of morphine. It provides rapid pain relief, but causes sedation, dysphoria, and may produce rebound headaches if overused.[42] The adverse side effect profile of butorphanol is sufficiently problematic to categorize this agent as an undesirable choice for migraine treatment. A study of optimal butorphanol dosing and safety revealed that intramuscular injections of 2-3 mg provided significantly greater analgesia than a 1 mg injection, but no significant difference in efficacy was observed between the 2 mg and 3 mg doses. No major adverse effects

Table 4. Migraine Triggers[19]

- Nitrites (processed meats and foods, nitroglycerin)
- Tyramine (wine, sausages, some cheese)
- Tyrosine
- Phenylalanine
- Phenylethamine (cheese, chocolate)
- 1-octopamine (citrus fruits)
- Aspartame
- Monosodium glutamate
- Alcohol
- Tobacco
- Overuse of caffeine, or caffeine withdrawal
- Too much or too little sleep
- Fasting
- Physical activity, or relaxation following activity/stress
- Hot, humid weather; or change in weather
- Menstruation, or estrogen-containing oral contraceptives
- Minor head trauma

occurred, although sedation, decrease in respiratory rate (of no clinical significance), and psychomimetic side effects (e.g., vivid dreams, hallucinations) were reported.[14] A study of transnasal butorphanol (TNB) use for migraine headaches in the ED found that 1 mg of TNB alone provided adequate relief in 60% of patients. Thirty-six percent reported side effects, although most were mild (drowsiness, dysphoria); 52% had some degree of headache recurrence within 48 hours.[28] As a result of these findings, butorphanol is not an ideal medication for migraine, although it can be used for patients with infrequent but severe migraine attacks for whom other treatments are either ineffective, inconvenient, or contraindicated.[30]

Lidocaine. Lidocaine nose drops have been recommended in one study as more effective than placebo in alleviating migraine headaches. One mg of 4% lidocaine may be instilled into the nostril ipsilateral to the head pain, with the head hyperextended 45 degrees and turned 30 degrees toward the headache side. Fifty percent of patients experience relief within minutes, but 50% of these headaches recur within one hour. This approach certainly is suboptimal for routine consideration.[42] On the other hand, about 80% of cluster headaches will resolve with 4% lidocaine (or cocaine hydrochloride[19]) administration into the sphenopalatine fossa. Lidocaine may, therefore, be considered in addition to 100% oxygen therapy for cluster headache.[20]

Corticosteroids. The use of corticosteroids in migraine is reserved for patients with a severe headache lasting more than 72 hours (status migrainosus). Chronic steroids should be reserved as a last resort for patients not responding to other measures, as they are less effective and more prone to side effects (hyperglycemia, hypertension, aseptic necrosis, GI bleeding, infection, cataracts, memory disturbances, etc.) than many other modalities.[42] Corticosteroids take several hours to produce clinical results, so additional medication for sleep may be given concomitantly. Antacids, H2-blockers, or other agents should also be considered for GI protection, and a sedating anti-emetic (hydroxyzine, prochlorperazine) may alleviate nausea, as well as insomnia caused by the corticosteroids.[42]

An ED study of corticosteroid use in migraine patients found that 72% of patients treated with meperidine 75-100 mg, promethazine 50 mg, and dexamethasone 8 mg reported significant relief. Only 37% of patients treated with DHE 1 mg and meperidine 75-100 mg obtained relief, and only 29% of patients treated with meperidine 75-100 mg and promethazine 50 mg. While the groups are not strictly comparable, patients receiving corticosteroids had a superior outcome.[24]

Multiple dosing regimens for corticosteroids have been cited in the literature. Intravenous hydrocortisone 100 mg three times a day may be used, but should be considered only in patients admitted for their refractory headaches. Burst therapy with 10 mg of dexamethasone, repeated the next day if necessary, or a one-week tapering dose of prednisone (60 mg for 3 days, 40 mg for 2 days, 20 mg for 2 days) also may be considered.[42] Other authors have recommended either dexamethasone acetate, 16-mg long-acting preparation, or methylprednisolone acetate 80-mg IM injection, but they caution against repeating this therapy in less than three weeks.[10] A third source reports a dosing regimen of dexamethasone 8-20 mg IM or IV, or methylprednisolone sodium succinate 100-250 mg IV, either with or without added narcotic and antiemetic.[30]

Special Considerations

Special mention should be made of recommendations for migraine patients who are pregnant, and for pediatric patients. As mentioned above, the ergots are contraindicated in pregnancy due to oxytocic effects, and the triptans have unproven safety profiles in pregnant patients. Steroids and NSAIDs also have known adverse effects in pregnancy, and should be avoided. Therefore, for pregnant patients with mild to moderate symptoms, simple analgesics, such as acetaminophen, are recommended. Patients with severe headaches or those who fail therapy with analgesics should be given a trial of narcotic medication, a last resort in most other patient populations.[27]

For pediatric migraine, initial therapy consists of rest, removal of triggering factors *(please see Table 4)*, and basic analgesics, such as acetaminophen 15-20 mg/kg. Some children may respond better to NSAIDs, and ibuprofen should therefore be considered. Aspirin should be avoided due to its association with Reye's syndrome. Second-line therapy includes addition of an antiemetic, such as promethazine, prochlorperazine, or metoclopramide. The antiemetics carry a higher risk of extrapyramidal side effects in children, however, and must be used with caution. Metoclopramide (0.1 mg/kg up to a maximum of 10 mg) has less propensity for causing these side effects, and therefore it is the antiemetic of choice in pediatric patients. For the rare child who does not respond to these measures, only IV DHE has been studied (in combination with metoclopramide) in children as young as 6 years. Because of associated side effects, however, this drug must be titrated carefully by a physician experienced in pediatric migraine treatment. Therefore, if headache is severe enough to mandate further abortive therapy beyond rest, reassurance, analgesics, and antiemetics, the emergency physician should consider consultation with a pediatric neurologist, or perhaps even admission for more intensive migraine therapy.[44]

Nonpharmacologic Therapy. Some nonpharmacologic adjuncts to migraine therapy have been found to be beneficial. Patient education should include a clear, definitive diagnosis of migraine once other causes of head pain have been ruled out. Reassurance that no other serious underlying etiology has been found can be an important component of initial therapy. Realistic goals of therapy should be addressed (the concept of control, rather than cure, of migraine). Recognition and avoidance of triggering factors is also important for prevention of future exacerbations, so patients should be educated about the common migraine triggers (please see Table 4) and, perhaps, encouraged to keep a headache diary to be reviewed in follow-up with the primary physician. Other nonpharmacologic modalities that have been assessed and shown as possibly valuable include cold or pressure application to the head, reduction of activity and sensory input in a quiet or dark environment, and sleep. Less proven therapies include relaxation therapy/biofeedback, psychotherapy, hypnosis, transcutaneous electrical stimulation, acupuncture, chiropractic, and occipital or supraorbital nerve blockade.[31] These are outside of the scope of routine ED treatment, but may be offered to patients in the outpatient setting.[20]

Migraine Prophylaxis. Although it is unlikely that preventive medications will be prescribed by the emergency physician,[20] these agents are mentioned because migraine patients may already be using these therapies or they may ask about their role in migraine treatment when they present for acute headache control. Propranolol is probably the most common prophylactic medication used for migraine. This beta-blocker has been shown to decrease headache frequency by about 31%.[30] Metoprolol has been shown to reduce attack frequency by 28-33% in three separate trials.[19,20] Beta-blockers are contraindicated in asthmatics.[30] Amitryptiline and other tricyclic antidepressants also have been used, although only amitryptiline has been tested in double-blind, placebo-controlled trials. This agent may reduce the frequency of attacks up to 40%, and is the preferred preventive medication for patients with down mood or insomnia. Valproic acid has reduced the frequency of migraine attacks 39-43% below that of control groups, but it has been associated with birth defects and hepatotoxicity.[30] Valproate has recently been shown to be as effective as propranolol for the prophylaxis of migraine without aura.[47] Methysergide is the oldest of the preventives, but can induce an inflammatory fibrosis in the retroperitoneum, lungs, and heart valves. Discontinuing the medication for one month out of every 4-6 months of use can prevent this complication. Verapamil, aspirin, and NSAIDs have been shown to be effective prophylactic medications in selected groups of migraine sufferers. Magnesium, cyproheptadine, fluoxetine (and other selective serotonin reuptake inhibitors), riboflavin (vitamin B_2), have all been suggested as preventive treatments for migraine, but definitive trials are lacking.

Disposition

The majority of patients with migraine headaches may be discharged from the ED after treatment and an appropriate observation period to ensure that adequate relief of headache and other symptoms has been achieved. It has been suggested that patients who leave the ED with residual headache have a much higher rate of headache persistence (61%) at 24 hours than the rate of headache recurrence in patients who leave the ED headache-free (31%), regardless of initial headache severity.[12] Therefore, it is prudent to observe patients and continue therapy until headache resolution, if possible. Obviously, this needs to be weighed against the reality of ED flow and resource availability.

Not all patients who still have residual headache after ED therapy require admission to the hospital. Nevertheless, some subgroups of patients may necessitate hospitalization for observation and continued therapy. Some indications for hospital admission might include: headache and concomitant nausea/vomiting persisting for several days with signs of dehydration; headache complicated by overuse of therapeutic medications; chronic daily headache not responding to outpatient management; headache accompanied by other medical/surgical problem; intractable cluster headache; suspicion for possible organic disease (e.g., subarachnoid hemorrhage, tumor, meningitis); or interruption of ability to carry out activities of daily living.[19]

Conclusion

Migraine headaches afflict as many as 10-20% of the population and are disabling in at least one-half of these individuals. Recent developments have illuminated the importance of dopaminergic and serotonergic modulation as pathophysiologic mechanisms for migraine therapy. The importance of intravenous hydration in a migraine sufferer who has been vomiting is very important and should not be overlooked. The use of phenothiazines and related antinauseants as first-line therapy for migraine has developed from this knowledge. Triptans are also considered to be first-line agents.

The best initial agent for migraine often is the analgesic that has provided relief for the individual patient in the past. For those patients who cannot identify an appropriate analgesic that has predictably produced pain relief, an antiemetic is the best first-line choice. Prochlorperazine and metoclopramide are both highly effective and safe in most patients. DHE or sumatriptan may be added if pain relief is inadequate after 30 minutes. Intravenous chlorpromazine may be safely tried in the patient with an IV access, and ketorolac is a reasonable choice for patients without an IV access. In selected patients, narcotics may be used, but should be considered a last resort, except in pregnancy or when other agents are contraindicated.[27,38] As much as possible, patients should be treated in the ED until their headaches are completely resolved, as patients not obtaining complete relief in the ED have a higher rate of headache persistence or recurrence than do those who leave the ED with no pain.[12] Nonpharmacologic and prophylactic therapy may assist in the management of migraine sufferers, but are best left for the primary care physician or neurologist to manage in the outpatient arena.

References

1. Akpunonu BE, Mutgi AB, Federman DJ, et al. Subcutaneous sumatriptan for treatment of acute migraine in patients admitted to the emergency department: A multicenter study. *Ann Emerg Med* 1995;25:464-469.
2. Barton CW. Evaluation and treatment of headache patients in the emergency department: A survey. *Headache* 1994;34: 91-94.
3. Becker WJ, Riess CM, Hoag, J. Effectiveness of subcutaneous dihydroergotamine by home injection for migraine. *Headache* 1996;36:144-148.
4. Cameron JD, Lane PL, Speechley M. Intravenous chlorpromazine vs intravenous metoclopramide in acute migraine headache. *Acad Emerg Med* 1995;2:597-602.
5. Carleton SC, Shesser RF, Pietrzak MP, et al. Double-blind, multicenter trial to compare the efficacy of intramuscular dihydroergotamine plus hydroxyzine versus intramuscular meperidine plus hydroxyzine for the emergency department

treatment of acute migraine headache. *Ann Emerg Med* 1998; 32:129-138.
6. Clark RF, Wei EM, Anderson PO. Meperidine: Therapeutic use and toxicity. *J Emerg Med* 1995;13:797-802.
7. Coppola M, Yealy DM, Leibold RA. Randomized placebo-controlled evaluation of prochlorperazine versus metoclopramide for emergency department treatment of migraine headache. *Ann Emerg Med* 1995;26:541-546.
8. Davis CP, Torre PR, Schafer NC, et al. Ketorolac as a rapid and effective treatment of migraine headache: Evaluations by patients. *Am J Emerg Med* 1993;11:573-575.
9. Davis CP, Torre PR, Williams C, et al. Ketorolac versus meperidine-plus-promethazine treatment of migraine headache: Evaluations by patients. *Am J Emerg Med* 1995; 13:146-150.
10. Diamond S, Diamond ML. Emergency treatment of migraine: Insights into current options. *Postgrad Med* 1997; 101:169-179.
11. Duarte C, Dunaway F, Turner L, et al. Ketorolac versus meperidine and hydroxyzine in the treatment of acute migraine headache: A randomized, prospective, double-blind trial. *Ann Emerg Med* 1992;21:1116-1121.
12. Ducharme J, Beveridge RC, Lee JS, et al. Emergency management of migraine: Is the headache really over? *Acad Emerg Med* 1998;5:899-905.
13. Edwards RJ, Fulde GWO, McGrath MA. Successful limb salvage with prostaglandin infusion: A review of ergotamine toxicity. *Med J Aust* 1991;155:825-827.
14. Elenbaas RM, Iacono CU, Koellner KJ, et al. Dose effectiveness and safety of butorphanol in acute migraine headache. *Pharmacotherapy* 1991;11:56-63.
15. Ellis GL, Delaney J, DeHart DA, et al. The efficacy of metoclopramide in the treatment of migraine headache. *Ann Emerg Med* 1993;22:191-195.
16. Fisher H. A new approach to emergency department therapy of migraine headache with intravenous haloperidol: A case series. *J Emerg Med* 1995;13:119-122.
17. Foley JJ. Pharmacologic treatment of acute migraine and related headaches in the emergency department. *J Emerg Nurs* 1993;19:225-229.
18. Hay E. Treatment of migraine with sumatriptan in the ED. *Am J Emerg Med* 1994;12:388-389.
19. Henry GL. Headache. In: Rosen P, et al., eds. *Emergency Medicine: Concepts and Clinical Practice.* 3rd ed. St. Louis: Mosby Year Book; 1992:1751-1766.
20. Hoffman GL. Headache and Facial Pain. In: Tintinalli JE, et al, eds. *Emergency Medicine: A Comprehensive Study Guide.* 4th ed. New York: McGraw Hill; 1996:1008-1013.
21. Jones EB, Gonzalez ER, Boggs JG, et al. Safety and efficacy of rectal prochlorperazine for the treatment of migraine in the emergency department. *Ann Emerg Med* 1994;24: 237-241.
22. Jones J, Pack S, Chun E. Intramuscular prochlorperazine versus metoclopramide as single-agent therapy for the treatment of acute migraine headache. *Am J Emerg Med* 1996;14: 262-265.
23. Kelly AM, Ardagh M, Curry C, et al. Intravenous chlorpromazine versus intramuscular sumatriptan for acute migraine. *J Accid Emerg Med* 1997;14:209-211.
24. Klapper J. The pharmacologic treatment of acute migraine headaches. *J Pain Symptom Manage* 1993;8:140-147.
25. Klapper J, Stanton J. Current emergency treatment of severe migraine headaches. *Headache* 1993;33:560-562.
26. Larkin GL, Prescott JE. A randomized, double-blind, comparative study of the efficacy of ketorolac tromethamine versus meperidine in the treatment of severe migraine. *Ann Emerg Med* 1992;21:919-924.
27. Lobo BL, Landy S. Recommendations for the emergency treatment of migraine headache. *J Tenn Med Assoc* 1994;87: 53-54.
28. Melanson SW, Morse JW, Pronchik DJ, et al. Transnasal butorphanol in the emergency department management of migraine headache. *Am J Emerg Med* 1997;15:57-61.
29. Peroutka SJ. Dopamine and migraine. *Neurology* 1997;49: 650-656.
30. Pryse-Phillips WEM, Dodick DW, Edmeads JG, et al. Guidelines for the diagnosis and management of migraine in clinical practice. *CMAJ* 1997;156:1273-1287.
31. Pryse-Phillips WEM, Dodick DW, Edmeads JG, et al. Guidelines for the nonpharmacologic management of migraine in clinical practice. *CMAJ* 1998;159:47-54.
32. Rowat BMT, Merrill CF, Davis A, et al. A double-blind comparison of granisetron and placebo for the treatment of acute migraine in the emergency department. *Cephalalgia* 1991; 11:207-213.
33. Salomone JA, Thomas RW, Althoff JR, et al. An evaluation of the role of the ED in the management of migraine headaches. *Am J Emerg Med* 1994;12:134-137.
34. Seim MB, March JA, Dunn KA. Intravenous ketorolac vs intravenous prochlorperazine for the treatment of migraine headaches. *Acad Emerg Med* 1998;5:573-576.
35. Shrestha M, Singh R, Moreden J, et al. Ketorolac vs. chlorpromazine in the treatment of acute migraine without aura: A prospective, randomized, double-blind trial. *Arch Intern Med* 1996;156:1725-1728.
36. Stiell IG, Dufour DG, Moher D, et al. Methotrimeprazine versus meperidine and dimenhydrinate in the treatment of severe migraine: a randomized, controlled trial. *Ann Emerg Med* 1991;20:1201-1205.
37. Stratton SJ. Sumatriptan: A clinical standard? *Ann Emerg Med* 1995;25:538-539.
38. Thomas SH, Stone CK. Emergency department treatment of migraine, tension, and mixed-type headache. *J Emerg Med* 1994;12:657-664.
39. Turkewitz LJ, Casaly JS, Dawson GA, et al. Self-administration of parenteral ketorolac tromethamine for head pain. *Headache* 1992;32:452-454.
40. Von Seggern RL, Adelman JU. Cost considerations in headache treatment, part 2: Acute migraine treatment. *Headache* 1996; 36:493-502.
41. Von Seggern RL, Adelman JU. Oral narcotic protocol to reduce narcotic injections in refractory migraine patients. *Headache* 1997;37:341-345.
42. Ward TN. Management of an acute primary headache. *Clin Neurosci* 1998;5:50-54.
43. Weisz MA, El-Raheb M, Blumenthal HJ. Home administra-

tion of intramuscular DHE for the treatment of acute migraine headache. *Headache* 1994;34:371-373.
44. Welborn CA. Pediatric migraine. *Emerg Med Clin North Am* 1997;15:625-636.
45. Witting MD. Renal papillary necrosis following emergency department treatment of migraine. *J Emerg Med* 1996;14: 373-376.
46. Kelly KM. Cardiac arrest following sumatriptan. *Neurology* 1995;45:1211-1213.
47. Kaniecki RG. A comparison of divalproex with propranolol and placebo for the prophylaxis of migraine without aura. *Arch Neurol* 1997;54:1141-1145.

Status Epilepticus

J. Stephen Huff, MD

Among the most challenging and life-threatening conditions that may face the physician is generalized convulsive status epilepticus (GCSE). It demands prompt etiological characterization and a logically sequenced approach to pharmacotherapeutic stabilization.

Not surprisingly, management of these patients frequently mandates a team approach. From a practical clinical perspective, the treating physician must put an end to the seizures, stabilize the patient's overall medical condition, identify an etiology for the epileptic episode, coordinate care with appropriate subspecialists, and develop a treatment plan to minimize the risk of recurrence.

Interventions must be aimed toward maximizing the opportunity for seizure cessation while minimizing the risks from complications of drug therapy and invasive procedures designed to control the airway. This balancing act requires clinical acumen, a thorough understanding of seizure pathophysiology and classification, and a measured assessment of the risk of medication-related adverse effects. Because unusual, multi-factorial, or chronic etiologies may be the precipitating factors in GCSE, comprehensive care of the patient inevitably involves the coordination with a number of specialists, including neurologists, neurosurgeons, internists, pediatricians, and intensivists.

There are three important questions facing the physician in identifying the cause of GCSE. First, what are the most common etiologies? Medication non-compliance, ischemia, and infection are among the most common. Second, what should be included in the work-up: STAT EEG and/or computerized tomography (CT) scanning? And, third, what are the appropriate treatment algorithms and drugs of choice for managing GCSE?

As might be expected, the literature on epilepsy is vast, and clinical trials cited in this review are oriented primarily to initial strategies for diagnosis and management. Also, due to space considerations, a targeting and clinically oriented approach to the diagnosis and management of GCSE will be directed to the adult patient.

Historical Features and Current Classification of Status Epilepticus

Baffled by the unusual and violent movements that characterize epilepsy, the ancients attributed SE to possession by spirits or demons. In fact, the earliest surviving reference to SE is found in Babylonian cuneiform stone tablets dating to the middle of the first millennium BC.[1] Interestingly, these tablets note the mortality associated with repeated seizures. Later, Hippocrates referred to epilepsy as "the sacred disease." The modern description of continuous seizure activity has been attributed to a French physician who published his obervations in 1824, with the term "status" appearing in an English translation of this work.[2] The first American descriptions of clinical SE date from the early 1900s. The syndrome of GCSE is clearly described in these reports, which emphasize the morbidity and mortality associated with this clinical syndrome.[3,4]

Current Classification. Currently, SE is a term that may be used to describe any continuing seizure acitvity regardless of its etiology. From a clinical perspective, an extremely useful approach to categorizing SE is to divide SE into classifications that are similar to those used for seizure disorders. As might be expected, these classifications are based on information and neuronal discharge patterns observed on video-electroencephalograms (VEEG).[5,6]

Simple Seizures. Using this scheme, the term "simple" implies that an isolated area of the cortex is involved. Clinically speaking, simple SE patterns will produce unremitting focal motor or sensory phenomena, with full preservation of consciousness. For example, the twitching of an extremity or small area of the body in the setting of preserved consciousness (and confirmatory electroencephalogram [EEG] evidence of focal electrical abnormality) would be categorized as a simple motor seizure.

Generalized Seizures. The term "generalized" indicates that abnormal electrical activity involves all areas of the cerebral cortex. In this case, generalized activity may spread from a single, focal area of electrical abnormality, or it may originate in all areas of the cortex simultaneously. When all cortical areas are observed (by EEG) to be involved at once, the condition is characterized as a primarily generalized seizure. This epileptic pattern may occur with petit mal seizures and in some (primary) generalized tonic-clonic seizures. Absence seizures (also known as petit mal) are a primarily generalized seizure type involving all cortical areas at once. If diffuse involvement of the cortex results from a localized or focal cortical area, this is "secondary generalization;" this spread may be observed at the bedside or by EEG. Accordingly, GCSE, refers to a continuing generalized seizure, regardless of its underlying eliptogenic trigger or pattern of electrical migration.

In adults, most generalized seizures originate from a focal area of abnormal electrical activity that then spreads through secondary generalization to involve all areas of the cortex. Often, this electrical migration occurs too rapidly to be observed clinically. On occasion, the typical aura of a generalized convulsive seizure will persist in the absence of any associated motor movements. It should be stressed that this aura represents ongoing seizure activity that is limited to a focal area of the cortex. In this case, however, the abnormal, localized electrical activity associated with the seizure does not spread or generalize to the entire cerebral cortex but remains circumscribed in one abnormal focus.

Complex Seizures. With respect to seizure classification, the term "complex" signifies that consciousness has been altered. For example, a simple motor seizure may evolve into a complex partial seizure with altered consciousness. Occasionally, this state may persist for hours or days with minimal or no associated motor activity. The terminology that applies to this clinical presentation is partial complex SE. Absence SE and complex partial SE are often grouped under the term "nonconvulsive status epilepticus" and are sometimes referred to as twilight or fugue states.

Nonconvulsive Status Epilepticus. The physician should be aware that there is controversy surrounding the term "nonconvulsive status epilepticus."[7] In the past, this term has been used to describe a state characterized by the absence of clinically apparent convulsive seizures in conjunction with EEG activity indicating that generalized seizures are continuing throughout the cortex.[8] Typically, this is a seizure disorder of childhood and produces a characteristic EEG pattern. At times, absence seizures persist with minimal motor movements and altered consciousness for as long as hours or days. Currently, the term nonconvulsive status epilepticus should be reserved for absence SE and partial complex SE. The term "subtle status epilepticus" is more correctly used to indicate patients that have evolved from GCSE or are in a comatose state with epileptiform activity.[9-13] *(See Table 1.)*

Table 1. Clinical Classification of Status Epilepticus*

OVERT GENERALIZED CONVULSIVE STATUS EPILEPTICUS

Continuous convulsive activity and intermittent convulsive activity without regaining full consciousness
- convulsive (tonic-clonic)
- tonic
- clonic
- myoclonic

SUBTLE GENERALIZED CONVULSIVE STATUS EPILEPTICUS

Coma following generalized convulsive status epilepticus with or without motor activity

SIMPLE STATUS EPILEPTICUS (CONSCIOUSNESS PRESERVED)
- simple motor status epilepticus
- sensory status epilepticus
- aphasic status epilepticus

NONCONVULSIVE STATUS EPILEPTICUS

Consciousness impaired; twilight or fugue state
- petit mal status
- complex partial status epilepticus

Note: There is no uniform or consensus of classification at this time. See text.

* Includes both primary and secondarily generalized seizures

The Electroencephalogram. Although a detailed discussion of EEG findings in in GCSE is not necessary, it should be stressed that some patients, in whom the diagnosis of SE is not clear on the basis of clinical findings alone, may require emergent EEG testing. In this vein, a predictable evolution of EEG patterns has been observed in clinical and experimental studies of GCSE, progressing from discrete EEG seizure activity to periodic epileptiform discharges on a flat background. These changes seem correlated to bedside observations in which continuous seizure activity evolves into subtle GCSE.[9,14,15]

Clinical Correlations. Clinical management of SE has been complicated by debate surrounding its precise definition, a universal consensus of which, unfortunately, has not been forthcoming. From a clinical perspective, there is an urgent need to clarify the relationship between seizure duration and the likelihood of self-termination. Generally speaking, seizures with a sufficiently short duration frequently cease on their own and require less aggressive intervention, whereas those lasting for longer periods are more resistant to self-termination and require more aggressive pharmacological intervention.

The World Health Organization (WHO), for example, defines SE as "a condition characterized by an epileptic seizure that is sufficiently prolonged or repeated at sufficiently brief intervals so as to produce an unvarying and enduring epileptic condition."[6] Typically, SE has been defined as 30 minutes of continuous seizure activity or a series of seizures without return to full consciousness between the ictal episodes.[16] Unfortunately, this definition is ambiguous and imprecise; therefore, academic clinicians in the area often use their own criteria. It should be noted that the WHO definitions are based on clinical observations rather than EEGs or any other physiologic monitoring.

In response to the WHO criteria, a number of experts have cited landmark pathophysiologic studies demonstrating that a shorter period (i.e., < 30 minutes) of seizure activity may be associated with neuronal injury, which makes seizure self-termination unlikely. They suggest that SE be defined as a continuous convulsion lasting 20 minutes or longer.[17] Another consensus panel states that aggressive treatment for GCSE should be initiated when a seizure has persisted for just 10 minutes or longer.[16] Other neurological investigators have noted that the likelihood that a seizure will self-terminate diminishes after only four minutes of seizure activity.[18]

To clarify the relationship between seizure duration and ictal self-termination, one study evaluated a series of patients with frequent secondarily generalized tonic-clonic seizures documented by VEEG monitoring.[19] This investigation revealed that the mean duration of such seizures was one minute, and seizures that ceased spontaneously usually terminated within a two-minute window. Based on these results, the authors of this study recommended intravenous anticonvulsant drug administration for generalized tonic-clonic seizures that last longer than two minutes.[19] Althugh a consensus has not been achieved, physicians require temporal end points to guide management of SE. Consequently, for purposes of this review, a duration of five minutes or greater of continuous generalized convulsive seizure activity will arbitrarily be used as the definition of GCSE and to initiate diagnostic and treatment pathways.

Epidemiology

As would be expected, epidemiologic study of SE presents formidable reporting problems, since a significant percentage of episodes of SE occur with an acute systemic or neurologic insult. Because in many hospitals, family physicians, internists, and intensivists care for patients with SE without neurologic consultation, epidemiologic studies that depend exclusively on neurologists for identification of SE by neurologists will underestimate the prevalence of this clinical syndrome.[20] Reporting also is complicated by the fact that epidemiologic investigators usually employ a seizure duration of 30 minutes to define SE, a time period that does not conform to all current expert definitions. The arbitrary 30-minute duration criterion employed in these studies clearly underestimates the clinical incidence of SE.

With these caveats and inclusionary criteria as possible disclaimers, one report estimates that SE occurs in approximately 50,000-60,000 individuals in the United States annually.[21] In contrast, another estimate generated by an ongoing, prospective study suggests that 126,000-195,000 cases occur each year.[20] Distribution of SE by age is bimodal, with the greatest number of cases occurring in children and in invividuals older than 60 years of age.[21] The overall mortality of SE in this study was 22%, with a 3% mortality rate in the pediatric group (excluding infants less than one month of age) and 26% in the adult group. The highest mortality rates were observed in the elderly patients in the setting of hypoxic, hemorrhagic, or ischemic insults.[20]

Etiologies: Triggers, Toxins, and Trauma

In a very broad sense, the "imperfect rule of thirds" applies to the etiology of SE. That is, about one-third of all episodes of SE occur in patients with known seizure disorders, about one-third of episodes occur in patients as the initial manifestation of a seizure disorder, and the remainder result from a myriad of other medical, toxicologic, neurologic, and neurosurgical conditions. Specific incidence rates vary among studies, as do age groups evaluated, inclusionary criteria, and definitions of specific etiologies.

Causative Factors. In a 10-year retrospective review of patients 14 years of age or older at an urban hospital, the causes of GCSE included, in descending order: discontinuation or irregularity of anticonvulsant drug regimen; alcohol-related seizures; cerebrovascular disease; drug overdose; metabolic disorders; cardiac arrest; and CNS infections, trauma, and cerebral tumors. A few patients had no discernible cause.[22] A similar review performed a decade later (1980-1990) at the same institution demonstrated that these incidence rates remained essentially unchanged.[23] *(Please see Table 2.)*

An initial report from another ongoing, prospective epidemiologic study in Richmond, VA, identified three major etiologies for SE in adults: low antiepileptic drug levels; remote (i.e., secondary symptomatic) etiologies associated with a previous CNS insult including stroke, hemorrhage, or tumor, and; other precipitants, including alcohol, hypoxia, and metabolic derangments. Almost half of the adult cases with SE were caused by acute or remote cerebrovascular disease.[20] The prognosis in adults was linked primarily to underlying medical conditions, among them anoxia (71%) and hypoxia (53%), which were associated with mortality rates in excess of 25%. In contrast, SE resulting from low or indaequate antiepileptic drug levels was associated with only a 4% mortality rate.[20]

Lacking consistency in study design and terminology, these studies highlight one of the problems with assigning an etiology to episodes of SE. For example, anticonvulsant drug irregularity or noncompliance is the terminology used for the most common cause of SE in one study,[22] anticonvulsant withdrawal is the most common assigned cause in another,[23] and low antiepileptic drug levels is used in another.[20] Without question, these studies are using different terminology to refer to seizures related to irregular medication use. What is clear from these studies, despite their inconsistencies, is that most patients presenting with SE who have been prescribed anticonvulsant medications have no detectable blood levels of anticonvulsants—as many as 75% in one study [23]—and that acute treatment in the majority of these patients will not need to be altered because of concerns about anticonvulsant drug toxicity.[23]

Toxins and Antidotes. Although an in-depth discussion of toxin-induced seizures is beyond the scope of this article, common etiologies encountered by the physician will be highlighted. In this regard, theophylline, isoniazid (INH), antidepressants, and sympathomimetics including cocaine are among the common ingestions that may precipitate seizures and SE. In particular, the physician must

Table 2. Etiology of SE *(Partial List)*

SE in a patient with a history of seizure disorder
- noncompliance with prescribed medical regimen
- withdrawal seizures from anticonvulsants
- breakthrough seizures

New onset seizure disorder presenting with SE

SE secondary to medical, toxicologic, or structural symptoms
- hypoxic injury
  - post-resuscitation
  - others
- stroke syndromes
  - ischemic
  - acute
  - delayed
- subarachnoid hemorrhage
- intracranial tumor
- trauma
- toxicologic
  - theophylline
  - cocaine
  - amphetamines
  - isoniazid
  - alcohol withdrawal
- metabolic
  - hyponatremia
  - hypernatremia
  - hypercalcemia
  - hepatic encephalopathy
- infectious
  - meningitis
  - brain abscess
  - encephalitis
  - CNS
  - cysticercosis

maintain a high index of suspicion for INH-induced seizures, inasmuch as a specific antidote is available for what might otherwise apprear to be intractable seizures: one-time administration of high-dose pyridoxine in a dose equivalent to the gram amount of isoniazid ingested is useful for preventing recurrent seizures.[24] All patients with toxin-induced, GCSE require aggressive supportive care, including endotracheal intubation. In addition, repetitive charcoal dosing or hemoperfusion may be useful for some ingestions. The reader is referred to recent reviews for more information.[25,26]

Neurological and Systemic Consequences of Status Epilepticus

The necessity for targeted and aggressive management of SE is best explained against the backdrop of neurological and systemic derangements that occur with prolonged seizure activity. Because GCSE can produce permanent neuronal damage, prompt and definitive treatment is mandatory. The extent to which, and the reasons for why brain tissue is damaged are not fully characterized, but extensive animal studies—as well as more limited pathologic studies in humans following GCSE—consistently demonstrate neuronal damage.[27,28] In fact, the causes of GCSE-mediated CNS damage have been under investigation for more than 25 years, and, recently, a clearer pathophysiological picture has emerged.

Systemic Derangements. First, it should be stressed that significant physiologic changes accompany GCSE, most of which can be corrected with treatment directed at the seizure disorder. Although body temperature varies among patients with SE, there is a clear tendency for hyperpyrexia, even when infectious causes are excluded. Temperature elevation is thought to follow vigorous muscle activity associated with SE, with elevations greater than 41°C commonly observed. Peripheral leukocytosis is common as CSF pleocytosis occurs, which must be distinguished from infectious causes.[22,29,30] Hypertension, tachycardia, cardiac arrhythmias, and hyperglycemia are among the systemic effects caused by a marked increase in catecholamines that accompany GCSE.[31]

An important diagnostic clue suggesting the presence of recent seizure activity, lactic acidosis commonly occurs following a single generalized motor seizure and resolves upon termination of the seizure.[32] In fact, profound metabolic acidosis in SE has been reported with a pH less than 7.1.[33] Many of these systemic responses are believed to result from catecholamine surges that follow seizure actvity and which also accompany GCSE.[34] As a rule, the aforementioned effects are seen early in the course.[31] Increased pulmonary transcapillary fluid flux may produce pulmonary edema, although this is thought to occur from mechanisms unrelated to the increased sympathomimetic activity.[35] Prolonged GCSE can produce a variety of other clinical consequences, including hypotension, hypoglycemia, rhabdomyolysis, and CNS damage, which results primarily from ischemia and other tissue-compromising factors.[31,35,36]

As would be expected, cerebral metabolic demand increases greatly with GCSE. Surprisingly, however, cerebral blood flow and oxygenation are thought to be preserved, or even elevated, early in the course of GCSE.[37] As long as compensatory hemodynamic responses are in place, cerebral oxygenation appears to be adequate to forestall neuronal damage. However, late-stage descompensation of cardiovascular hemostasis observed in GCSE, which usually is characterized by hypotension, can occur after hours of elevated catecholamine levels.[37] Experts believe that systemic hypotension that results from prolonged GCSE may contribute to the late development of cerebral ischemia, a period characterized by diminished perfusion at a time during which cellular energy demands remain high.[31] In other words, the transition from early to late status epilepticus is often characterized by a shift from adaptive to maladaptive mechanisms.[28,26]

A marker of brain injury, serum neuron-specific enolase, has been noted to be elevated in patients with SE and may serve as a marker of brain injury.[38] Morphologic changes in humans following severe SE have also been reported.[39] Moreover, experiments in paralyzed and artificially ventilated animals in which many of the systemic metabolic changes seen in GCSE have been artificially induced suggest that neuronal loss after focal or generalized SE is linked to the abnormal neuronal discharges and not simply to the systemic effects of GCSE.[40] In this regard, excitotoxic mechanisms involving glutamate and, possi-

Table 3. Differential Diagnosis of GCSE

Nonepileptic (psychogenic) seizures
Repetitive abnormal posturing (extensor, flexor)
Tetanus
Neuroleptic malignant syndrome
Rigors due to sepsis
Myoclonic jerks
Tremors
Hemiballism
Involuntary movements

bly, aspartate have been postulated, the end result of which is calcium entry into the neuron, followed by activation of calcium-dependent enzymes that produce irreversible neuronal damage. Finally, changes in membrane lipids, free radicals, second messengers, protein kinases, and immediate-gene expression are other mechanisms postulated to cause neuronal injury. The reader is referred to recent reviews for detailed information.[27,36,41-44]

Clinical Presentation and Differential Diagnosis

Although GCSE can usually be recognized by the clinician without difficulty at the bedside, there is a limited, but important, differential diagnosis that must be considered in the patient with SE. *(Please see Table 3.)* For example, on occasion, psychogenic seizures may be difficult to distinguish from GCSE by appearance alone. In this regard, one study has noted that when confronted by pseudoseizures, a significant percentage of physicians immediately assumed that a neurological emergency was present, and, in response, embarked on an aggressive course of pharmacotherapy. In many cases, important elements of the physical examination and historical information were neglected. In this study, unresponsiveness without movement was the most common presentation.[45]

Other presentations of psychogenic SE may include asynchronous extremity movement, forward pelvic thrusting, and geotropic eye movements, a physical finding in which the eyes point in a nonphysiologic manner toward the ground, whether the head is turned left or right.[46,47] The gold standard test is confirmatory EEG monitoring at the time of seizure activity. Another potentially confusing presentation is seen in patients with acute injuries or insults to the CNS who may demonstrate rapidly repeating extensor or flexor posturing, which may be confused with convulsive activity.[48]

Diagnostic Evaluation. The initial laboratory database for patients presenting with presumed GCSE should include a CBC, blood glucose level, serum electrolytes, anticonvulsant drug levels, and urinalysis. A lumbar puncture will be necessary if meningitis is suspected. Toxicologic screening and other blood work are indicated for specific situations. A CT scan is indicated if tumor, abscess, hemorrhage, or trauma is suspected, or if the patient has no prior history of seizures.

Electroencephalogram. Evidence is accumulating that rapid access to an EEG may be required on an individualized basis. For example, if the patient fails to awaken promptly after clinical termination of the seizures, or if there is evidence of subtle SE, arrangements should be made for a prompt EEG. CT scanning might also be conisidered if the history suggests an expanding intracranial lesion. The time frame for obtaining an EEG has not been formalized, but some authors recommend 20 minutes as a decision point. In one study, 37% of patients referred for emergency EEG had combined EEG and clinical evidence of SE that was not tonic-clonic in nature and that would have gone undetected without EEG.[11]

In the recent randomized investigation evaluating treatment for GCSE, an EEG was requested as soon as a patient was entered into the study. In this trial, more than 20% of patients had ictal activity on EEG, even though tonic-clonic motor movements had ceased.[49] Clearly, EEGs may be helpful in unmasking atypical presentations of GCSE. In this regard, delays in initiating treatment for GCSE have been noted in patients who present with an altered state of consciousness that is ascribed to a postictal state, when, in fact, these individuals are in an interictal state. In these cases, treatment was delayed until further seizures were observed. STAT EEGs are recommended for the aforementioned presentations as well as for nonconvulsive SE (absence or partial complex SE), which often goes unrecognized or is mistaken for behavioral disturbance.[15,50]

Current Management Standards and Sequenced Pharmacotherapy

The rationale for emergent and aggressive treatment of generalized convulsions is based on evidence reported in clinical trials and on the basis of clinical experience. *(Please see Table 4.)* First of all, that seizures beget more seizures is a well-accepted clinical axiom. Accordingly, it follows that early treatment of an seizure episode may play a role in the prevention of SE.

Despite the life- and brain-threatening consequences of GCSE, there is no universally accepted treatment algorithm. Although many recent reviews of SE have been published, each targeting a slightly different audience, [16,51-57] until recently, none represented findings gleaned from a double-blind, randomized, multicenter trial. In contrast, the recommendations for initial treatment of SE in this article are based on the definition of GCSE as presented above and on evidentiary findings reported in a recently completed, randomized, multicenter VA trial evaluating GCSE in adults.[49]

In this study, GCSE was defined as overt (i.e., two or more seizures without complete recovery of consciousness or continuous seizure activity for 10 minutes) or subtle (coma following seizures with epileptiform activity detected on EEG). Treatment success was judged on the basis of both clinical and EEG absence of seizure activity 20-60 minutes after medication administration. Importantly, four different intravenous drug regimens were evaluated in a blinded, randomized manner for the initial treatment of GCSE: phenytoin at 18 mg/kg; diazepam 0.15 mg/kg; phenobarbital 15 mg/kg; and lorazepam 0.1 mg/kg. Lorazepam was the most successful initial medication for halting SE (65% resolved with lorazepam alone). In addition, either lorazepam or diazepam followed by phenytoin was more effective than phenytoin alone in the initial treatment of GCSE.[49]

General Principles. Management of these patients must be systematic, logical, and sequential. After the differential diagnosis

Table 4. Rationale for Aggresive Treatment of Status Epilepticus

1. The longer GCSE persists, the harder it is to control.
2. Neuronal damage is primarily caused by continuous excitatory activity, not systemic complications of GCSE.
3. Systemic complications of seizure activity, particularly hyperpyrexia, may exacerbate neuronal damage.
4. Every seizure counts in terms of making GCSE more difficult to control and for causing neuronal damage.

of GCSE is considered, pertinent history from the patient's family is obtained, and a brief physical examination is performed, the type of SE should be determined. *(Please see Table 5.)* Initial stabilization consists of aggressive supportive care, including airway management, rapid glucose testing, intravenous access (ideally, a freely flowing catheter into a large vein), as well as cardiac and hemodynamic monitoring. The precise etiology of the GCSE must be considered as treatment commences. Rather than enumerate a deterministic time line for treatment, all options are presented on an "ASAP" basis, although intervals between different interventions will depend on the individual clinical presentation.

Initial Pharmacotherapy. After the diagnosis of GCSE is confirmed, clinical data and expert recommendations indicate that the initial medication should be lorazepam (0.1 mg/kg, or 8 mg for an 80 kg adult) infused at 2 mg/min. Higher doses are unlikely to be effective. *(Please see Table 6.)* Diazepam (0.15 mg/kg or 12 mg in an 80 kg adult) may be used if lorazepam is not available, as is sometimes the case in the prehospital setting. Some experts recommend a maximum diazepam dose of 20 mg/kg in the adult if seizures are not controlled.

If the seizures have not stopped within five minutes of benzodiazepine administration, a second drug should be administered. Current recommendations suggest that the next agent should be a phenytoin compound, either phenytoin or the pro-drug fosphenytoin. No data are available that suggest a clear preference of one drug over another. However, there are important differences between these two antiepileptic agents. Phenytoin (which contains a propylene glycol diluent and a high pH) is associated with soft tissue irritation, inflammation, and rarely, tissue loss. An equivalent dose of fosphenytoin may be administered at a more rapid rate and achieves a peak level in the therapeutic range more quickly. The clinical significance of these benefits is not entirely clear, although these features of fosphenytoin would seem to have advantages. In addition, soft tissue injury is less common with water-soluble fosphenytoin.

The favorable features of fosphenytoin must be weighed against its higher cost. In fact, access to fosphenytoin is limited at many institutions because of the cost alone (approximately $70 for 1000 mg fosphenytoin vs. $3 for generic phenytoin). Studies indicate that fosphenytoin may be administered safely at 150 phenytoin equivalents (PE)/min. The FDA has determined that fosphenytoin will be dosed

Table 5. Classification of SE According to Need for Aggressive Treatment

SE REQUIRING IMMEDIATE, AGGRESSIVE TREATMENT

- Continuous generalized convulsive activity with impaired consciousness lasting greater than five minutes*
- Serial seizures without return to full consciousness between seizures
- Subtle GCSE—Coma with minimal or no associated motor activity. † (Consider if post-ictal state is not improving in 20 minutes.* May evolve from generalized convulsive status epilepticus.)

SE THAT POSSIBLY BENEFITS FROM AGGRESSIVE TREATMENT

Evidence of CNS injury from seizures is not as clear.

- Complex partial status epilepticus (twilight or fugue state)†

SE REQUIRING TREATMENT

No data to suggest time of stopping is critical to prevent CNS damage.

- Absence status epilepticus (spike-wave status epilepticus)†
- Simple motor status epilepticus (epilepsia partialis continua)†

*time is arbitrary; see text for details
†EEG may be required for diagnosis

in PE; a loading dose for an 80 kg person (20 PE/kg) could be given in as little as 10 minutes and 40 seconds following these guidelines.[58,59] Phenytoin administered at that dose (20 mg/kg) at the maximum recommended rate of 50 mg/min would require 32 minutes to complete the infusion. Dextrose-containing solutions must be avoided with phenytoin; fosphenytoin may be administered in any common intravenous solution. Cardiac monitoring and blood pressure monitoring should be in place and the need for aggressive supportive care continually reassessed regardless of which agent is employed. Hypotension and cardiac arrhythmias may be encountered at rapid infusion rates and usually respond to slowing or halting the infusion.[60]

If seizures continue after a benzodiazepine has been administered and a phenytoin (or fosphenytoin) infusion has been given at a dose consistent with 20 mg(PE)/kg, many experts recommend additional phenytoin to achieve a total of 30 mg (or PE)/kg of body weight.[16] Although this seems like a reasonable recommendation, there are no data to support this recommendation. However, it is consistent with a general principle to push each drug to a maximum or ideal dose before adding additional medications.

Refractory Generalized Convulsive Status Epilepticus. Refractory GCSE is defined in various ways, but most often, is

Table 6. Drugs for Treatment of GCSE in Adults

REGIMENS*	GENERIC	PROPRIETARY	ROUTE	DOSE	RATE	COMMENTS
Initial drug of choice—a benzodiazepine administered IV	Lorazepam	Ativan	IV	0.1 mg/kg	2 mg/min	Doses higher than 8 mg likely ineffective
	Diazepam	Valium	IV	0.15 mg/kg	4 mg/min	20 mg maximum dose reconsidered by some
If IV route unavailable, alternative regimens for benzodiazepine administration	Midazolam	Versed	IM	10 mg		Case report in adult, limited clinical information
	Midazolam	Versed	Intranasal	10 mg		Case reports dose for adult
	Diazepam	Valium	P.R.	0.5 mg/kg		Return administration reported in children. Repeat dose of 0.25 mg/kg P.R. if seizure fails to stop
	Lorazepam	Ativan	P.R.	0.1 mg/kg		Limited case reports in children
Second Agent: A phenytoin. Administer if seizures fail to stop within five minutes of drug administration	Phenytoin	Dilantin	IV	20 mg/kg	50 mg/min	Must be administered in normal saline. Hypotension, arrhythmias may necessitate slowing administration rate further. Soft-tissue necrosis reported with extravasation. Cardiac and BP monitoring necessary.
	Fosphenytoin	Cerebyx	IV or IM	20 PE**/kg	150 PE/min	Increased cost ($70-$100). Soft-tissue reactions thought to be eliminated with near-physiologic pH. Cardiac and BP monitoring necessary
Third Agent: If seizures fail to stop after optimal dosing of a benzodiazepine and phenytoin, no clear pathway exists. A variety of agents are summarized here.	Phenytoin Fosphenytoin	Dilantin Lerebyx	IV	Increase to total 30 mg/kg or 30 PE/kg	*(Same as above)*	Consensus recommendation
	Midazolam	Versed	IV	0.2 mg/kg loading dose	0.1-0.4 mg/kg (max rate infusion is 4 mg/min)	Continuous intubation, pressure support ICU admission, and EEG monitoring†
	Phenobarbital		IV	20 mg/kg	Max rate is 100 mg/min	One recommendation: Additional 10 mg/kg every 30 minutes until seizures stop
	Pentobarbital			Loading dose 5-12 mg/kg	0.5 mg/kg/h (max rate of infusion is 50 mg/min)	*(Same as above)*
	Propofol	Diprivan	IV	Loading dose 0.2 mg/kg	Infusion 0.1-2.0 mg/kg/h	Doses as high as 7.5 mg/kg/h reported
	Lidocaine			1-1.5 mg/kg bolus		Anecdotal reports; Repeat dose once reported
	Etomidate			0.3 mg/kg bolus	Infusion 20 mcg/kg/min	

characterized as persistent epileptic seizures that fail to respond to recommended doses of benzodiazepine, phenytoin, and perhaps, phenobarbital.[61] For the purposes of this discussion, refractory SE is defined as a failure to halt clinical seizure activity at the termination of benzodiazepine and phenytoin administration, or, persistent seizure activity (clinical or EEG) persisting 60 minutes after the onset of seizure activity and after adequate doses of a benzodiazepine and a phenytoin have been administered. The treatment of repetitive myoclonus in a comatose patient following diffuse hypoxic brain injury is controversial, since the response to antiepileptic drugs is poor as is the prognosis. The physiologic origin of this syndrome may not be cortical. The myoclonus is usually limited in duration and often is not treated as aggressively as GCSE unless an epileptiform EEG pattern is present.[11,62,63]

Following benzodiazepine and phenytoin administration, many options have been recommended, even though there is no data confirming the relative advantage of one additional agent over another. If seizure activity persists through and/or following the maximal therapeutic doses of a benzodiazepine and phenytoin, the likelihood of stopping the seizures with any additional agent diminshes. Additional drugs may need to be administered to the point of coma and cessation of epileptiform EEG activity. Again, there are no controlled studies or data for this group of patients and all treatments are based on consensus opinion, personal statements, case series, or isolated case reports.

Supportive care is key. The patient will most likely require intubation at this point, if not already performed, and blood pressure support with fluids or pressors is likely to be needed. Arrangements should be in progress for transfer to an ICU or other appropriate facility. EEG monitoring may become necessary and is desirable since the end point may be EEG termination of electrical seizure activity in a paralyzed patient. Of course, the etiology of the GCSE should be investigated with consideration of electrolyte abnormalities, CNS infection, or mass lesion.

Second-Line Antiepileptic Therapy. Intravenous midazolam has been recommended by some as the next choice if seizures continue following optimal dosing of lorazepam and a phenytoin. A 0.2 mg/kg loading dose is administered followed by a continuous infusion of 0.1-0.4 mg/kg/h, as determined by clinical activity and EEG monitoring. Doses may have to be increased beyond this range.[64-67]Blood pressure and respiratory support will be required. Intravenous diazepam infusion has also been employed for refractory GCSE.[68]

Third-Line Antiepileptic Therapy. An intravenous barbiturate is often recommended as the additional drug following lorazepam and a phenytoin, or it may be useful following midazolam. The choice of many intensivists is pentobarbital (5-12 mg/kg followed by 0.5-5 mg/kg/h). EEG monitoring is necessary to monitor cortical activity; intubation and pressure support will be required as well.[51,64,69,70] Traditionally, phenobarbital has been the barbiturate of choice. Recommended initial loading dosage is 20 mg/kg (no faster than 100 mg/min); again, blood pressure support, ventilation support, and EEG monitoring will be necessary. Phenobarbital may be continued at an additional 10 mg/kg every 30 minutes until the seizures stop.[51]

Miscellaneous Antiepileptic Drugs. Intravenous propofol is reported as being successful in terminating GCSE in a handful of cases with tricyclic antidepressant overdose, stroke, acute brain injury, or encephalopathy.[71,72-74] In all cases, other anticonvulsants had been administered. A bolus dose of 0.2 mg/kg may be given initially followed by infusion of 0.1-2.0 mg/kg/h with the dose titrated to clinical and EEG response. Doses as high as 7.5 mg/kg/h have been reported. Significant volume and caloric loads will accrue at this dose; expense may range to greater than $1000/d for this dose. In one study, a patient was maintained on propofol infusion as well as other anticonvulsants for eight days with eventual good recovery.[74]

Etomidate infusion has been used in the setting of refractory GCSE to terminate convulsive activity. An initial bolus is given (0.3 mg/kg) followed by additional bolus administered empirically based on continuing seizure activity. Once seizure cessation has been achieved, an infusion (20 mcg/kg/min) can be administered, which is then adjusted with EEG monitoring. In a study evalutating etomidate, patients had a variety of neurologic and medical conditions and were receiving other anticonvulsants.[75]

Anecdotal reports of intravenous lidocaine terminating refractory GCSE are scattered in the literature; undoubtedly, many unreported cases exist.[73,74] The dose in an adult is typically 100 mg repeated once if necessary; other anticonvulsants typically have been administered in varying doses. Lidocaine toxicity may cause seizures and, therefore, some consider it contraindicated for use in SE.

Neuromuscular Blocking Agents. Traditional clinical axioms state that neuromuscular (NM) blocking agents are contraindicated in patients with SE. There is certainly no merit to this unqualified statement. Short-acting NM agents may be necessary for airway management and ventilation support. The use of longer-acting agents to control motor activity necessitates EEG monitoring to verify that SE with continuing epileptiform electroencephalograhic activity is not continuing.[17,61,65]

Alternative Treatment In The Absence of Intravenous Access. Occasionally, GCSE may be encountered in a patient in whom rapid intravenous access is not possible. A variety of approaches to this problem have been described, primarily in case reports. These options are offered for information only; no recommendations can be made regarding efficacy of one treatment over another.

Diazepam administered via the rectal route has been reported effective in a number of series involving pediatric patients.[78-79] Doses of 0.5 mg/kg with a repeat dose of 0.25 mg/kg in 10 minutes is recommended, if necessary, until intravenous access can be achieved. Administration through a soft rubber catheter or using a small syringe inserted 4-5 cm inside the rectum is the described technique. In another pediatric study, a small number of children received rectal lorazepam at a dose of 0.1 mg/kg; the protocol was to repeat the dose in 15 minutes if seizures did not stop, but this did not prove necessary because all seizures were clinically terminated in the children who received one dose of lorazepam by the rectal route.[81]

A 10 mg IM dose of midazolam has been reported to terminate seizures in adults.[82] Intranasal midazolam has recently been reported to terminate SE in two cases where intravenous access was problematic. The dose employed for an adult with a renal failure, diabetes, and a history of stroke was 10 mg; for a 2-year-old child with two episodes of GCSE, doses of 1.6 mg (repeated 5 minutes later when seizures recurred) and on another occasion 4.0 mg intranasally were employed. The child had a chronic seizure disorder and was on phenobarbital chronically.[83]

IM fosphenytoin may be safely administered with peak levels occurring about 30 minutes after injection. Cardiovascular monitoring is not a label requirement. The volume of injection will be large and some prefer to divide the injection into multiple sites.[84] Although no reports have evaluated fosphenytoin administered by the IM route for terminating SE, this route of administration can be considered.

Disposition. Patients with generalized convulsive status epilepticus should be admitted to a hospital unit where vigilant observation is available and rapid intervention is possible should seizures recur. Frequently, coexisting medical conditions or advanced supportive care will necessitate ICU admission. If SE cannot be stopped, or there is evidence or suspicion of subtle SE, the patient should receive neurologic consultation in the ICU, and an EEG should be ordered on a STAT basis.

Summary

The physician will maximize clinical outcomes by using an expanded definition of GCSE. In this regard, GCSE should be considered if continuous seizure activity is present for five minutes or longer and if the patient does not awaken between seizures. Historical information, including prehospital history, should be included in the timing of onset of GCSE. Experimental evidence suggests that the abnormal electrical activity and associated changes in CNS environment makes seizures more difficult to stop once duration extends beyond 5-10 minutes.

From a practical clinical perspective, GCSE is a brain-injuring emergency that demands aggressive treatment. Put simply, neuronal injury will occur if GCSE is not terminated. Overall prognosis is most closely related to the etiology of the seizure. Lorazepam is the most effective, first drug for terminating SE and should be followed by a phenytoin compound. No clear data exist for additional recommendations, although a course of action has been outlined. It should be emphasized that SE may be secondary to a systemic or new CNS precipitant, in which case, treatment of other medical conditions is necessary.

References

1. Wilson JVK, Reynolds EH. Translation and analysis of a Cuneiform text forming part of a Babylonian treatise on epilepsy. *Med Hist* 1990;34:185-198.
2. Calmeil J. De l'epilepsie, etudieè sous le rapport de son siege et de son influence sur la production de alienation mentale. Universitè de Paris. 1824.
3. Clark LP, Prout TP. Status epilepticus: A clinical and pathological study in epilepsy. *Am J Insanity* 1904;60:645-699.
4. Clark LP, Prout TP. Status epilepticus: A clinical and pathological study in epilepsy. *Am J Insanity* 1904;61:81-108.
5. Gastaut H. Classification of status epilepticus. *Adv Neurol* 1983;34:15-35.
6. Gastaut H. Dictionary of Epilepsy. Part I: Definitions. Geneva: World Health Organization; 1973.
7. Huff JS. Nonconvulsive status epilepticus in adults (letter). *Am J Emerg Med* 1989;7:44.
8. Fagan KJ, Lee SI. Prolonged confusion following convulsions due to generalized nonconvulsive status epilepticus. *Neurology* 1990;40:1689-1694.
9. Treiman DM, Walton NY, Kendrick C. A progressive sequence of electroencephalographic changes during generalized convulsive status epilepticus. *Epilepsy Res* 1990;5:49-60.
10. Rutecki P, Sutula T. Status epilepticus. In: Johnson RT, Griffin JW, eds. *Current Therapy in Neurologic Disease.* St. Louis: Mosby-Year Book, Inc.; 1997:41-46.
11. Privitera MD, Strawsburg RH. Electroencepahlographic monitoring in the emergency department. *Emerg Med Clin N Am* 1994;12:1089-1100.
12. Treiman DM, DeGiorgio CM, Salisbury S, et al. Subtle generalized convulsive status epilepticus. *Epilepsia* 1984;25:653.
13. Treiman DM. Epileptic emergencies and status epilepticus. In: Grotta JC, ed. *Management of the Acutely Ill Neurological Patient.* New York: Churchill Livingstone; 1993:111-121.
14. Treiman DM. Generalized convulsive status epilepticus in the adult. *Epilepsia* 1993;34:S2-S11.
15. Jordan KG. Status epilepticus: A perspective from the neuroscience intensive care unit. *Neurosurg Clin N Am* 1994;5: 671-686.
16. Epilepsy Foundation of America. Treatment of convulsive status epilepticus: Recommendations of America's Working Group on status epilepticus. *JAMA* 1993;270:854-859.
17. Bleck TP, Stefan H. Status epilepticus. In: Hacke W, Hanley DF, Einhäupl KM, et al, eds. *Neurocritical Care.* New York: Springer-Verlag; 1994:761-769.
18. Bleck TP. Unpublished data. 1997.
19. Theodore WH, Porter RJ, Albert P, et al. The secondarily generalized tonic-clonic seizure: A videotape analysis. *Neurology* 1994;44:1403-1407.
20. DeLorenzo RJ, Hauser WA, Towne AR, et al. A prospective population-based epidemiological study of status epilepticus in Richmond, Virginia. *Neurology* 1996;46:1029-1035.
21. Hauser WA. Status epilepticus: Epidemiologic considerations. *Neurology* 1990;40:9-13.
22. Aminoff MJ, Simon RP. Status epilepticus: Causes, clinical features and consequences in 98 patients. *Am J Med* 1980; 69:657-666.
23. Lowenstein DH, Alldredge BK. Status epilepticus at an urban public hospital in the 1980's. *Neurology* 1993;43:483-488.
24. Wasson S, et al. Single high-dose pyridoxine treatment for isoniazid overdose. *JAMA* 1981;246:1102-1104.
25. Kunisaki TA, Augenstein WL. Drug-and toxin-induced seizures. *Emerg Med Clin N Am* 1994;12:1027-1056.
26. Olsen KR, Kearney TE, Dyer JE, et al. Seizures associated with poisoning and drug overdose. *Am J Emerg Med* 1992; 11:565-568.
27. Fountain NB, Lothman EW. Pathophysiology of status epilepticus. *J Clin Neurophysiol* 1995;12:326-342.
28. Lothman E. The biochemical basis and pathophysiology of status epilepticus. *Neurology* 1990;40:13-23.
29. Schmidley JW, Simon RP. Postictal pleocytosis. *Ann Neurol* 1981;9:81-84.
30. Devinsky O, Nadi NS, Theodore WH, et al. Pleocytosis following simple, complex partial, and generalized tonic-clonic seizures. *Ann Neurol* 1988;23:402-403.
31. Walton NY. Systemic effects of generalized convulsive status epilepticus. *Epilepsia* 1993;34:S54-S58.
32. Orringer CE, Eustace JC, Wuncsh CD, et al. Natural history of lactic acidosis after grand mal seizures. *N Engl J Med* 1977;297:796-799.

33. Tawadros HH, Thiagarajan D, Mukherji BB. Life-threatening lactic acidosis in status epilepticus. *J Kansas Med Soc* 1980; 81:461-464.
34. Simon RP. Changes in plasma catecholamines after tonic-clonic seizures. *Neurology* 1984;34:255-257.
35. Simon RP. Physiologic consequences of status epilepticus. *Epilepsia* 1985;26:S58-S66.
36. Wasterlain CG, Fujikawa DG, Penix L, et al. Pathophysiological mechanisms of brain damage from status epilepticus. *Epilepsia* 1993;34:S37-S53.
37. Benowitz NL, Simon RP, Copeland JR: Status epilepticus: Divergence of sympathetic activity and cardiovascular response. *Ann Neurol* 1986;19:197-199.
38. DeGiorgio CM, Corrale JD, Gott PS, et al: Serum neuron-specific enolase in human status epilepticus. *Neurology* 1995;45:1134-1137.
39. DeGiorgio CM, Tomiyasu U, Gott PS, et al. Hippocampal pyramidal cell loss in human status epilepticus. *Epilepsia* 1992;33:23-27.
40. Meldrum BS. Metabolic factors during prolonged seizures and their relation to nerve cell death. *Adv Neurology* 1983;34: 261-275.
41. Young D, Dragunow M. Status epilepticus may be caused by loss of adenosine anticonvulsant mechanisms. *Neuroscience* 1994;58:245-261.
42. Represa A, Jorquera L, Le Gal La Salle G, et al. Epilepsy-induced collateral sprouting of hippocampal mossy fibers: Does it induce the development of ectopic synapses with granule cell dendrites? *Hippocampus* 1993;3:257-268.
43. Sloviter RS, Dean E, Sollas AL, et al. Apoptosis and necrosis induced in different hippocampal neuron populations by repetitive perforant path stimulation in the rat. *J Comp Neurol* 1996;366:516-533.
44. Lothman EW, Bertram EH. Epileptogenic effects of status epilepticus. *Epilepsia* 1993;34:S59-S70.
45. Young GB, Gilbert JJ, Zochodne DW. The significance of myoclonic status epilepticus in postanoxic coma. *Neurology* 1990;40:1843-1848.
46. Jagoda A, Richey-Klein V, Riggio S. Psychogenic status epilepticus. *J Emerg Med* 1995;13:31-35.
47. Chabolla DR, Krahn LE, Elson LS, et al. Psychogenic nonepileptic seizures. *Mayo Clin Proc* 1996;71:493-500.
48. Haines SJ. Decerebrate posturing misinterpreted as seizure activity. *Am J Emerg Med* 1988;6:173-177.
49. Treiman DM, Meyers PD, Walton NY, et al. Treatment of generalized convulsive status epilepticus: A randomized double-blind comparison of four intravenous regimens. *N Engl J Med* 1997; (in press).
50. Kaplan PW. Nonconvulsive status epilepticus in the emergency room. *Epilepsia* 1996;37:643-650.
51. Cascino GD. Generalized convulsive status epilepticus. *Mayo Clin Proc* 1996;71:787-792.
52. Delgado-Escueta AV, Bajorek JG. Status epilepticus: mechanisms of brain damage and rational management. *Epilepsia* 1982;23:S29-S41.
53. Walsh GO, Delagado-Escueta AV. Status epilepticus. *Neurolgic Clin* 1993;11:835-855.
54. Shepherd SM: Management of status epilepticus. *Emerg Med Clin N Am* 1994;12:941-961.
55. Chang CWJ, Bleck TP. Status epilepticus. *Neurologic Clin* 1995;13:529-548.
56. Ramsey RE. Treatment of status epilepticus. *Epilepsia* 1993; 34:S71-S81.
57. Runge JW, Allen FH. Emergency treatment of status epilepticus. *Neurology* 1996;46(supp 1):S20-S23.
58. Knapp LE, Kugler AR, Eldon MA. Fosphenytoin: pharmacokinetics and administration. *Emerg Med* 1996;28:9-16.
59. Ramsey RE, DeToledo J. Intravenous administration of fosphenytoin: options for management of seizures. *Neurology* 1996;46:S17-S19.
60. Earnest MP, Marx JA, Drury LR. Complications of intravenous phenytoin for acute treatment of seizures. *JAMA* 1983;249:762-765.
61. Jagoda A, Riggio S. Refractory status epilepticus in adults. *Ann Emerg Med* 1993;22:1337-1348.
62. Leis AA, Ross MA, Summers AK. Psychogenic seizures: Ictal characteristics and diagnostic pitfalls. *Neurology* 1992; 42:95-99.
63. Kumar A, Bleck T. Intravenous midazolam for the treatment of refractory status epilepticus. *Crit Care Med* 1992;20: 483-488.
64. Bleck TP. Refractory status epilepticus. *Neurol Chronicle* 1992;2:1-4.
65. Gavrilescu T, Otis JAD. Efficacy of midazolam in pentobarbital-resistant status epilepticus. *Neurology* 1995;45:A346.
66. Parent JM. Treatment of refractory status epilepticus with continuous infusion of midazolam. *Neurology* 1994;44: 1837-1840.
67. Bell HE, Bertino JS. Constant diazepam infusion in the treatment of continuous seizure activity. *Drug Intell Clin Pharm* 1984;18:965-970.
68. Lowenstein DH, Aminoff MJ, Simon RJ. Barbiturate anesthesia in the treatment of status epilepticus: Clinical experience in 14 patients. *Neurology* 1988;38:395-400.
69. Rashkin MC, Youngs C, Penovich P. Pentobarbital treatment of refractory status epilepticus. *Neurology* 1987;37:500-503.
70. Borgeat A, Wilder-Smith OH, Jallon P, et al. Propofol in the management of refractory status epilepticus. *Intensive Care Med* 1994;20:148-149.
71. Pitt-Miller P, Elcock BJ, Maharaj M. The management of status epilepticus with a continuous propofol infusion. *Anesth Analg* 1994;78:1193-1194.
72. Merigian KS, Browning RG, Leeper KV. Successful treatment of amoxapine-induced refractory status epilepticus with propofol (Diprivan). *Acad Emerg Med* 1995;2:128-133.
73. Huff JS, Bleck TP. Propofol and midazolam in status epilepticus (letter). *Acad Emerg Med* 1996;3:179.
74. Yeoman P, Hutchinson A, Byrne A, et al. Etomidate infusions for the control of refractory status epilepticus. *Intensive Care Med* 1989;15:225-259.
75. Pascual J, Sedano MJ, Polo JM, et al. Intravenous lidocaine for status epilepticus. *Epilepsia* 1988;29:584-589.
76. Aggarwal P, Wali JP. Lidocaine in refractory status epilepticus: a forgotten drug in the emergency department. *Am J Emerg Med* 1993;11:243-244.
77. Albano A, Reisdorff EJ, Wiegenstein JG. Rectal diazepam in

pediatric status epilepticus. *Am J Emerg Med* 1989;70: 168-172.
78. Seigler RS. The administration of rectal diazepam for acute management of seizures. *J Emerg Med* 1990;8:155-159.
79. Dieckmann RA. Rectal diazepam for prehospital pediatric status epilepticus. *Ann Emerg Med* 1994;23:216-224.
80. Appleton R, Sweeney A, Choonara I, et al. Lorazepam versus diazepam in the acute treatment of epileptic seizures and status epilepticus. *Dev Med Child Neuro* 1995;37:682-688.
81. Mayhue FE. IM midazolam for status epilepticus in the emergency department. *Ann Emerg Med* 1988;17:643-645.
82. Kendall JL, Reynolds MRG. Intranasal midazolam in patients with status epilepticus. *Ann Emerg Med* 1997;29:415-417.
83. Uthman BM, Wilder BJ, Ramsey RE. Intramuscular use of fosphenytoin: an overview. *Neurology* 1996;46:S24-S28.

Hypoglycemia

William J. Brady, MD, FACEP
Alan C. Dalkin, MD

Hypoglycemia is a metabolic disorder not infrequently encountered in the emergency department (ED). Up to 20% of patients with diabetes mellitus using insulin or oral hypoglycemic agents (OHA) will experience symptoms of hypoglycemia in their lifetimes, which often require ED evaluation and therapy.[1-3] If one considers all patients with altered mentation presenting to the ED, hypoglycemia is identified as the underlying process in approximately 7% of cases. In addition to the diabetic patient, numerous other clinical scenarios may involve hypoglycemia, including toxicologic, infectious, psychiatric, and metabolic syndrome presentations.[4,5]

Fortunately, hypoglycemia most often is diagnosed easily and is rapidly treated with satisfactory patient outcome in the ED. The classic presentation of hypoglycemia involves a diaphoretic patient with a history of diabetes mellitus who is found to have an altered mental status; the patient is subsequently found to have used insulin or OHA and taken relatively little oral nutrition. The patient's presentation and history, however, may lead the provider to believe that the condition is due to some other condition such as a cerebrovascular accident, status epilepticus, intoxication, sepsis, or traumatic injury.[6-10]

The purpose of this review is to outline current diagnostic and management approaches to the patient suspected of having hypoglycemia.

Introduction

The diagnosis of hypoglycemia is based on the presence of Whipple's triad, which consists of a low plasma glucose concentration, symptoms consistent with the diagnosis, and improvement of these symptoms following an increase in the plasma glucose level. This definition certainly has a number of problems when applied clinically. For example, diabetic patients may manifest hypoglycemic symptoms at normal or even elevated plasma glucose values due to the presence of altered glycemic thresholds. In the other extreme, apparently normal women may develop asymptomatic plasma glucose concentrations of fewer than 40 milligrams per deciliter (mg/dL) during a fast. The serum glucose value must not be considered the absolute criterion for hypoglycemia; rather, the serum sugar level must be correlated with the clinical picture.

Both the diagnosis and treatment of hypoglycemia are easily accomplished, assuming the clinician considers the possibility of such a metabolic derangement. It is imperative that the emergency physician consider hypoglycemia in all patients with any mental status abnormality, focal neurological deficit, or seizure activity—even when the findings seem to be explained initially by other etiologies. Blood glucose should be monitored in any patient with any degree of mental status abnormality, even if the altered mentation appears to be explained by other clinical findings or medical conditions. An estimate using a bedside glucose monitoring device is sufficient, with the understanding that these devices have greater error at the high and low extremes.

If bedside monitoring suggests hypoglycemia, laboratory levels should be determined, followed by rapid glucose replacement therapy. Significant medical harm to the patient and medicolegal risks for the emergency physician are issues to consider in cases involving misdiagnosis, incorrect therapy, and inappropriate disposition.[11] Although hypoglycemia is rarely fatal, significant, irreversible central nervous system (CNS) damage may occur if the blood glucose concentration is not rapidly corrected. Further, medical interventions such as neuromuscular blockade-assisted endotracheal intubation may be avoided with prompt normalization of the mental status abnormality by dextrose infusion.[8-10]

Clinical Pathophysiology

Blood glucose homeostasis is essential for maintenance of normal brain function, and involves a complex interaction of neural, metabolic, and hormonal factors. The brain requires approximately 150 grams/day of glucose, which must be continuously available.

Specific measurements of daily glucose requirements in the child are lacking; on the basis of animal studies, however, it appears that the necessary amount is two- to three-fold greater compared to the adult. The CNS depends upon glucose as its primary energy source, requiring a continuous supply of carbohydrate fuel for normal function; the CNS has a small reservoir of glucose that is sufficient for only a few minutes of normal brain function. Ketone bodies may be used by the CNS for metabolism if glucose is not available. In the acute setting, neuronal death due to hypoglycemia begins rapidly after the onset of significant mental status alteration, particularly if coma ensues. Despite these stringent demands, the body normally functions quite well in maintaining plasma glucose levels within a narrow range even with constant changes in glucose intake and/or utilization.

Glucoregulation. The primary glucoregulatory organs are the pancreas and the adrenal medulla and cortex and the pituitary gland. These organs maintain glucose control via the release and interaction of various hormonal agents, including insulin, glucagon, the catecholamines epinephrine and norepinephrine, cortisol, and growth hormone. Insulin is the major metabolic regulatory factor, acting predominantly in the liver, skeletal muscle, and adipose tissue. The secretion of insulin suppresses endogenous glucose production, stimulates glucose utilization, and increases glucose storage in the form of glycogen, thus lowering the plasma glucose concentration.

The first defense against the development of hypoglycemia is a decrease in insulin secretion. It has been clearly demonstrated, however, that additional counter-regulatory mechanisms are involved in a complex hierarchical fashion. Experimental studies have demonstrated that both glucagon and epinephrine are of primary importance in the acute protection against hypoglycemia. Both of these counter-regulatory hormones are the only agents capable of stimulating hepatic glucose production within minutes of their release into circulation, primarily via glycogenolysis (the release of glucose from its intracellular storage depot glycogen).

The effect of these two hormones, beyond the immediate period after their release, is felt predominately through their effect on gluconeogenesis (i.e., the de novo production of glucose from other metabolic substrates). Glucagon is thought to be the major counter-regulatory hormone, while epinephrine is important under certain conditions, especially during glucagon deficiency and in the generation of warning symptoms of hypoglycemia: the hyperepinephrinemic constellation of findings. Epinephrine also stimulates hepatic glucose production and limits glucose utilization. In contrast to glucagon and epinephrine, glucocorticoid and growth hormone responses to the presence of hypoglycemia are thought to be of minor importance in the acute setting; in fact, cortisol and growth hormone have been shown to be largely involved in the protection against prolonged hypoglycemia which can last days to weeks.

The fasting period describes the interval between feedings, beginning approximately four hours after eating and extending up to the next meal; blood glucose concentrations can begin to decline in as little as six hours when fasted. In the fasted individual, the maintenance of normal blood glucose levels are dependent on an adequate supply of endogenous gluconeogenic substrates (amino acids, glycerol, lactate), functionally intact hepatic and renal glycogenolytic and gluconeogenic enzymatic systems, and normal endocrinologic function for integrating and modulating these processes. Hypoglycemia may result if any part of this system is disrupted.

During fasting, relatively low insulin levels initiate the mobilization of these various stored fuels from host tissue sources. The most readily and rapidly available source of glucose is hepatic glycogen that is formed via glycogenolysis. The glycogen reserve is limited and will be depleted after 24-48 hours of fasting in the healthy patient and possibly earlier in the malnourished individual (e.g., chronic alcohol abuser or patient with end stage renal disease). With continuation of fasting (approximately 4-6 hours), gluconeogenesis becomes the primary source of blood glucose required for CNS metabolism and other bodily processes.

Gluconeogenesis, which takes place primarily in the liver, uses various metabolic substrates to generate this additional glucose supply. Amino acids represent one such source of metabolic substrate for gluconeogenesis and are mobilized from muscle tissue via proteolysis, which is facilitated by low insulin levels and mediated by both cortisol and glucagon. Lactate, from recycled glucose, and glycerol, from lipolysis, represent relatively minor yet important sources of substrate for gluconeogenesis. During overnight fasting, 90% of gluconeogenesis occurs via proteolysis with conversion of amino acids to glucose.

The adult human is capable of maintaining normal blood glucose levels even when totally deprived of caloric intake for weeks, or in the case of obese subjects, for several months. In the infant, this homoeostatic process is more complex. The normal term infant exhibits an immediate drop in serum glucose concentration during the first 4-6 hours of life; this reduction ranges from approximately 45 mg/dL to a level equal to the maternal concentration. The child must quickly assume the function of blood glucose homeostasis. In the fasting state, the normal neonate and infant exhibit a progressive fall in the blood glucose content to hypoglycemic levels when fasted for relatively short periods.

This response is in marked contrast to the adult who is capable of maintaining normal serum glucose values for prolonged periods without an exogenous supply of metabolic fuel. The specific reasons for this difference are unclear, yet it is obvious that the young individual, when fasted, is unable to supply sufficient glucose to meet the obligatory metabolic demands of the body. Similar issues are encountered in the malnourished adult who has fasted for greater than 12 hours; for example, the chronic alcoholic who is managed in an ED-based observation unit.

Symptoms and Responses to Hypoglycemia

Development of low serum sugar values without the physiologic ability to react places the individual at greater risk for coma and other neurologic sequelae; the patient with such a process will not recognize the complication until lower serum sugar levels are reached. Various issues contribute to an unawareness of hypoglycemia, including age, comorbidity, medication therapy, autonomic neuropathy, and the degree of serum sugar control. It has been suggested that the elderly patient is more likely to experience hypoglycemia without an awareness of the event; the presence of past CNS injury, such as stroke, in the older patient also increases the chance of unrecognized hypoglycemia.

Beta-adrenergic receptor antagonists block the effects of epinephrine, thereby contributing to a patient being unaware of hypoglycemia. Furthermore, patients with diabetes mellitus and autonomic neuropathy demonstrate blunted counter-regulatory responses to hypoglycemia—such a blunted response may result clinically in a patient's being unaware of hypoglycemia.[12] With increasingly rigid control of the serum sugar (i.e., a lower mean serum sugar level maintained over time), it has been demonstrated that patients with diabetes mellitus without neuropathy also have reduced responses of the counter-regulatory hormones—potentiating a lack of awareness of hypoglycemia.[13] This may result from either a lack of CNS recognition of hypoglycemia or impaired autonomic response to low serum sugar.

Etiology of Hypoglycemia: Common Syndromes

A number of clinical conditions that produce hypoglycemia are recognized and frequently encountered in the ED. Please see Table 1 for a listing of such syndromes relative to patient age. Perhaps the most frequent situation involves the patient with diabetes mellitus who is maintained on either insulin or OHA. Excessive medication use and/or lack of caloric intake naturally results in hypoglycemia. Acute ethanol intoxication, chronic alcohol abuse, chronic malnutrition, liver disease, sepsis, fasting, and endocrinopathies (hypothyroidism, hypoadrenalism, and insulinoma) also are common settings in which hypoglycemia develops. Unfortunately, the clinical manifestations noted on ED presentation are not predictive of the etiology of hypoglycemia; in many instances, the ultimate etiology is not discovered in the ED. The most common clinical scenarios producing hypoglycemia in patients presenting to an urban ED were noted to occur at the following frequencies: diabetic medical therapy, 54%; ethanol use, 48%; and sepsis, 12%.[4]

Pharmacologic therapy for diabetes mellitus is the most frequently cited reason for development of hypoglycemia managed in the ED.[4] Typically, the patient has a history of diabetes mellitus and is taking physician-supervised medications for treatment of the condition; at times, however, the patient without diabetes mellitus will present with hypoglycemia resulting from an adverse reaction to such medical therapy.

The various patient scenarios include the following: 1) the diabetic patient who correctly uses anti-diabetic medications yet consumes little oral nutrition with or without significant physical exertion; 2) a similar patient who develops hypoglycemia due to incorrect medication dosing or drug interactions; 3) the patient—with or without a history of diabetes—who knowingly injects insulin or ingests an OHA in a self-harm attempt; and 4) the child who is accidentally exposed to diabetic medications.

If one considers the long-term use of insulin or OHA in the management of diabetes mellitus, hypoglycemia will occur yearly in 15-20% of patients.[1,2,4] The characteristics of the diabetic patient who

Table 1. Potential Etiologies of Hypoglycemia Relative to Age

AGE GROUP	CAUSE/SYNDROME
NEONATE	
	Maternal diabetes mellitus
	Maternal toxemia
	Small size for gestational age
	Sepsis
	Malnutrition/fasting
	Hyperinsulinism
	Deficiency of glycogenolytic enzyme
	Deficiency of gluconeogenic enzyme
	Hormone deficiency
	Medication/toxin effect
	Idiopathic
INFANT	
	Sepsis
	Malnutrition/fasting
	Hyperinsulinism
	Deficiency of glycogenolytic enzyme
	Deficiency of gluconeogenic enzyme
	Hormone deficiency
	Medication/toxin effect
	Idiopathic
CHILD	
	Sepsis
	Malnutrition/fasting
	Ketotic hypoglycemia
	Islet cell adenoma
	Hormone deficiency
	Medication/toxin effect
	Idiopathic
ADOLESCENT	
	Sepsis
	Malnutrition/fasting
	Islet cell adenoma
	Hormone deficiency
	Medication/toxin effect
	Idiopathic
ADULT	
	Sepsis
	Malnutrition/fasting
	Medication/toxin effect

is more likely to experience hypoglycemia include male gender, both adolescent and very elderly age groups, African-American heritage, a history of hypoglycemia, "intensive" diabetic medical therapy, insulin use (compared to OHA therapy), polypharmacy (more than 5 agents), and recent hospitalization.[1-3]

Pharmacologic Precipitants. Several classes of oral hypoglycemic agents used in the treatment of diabetes can cause hypoglycemia.[14,15] The sulfonylureas act to increase endogenous insulin secretion and thereby increase hepatic glucose uptake and peripheral tissue glucose disposal. Thus, sulfonylurea treatment with reduced caloric intake can result in hypoglycemia. Sulfonylureas are both metabolized by the liver and cleared by the kidneys. Therefore, progressive renal insufficiency, as is seen with diabetic nephropathy, can prolong the half-life of certain sulfonylureas and result in prolonged hypoglycemia.

The thiazolidinediones are a newer class of agents that act to reduce insulin resistance in skeletal muscle, liver, and adipose tissue via peroxisome proliferator-activated receptors (PPAR). In so doing, they do not directly alter insulin secretion; therefore, their use as single agents is not associated with hypoglycemia. The introduction of the medication metformin, a biguanide, has added another medication to the list of agents encountered in the diabetic patient. Metformin improves the end-organ sensitivity to insulin and acts via a number of mechanisms in the diabetic patient, including a reduction in hepatic glucose output and enhanced peripheral glucose uptake. Metformin is considered an anti-hyperglycemia drug rather than a hypoglycemic agent such as the sulfonylureas and insulin; hypoglycemia is rarely encountered in patients using only metformin.

Notably, current approaches to treating patients with Type II diabetes mellitus include step-wise addition of medications as glycemic control worsens. In so doing, combinations of agents such as sulfonylureas and biguanides or thiazolidinediones are often utilized. While the biguanides or thiazolidinediones when used alone do not precipitate hypoglycemia, when used with an agent that increases insulin secretion (e.g., a sulfonylurea), hypoglycemia may become a significant problem.

From the perspective of drug-induced hypoglycemia, diabetic medical therapy is the most frequent etiologic factor in the hypoglycemic patient who presents to the ED; 54% percent of hypoglycemic patients presenting to the ED developed the complication due to such adverse medication effects.[4] Among patients experiencing symptomatic low blood sugar, insulin is the most frequent specific agent, and is reportedly responsible for hypoglycemia twice as often as OHA.[3] OHAs, both in diabetic patients using such therapy and in children accidentally exposed to the medication, represent another frequent drug-related etiology of hypoglycemia.[3,16,17] Seltzer showed that 220 (47%) of 473 patients exhibited exogenous hypoglycemia resulting from the use of OHA.[5] Additionally, ethanol was involved in 36% of cases. Three percent of these patients developed hypoglycemia due to salicylates. Interestingly, insulin was infrequently encountered as a cause of hypoglycemia in this study.

Another commonly used medication class that may be encountered in patients developing hypoglycemia is the adrenergic-blocking agents, particularly beta-blockers. Most often, the beta-adrenergic blocking agent is implicated as a co-instigator in the development of hypoglycemia, rather than the actual cause of lowered blood sugar levels. Such medications, particularly the nonselective beta-blocker agents, impair glycogenolysis and the hyperepinephrinemic response to lowered serum sugar levels, thus predisposing to hypoglycemia. Hypoglycemia resulting from the sole ingestion of such adrenergic-blocking agents is rare.[5]

Ethanol. Approximately 50% of patients treated for hypoglycemia in an urban ED were acutely intoxicated with ethanol or were chronic alcohol abusers.[4] Alcohol inhibits hepatic gluconeogenesis, which becomes problematic when the patient has not eaten for a prolonged period and the glycogen stores have been depleted by glycogenolysis. A 12-hour fast often is sufficient for alcoholics to become hypoglycemic due to pre-existing malnutrition. Hypoglycemia also has been produced in healthy adults by infusing 75 grams of alcohol after a 36-hour fast. The depressed level of consciousness found in the patient acutely intoxicated with ethanol can mask the clinical findings of hypoglycemia, making it essential for rapid bedside serum glucose determinations to be performed on all such patients with any degree of mental status abnormality or evidence of alcohol use.

Sepsis. Sepsis may cause hypoglycemia by inhibition of gluconeogenesis and/or by increased responsiveness to insulin. Systemic hypoperfusion, often associated with sepsis, increases peripheral glucose utilization, while metabolic acidosis decreases gluconeogenesis. The multiorgan failure associated with the sepsis syndrome not infrequently includes hepatic dysfunction and an increased potential for hypoglycemia.

Pediatric Patients. Considering the pediatric perspective, the vast majority of neonates developing hypoglycemia will have clinical markers (maternal diabetes mellitus or toxemia of pregnancy, small for gestational age, or prematurity) that immediately identify these patients as high-risk infants. Hypoglycemia in most newborns resolves spontaneously within hours to days of diagnosis. In that neonatal hypoglycemia is a relatively common, transient event, it is usually treated empirically without a detailed diagnostic evaluation. If hypoglycemia in the infant is persistent or severe, however, a diagnostic evaluation must be initiated. Despite the many known causes, an infant with persistent hypoglycemia is likely to have a disorder in one of four categories, including: hyperinsulinism, deficiency of a glycogenolytic or gluconeogenic enzyme, hormone deficiency, or idiopathic disorder. Similarly, the older child with an isolated, persistent finding of hypoglycemia is likely to have one of the following disorders producing primary hypoglycemia: ketotic hypoglycemia, hormone deficiency (growth hormone or glucocorticoid), or islet cell adenoma.

Secondary hypoglycemia in children has been seen in certain toxicologic syndromes (the various diabetic medical therapies, ethanol, salicylates, and beta-adrenergic blocking agents), sepsis, and fasting states. Excessive diabetic medication use and/or lack of caloric intake naturally results in hypoglycemia. In a study by Seltzer, 3% of these patients developed hypoglycemia due to salicylates;[5] of the cases involving salicylate-induced hypoglycemia, 87% were in children with a 39% death rate. Sixteen percent of hypoglycemic cases related to ethanol occurred in children, with a mortality rate of 25% in this subgroup.

Clinical Presentation and Evaluation

Patients with hypoglycemia may present to the ED with a range of symptoms and signs. (Please see Table 2 for a listing of the occurrence frequency of the symptoms and signs of the hypoglycemic patient seen in the ED.) The clinical manifestations of hypoglycemia can be divided into two broad categories: neuroglycopenic and hyperepinephrinemic (also known as the autonomic or sympathomimetic findings). As glucose is the main energy source for the CNS, it is not surprising that most episodes of symptomatic hypoglycemia present with neurologic dysfunction. With a decline in serum sugar, the brain quickly exhausts its reserve supply of carbohydrate fuel, resulting in CNS dysfunction, which is manifested most commonly by alterations in consciousness such as lethargy, confusion, and unresponsiveness.

Importantly, agitation and combativeness also are seen in these patients. Other neuroglycopenic manifestations include convulsive activity and the development of focal neurologic deficits. A review of 125 cases of hypoglycemia presenting to an urban ED showed that the neuroglycopenic findings predominated.[4] A depressed sensorium was noted in 52% of cases, with other mental status changes (e.g., agitation and combativeness) found in 30% of patients. Described less frequently, seizure activity and focal neurological findings were encountered in 7% and 2% of such ED patients, respectively.[4] In the absence of neuronal damage, these neurologic deficits should reverse with the administration of glucose and do not require aggressive evaluation such as the computed tomography (CT) scan of the head.

A rapid fall in blood glucose levels and/or the hypothalamic sensing of neuroglycopenia cause the release of the counter-regulatory hormones, primarily the catecholamines epinephrine and norepinephrine. The release of these counter-regulatory hormones is responsible for the hyperepinephrinemic findings, including anxiety, nervousness, irritability, nausea, vomiting, palpitations, and tremor. These findings result from the actions of the adrenergic nervous system (e.g., catecholamine release) that are triggered by hypoglycemia. Such signs and symptoms were noted in 8% of ED patients with hypoglycemia.[4] Stimulation of the cholinergic nervous system also occurs and may result in manifestations such as sweating, changes in pupillary size, bradycardia, and increased secretion of parotid saliva.The term "hyperepinephrinemic" is a misnomer in that cholinergic factors resulting from autonomic nervous system stimulation also are noted in certain patients.

The rapidity of onset of the hypoglycemic event in part determines the presentation. A gradual onset of hypoglycemia results from a relatively slow decrease in the serum glucose and the development of the neuroglycopenic signs and symptoms. Conversely, a sudden drop in the blood sugar level will produce anxiety, diaphoresis, tremor, and the other hyperepinephrinemic findings. In most cases of hypoglycemia, however, CNS dysfunction predominates with some degree of alteration in the level of awareness, and is accompanied by diaphoresis and tachycardia.

Children. Similar symptoms and signs are encountered in the pediatric setting, especially in the older child. Although the biochemical diagnosis of hypoglycemia is rather simple in the pediatric patient, clinical manifestations in the child can sometimes be misleading. In newborns and young infants, for example, hypoglycemia frequently presents with a number of nonspecific findings usually associated with other etiologies; these presentations include feeding difficulties, irritability, lethargy, cyanosis, tachypnea, and hypothermia. In fact, Losek has shown that approximately one in five children undergoing resuscitation have hypoglycemia requiring therapy.[18] Furthermore, hypoglycemia also has been reported in the child with dehydration of various causes as occurring approximately 10% of the time; this finding, of uncertain clinical significance, may only require appropriate therapy for the underlying illness—most often, viral gastroenteritis.[19] These signs and symptoms are in marked contrast to those encountered in the older child and the adult.

Table 2. Frequency of Presenting Signs and Symptoms in Hypoglycemia[4]

CLINICAL PRESENTATION	FREQUENCY (%)
Depressed sensorium	52
Other mental status changes	30
Hyper-epinephrinemic findings	8
Seizure	7
Focal neurologic findings	2

Differential Diagnosis. Unsuspected hypoglycemia may masquerade as neurologic, psychiatric, traumatic, or toxicologic disorders. Hypoglycemia has been misdiagnosed as cerebrovascular accident, transient ischemic attack, seizure disorder, traumatic head injury, brain tumor, narcolepsy, multiple sclerosis, psychosis, sympathomimetic drug ingestion, hysteria, and depression. A number of reports are found in the medical literature describing hypoglycemic patients who present with mental status abnormalities and focal neurological deficits, masquerading as cerebrovascular accidents (CVA).[6,7] These patients were initially suspected of having suffered a CVA; only later in the evaluation was the diagnosis of hypoglycemia discovered. Hypoglycemia also can masquerade as traumatic head injury with varying degrees of altered mentation,[10] as well as cardiac arrhythmia with bradycardia.[20]

Patients with hypoglycemia have been misdiagnosed with decompensated psychosis, as well as acute sympathomimetic ingestion.[8] Law enforcement officials also have detained, arrested, and eventually transported patients to the ED with unrecognized hypoglycemia; out-of-hospital information provided by police personnel should not dissuade the emergency physician from the consideration of hypoglycemia.[21] Other atypical presentations of hypoglycemia also are seen in the ED, including urticaria, night terrors in children, altered sleep patterns in adults, and orthopedic injuries, particularly posterior shoulder dislocation, which most often results from hypoglycemic convulsive activity.

Misdiagnosis. The importance of these various atypical clinical presentations is found in the initial impression of an alternative, more common explanation for the patient's abnormalities. Such an approach not infrequently leads to failure of blood glucose determination early in the evaluation. This approach also results in either a delayed or missed diagnosis, with associated morbidity due to CNS injury and/or unnecessary invasive procedures and therapies. It is imperative for emergency physicians to consider hypoglycemia as a potential cause of altered mentation and rapidly screen for this metabolic abnormality with a bedside determination followed by replacement therapy, regardless of the presumed reason for the patient's condition. The use of bedside testing is preferred in that the result is immediately available to the clinician; its result may alter therapeutic and diagnostic plans. Reliance on the clinical laboratory serum sugar result may expose the patient to prolonged, unrecognized hypoglycemia and unnecessary treatments, procedures, and investigations.[22]

Glucose Testing. Beyond serum glucose determination, the ability to evaluate hypoglycemia in the ED is limited. A thorough history, physical examination, selected radiographic investigations, and laboratory studies, such as random glucose, are the main tools available to the emergency physician. Obvious infectious, toxicologic, and metabolic issues should be investigated and ruled out as necessary. Other laboratory studies, such as measurement of the levels of serum insulin, insulin antibodies, and C peptides, should be obtained in conjunction with either the patient's primary physician or the health care provider charged with outpatient responsibility. Progressive renal insufficiency should be ruled out by an analysis of the blood urea nitrogen and serum creatinine; in that insulin is significantly metabolized by the kidney, reduced renal function will prolong its active life and cause hypoglycemia.

In most instances, the diagnosis of hypoglycemia is easily and rapidly accomplished in the ED. A bedside glucose test should be performed as soon as possible after the patient arrives to the ED if the patient has an abnormal mental status. The accuracy of these bedside reflectance tests is acceptable, though less reliable at the extremes of the spectrum, i.e., extremely low and high serum sugar levels. If possible, immediately prior to IV dextrose therapy, a serum sample should be obtained and sent to the lab for definitive analysis.

The serum glucose level at which individual patients develop symptoms varies as a function of age, sex, recent dietary intake, chronic nutritional status, emotional state, comorbidity, and medication use. Hence, a single definition which defines a level at which hypoglycemia occurs in all patients is not possible. Blood glucose levels do not predict symptoms;[4] in fact, the clinical state of the patient must be correlated with the glucose value made at the determination.[4] Patients may present with profound coma and demonstrate only modestly low serum glucose levels. Conversely, a serum sugar of 20 mg/dL may be measured in an alert patient who only complains of anxiety, weakness, and extreme hunger. In the nondiabetic patient (i.e., normal patient) with the plasma glucose value dropping to approximately 50 mg/dL, epinephrine release occurs with activation of the autonomic nervous system—and the development of the hyperepinephrinemic findings.

If the process continues without curative therapy, the serum sugar will continue to decline; neuroglycopenic signs may not occur until the serum sugar concentration reaches even lower levels in the range of 20 mg/dL. Diabetic patients with poorly controlled sugar levels appear to have higher symptomatic thresholds (i.e., higher serum glucose values) for the development of symptomatic hypoglycemia, whereas well controlled diabetics and nondiabetics have significantly lower thresholds (i.e., lower serum glucose values).[23] Anorexia nervosa and other chronic starvation states produce a lower fasting serum glucose at which patients develop symptomatic hypoglycemia.[24]

Furthermore, the definition of hypoglycemia in the infant and child differs from that commonly used in the adult. Infants and children generally become symptomatic when the blood glucose drops below a concentration of 40 mg/dL. Blood glucose concentrations below 20-30 mg/dL during the first three days of life are considered hypoglycemic in pre-term or small-for-date neonates and values below 30 mg/dL in term infants. Other investigators disagree with these limits, defining the lowest acceptable levels to be between 40 and 50 mg/dL for all age groups—children and adult. This recommendation seems reasonable for the emergency physician; such an approach will insure that all hypoglycemic patients receive appropriate therapy.

Interpretation. The serum glucose value, therefore, must not be considered the absolute criterion to define hypoglycemia. Rather, the serum sugar level must be correlated with the clinical picture and the particular patient with age and comorbidity considerations. Emergency physicians, however, must establish a numerical threshold below which prompt treatment is administered even in the absence of symptoms; a plasma glucose value below 50 mg/dL is significant and sufficient to make a diagnosis of hypoglycemia, prompting treatment. Such an approach appears reasonable in most instances in that this value represents the physiologic level at which counter-regulatory systems are activated.

When interpreting serum sugar results, it also is important to consider both the methods of sample collection and storage of the blood sample. It has been shown that the glucose values of whole blood are approximately 15% less than serum or plasma. This discrepancy is due to the relatively low glucose concentration in red blood cells—with storage, equilibriation occurs. Venous blood has been found to have a 10% lower glucose concentration when compared to either capillary or arterial blood. Finally, the collecting tube should contain fluoride to inhibit glycolysis in vitro before the sample is assayed.

Endocrine Evaluation

Having fulfilled the criteria of Whipple's triad (the presence of symptoms at the time of documented hypoglycemia with resolution of those symptoms following restoration of euglycemia), it is essential to establish a specific etiology for hypoglycemia.[25] As noted above, in the diabetic patient treated with either insulin or certain oral hypoglycemic agents, the sequence of events resulting in low blood glucose values may be readily apparent. However, it should be cautioned that in the well-controlled diabetic patient with previously rare hypoglycemia, the recent appearance of recurrent low blood sugars should alert the physician to consider additional medical conditions. For example, alteration in insulin levels and subsequent hypoglycemia may be observed in progressive renal failure or hypothyroidism. Similarly, the loss of a counter-regulatory hormone (see below), as seen in adrenal insufficiency, should be considered. Addison's disease may result from an unrelated adrenal process in patients with Type I diabetes or may be part of a polyglandular autoimmune syndrome.

Differential Diagnosis. Aside from the scenarios of exogenous insulin, oral hypoglycemic agents, alcohol intoxication, or overwhelming sepsis, identification of the cause for spontaneous hypoglycemia requires a careful and rigorous medical evaluation. Three broad categories encompass the most common causes of hypoglycemia: 1) an excess of glucose lowering hormones; 2) a deficit of glucose "stores" during fasting, usually related to depletion of glycogen stores (see above); and 3) a deficit of counter-regulatory hormones. While some physicians have grouped the various diagnoses into fasting and non-fasting patterns, the distinction between these two profiles are often blurred, and patients may have episodes of hypoglycemia that do not neatly fit into either category.

Insulinoma. Three peptide hormones retain the action of reducing blood glucose levels. This includes insulin as well as insulin-like growth factor (IGF) -I and -II. Insulinomas, islet cell tumors secreting insulin in a non-regulated fashion, are the most common tumor type resulting in hypoglycemia. These tumors usually present in patients older than age 40, with symptoms becoming apparent either with fasting or several hours after a meal. Hypoglycemia commonly occurs after exercise or alcohol ingestion. Forty percent of insulinomas are smaller than 1 cm in size, rendering it difficult to image these neoplasms. The distribution of islet cell neoplasms is generally equal between the head, body, and tail of the pancreas, though a rare tumor (< 1%) is ectopic to the pancreas. Eighty percent of insulinomas are single neoplasms, with 10% of cases having multiple adenomas (often associated with the multiple endocrine neoplasia syndromes).

As the initial step in documenting the presence of an insulinoma, it is mandatory to establish an inappropriate circulating insulin level in the presence of hypoglycemia. Moreover, hormonal evaluation should precede any attempt at imaging a possible tumor. In evaluating the relationship between insulin and glucose, this must be undertaken during a fast. Following caloric intake, patterned changes in glucose and then insulin are observed, and either high or low ratios of insulin to glucose are observed in normals as well as patients with endocrine tumors. As noted above, the prolonged fast is the gold standard test, with 30% of patients with insulinoma manifesting hypoglycemia within 12 hours, 70% within 24 hours, 92% within 48 hours, and 98% within 72 hours.

Due to the need for frequent sampling of insulin and glucose levels, as well as the severity of the hypoglycemia should it occur, these studies are routinely performed in the hospital setting. Generally, glucose and insulin values are obtained simultaneously every six hours and with any symptoms of hypoglycemia. While absolute blood glucose values at which to terminate the fast may differ between centers, we generally view values of less than 50 mg/dL in males and 40 mg/dL in females as the thresholds below which pathologic hypoglycemia is certain. However, the presence of "typical" hypoglycemic symptoms at a higher blood glucose value may be sufficient to terminate the fast.

For establishing pathologic hypoglycemia, the ratio of insulin to glucose is calculated. Simply, insulin (μU/mL) concentration is divided by glucose (mg/dL) concentration with normals having ratios less than 0.3. To improve specificity, the "amended" insulin to glucose ratio is more widely utilized and is calculated as: (insulin (μu/mL) x 100)/ (glucose (mg/dL) - 30). Normal individuals have an AIGR less than 50. During a fast, supporting evidence for an insulinoma also may include proinsulin levels greater than 22% and a failure to detect ketonuria (assessed daily), as ongoing insulin secretion will suppress ketone body production.

As a caution in interpreting insulin levels, either exogenous insulin or the administration of oral hypoglycemic drugs such as sulfonylureas will result in abnormal insulin to glucose ratios. In that light, we suggest that a serum sample for C-peptide and a urine sample be analyzed for sulfonylurea usage at the time of hypoglycemia. In a patient administering insulin, C-peptide levels are low while insulin levels are inappropriately high. Surreptitious use of sulfonylureas increases both insulin and C-peptide concentrations; hence, results may appear quite similar to those seen in a patient with an insulinoma.

Radiographic Studies. Localizing studies for pancreatic neoplasms in general and insulinomas in specific include CT scanning, magnetic resonance imaging (MRI), angiography, selective venous sampling, and octreotide scintigraphy. As many insulin-producing neoplasms are small, CT or MRI may fail to detect the tumor. Success with angiography is highly variable, with reports ranging from 30% to 90% sensitivity. Venous sampling also is difficult and carries a substantial risk in terms of complications. Recently, it has become clear that a substantial percentage of insulinomas express cell surface receptors for somatostatin. The somatostatin analog, octreotide, has therefore been used as a diagnostic (and therapeutic) tool. Radiolabled octreotide scanning has a detection rate that varies between 40% and 80%, which is likely related to the range of receptor expression in tumor tissues as well as the technical difficulty of the procedure.

Non-Islet Cell Tumors. Non-islet cell tumors also may result in hypoglycemia. While there exist a number of postulated mechanisms for low glucose concentrations, these tumors do not release insulin itself but rather produce insulin-like peptides. IGF-1 is produced primarily by the liver and is thought to be important in multiple facets of physiology, including tissue repair and linear growth. It is primarily regulated by pituitary growth hormone. While administration of IGF-1 can reduce glucose concentrations, no tumor associated with hypoglycemia that produces solely IGF-1 has been reported to date. Moreover, acromegaly with increased growth hormone and IGF-1 concentrations is associated with hyperglycemia and insulin resistance. In contrast, IGF-2 production has been associated with hypoglycemia. Physiologically, IGF-2 is thought to be involved in fetal growth and, as it is present in an array of adult tissues, function as an autocrine/paracrine signal. Neoplasms of embryonal (e.g., Wilm's tumor, nephroglastoma, rhabdomyosarcoma, hepatoblastoma) mesenchymal (fibrosarcoma, leiomyosarcoma, hemangiopericytoma, and liposarcoma), neuroendocrine (pheochromocytoma and neuroblastoma), and epithelial (colon, liver, and breast) derivation have been described to produce IGF-2.

Notably, only the mesenchymal tumors have been shown to be associated with hypoglycemia. Measurement of IGF levels is complex as the result of numerous circulating binding protein; therefore, a complete discussion is beyond the scope of this paper. However, when present, increased IGF-2 is associated with hypoglycemia and a suppressed insulin concentration. In that instance, rigorous imaging techniques are essential, as tumors such as hemangiopericytomas may be small and located in either the truncal region or in the extremities.

Four compounds are regarded as counter-regulatory hormones: glucagon, cortisol, epinephrine, and growth hormone. Practically, glucagon deficiency occurs only in the post-pancreatectomy setting and is, therefore, not a diagnostic challenge. Similarly, though beta blockade can reduce glucagon secretion and predispose a patient to hypoglycemia, true catecholamine deficiency is essentially never a clinical concern. Isolated growth hormone deficiency appears to have a minimal role in causing hypoglycemia. In contrast, pituitary insufficiency with loss of both growth hormone and adrenocorticotropic hormone clearly can present with hypoglycemia. Primary adrenal failure of any cause is associated with hypoglycemia and, as primary adrenal failure also includes the loss of aldosterone, hyperkalemia. In this regard, measurement of cortisol and growth hormone at the time of hypoglycemia may be indicated.

Management

As in any patient presenting in extremis, the emergency physician must perform a rapid, thorough review of the ABCs, insuring a stable airway and ventilatory status, as well as an adequate hemodynamic state. After stabilization of the patient with either suspected or known hypoglycemia, the next management goal involves glucose replacement therapy. In certain cases with adequate personnel in the resuscitation area, early bedside determination of the glucose status may occur in conjunction with correction of alterations in the ABC functions. Such treatment involves rapid glucose replacement using the oral, topical (mucosal), or parenteral route.

Patients who are cooperative, lack CNS abnormalities, and are able to take liquids by mouth can be treated with oral carbohydrates. Oral replacement therapy may take the form of glucose gel or various drinks (juice or soda); solid foods such as candy should only be given to the patient with an entirely normal level of consciousness. In the rare patient without IV access when glucagon therapy is not possible (i.e., not available), the emergency physician may apply a dextrose-rich solution to the buccal mucosa; extreme care must be exercised to avoid both iatrogenic aspiration by the patient and injury to the physician by accidental biting of the examiner's finger. Furthermore, the oral glucose route may be used in patients who initially received parenteral therapy and have normalized their mental status alteration yet require additional dextrose. Finally, fructose and other complex carbohydrates should not be used to correct hypoglycemia in that these sugars do not cross the blood-brain barrier effectively and/or require extensive metabolic conversion prior to internal consumption.

Glucose Replacement. Guidelines for oral glucose replacement therapy in the hypoglycemic patient suggest the initial use of 10-20 grams glucose, delivered in either 4 ounces of orange juice or 8 ounces of milk. Five grams is usually sufficient for an infant or toddler. Commercially available formulations will provide 5 grams of glucose per tablet. In addition, there are 3 grams of glucose in a Lifesaver candy, 4 grams per teaspoon of granulated table sugar, 10-15 grams of sugar per 120 mL of orange or apple juice, or 15 grams per application of glucose gel. The initial therapy should be followed by a laboratory determination of the glucose value and reassessment of the patient's condition within 15-30 minutes. If symptoms persist, additional oral therapy is indicated. If the patient should develop any mental status alteration during the oral replacement therapy, then parenteral treatment is required.

The adult patient with an altered level of consciousness including agitation, lethargy, or frank coma should receive a bolus of 25-50 grams of glucose as a 50% dextrose solution—the "one amp of D50" approach. The symptomatic infant and young child should be given intravenous glucose at 1 g/kg of body weight. The dilution of a 50% dextrose solution to a 25% concentration is recommended in the infant due to the possibility of tissue necrosis should accidental tissue infiltration occur. The use of 50% dextrose solution will provide 50 grams of glucose in a 100 milliliter treatment. The use of D5W intravenous fluid (a 5% dextrose solution) will provide 5 grams of glucose per liter.

A continuous infusion of at least a 10% dextrose solution is recommended in cases where hypoglycemia recurs after bolus therapy and the patient is not able to take oral carbohydrate. Such constant infusion treatment can be anticipated and empirically administered in cases of massive insulin overdose, hypoglycemia related to OHA therapy, sepsis, severe malnutrition, liver failure, profound malnutrition, prolonged fasting, and known enzyme disorder. The serum glucose level with the infusion running should be maintained at least 100 mg/dL or greater with frequent monitoring (initially every 30 minutes in the early phase of ED care). Persistent hyperglycemia, maintained by slow administration of dextrose, indicates that the infusion may be reduced and eventually withdrawn. The use of 10% dextrose solution will provide 10 grams of glucose per liter infused. Five percent dextrose infusions (i.e., D5W IV solution) provide little usable calories and, therefore, are not recommended as replacement therapy in the acute setting.

Failure to respond to parenteral glucose administration should prompt consideration for other causes of altered mental status. The emergency physician, however, must realize that profound or prolonged hypoglycemia may not respond immediately to replacement therapy; the recovery from such extreme hypoglycemia may require significantly longer periods of time, approaching 5-10 minutes.[10] Other etiologies of altered consciousness must be investigated in the interim.

Glucagon. If IV access is not possible, glucagon use should be considered. Glucagon can be administered intramuscularly, subcutaneously, or intravenously. In most cases, glucagon is given via the intramuscular route at a dose of 1 mg for the adolescent and adult; the infant and larger child doses of glucagon are 0.5 mg. Response to glucagon therapy is generally slower when compared to IV dextrose, requiring 7-10 minutes prior to normalization of mental status; additionally, the response to glucagon administration may be short-lived.[26,27] Glucagon acts by stimulating glycogenolysis in the liver and therefore may not be effective in malnourished patients with little to no hepatic glycogen reserve, such as the chronic ethanol abuser. Glucagon also may be given to hypoglycemic patients who have not responded to IV dextrose; if so, it is usually administered IV along similar dosing recommendations.

In patients developing sulfonylurea-related hypoglycemia, the theoretical risk of paradoxically worsening hypoglycemia is present, though such individuals not infrequently receive glucagon with favorable clinical response. Such an event may occur via inhibition of hepatic gluconeogenesis, which has been noted with chronic use of OHA. Glucagon also may potentiate insulin release in healthy patients as well as diabetics. Nonetheless, endocrinologists recommend the use of glucagon in addition to dextrose in the treatment of patients with hypoglycemia related to most etiologies including OHA ingestion.

Octreotide. Octreotide, a synthetic analogue of somatostatin, inhibits the release of insulin and has been used in the treatment of sulfonylurea-induced hypoglycemia. One recent report describes the use of octreotide in patients who ingested excessive amounts of sulfonylurea OHA.[28] These patients, prior to octreotide administration, had experienced recurrent hypoglycemia. Soon after the initiation of octreotide therapy, serum sugar levels stabilized with a significant reduction in recurrent hypoglycemia. It is administered subcutaneously at an initial dose of 50-125 mcg; both constant infusions (125 mcg/hr) and repeat dosing (50-100 mcg) at 6- to 12-hour intervals have been employed successfully. The optimal dose, frequency of administration, and duration of therapy have not been defined. Intravenous glucose is still the most appropriate therapy for hypoglycemia. Octreotide is only recommended after initial therapy has been initiated in the sulfonylurea ingestion. Its use primarily is designed to reduce the chance of recurrent hypoglycemia.

Thiamine. Administration of parenteral thiamine at a dose of 100 mg is required in conjunction with glucose therapy (delivered by any route) in cases of suspected ethanol abuse or other nutritional deficiency states to avoid acute development of Wernicke's encephalopathy.[29] The concern with administration of glucose-containing solutions in a thiamine deficient state centers on the fact that thiamine is a co-factor in glucose metabolism. If glucose is given before thiamine, this may lead to an exacerbation of thiamine deficiency and the development of an acute Wernicke's syndrome.

Acute precipitation of the classic syndrome has been reported in four patients; it is quite rare.[29] In each instance (an ethanol user with chronic gastritis and persistent emesis; a schizophrenic with colonic pseudo-obstruction; a patient with end-stage renal disease managed by chronic peritoneal dialysis; and a trauma victim receiving total parenteral nutrition), the patient was exposed to dextrose and rapidly developed manifestations of Wernicke's encephalopathy. Prompt administration of thiamine reversed the ophthalmoplegia, mental status abnormalities, and ataxia during the following 12-24 hours. The investigators theorize that by providing relatively large amounts of glucose to these patients with pre-existing thiamine deficiency, the classic findings of the syndrome appeared in a rapid manner as available supplies of thiamine were quickly depleted.

Table 3. Admission Indications in the Hypoglycemic Patient Presenting to the ED

Issue under Consideration	In-patient Location (non-critical care setting vs critical care setting*)	Indication (Relative/absolute)
Patient age: neonate/infant & very elderly	Variable	Relative
Medication etiology: non-short-acting insulins and all OHA	Variable	Absolute
Continued/recurrent mental status change	CCS	Absolute
Continued/recurrent hypoglycemia	Likely CCS	Absolute
Lack of "reactive" hyperglycemia despite adequate glucose replacement therapy	Variable	Relative
Requirement for frequent/continuous glucose administrations	CCS	Absolute
Etiology of event: sepsis, severe malnutrition, toxicologic response to ingestion with other body system failures	CCS	Absolute
Psychiatric (i.e., intentional ingestion) etiology	Variable	Absolute
Lack of: 1) responsible adult supervision, 2) motivated patient or caretaker, and 3) identified physician for outpatient care.	Variable	Absolute
Significant comorbidity	Variable	Relative
History of hypoglycemia	Variable	Relative

* CCS = Critical care setting

Thiamine acts as a co-enzyme in several reactions in intermediary metabolism, specifically in the conversions of pyruvate to acetyl CoA (linking glycolysis to the TCA cycle) and alpha-ketoglutarate to succinate (a reaction in the TCA cycle). As thiamine reserves disappear, the reactions halt, removing the central nervous system's main source of ATP and causing the acute development of Wernicke's syndrome.

Steroid administration should be considered in patients with hypoglycemia that is either resistant to aggressive glucose replacement therapy or associated with the signs of adrenal insufficiency. In addition to hypoglycemia, adrenal insufficiency is characterized by profound weakness, hypothermia, hypotension poorly responsive to crystalloid and vasopressor infusions, and various metabolic abnormalities (hyponatremia, hyperkalemia, and azotemia). Initial, ED steroid replacement includes the rapid administration of hydrocortisone via the IV route: 100-200 mg in the adult and 1-2 mg/kg in children.[35]

Potential Risks of Glucose Administration. The use of glucose replacement therapy is not without theoretical risk to the head injured patient, in both atraumatic and traumatic settings. Hyperglycemia at the time of hospital admission has been associated with poor neurologic recovery in stroke patients[30] and survivors of out-of-hospital cardiopulmonary arrest.[31] Similar concern has been voiced regarding the association with worsened neurologic outcome and hyperglycemia in patients with acute head injury.[32,33] These retrospective studies have proposed an association between hyperglycemia and worsened neurologic outcome; these same studies, however, have not established a cause and effect relationship.

It is theorized that hyperglycemia accentuates local tissue damage via continued or increased anaerobic metabolism, lactate production, and intracellular acidosis. This acidosis may trigger a cascade that includes calcium entry into cells, lipolysis, and cytotoxic fatty acid release, culminating in neuronal death. At the present time, no controlled, prospective studies have been performed examining these issues in the setting of acute ischemic stroke or head injury. It is a known fact, however, that hypoglycemia will worsen neurologic outcome in patients with and without CNS injury of any etiology. Hypoglycemia clearly must be avoided—the emergency physician must always consider hypoglycemia as a causative or contributing factor in patients with altered mentation—even if the etiology appears to be related to another process or event.

The empiric use of IV dextrose for the patient experiencing altered mentation in the out-of-hospital setting without prior documentation of hypoglycemia places the emergency physician in a difficult position. After the administration of dextrose by emergency medical services (EMS) personnel, the emergency physician must then interpret the post-intervention serum glucose value. Although the literature suggests that each ampule of glucose (50 grams of a 50% dextrose solution) will raise the serum sugar by 60 mg/dL,[34] this post-treatment correction does not consider the time interval from initial therapy to glucose determination; such a calculation probably does not adequately estimate the post-treatment serum glucose level. Other authorities have demonstrated that a marked variation in serum glucose values after administration of 50 grams of a 50% dextrose solution is encountered such that any prediction of post-treatment levels is impossible.[35]

Disposition. Disposition considerations must weigh a number of factors, including: 1) the patient's current mental status as well as the level of consciousness during observation in the ED; 2) serial determinations of the serum glucose; 3) both the timing and extent of the response to resuscitative therapy; 4) the need for additional replacement therapy; 5) the pathophysiology (i.e., etiology) of the hypoglycemic event; 6) any comorbidities; 7) the social situation of the particular individual; 8) any psychiatric issues; and 9) the agent ingested. These issues are listed in Table 3 along with the strength of the admission recommendation (relative vs absolute indication), as well as the suggested in-hospital destination.

Obviously, either continued or recurrent mental status alteration, recurrent hypoglycemia, or a downward trend in serial glucose values during ED observation despite adequate replacement therapy demands admission to the hospital. Also, any patient requiring large doses of dextrose in both bolus and infusion fashion should be admitted to the intensive care unit not only for ongoing therapy but also for close evaluation of the mental status and serial serum glucose samplings. An inpatient disposition in a critical care setting is likely warranted in cases involving the following etiologies: massive insulin or OHA ingestion, marked malnutrition, sepsis, acute liver failure, or any other event associated with the tendency toward profound hypoglycemia. Further, the patient without proper, outpatient supervision should be admitted to the hospital for observation.

The case suitable for outpatient observation is characterized by both a responsible adult who will monitor the patient's mental status every three hours and a motivated patient who will perform serum glucose determinations frequently; an absence of either of these features should prompt admission to the hospital. Obviously, the suspected or known intentional ingestion (i.e., the self-harm scenario) of either insulin or OHA must be admitted for ongoing medical and psychiatric care.

The particular medication ingested must be strongly weighed in disposition decisions. Short-acting insulin preparations do not always demand hospitalization; intermediate and long-acting preparations, however, likely will require admission for ongoing observation and, at times, continued supportive care. Care must be exercised in the large short-acting insulin ingestion in that the pharmacodynamics of such insulin preparations are altered in the massive exposure situation; the expected, relatively short half-life may not be encountered. OHAs also represent an indication for hospitalization due to relatively long serum half-life with a prolonged tendency toward the development of hypoglycemia. A single tablet ingestion in a child can produce significant hypoglycemia; additionally, low serum sugars may develop as much as 16 hours after ingestion, though the majority of patients will become symptomatic within eight hours of exposure.[16]

The ultimate outcome of recurrent, unrecognized hypoglycemia is catastrophic—both medically for the patient and legally/psychologically for the emergency physician;[11] if any doubt exists as to the need for inpatient observation in the hypoglycemic patient, the emergency physician should err on the cautious side and arrange for an admission for short-term observation. If an outpatient status is recommended, very close medical follow-up (i.e., within 12-24 hours) is needed for additional adjustments.

References

1. Hayward RA, Manning WG, Kaplan SH, et al. Starting insulin therapy in patients with type 2 diabetes: Effectiveness, complications, and resource utilization. *J Am Med Assoc* 1997;278: 1663-1669.
2. Anonymous. Hypoglycemia in the Diabetes Control and Complications Trial: The Diabetes Control and Complications Trial Research Group. *Diabetes* 1997;46:271-286.
3. Shorr RI, Ray WA, Daugherty JR, et al. Incidence and risk factors for serious hypoglycemia in older persons using insulin or sulfonylureas. *Arch Int Med* 1997;157:1681-1686.
4. Malouf R, Brust JCM. Hypoglycemia: Causes, neurological manifestations, and outcome. *Ann Neurol* 1985;17:421-430.
5. Seltzer HS. Drug-induced hypoglycemia: A review based on 473 cases. *Diabetes* 1972;21:955-966.
6. Wallis WE, Donaldson I, Scott RS, et al. Hypoglycemia masquerading as cerebrovascular disease (hypoglycemic hemiplegia). *Ann Neurol* 1985;18:510-512.
7. Foster JW, Hart RG. Hypoglycemic hemiplegia: Two cases and a clinical review. *Stroke* 1987;18:944-946.
8. Brady WJ, Duncan CW. Hypoglycemia masquerading as acute psychosis and acute cocaine intoxication. *Am J Emerg Med* 1999;17:318-319.
9. Luber S, Meldon S, Brady W. Hypoglycemia presenting as acute respiratory failure in an infant. *Am J Emerg Med* 1998;16: 281-284.
10. Luber S, Brady W, Brand A, et al. Acute hypoglycemia masquerading as head trauma: A report of four cases. *Am J Emerg Med* 1996;14:543-547.
11. Fink S, Chaudhuri TK. Iatrogenic hypoglycemia and malpractice claims. *South Med J* 1997;90:251-253.
12. Fanelli C, Pampanelli S, Lalli C, et al. Long-term intensive therapy of IDDM patients with clinically overt autonomic neuropathy: Effects on hypoglycemia awareness and counterregulation. *Diabetes* 1997;46:1172-1181.
13. Boyle PJ, Kempers SF, O'Connor AM, et al. Brain glucose uptake and unawareness of hypoglycemia in patients with insulin-dependent diabetes mellitus. *N Engl J Med* 1995;333: 1726-1731.
14. Mahler RJ, Adler ML. Type 2 diabetes mellitus: Update on diagnosis, pathophysiology and treatment. *J Clin Endocrinol Metab* 1999;84:1165-1171.
15. Davidson MB. An overview of metformin in the treatment of type 2 diabetes mellitus. *Am J Med* 1997;102:99-110.
16. Quadrani DA, Spiller HA, Widder P. Five year retrospective evaluation of sulfonylurea ingestion in children. *J Toxicol Clin Toxicol* 1996;34:267-270.
17. Spiller HA, Villalobos D, Krenzelok EP, et al. Prospective multi-center study of sulfonylurea ingestion in children. *J Pediatr* 1997;131:141-146.
18. Losek JD. Hypoglycemia and the ABC'S [sugar] of pediatric resuscitation. *Ann Emerg Med* 2000;35:43-46.
19. Losek JD, Reid S. Letter to the Editor. *Ann Emerg Med* 2000; 36:279.
20. Pollock G, Brady WJ, Hargarten S, et al. Hypoglycemia manifested by sinus bradycardia: A report of three cases. *Acad Emerg Med* 1996;3:700-707.
21. Shen F. Motorist in diabetic shock arrested in MD; Man's erratic behavior prompts beating, dog attack and multiple charges. *The Washington Post* June 22, 1998:B3.

22. Brady WJ, Butler K, Fines R, et al. Hypoglycemia in multiple trauma victims. *Am J Emerg Med* 1999;17:4-5.
23. Boyle PJ, Schwartz NA, Shah SD. Plasma glucose concentrations at the onset of hypoglycemic symptoms in patients with poorly controlled diabetes and in nondiabetics. *N Engl J Med* 1988;318: 1487-1492.
24. Rich LM, Caine MR, Findling JW, et al. Hypoglycemic coma in anorexia nervosa: Case report and review of the literature. *Arch Int Med* 1990;150:894-895.
25. Service FJ. Hypoglceic disorders. *N Engl J Med* 1995;332: 1144-1152.
26. Collier A, Steedman DJ, Patrick AW, et al. Comparison of intravenous glucagon and dextrose in treatment of severe hypoglycemia in an accident and emergency department. *Diabetes Care* 1987;10:712-715.
27. Patrick AW, Collier A, Hepburn DA, et al. Comparison of intramuscular glucagon and intravenous dextrose in treatment of hypoglycemic coma in an accident and emergency department. *Arch Emerg Med* 1990;7:73-77.
28. MacLaughlin SA, Crandell CS, McKinney PE. Octreotide: An antidote for sulfonylurea-induced hypoglycemia. *Ann Emerg Med* 2000;36:133-138.
29. Watson AJS, Walker GH, Tomkin MMR, et al. Acute Wernicke's encephalopathy precipitated by glucose loading. *Irish J Med Sci* 1981;150:301-303.
30. Pulsinelli WA, Levy DE, Sigsbee B, et al. Increased damage after ischemic stroke in patients with hyperglycemia with or without established diabetes mellitus. *Am J Med* 1983;74:540-544.
31. Longstreth WT, Inui TS. High blood glucose level on hospital admission and poor neurological recovery after cardiac arrest. *Ann Neurol* 1984;15:59-63.
32. Lam AM, Winn HR, Cullen BF, et al. Hyperglycemia and neurologic outcome in patients with head injury. *J Neurosurg* 1991;75:545-551.
33. Young B, Ott L, Dempsey R, et al. Relationship between admission hyperglycemia and neurologic outcome of severely brain-injured patients. *Ann Surg* 1989;210:466-473.
34. Hoffman RS, Goldfrank LR. The poisoned patient with altered consciousness: Controversies in the use of a "coma cocktail." *J Am Med Assoc* 1995;274:562-569.
35. Balentine JR, Gaeta TJ, Kessler D, et al. Effect of 50 milliliters of 50% dextrose in water administration on the blood sugar of euglycemic volunteers. *Acad Emerg Med* 1998;5:691-694.

Movement Disorders

Sid M. Shah, MD, FACEP

A slogan of neurologists, "everything that shakes is not seizure" strikes home in emergency departments (EDs). When confronted with abnormal movements of the body, the emergency physician must consider a differential diagnosis that is broader than seizure disorder. Movement disorders (MDs) typically are a symptom of a larger problem and may well be associated with serious illness. The emergency physician must determine whether or not the MD is a harbinger of an undiagnosed, critical condition.

Parkinsonism is one of the most common MDs. As the ED visits of elderly patients increase, emergency physicians will see more patients with parkinsonism. Elderly patients more often seek ED care for complications of parkinsonism or its therapy (such as orthostasis, causing falls) than for the symptoms of parkinsonian tremors. Other commonly seen MD drug-induced dystonias are a diagnostic challenge if the patient cannot provide a good history. Hemiballism is a MD that is important to recognize as a rare complication of stroke.

ED encounters with MDs are probably more common in the daily practice of emergency medicine than genuine "seizures." However, MDs often are not considered a major consequence unless they are associated with a complication. This issue is devoted to the often overlooked neurological condition (an MD) that can indeed be a symptom of a critical underlying neurological or a non-neurological disease process.

Introduction

MDs are abnormal motor activities that are not associated with primary dysfunction of the corticospinal tracts, cerebellum, sensory pathways, or peripheral nervous system. This term often is used as a synonym for basal ganglia disorders. However, some disorders that are classified as MDs, such as myoclonus and some forms of tremor, are not associated with basal ganglia pathology. MDs can be associated with an acute, primary neurological disease such as a cerebrovascular event, or a focal neurological disease such as a neoplasm. Some MDs are a manifestation of underlying systemic illness such as hepatic or renal failure or autoimmune disease. MDs, dystonia in particular, often are misdiagnosed as being hysterical or psychiatric in origin. The primary task of the emergency physician in evaluating a patient with a suspected MD is to identify the features of MD and determine if a critical underlying neurological or non-neurological condition exists that may need urgent attention. A thorough history and a focused neurological examination will yield clues that will help distinguish these conditions.

Pre-Hospital Care

MDs, especially acute dystonic reactions (ADRs), easily can be confused with focal or generalized seizure activity. Pre-hospital care providers are advised against pursuing aggressive measures when the diagnosis of ongoing seizure is uncertain. It is important to differentiate generalized tonic-clonic status epilepticus from a MD or other cause of involuntary movements. For conditions other than seizures, supportive measures usually suffice as long as the airway is not compromised and vital signs are stable. Information collected by pre-hospital care providers on conditions leading to falls or other acute events is very important in evaluating patients with suspected MDs. Drug ingestion, substance abuse, and exposure to environmental toxins such as carbon monoxide can be associated with several different types of MDs.

Emergency Department Evaluation

Assessment of vital signs and the adequacy of the airway are the first priority in the ED. A seizure disorder is distinguished from a MD on presentation by obtaining a thorough history and by performing a focused physical and neurological examination. *(Please see Table 1.)* Information from bystanders or family members is crucial for making a diagnosis of a seizure disorder. If a patient is unable to communicate, old medical records and a description of events as witnessed by pre-hospital care providers and others are most useful.

MDs usually are distinguished from seizure disorders on the basis of clinical evaluation. The patient history contributes the most to a diagnosis, with little additional information provided by laboratory and radiographic studies. Family, social, and psychiatric histories are reviewed. Use of psychotropic medications, particularly the use of antiemetics, is questioned. A careful physical examination can reveal signs of metabolic or endocrine derangements or toxic exposures.

A careful neurological examination with accurate characterization of the abnormalities will allow distinction of various types of MD. The character of the involuntary movement(s) is first assessed by observation of the patient's head, trunk, and limbs. Eye movements, tone (resistance of muscles/joints to passive manipulation), gait (casual, toe, heel, and tandem), and fine coordination (rapid finger tapping or alternating pronation and supination of the hands) are tested. Detection of neurological abnormalities other than the MD is essential in neuroanatomical localization of pathology and assists in generating differential diagnoses. Incoordination does not necessarily indicate the presence of a MD because it can result from injury to the corticospinal tracts, cerebellum, sensory pathways, or basal ganglia.

A laboratory evaluation, guided by results of the history and physical examination, can include basic serum chemistries, drug levels, and toxicological studies. If illicit drug use is suspected, urine can be tested for these substances.

The role of neuroimaging studies in the evaluation of MDs is limited. Some MDs occur acutely from focal structural lesions such as can occur from stroke. Typically, they are present in a localized body area or follow a "hemi-distribution," as in hemidystonia or hemiballism. Urgent brain imaging can be helpful following the acute onset of symptoms with a focal distribution.

Classification of Movement Disorders

MDs can be classified into four broad categories based on phenomenological features, clinical pharmacology, and neuropathology: 1) hypokinetic disorders, which are identical with the syndrome of parkinsonism; 2) hyperkinetic/choreic movement disorders; 3) tremors; and 4) myoclonus. *(Please see Table 2.)*

Table 1. Important Historical Questions for Evaluation of a Patient with Suspected MD

1. Manner and temporal nature of symptom onset
2. Location of symptoms; body parts most affected
3. Factors that alleviate or exacerbate the symptoms
4. Whether symptoms are present at rest, with sustained posture, with movement, or only during the execution of specific tasks
5. Exposure to toxins or environmental factors and medication use
6. History of premature birth, perinatal injury, or behavioral problems

Descriptive features of individual MDs are summarized in Table 3. In some cases, differentiating specific MDs can be difficult and at times unnecessary (e.g., distinguishing mild myoclonus from chorea). Chorea, athetosis, and ballism are appropriately viewed as part of a spectrum of involuntary movements with a common pathophysiology.

Hypokinetic MD (Parkinsonism)

Parkinsonism, a prototypical example of hypokinetic MD, is a syndrome caused by deficient dopaminergic effects within the striatum (caudate and putamen). Any process interfering with striatal dopaminergic function can cause parkinsonism. *(Please see Table 4.)* This frequently is a result of idiopathic dysfunction of dopamine innervation within the striatum, but also can occur as a result of side effects of certain drugs (e.g., phenothiazines). Parkinson's disease affects more than 1 million individuals in the United States. The incidence increases with age, resulting in a high prevalence in the elderly.

Important historical features useful in establishing a diagnosis of parkinsonism are: difficulty with initiating or halting movement, especially getting in or out of chairs; and a history of micrographia, the tendency for letter size to become progressively smaller during handwriting.

Clinical findings in parkinsonism often are asymmetrical, with onset and preponderance of symptoms on one side of the body. Incoordination, notably with fine motor tasks, is common. A loss of facial expression (masked facies) or loss of voice amplitude (hypophonia) also are common. Examination reveals stooped posture, masked facies, saccadic pursuit eye movements, low-volume voice, reduced blinking rates, and generalized slowing of movement. Gait often is slow and shuffling, with loss of associated arm swing and the need to take several steps to turn. Muscle tone is increased, with plastic (increased resistance throughout range of motion independent of velocity) or cogwheel (ratchet-like) quality. Postural reflexes are impaired, which can lead to falls. A characteristic resting tremor often is present in the hands, legs, or chin. *(Please see Table 5.)*

Parkinson's disease usually has an insidious onset and is slowly progressive. Patients do not present to the ED for initial evaluation of parkinsonian tremors, but rather for problems that arise from some complications of Parkinson's disease and its treatment. *(Please see Table 6.)*

Table 2. Classification of Movement Disorders

HYPOKINETIC MD/ PARKINSONISM	HYPERKINETIC/CHOREIC MOVEMENT DISORDERS
Parkinson's disease	Chorea
Drug-induced parkinsonism	Athetosis
Parkinsonian syndromes	Ballism (Hemiballism is more common)
	Dystonia
	Tics
TREMORS	**MYOCLONUS**
Resting tremors	Generalized
Postural tremors	Segmental
Kinetic tremors	Focal
Task-related tremors	

Used with permission from: Shah S, Albin R. Movement Disorders. In: Shah S, Kelly K, eds. *Emergency Neurology: Principles and Practice.* New York: Cambridge University Press; 1999.

Drug therapy with dopamine replacement and/or dopamine agonists provides excellent symptomatic relief for several years. Many patients experience progression of disease that results in poor response to medication or difficult-to-manage side effects. Many patients develop marked fluctuations in response to therapy, with periods of complex involuntary movements (dyskinesias). These dyskinesias have features of both dystonia and chorea occurring in close temporal association with periods of severe bradykinesia and rigidity. These fluctuations are difficult to manage and often require judicious manipulation of medications and dosage schedules over a long period of time for optimal control of symptoms. Choreic dyskinesias tend to occur at times when the effect of dopamine replacement therapy is at its peak. Choreic dyskinesias can be improved by decreasing medication doses or lengthening the dosing interval.

Nausea is another common problem associated with the use of carbidopa/L-dopa or dopamine agonists. Taking medications at the end of a meal to slow their absorption can reduce nausea. For patients taking carbidopa/L-dopa, an adequate amount of carbidopa must be taken to block the peripheral effects of L-dopa and reduce nausea. For an average-size person, 75 mg of carbidopa usually is sufficient to reduce peripheral side effects. Other peripheral side effects include flushing and orthostatic hypotension. Orthostatic hypotension is especially troublesome, and some patients with Parkinson's disease can have autonomic insufficiency independent of drug treatment. Orthostatic hypotension can lead to syncope and falls, with their attendant consequences.

All medications used in the treatment of Parkinson's disease can cause altered mental status. Hallucinations are a relatively common side effect of carbidopa/L-dopa and dopamine agonists, and can occur with the use of anticholinergics and amantadine. These hallucinations usually are visual, typically non-threatening in character, and commonly occur in the absence of other features of delirium. However, typical delirium also can occur. Hallucinations, delirium, and other mental status changes occur most frequently in the many patients with Parkinson's disease that develop dementia. In Parkinson's patients with changes in mental status, subdural hematoma is an important diagnostic consideration due to the high incidence of falls in these patients.

Many patients with Parkinson's disease can manifest varied symptoms caused by pain, such as muscle spasms, cramps, and burning paresthesias.[1-4] These painful symptoms have several causes. Painful muscle spasms and uncomfortable paresthesias of uncertain etiology are common in Parkinson's disease. Many patients with complex dyskinesias have a painful dystonic component to their involuntary movements. Severe, localized limb pain, chest pain, or abdominal pain in the patient with Parkinson's disease poses a diagnostic challenge in the ED.

Discontinuation of dopamine replacement therapy can cause neuroleptic malignant syndrome, which is a medical emergency.

Hyperkinetic Movement Disorders

Examples of hyperkinetic MDs include dystonia, chorea, hemiballism, and tics. The distinguishing feature of hyperkinetic MDs is the overwhelming presence of involuntary movements into the normal flow of movements of specific groups of muscles. Some overlap of the different hyperkinetic MD disorders is common.

Dystonia. Any voluntary muscle group in the body can be affected by dystonia. Some muscle groups more commonly are involved than others are. Dystonia is characterized by sustained (tonic), spasmodic (rapid or clonic), or patterned or repetitive muscular contractions that frequently result in a wide range of involuntary twisting, repetitive movements, or abnormal postures. Abnormal postures, such as neck torsion, forced jaw opening, or inversion and dorsiflexion of the foot, are characteristic of dystonia.

Certain specific tasks or postures can elicit dystonia. For example, dystonia can be elicited by writing (writer's cramp) but not by other fine coordinated movements. "Spasmodic dysphonia" (a type of laryngeal dystonia), can cause difficulty with speaking but not with singing. Commonly, patients discover postures or maneuvers that reduce dystonia. The most common of these "sensory tricks" is gentle stimulation of one side of the face to reduce torticollis.

Dystonia is a primary neurological disorder or a prominent manifestation of a neurological disorder due to metabolic derangement as occurs in Wilson's disease, Lesch-Nyhan syndrome, and mitochondrial cytopathies. Dystonia also is known to result from structural injury to the central nervous system (CNS). *(Please see Table 7.)*

With liberal use of phenothiazines in the ED, drug-induced dystonia probably is more common than is generally recognized. Drug-induced dystonia also is the most commonly observed dystonia in the ED. Many patients treated with phenothiazines report feeling "jittery" and "uneasy." Overt manifestations of a dystonic reaction, such as bizarre movements and postures, may not always be present.

Dystonia frequently can be misinterpreted as a psychiatric or hysterical condition because of several reasons, including:[5]

1) Bizarre movements and postures;
2) The finding of "action-induced dystonia" (the exacerbation of symptoms with stress and improvement with relaxation);
3) Diurnal fluctuations; and
4) Frequent effectiveness of various sensory tricks.

Selected Examples of Dystonia. Idiopathic torsion dystonia (dystonia musculorum deformans) is a familial (more common in Ashkenazi Jews) neurological disorder that has an autosomal domi-

Table 3. Phenomenology of Movement Disorders

MOVEMENT DISORDER	FEATURES	AREAS OF INVOLVEMENT	ANATOMIC LOCALIZATION
Parkinsonism	Bradykinesia, rigidity, often resting tremor, often postural instability, stooped posture, masked facies, hypophonia	Often asymmetric at onset, but can be generalized	Basal ganglia—Interruption of or interference with nigrostriatal dopaminergic neurotransmission
Dystonia	Sustained, spasmodic, repetitive contractions causing involuntary abnormal postures	Any voluntary muscle can be affected (usually head, neck, face, and limbs)	Presumed to be basal ganglia—Associated with putamen lesions in some cases.
Tremor	Involuntary, rhythmic and roughly sinusoidal movements: some are action-induced	Head, hands, limbs, and voice	In parkinsonian resting tremor—Basal ganglia Most other tremors may involve cerebelar dysfunction
Chorea	Involuntary, irregular, rapid, jerky movements without a rhythmic pattern; dance-like	Generally limbs, but any body part can be affected	Basal ganglia—Striatum or subthalamic nucleus
Athetosis	Akin to chorea but with distinct "writhing" movements	Limbs, but any body part can be involved	Identical to chorea
Myoclonus	Brief, rapid, shock-like jerks	Generally involves very small muscles	Can result from dysfunction at any level of central nervous system
Tics	Intermittent, brief, sudden, repetitive, stereotyped movements or sounds	Any body part can be affected; phonation/sounds	Presumed to be basal ganglia
Hemiballism	Uncontrollable, rapid, large amplitude flinging movements of a limb	Generally a limb	Basal ganglia—Subthalamic nucleus or striatum

Used with permission from: Shah S, Albin R. Movement Disorders. In: Shah S, Kelly K, eds. *Emergency Neurology: Principles and Practice.* New York: Cambridge University Press; 1999.

nant trait with variable penetrance.[6] Childhood-onset of primary dystonia is common. In the early stages, the abnormal movements are characterized by "action dystonia" and commonly start in one leg. With progression of the disease, dystonia often becomes generalized and is present at rest.

Focal dystonia refers to the involvement of a specific part of the body. A primary dystonia that begins in adulthood usually is focal (e.g., spasmodic torticollis). Torticollis can mimic a variety of orthopedic and neurological disorders that are important to recognize in the ED. *(Please see Table 8.)*

Blepharospasm, involuntary, periodic blinking of eyelids, is the second most common focal dystonia that is either isolated or associated with oromandibular dystonia, and is more common in women than in men. Approximately 15% of patients become functionally blind due to tonic closure of the eyelids. Blepharospasm can respond to sensory stimulation as occurs with talking, singing, and yawning.[7]

Oromandibular dystonia is characterized by forced mouth opening, occasionally with tongue protrusion, or involuntary jaw clenching that can result in mutilation of the lips and teeth. Blepharospasm-oromandibular dystonia syndrome commonly is referred to as Meige syndrome.

Spasmodic dysphonia is a form of laryngeal dystonia that causes spasm of the vocal cords. Patients generally are asymptomatic except for abnormalities of voice.

Writer's cramp is a focal "action dystonia," and is described as task-specific. As suggested by the name, dystonia of the hand and arm occurs only when attempting to write. A change in handwriting can be the presenting complaint. "Muscle ache" and dystonic spasms of the forearm musculature are common complaints in these patients.

Secondary dystonia is a term reserved for dystonia that results from identifiable metabolic disorders, CNS degenerative processes, or structural lesions of the CNS. There are no distinguishing clinical features of secondary dystonia. However, sudden onset, presence of dystonia at rest, rapid progression, or an unusual distribution such as hemidystonia in an adult suggests secondary dystonia. A thorough neurological examination usually reveals dysfunction of other parts of the CNS, including the cranial nerves, pyramidal system, cerebellar system, or the higher cortical functions. Hemidystonia suggests a focal lesion such as a mass, infarction, or hemorrhage of the basal ganglia. Secondary dystonia can have delayed onset of weeks to years following a cerebral injury such as stroke. The most frequent causes of delayed-onset dystonia are perinatal trauma or hypoxia.

Torticollis refers to dystonia-producing abnormal neck postures and it merits special attention in the ED because it has a more complicated differential diagnosis. Potentially life-threatening etiologies of torticollis, such as atlantoaxial subluxation or a posterior fossa tumor, must be considered before declaring dystonia as the cause of torticollis.[8] Causes of torticollis other than dystonia are listed in Table

Table 4. Forms of Parkinsonism

IDIOPATHIC PARKINSONISM
Involves basal ganglia but no discernible degenerative conditions
DRUG-INDUCED PARKINSONISM
Neuroleptics, phenothiazine, haloperidol, tricyclic anti-depressants, methyldopa, lithium, metoclopramide
NEURODEGENERATIVE DISORDERS
(Clinically indistinguishable from other forms of parkinsonism.) Involve basal ganglia. Discernible degenerative conditions

8. Direct or indirect trauma to the neck suggests atlantoaxial subluxation. Gradually progressive extremity paresthesias and weakness suggest a herniated cervical disc. Visual disturbance and headaches can be caused by a posterior fossa tumor. Cervical adenopathy can cause torticollis in children. Associated neck dystonia with an impaired level of consciousness or other symptoms suggests the possibility of seizures. Dystonic torticollis can produce neurological complications such as cervical myelopathy or radiculopathy due to persistent abnormal neck postures.

Evaluation and Management of Dystonia. The goal of ED evaluation is to identify 1) "secondary dystonia," which may have a treatable cause; and 2) complications of conditions responsible for primary dystonia. It is important to distinguish dystonia from focal seizures. Recent-onset twisting and repetitive abnormal movements in an adult that respond to sensory stimuli or abnormal movements that can be suppressed voluntarily favor the diagnosis of dystonia.

Management of most dystonias is difficult, and symptomatic therapy generally is prescribed. High doses of anticholinergic medications frequently are successful in relieving some symptoms of dystonia. The higher doses of phenothiazines are better tolerated in children than in adults. Specific drug therapy is available for Parkinson's disease and Wilson's disease and should be prescribed in consultation with the neurologist. Patients with blepharospasm, oromandibular dystonia (especially jaw closing), spasmodic torticollis, spasmodic dysphonia, and cases of focal limb dystonia should be referred for botulinum toxin therapy.

Chorea. Involuntary irregular, rapid, jerky movements without a rhythmic pattern, that are randomly distributed with a flowing "dance-like" quality, characterize chorea, the Greek term for dance. Chorea generally involves multiple body parts. Athetosis (writhing movement) and ballism are part of the spectrum of chorea, and appear to share a common pathophysiology, usually involving the striatum or subthalamic nucleus.

Many neurological and non-neurological disorders are associated with the development of chorea.[9] *(Please see Table 9.)* The non-neurological conditions capable of causing chorea include certain immunological, infectious, metabolic, degenerative, and drug- and toxin-induced disorders.

The use of the medication L-dopa, a commonly prescribed therapy for parkinsonism, is associated with the development of chorea and probably is the most commonly encountered chorea in the ED.[8] Titration of L-dopa dosing can minimize the choreiform movements often seen in patients with parkinsonism.

Table 5. Cardinal Features of Parkinsonism

BRADYKINESIA
Slowness of movement with a paucity of normal spontaneous movements such as arm swing when walking
RIGIDITY
Form of increased resistance to passive manipulation in which the increased tone has a "plastic" (constant resistance to passive manipulation) quality or "cogwheel" rigidity (in which resistance has a ratchet-like characteristic)
TREMOR
Typically a "resting tremor" of the hands/arms, legs, or chin that improves with use of the affected body part
IMPAIRMENT OF POSTURAL REFLEXES
Manifested by falls or near falls, and in difficulty in maintaining a stable stance when displaced gently backward on examination

Autoimmune causes of chorea include systemic lupus erythematosus (SLE) and primary antiphospholipid antibody syndromes.[10,11] However, only 2% of patients with SLE have chorea.[10] The cause of chorea in autoimmune disorders is not known but autoimmune-mediated injury to the basal ganglia has been postulated.[12] Chorea from autoimmune disorders can last from days to years and can be episodic and recurrent; this makes sufferers more likely to seek emergency care. Other neurological findings in SLE include migraine, stroke, seizures, cognitive impairment, peripheral neuropathy, and transient ischemic attacks. Antiphospholipid antibody syndrome is associated with recurrent vascular thrombosis, recurrent spontaneous abortions, and stroke. An antiphospholipid antibody titer is obtained in cases of chorea associated with these clinical situations. Imaging studies typically are normal.[12]

Structural lesions from cerebral infarctions involving the basal ganglia and thalamus can produce chorea. Stroke is likely the most common cause of hemichorea-hemiballismus.[13-15] Other causes include arteriovenous malformations, venous angiomas, metastatic tumors, or primary CNS neoplasms.

Thyroid dysfunction is a rare cause of chorea. Interestingly, both hyperthyroidism and hypothyroidism are known to be associated with chorea.[16] The pathophysiology is not well understood but is likely due to altered function of the basal ganglia, particularly the striatum.

Sydenham's chorea is a form of autoimmune chorea preceded by group A streptococcus infection, typically rheumatic fever. Unlike other manifestations of rheumatic fever, Sydenham's chorea occurs several months after the onset of acute streptococcal infection, usually affects patients between ages 5 and 15 years, and develops in girls more frequently than boys.[19] There appears to be a familial prevalence,

Table 6. Common ED Presentations of the Parkinsonian Patient

COMPLICATIONS OF PARKINSONISM

1. Falls due to impaired postural reflexes (consider subdural hematoma in a patient with mental status changes)
2. Orthostatic hypotension from autonomic instability resulting in syncope and falls
3. Painful muscle spasms
4. Paresthesias
5. Severe localized limb pain, chest pain, or abdominal pain[1-4]

COMPLICATIONS OR SIDE EFFECTS OF DRUG THERAPY FOR PARKINSONISM

1. Nausea: Common with carbidopa/L-dopa or dopamine agonists
2. Flushing and orthostasis resulting from the therapy
3. Mental status changes, particularly hallucinations, delirium, and dementia
4. Neuroleptic malignant syndrome can result from discontinuation of dopamine replacement therapy

suggesting hereditary susceptibility. It tends to occur abruptly, worsens over 2-4 weeks, and usually resolves spontaneously in 3-6 weeks. It occurs more commonly in children who lack appropriate antibiotic care. Outbreaks of Sydenham's chorea have occurred in the United States and other developed countries. Measurement of antistreptolysin-O titers can help detect recent streptococcal infection. Since Sydenham's chorea can occur as late as six months after the streptococcal infection, measurements of antistreptolysin-O and antistreptokinase antibody concentrations obtained later may not be useful.[17]

Chorea gravidarum refers to choreiform movements associated with pregnancy. Approximately one-third of patients with chorea gravidarum have had Sydenham's chorea, suggesting that previous injury to the basal ganglia predisposes to chorea when estrogens and progesterone levels are elevated.[17,18] The use of oral contraceptives in women is associated with the development of chorea, especially in patients with a history of Sydenham's chorea. Chorea also is associated with the use of numerous other medications.

Huntington's disease (HD), commonly associated with choreiform movement, is an autosomal dominant neurodegenerative disorder. In addition to chorea, athetosis, dystonia, dementia, and psychiatric problems are common in patients with HD. Neurobehavioral disturbances, such as personality changes, agitation, apathy, depression, obsessive-compulsive disorders, social withdrawal, and sometimes, features of psychosis can precede choreiform movements. Symptoms and signs of HD begin at any age, but commonly present in the fourth and fifth decades. Life expectancy is approximately 15-20 years after diagnosis.[8]

Patients with HD seek emergency care for complications caused by their underlying disease process. Swallowing dysfunction can lead to poor nutrition and/or aspiration pneumonia, and sometimes asphyxia. Falls are common. Cerebral atrophy associated with HD places these patients at a higher risk for subdural hematomas. Severe dysarthria, dysphagia, dementia, and loss of ambulation occur in the final stages of the disease. Psychiatric disorders are associated with a high rate of suicide.[8]

Assessing the underlying cause of chorea is important. Medications that reduce dopaminergic neurotransmission can lessen the severity of chorea. The dopamine receptor antagonist haloperidol is the medication most frequently used to achieve this effect. Dopamine-depleting agents, such as reserpine or tetrabenazine, also can be effective. In many patients, impairments of coordination or mentation result from the doses of dopamine antagonists needed to reduce chorea significantly. Management of chorea in the ED is providing supportive care. Chorea does not require emergent treatment unless it interferes with function.

Hemiballism. Hemiballism, a hyperkinetic MD, is considered to be an extreme form of "hemichorea." Uncontrollable, rapid, large-amplitude proximal flinging movements of a limb characterize hemiballism. Hemiballism refers to unilateral involvement, whereas rare bilateral involvement is called biballism. Typically, the face is not affected.[13] Hemiballism formerly was attributed solely to lesions of the subthalamic nucleus. It is now known that hemiballism can occur from lesions in other parts of the basal ganglia and the thalamus.

Stroke, generally a lacunar infarct in the subthalamic nucleus, is the most common cause of hemiballism. Hemiballism occurs most frequently in individuals older than 60 years of age who also have risk factors for stroke. Other causes of hemiballism are listed in Table 10. Common predisposing factors include hypertension, diabetes, thrombocytosis, or vasculitis.

Appropriate measures are taken to prevent injuries caused by violent hemiballistic movements. Disabling

Table 7. Etiologies of Selected Dystonias

DYSTONIA DUE TO DEGENERATIVE DISORDERS OF CNS	DYSTONIA DUE TO NON-DEGENERATIVE DISORDERS OF CNS
Parkinson's disease	Traumatic brain injury
Huntington's disease	History of perinatal anoxia
Progressive supranuclear palsy	Kernicterus
Other degenerative disorders of the basal ganglia and midbrain	Stroke (cerebral infarction)
	Arteriovenous malformation
Wilson's disease	Encephalitis
Storage diseases	Toxins (e.g., manganese)
GTP cyclohydrolase deficiency	Brain tumors
Lesch-Nyhan disease	Multiple sclerosis
Mitochondrial disorders	Drugs
Leigh's syndrome	Peripheral trauma

Used with permission from: Shah S, Albin R. Movement Disorders. In: Shah S, Kelly K, eds. *Emergency Neurology: Principles and Practice.* New York: Cambridge University Press; 1999.

Table 8. Disorders Simulating Dystonic Torticollis (Cervical Dystonia)

NEUROLOGICAL DISORDERS
Posterior fossa tumor
Focal seizures
Bobble-head syndrome (third ventricular cyst)
Syringomyelia
Congenital nystagmus
Extraocular muscle palsies
Arnold-Chiari malformation
MUSCULOSKELETAL/ STRUCTURAL
Herniated cervical disc
Rotational atlantoaxial subluxation
Congenital muscular or ligamentous absence, laxity, or injury
Bony spinal abnormalities: Degenerative; neoplastic; infectious
Cervical soft-tissue lesions: Adenitis; pharyngitis
Labyrinthine disease
Abnormal posture in utero

Adapted from: Wiener W, Lang A. *Movement Disorders: A comprehensive Survey.* Mount Kisco, NY: Futura Publishing Co.; 1989.

Table 9. Differential Diagnosis of Chorea

HEREDITARY CHOREAS	**CEREBROVASCULAR CHOREAS**
Huntington's disease (classic choreiform movement)	Basal ganglia infarction
Neuroacanthocytosis	Arteriovenous malformation
Wilson's disease	Venous angiomata
Benign familial chorea	Polycythemia
Inborn errors of metabolism	
Porphyria	**STRUCTURAL CHOREAS**
Ataxia-telangiectasia	Posttraumatic
Tuberous sclerosis	Subdural and epidural hematoma
METABOLIC CHOREAS	Tumor (primary CNS or metastatic)
Hyper- and hypothyroidism	
Hyper- and hypopara-thyroidism	**DRUGS/MEDICATIONS**
Hypocalcemia	Phenytoin
Hyper- and hyponatremia	Phenothiazines
Hypomagnesemia	Lithium
Hepatic encephalopathy	Amphetamines
Renal encephalopathy	Oral contraceptives
	Levodopa
INFECTIOUS OR IMMUNOLOGICAL CHOREAS	**TOXINS**
Sydenham's chorea (post rheumatic fever)	Mercury
Chorea gravidarum	Carbon monoxide
Systemic lupus erythematosus	**INFECTIONS**
Polycythemia vera	Neurosyphilis
Multiple sclerosis	Lyme's disease
Sarcoidosis	Subacute sclerosing panencephalitis
Viral encephalitis	
Tuberous meningitis	

Used with permission from: Shah S, Albin R. Movement Disorders. In: Shah S, Kelly K, eds. *Emergency Neurology: Principles and Practice.* New York: Cambridge University Press; 1999.

hemiballism requires immediate symptomatic relief even when the cause is not known. A neuroleptic medication such as haloperidol is most effective. Following a focused history and physical examination, ancillary tests should be directed toward diagnosing metabolic disorders, particularly a nonketotic hyperosmolar state. A history of medication use, including estrogens, oral contraceptives, phenytoin toxicity, and levodopa is sought. CT imaging may reveal evidence of a stroke.

Tics. Most common of all the MDs, tics are characterized by intermittent, sudden, repetitive, stereotyped movements (motor tics) or sounds (vocal tics). Tics can result from contraction of just one group of muscles, causing simple tics, which are brief, jerk-like movements or single, meaningless sounds. Complex tics result from a coordinated sequence of movements. Complex vocal tics can include linguistically meaningful utterances. Patients often admit that the tic occurs as an unavoidable but purposeful performance of the movement or sound. Tics can be suppressed temporarily and often wax and wane in type, frequency, and severity.

Tics can vary from a mild, transient disorder to a potentially devastating neurobehavioral disorder. Simple tics are extremely common and many people have some form of them. Tics rarely require emergent therapy. Several neurological and non-neurological disorders associated with tics are listed in the Table 11. Tics can be associated with stroke, head trauma, encephalitis, post-encephalitic syndrome of encephalitis lethargica, brain tumors, and carbon monoxide poisoning. They can occur as a result of long-term neuroleptic use (i.e., tardive tics).

Transient tic disorders (TTD) are tic disorders that are present in childhood for less than one year. They are extremely common among school-aged children, with an estimated prevalence of 5-24%.[19] An example of a TTD is a "chronic cough" that has not responded to medications.

Gilles de la Tourette's syndrome is the best known of all tic disorders. Tourette's syndrome (TS) is a disorder characterized by childhood onset of motor and vocal tics. Obsessive-compulsive disorder (OCD) and attention deficit hyperactivity disorder (ADHD) are strongly associated with TS. The established criteria for diagnosis of TS are onset before age 21 years, multiple motor tics, one or more vocal tics, and a fluctuating course and presence of tics for longer than one year. Males are affected more frequently than females, and there is a substantial genetic component.[20,21] Non-genetic factors such as maternal life stressors during pregnancy, gender of the child, and severe hyperemesis gravidarum are known to influence the form and severity of TS. The precise neuroanatomical location of a pathological lesion in TS is not known, although striatal abnormalities are hypothesized. The biochemical basis of TS is likely an increased activity of the dopaminergic system. TS frequently has a variable course, with waxing and waning of tics over several years. Tics tend to worsen in adolescence and abate in adulthood.

Table 10. Causes of Hemiballism

CAUSES	SUBTYPES
Cerebrovascular accidents	Ischemic, hemorrhagic Arteriovenous malformation Subarachnoid hemorrhage
Space occupying lesions	Metastatic cancer Subthalamic nucleus cyst
Infections	Tuberculous meningitis
Cerebral trauma	
Metabolic disorders	Non-ketotic hyperosmolar state
Multiple sclerosis	
Drugs	Phenytoin toxicity Oral contraceptives and estrogens Levodopa
Complications of stereotactic surgery	

Adapted from: Wiener WM J, Lang Anthony L, eds. Movement Disorders: A Comprehensive Survey. Mount Kisco, NY: Futura Publishing Co.; 1989.

Table 11. Etiological Classification of Tics

PRIMARY TIC DISORDERS

Tourette's syndrome
Various chronic tic disorders

SECONDARY TIC DISORDERS

Inherited: Huntington's disease
Neuroacanthocytosis
Torsion dystonia
Chromosomal abnormalities
Other

Acquired: *Drugs:* Neuroleptic, anticonvulsants, levodopa, stimulants
Trauma
Infections: Encephalitis, Creutzfeldt-Jakob disease, Sydenham's chorea
Developmental: Mental retardation, static encephalopathy, autism, pervasive developmental disorder
Stroke
Degenerative: Parkinsonism, progressive supranuclear palsy
Toxic: Carbon monoxide

Adapted from: Kurlan R, ed. *Treatment of Movement Disorders.* Philadelphia, PA: J.B.Lippincott Co.; 1995.

Haloperidol, a dopamine receptor antagonist, is most effective for control of tics. Haloperidol is used in doses ranging from 0.25 to 2.5 mg/day. Higher doses can be used in acute disorders. Clonidine, an alpha$_2$-adrenergic receptor agonist, can be useful in treating TS. New, atypical antipsychotics, such as risperidone, might have a role in the management of TS. Selective serotonin reuptake inhibitors, such as fluoxetine, are used widely to treat OCD, which frequently is associated with TS. Because of the possibilities of developing a tardive MD and other complications of neuroleptic use, these agents are reserved for disabling tics. Initial treatment with clonidine is preferred.

Tremors

Tremors are defined as involuntary, rhythmic, and roughly sinusoidal movements.[22] Tremors can be characterized as resting, postural, kinetic, or task-related. Resting tremor refers to tremor while a body part is relaxed without the influence of gravity. Postural tremor occurs during maintenance of steady body posture against gravity, which usually can be assessed by asking patients to extend their arms in front of them. Kinetic tremor occurs during goal-directed movements such as finger-to-nose testing. Task-related tremor occurs only during the performance of a specific task (e.g., a primary writing tremor). Intention tremor is an imprecise term generally used to describe wide oscillations that occur when a limb approaches a precise destination.

Selected Examples of Tremors. Physiological tremor is considered to be a normal phenomenon. Anxiety, fatigue, or stress exacerbates it. *(Please see Table 12.)* Hypoglycemia, hyperthyroidism, and pheochromocytoma all can enhance physiological tremors. Normal and enhanced physiological tremors are minimal at rest, present with posture, and worse with use of the affected limb. Many medications can cause tremor (please see Table 13), likely by exacerbating physiological tremor.

Essential tremor (ET) is a distinct neurological syndrome characterized by postural and kinetic tremor of the hands; isolated head tremor; and voice tremor with no identifiable cause, such as drugs or toxins; or other focal neurological findings. ET can begin at any age; however, it is more common in the elderly. The tremor of parkinsonism usually is a resting tremor, and patients with ET do not have other features of parkinsonism. Emotional stress, anxiety, thyrotoxicosis, caffeine, and other stimulants exacerbate ET. The pathophysiology of ET is unknown but is likely due to alterations in cerebellar function.

Propranolol in a dose of 240-320 mg/day is a widely used treatment for ET. Primidone and benzodiazepines have been used for ET with variable success.

Task-related tremor occurs during specific motor tasks. The most common is primary writing tremor. Benzodiazepines can be useful in treating these unusual tremors.

Orthostatic tremor is a rare but frequently misdiagnosed condition. It occurs more frequently in women, and the onset is typically in the sixth decade. It manifests as tremor of the legs that is triggered by standing.[23] Orthostatic tremor should be distinguished from ataxia, which is unrelated to orthostasis.

Cerebellar tremor is a common consequence of injury to the cerebellum or its outflow pathways. This type of tremor can have resting, postural, and kinetic components. It is commonly described as affect-

Table 12. Conditions that Can Enhance Physiologic Tremor

- **Mental state:** Anger, anxiety, stress, fatigue, excitement
- **Metabolic:** Fever, thyrotoxicosis, pheochromocytoma, hypoglycemia
- **Drugs and toxins**
- **Miscellaneous:** Caffeinated beverages, monosodium glutamate, nicotine

Adapted from: Weiner W, Lang A. In: Movement Disorders: A Comprehensive Survey. Mount Kisco, NY: Futura Publishing Company, Mount Kisco; 1989.

ing proximal muscles and invariably is associated with ataxia, dysmetria, and other signs of cerebellar dysfunction.

Psychogenic tremor is the typical hysterical MD. Marked fluctuation of the tremor is the hallmark of this tremor. Patients demonstrate marked tremor that improves significantly when they are distracted. Other signs of functional illness are nonphysiological sensory deficits, tunnel vision, and bizarre gait disturbance. *(Please see Table 14.)*

Table 13. Well-Known Causes of Tremor

PHYSIOLOGIC
PATHOLOGIC
Essential tremor
Parkinson's disease
Wilson's disease
Midbrain tremor
Peripheral neuropathy
Multiple sclerosis
Cerebellar infarction
Cerebellar degenerative disorders
PSYCHOGENIC TREMORS
DRUGS AND TOXINS
Neuroleptics
Lithium
Adrenocorticosteroids
Beta-adrenergic agonists
Theophylline
Ethanol
Calcium channel blockers
Valproic acid
Thyroid hormone
Caffeine
Nicotine
Tricyclic antidepressants

Used with permission from: Shah S, Albin R. Movement Disorders. In: Shah S, Kelly K, eds. *Emergency Neurology: Principles and Practice.* New York: Cambridge University Press; 1999.

Myoclonus

Myoclonus are brief, very rapid, sudden, and shock-like jerks that involve very small muscles or the entire body. Hiccup is a good example of "physiological myoclonus" that is called diaphragmatic myoclonus. Myoclonus is a descriptive term and not a diagnosis. Myoclonus does not indicate a specific neurological etiology.[24] These movements can be caused by active muscle contractions (positive myoclonus) or lapses in posture or muscle contractions (negative myoclonus or "asterixis"). Each jerk or sudden movement is a discrete, separate movement, in contrast to chorea, where dance-like, continual flow of movement occurs from one body part to another without interruption. Myoclonus differs from "tic syndromes" in that tics are stereotypic in quality and anatomical distribution, and generally can be suppressed with conscious effort by the patient.[25,26]

The four broad categories of myoclonus are 1) physiological; 2) essential or idiopathic; 3) epileptic; and 4) symptomatic.

Physiological Myoclonus. Physiological myoclonus occurs in normal people and includes sleep (hypnic) jerks, anxiety-induced myoclonus, exercise-induced myoclonus, and hiccup.

Essential Myoclonus. Essential myoclonus is a rare, possibly autosomal dominant hereditary disorder, which begins at a young age and generally has a benign course.

Epileptic Myoclonus. Epileptic myoclonus, as the term suggests, occurs in the setting of a chronic seizure disorder, and is a component of several different epileptic syndromes. Myoclonus can occur as a component of a seizure or as the sole manifestation of a seizure.

Symptomatic Myoclonus. Symptomatic myoclonus refers to myoclonic syndromes associated with an identifiable underlying neurological or non-neurological disorder. This is the most common cause of non-physiologic myoclonus. Associated neurological deficits include encephalopathy, dementia, ataxia, and pyramidal or extrapyramidal signs as dominant features of the illness. When recognized, clinical disorders responsible for this group of myoclonus may be treatable. Posthypoxic myoclonus resulting from global cerebral hypoxia from any cause is a well-known clinical entity.[27,28]

Symptomatic myoclonus resulting from metabolic derangements such as uremia, hepatic coma, hypercapnia, and hypoglycemia usually produces multifocal, arrhythmic myoclonic jerks predominantly affecting the face and proximal musculature. Changes in mental status are characteristic. The myoclonus caused by metabolic encephalopathy resolves as the encephalopathy is corrected. No specific therapeutic measure is required.

Asterixis, or negative myoclonus, was described originally in patients with hepatic encephalopathy, but also can occur in other metabolic or toxic disorders. Asterixis can occur in the recovery phase of general anesthesia, with sedative or anticonvulsant drug administration, and in normal drowsy individuals.[29-34]

Although rare, intractable myoclonus (as in viral encephalitis) can cause hyperthermia, hyperkalemia, hyperuricemia, systemic hypotension, and renal failure secondary to rhabdomyolysis.[35] Myoclonus can be a manifestation of serious underlying disease processes such as toxic or metabolic encephalopathies, or chronic epileptic disorders requiring urgent medical attention.

Table 14. Features of Psychogenic Tremor

1. History of many undiagnosed conditions
2. History of multiple somatization
3. Absence of significant finding on physical examination or imaging study
4. Presence of secondary gain (pending compensation or litigation)
5. Spontaneous remissions and exacerbations
6. Employment in the health care delivery field
7. History of psychiatric illness

Used with permission from: Shah S, Albin R. Movement Disorders. In: Shah S, Kelly K, eds. *Emergency Neurology: Principles and Practice.* New York: Cambridge University Press; 1999.

The focus of the examination in the ED is to determine possible correctable causes of the underlying illness causing myoclonus. Serum glucose levels, electrolytes, hepatic and renal function tests; drug and toxin screens; brain imaging; and urgent EEG can assist in diagnosing the most common metabolic and neurological derangements. Advanced studies such as evoked potentials, determination of enzyme activities (for storage disorders), DNA tests, tissue biopsy (for storage disorders and mitochondrial disease), or copper studies (for Wilson's disease) require referral to a neurologist.

Management of myoclonic movements in the ED is directed to specific management of the underlying illness in cases of symptomatic myoclonus. Valproic acid and clonazepam are effective for treating symptomatic myoclonus in many individuals.[36,37] Physiological myoclonus does not require specific treatment. Reassuring the patient is helpful. Standard antiepileptic drug (AED) therapy is used for myoclonus that is a component of an epileptic syndrome.

Movement Disorders Caused by Commonly Used Drugs

MD caused by the use of various medications is more common than generally is recognized. The cause-and-effect relationship between the drug and the MD is poorly understood, but pre-existing CNS pathology likely predisposes to the development of MDs. Many MDs improve after the offending medication is discontinued. The following groups of commonly prescribed medications are known to cause MDs: antiepileptics; neuroleptics; CNS stimulants; oral contraceptives; calcium channel blockers; antihistaminics and anticholinergics; and antidepressants.

Antiepileptics. Nystagmus, dysarthria, and ataxia commonly are associated with toxic levels of phenytoin and carbamazepine. Asterixis and spontaneous myoclonic jerks are common in the toxicity of phenytoin, phenobarbital, primidone, and carbamazepine. Chorea and dystonia are known to occur with the use of AEDs.[38,39] Chorea generally is associated with the chronic use of multiple antiepileptics. Initial use of an AED rarely results in chorea or dystonia. However, one exception is the development of chorea and dystonia with intravenous administration of phenytoin for status epilepticus.[40] This effect resolves gradually as the peak drug levels decrease.

Valproic acid is known to cause postural tremor (similar to benign essential tremor or enhanced physiological tremor) in approximately 20-25% of patients taking the medication.[41] Severity of tremor does not directly correlate with serum drug levels of valproate, but symptoms subside with decreasing drug levels.

Neuroleptics. The five major categories of MDs associated with the use of neuroleptic medications are listed in Table 15.

The time of onset of MD has some bearing on the type of MD seen with the use neuroleptic medications. ADR, akathisia, and parkinsonism generally occur early after treatment with neuroleptic medications is begun. Tardive disorders occur with prolonged use of neuroleptics. Neuroleptic malignant disorder (NMS) can occur at any time. The dopamine-blocking effects of neuroleptic medications likely are the pharmacological basis for the development of these MDs.

Acute Dystonic Reaction (ADR). Parenteral administration of phenothiazines is more likely to cause ADR than oral preparations, and the risk of ADR increases with the size of the dose. The risk of causing ADR after administration of phenothiazine is approximately 2-5%. ADR usually occurs at the initiation of therapy; 95% of ADR episodes occur within 96 hours of receiving the offending medication.[42] ADR is more common in children and young males. Females between the ages of 12 and 19 years are more prone to metoclopramide (Reglan)-induced ADR.[43] A history of ADR with neuroleptic therapy is an indicator for future risk of development of a MD.[44] Cocaine abuse increases the risk of a neuroleptic-induced ADR.[45] ADR typically involves cranial or truncal musculature. Children tend to have more generalized involvement, particularly in the trunk and extremities. Adults have a more restricted involvement of cranial, neck, and upper limb musculature. ADR is the most common cause of "oculogyric crisis," which consists of forced conjugate eye deviation upward or laterally, often accompanied by extension or lateral movements of the neck, mouth opening, and tongue protrusion. Blepharospasm, grimacing, trismus, forceful jaw opening, and tongue twisting are examples of involvement of other cranial musculature. Milder forms of muscle involvement can present as muscle cramps or tightness of jaw and tongue, leading to difficulty chewing, swallowing, and speaking. Respiratory stridor with resultant cyanosis can occur in patients with severe ADR.[46] ADR can result in extremely disabling dysarthria, dysphagia, jaw dislocation, compromised extremity function, and abnormal gait. ADR typically follows a varied course, with symptoms lasting from minutes to hours. ADR can be difficult to diagnose in the ED because abnormal movements can subside or fluctuate spontaneously, and can improve with reassurance of the patient.

The risk of developing ADR increases with the potency of the neuroleptic drugs and occurs more frequently with parenteral neuroleptics than with oral medications. The duration of symptoms depends on the half-life of the drug. Symptoms of ADR can be controlled quickly by parenteral administration of anticholinergics such as benztropine (Cogentin) or biperiden. The initial dose of benztropine is 2 mg given intravenously, with a maintenance dose of 1-2 mg orally twice daily for 7-14 days to prevent recurrence. Alternatively, diphenhydramine, which has antihistaminic and anticholinergic properties, can be given in a dose of 25-50 mg parenterally for rapid control of symptoms, and a maintenance dose of 25-50 mg orally 3-4 times daily for a few days. Some neurologists prescribe prophylactic use of amantadine for young males requiring neuroleptic therapy.

Table 15. Neuroleptic Medication-Induced MD

1. Acute dystonic reaction (ADR)
2. Akathisia
3. Drug-induced parkinsonism
4. Neuroleptic malignant disorder
5. Tardive disorders

Akathisia is a subjective sensation of restlessness commonly associated with the inability to remain seated.[47] Abnormal limb sensation; inner restlessness, dysphoria, and anxiety are the commonly described symptoms associated with akathisia. This disabling condition can be mistaken for psychiatric illness such as agitation, hyperactivity, or anxiety in patients with agitated depression or schizophrenia.[48] Symptoms abate when the responsible medication is withheld, but management of this disorder often is very difficult.

Drug-induced parkinsonism (DIP) is associated with the use of neuroleptic medications, anti-nausea medication (metoclopramide), and antihypertensive agents (reserpine). The features of DIP generally are indistinguishable from those of idiopathic parkinsonism. A rhythmic, perioral, and perinasal tremor mimicking a rabbit chewing, termed rabbit syndrome, is typical of DIP.[49] The risk of developing DIP is higher in females than in males. Other risk factors include the dose and potency of neuroleptic medications. Anticholinergics and amantadine frequently are used to treat DIP, and have variable success.

Tardive disorder occurs following prolonged use of neuroleptic medications in about 20% of patients treated with these drugs.[50] Tardive disorder often is precipitated or worsened when the dose of the neuroleptic medication is reduced or the drug is withdrawn. Increasing age increases the risk for developing tardive dyskinesia,[51] and the probability of spontaneous remission declines with advancing age. Involuntary stereotypical movements involving orofacial, neck, trunk, and axial muscles constitute the typical tardive dyskinesia. Patients commonly demonstrate pursing, smacking, chewing with frequent tongue protrusion, or pushing the tongue into the inner cheek.

Stimulants. Dextroamphetamine, methylphenidate (Ritalin), pemoline, and cocaine are all stimulant (dopaminomimetic) drugs with peripheral and central actions. Acute and chronic use of these drugs can result in chorea, orofacial dyskinesia, stereotyped movements, dystonia, and tics. Of these, stereotyped movements, comprising compulsive and complex activities, occur most often.

Oral Contraceptives. Chorea is the most frequently experienced MD caused by the use of oral contraceptives in otherwise healthy young females. It typically develops in a nulliparous woman who has been taking the contraceptive for nine weeks.[18] A unilateral distribution of chorea suggests the possibility of preexisting basal ganglia pathology. Symptoms generally abate within a few weeks following discontinuation of the contraceptive.

Antihistaminics and Anticholinergics. The use of chlorpheniramine and brompheniramine is associated with the development of orofacial dyskinesia, blepharospasm, tic-like movements, dystonia, and involuntary, semi-purposeful movements of the hands.[48] ADR with the use of diphenhydramine (Benadryl) has been reported.[52] The use of H_2-receptor blockers cimetidine and ranitidine is associated with the development of postural and action tremor, dystonic reactions, parkinsonism, confusion, and cerebellar dysfunction.[53] The movement abnormalities induced by these agents are generally short-lived and resolve after the responsible medication is discontinued.

Antidepressants. Although not common, tricyclic antidepressants such as amitriptyline, imipramine, and nortriptyline are known to cause choreiform movements, particularly orofacial dyskinesia.[54,55] The anticholinergic effects of tricyclic antidepressants are considered to be responsible for the development of chorea. The use of monoamine oxidase (MAO) inhibitors is associated with tremors and less often with myoclonic jerks.[56] As with MAO inhibitors, an overdose of tricyclic antidepressants is associated with myoclonus.

References

1. Quinn NP, Koller WC, Lang AE, et al. Painful Parkinson's disease. *Lancet* 1986;1:1366.
2. Goetz CG, Lance CM, Levy M, et al. Pain in idiopathic Parkinson's disease. *Mov Disord* 1986;1:45.
3. Koller WC. Sensory symptoms in Parkinson's disease. *Neurology* 1984;34:957.
4. Snider SR, Fahn S, Isgreen WP, et al. Primary sensory symptoms in parkinsonism. *Neurology* 1976;26:423.
5. Fahn S. The varied clinical expressions of dystonia. *Neurol Clin* 1984;2:541-554.
6. Zeman W, Dyken P. Dystonia musculorum deformans. Clinical, genetic and pathoanatomical studies. *Psychiatr Neurolog Neurochirurg* 1967;70:77-121.
7. Jankovic J, Orman J. Blepharospasm. Demographic and clinical survey of 250 patients. *Ann Ophthalmol* 1984;16:371.
8. Shah S, Albin R. Movement Disorders. In: Shah S, Kelly K, Eds. *Emergency Neurology: Principles and Practice.* New York: Cambridge University Press; 1999.
9. Shoulson I. On Chorea. *Clin Neuropharmacol* 1986;9:585.
10. Bruyn GW, Padberg G. Chorea and systemic lupus erythematosus—A critical review. *Eur Neurol* 1984;23:278-290.
11. Hughes GRV. Thrombosis, abortion, cerebral disease and the lupus anticoagulant. *Br Med J* 1983;297:1088.
12. Lahat E, Eschal G, Azizi E, et al. Chorea associated with systemic lupus erythematosus in children. A case report. *Isr J Med Sci* 1989;25:568.
13. Dewey RB, Jankovic J. Hemiballism-hemichorea. Clinical and pharmacologic findings in 21 patients. *Arch Neurol* 1989;46:862.
14. Klawans HL, Moses H, Nausieda PS, et al. Treatment and prognosis of hemiballism. *N Engl J Med* 1976;295:1348.
15. Johnson WG, Fahn S. Treatment of vascular hemiballism and hemichorea. *Neurology* 1977;27:634.
16. Logothetic L. Neurologic and muscular manifestations of hyperthyroidism. *Arch Neurol* 1961;5:533-544.
17. Nausieda PS, Bieliauskas LS, Bacon L, et al. Chronic dopaminergic sensitivity after Sydenham's chorea. *Neurology* 1983;31:750.
18. Nausieda PA, Koller WC, Weiner WJ, et al. Chorea induced by oral contraceptives. *Neurology* 1979;29:1605.
19. Riley D, Lang A. Movement disorders. In: Bradley W, Daroff R, Fenichel A, et al, eds. *Neurology in Clinical Practice.* Boston, MA: Butterworth-Heinemann; 1991.
20. Kurlan R, Lichter D, Hewitt D. Sensory tics in Tourette's syndrome. *Neurology* 1989;39:731.

21. Pauls DL, Leckman JF. The inheritance of Gilles de la Tourette's syndrome and associated behaviors. Evidence for autosomal dominant transmission. *N Eng J Med* 1986;315:993.
22. Elbe RJ, Koller WC. *Tremor*. Baltimore, MD: Johns Hopkins University Press; 1990.
23. Fitzgerald PM, Jankovic J. Orthostatic tremor: An association with essential tremor. *Mov Disord* 1991;6:60.
24. Caviness J. Myclonus. *Mayo Clin Proc* 1996;71:679-688.
25. Marsden CD, Obeso JA, Traub MM, et al. Muscle spasms associated with Sudek's atrophy after injury. *Br Med J* 1984;288:173-176.
26. Banks G, Nielsen VK, Short MP, et al. Brachial plexus myoclonus. *J Neurol Neurosurg Psychiatry* 1985;48:582-584.
27. Swanson PD, Luttrell CN, Magladery JW. Myoclonus—A report of 67 cases and review of literature. *Medicine* 1962;41:339.
28. Wolf P. Periodic synchronous and stereotyped myoclonus with postanoxic coma. *J Neurol* 1977;215:39.
29. Fahn S. Posthypoxic action myoclonus: Review of the literature and report of two new cases with response to valproate and estrogen. *Adv Neurol* 1979;26:49.
30. Fahn S. Posthypoxic action myoclonus: Literature review update. *Adv Neurol* 1986;43:157.
31. Marsden CD, Hallett M, Fahn S. The nosology and pathophysiology of myoclonus. In: Marsden CD, Fahn S, eds. *Movement Disorders*. London: Butterworth; 1982.
32. Kuzniecky R, Berkovic S, Anderman F, et al. Focal cortical myoclonus and rolandic cortical dysplasia: Clarification by magnetic resonance imaging. *Ann Neurol* 1988;23:317-325.
33. Young RR, Shahani BT. Asterixis: One type of negative myoclonus. *Adv Neurol* 1986;43:137.
34. Young RR, Shahani BT. Anticonvulsant asterixis. *Electroencephalogr Clin Neurophysiol* 1973;34:760a.
35. Langston JW, Ricci DR, Portlock C. Nonhypoxemic hazards of prolonged myoclonus. *Neurology* 1977;27:542.
36. Meldrum BS. Drugs acting on aminoacid neurotransmitters. *Adv Neurol* 1986;43:687-706.
37. Pranzatelli MR, Snodgrass SR. The pharmacology of myoclonus. *Clin Neuropharmacol* 1985;8:99-130.
38. Harrison MB, Lyons GR, Landow ER. Phenytoin and dyskinesias: A report of two cases and a review of the literature. *Mov Disord* 1993;8:19.
39. Bimpong-Buta K, Froescher W. Carbamazepine-induced choreoathetotic dyskinesia. *J Neurol Neurosurg Psychiatry* 1982;45:560.
40. Miyasaki JM, Lang AE. Treatment of drug induced movement disorders. In: Kurlan R, ed. *Treatment of Movement Disorders*. Philadelphia, PA: JB Lippincott Co.; 1995.
41. Karas BJ, Wilder BJ, Hammond EJ, et al. Valproate tremors. *Neurology* 1982;32:428-432.
42. Keepers GA, Clappison VJ, Casey DE. Initial anticholinergic prophylaxis for neuroleptic-induced extrapyramidal syndromes. *Arch Gen Psychiatry* 1983;40:113.
43. Bateman DN, Rawlins MD, Simpson JM. Extrapyramidal reactions with metoclopramide. *Br Med J* 1985;291:930.
44. Keepers GA, Casey DE. Use of neuroleptic-induced extrapyramidal symptoms to predict future vulnerability to side effects. *Am J Psychiatry* 1991;148:85.
45. Cardoso FEC, Jankovic J. Cocaine-related movement disorders. *Mov Disord* 1993;8:175.
46. Marsden CD, Tarsy D, Baldessarini RJ. Spontaneous and drug induced movement disorders in psychotic patients. In: Benson DF, Blumer D, eds. *Psychiatric Aspects of Neurological Disease*. New York, NY: Grune & Stratton; 1975.
47. Lang AE. Akathisia and the restless leg syndrome. In: Jankovic J, Tolosa E, eds. *Parkinson's Disease and Other Movement Disorders*. Baltimore, MD: Urban and Schwarzenberg; 1987.
48. Weiner WJ, Lang AE. *Movement Disorders: A Comprehensive Survey*. Mount Kisco, NY: Futura Publishing Co; 1989.
49. Villeneuve A. The rabbit syndrome: A peculiar extrapyramidal reaction. *Can Psychiatr Assoc J* 1972;17(suppl):SS69.
50. Kane JM, Smith JM. Tardive dyskinesia: Prevalence and risk factors, 1959-1979. *Arch Gen Psychiatry* 1982;39:473.
51. Kane JM, Woerner M, Lieberman J. Tardive dyskinesia: Prevalence, incidence and risk factors. *J Clin Psychopharmacol* 1988;8(suppl):52.
52. Lavenstein BL, Cantor FK. Acute dystonia. An unusual reaction to diphenhydramine. *JAMA* 1976;236:291.
53. Handler CE, Besse CP, Wilson AO. Extrapyramidal and cerebellar syndrome with encephalopathy associated with cimetidine. *Postgrad Med J* 1982;58:527.
54. Fann WE, Sullivan JL, Richman BW. Tardive dyskinesia associated with tricyclic antidepressants. *Br J Psychiatry* 1976;128: 490-493.
55. Woogen S, Graham J, Angrist B. A tardive dyskinesia-like syndrome after amitryptaline treatment. *J Clin Psychopharmacol* 1981;1:34-36.
56. Lieberman JA, Kane JM, Reife R. Neuromuscular effects of monoamine oxidase inhibitors. *Adv Neurol* 1986;43:231.

Part IV

Pulmonary Disorders

Chronic Obstructive Pulmonary Disease (COPD): Assessment of Acute Exacerbations

Charles L. Emerman, MD
Gideon Bosker, MD, FACEP

The clinical challenges of managing patients with acute exacerbations of chronic obstructive pulmonary disease (AECOPD) are well known to emergency physicians, pulmonologists, and primary care physicians. With their strenuous respiration, agitation, tachypnea, sputum production, and/or shortness of breath, these recurrent visitors are among the most difficult patients encountered in the acute-care setting.

Typically, patients with bacterial exacerbations of chronic obstructive pulmonary disease (COPD) present in acute distress that may be characterized by a worsening, productive cough, increasing dyspnea on exertion, and difficulty breathing. Not infrequently, these individuals will report a low-grade fever, a change in the color and tenacity of their sputum, and mild pleuritic chest pain. Difficult (but critical) decisions, including choice of stabilizing medical therapy, selection of an outcome-effective antibiotic, use of invasive vs. non-invasive ventilation techniques, and patient disposition, must be made promptly based on objective physical as well as historical information.

The construction of a safe, effective drug regimen is always an important consideration, both in patients requiring hospitalization and those deemed suitable for management as outpatients. Polypharmacy with such drugs as inhaled and systemic corticosteroids, antibiotics, and/or bronchodilators is the rule rather than the exception.

Combination drug therapy has the advantage of improving functional status, permitting outpatient management, and reducing frequency of exacerbations, but has the potential disadvantages of drug interactions, dose-related toxicity, and cost. Identifying therapeutic agents that maximize medication compliance, reduce duration of therapy, and decrease risk of drug-drug interactions is of paramount importance.

There is a general consensus that patients with AECOPD, who frequently suffer from other co-morbid conditions, can be difficult to diagnose and even more problematic to stabilize. In addition, it may be difficult to distinguish bacterial from non-bacterial (i.e., viral) exacerbations. Accordingly, to optimize clinical outcomes, evaluation of patients with AECOPD should focus on identifying inciting factors and accurate assessment of disease severity.

Unfortunately, universally accepted, consistent guidelines and critical pathways for managing patients with AECOPD are not available, primarily because long-term, prospective studies comparing the effectiveness of specific agents, including antibiotics, in well-matched subgroups have not been performed. Consequently, recommendations generated by consensus groups, national associations, and managed care organizations frequently differ in their approach to risk stratification and selection of antimicrobial therapy.

Most of the support for using antibiotics in patients with AECOPD has been derived from meta-analysis data, which have the limitation of comparing older agents under varying, region-specific conditions of antimicrobial resistance. Because these resistance patterns may have changed over time, new approaches to antimicrobial therapy may be warranted. Moreover, risk-stratification strategies have not been standardized in these studies, which has made it difficult to determine when intensification and amplification of coverage from one class of antibiotics (macrolides) to another (quinolones) are appropriate in specific patient subgroups.

Although experts in the field of emergency and pulmonary medicine agree that acute management should be directed toward reducing airflow obstruction, treating complications, decreasing frequency of future exacerbations, and preventing acute respiratory deterioration, the precise approach to patients with AECOPD is in evolution. What is clear, however, is that the clinical mission statement for patients with AECOPD is to identify a safe, effective regimen that will improve functional status and prevent future relapse.

With these considerations in mind, this chapter provides a practical, although detailed and comprehensive, approach for initial evaluation and treatment of patients with acute bacterial exacerbations of COPD. Providing specific clinical pathways and therapeutic strategies, this monograph emphasizes the importance of the history, physical examination, laboratory data, and radiologic modalities for maximizing clinical outcomes.

Overview

Chronic obstructive pulmonary disease is a leading cause of morbidity and mortality among smokers 55 years of age and older. It is estimated that this condition affects more than 20 million Americans,[2] and among Medicare patients, COPD accounts for about 150,000 hospitalizations per year.[3] While the overall in-hospital mortality rate from COPD has not changed dramatically over the past decade, an increasing number of patients require placement in extended care facilities.

From a disease categorization standpoint, COPD is occasionally referred to as chronic obstructive lung disease (COLD), and from a clinical perspective, this condition is composed of three distinct entities: 1) chronic bronchitis; 2) emphysema; and 3) peripheral airways disease.[4] It should be stressed that the diagnosis of chronic bronchitis or emphysema is not synonymous with irreversible airflow obstruction and that these patients can benefit from bronchodilators, steroids, antibiotics, and other therapeutic measures.

The greatest percentage of patients with COPD have evidence of chronic bronchitis, a diagnosis that is based on a history of productive cough for three months of the year for two successive years. Patients with chronic bronchitis have an increase in the number and size of submucosal glands in the bronchi and evidence of bronchiolar inflammation. In contrast, the diagnosis of emphysema is based on the presence of airway enlargement. Most patients with COPD and emphysema have enlargement in the respiratory bronchioles. Clinically, emphysema is manifested by an elongated, hyperresonant chest. Diaphragmatic flattening and increased radiolucency is seen on the chest x-ray. Finally, patients with peripheral airways disease have inflammation of the terminal bronchioles and abnormal pulmonary function tests.

Differential Diagnosis. Patients may have any combination of these three entities. In fact, some degree of chronic bronchitis, emphysema, and/or peripheral airways disease with chronic airflow limitation usually coexists in most patients. Further complicating the picture is the fact that asthma presents with many of the same signs and symptoms observed in COPD.[3-5] Differentiating between these two conditions can be difficult, and older patients may not have a clearly established diagnosis. Distinguishing between asthma and COPD is important in the emergency department because management strategies are different for each condition.

The clinical history, which must include a detailed inquiry into precipitating factors, a careful record of character and severity of previous exacerbations, response to pharmacotherapeutic agents, and features of the current episode, will usually guide the practitioner toward the most appropriate assessment and management pathway. For example, the diagnosis usually is straightforward when an older patient presents with the late adult onset of respiratory disease associated with a long history of cigarette smoke. Similarly, a younger adult with a life-long history of asthma and no smoking history will generally be treated as having an asthma exacerbation. But many cases will be more ambiguous and differentiation of these patients may require formal pulmonary function testing with possible histamine challenge by a pulmonologist.

The majority of patients with COPD will have either a history of cigarette smoking or exposure to second-hand cigarette smoke. Occasionally, patients will develop COPD from occupational exposure. A minority of patients develop emphysema as a result of alpha-1-protease inhibitor deficiency or intravenous drug abuse. These patients develop emphysema earlier in life than those who acquire COPD secondary to cigarette smoke.

Prognosis. COPD is associated with decreased long-term survival. A number of predicting factors have been linked with the increased mortality rates reported in patients with chronic airflow limitation.[5] In this regard, patients with a FEV_1 less than 40% or an FEV_1/FVC ratio less than 40% have decreased survival as do those with a baseline $Pa0_2$ less than 55 mmHg, CO_2 retention, cor pulmonale, and decreased diffusion capacity. Overall, these high-risk patients have a 12-year survival probability of about 40%.[5]

As might be expected, acute respiratory failure is associated with an increased risk of short-term mortality. Patients requiring intensive care unit admission for COPD have an inpatient mortality rate ranging between 10% and 30%.[5,6] In some studies, however, the need for mechanical ventilation did not imply an increased mortality rate among patients requiring intensive care unit admission.

Issues regarding the potential pitfalls of mechanical ventilation have been fiercely debated among intensivists, emergency physicians, and pulmonary specialists. From a prognostic perspective, however, decisions regarding mechanical ventilation for patients with COPD must be made on a patient-by-patient basis, using sound clinical judgment. Many clinicians may be concerned that a large percentage of intubated patients will go on to require chronic mechanical ventilation. However, the data appear to suggest that the majority of patients who require intubation for COPD can be successfully weaned from mechanical ventilation over the course of 7-14 days, even after severe, life-threatening exacerbations.[6-8]

Nevertheless, the mortality rate for these patients over the next 1-2 years is substantial, ranging between 40% and 60%.[6-8] In most studies, short-term survival following an acute exacerbation is related to age, pulmonary function, oxygenation, the presence of congestive heart failure (CHF), and evidence of cor pulmonale. Many patients with COPD have co-existing cardiac disease which, in the form of left ventricular dysfunction, also is predictive of an increased mortality rate.[8]

The likelihood that patients with COPD will require hospitalization for their condition depends on the number, frequency, and severity of their exacerbations. More than three acute exacerbations of COPD per four-month period is associated with an increased risk of hospitalization. Hence, from an emergency medicine and primary care perspective, the most important clinical goal is to provide definitive treatment that is sufficiently aggressive to produce resolution of acute exacerbation and prolong the period between exacerbations.

Patient Assessment

Patients who present to the emergency department with an acute exacerbation of COPD may arrive in varying degrees of clinical distress. The patient in extreme distress will require immediate therapy. Generally speaking, efforts to obtain a comprehensive history, conduct a physical examination, and perform diagnostic studies may need to be delayed pending the initiation of rapid treatment, which may include oxygen, bronchodilators, and invasive or non-invasive ventilation. In less severe cases, or as the patient improves with therapy, the individual with AECOPD should be questioned about historical features that may aid in the differential diagnosis and guide management.

Clinical Differentiation. Although the patient with AECOPD usually will complain of either cough, sputum production, and/or dyspnea, the emergency physician should attempt to elicit other symptoms that may help identify the etiology of this attack. For example, acute exacerbations may be precipitated by an infectious process, exposure to noxious stimuli, or environmental changes such as a change in ambient temperature, humidity, or air pollution. In addition, signs and symptoms of COPD may mimic those seen in other diseases, such as lung carcinoma, decompensated CHF, pneumonia, or pulmonary embolism.

Even in patients who carry a diagnosis of COPD, the astute clinician must consider other life-threatening causes of shortness of breath and chest pain, especially in elderly patients with known obstructive disease. In particular, when there is a history of change in sputum character and a long course of corticosteroids, the diagnosis of pneumonia should be considered. A chest x-ray will help confirm this suspicion. Ischemic heart disease, with or without CHF, also may be accompanied by shortness of breath or chest pain. All patients should be questioned about medication use and compliance, as well as social factors such as continued cigarette smoking. In addition, it is important to characterize and compare the current illness with the severity of previous episodes and to be aware of previous intubation or admissions to the ICU. Some individuals with longstanding COPD may even be aware of their baseline FEV_1 or arterial blood gases (ABGs).

The elderly patient may present special challenges, one of which is the difficulty in distinguishing between decompensated CHF and an acute bacterial exacerbation of COPD. The distinction can be especially difficult, most notably in patients who have a preexisting history of both conditions. Nevertheless, certain findings may help make this distinction. For example, a peak expiratory flow rate (PEFR) greater than 150 L/min may suggest the possibility of CHF[5,9] especially in the presence of jugular venous distention, hepatic congestion, or pedal edema. It should be stressed that jugular venous distension, hepatic congestion, and pedal edema can occur in cor pulmonale as well as CHF. Differentiation between asthma and COPD also can be problematic, since both conditions may respond favorably to acute administration of aerosolized beta-agonists.

Pulmonary embolism (PE) can be very difficult to confirm in patients with COPD on the basis of clinical evaluation alone.[6] The ventilation/perfusion scan is frequently indeterminate in patients with COPD. Evidence of calf swelling, tenderness, increased warmth, erythema, or the presence of a tender venous cord may suggest the diagnosis of deep venous thrombosis, which may be verified by impedance plethysmography, ultrasound, venography, or d-dimer.

When these symptoms are accompanied by typical manifestations of PE, this diagnosis is strongly suggested. Recent studies have suggested the utility of chest computed tomography to diagnose pulmonary embolism in the setting of COPD. However, this modality is not widely accepted and requires interpretation by a radiologist proficient in this particular test. The spiral CT scan has relatively good specificity for pulmonary embolism, but it still lacks adequate sensitivity to replace other established modalities (ventilation/perfusion scan and pulmonary angiography) whose utility in pulmonary embolism has been confirmed.[10]

Finally, with respect to the severity of an acute attack, the clinician should be aware that although physical findings can be misleading, they should nevertheless be documented. Cyanosis is a late and uncommon finding. The patient who is confused, combative, or agitated is probably severely hypoxemic, although relatively few patients present initially with this constellation of findings. Intercostal retractions, accessory muscle use, and an increase in the pulsus paradoxus usually suggest significant airway obstruction.[7] Wheezing is variably associated with airway obstruction. Biphasic wheezing tends to imply a more significant airway obstruction, although this is not universally true. Wheezing disappears when pulmonary function rises to 60% of the predicted normal value.[8,11]

Community-Acquired Pneumonia in COPD

Clinicians should note that patients with COPD also are at high risk for developing community-acquired pneumonia (CAP), a condition that always requires treatment with antibiotics when bacterial organisms are suspected or implicated. Unfortunately, the exact incidence of pneumonia in patients with obstructive lung disease is uncertain. Not surprisingly, the clinical presentation of acute bronchitis superimposed on chronic lung disease can be difficult to differentiate from bacterial pneumonia in the patient with COPD. Symptoms such as fever, sputum production, and abnormal lung sounds are findings common to both conditions. In addition, many patients with COPD have abnormal chest radiographs.[12] Furthermore, a variety of noninfectious conditions can mimic pneumonia in patients with COPD, including pulmonary infarction, CHF, drug reaction, pulmonary cancers, pulmonary hemorrhage, and chemical inhalation.[13] Nevertheless, the appearance of new radiographic abnormalities (lobar consolidation, atelectasis, infiltrates, pleural effusions, and other findings) in association with symptoms of acute pulmonary infection should probably prompt the emergency physician to treat the patient for bacterial pneumonia.

As is the case when CAP occurs in individuals without COPD, *Streptococcus pneumoniae* is the most common organism isolated from patients with CAP who have underlying COPD, although this organism is being demonstrated with decreasing frequency. *Hemophilus influenzae* and *Moraxella catarrhalis* also are commonly isolated from COPD patients with CAP; their frequency increases during the winter months. *Legionella pneumophila* can be encountered any time of the year and chronic lung disease is a risk factor for CAP caused by *Legionella pneumophila*. Pneumonia caused by this agent is associated with a variable clinical presentation ranging from a mild cough to life-threatening respiratory infection and ventilatory failure. *Pseudomonas aeruginosa* is a common organism isolated from the sputum of patients with COPD, and in a significant percentage of cases, isolation of this organism represents colonization of the respiratory tract. Although pseudomonas pneumonia is uncommon in ambulatory patients with COPD, it must be considered in patients with more severe presentations, especially as a nosocomial infection in the hospital environment.[21-24]

Staphylococcal pneumonia is not a common cause of CAP in patients with COPD. However, in patients with chronic lung disease, it appears that viral infection with influenza predisposes patients to subsequent bacterial pneumonia, including both streptococcal and staphylococcal disease. Studies using the influenza vaccine have shown an overall decreased mortality rate, although they have not been done exclusively on patients with COPD.[131] Pneumococcal vaccination has been shown to be cost-effective in high-risk patients, and most experts agree that Pneumovax 23 is indicated in the subset of patients with COPD.[14] At present, it seems reasonable and prudent to advocate use of pneumococcal and influenza vaccine for patients with COPD.

Infectious Precipitants of AECOPD

The role of bacterial and viral-mediated infection as precipitants of acute respiratory decompensation in the setting of COPD has been controversial. Certainly, numerous studies have confirmed the role of viral infection in acute exacerbations of COPD.[15-17] In one study, 32% of patients with an acute exacerbation had evidence of viral infection.[16] In these and other investigations evaluating the role of viral infection, the most common agents identified include influenza virus, parainfluenzae, and respiratory syncytial (RSV) virus.[15-19]

Interestingly, although many treatment guidelines for AECOPD do not mandate empirical antimicrobial coverage of atypical organisms, among them, *Mycoplasma pneumoniae*, *Chlamydia pneumoniae*, and legionella, for patients with AECOPD, studies show that atypical organisms such as mycoplasma or chlamydia may occasionally be associated with decompensation in patients with COPD. In fact, many patients with COPD have serologic evidence of previous Chlamydia infection. On the other hand, recent studies suggest that acute *Chlamydia pneumoniae* infection occurs in only about 5% of acute exacerbations of COPD.[17,18]

Epidemiology. The precise role of bacterial infection is more difficult to ascertain, and equally problematic to confirm in the individual patient. Nevertheless, it is clear that bacterial precipitants play an important etiologic role in AECOPD. In one Canadian study enrolling 1687 patients (80% of which had AECOPD), sputum cultures were obtained in 125 patients (7.4%). Normal flora was found in 76 of 125 sputum specimens (61%), and a pathogen was found in 49 (39%). Of all the patients having sputum cultures, *H. influenzae* was the most common pathogen, occurring in 24 cases (19%), followed by *Streptococcus pneumoniae* in 15 (12%) and *Moraxella catarrhalis* in 10 (8%).[20] Complicating confirmation of a linkage between acute bacterial infection and clinical deterioration in COPD is the fact that patients with COPD have chronic colonization of the respiratory tree with such organisms as *Streptococcus pneumoniae, Hemophilus influenzae*, and *Hemophilus parainfluenzae*.[19] In addition, *Moraxella catarrhalis* is being recognized with increasing frequency.

Role of Antibiotics. One way of delineating the precise role of bacterial infection in AECOPD is to evaluate the efficacy of antibiotics in producing symptomatic and functional improvement in patients during an acute exacerbation of COPD. A number of trials dating back to the 1950s have been performed to assess the relationships between antibiotic treatment and resolution of symptoms, many of them using tetracycline as the therapeutic agent.[15] Some of these studies demonstrated a role for antibiotics during the acute exacerbation, while others did not find a significant advantage.

However, a recent meta-analysis of nine studies performed between 1957 and 1992 confirms that there is a small, but statistically significant benefit when antibiotics are used for acute exacerbations of COPD.[21] The benefits are relatively greater for those patients with AECOPD who require hospitalization. It should be noted that these studies were performed prior to the availability of more potent, compliance-enhancing agents, many of which, such as azithromycin and the new-generation fluoroquinolones, are not only active against atypical organisms, but also against beta-lactamase-producing *H. influenzae* and *M. catarrhalis*. Furthermore, the failure rate of older antibiotics may be as high as 25%.[22,23]

Clinical studies of acute exacerbations of COPD are difficult to interpret because of the heterogeneous nature of COPD, diffuse symptoms that can vary spontaneously, and difficulties in defining clinical response both in the short and long term. Although the role of bacterial infection—and as a result, empiric use of antibiotics—in COPD is somewhat controversial, the most currently available evidence shows that bacterial infection has a significant role in acute exacerbations, but its role in disease progression is less certain. Moreover, based on the preponderance of published evidence, antibiotic therapy is recommended in all patients with AECOPD who present with infectious symptoms (i.e., increased sputum production, change in character of the sputum, increased coughing and shortness of breath) suggesting that antimicrobial therapy will produce a better outcome.[20,24-27]

Upper respiratory tract commensals, such as nontypable *Haemophilus influenzae*, cause most bronchial infections by exploiting deficiencies in the host defenses.[24] Some COPD patients are chronically colonized by bacteria between exacerbations, which represents an equilibrium in which the numbers of bacteria are contained by the host defenses but not eliminated. When an exacerbation occurs, this equilibrium is upset and bacterial numbers increase, which incites an inflammatory response. Neutrophil products can further impair the mucosal defenses, favoring the bacteria, but if the infection is managed, symptoms resolve. However, if the infection persists, chronic inflammation may cause lung damage. About 50% of exacerbations involve bacterial infection, but these patients are not easy to differentiate from those who are uninfected, which means that antibiotics should be given empirically to the majority of patients who present with AECOPD. Further research is needed to characterize those patients in whom bacterial infection may play a more important role and in whom more intensive antibiotic coverage is required.

Old vs. New Agents. The antibiotic arsenal available for treatment of acute bacterial exacerbations of COPD includes a wide range of older and newer agents representing several drug classes. Although many of the studies confirming efficacy of antibiotics in AECOPD were performed with such older agents as amoxicillin and tetracycline, usage patterns are changing in favor of newer agents such as macrolides with a broader spectrum of coverage and which also have compliance-enhancing features.

There is evidence-based justification for this evolution in prescribing practices.[20,24-26] In the past, antibiotics such as amoxicillin, ampicillin, tetracycline, erythromycin, and co-trimoxazole were widely employed. Many of the meta-analysis trials demonstrating the usefulness of antibiotics drew upon studies using these agents. But resistance patterns have changed.[24-29] In particular, during the last 10 years, there has been a steady rise in the frequency of β-lactamase production by *H. influenzae* and *M. catarrhalis*, and more recently, strains of penicillin-resistant pneumococci have emerged.[24-30]

Fortunately, these older antibiotics have been joined by newer agents with either a wider spectrum of activity in vitro, better pharmacokinetics, lower incidence of side effects, more convenient dosing, and/or a shorter duration of therapy. Among the antibiotics approved for acute bacterial exacerbations of COPD, and which also have evidence-based support for their efficacy in this condition, the azalide azithromycin and quinolones such as levofloxacin are playing an increasingly important role as first-line therapy.[26-31] In addition, β-lactamase inhibitors, including second- and third-generation cephalosporins, also are available.[24] A more detailed discussion of antibiotic therapy and the selection process are presented in subsequent sections of this review.

Antibiotic Outcome-Effectiveness and Total Cost of Therapy. Unfortunately, limited data exist to guide physicians in the cost-effective treatment of acute exacerbation of chronic bronchitis (AECOPD). One important study, however, attempted to determine the antimicrobial efficacy of various agents and compared total outcome costs for patients with AECOPD.[32] For the purpose of this analysis, a retrospective review was performed of 60 outpatient medical records of individuals with a diagnosis of COPD associated with acute episodes seen in the pulmonary clinic of a teaching institution.

The participating patients had a total of 224 episodes of AECOPD requiring antibiotic treatment. Before review, empirical antibiotic choices were divided into first-line (amoxicillin, co-trimoxazole, tetracyclines, erythromycin); second-line (cephradine, cefuroxime, cefaclor, cefprozil); and third-line (azithromycin, amoxicillin-clavulanate, ciprofloxacin) agents. The designations "first-line," "second-line," and "third-line" were based on a consensus of resident pulmonologists, and was not intended to indicate superiority of one group of drugs vs. another. The residents were asked, "What antibiotic would you choose to treat a patient with AECOPD on their initial presentation, on their second presentation, and on a subsequent presentation, if each episode was separated by 2-4 weeks?"[33]

The results have potentially interesting implications for antibiotic selection in the outpatient environment. In this study, patients receiving first-line agents (amoxicillin, co-trimoxazole, tetracyclines, erythromycin) failed significantly more frequently (19% vs 7%; $P < 0.05$) than those treated with third-line agents (azithromycin, amoxicillin-clavulanate, ciprofloxacin). Moreover, patients prescribed first-line agents were hospitalized significantly more often for AECOPD within two weeks of outpatient treatment as compared with patients prescribed third-line agents (18.0% vs 5.3% for third-line agents; $P < 0.02$). Time between subsequent AECOPD episodes requiring treatment was significantly longer for patients receiving third-line agents compared with first-line and second-line agents ($P < 0.005$).[32] The high failure rate with such older agents as amoxicillin, tetracycline, and erythromycin correlates well with recent reports of increasing antibiotic resistance.[33-35]

As might be expected, initial pharmacy acquisition costs were lowest with first-line agents (first-line U.S. $10.30 ± 8.76; second-line U.S. $24.45 ± 25.65; third-line U.S. $45.40 ± 11.11; $P < 0.0001$), but third-line agents showed a trend toward lower mean total costs of AECOPD treatment (first-line U.S. $942 ± 2173; second-line, U.S. $563 ± 2296; third-line, U.S. $542 ± 1946). The use of so-called third-line antimicrobials, azithromycin, amoxicillin-clavulanate, or ciprofloxacin, significantly reduced the failure rate and need for hospitalization, prolonged the time between AECOPD episodes, and were associated with a lower total cost of management for AECOPD. Well-designed, prospective studies are needed to confirm these findings and determine how critical pathways should be constructed to maximize outcome-effectiveness of antibiotics used for AECOPD.

Based on these results, the authors of this retrospective analysis suggest that these trends should be of interest to the following groups: 1) managed care decision-makers involved in the formulary selection process; 2) physicians whose objective is to optimize outcome-effectiveness of antibiotic therapy; and 3) to patients with AECOPD, since definitive treatment of the initial presentation is necessary to minimize work disability, to permit continuance of normal activities, to reduce hospitalizations requiring more intensive therapy, and to prevent further clinical deterioration from bronchitis to pneumonia.[33]

In addition, the reduction in hospitalization rate observed with second-line and third-line agents, when compared with first-line agents, may have potential impact on the mortality of patients with COPD. In a recent study of 458 patients with COPD who required admission to hospital for acute exacerbation of chronic bronchitis (AECB), mortality was 13% after a median length of stay of 10 days; mortality at 180 days was 35%.[36] The severity of ventilator-related impairment of lung function in patients with COPD is strongly related to death both from obstructive lung disease and from all causes.[36-37] Moreover, patients who experience frequent episodes of AECOPD are at risk for accelerated loss of lung function and effective antibiotic therapy may slow this decline. The use of third-line antibiotics in the outpatient setting could decrease the number of hospitalizations and the degenerative disease process, and thus prolong the survival of patients with COPD. Further evaluation of this hypothesis is required.[33,35-38]

Based on the data collected in this study, the use of azithromycin, amoxicillin-clavulanate, or ciprofloxacin for the treatment of AECB resulted in significantly fewer physician office visits and appeared to prevent hospitalizations when compared with first- or second-line antimicrobial therapy.[33] Whether there is any difference among these agents remains to be evaluated longitudinally. Additionally, the repetitive nature of return visits to the emergency department or outpatient clinic for AECOPD may assist in identifying patients who require initial treatment with more effective agents to prevent AECOPD-related hospital admissions and progression of the disease.

Diagnostic Testing

Although the physical examination and history provide important information for guiding therapy, it is nevertheless difficult to estimate the degree of airway obstruction and exclude conditions that can mimic AECOPD without ancillary diagnostic tests. Not infrequently, clinical findings can abate even though patients still may have moderate to severe obstruction. Signs typically associated with severe obstruction, such as pulsus paradoxus, cyanosis, or retractions, are seen in a minority of patients, and their absence does not rule out significant obstruction. Even experienced pulmonologists may be unable to accurately estimate pulmonary function. Studies in the emergency department setting suggest that clinicians are unable to accurately predict pulmonary function and, frequently, cannot determine whether patients, in fact, have had an objective improvement in expiratory airflow.[12,18,19,21-23,39] Because of the limitations based on physical assessment alone, it is important to make objective measurements of lung function.

Pulse Oximetry. The mainstay of acute, intra-departmental evaluation of patients with AECOPD, pulse oximetry is an inexpensive, noninvasive procedure for assessing oxygen saturation. Unlike blood gas sampling, pulse oximetry is noninvasive; in addition, results are available immediately and can be followed continuously, thereby permitting the physician to evaluate patient progress in response to therapy. Pulse oximetry measurements are based on the fact that oxyhemoglobin absorbs more light in the infra-red band (800-1000 nm) than reduced hemoglobin, which absorbs more light in the red band (600-750 nm).[40] Dynamic responsiveness depends on pulmonary oxygen stores, distribution of ventilation, blood transit times, and the electronics of the system.[41] Response time has been estimated at about six seconds plus the transit time of 20 seconds for blood to reach the finger (or about 15 seconds for it to reach the ear).[42] The response to resaturation is faster than response to desaturation.

As a general rule, oximetry is accurate to within 3-5% at saturations greater than 70%.[42] However, oximetry is less reliable at oxygen saturations less than 65-70%, because no empirical correlation exists.[40] The relationship between the PaO_2 and oxygen saturation is complex and varies depending on many factors, including the PO_2 and the acid-base status. Most importantly, however, the pulse oximetry provides a relatively rapid means of categorizing patients into mild, moderate, and severe respiratory impairment. In addition, time-dependent trends in the oxygen saturation provide important, objective information that reflects the efficacy of therapy. Capnometry can also be used as an adjunct to pulse oximetry in order to moniter evolving respiratory failure or response to treatment.

Arterial Blood Gases. Both hypercarbia and hypoxemia occur when pulmonary function falls below 25-30% of the predicted normal value.[43] Severe hypoxemia can occur in patients with acute exacerbations of COPD, even though their pulmonary function approaches 50% of the predicted normal value.[44] As is the case with asthma, severe hypercarbia generally occurs only with severe airway obstruction (i.e., when pulmonary function is below 25% of the predicted normal value).

Some clinicians routinely obtain ABGs on all patients with acute exacerbation of COPD upon arrival to the hospital. Comparison of ABG values during an acute exacerbation with baseline values can help establish the severity of an exacerbation and risk-stratify the patient. However, the practice of obtaining routine ABGs is not universal, especially since pulse oximetry can provide useful, accurate information about a patient's respiratory status, but it does not provide information about CO_2-dependent ventilatory drive. Unlike patients with acute asthma, the patient with COPD may develop acute respiratory failure due to administration of supplemental oxygen. It had been previously thought that acute respiratory acidosis occurs as a result of the diminished hypoxic drive when oxygen was administered. While this may occur, part of the explanation is that acute respiratory acidosis also occurs because of ventilation perfusion abnormalities and gas transfer between alveoli secondary to emphysematous changes.[45]

In the patient whose initial arterial blood gas does not demonstrate a life-threatening abnormality, the remainder of the ED course usually can be followed using pulse oximetry.[46] Patients who have significant abnormalities on the first arterial blood gas will require repeat analysis to confirm resolution of the abnormality and aid in disposition.

Pulmonary Function Tests. Pulmonary function testing is a useful means for assessing ventilatory function. Relatively inexpensive peak flow meters are available that can provide a quick assessment of expiratory function. It should be stressed that the peak expiratory flow meter is effort-dependent. In addition, most of the formulae used to derive expected peak flow have been derived from young, healthy patient populations. Furthermore, peak flow meters overestimate lung function in their midrange and lose accuracy after 200 examinations.

Portable spirometers also are readily available and are simple to operate. Fortunately, newer spirometers have eliminated many of the disadvantages that plagued the older, water-sealed devices. Modern spirometers are lightweight, portable, and computerized, permitting rapid calculation of critical clinical values. Furthermore, the spirometer provides for a graphic output, which permits the clinician to visually assess the adequacy of the effort. In addition, many spirometers will display a flow volume loop that can help differentiate between obstructive, restrictive, and proximal obstructive disease.

The spirometer has some advantages over the peak flow meter in that it is easily calibrated. The FEV_1 is less effort-dependent than the peak expiratory flow rate, and the spirometer provides a graphic output, which can be entered into the medical record. Additionally, the spirometer allows for the differentiation between restrictive, obstructive, and proximal airway disease. Many patients in acute respiratory distress will have a restrictive pattern because of inadequate forced expiratory maneuver, chest hyperexpansion, and chest wall discomfort. This pattern may resolve with therapy, giving more typical obstructive pattern.

Compared to the FEV_1, the peak expiratory flow rate tends to underestimate the degree of airway obstruction.[47] Although there is general correlation between the peak expiratory flow rate (PEFR) and the FEV_1 in COPD, significant differences may be seen between the two measurements. It appears that there are some advantages to performing spirometry in the emergency department. However, it should be emphasized that some measure of expiratory function is preferable even if it is limited to the peak expiratory flow rate.

Spirometry is useful because patients with COPD frequently have alterations of gas exchange. These patients have chronic airway obstruction and may have chronic CO_2 retention. In addition, there is impairment of pulmonary diffusion capacity and there are ventilation perfusion abnormalities that may lead to hypoxemia. In general, the results of pulmonary function testing help predict the presence of hypercarbia.[48] Significant hypercarbia is unlikely to occur with patients with a FEV_1 less than 35% of predicted normal.[48] On the other hand, patients may have severe hypoxemia even in the presence of moderate airway obstruction.

Various authors have advocated selective use of arterial blood gases in patients with AECOPD. While selective use of ABGs may reduce costs of care in some patients, it is not yet clear how patient outcomes might be affected by restricting the use of this modality. Based on these observations and recommendations, it appears reasonable and prudent to use a combination of techniques to identify patients with severe respiratory impairment. To this end, spirometry can help identify patients at risk for hypercarbia, and pulse-oximetry can be used to identify patients with oxygen desaturation. In patients with significant deviations from baseline based on spirometric and pulse oximetric data, ABGs can further elucidate the acuity of decompensation, the patient's acid-base status, and the need for urgent ventilatory support. However, this scheme has not been tested prospectively in a rigorous manner.

Chest Radiography. A significant percentage of patients with COPD will have abnormalities on their chest radiographs. From an emergency treatment perspective, new abnormalities must be distinguished from chronic changes, and the ability to identify patients with COPD who have community-acquired pneumonia is especially important. Some authors have tried to develop decision rules to increase the yield of chest radiographs. One proposed scheme suggests that a chest radiograph should be obtained in patients with a history of CHF, leukocytosis or a left-shift, or peripheral edema.[40] Unfortunately, these high-yield criteria have not been validated in subsequent studies,[12,13] and therefore, radiographs should be performed based on the severity of the clinical presentation.

Overall, about 15% of patients with acute exacerbation of COPD will have significant new abnormalities on chest radiography.[14] Given the extensive differential diagnosis in patients who present with symptoms typical of acute exacerbation of COPD (cough, sputum production, change in sputum character, fever, shortness of breath), routine chest radiography may be warranted.[14] In particular, the chest radiograph will permit identification of those individuals with pneumonia, pneumothorax, and decompensated CHF; on occasion, a new lung mass suggesting malignancy may be detected. Portable radiographs may be necessary for patients who are clinically unstable; studies suggest that portable radiographs will detect more than 90% of abnormalities detectable on a standard PA and posteriolateral radiograph.[14]

Laboratory Tests. Although a variety of laboratory tests may be obtained in patients with COPD, these studies should be tailored to the specific clinical situation. For example, patients with COPD may be at higher risk for acquiring coronary artery disease because of their history of cigarette smoking. In this subgroup, an ECG may be useful, particularly in patients who have a history of chest pain, syncope, palpitations, and when the differential diagnosis includes CHF.

As a general rule, the complete blood count (CBC) is not particularly useful as a routine test in patients with acute exacerbation of COPD unless pneumonia is suspected, in which case chest radiography is more sensitive and specific. Moreover, COPD patients with chronic, systemic corticosteroid use may have elevated white blood cell counts reflecting drug-induced changes. In addition, the hematocrit is frequently elevated as a result of chronic hypoxemia. Serum electrolytes are generally not required as a part of the routine assessment of these patients, although hypokalemia can result from aggressive use of beta-agonists, systemic corticosteroids, and thiazide diuretics.[41]

Table 1. Factors Affecting Clearance of Theophylline

INCREASE	DECREASE	
Smoking	Advanced age	Propafenone
Younger age	CHF	Mexiletine
High-protein, low-carbohydrate diet	Cor pulmonale	Tocainide
	Pneumonia/fever	Cimetidine
Phenobarbital	Erythromycin	Clarithromycin
Phenytoin	Allopurinol	Cirrhosis
Rifampin	Quinolones	Oral contraceptives

Both to guide therapy and avoid drug toxicity, a serum theophylline level should be obtained in patients who are taking theophylline on an outpatient basis.[49] Unfortunately, the theophylline level, which is frequently in the low therapeutic range, cannot be predicted on the basis of a medication history. The serum theophylline may vary because of comorbid illnesses, patient compliance, acute respiratory acidosis, or the concomitant administration of medications that impair its metabolism. *(Please see Table 1.)* Loading doses of aminophylline should not be given to patients until a serum theophylline level has been obtained. In general, each milligram per kilogram of aminophylline raises the serum theophylline level by 2 mcg/mL.

Pharmacotherapy for Patient Stabilization: A Multi-Modal Approach for Optimizing Clinical Outcomes

Optimizing outcomes in patients with AECOPD requires prudent but prompt administration of pharmacological agents directed at relieving bronchoconstriction and improving oxygenation. A multimodal approach to initial stabilization is the rule rather than the exception. As might be expected, pharmacological approaches for chronic maintenance therapy differ somewhat from those used for acute management. In both cases, it should be stressed that the response to various pharmacotherapeutic modalities may vary from one patient to another; hence, sequencing and combining therapy (using such agents as oxygen, beta-agonists, anticholinergics, and/or corticosteroids) according to previously documented patterns of clinical response may represent the most logical approach in the majority of patients. The role of antibiotic therapy is discussed in a separate section.

Oxygen. Patients with COPD may have hypoxemia due to structural lung abnormalities, impairment of diffusion capacity, or ventilation perfusion mismatch. In a small minority of patients, beta-agonist therapy may slightly worsen ventilation perfusion mismatch. Accordingly, patients in respiratory distress should receive supplemental oxygen therapy, the administration of which should be guided by pulse-oximetry and arterial blood gases when available.

Oxygen therapy usually is initiated by nasal cannula. The typical

Table 2. Technique for Using a Metered-Dose Inhaler

1. Invert inhaler so that opening pointed is downward after shaking briskly.
2. Hold inhaler about four finger-widths in front of open mouth.
3. Exhale normally to functional residual capacity.
4. Activate inhaler at beginning of inspiration.
5. Inhale slowly and deeply to total lung capacity.
6. Hold breath for 10 seconds.
7. Exhale slowly.

Table 3. Beta-Agonist Dosages

Albuterol (Proventil, Ventolin)	2-4 puffs q4h	0.5 cc (2.5 mg) in 2.5 cc NS
Bitolterol (Tornalate)	2 puffs q8h	0.5 cc (0.2% [1 mg]) in 2 cc NS
Isoetharine (Bronkosol)	4 puffs q4h	0.5 cc (0.25%) in 3 cc NS
Isoproterenol (Isuprel)	5-15 puffs (1:200) q4h	0.5 cc (0.5%) in 3 cc NS
Metaproterenol (Alupent, Metaprel)	2-3 puffs q3-4h	0.3 cc (1.5 mg) in 2.5 cc NS
Pirbuterol (Maxair)	2 puffs q4-6h	
Terbutaline (Brethine)	2 puffs q4-6h	
Salmeterol (Serevent)	2 puffs q12h	

target point is to maintain an O_2 saturation greater than 90%. Patients with hypercarbia may require controlled oxygen therapy using a Venturi mask in order to achieve more precise control of the FiO_2. Oxygen administered via nasal cannulae has a varying FiO_2, which is influenced by the respiratory rate and mouth breathing. FiO_2 administered via a Venturi mask is more predictable. Therapy can be initiated with one of these masks, with upward adjustment based on the arterial blood gas and subsequent monitoring by pulse oximetry.

Acute exacerbation of hypercarbia may, but does not invariably, occur when high flow oxygen therapy is administered to patients with chronic CO_2 retention. There is a common misconception that the increase in CO_2 retention occurs from the elimination of the hypoxemic stimulus to respiratory drive. In fact, this is a rare phenomenon inasmuch as studies have demonstrated that minute ventilation, cardiac output, and oxygen uptake remain relatively constant during supplemental oxygen therapy in spite of rising PaO_2 and PCO_2.[50-52] These findings suggest that the rise in PCO_2 that accompanies the correction of hypoxemia is due to the Haldane effect (a shift of the hemoglobin-CO_2 binding curve) and increases in CO_2 production, as well as changes in physiologic dead-space.[53]

From a practical perspective, the clinician will not be able to predict worsening hypercarbia by assessing the patients respiratory rate. Since the PCO_2 can rise in the absence of hypoventilation, the clinician must strike a balance between worsening hypercarbia and the significant benefits of relieving hypoxemia. In those patients in whom oxygen administration is accompanied rising PCO_2, the concept of "permissive hypercapnia" has been advocated. According to this strategy for patients with respiratory failure, it may be advantageous to tolerate slight increases in the PCO_2 for the purpose of maintaining adequate oxygenation as long as the pH remains greater than 7.26. Precise, sequential measurement of ABGs usually is required in this patient subgroup. There may be a role for measurement of end-tidal CO_2.

Beta-agonists. The majority of patients with COPD have airway obstruction that, to some degree, will show clinically significant reversibility in response to beta-agonist therapy. The effectiveness of beta-agonist-mediated airway expansion can be dramatic, with at least one study suggesting that the the response to bronchodilators acutely does not help to differentiate between patients with asthma and those with COPD.[11] Furthermore, in the setting of severe respiratory distress, even modest improvements in ventilatory resistance may be of significant clinical benefit.[54]

Beta-agonists may improve dyspnea and improve pulmonary functional status even in the absence of dramatic improvements in the peak expiratory flow rate. As a result, inhaled beta-agonists are considered to be first-line therapy for AECOPD. Beta-agonists can be administered via small volume nebulizers. Drug delivery is enhanced by dilution of the drug to 2-3 cc, with airflow in the range of 6-8 L/min. In addition, beta-agonists can be delivered by metered-dose inhalers which, in conjunction with a spacer, have been shown to be equivalent to the use of air driven, small volume nebulizers. *(Please see Table 2.)*

A variety of beta-agonists are available for use in patients with AECOPD. *(Please see Table 3.)* In general, the onset of action of inhaled beta-agonists is rapid, usually on the order of about 10 minutes. The various beta-agonist agents vary in terms of duration of action and relative beta-2 agonist selectivity. *(Please see Table 4.)* For example, isoproterenol and isoetharine are very rapid-acting agents, but they have limited beta-2 agonist selectivity. Their duration of action is on the order of 1-2 hours.

Metaproterenol, terbutaline, and albuterol are among the beta-2 selective agents; albuterol is probably the most widely used agent. These formulations achieve their peak effect at around one hour and have a duration of action that can be as long as six hours. Salmeterol is a very long-acting beta-2 selective agonist, which has duration of action on the order of 12 hours. Because it has a delayed peak effect, its use is not recommended for acute respiratory distress. In fact, patients who are on this agent for home therapy need to be warned about the lack of efficacy for acute exacerbations of COPD.

In theory, based on target receptor selectivity, the beta-2 selective agents should have fewer undesirable cardiovascular side effects than non-selective beta-agonists. There is evidence of a decreased incidence of hypotension, palpitations, hypokalemia, anxiety, tremulous, or vomiting. Nevertheless, these agents can lead to tachycardia and supraventricular arrhythmias, particularly in patients with pre-exist-

Table 4. Characteristics of Bronchodilators Delivered by Metered-Dose Inhalers

Medication	Dose (mg)/Puff	LEVEL OF ACTIVITY Beta-1-Agonist*	Beta-2-Agonist*	Anticholinergic*	TIME OF EFFECT Onset (Min)	Peak (Min)	Duration (Min)
Isoproterenol	0.08	+ + +	+ + +	-	3-5	5-10	60-90
Isoetharine	0.34	+ +	+ +	-	3-5	5-20	60-150
Metaproterenol	0.65	+	+ + +	-	5-15	10-60	60-180
Terbutaline	0.20	+	+ + + +	-	5-30	60-120	180-360
Albuterol	0.09	+	+ + + +	-	5-15	60-90	240-360
Bitolterol	0.37	+	+ + + +	-	5-10	60-90	300-480
Pirbuterol	0.20	+	+ + +	-	5-10	30-60	180-240
Salmeterol	0.04	+	+ + + +	-	10-20	180	720
Ipratropium	0.18	-	-	+ + + +	5-15	60-120	240-480

* The number of plus signs denotes the relative level of activity.

ing cardiac arrhythmias or hypoxemia.[55] Patients suffering from AECOPD, however, rarely deteriorate due to cardiac arrhythmias. In the acute exacerbation, there is little evidence conclusively establishing that any specific agent has superior efficacy as compared to others. However, there may be some advantages to the longer-acting agents in that there will be prolonged bronchodilation. Aside from these considerations, selection of beta-agonist, to a great degree, is a matter of personal preference.

Adrenergic agents also can be administered by injection. Although tradition has held that patients with COPD should receive terbutaline instead of epinephrine, one study has shown there are no differences in the side effect profile when these two agents are given to older patients with airway disease.[56] In theory, patients with significant bronchoconstriction may not achieve adequate delivery of drug to the distal airways when given by inhalation. Some have advocated initiating therapy with injectable agents followed by inhaled agents. This approach has not been demonstrated to lead to greater clinical efficacy.

Finally, there is a great deal of controversy regarding the timing and optimal dose of inhaled beta-agonists. Whereas these agents once were administered at a moderate dose every hour, there has been a trend toward increasing frequency and size of dosing for inhaled beta-agonists. One study failed to demonstrate a significant advantage by giving albuterol more frequently than once every 60 minutes.[57] Recommendations for management in patients with asthma include administration of an agent such as albuterol in a dose of 2.5-5 mg every 20 minutes. There is no evidence to suggest that this approach is necessary in patients with AECOPD.

Anticholinergic Agents. Anticholinergic therapy has been studied as an adjunct with beta-agonists in the treatment of acute exacerbation of COPD. Anticholinergic drugs produce preferential dilatation of the larger central airways, in contrast to beta-agonists, which affect the peripheral airways. Until recently, atropine was the primary anticholinergic agent used in nebulization. It acts more rapidly than ipratropium but has a shorter duration of action. Atropine is readily absorbed through the airway mucosa, leading to potential anticholinergic side effects such as tachycardia, flushing, dry mouth, blurred vision, and confusion. It can also precipitate glaucoma and acute urinary retention in susceptible patients. It should be emphasized that anticholinergic agents have a slower onset of action and take longer to reach peak effect than beta-agonists. The mechanism of action is thought to occur through inhibition of vagal stimulation on the bronchial tree, thereby blocking smooth-muscle contraction and bronchial gland secretion.

Generally speaking, the precise clinical role of anticholinergic compounds in the acute exacerbation of COPD is unclear, although these agents may have selective advantages for managing patients who respond poorly to beta-agonist therapy alone. Since these agents are relatively safe, their use should be considered in patients with severe respiratory distress or respiratory failure who fail to respond to usual measures.

Most studies using anticholinergic agents have used one of the quaternary ammonium compounds, since they have a better safety profile than nebulized atropine. In particular, glycopyrrolate is another quaternary ammonium compound with few atropine-like side effects.The drug has been used for a number of years to minimize secretions during operative procedures. There have been case reports of reversal of bronchospasm in patients with acute exacerbation of COPD when given intravenously.[58] It has recently been shown that the combination of glycopyrrolate and albuterol results in a greater improvement in pulmonary function than albuterol alone.[59]

Some studies have found a beneficial effect by using combination treatment with glycopyrrolate and either albuterol or metaproterenol.[60,61] Glycopyrrolate is commonly available in most hospitals since it is used in the operating room. In combination with metaproterenol, glycopyrrolate leads to greater peak effect, with maximal activity at around 2-3 hours.[60] Another study reported that in combination with albuterol, glycopyrrolate lead to a significantly greater improvement in FEV_1 among patients presenting to the emergency department with AECOPD.[62] Unfortunately, the typical pre-anesthetic dose of glycopyrrolate (0.2 mg) is far lower than the therapeutic dose required for an acute exacerbation of COPD (2.0 mg). If glycopyrrolate is not available in a multidose vial in a given hospital, it requires significant nursing effort in order to prepare an appropriate dose.

Some authors consider ipratropium to be one of the first-line therapeutic options for chronic, outpatient management of stable patients with COPD.[63-67] The margin of safety with ipratropium is wide, since more than 10 times the usual dose can be given before side effects are seen. When administered via metered-dose inhaler, the usual dose is 2-4 puffs every six hours. To maximize results, patients should be instructed in the proper use of the metered-dose inhaler. There have been about six studies comparing ipratropium in combination with beta-agonists for AECOPD. Most of these studies however, have found no particular added benefit to the addition of ipratropium to inhaled beta-agonists.[59,68] Consequently, the role of ipratropium in patients with an acute exacerbation is not clear and requires more investigation. Ipratropium is available both as a metered dose inhaler and as a solution for inhalation.

Corticosteroids. The administration of corticosteroids is part of the mainstay of treatment of patients with acute asthma. With contradictory results in COPD, their role in managing AECOPD is evolving but not yet fully elaborated.[69-71] In general, however, there is mounting evidence that rapidly tapering courses of corticosteroids, in combination with bronchodilators and antibiotics, when indicated, are effective in preventing relapses and maintaining longer symptom-free intervals in patients who have had AECOPD.

It should be stressed that the studies evaluating steroid therapy vary in design and to some extent, have produced conflicting results.[69-73] A small number of studies have demonstrated a role for corticosteroids in patients with AECOPD. For example, one study performed almost 20 years ago demonstrated improvement in pulmonary function among patients admitted for acute exacerbations of COPD when methylprednisolone was administered at a dose of 0.5 mg/kg.[72] Another study, however, found that the administration of steroids did not lead to a change in the short course of treatment in the emergency department.[73]

Several studies have suggested that patients with an acute exacerbation of COPD should receive steroids as a mainstay of outpatient therapy.[69,70] One trial reported improvement in both recovery of oxygenation and pulmonary function over the course of a nine-day tapering dose of prednisone.[70] Another trial found that the administration of steroids either in the emergency department or as an outpatient resulted in a significantly lower relapse rate among patients who were discharged from the emergency department for acute exacerbation of COPD.[69] A more recent study of hospitalized VA patients demonstrated that a two-week tapering course of prednisone decreased the rate of treatment failure for up to three months.[71] Among patients with stable COPD, the addition of inhaled steroids seems to result in improved pulmonary function and decreased beta-agonist use in about 25% of patients.[74] There does not appear to be a role for inhaled corticosteroids in the treatment of acute exacerbations.

Theophylline. Methylxanthines, including theophylline and aminophylline, are still used in the treatment of COPD, but their role remains controversial. In fact, many experts feel there is little if any role for theophylline as part of multi-modal therapy in the setting of AECOPD. The exact mechanism of action of theophylline in clinical doses for acute airway obstruction remains controversial. Although it was postulated that theophylline produced salutory effects by inhibiting phosphodiesterase, other actions, including alteration of calcium flux, interference of prostaglandin synthesis, or inhibition of adenosine receptors, probably also play a role. In addition, theophylline may also improve diaphragmatic muscle strength.

Relatively few studies have been performed on the clinical effect of theophylline in acute exacerbations of COPD. Of the two larger studies that have been performed, the results were contradictory.[75,76] It should be stressed that the medication history is an inaccurate guide to drug levels for patients with COPD. Theophylline has a relatively narrow therapeutic index with side effects that range from minor, such as nausea, vomiting, and tremor, up to more serious side effects, including intractable seizures and ventricular arrhythmias. A theophylline level should be measured prior to administering theophylline in patients on chronic therapy.

There is insufficient evidence at this time to conclusively determine whether aminophylline has any role in the ED management of acute exacerbation of COPD. Although some authors suggest this agent should be considered in patients who are unresponsive to other therapies, others maintain there is no role for its use at the present time.[74-76]

Magnesium. Magnesium has been studied in several series, most of which have evaluated its effectiveness in the setting of acute asthma. Magnesium presumably acts by opposing calcium-induced bronchoconstriction. One recent study demonstrated a significant improvement in pulmonary function in patients given magnesium during an acute exacerbation of COPD.[77] Given at a dose of 1-2 gm over 20 minutes, magnesium significantly improved peak expiratory flow, although there was a nonsignificant decrease in the hospitalization rate. At these doses, magnesium is relatively safe. Adverse effects can include flushing sensation, transient hypotension, and at higher doses, cardiac conduction delays. Magnesium levels may be elevated in patients with renal insufficiency.

Heliox. Helium/oxygen mixtures have been found to decrease dyspnea in patients with COPD by minimizing the risks of gas flow, since helium is only 14% as dense as nitrogen. This decrease in expiratory resistance has been thought to enhance ventilation and lower PCO_2. There have been anecdotal reports of beneficial effects in improving peak expiratory flow. There are no large-scale studies evaluating the use of helium/oxygen mixtures in patients with acute exacerbation of COPD. Its use should probably be limited to experimental studies or as a last alternative for patients in extremis.

Summary of Therapeutic Approaches. Patients with an acute exacerbation of COPD should receive oxygen therapy, guided by pulse oximetry. Patients with baseline hypercarbia or severe airway obstruction (less than 35% of predicted normal) should have arterial blood gases in order to insure that oxygen therapy is not leading to a worsening of hypercarbia and acute systemic, respiratory acidosis; controlled flow oxygen masks may be needed in patients at risk for hypercarbia.

Beta-agonist therapy, using any of the available rapid-onset agents administered by small volume nebulizer or meter dose inhaler with spacer, should be initiated promptly. The timing and dose have not been well established, but a reasonable regimen would be to initiate therapy with albuterol at a dose of 2.5 mg every 20 minutes. In patients who are not responding to these pharmacological maneuvers, consideration may be given to adding ipratropium to the aerosolization.

In those individuals who still fail to respond, the clinician can consider administration of intravenous theophylline (after measuring the theophylline level), or magnesium at a dose of 2 gm over 20 minutes. Oral or parenteral steroids can be administered at the time of the exacerbation, although acute clinical benefits may not be evident. As a rule, these agents should be considered in patients who are deteriorating in spite of adequate beta-agonist therapy.

References

1. Bosker G. *Pharmatecture: Minimizing Medications To Maximize Results*. St. Louis: Facts and Comparisons; 1999.
2. Statistics VaH. Current Estimates from the National Health Interview Survey. NHS Publication. 1990:1643.
3. Cydulka R, McFadden E, Emerman C, et al. Patterns of hospitalization in elderly patients with asthma and chronic obstructive pulmonary disease. *Am J Respir Crit Care Med* 1997;156:1807-1812.
4. Celli BR, Snider GL, Heffner J. Standards for the diagnosis and care of patients with chronic obstructive pulmonary disease. *Am J Respir Crit Care Med* 1995;152:S77-S120.
5. Kanner RE, Renzetti AD, Jr., Stanish WM, et al. Predictors of survival in subjects with chronic airflow limitation. *Am J Med* 1983;74:249-255.
6. Seneff MG, Wagner DP, Wagner RP, et al. Hospital and 1-year survival of patients admitted to intensive care units with acute exacerbation of chronic obstructive pulmonary disease. *JAMA* 1995;274:1852-1857.
7. Connors AF, Jr., Dawson NV, Thomas C, et al. Outcomes following acute exacerbation of severe chronic obstructive lung disease. The SUPPORT investigators (Study to Understand Prognoses and Preferences for Outcomes and Risks of Treatments) *Am J Respir Crit Care Med* 1996;154: 959-967.
8. Fuso L, Incalzi RA, Pistelli R, et al. Predicting mortality of patients hospitalized for acutely exacerbated chronic obstructive pulmonary disease. *Am J Med* 1995;98:272-277.
9. McNamara RM, Cionni DJ. Utility of the peak expiratory flow rate in the differentiation of acute dyspnea. Cardiac vs. pulmonary origin. *Chest* 1992;101:129-132.
10. Drucker EA, Rivitz SM, Shepard JA, et al. Acute pulmonary embolism: Assessment of helical CT for diagnosis. *Radiology* 1998;209:235-241.
11. Kesten S, Rebuck AS. Is the short-term response to inhaled beta-adrenergic agonist sensitive or specific for distinguishing between asthma and COPD? *Chest* 1994;105: 1042-1045.
12. Emerman CL, Cydulka RK. Evaluation of high-yield criteria for chest radiography in acute exacerbation of chronic obstructive pulmonary disease. *Ann Emerg Med* 1993;22: 680-684.
13. Griffith DE, Mazurek GH. Pneumonia in chronic obstructive lung disease. *Infect Dis Clin North Am* 1991;5:467-484.
14. Sisk JE, Moskowitz AJ, Whang W, et al. Cost-effectiveness of vaccination against pneumococcal bacteremia among elderly people. *JAMA* 1997;278:1333-1339.
15 Fagon JY, Chastre J. Severe exacerbations of COPD patients: The role of pulmonary infections. *Semin Respir Infect* 1996; 11:109-118.
16. Gump DW, Philips CA, Forsyth BR. Role of infection in chronic bronchitis. *Am Rev Respir Dis* 1976;113:465-474.
17. Blasi F, Legnani D, Lombardo VM, et al. *Chlamydia pneumoniae* infection in acute exacerbations of COPD. *Eur Respir J* 1993;6:19-22.
18. Beaty CD, Grayston JT, Wang SP, et al. *Chlamydia pneumoniae,* strain TWAR, infection in patients with chronic obstructive pulmonary disease. *Am Rev Respir Dis* 1991;144: 1408-1410.
19. Eller J, Ede A, Schaberg T, et al. Infective exacerbations of chronic bronchitis: Relation between bacteriologic etiology and lung function. *Chest* 1998;113:1542-1548.
20. Salit IE, Mederski B, Morisset R, et al. Azithromycin for the treatment of acute LRTIs: A multicenter, open-label study of infections in medicine. *Infect Med* 1998;15:773-777.
21. Saint S, Bent S, Vittinghoff E, et al. Antibiotics in chronic obstructive pulmonary disease exacerbations. A meta-analysis [see comments]. *JAMA* 1995;273:957-960.
22. Ball P, Harris JM, Lowson D, et al. Acute infective exacerbations of chronic bronchitis. *QJM* 1995;88:61-68.
23. Macfarlane JT, Colville A, Guion A, et al. Prospective study of etiology and outcome of adult lower-respiratory-tract infections in the community. *Lancet* 1993;341:511-514.
24. Wilson R. The role of infection in COPD. *Chest* 1998;113: 242S-248S.
25. Shu D, et al. A controlled randomized multicenter trial comparing 5 days of azithromycin to 10-14 days of clarithromycin for the treatment of acute bacterial exacerbations of chronic bronchitis. In: American Society for Microbiology, ed. *37th Interscience Conference on Antimicrobial Agents and Chemotherapy*; 1997 Sept.-Oct. 28-1; Toronto, Ont. Washington, D.C.; 1997:372
26. Rosen MJ. Treatment of exacerbations of COPD. *Am Fam Phys* 1992;45:693-697.
27. Rodnick JE, Gude JK. The use of antibiotics in acute bronchitis and acute exacerbations of chronic bronchitis. *West J Med* 1988;149:347-351.
28. Wallace RJ, Jr. Newer oral antimicrobials and newer etiologic agents of acute bronchitis and acute exacerbations of chronic bronchitis. *Semin Respir Infect* 1988;3:49-54.
29. Wallace RF Jr, Steele LC, Brooks DL, et al. Amoxicillin/clavulanic acid in the treatment of lower respiratory tract infections caused by b-lactamase-positive *Haemophilus influenzae* and *Branhamella catarrhalis*. *Antimicrob Agents Chemother* 1985;27:912-915.
30. Hopkins SJ. Clinical toleration and safety of azithromycin in adults and children. *Rev Contemp Pharmacother* 1994;5: 383-389.
31. Nightingale CH, Belliveau PP, Quintiliani R. Cost issues and considerations when choosing antimicrobial agents. *Infect Dis Clin Pract* 1994;3:8-11.
32. Destache CJ, Dewan N, O'Donohue WJ. et al Clinical and economic considerations in the treatment of acute exacerbations of chronic bronchitis. *J Antimicrob Chemother* 1999;43:A107-A113.
33. Davies. J. Inactivation of antibiotics and the dissemination of resistance genes. *Science* 1994;264:375-382.
34. Jorgensen JH, Doern GV, Maher LA, et al. Antimicrobial resistance among respiratory isolates of *Haemophilus influenzae, Moraxella catarrhalis,* and *Streptococcus pneumoniae* in the United States. *Antimicrob Agents Chemother* 1990;34:2075-2080.
35. Doern GV. Trends in antimicrobial susceptibility of bacterial pathogens of the respiratory tract. *Am J Med* 1995;99:3S-7S.

36. Knaus WA, Harrell FEJ, Lynn J, et al. The SUPPORT Program prognostic model. Objective estimates of survival for seriously ill hospitalized adults. Study to understand prognosis and preferences for outcomes and risks of treatments. *Ann Intern Med* 1995:122:191-203.
37. Lange P, Nyboe J, Appleyard M, et al. Relationship of ventilatory impairment and of chronic mucous secretion to mortality from chronic obstructive lung disease and from all causes. *Thorax* 1990;45:579-585.
38. Sherman CB, Zu X, et al. Longitudinal lung function decline in subjects with respiratory symptoms. *Am Rev of Resp Dis* 1992:146;855-859.
39. Emerman CL, Lukens TW, Effron D. Physician estimation of FEV_1 in acute exacerbation of COPD. *Chest* 1994;105: 1709-1712.
40. Kelleher J. Pulse oximetry. *J Clin Monitor* 1989;5:37-62.
41. Tobin M. Respiratory monitoring. *JAMA* 1990;264:244-251.
42. Wiedemann H, McCarthy K. Noninvasive monitoring of oxygen and carbon dioxide. *Clin Chest Med* 1989;10: 239-254.
43. Nowak RM, Tomlanovich MC, Sarkar DD. Arterial blood gases and pulmonary function testing in acute bronchial asthma. *JAMA* 1983;249:2043-2046.
44. Emerman CL, Connors AF, Lukens TW, et al. Relationship between arterial blood gases and spirometry in acute exacerbations of chronic obstructive pulmonary disease. *Ann Emerg Med* 1989;18:523-527.
45. West JB. Causes of carbon dioxide retention in lung disease. *N Engl J Med* 1971;284:1232-1236.
46. Young GP. Ability of spirometry and oximetry to guide use of arterial blood gases in acute exacerbations of chronic obstructive pulmonary disease. *Ann Emerg Med* 1990; 19:481.
47. Emerman CL, Cydulka RK. Use of peak expiratory flow rate in emergency department evaluation of acute exacerbation of chronic obstructive pulmonary disease. *Ann Emerg Med* 1996;27:159-163.
48. Emerman CL, Connors AF, Lukens TW, et al. Relationship between arterial blood gases and spirometry in acute exacerbations of chronic obstructive pulmonary disease. *Ann Emerg Med* 1989;18:523-527.
49. Emerman CL, Connors AF, Lukens TW, et al. Theophylline concentrations in patients with acute exacerbation of COPD. *Am J Emerg Med* 1990;8:289-292.
50. West JB. Causes of carbon dioxide retention in lung disease. *N Engl J Med* 1971;284:1232-1236.
51. Gilbert R, Keighley J, Auchingloss Jr. JH. Mechanisms of chronic carbon dioxide retention in patients with obstructive pulmonary disease. *Am J Med* 1965;38:217-225.
52. Tardif C, Bonmarchand G, Gibon JF, et al. Respiratory response to CO_2 in patients with chronic obstructive pulmonary disease in acute respiratory failure. *Eur Respir J* 1993;6:619-624.
53. Hanson CW, 3rd, Marshall BE, Frasch HF, et al. Causes of hypercarbia with oxygen therapy in patients with chronic obstructive pulmonary disease. *Crit Care Med* 1996;24: 23-28.
54. Kuhl DA, Agiri OA, Mauro LS. Beta-agonists in the treatment of acute exacerbation of chronic obstructive pulmonary disease. *Ann Pharmacother* 1994;28:1379-1388.
55. Cazzola M, Imperatore F, Salzillo A, et al. Cardiac effects of formoterol and salmeterol in patients suffering from COPD with preexisting cardiac arrhythmias and hypoxemia. *Chest* 1998;114:411-415.
56. Cydulka R, Davison R, Grammer L, et al. The use of epinephrine in the treatment of older adult asthmatics. *Ann Emerg Med* 1988;17:322-326.
57. Emerman CL, Cydulka RK. Effect of different albuterol dosing regimens in the treatment of acute exacerbation of chronic obstructive pulmonary disease. *Ann Emerg Med* 1997;29:474-478.
58. Rebuck AS, Chapman KR, Abboud R, et al. Nebulized anticholinergics and sympathomimetic treatment of asthma and COPD in the emergency room. *Am J Med* 1987;82: 59-64.
59. O'Driscoll BR, Taylor RJ, Horsley MG, et al. Nebulized salbutamol with and without ipratropium bromide in acute airflow obstruction. *Lancet* 1989;1:1418-1420.
60. Tzelepis G, Komanapolli S, Tyler D, et al. Comparison of nebulized glycopyrrolate and metaproterenol in chronic obstructive pulmonary disease. *Eur Respir J* 1996;9:100-103.
61. Shrestha M, O'Brien T, Haddox R, et al. Decreased duration of emergency department treatment of chronic obstructive pulmonary disease exacerbations with the addition of ipratropium bromide to beta-agonist therapy. *Ann Emerg Med* 1991;20:1206-1209.
62. Cydulka RK, Emerman CL. Effects of combined treatment with glycopyrrolate and albuterol in acute exacerbation of chronic obstructive pulmonary disease. *Ann Emerg Med* 1995;25:470-473.
63. Ferguson GT, Cherniack RM. Management of COPD. *N Engl J Med* 1993;328:1017-1022.
64. Colice GL. Nebulized bronchodilators for outpatient management of stable chronic obstructive pulmonary disease. *Am J Med* 1996;100:11S-18S.
65. Gross NJ, Petty TL, Friedman M, et al. Dose response to ipratropium as a nebulized solution in patients with chronic obstructive pulmonary disease. A three-center study. *Am Rev Respir Dis* 1989;139:1188-1191.
66. Karpel JP, Kotch A, Zinny M, et al. A comparison of inhaled ipratropium, oral theophylline plus inhaled beta-agonist, and the combination of all three in patients with COPD. *Chest* 1994;105:1089-1094.
67. Braun SR, McKenzie WN, Copeland C, et al. A comparison of the effect of ipratropium and albuterol in the treatment of chronic obstructive airway disease. *Arch Intern Med* 1989; 149:544-547.
68. Rebuck AS, Chapman KR, Abboud R, et al. Nebulized anticholinergic and sympathomimetic treatment of asthma and chronic obstructive airways disease in the emergency room. *Am J Med* 1987;82:59-64.
69. Murata GH, Gorby MS, Chick TW, et al. Intravenous and oral corticosteroids for the prevention of relapse after treatment of decompensated COPD. Effect on patients with a history of multiple relapses. *Chest* 1990;98:845-849.
70. Thompson WH, Nielson CP, Carvalho P, et al. Controlled

trial of oral prednisone in outpatients with acute COPD exacerbation. *Am J Respir Crit Care Med* 1996;154:407-412.

71. Niewoehner D, Erbland M, Deupree R, et al. Effect of systemic glucocorticoids on exacerbations of chronic obstructive pulmonary disease. *N Engl J Med* 1999;340: 1941-1947.
72. Albert RK, Martin TR, Lewis SW. Controlled clinical trial of methylprednisolone in patients with chronic bronchitis and acute respiratory insufficiency. *Ann Intern Med* 1980;92: 753-758.
73. Emerman CL, Connors AF, Lukens TW, et al. A randomized controlled trial of methylprednisolone in the emergency treatment of acute exacerbations of COPD. *Chest* 1989;95: 563-567.
74. Weiner P, Weiner M, Azgad Y, et al. Inhaled budesonide therapy for patients with stable COPD. *Chest* 1995;108: 1568-1571.
75. Rice KL, Leatherman JW, Duane PG, et al. Aminophylline for acute exacerbations of chronic obstructive pulmonary disease. A controlled trial. *Ann Intern Med* 1987;107: 305-309.
76. Wrenn K, Slovis CM, Murphy F, et al. Aminophylline therapy for acute bronchospastic disease in the emergency room. *Ann Intern Med* 1991;115:241-247.
77. Skorodin MS, Tenholder MF, Yetter B, et al. Magnesium sulfate in exacerbations of chronic obstructive pulmonary disease. *Arch Intern Med* 1995;155:496-500.

Chronic Obstructive Pulmonary Disease (COPD): Antibiotic Therapy and Management of Acute Exacerbations

Charles L. Emerman, MD
Gideon Bosker, MD FACEP

Acute bacterial exacerbations of chronic obstructive pulmonary disease (ABE/COPD) are common, costly, and, above all, complex to manage. In fact, few conditions produce such a broad range of outcomes, require such customized approaches, or present so many options for treatment.

Although there have been important advances in patient assessment techniques and therapeutics—including pulmonary function testing, capnometry, pulse oximetry, disposition support tools, and antimicrobial therapy—ABE/COPD continues to be a leading cause of morbidity and mortality in the United States. From patient disposition to antimicrobial selection, optimizing management of these patients requires the clinician to integrate a number of clinical, laboratory, radiologic, and etiologic factors, and then initiate a course of action that accounts for all the risks, costs, and benefits of an individualized treatment plan.

Despite the plethora of guidelines and the availability of new, targeted spectrum antibiotics, the management of ABE/COPD remains extremely challenging. More than ever, it requires a multifactorial analysis of myriad clinical, historical, and laboratory parameters that predict success or possible failure for each individual case. In this regard, clinical decision-making in ABE/COPD can be treacherous for the emergency physician.

Achieving optimal patient outcomes for this potentially life-threatening condition requires the clinician to consider several features of each individual case. Factors that must be considered include the patient's age, response to medical therapy, overall pulmonary function, character and severity of previous exacerbations, bacterial colonization status of the patient, previous requirements for mechanical ventilation, and local antimicrobial resistance patterns. With this in mind, a Severity-of-Exacerbation and Risk Factor (SERF) pathway can be employed to help guide patient disposition, empiric antibiotic selection, and necessity for additional diagnostic investigation.

The antibiotic selection process for ABE/COPD is especially daunting. Currently, the pathogens most often responsible for causing "uncomplicated and typical" cases of ABE/COPD that can be treated in the outpatient environment include the bacterial organisms, *S. pneumoniae*, *H. influenzae*, and *M. catarrhalis*. Because it may be difficult, if not impossible, to identify a specific pathogen at the time of initial patient assessment, empiric antimicrobial coverage against all expected pathogens may be necessary to minimize treatment failures. Patients with advanced disease and multiple risk factors may have exacerbations caused by *Klebsiella spp*., *Pseudomonas aeruginosa*, and other gram-negative species.

In this vein, the development of advanced generation macrolides, such as azithromycin as well as extended spectrum quinolones, has made it possible to treat most patients using monotherapy. Finally, because there is a growing incidence of resistance among common bacterial agents that cause community acquired pneumonia (CAP) (in some areas of the United States, intermediate-to-complete resistance to penicillin among *Streptococcus pneumoniae* is reported to be greater than 25%), antibiotic selection must be guided by local and/or regional resistance patterns.

The purpose of this comprehensive review is to provide a state-of-the-art clinical resource outlining, in precise and practical detail, clinical protocols for acute management of ABE/COPD. To achieve this goal, all of the critical aspects entering into the equation for maximizing outcomes, while minimizing costs, including systematic patient evaluation, disposition decision trees, and outcome-effective antibiotic therapy, will be discussed in detail. Pharmacotherapy for patient stabilization in the ED, multi-modal approaches to optimizing clinical outcomes, and approaches to acute ventilatory management are discussed in detail.

In addition, because appropriate disposition of patients with ABE/COPD has become essential for cost-effective patient management, this chapter includes critical pathways and treatment tables that incorporate risk stratification protocols and intensification-of-treatment trigger (IOTT) criteria that can be used to identify those patient subgroups that are suitably managed in the outpatient setting, and those more appropriately admitted to the hospital for more intensive care.

Antibiotic Therapy: The SERF Pathway for Outcome-Effective Drug Selection

Patients in whom exacerbation of chronic obstructive pulmonary disease (COPD) is associated with acute respiratory infection are at high risk for relapse unless treated.[1] Patients with acute bronchitis that is unrelated to COPD probably do not benefit from antibiotic therapy. It should be noted, however, that in patients with COPD, antibiotics appear to have a role in the treatment of exacerbations caused by bacterial bronchitis (i.e., ABE/COPD). The patient with an increase in sputum quantity and/or a change in character or color, especially if accompanied by increasing cough and dyspnea, should be treated with antibiotics upon discharge from the emergency department or clinic. It should be stressed that many patients with COPD have colonization of their tracheal tract with *Streptococcus pneumoniae, Haemophilus influenzae,* or *Moraxella catarrhalis*. Other organisms, such as *Klebsiella* species, *Mycoplasma pneumoniae, Pseudomonas, Staphylococcus aureus, Proteus* species, or *Chlamydia* TWAR also may be seen. Unfortunately, making an etiologic bacteria-specific diagnosis in ABE/COPD is usually not possible. Consequently, most patients will require empiric therapy directed at the most likely etiologic organisms.

Although a number of clinical decision support tools, consensus guidelines, and recommendations have been issued, none has universal support. In large part, this is because the etiologic agents responsible for ABE/COPD, the outcome-effectiveness of various antibiotics, and risk-stratification parameters are not as thoroughly elaborated as they are for CAP. Consequently, several authors have argued that there is an immediate need for guidelines on antibiotic use in COPD.[1,4,12,17] Several attempts to formulate such protocols have resulted in broadly similar recommendations. Although the guidelines inevitably have been hampered by the lack of well-designed prospective studies, they have taken a practical approach that seems to be logical and can be used in the emergency department and primary care setting. *(Please see Tables 1 and 2.)* It must be emphasized, however, that the concepts on which the guidelines are based have not yet been verified by prospective clinical trials.[2-4]

Antibiotics. A number of relatively inexpensive, well-tolerated antibiotics are available, including amoxicillin, trimethoprim-sulfamethoxazole, doxycycline, and tetracycline. Antimicrobial resistance, particularly involving *H. influenzae, M. catarrhalis,* and *S. pneumoniae*, has been a problem with many of these agents, specifically with older members of each of these drug classes. There is an increase amoxicillin-resistant, beta-lactamase-producing *H. influenzae*. New agents are providing solutions to these difficulties. The azalide antibiotic azithromycin has the advantage of an appropriate spectrum of coverage, an excellent safety profile, reasonable cost, and a patient-dosing schedule that improves patient compliance. The new fluoroquinolone levofloxacin also is advantageous when gram-negative bacteria predominate; ciprofloxacin is suitable in this subgroup of patients with ABE/COPD but is not the agent of choice when the bacterial exacerbation is suspected to be caused by *S. pneumoniae*. Amoxicillin-clavulanate also has in vitro activity against beta-lactamase-producing *H. influenzae* and *M. catarrhalis*; moreover, the agent's clinical efficacy in lower respiratory tract infection attributable to enzyme-producing strains has been demonstrated.

Severity of Exacerbation and Risk Factors Pathway. The Severity of Exacerbation and Risk Factors (SERF) pathway for antibiotic selection in patients with ABE/COPD is a clinical decision, consensus-driven support tool based on epidemiology, efficacy, and prognostic data generated by many published clinical trials.[3-21] In general, the need for intensification and amplification of antimicrobial coverage in patients with acute exacerbations of chronic obstructive lung disease (ABE/COPD) depends on the likelihood of infection with gram-negative enterobacteria, colonization status, the patient's history of exacerbations and antimicrobial treatment response record, the ability of the patient to tolerate a treatment failure given his or her respiratory status, and other factors.

The SERF Pathway *(Please see Table 3)*, which is based on evidence-based trials and consensus opinion, is designed as a clinical support tool to help guide empiric antibiotic therapy for outpatients with ABE/COPD. Final decisions regarding drug selection should be made by the clinician on a patient-by-patient basis using a comprehensive database including history, physical examination, and other diagnostic information. Specifically, the SERF pathway identifies a number of intensification-of-treatment trigger (IOTT) criteria that have been generated from consensus reports, reviews, and prospective trials in acute exacerbations of chronic obstructive pulmonary disease (AECOPD). These factors should be considered when selecting an antibiotic for empiric outpatient treatment of ABE/COPD. When at least 2-3 IOTT criteria are present (or any single IOTT criterion is of such severity as to predict a poor outcome) in any individual patient, clinicians should consider newer agents with evidence-based support as indicated, and recognize possible limitations of older agents such as sulfonamides, penicillins, and tetracyclines. *(Please see Table 4.)*

There is ample support in the medical literature for the SERF pathway and IOTT criteria proposed in Tables 3 and 4. Approximately one-half of all exacerbations of COPD can be attributed to bacterial infection, and antibiotic therapy has been demonstrated to improve clinical outcomes and accelerate clinical and physiologic recovery. The major pathogen continues to be *H. influenzae*, and resistance to beta-lactam antibiotics such as ampicillin can be expected in 20-40% of isolated strains.[22] Certain high-risk patients, in whom the cost of clinical treatment failure is high, can be identified by simple clinical criteria.

Studies suggest, for example, patients with significant cardiopulmonary comorbidity, frequent purulent exacerbations of COPD, advanced age, generalized debility, malnutrition, chronic corticosteroid administration, long duration of COPD, and severe underlying lung function may be more likely to fail therapy with older drugs, such as ampicillin, and that early relapse can be expected.[22] Treatment directed toward resistant pathogens using appropriate agents may be expected to lead to improved clinical outcomes and overall lower costs, particularly if hospital admissions and respiratory failure can be prevented. Future studies examining the role of antibiotics should enroll these high-risk patients to determine if new therapies have significant clinical, quality-of-life, and economic advantages over older agents.[22]

Table 1. Recommended Dosing and Duration of Antibiotic Therapy for Acute Exacerbation of COPD (ABE/COPD)

FIRST-LINE AGENTS WITH CLINICALLY ACCEPTABLE COVERAGE FOR ABE/COPD CAUSED BY *H. INFLUENZAE*, *M. CATARRHALIS*, OR *S. PNEUMONIAE* §

Macrolides/Azalides

- Azithromycin (Zithromax): 500 mg on 1st day, 250 mg qd × 4 days. Five-day total course of therapy (preferred agent based on Pharmatectural and PPD criteria:† cost, compliance, coverage, drug interaction, and side-effect profiles).

Penicillins

- Amoxicillin/clavulanate (Augmentin):500 mg tid × 10 days (bid therapy is also an option)

Fluoroquinolones

- Levofloxacin (Levaquin): 500 mg qd × 7-14 days

FIRST-LINE AGENTS WITH CLINICALLY ACCEPTABLE COVERAGE FOR ABE/COPD CAUSED BY *H. INFLUENZAE*, *M. CATARRHALIS*, OR *S. PNEUMONIAE*, PLUS ACCEPTABLE COVERAGE OF SOME GRAM-NEGATIVE SPECIES KNOWN TO CAUSE ABE/COPD IN PATIENTS WHO HAVE BEEN RISK-STRATIFIED TO A MORE SEVERE DISEASE CATEGORY §

Fluoroquinolones

- Levofloxacin (Levaquin): 500 mg qd × 7-14 days
  Indicated for acute bacterial exacerbations of chronic bronchitis caused by *H. parainfluenzae*, *M. catarrhalis*, *H. influenzae*, *S. pneumoniae*, and *S. aureus*
- Ciprofloxacin (Cipro): 500 mg bid × 10 days
  Although effective in clinical trials, ciprofloxacin is not considered the agent of first choice when ABE/COPD is secondary to *S. pneumoniae* infection

ALTERNATIVE, SECOND-LINE AGENTS WITH CLINICALLY ACCEPTABLE COVERAGE OF ABE/COPD CAUSED BY *H. INFLUENZAE*, *M. CATARRHALIS*, OR *S. PNEUMONIAE* §

Second-Generation Macrolide

- Clarithromycin (Biaxin): 250 mg bid (for *S. pneumoniae/M. catarrhalis*); 500 mg bid (for above *plus H. influenzae*) × 7-14 days
- Dirithromycin (Dynabac): 500 mg qd × 7 days

Cephalosporins

- Cefixime (Suprax): 400 mg qd × 10 days
- Cefprozil (Cefzil): 500 mg bid × 10 days
- Cefuroxime (Ceftin): 500 po bid × 10 days

ALTERNATIVE AGENTS WITH CLINICALLY ACCEPTABLE COVERAGE FOR ABE/COPD CAUSED BY *H. INFLUENZAE* OR *M. CATARRHALIS* (LOMEFLOXACIN), OR *S. PNEUMONIAE* OR *H. INFLUENZAE* (OFLOXACIN)

Quinolones

- Ofloxacin (Floxin): 400 mg bid × 10 days
  Not indicated for ABE/COPD caused by *M. catarrhalis*
- Lomefloxacin (Maxaquin): 400 mg qd × 10 days
  Indicated for ABE/COPD caused by *H. influenzae* or *M. catarrhalis*, but not indicated for the empiric treatment of ABE/COPD when *S. pneumoniae* is the causative organism

ALTERNATIVE AGENTS (GENERIC PREPARATIONS) FOR TREATMENT OF UNCOMPLICATED, ACUTE EXACERBATIONS OF CHRONIC BRONCHITIS ¶

- Trimethoprim-sulfamethoxazole (Bactrim, Septra): 1 DS tab po bid 7-14 days
- Amoxicillin (Amoxil, Wymox): 500 mg tid × 7-14 days
- Tetracycline: 500 mg qid × 7-14 days
- Doxycycline (Doryx, Vibramycin): 100 mg bid × 7-14 days

§ Possible β-lactam resistance may be encountered, especially among *H. influenzae* and *M. catarrhalis*; therefore, these first-line agents include specific antimicrobials likely to be active against such species.)

¶ Emerging, clinically significant resistance among *S. pneumoniae* to sulfonamides, penicillins, and tetracyclines (as well as incidence of β-lactamase-producing species) has the potential to compromise clinical efficacy of these agents in ABE/COPD. Not recommended as first-line therapy.

† Bosker G. *Pharmatecture: Minimizing Medications to Maximize Results.* St. Louis: Facts and Comparisons; 1999.

Other authors have proposed different classification schemes. There is general agreement that acute exacerbations of chronic bronchitis (AECB) can be defined as the presence of increases in cough/sputum, sputum purulence, and dyspnea. However, recent investigations suggest that the severity of AECB also may be divided into three stages based on the history of the patient: 1) previously healthy individuals; 2) patients with chronic cough and sputum and infrequent exacerbations; and 3) persons with frequent exacerbations or more severe chronic airflow limitation.

Recent Trials of Antibiotic Efficacy in Acute Bacterial Exacerbations of COPD. The goals of therapy for ABE/COPD are to resolve the infection expeditiously, maintain an infection-free

Table 2. Antibiotic Treatment of Acute Infectious Exacerbations of COPD

	SERF† PATHWAY AND IOTT CRITERIA/RISK FACTORS§	PATHOGENS	ANTIBIOTIC TREATMENT‡
Acute tracheobronchitis			
	No underlying structural disease	Usually viral	None, if viral infection is suspected. Azithromycin if bacterial etiology and ABE/COPD are likely
Acute bacterial exacerbation of chronic bronchitis			
	FEV_1 > 50%; two of three of the following are present: increased sputum volume, increased purulence, or increased cough	*H. influenzae, M. catarrhalis, S. pneumoniae* (possible β-lactam-resistant species can be encountered, especially among *H. influenzae* and *M. catarrhalis*)	Azithromycin, amoxicillin-clavulanate
Acute bacterial exacerbation of *complicated* chronic bronchitis			
	FEV_1 < 50%, advanced age, (four exacerbations/year; co-morbidity)	*H. influenzae, M. catarrhalis, S. pneumoniae* (possible β-lactam-resistant species can be encountered, especially among *H. influenzae* and *M. catarrhalis*). In addition, likelihood of infection with gram-negative organisms may be increased	Fluoroquinolone (levofloxacin, ciprofloxacin) if gram-negative enterobacteriaceae are strongly suspected; second-generation macrolide (azithromycin), if *H. influenzae, M. catarrhalis*, or *S. pneumoniae* are suspected; or second-line alternative: cephalosporin.
Chronic bronchial infection			
	Advanced disease with continuous sputum throughout year	*H. influenzae, M. catarrhalis, S. pneumoniae*, plus *Enterobacteria, P. aeruginosa*	Quinolones

‡ Authors' recommended antibiotics appearing in this table are based on pharmatectural criteria of convenience of dosing, cost, side effects, spectrum of coverage, and risk of drug-drug interactions (See Bosker, G. *Pharmatecture: Minimizing Medications To Maximize Results.* St. Louis: *Facts and* Comparisons; 1999.)

† SERF = Severity of Exacerbation and Risk Factors

§ IOTT= Intensity of Treatment Trigger

Framework adapted with permission from: Grossman RF. *Chest* 1997;112:3105-3125.

interval for as long as possible, and select an antibiotic with the fewest adverse effects and most favorable compliance profile. Because patients with COPD frequently are on complicated, multimodal drug therapy—consumption of many medications with a complicated dosing schedule is not uncommon—identifying effective, compliance-enhancing regimens for ABE/COPD is an important clinical objective. Moreover, because the key meta-analysis study supporting the efficacy of antibiotics in ABE/COPD was based on older trials with "older" agents, it is important that practitioners are aware of more recent studies evaluating effectiveness of newer antibiotics for this condition.

Many excellent studies are now available. One randomized, multicenter, investigator-blinded, parallel-group study compared a five-day, once-daily course of azithromycin (two 250 mg capsules on day 1, followed by one 250 mg capsule on days 2-5) with a 10-day, three-times-daily course of amoxicillin-clavulanate (one 500 mg tablet tid) in 70 patients with acute bacterial exacerbations of chronic obstructive pulmonary disease (ABE/COPD).[20] At the end of therapy, all 29 (100%) efficacy-assessable patients treated with azithromycin were cured or improved, compared with 25 (93%) of 27 assessable patients given amoxicillin-clavulanate (P = NS). Bacteriologic eradication rates were 86% (25 of 29 isolates) with azithromycin and 87% (20 of 23 isolates) with the comparative agent. Azithromycin was well tolerated; adverse events considered related or possibly related to treatment were reported in 28% of azithromycin recipients, compared with 39% of amoxicillin-clavulanate recipients (P = NS). The authors concluded that the five-day, once-daily regimen of azithromycin is comparable to a standard agent in the treatment of patients with ABE/COPD.[20]

The results of this study indicated that the administration of azithromycin once daily for five days is comparable to amoxicillin-clavulanate in the treatment of patients with ABE/COPD. The dosing schedule of azithromycin described in this trial is the shortest and simplest of the commonly prescribed oral antibiotics for ABE/COPD. Because reduced frequency of dosing and shorter therapy duration may improve patient compliance, and potentially,

Table 3. The SERF Risk-Stratification Pathway for Antibiotic Selection in ABE/COPD

SEVERITY OF EXACERBATION AND RISK FACTOR (SERF) SUPPORT TOOL

RATIONALE

The need for intensification and amplification of antimicrobial coverage in patients with acute exacerbations of chronic obstructive lung disease (ABE/COPD) depends on:

- Likelihood of infection with gram-negative enterobacteria
- Colonization status
- Patient's history of exacerbations and antimicrobial treatment response record
- Ability of patient to tolerate a treatment failure given his or her respiratory status
- Other factors requiring sound clinical judgment.

THE SERF PATHWAY

- Based on evidence-based trials and consensus opinion
- Designed as a clinical decision support tool to help guide empiric antibiotic therapy for outpatients with ABE/COPD.

Final decisions regarding drug selection should be made by the clinician on a patient-by-patient basis using on a comprehensive database including history, physical examination, and other diagnostic information.

Table 4. SERF Pathway: Intensification of Treatment Trigger (IOTT) Criteria for Risk-Stratification in ABE/COPD

INTENSIFICATION-OF-TREATMENT TRIGGER (IOTT) CRITERIA SHOULD BE CONSIDERED WHEN SELECTING AN ANTIBIOTIC FOR EMPIRIC OUTPATIENT TREATMENT OF ABE/COPD.

WHEN IOTT CRITERIA ARE PRESENT, CLINICIANS SHOULD CONSIDER NEWER AGENTS WITH EVIDENCE-BASED SUPPORT AS INDICATED AND RECOGNIZE POSSIBLE LIMITATIONS OF OLDER AGENTS SUCH AS SULFONAMIDES, PENICILLINS, AND TETRACYCLINES.

IOTT criteria include the following:

- History of multiple bacterial exacerbations of COPD within a short time period (more than 3 exacerbations in < 4 months)
- Multiple antimicrobial treatment exposures
- Documentation of gram-negative (enterobacteria, pseudomonas, Klebsiella, etc.) respiratory tract colonization
- History of requiring mechanical ventilation after treatment failure of ABE/COPD
- History of gram-negative nosocomial lower respiratory tract infection
- Chronic, systemic corticosteroid use
- Multiple emergency department visits with relapse within a 10-day period
- Supplemental home oxygen
- Smoking
- High prevalence (documented) *S. pneumoniae* resistance to penicillin
- Chronic alcoholism associated with history of gram-negative (*Klebsiella*) lower respiratory tract infection
- Serious co-morbidity (immunosuppression, HIV, underlying malignancy, etc.)

outcomes, practitioners should be aware of differences among effective agents as they relate to these compliance-sensitive parameters. Another Italian study comparing dirithromycin and azithromycin for the treatment of acute bacterial exacerbations of chronic bronchitis showed both drugs to be equally effective with cure or improvement at the immediate post-therapy period in the 90-92% range for both agents.[21]

An extended elimination half-life and good tissue penetration permit oral azithromycin to attain high and prolonged concentrations in infected tissues, yielding high antibacterial activity in vivo. However, there has been speculation among some authors, who have suggested that prolonged subinhibitory concentrations of azithromycin from two to four weeks after acute therapy may lead to the emergence of azithromycin resistance in vivo, compared with other macrolide antibiotics.[24-26]

This analysis is not universally accepted. In fact, data from two types of in vitro susceptibility studies, an animal tissue infection model, and a clinical pediatric study, demonstrated that prolonged tissue concentrations of azithromycin are unlikely to lead to the emergence of resistance in the clinical setting. Induction of resistance to macrolides in the laboratory is difficult, even with serial subculture and long-term experiments. Moreover, susceptibility testing of *S. pneumoniae* in one of the studies[25] was performed using the E-test method. Other studies reviewed indicate that use of CO_2 incubation can significantly overestimate the MIC values of bacterial strains exposed to macrolides, compared with standard and approved methodologies. This effect is particularly marked in the case of azithromycin. As a result, caution should be exercised when interpreting results generated by the E-test method when testing organisms such as *S. pneumoniae*, which require incubation in the presence of CO_2.[24-28]

In another prospective, multicenter, double-blind study, the efficacy of ciprofloxacin was compared with that of clarithromycin as therapy for patients with acute bacterial exacerbations of chronic bronchitis (ABE/COPD) from whom a pretherapy pathogen was isolated; the efficacy was measured by the infection-free interval. Patients randomly received either ciprofloxacin or clarithromycin (500 mg twice a day for 14 days). Three hundred seventy-six patients with acute exacerbations of chronic bronchitis were enrolled in the study, 234 of whom had an ABE/COPD. Clinical resolution was observed in 90% (89 of 99) of ciprofloxacin recipients and 82% (75 of 91) of clarithromycin recipients for whom efficacy could be evaluated. The median infection-free interval was 142 days for ciprofloxacin recipients and 51 days for clarithromycin recipients ($P = 0.15$). Bacteriologic eradication rates were 91% (86 of 95) for ciprofloxacin recipients and 77% (67 of 87) for clarithromycin recipients ($P = 0.01$). The investigators concluded that compared with clarithromycin, treatment of ABE/COPD with ciprofloxacin was associated with a trend toward a longer infection-free interval and a statistically significantly higher bacteriologic eradication rate.[29]

Ventilatory Assistance

Despite appropriate and aggressive pharmacological treatment of AECOPD, some patients may require assisted ventilation in the emergency department. In the past, there may have been a reluctance to intubate these patients because of fear that once intubated, patients become ventilator-dependent. Most patients with COPD will survive an initial episode of acute respiratory failure, although the mortality rate over the next several years is high. On average, patients who survive an episode of acute respiratory failure are intubated for an average of about 10 days.[31-33]

The decision to use ventilatory assistance should be made on the basis of both clinical and laboratory parameters. A single arterial blood gas is generally not adequate to judge whether a patient requires artificial ventilation. The significance of the PCO_2 is dependent on a number of factors, including evidence of chronic retention and the effects of oxygen administration. Patients with poor nutritional status or elevated APACHE II scores are likely to require intubation.[34] Many patients will tolerate moderate hypercarbia, as long as pH above 7.26 and adequate oxygenation are maintained.

Nevertheless, patients with extreme dyspnea, discordant breathing, fatigue, inability to speak, or deteriorating mental status in the face of adequate therapy may require ventilatory assistance. Hypoxemia that does not respond to oxygen therapy or worsening of acid-base status in spite of controlled oxygen therapy may also indicate the need for ventilatory assistance. Once intubated, care should be taken to avoid precipitous drops in the PCO_2 since this may lead to severe respiratory alkalosis.

Noninvasive Ventilation. One of the most important developments in the treatment of AECOPD over the past few years has been the acceptance of noninvasive, nasal, bilevel positive airway pressure (BiPAP). Studies conducted in the late 1980s have demonstrated the safety and efficacy of this approach. Patients with COPD have an intrinsic positive end expiratory pressure (PEEP) that significantly increases the inspiratory workload.[35] By applying external positive airway pressure, this intrinsic PEEP can be overcome, improving the work of breathing. In addition, applying inspiratory, positive-pressure ventilation reduces diaphragmatic work and improves gas exchange.[36] Noninvasive ventilation leads to improvement in respiratory rate, tidal volume, and minute ventilation. Mask ventilation decreases venous return and reduces left ventricular transmural pressure, which may lead to a drop in cardiac output and in systemic blood pressure.

Invasive ventilation can be associated with significant complications before, during, and after tube placement. This includes adverse events associated with intubation, including airway trauma, cardiac arrhythmias, transient hypoxemia, and aspiration of gastric contents. Post-intubation, the patient is at risk for tracheal stenosis, sinusitis, nosocomial pneumonia, and inadvertent extubation. Noninvasive positive pressure ventilation (NPPV) has a lower incidence of infection. Mask ventilation can be complicated by local skin irritation, aerophagia with subsequent emesis, and reduced cardiac output at high pressures. The advantages, however, are that patients are able to talk, swallow, and expectorate.

Overall, noninvasive ventilation is successful in about two out of three of patients[37] and decreases ICU stay and overall mortality rate. Patients successfully treated with noninvasive ventilation have a lower incidence of pneumonia and sinusitis.[38] The response to noninvasive ventilation is usually seen within the first hour. Patients who do not demonstrate improvement within the first hour will probably require mechanical ventilation over the course of several hours.

Nasal BiPAP. Nasal BiPAP requires a cooperative patient. The technique cannot be used in the apneic or comatose patient. Patients at high risk for aspiration may require intubation, although there are significant risks with this procedure as well. Patients requiring frequent suctioning may require intubation. Very obese patients (i.e., > 135 kilograms) may not obtain an adequate seal with the available masks.

The initial setup and monitoring techniques are time consuming. During the initiation of nasal BiPAP, a caregiver will probably be required at the bedside for some period of time. Nasal BiPAP is initiated with an explanation of the procedure to the patient. Expiratory pressure levels beginning around 3 cm H_2O with inspiratory pressure of around 8 cm of H_2O are typical settings. The inspiratory positive airway pressure (IPAP) is increased in 2-cm increments to titrate the PCO_2, while the expiratory positive airway pressure (EPAP) is increased to titrate the PO_2. The IPAP must be maintained above the EPAP.

The expiratory and inspiratory pressures are increased rapidly over the course of 15 minutes to achieve targeted oxygenation and CO_2 levels. If a patient does not improve within 1-2 hours of initiation of nasal BiPAP, then intubation may be required. Most patients started on nasal BiPAP will require ventilatory support for 1-2 days before weaning. Randomized trials have demonstrated that a majority of patients started on noninvasive ventilation will have improvement in oxygenation and a decrease in hypercarbia.[36-40] Patients successfully treated with nasal BiPAP have a decrease in complication rate with a markedly lower rate of sinusitis or pneumonia. In addition, patients treated with noninvasive ventilation have a decreased length of stay in the ICU and a lower total hospital ICU stay. In fact, one small case series has demonstrated that patients who have been treated with invasive ventilation on some occasions may respond on subsequent admissions to noninvasive ventilation.[37-38]

It should be emphasized that not all studies have demonstrated efficacy with nasal BiPAP.[39] Patients who fail nasal BiPAP tend to have a greater severity of illness, are unable to minimize mouth leak because of lack of teeth or increased oral secretions, and have difficulty coordinating with the ventilator.[40]

Disposition, Triage, and Outpatient Treatment Protocols

A number of factors are used to determine the disposition of patients treated in the emergency department with an acute exacerbation of COPD. These include the patient's overall respiratory status post treatment, as determined by the respiratory rate, respiratory effort, oxygen saturation, and pulmonary function. In addition, factors such as the patient's home living conditions, mental status, and concomitant illnesses may play a role in the decision to admit or discharge a patient. It should be noted that there is a high rate of relapse, ranging from 15% to 30% following discharge from the emergency department.[41,42] Interestingly, patients are at higher risk of relapse if they have nighttime ED visits, if they have a component of "asthma" as part of the chronic obstructive disease, or if they have weekend visits.[6,41,42] The results of pulmonary function testing in association with patient assessment of respiratory distress may be useful in predicting the risk of relapse.

Unlike patients with asthma, who tend to have normal or near-normal pulmonary function between attacks, patients with COPD may have chronic airflow limitation. Therefore, the post-treatment pulmonary function compared to documented baseline function should be considered along with the patient's self-assessment of respiratory distress.[42] From a relapse perspective, patients with a post-treatment FEV_1 less than 40% of predicted normal will have a significant relapse rate, even when the patient reports minimal respiratory distress. In contrast, patients with a post-treatment FEV_1 greater than 40% of predicted normal can usually be treated successfully at home, especially when the patient has only mild residual respiratory distress.

The results of arterial blood gas testing are not particularly useful in predicting the risk of relapse, although patients with severe hypoxemia or respiratory acidosis will require admission. In addition, patients are more likely to relapse if they have had a shorter duration of dyspnea, have a lower FEV_1, require a greater number of treatments with nebulized bronchodilators, require parenteral adrenergic drugs, or have a history of frequent relapses.[42]

Home-Based Treatment Plan

On discharge from the emergency department, several adjustments to the patient's outpatient medical regimen may be considered.

Oxygen. First, patients with severe COPD may be eligible for home oxygen therapy. Although this is generally not initiated as part of the emergency department treatment, patients may benefit from a referral for subsequent consideration for home oxygen therapy. Patients with a PaO_2 less than 55 mmHg at rest or PaO_2 between 55-60 mmHg with evidence of cor pulmonale may meet Medicare criteria for reimbursable oxygen supplementation. It has been shown that home oxygen therapy prolongs survival, reduces polycythemia, decreases the risk of pulmonary hypertension, and reduces the risk of right ventricular failure. Accordingly, patients who meet these criteria should be referred to appropriate providers who can arrange for home oxygen supplementation

Bronchodilators. Long-term management of the patient with COPD almost always requires use of various bronchodilating agents. Studies have shown that most patients with COPD respond to bronchodilators.[43,44] Significant improvements in pulmonary function may occur in response to inhaled beta-agonists, inhaled anticholinergic agents, and oral methylxanthines. Accordingly, patients should be discharged on bronchodilators, beginning with either inhaled beta-agonists or inhaled anticholinergics. Although the older, nonselective beta-agonists are effective in COPD, when used for long-term therapy, patients should be on one of the newer, longer acting, beta-2 selective agonists such as metaproterenol, albuterol, terbutaline, or bitolterol. For long-term maintenance, these agents are typically used in a dose of two puffs up to 4 times a day by metered dose inhaler. Some patients, however, may require larger doses, and studies in patients with chronic disease have found dose-related improvements up to 1600 mcg.[45]

In large studies, albuterol has been found to improve pulmonary function for stable patients with COPD.[45] The effectiveness, however, decreases over time. Albuterol is safe for the long-term management of COPD, as the incidence of drug-related adverse events are low. Patients with COPD tend to be older, and as such, have decreased sensitivity to adrenergic compounds. Some authors have found that the response to anticholinergic compounds in chronic therapy may be superior to beta-agonists for routine use.

Anticholinergic Agents. Anticholinergics should probably be used for routine maintenance in most patients with COPD. Inhaled quaternary ammonium anticholinergic agents have been found in some studies to lead to greater bronchodilation than beta-agonists or theophylline. Since older patients have a decrease in responsiveness to the adrenergic receptors, the cholinergic receptors become even more important in the older patients with COPD. Ipratropium is the primary agent used by metered-dose inhaler in this country. It is relatively safe, with side effects generally limited to dry mouth or the sensation of a "metallic" taste in the mouth. Again, this agent leads to increasing bronchodilation as the dose increases up to 600 mcg. Ipratropium is available in 500 mcg doses by metered-dose inhaler.

A meta-analysis of seven long-term studies comparing ipratropium with beta-agonists demonstrated that ipratropium leads to greater improvement in FEV_1 and even greater improvements in force vital capacity over the course of 90 days. Ipratropium leads to greater improvements in quality-of-life measurements. The improvements in pulmonary function are greatest in patients who have stopped smoking compared to current smokers. Furthermore, patients using ipratropium are less likely than patients using beta-agonists to develop a decreased response over time.[46] Ipratropium has minimal side effects that primarily are related to dry mouth or leaving a bad taste in the mouth.

Inhalers. Prior to discharge, patients should be taught the proper means of using meter-dose inhalers. Many patients will benefit from the use of a spacer device. A typical discharge regimen will include albuterol by meter dose inhaler either on an as needed basis for rescue therapy or for chronic maintenance therapy.[47,48] In addition, most patients with COPD should be using ipratropium by meter-dose inhaler for chronic maintenance therapy. These drugs are available as combination therapy in meter-dose inhalers. Patients who have prominent nighttime symptoms may benefit from a long-acting beta-agonist such as salmeterol. Patients should be counseled, however, that salmeterol should not be used for rescue therapy.

Theophylline. Theophylline does have dose-related effects on pulmonary function in patients with stable COPD. This drug may be used for patients who cannot or will not use meter-dose inhalers, patients who are not responding to otherwise maximal therapy, or patients who have prominent nighttime symptoms. Therapy is usually initiated at a dose of 300 mg twice a day with monitoring of the theophylline level. Therapeutic theophylline levels are considered to be between 10 and 20 micrograms per cc, although the FDA has changed labeling requirements for these drugs to suggest that consideration be given to maintain the level between 10 and 15 micrograms per cc. Theophylline metabolism is affected by a number of factors and patients should be cautioned not to increase their dose without seeking medical advice.

Corticosteroids. About 25% of patients with COPD will respond to oral steroids. Patients with a significant degree of reversibility of pulmonary function on baseline testing are most likely to respond to steroids.[49] It seems reasonable to initiate a two-week trial of oral steroids for patients with COPD. Limited studies indicate that there may be a role for inhaled corticosteroids in patients with COPD. In this regard, one study found that the addition of inhaled corticosteroids over the course of two years decreased morbidity and improved airway obstruction when used in conjunction with an inhaled beta-2 agonist.[50] A more recent study found a short-term improvement in lung function in smokers with COPD treated with inhaled steroids, but this then was followed by continued deterioration in lung function.[51]

Antibiotics. While many episodes of acute exacerbation of COPD are caused by viral infection, the weight of evidence seems to indicated that patients respond to oral antibiotics; especially, when the exacerbation is associated with signs and symptoms of acute, bacterial bronchitis that is superimposed on COPD with a presentation characterized by fever, dyspnea, increase in sputum production, or change in the color of sputum.[52] Available antibiotics with evidence-based support for their efficacy and which have indications for ABE/COPD have been discussed in detail.

Patients with ABE/COPD who are deemed suitable for oral, outpatient therapy and who do not have IOTT criteria in the SERF pathway *(please see Table 4)* that suggest the need for more extensive gram-negative coverage, should be discharged with a compliance-sensitive antibiotic that provides adequate coverage of *S. pneumoniae*, *H. influenzae*, and *M. catarrhalis*. *(Please see Table 1.)*

Based on evidence-based trials and pharmatectural criteria (duration of therapy, reduced dosing frequency, drug interaction profile, cost, and spectrum of coverage), azithromycin should be considered a first-line agent in patients with ABE/COPD who, on the basis of clinical judgement, are likely to be infected with *S. pneumoniae, H. influenzae*, or *M. catarrhalis*.[3-4,12-15,53-55] Other advanced generation macrolides, as well as penicillin derivatives such amoxicillin-clavulanate, also are available and effective, although these agents require more frequent dosing and have a longer course of therapy.

It should be stressed that some of the advanced macrolides also have the advantage of a simplified dosing schedule, especially azithromycin, which is given once daily for only five days (500 mg po on day 1 and 250 mg po qd on days 2-5). Azithromycin (500 mg on day 1 and 250 mg on days 2-5) did not affect the plasma levels or pharmacokinetics of theophylline administered as a single intravenous dose. However, because the effect of azithromycin on plasma levels or pharmacokinetics of theophylline is not known, until further data are available, prudent medical practice dictates careful monitoring of plasma levels of theophylline in COPD patients receiving azithromycin and theophylline concomitantly. The same precaution should be applied to patients receiving warfarin and azithromycin concomitantly. Other macrolides generally require a similar monitoring strategy.

Clarithromycin, another advanced generation macrolide, requires a longer course of therapy and, as a 10-day course (500 mg bid) is more expensive ($58-$72 for a 10-day course) than a five-day course of azithromycin. Dirithromycin, a semi-synthetic macrolide is indicated for acute bacterial exacerbations of chronic bronchitis due to *S. pneumoniae*, *H. influenzae*, or *M. catarrhalis*. In general, the decision to use a macrolide such as azithromycin is based on consideration of its generally acceptable cost ($39-$44 for a five-day treatment regimen), as well as its real-world advantages, which include convenient, once-daily dosing, a correct spectrum of coverage, its favorable drug interaction profile, and toleration data (gastrointestinal side effects occur in about 3-5% of patients taking a five-day, multiple-dose regimen). The oral tablet formulation permits consumption of the antibiotic without regard to food ingestion.

Patients who are macrolide treatment failures, who are suspected of gram-negative infection with enterobacteria, and/or who present with multiple IOTT points on the SERF pathway may be effectively served by a fluoroquinolone such as levofloxacin or ciprofloxacin, the latter of which is not recommended when *S. pneumoniae* is the presumed causative agent. Levofloxacin is well-tolerated, with the most common side effects, including nausea, diarrhea, headache, and constipation. Food does not affect the absorption of the drug, but it should be taken at least two hours before or two hours after antacids containing magnesium or aluminum, as well as sucralfate, metal cations such as iron, and multivitamin preparations with zinc. Dosage adjustment for levofloxacin is recommended in patients with impaired renal function (clearance < 50 mL/min).

Although no significant effect of levofloxacin on plasma concentration of theophylline was detected in 14 health volunteers studied, because other quinolones have produced increases in patients taking concomitant theophylline, theophylline levels should be closely monitored in patients on levofloxacin and dosage adjustments made as necessary. Monitoring patients on warfarin also is recommended in patients on quinolones. All quinolones have been associated with cartilage damage in animal studies, and therefore, they are not recommended for use in children, adolescents, and pregnant and nursing women. Cephalosporins are also available and effective for treatment of ABE/COPD.

Patients with a greater risk of respiratory failure are more likely to benefit from antibiotic therapy. This would include patients of advanced age and patients with significant lung impairment, impairment due to other co-morbid conditions, frequent exacerbations, or steroid use. Accordingly, these patients may require intensification and amplification of antibiotic therapy (i.e., the movement from azithromycin to a fluoroquinolone) to cover gram-negative organisms in addition to the three common offenders cited above.

Less expensive and still widely used in certain institutions and health plans, many of the older agents (sulfa-derivatives, tetracyclines, and amoxicillin) are becoming resistant to *S. pneumoniae* or do not cover beta-lactamase-producing organisms and, as a result, may no longer represent the best choice for empiric therapy of ABE/COPD.[3,4,11-13,55,56] The finding in one retrospective study that such antimicrobials as azithromycin, amoxicillin-clavulanate, or ciprofloxacin significantly reduced the failure rate and need for hospitalization, prolonged the time between AECOPD episodes, and were associated a lower total cost of management for AECOPD compared to the older agents is extremely provocative and requires further investigation.[55]

Even until clarification of outcome-effectiveness is forthcoming, clinicians should be aware that a number of newer antibiotic agents are available, including advanced generation macrolides and quinolones, which have the advantage of a broader spectrum of activity, simplified dosing regimens, and lower resistance rates.[57] These agents, however, have not been demonstrated to have greater clinical efficacy than less expensive agents in controlled clinical trials. One such stratification scheme has been proposed although it has not been rigorously tested.[58]

Pneumonia in COPD. The development of pneumonia in a patient with COPD will frequently provide an indication for admission. However, there are younger patients with very mild COPD who have good ventilatory status and who do not have other concomitant medical diseases who, on the basis of clinical judgement, may be given a trial of outpatient antibiotic therapy. Protocols for treatment of CAP are widely published. However, most patients with COPD complicated by pneumonia will require admission.

The small percentage of patients who are discharged, and therefore judged appropriate for outpatient treatment, should be treated for the most common causative agents, which include *S. pneumoniae, H. influenzae, M. catarrhalis, M. pneumoniae*, and *C. pneumoniae.* Given the spectrum of organisms encountered, it is probably preferable to initiate therapy with either a macrolide such as azithromycin or a quinolone such as levofloxacin. If amoxicillin/clavulanic acid or a third-generation cephalosporin is used to treat CAP, the authors recommend mandatory co-treatment with an agent (usually an advanced generation macrolide such as azithromycin) providing coverage of atypical organisms.

Patient Counseling

Long-term studies have demonstrated that smoking cessation, even when undertaken in later years, leads to moderation of the decline in pulmonary function that occurs with chronic cigarette use. Patients who stop smoking do not return to predicted pulmonary function, however, their rate of decline in pulmonary function begins to mirror those of patients who have never smoked. In addition to the beneficial pulmonary effects of smoking cessation, within 3-4 years a decrease in the risk of cardiovascular disease also is observed. Prior to discharge, the patient's ability to correctly use his or her metered-dose inhaler should be verified. Patients with COPD are at risk for streptococcal pneumonia. Patients should be counseled, therefore, about the need for anti-pneumococcal vaccinations and for annual influenza vaccination.

Summary

Assessment of the patients with acute exacerbation of COPD should include a systemic approach to distinguishing among many entities that may produce a similar clinical picture. These include congestive heart failure, pulmonary embolism, bacterial pneumonia, and pneumothorax. Once the diagnosis of ABE/COPD is verified, stabilization therapy should be initiated with oxygen and beta-agonists. Other pharmacologic intervention such as anticholinergic agents, theophylline, steroids, or magnesium should be considered only in patients with impending respiratory failure, those who have failed standard therapy, and those individuals considered for admission. Patients with unresponsive respiratory failure may be considered for a trial of nasal BiPAP before invasive ventilation.

Patients who on the basis of risk-stratification criteria are eligible for discharge may require modification of their outpatient regimen. When patients with COPD present with two or more of the following symptoms (increase in sputum production, increase in sputum purulence, increasing cough or dyspnea), outpatient antibiotic therapy has been shown improve clinical outcomes, including time to resolution, decrease in relapse rate, and improvement in functionality as measured by FEV_1 and other respiratory parameters. The SERF pathway can be used to identify IOTT criteria to aid in antibiotic selection.

References

1. Anthonisen NR, Manfreda J, Warren CP, et al. Antibiotic therapy in exacerbations of COPD. *Ann Intern Med* 1987;106: 196-204.
2. Wilson R. The Role of Infection in COPD. *Chest* 1998;113: 242S-248S.
3. Shu D, et al. A Controlled Randomized Multicenter Trial Comparing 5 Days Of Azithromycin to 10-14 Days of Clarithromycin for the Treatment of Acute Bacterial Exacerbations of Chronic Bronchitis. In: American Society for Microbiology, ed. 37th Interscience Conference on Antimicrobial Agents and Chemotherapy; Sept. 28-Oct. 1, 1997; Toronto, Ont. Washington, D.C.; pg. 372
4. Rosen MJ. Treatment of exacerbations of COPD. *Am Fam Phys* 1992;45:693-697.
5. Cydulka R, McFadden E, Emerman C, et al. Patterns of hospitalization in elderly patients with asthma and chronic obstructive pulmonary disease. *Am J Respir Crit Care Med* 1997;156:1807-1812.
6. Celli BR, Snider GL, Heffner J. Standards for the diagnosis and care of patients with chronic obstructive pulmonary disease. *Am J Respir Crit Care Med* 1995;152:S77-S120.
7. Kanner RE, Renzetti AD, Jr., Stanish WM, et al. Predictors of survival in subjects with chronic airflow limitation. *Am J Med* 1983;74:249-255.
8. Gump DW, Philips CA, Forsyth BR. Role of infection in chronic bronchitis. *Am Rev Respir Dis* 1976;113:465-474.
9. Blasi F, Legnani D, Lombardo VM, et al. *Chlamydia pneumoniae* infection in acute exacerbations of COPD. *Eur Respir J* 1993;6:19-22.
10. Beaty CD, Grayston JT, Wang SPP, et al. *Chlamydia pneumoniae,* strain TWAR, infection in patients with chronic obstructive pulmonary disease. *Am Rev Respir Dis* 1991;144: 1408-1410.
11. Rodnick JE, Gude JK. The use of antibiotics in acute bronchitis and acute exacerbations of chronic bronchitis. *West J Med* 1988;149:347-351.
12. Wallace RJ Jr. Newer oral antimicrobials and newer etiologic agents of acute bronchitis and acute exacerbations of chronic bronchitis. *Semin Respir Infect* 1988;3:49-54.
13. Wallace RF Jr, Steele LC, Brooks DL, et al. Amoxicillin/clavulanic acid in the treatment of lower respiratory tract infections caused by b-lactamase-positive *Haemophilus influenzae* and *Branhamella catarrhalis*. *Antimicrob Agents Chemother* 1985;27:912-915.
14. Hopkins SJ. Clinical toleration and safety of azithromycin in adults and children. *Rev Contemp Pharmacother* 1994;5: 383-389.
15. Nightingale CH, Belliveau PP, Quintiliani R. Cost issues and considerations when choosing antimicrobial agents. *Infect Dis Clin Pract* 1994;3:8-11.
16. Eller J, Ede A, Schaberg T, et al. Infective exacerbations of chronic bronchitis: Relation between bacteriologic etiology and lung function. *Chest* 1998;113:1542-1548.
17. Knaus WA, Harrell FEJ, Lynn J, et al. The SUPPORT Program prognostic model. Objective estimates of survival for seriously ill hospitalized adults. Study to understand prognosis and preferences for outcomes and risks of treatments. *Ann Intern Med* 1995:122:191-203.
18. Lange P, Nyboe J, Appleyard M, et al. Relationship of ventilatory impairment and of chronic mucous secretion to mortality from chronic obstructive lung disease and from all causes. *Thorax* 1990:45:579-585.
19. Sherman CB, Zu X, et al. Longitudinal lung function decline in subjects with respiratory symptoms. *Am Rev of Resp Dis* 1992:146:855-859.
20. Warren Whitlock on behalf of the Multicenter Chronic Obstructive Pulmonary Disease Study Group. Multicenter comparison of azithromycin and amoxicillin/clavulanate in the treatment of patients with chronic obstructive pulmonary disease. *Curr Therapeutic Res* 1995;56:10.
21. S. Maugeri Foundation, Institute of Care and Research, Medical Center of Rehabilitation, Clinical Pharmacology Unit and Respiratory Pharmacology Center, Veruno (NO), Italy. Comparative study of dirithromycin and azithromycin in the treatment of acute bacterial exacerbations of chronic bronchitis. *J Chemother* 1999;11:119-125.
22. Grossman RF. The value of antibiotics and the outcomes of antibiotic therapy in exacerbations of COPD. *Chest* 1998;113: 249S-255S.
23. Ball P, Make B. Acute exacerbations of chronic bronchitis: An international comparison. *Chest* 1998;113:199S-204S.
24. Bauernfreind A., Jungwirth R., Eberlein E. Comparative pharmacodynamics of clarithromycin and azithromycin against respiratory pathogens. *Infection* 1995;23:316-321.
25. Guggenbichler JP, Kastner H. The influence of macrolide antibiotics on the fecal and oral flora. *Infect Medicate* 1998;15(Suppl D):17-25.
26. Adam D, Grimm H, Lode H, et al. Comparative pharmacodynamics of clarithromycin and azithromycin against respiratory pathogens. *Infection* 1996;24:270.
27. Retsema JA. Susceptibility and resistance emergence studies with macrolides. *Int J Antimicrob Agents* 1999;11:S15-S21.
28. Girard AE, Cimochowski CR, Faiella JA. Correlation of increased azithromycin concentrations with phagocyte infiltration into sites of localized infection. *J Antimicrob Chemother* 1996;37(Suppl C):9-19.
29. Chodosh S, Schreurs A, Siami G, et al. Efficacy of oral ciprofloxacin vs. clarithromycin for treatment of acute bacterial exacerbations of chronic bronchitis. The Bronchitis Study Group. *Clin Infect Dis* 1998;27:730-738.
30. Chodosh S, McCarty J, Farkas S, et al. Randomized, double-blind study of ciprofloxacin and cefuroxime axetil for treatment of acute bacterial exacerbations of chronic bronchitis. The Bronchitis Study Group. *Clin Infect Dis* 1998;27: 722-729.

31. Seneff MG, Wagner DP, Wagner RP, et al. Hospital and 1-year survival of patients admitted to intensive care units with acute exacerbation of chronic obstructive pulmonary disease. *JAMA* 1995;274:1852-1857.
32. Connors AF, Jr., Dawson NV, Thomas C, et al. Outcomes following acute exacerbation of severe chronic obstructive lung disease. The SUPPORT investigators (Study to Understand Prognoses and Preferences for Outcomes and Risks of Treatments). *Am J Respir Crit Care Med* 1996;154:959-967.
33. Fuso L, Incalzi RA, Pistelli R, et al. Predicting mortality of patients hospitalized for acutely exacerbated chronic obstructive pulmonary disease. *Am J Med* 1995;98:272-277.
34. Vitacca M, Clini E, Porta R, et al. Acute exacerbations in patients with COPD: Predictors of need for mechanical ventilation. *Eur Respir J* 1996;9:1487-1493.
35. Ranieri VM, Giuliani R, Cinnella G, et al. Physiologic effects of positive end-expiratory pressure in patients with chronic obstructive pulmonary disease during acute ventilatory failure and controlled mechanical ventilation [see comments]. *Am Rev Respir Dis* 1993;147:5-13.
36. Goldberg P, Reissmann H, Maltais F, et al. Efficacy of noninvasive CPAP in COPD with acute respiratory failure. *Eur Respir J* 1995;8:1894-1900.
37. Brochard L, Mancebo J, Wysocki M, et al. Noninvasive ventilation for acute exacerbations of chronic obstructive pulmonary disease [see comments]. *N Engl J Med* 1995;333: 817-822.
38. Antonelli Ma, Conti Ga, Rocco Ma, et al. A Comparison of noninvasive positive-pressure ventilation and conventional mechanical ventilation in patients with acute respiratory failure. *N Engl J Med* 1998;339:429-435.
39. Wysocki M, Tric L, Wolff MA, et al. Noninvasive pressure support ventilation in patients with acute respiratory failure. A randomized comparison with conventional therapy. *Chest* 1995;107:761-768.
40. Soo Hoo GW, Santiago S, Williams AJ. Nasal mechanical ventilation for hypercapnic respiratory failure in chronic obstructive pulmonary disease: determinants of success and failure. *Crit Care Med* 1994;22:1253-1261.
41. Emerman CL, Effron D, Lukens TW. Spirometric criteria for hospital admission of patients with acute exacerbation of COPD. *Chest* 1991;99:595-599.
42. Murata G, Gorby M, Chick T, et al. Treatment of decompensated chronic obstructive pulmonary disease in the emergency department: Correlation between clinical features and prognosis. *Ann Emerg Med* 1991;20:125-129.
43. Tashkin DP, Bleecker E, Braun S, et al. Results of a multicenter study of nebulized inhalant bronchodilator solutions. *Am J Med* 1996;100:62S-69S.
44. Cazzola M, Di Perna F, Noschese P, et al. Effects of formoterol, salmeterol or oxitropium bromide on airway responses to salbutamol in COPD. *Eur Respir J* 1998;11:1337-1341.
45. Corris PA, Neville E, Nariman S, et al. Dose-response study of inhaled salbutamol powder in chronic airflow obstruction. *Thorax* 1983;38:292-296.
46. Colice GL. Nebulized bronchodilators for outpatient management of stable chronic obstructive pulmonary disease. *Am J Med* 1996;100:11S-18S.
47. Rennard Sa, Serby Ca, Ghafouri Ma, et al. Extended therapy with ipratropium is associated with improved lung function in patients with COPD. *Chest* 1996;110:62-70.
48. Friedman M. A multicenter study of nebulized bronchodilator solutions in chronic obstructive pulmonary disease. *Am J Med* 1996;100:30S-39S.
49. Chanez P, Vignola AM, O'Shaugnessy T, et al. Corticosteroid reversibility in COPD is related to features of asthma. *Am J Respir Crit Care Med* 1997;155:1529-1534.
50. Kerstjens Ha, Brand Pa, Hughes Ma, et al. A comparison of bronchodilator therapy with or without inhaled corticosteroid therapy for obstructive airways disease. *N Engl J Med* 1992; 327:1413-1419.
51. Pauwels R, Claes-Goran L, Laitinen L, et al. Long-term treatment with inhaled budesonide in persons with mild chronic obstructive pulmonary disease who continue smoking. *N Engl J Med* 1999;340:1948-1953.
52. Saint S, Bent S, Vittinghoff E, et al. Antibiotics in chronic obstructive pulmonary disease exacerbations. A meta-analysis [see comments]. *JAMA* 1995;273:957-960.
53. Bosker G. *Pharmatecture: Minimizing Medications To Maximize Results*. St. Louis: Facts and Comparisons; 1999.
54. Salit IE, Mederski B, Morisset R, et al. Azithromycin for the treatment of acute LRTIs: A multicenter, open-label study. *Infect Med* 1998;15:773-777.
55. Destache CJ, Dewan N, O'Donohue OJ, et al. Clinical and economic considerations in the treatment of acute exacerbations of chronic bronchitis. *J Antimicrob Chemother* 1999; 43:107-113.
56. Davies J. Inactivation of antibiotics and the dissemination of resistance genes. *Science* 1994;264:375-382.
57. Schentag JJ, Tillotson GS. Antibiotic selection and dosing for the treatment of acute exacerbations of COPD. *Chest* 1997;112: 314S-319S.
58. Grossman R. Guidelines for the treatment of acute exacerbations of chronic bronchitis. *Chest* 1997;112:310S-313S.
59. Emerman CL, Bosker G, Miller LA. Outpatient and in-hospital management of community-acquired pneumonia: Prediction rules for patient disposition and outcome-effective antibiotic selection. *Emerg Med Rep* 1998;19:219-238.

Pulmonary Embolism: Etiology and Clinical Features

Stephen A. Colucciello, MD, FACEP

It is ironic that the diagnosis of pulmonary embolism (PE), a major cause of death in the United States, often remains elusive. Controversies abound regarding which patients require evaluation for PE, as well as which diagnostic tests to pursue. A preponderance of hospitalized patients and a paucity of emergency department (ED) patients have skewed the medical literature away from the ambulatory setting. Research that relies on ventilation/perfusion (V/Q) scans as the gold standard for the diagnosis of PE handicaps many investigations. A diagnosis based on angiography or autopsy characterizes the best research in this field. Many current recommendations evolved from the Prospective Investigation of Pulmonary Embolism Diagnosis (PIOPED) study.[1] This study prospectively evaluated 755 patients in six clinical centers who underwent angiography during the workup for PE.

PE is a manifestation of the larger disease process of thromboembolism. While frequent, it is notoriously difficult to recognize, and its presentation is often nonspecific.[2] PE may be silent, and up to 40% of patients with deep venous thrombosis suffer clinically occult PE.[3,4] Physicians often fail to consider the diagnosis of PE in patients with prior cardiac or pulmonary disease.[5] The possibility of PE is frequently ignored in such patients who present with shortness of breath—the physician usually attributes the acute symptoms to the comorbid disease instead of suspecting PE. The emergency physician must have a heightened awareness of the risk factors and a ready suspicion for the diagnosis.[6]

At least 12% of patients with PE do not have associated risk factors detected by a careful history.[7] Unfortunately, most readily available tests in the ED setting, such as chest x-ray, electrocardiogram, and arterial blood gas cannot distinguish between PE and other conditions. Ancillary tests, including V/Q scan, angiography, D-dimer, dead space analysis, transesophageal echocardiography, helical CT, and MRI, all have potential roles in the diagnosis of PE. Clinical algorithms are useful to direct the evaluation of patients with suspected PE, and serve to limit complications, control costs, and improve diagnosis.[9]

The recognition and management of PE poses significant challenges for the emergency physician. This chapter will attempt to simplify the often frustrating conundrum of PE.

Epidemiology

PE is the most common preventable cause of hospital death and, paradoxically, the most common undiagnosed cause of hospital death. Most cases of PE are recognized by the true expert in this field—the pathologist. Seventy percent of all diagnoses are made postmortem.[10,11]

There are an estimated 650,000 cases per year in the United States and 200,000 deaths.[12] Despite improved prophylaxis of high-risk patients, the incidence has remained stable over the past three decades.[13] Epidemiologists underestimate the true incidence of

Table 1. Risk Factors for Thromboembolic Disease

STASIS	**INCREASED ESTROGEN**
Immobility	Pregnancy
Four days' bed rest	Post-partum < 3 months
Long plane ride (economy-class syndrome)	Therapeutic abortion
Train or car ride	Oral contraceptives
Paralysis—stroke, spinal cord injury, cast	
HYPERCOAGULABILITY	**INTIMAL DAMAGE**
Malignancy	IV drug abuse
Previous thromboembolic disease	Trauma
Inflammatory conditions (SLE, IBD, PVD)	Recent surgery
Nephrotic syndrome (loss of antithrombin III)	Central lines
Sepsis	**MULTIFACTORIAL**
Coagulation disorders—inheritable vs. acquired	Trauma
Protein S deficiency	Recent surgery
Protein C deficiency	Age > 60
Antithrombin III deficiency	Cardiac disease
Disorders of fibrinogen or plasminogen	Obesity
Lupus anticoagulant	Heart failure
Antiphospholipid antibodies (lupus anticoagulant and anticardiolipin)	

thromboembolism because of the often silent nature of the disease and the falling number of autopsies.[14] It is especially difficult to determine the frequency of PE in the ED. Two disturbing studies from the 1980s have shown that 21% of all ED patients with pleuritic chest pain have pulmonary emboli proved by angiography.[15,16]

Mortality. The morbidity of thromboembolic disease increases with advancing age and male sex.[17,18] Most patients who die of PE succumb in the first hour; however, a large number also die of subsequent emboli. Acute mortality correlates with right ventricular function, while long-term mortality relates to comorbid disease.[19] Patients with PE who have cancer, congestive heart failure (CHF), or chronic obstructive pulmonary disease (COPD) have the highest one-year mortality rate.[20] Massive or "saddle" emboli that obstruct major branches of the pulmonary artery cause most deaths, but small emboli produce significant morbidity and mortality in patients with limited cardiopulmonary reserve. Patients younger than 40 have only a 2.5% mortality compared to older adults, 18% of whom die from their PE.[21] Geriatric patients are at particular risk. In the elderly, the one-year mortality rate associated with PE is 39% despite treatment.[22] Fatal thromboembolism in young women is linked to a history of major illness, especially prior thrombosis, recent surgery, and trauma.[23] Surprisingly, there does not appear to be an excess of oral contraceptive use in young women with fatal PE.[23] Recognition and aggressive treatment of PE saves lives. There is a 30% mortality in untreated patients, which drops to 5% in those placed on heparin.[24]

Most cases of PE occur in adults older than 40, and the risk rises gradually with increasing age. While PE in infants is rare, children and especially teens are not immune to thromboembolic disease.[25,26] One out of every 1000 admissions in children may be for thromboembolic disease.[25,26]

Etiology

Ninety percent of all pulmonary emboli arise from the deep venous system, usually from the lower extremities.[27,28] During the 19th century, Virchow elucidated his famous triad that produces venous thrombosis. These include: 1) intimal damage to a blood vessel; 2) venous stasis; and 3) hypercoagulability.[29] At least 80-90% of patients with PE have one or more risk factors that relate to this triad.[30] *(Please see Table 1.)*

Immobility produces venous stasis, and several days of bed rest or prolonged travel can precipitate thrombosis in susceptible individuals.[31] A major cause of death of arriving passengers at Heathrow Airport is PE. The "economy-class syndrome" describes PE caused by the cramped quarters on transatlantic flights.[32] Paralysis from stroke, spinal cord injury, or external immobilization from a cast predispose to thromboembolic disease.[33] Spinal cord injury leads to pathological thrombosis in children and adults. More than 50% of all patients in the PIOPED study were immobilized in the three months before their PE.[34]

Trauma and surgery cause up to 40% of thromboembolic disease through multiple mechanisms.[17,35] They can produce immobility, intimal damage to the veins of the lower extremities, and trigger a hypercoagulable state. Orthopedic surgery to the lower extremities is notorious for causing DVT and subsequent PE.[36] Other causes of inti-

Table 2. Important Patient History Questions in Those Suspected of Having PE

1. Have you or anyone in your family ever had a blood clot in their leg or lung?
2. Have you been on a long trip—car, plane, etc.?
3. Have you recently been bedridden for more than three days?
4. Have you had surgery or trauma in the last 2-3 months?
5. Have you been pregnant in the last three months (therapeutic abortion, miscarriage, current pregnancy)?
6. Are you on birth control pills and do you smoke?
7. Do you have any medical problems (malignancy, SLE, CHF)?
8. Have you had chest pain or shortness of breath?

mal damage include IV drug use and central lines. Up to 15% of catheter-related upper-extremity thrombosis result in PE—sometimes with fatal results.[37,38] Central lines are a significant cause of venous thrombosis in children and are responsible for 20-30% of all pediatric thrombosis.[26,39]

Coagulation disorders may be inherited or acquired. Careful attention to family history will raise suspicion of inherited thrombophilia.[40] Resistance to activated protein C (APC), a genetic defect seen in familial venous thrombophilia, is the most common inherited hypercoagulable state.[41] Other relatively common disorders include deficiencies of protein S, protein C, and antithrombin-III.[42,43] Once heparin or coumadin is started, serum tests for these disorders are unreliable. Therefore, setting aside blood samples before initiating anticoagulation treatment can be helpful later. In children and young adults, antiphospholipid antibodies, such as the lupus anticoagulant and anticardiolipin, precipitate thromboembolism.[44] The rare disorders of fibrinogen or plasminogen play a small role in venous thrombosis and PE.

Acquired thrombophilia occurs with malignancy and a variety of inflammatory conditions, such as systemic lupus erythematosus, other collagen vascular diseases, and inflammatory bowel disease.[45] Since neoplasms are responsible for at least 4% of thromboembolic disease, it is not surprising that up to 9% of patients with apparently idiopathic PE subsequently develop cancer.[17,46,47] The nephrotic syndrome accelerates thrombosis through loss of antithrombin III or protein S in the urine.[48]

Increased estrogen from any cause also leads to urinary loss of antithrombin III or protein S. Estrogens also induce increased hepatic protein synthesis, including that of coagulation factors. This can accentuate any underlying tendency toward a hypercoagulable state. Low estrogen and progesterone pills, implants, or injections slightly increase the risk of thrombosis. Therapeutic abortion places the adolescent female in real danger of PE. Cigarette smoking and surgery predispose to thromboembolism in all high-estrogen states.[49]

Pathophysiology

Once a clot forms in the deep venous system, all or part of it can break off and embolize to the lung. Certain clots are more likely to embolize than others. Patients with prior pulmonary emboli are more likely to have future emboli than those with a history of isolated DVT.[51] Clots that have a free-floating "tail" seen on venography or ultrasound are particularly dangerous. While large clots in the deep venous system of the thigh and pelvis are ominous, calf vein clots also pose a significant and occasionally fatal risk.[52] Thrombi that form below the popliteal vein are small and rarely cause significant morbidity if they embolize. However, 20% of these clots propagate and subsequently embolize, leading to respiratory distress or even death.[135-137] It is a perilous myth that clots in the upper extremities are too small to be dangerous. DVT of the upper extremities can lead to fatal PE, particularly in children.[138]

Once a clot embolizes to the lungs, a variety of physiologic responses occur. Large clots, particularly if they obstruct the main pulmonary artery or sit like a "saddle" over two major branches, can produce right heart strain and acute cor pulmonale. Pulmonary artery hypertension results, and the patient develops a ventilation perfusion mismatch and subsequent hypoxia.[53] There are a variety of neurohumoral factors triggered by pulmonary emboli.[54] These lead to pulmonary vasoconstriction and occasionally wheezing. Some lung units become overventilated relative to perfusion. This increases the dead space and dilutes the expired CO_2.[54]

After embolization, the body's endogenous fibrinolytic system begins to dissolve the clot. Plasmin works to degrade the clot, fibroblasts infiltrate, and the thrombus retracts. Recanalization of the vessel may result in intraluminal bands and webs.[55] Several weeks later, most patients show significant clot lysis and retraction on pulmonary angiography. However, pulmonary hypertension and impaired lung function may persist. In less than 1% of patients, persistent pulmonary hypertension ensues, producing "chronic pulmonary embolism."[56]

Clinical Features

During the interview, assess the patient for risk factors. *(Please see Table 2.)* While there appears to be a "laundry list" of important historical questions, the physician should never forget the most obvious: "Have you ever had a blood clot in your leg or lung before?" Nearly 20% of all patients with thromboembolic disease report a prior episode.[50]

The emergency physician may not recognize PE because the manifestations are protean.[49,57,58] *(Please see Table 3.)* The "classic" triad of hemoptysis, dyspnea, and pleuritic chest pain is actually rare, especially in fatal cases.[7] Young adults (under 40) with PE are problematic because up to 28% have no known risk factors and nearly 60% have normal vital signs.[21] The elderly and those with spinal cord injury may present in unusual ways. Geriatric patients may exhibit acute confusion secondary to hypoxia.[59] Some paraplegics have isolated supraventricular tachycardia (SVT), acute disturbances of behavior, unexplained fever, or other nonspecific findings.[60-62]

Fortunately, some combination of dyspnea, tachypnea, or pleuritic chest pain occurs in 97% of patients with clinically apparent PE.[34,63] Dyspnea is the most frequent complaint, followed by pleuritic chest pain. Up to 10% of patients have syncope.[34,64] Such patients

Table 3. Presentation of PE

SYMPTOMS		SIGNS	
Dyspnea	73%	Respiratory rate ≥ 20	70%
Pleuritic pain	66%	Rales	51%
Cough	37%	Tachycardia	30%
Leg swelling	28%	Accentuated P_2	23%
Hemoptysis	13%	Circulatory collapse	8%
Wheezing	9%		
Angina-type pain (radiation to jaw or arms is rare)	4%		

Adapted from: Quinn DA, Thompson BT, Terrin ML, et al. A prospective investigation of pulmonary embolism in women and men. *JAMA* 1992;268:1689-1696.

are frequently hypotensive and demonstrate right heart failure. Other patients complain of cough or, more rarely, isolated leg swelling.

There are three main syndromes associated with PE. Pulmonary hemorrhage/infarction is the most common.[63] This syndrome is frequently associated with chest pain, rales, and an abnormal chest x-ray. Unexplained dyspnea is the next most common complaint. Because such patients have submassive emboli, the ECG and chest x-ray are often normal while the PO_2 may be low. The most dramatic and fortunately least common scenario is cor pulmonale. This occurs when 60-70% of the pulmonary vasculature is obstructed, and patients present in extremis. It is characterized by shock, marked respiratory distress, or syncope. The chest x-ray, ECG, and ABG are frequently abnormal.

Physical Examination

The physical examination of the patient with PE is often nonspecific. A significant number of patients will have normal vital signs. Those who are diaphoretic on arrival are likely to have serious pathology. While patients may be febrile, the temperature is rarely greater than 102°F. Tachypnea is frequent, but the respiratory rate is less than 20 in 30% of patients.[34] The heart rate is normal in 70% of patients.[34]

Target the pulmonary and circulatory systems for intense scrutiny. Look for elevated neck veins. A paradoxical distension of the neck veins during inspiration (Kussmaul's sign) reflects elevated right ventricular pressure. Cardiac tamponade, tension pneumothorax, and right ventricular infarct may also produce this finding. The hyperdynamic state associated with large emboli may result in a parasternal heave. Pulmonary hypertension accentuates the P2 during cardiac auscultation, but this finding is rarely appreciated in a noisy ED. Ask patients to point where they hurt, and listen to the lungs over this area of maximal pain to hear the occasional friction rub. Recognize that rales are frequent in PE. The "classic" presentation of a clear chest exam with PE is actually uncommon. An examination of the extremities is routine but rarely helpful. Never exclude PE based on the presence of a normal extremity exam. Calf swelling, tenderness, and asymmetry cannot distinguish between those with PE and those without thromboembolic disease.[65] The presence of a cord should increase the suspicion of PE. Homans's sign, pain in the posterior calf with forced dorsiflexion of the foot, is no more accurate than a coin toss. Patients with superficial thrombophlebitis are also at risk for PE, as the superficial clot propagates into the deep system in 20% of cases.[66] In general, physical examination is rarely definitive in the diagnosis of PE.

Diagnostic Studies

The patient with suspected PE often undergoes a variety of ED tests before the physician decides to order a lung scan. However, tests such as chest x-ray, ECG, and ABG are usually nondiagnostic for PE.[1] *(Please see Table 4.)* They are more helpful to make or eliminate other potential diagnoses (e.g., AMI, pneumonia). Most clinical and laboratory tests only suggest the need for further studies such as V/Q scans or angiography.

The emergency physician should order a chest x-ray on every patient suspected of PE.[67] It can exclude conditions that clinically mimic PE, such as pneumothorax, rib fracture, or bony lesion. Chest x-rays also aid the interpretation of lung scans. They are abnormal in 84% of patients with PE. The most frequent abnormalities include atelectasis, blunting of the costophrenic angle (which represents small pleural effusion), and elevated hemidiaphragm on the side of the embolus.[67] Chest x-rays may also show embolism-related infiltrates that are indistinguishable from pneumonia.

There are several eponyms that define supposedly classic findings in PE. Hampton's hump is a wedge-shaped, pleural-based infiltrate that represents an area of lung infarction. Westermark's sign is peripheral oligemia caused by a clot interrupting blood flow. It is characterized by an increased lucency on chest x-ray. A large, sausage-shaped pulmonary artery marks the Fleischner sign. Unfortunately, none of these signs are good predictors of PE.[67] Except when it demonstrates a pneumothorax, acute rib fracture, or other diagnoses, a chest x-ray can neither confirm nor eliminate the diagnosis of PE.

ECG. ECG is primarily used to exclude AMI or pericarditis. The ECG changes of PE are not specific but may reflect signs of right ventricular strain. These include new onset of right bundle branch block, right axis deviation, shift in the transition zone to V5, and variations of the S1 Q3 T3 pattern.[68] This frequently discussed pattern is found more often in articles on PE than in patients with the disease and is helpful only when of new onset. Twenty to thirty percent of patients will have a normal ECG, and fifty percent will have nonspecific ST-T wave changes. Electrical alternans or T-wave inversions occur along with a variety of atrial dysrhythmias.[69] The differential diagnosis of new-onset atrial fibrillation must include PE. In general, although frequently obtained, the ECG is not mandatory to evaluate PE unless a primary cardiac problem is suspected.

Arterial Blood Gas. The arterial blood gas may be normal or near-normal in a significant percent of patients. Over one-quarter of all patients with PE will have a room air PO_2 of greater than 80 mmHg.[70] Some patients may even have a PO_2 of greater than 100 mmHg on room air. While a high PO_2 makes PE less likely, it does not exclude the diagnosis. A high PO_2 reflects a large pulmonary reserve and greater tolerance of embolic insult. Some authors suggest that a normal arterial-alveolar gradient (A-a) makes PE very unlikely.[71,72] Quickly estimate the A-a gradient at sea level by the formula:

Table 4. Features of Diagnostic Testing for PE

CHEST X-RAY

84% abnormal

Atelectasis, pleural effusion, elevated hemidiaphragm (most common)

Infiltrate occasionally present

Hampton's hump—pleural based wedge shaped infiltrate (rare)

Westermark sign—peripheral oligemia (rare)

ECG

Normal 20-30%

Nonspecific ST-T changes 50%

S1 Q3 T3, electrical alternans (rare)

Atrial dysrhythmias common, including atrial fibrillation

ARTERIAL BLOOD GAS (ROOM AIR)

PO_2 > 80 mmHg: 26%

PO_2 > 100 mmHg: 3%

Normal A-a gradient: 10%[70]

D-DIMER

Very sensitive, not specific

ALVEOLAR DEAD SPACE ANALYSIS

Promising new technology

Negative predictive value 96%

ECHOCARDIOGRAPHY

TEE more accurate than transthoracic

Useful for the unstable patient

CT

May detect clinically significant PE, but insensitive to peripheral emboli

MRI

Useful to distinguish pneumonia from embolism

Useful for the diagnosis of PE in pregnancy

V/Q SCAN

Must combine with clinical suspicion to be useful

ANGIOGRAPHY

Gold standard for diagnosis of PE—underutilized

COLOR-FLOW DOPPLER OF LOWER EXTREMITIES

Useful in patients with nondiagnostic lung scans

Specific but not sensitive

150 - 1.25 PCO_2 - PO_2. Because the A-a gradient increases with age, use the formula: (patient age / 4) + 4 to determine normal limits. The PIOPED study revealed that 8-10% of patients with angiographically proven PE have a normal A-a gradient.[70] Consideration of both the A-a gradient and the room air PCO_2 will increase the sensitivity of the ABG.[71] A normal gradient and a PCO_2 of greater than 36 mmHg yields a 98% negative predictive value for PE.[72] While low-risk ED patients with a normal A-a gradient and a normal PCO_2 may not require further work-up for embolism, very few patients meet these strict criteria. In summary, an elevated A-a gradient is nonspecific and a normal gradient does not eliminate the diagnosis.[73] Because it is insensitive to changes in PO_2 in the normal range, and cannot measure the A-a gradient, do not use pulse oximetry to exclude the diagnosis of PE.

D-dimer. Clot formation activates the endogenous fibrinolytic system. Fibrin breakdown produces a variety of degradation products, the most clinically useful of which is the D-dimer. Patients with thromboembolic disease frequently show elevations in D-dimer. The laboratory measures these levels by a variety of methods. These include the more sensitive but time-consuming (up to 17 hours) enzyme-linked immunoabsorbent assay (ELISA) and the rapid but less-sensitive latex agglutination.[74] Bedside latex agglutination tests take less than five minutes,[75] but limited sensitivity undermines their value.[76] The many tests for D-dimer vary in sensitivity, so a single "cut off" value to exclude PE does not exist.[76] D-dimer is 85-100% sensitive for PE[77,78] and is elevated for a week after the acute event.[78] It is also inexpensive, costing the patient about $45. Its greatest drawback is a poor specificity (range, 15-38%).[76,78-81] The specificity of D-dimer increases when no comorbid disease is present,[75] and one small study showed a specificity of 77%.[77] In one of the best-designed trials, a D-dimer of 500 ng/mL or more, using a monoclonal antibody assay, was 93% sensitive and 25% specific for PE.[80] A negative D-dimer coupled with a low clinical suspicion may obviate the need for an extensive work-up. Most research shows that a normal D-dimer has a negative predictive value of 92-98% for PE.[75,78,80,82] However, many authorities suggest that the D-dimer should be considered in conjunction with the V/Q scan to decide the likelihood of PE.

Alveolar Dead Space Analysis. When a clot interrupts pulmonary blood supply, the alveolar dead space increases and the amount of carbon dioxide in the exhaled breath drops; the larger the emboli, the greater the impact on dead space.[83] Analysis of dead space is simple and widely available. Not only can it detect PE in patients with normal lungs, but it can distinguish PE from other lung pathology such as COPD or interstitial lung disease.[84] Analyze dead space with an end-tidal CO_2 detector in conjunction with the arterial blood gas. Measure the alveolar dead space by the equation V_D/V_T = ($PaCO_2$ - $P_{et}CO_2$) / Pa CO_2, where V_D/V_T equals dead space and $P_{et}CO_2$ represents the end-tidal CO_2. A dead space less than 0.4 in association with a normal spirogram has a negative predictive value of 96% for PE.[85] Dead space analysis detects very small changes in pulmonary artery flow and can identify emboli as small as 1 mm.[86]

Echocardiography. Early investigations indicate that transthoracic echocardiography may be valuable in the diagnosis of massive and submassive pulmonary emboli and is up to 85% sensitive for large pulmonary insults.[89,90] Transesophageal echocardiography (TEE) is even more accurate, being 90% sensitive for hemodynamically significant emboli and 100% specific in one study.[87] In another study of critically ill patients initially diagnosed with congestive heart failure, cardiogenic shock, or pneumonia, TEE showed several cases of unsuspected PE.[88]

While an echocardiogram may visualize clot in the central pulmonary artery, it is more likely to demonstrate secondary cardiac effects associated with right ventricular overload. The echocardiogram detects increases in right ventricular end diastolic volume, tricuspid regurgitation, right ventricular asynergy, and abnormal septal movement associated with PE.[89,90] As ED use of echo becomes more routine, it may be useful to screen patients to determine the need for further studies. Currently, echocardiography is most valuable in the patient in shock who is too unstable for V/Q scanning as a supplement to color Doppler of the lower extremities.[91]

Transthoracic echocardiography can also visualize pulmonary infarction by sonographic changes in lung tissue. Using an intercostal sonographic window, hypoechoic lesions with a pleural base identify PE with 90% accuracy.[92] Further studies will better define its role in the ED.

Computed Tomography. CT has variable accuracy in the diagnosis of PE. It is more sensitive for large central than small peripheral emboli. The sensitivity of helical CT is 86% for central embolism, but only 63% for clot in the subsegmental vessels.[93] Ultra-fast CT has the potential to detect experimental emboli in the second through fourth division pulmonary vessels.[94] Contrast-enhanced electron beam CT accurately images "clinically significant" PE. While some authorities believe that it is more sensitive and specific than V/Q scanning, most do not.[95,96] Because it can detect other causes of lung pathology, such as tumor or aneurysm, CT has an advantage over nuclear medicine studies when the chest x-ray suggests these conditions. Despite its future promise, CT is not yet a first-line test for PE.[93]

Magnetic Resonance Imaging. Like CT, MRI is sensitive for proximal but not peripheral clot. MRI is 90% sensitive to central embolism and 80% specific.[97] MR angiography may be 92-100% sensitive and 62% specific for the detection of PE.[98] Because of the different properties of infarcted tissue and pneumonic infiltrate, MRI can distinguish between these conditions.[97] Because V/Q scans are rarely helpful in such cases, MRI is useful in patients who have an infiltrate on chest x-ray and absolute contraindications to angiography.[99] In the near future, it may become a major diagnostic tool for suspected thromboembolic disease during pregnancy. It is 97% sensitive and 95% specific for DVT and can detect leg, pelvis, and pulmonary thrombi.[100,101] A single examination images both arterial and deep venous clot.[98] While it is not currently recommended by the American College of Obstetricians and Gynecologists during the first trimester, experts consider it safe in all stages of pregnancy, making it potentially of greater value than V/Q scan or CT in that setting.[102]

Ventilation Perfusion Scanning. V/Q scans are the principal screening tests for PE. The technician injects ^{99m}Technetium-labeled macroaggregated albumin into a peripheral vein. Areas of decreased lung perfusion appear as defects on a gamma camera. Defects in perfusion are either matched or unmatched by defects in ventilation. The total number of mismatched defects is a powerful tool in assessing risk of PE.

Scans are divided into normal or near-normal, low-probability, intermediate-probability, and high-probability scans. This classification system is often misleading, since a significant number of patients with low-probability scans may have PE, while a similar number of patients with high-probability scans do not have PE. Several authorities suggest that scans be divided into "diagnostic" and "nondiagnostic" studies.[105] Patients with normal or near-normal scans, as well as those with high-probability scans, are usually considered to have diagnostic studies. A normal or near-normal scan defines a population with a 4% incidence of PE.[103,104] Low-probability and intermediate-probability scans are considered nondiagnostic. It is important to recognize that the majority of patients with PE *do not* have high-probability scans. Only 40% of patients with proven PE have high-probability scans, 40% have intermediate scans, and 20% have low-probability scans.[105] A low-probability scan does not rule out the possibility of PE. At least 12% of patients with low-probability scans have PE. In cases of high clinical suspicion, as many as 40% of patients with low-probability scans may have emboli.[106] Patients with a history of immobilization, trauma to the lower extremities, recent surgery, or central venous catheterization are most likely to have PE despite a low-probability scan.[107]

Conversely, patients with a high-probability scan may not have a PE. At least 12% of patients with high-probability scans do not have PE.[1]

While there are many different scoring systems for interpretation of V/Q scans, the modified PIOPED criteria are the most widely accepted.[108,109] Although the modified PIOPED criteria are more reliable than the original system, the "gestalt" of an experienced reader is the most accurate means of assigning a probability estimate to a V/Q scan.[110]

V/Q scans are not significantly limited by prior cardiac or pulmonary disease, although prior PE leads to a slight loss of sensitivity.[111,112] On the other hand, healthy patients are at higher risk for PE in the presence of minor perfusion abnormalities.

The emergency physician must recognize the very real limitations of these nuclear medicine studies. Scans are highly reader-dependent and there may be marked variation between initial reading and the "next-day" reading by a nuclear medicine specialist. Radiologists disagree over interpretations 20% of the time.[113] Disagreement is particularly high when scans are nondiagnostic (intermediate- or low-probability).[105] In addition to variation in reading, there is a wide disparity in the language used to report lung scan results.[114] There is no such thing as an "OK" scan. The emergency physician should insist on language that uses a normal, low-, intermediate-, or high-probability classification system when taking report from the radiologist.

The emergency physician must combine the results of the V/Q scan with his or her clinical assessment to estimate the likelihood of PE.[8] *(Please see Table 5.)* A clinical assessment that agrees with the V/Q scan is called concordant, while an assessment that disagrees is discordant (i.e., low clinical suspicion and low-probability V/Q scan is concordant; low-probability V/Q scan with high suspicion is discordant). It is important for the physician to commit to a level of clinical suspicion for PE (low, moderate, or high), *prior* to receiving the results of the V/Q scan. A high clinical suspicion combined with

Table 5. The Utility of the V/Q Scan for Diagnosing PE

	LOW-PROBABILITY SCAN	INTERMEDIATE-PROBABILITY SCAN	HIGH-PROBABILITY SCAN
Low clinical suspicion*	4% PE	16% PE	56% PE *
High clinical suspicion*	40% PE	66% PE	96% PE *
Comorbid disease†	8% mortality		
No comorbid disease†	0.15% mortality		

* Stein PD, et al. Strategy for diagnosis of patients with suspected acute pulmonary embolism. *Chest* 1993;103:1553.
† Hull RD, et al. The low-probability lung scan. A need for change in nomenclature. *Arch Intern Med* 1995;155:1845-1851.

a high-probability scan increases the positive predictive value from 88% to 96%. Similarly, a low clinical suspicion combined with a low probability scan increases the negative predictive value from 88% to 96%.[1] Unfortunately, there is no widely accepted scoring system that can objectively determine this clinical score.[108,109]

The limitations of V/Q scanning are often not recognized by the practicing emergency physician. *Lung scanning substantiates or excludes PE in only half of all patients with PE.* V/Q scanning is often an initial step in the evaluation of patients with suspected thromboembolic disease. A scan that is nondiagnostic usually requires further work-up. Despite this frequently published recommendation, the majority of patients with inconclusive lung scans have no further evaluation for PE.[115] Angiography is clearly underutilized. As stated by the PIOPED investigators, "for a majority of patients, angiography is required for definitive diagnosis of pulmonary embolism."[1]

Evaluation of the Venous System. Because thromboembolic disease is a continuum from venous thrombosis to PE, it is reasonable to assume that the evaluation of the deep venous system could serve as an adjunct to direct lung imaging. A patient with documented DVT and chest pain is generally treated the same as a person with DVT alone. While venography accurately images the venous system, noninvasive studies such as color-flow duplex ultrasound cause less morbidity. Impedance plethysmography (IPG) is no longer considered a first-line study since it is only 65% sensitive for proximal thrombosis.[116] Recent studies demonstrate that color-flow duplex scans are as reliable as venography in the diagnosis of proximal DVT.[117]

Unfortunately, only 10-60% of patients with angiographically proven pulmonary emboli have venous pathology documented by ultrasound or venography.[118,119] This is due to a variety of reasons. In some patients, the entire clot may dislodge from the leg and travel to the lung, leaving no residual thrombus. Some clots arise from pelvic vessels, renal veins, inferior vena cava, or even the heart. Thrombus in these areas is rarely detected by venography or ultrasound. Because of its limited sensitivity, venous evaluation plays a secondary role in the diagnosis of PE. It is best used after a nondiagnostic V/Q scan. In one study, over half the patients with intermediate-probability V/Q scans had leg thrombi by ultrasound and were spared angiography.[120] If angiography is ordered only on patients with nondiagnostic V/Q scans and negative leg studies, costs could be reduced by 9%.[121] This is in comparison to the more expensive strategy of obtaining angiography on all patients with nondiagnostic V/Q scans. Serial noninvasive leg studies may be another safe way to avoid angiography. Patients with an adequate cardiopulmonary reserve, nondiagnostic lung scan, and negative initial leg ultrasound may undergo serial noninvasive leg studies over a two-week period without anticoagulation.[118,122] About 3% of patients undergoing serial studies demonstrate proximal venous thrombosis. However, this strategy may miss an additional 2% of patients who go on to develop thromboembolism despite negative leg studies. Serial examinations require tremendous compliance on the part of the patient who needs to return to the hospital seven more times in a two-week period for repeat ultrasounds. The cost of this approach is also considerable.

Angiography. Angiography is the most accurate means, premorbid, to diagnose PE. A normal angiogram almost excludes the diagnosis of PE. While the false-negative rate is 1.6%, there is significant interobserver variation in angiogram readings.[123] In addition, up to 3% of angiograms may be nondiagnostic.[124] Intravenous digital subtraction angiography (DSA), while less invasive, is inaccurate and should not be used.[123] Intra-arterial pulmonary DSA is safe and provides good-to-excellent images.[125]

There is considerable reluctance on the part of emergency physicians to order, and radiologists to perform, angiography. In the United Kingdom, doctors order approximately 100 V/Q scans for every angiogram.[126] Yet, angiography is a safe procedure with low morbidity and mortality. The morbidity associated with angiography is dwarfed by the complications associated with unnecessary anticoagulation. Angiographic morbidity ranges from 1% to 2%, while chronic anticoagulation has a morbidity of 1.5-20% per year. There is a 0.1-0.5% mortality rate with angiography, but most deaths occur in unstable patients or in those with severe cardiopulmonary disease.[124] Complications include bleeding, dye reaction, pulmonary artery rupture, and cardiac arrest. Renal dysfunction secondary to contrast load is most likely in the elderly but can be reduced through the use of low-osmolar agents.[127]

The Future of Diagnostic Testing. New tests will soon change our practice. Radiolabeled, inactivated tissue-type plasminogen activator (tPA) detects experimental pulmonary emboli in dogs.[128] Radiolabeled platelets can also be incorporated into clot.[129] In the future, such substances injected into patients suspected of PE will "tag" the emboli. These tagged emboli will glow on single-photon emission CT or planar imaging.

Advances in CT and MRI may make V/Q scans obsolete.[95,130] Although fast CT is more rapid and less expensive than MRI,[130] MRI

Table 6. Pitfalls in the Diagnosis of PE

1. Inappropriately high suspicion for PE in young, healthy women on birth control pills, compared to inappropriately low suspicion in older patients with comorbid disease.
2. Relying on normal vital signs or normal physical exam to rule out PE.
3. Relying on pulse oximetry to rule out PE.
4. Making the diagnosis of pleurisy without the use of objective tests.
5. Ignoring the role of clinical suspicion and using the V/Q scan alone to rule out PE.
6. Failure to perform additional studies for patients with high clinical suspicion and indeterminate V/Q scans.

can visualize the deep venous system as well as the pulmonary circulation.[131]

Progress in ultrasound technology also appears promising. Intravascular ultrasound rapidly confirms the presence of large proximal emboli in early studies performed.[132]

Dead-space analysis may become routine in the work-up of PE. Patients can be rapidly and inexpensively screened by using a room air blood gas and an end-tidal CO_2 detector. Combining a very specific test like dead space analysis with a very sensitive test such as the D-dimer would select those individuals requiring further study.

Innovations in computer technology will allow physicians to manipulate clinical and diagnostic information. Neural networks using clinical data predict the likelihood of PE with an accuracy comparable to experienced clinicians.[133] Other neural networks utilize V/Q scans and chest x-ray information to outperform physicians in PE diagnosis.[134]

Summary

PE must remain high in the differential diagnosis of many patients who present to the ED. Classic presentations are, in reality, rather uncommon, and reliance on these leads to many pitfalls. *(Please see Table 6.)* Despite a multitude of diagnostic tests, patients are best served by the astute clinician with a keen clinical awareness of the subtleties by which PE may present.

References

1. PIOPED Investigators. Value of the ventilation/perfusion scan in acute pulmonary embolism. Results of the prospective investigation of pulmonary embolism diagnosis, PIOPED. *JAMA* 1990;263:2753-2759.
2. Miller GH, Feied CF. Suspected pulmonary embolism. The difficulties of diagnostic evaluation. *Postgrad Med* 1995;97: 51-58. Review.
3. Nielsen HK, Husted SE, Krusell LR, et al. Silent pulmonary embolism in patients with deep venous thrombosis. Incidence and fate in a randomized, controlled trial of anticoagulation versus no anticoagulation. *J Intern Med* 1994;235:457-461.
4. Moser KM, Fedullo PF, LitteJohn JK, et al. Frequent asymptomatic pulmonary embolism in patients with deep venous thrombosis. *JAMA* 1994;271:223-225.
5. Robin ED. Overdiagnosis and overtreatment of pulmonary embolism: The emperor may have no clothes. *Ann Intern Med* 1977;87:775.
6. Gray BH, Graor RA. Deep venous thrombosis and pulmonary embolism. The importance of heightened awareness. *Postgrad Med* 1992;91:207-211, 213-214, 217-220. Review.
7. Morgenthaler TI, Ryu JH. Clinical characteristics of fatal pulmonary embolism in a referral hospital. *Mayo Clin Proc* 1995;70:417-424.
8. Stein PD, Henry JW, Gottschalk A. The addition of clinical assessment to stratification according to prior cardiopulmonary disease further optimizes the interpretation of ventilation/perfusion lung scans in pulmonary embolism. *Chest* 1993;104:1472-1476.
9. Henschke CI, Whalen JP. Evaluation of competing diagnostic tests: sequences for the diagnosis of pulmonary embolism, Part II. *Clin Imag* 1994;18:248-254.
10. Rosenow EC. Venous and pulmonary thromboembolism: An algorithmic approach to diagnosis and management. *Mayo Clin Proc* 1995;70:45-49. Review.
11. McKelvie PA. Autopsy evidence of pulmonary thromboembolism. *Med J Aust* 1994;160:127-128.
12. Dalen JE, Alpert JW. Natural history of PE. *Prog Cardiovasc Dis* 1975;17:259.
13. Lindblad B, Sternby NH, Bergqvist D. Incidence of venous thromboembolism verified by necropsy over 30 years. *BMJ* 1991;302:709-711.
14. Anderson FA, Jr., Wheeler HB, Goldberg RJ, et al. A population-based perspective of the hospital incidence and case-fatality rates of deep vein thrombosis and pulmonary embolism. The Worcester DVT Study. *Arch Intern Med* 1991;151:933-938.
15. Branch WT, McNeil BJ. Analysis of the differential diagnosis and assessment of pleuritic chest pain in young adults. *Am J Med* 1983;75:671-679.
16. Hull RD, Raskob GE, et al. Pulmonary embolism in outpatients with pleuritic chest pain. *Arch Intern Med* 1988; 148:838-844.
17. Giuntini C, Di Ricco G, Marini C, et al. Pulmonary embolism: Epidemiology. *Chest* 1995;107(1 Suppl):3S-9S.
18. Lilienfeld DE, Godbold JH. Geographic distribution of pulmonary embolism mortality rates in the United States, 1980 to 1984. *Am Heart J* 1992;124:1068-1072.
19. Heit JA. An analysis of current pulmonary embolism therapy. *Int Angiol* 1992;11:57-63. Review.
20. Carson JL, Kelley MA, Duff A, et al. The clinical course of pulmonary embolism. *N Engl J Med* 1992;326:1240-1245.
21. Green RM, Meyer TJ, Dunn M, et al. Pulmonary embolism in younger adults. *Chest* 1992;101:1507-1511.
22. Kniffin WD, Jr., Baron JA, Barrett J, et al. The epidemiology of diagnosed pulmonary embolism and deep venous thrombosis in the elderly. *Arch Intern Med* 1994;154: 861-866.

23. Thorogood M, Mann J, Murphy M, et al. Risk factors for fatal venous thromboembolism in young women: A case-control study. *Int J Epidemiol* 1992;21:48-52.
24. Goldhaber SZ, Morpurgo M. Diagnosis, treatment, and prevention of pulmonary embolism. Report of the WHO/International Society and Federation of Cardiology Task Force. *JAMA* 1992;268:1727-1733. Review.
25. Champ C, Byard RW. Pulmonary thromboembolism and unexpected death in infancy. *J Paediatr Child Health* 1994;30:550-551. Review.
26. Andrew M, David M, Adams M, et al. Venous thromboembolic complications (VTE) in children: First analyses of the Canadian Registry of VTE. *Blood* 1994;83: 1251-1257.
27. Browse NL, Thomas ML. Source of nonlethal pulmonary emboli. *Lancet* 1974;1:258.
28. Havig GO. Source of pulmonary emboli. *Acta Chir Scand* 1977;478(Suppl):42.
29. Virchow R. Ein Vortag uber die Thrombose von Jahre 1845. In: Virchow R, ed. *Gesammelte Abhandlungen zur wissenschaftlichen Medizin.* Frankfurt: Meidinger; 1856: 478-486.
30. Hastings GE, Seery DS, Vine DL. Recent developments in the diagnosis, treatment, and prevention of pulmonary embolism. *Arch Fam Med* 1993;2:655-669. Review.
31. Milne R. Venous thromboembolism and travel: Is there an association? J *R Coll Physicians London* 1992;26:47-49. Review.
32. Sahiar F, Mohler SR. Economy class syndrome. *Aviat Space Environ Med* 1994;65:957-960.
33. Clarke AM, Winson IG. Does plaster immobilization predispose to pulmonary embolism? *Injury* 1992;23:533-534.
34. Stein PD, Terrin ML, Hales CA, et al. Clinical, laboratory, roentgenographic, and electrocardiographic findings in patients with acute pulmonary embolism and no pre-existing cardiac or pulmonary disease. *Chest* 1991;100:598-603.
35. Geerts WH, Code KI, Jay RM, et al. A prospective study of venous thromboembolism after major trauma. *N Engl J Med* 1994;331:1601-1606.
36. Anderson FA, Jr., Wheeler HB. Venous thromboembolism. Risk factors and prophylaxis. *Clin Chest Med* 1995;16:235-251. Review.
37. Monreal M, Raventos A, Lerma R, et al. Pulmonary embolism in patients with upper extremity DVT associated to venous central lines—a prospective study. *Thromb Haemost* 1994;72:548-550.
38. Monreal M, Lafoz E, Ruiz J, et al. Upper-extremity deep venous thrombosis and pulmonary embolism. A prospective study. *Chest* 1991;99:280-283.
39. Nuss R, Hays T, Manco-Johnson M. Childhood thrombosis. *Pediatrics* 1995;96:291-294.
40. Briet E, van der Meer FJ, Rosendaal FR, et al. The family history and inherited thrombophilia. *Br J Haematol* 1994;87: 348-352.
41. Svensson P, Dahlback B. Resistance to activated proteinC as a basis for venous thrombosis. *N Engl J Med* 1994;330:517.
42. Melissari E, Monte G, Lindo VS, et al. Congenital thrombophilia among patients with venous thromboembolism. *Blood Coag Fibrinol* 1992;3:749-758.
43. Demers C, Ginsberg JS, Hirsh J, et al. Thrombosis in antithrombin-III-deficient persons. Report of a large kindred and literature review. *Ann Intern Med* 1992;116:754-761. Review.
44. Ginsberg KS, Liang MH, Newcomer L, et al. Anticardiolipin antibodies and the risk for ischemic stroke and venous thrombosis. *Ann Intern Med* 1992;117:997-1002.
45. Montes de Oca MA, Babron MC, Bletry O, et al. Thrombosis in systemic lupus erythematosus: A French collaborative study. *Arch Dis Child* 1991;66:713-717.
46. Monreal M, Casals A, Boix J, et al. Occult cancer in patients with acute pulmonary embolism. A prospective study. *Chest* 1993;103:816-819.
47. Gore JM, Appelbaum JS, Greene HL, et al. Occult cancer in patients with acute pulmonary embolism. *Ann Intern Med* 1982;96:556-560.
48. Zimmerman RL, Novek S, Chen JT, et al. Pulmonary thrombosis in a 10-year-old child with minimal change disease and nephrotic syndrome. A clinical, radiologic, and pathologic correlation with literature review. *Am J Clin Pathol* 1994;101:230-236.
49. Quinn DA, Thompson BT, Terrin ML, et al. A prospective investigation of pulmonary embolism in women and men. *JAMA* 1992;268:1689-1696.
50. Anderson FA, Jr., Wheeler HB. Physician practices in the management of venous thromboembolism: A community-wide survey. *J Vasc Surg* 1992;15:707.
51. Monreal M, Ruiz J, Olazabal A, et al. Deep venous thrombosis and the risk of pulmonary embolism. A systematic study. *Chest* 1992;102:677-681.
52. Saeger W, Genzkow M. Venous thromboses and pulmonary embolisms in post-mortem series: Probable causes by correlations of clinical data and basic diseases. *Pathol Res Pract* 1994;190:394-9. Review.
53. Santolicandro A, Prediletto R, Fornai E, et al. Mechanisms of hypoxemia and hypocapnia in pulmonary embolism. *Am J Respir Crit Care Med* 1995;152:336-347.
54. Elliott CG. Pulmonary physiology during pulmonary embolism. *Chest* 1992;101:163S-171S. Review.
55. Wagenvoort CA. Pathology of pulmonary thromboembolism. *Chest* 1995;107:10S-17S. Review.
56. Fedullo PF, Anger WR, Charrick C, et al. Chronic thromboembolic pulmonary hypertension. *Clin Chest Med* 1995;16:353.
57. Hoffman JM, Lee A, Grafton ST, et al. Clinical signs and symptoms in pulmonary embolism. A reassessment. *Clin Nucl Med* 1994;19:803-808.
58. Stein PD, Saltzman HA, Web J. Clinical characteristics of patients with acute pulmonary embolism. *Am J Cardiol* 1991;68:1723-1724.
59. Shaw JE, Belfield PW. Pulmonary embolism: A cause of acute confusion in the elderly. *Postgrad Med J* 1991;67: 560-561.
60. Frisbie JH, Sharma GV. Pulmonary embolism manifesting as acute disturbances of behavior in patients with spinal cord injury. *Paraplegia* 1994;32:570-572.
61. Zwecker M, Heim M, Azaria M, et al. Supraventricular

tachycardia as a presenting sign of pulmonary embolism in paraplegia. Case report and review. *Paraplegia* 1995;33: 278-280.

62. Stallman JS, Aisen PS, Aisen ML. Pulmonary embolism presenting as fever in spinal cord injury patients: Report of two cases and review of the literature. *J Am Paraplegia Soc* 1993;16:157-159. Review.
63. Stein PD. Acute pulmonary embolism. *Dis Month* 1994;40:467-523. Review.
64. Thames MD, Alpert JS, Dalen JE. Syncope in patients with pulmonary embolism. *JAMA* 1977;238:2509-2511.
65. Stein PD, Henry JW, Gopalakrishnan D, et al. Asymmetry of the calves in the assessment of patients with suspected acute pulmonary embolism. *Chest* 1995;107:936-939.
66. Grant BJB, El-Solh AA. Thromboembolic disease, optimizing recognition. *Hosp Med* 1995;31:14-24.
67. Worsley DF, Alavi A, Aronchick JM, et al. Chest radiographic findings in patients with acute pulmonary embolism: Observations from the PIOPED Study. *Radiology* 1993;189: 133-136.
68. Sreeram N, Cheriex EC, Smeets JL, et al. Value of the 12-lead electrocardiogram at hospital admission in the diagnosis of pulmonary embolism. *Am J Cardiol* 1994;73:298-303.
69. Lui CY. Acute pulmonary embolism as the cause of global T wave inversion and QT prolongation. A case report. *J Electrocardiol* 1993;26:91-95.
70. Stein PD, Goldhaber SZ, Henry JW. Alveolar-arterial oxygen gradient in the assessment of acute pulmonary embolism. *Chest* 1995;107:139-143.
71. Cvitanic O. Improved use of arterial blood gas analysis in suspected pulmonary embolism. *Chest* 1989;95:48.
72. McFarlane MJ, Imperiale TF. Use of the alveolar-arterial oxygen gradient in the diagnosis of pulmonary embolism. *Am J Med* 1994;96:57-62.
73. Jones JS, VanDeelen N, White L, et al. Alveolar-arterial oxygen gradients in elderly patients with suspected pulmonary embolism. *Ann Emerg Med* 1993;22:1177-1181.
74. de Moerloose P, Minazio P, Reber G, et al. D-dimer determination to exclude pulmonary embolism: A two-step approach using latex assay as a screening tool. *Thromb Haemost* 1994;72:89-91.
75. Ginsberg JS, Wells PS, Brill-Edwards P, et al. Application of a novel and rapid whole blood assay for D-dimer in patients with clinically suspected pulmonary embolism. *Thromb Haemost* 1995;73:35-38.
76. van Beek EJ, van den Ende B, Berckmans RJ, et al. A comparative analysis of D-dimer assays in patients with clinically suspected pulmonary embolism. *Thromb Haemost* 1993;70:408-413.
77. Pappas AA, Dalrymple G, Harrison K, et al. The application of a rapid D-dimer test in suspected pulmonary embolus. *Arch Pathol Lab Med* 1993;117:977-980.
78. Bounameaux H, Cirafici P, de Moerloose P, et al. Measurement of D-dimer in plasma as diagnostic aid in suspected pulmonary embolism. *Lancet* 1991;337:196-200.
79. Ginsberg JS, Brill-Edwards PA, Demers C, et al. D-dimer in patients with clinically suspected pulmonary embolism. *Chest* 1993;104:1679-1684.
80. Goldhaber SZ, Simons GR, Elliott CG, et al. Quantitative plasma D-dimer levels among patients undergoing pulmonary angiography for suspected pulmonary embolism. *JAMA* 1993;270:2819-2822.
81. Harrison KA, Haire WD, Pappas AA, et al. Plasma D-dimer: A useful tool for evaluating suspected pulmonary embolus. *J Nucl Med* 1993;34:896-898.
82. Demers C, Ginsberg JS, Johnston M, et al. D-dimer and thrombin-antithrombin III complexes in patients with clinically suspected pulmonary embolism. *Thromb Haemost* 1992;67:408-412.
83. Hatle L, Rokseth R. The arterial to end expiratory carbon dioxide tension gradient in acute pulmonary embolism and other cardiopulmonary diseases. *Chest* 1974;66:352-357.
84. Eriksson L, Wollmer P, Olsson CG, et al. Diagnosis of pulmonary embolism based upon alveolar dead space analysis. *Chest* 1989;96:357-362.
85. Burki NK. The dead space to tidal volume ratio in the diagnosis of pulmonary embolism. *Am Rev Respir Dis* 1986; 133:679-685.
86. Carroll GC. Capnographic trend curve monitoring can detect 1 mL pulmonary emboli in humans. *J Clin Monit* 1992;8: 101-106.
87. Pruszczyk P, Torbicki A, Kuch-Wocial A, et al. Transoesophageal echocardiography for definitive diagnosis of haemodynamically significant pulmonary embolism. *Eur Heart J* 1995;16:534-538.
88. Patel JJ, Chandrasekaran K, Maniet AR, et al. Impact of the incidental diagnosis of clinically unsuspected central pulmonary artery thromboembolism in treatment of critically ill patients. *Chest* 1994;105:986-990.
89. Nazeyrollas P, Metz D, Chapoutot L, et al. Diagnostic accuracy of echocardiography-Doppler in acute pulmonary embolism. *Int J Cardiol* 1995;47:273-280.
90. Cheriex EC, Sreeram N, Eussen YF, et al. Cross sectional Doppler echocardiography as the initial technique for the diagnosis of acute pulmonary embolism. *Br Heart J* 1994;72:52-57.
91. Johnson ME, Furlong R, Schrank K. Diagnostic use of emergency department echocardiogram in massive pulmonary emboli. *Ann Emerg Med* 1992;21:760-763.
92. Mathis G, Metzler J, Fussenegger D, et al. Sonographic observation of pulmonary infarction and early infarctions by pulmonary embolism. *Eur Heart J* 1993;14:804-808.
93. Goodman LR, Curtin JJ, Mewissen MW, et al. Detection of pulmonary embolism in patients with unresolved clinical and scintigraphic diagnosis: helical CT versus angiography. *AJR Am J Roentgenol* 1995;164:1369-1374.
94. Stanford W, Reiners TJ, Thompson BH, et al. Contrast-enhanced thin slice ultrafast computed tomography for the detection of small pulmonary emboli. Studies using autologous emboli in the pig. *Invest Radiol* 1994;29:184-187.
95. Teigen CL, Maus TP, Sheedy PF, et al. Pulmonary embolism: Diagnosis with contrast-enhanced electron-beam CT and comparison with pulmonary angiography. *Radiology* 1995;194:313-319.
96. Teigen CL, Maus TP, Sheedy PF, et al. Pulmonary embolism: Diagnosis with electron-beam CT. *Radiology* 1993;188:

839-845.

97. Erdman WA, Peshock RM, Redman HC, et al. Pulmonary embolism: Comparison of MR images with radionuclide and angiographic studies. *Radiology* 1994;190:499-508.
98. Grist TM, Sostman HD, MacFall JR, et al. Pulmonary angiography with MR imaging: Preliminary clinical experience. *Radiology* 1993;189:523-530.
99. Goldberg SN, Palmer EL, Scott JA, et al. Pulmonary embolism: Prediction of the usefulness of initial ventilation-perfusion scanning with chest radiographic findings. *Radiology* 1994;193:801-805.
100. Spritzer CE, Norconk JJ, Jr., Sostman HD, et al. Detection of deep venous thrombosis by magnetic resonance imaging. *Chest* 1993;104:54-60.
101. Evans AJ, Sostman HD, Knelson MH, et al. 1992 ARRS Executive Council Award. Detection of deep venous thrombosis: prospective comparison of MR imaging with contrast venography. *AJR Am J Roentgenol* 1993;161: 131-139.
102. Spritzer CE, Evans AC, Kay HH. Magnetic resonance imaging of deep venous thrombosis in pregnant women with lower extremity edema. *Obstet Gynecol* 1995;85:603-607.
103. van Beek EJ, Kuyer PM, Schenk BE, et al. A normal perfusion lung scan in patients with clinically suspected pulmonary embolism. Frequency and clinical validity. *Chest* 1995;108:170-173.
104. Hull RD. Clinical validity of a normal perfusion lung scan in patients with suspected pulmonary embolism. *Chest* 1990; 97:23.
105. Ralph DD. Pulmonary embolism. The implications of prospective investigation of pulmonary embolism diagnosis. *Radiol Clin North Am* 1994;32:679-687.
106. McCabe JL, Grossman SJ, Joyce JM. Ventilation-perfusion scintigraphy. *Emerg Med Clin North Am* 1991;9:805-825. Review.
107. Worsley DF, Palevsky HI, Alavi A. A detailed evaluation of patients with acute pulmonary embolism and low- or very-low-probability lung scan interpretations. *Arch Intern Med* 1994;154:2737-2741.
108. Freitas JE, Sarosi MG, Nagle CC, et al. Modified PIOPED criteria used in clinical practice. *J Nucl Med* 1995;36: 1573-1578.
109. Gottschalk A, Juni JE, Sostman HD, et al. Ventilation-perfusion scintigraphy in the PIOPED study. Part I. Data collection and tabulation. J Nucl Med 1993;34:1109-1118.
110. Sostman HD, Coleman RE, DeLong DM, et al. Evaluation of revised criteria for ventilation-perfusion scintigraphy in patients with suspected pulmonary embolism. *Radiology* 1994;193:103-107.
111. Lesser BA, Leeper KV, Jr., Stein PD, et al. The diagnosis of acute pulmonary embolism in patients with chronic obstructive pulmonary disease. *Chest* 1992;102:17-22.
112. Stein PD, Coleman RE, Gottschalk A, et al. Diagnostic utility of ventilation/perfusion lung scans in acute pulmonary embolism is not diminished by pre-existing cardiac or pulmonary disease. *Chest* 1991;100:604-606.
113. van Beek EJ, Tiel-Van Buul MM, Hoefnagel CA, et al. Reporting of perfusion/ventilation lung scintigraphy using an anatomical lung segment chart: A prospective study. *Nucl Med Comm* 1994;15:746-751.
114. Gray HW, McKillop JH, Bessent RG. Lung scan reporting language: what does it mean? *Nucl Med Comm* 1993;14: 1084-1087.
115. Schluger N, Henschke C, King T, et al. Diagnosis of pulmonary embolism at a large teaching hospital. *J Thorac Imag* 1994;9:180-184.
116. Ginsberg JS, Wells PS, Hirsh J, et al. Reevaluation of the sensitivity of impedance plethysmography for the detection of proximal deep vein thrombosis. *Arch Intern Med* 1994;154:1930-1933.
117. Labropoulos N, Leon M, Kalodiki E, et al. Colour flow duplex scanning in suspected acute deep vein thrombosis; experience with routine use. *Eur J Vasc Endovasc Surg* 1995; 9:49-52.
118. Kearon C, Hirsh J. The diagnosis of pulmonary embolism. *Haemostasis* 1995;25:72-87. Review.
119. Smith LL, Iber C, Sirr S. Pulmonary embolism: Confirmation with venous duplex US as adjunct to lung scanning. *Radiology* 1994;191:143-147.
120. Bradley MJ, Alexander L. The role of venous colour flow Doppler to aid the non-diagnostic lung scintigram for pulmonary embolism. *Clin Radiol* 1995;50:232-234.
121. Beecham RP, Dorfman GS, Cronan JJ, et al. Is bilateral lower extremity compression sonography useful and cost-effective in the evaluation of suspected pulmonary embolism? *AJR Am J Roentgenol* 1993;161:1289-1292.
122. Hull RD, Raskob GE, Ginsberg JS, et al. A noninvasive strategy for the treatment of patients with suspected pulmonary embolism. *Arch Intern Med* 1994;154:289-297.
123. Henry JW, Relyea B, Stein PD. Continuing risk of thromboemboli among patients with normal pulmonary angiograms. *Chest* 1995;107:1375-1378.
124. Stein PD, Athanasoulis C, Alavi A, et al. Complications and validity of pulmonary angiography in acute pulmonary embolism. *Circulation* 1992;85:462-468.
125. van Rooij WJ, den Heeten GJ, Sluzewski M. Pulmonary embolism: Diagnosis in 211 patients with use of selective pulmonary digital subtraction angiography with a flow-directed catheter. *Radiology* 1995;195:793-797.
126. Cooper TJ, Hayward MW, Hartog M. Survey on the use of pulmonary scintigraphy and angiography for suspected pulmonary thromboembolism in the UK. *Clin Radiol* 1991; 43:243-245.
127. Stein PD, Gottschalk A, Saltzman HA, et al. Diagnosis of acute pulmonary embolism in the elderly. *J Am Coll Cardiol* 1991;18:1452-1457.
128. De Bruyn VH, Bergmann SR, Keyt BA, et al. Visualization of thrombi in pulmonary arteries with radiolabeled, enzymatically inactivated tissue-type plasminogen activator. *Circulation* 1995;92:1320-1325.
129. King MA, Bergin CJ, Yeung DW, et al. Chronic pulmonary thromboembolism: Detection of regional hypoperfusion with CT. *Radiology* 1994;191:359-363.
130. Matsumoto AH, Tegtmeyer CJ. Contemporary diagnostic approaches to acute pulmonary emboli. *Radiol Clin North Am* 1995;33:167-183. Review.

131. Greenspan RH. Pulmonary angiography and the diagnosis of pulmonary embolism. *Prog Cardiovasc Dis* 1994;37:93-105. Review.

132. Tapson VF, Gurbel PA, Witty LA, et al. Pharmacomechanical thrombolysis of experimental pulmonary emboli. Rapid low-dose intraembolic therapy. *Chest* 1994;106:1558-1562.

133. Patil S, Henry JW, Rubenfire M, et al. Neural network in the clinical diagnosis of acute pulmonary embolism. *Chest* 1993; 104:1685-1689.

134. Tourassi GD, Floyd CE, Sostman HD, et al. Acute pulmonary embolism: artificial neural network approach for diagnosis. *Radiology* 1993;189:555-558.

135. Philbrick JT, Becker DM. Calf deep venous thrombosis. A wolf in sheep's clothing? *Arch Intern Med* 1988;148: 2131-2138.

136. Saeger W, Genzkow M. Venous thromboses and pulmonary embolisms in post-mortem series: Probable causes by correlations of clinical data and basic diseases. *Pathol Res Pract* 1994;190:394-399. Review.

137. Giachino A. Relationship between deep vein thrombosis in the calf and fatal pulmonary embolism. *Can J Surg* 1988;31: 129-130.

138. Black MD, French GJ, Rasuli P, et al. Upper extremity deep venous thrombosis. Underdiagnosed and potentially lethal. *Chest* 1993;103:1887-1890.

Pulmonary Embolism: Diagnosis and Management

Stephen A. Colucciello, MD, FACEP

Pulmonary embolism (PE), a common diagnostic consideration in patients presenting to emergency departments (EDs), remains a frequent cause of death in the United States. PE can be quite difficult to recognize and diagnose even when considered by the astute clinician. It is especially important to appreciate that PE may cause shortness of breath in patients with underlying cardiorespiratory disease.

In this chapter the extensive diagnostic considerations for PE patients are reviewed, and specific recommendations are provided based on the medical literature. Discussions on the treatment of the moribund patient suspected of PE are highlighted, as well as the potential future role of low molecular weight heparins, thrombolytic therapy, and the evaluation and management of PE in the pregnant patient.

Differential Diagnosis

The differential diagnosis of PE is astoundingly broad. *(Please see Table 1.)* It can encompass any condition that produces chest pain, shortness of breath, cough, wheezing, or syncope. The emergency physician should assess risk factors for thromboembolic disease in such patients. Physical findings, such as a palpable cord or Kussmaul's sign, occasionally provide a clue to PE.

The differential diagnosis of massive PE includes any significant cardiopulmonary insult that results in shock, such as acute myocardial infarction (MI), congestive heart failure, aortic dissection, volume loss, sepsis, or drug reaction. Crushing, anginal-type chest pain occurs in 4% of PE patients, but in the PIOPED study no patient had radiation of pain to the arms or jaw.[1] Evaluate patients who may have acute MI or aortic dissection with ECG and chest x-ray. The ECG also can detect pericarditis, while a normal chest x-ray excludes pneumothorax.

Emergency physicians frequently misdiagnose PE as chest wall syndrome, pleurisy, pneumonia, or anxiety attack. Recognize that patients with PE may have chest wall tenderness and pain with chest torsion. Clinical response to nonsteroidal anti-inflammatory drugs (NSAIDs) in this setting certainly *does not* rule out PE. Pleurisy often is clinically indistinguishable from PE. Both produce pleuritic chest pain. Clues to PE may include tachycardia, tachypnea, widened A-a gradient, and abnormal chest x-ray. While a friction rub sometimes occurs with pleurisy, a rub is more common with PE. Liberal use of V/Q scans best distinguishes pleurisy from PE.

PE also masquerades as acute pneumonia. Patients with PE may have a low-grade fever, a cough productive of purulent

Table 1. Differential Diagnosis of Pulmonary Embolism

- Pleurisy
- Pneumothorax/Pneumomediastinum
- Pneumonia
- Cocaine abuse
- Chest wall syndrome/Costochondritis
- Drug reaction
- Anxiety attack
- Sepsis
- Acute myocardial infarction
- Unusual emboli (fat, air, missile, tumor)
- Pericarditis
- Asthma
- Aortic dissection
- Congestive heart failure
- Metabolic acidosis

Table 2. Management of the Moribund Patient with Suspected Pulmonary Embolism

1. High-flow O_2—intubate as needed.
2. Repeat small boluses of crystalloid—evaluate for response.
3. Vasopressors as indicated (norepinephrine or epinephrine drip).
4. Chest x-ray and ECG.
5. Transesophageal echo or transthoracic echo if available.
6. Thrombolytics for PE based upon echo or strong clinical suspicion.
7. Open-chest CPR as indicated.

sputum, shortness of breath, and an infiltrate on chest x-ray.[1] The time course of the disease provides some clue, as the onset of PE is often more abrupt. While many patients with PE are febrile, temperatures are rarely higher than 102°F. Entertain the diagnosis of PE in patients with apparent pneumonia, and if multiple risk factors for thromboembolic disease are present, consider further testing. Patients with an infiltrate on chest x-ray usually have a nondiagnostic V/Q scan consisting of a matched defect. Angiography often is necessary to differentiate such cases. MRI distinguishes parenchymal consolidation from pulmonary infarction and may play an increasing role in the future.

Chest pain associated with crack cocaine use also can mimic PE. Pulmonary vasoconstriction secondary to cocaine produces V/Q scans compatible with embolism. A clinical history of cocaine use or a positive toxicology screen is essential for this diagnosis.

Not all emboli are fibrin clots. Atrial myxoma can produce recurrent emboli of tumor fragments.[2] Similarly, dyspnea or chest pain in a cancer patient may be associated with tumor emboli. Scuba diving accidents, blunt or penetrating chest trauma, and central line insertions generate air emboli. An unusual form of air embolism results from blowing air into the vagina of a pregnant woman during cunnilingus. Amniotic fluid embolism is a rare event that occurs only during pregnancy and is isolated to labor or immediately after significant trauma. In the first 24-48 hours after a long bone fracture, fat emboli develop, which can lead to altered mental status and petechiae.[3] Occasionally reported is missile embolus, which occurs when a foreign body, usually a bullet, enters a blood vessel and travels to the lung.[4] All of these unusual conditions involve a very distinct clinical scenario.

Diagnosis and Management

Up to 8% of patients with PE may present in extremis.[5,6] Such patients require airway management, high-flow O_2, and, frequently, intubation.[5] Rapidly obtain venous access and give 250-500 cc of crystalloid. If the blood pressure rises, titrate additional fluid as needed. Excessive fluid may be counterproductive in massive PE and has been reported to worsen hypotension.[7] Consider vasopressors such as norepinephrine or epinephrine to support the circulation.[8] Streamline the diagnostic work-up of patients who arrive in profound distress. Such patients require an ECG to rule out acute MI and a chest x-ray to exclude tension pneumothorax, thoracic dissection, and other catastrophes. While bedside transthoracic or transesophageal echocardiography may provide rapid diagnosis of PE, such technologies are not available in all EDs. If patients leave the department for V/Q scan or angiography, recognize the potential for decompensation. Patients with a strong clinical likelihood of PE who present in extremis may be treated empirically with heparin.[9] Thrombolytics are especially useful for patients who present in shock with a clinical picture compatible with massive PE. They may be lifesaving when PE is the cause of cardiac arrest.

Closed-chest CPR is usually ineffective when cardiac arrest is caused by massive embolus. In other cases, CPR may break up clots and save patients with "saddle" embolus. If thrombolytics are unavailable, further resuscitation (if indicated) could include ED thoracotomy and manual compression of the heart.[7] "Milking" the pulmonary artery has been reported to disintegrate or advance the clot, while clot removal is possible via

Figure 1. Workup of Suspected Pulmonary Embolism

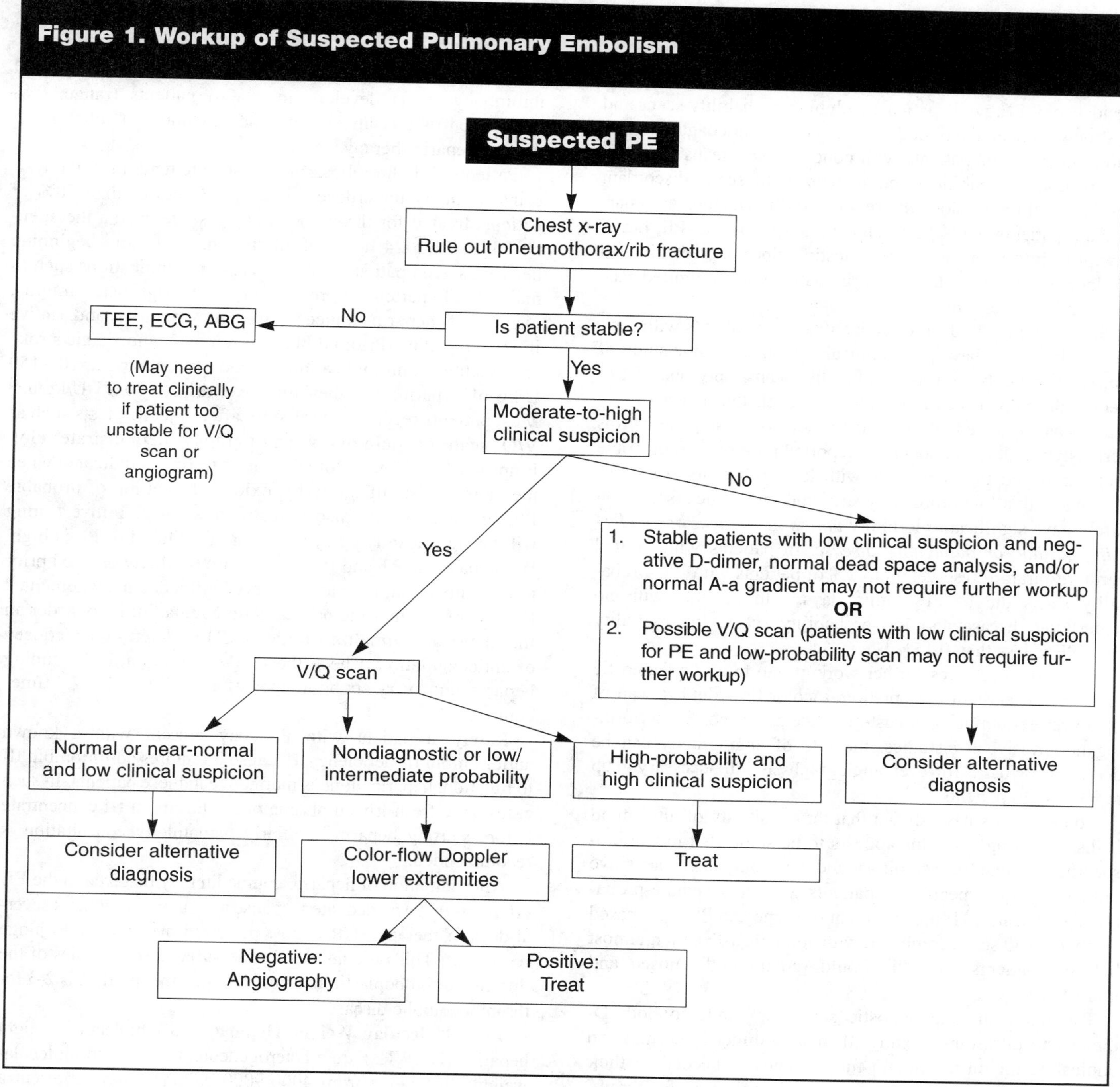

open thrombectomy. Emergency femoral-femoral bypass may be lifesaving but is rarely available in the ED.[10] *(Please see Table 2.)*

Fortunately, most ED patients with PE are not moribund. Some may be dyspneic, and pulse oximetry in conjunction with physical examination rapidly identifies patients who require oxygen. Arterial blood gases, while frequently helpful, are not mandatory as part of the workup of PE. All patients suspected of PE require chest radiography. Obtain an ECG in patients who are unstable or who may have a cardiac etiology for their chest pain.

Decision-Making. *(Please see Figure 1.)* If clinical suspicion for PE is low, a combination of chest x-ray and blood tests may obviate the need for V/Q scanning. In the stable patient with minimal or no risk factors for thromboembolic disease, a normal A-a gradient, and a negative D-dimer by ELISA makes PE very unlikely. This strategy, however, is not foolproof. The A-a gradient may be normal in 8-10% of patients with PE,[11] and the D-dimer by latex agglutination may be normal in 5-10%.[12-14] Whether the D-dimer would pick up cases missed by A-a gradient and vice versa requires further study. Patients with unexplained shortness of breath and/or pleuritic chest pain require V/Q scans. In general, the management of patients with diagnostic scans is straightforward. Patients with normal or near-normal scans and a low clinical suspicion have a very low incidence of PE, while patients with high-probability scans and a strong clinical likelihood of PE require anticoagulation or thrombolysis. It is patients with nondiagnostic scans (low and intermediate probability) and patients with scans discordant with clinical impression who require additional studies. In particular, patients with high clinical suspicion of PE but a low-probability scan need further testing. Special precautions to exclude PE may be necessary in patients with limited cardiopulmonary reserve.

It is of some comfort to realize that most patients with low-probability scans have good clinical outcomes. In one study of untreated patients with low-probability scans, only one of 173 people developed recurrent PE.[15] However, the power of this study was weakened by the fact that none of these patients was seriously ill. Other authors have reported poor or fatal outcome from untreated PE in patients with low-probability scans.[16,17] Patients with a low-probability scan and low clinical suspicion rarely have significant morbidity *unless the patient has underlying cardiac or pulmonary disease.* In patients with limited cardiorespiratory reserve, up to 8% of patients with low-probability scans die of PE within days.[18] In patients with no underlying disease and low-probability scans, the mortality from PE is less than 0.15%.[18]

If a patient requires further workup due to a nondiagnostic scan or a discordant presentation, a color-flow duplex scan of the lower extremities is a cost-effective approach. By performing noninvasive leg studies, the rate of angiography can be decreased by half. However, angiography is still necessary in up to 33% of all patients.[19-21]

Some authors have shown that the sensitivity of ultrasound is disappointing. Its value appears to be somewhat institution-specific. In one series, ultrasound was only 13% sensitive (although 100% specific) in patients with intermediate-probability V/Q scans.[22] If the treatment of suspected PE were based solely on V/Q scans combined with color-flow Doppler, almost half the patients with PE would remain undiagnosed and untreated.[23]

Patients with nondiagnostic scans can undergo both D-dimer and ultrasound testing. If their D-dimer is normal and clinical suspicion is low, no further study is needed. If their ultrasound is positive, the patient requires therapy for thromboembolic disease. This strategy can decrease pulmonary angiography by at least one-third.[24] If the clinical suspicion for PE is very high, neither a negative D-dimer nor a normal ultrasound can effectively rule out PE. Such patients require angiography.[22]

Therapy

The ED management of the stable patient with PE centers on prevention of recurrent embolism. Heparin is the mainstay of treatment. Heparin prevents the conversion of fibrinogen to fibrin through the activation of antithrombin III and inhibits factors XIIa, XIa, IXa, and Xa.[25] Significant bleeding can result with heparin, but rarely during the ED loading phase. Seven to thirty percent of patients ultimately bleed, and complications occur at a rate of 1-3% per day.[26] Heparin-induced thrombocytopenia develops in 3% of patients (range, 0.8-26.0%), but is a relatively late phenomenon that follows 3-5 days of heparin therapy.[27,28]

Patients with thrombosis are resistant to heparin, and physicians routinely underdose this drug.[29,30] Fewer than 50% of patients treated for thromboembolic disease have a therapeutic PTT within 24 hours of admission.[31,32] Before beginning heparin, screen patients for absolute contraindications such as malignant hypertension, recent surgery or significant trauma, history of heparin-induced thrombocytopenia, and active internal bleeding. Prior GI bleed or remote hemorrhagic stroke are relative contraindications. Load patients with 100-150 U/kg of heparin, and then initiate a drip at 20-25 U/kg/h.[33] Most patients receive heparin only after objective tests such as V/Q scan or pulmonary angiography demonstrate clot. Empiric ED loading before definitive testing is indicated when the patient is significantly hypoxic in the setting of probable PE. Empiric loading also is justified when definitive testing will be significantly delayed and the likelihood of PE is high. While baseline PT and PTT values are routinely ordered prior to heparinization, they almost never influence management.[34] Document whether the patient is on coumadin; if so, order an International Normalized Ratio (INR) to determine adequacy of anticoagulation. Check the PTT six hours after beginning heparin, and every six hours thereafter until it is 1.5-2.5 times control.[35,36]

Rarely, a patient with PE may present with a known antithrombin III deficiency. Because it requires antithrombin III to function, heparin alone is ineffective in these patients. In such cases, give fresh frozen plasma or antithrombin III concentrate before starting heparin.[37,38] Early hematology consultation is recommended.

After initiation of heparin, coumadin may be given in the ED (10 mg po).[39] An adequate response to coumadin requires several days of therapy. INR is now preferred over the PT to judge response.[40] This ratio adjusts for the variable sensitivities of the different thromboplastin reagents.[41] A therapeutic INR is 2-3 for thromboembolic disease.[36]

Low Molecular Weight Heparin. Low molecular weight heparins (LMWHs) are a heterogeneous family with molecular weights that range from 4000-9000 daltons. They represent a significant advance in the treatment of thromboembolic disease. While most studies on LMWH involve DVT, one study showed that subcutaneous LMWH was superior to IV unfractionated heparin in the treatment of submassive PE.[42]

Subcutaneous LMWH has greater antithrombotic effects and fewer adverse consequences than IV heparin.[43-45] Because they are more bioavailable and have a longer half-life than unfractionated heparin, LMWHs are given subcutaneously once or twice a day. Unlike unfractionated heparin, LMWH has little effect on thrombin or platelet aggregation, so hemorrhagic complications are rare and there is less tendency to develop thrombocytopenia.[46] Because these drugs primarily inhibit factor Xa and do not elevate the PTT, laboratory studies

Table 3. FDA-Approved Regimens for Thrombolysis of Pulmonary Embolism

- t-PA 100 mg IV over two hours
- Urokinase 4400 U/kg IV over 10 minutes, then 4400 U/kg/h for 12-24 hours
- Streptokinase 250,000 units IV over 30 minutes, then 100,000 units per hour for 24 hours

Heparin can be initiated once infusion is complete and PTT is less than 80. No loading dose is necessary.

are not necessary to determine adequate anticoagulation. The dose is either fixed or based on the patient's weight and is not adjusted according to the PTT. Due to its safety and ease of use, LMWH may someday treat PE in outpatients.

LMWH is currently approved in the United States for prophylaxis after orthopedic surgery to the lower extremities. It awaits FDA licensing for the treatment of DVT and PE. Heparinoids such as danaparoid are closely related to LMWH and may have similar advantages over unfractionated heparin in the treatment of venous thromboembolism.[44]

Thrombolysis. Fewer than 10% of patients in the United States receive thrombolysis for PE.[47] *(Please see Table 3.)* However, thrombolysis represents a significant advance in the treatment of PE.[48] While thrombolytics produce rapid resolution of emboli and early improvement in hemodynamics,[49] no one has ever shown that lytic agents decrease mortality.[50] After one week, patients treated with heparin have equivalent cardiovascular and pulmonary parameters to those of patients treated with thrombolytics. Early trials of thrombolytics such as UPET showed a 45% complication rate and a 100% increase in intracranial bleeds compared to heparin alone. However, most bleeding complications were related to the use of invasive procedures and aggressive diagnostic phlebotomy.[50] Since the 1970s, greater experience and newer agents have decreased complications and introduced a new era of thrombolysis in acute PE. Major bleeds occur in only 4% of patients treated with t-PA, and intracranial bleeds develop in less than 1%. In the elderly, t-PA causes no additional bleeding compared to younger patients.[51] While surgery within two weeks is considered a contraindication for thrombolysis, urokinase infused into the pulmonary artery safely dissolved pulmonary emboli without adverse effects in 13 postoperative patients.[52] In a compelling trial of t-PA plus heparin vs. heparin alone, right ventricular function improved in 34% with t-PA compared to 17% with heparin. Pulmonary perfusion increased 15% with t-PA and only 2% with heparin.[53] Surprisingly, the group treated with heparin alone had more adverse effects, including recurrent PE.

In the past, some authorities recommended intrapulmonary lytics.[54] It is important for the emergency physician to realize that IV t-PA is as effective as an intrapulmonary infusion of the drug.[54] While bolus administration may be helpful during CPR, there is no advantage in bolus t-PA over the standard two-hour infusion for patients who still have a pulse.[55] A two-hour t-PA infusion dissolves clot more rapidly than the standard 12- or 24-hour urokinase protocol, with fewer complications.[56] The approved urokinase infusion takes 12-24 hours; however, an accelerated dose of 3 million units over two hours (with the initial 1 million units given over 10 minutes) has been shown to be safe and effective.[57]

Thrombolysis is no longer considered a heroic therapy in PE. Initiate thrombolysis when the patient is in shock or in marked respiratory distress.[58] Screen carefully for contraindications before giving thrombolytics, being mindful that contraindications are relatively common in this patient population. Lytic agents may be life-saving for patients with suspected PE who present in cardiac arrest. Case series reveal a 55-100% survival rate following a lytic bolus to patients with PE receiving CPR.[58] Most reports used a bolus of 2 million units of urokinase, although t-PA would be a reasonable alternative.[59] In contrast to the narrow time limits associated with thrombolysis in acute MI, there is a two-week window in which to use thrombolytics in PE. The only laboratory tests necessary to initiate thrombolysis are a hemoglobin level and a type and screen.[47] Angiographic proof of PE is not necessary in all cases. A high-probability V/Q scan coupled with a high clinical suspicion provides an adequate level of certainty.[60] In the truly unstable patient, a strong clinical suspicion alone may be sufficient.

Begin heparin only after the lytic infusion is complete. Heparin infusion should be started without a bolus when the PTT is less than 80.[47] Because 20% of patients with massive PE re-embolize during lytic therapy, some authorities suggest placement of a temporary caval umbrella.[61]

Mechanical Barriers. Vena caval filters are indicated in patients with strong contraindications to anticoagulation and in patients who develop recurrent thromboembolism despite adequate anticoagulation.[62] Up to 7% of patients develop recurrent pulmonary emboli while on adequate doses of IV heparin and thus require a filter.[63] Some authorities recommend these "umbrellas," instead of heparin, as primary therapy in patients with cancer and thromboembolic disease.[64] The efficacy and complication rate of vena caval filters compare favorably to anticoagulation. Procedural morbidity is small, although DVT may occasionally occur at the puncture site.[65] Commonly used devices include the stainless steel Greenfield filters, titanium Greenfield filters with modified hook, the Vena Tech filter, Simon Nitinol filter, and the bird's nest filter. Complications appear most often with the bird's nest filter, which has a 15% symptomatic caval thrombosis associated with significant mortality.[66] Recurrent PE occurs in only 4% of patients with the stainless steel Greenfield filter.[67] The long-term caval patency of this filter is 96%, and it is associated with minimal to no excess mortality.[66] Vena caval interruption only prevents further emboli and does not treat an acute clot.

Embolectomy. Patients who are not candidates for anticoag-

Table 4. Workup of Suspected Pulmonary Embolism During Pregnancy

1. Chest x-ray (shield uterus)
2. Consider color-flow duplex ultrasound of lower extremities (false-positives after 20 weeks' gestation)*
3. Reduced-dose perfusion scan after Foley catheter and brisk hydration
4. Perform ventilation scan only if perfusion is abnormal
5. Perform limited pulmonary angiogram with shielding if V/Q scan is nondiagnostic

* Many authorities recommend V/Q scanning prior to duplex ultrasound.

ulation and are acutely unstable may be candidates for an invasive procedure, such as embolectomy. Mortality for embolectomy is high, as only the most unstable patients undergo the procedure. However, embolectomy may be the only option for the moribund patient with absolute contraindications to anticoagulation or thrombolysis.[68] Techniques include both open and percutaneous approaches. Transvenous catheter embolectomy done under local anesthesia provides a relatively safe and effective alternative to open embolectomy, which requires cardiopulmonary bypass. Percutaneous embolectomy may save 70% of patients with major or massive PE, a figure equivalent to lytic therapy.[69,70] Suction devices introduced into the pulmonary artery may pull the clot out, but clot fragmentation by laser has also been reported.[71] A simple pulmonary artery catheter can also break up clot.[72] In rare circumstances, a percutaneously introduced pulmonary artery stent may be life-saving.[73]

Additional Aspects

Pulmonary Embolism in Pregnancy. PE is common in pregnancy *(please see Table 4)* and occurs in one out of every 2000 pregnant women.[74-76] It is a leading cause of pregnancy-related mortality in the United States.[74] and is responsible for approximately 15% of all deaths among pregnant women.[75] For years, experts believed that thromboembolic disease was isolated to the third trimester, but recent data show that the risk is increased throughout pregnancy.[77] Age older than 30, obesity, multiparity, prolonged bed rest, and cesarean section all predispose to embolism.[78,79] It is ironic that while PE is so common and dangerous during pregnancy, physicians are reluctant to order the tests necessary to make the diagnosis. The danger of fetal death secondary to maternal PE *far* outweighs the risk of radiation involved in V/Q scanning or the risks of unnecessary anticoagulation.[33,76,79] Mortality of untreated PE in pregnancy is 12.8%; this drops to 0.7% with therapy.[80] While consultation with an obstetrician is not inappropriate, the emergency physician *must* order the necessary studies if clinical suspicion exists.

Interpret ABGs in light of the altered physiology of pregnancy. Pregnant women normally have a compensated respiratory alkalosis and a widened A-a gradient. Because the PO_2 drops 15 mm in the supine position during pregnancy, obtain the ABG while the patient is sitting or standing.

A chest x-ray is necessary to exclude pneumothorax and other acute thoracic disorders. Place a lead shield over the uterus to decrease fetal radiation exposure. A color-flow duplex scan of the lower extremities is a reasonable initial test in a pregnant woman suspected of PE. While duplex scans are very sensitive for proximal DVT, they are inadequate to rule out PE. Patients with a negative scan will require further workup. After 20 weeks' gestation, duplex scans are more difficult to interpret and may be falsely abnormal.[81] This is due to altered venous return associated with vena cava compression by the uterus. MRI is very sensitive and specific for DVT and may play a role in the evaluation of pregnant women. However, the American College of Obstetricians and Gynecologists does not recommend MRI during the first trimester due to lack of sufficient data.[82]

Most authorities recommend V/Q scans as the diagnostic test of choice for pregnant women suspected of PE. There are no reports of adverse fetal outcomes secondary to V/Q scanning. A reduced dose perfusion scan results in small radiation exposure to the fetus (0.006-0.14 rads)—less radiation than a standard chest x-ray.[83,84] Fetal exposures of less than 5 rads are considered safe.[83] A normal perfusion scan would essentially rule out PE. Perform a ventilation scan only if the perfusion component is abnormal. There is good evidence from the PIOPED study that the ventilation component of the V/Q scan adds very little compared to the perfusion scan alone.[85] During the V/Q scan, 85% of fetal radiation exposure comes from the ventilation agent, which collects in the maternal bladder.[86] By hydrating the woman and placing a Foley catheter, fetal exposure is reduced. A complete V/Q scan yields a maximum fetal exposure of about 0.050 rads. If pulmonary angiography is necessary, arrange for a limited study with non-ionic contrast performed with a shielded uterus. A unilateral, selective angiogram with shielding results in an acceptable fetal exposure.[84]

Pregnant women with thromboembolism require intravenous heparin for 4-5 days, with subsequent administration of subcutaneous heparin after discharge. LMWH is safe and effective in pregnancy, and in the near future should replace unfractionated heparin. Coumadin is contraindicated during pregnancy due to its teratogenic effects. Authorities have long considered pregnancy a contraindication to thrombolytics, but lytics have been safely used in a pregnant woman with life-threatening PE.[87] They have even been used during labor, although massive transfusions were required.[88] Consider embolectomy, if rapidly available, for the treatment of pregnant women with acute, life-threatening PE.

Management of the Patient on Coumadin. Recurrent thromboembolism occurs in 10-20% of adequately anticoagulated patients.[89] Measure the INR in patients on coumadin

Table 5. Pitfalls in the Management of Pulmonary Embolism

1. Failure to aggressively treat and diagnose the moribund patient. Such patients require empiric thrombolytics if clinical suspicion for PE is strong and no contraindications exist.
2. Failure to use thrombolytics in patients with hypotension or significant respiratory distress.
3. Failure to adequately load with heparin.
4. Failure to load with heparin if clinical suspicion is strong and diagnostic studies will be delayed.
5. Waiting for results of PT/PTT before beginning heparin (if patient is not on coumadin).
6. Failure to arrange for placement of IVC filter in patients with absolute contraindications to anticoagulation.
7. Failure to order IVC filter in patients with recurrent thromboembolism despite adequate anticoagulation.
8. Failure to aggressively diagnose PE during pregnancy.
9. Failure to insist upon immediate V/Q scans for patients with contraindications to anticoagulation.

suspected of PE. Patients who have an INR of less than 2 are inadequately anticoagulated. If objective tests demonstrate PE, give intravenous heparin and increase their coumadin. When a patient has PE despite an INR of greater than 2, aggressive therapy is indicated. Start heparin in the ED and consult a specialist to place a vena caval filter. While some authorities add aspirin or other antiplatelet therapy to coumadin, definitive treatment is vena cava interruption.

Limited Resources. The diagnosis of PE may be limited by hospital resources. Some hospitals may not have V/Q or angiographic capabilities, and even the largest hospitals have limited resources at night. Patients with good cardiopulmonary reserve who have a low clinical suspicion for PE may await studies in the morning without receiving heparin in the interim. Scoring systems may help the clinician identify patients who require empiric therapy prior to radiologic studies.[90,91] A negative D-dimer test by ELISA would further decrease the likelihood of significant PE. If patients have a strong clinical probability of PE and no contraindications, begin heparin while awaiting V/Q scan. However, in one study, 7% of patients who ultimately proved *not* to have PE suffered major bleeding complications with this strategy.[92] Empiric heparin is not likely to be dangerous if there are no contraindications and V/Q scanning is performed immediately the following day. Patients with a strong clinical likelihood of PE who have contraindications to heparin pose the greatest nighttime quandary. In these cases, the emergency physician must mobilize the full resources of the hospital. This includes calling in necessary technicians and radiologists for appropriate diagnostic evaluation.

The Clinically Insignificant Embolus. It is very expensive to detect and treat every patient with PE. But what if some emboli are clinically insignificant and require neither diagnosis nor treatment? If this is true, resources could be redirected to patients at highest risk of death or disability. One study reviewed PIOPED patients who had initial negative angiograms and were consequently not treated for PE.[93] Angiograms were later reviewed by an expert panel, who determined that 20 patients had missed emboli restricted to small or peripheral branches of the pulmonary arteries. There was no difference in the number of fatal PEs between patients with small untreated emboli and treated controls. Unfortunately, the small numbers in this study limit its statistical power. Other authors suggest that small pulmonary emboli have epidemiologic but no clinical import. If treatment is not indicated for these small emboli, extensive investigation is also unwarranted.[94] In a prospective study, 92 patients with pleuritic chest pain underwent very limited evaluation. Chest x-rays were performed in 91%, ABGs in 23%, V/Q scans in 17%, and Doppler scans in 3%. Only one patient was diagnosed with PE and none required subsequent hospital admission.[95] Whether many more patients had minor PE that would have been diagnosed by angiography remains unknown. Clearly, this small study cannot be extrapolated to populations in whom the risk of fatal or recurrent PE is high.

Some authorities believe that a nondiagnostic V/Q scan combined with a negative noninvasive leg study ends the workup for PE.[96] They feel that such patients do not need angiography despite strong clinical suspicion. They argue that emboli discovered only by angiography are clinically benign, and in the absence of venous disease do not require treatment. This is a minority opinion. Patients with a low-probability scan who have a high clinical likelihood for PE *and comorbidity* remain at risk for fatal PE. They should undergo angiography even if noninvasive studies are negative. There are many reports in the literature of patients with low-probability V/Q scans who later die of PE.

Disposition

Admit patients with PE to the hospital. Those with hemodynamic or respiratory compromise require thrombolytics and intensive care. Internal medicine physicians will manage most patients admitted with PE. Consult specialists able to insert a vena caval filter when the patient has absolute contraindications to heparin, or if emboli occur in adequately anticoagulated patients. Expanded FDA approval of LMWH may make outpatient therapy of DVT, and even PE, a cost-effective alternative for stable patients.

Summary

The detection of PE hinges upon clinical suspicion. The physician must assess risk factors and estimate the patient's cardiopulmonary reserve. Physical examination, chest-ray, and ABG can rarely exclude PE but can suggest whether clinically significant embolism is likely. V/Q scan together with clinical judgment are the main tools in the diagnosis of PE. Further testing is necessary if the scan is nondiagnostic or if the clinical suspicion conflicts with scan results. Since the publication of the PIOPED data, physicians order significantly more ultrasound studies of the lower extremities and fewer angiograms.[97] In the future, combinations of dead space analysis and D-dimer may effectively identify high- and low-risk patients. As technology improves, CT or MRI may replace V/Q scans as the primary imaging modality. An important research goal will be to identify those patients with clinically significant emboli. This will limit intensive investigation to those who need it.[98]

The treatment of most pulmonary emboli requires adequate doses of unfractionated IV heparin, but thrombolytics are expected to play a growing role. *(Please see Table 5.)* In the near future, subcutaneous LMWH will provide a safer and more effective treatment than unfractionated heparin. Due to these advances, the use of vena caval filters and embolectomy will remain select interventions for a minority of patients.

References

1. Stein PD, Terrin ML, Hales CA, et al. Clinical, laboratory, roentgenographic, and electrocardiographic findings in patients with acute pulmonary embolism and no pre-existing cardiac or pulmonary disease. *Chest* 1991;100:598-603.
2. Miyauchi Y, Endo T, Kuroki S, et al. Right atrial myxoma presenting with recurrent episodes of pulmonary embolism. *Cardiology* 1992;81:178-181.
3. Fulde GW, Harrison P. Fat embolism—a review. *Arch Emerg Med* 1991;8:233-239.
4. John LC, Edmondson SJ. Bullet pulmonary embolus and the role of surgery. *Thorac Cardiovasc Surg* 1991;39:386-388.
5. Tapson VF, Hull RD. Management of venous thromboembolic disease. The impact of low-molecular-weight heparin. *Clin Chest Med* 1995;16:281-294.
6. Stein PD. Acute pulmonary embolism. *Dis Month* 1994;40:467-523. Review.
7. Handler JA, Feied CF. Acute pulmonary embolism. Aggressive therapy with anticoagulants and thrombolytics. *Postgrad Med* 1995;97:61-62, 65-68, 71-72.
8. Boulain T, Lanotte R, Legras A, et al. Efficacy of epinephrine therapy in shock complicating pulmonary embolism. *Chest* 1993;104: 300-302.
9. Mohindra SK, Udeani GO. Treatment of massive pulmonary embolism with centrally administered tissue-type plasminogen activator. *Ann Emerg Med* 1993;22:1349-1352.
10. Phillips SJ. Resuscitation for cardiogenic shock with extracorporeal membrane oxygenation systems. *Sem Thorac Cardiovasc Surg* 1994;6:131-135.
11. Stein PD, Goldhaber SZ, Henry JW. Alveolar-arterial oxygen gradient in the assessment of acute pulmonary embolism. *Chest* 1995; 107:139-143.
12. Pappas AA, Dalrymple G, Harrison K, et al. The application of a rapid D-dimer test in suspected pulmonary embolus. *Arch Pathol Lab Med* 1993;117:977-980.
13. Bounameaux H, Cirafici P, de Moerloose P, et al. Measurement of D-dimer in plasma as diagnostic aid in suspected pulmonary embolism. *Lancet* 1991;337:196-200.
14. Goldhaber SZ, Simons GR, Elliott CG, et al. Quantitative plasma D-dimer levels among patients undergoing pulmonary angiography for suspected pulmonary embolism. *JAMA* 1993;270:2819-2822.
15. Smith R, Maher JM, Miller RI, et al. Clinical outcomes of patients with suspected pulmonary embolism and low-probability aerosol-perfusion scintigrams. *Radiology* 1987;164:731-733.
16. Hull RD, et al. The low-probability lung scan. A need for change in nomenclature. *Arch Intern Med* 1995;155:1845-1851.
17. Bone RC. The mow-probability lung scan. A potentially lethal reading. *Arch Intern Med* 1993;153:2621-2622.
18. Hull RD, Raskob GE, Pineo GF, et al. The low-probability lung scan. A need for change in nomenclature. *Arch Intern Med* 1995;155:1845-1851.
19. Bradley MJ, Alexander L. The role of venous colour flow Doppler to aid the non-diagnostic lung scintigram for pulmonary embolism. *Clin Radiol* 1995;50:232-234.
20. Beecham RP, Dorfman GS, Cronan JJ, et al. Is bilateral lower extremity compression sonography useful and cost-effective in the evaluation of suspected pulmonary embolism? *AJR Am J Roentgenol* 1993;161:1289-1292.
21. Hull RD, Raskob GE, Ginsberg JS, et al. A noninvasive strategy for the treatment of patients with suspected pulmonary embolism. *Arch Intern Med* 1994;154:289-297.
22. Quinn RJ, Nour R, Butler SP, et al. Pulmonary embolism in patients with intermediate probability lung scans: diagnosis with Doppler venous US and D-dimer measurement. *Radiology* 1994;190:509-511.
23. Killewich LA, Nunnelee JD, Auer AI. Value of lower extremity venous duplex examination in the diagnosis of pulmonary embolism. *J Vasc Surg* 1993;17:934-938; discussion 938-939.
24. Perrier A, Bounameaux H, Morabia A, et al. Contribution of D-dimer plasma measurement and lower-limb venous ultrasound to the diagnosis of pulmonary embolism: a decision analysis model. *Am Heart J* 1994;127:624-635.
25. Olson ST, Bjork I. Regulation of thrombin activity by antithrombin and heparin. *Sem Thromb Hemostasis* 1994;120:373-409.
26. Hirsh J, Dalen JE, Deyken D, et al. Heparin: Mechanism of action, pharmacokinetics, dosing considerations, monitoring, efficacy and safety. *Chest* 1992;104:337S-51S.
27. Workentin TE, Levine MN, Hirsch JH, et al. Heparin-induced thrombocytopenia in patients treated with low molecular weight heparin or unfractionated heparin. *N Engl J Med* 1995;332:1330-1335.
28. Chong. Heparin induced thrombocytopenia. *Br J Haematol* 1995; 89:431-439.

29. Tan G, Cohen H, Taylor F, et al. Audit of start of anticoagulation treatment in inpatients. *J Clin Pathol* 1993;46: 67-71.
30. Hirsh J. Antithrombotic therapy in deep vein thrombosis and pulmonary embolism. *Am Heart J* 1992;123: 1115-1122.
31. Wheeler AP, Jaquiss RD, Newman JH. Physician practices in the treatment of pulmonary embolism and deep venous thrombosis. *Arch Intern Med* 1988;148:1321-1325.
32. Israeli D, Kalhorn A, Menzoian JO. Physicians' practices in the diagnosis and management of patients with pulmonary embolism. *Ann Vasc Surg* 1991;5:337-344.
33. Hirsh J. Venous thrombosis and pulmonary embolism: diagnosis during pregnancy. *Emerg Dec* 1988;4:18-20.
34. McKinley L, Wrenn. Are baseline prothrombin time/partial thromboplastin time values necessary before instituting anticoagulation? *Ann Emerg Med* 1993;22:697-702.
35. Bolan CD, Alving BM. Recurrent venous thrombosis in hypercoagulable states. *Am Fam Physician* 1991;44: 1741.
36. Hirsh J, Poller L, Deykin D, et al. Optimal therapeutic range for oral anticoagulants. *Chest* 1989;95(suppl 2):5S.
37. Humphries JE. Acquired antithrombin-3 deficiency replacement with antithrombin-3 concentrates in a patient with protein S deficiency accelerates response to therapy. *Acta Hematologica* 1993;90:151-154.
38. Buller HR, Tencate JW. Acquired antithrombin-3 deficiency. Laboratory diagnosis, incidence, clinical implications and treatment with antithrombin-3 concentrate. *Am J Med* 1989;87 S3-B:44-48.
39. Zamorski MA, Opdycke RA. Advances in the prevention, diagnosis and treatment of deep venous thrombosis. *Am Fam Physician* 1993;47:457-469.
40. Stein PD. Acute pulmonary embolism. *Dis Month* 1994;40:467-523.
41. Hirsh J, Poller L. The International Normalized Ratio. A guide to understanding and correcting its problems. *Arch Intern Med* 1994; 154:282-288.
42. Thery C, Simonneau G, Meyer G, et al. Randomized trial of subcutaneous low-molecular-weight heparin CY 216 (Fraxiparine) compared with intravenous unfractionated heparin in the curative treatment of submassive pulmonary embolism. A dose-ranging study. *Circulation* 1992;85:1380-1389.
43 Hull RD, Raskob GE, Pineo GF, et al. Subcutaneous low-molecular-weight heparin compared with continuous intravenous heparin in the treatment of proximal-vein thrombosis. *N Engl J Med* 1992;326:975.
44. de Valk HW, Banga JD, Wester JW, et al. Comparing subcutaneous danaparoid with intravenous unfractionated heparin for the treatment of venous thromboembolism. A randomized controlled trial. *Ann Intern Med* 1995;123: 1-9.
45. Leizorovicz A, Simonneau G, Decousus H, et al. Comparison of efficacy and safety of low molecular weight heparins and unfractionated heparin in initial treatment of deep venous thrombosis: a meta-analysis. *BMJ* 1994; 309:299-304.
46. Nurmohamed MT, Verhaeghe R, Haas S, et al. A comparative trial of a low molecular weight heparin (enoxaparin) versus standard heparin for the prophylaxis of postoperative deep vein thrombosis in general surgery. *Am J Surg* 1995;169:567-571.
47. Goldhaber SZ. Contemporary pulmonary embolism thrombolysis. *Chest* 1995;107:45S-51S.
48. Goldhaber SZ. Thrombolytic therapy in venous thromboembolism. Clinical trials and current indications. *Clin Chest Med* 1995; 16:307-320.
49. Dalla-Volta S, Palla A, Santolicandro A, et al. PAIMS 2: alteplase combined with heparin versus heparin in the treatment of acute pulmonary embolism. Plasminogen activator Italian multicenter study 2. *J Am Coll Cardiol* 1992;20: 520-526.
50. Anderson DR, Levine MN. Thrombolytic therapy for the treatment of acute pulmonary embolism. *Can Med Assoc J* 1992;146:1317-1324.
51. Meneveau N, Bassand JP, Schiele F, et al. Safety of thrombolytic therapy in elderly patients with massive pulmonary embolism: A comparison with nonelderly patients. *J Am Coll Cardiol* 1993; 22:1075-1079.
52. Molina JE. Thrombolytic therapy for post-operative pulmonary embolism. *Am J Surg* 1992;163:375.
53. Goldhaber SZ, Haire WD, Feldstein ML, et al. Alteplase versus heparin in acute pulmonary embolism: randomised trial assessing right-ventricular function and pulmonary perfusion. *Lancet* 1993; 341:507-511.
54. Verstraete M. Intravenous and intrapulmonary recombinant tissue-type plasminogen activator in the treatment of acute massive pulmonary embolism. *Circulation* 1988;77: 353.
55. Goldhaber SZ, Agnelli G, Levine MN. Reduced dose bolus alteplase vs conventional alteplase infusion for pulmonary embolism thrombolysis. An international multicenter randomized trial. The Bolus Alteplase Pulmonary Embolism Group. *Chest* 1994;106:718-724.
56. Meyer G, Sors H, Charbonnier B, et al. Effects of intravenous urokinase versus alteplase on total pulmonary resistance in acute massive pulmonary embolism: A European multicenter double-blind trial. The European Cooperative Study Group for Pulmonary Embolism. *J Am Coll Cardiol* 1992; 19:239-245.
57. Goldhabert SZ, Kessler CM, Heit JA, et al. Recombinant tissue-type plasminogen activator versus a novel dosing regimen of urokinase in acute pulmonary embolism: a randomized controlled multicenter trial. *J Am Coll Cardiol* 1992;20:24-30.
58. Witty LA, Krichman A, Tapson VF. Thrombolytic therapy for venous thromboembolism. Utilization by practicing pulmonologists. *Arch Intern Med* 1994;154:1601-1604.
59. Bottiger BW, Reim SM, Diezel G, et al. High-dose bolus injection of urokinase. Use during cardiopulmonary resuscitation for massive pulmonary embolism. *Chest* 1994;106:1281-1283.
60. Stein PD, Hull RD, Raskob G. Risks for major bleeding from

thrombolytic therapy in patients with acute pulmonary embolism. Consideration of noninvasive management. *Ann Intern Med* 1994; 121:313-317.

61. Gulba DC, Schmid C, Borst HG, et al. Medical compared with surgical treatment for massive pulmonary embolism. *Lancet* 1994;343: 576-577.
62. Ballew KA, Philbrick JT, Becker DM. Vena cava filter devices. *Clin Chest Med* 1995;16:295-305.
63. Monreal M, Lafoz E, Olive A, et al. Comparison of subcutaneous unfractionated heparin with a low molecular weight heparin (Fragmin) in patients with venous thromboembolism and contraindications to coumarin. *Thromb Haemost* 1994;71:7-11.
64. Cohen JR, Grella L, Citron M. Greenfield filter instead of heparin as primary treatment for deep venous thrombosis or pulmonary embolism in patients with cancer. *Cancer* 1992;70:1993-1996.
65. Ferris EJ, McCowan TC, Carver DK, et al. Percutaneous inferior vena caval filters: Follow-up of seven designs in 320 patients. *Radiology* 1993;188:851-856.
66. Mohan CR, Hoballah JJ, Sharp WJ, et al. Comparative efficacy and complications of vena caval filters. *J Vasc Surg* 1995;21:235-245; discussion 245-246.
67. Greenfield LJ, Proctor MC. Twenty-year clinical experience with the Greenfield filter. *Cardiovasc Surg* 1995;3: 199-205.
68. Meyns B, Sergeant P, Flameng W, et al. Surgery for massive pulmonary embolism. *Acta Cardiologica* 1992;47: 487-493.
69. Greenfield LJ, Proctor MC, Williams DM, et al. Long-term experience with transvenous catheter pulmonary embolectomy. *J Vasc Surg* 1993;18:450-457; discussion 457-458.
70. Boulafendis D, Bastounis E, Panayiotopoulos YP, et al. Pulmonary embolectomy (answered and unanswered questions). *Int Angiol* 1991;10:187-194.
71. Silverman JM, Julien PJ, Adler L, et al. Use of laser energy to treat central pulmonary emboli: A preliminary report. *Lasers Surg Med* 1993;13:553-558.
72. Brady AJ, Crake T, Oakley CM. Percutaneous catheter fragmentation and distal dispersion of proximal pulmonary embolus. *Lancet* 1991;338:1186-1189.
73. Haskal ZJ, Soulen MC, Huettl EA, et al. Life-threatening pulmonary emboli and cor pulmonale: Treatment with percutaneous pulmonary artery stent placement. *Radiology* 1994;191:473-475.
74. Kaunitz AM, Hughes JM, Grimes DA, et al. Causes of maternal mortality in the USA. *Obstet Gynecol* 1985;65: 605-610.
75. Rochat RW, Koonin LM, Atrash HK, et al. Maternal mortality in the United States. Report from the maternal mortality collaborative. *Obstet Gynecol* 1988;72:91.
76. Demers C, Ginsberg JS. Deep venous thrombosis and pulmonary embolism in pregnancy. *Clin Chest Med* 1992;13:645-656.
77. Bergqvist D, Hedner U. Pregnancy and venous thromboembolism. *Acta Obstet Gynecol Scand* 1983;62: 449-453.
78. Jeffries WS, Bochner F. Thromboembolism and its management in pregnancy. *Med J Aust* 1991;155:253-258.
79. Rutherford SE, Phelan JP. Clinical management of thromboembolic disorders in pregnancy. *Crit Care Clin* 1991;7:809-828.
80. Villa Santa U. Thromboembolic disease in pregnancy. *Am J Obstet Gynecol* 1965;93:142.
81. Douketis JD, Ginsberg JS. Diagnostic problems with venous thromboembolic disease in pregnancy. *Haemostasis* 1995;25:58-71.
82. American College of Obstetricians and Gynecologists. Guidelines for Diagnostic Imaging During Pregnancy. Committee Opinion. 1995;156.
83. Ginsberg JS, Hirsh J, Rainbow AJ, et al. Risks to the fetus of radiologic procedures used in the diagnosis of maternal venous thromboembolic disease. *Thromb Haemost* 1989;61:189-196.
84. Fields CL, Magee SE, Exparza E, et al. Double jeopardy: The diagnosis and treatment of pulmonary thromboembolism in pregnancy. *KMA Journal* 1989;87:554-559.
85. Stein PD, Terrin ML, Gottschalk A, et al. Value of ventilation/perfusion scans versus perfusion scans alone in acute pulmonary embolism. *Am J Cardiol* 1992;69:1239-1241.
86. Marcus CS, Mason GR, Kuperus JH, et al. Pulmonary imaging in pregnancy. Maternal risk and fetal dosimetry. *Clin Nucl Med* 1985;1:1-4.
87. Kramer WB, Belfort M, Saade GR, et al. Successful urokinase treatment of massive pulmonary embolism in pregnancy. *Obstet Gynecol* 1995;86:660-662.
88. Fagher B, Ahlgren M, Astedt B. Acute massive pulmonary embolism treated with streptokinase during labor in the early puerperium. *Acta Obstet Gynecol Scand* 1989;68: 267-270.
89. Hull R, Hirsh J, Jay R. Different intensities of anticoagulation in the long-term treatment of proximal vein thrombosis. *N Engl J Med* 1982;307:1676.
90. Manganelli D, Palla A, Donnamaria V, et al. Clinical features of pulmonary embolism. Doubts and certainties. *Chest* 1995;107:25S-32S.
91. Palla A, Petruzzelli S, Donnamaria V, et al. The role of suspicion in the diagnosis of pulmonary embolism. *Chest* 1995;107:21S-24S.
92. van Beek EJ, Kuyer PM, Schenk BE, et al. A normal perfusion lung scan in patients with clinically suspected pulmonary embolism. Frequency and clinical validity. *Chest* 1995;108:170-173.
93. Stein PD, Henry JW, Relyea B. Untreated patients with pulmonary embolism. Outcome, clinical, and laboratory assessment. *Chest* 1995;107:931-935.
94. Miller GH. Pulmonary embolism. In: Weatherall DS, Leningham JGG, Warreli DA, eds. *Oxford Textbook of Medicine.* Oxford: Oxford University Press; 1996: 13-355.
95. Thomas L, Reichl M. Pulmonary embolism in patients attending the accident and emergency department with pleuritic chest pain. *Arch Emerg Med* 1991;8:48-51.
96. Juni JE, Alavi A. Lung scanning in the diagnosis of pul-

monary embolism: The emperor redressed. *Semin Nucl Med* 1991;21:281-296.

97. Henschke CI, Mateescu I, Yankelevitz DF. Changing practice patterns in the workup of pulmonary embolism. *Chest* 1995;107:940-945.
98. Matsumoto AH, Tegtmeyer CJ. Contemporary diagnostic approaches to acute pulmonary emboli. *Radiol Clin North Am* 1995;33:167-183.

Allergic Disease Update

Michael Lynn, MD
Eric Snoey, MD
Gideon Bosker, MD, FACEP

Whether the symptoms are mild or severe, the therapeutic mission statement is always the same—to get the red out. Most importantly, to get the red out quickly and to keep it out, with the hope of making misery a memory for the patient, preferably with medications that work rapidly and that produce as few side effects as possible. Although, except in the case of anaphylaxis, allergy-mediated diseases rarely produce life-threatening illness, the spectrum of conditions associated with allergic complaints frequently brings patients into the ED.

Among allergic conditions bringing patients to the ED—which are then not infrequently triaged into fast-track or immediate-care ambulatory settings—are seasonal allergic rhinitis, perennial allergic rhinitis, acute and chronic urticaria, and anaphylaxis. Symptom-ameliorating measures will almost always include pharmacotherapeutic intervention, which can range from antihistamines, decongestants, and nasal steroids in less severe cases to epinephrine and systemic steroids in life-threatening cases. Outcomes will be optimized if physicians are able to distinguish among available medications—in particular, by placing special emphasis on rapidity of onset of action, side effects, and efficacy of symptom relief.

Characterized by rhinorrhea, sneezing, and nasal congestion, allergic rhinitis—whether of the seasonal or perennial variety—requires selecting medications that work as quickly as possible, have low discontinuation rates, make patients comfortable enough to resume or maintain their customary work, sleep, and recreational activities, and which are associated with minimal side effects. In the majority of cases, systemic oral therapy with second-generation H-1 receptor antagonists will constitute the primary bulwark of defense for initial treatment of acute symptoms; this may be followed by nasal corticosteroids for long-term suppression of symptoms. Patients with idiopathic urticaria require medications that reduce wheal and erythema, whereas individuals who present with anaphylaxis usually require multi-modal therapy linked to epinephrine and fluid administration as the cornerstone of treatment.

With these issues in focus, the following review presents a clinically useful classification of common allergic diseases encountered by the emergency and ambulatory care practitioner. A detailed comparison-analysis of medications used for these conditions is provided, and strategies for optimizing outcomes are presented.

Introduction

Ranging from mild nasal congestion and uncomfortable skin rashes to life-threatening anaphylaxis, allergic reactions have a dramatic impact on peoples' lives. An allergic reaction is defined by a hypersensitive state acquired after exposure to a particular allergen.[1] In broad clinical terms, allergic reactions include such conditions as rhinitis, urticaria, angioedema, and anaphylaxis. Allergic rhinitis has a prevalence rate ranging from 5-22% and is the sixth most common

Table 1. Signs and Symptoms of Allergic and Other Types of Rhinitis

NASAL MUCOSAL DISORDER	SIGNS AND SYMPTOMS
Seasonal allergic rhinitis	Watery rhinorrhea, sneezing, and pruritus of nose, eyes, ears, throat
Perennial allergic rhinitis	Chronic nasal obstruction
Infectious rhinitis	Beet-red nasal mucosa, neu trophilic nasal secretions, fever, sore throat
Rhinitis medicamentosa	Rebound nasal congestion

Adapted from: Pedinoff AJ. Approaches to the treatment of seasonal allergic rhinitis. *South Med J* 1996;89:1130-1139.

chronic condition in the United States, even outranking heart disease.[2] Up to 30 million Americans suffer from the disorder, and, while the disease may begin at any age, children and adolescents are most commonly afflicted.[2] An estimated 1.5 million school days and 3.4 million work days are lost each year due to allergic rhinitis. In addition, allergy sufferers who stay on the job report a 25% reduction in productivity secondary to the disease itself or sedation from drugs used to treat their symptoms.[3,4] The combination of lost productivity, physician visits, and medication costs has an estimated economic impact of $1.8 billion per year.[4] Clearly, allergic rhinitis has far-reaching implications.

Urticaria and angioedema also represent part of the spectrum of allergic reactions. In fact, up to 20% of the general population will develop urticaria or angioedema at some point in their lives.[5] Although generally not life-threatening, urticaria and angioedema are distressing to patients and may be associated with significant morbidity. Anaphylaxis, on the other hand, is acutely life-threatening, often unpredictable, and demands immediate assessment and intervention.[6,7-13]

Rhinitis

Clinical Categories. The term rhinitis refers to diseases characterized by inflammation of the nasal mucosa. Symptoms include variable periods of nasal discharge, congestion, and sneezing, that classically persist for at least one-half hour per day.[14] Rhinitis can be broadly categorized based on infectious and non-infectious etiologies. Infectious rhinitis is best exemplified by the common cold, with its constellation of viral symptoms, including low-grade fever and cloudy nasal secretions. This review is limited to the non-infectious allergic variety of rhinitis. *(Please see Table 1.)*

Non-infectious rhinitis can be further subdivided into seasonal allergic rhinitis and perennial allergic rhinitis. Patients with non-infectious—so-called allergic rhinitis—have clear nasal discharge, often with large numbers of eosinophils.[14] Fever typically is not present.[15] Seasonal rhinitis and perennial allergic rhinitis are similar in their clinical manifestations. The fundamental difference is that perennial rhinitis has no seasonal variation. Although subtle differences in etiology and clinical manifestations exist, management of these disorders is similar.

Allergic Rhinitis. Allergic rhinitis may begin at any age, but it most often affects children and adolescents. An estimated 20-30% of adolescents suffer from this disorder.[14] It is thought that infants are only rarely affected because a minimum of two seasons of exposure to new antigens are required before the disease can manifest itself. The need for prolonged, repeated exposure may also explain why patients without a history of allergic rhinitis may develop symptoms several years after moving to a new location that harbor different allergens. Allergic rhinitis afflicts men and women equally, and there is no ethnic or racial predominance. Once the disease begins, it tends to persist indefinitely, although spontaneous remissions have occurred.[14]

Etiology. The most common allergens implicated in seasonal allergic rhinitis are molds and pollens. Contrary to popular belief, plants that rely on insects for pollination (e.g., roses, dandelions) do not cause allergic rhinitis unless patients are continually in close contact with these plants. Rather, vegetation that depends on wind for cross-pollination (e.g., most grasses, trees, and weeds) are the more common precipitants of allergic rhinitis. In this regard, ragweed pollen appears in the northeastern and midwestern United States from mid-August through September. Sage brush is common in the western United States. Grass pollens occur throughout the nation in spring and summer months. These pollens contribute little; however, to symptoms of perennial allergic rhinitis. In perennial disease, house dust, animal dander, and molds are the most likely responsible allergens.[14] This explains why perennial rhinitis generally does not vary with the seasons, although seasonal exacerbations may occur in patients with concomitant pollen allergy.

Pathophysiology. Allergic rhinitis requires two predisposing conditions to produce overt clinical disease: genetic predisposition and exposure to allergens.[15] From a pathophysiological perspective, antigens such as pollens, molds, grains, and animal dander infiltrate the respiratory mucosa where Langerhans cells process and present them to T-lymphocytes. T-lymphocytes, in turn, release cytokines and granulocyte-macrophage colony-stimulating factor, which stimulate B-lymphocytes to produce IgE. IgE binds to receptors on mast cells in the nasal mucosa,[16] and remains there until re-exposure to the allergen. At this point, the nasal mucosa is considered "sensitized" to that particular allergen. Interestingly, the nasal mucosa of people with allergic rhinitis has significantly more mast cells than that of non-affected people.[17] Repeated exposure of IgE to the same allergen triggers an explosive release of a variety of vasoactive mediators from mast cells. This release is postulated to be the critical initiating event in the development of allergic symptoms. Mediators include histamine, leukotrienes, bradykinin, and prostaglandins. Histamine, which is the most important mediator, binds specifically to H-1 receptors in the nasal mucosa, inducing rhinorrhea, mucus production, and sneezing symptoms typical of allergic rhinitis.[17]

The mechanism of allergic rhinitis has been shown to involve both an immediate phase and a late phase. Immediate phase refers to the release from mast cells of preformed mediators such as histamine and leukotrienes that produce such clinical symptoms as rhinorrhea and sneezing within 30-60 minutes of exposure. Late-phase symptoms occur 4-24 hours after mast cell degranulation and are thought to be secondary to inflammatory cell infiltration of the nasal mucosa. The late phase differs from immediate phase in that nasal congestion and obstruction, rather than rhinorrhea, predominate.[3] The distinction between immediate and late phase has significant therapeutic implications.

Table 2. Relative Effectiveness of Medication Classes on Symptoms of Allergic Rhinitis

MEDICATION	SNEEZING	RHINORRHEA	ITCHING	NASAL CONGESTION
Antihistamines	++	++	++	0
Decongestants	0	0	0	++
Nasal Steroids	++	++	++	++
Cromolyn	+	+	+	+
Anticholinergics	0	+	0	0

Adapted from: Graft DF. Allergic and nonallergic rhinitis. *Postgrad Med* 1996;100:64-69.

Clinical Symptoms and Signs. Rhinorrhea, nasal congestion, sneezing, and palatal itching are classic symptoms of allergic rhinitis. Sneezing may include paroxysms of as many as 10-20 sneezes, most commonly in the morning, when windborne pollens are released in greatest numbers.[14] Rhinorrhea is often profuse and sustained, and, usually, is thin and watery. Purulent rhinorrhea may indicate secondary bacterial infection. Swollen nasal turbinates frequently cause bothersome nasal congestion that, initially, is intermittent early in the season, but often becomes constant as the allergy season progresses. Headache and earache may accompany nasal congestion, and sustained obstruction may even lead to alteration or loss of smell and taste. Persistent oropharyngeal drainage of nasal secretions causes an irritating sensation in the throat and, oftentimes, a chronic non-productive cough.[14] Bronchial irritation may exacerbate reactive airway disease and present with typical symptoms of asthma.[18] In fact, studies suggest that up to 38% of patients with allergic rhinitis have asthma, compared to 3-5 % in the general population.[19]

Once symptoms of allergic rhinitis develop, they usually recur at approximately the same time each year. Acutely sensitive patients develop symptoms early in the pollen season. As pollen concentrations increase, symptoms generally worsen. At the end of the season, symptoms gradually abate. Interestingly, in some individuals, symptoms may persist up to three weeks following the end of pollen season. This is thought to be secondary to a form of increased reactivity termed the "priming effect." Patients have a "primed" nose from a season of allergic symptoms and subsequently react to irritants that would not normally affect them. This "priming effect" generally abates within 2-3 weeks.[14]

On physical examination, a patient often has red, irritated skin in the area of the midface from rubbing or blowing the nose. Nasal turbinates are pale and edematous and may completely obstruct the nasal passages. Eyes usually demonstrate injected conjunctiva. Dark edematous circles under the eyes, common to atopic individuals, are the result of venous obstruction in the inferior orbital area due to nasal congestion. The posterior pharynx usually is normal, although lymphoid hyperplasia may be evident.[15] Chest exam is unremarkable except in patients with concomitant reactive airway disease.

Drug Therapy for Allergic Rhinitis

Patients with allergic rhinitis should be treated in order to alleviate immediate symptoms and, with the objective of avoiding more problematic sequelae such as chronic sinusitis, inner-ear dysfunction, and sleep apnea. Not surprisingly, treatment options are variable and can be complex, and the emergency physician is faced with a wide range of pharmacotherapeutic alternatives. *(Please see Tables 2 and 3.)* In this regard, the type and etiology of allergic rhinitis, the patient's age, occupation, and underlying co-morbid conditions will all affect management decisions. For example, sedating antihistamines must be used with caution in children as well as adults who cannot tolerate daytime sleepiness. Anticholinergic side effects may adversely affect urinary flow in men with benign prostatic hypertrophy. Drug-drug interactions are known to cause a fatal torsades des pointes in patients taking terfenadine or astemizole together with certain antimicrobial medications. Basic knowledge of the mechanism of pharmacologic agents used in allergic rhinitis clarifies the most suitable treatment options.

Antihistamines. Antihistamines have been available for 50 years, but remain the most commonly used medication in the treatment of patients with allergic rhinitis. Currently, there are approximately 100 different antihistamines on the market, reflecting a wide range of pharmacological and clinical effects.[3] When histamine is released from mast cells, it acts on three receptors: H-1, H-2, and H-3. H-1 receptor activation stimulates smooth muscle contraction and increases vascular permeability. Mucus production increases and sensory nerves are activated causing nasal pruritus and sneezing. H-2 receptor activation causes blood vessel dilation and gastric acid secretion. Finally, H-3 receptors, located in the brain, play a role in regulating the production and release of histamine from nerve tissue.[2,6] Although histamine binds to all three receptors, only its effect on H-1 receptors is clinically important in allergic rhinitis. Antihistamine agents essentially work through competitive inhibition of these H-1 receptors.[20] By blocking H-1 receptors, immediate phase symptoms are blunted. In contrast, H-2 antagonists, such as cimetidine and ranitidine, have little effect on H-1 receptors and, consequently, have not been shown to be clinically effective in the management of allergic rhinitis.[2]

First-generation antihistamines, such as diphenhydramine (Benadryl) and chlorpheniramine (Chlor-Trimeton), are highly lipophilic and penetrate the blood brain barrier. This results in unacceptable sedation and disruption of motor skills in up to 25% of patients.[20-22] Because of their sedation profile, several first-generation antihistamines are approved for use as sleeping medications.[2] Due to sedation side effects, first-generation antihistamines usually are not recommended in school-aged patients nor should they be the daytime drugs of choice for adults who need to be truly alert (i.e., those who drive or operate heavy machinery.)[21] These antihistamines also can produce profound anticholinergic side effects such as urinary retention, constipation, dry eyes, narrow-angle glaucoma,[23] and tachycardia, which may preclude their use in the elderly or patients with comorbid conditions. Furthermore, first-generation antihistamines are contraindicated in pilots within 24 hours of flight because of sedation and changes in reflexes and depth perception.[3]

Some of the second-generation antihistamines—among them, terfenadine (Seldane), loratadine (Claritin), astemizole (Hismanal),

Table 3. Treatment Strategies for Managing Allergic Rhinitis

CONDITION SEVERITY	TREATMENT
Mild	• Avoid allergen if possible • Non-sedating antihistamine
Moderate	• Non-sedating antihistamine • Nasal steroids, beginning early in season • Oral decongestant until nasal steroids become effective
Severe	• Non-sedating antihistamine • Nasal steroids, beginning early in season • Topical decongestant for less than five days, then oral decongestant • Consider systemic steroids • Referral to allergist

cetirizine (Zyrtec), and fexofenadine (Allegra)—have been available in either U.S. or non-U.S. markets for up to 10 years and represent a significant advance in the therapy of allergic rhinitism. *(Please see Table 4.)* In contrast to first-generation antihistamines, these drugs are far less sedating because they are more lipophobic[20] and, therefore, are less likely to penetrate the blood brain barrier. Additionally, second-generation antihistamines have few, if any, anticholinergic side effects. A placebo-controlled, double-blinded study of 15 pediatric patients with allergic rhinitis found a significantly lower incidence of sedation and cognitive impairment in patients receiving terfenadine compared with the first-generation antihistamine chlorpheniramine.[24] In a second study evaluating loratadine and diphenhydramine, 12 performance tests were administered that evaluated such skills as mathematical reasoning and memory before and after drug administration. The loratadine group performance was similar to placebo, but diphenhydramine lowered performance in two-thirds of the tests.[18]

The five low non- and/or minimally sedating second-generation antihistamines differ largely in terms of their half-lives, onset of action, and toxicity. Fexofenadine and terfenadine have a relatively short half-life, and therefore, require bid administration that may represent an inconvenience in a significant percentage of patients. Astemizole and loratadine have longer half-lives, permitting once-daily dosing, which may improve patient compliance. Cetirizine (Zyrtec) also has a long half-life similar to loratadine and astemizole, but its sedation profile is slightly different. Compared to the other previously mentioned second-generation antihistamines, which in placebo-controlled trials produce drowsiness in about 1-2% percent of patients, cetirizine produces symptoms such as drowsiness and/or sedation in an additional 7-8% of patients *above* the number of those reporting such symptoms in the placebo arm. (Overall, about 14% of patients taking cetirizine reported somnolence-related side effects in placebo-controlled studies.) From a clinical perspective, then, cetirizine, as *compared* to loratidine or fexofenadine, can be expected to produce drowsiness or sedation in only an additional six or seven patients out of 100 individuals receiving these medications.[7-13] This difference must be weighed against the potential advantages demonstrated by cetirizine, in particular, its rapid onset of action as compared to other agents, its lower cost among the second-generation antihistamine class, efficacy, and the fact it has FDA approval for seasonal allergic rhinitis, perennial allergic rhinitis, and chronic urticaria.[6-12]

Multiple studies have compared the effectiveness of second-generation antihistamines to each other and to placebo. Two studies comparing loratadine, terfenadine, and placebo in patients with seasonal allergic rhinitis found a significant reduction of symptoms in the drug-treated group, with no difference in efficacy or side effects.[26,27] A comparison study of cetirizine and terfenadine found both to be effective in reducing symptoms of perennial allergic rhinitis, but cetirizine caused slightly more sedation.[28] Likewise, fexofenadine has been shown to be more effective than placebo, but there are no published studies comparing this antihistamine with other H-1 receptor antagonists.[29-32]

Although all second-generation antihistamines have similar efficacy, two have a rare but important side effect that, for all practical purposes, makes them less desirable than the others. Terfenadine and astemizole were recently linked to fatal cardiac arrhythmias, in particular torsades des pointes. A common pathway appears to be the prolongation of the Q-T interval.[22,36] Independent risk factors are high serum drug levels[22], interactions with macrolide antibiotics and antifungals,[29,33-35] liver disease, or intrinsic cardiac disease.[15] Concomitant use of Type 1a antiarrhythmic agents, thioridazine, and the selective serotonin re-uptake inhibitors fluvoxamine (Luvox) and neferzodone (Serzone) also have been implicated.[3] In addition, patients at risk for hypokalemia and hypomagnesemia should have other antihistamines prescribed for them, such as loratadine, fexofenadine, or cetirizine, all of which have no effect on the Q-T interval.[22,26-28]

Antihistamine Selection: Getting The Red Out. From an emergency medicine—as well as primary care—perspective one of the most important considerations when choosing an antihistamine for an acutely symptomatic patient is the onset of action of the drug and its efficacy. Comparing efficacy and rapidity of symptomatic relief requires head-to-head studies involving all available antihistamines that, until recently, have been lacking, especially for the newer, selective, peripheral histamine H-1-receptor antagonists. The lack of definitive studies comparing this class of medications has fueled considerable debate among emergency and primary care specialists as to which antihistamine is best-suited as initial therapy, especially for patients requiring definitive, prompt relief of discomforting or disabling symptoms caused by seasonal allergic or perennial allergic rhinitis.

Recently, however, an important study that attempted to rank such medications as cetirizine, loratidine, astemizole, and terfenadine according to their ability to produce relief of symptoms of allergic rhinitis has been published.[36] In this well-designed investigation (financially supported, in part, by Nordic Merrell Dow, which markets terfenadine) that has important implications for initial selection of antihistamines, 111 ragweed-sensitive subjects were primed with pollen in an Environmental Exposure Unit. Individuals who were evaluated included those with sufficient symptoms produced over a three-hour exposure to 5000 +/- 300 grains/m^3 of ragweed pollen. When subjects had been sufficiently symptomatic after at least a 60-minute exposure, they were then given a single dose of either terfenadine (60 mg), astemizole (10 mg), cetirizine (10 mg), lorati-

Table 4. Comparison Table of Antihistamines

ANTIHISTAMINE	DOSE (MG)	ROUTE	ONSET OF ACTION†	SEDATION	THREE APPROVED INDICATIONS	ANTICHOLINERGIC SIDE EFFECTS	TORSADES DE POINTES RISK	COST 1 MONTH
Fexofenadine	60 bid	po	+++	0	No	0	No	$51.56
Terfenadine	60 bid	po	+++	0	No	0	Yes	$58.61
Astemizole	10 qd	po	+	0	No	0	Yes	$57.66
Loratadine	10 qd	po	++	0	No	0	No	$60.67
Cetirizine	10 qd	po	++++	++	Yes	0	No	$51.41
Diphenhydramine	50 q4	po/IM/IV	++	+++	No	+++	No	$2.03
Hydroxyzine	25 q8	po/IM	++	+++	No	+++	No	$3.11

† Onset of action (++++/fastest, +/slowest)
*Approved for seasonal allergic rhinitis, perennial allergic rhinitis, and chronic urticaria.
Adapted from: Fexofenadine. *Med Lett Drugs Ther* 1996;38:95-96; Cetirizine: A new antihistamine. *Med Lett Drugs Ther* 1996;38:21-23.

dine (10 mg), or placebo. During treatment, the allergen levels were maintained and the patients symptoms recorded every 30 minutes.

The percentage of patients who demonstrated clinically important relief (defined as "marked relief" or "complete relief" at three consecutive time points) were greatest in the cetirizine group (69.6%), followed by terfenadine (54.5%), loratidine (50.0%), astemizole (40.9%), and placebo (31.8%), but these differences were not different among the treatment groups (P = 0.119). Analysis, however, did demonstrate that cetirizine was different from placebo (P = 0.025). Interestingly, while the antihistamines did not differ significantly with respect to clinically important relief, when investigators examined the times to onset of relief and the proportion of individuals who achieved definitive relief of symptoms caused by allergic rhinitis, significant differences were detected among the four treatment groups tested with the second-generation antihistamines. Definitive relief, which represents a clinically desirable extension of "marked relief," was defined as "marked relief" or "complete relief" without being followed by such subsequent patient assessments as "moderate, slight, or no relief" on the effectiveness scale.

The percentage of patients reporting definitive relief in the various treatment groups were: 65.2% in the cetirizine group; 45.5% in the terfenadine group; 31.8% in the loratidine group; 27.3% in the placebo group; and 22.7% in the astemizole group (P = 0.023). These differences were statistically significant. In addition, the times to onset of definitive relief for seasonal allergic rhinitis were statistically significant among the five groups (P = 0.010). The ranking from quickest to slowest was cetirizine, terfenadine, loratidine, astemizole, respectively. Finally, a "global" evaluation, in which the patients express their willingness to take the study medication again, yielded the following percentages: cetirizine (82.6%), terfenadine (66.7%), astemizole (63.6%), loratidine (40.9%), and placebo (36.4%) (P = 0.036). Based on these studies, the investigators concluded that cetirizine and terfenadine continuously ranked higher in terms of onset of action and efficacy, while loratidine and astemizole ranked lower.

Unfortunately, fexofenadine was not evaluated in this study, and therefore, head-to-head comparisons between this drug and others are not available. However, based on these study results, and the ongoing concern over drug interactions with terfenadine (which the FDA has recommended removing from the market), it would appear as if cetirizine currently represents an excellent initial antihistamine of choice for allergic or perennial rhinitis patients encountered in the ED or primary care setting. It should be stressed that because of the rapid onset of action of cetirizine, some patients—especially those with unpredictably waxing and waning symptoms—may be able to achieve adequate relief by taking the medication on a once-daily, "as-needed" basis, and may be especially attractive in cost-conscious managed care settings. This approach can substantially reduce overall costs of antihistamine therapy. Finally, if patients on cetirizine subsequently complain of drowsiness or sedation, they can be switched to another second generation antihistamine.[36]

Very few other side effects have been found with second-generation antihistamines. Several reports of mechanical upper gastrointestinal tract obstruction in patients taking a loratadine/decongestant combination (Claritin-D 24 hour) suggest caution in prescribing this medicine to patients with known dysphagia or gastrointestinal anatomic abnormalities.[37] Patients taking astemizole have reported weight gain.[38] The single overall drawback of second-generation antihistamines is their expense. Loratadine, for example, has a wholesale cost of $58.08 for a one-month supply, compared to $2.03 for diphenhydramine.[39]

Decongestants. Because numerous non-histaminergic mediators also are involved, antihistamines alone may not adequately control symptoms of allergic rhinitis.[18] For example, late-phase symptoms of allergic rhinitis, such as nasal congestion and construction, may be attenuated by decongestants.[3,18,20,23] Decongestants are sympathomimetics that produce clinical relief by stimulating alpha receptors in the nasal mucosa, causing a reduction in edema and blood flow.[22] Topically administered decongestants control symptoms more rapidly and selectively than orally administered ones, with few systemic side effects.[2] Common topical agents include phenylephrine (Neosynephrine) and oxymetazoline (Afrin), both of which are equally effective and have a duration of action between one and eight hours, respectively.[22] Importantly, topical agents can only be used safely for a maximum of five days before risking "rhinitis medicamentosa", a form of rebound nasal congestion.[20,22] This prospect significantly limits the role of these agents to intermittent, PRN use; accordingly, prolonged use is ill-advised.

Oral decongestants (e.g., pseudoephedrine [Sudafed], and phenylpropanolamine) are commonly combined with antihistamines to enhance control of both nasal congestion and rhinorrhea. Combinations of pseudoephedrine with loratadine (Claritin-D) or terfenadine (Seldane-D) are typical examples. A randomized, triple-blinded study comparing loratadine/pseudoephedrine with chlorpheniramine/pseudoephedrine demonstrated symptomatic improvement in both groups. However, there were significantly fewer complaints of sedation and dry mouth in the loratadine/pseudoephedrine group.[40] Unfortunately, all forms of oral decongestants may be associated with systemic side effects such as tachycardia, irritability, and "agitated sedation."[3,20,22] These side effects can be significant. Interestingly, the sense of agitated sedation may occur even when oral decongestants are combined with sedating first-generation antihistamines such as chlorpheniramine.[3] Cautious use of phenylpropanolamine-containing compounds is mandatory, especially in patients with hypertension. Consequently, combination agents are generally not advised as first-time therapy, unless non-combination agents fail to produce desired clinical effects.

Table 5. Comparison Table of Nasal Sprays

NASAL STEROID	DOSE PER NOSTRIL	PUFFS PER BOTTLE	COST PER MONTH
Steroids			
Beclomethasone diproprionate			
Beconase	1-2 puffs bid	200	$19.67
Vancenase	1-2 puffs bid	200	$19.67
Budenoside			
Rhinacourt	2 puffs bid	200	$18.75
Dexamethasone sodium phosphate			
Dexacourt Turbinaire	1-2 puffs bid	170	$22.78
Flunisolide			
Nasalide	1-2 puffs bid	200	$16.55
Nasarel	1-2 puffs bid	200	$20.88
Fluticasone propionate			
Flonase	1-2 puffs qd	120	$20.31
Triamcinolone acetonide			
Nasacort	2 puffs qd	100	$25.30
Other			
Cromolyn sodium			
Nasalcrom	1 puff qid	200	$14.89-29.68
Ipatropium bromide			
Atrovent (0.03%)	2 puffs tid	345	$23.40-35.10

Adapted from: Ferguson BJ. Allergic rhinits. Options for pharmacotherapy and immunotherapy. *Postgrad Med* 1997;101;124-125.

Topical Corticosteroids. In patients who can tolerate them, nasal steroids have become a cornerstone of treatment for allergic rhinitis.[3,10,16] *(Please see Table 5.)* These agents decrease nasal mast cell density,[17] inhibit multiple steps in the inflammatory process, and decrease capillary permeability.[22] In contrast to many antihistamines and decongestants, nasal steroids act on both immediate (e.g., rhinorrhea) and late (e.g., nasal congestion) phase reactions. This permits control of all aspects of allergic rhinitis.[23] An estimated 90% of patients with allergic rhinitis have significant symptomatic relief when treated with nasal steroids;[2] the efficacy of these agents has been shown in multiple studies.[2,41,42] Comparison studies of steroids with placebo demonstrate significant improvement in symptoms and fewer lost days from work.[42]

Nasal steroids are non-sedating and can be combined with antihistamines/decongestants in patients who have symptoms that are difficult to control. Adverse effects are usually minimal and include nasal irritation and mild epistaxis, the most commonly reported problems. Nasal *Candida albicans* has not been reported.[22] Adverse systemic effects of nasal steroids are controversial but may include reversible open-angle glaucoma in patients over age 60 and cataract formation.[23] A recent Canadian study, however, did not find any association between glaucoma and extended use of nasal steroids.[43] It is prudent, however, for the ED or primary care physician to suggest glaucoma and cataract screening within three months of beginning steroid therapy.[23]

An important drawback to these agents is the need for at least three days of regular use before a noticeable clinical response, which is in contrast to the rapid onset of antihistamines such as cetirizine. Since allergen exposure typically is unanticipated, patients often require "rescue" from their misery with a short course of antihistamines until the nasal steroids take effect.[3]

Systemic therapy with steroids is rarely indicated in the treatment of allergic rhinitis. Their use should be limited to patients with complete nasal obstruction refractory to decongestant and antihistamine therapy, since these patients may progress to develop inner-ear disorders or sleep apnea. A short 10-day tapering regimen course is suggested.[2]

Cromolyn Sodium. Cromolyn nasal preparations are effective in reducing symptoms of allergic rhinitis through suppression of mast cell degranulation. Like antihistamines, cromolyn is more effective in alleviating immediate-phase symptoms such as sneezing, rhinorrhea, and nasal pruritus but does not attenuate nasal congestion or other late-phase symptoms.[44] Cromolyn requires prophylactic administration, 4-6 times per day, and may take from 1-4 weeks before producing symptomatic relief.[3,22] In some patients, cromolyn may be ineffective if started after onset of symptoms. Due to its very favorable side-effect profile, it is especially suitable for children and the elderly, although compliance with its frequent use may be a limiting factor.

Anticholinergics. In 1996, ipatropium bromide (Atrovent) nasal spray became available for use in the treatment of allergic rhinitis. Although it has yet to gain widespread use, this anticholinergic medicine effectively controls rhinorrhea. Ipatropium bromide reduces the volume of nasal secretions by inhibiting parasympathetic stimulation of nasal tissue. At therapeutic levels, rhinorrhea has been shown to decrease significantly. It has no effect on sneezing and nasal pruritus, nor does it relieve nasal congestion.[22,23] Ipatropium bromide does not cross the blood brain barrier, and it has no systemic anticholinergic effects.[45] Similarly, long-term adverse effects, as well as tolerance to its therapeutic effects, do not occur. Epistaxis and nasal dryness are the most common reported side effects.[22,46]

Table 6. Selected Causes of Urticaria, Angiodema, and Anaphylaxis

URTICARIA AND ANGIOEDEMA	ANAPHYLAXIS
Drugs (penicillin, ACE-inhibitors)	Antibiotics (especially parenteral)
Foods	*Hymenoptera* venom
Hymenoptera	Contrast media
Contactants	Foods (nuts, shellfish, eggs)
Inhalents	NSAIDs, ASA
C1 esterase deficiency	Blood products
Systemic disease: (SLE, malignancy, infections)	

Immunotherapy. Although not a treatment option in the acute ambulatory or emergency setting, patients may inquire about "allergy shots." The principal behind this therapeutic option is to repeatedly inject tiny amounts of a specific allergen in order to gradually reduce the body's immunologic response to this allergen. Symptom relief takes between three months and two years, and therapy must be continued for several years after the cessation of symptoms. Immunotherapy may help allergic symptoms to a specific allergen, but it will not affect concomitant allergies to other allergens. Thus, continued use of adjunctive pharmacotherapy is often necessary. Finally, immunotherapy poses a small but significant risk of anaphylactic reaction to the injected allergen. It should only be administered by specialists with resuscitative equipment at hand. Immunotherapy is contraindicated in patients on beta-blockers (which may render the patient refractory to standard anaphylactic treatment), severe asthma, or severe atopic dermatitis. Despite the risks, immunotherapy may be useful in patients who cannot avoid allergens (e.g., veterinarians who develop animal dander allergies),or who prove refractory to standard pharmacotherapy.[3,47]

Urticaria and Angiodema

Clinical Background. Urticaria and angioedema affect up to 20% of the population at some point in their lives.[48] These disorders are usually acute and self-limited, although chronic forms do exist. Both disorders represent cutaneous or subcutaneous manifestations of mediators released from cells that have been stimulated by allergens. Urticaria is characterized by erythematous, well-circumscribed edematous lesions that are often evanescent and pruritic. The distribution of urticarial lesions is highly variable but most commonly involves the trunk.[48] Angioedema represents a similar pathological reaction to urticaria, but the reaction is located in the deep dermis and subcutaneous tissue rather than in the superficial skin layers, where there are few sensory nerve endings, the lesions tend to be non-pruritic and the skin itself may appear normal.[5] Angioedema most often involves the face, eyelids, and tongue, where it may produce findings ranging from mild edema to massive lingual and pharyngeal swelling. Angioedema co-exists with urticaria in approximately 50% of patients.[5] It is unclear why some patients develop urticaria, some develop angioedema, and others manifest both.

Pathogenesis. The pathogenesis of urticaria and angioedema involve multiple mediators and pathways, some of which remain poorly understood. The most important mechanism is similar to that of allergic rhinitis: an allergen stimulates production of IgE, which then binds to mast cells (and other cells as well). Histamine and other mediators (e.g., leukotrienes) are released from mast-cell granules. These mediators cause vasodilation (erythema) and increased vascular permeability (edema). A second pathway involves the complement cascade. Specifically, C3a, C4a, and C5a interact directly with the mast-cell surface to induce histamine release. Another pathway involves activation of Hageman factor that, via the coagulation cascade, initiates the formation of mediators such as kallikrein and bradykinin.[5]

Etiology. The etiology of urticaria and angioedema is often idiopathic.[41] *(Please see Table 6.)* In general, allergens that have been ingested or are in direct contact with skin are most likely to be the responsible agents. This is in contrast with inhaled allergens, which are more likely to cause nasal or respiratory symptoms.[5] Of the identifiable causes of urticaria and angioedema, drugs are most commonly responsible.[48] Virtually any drug may induce an allergic reaction, but several medicines are uniquely capable of directly activating mast cells. These drugs include morphine, codeine, vancomycin, and radiocontrast agents, among others. Penicillin is also well-known for causing urticaria, although through an IgE-mediated mechanism rather than direct mast-cell stimulation. Angiotensin-converting enzyme (ACE) inhibitors cause angioedema through a mechanism that is thought to involve production of bradykinin.[49] Likewise, foods such as nuts and shellfish are frequently implicated in allergic reactions. Insect bites and stings, exercise, latex gloves, and even semen are known to induce urticaria and angioedema.[50-53] Uncommon and poorly defined syndromes related to cholinergic sensitivity, cold, sun, water, and dermatographism also have been described.[5]

There also are chronic and hereditary forms of these disorders. Chronic urticaria is arbitrarily defined as a reaction that lasts longer than six weeks. It is usually idiopathic, although autoimmune disorders such as systemic lupus erythematosus (SLE) and rheumatoid arthritis may occasionally be responsible. Seven percent of patients with SLE develop hives at some point in their illness.[48] Other systemic disorders such as infection, malignancy, and endocrine dysfunction may also involve chronic urticaria.[48] Hereditary angioedema is caused by a deficiency in C-1 esterase inhibitor, which results in repeated episodes of idiopathic angioedema.[49] Attacks are typically mild and infrequent but can, in rare patients, become a daily, debilitating event.[54] Interestingly, inciting allergens or events leading to attacks of hereditary angioedema often cannot be identified. A family history of angioedema is suggestive of this disorder.

Signs and Symptoms. Patients with acute urticaria will complain of intense pruritus; hives typically will be evident on physical exam. Individuals with chronic urticaria generally have less pruritus, and hives may be less prominent. Patients with angioedema generally have non-pruritic edema of the affected area. Edema usually is moderate and self-limited, but lingual and pharyngeal swelling is massive at times and may result in airway obstruction. Stridor, hoarseness, dysphagia, and drooling are typical signs of impending airway compromise.

Laboratory Work-up and Treatment. Unless an underlying illness is suspected, laboratory tests play no role in the acute management of urticaria and angioedema. Treatment of these disorders ideally involves avoidance of the inciting allergen. However, since allergens usually are unknown or have already caused symptoms, drug therapy plays a key role. Antihistamines are a mainstay of therapy. In acute urticaria, a short course will block histamine-mediated effects such as pruritus. Patients with chronic urticaria benefit from taking antihistamines prophylactically. In mild reactions or chronic forms of these disorders, oral antihistamines are given. The second-generation cetirizine, which is approved for use in patients with chronic urticaria, has the advantage of rapid onset of action time (usually, within 60 minutes) and less sedation than such classically used agents as hydroxyzine (Atarax) and diphenhydramine (Benadryl). No difference in efficacy has been found in clinical trials comparing first- and second-generation antihistamines to each other.[55,56] Patients with severe urticaria or angioedema should receive SQ epinephrine and parenteral diphenhydramine (1 mg/kg up to 50 mg). Non-sedating antihistamines are not available in parenteral form.

H-2 blockers such as cimetidine (Tagamet) and ranitidine (Zantac) can be particularly useful in urticaria, especially when combined with H-1 blockers.[5] The rationale for use of H-2 blockers reflects the presence of a small number of H-2 receptors in skin, in addition to large numbers of H-1 receptors located there. By blocking both receptors, antihistamines potentially have a greater effect. H-2 blockers have also been proposed for use in treating acute angioedema, but clinical trials have not shown improved outcomes.

Steroid creams and ointments are not beneficial in the management of either urticaria or angioedema. Oral and IV steroids, however, are effective in reducing oropharyngeal inflammation in angioedema or urticaria,[49] although clinical effects may take several hours to become apparent. In a prospective, randomized, double-blinded study of patients with acute urticaria, patients who received prednisone for four days improved more rapidly than those who received placebo.[57] Similarly, patients with oropharyngeal angioedema should receive a short tapering course of oral steroids as outpatients.

Patients who have signs or symptoms of airway obstruction should be treated similarly to patients with systemic anaphylaxis. They should receive incremental doses of epinephrine 0.3 mg SQ q 20 minutes.[5,58] In addition, nebulized racemic epinephrine should also be considered. Patients in extremis may require IV epinephrine. For reasons that are unclear, patients with hereditary angioedema or ACE-inhibitor induced angioedema may be less responsive to epinephrine, H-1 and H-2 blockers, and steroids.[54,59] Definitive airway management with endotracheal intubation or crichothyroidotomy may be necessary.

Anaphylaxis

Inasmuch as true anaphylaxis represents a life-threatening allergic reaction demanding immediate action, a brief review is warranted, with emphasis on management techniques.

The first fatal anaphylactic reaction was described over 4000 years ago following a *Hymenoptera* sting. In the modern era, however, iatrogenic causes have eclipsed *Hymenoptera* stings as causes of severe or fatal anaphylactic reactions.[60-67] Horse serum used in diphtheria and tetanus antitoxins was an early culprit. In hospitalized patients today, radiocontrast dyes and beta-lactam antibiotics account for an estimated 500 fatalities annually.[67] Penicillin, which became widely available after World War II, caused its first-reported anaphylactic death in 1949.[61] Anaphylactic reactions to beta-lactam antibiotics occur in 1-5 per 10,000 administrations. About 10% of these are life-threatening, and 1% are fatal. Importantly, the vast majority of these reactions stem from intravenous or intramuscular administrations rather than oral therapy.[60] *Hymenoptera* venom (yellow jackets, hornets, honeybees, bumblebees, wasps, and fire ants) causes an estimated 50 deaths per year in the United States,[63,64] far outnumbering deaths from snake bites. Interestingly, only 9-25% of fatal stings report previous hymenoptera allergy.[65] Anaphylactic reactions to foods, such as shellfish, nuts, and eggs, can also occur.

The pathophysiology of anaphylaxis involves an IgE-mediated hypersensitivity reaction. First, IgE, formed in response to a specific allergen, binds to mast cells. Upon re-exposure to the allergen, the IgE cross stimulates the release of preformed mediators such as histamine. In contrast, anaphylactoid reactions are non-IgE mediated but are clinically indistinguishable from true anaphylaxis. Importantly, while anaphylaxis requires previous exposure to the allergen, anaphylactoid reactions require no immunologic memory; in this case, degranulation of mast cells thus may occur on first exposure to the allergen.[60]

Clinical Features. Patients vary greatly in terms of the presentation, onset, and course of anaphylaxis, but clinical manifestations usually occur within seconds to minutes.[61] A small subset of patients may remain relatively asymptomatic for an hour or more before developing severe symptoms.[68] Most patients have a predictable, uniphasic course where they develop signs and symptoms of anaphylaxis early, respond to therapy, and remain asymptomatic thereafter.[60] About 20% of patients, however, have biphasic reactions characterized by a second episode of anaphylaxis up to eight hours following apparent recovery from the initial event.[61,69] Rarely, anaphylaxis will be protracted, with symptoms persisting up to three weeks.[68] Unfortunately, no particular test or spectrum of clinical symptoms allows prediction of which patients will have biphasic or protracted responses.

Airway obstruction and cardiovascular collapse are the leading causes of death from anaphylaxis. These may be early events, occurring within seconds of exposure to inciting allergen, or they may develop more gradually. Patients with a history of asthma, or those with cardiac disease and using beta-blockers, are at greatest risk for severe reaction.[60] The vast majority of patients will have pruritus (especially of hands, feet, groin, and palatal and nasal areas[61]), urticaria, or angioedema. Laryngeal edema may manifest as hoarseness, stridor, or a "lump in the throat," while wheezing and chest tightness signify lower airway obstruction. Hypotension, chest pain, arrhythmias, and shock represent cardiovascular involvement.[60] Myocardial infarction secondary to anaphylaxis has been reported.[70] Nausea, vomiting, diarrhea, anxiety, and a sense of impending doom also are common, as are confusion, dizziness, and seizures, which probably reflect cerebral hypoperfusion.[61]

Principles of Management. It is critical to think of anaphylaxis as one end of a spectrum of clinical disorders that includes asthma, urticaria, and angioedema. Although anaphylaxis implies systemic collapse, clinically it may include aspects of bronchospasm, skin disorders, and laryngeal edema. Distinguishing whether a patient technically is suffering from angioedema rather than anaphylaxis is clinically unimportant in the acute setting; ultimately, initial management is identical.

Patients with suspected anaphylactic reactions must be triaged to a treatment area immediately. Since there is no way to predict how rapidly a reaction will progress, all patients should receive an immediate assessment of the stability of their ABCs. Voice changes, shortness of breath, lingual or oropharyngeal angioedema suggest impending airway obstruction and warrant immediate pharmacotherapy and preparation for intubation. All patients with symptoms of a systemic reaction should undergo close blood pressure monitoring, have two large-bore IVs started, and have intubation and cricothyroidotomy equipment at the bedside. If there are no immediate signs of airway obstruction or cardiovascular collapse, patients should be questioned about inciting allergens and previous history of similar reactions. If the etiology is known, exact time from exposure to symptom onset should be obtained.

First-Line Therapy—Epinephrine. Epinephrine is the drug of choice for treatment of systemic anaphylaxis.[50,58,60,61,71] Both the alpha and beta-agonist effects of epinephrine counteract the multiple actions of vasoactive mediators. Alpha-agonist activity reverses peripheral vasodilation and increases both systolic and diastolic blood pressure. Angioedema and urticaria, which often accompany anaphylaxis, also are reduced through alpha-mediated peripheral vasoconstriction. Epinephrine's beta-agonist activity promotes bronchodilation and enhances cardiac inotropy and chronotropy. Beta-agonist actions also facilitate production of cAMP, which is thought to further decrease mediator release.[58]

Unfortunately, the same mechanisms of action that make epinephrine so useful in the treatment of anaphylaxis can be potentially associated with serious side-effects. Excessive stimulation of alpha-receptors with subsequent peripheral vasoconstriction may precipitate a hypertensive crisis, causing cerebral hemorrhage, pulmonary edema, or other sequelae. Similarly, overstimulation of beta-receptors may induce arrhythmias or myocardial ischemia secondary to increased myocardial oxygen demand.[58,70] However, the adverse side effects of epinephrine can be largely mitigated by employing proper dose and route of administration, even in those with relative contraindications (e.g., cardiovascular disease, pregnancy, elderly). Ultimately, epinephrine is warranted in any life-threatening reaction that is refractory to other treatments. In a case study of 13 children who had fatal or near-fatal food-induced anaphylaxis, none of the fatalities received epinephrine prior to onset of severe respiratory symptoms; however, all patients who survived received epinephrine before or within five minutes of onset of respiratory symptoms. Interestingly, even the survivors (who received early epinephrine) eventually required intubation.[68]

Dose and Route. Indications for epinephrine, and its preferred route of administration, are based on the severity of the anaphylactic reaction. *(Please see Table 7.)* Although a very small percentage of adults may be managed with agents other than epinephrine, SQ epinephrine is recommended, even in patients with mild presentations. However, all patients with more severe reactions (e.g., laryngeal edema, hypotension) should receive 0.3 mg to 0.5 mg subcutaneously q 15-20 minutes until symptoms abate. The pediatric dose is 0.01 mg/kg at the same dosing frequency.[58] Intramuscular injection of epinephrine is warranted in both pediatric and adult patients who exhibit signs of impending airway obstruction, hypotension, or poor response to the subcutaneous route.[60] A systolic blood pressure of 60 mmHg is sufficient to absorb IM or SQ epinephrine.[50] Racemic epinephrine 2.25% diluted in 2.5 cc of normal saline also should be used in patients with signs or symptoms of airway compromise.[49,60] Nebulized albuterol may improve symptoms of bronchospasm.

Intravenous Epinephrine. Patients with airway obstruction, severe bronchospasm, or hypotension refractory to IM and racemic epinephrine may require IV epinephrine. The dose of IV epinephrine is somewhat controversial, and no studies have established a definitive dose that is both safe and therapeutic in systemic anaphylaxis. However, pharmacological studies suggest that slow, low-dose infusion rates stimulate beta-receptors more than alpha-receptors, thus producing bronchodilation and modest increase in systolic blood pressure. Fast, high-dose infusions appear to preferentially stimulate alpha-receptors, causing severe hypertension, arryhthmias, and myocardial ischemia. The American Heart Association's Advanced Cardiac Life Support (ACLS) protocol for IV epinephrine in adults is an initial dose of 1 mcg/min, titrated to 4 mcg/min if symptoms persist.[72] Other authors recommend a 100 mcg bolus at 10 mcg/min.[58] These concentrations are obtained by mixing 1 mg of epinephrine in 100 cc normal saline, to give a concentration of 10 mg/cc. In pediatric patients, the infusion rate begins at 0.1 mcg/kg/min, increasing to a maximum of 1.5 mcg/kg/min. This solution is prepared as above.[58]

Fluids. Hypotension should be treated with IV fluids since profound plasma volume loss (up to 50% in 10 minutes) has been reported.[73] Anaphylactic shock that remains refractory to volume replacement should be treated with dopamine or other pressors. These patients may also require central venous pressure monitoring or pulmonary artery catheterization for more precise fluid management.

Antihistamines. Antihistamines will not reverse end-organ effects, hypotension, or fluid loss in patients with anaphylaxis. Nevertheless, antihistamines remain an important adjunctive therapy by blocking further release of histamine and providing symptomatic relief in anaphylactic reactions accompanied by urticaria. As previously mentioned, H-2 agents probably have no direct effect when given alone, but may act synergistically with H-1 blockers.[74] Diphenhydramine 1 mg/kg up to a maximum 50 mg q 6 h, and cimetidine 4 mg/kg have been proposed.[64] There is no evidence of superiority of a 25 mg vs. 50 mg dosage of diphenhydramine.

Second-Line Therapy—Glucagon. The use of glucagon in anaphylaxis is largely anecdotal. However, patients on beta-blockers or those who have contraindications to epinephrine may benefit from a trial of this naturally occurring hormone. Glucagon is produced by the pancreas and serves a variety of functions including the stimulation of cyclic AMP. Increased levels of cardiac cyclic AMP may enhance contractility and cardiac output in patients with hypotension due to anaphylaxis. Patients on beta-blockers who experience anaphylaxis present a special challenge. When epinephrine is given for symptoms of anaphylaxis, peripheral beta-blockage results in unopposed alpha stimulation, possibly leading to malignant hypertension with serious consequences. Glucagon represents a safer alternative since the adrenergic receptors are bypassed.[58,75-77] Patients who may benefit from glucagon should receive an initial 1 mg IV bolus.[64,76,77] Because of its short half-life, repeat doses often are required, and can be given q 5 min.[78] Glucagon is generally well-tolerated.

Steroids. Steroids play no role in the immediate reversal of ana-

Table 7. Management of Anaphylaxis

First-Line Therapy - Epinephrine			
REACTION SEVERITY	**ROUTE**	**ADULT DOSE**	**PEDIATRIC DOSE**
Mild (urticaria, bronchospasm)	SQ	0.3 mg	0.01 mg/kg
Moderate (angioedema, hypotension)	SQ/IM	0.3-0.5 mg	0.01 mg/kg
Severe (laryngeal edema, respiratory failure, hypotension refractory to fluids and IM epinephrine)	IV 1-10 mcg/min	1 mg in 100 cc NS 0.1-1.5 mcg/kg/min	1 mg in 100 cc NS
Second-Line Therapy - Glucagon			
INDICATIONS	**ROUTE**	**ADULT DOSE**	**PEDIATRIC DOSE**
Consider use in patients with relative contraindications to epinephrine, e.g, patients with coronary artery disease, severe hypertension, patients on beta-blockers, pregnant patients, or those refractory to epinephrine therapy.	IV	1-5 mg bolus 2-5 mg/h	0.5-2.0 mg bolus 1-2 mg/h
Second-Line Therapy - Others			
MEDICATION	**ROUTE**	**ADULT DOSE**	**PEDIATRIC DOSE**
Diphenhydramine	IV	25-50 mg	1 mg/kg
Cimetidine	IV	300 mg	5-10 mg/kg
or			
Ranitidine	IV	50 mg	0.5 mg/kg
Methylprednisolone	IV	125 mg	1-2 mg/kg
Racemic epinephrine	Nebulized	0.5 cc in 2.5 cc NS	0.5 cc in 2.5 cc NS
Albuterol	Nebulized	0.5 cc in 2.5 cc NS	0.01 cc/kg
Methylene Blue (repeat in 90 min)	IV	2 mg/kg over 15min	Unknown

phylaxis since the onset of action may be delayed as much as 4-6 hours. However, steroids can inhibit or lessen biphasic and protracted anaphylactic reactions (especially bronchospasm) and should be administered. Methylprednisolone (SoluMedrol) 125 mg IV, or prednisone 60 mg po are common formulations.[60]

Experimental Treatment. Recently, methylene blue was shown anecdotally to reverse anaphylactic shock in several patients refractory to epinephrine.[48]

Disposition. All patients with systemic anaphylaxis should be observed for at least 6-8 hours, even if they have had prompt reversal of all symptoms and signs with standard therapy. The majority of biphasic reactions occur within this time period.[50] Patients with more severe reactions (e.g., hypotension or airway obstruction) must be observed for 24-48 hrs, even in the absence of persistent symptoms. Approximately 10% of patients with severe anaphylaxis will need repeated administration of epinephrine, even if they had complete resolution of symptoms between injections.[79] In one study, 28% of patients who responded to initial therapy had life-threatening recurrences, up to eight hours after apparent remission.[69] Elderly patients, those with asthma or underlying cardiac disease, and those on beta blockers also should be considered for admission even with mild reactions. Keep in mind that patients may have deceptively mild symptoms for two hours or more before severe compromise occurs.[68] All patients should receive a self-injectable kit (Epi-pen, Ana-kit) and be instructed in its use. ED physicians are often remiss in prescribing these epinephrine kits. In one study, 40% of children with hymenoptera allergy did not receive an epinephrine prescription.[80]

References

1. *Dorland's Pocket Medical Dictionary.* 24th ed. Philadelphia: W.B. Saunders Co; 1989.
2. Naclerio RM. Allergic rhinitis. *N Engl J Med* 1991;325: 860-869.
3. Pedinoff AJ. Approaches to the treatment of seasonal allergic rhinitis. *South Med J* 1996;89:1130-1139.
4. McMenamin P. Costs of hay fever in the United States in 1990. *Ann Allergy* 1994;73:35-39.
5. Kaplan AP. Urticaria and angioedema. In: Middleton EM Jr, Reed CE, Ellis EF, et al., eds. *Allergy: Principles and Practice.* 4th ed. St. Louis: Mosby-Year Book Inc; 1993: 1553-1580.
6. Aaronson DW. Comparative efficacy of H-1 antihistamines. *Ann Allergy* 1991;67:541-547.
7. Cetrizine. Pfizer package insert.
8. Terfenadine. Pfizer package insert.
9. Loratidine. Schering Plough package insert.
10. Fexofenadine. Schering Plough package insert.
11. Aztemizole. Schering Plough package insert.
12. Olin B, ed. *Drug Facts and Comparisons.* St. Louis: Mosby-Year Book, Inc.; 1997.
13. *Physicians Desk Reference.* Montvale, NJ: Medical Economics Co.; 1997.
14. Ricketti AJ. Allergic rhinitis. In: Patterson R, ed. *Allergic Diseases: Diagnosis and Management.* 3rd ed. Philadelphia: J.B. Lippincott Co; 1985:207-231.

15. Ferguson BJ. Allergic rhinitis. Recognizing signs, symptoms, and triggering allergens. *Postgrad Med* 1997;101:110-116.
16. Raphael GD, Igarashi Y, White MV, et al. The pathophysiology of rhinitis. *J Allergy Clin Immunol* 1991; 88:33-42.
17. Baraniuk JN. Pathogenesis of allergic rhinitis. *J Allergy Clin Immunol* 1997;99:S763-772.
18. Graft DF. Allergic and nonallergic rhinitis. Directing medical therapy at specific symptoms. *Postgrad Med* 1996;100:64-69.
19. Corren J. Allergic rhinitis and asthma: How important is the link? *J Allergy Clin Immunol* 1997;99:S781-786.
20. Parikh A, Scadding GK. Seasonal allergic rhinitis. *BMJ* 1997; 314:1392-1395.
21. Kemp JP. Special considerations in the treatment of seasonal allergic rhinitis in adolescents: The role of antihistamine therapy. *Clin Pediatr* 1996;358:383-389.
22. Meltzer EO. An overview of current pharmacotherapy in perennial rhinitis. *J Allergy Clin Innumol* 1995;95:1097-1110.
23. Ferguson BJ. Allergic rhinitis. Options for pharmacotherapy and immunotherapy. *Postgrad Med* 1997;101:117-120,123-126, 131.
24. Simons FER, Reggin JD, Roberts JR, et al. Benefit/risk ratio of the antihistamines (H-1-receptor antagonists) terfenadine and chlorpheniramine in children. *J Pediatr* 1994;124: 979-983.
25. Adelsberg BR, D'Amico-Beadon A. The effects of loratadine, diphenydramine and placebo on worker productivity: Results of a double-blind trial. [Abstract] *J Allergy Clin Immunol* 1990;85:296.
26. Gutkowski A, Bedard P, Del Carpio J, et al. Comparison of the efficacy and safety of loratadine, terfenadine, and placebo in the treatment of seasonal allergic rhinitis. *J Allergy Clin Immunol* 1988;81:902-907.
27. Del Carpio J, Kabbash L, Turrene Y, et al. Efficacy and safety of loratadine (10 mg once daily), terfenadine (60 mg twice daily), and placebo in the treatment of seasonal allergic rhinitis. *J Allergy Clin Immunol* 1989;84:741-746.
28. Renton R, Fidler C, Rosenberg R. Multicenter, crossover study of the efficacy and tolerability of terfenadine, 120 mg, vs. cetirizine, 10 mg, in perennial allergic rhinitis. *Ann Allergy* 1991;67:416-420.
29. Fexofenadine. *Med Lett Drugs Ther* 1996;38:95-96.
30. Day JH, Briscoe MP, Welsh A, et al. Onset of action, efficacy and safety of a single dose of 60 mg and 120 mg fexofenadine HCl for ragweed (RW) allergy using controlled antigen exposure in an environmental exposure unit (EEU). [Abstract] *J Allergy Clin Immunol* 1996;97:434.
31. Tinkelman D, Falliers C, Bronsky E, et al. Efficacy and safety of fexofenadine HCl in fall seasonal allergic rhinitis. [Abstract] *J Allergy Clin Immunol* 1996;97:435.
32. Bernstein D, Schoenwetter W, Nathan R, et al. Fexofenadine: A new nonsedating antihistamine is effective in the treatment of seasonal allergic rhinitis. [Abstract] *J Allergy Clin Immunol* 1996;97:435.
33. Nightingale CH. Treating allergic rhinitis with second-generation antihistamines. *Pharmacotherapy* 1996;16: 905-914.
34. Affrime MB, Lorber R, Danzig M, et al. Three month evaluation of electrocardiographic effects of loratadine in humans. [Abstract] *J Allergy Clin Immunol* 1993;91:259.
35. Sale ME, Woosley RL, Barby JT, et al. Lack of electrocardiographic effects of cetirizine in healthy humans. [Abstract] *J Allergy Clin Immunol* 1993;91:258.
36. Day, JH, Briscoe, MP, Clark, RH, et al. Onset of action and efficacy of terfenadine, astemizole, cetirizine, and loratidine for the relief of symptoms of allergic rhinitis, *Ann Allergy Asthma Immunol* 1997;79:163-172.
37. Claritin-D. Schering Corporation, Kenilworth NJ, Feb. 1997. Product information labeling change.
38. Chervinsky P, Georgitis J, Banov C, et al. Once daily loratadine vs. astemizole once daily. *Ann Allergy* 1994;73: 109-113.
39. Cetirizine: A new antihistamine. *Med Lett Drugs Ther* 1996; 38:21-23.
40. Prevost M, Turenne Y, Moote DW, et al. Comparative study of SCH 434 and CTM-D in the treatment of seasonal allergic rhinitis. *Clin Ther* 1994;16:50-56.
41. Davies RJ, Nelson HS. Once-daily mometasone furoate nasal spray: Efficacy and safety of a new intranasal glucocorticoid for allergic rhinitis. *Clin Ther* 1997;19:27-38.
42. Mackowiak JI. Fluticasone propionate aqueous nasal spray (FP) improves rhinitis quality of life and reduces lost labor costs. [Abstract] *Ann Allergy* 1994;72:99.
43. Inhaled and nasal steroids and the risk of glaucoma. *Emerg Med* 1997;29:32-33.
44. Druce HM. allergic and nonallergic rhinitis. In: Middleton EM Jr, Reed CE, Ellis EF, et al, eds. *Allergy: Principles and Practice.* 4th ed. St. Louis: Mosby-Year Book Inc; 1993: 1433-1453.
45. Bronsky EA, Druce H, Findlay SR, et al. A clinical trial of ipratropium bromide nasal spray in patients with perennial nonallergic rhinitis. *J Allergy Clin Immunol* 1995;95: 1117-1122.
46. Milford CA, Mugliston TA, Lund VJ, et al. Long-term safety and efficacy study of intranasal ipratropium bromide. *J Laryngol Otol* 1990;104:123-125.
47. Norman PS. Current status of immunotherapy for allergies and anaphylactic reactions. *Adv Intern Med* 1996;41:681-713.
48. Hobbs KF, Schocket A. Urticaria and angioedema. In: Bierman WC, Perlman DS, Shapiro GG, et al, eds. *Allergy, Asthma, and Immunology from Infancy to Adulthood.* 3rd ed. Philadelphia: W.B. Saunders Co; 1996:643-652.
49. Goldberg R, Lawton R, Newton E, et al. Evaluation and management of acute uvular edema. *Ann Emerg Med* 1993; 22:251-255.
50. Jerrard DA. ED management of insect stings. *Am J Emerg Med* 1996;14:429-433.
51. Volcheck GW, Li JTC. Exercise-induced urticaria and anaphylaxis. *Mayo Clin Proc* 1997;72:140-147.
52. Kam PCA, Lee MSM, Thompson JF. Latex allergy: An emerging clinical and occupational health problem. *Anaesthesia* 1997;52:570-575.
53. Ebo DG, Stevens WJ, Bridts CH, et al. Human seminal plasma anaphylaxis (HSPA): Case report and literature review. *Allergy* 1995;50:747-750.
54. Pruet CW, Kornblut AD, Brickman C, et al. Management of

the airway in patients with angioedema. *Laryngoscope* 1983; 93:749-755.

55. Goldsmith P, Dowd PM. The new H-1 antihistamines. Treatment of urticaria and other clinical problems. *Dermatol Clin* 1993;11:87-95.
56. Monroe EW. Nonsedating H-1 antihistamines in chronic urticaria. *Ann Allergy* 1993;71:585-591.
57. Pollack CV Jr, Romano T. Outpatient management of acute urticaria: The role of prednisone. *Ann Emerg Med* 1995; 26:547-551.
58. Barach EM, Nowak RM, Tennyson GL, et al. Epinephrine for treatment of anaphylactic shock. *JAMA* 1984;251:2118-2122.
59. Thompson T, Frable MAS. Drug-induced, life-threatening angioedema revisited. *Laryngoscope* 1993;103:10-12.
60. Heilpern KL. The treacherous clinical spectrum of allergic emergencies: diagnosis, treatment, and prevention. *Emerg Med Rep* 1994;15:211-222.
61. Marquardt DL, Wasserman SI. Anaphylaxis. In: Middleton EM Jr, Reed CE, Ellis EF, et al, eds. *Allergy: Principles and Practice.* 4th ed. St. Louis: Mosby-Year Book Inc; 1993: 1525-1536.
62. Tintinalli JE, Ruiz E, Krome RL, eds. *Emergency Medicine: A Comprehensive Study Guide.* 4th ed. New York: McGraw Hill; 1996.
63. Civetta JM, Taylor Rw, Kirby RR. *Critical Care.* 3rd ed. Philadelphia: Lippincott-Raven; 1997.
64. Wittbrodt ET, Spinler SA. Prevention of anaphylactoid reactions in high-risk patients receiving radiocontrast media. *Ann Pharmacother* 1994;28:236-241.
65. Charpin D, Birnbaum J, Vervloet D. Epidemiology of *Hymenoptera* allergy. *Clin Exp Allergy* 1994;24:1010-1015.
66. Van der Klauw MM, Wilson JHP, Stricker BH. Drug-associated anaphylaxis: 20 years of reporting in The Netherlands (1974-1994) and review of the literature. *Clin Exp Allergy* 1996;26:1355-1363.
67. Kemp SF, Lockey RF, Wolf BL, et al. Anaphylaxis: A review of 26 cases. *Arch Intern Med* 1995;155:1749-1754.
68. Sampson HA, Mendelson L, Rosen JP. Fatal and near-fatal anaphylactic reactions to food in children and adolescents. *N Engl J Med* 1992;327:380-384.
69. Stark BJ, Sullivan TJ. Biphasic and protracted anaphylaxis. *J Allergy Clin Immunol* 1986;78:76-83.
70. Vaswani SK, Plack RH, Norman PS. Acute severe urticaria and angioedema leading to myocardial infarction. *Ann Allergy Asthma Immunol* 1996;77:101-104.
71. Friday GA Jr, Fireman P. Anaphylaxis. *Ear Nose Throat J* 1996;75:21-24.
72. Advanced Cardiac Life Support (ACLS) guidelines. American Heart Association, 1994.
73. Yocum MW, Khan DA. Assessment of patients who have experienced anaphylaxis: A three-year survey. *Mayo Clin Proc* 1994;69:16-23.
74. Yarbrough JA, Moffitt JE, Brown DA, et al. Cimetidine in the treatment of refractory anaphylaxis. *Ann Allergy* 1989;63: 235-238.
75. Wyatt R. Anaphylaxis: How to recognize, treat, and prevent potentially fatal attacks. *Postgrad Med* 1996;100:87-98.
76. Javeed N, Javeed H, Javeed S, et al. Refractory anaphylactoid shock potentiated by beta-blockers. *Cathet Cardiovas Diagn* 1996;39:383-384.
77. Zaloga GP, Delacey W, Holmboe E, et al. Glucagon reversal of hypotension in a case of anaphylactoid shock. *Ann Int Med* 1986;105:65-66.
78. Pollack CV Jr. Utility of glucagon in the emergency department. *J Emerg Med* 1993;11:195-205.
79. Fisher M. Treatment of acute anaphylaxis. *BMJ* 1995;311: 731-733.
80. Moffitt JE, Yates AB, Price W, et al. ER survey of hymenoptera (HM) stings in children. [Abstract] *Ann Allergy* 1992;68:81.

Part V

Cardiovascular and Thrombosis-Related Conditions

Preventive Cardiology in the Office, Part I

James J. Maciejko, MS, PhD, FACC

Although mortality rates for coronary heart disease (CHD) have been declining in recent years, CHD still remains the No. 1 cause of death and disability in the United States. The cost of our interventional procedures and drugs to manage symptomatic CHD (e.g., balloon angioplasty, stents, low-molecular-weight heparins, glycoprotein IIb-IIIa inhibitors, and bypass surgery) should lead us to pause and reconsider the benefits of prevention and risk stratification. This chapter and the next will explore the identification of these risk factors and our better understanding of them and provide the primary care physcian effective strategies for intervention. The next chapter will highlight Category II, III, and IV risk factors and provide a summary of the recommendations in order of importance.

Introduction

Control or cure of most infectious diseases in the industrialized countries has led to chronic illnesses, becoming the major health problems in those nations. Although a decline in rates has been observed over the past 30 years,[1,2] cardiovascular diseases remain the leading cause of death and disability in the United States. Approximately 75% of cardiovascular disease deaths are the result of atherosclerosis, which causes coronary heart, cerebral vascular, and peripheral vascular diseases. Forty percent of first major CHD episodes result in death within 30 days,[3] and survivors of a first myocardial infarction (MI) have a several-fold increase in the probability of death during the next 5-10 years compared to the risk for persons without a prior history of CHD.[4] These facts highlight the importance of primary prevention as a major clinical strategy for better control of this epidemic. This does not suggest that prevention to reduce reoccurrence of clinical events for those already afflicted with CHD is not of value (i.e., secondary prevention), rather, it emphasizes that secondary prevention, emergency service, and long-term medical and surgical interventions alone are not sufficient to reduce this healthcare burden. A major challenge of healthcare professionals is to control and significantly reduce atherosclerotic cardiovascular disease (ASCVD) in the United States.

Implementation of a strategy combining public health efforts for the general population and specific clinical efforts for persons and families at high risk for ASCVD are necessary. An essential component of this approach involves efforts beginning early in life that promote healthy habits in children. Physicians can contribute to this prevention effort by effectively interacting with their patients and families.

People who develop ASCVD have common predisposing characteristics. These characteristics are called risk factors and are reliable predicators of an individual's likelihood of developing ASCVD. Risk factors have been categorized in several ways including modifiable vs. nonmodifiable, acquired vs. biochemical/physiological, causal vs. associative, and chronic vs. acute. The 27th Bethesda Conference held

Table 1. Risk Factors for Atherosclerosis Based on Priority

CATEGORY	I	II	III	IV
Risk Factors	Smoking	Diabetes mellitus	Psychosocial factors	Age
	Hypercholesterolemia	Sedentary lifestyle	Hypertriglyceridemia	Gender
	Hypertension	Hypoalpha-lipoproteinemia	Hyper-Lp(a)-lipoproteinemia	Positive family history
	Hypercoagulability	Obesity	Hyperhomocystemia	
		Postmenopause	Oxidative stress	
		Excess alcohol consumption		

Adapted from: Pasternak RC, et al. Task Force 3. Spectrum of risk factors for coronary heart disease. *J Am Coll Cardiol* 1996;27:979-990.

in 1995 ("Matching the Intensity of Risk Factor Management with the Hazard for Coronary Disease Events") classified ASCVD risk factors according to "descending levels of evidence to support direct management."[5,6] This format allows for prioritization of ASCVD risk factors relative to their significance. Four risk factor categories have been proposed: 1) risk factors for which interventions have been proved to reduce the incidence of coronary artery disease (CAD) events; 2) risk factors associated with increased CAD risk that, if modified, will likely reduce the incidence of CAD events; 3) risk factors associated with increased CAD risk that, if modified, might reduce the incidence of CAD events; and 4) risk factors associated with increased CAD risk that cannot be modified or whose modification would be unlikely to change the incidence of CAD events (please *see Table 1*). This categorization format allows the primary care physician to focus on those risk factors for which there is evidence that their modification favorably affects outcome.

Category I Risk Factors (Highest Priority)

Cigarette Smoking. Cigarette smoking is the single most obvious and important risk factor for CAD and other atherosclerotic vascular diseases.[7,8] Smoking accelerates atherosclerosis[9] and leads to abnormalities of coronary arterial tone,[10] of thrombogenesis,[11] and of lipoprotein metabolism.[12,13] The net consequence of smoking is an increased incidence of all clinical CAD sequelae including MI,[14] unstable angina pectoris,[15] sudden death,[16] and ventricular dysfunction.[17]

The incidence of CHD in men by smoking status was examined in five prospective cardiovascular epidemiological studies in the United States as part of the National Cooperative Pooling Project.[18] All of the studies documented higher incidences of CHD in smokers than in nonsmokers. Additionally, a definitive dose-response relationship between the amount smoked and CHD risk in current smokers also was apparent. A study in women indicated a distinct relation between smoking and CHD mortality, with smoking accounting for half of all cardiovascular deaths.[19] This study also demonstrated that casual women cigarette smokers were at enhanced risk of CHD.

Clinical data have shown that smoking cessation produces a substantial and prompt reduction in CHD death rates.[20,21] Prospective smoking cessation studies demonstrate that CAD events decline more rapidly than overall death from CHD, with the greatest proportion of risk reduction occurring in the first several months after smoking cessation.[8] Patients who continue to smoke after acute MI have an increase in the risk of death from reinfarction that is, on average, 33% higher than in patients who terminate smoking.[22]

Exposure to second-hand (passive) smoke also may increase risk. Second-hand smoke may be the third leading cause of preventable death in this country. It is estimated that passive smoking accounts for about 40,000 CHD deaths annually in this country.[23]

Healthcare professionals should set an example by not smoking and should take an active role in programs designed to dissuade all individuals, especially teenagers, from starting to smoke. A smoking history should be routinely obtained, and all patients should be informed that cigarette smoking causes ASCVD and lung cancer. All patients who smoke should be counseled to quit and should receive personal assistance both to stop smoking and to maintain an ex-smoker status. Patients with ASCVD and chronic obstructive pulmonary disease (COPD), as well as asymptomatic patients at high CHD risk, should receive special attention. Patients who are candidates for coronary artery bypass graft surgery (CABG) or arterial reconstructive surgery of the lower extremities should be advised of smoking-related surgical risks. Patients receiving oral contraceptives and a wide variety of cardiopulmonary medications should be instructed about possible adverse interactions between cigarette smoking and these medications.

Hypercholesterolemia. Hypercholesterolemia (i.e., elevated low-density lipoprotein [LDL]-cholesterol concentrations) is causally related to the development of atherosclerosis. The evidence linking an elevated LDL-cholesterol and ASCVD is derived from extensive epidemiologic and clinical trial data. The landmark epidemiologic (observational) studies are the Framingham Heart

Table 2. Primary and Secondary Prevention Lipid-Lowering Trials

	INTERVENTION	% LDL-C LOWERING	% REDUCTION IN NONFATAL MI/CAD DEATH
Primary Prevention Trials			
LRC-CPPT	cholestyramine	20%	19%
WOSCOPS	pravastatin	26%	31%
AF/Tex CAPS	lovastatin	25%	36%
Secondary Prevention Trials			
CDP	nicotinic acid	20%	15%
POSCH	partial ileal bypass	38%	35%
4(S)	simvastatin	35%	36%
CARE	pravastatin	28%	24%
Post-CABG	lovastatin	39%	30%
LIPID	pravastatin	25%	23%

Key:

LRC-CPPT: Lipid Research Clinics-Coronary Primary Prevention Trial[27]
WOSCOPS: West of Scotland Coronary Prevention Study[28]
AF/TexCAPS: Air Force/Texas Coronary Atherosclerosis Prevention Study[29]
CDP: Coronary Drug Project[30,31]
POSCH: Program on the Surgical Control of the Hyperlipidemias[32]
4S: Scandinavian Simvastatin Survival Study[33]
CARE: Cholesterol and Recurrent Events Study[34]
Post-CABG: Post Coronary Artery Bypass Graft Study[35]
LIPID: Long-Term Intervention with Pravastatin in Ischemic Disease[36]

Study,[24] the Seven Countries Study,[25] and the PROCAM Study.[26] These epidemiologic studies indicated a 2% increase in risk for CHD per 1% increase in the plasma LDL-cholesterol concentration.

Extensive interventional data from both primary- and secondary-prevention trials have demonstrated that lowering total and LDL-cholesterol concentrations reduces coronary events (unstable angina pectoris, acute MI), coronary mortality, and total mortality *(please see Table 2)*.[27-36] The clinical benefit appears to be related to the degree of LDL-cholesterol reduction.[35]

Recently, three landmark trials with clinical end points, each using an HMG-CoA Reductase Inhibitor (i.e., statin) in conjunction with dietary therapy, have been completed and extend the evidence demonstrating that lowering LDL-cholesterol can increase overall survival in secondary and primary prevention, and can reduce CHD risk in patients without hypercholesterolemia. The Scandinavian Simvastatin Survival Study (4S),[33] the West of Scotland Coronary Prevention Study (WOSCOPS),[28] and the Cholesterol and Recurrent Events Study (CARE)[34] collectively enrolled more than 15,000 patients. The 4S provided the first evidence that aggressive LDL-cholesterol lowering can significantly reduce all-cause mortality (30%) in patients with CHD. The risk of all-cause mortality was also reduced by 22% in the WOSCOP primary prevention study. Additionally, both of these studies demonstrated significant reductions in nonfatal MI and CHD death rate, the need for revascularization procedures, and stroke. The beneficial effect on nonfatal MI and CHD death applied to all subgroups including patients 55 years and older, patients 54 years and younger, and patients with and without multiple CHD risk factors (i.e., smokers, hypertensives, diabetics).

The CARE trial[34] was a secondary prevention study in survivors of MI with average plasma levels of cholesterol (mean LDL-cholesterol, 137 mg/dL). The results from CARE indicated that LDL-cholesterol lowering can reduce coronary morbidity and mortality rates in CHD patients without hypercholesterolemia.

Although some of the lipid-lowering interventional trials were conducted in men only, treatment of women with hypercholesterolemia is also warranted. The Air Force/Texas Coronary Artery Prevention Study (AF/Tex CAPS)[29] demonstrated that the effect of treatment with lovastatin on the rate of first acute major coronary events was greater in women than in men (46% vs 37% reduction in relative risk). 4S[33] found that the reduction in risk of CHD morbidity and mortality from LDL-cholesterol lowering by simvastatin was equal in both genders.

Treatment of hypercholesterolemia in patients older than 70 years and without clinical evidence of atherosclerosis remains controversial. Although total cholesterol levels are slightly lower in older age groups, as compared to younger people, the prevalence of hypercholesterolemia in the elderly is substantial. Treatment of elevated total cholesterol or LDL-cholesterol levels is often advocated to prevent CHD, which is a leading cause of mortality and morbid-

Table 3. Classification of Blood Pressure for Adults 18 Years and Older

Classification	Systolic Blood Pressure (mmHg)		Diastolic Blood Pressure (mmHg)
Optimal	< 120	and	< 80
Normal	< 130	and	< 85
High-normal	130-139	or	85-89
Hypertension:			
Stage 1	140-159	or	90-99
Stage 2	160-179	or	100-109
Stage 3	≥ 180	or	≥ 110

Note: Based on the average of two or more readings taken at each of two or more visits after the initial screening.

Adapted from: National Heart, Lung, and Blood Institute. Sixth Report of the Joint National Committee on Prevention, Detection, and Treatment of High Blood Pressure; Bethesda, MD: U.S. Department of Health and Human Services. National Institutes of Health, 1997.

Table 4. Recommendations for Treating High Blood Pressure Based on Risk

Blood Pressure Stages	Group A (no risk factors or TOD/CCD)*	Group B (at least 1 risk factor, not including diabetes; no TOD/CCD)	Group C (TOD/CCD and/ or diabetes, with or without other risk factors)
High-normal	Lifestyle modification	Lifestyle modification	Drug therapy†
Stage 1	Lifestyle modification (up to 12 months)	Lifestyle modification‡ (up to 6 months)	Drug therapy
Stages 2 or 3	Drug therapy	Drug therapy	Drug therapy

Note: Lifestyle modification should be adjunctive therapy for all patients recommended for pharmacologic therapy.

* TOD/CCD, target organ disease/clinical cardiovascular disease

† For patients with heart failure, renal insufficiency, or diabetes mellitus

‡ For patients with multiple risk factors, physicians should consider pharmacologic agents as initial therapy with lifestyle modifications.

ity in this population. A current study, the Antihypertensive and Lipid Lowering Treatment to Prevent Heart Attack (ALLHAT), is designed to address this issue by recruiting men and women older than 65 years of age.[37] The results of the Established Populations for Epidemiologic Studies of the Elderly (EPESE)[38] indicated that low high-density lipoprotein (HDL)-cholesterol predicts CHD mortality and occurrence of new CHD events in persons older than 70 years. The EPESE results suggest that lipid-lowering therapy should be considered in hyperlipidemic elderly patients with low HDL-cholesterol concentrations (< 35 mg/dL).

Approximately 35% of all American adults have a total cholesterol level that is associated with an increased risk of developing CHD. Initially, most individuals are candidates for lifestyle and dietary modifications. However, if such measures fail to improve LDL-cholesterol levels adequately, then combined diet and drug treatment should be considered.

A number of cholesterol-modifying drugs, including bile acid sequestrants, niacin, and statins, are effective in lowering LDL-cholesterol and have been shown to prevent coronary events. Statins have the advantage of a low side-effects profile and high compliance rate.

Current evidence indicates that cholesterol lowering is underused in patients with established CHD because of confusion over the degree of benefit they provide in patients with and without established CHD.[39,40] Given the conclusive evidence of the benefits of cholesterol lowering in patients with established ASCVD, withholding cholesterol-lowering medication in such patients is irrational and dangerous. It is imperative that monitoring of cholesterol levels be incorporated into the management of patients with established CHD and that treatment be prompt and effective. The National Cholesterol Education Program (NCEP) provides guidelines for the selection of individuals for diet and pharmacologic therapy for hypercholesterolemia.[41]

Hypertension. Elevated blood pressure (BP) is a significant risk factor for ASCVD. Numerous studies have indicated a continuous relationship between systolic and diastolic arterial blood pressures and ASCVD risk.[42,43] The Joint National Committee (JNC) VI report defines hypertension as a systolic BP of 140 mmHg or greater or a diastolic BP of 90 mmHg or greater.[44] The diagnosis of hypertension is based on an average of two or more readings taken at two or more visits after an initial screening visit *(please see Table 3)*.

Lifestyle modifications (e.g., weight reduction, smoking cessation, exercise) to reduce BP are highly encouraged with medications used as necessary to normalize BP. One of the new features of the JNC VI report is the use of risk stratification.[44] It was reasoned that the risk of cardiovascular disease in hypertensive patients is related not only to the level of BP but also to the presence of additional risk factors, and target organ damage or clinical cardiovascular disease. The need for pharmacologic therapy is determined according to the components of risk stratification and the level of blood pressure *(please see Table 4)*. Risk group A is associated with no risk factors other than an elevation in BP and no target organ damage or clinical signs of cardiovascular disease. Risk group B has at least one risk factor (not including diabetes mellitus), in addition to hypertension, and no target organ damage or clinical cardiovascular disease. Risk group C has target organ damage or clinical cardiovascular disease and/or diabetes mellitus with or without other cardiovascular risk factors. Patients with proteinuria greater than 1 g/d should be treated to a goal BP of 125/75 mmHg. Diabetics and patients with renal insufficiency and less than 1 g/d of proteinurea should be treated to a goal BP of 130/85 mmHg.[44]

Lifestyle modifications including weight loss, sodium restriction (< 2.4 g sodium/d), smoking cessation, increase in aerobic activity, and reduction in alcohol intake should always be included in the treatment of hypertension. For patients with uncomplicated conditions, diuretics or beta blockers are preferred as initial therapy.

Certain clinical situations require specific anti-hypertensive medications. MI requires beta-blocker therapy without intrinsic sympathomimetic activity and angiotensin-converting enzyme (ACE) inhibitors when systolic dysfunction is present. Patients with Type 1 diabetes mellitus and proteinurea would benefit from ACE inhibitors. For congestive heart failure, ACE inhibitors and diuretics are preferred. Diuretics are suggested for older patients with isolated systolic hypertension, although long-acting dihydropyridine calcium antagonists may be used.[44]

There is evidence that reducing BP decreases the development of cardiovascular disease including CAD, cerebralvascular disease, and heart failure.[45,46] Although the reduction in coronary events in some of these studies was less than expected from the magnitude of BP reduction,[45] this observation should not diminish acceptance of the role of hypertension in the production of ASCVD or the importance of its treatment.[5]

It is essential to recognize, evaluate, and treat every patient with an elevated arterial pressure. Lowering BP reduces the risk of complication from hypertension, stroke, and CHD, and decreases the occurrence of cardiovascular morbidity and mortality. In future years, newer and improved therapies should become available and they will likely be associated with even lower morbidity and mortality from hypertension. However, this cannot be achieved without constantly screening for new patients with unrecognized hypertension.

Thrombogenic Factors. Acute MI generally follows occlusion of a coronary artery by a thrombus. Aspirin has been documented to reduce both primary and secondary CHD events, affirming that reduction of thrombogenic potential improves outcome.[47] A number of prothrombotic factors have been identified and quantified, and these factors have been shown to be associated with increased CHD risk and events. However, treatment of any single thrombogenic variable has not yet been adequately shown to significantly lower CHD risk.

Low-dose aspirin therapy is a useful pharmacologic intervention for the prevention and treatment of acute thrombotic events. Aspirin irreversibly inhibits platelet cyclooxygenase and thromboxane A_2 production, resulting in an inhibition of platelet aggregation. This inhibition of platelet function dramatically reduces the risk of acute thrombosis, an effect that can be achieved with a dose of 80 mg aspirin each day (i.e., "baby" aspirin).[48]

Randomized clinical trials have demonstrated the benefit of aspirin in both the secondary and primary prevention of cardiovascular disease. In a recent overview of 25 trials of antiplatelet therapy among patients with established vascular disease, the use of aspirin was associated with a 32% overall reduction in subsequent nonfatal MI, a 27% reduction in subsequent nonfatal stroke, and a 15% reduction in total cardiovascular mortality.[49] Among subjects with unstable angina, aspirin therapy has been associated with a 37% reduction in cardiovascular death.[50,51] The Second International Study of Infarct Survival (ISIS-2) demonstrated that aspirin therapy reduced nonfatal reinfarction by 50%, reduced nonfatal stroke by 46%, and reduced total cardiovascular mortality by 23%.[52]

Aspirin has been shown to reduce the risk of a first acute MI in people without ASCVD. Two randomized trials of the primary prevention of occlusive vascular disease have been reported—the Physicians' Health Study[53] and the British Doctors' Trial.[54] The Physicians' Health Study, which included 22,000 males, demonstrated a 44% reduction in the incidence of MI in the physicians (ages 40-84 years) receiving aspirin (325 mg every other day) compared to the physicians taking a placebo. However, the British Doctor's Trial of 5000 male physicians found no difference in MI or cardiovascular death between the group taking aspirin (500 mg/d) and the group not taking aspirin. There was a very small increase in disabling strokes in the aspirin-treated group.[54] Based on the current data, the United States Preventative Services Task Force recommends that physicians consider aspirin therapy to prevent a first MI among men at heightened risk.[55] Although no randomized trial data of aspirin therapy in women are available, epidemiologic studies have suggested similar benefit.[56]

There are several disease states that are associated with hypercoagulability and increased incidence of thrombosis *(please see Table 5)*. Although the number of patients with these disorders is small, it is important to consider them since early identification can lead to significant improvements in clinical care.

Table 5. Clinical States Associated with Hypercoagulability and Increased Risk of Thrombosis

Primary abnormalities of coagulation and fibrinolysis
- Antithrobin III deficiency
- Protein C or protein S deficiency
- Hypoplasminogenemia
- Abnormal plasminogen activation and inhibition
- Lupus anticoagulants

Secondary abnormalities of coagulation and fibrinolysis
- Malignant neoplasm
- Pregnancy
- Oral contraceptive use
- Nephrotic syndrome

Abnormalities of platelet function
- Myeloproliferative disorders
- Paroxysmal nocturnal hemoglobinuria
- Hyperlipidemia
- Diabetes mellitus
- Spontaneous platelet aggregation

Abnormalities of blood vessels and rheology
- Venous stasis
- Vascular prostheses
- Vasculitis
- Homocystinuria
- Hyperhomocysteinemia
- Hyperviscosity
- Polycythemia
- Insulin resistance
- Abnormal renin profile

References

1. Gillum R. Trends in acute myocardial infarction and coronary heart disease in the United States. *J Am Coll Cardiol* 1994;23:1273-1277.
2. Rosamon WD, et al. Trends in the incidence of myocardial infarction and in mortality due to coronary heart disease, 1987 to 1994. *N Engl J Med* 1998;339: 861-867.
3. Stamler J, Foreword, in Pearson, TA, Criqui, MH, Luepker, RV, Oberman, A, Winston, M. (eds.): *Primer in Preventative Cardiology*. Dallas, American Heart Association, 1994; i-iv.
4. Kannel WB, et al. Prognosis after initial myocardial infarction: The Framingham Study. *Am J Cardiol* 1979;44:53-59.
5. Pasternak RC, et al. Task Force 3. Spectrum of risk factors for coronary heart disease. *J Am Coll Cardiol* 1996; 27:978-990.
6. Furberg CD, et al. Task Force 2. Clinical epidemiology: The conceptual basis for interpreting risk factors. *J Am Coll Cardiol* 1996;27:976-978.
7. Holbrook JH, et al. Cigarette smoking and cardiovascular diseases. A statement for health professionals by a task force appointed by the steering committee of the American Heart Association. *Circulation* 1984;70:114A-1117A.
8. *The Health Consequence of Smoking: Cardiovascular Disease. A Report of the Surgeon General*, publication DHHS (PHS) 84-50204. U.S. Department of Health and Human services, Public Health Services, Office on Smoking and Health. Rockville, Md, 1983.
9. Moise A, et al. Factors associated with progression of coronary artery disease in patients with normal and minimally narrowed coronary arteries. *Am J Cardiol* 1985; 56:30-34.
10. Fried LP, et al. Long-term effects of cigarette smoking and moderate alcohol consumption on coronary artery diameter. *Am J Med* 1986;80:37-44.
11. Folts JD, Bonebrake FC. The effects of cigarette smoke and nicotine on platelet thrombus formation in stenosed dog coronary arteries: Inhibition by phentolamine. *Circulation* 1982;65:465-470.
12. Stamford BA, et al. Cigarette smoking, exercise and high density lipoprotein cholesterol. *Atherosclerosis* 1984;52:73-83.
13. Fortmann SP, et al. Changes in plasma high density lipoprotein cholesterol after changes in cigarette use. *Am J Epidemiol* 1986;317:1303-1309.
14. Hartz AJ, et al. Smoking, coronary artery occlusion, and nonfatal myocardial infarction. *JAMA* 1981;246:851-853.
15. Ouyant P, et al. Variables predictive of successful medical therapy in patients with unstable angina; selection by multivariate analysis from clinical electrocardiographic, and angiographic evaluations. *Circulation* 1984;70:367-376.
16. Hallstrom AP, et al. Smoking as a risk factor for recurrence of sudden death. *N Engl J Med* 1986;314: 271-275.
17. Hartz AJ, et al. The association of smoking with cardiomyopathy. *N Engl J Med* 1984;311:1201-1206.
18. Pooling Project Research Group: Relationship of blood pressure, serum cholesterol, smoking habit, relative weight and ECG abnormalities to incidence of major coronary events: Final report of the Pooling Project. *J Chronic Dis* 1978;31:201-306.
19. Willet WC, et al. Relative and absolute excess risks of coronary heart disease among women who smoke cigarettes. *N Engl J Med* 1987;317:1303-1309.
20. Hermanson B, et al. Beneficial six year outcome of smoking cessation in older men and women with coronary artery disease. Results from the CASS registry. *N Engl J Med* 1988;319:1365-1369.
21. Rosenberg L, et al. The risk of myocardial infarction after quitting smoking in men under 55 years of age. *N Engl J Med* 1985;313:1511-1514.
22. Friedman GD, et al. Mortality in cigarette smokers and quitters. Effects of base-line differences. *N Engl J Med* 1981;304:1407.
23. Glantz SA, Parmley WW. Passive smoking and heart disease. Mechanisms and risk. *JAMA* 1995;273:1047-1053.
24. Kannel WP, et al. Serum cholesterol, lipoproteins, and the risk of coronary heart disease: The Framingham Study. *Ann Intern Med* 1971;74:1-12.
25. Keys A (ed): Coronary heart disease in seven countries. *Circulation* 1970;41(suppl 1):1-198.
26. Assmann G, Schulte H. Relation of high-density lipoprotein cholesterol and triglycerides to incidence of atherosclerotic coronary artery disease (the PROCAM experience). *Am J Cardiol* 1992;70:733-737.
27. Lipid Research Clinics coronary Primary Prevention Trial Results. I. Reduction in incidence of coronary heart disease. *JAMA* 1984;251:351-364.
28. Shepherd J, et al. For the West of Scotland Coronary Prevention Study Group. Prevention of coronary heart disease with pravastatin in men and hypercholesterolemia. *N Engl J Med* 1995;333:1301-1307.
29. Downs JR, et al. For the Air Force/Texas Coronary Atherosclerosis Prevention Study Group. Primary prevention of acute coronary events with lovastatin in men and women with average cholesterol levels. *JAMA* 1998;279:1615-1622.
30. The Coronary Drug Project Group. Clofibrate and niacin in coronary heart disease. *JAMA* 1975;231:360-381.
31. Canner PL, et al. Fifteen year mortality in the coronary drug project patients: Long-term benefit with patients. *J Am Coll Cardiol* 1988;8:1245-1255.
32. Buchwald H, et al. Effects of partial ileal bypass surgery on mortality and morbidity from coronary

heart disease in patients with hypercholesterolemia: Report of the Program on the Surgical Control of the Hyperlipidemias (POSCH). *N Engl J Med* 1990;323: 946-955.

33. Scandinavian Simvastatin Survival Study Group. Randomized trial of cholesterol lowering in 4444 patients with coronary heart disease: The Scandinavian simvastatin Survival Study (4S). *Lancet* 1994; 344: 1383-1389.
34. Sacks FM, et al. The effect of pravastatin on coronary events after myocardial infarction in patients with average cholesterol levels. *N Engl J Med* 1996;335: 1001-1009.
35. Post Coronary Artery Bypass Graft Trial Investigators. The effect of aggressive lowering of low-density lipoprotein cholesterol levels and low-dose anticoagulation on obstructive changes in saphenous-vein coronary-artery bypass grafts. *N Engl J Med* 1997;336:153-162.
36. The Long-Term Intervention with Pravastatin in Ischemic Disease (LIPID) Study Group. Prevention of cardiovascular events and death with pravastatin in patients with coronary heart disease and a broad range of initial cholesterol levels. *N Engl J Med* 1998;339: 1349-1357.
37. Davis BR, et al. Rationale and design for the Antihypertensive and Lipid Lowering Treatment to Prevent Heart Attack Trial (ALLHAT). *Am J Hypertens* 1996;9:342-360.
38. Corti MC, et al. HDL-cholesterol predicts coronary heart disease mortality in older persons. *JAMA* 1995; 274:539-544.
39. Clinical Quality Improvement Network (CQIN) Investigators. Low incidence of assessment and modification of risks in acute care patients at high risk for cardiovascular events, particularly among females and the elderly. *Am J Cardiol* 1995;76:570-573.
40. Shepherd J, Pratt M. Prevention of coronary heart disease in clinical practice: a commentary on current treatment patterns in six European countries in relation to published recommendations. *Cardiology* 1996;87:1-5.
41. National Cholesterol Education Program Expert panel. Summary of the second report of the National Cholesterol Education Program (NCEP) Expert Panel on Detection, Evaluation, and Treatment of High Blood Cholesterol in Adults (Adult Treatment Panel II). *JAMA* 1993; 269:3015-3023.
42. McGill HC, et al. General findings of the International Atherosclerosis Project. *Lab Invest* 1968;18:498-502.
43. MacMahon S, et al. Blood pressure, stroke, and coronary heart disease. Part I, prolonged differences in blood pressure: Prospective, observational studies corrected for the regression dilution bias. *Lancet* 1990;335:765-774.
44. National Heart, Lung, and Blood Institute. Sixth Report of the Joint National Committee on Prevention, Detection, and Treatment of High Blood Pressure. Bethesda, MD: U.S. Department of Health and Human Services. National Institutes of Health. 1997.
45. Collins R, et al. Blood pressure, stroke, and coronary heart disease. Part II, short-term reductions in blood pressure: Overview of randomized drug trials in their epidemiological context. *Lancet* 1990;335:827-838.
46. Cutler JA, et al. Public Health Issues in Hypertension Control; What has Been Learned from Clinical Trials. In: Laragh JH, Brenner BM, eds. *Hypertension: Pathophysiology, Diagnosis Management*. 2nd ed. NY: Raven Press, 1995:253-270.
47. Hennekens CH, et al. Aspirin and other antiplatelet agents in the secondary and primary prevention of cardiovascular disease. *Circulation* 1989;80:746-756.
48. Ridker PM, Hennekens CH. Risk factors for acute thrombosis, in Pearson TA, Criqui MH, Luepker RV, Oberman A, Winston M (eds.): *Primer in Preventative Cardiology*. Dallas, American Heart Association, 1994; 205-216.
49. Antiplatelet Trialists' Collaboration: Secondary prevention of vascular disease by prolonged antiplatelet therapy. *Br Med J* (Clin Res Ed) 1988; 291:320-331.
50. Lewis HD, Jr., et al. Protective effects of aspirin against acute myocardial infarction and death in men with unstable angina. *N Engl J Med* 1983;309:396-403.
51. Cairns JA, et al. Aspirin, sulfinpyrazone, or both in unstable angina: Results of a Canadian multicenter trial. *N Engl J Med* 1985;313:1369-1375.
52. ISIS-2 (Second International Study of Infarct Survival) Collaborative Group: Randomized trial of intravenous streptokinase, oral aspirin, both, or neither among 17,187 cases of suspected acute myocardial infarction: ISIS-2. *Lancet* 1988;2:349-360.
53. Steering Committee of the Physicians' Health Study Research Group: Final report on the aspirin component of the ongoing Physicians' Health Study. *N Engl J Med* 1989;321:129-135.
54. Peto R, et al. A randomized trial of prophylactic daily aspirin in British male doctors. *Br Med J* (Clin Res Ed) 1988;29:313-316.
55. U.S. Preventive Services Task Force. Aspirin Prophylaxis. In: *Guide to Clinical Preventive Services: An Assessment of the Effectiveness of 169 Interventions.* Report of the U.S. Preventive Services Task Force. Baltimore, William and Wilkins, 1989.
56. Manson JE, et al. A prospective study of aspirin use and primary prevention of cardiovascular disease in women. Presented at 31st Annual Conference on Cardiovascular Epidemiology, March 14-16, Orlando, FL. 1992.

Preventive Cardiology in the Office, Part II

James J. Maciejko, MS, PhD, FACC

Although mortality rates for coronary heart disease (CHD) have been declining in recent years, CHD still remains the No. 1 cause of death and disability in the United States. The cost of our interventional procedures and drugs to manage symptomatic CHD (e.g., balloon angioplasty, stents, low-molecular-weight heparins, glycoprotein IIb-IIIa inhibitors, and bypass surgery) should lead us to pause and reconsider the benefits of prevention and risk stratification. This chapter is the second of two chapters exploring the identification of these risk factors and our better understanding of them and providing the primary care physcian effective strategies for intervention. Part two highlights Category II, III, and IV risk factors and provides a summary of the recommendations in order of importance.

Category II Risk Factors

Category II risk factors are those for which interventions are likely to reduce the incidence of coronary artery disease (CAD) events. As with category I risk factors (*See Preventative Cardiology in the Office, Part I*), they are useful for atherosclerotic cardiovascular disease (ASCVD) risk assessment and should be considered and evaluated. They should also be treated as part of an optimal risk reduction program.

Diabetes Mellitus. People with diabetes mellitus (both type I and type 2) are at increased risk for ASCVD. In the United States, about 90% of all diabetic deaths are due to ASCVD, with 75% occurring as a result of CAD alone.[1,2] Recently, Haffner and colleagues reported the results of a Finnish study examining the risk of myocardial infarction (MI), over a seven-year period, in nondiabetic and Type 2 diabetic individuals.[3] Nondiabetic people without a prior history of MI had a 3.5% incidence of MI. Nondiabetic individuals with a prior history of MI had an 18.8% incidence of a subsequent event. Type 2 diabetic subjects without a prior history of CHD had a 20.2% incidence of MI, and diabetics with a prior history of CHD had a 45% incidence of a subsequent event. This study clearly demonstrates that Type 2 diabetics without clinical evidence of CHD are at risk of having an MI approximately equal to the risk of a recurrent event in a nondiabetic with CHD. The study also suggests that relative to risk stratification, diabetic patients belong in the same category as patients with existing CHD and should be treated as aggressively in terms of risk reduction.

There also are good data showing that diabetic patients who suffered a MI may benefit more from lipid-lowering therapy than nondiabetic individuals. The results of a post-hoc analysis based on a 5.4 year follow-up of 202 diabetic patients with CHD from the Scandinavian Simvastatin Survival Study (4S) shows a 55% reduction in CHD events in the treatment group.[4] This reduction in risk was greater than observed in the nondiabetic population (risk reduction [RR], 32%; $P < 0.0001$).

Whether improved control of hyperglycemia in diabetics reduces risk of ASCVD is somewhat controversial. However, the results of the Diabetes Control and Complications Trial (DCCT)[1] and, in particular, the United Kingdom Prospective Diabetes Study (UKPDS)[5] have provided some evidence demonstrating the importance of glycemic control for reducing ASCVD risk. DCCT participants were Type 1 diabetics and UKPDS were Type 2 diabetics.

Over a nine-year period, the DCCT looked at 1441 individuals with Type 1 diabetes who were between 13 and 39 years of age. At the beginning of the study, the participants had no significant complications other than background retinopathy. The patients were randomized into two groups. One group received standard care (1 or 2 injections of insulin daily) and achieved a HbAlc on average of 9%. The other group received intensive care (several small-dose injections of insulin throughout the day) and achieved a HbAlc on average of 7%. The more tightly controlled group recorded a 76% reduction in the onset of diabetic retinopathy, a 69% reduction in neuropathy, and a 44% reduction in nephropathy compared to the standard care treatment group.[1]

UKPDS was a randomized controlled trial that compared the effects of intensive blood glucose control (achieved with either sulphonylurea derivatives or insulin) with conventional treatment on the risk of microvascular and macrovascular complications of diabetes. UKPDS started in 1977 and continued for 20 years. The participants were 3867 newly diagnosed Type 2 patients (median age, 54 years) who, after three months of dietary treatment, had a fasting plasma glucose of 6.1-15 mmol/L. Only 0.3% of participants received lipid-lowering treatment and 11.6% were receiving antihypertensive treatment.

End points of this study were any diabetes-related end point (sudden death, death from hyperglycemia or hypoglycemia, fatal or nonfatal MI, angina, heart failure, stroke, renal failure, amputation, vitreous hemorrhage, retinopathy requiring photocoagulation, blindness in one eye, or cataract extraction) and all-cause mortality. During the trial, the HbAlc was reduced by 11% (from 7.9 to 7.0) in the intensive treatment group compared to conventional treatment and there was a 12% decrease in the risk for any diabetic end point (P = 0.029). RR was 0.84 (95% confidence limits 0.781-1.00; P = 0.052). This included combined fatal and nonfatal MI and sudden death. There was no effect on allcause mortality, and the incidence of stroke was not affected (RR =1.11 [0.81-1.51; P = 0.52]). Likewise, there was no effect on the incidence of limb amputations or death from peripheral vascular disease (RR 0.65 [0.36-1.18; P = 0.14]). Similar to the DCCT, there was an increased incidence of hypoglycemia in the intensive treatment group. Major hypoglycemic episodes occurred on treatment with sulfonylureas in 1.4% of participants, with insulin in 1.8% and on diet alone in 0.7% of participants. Minor hypoglycemic episodes were much more common, occurring in 15-21% of patients treated with sulphonylurea derivatives, in 28% of patients treated with insulin, and in 10% of individuals treated with diet alone. There was more weight gain in the intensive treatment group.

Diabetes mellitus is a major ASCVD risk factor and is associated with changes in other cardiovascular risk factors, including lipids, blood pressure, fibrinogen, platelet activity, and insulin. The clinician should be aware of these risk factors and treat them by diet, improved glycemic control, and drug therapy. Evidence suggests that correction of lipoprotein abnormalities, raised blood pressure (BP), and smoking is beneficial.[1,5]

Sedentary Lifestyle. The concept that inactivity leads to an increased risk of ASCVD has become generally accepted by healthcare professionals and the public. This has led to physical inactivity becoming a major target for preventative medicine in the United States. It is estimated that 12% of all mortality in the United States may be related to lack of regular physical activity.[6] However, no single study provides significant evidence of a causal relation between physical inactivity and ASCVD risk.

During the past half century, approximately 50 studies have suggested an association between physical inactivity and the prevalence or incidence of initial clinical manifestations of CHD, especially MI and sudden cardiac death.[7] The diversity in the protocols used in these various studies preclude the collating of the data into a single summary statement. Several findings occurred frequently enough to allow for the formulation of preliminary conclusions. These include: 1) more active people appear to be at lower risk of cardiovascular disease; and 2) moderate amounts of exercise may be beneficial.

Exercise probably exerts its beneficial effect through a variety of mechanisms.[8] Physical training improves the myocardial supply/demand relationship, lowers plasma triglycerides, raises HDL-cholesterol, reduces BP, and decreases platelet aggregation. Although no single trial of physical activity in patients with CAD has had sufficient power to convincingly demonstrate a risk reduction, intermediate end points (e.g., HDL-cholesterol and BP) are regularly improved and several meta-analyses of randomized trials support a reduction (20-30%) in coronary disease death with regular aerobic exercise.[9,10]

Hypoalphalipoproteinemia. There is a strong inverse epidemiologic association between plasma HDL-cholesterol concentrations and ASCVD risk. This relationship is sustained over a wide range of HDL-cholesterol plasma concentrations, and it is estimated that for every 1 mg/dL decrease in HDL-cholesterol, the relative risk for CAD events increases by 2-3%.[11] The relationship appears to be equally strong in men, women, and among asymptotic individuals as well as patients with established CHD.

HDL is secreted by the intestine, the liver, and cholesteryl ester-enriched macrophages. The initial form, referred to as nascent HDL, is a precursor to the mature lipoprotein. The particle matures as it acquires unesterified cholesterol from cell membranes during cell renewal or death. The cholesterol obtained is esterified by plasma: lecithin cholesterol acyltranasferase (LCAT), and, as the lipid content rises, nascent HDL become the small HDL_3 particles and, eventually, HDL_2 particles. The increased cholesterol-carrying capacity of HDL_2 particles is thought to be crucial to the process of reverse cholesterol transport, by which HDL particles carry cholesterol from peripheral tissues to the liver for excretion.

HDL-cholesterol concentrations are influenced by family history and by certain lifestyle factors that are also risk factors (cigarette smoking, obesity, physical inactivity). Frequently, low HDL-cholesterol concentrations are accompanied by high levels of triglycerides due to the metabolic relationship involving cholesterol ester transfer between HDL particles and triglyceride-rich lipoproteins.

Many lipid-altering agents and lifestyle factors affect several lipoproteins concurrently, and, therefore, it has been difficult to demonstrate that an independent increase in HDL-cholesterol reduces CHD risk. The HDL Intervention Trial (HIT)[12] evaluated the effect of independently raising HDL-cholesterol on recurrence of coronary events in a group of men with CAD, having isolated low levels of HDL-cholesterol, and normal LDL-cholesterol and triglyceride levels. A total of 2500 men were randomized to gemfibrozil (1200 mg/d) or placebo and were followed for seven years. An 8% increase in HDL-cholesterol in the men receiving gemfibrozil was associated with a 22% reduction in the incidence of CHD death and nonfatal MI and a 26% reduction in stroke. HIT demonstrated that raising a low HDL-cholesterol level independent of lowering LDL-cholesterol is important for reducing ASCVD risk. The observation of the Helsinki Heart Study[13] demonstrating that a reduction in CAD with gemfibrozil exceeded that expected from the LDL-cholesterol lowering alone, has also been interpreted by some to indicate a therapeutic benefit from raising HDL-cholesterol concentrations.

Nonpharmacologic methods for raising plasma HDL-cholesterol concentrations include exercise, weight reduction, and smoking cessation. Diets rich in mono-unsaturated fats (e.g., olive and canola oils) also raise HDL-cholesterol levels. The most effective pharmacologic agents are nicotinic acid, fibric acid derivatives, and estrogens.

Obesity. Obesity (weighing 40% more than the desirable weight range) is one of the most prevalent health problems in this country. About 30% of the U.S. population is obese.[14,15] Epidemiologic studies have observed an increase in mortality from both CHD and stroke with increasing obesity.[16,17] Obesity is associated with other ASCVD risk factors including low HDL-cholesterol concentration, diabetes mellitus, hypertension, and increased triglyceride concentration. It is probable that much of the increased ASCVD risk associated with obesity is mediated by these other metabolic abnormalities.

Visceral or central obesity, which can be quantified by the waist-to-hip ratio, is a common form of obesity associated with a particular metabolic syndrome of insulin resistance, low HDL-cholesterol, elevated triglycerides, LDL subclass pattern B, and hypertension. This cluster of related abnormalities is referred to as Syndrome X. The constellation of lipid abnormalities in Syndrome X is designated as the Atherogenic Lipoprotein Phenotype (ALP). ALP has been shown to increase CAD risk.[18] A desirable waist-to-hip ratio for men is less than 0.9 and less than 0.8 for women. No study has specifically examined the effect of weight loss or the type of weight loss on CAD events. Obesity is included as a class II risk factor because of the probability that weight reduction will beneficially alter other important risk factors (e.g., lipoprotein abnormalities) that are associated with obesity.

Support, advice, encouragement, and interest from the primary care physician is important for a patient's success in reducing weight. Changing behavior is difficult and does not occur quickly. Comprehensive behavioral approaches to weight loss can provide significant effect.

Postmenopausal State. CHD is the leading cause of death in adult U.S. women. Annually, there are more than 250,000 deaths from CHD. Lack of estrogen has been implicated as a risk factor for CAD, since the association between surgical or natural menopausal status and CAD was demonstrated.[19,20]

Most of the population-based studies on hormone replacement therapy (HRT) have demonstrated a 30-50% reduction in cardiovascular and all-cause mortality in current users of estrogen. It has been shown repeatedly both in population-based[21,22] and angiographic[23] studies that HRT in women with known CAD or with coronary risk factors tend to benefit much more than healthy postmenopausal women without HRT.

After 8.5 years, the Lipid Research Clinic Follow-Up Study found that there was almost a five-fold reduction in death among estrogen users with known CAD at baseline, compared with a two-fold reduction in death among estrogen users without baseline CAD.[24] The Nurses' Health Study (NHS) found that users of HRT who had one or more cardiovascular risk factors had a 50% reduction in all-cause mortality compared with an 11% reduction in HRT users without risk factors.[22] In addition, angiographic studies have shown less CAD at baseline in users of HRT[25] and lower mortality rates after 10 years of follow-up, with particularly significant findings in women with the more severe CAD at baseline.[23] Women who have undergone percutaneous or surgical coronary revascularization also appear to benefit from HRT. Improved long-term survival has been shown for HRT users who have undergone coronary artery bypass grafting[26] or percutaneous transluminal coronary angioplasty (PTCA).[27] These studies strongly suggested that HRT may be an important issue for the secondary prevention of CAD or in patients with known coronary risk factors.

Despite these observational study data, prospectively randomized trials to address the effectiveness and safety of HRT for the primary and secondary prevention of CAD in postmenopausal women have just been initiated within the past several years. Results from the primary prevention study (Women's Health Initiative) will become available during the next several years. The results of the secondary prevention study (Heart and Estrogen/progestin Replacement Study [HERS]) were recently published by Hulley and associates.[28]

The HERS randomized 2763 postmenopausal women with CHD (younger than 80 years), and intact uteri to either 0.625 mg of conjugated equine estrogen plus 2.5 mg of medroxyprogesterone acetate in one tablet daily or to placebo. The women were followed for an average of 4.1 years, and the primary outcome was the occurrence of nonfatal MI or CHD death. Secondary cardiovascular outcomes included coronary revascularization, unstable angina, congestive heart failure, stroke or transient ischemic attack, and peripheral arterial disease. Overall, there were no significant differences between groups in the primary or secondary outcomes. The lack of an overall effect occurred despite a net 11% lower LDL-cholesterol level and a 10% higher HDL-cholesterol level in the hormone group compared with the placebo group ($P < 0.001$). Within the overall null effect, there was a statistically significant time trend, with more CHD events in the hormone group than in the placebo group in year one and fewer in years four and five. More women in the hormone group than in the placebo group experienced venous thromboembolic events (including MI) and gallbladder disease.[28]

Based on this finding of no overall cardiovascular benefit and a pattern of early increase in risk of CHD events, it was not recommended to initiate HRT for secondary prevention of CHD. Hulley et al suggested that given the favorable pattern of CHD events after several years of treatment, HRT could be appropriate for women currently receiving this treatment to continue.[28] While HRT is not recommended for the secondary prevention of ASCVD, no general recommendations can be given relative to primary prevention until the results of the Women's Health Initiative Study are completed. Over the next decade, research must be aggressive in defining the optimal timing and duration of HRT, the lowest effective estrogen dose (for cardiovascular risk reduction), and further identification of patients who will benefit most from this therapy. It will be imperative for all physicians, particularly cardiologists, to remain current with the outcomes of pertinent trials and to be cognizant of the rapidly changing pharmacotherapy in this field.

Category III Risk Factors

Category III risk factors are those that are associated with an increased risk of ASCVD, which, if modified, might lower the incidence of cardiovascular events. Primary care physicians should place less emphasis on these risk factors than Category I or II risk factors. Several of the Category III risk factors accompany Category I and II risk factors.

Psychosocial and Behavioral Factors. Many behavioral and psychosocial factors are associated with increased ASCVD risk *(please see Table)*. There is increased prevalence of CHD in men, African-Americans, Hispanics, Native Americans, people with less education or income, and single people (particularly those who are divorced or separated).

The mechanism through which psychological and social issues may influence ASCVD can be divided into two general categories: 1) direct mechanisms exerting their influence through neural endocrine effects; and 2) indirect mechanisms influencing the patient's adherence to preventative therapeutic strategies. Interventions to improve psychosocial traits can improve adherence to medical regimens and enhance an individual psychological state. Health education programs that are targeted to the specific needs of each patient can improve adherence to risk factor modification strategies (e.g., smoking cessation, improvement in dietary habits). These programs generally consist of three phases; 1) instruction on CHD risk and importance of modification through specific intervention(s); 2) follow-up and support on an individual basis; and 3) small group discussions with peer support. This intervention approach has been successful for improving adherence to treatments for hypertension, smoking, hyperlipidemia, and CAD risk factor reduction.

Hypertriglyceridemia. Despite decades of interest and numerous clinical and epidemiological investigations, the status of the elevated serum triglyceride concentration as a risk factor for CHD remains controversial.[29-31] Many prospective studies have identified hypertriglyceridemia (HTG) as a risk factor in univariate analysis, although after adjustment in multivariate analysis for HDL-cholesterol or Apo B, the association is diminished.[32-35] High triglycerides are often associated with a low HDL-cholesterol concentration, suggesting that this may be responsible for the increase in CAD risk from HTG. Additionally, HTG also is associated with small, dense LDL particles and high Apo B concentrations. Small dense LDL particles and high Apo B are independent risk factors for CAD.[36] HTG is also a common finding in the insulin resistance syndrome (Metabolic Syndrome X).

Reduction of serum triglycerides is correlated with a decrease in CHD risk. In the Stockholm Ischemic Heart Disease Secondary Prevention Study,[37] the group treated with clofibrate and nicotinic acid had a significant reduction in the rate of mortality from CHD, which was significantly correlated with the reduction in total triglyceride levels and not with the reduction in cholesterol levels. HTG was the most common lipid abnormality in this study, occurring in 50% of the patients, whereas hypercholesterolemia was present in only 13%. In the Helsinki Heart Study,[13] the reduction in CHD resulting from gemfibrozil therapy was largely localized to the subgroup with a triglyceride level of more than 204 mg/dL and a ratio of LDL-cholesterol to HDL-cholesterol of more than five.

Since HTG is commonly associated with low HDL-cholesterol, LDL pattern B (small, dense LDL) and hyperinsulinemia, management of elevated triglycerides should also focus on correcting these accompanying metabolic derangements. Lowering triglycerides will generally raise HDL-cholesterol and convert LDL pattern B to LDL pattern A (normal sized LDL).[38,39] Measuring a fasting insulin level, particularly in HTG subjects with obesity and normal fasting glucose levels, can be considered. An elevated fasting insulin level in normoglycemia suggests intervention that will increase insulin sensitivity along with reducing triglycerides. Weight reduction, exercise, and diets lower in carbohydrates (i.e., < 45% of calories) and higher in protein (i.e., 20-25% of calories) can be considered. Certainly, with more marked elevations of triglycerides (> 500 mg/dL), pharmacologic therapy may be necessary and would include fibric acid derivatives, and in nondiabetic, nonhyperinsulinemic individuals, nicotinic acid may be considered.

The 1993 National Cholesterol Education Program (NCEP) guidelines[40] define a favorable triglyceride as less than 200 mg/dL with 200-400 mg/dL as borderline-high triglycerides, 400-1000 mg/dL as high triglycerides, and greater than 1000 mg/dL as very high triglycerides. High triglyceride concentrations (i.e., ≥ 1000 mg/dL) are associated with an increased risk of pancreatitis. Recently, Miller and associates suggested that the NCEP definition of "elevated" triglyceride levels be lowered to reflect the growing concern about the health effects of elevated lipid levels in general.[41] Their research uncovered three independent predictors of CAD events: diabetes mellitus; low HDL-cholesterol levels (< 35 mg/dL); and triglyceride levels greater than 100 mg/dL. Based on their retrospective cohort study of 740 heart disease patients, the researchers emphatically state that "triglyceride levels previously considered normal are predictive of new CAD events. The cutpoints established by the National Cholesterol Education Program for elevated triglycerides (> 200 mg/dL) may need to be refined."

Lipoprotein(a). Lipoprotein(a) (Lp[a]) is a lipoprotein particle consisting of an LDL particle attached to an additional protein molecule called Apo (a).[42] Numerous studies in which quantitative immunochemical methods have been used to measure Lp(a) have established that Lp(a) plasma concentrations (range, < 0.1 mg/dL to > 250 mg/dL) are strongly influenced by genetic factors.[43,44] Lp(a) concentrations also vary considerably among ethnic groups. The frequency distribution in whites is skewed toward lower concentrations, while the median Lp(a) concentration in blacks is three times as high as in whites.[45] Lp(a) concentrations increase by about 8% in women after menopause and estrogen replacement therapy reduces the concentration.[42]

Observational studies have generally observed that elevated Lp(a) concentrations are associated with CHD,[46-51] CAD progression,[52,53] restenosis after PTCA,[54,55] cerebrovascular disease,[56-58] and intermittent claudication.[59-61] In a study of MI survivors with Lp(a) concentrations greater than 30 mg/dL, the relative risk was 1.75-fold higher than in subjects with Lp(a) concentrations less than 30 mg/dL.[62] Recently, one study did not observe an association between Lp(a) concentrations and risk of MI in men.[63]

Table. Pyschosocial and Behavioral Factors Associated with Increased Risk of Atherosclerotic Cardiovascular Disease

Behavioral factors
- Adherence behavior
- Type A behavior

Psychosocial interactive factors
- Excess demand, strain, stress
- Social isolation
- Social support

Sociodemographic factors
- Age
- Race
- Gender
- Socioeconomic status
- Marital status

The evidence that Lp(a) is a risk factor for ASCVD is based largely on observational studies. These findings, combined with laboratory investigations demonstrating a variety of proatherogenic effects for this lipoprotein, have led to widespread interest in its concentration and as an important risk factor. Only one study has examined the usefulness of lowering Lp(a) on angiographic CAD progression. Thompson and colleagues reported that decreasing Lp(a) levels by 35% with LDL-apheresis over a two-year period did not affect CAD.[64] No benefit from reducing Lp(a) was observed on angiographic progression or regression of CAD. Among conventional lipid-lowering drugs, only nicotinic acid consistently reduces Lp(a) concentrations (20-25% reduction).[65]

It is clear that additional studies of Lp(a) are required before its role in CHD risk can be resolved. At the present time, screening for Lp(a) is cautiously recommended and only for patients with, or with a family history of, premature ASCVD. Management of patients with elevated Lp(a) concentrations (i.e., ≥ 30 mg/dL) should be directed at more aggressively lowering LDL-cholesterol and/or triglyceride concentrations.

Homocysteine. Homocystinuria refers to a group of rare inborn errors of metabolism resulting in high concentrations of plasma homocysteine (> 100 mcg/mol/L) and urinary homocysteine. A characteristic in patients with homocystinuria is premature vascular disease. Plasma homocysteine concentrations can be increased by deficiencies of vitamins B_6 and B_{12}, or folic acid.[66,67]

More than 75 clinical and epidemiologic studies have shown a relation between total homocysteine levels and CAD, peripheral vascular disease, stroke, or venous thrombosis.[69-73] The Physician's Health Study reported that an elevated homocysteine concentration was associated with a 3.4-fold increase in five-year MI risk.[74] A recent study examined the relationship between CHD and homocysteine in a prospective cohort of 769 individuals enrolled in the Atherosclerosis Risk in Communities (ARIC) study.[75] The participants were originally evaluated during a three-year span (1987-1989) and were followed for an average of 3.3 years. After controlling for a variety of CHD risk factors, only vitamin B_6 was independently associated with risk of CHD. The implication of these results is that homocysteine may not be as important as prior research suggests, and more studies are needed to clarify how homocysteine, B vitamins, and ASCVD are linked.

Although elevated plasma homocysteine levels (i.e., ≥ 15 mcg/mol/L) have been associated with ASCVD risk, there are no prospective interventional data. However, Rimm and associates[68] reported that intake of folic acid and vitamin B_6 above the current recommended dietary allowance (400 mg/d and 3 mg/d, respectively) may be important in the primary prevention of CHD in women. Based on the observational data from the Nurses Health Study,[68] it would appear that a prudent, healthy diet should contain at least 400 mcg/d of folic acid and 3 mg/d of vitamin B_6.

Oxidative Stress. Extensive laboratory data indicate that oxidation of LDL particles accelerates the atherogenic process. Oxidized LDL may facilitate atherosclerotic disease by recruiting T-lymphocytes, circulating monocytes, and stimulating autoantibodies into the subendothelial space of medium- and large-sized arteries.[76]

There have been a number of recent reports that provide strong evidence that high dietary intakes of antioxidant vitamins can significantly reduce the production of atherogenic oxidized LDL particles and significantly lower CHD incidence. A study by Regnstrom and colleagues[77] indicated that there is an inverse relationship between the concentration of plasma LDL vitamin E and the severity of CHD. In 64 male survivors of MI, the lipid-adjusted serum and LDL vitamin E concentrations were significantly lower than in an age-matched control population. Based on the analysis of coronary angiograms to determine stenotic lesions, Regnstrom et al concluded that a low LDL vitamin E content may play a role in the development of stenoses of the coronary arteries and clinical CHD.

Niki and associates[78] investigated the interactive effects of three antioxidants (ascorbid acid, alpha-tocopherol, and beta-carotene) and reported that vitamins C and E are the most important hydrophilic and hydrophobic antioxidants that synergistically act against oxidative stress induced by free radicals and active oxygen species. Whereas vitamin E is more effective than vitamin C in scavenging free radicals in lipoproteins, vitamin C reduces the resulting vitamin E radical, thereby breaking the free radical chain reaction. Vitamins E and C are localized in different domains of body tissues and appear to interact at the interface between the lipoprotein and water to protect the lipoprotein from oxidative damage.

The Cambridge Heart Antioxidant Study (CHAOS)[79] was a prospective study designed to test the hypothesis that treatment with vitamin E would reduce the risk of MI in patients with angiographic evidence of CAD. In this double-blind, placebo-controlled study, 2002 patients were randomized to receive vitamin E (800 IU/d or 400 IU/d) or placebo. After a follow-up of 510 days (median range, 3-981 days), vitamin E treatment resulted in a reduced rate (47%) of nonfatal and fatal MI. Vitamin E did not affect serum cholesterol concentrations.

These reports add to the building of a substantial scientific basis for the antioxidant hypothesis of CHD. The results from epidemiological and basic research combine to provide strong support for this hypothesis. While no firm recommendations can be given at this time, it appears prudent to supplement the diets of individuals at high risk of CHD with vitamin E (e.g., 200-400 units/d).

Alcohol Consumption. Individuals reporting moderate amounts of alcohol intake have a 50% reduction in CAD risk compared to individuals who do not consume alcohol.[80-82] Excessive consumption of alcohol is associated with increased CHD, possibly resulting from misclassification of alcoholic cardiomyopathy as CHD disease or from alcohol's ability to produce hypertension and increase cardiac arrhythmias.[83] Excessive alcohol consumption also intake produces other medical problems that can outweigh its beneficial effects on CHD risk.[84] It has been suggested that the reduction in CHD risk associated with alcohol is due to the effect of alcohol alone. For example, alcohol consumption increases levels of HDL-cholesterol and Apo A-I.[85,86] More important, alcohol affects several clotting mechanisms including decreasing platelet aggregation,[87] lowering fibrinogen levels, and increasing fibrinolytic activities. Through reducing the coagulability of blood, alcohol may be more consequential in mitigating the risk of cardiovascular events (e.g., MI) than the risk of atherogenesis.

Among populations with high cholesterol and saturated fat diets, wine consumption is more strongly related to reduced risk of CHD than total alcohol consumption, and wine intake might explain some of the decrease rate of CHD among the French despite their high saturated fat intake.[88] Bioflavonoids have been found in high concentration in red grapes and may provide an antioxidant effect and, therefore, influence CAD risk.[89]

Identification of patients with a current or potential alcohol problem is an important component of good preventative medicine. A small amount of alcohol (e.g., 1 glass of wine/d or 1 glass of beer/d) may have some protective effects against heart attack. Unfortunately, alcohol can be abused, and it is not possible to reliably predict who is at risk and when a person might suffer acute adverse effects (including accidents) from alcohol consumption. The challenge is to weigh potential benefits against risks for any individual. A blanket recommendation to increase alcohol intake to reduce the risk of heart attack is unwarranted.

Category IV Risk Factors

Although gender, age, and family history are not modifiable, these factors exert their influence on CAD risk, at least in part, through other risk factors previously discussed. CAD risk increases nearly linearly with age and is greater in men compared to women until approximately age 75 when the prevalence is nearly equal in most westernized populations. Below 55 years of age, the incidence of CHD among men is about three times higher than in women. After age 55, the rate of increase in men declines and that in women continues to increase so that the incidence rates in men and women become similar in older people.[90]

CAD clusters in families, and, therefore, a family history of premature CHD is a definite risk factor. With increasing numbers of elderly patients, the high prevalence of CHD, and increasing levels of therapeutic intervention in older patients, it is important to define premature in relation to the development of CHD. Although age is a continuous variable, cut points are useful and for the purpose of the NCEP, family history of premature CHD is defined as an MI or sudden death before 55 years of age in a father or other first-degree male relative or before 65 years of age in a mother or other first-degree female relative.[40]

Summary

CHD is extremely prevalent and is preventable. Coronary risk factors are involved in the genesis of atherosclerosis and the occurrence of cardiovascular events. The primary care physician must recognize these risk factors and institute treatment to eliminate or control these factors. The treatment goals for the prevention of CHD and other ASCVD should include (in order of intensity):

- Smoking cessation;
- Reduction of LDL-cholesterol;
  < 100 mg/dL (secondary prevention)
  < 130 mg/dL (primary prevention)
- Control of BP (< 140/90 mmHg);
- Aspirin 80-325 mg/d;
- Control of diabetes mellitus (hemoglobin A1c < 7%);
- Physical exercise (30 minutes, 3-5 times/week);
- Increase HDL-cholesterol (> 35 mg/dL);
- Weight reduction (body mass index < 25 kg/m^2);
- Consider HRT for postmenopausal women without clinical evidence of CHD;
- Reduce triglycerides (< 200 mg/dL);
- Limitation of alcohol intake;
- Consider supplementing diet with vitamin E (200-400 units/d) and folic acid (400 mcg/d).

For post-MI patients, in addition to the aforementioned recommendations, consider:

- Beta-blocker therapy;
- ACE-inhibitor therapy, particularly for patients with left ventricular ejection fractions < 40%.

References

1. The Diabetes Control and Complications Trial Research Group. The effect of intensive treatment of diabetes on the development and progression of long-term complications in insulin-dependent diabetes mellitus. *N Engl J Med* 1993; 329:997-986.
2. Getz GJ. Report on the workshop on diabetes and mechanisms of atherogenesis. September 17th and 18th, 1992, Bethesda, MD. *Atheroscler Thromb* 1993;13:459-464.
3. Haffner SM, et al. Mortality from coronary heart disease in subjects with type 2 diabetes and in nondiabetic subjects with and without prior myocardial infarction. *N Engl J Med* 1998; 339:229-234.
4. Pyorala K, et al. Cholesterol lowering with simvastatin improves prognosis of diabetic patients with coronary heart disease. *Diabetes Care* 1997;20:614-620.
5. UK Prospective Diabetes Study (UKPDS) Group. Intensive blood-glucose control with sulphonylureas or insulin compared with conventional treatment and risk of complications in patients with type 2 diabetes (UKPDS 33). *Lancet* 1998;352:837-853.
6. Pate RR, et al. Physical activity and public health. A recommendation from the Centers for Disease Control and Prevention and the American College of Sports Medicine. *JAMA* 1995;273:402-407.
7. Powell KE, et al. Physical activity and the incidence of

coronary heart disease. *Ann Rev Public Health* 1987;8: 253-287.

8. NIH Consensus Development Panel on Physical Activity and Cardiovascular Health. Physical activity and cardiovascular health. *JAMA* 1996;276:241-246.
9. O'Connor GT, et al. An overview of randomized trials of rehabilitation with exercise after myocardial infarction. *Circulation* 1989;80:234-244.
10. Oldridge NB, et al. Cardiac rehabilitation after myocardial infarction. Combined experience of randomized clinical trials. *JAMA* 1988;260:945-950.
11. Gordon DJ, et al. High-density lipoprotein cholesterol and cardiovascular disease: Four prospective American studies. *Circulation* 1989;79:8-15.
12. Rubins H. AHA Plenary Session XII. November 11, 1998, American Heart Association Annual Meeting; Anaheim, CA.
13. Manninen V, et al. Lipid alterations and a decline in the incidence of coronary heart disease in the Helsinki Heart Study. *JAMA* 1988;260:641-651.
14. Williamson DF, et al. The 10-year incidence of overweight and major weight gains in U.S. adults. *Arch Intern Med* 1990;150:665-672.
15. Harlan WR, et al. Secular trends in body mass in the United States, 1960-1980. *Am J Epidemiol* 1988;128:1065-1074.
16. Berg FM. Health Risks of Obesity; 1993 Special Report. Hettinger ND, Obesity & Health, 1992.
17. Manson JE, et al. A prospective study of obesity and risk of coronary heart disease in women. *N Engl J Med* 1990;322: 882-889.
18. Havel RJ, Rapaport E. Management of primary hyperlipidemia. *N Engl J Med* 1995;332:1491-1498.
19. Wuerst JH, Jr., et al. The degree of coronary atherosclerosis in bilaterally oophorectomized women. *Circulation* 1953; 7:801.
20. Lerner DJ, Kannel WB. Patterns of coronary heart disease morbidity and mortality in the sexes: 26-year follow-up of the Framingham population. *Am Heart J* 1986;113:383-390.
21. Bush TL, et al. Cardiovascular mortality and noncontraceptive use of estrogen in women: Results from the Lipid Research Clinics Program follow-up study. *Circulation* 1987;75:1102-1109.
22. Grodstein F, et al. Postmenopausal hormone therapy and mortality. *N Engl J Med* 1997;336:1769-1775.
23. Sullivan JM, et al. Estrogen replacement and coronary artery disease: Effect on survival in postmenopausal women. *Arch Int Med* 1988;108:358-363.
24. Bush TL, et al. Cardiovascular and noncontraceptive use of estrogen in women: Results from the Lipid Research Clinic Program Follow-Up Study. *Circulation* 1987;75:1102-1109.
25. Gruchow HW, et al. Postmenopausal use of estrogen and occlusion of coronary arteries. *Am Heart J* 1988;115: 954-963.
26. Sullivan JM, et al. Effects on survival of estrogen and occlusion of coronary artery bypass grafting. *Am J Cardiol* 1997;79:847-850.
27. Kim SC, et al. Estrogen improves long-term outcome after coronary angioplasty. *Circulation* 1995;92(suppl I):I-674.
28. Hulley S, et al. For the Heart and Estrogen/progestin Replacement Study research group. Randomized trial of estrogen plus progestin for secondary prevention of coronary heart disease in post-menopausal women. *JAMA* 1998;280:605-613.
29. Hulley SB, et al. Epidemiology as a guide to clinical decisions: The association between triglyceride and coronary heart disease. *N Engl J Med* 1980;302:1383-1389.
30. Nestel PJ. Is serum triglyceride an independent predictor of coronary artery disease? *Pract Cardiol* 1987;13:96-101.
31. Austin MA. Plasma triglyceride as a risk factor for coronary heart disease: The epidemiologic evidence and beyond. *Am J Epidemiol* 1989;129:249-259.
32. Wilhelmsen L, et al. Multivariate analysis of risk factors for coronary heart disease. *Circulation* 1973;48:905-908.
33. Salonen JT, Puska P. Relationship of serum cholesterol and triglycerides to the risk of acute myocardial infarction, cerebral stroke and death in eastern Finnish male population. *Int J Epidemiol* 1983;12:26-31.
34. Cambien F, et al. Is the level of serum triglyceride a significant predictor of coronary death in "normocholesterolemic" subjects? A Paris prospective study. *Am J Epidemiol* 1986; 124:624-632.
35. Pocock SJ, et al. Concentrations of high density lipoprotein cholesterol, triglycerides, and total cholesterol in ischaemic heart disease. *Br Med J* 1989;298:998-1002.
36. Austin MA, et al. Low density lipoprotein subclass patterns and risk of myocardial infarction. *JAMA* 1988;260: 1917-1921.
37. Carlson LA, Rosenhamer G. Reduction of mortality in the Stockholm Ischemic Heart Disease Secondary Prevention Study by combined treatment with clofibrate and nicotinic acid. *Acta Med Scand* 1988;223:405-418.
38. Dachet C, et al. Effect of gemfibrozil on the concentration and composition of very low density and low density lipoprotein subfractions in hypertriglyceridemic patients. *Atherosclerosis* 1995;113:1-9.
39. Franceschini G, et al. Effect of gemfibrozil treatment in hypercholesterolemia on low density lipoprotein (LDL) subclass distribution and LDL-cell interaction. *Atherosclerosis* 1995; 114:61-71.
40. National Cholesterol Education Program Expert panel. Summary of the second report of the National Cholesterol Education Program (NCEP) Expert Panel on Detection, Evaluation, and Treatment of High Blood Cholesterol in Adults (Adult Treatment Panel II). *JAMA* 1993;269: 3015-3023.
41. Miller M, et al. Normal triglyceride levels and coronary artery disease events: The Baltimore Coronary Observational Long-term Study. *J Am Coll Cardiol* 1998;31:1252-1257.
42. Scanu AM, Fless GM. Lipoprotein(a): Heterogeneity and biological relevance. *J Clin Invest* 1990;85:1709-1715.
43. Berg K. Twin research in coronary heart disease. In: Gedda L, Parisi P, Nance WE, eds. *Twin Research 3: Epidemiological and Clinical Studies*. New York, NY: Alan R. Liss, Inc; 1981:117-130.
44. Lamon-Fava S, et al. The NHLBI twin study: Heritability of apolipoprotein A-I, B, and low density lipoprotein subclasses and concordance for lipoprotein(a). *Atherosclerosis* 1991;

91:97-106.
45. Guyton JR, et al. Relationship of plasma lipoprotein Lp(a) levels to race and to apolipoprotein B. *Atherosclerosis* 1985; 5:265-272.
46. Rosengren A, et al. Lipoprotein(a) and coronary heart disease: A progressive case-control study in a general population sample of middle-aged men. *Br Med J* 1990; 301:1248-1251.
47. Jauhiainen M, et al. Lipoprotein(a) and coronary heart disease risk, a nested case-control study of the Helsinki Heart Study participants. *Atherosclerosis* 1991;89:59-67.
48. Sigurdsson G, et al. Predictive valve of apolipoproteins in a prospective survey of coronary artery disease in men. *Am J Cardiol* 1992;69:1251-1254.
49. Sandholzer C, et al. Apolipoprotein(a) phenotypes, Lp(a) concentration and plasma lipid levels in relation to coronary heart disease in a chinese population: Evidence for the role of the apo(a) gene in coronary heart disease. *J Clin Invest* 1992;89:1040-1046.
50. Schaefer EJ, et al. Lipoprotein(a) levels and risk of coronary heart disease in men: The Lipid Research Clinics Coronary Primary Prevention trial. *JAMA* 1994;271:999-1003.
51. Rader DJ, et al. Quantitation of plasma apolipoproteins in the primary and secondary prevention of coronary artery disease. *Ann Intern Med* 1994;120:1012-1025.
52. Tamura A, et al. Serum lipoprotein(a) concentrations are related to coronary disease progression without new myocardial infarction. *Br Heart J* 1995;74:365-369.
53. Terres W, et al. Rapid angiographic progression of coronary artery disease in patients with elevated lipoprotein(a). *Circulation* 1995;91:948-950.
54. Desmarais RL, et al. Elevated serum lipoprotein(a) is a risk factor for clinical recurrence after balloon coronary angioplasty. *Circulation* 1995;91:1403-1409.
55. Yamamoto H, et al. Risk factors for restenosis after percutaneous transluminal coronary angioplasty: Role of lipoprotein(a). *Am Heart J* 1995;130:1168-1173.
56. Koltringer P, Jurgens G. A dominant role of lipoprotein(a) in the investigation and evaluation of parameters indicating the development of cervical atherosclerosis. *Atherosclerosis* 1985;58:187-198.
57. Murai A, et al. Lp(a) lipoprotein as a risk factor for coronary heart disease and cerebral infarction. *Atherosclerosis* 1986; 59:199-204.
58. Zenker G, et al. Lipoprotein(a) as a strong indicator for cerebrovascular disease. *Stroke* 1986;17:942-945.
59. Molgaard J, et al. Significant association between low-molecular-weight apolipoprotein(a) isoforms and intermittent claudication. *Atheroscler Thromb* 1992;12: 895-901.
60. Valentine RJ, et al. Lp(a) lipoprotein is an independent, discriminating risk factor for premature peripheral atherosclerosis among white men. *Arch Intern Med* 1994;154:801-806.
61. Cantin B, et al. Lp(a) distribution in a French Canadian population and its relation to intermittent claudication (the Quebec Cardiovascular Study) *Am J Cardiol* 1995;75: 1244-1248.
62. Rhoads GG, et al. Lp(a) lipoprotein as a risk factor for myocardial infarction. *JAMA* 1986;256:2540-2544.
63. Cantin B, et al. Is lipoprotein(a) an independent risk factor for ischemic heart disease in men? The Quebec Cardiovascular Study. *J Am Coll Cardiol* 1998;31:519-525.
64. Thompson GR, et al. Familial hypercholesterolemia regression study. A randomized trial of low density lipoprotein apheresis. *Lancet* 1995;345:811-816.
65. Guraker A, et al. Levels of lipoprotein Lp(a) decline with neomycin and niacin treatment. *Atherosclerosis* 1985;57: 293-301.
66. Selhub J, et al. Vitamin status and intake as primary determinants of homocysteinemia in an elderly population. *JAMA* 1993;270:2693-2698.
67. Ubbink JB, et al. Vitamin B_{12}, vitamin B_6, and folate nutritional status in men with hyperhomocysteinemia. *Am J Clin Nutr* 1993;57:57-53.
68. Rimm EB, et al. Folate and vitamin B_6 from diet and supplements in relation to risk of coronary heart disease among women. *JAMA* 1998;279:359-364.
69. Ueland PM, et al. Plasma homocysteine and cardiovascular disease. In: Francis RB, Jr., ed. *Atherosclerotic Cardiovascular Disease, Hemostasis, and Endothelial Function*. New York: Marcel Dekker; 1992:183-236.
70. Boushey CJ, et al. A quantitative assessment of plasma homocysteine as a risk factor for vascular disease: Probable benefits of increasing folic acid intakes. *JAMA* 1995;274: 1049-1057.
71. Verhoef P, Stampfer MJ. Prospective studies of homocysteine and cardiovascular disease. *Nutr Rev* 1995; 53:283-288.
72. Brattstrom L. Vitamins as homocysteine-lowering agents. *J Nutr* 1996;126(Suppl):1276S-1280S.
73. den Heijer M, et al. Hyperhomocysteinemia as a risk factor for deep-vein thrombosis. *N Engl J Med* 1996;334:759-762.
74. Stampfer MJ, et al. A prospective study of plasma homocysteine and risk of myocardial infarction in U.S. physicians. *JAMA* 1992;268:877-881.
75. Kuller LH, Evans RW. Homocyseine, vitamins and cardiovascular disease. *Circulation* 1998;98:196-199.
76. Libby P. Molecular basis of acute coronary syndromes. *Circulation* 1995;91:2844-2850.
77. Regnstrom J, et al. Inverse relation between the concentration of low-density lipoprotein vitamin E and severity of coronary artery disease. *Am J Clin Nutr* 1996; 63:377-385.
78. Niki E, et al. Interaction among vitamin C, vitamin E, and beta-carotene. *Am J Clin Nutr* 1995;62(suppl):1322S-1326S.
79. Stephens NG, et al. Randomized controlled trial of vitamin E in patients with coronary disease: Cambridge Heart Antioxidant Study (CHAOS). *Lancet* 1996;347:781-786.
80. Boffetta P, Garfinkel L. Alcohol drinking and mortality among men enrolled in an American Cancer Society prospective study. *Epidemiology* 1990;1:342-348.
81. Klatsky AL, et al. Risk of cardiovascular mortality in alcohol drinkers, ex-drinkers and nondrinkers. *Am J Cardiol* 1990;66:1237-1242.
82. Colditz GA. A prospective assessment of moderate alcohol

intake and major chronic diseases. *Ann Epidemiol* 1990;1: 167-177.

83. Criqui MH. The roles of alcohol in the epidemiology of cardiovascular disease. *Acta Med Scand* 1987;717(Suppl): 73-85.
84. Regan TJ. Alcohol and the cardiovascular system. *JAMA* 1990;264:377-381.
85. Gordon T, et al. Alcohol and high-density lipoprotein cholesterol. *Circulation* 1981;64(Suppl III):63-67.
86. Miller GJ, Miller NE. Plasma-high-density-lipoprotein concentration and development of ischemic heart disease. *Lancet* 1976;1:16-19.
87. Meade TW, et al. Effects of changes in smoking and other characteristics of clotting factors and the risk of ischemic heart disease. *Lancet* 1987;2:986-988.
88. Renaud S, deLorgeril M. Wine, alcohol, platelets and the French paradox for coronary heart disease. *Lancet* 1992; 339:1523-1526.
89. Hertog MGL, et al. Content of potentially anticarcinogenic flavonoids of tea infusions, wines and fruit juices. *J Agric Food Chem* 1992;40:2379-2383.
90. Blackburn H. The concept of risk. In: Pearson TA, Criqui MH, Luepker RV, Oberman A, Winston M, eds. *Primer in Preventative Cardiology*. Dallas, TX: American Heart Association; 1994:25-41.

Vascular Screening

J. Crayton Pruitt, MD, FACS

Appropriately targeted screening programs are one of the most cost-effective modalities we have for preventing disease or detecting disease at an early, treatable stage. Because cardiovascular disease (CVD) remains the number one cause of death and morbidity in this country, it would seem reasonable that screening for CVD would be a productive exercise. We already routinely screen for high blood pressure, cholesterol, and diabetes. The conundrum for clinicians is that screening procedures often are insufficiently reimbursed or not reimbursed at all. The current article describes the rationale for expanding the role of CV screening in selected populations and discusses some of the methodological challenges.

It has become increasingly apparent that the most efficient method of diagnosing some medical problems involves screening those persons most at risk for the condition. Screening can be defined as "a mass examination of the population to detect the existence of a particular disease."[1] *(Please see Table 1.)*

This chapter deals with vascular screening only and includes a discussion of recording of pertinent medical history, risks, patient education, notification of results, sensitivity, specificity and predictive value. *(Please see Table 2.)*

Obtaining History

The necessary history to be obtained and recorded when screening for vascular conditions should include questions providing information concerning risk factors and symptoms suggestive of the conditions. (*Please see Table 3.*)

Risk Factors for Carotid Stenosis, Abdominal Aortic Aneurysms, and Peripheral Arterial Insufficiency

The most common cause of carotid stenosis, abdominal aortic aneurysm, and peripheral arterial insufficiency is atherosclerotic vascular disease. So risk factors for these three conditions are similar. Those risk factors include:

- **Family history.** Relatives who have suffered strokes or had peripheral arterial insufficiency or abdominal aortic aneurysms may mean increased risk.
- **Age.** The risk of vascular problem increases with advancing age.
- **Gender.** Males are more likely to develop carotid stenosis, abdominal aortic aneurysms, and peripheral arterial insufficiency than females, although all three conditions also occur in females.
- **Hypertension.** High blood pressure damages the wall of the arteries and causes an acceleration of the atherosclerotic process.
- **Previous symptoms.** Transient neurologic deficits or intermittent claudication may indicate carotid stenosis or peripheral arterial insufficiency.

- **Previous stroke.** A previous stroke increases the likelihood that the problem will recur.
- **Ulcerated plaque.** Ulcerated plaque in the carotid artery increases the danger of emboli or thrombosis.
- **Diabetes mellitus.** Predisposes to early atherosclerotic disease.
- **Myocardial infarction.** Previous history of myocardial infarction is a warning sign that the patient has an increased likelihood of developing carotid stenosis or peripheral arterial insufficiency.
- **Hyperlipidemia.** The elevation of serum cholesterol or triglycerides increases the risk of the atherosclerotic process and intermittent claudication. Pain in the legs often indicates arterial insufficiency and patients with arterial insufficiency in the legs also frequently get abdominal aortic aneurysms or carotid stenosis.

Vascular Conditions for Which Screening may be Helpful: Hyperlipidemia

To screen for hypercholesterolemia or hyperlipidemia a lipid profile is ordered, which is a series of blood tests involving measurement of fatty material in the blood. Two types of lipids are measured, cholesterol and triglycerides. They are measured in milligrams per deciliter (mg/dL). The total cholesterol represents the total number of cholesterol particles in your blood. Total cholesterol should be 200 mg/dL or less. The total cholesterol is made up of high-density lipoprotein (HDL), which is considered a good type of cholesterol, and low-density lipoprotein (LDL), which is considered a bad type of cholesterol. The HDL value should be 35 mg/dL or more. The total cholesterol/HDL ratio compares the amount of good cholesterol to your total cholesterol level. A TC/HDL ratio of 4.5 or less is desirable.[7]

LDL cholesterol is considered undesirable cholesterol. An LDL value of 130 mg/dL or less is normal.

Triglycerides in the blood should measure 250 mg/dL or less.

Blood glucose levels help to determine if one needs to be evaluated for diabetes mellitus. A glucose value of less than 120 mg/dL is normal and more than 120 mg/dL is abnormal.

Carotid Stenosis

Although there are at least 20 different conditions that can lead to stroke, almost 90% of strokes are caused by carotid stenosis, atrial fibrillation with emboli to the brain, and hypertension with hemorrhage into the brain. It should be possible to screen for the three conditions to find those most at risk and, with treatment, significantly reduce the incidence of stroke. This should be done because in spite of our current knowledge of the causes of stroke, it is estimated that in 1998 there were 730,000 strokes in the United States alone.[8] More than 4 million persons die each year worldwide of strokes.

The primary cause of stroke is carotid stenosis. About 50% of people who have a stroke do not have any symptoms before they have the stroke, so in order to identify the asymptomatic patients at risk for stroke screening is the most efficient way. National and international cooperative studies, which were double-blind carefully monitored studies, have now provided information on which groups of patients with carotid stenosis should be treated medically and which groups should be treated by carotid endarterectomy.

Table 1. Common Medical Conditions for Which Screening Tests are Frequently Recommended

- PAP smear for carcinoma of the cervix.[2]
- Mammography for carcinoma of the breast.[3]
- Chest x-ray for carcinoma of the lung.[4]
- Bone density for osteoporosis.[5]
- ECG rhythm strip for atrial fibrillation.[6]

Those national and international cooperative studies include:

- The North American Symptomatic Carotid Endarterectomy Trial (NASCET). The NASCET study reported February 21, 1991, and indicated that carotid endarterectomy was highly beneficial for patients with recent hemispheric transient ischemic attacks with ipsilateral 70-99% stenosis.[9]
- The European Carotid Surgery Trial (ECST) also was reported in 1991, confirming surgery was better than medical management for patients with 70-99% unilateral carotid stenosis who were symptomatic.[10]
- The VA Symptomatic Carotid Endarterectomy Trial reported also in 1991 that surgery was better than medical management for patients with 70% stenosis in one carotid artery who were symptomatic.[11]
- The Asymptomatic Carotid Atherosclerosis Study (ACAS) was a study of asymptomatic patients with 60% stenosis of one carotid artery. Results were reported on May 10, 1995. Results indicated that when carotid endarterectomy in these patients was performed in medical centers with documented combined perioperative morbidity mortality rates of less than 3%, surgery was better than medical management.[12]

To significantly reduce the 730,000 strokes that occur in the United States each year it will be necessary to screen those patients at risk for carotid stenosis in order for them to be treated before the actual stroke occurs. At the present time it is probably wise to recommend carotid endarterectomy for prevention of stroke in patients who have 60% or greater stenosis if there are no serious medical contraindications.

Risk Factors for Stroke Identified in the NASCET Study and the European Carotid Surgery Trial:

- Age older than 80 years;
- Male gender;
- Systolic blood pressure above 160 mm Hg;
- Diastolic blood pressure above 90 mm Hg;
- Transient ischemic attacks occurring within the previous 31 days;
- Previous completed stroke;
- Greater than 80% carotid stenosis;
- Plaque ulcer;
- History of smoking;
- Myocardial infarction;
- Congestive heart failure;
- Diabetes;
- Hyperlipidemia;
- Intermittent claudication; and
- High blood pressure.

The odds of having a stroke within two years in the medically treated patients increased with the number of risk factors.

Screening for Carotid Stenosis

If everyone who were going to have a stroke had a symptom first, then there would not be a problem in diagnosing this condition before the stroke occurred. It is true, however, that at least half of the people who have a stroke do not have any prior transient ischemic attacks. The stroke is the first event. Therefore, it is necessary to perform some type of screening test to determine which patients are at risk. Many patients with significant carotid stenosis have a bruit but a large number of patients with significant carotid stenosis do not have a bruit. Some of those patients have more than 90% stenosis and still do not have a bruit. Therefore, listening with a stethoscope or even a handheld Doppler device is not adequate. It is necessary to do an ultrasound screening test to rule out asymptomatic carotid stenosis. The test is painless, harmless, and inexpensive. The National Stroke Association has recommended a program for screening for carotid artery stenosis, atrial fibrillation, and hypertension in all persons older than 50 years of age.[13] Organizations, which recommend screening of the carotid artery, have recommended screening methods varying from simply listening to the carotid artery with a stethoscope or listening to the carotid artery with a handheld Doppler to performing an abbreviated color flow duplex ultrasound test.[14] The most accurate method of screening is an abbreviated color flow duplex ultrasound test. If a person is screened and found to have no atherosclerotic plaques in the carotid arteries, another screening test is not necessary for about three years. If he or she is found to have a mild amount of atherosclerotic plaque, another test should be done in two years. If a mild to moderate amount of plaque is reported, another test should be done in one year and if a moderate to severe amount of plaque or a severe amount of plaque is reported, instructions should be included with the report advising that an appointment be made with his or her personal physician. Usually at that time the physician will suggest ordering a more complete ultrasound test at an accredited vascular laboratory. Whether treatment is necessary will depend on the confirmation of significant stenosis by the more complete test. Some physicians will prefer to have a digital carotid arteriogram rather than another ultrasound test, and some will recommend a magnetic resonance angiogram.

Cost-Effectiveness of Screening

There are many screening organizations in the United States that do abbreviated ultrasound screening of the carotid arteries for carotid stenosis. Most charge about $35 for a screening test. Those patients who have moderately severe or severe stenosis on the screening test are sent certified letters advising them to see their physician to be considered for further diagnostic testing. Several articles have appeared in the literature recently recommending screening for asymptomatic carotid stenosis.[15-20] "Cost-Effectiveness of Screening for Asymptomatic Carotid Stenosis" was addressed and confirmed by several authors.[21-24] Patients older than 65 were 4.1 times more likely to have significant stenosis than those younger than 65.

Table 2. Vascular Conditions for Which Screening may be Helpful

- Hypercholesterolemia or lipidemia
- Carotid stenosis
- Abdominal aortic aneurysms
- Peripheral arterial insufficiency
- Atrial fibrillation
- Hypertension

Abdominal Aortic Aneurysm

Abdominal aortic aneurysm is a fairly common condition, which is a major cause of sudden death if not diagnosed before rupture occurs.[25] Abdominal aortic aneurysms increase in incidence with advancing age. They usually occur just below the renal arteries, although aneurysms also can involve the renal artery segment and also the thoracic aorta. Most abdominal aortic aneurysms are secondary to atherosclerosis. Surgical removal of the aneurysm with insertion of a Dacron or gortex graft is the conventional method of treating abdominal aortic aneurysms. At least 95% of abdominal aortic aneurysms can be successfully treated if operated on electively. It is for that reason that it is extremely important to detect the aneurysm before rupture. Risk factors include age, smoking, elevated serum cholesterol levels, hypertension, and coronary artery disease. Family history is important and some aneurysms are thought to have a hereditary component. Often an abdominal aortic aneurysm can be suspected or diagnosed by physical exam. A pulsating mass is sometimes palpable.[26] If not diagnosed and treated by grafting, 33% will rupture within one year and 81% will rupture within five years. Most aneurysms are asymptomatic until rupture.

Screening for abdominal aneurysms is usually accomplished by duplex ultrasound, which is noninvasive and painless and inexpensive.[27] Most screening facilities charge approximately $35 for an aortic ultrasound screen to discover the presence of an abdominal aortic aneurysm. Recent statistics from a leading screening organization revealed that 1.84% of all patients screened were positive for abdominal aortic aneurysms. The prevalence of abdominal aortic aneurysms in older adults (age 65-80 years) varies from 4-7%.[28,29] An abdominal aorta is considered to be aneurysmal if its diameter is greater than 3.0 cm.[30] Some aneurysms can be repaired by endovascular stent grafts.[31-34] Additional papers concerning aortic aneurysm screening are given.[35-37] One group thought screening was a bad idea.[38]

Peripheral Arterial Insufficiency

Peripheral arterial insufficiency is most often caused by atherosclerotic vascular disease, and risk factors include hyper-cholesterolemia, smoking, hypertension, diabetes mellitus, age, and heredity. These are essentially the same risk factors as those causing atherosclerosis in the coronary vessels and the extracranial vessels, so if a patient is found to have peripheral arterial insufficiency a physician should suspect that the patient might

Table 3. Obtaining Patient History

Screening for vascular conditions should include the following questions:

1. Have you ever had a stroke or have you ever had a sudden temporary weakness or numbness of the face, arms, or legs?
2. Have you had a sudden loss of speech or trouble understanding speech?
3. Have you had a sudden transient memory loss?
4. Have you had a sudden loss or shading of your vision, either temporary or permanent?
5. Have you had severe dizzy spells?
6. Have you had a recent change in personality?
7. Have you ever been told that you had carotid artery disease?
8. Have you been told that you have atherosclerosis or hardening of the arteries?
9. Have you ever had a ministroke?
10. Have you had an aortic ultrasound test in the past?
11. Has anyone in your family had a stroke?
12. Has anyone in your family had heart disease?
13. Has anyone in your family had diabetes mellitus?
14. Has anyone in your family had an abdominal aortic aneurysm?
15. Have you ever been told that you have a high cholesterol level in your blood? What was your cholesterol when last tested?
16. Have you ever been told that you have a high triglyceride level?
17. Are you currently taking medication for high cholesterol? If yes, what is the name of the medication?
18. Do you have leg pain during exercise, which is relieved by rest?
19. Do you have constant leg pain?
20. Do you have numbness or loss of sensation in your feet?
21. Do you have hair loss from your toes and feet?
22. Do minor scratches and injuries heal properly?
23. Do your legs and feet feel cold all the time?
24. Have you ever had an ultrasound test of your abdominal aorta? If so, when? Results?
25. Have you ever had a carotid ultrasound test? When? Results?
26. Do you smoke?
27. Have you ever smoked? How long? How many packs per day? When did you quit smoking?
28. How far can you walk without leg pain?
29. Have you ever been told that your blood pressure was elevated?

also have coexisting atherosclerosis in the coronary arteries or extracranial vessels. Some of these risk factors are treatable to slow down the formation of the atherosclerotic process. Those include hypercholesterol or lipidemia, hypertension, smoking, and diabetes mellitus. Screening for arterial insufficiency involves obtaining Doppler blood pressures in the upper arm and in the ankles bilaterally. An ankle/brachial index is calculated and if the ankle/brachial index is less than 0.90 the person is considered to have a positive screening test and is advised to have further evaluation by his or her physician. The calculation of the ankle/brachial index is easy to do and it is a reliable test for peripheral arterial insufficiency.[39-41] Diabetic patients frequently have increased arterial wall stiffness and the vessels are not easily compressible, resulting in high-pressure readings. In cases of high-pressure readings because of non-compressibility, diabetes mellitus needs to be ruled out. Lifeline screening recently reported an incidence of 5.74% of patients screened who were found to have abnormal ankle/brachial indices.[42] The usual charge for screening for peripheral arterial insufficiency is about $35.

Atrial Fibrillation

Atrial fibrillation is a condition occurring when the two upper chambers of the heart contract in a rapid but irregular and inefficient manner. The rhythm is not capable of pumping the blood in a meaningful way so blood remains static in the upper heart chambers long enough to form thrombi. Some of the thrombi may break loose from the left atrium and travel through the blood vessels to the brain, causing stroke, or they may travel to other organs, causing sudden ischemia to the kidney or legs depending upon their ultimate resting place. More than 2 million adults in the United States have atrial fibrillation and the incidence increases with increasing age.[43]

Risk Factors for Atrial Fibrillation

Risk factors include history of rheumatic fever, history of hypertension, and history of ischemic heart disease. When any of those conditions cause congestive heart failure the risk of atrial fibrillation is increased.

Structural heart disease is present in 85-90% of patients with atrial fibrillation. Atrial fibrillation affects approximately 4% of the population older than age 60 and 10% of persons older than age 80.[44]

Large cooperative trials performed in a prospective manner have definitively demonstrated that long-term anticoagulant use can safely reduce the risk of stroke due to atrial fibrillation for those patients who cannot be cardioverted successfully and monitored in a normal sinus rhythm. The anticoagulant treatment helps to prevent the formation of blood clots and therefore reduces emboli to the brain. At the present time, fewer than half of the appropriate patients with atrial fibrillation are actually on long-term anticoagulation treatment.[45,46]

Atrial fibrillation is not difficult to diagnose. It can usually be discovered with a screening test using a rhythm strip obtained from an electrocardiograph machine and interpreted by a physician. *(Please see Figure 1.)*

Approximately 15% of strokes are caused by atrial fibrillation with thrombi formation and emboli to the brain.[47] If efficient screening methods were used and those patients with atrial fibrillation were diagnosed and cardioverted or placed on anticoagulant therapy most of these strokes could be prevented.[48,49]

Hypertension

Hypertension or abnormal high blood pressure over time injures key organs and blood vessels in many parts of the body. Damage to these blood vessels often leads to atherosclerosis, increasing the risk of heart disease and stroke. More than 62 million Americans are hypertensive and nearly half of them do not realize they are hypertensive and are not controlling the problem.[50] Usually hypertension causes no symptoms and people may be hypertensive for many years without realizing it. Screening for hypertension is easy, requiring only a blood pressure measurement on several occasions to confirm consistent elevation of the pressure above 140/90 mm Hg. If a screening test reveals hypertension, the patient should be referred to his or her physician in order that additional testing may be performed to determine that the blood pressure persistently remains above 140/90 mm Hg and so additional testing can be performed to determine why the patient has hypertension. The hypertension most often is essential hypertension but sometimes it is due to kidney disease or renal artery stenosis or coartation of the aorta or an adrenal tumor. Risk factors include:

1. Age. Hypertension increases with increasing age.
2. Race. African Americans, Asians, Puerto Ricans, Cuban Americans, and Hispanics are more often hypertensive than other groups.
3. Pregnancy. Pregnant women are at greater risk of becoming hypertensive than other women.

If a person is diagnosed as having hypertension it is extremely important that the hypertension is treated to prevent the complications of persistent hypertension.

Education

The screening event for all the above conditions should be considered an opportunity to better educate potential candidates about the conditions for which they are being screened. Literature pointing out the prevalence of the conditions, the risk factors, and the symptoms of the conditions should be provided and the likely outcome with and without treatment should be discussed. The group being screened should be made aware of the accuracy of the screen and when or if another screen should be done at a later time and, if so, at what time interval. Companies providing screening tests need to be aware that recommendations for screening too often and screening persons who are not at risk open the companies to criticism for overuse.

Notification of Results

It should be made clear to the person being screened how soon results will be available and how he or she will receive those results. Results should be available within two weeks and preferably results should be mailed to each individual. If the screening test is positive, it is preferable to send the results by certified mail. The individual should be advised in writing to take the written result to their physician so their physician may decide if any further testing or treatment is necessary. Positive screening tests usually require additional testing for confirmation before a definitive diagnosis can be established.

Sensitivity, Specificity, and Predictive Value

Sensitivity. The specificity, sensitivity, and predictive value of the test performed should be calculated and provided to all interested parties. There is a trade-off between sensitivity and specificity with any screening tests. To avoid missing those who are "true positive" and increase the specificity, one must allow for a decrease in the sensitivity.

The sensitivity of a screening test equals the probability that if the screening test is positive, the diagnostic test is also positive. The ratio is sensitivity = screening test +/diagnostic test +.

In other words, in the case of carotid stenosis when we desire to locate all the persons with a carotid stenosis of 60% or greater the screening tests would be reported positive at 60% stenosis, meaning that person should have an additional diagnostic test to confirm. We need to know what is the probability that the diagnostic test (either a complete ultrasound study in a certified vascular laboratory or a carotid angiogram) will actually confirm the 60% stenosis seen on the screening test.

Specificity. The specificity of the test equals probability that if the screening test is negative, the diagnostic test would also be negative. In the case of carotid screening, the screening ultrasound test reported less than 60% stenosis and on the report the category sent out was "does not need follow-up testing." If one performed a diagnostic test anyway on that person (either a complete carotid ultrasound test in an accredited vascular laboratory or a carotid angiogram), what is the probability that the diagnostic test would also be negative? This would only be done at some expense because insurance companies and Medicare could not be expected to pay for these expensive tests to confirm negative screening tests.

By increasing the threshold velocity in the internal carotid required to call a stenosis significant we can increase the likelihood of the diagnostic tests confirming a positive screening test (sensitivity). However, we at the same time would be increasing the possibility of missing some individuals who actually had a 60% stenosis but were classified as "does not need follow-up diagnostic test."

Predictive Value. The predictive value of a positive test is equal to probability of the diagnostic test being positive divided by the screening test being positive.

The predictive value of a positive test is the percentage of persons reported positive on a diagnostic test divided by the percentage of persons reported positive on a screening test.

The predictive value of a negative screening test equals the probability of diagnostic tests being negative divided by the screening test being negative.

References

1. *Dorlands Illustrated Medical Dictionary*. 24th ed. Philadelphia, Pa; London, England: W.B. Saunders and Company; 1968.
2. Eady DM. *Primary Care Reports*. 123.
3. Hayward RP. *Primary Care Reports*. 123.
4. National Cancer Institute PDQ Website. http://cancernet.NCI.NIHgov/cancer/inks. 01/2000.

5. Osteoporosis. http://www.crha-health.ab.ca/hlthconn/items.osteo.htm
6. Patient Outcomes Research Team. "Secondary and Tortuary Prevention of Stroke." Agency for Healthcare and Policy Research publication no. 950051 (Sept. 1995).
7. Caplan LR, et al. *American Heart Association Family Guide to Stroke: Treatment, Recovery, and Prevention*. New York: Times Books; 1994:69.
8. National Stroke Association Home Page: www.stroke.org (1998).
9. North American Symptomatic Carotid Endarterectomy Trial Collaborators. Beneficial effect of carotid endarterectomy in symptomatic patients with high-grade carotid stenosis. *N Engl J Med* 1991;325:445-453.
10. European Carotid Surgery Trialists' Collaborative Group. MRC European Carotid Surgery Trial: Interim results for symptomatic patients with severe (70-99%) or with mild (0-29%) carotid stenosis. *Lancet* 1991;337:1235-1243.
11. Mayberg MR, et al. Carotid endarterectomy and prevention of cerebral ischemia in symptomatic carotid stenosis. *JAMA* 1991;266:3289-3294.
12. ACAS. Endarterectomy for asymptomatic carotid artery stenosis. *JAMA* 1995;273:1421-1428.
13. Be Stroke Smart. National Stroke Association Newsletter 11, no. 2 (1994): 3.
14. Lavenson GS Jr. Carotid screening: Preparing for the future. *Vasc US Today* 1997;2:61-72.
15. Bluth EL, et al. A screening test for carotid stenosis: A preliminary feasibility study. RSNA: Session 1706: Nov. 28, 1997.
16. Lavenson GS Jr. Carotid screening: Preparing for the future. *Vasc US Today* 1997;2:61-72.
17. Smith JK, et al. Assessment of new criteria for the duplex Doppler ultrasound detection of clinically significant carotid artery stenosis. RSNA: Session 1703; Nov. 28, 1997.
18. Brown JJ, Pruitt JC. The efficiency of screening for carotid artery stenosis in the asymptomatic population: A historical and clinical perspective. Educational pamphlet for Lifeline Screening, Inc. 1998.
19. Obuchowski NA, et al. Assessment of the efficacy of noninvasive screening for patients with asymptomatic neck bruits. *Stroke* 1997;28:1330-1339.
20. Fujitani RM, Kafie F. Screening and preoperative imaging of candidates for carotid endarterectomy. *Semin Vasc Surg* 1999;12:261-274.
21. Yin D, Carpenter JP. Cost-effectiveness of screening for asymptomatic carotid stenosis. *J Vasc Surg* 1998;27:245-255.
22. Carsten CG III, et al. Use of limited color-flow duplex for a carotid screening project. *Am J Surg* 1999;178:173-176.
23. Lavenson GS Jr, Sharma D. Cost savings of carotid endarterectomy: Value of one vascular surgeon in one year. *Perspect Vasc Surg* 1994;7.
24. Brown JJ, Pruitt JC. The efficiency of screening for carotid artery stenosis in the asymptomatic population: A historical and clinical perspective. Educational pamphlet for Lifeline Screening, Inc. (1998).
25. Estes JE, Jr. Abdominal aortic aneurysm: A study of one hundred and two cases. *Circulation* 1950;2:258.
26. Pysklywec M, Evans MF. Diagnosing abdominal aortic aneurysm. How good is the physical examination? *Can Fam Physician* 1999;45:2069-2070.
27. Wong JG. Appropriate abdominal aortic aneurysm screening. *Postgrad Med* 2000;107:21-22.
28. Lifeline Screening, Inc; Personal communication, 4-1-00.
29. Kyriakides C, et al. Screening of abdominal aortic aneurysm: A pragmatic approach. *Ann R Coll Surg Engl* 2000;82:59-63.
30. Vardulaki KA, et al. Incidence among men of asymptomatic abdominal aortic aneurysms: Estimates from 500 screen detected cases. *J Med Screen* 1999;6:50-54.
31. Allen RC, et al. What are the characteristics of the ideal endovascular graft for abdominal aortic aneurysm exclusion? *J Endovasc Surg* 1997;4:195-202.
32. Moore WS. The EVT tube and bifurcated endograft systems: Technical considerations and clinical summary. *J Endovasc Surg* 1997;4:182-194.
33. Thompson MM, et al. Aortomonoiliac endovascular grafting: Difficult solutions to difficult aneurysms. *J Endovasc Surg* 1997;4:174-181.
34. Manord JD, et al. Endovascular treatment of abdominal aortic aneurysm: Case report and review of literature. *J La State Med Soc* 1997;149:334-337.
35. Beebe HG, Kritpracha B. Screening and preoperative imaging of candidates for conventional repair of abdominal aortic aneurysm. *Semin Vasc Surg* 1999;12:300-305.
36. Lindholt JS, et al. Mass or high-risk screening for abdominal aortic aneurysm. *Br J Surg* 1997;84:40-42.
37. Cole CW. Prospects for screening for abdominal aortic aneurysms. *Lancet* 1997;349:1490-1491.
38. Shiralkar S, et al. The case against a national screening programme for aortic aneurysms. *Ann R Coll Surg Engl* 1997;79:385-386.
39. Ray SA, et al. Reliability of ankle: Brachial pressure index measurement by junior doctors. *Br J Surg* 1994;81:181-190.
40. Stoffers HE. Peripheral arterial occlusive disease in general practice: The reproducibility of ankle:arm systolic pressure ratio. *Scand J Primary Health Care* 1991;9:109-114.
41. Fowkes FGR, et al. Variability of ankle and brachial systolic pressures in the measurement of atherosclerotic peripheral arterial disease. *J Epidemiol Commun Health* 1988;42:128-133.
42. Lifeline Screening, Inc., personal communication, April 1, 2000.
43. Wiener DH. Atrial fibrillation: Comprehensive management in the primary care setting. Monograph from the Temple University School of Medicine; 1995:1-11.
44. Wolf PA, et al. Atrial fibrillation as an independent risk factor for stroke: The Framingham Study. *Stroke* 1991;22:983-988.
45. Albers GW, et al. Status of antithrombotic therapy for patients with atrial fibrillation in university hospitals. *Arch Intern Med* 1996;156:2311-2316.
46. Stafford RS, Singer DE. National patterns of warfarin use in atrial fibrillation. *Arch Intern Med* 1996;156:2537-2541.
47. Kannel WB, et al. Epidemiologic features of chronic atrial fibrillation: The Framingham Study. *N Engl J Med* 1982;306:1018-1022.

48. Patient Outcomes Research Team. Secondary and tertiary prevention of stroke. Agency for Healthcare and Policy Research publication no. 95-0091 (Sept. 1995).
49. Stafford RS, Singer DE. National patterns of warfarin use in atrial fibrillation. *Arch Intern Med* 1996;156:2537-2541.
50. Caplan LR, et al. *American Heart Association Family Guide to Stroke, Treatment, Recovery and Prevention*. New York: Times Books; 1994:54-55, 58-59.

Electrocardiographic Diagnosis: Evaluating Patients With Chest Pain

William J. Brady, MD

The 12-lead electrocardiogram is arguably the most powerful, least invasive, most cost-effective, and predictive tool in our diagnostic armamentarium. In recent years especially, the widely recognized benefits of early diagnosis and rapid revascularization of AMI have cast into focus the urgency of clinical competence in bedside electrocardiographic (ECG) assessment. The emergency physician is frequently the first in-hospital clinician to evaluate patients with chest pain. In this regard, he or she is charged with the responsibility of making a rapid, precise diagnosis and then initiating or recommending appropriate mortality-reducing and myocardium-sparing pharmacotherapeutic and invasive interventions.

As a general rule, the clinical pathway in chest-pain patients bifurcates in two directions. In the case of documented AMI with ST segment elevation (STE) on the ECG, revascularization therapies and other interventions should be considered. To maximize the benefits of such therapy, pharmacotherapeutic or surgically mediated interventions to establish coronary artery patency must be delivered soon after the onset of infarction. In contrast, when patients with chest pain demonstrate STE that is associated with a noninfarction syndrome—pericarditis, bundle branch block, CNS event—a different management pathway should be followed that will not only improve outcomes in this subgroup but also avoid unnecessary application of potentially dangerous and/or invasive therapies such as thrombolysis or angioplasty.

Because these are critical clinical decisions, with both financial and outcome implications, the emergency physician must become proficient in ECG interpretation, which is often pivotal to the clinical management of patients with chest pain. Unfortunately, the ECG has numerous shortcomings when it is used for evaluation of the chest-pain patient. Whereas some patients with chest pain present with STE that is due to an AMI, other patients present with confounding patterns and/or masquerading syndromes. In many cases, perhaps the majority, STE caused by AMI is readily appreciated. However, confounding patterns such as left bundle-branch block (LBBB), ventricular paced rhythms (VPR), and left ventricular hypertrophy (LVH) may obscure the typical electrocardiographic findings of AMI as well as produce noninfarctional STE that may lead the uninformed emergency physician astray.

With these issues in mind, the following chapter focuses on strategies for evaluating the chest-pain patient with STE. The differential diagnosis of these patients is reviewed in detail, and strategies for confirming a coronary ischemia-related condition are outlined. Finally, comprehensive sets of electrocardiographic tracings are provided to enhance the evaluation of ECGs at the bedside.

ECG Diagnosis: Pearls and Pitfalls

Despite the attention that is given to the diagnosis and management of AMI, fewer than 5% of ED visits are precipitated by the

Table 1. Syndromes that May Cause STE

MI
Variant angina
Acute pericarditis
Benign early repolarization
Left ventricular hypertrophy
Bundle branch block
Cardiomyopathy
Acute myocarditis
Left ventricular aneurysm
Pre-excitation syndromes
Hyperkalemia
Hypothermia
CNS events
Acute abdominal disorder

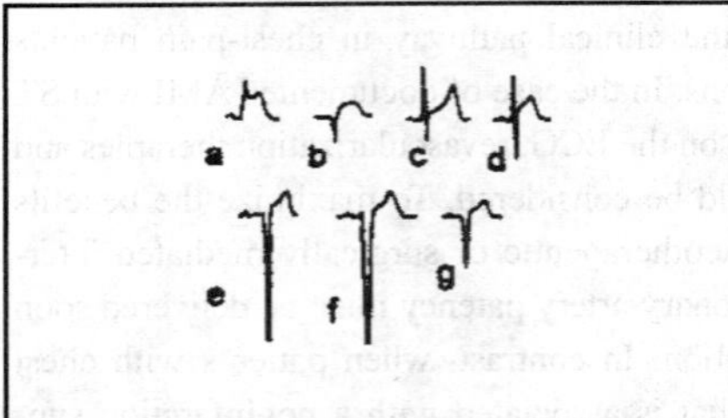

Figure 1

Examples of STE among chest pain patients; lead V_3 is depleted. **[a]** AMI with obliquely flat STE. **[b]** AMI with convex STE. **[c]** Benign early repolarization. **[d]** Acute pericarditis. **[e]** Left ventricular hypertrophy. **[f]** LBBB. **[g]** Left ventricular aneurysm.

chief complaint of chest discomfort.[1-3] However, depending upon the patient population encountered, as many as one-fifth of these patients will experience an AMI; a much higher proportion may be diagnosed with unstable angina pectoris, while the remainder will be found to have a non-coronary source of chest discomfort.[4,5]

To distinguish among these etiologies, the emergency physician typically relies upon three principle evaluation strategies: a complete history of the event; the 12-lead ECG; and cardiac enzyme levels and other serum markers of myocardial injury. While the clinical history of the discomfort and its associated issues are of major importance, the ECG remains a powerful clinical tool for evaluation of these patients. Moreover, the ECG is essential for directing the emergency physician toward proper therapy, especially treatments aimed at interrupting the ischemic cascade and restoring coronary perfusion as well as securing an adequate disposition.[6-9]

Consequently, accurate interpretation of the ECG and confirming a diagnosis of AMI among the numerous causes of STE is a mandatory skill for the emergency physician. Complicating this assessment, however, is the fact that syndromes causing non-AMI STE are frequently misdiagnosed as acute infarction. For example, one study notes that 11% of patients receiving a thrombolytic agent were not experiencing an AMI. The electrocardiographic syndromes producing this pseudo-infarct STE included benign early repolarization (30%), LVH (30%), and various intraventricular conduction abnormalities (30%).[10] Incorrect electrocardiographic interpretations by emergency physicians have been noted in other reviews as well.[11-13] *(Please see Table 1 and Figure 1.)*

Table 2. Causes of STE Among Chest Pain Patients in the ED

Causes of ST segment elevation among ED chest-pain patients. 902 patients presented with chest pain; 202 (22%) patients demonstrated STE on ECG; the responsible etiologies are listed below.[12]

Syndrome	% of Patients
LVH	25
LBBB	15
AMI	15
BER	12
RBBB	5
IVCD*	5
Aneurysm	3
Pericarditis	2
Undefined	18

* IVCD = Intraventricular conduction delay

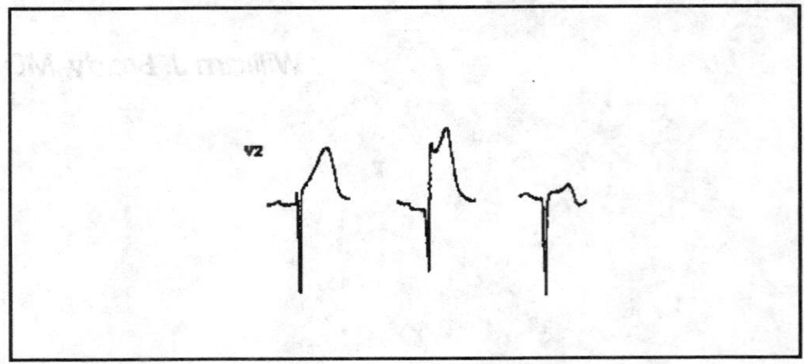

Figure 2

The electrocardiographic evolution of AMI. **Left panel**—hyperacute T wave 15 minutes after onset of chest discomfort. **Middle panel**— marked STE with prominent Q wave three hours into AMI. **Right panel**—persistent STE with Q wave six weeks after AMI, indicative of an aneurysm.

Generally speaking, ST segment elevation is the most "challenging" electrocardiographic feature encountered in the chest-pain patient—challenging because its presence must be explained and, if the clinical history suggests AMI, urgent therapeutic decisions must be made. Unfortunately, STE also is seen in other noninfarction syndromes, reinforcing the point that STE is an insensitive marker of AMI.[14]

Underscoring this observation is a prehospital study of adult chest pain patients that demonstrates that the majority of patients manifesting STE on the ECG did not have AMI as their final hospital diagnosis. Instead, LVH and LBBB accounted for the majority of the cases.[15] Furthermore, in another review of adult ED chest-pain patients with STE on the ECG, the STE resulted from AMI in only 15% of this population; LVH, which was seen in 30% of adult chest-pain patients, was the most frequent cause of this STE in this group of patients.[16] Finally, in the coronary care unit population, another study demonstrated that STE was diagnostic for acute infarct in only half of patients with a history of ischemic heart disease who had characteristic ST segment changes.[17] *(Please see Table 2.)*

The ECG in AMI

Depending upon the patient population and the associated prevalence of ischemic heart disease, the ECG will be diagnostic for AMI in only 25-50% of all patients with proven infarction.[5-7] Moreover, it should be stressed that AMI is not the most common diagnosis in adult chest-pain patients with STE. Consequently, a comprehensive understanding of ECG patterns in AMI—which can range from subtle and confusing to classical and unequivocal—is essential for detecting patients with suggestive historical features who can benefit from mortality-reducing interventions.

ST Segment Elevation (STE). AMI-related STE is said to occur when the ST segment is elevated at least 1 mm (0.1 mv) at a distance measured 0.08 seconds from the J point of the QRS complex. STE in AMI is caused by the electrical current of injury associated with cellular compromise and/or death. In the presence of myocyte dysfunction, leakage of predominantly negatively charged ions from the intracellular space into the extracellular space alters the electrical charge across the cellular membrane. As a result, myocardial cells are no longer able to maintain a normal resting membrane potential during electrical diastole. The relative difference in membrane potentials between injured and normal cells produces the current of injury that manifests as STE on the surface ECG.

Temporal Evolution. The ECG undergoes a well-established temporal evolution following the onset and continuing presence of coronary artery occlusion. *(Please see Figure 2 and Figure 3a through Figure 3c for ECGs of evolving AMI.)* The earliest electrocardiographic finding associated with AMI is the hyperacute T wave, which may appear minutes after the interruption of blood flow to the myocardium; the R wave also increases in amplitude at this stage. Accordingly, the differential diagnosis of the hyperacute T wave includes both transmural AMI and hyperkalemia.

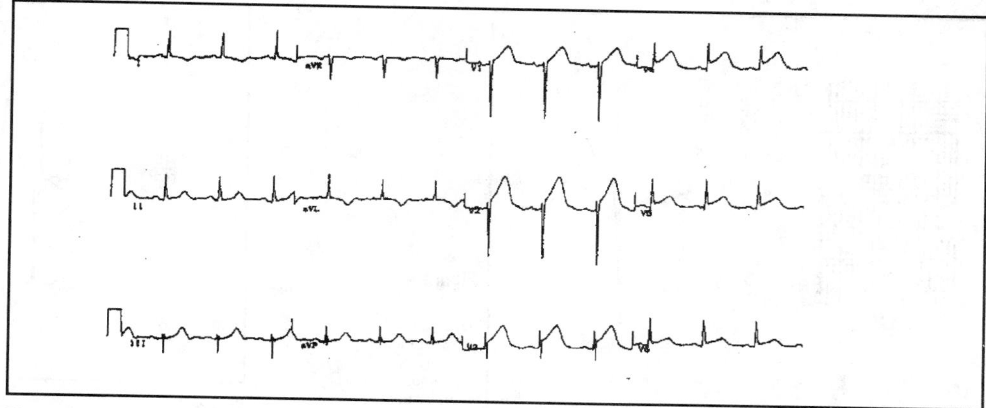

Figure 3a

12-lead ECG obtained 20 minutes after the onset of chest pain depicting hyperacute T waves in leads V_1 and V_2 and minimal STE in leads V_3 to V_6, indicative of an early anterolateral AMI.

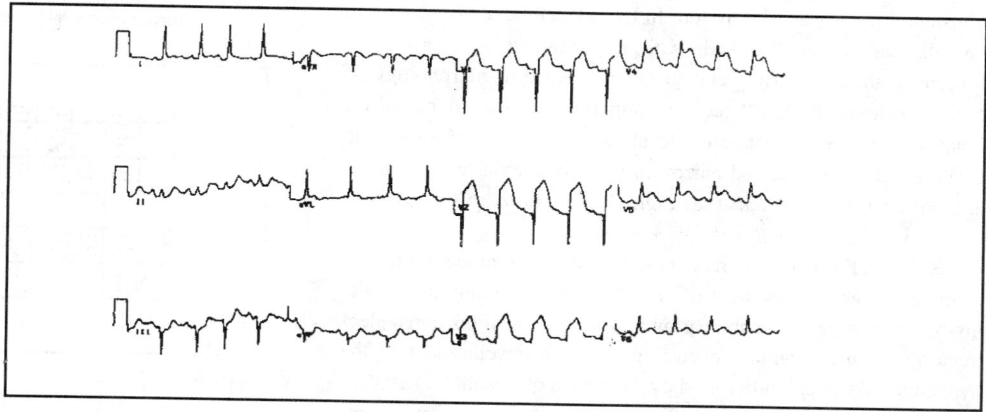

Figure 3b

ECG obtained 2.5 hours after onset of chest pain showing STE in anterolateral distribution. Note the prominent Q wave with marked STE at this early stage of AMI. Giant R waves are seen in leads V_3 and V4; STD (reciprocal change) is also seen in inferior leads.

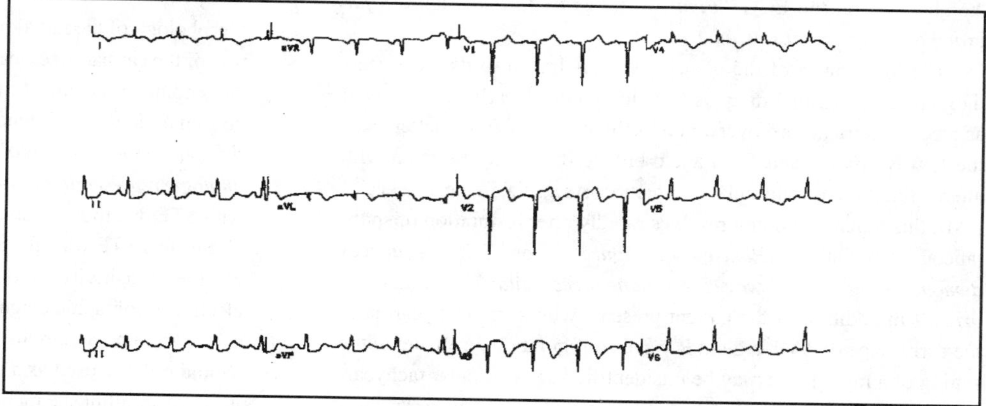

Figure 3c

Persistent STE approximately seven weeks after extensive AMI indicates left ventricular aneurysm.

Hyperacute T Wave. In the case of AMI, the hyperacute T wave is noted as early as 30 minutes after the onset of coronary occlusion and transmural infarction. It tends to be a short-lived phenomenon that evolves rapidly to STE. The hyperacute T wave of early AMI is often asymmetric with a broad base. Not infrequently, these T waves are with reciprocal ST segment depression in other ECG leads. *(Please see Figure 2, the left panel in Figure 3a, and Figure 4 for examples of hyperacute T waves associated with AMI.)*

T waves of large magnitude also are seen in patients with hyperkalemia. Because this T wave morphology also is described as

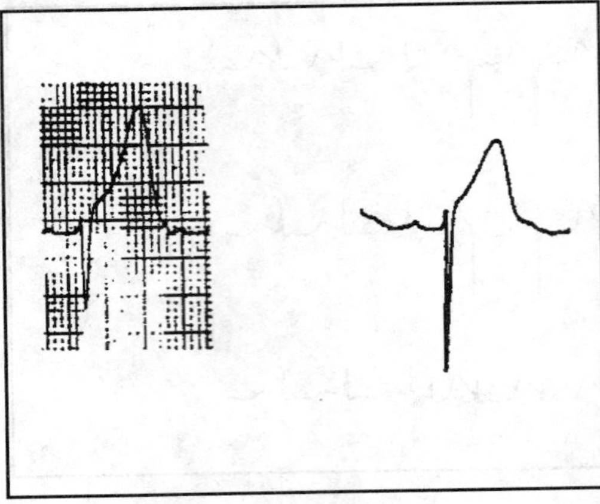

Figure 4

Hyperacute T waves of early AMI are often asymmetric with a broad base.

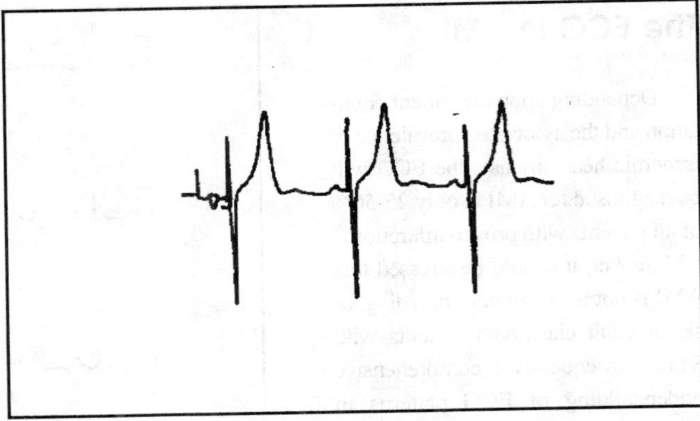

Figure 5

Hyperkalemic T waves tend to be tall, narrow, and peaked with prominent or sharp apex. Also, these T waves tend to be symmetric in morphology; if "split down the middle," the resulting portions would be mirror images. As the serum potassium level increases, the T waves tend to become taller, peaked, and narrowed in a symmetric fashion in the anterior distribution. This T wave morphology may be confused with the hyperacute T wave of early transmural myocardial infarction.

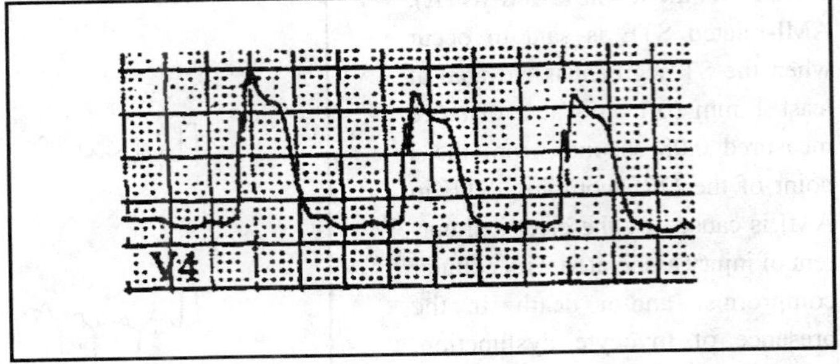

Figure 6

The giant R wave is formed when the ST segment elevates and combines with the prominent R wave particularly in the anterior distribution; the giant R wave has also been referred to as a "tombstone" on the ECG as seen here. The giant R wave is best described as an intermediate electrocardiographic structure in the AMI setting, occurring after the development of the hyperacute T wave and before the appearance of typical STE.

"hyperacute," it may be confused with the hyperacute T wave of early transmural myocardial infarction. In hyperkalemia, T waves tend to be tall, narrow, and peaked, with a prominent or sharp apex. Moreover, these T waves tend to be symmetric in morphology; if "split down the middle," the resulting portions should be mirror images. As the serum potassium level increases, the T waves tend to become taller, peaked, and narrowed in a symmetric fashion in the anterior distribution. *(Please see Figure 5 for an example of a hyperacute T wave associated with hyperkalemia.)*

R Wave. From a temporal perspective, a large (some refer to it as a "giant") R wave is the next ECG finding in continuing myocardial infarction. It is best described as an intermediate or transitional electrocardiographic structure, occurring after the development of the hyperacute T wave, but before the appearance of typical STE.

In fact, this structure is not often seen, inasmuch as it is very transient in nature. The giant R wave is formed when the ST segment elevates and combines with the prominent R wave, particularly in the anterior distribution. The giant R wave also has been referred to as a "tombstone" on the ECG. *(Please see Figure 3b and Figure 6 for examples of the giant R wave.)*

The importance of the giant R wave is linked to its electrocardiographic differential diagnosis, which includes early AMI as well as recent electrical cardioversion of arrhythmia.[18,19] In the latter case, the R wave may result from acute bundle branch dysfunction with altered, inefficient ventricular conduction. As a rule, in the absence of AMI, this transient finding resolves rapidly after restoration of spontaneous circulation. *(Please see Figure 7 for ECG sequences demonstrating giant R waves in a patient resuscitated from cardiac arrest.)* In addition, if the patient presents with sinus tachycardia in the early stage of AMI, a giant R wave configuration occurring in the setting of a rapid pulse may be misidentified as ventricular tachycardia. *(Please see Figure 8 for an example of a patient with sinus tachycardia and inferior wall AMI who was misdiagnosed initially as having ventricular tachycardia.)*

ST Segment Elevation. As myocardial infarction progresses, the STE assumes a more typical morphology. The initial upsloping portion of the ST segment usually is either convex or flat; if the ST segment is flat, it may be either horizontally or oblique to baseline. *(Please see Figure 9 for examples of STE morphologies in encountered in AMI.)*

Not infrequently, an analysis of the ST segment waveform may help distinguish among the various causes of STE and, therefore, assist in identifying the patient with the AMI. This technique evaluates the morphology of the initial portion of the ST segment/T wave. This portion of the cardiac electrical cycle is defined as beginning at the J point and ending at the apex of the T wave. The waveform of patients with non-infarctional STE tends to be concave. *(Please see Figures 1c through 1g for examples of STE with a concave initial ST segment morphology, representing non-infarction syndromes.)* Conversely, patients with STE due to AMI have either obliquely flat or convex waveforms. Use of this STE waveform analysis in ED chest-pain patients increases the sensitivity and positive predictive value for correct electrocardiographic diagnosis of AMI markedly.[16]

It should be emphasized that these morphologic distinctions should only be used as a general guideline. As with most guidelines, it is not infallible. Patients with ST segment elevation due to AMI may demonstrate concavity of this portion of the waveform.[20] *(Please see Figure 10a through Figure 10c for examples of patients with documented AMI and concave ST segment waveforms.)* On the other hand, patients with acute pericarditis may present with STE characterized as obliquely flat. *(Please see Figure 1d.)* The total height of the STE is usually greater in the anterior leads compared to all others; the evolution of the electrocardiographic features noted above also occurs more rapidly in anatomic segments other than the anterior wall. Following maximum STE, the ST segment gradually returns to its baseline location over 12-24 hours.[21-23] This is accompanied by T wave inversion.

Q Wave. Eventually, the R wave diminishes and may disappear entirely with the development of the Q wave. In general, Q waves represent myocardial necrosis and completed infarction. Although Q waves may be encountered in the initial, early stages of transmural AMI, they usually are not fully developed until 12 hours after infarction ensues. In patients who present to the ED with an ECG demonstrating characteristic Q waves, the benefits of thrombolytic therapy are uncertain. In this regard, it should be noted that a small percentage of patients with AMI will develop Q waves as early as two hours after the onset of transmural AMI.[21-23] *(Please see Figure 2 [middle panel], Figure 3b, and Figure 11.)* Consequently, an accurate history confirming two hours of chest discomfort in a patient with STE accompanied by prominent, simultaneous Q waves in the same anatomic distribution does not preclude the patient from being considered for acute revascularization therapy.[20]

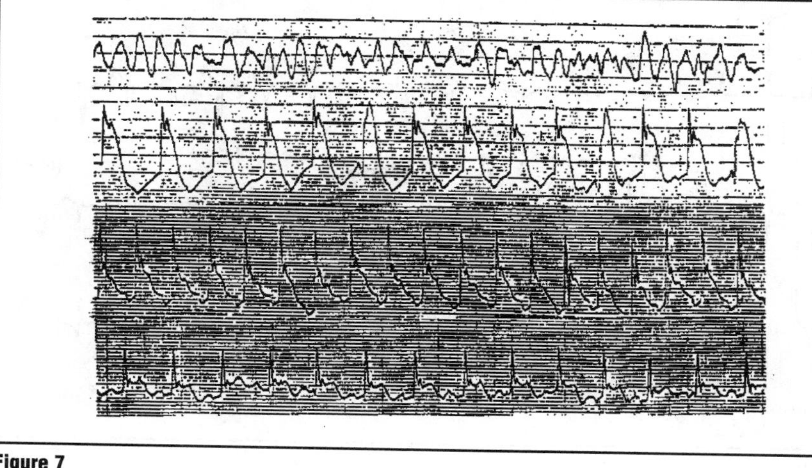

Figure 7

The importance of the giant R wave lies in the consideration of its electrocardiographic differential diagnosis that includes early AMI as well as recent electrical cardioversion of arrhythmia. Depicted here is the sequential example of a patient resuscitated from a ventricular fibrillation cardiac arrest who initially revealed the giant R wave configuration on the rhythm strip; this patient was not experiencing an AMI.

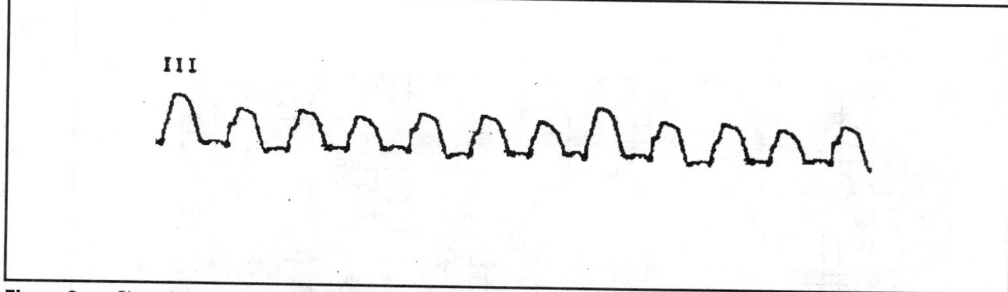

Figure 8 Shown here is the example of a patient with sinus tachycardia and inferior wall AMI manifested by the giant R wave who was misdiagnosed initially as having ventricular tachycardia.

Reciprocal ST Segment Depression. Reciprocal ST segment depression (STD), also known as reciprocal change, is defined as STD in leads that are separate and distinct from leads manifesting STE. The STD is either horizontal *(please see Figure 12, upper panel)* or downward-sloping *(please see Figure 12, lower panel)*. The cause(s) of reciprocal change remain(s) unknown but may involve displacement of the injury current vector away from the infarcting myocardium, co-existing distant ischemia, and/or it may be a manifestation of infarct extension.

Regardless of its cause, reciprocal changes in the setting of transmural AMI identify a subset of patients with an increased chance of poor outcome and, therefore, patients who may benefit from a more aggressive approach in the ED. Furthermore, its presence on the ECG supports the diagnosis of AMI with very high sensitivity and positive predictive values greater than 90%.[15,16]

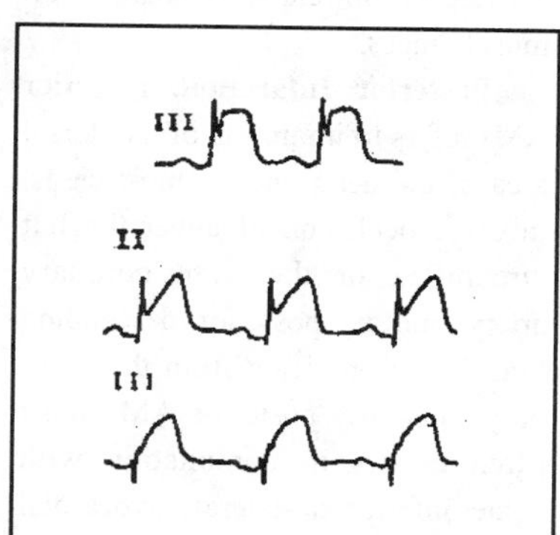

Figure 9

An analysis of the ST segment waveform (from the beginning at the J point to the end at the apex of the T wave) may be particularly helpful in distinguishing among the various causes of STE and identifying the AMI case. The initial upsloping portion of the ST segment usually is either flat (horizontally or obliquely) or convex in the AMI patient.

The use of reciprocal change in both prehospital and ED chest-pain patients retrospectively increased the diagnostic accuracy in the electrocardiographic recognition of AMI.[15,16] It is perhaps most useful in patients with chest pain and STE of uncertain etiology. The presence of reciprocal STD in these cases strongly suggests AMI. Its absence, unfortunately, cannot be used to rule-out AMI in that reciprocal change is not encountered in all patients with acute infarction. Patients with inferior wall AMI manifest reciprocal changes in approximately 75% of cases, whereas anterior wall myocardial infarcts demonstrate such STD in no more than one-third of patients. Moreover, the combination of ST segment waveform analysis and reciprocal changes in ED chest-pain patients does not appear to increase the diagnostic accuracy of the ECG for AMI beyond the use of each strategy independently.[16]

Premature Ventricular Contractions (PVCs). Premature ventricular contractions (PVCs) occur frequently in patients with acute coronary ischemia. In most cases of PVC, the "rule of appropriate discordance" describes the normal and benign relationship of the terminal portion of the QRS complex to the ST segment/T wave. The same principles that are applied in the LBBB and VPR situations may be used. For example, the observation of a PVC with a concordant ST segment may suggest AMI. In most cases, other sinus beats on the ECG should support such a diagnosis. Certain cases, however, may involve questionable STE, in which case confirmation of AMI may be made by observing a PVC with concordant ST segment changes. *(Please see Figure 13, which shows a series of PVCs in the right precordial leads V_1 top to V_3 bottom.)* The PVCs in leads V_1 and V_2 demonstrate concordant STE that is not the expected waveform morphology; the correct waveform morphologic relation-

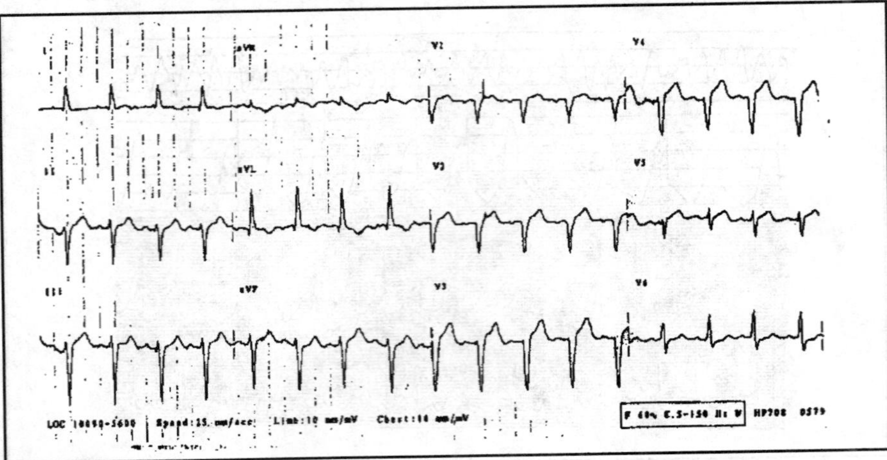

Figure 10a

The initial upsloping portion of the ST segment usually is either flat or convex in the AMI patient. This morphologic observation, however, should only be used as a guideline—it is not infallible. Patients with ST segment elevation due to AMI may demonstrate concavity of this portion of the waveform, as seen in examples **[a]** anterior wall AMI, **[b]** anterior wall AMI, and **[c]** inferior wall AMI.

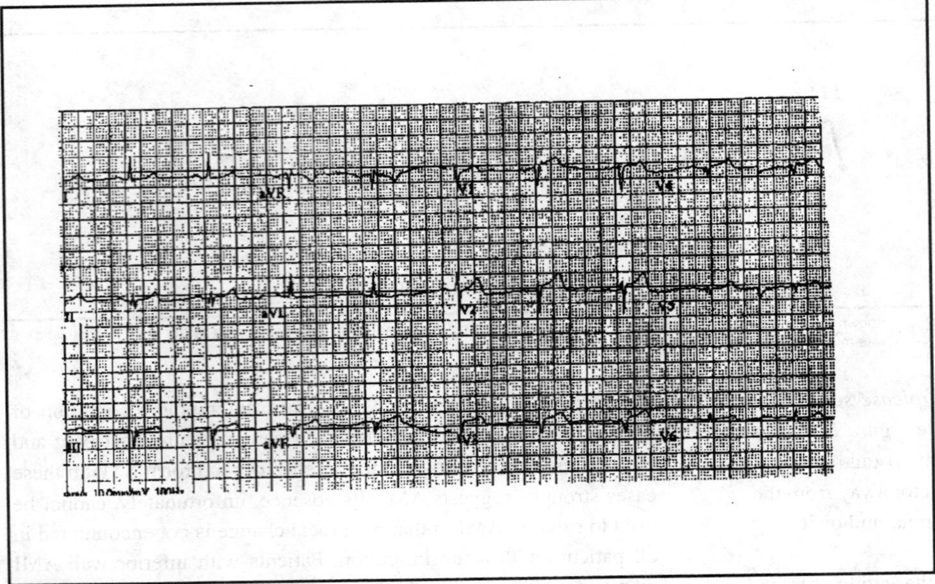

Figure 10b

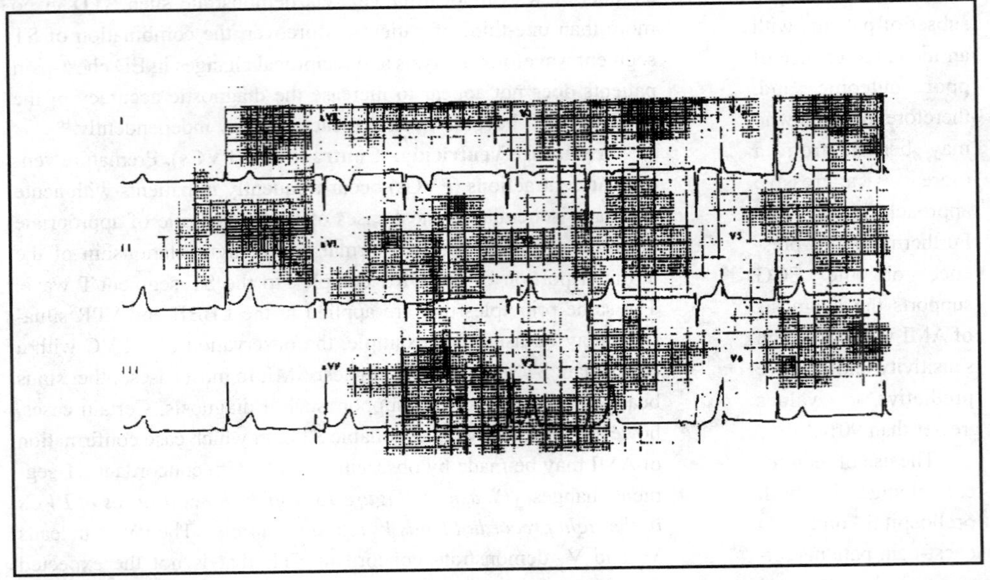

Figure 10c

ship is seen in lead V_3 —it is one of discordance with the terminal portion of the QRS complex.

Additional Leads. Additional lead ECGs are used to better define the extent of myocardial injury, particularly in cases involving the right ventricle (RV) and the posterior wall of the left ventricle. The 15-lead ECG technique uses three additional leads to investigate the right ventricle (lead RV_4) and the posterior wall (leads V_8 and V_9). The standard 12-lead ECG does not define either area well. Right ventricular infarction complicates approximately 25% of inferior wall AMI. Patients with inferior wall infarction present with hypotension resulting from acute right-sided heart failure and reduced preload from either pre-existing volume depletion or nitrate-induced venodilation.

Right Ventricular Infarction (RV). In right ventricular infarction, the 12-lead ECG reveals typical STE in the inferior leads as well as STE in the right precordial leads, especially lead V_1. In contrast to the anteroseptal AMI, which is characterized by increasing STE as one moves from right to mid-precordial leads, in RV AMI, decreasing magnitude of ST segment elevation in the V_1 to V_4 distribution is noted. Additional lead applications can be used to define RV injury, including a complete reversal of the standard left-sided precordial leads (resulting in RV_1 through RV_6, *please see Figure 14*) or a simplified approach, using only RV_4. *(Please see Figure 15.)* In either case, the degree of STE in the right-sided leads may be of smaller magnitude than that observed in anterior MI due to the relatively smaller RV muscle mass.

Posterior Infarction. Posterior AMI refers to infarction of the dorsal area of the heart and, in most cases, involves occlusion of either the left circumflex or the right coronary artery and its posterior descending branch. As predicted from the coronary anatomy, posterior AMI most often occurs in conjunction with acute inferior or lateral myocardial infarction. Although true, isolated posterior AMI does occur, it is rare.[24]

The emergency physician may employ additional-lead ECGs in select cases, looking for involvement of the posterior wall in patients with co-existing inferior or lateral acute infarct. Alternatively, in a chest-pain patient with a high clinical suspicion for AMI, but in whom only STD is noted in the right precordial leads, an additional-lead ECG may reveal posterior AMI. Identification of a larger infarct, as with the case of extension to posterior MI, may not have an impact on therapy. On the other hand, identifying a patient with an isolated posterior AMI, however uncommon, which may have escaped detection using standard electrocardiography, may alter therapeutic decisions and clinical outcome.

Additional Lead ECG. Using additional-lead ECGs in all adult chest pain patients encountered in the ED does not appear to have therapeutic or diagnostic benefits.[25] However, when considering a high-risk population of patients, such as coronary care unit admissions, additional lead ECGs have been shown to improve the rate of diagnosis of posterior AMI.[26]

Because the endocardial surface of the posterior wall faces the precordial leads, the electrocardiographic changes resulting from AMI will be reversed. An R wave with increased voltage in the right precordial leads (V_1 to V_3) is the major electrocardiographic feature associated with posterior AMI. An R/S wave ratio greater than 1.0 in leads V_1 or V_2 is another suggestive finding.[24] *(Please see Figure 15.)* Moreover, ST segment depression with a prominent, upright T wave in a similar distribution are highly correlated with posterior AMI.

If one considers the "reverse nature" of these electrocardiographic abnormalities when applied to the posterior wall, the findings assume a more recognizable, ominous meaning. The tall R wave is actually a significant Q wave while the ST segment/T wave abnormalities represent ST segment elevation with inverted T wave. When interpreting the ECG in an appropriate patient, the finding of STD in the right precordial leads should suggest either anterior wall ischemia or acute posterior wall myocardial infarction. Greater than 1 mm ST segment elevation in the posterior leads, V_8 and V_9, confirms the presence of posterior AMI and are felt to be more accurate in confirming the diagnosis as compared to the findings noted in leads V_1 through V_3.[26] *(Please see Figure 15 for an example of an infero-latero-posterior AMI diagnosed via a 15-lead ECG.)*

Variant Angina. Prinzmetal's angina, also known as variant angina, presents with chest discomfort and ST segment abnormalities; the basic pathophysiologic lesion is felt to be vasospasm. The actual ST waveform encountered in such cases depends upon the size of the vessel involved—large vessel involvement produces STE while smaller caliber vessels in spasm cause STD. Most commonly, the electrocardiographic manifestation is STE. Classically, the chest discomfort occurs at rest and resolves with traditional antianginal therapy or calcium antagonist treatment. If the episode is prolonged, AMI may occur. The ST segment elevation in variant angina is difficult, if not impossible, to distinguish from that associated with AMI.

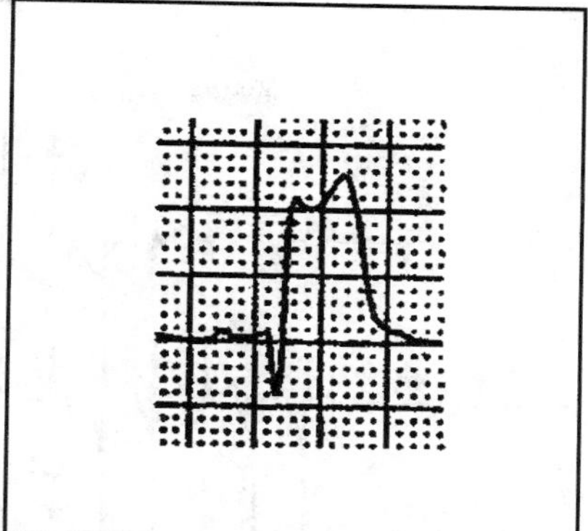

Figure 11

Prominent Q wave with marked STE in a patient with AMI. The chest discomfort started approximately three hours prior to presentation.

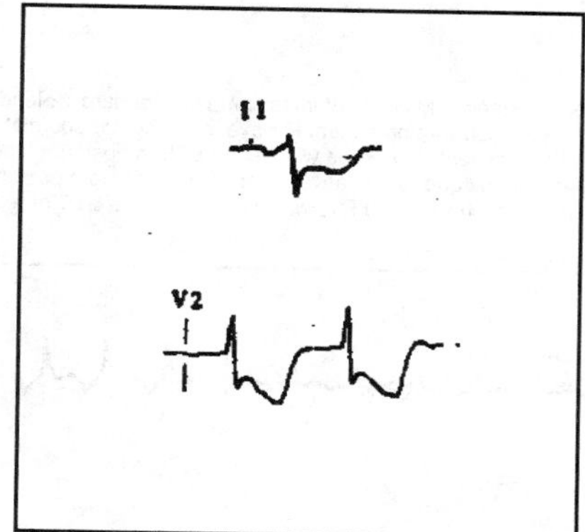

Figure 12

Reciprocal ST segment depression, also known as reciprocal change, is defined as ST segment depression in leads separate and distinct from leads reflecting STE. The ST segment depression is either horizontal (upper panel) or down-sloping (lower panel). Reciprocal ST segment depression in the setting of STE on other electrocardiographic leads strongly supports the diagnosis of AMI.

Figure 13

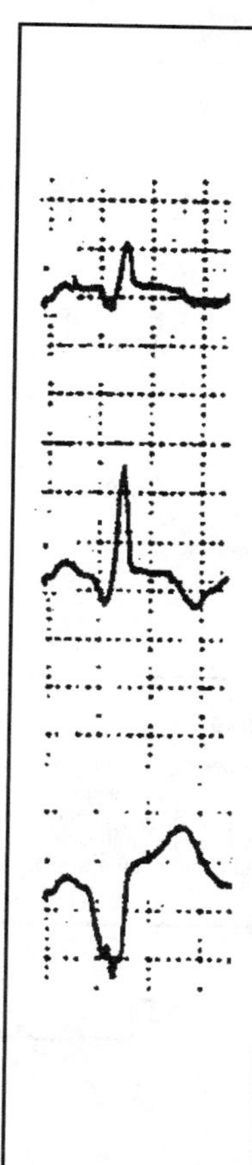

In most cases of PVC, the rule of appropriate discordance once again describes the relationship of the terminal portion of the QRS complex to the ST segment / T wave—the same principle as applied in the LBBB and VPR situations. The observation of a PVC with a concordant ST segment may suggest AMI, as seen in leads V_1 (top) and V_2 (middle).The correct waveform morphologic relationship is seen in lead V_3 (bottom)— one of discordance with the terminal portion of the QRS complex.

18-lead ECG revealing an inferolateral AMI with RV infarction. This ECG will reveals the typical STE in the inferior and lateral leads as well as STE in the right-sided chest leads (i.e., a complete reversal of the standard left-sided precordial leads resulting in RV1 through RV_6). As evidenced in this example, the degree of STE in leads RV_3 to RV_6 is less pronounced than that seen in the inferior distribution due to the relatively smaller RV muscle mass.

Figure 14

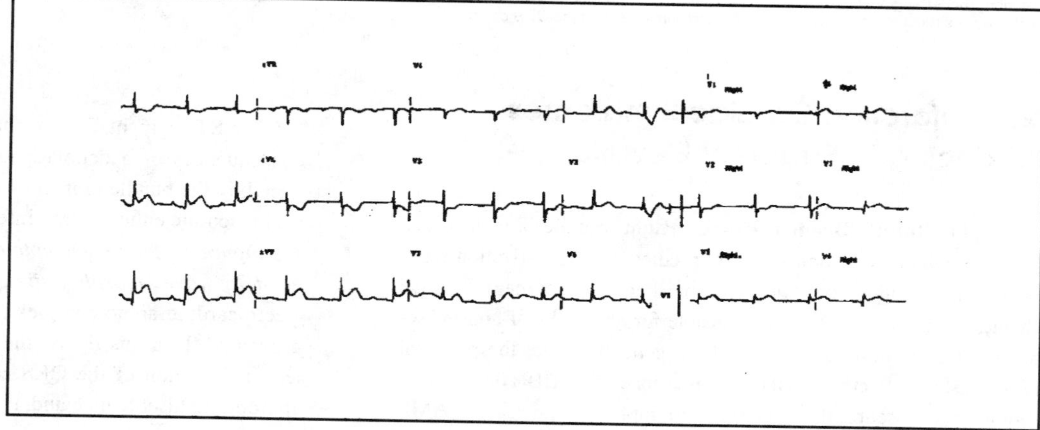

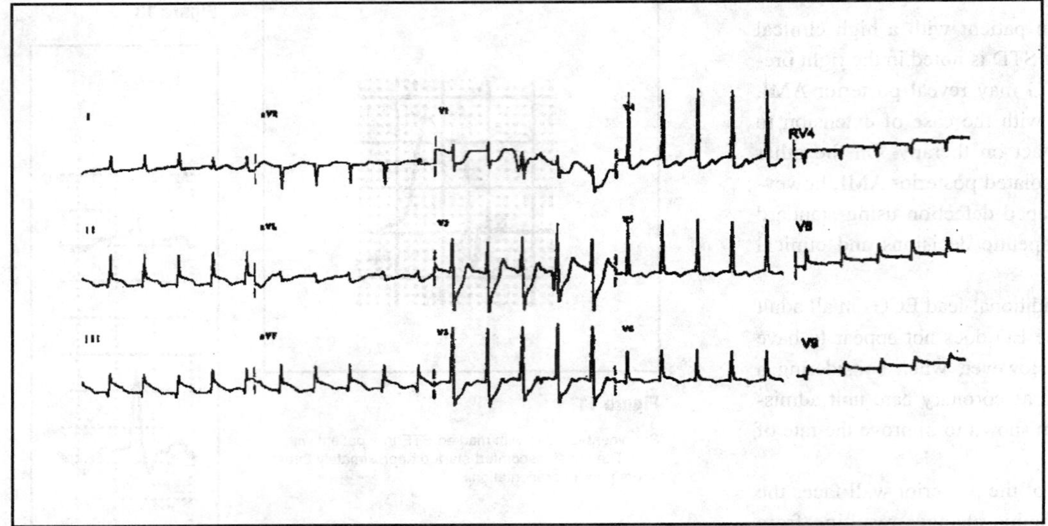

Figure 15

15-lead ECG revealing an infero-latero-posterior AMI with RV infarction. The standard 12-lead ECG will reveal the typical STE in the inferior and lateral leads as well as ST segment depression with prominent R wave in the right precordial leads. Posterior AMI is indicated by both the right precordial ST segment depression with prominent R wave as well as the STE in posterior leads V_8 and V_9. Note that the degree of STE is less pronounced than that seen in the inferior leads due to a relatively longer distance from posterior epicardium to surface leads. The RV infarction is noted in this case using the simplified approach with only RV_4 which demonstrates STE of relatively small magnitude.

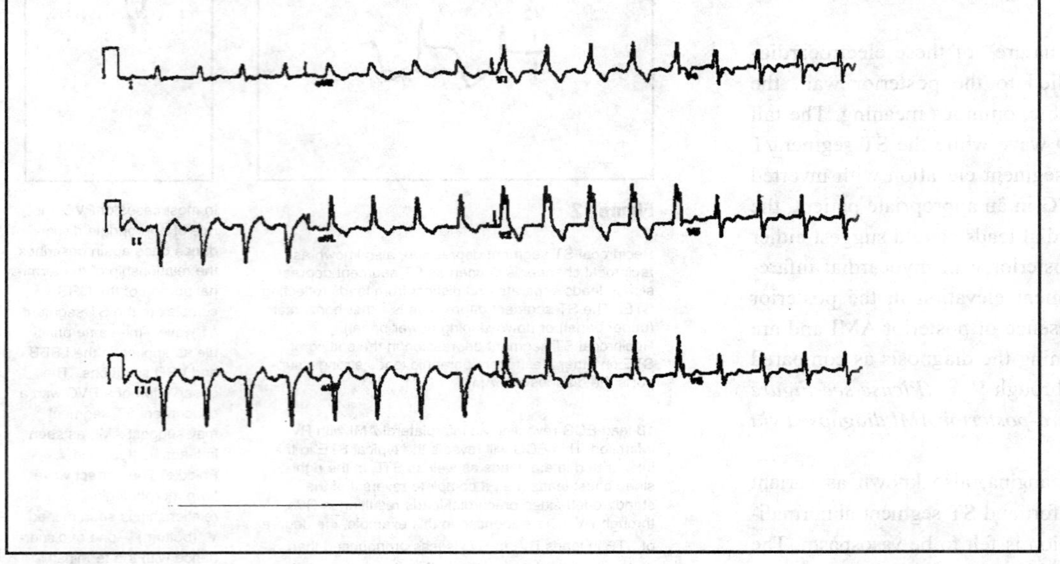

Figure 16

Right bundle branch block with its associated ST segment/T wave changes. Marked ST segment changes are seen and are the new "norm" in the patient with RBBB. The right precordial leads with the predominantly positive forces are associated with ST segment depression and T wave inversion. The ST segment in the inferior is elevated with an upright T wave. As predicted by the rule of appropriate discordance, the ST segment/T wave structure is directed opposite the terminal portion of the QRS complex.

Non-Infarction Cardiac Syndromes Producing ST Segment Elevation

Right Bundle-Branch Block. Right bundle-branch block (RBBB), which is accompanied by predictable depolarization-repolarization changes, can produce marked ST segment/T wave changes.[20] In fact, RBBB is responsible for about 5% of non-infarctional STE in chest pain patients.[16] In general, unlike the potential AMI-masking effect of a LBBB, the presence of a RBBB on the ECG should not obscure the electrocardiographic diagnosis of AMI, although it can suggest an incorrect diagnosis to the uniformed observer. False-positive diagnoses will not occur if the clinician is well versed in the electrocardiographic characteristics—including variations and morphologies—of RBBB and its associated ST segment/T wave abnormalities.

In RBBB, the deflection representing right ventricular activation is delayed and becomes very prominent, resulting in a broad R wave in lead V_1. This broadened R wave may take any of the following morphologies: monophasic R, biphasic RSR, or qR formation. In lead V_6, early intrinsicoid deflection and either a wide S or RS complex wave are seen. QS complexes are encountered in the inferior leads. The QRS complex duration is prolonged (i.e., it is usually greater than 0.12 seconds).

In addition, pronounced ST segment changes are seen and, in fact, are the "norm" in the patient with RBBB.[21] The right precordial leads, which reflect predominantly positive forces, are usually associated with STE and T-wave inversion. The ST segment in the inferior and left precordial leads is frequently elevated with an upright T wave; the degree of STE is usually greater in the inferior distribution. As predicted by the rule of appropriate discordance, the ST segment/T wave structure is directed opposite the terminal portion of the QRS complex.

The ST segment/T wave changes noted above are the expected consequences of a depolarization-repolarization disturbance produced by the bundle branch block. Accordingly, the RBBB pattern may resemble either lateral, inferior, or posterior wall AMI. *(Please see Figure 16 for an example of RBBB with the expected ST segment/T wave morphologies.)* Figure 17a shows a single electrocardiographic complex (lead V_1) in a patient with enzyme-proven AMI. In this figure, the ST segment is concordant with the terminal portion of the QRS complex—a violation of the rule of appropriate discordance and, therefore, strong electrocardiographic

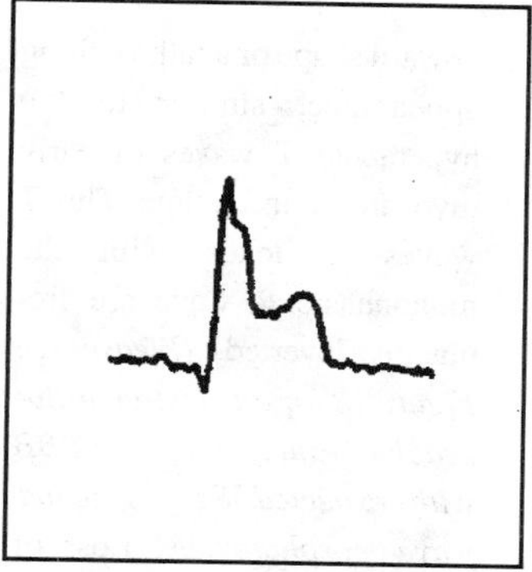

Figure 17a

A single electrocardiographic complex (lead V_1) in a patient with enzyme-proven AMI. The ST segment is elevated and concordant with the terminal portion of the QRS complex—a violation of the rule of appropriate discordance and a strong electrocardiographic suggestion of AMI in a patient with RBBB.

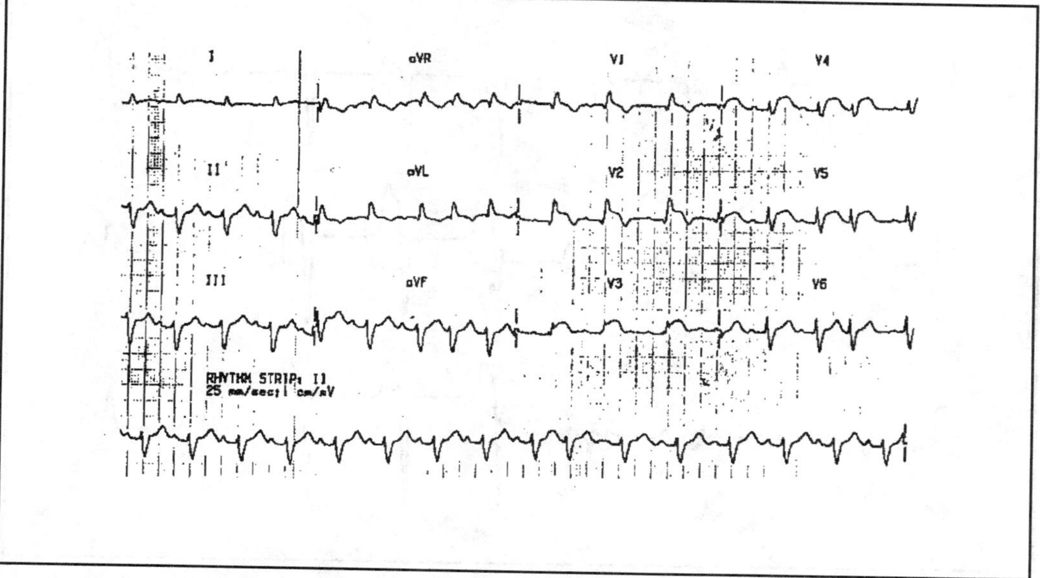

Figure 17b 12-lead ECG with RBBB and AMI with concordant STE in the right precordial leads.

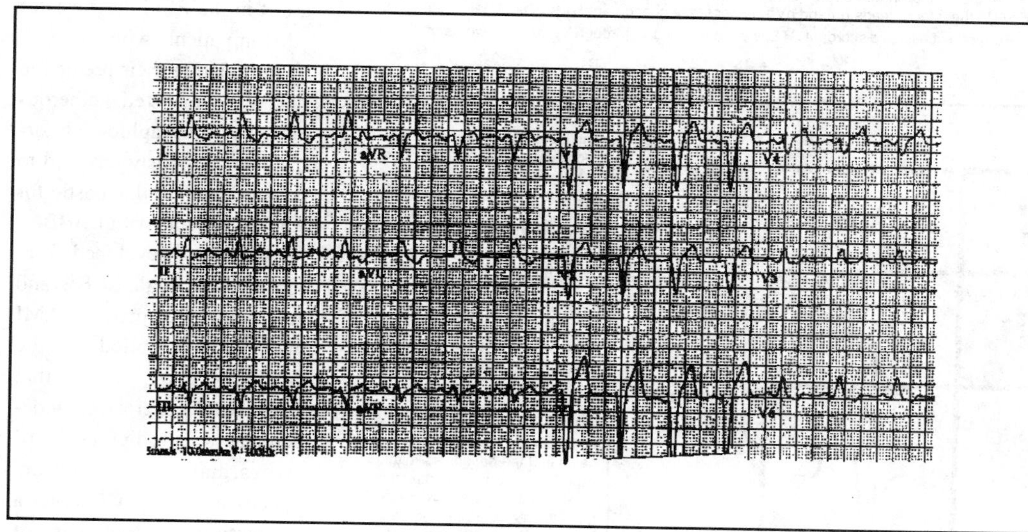

Figure 18

In the patient with LBBB, the anticipated or expected ST segment/T wave configurations are discordant, directed opposite from the terminal portion of the QRS complex and called QRS complex/T wave axes discordance. As such, leads with either QS or rS complexes may have markedly elevated ST segments, mimicking AMI. Leads with a large monophasic R wave demonstrate ST segment depression. The T wave, especially in the right to mid precordial leads, has a convex upward shape or a tall, vaulting appearance, similar to the hyper-acute T wave of early myocardial infarction. The T waves in leads with the monophasic R wave are frequently inverted.

evidence of AMI. Figure 17b represents a 12-lead ECG in a patient with RBBB and AMI; again, the STE is concordant in the right precordial leads, which is strongly suggestive of AMI.

Left Bundle-Branch Block (LBBB). In contrast to RBBB, LBBB markedly reduces the diagnostic power of the ECG. With this finding, the associated and expected ST segment-T wave abnormalities of LBBB can mimic both acute and chronic ischemic changes.[20,24,27,28] Of special concern is the fact that these morphological abnormalities have the potential of suggesting an incorrect diagnosis of MI. Furthermore, such changes also can mask the classic electrocardiographic findings of AMI. One recent study of out-of-hospital chest pain patients undergoing 12-lead ECG analysis revealed that 51% of patients with 1 mm or greater ST segment elevation in two anatomically contiguous leads (i.e., electrocardiographic thrombolytic agent criteria) had non-myocardial infarction conditions for their final hospital diagnosis.[15] LBBB was the second most frequently encountered electrocardiographic pattern responsible for this non-infarction ST segment elevation.

If one considers the ED chest pain population, LBBB was responsible for 15% of STE syndromes; as in the prehospital chest pain population, LBBB represents the second most often seen pattern causing non-AMI STE in the ED.[16] The ST segment/T wave abnormalities encountered with LBBB are the most frequently misinterpreted pseudoinfarct pattern in practice today.[24]

As every physician knows, the electrocardiographic abnormalities associated with AMI may be masked by altered patterns of ventricular conduction observed in patients with LBBB. This situation, however, is far from hopeless. Although common medical opinion holds that the electrocardiographic diagnosis of AMI is virtually impossible in the presence of LBBB, in fact, the diagnosis of MI, even in the presence of LBBB, is often straightforward and considered "disarmingly easy" by several authorities.[29] In this regard, a recent study by Sgarbossa and his group[30] successfully addresses this clinical misconception. Their approach has been to develop a clinical prediction rule that can be used quickly and easily in ED patients with suspected acute myocardial infarction and concomitant LBBB.

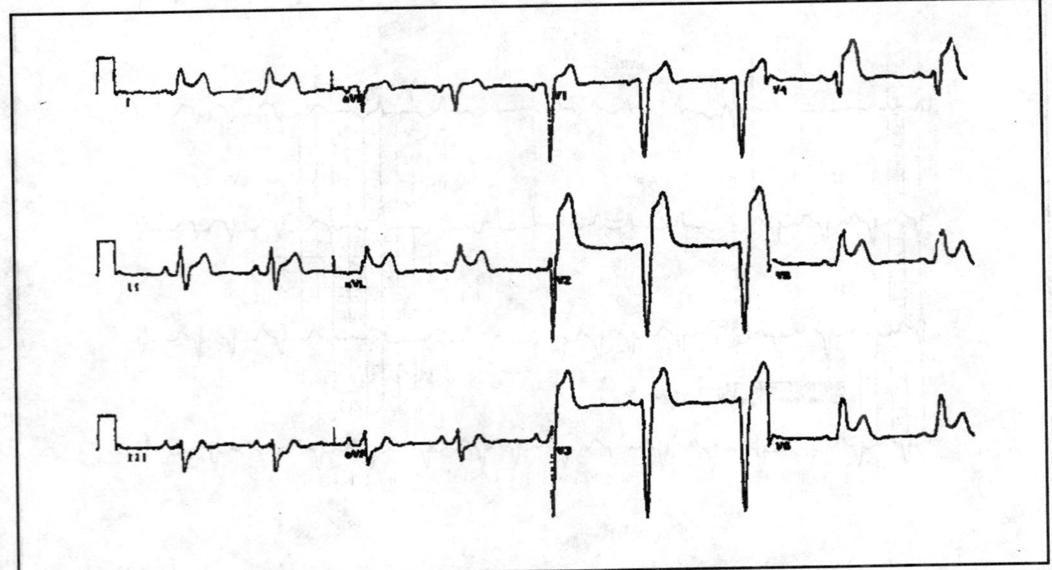

Figure 19

Anterolateral AMI in a patient with pre-existing LBBB. The rule of appropriate discordance is violated in a number of leads in this example. The lateral leads (I, aV_l, V_5, and V_6) reveal concordant STE while the inferior leads (III and aVf) demonstrate concordant ST segment depression—both features which suggest acute coronary ischemia. Further, excessive discordant STE is seen in leads V_2 through V_4, another worrisome feature for AMI.

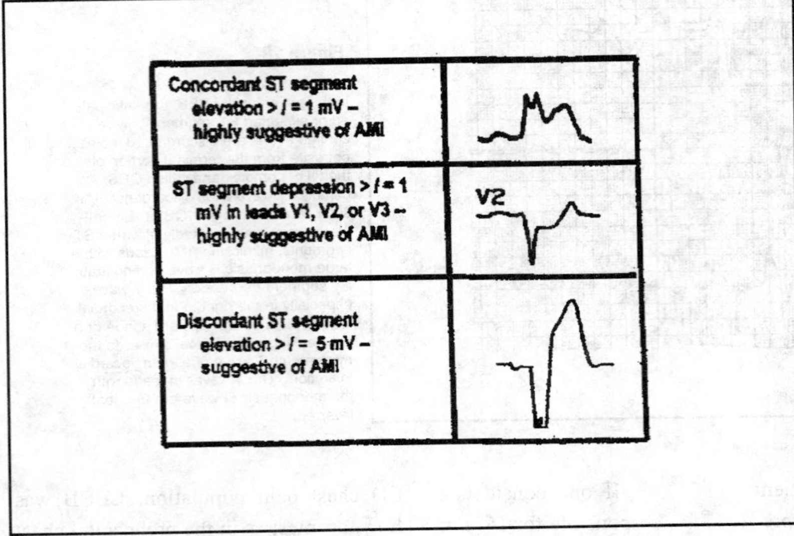

Figure 20

The electrocardiographic criteria suggesting a diagnosis of acute myocardial infarction according to Sgarbossa et al,[28] include in the upper panel [1] ST segment elevation greater than one millimeter which is concordant with the QRS complex (score of 5); in the middle panel [2] ST segment depression greater than one millimeter in leads V_1, V_2, or V_3 (score of 3); and in the lower panel [3] ST segment elevation greater than five millimeters which is discordant with the QRS complex (score of 2). A total score of three or more suggests that the patient is likely experiencing an acute infarction based on the electrocardiographic criteria. With a score less than three, the electrocardiographic diagnosis is less assured, requiring additional evaluation.

In the patient with LBBB,[20,29] the 12-lead ECG records abnormal ventricular activation as it moves from right to left, producing a broad, mainly negative QS or rS complex in lead V_1. In lead V_6, late intrinsicoid deflection is noted, resulting in a positive, monophasic R wave; similar structures are frequently found in leads I and aV_l. Poor R wave progression or QS complexes are noted in the right to mid precordial leads, rarely extending beyond leads V_4 or V_5. QS complexes also may be encountered in leads III and aVf. The anticipated or expected ST segment-T wave configurations are discordant (i.e., they are directed opposite from the terminal portion of the QRS complex); this is called QRS complex-T wave axis discordance. As such, leads with either QS or rS complexes may have markedly elevated ST segments, mimicking acute myocardial infarction. Leads with a large monophasic R wave demonstrate ST segment depression. The T wave, especially in the right to mid precordial leads, has a convex upward shape or a tall, vaulting appearance, similar to the hyperacute T waves of early myocardial infarction. The T waves in leads with the monophasic R wave are frequently inverted. *(Please see Figure 18 for an electrocardiographic example of a LBBB with expected ST segment/T wave morphologies.)* Loss of this normal QRS complex-T wave axis discordance in patients with LBBB may imply an acute process, such as acute myocardial infarction.

Using specific electrocardiographic findings, the Sgarbossa group has developed a clinical prediction rule to assist in the ECG diagnosis of AMI in patients with LBBB.[30] In formulating their prediction rule, they analyzed numerous electrocardiographic abnormalities previously reported to be suspicious or diagnostic for AMI in patients with LBBB.

The rule, developed from 131 patients with LBBB and enzymatically proven AMI who were enrolled in the GUSTO-I trial, states that three ECG criteria are independent predictors of myocardial infarction. Specifically, the ECG criteria suggesting a diagnosis of AMI, ranked with a scoring system based on the probability of such a diagnosis, include: ST segment elevation greater than 1 mm that is concordant with the QRS complex (score of 5) *(Please see Figure 19—leads I, aV_l, V_5, and V_6)*; ST segment depression greater than 1 mm in leads V_1, V_2, or V_3 (score of 3); and ST segment elevation greater than 5 mm that is discordant with the QRS complex (score of 2). *(See Figure 19—leads V_2 through V_4.)*

A total score of three or more suggests that the patient is likely to have an AMI, based on the ECG criteria. In chest pain patients with a score less than three, the electrocardiographic diagnosis is less assured, and the patient will require additional clinical evaluation. *(Please refer to Figure 20 for elucidation of these criteria and an accompanying ECG supporting the electrocardiographic diagnosis of AMI.)* The usefulness of this clinical prediction instrument emphasizes the importance of becoming familiar with associated, or anticipated, ST segment/T wave changes caused by abnormal ventricular conduction patterns observed in LBBB.

Ventricular Paced Rhythms (VPR). In right ventricular-paced rhythms, the ventricular depolarization pattern is abnormal (i.e., activation of the ventricles proceeds from the right to the left which, in most cases, resembles a LBBB pattern). This produces a broad, mainly negative QS or rS complex in leads V_1 to V_6, with either poor R wave progression or QS complexes. A large monophasic R wave is encountered in leads I and aVL and, on occasion, in leads V_5 and V_6. QS complexes may also be encountered in leads II, III, and aVf. The anticipated ST segment-T wave configurations are discordant (i.e., they are directed opposite of the terminal portion of the QRS complex). This illustrates the rule of appropriate discordance and is similar to the electrocardiographic principles applied in the setting of LBBB.[20,27] *(Please see Figure 21a for the appropriate discordant QRS complex-ST segment/T wave relationship.)*

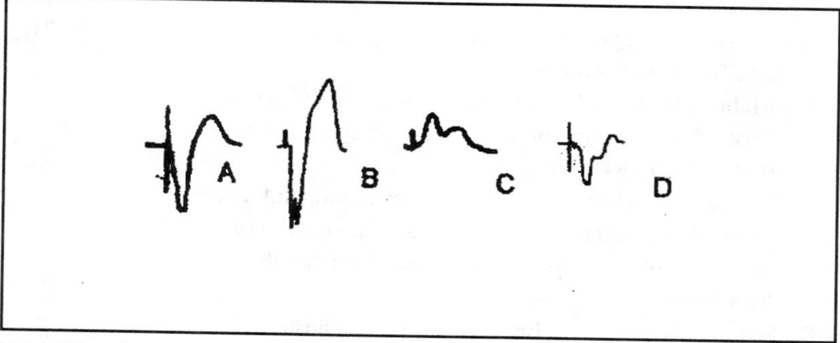

Figure 21

Characteristic electrocardiographic changes associated with AMI according to Sgarbossa et al.[31] **[a]** Normal, or expected, discordant relationship of the terminal portion of the QRS complex and the ST segment. **[b]** Discordant STE > 5 mm. **[c]** Concordant STE > 1 mm. **[d]** ST segment depression > 1 mm in leads V_1, V_2, or V_3.

As a result, leads with QS complexes may have marked STE, mimicking AMI. Leads with a large monophasic R wave demonstrate STD. The T wave, especially in the right to mid precordial and inferior leads, has a convex upward shape or a tall, vaulting appearance similar to the hyperacute T wave of early myocardial infarction. The T waves in leads with the monophasic R wave are frequently inverted. The ECGs in patients with VPR should be inspected for a loss of this QRS complex/T-wave axes discordance. Loss of this normal QRS complex/T wave axes discordance in patients with VPR may imply an acute process, such as AMI.[31,32]

In a report similar to one they published on LBBB, the Sgarbossa group published a report detailing the electrocardiographic changes encountered in patients with VPR with confirmed AMI.[30,33] Of 41,021 patients with enzymatically confirmed AMI entered in the GUSTO trial, 32 patients with VPR (0.1%) were encountered and enrolled in this study. Fifteen patients were excluded due to the presence of native rhythm or other non-right ventricular paced rhythms, leaving 17 cases (6 single- and 11 dual-chamber ventricular pacemakers) that were used for analysis.[1,10] These study patients were compared to a similar number of randomly selected, age-matched control subjects with known, stable coronary artery disease and permanent right-ventricular pacing.

Classic ECG criteria for myocardial infarction in the setting of ventricular pacing were assessed between the two groups.[34-36] Three ECG criteria were found to be useful in the early diagnosis of AMI, including: discordant STE greater than or equal to 5 mm *(please see Figure 21b)*; concordant STE greater than or equal to 1 mm *(please see Figure 21c)*; and ST segment depression greater than or equal to 1 mm in leads V_1, V_2, or V_3.[32,33] *(Please see Figure 21d.)* Interestingly, no criteria involving QRS-complex or T-wave morphologies alone were found to be useful. This article, in contrast to much of the existing cardiology literature, distinguishes between past myocardial infarction and AMI; it furthers provides electrocardiographic, interpretative tools for making the early electrocardiographic diagnosis of AMI.[34,36] It should be stressed that these ST segment changes are only suggestive of AMI in patients with complicated ECGs; they are not diagnostic of AMI. Furthermore, their absence does not rule out the possibility of AMI.

Another strategy also is available for improving accuracy of interpretation of the ECG in patients with permanent ventricular pacemakers—the clinician may perform an analysis of the native, underlying rhythm. In this case, the pacemaker may be deactivated temporarily, but only if the underlying rhythm is able to sustain adequate perfusion and the emergency physician has the equipment and expertise for such a maneuver. Alternatively, some patients may experience intermittent periods of the native rhythm. Assuming that the focus is supraventricular in origin and the intraventricular conduction is normal, information may be obtained from this brief glimpse.[37] Unfortunately, this approach will not be useful in most patients with AMI and VPR.

Summary

Patients who have chest pain and ST segment elevation (STE) on the 12-lead electrocardiogram and are experiencing AMI may be candidates for urgent coronary revascularization, with either thrombolysis or primary angioplasty. Other chest-pain patients with electrocardiographic STE may be suffering from a non-coronary chest discomfort syndrome. Correct identification of these patients is required to offer the most appropriate treatments and to avoid potentially dangerous therapies.

References

1. Hedges JR, Kobernick MS. Detection of myocardial ischemia/infarction in the emergency department patient with chest discomfort. *Emerg Med Clin North Am* 1988;6: 317-340.
2. Hedges JR, Rouan GW, Toltzis R, et al. Use of cardiac enzymes identifies patients with acute myocardial infarction otherwise unrecognized in the emergency department. *Ann Emerg Med* 1987;16:248-253.
3. Rouan GW, Hedges JR, Toltzis R, et al. A chest pain clinic to improve the follow-up of patients released from an urban university teaching hospital emergency department. *Ann Emerg Med* 1987;16:1145-1150.
4. Aufderheide TP, Hendley GE, Woo J, et al. A prospective evaluation of prehospital 12-lead ECG application in chest pain patients. *J Electrocardiol* 1992;24(suppl):8-13.
5. Aufderheide TP, Keelan MH, Hendley GH, et al. Milwaukee prehospital chest pain project: Phase I. Feasibility and accu-

racy of prehospital thrombolytic candidate selection. *Am J Cardiol* 1992;69:991-996.

6. Muller DW, Topol EJ. Selection of patients with acute myocardial infarction for thrombolytic therapy. *Ann Intern Med* 1990;113:949-960.
7. Kleiman NS, White HD, Ohman EM, et al. Mortality within 24 hours of thrombolysis for myocardial infarction: The importance of early reperfusion. *Circulation* 1994;90: 2658-2665.
8. Lee TH, Weisberg MC, Brand DA, et al. Candidates for thrombolysis among emergency room patients with acute chest pain: Potential true-and false-positive rates. *Ann Intern Med* 1989;110:957-962.
9. The GUSTO Investigators: An international randomized trial comparing four thrombolytic strategies for acute myocardial infarction. *N Engl J Med* 1993;329:673-682.
10. Sharkey SW, Berger CR, Brunette DD, et al. Impact of the electrocardiogram on the delivery of thrombolytic therapy for acute myocardial infarction. *Am J Cardiol* 1994;73:550-553.
11. Chapman GD, Ohman M, Topol EJ, et al. Minimizing the risk of inappropriately administering thrombolytic therapy (Thrombolysis and angioplasty in myocardial infarction [TAMI] study group). *Am J Cardiol* 1993;71:783-787.
12. Blankenship JC, Almquist AK. Cardiovascular complications of thrombolytic therapy in patients with a mistaken diagnosis of acute myocardial infarction. *J Am Coll Cardiol* 1989;14: 1579-1582.
13. Larsen GC, Griffith JL, Beshansky JR, et al. Electrocardiographic left ventricular hypertrophy in patients with suspected acute cardiac ischemia—Its influence on diagnosis, treatment, and short-term prognosis. *J Gen Intern Med* 1994;9:666-673.
14. Rude RE, Poole WK, Muller JE, et al. Electrocardiographic and clinical criteria for recognition of acute myocardial infarction based on analysis of 3,697 patients. *Am J Cardiol* 1983; 52:936-942.
15. Otto LA, Aufderheide TP. Evaluation of ST segment elevation criteria for the prehospital electrocardiographic diagnosis of acute myocardial infarction. *Ann Emerg Med* 1994;23:17-24.
16. Brady WJ. Causes of ST segment elevation in emergency department chest pain patients. Abstract presented at the International Emergency Medicine Conference, Vancouver, British Columbia, March 26, 1998.
17. Miller DH, Kligfield P, Schreiber TL, et al. Relationship of prior myocardial infarction to false-positive electrocardiographic diagnosis of acute injury in patIents with chest pain. *Arch Int Med* 1987;147:257-261.
18. Van Gelder IC, Crijns HJ, Van Der Laarse A, et al. Incidence and clinical significance of ST segment elevation after electrical cardioversion of atrial fibrillation and atrial flutter. *Am Heart J* 1991;12:51-56.
19. Madias JE, Krikelis EN. Transient giant R waves in the early phase of acute myocardial infarction: Association with ventricular fibrillation. *Clin Cardiol* 1981;4:339-349.
20. Aufderheide TP, Brady WJ. Electrocardiography in the patient with myocardial ischemia or infarction. In: Gibler WB, Aufderheide TP eds. *Emergency Cardiac Care.* 1st ed. St. Louis: Mosby; 1994:169-216.
21. Fesmire FM, Percy RF, Wears RL, et al. Risk stratification according to the initial electrocardiogram in patients with suspected acute myocardial infarction. *Arch Intern Med* 1989; 149:1294-1299.
22. Hackworthy RA, Vogel MB, Harris PJ. Relationship between changes in ST-segment elevation and patency of the infarct-related coronary artery in acute myocardial infarction. *Am Heart J* 1986;112:279-288.
23. Cohen M, Hawkins L, Greenberg S, et al. Usefulness of ST-segment changes in >/= leads on emergency room electrocardiogram in either unstable angina pectoris or non-Q-wave myocardial infarction in predicting outcome. *Am J Cardiol* 1991;67:1368-1377.
24. Goldberger A. *Myocardial Infarction: Electrocardiographic Differential Diagnosis.* 4th ed, St. Louis: Mosby; 1991.
25. Brady WJ, Chang N, Hwang V, et al. The 15-lead electrocardiogram in emergency department chest pain patients: Comparison to the 12-lead electrocardiogram. *Ann Emerg Med* 1997;30:281.
26. Zalenski RJ, Cook D, Rydman R. Assessing the diagnostic value of an ECG containing leads V_4R, V_8, and V_9: The 15-lead ECG. *Ann Emerg Med* 1993;22:786-791.
27. Brady WJ, Aufderheide TP. Left bundle block pattern complicating the evaluation of acute myocardial infarction. *Acad Emerg Med* 1997;4:56-62.
28. Rosner MH, Brady WJ. The electrocardiographic diagnosis of acute myocardial infarction in the presence of left bundle branch block: A report of two illustrative cases. *Am J Emerg Med* (1998 accepted/publication pending).
29. Marriott HJL. Myocardial infarction. In: Marriott HJL, ed. *Practical Electrocardiography.* 8th ed. Baltimore, MD: Williams and Wilkins; 1988:419-450.
30. Sgarbossa EB, Pinski SL, Barbagelata A, et al. Electrocardiographic diagnosis of evolving acute myocardial infarction in the presence of left bundle branch block. *N Engl J Med* 1996;334:481-487.
31. Kozlowski FH, Brady WJ, Aufderheide TP, et al. The electrocardiographic diagnosis of acute myocardial infarction in patients with ventricular paced rhythms. *Acad Emerg Med* 1998;5:52-57.
32. Rosner MH, Brady WJ. The electrocardiographic diagnosis of acute myocardial infarction in patients with ventricular paced rhythms. *Am J Emerg Med* (1998 accepted/publication pending).
33. Sgarbossa EB, Piniski SL, Gates KB, et al. Early electrocardiographic diagnosis of acute myocardial infarction in the presence of ventricular-paced rhythm. *Am J Cardiol* 1996;77: 423-424.
34. Barold SS, Falkolff MD, Ong LS et al. Electrocardiographic diagnosis of myocardial infarction during ventricular pacing. *Cardiol Clin* 1987;5:403-417.
35. Barold SS, Wallace WA, Ong LS, et al. Primary ST and T wave abnormalities in the diagnosis of acute anterior myocardial infarction during permanent ventricular pacing. *J Electrocardiol* 1976;9:387-390.
36. Niremberg V, Amikam S, Roguin N, et al. Primary ST changes. diagnostic aid in patients with acute myocardial infarction. *Br Heart J* 1977;39:502-507.

37. Brady WJ. Cases in electrocardiography—The electrocardiographic diagnosis of acute myocardial infarction in patients with ventricular-paced rhythms: Value of the native rhythm. *Am J Emerg Med* 1998;16:85-86.

Electrocardiographic Diagnosis: Specific Clinical Syndromes

William J. Brady, MD

The differential diagnosis of ST elevation (STE) frequently presents a diagnostic challenge in patients who present to the emergency department (ED) with chest pain. This chapter provides detailed discussions of STE and its associated features in a wide range of cardiovascular conditions, including left ventricular hypertrophy, benign early repolarization, and left ventricular aneurysm. A comprehensive glossary of ECG strips is provided to assist with morphological identification.

ECG Changes Associated with Non-MI Syndromes

Left Ventricular Hypertrophy (LVH). Electrocardiographic changes consistent with LVH and associated repolarization changes are commonly encountered in the ED chest-pain patient. LVH is seen frequently in prehospital chest-pain patients and is the leading cause of noninfarctional ST segment change.[1] Among ED patients with the chief complaint of chest discomfort, LVH is responsible for approximately 25% of noninfarctional ST segment elevation (STE).[2] Its presence on the ECG, especially the repolarization changes that alter the morphology of the ST segment and/or the T wave, may complicate early ED evaluation of the chest pain patient.

One group has shown that the electrocardiographic pattern consistent with LVH is encountered in approximately 10% of adult chest pain patients initially diagnosed in the ED with acute ischemic heart disease.[3] After hospital admission and more extensive evaluation, only 26% of these patients were found to have unstable angina or AMI. Of the remainder of the patients, the vast majority were ultimately diagnosed with non-ischemic syndromes. The physicians caring for the patients in this study incorrectly interpreted the ECG more than 70% of the time. In particular, they frequently failed to identify the LVH pattern and, therefore, attributed the ST segment/T wave changes to ischemia or infarction. In fact, the observed ST segment/T wave changes resulted from repolarization abnormality associated with LVH.[3]

In patients with LVH, ST segment/T wave changes result from altered repolarization of the ventricular myocardium.[4] These ST segment/T wave abnormalities are the new "norm" in many patients with LVH and may mask and/or mimic findings that are consistent with early AMI. These effects, however, occur less often than they do in LBBB and VPR situations.[5] In particular, LVH is associated with poor R-wave progression and loss of the septal R wave in the right-to-mid-precordial leads, most commonly producing a QS pattern. In general, these QS complexes are located in leads V_1 and V_2, rarely extending beyond lead V_3.

As predicted by the rule of appropriate discordance (that is, the terminal portion of the QRS complex and ST segment/T wave are located on opposites sides of the iso-electric baseline), ST segment elevation is encountered in this distribution along with prominent,

Table 1. Four Stages of ECG Findings in Pericarditis

STAGE 1	Characterized by STE
STAGE 2	Resolution of STE
STAGE 3	T wave inversion
STAGE 4	Normalization and a return to the baseline ECG

Table 2. ECG Features of Acute Pericarditis

Feature
STE
Prominent Q waves
PR segment depression
PR segment-ST segment discordant ratio greater than 0.25

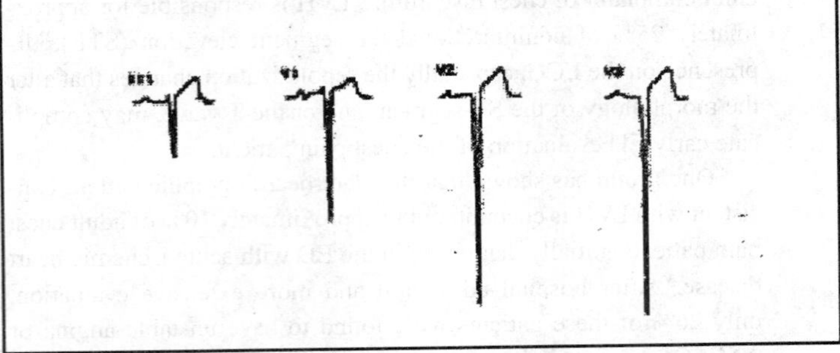

Figure 22
Various electrocardiographic leads demonstrating LVH-related STE.

"hyperacute" T waves. The ST segment elevation seen in this distribution may be greater than 5 mL in height *(please see Figures 22 and 23)* and is difficult to distinguish from that associated with AMI. The initial, up-sloping portion of the ST segment-T wave complex is frequently concave in LVH compared to either the flattened or convex pattern observed in the AMI patient.[5] However, this morphologic feature is imperfect; early AMI may reveal such a concave feature.

Another feature of LVH-related ST segment/T wave change is its relative permanence. The electrocardiographic changes resulting from acute coronary ischemia are dynamic in nature; they are likely to change over the short-term in the early phase of evaluation in the ED. Conversely, the ST segment/T wave abnormalities related to LVH are relatively constant or fixed; these changes are unlikely to change during initial ED evaluation. This difference in the longevity of the ST segment/T wave changes in the two syndromes lends itself to differentiation using either serial electrocardiographic monitoring or ST segment trend analysis.

One last point should be emphasized. LVH with the related repolarization changes represents a particular patient's "normal" or baseline electrocardiographic pattern. Its presence, like the normal or nondiagnostic ECG in the case without LVH, does not rule out the possibility of an early acute coronary ischemic event in a patient experiencing chest pain or other anginal equivalent complaints.[5,6]

Acute Pericarditis. Acute pericarditis, which may be caused by a number of infectious agents, various rheumatologic and malignant syndromes, and uremia, produces diffuse inflammation of the superficial epicardium. Ventricular inflammation produces a current of injury that is manifested, initially, by STE on the ECG, while PR segment depression is indicative of similar irritation of the atrial epicardium. The electrocardiographic changes caused by pericarditis evolve through four classic stages. The first stage is characterized by STE, which is followed by resolution of the elevation in the second stage. The third stage is characterized by T wave inversion, which is followed by normalization and a return to the baseline ECG in stage four. Q waves are not encountered in patients with pericarditis. *(Please see Table 1.)*

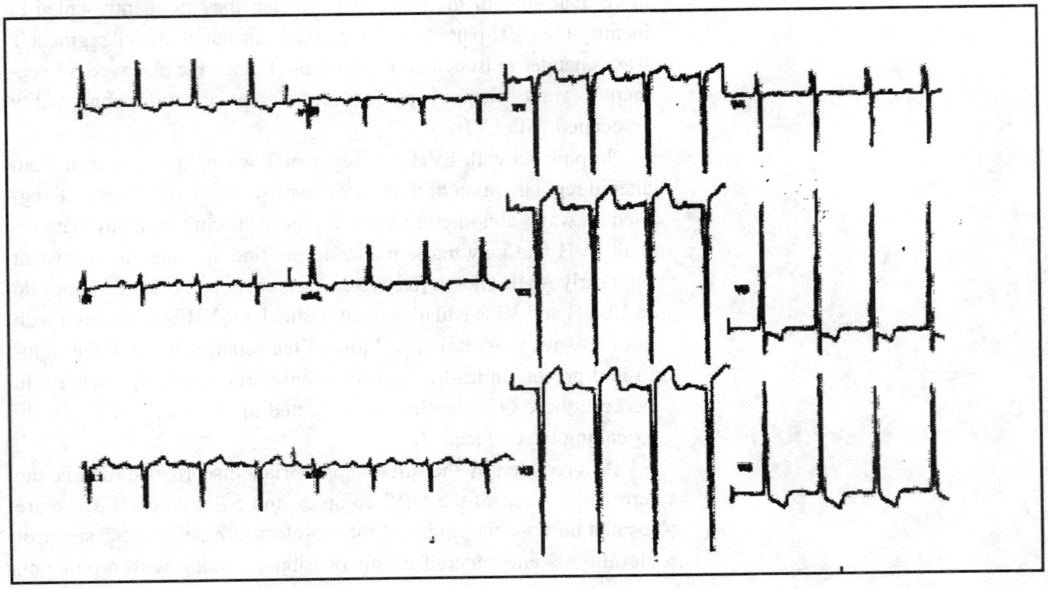

Figure 23
LVH is associated with poor R wave progression and loss of the septal R wave in the right to mid-precordial leads, most commonly producing a QS pattern in leads V_1 and V_2, rarely extending beyond lead V_3. As predicted by the concept of appropriate discordance, ST segment elevation is encountered in this distribution along with prominent, "hyperacute" T waves. The ST segment elevation seen in this distribution may be greater than 5 millimeters in height and is difficult to distinguish from that associated with AMI. The initial, up-sloping portion of the ST segment/T wave complex is frequently concave in LVH compared to the either flattened or convex pattern observed in the AMI patient.

The temporal evolution of these electrocardiographic stages occurs in a very unpredictable manner when compared to AMI. In general, stages one through three are seen over hours to days, while stage four may not be observed for several weeks. Furthermore, patients may not manifest all characteristic electrocardiographic features of pericarditis (i.e., the chest pain patient may present with stage 1 findings and progress directly to stage 4).

STE seen in patients with stage 1 pericarditis is usually less than 5 mm in height, it is observed in numerous leads, and is characterized by a concavity in its initial upsloping portion. *(Please see Figures 24 and 25, upper and middle panels, for examples of acute pericarditis.)* In some cases, the STE may be obliquely flat; convexity of the ST segment elevation, however, strongly suggests AMI. The STE due to acute pericarditis is usually noted in the following electrocardiographic leads: I, II, III, aV_l, aVf, and V_2-V_6—essentially, all leads except V_1; reciprocal ST segment depression (STD) also is seen in lead aVr and occasionally in lead V_1. *(Please see Figure 24 in lead aVr and Figure 25, lower panel.)* The STE is most often seen in many leads simultaneously, though it may be limited to a specific anatomic segment. If the process is focal, the inferior wall is often involved, in which case leads II, II and aVf, are most often affected.

Several electrocardiographic features will help identify pericarditis-related STE. The absence of Q waves in the setting of STE is not particularly helpful. Conversely, the presence of Q waves suggests an alternative diagnosis of either myocarditis or AMI. However, an inflammatory process producing pericarditis also may affect the myocardium,

Table 3. ECG Features Distinguishing AMI from BER

BER
Initial, up-sloping portion of the ST segment/T wave complex is concave
Absence of reciprocal changes
AMI
Initial, up-sloping portion of the ST segment/T wave complex is convex or flattened
Presence of reciprocal changes
Presence of Q waves

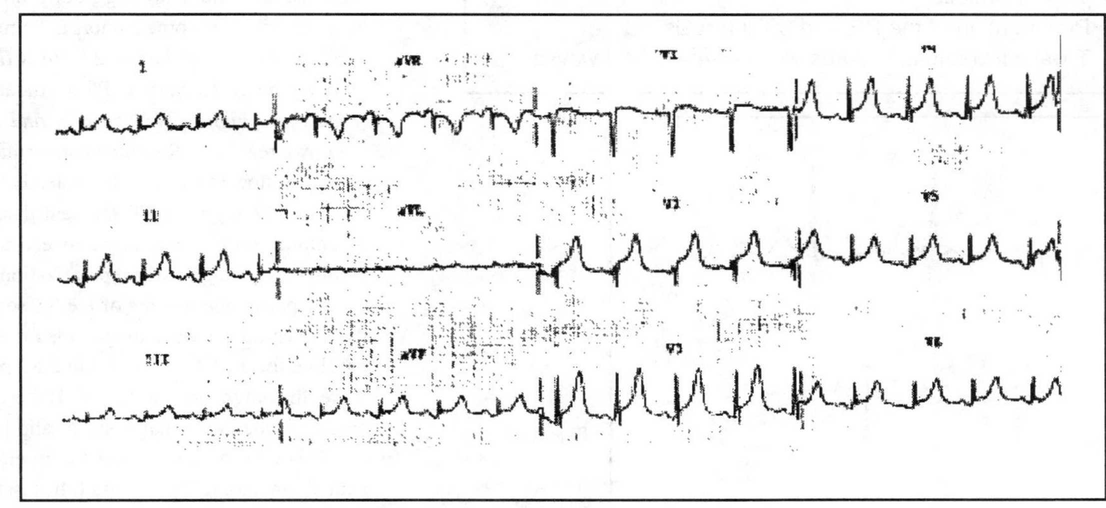

Figure 24

12-lead ECG of a patient with acute pericarditis showing STE in the antero-infero-lateral leads with reciprocal ST segment depression (aVr), PR segment depression (II and V_3-V_6), and PR segment elevation (lead aVr).

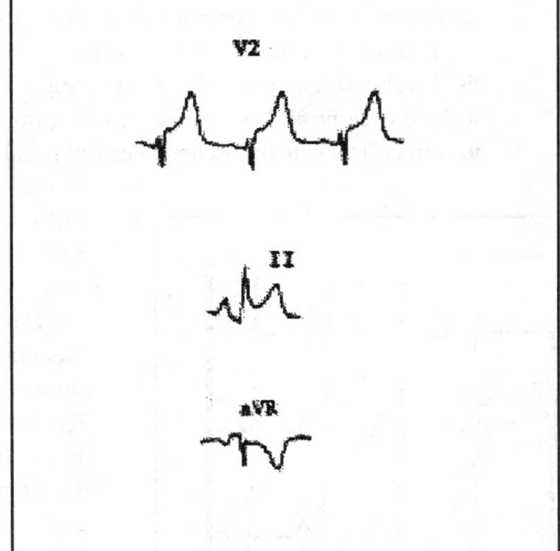

Figure 25

Representative electrocardiographic complexes of acute pericarditis. **Upper panel**, STE in lead V2; **middle panel,** STE with PR segment depression in lead II; **lower panel,** reciprocal ST segment depression with PR elevation in lead aVr.

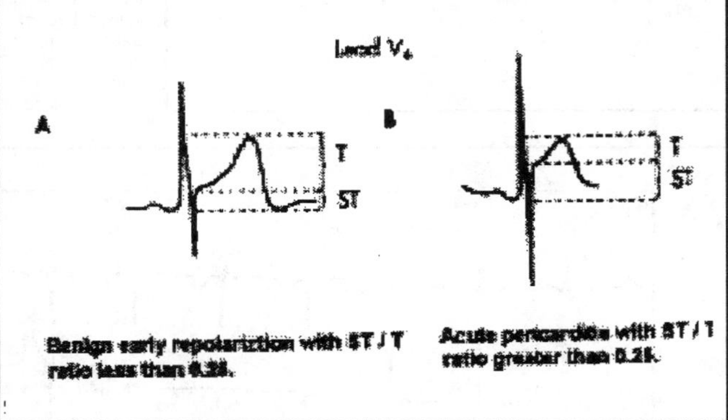

Figure 26

This PR segment-ST segment discordant ratio may also be helpful in discriminating between the STE resulting from BER and acute pericarditis. It is objectively assessed by comparing the heights of the ST segment and T wave in lead V_6—the ST segment/T wave magnitude ratio. Using the PR segment as the baseline for the ST segment and the J point as the beginning of the T wave, the heights are measured with calculation of the ratio. If the ratio is greater than 0.25, pericarditis is the likely diagnosis; with results less than 0.25, one should consider BER.

Table 4. ECG Signs of Hyperkalemia

Presence of tall, symmetric T waves
Shortened QT interval
Prolonged PR interval
Widening QRS complex

Table 5. ECG Signs of Hypothermia

J point and the adjacent ST segment that appear to have lifted off the iso-electric baseline
Bradycardia
Tremor artifact
Prolongation of the PR and QT intervals
T wave inversions in leads with pre-eminent J waves

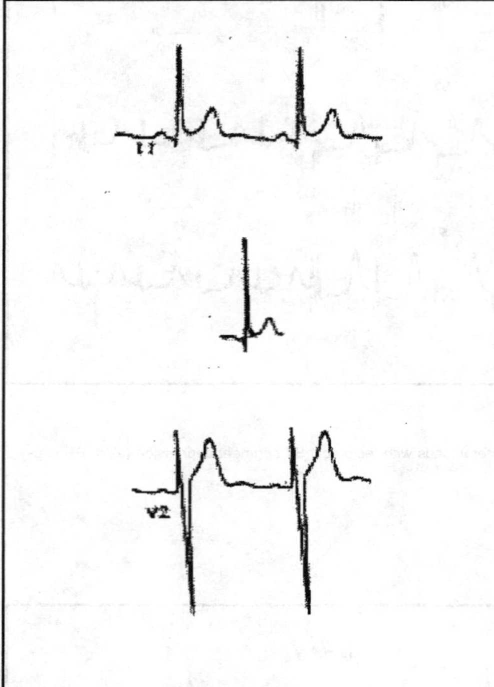

Figure 27

Various electrocardiographic leads demonstrating BER-related findings. **Upper panel,** STE with concavity of the initial segment and prominent T wave in lead II; **middle panel,** STE with notching of the J point in lead II; **lower panel,** prominent T waves with STE in a precordial lead.

hence, myopericarditis can develop. Patients with acute myopericarditis, therefore, may present with electrocardiographic features involving both processes, including STE, prominent Q waves, and other findings as described in the "acute myocarditis" section below.

Reciprocal STD strongly supports the electrocardiographic diagnosis of AMI; in fact, the presence of reciprocal STD on the ECG has a positive predictive value for the diagnosis of AMI in the 90-95% range.[1,2] Reciprocal changes noted in AMI usually are observed in the inferior, lateral, and right precordial leads. Recall that reciprocal STD may be seen in leads aVr and V_1 in acute pericarditis. The relatively static nature of STE in patients with pericarditis also may help distinguish ST segment changes from AMI; the use of either ST segment trend monitoring or serial ECGs as well as a comparison with past electrocardiograms also can be useful in these settings.

PR segment depression associated with pericarditis is perhaps the most useful feature for suggesting this diagnosis. This finding has been described by some authors as "almost diagnostic" for acute pericarditis. *(Please see Figure 24, leads II and V_3 to V_6, and Figure 25, middle panel.)*[5] Reciprocal PR segment elevation is seen in lead aVr. *(Please see Figure 24, lead aVr, and Figure 25, lower panel.)* For unknown reasons, PR segment abnormalities are best seen in leads V_5 and V_6, followed by the inferior leads.

This PR segment-ST segment discordant relationship may also be helpful in discriminating between the STE caused by acute pericarditis and benign early repolarization (BER). This can be assessed by comparing the heights of the ST segment and T wave in lead V_6: the ST segment/T wave magnitude ratio. Using the PR segment as the baseline for the ST segment and the J point as the beginning of the T wave, the heights are measured. If the ratio is greater than 0.25, pericarditis is the likely diagnosis; a ratio less than 0.25 suggests BER.

This ratio may be calculated in electrocardiographic leads other than V_6, including V_5, V_4, and I. In essence, this ratio reflects the conduction differences in the two syndromes. In BER, the J point is elevated minimally with a prominent T wave. In pericarditis, the J point is elevated to a significantly greater extent, with a less prominent T wave; furthermore, PR segment depression only increases the STE contribution to this ratio. *(Please see Figure 26, in which this discordance ratio is used to distinguish BER from acute pericarditis.)*[5,7,8]

Pericardial effusion also may be seen in patients with pericarditis. Electrocardiographic observations suggestive of this diagnosis include widespread low voltage (resulting from increased resistance to current flow with the accumulated fluid) and electrical alternans (a beat-to-beat alteration in QRS complex size due to shifting fluid in the pericardium).

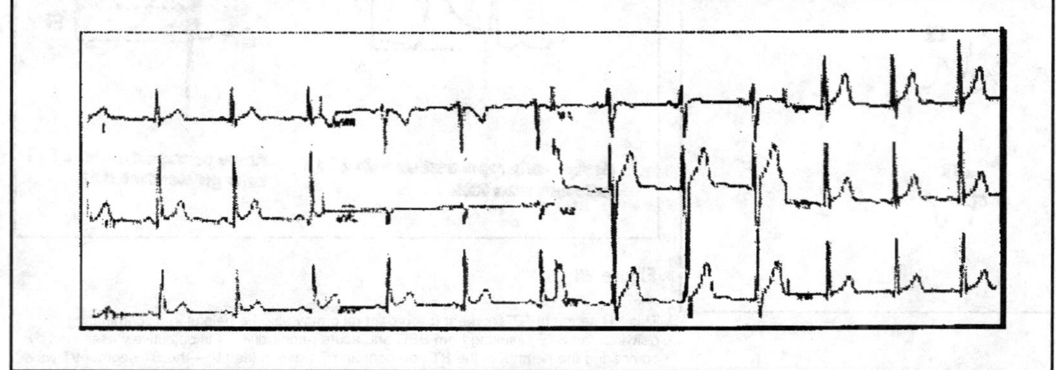

Figure 28

12-lead ECG of a patient with BER and widespread STE with prominent T waves.

Benign Early Repolarization. The syndrome of benign early repolarization, first described in 1936 by Shipley and Hallaran,[9] is felt to be a normal variant and is not indicative of underlying cardiac disease. BER has been reported in men and women of all age groups and in people of varying ethnic background. About 1% of the general population will have early repolarization on their ECG, with an increased incidence among younger individuals. Among adult ED chest pain patients, BER is seen at an increased frequency and is encountered in 12% of such cases.[2] BER is seen on the ECG in 23-48% of adult ED chest pain patients who have used cocaine.[10]

In a large population-based study of BER, the mean age of patients with this ECG finding was 39 years, with an age range of 16-80. The syndrome was seen predominantly in patients younger than 50 years of age and was rarely encountered in individuals older than 70 (3.5%).[11] Men manifest BER significantly more often than women. And, for unknown reasons, BER is more often encountered in black males between the ages of 20-40 years,[12] although some authors dispute this observation.[11]

Recall that the ST segment of the cardiac electrical cycle represents the period between depolarization and repolarization of the left ventricle. Characteristically, the ST segment is isoelectric, meaning that it is neither elevated nor depressed relative to the TP segment. The electrocardiographic definition of BER includes the following characteristics: ST segment elevation; upward concavity of the initial portion of the ST segment; notching or slurring of the terminal QRS complex; symmetric, concordant T waves of large amplitude; widespread or diffuse distribution of STE on the ECG; and relative temporal stability.[13,14]

The STE begins at the "J" (or junction) point (i.e., the portion of the electrocardiographic cycle where the QRS complex ends and the ST segment begins). The degree of J-point elevation is usually less than 3.5 mm.[13] Morphologically, the STE appears as if the ST segment has been evenly lifted upward from the isoelectric baseline at the J point.[42] This elevation results in a preservation of the normal concavity of the initial, up-sloping portion of the ST segment-T wave complex. This is an important electrocardiographic feature that is used to distinguish between BER-related STE from STE associated with AMI.

The STE elevation encountered in BER is usually less than 2 mm, but may approach 5 mm in certain individuals. Overall, 80-90% percent of individuals demonstrate STE that is less than 2 mm in the precordial leads and less than 0.5 mm in the limb leads; only 2% of cases of BER manifest STE greater than 5 mm.[13,15] The greatest degree of STE related to BER is usually

Table 6. ECG Signs of CNS Disorders
Diffuse, deep inversion of T wave
Prominent U waves of either polarity
QT prolongation that can exceed 60% of normal value

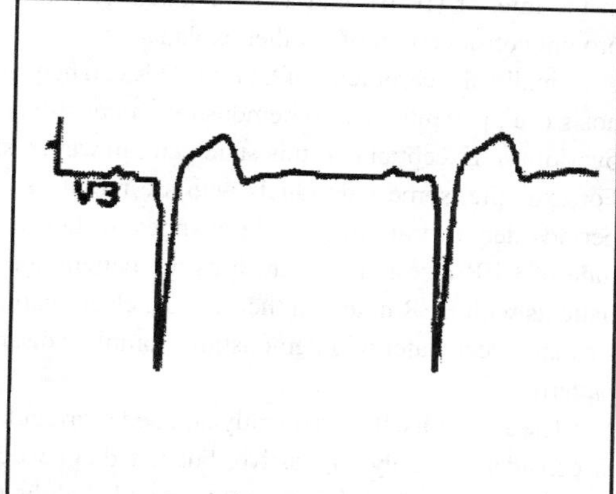

Figure 29

Prominent STE in lead V_3 in a patient with known LVA.

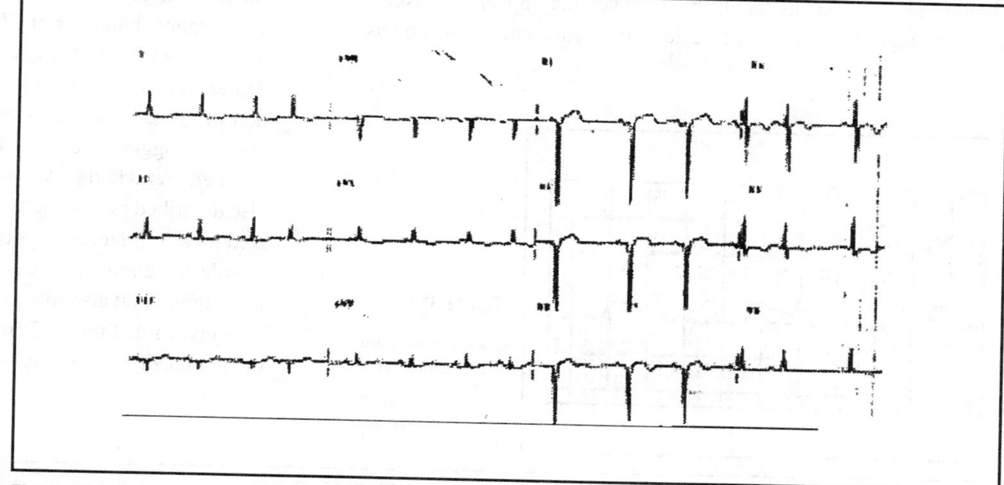

Figure 30

12-lead ECG demonstrating STE and prominent Q waves in the anterior distribution. The patient had experienced an extensive anterior myocardial infarction three months ago. The persistent STE resulted from a LVA confirmed by echocardiography.

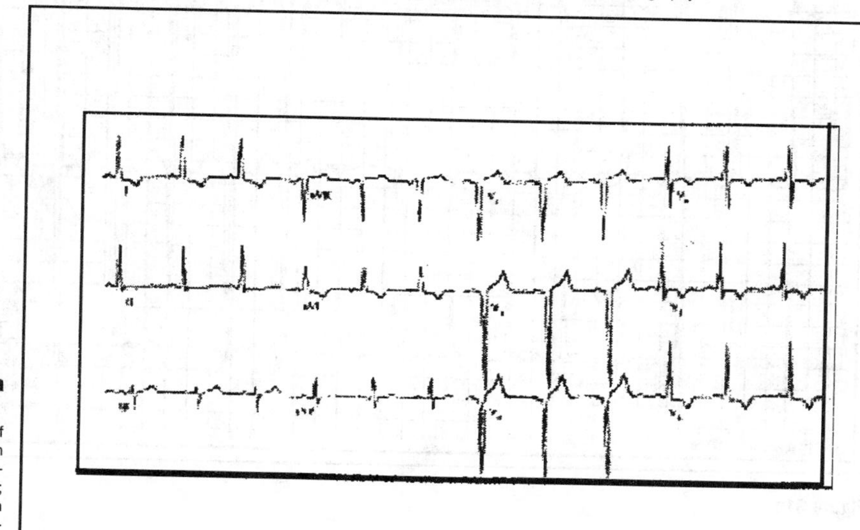

Figure 31a

12-lead ECG of a patient with hypertrophic cardiomyopathy; STE is seen in the right precordial leads.

observed in the mid- to left precordial leads (leads V_2 to V_5). The ST segments in other electrocardiographic leads tend to be less elevated than those in leads V_2 through V_5. The limb leads (I, II, III, aV_l, and aVf) demonstrate STE even less frequently. In one large series, limb leads revealed STE in only 45% of cases with BER.[13-15] In this regard, "isolated" BER in the limb leads (i.e., with no precordial STE) is a very rare find. In addition, the presence of "isolated" STE in the inferior (II, III, and aVf) or lateral (I and aV_l) leads should prompt consideration of another explanation.

Finally, the chronicity of STE in BER can help confirm the diagnosis (i.e., patients tend to demonstrate a consistent pattern of STE over time). Exceptions to this statement, however, should be noted. For example, some individuals who are monitored over prolonged periods demonstrate magnitude changes in their STE. The magnitude of BER also may diminish as the patient ages. In 25-30% of patients with BER noted on their ECGs, electrocardiographic analysis many years later will demonstrate complete disappearance of the pattern.[11,13,15]

The J point itself is frequently notched or irregular in contour and is considered highly suggestive, but not diagnostic, of BER.[16,11,15] Prominent T waves of large amplitude and slightly asymmetric morphology also are encountered; the T waves may appear "peaked," whch is suggestive of the hyperacute T wave encountered in patients

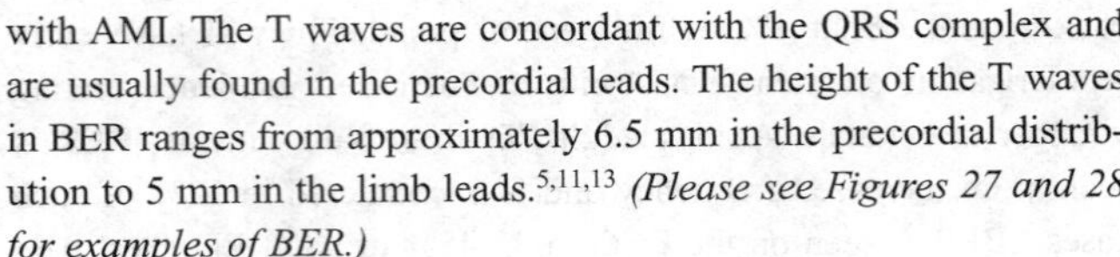
with AMI. The T waves are concordant with the QRS complex and are usually found in the precordial leads. The height of the T waves in BER ranges from approximately 6.5 mm in the precordial distribution to 5 mm in the limb leads.[5,11,13] *(Please see Figures 27 and 28 for examples of BER.)*

In the setting of STE, several electrocardiographic features help distinguish BER from AMI. Especially useful for making this distinction is analysis of the ST segment/T wave complex waveform, the presence of reciprocal changes, and evolutionary changes. At times, however, making this distinction can be difficult, as is suggested by one study noting that 30% of patients who incorrectly received thrombolytic therapy for presumed AMI actually had BER (a non-infarction chest pain syndrome) on the ECG.[17] *(Please see Table 3.)*

First, the initial, up-sloping portion of the ST segment/T wave complex is concave in BER, as compared to being either flattened or convex in the AMI patient. This morphologic observation should only be used as a guideline. Reciprocal changes, defined as ST segment depression in leads distant from the area of acute infarction, is a very useful electrocardiographic finding suggestive of MI.[1] Reciprocal changes are not encountered in patients with BER; the electrocardiographic finding of ST segment depression greater than 1 mm in a patient with STE on the ECG should suggest the possibility of AMI.[7] The combined findings of ST segment elevation greater than 1 mm in two anatomically contiguous leads and reciprocal ST segment depression increase diagnostic accuracy for AMI to 90%.[1,2] The addition of Q waves to the findings of reciprocal change and STE also strongly suggests the possibility of AMI.[7]

Left Ventricular Aneurysm. Left ventricular aneurysm (LVA), also described as dyskinetic ventricular segment, is defined as a localized area of infarcted myocardium that bulges outward during both systole and diastole. LVA is most often noted after large anterior wall infarction, but it also may be encountered after inferior and posterior wall myocardial injury. In most cases, LVA is manifested electrocardiographically by varying degrees of STE, which may be difficult to distinguish from ST segment changes due to AMI.[5,18] STE associated with LVA probably results from either an injury current originating from viable, but ischemic, myocytes in the aneurysm, or alternatively, from mechanical wall stress caused by traction on the normal, adjacent myocardium.

Electrocardiographically, LVA is characterized by persistent STE that develops several weeks after AMI. Because LVA is frequently anterior in location, STE is usually observed in

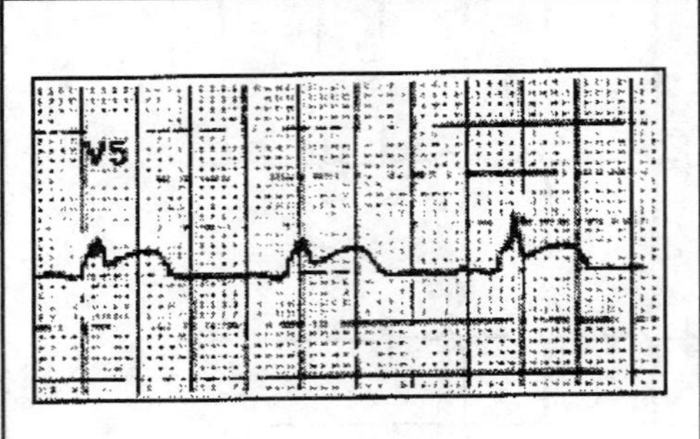

Figure 31b

Lead V_5 of a patient with hypertrophic cardiomyopathy, showing marked STE very suggestive of AMI.

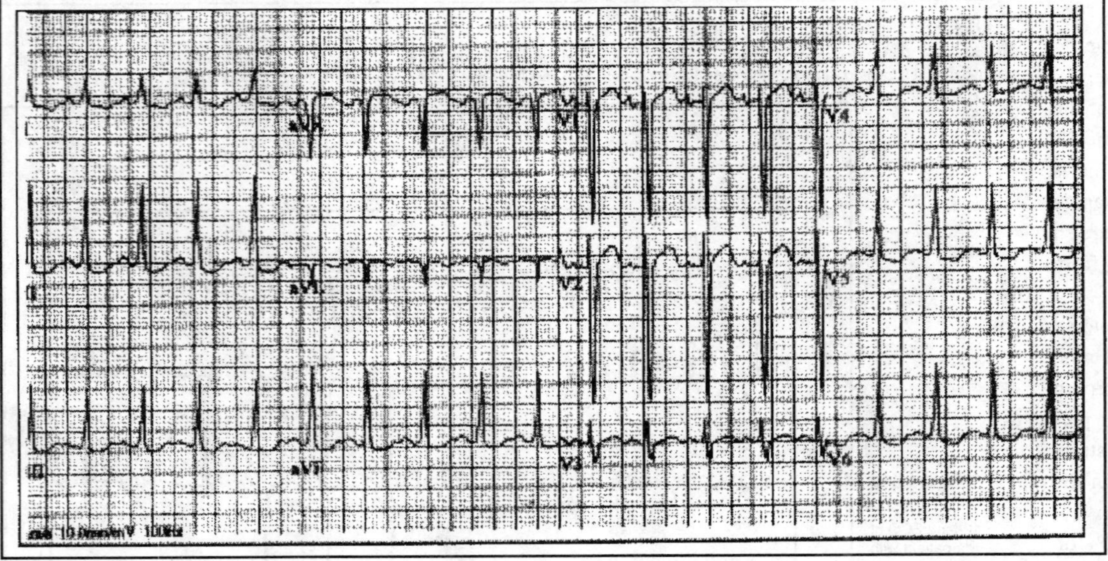

Figure 31c

12-lead ECG of a patient with idiopathic cardiomyopathy. STE is seen in leads V_1 to V_3, once again strongly suggestive of AMI.

leads I, aV_l, and V_1-V_6. As would be expected, the surface ECG of inferior wall LVA is characterized by STE in the inferior leads; in these locations, STE is usually less pronounced than the ST segment changes seen in the anterior leads. The actual ST segment abnormality due to the LVA may present with varying morphologies, ranging from obvious, convex STE to minimal, concave elevations. Consequently, distinguishing LVA-mediated STE from AMI may be difficult.[5]

When present, reciprocal change—an electrocardiographic feature of AMI—strongly suggests that ST segment changes, at least in part, are the result of acute infarction. Patients with LVA, which is usually the result of extensive anterior wall infarction, also may have significant Q waves. In contrast, the simultaneous appearance of a Q wave is not a feature that unquestionably supports the electrocardiographic diagnosis of LVA. The dynamic nature of AMI-related STE compared to the often static ST segment character in LVA means that a review of previous ECGs, serial ECGs, or ST segment trend monitoring can be of considerable diagnostic value. *(Please see Figures 3c, 29, and 30 for examples of LVA. Figure 3c is in the previous chapter of this textbook.)*

Cardiomyopathies. Cardiomyopathies also can produce electrocardiographic patterns that simulate findings associated with ischemic heart disease.[5,18] These findings include significant Q waves, ST segment changes, and T wave abnormalities; moreover, these patients also may present with LVH and bundle branch block patterns.

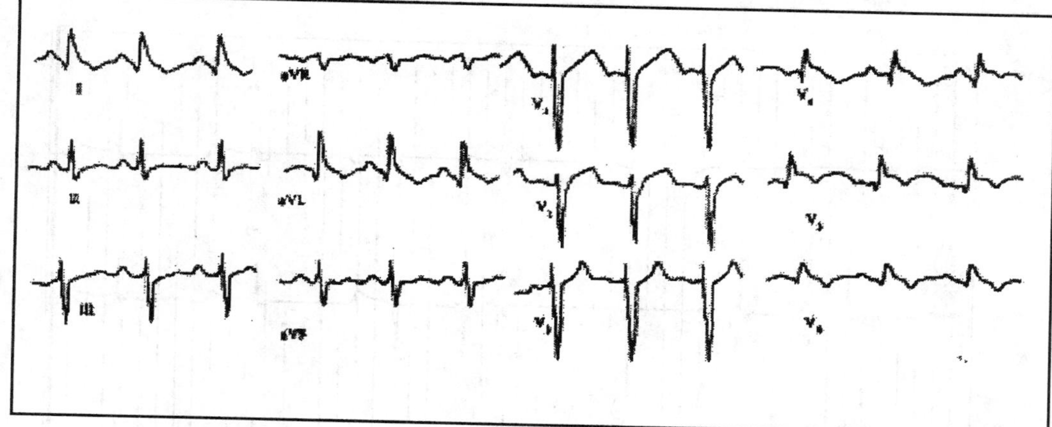

Figure 32 ECG of a patient with acute myocarditis demonstrating STE in leads I, aVl, V_1, and V_2 as well as V_4 through V_6. The STE in the anterolateral distribution certainly is suggestive of AMI.

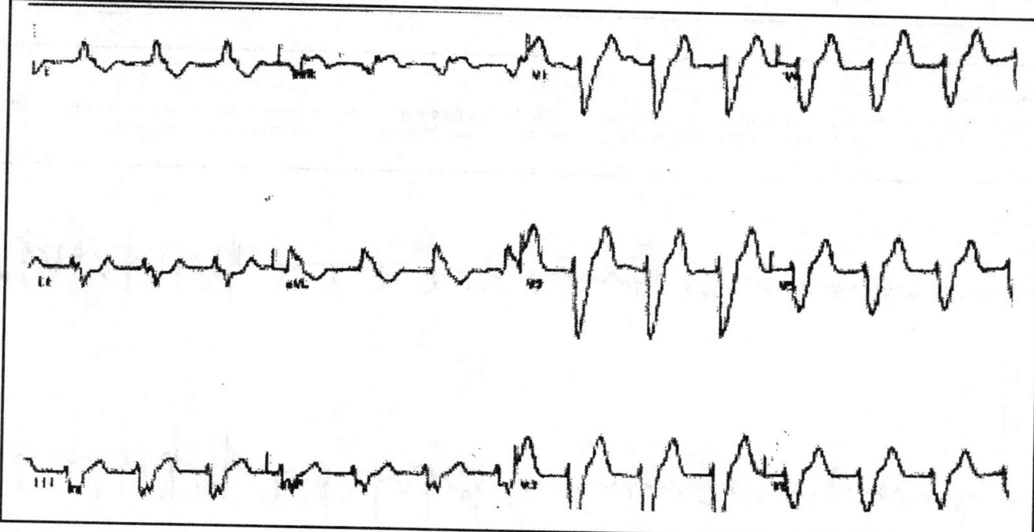

Figure 33 Widened QRS complex associated with profound hyperkalemia. In this example, STE is seen in the anterior, lateral, and inferior leads. The J point is elevated with an initial concavity to the ST segment - features suggestive of hyperkalemia.

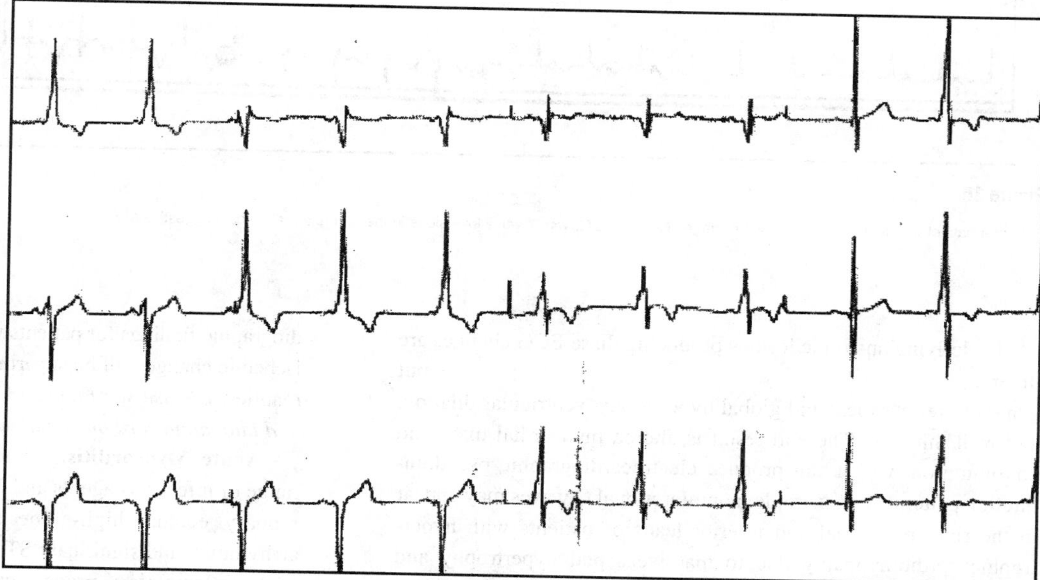

Figure 34 This ECG demonstrates STE in the inferior leads in a patient with the classic triad of WPW findings, including PR interval shortening, a Delta wave, and QRS complex widening. Other findings potentially suggestive of ischemic heart disease include Q waves (III and aVf) and T wave inversions (I, aVl, and V_1 through V_6).

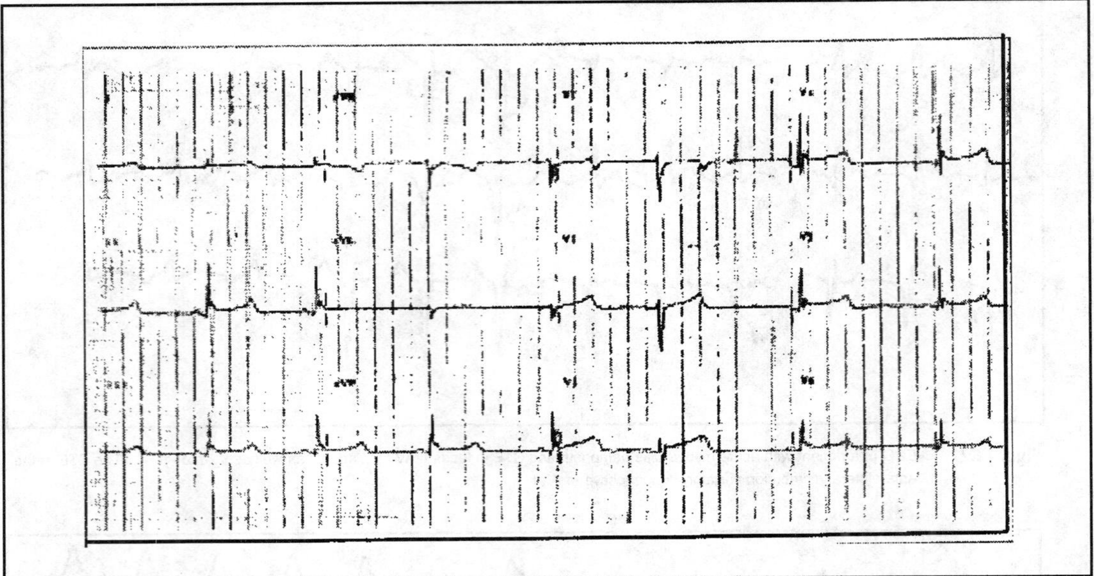

Figure 35

ECG of a patient with body temperature 28°C. The J point and the immediately adjacent ST segment appears to have been unevenly elevated off the iso-electric baseline lifted off the baseline, producing the J wave of hypothermia, also know as the Osborn wave and Osborn J wave.

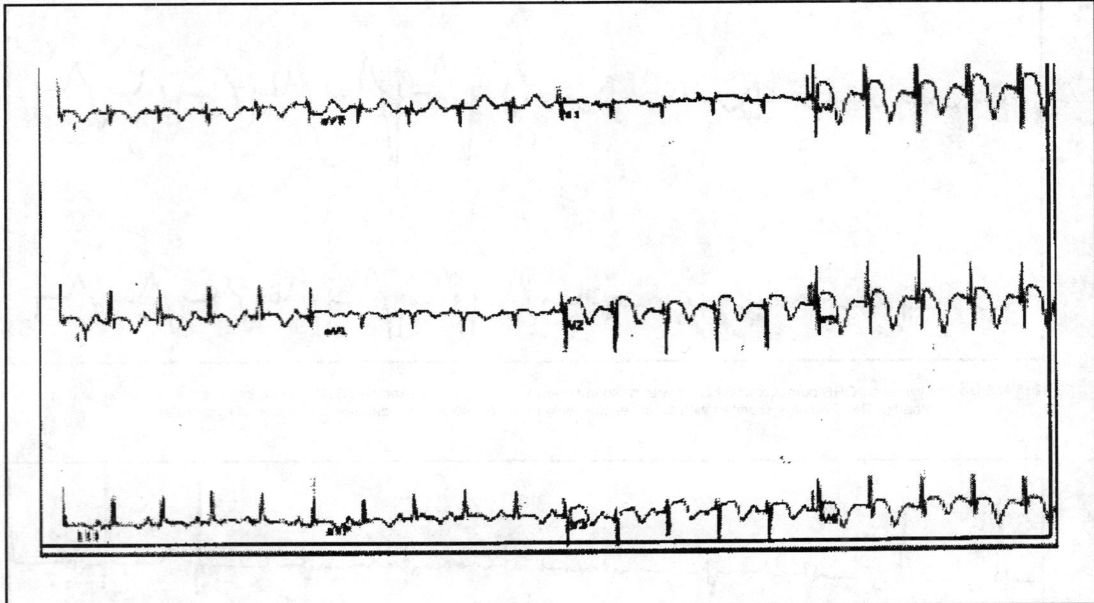

Figure 36

ECG of a patient with a subarrachnoid hemorrhage. Note the STE with T wave inversions in the anterolateral leads, suggestive of AMI.

changes that, at times, can mimic AMI.

Cardiomyopathies also may produce significant Q waves in the inferior and right precordial distributions; in some cases, these Q waves may be seen across the precordium and involve the entire anterolateral region of ECG. As is true with LBBB, VPR, and LVH, those leads with Q waves may display STE with prominent T waves. Once again, the rule of appropriate QRS complex-ST segment/T wave discordance is a useful guide for predicting expected morphologies. The STE seen in these leads is usually less than 5 mm in height; the initial upsloping portion of the ST segment/T wave complex is concave in appearance compared to the either obliquely flat or convex structure of AMI.

In most cases of cardiomyopathy with noninfarctional STE, the STE is atypical in appearance for AMI. Certain examples of STE seen in patients with cardiomyopathy may be impossible to distinguish from AMI. In other instances, the ED physician must realize that such patterns are the new normal electrocardiographic findings for patients with cardiomyopathy; as such, actual ischemic change will be superimposed upon these "baseline" abnormalities. *(Please see Figures 31a-31c for examples of hypertrophic and idiopathic cardiomyopathies with STE.)*

Underlying anatomic lesions producing these ECG changes are diverse, but generally reflect focal and global hypertrophy, ventricular dilation, and wall thinning. The end result is altered myocardial mass and configuration, which can produce electrocardiographic pseudoinfarction patterns. For example, noninfarctional Q waves may appear in the right precordial and inferior leads of patients with hypertrophic cardiomyopathy due to massive septal hypertrophy and associated altered depolarization vector. Altered ventricular activation, which is seen in patients with both hypertrophic and idiopathic cardiomyopathies, may produce marked ST segment/T waves

Acute Myocarditis. Acute myocarditis can be caused by a range of infectious agents and it frequently presents with acute pulmonary edema, high-grade atrioventricular block, ventricular arrhythmia, and significant ST segment/T wave abnormalities. The acute inflammatory process can lead to myocardial necrosis and marked, permanent ventricular dysfunction. The ST segment/T wave abnormalities include ST segment changes—both elevation

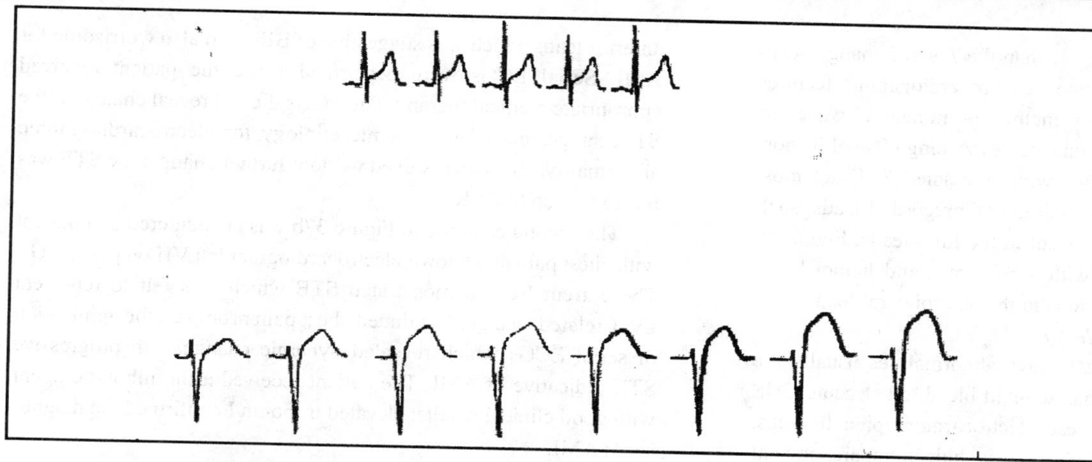

Figure 37

[a] (top figure) Serial ECGs performed (lead V_3 is presented) of a patient with cocaine-related chest pain. The initial and subsequent ECGs demonstrated STE which did not progress. The lack of dynamic change as well as the waveform morphologies suggested a non-AMI diagnosis responsible for the STE. In this case, BER. **[b] (bottom figure)** Serial ECGs performed (lead V_3 is presented) of a patient with chest pain and known electrocardiographic LVH. The current ECG demonstrated STE which was felt to represent LVH-related change. Continued chest pain prompted the application of serial ECGs which revealed dynamic change with progressive STE indicative of AMI.

and depression—as well as numerous T wave morphologies. These changes may reflect an associated bundle branch block. Q waves also may be encountered.

Although acute myocarditis may be found in patients of all ages, this clinical entity may be difficult to distinguish from AMI complicated by ventricular arrhythmia and pulmonary edema.[5,18] Figure 32 presents the ECG of a 45-year-old male who presented with ventricular tachycardia and pulmonary edema. Although the patient's initial presentation and electrocardiographic findings suggested anterolateral AMI, the entire picture resulted from acute myocarditis.

Other Syndromes Producing STE

Hyperkalemia. The earliest sign of potassium intoxication (i.e., hyperkalemia) is the appearance of tall, symmetric T waves. Typically, this T wave morphology is described as "hyperacute" and may be confused with the hyperacute T wave of early transmural myocardial infarction.[5] As the serum potassium level increases, the T waves tend to become taller, peaked, and narrowed in a symmetric fashion in the anterior distribution. The QT interval also may become shortened at this point. With additional increases in serum potassium concentration, the PR interval is prolonged and eventually is followed by QRS complex widening, an ominous sign. *(Please see Figure 33.)*

In early stages of QRS complex widening, the ST segment may appear elevated, a source of possible confusion. In general, this pseudo-STE associated with hyperkalemia is characterized by J point elevation and prominent, hyperacute T waves. The initial, upsloping portion of the ST segment is concave rather than the flat or convex patterns seen in the AMI patient with STE. *(Please see Figure 33 for an example of sinus rhythm with a markedly widened QRS complex.) (Please also see Table 4.)*

Pre-excitation Syndromes. Pre-excitation syndromes, which usually involve Wolff-Parkinson-White syndrome (WPW), frequently present with either evidence of ventricular pre-excitation or arrhythmias. Evidence of pre-excitation includes the classic electrocardiographic triad of PR interval shortening, a Delta wave, and QRS complex widening. The patient may present with "typically appearing" paroxysmal supraventricular tachycardia, rapid, bizarre atrial fibrillation, broad-complex tachycardia, or sudden cardiac death. Regardless of the presentation, the classic triad may be apparent following stabilization and restoration of sinus rhythm.

Also of concern are various pseudo-infarction findings that, if not recognized, may lead to the wrong diagnosis and inappropriate therapy.[5] For instance, Q waves may be seen in leads II, III, and aVf, which may mimic previous inferior myocardial infarction; tall R waves in the right precordial leads are suggestive of a posterior wall AMI. The ED physician must not only recognize the pseudo-infarction pattern of the WPW but also realize that such patterns may initially conceal early findings of AMI. Figure 34 demonstrates STE in the inferior leads in a patient with the classic triad of WPW findings, including PR interval shortening, a Delta wave, and QRS complex widening.

Hypothermia. When core body temperature approaches 32°C, hypothermia produces alterations in the ECG that might be mistaken for AMI. Most often, hypothermia-related electrocardiographic changes are observed at the junction between the terminal portion of the QRS complex and the initial ST segment (i.e., the J point). The J point and the adjacent ST segment appears to have lifted off the isoelectric baseline. Unlike the J point elevation seen in BER, in which the J point and ST segment are uniformly lifted upward, the J point and adjoining ST segment in hypothermia are unevenly elevated off the baseline. The resulting configuration produces the J wave, also know as the Osborn wave, or the Osborn J wave. *(Please see Figure 35 for an example of an ECG depicting the J wave in a hypothermic patient.) (Please also see Table 5.)*

In the typical situation, the J wave and related STE are most prominent in the mid-precordial and lateral precordial leads; it is seen to a lesser extent in the limb leads. In general, the amplitude of the J wave is inversely proportional to the degree of hypothermia; the J wave will increase in amplitude as the core temperature continues to drop and, conversely, will lessen as successful rewarming progresses. Other electrocardiographic features associated with hypothermia include: bradycardia; tremor artifact; prolongation of the PR and QT intervals; T wave inversions in leads with prominent J waves; and arrhythmias such as atrial fibrillation and ventricular fibrillation.[5]

Central Nervous System (CNS) Disorders. Certain intracranial disasters may produce significant ST segment-T wave changes.[5] Most often, these alterations involve the T wave with diffuse, deep inversion. In the setting of a CNS event, relatively minor degrees of STE have been reported in leads with obviously abnormal T waves. The amplitude of the T wave inversion is impressive, approaching 15 mm in some cases. Morphologically, the T wave is asymmetric with a characteristic outward bulge in its ascending portion.

STE frequently is less noticeable than the T wave changes-usually, it is less than 3 mm. Other electrocardiographic features associated with acute CNS injury include prominent U waves of either polarity and QT prolongation often exceeding 60% of its normal value. The T wave inversions with associated STE are most pronounced in the mid-precordial and lateral precordial leads; such findings also are noted to a less extent in the limb leads. Figure 36 presents the ECG of a patient with a subarrachnoid hemorrhage; note the STE with T wave inversions in the anterolateral leads, suggestive of AMI. *(Please see Table 6.)*

Although these ST segment/T wave abnormalities usually are encountered in patients with subarrachnoid bleed, other acute CNS events also may present with these electrocardiographic findings. Other conditions causing ECG changes include intraparenchymal hemorrhage, thromboembolism with infarction, cerebral artery occlusion, and CNS mass lesion with edema. Overall, 60% of patients with subarrachnoid hemorrhage will manifest an electrocardiographic abnormality. The pathophysiologic explanation for such electrocardiographic findings is controversial but may involve either CNS-mediated increases in sympathetic and vagal tone as well as actual myocardial damage called, "contraction band necrosis."

Acute Abdominal Disease. Acute abdominal disorders (e.g., pancreatitis, cholecystitis, hepatitis, and peritonitis) have been reported to cause electrocardiographic abnormalities ranging from Q waves to ST segment abnormalities.[19] STE, which has been observed in patients with gastrointestinal emergencies, may be difficult to distinguish from from AMI. For example, the elderly diabetic patient presenting with epigastric pain and emesis who manifests STE on the ECG will almost certainly be diagnosed with AMI.

The majority of such patients will, in fact, have AMI, while a minority will experience non-cardiac discomfort with an abdominal etiology. The pathophysiologic mechanism for ECG changes in abdominal disease is poorly understood but may involve direct transdiaphragmatic epicardial irritation or electrocardiographic detection of the visceral inflammatory process; either process can generate a current of injury manifested by STE. The STE may take many forms, ranging from minimal and concave to pronounced and convex.

Clinical Strategies for ECG Diagnosis: A Summary

Several strategies are available to facilitate accurate interpretation of electrocardiographic patterns in patients with chest pain. First, a knowledge of the associated, or anticipated, ST segment/T wave changes resulting from the confounding and mimicking patterns is a prerequisite for clinical management. Abnormalities of the ST segment/T wave complex that are not consistent with the altered patterns should alert the physician to the possibility of acute ischemic electrocardiographic change.[5,22] Use of the rule of appropriate discordance is of considerable use in patients with LBBB, VPR, and other situations.

In other cases, serial ECGs may demonstrate the dynamic electrocardiographic changes usually encountered in acutely ischemic patients.[20,21] For example, refer to Figures 37a and 37b for two examples of the serial ECG technique, both in lead V_3. In the first example (Figure 37a), a 40-year-old male presented to the ED with chest discomfort after using cocaine. The ECG revealed STE in the anterior leads which was suggestive of BER and also worrisome for AMI. Serial ECGs were performed while the patient received appropriate medical therapy. The ECGs did not reveal change of the STE, suggesting a nonischemic etiology for electrocardiographic abnormality. His pain resolved without further change; the STE was felt to be due to BER.

The second example in Figure 37b was encountered in a patient with chest pain and known electrocardiographic LVH on past ECGs. The current ECG demonstrated STE which was felt to represent LVH-related change. Continued chest pain prompted the application of serial ECGs which revealed dynamic change with progressive STE indicative of AMI. The patient received a thrombolytic agent with good clinical results; elevated troponin I confirmed the diagnosis of AMI.

References

1. Otto LA, Aufderheide TP. Evaluation of ST segment elevation criteria for the prehospital electrocardiographic diagnosis of acute myocardial infarction. *Ann Emerg Med* 1994;23:17-24.
2. Brady WJ. Causes of ST segment elevation in emergency department chest pain patients. Abstract presented at the International Emergency Medicine Conference, Vancouver, British Columbia, March 26, 1998.
3. Larsen GC, Griffith JL, Beshansky JR, et al. Electrocardiographic left ventricular hypertrophy in patients with suspected acute cardiac ischemia—It's influence on diagnosis, treatment, and short-term prognosis. *J Gen Intern Med* 1994;9:666-673.
4. Huwez FU, Pringle SD, Macfarlane FW. Variable patterns of ST-T abnormalities in patients with left ventricular hypertrophy and normal coronary arteries. *Brit Heart J* 1992;67:304-347.
5. Aufderheide TP, Brady WJ. Electrocardiography in the patient with myocardial ischemia or infarction. In: Gibler WB, Aufderheide TP, eds. *Emergency Cardiac Care*, 1st ed., St. Louis: Mosby; 1994:169-216.
6. Brady WJ. Electrocardiographic left ventricular hypertrophy in chest pain patients: Differentiation from acute coronary ischemic events. *Am J Emerg Med* (1998 accepted/pending).
7. Spodick DH. Differential diagnosis of the electrocardiogram in early repolarization and acute pericarditis. *N Engl J Med* 1976;295:523-526.
8. Glinzton LE, Laks MM. The differential diagnosis of acute pericarditis from the normal variant: New electrocardiographic criteria. *Circulation* 1982;65:1004-1009.
9. Shipley RA, Hallaran WR. The four-lead electrocardiogram in two hundred normal men and women. *Am Heart J* 1936;11: 325-45.
10. Hollander JE, Lozano M, Fairweather P, et al. "Abnormal" electrocardiograms in patients with cocaine-associated chest pain are due to "normal" variants. *J Emerg Med* 1994;12: 199-205.
11. Mehta MC, Jain AC. Early repolarization on scalar electrocardiogram. *Am J Med Sci* 1995;309:305-311.
12. Thomas J, Harris E, Lassiter G. Observations on the T wave

and S-T segment changes in the precordial electrocardiogram of 320 young negro adults. *Am J Cardiol* 1960;5:468-474.
13. Wasserburger RM, Alt WJ, Lloyd C. The normal RS-T segment elevation variant. *Am J Cardiol* 1961;8:184-192.
14. Brady W. Benign early repolarization: Electrocardiographic manifestations and differentiation from other ST segment elevation syndromes. *Am J Emerg Med* (1998 accepted/ pending).
15. Kabara H, Phillips J. Long-term evaluation of early repolarization syndrome (normal variant RS-T segment elevation). *Am J Cardiol* 1976;38:157-161.
16. Aufderheide TP, Brady WJ. Electrocardiography in the patient with myocardial ischemia or infarction. In: Gibler WB, Aufderheide TP eds. *Emergency Cardiac Care.* 1st ed. St. Louis: Mosby; 1994:169-216.
17. Sharkey SW, Berger CR, Brunette DD, et al. Impact of the electrocardiogram on the delivery of thrombolytic therapy for acute myocardial infarction. *Am J Cardiol* 1994;73: 550-553.
18. Hackworthy RA, Vogel MB, Harris PJ. Relationship between changes in ST-segment elevation and patency of the infarct-related coronary artery in acute myocardial infarction. *Am Heart J* 1986;112:279-288.
19. Ryan ET, Pak PH, DeSanctis RW. Myocardial infarction mimicked by acute cholecystitis. *Ann Int Med* 1992;116: 218-220.
20. Fesmire FM. ECG diagnosis of acute myocardial infarction in the presence of left bundle branch block in patients undergoing continuous ECG monitoring. *Ann Emerg Med* 1995;26:69-82.
21. Fesmire FM, Percy RF, Bardoner JB, et al. Usefulness of automated serial 12-lead ECG monitoring during the initial emergency department evaluation of patients with chest pain. *Ann Emerg Med* 1998;31:3-11.
22. Brady WJ, Aufderheide TP: Left Bundle Block Pattern Complicating the Evaluation of Acute Myocardial Infarction. *Acad Emerg Med* 1997;4:56-62.

Diabetes Management and Insulin Pump Therapy

Jeffrey R. Unger, MD
Linda P. Fredrickson, MD, RN, CDE

The primary care physician often treats patients with insulin-dependent diabetes mellitus who use conventional insulin therapy (1-2 injections per day with minimal blood glucose testing). The publication in 1993 of a landmark 10-year study funded by the National Institutes of Health[1] demonstrated that improved glucose levels significantly reduced the incidence and progression of diabetic complications. Since then, more and more physicians and patients are practicing intensive diabetes management (≥ 3 injections per day or insulin pump therapy with blood glucose testing 4 times daily) to improve glucose control. The role of the primary care physician is explained in this issue relating to the benefits and use of intensive diabetes management therapies and, in particular, insulin pump therapy. Practical guidelines are given for pump therapy (i.e., the "nuts and bolts" of how a pump works), as well as formulas for starting pump dosages and guidelines for the prevention of adverse events. In addition, guidelines are given for carbohydrate counting, exercising, the use of the pump during pregnancy, and candidate selection.

Introduction to Insulin Pump Therapy

Between 750,000 and 1 million Americans have insulin-dependent diabetes mellitus (IDDM), with 30,000 new cases diagnosed each year.[2] It has been proven that the long-term complications of diabetes can be significantly delayed and/or prevented by maintaining glycemic control as close to the normal range as possible throughout the patient's lifetime. People with diabetes are usually unable to achieve ideal blood glucose control unless they are intensively managed. *(Please see Table 1.)* Insulin pump therapy, or continuous subcutaneous insulin infusion (CSII), evolved in 1974 from the desire to develop insulin delivery that simulates normal pancreatic function for people with IDDM.[3] Through a continuous "basal" insulin infusion and incremental, or "bolus," insulin administration at meal times, CSII provides a more normal physiological insulin delivery than possible with conventional injection therapy.[4]

The acceptance of insulin pump therapy increased following the Diabetes Control and Complication Trial (DCCT), the 10-year study funded by the NIH and published in 1993. The DCCT demonstrated that improvement in glycemic control can significantly reduce by 60% the incidence of microvascular complications (retinopathy, neuropathy, and nephropathy).[1] In the DCCT, patients achieved intensive control either with three or more injections daily or with the use of an insulin pump. At the end of the study, 42% of all the intensively managed

Table 1. Components of Intensive Diabetes Management

- Physician and patient understand pharmacology of insulin
- Patient has ability to determine proper insulin dosage adjustments
- Patient understands effects of exercise on insulin usage
- Patient understands principles involved in flexible meal planning and carbohydrate counting
- Patient is able to use home blood glucose monitoring
- Patient is able to implement treatment protocols for hypo- and hyperglycemia
- Patient understands protocol for sick day insulin regimen
- Patient has demonstrated ability to maintain close communication with health care profilers so that all aspects of diabetes care can be monitored and continually updated

Figure 1. Insulin Pump Usage in the United States, 1990-1996

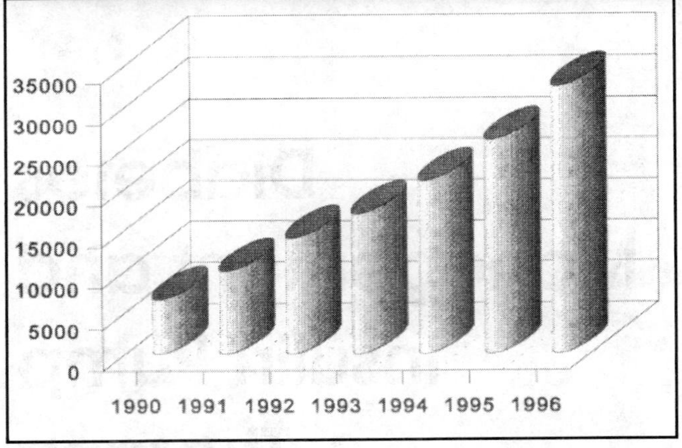

patients were using pump therapy.[5] Currently, 3% (32,500) of U.S. patients with IDDM are treated with CSII. *(Please see Figure 1.)* As shown, this number has been steadily increasing, which indicates that more and more physicians and patients are accepting insulin pump therapy as an option for intensive diabetes management.

Most patients with diabetes are treated by primary care physicians whose speciality is not diabetes or endocrinology.[6] Patients who use CSII are usually knowledgeable about diabetes and insulin pump therapy. When these patients move or join new insurance providers, they frequently encounter a physician who has limited or no knowledge of CSII. These patients may be told that "insulin pump therapy will not work," or "insulin pumping is just a fad." However, very few patients are willing to give up pump therapy to return to multiple daily injections. As a result, many pump patients stop seeing these healthcare providers who are not familiar with pump therapy. Therefore, it is becoming more important for the primary care physician to know the mechanics and principles of insulin pump therapy and of intensive diabetes management.

Benefits of Continuous Insulin Infusion

With injection therapy, absorption from the injection site with the use of intermediate- and long-acting insulins does not provide a constant basal rate due to their highly variable absorption, which ranges from 10% to 52% of the injected daily dose.[7] Variable insulin absorption is responsible for up to 80% of the day-to-day fluctuation in blood glucose concentrations in persons using injection-based therapy.[8] With CSII, patients use only regular insulin, in which there is far more predictable absorption, varying by less than 2.8% from the administered 24-hour dose.[7] CSII provides the greatest day-to-day reproducibility in insulin availability and the least unexpected fluctuation in glycemic control.

In the past, insulin pump use was contraindicated in individuals with severe, recurrent hypoglycemia. However, pump therapy, with its more predictable delivery of insulin, has been shown to reduce the incidence of severe hypoglycemia.[9-12] Newer studies have shown that CSII should be considered as an important indication for patients with frequent severe hypoglycemia.[12-14]

Another indication for insulin pump therapy is extreme insulin sensitivity (total daily dose < 20 units per day).[15] The pump permits convenient administration of fractional insulin units (in 0.1 unit increments), a level of precision not available with injections.

Pump therapy allows individuals to lead a more normal lifestyle. Pump users are able to experience a degree of freedom in the timing of meals, work, sleep, and physical activity not possible with the conventional treatment of multiple daily injections (MDI). Diabetes treatment protocols that rely on rigid dieting and activity schedules are unrealistic and inconvenient for most people. Having that freedom without loss of diabetes control is thought to be a major reason for the decreased depression and greater perception of self-efficacy found among pump users.[16]

How Does the Pump Work?

Although the original pumps were quite large and weighed close to 2 pounds, patients with diabetes were still able to master this form of therapy and achieve near normal glycemic

Figure 2. Infusion Site of Typical Insulin Pump

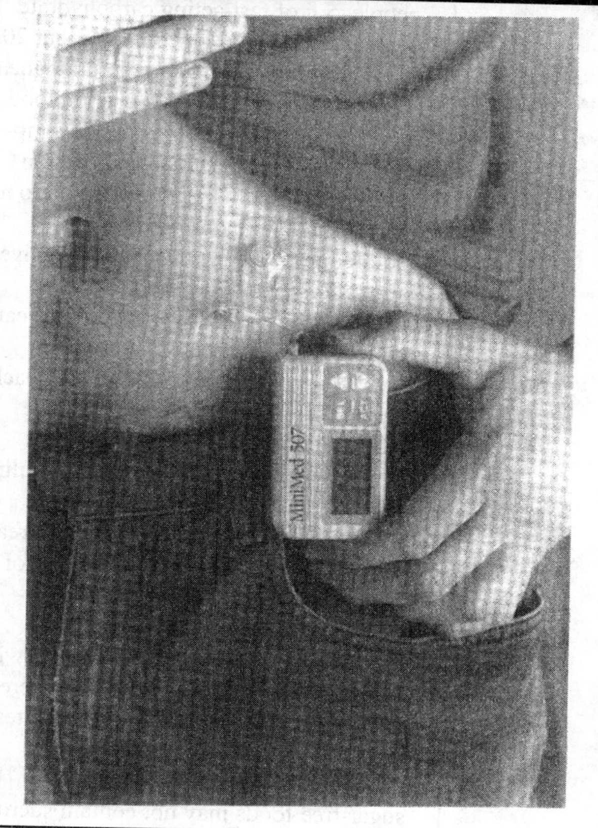

control.[17,18] Today's insulin pumps weigh only 4 ounces and are about the size of a beeper. *(Please see Figure 2.)*

Insulin pumps use a flexible infusion set with catheter lengths of 24 or 42 inches to facilitate placement inside or outside clothing. A 24-gauge soft catheter or 27-gauge bent needle is located at the far end of the plastic tubing. The insertion site is cleaned with alcohol or Hibiclens before inserting the needle into the chosen infusion site. The majority of pump wearers use the abdomen as the infusion site, although the buttocks or arms can be used. *(Please see Figure 2.)* The newer catheters have a Quick Release (MiniMed, Inc., Sylmar, CA) feature, which allows the patient to separate the catheter from the insulin syringe/reservoir located within the pump for bathing, exercise, or intimate activities. The insulin is located within a 3 cc syringe/reservoir on the pump. The syringe and infusion set must be filled and changed every 2-3 days by the patient. Prolonged use of the infusion set at a single site could result in irritation at the infusion site or the formation of a superficial abscess requiring surgical drainage in the office.[15] The pump is powered by disposable batteries which last approximately eight weeks.

The physician sets and programs the pump infusion parameters into the pump's memory. Each pump comes with specified built-in alarms to prevent inadvertent insulin delivery or to warn the patient if the infusion set becomes clogged or dysfunctional.[19]

Principles of Insulin Pumping

1. Establishing the pump parameters. *(Please see Figure 3.)* When initiating any form of intensive diabetes management, the physician must first determine the total daily dose of insulin that the patient will require. Because many patients need less insulin when beginning CSII,[14] the prepump total daily dose is reduced by 10-25%. Approximately 50% of the adjusted total daily dose of insulin is used as "basal insulin," and the other 50% is given prior to meals as "bolus insulin."[20] CSII uses basal insulin to maintain hepatic glucose output equivalent to peripheral basal glucose utilization.[19] Insulin given as a bolus prior to eating will control postprandial hyperglycemia.

Basal Rate. To program the basal rate, 50% of the reduced total daily insulin dose is divided by 24 hours. The patient with a prepump total daily dose of 54 units would have a basal rate equal to 50% of the reduced total daily dose of 40 units, or 20 units. This rate is then divided by 24 hours, for an hourly rate of 0.8 units. The most commonly used insulin pumps have the capability of programming 12 different basal rates. However, the majority of patients require only 2-3 basal rates.[14] If a patient has significant early morning hyperglycemia, a second basal rate can be programmed to counter the "dawn phenomenon," which occurs due to the production of growth hormone and cortisol, both of which raise fasting blood glucose levels and result in insulin resistance.[21] By increasing the basal rate 0.2-0.4 units per hour beginning 2-3 hours prior to rising, patients will be able to arise with normal blood glucose levels.[21]

Bolus Dosages. Premeal insulin bolus doses should be determined according to: a) the preprandial blood glucose levels; b) estimation of the grams of carbohydrates that will be consumed during that meal; and c) anticipated activity level after eating.[22]

2. Meal Planning. Diabetes interferes with the metabolism of carbohydrates. Therefore, the more carbohydrates consumed in a meal, the higher the anticipated rise in postprandial blood glucose, since carbohydrates are completely metabolized into glucose. Bolus insulin can be determined as demonstrated in Figure 3.

Correcting High Blood Glucoses. Supplemental insulin can also be given with the routine preprandial bolus to correct any high blood glucose levels that are present before eating. The supplemental insulin dose is based on the "1500 rule."[14,23] This rule calculates the patient's insulin sensitivity factor and allows the patient to predict how much 1.0 unit of insulin will lower the blood glucose. The formula is depicted in Table 2. Using the example in Table 2, for a patient whose TDD is 50 units, 1.0 unit of insulin will drop blood glucose by 30 mg/dL. Therefore, a blood glucose level of 160 mg/dL would require a 2.0 unit supplement of insulin to reach the preprandial target of 100 mg/dL. The 2.0 unit supplement would be added to the normal meal bolus used to cover the carbohydrates in the meal.

Determining insulin sensitivity is particularly important in assisting patients to avoid extremely labile swings in blood glucose (i.e., over-correcting for an increased blood glucose and then becoming hypoglycemic several hours later). Meal plan-

Figure 3. Establishing Pump Parameters

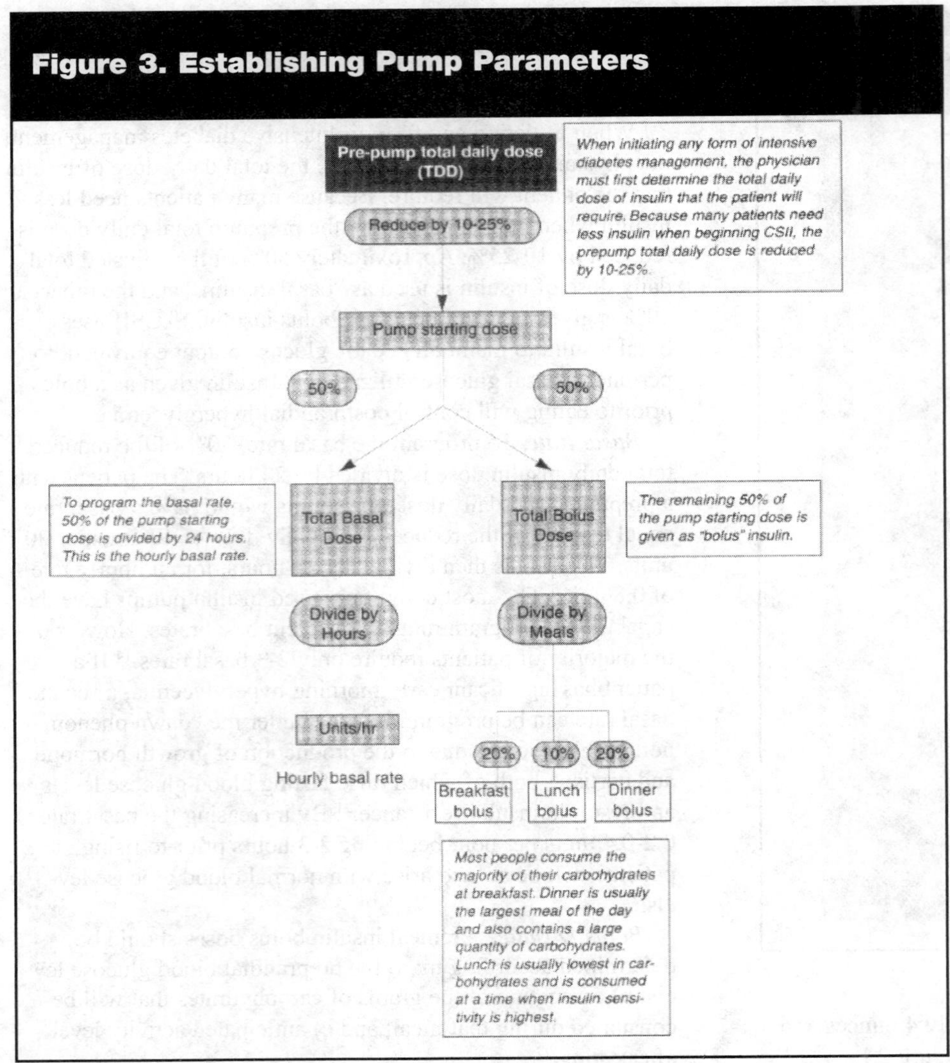

ning for patients with IDDM is an essential aspect of intensive diabetes management; many are often frightened by the term "diet." Physicians all too often prescribe the standard "1800-calorie American Diabetes Association diet" for all patients with diabetes regardless of age, weight, activity level, or total daily insulin requirements. People with diabetes require a careful balance of food intake, activity level, and insulin dosage. When patients learn the influence of various foods and activities on glycemic levels, they are able to balance these components of diabetes management at an optimum level.

Counting Carbohydrates. When discussing meal planning with the patient, physicians should emphasize the importance of sound nutritional practices, including avoiding excess intake of saturated fats and cholesterol, limiting salt consumption, and avoiding foods that have a high glycemic index, which could result in a rapid rise in plasma-glucose levels.[24] Unless the patient is overweight, there is no need to limit calorie consumption. Recently, health care professionals have begun teaching intensively treated IDDM patients how to count carbohydrates.[25] This simple concept requires that the patient learn to dose insulin according to the amount of carbohydrates consumed.

To successfully count carbohydrates, patients must be familiar with the effects of carbohydrate consumption. For most people, 5 g of fast-acting carbohydrate will raise the blood glucose by about 20 mg/dL.[26] Thus, a 30 g carbohydrate meal will result in a 120 mg/dL rise in blood glucose within 90 minutes of consumption. Next, the patient can be given an insulin-to-carbohydrate coverage ratio to help calculate the dose of insulin required to cover the ingestion of a given amount of carbohydrate. One unit of insulin will usually cover 10-15 g of carbohydrate.[27] However, this ratio will have to be individually adjusted for each patient. In general, patients who have smaller body size and are extremely insulin-sensitive will require less insulin and more precise calculations.[28]

Patients should be encouraged to read food labels and estimate the amount of insulin required to cover the carbohydrate load contained within a meal. Eating a meal high in carbohydrates will require an increased meal bolus, whereas eating a small amount of carbohydrates requires bolusing less insulin. The patient should also understand that sugar-free foods may not contain sucrose but might contain other forms of carbohydrate that would require the use of insulin. Snacks will also require bolus insulin. A patient who goes to a movie and eats a box of popcorn will need to take insulin, or blood glucose will rise substantially. Therefore, patients need to be aware that all carbohydrate consumption must be matched with appropriate insulin boluses.

With practice, carbohydrate counting becomes commonplace. During the initiation phase, patients must learn to check postprandial blood glucose levels 1-2 hours after the meal to see if they fall within a target range. *(Please see Table 3.)* If the blood glucose levels fall outside of the target range, adjustments must be made to the amount of insulin taken as a bolus prior to consuming that same amount of carbohydrates next time a similar meal is eaten. Patients who fail to achieve normal glycemic control following a given meal are advised to eat the same meal the following day and attempt to make the appropriate insulin adjustments. Using standard meals will decrease the variability encountered during the evaluation or reevaluation phase of CSII. Once the target goal is attained, teach the patient to remember how much insulin is required for commonly consumed meals. Food diaries containing information on matching insulin dosing with commonly eaten foods are especially helpful.

Intensively managed patients must ask the following five questions prior to preprandial bolus dosing of insulin:

Table 2. Calculating Insulin Sensitivity for Supplemental Boluses

GENERAL PRINCIPLES	"1500 RULE"	EXAMPLES TDD	1.0 unit of insulin lowers BG mg/dL
1. Determine the amount of blood glucose (BG) reduction for 1.0 unit of insulin in every patient	Divide 1500 by Total daily dose (TDD)	15	100
	Example: TDD is 50 units	25	60
		30	50
2. The value varies depending on the insulin requirement	• 1500/50 = 30 mg/dL drop per 1.0 unit of insulin	40	40
		50	30
		60	25
3. The "1500 rule" is used to estimate BG drop per 1.0 unit of insulin	• If BG target midpoint is 100 and BG is 160, 2.0 extra units needed	75	20
		100	15

1. What is my blood glucose now?
2. What type of food will I be eating, and is the meal high in carbohydrates?
3. How much insulin do I need to cover this meal?
4. What happened to my blood glucose the last time I gave this dose of insulin for this amount of food?
5. Is there any anticipated postmeal exercise planned?

3. Exercising with the Insulin Pump. A regular exercise program can potentially improve glycemic control in nearly all diabetic individuals. Clear-cut cardiovascular benefits accrue to patients who participate in a program of regular exercise.[29] The effect of exercise is dependent on several factors: 1) intensity and duration of exercise; 2) degree of physical conditioning of the individual; 3) preexercise diet; 4) dosage and timing of insulin taken prior to exercise; and 5) duration of the diabetes. Nearly all people can perform some type of exercise including walking, biking, aerobics, weight training, swimming, running, or chair exercises. Caloric expenditure of 500-3500 calories weekly will result in increased longevity, improved glycemic control, and weight maintenance. Walking for 20 minutes four times weekly is sufficient exercise for most people with diabetes. Exercise can also improve an individual's sense of well-being and quality of life.[30]

General Health Status. Prior to beginning an exercise program, a physician must evaluate the patient for evidence of eye, kidney, nerve, or cardiovascular problems that might prohibit certain types of exercise. Loss of sensation in the feet can result in weakened arches, increased callous formation, joint damage, and pressure ulceration. Patients with neuropathy should perform low-impact, high-intensity exercise such as swimming and biking. Running is contraindicated in patients with neuropathy due to loss of proprioception and balance mechanisms. Patients with proliferative retinopathy should avoid resistance weight training because of an increase risk of retinal detachments. An exercise-stress ECG is recommended for all patients over 35 years of age. This test will help identify silent heart disease and may identify patients who have an exaggerated hypertensive response to exercise and/or may develop postexercise orthostatic hypotension.[30]

Blood Glucose Goals. Patients with IDDM should begin exercise within a target blood glucose of 120-180 mg/dL. Intensive exercising below 120 mg/dL may result in hypoglycemia. The symptoms of hypoglycemia are similar to those seen commonly with exercise—palpitations, sweating, dizziness, and fatigue. If the blood glucose is below 120 mg/dL prior to exercise participation, the patient can consume 15-25 g of carbohydrates such as a fruit or a carbohydrate-enhanced "power bar" in order to elevate the blood glucose to the target range. An absolute deficiency of insulin will result in impaired glucose uptake, hyperglycemia, and ketosis;[31] therefore, patients should not exercise if the blood glucose is above 240 mg/dL. At this level, exercise will cause insulin levels to drop, with a consequent rise in blood glucose levels that can cause ketosis.

Temporary Basal Rate. During exercise, the insulin pump offers several advantages over multiple daily injections. In anticipation of exercise, the pump can be stopped or slowed down using a temporary basal rate (TBR).[32] A TBR allows the patient to bypass the programmed basal rate in favor of one that is either decreased or increased. Thus, a lower TBR can be set prior to the anticipated exercise start time so that circulating exogenous insulin levels begin to fall. The TBR should be continued throughout the exercise period as well as several hours after exercise is completed in order to avoid postexercise hypoglycemia.[33]

A well-conditioned athlete who is performing the same level of intense exercise on a routine basis may not have to alter his insulin delivery rate at all. However, if an athlete is poorly conditioned, the blood glucose will drop rapidly and remain low in the fasting state for up to 12 hours after exercising.[33,34] The guidelines for exercising with an insulin pump are summarized in Table 4.[35]

Table 3. Target Blood Glucose Levels for Patients with IDDM

	Ideal	Acceptable
Premeal	70-105	70-130
1 hour postprandial	100-160	100-180
2 hours postprandial	80-120	80-150
2:00 am-4:00 am	80-120	100-140

Risk Assessment and Prevention

Any diabetes treatment plan carries potential risks to the patient. Proper education, close monitoring, and adherence to recommended guidelines are the cornerstones to dealing with problems unique to pump therapy and preventing minor problems from escalating into adverse events.

Hypoglycemia. Patients undergoing intensive diabetes management are at increased risk for developing hypoglycemia. During the DCCT, severe hypoglycemia, defined as a hypoglycemic episode requiring assistance of another person, was increased threefold in the intensive therapy group in comparison to the conventional group.[36] Of severe hypoglycemic episodes, 53% occurred during sleep, and 35% occurred without warning symptoms while patients were awake. Patients who have had IDDM for more than five years often lose their counterregulatory mechanism for identifying and metabolically reversing hypoglycemia.[37] These patients often develop "hypoglycemic unawareness,"[38] functioning fairly well with blood glucoses as low as 40 mg/dL. The most dangerous consequences of hypoglycemia are impaired cognitive and disordered intellectual functioning, making self-medication and reversal of hypoglycemia impossible.[39] This could be very dangerous if hypoglycemia occurs at a time when concentration and cognitive thinking are essential, such as while driving a car, working in the operating room, or taking care of small children. Strategies to prevent hypoglycemia include the following:

Setting higher target glucose goals. Insulin pump therapy offers several advantages in preventing hypoglycemia. If the patient on multiple daily injections is experiencing frequent wide glycemic swings including hypoglycemia on a daily basis, placing the patient on an insulin pump will permit the physician to aim for higher target blood glucose levels.[14] Setting a lower than normal basal rate, the blood glucose levels will rise, and the patient will experience fewer episodes of hypoglycemia. Blood glucose targets can be set in the range of 120-180 mg/dL instead of 70-130 mg/dL. After resetting the target blood glucose range and maintaining that target for 6-8 weeks, the basal rate can be increased once again, allowing the physician to lower the target blood glucose range closer to normal. Hypoglycemic awareness has been reported to be reestablished in patients using this technique to avoid hypoglycemia.[40,41]

Hypoglycemia Treatment Guidelines. Patients with frequent hypoglycemia who eat to raise blood glucoses will often gain weight and require even more insulin to control their glucose levels. CSII allows the patient to avoid "eating their way out of hypoglycemia" by decreasing the basal rate when hypoglycemia occurs. Hypoglycemia that does not improve with these modalities can be treated with glucose tablets that contain 5 g of carbohydrates. *(Please see Table 5.)* All people with diabetes should have access to glucagon for the treatment of severe hypoglycemia, and their family members or significant others should know how to administer the injection.

Blood Glucose Monitoring Guidelines. Many patients using intensive diabetes management do so in the hope of avoiding the long-term diabetes complications. They may not view a low blood glucose value as dangerous as a high blood glucose value. Physicians need to educate patients on the two problems caused by repeated episodes of hypoglycemia. First, repeated episodes blunt hormonal defense mechanisms that prevent hypoglycemia; second, they lower the level at which early hypoglycemic symptoms are perceived. Understanding the principle that hypoglycemia begets more hypoglycemia,[42] patients must be taught how to be their own "glucose sensor" based on frequent self-monitoring of blood glucose (SMBG) levels.[43] Blood glucose levels should be monitored at least four times per day in all patients—before each meal, at bedtime, prior to driving and before exercising. In addition, once a week a blood glucose test should be performed three hours after going to bed in order to detect nocturnal hypoglycemia.

Skin Infections. Skin irritations and skin infections may appear at the infusion site. Occasionally, an abscess may occur and must be surgically drained. Most infections are caused by coagulase-positive Staphylococcus aureus.[44] Infections usually occur because the patient fails to change the infusion set at the appropriate interval. Infusion sets with the soft cannula (Sof-set) can be changed every three days. Bent needle sets must be changed more frequently (i.e., every 2 days). If pain and redness appear at the infusion site, the infusion set and site need to be changed immediately to prevent development of a skin infection.

Unexplained Hyperglycemia. Unexplained hyperglycemia is a high blood glucose level that persists for more than 2-4 hours for no obvious reason. Usually the patient is not ill but performs a routine blood glucose test only to be surprised that the reading is in the 300-400 mg/dL range.

There are several potential causes of unexplained hyperglycemia, which, when present, requires a systematic investigation of the pump, syringe, infusion set, infusion site, and insulin vial to identify the cause. *(Please see Table 6.)* Since pump therapy uses only rapid-acting insulin, even a minor interruption of insulin delivery will result in hyperglycemia. Diabetic ketoacidosis (DKA) can occur in 4-6 hours after the insulin infusion is interrupted.[15,45]

As soon as the patient determines the presence of unexplained hyperglycemia, a bolus of insulin should be administered via the pump. The supplemental dose of insulin should be determined by the "1500 Rule,"[14] which is used to determine an individual's sensitivity to insulin. When properly

Table 4. Exercise Guidelines for Patients on Insulin Pump Therapy

	EXERCISE INTENSITY								
	MILD			MODERATE			INTENSE		
Duration	CHO	Bolus	Basal	CHO	Bolus	Basal	CHO	Bolus	Basal
15 min	—	—	—	—	—	—	↑	—	—
30 min	—	—	—	↑	—	—	↑	↓30%	—
45 min	↑	—	—	↑	↓30%	—	↑	↓50%	—
60 min	↑	↓30%	—	↑	↓30%	↓20%	↑↑	↓50%	↓20%
120 min	↑	↓30%	—	↑↑	↓50%	↓20%	↑↑	↓50%	↓40%
240 min	↑↑	↓30%	—	↑↑	↓50%	↓20%	↑↑↑	↓50%	↓40%

calculated, the supplemental dose should return the blood glucose to the target blood glucose range. Two hours after administering the bolus, the blood glucose should be checked again. If the glucose remains high, an injection of insulin should be given using a regular insulin syringe. The infusion set should be changed, which should restore normal glycemic levels. However, if blood glucose remains high, the patient should discontinue CSII and initiate an emergency protocol during which routine insulin injections are administered every four hours based upon the blood glucose levels and carbohydrate counting at meal times.

If nausea or vomiting develops in the presence of unexplained hyperglycemia, a subcutaneous injection of insulin should be administered immediately. It is imperative for a pump user to understand that high blood glucose levels can lead to DKA and must be treated immediately. The cause of the high blood glucose must be treated subsequently.[46]

Weight Gain. Weight gain has been associated with intensive insulin regimens. In the DCCT, subjects using intensive diabetes management gained an average of 5.1 kg over the whole study (average, 6.5 years per patient) compared with an average weight gain of 2.4 kg in conventionally treated subjects.[47] The largest weight gain was associated with the greatest decreases in glycosylated hemoglobin levels and increased frequency of severe hypoglycemia. The weight gain occurred despite a reduction in caloric intake from baseline.

This weight gain, which occurs when blood glucose control is improved, is due to a reduction of caloric loss in the form of glycosuria. Frequent episodes of over-treatment of hypoglycemia may also be a factor. Weight reduction may be facilitated with CSII since patients do not need to eat as frequently or to eat between meal snacks, and can often skip meals without loss of glycemic control.[22]

Can a Pump be Used During Pregnancy?

In no individual is excellent blood glucose control more important than in the pregnant diabetic patient.[48] Hyperglycemia in pregnancy can result in congenital abnormalities including intrauterine growth delay, macrosomia, neonatal hypoglycemia, respiratory distress syndrome, and neonatal jaundice.[29,49,50] The intrauterine mortality associated with DKA approaches 50%.[51]

CSII is best initiated before conception but can also be started during the pregnancy. The basal and bolus parameters will need to be updated frequently as the pregnancy progresses due to the accelerated catabolism, increasing insulin demand, and intensified production of counterregulatory hormones that oppose the actions of insulin during pregnancy. The target blood glucose levels during pregnancy are 70-110 mg/dL fasting and < 120 mg/dL two hours postprandially. Also, as the skin stretches during pregnancy, abdominal sites become less comfortable. Therefore, most pregnant pump users choose the upper arm or hip as the infusion site.

Special precautions and protocols must be used during pregnancy to prevent DKA. Due to the high rate of fetal mortality associated with DKA, a small supplemental bedtime dose of NPH or Lente insulin (0.2 u/kg) is recommended in addition to the normal or reduced nighttime basal rate.[48] This NPH or Lente supplement reduces the likelihood that DKA will occur if the infusion of insulin is interrupted for any reason while sleeping.

What Types of Insulin Are Used?

Currently, only regular buffered insulin (Velosulin BR, Novo Nordisk, Princeton, NJ) is labeled for pump use. A new fast-acting insulin, insulin lispro (Humalog for injection) has been approved by the FDA and is now available for injection therapy. It is manufactured by Eli Lilly (Indianapolis, IN) and requires a doctor's prescription. Insulin lispro is not yet labeled for use for pump therapy; however, tests using lispro in pumps are currently being conducted at three U.S. centers. Bench tests with pumps and infusion systems have demonstrated the stability of the insulin.[52]

In Canada, 30 Type I patients participated in a study using lispro and the pump.[53] Both physician and participant were blinded as to whether they were taking lispro or regular insulin by pump for a three-month period. Participants were then "crossed over" to the alternate insulin for an additional three months. The authors reported significantly lower glycosylated hemoglobin (HbA1c) in the lispro group compared to the regu-

Table 5. Treatment of Hypoglycemia

1. All patients should carry some form of fast-acting glucose while away from home, driving, or exercising
2. Recheck BG in 15 minutes. If BG is below 60, a second or third tablet is needed.
3. Honey is readily absorbed and fast-acting antidote for hypoglycemia. Two to four reaspoons of honey will usually raise the blood sugar into the target range.
4. A half-can of regular cola will raise the blood sugar approximately 80 points.
5. Administer 1 mg of glucagon intramuscularly or subcutaneously for severe hypoglycemia.

lar group (7.65% vs 7.99%; $P = 0.0041$) without an increase in the number of hypoglycemic episodes. Specific guidelines/algorithms for pump use are not expected until the results of the multi-center trial in the United States is completed. Studies (without the pump) have shown that the glucose-lowering action of lispro begins within five minutes of injection and that the duration of action is shorter.

Because insulin lispro has a shorter duration of action than regular insulin, it is more rapidly cleared from the body. Therefore, when it is approved for pump use, patients must be aware of the increased potential for more rapid onset of high blood glucose and diabetic ketoacidosis (DKA) if insulin delivery is interrupted. Extra attention should be given to self-monitoring of blood glucose and DKA prevention guidelines. In addition, it may be particularly important to adhere to the recommended infusion set change interval of every 2-3 days to be certain that interruption of flow does not occur.

Choosing Pump Therapy

The indications for CSII include the need for improved glycemic control and a patient's desire to lead a more normal life, especially when daily schedules are erratic. Appropriate candidate selection is essential to the success of pump therapy. *(Please see Table 7.)*[54] Pump therapy requires that patients possess certain physical, intellectual, and motivational abilities to ensure the optimum benefit and to reduce risks. Physical abilities are needed to accurately perform blood glucose monitoring and to carry out the technical components of insulin pump use. It is essential that a pump user understands the components of the pump regimen as well as troubleshooting the pump and infusion system if a problem should arise. The patient must be willing to comply with professional recommendations and to aggressively self-monitor blood glucose levels, to anticipate insulin needs for changing circumstances, and to make purposeful decisions and evaluate actions taken. Patients who take an active role in using pump therapy will have the best short- and long-term outcomes. When patients

Table 6. Potential Causes of Unexplained Hypoglycemia

1. Insulin pump
   - Basal rate programmed incorrectly
   - Pump malfunction; syringe is not advancing
2. Syringe
   - Improper placement in pump
   - Empty syringe (insulin depleted)
   - Syringe not primed in pump
   - Insulin is leaking in the pump
3. Infusion set/needle
   - Insulin leakage
   - Needle has become dislodged from infusing site
   - Air/blood is in infusion set
   - Needle has been placed in scar tissue; insulin cannot be delivered, and high pressure alarm will sound
   - Kinked tubing
   - Insulin occlusion due to non-buffered insulin usage
4. Infusion site
   - Redness, irritation, inflammation
   - Discomfort
   - Area of friction or near the belt time
5. Insulin
   - Insulin has been exposed to extreme temperatures
   - Insulin has expired

see the benefit of the increased effort, they are willing to work harder to achieve that goal.

Summary

Insulin pump therapy is an integral part of a complete intensive diabetes management program. As the number of patients being placed on CSII is increasing each year, physicians are often introduced to the pump when patients already using CSII are transferred to a new clinic. If the health care provider is unfamiliar with CSII, active participation in the patient's daily pump management will enhance their ability to provide support and education for this intensively managed group of patients. Physicians must be knowledgeable in all aspects of intensive diabetes management in order to manage pump patients. Health care providers should attend professional pump programs where they may "mentor" and network with more experienced providers. Also, pump manufacturer representatives can provide instructional materials, operation manuals, tutorials, and videos to pump candidates and physicians.

As physicians and health care providers, we are challenged to design for the patient an insulin regimen that promotes both short- and long-term well-being. Each patient should have an

Table 7. Candidate Selection for Insulin Pump Therapy

PREREQUISITES

- Patient has demonstrated ability to self-monitor blood glucose levels at least four times a day; and
- Patient is motivated to achieve and maintain improved glycemic control

WITH ONE OR MORE OF THE FOLLOWING:

- Glycosylated hemoglobin (HbA_{1c}) level greater than 7.0%
- History of severe glycemia excursions (commonly associated with hypoglycemic unawareness, nocturnal hypoglycemia, extreme insulin sensitivity, and/or very low insulin requirements)
- Wide fluctuations in blood glucose before mealtime (e.g., preprandial blood glucose level commonly exceeds 150 mg/dL)
- Dawn phenomenon, where fasting blood glucose level often exceeds 200 mg/dL
- Day-to-day variations in work schedule, mealtimes, and/or activity level, which confound the degree of regimentation required to self-manage glycemia with multiple insulin injections
- Preconceptions or pregnancy with a history of suboptimal glycemic control
- Suboptimal glycemic and metabolic control post-renal transplant

individualized treatment regimen so that the patient's potential for achieving optimal health and personal freedom is enhanced. Insulin pump therapy is an exciting option for the patient striving for improved diabetes self-care and a more normal lifestyle.

References

1. DCCT Research Group. The effect of intensive treatment of diabetes on the development and progression of long-term complications in insulin-dependent diabetes mellitus. *N Engl J Med* 1993;329:977-986.
2. LaPorte RE, et al. Prevalence and incidence of insulin-dependent diabetes. In: Diabetes in America, 2nd edition. Harris MI, et al (eds). National Institutes of Health; 1995:37.
3. Slama G, et al. One to five days of continuous intravenous insulin infusion on seven diabetic patients. *Diabetes* 1974;23:732-738.
4. Hirsch IB, et al. Intensive insulin therapy for treatment of type I diabetes. *Diabetes Care* 1990;13:1265-1283.
5. DCCT Research Group. Implementation. *Diabetes Care* 1995.
6. Harris, et al. The DCCT and Medical Care for Diabetes in the U.S. *Diabetes Care* 1994;17:761-764.
7. Lauritzen T, et al. Pharmacokinetics of continuous subcutaneous insulin infusion. *Diabetologia* 1983;24:326-329.
8. Binder C, et al. Insulin pharmacokinetics. *Diabetes Care* 1984; 7:188-200.
9. Ronn B, et al. Evaluation of insulin pump treatment under routine conditions. *Diabetes Res Clin Pract* 1989;3:191-196.
10. Eichner HL, et al. Reduction of severe hypoglycemic events in type I (insulin-dependent) diabetic patients using continuous subcutaneous insulin infusion. *Diabetes Res* 1989;8:189-193.
11. Bell DSH, et al. The feasibility of long-term treatment of diabetes with continuous subcutaneous insulin infusion. *Diab Nutr Metab* 1993;6:57-60.
12. Hirsch IB, et al. Continuous subcutaneous insulin infusion for the treatment of diabetic patients with hypoglycemia unawareness. *Diab Nutr Metab* 1991;4:41-43.
13. Farkas-Hirsch R, Hirsch IB. Continuous subcutaneous insulin infusion: A review of the past and its implementation for the future. *Diabetes Spectrum* 1994;7:80-138.
14. Bode BW, et al. Reduction in severe hypoglycemia with long-term continuous subcutaneous insulin infusion in type I diabetes. *Diabetes Care* 1996;19:324-327.
15. Mecklenberg RS, et al. Acute complications associated with insulin infusion pump therapy. Report of experience with 161 patients. *JAMA* 1984;252:3265-3269.
16. Shapiro J, et al. Personality and family profiles of chronic insulin-dependent diabetic patients using portable insulin infusion pump therapy: A preliminary investigation. *Diabetes Care* 1984;7:137-142.
17. Pickup JC, et al. Continuous subcutaneous insulin infusion: An approach to achieving normoglycemia. *BMJ* 1978;1:204-207.
18. Tamborlane WV, et al. Reduction to normal of plasma glucose in juvenile diabetes by subcutaneous administration of insulin with a portable infusion pump. *N Engl J Med* 1979;300:573-578.
19. Skyler JS. Continuous subcutaneous insulin infusion (CSII) with external devices: Current status. In: *Update in Drug Delivery Systems.* Ensminger WD, Selam JL (eds). Mount Kisco, NY: Futura; 1989:163-183.
20. Bode BW. Establishing and verifying basal rates. In: *The Insulin Pump Therapy Book: Insights from the Experts.* Fredrickson L (ed). Sylmar, CA: MiniMed, Inc.; 1995:49-56.
21. Koivisto VA, et al. Pathogenesis and prevention of dawn phenomenon in diabetic patients treated with CSII. *Diabetes* 1985;35:78-82.
22. Strowig SM. Initiation and management of insulin pump therapy. *Diabetes Educator* 1993;18:50-59.
23. Davidson PC. Bolus and supplemental insulin. In: *The Insulin Pump Therapy Book: Insights from the Experts.* Fredrickson L (ed). Sylmar, CA: MiniMed; 1995:59-71.
24. American Diabetes Association. Position statement. Nutrition recommendations and principles for people with diabetes mellitus. *Diabetes Care* 1996;19:S16-S19.
25. Brackenridge BP. Carbohydrate gram counting: A key to accurate mealtime boluses in intensive therapy. *Practical Diabetology* 1992; 11:22-28.
26. Hirsch IB, Polansky WH. Hypoglycemia and its prevention. In: *The Insulin Pump Therapy Book: Insights from the Experts.* Fredrickson L (ed). Sylmar, CA: MiniMed, Inc.; 1995:129-142.
27. American Diabetes Association. Insulin infusion pump therapy. In: *Intensive Diabetes Management.* Farkas-Hirsch R (ed). Alexandria, VA: American Diabetes Association; 1994:65-78.
28. Brackenridge BP, Reed JH. Counting carbohydrates: The key to proper bolusing. In: *The Insulin Pump Therapy Book: Insights from the Experts.* Fredrickson L (ed). Sylmar, CA: MiniMed, Inc.;

1995:73-83.

29. American Diabetes Association. *Medical Management of Insulin-Dependent Type I Diabetes,* 2nd ed. Santiago JV (ed). Alexandria, VA: American Diabetes Association; 1994:67-72.
30. American Diabetes Association. *Therapy for Diabetes Mellitus and Related Disorders,* 2nd ed. Lebonitz HE (ed). Alexandria, VA: American Diabetes Association; 1994;107-115.
31. Zinman B. Exercise and the pump. In: *The Insulin Pump Therapy Book: Insights from the Experts.* Fredrickson L (ed). Sylmar, CA: MiniMed, Inc.; 1995.
32. Unger J. Principles of intensive insulin therapy. *Hospital Physician* 1994;11:8-20.
33. Sonnenberg GE, et al. Exercise in type I (insulin-dependent) diabetic patients treated with continuous subcutaneous insulin infusion. *Diabetologia* 1990;33:696-703.
34. Campaigne BN, et al. Glucose and insulin response in relation to insulin dose and caloric intake 12 hours after acute physical exercise in men with IDDM. *Diabetes Care* 1987;10:716-721.
35. Walsh J, Roberts R. *Insulin Pump Therapy Handbook.* Sylmar, CA: MiniMed, Inc.; 1992:34.
36. DCCT Research Group. The effect of intensive treatment of diabetes on the development and progression of long-term complications in insulin-dependent diabetes mellitus. *N Engl J Med* 1993;329:977-986.
37. Cryer PE, et al. Hypoglycemia. Diabetes Care 1994;17:734-755.
38. Cryer PE. Hypoglycemia unawareness in IDDM. *Diabetes Care* 1993;16 (Suppl 3):40-47.
39. White NH. Hypoglycemia: A limiting factor in implementing intensive therapy. *Clinical Diabetes* 1994;12:101-105.
40. Fanelli CG, et al. Meticulous prevention of hypoglycemia normalizes the glycemic threshold and magnitude of most of neuroendocrine responses to, symptoms of, and cognitive function during hypoglycemia in intensively treated patients with short-term IDDM. *Diabetes* 1993;42:1683-1689.
41. Fanelli C, et al. Long-term recovery from unawareness, deficient counterregulation and lack of cognitive dysfunction during hypoglycemia, following institution of rational, intensive insulin therapy in IDDM. *Diabetologia* 1994;37:1265-1276.
42. Cryer PE. Hypoglycemia begets hypoglycemia in IDDM. *Diabetes* 1993;42:1691-1693.
43. Farkas-Hirsch R, Hirsch IB. Continuous subcutaneous insulin infusion: A review of the past and its implementation for the future. *Diabetes Spectrum* 1994;7:80-138.
44. Mecklenburg R. Acute complications associated with the use of insulin infusion pumps. *Diab Educ* 1989;15:40-43.
45. Bending JC, et al. Eight-month correction of hyperglycemia in insulin-dependent diabetes mellitus is associated with a significant and sustained reduction of urinary albumin excretion rates in patients with microalbuminuria. *Diabetes* 1985;34:69-73.
46. Fredrickson L. Insulin Pump Safety, Certified Pump Trainer Manual. Sylmar, CA: MiniMed, Inc.; 1996:65-75.
47. DCCT Research Group. Weight gain associated with intensive therapy in the Diabetes Control and Complications Trial. *Diabetes Care* 1988;11:567-573.
48. Marcus AO, Fernandez M. Insulin pump therapy; acceptable alternative to injection therapy. *Postgraduate Med* 1996;3:125-143.
49. Pedersen JF, Molsted-Pedersen L. Early growth retardation in diabetic pregnancy. In: Jovanovic L, et al (eds). *Diabetes and Pregnancy,* 1st ed. New York: Praeger; 1986.
50. Jovanovic L, et al. Effect of euglycemia on the outcome of pregnancy in insulin-dependent diabetic women as compared with normal control subjects. *Am J Med* 1981;71:921-927.
51. Kitzmiller JL. Diabetic ketoacidosis and pregnancy. In: Queenan JT (ed). *Managing OB-Gyn Emergencies,* 2nd ed. Oradell, NJ: Medical Economics; 1983:44-55.
52. Lougheed WD, et al. Chemical stability of insulin lispro in insulin infusion systems. *Diabetes* 1996;45:28A#1058.
53. Zinman B, et al. Insulin lispro in CSII: Results of a double-blind, crossover study. *Diabetes* 1996;45:28A#98.
54. Tanenberg RJ. Candidate selection. In: *The Insulin Pump Therapy Book: Insights from the Experts.* Fredrickson L (ed). Sylmar, CA: MiniMed, Inc.; 1995:21-30.

Gestational Diabetes

Robin M. Clemons, MD

Gestational diabetes is defined as a carbohydrate intolerance of variable severity with onset or first recognition during pregnancy.[1-4] It is an asymptomatic state.[5] This definition includes patients who had diabetes but who weren't previously screened or diagnosed. Diabetes also can be pre-existing or pregestational.[6] There is type 1 (formerly known as insulin-dependent diabetes mellitus), and type 2 (noninsulin-dependent diabetes mellitus).[6] About 90% of pregnancies complicated by diabetes fall into the category of gestational diabetes.[7]

The prevalence of gestational diabetes mellitus ranges from 1.4% to 12.3% in the United States, depending on the population being studied.[1,7-10] The incidence of type 1 diabetes in pregnancy is 0.2%, and type 2 diabetes in pregnancy is 0.3%.[1,8]

Risk factors that influence the frequency of gestational diabetes include increasing maternal age (> 30); maternal obesity (> 90 kg or 200 lbs); a family history of either type 1, type 2, or gestational diabetes; and race/ethnicity (particularly Latinos, Native Americans, Indians, and southeast Asians).[11] *(Please see Table 1.)* Other risk factors include multiparity, and having an abnormal history in previous pregnancies of problems such as macrosomia, unexplained fetal demise, congenital anomalies, and multiple spontaneous abortions.[11]

Although most primary care providers do refer their patients with gestational diabetes for management, there are many instances where co-management and management with consultation are the only treatment options. Hence, primary care providers need this information. Management strategies include diet, exercise, and in some cases, insulin therapy.

Morbidity of Gestational Diabetes

Gestational diabetes is a known risk factor for adverse pregnancy outcomes. Pregnancies complicated with gestational diabetes have an increased risk of maternal and perinatal complications, long-term maternal morbidity, and morbidity to the offspring. Perinatal morbidity and mortality are higher in pregnancies complicated by gestational diabetes. Although the rate of congenital defects is high in patients with pregestational diabetes, in pregnancies complicated by gestational diabetes the rate of congenital defects appears to be similar to the normal pregnant population.[1] This has been hypostulated to be secondary to women with gestational diabetes having normal glucose tolerance during the first trimester when important organogenesis occurs in the fetus.

The causes of perinatal morbidity are neonatal hypoglycemia, hyperbilirubinemia, hypocalcemia, polycythemia, macrosomia, birth weight more than 9 lbs (or 4 kg), and with that the problem shoulder dystocia, an abnormal apgar score, and Erb's palsy (please see Table 2).[1]

Table 1. Risk Factors for Gestational Diabetes

- Maternal age older than 30 years
- Pregravid weight more than 90 kg
- Family history of diabetes
- Race
- Multiparity
- Macrosomia

Table 2. Causes of Perinatal Morbidity

- Neonatal hypoglycemia
- Hyperbilirubinemia
- Hypocalcemia
- Polycythemia
- Macrosomia
- Shoulder dystocia
- Abnormal APGAR
- Erb's palsy

The causes of maternal morbidity in pregnancies complicated by gestational diabetes are an increased rate of c-section, and with it increased complications from that procedure such as postpartum endometritis, pain, postpartum hemorrhage, and an increased number of days off work.[12] *(Please see Table 3.)* In addition, there has been a correlation with an increased incidence of pre-eclampsia and hypertensive disorders, as well as polyhydramnios.[11,12]

Long-term studies of patients with gestational diabetes show that these women are at risk of developing type 2 diabetes later in life.[11,12] O'Sullivan, in a 20-year follow-up study, showed that 40% of women diagnosed with gestational diabetes develop type 2 diabetes mellitus.[14] Other studies of patients carried out for five years postpartum by Mestman found an incidence of 55% of these women developing diabetes. In another study carried out 15 years after the diagnosis of gestational diabetes, the incidence went up to 60%.[15]

There are some exciting studies on long-term follow-up of the offspring of these mothers, particularly looking at the development of diabetes, hypertension, and obesity in these children, their neuropsychological development, and correlating these data with the degree of maternal glycemic control and lipid metabolism.[6,16] It appears that childhood obesity, higher blood pressure, glucose intolerance, and lower than expected intellectual and psychomotor development are related to the metabolic control of diabetes in both gestational and pregestational diabetics during pregnancy.[16]

Determinants of Gestational Diabetes

The causes of this condition are believed to be multifactorial. In normal nonobese women, pregnancy produces a greater than normal sensitivity to insulin during the first trimester in comparison to the second and third.[2,17] Other studies confirmed these findings and, in addition, showed an increase in insulin secretion during glucose tolerance testing. This may be due to hormonal factors such as increased plasma estrogen levels.[2,17] Increased insulin with normal to increased tissue sensitivity produces increased lipogenesis.[2] Other hormonal changes that are known to occur during early pregnancy include increases in serum cortisol and progestins, which, in addition to estrogen, encourage fat accumulation.[2] This could be a preparation for the increased energy needs of the second and third trimesters.[2]

Later in pregnancy the situation changes. Fetal growth is accelerated. The hormonal milieu changes so that human chorionic somatomammotropin (fetal placental lactogen) increases and, along with it, the tissue response to insulin decreases.[2] Although insulin output has been shown to increase from hepatic tissue, insulin resistance increases as much as 50% in muscle tissue.[2] These changes could be due to increases in prolactin, human chorionic somatomammotropin, cortisol, progesterone, estrogen, and the hyperplasia of pancreatic islet cells that occurs during late pregnancy.[2,17,18] This, along with proliferating nutrition demands by increasing fetal growth, leads to the continuous withdrawal of nutrients from the maternal circulation.[2]

In summary, the hormonal changes in early and late pregnancy are designed to provide a constant supply of glucose for the fetus.

Because of increased fetal needs, gluconeogenesis needs to be enhanced during late pregnancy. This cannot be fueled by protein stores from muscle, as they are low in the maternal circulation during this time.[2] So, gluconeogenesis is fueled by fat metabolism.[2]

Metabolic, islet cell, and hormonal changes during pregnancy, age, race/ethnicity, body habitus, plus genetically determined insulin resistance combine to produce gestational diabetes.[2,17] Insulin resistance, insulin secretion, and hyperglycemia are all increased in the second and third trimesters in gestational diabetes when compared to normal pregnant women.[2] Increases in serum glucose develop from hepatic glucose production (gluconeogenesis) as well as peripheral insulin resistance.[2]

Islet cell antibodies may play a role in the development of this condition. In a study from Spain, women diagnosed as having gestational diabetes were more likely to have islet cell antibodies (13%) than women from the general population. This subset of women also were at greater risk of developing type 1 diabetes later in life.[17,19]

Also, there are certain nutrients needed to facilitate pancreatic function, which can become depleted during pregnancy. Chromium, magnesium, potassium, and pyridoxine help to preserve pancreatic function and increase insulin sensitivity. Supplementation of these nutrients as a means of reduction of symptoms, treatment, or prevention of gestational diabetes needs to be analyzed in large-scale studies.[20]

Diagnosis of Gestational Diabetes

There are no internationally accepted criteria for diagnosing gestational diabetes mellitus. The diagnosis of gestational diabetes

Table 3. Causes of Maternal Morbidity

- NIDDM
- C-Section
- Complications from instrumented deliveries

Table 4. Screening for Gestational Diabetes

- One-hour glucola
- Patients do not have to be fasting
- One screening should be performed between 24 and 28 weeks
- Patients are given 50 g of glucose orally
- A blood glucose is drawn at one hour
- A blood sugar of 140 mg/dL or greater is considered positive

Note: It may be beneficial to screen high-risk women earlier in pregnancy

is usually accomplished early in the third trimester of pregnancy. This is because the problem is not easily diagnosed before the 24th week of gestation. The data in the figure are from a study on 84 pregnant diabetic women.[15] Their amniotic fluid was analyzed for insulin content from 16-40 weeks of gestation. The insulin content of the amniotic fluid started to increase between the 24th and 28th weeks of gestation. From these data, it is apparent that the carbohydrate intolerance or insulin resistance worsens around 24-28 weeks.[15]

A number of organizations offer differing recommendations on how to diagnose gestational diabetes. In the United States we use the one-hour glucola test as a screening test (please see table 4).

Nonfasting women are given 50 grams of glucose in a flavored solution, and their blood is taken one hour after ingestion. If the blood sugar equals or exceeds 140 mg/dL, then women are asked to take a three-hour glucose tolerance test (GTT) (please see Tables 5 and 6).[4]

For the three-hour GTT, women are advised to consume an unrestricted diet containing at least 150 grams of carbohydrates daily three days prior to testing. They are asked to fast for 10-14 hours prior to testing. All tests are performed in the morning. Women are asked to refrain from activity during the test, and not to smoke. Blood is drawn fasting and at 1, 2, and 3 hours postingestion of a 100-gram glucose-containing solution. If any two (out of 4) or more results are abnormal, then they are diagnosed as having gestational diabetes (please see table 5).[4]

The importance of the three days of unrestricted diet has to be stressed. Starvation has been shown to produce a decreased tolerance to glucose in studies that demonstrated this in human and animal subjects.[21,22,23] These subjects were given a three-hour GTT

Figure. Amniotic-Fluid Insulin Content

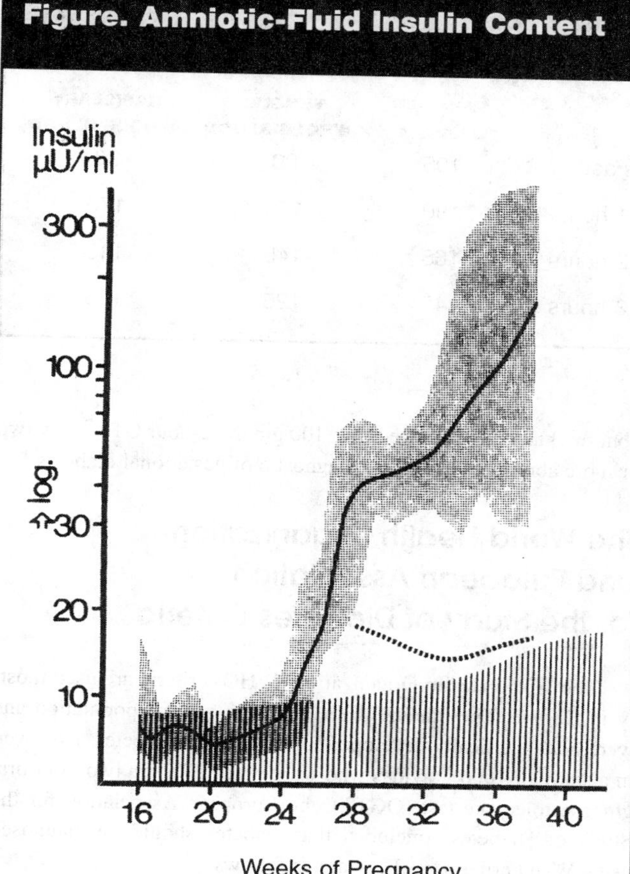

Amniotic-fluid insulin content in 84 diabetic women (White-Class A-R) during conventional insulin therapy. Solid line: mean, dotted area: zone of dispersion; hatched zone: normal range of the amniotic-fluid insulin content between the 3rd and 97th percentile (Weiss et al, 1984). Broken line: mean amniotic-fluid insulin content in 91 metabolically healthy women during tocolytic therapy (ritodrine).

Reprinted with permission from: Weiss PAM, Coustan DR, (eds). *Gestational Diabetes*. New York, NY: Springer Verlag; 1988.

after receiving diets low in carbohydrates. Then, after they were given a 150-mg carbohydrate diet daily for four or five days, the test was repeated. When the individual test results were compared, the low carbohydrate diet impaired glucose tolerance to diagnostic levels. More patients had abnormal tests after starvation, which subsequently improved on refeeding.[21,23]

The following are the criteria for diagnosis of gestational diabetes and the organizations that recommend them.

ADA and ACOG Criteria

Screening of pregnant women at 24-28 weeks gestation with a 50 gm one-hour glucose screening test (1-hour glucola).[3,24] Values of 140 mg/dL (7.8 mmol/L) or greater are considered abnormal. All

Table 5. Three-Hour Glucose Tolerance Test

	VENOUS PLASMA	VENOUS WHOLE BLOOD	CAPILLARY WHOLE BLOOD
Fasting	105	90	90
1 hour	190	170	170
2 hours	165	145	145
3 hours	145	125	125

abnormal tests are followed by a 100 gm three-hour GTT.[3] Any two or more abnormal values are diagnostic of gestational diabetes.[3]

The World Health Organization and European Association for the Study of Diabetes Criteria

The World Health Organization (WHO) criteria are used mostly in Europe. They define diabetes in the general population and were not specifically developed for gestational diabetes. However, in a study of 1000 gravidas who were given a 75 gm two-hour oral glucose tolerance test (OGTT), the European Association for the Study of Diabetes concluded that diabetes should be diagnosed using WHO criteria.[4,17] They are as follows:

The patient is given a 75 gm OGTT. Venous blood is then sampled at one and two hours after ingestion. A fasting blood sugar of 140 mg/dL (7.8 mmol/L) or a two-hour postprandial blood sugar of 200 mg/dL (11.1 mmol/L) is diagnostic of gestational diabetes.

National Diabetes Data Group Criteria

The National Diabetes Data Group criteria are based on the patient receiving a 100 gm three-hour GTT.[3] Results are derived from plasma or serum glucose determined by the glucose oxidase method. They are as follows:[3,4]

Fasting	5.83 mmol/L	(105 mg/dL)
1 hour	10.56 mmol/L	(190 mg/dL)
2 hour	9.17 mmol/L	(165 mg/dL)
3 hour	8.06 mmol/L	(145 mg/dL)

Any two or more abnormal results are diagnostic of gestational diabetes.

Management

The goal of management in this condition is to reduce perinatal morbidity and mortality through controlling the blood sugar level of the prenatal patient with gestational diabetes. Management of gestational diabetes is best accomplished using a team approach. This team could consist of physicians (obstetrician, endocrinologist, perinatologist), diabetes educators, nutritionists, nurses, midwives, or nurse practitioners and, in some cases, a pharmacist.[25]

When patients are first told that they may have gestational diabetes they may experience some denial; others avoid further testing as a way of postponing or avoiding what they consider obnoxious treatments. A team approach can help these patients accept their diagnosis and receive treatment promptly (just because they hear the information from more than one authoritative source).

Table 6. Three-Hour Glucose Tolerance Test

- The patient should have an unrestricted diet of at least 150 g of carbohydrates for three days preceding the test
- Test in the morning
- Fast for 10-14 hours before the test
- Patients are seated (and not smoking) during the test
- A blood glucose is drawn fasting, at 1 hour, at 2 hours, and at 3 hours

Patient Education

Educating the patient about her condition and its management, without alarming her, can go a long way to improve compliance. Your patient needs to understand what gestational diabetes is, and why it is important to her and her baby's health. She needs to understand what the dietary and exercise recommendations are, and how to implement these into her daily life. She also needs to know how to perform glucose monitoring, when to check her blood sugar, as well as when and how these results should be communicated to you. She also may need to learn how to give herself insulin injections, how to prevent hyper- and hypoglycemia, and what to do should these problems occur.[25] Organizations such as the March of Dimes, ACOG, AAFP, and the ADA have produced patient education materials that you may wish to review for your patient's use.

Dietary Management

There is a great deal of controversy about what constitutes the ideal diet for women with gestational diabetes. The number of calories and the composition of these calories into macronutrients such as percentage of protein, percentage of carbohydrate, and percentage of fat are described in Tables 7 and 8. However, how many meals per day and how many snacks per day that these calories should be optimally divided into to promote euglycemia and prevent the complications of gestational diabetes has yet to be determined.

There is some evidence that having your patient consume some calories on an hourly basis can lead to her needing less insulin over 24 hours (thereby decreasing insulin resistance).[2] Your patient will probably appreciate this in late pregnancy, when her stomach capacity is diminished and there is decreased gastric emptying due to the enlarging uterus.[7] However, the long-term studies to demonstrate that this dietary plan leads to fewer complications for the mother and infant have yet to be accomplished. What seems better tolerated by patients is a meal schedule that looks somewhat like the one they use in the nonpregnant state, which would consist of

Table 7. Nutrients

Carbohydrates	38-45%
Protein	20-25%
Fat	30-40%

three meals a day with one or two snacks interspersed as well as a snack after dinner.[27]

Nutritional goals are to achieve normal blood sugar levels while providing adequate caloric intake for normal growth and development, without hyperglycemia or ketonemia.[26] This is best done by consulting a nutritionist who is familiar with the patient's cultural (and culinary) milieu.[28,29] Goal attainment is monitored by glucose monitoring, following the patient's pattern of weight gain, as well as dietary reassesment in order to determine if the nutritional needs of pregnancy are being met.[13,28]

Specific dietary prescriptions depend on the patient's pre-pregnancy weight (whether she is under, normal, or overweight), her height, activity level, as well as her individual dietary and exercise habits.[13,28] It is a good idea to have your patient start a diet diary prior to seeing the nutritionist (if this does not delay therapy).

Initial dietary recommendation should consist of a dietary intake of 35 kcal/kg of ideal body weight for most nonunderweight, nonobese patients (please see Table 8).[7,29] It is not recommended that obese patients lose weight during pregnancy; however, excessive weight gain should be avoided. Generally a diet consisting of complex carbohydrates (as opposed to simple sugars), soluble fiber, low in fat, while reduced in saturated fats, is recommended.[1,12,30] Other researchers state that because gestational diabetes is a short-term disease, restriction of fats and protein to prevent long-term heart and kidney complications (as we do in treatment of diabetes in the nonpregnant population) is unnecessary.[7]

Although the proportion of nutrients remains controversial, one consistent recommendation is to limit carbohydrates during the morning meal because glucose tolerance is diminished in the early morning hours.[7,29] Control of blood sugar in gestational diabetes is correlated to the percentage of calories from carbohydrates ingested.[1] A handout for your patients describing dietary recommendations for this condition is found at the end of this chapter.

Exercise Management

Nonweight-bearing aerobic exercise is recommended for pregnant diabetics. The activity should be one that the patient enjoys, such as walking, bicycling, or swimming. It should be gradually added to your patient's schedule, starting slowly for 5-10 minutes a session, and gradually increased in length. Each session is preceded with a 5-10 minute warm-up and ended with a 5-10 minute cool-down period. During the warm-up and cool-down periods, the patient should perform slow aerobic activity such as strolling or walking. Slow movements, such as pedaling slowly for bicycling or gliding for swimming activities, also are acceptable. The cool-down period is usually ended with stretching the muscles in long, slow movements.

The theory behind exercise therapy is that it uses the glucose, controls weight gain, alters hyperlipidemia, and alters the tissue sensitivity to endogenous insulin.[7,9] Exercise also has important psychological benefits as well.[7]

The ideal exercise goals for women with gestational diabetes have not yet been determined. How much of what activities, to what intensity, for what length of time that will normalize blood glucose and reduce macrosomia, without leading to hypoglycemic events, is still being studied.

The controversy regarding exercise in pregnancy concerns possible fetal distress as measured by fetal heart rate, maternal uterine activity and blood flow, and infant birth weight.[1]

However, since exercise is recommended for diabetic control in the nonpregnant state and has been shown to decrease tissue insulin resistance, the current recommendation is to not discourage currently active women. Regular cardiovascular exercise should be continued (as opposed to sporadic exercise activities), as long as these activities are not contraindicated (please see Table 9).[13,39,40] Activities studied in pregnant diabetics in the past are recumbent bicycling and arm ergometer training.[9,28]

Participation in aerobic activities three to four days per week for 15-30 minutes per session may be beneficial. Intensity should

Table 8. Energy Requirements

PREGRAVID WEIGHT CATEGORY	% IDEAL BODY WEIGHT	PREGRAVID BODY MASS INDEX	RECOMMENDED KCAL/KG	RECOMMENDED WEIGHT GAIN
Underweight	< 80%	< 19.8	35-40	28-40 lbs
Normal weight	80-120%	19.8-26	30-35	25-35 lbs
Overweight	121-150%	26-29	25-35	15-25 lbs
Obese	> 151%	> 29	25-35	at least 15 lbs

Reprinted with permission from: the National Academy of Sciences. *Nutrition During Pregnancy.* Washington, DC: National Academy Press; 1990.

Table 9. Contraindications for Exercise in Pregnancy

- Placenta previa
- Risk of premature labor
- Vaginal bleeding during pregnancy
- Pregnancy induced hypertension
- Incompetent cervix/cerclage
- Intrauterine growth retardation
- Malpresentation in the third trimester
- Pulmonary disease
- Cardiac disease
- Thyroid disease
- Vascular disease

Adapted from: Artal R. Exercise: An alternative therapy for gestational diabetes. *Phys Sportsmed* 1996;24. http://www.physsportsmed.com/issues/mar_96/artal.htm.

be monitored by having the patient take her pulse frequently. This should not exceed 70-80% of her maximal heart rate adjusted for her age (target heart rate = [220 - age] × 70%).[27] This will be between 130-150 for most prenatal patients.

Insulin and Other Medications

The criteria for insulin therapy are failure of dietary and exercise management. If the fasting blood sugar is greater than 95, if the one-hour postprandial blood sugar is equal to or greater than 140, or if the two-hour postprandial blood sugar is equal to or greater than 120, then the patient needs tighter control of the blood sugar.

Human insulin is the drug of choice for treatment of gestational or pregestational diabetes.[7,29] Oral hypoglycemic agents have been contraindicated for use in pregnancy due to possible teratogenic effects and prolonged fetal hyperinsulinemia.[10] Insulin dosing of 0.7-1.0 U/kg, depending on the patient's week of gestation (longer gestation usually requiring the higher dose), also is commonly recommended.[10,27] Your patient may require multiple doses of short-acting or regular insulin before meals, or a combination of long-acting NPH with regular insulin.[10,29] Insulin doses are adjusted frequently to achieve treatment goals (please see Table 10). An evening dose of long-acting NPH may be helpful for persistent fasting hyperglycemia.

Glycosylated Hemoglobin

HbA_1C, or glycosylated hemoglobin levels, have not been useful in following gestational diabetics.[8] This is probably due to the level of control necessary to prevent complications of gestational diabetes, which differs from the control in nonpregnant diabetics.[8]

Other reasons include that the normal level for fasting blood sugar as well as postprandial blood sugar are different than in nonpregnancy diabetics (fasting values are lower in the pregnant state).[8] There is increased erythropoesis in pregnancy that also changes glycosylated hemoglobin values.[8] Apparently the glucose impairment from gestational diabetes happens only during a short period (24 weeks gestation and beyond), making a two- to three-month average in HbA_1C less practical.[8]

Blood Glucose Monitoring

In gestational diabetes the blood sugar should be checked at least four times daily.[1] Patients should be encouraged to obtain and taught to use a home glucometer. The fasting blood sugar should not exceed 95 mg/dL and the two-hour postprandial blood sugar should not exceed 120 mg/dL.[1,31]

Home blood glucose monitoring, even in diet-controlled patients, can be advantageous because it makes our patients more mindful of the effect of their behavior on their blood sugar, thereby improving compliance with nonpharmacologic recommendations for glucose control.[26] This gives you, the provider, a clear look into the patient's level of glucose control over the past 24 hours, and allows you to make adjustments in diet, exercise, or medication as necessary to keep control of blood sugar as tight as possible.[26]

Fetal Surveillance

Controversy surrounds when testing for fetal well-being should commence. Some recommend as early as 28 weeks, others start at 36 weeks.[31] Some recommend starting at the earlier date in diabetics with poor control or those with co-morbidities such as vascular or hypertensive disease, or a history of previous stillbirth.[25] In a meta-analysis looking at the effectiveness of fetal surveillance in predicting adverse outcomes in diabetic pregnancies, Fuentes and Chez concluded that there were insufficient data to support a specific time in pregnancy to begin fetal surveillance testing in patients with well-controlled diabetes class A through D without other obstetric complications.[32]

This lack of consensus allows us to use a more flexible, individualized approach to the third trimester evaluation of our patients. It also reflects the uncertainty of scientific evidence that should be shared with the patient. Perinatal complications in diabetic pregnancies can be prevented with a combination of early detection and strict metabolic control.[33] Detecting macrosomia, early induction of labor (based on ultrasonic and clinical estimation of fetal weight), and use of c-section (when induction fails) may help to avoid traumatic birth in these pregnancies.[34] The possibility of c-section should be discussed with your patient and their family early to avoid conflict near the end of gestation or during labor.

Opinions on how to test for fetal well-being also vary. Some do simple kick counts, others nonstress tests, and still others recommend biophysical profiles.

Kick counts, started as early as 28 weeks gestation, are a simple low-tech, inexpensive way of measuring fetal well-being. After experiencing a stillbirth, most mothers recant a history of decreased or absent fetal movement prior to the event. If medical intervention can occur quickly during this period of decreased fetal movement, perhaps this tragic outcome could be prevented. Kick counts are

Table 10. Treatment Goals for Gestational Diabetes Mellitus

TIME	BLOOD SUGAR[1]	BLOOD SUGAR[1]
Fasting	95 mg/dL	< 5.3 mmol/L
1 hr PP[2]	140 mg/dL	< 7.8 mmol/L
2 hr PP	120 mg/dL	< 6.7 mmol/L

[1]Serum
[2]PP = Postprandial

usually done after a meal or snack. Your patient lies on her left side and counts the number of fetal movements over a one-hour period. When she gets to 10 movements or kicks, she has accomplished a reassuring test of fetal well-being (and can now get up and do something else with her time).

Ultrasonography is particularly useful in diagnosing abnormalities in fetal growth (such as macrosomia, intrauterine growth retardation, or polyhydramnios) and may be a useful tool where these conditions are suspected. Scanning the crown rump length in the first trimester can confirm your patient's dates. Other physicians advocate scanning between 16-22 weeks gestation to confirm dates and exclude any major congenital malformations (thereby eliminating doing 2).[10,30]

Fetal ultrasonography used in the third trimester can give you an estimated fetal weight and allow measurement of the abdominal circumference. Abdominal circumference below the 90th percentile for gestational age between 29-33 weeks gestation has been correlated with a less than 5% risk of delivering a large for gestational age (LGA) infant in patients with good dietary control.[35]

A maternal serum alpha-fetal protein level is important at 16-18 weeks because of the increased incidence of open neural tube defects in diabetic pregnancies.[10]

Nonstress testing is also used to evaluate fetal well-being of pregestational or gestational diabetic pregnancies. The antepartum fetal heart rate is monitored in response to spontaneous contractions, noise, and cervical stimulation. Two accelerations of the heart rate from the baseline over a 20-minute period of monitoring is a favorable response.[10]

Biophysical profiles are helpful because they combine ultrasonography with nonstress testing. This allows evaluation of amniotic fluid volume as well as abnormalities in fetal growth or development that may have gone undetected earlier in pregnancy.[10] A score is derived from observing fetal activity, tone, breathing, and amniotic fluid. A score of 8 or above is reassuring.

Labor and Delivery

Timing of delivery is important. Delivery before term can lead to respiratory distress syndrome in the newborn, and should be avoided. Delivery after 38 weeks increases the probability of the infant developing macrosomia. Unless the pregnancy is complicated by macrosomia, polyhydramnios, poor control of diabetes, or other obstetrical indications (such as pre-eclampsia or intrauterine growth retardation), delivery at term is recommended.[25]

The policy of premature delivery in women with diabetes developed because of the association of gestational diabetes and late fetal demise. Current studies performed on women with pregestational and gestational diabetes have shown that the critical factor in deciding the timing of delivery was the degree of diabetic control (macrosomia and polyhydramnios being indicators of suboptimal control).[6] Your patients with gestational diabetes can be allowed to deliver at term without increased perinatal and maternal risk, provided that the diabetes is well controlled, intensive fetal surveillance is reassuring, and there are no other obstetric indications for early delivery.

If delivery is decided on prior to 38 weeks, the need for amniocentesis to evaluate lung maturity will depend on the urgency for delivery. A lecithin to sphingomyelin (L/S) ratio of 2 or greater along with the presence of phosphatidylglycerol is what is recommended as being indicative of lung maturity for elective delivery before 38 weeks.[6,30] After 38 weeks, if your patient has good dates and had a first or second trimester ultrasound that confirms the gestational age, an amniocentesis does not need to be performed.

With good diabetic control and no other obstetric complications, your patient with gestational diabetes should be able to continue her pregnancy to term, and may be able to avoid c-section. There is some evidence that prolonging pregnancy beyond 40 weeks may be detrimental.[30]

Inform your patient of the benefits of induction if she does not spontaneously go into labor between 39 and 40 weeks.[31] At 40 weeks if her cervix is unfavorable, prostaglandin agents may be necessary to help ripen her cervix.[31]

Diabetes management during labor requires good control of blood sugar while avoiding hypoglycemia. Commonly your patient in labor is only taking in liquids, yet using energy during labor. Because of this, her insulin requirements are diminished. Many patients require no insulin during labor.[31] Blood sugar should be checked every 1-2 hours during labor.[24,31] Dextrose will need to be given intravenously if your patient's blood sugar falls below 70 mg/dL (4.0 mmol/L). Short-acting regular insulin may need to be given intravenously for blood sugars rising above 140 mg/dL (7.8 mmol/L).[31]

Fetal monitoring should be performed as well as fetal blood sampling if indicated.[30] You may want the extra skill of a neonatologist or pediatrician to help with neonatal resuscitation if necessary.[25]

Postpartum Care

Insulin requirements decrease after the placenta has been delivered. If the patient was on an insulin infusion during labor the dose should be cut in half at this time. Also, breast feeding may reduce your patient's insulin requirements by 25%.[30] For patients with pregestational diabetes you can reinstitute the prepregnancy insulin dose as the patient is able to eat. Your patient needs the additional caloric requirements of breast feeding to be included in her diet postpartum, as hypoglycemia decreases milk production.[31]

It is important to stress the long-term complications of gestational diabetes with your patients. They need to know the importance of proper diet (low in concentrated sweets, high in fiber), exercise, controlling their weight, and controlling their lipids in prevention or delaying the onset of type 2 diabetes, as well as reducing cardiovascular risk in the future.[5,6,26] Your patients also need to be educated about the symptoms of diabetes so that they can present themselves for screening and treatment early.[36] Some authors recommend routine screening of postpartum women for diabetes at six weeks and at regular intervals (every 2 years in low-risk patients).[25,36,37]

Although your patients are probably counseled on birth control options during prenatal visits, postpartum is the time when these plans are implemented. Barrier methods are good alternatives for motivated couples, but may not be well suited to the lifestyles of the majority of your patients.[37] Intrauterine devices can be used by your patient using the same indications and precautions as you would in other individuals (parous women in monogamous, stable relationships).[37] Oral contraceptives tend to decrease insulin sensitivity and compromise insulin secretion in women with a history of gestational diabetes.[37] However, subsequent pregnancy in women with a prior history of gestational diabetes also increases the risk of developing type 2 diabetes.[5] The progesterone-only pill has no significant effect on carbohydrate or lipid metabolism and can be used during breast feeding and beyond.[30] You may want to advise your patients who desire to use combination oral contraceptives of the increased risk of cardiovascular complications in women older than 35 years of age with a history of smoking, hypertension, or other vascular disease.[2,37]

Your patient also should know that having gestational diabetes in one pregnancy is a risk factor for the development of this condition in subsequent pregnancies. She needs to understand the benefits of preconceptional counseling and early prenatal care for her future pregnancies.[31] It could even be stated that preconceptional counseling for subsequent pregnancies should begin in the postpartum period.[37] Since a prepregnancy weight of more than 90 kg is not only a risk factor for gestational diabetes, but for macrosomia as well, it is important to stress the continued importance of diet and exercise for the health of your patient, and the well-being of any future pregnancies.[38]

Management of the Newborn

Infants born from pregnancies complicated by gestational diabetes can have the complications of infants of mothers with pregestational diabetes. They need to have their blood glucose monitored for hypoglycemia. Also, you will want to evaluate their blood count for polycythemia and its accompanying problem of hyperbilirubinemia. These newborns need to be observed closely for respiratory distress. If the neonates are macrosomic (> 4000 g), they need to have their calcium and magnesium levels checked.

Breast feeding should be encouraged; babies should be offered the breast within their first hours of life.[25,30] This can be difficult in the setting of cesarean section, separation from the mother for frequent examination and testing, as well as possible dietary supplementation for hypoglycemia.[30] Antenatal breast feeding education, support, and counseling should help your patients get over this period of initial discouragement.[30]

Conclusion

Gestational diabetes is defined as carbohydrate intolerance of variable severity with onset or first recognition during pregnancy. It has serious perinatal and maternal consequences and multiple risk factors. Universal screening for gestational diabetes mellitus with a 50 gm glucose challenge test (or 1-hour glucola) is recommended for all pregnant women between 24 and 28 weeks gestation. A result greater than or equal to 140 is abnormal. Patients with abnormal results should have a three-hour GTT performed. If any two values are abnormal, the diagnosis of gestational diabetes is made.

Management of gestational diabetes is best accomplished using a team approach. Diet therapy is the mainstay of treatment. Ideally, the blood sugar should be checked at least four times daily to monitor treatment goals. The fasting blood sugar should not exceed 95mg/dL and the two-hour postprandial blood sugar should not exceed 120 mg/dL. Insulin therapy should be instituted in a timely manner for patients who are not controlled with diet and/or exercise.

References

1. Bevier WC, et al. Pancreatic disorders of pregnancy. Diagnosis, management, and outcome of gestational diabetes. *Endocrinol Metab Clin North Am* 1995;24: 103-138.
2. Boden G. Fuel metabolism in pregnancy and in gestational diabetes mellitus. *Obstet Gynecol Clin North Am* 1996; 23:1-10.
3. Coustan DR. Screening and testing for gestational diabetes mellitus. *Obstet Gynecol Clin North Am* 1996;23:125-136.
4. Coustan DR, Carpenter MW. The diagnosis of gestational diabetes. *Diabetes Care* 1998;21(S2):B5-8.
5. Kjos SL, et al. Hormonal choices after gestational diabetes. Subsequent pregnancy, contraception, and hormone replacement. *Diabetes Care* 1998;21(S2):B50-B57.
6. Oats JN. Diabetes. *Baillieres Clin Obstet Gynaecol* 1995; 9(3):481-495.
7. Sullivan BA, et al. Gestational diabetes. *J Am Pharm Assoc* 1998;38:364-373.
8. Homko CJ, Khandelwal M. Glucose monitoring and insulin therapy during pregnancy. *Obstet Gynecol Clin North Am* 1996; 23:47-74.
9. Bung P, Artal R. Gestational diabetes and exercise: A survey. *Semin Perinatol* 1996;20:328-333.
10. Homko CJ, Reece EA. Ambulatory care of the pregnant woman with diabetes. *Clin Obstet Gynecol* 1998;41: 584-596.
11. Johnston DG, et al. Aspects of metabolism in normal and gestational diabetic pregnancy. *Biochem Soc Trans* 1995; 2(S):512-516.
12. Weller KA. Diagnosis and management of gestational diabetes. *Am Fam Physician* 1997;55(5):2053-2057; 2061-2062.
13. Fagen C, et al. Nutritional management in women with gestational diabetes: A review by ADA's diabetes care and education dietetic practice group. *J Am Diet Assoc* 1995; 95:460-467.
14. O'Sullivan JB. Diabetes mellitus after GDM. *Diabetes* 1991;40(2S):131-135.
15. Mestman JH. Follow-up studies in women with gestational diabetes mellitus. The experience at Los Angeles

County/University of Southern California Medical Center. In: Weiss PAM, Coustan DR, eds. *Gestational Diabetes.* New York, NY: Springer Verlag; 1988:191-198.
16. Silverman BL, et al. Long-term effects of the intrauterine environment. *Diabetes Care* 1998;21(S2):B142-B149.
17. Linn T, Bretzel RG. Diabetes in pregnancy. *Eur J Obstet Gynecol Reprod Biol* 1997;75:37-41.
18. Jovanovic L. American Diabetes Association's fourth international workshop—Conference on gestational diabetes mellitus: Summary and discussion. *Diabetes Care* 1998; 21(2S):B131-B137.
19. Mauricio D, et al. Islet cell autoimmunity in women with gestational diabetes and risk of progression to insulin-dependent diabetes mellitus. *Diabetes Metab Rev* 1996; 12:275-285.
20. Jovanovic-Peterson L, Petterson CM.Vitamin and mineral deficiencies which may predispose to glucose intolerance of pregnancy. *J Am Coll Nutr* 1996;15:14-20.
21. Wilkerson H, et al. The effect of prior carbohydrate intake on the oral glucose tolerance test. *Diabetes* 1960;9:386-391.
22. Fujita Y, et al. Influence of antecedent carbohydrate intake on the biphasic insulin response to intravenous glucose. *Diabetes* 1975;24:1072-1080.
23. Conn JW. Interpretation of the glucose tolerance test. The necessity of a standard preparatory diet. *Am J Med Sci* 1940;199:555-564.
24. American College of Obstetrics and Gynecology Diabetes and Pregnancy. Technical bulletin no. 200. ACOG Washington, DC; 1994:200.
25. Hoffman L, et al. Gestational diabetes mellitus-management guidelines. *Med J Aust* 1998;169:93-97.
26. Gunderson EP. Intensive nutrition therapy for gestational diabetes. *Diabetes Care* 1997;20:221-226.
27. Jovanovic-Peterson L, Peterson CM. Review of gestational diabetes mellitus and low-calorie diet and physical exercise as therapy. *Diabetes Metab Rev* 1996;12:287-308.
28. Langer O, Hod M. Management of gestational diabetes mellitus. *Obstet Gynecol Clin North Am* 1996;23:137-159.
29. Davidson JA, Roberts VL. Gestational diabetes: Ensuring a successful outcome. *Postgrad Med* 1996;99:165-172.
30. Brown CJ, et al. Report of the pregnancy and neonatal care group. *Diabet Med* 1996;13:S43-S53.
31. Pasuai K, McFarland KF. Management of diabetes in pregnancy. *Am Fam Phys* 1997;55:2731-2738, 2742-2744.
32. Fuentes A, Chez RA. Role of fetal surveillance in diabetic pregnancies. *J Matern Fetal Med* 1996;5:85-88.
33. Langer O. Maternal glycemic criteria for insulin therapy in gestational diabetes mellitus. *Diabetes Care* 1998;21(2S): B91-B98.
34. Hod M, et al. Antepartum management protocol. Timing and mode of delivery in gestational diabetes. *Diabetes Care* 1998; 21(S2):B113-B117.
35. Buchanan TA, et al. Utility of fetal measurements in the management of gestational diabetes mellitus. *Diabetes Care* 1998; 21(S2):B99-B106.
36. Dornhorst A, Rossi M. Risk and prevention of type 2 diabetes in women with gestational diabetes. *Diabetes Care* 1998;21(S2): B43-B49.
37. Petersen KR, et al. Contraception guidance in women with pre-existing disturbances in carbohydrate metabolism. *Euro J Concep Reprod Health Care* 1996;1:53-59.
38. Catalano PM, et al. Effect of maternal metabolism on fetal growth and body composition. *Diabetes Care* 1998;21: B85-B90.
39. American College of Obstetrics and Gynecology. Exercise during pregnancy and the postpartum period. Technical bulletin no. 189. ACOG. Washington DC; 1994:189.
40. Artal R. Exercise: An alternative therapy for gestational diabetes. *Phys Sportsmed* 1996;24. http://www.physsportsmed.com/issues/ mar_96/artal.htm.
41. Jovanovic-Peterson L, ed. *Medical Management of Pregnancy Complicated by Diabetes*. 2nd ed. Alexandria, VA: American Diabetes Association; 1995.

Pericardial Disease

Gary D. Hals MD, PhD
Steven C. Carleton, MD, PhD

"There's a patient in the resuscitation room with chest pain." This statement is made daily in virtually every emergency department (ED) in the country, and the classic six life-threatening causes of chest pain (myocardial infarction [MI], unstable angina, aortic dissection, tension pneumothorax, pericarditis with tamponade, and pulmonary embolus) typically run through the emergency physician's mind. Pericarditis with tamponade is probably one of the least commonly encountered entities on this list and one of the more difficult to diagnose. There are several reasons for this. Cardiac tamponade results from pericardial effusion, and patients with pericardial effusion may have acute chest pain and dyspnea, or they may be asymptomatic. Cardiac tamponade may arise acutely from penetrating chest trauma, as a sudden complication of cardiac surgery (1.9% incidence in one series), or as a complication of pericarditis.[1] Since pericardial diseases are much less common than heart disease from coronary artery disease, hypertension, or valvular disorders, nontraumatic tamponade often is not recognized or is considered and treated too late. The oft-quoted Sir William Osler's statement still applies today: "Probably no serious disease is so frequently overlooked by the practitioner. Postmortem experience shows how often pericarditis is not recognized, or goes on to resolution and adhesion without attracting notice." [2]

Pericardial disease has a wide spectrum of manifestations, from occult to life-threatening. Its causes are equally diverse, ranging from infection, trauma, malignancy, and drug reactions to iatrogenic. It can appear in conjunction with myocarditis or as a complication of myocardial infarction, thoracic surgery, renal failure, or connective tissue diseases. The chest pain and electrocardiogram (ECG) changes associated with acute pericarditis may be misdiagnosed as acute MI. This can result in serious complications (i.e., hemorrhagic pericardial effusion progressing to tamponade after thrombolytic therapy). Constrictive pericarditis presents in a similar fashion to congestive heart failure (CHF), but treatment for CHF will worsen symptoms associated with constrictive pericarditis. For all these reasons, the ED management of pericardial diseases is especially challenging.

This chapter discusses the common causes of pericardial disease and their management in the ED. Emphasis is placed on differentiating acute pericarditis from ischemic heart disease, and the complication of tamponade is discussed in terms of pathophysiology, diagnosis, and ED treatment options. Finally, constrictive pericarditis will be discussed and contrasted with CHF.

Background

There are three principal manifestations of diseases that affect the pericardium: pericarditis, pericardial effusion, and cardiac tamponade. Pericarditis is the nonspecific term for an inflammatory process involving the pericardium and is rarely a medical emergency. Pericardial effusion signifies accumulation of fluid in the pericardial

Table 1. Pericarditis vs. Ischemia/Infarction: Comparison of Pain Features and ECG Changes

FEATURE	PERICARDITIS	ISCHEMIA/INFARCTION
Pain location	Precordium, left trapezius ridge	Retrosternal, left shoulder, arm
Pain quality	Pleuritic or positional	Pressure, tightness, burning
Thoracic-motion exacerbation	Worse with breathing, rotating thorax	No effect
Duration	Hours to days	Possible history of 1-15 minutes of similar exertional pain
Posture	Leaning forward for relief, worse with recumbency	No effect
Associated symptoms	Shortness of breath, diaphoresis, but typically no nausea or vomiting	Nausea, vomiting, diaphoresis, and shortness of breath
Vital signs	Often febrile	High fever rare
ECG: ST elevation	Diffuse, concave slope	Localized, convex shape
ST changes	No reciprocal changes	Has reciprocal changes
PR segment	Depression pathognomonic	No PR segment depression
Q-T prolongation	Rarely seen in absence of myocarditis	More commonly seen
Evolution	Normalization in Stage 2	Typical MI progression with development of Q waves
Electrical alternans	Present with tamponade	Absent

space; this fluid may be serous, purulent, fibrinous, or hemorrhagic. Patients with effusions require close observation for evidence of tamponade. Cardiac tamponade is a medical emergency that occurs when there is impairment of ventricular filling due to accumulation of pericardial fluid or thickening of the pericardium.

Pericardial Physiology. The normal pericardium is composed of a dense, outer parietal layer, and a thin, visceral layer closely applied to the epicardial surface of the myocardium. The parietal pericardium is attached to the sternum, diaphragm, and mediastinum by fibrous extensions and adventitia. Since the major component of the parietal layer is collagen, it is relatively stiff and inelastic, a contributory feature in the development of tamponade. A potential space exists between the visceral layer and the parietal, the location of fluid in pericardial effusion. Between 15 and 60 mL of fluid are normally contained in the pericardial space.[3] The functions of pericardial fluid may include reduction of friction between the surface of the heart and adjacent structures, prevention of the spread of infection from adjacent thoracic structures, augmentation of atrial filling, and maintenance of normal pressure-volume relationships of the cardiac chambers. Still, no significant hemodynamic consequences are apparent in either surgical removal, or congenital absence, of the pericardium.[4] The pericardium receives parasympathetic innervation via the vagus and left recurrent laryngeal nerves, and sympathetic innervation from the stellate and first thoracic ganglia. There is little direct somatic sensory innervation, which accounts for the visceral nature of chest pain in pericarditis.

Myocardial Ischemia vs. Acute Pericarditis. Some cases of acute pericarditis are nearly impossible to differentiate from ischemic pain in the ED. Both may present with sudden onset of pain with or without shock. Nevertheless, there are several key features of the symptoms, signs, and ECG that bear summary. *(Please see Table 1.)* The most important difference in symptoms is the effect of motion on pain. The pain of pericarditis is typically relieved by sitting forward and aggravated by motions of the chest wall including; lying down, deep breathing, and turning in bed. Ischemic pain often has an exertional component and is typically not related to position. On occasion, however, patients may present with angina decubitus, anginal pain secondary to increased myocardial workload from augmented venous return due to the supine position. Furthermore, pericardial pain may be present continually for days before presentation to the ED. This is seldom the case in myocardial ischemia. While a normal temperature is not useful to distinguish these entities, the presence of fever is more indicative of acute pericarditis. Helpful points on the ECG are a nonanatomic distribution of ST-T wave changes in acute pericarditis, and a lack of reciprocal changes. Upright T waves with ST-segment elevation are seen in pericarditis, while ST-segment elevation is commonly accompanied by T-wave inversion in acute MI. Also, in acute transmural MI, subsequent tracings will evolve into the expected MI pattern with appearance of Q waves.

Pericarditis

Etiology. The causes of pericarditis are numerous and varied, and the actual incidence is unknown. *(Please see Table 2.)* Nearly all forms of pericarditis can occur with or without effusion and can progress to cardiac tamponade or constrictive pericarditis if untreated. Given the various etiologies of pericardial disease, its definitive, causal diagnosis may be daunting. Emergency physicians will generally encounter pericardial disease in one of the following syndromes: viral, bacterial, traumatic, malignant, post-irradiation, post-MI, drug-induced, or secondary to collagen vascular disease. The next sections review each of these categories.

Viral Pericarditis. Viral infection is cited as the most common cause of acute pericarditis in the general population,[5] whether adult or pediatric.[6] Many cases of idiopathic pericarditis also are thought to be viral in origin, but can only be inferentially related to a viral etiology by history.[7] While many viruses can cause acute pericarditis, the principal offenders are the enteroviruses (coxsackie A and B, and echovirus). *(Please see Table 2.)* It is important to note that while AIDS-associated pericarditis often results from mycobacterial infection, it has been shown that HIV infection can affect the pericardium primarily.[7]

Signs and Symptoms. The typical syndrome of viral pericarditis consists of chest pain, a pericardial friction rub, and fever. The syndrome often develops 2-4 weeks after an antecedent influenza-like illness (delayed) but also may occur during the acute viremic stage of the illness (immediate). It remains unclear whether the pathogenesis of viral pericarditis results from direct viral cytotoxicity or indirect antibody-mediated effects. It has been suggested that immediate pericarditis results from direct viral injury, and delayed pericarditis results from antibody-mediated injury.[8]

The chest pain of pericarditis is usually precordial and may radiate to the left trapezius muscle and left scapula. It is classically pleuritic or "sharp" and increases with inspiration. It is relieved by sitting forward and aggravated by rotating the thorax or lying supine. The pain may be of sudden onset and mimic that of myocardial infarction. The patient may present in varying degrees of acute distress, with fever, tachycardia, tachypnea, dyspnea, and diaphoresis. The classic physical finding is a friction rub. The rub is best heard with the diaphragm of the stethoscope over the mid to lower left sternal border, where the least amount of lung tissue intervenes. Having the patient sit forward often increases the rub, and listening with breath held will increase the chance of detection. The rub is often described as "scratchy" and seems closer to the skin than the heart sounds. Although classically the rub is triphasic, consisting of presystolic, systolic, and diastolic components, it may only consist of one or two of these.[9] A rub with only one component is easily confused with various systolic murmurs, and care must be taken to differentiate a two-component rub from the murmur of aortic stenosis with regurgitation. The rub may be inconsistent, vary in intensity and location over time, and its presence may wax and wane during the ED stay. It may disappear as the volume of the pericardial effusion increases, or it may persist despite a large effusion.[10] This suggests that the origin of the rub is more complicated than physical abrasion of the epicardium against the visceral pericardium.

Diagnostic Findings. The ECG in acute viral pericarditis typically shows changes that evolve over a period of 3-4 weeks through four stages (although only about 50% of patients with pericarditis demonstrate all four phases):

Stage 1. Diffuse ST-segment elevation is seen in virtually all leads. *(Please see Figure 1.)* ST segments are concave upward, with no distinct J point, and there are no T-wave inversions at this stage. Up to 82% of patients have coexisting depression of the PR segment in this stage.[11] This is in contrast to the ECG in MI, where T-wave inversions may occur in the setting of an upwardly convex, elevated ST segment, and changes in the PR segment are absent. The ST-segment elevation in pericarditis is thought to result from subepicardial injury of the ventricular myocardium, while the PR segment depression is thought to be from injury to the atria. According to several authors, the most difficult ECG to differentiate from the stage 1 ECG of acute pericarditis is that of early repolarization, as both will have elevated ST segments with upward concavity. Indistinct J points, and presence of PR depression help identify acute pericarditis. Early repolarization is most commonly encountered in young males. Diffuse ST-segment elevations in other populations should increase the suspicion for pericarditis. Changes should be present on previous ECGs, if available for comparison, to support the diagnosis of early repolarization.

Stage 2. The ECG may appear essentially normal. ST and PR segments transiently return toward baseline. T-wave flattening may be present.

Stage 3. Stage 3 is characterized by deep, uniform inversion of T waves.

Stage 4. Electrocardiographic resolution with return to normal. While the ECG can be very useful in diagnosing acute viral pericarditis, most blood tests are only helpful in ruling out other differential diagnoses. Though quite nonspecific, the erythrocyte sedimentation rate (ESR) is typically elevated in viral pericarditis, and a normal ESR helps make this diagnosis less credible. Leukocytosis often is present, but is not a specific finding. Elevations in creatine kinase (and CK-MB isoenzyme) often are present, but at low levels as they are thought to result from damage to a superficial layer of subepicardial myocardium.[12] However, larger elevations in CK-MB isoenzymes may still be consistent with pericarditis when it occurs in concert with myocarditis.[13] Echocardiogram is useful if a pericardial effusion is seen, but absence of effusion does not rule out pericarditis. Pericardial effusion also may be seen on chest radiography, but most often the chest x-ray is normal.

Treatment and Disposition. While viral pericarditis rarely progresses to cardiac tamponade, all patients with an effusion require observation to monitor for possible additional fluid accumulation.[14] Effusion should be suspected in patients with dyspnea, easy fatiguability, or findings consistent with early tamponade. Presence of an effusion introduces the need to distinguish between purulent pericarditis and pericarditis of viral etiology. The need for diagnostic pericardiocentesis to settle this issue should be discussed with the consulting cardiologist before the patient leaves the ED. In the absence of pericardial effusion, treatment for acute viral pericarditis revolves around symptom control. Nonsteroidal anti-inflammatory drugs (NSAIDs), such as aspirin, ibuprofen, and indomethicin, in typical doses often provide good relief from pain and fever. Recently, colchicine 1-2 mg po each day has been shown to be helpful.[15] Steroids are reserved for cases resistant to NSAIDs. Patients should be admitted when MI cannot be ruled out, or when pain control with enteral medications is insufficient.

Bacterial Pericarditis. While occurring less frequently than viral pericarditis, bacterial infection remains an important cause of pericardial disease, especially in Asia, Africa, and developing countries.[16,17] Purulent pericarditis generally carries a higher mortality

Table 2. Six Causes of Pericarditis

INFECTION
Viral: Coxsackie virus A and B, echovirus, adenovirus, mumps virus, Epstein-Barr virus, varicella zoster virus, hepatitis B virus, influenza virus, HIV
Bacterial: Staphylococci, Pneumococci, Meningococci, Streptococci, *H. influenzae, Legionella pneumophilia, Salmonella*, psittacosis, tuberculosis
Other: Fungal, rickettsia, amebiasis, Lyme disease, aspergillosis, toxoplasmosis
TRAUMA
Penetrating chest injury
Blunt chest injury
Perforation of RV by catheter placement
Pericardiotomy
Pacemaker implantation
Dissecting aneurysm
Cardiac surgery
MALIGNANCY
Primary: Mesothelioma sarcoma
Metastatic: Brochogenic carcinoma, breast carcinoma, lymphoma, leukemia
SYSTEMIC ILLNESS
Connective tissue disease
Rheumatic fever
Lupus erythematosus
Sarcoidosis
Myxedema
Inflammatory bowel disease
Scleroderma
Polyarteritis nodosa
MYOCARDIAL INFARCTION
Acute MI
Dressler syndrome
DRUG RELATED
Anticoagulants
Procainamide
Hydralazine
Isoniazid
Doxorubicin

rate than viral pericarditis and is more commonly associated with cardiac tamponade.[6] While the causative organisms are most commonly *Streptococcus* species, particularly *Pneumococcus,* infections with coagulase-positive *Staphylococcus,* gram-negative, and anaerobic organisms are increasing in incidence.[18] Cases secondary to tuberculous infection and Lyme disease also may be encountered.[19] The syndrome caused by bacterial pericarditis is similar to that of viral pericarditis, with a friction rub, fever, and chest pain. Typical ECG changes fail to differentiate the two. Pnemonia and empyema commonly coexist and serve as predisposing conditions. In one series, the classic findings of pericarditis were often absent, and the diagnosis was not made until the development of tamponade or at autopsy.[20] Antibiotics tailored to the likely etiologic agent should be instituted in the ED, after appropriate cultures are obtained, whenever bacterial pericarditis is suspected. The actual diagnosis is often not made until pericardiocentesis is performed, and cultures grow the offending organism from pericardial fluid. All patients with the tentative diagnosis of purulent pericarditis should be admitted to an intensive care unit (ICU) setting. In complicated cases, partial surgical resection of the pericardium may be required to prevent progression to constrictive pericarditis.

Uremic Pericarditis. Uremic pericarditis may occur as a manifestation of untreated end-stage renal disease (ESRD), but underdialysis often is the cause. Although the exact mechanism remains unknown, it is thought to be due in part to the hemorrhagic diathesis of uremia. Most patients have bloody pericardial effusions. Furthermore, uremic pericarditis has a relatively high association with tamponade.[21] The ED physician must remember that hemodialysis patients have decreased immune function, and that infectious causes must be considered in these patients when they present with symptoms of pericarditis. The chest radiograph may suggest effusion if an increase in cardiac size is noted in comparison to old films. Since cardiomegaly and fluid overload are common in ESRD, echocardiography is the single best test to establish the presence of pericardial effusion. The ECG often is normal in uremic pericarditis, as the epicardium is less involved than in infectious pericarditis.

Treatment consists of admission to an ICU setting for more frequent dialysis. Use of NSAIDs for pain must be judicious to prevent the complication of increased bleeding in uremia. Steroids are effective but take 1-2 weeks for effect.[22] Even though left ventricular failure is a common cause of hemodynamic compromise in ESRD patients, tamponade must be considered and ruled out when hypotension is present. Unfortunately, pericardial effusions are often loculated in uremia; and therefore, pericardiocentesis may not be as effective as in other causes of tamponade. Other alternative treatments for tamponade include a surgical "window" or pericardiectomy, neither of which is within the purview of the emergency physician. Rapid consultation with a cardiothoracic surgeon is recommended.

Post-MI Pericarditis. Pericarditis may occur within days of acute MI, or may appear weeks to months after as Dressler's syndrome. In the past, these have been regarded as two separate entities, but now are felt to be a continuum of the same disorder.[23] Pericarditis early after acute MI often presents as a different character chest pain 2-4 days post-infarction. Care is needed to distinguish this pain from that of reinfarction. A friction rub may be present but is highly variable and difficult to detect. Post-MI pericarditis is found only in patients who have suffered transmural injury. While the clinical incidence in these patients is reported at 7-16%, autopsy findings show changes consistent with pericarditis in 28-32% of patients.[23] The symptoms are self-limited, and resolve in days with NSAIDs for pain control.

In 1956, Dressler described a syndrome of fever, chest pain, leukocytosis, pleuritis, and pericardial or pleural effusion on chest radiograph occurring in patients several weeks post-MI. These findings are more common in patients with large, complicated MIs.

Figure 1. ECGs of Pericarditis, Acute MI, and Early Repolarization

A

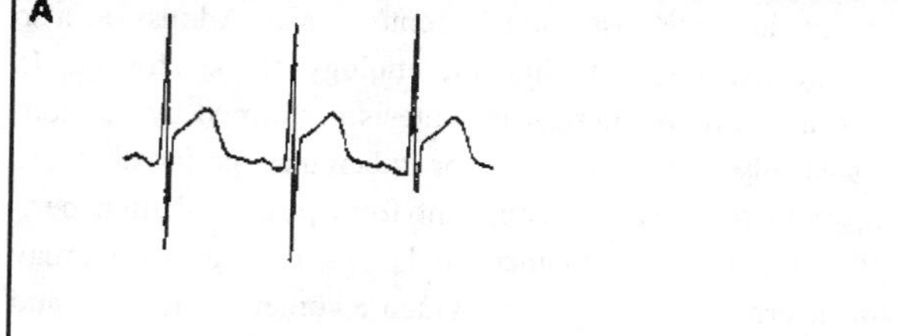

B

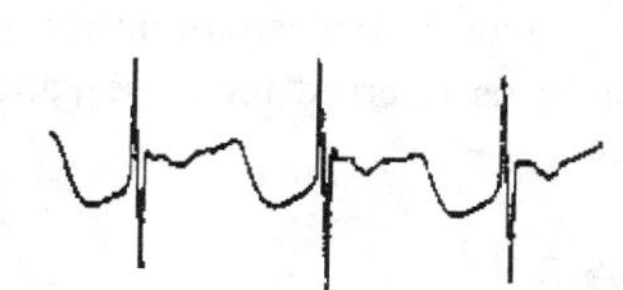

A—Concave upward ST-segment elevation in stage 1 of pericarditis. B—Convex upward ST-segment elevation with T-wave inversion in AMI.

C

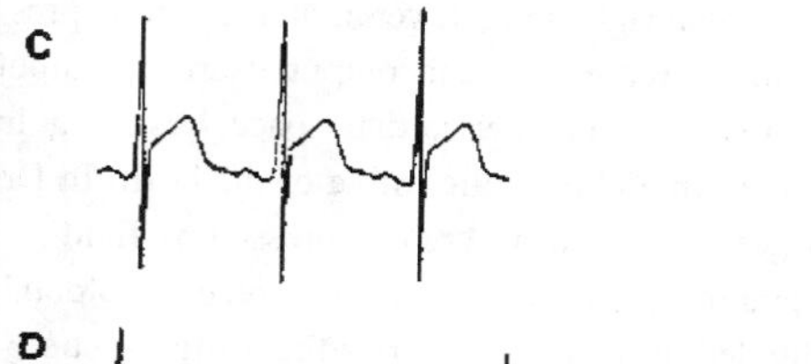

D

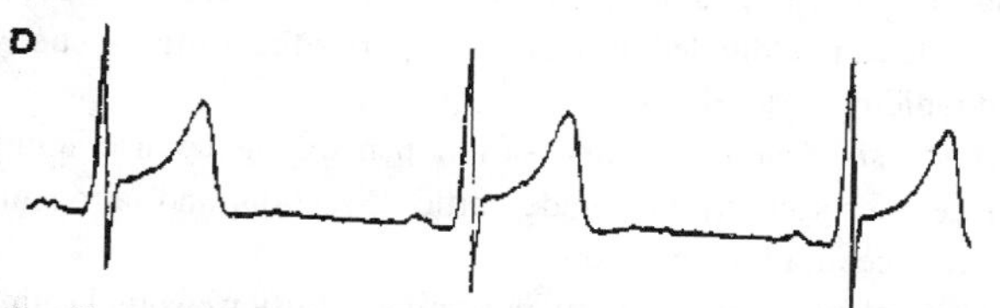

C—Concave upward ST-segment elevation in stage 1 of pericarditis. D—Concave upward ST-segment elevation in benign early repolarization.

Used with permission: Gibler WB, Aufderheide TP, eds. *Emergency Cardiac Care.* St. Louis: CV Mosby Co; 1992:470.

While the mechanism for this syndrome remains unclear, autoimmune reactions and slow hemorrhage into the pericardial space have been suggested as causes. As with early post-MI pericarditis, ruling out recurrent ischemia takes precedence. Treatment is with NSAIDs for pain and fever. Most cases are self-limited, and steroids are reserved for resistant cases.

Collagen Vascular Disease Pericarditis. While pericarditis is found in many collagen vascular diseases and autoimmune disorders *(please see Table 1)*, the current discussion is limited to rheumatoid arthritis (RA) and systemic lupus erythematosus (SLE). RA is the leading cause of pericarditis secondary to systemic disease, with autopsy showing pericardial involvement in 30-50% of cases.[24] Fortunately, the vast majority of cases are clinically silent.[24] Although there are often no findings on ECG or chest radiograph, pericardial disease must be suspected in any patient with RA who presents with symptoms of right-sided CHF. Patients with pericarditis secondary to RA may develop pericardial effusion and require pericardiocentesis. Unfortunately, as with uremia, effusions can be loculated and difficult to drain. RA-associated pericarditis may be further complicated by progression to constrictive pericarditis.

SLE is commonly associated with pericardial disease. Autopsy numbers show at least 50% of patients with SLE chronically treated with steroids develop pericarditis. [25] These patients also may progress to constrictive pericarditis. For both RA and SLE-associated pericarditis, corticosteroid treatment is used for symptomatic relief.

Malignant Pericarditis. While primary tumors of the pericardium are rare, metastatic disease involving the pericardium is not. The incidence of malignant pericardial effusion is approximately 10% in cancer patients, with most cases originating from lung or breast cancer, followed by lymphoma, leukemia, and malignant melanoma.[26] Pericardial involvement by Kaposi's sarcoma has been noted in HIV-positive patients.[27] In children, the most common malignancies causing pericarditis are Hodgkin's disease, lymphosarcoma, and leukemia. While pericardial metastases are most often associated with advanced disease, pericarditis can be the initial presentation of bronchogenic lung cancer. Metastases spread to the pericardium via passage from mediastinal lymph nodes. Drainage of the cardiac lymphatics at the root of the aorta may be disrupted, resulting in malignant pericardial effusion.

Presentation varies from incidental findings to dyspnea, diffuse chest pain, fatigue, and malaise. Malignant pericardial effusion also can present with signs of acute right heart failure. Nearly 50% of patients with malignant effusions have other potential causes of pericardial disease, such as post-irradiation, idiopathic, autoimmune, hypothyroidism, or medications.[28] Malignant pericarditis may be accompanied by ECG findings, including AV block, indicating likely invasion of the conducting system by tumor spread. Physical findings are similar to cardiac effusion and tamponade by other causes. Malignant pericardial effusions, compared to effusions secondary to other causes, progress to tamponade in 50-85% of cases.[29,30] Even though the underlying pathology is usually incurable, prompt treatment of tamponade in these patients can lead to significant prolongation of life. The appropriateness of aggressive therapy should be discussed with the patient and next of kin. Pericardiocentesis with fluid cytology establishes the definitive diagnosis and is a more sensitive test for pericardial involvement than direct biopsy.[31]

Post-Irradiation Pericarditis. Irradiation of the pericardium has both early and late complications. In the first days to months of radiation treatment, pericardial effusions can develop. The likelihood of developing an effusion directly correlates with the dosage. Effusions may be transient. When pericardial effusion occurs in the setting of radiation therapy for cancer, post-irradiation pericarditis must be distinguished from malignant effusion arising from tumor spread. While the most common presenting symptom early in treatment is shortness of breath with exertion, early post-irradiation pericarditis may present similar to infectious pericarditis, with fever, chest pain, and friction rub.[32] Therapy for post-irradiation pericarditis is similar to that for viral pericarditis: NSAIDs for pain and steroids for resistant cases. Effusion, if present, may require pericardiocentesis, but early post-irradiation pericarditis often resolves spontaneously. In some cases, however, the condition may persist up to two years. The later effects of radiation on the pericardium often present as constrictive pericarditis, and may not become obvious until 20 years or more after treatment. Often the connection between the radiation treatment and the symptoms will not be made at initial presentation unless specifically inquired about. Post-irradiation constrictive pericarditis often requires pericardiectomy for symptomatic resolution.

Drug-Induced Pericarditis. Procainamide, hydralazine, isoniazid, methyldopa, and reserpine all can produce a lupus-like syndrome that may lead to acute pericarditis. This usually occurs with chronic use of these drugs. Penicillin and cromolyn sodium may induce pericarditis via a hypersensitivity reaction. Methysergide, used in the treatment of migraine headaches, can cause chronic constrictive pericarditis as a component of generalized mediastinal fibrosis. Doxorubicin, a chemotherapeutic agent, may result both in a cardiomyopathy and pericarditis.[26] Therapy for drug-induced pericarditis involves cessation of the causative agent and symptomatic treatment. Tamponade is a rare complication in pericardial disease induced by drug reactions.

Pericardial Effusion

A pericardial effusion is an abnormal increase in the amount of pericardial fluid. Effusions often appear as a result of acute pericarditis and can be benign or life-threatening. Most effusions result from pericarditis of viral, uremic, malignant, and post-irradiation origins. In the setting of trauma, hemorrhagic effusions can occur and rapidly progress to cardiac tamponade. Proximal progression of an aortic dissection also may result in hemorrhagic effusion with tamponade.[33] Hemorrhagic effusions from wall rupture following MI are rare, occur several days post MI, and are rarely encountered in the ED. As many pericardial effusions are clinically silent in their early course, the key to diagnosis is a healthy suspicion. Diseases in which pericardial effusion is common must be recognized: renal failure, certain cancers, or acute infectious pericarditis. Classic physical findings of "distant heart sounds" and "percussed dullness beyond the cardiac apex" are very subjective and cannot necessarily be relied upon in the ED. Chest radiography may assist in diagnosis when an acute enlargement of the cardio-pericardial silhouette is seen, but readers should be aware that 200-250 mL of pericardial fluid may be needed to produce an enlargement visible on chest x-ray.[10] ECG findings also are insensitive indicators but may include generalized low voltage (R-wave height < 1 cm in all leads), and electrical alternans (beat-to-beat variation in height of ECG complexes corresponding to to-and-fro motion of heart in pericardial fluid). The diagnostic gold standard is two dimensional (2D) rather than motion mode (M-mode) echocardiography. This is especially true in the ED, since 2D echos are more easily interpreted by ED physicians, and less prone to diagnostic errors.[34]

2D echo is useful in evaluating pericardial effusion because it can provide a rough estimate of the size of the effusion and provide an early suggestion of cardiac tamponade. It also can show whether the effusion is loculated, a particularly common finding after cardiac surgery. Echocardiography also provides a quick evaluation on general heart function (i.e., valve disease and wall motion abnormalities). Serial echocardiography is the technique of choice to follow patients with asymptomatic pericardial effusions and to watch for signs of progression to tamponade. CT scans also show pericardial effusions, but hemopericardium can be difficult to diagnose by CT, since blood presents a similar density as the myocardium. Furthermore, CT scans cannot provide the information on cardiac function seen with 2D echos.

All patients with acute, symptomatic pericardial effusion should be admitted to an ICU setting for serial 2D echos to follow progression of the effusion and assess risk for cardiac tamponade. Most patients with known chronic effusions have minimal symptoms, and the risk of tamponade is exceedingly small.[35] Pericardioectomy is the only treatment in these cases and is controversial. Admission also should be directed toward finding the etiology of the effusion. In some cases, this involves pericardiocentesis performed by the consultant, especially when bacterial or tubercular pericarditis are suspected, or to differentiate malignant from post-irradiation pericarditis. Pericardial fluid is obtained for diagnostic purposes and may be sent for determination of protein, glucose content, cell count and differential, hematocrit, or for cytology, Gram and acid-fast stains, fungal smears, and appropriate cultures. Pericardiocentesis performed by the emergency physician is reserved for those patients with significant hemodynamic compromise.

Cardiac Tamponade

Definition. Cardiac tamponade was first described in 1669 by Richard Lower.[36] It is defined as the progressive elevation of pressure in the pericardial space (typically from fluid accumulation) that leads to equilibration of pericardial right and left ventricular diastolic pressures, which results in decreased cardiac output. Cardiac output slows as fluid accumulates in the pericardial space, resulting in impairment of venous return and diastolic filling of the heart. In Dr. Lower's words, "The walls of the heart are compressed by fluid . . . so that the heart cannot dilate sufficiently to receive blood". Tamponade can be divided into three categories that differ in etiology and rapidity of development:

1. *Acute surgical tamponade*—from penetrating cardiac injury (see later section), antegrade aortic dissection, and iatrogenic (from central line insertion).
2. *Medical tamponade*—from pericardial effusions complicating acute pericarditis, malignant pericarditis, or renal failure/dialysis.
3. *Low-pressure tamponade*—also a more chronic, medical cause, seen where left heart pressure is lowered to equilibrate with right heart pressure—seen in severely dehydrated patients.

Pathophysiology. As pericardial fluid accumulates, several factors influence whether or not it will become clinically apparent as tamponade. Both the volume of pericardial fluid and the time over which it accumulates can influence whether tamponade will develop. If an effusion develops over minutes, volumes as small as 200 mL may produce a significant reduction in cardiac output.[36] If an effusion accumulates over days, the parietal pericardium can stretch to accommodate a similar volume with little or no evidence of cardiac tamponade. The thickness of the parietal pericardium varies between individuals, and will influence its ability to stretch. Tamponade will present at lower volumes of effusion with a thick, noncompliant parietal pericardium. Ventricular wall thickness also may influence the volume of effusion required to produce tamponade. Higher volume effusions are necessary to compress thicker ventricles. Lastly, intravascular volume can influence the development of tamponade. Higher central venous pressure renders the right ventricle resistant to external compression by elevated intrapericardial pressure.

Normal diastolic pressures are 3-4 mmHg for right ventricular (RV) pressures and ~ 10 mmHg for left ventricular (LV) pressures. Intrapericardial pressures are lower still at -3 mmHg.[36] As intrapericardial pressure increases, it first equilibrates with the RV diastolic pressure. Physiologic compensation for increasing intrapericardial pressure involves increasing central venous tone and right atrial pressure by constriction of capacitance vessels to maintain diastolic filling. Although the patient is generally asymptomatic at this point, jugular venous distention will be apparent on physical exam, and chest x-ray may show cardiomegaly if fluid accumulation was not immediate. As intrapericardial pressure increases further, cardiac output is compromised, and heart rate increases. Indeed, tachycardia is one of the earliest signs of clinically significant tamponade. Further vasoconstriction occurs to maintain the elevated venous pressure needed for adequate RV filling. These benefits are not without cost; vasoconstriction increases afterload, which increases the pressure-work of the heart, and higher heart rates decrease time for diastolic filling, limiting end-diastolic volume and beat-to-beat compensation via the Frank-Starling mechanism. As pressure increases still higher, intrapericardial, RV diastolic, and LV diastolic pressures will all equalize at ~ 10 mmHg. Moderate symptoms of cardiac tamponade will be evident. In the case of pre-existing LV failure, where LV end-diastolic pressure is already elevated, tamponade will be clinically evident before equalization of all three pressures occurs. Further increases in intrapericardial pressure to 15-20 mmHg will produce severe symptoms of tamponade, with failure of compensatory mechanisms, reduction of cardiac output, and hypotension. At this stage, death is likely to occur in the absence of prompt intervention. Thus, hypotension is a late finding of cardiac tamponade and may occur precipitously with small increases in pericardial volume at this stage.

As tamponade develops, forward venous flow ceases in early diastole as no gradient is present between the central venous, right atrial (RA), and RV diastolic pressures. At this point, pulsus paradoxus will be apparent. Pulsus paradoxus is defined as a greater than 10 mmHg fall in systolic blood pressure (SBP) with inspiration. This sign was originally described by Kussmaul, and was "paradoxical" to him because arterial pressure decreased without a decrease in auscultated heart sounds, not because SBP does not normally drop in inspiration. Though seen in severe asthma, tension pneumothorax, and RV infarct in the appropriate clinical setting, pulsus paradoxus is pathognomonic of advanced cardiac tamponade. However, it may be absent with tamponade in patients with simultaneous LV failure

Paradoxical pulse occurs through the following mechanism. Inspiration transiently lowers intrathoracic pressure in comparison to central venous pressure. This augments right heart filling by increasing the pressure gradient between the central veins and the right atrium. In the setting of tamponade, the increase in RV filling mediated by inspiration increases RV end-diastolic pressure over LV end-diastolic pressure. Because fluid in the pericardium limits the distensibility of the free walls of the RV, the diastolic pressure mismatch between the ventricles causes the interventricular septum to bow, or shift into the LV cavity, which can be seen by echo. This reduces LV end-diastolic volume. LV end-diastolic volume is further reduced during inspiration by pooling of blood in the pulmonary veins. In aggregate these effects reduce stroke volume, cardiac output, and systolic pressure. In the setting of LV failure, the mechanism producing paradoxical pulse in tamponade is overcome by pathologically elevated LV end-diastolic pressures. Pulsus paradoxus also may be absent during tamponade in the presence of positive-pressure ventilation, large atrial septal defects or severe aortic insufficiency, or profound hypotension.[37]

Cardiac tamponade can occur at normal central venous and RV diastolic pressures when LV diastolic pressure is pathologically lowered. This phenomenon is called "low pressure tamponade." [38] Low pressure tamponade is rare but can occur when pericardial effusion occurs in concert with hypovolemeia or dilation of venous capacitance vessels. This may occur with dehydration, hemorrhage, overzealous diuresis or dialysis, or nitrate therapy.

Signs and Symptoms. Acute cardiac tamponade can present in a variety of ways. Rapid onset of tamponade, most commonly seen in trauma and proximal aortic dissection, quickly leads to shock. The patient will be combative to obtunded, hypotensive, and exhibit poor peripheral perfusion. Medical cases of tamponade can suddenly decompensate and present in a similar fashion. Patients presenting in shock must have other causes of hypotension ruled out, such as MI, PE, sepsis, leaking thoracic or abdominal aneurysm, GI bleeding, toxins, or severe dehydration.

Most patients with medical tamponade do not present in frank shock. However, medical tamponade may mimic the presentation of acute CHF, with patients complaining of shortness of breath, chest pain/tightness, pedal edema, dyspnea with exertion, possible altered mental status, and weight gain. The physical exam can often help differentiate these two entities if pulsus paradoxus can be elicited, but pulsus is not specific for cardiac tamponade. Paradoxical pulse also can be seen in COPD, PE, RV infarct, and cardiogenic shock. Beck's triad of hypotension, increased jugular venous distention, and muffled heart sounds is helpful when present but is an extremely late finding.[39] Pericardial friction rubs are not reliable to diagnose tamponade because they are often absent with large effusions. Kussmaul's sign, distension of neck veins with inspiration, may provide an early clue to the diagnosis. This sign may be seen with other disorders, however, including RV infarct, tension pneumothorax, PE, and cardiac contusion. Ultimately, the diagnosis of tamponade cannot be made on clinical signs alone.

Ancillary Studies. Chest radiography, ECG, CVP measurement, cardiac catheterization, and echocardiography are all useful tests in the diagnosis of tamponade. Chest x-ray can show signs of a pericardial effusion, acute increase in cardiac size without pulmonary vascular redistribution, but will be normal with acute development of tamponade. The ECG finding of electrical alternans is considered diagnostic of effusion, but it is not specific for tamponade and also can be seen in supraventricular tachycardia. Electrical alternans consists of alternating levels of P wave, QRS complex, and T-wave voltage, and is thought to result from the heart "swinging" in a large pericardial effusion. Elevated CVPs of greater than 12-14 mmHg are suggestive of tamponade, especially when seen in combination with systemic hypotension. However, CVP may be normal in hypovolemic patients with tamponade. While measurement of intracardiac pressures by cardiac cath is possible, this is not readily available in the ED. This leaves echocardiography as the diagnostic procedure of choice.

Echocardiography is especially useful when the diagnosis of cardiac tamponade is being considered, because it can definitively establish the presence, size, and effects of an effusion. After finding the effusion with the echo, the diagnostic signs of cardiac tamponade can then be sought out. These include:

1. *RV diastolic collapse*—length of time RV collapse persists in diastole directly correlates with severity of tamponade. This is not seen with RV hypertrophy.
2. *RA compression*—not seen in pulmonary hypertension, heart failure, or tricuspid valve disease.

3. *Bowing of septum into LV with inspiration*—normally the RV's volume increases with increasing venous return on inspiration; but, as the intra-pericardial pressure opposes free-wall expansion of the RV, the increased venous return forces the septum towards the LV.

Other, less diagnostic signs exist, including pseudomitral valve prolapse, and a pendular motion of the heart in cases with large pericardial effusions. While the echocardiographic signs of tamponade are very useful, they must be correlated with clinical findings. Patients can have classical clinical findings without echocardiographic evidence and vice versa.[40] Lower effusion volumes may produce symptoms in patients with pre-existing heart disease, and false-positive RV compression may be seen. The decision to perform invasive therapeutic procedures should never be based on echocardiographic findings alone without clinical correlation.

Treatment and Disposition. Consistent with the theme of pericardial disease, the treatment of cardiac tamponade can vary from direct ED thoracotomy to hospital admission for observation and serial 2D echocardiography. All patients require admission to an ICU setting because of the potential for rapid hemodynamic decompensation. Patients with severe hemodynamic instability from cardiac tamponade on initial presentation require urgent pericardial decompression. Patients without any evidence of cardiovascular compromise, where tamponade is noted primarily on echo, may be admitted for expectant observation without acute intervention. Since the majority of patients with cardiac tamponade will present with moderate-to-severe but not preterminal symptoms, the decision of when and how to intervene should be approached on a case-by-case basis after appropriate consultation. In cases of life-threatening tamponade, intervention and pericardiocentesis may need to precede consultation.

When tamponade is accompanied by hemodynamic compromise, pericardiocentesis and surgical pericardiectomy are recommended unless an ED thoracotomy is performed in treatment of trauma. ED pericardiocentesis may be deferred if better facilities (i.e., cath lab) are readily available and the patient can tolerate transport. Prior to ED pericardiocentesis, medical interventions should be instituted to help stabilize the patient by augmenting filling pressures and contractility to increase cardiac output. These include volume expansion with crystalloid and/or blood, and treatment with positive inotropic agents. Dobutamine is the preferred agent if blood pressure is adequate. Although afterload reduction (i.e., nitroprusside) makes physiological "sense" as an additional treatment to increase cardiac output, studies have failed to confirm benefit, and the use of vasodilators should be avoided in tamponade because of potential deleterious effects on blood pressure.[41] Because in tamponade there is a steep slope in the pericardial pressure-volume curve, removal of even 10-20 ccs can be therapeutic. Pericardiocentesis is best performed with the aid of 2D echo to help guide the needle away from vital structures but can be done without imaging if echo is not readily available. Three accepted approaches exist: subxiphoid, parasternal, and apical.

The subxiphoid approach is the preferred technique. Contrary to the parasternal and apical approaches, it directs the needle away from the coronary arteries. Furthermore, pneumothorax is less common than with the apical approach. Before starting, equipment should be prepared in advance; this includes a cardiac defibrillator. The procedure should be performed with the patient sitting at a 45° angle to move the heart farther from the anterior chest wall. In the ED setting, where hemodynamic compromise is likely, the procedure must be performed in the supine position. Liberal use of local anesthetic is necessary for awake patients, as the pericardium is sensitive to pain. A 16-18 gauge spinal needle is inserted between the xiphod process and the left costal margin at a 30-45° angle to the skin. Alternatively, a catheter over a needle can be used, and the catheter left in place for repeated aspiration of pericardial fluid. The needle is directed toward the left shoulder. The V-lead of an ECG monitor electrode can be attached to the needle to detect epicardial contact and the potential for ventricular puncture. With epicardial contact, ST elevation indicating a "current of injury" will occur. The needle should not be advanced further, as this will increase the risk of ventricular puncture and coronary artery laceration. As much fluid as possible should be aspirated, with samples sent for Gram's stain, culture, and cytology where appropriate.

Cardiac Tamponade in Trauma. While the most common traumatic causes of pericardial injury are stab and gunshot wounds, several iatrogenic causes also have been reported. *(Please see Table 2.)* Placement of central venous pressure (CVP) lines, pacemaker insertion, and pericardiocentesis have been associated with cardiac or pericardial injury leading to cardiac tamponade.[42] When blunt trauma is the cause of pericardial injury, the mechanism of injury is typically a severe deceleration impact. Cardiac rupture is more commonly the cause of tamponade in blunt trauma than isolated pericardial injury. When cardiac rupture is present, the pericardium is only lacerated in about 10% of cases.[43] Patients with cardiac rupture and pericardial laceration arrest secondary to exsanguination. In patients in whom the pericardium is intact, cardiac rupture leads to acute tamponade. In such cases, mortality is extremely high.

Cardiac tamponade resulting from chest trauma deserves special attention. Traumatic tamponade generally develops rapidly, results from smaller pericardial effusions than from nontraumatic etiologies, and leaves the body little time for physiologic compensation. Urgent pericardiocentesis can be life-saving. Cardiac tamponade from trauma can be divided into three groups: [44]

1. *Early tamponade*—mildly increased CVP and heart rate; cardiac output remains normal or is mildly elevated, occurs with < 200 cc of blood in the pericardium of adults.
2. *Moderate tamponade*—tachycardia and moderately elevated CVP, cardiac output now begins to fall as compensatory mechanisms fail. SBP begins to fall, seen with ~ 200 cc blood in pericardium.
3. *Severe tamponade*—markedly depressed cardiac output, high CVP, and severe hypotension. Central venous pressure may be low if significant blood loss has occurred. Bradycardia may be seen; occurs with > 200 cc blood in the pericardium.

The reported incidence of cardiac tamponade from chest trauma is low, occurring in less than 2% of penetrating trauma cases and even less frequently with blunt chest trauma.[45] In the setting of actual penetrating injury to the heart, tamponade is very common. It is reported that 80-90 % of stab wounds (SW), and 20% of gunshot wounds (GSW) to the heart result in acute cardiac tamponade.[46] The low overall incidence of cardiac tamponade with penetrating chest trauma simply suggests that most penetrating chest injuries actually miss the heart. Though rare, delayed cardiac tamponade has been seen as a feature of SWs to the chest occurring up to two weeks after the original injury.[47] Be aware that patients with only small myocardial lacerations may present in a subtle manner, with tamponade developing slowly.

SWs more commonly cause tamponade than GSWs, because they produce smaller injuries to the pericardium that often self-seal. As the right heart comprises the majority of the anterior surface of the heart, it is most often injured with penetrating chest trauma (RA, 14 %, RV, 43 %).[46] The thin-walled right ventricle often is not able to seal spontaneously and may continue to bleed into the "sealed" pericardium and cause tamponade. Tamponade seen with GSWs is most often associated with low-velocity weapons, as the zone of injury to the pericardium is smaller than with high-velocity projectiles. It has been suggested that a moderate component of cardiac tamponade can be protective in penetrating cardiac injury by decreasing hemorrhage into the chest.[48]

Cardiac tamponade should be suspected in every patient with penetrating injury to the chest, axilla, neck, back, or upper abdomen. Suspicion should be even higher when these patients are hypotensive. Clinically, patients present with signs of shock (hypotension, tachycardia, cool/clammy skin, cyanosis), dyspnea, distended neck veins, and muffled heart sounds. Beck's triad of hypotension, distended neck veins, and a small, quiet heart is the reported "classical" presentation. Be warned that penetrating chest trauma patients can present with relatively normal vital signs and no significant findings only to have tamponade suddenly develop later during the ED stay.[49] At first, it would appear that measurement of CVP is all that is needed to diagnose cardiac tamponade in trauma; CVP greater than 15 mmHg with hypotension and tachycardia is diagnostic.[45] Unfortunately, it is not that straightforward. CVP can vary in the trauma patient with intoxication, Valsalva maneuver, guarding, peritoneal or pleural irritation, or with malposition of the catheter.[46] In addition, tamponade may not be apparent until after volume resuscitation has been given. Further, tamponade can be intermittently present with blood clots stopping blood flow out of a lacerated pericardium. Pulsus paradoxus (nonspecific), chest x-ray (unreliable, often poor quality portable films), and ECG (useful signs only common in more chronic effusions), also are of limited use in diagnosing tamponade in the trauma setting. Transthoracic echocardiography is currently the best diagnostic test in these patients, but it is often not available quickly enough for realistic benefit. Transesophageal echocardiography is being studied as a more reliable test for penetrating cardiac injury. A recent study reported accuracies of 100% with a single exam, while the transthoracic method needs serial exams to reach comparable results.[50]

Treatment in trauma patients in whom cardiac tamponade is suspected should be rapid and directed. Cardiothoracic surgery consultation should be sought immediately. If tamponade is suspected, and the patient remains hemodynamically unstable after volume loading, pericardiocentesis is indicated. This procedure is not without risks (dysrhythmia, false negatives, ventricular puncture tamponade), but the ED physician must be able to perform it when indicated. A catheter may be placed into the pericardium to provide a continuous drainage when definitive thoracotomy is not readily available. It is important to remember that the majority of blood in the pericardial space may be clotted, and that pericardiocentesis may not be very helpful. A "negative tap" in the setting of clotted blood can be dangerously misleading. If the patient arrests at any time in the ED, lateral thoracotomy should be performed by the ED physician if surgical consultants are not at the bedside. Roberts and Hedges provide recent discussions on the procedure.[51] The goals of thoracotomy are fourfold: First, pericardiotomy to relieve tamponade; second, cross-clamp of the aorta to preserve cardiac and cerebral perfusion; third, repair (even if temporary) of the myocardial injury; and fourth, direct cardiac massage to permit effective CPR.[52]

Constrictive Pericarditis

Definition. Constrictive pericarditis results when the pericardium, in response to a prior insult, forms diffuse fibrous adhesions to the epicardium. This causes loss of its normal compliance and can impair diastolic filling and stroke volume as in cardiac tamponade secondary to effusion. Although the pathophysiological changes are similar to those of tamponade, constrictive pericarditis is typically subacute or chronic. Constrictive pericarditis and tamponade can be distinguished by the presence of pulsus paradoxus in tamponade. This is not seen in constrictive pericarditis, because intrathoracic pressure changes are not transmitted to the right side of the heart by scarred pericardium. In contrast to cardiac tamponade, auscultatory findings of constrictive pericarditis are characterized by normal (not distant) heart sounds and the possible occurrence of an early diastolic knock.

Although any form of acute pericarditis can lead to constrictive pericarditis, the most common causes, in decreasing order of frequency, include: neoplasm, post-irradiation changes, ESRD, prior thoracic trauma, infections, and collagen vascular diseases.[53] Prior to the development of effective pharmacotherapy, tuberculosis was the most common cause of constrictive pericarditis. It remains so in developing countries.

Clinical Findings and Diagnosis. Constrictive pericarditis typically presents with symptoms of right heart failure: dyspnea, fatigue, weight gain, hepatomegaly, ascites, and peripheral edema. Chest pain is notably absent. A key diagnostic finding on cardiac auscultation is an early diastolic knock. This is caused by the abrupt termination of ventricular filling by a noncompliant pericardium. Friction rubs may be heard. Pleural effusions may be present, resulting in decreased breath sounds and dullness to percussion. Although often quoted as a finding, Kussmaul's sign (paradoxical increase in jugular venous pressure with inspiration) is rarely elicited in symptomatic patients.[54] Dyspnea frequently prevents the patient from taking the long, slow, deep breaths needed to demonstrate this finding. Blood tests are of limited use but may show evidence of enzymatic abnormalities associated with hepatic congestion. Chest radiography often reveals normal heart size, but calcification of the pericardium may be evident, and is pathognomonic. ECG shows low QRS voltage, nonspecific ST-T wave changes, and often atrial fibrillation.[55] Echocardiography is useful in diagnosing constrictive pericarditis, but is not useful as a guide to therapy once the diagnosis is established. Calcification and thickening of the pericardium are best seen on chest CT.

Because of the similarity of presenting symptoms, constrictive pericarditis is often confused with liver disease and CHF. Constrictive pericarditis and CHF can be differentiated from liver disease by the presence of jugular venous distention. The distinction between CHF and constrictive pericarditis is less obvious, but critical, as reduction of intravascular volume with diuretics in constrictive pericarditis can further decrease cardiac output and worsen symptoms. Important clues to aid in distinguishing CHF and constrictive pericarditis center on the common finding of normal LV function in constrictive pericarditis, and include:

1. absence of pulmonary edema;
2. normal heart size on chest radiograph;
3. no significant cardiac murmurs;
4. normal LV function demonstrated on echocardiography; and
5. absence of bundle branch blocks or hypertrophy on ECG.

While these points may help, the distinction can be difficult, and final diagnosis may not be made until the patient undergoes cardiac catheterization. It is important to remember the possibility of constrictive pericarditis whenever symptoms suggesting CHF do not respond to usual treatment measures.

Treatment and Disposition. Constrictive pericarditis is a late complication of acute pericarditis; the progression of the disease is relatively slow. When pericardial calcifications are noted incidentally on chest radiograph, the asymptomatic patient can be referred to his or her primary physician for follow-up with detailed instructions on symptoms that should prompt immediate return to the ED. When patients are symptomatic from constrictive pericarditis, admission is indicated. The only definitive treatment is surgical pericardiectomy, which often provides striking improvement in symptoms. In comparison to cardiac tamponade, patients with constrictive pericarditis do not routinely need emergent surgical intervention, and acute hemodynamic instability is uncommon. When hemodynamic compromise is present, however, urgent consultation and intervention are mandatory.

Summary

Pericardial disease and tamponade can be very challenging for the ED physician to diagnose and manage. The key in most cases is to recognize the clinical presentations and common causes of these entities. In the absence of effusion, tamponade, or constrictive pericarditis with hemodynamic compromise, symptomatic treatment and referral for follow-up are sufficient. All effusions (unless asymptomatic and documented to be chronic) require admission to an ICU setting for surveillance of signs of cardiac tamponade. Finally, the ED physician must be comfortable with pericardiocentesis as a lifesaving treatment for acute cardiac tamponade and know when the procedure is indicated.

References

1. Bruyn GA, DeKoning J, Reijoso FJ, et al. Lyme pericarditis leading to tamponade. *Brt J Rheumatol* 1994;33:852.
2. Osler W. *The Principles and Practice of Medicine.*New York: Appleton & Co; 1892.
3. Holt JP. The normal pericardium.*Am J Cardiol* 1970;26:455.
4. Shabetai R. Function of the pericardium. In: Fowler, NO, ed. *The Pericardium in Health and Disease.*Mt. Kisco, NY: Furtura; 1985:19-50.
5. Rosen P, Barkin RM, Levy RC, eds. *Emergency Medicine: Concepts and Clinical Practice.* 3rd ed. St. Louis: CV Mosby Co; 1992:1305.
6. Gewitz MH, Vetter VL. Cardiac emergencies. In: Fleisher GR, Ludwig S, eds. *Textbook of Pediatric Emergency Medicine.* Baltimore, MD: Williams & Wilkins; 1993:559.
7. Shabetai R, Etiology, pathophysiology, clinical recognition, and treatment (of pericardial disease). In: Hurst JW, Schlant RC, eds. *The Heart, Arteries and Veins.* 8th ed. New York: McGraw-Hill; 1995:1012-1013.
8. Bates B, Bickley L, Hockelman R. *A Guide to Physical Examination and History Taking.* Philadelphia: J.B. Lippincott Co; 1995:312.
9. Houghton, Houghton JL. Pericarditis and myocarditis. *Postgrad Med* 1992;91:273-282.
10. Spondick DH. Pericarditis, pericardial effusion, cardiac tamponade and constriction. *Crit Care Clin* 1989;5:455.
11. Spondick DH. Diagnostic electrocardiographic sequences in acute pericarditis—significance of PR segment and PR vector changes. *Circulation* 1973;48:575.
12. Karjalainen J, Heikkila J. Acute pericarditis: Myocardial enzyme release as evidence of myocarditis. *Am Heart J* 1986; 111 546.
13. Houghton JL. Pericarditis and myocarditis. *Postgrad Med* 1992;91:273-282.
14. Debehnke DJ. Cardiac-related acute infectious disease. In: Gibler WB, Aufderheide TP, eds. *Emergency Cardiac Care.* 1st ed. St. Louis: Mosby Co; 1994:464.
15. Guindo J, de la Serna AR. Recurrent pericarditis: Relief with colchicine. *Circulation* 1990;82:1117-1120.
16. Park S, Bayer, AS. Purulent pericarditis. *Curr Clin Top Infect Dis* 1992;12:56.
17. Dupuis C, Gronnier P, Kachaner J, et al. Bacterial pericarditis in infancy and childhood. *Am J Caridol* 1994;74:807-809.
18. Demey HE, Eycken M, Vandermast M, et al. Purulent pericarditis due to methicillin-resistant *Staphylococcus aureus. Acta Cardiol* 1991;46:485.
19. Sagrista-Sauleda J, Barrabes J, Permanyer-Miralda G, et al. Purulent pericarditis: Review of a 20-year experience in a general hospital. *J Am Coll Cardiol* 1993;22:1661.
20. Isselbacker EM, Cigarroa JE, Eagle KA. Cardiac tamponade complicating proximal aortic dissection—is pericardiocentesis harmful? *Circulation* 1994;90:2375.
21. Shabetai R. Pericardial disease. In: Hurst JW, Schlant RC, eds. *The Heart*. 7th ed. New York: McGraw-Hill; 1990.
22. Rosen P, Barkin RM, Levy, RC, eds. *Emergency Medicine: Concepts and Clinical Practice.* 3rd ed. St. Louis: CV Mosby Co; 1992:1396.
23. Gregoratos G. Pericardial involvement in acute myocardial infarction. *Cardiol Clin* 1990;8:601-608.
24. Rosen P, Barkin RM, Levy RC, eds. *Emergency Medicine: Concepts and Clinical Practice.* 3rd ed. St. Louis: CV Mosby Co; 1992:1399.
25. Rosen P, Barkin RM, Levy RC, eds. *Emergency Medicine:* Concepts and Clinical Practice. 3rd ed. St. Louis; Mosby Co: 1992:1399.
26. Sternbach GL. Pericarditis. *Ann Emerg Med* 1988;17: 214-220.
27. Dacso CC. Pericarditis in AIDS. *Cardiol Clin* 1990;8: 697-699.
28. Posner MR, Cohen GI, Skarin, AT. Pericardial disease in patients with cancer—the differentiation of malignant from idiopathic and radiation-induced pericarditis. *Am J Med* 1981;71:407.
29. Vaitkus PT, Herrmann, HC, LeWinter, MM. Treatment of malignant pericardial effusion. *JAMA* 1994;272:59.

30. Rosen P, Barkin RM, Levy RC, eds. *Emergency Medicine: Concepts and Clinical Practice.* 3rd ed. St. Louis: CV Mosby Co; 1992: 1398.
31. Chen KTK. Extracardiac malignancy presenting with cardiac tamponade. *J Surg Oncol* 1983;23:67.
32. Schneider, JS, Edwards JE. Irradiation-induced pericarditis. *Chest* 1979;75:560.
33. Pepi M, Muratori M, Barbier P, et al. Pericardial effusion after cardiac surgery: Incidence, site, size, and haemodynamic consequences. *Br Heart J* 1994; 72:327.
34. Hauser AM. The emerging role of echocardiography in the emergency department. *Ann Emerg Med* 1989;18:1298.
35. Shabetai R. Etiology, pathophysiology, clinical recognition, and treatment (of pericardial disease). In: Hurst JW, Schlant RC, eds. *The Heart, Arteries and Veins.* 8th ed. New York: McGraw-Hill; 1995:1016.
36. Shabetai R. *The Pericardium.* New York: Grune & Stratton; 1981.
37. Kronzon I, Cohen ML, Winer HE. Contribution of echocardiography to the understanding of the pathophysiology of cardiac tamponade. *J Am Coll Cardiol* 1983;1:1180.
38. Antman, EM, Cargil V, Grossman W. Low-pressure cardiac tamponade. *Ann Intern Med* 1979;91:403.
39. Debehnke DJ. Cardiac-related acute infectious disease. In: Gibler WB, Aufderheide TP, eds. *Emergency Cardiac Care.* 1st ed. St. Louis: Mosby Co; 1994.
40. Shabetai R. Etiology, pathophysiology, clinical recognition, and treatment (of pericardial disease). In: Hurst JW, Schlant RC, eds. *The Heart, Arteries and Veins.* 8th ed. New York: McGraw-Hill; 1995:1020.
41. Kerber RE. Hemodynamic effects of volume expansion and nitroprusside compared with pericardiocentesis in patients with acute tamponade. *N Engl J Med* 1982;307:929.
42. Edwards H, King TC. Cardiac tamponade from central venous catheter. *Arch Surg* 1982;117:965.
43. Martin TD, Flynn TC, Rowlands BJ, et al. Blunt cardiac rupture. *J Trauma* 1984;24:4.
44. Shoemaker WC, Carey S, Yao ST, et al. Hemodynamic monitoring for physiologic evaluation, diagnosis, and therapy of acute hemopericardial tamponade from penetrating wounds. *J Trauma* 1973;13:36.
45. Rosen P, Barkin RM, Levy RC, eds. *Emergency Medicine: Concepts and Clinical Practice.* 3rd ed., St. Louis: CV Mosby Co. 1992:445.
46. Karrel R, Shaffer KR, Franaszek JB. Emergency diagnosis, resuscitation, and treatment of acute penetrating cardiac trauma. *Ann Emerg Med* 1982;11:504.
47. Aaland MO, Sherman RT. Delayed pericardial tamponade in penetrating chest trauma: case report. *J Trauma* 1991;31(11): 1563-1565.
48. Wilson RF. Thoracic trauma. In: Tintinalli JE, Ruiz E, Krome RL, eds. *Emergency Medicine: A Comprehensive Study Guide.* 4th ed. New York: McGraw-Hill; 1996:465.
49. Bolton JW, Bynoe RP, Lazar HL, et al. Two-dimensional echocardiography in the evaluation of penetrating intrapericardial injuries. *Ann Thorac Surg* 1993;56:3.
50. Skoularigis J, Essop MR, Sareli P. Usefulness of transesophageal echocardiography in the early diagnosis of penetrating stab wounds to the heart. *Am J Cardiol* 1994; 73:5.
51. Roberts JR, Hedges JR. *Clinical Procedures in Emergency Medicine.* 2nd ed. Philadelphia: WB Saunders; 1992:210-228, 236-252.
52. Rosen P, Barkin, RM, Levy RC, eds. *Emergency Medicine: Concepts and Clinical Practice.* 3rd ed., St. Louis: CV Mosby Co; 1992:448.
53. Shabetai R. Etiology, pathophysiology, clinical recognition, and treatment (of pericardial disease). In: Hurst JW, Schlant RC, eds. *The Heart, Arteries and Veins.* 8th ed. New York: McGraw-Hill; 1995:1028.
54. Meyer TE. Mechanism underlying Kussmaul's sign in chronic constrictive pericarditis. *Am J Cardiol* 1989;64:1069.
55. Shabetai R. Etiology, pathophysiology, clinical recognition, and treatment (of pericardial disease). In: Hurst JW, Schlant RC, eds. *The Heart, Arteries and Veins.* 8th ed. New York: McGraw Hill; 1995:1030.

Acute Myocardial Infarction: Laboratory Assessment and Stabilization

Gideon Bosker, MD, FACEP
David J. Robinson, MD, MS
David A. Jerrard, MD, FACEP
Dick C. Kuo, MD

Acute myocardial infarction (AMI) is the leading cause of death in the United States and most Western industrialized nations.[1] In 1998, there were more than 1.6 million cases of AMI in the United States, and almost 500,000 associated deaths. Forty-six percent of AMIs occurred in those younger than age 65. AMI most commonly occurs from a sudden thrombotic occlusion at the site of a ruptured or fissured atherosclerotic plaque.[2] The coronary artery occlusion leads to characteristic chest pain and impending infarction. Preservation of functional myocardium correlates best with future morbidity and mortality.

Few argue that early identification of AMI, prevention of evolving infarction, and, if possible, restoration of coronary perfusion improve outcomes in patients with AMI. A 1994 study of 205,000 AMIs demonstrated significant improvements in mortality and morbidity with early, aggressive management.[3] Clearly, the ED physician must be prepared to recognize indications for emergent, mortality-reducing interventions such as t-PA in eligible patients with AMI. Prompt execution of appropriate treatment strategies will preserve myocardium, reduce complications, and produce significant reductions in mortality and morbidity.

With these clinical issues in clear focus, this review provides an overview of current diagnostic and therapeutic approaches to AMI.[4-7] The objectives are to provide a systematic approach to patient assessment, identify the clinical advantages of newer enzymatic tests for confirming the diagnosis of acute coronary ischemia, and review, in detail, the mortality reduction techniques—including pharmacotherapeutic and invasive procedures—supported by evidentiary clinical trials.[8,9] Finally, a clinical algorithm outlining outcome-enhancing strategies for this life-threatening condition is presented.

Overview of Clinical Principles: Diagnostic Criteria

In 1996, the American Heart Association and American College of Cardiology (AHA/ACC Guidelines) outlined three components necessary to establish the definitive diagnosis of AMI.[10] This triad consists of chest pain suggestive of cardiac disease, an ECG with characteristic changes suggesting myocardial infarction, and cardiac-specific biochemical markers exceeding the standard reference ranges in a pattern consistent with AMI. Two of the three findings are necessary to diagnose AMI. Presently, this group of findings is considered the "gold standard" for diagnosis.

History. Chest pain is present in 65-69% of patients with AMI and is characteristically ischemic in nature, although a large number of patients report "atypical" chest pain with known ischemic disease. Atypical pain presentations in AMI include pleuritic, sharp, burning, or reproducible chest pain, as well as pain referring to the back,

Figure 1. Facts about Diagnosis and Misdiagnosis of AMI

- Approximately 25% of all AMIs go undetected ("silent heart attacks"), leaving patients at a higher risk of dying from a subsequent AMI.
- Approximately 27% of all patients who suffer AMIs die within one hour of the event ("sudden death"), usually before reaching an emergency room.
- Approximately 36% of AMI patients die immediately or within several days following onset of AMI.
- Each year, approximately 5 million people present in emergency rooms with chest pain; only 5-10% of these patients are actually experiencing an AMI.
- Only about one-half of patients who experience an AMI are actually diagnosed in time to permit meaningfully therapeutic intervention.
- Estimates are that more than 35,000 patients per year are wrongly discharged from emergency rooms because of failure to diagnose AMI; 8750 (about 25%) of these patients die or suffer life-threatening outcomes within 24 hours following discharge.
- Fewer than 25% of patients admitted to the hospital with ischemic-type chest discomfort are subsequently diagnosed as having had an AMI, adding significant costs to the health care system.
- Emergency department cases account for approximately 17% of all medical malpractice claims made; about 20% of these cases are attributable to failure to diagnose AMI.

Source: American Heart Association; Decision Resources, Inc.

Table 1. Killip Classification

CLASS I
No clinical heart failure, < 5% mortality
CLASS II
Rales bilaterally in up to 50% of lung fields, isolated S_3, good prognosis
CLASS III
Rales in all lung fields, acute mitral regurgitation, aggressive management required
CLASS IV
Cardiogenic shock: stuporous, systolic BP < 90, decreased urine output, pulmonary edema, and cold clammy skin; mortality near 80%

abdomen, neck, or arm. Atypical or nonspecific pain or anginal equivalents such as dyspnea, nausea, vomiting, palpitations, syncope, stroke, or depressed mental status may be the only complaints in those presenting with AMI, especially in the elderly. *(Please see Figure 1.)* Atypical presentations for AMI may fail to satisfy the AHA/ACC criteria for the diagnosis of AMI. In these patients, repeat ECGs and enzymes can assist in establishing diagnosis.

Risk Factors. Significant cardiac risk factors include hypertension, hyperlipidemia, diabetes, smoking, and a strong family history, which means a history of coronary artery disease (CAD) in early or mid-adulthood in a first-degree relative. It is well-known that cocaine use also presents some degree of risk for AMI due to its association with coronary vasospasm. Other minor risk factors may include type A personality, obesity, male sex, and a sedentary lifestyle. However, several studies have failed to confirm some of these factors as independent variables significantly contributing to AMI, except a history of infarction or angina.[6-8]

Physical Examination. Physical examination of the patient with AMI reveals such abnormal signs as a tachy- or bradycardia, other arrhythmias, hyper- or hypotension, and tachypnea. Diaphoresis strongly suggests cardiac chest pain and is considered an independent variable for AMI.[7] Up to 60% of patients with AMI present with diaphoresis.[9]

The Killip classification provides a quantitative assessment of cardiopulmonary function by correlating physical findings with patient outcomes in AMI. It is useful for predicting future morbidity and mortality and may help guide medical management. *(Please see Table 1.)*

Inspiratory rales and an S_3 gallop are associated with left-sided failure. Jugulovenous distentions (JVDs), hepatojugular reflux, and peripheral edema suggest right-sided failure. An S_4 denotes decreased left ventricular compliance and possible pump failure. A systolic murmur may indicate ischemic mitral regurgitation or ventricular septal defect (VSD).

Electrocardiogram (ECG). Although the ECG is highly specific for diagnosis of AMI, the initial ECG reveals diagnostic ST elevations in only 40% of patients who eventually have a confirmed AMI. AHA/ACC guidelines state that "ST-segment elevation (equal to or greater than 1 mV) in contiguous leads provides strong evidence of thrombotic coronary arterial occlusion and makes the patient a candidate for immediate reperfusion therapy, either by fibrinolysis or primary percutaneous transluminal coronary angioplasty (PTCA). Symptoms consistent with AMI and new left bundle-branch block (LBBB) should be managed like ST-segment elevation. In contrast, the patient without ST-segment elevation should not receive thrombolytic therapy. The benefit of primary PTCA in these patients remains uncertain."[10]

Although confirming AMI in the presence of LBBB can be difficult, certain findings can be useful for suggesting the diagnosis. For example, ongoing ischemia and infarction may be detected in the presence of LBBB.[11,12] Either a deflection of the J point (and ST segment) in the direction of the major QRS complex or an elevation of the ST segment of more than 7-8 mm opposite the direction of the major QRS complex suggests AMI. These findings have a sensitivity of greater than 50% and are about 90% specific for detecting acute myocardial injury.[12] The presence of Q waves in leads I, AVL, V_5, and V_6 is also a reliable sign of AMI in LBBB.

The diagnosis of myocardial injury in patients with artificial ventricular pacemakers can be difficult due to the abnormal sequence of ventricular excitation. In this subgroup of patients, the presence of new ST and T wave changes in the presence of a paced ventricular rhythm should be considered abnormal until proven otherwise.

Table 2. Common Markers Used to Identify Acute Myocardial Infarction

MARKER	INITIAL ELEVATION AFTER AMI	MEAN TIME TO PEAK ELEVATIONS	TIME TO RETURN TO BASELINE
Myoglobin	1-4 h	6-7 h	18-24 h
CTnI	3-12 h	10-24 h	3-10 d
CTnT	3-12 h	12-48 h	5-14 d
CKMB	4-12 h	10-24 h	48-72 h
CKMBiso	2-6 h	12 h	38 h
LD	8-12 h	24-48 h	10-14 d

CTnI, CTnT = troponins of cardiac myofibrils; CPK-MB, MM = tissue isoforms of creatine kinase; LD = lactate dehydrogenase.

Adapted from: Adams JE III, Abendschein DR, Jaffee S. Biochemical markers of myocardial injury: Is MB creatine kinase the choice for the 1990s? *Circulation* 1993;88:750-763.

Common patterns of ECG-lead ST elevations help identify the location of the myocardial damage. For example, ST-T wave elevations in I, AVL, and V_1-V_3 suggest anterior infarction, depressed ST segments in V_1 and V_2 suggest posterior-wall MI or an inferior-wall AMI with posterior extension, and ST elevations leads II, III, and AVF characteristically suggest inferior-wall infarction. ST segments may be falsely elevated in many conditions including myocarditis, ventricular aneurysms, LVH, LBBB, early repolarization, hypothyroidism, and hyperkalemia.

Laboratory Markers: Diagnostic and Prognostic Indications

General Principles. Enzyme markers are routinely used for the detection and management of AMI. Serum markers enhance the sensitivity for early detection of myocardial necrosis and ischemia as compared with the ECG. They also help determine the time of cardiac injury, especially when used in combination with other cardiac markers. It should be stressed that enzyme- and muscle-based cardiac markers vary in their performance characteristics, sensitivity, and specificity. *(Please see Table 2.)* To maximize the usefulness of these assays, the emergency physician must be aware of the specificity of cardiac markers for myocardial tissue, its release pattern, its half-life in plasma, and the period of time after release during which the marker remains detectable in serum. Analyzing temporal patterns of multiple markers can improve detection of myocardial ischemia and/or infarction and can help characterize the time of onset, progression, and extent of myocardial damage.

Although creatine kinase (CK)—in particular, the MB fraction of CK (CK-MB)—remains the most widely used enzyme marker and is still sine qua non for the diagnosis of AMI, other cardiac markers have received considerable attention. Among the most clinically promising in this regard are troponin I and troponin T, which exhibit both sensitivity and specificity for the diagnosis of AMI. At present, these protein markers should not be considered replacements for CK-MB for the identification and management of AMI, but they are extremely useful adjuncts and can provide considerable information that helps quantify and prognosticate a patient's risk for complications, morbidity, and mortality associated with AMI.

Creatine Kinase (CK). CK is an ubiquitous enzyme found in nearly all tissues. The cardiac-specific dimer, CK-MB, however, is present almost exclusively in myocardium, although it represents only 15-30% of total cardiac enzyme activity.[4,13] The most common causes for serum increases in total creatine kinase (TCK) remain non-cardiac in nature and include trauma, rhabdomyolysis, hyperthermia, vigorous physical activity, renal or endocrine disease, systemic infections, or any disease state causing destruction to muscle tissue. However, in the setting of chest pain in the absence of trauma, an elevated TCK level increases the likelihood that myocardial necrosis is present.

The majority of CK enzymes detected from myocardial injury result from CK-MM (isoenzyme of CK with muscle subunits) released from damaged cells. Accordingly, TCK, which is the measured sum of CK-MM, -MB, and -BB (found predominantly in brain tissue), is often elevated in MI. General reference ranges for normal TCK levels are less than 70 U/L. For AMI, the mean time required to exceed the reference range is 4.75 hours (range, 3.50-5.25 h) due to its large size and slow release ratio. Consequently, TCK is not sensitive for the early diagnosis of AMI. At four hours, the sensitivity of TCK is only 44%, while the specificity is 82%.[14] Specificity improves to nearly 100% by 10 hours. TCK levels peak at about 13 hours (range, 11.5-15.8 h) and remain elevated for 72 hours (range, 50-96 h).[14]

Conversely, insufficient TCK elevations should not be used to exclude the diagnosis of AMI. In fact, patients with small muscle mass (i.e., an elderly female with small muscle mass or a non Q-wave MI) may not release sufficient quantities of CK to exceed the laboratory reference range. Therefore, in the presence of suspected AMI, the ED physician should not rely on normal TCK values to exclude AMI.[15] Instead, a ratio of serum CK-MB to TCK (CK-MB/ TCK $\times$ 100%) should be calculated. A "cardiac index" ratio exceeding 3-5% (or a CK-MB mass assay/TCK ratio of 2.5% or greater) represents a disproportionately high concentration of CK-MB isoenzyme in the blood, which, in turn, suggests cardiac necrosis.[5] High levels of TCK released from muscle after trauma or rhabdomyolysis can also release large amounts of CK-MB, producing false-positive CK-MB interpretations. In this scenario, a cardiac index less than the cutoff value supports a non-cardiac etiology for elevated TCK. Regardless, an elevated cardiac index in a patient presenting with non-traumatic chest pain or with ECG changes suggesting cardiac involvement, confirms AMI by the WHO criteria.

CK-MB Subunits. Subunits of CK, CK-MB, -MM, and -BB, are high molecular-weight (86,000 D) markers associated with a slow release into the blood from damaged cells. Although CK-MB is produced almost exclusively in the myocardium, trace amounts of activity are also found in the small intestine, tongue, diaphragm, uterus, and prostate.[13,16] Elevated CK-MB enzyme levels are observed in the serum 2-6 hours after MI, but may not be detected until up to 12 hours after the onset of symptoms. The mean time to exceed reference standard is about 4.5 hours, which reflects the slow release kinetics of this enzyme. Peak CK-MB levels are observed from 12-24 hours (mean, 18 h) after AMI, and the enzyme is cleared from the bloodstream within 48-72 hours.

Various laboratory techniques are used to separate and identify cardiac specific CK-MB subforms from the non-specific CK-MM and -BB isoforms. The laboratory directly or indirectly measures CK-MB release. Indirect calculations of the amount of CK-MB enzymatic activity in the presence of substrate are reported in units of activity per liter (IU/L). This technique uses electrophoresis and is referred to as CK-MB activity. Monoclonal antibody techniques have greatly improved both specificity and sensitivity for detection of AMI by providing direct measurements of CK-MB mass. Mass assays are reported in mcg/L. Generally, the mass assay is more sensitive for detection of AMI and should be requested from the laboratory service. Both processes are limited by delayed enzyme release from damaged myocardial cells. Sensitivity for detection of AMI approaches 100% at 10-12 hours, but is only about 57% for the mass assay and about 32% for CK-MB activity during the first four hours.[14]

Assays of CK-MB isoforms, $CK\text{-}MB_1$ and $CK\text{-}MB_2$, separate two isoelectric forms of CK-MB. $CK\text{-}MB_2$ values greater than 2.6 IU/L and $CK\text{-}MB_2$ to $CK\text{-}MB_1$ ratios greater than 1.7 are indicative of myocardial necrosis. These isoforms are released simultaneously into the blood at 2-6 hours following AMI. However, increased isoform ratios can be detected in the serum earlier than CK-MB isoenzyme alone, increasing the sensitivity for early AMI detection and identification over standard CK-MB assays (at 6 hours, 91% sensitivity for subunits vs 62% for CK-MB).[17] Unfortunately, these assays are not available at all institutions, and are technically difficult tests requiring special equipment.

Other enzymes and/or enzyme panels, including such markers as myoglobin and troponin T and I, are often employed to enhance detection of early AMI until confirmatory levels of CK-MB are achieved. Accordingly, it is not advisable to discharge a patient with suspected cardiac chest pain until the CK-MB measurements supercede the duration of chest pain symptoms by at least nine hours (longer if the patient has ongoing chest pain). This corresponds to the expected peak CK-MB level. Given these kinetics, patients who have a discrete episode of chest pain, followed by a pain-free course of at least nine hours and who also have normal CK-MB measurements throughout this period do not have AMI. However, this "rapid rule out" does not exclude the presence of acute cardiac/coronary ischemia. Admission for stress testing or direct coronary angiography may be necessary in those with continued atypical chest pain suspicious for a cardiac etiology, regardless of CK-MB levels.

Troponin T and I. Acute coronary syndromes reflect a continuum of ischemic syndromes that range from silent ischemia to unstable angina and non Q-wave MI, and, finally, AMI.[18] Some of these syndromes represent reversible myocardial insult. For example, unlike AMI, acute cardiac ischemia (ACI), if it is detected in its early stages, may be amenable to medical or surgical management. In other words, interventions that successfully prevent evolution from ischemia to completed myocardial infarction may be pressed into service to reduce morbidity and mortality.

Not surprisingly, new techniques that can detect and confirm ischemic myocardial insult prior to irreversible damage are being given high priority in emergency medicine. In this regard, protein subunits derived from muscle tissue have gained recognition as promising markers. During muscle contraction, thick filaments of myosin and thin filaments of actin slide across each as a result of calcium-mediated, ATP-dependent contraction. Released calcium binds to a "complex" of three proteins on the tropomyosin filament, troponin C, T, and I, which regulates muscle contraction.

Proteins of troponin T and I have been purified from myocardial tissue, allowing the development of cardiac specific immunoassays.[19] Because the amino acid sequence for troponin C is identical in all tissues, it is not useful as a cardiac marker. Unlike CK-MB or myoglobin, the troponins T and I are cardiac-specific structural proteins, and, therefore, are not normally detectable in blood without myocardial insult. False-positive results do not occur with skeletal muscle disease, exercise, non-cardiac trauma, or renal failure, as they would would with creatine kinase.

Cardiac-specific troponin T (cTnT) is a qualitative assay with a turnaround time of 30 minutes; it also is available as a rapid bedside assay. Cardiac troponin I (cTnI) is a quantitative assay with a processing time of about one hour. Troponin assays require only a single test, whereas two tests are required to interpret elevated creatine kinase, total creatine kinase, and CK-MB.[18] Also, since cTnT remains elevated in serum up to 14 days (more than 5 times longer than CK-MB), and cTnI for 3-7 days after infarction, normal troponin results can provide information during the evaluation of patients with sustained chest pain.

Sensitivity and Specificity. Detection of cTnT or cTnI should be considered a positive finding. However, small measured quantities may suggest a "microinfarction," or even unstable angina, rather than a significant MI. After myocardial damage, cTnT and cTnI are released in a temporal fashion similar to that of CK-MB.[19,20] Initial troponin levels are usually first detected at 2-4 hours after AMI. The sensitivity of cTnT for AMI detection at two, four, eight, and greater than eight hours is 33%, 50%, 75%, and 86%, respectively. In contrast, specificity of cTnT between four and eight hours post AMI was 100%; it is 95% at two hours and 86% after eight hours.[21] In another trial, the sensitivity and specificity for AMI detection with CK-MB was 99% and 72%, vs. 100% and 69% for cTnT, respectively.[22] However, troponin assays may have a lower specificity than CK-MB for "true" AMI, since significant amounts of troponins can be detected with small myocardial insults, now referred to as ACI.[19]

Recent studies have focused on the high sensitivity of cTnT for detecting minimal myocardial damage and on its role as a tool for risk stratification prior to completed MI.[21,23-25] The GUSTO-IIa subtrial of 755 patients evaluated patients with chest pain and attempted to characterize those with AMI vs. ACI.[18] With a mean symptom-to-initial-sampling time of 3.5 hours, 36% of patients had cTnT elevations compared to 32% with elevated CK-MB. The 30-day mor-

Figure 2. Management of AMI

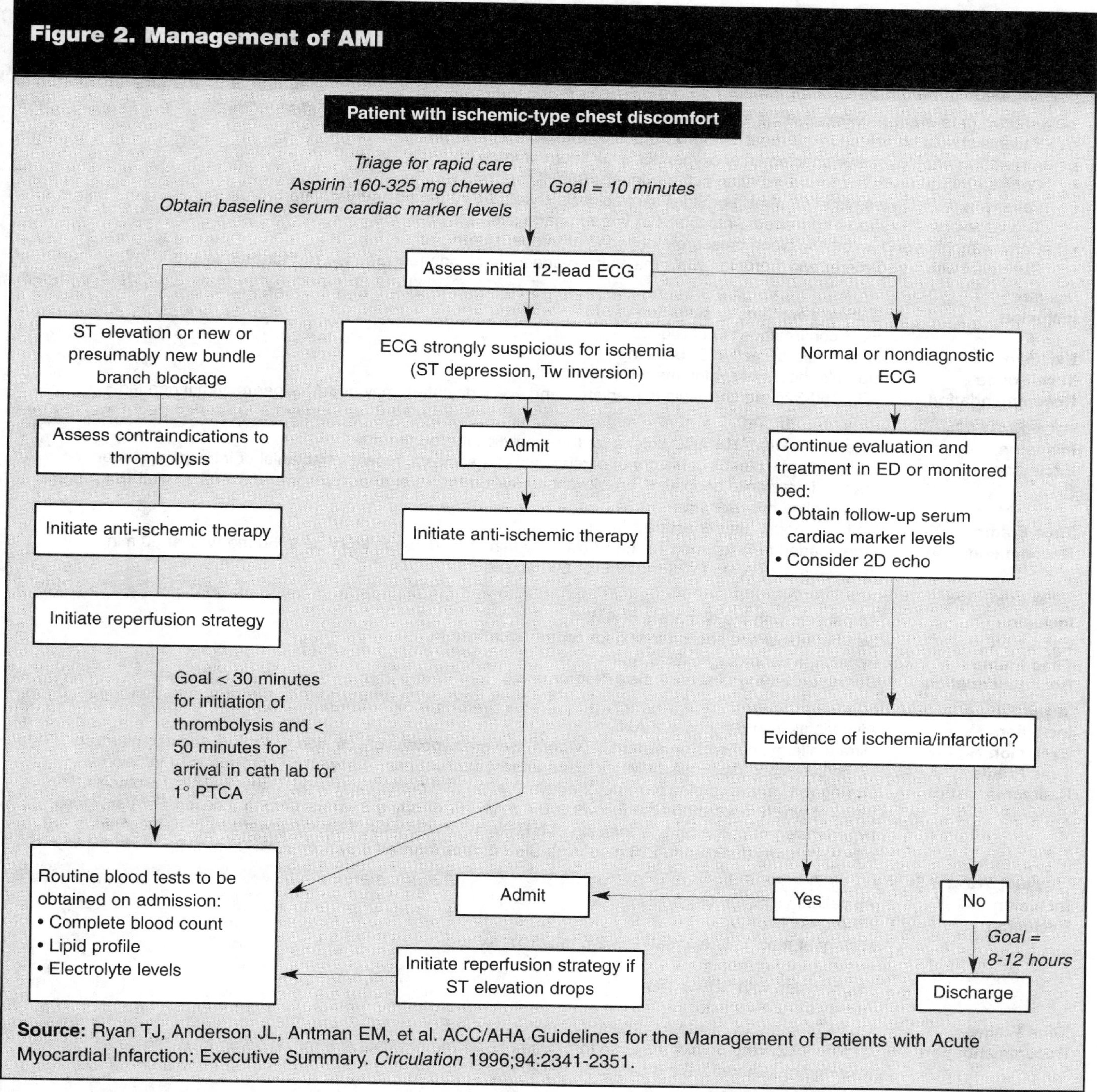

Source: Ryan TJ, Anderson JL, Antman EM, et al. ACC/AHA Guidelines for the Management of Patients with Acute Myocardial Infarction: Executive Summary. *Circulation* 1996;94:2341-2351.

tality of those with elevated cTnT greater than 0.1 ng/mL was 11.8% vs. 3.9% in the negative cTnT group.[18] This study suggests that cTnT may help stratify post-AMI patients into those at high risk for cardiac-related mortality.

Other studies involving ACI suggest that elevated cTnT more closely correlates with 30-day mortality than CK-MB or ECG. In a trial of 183 unstable angina patients with cTnT levels drawn 12 and 24 hours after admission, increased rates of cardiac death and angioplasty during the two-year follow-up period were reported in patients in the positive cTnT group.[24] Also, patients with a positive cTnT who have had AMI ruled by traditional criteria appear at greater risk for short-term adverse events, including cardiac arrest, AMI, arrhythmia, and recurrent angina, than those with a negative cTnT.[25] Finally, patients with negative troponin I results and normal ECGs during their chest pain evaluation have significantly lower risk for future adverse cardiac events than those with abnormal cTnI.[26] These trials suggest that cTnT and cTnI may be reliable prognostic markers for myocardial insult, and may be useful in risk stratifying those non-AMI patients with unstable angina.[24-26]

Because ACI is on the continuum that terminates in AMI, the value of troponin markers for the management of AMI is in evolu-

Table 3. Treatment Recommendations for AMI

SUPPORTIVE CARE WITH MANAGEMENT OF CHEST PAIN

- Patients should be placed in the most comfortable position, usually sitting up.
- All patients should receive supplemental oxygen for a minimum of three hours.
- Continue oxygen with titration to maintain pulse oximetry, 95% if hypoxic.
- Patients with PaO_2 less than 60 mmHg or significant acidosis should be intubated and ventilated.
- Two large-bore IVs should be placed. Antecubital or large forearm sites are preferred.
- Cardiac monitor and automatic blood pressure monitoring at frequent intervals.
- Pain relief with nitroglycerin and morphine while maintaining adequate blood pressure (see text for precautions).

ASPIRIN	
Inclusion	Clinical symptoms or suspicion of AMI ECG confirmation is not required
Exclusion	Aspirin allergy, active GI bleeding
Time Frame	Up to 24 hours of symptoms onset
Recommendation	ASA 160-325 mg chewable immediately and every day after; may use ASA per rectum if needed
THROMBOLYTICS	
Inclusion	All patients with AHA/ACC criteria for thrombolytic infusion therapy
Exclusion	Active internal bleeding; history of cerebrovascular accident; recent intracranial or intraspinal surgery or trauma; intracranial neoplasm, arteriovenous malformation, or aneurysm; known bleeding diathesis; severe, uncontrolled hypertension
Time Frame	Up to six hours after chest pain begins
Recommendation	Front-loaded t-PA regimen 15 mg IV over 1-2 min, then 0.75 mg/kg IV up to 50 mg IV over 30 min, then 0.5 mg/kg IV up to 35 mg IV over 60 minutes
BETA-BLOCKADE	
Inclusion	All patients with the diagnosis of AMI
Exclusion	See beta-blockade section in text for contraindications
Time Frame	Immediate upon diagnosis of AMI
Recommendation	Dosing according to specific beta-blocker used
NITRATES	
Inclusion	All patients with diagnosis of AMI
Exclusion	Nitrate allergy; patients on sildenafil (Viagra); severe hypotension; caution in right ventricular infarction
Time Frame	Immediate upon diagnosis of MI for management of chest pain, followed by continuous IV infusion
Recommendation	Dosing will vary according to route of administration and preparation used. Consult clinical protocols, many of which recommend the following: 0.4 mg NTG initially q 5 minutes, up to 3 doses. For persistent hypertension or chest pain, IV infusion of NTG at 10-20 mcg/min, titrating upward by 5-10 mcg/min q 5-10 minutes (maximum, 200 mcg/min). Slow or stop infusion if systolic BP < 90 mmHg
ACE INHIBITORS	
Inclusion	All patients with the diagnosis of AMI
Exclusion	Killip class III or IV History of renal failure, creatine > 2.5 mg/dL or hx Renal artery stenosis Hypotension with SBP < 100 Allergy to ACE inhibitor
Time Frame	Up to 24 hours to initiate treatment, not necessary in ED
Recommendation	Captopril 12.5 mg po bid, may use test dose of 6.25 mg or lisinopril 5 mg po qd up to 10 mg qd as tolerated or lisinopril 2.5 mg po if SBP < 120
HEPARIN	
Inclusion	Those patients receiving t-PA or those patients not receiving ASA
Exclusion	Hypersensitivity Active internal bleeding Prolonged CPR Recent head trauma/CNS surgery/known intracranial neoplasm Hemorrhagic ophthalmic condition
Time Frame	To be given concomitantly with t-PA
Recommendation	• With t-PA administration, begin weight-based IV heparin protocol to maintain a PTT at 1.5 to 2.0 × control for the next 48 hours • Treatment beyond 48 hours is recommended only for those patients with a high risk for systemic or venous thromboembolism • In patients not receiving t-PA, weight-based heparin only for patients with high risk systemic emboli (large or anterior AMI, a-fib, previous embolus or known LV thrombus) for 48 hours to maintain a PTT at 1.5-2.0 × control

tion. Both markers are as reliable as CK-MB for detection of AMI, but also may be positive in acute coronary syndromes—what some call a "preinfarction state." At present, it does not appear that cTnT or cTnI should supplant CK-MB assay for identification of AMI, but these markers should help risk stratify those not identified for AMI by traditional means. Since AMI represents only a small percentage of patients presenting with chest pain, the utility of troponin in this setting requires more thorough evaluation.

Guidelines for Mortality Reduction: Non-thrombolytic Agents

The goal of management in AMI is to prevent evolution of infarction, reduce myocardial necrosis, minimize complications, and ultimately reduce short- and long-term mortality. *(Please see Figure 2.)* Diagnostic confirmation should be followed promptly by reperfusion whenever possible. Inclusionary and exclusionary criteria for thrombolysis should be assessed by the ED physician as soon as possible, and this intervention should be integrated with all aspects of care in a concise and effective manner. *(Please see Table 3.)*

Supportive Care. Oxygen should be administered at a flow rate of at 2 L/min as required and continued if pulse oximetry is less than 90%.[26] The patient should be placed on a cardiac monitor and blood drawn for baseline laboratory studies. At least two IVs are helpful, especially if the patient is eligible and requires thrombolysis. Blood pressure should be monitored every 15 minutes until stable and then at least every four hours. Strict bedrest is advised.[27]

Pain Control. Administer morphine sulfate 2-4 mg IV every 5-10 minutes to blunt the sympathetic response to pain and anxiety. Doses approaching 25-30 mg may be necessary to achieve adequate pain relief.[28] Morphine-induced hypotension typically occurs in volume-depleted patients but is uncommon in patients who remain in the supine position.[28] Some cardiologists feel that morphine may mask ischemic pain and prefer to use nitrates or procedural interventions for pain management.

Nitroglycerin. Sublingual nitroglycerin (NTG) may improve ischemic chest pain but also can cause headaches. Initially, give up to three doses of 0.4 mg sublingual NTG every five minutes.

Nitroglycerin also is indicated for persistent hypertension and congestive heart failure. NTG should be used with caution in patients with inferior-wall MI that is accompanied by right ventricular (RV) infarction, hypovolemia, or hypotension. For persistent hypertension, start an infusion of intravenous NTG at 10-20 mcg/min, titrating upward by 5-10 mcg/min every 5-10 minutes (maximum, 200 mcg/min). Titrate to decrease the mean arterial pressure by 10% in normotensive patients and by 30% in those with hypertension. Slow or stop the infusion when the SBP drops below 90.[27] If clinically significant hypotension occurs with IV NTG administration, discontinue the drug, drop the head of the bed, and administer fluids as needed. Atropine may be appropriate if severe hypotension persists.[27]

Aspirin. The benefits of aspirin therapy for reducing mortality after MI and in the setting of unstable angina are substantiated by numerous trials. The largest, the second International Study on Infarct Survival (ISIS-2), demonstrated a 20% reduction in mortality ($P < 0.001$), which resulted in prevention of 25 early deaths for every 1000 patients with suspected AMI.[29] Those individuals who were treated with aspirin for one month following AMI experienced nearly twice the reduction from further deaths, reinfarctions, and strokes than the group randomized to placebo. These benefits were independent of thrombolytic or heparin administration, and do not appear dose dependent (initial dose of at least 160 mg/d).

The benefits of aspirin, which is most efficacious if given in the first four hours, are very substantial, as was demonstrated in more than 17,000 patients in the ISIS-2 trial. In the absence of contraindications (allergy, active GI bleeding, or recent intracranial hemorrhage), aspirin should be administered to all patients presenting with cardiac chest pain in the ED. A dose of 160-325 mg should be given on day 1 of AMI and continued indefinitely on a daily basis thereafter.[10] For the rare patient with a contraindication to aspirin, another antiplatelet drug, such as ticlopidine, should be administered. Newer agents that block the final common pathway for platelet aggregation (IIb/IIIa inhibitors) are a promising substitute for aspirin.

Beta Blockade. Beta-blockers have been shown to decrease mortality and to reduce infarct size in several clinical trials.[30-32] The First International Study on Infarct Survival (ISIS-1) and the Metoprolol in Acute Myocardial Infarction (MIAMI) trial are the most important trials showing benefits from this intervention. In ISIS-1, 16,027 patients were randomized to receive IV atenolol or placebo. There was a significant, relative decrease in mortality rates (3.89% mortality rate in the drug group vs 4.57% placebo) in the first week and at one year (10.7% vs 12%) following AMI. Overall, beta-blocker use during AMI can be expected to produce about an 11% reduction in mortality.[30] The MIAMI trial included 5778 patients; a definitive AMI was confirmed in 4127 patients. Oral metoprolol was administered in doses ranging from 15-200 mg daily for 15 days. The metoprolol group had a mortality rate of 4.3% vs. 4.9% for the placebo group, demonstrating a 13% relative decrease in mortality. High-risk patients had a 29% lower mortality rate than control.[31] Beta-blockers also decrease recurrent ischemia and nonfatal reinfarction in patients treated with tissue plasminogen activator (t-PA).[35] Contraindications to beta-blockade include allergy, significant bronchial hyperreactivity, bradycardia, hypotension, PR interval greater than 0.24 s, second- or third-degree AV block, pulmonary edema, insulin-dependent diabetes mellitus, severe peripheral vascular disease, or hypoperfusion.[26]

Heparin. The AHA/ACC criteria for using heparin are as follows:

- *Class I:*
  - Patients undergoing percutaneous or surgical revascularization.
- *Class IIa:*
  - Intravenously in patients undergoing reperfusion therapy with alteplase;
  - Subcutaneously (7500 U bid) (intravenous heaprin is an acceptable alternative) in all patients not treated with thrombolytic therapy who do not have a contraindication to heparin. In patients who are at high risk for systemic emboli (large or anterior MI, atrial fibrillation [AF], previous embolus, or known LV thrombus), intravenous heparin is preferred;
  - Intravenously in patients treated with nonselective thrombolytic agents (streptokinase, anistreplase, urokinase) who are at high risk for systemic emboli (large or anterior MI, AF, previous embolus, or known LV thrombus).

Choosing a Thrombolytic Agent

Myocardial infarction (MI) is the direct consequence of thrombotic occlusion of a coronary artery. Therapeutic strategies focus on the rapid identification of the patient suffering acute coronary artery thrombosis, optimal reperfusion of the occluded artery, and prevention of subsequent complications, including reinfarction, bleeding, stroke, arrhythmic death, and heart failure.

Nine large placebo-controlled, randomized, clinical trials of more than 58,000 patients clearly demonstrated that intravenous fibrinolytic therapy confers a significant morbidity and mortality benefit in the treatment of patients with acute MI with ST elevation or bundle branch block.[1] Despite an increased risk of hemorrhagic complications and stroke, this net benefit extended across all patient subgroups and was independent of all other outcome determinants. The clinical benefit also was more prominent the earlier treatment began. As a result, intravenous fibrinolytic therapy is the standard-of-care to which newer strategies are compared.

Subsequent studies have compared the effects of several available plasminogen activators, particularly recombinant tissue plasminogen activator (t-PA, alteplase) and streptokinase (SK). The GUSTO-1 trial ushered in the current era of intravenous fibrinolytic therapy by demonstrating a significant mortality benefit of the accelerated infusion of t-PA over SK.[2]

DETERMINANTS OF OUTCOME IN ACUTE MI

The primary determinants of outcome in acute MI are the baseline risk characteristics of the patient, the adequacy of flow in the reperfused artery, speed of reperfusion, the incidence of reocclusion of the infarct-related coronary artery, and the direct complications of the therapeutic intervention.

In a multivariate regression analysis of the data from the 41,021 patients in the GUSTO-1 trial, Lee and colleagues identified 16 baseline patient characteristics and their relative weights as independent predictors of 30-day mortality: age, systolic blood pressure, Killip class (degree of heart failure), heart rate, site of current infarction, prior infarction, the interaction of age with Killip class, height, time-to-treatment, diabetes, weight, smoking status, type of thrombolytic therapy, prior bypass surgery, hypertension, and prior cerebrovascular disease.[3] Califf and associates then developed a model using a reduced set of these determinants that retained 90% of the predictive value of the original model.[4] The most powerful variables predictive of 30-day mortality were as follows:

Although the other factors such as time-to-treatment or prior cerebrovascular disease may affect the physiologic status of the patient, the independent contribution is relatively small. The impact of age is nearly two orders of magnitude greater than the choice of lytic agent.

The patency of the infarct-related artery is an important determinant of outcome. Infarct-artery patency is described using angiographic criteria from the early Thrombolysis in Myocardial Infarction (TIMI) trials. TIMI grade 3 flow is essentially normal flow. TIMI grade 2 flow is reduced flow but considered adequate to prevent immediate cell death. TIMI grades 0 and 1 flow reflect either no or inadequate perfusion, respectively.

A substudy in the GUSTO-1 trial randomized 2431 patients to evaluate the angiographic determinants of out-

- *Class IIb:*
  - Patients treated with nonselective thrombolytic agents, not at high risk, subcutaneous heparin, 7500-12,500 U bid until completely ambulatory.
- *Class III:*
  - Routine intravenous heparin within six hours to patients receiving a nonselective fibrinolytic agent (streptokinase, anistreplase, urokinase) who are not at high risk for systemic embolism.[10]

ACE Inhibitors. Both the ISIS-4 trial[33] and the GISSI-3 trial[34-35] have shown increased survival in patients with AMI who are given an oral ACE inhibitor within the first 24 hours. In the GISSI-3 trial, which consisted of 19,394 patients, patients were randomized to lisinopril or placebo for six weeks after AMI. Patients were followed and evaluated for death or severe ventricular dysfunction for six months after their AMI. ACE-inhibitors reduced the incidence of combined end points from 19.3% (placebo) to 18.1% (treatment group). ISIS-4 enrolled 58,050 patients and compared mortality rates for oral captopril, oral mononitrate, and IV magnesium. Captopril was given as a 6.25 mg initial dose and titrated up to 50 mg po bid for one month. Mortality rates at five weeks were significantly better with ACE-inhibitors (7.19%) than with placebo (7.69%). ACE-inhibitors are recommended within the first 24 hours of AMI, but are not necessarily required for the initial ED management of AMI.

Magnesium. Intravenous magnesium was shown to be beneficial in the LIMIT-2 study of 2316 patients, as well as in a meta-analysis trial consisting of seven other smaller trials that analyzed 3566 patients.[36,37] In the LIMIT-2 trial, mortality reduction was 24% in the magnesium-treated group.[36,37] The overall mortality rates for AMI were 7.8% in the magnesium group vs. 10.3% in the placebo group. However, magnesium failed to reduce AMI mortality in the large, prospective and randomized ISIS-4 trial.[33] Enrolling 58,050 patients, ISIS-4 failed to confirm mortality-reducing benefits associated with magnesium.

These differences may be attributed to variations in magnesium dosages and to the acuity of its administration. In the ISIS-4 trial, magnesium was not administered until the completion of thrombolytic therapy. In light of the inconsistencies between available studies, other trials may still be indicated. Hypermagnesemia should be avoided and magnesium should not be administered when the serum creatine is above 3 or in patients with heart block. Despite that magnesium appears to be a relatively benign drug, it is not recommended by most authorities for routine administration in AMI at this time.

come.[5] Left ventricular (LV) function was strongly correlated with the 90-minute infarct-related artery patency. The patients with TIMI-3 flow had better LV function and myocardial wall motion at 90 minutes and seven days. The 30-day mortality for patients with TIMI-3 flow in the infarct-related artery was 4.4%, while the mortality in the patients with TIMI-2 flow was 7.4%.

A pooled analysis by Barbagelata and associates of angiographic studies performed after thrombolysis confirmed the findings of the GUSTO angiographic investigators.[6] TIMI-3 flow is associated with a substantially lower rate of congestive heart failure, lower rate of recurrent ischemia, better LV function, and 30-50% lower mortality compared to TIMI-2 flow, which is in turn better than TIMI-0 or -1 flow.

T-PA VS. SK

Mortality. The GUSTO-1 trial (1993) used a new approach to the administration of t-PA by "accelerating" the administration of the fibrinolytic (using a weight-adjusted dose) over 90 minutes instead of the "standard" 180 minute t-PA dosage regimen and by giving intravenous heparin immediately. A significant mortality benefit of "accelerated" t-PA over streptokinase regimens was evident throughout all treatment groups. An analysis by Califf et al demonstrates that the absolute mortality benefit of t-PA vs. SK increases with increasing mortality risk.[4] As a result, despite higher risks of treatment, the net mortality benefit of t-PA for the high-risk patient (e.g., elderly patient, anterior MI, and CHF) was predictably greater than for the low-risk patient (e.g., young patient with inferior MI without heart failure). The higher the risk, the greater the absolute mortality benefit of t-PA vs. SK. The mortality benefit of accelerated t-PA over SK is attributed to the higher rate of early infarct-related artery patency.

The angiographic substudy of GUSTO-1 revealed that accelerated t-PA produced a significantly higher rate of open vessels (TIMI 2 and 3 combined) of 81% and complete reperfusion (TIMI 3) of 54% at 90 minutes, compared to SK rates of 60% and 41%, respectively. The patency rates were not significantly different at 180 minutes between t-PA and SK. Most of the survival benefit of accelerated t-PA over SK in the GUSTO-1 trial appears to be largely due to this advantage of early patency.

SUMMARY

Intravenous fibrinolytic therapy is the standard of care for eligible acute MI patients with ST elevation or bundle branch block. Treatment with the weight-adjusted accelerated t-PA protocol of GUSTO-1 provides a net absolute mortality benefit in all treatment groups as compared to SK.

REFERENCES

1. Fibrinolytic Therapy Trialists' Collaborative Group. *Lancet* 1994;343:311-322.
2. The GUSTO Investigators. *N Engl J Med* 1993;329: 673-682.
3. Lee KL, et al. *Circulation* 1995;91:1659-1668.
4. Califf RM, et al. *Am Heart J* 1997;133:630-639.
5. The GUSTO Angiographic Investigators. *N Engl J Med* 1993;329:1615-1622.
6. Barbagelata NA, et al. *Am Heart J* 1997;133:273-282.

Author: William E. Davis, MD

Calcium Channel Blockers. No benefits have been attributed to calcium channel blockers for acute management of AMI. In fact, significant increases in mortality have been reported in patients with heart failure or depressed left ventricular function, especially with short-acting calcium channel blockers. This class of drugs is not recommended in AMI.

References

1. Gillum RF. Trends in acute myocardial infarction and coronary heart disease in the United States. *J Am Coll Cardiol* 1994;23:1273-1277.
2. Davies MJ, Thomas AC. Plaque fissuring—The cause of acute myocardial infarction, sudden ischemic death and crescendo angina. *Br Heart J* 1985;53:363-373.
3. McClellan M, McNeill BJ, Newhouse JP, et al. Does more intensive treatment of acute myocardial infarction in the elderly reduce mortality? Analysis using instrument variables. *JAMA* 1994;272:859-866.
4. Gillum RF, Formann SP, Prineas RJ, et al. International diagnostic criteria for acute myocardial infarction and stroke. *Am Heart J* 1984;108:150-158.
5. Apple FS. Acute myocardial infarction and coronary reperfusion: Serum cardiac markers for the 1990s. *Am J Clin Pathol* 1992;97:217-226.
6. Goldman L, Cook EF, Brand DA, et al. A computer protocol to predict myocardial infarction in emergency department patients with chest pain. *N Engl J Med* 1988;318:797-803.
7. Tierney WM, Roth BJ, Psaty B, et al. Predictors of myocardial infarction in emergency room patients. *Crit Care Med* 1985;13:526-531.
8. Pozen MW, D'Agostino RB, Selker HP, et al. A predictive instrument to improve coronary care unit admission practices in acute ischemic heart disease: A prospective multicenter clinical trial. *N Engl J Med* 1984;310:1273-1278.
9. Gruppo Italiano per lo Studio della Sopravivenza nell' Infarcto Miocardico. Comparison of frequency, diagnosis, and prognostic significance of pericardial involvement in acute myocardial infarction treated with and without thrombolytics. *Am J Cardiol* 1993;71:1377-1381.
10. Ryan TJ, Anderson JL, Antman EM, et al. ACC/AHA guidelines for the management of patients with acute myocardial infarction: Executive summary. *Circulation* 1996;94: 2341-2350.
11. Rouan GW, Lee TH, Cook EF, et al. Clinical characteristics and outcome of acute myocardial infarction in patients with initially normal or nonspecific electrocardiograms (a report from the Multi-center Chest Pain Study). *Am J Cardiol* 1989; 64:1087-1092.

12. Fesmire F. ECG diagnosis of acute myocardial infarction in the presence of left bundle branch block in patients undergoing continuous ECG monitoring. *Ann Emerg Med* 1995;26: 69-72.
13. Howanitz JH, Howanitz PJ, eds. *Laboratory Medicine: Test Selection and Interpretation.* New York; Churchill Livingstone; 1991:25-39.
14. Mair J, Artner-Dworzak E, Dienstl A, et al. Early detection of acute myocardial infarction by measurement of mass concentration of creatine kinase-MB. *Am J Cardiol* 1991;68: 1545-1549.
15. Hong RA, Licht JD, Wei JY, et al. Elevated CK-MB with normal total creatine kinase in suspected myocardial infarction: Associated clinical findings and early prognosis. *Am Heart J* 1986;111:1041-1046.
16. Selker HP, Zalenski RJ, Antman EM, et al. An evaluation of technologies for identifying acute cardiac ischemia in the emergency department: Executive summary of a National Heart Attack Alert Program Working Group Report. *Ann Emerg Med* 1997;29:59-63.
17. Puleo PR, Guadagno PA, Roberts R, et al. Early diagnosis of acute myocardial infarction based on assay for subforms of creatine kinase-MB. *Circulation* 1990;82:759-764.
18. Ohman EM, Armstrong PW, Christenson RH, et al. Cardiac troponin T levels for risk stratification in acute myocardial ischemia. *N Engl J Med* 1996;335:1333-1341.
19. Christenson RH, Newby LK, Ohman EM. Cardiac markers in the assessment of acute coronary syndromes. The strategy of the chest pain units (in emergency departments) in the war against heart attacks: Proceedings from the first Maryland Chest Pain Center Research Conference. *Maryland Med J* 1997:Suppl 12;18-25.
20. deWinter RJ, Koster RW, Sturk A, et al. Value of myoglobin, troponin T, and CK-MB mass in ruling out an acute myocardial infarction in the emergency room. *Circulation* 1995;92: 3401-3407.
21. Antman EM, Grudzien C, Sacks DB. Evaluation of a rapid bedside assay for detection of serum cardiac troponin T. *JAMA* 1995;273:1279-1282.
22. Ravkilde J, Horder M, Gerhart W, et al. Diagnostic performance and prognostic value of serum troponin T in suspected acute myocardial infarction. *Scan J Clin Lab Invest* 1993;53: 677-685.
23. Wu Ah, Abbas SA, Green S, et al. Prognostic value of cardiac troponin T in unstable angina pectoris. *Am J Cardiol* 1995;76: 970-972.
24. Stubbs P, Collinson P, Moseley D, et al. Prospective study of the role of cardiac troponin T in patients admitted with unstable angia. *BMJ* 1996;313:262.
25. Green GG, Beaudreau RW, Chan DW. Use of troponin T and creatine kinase-MB subunit levels for risk stratification of emergency department patients with possible myocardial ischemia. *Ann Emerg Med* 1998;31:19-29.
26. Hamm CW, Goldmann BU, Heeschen C, et al. Emergency room triage of patients with acute chest pain by means of rapid testing for cardiac troponin T or troponin I. *N Engl J Med* 1997;337:1648-1653.
27. Ryan TJ, Anderson JL, Antman EM, et al. ACA/AHA Guidelines for the management of patients with acute myocardial infarction. A report of the American College of Cardiology/American Heart Association Task Force on Practice Guidelines (Committee on Management of Acute Myocardial Infarction). *J Am Coll Cardiol* 1996;28: 1328-1428.
28. Antman EM. General hospital management. In: Julian DG, Braunwald E, eds. *Management of Acute Myocardial Infarction.* London, England; WB Saunders Co. Ltd; 1994: 42-44.
29. ISIS-2 (Second International Study of Infarct Survival) Collaborative Group. Randomized trial of intravenous streptokinase, oral aspirin, both or neither among 17,187 cases of suspected acute myocardial infarction: ISIS-2. *Lancet* 1988;2: 349-360.
30. ISIS-1 (First International Study of Infarct Survival) in Collaborative Group. Randomised trial of intravenous atenolol among 16027 cases of suspected acute myocardial infarction. *Lancet* 1986;2:57-66.
31. The MIAMI Trial Research Group. Metoprolol in acute myocardial infarction (MIAMI). A randomized placebo-controlled international trial. *Eur Heart J* 1985;6:199-226.
32. The TIMI Study Group. Comparison of invasive and conservative strategies after treatment with intravenous tissue plasminogen activator in acute myocardial infarction: Results of the Thrombolysis in Myocardial Infarction (TIMI) Phase II Trial. *N Engl J Med* 1989;320:618-627.
33. ISIS-4 Collaborative Group. A randomized factorial trial assessing early oral captopril, oral mononitrate and intravenous magnesium sulphate in 58,050 patients with suspected acute myocardial infarction. *Lancet* 1995;345:669-682.
34. Gruppo Italiano per lo Studio della Sopravivenza nell' Infarcto Miocardico. GISSI-3: Effects of lisinopril and transdermal glyceryl trinitrate singly and together on six-week mortality and ventricular function after acute myocardial infarction. *Lancet* 1994;343:1115-1122.
35. GISSI-3 Investigators. Six month effects of early treatment with lisinopril and transdermal glyceryl trinitrate singly and together withdrawn six weeks after acute myocardial infarction: The GISSI-3 trial. *J Am Coll Cardiol* 1996;27:337-344.
36. Woods KL, Fletcher S, Roffe C, et al. Intravenous magnesium sulphate in suspected acute myocardial infarction: Results of the second Leicester Intravenous Magnesium Intervention Trial (LIMIT-2). *Lancet* 1992;339:1553-1558.
37. Woods KL, Fletcher S. Long-term outcome after intravenous magnesium sulphate in suspected acute myocardial infarction: The second Leicester Intravenous Magnesium Intervention Trial (LIMIT-2). *Lancet* 1994;343:816-819.

Acute Myocardial Infarction: Thrombolysis and Procedural Revascularization

Gideon Bosker, MD, FACEP
David J. Robinson, MD, MS
David A. Jerrard, MD, FACEP
Dick C. Kuo, MD

Emergency management of acute myocardial infarction (AMI) is evolving at an extremely rapid pace. What nearly all mortality-reducing strategies have in common is prompt restoration of blood flow to ischemic myocardium that has been compromised by intracoronary thrombosis. Although the precise relationship between the degree of coronary patency/flow and clinical outcomes may be debated, all experts agree that "time is muscle." Moreover, regardless of whether pharmacological (thrombolysis) or procedural interventions (angioplasty, stent, or coronary artery bypass) are employed, short- and long-term prognosis is optimized when blood flow to injured tissue is restored as quickly as possible.

Although the mandate to restore coronary perfusion is well-accepted, approaches to myocardial salvage vary from one institution to another. For example, in those emergency departments (EDs) where access to coronary angiography is limited, thrombolytic therapy with such agents as t-PA will be the anchor agent for pharmacologic therapy, which, along with aspirin, also may include a mortality-reducing cocktail of beta-blockers, nitrates, and anticoagulants. In contrast, other institutions may be intervention intensive, in which case the majority of patients with AMI will be catheterized on an emergent basis, and, depending upon the anatomic lesions encountered, angioplasty and/or stent insertion will be the procedures of choice. Complicating approaches to patient management is the emergence of data from recent studies suggesting that some combination of thrombolytic and procedural intervention may be better than either technique alone.

The purpose of this chapter is to review current strategies for myocardial salvage, with an emphasis on recent advances and controversies in thrombolytic therapy. In addition, new developments in combined pharmacologic and procedural approaches to AMI are discussed. Finally, future strategies for mortality reduction in AMI are highlighted.

Thrombolytics: Mortality-Reducing Options

Introduction. Plasmin is the complex that facilitates lysis of a coronary thrombus that precipitates AMI. Thrombolytic therapy enhances the conversion of plasminogen to plasmin, thereby inducing clot lysis. Plasminogen is an inactive proteolytic enzyme that is found in plasma and bound to fibrin in thrombi.[1] Tissue plasminogen activator (t-PA) essentially induces clot-specific lysis by cleaving bound plasminogen to the active form, plasmin, which then degrades fibrin to degradation products. These degradation products have antiplatelet and anticoagulant effects and also reduce viscosity. All t-PA variants can be compared regarding risks and benefits *(please see Table 1),* and all have the same contraindications. *(Please see Table 2.)* The major limitation of all available plasminogen activators is that they generate active thrombin and stimulate platelet aggregation,

Table 1. Benefits and Risks of Thrombolytics

ALTEPLASE (t-PA, rt-PA, ACTIVASE)	
Benefits:	> 10 yrs clinical experience > 1 million patients treated Fibrin specificity Weight-dosed regimen
30 day mortality:	6.3% (GUSTO I)
ICH rate:	0.7% (GUSTO I)
RETEPLASE (RPA, RETAVASE)	
Benefits:	Double bolus dosing
30 day mortality:	7.47% (GUSTO III)
ICH rate:	0.91% (GUSTO III)
STREPTOKINASE (SK, STREPTASE)	
Benefits:	Less expensive than t-PA
30 day mortality:	7.3% (GUSTO I)
ICH rate:	0.6% (GUSTO I)
PTCA	
Benefits:	Fewer bleeding complications than thrombolysis Successful if performed in timely fashion
In-hospital mortality:	2.6% (PAMI)
ICH rate:	0% (PAMI)

Table 2. Contraindications to Thrombolytic Therapy

CONTRAINDICATIONS

- Active internal bleeding
- History of cerebrovascular accident
- Recent intracranial or intraspinal surgery to trauma. *(See Warnings.)*
- Intracranial neoplasm, arteriovenous malformation, or aneurysm
- Known bleeding diathesis
- Severe uncontrolled hypertension

WARNINGS

- Recent major surgery (e.g., coronary artery bypass graft, obstetrical delivery, organ biopsy, previous puncture of noncompressible vessels)
- Cerebrovascular disease
- Recent gastrointestinal or genitourinary bleeding
- Recent trauma
- Hypertension: systolic BP ≥ 180 mmHg and/or diastolic BP ≥ 110 mmHG
- High likelihood of left heart thrombus (e.g., mitral stenosis with atrial fibrillation)
- Acute pericarditis
- Subacute bacterial endocarditis
- Hemostatic defects including those secondary to severe hepatic or renal disease
- Significant hepatic dysfunction
- Pregnancy
- Diabetic hemorrhagic retinopathy or other hemorrhagic ophthalmic conditions
- Septic thrombophlebitis or occluded AV cannula at seriously infected site
- Advanced age (e.g., older than 75 years)
- Patients currently receiving oral anticoagulants (e.g., warfarin sodium)
- Any other condition in which bleeding constitutes a significant hazard or would be particularly difficult to manage because of its location

which necessitates therapy with antithrombin and antiplatelet drugs to maintain arterial patency.

Streptokinase. Streptokinase (SK) is produced from β-hemolytic Streptococci cultures. Intravenous SK acts on circulating inactive plasminogen to produce the active enzyme plasmin. This, in turn, leads to fibrin lysis and thrombus dissolution, but is not clot-specific.[2] Reports of IV and intracoronary SK use were first published in 1958 and 1976, respectively.[2,3] It was demonstrated in the early 1980s that SK could recanalize an acutely occluded coronary artery in a living patient.[4] European, placebo-controlled megatrials, such as GISSI-1 and ISIS-2, showed that mortality in patients with AMI could be reduced 23% and 30%, respectively, by administering IV SK within six hours of the onset of chest pain.[5,6]

The current recommended dose of IV SK is 1.5 million units given over 60 minutes. A drawback to SK is its antigenicity. In the GUSTO trial, 5.7% of patients developed allergic reactions and 13% had sustained hypotension. Because of this potential, it is not recommended for use in those with recent Streptococcal throat infection or readministration to those who have had previous use in the prior 12 months. In these individuals, the use of a nonantigenic thrombolytic agent, such as t-PA, is recommended.[7]

Tissue Plasminogen Activator. The first reported clinical use of t-PA was in 1984.[8,9] Tissue plasminogen activator is a naturally occurring enzyme found in vascular endothelial cells. This agent converts plasminogen to plasmin. At low doses, t-PA is characterized as clot-specific because of its propensity to bind to any new thrombus within the coronary artery lumen. Activase was proven to be superior to streptokinase in the GUSTO I trial (1993).[10,11] Thirty-day mortality rates for accelerated Activase with IV heparin were 6.3%, compared with 7.3% for streptokinase with heparin—a statistically significant difference. The mortality reduction was sustained at one year and was consistent in all major subgroups; as a result, this 1% mortality difference has become a standard threshold for improvement when new thrombolytics are compared.

The GUSTO III trial (1997) was a 15,000-patient study designed to prove the superiority of Retavase over Activase.[12] The trial failed to show superiority of Retavase; 30-day mortality rates were 7.47% and 7.24% for Activase. Ninety-five percent confidence intervals ranged from -1.11 to 0.66, implying that Retavase could be up to 1.11% worse than Activase, or 0.66% better than Activase.

Weight-Adjusted Dosing of Alteplase: Maximizing Benefit/Risk Ratio

A recent study examined the frequency of risk factors for intracranial hemorrhage with t-PA in patients treated for AMI.[13] The study was performed retrospectively by collecting data on 71,703 AMI patients entered in the National Registry of Myocardial Infarction (NRMI-2) who received treatment with t-PA as the initial reperfusion strategy. The main outcome measure was occurrence of intracranial hemorrhage, confirmed by computed tomography or magnetic resonance imaging.

The study found that 673 patients (0.95%) suffered intracranial hemorrhage (ICH) during hospitalization for acute MI; 625 patients (0.88%) had the event confirmed by CT imaging or MRI. Of these 625 patients, 331 (52.9%) died during the hospitalization. Risk factors significantly associated with the occurrence of ICH were older patients, female gender, black race, systolic blood pressure higher than 140 mmHg, diastolic blood pressure higher than 100 mmHg, history of previous stroke, t-PA dose greater than 1.50 mg/kg, and lower body weight.

It was noted that the occurrence of intracranial hemorrhage in the study was somewhat higher than that observed in the clinical trial setting. For example, the incidence rate of ICH in the GUSTO-I trial was 0.70%, compared with 0.88-0.95% observed in this study of registry patients. The authors suggest that variances were due to differing characteristics in the two patient populations; for example, the NRMI-2 population included a greater percentage of women than did GUSTO-I, the average systolic blood pressure among registry patients was substantially higher than in the GUSTO-I population, and participants in the GUSTO-I trial did not receive doses of t-PA greater than 1.50 mg/kg.

Specific differences in patient management patterns among different thrombolytic trials can be highlighted to give emergency physicians a framework for how to maximize benefits of t-PA therapy. For example, in GUSTO I, patients were administered t-PA according to a weight-dosing protocol to which physicians strictly adhered. In the Gurwitz study, 15% of patients received a dose of 1.5 mg/kg—a factor that was found to be associated more commonly with ICH.[13] Moreover, a history of stroke was an exclusion criterion for the GUSTO I trial, whereas this analysis reveals that 3% of patients treated with t-PA were found to have a history of stroke, a factor significantly associated with ICH. In addition, the study population differed from that of GUSTO I in that it included a greater percentage of women, a history of diabetes mellitus and hypertension were more common, and median systolic blood pressure was higher (140 mmHg) than in GUSTO I (130 mmHg). Based on this analysis, there is a suggestion that lower body weight patients may benefit from weight-adjusted dosing of thrombolytic therapy in terms of less bleeding complications.

This NRMI-2 study only reinforces the need to weigh the potential benefits of thrombolysis against the potential risks on a patient-by-patient basis. Moreover, it illustrates the importance of individual risk assessment for intracranial hemorrhage in AMI patients being considered for thrombolysis. These findings emphasize the critical importance of weight-adjusted dosing of t-PA, especially in light of the fact that the authors found a strong inverse relationship between body weight and intracranial hemorrhage, and that a t-PA dose greater than 1.50 mg/kg was associated more commonly with ICH than lower doses (< 1.50 mg/kg). From a risk management and quality assurance perspective, it should be emphasized that more than 15% of NRMI-2 study patients received this higher dose of t-PA, which may have contributed to the excessive ICH rate observed in this trial as compared with previous clinical trials.

This retrospective analysis should be considered cautionary and stresses the importance of ensuring that all patients with MI who are treated with t-PA are dosed according to weight and in compliance with the manufacturer's prescribing information. What is the appropriate, weight-adjusted dose? For patients weighing more than 67 kg, the recommended dose administered is 100 mg as a 15 mg intravenous bolus, followed by 50 mg infused over the next 30 minutes, and then 35 mg infused over the next 60 minutes. For patients weighing less than or equal to 67 kg, the recommended dose is administered as a 15 mg intravenous bolus, followed by 0.75 mg/kg infused over the next 30 minutes not to exceed 50 mg, and then 0.5 mg/kg over the next 60 minutes not to exceed 35 mg. Total dose should not exceed 100 mg.

Reteplase. Reteplase (r-PA) is a non-glycosylated deletion mutant of wild-type t-PA. Reteplase is administered as a double bolus infusion of 10 megaunits (10 MU) 30 minutes apart. In INJECT, r-PA was compared to SK, and demonstrated equivalence but not superiority. Mortality rates at 35 days were 9.0% for r-PA and 9.5% for streptokinase (P = NS). Outcomes data from the large GUSTO-III trial support its efficacy.[12] It is important to note that the magnitude of clinical experience is an important determinant in selecting a thrombolytic agent.

Combination Therapy with t-PA and Antiplatelet GP IIb/IIIa Inhibitors: Evolving Cocktails for Mortality Reduction

Optimal outcome in acute treatment of MI is now defined by how the most effective thrombolytic is combined with the best mix of platelet inhibitors and anticoagulants. The goal is to speed restoration of blood flow and keep the artery open, with minimal bleeding complications. According to Eric J. Topol, MD, Cleveland Clinic Foundation, Cleveland, OH, "rapid reperfusion is the standard of care, but patency at 90 minutes is not the whole story. Even the most potent thrombolytic therapies do not restore complete coronary blood flow in all patients."[14] He suggested that the new goals of therapy are emerging in the types of regimens used in the recently completed TIMI-14 (the 14th study in the Thrombolysis in Myocardial Infarction trial series) and SPEED trials. Because each of these trials involve a reduced dose of the thrombolytic agent, it is conceivable that the risk of hemorrhagic complications may be reduced.

In each of these trials, abciximab was combined with different reduced doses of thrombolytics. Initial results suggest that the efficacy of this combination may be greatest when abciximab is combined with t-PA.

The abciximab/t-PA combination was evaluated in the first part of the TIMI-14 study, with the best regimen (full-dose abciximab plus half-dose t-PA) showing TIMI-3 patency (indicating a fully open vessel) at 60 minutes in 73% of patients and at 90 minutes in 77% of patients. These results compare favorably with those seen with full-dose t-PA alone (which gave TIMI-3 flow rates of 43% at 60 minutes and 62% at 90 minutes in this study).

In contrast, results from the second phase of TIMI-14 testing abciximab with r-PA (reteplase, Retavase) demonstrate a TIMI-3 flow rate at 90 minutes of 70% with the arm chosen for further study (full-dose abciximab plus half-dose r-PA given as two 5 mg bolus doses 30 minutes apart). Efficacy more in line with the abciximab/t-PA combination has been seen when the r-PA dose is increased to 10 mg plus 5 mg. The SPEED trial also tested r-PA (5 mg + 5 mg) with abciximab, and TIMI-3 flow rates at 60-90 minutes were 62%.

Percutaneous Coronary Angioplasty. One of the most important debates in emergency medicine is whether pharmacologic therapy (thrombolysis) or mechanical therapy (PTCA) is the preferred strategy for achieving reperfusion with AMI. In this regard, the Primary Angioplasty in Myocardial Infarction (PAMI) Study Group reported a lower combined incidence of reinfarction and death in the hospital in those treated with percutaneous transluminal coronary angioplasty (PTCA) vs. patients treated with thrombolytic therapy.[15] Patients who received PTCA also had a lower incidence of intracranial bleeding (0% vs 2%).

However, preliminary results from GUSTO II-b revealed that there was no statistical difference in mortality rates after 30 days. These differences may reflect heterogeneity in door-to-balloon time. In PAMI, 60 minutes was the usual time from door to balloon. In GUSTO II-b, the time was 114 minutes. The Myocardial Infarction Triage and Intervention (MITI) trial reported no difference in mortality, either in hospital or in the long-term.[16] Because 14 of the 19 hospitals in this study were community based, it is quite possible that the data didn't properly reflect the "high-volume expert centers." Outcomes may vary considerably secondary to the expertise of the interventionist. In 1997, it was concluded that in New York, at least, both hospital and cardiologist PTCA volume are inversely related to in-hospital mortality rate and same stay CABG surgery rate. The lowest same-stay CABG surgery rates were achieved with annual cardiologist PTCA volumes of 75 or more and annual hospital PTCA volumes between 600 and 999.[17]

PTCA is an alternative to thrombolytic therapy only if performed in a timely fashion by individuals skilled in the procedure (those who perform more than 75 PTCA procedures per year) and supported by the experienced personnel in high-volume centers. Current recommendations that favor PTCA over thrombolytic administration include the ability to perform PTCA within 60-90 minutes of AMI. It also is recommended in patients at high risk for intracranial bleeding and in individuals who fail to qualify for thrombolytic therapy. In those situations where PTCA will not be available for more than 60-90 minutes, thrombolytics should be considered the primary mortality-reducing intervention. In the hands of experienced operators, PTCA may provide superior, short-term outcomes and is highly recommended in those patients with cardiogenic shock. It would appear that the success of PTCA is very much dependent on the volume of procedures that is performed by the hospital or operator. Recent data suggest that the lowest mortality rates of patients undergoing PTCA are reported when the center and the cardiologist perform in excess of 400 and 200 cases, respectively, each year.[17]

Generally speaking, either angioplasty or thrombolytic agents are used for mortality reduction in AMI. However, studies are currently evaluating protocols using a combined approach, in which patients are given a lower dose of a thrombolytic, which is followed immediately by angioplasty. Early results suggest that outcomes may be improved with this combined approach. The rationale is that a lower dose of the thrombolytic agent may prevent bleeding complications associated with a procedural intervention, while at the same time promoting early patency, until the procedure can be performed. Until more definitive comparative data become available, the goal should be to maximize the speed and efficiency of both approaches.

Complications of Thrombolysis

Bleeding is the most common adverse effect associated with thrombolysis.[18,19] Most complications occur at vascular access sites and rarely require transfusions. Other sites include gastrointestinal, genitourinary, and intracranial locations. (Contraindications to thrombolytics are listed in Table 2.)[20] Intracranial hemorrhage is the most serious complication of thrombolytic therapy; standard ICH rates are listed in Table 1.

Despite the increased incidence of hemorrhagic stroke after thrombolytic therapy, the overall incidence of stroke is similar whether or not thrombolytic therapy is administered. The difference, of course, is that most strokes in AMI patients who have not received thrombolytics are of the nonhemorrhagic variety.[19,21] The risk of intracranial hemorrhage with t-PA use is greater in patients older than 65 years, those with hypertension, or who weigh less than 70 kg. Focal neurologic deficits mandate immediate CT scan. If positive, thrombolytic therapy and heparin should be discontinued.

Adverse effects may occur in patients treated with SK. Hypotension may occur, but it is usually responsive to IV fluids and may not necessitate halting the SK infusion.[22] Bronchospasm, urticaria, and serum sickness may occur in up to 20% of patients.[23] Since anaphylactic reactions are rare, pretreatment with antihistamines and corticosteroids may not be necessary. Systemic bleeding has been noted to occur slightly more frequently with SK vs. t-PA, but t-PA is associated with a higher incidence of intracranial hemorrhage than SK.[24]

Punctured vessels that bleed secondarily to thrombolytics usually respond to direct pressure. It may occasionally be necessary to stop the anticoagulant and thrombolytic if bleeding from these vessels continues unabated or worsens. Transfusion may be required. Protamine sulfate, in a dose of 1 mg per 100 units of heparin, may be given to shorten the half-life of heparin. Cryoprecipitate (10-15 bags) may be employed as well if bleeding does not respond. Continuing hemorrhage would require fresh frozen plasma (2-6 units). Platelets also may be administered to gain control of hemorrhage.

Selecting Patients for Thrombolysis

ECG Criteria. Traditionally, ST elevation in limb and chest leads has been an essential criterion for initiating thrombolytic therapy. The AHA/ACC criteria for using thrombolysis are as follows:[25]

- *Class I:*
  - ST Elevation (greater than 0.1 mV, two or more contiguous leads), time to therapy 12 hours or less, age younger than 75 years.

- Bundle branch block (obscuring ST-segment analysis) and history suggesting acute MI.
- *Class IIa:*
  - ST elevation, age 75 years or older.
- *Class IIb:*
  - ST Elevation, time to therapy greater than 12-24 hours.
  - Blood pressure on presentation greater than 180 mmHg systolic and/or greater than 110 mmHg diastolic associated with high-risk MI.
- *Class III:*
  - ST elevation, time to therapy greater than 24 hours, ischemic pain resolved.
  - ST-segment depression only.

Hypertension. Historically, acute hypertension was considered a contraindication to thrombolytic use because elevated blood pressure is associated with a higher rate of hemorrhagic CVA. Studies have supported this rationale.[26] The risk of ICH is significantly greater when the presenting BP at time of AMI is 180/110 mmHg or greater. The TIMI-2 trial observed that aggressive reduction in blood pressure with beta-blockade therapy decreased the incidence of hemorrhagic CVA in patients with AMI in whom t-PA was administered.[20] Those with anterior AMI are most likely to experience hypertension and might benefit from IV beta-blockade. However, paradoxical blood pressure depression is more commonly seen after administration of nitroglycerine and morphine. Elderly patients presenting with AMI and hypertension are at high risk for intracranial hemorrhage (ICH).[27] A benefit to risk ratio must be considered when administering thrombolytics in all populations.

CPR. A number of studies have touted the safety of thrombolysis in patients who have received CPR.[28,29] A 1991 report was more cautious in its recommendation. The authors suggest a possible increase in major bleeding episodes.[30] The benefit to risk ratio must be calculated on an individual basis. More recent recommendations suggest that thrombolytics may be administered if CPR was performed for less than 10 minutes.[31] Musculoskeletal trauma such as broken ribs may complicate thrombolytic therapy after prolonged CPR and should be considered a risk factor for continued bleeding.

Patient Age. Despite higher morbidity and mortality as compared to younger patients who receive thrombolytics, the number of lives saved in those older than 75 years of age is greater than those younger than age 75.[32] However, many comorbid conditions in this age group can preclude or diminish the attractiveness of thrombolytic use in the elderly. *(Please see Table 2.)* Age older than 65 increases the odds of intracranial hemorrhage,[33,34] as well as that of nonhemorrhagic stroke. But absolute mortality reductions, nevertheless, favor treatment of the elderly. AHA/ACC guidelines suggest that "thrombolysis benefits the patient irrespective of age."

Treatment Time. A number of studies have shown that mortality rates drop precipitously when thrombolytic agents are given as soon as possible after coronary artery occlusion. The prehospital MITI trial group noted early thrombolytic treatment within 70 minutes reduced mortality to 1.2%, compared to 9% for those patients who waited for more than 70 minutes to begin treatment.[35] GISSI-1 demonstrated a mortality reduction of 50% when thrombolytic therapy was given one hour or less after onset of symptoms.[36] A meta-analysis of 60,000 patients by the Fibrinolytic Therapy Trialists Collaborative Group reported an increase of 1.6 lives/1000 lost with each hour delay.[37]

At one time, it was felt that thrombolytics might confer no benefit if given beyond six hours of symptom onset. GISSI-1 revealed no benefit in mortality reduction beyond six hours with SK.[38] However, ISIS-2, the LATE trial, and the EMRAS trial[5,39] demonstrated mortality benefits if thrombolytics were administered within 12 hours. Only ISIS-2 suggested any benefit beyond this 12-hour window. AHA/ACC guidelines mention that "the greatest benefit occurs when thrombolysis is initiated within six hours of symptom onset, although it exerts definite benefit when begun within 12 hours."[25]

Thrombolysis vs. PTCA. Survival and LV function are clearly improved with early administration of IV thrombolytics such as t-PA. This likely equates with a greater reduction in AMI-associated mortality. Front-loaded regimens of t-PA provide better patency rates and are now supported as the regimen of choice by most institutions.

Although the debate still persists, experts agree that too few AMI patients receive reperfusion or receive it quickly enough. The time from onset of symptoms to definitive management has not changed in the last seven years.

Studies support PTCA as the most effective therapy in cardiogenic shock and in patients in whom attempts with thrombolysis are not successful. Debate continues as to which modality, primary PTCA or thrombolytics, is the best first-line treatment for other patients AMI. Primary PTCA may be favored over thrombolytics assuming the hospital and interventional cardiologist have adequate experience and PTCA can be initiated within 60 minutes of arrival to the hospital. However, since fewer than 20% of U.S. hospitals have an angioplasty suite or the capability to staff one in rapid fashion, thrombolysis with t-PA remains a primary modality in the majority of hospital EDs.

Managing Complications of AMI

Arrhythmias. ACLS protocols are readily available for the management of arrhythmias encountered in the setting of AMI. Immediate defibrillation is the treatment of choice for V-fib or hemodynamically unstable ventricular tachycardia (VT). Ventricular ectopy is common in the setting of AMI and should not be routinely treated. Lidocaine may be used for the treatment of frequent (5/minute) ventricular premature depolarizations (VPDs), multifocal VPDs, or those that may induce VT or V-fib. Procainamide may be used if lidocaine is ineffective, although hypotension and widening of the QRS complex may be observed.

Accelerated idioventricular rhythm (AIVR) often occurs after thrombolysis has produced coronary reperfusion. This wide complex escape rhythm may occur when the sinus rate falls to less than 60. This rhythm usually requires no specific treatment and lidocaine should be avoided, inasmuch as ventricular suppression may lead to symptomatic bradycardia or asystole. If there is hemodynamic instability or if this rhythm is associated with VF or VT, atropine or overdrive pacing may be used.

Supraventricular rhythms also are encountered. Persistent sinus tachycardia may suggest a poor prognosis. The underlying causes (fever, pain, anxiety, hypovolemia, CHF) should be treated and, if necessary, treatment with judicious amounts of a beta-blocker is indicated. Paroxysmal supraventricular tachycardia (PSVT) is uncommon but should be treated with synchronized cardioversion if the patient is unstable. Stable patients may require standard pharmacologic management as appropriate. Atrial fibrillation and flutter may be treated with IV diltiazem, verapamil, or propranolol, but if the patient is unstable, synchronized cardioversion is the treatment of choice. Atrial fibrillation with a rapid ventricular rate also should be cardioverted. Unstable atrial fibrillation with ventricular rates below 100 may require transvenous pacing before cardioversion to prevent asystole.

Sinus bradycardia is associated with inferior MI and should be treated with atropine if associated with symptoms of decreased cardiac output. Temporary pacing is indicated for any unstable patient who fails to respond to atropine or develops a high grade heart block. Mobitz type II requires pacing regardless of symptoms and third-degree AV block requires emergent transvenous pacing, as these patients may readily progress to asystole.

Pump Failure. Pump failure is usually the result of decreased left ventricular systolic function or decreased compliance of the left ventricle. Acute mitral regurgitation, VSD, or exacerbation of existing valvular disease also may result in pulmonary edema or shock. Mild heart failure may be treated with furosemide but hypovolemia and hypotension should be avoided. Topical or low-dose IV nitrates may be of some benefit by reducing left ventricular filling pressures. ACE inhibitors may be used in patients with heart failure, but hypotension must be avoided. Initially, hypovolemia should be treated with fluids. These patients will have a low pulmonary capillary wedge pressure (PCWP) and a low cardiac index. Patients with volume overload or decreased left ventricular compliance can be treated with diuretics or nitrates. Swan-Ganz catheters are helpful in the management of patients with pump failure to measure CI and PCWP, but are rarely available in the ED. Advanced management in the critical care unit is recommended in patients with pump dysfunction in the setting of AMI.

The mortality of patients with cardiogenic shock is greater than 75%. Cardiogenic shock usually reflects infarction involving more than 50% of left ventricular mass. This may reflect an acute event or cumulative old and new infarctions. Left ventricular dysfunction, typically associated with decreased cardiac output and elevated PCWP, might temporarily benefit from alpha and beta agonists. Intravenous dopamine starting at 0.5-1.0 mcg/kg/min is helpful in cases of severe shock (< 80 mmHg sbp). Doses higher than 10 mcg/kg/min may induce vasoconstriction, which is deleterious to ischemic or infarcting tissue. Dobutamine is most effective when hypertension is secondary to low cardiac output. Dobutamine at 2.5 to 15.0 mcg/kg/min primarily affects b-1 receptors, but also has smaller affects on peripheral b-2 and a-receptors. Dobutamine increases cardiac output, decreases peripheral resistance and increases perfusion. Unsuccessful use of vasopressors may dictate the need for an intra-aortic balloon pump. This may provide temporary left ventricular assistance.

Right Ventricular Infarction (RVI). RVI occurs in approximately 30-50% of posterior-inferior infarctions.[40] Hypotension, low PCWP, and intolerance to nitrates characterize decreased right ventricular propulsion. Right-sided precordial leads such as V4R exhibiting ST segment elevation indicate RVI. In RVI, a high right ventricular filling pressure must be supported by administration of fluids to maintain adequate left ventricular filling pressures. Clinically, RVI is usually recognized by evidence of impedance to right ventricular filling (elevated neck pains, quiet lung fields). Rarely, patients with RVI may present with cardiogenic shock reflecting concomitant left ventricular dysfunction. Use of Swan-Ganz monitoring techniques may be required to distinguish left ventricular forward failure or cardiogenic shock from hypovolemia or RVI. Dobutamine may be needed for inotropic augmentation in selected cases.

Table 3. TNK-tPA vs. t-PA

	TNK-tPA	t-PA	
30-day mortality	6.17%	6.15%	
ICH	0.93	0.94%	
Severe bleed	0.83%	1.05%	
Mild and moderate bleed	26.0%	28.1%	p = 0.002
Units transfused			p = 0.001
	None (%)	95.8%	94.5%
	1-2 (%)	2.59%	3.2%
	> 2 (%)	1.66%	2.2%

Advanced Generation Thrombolytics

Although thrombolytic therapy has greatly advanced the management of AMI, the currently available agents are subject to several limitations. The ideal thrombolytic therapy would offer enhanced fibrin specificity and resistance to plasminogen activator inhibitor-1, resulting in more complete and rapid reperfusion; a prolonged half-life, allowing for single-bolus dosing; limited activation of the fibrinolytic system, reducing the risk of bleeding complications; better compatibility with potent antiplatelet/antithrombin therapies, increasing potency and reducing the risk of reocclusion; a lack of antigenicity, permitting repeat administration; and reasonable cost. Some of these goals may be achieved by newer thrombolytic therapies currently under development. TNK-tPA has been specifically bioengineered to have an extended half-life that allows for single-bolus dosing, enhanced resistance to plasminogen activator inhibitor-1 (PAI-1), and a high degree of fibrin specificity and potency, with minimal systemic anticoagulation activity. In large dose-finding trials, TNK-tPA has been associated with high patency rates and a low incidence of bleeding complications.[41-44]

In the phase II Thrombolysis in Myocardial Infarction (TIMI) 10B study, patients with AMI presenting within 12 hours of symptom onset (n = 886) were randomized in an open-label design to one of three treatment arms: 30 mg TNK-tPA as a single 5- to 10-second bolus; 50 mg TNK-tPA (replaced with a 40-mg dose early in the trial) as a single 5- to 10-second bolus; or 100 mg t-PA (90-minute infusion, accelerated dosing).[27] The efficacy of TNK-tPA was comparable to that of t-PA. No significant difference in 90-minute TIMI grade 3 flow was seen between t-PA and 40 mg or 50 mg TNK-tPA.

A large, international double-dummy, double-blind Phase III mortality trial, called ASSENT II, has been completed. The objective of the trial was to demonstrate equivalence in 30-day mortality between bolus administration of TNK-tPA and accelerated t-PA. In 16,505 eligible, randomized patients, results showed that TNK-tPA is equivalent to accelerated t-PA in reducing 30-day mortality rates. *(Please see Table 3.)* Results were presented at the March 1999 American College of Cardiology meeting.

In addition, TNK-tPA showed a significant reduction in bleeding complications compared with Activase. Investigators at the ACC meeting suggested a possible link between fibrin specificity and safety (i.e., fewer bleeds).

Summary

Aggressive methods to detect and treat AMI are imperative to reduce mortality among the 1.5 million patients with AMI each year. The history and physical exam can be invaluable in aiding diagnosis. The electrocardiogram and serum enzyme markers (CK-MB) continue to be the mainstay in AMI detection, although newer cardiac markers show promise as ancillary aids.

Once diagnosis of AMI is confirmed, management should be aggressive and systematic. Thrombolytic agents such as t-PA (front-loaded) can reduce mortality significantly and should be administered promptly in eligible candidates. Adjunctive agents such as beta blockers, ACE-inhibitors, and aspirin also have been shown to decrease mortality. Mechanical means to open obstructed coronary arteries should be given preferential consideration provided the facility has significant PTCA experience and can perform this procedure in an expedient manner. Next generation thrombolytic agents offer significant hope for improvement in AMI patient care.

References

1. Marder V. Relevance of changes in blood and coagulation parameters during thrombolytic therapy. *Am J Med* 1987; 83:15.
2. Fletcher A, Alkajaerstig N, Smyrniotis F. The treatment of patients suffering from early myocardial infarction with massive and prolonged streptokinase therapy. *Trans Assoc Am Phys* 1958;71:287.
3. Chazav E, Matteeva L, Mazadev A. Intracoronary administration of fibrinolysis in acute myocardial infarction. *Ter Arkh* 1976;48:8.
4. Rentrop P, Blanke H, Karsch K. Selective intracoronary thrombolysis in acute myocardial infarction and unstable angina pectoris. *Circulation* 1981;63:307.
5. ISIS-2 (Second International Study of Infarct Survival) Collaborative Group. Randomized trial of intravenous streptokinase, oral aspirin, both or neither among 17187 cases of suspected acute myocardial infarction: ISIS-2. *Lancet* 1988;2:349-360.
6. ISIS-1 (First International Study of Infarct Survival) in Collaborative Group. Randomized trial of intravenous atenolol among 16027 cases of suspected acute myocardial infarction. *Lancet* 1986;2:57-66.
7. Dykewicz, M, McGrath K, Davison R. Identification of patients at risks for anaphylaxis due to streptokinase. *Arch Intern Med* 1986;146:305-307.
8. Vandewerf, Ludbrook P, Bergman S. Coronary thrombolysis with tissue plasminogen activator in patients with evolving myocardial infarction. *N Engl J Med* 1984;310:609-613.
9. Rao A, Pratt C, Berke A. Hemorrhagic manifestations and changes plasma fibrinolytic system in patients treated with tissue plasminogen activator and streptokinase. *J Am Coll Cardiol* 1988;11:1.
10. The GUSTO Investigators. An international randomized trial comparing four thrombolytic strategies for acute myocardial infarction. *N Engl J Med* 1993;329:673-682.
11. The GUSTO Angiographic Investigators. The effects of tissue plasminogen activator, streptokinase, or both on coronary artery patency, ventricular function and survival after acute myocardial infarction. *N Engl J Med* 1993;329: 1615-1622.
12. Recent Developments in Coronary Intervention: GUSTO-III and other Highlights from ACC '97. Roberts R, McCabe JB, eds. In: *Clinical Challenges in Acute Myocardial Infarction*. 1997;7:1-11.
13. Gurwitz JH, Gore JM, et al. Risk for intracranial hemorrhage after tissue plasminogen activator treatment for acute myocardial infarction. *Ann Intern Med* 1998;129:597-604.
14. Ferguson JJ. Meeting highlights: XIXth Congress of the European Society of Cardiology. *Circulation* 1997;96: 3818-3821.
15. Grines C, Browne K, Marco J, et al. A comparison of immediate angioplasty with thrombolytic therapy for acute myocardial infarction. *N Engl J Med* 1993;328:673-679.
16. Every N, Parsons L, Hlatky M, et al. A comparison of thrombolytic therapy with primary coronary angioplasty for acute myocardial infarction. *N Engl J Med* 1996;335: 1253-1262.
17. Hannan E, Racz M, Ryan T, et al. Coronary angioplasty volume-outcome relationships for hospitals and cardiologists. *JAMA* 1997;277:892-898.
18. Blankenship J, Almquist A. Cardiovascular complications of thrombolytic therapy in patients with a mistaken diagnosis of acute myocardial infarction. *J Am Coll Cardiol* 1989;14: 1579-1582.
19. Eleff S, Borel C, Bell W. Acute management of intracranial hemorrhage in patients receiving thrombolytic therapy case reports. *Neurosurgery* 1990;26:867-869.
20. Bovill E, Terrin M, Stump D, et al. Hemorrhagic events during therapy with tissue plasminogen activator, heparin and aspirin for acute myocardial infarction: Results of the TIMI, phase II trial. *Ann Intern Med* 1991;115:256-265.
21. Maggioni A, Franzosi M, Santoro E, et al. The risk of stroke in patients with acute myocardial infarction after thrombolytic and antithrombotic treatment. *N Engl J Med* 1992;327:1-6.
22. Bednarczyk E, Sherlock S, Farah M, et al. Anaphylactic reaction to streptokinase with first exposure: Case report and review of the literature. *Ann Pharmacother* 1989;23:869.
23. Schweitzer D, vander Wall, Bosker H. Serum sickness-like illness as a complication after streptokinase therapy for acute myocardial infarction. *Cardiology* 1991;78:68-71.
24. GISSI-2. A factorial randomized trial of alteplase versus streptokinase and heparin versus no heparin among 12490 patients with acute myocardial infarction. *Lancet* 1990;336: 65-71.

25. Ryan TJ, Anderson JL, Antman EM, et al. ACC/AHA guidelines for the management of patients with acute myocardial infarction: Executive summary. *Circulation* 1996;94:2341-2350.
26. Anderson J, Karagounis L, Allen A, et al. Older age and elevated blood pressure are risk factor for intracerebral hemorrhage after thrombolysis. *Am J Cardiol* 1991;68: 166-170.
27. The TIMI Study Group. Comparison of invasive and conservative strategies after treatment with intravenous tissue plasminogen activator in acute myocardial infarction: Results of the thrombolysis in myocardial (TIMI) phase II trial. *N Engl J Med* 1989;320:618-627.
28. Cross S, Lee H, Rawles J, et al. Safety of thrombolysis in association with cardiopulmonary resuscitation. *BMJ* 1991; 303:1241-1242.
29. Scholz K. Frequency of complications of cardiopulmonary resuscitation after thrombolysis during acute myocardial infarction. *Am J Cardiol* 1992;69:724-728.
30. Tenaglia A, Califf R, Candela R, et al. Thrombolytic therapy in patients requiring cardiopulmonary resuscitation. *Am J Cardiol* 1991;68:15.
31. Habib G. Current status of thrombolysis in acute myocardial infarction. *Chest* 1995;107:528-534.
32. Krumholz H, Pasternak R, Weinstein M, et al. Cost-effectiveness of thrombolytic therapy with streptokinase in elderly patients with suspected acute myocardial infarction. *N Engl J Med* 1992;327:7-13.
33. Simoons ML, Maggioni AP, Knatterud G, et al. Individual risk assessment for intracranial hemorrhage during thrombolytic therapy. *Lancet* 1993;342:1523-1528.
34. De Jaegere PP, Arnold AA, Balk AH, et al. Intracranial hemorrhage in association with thrombolytic therapy: Incidence and clinical predictive factors. *J Am Coll Cardiol* 1992;19:289-294.
35. Weaver W, Cerqueira M, Hallstrom A, et al. Prehospital initiated vs. hospital-initiated thrombolytic therapy: The Myocardial Infarction Triage and Intervention Trial. *JAMA* 1993;270:1211-1216.
36. Tierney WM, Roth BJ, Psaty B, et al. Predictors of myocardial infarction in emergency room patients. *Crit Care Med* 1985;13:526-531.
37. Fibrinolytic Therapy Trialists Collaborative Group. Indications for fibrinolytic therapy in suspected acute myocardial infarction: Collaborative overview of early mortality and major morbidity results from all randomized trials of more than 1000 patients. *Lancet* 1994;343:311-321.
38. GISSI. Effectiveness of intravenous thrombolytic treatment in acute myocardial infarction. *Lancet* 1986;1:397-402.
39. EMERAS Collaborative Group. Randomized trial of late thrombolysis in patients with suspected acute myocardial infarction. *Lancet* 1993;342:767.
40. Zehender M, Kasper W, Kander E, et al. Right ventricular infarction as an independent predictor of prognosis after acute inferior infarction. *N Engl J Med* 1993;328:982-988.
41. Cannon CP, McCabe CH, Gibson M, et al. TNK-tissue plasminogen activator in acute myocardial infarction. *Circulation* 1997;95;351-356.
42. Cannon CP, McCabe CH, Gibson M, et al. TNK-tissue plasminogen activator compared with front-loaded tissue plasminogen activator in acute myocardial infarction: primary results of the TIMI I 10B trial. *Circulation* 1997;96:1-206.
43. Gibson M, Cannon CP, van de Werf FJ, et al. A randomized prospective comparison of T-PA with TNK using the TIMI frame count: Results of TIMI 10B. *Circulation* 1997; 96(suppl):1-330.
44. Keyt BA, Paoni NF, Refino CJ, et al. A faster-acting and more potent form of tissue plasminogen activator. *Proc Natl Acad Sci USA* 1994;91:3670-3674.

Recommended Reading

- Bode C, Smalling R, Berg G. Randomized comparison of coronary thrombolysis achieved with double-bolus reteplase (recombinant plasminogen activator) and front-loaded, accelerated alteplase (recombinant tissue plasminogen activator) in patients with acute myocardial infarct. *Circulation* 1996;94:891-898.
- Jugduff BL, Warnica JW. Intravenous nitroglycerin therapy to limit myocardial infarct size, expansion, and complications. Effect of timing, dosage, and infarct location. *Circulation* 1988;78:906-919.
- Yusuf S, Collins R, MacMahon S, et al. Effect of intravenous nitrates on mortality in acute myocardial infarction: An overview of the randomized trials. *Lancet* 1988;1:1088-1092.
- HART. A comparison between heparin and low-dose aspirin as adjunctive therapy with tissue plasminogen activator for acute myocardial infarction. Heparin Aspirin Reperfusion Trial. *N Engl J Med* 1990;323:1433-1437.
- SCATI. Randomized controlled trial of subcutaneous calcium-heparin in acute myocardial infarction. Studio Sella Cacipamina nell Angina enella Trombosi Venticolare nell Infarcto. *Lancet* 1989;2:182-186.
- SIS-3 (Third International Study of Infarct Survival) Collaborative Group. ISIS-3: A randomized comparison of streptokinase vs. tissue plasminogen activator vs. anistreplase and of aspirin plus heparin vs. aspirin alone among 41,299 cases of suspected acute myocardial infarction. *Lancet* 1992;339:753-770.
- GUSTO investigators: The effects of tissue plasminogen activator, streptokinase, or both on coronary artery patency, ventricular function, and survival after acute myocardial infarction. *N Engl J Med* 1993;329:1615-1622.
- Brett J. Late assessment of thrombolytic efficacy with alteplase (rt-Pa) six-24 hours after onset of acute myocardial infarction. *Aust N Z J Med* 1993;23:745-748.
- Granger C, White H, Bates E. A pooled analysis of coronary artery patency and left ventricular function after intravenous thrombolysis for acute myocardial infarction. *Am J Cardiol* 1994;74:1220-1226.
- Newhaus K, von Essen R, Tebbe U. Improved thrombolysis in acute myocardial infarction with front-loaded administration of alteplase: Results of the rt-Pa - APSAC patency study (TAPS). *J Am Coll Cardiol* 1992;19:885-891.
- O'Neill W, Weintraub R, Grines C. et al. A prospective

placebo-controlled randomized trial of intravenous streptokinase and angioplasty therapy of acute myocardial infarction. *Circulation* 1992;86:1710-1717.

- Ridker P, O'Donnell C, Marder V, et al. A response to "holding GUSTO up to the light." *Ann Intern Med* 1994;120:882-888.
- Maggioni A, Franzosi M, Farina M, et al. Cerebrovascular events after myocardial infarction: Analysis of the GISSI trial. *BMJ* 1991;302:1428-1431.
- Risenfors M, Zukauskiene I, Albertsson P, et al. Early thrombolytic therapy in suspected acute myocardial infarction-role of electrocardiogram: Results from the TEAHAT Study. *J Intern Med* 1991;734(Suppl):19-25.
- Cannon CP, McCabe CH, Diver DJ, et al. Comparison of front-loaded recombinant tissue-type plasminogen activator, anistreplase and combination thrombolytic therapy for acute myocardial infarction: results of the Thrombolysis in Myocardial Infarction (TIMI) 4 trial. *J Am Coll Cardiol* 1994;24:1602-1610.

Non-Myocardial Infarction Chest Pain

Sandra M. Schneider, MD

It has become a familiar refrain: "Well, it's not your heart," the emergency physician reassuringly tells his or her patient. Every day, in fact, thousands of patients hear this "diagnosis of exclusion," and sometimes they are discharged from the emergency department (ED) without a clear understanding of what the underlying cause of their chest pain really is. Uncertainty, coupled with fear, especially in the company of concerned family members, can produce even more anxiety. As might be expected, identifying and communicating the precise cause of chest discomfort is an essential component of patient management. Unfortunately, confirming a specific diagnosis in the emergency setting can be extremely difficult.

Important nonischemic causes of chest pain include pneumothorax, perforated peptic ulcer, and acute biliary colic. Not surprisingly, chest pain from any cause may carry with it a psychological fear, and the secondary physiological response to that fear—palpitations, anorexia, or a "sick" feeling—exacerbates the feeling of crisis for the patient.

With these concerns in mind, this chapter reviews current diagnostic and therapeutic approaches to chest pain that is not precipitated by acute or chronic coronary ischemia. Highlighting a wide range of nonischemic causes of chest pain—as well as esophageal, aortic, and musculoskeletal etiologies—this article discusses essential elements of the physical examination and history that will help identify specific causes for non-cardiac chest pain and that will direct the clinician toward an appropriate disposition and treatment plan.

Background

Attempting to identify the cause of chest pain is one of the most important clinical priorities in emergency medicine. Unfortunately, precise delineation of this symptom is frequently problematic. In the ambulatory clinic setting, for example, only a small percentage of patients with chest pain are provided a definite organic diagnosis.[1] In the ED, although the percentage of patients with a confirmed diagnosis of acute myocardial infarction or coronary ischemia is much higher,[7] a significant percentage of patients are discharged without a precise, nonischemic etiology.

Many patients with noncardiac chest pain have symptoms that mimic those see in acute coronary ischemia. In this regard, 10-30% of all patients undergoing coronary angiography will have normal arteries.[2,3] Moreover, less than 40% of patients given a diagnosis of atypical or noncardiac chest pain in the ED believe the diagnosis.[4] Even those individuals with a subsequent negative exercise test often believe they have organic disease.[5]

Psychological uncertainties surrounding chest pain can lead to missed employment and medical costs associated with unnecessary invasive tests required to convince the patient of the absence of coronary disease. One study shows that after a cardiac catheterization

Table 1. Causes and Typical Presentations of Chest Pain

CAUSE	QUALITY OF PAIN	RADIATION	SPECIAL FEATURES
Cardiac	Tightness, aching, pressure, squeezing. Can be burning or pleuritic.	Neck, shoulder, back, jaw, arm (medial aspect)	Associated with nausea, vomiting, dyspnea, orthopnea, diaphoresis, tachycardia, or bradycardia
Pericarditis	Sharp, pleuritic, retrosternal	Neck, back, left shoulder, left arm, epigastrium, trapezius ridge	Aggravated in the supine position, can occur with each heartbeat
Hypertrophic cardiomyopathy	Tightness, pressure, aching, squeezing		Syncope, sudden death, lightheadedness, increased pain with nitroglycerin, relieved by squatting, systolic murmur increases with Valsalva maneuver
Mitral valve prolapse	Brief, stabbing		Pain at rest, lightheadedness, palpitation, mid-systolic click
Dissecting thoracic aortic aneurysm	Tearing, sudden onset	Anterior to back, neck, flank, legs	Sudden onset, refractory to narcotics and nitroglycerin. Syncope, aortic insufficiency, murmur, blood pressure difference
Respiratory	Pleuritic		Fever, cough, rales in chest
Pulmonary embolism	Pleuritic, sudden onset		Dyspnea greater than pain, sudden onset, friction rub, tachycardia, hypoxemia
Esophageal spasm	Anginal	Diffuse thoracic distribution, radiation to arms	Precipitated by swallowing, relieved by nitroglycerin, dysphagia, odontophagia
Esophageal reflux	Burning or anginal		No relation to exertion, comes when lying down
Musculoskeletal	Sharp or dull, pleuritic		Tenderness to palpation, increases with movement of the arms or shoulders, increases with exertion
Psychogenic	Sharp stabbing or heaviness	Neck, back, shoulders	Relief with nitroglycerin takes more than five minutes, history of normal coronary arteries, history of panic disorder, hyperventilation causes recurrent pain

demonstrating normal arteries, more than 50% of patients continue to curtail activity, becoming cardiac cripples.[2,3] Perhaps if patients are convinced that they have a noncardiac diagnosis at the *initial* medical encounter, it is possible that expensive diagnostic procedures and disabling behavior can be prevented.[4]

Finally, because patients often forget what they are told in the busy, anxiety-provoking atmosphere of the ED, it is important to communicate effectively—preferably in writing—a diagnosis of noncardiac chest pain. Interestingly, nearly 35% of patients diagnosed with an esophageal etiology for their chest pain did not remember being provided with this information during their clinical encounter.[6]

Pathophysiology and Clinical Correlation

Cardiac chest pain is transmitted through the afferent nerves C8-T4. These nerves also innervate the great vessels, esophagus, pleura, and chest wall. Pain associated with myocardial ischemia is caused by abnormal stretching of the ventricles. Pain emanating from the great vessels is generated from acute distention, whereas pain from the esophagus originates from spasm or irritation. Because of shared innervations and the diffuse nature of visceral chest pain, many etiologies produce similar pain. For example, nearly half of patients with typical crushing, heavy substernal chest pain will have *noncardiac* pain.[7,8] Conversely, burning chest pain, typical of esophagitis, occurs in more than 40% of patients with myocardial infarction or unstable angina.[7,8] *(Please see Table 1.)*

Because of similarities and overlap in chest pain syndromes, various bedside maneuvers have been evaluated for their ability to distinguish among specific etiologies. For example, antacids are often administered to distinguish between the pain of esophagitis and myocardial infarction. Although many physicians rely on this provocative maneuver, one study has demonstrated that 7% of all patients with confirmed myocardial ischemic pain will have complete relief of pain with antacid administration.[9] Furthermore, even viscous lidocaine, when administered orally with or without antacids, can give prompt relief not only to patients with esophagitis, but to patients with cardiac ischemia.[10] Consequently, the use of antacids as a diagnostic maneuver is not reliable and should be avoided. Other strategies for improving diagnostic accuracy have also proven less than reliable. For example, some patients with proven myocardial infarction will have notable chest wall tenderness, with one study reporting that eight of 104 patients with acute infarction had their chest pain reproduced either partially or fully by chest wall palpation.[8]

Life-Threatening Causes of Chest Pain

Thoracic Aortic Aneurysm. Not surprisingly, the pain associated with dissecting thoracic aortic aneurysm can easily be confused with symptoms caused by myocardial ischemia. The pain is usually of acute onset, severe, and often described as "tearing" and radiating into the back. However, it also can radiate to the neck, flank, or legs. The pain is often refractory to large doses of narcotics. From a historical perspective, it should be stressed that the typical patient with dissecting thoracic aortic aneurysm will have a history of hypertension. In addition, other predisposing conditions for dissection include disorders of collagen integrity, such as Ehlers-Danlos syndrome and Turner's syndrome, as well as trauma and pregnancy.

Physical examination may disclose a blood pressure difference between the right and left arm (involvement of the innominate artery), between the arms and legs, or occasionally the murmur of aortic insufficiency (involvement proximally into the aortic valve). Syncope at the onset of pain is an important clue to the diagnosis. Patients may develop hemiparesis or hemianesthesia. The diagnosis is suggested by a chest x-ray demonstrating an enlarged mediastinum. Confirmation with an echocardiogram (transesophageal echo is especially useful), CT scan, or MRI is almost always necessary.

Untreated dissecting aortic aneurysms are generally fatal; 24% of patients with a confirmed diagnosis die within 24 hours, 50% die within one week; and 90% will die within one year.[11] Initial medical therapy includes IV nitroprusside with beta-blockers to reduce both blood pressure and shear forces on the aorta (dP/dT). Temporary stabilization will usually permit time for imaging and consultation. Therapy should be initiated at low doses and raised to maintain the diastolic blood pressure below 100 mmHg and systolic blood pressure below 120 mmHg. Relief of pain may indicate cessation of dissection. Although surgical mortality and morbidity are high, 60% of patients recover to live a normal life span.[11]

Pulmonary Embolism. Pulmonary emboli can present with myriad symptoms, ranging from shortness of breath and lightheadedness to syncope and sudden death. Although the true incidence of pulmonary embolism (PE) is very speculative, one study estimated an annual incidence between 650,000 and 700,000 cases, with an acute mortality rate of about 10%.[12]

Pulmonary emboli primarily originate in deep venous vessels above the knee and occasionally from the pelvic and hepatic circulation or the right heart. Risk factors for PE are listed in Table 2. Although thrombotic emboli are the most common, pulmonary emboli also can arise from fat (after long bone fractures), air, amniotic fluid, foreign bodies, and infected vegetations.

Pathophysiologically, emboli obstruct blood flow to one or more segments of lung while ventilation remains unimpaired. Pulmonary artery and right ventricular pressures increase. Blood flow decreases in some areas of the lung and increases in others, creating a ventilation/perfusion mismatch. Some blood gets shunted through unventilated areas and thus reduces the PO_2. This leads to the anxiety and feeling of doom that often accompany the event. Hypoxemia has been observed in up to 85% of patients with emboli obstructing two or more lung segments.[13] Later in the course of the illness, surfactant production falls, and atelectasis accounts for prolonged hypoxemia lasting days after the initial event.

Table 2. Risk Factors for Pulmonary Embolism

- Immobilization (including postoperative period)
- Deep venous thrombosis
- Heart disease (including congestive heart failure)
- Trauma to pelvis, hips, lower extremities
- Obesity
- Burns
- Previous pulmonary embolism
- Hypercoagulable state (Protein C or S deficiency, antithrombin III deficiency, malignancy)
- Pregnancy/post partum
- Oral contraceptives and estrogen intake
- Polycythemia

Patients with classic pulmonary infarction present with sudden onset of severe pleuritic chest pain and shortness of breath. Although these symptoms can also be suggestive of pneumonia, sudden onset of pain should raise clinical suspicion for a PE. The pain associated with PE can be sharp and pleuritic or heavy substernal or simply chest wall tenderness (if the underlying pleura is inflamed). In about 5% of patients, the pain may be anginal in character.[14] Atypical presentations may be even more confusing. Patients can present with fever, abdominal pain (hepatic congestion), disseminated intravascular coagulation, or new-onset asthma. Overall, the "classical" symptoms of hemoptysis, dyspnea, and chest pain are present in less than 20% of patients.[15] Recurrent emboli can cause a particularly deceiving presentation characterized by behavioral abnormalities and mental status changes.

Patients with submassive emboli can present with dyspnea either on exertion or at rest—a presentation that may mimic such conditions as pneumonia, congestive heart failure, asthma, or psychogenic hyperventilation. Large saddle emboli cause sudden death, syncope, or severe dyspnea and hypotension. These patients may have signs of acute right ventricular failure with right ventricular gallop and heave, as well as a loud pulmonary component of the second heart sound. This presentation may be difficult to distinguish from myocardial infarction, hypovolemia, or septic shock.

Patients should be suspected of PE if symptoms of dyspnea and/or tachycardia have no other explanation. The diagnosis is supported by the finding of abnormalities on an arterial blood gas. Although a low oxygen saturation on pulse oximetry may suggest a PE, generally speaking, it is neither sensitive nor specific enough for diagnostic purposes. And, although uncommon, it is possible for the PO_2 to be normal in patients with acute pulmonary emboli. Because of these limitations, a more sensitive diagnostic approach is to use the A-a gradient, which can detect a ventilation/perfusion mismatch suggestive of PE. The A-a O_2 gradient can be calculated in the following way:

$$\textbf{A-a } O_2 \textbf{ gradient} = 150 - (PaO_2 + [PCO_2/0.8])$$

with a normal score being 3-4 in patients younger than 20 and age/10 + 10 in patients older than 20.

Although nonspecific and insensitive, the chest x-ray may demonstrate an infiltrate, pleural effusion, atelectasis, or an elevated hemidiaphragm. Hampton's hump is a pleural-based infiltrate, usually at the costophrenic junction, that appears to point to the hilum. More subtle, Westermark's sign represents congestion of pulmonary vessels that are sharply cut off at the area of the embolus. These signs are rare but, when present, can be quite specific. ECG changes are common but nonspecific. The sudden appearance of P pulmonale, right bundle-branch block, or S1 Q3 T3 is certainly suggestive of the diagnosis.

If there is a clinical suspicion of pulmonary emboli, screening tests for either emboli (such as ventilation and perfusion lung scan) or venous thrombosis (such as venous duplex Doppler studies) are mandatory.[16] If these tests yield clearly positive results, the patient should be acutely anticoagulated with heparin, unless there are contraindications to such therapy. If these tests yield equivocal results, or if there are contraindications to anticoagulation, then pulmonary angiography is used as the standard for definitive diagnosis.

Pericarditis. Pericarditis, inflammation of the pericardium, is usually due to viral infection (*Coxsackie* or ECHO), uremia, connective tissue disease, tuberculosis, malignancy, or drugs (procainamide, hydralazine, methyldopa). It can occur after cardiac trauma, cardiac surgery, or after an acute MI. Often, the cause is unknown. Typically, the pain is retrosternal, sharp, or knife-like, and frequently there is a pleuritic component. Aggravated by deep breathing or twisting of the chest wall, the pain can radiate to the neck, back, shoulders, arm, or epigastrium, and patients generally prefer to sit forward; lying supine increases the pain. At times, the pain can occur with each heartbeat or with swallowing.

The physical exam reveals a one- to three-component friction rub, which often is intermittent and is usually heard over the sternum during expiration. Low-grade fever is common. The diagnosis may be suggested by ECG changes of diffuse ST elevation or downward sloping of the PR segment. The major complication of pericarditis is pericardial tamponade. Echocardiography is particularly useful for evaluating the presence of a pericardial effusion and should be employed in patients with signs of diminished cardiac output and pulsus paradoxus. Treatment is directed at the cause. Symptoms can be relieved with IV steroids or nonsteroidal anti-inflammatory drugs, which may be given with more specific therapy when indicated (e.g., anti-tuberculosis therapy).

Acute Chest Syndrome in Sickle Cell Disease. Although many patients with sickle cell anemia have painful crises involving chest pain, the findings of cough, dyspnea, fever, and pulmonary infiltrates suggest the presence of a far more serious syndrome. The etiology of this syndrome is not entirely clear, although there is evidence that some patients have pulmonary thrombosis (in situ or thromboembolic), while others have bone marrow embolization or infection (*Haemophilus influenzae* or *Staphylococcus aureus* are common isolates). Nearly all patients have chest pain, usually pleuritic, and bibasilar rales or a friction rub. Leukocytosis is common but is also seen in painful crisis. Many patients will be hypoxemic.

Admission is indicated in all patients. Supportive treatment with hydration and supplemental oxygen is helpful. Definite treatment is directed at the underlying etiology.

Non-Life-Threatening Causes of Chest Pain

Chronic Pulmonary Hypertension. Chronic pulmonary hypertension, which may accompany mitral stenosis or congenital heart disease, can produce angina-like pain. The pain is often caused by underlying myocardial ischemia associated with reduced cardiac output.

Mitral Valve Prolapse. Mitral valve prolapse is a common defect occurring primarily in women. Some patients experience sharp, stabbing pain that often occurs at rest. Hyperventilation, anxiety, palpitations, and depression are common. The finding of a mid-systolic click supports the diagnosis. The mid-systolic click will move earlier in systole during the strain phase of the Valsalva maneuver or with the administration of amyl nitrite.

Hypertrophic Cardiomyopathy. Patients with hypertrophic cardiomyopathy (idiopathic hypertrophic subaortic stenosis) usually present with angina-like pain accompanied by syncope, lightheadedness, and dyspnea. Some patients with hypertrophic cardiomyopathy may have sudden death as their presentation, without previous warning symptoms. The typical systolic crescendo-decrescendo murmur is loudest with Valsalva maneuver and fades with squatting. There may be a family history of the disorder. It also occurs in patients with Friedrich's ataxia.

Aortic Stenosis. Aortic stenosis typically causes ischemic chest discomfort that may be associated with exertional dyspnea and syncope. This pain is due to a decrease in cardiac output and an increase in oxygen consumption. Many patients will have coexisting coronary disease. Most patients present with chest pain during the fifth to seventh decades of life. The characteristic systolic crescendo-decrescendo murmur and the finding of a decreased and delayed carotid upstroke help confirm the diagnosis.

Esophageal Disease. Chest pain of esophageal origin is common, occurring in 25,000-75,000 patients each year.[17] These patients are frequent visitors to EDs and primary care providers. As a group, they account for total annual medical costs in excess of $40 million.[18]

Pain from the esophagus arises from distention, spasm, or frequent contractions of the esophagus. Pain due to heat or acid stimuli is felt through sensory receptors and carried from the glossopharyngeal, superior laryngeal, recurrent laryngeal, and sympathetic nerves via the dorsal roots of T3-T12. Tight, vice-like pain occurs in 91% of patients with esophageal disease. Pain radiating to the left arm, shoulder, or neck is reported in 79% of patients.[18] Postprandial pain, pain on recumbency, and prolonged pain unrelated to exertion should suggest an esophageal origin.

Infection. Pain associated with swallowing suggests an inflammatory esophageal disorder caused by infection (*Herpes simplex, Candida, Varicella zoster*), malignancy, reflux, obstruction, or radiation. In severe cases, or with chemical ingestions, esophagoscopy can be helpful. Treatment is directed at the cause. When indicated, infections can be treated with antifungal therapy (e.g., nystatin, fluconazole, ketoconazole) or antiviral agents (acyclovir or ganciclovir). Viscous xylocaine can provide symptomatic relief.

Esophageal Reflux. Burning, substernal pain is often suggestive of reflux esophagitis. In fact, almost 35% of the "normal" population experiences heartburn at least once a month.[19] Pregnant women may experience heartburn daily. Reflux occurs when there is a decrease in lower esophageal sphincter tone, impaired acid clearance, or poor gastric emptying. Hiatal hernia is a major cause of reflux. Although pain is generally burning in nature, some individuals experience a heavy or sharp pain.

Symptoms may resolve with a dose of antacids, which also relieve pain in 7% of patients with myocardial ischemia.[18] Use of viscous xylocaine with antacids has been described and was felt to be specific for reflux esophagitis. However, many patients with acute cardiac pain also respond to this "cocktail."[18,19]

Histamine-2 antagonists (H_2 blockers) are the cornerstone of chronic therapy. Although proton-blockers such as omeprazole may be more effective, long-term safety has not been established definitively. All liquid antacids are equally effective. H_2 blockers are effective in decreasing nocturnal acid secretion. Although symptoms should be controlled in one week, prolonged therapy for up to three months may be necessary. Modifications in lifestyle are often required, including frequent, small meals and raising the head of the bed 15 cm. *(Please see Table 3.)*

The diagnosis of esophagitis should be suspected when a patient presents with burning substernal chest pain. The Bernstein test (acid perfusion of the esophagus) is sensitive for the presence of esophagitis. When the diagnosis is in doubt, endoscopic examination or pH monitoring can helpful.[20,21] In most patients, however, a therapeutic trial of antacids with or without H_2 blockers is cheaper and less invasive. Finally, a clue to the presence of gastroesophageal reflux is chronic nocturnal cough, which may indicate recurrent aspiration. These patients can develop lung abscess as their initial presentation.

Esophageal Spasm. Pain associated with esophageal spasm is thought to occur from contraction of smooth muscle and is transmitted along the same innervation as that of esophagitis and myocardial ischemia. The pain is felt as a tightness in the substernal region. Nitrates relieve the pain of both esophageal spasm and myocardial ischemia, although pain relief is often delayed more than five minutes in esophageal spasm. The presence of dysphagia is very useful because this symptom points to the esophagus as the cause of the pain.

Achalasia is a severe form of esophageal spasm. The lower esophageal sphincter tone is increased, and there are abnormal contractions of the esophageal musculature. The defect is in the innervation of the smooth muscles of the esophagus and of the lower esophageal sphincter. Patients complain of dysphagia of both solids and liquids that is made worse with stress. Chest pain is generally described as tight or dull, often suggestive of cardiac etiology. Regurgitation is common, and pulmonary aspiration can occur. Chest x-ray will show the absence of the gastric air bubble and, at times, an air/fluid level in the mediastinum. The diagnosis is confirmed by manometry, which shows normal or elevated lower esophageal sphincter pressure. Endoscopy is performed to rule out a secondary cause such as gastric carcinoma.

Diffuse Esophageal Spasm. More common is diffuse esophageal spasm, which goes by a number of names (e.g., nutcracker esophagus, corkscrew esophagus), according to observed manometric patterns. Patients present with classic chest pain (dull, substernal) that, in many cases, is accompanied by dysphagia.

Diffuse esophageal spasm is poorly understood. Collagen vascular disease, diabetic neuropathy, reflux esophagitis, irradiation esophagitis, and cholinergic and anticholinergic drugs all can cause esophageal motor abnormalities. Although many patients have motility disorders when evaluated with 24-hour manometry, many motility abnormalities occur without causing chest pain.[20,21] Pain may be perceived before the abnormal contraction is initiated, suggesting that the pain may trigger the spasm.[22]

Table 3. Foods and Drugs Associated with Esophageal Reflux
Chocolate
Spearmint
Peppermint
Citrus juices
Tomatoes
Alcohol
Caffeine
Theophylline
Prostaglandin E_1 and E_2
Calcium-channel blockers
Beta-blockers
Nitroglycerin
Smoking

The gold standard for diagnosis of esophageal motility disorders is manometry, preferably a 24-hour study with symptom diary. Up to 50% of patients with noncardiac chest pain have esophageal dysfunction on testing.[23] The pain of esophageal spasm can be relieved with nitroglycerin,[24,25] adding confusion to a presentation where cardiac disease is still a consideration. Pain relief, when it does occur, generally takes longer than five minutes, a fact that may help distinguish cardiac pain from that of an esophageal origin.[9] Relief with nitroglycerin will last one hour, and with long-acting forms, up to four hours.[24] Muscle relaxants and anticholinergic medications also are helpful. Despite their ability to relax smooth muscle, calcium-channel blockers have not been effective in relieving symptoms.[26]

Chest Wall Syndrome. Tietze's syndrome is characterized by the presence of point tenderness of one or more costal cartilages associated with nonsuppurative swelling. Pathologically, the area shows only minimal inflammatory changes.[27] Tietze's syndrome, along with other musculoskeletal disorders (e.g., acute costochondritis, painful rib, slipping rib, traumatic muscle pain, precordial catch, myalgia, firositis), accounts for 10-69% of patients presenting with chest pain.[28,29]

Musculoskeletal chest pain usually occurs in the center of the chest, typically after exertion, and lasts for 30-120 minutes. The pain is often continuous but may be punctuated by acute exacerbations. Usually dull and aching, the pain also may be sharp or stabbing and is aggravated by movement of the left arm. Radiation does not occur outside the thorax. Occasionally, the pain is persistent or recurring, incapacitating the patient for months.

On physical examination, there is characteristic point tenderness of the chest wall, most commonly at a costochondral junction. It should be stressed that this syndrome can occur in patients with coexisting documented cardiac disease. In fact, chest wall tenderness has been described in patients with acute myocardial infarction, pneumonia, and pulmonary emboli.[30] Patients recovering from an acute myocardial infarction can have chest wall tenderness.

Patients can generally pinpoint a specific area of intense pain (i.e., the trigger point). Palpation of this area reproduces the pain.

Table 4. Procedure for Injection of Costochondral Trigger Point

- Locate the point of maximal tenderness—it should be over a rib (costochondral junction). Occasionally there may be a second point.
- Clean the area with antiseptic. Place a finger on each side of the rib to assure that you do not enter the pleura.
- Inject the area with 2-10 cc of 1% lidocaine. Pain relief should occur in 2-25 minutes

Injection of the site with local anesthetic may be painful initially but will quickly eliminate the pain. *(Please see Table 4.)* Total elimination of the pain with local injection is highly supportive of the diagnosis of chest wall syndrome and helps to relieve anxiety. Nitroglycerin typically does not relieve the pain.

Post-Sternotomy Chest Pain. Following sternotomy, many patients have recurrent pain over their incision. Rarely, this is due to serious causes such as nonunion of the sternum, infection, or fractured ribs. In some patients, it may be due to sternal wires. Up to 10% of females and 2% of males are sensitive to nickel. Pain is localized over the sternal wire(s). Removal may provide relief.

Herpes Zoster. H. zoster involves the thoracic roots in 50% of cases. A sharp, severe pain along one or more dermatomes may be present a few days before the characteristic vesicular eruption. Acyclovir may decrease the duration of pain, but opioids are often needed for acute analgesia.

Thoracic Outlet Syndrome. Thoracic outlet syndrome is caused by compression of the brachial plexus or artery by the first rib, cervical rib, or scalene muscle. It commonly causes dull or aching pain and/or paresthesias in the ulnar distribution of the arm or neck. In some cases, the pain is in the anterior chest. Pain generally begins spontaneously, although in some cases, it is initiated or exacerbated by trauma to the chest.

This is generally a benign syndrome that causes pain only, but in some cases, arterial obstruction from thrombosis or thromboembolism can occur. The pain is made worse with movement. Several maneuvers are used to reproduce the pain and support the diagnosis. The Adson test involves having the patient take a deep breath with lifting the chin and turning the head to the affected side. The radial pulse is palpated before and during this maneuver. The test is positive if the radial pulse diminishes or is absent. Unfortunately, this maneuver is associated with a 50% false-positive rate.[31]

A second test involves raising both hands over the head while the radial pulse is palpated. Again, a decrease in pulse suggests the presence of thoracic outlet syndrome. This procedure has about the same accuracy as the Adson test. The elevated arm stress test (EAST) is performed by having the patient sit with the arms abducted 90° from the thorax and elbows flexed to 90°.[32] The patient then opens and closes his fists slowly. This maneuver is continued for three minutes. Patients with thoracic outlet syndrome will develop numbness of the hand and aching in the arm and shoulders.

Patients thought to have thoracic outlet obstruction should be referred for physical therapy to strengthen the shoulder girdle muscles. In severe cases, surgical resection of the rib is indicated.

Rib Fracture. Most patients with rib fractures present with a history of direct trauma, which makes the diagnosis relatively easy. In these patients, a cardiac cause is rarely considered. However, pathologic fractures or fractures induced by coughing may occur. The pain occurs from irritated intercostal nerves and intercostal muscle spasm, which produces splinting and reduces respiratory function. The pain is generally sharp and located to a specific rib area. The pain is often pleuritic, made worse by deep inspiration. Palpation of the area reveals point tenderness, and, occasionally, swelling and abnormality of the underlying structure can be appreciated.

Radiographs are indicated in patients in whom pathologic fracture is suspected (fracture that occurs with little or no trauma or minimal coughing), and to rule out an underlying pneumothora. Because treatment of a fractured rib is similar to that employed for a contusion, detailed x-rays are a costly test that do not change therapy. In general, a PA chest film is all that is required. Lateral films and rib series do not affect routine management of patients with suspected rib fracture, especially if there is no evidence of pneumothorax, hemothorax, or pulmonary contusion on the PA film.

Nonsteroidal anti-inflammatory medications provide some relief, but often opioids are required for the first few days. Rib belts and circumferential taping of the chest enhance pain control but increase splinting, decrease respiratory function, increase atelectasis, and potentially increase the possibility of pneumonia. Local anesthetic can be injected into the area over and around the fracture site (hematoma block) allowing for a decrease in pain and splinting. This technique is done exactly as described above for costochondral block only over the rib itself. Up to 12 hours of pain relief can be obtained from a single injection, which can be repeated if necessary. Intercostal nerve blocks also can be used to provide analgesia and reduce splinting. This is particularly useful when more than one rib is fractured.

Admission is indicated when more than three ribs are fractured (especially in the elderly), when a flail chest is identified, or when there is significant trauma (e.g., underlying pulmonary contusion, hemothorax) that may predispose to serious complications.

Psychogenic or Idiopathic Chest Pain. Panic attacks and depression are common psychogenic disorders associated with chest pain. Panic attacks are precipitated by recurrent episodes of sympathetic stimulation that cause the patient to feel alarmed and uneasy. In most cases, there is *no* precipitating stressful event. Physical symptoms include shortness of breath, dizziness, palpitations, choking, abdominal pain, and substernal chest tightness.

Most often, chest pain is felt over the left mammary area. Pain is often stabbing and fleeting, though it can feel like a tightness. It typically begins after exertion. These physical symptoms add to the psychological component. Many patients will express a fear of imminent death ("angor animi"). It is important to remember that panic symptoms also can occur in patients with myocardial ischemia and PE. In a panic attack, the ECG will be normal, with the exception of tachycardia. Nitroglycerin may relieve the pain, but rarely within five minutes; more commonly, relief will require 30 minutes or more.

Hyperventilation syndrome is usually encountered in individuals 40 years of age or younger. Patients present with tachycardia, shortness of breath, and tachypnea. Often the syndrome is precipitated by a stressful event. Patients have substernal chest heaviness, palpitations, and occasionally paresthesias and dizziness. Carpal-pedal spasm is common, adding to the patient's anxiety. Voluntary hyperventilation replicates the symptoms. Patients often display an increased awareness of body sensations.

Hyperventilation syndrome may be a variant of panic disorder. Using a rebreathing mask or a simple paper bag will usually raise the PCO_2 and break the recurrent cycle of breathing. Caution should be used in patients in whom the diagnosis is in doubt. Raising the PCO_2 in a patient with pulmonary emboli could be disastrous.

Patients with a psychogenic cause of chest pain usually benefit from cognitive/behavior therapy. In severe cases characterized by disabling symptoms, short-term treatment with a short-acting benzodiazepine can be initiated in the ED. In general, a prescription for no more than five days of benzodiazepine is appropriate, and follow-up should always be arranged. Antidepressants such as imipramine and selective serotonin reuptake inhibitors may provide long-term relief for patients with recurrent panic attacks.

Chest Pain in the Pediatric Population. Chest pain is the third leading nontraumatic complaint in the pediatric outpatient population, following headache and abdominal pain.[33] The vast majority of chest pain in children is non-cardiac in etiology, although there are some infrequent cardiac causes that may produce chest pain. Cardiac disease in pediatric patients may be associated with congenital heart defects. Ischemic syndromes, however, can be seen in children with anomalous left coronary artery, polyarteritis nodosa, Kawasaki disease, or type IIA homozygous hyperlipidemia. As with adults, cocaine use causes coronary artery spasm and local myocardial damage. Gastrointestinal disorders, respiratory causes (coughing, asthma), and musculoskeletal causes each account for 10-20% of cases.[34] Presentation and diagnosis are similar to the adult population.

Children with rapid growth spurts often complain of pain (dull or sharp) located over the precordium. This syndrome is more common in females and is always benign. Many of these patients become frequent users of the health care system. Reassurance of both the child and the parent is essential and should commence with the first presentation. Repeated testing often accentuates the behavior and validates the idea that "something must be wrong."

Summary

Patients with recurrent noncardiac chest pain can become frequent visitors to the ED, especially when anxiety and uncertainty characterize the clinical picture. Because of medicolegal concerns and overlapping presentations, these patients can present a formidable clinical challenge. Often, a comprehensive ED evaluation to exclude ischemic origins will be followed by extensive follow-up workups to assure patients that they do not have cardiac disease. Even when the assessment process is thorough and reassurance is provided, fewer than 40% of patients who are seen in the ED and given a diagnosis of noncardiac chest pain believe the diagnosis.[4]

Excluding serious ischemic, embolic, and vascular causes of chest pain remains a priority for the emergency physician. Once these entities are excluded, a systematic approach to the differential diagnosis will frequently yield a diagnosis. Prompt relief of pain in the ED accompanied by an explanation of the diagnosis and likely prognosis can reduce the possibility of recurrent visits for the same condition. When appropriate, reassurance is an important component of patient management.

References

1. Kroenke K, Mangelsdorff DA. Common symptoms in ambulatory care: Incidence, evaluation, therapy, and outcome. *Am J Med* 1989;86:262-266.
2. Kemp HG, Bokonas PS, Cohn PF, et al. The anginal syndrome associated with normal coronary arteriograms: Report of a six-year experience. *Am J Med* 1973;54:735-742.
3. Katon W, Hall ML, Russo J, et al. Chest pain: Relationship of psychiatric illness to coronary arteriographic results. *Am J Med* 1988;84:1-9.
4. Roll M, Kollind M, Theorell T. Clinical symptoms in young adults with atypical chest pain attending the emergency department. *J Intern Med* 1991;230:271-277.
5. Channer KS, James MA, Papouchado M, et al. Failure of a negative exercise test to reassure patients with chest pain. *Q J Med* 1987;240:315-322.
6. Ward BC, Wu WC, Richter JE, et al. Long-term follow-up of symptomatic status of patients with noncardiac chest pain: Is diagnosis of esophageal etiology helpful? *Am J Gastroenterol* 1987;82:215-218.
7. Goldman L. Acute chest pain: Emergency room evaluation. *Hosp Pract* 1986;(July):94A-94T.
8. Lee TH, Cook EF, Weisberg M, et al. Acute chest pain in the emergency room: Identification and examination of low-risk patients. *Arch Intern Med* 1985;145:65-69.
9. Bennett JR, Atkinson M. The differentiation between oesophageal and cardiac pain. *Lancet* 1966;2:1123-1127.
10. Servi RJ, Skiendzielewski JJ. Relief of myocardial ischemia pain with a gastrointestinal cocktail. *Am J Med* 1985;3: 208-209.
11. Goldman AP, Kotler MN, Scanlon MH, et al. Magnetic resonance imaging and two dimensional echocardiography: Alternative approach to aortography in the diagnosis of aortic dissecting aneurysm. *Am J Med* 1986;80:1225-1229.
12. Frieman DG, Suyemoto J, Wessler S. Frequency of pulmonary thromboembolism in man. *N Engl J Med* 1965;272:1270.
13. American Heart Association. The Urokinase Pulmonary Embolism trial: A national cooperative study. American Heart Association Monograph No. 39. *Circulation* 1973;47:1-108.
14. Dreyfuss AI, Weiland DS. Chest wall tenderness as a pitfall in the diagnosis of acute pulmonary embolism. *Arch Intern Med* 1984;144:2057.
15. Wenger NK, Stein PD, Willis PW III. Massive acute pulmonary embolism. The deceivingly non-specific manifestations. *J Am Med Assoc* 1972;220:843-844.
16. Dunmire SM. Pulmonary embolism. *Emerg Med Clin North Am* 1989;7:339-354.
17. Richter JE, Castell DO. Diffuse esophageal spasm: A reappraisal. *Ann Intern Med* 1984;100:242-245.
18. Richter JE. Gastroesophageal reflux disease as a cause of chest pain. *Med Clin North Am* 1991;75:1065-1080.
19. Nebel OT, Fornes MF, Castell DO. Symptomatic gastroesophageal reflux. Incidence and precipitating factors. *Dig Dis Sci* 1976;21:953-956.
20. Clouse RE, Starano A, Landau DW, et al. Manometric findings during spontaneous chest pain with presumed esophageal

"spasms." *Gastroenterology* 1983;85:395-402.

21. Hewson EG, Sinclair JW, Dalton CB, et al. Twenty-four-hour esophageal pH monitoring: The most useful test for evaluating noncardiac chest pain. *Am J Med* 1991;90:576-583.
22. The oesophagus and chest pain of uncertain cause. *Lancet* 1992;339:583-584. Editorial.
23. Gillebert G, Janssens J, Vantrappen G, et al. Ambulatory 24-hour intraoesophageal pH and pressure recordings vs. provocative tests in the diagnosis of chest pain of esophageal origin. *Gut* 1990;31: 738-744.
24. Parker WA, MacKinnon GL. Nitrates in the treatment of diffuse esophageal spasm. *Drug Intell Clin Pharmacol* 1981;15: 806-807.
25. Orlando RC, Bozymski EM. Clinical and manometric response to nitroglycerin in diffuse esophageal spasm. *N Engl J Med* 1973;289:23-25.
26. Richter JE, Dalton CB, Bradley LA, et al. Oral nifedipine in the treatment of noncardiac chest pain in patients with the nutcracker esophagus. *Gastroenterology* 1987;93:21-28.
27. Landon J, Malpas JS. Tietze's syndrome. *Ann Rheum Dis* 1959;62:223-225.
28. Wolf E, Stern S. Costosternal syndrome: Its frequency and importance in differential diagnosis of coronary heart disease. *Arch Intern Med* 1976;136:189-191.
29. Wise CM, Semble EL, Dalton CB. Musculoskeletal chest wall syndromes in patients with noncardiac chest pain: A study of 100 patients. *Arch Phys Med Rehabil* 1992;73:147-149.
30. Prinzmetal M, Massumi RA. The anterior chest wall syndrome—chest pain resembling pain of cardiac origin. *JAMA* 1955;159:177.
31. Gage M, Parnell H. Scalene anticus syndrome. *Am J Surg* 1947;73:252-268.
32. Roos DB. Congenital anomalies associated with thoracic outlet syndrome. Anatomy, symptoms, diagnosis, and treatment. *Am J Surg* 1976;132:771-778.
33. Coleman WL. Recurrent chest pain in children. *Pediatr Clin North Am* 1984;31:1007-1026.
34. Selbst SM, Ruddy R, Clark BJ. Chest pain in children. *Clin Pediatr* 1990;29:374-377.

Reperfusion and Revascularization Therapies

*The CTAP Panel**

Over the past decade, impressive reductions in mortality, length, reinfarction, and length of hospital stay have been reported in large-scale studies of patients with acute myocardial infarction (AMI). Despite these advances, substantial challenges remain in identifying the precise combination and dosing of therapeutic agents (e.g., fibrinolytics, low-molecular weight heparins [LMWHs], unfractionated heparin [UFH], and glycoprotein [GP] IIb/IIIa inhibitors) that will maximize outcomes while minimizing drug-related adverse events in patients with ST-elevation MI.

When one adds the various pharmacological options; possible drug combinations; and the myriad percutaneous, interventional approaches (angioplasty and stenting) available for establishing coronary reperfusion, the decision-making process for hospital pharmacists, cardiologists, emergency physicians, and intensivists becomes even more difficult. Regardless of the modality used to establish reperfusion, there are a number of pathophysiological and clinical issues that must be factored into the efficacy and safety equation evaluating optimum medical approaches to AMI management, including: suboptimal macroperfusion and microperfusion, recurrent ischemia, reinfarction, and intracranial hemorrhage.

Is also is clear that antithrombin agents, especially low molecular weight heparins (LMWHs), have continued to play a central—and based on the results of recent clinical trials, an increasingly important—role in pharmacological reperfusion therapy for AMI. Until recently, UFH and aspirin, along with a fibrinolytic agent, were routinely administered to most patients with acute coronary ischemia. However, recent trials (ASSENT-3, HART II, and ENTIRE) support a pivotal role for the low-molecular-weight heparin enoxaparin in the setting of fibrinolysis.[1] Unlike UFH, enoxaparin has more predictable kinetics, is less protein-bound, has less potential for platelet activation, and requires no monitoring; this is a combination of benefits that provides a strong rationale for achieving potentially better outcomes when this LMWH is given in combination with fibrinolytic agents.

The track record of enoxaparin's success—and compared to UFH, its superiority—in unstable angina and non-ST elevation MI (NSTEMI) has been impressive; therefore, the rapidly evolving story of its outcome-enhancing role in ST-elevation MI should come as no surprise to clinicians who follow reperfusion strategies. Most previous studies comparing enoxaparin to UFH in unstable angina have demonstrated either less reocclusion, enhanced late patency of the infarct-related vessel, or a reduction in reinfarction rate when compared with UFH. The superior outcomes with enoxaparin vs. UFH across the entire spectrum of acute coronary sydromes (ACS), including its most recent value in ST-elevation MI as reported in ASSENT-3, have elevated this antithrombin agent to a prominent, unique position among pharmacological modalities used to manage acute coronary ischemia.

As would be expected, GP IIb/IIIa inhibitors also have undergone intense scrutiny, and in the case of this therapeutic class, the results have been mixed in patients not requiring percutaneous coronary intervention (PCI), but very favorable in patients with PCI, especially in the case of coronary stent insertion. Pilot studies with platelet GP IIb/IIIa inhibitors and reduced-dose fibrinolytic agents have shown enhanced patency of the epicardial infarct-related artery, and signs of improved tissue reperfusion. Use of clopidogrel for pretreatment of patients both with and without PCI also have been encouraging.

The phase III Global Use of Strategies to Open Occluded Coronary Arteries (GUSTO)-V trial demonstrated a reduction in ischemic complications of AMI with half-dose reteplase and abciximab, as compared with full-dose reteplase. The GUSTO-V trial, however, failed to show a significant reduction in 30-day mortality, and there was a significant increase in non-cerebral bleeding complications, thereby offsetting potential benefits and dampening enthusiasm for an imminent paradigm shift that would routinely include abciximab as a required agent in fibrinolytic protocols in the absence of PCI.

Although fibrinolysis is widely available and has demonstrated its ability to improve coronary flow, limit infarct size, and improve survival in AMI patients, many individuals with acute infarction are not considered suitable candidates for such treatment. Patients with absolute or relative contraindications to fibrinolytic therapy, cardiogenic shock, NSTEMI, and/or unstable angina may be ineligible for fibrinolytic therapy. The requirement of administering prompt reperfusion therapy to these patients, as well as the other limitations of fibrinolytic therapy, have led many clinicians to advocate PCI as the primary therapy and treatment of choice for AMI.

PCI, which may include percutaneous transluminal coronary angioplasty/PTCA or coronary stenting, has many theoretical and practical advantages over fibrinolysis and is becoming the preferred strategy for most patients with AMI. First, there is a larger patient eligibility pool for PCI, a lower risk of intracranial bleeding, and a significantly higher initial reperfusion rate. This strategy always affords earlier definition of coronary artery anatomy and the ability to risk stratify patients, thereby permitting rapid triage to surgical intervention when indicated.

Several trials of varying sizes comparing primary PCI with fibrinolysis have been reported in the past 10 years. Interventions in the early trials were performed using PTCA, prior to the current widespread use of coronary stents. Despite a clear and consistent benefit of primary PTCA in restoring patency of the infarct-related artery, differences in mortality in the individual trials have been difficult to evaluate due to small sample sizes and differences in study design, patient selection, and medical therapy. However, recent trials comparing coronary stenting to fibrinolysis have been more definitive in clarifying the superiority of invasive techniques in the management of appropriately risk-stratified patients with acute coronary syndromes.

With these clinical controversies and treatment options in clear focus, the authors of this landmark review and its accompanying protocols critically evaluate recent clinical trials and outline an evidence-based strategy that employs pharmacological and/or invasive interventions as indicated based on risk-group stratification for maximizing outcomes in patients with ST-elevation AMI.

Introduction

A wide range of mechanical and pharmacological options are available for restoring perfusion in coronary arteries that have been occluded by thrombosis in the setting of AMI. These include: 1) PCI (intracoronary stenting and/or angioplasty); 2) fibrinolysis which may include some combination of a fibrinolytic agent, an anticoagulant, and aspirin; or 3) fibrinolysis-facilitated mechanical reperfusion (i.e., pretreatment with a fibrinolytic agent or some combination of a fibrinolytic agent and GP IIb/IIIa platelet antagonist followed by PCI).

Determining which of the aforementioned approaches is appropriate for any given patient can be difficult, and requires a multi-factorial assessment. In this regard, the optimal approach for establishing coronary reperfusion after myocardial infarction depends on a number of clinical factors, among them: patient eligibility for specific interventions (medical vs invasive) based on risk stratification; adherence to risk-stratification protocols; availability of institutional resources for performing interventional techniques; availability of cardiologists with sufficient experience in transcutaneous coronary reperfusion techniques; the ability to provide prompt transfer to another hospital for patients who may require PCI; and the presence of exclusionary and inclusionary factors that determine patient eligibility for fibrinolysis.

The key point is that selection of a reperfusion strategy is a fluid process that must account for myriad patient, institutional, and risk factors to yield optimal outcomes. *(Please See Figures 1-4, in which protocols for managing the spectrum of acute coronary syndromes [UA, NSTEMI, STEMI] are presented.)*

Although the guidelines presented in this comprehensive review prioritize some strategies and agents over others, the dominant approach for a particular patient type identified in the guidelines may not always be the most suitable strategy if institutional, timing, or physician factors are not synchronized with the implementation of a specific intervention. Accordingly, clinical judgement should prevail when applying guidelines articulated in this review.

Fibrinolytic Therapy—The Current Landscape

In appropriately selected patients with AMI, early administration of fibrinolytic agents reduces mortality and is associated with improved short- and long-term clinical outcomes. From a pathophysiological perspective, prompt restoration of patency in the infarct-related artery reduces infarct size and minimizes the extent of myocardial damage, preserves left ventricular function, reduces morbidity, and prolongs survival. Compared to standard therapy, fibrinolysis is associated with a 21% reduction in 30-day mortality.[2] However, these agents also are associated with intracranial hemorrhage in about 0.5-0.9% of patients. In addition, only 30-60% of patients achieve TIMI 3 (normal) flow in the affected epicardial artery within 90 minutes.[2] Because of these drawbacks, safer and more effective fibrinolytic therapies have been developed through bioengineering techniques on the t-PA molecule. In addition, the role of combination therapy with adjunctive agents, such as enoxaparin and GP IIb/IIIa inhibitors, is emerging.

Mechanism and Efficacy. From an outcome-effectiveness perspective, it should be stressed that mortality is affected by factors other than epicardial vessel flow. In this regard, reperfusion at the tissue level may be a critical factor in myocardial salvage and this does not necessarily correlate with epicardial vessel flow. Patients with documented TIMI 3 epicardial flow, but poor TIMI myocardial perfusion (TMP) grades (TMP 0 or 1), had a higher mortality rate (5.4%) than those patients with adequate (TMP grade 2 flow) or complete tissue perfusion (TMP grade 3 flow), 2.9% and 0.7%, respectively.[3] Therefore, while survival in studies has been correlated with epicardial vessel flow, there is still much to decipher about perfusion characteristics and predictors of mortality.

The ideal fibrinolytic agent provides rapid lysis, enhances tissue-level perfusion, has low (< 1%) intracranial and systemic hemorrhage rates, has a long half-life enabling single-bolus administration, has no antigenicity, and has a low reocclusion rate. Enhanced fibrin specificity also is desirable because it permits preferential activation of fibrin-bound plasminogen at the clot surface; this has the potential to increase patency and produce higher initial patency rates, and may be associated with fewer bleeding complications. Greater fibrin specificity also decreases activation of circulating plasminogen and degradation of fibrinogen, resulting in less bleeding and a reduced need for transfusion.

Outcome-Optimizing Pharmacological Combinations. Fibrinolytic therapy unequivocally improves survival in patients presenting with ST segment elevation AMI. Re-establishing perfusion in the infarct-related coronary artery with the use of fibrinolytic therapy—in essence, reopening the infarct-related artery—increases the opportunity for salvage of the ischemic myocardium and, consequently, reduces morbidity and mortality.

Three megatrials comparing alteplase to streptokinase have been published. The GISSI-2 trial[4] and the closely related International Study[5] compared a 100 mg infusion of alteplase over three hours to streptokinase with or without heparin. The GISSI-2 was the first large-scale mortality trial directly comparing alteplase and streptokinase in patients with AMI. The investigators found no difference in mortality between the two treatment groups. More strokes were reported with alteplase than with streptokinase (1.3% vs 1%) in the International Study, yet the frequency of confirmed hemorrhagic stroke was similar for both agents. Similar results were found in the ISIS-3 trial,[6] the next fibrinolytic megatrial, which compared alteplase, streptokinase, and anistreplase in approximately 40,000 patients. In marked contrast to current practice, the inclusion criteria allowed both entry up to 24 hours after symptom onset and did not require diagnostic electrocardiographic change. A significant difference in both 35-day mortality and ICH was not found.[6]

Vascular Patency and Outcomes. Current fibrinolytic practice was highly affected by the results of the Global Use of Streptokinase and alteplase for occluded coronary arteries (GUSTO-I) trial.[7] The purpose of the GUSTO-I trial was to test the hypothesis that early and sustained infarct-vessel patency was associated with better survival rates in patients with AMI.[7] More than 41,000 patients were randomized to four different fibrinolytic strategies: accelerated alteplase given over 90 minutes plus IV heparin, a combination of streptokinase plus a reduced-dose of alteplase along with IV heparin, and two control groups (streptokinase plus subcutaneous heparin and streptokinase plus IV heparin). Unlike previous trials, alteplase was given in a more aggressive, front-loaded, 90-minute infusion, which was referred to as the "accelerated" regimen.

In addition to the primary end point of 30-day mortality, the GUSTO investigators explored the relationship between coronary artery patency and degree of normalization of flow in an angiographic substudy; this portion of the larger trial was designed to determine the relationship between early coronary artery patency and outcome. In this trial, accelerated alteplase, administered with intravenous heparin, was shown to significantly reduce 30-day mortality by 15% as compared to streptokinase with either form of heparin, or the combination of alteplase and streptokinase with intravenous heparin. However, ICH was significantly higher in the accelerated alteplase group (0.72 vs 0.54 for streptokinase plus UFH, P = 0.03). The benefit was most consistent among patients with AMI; this difference remained significant at one year of follow-up.

The angiographic substudy[4] demonstrated a strong relationship between TIMI flow and outcome. Patients with strong forward flow (i.e., TIMI grade 3 flow) at 90 minutes had significantly lower mortality rates compared with patients with little to no flow. The mechanism for this benefit was found to be earlier, more complete infarct vessel patency with accelerated alteplase; this early alteplase patency advantage over other agents was lost by 180 minutes after symptom onset. As would be expected, the patients with the higher risk derived the most substantial benefit from accelerated alteplase compared to streptokinase in this large study. Patients who received accelerated alteplase did suffer more hemorrhagic strokes compared to those who received streptokinase, but the combined end point of death and disabling stroke still favored the accelerated alteplase regimen.

Fibrin Specificity. A more recent addition to the fibrinolytic agent literature includes the GUSTO-III investigation.[8] This study compared accelerated alteplase to reteplase. In this very large trial, reteplase was found to similar to accelerated alteplase, with 30-day mortality rates of 7.47% and 7.24%, respectively. There has been some debate about the implications of this study, however, with some reviewers arguing that it was designed as a superiority trial, not an equivalence trial, and that as such, it did not have the power to prove equivalence. The primary conclusion most experts agree upon is that alteplase and reteplase are similar in their clinical outcomes.[8] Reteplase is a mutant form of alteplase that allows it to be administered in a fixed double-bolus dose, with no adjustment required for weight, thus simplying administration.

The ASSENT-2 trial investigated the use of tenecteplase, another mutant of wild-type alteplase. Tenecteplase has several interesting characteristics and associated potential benefits, including: 1) its longer half-life allows it to be administered as a single bolus; 2) it is 14 times more fibrin-specific than alteplase and even more so than reteplase; and 3) it is 80 times more resistant to PAI-1 than alteplase. The ASSENT-2 trial[9] randomized approximately 17,000 patients with AMI to single-bolus tenecteplase (30-50 mg based upon body weight) or accelerated alteplase (100 mg total infusion); the primary outcome variable was 30-day all-cause mortality. This was a weight-based, tiered dose infusion since not all patients received 100 mg. The investigators found no differences in mortality or ICH.[9]

In a reported subgroup analysis, a lower 30-day mortality was noted among patients who presented greater than four hours after onset of symptoms; furthermore, fewer non-intracranial major bleeding episodes were encountered in the tenecteplase group. However, the subgroup analysis for those presenting at greater than four hours has been more carefully scrutinized and its conclusions have been called into question by an FDA statistics reviewer. CBER performed a multivariate analysis for the four- to six-hour time to treatment sub-group, using the same cofactors utilized for the primary end point (age, Killip class, heart rate, systolic blood pressure, and infarct location. This group encompassed approximately 22% of the total study population. The mortality advantage of tenecteplase was not statistically significant when the cofactors were included in the analyses. Moreover, there were important imbalances between treatment groups with resect to baseline heart rate and age favoring prognosis in the TNK group.[10]

Based on these results, it can be concluded that tenecteplase was equally effective, particularly in late presenters, although only 22% of patients presented after four hours. As far as adverse reactions, tenecteplase also appeared to be modestly safer than accelerated alteplase. Finally, due to its single bolus administration, tenecteplase is easy to use in the emergency department (ED) and other settings, such as the air and ground prehospital environments. Following-up on these observations, the ASSENT-3 trial compared tenecteplase regimens combined with enoxaparin or abciximab vs. a standard tenecteplase/UFH.[1]

Candidacy for Fibrinolysis: Patient Screening, Relative and Absolute Contraindications, and Risk Stratification

Optimizing outcomes in patients with ACS requires matching patients with strategies that will produce the best results in specific clinical subgroups. Identifying those patients who represent ideal candidates for fibrinolysis, and who are likely to have outcomes at least as favorable as they would with percutaneous interventions, has become an area of intense focus among cardiologists and emergency physicians. A number of factors that should be considered when assessing patients with AMI for either percutaneous or fibrinolytic therapy are discussed in the following sections.

Patient Age. In general, published trials do not provide evidence to support withholding fibrinolytic therapy on the basis of a patient's age alone. In fact, the FTT Collaborative Group[11] concluded that, "clearly, age alone should no longer be considered a contraindication to fibrinolytic therapy." At the same time, it must be recognized that patients older than age 75 do have a higher incidence of hemorrhagic stroke than younger patients. Moreover, the recent GUSTO-V Trial suggested inferior outcomes when abciximab was combined with UFH and tenecteplase in patients older than age 75.

Time from Chest Pain Onset—The Therapeutic Window. The generally accepted therapeutic time window for administration of a fibrinolytic agent after the onset of ST segment elevation AMI is 12 hours. Considerable data support this time period.[7,12-19] Without question, the earlier the treatment is initiated, the greater the likelihood that the patient will experience a good outcome. This is the case in patients who present within the first six hours of AMI. Delayed administration (i.e., those occurring between 6 and 12 hours after AMI onset) also confers benefit, although of a lesser magnitude.[20]

The Late Assessment of Fibrinolytic Efficiency (LATE) trial, which compared fibrinolytic therapy with placebo, found a significant 26% decrease in 35-day mortality in patients treated with alteplase, heparin, and aspirin 6-12 hours after the onset of symptoms.[21] There is no significant decrease in mortality among patients treated 12-24 hours after symptom onset. These studies, then, clearly establish benefit from treatment at 0 to 12 hours in patients who are otherwise appropriate candidates for fibrinolytic therapy. Treatment beyond that time is not supported by results of currently available trials. The single exception may be a patient with a "stuttering" pattern of chest pain between 12 and 24 hours after symptom onset. This emphasized the importance of an adequate history. If there is evidence of marked ST segment elevation on a 12-lead ECG, the patient should be considered a potential fibrinolytic candidate.

Previous Myocardial Infarction or Coronary Artery Bypass Grafting. In the setting of AMI, a previous MI should not preclude consideration for treatment with fibrinolytic agents, although there is evidence that PCI may be preferable.[19] Without treatment, there is a potential for greater loss of function in the newly infarcting region of the myocardium. Although the GISSI-1 trial[22] shows no treatment benefits with fibrinolytic therapy in patients with previous MI, the ISIS-2 trial demonstrates a 26% relative mortality rate reduction for patients with previous MIs treated with fibrinolytic therapy.[12] The FTT (Fibrinolytic Therapy Trialist's Collaborative Group) meta-analysis further demonstrates that patients with a history of past MI who receive fibrinolytic therapy for recurrent acute infarction have a mortality rate of 12.5%, compared with 14.1% among control patients.[19]

Many studies have reported successful fibrinolysis in AMI patients with prior coronary artery bypass graft (CABG). Complete thrombotic occlusion of the bypass graft is the cause of AMI in approximately 75% of cases, as opposed to native vessel occlusion. It has been suggested that because of the large mass of thrombus and absent flow in the graft, conventional fibrinolytic therapy may be inadequate to restore flow. Because patients who have undergone CABG may be relatively resistant to fibrinolytic therapy, they should be considered for direct angioplasty or combined fibrinolysis and rescue angioplasty.[23]

Stroke. A history of previous stroke or transient ischemic attack (TIA) is a major risk factor for hemorrhagic stroke after treatment with fibrinolytic therapy. A history of previous ischemic stroke should remain a strong relative contraindication to fibrinolytic therapy. A history of previous hemorrhagic stroke within one year should remain an absolute contraindication. American College of Cardiology (ACC) Guidelines should be consulted for additional information and specific exclusionary criteria.[24,25]

Recent Surgery and Trauma. Recent surgery or trauma is considered a relative contraindication to fibrinolytic therapy. The term recent has been variably interpreted, however, in fibrinolytic therapy trials. In the GISSI-1 trial,[22] patients were excluded if they had surgery or trauma within the previous 10 days. In the ASSET trial, patients were excluded for surgery or trauma within the previous six weeks.[26] Other fibrinolytic therapy trials have not defined "recent surgery or trauma." It is prudent to consider alternative interventions such as angioplasty, if available, in patients with AMI with recent (within 2-4 weeks for all surgical procedures, and < 3 weeks for major surgey) surgery or significant trauma.

Elevated Blood Pressure. Current evidence indicates that patients with a history of chronic hypertension should not be excluded from fibrinolytic therapy if their blood pressure is under control at the time of presentation or if it can be predictably lowered to acceptable levels using standard therapy for ischemic chest pain. In this regard, the admission blood pressure also is an important indicator of risk of intracerebral hemorrhage.

The FTT meta-analysis[19] demonstrates that the risk of cerebral hemorrhage increases with systolic blood pressure greater than 150 mmHg on admission and further increases when systolic blood pressure is 175 mmHg or greater. Despite an increased mortality rate during days 0 and 1, the FTT meta-analysis demonstrates an overall, long-term benefit of 15 lives saved per 1000 for patients with systolic blood pressures greater than 150 mmHg and 11 lives saved per 100 for patients with systolic blood pressures of 175 mmHg or greater.[19] Although the FTT meta-analysis appears to indicate an acceptable risk-benefit ratio for patients with substantially increased systolic blood pressure, a persistent blood pressure greater than 180/110 mmHg generally is considered an absolute contraindication to fibrinolytic therapy. The American Heart Association (AHA)/ACC recommends that a blood pressure of greater than 180/110 is a relative contraindication; this is derived from the TIMI-II trial, in which intracranial hemorrhage occurred in 9.1% (n = 22 patients) with a systolic blood pressure of greater than 180 or diastolic blood pressure of greater than 110 before receiving thrombolytic therapy compared with 1.4% (n = 9) of patients without an elevated blood pressure.[24,25,27]

Hypotension. The benefit of fibrinolytic therapy in patients with hypotension remains controversial. The FTT meta-analysis, however, does not support this hypothesis.[19] In its meta-analysis, patients with an initial systolic blood pressure of less than 100 mmHg who were not treated with fibrinolytic therapy had a very high risk of death (35.1%), and those who were treated with fibrinolytic therapy had the largest absolute benefit (60 lives saved per 1000 patients).[19] Based on this evidence, the FTT Collaborative Group suggests that hypotension, heart failure, and perhaps even shock should not be contraindications to fibrinolytic therapy.[19] The value of PCI in these patients also has been established. Overall, the data support immediate treatment directed to myocardial reperfusion, regardless of the method, PCI or fibrinolysis, as indicated by clinical judgement.

Menstrual Bleeding. Experts have debated whether actively menstruating women with AMI are candidates for fibrinolysis. There has been previous concern regarding whether menstruating women with AMI should be considered candidates for fibrinolytic therapy. Because natural estrogen is cardioprotective, there has been little experience with fibrinolysis among premenopausal women. Significant adverse effects, however, have not been reported by clinicians who administer fibrinolytic therapy to such patients. Gynecologists indicate that any excessive vaginal bleeding that may occur after receiving fibrinolytic therapy should be readily controlled by vaginal packing; therefore, it can be considered a compressible site of bleeding.

The Electrocardiogram. Combined with the patient's history and physical examination, the 12-lead ECG is the key determinant of eligibility for fibrinolysis. The electrocardiographic findings include two basic issues: 1) ST segment elevation of 1 mm or more in two or more anatomically contiguous standard limb leads and 2 mm or more elevation in two or more contiguous precordial leads; or 2) new or presumed new left-bundle branch block (LBBB). No evidence of benefit from fibrinolytic therapy is found in patients with ischemic chest pain

Figure 1. Guidelines for Effective Acute Coronary Syndrome Management

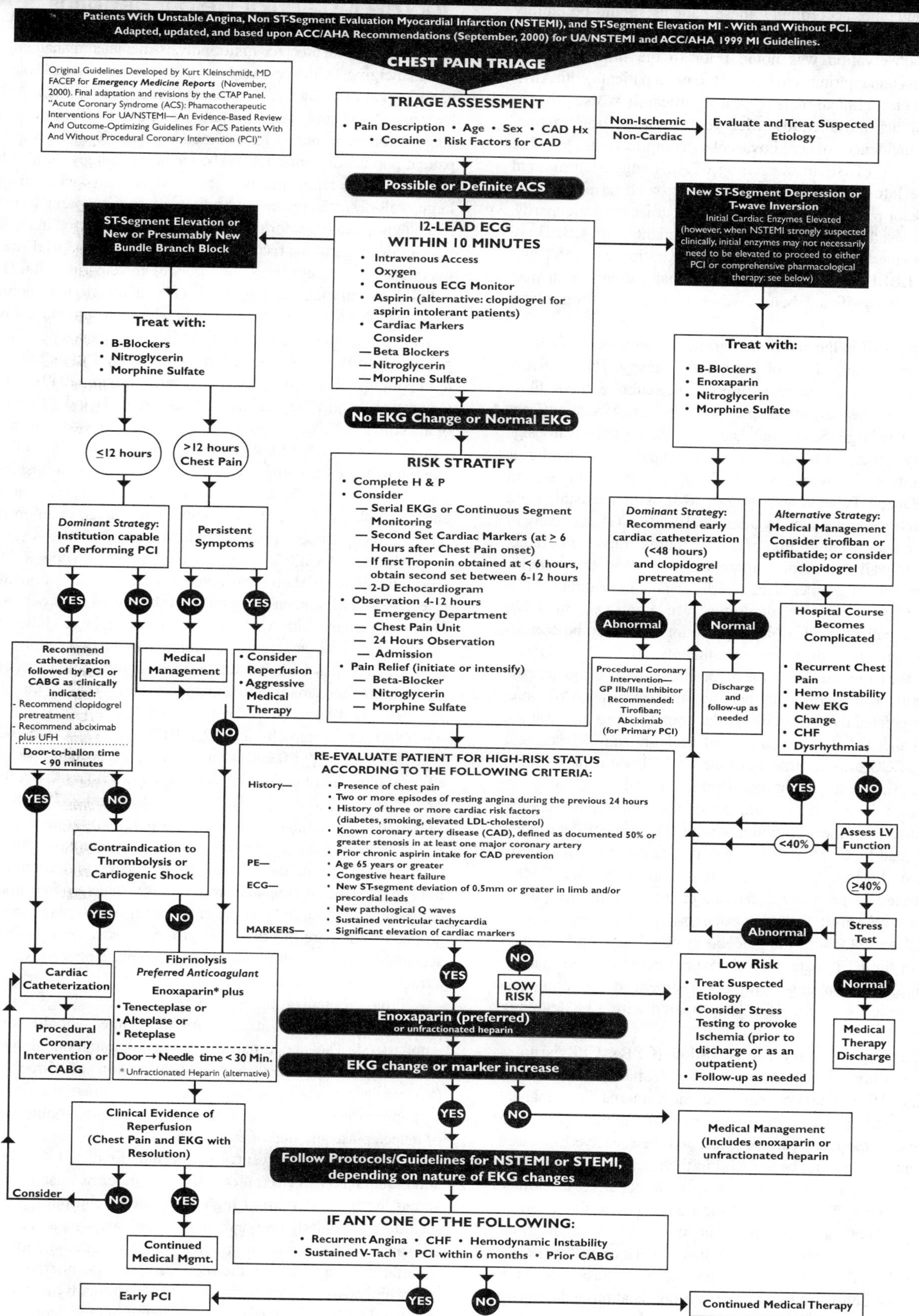

who lack either appropriate ST-segment elevation or the new development of LBBB.

Patients with LBBB and AMI are at an increased risk of experiencing a poor outcome; accordingly, these patients should be rapidly and aggressively managed in the ED with appropriate reperfusion therapies.[19,27] This observation was noted prior to the introduction of fibrinolytic agents and continues to be true today. In patients with AMI, new-onset LBBB is a clinical marker for a significantly worse prognosis in terms of higher mortality, lower left ventricular ejection fraction, and increased incidence of cardiovascular complications.[19,27] The development of new LBBB in the setting of AMI suggests proximal occlusion of the left anterior descending artery; such an obstruction places a significant portion of the left ventricle in ischemic jeopardy. Despite this increased risk of a poor outcome, patients with LBBB are less likely to receive fibrinolytic agents than are patients with ST-elevation without LBBB. It should be stressed that patients with new onset LBBB show significant benefit when treated with fibrinolytic therapy.[19]

Patients with AMI in the anterior, inferior, or lateral anatomic locations benefit from administration of fibrinolytic therapy. The relatively favorable prognosis associated with inferior infarction without fibrinolytic therapy requires larger sample sizes to detect a significant survival benefit. The large ISIS-2 trial[12] demonstrated a statistically significant mortality benefit for fibrinolytic therapy in patients with inferior AMI: the mortality at five weeks is 6.5% for streptokinase plus aspirin vs. 10.2% for placebo. Patients with inferior AMI, with coexisting right ventricular infarctions as detected by additional-lead ECGs, are likely to benefit because a significant portion of myocardium is onvolved. Acute, isolated posterior wall myocardial infarction, diagnosed by posterior leads, may represent yet another electrocardiographic indication for fibrinolysis. Although improved outcomes are unproven in large fibrinolytic trials, patients with isolated posterior AMI may be considered as possible candidates for reperfusion therapy.

In general, the larger the size of the myocardial infarct, the greater the mortality reduction with fibrinolytic therapy. The size of an AMI—and therefore, the associated risk of cardiovascular complications and death—is reflected by either the absolute number of leads showing ST segment elevation on the ECG or a summation of the total ST segment deviation from the baseline (i.e., both ST segment depressions and elevations).

The current evidence strongly indicates that fibrinolytic therapy should not be used routinely in patients with ST-segment depression only on the 12-lead ECG. Mortality rate may actually be increased by administration of fibrinolytics in this patient subgroup. The TIMI-3 trial[28] demonstrated a significant difference in outcome in fibrinolytic-treated patients with only ST segment depression: 7.4% incidence of death compared with 4.9% in the placebo group. These findings also are supported in the FTT meta-analysis, which demonstrated that the mortality rate among patients with ST segment depression who received fibrinolytic therapy is 15.2%, compared with 13.8% among controls.[19]

Recent Cardiopulmonary Resuscitation (CPR). CPR is not a contraindication to fibrinolytic therapy unless CPR has been prolonged (i.e., greater than 10 minutes) or extensive chest trauma from manual compression is evident.[93] Although in-hospital mortality rate is higher in AMI patients who experience cardiac arrest and then receive ED-based fibrinolytic agents, no difference is found in the rates of bleeding complications. No hemothorax or cardiac tamponade occurred in cardiac arrest patients receiving fibrinolytics.[29] One study reported that up to 25 minutes of CPR did not place patients at increased risk for complications of fibrinolysis. Although prolonged CPR that is performed for greater than 20 minutes is not an absolute contraindication to thrombolysis, it should, perhaps, be considered a relative contraindication and primary PCI may be preferred in this subgroup.[30,31]

ST-Elevation Myocardial Infarction (STEMI)—Fibrinolytic Strategies: New Considerations for Low Molecular Weight Heparins

An important advance in fibrinolysis-mediated management of AMI is the emerging, evidence-based support defining a pivotal role for enoxaparin as part of a tenecteplase-based, fibrinolytic regimen. Although the largest body of published literature evaluating LMWH in the setting of acute coronary ischemia has focused on the role of enoxaparin in this patient population, other LMWHs, including dalteparin, also have been evaluated.[32-34] Because the most recent, significant data to emerge from a large, well-designed prospective trail involves enoxaparin, its role in pharmacological strategies for reperfusion will be discussed in detail.

In this regard, the recently published ASSENT-3 trial was designed to compare the effectiveness and safety of enoxaparin vs. UFH as part of a full-dose tenecteplase regimen.[1] This landmark trial enrolled 6095 patients with AMI of less than six hours duration, and randomly assigned patients to one of three regimens: 1) full-dose tenecteplase plus enoxaparin (30 mg IV bolus followed immediately by 1 mg/kg SC q12 hr) for a maximum of seven days (enoxaparin group, 2040); 2) half-dose tenecteplase with weight-adjusted, low-dose UFH and a 12-hour infusion of abciximab (abciximab group, 2017); and 3) full-dose tenecteplase with weight-adjusted, UFH for 48 hours (UFH group, n = 2038). The primary end points were the composites of 30-day mortality, in-hospital reinfarction, or in-hospital refractory ischemia (efficacy end point); and the above end point plus in-hospital intracranial hemorrhage or in-hospital major bleeding complications (efficacy plus safety end point).

Although ASSENT-3 was not empowered to show a difference in mortality alone, it should be noted that the combination of full-dose tenecteplase plus enoxaparin produced the lowest 30-day mortality rates (5.4%) in patients with AMI reported in similar, large clinical trials evaluating fibrinolytic strategies in similar patient populations. Consistent with this finding is the fact that there were significantly fewer efficacy end points in the enoxaparin and abciximab groups than in the UFH group: 233/2037 (11.4%) vs. 315/2038 (15.4%; RR 0.74 [95% CI, 0.63-0.87], P = 0.0002) for enoxaparin, and 223/2017 (11.1%) vs. 315/2038 (15.4%; 0.72 [0.61-0.84], P < 0.0001) for abciximab. The same was true for the efficacy plus safety end point: 280/2037 (13.7%) vs. 347/2036 (17.0%; 0.81 [0.70-0.93], P = 0.0037) for enoxaparin, and 287/2016 (14.2%) vs. 347/2036 (17.0%; 0.84 [0.72-0.96], P = 0.01416) for abciximab.

The investigators concluded that the tenecteplase plus enoxaparin or abciximab regimens reduced the frequency of ischemic complications in AMI, producing an overall relative reduction in primary adverse end points of about 26% in the enoxaparin-tenecteplase and abciximab groups as compared to the UFH group. Its ease of administration and acceptable safety profile make the tenecteplase plus enoxaparin arm an attractive reperfusion regimen.

From a practical, time-to-treat myocardial salvage perspective, the convenience factor of the enoxaparin regimen should not be underemphasized. The abciximab arm required initiation of two infusions (abciximab plus UFH) and administration of three IV boluses (tenecteplase, abciximab, and heparin). In contrast, the enoxaparin arm was appropriately convenient, requiring two simple bolus infusions, one of tenecteplase and one of enoxaparin.

These practical advantages, combined with a lower bleeding rate and maintenance of overall effectiveness in terms of safety and efficacy across the full-spectrum of high risk patient subgroups with AMI (i.e., including the elderly and diabetic subsets) supports a paradigm shift to enoxaparin/tenecteplase or enoxparin in combination with other fibrin-specific thrombolytics, as the preferred pharmacotherapeutic approach to fibrinolysis-mediated therapy of AMI. Although the ASSENT-3 trial evaluated a fibrinolytic regimen consisting of tenecteplase, it is reason-

Figure 2. Guidelines for Effective Management of Unstable Angina

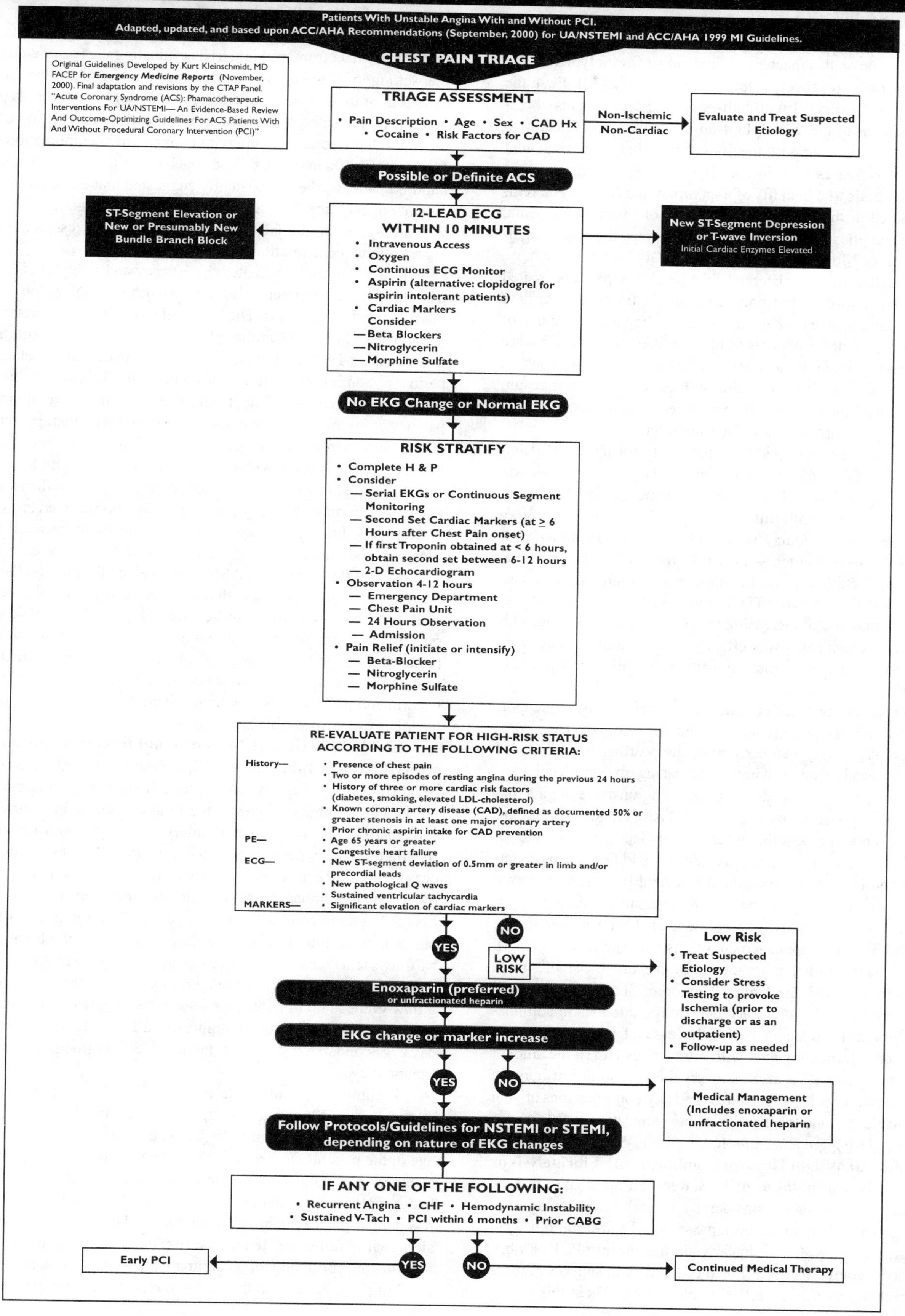

able to suggest that enoxaparin also should be the preferred anticoagulant agent, over UFH, when used in combination with other fibrinolytic agents such as alteplase and reteplase. However, at present, these data are lacking.

There are several findings that support the important role of enoxaparin in combination with tenecteplase and other fibrinolytics as the optimal regimen for appropriately selected patients with AMI. First, the results obtained in ASSENT-3 with half-dose tenecteplase plus abciximab are very similar to those with half-dose reteplase and abciximab seen in GUSTO-V, and support the hypothesis that a more potent antiplatelet agent increases flow in the infarct-related coronary artery. However, in both trials, the benefits of abciximab in a fibrinolytic regimen were obtained at the cost of a higher rate of thrombocytopenia, major bleeding complications, and blood transfusions, thereby mitigating its attractiveness. Moreover, as is the case in GUSTO-V, no benefit, and perhaps even harm, was observed in ASSENT-3 patients treated with the abciximab/half-dose fibrinolytic regimen who were older than age 75, which the reinforces the need for caution regarding the use of this combination in elderly patients. Although these observations are made on the basis of subgroup analysis, and its inherent limitations, in contrast to GUSTO-V, ASSENT-3 also suggested an inferior result, compared to heparin, for the abciximab regimen in diabetic patients, a finding that should prompt additional investigation.

Further support for enoxaparin's safety and efficacy in AMI has been forthcoming from the second trial of Heparin and Aspirin Reperfusion Therapy (HART II) in which 400 patients with AMI compared enoxaparin (30 mg intravenous bolus then 1 mg/kg subcutaneously every 12 hours) with UFH intravenous infusion as adjunct to a 90-minute regimen with a maximum of 100 mg human recombinant alteplase and aspirin. Enoxaparin was found to be at least as effective as UFH for achieving TIMI grades 3 and 2 flow, and in preventing reocclusion, without increasing the risk of major bleeding. This study showed that enoxaparin was effective and safe in patients with AMI and that it may be a convenient substitute for UFH in conjunction with fibrinolytics in this indication.[35]

Pharmacoeconomic Implications. A number of studies support the observation that enoxaparin reduces the incidence of adverse cardiovascular end points, among them: recurrent myocardial infarction and the need for revascularization without increasing major bleeding in patients with acute coronary syndromes, including unstable angina and acute ST-elevation myocardial infarction.[1,36-38] These clinical benefits are associated with economic benefits in terms of reduced expenditure on revascularisation procedures, the requirement for additional drug therapies and drug administration. Accordingly, several pharmacoeconomic analyses have been conducted on the use of enoxaparin in ACS.[39-42]

Enoxaparin has been shown to be associated with a cost saving compared with UFH in the management of unstable angina and non-ST segment elevation myocardial infarction in health economic studies from Canada, the United States, the United Kingdom, South America, and France.[39-42] These cost savings are accrued from reductions in administration costs (primarily associated with the ease of administration of subcutaneous enoxaparin compared with intravenous UFH); the amount of nursing time required (that also increases the availability of nurses); the need for revascularization procedures (and any complications arising from these procedures); and the duration of hospitalization.[41] *(Please see Table 1 for drug dosing guidelines in ACS.)*

Low Molecular Weight Heparin Combined with Fibrinolysis or PCI Plus a GP IIb/IIIa Inhibitor in ACS. Recent trials suggest that the LMWH enoxaparin now can be considered a pivotal, important agent in reperfusion regimens. Heparin has been the standard anti-thrombin agent in the management of AMI, particularly during the pre-PCI or fibrinolytic phase of therapy. However, much of the data in support of it are non-randomized and retrospective.[43] The role of LMWHs in this setting is now being intensively explored. Because of their prolonged half-life and the risk of possible hemorrhage during mechanical reperfusion, there has been concern about performing PCI in patients who have already been treated with LMWH for unstable angina or NSTEMI.

These concerns are now being allayed as new study data emerge. Preliminary data from multiple trials evaluating the use of enoxaparin in the setting of fibrinolysis or PCI were released at the Year 2000 Congress of the European Society of Cardiology. These trials primarily focused on the safety of enoxaparin in these clinical settings. Some of the trials also assessed the safety of enoxaparin in combination with different GP IIb/IIIa inhibitors. While each of the trials involved only a few hundred patients, they consistently suggested that enoxaparin is safe in patients undergoing PCI, as well as in those undergoing fibrinolysis or who are treated with a GP IIb/IIIa inhibitor. These results are undergoing additional confirmation in larger trials.

Two recent trials evaluated the efficacy and safety of enoxaparin in patients with ST-segment elevation myocardial infarction who were managed with fibrinolysis. The HART-II trial compared enoxaparin with heparin as adjunctive antithrombin therapy in 400 patients receiving front-loaded t-PA for ST-segment elevation AMI.[44] In this study, enoxaparin was administered intravenously (30 mg), followed by the standard subcutaneous regimen. The primary end points were infarct-related patency at 90 minutes after initiation of fibrinolytic therapy, reocclusion at 5-7 days, and safety. The TIMI grade 2 or 3 flow was comparable between groups, 80.1% with enoxaparin and 75.1% with heparin.

Reocclusion within one week occurred in 9.1% of the patients who received heparin and in only 3.1% of those who received enoxaparin (P = 0.1). Bleeding complications were comparable between groups.[44] Menown and others assessed the efficacy and safety of enoxaparin vs. heparin in 300 patients with AMI who received fibrinolytic therapy. The enoxaparin group received a 40 mg intravenous bolus followed by subcutaneous injections, while the heparin group received a 5000 unit bolus plus 30,000 units per 24 hours with adjustment to maintain an appropriate aPTT. The triple end point of death, AMI, or readmission with unstable angina at three months occurred in 36% of those who received heparin and in 26% of those who received enoxaparin (P = 0.04). Major bleeding was comparable between groups.[44]

ENTIRE STUDY (ENoxparin and tenecteplase with or without GP IIb/IIIa Inhibitor as REperfusion strategy in ST-elevation MI). The ENTIRE Study was a phase II stratified, randomized, open-label, angiographic trial conducted to assess the safety and efficacy of enoxaparin as an adjunct to fibrinolytic therapy, with or without GP IIb/IIIa therapy, in patients with ST elevation MI.[45] It should be pointed out that ENTIRE has been presented in abstract form and has a relatively small number of patients in its treatment arms. Specifically, ENTIRE attempted to determine the dose of enoxaparin that 1) in combination with full dose tenecteplase; and 2) in combination with a half-dose tenecteplase (0.27 mg/kg) and a full-dose of abciximab (bolus 0.25 mg/kg, infusion 0.125 mg/kg/min x 12h) is associated with a TIMI 3 flow grade at 60 minutes in at least 60% of patients. The primary end point was TIMI 3 flow at 60 minutes, and TIMI major hemorrhage at 30 days. Secondary end points included ST segment restoration and ischemic events.

Preliminary results were reported for 461 patients (456 patients treated, with 30-day follow-up available for 424 patients) at the European Society for Cardiology (Sept. 2, 2001, Stockholm). Average age of the patients studied was 58 years, 80% were males, and 34% had an anterior MI. Study patients included those with ST-elevation MI who had symptoms for 30 minutes or longer but for less than six hours. After receiving aspirin, patients were randomized to receive standard reperfusion with full-dose tenecteplase (0.53 mg/kg) or combination reperfusion consisting of abciximab plus one-half dose tenecteplase (0.27 mg/kg). Patients in the standard reperfusion group were then randomly assigned to receive either UFH (60 U/kg bolus; infusion 1 U/kg/h) or enoxaparin for up to eight days of therapy. In the combination reperfusion group, patients were randomized to receive either UFH (40 U/kg; infusion 7 U/kg/h) or enoxaparin for up to eight days of therapy. Subjects then underwent angiography and PCI, as indicated. Sheath removal following angiogram was performed four hours after PCI (or ACT < 180 seconds) in the heparin group, eight hours after the last subcutaneous dose of enoxaparin in the standard reperfusion group, and eight hours after the last subcutaneous dose or four hours past the last IV dose of enoxaparin.

Results of the study indicate that in angiographically evaluable patients, there were no significant differences in TIMI 2 and 3 blood flow at 60 minutes among the treatment arms, and in particular, no differences between UFH and enoxaparin. With respect to TIMI major hemorrhage at 30 days, there was a greater risk of hemorrhage in the combination (half-dose tenecteplase plus abciximab) group than in the full-dose tenecteplase group, and no significant differences between the UFH and enoxaparin subsets within this treatment arm. Among all patients undergoing PCI (n = 181), TIMI major hemorrhage occured in 2.5% of enoxaparin treated patients and in 6.7% of patients treated with UFH. At 30 days, the death/MI rate in the full-dose tenecteplase group was 4.4% in the enoxaparin group and 14.9% in the UFH group (P = 0.005). Although there was a relatively small number of patients with which to evaluate clinical outcomes, the death/MI/major hemorrhage triple end point rate in the full-dose tenecteplase group was 16.2% in patients treated with UFH and 6.3% in the enoxaparin group (P = 0.015).

Overall, the preliminary results of ENTIRE suggest that, regardless of whether full-dose fibrinolysis with tenecteplase or combination therapy is employed for facilitated reperfusion in the setting of cardiac catheterization and/or PCI, the anticoagulant enoxaparin is at least as effective and safe as UFH in all patient subsets. And moreover, if preliminary results and trends are confirmed in larger clinical trials, patients treated with enoxaparin plus full-dose tenecteplase may have better clinical outcomes than patients treated with full-dose fibrinolysis plus UFH. In addition, enoxaparin may be associated with a lower risk of hemorrhage than UFH in patients treated with half-dose tenecteplase plus abciximab.[45]

In combination with the results reported in the ASSENT-3 and NICE-3 trials (see below), enoxaparin's safety and efficacy in ACS patients treated with fibrinolysis either in the setting of medical (non-PCI) management or in the setting of interventional (PCI/catheterization) approaches in NSTEMI has been confirmed in well-designed, randomized trials. Because of superior clinical outcomes as compared to UFH in specific patient subgroups—STEMI (medical management, ASSENT-3), lower triple-end point (death/MI/major hemorrhage) rates in ENTIRE in the full-dose tenecteplase treatment arm—enoxaparin should be considered the anticoagulant of choice for the entire spectrum of patients with NSTEMI, whether they are treated with fibrinolytic regimens and/or GP IIb/IIIa antagonists, in those both with and without PCI. The role of enoxaparin in PCI patients with STEMI cannot be fully assessed until additional trials focusing on this issue are published, although a number of centers are using enoxaparin in this setting.

ST-Elevation Myocardial Infarction: Primary Percutaneous Coronary Interventions

Although fibrinolysis is widely available and has been documented to improve coronary flow, limit infarct size, and improve survival in AMI patients, many individuals with acute infarction simply are not considered suitable candidates for such treatment. In this regard, patients with absolute contraindications to fibrinolytic therapy, multiple relative contraindications, cardiogenic shock, and/or unstable angina may be ineligible to receive fibrinolytic therapy.

The mandate to implement prompt reperfusion therapy in these patients, as well as the other limitations of fibrinolytic therapy, have encouraged many clinicians to advocate PTCA, and more recently another PCI and intracoronary stenting, as the primary treatment modality for the majority of patients with AMI. Indeed, PCI has many theoretical advantages over fibrinolysis, including a greater pool of potentially eligible patients, a lower risk of intracranial bleeding, a significantly higher initial reperfusion rate, earlier delineation of coronary artery architecture with rapid triage to surgical intervention, and more precise risk-stratification, which may facilitate safe and earlier hospital discharge.

Several trials of varying sizes comparing primary PTCA with fibrinolysis have been reported in the past 10 years. Interventions in the early trials were performed using PTCA (i.e., they were performed prior to the current widespread use of coronary stents, the current PCI of choice). Despite a clear and consistent benefit of primary PTCA in restoring patency of the infarct-related artery, differences in mortality in the individual trials were difficult to evaluate due to the smaller sample sizes in the studies.

The PAMI trial[46] enrolled 395 patients who were randomly assigned to undergo primary PTCA or to receive alteplase. Compared with standard-dose alteplase, primary PTCA reduced the combined occurrence of nonfatal reinfarction or death, was associated with a lower rate of intracranial hemorrhage, and resulted in a similar left ventricular function. The results of the Netherlands trial indicated that primary angioplasty was associated with a higher rate of patency of the infarct-related artery, a less severe residual stenotic lesion, better left ventricular function, and less recurrent myocardial ischemia and infarction than was streptokinase.[47]

In a substudy of the GUSTO IIb trial,[48] the authors randomly assigned 1138 patients with AMI to either primary PTCA or accelerated alteplase. The composite end point of the study included death, nonfatal reinfarction, and nonfatal disabling stroke, all occurring within 30 days of the AMI. Of those patients assigned to primary PTCA therapy, 83% were candidates for such treatment and underwent angioplasty 1.9 hours after ED arrival for a total elapsed time from chest pain onset to therapy of 3.8 hours. Ninety-eight percent of the patients assigned to fibrinolytic therapy received alteplase 1.2 hours after hospital arrival. The occurrence of the composite end point was encountered significantly less often in the PTCA group (9.6%) compared to the alteplase group (13.7%) at 30 days.

When the individual components of the composite end point at 30 days were considered separately, the incidence of death (5.7% vs 7%), infarction (4.5% vs 6.5%), and stroke (0.2% vs 0.9%) occurred at statistically similar rates for both treatment groups: PTCA and alteplase, respectively. Additional evaluation in the form of a meta-analysis by Weaver et al[49] reviewed 10 major studies that compared fibrinolysis vs. primary PTCA in more than 2600 patients. The 30-day mortality was found to be significantly lower in the PTCA group, 4.4%, vs. 6.5% in the patients treated with fibrinolytics. Primary PTCA also was associated with a significant reduction in total stroke and hemorrhagic strokes.

The longer-term results of primary PTCA, however, are less clear. The GUSTO IIb study[48] showed no overall mortality advantage of primary PTCA at six months; conversely, two-year follow-up from the PAMI trial[46] found a significant reduction in hospital readmission, recurrent ischemia, target vessel revascularization, and reinfarction, with a trend toward a reduction in mortality in the PTCA group whencompared to treatment with fibrinolysis. Much of the previous literature comparing the acute reperfusion therapies in the AMI patient does not include or evaluate the use of coronary stenting as the PCI of choice. However, more recent studies suggest the introduction of intracoronary stenting likely will favorably alter the outcomes of AMI patients, making stent placement a superior method of management for appropriately selected patients at institutions where physicians are experienced in this procedure.

Figure 3. Guidelines for Effective Management of ST-Elevation Myocardial Infarction

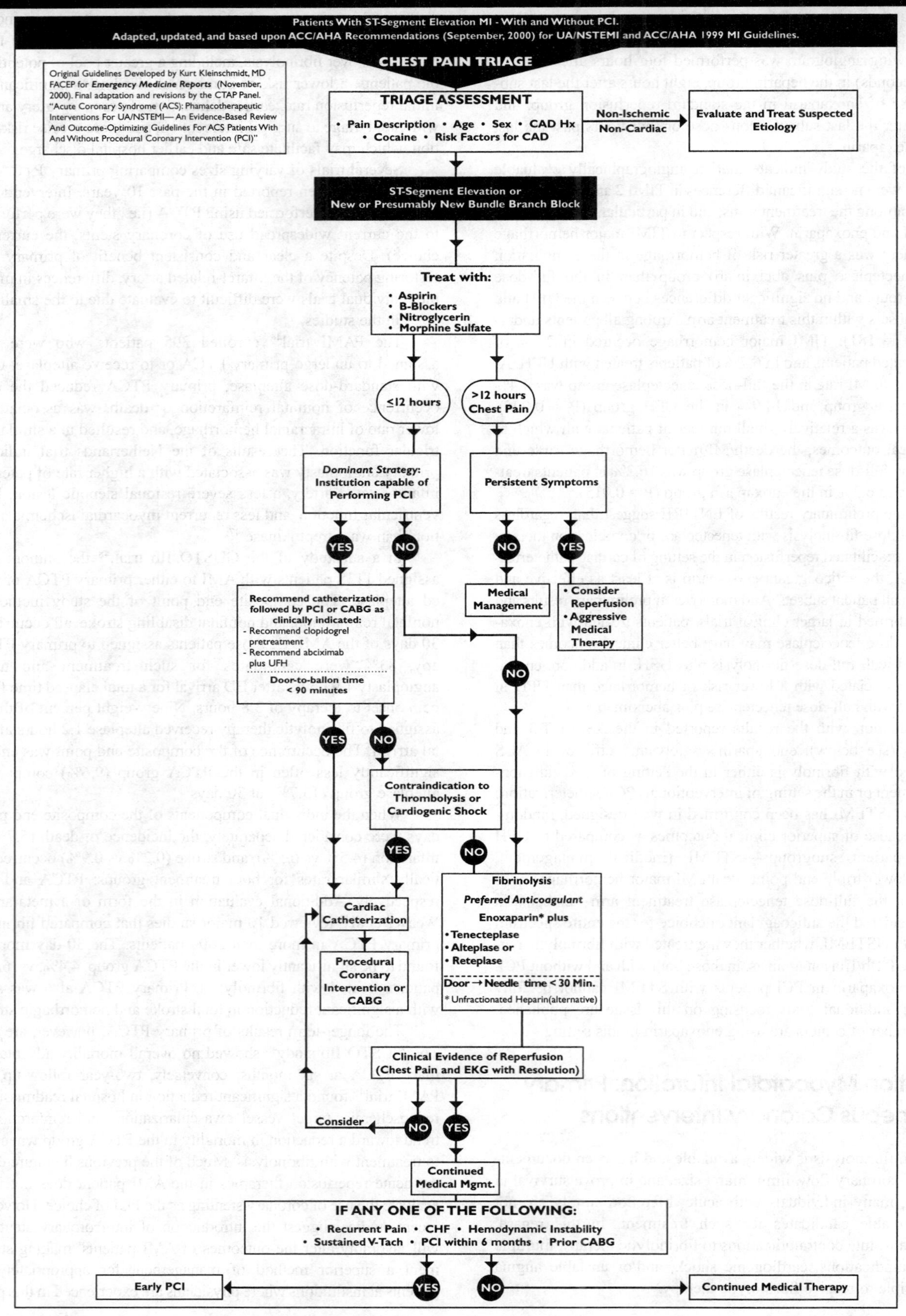

Figure 4. Guidelines for Effective Management of Non ST-Elevation Myocardial Infarction

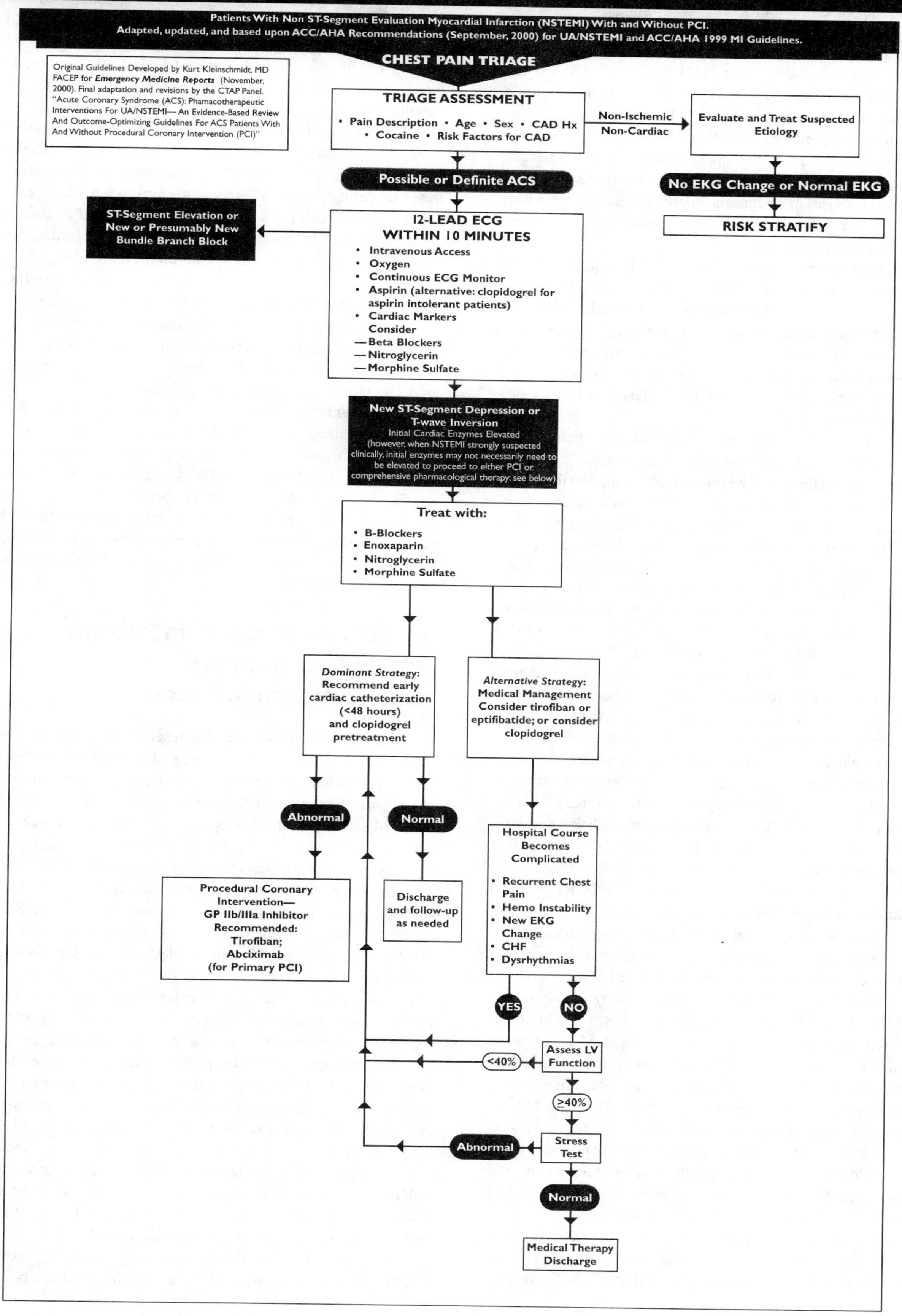

Intracoronary Stenting. A significant development in the use of PCI for managing patients with AMI involves intracoronary stents. In the recent past, early use of stenting in the AMI patient was considered problematic due to the real possibility of stent thrombosis. With the introduction of aggressive antiplatelet therapy using aspirin, ticlopidine, or clopidogrel, the rates of stent thrombosis have significantly decreased. Exploring early stent placement in the AMI patient, the PAMI-stent trial[50] compared urgent treatment with PTCA with or without stenting in 900 patients. Stenting significantly reduced both stenosis and re-occlusion at six months. No differences in death, reinfarction, or stroke at six months, however, was noted. Thus, it appears that in selected patients with AMI, primary stenting can be applied safely and effectively, resulting in a lower incidence of recurrent infarction and a significant reduction in the need for subsequent target-vessel revascularization compared with balloon angioplasty.

Support for the primary—and based on recent data, superior—role of coronary stenting in patients with STEMI comes from investigators involved in the Stent versus Thrombolysis for Occluded Coronary Arteries in Patients with Acute Mycoardial Infarction Study (STOPA-MI).[51] The purpose of this study was to assess whether coronary stenting combined with blockade of platelet GP IIb/IIIa produces a greater degree of myocardial salvage than fibronolysis with an accelerated infusion of alteplase.

In this study, a total of 140 patients with STEMI were enrolled in a randomized trial, with 71 assigned to receive a stent plus abciximab, and 69 to receive intravenous alteplase. The primary end point was the degree of myocardial salvage, determined by means of serial scintigraphic studies, and the secondary end point was a composite of death, reinfarction, and stroke within six months after randomization. In the group that received a stent plus abciximab, the median size of the final infarct was 14.3% of the left ventricle, as compared with a median of 19.4% in the alteplase group. The cumulative incidence of death, reinfarction, or stroke at six months was lower in the stent group than in the alteplase group (8.5 vs 23.2%, P = 0.02, RR, 0.34; 95% CI, 0.13-0.88).[51] The investigators concluded that in patients with AMI, coronary stenting plus abciximab produces a greater degree of myocardial salvage and a better clinical outcome than does fibrinolysis with a tissue plasminogen activator.

Recent research has evaluated the use of therapeutic combinations, including glycoprotein inhibition with both PCI and fibrinolysis, low-dose fibrinolysis followed by primary angioplasty, and intracoronary stent placement during PCI. As emphasized, reperfusion with primary PCI may be improved with the use of GP IIb/IIIa inhibitors, although there are conflicting results regarding their use in non-PCI patients. Abciximab with intracoronary stenting in AMI has been studied in the RAPPORT,[52] the ADMIRAL,[53] and the CADILLAC trials.[54] In the RAPPORT trial,[52] a significant reduction in the combined end point of death, MI, and urgent need for revascularization was noted at 30 days; no significant differences, however, were seen at six months. An increase in major bleeding episodes and the need for transfusions was encountered in the abciximab group, which was likely due to high-dose heparin therapy.

The ADMIRAL trial[53] reported a significantly lower rate of occurrence of the combined end point of death, recurrent MI, and target vessel revascularization at 30 days in the treatment group. In addition, lower doses of heparin were given to patients in the abciximab group, and no increase in major bleeding was observed. The CADILLAC trial[54] randomized primary PCI patients with AMI to stenting and abciximab vs. placebo. Preliminary results suggest that the abciximab-treated patients appeared to have had a modest reduction in acute events. The use of glycoprotein inhibitors in the setting of AMI treated with PCI appears to benefit the appropriately selected patients.

Perhaps the most interesting and controversial arena involves a "combination therapy" approach to the AMI patient, using a fibrinolytic agent and glycoprotein inhibitor. The IMPACT-AMI study[55] examined patients with AMI and randomly assigned them to receive either eptifibatide or placebo. In addition, patients received aspirin, heparin, and tissue plasminogen activator. Thus, this study looked at the role of a GP IIb/IIIa inhibitor (eptifibatide) in conjunction with a fibrinolytic agent in AMI; this was a departure from studies of unstable angina with or without catheter-mediated revascularization. The highest dose of eptifibatide studied achieved higher 90-minute patency rates than placebo, but similar rates of in-hospital death, stroke, reinfarction, vascular procedures, and new heart failure.

The PARADIGM trial[56] was designed to assess the safety and efficacy of combination therapy involving the platelet GP IIb/IIIa inhibitor lamifiban when given with fibrinolytic agents (alteplase or streptokinase) to patients with ST segment elevation AMI. A composite of angiographic, continuous electrocardiographic and clinical markers of reperfusion was the primary efficacy end point; bleeding was the primary safety end point. Lamifiban induced more rapid reperfusion, though a higher rate of bleeding was noted as well (transfusions in 16.1% lamifiban-treated vs. 10.3% placebo-treated patients). This trial, while small, suggests that such combination therapy may hasten clinical improvement and favorably alter outcome; additional, large trials are required to further explore this issue.

The use of a reduced-dose fibrinolytic agent in the AMI patient who is a candidate for primary PCI also has been explored. The PACT trial[57] randomized patients in the ED to either reduced-dose alteplase (50 mg) or placebo in preparation for primary angioplasty. Fibrinolytic-managed patients demonstrated higher rates of infarct vessel patency and TIMI grade 3 flow, with similar rates of adverse effect, suggesting that reperfusion can be enhanced prior to immediate PCI. This approach, called "facilitated percutaneous coronary intervention," suggests that early reperfusion therapy prior to catheterization not only is safe but also is effective.

Primary Angioplasty in Patients with Failed Fibrinolysis and Cardiogenic Shock

Current trial data suggest that rescue angioplasty may be advantageous in patients whose infarct-related arteries fail to reperfuse after fibrinolytic therapy.[58] Some centers routinely catheterize patients after fibrinolytic therapy to determine whether successful reperfusion has occurred and to perform angioplasty if necessary and anatomically feasible. Clinicians should be aware of signs and symptoms of failed reperfusion, including persistent ST-T wave elevation on the ECG at 30-45 minutes, as well as ongoing or recurrent chest pain. Other centers catheterize patients after fibrinolytic therapy only if there is clinical evidence that the infarct-related artery has failed to open, such as continued chest pain or persistent ST-segment elevation. The GISSI-1 and GISSI-2 trials show no apparent reduction of mortality rate with fibrinolytic therapy among patients classified in either Killip class III or IV.[14,22] These findings have led to the previous claim that primary angioplasty, not fibrinolytic therapy, should be used in patients with cardiogenic shock.

Patients with AMI who present with cardiogenic shock, which occurs in up to 10% of cases, demand special attention because this population has a mortality rate of almost 80%.[22] Fibrinolysis appears to be less effective in this subgroup of AMI patients, most likely due to a significantly lower coronary perfusion pressure; in the shock state, it is felt that the occlusive thrombus is not adequately exposed to the fibrinolytic agent, which may account for the clinical failure of the drug. In reviewing large fibrinolytic trials such as GISSI-1[22] and ISIS-2,[12] AMI patients presenting in cardiogenic shock did not benefit from fibrinolysis. Conversely, primary PCI has been investigated in more than 600 patients in several small studies; a cumulative analysis of this data revealed a significantly lower mortality rate (45%) compared to placebo and/or historical controls.[59]

The SHOCK trial[60] compared the outcomes of AMI patients presenting in cardiogenic shock; patients were randomly assigned to emergency revascularization (primary PTCA without stenting, or emergent CABG) or initial medical stabilization including fibrinolysis. The primary end point was mortality from all causes at 30 days; six-month survival was the secondary end point. Overall mortality at 30 days did not differ significantly between the revascularization and medical therapy groups (46.7% vs 56%, respectively). Six-month mortality was lower in the revascularization group than in the medical therapy group. The authors concluded that in AMI patients with cardiogenic shock, emergency revascularization did not significantly reduce overall mortality at 30 days. After six months, however, there was a significant survival benefit. The pre-specified subgroup analysis of patients younger than age 75 showed an absolute reduction of 15.4% in 30-day mortality and 21.4% in six-month mortality in the revascularization group. Therefore, when catheterization facilities are not available in patients with cardiogenic shock, fibrinolytic therapy should be given to eligible patients, and urgent transfer to a facility with interventional capabilities should be strongly considered.[60]

Primary PCI Versus Fibrinolytic Reperfusion Therapies for STEMI—Options, Logistics, System Issues, and Patient Outcomes

It is widely accepted that the early restoration of perfusion in the AMI patient limits myocardial damage, preserves left ventricular function, and reduces mortality; such restoration may be accomplished by either administration of a fibrinolytic agent or PCI. The rapid application of reperfusion therapy is mandatory in the patient with ST-elevation AMI. Naturally, a number of factors must be considered by clinicians regarding reperfusion treatment decisions when managing the AMI patient. Among the most important issues are time to application of the intervention and the level of experience of the invasive cardiologist.

Although primary angioplasty, in appropriately selected patients, may offer improved outcome over fibrinolysis, PTCA or other forms of PCI (stenting) must be instituted as early as possible without prolonged delay. In fact, a recent investigation demonstrated that the time to reperfusion in the patient with AMI treated with PTCA is related to outcome; in this study, mortality in AMI patients was decreased in the patient subgroup treated within two hours as compared to those individuals managed with angioplasty after two hours of infarct onset. Consequently, if a delay in activation of the catheterization laboratory is anticipated or actually occurs, the physician must proceed with fibrinolysis if the patient is an appropriate candidate.[61,62]

It should be stressed that restoration of perfusion does not occur immediately or soon after administration of the fibrinolytic agent. In fact, a "full fibrinolytic state" is not reached for at least 45-60 minutes after administration of the fibrinolytic agent. As a result, if one considers a time-line regarding various treatment options and the time to expected full benefit, actual reperfusion may not occur for at least 75-90 minutes in the fibrinolytic-managed patient, assuming a 30-minute door-to-needle time.

In addition to the door-to-balloon time parameter, technical expertise and hospital volume should be considered. In the GUSTO-IIb trial,[48] the majority of partcipating physicians performed at least 75 procedures per year; these results may not generalize to smaller-volume centers with less-experienced operators (i.e., < 50 cases per year). Another study addressed these issues, i.e., hospital volume and physician experience relative to patient outcome in the PCI-managed individual.[63] Primary angioplasty was found to offer a greater chance of positive outcomes in high-volume angioplasty with physicians performing more procedures on a regular basis. Another investigation[64] considered hospital volume in a comparison of fibrinolysis and primary angioplasty in patients with AMI. They found high-volume centers (i.e., performing frequent primary angioplasties) were associated with improved outcomes in the PCI group compared to the fibrinolytic group.[62] Interestingly, lower volume PCI centers demonstrated similar outcomes in the two treatment groups.

Another systems-related issue regarding time-to-arrival in the catheterization laboratory also must be considered. In certain centers, PCI may not be available, necessitating rapid transfer to another facility. Indications for transfer of a patient with AMI to a regional, tertiary care facility with PCI and cardiovascular surgery capabilities include patients with contraindications to fibrinolytic therapy who may benefit from PCI or CABG, persistent hemodynamic instability, persistent ventricular dysrhythmias, or postinfarction or post-reperfusion ischemia. Hospital transfer for primary PCI is required in patients with fibrinolytic agent contraindications. The urgent transfer of a fibrinolytic-eligible AMI patient for primary PCI to another institution is not recommended until fibrinolytic therapy is initiated; the delay in restoring perfusion in such a patient is not acceptable in most instances. If the patient is an acceptable candidate for fibrinolysis, the fibrinolytic agent should be started before or during transport to the receiving hospital.

Prior agreement between the ED and the inpatient physicians at institutions both with and without PCI capability must be obtained so that PCI consideration will not introduce further delays in fibrinolytic drug administration; such cooperation has been shown to limit additional delays in the administration of fibrinolytic agents in patients who are considered for PCI in AMI.[65] If performed without a time delay by experienced hands, PCI appears to produce improved outcomes in the urgent management of AMI. It must be stressed that, while PCI is felt to be superior in the treatment of AMI, it must be initiated within 90-120 minutes of arrival to the hospital ED.[24,66,67]

If the time required to mobilize staff and arrange for PCI is prolonged (i.e., greater than approximately 2 hours to balloon catheter inflation or stenting across the culprit coronary lesion), then fibrinolysis is preferred.[61] Delays beyond this time period are unacceptable if the patient originally was a fibrinolytic candidate. These various time periods are suggestions; individual patient and system issues must be considered in the treatment decisions.

Finally, PCI was associated with a documented clinical success rate with Thrombolysis in Myocardial Infarction (TIMI) II through III flow attained in more than 90% of patients without emergency CABG, stroke, or death; emergency CABG rate less than 5% among all patients undergoing the procedure; and actual performance of angioplasty in a high percentage of patients (85%) brought to the laboratory. Otherwise, the focus of treatment should be the early use of thrombolytic therapy, although the data support utilization of PCI in an "appropriate laboratory setting," of which high-volume centers provide more consistent documentation of benefit.[61]

Non-ST Elevation Acute Coronary Syndromes—Current Management Options

Perhaps one of the most important aspects of managing patients with acute coronary ischemic syndromes is the ability to risk-stratify patients into those imdividuals who will benefit most from either pharmacological or percutaneous strategy-mediated reperfusion. It has been difficult to generate a deterministic patient selection process that will guarantee an optimal outcome for each individual case. Although a number of risk-stratification tools have been suggested by clinical experts and associations, the TIMI risk factor analysis has emerged as one of the most widely accepted approaches for identifying patients who are most likely to benefit from specific strategies.[68]

TIMI Risk Factor Stratification. The following factors are among those included in the TIMI risk-stratification scheme: 1) presence of chest pain; 2) significant elevation of cardiac markers; 3) history of three or more cardiac risk factors (i.e., diabetes, smoking, elevated LDL-cholesterol, etc.); 4) ages 65 or older; 5) known coronary artery disease (CAD), defined as documented 50% or greater stenosis in at least one major coronary artery; 6) prior chronic aspirin intake for CAD prevention; 7) two or more episodes of resting angina during the previous 24 hours prior to presentation; and 8) new ST-segment deviation of 0.5 mm or greater in limb and/or precordial leads.

As the number of risk factors increases from 0/1 to 6/7, the risk of death, MI, or urgent revascularization within 14 days increases from 4.7% to 40.9% in a graded fashion. Many institutions are utilizing the risk score, which is available on-line at clinicaltrialresults.org, in therapeutic decision making for the patient presenting with non-ST elevation acute coronary syndromes.

GP IIb/IIIa Inhibitors. In patients receiving PCI, among the GP IIb/IIIa inhibitors, abciximab has demonstrated consistent benefit. In contrast, neither eptifibatide nor tirofiban significantly decreased ischemic events after PCI in the RESTORE and IMPACT II trials, respectively. Integrilin did significantly decrease ischemic events in ESPRIT.

In the EPIC, EPILOG, and EPISTENT trials, abciximab produced 4.5-6.4% absolute reductions in the 30-day composite end point and these benefits persisted at six months in the EPIC and EPILOG trials (EPISTENT did not assess 6-month outcomes). The benefits also persisted at more extended follow-up. At one-year, patients in the EPILOG trial had a significant reduction of the composite end point from 16.1% in the placebo group to 9.6% in the abciximab groups ($P < 0.001$).[69] At three years, patients in the EPIC trial also had a significant reduction of the composite end point from 47.2% in the placebo group to 41.1% in the abciximab bolus plus infusion group ($P = 0.009$).[70] In the EPISTENT trial, the composite end point of mortality or AMI at one-year was significantly reduced in the stent plus abciximab group (5.3%) compared to the stent plus placebo group (11.0%; $p < 0.001$).[71] EPISTENT demonstrated a significant mortality benefit at one year (2.4% stent vs 1.0% stent plus abciximab).

The CAPTURE trial, which evaluated abciximab and mandatory PCI, found significant benefit at 30 days but not at six months. Various factors may be responsible for the lack of enduring benefits. Patients received abciximab for only one hour after PCI in the CAPTURE trial vs. for 12 hours after PCI in both the EPIC and EPILOG trials. The 12-hour administration period post-procedure may be very important for establishing the long-term (6 months to three years) benefit of abciximab. This difference supports the concept of arterial passivation, in which the agent affects the vessel wall surface so as to inhibit further platelet-thrombin deposition. The significance of the pharmacologic differences between abciximab and the small molecule agents is unclear; however, they might contribute to the potential passivation associated with abciximab.

The prolonged, platelet-bound biologic half-life of abciximab might account for its prolonged effect on platelet function. The longer duration of action may have been the reason for abciximab's success with a 12-hour infusion vs. the 20- to 72-hour infusions used with eptifibatide or tirofiban. The highest risk for thrombotic events after PCI is within 48 hours. The prolonged and tapered effect of abciximab neutralizes platelets while the vessel heals itself, providing "artificial" passivation when the patient's thrombosis risk profile gradually progresses from high-risk to low-risk.[72]

The role of GP IIb/IIIa inhibitors in patients who are not necessarily having a PCI is controversial. It is important to note that the patient populations treated in these trials were very sick. Entry into these trials required either ECG changes or cardiac enzyme or marker elevation. All of the trials (PURSUIT, PRISM, PRISM-Plus, and PARAGON) included patients who did and did not receive PCI and, importantly, the use of PCI was not randomized. Differentiating the outcomes of patients who received only medical therapy vs. those having a PCI is not easy. These groups were not differentiated in the PARAGON trial and no differences were found between the groups in the PURSUIT trial. As noted above, the PURSUIT trial also was interesting because the benefit among geographic locations varied directly with the frequency of catheterizations performed in the locations, supporting the concept that GP IIb/IIIa inhibitors might be optimal in the PCI population.[73-75]

The data on tirofiban from the PRISM and PRISM-PLUS trials are very interesting. Note that these trials were published together in the same journal issue. The PRISM trial noted a significant reduction in the combination of death and AMI at 30-days in those treated only medically with tirofiban (vs only with heparin). There was no difference in these same outcomes in patients who also underwent PCI. Conversely, in the PRISM-PLUS trial, the trial arm that used tirofiban alone was terminated early because of increased mortality. This is the same arm that demonstrated an improved outcome in PRISM. Another problem is that the authors in PRISM-PLUS report, in patients treated only medically, that the tirofiban plus heparin arm resulted in improved mortality and myocardial infarction outcomes compared to the heparin-alone arm. However, the data were not statistically significant because the confidence intervals crossed one. Once again, the data pertaining to those treated only medically were very limited.

The role of abciximab in medically managed patients with UA/NSTEMI also is not clear. The CAPTURE trial, despite having mandated PCI, did start with an 18-24 hour infusion of abciximab before PCI. During this "medical only treatment" phase of the study, the AMI rate was reduced from 2.1% to 0.6% in the abciximab arm. However, the GUSTO-IV-ACS trial of 7800 patients with UA/NSTEMI found that abciximab provided no benefit beyond standard therapy. Patients all received aspirin and heparin and were randomized to placebo or to one of two abciximab infusion regimens. Like the previous trials in this population, this was a very sick population, with all patients having ECG changes or marker elevations. At 30 days, death and myocardial infarction were comparable among groups.

LWMH in NSTEMI. The approach to patients with unstable angina (UA) and NSTEMI continues to undergo refinement. New studies, however, increasingly support a paradigm shift toward enoxaparin to a central role in patients with ACS, whether treated with medical or percutaneous interventions. An institutional analysis from a single center was reported at the American College of Cardiology Scientific Assembly in March 2001. Conducted by investigators at the Royal Infirmary of Edinburgh, the study demonstrated that enoxaparin is superior to UFH in patients with unstable angina (UA)/non-ST-segment elevation myocardial infarction (MI): 7.1% vs. 8.6% ($P = 0.02$) death/MI at 43 days. Decisions to proceed to revascularization were independent of trial randomization.

The group analyzed a population comprising 6098 patients for death or MI at 43 days using chi-squared tests; 983 patients undergoing coronary artery bypass grafting were excluded. Clinicians were blinded to enoxaparin vs. UFH. PCI was not randomized but was performed at the discretion of the treating physician. The authors concluded that patients undergoing PCI (compared with those who were not) sustained more events, including events prior to PCI, which was consistent with a higher risk population. Enoxaparin treatment, when compared with UFH treatment, benefited both patients treated solely medically and those patients who underwent PCI following an initial period of medical stabilization.

Table 1. Drug Dosing Guidelines for ACS

Drug	Dosing
Aspirin	Initial 162.5-325 mg (non-enteric coated) po followed by 81-325 mg po per day
IV nitroglycerin:	Initial dose 5 mg/min IV; increase dose by 5-10 mg/min until relief of ischemic chest pain, or mean arterial pressure decreased by 30% if hypertensive (but never a systolic blood pressure < 90 mm Hg; utilize for approximately 24 hrs
Metoprolol (Lopressor):	5 mg IV q 5 min x 3 followed in 15 min by 25-50 mg po q6 hr x 24 hrs, titrate dose to HR/BP; switch to twice daily or qd (extended-release formulation) regimen prior to hospital discharge
Unfractionated heparin:	60 U/kg IV bolus (maximum 4000 U) followed by 12 U/kg/hr (maximum 1000 U/hr); measure aPTT at 4-6 hrs and titrate dose to aPTT of 50-70 sec (or titration specific range) using a weight-based dosing nomogram.
Enoxaparin (Lovenox):	**Dose for NSTE/ACS:** 1 mg/kg sc q12 hr **Dose for STE/ACS:** 30 mg IV bolus followed immediately by 1 mg/kg sc q12 hr **Dose for PCI in patients with NSTE/ACS:** If last dose administered < 8 hrs, no supplemental enoxaparin (or unfractionated heparin) dose needed; if last dose administered more than 8 hours (and less than 12 hrs), administer 0.3 mg/kg IV bolus Avoid in patients with CrCL < 30 mL/min
Morphine sulfate:	2-4 mg IV bolus; repeat and titrate if necessary for complete pain relied
Alteplase (tPA)*:	15 mg bolus followed by 0.75 mg/kg IV over 30 min (max 50 mg) followed by 0.5 mg/kg (max 35 mg) over 60 min (Max dose = 100 mg)
Reteplase (rPA, Retavase)*:	10 U IV bolus x 2, 30 min apart
Tenecteplase (TNKase)*:	< 60 kg = 30 mg IV bolus 60-69.9 kg = 35 mg IV bolus 70-79.9 kg = 40 mg IV bolus 80-89.9 kg = 45 mg IV bolus ≥90 kg = 50 mg IV bolus
Clopidogrel (Plavix):	Initial dose—300 mg (4, 75 mg tablets) po then 75 mg po qd beginning Day 2; For NSTE/ACS in aspirin intolerant patients, administer 75 or 300 mg as initial dose followed by 75 mg po qd.
Abciximab (ReoPro):	**Dose for PCI and STE/ACS:** 0.25 mg/kg IV bolus followed by 0.125 mg/kg/min, max 10 mg/min x 12 hrs; no dosage adjustment in renal insufficiency; not recommended for medical management of NSTE/ACS
Tirofiban (Aggrastat):	**Dose for PCI:** 10 mg/kg IV bolus over 3 min followed by 0.15 mg/kg/min x 18-24 hrs **Dose for NSTE/ACS:** 0.4mg/kg IV bolus over 30 min followed by 0.1 mg/kg/min x 48-72 hrs Not recommended for STE/ACS; for patients with CrCL < 50 mL/min, decrease maintenance and infusion rates by 50%
Eptifibatide (Integrilin):	**Dose for PCI and NSTE/ACS:** 180 mcg/kg IV bolus, followed by an infusion of 2 mcg/kg/min with a second 180 mcg/kg IV bolus administered 10 min after the first bolus; continued infusion for x 18-48 hrs; Limited data suggests reducing the maintenance infusion to 1 mg/kg/min for patients with SCr 2.0-4.0 mg/dL; Avoid in patients with SCr > 4.0 mg/dL.

*These recommended doses are for full-dose fibronlytic therapy and are not for use with GP IIb/IIIa receptor blocker as initial therapy.

Another investigative cardiology group from Greece reported the results of a trial comparing enoxaparin vs. tinzaparin in the management of unstable coronary artery disease (EVET Study). The researchers noted that LMWHs are rapidly emerging as an alternative form of antithrombotic therapy to the standard UFH. Despite similarities in origin, synthesis, and structure, the LMWHs have different pharmacokinetic and pharmacodynamic characteristics and possibly elicit different efficacies.

The aim of EVET was to compare head-to-head the efficacy of enoxaparin vs. tinzaparin in the management of acute coronary syndromes. In a prospective study, 438 patients with unstable angina or non-Q wave myocardial infarction were randomized to receive either subcutaneous injections of 100 mg/kg enoxaparin twice daily (n = 220) or 175 UI/Kg tinzaparin once daily (n = 218) for seven days. The primary end points were death, myocardial infarction, refractory angina, and recurrence of unstable angina. Secondary end points were rehospitalization due to unstable angina or myocardial infarction, death, and need for revascularization at 30 days.

At seven days, recurrence of unstable angina occurred less frequently in the enoxaparin than in the tinzaparin group (24/220 vs 41/218, P = 0.029). No statistically significant differences were observed between these two groups with respect to death, myocardial infarction, or refractory angina at seven days. At 30 days there were no differences between the two groups regarding rehospitalization and death. The need for revascularization at 30 days was significantly less frequent in the patients assigned to enoxaparin (36/220 vs 57/218, P = 0.019). Bleeding complication rates were similar in the two groups. These investigators concluded that antithrombotic treatment with enoxaparin for seven days was more effective than tinzaparin for reducing the incidence of recurrent angina in patients with unstable angina or non-Q wave myocardial infarction in the early phase. Enoxaparin recipients also had significantly reduced need for revascularisation at 30 days. This benefit was achieved without an increase in bleeding complications.

Invasive vs. Medical Therapy. The syndrome of unstable angina and myocardial infarction without ST-elevation accounts for about 1.4 million hospital admissions annually in the United States. As discussed in previous sections, until recently, therapy has focused primarily on medical management using a combination of antianginal agents, and anti-thrombotic agents, including aspirin and LMWH. The most current studies have attempted to evaluate and compare early invasive and conservative strategies in patients with unstable coronary syndromes treated with GP IIb/IIIa inhibitors such as tirofiban.[76]

This group of investigators (the TACTICS-Thrombolysis in Myocardial Infarction 18 investigators [TACTICS TIMI 18]) enrolled 2220 patients with unstable angina and myocardial infarction without ST-segment elevation who had electrocardiographic evidence of changes in the ST segment or T wave, elevated levels of cardiac markers, a history of coronary artery disease, or all three findings. All patients were treated with aspirin, heparin, and the GP IIb/IIIa inhibitor tirofiban. Patients were randomly assigned to an early invasive strategy, in which routine catherization was performed no later than 48 hours after presentation and revascularization was performed as appropriate, or to a more conservative (selectively invasive) strategy, in which catheterization was performed only if the patient had objective evidence of recurrent ischemia or an abnormal stress test. The primary end point was a composite of death, nonfatal myocardial infarction, and rehospitalization for an acute coronary syndrome at six months.

At six months, the rate of the primary end point was 15.9% with the use of the early invasive strategy and 19.4% with the use of the conservative strategy (OR 0.78; 95% CI, 0.62-0.97; P = 0.025). The rate of death or non-fatal myocardial infarction at six months was similarly reduced (7.3% vs 9.5%; OR, 0.74; 95% CI, 0.54-1.00; P < 0.05). The economic analysis suggested a neutral cost for this added benefit.

The economic analysis from TACTICS TIMI 18 was presented at the AHA 2000 Scientific Assembly. The results were as follows: Mean hospital costs for the invasive arm were $14,660 and $12,667 for the conservative arm, with a difference in groups of $1994 (CI $6888-3329). Mean six-month follow-up costs were $6,063 in the invasive patients and $7203 in the conservative patients; difference -1140 (CI -2165- -50). The primary end point was total costs, which were $629 more in the conservative group with CI of -1273-2465; therefore, the two arms were cost-neutral.[25]

Based on these results, the investigators concluded that in patients with unstable angina and myocardial infarction without ST-segment elevation who were treated with the GP IIb/IIIa inhibitor tirofiban, the use of an early invasive strategy significantly reduced the risk of major cardiac events.

LMWH in PCI. Recent trials also have assessed the safety of enoxaparin in the setting of PCI not associated with ST-segment elevation myocardial infarction. The NICE-3 trial evaluated the incidence of bleeding while performing catheterization in 661 patients with ACS, all of whom received enoxaparin plus a GP IIb/IIIa inhibitor (either abciximab, eptifibatide, or tirofiban).[77] At the time of catheterization, enoxaparin (0.3 mg/kg IV) was administered if it had been more than 8 hours since the last subcutaneous dose. The combination of enoxaparin with different GP IIb/IIIa inhibitors resulted in similar clinical outcomes and bleeding frequency in comparison to those seen in the large GP IIb/IIIa inhibitor trials.[77]

The NICE-4 trial combined enoxaparin with abciximab during PCI. Enoxaparin was given as a 0.75 mg/kg intravenous bolus, while abciximab was administered in its usual fashion. Data from the first 310 patients who received enoxaparin and abciximab revealed that the incidence of major non-CABG bleeding and transfusion in this group was 0.6%, which compared favorably with an incidence of 2.7% occurring in patients receiving abciximab and low-dose heparin in the EPILOG trial.[69] Another group assessed the safety and outcomes in patients with unstable angina or NSTEMI. Of the 451 patients, a non-randomized 293 underwent catheterization within eight hours of the morning enoxaparin injection, which was followed by immediate PCI in 132 patients (28%). The procedures were done without additional heparin or enoxaparin. Major bleeding occurred in 0.8% of those who received catheterization, comparable to the 1.2% in those who were not studied.[78]

In 200 patients receiving elective PCI after three days of aspirin and tirofiban, another group performed a randomized comparison of peri-procedural heparin vs. enoxaparin. Clinical outcomes and major bleeding were comparable between the groups at 30 days.[79] While not a study in the setting of PCI, the pharmacokinetics, pharmacodynamics, and safety of the combination tirofiban with enoxaparin vs. heparin in non-Q wave myocardial infarction was addressed in a 55 patient series. As with most studies, more minor bleeding occurred with the enoxaparin combination, while major bleeding was comparable. The combination of tirofiban and enoxaparin resulted in a more consistent inhibition of platelet aggregation and lower adjusted bleeding time than did the combination with heparin.[36] One study measured anti-Xa levels in patients undergoing angiography with or without PCI using the NICE-3 enoxaparin regimen and found stable levels. This investigation evaluated anti-Xa levels with enoxaparin in patients undergoing coronary angiography with or without PCI. The levels averaged 0.99 + 0.02 IU/mL in patients undergoing coronary angiography (n = 293) and 0.98 + 0.03 IU/mL in PCI patients, demonstrating remarkable reproducibility with little (< 3%) variation in a large population of patients.[88]

The FRISC II trial assessed the role of three months of dalteparin therapy after the use of PCI in patients with unstable angina or NSTEMI or after the use of fibrinolysis in AMI. While the initial randomization compared three months of dalteparin vs. placebo, a second randomization, in a 2-by-2 design, compared the use of early PCI with its more conservative use. At six months, the composite of death or AMI was decreased by early PCI from 12.1% to 9.4% in those with less aggressive use (P = 0.031).[80] Dalteparin decreased adverse coronary events during the three-month administration primarily in patients who received conservative use of PCI. It also was observed that there was no benefit from the three-month dalteparin administration in patients who were in the non-invasive segment of the study.

The Role of Enoxaparin in ACS. The use of enoxaparin in non-STEMI ACS is supported by data from the ESSENCE and TIMI 11B clinical studies.[81,82] In the ESSENCE study, the need for revascularization procedures at 30 days was significantly less frequent with enoxaparin compared with UFH (27.0% compared with 32.2%; P = 0.001). In the TIMI 11B study, urgent revascularisation was required in 10.7% of patients who received enoxaparin and 12.6% of patients who received UFH at 43 days (P = 0.05). The incidence of cardiac and hemorrhagic events in patients undergoing PCI in the ESSENCE and TIMI 11B clinical studies was similar irrespective of the initial type of anticoagulation (enoxaparin or UFH) and the timing of the intervention (PCI on treatment/within 12 hours of the final dose or at any time during initial hospitalization).[81,82]

The ACC/AHA guidelines for unstable angina and NSTEMI present a somewhat mixed message in their prioritization of LMWHs vs. UFH.[83] First, although the document provides figures demonstrating superiority data for enoxaparin in UA and NSTEMI, when issuing recommendations for use of LMWH in ACS, the guidelines lumped all LMWHs together. Specifically, the ACC/AHA guidelines suggest that heparin or a LMWH (in this order) may be used in high-risk patients. However, within the text of the document, they state that a "LMWH can be substituted advantageously" for heparin. The term "advantageously" would seem to reflect superiority data, despite their recommendation that heparin be used over LMWHs.

The guidelines appropriately indicate that it is somewhat difficult to draw conclusions about the relative efficacy of one LMWH vs. the others, and that head-to-head trials are the only conclusive way to settle this issue. However, the ESSENCE and TIMI-11B data, in the defined high-risk populations they studied, both clearly demonstrated superiority of enoxaparin over heparin for the composite end points of death, AMI, and recurrent angina. It has been argued the reason enoxaparin trials demonstrated superiority, as opposed to the FRIC and FRAXIS trials which did not show superiority of other LMWHs over UFH, is because of differences in trial populations and study designs. For example, it is argued that the ESSENCE and TIMI-11B populations were at higher risk than in the other trials and that the magnitude of benefit in randomized trials is generally greater in patients at high risk compared with those at low risk. Patients in these trials were at higher risk because: 1) they had to present within 24 hours of the chest pain episode, while those in FRIC and FRAXIS presented in 72 and 48 hours, respectively; and; 2) the definition of AMI was softer than in FRIC and FRAXIS.

However, patients with chest pain and a history or previous coronary artery disease were included in ESSENCE and TIMI-11B. Many of the patients in these trials did not have elevation of markers or ECG changes. Conversely, patients in the FRIC and FRAXIS trials had to have ECG changes, which could reflect a higher risk group. The point is that while arguments relative to design and population are endless, the data for the high risk population defined in the ESSENCE and TIMI-11B trials clearly reflect enoxaparin superiority as compared to heparin.[25]

Interestingly, in their analysis of the LMWHs, the ACC/AHA guidelines for AMI, state that "enoxaparin for the acute management of patients with unstable angina/non-Q wave MI has been shown to be superior to heparin for reducing death and serious cardiac ischemic events. This superiority is achieved without an increase in the rate of either spontaneous or instrumented major hemorrhage." Consequently, from a practical, clinical perspective, enoxaparin, specifically and uniquely, can and should be substituted "advantageously" for heparin in unstable angina and NSTEMI. Data for substituting other LMWHs "advantageously" for heparin simply do not exist, and it is somewhat curious that this distinction was not emphasized in the "advantageous" designation advocating LMWH substitution for UFH

Despite the evidence-based support of enoxaparin superiority, the ACC/AHA guidelines issues a potential cautionary note concerning use of LMWHs in the setting of PCI because of the theoretical risk of increasing bleeding complications that may be associated with prolonged anticoagulation. The authors of the ACC/AHA document appropriately noted that enoxaparin was stopped 6-12 hours prior to PCI in ESSENCE and TIMI-11B, and therefore, it was difficult to draw conclusions regarding its safety in the PCI patient population.

Publication of the NICE-3 study supported the safety and efficacy of enoxaparin in the setting of PCI. Safety end points included major hemorrhage compared with historical controls, minor bleeding and platelet counts to seven days, efficacy end points included death, myocardial infarction, and urgent revascularization. The combination of enoxaparin and a GP IIb/IIIa antagonist did not result in an excess of non-CABG major bleeding (0.7-3.2% of patients), and clinical outcomes were comparable with those in earlier studies. The NICE-3 study concluded that patients on combination therapy that included enoxaparin and a GP IIb/IIIa antagonist can safely undergo PCI.[83] In the NICE-4 study, an intravenous bolus of enoxaparin 0.75 mg/kg plus abciximab 0.25 mg/kg bolus and 0.125 mg/kg/min infusion for 12 hours was administered during PCI in 826 patients. There was a low incidence of minor and major bleeding and transfusion, and infrequent major cardiac events to 30 days follow-up. Enoxaparin with concomitant abciximab was concluded to provide safe, well-tolerated and effective anticoagulation in PCI. [84]

In summary, the most recent clinical trial data confirm enoxaparin as the LWMH of choice in patients with ACS—and in most cases, as the preferable substitute for UFH. Moreover, they also provide increasing evidence that patients with PCI can be safely and effectively managed using a combination of enoxaparin and a IIb/IIIa antagonist. *(Please See Figures 1-4, in which protocols for managing a spectrum of acute coronary syndromes [UA, NSTEMI, STEMI] are presented.)*

Oral Platelet Antagonists—The Role of Clopidogrel Pretreatment. The Clopidogrel in Unstable Angina to Prevent Recurrent Events (CURE) trial was designed to compare the efficacy and safety of the early and long-term use of clopidogrel plus aspirin with those of aspirin alone in patients with acute coronary syndromes and no ST-segment elevation.[85] In the CURE trial, 12,562 patients who had presented within 24 hours after the onset of symptoms were randomly assigned to receive either clopidogrel (300 mg immediately, followed by 75 mg once daily) or placebo, in addition to aspirin, for 3-12 months.

The first primary outcome (a composite of death from cardiovascular causes, nonfatal myocardial infarction, or stroke) occurred in 9.3% of the patients in the clopidogrel group and 11.4% of the patient in the placebo group (RR with clopidogrel as compared with placebo, 0.80; 95% CI, 0.72-0.90; P < 0.001). The second primary outcome—the first primary outcome or refractory ischemia—occurred in 16.5% of the patients treated with clopidogrel and 18.8% of the patients in the placebo group (RR, 0.86 P < 0.001). The percentage of patients with major bleeding was greater in the clopidogrel group (RR, 1.38), although the percentage of patients with life-threatening bleeding was not greater.[85] Among 2568 patients receiving PCI in the CURE study, pretreatement with clopidogrel also was beneficial in those patients undergoing mechanical revascularization.[86] A clopidogrel loading dose for appropriately selected patients is recommended in the setting of ACS based on a study which demonstrates an onset of effect within two hours compared to greater than six hours without the loading dose.[87]

It should be emphasized that not all patients are appropriate candidates for clopidogrel. Transfusions are increased, and in PCI there was no benefit beyond 30 days. The benefit was limited to recurrent MI reduction only, and there was no concomittant use of GP IIb/IIIa blockers in this trial.

Summary

It is widely accepted that the early restoration of perfusion in the AMI patient limits myocardial damage, preserves left ventricular function, and reduces mortality; such restoration may be accomplished by either administration of a fibrinolytic agent or stent insertion; in the rare case, emergent coronary artery bypass grafting is a third revascularization method.

The rapid application of reperfusion therapy is mandatory in the patient with ST-elevation AMI. Many factors must be considered by both emergency and cardiovascular physicians regarding the early reperfusion treatment decisions when managing the AMI patient. While primary angioplasty may offer improved outcome over fibrinolysis, PTCA must be applied early without prolonged delay. Should catheterization laboratory activation delay either be anticipated or occur, the treating physician must proceed with fibrinolysis if the patient is an appropriate candidate. Prior agreement between the ED and the cardiovascular physicians at institutions with angioplasty capability must be obtained so that consideration of PTCS will not introduce further delays in fibrinolytic drug administration; such cooperation has been shown to limit additional delays in the administration of fibrinolytic agents in patients who are considered for PTCA in AMI.

If applied without time delay in experienced hands, the data suggest that PCI can produce improved outcomes in AMI. It must be stressed, however, that although PCI is felt to be superior in the treatment of AMI, this procedure must be initiated within 90 minutes of patient arrival to the hospital ED.[32] If the time required to mobilize staff and arrange for PTCA is prolonged (i.e., > 90 minutes to balloon catheter inflation across the culprit coronary lesion), then fibrinolysis is the preferred mode of therapy.[33] Delays beyond this time period are unacceptable if the patient originally was considered to be fibrinolytic candidate.

When fibrinolysis is employed, the most recent evidence suggests a therapeutic paradigm shift toward a regimen that combines enoxaparin with full-dose tenecteplase. Compared to a more traditional UFH/tenecteplase combination, the substitution of UFH with enoxaparin produces a relative reduction of 26% in the frequency of ischemic complications of AMI. In light of its ease of administration, predictable anti-thrombin activity, and improved outcomes, a tenecteplase-plus-enoxaparin reperfusion regimen currently must be considered the pharmacological cocktail of choice.

Several issues must be considered by the physician when evaluating the relative desirability of various therapeutic options. First, the literature base for answering questions related to therapeutic options is somewhat heterogeneous in construction (e.g., differing therapies, study sites, outcome measures, etc.). Therefore, making absolute, all-encompassing recommendations is impossible.

The CTAP Panel*

Sarah A. Spinler, Pharm.D., FCCP, CTAP Scientific Panel Co-Chairperson and Co-Moderator, Philadelphia College of Pharmacy, University of the Sciences in Philadelphia; **Gideon Bosker, MD FACEP**, CTAP Scientific Panel Co-Chairperson and Co-Moderator, Yale Universiy School of Medicine; **William J. Brady, MD FACEP**, Department of Emergency Medicine, University of Virginia Health Sciences Center; **Judy Cheng, Pharm.D., BCPS**, Long Island University Clinical Pharmacy, Mount Sinai Medical Center; **Paul P. Dobesh, Pharm.D., BCPS**, Division of Pharmacy Practice St. Louis College of Pharmacy; **Charles L Emerman, MD FACEP**, Department of Emergency Medicine, Cleveland Clinic Foundation; **Kurt Kleinschmidt, MD FACEP**, Department of Emergency Medicine, University of Texas Southwestern Medical School; **Jean Nappi, Pharm.D.**, Department of Pharmacy, Medical University of South Carolina, Columbia, South Carolina; **John Pieper, Pharm.D., FCCP, BCPS**, School of Pharmacy, University of North Carolina; **Ian J Sarembock MB, ChB, MD**, Cardiovascular Division, University of Virginia Health System; **Kathleen A. Stringer, PharmD, FCCP**, School of Pharmacy,University of Colorado Health Sciences Center; **Robert Talbert, Pharm.D., FCCP, BCPS**, Professor and Chair, Clinical Pharmacy Program, University of Texas at Austin; **Gregory Volturo, MD FACEP**, Department of Emergency Medicine, University of Massachusetts Medical School; **Ann Wittkowsky, Pharm.D.**, Department of Pharmacy Practice, University of Washington.

*** CTAP—Current Cardiovascular Therapy And Protocols for Pharmacists and Physicians**

References

1. ASSENT-3. *Lancet* Aug. 28, 2001.
2. Hayes OW. Emergency management of acute myocardial infarction. *Emerg Med Clin North Am* 1998;16:542-563.
3. Mukherjee D, Moliterno D. Achieving tissue-level perfusion in the setting of acute myocardial infarction. *Am J Cardiol* 2000;85: 39C-46C.
4. GISSI-2: A factorial randomised trial of alteplase versus streptokinase and heparin versus no heparin among 12,490 patients with acute myocardial infarction. *Lancet* 1990;336:65.
5. The International Study Group. In-hospital mortality and clinical course of 20,891 patients with suspected acute myocardial infarction randomized between alteplase and streptokinase with or without heparin. *Lancet* 1990;336:71.
6. ISIS-3. A randomised comparison of streptokinase vs tissue plasminogen activator vs anistreplase and or aspirin plus heparin vs aspirin alone among 41,299 cases of suspected acute myocardial infarction. *Lancet* 1992;339:753.
7. The GUSTO Angiographic Investigators. The effects of tissue plasminogen activator, streptokinase, or both on coronary-artery patency, ventricular function, and survival after acute myocardial infarction. *N Engl J Med* 1993;329:1615.
8. The GUSTO-III Investigators. An international, multicenter, randomized comparison of reteplase with alteplase for acute myocardial infarction. *N Engl J Med* 1997;337:1118.
9. Single-bolus tenecteplase compared with front-loaded alteplase in acute myocardial infarction: The ASSENT-2 double-blind randomized trial. *Lancet* 1999;354:716.
11. Fibrinolytic Therapy Trialist's (FTT) Collaborative Group: Indications for fibrinolytic therapy in suspected acute myocardial infarction: Collaborative overview of early mortality and major morbidity results form all randomised trials of more than 1000 patients. *Lancet* 1994;343:311.
12. ISIS-2 (Second International Study of Infarct Survival) Collaborative Group. Randomized trial of intravenous streptokinase, oral aspirin, both, or neither amount 17,187 cases of suspected acute myocardial infarction: ISIS-2. *Lancet* 1988;2:349.
13. Weaver WD for the Myocardial Infarction Triage and Intervention Project Group: Prehospital-initiated vs hospital-initiated fibrinolytic therapy: The Myocardial Infarction Triage and Intervention trial. *JAMA* 1993;270:1211.
14. GISSI-2: A factorial randomised trial of alteplase versus streptokinase and

heparin versus no heparin among 12,490 patients with acute myocardial infarction. *Lancet* 1990;336:65.

15. The International Study Group: In-hospital mortality and clinical course of 20,891 patients with suspected acute myocardial infarction randomized between alteplase and streptokinase with or without heparin. *Lancet* 1990;336:71.
16. ISIS-3: A randomised comparison of streptokinase vs tissue plasminogen activator vs anistreplase and or aspirin plus heparin vs aspirin alone among 41,299 cases of suspected acute myocardial infarction. *Lancet* 1992;339:753.
17. The GUSTO-III Investigators: An international, multicenter, randomized comparison of reteplase with alteplase for acute myocardial infarction. *N Engl J Med* 1997;337:1118.
18. Single-bolus tenecteplasecompared with front-loaded alteplase in acute myocardial infarction: The ASSENT-2 double-blind randomized trial. *Lancet* 1999;354:716.
19. Fibrinolytic Therapy Trialist's (FTT) Collaborative Group: Indications for fibrinolytic therapy in suspected acute myocardial infarction: Collaborative overview of early mortality and major morbidity results form all randomised trials of more than 1000 patients. *Lancet* 1994;343:311.
20. Estudio Multicentrico Estreptoquinas Republicas de America del Sur (EMERAS) Collective Group: Randomised trial of late fibrinolysis in patients with suspected acute myocardial infarction: EMERAS. *Lancet* 1993;342:767.
21. LATE Study Group: Late assessment of fibrinolytic efficacy (LATE) study with alteplase 6-24 hours after onset of acute myocardial infarction. *Lancet* 1993;342:759.
22. Gruppo Italiano per lo Studio della Streptochinasi nell'Infarto Miocardico (GISSI): Effectiveness of intravenous fibrinolytic treatment in acute myocardial infarction. *Lancet* 1986;8478:397.
23. Grines CL, Browne KF, Marco J, et al: A comparison of immediate angioplasty with fibrinolytic therapy for acute myocardial infarction. *N Engl J Med* 1993;328:673.
24. Ryan TJ, Anderson JL, Antman EM, et al. 1999 Update: ACC/AHA guidelines for the management of patients with acute myocardial infarction. *J Am Coll Cardiol* 1999;34:890.
25. Antman EM, Beasley JW, Califf RM, et al. ACC/AHA guidelines for the management of patients with unstable angina and non-ST-segment elevation myocardial infarction. *J Am Coll Cardiol* 2000;36:970-1062.
26. Wilcox RG, von der Lippe G, Olsson CG, et al. For the ASSET Study Group: Trial of tissue plasminogen activator for mortality reduction in acute myocardial infarction: the Anglo-Scandinavian Study of Early Fibrinolysis (ASSET). *Lancet* 1988;2:525.
27. Sgarbossa EB, Pinski SL, Barbagelata A, et al. Electrocardiographic diagnosis of evolving acute myocardial infarction in the presence of left bundle branch block. *N Engl J Med* 1996;334:481.
28. The TIMI-IIIB Investigators: Effects of tissue plasminogen activator and a comparison of early invasive and conservative strategies in unstable angina and non-Q-wave myocardial infarction: Results of the TIMI-IIIB trial. *Circulation* 1994;89:1545.
29. Tenaglia AN, Califf EM, Candela RJ, et al. Fibrinolytic therapy in patients requiring cardiopulmonary resuscitation. *Am J Cardiol* 1991;68:1015.
30. van Campen LCMC, Leeuwen GR, Verheugt FWA. Safety and efficacy of thrombolysis for acute myocardial infarction in patients with prolonged out-of-hospital cardiopulmonary resuscitation. *J Cardiol* 1994;73:953-955.
31. Bottiger BW, Bode C, Kern S, et al. Efficacy and safety of thrombolytic therapy after initially unsuccessful cardiopulmonary resuscitation: A prospective clinical trial. *Lancet* 2001;357:1583-1585.
32. Wallentin L, Delborg DM, Lindahl B, et al. The low molecular weight heparin daleparin as adjuvant therapy in acute myocardial infarction: The ASSENT PLUS study. *Clin Cardiol* 2001;24:12.
33. Kakkar VV, Iyengar SS, et al. Low molecular weight heparin for the treatment of acute myocardial infarction (FAMI): Fragmin (dalteparin) in acute myocardial infarction. *Indian Heart J* 2000;52:533-539.
34. Chamuleau SAJ, de Winter RJ, et al. Low molecular weight heparin as an adjunct to thrombolysis for acute myocardial infarction. The FATIMA study. *Heart* 1998;80:35-39.
35. Ross AM, Molhoek GP, Knudtson ML, et al. A randomized comparison of low-molecular-weight heparin and unfractionated heparin adjunctive to t-PA thrombolysis and aspirin (HART-II) [Abstract]. *Circulation* 2000;102(Suppl 18):II-600.
36. Cohen M. Low molecular weight heparins in the management of unstable angina/non-Q-wave myocardial infarction. *Thrombo Haemosta* 1999;25(Suppl 3):113-121.
37. Antman EM, McCabe CH, Gurfinkel EP, et al. Enoxaparin prevents death and cardiac ischemic events in unstable angina/non-Q-wave myocardial infarction. *Circulation* 1999;100:1593-1601.
38. Wallentin L. Efficacy of low-molecular-weight heparin in acute coronary syndromes. *Am Heart J* 2000;139(2 Part 2):S29-S32.
39. Balen RM, Marra CA, Zed PJ, et al. Cost-effectiveness analysis of enoxaparin versus unfractionated heparin for acute coronary syndromes: A Canadian hospital perspective. *Pharmacoeconomics* 1999;16(5 II):533-542.
40. Mark DB, Cowper PA, Berkowitz SD, et al. Economic assessment of low molecular weight heparin (enoxaparin) versus unfractionated heparin in acute coronary syndrome patients. Results from the ESSENCE randomized trial. *Circulation* 1998;97:1702-1707.
41. Fox KAA, Bosanquet N. Assessing the UK cost implications of the use of low molecular weight heparin in unstable coronary artery disease. *Br J Cardiol* 1998;5:92-105.
42. Detournay B, Huet X, Fagnani F, et al. Economic evaluation of enoxaparin sodium versus heparin in unstable angina. *Pharmacoeconomics* 2000;18:83-89.
43. Kereiakes D, Fry E, Matthai W, et al. Combination enoxaparin and abciximab therapy during percutaneous coronary intervention: "NICE guys finish first". *J Invas Cardiol* 2000;12(Suppl A):1A-5A.
44. Ross A. A randomized comparison of low molecular weight heparin and unfractionated heparin adjunctive to T-PA fibrinolysis and aspirin. 4th Annual Session American College Cardiology Anaheim 2000.
45. ENTIRE Study. Preliminary data reported at European Society of Cardiology, Sept. 2-4, 2001, Stockholm.
46. Grines CL, Browne KF, Marco J, et al. A comparison of immediate angioplasty with fibrinolytic therapy for acute myocardial infarction. *N Engl J Med* 1993;328:673.
47. Zijlstra F, de Boer MJ, Hoorntje JCA, et al. A comparison of immediate coronary angioplasty with intravenous streptokinase in acute myocardial infarction. *N Engl J Med* 1993;328:680.
48. The GUSTO IIb Angioplasty Substudy Investigators: A clinical trial comparing primary coronary angioplasty with tissue plasminogen activator for acute myocardial infarction. *N Engl J Med* 1997;336:1621.
49. Weaver WD, Simes RJ, Betriu A, et al. Comparison of primary coronary angioplasty and intravenous fibrinolytic therapy for acute myocardial infarction: A quantitative review. *JAMA* 1997;278:2093.
50. Suryapranata H, van't Hof AWJ, Hoorntje JCA, et al. Randomized comparison of coronary stenting with balloon angioplasty in selected patients with acute myocardial infarction. *Circulation* 1998;97:2502.
51. Schomig, A, Kastrati, A, et al. Coronary stenting plus platelet glycoprotein

GP IIb/IIIa blockade compared with tissue plasminogen activator in acute myocardial infarction. *N Engl J Med* 2000;343:10.

52. Brener SJ, Barr LA, Burchenal JE, et al. Randomized, placebo-controlled trial of platelet glycoprotein GP IIb/IIIa blockade with primary angioplasty for acute myocardial infarction. ReoPro and Primary PTCA Organization and Randomized Trial (RAPPORT) Investigators. *Circulation* 1998;98:734.
53. Montalescot G, Barragan P, Beauregard P, et al. Abciximab associated with primary angioplasty and stenting in acute myocardial infarction: The ADMIRAL study, 30 day final results. *Circulation* 1999;100:I-87.
55. Ohman EM, Kleiman NS, Gacioch G, et al. Combined accelerated tissue-plasminogen activator and platelet glycoprotein GP IIb/IIIa integrin receptor blockade with Integrilin in acute myocardial infarction. Results of a randomized, placebo-controlled, dose-ranging trial. IMPACT-AMI Investigators. *Circulation*. 1997;95:846.
56. Anonymous. Combining fibrinolysis with the platelet glycoprotein GP IIb/IIIa inhibitor lamifiban: Results of the Platelet Aggregation Receptor Antagonist Dose Investigation and Reperfusion Gain in Myocardial Infarction (PARADIGM) trial. *J Am Coll Cardiol* 1998;32:2003-2010.
57. Ross AM, Coyne KS, Reiner JS, et al. A randomized trial comparing primary angioplasty with a strategy of short-acting fibrinolysis and immediate planned rescue angioplasty in acute myocardial infarction: the PACT trial. *J Am Coll Cardiol* 1999;34:1954.
58. Califf RM, Topol EJ, Stack RS, et al. Evaluation of combination fibrinolytic therapy and timing of cardiac catheterization in acute myocardial infarction: results of fibrinolysis and angioplasty in myocardial infarction phase 5 randomized trial. *Circulation* 1991;83:1543.
59. Goldberg RJ, Gore JM, Alpert JS, et al. Cardiogenic shock after acute myocardial infarction: Incidence and mortality from a community-wide perspective, 1975 to 1988. *N Engl J Med* 1991;325:1117.
60. Hochman JS, Sleeper LA, Webb JG, et al. Early revascularization in acute myocardial infarction complicated by cardiogenic shock. *N Engl J Med* 1999;341:625.
61. Cannon CP, Gibson CM, Lambrew CT, et al. Relationship of symptom-onset-to-balloon time and door-to-balloon time with mortality in patients undergoing angioplasty for acute myocardial infarction. [see comments]. *JAMA* 2000;283:2941-2947.
62. Canto JG, Every NR, Magid DJ, et al. The volume of primary angioplasty procedures and survival after acute myocardial infarction. National Registry of Myocardial Infarction 2 Investigators. [see comments]. *N Engl J Med* 2000;342:1573-1580.
63. Reference #1 JAMA 2000
64. Reference #2 JAMA 2000
65. Brady WJ, Esterowitz D, Syverud S. Consideration of primary angioplasty in AMI: Effect on door-to-drug time in fibrinolytic candidates. *Am J Emerg Med* 2001;19:15-18.
66. Cannon CP, et al. JAMA 2000.
67. Ryan TJ, Anderson JL, Antman EM, et al. ACC/AHA: ACC/AHA guidelines for the management of patients with acute myocardial infarction: Executive summary. *Circulation* 1996;94:2341.
68. Antman EM, Cohen M, Bernink PJLM, et al. The TIMI Risk Score for unstable angina/non-ST elevation MI, a method for prognostication and therapeutic decision-making. *JAMA* 2000;284:835-842.
69. Lincoff AM, Tcheng JE, Califf RM, et al. Sustained suppression of ischemic complications of coronary intervention by platelet GP GP IIb/IIIa blockade with abciximab: One year outcome in the EPILOG trial. *Circulation* 1999;99:1951-1958.
70. Topol EJ, Ferguson JJ, Weisman HF, et al. Long-term protection from myocardial ischemic events in a randomized trial of brief integrin beta3 blockade with percutaneous coronary intervention. *JAMA* 1997;278:479-484.
71. Topol EJ, Mark DB, Lincoff AM, et al. Outcomes at 1 year and economic implications of platelet glycoprotein GP IIb/IIIa blockade in patients undergoing coronary stenting: results from a multicentre randomized trial. *Lancet* 1999;354:2019-2024.
73. The PARAGON Investigators. International, randomized, controlled trial of lamifiban (A platelet glycoprotein IIb/IIIa inhibitor), Heparin, or both in unstable angina. *Circulation* 1998;97: 2386-2395.
74. PRISM-PLUS Study Investigators. Inhibition of the platelet glycoprotein IIb/IIIa receptor with tirofiban in unstable angina and Non-Q-Wave myocardial Infarction. *N Engl J Med* 1998;338: 1488-1497.
75. PRISM Study Investigators. A Comparison of aspirin plus tirofiban with aspirin plus heparin for unstable angina. *N Engl J Med* 1998; 338:1498-1505.
76. Cannon C, Weintraub W, Demoupoulos L, et. al. Comparison of early invasive and conservative strategies in patients with unstable coronary syndromes treated with glycoprotein IIb/IIIa inhibitors tirofiban. *N Engl J Med* 2001;344:1879-1887.
77. Ferguson JJ. NICE-3 prospective, open label, non-randomized observational safety study on the combination of LMW heparin with the clinically available GP IIb/IIIa antagonists in 600 patients with acute coronary syndromes. *Eur Heart J* 2000;21:599.
78. Collet JP, Montalscot G, Lison L, et al. Percutaneous coronary intervention in unstable angina patients pretreated with subcutaneous enoxaparin. *Eur Heart J* 2000;21:599.
79. Dudek D, Zymek P, Bartus S, et al. Prospective randomized comparison of enoxaparin versus unfractionated heparin for elective percutaneous coronary interventions among ticlopidine-pretreated patients. *Eur Heart J* 2000;21:381.
80. FRISC II Investigators. Invasive compared with non-invasive treatment in unstable coronary-artery disease: FRISC-II prospective randomized multicentre study. *Lancet* 1999;354:708-715.
81. Cohen M, Demers C, Gurfinkel EP, et al. A comparison of low-molecular-weight heparin with unfractionated heparin for unstable coronary artery disease. *N Engl J Med* 1997;337:447-452.
82. Antman EM, McCabe CH, Gurkinkel EP, et al. Enoxaparin prevents death and cardiac ischaemic events in unstable angina/non-Q-wave myocardial infarction. Results of the thrombolysis in myocardial infarction (TIMI) 11B trial. *Circulation* 1999;100:1593-1601.
83. Fergusson JJ, Antman EM, Bates ER, et al. The use of enoxaparin and GP IIb/IIIa antagonists in acute coronary syndromes, including PCI: Final results of the NICE 3 study. *J Am Coll Cardiol* 2001;37(2 Suppl A):365A.
84. Kereiakes DJ, Grines C, Fry E, et al. Enoxaparin and abciximab adjunctive pharmacotherapy during percutaneous coronary intervention. *J Invasive Cardiol* 2001;13:272-278.
85. The Clopidogrel in Unstable Angina To Prevent Recurrent Events Trial Investigators. Effects of Clopidogrel in addition to aspirin in patients with acute coronary syndromes without ST-segment elevation. *N Engl J Med* 2001;345:494-502.
86. Mehta S, Yusuf S, Peters R, et al. Effects of pretreatment with clopidogrel and aspirin followed by long-term therapy in patients undergoing percutaneous coronary intervention: The PCI-CURE study. *Lancet* 2001;358:527-533.
87. Helft G, Osende JI, Worthley SG, et al. Acute antithrombotic effect of a front-loaded regimen of clopidogrel in patients with atherosclerosis

on aspirin. *Arterioscler Thromb Vasc Biol* 2000;20:2316-21.

88. Collet JPh, Motalescot G, Lison L, et al. Percutaneous coronary intervention after subcutaneous enoxaparin pretreatment in patients with unstable angina pectoris. *Circulation* 2001;103:658-662.

Acute Coronary Syndromes: Clinical Pathophysiology

Kurt Kleinschmidt, MD, FACEP

Perhaps no aspect of emergency medicine is evolving more rapidly than the pharmacological and procedural landscape devoted to the management of patients with acute coronary syndromes (ACS). As every emergency physician and cardiologist understands, making the right choice—whether it is drug therapy, a procedural coronary intervention (PCI), or some combination of both strategies—can make the difference between a favorable and an unfavorable outcome.

From an acute, clinical perspective, the challenge of formulating a management action plan that predictably yields optimal outcomes is compromised because there are many classes of agents (antiplatelet drugs, glycoprotein [GP] IIb/IIIa inhibitors, low molecular weight heparins [LMWHs], fibrinolytics), and many individual agents within those classes. More often than not, the trials evaluating the efficacy of specific pharmacotherapeutic interventions are difficult to compare, and the number of head-to-head studies contrasting the risks and benefits of individual agents within a class are almost nonexistent.

Complicating application of the trial data, some drugs may be more or less beneficial for a patient with ACS depending on whether a PCI is likely to be part of the treatment plan.

The multiplicity of interpretations regarding clinical trials, the variations among institutional protocols, proficiency or propensity for performing PCI, and personal preferences among physicians have produced a less-than-consistent approach to managing PCI patients. What's more, even consensus guidelines, such as those recently issued by the American Heart Association and American College of Cardiology for Unstable Angina/Non-ST Elevation Myocardial Infarction (UA/NSTEMI), provide a range of options that are amenable to interpretation and drug substitutions.

Despite these limitations, evidentiary trials continue to support an aggressive approach to managing patients with ACS—an approach that is multi-modal, algorithmic, and risk-stratification driven, and that typically requires sequential administration of such agents as aspirin, beta-blockers, enoxaparin (or UFH), GP IIb/IIIa inhibitors, and/or fibrinolytic therapy. When PCI intervention is contemplated, the pharmacological cocktail for ACS may be modified as required, depending on whether a specific drug has demonstrated safety and efficacy in this setting. Outcome-effective management of patients with acute coronary ischemia requires prompt and accurate risk-stratification, followed by a benefit-maximizing, risk-reducing combination of pharmacological and procedural interventions.

With these issues in clear focus, the purpose of this landmark review of ACS is to present a set of evidence-based guidelines and recommendations that emergency physicians and cardiologists can use to establish critical pathways for their institutions. Given the multiplicity of options and the profusion of recent literature on this subject, objectives of this three-part series include establishing an evidentiary infrastructure, presenting trial-based pathways, and providing an analysis base that can bring emergency physicians and their cardiology colleagues together on how best to manage life-threatening disorders characterized by acute coronary ischemia. To translate data and information into the world of practical, day-to-day

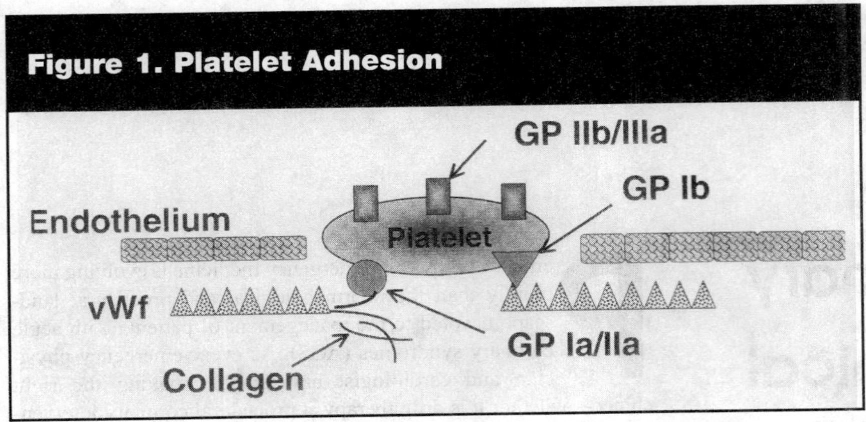

clinical application, an evidence-based critical pathway for ACS has been generated for reader, academic, and institutional use.

Definition

Ischemic heart disease encompasses a wide spectrum of conditions, ranging from silent ischemia to acute myocardial infarction (AMI). Coronary ischemic syndromes have been classified into distinct diagnostic categories, including stable angina, unstable angina (UA), non-Q wave myocardial infarction (MI), and Q wave MI. Not surprisingly, the terminology for these conditions has evolved as new studies have shed light on the pathophysiology and natural history of these conditions.

On Sept. 8, 2000, The American College of Cardiology and American Heart Association (ACC/AHA) issued their Year 2000 ACC/AHA Guidelines for the Management of Patients with Unstable Angina and Non-ST-Segment Elevation Myocardial Infarction. The guidelines have replaced the commonly used category, non-Q wave MI, with the clinical designation, Non-ST-segment Elevation Myocardial Infarction (NSTEMI). This change in terminology reflects the fact that among patients with MI, the presence or absence of ST-segment elevation does not always correlate with Q wave or non-Q wave MI, respectively. In other words, not all patients with ST-segment elevation develop Q waves, whereas some patients without ST-segment elevation on presentation eventually do develop Q waves.

From a practical perspective, this terminology also reflects that initial management of a patient with an ACS is based on the presence or absence of ST-segment elevation. While this review uses the new terminology, it must be recognized that most of the literature uses the term Q wave. UA includes many subtypes, including angina at rest, new-onset exertional angina, recent acceleration of angina, variant angina, and post-MI angina.[1] The term acute coronary syndrome (ACS) refers to conditions that share similar pathophysiology. These include UA, NSTEMI, and ST-segment elevation MI (STEMI).[1,2]

Epidemiology

Coronary artery disease (CAD) is present in more than 7 million Americans and is the cause of more than 500,000 deaths annually.[2] More than 1 million Americans have an AMI annually, and approximately 25% of all deaths are due to AMI.[2] In 1996 there were 750,000 admissions for AMI, approximately one-half of which had ST-segment elevation and one-half of which did not.[1,2]

UA is one of the leading causes of hospital admission for patients with CAD, with more than 1 million hospitalizations annually in the United States.[2,3] First year, direct medical costs associated with UA and AMI have been estimated at more than $12,000 per patient, which translates to an estimated national expenditure exceeding $16 billion.[3] Among patients with UA who receive treatment, about 1-5% die and 2-10% experience an AMI within the first 28 days after hospital admission.[4]

Clinical Pathophysiology

Our understanding of the underlying lesions, pathophysiology, and natural history of ACS has evolved considerably during the past 25 years. It was hypothesized in the 1970s and early 1980s that the degree of vessel stenosis affected the frequency of ACS. However, it was later noted that the extent of luminal narrowing and severity of coronary stenonsis on angiography did not consistently correlate with the risk of thrombotic complications or the location of subsequent coronary artery occlusions.[5]

By the late 1980s, the concept of vulnerable atherosclerotic plaque had evolved, and it was observed that the presence of vulnerable lesions, some of which were associated with only minimal occlusion of the vessel, correlated with the development of ACS.[5] Subsequently, intravascular ultrasound techniques have revealed that arteries accommodate plaque growth through outward displacement of the vessel wall, thereby preserving much of the patency of the vessel lumen. Most MIs result from coronary artery occlusions associated with a degree of stenoses of less than 50% on angiography.[5] The unpredictable and episodic progression of plaques likely results from plaque disruption and subsequent thromboses, causing changes in plaque geometry and growth and intermittent ACS events.[1]

The natural history of ACS confirms that the pathogenesis of ischemic cardiovascular conditions is a complex process that is neither linear nor predictable. However, characteristic, pathologic phases that occur as part of the natural history of ACS include plaque formation (atherogenesis), plaque disruption (rupture or fissuring) or endothelial erosion, and thrombosis following plaque disruption. Inflammation contributes to the pathogenesis of ACS, as suggested by the fact that excised plaques from culprit lesions in UA patients have more inflammatory cell infiltration than do plaques from patients with stable angina.[6]

Atherogenesis. Atherogenesis frequently is initiated by endothelial cell changes, which may result from enhanced expression of adhesion molecules in intact cells. Factors that may initiate these changes include hypercholesteremia and certain constituents of cigarette smoke. It is postulated that endothelial cell changes permit blood monocytes to adhere to the altered endothelium and then enter the subendothelium. There, low-density lipoproteins (LDL-cholesterol) undergo oxidation, collect within the extracellular space, and bind to the macrophage receptors. This is the precursor phase to LDL sequestration by macrophages, which accumulate the LDLs (a process that results in the formation of foam cells).

Foam-laden macrophages and endothelial cells then secrete growth factors, resulting in smooth muscle cell proliferation. Subendothelial lipids eventually coalesce and form the lipid core of growing atherosclerotic plaques. Additional toxic products (among them, free radicals released by macrophages) produce local cell injury and denuding of endothelium. Platelets adhere to endothelial cell injury sites and release additional growth factors that result in more proliferation of intimal smooth muscle cells, promoting plaque growth. Smooth muscle cells also stimulate development of an extracellular matrix through collagen formation. This matrix consists of a fibrous cap that becomes an interface between the lipid core and the endothelium.

Upon analysis of excised plaques, angiographically-demonstrated lesions may consist primarily of smooth muscle proliferation. However, many plaques also have a thrombus incorporated within their matrix. It is postulated that thrombi are a potent stimulus for smooth muscle cell proliferation, as are cytokines or growth factors released from inflammatory cells. Other stimuli, including such infectious agents as *Chlamydia pneumoniae* and cytomegalovirus also have been identified as precipitants of atherogenesis.[6]

Plaque accretion and instability can result from disruptions to its various components. For example, a minor disruption might produce a small thrombus that becomes organized and may eventually lyse or, alternatively, be replaced by the vascular repair response. It should be emphasized that vascular repair can produce rapid plaque growth.[1,5] In this regard, serial angiograms performed before and after an episode of UA, without an intervening coronary intervention, have shown progression of CAD in about 75% of patients.[6]

Figure 2. Affectors of Platelet Aggregation

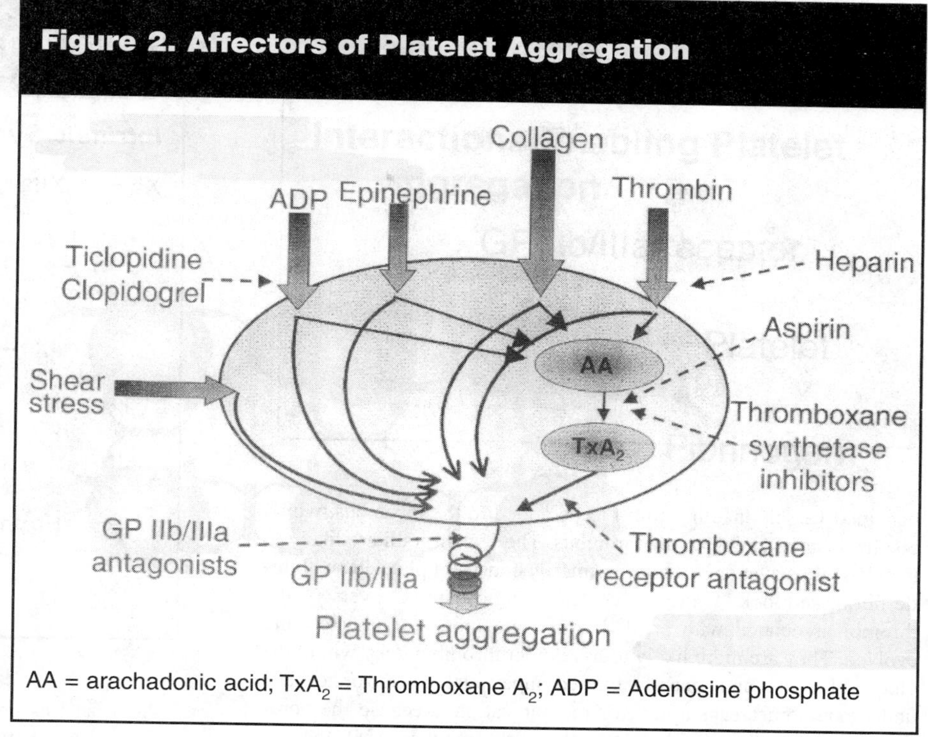

AA = arachadonic acid; TxA_2 = Thromboxane A_2; ADP = Adenosine phosphate

Atherosclerotic plaques may be stable or vulnerable (i.e., prone to rupture). Vulnerable plaques often have a thin fibrous cap, a large lipid core, soft cholesterol ester lipids (rather than free cholesterol monohydrate), and an inflammatory cell infiltrate.[5,7] The arterial lumen may be well preserved at the site of a vulnerable plaque. Cap thickness results from the balance between new collagen production by smooth muscle cells and degradation secondary to inflammatory activity of macrophages.

Plaque Disruption. A number of mechanisms may cause plaque disruption. Plaques rich in extracellular matrix and smooth muscle cells may not necessarily be vulnerable or lipid rich, but they may, nevertheless, simply erode over time.[1] Passive or active forces may disrupt vulnerable plaques. Propensity to rupture depends on circumferential wall stress or cap "fatigue"; location, size, and consistency of the atheromatous core; and blood flow characteristics, especially the effect of flow on the proximal aspect of the plaques (i.e., configuration and angulation of the plaque).[1]

Passive physical forces typically cause disruption at the shoulder of the plaque, between the plaque and the adjacent vessel wall. The cap is weakest at the shoulder because it is thinner and more infiltrated with foam cells. Disruption may be triggered by myriad events, such as emotional stress or physical activity. A surge in sympathetic activity, with an increase in blood pressure, heart rate, force of cardiac contraction, and coronary blood flow, may lead to plaque disruption.[1] Vasospasm due to any cause may compress a plaque, causing rupture. Macrophages may induce active disruption. They degrade extracellular matrix by phagocytosis, and they secrete proteolytic enzymes such as plasminogen activators and matrix metalloproteinases (collagenases, gelatinases, and stromelysins) that may weaken the fibrous cap, predisposing it to rupture.[1]

Thrombosis. Initiated by plaque disruption or injury, thrombosis is a complicated process mediated by thrombin and platelets. The size of the thrombosis, and therefore, the degree of occlusion and clinical outcome, are affected by many factors. Thrombosis size is decreased by minor plaque disruption, high vessel blood flow, and increased fibrinolytic activity. Thrombosis is enhanced by larger plaque disruptions, low blood flow, hypercoagulable (such as increased fibrinogen) or hypofibrinolytic states, and increased platelet reactivity.[1,5,7] Thrombi may be labile, resulting in recurrent episodes of occlusion. Thrombosis may be intramural alone or may occlude the arterial lumen to varying extents.

After a plaque is disrupted, platelets adhere to denuded endothelium and form a monolayer. Platelets adhere via their GP Ia/IIa receptors binding to subendothelial collagen and their GP Ib receptors binding to the von Willebrand factor. *(Please see Figure 1.)* The process of adhesion and thrombin formation both activate the adhered platelets, resulting in the secretion of adenosine diphosphate (ADP), thromboxane A2, and serotonin. These mediators, along with local shear forces, attract and activate other platelets.[1] *(Please See Figure 2.)* Platelet activation includes activation of their GP IIb/IIIa receptors, one of the most densely expressed receptors known. Platelet activation results in a conformational change of the GP IIb/IIIa receptors, increasing their affinity for fibrinogen. Once adjacent platelets have activated GP IIb/IIIa receptors, fibrinogen can bridge between the platelets, and aggregation occurs. *(Please see Figure 3)* This is the "final common pathway" for platelet aggregation, resulting in a platelet plug at the subendothelial disruption site.

In addition to the aforementioned platelet-related events, plaque disruption also results in the release of tissue factor from foam cells, activating factor VII and the extrinsic coagulation pathway. *(Please see Figure 4.)* Activation of the extrinsic coagulation pathway results in the production of thrombin and fibrin, which stabilize the platelet plug. Activated factor VII and tissue factor combine to also activate factor IX within the intrinsic pathway, initiating further production of thrombin and fibrin. *(Please see Figure 4.)* In addition to converting fibrinogen to fibrin, thrombin also amplifies the coagulation cascade by activating factors V and VIII and is a powerful platelet agonist.[8]

Coronary artery thrombi vary both in content and location within the vessel and can be described in many ways, including being mural, occlusive, platelet-rich, fibrin-rich, organized, multi-layered, or re-endothelialized.[7] The differences in thrombi content may explain why fibrinolytic drugs benefit patients with MI but fail those with UA. Thrombus formation results in decreased blood flow through the

Figure 3. Interactions Enabling Platelet Aggregation

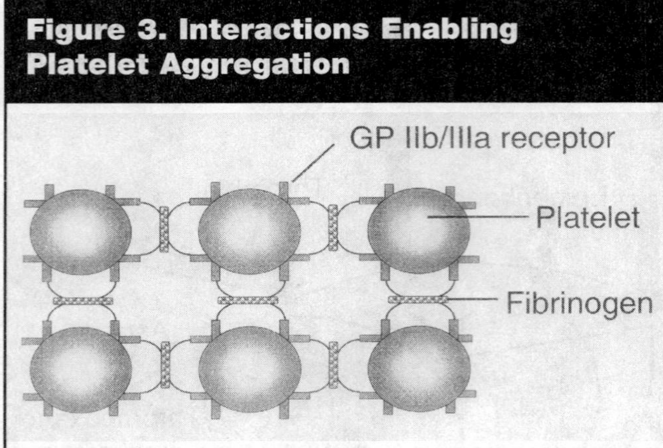

Figure 4. The Coagulation Cascade

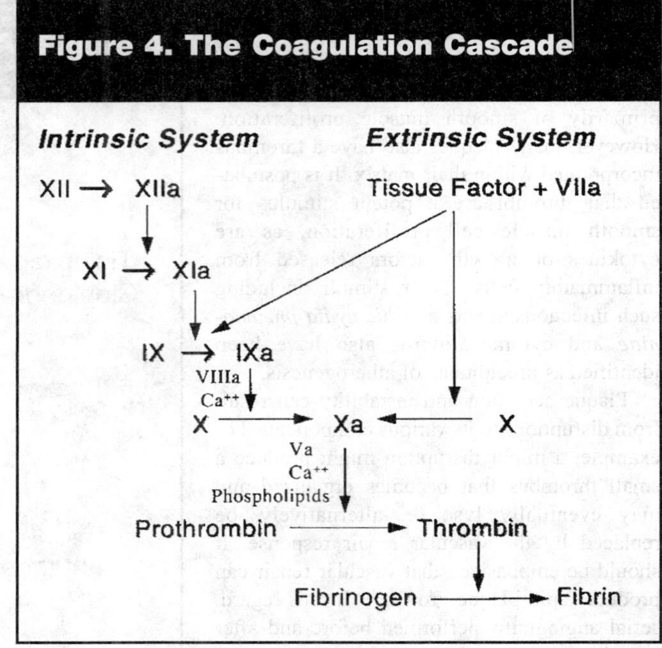

occluded vessel, enabling fibrin to be added to the thrombus, which results in stabilization of the thrombus. The UA thrombi are likely to be relatively newer and smaller; primarily consist of platelets, with little fibrin; and look "white" on coronary angioscopy. Conversely, the thrombi associated with an AMI often are more complicated and evolved. They are more likely to have older thrombin deep within the clot, with loose and recently formed superficial layers, or to have undergone some reabsorption or reorganization. Because the coronary artery usually is occluded totally by thrombus in AMI, there is significant stasis of blood flow.

This stasis permits fibrin and red blood cells to become superimposed on the original platelet-rich thrombus. On angioscopy, the thrombi of AMI appear red because of the trapped red cells and fibrin.[6] Fibrinolytic agents target fibrin within the thrombus. The varied complexity and content of the thrombi associated with AMI likely reflects why normal (TIMI grade III) blood flow is achieved in only 50-60% of patients who receive fibrinolytics.[7] Within a thrombus is a catalytically active thrombin called clot-bound thrombin, which is likely of great importance. Thrombolysis re-exposes "clot-bound thrombin" to the circulation, reinitiating thrombosis by activating both platelets and thrombin. This process may contribute significantly to the vessel reocclusion that occurs after thrombolysis.

Clinical Presentation

Pathogenesis of CAD is linked to progression of atherosclerosis and, more specifically, to factors precipitating plaque disruption and subsequent thrombosis formation. Symptoms of ischemia, on the other hand, reflect an imbalance between myocardial blood (oxygen) supply and oxygen demand. Accordingly, ischemic coronary pain at rest can result from transient decreases in oxygen supply secondary to 1) thrombus formation; 2) embolization; or 3) transient increases in vasomotor tone producing diminished blood flow to the myocardium.

As principal mediators of ACS, activated platelets release several vasoactive substances that, in the presence of endothelial dysfunction (impaired vasodilation), can result in vasoconstriction near the lesion and a transient decrease in blood flow. Patient symptoms depend on many factors, including the degree of occlusion and the presence of collateral circulation. Plaque disruption, accompanied by isolated mural thrombosis formation, but without clinical symptoms, may be more common than once suspected. Patients with stable CAD may have angina or silent ischemia that results from increases in myocardial oxygen demand that outstrip the ability of a stenosed coronary artery to deliver the required oxygen load.

ACS patients present with variable symptomatology somewhere on the disease continuum that typically results from an abrupt reduction in coronary artery flow secondary to acute thrombosis. UA patients may have small erosions or fissuring on the plaques with small changes in plaque structure or small thromboses. Arterial occlusions, and accordingly, patient symptoms, may be transient if the thrombi are labile. NSTEMI may result from more severe plaque damage and a more persistent thrombotic occlusion. Patients with NSTEMI likely have high rates of spontaneous reperfusion as reflected by the fact that only 25% of this subgroup have complete coronary occlusions on early angiography. STEMI, with transmural necrosis of the involved myocardium, may be attenuated by spontaneous thrombolysis, resolution of vasoconstriction, or the presence of collateral circulation. Acute STEMI most likely results from larger plaque fissures and the formation of fixed and persistent thrombi.[1]

Acute Management

Overview. The goals of acute management of ACS are to relieve symptoms; prevent progression of the disease to AMI; minimize loss of myocardial muscle and function; reduce mortality; and treat specific complications of ischemia, such as dysrhythmias or pulmonary edema. Acute pharmacotherapeutic interventions aimed at minimizing or aborting pathogenic processes producing ischemic coronary events usually will require a multi-modal, "cocktail" approach—a polypharmacy strategy that addresses the complex pathogenesis of ACS. Accordingly, multiple agents will be required, each reflecting activity against a distinct precipitant of plaque disruption, thrombosis formation, or coronary vasoconstriction. This will include agents directed at thrombin generation, platelet aggregation, fibrin deposition, and inflammation.

Aspirin, heparin, and increasingly, LMWHs such as enoxaparin, routinely are used in the treatment of these syndromes. The need to target multiple pathogenic end points has stimulated the development of new antithrombotic drugs. Several new agents have been evaluated, particularly for the treatment of ACS. *(Please see Table 1)* Many trials have been conducted to evaluate these agents, used as monotherapy and in combination. Unfortunately, sorting out these trials and their implications for clinical practice has been difficult because the trial names lead to an "alphabet soup" of confusion, and they have reported on different patient groups evaluated with different protocols. *(Please see Table 2.)* The relationships of some of these trials relative to different treatment modalities are summarized in Figure 5.

Antiplatelet Therapy

Overview. Platelet activation and aggregation involve multiple steps, each of which is a potential target for pharmacotherapeutic inhibition. Another goal of therapy is "passivation," which refers to the conversion of platelets that are already activated, highly reactive, and thrombogenic—to a non-reactive, non-thrombogenic state. Passivation occurs in approximately eight hours in a normal artery; however, an artery with atherosclerotic disease may require days or longer.[7] Aspirin has been the primary antiplatelet agent used in ACS. Other antiplatelet agents include inhibitors of GP IIb/IIIa receptors, ADP, and thromboxane synthetase.

Aspirin. Aspirin is the mainstay of ACS therapy. No other antiplatelet agent has a more impressive risk-benefit ratio and costs so little. Aspirin acts rapidly, achieving platelet inhibition within one hour. Aspirin dosages have varied among clinical trials, with 81-325 mg being the usual range. Clinicians should avoid enteric-coated aspirin in the setting of ACS because its onset of action is delayed 3-4 hours. Aspirin permanently inactivates the platelet enzyme cyclooxygenase for the eight- to 10-day life of the platelet. This results in decreased production of thromboxane A2, which is pro-aggregatory and causes vasoconstriction. However, by blocking thromboxane A2 production at the cyclooxygenase level, prostacyclin (a vasodilator, platelet inhibitor, and protector of gastrointestinal mucosa integrity) synthesis also is inhibited.

The importance of platelet inhibition in MI was confirmed in ISIS-2, in which aspirin produced a 23% reduction in mortality and reduced the rate of hospital reinfarction from 2.9% to 1.9%.[9] Other trials also have demonstrated that aspirin decreases death and MI following UA by 31-50%.[10-12] In patients at high risk for atherosclerotic disease, regular aspirin use reduces eventual nonfatal MI by 30%, nonfatal stroke by 30%, and vascular deaths by 17%.[13]

Despite its great benefits, aspirin has its limitations. It is a weak antiplatelet agent and does not inhibit platelet aggregation caused by thromboxane A2-independent pathways (e.g., via ADP or collagen stimulation). Aspirin has no effect on thrombin, which likely plays a major role in platelet activation in acute ischemic syndromes. Aspirin also does not inhibit platelet adhesion or suppress platelet secretion of thrombogenic mediators. In addition, there are individual differences in patient response. Finally, aspirin, like most antiplatelet agents, increases the risk of bleeding complications.

Thromboxane Synthetase Inhibitors. Ridogrel selectively inhibits thromboxane synthetase, thereby limiting thromboxane production without affecting prostacyclin. Since inhibition of prostacylin synthesis has the potential to promote thrombogenesis, these more selective agents should, in theory, be more effective than aspirin. The effectiveness of ridogrel and aspirin for ACS were compared in the Ridogrel vs. Aspirin Patency Trial (RAPT).[14] All patients received streptokinase. The primary end point was arterial patency between seven and 14 days and secondary end points were clinical markers of reperfusion and safety. No differences in efficacy or safety were observed.[14]

Adenosine Diphosphate Inhibitors. ADP is secreted by activated platelets and stimulates additional platelet activation and aggregation via the platelet P2T cell surface receptor. Ticlopidine (Ticlid) and clopidogrel (Plavix) are structurally similar to P2T antagonists. These agents selectively and irreversibly inhibit ADP binding to the P2T cell surface receptor, stopping platelet activation via this route. However, they also interfere with a specific ADP-dependent step of GP IIb/IIIa complex activation, resulting in less platelet aggregation and, ultimately, less thrombus formation.[4] As a result, these agents provide broader inhibition of platelet aggregation than aspirin because they not only limit ADP-receptor stimulated aggregation but also aggregation triggered by a number of other stimuli. However, they are similar to aspirin in that their effect on platelet aggregation is incomplete and aggregation still occurs.[4]

The first ADP antagonist introduced, ticlopidine, has been shown to be better than placebo for reducing the risk of stroke, AMI, and vascular death in patients with atherosclerotic disease.[13] It is comparable to aspirin for reducing risk of stroke, MI, and vascular death.[13]

The Clopidogrel vs. Aspirin in Patients at Risk of Ischemic Events (CAPRIE) trial involved 19,185 patients in a randomized, double-blinded assessment of safety and efficacy.[15] Patients with ischemic stroke, AMI, or symptomatic atherosclerotic peripheral arterial disease were randomly assigned to receive aspirin or clopidogrel for 1-3 years. The combined end point of ischemic stroke, AMI, or vascular death occurred in 5.3% of the clopidogrel patients and in 5.8% of aspirin-treated cohort, a relative risk reduction of 8.7% ($P = 0.043$) in favor of the clopidogrel group.

Table 1. Antithrombin and Antiplatelet Agents

ANTITHROMBIN AGENTS

- AT III dependent
  - Heparin
  - LMWH
    - Dalteparin (Fragmin)
    - Enoxaparin (Lovenox)
    - Nadroparin (Fraxiparine)
- AT III independent
  - Hirudin
  - Hirulog

ANTIPLATELET AGENTS

- Cyclooxygenase inhibitor
  - Aspirin
- GP IIb/IIIa inhibitors
  - Abciximab (Reopro)
  - Eptifabitide (Integrilin)
  - Tirofiban (Aggrastat)
- ADP inhibitors
  - Ticlopidine (Ticlid)
  - Clopidogrel (Plavix)
- Thromboxane synthetase inhibitor
  - Ridogrel

THROMBOLYTIC AGENTS

- Alteplase (t-PA)
- Reteplase (r-PA)
- Streptokinase
- Tenecteplase (TNK-tPA)

Table 2. Abbreviations and Acronyms of Major Trials Involving GP IIb/IIIa Inhibitors or Low Molecular Weight Heparins

Acronym		Full name
ADMIRAL	=	Abciximab before Direct angioplasty and stenting in acute Myocardial Infarction Regarding Acute and Long-term follow-up
ASSENT	=	ASsessment of the Safety and Efficacy of a New Thrombolytic agent
ASSET	=	Anglo-Scandinavian Study of Early Thrombolysis
CADILLAC	=	Controlled Abciximab and Device Investigation to Lower Late Angioplasty Complications
CAPTURE	=	C7E3 AntiPlatelet Therapy in Unstable angina REfractory to standard treatment
ECSG	=	European Cooperative Study Group
EPIC	=	Evaluation of c7E3 for Prevention of Ischemic Complications
EPILOG	=	Evaluation in PTCA to Improve Long-term Outcome by GP IIb/IIIa receptor blockade
EPISTENT	=	Evaluation of Platelet Inhibition in STENTing
ESSENCE	=	Efficacy and Safety of Subcutaneous Enoxaparin in Non-Q wave Coronary Events
FRAXIS	=	FRAXiparin in Ischemic Syndromes
FRIC	=	FRagmin In Coronary artery disease
FRISC	=	FRagmin during InStability in Coronary artery disease
GISSI	=	Gruppo Italiano per lo Studio della Streptochinasi nell' Infarcto miocardico
GUSTO	=	Global Utilization of Streptokinase and T-PA in Occluded arteries
HART	=	Hypertension Audit of Risk factor Therapy
IMPACT	=	Integrilin to Minimize Platelet Aggregation and Coronary Thrombosis
NICE	=	National Investigators Collaborating on Enoxaparin
PACT	=	Plasminogen activator and Angioplasty Compatibility Trial
PAMI	=	Primary Angioplasty in Myocardial Infarction
PARADIGM	=	Platelet Aggregation Receptor Antagonist Dose Investigation for reperfusion Gain in Myocardial infarction
PARAGON	=	Platelet IIb/IIIa Antagonism for the Reduction of Acute coronary syndrome events in the Global Organization Network
PRISM	=	Platelet Receptor Inhibition in ischemic Syndrome Management
PRISM PLUS	=	PRISM in Patients Limited by Unstable Signs
PURSUIT	=	Platelet IIb/IIIa in Unstable angina: Receptor Suppression Using Integrilin Therapy
RAPPORT	=	Reopro And Primary PTCA Organization and Randomized Trial
RESTORE	=	Randomized Efficacy Study of Tirofiban for Outcomes and REstenosis
SPEED	=	Strategies to Promote Early reperfusion in the Emergency Department
SWIFT	=	Should We Intervene Following Thrombolysis
TAMI	=	Thrombolysis and Angioplasty in Myocardial Infarction
TIMI	=	Thrombolysis In Myocardial Infarction
VANQWISH	=	Veterans Affairs Non-Q Wave Infarction Strategies in Hospital

Patients with peripheral arterial disease had particularly good benefit. Aspirin was associated with significantly more gastrointestinal hemorrhage, while clopidogrel caused significantly more rash. Severe neutropenia occurred in 0.1% of both treatment groups.[15] The CAPRIE trial suggested that clopidogrel is at least as effective as aspirin, if not more effective, for the secondary prevention of ischemic events. However, the efficacy of ADP-inhibitors for ACS is inferior to that of aspirin. Accordingly, clopidogrel should be used as a second-line agent for antiplatelet therapy, particularly in patients unable to tolerate aspirin therapy.

Thromboxane A2 receptor antagonists have numerous limitations. Compared to aspirin, these agents are relatively costly at $1 to $3 per tablet.[16] Moreover, ticlopidine requires 3-5 days for onset of action and, therefore, is not useful for ACS. Clopidogrel's onset is two hours, still slower than the 30-60 minute onset for aspirin. Complications with ticlopidine include diarrhea, pruritis, urticaria, and skin rash. Hepatocellular enzyme elevation occurs in as many as 8% of patients. Most significant are the hematologic side effects, particularly neutropenia. An absolute neutrophil count (ANC) of fewer than 1200 occurs in 2.4% of patients and an ANC of fewer than 450 in 0.8% of patients. While the neutropenia typically occurs between three weeks and three months after initiation of therapy, it may occur later and its onset may be sudden. Thrombocytopenia may occur and can present like immune thrombocytopenia or thrombotic thrombocytopenic purpura (TTP). Clopidogrel's side effect profile is safer and comparable to that of aspirin. Abdominal discomfort and rash each occur in approximately 4% of patients, while hematologic complications are rare.[16]

Glycoprotein IIb/IIIa Inhibitors: Pharmacology, Actions, and Side Effects

Overview. Many substances can activate platelet aggregation, especially GP IIb/IIIa receptors, which mediate the obligatory last step, or final common pathway, for platelet aggregation. GP IIb/IIIa receptors are platelet-specific, and there are approximately 50,000 per platelet.[17,18] Platelet activation causes these receptors to become activated and exteriorized, and to undergo a conformational change. The GP IIb/IIIa receptor is a functional receptor for such adhesive macromolecules as fibrinogen, fibronectin, vitronectin, and vWF. Each of these molecules can interact with multiple platelets via GP IIb/IIIa receptors.

Molecules that interact with GP IIb/IIIa receptors contain the arginine-glycine-aspartic acid (RGD) sequence, which serves as the minimal recognition sequence for the receptor. Fibrinogen contains this RGD sequence on each of its a-chains, as well as a dodecapeptide on its g-chain that also is capable of binding to the receptor. However, whereas the RGD sequence is recognized by many other integrin receptors, the dodecapeptide is specific for fibrinogen binding to platelets. During clot formation, activated platelets, with active GP IIb/IIIa receptors, recognize the RGD sequence in fibrinogen. Platelets and fibrinogen bind, initiating platelet aggregation, resulting in a hemostatic plug.[17,18] *(Please see Figure 3.)*

Figure 5. Triple Pharmacotherapy for Acute Myocardial Infarction*

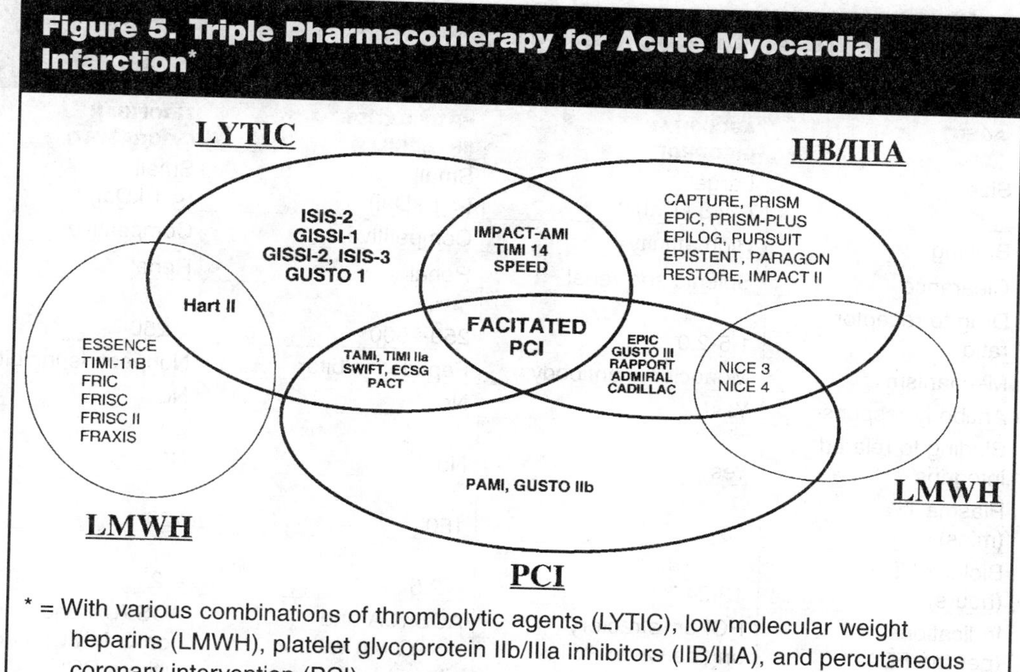

* = With various combinations of thrombolytic agents (LYTIC), low molecular weight heparins (LMWH), platelet glycoprotein IIb/IIIa inhibitors (IIB/IIIA), and percutaneous coronary intervention (PCI).

Virtually all platelet aggregation can be stopped by inhibition of 80% of the GP IIb/IIIa receptors.[19] GP IIb/IIIa receptor antagonists—all of which contain the RGD sequence—include abciximab (ReoPro), tirofiban (Aggrastat), eptifibatide (Integrilin), and lamifiban. The first three have received FDA approval, while lamifiban has been used in Canada.

The GP IIb/IIIa receptor is an excellent target for inhibition of platelet aggregation because it is specific for platelets and it is the "final common pathway" for platelet aggregation, regardless of the specific mechanism responsible for platelet activation.[20] However, inhibition of the GP IIb/IIIa receptor does not abolish other platelet functions such as adhesion, activation, or secretion. These agents also do not block thrombin generation occuring on the surface of activated platelets. Consequently, IIb/IIIa antagonists may work best in combination with agents that block thrombin generation. They also do not affect tissue factor induced coagulation, and they do not prevent inflammation.[17,20]

From a clinical and pathophysiological perspective, early use of GP IIb/IIIa inhibitors *(please see Table 3)* prevents disrupted coronary arterial surfaces from supporting platelet deposition. This clinically advantageous event has been termed passivation. Heightened platelet activity associated with ACS is known to be associated with abrupt closure after angioplasty and coronary reocclusion after thrombolysis. Passivation may include limiting production of platelet-derived vasoconstrictors in the short term and growth factors in the long term. Decreased platelet aggregation may enable arterial surfaces to heal more favorably, reducing the likelihood of (re)infarction.[21]

Abciximab. *Pharmacology and Antiplatelet Effects.* Abciximab is a recombinant monoclonal antibody fragment (Fab) that blocks IIb/IIIa receptors. It has a high affinity for the GP IIb/IIIa receptor and, consequently, binds rapidly and irreversibly to platelets. Because of its large size, the unbound plasma fraction is rapidly cleared by the reticuloendothelial system. The rapid binding and clearance of abciximab results in a very short serum half-life and, therefore, it must be given as a continuous intravenous infusion. Maximum receptor blockade and inhibition of aggregation occurs two hours after a bolus injection and returns toward normal within 12 hours. However, because of its high affinity for the receptor, it has a long biologic half-life and aggregation may return toward baseline as late as 12-36 hours after discontinuation of the infusion.[20]

Abciximab undergoes gradual redistribution after administration, with antibody redistributing to newly produced platelets, prolonging the antihemostatic effect.[4] GP IIb/IIIa receptor occupancy by abciximab exceeds 30% at eight days and 10% at 15 days, and it has been found on receptors as far out as 21 days.[19,20] Recovery in platelet aggregability is gradual and smoothly transitioned after abciximab therapy. It is relatively rapid after tirofiban or eptifibatide discontinuation. The gradual tapering of antiplatelet effect theoretically could attenuate the propensity for rebound.

The pharmacology of abciximab could result in less of it being available to bind additional GP IIb/IIIa receptors expressed on platelet surfaces from the alpha granule storage pool. This may explain the erosion in the magnitude and the dispersion in consistency of platelet inhibition during a continuous 12-hour infusion of abciximab. Indeed, although greater than 95% of patients will exhibit more than 80% GP IIb/IIIa receptor inhibition after the bolus dose of abciximab, approximately 15% will be less than 80% inhibited at 8-10 hours into the continuous infusion.[20] However, despite this loss of receptor inhibition over time, the clinical benefit of adjunctive abciximab therapy during PCI is quite robust. This suggests that the benefit of abciximab might not be solely explained by the degree of GP IIb/IIIa platelet inhibition, but also may be related to other differences in pharmacodynamics such as the gradual redistribution or the nonspecific receptor affinity.

Abciximab is not very specific because it inhibits the GP IIb/IIIa receptor simply because of its size. In fact, it not only inhibits the b3 chain of the GP IIb/IIIa receptor, but also the receptor avb3 (vitronectin) and the leukocyte receptor MAC-1. The vitronectin receptor is found not only on platelets, but also on smooth muscle cells, endothelial cells (including those that overlie an atherosclerotic plaque) monocytes, and polymorphonuclear leukocytes.[20,22] Of special interest, the vitronectin receptors on smooth muscle cells have been associated with an intimal hyperplasia response that follows vascular injury, including that associated with PCI.

As a result, it has been proposed that the vitronectin receptor may contribute to restenosis,[20] although it is uncertain whether inhibition

Table 3. Comparison of Parenteral GP IIb/IIIa Inhibitors

AGENT		ABCIXIMAB (REOPRO)	EPTIFIBATIDE (INTEGRILIN)	TIROFIBAN (AGGRASTAT)
Size		Large (~ 48 kDal)	Small (< 1 kDal)	Small (< 1 kDal)
Binding		High affinity	Competitive	Competitive
Clearance		Splenic and renal	Renal	Renal
Drug to receptor ratio		1.5-2.0	250-2500	> 250
Mechanism		Monoclonal antibody	Peptide inhibitor	Nonpeptide inhibitor
Antibody response		Yes	No	No
Binding to related integrins		Yes	No	No
Plasma T½ (mins)		10	150	120
Biologic[1] T½ (hours)		12-24	~ 2.5	~ 2
Indications (per the FDA)		PCI or refractory angina when PCI is planned within 24 hr	ACS (UA and non-Q MI) with or without PCI	ACS (UA and non-Q MI) with or without PCI
FDA approved dose	PCI	0.25 mg/kg bolus before PCI; 0.125 mcg/kg/min (max, 10 mcg/min) infusion × 12 hr after PCI	135 mcg/kg bolus, 0.5 mcg/kg/min infusion for 20-24 hr (IMPACT II dose)[3]	0.4 mcg/kg/min × 30 min, then 0.1 mcg/hg/min × 48-108 hr
	UA	0.25 mg/kg bolus and then 10 mcg/min infusion × 18-24 hr before PCI, continued 1 hr after PCI[2]	180 mcg/kg bolus, 2.0 mcg/kg/min infusion × 72-96 hr (PURSUIT dose)	

UA = unstable angina; NQMI = non-Q wave myocardial infarction; PCI = procedural coronary intervention; T½ = half-life

[1] Is the platelet-bound half-life

[2] This approval is for patients who are not responding to conventional medical therapy when PCI is planned within 24 hours.

[3] FDA approved dose may not be optimal. The larger dose of eptifibatide used in the PURSUIT trial is recommended for use in the setting of PCI.

monoclonal antibodies or after blockade by eptifibatide or tirofiban in combination with heparin.[20]

Abciximab also binds and inhibits the leukocyte MAC-1 (amb3) receptor, recognizing the am subunit. Activation of this receptor increases the intensity of interactions among white blood cells (WBCs) and platelets, thereby accelerating the inflammatory response to vessel injury. Following stent deployment, adhesion of WBCs is significantly reduced by abciximab, as is leukocyte accumulation in balloon-damaged blood vessels. These inflammation-reducing effects may decrease the restenosis rate in patients undergoing PCI.[20,22]

Tirofiban and Eptifibatide. *Pharmacology and Antiplatelet Effects.* Other GP IIb/IIIa receptor inhibitors, eptifibatide and tirofiban, are peptide and nonpeptide agents, respectively. Unlike abciximab, they are small molecules that competitively, and specifically, inhibit the RGD sequence of the GP IIb/IIIa receptor. They do not affect other receptors such as vitronectin. Because the GP IIb/IIIa receptor affinity of these agents is lower than that of abciximab, they have a short duration of action at the platelet target receptor, a short biologic half-life, and their antiplatelet effect is readily reversible. They dissociate from the receptors within seconds (vs hours for abciximab). They also undergo slow hepatic and renal clearance. Because of their low affinity and their slow clearance, they have a relatively long plasma half-life.[20,22]

In vitro experiments have shown that tirofiban and eptifibatide, but not abciximab, enhance leukocyte-platelet aggregation in whole blood. Because leukocyte-platelet interactions affect atherogenesis, restenosis, and reperfusion injury, these agents may elicit a potentially deleterious cellular response despite their ability to inhibit platelet aggregation.[22] Eptifibatide is derived from the venom of the Southeastern pygmy rattlesnake while tirofiban is obtained from the venom of an African saw-scaled viper. Receptor inhibition is achieved within 15 minutes for eptifibatide and 5 minutes for tirofiban. Once the infusion is stopped, platelet aggregation function returns toward baseline within 30 minutes to 4 hours, much more rapidly than is the case with abciximab.[19] As expected, these agents require much larger molar concentrations (drug-to-receptor dose) to maintain receptor blockade than does abciximab.[18]

of vitronectin contributes to the effectiveness of abciximab in humans. Animal studies demonstrate that vitronectin receptor inhibition can prevent intimal hyperplasia and the late vessel lumen loss after balloon angioplasty or stenting.[20] In laboratory animals, vitronectin blockade attenuates injury-induced smooth muscle migration and neointimal hyperplasia. Vitronectin receptors upregulate upon activation of smooth muscle and endothelial cells. These receptors may affect cell attachment, proliferation, migration, and survival; therefore, they may affect intimal hyperplasia and angiogenesis. These effects may play a role in new plaque formation and restenosis.[22]

Vitronectin receptors on activated platelets also have been implicated in both platelet adhesion to osteopontin (which is present in atherosclerotic plaques) and platelet-mediated thrombin generation. As a result, dual receptor blockade (GP IIb/IIIa and vitronectin) has been demonstrated to provide more potent inhibition of platelet-supported thrombin generation than monoreceptor blockade by specific

Oral agents in the GP IIb/IIIa inhibitor class also are being developed, among them xemilofiban, orbofiban, and sibrafiban. The clinical focus of these agents has been long-term therapy for the secondary prevention of ACS. Unfortunately, thus far, phase III trials have not demonstrated clinically significant efficacy; as a result, they have no role in the management of ischemic syndromes.[3]

Complications and Adverse Effects. The most important complications associated with GP IIb/IIIa inhibitors are bleeding, thrombocytopenia, and reactions to readministration. Abciximab is designated as a Pregnancy Class C agent, while eptifibatide and tirofiban are designated as Class B agents.

Major bleeding was doubled in patients receiving GP IIb/IIIa inhibitors in the EPIC and CAPTURE trials. However, vascular sheaths were left in for hours after the trial drug infusions were stopped, venous access site management was not optimal, and weight-based heparin dosing was not used. Subsequent trials that corrected for the aforementioned problems demonstrated major bleeding rates comparable to placebo, ranging from 0.4-7.8%. Mild bleeding generally is slightly more common with the use of GP IIb/IIIa inhibitors.[23]

Prompt reversal of the effects of GP IIb/IIIa inhibitors may be required in patients who develop a bleeding diathesis and in those individuals who require immediate coronary artery bypass graft (CABG) surgery.[24] Eptifibatide and tirofiban have short biologic, but long plasma half-lives; they are cleared by the kidney. Normal hemostasis should return within hours of stopping an infusion of these agents if renal function is good. Hemodialysis may reverse the hemostasis defect, although this has not been tested. Platelet transfusion is of no benefit because the number of drug molecules overwhelms the number of GP IIb/IIIa receptors. Conversely, abciximab's long biologic and short plasma half-life results in slow elimination. Platelet transfusions may reverse the hemostatic defect despite the redistribution of drug onto the new platelets. This is because there are relatively few abciximab molecules and their effects will be diluted by the large number of new platelets that are introduced.[24]

In the GP IIb/IIIa trials, mild thrombocytopenia (< 100,000 platelets/mm^3) occurred in approximately 5% of patients, while moderate thrombocytopenia (< 50,000 platelets/mm^3) occurred in 2% of the abciximab patients and in less than 1% of the eptifibatide and tirofiban patients. Severe thrombocytopenia (< 20,000 platelets/mm^3) rarely occurred with eptifibatide or tirofiban, but it did affect 0.7% of patients receiving abciximab. It has been proposed that abciximab is more likely to cause thrombocytopenia because it may have a complex interaction with heparin, leading to thrombocytopenia.[24]

The chimeric antibody fragments of abciximab are immunogenic. Low titers of antichimeric antibody develop in approximately 6-7% of patients receiving abciximab.[4,24] Titers peak one week to one month after administration and then gradually decline. Immunoglobulin G antibodies do not interfere with efficacy and are not associated with anaphylactic reactions. The significance of the antibody is unclear. Readministration of abciximab is not associated with an increased risk of anaphylaxis or altered benefit. However, severe thrombocytopenia has occurred in 2.4% of patients upon readministration of abciximab.[24]

Cost. Despite significant acquisition costs, GP IIb/IIIa inhibitors may be cost-effective by reducing the need for revascularization and/or hospital stay. Economic analyses are just being released. The acquisition costs for 24-72 hour infusions of these medications range from \$1260 to \$2160. Abciximab costs approximately \$1400 per patient for a standard 12-hour infusion. The infusion time for eptifibatide and tirofiban is variable and cost varies according to infusion time. Many trials have used 48- to 96-hour infusions, and the procurement cost is more than \$1000 for these agents.[25]

Investigators have performed pharmacoeconomic analyses of GP IIb/IIIa inhibitors used in various PCI and ACS trials. In the PCI setting, the cost savings are secondary to reduced cardiac events with abciximab and tirofiban and partially offset drug acquisition costs. In general, it was concluded that only the very high-risk patients (elevated cardiac markers, persistent angina, etc.) have cost-effectiveness ratios that would be considered acceptable.[25]

GP IIb/IIIa Inhibitor Trials of Unstable Angina or NSTEMI With Mandated Procedural Coronary Intervention

The role of GP IIb/IIIa inhibitors in the setting of PCI has been established by seven randomized, blinded, placebo-controlled trials involving a total of approximately 15,000 patients. The six larger trials are summarized in Table 4. All patients in these trials received aspirin and heparin. Except for CAPTURE, all trials administered the study drug or placebo as a bolus immediately before PCI, followed by infusions of variable durations. The rapidly reversible, small molecules, eptifibatide and tirofiban, were infused for 24 hours or 36 hours, respectively. Conversely, the slowly reversible abciximab was infused for only 12 hours. In the CAPTURE trial, the study drug was infused for 20-24 hours before angioplasty and one hour after. In EPISTENT, patients received ticlopidine for four weeks after stenting, according to standard practice for stent implantation.

EPIC Trial. The EPIC trial was the first major study evaluating the effectiveness and safety of a GP IIb/IIIa inhibitor. Its design was based on the concept that platelet aggregation may be triggered by revascularization procedures inasmuch as reocclusion is common following percutaneous transluminal coronary angioplasty (PTCA). The purpose of the EPIC trial was to determine if abciximab could reduce reocclusion following PTCA.[26] It included 2099 patients at high risk for vessel closure (UA, unfavorable coronary artery lesion morphology, AMI within 12 hours that needed rescue percutaneous intervention, or early postinfarction angina). Many of these patients did not have acute coronary ischemia. Patients were randomized to one of three treatment arms: 1) abciximab bolus without infusion; 2) abciximab bolus plus infusion; or 3) placebo bolus plus placebo infusion. Study drugs were initiated just prior to PCI and administered for 12 hours after the procedure. The primary end point was the composite of death, AMI, or need for revascularization at 30 days.

The absolute reduction (4.5%) in the composite end point by abciximab bolus plus infusion was significant compared to placebo.[26] The reduction in the composite end point was still evident at six months and at three years.[26,27] It should be noted that in the EPIC study, a doubling of major hemorrhage was observed with abciximab, primarily during CABG surgery or at the femoral puncture site. There was no difference in intracranial hemorrhage. Bleeding was more severe in patients who received relatively more of the fixed heparin dose. It was felt that bleeding resulted from the lack of weight-based heparin dosing, inadequate venous access care, and leaving the access sheath in place for several hours after the infusion had been completed.

EPILOG Trial. The purpose of the EPILOG trial was to see whether the efficacy of abciximab could be maintained while reducing the rate of major bleeding complications as compared to the results of EPIC.[28] To decrease hemorrhage, patients received weight-based heparin, meticulous access site care, and early sheath removal. Patients were less ill than in the EPIC trial because it was felt that the benefit of abciximab in those with more acute ischemic syndromes had already been demonstrated. As with EPIC, both elective and urgent PCIs were studied. Patients received one of the following three regimens: 1) placebo plus standard-dose heparin (100 units per kilo-

Table 4. Trials Using GP IIb/IIIa Inhibitors in Non-ST-Segment Elevation Acute Coronary Syndromes with Mandated PCI

TRIAL	EPIC	EPILOG	EPISTENT	CAPTURE	IMPACT II	RESTORE
Agent	Abciximab	Abciximab	Abciximab	Abciximab	Eptifibatide	Tirofiban
Entry Criteria	Elective to emergent: MI w/i 12 hrs requiring rescue, early post-MI angina, UA w/i 24 hrs, or vessels at high risk for closure	Elective or urgent PCI pts w/ a stenosis of ≥ 60% (Not pts with acute ischemia)	Elective or urgent PCI pts w/ a stenosis of ≥ 60% (Not pts with acute ischemia)	Refractory UA defined as: CP + EKG Δ on admission, then more CP *or* EKG Δ despite medical Rx	Elective, urgent, or emergent PCI pts	Pts undergoing PCI w/i 72 hrs of presentation w/ UA, NQMI, or MI with ST ↑
Patient Number	2099	2792	2399	1265	4010	2141
Primary End Point	Death, MI, CABG, repeat emergent PCI, *or* stenting at 30 d	Death, MI, *or* urgent revasc (CABG or PCI) at 30 d	Death, MI, *or* urgent revasc (CABG or PCI) at 30 d	Death, MI, *or* urgent revasc (CABG or PCI) at 30 d	Death, MI, *or* urgent revasc (CABG or PCI) at 30 d	Death, MI, *or* any revasc (CABG or PCI) at 30 d
Drug Dosing	Abcix bolus (0.25 mg/kg) and inf (10 mcg/min)	Abcix bolus (0.25 mg/kg) and inf (0.125 mcg/kg/min to max of 10 mcg/min)	Abcix bolus (0.25 mg/kg) and inf (0.125 mcg/kg/min to max of 10 mcg/min)	Abcix bolus (0.25 mg/kg) and inf (10 mcg/min)	Eptif 135 mcg/kg bolus, then inf at: LD: 0.5 mcg/kg/min HD: 0.75 mcg/kg/min	Tirofiban bolus (10 mcg/kg) and inf (0.15 mcg/kg/min)
Drug Duration	12 hrs (started w/i 1 hr of PCI)	12 hrs (started w/i 1 hr of PCI)	12 hrs (started w/i 1 hr of PCI)	18-24 hrs *before* PCI then 1 hr after PCI	20-24 hrs beginning after access established	36 hrs after angioplasty guidewire was across the lesion
Vase Sheaths	Removed 6 hrs after end of inf.	Early removal and meticulous wound care	Early removal and meticulous wound care	Removed 4-6 hrs after end of inf. Meticulous site care.	Removed 4-6 hrs after end of PCI	Early removal
Randomized Groups	Three Arms: Abcix bolus + abcix inf Abcix bolus + placebo inf Placebo bolus + placebo inf	Three Arms: Placebo + stand UFH Abcix + stand UFH Abcix + LD UFH	Three Arms: ST + placebo ST + abcix Angio + abcix	All with early angiography and had culprit lesions. Then, two arms: Abcix bolus + abcix inf Placebo bolus + placebo inf Then, PCI performed	Three Arms: LD Ept infusion HD Ept infusion Placebo bolus + placebo inf	Two Arms: Tiro bolus + tiro inf Placebo bolus + placebo inf
1° End Point (30 d) IIb/IIIa Placebo	 8.3*[3] 12.8	 5.3* (Both abcix groups) 11.7		 11.3* 15.9	 LD: 9.2, HD: 9.9 11.4	 10.3, 8.0[3] 12.2, 10.5[5]
2° End Point (6 m)[2] IIb/IIIa Placebo	 27.0* 35.1	 22.8 (stand); 22.3* (LD) 25.8		 31 30.8	 LD: 10.5, HD: 10.1 11.6	
1° End Point (30 d)[1] ST + Placebo ST + IIb/IIIa Angio + IIb/IIIa			 10.8 5.3* 6.9*			
Major/Intermediate Bleeding[4] IIb/IIIa Placebo	 14* 7	 3.5 (stand); 2.0 (LD) 3.1	 1.5 (ST + angio groups) 2.2	 3.8* 1.9	 LD: 5.1, HD: 5.2 4.8	 2.4 2.1

Key: PCI (percutaneous coronary intervention) includes angioplasty, directional atherectomy, and/or stenting; CABG, coronary artery bypass grafting; MI, myocardial infarction; Abcix, abciximab; Ept, eptifibatide; Tiro, tirofiban; inf, infusion; LD, low-dose; HD, high-dose; pts, patients; Angio, angioplasty; ST, stent; Vasc, vascular; Rx, treatment; UFH, unfractionated heparin; d, day(s); m, months; w, with; w/i, within; hrs, hours.

‡ All patients in the trials received aspirin and heparin.

* $P < 0.05$

1 Death, MI, or urgent revascularization.

2 Death, MI, or any revascularization (except IMPACT II which was only death or MI).

3 Data for abciximab bolus plus infusion group. The abciximab bolus only group was not different from placebo.

4 Major bleeding defined by TIMI criteria for all reported trial results.

5 These numbers reflect the combined end point when only emergent or urgent PTCA was considered ($P = 0.052$).

gram with a maximum of 10,000 units); 2) abciximab with standard-dose heparin; or 3) abciximab plus low-dose heparin (70 units per kilogram with a maximum of 7000 units). Study drugs were started just before the PCI and infused for 12 hours after the procedure. The composite end point included death, AMI, and need for urgent revascularization.

The trial was suspended after enrolling only 2792 of the planned 4800 patients because both clinically significant superiority was demonstrated in both abciximab treatment arms. There was a significant reduction of the composite end point at both 30 days and 6 months. *(Please see Table 4.)* Of special clinical significance was the finding that major bleeding was comparable between the placebo group and both of the abciximab groups.[28]

EPISTENT Trial. The EPISTENT trial was performed to determine whether GP IIb/IIIa inhibitors would be beneficial in patients receiving intracoronary stents (metal scaffolding devices inserted angiograpgically in vessel lumens).[29] Patients in the EPISTENT trial were similar to those in EPILOG (i.e., they were not having an acute ischemic event, but were about to receive elective or urgent PCI).

In this trial, 2399 patients were randomized to receive one of the following three PCIs and pharmacotherapeutic agents: 1) stent plus placebo; 2) stent plus abciximab; or 3) angioplasty plus abciximab. The primary end point was death, AMI, or the need for urgent revascularization within the first 30 days. All patients also received ticlopidine for four weeks after stenting, according to contemporary post-interventional practice. The groups receiving abciximab reached the composite, morbid end point in significantly fewer patients *(please see Table 4)* without a significant increase in major bleeding.[29]

CAPTURE Trial. The CAPTURE trial was unique among the abciximab trials for several reasons.[30] First, unlike other abciximab evaluations, all patients in CAPTURE presented with active UA within the previous 72 hours. This study assessed the effect of 18-24 hours of medical stabilization with abciximab prior to PTCA. Abciximab was given before PCI and continued for only one hour after the procedure was completed. All patients underwent angiography upon presentation and had significant CAD with a "culprit" lesion deemed suitable for angioplasty. However, angioplasty was not done at the time of the original angiography. Patients were randomized within 24 hours of angiography to receive placebo or abciximab during the 18-24 hours before angioplasty was performed and for 1 hour after the procedure. The primary end point was a composite of death due to any cause, AMI, or need for urgent revascularization at 30 days.

The end points were significantly improved in the abciximab group at 30 days, but the difference was not maintained at 6 months.[30] *(Please see Table 4.)* The decreased long-term efficacy in comparison to the EPIC trial may have resulted from the lack of post-procedural abciximab infusion. During the 18-24 hour infusion of drug prior to PCI, those who received abciximab had 67% fewer patients progress to AMI than did patients receiving placebo (2.1% vs 0.6%; $P = 0.029$). In comparison to placebo, major bleeding occurred twice as often in the abciximab group. *(Please see Table 4.)* However, major bleeding was less common in the CAPTURE trial than in the EPIC trial. This may have resulted from using a lower heparin dose and more meticulous access site care than that reported in the EPIC trial. Bleeding may have been reduced further in the CAPTURE trial by removing the sheath early. The authors recommended that the heparin dose be restricted to 70 IU/kg during PTCA.[30]

IMPACT-II Trial. The IMPACT-II trial assessed the role of eptifibatide in 4010 patients undergoing elective, urgent, or emergent PCI.[31] The trial included three arms: 1) bolus plus high-dose infusion; 2) bolus plus low-dose infusion; and 3) placebo. The primary end point was the composite of death, AMI, or need for urgent revascularization within the first 30 days. Although there was a significant reduction in coronary events at the end of the 24-hour infusion in the eptifibatide groups, there were no significant differences at 30 days.[31] *(Please see Table 4.)* The authors suggest that the lack of efficacy may have resulted from inadequate eptifibatide dosing or insufficient duration of infusion. There are, in fact, data suggesting that the dose may have achieved only 30-50% of platelet inhibition vs. the 80% required.[31]

RESTORE Trial. The RESTORE trial assessed the role of tirofiban in 2141 patients with ACS of 72 hours duration or less.[32] *(Please see Table 4.)* Patients were randomized to receive tirofiban or placebo for 36 hours after PCI. The primary end point was the composite of death, AMI, or need for urgent revascularization in the first 30 days. There was a significant reduction in coronary events at 2 and 7 days, but no significant difference at 30 days.[32] *(Please see Table 4.)* Major hemorrhage was comparable between groups. The authors indicated that the lack of efficacy at 30 days, as compared to abciximab in EPIC, may have resulted from different end point definitions between the trials. The composite end point in the EPIC trial included only emergency revascularization procedures, whereas the RESTORE trial considered all revascularizations ascribed to ischemia during the 30-day post-infusion period.[32]

GP IIb/IIIa Inhibitor Trials of Unstable Angina or Non-Q wave MI with Procedural Coronary Intervention not Mandated

The data for GP IIb/IIIa inhibitors in patients without PCI also suggest some possible advantages for one agent vs. another. The following trials (also known as the "Four Ps") targeted patients with ACS who did not have permanent ST-segment elevation. *(Please see Table 5.)* The objective of these investigations was to assess the role of the GP IIb/IIIa inhibitors in high-risk patients who were not necessarily going to have a PCI performed. One of the principal challenges when reviewing these studies is determining the outcome of patients who had PCI performed vs. those who did not. The use of PCI in these studies was not randomized. The preliminary results of GUSTO 4 ACS also address this issue.

PARAGON Trial. The PARAGON trial involved 2282 patients with UA, NSTEMI, or temporary ST-segment elevation who presented within 12 hours of onset and had ECG changes.[21] The five arms included a placebo group plus groups receiving lamifiban at both low and high doses, with or without heparin for 3-5 days of treatment. Percutaneous coronary intervention was discouraged during the first 48 hours. The primary end point was the composite of death due to all causes, AMI, or reinfarction within 30 days. There was no difference between groups at 30 days. *(Please see Table 5.)* However, at six months, low-dose lamifiban yielded a significantly lower composite end point than did placebo. Major bleeding occurred significantly more in patients who received heparin plus any dose of lamifiban. *(Please see Table 5.)* It was surprising that a very short-acting drug provided no benefits at 30 days but there was a significant difference at six months.[21]

PURSUIT Trial. The PURSUIT trial assessed the role of eptifibatide in 10,948 patients with ACS who presented with chest pain accompanied by either ECG changes or elevated markers.[33] Patients received either placebo, eptifibatide bolus plus a high-dose infusion, or eptifibatide bolus plus a low-dose infusion. Percutaneous coronary intervention was used at the discretion of the physicians. The primary end point was the composite of death or AMI at 30 days. The out-

Table 5. Trials Using GP IIb/IIIa Inhibitors in Non-ST-Segment Elevation Acute Coronary Syndromes (PCI Not Mandated)‡

TRIAL	PARAGON	PURSUIT	PRISM	PRISM-PLUS
Agent	Lamifiban	Eptifibatide	Tirofiban	Tirofiban
Entry criteria	CP w/i 12 hrs + EKG Δ (ST temp ↑ or ↓ or T ↓)	CP w/i 24 hrs + [EKG Δ (ST temp ↑ or ↓ or T ↓) *or* enzyme ↑]	CP w/i 24 hrs + [EKG Δ (ST temp ↑ or ↓ or T ↓) *or* enzyme ↑ *or* evidence prior CAD]	CP w/i 12 hrs + [EKG Δ (ST or T ↓) or enzyme ↑]
Patients				
Number	2282	10948	3232	1915
EKG Δ (%)	100	92	75	90
Enzyme ↑ (%)	36	45	25	45
Revascularized	25	38	38	54
Primary end point	Death *or* nonfatal MI at 30 d	Death *or* nonfatal MI at 30 d	Death, MI, *or* refractory ischemia at 48 hrs	Death, MI, *or* refractory ischemia at 7 d[4]
Drug therapy	3-5 d[2]	≤ 72 hrs[2]	48 hrs	48 hrs[2]
Randomized groups	Five arms: Placebo; Lam (LD or HD) (w/ or w/o UFH)	Three arms: Placebo; HD or LD Ept; (UFH)[3]	Two arms: Tiro; UFH	Three arms: Tiro[5]; UFH; Tiro + UFH
Invasive procedures[1]	Discourages × 48 hours	Physician discretion	Discouraged during 48 hour infusion	Discouraged during 48 hour infusion. Encouraged 48-96 hours
Outcome (primary end point) (%)	30 d: No difference; 6 m: LD Lam ± UFH 13.7*, Placebo 17.9	30 d: HD Ept 14.2*, Placebo 15.7 (No difference between groups in those with only medical Rx)	2 d: Tiro 3.8, UFH 5.6; 30 d: Tiro 15.9, UFH 17.1	7 d: Tiro + UFH 12.9, UFH 17.9; 30 d: Tiro + UFH 18.5*, UFH 22.3; 6 m: Tiro + UFH 27.7*, UFH 32.1
Major/intermediate bleeding (%)	UFH 5.9*; Lam 7.8; UFH + Lam 10.5	Ept 10.6; Placebo 9.1*	Tiro 0.4; Heparin 0.4	Tiro + UFH 4; UFH 3

Key: PCI (percutaneous coronary intervention) includes angioplasty, directional atherectomy, and/or stenting; CP, chest pain; MI, myocardial infarction; CAD, coronary artery disease; LD, low-dose; HD, high-dose; w/, with; w/o, without; w/i, within; UFH, unfractionated heparin; Ept, eptifibatide; Lam, Lamifiban; Tiro, Tirofiban; hrs, hours; d, day(s); m, months; temp, temporary; Rx, treatment.

‡ All trials included aspirin for all patients and all contained patients with non-Q-MI. Some trials permitted patients who had temporary ST-segment elevation. PCI (percutaneous coronary intervention) includes angioplasty, directional atherectomy, and/or stenting.

* $P < 0.05$

[1] Includes diagnostic catheterization, PCI, CABG.

[2] If intervention was performed at end of drug therapy, the study drug could be infused for an additional 24 hours (PURSUIT), 48 hours (PRISM PLUS), or 12-24 hours (PARAGON) after the procedure.

[3] Heparin was optional.

[4] The 30-day and 6-month end points also included rehospitalization.

[5] Tirofiban alone arm dropped early in study because of increased adverse effects.

comes of patients who received only medical therapy vs. those who had PCI performed were difficult to differentiate. At 30 days, there was a significant reduction of the composite end point within the high-dose eptifibatide group. *(Please see Table 5.)*

It should be stressed, however, that outcomes were different among different regions of the world in this multinational trial. Patients enrolled in Latin America or Eastern Europe derived less benefit than those enrolled in Western Europe or the United States. The difference may have resulted from regional differences in the use of PCI. Patients had catheterization performed 79% of the time in North America, 58% in Europe, 46% in Latin America, and 20% in Eastern Europe. The observed treatment benefit varied directly with the frequency of catheterization. This suggests that the greatest benefits of eptifibatide were experienced by patients undergoing a PCI. More bleeding and more transfusions were required in the eptifibatide group, albeit most occurred at the femoral access site. Most major bleeding occurred in patients undergoing a CABG.[33]

PRISM Trial. The PRISM trial evaluated 3232 patients who were randomized to receive a 48-hour infusion of tirofiban or heparin.[34] Patients had onset of chest pain within 24 hours and either ECG changes, enzyme elevation, or prior documentation of CAD. PCI was discouraged during the 48-hour infusion. The primary end point was the composite of death, AMI, or refractory ischemia at two days. There was a significant reduction of the composite end point at 2 days; however, the difference was not maintained at 30 days. *(Please see Table 5.)* For patients who were treated with medical therapy alone, the rate of death or AMI was reduced from 6.2% in the heparin group to 3.6% in the tirofiban group at 30 days ($P < .01$). Bleeding complications were comparable between groups.[34]

PRISM PLUS Trial. The PRISM PLUS trial evaluated 1915 patients with very high-risk ACS without ST elevation, even more so than the patients in the PRISM trial.[35] Patients presented within 12 hours of symptom onset and were randomized to receive a 48-hour infusion of tirofiban, heparin, or of both. PCI was discouraged during the 48-hour infusion period but was encouraged thereafter. The study drug was used during interventions, unlike in PRISM. The primary end point was the composite of death from any cause, AMI, refractory ischemia at 7 days, or rehospitalization at 7 days, 30 days, or 6 months. The tirofiban-alone arm was discontinued early because of excess events (5% died during the first 7 days). The composite end point was significantly improved in the tirofiban plus heparin group vs. the heparin alone group at 7 and 30 days and at 6 months. *(Please see Table 5.)*

The primary difference between the groups was the occurrence of refractory ischemia. Among patients who were treated with medical management, those who received tirofiban and heparin had a lower composite end point at 30 days (14.8%) than did those treated with heparin alone (16.8%). Bleeding complications were comparable between groups.[35] The tirofiban-alone arm was stopped early because of excess mortality. This mortality was surprising because no such excess was observed in the composite end point or in refractory ischemia. In addition, the PRISM trial also had a tirofiban-alone arm that had a significant reduction in the composite end point at two days.

GUSTO 4 Trial. Initial data from the GUSTO 4 trial were presented August 2000 at the European Society of Cardiology Congress.[36] The trial involved 7800 patients with UA or NSTEMI, without a planned PCI, who were randomized to receive: 1) a 24-hour infusion of abciximab; 2) a 48-hour infusion of abciximab; or 3) placebo. The primary outcome was the composite of death or AMI at 30 days. There was no significant difference between groups, with the primary outcome occurring in 8.2%, 9.1%, and 8.0%, respectively. Major bleeding was comparable between groups (0.6%, 1.0%, and 0.3%, respectively).[36]

Management of Unstable Angina and NSTEMI: Summary of Benefits Using GP IIb/IIIa Inhibitors

The aforementioned trials provide evidence-based support for management of subgroups of patients with ACS. In patients receiving PCI, abciximab has demonstrated consistent benefit. In contrast, neither eptifibatide nor tirofiban significantly decreased ischemic events after PCI in the RESTORE and IMPACT-II trials, respectively. In the EPIC, EPILOG, and EPISTENT trials, abciximab produced 4.5-6.4% absolute reductions in the 30-day composite end point, and these benefits persisted at 6 months in the EPIC and EPILOG trials (EPISTENT did not assess 6-month outcomes). The benefits also persisted at more extended follow-up. At one-year, patients in the EPILOG trial had a significant reduction of the composite end point from 16.1% in the placebo group to 9.6% in the abciximab groups ($P < .001$).[37] At three years, patients in the EPIC trial also had a significant reduction of the composite end point from 47.2% in the placebo group to 41.1% in the abciximab bolus plus infusion group ($P = 0.009$).[27] In the EPISTENT trial, the composite end point of mortality or AMI at one year was significantly reduced in the stent plus abciximab group (5.3%) compared to the stent plus placebo group (11.0%; $P < 0.001$).[38]

The CAPTURE trial, which evaluated abciximab and mandatory PCI, found significant benefit at 30 days but not at 6 months. Various factors may be responsible for the lack of enduring benefits. Patients received abciximab for only one hour after PCI in the CAPTURE trial vs. for 12 hours after PCI in both the EPIC and EPILOG trials. The 12-hour administration period post-procedure may be very important for establishing the long-term (6 months to 3 years) benefit of abciximab. This difference supports the concept of arterial passivation, in which the agent affects the vessel wall surface so as to inhibit further platelet-thrombin deposition. The significance of the pharmacologic differences between abciximab and the small molecule agents is unclear *(please see Table 3)*; however, they might contribute to the potential passivation associated with abciximab.

The GP IIb/IIIa inhibitors work comparably during the 12- to 36-hour intravenous infusions. The prolonged platelet-bound biologic half-life of abciximab might account for its prolonged effect on platelet function. The longer duration of action may have been the reason for abciximab's success with a 12-hour infusion vs. the 20- to 72-hour infusions used with eptifibatide or tirofiban. The highest risk for thrombotic events after PCI is within 48 hours. The prolonged and tapered effect of abciximab neutralizes platelets while the vessel heals itself, providing "artificial" passivation when the patient's thrombosis risk profile gradually progresses from high risk to low risk.[7]

The role of GP IIb/IIIa inhibitors in patients who are not necessarily having a PCI is controversial. All of the trials (PURSUIT, PRISM, PRISM-PLUS, and PARAGON) included patients who did and did not receive PCI and, importantly, the use of PCI was not randomized. Differentiating the outcomes of patients who received only medical therapy vs. those having a PCI is not easy. These groups were not differentiated in the PARAGON trial and no differences were found between the groups in the PURSUIT trial. As noted above, the PURSUIT trial also was interesting because the benefit among geographic locations varied directly with the frequency of catheterizations performed in the locations, supporting the concept that GP IIb/IIIa inhibitors might be optimal in the PCI population.

The PRISM trial noted a significant reduction in the combination of death and AMI at 30 days in those treated only medically with tirofiban. However, the data presented on the population receiving only medical therapy were limited. Patients treated with tirofiban and heparin, without PCI, had an improved 30-day composite outcome compared to those treated with only heparin in the PRIME-PLUS trial. Once again, the data pertaining to those treated only medically were limited. The CAPTURE trial, despite having mandated PCI, did start with an 18- to 24-hour infusion of abciximab before PCI. During this medical only treatment phase of the study, the AMI rate was reduced from 2.1% to 0.6% in the abciximab arm.

The GP IIb/IIIa inhibitors have not been compared directly in any trials. The first one planned is the Do Tirofiban and Abciximab for Revascularization Give Equivalent outcomes Trial (TARGET). It will be a randomized, double-blind comparison of these agents during PCI. Concerns exist that it may be too small to attain statistical power. In addition, there is a question that a 30-day end point may not be long enough to adequately assess the extended benefits noted in previous trials with abciximab. Indeed, benefits with tirofiban and eptifibatide have not been demonstrated at 30 days, let alone at six months, in trials involving mandated PCI.[20]

Major bleeding has not been a significant problem in most of the studies, except the EPIC and CAPTURE trials. However, these trials did not use the same safety considerations applied in later trials, such as stopping the heparin infusion after the PCI, pulling the vascular sheaths early, and performing meticulous access site care.

It must be emphasized that trials involving GP IIb/IIIa inhibitors have involved high-risk patients, many of whom had ischemic ECG changes or positive cardiac enzymes. This point applies especially to the four-P trials of patients without mandated PCI. Even if one felt there was evidence suggesting that patients not receiving PCI would benefit from treatment with GP IIb/IIIa inhibitors, many patients admitted to the emergency department with ACS would not be eligible for these agents according to the entry criteria of the trials.

References

1. Theroux P, Fuster V. Acute coronary syndromes: Unstable angina and non-Q-wave myocardial infarction. *Circulation* 1998;97: 1195-1206.
2. Yun DD, Alpert JS. Acute coronary syndromes. *Cardiology*. 1997;88:223-237.
3. Braunwald E, Califf RM, Cannon C, et al. Redefining medical treatment in the management of unstable angina. *Am J Med* 2000;108:41-53.
4. Weitz JI, Bates S. Beyond heparin and aspirin. *Arch Intern Med* 2000;160:749-758.
5. Kull IJ, Edwards WD, Schwartz RS. Vulnerable plaque: Pathobiology and clinical implications. *Ann Intern Med* 1998;129: 1050-1060.
6. Ambrose JA, Dangas G. Unstable angina: Current concepts of pathogensesis and treatment. *Arch Intern Med* 2000;160:25-37.
7. Arbustini E, Morbini P, DalBello B, et al. From plaque biology to clinical setting. *Am Heart J* 1999;138(2 Pt 2):S55-S60.
8. Hirsh J, Warkentin TE, Raschke R, et al. Heparin and low-molecular-weight heparin: Mechanisms of action, pharmacokinetics, dosing considerations, monitoring, efficacy, and safety. *Chest* 1998;114:489S-510S.
9. ISIS-2. Randomized trial of intravenous, oral aspirin, both, or neither among 17,187 cases of suspected acute myocardial infarction: ISIS-2. *Lancet* 1988;2:349-360.
10. The RISC Group. Risk of myocardial infarction and death during treatment with low dose aspirin and intravenous heparin in men with unstable coronary artery disease. *Lancet* 1990;336:827-830.
11. Lewis H, Davis JW, Archibald D, et al. Protective effects of aspirin against acute myocardial infarction and death in men with unstable angina. *N Engl J Med* 1983;309:396-403.
12. Cairns J, Gent M, Singer J, et al. Aspirin, sulfinpyrazone, or both in unstable angina. *N Engl J Med* 1985;313:1369-1375.
13. Antiplatelet Trialist' Collaboration. Collaborative overview of randomized trials of antiplatelet therapy-I: Prevention of death, myocardial infarction, and stroke by prolonged antiplatelet therapy in various categories of patients. *BMJ* 1994;308:81-106.
14. RAPT. Randomized trial of ridogrel. A combined thromboxane A2 synthase inhibitor and thromboxane A2/prostaglandin endoperoxide receptor antagonist, versus aspirin as adjunct to thrombolysis in patients with acute myocardial infarction. *Circulation* 1994;89: 588-595.
15. CAPRIE Steering Committee. A randomized, blinded, trial of clopidogrel versus aspirin in patients at risk of ischaemic events (CAPRIE). *Lancet* 1996;348:1329-1339.
16. Patrono C, Coller BS, et al. Platelet-active drugs: The relationships among dose, effectiveness, and side effects. *Chest* 1998;114 (Suppl 5):470S-488S.
17. Coller BS. Blockade of platelet GP IIb/IIIa receptors as an antithrombotic strategy. *Circulation* 1995;92:2373-2380.
18. Kleiman NS. Pharmacokinetics and pharmacodynamics of glycoprotein IIb-IIIa inhibitors. *Am Heart J* 1999;138:S263-S275.
19. Lincoff AM, Califf RM, Topol EJ. Platelet glycoprotein IIb/IIIa receptor blockade in coronary artery disease. *J Am Coll Cardiol* 2000;35:1103-1115.
20. Kereiakes D, Runyon J, Broderick T, et al. IIb's are not IIb's. *Am J Cardiol* 2000;85:23c-31c.
21. The PARAGON Investigators. International, randomized, controlled trial of lamifiban (A platelet glycoprotein IIb/IIIa inhibitor), heparin, or both in unstable angina. *Circulation* 1998;97:2386-2395.
22. Coller BS. Potential non-glycoprotein IIb/IIIa effects of abciximab. *Am Heart J* 1999;138(1 Part 2):S1-S5.
23. Blankenship JC. Bleeding complications of glycoprotein IIb/IIIa receptor inhibitors. *Am Heart J* 1999;138:S287-S296.
24. Tcheng JE. Clinical challenges of platelet glycoprotein IIb/IIIa receptor inhibitor therapy: Bleeding, reversal, thrombocytopenia, and retreatment. *Am Heart J* 2000;139(2 Part 2):S38-S45.
25. Hillegass WB, Newman AR, Raco DL. Economic issues in glycoprotein IIb/IIIa receptor therapy. *Am Heart J* 1999;138(2 Pt 1):S24-S32.
26. The EPIC Investigators. Use of a monoclonal antibody directed against the platelet glycoprotein IIb/IIIa receptor in high risk coronary angioplasty. *N Engl J Med* 1994;330:956-961.
27. Topol EJ, Ferguson JJ, Weisman HF, et al. Long-term protection from myocardial ischemic events in a randomized trial of brief integrin beta3 blockade with percutaneous coronary intervention. *JAMA* 1997;278:479-484.
28. The EPILOG Investigators. Platelet glycoprotein IIb/IIIa receptor blockade and low-dose heparin during percutaneous coronary revascularization. *N Engl J Med* 1997; 336:1689-1696.
29. The EPISTENT Investigators. Randomized placebo-controlled and balloon angioplasty controlled trial to assess safety of coronary stenting with use of platelet glycoprotein IIb/IIIa blockade. *Lancet* 1998;352:87-92.
30. The CAPTURE Investigators. Randomized placebo controlled trial of abciximab before and during coronary intervention in refractory

unstable angina: The CAPTURE study. *Lancet* 1997;349:1429-1435.

31. The IMPACT-II Investigators. Randomized placebo-controlled trial of effect of eptifibatide on complications of percutaneous coronary intervention: IMPACT-II. *Lancet* 1997;349:1422-1428.
32. The RESTORE Investigators. Effects of platelet glycoprotein IIb/IIIa blockade with tirofiban on adverse cardiac events in patients with unstable angina or acute myocardial infarction undergoing coronary angioplasty. *Circulation* 1997;96:1445-1453.
33. The PURSUIT Trial Investigators. Inhibition of platelet glycoprotein IIb/IIIa with eptifibatide in patients with acute coronary syndromes. *N Engl J Med* 1998;339:436-443.
34. PRISM Study Investigators. A comparison of aspirin plus tirofiban with aspirin plus heparin for unstable angina. *N Engl J Med* 1998;338:1498-1505.
35. PRISM-PLUS Study Investigators. Inhibition of the platelet glycoprotein IIb/IIIa receptor with tirofiban in unstable angina and non-Q-wave myocardial infarction. *N Engl J Med* 1998;338:1488-1497.
36. Simoons M, Wallentin L. GUSTO 4 acute coronary syndromes. Presentation: European Society of Cardiology Congress, 2000.
37. Lincoff AM, Tcheng JE, Califf RM, et al. Sustained suppression of ischemic complications of coronary intervention by platelet GP IIb/IIIa blockade with abciximab: One year outcome in the EPILOG trial. *Circulation* 1999;99:1951-1958.
38. Topol EJ, Mark DB, Lincoff AM, et al. Outcomes at 1 year and economic implications of platelet glycoprotein IIb/IIIa blockade in patients undergoing coronary stenting: Results from a multicenter randomized trial. *Lancet* 1999;354:2019-2024.

Acute Coronary Syndromes: Antithrombin Therapy

Kurt Kleinschmidt, MD, FACEP

Coronary heart disease (CHD) remains the most important cause of mortality in the United States. Among acute coronary ischemic syndromes (ACS), acute myocardial infarction (AMI) remains the leading single cause of death, with more than 1.5 million cases and more than 500,000 associated deaths per year. Of the more than 95 million annual visits to emergency departments (EDs) in the United States each year, nearly 8 million (8.4%) are due to chest pain. Not all of these patients, however, suffer from AMI; in fact, approximately 3 million of these individuals will have a noncardiac diagnosis. Of the 5 million patients with a probable cardiac etiology, 20% will have an AMI, 16% will have unstable angina (UA), and 6% will die suddenly from a variety of causes.[1]

The principal focus of this issue is on anti-thrombin agents—direct thrombin inhibitors, standard (unfractionated) heparin (UFH), and low molecular weight heparins (LMWHs). Although both types of heparin are currently used for managing ACS, there is mounting evidence that superior outcomes can be achieved with the use of certain LMWHs in patients with unstable angina.

In addition, it should be stressed that UFH has several disadvantages as an antithrombotic agent. At therapeutic levels, UFH can lead to thrombin formation by activating platelets. Thrombin generation also has been reported after discontinuation of UFH. UFH is difficult to administer, requiring continuous intravenous infusions and frequent monitoring of aPTT. Finally, the incidence of heparin-induced thrombocytopenia is significant, and is greater in patients receiving GP IIb/IIIa antiplatelet receptor inhibitors.

To circumvent the limitations and pitfalls of UFH—and to evaluate the possibility of improving patient outcomes in ACS—low molecular weight heparins (LMWHs) such as enoxaparin have been intensively studied as an evidence-based replacement for UFH in patients with unstable angina and other acute coronary ischemic syndromes, including non-ST elevation myocardial infarction (NSTEMI).

From a pathophysiological perspective, LMWHs are more potent inhibitors of thrombin generation than UFH and they are resistant to inhibition by activated platelets. Other benefits associated with LMWHs as compared to UFH include relatively simple dosing, ease of administration, limited requirements for further blood monitoring, and a more predictable anticoagulant effect.[2-4] Finally, the rationale for use of LMWHs in acute coronary ischemic syndromes is supported by a number of evidentiary trials.

With these clinical issues in focus, the purpose of this guideline statement is to examine the role of anti-thrombin agents in the management of ACS. Finally, this chapter presents outcome-based strategies for using LMWHs and UFH in appropriately risk-stratified subgroups of patients with ACS.

Anti-thrombin Agents: Centerpiece Drugs for Management of Acute Coronary Syndromes

Overview. Anti-thrombin agents are a mainstay of therapy for patients with ACS. A number of antithrombin agents are available and they typically are differentiated according to their dependence upon antithrombin (AT) III. Both standard, unfractionated heparin and LMWHs depend upon AT III for their activity and are referred to as indirect thrombin inhibitors. Conversely, AT III-independent agents inhibit thrombin directly and do not require AT III for their activity.

Direct Thrombin Inhibitors. Hirudin is the most potent, naturally occurring, specific inhibitor of thrombin. Natural hirudin (from leech saliva), recombinant hirudin, and hirulog, a synthetic analog, are direct thrombin inhibitors. Each of these molecules binds directly and reversibly to thrombin at a 1:1 ratio both at the active site and to the fibrinopeptide-binding region of thrombin. Hirudin's plasma half-life is 40 minutes following intravenous administration and approximately 120 minutes after subcutaneous injection.[4] Hirulog has a plasma half-life of 24 minutes after intravenous infusion.[5] Hirudin is approved for management of patients with heparin-induced thrombocytopenia and for ongoing anticoagulant therapy; however, it has not received an indication for ACS. In the setting of ACS, hirudin has been evaluated in patients with unstable angina and NSTEMI; hirulog has been assessed primarily in patients undergoing PTCA.

Direct thrombin inhibitors have some theoretical advantages over indirect-acting heparins. These agents inhibit thrombin activity without affecting AT III, and they also suppress positive feedback mechanisms that promote further thrombin generation; in addition, they are not inactivated by platelet factor 4.[6,7] These agents inactivate not only circulating thrombin but, unlike heparin, they also inhibit fibrin (clot)-bound thrombin. Because direct thrombin inhibitors do not bind endothelial cells and other plasma proteins—as does standard heparin—they have a more consistent dose-response and yield more predictable activated partial thromboplastin times.[6,8] Unlike LMWHs, their use requires monitoring of the activated partial thromboplastin time.[7]

Two studies have evaluated and compared clinical outcomes of hirudin vs. heparin in patients with ACS not undergoing PCI. They are: 1) the Global Utilization of Streptokinase and Tissue Plasminogen Activator for Occluded Coronary Arteries (GUSTO)-IIb; and 2) the Organization to Assess Strategies for Ischemic Syndromes (OASIS) II trials. The GUSTO-IIb trial evaluated 12142 patients with an ACS. There was no significant difference in the primary end point of death or AMI at 30 days between patients treated with heparin and hirudin who did not have ST-segment elevation (9.1% vs 8.3%; $P = 0.22$).[42] The OASIS II study included 10141 patients with unstable angina or NSTEMI who were randomized to receive hirudin (0.4 mg/kg bolus, followed by a 0.15 mg/kg per hour infusion) or heparin (5000 U bolus followed by a 15 U/kg/hour infusion). Drug dosages were adjusted to maintain a therapeutic activated partial thromboplastin time. At 72 hours and at seven days there was a non-statistically significant trend toward less cardiovascular death or new AMI in the hirudin group.[10]

Direct thrombin inhibitors have been compared with heparin during angioplasty in the Hirulog Angioplasty Trial[11] and the Hirudin Trial (HELVETICA).[12] The Hirulog Angioplasty Trial was a randomized, double-blind comparison of heparin (175 U/kg bolus followed by an 18-24 hour infusion at 15 U/kg/hour) with hirulog (1.0 mg/kg bolus followed by a 4 hour infusion at 2.5 mg/kg/hour and then a 14-20 hour infusion at 0.2 mg/kg/hour infusion).[11] All patients received aspirin.

The incidence of the composite primary end points of in-hospital death, AMI, abrupt vessel closure, or rapid clinical deterioration of cardiac origin was comparable between groups (11.4% for hirulog, 12.2% for heparin; $P = 0.44$). Major bleeding was significantly less frequent in those receiving hirulog compared with those receiving heparin (3.5% and 9.8%, respectively; $P < 0.001$).[11] In the HELVETICA trial, hirudin therapy decreased the incidence of adverse clinical events at 96 hours after angioplasty vs. heparin therapy. However, there was no difference between the groups in the incidence of recurrent symptoms, clinical events, or restenosis at seven months.[12]

Standard Heparin (UFH)—Pharmacokinetics. Standard (unfractionated) heparin (UFH) is a highly sulfated glycosaminoglycan found in mast cells of such animal tissues as lung, liver, and intestines. It is a mixture of polysaccharides with molecular weights between 5,000-30,000 Daltons (average 12,000-15,000). It has been the mainstay of anticoagulant therapy and its clinical uses include prophylaxis against venous thromboembolism, acute management of thromboembolic disease, and as an integral component of multimodal therapy for ACS.

Unfortunately, heparin UFH has several shortcomings. Its use for acute thromboembolic disease or ACS requires admission to the hospital for intravenous administration. In addition, the pharmacokinetic properties of heparin make it difficult to achieve and maintain therapeutic levels; this may result in inadequate anticoagulation or over-anticoagulation with hemorrhagic complications. Heparin is neutralized by platelet factor 4, large quantities of which are released from platelets activated at sites of plaque rupture.

It should be pointed out that heparin does not inactivate activated factor X (factor Xa), which is bound to activated platelets trapped within the thrombus. From a thrombosis perspective, factor Xa activates prothrombin, and the resulting thrombin then binds to fibrin, where it also is protected from inactivation by heparin. As a result, fibrin- or clot-bound thrombin remains enzymatically active and accelerates thrombus growth through activation of local platelets and amplification of the coagulation system.[2] As would be expected, frequent laboratory monitoring of the activated partial thromboplastin (aPTT) time is necessary to avoid these potential problems, which may contribute to increased cost of care and increased risks for patients.

Unstable Angina and Non-ST Elevation Myocardial Infarction (NSTEMI). Heparin has been a mainstay of therapy for unstable angina, NSTEMI, and ST-segment elevation AMI. Its benefit has been demonstrated in various trials comparing it to, and evaluating its efficacy in combination with aspirin therapy.[3,13,14] One study showed that heparin was superior to aspirin therapy in reducing cardiac events, particularly refractory angina, whereas others suggested it was at least as good as aspirin therapy. However, with heparin therapy alone, one study found rebound unstable angina within the first 12 hours of cessation of heparin administration.[15] This rebound phenomenon, which also is seen with other antithrombin agents, could be prevented by pretreatment with aspirin.

Based on these findings, it is now routine to treat patients early with a combination of aspirin and heparin—or LMWH (see below)—

unless there is a contraindication. One double-blinded, randomized, placebo-controlled study compared aspirin, heparin, and aspirin plus heparin in 479 patients.[3] Major end points included recurrent angina, MI, or death. All three arms had better outcomes than placebo. Patients receiving heparin had twice the bleeding compared to those treated with aspirin. Outcomes were similar among the three arms, with a trend toward heparin being better than aspirin alone.[3]

Unfractionated heparin has become a standard part of the management of unstable angina. A number of randomized trials have suggested that heparin adds therapeutic benefit to aspirin in unstable angina.[3,13,16,19] However, the evidence is still not conclusive. The trials were small, only two were double-blind, and the confidence intervals were large. As is the case with GP IIb/IIIa trials, the populations in these heparin trials were sicker than many acute chest pain patients admitted to the hospital through the emergency department.

One group performed a meta-analysis of six small, unstable angina studies that randomized patients to aspirin or a combination of aspirin and heparin. Pooled data from 1353 patients found a 33% reduction in progression to AMI or death with the addition of heparin, but this was of marginal statistical significance (P = 0.06).[20] In these trials, heparin was associated with more major bleeding events (e.g., intracranial hemorrhage) requiring transfusion. The risk/benefit ratio must be considered before heparin is used in patients with unstable angina. In today's environment, heparin should be used in moderate or high-risk patients. Data do not support the routine use of heparin in low-risk patients.

Table 1. Comparison of UFH and LMWH

EFFECT	UFH	LMWH	SIGNIFICANCE OF DIFFERENCE ON LMWH
Mean molecular weight	12,000-15,000 Daltons	4000-6500 Daltons	
Mean saccharide units	40-50	13-22	
Anti-Xa:Antithrombin activity	1:1	2-4:1	
Nonspecific protein binding	Much	Minimal	↑ Bioavailability ↑ Antithrombin potency
Neutralization by Platelet factor 4	Yes	Minimal	↑ Antithrombin potency
Inhibition of fibrin-bound thrombin	No	Yes	↑ Antithrombin potency
Binding to endothelium	Yes	Minimal	↑ Bioavailability ↓ Bleeding[1]
Binding To macrophages	Yes	Minimal	↑ Bioavailability ↑ Half-life[2]
Inactivation of platelet-bound Xa	Weak	Strong	↑ Antithrombin potency
Inhibition of platelet function	++++	++	↓ Bleeding
Interaction with platelets	More	Less	↑ Bioavailability
Causes thrombocytopenia	Not rare	Very rare	↓ Bleeding
Dose response	Poor	Fair	↑ Safety and consistency
Bioavailability	~ 30%	> 90%	↑ Safety and consistency

UFH, Unfractionated heparin; LMWH, Low molecular weight heparin; SC, Subcutaneous

1 = Interaction with endothelial cells causes increased vascular permeability, resulting in potentially increased bleeding.

2 = Hepatic macrophage uptake of an agent results in increased hepatic metabolism

Reprinted with permission from: Garrison R, Kleinschmidt K. Use of Low molecular weight heparins. *Crit Decis Emerg Med* 1999;13:11-19.

Low Molecular Weight Heparin (LMWH)—The New Standard for ACS

In the late 1970s, it was recognized that it might be possible to dissociate the beneficial antithrombotic effects of heparin from its hemorrhagic anticoagulant effects. This insight provided the impetus to fractionate heparin and isolate the antithrombotic effects in the form of LMWHs. Compared with UFH, LMWHs have superior absorption and pharmacokinetic profiles, similar antithrombotic activities, and potentially fewer hemorrhagic complications. *(Please see Table 1.)* Moreover, low molecular weight heparins are proving to be at least as effective as heparin in a number of clinical settings, and they are revolutionizing the management of acute deep venous thrombosis by permitting home-based therapy.

Pharmacokinetics and Mechanisms of Action. Low molecular weight heparins are fractions or fragments of heparin with molecular weights between 4,000-6,500 Daltons. All are produced by the fractionation of heparin molecules by controlled chemical or enzymatic depolymerization. Various depolymerization methods are used, resulting in many commercial LMWHs. It is important to recognize that each LMWH preparation has a distinct mean molecular weight, pharmacokinetic spectrum, and pharmacologic activity. The clinical relevance of these differences is not entirely clear, and randomized trials comparing the different LMWH preparations have yet to be done. However, regulatory authorities consider each LMWH preparation to be a distinct molecule requiring its own documentation and FDA approval for specific clinical indications. Accordingly, the efficacy and safety features of one LMWH cannot be extrapolated to another, and each agent should be used according to evidence-based support and approved indications.

A number of LMWHs have been developed and approved for human use over the past decade. Interestingly, clinical use of LMWHs in the United States is relatively new, with four agents having received FDA approval: ardeparin (Normiflo®; Wyeth-Ayerst Laboratories), dalteparin (Fragmin®; Pharmacia & Upjohn), tinzaparin (Innohep®; Dupont); and enoxaparin (Lovenox®; Aventis Pharmaceuticals). All four agents have been approved for management, prophylaxis, and/or treatment of venous thromboembolism. Enoxaparin is the only LMWH approved for prophylaxis, inpatient and outpatient treatment of venous thromboembolism, and acute management of ACS.[4]

Some generalizations can be made about the pharmacokinetics and metabolism of the different LMWHs. *(Please see Table 1.)* They are readily absorbed from the subcutaneous tissue, they are rapidly distributed to most organs and tissues, and they attain antithrombotic levels within 30 minutes of administration. Of special importance is the fact that LMWHs have greater than 90% bioavailability, vs. approximately 30% for heparin. This difference in bioavailability is primarily related to heparin's increased binding to plasma proteins, macrophages, and endothelial cells. Once bound, heparin's antithrombotic activity is decreased because it can't interact with the coagulation cascade proteinases. In addition, heparin binding is inconsistent, resulting in unpredictable activity.

The plasma half-life of LMWHs is two to four times longer than that of heparin, a feature that permits only once- or twice-daily administration. Elimination of heparin involves a rapid, saturable hepatic phase and a slower, renal clearance phase. The hepatic phase is dose-dependent, resulting in inconsistent elimination. In contrast, LMWHs undergo primarily slower renal elimination, which results in a longer half-life and more consistent elimination. The relative lack of platelet reactivity compared to heparin may result in less platelet activation and/or aggregation during an ACS. *(Please see Table 1.)*

Laboratory Monitoring. Antithrombotic and anticoagulant effects are different concepts. The beneficial antithrombotic properties reflect a molecule's ability to prevent formation of a new thrombus or propagation of an existing thrombus. While it would be desirable to measure antithrombotic activity, there is no simple test for assessing antithrombotic activity. The anticoagulant effect of a substance reflects its ability to inhibit hemostasis, which may result in excessive bleeding. Anticoagulation activity can be indirectly measured by the activated aPTT, the test used to monitor the effect of heparin therapy. Unfortunately, the variable responsiveness of thromboplastin reagents used in the aPTT test can cause inconsistent results despite equivalent degrees of anticoagulation. Similar problems occurred with the use of prothrombin time ratios for the monitoring of oral anticoagulant therapy. This problem was overcome by standardizing the thromboplastin reagents and adapting the international normalized ratio (INR) system of reporting. However, no similar standardization for aPTT reagents is currently available.

The inaccuracy of the aPTT test for determining the anticoagulant effect of heparin is a problem because heparin's dose-response is inconsistent. The inconsistent dose-response results from heparin's low bioavailability and from its irregular elimination. Maintenance of therapeutic levels of heparin is difficult. Conversely, low molecular weight heparin's high and consistent bioavailability and dose-independent clearance result in a predictable anticoagulant response and, therefore, laboratory monitoring is not needed in most patients. This is fortunate because the degree of anticoagulation induced by LMWH is generally too small to be detectable by the aPTT test. Anticoagulation should be monitored in patients receiving LMWHs who have renal insufficiency or those at the extremes of weight. This monitoring is done by a special test for anti-Xa activity.

Complications. Hemorrhage is the main complication of LMWH therapy. Bruising at the site of subcutaneous administration may occur, but this does not require alterations in therapy. While LMWH resulted in less hemorrhage than heparin in some early clinical trials, recent studies have revealed comparable hemorrhage rates. Caution must be used before giving LMWHs to patients at risk of hemorrhage. Neuroaxial hematomas have been reported in patients with the concurrent use of enoxaparin and spinal/epidural anesthesia. However, many of these events occurred prior to initiation of guidelines to decrease events.

Concomitant administration of LMWHs and other agents that impair hemostasis should be avoided. If a patient develops major bleeding complications secondary to a LMWH, protamine sulfate provides some but not complete neutralization of the anti-thrombin effect. In-vitro studies have reflected that neutralization of anti-thrombin activity of LMWHs is virtually 100% while that for anti-Xa ranges from 30-60% when protamine is used on a milligram per milligram basis.[21] Little clinical information exists about the relative efficacy of protamine for stopping LMWH-related hemorrhage. One case report found reversal to be poor in a patient with a subdural hemorrhage who was inadvertently given enoxaparin 1 mg/kg bid for a period of four days. However, the protamine doses were only 20 mg; he eventually received a total dose of 100 mg total.[22]

Both heparin and LMWHs may result in a transient decrease in platelet counts early in the course of therapy. Programs using LMWHs typically assess platelet counts every 2-3 days during therapy.[23] One prospective series found a mild decrease in platelets in 28% of the patients receiving either heparin or LMWHs. This mild thrombocytopenia resolved in 99% of the patients within three days despite continuation of heparin or LMWH therapy.[24] If the platelet count decreases to less than 100,000/mm^3, LMWH therapy should be discontinued.[4]

Heparin-induced thrombocytopenia (HIT) is a more serious platelet-heparin interaction. This process is a progressive, immune-mediated phenomenon typically occurring after 7-10 days of heparin therapy. It paradoxically results in hyperthrombosis and is associated with significant morbidity and mortality. Venous or arterial thromboses may occur, resulting in myocardial infarction, pulmonary emboli, and cerebrovascular accidents. Heparin-induced thrombocytopenia is less commonly associated with LMWHs than with heparin.[24,25]

One large series of 665 patients found that 2.7% of heparin-treated patients developed heparin-induced thrombocytopenia while no cases occurred in those treated with LMWHs. The general consensus is that severe thrombocytopenia is much more rare with LMWHs than with UFH. Some of the patients treated with LMWHs did develop anti-platelet antibodies, reflecting the potential for developing heparin-induced thrombocytopenia.[25] Both heparin and LMWH are contraindicated in patients who have previously had heparin-induced thrombocytopenia.

Up to 5% of patients receiving heparin or LMWHs have small, asymptomatic elevations of aspartate and alanine aminotransferases that reverse upon discontinuation of drug therapy. No monitoring guidelines exist for these aminotransferases. Low molecular weight heparin has limited transfer through the placenta and teratogenic effects have not been noted. They are listed as category B drugs. It is unknown if LMWHs are excreted within the breast milk and caution should be exercised when treating nursing women.

Comparison of LMWH with Standard Heparin. The differences in action between heparin and LMWH are better understood if

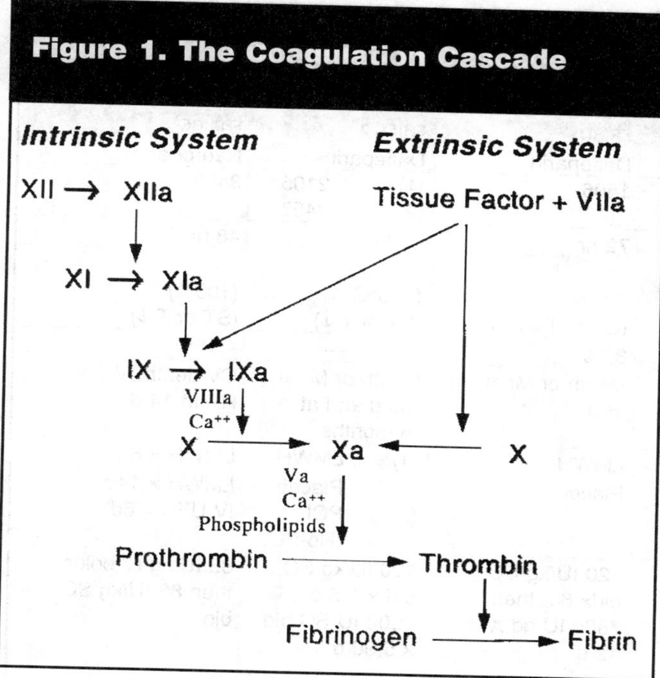

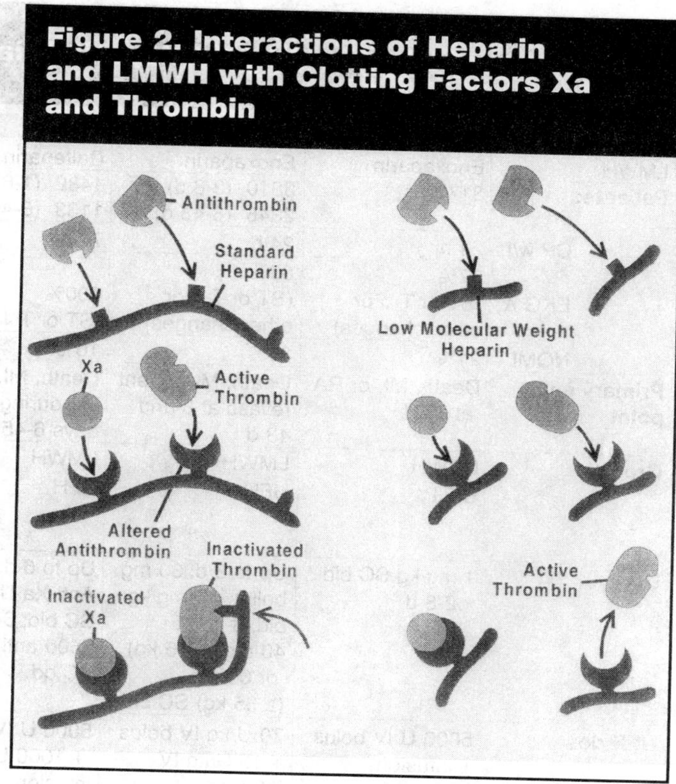

the coagulation cascade *(please see Figure 1)* is first reviewed. The cascade is a sequential, proteolytic activation of coagulation factor precursors (zymogens) into their active enzyme forms. Factors V and VIII serve as cofactors in the cascade. Most coagulation occurs via the extrinsic pathway, which is started by the interaction of factor VIIa with tissue factor, a plasma membrane protein on many cells. Tissue injury exposes tissue factor to VIIa, leading to the conversion of zymogen X to its active Xa form.

Tissue factor also activates zymogen IX, initiating the intrinsic pathway. Both the extrinsic and intrinsic pathways culminate in the activation of factor X and the formation of the prothrombinase complex on the platelet membrane. This prothrombinase complex contains calcium, phospholipids, active factor Xa, and cofactor Va. The complex converts prothrombin to thrombin, which converts fibrinogen to fibrin. While thrombin further supports thrombosis by activating platelets, it also counterbalances coagulation by facilitating the creation of antithrombin III and Protein C, the principle anticoagulants.

Heparin's anticoagulant activity requires antithrombin III. *(Please see Figure 2.)* Antithrombin III is the primary inhibitor of thrombin and the other proteinases IXa, Xa, XIa, and XIIa. Heparin binds antithrombin III, producing a conformational change in the latter that potentiates its ability to rapidly inhibit the proteinases. Antithrombin III most easily suppresses thrombin (factor IIa) while factor Xa is the most difficult factor for antithrombin III to inhibit because it is protected when bound within the prothrombinase complex.

The primary difference between heparin and LMWH is their interaction with thrombin *(please seeFigure 2)*. Most heparin molecules are long, with virtually all of these molecules being greater than 18 saccharide units in length. The long molecules can form a tertiary complex with antithrombin III and thrombin. When bound in this complex, thrombin is inactivated. Heparin molecules shorter than 18 saccharide units cannot form the tertiary complex and do not effectively inactivate thrombin. Because only 25-50% of LMWH molecules are more than 18 units long, LMWH does not inactivate thrombin as well as heparin. Conversely, factor Xa needs only a very short segment of heparin plus antithrombin III to be inactivated and it is equally inactivated by LMWH or by heparin. Thus, the anti-Xa to anti-thrombin inhibition ratio for heparin is 1:1 while it is 2-4:1 for LMWHs.

Differences also exist among the LMWHs. Comparisons are difficult because no standardization exists and their activities likely result from multiple mechanisms. The most prominent difference is that the anti-Xa to anti-thrombin ratio varies among the LMWHs. However, the significance of this variation is not known. Head-to-head trials comparing the different LMWHs have not been performed.

LMWHs for Unstable Angina and NSTEMI: Clinical Trials and Comparative Outcomes

Several trials have assessed the efficacy and safety of LMWHs in the management of patients with unstable angina and NSTEMI. *(Please see Table 2.)*[19,26,27] These trials have compared various combinations of aspirin, heparin, and LMWH. Indications for LMWHs in ACS are similar to those of heparin; both enoxaparin and dalteparin have received FDA approval for the management of ACS.

Nadroparin. The first trials comparing LMWH to standard, heparin-based regimens were small and open-label,[19] and employed a randomized, single-blinded, study of 219 patients with underlying ischemic heart disease who presented with unstable angina.[19] Patients were randomized to receive intravenous heparin plus aspirin, once-daily subcutaneous nadroparin plus aspirin, or aspirin alone. The primary end point was the composite of death, AMI, or recurrent angina. Nadroparin plus aspirin reduced the number of patients with

Table 2. Low Molecular Weight Heparin Trials in Acute Coronary Syndromes

TRIALS	ESSENCE	TIMI IIB	FRIC	FRISC	FRISC II	FRAXIS
LMWH	Enoxaparin	Enoxaparin	Dalteparin	Dalteparin	Dalteparin	Nadroparin
Patients: #	3171	3910 (3-8 d) 2346 (8-43 d)	1482 (1-6 d) 1133 (6-45 d)	1506	(1) 2105 (2) 2457	3468
CP w/i	24 hr	24 hr	72 hr	72 hr	72 hr	48 hr
EKG Δ	57% (ST or T ↓ or other changes)	83% (ST or T ↓ or other changes)	100% (ST or T ↓)	100% (ST or T ↓)	(100%) (ST or T ↓)	(100%) (ST or T ↓)
NQMI	21%	34%	16%	38%	—	~ 16%
Primary end point	Death, MI, or RA at 14 d	Death, MI, urgent revasc at 8 and 43 d	Death, MI, or RA during days 6-45	Death or MI at 6 d	Death or MI at 30 d and at 6 months	CV death, MI, or RA at 14 d
Groups	LMWH UFH	LMWH UFH	LMWH UFH	LMWH Placebo	(1) LMWH Placebo (2) PCI No-PCI	LMWH × 6d LMWH × 14d IV UFH × 6d
Dose	1 mg/kg SC bid × 2-8 d	Up to 8 d: 30 mg bolus + 1 mg/kg bid; 8-43 d: 40 mg (< 65 kg) or 60 mg (≥ 65 kg) SC bid	Up to 6 d: 120 Anti-Xa U/kg SC bid; 6-45 d; 7500 anti-Xa SC qd	120 IU/kg SC bid× 6 d then 7500 IU qd X 42 d	120 IU/kg SC bid × 1-5 d + 7500 IU SC bid × 5-90 d	86 IU/kg IV bolus then 86 IU/kg SC bid
UFH dose	5000 U IV bolus + infusion	70 U/kg IV bolus + 15 U/kg IV infusion	5000 U IV bolus + 1000 U/hr infusion	UFH only used as a rescue drug[3]	UFH only used as a rescue drug[3]	5000 U IV bolus + 1250 U infusion
Death MI (%) LMWH	—	—	—	6 d: 1.8* 40 d: 8.0	30 d: 3.1 90 d: 6.7*	—
Placebo				6 d: 4.8 40 d: 10.7	30 d: 5.9 90d: 8.0	
Death MI RA (%) LMWH	14 d: 16.6*[1] 30 d: 19.8*[1]	8 d: 12.4* 43 d: 17.3*[1]	6 d: 9.3 6-45 d: 12.3	—	—	14 d: (6 d R_X - 17.8) (14 d R_X - 20.0)
UFH	14 d: 19.8 30 d: 23.3	8 d: 14.5 43 d: 19.7	6 d: 7.6 6-45 d: 12.3	—	—	14 d: 18.1
Major Bleed[2] (%) LMWH	30 d: 7.0	8 d: 1.5 43 d: 2.9*	6 d: 1.1 6-45 d: 0.5	6 d: 0.8 40 d: 0.3	90 d: 3.3	6 d & 14 d nadro at 6 d: 1.0 6 d nadro at 14 d: 1.5 14 d nadro at 14 d: 3.5*
UFH	30 d: 6.5	8 d: 1.0 43 d: 1.5	6 d: 1.0 6 d-45 d: 0.4	—	—	6 d UFH at 6 d: 1.0 6 d UFH at 14 d: 1.6
Placebo	—	—	—	6 d: 0.5 40 d: 0.3	90 d: 1.5	—

d, day(s); RA, recurrent angina; UFH, unfractionated heparin; NQMI, non-Q wave MI; Revasc, revascularization (PTCA, CABG); CV, cardiovascular; w/i, within; NA, not applicable; SC, subcutaneous; nadro, nadroparin; LMWH, low molecular weight heparin; CP, chest pain.

* $P < 0.05$

1 = Difference primarily due to need for fewer revascularization procedures.

2 = Major hemorrhage defined: FRISC: ↓ hemoglobin of 20 g/L, required transfusion, was intracranial, or caused death or cessation of study treatment. In ESSENCE & TIMI IIB: bleeding resulting in death, transfusion of ≥ 2 units of blood, a ↓ hemoglobin of 30 g/L, or a retroperitoneal, intracranial, or intraocular hemorrhage. In FRAXIS: symptomatic bleeding associated with a ↓ hemoglobin > 2g/dL, retroperitoneal or intracranial hemorrhage, or if transfusion required or death caused.

3 = UFH also was used, but the trial was not designed to compare UFH with a LMWH.

the end point from 59% in the aspirin group and 63% in the aspirin-plus-heparin group to 22% (P = 0.001).[19]

The FRAXIS trial compared nadroparin with heparin in 3468 patients with unstable angina or NSTEMI.[28] Patients were randomized to receive intravenous heparin for six days or twice-daily subcutaneous nadroparin for six days or for 14 days. The primary end point was the composite of cardiovascular death, AMI, or recurrent/refractory angina at 14 days. No difference in outcome was found between the treatment groups. While the 14-day regimen of nadroparin resulted in significantly more bleeding than did heparin (3.5% vs 1.6%), six days of therapy with nadroparin resulted in major bleeding in only 1.5% *(Table 2)*. At 3 months, the patients who received nadroparin for 14 days had a significantly increased incidence of cardiac events (26.2% vs 22.2% with heparin) as well as increased hemorrhage (4.0% vs 2.4% with heparin).[28]

Dalteparin (Fragmin®). Dalteparin was the first LMWH to receive an indication for use in ACS in Europe. These trials [26,29,30] used prolonged anticoagulant therapy (up to 90 days) because the risk of recurrent ischemia remains high for 6-12 weeks and because coagulant activity and thrombin generation are also increased for months after an acute event.[26] This approach targeted the "rebound" or reactivation of the thrombotic process that may occur after heparin is discontinued in patients with ACS. The "rebound" may result from incomplete healing of damaged endothelial barrier at the time that heparin is stopped.[31] It is debatable whether the events are a true rebound or just incomplete therapy for a continuing process. It was hoped that "chronic" administration of dalteparin would confirm that low-dose, daily injections could reduce the incidence of "rebound."

FRISC Trial. The FRISC trial was a randomized comparison of dalteparin with placebo in 1,506 patients who presented within 72 hours of the onset of unstable angina or NSTEMI.[26] Unlike many of the other LMWH trials, there was no comparison with heparin. The primary end point was the composite of death or AMI at six days. A secondary goal was to determine whether long-term anticoagulant therapy would provide additional benefit beyond that obtained with anticoagulation only during the acute phase.

The dalteparin group received 120 IU/kg twice-daily during the "acute" phase. Patients who received dalteparin during the acute phase also received once-daily subcutaneous dalteparin (7500 IU) during the 35- to 45-day "chronic" phase. Dalteparin significantly reduced the frequency of death or AMI from 4.8% to 1.8% (P = 0.001) at six days; however, the difference was no longer significant at 40 days. *(Please see Table 2.)* The composite end point (death, myocardial infarction, revascularization, or use of intravenous heparin) also was significantly decreased in the dalteparin group at 40 days. However, no significant differences between groups existed by 150 days, reflecting that long-term, once-daily dosing was inadequate for ACS.[26] There was no significant difference in bleeding between groups.

FRIC Trial. The FRIC trial was a randomized comparison of dalteparin with heparin in 1482 patients who presented within 72 hours of the onset of unstable angina/NSTEMI.[30] It is the only trial that directly compared dalteparin with heparin. The primary end point was the composite of death, AMI, or recurrent ischemia. The dalteparin group received 120 IU/kg twice-daily during the six day "acute" phase. Patients who received dalteparin during the acute phase received once-daily subcutaneous dalteparin (7500 IU) during the 35-45 day "chronic" phase. In summary, there was no significant difference in the composite outcome between the patient groups at six days *(please see Table 2)*.[30] Both groups had a composite outcome of 12.3% at 45-days.[30] Of note is that the composite end point was actually more common in those who received dalteparin. In fact, six-day mortality was significantly increased in the dalteparin group compared to the heparin group (1.5% vs. 0.4%; p = 0.05). Bleeding complications were similar among groups.

FRISC II Trial. The FRISC II trial assessed the efficacy of long-term treatment with dalteparin, vs. placebo, in a double-blinded, randomized comparison of 2267 patients who received either dalteparin or placebo for three months. *(Please see Table 2.)*[29] As with FRISC, this trial was not a comparison with heparin. The dalteparin group received 120 IU/kg twice daily during the "acute" phase and 7500 IU twice daily (5000 IU for smaller patients) during the remaining three months. The primary end point was the composite of death or AMI at six months. There was a non-significant decrease in the primary composite end point of 6.7% and 8.0% in the dalteparin and placebo groups, respectively (P = 0.17). The difference was significant at 30 days; 3.1% vs. 5.9%, respectively (P = 0.002). There also was a decrease in death, AMI, or need for revascularization from 33.4% to 29.1% in the dalteparin group (P = 0.031). The differences were not sustained at six-month follow-up. Treatment with dalteparin was associated with an increased risk of major bleeding (3.3% vs 1.5%) and more hemorrhagic strokes (8 vs 0 events).[29]

GUSTO-4 Trial. Dalteparin was compared with heparin in a substudy of the GUSTO 4 Trial where 974 (13%) of the 7800 total patients received dalteparin instead of heparin. The focus of this trial was the comparison of a 24-hour infusion of abciximab, a 48-hour infusion of abciximab, and a placebo infusion in patients with non-ST-segment elevation ACS. Patients who received dalteparin were spread evenly among the three arms of the trial. There was no difference in the primary end point of the composite of death or AMI at 30 days among dalteparin patients in any of the three treatment arms. Major bleeding and other adverse events were comparable between the dalteparin-plus-abciximab group and the dalteparin alone group. The data from this major trial were just presented at the European Society of Cardiology Congress and the full paper has not yet been published.[32]

Enoxaparin (Lovenox®). Enoxaparin was the first LMWH to receive FDA approval for the management of ACS. This approval was based upon two positive trials in comparison with heparin (unlike the trials vs placebo as was the case for dalteparin).

The ESSENCE trial was a randomized, double-blinded study of 3171 patients with unstable angina or NSTEMI who presented within 24 hours of symptom onset. *(Please see Table 2.)*[27] Groups were treated up to eight days with either subcutaneous enoxaparin 1 mg/kg twice daily or intravenous heparin. The primary end point was the composite of death, AMI, or recurrent angina at 14 days.

Enoxaparin resulted in a significant reduction of the end point from 19.8% to 16.6% (P = 0.02) at 14 days and from 23.3% to 19.8% (p = 0.02) at 30 days. The most significant reduction was in the recurrence of angina. The need for urgent revascularization (coronary artery bypass or PTCA) during the 30-day study period was relatively reduced by 16% in the enoxaparin arm (from 32.2% to 27.0%; P = 0.001). The groups had comparable major bleeding events.[27]

This was the first major trial using a LMWH that reflected significant superiority over heparin. One-year follow-up data for 2915 of the patients (92%) found that the combined end point of death, AMI, or recurrent angina was lower in enoxaparin-treated than heparin-treated patients (32.0% vs 35.7%; P = 0.02).[33]

The TIMI-11B trial was a randomized comparison of 3910 patients with unstable angina or NSTEMI. *(Please see Table 2.)*[34] Patients were initially eligible if they had a significant history of CAD, EKG changes, or cardiac marker elevation. However, after 1800 patients had been enrolled, the focus was changed to include higher-risk patients by requiring that all patients have either ST-segment deviation or positive serum markers. Patients received up to eight days of weight-adjusted intravenous heparin followed by placebo or enoxaparin (30 mg bolus, then twice-daily 1 mg/kg subcutaneous injections up to eight days, then up to 43 days of low-dose therapy).[34] The primary end point was the composite of death, AMI, or need for urgent revascularization at eight and 43 days.

Patients receiving enoxaparin had significantly fewer end point events at eight days (12.4% vs 14.5%; P = 0.048) and at 14 days (14.2% vs 16.7%; P = 0.03). At 43 days, the beneficial effect of enoxaparin proved to be durable (end points: 17.3% vs 19.7%; P = 0.05); however, no further relative decrease in events was observed.[34] Major hemorrhage was similar between groups during the acute phase; however, by day 43, it had occurred in 2.9% of those treated with enoxaparin compared with 1.5% in the placebo arm (P = 0.02).[34] As was the case in ESSENCE, enoxaparin proved to be superior to heparin in TIMI-11B. However, administration of enoxaparin beyond the hospitalization phase cannot be recommended because no incremental benefit was achieved by continuing the enoxaparin treatment beyond the initial hospitalization and because of the increased risk of hemorrhage in the outpatient setting.

A meta-analysis of the ESSENCE and TIMI-11B trials found that, in comparison to heparin, enoxaparin treatment is associated with a 20% relative reduction in clinical events in patients with unstable angina or NSTEMI. The reduction was achieved without a significant increase in the rate of major hemorrhage during the acute phase of therapy. These data support preferential use of enoxaparin over heparin and other LMWHs as the foundation anti-thrombin agent for patients with UA and NSTEMI. *(See ACS Treatment Pathway.)*

LMWH Costs. Evidence currently supports the cost benefit of LMWHs over heparin for ACS. Cost efficacy in CAD was addressed by a pharmacoeconomic analysis of the ESSENCE trial.[35] These investigators found that the use enoxaparin vs. heparin saved $763 by hospital discharge and $1172 at 30 days. The greatest change in resource use was a decrease in coronary angioplasty. This analysis did not consider the nursing and pharmacy labor costs associated with the use of these agents, which would likely have resulted in even further savings with enoxaparin therapy.[35]

Figure 3. Low Molecular Weight Heparins: Effect on Triple End Points in Comparison to Heparin

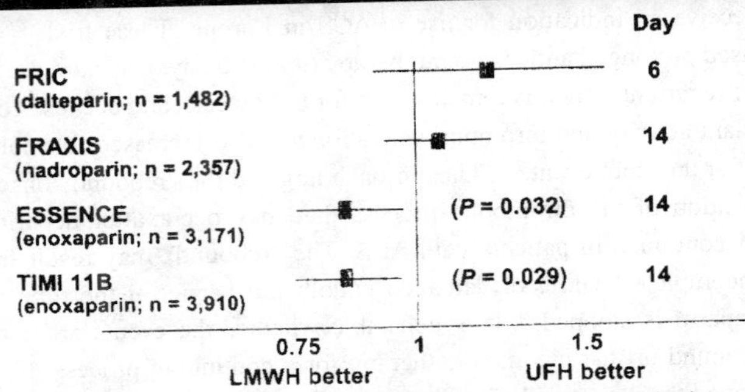

* Triple endpoint: death, MI, recurrent ischemia ± urgent revascularization.

The use of LMWH in unstable angina/NSTEMI on the triple end point of death, AMI, and recurrent Ischemia with or without revascularization. Early (6 day) and intermediate outcomes of the four trials that compared LMWH and heparin: ESSENCE, TIMI IIB, FRIC, and FRAXIS. Nadroparin in FRAXIS was given for 14 days. Reproduced with permission from: Braunwald E, Antman EM, Beasley JW, et al. The ACC/AHA Guidelines for Unstable Angina. *J Am Coll Cardiol* 2000;36:1055.

Management of ACS and NSTEMI With LMWHs—Summary of Current Guidelines

Comparing the different LMWHs is difficult. Outcomes of the trials varied either because of dissimilar pharmacologic properties of the LMWHs or because the trial designs differed as to patient selection, relative doses of medication, active treatment duration, and/or the definition and assessment of end points. In addition, the trials used different durations of therapy and drug doses for both the LMWH and for heparin. Another difference among trials is that the last episode of chest pain was within 72 hours in the FRISC and FRIC trials using dalteparin, whereas chest pain was within 24 hours of onset in the enoxaparin trials, ESSENCE and TIMI-11B. This is actually not likely to be significant because more than 90% of the patients in the dalteparin trials were actually enrolled in less than 24 hours.

Although antithrombotic therapy is used for less than a week in patients with unstable angina/NSTEMI, there is a rationale for more prolonged treatment, since a coronary lesion thrombus lasts for several months and coagulation activity is elevated for at least three months.[36] Five of the six LMWH trials *(please see Table 2)* addressed this issue by using the agent for between 8 and 90 days. Neither FRIC (dalteparin) or FRAXIS (nadroparin) found the LMWH to be superior to heparin at any primary end point, let alone any extended period. The FRISC trial (dalteparin) found no benefit to use beyond the acute study period.[26] The FRISC II (dalteparin) trial did find superiority for the LMWH over heparin at 30 days, but it is unclear whether this occurred because of the acute phase therapy or from the chronic phase therapy.

TIMI-11B found enoxaparin to be superior to heparin at 43 days, and there was no incremental benefit over that which existed at 14 days. Interestingly, the ESSENCE trial, which used enoxaparin only during the acute phase, found continued benefit at 30 days. However, as with TIMI 11B, there was not incremental benefit beyond that which existed at 14 days. Prolonged administration of a LMWH resulted in more major hemorrhage in three (FRAXIS, FRISC II, TIMI 11B) of the five trials that used chronic phases of administration of drug. Most of the trials had increased minor bleeding in the LMWH groups. These were mostly ecchymoses at injection sites and hematomas at vascular access sites.

Despite the difficulty in making certain comparisons among the LMWHs, some clinically relevant conclusions can be made. The first point is that all of the LMWH trials involved very high-risk patients, virtually all of which had either ECG changes or NSTEMI. Nadroparin was superior to placebo in one trial[19] and dalteparin was superior to placebo in both FRISC[26] and FRISC II.[29] This data, in addition to the finding that heparin was superior to placebo, reflects the second point: that high-risk patients should receive some heparin product, and the preferred agent is enoxaparin.

Of the four large randomized clinical trials, that compared a LMWH with heparin (FRIC, ESSENCE, TIMI-11B, and FRAXIS trials), only two trials, both using enoxaparin (ESSENCE and TIMI-11B), reflected superiority over heparin *(please see Figure 3)*. Therefore, the third point is that only enoxaparin has been shown to be superior to heparin in the management of patients with unstable angina/NSTEMI. The fourth point is that there are not enough data to support the administration of any LMWH beyond the acute hospital phase and that chronic administration is associated with increased major hemorrhage.

Many factors will affect the future use of LMWHs for ACS. Some cardiologists are concerned about using the long-acting LMWHs at the time of PCI. Another factor is the increased use of antiplatelet agents including the glycoprotein IIb/IIIa inhibitors, thromboxane synthetase inhibitors (ridogrel), and ADP binding inhibitors (ticlopidine and clopidogrel). The interaction between these agents is unclear. Even with the rapidly expanding uses of the GP IIb/IIIa inhibitors, anticoagulation with an anti-thrombin agent remains mandatory in the current management of ACS. This was dramatically demonstrated in the PRISM-PLUS trial. Although the combination of low-dose tirofiban combined with heparin produced a significant reduction in death, AMI, or refractory ischemia at seven days, the tirofiban arm was discontinued by the safety monitoring committee because of excessive mortality rate in comparison to the tirofiban-heparin or heparin-alone arms.

The sequencing, indications, and entry points for use of LMWHs and anti-platelet agents is summarized on the ACS Treatment Pathway. *(Please see Figure 4.)*

Management Summary and Critical Pathway: Acute Coronary Syndromes

Optimizing future management of ACS will consist of identifying the highest-benefit, lowest-risk combination of pharmacotherapeutic agents, in conjunction with mechanical revascularization techniques. Outcome-enhancing choices among the myriad pharmacotherapeutic options for ACS are evolving at an extremely rapid pace. Unfortunately, even in the face of new investigational data, it is frequently difficult to compare clinical trials, because trigger points for PCI and entry criteria for specific treatment modalities differ slightly among the trials, and head-to-head comparisons may be lacking. Moreover, because so many combinations of LMWH, GP IIb/IIIa inhibitors, fibrinolytic agents—with and without PCI—are possible for any ACS syndrome, it is unlikely that a "definitive" combination of specific agents will emerge that can conclusively be shown to provide the best results. In addition, each subgroup of patients with ACS—those with NSTEMI, UA, or T-segment elevation AMI—may eventually have a unique cocktail of anti-thrombin, anti-platelet, and anti-fibrin agents best suited for a specific patient population.

With these limitations in mind, a practical, heat-of-battle critical pathway of care for patients with acute coronary syndromes is presented in the Acute Coronary Syndrome Pathway. *(Please see Figure 4.)* Although this pathway is based primarily upon the ACC/AHA guidelines, some modifications, updates, and refinements have been made, particularly as they relate to the role of the LMWH enoxaparin vs. unfractionated heparin and the relative indications of specific GP IIb/IIIa inhibitors. As would be expected, the standard, time-honored, clinically proven agents used for management of ACS—among them, aspirin, beta-blockers, NTG, and analgesics—have been incorporated into the pathway.

Certain components of ACS management are, put simply, mandatory. For example, it is extremely important to give aspirin as soon as a patient is determined to have a possible or definite ACS. This occurs at the very beginning of our critical pathway. It also is important that patients with a possible or definite ACS have an ECG immediately upon arrival in the emergency department. Major treatment decisions and the critical pathways to be followed are based upon the results of the ECG. Risk stratification using observation, cardiac monitoring, serial ECGs, cardiac markers, and clinical response must be done for patients who don't have initial ECG changes. This evaluation can be performed in various settings, including the emergency department itself.

It is recognized that many treatment decisions will be done by local consultants, particularly relative to the role of PCI. However, emergency medicine providers must be aware of the general approach to management to be able to provide the most optimal initial care. It also is recognized that the use and timing of PCI in the setting of unstable angina and NSTEMI is very controversial and that the decision will often vary with the institutions and cardiologists involved. The same can be said for the role of PCI vs. thrombolysis in patients with ST-segment elevation myocardial infarction. Depending on the setting, assessment of ventricular function and/or stress testing could be done by emergency medicine providers as a part of a local comprehensive program.

Low Molecular Weight Heparins (LMWHs): Enoxaparin. The use and potential advantage of LMWHs in patients with ACS is a somewhat controversial area that is in a state of flux. In this vein, the ACC/AHA guidelines for unstable angina and NSTEMI present a somewhat mixed message in their prioritization of LMWHs vs. UFH. First, although the document provides figures demonstrating superiority data for enoxaparin in UA and NSTEMI, when issuing recommendations for use of LMWH in ACS, the guidelines lump all LMWHs together. Specifically, the guidelines suggest that heparin or a LMWH (in this order) may be used in high-risk patients. However, within the text of the document, they state that a "LMWH can be substituted advantageously" for heparin. The term "advantageously" would seem to reflect superiority data, despite the recommendation that heparin be used over LMWHs.

The guidelines appropriately indicate that it is somewhat difficult to draw conclusions about the relative efficacy of one LMWH vs. the others, and that head-to-head trials are the only conclusive way to settle this issue. However, the ESSENCE and TIMI-11b data, in the defined high-risk populations they studied, both clearly demonstrated superiority of enoxaparin over heparin for the composite endpoints of death, AMI, and recurrent angina. It has been argued that the reason the enoxaparin trials demonstrated superiority, as opposed to the FRIC and FRAXIS trials which did not show superiority of other LMWHs over UFH, is because of differences in trial populations and study designs. For example, it is argued that the ESSENCE and TIMI-11b populations were at higher risk than those in the other trials and that the magnitude of benefit in randomized trials is generally greater in patients at high risk compared with those at low risk. Patients in these trials were at higher risk because: 1) they had to present within 24 hours of the chest pain episode while those in FRIC and FRAXIS presented in 72 and 48 hours, respectively; and 2) the definition of AMI was softer than in FRIC and FRAXIS.

However, patients with chest pain and a history of CAD were included in ESSENCE and TIMI-11b. Many of the patients in these trials did not have elevation of markers or ECG changes. Conversely, patients in the FRIC and FRAXIS trials had to have ECG changes, which could reflect a higher-risk group. The point is that while argu-

Figure 4. Guidelines for Outcome-Effective Treatment of Acute Coronary Syndromes

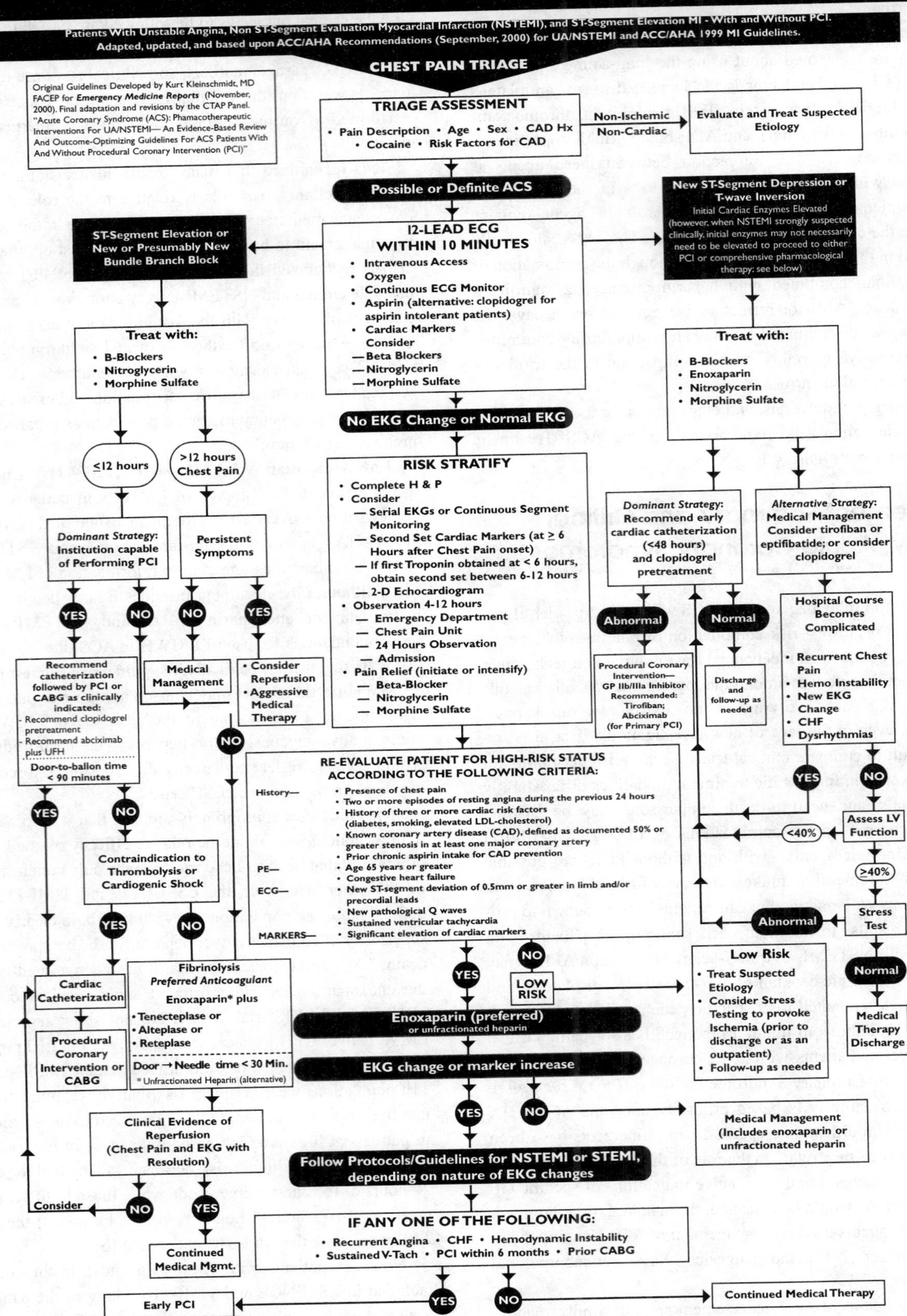

ments relative to design and population are endless, the data for the high-risk population defined in the ESSENCE and TIMI-11b trials clearly reflect enoxaparin superiority to heparin. Interestingly, in their analysis of the LMWHs, the ACC/AHA guidelines for AMI state that "enoxaparin for the acute management of patients with unstable angina/non-Q-wave MI has been shown to be superior to heparin for reducing death and serious cardiac ischemic events. This superiority is achieved without an increase in the rate of either spontaneous or instrumented major hemorrhage." Consequently, from a practical, clinical perspective, enoxaparin, specifically and uniquely, can and should be substituted "advantageously" for heparin in unstable angina and NSTEMI. Data for substituting other LMWHs "advantageously" for heparin simply do not exist, and it is somewhat curious that this distinction was not emphasized in the "advantageous" designation advocating LMWH substitution for UFH.

Despite the evidence-based support of enoxaparin superiority, the ACC/AHA guidelines issue a potential cautionary note concerning use of LMWHs in the setting of PCI because of the theoretical risk of increasing bleeding complications that may be associated with prolonged anticoagulation. The authors of the ACC/AHA document appropriately noted that enoxaparin was stopped 6-12 hours prior to PCI in ESSENCE and TIMI-11b, and therefore it was difficult to draw conclusions regarding its safety in the PCI patient population.

In this regard, it should be stressed that the recommendations of the ACC/AHA document were generated prior to very recent studies, all of which suggest that enoxaparin can be used safely, without a heparin window, in the peri-PCI setting. The NICE-3 trial assessed the incidence of bleeding while performing catheterization in 661 patients with ACS, all of whom received enoxaparin plus a GP IIb/IIIa inhibitor (either abciximab, eptifibatide, or tirofiban).[37] At the time of catheterization, enoxaparin (0.3 mg/kg intravenously) was administered if more than eight hours had elapsed since the last subcutaneous dose. NICE-3 provides compelling data that enoxaparin in combination with the different GP IIb/IIIa inhibitors produces similar clinical outcomes and bleeding frequency when compared to these end points reported in the large GP IIb/IIIa inhibitor trials.[37] Put simply, NICE-3 suggests enoxaparin plus GP IIb/IIIa inhibitors is as safe as UFH plus GP IIb/IIIa inhibitors in the setting of ACS and PCI, a finding that should be applied clinically as indicated.

In addition, the NICE-4 trial combined enoxaparin with abciximab during PCI. Enoxaparin was given as a 0.75 mg/kg intravenous bolus while abciximab was administered in its usual fashion. Data from the first 310 patients reveal the incidence of major non-CABG bleeding and transfusion to be 0.6%, which compared favorably with the 2.7% occurring in patients receiving abciximab and low-dose heparin in the EPILOG trial.[38] It must be recognized that minor, but not major bleeding, does occur more frequently with enoxaparin. Based on enoxaparin superiority in UA/NSTEMI as compared to heparin as well as recent confirmation of safety as it relates to bleeding complications (NICE-3 and NICE-4) in PCI, the guidelines in this review prioritize enoxaparin as the preferred anti-thrombin agent in UA/NSTEMI patients, including those with PCI.

References

1. ACC/AHA Taskforce on practice guidelines (Committee on management of Acute Myocardial Infarction). *J Am Coll Cardiol* 1996; 28:1328-1428.
2. Weitz JI, Bates S. Beyond heparin and aspirin. *Arch Inter Med* 2000;160:749-758.
3. Theroux P, McCans J, McCans J, et al. Aspirin, heparin, or both to treat acute unstable angina. *N Engl J Med* 1988;319:1105-1111.
4. Lovenox. Enoxaparin Insert. Lovenox Package Insert 1999;1-1.
5. Fox I, Dawson A, Loyonds P. Anticoagulant activity of Hirulog, a direct thrombin inhibitor, in humans. *Thrombo Haemosta* 1993;69: 157-163.
6. Ambrose JA, Dangas G. Unstable angina: Current concepts of pathogensesis and treatment. *Arch Inter Med* 2000;160:25-37.
7. Hull RD, Pineo GF. Hirudin vs. heparin and low-molecular-weight heparin: And the winner is... *J Lab Clin Med* 1998;132:171-174.
8. Cannon C, Braunwald E. Hirudin: Initial results in acute myocardial infarction, unstable angina and angioplasty. *JACC* 1995;25: 30S-37S.
9. GUSTO IIb Investigators. A comparison of recombinant hirudin with heparin for the treatment of acute coronary syndromes. *N Engl J Med* 1996;335:775-782.
10. OASIS-2 Investigators. Effects of recombinant hirudin (lepirudin) compared with heparin on death, myocardial infarction, refractory angina, and revascularization procedures in patient with acute myocardial ischemia without ST elevation: A randomized trial. *Lancet* 1999;353:423-424.
11. Bittl JA, Strony J, Brinker JA, et al. Treatment with bivalirudin (HIRULOG) as compared with heparin during coronary angioplasty for unstable or postinfarction angina. *N Engl J Med* 1995; 333:764-769.
12. Serruys PW, Herrmann H, Simon RP, et al. A comparison of hirudin with heparin in the prevention of restenosis after coronary angioplasty. *N Engl J Med* 1995;333:757-763.
13. The RISC Group. Risk of myocardial infarction and death during treatment with low dose aspirin and intravenous heparin in men with unstable coronary artery disease. *Lancet* 1990;336:827-830.
14. Theroux P, Waters D, Qiu S. Aspirin vs. heparin to prevent myocardial infarction during the acute phase of unstable angina. *Circulation* 1993;88:2045-2048.
15. Theroux P, Waters D, Lam J, et al. Reactivation of unstable angina after the discontinuation of heparin. *N Engl J Med* 1992;327: 141-145.
16. Cohen M, Adams P, Hawkins L, et al. Usefulness of antithrombotic therapy in resting angina pectoris or non-Q-wave myocardial infarction in preventing death and myocardial infarction (a pilot study from the Antithrombotic Therapy in Acute Coronary Syndromes Study Group). *Am J Cardiol* 1990;66:1287-1292.
17. Cohen M, Adams P, Parry G. Combination antithrombotic therapy in unstable rest angina and non-Q-wave infarction in non-prior aspirin users: Primary end points analysis from the ATACS Trial. *Circulation* 1994;89:81-88.
18. Holdright D, Patel D, Cunningham D. Comparison of the effect of heparin and aspirin vs. aspirin alone on transient myocardial ischemia and in-hospital prognosis in patients with unstable angina. *J Am Coll Cardiol* 1994;24:39-45.
19. Gurfinkel EP, Manos EJ, Mejail RI, et al. Low molecular weight heparin versus regular heparin or aspirin in the treatment of unstable angina and silent ischemia. *JACC* 1995;26:313-318.
20. Oler A, Whooley MA, Oler J, et al. Adding heparin to aspirin reduces the incidence of myocardial infarction and death in patients with unstable angina. *JAMA* 1996;276:811-815.
21. Fareed J, Jeske W, Hoppensteadt D, et al. Low-molecular-weight heparins: Pharmacologic profile and product differentiation. *Am J Cardiol* 1998;82:3L-10L.
22. Makris M, Hough RE, Kitchen S. Poor reversal of low molecular weight heparin by protamine. *British J Haematol* 2000;108:

884-885.
23. Hickey A. Personal conversation with Amy D. Hickey, RN, Clinical Nurse Specialist. Personal communication, 1998.
24. Warkentin TE, Levine MN, Hirsh J, et al. Heparin-induced thrombocytopenia in patients treated with low-molecular-weight heparin or unfractionated heparin. *N Engl J Med* 1995;332:1330-1335.
25. Warkentin TE, Kelton JG. A 14-year study of heparin-induced thrombocytopenia. *Am J Med* 1996;101:502-507.
26. FRISC study group. Low-molecular-weight heparin during instability in coronary artery disease. *Lancet* 1996;347:561-568.
27. Cohen M, Demers C, Gurfinkel EP, et al. A comparison of low-molecular-weight heparin with unfractionated heparin for unstable coronary artery disease. *N Engl J Med* 1997;337:447-452.
28. The FRAXIS Study Group. Comparison of two treatment durations (6 days and 14 days) of a low molecular weight heparin with a 6 day treatment of unfractionated heparin in the initial management of unstable angina or non-Q-wave myocardial infarction: FRAXIS (FRAxiparine in Ischaemic Syndrome). *Eur Heart J* 1999;20:1553-1562.
29. FRISC II Investigators. Long-term low-molecular mass heparin in unstable coronary-artery disease: FRISC II prospective randomized multicentre study. *Lancet* 1999;354:701-707.
30. Klein W, Buchwald A, Hillis SE, et al. Comparison of low-molecular-weight heparin with unfractionated heparin acutely and with placebo for 6 weeks in the management of unstable coronary artery disease. *Circulation* 1997;96:61-68.
31. Granger CB, Miller JM, Bovill EG, et al. Rebound increase in thrombin generation and activity after cessation of intravenous heparin in patients with acute coronary syndromes. *Circulation* 1995;91:1929-1935.
32. Simoons M, Wallentin L. GUSTO 4 acute coronary syndromes. Presentation: European Society of Cardiology Congress, 2000.
33. Goodman S, Bigonzi F, Radley D, et al. Antithrombotic therapy in acute coronary syndromes. *Eur Heart J* 1998;199(Suppl):477.
34. Antman EM, McCabe CH, Gurfinkel EP, et al. Enoxaparin prevents death and cardiac ischemic events in unstable angina/non-Q wave myocardial infarction. *Circulation* 1999;100:1593-1601.
35. Mark DB, Cowper PA, Berkowitz SD, et al. Economic assessment of low-molecular-weight heparin (enoxaparin) versus unfractionated heparin in acute coronary syndrome patients results from the ESSENCE randomized trial. *Circulation* 1998;97:1702-1707.
36. Wallentin L. Efficacy of low-molecular-weight heparin in acute coronary syndromes. *Am Heart J* 2000;139(2 Part 2):S29-S32.
37. Ferguson JJ. NICE-3 prospective, open label, non-randomized observational safety study on the combination of LMW heparin with the clinically available IIb/IIIa antagonists in 600 patients with acute coronary syndromes. *Eur Heart J* 2000;21:599.
38. Kereiakes D, Fry E, Matthai W, et al. Combination enoxaparin and abciximab therapy during percutaneous coronary intervention: "NICE guys finish first". *J Invas Cardiol* 2000;12(Suppl A): 1A-5A.

Acute Coronary Syndromes: Treatment Guidelines

Kurt Kleinschmidt, MD, FACEP

If one could only go with the flow. But no such luck. The appropriate strategy for managing patients with acute coronary syndromes (ACS) seems to change as rapidly as any therapeutic area in the field of acute care medicine. Part of the problem in identifying the outcome-optimizing approach to managing patients with unstable angina (UA), non-ST elevation myocardial infarction (NSTEMI), and ST-elevation myocardial infarction is the sheer number, and combinations, of pharmacological and procedural options available for reducing morbidity and mortality in ACS.

Complicating both the development and application of national guidelines is the fact that not every institution is equipped to apply the interventional strategies that clinical trials suggest represent the best approach to managing these patients. In particular, landmark studies conducted at teaching institutions confirm the value of using percutaneous transluminal angioplasty (PTCA) or stent insertion in patients with ST-elevation MI. However, the majority of American hospitals do not have the human or technical resources for managing patients using these techniques, which require prompt application—i.e., no more than 90 minutes from presentation to balloon catheter inflation across the culprit coronary lesion—to maximize clinical outcomes. In such institutions, clinicians may have to "default" to thrombolytic therapy as the mortality-reducing procedure of choice.

Then again, recent trials have demonstrated the potential value of using procedural coronary intervention (PCI) in combination with other pharmacological modalities, including GP IIb/IIIa inhibitors, thrombolytics, and low molecular weight or unfractionated heparins. The strategy of combining the two modalities is characterized as "facilitated" perfusion. The combination may be cost-effective if a pharmacologic regimen decreases the need for early mechanical intervention, or improves the results of PCI. Moreover, patients may be more stable in the catheterization lab after thrombolysis. In particular, patients arriving with more patent arteries due to earlier reperfusion are less likely to be in shock or to suffer dysrhythmias. Finally, the technical success of the procedure may be enhanced by the ability to better visualize distal vessels. Even when pharmacological therapy is the foundation of management, newer trials are assessing the efficacy and safety of using multi-modal approaches—a cocktail of anti-thrombotic, antiplatelet, and fibrionolytic agents administered in less than full doses—to improve patient outcomes.

Against the backdrop of rapid change and new data is the emergence of paradigm shifts within therapeutic classes. Studies suggest, for example, that new thrombolytics such as tenecteplase (TNK/t-PA) may reduce the rate of non-cerebral hemorrhage and transfusion requirements following thrombolysis; that enoxaparin is superior to heparin for patients with unstable angina and NQMI, and can be safely used as an anti-thrombin agent in the setting of PCI; and that abciximab may produce better results in patients who are destined to have PCI.

The purpose of this evidence-based chapter is to evaluate the latest efficacy and safety trials that have been designed to measure the cardioprotective benefits of acute procedural and pharmacological interventions in patients with ACS. Then, based on a comparative assessment of such trials—and with the AHA/ACC recommendations for UA and NSTEMI as a platform—the author generates a detailed, practical, and evidence-based set of treatment guidelines that can be applied by emergency physicians and cardiologists in the heat of battle to maximize clinical outcomes in patients with ACS.

Thrombolytic Therapy

In appropriately selected patients with acute mycoardial infarction (AMI), early administration of thrombolytic agents reduces mortality and is associated with improved short- and long-term clinical outcomes. From a pathophysiological perspective, prompt restoration of patency in the infarct-related artery reduces infarct size and minimizes the extent of myocardial damage, preserves left ventricular function, reduces morbidity, and prolongs survival. Compared to standard therapy, thrombolysis is associated with a 21% reduction in 30-day mortality.[1] However, these agents also are associated with intracranial hemorrhage in about 0.5-0.9% of patients. In addition, only 30-60% of patients achieve TIMI 3 (normal) flow in the affected epicardial artery within 90 minutes.[1] Because of these drawbacks, safer and more effective fibrinolytic therapies have been developed through bioengineering techniques on the t-PA molecule. In addition, the role of combination therapy with adjunctive agents such as GP IIb/IIIa inhibitors is emerging.

Mechanism and Efficacy. From an outcome point of view, it should be stressed that mortality is affected by factors other than epicardial vessel flow. In this regard, reperfusion at the tissue level may be a critical factor in myocardial salvage and this does not necessarily correlate with epicardial vessel flow. Patients with documented TIMI 3 epicardial flow, but poor TIMI myocardial perfusion (TMP) grades (TMP 0 or 1), had a higher mortality rate (5.4%) than those patients with adequate (TMP grade 2 flow) or complete tissue perfusion (TMP grade 3 flow), 2.9% and 0.7%, respectively.[2] Therefore, while survival in studies has been correlated with epicardial vessel flow, there is still much to be deciphered about perfusion characteristics and predictors of mortality.

The ideal fibrinolytic agent provides rapid lysis, enhances tissue-level perfusion, reduces intracranial and systemic hemorrhage, has a long half-life enabling single-bolus administration, has no antigenicity, and has a low reocclusion rate. Enhanced fibrin specificity also is desirable because it permits preferential activation of fibrin-bound plasminogen at the clot surface; this has the potential to increase patency and produce higher initial patency rates, and may be associated with fewer bleeding complications. Greater fibrin specificity also decreases activation of circulating plasminogen and degradation of fibrinogen, resulting in less bleeding and reducing the need for transfusion. Plasminogen activator inhibitor-1 (PAI-1) inhibits thrombolysis. Greater resistance to the action of PAI-1 would increase the potency of fibrinolytic agents.

Streptokinase. Streptokinase was the first fibrinolytic to be extensively used in the setting of AMI. The benefits associated with intravenous streptokinase were clear, as established by the GISSI-1 and ISIS-2 trials. These trials demonstrated a mortality reduction of 23% and 30%, respectively, in patients with AMI who received this therapy within six hours of symptom onset compared with placebo.[1] The current dose is 1.5 million units given intravenously over 60 minutes. Streptokinase can cause allergic reactions and it is recommended that this fibrinolytic not be adminsitered to patients with a history of recent streptococcal pharyngitis or to those who have received streptokinase within 12 months.[1] This has been associated with a lower risk of intracranial hemorrhage than other thrombolytics.

Alteplase. Alteplase (recombinant t-PA) is cloned from endogenous human t-PA and it has become a standard against which other agents are compared. It has a short, 4-8 minute half-life, it is administered as an initial intravenous bolus followed by a 90-minute intravenous infusion (accelerated regimen), it is a direct activator of plasminogen, and it is non-immunogenic. Alteplase yields patency (TIMI 2/3 flow) rates of 70-85% at 90 minutes.[1] It has been shown to reduce mortality in various trials, including: vs. placebo in the Anglo-Scandinavian Study of Early Thrombolysis (ASSET-1)[3]; and vs. streptokinase in the Global Utilization of Streptokinase and t-PA in Occluded Arteries (GUSTO-I) trial.[4] Its clinical benefit is evident even when administered up to 12 hours following symptom onset.[5]

Reteplase. The first fibrinolytic to be bioengineered from the t-PA molecule, r-PA, like alteplase, is a direct plasminogen activator and is non-immunogenic. However, its longer half-life permits administration as two bolus injections given 30 minutes apart.[1] Its efficacy in comparison to alteplase was demonstrated in the GUSTO-III trial.[6] In this trial, r-PA and t-PA had similar 30-day mortality rates (7.5% and 7.2%, respectively).

Tenecteplase. Tenecteplase (TNK-tPA) has been bioengineered to have a relatively long half-life of approximately 20 minutes, enabling it to be administered as a single bolus injection. Unlike t-PA and r-PA, its administration is weight-based. It has a 14-fold greater fibrin specificity than t-PA in in-vitro testing, which yields more potent fibrinolytic activity at the site of the clot and reduces systemic plasmin generation, potentially enhancing the speed to patency. It also is more resistant to PAI-1 compared with t-PA; this permits longer association of TNK-tPA with the fibrin-rich clot. It also may be associated with less procoagulant effects than seen with other thrombolytics.

The ASSENT-2 trial compared the 30-day mortality of accelerated t-PA with TNK-tPA. Mortality rates were similar (6.15% and 6.18%, respectively) as were intracranial hemorrhage rates (0.94% and 0.93%, respectively).[7] Interestingly, the rate of noncerebral bleeding was significantly lower for TNK-tPA compared with t-PA (26.4% vs 29%; $P < 0.0003$) as was the need for blood transfusion (4.25% vs 5.49%; $P < 0.0002$). The lower rate of noncerebral bleeding might be attributed to the higher fibrin specificity of the TNK-tPA. The greater fibrin specificity also may lead to enhanced dissolution of older fibrin clots, which may produce a better clinical outcome in patients who present late (i.e., after 3 or 4 hours of chest pain) in the clinical course of AMI.[7] It also was noted that patients who were treated more than four hours after symptom onset exhibited a statistically better outcome (30-day mortality) with TNK-tPA compared with t-PA ($P = 0.018$).[7]

Primary Percutaneous Transluminal Coronary Angioplasty (PTCA)

ST-Segment Elevation Myocardial Infarction. "Primary" PTCA is the use of standard balloon angioplasty as the initial approach to coronary reperfusion. The main benefits as compared with thrombolysis include the potential for improved patency with avoidance of life-threatening hemorrhagic complications. There are no randomized controlled trials comparing primary PTCA with no reperfusion. Primary PTCA has been compared with thrombolysis in several small, randomized studies. Most trials reflect that PTCA results in either a statistically significant improvement or at least a trend toward enhancement of in-hospital or 30-day mortality, while reducing hemorrhage and stroke.[8,9]

Other studies have shown that primary PTCA is at least as cost-effective than thrombolysis because it reduces early and late recurrent ischemic events and, as a result, facilitates earlier discharge.[8] It must be recognized that trials comparing PTCA with thrombolysis do not include patients who have contraindications to thrombolysis. Moreover, from a "real world" perspective, thrombolysis will continue to be the workhorse strategy for dissolving clots and establishing coronary artery patency in the setting of AMI because only approximately 20% of U.S. hospitals maintain catheterization capabilities and a smaller percentage have the resources required to perform PTCA.[10]

The authors of the 1999 ACC/AHA guidelines outlining management of patients with acute myocardial infarction expressed "serious concern" that PTCA should only be done by physicians and teams that are very experienced and in facilities where many such interventions performed. They recognized that the PTCA trials were generally conducted by physicians with special interest and skills in PCI and that the results may not be extrapolatable to all institutions. They stressed that thrombolysis should not be delayed for the purpose of enabling transfer of patients to a facility that can perform a PCI.[10]

Despite the advantage of mechanical perfusion, angioplasty is associated with restenosis in up to 50% of vessels and the need for repeat target-vessel revascularization in 20% of patients. Intracoronary stents appear to reduce restenosis and advances in antiplatelet therapy prevent subacute thrombosis. Three small trials in patients with AMI with vessels suitable for stenting have demonstrated a significant reduction with stenting in early (in-hospital or less than one month) recurrent ischemic events and in a late composite end point of death, recurrent AMI or repeat target-vessel revascularization by six months.[8,9] Another recent trial, and the largest to date, was the PAMI stent trial. The rate of death, recurrent AMI, and target-vessel revascularization was reduced from 20% with PTCA to 13% with stent implantation in 900 patients.[11] It appears, therefore, based on early data with primary stent implantation, that this technique may emerge as the PCI of choice in a large subset of patients. Optimization of this technique will require an appropriate—and as yet to be defined—combination of antiplatelet and antithrombin therapy.

Unstable Angina or NSTEMI. Various trials have compared the benefit of conservative (medical management) vs. early cardiac catheterization to determine the appropriate mode of revascularization (PCI or CABG). Data from the three primary trials have reflected mixed results.

The TIMI IIIB trial assessed the effects of thrombolysis with t-PA followed by randomization to conservative medical therapy vs. early invasive therapy in patients with unstable angina or NSTEMI.[12] There were no significant differences in the rates of death or recurrent AMI at six weeks among the 1473 patients with ACS or in the subgroup of 476 patients with NSTEMI who were randomly assigned to an invasive (18 events) or to a conservative strategy (22 events).[12] The authors concluded that the two approaches were comparable. It must be noted that this trial was performed before the use of GP IIb/IIIa inhibitors, LMWHs, or stent implantation.

The VANQWISH trial randomized 920 patients with non-Q-wave MI to either early conservative or early invasive management. The incidence of death or AMI during the median follow-up of 23 months was comparable between groups (26.9% in early medical therapy arm vs 29.9% in the early invasive arm; P = 0.35).[13] As with TIMI IIIB, the trial was mostly conducted before the widespread use of GP IIb/IIIa inhibitors, LMWHs, or stents. Because the early invasive group had more deaths and recurrent myocardial infarctions at one year and the outcomes at the end of the follow-up period were comparable, the authors concluded that an initial medical-therapy approach was appropriate in patients with non-Q-wave MI and that an early invasive approach may be dangerous.[13]

The FRISC II trial, in addition to comparing chronic dalteparin administration vs. placebo as noted above, also compared an early invasive with a noninvasive treatment strategy in 2457 patients with unstable angina or NSTEMI.[14] The primary end point was the composite of death or AMI at six months. The early invasive and early medical management groups had angiography performed in 96% and 10% of the patients within seven days and revascularization performed in 71% and 9% within 10 days, respectively. At six months, the composite end point was decreased from 12.1% in the noninvasive group to 9.4% in the early invasive group, P = 0.031. The greatest advantages were seen in patients who were at high risk with electrocardiographic changes and/or elevated biochemical markers of myocardial damage.[14]

In summary, the three trials produced somewhat conflicting, inconsistent results, which might be explained by the variation in study design and the proportion of each group that actually underwent revascularization. In this regard, the FRISC II trial used more modern catheterization techniques, including stents and GP IIb/IIIa inhibitors. Even though the trials designated some patients to undergo early catheterization, patients from both early catheterization and early medical management underwent revascularization. Interestingly, in the TIMI IIIB and VANQWISH trials, the difference between the groups in those undergoing revascularization was only 6% and 11%, respectively. Conversely, 38% more patients in the early invasive group in the FRISC II trial underwent revascularization.

Combinations of PCI, Thrombolysis, GP IIb/IIIa Inhibitors, and Low Molecular Weight Heparins

At the same time that the advantages of primary angioplasty and/or stenting were becoming more apparent, the benefit of aggressive antiplatelet and antithrombin therapy during these procedures also was emerging. Put simply, mechanical recanalization or surgical revascularization will only provide optimal efficacy and safety if combined with appropriate pharmacotherapy. Medical management may be best used to stabilize lesions until revascularization can be performed or to treat the most significant complications of angioplasty—acute and subacute vessel closure and restenosis. The full range of synergies between pharmacotherapeutic and procedural interventions is still being defined through many ongoing studies.

Primary PTCA vs. Thrombolysis in AMI with ST-Segment Elevation. The benefits of primary PTCA as compared with thrombolysis in AMI characterized by ST-segment elevation include the potential for improved patency and fewer hemorrhagic complications. However, primary PTCA is available in only a minority of U.S. hospitals. Numerous comparisons of PTCA with thrombolysis have been performed and most suggest that PTCA is superior relative to reinfarction rates, stroke rates, 30-day mortality, and long-term benefits.[9]

Despite the apparent advantage of mechanical reperfusion, primary PTCA is associated with angiographic restenosis in up to 50% of vessels and the need for repeat target-vessel revascularization in 20% of patients.[8] It appears that stents reduce restenosis and new antiplatelet therapy prevents subacute thrombosis. Thus, recent trials have compared PTCA with stenting. Various small trials have demonstrated that stenting reduced early (in-hospital or less than one month) recurrent ischemic events and the late composite end point of death, recurrent AMI, or repeat target-vessel revascularization by six months.[9]

The largest trial of these trials was the PAMI stent trial. The rate of death, recurrent AMI, and target-vessel revascularization was reduced from 20% with PTCA to 13% with stent implantation in 900 patients.[11] The benefit of stents was further evidenced by the STOP-AMI trial where 140 patients were randomized to receive thrombolysis or primary stenting plus abciximab. The stent-plus-abciximab group developed a significantly smaller infarct than did the thrombolysis group (14.3% vs 19.4% of the left ventricle, P = 0.02). The cumulative incidence of death, reinfarction, or stroke at six months was lower in the stent group than in the alteplase group (8.5% vs 23.2%, P = 0.02).[15]

Thrombolysis Combined with PTCA (Facilitated PCI). Clinical trials in the 1980s that evaluated the efficacy of early PTCA followed by full-dose thrombolysis included TAMI,[16] ECSG,[17] and TIMI IIb.[18] These trials found that PTCA after thrombolysis offered no advantage over t-PA alone and suggested that the combination may be harmful. At that time, these approaches were then viewed upon as being competitive and mutually exclusive.

However, medical management of AMI has changed significantly since, the 1980s, especially with the introduction of antiplatelet agents, new dosing schedules, and multi-modal options for thrombosis management. For example, thrombolytics are no longer given as extended infusions, aspirin is now regularly used, anticoagulation is better monitored within the catheterization lab, and new adjunctive agents are available. It also has been recognized that the success of PTCA directly correlates with vessel patency before the procedure begins; that is, patients with vessels with initial TIMI 2-3 flow have better outcomes than those with vessels with starting TIMI 0-1 flow.[19]

Accordingly, the strategy of combining the two modalities has been rekindled and is referred to as "facilitated" perfusion. The combination may be cost-effective if an improved pharmacologic regimen decreases the need for early mechanical interventions. In addition, patients may be more stable in the catheterization lab after thrombolysis. In particular, patients arriving with more patent arteries due to earlier reperfusion are less likely to be in shock or to suffer dysrhythmias. Finally, the technical success of the procedure may be enhanced by the ability to better visualize distal vessels.[19]

To evaluate these possibilities, the recent PACT trial randomized 606 patients to reduced-dose thrombolysis (tissue plasminogen activator, 50 mg) or placebo followed by immediate angiography with PTCA if needed.[20] Patency was higher with fibrinolytic administration and ejection fraction was highest with either successful thrombolysis or early PTCA. Most importantly, unlike the earlier trials, this trial demonstrated no adverse risk associated with early intervention.[20]

Thrombolysis Combined with a GP IIb/IIIa Inhibitor. The concept of combining more effective antiplatelet therapy with thrombolysis is attractive because platelet activation and aggregation are increased during an ACS. Various studies investigated the combination of GP IIb/IIIa inhibitors with full-dose thrombolysis including TAMI-8,[21] IMPACT-AMI,[22] and PARADIGM.[23] The TAMI 8 trial involved 70 patients in a dose-escalation study using abciximab in combination with full-dose t-PA. The infarct-related coronary artery was patent in five of nine (56%) of the control patients and in 34 of 37 (92%) of the patients who received abciximab. Major bleeding was comparable between groups.[21]

The IMPACT-AMI trial evaluated 132 patients who received full-dose, accelerated t-PA plus placebo or one of several different doses of eptifibatide. Sixty-six percent of the patients in the highest-dose eptifibatide group had 90 minute TIMI 3 flow vs 39% of the placebo group (P = 0.006).[22] Severe bleeding complications also were equal among groups.[22] Patients in the PARADIGM trial all received full-dose t-PA or streptokinase and were randomized to receive lamifiban or placebo. The time to resolution of the ST-segment elevation, a clinical marker of reperfusion, was significantly decreased in those who received lamifiban. More major bleeding occurred in the lamifiban group.[23] These trials were not powered to enable determination of clinical outcomes. In addition, there was an overall trend toward increased bleeding in the GP IIb/IIIa groups. However, the combination of GP IIb/IIIa inhibitors with thrombolytics resulted in significantly more rapid and more complete reperfusion than with thrombolysis alone.

The TIMI-14 trial was a phase 2 trial with 888 patients randomized within 12 hours to receive either t-PA alone, abciximab alone, half-dose t-PA with abciximab, or half-dose streptokinase with abciximab.[24] The group treated with reduced-dose streptokinase and abciximab showed only a modest improvement in TIMI 3 flow at 90 minutes as compared with abciximab alone, with an increase in bleeding complications. However, in patients given t-PA and abciximab, TIMI 3 flow was achieved in 77% of patients at 90 minutes as compared with 62% with t-PA alone (P = 0.02). Rates of major hemorrhage were 6% in patients receiving alteplase alone, 3% with abciximab alone, 10% with streptokinase plus abciximab, and 7% with 50 mg of alteplase plus abciximab and low-dose heparin, and 1% with 50 mg of alteplase plus abciximab with very-low-dose heparin. Another phase of TIMI-14 used either full-dose, double-bolus reteplase or half-dose, double-bolus of reteplase plus abciximab. While not reaching statistical significance, a trend toward higher TIMI 3 flow was observed in the reteplase plus abciximab group.[24]

The SPEED trial functioned as a pilot trial for the GUSTO 4 AMI trial. It enrolled 530 patients with AMI to receive either abciximab alone or abciximab and single or double boluses or r-PA. The primary end point was TIMI 3 flow at the 60-90 minute catheterization. The first phase of the study determined the appropriate dose of r-PA to be 5 units followed by another 5 units plus abciximab. In the second phase of the trial, 54% of those who received half-dose reteplase plus abciximab attained TIMI 3 flow vs. 47% of those who received full-dose reteplase alone. Flow rates were improved by using a 60 u/kg heparin bolus vs. a lower dose. Major bleeding rates were comparable between groups.[25]

Results from the SPEED and TIMI 14 trials, along with the three smaller studies noted above, suggest improved TIMI 3 perfusion when abciximab is combined with a fibrinolytic agent in patients with AMI. While none of the studies was powered to examine major bleeding complications, more minor bleeding and venous access site bleeding occurred with the combination therapies. Full-dose streptokinase with abciximab produced an unacceptably high rate of major hemorrhage.[24] Clinical outcomes will be compared in the GUSTO 4 AMI trial, a phase III study that will randomize more than 16,000 patients to receive full-dose reteplase or reduced-dose reteplase and abciximab.

Thrombolysis Plus a IIb/IIIa Inhibitor Followed by PCI. The few data that exist on this combination have been pulled from the PCI subsets of the TIMI 14 and SPEED trials. In TIMI-14, PCI was discouraged and was done in only 133 patients (11%) after the 90-minute angiograms. In patients who received PCI after lysis, resolution of ST-segment elevation increased from 8% in patients treated with either alteplase or reteplase to 49% in patients treated with a combination of fibrinolytic and abciximab (P = 0.002). This difference was most prevalent in patients who had attained TIMI 3 flow before PCI.[24] In the SPEED trial, early PCI was encouraged and was done in 323 patients (61%) at a median of 62 minutes after reperfusion therapy began. Patients receiving early PCI had fewer ischemic events and bleeding complications (15%) than patients not undergoing early PCI (30%, P = 0.001). Patients receiving abciximab with reduced-dose reteplase (5U double bolus) had the highest TIMI 3 flow on initial angiography compared with other treatment regimens, and achieved 86% TIMI 3 flow at 90 minutes with a trend toward improved clinical outcomes.[25]

PTCA Combined with a GP IIb/IIIa Inhibitor in AMI. While numerous trials have assessed the efficacy of combining a GP IIb/IIIa inhibitor with PTCA in the setting of unstable angina or NSTEMI, little information exists on this combination in the patients with AMI. The RAPPORT trial randomized 483 patients with acute MI to abciximab or placebo before PTCA.[26] The primary end point was the composite of death, reinfarction, or any (urgent or elective) target vessel revascularization at six months. There was no significant difference between groups relative to this composite end point. However, abciximab did significantly reduce the composite of death, reinfarction, or need for urgent revascularization at six months (from 17.8% to 11.6%; P = 0.05).[26] A similar 52% reduction in a combined end point was observed in the ADMIRAL trial, which also allowed stent implantation.[27]

Low Molecular Weight Heparins Combined with Thrombolysis or PCI Plus a GP IIb/IIIa Inhibitor in ACS. Heparin has been the standard anti-thrombin agent in the management of AMI, particularly in the peri-PCI or thrombolytic period. However, much of the data in support of it are non-randomized and retrospective.[28] The role of LMWHs in this setting is now being intensively explored. There has been concern about performing PCI with in patients treated with LMWH for unstable angina or NSTEMI. The concerns are now being allayed as new study data emerge. Preliminary data from multiple trials evaluating the use of enoxaparin in the setting of thrombolysis or PCI were released at the 2000 Congress of the European Society of Cardiology. These trials primarily focused on the safety of enoxaparin in these clinical settings. Some of the trials also assessed the safety of enoxaparin in combination with different GP IIb/IIIa inhibitors. While each of the trials involved only a few hundred patients, they consistently suggested that enoxaparin was safe in patients undergoing PCI as well as in those undergoing thrombolysis, or treated a GP IIb/IIIa inhibitor. These results are undergoing additional confirmation in larger trials.

Two of the recent trials evaluated the efficacy and safety of enoxaparin in patients with ST-segment elevation myocardial infarction who were managed with thrombolysis. The HART-II trial compared enoxaparin with heparin as adjunctive antithrombin therapy for 400 patients receiving front-loaded t-PA for ST-segment elevation AMI.[29] In this study, enoxaparin was administered intravenously (30 mg), followed by the standard subcutaneous regimen. The primary end points were infarct-related patency at 90 minutes after initiation of thrombolytic therapy, reocclusion at 5-7 days, and safety. The TIMI grade 2 or 3 flow was comparable between groups, 80.1% with enoxaparin and 75.1% with heparin. Reocclusion within one week occurred in 9.1% of the patients who received heparin and in only 3.1% of those who received enoxaparin (P = 0.1). Bleeding complications were comparable between groups.[29] Menown and others assessed the efficacy and safety of enoxaparin vs. heparin in 300 patients with AMI who received thrombolytic therapy. The enoxaparin group received a 40 mg intravenous bolus followed by subcutaneous injections, while the heparin group received a 5000 unit bolus plus 30,000 units per 24 hours with adjustment to maintain an appropriate aPTT. The triple end point of death, AMI, or readmission with unstable angina at three months occurred in 36% of those who received heparin and in 26% of those who received enoxaparin (P = 0.04). Major bleeding was comparable between groups.[30]

In addition, five recent trials assessed the safety of enoxaparin in the setting of PCI not associated with ST-segment elevation myocardial infarction. The NICE-3 trial evaluated the incidence of bleeding while performing catheterization in 661 patients with ACS, all of whom received enoxaparin plus a GP IIb/IIIa inhibitor (either abciximab, eptifibatide, or tirofiban).[100] At the time of catheterization, enoxaparin (0.3 mg/kg intravenously) was administered if it had been more than eight hours since the last subcutaneous dose. The combination of enoxaparin with different GP IIb/IIIa inhibitors resulted in similar clinical outcomes and bleeding frequency in comparison to those seen in the large GP IIb/IIIa inhibitor trials.[31]

The NICE-4 trial combined enoxaparin with abciximab during PCI. Enoxaparin was given as a 0.75 mg/kg intravenous bolus while abciximab was administered in its usual fashion. Data from the first 310 patients who received enoxaparin and abciximab revealed that the incidence of major non-CABG bleeding and transfusion in this group was 0.6%, which compared favorably with an incidence of 2.7% occurring in patients receiving abciximab and low-dose heparin in the EPILOG trial.[28] Another group assessed the safety and outcomes in patients with unstable angina or NSTEMI. Of the 451 patients, a non-randomized 293 underwent catheterization within eight hours of the morning enoxaparin injection, which was followed by immediate PCI in 132 patients (28%). The procedures were done without additional heparin or enoxaparin. Major bleeding occurred in 0.8% of those who received catheterization, comparable to the 1.2% in those who were not studied.[32]

In 200 patients receiving elective PCI after three days of aspirin and tirofiban, another group performed a randomized comparison of peri-procedural heparin vs. enoxaparin. Clinical outcomes and major bleeding were comparable between the groups at 30 days.[33] While not a study in the setting of PCI, the pharmacokinetics, pharmacodynamics, and safety of the combination tirofiban with enoxaparin vs. heparin in non-Q-wave myocardial infarction was addressed in a 55-patient series. As with most studies, more minor bleeding occurred with the enoxaparin combination while major bleeding was comparable. The combination of tirofiban and enoxaparin resulted in a more consistent inhibition of platelet aggregation and lower adjusted bleeding time than did the combination with heparin.[34]

The FRISC II trial assessed the role of three months of dalteparin therapy after the use of PCI in patients with unstable angina or NSTEMI or after the use of thrombolysis in AMI. While the initial randomization compared three months of dalteparin vs. placebo, a second randomization, in a 2-by-2 design, compared the use of early PCI with its more conservative use. At six months, the composite of death or AMI was decreased by early PCI from 12.1% to 9.4% in those with less aggressive use ($P = 0.031$).[14] Dalteparin decreased adverse coronary events during the three-month administration primarily in patients who received conservative use of PCI. It also was observed that there was no benefit from the three-month dalteparin administration in patients who were in the noninvasive segment of the study.

Basic Management Principles in ACS

The American College of Cardiology/American Heart Association (ACC/AHA) have released clinical practice guidelines for the management of AMI,[18] for unstable angina, and for NSTEMI.[35] They have been incorporated into the overall management of ACS. *(Please see Figure 1.)* The following is an abridged summary of some of the recommendations from both of these clinical practice guidelines. The customary ACC/AHA classifications are used. Class I refers to conditions for which there is evidence and/or general agreement that a given procedure or treatment is useful and effective. Class II refers to conditions for which there is conflicting evidence and/or a divergence of opinion about the usefulness/efficacy of a procedure or treatment. For Class IIa, the weight of evidence/opinion is in favor of usefulness/efficacy while Class IIb is less well established by evidence/opinion.

• Supplemental oxygen, intravenous access, and continuous electrocardiographic monitoring should be established (Class I).

• **Oxygen:** This is recommended for pulmonary congestion, arterial oxygen desaturation ($SaO_2 < 90\%$), cyanosis, or respiratory distress (Class I). It may be administered to patients with uncomplicated AMI during the first 2-3 hours (Class IIa).

• **Aspirin:** All patients should receive 160-325 mg (Class I). However, those with an aspirin allergy should receive dipyridamole, ticlopidine, or clopidogrel (Class IIb recommendation).

• **Nitroglycerin:** Sublingual tablet or spray is appropriate initial therapy. In the setting of AMI, intravenous nitroglycerin is recommended for the first 24-48 hours in patients with AMI and CHF, large anterior infarction, persistent ischemia, or hypertension (Class I). It is only a Class IIb recommendation for patients with uncomplicated AMI. It should be used with extreme caution in patients with suspected right ventricular infarction. Nitroglycerin should be avoided in patients with hypotension, bradycardia, or tachycardia (Class I); and in those who have had sildenafil (Viagra) within 24 hours (Class III).

• **Morphine Sulfate:** This is recommended intravenously when symptoms are not immediately relieved with nitroglycerin or when acute pulmonary congestion and/or severe agitation is present (Class I).

• **Thrombolysis:** Thrombolysis is recommended if there is ST-segment elevation (> 0.1 mV, ≥ 2 contiguous leads), the time to therapy is ≤ 12 hours, and the age is < 75 years; or if there is a bundle branch block and a history suggesting an AMI (Class I). It also can be used in those ages ≥ 75 years (Class IIa) or if the time of chest pain is between 12 and 24 hours (Class IIb). It is not recommended if the time to therapy is > 24 hours, the pain has resolved, or if there is only ST-segment depression. The guidelines state that there was a serious concern that a "routine" policy for PTCA would result in unacceptable delays for many patients or in the procedure being done by less experienced personnel.

• **Primary Percutaneous Transluminal Coronary Angioplasty:** This is recommended as an alternative to thrombolytic therapy if it can be done within 12 hours of onset of symptoms, performed in a timely fashion, done by people skilled in the procedure, and supported by experienced personnel in an appropriate laboratory environment. It also is recommended if ischemic symptoms persist (Class I). It also may be used as a reperfusion strategy in reperfusion candidates who have a contradiction to thrombolytic therapy (Class IIa). It was reasonable to further explore the combination of thrombolysis with PTCA.

It is widely accepted that the early restoration of perfusion in the AMI patient limits myocardial damage, preserves left ventricular function, and reduces mortality; such restoration may be accomplished by either administration of a thrombolytic agent or performance of PTCA; in the rare case, emergent coronary artery bypass grafting is a third revascularization method.

Optimizing Outcomes. The rapid application of reperfusion therapy is mandatory in the patient with ST-elevation AMI. Many factors must be considered by both emergency and cardiovascular physicians regarding the early reperfusion treatment decisions when managing the AMI patient. While primary angioplasty may offer improved outcome over thrombolysis, PTCA must be applied early without prolonged delay. Should catheterization laboratory activation delay either be anticipated or occur, the treating physician must proceed with thrombolysis if the patient is an appropriate candidate. Prior agreement between the ED and the cardiovascular physicians at institutions with angioplasty capability must be obtained so that consideration of PTCS will not introduce further delays in thrombolytic drug administration; such cooperation has been shown to limit additional delays in the administration of thrombolytic agents in patients who are considered for PTCA in AMI.

If applied without delay in experienced hands, the data suggest that PTCA can produce improved outcomes in AMI. It must be stressed, however, that although PTCA is felt to be superior in the treatment of AMI, this procedure must be initiated within 90 minutes of patient arrival to the hospital ED.[36] If the time required to mobilize staff and arrange for PTCA is prolonged (i.e., greater than 90 minutes to balloon catheter inflation across the culprit coronary lesion), then thrombolysis is the preferred mode of therapy.[37] Delays beyond this time period are unacceptable if the patient originally was considered to be thrombolytic candidate.

Several issues must be considered by the emergency physician when evaluating the relative desirability of various therapeutic options. First, the literature base for answering questions related to therapeutic options is somewhat heterogeneous in construction (e.g., differing therapies, study sites, outcome measures, etc.). Therefore, making absolute, all-encompassing recommendations is impossible.

Second, the question of technical expertise in performing PCI must be considered. In the GUSTO-IIb trial[38] the vast majority of physicians performed at least 75 procedures per year; these results may not be generalizable to smaller-volume centers with less experienced operators (i.e., less than 50 cases per year). Third, another systems issue regarding time-to-arrival in the catheterization laboratory must be considered.

PTCA Availability and Patient Transfer. In certain centers, PTCA may not be available, necessitating rapid transfer to another facility; alternatively, in centers with PTCA capability, the catheterization laboratory may not be in operation at the time of the patient's arrival; this is likely to be a consideration at night and during weekends.

Indications for transfer of a patient with AMI to a regional tertiary care facility with angioplasty and cardiovascular surgery capability include patients with thrombolytic therapy contraindications who may benefit from PTCA or CABG, persistent hemodynamic instability, persistent ventricular dysrhythmias, or postinfarction or postreperfusion ischemia. Hospital transfer for primary PTCA is required in patients with thrombolytic agent contraindications. The urgent transfer of a thrombolytic-eligible AMI patient for primary PTCA to another institution is not recommended until thrombolytic therapy is initiated; the delay in restoring perfusion in such a patient is not acceptable in most instances.

• **Beta-Adrenergic Blocking Agents:** They are recommended in patients without a contraindication if they are treated within 12 hours of onset of infarction, irrespective of administration of concomitant thrombolytic therapy or performance of primary PTCA. Beta-blockers also are recommended for patients with continuing or recurrent ischemic pain or those with tachydysrhythmias (Class I). They can be used in patients with moderate left ventricular failure or with other contraindications if they can be monitored closely (Class IIb). Agents without intrinsic sympathomimetic activity are preferable. The recommendation for their use in high-risk patients with evolving pain is based on the demonstrated benefit in AMI patients.

• **Angiotensin-Converting Enzyme Inhibitors (ACEIs):** In the setting of AMI, they are recommended in patients within the fist 24 hours of a suspected AMI with ST-segment elevation in two or more anterior precordial leads or with clinical heart failure in the absence of hypotension. They also are recommended for those with AMI and left ventricular ejection fraction of less than 40% or patients with clinical heart failure on the basis of systolic pump dysfunction (Class I). In the setting of unstable angina/NSTEMI, they are recommended if hypertension persists despite treatment with nitroglycerin and a beta-blocker and in patients with left ventricular systolic dysfunction or congestive heart failure and in ACS patients with diabetes (Class I).

• **Calcium Channel Blockers:** Verapamil or diltiazem may be given to patients in whom beta-adrenoceptor blockers are ineffective or contraindicated (i.e., bronchospastic disease) for relief of ongoing ischemia or control of a rapid ventricular response with atrial fibrillation after AMI in the absence of congestive heart failure, left ventricular dysfunction, or atrio-ventricular block (Class IIa). Nifedipine is generally contraindicated because of its negative inotropic effect and the reflex sympathetic activation associated with its use. All calcium blockers are all contraindicated in the setting of MI and associated left ventricular dysfunction or CHF. They have not been shown to reduce mortality after AMI.

• **Intra-aortic balloon pump:** Counter pulsation is recommended for severe ischemia that is continuing or recurs frequently despite intensive medical therapy or for hemodynamic instability in patients before or after coronary angiography (Class IIa).

• **Early Invasive Strategy in Patients with Unstable Angina/NSTEMI:** This is recommended in patients who have any one of the following high-risk indicators (Class I):

— recurrent angina/ischemia at rest or with low-level activities despite intensive medical management;

— recurrent angina/ischemia with symptoms or CHF or new or worsening mitral regurgitation;

— depressed left ventricular systolic function (ejection fraction < 40%);

— hemodynamic instability;

— PCI within six months;

— prior CABG.

Management Summary and Critical Pathways: Acute Coronary Syndromes

Overview of Strategies. Optimizing future management of ACS will consist of identifying the highest-benefit, lowest-risk combination of pharmacotherapeutic agents, in conjunction with mechanical revascularization techniques. Outcome-enhancing choices among myriad pharmacotherapeutic options for ACS are evolving at an extremely rapid pace. Unfortunately, even in the face of new investigational data, it is frequently difficult to compare clinical trials, because trigger points for PCI and entry criteria for specific treatment modalities differ slightly among the trials, and head-to-head comparisons may be lacking.

Moreover, because so many combinations of LMWH, GP IIb/IIIa inhibitors, fibrinolytic agents—with and without PCI—are possible for any ACS syndrome, it is unlikely that a "definitive" combination of specific agents will emerge that can conclusively be shown to provide the best results. In addition, each subgroup of patients with ACS—those with NSTEMI, UA, or T-segment elevation AMI—may eventually have a unique cocktail of anti-thrombin, anti-platelet, and anti-fibrin agents best suited for a specific patient population.

With these limitations in mind, a practical, heat-of-battle critical pathway of care for patients with acute coronary syndromes is presented in the ACS Treatment Pathway. *(Please see Figure 1.)* Although this pathway is based primarily upon the ACC/AHA guidelines, some modifications, updates, and refinments have been made, particularly as they relate to the role of the LMWH, enoxaparin, vs. unfractionated heparin (UFH) and the relative indications of specific GP IIb/IIIa inhibitors. As would be expected, the standard, time-honored, clinically proven agents used for management of ACS—among them, aspirin, beta-blockers, NTG, and analgesics—have been incorporated into the pathway.

Certain components of ACS management are, put simply, mandatory. For example, there is little debate about the importance of giving aspirin as soon as a patient is felt to have a possible or definite ACS. This occurs at the very beginning of our critical pathway. It also is important that patients with a possible or definite ACS have an ECG immediately upon arrival. Major treatment decisions and the critical pathways to be followed are based upon the results of the ECG. Risk stratification using observation, cardiac monitoring, serial ECGs, cardiac markers, and clinical response must be done for patients who don't have initial ECG changes. This evaluation can be performed in various settings, including the emergency department.

It is recognized that many treatment decisions will be made by local consultants, particularly relative to the role of PCI. However, emergency medicine providers must be aware of the general approach to management so optimal initial care is provided. It also is recognized that the use and timing of PCI in the setting of unstable angina and NSTEMI is very controversial and that the decision will often vary among the institutions and cardiologists involved. The same can be said for the role of PCI vs. thrombolysis inpatients with ST-segment elevation myocardial infarction. Depending on the setting, assessment of ventricular function and/or stress testing could be done by emergency medicine providers as a part of a local comprehensive program.

Low Molecular Weight Heparins—Enoxaparin. The precise indications for and potential advantage of LMWHs in patients with ACS is a somewhat controversial area that is in a state of flux. In this vein, the ACC/AHA guidelines for unstable angina and NSTEMI present a somewhat mixed message in their prioritization of LMWHs vs. UFH. First, although the document provides figures demonstrating superiority data for enoxaparin in UA and NSTEMI, when issuing recommendations for use of LMWH in ACS, the guidelines lump all LMWHs together. Specifically, the ACC/AHA guidelines suggest that heparin or a LMWH (in this order) may be used in high-risk patients. However, within the text of the document, they state that a "LMWH can be substituted advantageously" for heparin. The term "advantageously" would seem to reflect superiority data, despite their recommendation that heparin be used over LMWHs.

The guidelines appropriately indicate that it is somewhat difficult to draw conclusions about the relative efficacy of one LMWH vs. the others, and that head-to-head trials are the only conclusive way to settle this issue. However, the ESSENCE and TIMI-11b data, in the defined high-risk populations they studied, both clearly demonstrated superiority of enoxaparin over heparin for the composite end points of death, AMI, and recurrent angina. It has been argued the reason enoxaparin trials demonstrated superiority, as opposed to the FRIC and FRAXIS trials that did not show superiority of other LMWHs over UFH, is because of differences in trial populations and study designs. For example, it is argued that the ESSENCE and TIMI-11b populations were at higher risk than in the other trials and that the magnitude of benefit in randomized trials is generally greater in patients at high risk compared with those at low risk. Patients in these trials were at higher risk because: 1) they had to present within 24 hours of the chest pain episode while those in FRIC and FRAXIS presented in 72 and 48 hours, respectively; and 2) the definition of AMI was softer than in FRIC and FRAXIS.

However, patients with chest pain and a history of CAD were included in ESSENCE and TIMI-11b. Many of the patients in these trials did not have elevation of markers or ECG changes. Conversely, patients in the FRIC and FRAXIS trials had to have ECG changes, which could reflect a higher risk group. The point is that while arguments relative to design and population are endless, the data for the high-risk population defined in the ESSENCE and TIMI-11b trials clearly reflect enoxaparin superiority to heparin. Interestingly, in their analysis of the LMWHs, the ACC/AHA guidelines for AMI state that "enoxaparin for the acute management of patients with unstable angina/non-Q wave MI has been shown to be superior to heparin for reducing death and serious cardiac ischemic events. This superiority is achieved without an increase in the rate of either spontaneous or instrumented major hemorrhage." Consequently, from a practical, clinical perspective, enoxaparin, specifically and uniquely, can and should be substituted "advantageously" for heparin in unstable angina and NSTEMI. Data for substituting other LMWHs "advantageously" for heparin simply do not exist, and it is somewhat curious that this distinction was not emphasized in the "advantageous" designation advocating LMWH substitution for UFH

Despite the evidence-based support of enoxaparin superiority the ACC/AHA guideline issues a potential cautionary note concerning use of LMWHs in the setting of PCI because of the theoretical risk of increasing bleeding complications that may be associated with prolonged anticoagulation. The authors of the ACC/AHA document appropriately noted that enoxaparin was stopped 6-12 hours prior to PCI in ESSENCE and TIMI-11b, and therefore, it was difficult to draw conclusions regarding its safety in the PCI patient population.

Enoxaparin Safety in PCI. It should be stressed that the recommendations of the ACC/AHA document were generated prior to very recent studies, all of which suggest that enoxaparin can be used safely, without a heparin window, in the peri-PCI setting. As previously mentioned, the NICE-3 trial assessed the incidence of bleeding during catheterization in 661 patients with ACS, all of whom received enoxaparin plus a GP IIb/IIIa inhibitor (either abciximab, eptifibatide, or tirofiban).[31] At the time of catheterization, enoxaparin (0.3 mg/kg intravenously) was administered if more than eight hours had elapsed since the last subcutaneous dose. NICE-3 provides compelling data that enoxaparin in combination with the different GP IIb/IIIa inhibitors produces similar clinical outcomes and bleeding frequency when compared to these end points reported in the large GP IIb/IIIa inhibitor trials.[31] Put simply, NICE-3 suggests enoxaparin plus GP IIb/IIIa inhibitors is as safe as UFH plus GP IIb/IIIa inhibitors in the setting of ACS and PCI, a finding that should be applied clinically as indicated.

In addition, the NICE-4 trial combined enoxaparin with abciximab during PCI. Enoxaparin was given as a 0.75 mg/kg intravenous bolus while abciximab was administered in its usual fashion. Data from the first 310 patients reveal the incidence of major non-CABG bleeding and transfusion to be 0.6%, which compared favorably with the 2.7% occurring in patients receiving abciximab and low-dose heparin in the EPILOG trial.[28] It must be recognized that minor, but not major bleeding, does occur more frequently with enoxaparin. Based on enoxaparin superiority in UA/NSTEMI as compared to heparin, as well as recent confirmation of safety as it relates to bleeding complications (NICE-3 and NICE-4) in PCI, the guidelines in this review prioritize enoxaparin as the preferred anti-thrombin agent in UA/NSTEMI patients, including those with PCI.

In the setting of ST-segment elevation myocardial infarction, the ACC/AHA AMI guidelines recommend heparin for patients undergoing PCI or surgical revascularization or for patients undergoing reperfusion therapy with alteplase. However, the preliminary results of 700 patients in the HART II and Menown trials reflected excellent efficacy and safety of enoxaparin in comparison to heparin. In addition, more than 1600 patients were involved in trials discussed above involving peri-procedural use of enoxaparin in ACS, also reflecting efficacy and safety. Our guidelines reflect that enoxaparin can be used as an alternative in patients with ST-segment elevation myocardial infarction who are receiving thrombolysis or a PCI.

GP IIb/IIIa inhibitors. The GP IIb/IIIa inhibitors are recommended for all patients with high-risk unstable angina/NSTEMI by the ACC/AHA guidelines. Our guidelines reflect a more specified

Figure 1. Guidelines for Outcome-Effective Treatment of Acute Coronary Syndromes

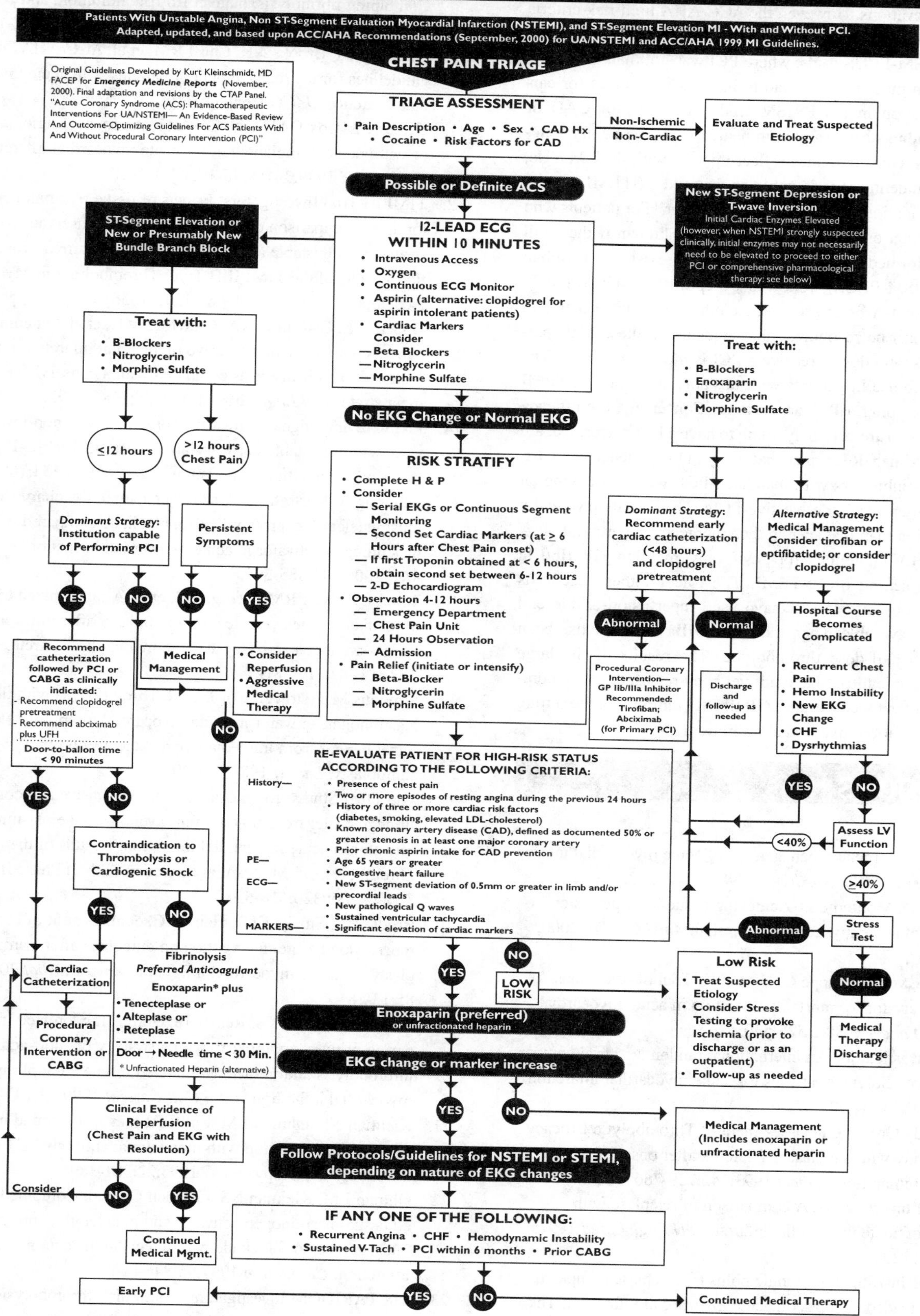

population. According to the ACC/AHA guidelines, patients can be high-risk because of either previous history of CAD, physical exam evidence of heart failure in the setting of ischemia, ECG changes, or cardiac marker elevations. However, the ACC/AHA high-risk criteria were not the inclusion criteria for the the PURSUIT, PARAGON, PRISM, and PRISM-PLUS trials, where PCI was not mandated.

The patients in these trials all had to have ECG changes (or cardiac marker elevation in the PRISM trial). A history of CAD or physical exam findings consistent with heart failure were entry criteria for these trials. Our guidelines reflect this. As with the LMWHs, the ACC/AHA guidelines for unstable angina and NSTEMI use the generic recommendation of a "GP IIb/IIIa inhibitor." For patients who have unstable angina or NSTEMI, where it is unknown if they will have a PCI performed, the best efficacy data exist for tirofiban (PRISM and PRISM-PLUS), followed by eptifibatide (PURSUIT). These are the patients who are seen in the emergency department.

However, it must be recognized that evidence in these trials pertaining to patients who do not receive a PCI is much less robust. The data for abciximab use in patients with unstable angina or NSTEMI who are not undergoing a PCI are lacking. Conversely, the efficacy data, for patients who are definitely going to have a PCI performed, are excellent for abciximab. Recognize that many of the patients, in the trials of GP IIb/IIIa inhibitors with mandated PCI, were not having an ACS and were often receiving elective PCIs. These trials involved a different population than that seen in the emergency department.

The ACC/AHA guidelines for AMI only mention GP IIb/IIIa inhibitors in the setting of NSTEMI. The role for these agents is evolving. Data from studies that have used reperfusion as the end point have been favorable when the GP IIb/IIIa inhibitor has been combined with a half-dose thrombolytic. The results of the large GUSTO 4 AMI clinical trial have not yet been released. Our recommendations do not yet incorporate a GP IIb/IIIa inhibitor in the setting of ST-segment elevation myocardial infarction.

References

1. Hayes OW. Emergency management of acute myocardial infarction. *Emerg Med Clin North Am* 1998;16:542-563.
2. Mukherjee D, Moliterno D. Achieving tissue-level perfusion in the setting of acute myocardial infarction. *Am J Cardiol* 2000; 85:39C-46C.
3. Wilcox RG, von der Lippe G, Olsson G. Trial of tissue plasminogen activator for mortality reduction in acute myocardial infarction. *Lancet* 1988;2:525-530.
4. GUSTO Investigators. An international randomized trial comparing four thrombolytic strategies for acute myocardial infarction. *N Engl J Med* 1993;329:673-682.
5. LATE Study Group. Late assessment of Thrombolytic Efficacy (LATE) study with alteplase 6-24 hours after onset of acute myocardial infarction. *Lancet* 1993;342:759-766.
6. GUSTOIII Investigators. A comparison of reteplase with alteplase for acute myocardial infarction. *N Engl J Med* 1997; 337:1118-1123.
7. ASSENT-2 Investigators. Single bolus tenecteplase compared with front-loaded alteplase in acute myocardial infarction: The ASSENT-2 double-blind randomized trial. *Lancet* 1999;354: 716-722.
8. Stone GW. Primary stenting in acute myocardial infarction. *Circulation* 1998;97:2482-2485.
9. Herrmann H. Triple therapy for acute myocardial infarction: Combining fibrinolysis, platelet IIb/IIIa inhibition, and percutaneous coronary intervention. *Am J Cardiol* 2000;85:10c-16c.
10. Antman EM, Brooks NH, Califf RM, et al. ACC/AHA Guidelines for the management of patients with acute myocardial infarction. *JACC* 1999;34:890-911.
11. Grines CL, Cox DA, Stone GW, et al. Coronary angioplasty with or without stent implantation for acute myocardial infarction. *N Engl J Med* 1999;341:1949-1956.
12. TIMI III Trial Investigators. Effects of tissue plasminogen activator and a comparison of early invasive and conservative strategies in unstable angina and non-Q-Wave myocardial infarction: results of the TIMI IIIB Trial: Thrombolysis in Myocardial Ischemia. *Circulation* 1999;89:1545-1556.
13. Boden WE, O'Rourke RA, Crawford MH, et al. Outcomes in patients with acute non-Q-wave myocardial infarction randomly assigned to an invasive as compared with a conservative management strategy. *N Engl J Med* 1998;338:1785-1792.
14. FRISC II Investigators. Invasive compared with non-invasive treatment in unstable coronary-artery disease: FRISC-II prospective randomized multicentre study. *Lancet* 1999;354:708-715.
15. Schomig A, Kastrati A, Dirschinger J, et al. Coronary stenting plus platelet glycoprotein IIb/IIIa blockade compared with tissue plasminogen activator in acute myocardial infraction. *N Engl J Med* 2000;343:385-391.
16. Topol EJ, Califf RM, George BS, et al. A randomized trial of immediate vs. delayed elective angioplasty after intravenous tissue plasminogen activator in acute myocardial infarction. *N Engl J Med* 1987;317:581-588.
17. Simoons M, Betriu A, Col J, et al. Thrombolysis with tissue plasminogen activator in acute myocardial infarction: No additional benefit from immediate percutaneous coronary angioplasty. *Lancet* 1988;197-202.
18. The TIMI Study group. Comparison of invasive and conservative strategies after treatment with intravenous tissue plasminogen activator in acute myocardial infarction: Results of the Thrombolysis in Myocardial Infarction (TIMI) Phase II. *N Engl J Med* 1989;320:618-627.
19. Brodie BR, Stuckey TD, Hansen C, et al. Benefit of coronary reperfusion before intervention on outcomes after primary angioplasty for acute myocardial infarction. *Am J Cardiol* 2000; 85:13-18.
20. Ross AM, Coyne KS, Reiner JS, et al. A randomized trial comparing primary angioplasty with a strategy of short-acting thrombolysis and immediate planned rescue angioplasty in acute myocardial infarction. *J Am Coll Cardiol* 1999;34:1954-1962.
21. Kleiman NS, Ohman EM, Califf RM, et al. Profound inhibition of platelet aggregation with monoclonal antibody 7E3 fab after thrombolytic therapy. *JACC* 1993;22:381-389.
22. Ohman EM, Kleiman NS, Gacioch G, et al. Combined accelerated tissue-plasminogen activator and platelet glycoprotein IIb/IIIa integrin receptor blockade with integrilin in acute myocardial infarction. *Circulation* 1997;95:846-854.
23. The PARIDGM Investigators. Combining thrombolysis with the platelet glycoprotein IIb/IIIa inhibitor lamifiban: Results of the Platelet Aggregation Receptor Antagonist Dose Investigation and

Reperfusion Gain in Myocardial Infarction (PARIDGM) trial. *J Am Coll Cardiol* 1998;32:2003-2010.

24. Antman EM, Giugliano RP, Gibson CM, et al. Abciximab facilitates the rate and extent of thrombolysis. *Circulation* 1999; 2720-2732.
25 SPEED Group. Trial of abciximab with and without low-dose reteplase for acute myocardial infarction. *Circulation* 2000;2788-2794.
26. Brener SJ, Barr LA, Burchenal JEB, et al. Randomized, placebo-controlled trial of platelet glycoprotein IIb/IIIa blockade with primary angioplasty for acute myocardial infarction. *Circulation* 1998;98:734-741.
27. Montalscot G, Barragan P, Wittenberg O, et al. Abciximab associated with primary angioplasty and stenting in acute myocardial infarction: The ADMIRAL study, 30-day final results. *Circulation* 1999;100(Suppl I):1-87.
28. Kereiakes D, Fry E, Matthai W, et al. Combination enoxaparin and abciximab therapy during percutaneous coronary intervention: "NICE guys finish first". *J Invas Cardiol* 2000;12(Suppl A):1A-5A.
29. Ross A. A randomized comparison of low molecular weight heparin and unfractionated heparin adjunctive to T-PA thrombolysis and aspirin. 4th Annual Session American College Cardiology. Anaheim, 2000.
30. Menown I, Baird SH, McBride SJ, et al. Evaluation of low-molecular-weight heparin in patients receiving fibrinolytic therapy for acute myocardial infarction. *Eur Heart J* 2000;21:599-599.
31. Ferguson JJ. NICE-3 prospective, open label, non-randomized observational safety study on the combination of LMW heparin with the clinically available IIb/IIIa antagonists in 600 patients with acute coronary syndromes. *Eur Heart J* 2000;21:599.
32. Collet JP, Montalscot G, Lison L, et al. Percutaneous coronary intervention in unstable angina patients pretreated with subcutaneous enoxaparin. *Eur Heart J* 2000;21:599-599.
33. Dudek D, Zymek P, Bartus S, et al. Prospective randomized comparison of enoxaparin vs. unfractionated heparin for elective percutaneous coronary interventions among ticlopidine-pretreated patients. *Eur Heart J* 2000;21:381-381.
34. Cohen M. Low molecular weight heparins in the management of unstable angina/non-Q-wave myocardial infarction. *Thrombo Haemosta* 1999;25(Suppl 3):113-121.
35. Antman EM, Beasley JW, Califf RM, et al. ACC/AHA guidelines for the management of patients with unstable angina and non-ST-segment elevation myocardial infarction. *J Am Col Cardiol* 2000; 36(3):970-1062.
36. Ryan TJ, Anderson JL, Antman EM, et al. 1999 Update: ACC/AHA guidelines for the management of patients with acute myocardial infarction. *J Am Coll Cardiol* 1999;34:890.
37. Ryan TJ, Anderson JL, Antman EM, et al. ACC/AHA: ACC/AHA guidelines for the management of patients with acute myocardial infarction: Executive summary. *Circulation* 1996; 94:2341.
38. The GUSTO IIb Angioplasty Substudy Investigators: A clinical trial comparing primary coronary angioplasty with tissue plasminogen activator for acute myocardial infarction. *N Engl J Med* 1997;336:1621.

Diagnosis and Management of Decompensated Heart Failure

Santosh G. Menon, MD
Roger M. Mills, Jr., MD

Congestive heart failure (CHF) is one of the top discharge diagnoses from acute hospitals in this country. It also accounts for a large percentage of readmissions to the hospital. In the elderly populations seeing primary care physicians, CHF is a common condition and is associated with significant morbidity and mortality. This chapter deals with the major pharmacological and surgical interventions found to be useful in the management of CHF and ranks these interventions in light of recent scientific clinical studies. Although not specifically addressed in this issue, patient compliance with salt and fluid restriction has always been a hallmark of treatment. One modality that has been rediscovered to help reduce the readmission rate to the hospital is daily weights. One U.S. hospital with arguably the lowest readmission rates for CHF employed a simple and inexpensive strategy—it provided easily readable scales for its CHF patients. The patients were carefully instructed to record morning weights and were empowered to take certain actions when the targeted dry weight ranges were exceeded. Readmission rates were dramatically reduced—a happy outcome for patient, physician, and managed care.

Definition of the Problem

Every year nearly 400,000 people in the United States experience the onset of congestive heart failure (CHF).[1] Of the 4.7 million people with CHF (1.5% of the total U.S. population), 900,000 will be hospitalized each year for exacerbation of their CHF. The cost of caring for these patients exceeds $6 billion annually. The total expenditure for heart failure treatment (DRG127) is nearly 5% of the total clinical expenditures of Health Care Financing Administration (HCFA).[8] In patients older than 65 years, CHF is the most common diagnosis-related group (DRG). It is the fourth leading cause of hospitalizations in U.S. adults.[7]

Heart failure is a syndrome associated with aging. As the U.S. population ages, both the incidence and prevalence of CHF will increase. The prevalence of CHF in those older than age 75 years is nearly 10%,[6] and chronic heart failure is characterized by a markedly reduced life expectancy.[2] In the face of these vast numbers, the present number of 2000 heart transplants in the United States per year cannot offer any meaningful effect, no matter how successful it may be for individual patients. Cardiologists deliver only a small fraction of heart failure care; most patients with heart failure see general internists or family physicians for management. The enormous expense, intense regulatory interest, and dire prognosis of CHF have prompted us to review state-of-the-art management of CHF for primary care physicians. First, we will briefly review the pathophysiology. We will then comment on newer diagnostic studies in patients with coronary artery disease. Finally, we will look at new and established pharmacologic strategies for management.

Pathophysiology of Congestive Heart Failure

Congestive heart failure occurs when the heart is unable to generate an adequate forward cardiac output to meet the metabolic needs of the body at normal filling pressures. When the cardiac output is limited due to left ventricular dysfunction, several neurohormonal mechanisms respond in an attempt to restore or maintain blood flow to meet the metabolic demand. This neurohormonal activation of this system is not only compensatory in nature, but also detrimental.

Neuroendocrine Activation: During the early stages of CHF, a complex sequence of neurohormonal changes takes place. Activation of peripheral receptors by the hypoperfusion due to the inadequate intravascular volume is characteristic of systolic heart failure. Initially, these compensatory mechanisms include activation of the renin-angiotensin-aldosterone axis, heightened adrenergic drive, and augmented release of vasopressin; these mechanisms help to maintain perfusion to vital organs and increase the reduced intra-arterial volume. The extravascular volume expansion, increased peripheral vascular resistance, and tachycardia produced by the neurohormonal response translates into: 1) hemodynamic abnormalities including elevated filling pressures, increased pulmonary artery pressures, and increased pulmonary capillary wedge pressure; and 2) remodeling of the heart with hypertrophy, dilatation, compensatory mitral regurgitation, and increased wall tension. As heart failure becomes chronic, these compensatory mechanisms are deleterious in that they cause excessive vasoconstriction, increased afterload, arrhythmias, sodium and fluid retention, and electrolyte abnormalities. Some of these effects are counteracted by release of atrial and ventricular naturetic peptides (ANP and VNP) in response to cardiac distention. The naturetic peptides, however, usually do not restore the situation to normal. Increased sympathetic activity is documented by the elevation of plasma and urine adrenergic norepinephrine (NE) in patients with CHF. Plasma levels in CHF patients at rest are two- to three-fold higher than in normal subjects at rest.[9] Twenty-four hour urinary NE excretion also is markedly elevated in patients with CHF.[10] The elevated NE levels result from a combination of increased release of NE from adrenergic nerve endings and the consequent "spillover" into plasma. The increased spillover of NE into the plasma from cardiac tissue is attributable to increased rates of sympathetic nerve firing. The severity of the left ventricular dysfunction correlates directly with the plasma NE level.[9] Ventricular tissue NE, conversely, is decreased in patients with CHF and correlates inversely with the plasma norepinephrine level.

In the milieu of elevated circulating catecholamines, Camici and associates confirmed down-regulation of beta-adrenergic receptors in the heart. They showed that the degree of down regulation was proportional to the severity of the heart failure.[13] Of the two types of beta-receptors in the heart (beta-1 and beta-2), beta-1 receptor down-regulation is most evident possibly because of the local action of elevated plasma NE levels.

As outlined above, impaired cardiac output leads to the activation of the renin-angiotensin system. The major stimulus for the release of renin from the juxtaglomerular apparatus appears to be stimulation of beta-1 adrenoreceptors by the elevated plasma NE levels. Reduction in renal flow also activates baroreceptors in the kidney, which leads to release of renin. Elevated plasma renin activity (PRA) can be demonstrated in most patients with CHF, leading to elevations in Angiotensin II, a potent vasoconstrictor. Importantly for preventive strategies, both symptomatic and asymptomatic CHF patients show elevated Angiotensin-II levels.[13] Angiotensin II increases afterload by its vasoconstrictor action; it also enhances the release of NE and facilitates sodium and water retention.

Arginine vasopressin (AVP) is a pituitary hormone that regulates free water clearance and plasma osmolality. Patients with CHF, especially those who develop CHF after an acute myocardial infarction, have elevated levels of AVP. Levels are higher in more symptomatic patients as compared to levels in asymptomatic patients. In contrast to normal physiology, secretion of AVP is not inhibited by a reduction in osmolality in CHF patients. This altered regulatory physiology may contribute to the inability to excrete free water in advanced heart failure, perhaps accounting for the serum hypo-osmolarity in some patients.

Although neurohormonal activation initially counteracts the effect of a low cardiac output by maintaining perfusion to the vital organs, chronic vasoconstriction and fluid retention has deleterious effects that tend to make the heart failure worse. Several changes take place in the myocardium in patients with CHF, such as apoptosis, which can be initiated by several factors, including: increased cytosolic free calcium levels, hypoxia, and muscle stretch. This process may play a crucial role in the development of CHF. Genetic studies have shown that 20% of dilated cardiomyopathy cases are familial.[39] Modern pharmacotherapy of CHF has shifted from dealing with the consequences of neurohormonal activation to blocking these neurohormonal effects with drugs such as angiotensin converting enzyme inhibitors (ACEIs), angiotensin II receptor blockers, and beta-blockers. Table 1 lists non-ischemic causes of CHF.

Work-Up of a Patient with CHF

Before initiating therapy, physicians must recognize that CHF is a non-specific syndrome that requires careful evaluation to: a) confirm that CHF is present; and b) clarify the etiology. Steps for evaluating a patient are outlined below.

History and Physical Examination: This is a vital part of the evaluation of any patient who presents with CHF.

Exercise intolerance, primarily manifested by subjective dyspnea, is the hallmark of heart failure and is often the first symptom. It is very important to differentiate dyspnea due to CHF from other causes of shortness of breath such as COPD, asthma, etc. Other, more advanced symptoms of CHF include orthopnea, paroxysmal nocturnal dyspnea, edema (which usually indicates the presence of right heart failure but also may be secondary to medications [e.g., calcium channel blockers]), cough (which may be secondary to CHF or due to side-effects of the medications including ACEI), fatigue and weakness usually due to a low flow state, nocturia, and oliguria caused by the redistribution of blood flow with an increase in the renal blood flow in the supine position. Chest pain, which may indicate obstructive coronary artery disease (CAD), also may occur in the absence of obstructive CAD in patients with pulmonary hypertension, valvular heart disease, or cardiomyopathy. Gastrointestinal complaints, including vomiting, malabsorption, protein-losing enteropathy, and hepatic dysfunction, usually occur with right heart failure. Neurologic symptoms include faintness and syncope, which may reflect hypotension or arrhythmias.

The physical examination should assess the severity and possibly the cause of the heart failure. Resting tachycardia, elevated jugular venous pressure, an S_3 gallop, rales, and peripheral edema suggest severe CHF with total body fluid overload. Other signs of severe compromise often overlooked include cool extremities caused by a low cardiac output and subsequent peripheral vasoconstriction and mild confusion (especially in the elderly). When the heart failure is longstanding and severe, patients may become cachectic. Cardiac cachexia also may be mistaken for malignancy. Protein-losing enteropathy, reduced caloric intake, increased caloric expenditure due to the excessive work of breathing, and markedly increased tumor necrosis factor (TNFα) levels may all play a role in the pathogenesis of cachexia.

Ancillary Testing: Table 2 lists a number of useful initial diagnostic tests for patients with CHF. Two-dimensional and Doppler echocardiography provide a tremendous amount of information. Routine echocardiography will demonstrate conditions, such as valvular heart disease or hypertrophic cardiomyopathy (IHSS), which may be the cause of the CHF. Transesophageal echcocardiography (TEE) is usually reserved for those patients in whom an initial transthoracic study was sub-optimal. However, identification of valvular vegetations or intracardiac thrombus can be done with much greater accuracy with TEE. Radionuclide angiography (first-pass and gated equilibrium) allows quantification of ejection fractions (EF) but does not give the wealth of physiologic information available from a carefully performed echocardiogram. Other diagnostic studies that should be done in patients with CHF include: complete blood count (CBC); iron studies, especially in patients who have dilated cardiomyopathy; a urinalysis to look for the presence of nephrotic syndrome; serum electrolytes; TSH (especially in patients with atrial fibrillation and CHF); and ECG. As indicated below, patients with angina or large areas of ischemic or hibernating myocardium, cardiac catheterization is warranted.[19] Right heart catheterization will help in tailoring the management. Right ventricular endomyocardial biopsy can be used to confirm the presence of infiltrative diseases such as amyloid, sarcoid, hemochromatosis, or acute myocarditis, but it is rarely indicated otherwise.[19] Twenty-four-hour Holter monitoring can be done to look for arrhythmias or silent myocardial ischemia. To help differentiate a cardiac cause from a pulmonary cause of shortness of breath, a VO_{2max} (O_2 consumption) can be done.

CHF due to Coronary Artery Disease (CAD)

CHF Secondary to Coronary Artery Disease. In the United States, probably 40% of all CHF patients have CAD, and patients who develop CHF secondary to coronary artery disease have a significantly worse prognosis when compared to patients who have a non-ischemic cause of their heart failure, despite appropriate medical treatment with vasodilators, beta-blockers, etc.

Ischemia due to inadequate coronary blood flow results in myocellular hypoxia. This hypoxia leads to cellular and biochemical damage to the myocyte. Coronary flow occurs mostly in diastole. When the left ventricular end diastolic pressure (LVEDP) is elevated, the diastolic flow is reduced and further worsens myocardial ischemia. Diastolic dysfunction appears to be the most sensitive to ischemia. Myocardial relaxation can be impaired within 20 seconds of coronary occlusion, making it one the first manifestations of myocardial ischemia.

Table 1. Non-Ischemic Causes of CHF

1. Hypertension
2. Familial idiopathic
3. Diabetes mellitus
4. Longstanding hypothyroidism
5. Pheochromocytoma
6. Chronic alcohol abuse
7. Heavy metals:
   - Iron (hemochromatosis)
   - Arsenic
   - Lead
   - Cobalt
8. Infectious/Post-infectious:
   - Viral: coxsackievirus, adenovirus
   - Bacterial: tuberculosis
   - Rickettsia: typhus, Q-fever
   - Protozoal: Chagas, malaria
   - Post-streptococcal infection/Rheumatic fever and valvular disease
   - Pulmonary hypertension and right heart failure secondary to schistosomiasis
9. Neuromuscular disease:
   - Fredriech's ataxia
   - Myasthenia gravis
   - Limb-girdle dystrophy of Erb
   - Duchenne muscular dystrophy
10. Toxins:
    - Carbon monoxide
    - Amphetamines
    - Cocaine
    - Anthracyclines
    - Cyclophospamide
    - Radiation (can cause valvular lesions, pericardial disease, and severe epicardial coronary artery disease)
11. Miscellaneous acquired:
    - Peripartum cardiomyopathy
    - Obesity
    - Prolonged tachycardia
    - Giant cell myocarditis

Myocardial Stunning. Myocardial stunning occurs after either a single or multiple brief episodes of coronary insufficiency. There is essentially a downregulation of myocardial function in response to the low blood flow. The stunned myocardium contracts normally when stimulated with inotropes. Also, following lytic therapy, there is a latent period of a few days to a few weeks after which the stunned myocardium will recover function. Over time, stunned myocardium will recover function without any sort of intervention.

Hibernating Myocardium. Hibernating myocardium occurs when there is a reduction of coronary perfusion, which leads to persistent left ventricular dysfunction. Studies have shown that ventricular function can be improved by restoring flow. The reduction in myocardial function is thought to be secondary to reduced tissue oxygen

Table 2. Recommended Tests for Patients with Suspected CHF

1. Electrocardiogram†
2. Complete blood count (CBC)‡
3. Urinalysis±
4. Serum creatinine@
5. Serum albumin§
6. T4 and TSH*
7. Echocardiogram
8. Right and left heart catheterization (if indicated)

† Look for: myocardial ischemia/old myocardial infarction, arrhythmias (atrial fibrillation—look for thyroid disease) left ventricular hypertrophy (consider diastolic dysfunction).

‡ Look for: anemia (reduced oxygen carrying capacity, which may worsen CHF)

± Proteinuria—suggestive of nephrotic syndrome

@ Volume overload may be due to renal failure

§ Hypoalbuminemia may worsen peripheral edema due to excess extravascular volume

* Hypo- as well as hyperthyroidism may cause or exacerbate CHF

delivery. Other features of hibernating myocardium may include remodeling without necrosis, as demonstrated by Smart et al.[15]

Evaluation for Hibernating Myocardium. Heart failure patients with coronary artery disease must be evaluated for possible myocardial viability in areas of hypoperfusion. A search for a history of ongoing angina or angina-equivalent (i.e., shortness of breath, dyspnea on exertion) is vital when evaluating a patient with CHF thought to be secondary to coronary artery disease. Patients with severe left ventricular dysfunction (ejection fractions < 20%) may show significant improvement in functional status and ejection fraction after revascularization of hibernating myocardium, either with CABG or balloon angioplasty (PTCA).[18]

Thallium (^{201}TI) scintigraphy and dobutamine echocardiography (DSE) are widely available and useful for identifying viable myocardium in patients with CHF secondary to coronary artery disease.[16-17] However, 23% of dysfunctional segments showing severely reduced ^{201}Tl uptake at four-hour redistribution improve after revascularization. Thus, a four-hour redistribution study may not be adequate to detect hibernating myocardium, but a 24-hour study may be able to detect viable myocardium in those patients who initially had fixed defects at four hours. Both the thallium uptake and dobutamine echo are of comparable sensitivity and specificity for the diagnosis of hibernating myocardium. The "gold standard" for detecting hibernating myocardium is positron emission tomography (PET scan), which is costly and not widely available, due to the expense of the equipment. Technetium -99m sestamibi is of value in measuring ventricular function and detecting ischemia but appears to be of lesser value in assessing myocardial viability.

Treatment of CHF

Once the diagnosis of CHF has been made and the severity of heart failure ascertained, then treatment should be begun immediately. The following discussion will be divided into the medical and surgical managements of CHF.

Medical Management of CHF

ACE Inhibitors. These are the first-line drugs in patients with CHF. Most, if not all, patients with symptomatic or asymptomatic left ventricular dysfunction should be started on ACE inhibitors unless contraindicated. In clinical trials in patients with symptomatic and asymptomatic CHF, ACEIs have been shown to reduce morbidity and mortality, improve quality of life, decrease hospitalizations, and prevent progression to a more severe disease. The Cooperative North Scandinavian Enalapril Survival Study (CONSENSUS) showed improved survival in patients treated with enalapril for advanced CHF (NYHA Class IV).[20] There was no significant reduction in mortality from sudden death. The improvement in mortality of 28% was due to a reduction in the progression of the heart failure. This study was terminated before completion because of the significant benefit of enalapril on survival, and it was felt to be unjustified to continue the study for ethical reasons.

In patients who are asymptomatic (Class I NYHA), enalapril has been shown to reduce hospitalizations for heart failure and shows a trend toward reduced mortality from CHF. Enalapril had no effect on sudden death when compared to placebo.[21]

When compared to the vasodilator combination of hydralazine-isosorbide dinitrate, enalapril decreased mortality by 11%. The benefit was greatest during the first two years of therapy.[22] The benefit during the first two years was thought to be secondary to a reduction in the risk of sudden death in patients treated with enalapril. This was seen mostly in patients who were mildly symptomatic or those who had asymptomatic left ventricular dysfunction (NYHA Class I, II). The hydralazine/isosorbide dinitrate combination resulted in a significantly greater improvement in ejection fraction during the initial 13 weeks.

Ramapril, in the AIRE study, showed a 27% reduction in mortality when compared to placebo in patients with symptomatic heart failure following an acute myocardial infarction.[23] The Survival and Ventricular Enlargement (SAVE) trial was a study that tested captopril vs. placebo in patients with LV systolic dysfunction following acute myocardial infarction.[24] Those patients who were randomized to captopril experienced a 19% reduction in the risk of death from all causes and a 22% reduction in the risk of hospitalization for heart failure. Trandolapril, in the TRACE study, was found to reduce all-cause mortality by 22% and sudden death by 24%.[25]

ACEI may be started concomitant with diuretics for volume overload. Patients should not be volume depleted due to over-diuresis (orthostatic hypotension, prerenal azotemia, or metabolic alkalosis). If this occurs, then it would prudent to stop the diuretics for 24-48 hours prior to starting ACEI. Patients should be monitored closely for first-dose hypotension. This is more common in the elderly and those who have a low serum sodium. These patients should be given a smaller starting dose and titrated up slowly. Patients should be followed closely once an ACEI has been initiated. Serum potassium should be checked within one week of initiation; if the level is greater than 5.5 mEq/L, then the ACEI may need to be stopped. Some patients will have an increase in their serum creatinine after being started on ACEI. If the serum creatinine increases by more than 0.5 mg/dL, stopping the ACEI should be considered. Those patients who do not tolerate ACEI should be tried on the combination of hydralazine and isosorbide dinitrate. Changing therapeutic regimens should be seriously considered in patients who develop hyperkalemia or significant elevation in the creatinine. The dose of ACEI should be titrated up over 2-3 weeks, with the goal of reaching the doses used in large-scale clinical trials.[26] In patients who become hypovolemic as a result of diuresis, the diuretic dose should be reduced, and, if the ACEI had been stopped, it should be restarted. If a patient fails a rechallenge with ACEI, then other vasodilators should be tried. Patients who develop a cough while on ACEI should be evaluated to see if the cough is due to heart failure before discontinuing the ACEI. In the SOLVD study, 37% of patients on ACEI developed cough,[21] but 31% of patients in the placebo group also developed cough. Patients also may develop angioedema from the ACEI, which mandates stoppage of the drug and is an absolute contraindication to further use of ACEI.

Angiotensin II Receptor Antagonists. Combination therapy of AT1 receptor antagonists and ACEI would, theoretically, lead to a more complete suppression of the renin-angiotensin system. In the ELITE study, Pitt et al compared losartan and captopril in elderly patients with CHF.[38] They found that there was a reduction in mortality and that losartan was better tolerated than captopril, in that fewer patients discontinued therapy in the losartan group. There was no difference in the incidence of renal dysfunction. Present guidelines do not recommend AT1 receptor antagonists as first-line therapy for CHF. They should be used as an additional vasodilator in patients already on maximal doses of ACEI. Studies are under way to look at the long-term benefits of this class of drugs.

Diuretics. Patients with symptoms and signs of significant fluid overload such as dyspnea on exertion (and, in severe cases, at rest), paroxysmal nocturnal dyspnea, and orthopnea with physical signs such as pulmonary rales, an S_3, jugular venous distension, and pulmonary edema on chest x-ray should receive diuretics immediately. Those with only mild signs and symptoms of CHF can be managed with thiazide diuretics, which have a less acute diuretic effect when compared to furosemide. Hydrochlorthiazide (HCTZ) should be given initially at a dose of 25-50 mg/d. If patients continue to have significant fluid overload despite 50 mg HCTZ, they should be switched to a loop diuretic such as furosemide. Furosemide should be started at a dose of about 20-40 mg daily, with a lower dose in elderly adults. Initial outpatient dosing of HCTZ should be once a day, and, if the patient does not have a significant response with improvement in symptoms, the dose should be doubled instead of adding a second dose.

When patients have signs and symptoms of marked fluid overload, they should be given intravenous furosemide. There is no standard dose of IV furosemide; it should be titrated to the volume status of the patient. Maximum dose of IV furosemide should be 240 mg/d; above this, a second diuretic should be added. Continuous infusion of furosemide at a dose of 4-16 mg/h after a loading dose can achieve greater diuresis in patients with severe CHF when compared to intermittent intravenous dosing.[18]

Diuretics can deplete serum potassium and occasionally magnesium. This effect is usually counteracted when patients are on ACEI, which tends to increase the serum potassium. Serum potassium should be checked every three days or so after initiation of therapy until the level stabilizes. A low serum potassium can aggravate ventricular arrhythmias. Serum potassium is not a very accurate indicator of total body potassium; therefore, patients with serum potassium less than 4.0 mEq/L should be given supplements or put on a potassium-sparing agent.[19] A rise in serum BUN disproportional to the creatinine usually indicates intravascular depletion and can be corrected by reducing the dose of the diuretic. In patients who are or become diuretic-resistant, a combination of diuretics can be tried (e.g., metolazone with a loop diuretic such as furosemide).

Diuretics have not shown to improved survival in CHF patients. They are ideally reserved for patients who are clinically volume overloaded. Side effects of these drugs include elevation of the renin, aldosterone, and angiotensin-II levels, gout, hyperglycemia, and dyslipidemias.

Digoxin. Cardiac glycosides are a group of drugs used for heart failure for nearly 200 years. Digoxin has been shown to improve symptoms in most patients with heart failure. Patients with mild or moderate CHF who are taken off of digoxin tended have a deterioration in exercise capacity and a reduction in the ejection fraction, when compared to similar patients who were left on the drug.[27] In the DIG trial (Digitalis Investigation Group), the investigators found that digoxin did not reduce mortality, but the drug did produce a reduction in hospitalizations and a trend toward a decrease in the risk of death attributed to worsening heart failure.[28] Digoxin, if not contraindicated, should be considered for all patients with CHF and atrial fibrillation, and most, if not all, in normal sinus rhythm. Loading doses of digoxin are not needed. If renal function is normal, a dose of 0.25 mg po daily can be started. In those patients who have renal insufficiency or in the elderly, a lower dose of 0.125 mg daily can be used. Patients should be monitored closely for symptoms of toxicity (e.g., nausea and vomiting). In symptomatic patients, digoxin should be started along with ACEI and diuretics. It is unclear if digoxin is beneficial in asymptomatic patients, since no benefit has been shown toward survival. Levels of digoxin need not be checked regularly unless there is deterioration of heart failure symptoms, worsened renal function, suspicion of toxicity, or a new medication has been added that may alter the bioavailability.

Beta-Blockers. Due to the excessive neurohormonal activation in CHF, there is uncoupling of the Beta receptors (B_1 and B_2) in the heart, with a 60-70% reduction in B_1 receptor density in patients with idiopathic dilated cardiomyopathy (IDC). In patients with post-infarction cardiomyopathy, the down-regulation of the B_1 receptors is not as severe. The changes in the adrenergic activity are seen mostly in the heart and kidney and minimally in the lungs or skeletal muscle. This excessive neurohormonal activation can have deleterious effects on the heart, including myocyte necrosis, ischemia, and lowering the arrhythmia threshold.[29] Recent studies have shown that beta-blockers are beneficial both in terms of survival and improvement in symptoms. Beta-adrenergic blockers blunt the effects of excessive neurohormonal activation on the heart and cause an up-regulation of the B_1 receptors. Beta-blockers have several beneficial effects in patients with IDC, including improved ventricular diastolic function, reduction in sudden death, reduction in heart rate, and reduction in afterload by its actions on renin.

Metoprolol was evaluated in the Metoprolol in Dilated Cardiomyopathy trial (MDC).[31] In this study, patients with IDC who were already on digitalis, diuretics, and an ACEI were randomized to receive metoprolol. Metoprolol was found to reduce the need for cardiac transplantation listing by 34%, but it had no effect on the primary end point—survival. Hospital readmissions for heart failure or arrhythmias were significantly lower in the metoprolol-treated group. There was also a significant increase in the ejection fraction and exercise tolerance in patients randomized to metoprolol.

The Cardiac Insufficiency Bisoprolol Study (CIBIS) evaluated the effect of the beta-blocker bisoprolol on mortality in patients with chronic heart failure.[32] The study found that bisoprolol improved survival in patients with IDC, when compared to placebo. There was no difference in sudden death or the incidence of ventricular tachycardia or fibrillation.

Carvedilol is a nonselective beta-adrenoreceptor antagonist with peripheral vasodilatory activity due to its adrenergic blocking activity. It also has an additional antioxidant activity, which may be beneficial in coronary ischemia syndromes. In the Multi-center Oral Carvedilol Heart Failure Assessment trial (MOCHA), low-dose (6.25 mg twice daily), medium-dose (12.5 twice daily), and high-dose (25 mg twice daily) carvedilol therapy was given to patients with moderate heart failure.[33] Carvedilol had no effects on the primary end point, submaximal exercise. The U.S. Carvedilol Heart Failure StudyGroup (US-CHF) evaluated the effects of carvedilol in patients with CHF in four various protocols.[34] Analyses of the data from this study found a 65% overall mortality reduction in the carvedilol group when compared to placebo. This led to the early termination of the study. Carvedilol, in other studies, has been reported to improve LV ejection fraction and LV end-diastolic and end-systolic dimensions, but it did not show any clear-cut improvement in symptoms of CHF.

In CHF patients who are decompensated, addition of beta-blockers may initially worsen their symptoms. Carvedilol was recently approved for the treatment of chronic heart failure, but the drug should be started when the heart failure is compensated. Standard CHF medications, including ACEI, diuretics, and digoxin should be maximized prior to initiating beta-blockers, and the lowest dose should be started (e.g., carvedilol 3.125 mg twice daily with meals). The initial dose of the drug should be given under supervision and blood pressure checked every 15 minutes for two hours. The drug can be up-titrated every two weeks, as tolerated. There may be an initial worsening of symptoms, followed by long-term improvement. Beta-adrenergic blockers should be combined with ACEI in all patients with left ventricular systolic dysfunction. If a patient decompensates while being up-titrated, then the dose of the beta-blocker can be reduced or stopped. Metoprolol should be initiated at very low doses (i.e., 6.25 mg twice daily) and titrated up over several weeks. The patient should be seen by the physician every time the drug dose is increased. Beta-blockers should be used cautiously, if at all, in patients with reactive airway disease, insulin-dependant diabetes mellitus, or peripheral vascular disease.

Positive Inotropic Agents. Oral inotropic agents, overall, have been disappointing. Enoximone, a phospodiesterase inhibitor, in the Enoximone Multicenter Trial (EMT), was found to increase mortality in patients with moderate-to-severe congestive heart failure. The drug had no effect on symptoms or exercise capacity. Milrinone, another phospho-diesterase inhibitor, in the PROMISE trial (Prospective Randomized Milrinone Survival Evaluation) was found to increase all-cause mortality by 28% and increased cardiovascular mortality by 34%.[35] This effect was greater in patients with Class IV CHF. Pimobendan, a positive inotropic agent, also was evaluated and found to increase mortality by 1.8 times when compared to placebo. Vesnarinone, a quinolone derivative, also was found to increase mortality significantly at a dose of 120 mg/d (high-dose), and this led to premature termination of the study. Ibopamine, a dopaminergic agonist, reduced plasma norepinephrine levels, and decreased renin activity; it also was found to increase mortality.

Intravenous inotropic agents including dobutamine and milrinone are useful in patients with chronic heart failure that is refractory to therapy. Current practice is to initiate intravenous inotropes on admission for most patients with decompensated CHF. Benefits of these medications include increase in diuresis and increased tolerance for higher doses of ACEI and beta-blockers. Long-term, low dose dobutamine or milrinone infusion via a central venous catheter may help improve the patient's symptoms.[40] Continuous intravenous therapy is most useful in patients who are difficult to wean off of inotropes. Milrinone, with its vasodilating activity is useful in patients with pulmonary hypertension and CHF. The advantage of milrinone over dobutamine is that rarely does a patient develop tolerance to the drug. Intermittent outpatient or inpatient therapy with IV inotropes for 24-48 hours also may improve symptoms in patients with refractory CHF who are admitted repeatedly for exacerbations.

Calcium Channel Blockers (CCBs). In theory, CCBs have the ability to reduce afterload and have anti-ischemic effects. In clinical trials, however, both diltiazem and nifedipine exacerbated CHF and possibly increased mortality in post-infarction patients with pulmonary edema or ejection fraction less than 40%.[36,37] In the PRAISE trial, amlodipine, a longer-acting dihydropyridine CCB had a survival benefit in patients with CHF. In patients with heart failure secondary to coronary artery disease, amlodipine produced neither benefit nor detriment. Mortality trials are under way to test the hypothesis that amlodipine reduces mortality in patients with idiopathic dilated cardiomyopathy. The MACH-1 trial with mibefradil, a nonvoltage regulator T-channel calcium antagonist, is currently evaluating the use of this drug in heart failure patients.[30]

On the basis of currently available evidence, amlodipine is the only CCB that might have a role in therapy of patients with CHF. The drug may be used as an adjunctive measure in addition to standard therapy to help control hypertension or otherwise intractable ischemia.

Anticoagulation. Routine anti-coagulation is not recommended for heart failure.[26] Patients who have a history of systemic embolism, pulmonary embolism, atrial fibrillation, or a mobile left-ventricular thrombi should be placed on warfarin. The prothrombin time should be 1.2-1.8 times each laboratory control (INR of 2.0-3.0).

Summary of Medical Management of CHF

Patients with CHF who are either symptomatic or asymptomatic should be started on an ACE inhibitor. Diuretics should be added if there are signs and symptoms of fluid overload. Digoxin, is most likely also beneficial in terms of improving symptoms. Angiotensin II receptor antagonists may have a role in patients who are not tolerant of ACEI due to a class-specific side-effect or in addition to ACEI. Anticoagulation with warfarin should be limited to patients with atrial fibrillation with CHF, those with documented left ventricular or left atrial clot, and those with a history of embolic stroke. Antiarrhythmics, especially amiodarone, may be beneficial in patients with a history of sudden death, syncope secondary to an arrhythmia, and documented ventricular tachycardia, but its role as prophylaxis in CHF patients remains unclear.

Newer Agents. Toborinone, an analogue of vesnarinone for parenteral use, has potent positive inotropic effects and may have a role in short-term in-patient management of CHF.

Surgical Management of CHF

In several trials, patients with moderate-to-severe LV dysfunction, angina, and multivessel disease enjoyed better survival after CABG.[41] "Stunned" or "hibernating" viable myocardium will regain function with successful revascularization.

The role of percutaneous transluminal coronary angioplasty (PTCA) in heart failure management remains unclear, but almost certainly PTCA will be employed in more patients as stent technology and antiplatelet drugs improve.

Other surgical procedures that remain experimental include ventricular volume reduction surgery with repair of the mitral valve (the "Batista" procedure), dynamic cardiomyoplasty, TMR, and chronic ventricular assist devices (VADs). A number of trials are being conducted to evaluate the safety and efficacy of these procedures.

References

1. Mark DB. Economics of treating heart failure. *Am J Cardiol* 1997;80(8B):33H-38H.
2. Massie BM, Conway M. Survival of patients with congestive heart failure: Past, present and future prospects. *Circulation* 1987;7 5(suppl IV):11-19.
3. Cohn JN, Johnson G, Ziesche S, et al. A comparison of enalapril with hydralazine-isosorbide dinitrate in the treatment of chronic congestive heart failure. *N Engl J Med* 1991;325:303-310.
4. The SOLVD investigators. Effect of enalapril on survival in patients with reduced left ventricular ejection fractions and congestive heart failure. *N Engl J Med* 1991;325:293-302.
5. Paul SD, et al. Costs and effectiveness of angiotensin converting enzyme inhibition in patients with congestive heart failure. *Arch Intern Med* 1994;154:1143-1149.
6. Kannel WB. Epidemiological aspects of heart failure. *Cardiol Clin* 1989;7:1-9.
7. Ghali JK, Cooper R, Ford E. Trends in hospitalization for heart failure in the United States, 1973-1986: Evidence for increasing population prevalence. *Arch Intern Med* 1990;150:769-773.
8. O'Connell JB, Bristow MR. Economic impact of heart failure in the United States: Time for a different approach. *J Heart Lung Transplant* 1994;13:107-112.
9. Thomas JA, Marks BH. Plasma norepinephrine in congestive heart failure. *Am J Cardiol* 1978;41:233.
10. Chidsey CA, Braunwald E, Morrow AG. Catecholamine secretion and cardiac stores of norepinephrine in congestive heart failure. *Am J Med* 1965;39:442.
11. Fowler MB, Laser JA, Hopkins GL, et al. Assessment of the beta-adrenergic receptor pathway in the intact failing human heart. *Circulation* 1986;74:1290.
12. Francis GS, Benedict C, Johnstone DE, et al. Comparison of neuroendocrine activation in patients with left ventricular dysfunction with and without congestive heart failure. A substudy of the left ventricular dysfunction (SOLVD). *Circulation* 1994;82:1724.
13. Camici PG, William W, et al. Pathophysiological mechanisms of chronic reversible left ventricular dysfunction due to coronary artery disease (Hibernating Myocardium). *Circulation* 1997;96: 3205-3214.
14. Iskandrian AS, Hakki A, et al. Rest and redistribution thallium-201 myocardial scintigraphy to predict improvement in left ventricular function after coronary artery bypass grafting. *Am J Cardiol* 1983;51:1312-1316.
15. Smart SC, Sawada S, et al. Low-dose dobutamine echocardiography detects reversible dysfunction after thrombolytic therapy of acute myocardial infarction. *Circulation* 1993;88:405-415.
16. Elefteriades JA, Tolis G Jr, et al. Coronary artery bypass grafting in severe left ventricular dysfunction: Excellent survival with improved ejection fraction and functional state. *J Am Coll Cardiol* 1993;22:1411-1417.
17. William JF, Bristow MR, Fowler MB, et al. Guidelines for the evaluation and management of heart failure: Report of the American College of Cardiology/American Heart Association task force on practice guidelines (Committee on evaluation and management of heart failure). *J Am Coll Cardiol* 1995;26:1376-1398.
18. Lahav M, Regev A, Ra'anani P, Theodor E. Intermittent administration of furosemide vs. continuous infusion preceded by a loading dose for congestive heart failure. *Chest* 1992;102:725-731.
19. Edmonds CJ, Jasani B. Total-body potassium in hypertensive patients during prolonged diuretic therapy. *Lancet* 1972;2:8-12.
20. The CONSENSUS Trial study group. Effects of enalapril on mortality in severe congestive heart failure: Results of the Cooperative North Scandanavian Enalapril Survival Study (CONSENSUS). *N Engl J Med* 1987;316:1429-1435.
21. The SOLVD investigators. Effect of enalapril on mortality and the development of heart failure in asymptomatic patients with reduced left ventricular ejection fractions. *N Engl J Med* 1992;327:685-691.
22. Cohn JN, Johnson G, et al. A comparison of enalapril with hydralazine-isosorbide dinitrate in the treatment of chronic congestive heart failure. *N Engl J Med* 1991;325:303-310.
23. The Acute Infarction Ramipril Efficacy (AIRE) Study Investigators. Effect of ramipril on mortality and morbidity of survivors of acute myocardial with clinical evidence of heart failure. *Lancet* 1993;342:821-828.
24. Peffer MA, Brauwald E, et al. Effect of captopril on mortality and morbidity in patients with left ventricular dysfunction after myocardial infarction: Results of the Survival and Ventricular Enlargement Trial. *N Engl J Med* 1992;327:669-677.
25. Købel L, Torp-Pederson C, et al. A clinical trial of the angiotensin-converting-enzyme inhibitor trandolapril in patients with left ventricular dysfunction after myocardial infarction. *N Engl J Med* 1995;333:1670-1676.
26. Konstam MA, Dracup K, Baker DW, et al. *Heart Failure: Evaluation and Care of Patients with Left-Ventricular Systolic Dysfunction.* 1994. AHCPR Publication No. 94-0612.
27. Adams KF Jr, Gheorghiade M, et al. Patients with mild heart failure worsen during withdrawal from digoxin therapy. *J Am Coll Cardiol* 1997;30:42-48.
28. Garg R, Gorlin R, and The Digitalis Investigation Group. The effect

of digoxin on mortality and morbidity in patients with heart failure. The Digitalis Investigation Group. *N Engl J Med* 1997;336: 525-533.

29. Packer M. The neurohormonal hypothesis: A theory to explain the mechanism of disease progression in heart failure. [Editorial] *J Am Coll Cardiol* 1992;20:248-254.
30. Levine TB. The design of the Mortality Assessment in Congestive Heart Failure Trial (MACH-1, mibefradil) *Clin Cardiol* 1997;4:320-326.
31. Waagstein F, Bristow MR, Swedberg K, et al. Beneficial effects of metoprolol in idiopathic dilated cardiomyopathy. *Lancet* 1993;342:1441-1446
32. CIBIS Investigators and Committees. A randomized trial of blockade in heart failure. The Cardiac Insufficiency Bisoprolol Study (CIBIS). *Circulation* 1994;90:1765-1773.
33. Bristow MR, Gilbert EM, Abraham WT, et al. Carvedilol produces dose-related improvements in left-ventricular function and survival in subjects with chronic heart failure. *Circulation* 1996;94: 2807-2816.
34. Packer M, Bristow MR, Cohn JW, et al. The effect of carvedilol on morbidity and mortality in patients with chronic heart failure. *N Engl J Med* 1996;334:1349-1355.
35. Packer M, Carver JR, Rodeheffer RJ, et al. Effect of oral milrinone on mortality in severe chronic heart failure. *N Engl J Med* 1991; 325:1468-1475.
36. Elkayam U, Amin J, Mehra A, et al. A prospective, randomized, double-blind, crossover study to compare the efficacy and safety of chronic nifedipine therapy with that of isosorbide dinitrate and their combination in the treatment of chronic congestive heart failure. *Circulation* 1990;82:1954-1961.
37. Goldstein RE, Boccuzzi SJ, Cruess D, et al. Adverse Experience Committee, Multicenter Diltiazem Postinfarction Research Group. Diltiazem increases late onset congestive heart failure in postinfarction patients with early reduction in ejection fraction. *Circulation* 1991;83:52-60.
38. Pitt B, Segal R, Martinez FA, et al. Randomized trial of losartan versus captopril in patients over 65 with heart failure (Evaluation of Losartan in the Elderly Study, ELITE). *Lancet* 1997;349:747-752.
39. Michels VV, Moll PP, Miller FA, et al. The frequency of familial dilated cardiomyopathy in a series of patients with idiopathic dilated cardiomyopathy. *N Engl J Med* 1992;326:77-82.
40. Miller LW, Mirkle EJ, Hermann V. Outpatient dobutamine for end-stage congestive heart failure. *Crit Care Med* 1990;18(Pt. 2): 530-533.
41. Alderman EL, Fisher LD, Litwin P, et al. Results of coronary artery surgery in patients with poor left ventricular function (CASS). *Circulation* 1983;68:785-795.

Congestive Heart Failure: Initial Assessment and Stabilization

David J. Robinson, MD
Rob Rogers, MD

From an emergency medicine perspective, the clinical presentation is well known: shortness of breath, weakness, fatigue, with or without ischemic symptoms, and a clinical severity profile that ranges from irritative symptoms to life-compromising pulmonary edema. Whether characterized by exercise intolerance, shortness of breath, peripheral edema, or pulmonary congestion, congestive heart failure (CHF) is one of the most important cardiovascular diseases amenable to emergency therapy. It affects approximately 1.5% of the U.S. adult population, causing a dramatic decline in quality of life and a shortened life expectancy among those who suffer from this condition.[1]

It is estimated that approximately 3 million people in the United States are afflicted with CHF. Because of the high morbidity, mortality, and cost associated with the disease, CHF is likely to remain a significant public health concern, with increasing emergency department (ED) encounters over time.

The most significant complication of ischemic cardiovascular disease, CHF is the most common hospital discharge diagnosis in patients older than age 65, and the fourth most common discharge diagnosis overall. In the United States alone, more than 400,000 new cases of heart failure are diagnosed annually, and CHF is the only major cardiovascular disease for which the incidence is increasing. As might be expected, the prognosis for patients with CHF is poor. Data from large clinical trials indicate that patients with CHF have a five-year mortality rate of approximately 50% and that patients with the most severe symptoms (NYHA Classes III-IV) have approximately a 50% one-year mortality.[2-5]

The economic impact of CHF, where most cases emerge as a consequence of ischemic heart disease, also is significant. In the United States, annual expenditures for the diagnosis and treatment of CHF exceed $10 billion. Of this amount, approximately $230 million is spent on drug therapy and $7.5 billion on hospitalization. The remainder is spent on nursing home days ($1.9 billion) and physician office visits ($690 million). The average length of hospitalization for CHF is approximately nine days, at an average cost of more than $12,000. These patients frequently require recurrent hospitalizations, multiple visits to the ED, and many different medications to maintain their functional status.

Therefore, innovations in the medical management of CHF should be evaluated for their ability to ameliorate symptoms, prevent hospitalizations, reduce medical costs, and increase life span. Recent trials with angiotensin-converting-enzyme inhibitors (ACEIs) and beta-blockers have documented progress toward these goals.

More than ever before, the role of the emergency physician caring for patients with CHF has expanded to include drug-based interventions with intravenous and oral agents, including: ACE inhibitors, beta-blockers, digoxin, diuretics, and oxygen. Fortunately, many patients who present to the ED with mild symptoms of heart failure, but without evidence of decompensation or acute, life-threatening complications (e.g., ischemia, hypoxia, hypotension, or arrhythmias) may be managed in the ED. However, almost without exception, stabilization and acute management of such patients will require pharmacotherapeutic intervention, using medications that decrease preload, reduce afterload, and/or prevent ischemia. These medications frequently can be initiated and/or titrated in the ED, in consultation with the patient's primary care physician or cardiologist. Consequently, familiarity with these drug classes is essential for optimizing patient outcomes.

This chapter outlines a systematic approach for evaluating and stabilizing patients with CHF. The authors emphasize the importance of identifying treatable conditions leading to left ventricular dysfunction, performing a detailed medication review to ensure that patients receive optimal therapy, and using adjunctive measures, when indicated, to stabilize respiratory status. In addition, the extensive differential diagnosis of CHF, which includes a diverse range of precipitating factors from acute myocardial infarction and drug-induced suppression of myocardial pump function to valvular insufficiency and inadequate medication therapy, requires the emergency physician to interpret an extended laboratory and radiographic data base to pinpoint inciting factors.

Introduction

One of the most common disease entities encountered in the ED, congestive heart failure (CHF) encompasses a broad category of conditions that culminate in the heart's inability to meet the metabolic and nutritional demands of the body. Heart failure can be characterized as a symptom complex that includes fatigue, shortness of breath and dyspnea on exertion, as well as other symptoms of congestion, and represents a clinically significant impairment in either the heart's ability to pump, fill adequately, or both.[2] As might be expected, CHF ranges in its severity from mild symptoms of volume overload to the severe symptoms of pulmonary edema and cardiogenic shock. Accordingly, it is essential that emergency physicians promptly intervene in patients with clinical decompensation, recognize medication side effects, be familiar with new trends in the treatment of heart failure, and develop a management plan that is customized for the patient's presentation.

As the population in the United States ages, the prevalence of CHF predictably will increase over the next several years.[6] In fact, it is estimated that the number of cases of heart failure will double over the next 40 years. Currently, CHF is the most common, "first-listed" diagnosis among hospitalized patients. From an emergency perspective, ED physicians must be capable of managing the increasing number of elderly patients with CHF who present to the ED not only with evidence of heart failure-mediated decompensation, but who also are taking new and experimental medications to treat this condition. Moreover, physicians must be aware of both typical and atypical presentations of CHF, they must remain current with the rapidly evolving therapeutic landscape in CHF, and they must be prepared for aggressive management modalities, including airway management and invasive hemodynamic monitoring.

Epidemiology

CHF is a common clinical entity, and the number of deaths attributable to heart failure has markedly risen during the past several decades.[1-4] These mortality and prevalence patterns are in stark contrast to the decrease in mortality from coronary disease and cerebrovascular disease over the same period. Put another way, many patients are surviving coronary events and hypertension only to develop CHF as their terminal event.[7] Advances in the treatment of other chronic conditions, such as end-stage renal disease, also have indirectly led to the increasing incidence and prevalence of heart failure.[6]

As might be expected, CHF has made a substantial effect on health care costs and quality of life. It is estimated that approximately 75% of patients with heart failure are older than 65-70 years of age. As the leading cause of hospitalization in the geriatric age group, it is estimated that 8% of patients between the ages of 75 and 86 have heart failure.[8,9] Currently, our country spends about $10 billion per year on the diagnosis and management of CHF. The presence of CHF more than doubles the age- and sex-adjusted risk of death from all causes.[6] In the previous decade, the number of admissions for heart failure rose from 577,000 to 871,000.[10] Moreover, those patients requiring hospitalization for CHF have an increased risk of mortality, a higher readmission rate, and a clinical course characterized by more precipitous functional decline.[11] Consequently, although it is not yet clear whether outcomes can be affected by outpatient care, measures aimed at preventing hospital admission for CHF should be pursued aggressively, especially for low-risk patients. Finally, there are powerful clinical and cost incentives for developing improved prevention and treatment strategies for patients with CHF.[6]

Etiology

The etiology of CHF is diverse and ranges from ischemic heart disease and valvular dysfunction to myocarditis and infectious endocarditis. Broadly speaking, CHF can result from any disorder that decreases the ability of the ventricles to eject blood.[7] Among the most common causes of CHF encountered by the ED physician are coronary artery disease, hypertension, and alcoholic cardiomyopathy. *(Please see Table 1.)* Valvular diseases such as aortic stenosis and mitral regurgitation, are also very common etiologies,[15] which often coexist with ischemia-mediated causes, especially in the elderly. In addition, elderly patients appear to be at higher risk for acquiring iatrogenic heart failure, which may be caused by medication-related bradyarrhythmias, myocardial suppression, or other drug-related complications. Iatrogenic heart failure may occur even when coexistent heart disease is not apparent.[11]

From a practical perspective, coronary artery disease is the etiology of heart failure in about two-thirds of patients with left ventricular dysfunction. Accordingly, in both the ED and primary care setting, heart failure should be presumed to be of ischemic origin until proven otherwise.[12] A common clinical entity that frequently is not recognized by the ED physician, diastolic heart failure is most often caused by chronic, uncontrolled hypertension, in which the ventricle is unable to relax and fill adequately for pumping blood to the periphery.[7] Other etiologies the ED physician must consider in the differential diagnosis include hypertrophic cardiomyopathy, pericardial disease, and myocardial toxins, most notably, chemotherapeutic agents such as donarubicin, myocardium-suppressing calcium channel blockers, and alcohol, which is a significant myocardial toxin and can induce dilated cardiomyopathy in individuals who suffer from chronic alcohol abuse.[13]

Table 1. Etiology of Congestive Heart Failure

- Coronary artery disease (acute, chronic)
- Hypertension
- Valvular disease (aortic stenosis, mitral regurgitation)
- Hyperthyroidism
- Idiopathic dilated cardiomyopathy
- Hypertrophic obstructive cardiomyopathy
- Pericardial disease (constrictive pericarditis)
- Post-partum cardiomyopathy
- Myocardial toxins (alcohol, donarubicin, cocaine, sympathomimetics)
- Infiltrative myocardial disease (amyloidosis, sarcoidosis, hemochromatosis)
- Tachycardia-induced cardiomyopathy
- High output failure (Paget's disease, AV fistula)
- Medications (calcium channel blockers, etc.)
- Thiamine deficiency

Clinical Presentation

Although the clinical pathophysiology of CHF is complex, it is most clearly understood as a state in which the heart is not able to meet the metabolic requirements of the body. In broad terms, heart failure is a syndrome characterized by inadequate cardiac output and elevated left ventricular filling pressures.[7] Moreover, it is clinically useful to characterize the signs and symptoms of CHF in terms of left vs. right heart failure. Left heart failure, regardless of the precipitating etiology, produces a constellation of signs and symptoms attributable to increased left ventricular filling pressures, which include dyspnea secondary to increased pulmonary capillary wedge pressure and fatigue associated with a decreased forward flow. Right heart failure, the most common cause of which is left ventricular failure, leads to lower extremity edema, ascites, congestive hepatomegaly, and jugular venous distension.[14]

Forward and backward symptoms refer to the predominant constellation of symptoms reported in any given patient with heart failure. For example, the major complaint in individuals with forward symptoms is fatigue, a consequence of inadequate ejection fraction. In contrast, backward symptoms are dominated by pulmonary congestion and include dyspnea, orthopnea, and paroxysmal nocturnal dyspnea. Elevated ventricular filling pressures lead to a symptom complex of dyspnea and fatigue. Although most cases of CHF are due to systolic dysfunction, a growing number of patients with heart failure maintain normal systolic function, but have a problem with left ventricular diastolic filling.

In approximately 80-90% of patients with CHF, clinical impairment is characterized by left ventricular systolic dysfunction, which is defined as an ejection fraction (EF) of less than 40%. As emphasized, diastolic heart failure is increasing in incidence and currently may account for as many as 40% of all inpatient hospitalizations for heart failure.[15] Occult valvular disease and chronic ischemic heart disease also should be considered in patients with normal or preserved left ventricular function and signs of diastolic dysfunction.

Specific disease states that induce diastolic heart failure include coronary ischemia, ventricular hypertrophy secondary to hypertension, infiltrative myocardial disease (such as amyloidosis), pericardial disease, hypertrophic cardiomyopathy, and aging.[7]

Drug Therapy in Congestive Heart Failure: The Neurohormonal Model

Targeted, outcome-effective drug therapy for CHF is based on a thorough understanding of the neurohormonal and hemodynamic models of cardiac decompensation. In fact, both acute and chronic drug-based therapy for CHF, including interventions or therapeutic modifications initiated in the ED, require selection of medications that affect the hormonal, compensatory responses to declining heart function, and that reduce cardiac workload in patients with impaired left ventricular function.

In the setting of clinically significant CHF, the failing myocardium activates several neurohormonal feedback loops that, over time, exacerbate the degree of cardiac decompensation and lead to progressive hemodynamic deterioration. In the setting of reduced pumping capacity, the heart initially attempts to maintain adequate systolic function by increasing heart rate and peripheral vascular resistance. These compensations are accomplished through activation of both the sympathetic nervous system and the renin-angiotensin-aldosterone system. Initially, these mechanisms are principally compensatory and can successfully maintain—and even augment—cardiac output. Eventually, however, these compensatory mechanisms can lead to cardiac decompensation requiring drug therapy.

Renin-Angiotensin II-Aldosterone System. The two most important systems activated by left ventricular dysfunction are the renin-angiotensin-aldosterone system and the sympathetic nervous system. Induction of renin release, production of angiotensin II, and release of norepinephrine lead to increased afterload, as well as salt and water retention, which leads to increased preload and afterload.[15] Because of these neurohormonal responses, it is becoming widely accepted that definitive treatment of CHF should not be based exclusively on altering hemodynamic derangements caused by left ventricular dysfunction, but also should use pharmacotherapeutic approaches that inhibit and/or modulate pathways that lead to cardiac decompensation.

This neurohormonal model is supported by the observation that in heart failure, such hormonal regulators as angiotensin II and norepinephrine are elevated. Their end-organ effects include vasoconstriction accompanied by increased blood volume, heart rate, and myocardial contractility. The pathogenesis of CHF centers around the neurohormonal model.[16] In this scheme, and initial insult to the myocardium, such as long-standing hypertension, acute myocardial infarction (AMI), or myocarditis, causes ventricular dysfunction, which then leads to cardiac remodeling and further reductions in EF and worsening of clinical symptoms such as arrhythmias and pump failure. Thus, the initial event damages functional myocytes and decreases the pumping ability of the heart.[17] Myocardial remodeling is probably the most important mediator in the progression of heart failure and can be identified through changes in ventricular shape and dimension.

Sympathetic Nervous System. Increased sympathetic activity and plasma norepinephrine levels, both of which are elevated in chronic heart failure, over time, may exert deleterious effects on myocardial structure and function. Initially, activation of these systems restore and maintain cardiac output, but, over time, can lead to cardiac decompensation.[16] In addition, mediators released when the renin-angiotensin-aldosterone system is activated can cause fibrosis and cardiac remodeling. It has been shown in animal models that stimulation of the beta-adrenergic receptors may induce myocyte apoptosis or programmed cell death. Activation of the sympathetic nervous system seems to play a central role in the development of myocyte necrosis and cardiac remodeling.[18] Accordingly, drug-based therapies, such as beta-blockers, that block adrenergic pathways, have been found to be effective in the treatment of heart failure.

Clinical-Therapeutic Correlations. Other chemical mediators implicated in the neurohormonal cascade of CHF include renin, arginine vasopressin, atrial natriuretic peptide, and endothelin. In one study, combined use of clonidine and captopril (by inhibiting activated neurohormonal mechanisms) caused significant improvement in preload and afterload.[19] Another model that has been invoked to explain clinical findings in patients with CHF is the cardiorenal model.[20] This sequence is based on the pathophysiology of heart failure and decreased forward flow. According to this scheme, decreased renal blood flow—an almost universal phenomenon in chronic heart failure—activates a cascade of events that eventually leads to the production of renin, angiotensin I, angiotensin II, aldosterone, norepinephrine, and endothelin; all of which act together to increase blood pressure, produce salt and water retention, and possibly, cardiac toxicity, as described in the neurohormonal model of CHF.[10] Drugs such as beta-blockers and ACE inhibitors target (inhibit) these critical pathways and prevent further deterioration.[21,22]

Diagnostic Challenges in Heart Failure

Patients who present to the ED with symptoms suggestive of CHF frequently suffer from other medical conditions that may confuse or mask the diagnosis, making it difficult to distinguish CHF from these other disease states. Perhaps, patients with chronic obstructive pulmonary disease (COPD) present the greatest diagnostic challenge since they frequently are elderly, have risk factors for heart disease, and present with such symptoms as shortness of breath, weakness, fatigue, and tachypnea. Other pulmonary processes also can present with symptoms compatible with heart failure, as can such conditions as obesity, coronary disease, and chronic conditions, including sleep apnea. Symptoms such as exertional dyspnea and orthopnea may suggest almost any chronic pulmonary disease, including thromboembolic disease, pulmonary hypertension, and lower respiratory tract infection.[23]

A thorough and detailed search for a precipitant should be sought in every case of CHF to avoid missing a potentially life-threatening and/or reversible condition. In this regard, the diagnosis of thyrotoxicosis should be considered in the patient who has tachycardia, is hypertensive, and has no previous history of heart failure. In contrast, hypothyroidism should be considered in the myxedematous patient with a history of thyroid rugery. Reversible causes of CHF include arrhythmias, such as atrial fibrillation, valvular disease, and pericardial disease. Cardiac ischemia always requires strong consideration in the differential diagnosis, especially in the elderly or diabetic patient at risk for silent ischemia.

As a general rule, the physician should assume that coronary ischemia is the precipitant of heart failure until it is proven otherwise. One of the most common precipitants in patients receiving appropriate therapy for CHF is failure of patients to maintain fluid balance.[24] In a recent study, 59% of admissions attributable to heart failure decompensation were due to excessive sodium retention which, in turn, lead to volume overload.[25] As with many other illnesses, CHF seems to be triggered by a number of well-characterized, precipitating factors. These include anemia, thyrotoxicosis, pregnancy or the post-partum state, hypoxia, and ischemia. Early and aggressive management of these precipitants and comorbid conditions is essential and can have a favorable effect on morbidity and mortality. *(Please see Table 2.)*

Table 2. Precipitants of Congestive Heart Failure[49,50]

- Myocardial ischemia or infarction
- Atrial fibrillation—new onset or rapid ventricular response
- Worsening valvular disease—mitral regurgitation
- Pulmonary embolism
- Hypoxia
- Severe, uncontrolled hypertension
- Thyroid disease
- Pregnancy
- Anemia
- Infection
- Tachycardia or bradycardia
- Alcohol abuse
- Medication or dietary noncompliance

History and Physical Examination

Whenever possible, a detailed, comprehensive history should be performed on all patients presenting with signs and symptoms suggestive of CHF. In particular, patients should be evaluated for the presence of coronary artery disease, hypertension, or valvular dysfunction. In addition, patients should be questioned regarding use of alcohol, chemotherapeutic agents such as donarubicin, negative inotropic agents, and symptoms suggestive of a recent viral syndrome. An assessment of conditions known to cause cardiac infiltrative disease, such as sarcoidosis and amyloidosis, should be sought in patients whose heart failure appears to be of unknown etiology. In all cases, a thorough differential diagnosis should be formulated, and such entities as pulmonary embolism, myocardial infarction (MI), and underlying pulmonary disease should be considered. It should be stressed that the findings of edema, rales, and dyspnea are nonspecific, and, in the patient with normal left ventricular function, these symptoms may reflect an alternative diagnosis.[7]

Patient's with CHF can present with myriad complaints, including shortness of breath, dyspnea on exertion, paroxysmal nocturnal dyspnea, orthopnea, nocturia, and cough. Exertional dyspnea is extremely common in patients with heart failure. The most common symptoms, dyspnea and orthopnea, reflect elevated filling pressures and pulmonary congestion.[24] Atypical presentations are quite common and include symptoms such chronic cough, fatigue, and insomnia. Patients also can present with ascites, right upper quadrant pain (from hepatic congestion), and weakness.

It is common for elderly patients to present in atypical fashion, which may include absence of dyspnea or orthopnea. The geriatric group—much like diabetics—is more likely to develop silent ischemia and MI as a precipitant of CHF. Consequently, all older patients who present to the ED with new onset or exacerbation of CHF require a work-up to determine whether coronary ischemia, either acute, unstable, or progressive, is the cause for myocardial pump dysfunction. Older patients in particular may present a diagnostic dilemma for emergency physicians because they may lack typical signs, symptoms, and physical findings.[26] For example, older patients may be less likely to report exertional dyspnea secondary to their sedentary lifestyle. Decreased exercise tolerance, fatigue, and unexplained confusion in the elderly also may be among the primary complaints in patients with CHF.[23] Pulmonary disease may complicate the diagnosis.[27] Older patients also may present to the ED with occult cardiogenic shock or ileus as the initial manifestation of heart failure.[28]

Physical Examination. One of the principal functions of the physical examination is to identify subtle signs and symptoms—lid lag, goiter, medication use, murmurs, abnormal heart rhythms—that suggest a treatable underlying disease. Patients with CHF may present with a wide range of findings, including resting tachycardia, jugular venous distension, a third heart sound, rales, lower extremity edema, a laterally displaced apical impulse, or they may present with only shortness of breath and weakness. Poor capillary refill, cool extremities, or an altered level of consciousness also may be present.[23] A third heart sound is considered one of the most reliable indicators of CHF. However, it is important to remember that some patients with severe systolic dysfunction who are currently taking digoxin and diuretics may lack a third heart sound, cardiomegaly, on chest x-ray, or edema.[29] Consequently, CHF cannot be excluded in patients who have a normal-sized heart on chest x-ray and absence of extremity edema or pulmonary rales.[2]

Pulmonary rales frequently are absent on physical examination, although, when present, they are strongly suggestive of cardiac decompensation.[24] Physical exam findings are not a sensitive indicator of heart failure.[30] Physical exam findings suggesting an alternate diagnosis, such as barrel-chest and diminished air movement, should be sought out to narrow the differential diagnosis. It should be stressed that wheezing may be secondary to bronchial wall edema and may be a manifestation of cardiac asthma, especially in patients with no history of COPD or asthma.

Assessment in the ED. Because the physical examination is not predictably sensitive or specific for the diagnosis of CHF, adjunctive diagnostic and radiographic procedures usually are required to establish the diagnosis, suggest a course for initial stabilization, generate a definitive treatment plan, and guide the triage decision. Every patient with symptoms suggestive of CHF should have a 12-lead ECG and should be placed on a cardiac monitor. Arrhythmias such as atrial fibrillation or signs of ischemia can give important clues to precipitants and comorbid conditions, such as left ventricular hypertrophy (LVH). Older patients with electrocardiographic evidence of LVH tend to have a higher incidence of new CHF and develop it earlier compared to patients without evidence of LVH.[31] A chest x-ray should be performed to identify pleural effusions, pneumothorax, pulmonary edema, or infiltrates.

Pulmonary edema secondary to left ventricular dysfunction initially begins as cephalization of pulmonary blood flow and proceeds to form the classic "bat wing" pattern. Patients in whom a diagnosis of cardiac ischemia or infarction is suspected should have cardiac enzymes drawn. A complete blood count, electrolytes, and digoxin level, if applicable, also are mandatory. Patients with suspected hyperthyroidism should have thyroid function studies drawn. Echocardiography has revolutionized the evaluation of cardiac disease and can be used in the ED to evaluate for the presence of pericardial effusion, tamponade, valvular regurgitation, or wall motion abnormalities. If an acute process such as a ruptured aortic valve from endocarditis or acute cardiac tamponade in a dialysis patient is suspected, echocardiography should not be delayed.

Patient Stabilization

Rapid, efficient assessment of patients with heart failure should always take priority so that appropriate interventions can be made expeditiously based on objective clinical data. Without exception, patients should be placed on a cardiac monitor, they should have a pulse oximeter attached, and intravenous access should be established. Patients also should be placed on oxygen to maintain adequate oxygen saturation. In patients with severe symptoms (i.e., individuals with acute heart failure and pulmonary edema), other measures such as continuous positive airway pressure (CPAP) and endotracheal intubation (ETI) may be employed when indicated to assure adequate oxygenation and ventilation.

Non-invasive ventilation (NIV) is defined as the administration of ventilatory support by noninvasive means, most commonly by face mask. In contrast, ETI is not a benign procedure and may be complicated by misplacement of the ET tube as well as increased sympathetic drive, which has the potential for exacerbating cardiac ischemia in susceptible patients. Moreover, ETI can increase intracranial pressure; the procedure is uncomfortable and prevents speaking and eating. Given these limitations, the use of NIV by way of CPAP or with BiPAP has gained growing popularity over the last few years. Supporting the patient's airway with NIV provides a valuable adjunct and may prevent more invasive interventions such as ETI. Nocturnal nasal CPAP (N-PAP) has been shown to eliminate recurrent episodes of severe cardiopulmonary disease, including pulmonary edema.[32]

Despite growing interest in assessing the benefits and risks of noninvasive ventilatory techniques for patients with CHF, COPD, and asthma, it should be stressed that there currently is considerable controversy surrounding the use of noninvasive ventilation in the ED. Its precise role for patients with CHF and ventilatory failure requires more evaluation before definitive recommendations can be made. At present, these ventilatory approaches are used most commonly for exacerbations of COPD and asthma, although they are being used more frequently in patients with CHF exacerbations, including those complicated by pulmonary edema.[33]

In this regard, one important study concluded that CPAP therapy delivered by face mask for the treatment of pulmonary edema is safe and effective.[34] In fact, there is a growing number of trials that suggest CPAP carries a favorable benefit-to-risk ratio. A trend toward lower mortality rates has been reported with the use of CPAP, and this technique, when used, appears to decrease the rate of intubations.[35] NIV appears to alleviate respiratory fatigue by significantly decreasing the work of breathing, which is a salutary effect in patients with fluid overload and pulmonary edema.

Moreover, NIV can be used as a temporizing measure while other therapeutic pharmacotherapeutic measures are undertaken, such as diuresis and preload reduction.[36] NIV increases alveolar recruitment, improves oxygenation, and decreases intrapulmonary shunting. Potential complications of NIV include gastric distension, pulmonary aspiration, and barotrauma.[34] Use of NIV requires a cooperative patient and should only be performed in appropriate clinical situations since NIV does not provide a definitive airway and should not be used if severe respiratory deterioration is anticipated. In a randomized, prospective trial of BiPAP vs. CPAP in pulmonary edema, one study found that BiPAP improves ventilation and vital signs more rapidly than CPAP.[37]

Despite the reported clinical utility of NIV, unfortunately, there is a lack of randomized, controlled trials that can provide definitive conclusions regarding its safety and efficacy in patients with respiratory compromise in the clinical setting of acute CHF. At least one report that NIV may worsen ischemia and increase the risk of MI in patients with pulmonary edema further clouds the issue.[33] Additionally, the use of NIV in some studies was found to actually increase the in-hospital mortality rate when used in patients with respiratory distress that is linked to multiple etiologies, including cardiogenic pulmonary edema.[32] Clearly, further studies are needed on the efficacy and safety of NIV before the administration of CPAP (NIV) can be routinely recommended in this patient population.[35]

Finally, other measures to improve gas exchange are currently under investigation, including the use of inhaled nitric oxide. Use of conventional vasodilators improve pulmonary hypertension and congestion but lead to a mismatch in ventilation-perfusion and actually worsen gas exchange in patients with CHF. However, recent studies suggest that the use of inhaled nitric oxide may decrease ventilation-perfusion mismatches and improve gas exchange.[1,38]

Drug-Based Management of Chronic Heart Failure: Initiation, Evaluation, and Titration of Oral Agents in the ED

From the emergency perspective, medical management of patients with CHF can include any one or more of the following interventions or assessments: 1) administering medications to treat hemodynamic derangements; 2) evaluating and ruling out such precipitants to CHF as coronary ischemia, thyrotoxicosis, infection, and anemia; 3) aggressive airway and respiratory management to treat hypoxia; 4) controlling a compromised airway; and 5) generating a disposition based on the stability of the patient.

Fortunately, many patients who present to the ED with mild symptoms of heart failure but without evidence of decompensation or acute, life-threatening complications (e.g., among them, ischemia, hypoxia, hypotension, or arrhythmias) may be managed in the ED. Almost without exception, stabilization and acute management of such patients will require pharmacotherapeutic intervention using medications that decrease preload, reduce afterload, and/or prevent ischemia. These medications frequently can be initiated and/or titrated in the ED, in consultation with the patient's primary care physician or cardiologist.

Measures to reduce volume overload, decrease afterload, improve left ventricular function, and inhibit the neurohormonal cascade associated with heart failure include administration of diuretics, ACE inhibitors, inotropic agents, and beta-blockers. It is mandatory that changes to drug dosages or the decision to add a medication to an existing regimen be discussed with the patient's primary care physician or cardiologist if possible. Many of these medications should only be added or have their dose increased in stable, euvolemic patients with no evidence of significant cardiac decompensation. Close follow-up after discharge from the ED should be arranged.

Beta-Blockers. Increasingly, beta-blockers have emerged as foundation drugs for the treatment of CHF, which means this class now has a dual role for management of chronic CHF and for use as cardioprotective agent following AMI. The emergency physician must be aware that the presence of CHF, even in the setting of MI, no longer represents an absolute contraindication to beta-blocker use, and that clinical judgement should dictate which patients might benefit from low-dose, gradual titration of a beta-blocker in this setting.

Numerous studies published in the last few years have validated the use of beta-blockers for the management of chronic CHF. The benefits of beta-blockers to prevent recurrent MI has been well established. Despite their effectiveness as cardioprotective agents, this medication class is underused in post-MI patients, with one study indicating that only 35-65% of eligible patients currently enrolled in managed care plans are currently receiving beta-blockers following their MI. This is unfortunate, because post-MI studies in the pre-thrombolytic era, as well as recent studies in the setting of thrombolysis, continue to show a benefit for beta-blockers.

Overall, studies with atenolol and propranolol show a 27% reduction in recurrent MI over a two-year period, if beta-blockers are started at the time of AMI and continued on an oral basis thereafter. Beta-blockers are useful for suppressing silent myocardial ischemia, they have a modest anti-arrhythmic effect, and when used carefully, especially in low doses with incremental titration, they also appear to be beneficial in heart failure and may prevent adverse remodeling of the left ventricle, as well as improve survival. Beta-blockers improve survival post-MI especially in patients with large MIs and LV dysfunction, but the mechanism for these salutary effects has not been established.

Two recent studies from Yale and the University of Maryland have again demonstrated the value of beta-blockers after MI. The Yale study evaluated more than 45,000 cases of AMI in patients 65 years of age or older. In this retrospective cohort study, half of the patients were given a beta-blocker at discharge. Beta-blocker use was associated with a 14% lower risk of mortality at one year post discharge. The Maryland study also was a retrospective study of more than 200,000 patients with MI. Thirty-four percent of these patients were given beta-blockers, and various subgroups were analyzed, including those with CHF, COPD, renal insufficiency, and diabetes. Mortality was lower in every subgroup of patients treated with beta-blockers compared with untreated patients. In otherwise healthy patients with no complications or comorbid conditions, mortality was reduced by 40% in the beta-blocker group. Both studies concluded that beta-blockers are underused post MI, especially in the elderly and in subgroups of patients who might not be considered candidates for beta blockade because of pre-existing conditions.

It is possible that the beta-blocker carvedilol, a non-selective beta-blocker with alpha-one mediated vasodilator properties as well as antioxidant activity, may play an important role not only for its approved indications (i.e., for hypertension and mild CHF) but also as a post-MI cardioprotective agent. A British study evaluated the role of carvedilol in AMI, in which the drug was intravenously administered to patients, after which subjects were converted to oral therapy. The six-month end points consisted of all major cardiovascular events. Results of the study demonstrated a significant (42%) reduction in serious cardiac events in the carvedilol group. Of the 30% of patients who had an EF less than 30% associated with their MI, at three months the group randomized to carvedilol treatment had a smaller chamber size, a trend toward increased EF, and improved wall motion score. Adverse cardiac events, including reinfarction, unstable angina, and need for urgent revascularization, also were reduced in this group, confirming that not only did post-MI patients with CHF on carvedilol not suffer adverse events from the drug but also achieved a significant remodeling benefit.

Of special note is the fact that about two-thirds of these MI patients received thrombolytic therapy, suggesting, but not proving conclusively, that improved survival benefits with beta-blockers such as carvedilol extend to patients who undergo clot lysis. Further studies are likely to be forthcoming. However, it appears as if carvedilol is safe to use after AMI with or without associated heart failure. But whether this agent is different than other beta-blockers with established track records in long-term cardio-protection cannot be answered from this small trial. Moreover, whether the remodeling benefits demonstrated in this study can be extended to other beta-blockers cannot be answered at the present time. Although the jury remains out on whether, or to what degree, carvedilol may be safer and more effective than other beta-blockers, it does appear to be an appropriate addition to the cardioprotective cocktail for patients with MI and associated heart failure.

Beta-blockers exert their salutary effects on CHF by inhibiting the neurohormonal cascade as mediated by the sympathetic nervous system and the renin-angiotensin-aldosterone system.[20] Cardiac adrenergic drive, a catecholaminergic state that has a direct depressant effect on cardiac myocytes, is increased in the failing myocardium, which leads to significant progression of left ventricular dysfunction.[12,39]

A plethora of well-designed, randomized studies have shown that beta-blockers not only improve symptoms of CHF, they improve left ventricular function and reverse altered hemodynamics. Long-term treatment of heart failure with beta-blockers can produce significant benefits.[40,41] In more than 20 studies evaluating more than 10,000 patients using beta-blockers in the setting of CHF, beta-blockers have been shown to increase EF and decrease the combined risk of death and hospitalization of CHF. Patients with class II-III heart failure of ischemic etiology on beta-blockers have been found to have an approximately 38% reduction in all-cause mortality, accompanied by a reduction of severity of symptoms linked to heart failure.[3,12] One meta-analysis demonstrated a 30% reduction in the mortality rate in patients on beta-blockers.[40]

The Cardiac Insufficiency Bisoprolol Study II (CIBIS-II) confirmed significant clinical benefits using the beta blocker, bisoprolol (a beta-1 selective adrenoceptor blocker) in patients with stable heart failure patients (class II & III) who did not have clinical evidence of severe class IV symptoms and recent instability. The CIBIS-II study showed a 32% reduction in all-cause mortality, a 45% reduction in sudden death, a 30% reduction in hospitalization for CHF, and a 15% reduction in all-cause hospitalization.[42] The Metoprolol in Dilated Cardiomyopathy (MDC) Trial , the first major placebo-controlled trial of a beta-blocker in heart failure, showed a 34% reduction in mortality. A three-year follow-up of the MDC trial continues to show a significant reduction in mortality.[43]

Future trials currently in progress are investigating what type of beta blocker (i.e., selective, non-selective, or vasodilating) will show the most significant effect in CHF, or whether clinical outcomes are equivalent. These trials include the Carvedilol or Metoprolol European Trial (COMET) and CIBIS-II. The COMET will compare the effects of carvedilol vs. metoprolol on all-cause mortality.[44] Currently, carvedilol, a beta 1, 2 and alpha 1-adrenergic antagonist and a vasodilator, is the only approved beta-blocker for treatment of CHF, although there are ongoing trials designed to evaluate such beta-blockers as metoprolol and bucindolol.[45] Carvedilol, in particular, has been shown to increase both left and right ventricular function in patients with systolic dysfunction.[46] Two trials, the PRECISE (Prospective Randomized Evaluation of Carvedilol on Symptoms and Exercise) and the MOCHA (Multicenter Oral Carvedilol Heart Failure Assessment study) trials have shown that beta-blocker therapy with carvedilol in patients with heart failure significantly reduces the risk of death and of hospitalizations.[7,12,16]

The PRECISE trial evaluated 278 patients with ischemic or non-ischemic cardiomyopathy. Patients were randomized to placebo or carvedilol at a dose of 50-100 mg/d, which was added to diuretic and other therapies. In this study, carvedilol produced a 39% reduction in combined risk of death or all cause hospitalization and a 46% reduction in risk of hospitalization for CHF and other cardiovascular reasons.[12,47]

As a rule, beta-blockers should not be used in the setting of acute pulmonary edema or decompensated heart failure, because there is a risk of inducing rapid deterioration. Concern that beta-blockers may lead to acute deterioration in patients with significantly depressed EFs has been a deterrent to their routine use in the ED in the setting of CHF. Accordingly, they are currently contraindicated in patients with hypervolemia and significant clinical signs of decompensation because of their negative inotropic effect. Typically, beta-blockers are most prudently initiated in the hemodynamically stable patient who has been deemed euvolemic and at low risk of decompensation.

It should be stressed that clinical trials evaluating beta-blockers have been performed only in stable patients, excluding patients with brittle or acute, severe CHF. Moreover, because ACE inhbitors constitute primary therapy for treatment of CHF, beta-blockers should be considered add-on or adjunctive therapy in patients already being treated with ACE inhibitors. In summary, more data are needed before this class can be recommended for routine use in patients with any significant degree of deterioration.[12] The COPERNICUS trial, the results of which will not be available until 2001, will evaluate the use of beta-blockers in this patient group. At present, in the ED, beta-blockers should not be used in the patient with decompensated CHF (stage IV NYHA functional class) inasmuch as there is no evidence to support their use in this unstable patient population.

Beta-blockers can be used safely in patients with stable CHF and, these agents do not prevent patients from deriving benefit from physical training.[48] Most patients with class II-III CHF should be started on a beta-blocker unless they are unable to tolerate it or have the appearance of side effects. Side effects include hypotension and fluid retention, as well as worsening heart failure, bradycardia, and heart block. Patients with asthma, underlying heart block, or bradycardia should not receive beta-blocker therapy.[12] As with most medication

Table 3. Carvedilol, Metoprolol, and Bisoprolol—Dosages and Side Effects

- Carvedilol—start at 3.125 mg bid and titrate up slowly, reduce or discontinue if patient decompensates
- Metoprolol—start at 12.5 mg bid
- Bisoprolol—start at 1.25 mg qd

Caution should be exercised in patients with clinical decompensation until further data are available. Do not start beta-blocker therapy unless patient is near euvolemic.

Table 4. Beta-Blockers' Effect on CHF—Mortality Benefit[39,60]

- Increase ejection fraction
- Decrease all-cause mortality
- Decrease mortality secondary to heart failure
- Prevent fatal arrhythmias
- Prevent ischemia

classes, beta-blockers should be started at very low doses and titrated up. Carvedilol, one of the drugs approved for use in heart failure, is generally started at 3.125 mg bid and titrated up slowly over weeks to 6.25 mg bid, 12.5 mg bid, 25 mg bid, and so forth. Diuretics may need to be titrated if decompensation and congestive symptoms increase before beta-blocker therapy is stabilized at a steady dose. *(Please see Tables 3 and 4.)*

ACE Inhibitors. ACE inhibitors (ACEIs) continue to be workhorse drugs for management of CHF. These agents exert their clinical effects by inhibiting the enzyme responsible for the conversion of angiotensin I to angiotensin II, a potent vasoconstrictor.[12] As a general rule, all patients with CHF should be prescribed an ACEI unless this class is contraindicated in the patient or the drug is poorly tolerated. Elderly patients with CHF not treated with an ACEI have an increased mortality rate compared to those on placebo.[4]

Numerous trials, including the Cooperative North Scandinavian Enalapril Survival Study (CONSENSUS), the Veteran's Administration Cooperative Vasodilator-Heart Failure Trial (V-HeFT I), the Studies of Left Ventricular Dysfunction (SOLVD), and the Survival and Ventricular Enlargement Trial (SAVE), have confirmed that ACEIs significantly reduce morbidity and mortality in CHF.[51] The Randomized Evaluation of Strategies for Left Ventricular Dysfunction Study (RESOLVD) is a trial evaluating the combination neurohormonal blockade regimen using an angiotensin II antagonist (eandesartan), an ACEI (enalapril), and a beta-blocker (metoprolol) in patients with heart failure. Although results from this study are not currently available, they will be used to design a large scale mortality trial and will aid in the understanding of the importance of neurohormonal blockade in CHF.[52,53]

Several studies also are in progress that will investigate the use of ACEIs in the progression of atherosclerotic disease. They include the Heart Outcome Prevention Evaluation (HOPE), the Study of Evaluate Carotid Ultrasound with Ramipril and Vitamin E (SECURE), the Quinapril Ischemic Event Trial (QUIET), and the Simvastatin and Enalapril Coronary Atherosclerosis Trial (SCAT).

Not only do ACEIs help improve symptoms of CHF, including fatigue and improving exercise tolerance, they also significantly decrease morbidity and mortality associated with the post-infarction state.[50] Several trials have confirmed the benefit of ACEIs in patients who have sustained a MI. In addition, however, ACEI therapy is associated with improved left ventricular function in patients sustaining myocardial damage during infarction and numerous studies have shown that ACEIs confer a substantial survival benefit to patients with CHF following MI.[54] The Survival and Ventricular Enlargement (SAVE) trial randomized 2231 patients with a recent MI and EF less than 40% to placebo vs. captopril (target dose 150 mg/d). Treatment with the ACEI decreased mortality by 19% and subsequent risk of developing moderate to severe heart failure by 22%. Other studies that have shown similar benefits with ACEI therapy in CHF include the Acute Infarction Ramipril Efficacy (AIRE) trial, the Trandolapril Cardiac Evaluation (TRACE) study, Studies of Left Ventricular Dysfunction (SOLVD) trial, and Fosinopril in Acute Myocardial Infarction Study (FAMIS). In most trials evaluating ACEIs in heart failure, dyspnea is relieved and exercise tolerance is improved.[12,55]

It should be stressed that despite proven benefits, this class of drugs is commonly underprescribed, especially in the elderly population, and therefore, ED physicians evaluating patients with CHF in the ED should ensure that eligible patients have not been denied the benefits of ACEIs. Moreover, older patients may be on lower than optimal doses, which places them at a higher risk for future clinical deterioration.[56] Some physicians are reluctant to use ACEIs because of their side effects, which include cough, worsening renal function, hyperkalemia, hypotension, and the risk of angioedema.[50,15] These must be weighed against the potential benefits in the individual patient.

Currently, five ACEIs are approved for the use in patients with CHF: They include: captopril, enalapril, lisinopril, quinapril, and fosinopril. ACEIs should be started at a very low dose and titrated up gradually over several weeks to achieve clinical end points (i.e., relief of fatigue, shortness of breath, and weakness) while avoiding side effects. Renal function should be followed very carefully, especially during initial titration, to avoid precipitating hyperkalemia and/or renal insufficiency. Renal function should be checked within 1-2 weeks of initiating therapy. Close monitoring of renal function and electrolytes should occur on a regular basis. *(Please see Table 5.)*

The Assessment of Treatment with Lisinopril and Survival (ATLAS) study established what dose (higher vs lower) of lisinopril, would be more beneficial in reducing hospitalization and mortality. Approximately 3500 patients from 287 centers in 19 different countries with class III and IV (and some hospitalized class II patients) heart failure were investigated. All-cause mortality and hospitalization was significantly lower in patients randomized to the higher dose of lisinopril. Importantly, there was no major difference in the side effect profile.[15] This study, however, did not show dramatic difference in all-cause mortality, although it did demonstrate a decrease in death, all-cause hospitalizations, and hospitalizations for heart failure in patients taking the higher dose lisinopril. A similar study, the NETWORK study, which evaluated enalapril dosing, did not show a significant benefit of high vs. low-dose enalapril. It seems reasonable to prescribe the highest dose of an ACEI tolerable until long-term,

Table 5. ACE Inhibitors and Dosage

DRUGS AND DOSAGES APPROVED FOR TREATMENT OF HEART FAILURE

- Captopril (Capoten)—start 6.25-12.5 mg po tid, usual dose 50-100 mg tid
- Enalapril (Vasotec)—start 2.5 mg po qd/bid, usual 2.5-10 mg tid
- Lisinopril (Prinivil, Zestril)—start 5 mg po qd, usual 5-20 mg/d
- Quinapril (Accupril)—start 5 mg po bid, usual 20-40 mg/d
- Fosinopril (Monopril)—start 10 mg po qd, usual 20-40 mg/d
- Ramipril (Altace) approved for use post-infarction—start 2.5 mg po bid, usual 10 mg/d

(BUN, Creatinine, and Potassium should be checked within 1-2 weeks starting therapy)

randomized trial results are available.[57] The ongoing ACHIEVE trial will investigate 10,500 patients with respect to high- vs. low-dose quinapril.

Even at target dosages, some patients will not respond as well, especially if they are taking NSAIDS or ASA. A subgroup analysis of the Cooperative New Scandinavian Enalapril Survival Study II (CONSENSUS II study) found evidence to suggest a significant interaction of the between the ACEI, enalapril, with aspirin. In this study, the favorable hemodynamic effects of enalapril were much less pronounced in patients taking aspirin compared to patients not taking aspirin.[58] Further ongoing studies are now being conducted to clarify this important issue.

The overall results from multiple trials suggest that emergency physicians should make every effort to use ACEIs at the dose proven in clinical trials unless impeded by side effects or poor patient tolerance. CHF readmission rates seem to be lower if patients are maintained on higher doses of ACEIs.[59]

References

1. Matsumoto, Momomura, Sugiura, et al. Effect of inhaled nitric oxide on gas exchange in patients with congestive heart failure. *Ann Intern Med* 1999;130:40-44.
2. Cohn JN. The management of chronic heart failure. *N Engl J Med* 1996;335:490-498.
3. Haim, Shotan, Boyko, et al. Effects of beta-blocker therapy in patients with coronary disease in New York Heart Association Classes II and III. *Am J Cardiol* 1998;81:1455-1460.
4. Havranek, Abrams, et al. Determinants of mortality in elderly patients with heart failure. *Arch Intern Med* 1998;158: 2024-2028.
5. Philbin, Rocco. Use of angiotensin-converting enzyme inhibitors in heart failure with preserved left ventricular systolic function. *Am Heart J* 1997;134:188-195.
6. Rich MW. Epidemiology, pathophysiology, and etiology of congestive heart failure in older adults. *J Am Geriatr Soc* 1997;45:968-974.
7. Dauterman, Massie, et al. Heart failure associated with preserved systolic function: A common and costly clinical entity. *Am Heart J* 1998;135:S310-S319.
8. Schulman, Mark, Califf. Outcomes and costs within a disease management program for advanced congestive heart failure. *Am Heart J* 1998;135:S285-S292.
9. Kupari, et al. Congestive heart failure in old age: Prevalence, mechanisms and 4-year progress in the Helsinki Aging Study. *J Int Med* 1997;241:387-394.
10. Haldeman, Croft, Giles, et al. Hospitalization of patients with heart failure: National hospital discharge survey, 1985 to 1995. *Am Heart J* 1999;137:352-360.
11. Rich, Shah, et al. Iatrogenic congestive heart failure in older adults: Clinical course and prognosis. *J Am Geriatr Soc* 1996;44: 638-643.
12. Packer, Cohn. Concensus recommendations for the management of chronic heart failure. *Am J Cardiol* 1999;83:1A-38A.
13. Sigurdsson, Swedberg. The role of neurohormonal activation in chronic heart failure and postmyocardial infarction. *Am Heart J* 1996;132:229-234.
14. Goldsmith, Dick. Differentiating systolic from diastolic heart failure: Pathophysiologic and therapeutic considerations. *Am J Med* 1993;95:645-655.
15. Gheorghiade, Cody, Francis, et al. Current medical therapy for advanced heart failure. *Am Heart J* 1998;135:S231-S248.
16. Baig, Mahon, McKenna, et al. The pathophysiology of advanced heart failure. *Am Heart J* 1998;135:S216-S230.
17. Kurrelmeyer, Karla, et al. Cardiac remodeling as a consequence and cause of progressive heart failure. *Clin Cardiol* 1998; 21(supp I):I14-I19.
18. Colucci WS. The effects of norepinephrine on myocardial biology: Implications for therapy of heart failure. *Clin Cardiol* 1998;21(supp I):I20-I24.
19. Manolis, Olympios, et al. Combined sympathetic suppression and angiotensin-converting enzyme inhibition in congestive heart failure. *Hypertension* 1997;29:525-530.
20. Pepper, Lee. Sympathetic activation in heart failure and its treatment with beta blockade. *Arch Intern Med* 1999;159: 225-234.
21. Mazayev, Fomina, Sulimov, et al. Valsartan in heart failure patients Previously untreated with an ACE inhibitor. *Int J Cardiol* 1998;65:239-246.
22. Levin. Evidence-based contemporary heart failure management. *Resid Staff Physician* 1999.
23. Bales, Sorrentino. Causes of congestive heart failure—Prompt diagnosis may affect prognosis. *Postgrad Med* 1997;101: 44-49,54-56.
24. Stevenson LW, et al. Optimizing therapy for complex or refractory heart failure: A management algorithm. *Am Heart J* 1998;135:S293-S309.
25. Bennett, Huster, Baker, et al. Characterization of the precipitants of hospitalization for heart failure decompensation. *Am J Crit Care* 1998;7:168-174.
26. Aronow, Tresch. The clinical diagnosis of heart failure in older patients. *J Am Geriatr Soc* 1997;45:1252-1257.

27. Emmet. Nonspecific and atypical presentation of disease in the older patient. *Geriatrics* 1998;53:50-60.
28. Minezaki, Okubo, Kamiishi, et al. Ileus, A clinical sign of congestive heart failure. *J Am Geriatr Soc* 1999;47:258-259.
29. Al-Khadra, Salem, et al. Antiplatelet agents and survival: A cohort analysis from the Studies of Left Ventricular Dysfunction (SOLVD) Trial. *J Am Coll Cardiol* 1998;31:419-425.
30. Clinical practice guidelines—Heart failure: Evaluation and treatment of patient's with left ventricular systolic dysfunction. *J Am Geriatr Soc* 1998;46:525-529.
31. Aronow, Ahn. Association of electrocardiographic left ventricular hypertrophy with the incidence of new congestive heart failure. *J Am Geriatr Soc* 1998;46:1280-1281.
32. Wood, Lewis, Von Harz, et al. The use of noninvasive positive pressure ventilation in the emergency department: Results of a randomized clinical trail. *Chest* 1998;113:1139-1346.
33. Hotchkiss, Marini. Noninvasive ventilation: An emerging supportive technique for the emergency department. *Ann Emerg Med* 1998;32:470-479.
34. Kelly, Georgakas, Bau, et al. Experience with the Use of Continuous Positive Airway Pressure (CPAP) therapy in the emergency management of acute severe cardiogenic pulmonary edema. *Aust N Z J Med* 1997;27:319-322.
35. Pang, Keenan, Cook, et al. The effect of positive pressure airway support on mortality and the need for intubation in cardiogenic pulmonary edema. *Chest* 1998;114:1185-1192.
36. Sacchetti, Harris. Acute cardiogenic pulmonary edema—What's the latest in emergency treatment? *Postgrad Med* 1998;103:145-147,153-154,160-162.
37. Mehta, Jay, Woolard, Hipona, et al. Randomized, prospective trial of bilevel versus continuous positive airway pressure in acute pulmonary edema. *Crit Care Med* 1997;25:620-628.
38. Koelling, Kirmse, Di Salvo, et al. Inhaled nitric oxide improves exercise capacity in patients with severe heart failure and right ventricular dysfunction. *Am J Cardiol* 1998;81:1494-1497.
39. Bristow. Mechanism of action of beta-blocking agents in heart failure. *Am J Cardiol* 1997;80(11A):26L-40L.
40. Lechat, Packer, et al. Clinical effects of beta adrenergic blockade in chronic heart failure—A meta-analysis of double-blind, placebo-controlled, randomized trials. *Circulation* 1998;98: 1184-1191.
41. Constant J. A review of why and how we may use beta-blockers in congestive heart failure. *Chest* 1998;113:800-808.
42. The Cardiac Insufficiency Bisoprolol Study II (CIBIS II): A random trial. *Lancet* 1999;3539-3513.
43. The Metoprolol in Dilated Cardiomyopathy Trial (MDC) Study Group—Three-year follow-up of patients randomized to the trial. *Lancet* 1998;351:1180-1181.
44. Francis G. Emerging data from heart failure trials: Clinical application. *Can J Cardiol* 1998;14;27D-29D.
45. Bristow, Roden, Lowes, et al. The role of third-generation beta blocking agents in chronic heart failure. *Clin Cardiol* 1998;12: I3-I13.
46. Quaife, Christian , et al. Effects of carvedilol on right ventricular function in chronic heart failure. *Am J Cardiol* 1998;81:247-250.
47. Packer M, et al. Double-blind, placebo-controlled study of the effects of carvedilol in patients with moderate to severe heart failure—The PRECISE Trial (Prospective Randomized Evaluation of Carvedilol on Symptoms and Exercise). *Circulation* 1996;94:2793-2799.
48. Demopoulos, Yeh, et al. Nonselective beta-adrenergic blockade with carvedilol does not hinder the benefits of exercise training in patients with congestive heart failure. *Circulation* 1997;95: 1764-1767.
49. O'Connor, Carson, Miller, et al. Effect of amlodipine on mode of death among patients with advanced heart failure in the PRAISE trial. *Am J Cardiol* 1998;82:881-887.
50. Rich, Brooks, et al. Temporal trends in pharmacotherapy for congestive heart failure at an academic medical center. *Am Heart J* 1998;135:367-372.
51. Parmley. Evolution of angiotensin-converting enzyme inhibition in hypertension, heart failure, and vascular protection. *Am J Med* 1998;105:27S-31S.
52. Tsuyuki, Yusef, Rouleau, et al. Combination neurohormonal blockade with ACE inhibitors, angiotensin II antagonists, and beta-blockers in patients with congestive heart failure: Design of the Randomized Evaluation of Strategies for Left Ventricular Dysfunction (RESOLVD) Pilot Study. *Can J Cardiol* 1997;13: 1166-1174.
53. Yusef, Maggioni, Held, et al. Effects of Candesartan, Enalapril or Their Combination on Exercise Capacity, Ventricular Function, Clinical Deterioration and Quality of Life in Heart Failure: Randomized Evaluation of Strategies for Left Ventricular Dysfunction (RESOLVD). (Abstract) *Circulation* 1997;96(supp):I-452
54. Foster, Johnson, et al. Changes in left ventricular mass and volumes in patients receiving angiotensin-converting enzyme inhibitor therapy for left ventricular dysfunction after Q-wave myocardial infarction. *Am Heart J* 1998;136:269-275.
55. Borghi, Marino, Zardini, et al. Short and long-term effects of early fosinopril administration in patients with acute anterior myocardial infarction undergoing intravenous thrombolysis: Results from the Fosinopril in Acute Myocardial Infarction Study (FAMIS). *Am Heart J* 1998;136:213-225.
56. Gattis, Larsen, Hasselblad, et al. Is optimal angiotensin enzyme inhibitor dosing neglected in elderly patients with heart failure? *Am Heart J* 1998;136:43-48.
57. O'Connor, Gattis, Swedberg, et al. Current and novel pharmacologic approaches in advanced heart failure. *Am Heart J* 1998;135:S249-S263.
58. Nguyen, Aursnes, Kjekshus. Interaction between enalapril and aspirin after acute myocardial infarction: Subgroup analysis of the Cooperative New Scandinavian Enalapril Survival Study II (CONSENSUS II). *Am J Cardiol* 1997;79:115-119.
59. Bown, Luzier, Forrest, et al. Impact of angiotensin-converting enzyme inhibitor underdosing on rehospitalization rates in congestive heart failure. *Am J Cardiol* 1998;82:465-469.

Congestive Heart Failure: Targeted Therapy and Invasive Interventions

David J. Robinson, MD
Rob Rogers, MD

As every emergency physician knows, congestive heart failure (CHF) is characterized by an extraordinary range of clinical presentations. Moreover, few conditions present with a more unstable triad of hemodynamic, respiratory, and metabolic parameters. In some cases, patients are very ill, unstable, and frequently, teetering on the cusp of precipitous clinical deterioration. In contrast, another subgroup may present with little more than mild dyspnea, fatigue, and limitations on physical exertion. Managing each of these populations requires a customized approach that can range from evaluation, titration, or addition of oral medication(s) used to improve cardiac function and CHF symptoms to, in cases of acute pulmonary edema, heat-of-battle, life-saving interventions with intravenous diuretics, morphine, oxygen, endotracheal intubation, and myocardial pump support.

Because of the diversity of presentations and the multiplicity of treatment and triage options in CHF, the emergency physician is faced with the challenge of managing some patients using a primary care model (i.e., making medication adjustments and evaluating suitability of the chronic treatment plan) and others from the perspective of an intensivist. Providing such a broad range of clinical services for a disease state as complicated as CHF is difficult at best, especially when the emergency department (ED) physician is seeing only a clinical snapshot of the patient at any point in time.

Complicating evaluation, stabilization, and disposition of patients with CHF is the fact that these individuals tend to be on complicated drug regimens that may include digoxin, ACE inhibitors, diuretics, and beta-blockers; therefore, a thorough understanding of drug interactions, evidence-based trials, and drug-based treatment strategies for CHF is essential. The ED physician can play a critical role in improving outcomes by making refinements in the patient's chronic drug regimen, and, especially, recognizing undertreatment in patients with CHF.

In this chapter, the authors continue to focus on drug-based strategies for both chronic and acute management of CHF, including life-threatening manifestations such as pulmonary edema and cardiogenic shock. The role of revascularization, pump support, and inotropic enhancement is discussed in detail, with a special emphasis on improving outcomes through multi-modal interventions.

Drug Therapy for CHF: Acute vs. Chronic Interventions

Successful management of the patient who presents to the ED with CHF requires careful evaluation of the patient's acute clinical status, prediction of the patient's propensity for clinical deterioration, and meticulous management of the oral drug regimen. In the setting of severe, acute CHF, pharmacologic management in the ED will focus on maintaining oxygenation (with oxygen and airway control),

Table 1. Angiotensin II Receptor Antagonist[5]

- Consider using in patients intolerant to ACEI
- Should not be a substitute in patients who have not been treated with ACEIs
- Currently, these agents are not approved by the FDA for therapeutic use in CHF

normalizing blood pressure, and usually, appropriate reduction of preload and afterload with such agents as diuretics and drugs that decrease peripheral vascular resistance. Other interventions also may be required.

In patients considered safe for discharge after ED evaluation and stabilization, the approach is markedly different. The ED physician will be required to review the medication regimen and determine whether CHF-ameliorating agents such as ACE inhibitors (ACEIs), beta-blockers, angiotensin II receptor blockers, oral diuretics, and/or digoxin require modification in dose, or whether some drugs should be deleted or added. Even if the patient with mild-to-moderate CHF is stabilized in the ED, the best clinical outcomes result when the patient's current drug regimen, in consultation with the primary care physician or cardiologist, is refined to maximize the benefits of drug therapy.

Angiotensin II Receptor Blockers (ARBs). Although angiotensin II receptor blockers (ARBs) currently do not carry formal FDA approval for treatment of CHF, these drugs have been studied for their therapeutic efficacy in CHF, and clinicians concur that they are especially useful in patients intolerant to ACEIs. Angiotensin II, a potent vasoconstrictor, has been implicated as an important mediator of increased afterload in patients with heart failure.[1] In addition, angiotensin II stimulates release of aldosterone, which increases salt and water retention and has growth-promoting effects in the myocardium and arterial wall. ARBs inhibit most of the effects of angiotensin II, whereas inhibition of the conversion of angiotensin I to angiotension II does not produce complete angiotensin II blockade, in large part, because angiotensin II still can be formed by other pathways during ACE inhibition. *(Please see Table 1.)*

The Evaluation of Losartan in the Elderly (ELITE) trial evaluated 722 patients with class II-IV heart failure. Patients were randomized to receive losartan or captopril for 48 weeks. Rates of hospital admission for heart failure were the same in both groups; however, significantly fewer patients discontinued therapy due to side effects.[2] A larger study, the ELITE II study, is in progress to compare effects on morbidity and mortality with losartan vs. captopril.

The Randomized Evaluation of Strategies for Left Ventricular Dysfunction (RESOLVD) trial studied 768 patients with either ischemic or nonischemic dilated cardiomyopathy and mild-to-moderate heart failure.[3] Patients were randomized to candesartan (up to 16 mg/d), enalapril (up to 20 mg/d), or both in combination added to conventional therapy, such as digoxin and diuretics. At the midpoint of the trial, patients were randomly assigned to metoprolol or placebo. In the first phase of the trial, no significant differences were found among the three treatments, suggesting, on a preliminary basis, that ARBs are as effective as ACEIs in managing patients with mild-to-moderate CHF.

At present, despite studies supporting its efficacy in managing mild-to-moderate CHF, ARBs, which are widely used and approved for treatment of high blood pressure, do not carry FDA approval for therapeutic use in patients with CHF. Consequently, this class of drugs has been positioned by many practitioners as a substitute for or alternative therapy in patients with CHF who are intolerant of ACEIs. Additional trials, including ELITE II, valsartan-HeFT, and the CHARM trial, are underway to study the benefits of using this class of medications in heart failure. Preliminary studies report that valsartan is generally well-tolerated and effective for this condition.[4]

As a general rule, ARBs should be used as initial agents for treatment of CHF only in patients who are intolerant to ACEIs because of cough or angioedema, and who require angiotensin II suppression as part of their CHF treatment plan. Typically, they are not to be used as the initial class of choice in patients who have not had a previous trial with ACEIs, or in patients who are tolerating ACEIs without side effects.[5] Reserving ARBs as back-up therapy, however, is subject to clinical judgment and may change with reports from ongoing trials and labeling changes regarding ARBs.

In fact, some trials are beginning to suggest additional benefits from combined use of ACEIs and ARBs. For example, the addition of the angiotensin II receptor blocker, losartan, to existing ACEI therapy appears to produce additional decreases in afterload with few side effects.[6] The Randomized Angiotensin Receptor Antagonist-Angiotensin-Converting Enzyme Inhibitor Study (RAAS) currently in progress will examine the possible advantages of combining an ACEI with an ARB. Another investigation, the Optimal Therapy in Myocardial Infarction with the Angiotensin II Antagonist Losartan (OPTIMAAL) trial, is an ongoing multicenter, double-blinded, randomized, parallel, captopril-controlled trial investigating the use of losartan in patients sustaining a myocardial infarction.[7,8]

Spironolactone (Aldactone). In the past few years, there has been renewed interest in the aldosterone antagonist, spironolactone. Currently, it is thought that patients may not achieve maximal suppression by taking ACEIs or ARBs and that the addition of spironolactone may contribute additional aldosterone suppression that may be useful in CHF management. Aldosterone not only promotes potassium loss, it also causes ventricular fibrosis and sodium retention, and it is speculated that by using an aldosterone antagonist such as spironolactone, sodium retention and myocardial fibrosis may be decreased.

To examine these issues, the RALES study evaluated the use of spironolactone in patients with CHF. Focusing primarily on all-cause mortality, the study enrolled 1600 patients with class III-IV heart failure who were already on ACEIs and diuretics and then had spironolactone added to their regimen. The study was terminated prematurely after demonstrating a significant benefit in the aldactone arm of the study.[5] It should be stressed that hyperkalemia can occur with spironolactone, and this adverse consequence of drug therapy is more likely to occur in patients already taking ACEIs. Based on this study, spironolactone is reserved primarily as adjunctive therapy in patients with stage IV heart failure; additional trials are needed to clarify its effectiveness for class II-III failure. Although spironolactone is not formally approved for use in heart failure, it can be used in selected patients, especially those who are refractory to other therapies.

Calcium Channel Blockers. Calcium channel blockers (CCBs) induce arterial dilatation in the coronary and systemic vascular beds.

The rationale for using these agents in CHF has been to improve cardiac performance by decreasing myocardial ischemia and afterload. The role of CCBs in CHF has undergone intensified investigation over the past decade. Numerous CCBs have been studied in this regard, among them verapamil (Calan, Covera, Isoptin), diltiazem (Cardizem, Dilacor, Tiazac), and nifedipine (Adalat, Procardia XL). Newer agents, including amlodipine (Norvase) and felodipine (Plendil), also have been evaluated in recent clinical trials. Although small, clinically significant benefits have been demonstrated in several randomized trials, CCBs do not carry formal approval for use as therapeutic agents to improve symptoms or outcomes in patients with CHF.[5]

In the Prospective Randomized Amlodipine Survival Evaluation (PRAISE-1), 1153 patients with class III-IV ischemic or nonischemic cardiomyopathy were randomized to placebo vs. amlodipine (up to 10 mg/d), which was added to conventional therapy. Amlodipine had no effect on the combined risk of death and hospitalization for cardiovascular events. Amlodipine did, however, decrease all-cause mortality, and it was found to lower the risk of death by 45% in patients with nonischemic cardiomyopathy; it had no adverse outcome on survival. This benefit was found only in the nonischemic myocardiopathic subgroup of the study. More data will need to be generated before a firm conclusion can be reached.[9]

What is known is that amlodipine is safe for use in patients with CHF who require CCB treatment for such other indications as hypertension or angina, especially when beta-blockers or nitrates have not been effective.[10] The possible benefits of amlodipine in patients with non-ischemic CHF currently is being evaluated in the PRAISE-2 Trial, which should shed more conclusive evidence on the value of adding amlodipine to triple drug therapy (ACEIs, digoxin, and diuretics) in patients whose LV dysfunction is non-ischemic in nature. Currently, however, amlodipine appears as if it can be used safely in patients with all stages of CHF, if they require calcium blocker therapy for clinical reasons.[11] *(Please see Table 2.)*

Felodipine, another dihydropyridine, has been evaluated in patients with stable Class II-III heart failure, but not Class IV. Felodipine was evaluated in the third Vasodilator Heart Failure Trial (V-HeFT III). In this trial, 450 patients with mild-to-moderate ischemic or nonischemic cardiomyopathy were randomized to sustained-release felodipine (10 mg/d) vs. placebo. Each was added to conventional therapy. Felodipine had no effect on exercise tolerance or all-cause mortality.[12] An absence of deleterious effects with CCB therapy also was shown in the Survival and Ventricular Enlargement Trial (SAVE), in which the incidence of all-cause mortality, cardiovascular death, severe heart failure, and recurrent myocardial infarction was evaluated in 940 patients taking CCBs and 1180 patients not taking CCBs 24 hours before randomization to placebo vs. captopril. The use of CCB in this study did not lead to clinical deterioration or improvement with respect to further cardiac events.[13]

Of the clinically available CCBs, only amlodipine and felodipine have long-term safety trials to support their permissive, but not therapeutic, use in patients with CHF. There is substantial evidence that they do not adversely affect outcome in patients with CHF. Based on labeling and clinical trials, amlodipine is the preferred CCB because it has been evaluated for safe use in all classes of CHF, including NYHA functional class IV, whereas felodipine has not. *(Please see Table 2.)* The results of further studies such as PRAISE-2 are needed to clarify whether CCBs will become part of the armamentarium for treatment of heart failure.

Table 2. Calcium Channel Blockers with Available, Long-Term Safety Data

(Not indicated for treatment of CHF)

- Amlodipine—start at 2.5 mg/d and titrate to 10 mg/d over weeks to months
- Felodipine—start at 2.5 mg/d and titrate up to 10 mg/d over weeks to months

Digoxin. Digitalis has remained an adjunct for the treatment of chronic CHF for more than 200 years and remains one of the most commonly prescribed drugs in the world. Despite its widespread use for treating patients with CHF, there are no conclusive data confirming its ability to reduce mortality and prolong life in patients with CHF. To clarify this issue, The National Heart, Lung, and Blood Institute, in conjunction with The Department of Veteran's Affairs, conducted a large clinical trial—the Digitalis Investigation Group (DIG) study—to investigate the benefits of digoxin in heart failure.

The DIG study was a randomized, double-blinded, collaborative, international trial of approximately 8,000 patients with CHF. The largest portion of the trial involved 6,800 patients with class I-IV heart failure with an ejection fraction (EF) less than 45%; 84% of the patients had class II and III heart failure. The primary end point was mortality, with the secondary end points including death from cardiovascular causes, death from worsening heart failure, hospitalization for worsening heart failure, and hospitalization for other causes. Ninety-five percent of the patients were taking an ACEI, 82% were being treated with diuretics, and 44% had been treated previously with digoxin. Patients were randomly assigned to placebo or digoxin and were followed for two years.

Importantly, digoxin had no effect on all-cause mortality, which was 35% for both groups. However, digoxin did reduce the risk of hospitalization over the study period; specifically, patients receiving digoxin had a 26.8% chance of hospitalization whereas patients taking placebo had a 34.7% chance of hospitalization.[14] These salutary effects related to reduced hospitalization rates are significant, but because digoxin did not demonstrate improved survival rates in CHF (as do ACEIs), this agent should not be used as exclusive, first-line treatment for CHF. It may be added to a regimen of ACEIs and diuretics if symptoms of heart failure persist despite treatment with these agents, and it may be considered early in the natural history of atrial fibrillation, especially when ventricular rate control is required in the setting of CHF or left atrial enlargement secondary to increased left ventricular end diastolic pressures.

Although life prolongation and mortality-reduction data are lacking, patients with severe CHF may derive unique benefits from digoxin because studies do show this agent can increase exercise tolerance, improve symptoms of CHF, and decrease the risk of hospitalization. The importance of these clinical benefits should not be underestimated. However, digoxin should be used with caution in patients with renal insufficiency and in patients currently taking amiodarone. In addition, digoxin levels should be measured in all patients presenting to the ED with cardiac symptoms, rhythm abnormalities, deterioration in CHF, or unexplained clinical findings suggestive of possible drug toxicity.

Table 3. Digoxin Dosing

- Start at 0.125 mg/d if renal function impaired. May need qod dosing
- 0.250 mg/d with near normal renal function
- Careful dosing in the elderly, impaired renal function, and patients taking amiodarone (may need dose reduction)
- Toxicity exacerbated by hypokalemia
- Frequent drug levels

Table 4. Diuretic Therapy in Congestive Heart Failure

LOOP DIURETICS

- Furosemide (Lasix)—20-200 mg daily or bid
- Bumetanide (Bumex)—0.5-4.0 mg daily or bid
- Torsemide (Demadex)—5-100 mg daily

LONG-ACTING THIAZIDE DIURETICS

- Metalazone 2.5-10.0 mg qd bid
- Hydrochlorothiazide 25 mg qd

Data from two other trials, the Randomized Assessment of Digoxin on Inhibitors of the Angiotensin-Converting Enzyme (RADIANCE) trial and the Prospective Randomized Study of Ventricular Failure and the Efficacy of Digoxin (PROVED) trial, also suggest benefits from chronic digoxin therapy in patients with class III-IV heart failure and increased heart size on chest x-ray.[15] Once again, however, it should be stressed that digoxin's primary role consists of add-on therapy to patients already on ACEIs and diuretics who require additional symptomatic relief, improvements in left ventricular function, or quality-of-life (i.e., functional class upgrades) enhancement in the setting of moderate-to-advanced heart failure. *(Please see Table 3.)* In this patient population, during consultation with the patient, the emergency physician may need to reinforce a preexisting regimen containing ACEIs and diuretic with the addition of digoxin to the regimen.

Diuretics. In the setting of CHF, diuretics induce peripheral vasodilation, reduce cardiac filling pressures, and prevent fluid retention.[16,17] Diuretics have been proven to be useful for symptomatic improvement in patients with heart failure, especially in those individuals with evidence of congestion, including dyspnea on exertion, edema, and orthopnea. In severe CHF, the most commonly used agents are loop diuretics, including furosemide (Lasix), torsemide (Demadex), and bumetanide (Bumex). In mild-to-moderate CHF, hydrochlorothiazide diuretics continue to play a pivotal role in symptom control. Furosemide is used most often for treatment of acute exacerbations and long-term maintenance therapy in patients with severely compromised left ventricular dysfunction. As a general rule, diuretics should be prescribed for the overwhelming majority of patients with heart failure who have symptoms of volume overload. Typically, these agents should be used in conjunction with ACEIs, which, unlike diuretics, prolong long-term survival in the patient with CHF.

Diuretics are effective for controlling edema and volume overload symptoms;[18] therefore, addition of these agents to a chronic regimen may be required in the ED in patients with worsening CHF symptoms. As such, the main goal of diuretic therapy is to alleviate signs and symptoms of fluid overload, which are assessed clinically by evaluating patients for the presence of jugular venous distension and peripheral edema. Therapy with diuretics should be continued until these signs and symptoms are well controlled. In patients with severe LV pump dysfunction, alleviation of fluid overload, pulmonary congestion, and edema may require aggressive diuretic therapy, even to the point of producing pre-renal azotemia, with significantly elevated BUN and creatinine levels. As long as the patient is asymptomatic and diuresis is controlling symptoms of overload, some degree of prerenal azotemia is permissible.[5]

Diuretic therapy can be titrated until there is evidence of orthostatic hypotension, acceptable azotemia, and/or reduction of jugular venous distension.[15] *(Please see Table 4.)* Potential side effects of administration of diuretics may include: 1) electrolyte abnormalities, especially potassium depletion, which may be a more pronounced loss if more than one diuretic is necessary for control (follow electrolytes vigilantly in patients on digoxin therapy); 2) activation of the neurohormonal cascade, which is known to be deleterious in patients with heart failure; and 3) pre-renal azotemia and hypotension, which are usually secondary to overdiuresis or progression of heart failure associated with decreased renal perfusion. This may produce a contraction alkalosis, accompanied by hypokalemia, and elevated serum bicarbonate concentration.

Although many controlled trials have been performed to evaluate the benefits of diuretic therapy in patients with CHF, none has conclusively shown long-term morbidity and mortality advantages. Therapy is generally initiated with a once-daily dose of a loop or thiazide diuretic, beginning at lower doses and titrating until signs and symptoms of volume overload are controlled.[19] In some patients, a second diuretic agent with a second site of action (e.g., a proximal tubule diuretic [thiazide] may be added to a loop [furosemide] diuretic, or a distal tubule diuretic [spironolactone] may be added to a loop or proximal tuble agent) may be added to provide better diuresis. This strategy may be necessary in patients with a decreased glomerular filtration rate and who, therefore, have decreased delivery of loop diuretics to their site of action.[20]

It should be stressed that resistance to diuresis also may be seen in patients taking nonsteroidal anti-inflammatory drugs (NSAIDs).[5] In fact, worsening symptoms of CHF, increasing peripheral edema, poorly controlled hypertension, azotemia, and/or hyperkalemia may be seen as a consequence of NSAID therapy in patients with CHF; these findings may require discontinuation of NSAID therapy. Some patients with relatively resistant edema may require twice daily dosing of their diuretic. When daily doses of furosemide exceed 80 mg, a bid dosing schedule can be used. Diuretic therapy should be accompanied by a dietary program characterized by avoidance of excessive sodium intake. Potassium levels and renal function should be measured frequently in patients taking diuretics

Table 5. Recommended Dosages of Hydralazine and Isordil

- Hydralazine—start at 10 mg po qid, target dose 75-100 mg/d, max 300 mg/d
- Isordil—start 10 mg po tid, target 40 mg tid

(Recommended is a nitrate free interval pm-am)

to avoid precipitating renal insufficiency and hypokalemia-mediated cardiac arryhthymias.[19]

Hydralazine and Isordil. Combination treatment with hydralazine and Isordil has remained an attractive alternative for afterload reduction, especially in patients who are intolerant to conventional afterload reduction with ACEIs. This combination of drugs should not be used in the treatment of heart failure in patients who have not first been given a trial with ACEIs. Although there is currently little evidence to support the use of either drug alone as therapy for CHF, two large trials have evaluated the long-term effects of combination hydralazine and Isordil. *(Please see Table 5.)*

In the first trial, the Vasodilator Heart Failure Trial (V-HeFT I), combination hydralazine and Isordil significantly improved EF and decreased mortality by 25-30% compared to prazosin. In the second trial, V-HeFT II, the vasodilator combination increased EF and exercise tolerance more than did the ACEI, enalapril. In other studies, combination therapy has been shown in some studies to work as well as ACE inhibition. There is no data showing additional benefits that may accrue from adding combination therapy to patients already on an ACEI or beta-blocker.[5,10]

Inotropic Support

Inotropic support of patients with CHF remains an important treatment option for patients with severe CHF, although its efficacy and safety in patients with class II-III heart failure is less well established. Parenterally administered positive inotropic therapy increases cardiac output and decreases symptoms of congestion. Despite the potential advantages of these agents in decompensated heart failure, some of these agents have been associated with an increased mortality rate in clinical trials, perhaps, in part, because inotropic agents are known to increase myocardial oxygen demand and may activate neurohormonal mechanisms.[5]

Parenteral inotropic agents can be administered continuously to patients admitted to the hospital with exacerbations of heart failure. These agents can be administered in the hospital or continuously at home with an infusion pump. Home inotropic therapy was shown in one study to reduce hospital admission length of stay and improve functional heart failure classes (I-IV).[21] In some patients, positive inotropic therapy may be necessary as a therapeutic bridge to transplantation.[22] Long-term outpatient use of positive inotropic agents has been discouraged due to reported increased mortality rates in some trials and lack of consensus on what agent should be used. For example, The Vesnarinone Evaluation of Survival Trial (VEST) found an increased mortality with the use of 60 mg/d of vesnarinone.[15,23] Another trial evaluating intravenous dobutamine was terminated because of an increased mortality rate.

Two different types of positive inotropes have been advocated for use in congestive heart failure: beta-adrenergic agonists such as dobutamine and phosphodiesterase inhibitors such as milrinone.[5] Both classes of agents work by increasing myocardial contractility. The American College of Cardiology and the American Heart Association recommend the use of dobutamine and milrinone for patients with refractory congestive heart failure requiring hospital admission or in patients with severe refractory heart failure at home. In other words, these drugs should only be used in patients who have failed to respond to maximal therapy with established and or/approved strategies such as ACEIs, diuretics, digoxin, and other agents.

When indicated, patients seen and admitted to the hospital through the ED can be started on these inotropic agents if their clinical condition has been refractory to other agents. It is recommended that dobutamine be started at a low dose (2-5 mcg/kg/min) to avoid arryhthymias, tachycardia, and exacerbation of myocardial ischemia. Milrinone may also be used; it should be started using a loading dose of 50 mcm/kg followed by a continuous infusion of 0.375-0.75 mcm/kg/min. Patients who respond to dobutamine may be transitioned to a chronic long-term basis at home.

In summary, there are few data demonstrating the safety and efficacy of using inotropic therapy in decompensated heart failure. The Outcome of a Prospective Trial of Intravenous Milrinone for Exacerbations of Chronic Heart Failure trial (OPTIME CHF) is a multicenter, randomized, placebo-controlled trial that is ongoing and will evaluate patients with heart failure. Currently, recommendations of the American College of Cardiology and the American Heart Association are to administer inotropic agents only to patients with severe or refractory heart failure. Positive inotropic therapy should be used with caution in patients with coronary artery disease and ischemic cardiomyopathy.

Anticoagulation in CHF

Oral anticoagulation with warfarin (Coumadin) for managing patients with CHF is controversial. The argument for anticoagulation stems from the observation that patients with severely depressed left ventricular function (EF < 35%) appear to be at higher risk for thromboembolic events. In particular, there does appear to be a propensity to form thromboemboli following large anterior wall myocardial infarction that is accompanied by a severely depressed EF. Accordingly, some experts recommend warfarin anticoagulation in individuals who have sustained a large, anterior wall myocardial infarction (AWMI) and have documentation of low EF. It is known that patients who have sustained a large anterior myocardial infarction benefit from warfarin anticoagulation.[24]

The use of warfarin in the setting of CHF in the absence of a history of recent AWMI is much more controversial. It is speculated that patients with dilated cardiomyopathy and reduced EF are more prone to intracardiac thrombus and emboli because of dilated ventricular chambers, atrial fibrillation, and the presence of wall motion abnormalities.[24,25] However, given that there are conflicting studies regarding the use of anticoagulation in congestive heart failure (dilated cardiomyopathy), it is unclear at this time which patients would best be served with warfarin vs. aspirin therapy.[5]

Several clinical trials in heart failure help shed some light on this difficult topic. In a cohort analysis from the Studies of Left

Ventricular Dysfunction (SOLVD) trial, patients with left ventricular dysfunction who were on warfarin had improved survival and reduced mortality.[26] However, patients in this study were not randomized to warfarin. An unexpected finding from this trial was that women were at a higher risk of thromboembolic events compared to men. Furthermore, a 10% reduction in EF in women was associated with an approximately 53% increased risk of thromboembolic disease. This effect was not observed in men.

The Survival and Ventricular Enlargement (SAVE) trial showed that patients with an EF less than 28% had a nearly two-fold increase in relative risk of stroke compared to patients with an EF greater than 28%. Based on data from the V-HeFT trials, there appears to be no difference in rate of thromboembolic event in patients with nonischemic cardiomyopathy compared to ischemic cardiomyopathy. The problem with these studies is that none corrects for well-known risks for thromboembolic disease, such as that seen with atrial fibrillation. The V-HeFT studies do not show a benefit of anticoagulation, while the SAVE trial had an 80% risk reduction of stroke in patients who received warfarin anticoagulation. Aspirin reduced the risk by 56%. It is important to note that anticoagulation therapy was not randomized or controlled. These trials consistently show a benefit of aspirin therapy in preventing thromboembolic disease in patients with dilated cardiomyopathy.[26] Complications of anticoagulation therapy are obvious and include serious intracranial hemorrhage and gastrointestinal bleeding.

Based on these studies, it seems reasonable to initiate warfarin anticoagulation in patients who have severe CHF (EF < 30%) that is accompanied by atrial fibrillation, previous TIA or thromboembolic events, a history of a left ventricular thrombus, or recent AWMI. Unless this constellation of risk factors and clinical findings are present, it seems prudent to opt for daily aspirin therapy (325 mg/d), since studies show benefits using this agent. Patients who take warfarin for the triad of CHF, low EF, and post-anterior MI should be carefully followed in anticoagulation clinics. Such drugs as trimethoprim-sulfa and fluoroquinolones can interfere with warfarin metabolism and potentiate the effects of warfarin. In summary, additional studies are needed before warfarin can be recommended routinely for most patients with CHF.

Severe CHF and Acute Pulmonary Edema: Emergency Intervention

Because of the increasing prevalence of CHF, ED physicians can expect to encounter more and more patients with decompensated CHF, pulmonary edema, and cardiogenic shock.[27] It is well documented that CHF can occur suddenly in patients as a consequence of acute coronary ischemia, myocardial infarction, arrhythmia, bacterial endocarditis, and, for a variety of reasons, in patients with chronically compensated heart failure.[28] If pharmacologic measures are instituted early in the patient's ED course, however, these usually are treatable conditions, and endotracheal intubation and other invasive procedures usually can be avoided. Moreover, early identification and aggressive management may prevent progression of mild, decompensated heart failure to overt pulmonary edema.

Etiology. Conditions that most commonly lead to the development of pulmonary edema (i.e., cardiogenic pulmonary edema) include myocardial ischemia, fluid excess and volume overload, medication noncompliance, arrhythmias such as atrial fibrillation, and hypertensive crisis. If myocardial infarction or ischemia is suspected, it is important to differentiate right ventricular from left ventricular dysfunction, because therapy for each entity is different. Left heart failure secondary to left ventricular ischemia or infarction may require aggressive diuresis and afterload reduction, whereas, right ventricular failure may require intravenous fluids to increase preload. Establishing whether the presentation is secondary to myocardial ischemia/infarction is a top priority since emergent reperfusion therapy, as well as other mortality-reducing interventions, may salvage myocardium and improve survival.[29]

Presentation. Typically, patients with pulmonary edema present in extremis with tachypnea, anxiety, shortness of breath, and diaphoresis, and may have classic "pink, frothy" sputum. Patients also may present with jugular venous distension, peripheral edema, hepatojugular reflex, and ascites. Many individuals with pulmonary edema will be hypertensive secondary to a hypercatacholaminergic state, or, alternatively, they may be hypotensive if cardiogenic shock is present. As with any other critical illness, airway management should always take precedence. This includes assuring adequate oxygenation and ventilation.

Medical Management. Management of the patient with pulmonary edema is complex and requires multi-modal drug therapy and frequent reassessments of the patient's clinical status. Patients should be placed in the upright position, placed on a monitor and pulse oximeter, and supplemental oxygen should be administered. An arterial blood gas is essential for guiding respiratory management. A Foley catheter should be inserted to follow urinary output and response to diuretic therapy. Medical management will focus around four essential principles and strategies: 1) Oxygen administration and proper airway management; 2) diuresis; 3) preload reduction and; 4) afterload reduction. *(Please see Tables 6 and 7.)*

Morphine. Anxiety and preload reduction can be accomplished by administering morphine sulfate at a dose of 2-4 mg IV, titrating up to 10 mg IV as required; blood pressure, mental status, and respiratory status should be monitored vigilantly. Morphine sulfate probably also decreases plasma catecholamine levels, thereby reducing afterload and decreasing risk of fatal arrhythmias. Blood pressure must be monitored carefully, especially in the setting of suspected inferior wall infarction, in patients with severely depressed left ventricular function, and in patients who have a tenuous airway or altered mental status.

Diuretics. Diuretics remain one of the most important and rapidly effective treatment modalities for management of cardiogenic pulmonary edema. Furosemide (Lasix), the most commonly used diuretic, also acts as a venodilator, which may have an additive effect in conjunction with other modalities that reduce preload. Furosemide produces rapid venodilation and, as a result, decreases left and right ventricular pressures.[30] Depending on the patient's clinical condition, state of hydration, and previous use of diuretics, an initial dose of 20-80 mg IV is administered. It should be stressed, however, that in patients with moderate to severe reduction in EF, only a small portion of the diuretic reaches its site of action in the renal tubules.[20]

Controversy in the literature continues over the relative efficacy of intravenous bolus furosemide vs. continuous infusion. One study found that continuous infusion was superior to bolus administration in patients with refractory congestive heart failure; however, other studies conclude that bolus furosemide is equally effective for achieving maximal diuresis.[31,32]

Table 6. Treatment of Pulmonary Edema[26]

- Oxygen therapy
- Nitroglycerin, IV or other route (can administer sublingual or spray while IV access being obtained)
- Intravenous diuretic
- Morphine sulfate
- Cardiovascular support medications—including dobutamine, dopamine, nitroprusside
- Thrombolytic therapy or revascularization for AMI
- Airway management—invasive and noninvasive
- Correction of underlying etiology—valve repair, etc.

Nitroglycerin. Nitroglycerin remains a foundation of medical management. Some patients who present in acute pulmonary edema may require redistribution of, rather than reduction in, circulating volume, and this is rapidly accomplished with nitrates.[33] As a general rule, nitroglycerin is administered in sublingual, spray, paste, or intravenous form. The sublingual or spray route of administration may suffice while venous access is being obtained. Once intravascular access is established, intravenous nitroglycerin (Tridil) is the preferred route of administration for lowering preload and increasing venous capacitance.

Nitroglycerin should be administered as an initial IV dose of 10-20 mcg/min and titrated to maintain arterial systolic pressure higher than 100 mmHg. It is the treatment of choice for patients with coronary disease and concomitant hypertension or pulmonary edema. In one study, intravenous nitrate therapy given in the prehospital setting was shown to improve short-term prognosis in patients with acute pulmonary edema.[34] Alternatively, intravenous afterload reduction with nitroprusside can be used for patients with little to no response to nitrates, in patients with acute aortic or mitral regurgitation, and in those with severe hypertension as a precipitating factor in pulmonary edema.[29]

ACE Inhibitors. Another approach that has gained favor in recent years is the administration of sublingual or intravenous ACEI therapy. ACEI therapy, specifically with captopril, or IV enalapril (Vasotec), decreases afterload and improves left ventricular function. In one study, sublingual captopril added to conventional therapy of oxygen, morphine, diuretics, and nitroglycerin produced more rapid clinical improvement. Furthermore, intravenous captopril has been shown to be effective in CHF by improving cardiac wall motion and left ventricular function.[35]

Accordingly, a combined approach of diuresis, preload, and afterload reduction is favored in most critically ill patients.[28] Patients with severe cardiogenic pulmonary edema also may benefit from intra-aortic ballon counterpulsation (IABCP). Placement of a pulmonary artery catheter should be considered in patients not responding to intensive medical therapy and those with worsening clinical parameters. Echocardiography should be performed immediately in most patients if it is available, unless an obvious etiology or precipitant has been identified. Such precipitating conditions as a ruptured chordae tendinae, endocarditis, or aortic dissection may be more clearly defined by echocardiography.[29,36]

Table 7. Treatment Modalities of Acute Heart Failure/Pulmonary Edema, Medication Dosages

- Lasix 20-80 mg IV (patients already on outpatient dose may require more), or
- Bumex 0.5-1 mg IV (1 mg of Bumex is roughly equivalent to 40 mg Lasix), or
- Demadex 5-20 mg IV
- Tridil start at 10-20 mcg/min and titrate to BP (use with caution if inferior/right ventricular infarction suspected)
- Sublingual nitroglycerin 0.4 mg
- Nitroglycerin spray
- Captopril: Captopril 25 mg SL, IV Vasotec (more studies needed before routine clinical practice)
- Morphine sulfate 2-4 mg IV. Avoid if inferior wall MI suspected or if hypotensive or presence of tenuous airway

Cardiogenic Shock Drug Therapy and Adjunctive Treatment Strategies

Cardiogenic shock represents a life-threatening—and frequently terminal—condition of the heart failure spectrum. Cardiogenic shock is defined as hypotension in the presence of pulmonary edema secondary to severe left ventricular systolic dysfunction accompanied by the inability of the heart to meet the metabolic demands of the body. Treatment often requires invasive hemodynamic monitoring by means of a Swan-Ganz catheter and insertion of an intra-arterial line for blood pressure monitoring.

Multiple etiologies can produce cardiogenic shock, among them: acute myocardial ischemia and infarction; aortic dissection; acute aortic regurgitation and insufficiency; pericardial tamponade; and right-ventricular infarction. Cardiogenic shock is caused most often by myocardial infarction, in which the ischemic insult has been severe enough to make at least 40% of the myocardium nonfunctional. Occurring in approximately 7.5-8% of all myocardial infarctions,[37] the presence of cardiogenic shock should be suspected in individuals with low systolic blood pressure (< 90 mmHg), altered mental status, oliguria, clammy or cyanotic skin in the setting of coronary artery disease, or suspected ischemia or infarction. Elderly patients with congestive heart failure and shock often do not present with classical findings.

Emergency physicians should have a high index of suspicion of cardiogenic shock, which usually occurs by four mechanisms: 1) left ventricular systolic dysfunction; 2) mechanical complications includ-

Table 8. Inotropic Agents Used in the Treatment of Cardiogenic Shock Dosages and Precautions

- Dopamine—start at 2-5 mcg/kg/min and titrate upward
- Dobutamine—start at 2-3 mcg/kg/min and titrate upward
- Norepinephrine—start at 2-4 mcg/min and titrate upward

ing ruptured ventricular aneurysm and acute mitral regurgitation from ischemic papillary muscle; 3) right ventricular infarction; and 4) drug effects and hypovolemia. Therapy for cardiogenic shock will require several different approaches including use of positive inotropic agents for blood pressure and tissue perfusion support, use of IABCP, and urgent revascularization by PTCA, thrombolysis, or CABG. In the cardiogenic shock and acute MI, emergency revascularization is the mainstay of therapy.

IABCP has been available for the treatment of cardiogenic shock since 1970. It is generally considered a bridging device until definitive revascularization with CABG, PTCA, and/or thrombolytics can be implemented. No studies to date have shown a definite mortality benefit from IABCP. However, this approach seems to be most effective when used in conjunction with revascularization. IABCP works primarily by "unloading" the heart during systole and augmenting coronary and cerebral flow during diastole.

Revascularization remains an attractive approach for the patient in cardiogenic shock secondary to myocardial infarction and treatable lesions in the coronary artery tree. Cardiogenic shock is the leading cause of death in patients hospitalized for myocardial infarction, with many nonrandomized studies suggesting that revascularization reduces mortality.[38] The first randomized study evaluating revascularization using CABG or PTCA, the Should we emergently revascularize Occluded Coronaries for Cardiogenic Shock (SHOCK) study, is currently in progress. This multicenter, randomized, unblinded study will evaluate the possible benefits of emergent revascularization for cardiogenic shock associated with acute MI. Patients are being randomized to two revascularization strategies: emergency PTCA or CABG vs. initial stabilization to include thrombolytic therapy and/or IABP followed by delayed revascularization.[37]

Revascularization with PTCA or CABG has a number of potential benefits that include reversal of myocardial ischemia associated with the shock state. Studies suggest that the benefit of coronary angioplasty in cardiogenic shock is observational, however, and are subject to selection bias. Moreover, some studies have shown no benefit from PTCA for cardiogenic shock. Until the SHOCK study generates definitive data and other studies address other aspects of this issue, it is unclear which approach is best.[5]

Thrombolytic therapy for acute myocardial infarction associated with cardiogenic shock also is controversial. It is thought by some experts that thrombolytic therapy may be less effective in patients with cardiogenic shock due to myocardial infarction. Data from the

Table 9. Clinical Pearls in the Management of Congestive Heart Failure[48]

- Avoid NSAIDs in patients with congestive heart failure if possible
- Never assume that lack of rales or x-ray evidence of edema means left-sided failure is not present
- Elderly patients can and often do present atypically without classic signs and symptoms such as increasing dyspnea, orthopnea, and PND.
- Patients presenting with heart failure are ischemic or infarcting until proven otherwise
- Avoid aggressive diuresis if inferior/right ventricular infarction suspected
- Avoid nitroglycerin if inferior/right ventricular infarction suspected
- If patients are not on what is deemed appropriate therapy, find out why and discuss management issues with their primary care physician to prevent ED visits and hospitalizations. This is especially true for ACE inhibitors
- Watch for hyperkalemia in patients on ACEI, Aldactone, and patients being heparinized, receiving Bactrim, NSAIDs.
- Patients receiving beta-blocker therapy may need dose reduction or discontinuance if clinically significant decompensation develops. Decompensation on beta-blocker therapy many times warrants a temporary increase in diuretic dose
- *Always* ascertain history of high sodium intake or medication noncompliance
- Consider thromboembolic disease in patients who present with a history of a large myocardial infarction and reduced ejection fraction
- Some patients with heart failure may need to have pre-renal indices (BUN 50, creatinine 3.0) to prevent congestive symptoms
- The precipitant for heart failure should be diligently pursued

Gruppo Italiano per lo Studio della Sopravvivenza nell' Infarto Miocardico (GISSI-I Trial) suggest that hospital mortality rates for patients with class IV heart failure were high. There were no significant differences between control patients and those treated with streptokinase (69.9% vs 70.1%, respectively). Although there are no randomized trials showing benefit of angioplasty (PTCA), the GISSI-I trial concluded that PTCA should be considered preferable to thrombolysis in this patient subgroup.

Table 10. Admission Criteria Chart[11,28]

- ❑ Hypoxia (oxygen saturation < 90%)
- ❑ Myocardial ischemia
- ❑ Poor social support
- ❑ Comorbid conditions such as COPD, anemia, hyperthyroidism
- ❑ Tachycardia
- ❑ Patients on numerous medications needing in-hospital titration
- ❑ Pulmonary edema or respiratory distress
- ❑ Comorbid medical problems (renal failure, pneumonia)
- ❑ Anasarca
- ❑ Syncope or hypotension

Table 11. Patient Discharge Criteria[11]

- ❑ Stable fluid balance
- ❑ Relatively free from congestion—orthopnea, edema, ascites
- ❑ Stable blood pressure
- ❑ Heart rate > 50 and < 100
- ❑ No evidence of angina of unstable pattern
- ❑ No symptomatic arrhythmias
- ❑ Able to perform activities of daily living
- ❑ Stable renal function, generally Cr < 2.5 and BUN < 50
- ❑ Stable serum sodium, generally > 133
- ❑ Worsening anemia not present

If PTCA is not available, a non-fibrin specific lytic agent, such as streptokinase, should be used.[39] Data from the APSAC Intervention Mortality Study (AIMS) trial showed an approximate 35% reduction in mortality at one month in hypotensive patients treated with lytic therapy. It also showed a 50% reduction in mortality at one year in this same patient population.[37] Pooled data from European thrombolytic trials have shown a statistically significant benefit of lytic therapy in patients with both a heart rate greater than 100 and a systolic blood pressure less than 100.[37] Conclusions drawn are that thrombolytic therapy both prevents the development of cardiogenic shock and may benefit patients who present in cardiogenic shock. Three placebo-controlled trials of thrombolysis have studied the development of cardiogenic shock after thrombolytic therapy. These include AIMS, Anglo-Scandinavian Study of Early Thrombolysis (ASSET), and the German Anisoylated Plasminogen Streptokinase Activator Complex (APSAC) trial. All three of these trials showed a reduction in the incidence of cardiogenic shock to less than 4% of the population studied.

The Global Utilization of Streptokinase and Tissue Plasminogen Activator for Occluded Coronary Arteries (GUSTO-I) trial showed that t-PA was the most successful lytic agent for reducing the incidence of cardiogenic shock; therefore, t-PA should be considered the drug of choice in patients suitable for thrombolytic therapy. Furthermore, early prehospital thrombolysis has been shown to significantly reduce frequency of CHF symptoms post myocardial infarction.[10] However, in one study, thrombolytic therapy for acute myocardial infarction (AMI) improved prognosis and prolonged life but increased the prevalence of CHF in the older population.[40] Predictors of the development of congestive heart failure include: 1) large anterior wall MI; 2) increased age; 3) diabetes; and 4) presence of rales on admission to the hospital.[41]

Drug therapy for cardiogenic shock consists of parenteral administration of positive inotropic agents to increase cardiac output and reduce pulsmonary wedge pressure. *(Please see Table 8.)* Agents used include dopamine, dobutamine, and norepinephrine. In patients with severe hypotension (less than 80 systolic), dobutamine should be avoided as it can cause vasodilation and further drops in mean arterial pressure because of its effect on peripheral beta-adrenergic receptors.[29] Invasive hemodynamic monitoring using a pulmonary artery catheter (Swan-Ganz) and echocardiography may be necessary in many cases. In cases in which shock persists despite dopamine doses in excess of 15 mcg/kg/min, IABP counterpulsation can be used as an adjunctive measure. Alternatively, norepinephrine can be added to dopamine if IABP is not readily available.

Disposition

The decision to admit or discharge the patient with CHF from the ED should be made as early as possible in the patient's course. *(Please see Table 9.)* Clearly, patients with arrhythmias (e.g., rapid atrial fibrillation, unstable ventricular rhythms, symptomatic bradycardia), evolving ischemia, infarction, syncope, evidence of shock, and/or hypoxia should be admitted for more intensive management and are not disposition dilemmas. Some hemodynamically stable patients with mild decompensation can be treated in the ED with diuresis and other measures—usually augmentation or modification of their anti-CHF drug regimen—and discharged with close follow-up with their physician. *(Please see Tables 10 and 11.)*

The ED physician should consider admitting symptomatic patients who have made numerous visits to their physician or clinic with similar complaints and in patients renal insufficiency. Evidence of congestion and hypoperfusion, development of ascites or anasarca, and decompensated heart failure coexisting with other renal or pulmonary diseases should warrant urgent hospitalization. Immediate hospitalization also should be considered in patients with pulmonary edema, evidence of arterial desaturation, tachycardia, hypotension, and changed mental status. Patients who take multiple medications and have severe class IV heart failure may need hospital admission for refinement and reinforcement of their drug regimen with agents known to be effective in CHF.

A large percentage of patients who are deemed to be at low risk for complications can be admitted to a general medical bed. In fact, one study suggests that a significant number of patients with heart failure exacerbations are at low risk for complications and do not need acute care hospitalization. These patients can potentially be treated at home with medication adjustment and with follow-up care delivered under the auspices of home health nursing. Low-risk patients in this study were defined as individuals with mild-to-moderate decompensation of chronic CHF or mild heart failure presenting for the first time.[42]

Another cost-effective strategy is intensive home-care surveillance of patients. This has been shown to prevent hospitalization and improve morbidity rates in older patients with severe heart failure.[43] Close telephone monitoring from heart failure experts also can prevent hospitalization in patients with severe disease.[11] In an important study, hospitalization for heart failure was significantly related to preventable factors, such as sodium retention.[44] Patient self-monitoring of weight, dyspnea, and edema plays an important role in the prevention of recurrent admission.

Accordingly, patient education in the ED is essential in patients seen for CHF. Patients who are referred to a multidisciplinary heart failure team have been shown to have lower hospitalization rates. In fact, patients with chronic heart failure are probably best served by these specialized teams.[10] For example, patients who are not on appropriate, outcome-maximizing medical therapy should have should be seen by specialized providers. ACEIs, which are considered an essential ingredient in the CHF treatment cocktail,[45] are underused in this population. Consideration also should be given to adding digoxin to the medical regimen of eligible patients since it has been shown to decrease the risk of hospitalization.[46] Noncompliance with medications or diet should be discussed with the patient, family members, and, in some cases, case managers to prevent recurrent hospital admissions.[29]

Summary

CHF is a common clinical entity, the prevalence of which can be expected to increase as our society ages.[47] Hence, emergency physicians must be prepared to meet the challenge of managing an increasing number of patients afflicted with this disorder. Important advances and studies in pharmacologic therapy have intensified treatment strategies. ED physicians must remain up-to-date not only with current treatments for heart failure, but also with strategies for decreasing morbidity and mortality and decreasing hospitalization rates for this condition. In conclusion, the care of the patient with heart failure is complex, and should be multidisciplinary, involving emergency physicians, primary care physicians, cardiologists, and specialized "heart failure teams."

References

1. Newby, Goonfield, Flapan, et al. Regulation of peripheral vascular tone in patients with heart failure: Contribution of angiotensin II. *Heart* 1998;80:134-140.
2. Pit B, Konstam. Overview of angiotensin II-receptor antagonists. *Am J Cardiol* 1998;8:475-495.
3. Tsuyuki, Yusef, Rouleau, et al. Combination neurohormonal blockade with ACE inhibitors, angiotensin II antagonists, and beta blockers in patients with congestive heart failure: Design of the Randomized Evaluation of Strategies for Left Ventricular Dysfunction (RESOLVD) Pilot Study. *Can J Cardiol* 1997;13: 1166-1174.
4. Ander, Jaggi, Rivers, et al. Undetected cardiogenic shock in patients with congestive heart failure presenting to the emergency department. *Am J Cardiol* 1998;82:888-891.
5. Packer, Cohn. Consensus recommendations for the management of chronic heart failure. *Am J Cardiol* 1999;83:1A-38A.
6. Hamroff G, Blaufarb, Mancini, et al. Angiotensin II-receptor blockade further reduces afterload in patients maximally treated with angiotensin-converting enzyme inhibitors for heart failure. *J Cardiovasc Pharmacol* 1997;30:533-536.
7. O'Connor CM, Gattis, Swedberg, et al. Current and novel pharmacologic approaches in advanced heart failure. *Am Heart J* 1998;135:S249-S263.
8. Kupari, et al. Congestive heart failure in old age: Prevalence, mechanisms and 4-Year progress in the Helsinki Aging Study. *J Int Med* 1997;241:387-394.
9. O'Connor, Carson, Miller, et al. Effect of amlodopine on mode of death among patients with advanced heart failure in the PRAISE trial. *Am J Cardiol* 1998;82:881-887.
10. Stevenson LW, Massie, Francis, et al. Optimizing therapy for complex or refractory heart failure: A management algorithm. *Am Heart J* 1998;135:S293-S309.
11. Shah NB, Der, Ruggerio, et al. Prevention of hospitalizations for heart failure with an interactive home monitoring program. *Am Heart J* 1998;135:373-378.
12. Levin. Evidence-based contemporary heart failure management. *Resid Staff Physician* 1999;2:59-67
13. Hager WD, Davis, Riba, et al. Absence of a deleterious effect of calcium channel blockers in patients with left ventricular dysfunction after myocardial infarction: The SAVE study experience. *Am Heart J* 1998;135:406-413.
14. Hobbs RE. Digoxin's effect on mortality and hospitalization in heart failure: Implications of the DIG study. *Cleve Clin J Med* 1997;64:234-237.
15. Gheorghiade, Cody, Francis, et al. Current medical therapy for advanced heart failure. *Am Heart J* 1998;135:S231-S248.
16. Cody, Kubo, Pickworth, et al. Diuretic treatment for the sodium retention of congestive heart failure. *Arch Intern Med* 1994;154: 1905-1914.
17. Morrison RT, et al. Edema and principles of diuretic use. *Med Clin N Am* 1997;81:689-704.
18. Haim, Shotan, Boyko, et al. Effects of beta-blocker therapy in patients with coronary disease in New York Heart Association Classes II and III. *Am J Cardiol* 1998;81:1455-1460.
19. Cohn JN. The management of chronic heart failure. *N Engl J Med* 1996;335:490-498.
20. Brater. Diuretic therapy. *N Engl J Med* 1998;339:387-395.
21. Harjai, Mehra, Ventura, et al. Home inotropic therapy in advanced heart failure—Cost analysis and clinical outcomes. *Chest* 1997;112:1298-1303.
22. Leier, Binkley. Parenteral inotropic support for advanced congestive heart failure. *Prog Cardiovasc Dis* 1998;41:207-224.
23. Scherrer-Crosbie, Cocca-Spofford, et al. Effect of vesnarinone on cardiac function in patients with severe congestive heart failure.

Am Heart J 1998;136:769-777.

24. Koniaris LS, Goldhaber. Anticoagulation in dilated cardiomyopathy. *J Am Coll Cardiol* 1998;31:745-748.
25. Garg, Gheorghiade, Syed. Antiplatelet and anticoagulation therapy in the prevention of thromboemboli in chronic heart failure. *Prog Cardiovasc Dis* 1998;41:225-236.
26. Al-Khadra AS, Salem, et al. Warfarin anticoagulation and survival: A cohort analysis from the studies of left ventricular dysfunction. *J Am Coll Cardiol* 1998;31:749-753.
27. Fromm, Varon, Gibbs. Congestive heart failure and pulmonary edema for the emergency physician. *J Emerg Med* 1995;13:71-87.
28. Levin. Acute congestive heart failure—The need for aggressive therapy. *Postgrad Med* 1997;101:97-100
29. Guidelines for the Evaluation and Management of Heart Failure-Report of the American College of Cardiology/American Heart Association Task Force on Practice Guidelines (Committee on Evaluation and Management of Heart Failure). *Circulation* 1995;92:2764-2784.
30. Pickkers, Dormans, Smits, et al. Direct vasoactivity of furosemide. *Lancet* 1996;347:1338-1339.
31. Aeser, Gullestad, et al. Effect of bolus injection versus continuous infusion of furosemide on diuresis and neurohormonal activation in patients with severe congestive heart failure. *Scand J Clin Lab Invest* 1997;57:361-367.
32. Pivac, Rumboldt, Sardelic, et al. Diuretic effects of furosemide infusion versus bolus injection in congestive heart failure. *Int J Pharmacologic Res* 1998;18:121-128.
33. Gammage M. Commentary—Treatment of acute pulmonary edema: Diuresis or vasodilatation? *Lancet* 1998;351:382-383.
34. Bertini G, Giglioli, et al. Intravenous nitrates in the prehospital management of acute pulmonary edema. *Ann Emerg Med* 1997;30:493-499.
35. Arcidiacono, Asmundo, et al. Left ventricular performance after intravenous infusion of captopril in patients with congestive heart failure. *Minerva Cardioangiol* 1995;43:481-484.
36. Sacchetti AD, Harris. Acute cardiogenic pulmonary edema—What's the latest in emergency treatment? *Postgrad Med* 1998;103:145-147,153-154,160-162.
37. Barry, Sarembock. Cardiogenic shock: Therapy and prevention. *Clin Cardiol* 1998;21:72-80.
38. Hochman, Sleeper, Godfrey, et al. Should we emergently revascularize occluded coronaries for cardiogenic shock: An international randomized trial of emergency PTCA/CABG-trial design. *Am Heart J* 1999;137:313-321.
39. White, Van de Werf, et al. Thrombolysis for acute myocardial infarction. *Circulation* 1998;97:1632-1646.
40. Gotsman, Admon, Zahger, et al. Thrombolysis in acute myocardial infarction improves prognosis and prolongs life but will increase the prevalence of heart failure in the geriatric population. *Int J Cardiol* 1998;65:S29-S35.
41. O'Connor CM, Hathaway, Bates, et al. Clinical characteristics and long-term outcome of patients in whom congestive heart failure develops after thrombolytic therapy for acute myocardial infarction: Development of a predictive model. *Am Heart J* 1997;133:663-673.
42. Butler, Hanumanthu, Chomsky, et al. Frequency of low-risk hospital admissions for heart failure. *Am J Cardiol* 1998;81:41-44.
43. Kornowski. Intensive home-care surveillance prevents hospitalization and improves morbidity rates among elderly patients with severe congestive heart failure. *Am Heart J* 1995;129:762-766.
44. Bennett, Huster, Baker, et al. Characterization of the precipitants of hospitalization for heart failure decompensation. *Am J Crit Care* 1998;7:168-174.
45. Lowe, Candlish, Henry, et al. Management and outcomes of congestive heart failure: A prospective study of hospitalized patients. *Med J Australia* 1998;168:115-118.
46. Mark DB. Economics of treating heart failure. *Am J Cardiol* 1997;80:33H-38H.
47. Uretsky BF, Pina, Quigg, et al. Beyond drug therapy: Nonpharmacalogic care of the patient with advanced heart failure. *Am Heart J* 1998;135:S264-S284.
48. Feenstra, Grobbee, Mosterd, et al. Adverse cardiovascular effects of NSAIDs in patients with congestive heart failure. *Drug Safety* 1997;17:166-180.

Angiotensin Receptor Blockers

John A. Brose, DO, FAAFP

Phone calls and clinic visits for antihypertensive medication side effects are a part of every primary care physician's life. Fatigue, cough, cold feet, loss of exercise tolerance, sexual dysfunction—the list of patient complaints is all too familiar. Patients now rightfully demand medications that are both effective and do not interfere with their quality of life.

Treatment decisions in hypertensive therapy also are influenced by the presence of coexisting diseases. Primary care physicians have long noted the association of hypertension with disorders such as hyperlipidemia, obesity, and glucose intolerance. When these disorders occur along with hypertension, choosing a medication becomes complicated. If the patient has heart failure, what is the inotropic effect of the antihypertensive? If the patient has diabetes, is the medication also going to protect the kidneys? If the patient has hyperlipidemia, is the medication going to raise the lipid levels?

A class of antihypertensives called angiotensin receptor blockers (ARBs), introduced recently and boasting a side effect profile similar to placebo, provides some possible answers to these concerns. For 30 years, animal studies have been suggesting that the renin-angiotensin system is intimately related to hypertension, heart failure, and kidney disease. Building upon these studies, scientists developed angiotensin converting enzyme (ACE) inhibitors to block formation of angiotensin II. Clinical benefits of angiotensin converting enzyme (ACE) inhibitors in heart and kidney failure have further indicted the renin-angiotensin system in these diseases. The ACE inhibitors, while highly effective, not only block the formation of angiotensin II but also increase bradykinin. This fact has both positive and negative consequences. Now there is preliminary evidence suggesting that the angiotensin receptor blockers may share some of the positive effects of ACE inhibitors, while lacking some of the troubling side effects.

In 1995, the first oral angiotensin II receptor blocker, losartan, was introduced. The ARB class provides a more complete blockade of angiotensin II than ACE inhibitors but lack the effects on bradykinin. Is this group of medications equally effective to other antihypertensive classes? Do they currently have a place in the treatment of heart failure and nephropathy? Are there situations in which they should not be used? Can they be safely used with other hypertensives?

To answer these questions, an understanding of the renin-angiotensin system and the mechanism of action of angiotensin II receptor blockers is required. This article provides an overview of the renin-angiotensin system and examines the mechanism of action of the ARBs. It will contrast the ARBs to each other and look at their efficacy compared to other drug classes. While the ARBs are currently indicated only for hypertension, this chapter reviews growing evidence that the class may eventually prove useful in heart failure and diabetic nephropathy.

Table 1. Side Effects of Commonly Used Antihypertensives

DIURETICS	BETA BLOCKERS	CALCIUM CHANNEL BLOCKERS	ALPHA BLOCKERS	ACE INHIBITORS
Glucose intolerance	Decreased exercise tolerance	Peripheral edema	Dizziness	Cough
Sexual dysfunction	Depression	Constipation	Orthostatic hypotension	Angioneurotic edema
Increased uric acid	Sexual dysfunction	Headache		Weakness
Hypokalemia	Cold extremities	Heart rhythm abnormalities		
Low magnesium	Exacerbated bronchospasm	Dizziness		

Angiotensin II receptor blockers provide a new and specific approach to the treatment of hypertension. Their efficacy, specificity, and safety profile provide primary care physicians with a new alternative for first-line hypertensive therapy.

Introduction

Hypertension is the most prevalent cardiovascular diseases in the United States. One in four American adults has hypertension, defined as either a diastolic blood pressure of 90 mmHg or greater or a systolic blood pressure of 140 mmHg or higher.[1]

Both the risks of hypertension and the benefits of improved recognition and treatment are clear. After adjusting for age, blood cholesterol, and smoking, a 7.5 mmHg difference in usual diastolic blood pressure is associated with a 46% difference in the risk of stroke and a 29% difference in the risk of coronary heart disease.[2] The public campaign to lower blood pressure has clearly affected the sequelae of hypertension. With aggressive public and professional awareness programs, increased attention to lifestyle issues, and improved medications, the age-adjusted death rates from stroke and coronary artery disease declined by nearly 60% and 53%, respectively.[3]

The identification and treatment of patients with hypertension also are improving. Public awareness programs, continuing medical education for physicians, and improved blood pressure lowering medications have each had a positive effect on the treatment of this disease. Contrasting data from 1976-1980 to 1988-1991, The National Health and Nutrition Examination Survey (NHANES) demonstrated an increase in patients' awareness of their hypertension from 51% to 73%. The treatment percentage of Americans with hypertension increased during that same period from 31% to 55%, and the number of hypertensive patients with blood pressure controlled to below 140/90 mmHg increased from 10% to 29%.[2,4]

Changing Goals of Treatment

With the availability of highly effective medications and an improved understanding of the long-term effects of hypertension, the goals of therapy have changed. While previous therapy was aimed almost entirely at reducing blood pressure to target levels, physicians are now equally concerned with issues of compliance, cost, and prevention of target organ damage. In addition, the focus is on using a single medication to treat more than one disease at a time. Thus, the cookbook method of attacking hypertension has been replaced by tailored medication choices matching individual patient characteristics. Antihypertensive medications previously available only partially met these goals. They often exhibited unwanted side effects, drug interactions, or other adverse effects. *(Please see Table 1.)* The ideal antihypertensive would be cost-effective, have minimal side effects, avoid drug interactions, and provide end organ protection.

A relatively recent class of antihypertensive medications, the angiotensin II receptor blockers (also known as angiotensin II receptor antagonists), attempts to address the new treatment paradigms. Until recently, many physicians viewed this class of medications as useful primarily in patients who cannot tolerate angiotensin converting enzyme inhibitors. The Joint National Committee's sixth report (JNC6) supports this view for patients with concurrent heart failure and diabetes.[3] However, the ARBs may offer some unique advantages over other classes of antihypertensive medications. If future studies confirm their theoretical advantages, this drug class may emerge as a preferred first-line antihypertensive therapy.

This discussion will review the mechanism of action, existing indications, and potential future uses of the angiotensin receptor blocking agents (ARBs). The ARBs currently available will be contrasted with each other and with other classes of antihypertensive medications.

The Renin-Angiotensin System (RAS)

While the exact etiology of essential hypertension remains unclear, important contributors have been identified. One of these is the renin-angiotensin system (RAS). It is well recognized that pharmacological interference with the RAS system can significantly improve hypertension. To fully understand the proven and potential benefits of medications that affect this system, a basic knowledge of RAS physiology and the vasoconstrictor angiotensin II is necessary.

The Case Against Angiotensin II

The primary vasoactive substance in the RAS relating to blood pressure is angiotensin II. This octapeptide activates receptors in the vascular endothelium, kidney, lung, heart, liver, brain, adrenal glands, and pituitary gland.[5] It has diverse effects, including induction of cell hypertrophy and/or hyperplasia and stimulation of hormone synthesis and ion transport in the heart, kidney, and adrenal gland.[6] Two main subtypes of angiotensin II receptors have been described. These are referred to as AT1 and AT2. The pharmacological effects of angiotensin II are primarily mediated by the AT1 receptor.[7]

Angiotensin elevates blood pressure directly and indirectly. Activation of receptors in blood vessel smooth muscle cells causes vasoconstriction and increases in peripheral resistance. Sodium and water are reabsorbed by the direct action of angiotensin II on AT1 receptors in the cells of the proximal tubules. Adding to the resulting volume overload, angiotensin II stimulates vasopressin release and initiates the thirst reflex.[8] In addition, it causes the adrenal cortex to increase the production and secretion of aldosterone, which in turn, causes sodium retention and secretion of potassium and hydrogen ions.[9]

Another effect of angiotensin II that has attracted a good deal of recent attention is cardiovascular remodeling (redistribution of mass). One mechanism for this involves an increase in blood volume and peripheral resistance resulting in increased cardiac workload. This can lead to cardiac hypertrophy, fibrosis, thickening of the intimal surface of the blood vessel wall, and increased wall-to-lumen ratio in the blood vessels. In addition, angiotensin II stimulates proliferation and hypertrophy of cardiac myocytes through its action on AT1 receptors in these cells.[9] Smooth muscle growth and migration is stimulated, resulting in synthesis of extracellular matrix protein by fibroblasts.[10] These changes may contribute to the cardiac sequelae associated with hypertension. *(Please see Figure 1.)*

Other problems result from these changes in morphology, as well. First, the reduction in the size of the lumen in blood vessels increases the wall sheer stress.[10] This may be critical in the development of atherosclerosis. Second, angiotensin II activates macrophages. During plaque formation, these macrophages produce even more local angiotensin II. Angiotensin at the tissue level may then increase the risk of thrombosis by preventing thrombolysis and taking part in platelet activation and aggregation.[11]

The resulting remodeling of blood vessels increases peripheral resistance, increases blood pressure, and may lead to atherosclerosis and thrombosis. In this way, a dangerous cycle of increasing hypertension and remodeling occurs, with each worsening the other. *(Please see Figure 2.)*

Finally, angiotensin II has an important role in the development of diabetic nephropathy. There is evidence that it acts synergistically with hyperglycemia to promote cellular injury in the kidney.[12] This will be discussed later in more detail.

The Production of Angiotensin II

The primary pathway for the production of angiotensin II begins with renin, which is released from the renal juxtaglomerular cells in response to hemodynamic and sympathetic stimuli. Renin is a protease that bonds in angiotensinogen, an abundant circulating alpha2-globulin produced in the liver. The result is a weak vasodilator called angiotensin I. Angiotensin I, in turn, is converted to angiotensin II by angiotensin converting enzyme (ACE), found in plasma, pulmonary endothelium, and other tissues. While angiotensin I has weak vasoconstrictive capabilities (< 1% as potent as angiotensin II), angiotensin II is a powerful vasoconstrictor with multiple actions. ACE is identical to kininase II, which is responsible for inactivating bradykinin and other potent vasodilator peptides.[9] This characteristic accounts for the increase in bradykinin levels seen in patients using ACE inhibitors. Increased bradykinin levels can have both positive and negative effects, as discussed below.

Figure 1. Effects of Angiotensin II

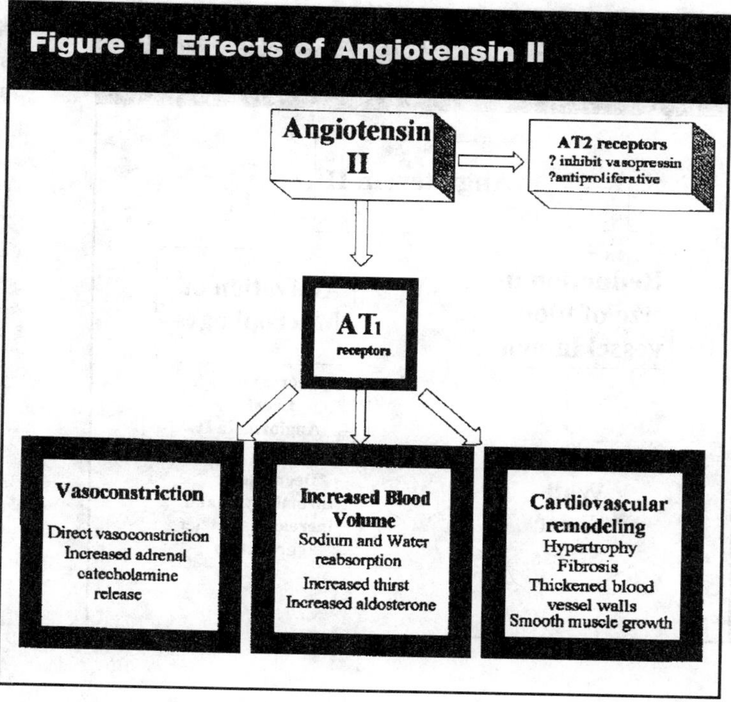

Why Block the AT1 Receptors? The Non-Renin Production of Angiotensin II

In addition to production through the renin-angiotensin system, angiotensin II is produced through alternative enzymatic pathways. Angiotensin-processing enzymes exist in some tissues that can convert angiotensinogen either to angiotensin I or directly to angiotensin II. While the significance of this production is still being determined, alternative pathways may be important at the local tissue (endothelial) level. Enzymes other than ACE that catalyze the conversion of angiotensin I to angiotensin II include cathepsin G, chymostatin-sensitive A II-generating enzyme (CAGE), and heart chymase.[9]

Feedback Mechanisms

Angiotensin II self regulates in two ways. First, it acts directly upon receptors found in the renal juxtaglomerular cells to inhibit the production of renin. Second, raising the blood pressure provides negative feedback by restricting renin production.[9] A properly functioning feedback mechanism is essential in maintaining normal blood pressure.

Other Angiotensins

In addition to its conversion to angiotensin II, angiotensin I can be cleaved to angiotensin 1-7, which may have vasodilatory properties. Similarly, angiotensin II catabolism yields angiotensin III.[13] Research is currently underway to determine the significance of these other forms of angiotensin. The roles of other types of

Figure 2. Role of Angiotensin II in Atherosclerosis

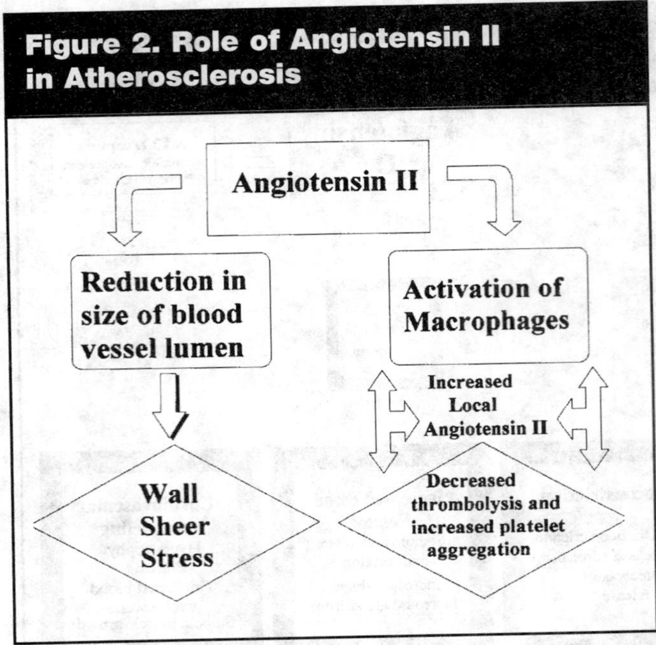

angiotensin and the AT2 receptors in the feedback mechanism are currently under investigation.

Attack on Angiotensin II: The ACE Inhibitors

As a better understanding of the renin-angiotensin system developed, researchers sought medications that could interfere in the production of angiotensin II. While beta-blockers were known to have some effects on the renin-angiotensin system, a medication to act more specifically on angiotensin II was required. In the 1960s, venom from pit vipers was found to contain factors that intensified response to bradykinin. This led to the synthesis of the first ACE inhibitor, teprotide. This medication lowered blood pressure and had positive effects on heart failure in humans, but it had to be administered parenterally. The search then ensued for an orally active ACE inhibitor. A group of compounds was found, the most active of which was captopril.[9]

ACE inhibitors lower the blood pressure by several mechanisms. First, they block the conversion of angiotensin I to angiotensin II by the competitive inhibition of ACE. As noted previously, however, tissues synthesize angiotensin II using enzymes unassociated with angiotensin converting enzyme. This inhibition of angiotensin II is, therefore, incomplete.

A second mechanism for blood pressure reduction with ACE inhibitors involves impeding the degradation of bradykinin and substance P, which, in turn, stimulates prostaglandin biosynthesis. ACE is identical to kininase II, which is responsible for degrading bradykinin. By blocking ACE, the ACE inhibitors also are increasing bradykinin levels. Bradykinin is a potent vasodilator and may be a significant contributor to the efficacy of ACE inhibitors.

Unfortunately, bradykinin and substance P also may be partially responsible for the side effects seen with ACE inhibitor use, including cough.[14] Cough is seen in 5-20% of patients on ACE inhibitor therapy. It is usually dry, persistent, and tends to linger for the duration of therapy. Over time, it can change the tone of the voice; when severe, it can result in vomiting. The cough tends to be resistant to antitussive agents and is a significant reason for discontinuation of ACE inhibitor therapy.[9]

While the exact mechanism of ACE inhibitor cough is not known, bradykinin is strongly suspected as a major factor. Bradykinin can induce cough by activating sensory C fibers. It also can increase the production of prostaglandins and leukotrienes, resulting in irritation of the lung. Finally, ACE inhibitors potentiate a neuropeptide known as substance P (tachykinin), which may increase sensitivity to the cough reflex.[14]

Thus, a search began for medications that prevent the detrimental effects of angiotensin II but that spare patients from the side effects associated with increased bradykinin levels.

The Angiotensin II Receptor Blockers

Alternative metabolic pathways of angiotensin production and the side effects of ACE inhibitors lead to a search for an alternative method of blocking angiotensin II. Since all known pressor effects of angiotensin II are mediated through the AT1 receptor, a medication that blocked these receptors would theoretically share therapeutic effects of the ACE inhibitors. This new approach yielded the angiotensin II receptor blockers (ARBs). The first blockade of the angiotensin II receptors was achieved in the 1970s with saralasin acetate, which had a short duration and had to be given parenterally. Losartan, the first orally administered angiotensin II type 1 receptor blocker, became available in 1995.

ARBs lower blood pressure by interfering with the action of angiotensin II, blockading the AT1 receptor site. This obstructs the

Figure 3. ARBs and the Renin-Angiotensin System

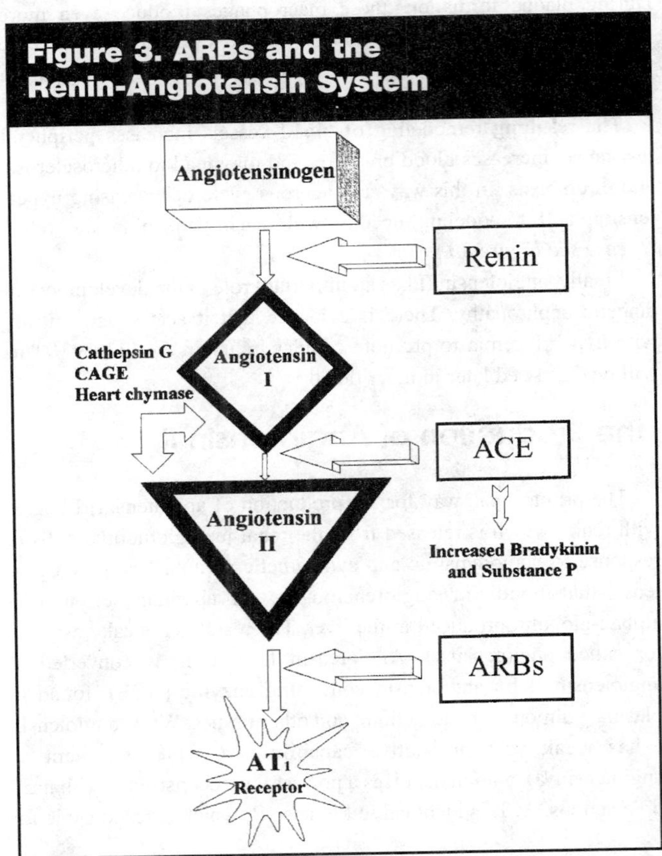

action of angiotensin II regardless of its site or mechanism of production. *(Please see Figure 3.)* ARBs do not interfere with ACE; therefore, they do not result in increased bradykinin or substance P. They have no effect on glomerular filtration rate, triglycerides, total or HDL cholesterol, or fasting glucose concentrations.[15]

Treatment with ARBs has a number of beneficial effects. By blocking the AT1 receptor site, ARBs decrease all of angiotensin II's known effects, including slow and fast pressor responses, sympathetic nervous system stimulation, CNS effects including thirst, release of adrenal catecholamines, secretion of aldosterone, direct and indirect effects on the kidneys, and growth-promoting actions.[9]

Unlike the ACE inhibitors, ARBs do not decrease the levels of angiotensin II. Indeed, because ARBs disrupt the negative feedback mechanism of angiotensin II synthesis, renin and angiotensin II levels increase. Because the ARBs are specific for the AT1 receptors only, the AT2 receptors are increasingly activated by the rise in angiotensin II. While the exact physiologic role of AT2 receptors is not known, animal studies suggest that stimulation may inhibit vasopressin release, counteract angiotensin II's pressor effects, and mediate an antiproliferative mechanism.[16-19] *(Please see Table 2.)*

Table 2. Benefits of Angiotensin II Receptor Blockers

- Block all of angiotensin II's known effects, including:
  - Pressor responses
  - Sympathetic nerve stimulation
  - CNS effects including thirst
  - Secretion of aldosterone
  - Direct effects on the kidneys
  - Growth promoting actions
- No effects on bradykinin or substance P
- Block angiotensin II regardless of the site of production
- Side effect profile similar to placebo

Currently Available ARBs

At the time of writing, three angiotensin II receptor blockers were available. At least several others will probably receive FDA approval this year.

Losartan (Cozaar) was the first available orally active ARB. It is available alone or in combination with low-dose hydrochlorothiazide (Hyzaar). Subsequently, valsartan (Diovan) was brought out in 1996 and irbesartan (Avapro) in 1997. Many other ARBs are in various stages of clinical development. The most important part of each structure is the biphenyl tetrazole moiety, which is necessary for AT1 receptor binding.[7] Variance in molecular structure causes differences primarily in the bioavailability and pharmacokinetics of the medications.

ARBs and Hypertension

All of the currently available ARBs have been shown to be clinically effective in hypertension. Since losartan was the first ARB introduced, it is the most extensively studied. Multiple clinical trials have demonstrated losartan's efficacy in hypertension.[20-25] Losartan has both an active parent and an active metabolite. Dosage in otherwise healthy patients is started at 50 mg/d and can be increased to 100 mg daily in a single or twice daily dose. Because there is little proven advantage to increasing the dose of losartan above 50 mg, it is often advantageous to add low-dose hydrochlorothiazide when increased efficacy is required. Losartan can be given with or between meals, as food has only minimal effects on bioavailability. A small uricosuric effect with chronic oral administration that is due to losartan's active parent.[26]

Valsartan has demonstrated effectiveness in hypertension in at least seven placebo-controlled, randomized clinical trials with more than 2000 patients.[27-29] The dose of valsartan is started at 80 mg once daily and can be titrated to 320 mg/d. Adding a low-dose diuretic such as hydrochlorothiazide to valsartan improves efficacy more than increasing dose above 80 mg. Although food decreases the peak plasma concentration by about 50%, it can be taken with or without food.[30]

The efficacy of irbesartan, the newest ARB, has been demonstrated in seven randomized, double-blind, placebo-controlled trials with more than 1900 patients. Irbesartan has a dose-dependent reduction in blood pressure at doses of 75 mg qd and greater that plateaus at doses of more than 300 mg.[31] The dose of irbesartan is generally started at 150 mg, then titrated to 300 mg once daily if necessary. Like the other ARBs, irbesartan demonstrates a significant increase in efficacy when combined with low-dose hydrochlorothiazide.[32] Taking irbesartan with food has no effect on bioavailability.[15]

Unlike the ACE inhibitors, cough is not a major problem with the ARB drug class. Three studies have compared ARBs with the ACE inhibitor enalapril. Comparing the incidence of cough in patients treated with losartan to those treated with enalapril, Tikkanen found a 3% incidence of cough with losartan compared to a 15.1% incidence with enalapril.[33] Larochelle found a 2.5% incidence with irbesartan compared to 13.1% for enalapril, and Holwerda found a 0.7% incidence in valsartan compared to 4.3% in enalapril.[27,34]

There is some indication that ARBs may not be as effective in African American patients as in Caucasian patients.[35,36] Patients older than age 65 generally respond well to the ARBs.[20,24,36]

Several unpublished trials suggest that there may be some differences in efficacy, response rate, and side effect profile among the three currently available ARBs.[23,37] However, to date there are insufficient data to conclude that one ARB is clearly superior to the others for controlling hypertension. *(Please see Table 3.)*

Comparison of ARBs to Other Drug Classes in Hypertension

Currently available ARBs have been compared in head-to-head studies against drugs in other antihypertensive classes. Attention has focused on comparisons with ACE inhibitors due to hope that the ARBs will share ACE inhibitors' positive effects in hypertension, congestive heart failure, and nephropathy.

Losartan vs. Enalapril, Atenolol, Nifedipine, Amlodipine, and Hydrochlorothiazide. In a study by Tikkanen, losartan was compared to enalapril after 12 weeks of treatment. The difference in blood

Table 3. Currently Available ARBs

	LOSARTAN	VALSARTAN	IRBESARTAN
Usual dose	50-100 mg/d	80-320 mg/d	150-300 mg/d
Clinical experience	Approved 1995	Approved 1996	Approved 1997
Side effects	Similar to placebo	Similar to placebo	Similar to placebo
Dosing	QD or BID	QD	QD
Effect of food	Minimal	50% decreased peak plasma concentration	None
Dosage adjustment for renal failure	None	Use carefully	None
Use with liver failure	With caution	With caution	No difference in pharmacokinetics

pressure response between the two medications was not significant.[33] In two other studies, losartan (up to 100 mg) and atenolol (up to 100 mg) had comparable blood pressure response rates.[22,36] Two trials compared losartan (with or without hydrochlorothiazide) to nifedipine and amlodipine and found that, particularly when combined with hydro-chlorothiazide, losartan and these calcium channel blockers had comparable efficacy.[20,24]

Valsartan vs. Lisinopril, Enalapril, Amlodipine. Black et al compared valsartan 80 mg once daily, titrated to 160 mg once daily if necessary, to lisinopril 10 mg, titrated if necessary to 20 mg once daily. No significant differences in efficacy at 12 weeks were found.[28] In another study, 80 mg of valsartan was compared to enalapril 20 mg once daily over an eight-week period; the two drugs showed no statistical difference in blood pressure response.[27] Corea et al compared valsartan to amlodipine and found no statistical difference in blood pressure control at 12 weeks.[38]

Irbesartan vs. Enalapril, Atenolol, Hydrochlorothiazide. In a study by Mimran et al, irbesartan, titrated over 12 weeks to 300 mg if necessary, was compared to enalapril, titrated to 40 mg if necessary. At week 12, reduction in diastolic blood pressure was not statistically different between the two medications.[39] Stumpe, in a recent trial of irbesartan vs. atenolol, showed similar efficacy of 150 mg of irbesartan to 100 mg of atenolol.[40] Kochar et al, comparing irbesartan to hydrochlorothiazide, found that irbesartan lowered diastolic blood pressure by a mean of 10.2 mmHg compared to 8.3 mmHg of hydrochlorothiazide.[32]

The Use of ARBs in Diseases Other than Hypertension

Currently, the ARBs are only indicated for treatment of hypertension. However, there is increasing evidence that they also may be effective in the treatment of other disorders, particularly congestive heart failure and diabetic nephropathy. Because losartan has been available the longest, most of the available studies were done with this medication.

ARBs and Heart Failure. Between one and two million adults in the United States are affected by heart failure.[41] Based on strong evidence citing improvement in heart failure with ACE inhibitors, JNC 6 recommends using angiotensin II receptor blockers for patients in whom ACE inhibitors are indicated but who are unable to tolerate them. Studies showing a similar benefit of ARBs to ACE inhibitors are accumulating but are as yet inconclusive.

ACE inhibitors are beneficial for decreasing symptoms and increasing survival in heart failure. Their mechanism of that protection, however, is not completely understood.[42,43] Some authorities have postulated that part of the positive effect of ACE inhibitors may be due to the increased effects of bradykinin. Since ARBs do not raise bradykinin levels, they theoretically may lack some of the efficacy seen with ACE inhibitors.[44,45] The significance of elevated bradykinin levels and their potential benefit is not yet clear.

Recent studies suggest that losartan can improve hemodynamics and exercise performance in patients with heart failure to a similar extent as ACE inhibitors.[25,46,47] In the Evaluation of Losartan in the Elderly trial (ELITE) study, 722 patients with NYHA class II-IV heart failure and ejection fractions of 40% or less were placed on losartan (352 patients) or captopril (370 patients). End points were persisting increase in serum creatinine on therapy, death and/or hospital admission for heart failure, total mortality, admission for heart failure, NYHA class, and admission for myocardial infarction or unstable angina. Results showed that persisting increases in serum creatinine were the same in both groups (10.5%), and fewer losartan patients discontinued therapy for adverse experiences. Death and/or hospital admission for heart failure was 9.4% in the losartan group compared to 13.2% in the captopril patients, primarily due to a reduction in all-cause mortality (4.8% vs 8.7%). Admissions with heart failure were the same for both groups, as was the improvement in NYHA functional class. The authors concluded that losartan was associated with an unexpected lower mortality rate than captopril and that losartan was generally better tolerated.[48] Further studies evaluating morbidity and mortality are ongoing, and additional evidence is required before recommending the use of ARBs for heart failure. In addition, specific drug studies are required to determine whether any beneficial effects are unique to losartan or common to the entire class of ARBs.

An interesting concept currently under study is the combination of an ARB with an ACE inhibitor. As mentioned earlier, some investigators feel that the beneficial effects of ACE inhibitors on heart failure are not only from angiotensin II inhibition, but also from the increase in bradykinin. Combining an ARB with an ACE inhibitor would theoretically block both the ACE- and non-ACE-dependent systems of angiotensin II formation. In addition, the increase in bradykinin caused by the ACE inhibitor would be preserved. This raises speculation that combining the two medications might be more effective for heart failure than either drug alone. Trials are currently underway to evaluate this hypothesis.[49]

Finally, ARBs also are being evaluated in hypoxemic cor pulmonale, and early results suggest that they may play a future role in therapy.[50]

ARBs and Diabetic Nephropathy. Diabetic nephropathy is the major cause of end-stage renal failure in the Western world. It is a major cause of morbidity and mortality in patients with diabetes. Roughly 40% of all diabetics, whether insulin-dependent or not, develop diabetic nephropathy.[51] ACE inhibitors, calcium antagonists, and low-dose diuretics (JNC 6) have emerged as preferred drugs in the hypertensive diabetic patient.[3,51,52] In addition, data support the use of ACE inhibitors or nondihydropyridine calcium-channel antagonists in nonhypertensive diabetics with proteinuria.[53]

Recent studies have implicated the renin-angiotensin system as an important contributor to renal disease and diabetic nephropathy.[12,54] It has been shown that antagonism of angiotensin II improves the hemodynamics of the glomerular capillary and modulates cellular components, resulting in preservation of the glomerular capillary cell wall function.[55] The protective effects of inhibition of the RAS also correlate with the suppression of transforming growth factor-ß production, which may induce renal fibrosis.[56]

ACE inhibitors have been shown to reduce proteinuria in a variety of proteinuric renal diseases, primarily mediated through a reduction of glomerular capillary pressure.[57] There is experimental evidence that the positive effect of ACE inhibitors in preventing diabetic nephropathy is directly related to effects on angiotensin II, rather than their effects on bradykinin.[58-60] Since ARBs appear to have similar effects on renal vasculature to ACE inhibitors, it seems reasonable that they may have a similar protective effect for preventing nephropathy, particularly in diabetic patients.[61] Preliminary animal and human studies support this hypothesis.

In diabetic rats treated either with insulin alone or insulin with losartan, losartan significantly prevented proteinuria and glomerulosclerosis. This effect seems to be a direct result of angiotensin II inhibition.[62,63] In a small study from Hong Kong, 12 elderly hypertensive patients with Type 2 diabetes were placed on either losartan or felodipine. Urinary albumin excretion was reduced by 27% in the losartan group, compared to no change in the felodipine-treated group.[64] While initial results are promising, further studies of ARBs are required before recommending their use to prevent diabetic nephropathy. As in the treatment of heart failure, it is currently unclear whether these beneficial effects are unique to losartan or are common to the entire ARB class.

Side Effects and Precautions for ARBs

One of the most notable benefits of the angiotensin II receptor blockers is their side effect profile. In non-pregnant patients with normal hepatic and renal function, multiple trials have shown the ARBs to have a side effect profile equal to or better than placebo.[27,33,34] ARBs have a neutral effect on levels of serum lipids and lipoproteins.[65] As discussed previously, ARBs are not associated with cough, an advantage over ACE inhibitors.

Despite an excellent side effect profile, there are some precautions for specific ARBs. Losartan and valsartan should be used with caution in patients with liver failure. The manufacturer of losartan recommends consideration of a decreased starting dose in patients with impaired liver function.[66] In seven-day studies, healthy subjects and patients with hepatic cirrhosis placed on irbesartan showed no significant differences in pharmacokinetics.[35]

When possible, volume depletion should be corrected prior to starting ARBs. Patients with severe renal failure should followed very carefully when started on valsartan; no dosage adjustment is necessary with irbesartan or losartan.

Like the ACE inhibitors, none of the ARBs should be used during pregnancy and should be discontinued as soon as possible if a patient becomes pregnant while taking the medication. When used during pregnancy, they can cause serious fetal problems, including renal failure and death.[67]

ACE inhibitors have been shown to markedly reduce renal perfusion in patients with bilateral renal artery stenosis or in patients with a single kidney renal artery stenosis.[70] Since there is a similar effect on the renal vasculature with ARBs, these medications must be monitored in a similar fashion.[3] If there is a persistent elevation in potassium or creatinine after starting an ARB, the diagnosis of renal artery stenosis should be entertained and the medication discontinued. Angioedema rarely has been reported with ARB use.[66]

Drug interactions are rare with the ARB class. There are no clinically significant interactions with digoxin or warfarin. They can be used with other antihypertensive medications with careful monitoring of the blood pressure. Levels of losartan are increased with cimetidine and decreased with phenobarbital, but the clinical effect is unclear.[53]

There are very few available data on overdosage with the ARBs. Treatment for overdosage is supportive, as they cannot be removed by hemodialysis.[53]

Studies have compared the side effects of ARBs with other classes of antihypertensives. These studies consistently demonstrated that ARBs have a side effect profile that is equal to or better than any other antihypertensive drug class.[20-22,27,28,32-34,38-40]

The treatment costs of ARBs have not yet been defined. While the cost of antihypertensive therapy was once based solely upon the cost of medication, it is now recognized that many other economic factors must be considered.[69] Clinic visits related to medication changes, treatment of side effects, and monitoring end organ effects greatly add to the cost of treatment. Similarly, laboratory testing to monitor glucose, lipids, electrolytes, uric acid, etc., can escalate the hidden costs of medication. Finally, the economic effect of non-compliance to treatment regimens is significant.[70] The excellent side effect profile, lack of metabolic effects, and preliminary evidence of end organ benefit in the ARB class suggest that the long-term cost of these medications will compare favorably to other antihypertensive agents. This is only speculative, however, and studies examining many of these issues are underway.

Summary

The goals of treatment in hypertension have been expanded to include control of blood pressure, protection against end-organ damage, limitation of medication adverse effects and drug interactions, and simultaneous treatment of other diseases. While a great deal more study is needed, angiotensin receptor blockers may address many of these goals. Angiotensin II receptor blockers interfere with the action of angiotensin II at the AT1 receptor, but they do not affect ACE or bradykinin.

For treatment of hypertension, ARBs have an efficacy similar to other drug classes but a side effect profile similar to placebo. If necessary, adding a low dose of hydrochlorothiazide can potentiate the antihypertensive effects of ARBs with minimal adverse effects. ARBs should not be used in pregnant patients, or in patients with suspected renal artery stenosis.

While early studies indicate that they may share ACE inhibitors' beneficial effects in heart failure and diabetic nephropathy, more studies are needed before use in for these indications can be recommended.

Because of their efficacy, specificity, and safety profile, angiotensin II receptor blockers provide an alternative as first-line therapy for the treatment of patients with hypertension.

References

1. Burt VL, Whelton P, Rocella EJ, et al. Prevalence of hypertension in the U.S. adult population: Results from the third National Health and Nutrition Examination Survey, 1988-1991. *Hypertension* 1995;25:305-313.
2. MacMahon S, Peto R, Cutler J, et al. Blood pressure, stroke, and coronary heart disease: Part 1, Prolonged differences in blood pressure: Prospective observational studies corrected for the regression dilution bias. *Lancet* 1990;335:765-774.
3. Sheps SG, et al. National Institutes of Health, National Heart, Lung, and Blood Institute, National High Blood Pressure Education Program. *The Sixth Report of the Joint National Committee on Prevention, Detection, Evaluation, and Treatment of High Blood Pressure.* NIH Publication No. 98-4080. 1997: 3-48.
4. Burt VL, Cutler JA, Higgins M, et al. Trends in the prevalence, awareness, treatment and control of hypertension in the adult U.S. population: Data from the health examination surveys, 1960-1991. *Hypertension* 1995;26:60-69.
5. Timmermans PBMWM, Wong PC, Chiuf AT. Angiotensin II receptors and angiotensin II receptor antagonists. *Pharmacol Rev* 1993;45:205-251.
6. Matsusaka T, Ichikawa I. Biological functions of angiotensin and its receptors. *Ann Rev Physiol* 1997;59:395-412.
7. Griendling KK, Lassegue B, Alexander RW. Angiotensin receptors and their therapeutic implications. *Ann Rev Pharmacol Toxicol* 1996;36:281-306.
8. Awan NA, Mason DT. Direct selective blockade of the vascular angiotensin II receptors in therapy for hypertension and severe congestive heart failure. *Am Heart J* 1996;131:177-185.
9. Jackson E, Garrison J. Renin and angiotensin. In: Goodman L, Gilman A, Hardman J, et al, eds. *The Pharmacological Basis of Therapeutics.* New York: McGraw-Hill; 1996:733-754.
10. Gibbons GH, Dzau VJ. The emerging concept of vascular remodeling. *N Engl J Med* 1994;330:1431-1438.
11. Dzau VJ, Pratt R, Gibbons GH. Angiotensin as local modulating factor in ventricular dysfunction and failure due to coronary artery disease. *Drugs* 1994;47(suppl 4):1-13.
12. Kennefick TM, Anderson S. Role of angiotensin II in diabetic nephropathy (review). *Semin Nephrol* 1997;17:441-447.
13. Benter IF, Ferrario CM, Morris M, et al. Antihypertensive actions of angiotensin-(1-7) in spontaneously hypertensive rats. *Am J Physiol* 1995;269:H313-H319.
14. Lacourciere Y, Lefebvre J. Modulation of the renin-angiotensin-aldosterone system and cough. *Can J Cardiol* 1995;11(suppl F):33F-39F.
15. Cziraky MJ, Mehra IV, Wilson MD, et al. Current issues in treating the hypertensive patient with diabetes: Focus on diabetic nephropathy. *Ann Pharmacother* 1996;30:791-801.
16. Nakajima M, Hutchinson, HG, Gujinaga M, et al. The angiotensin II type 2 (AT2) receptor antagonizes the growth effects of the AT1 receptor: Gain-of-function study using gene transfer. *Proc Natl Acad Sci USA* 1995;92:10663-10667.
17. Hein L, Barsh GS, Pratt RE, et al. Behavioral and cardiovascular effects of disrupting the angiotensin II type-2 receptor in mice. *Nature* 1995;377:744-747.
18. Hohle S, Culman J, Boser M, et al. Effect of angiotensin AT2 and muscarinic receptor blockade on osmotically induced vasopressin release. *Eur J Pharmacol* 1996;300:119-123.
19. Dahlof B. Effect of angiotensin II blockade on cardiac hypertrophy and remodeling: A review. *J Hum Hypertens* 1995;9:S37-S44.
20. Oparil S, Barr E, Elkins M, et al. Efficacy, tolerability, and effects on quality of life of losartan, alone or with hydrochlorothiazide, versus amlodipine, alone or with hydrochlorothiazide, in patients with essential hypertension. *Clin Therapeutics* 1996;18(4).
21. Gradman A, Arcuri K, Goldberg A, et al. A randomized, placebo-controlled, double-blind, parallel study of various doses of losartan potassium compared with enalapril maleate in patients with essential hypertension. *Hypertension* 1995;25:1345-1350.
22. Dahlof B, Keller SE, Makris L, et al. Efficacy and tolerability of losartan potassium and atenolol in patients with mild to moderate essential hypertension. *Am J Hypertens* 1995;8:578-583.
23. Oddou-Stock P, Gatlin M, Kobi P, et al. Comparison of the efficacy of two angiotensin II antagonists, valsartan and losartan, in essential hypertension. Poster presentation at the 12th Scientific Meeting of the American Society of Hypertension, San Francisco, CA, May 27-31, 1997.
24. Weir M, Elkins M, Liss C, et al. Efficacy, tolerability, and quality of life of losartan alone or with hydrochlorothiazide, versus nifedipine GITS in patients with essential hypertension. *Clin Therapeutics* 1996;18(3).
25. Crozier I, Ikram H, Awan N, et al. Losartan in heart failure. Hemodynamic effects and tolerability. Losartan Hemodynamic Study Group. *Circulation* 1995;91:691-697.
26. Data on file. Merck & Company, Inc.
27. Holwerda NJ, Fogari R, Angeli P, et al. Valsartan, a new angiotensin II antagonist for the treatment of essential hypertension: Efficacy and safety compared with placebo and enalapril. *J Hypertens* 1996;14:1147-1151.
28. Black, HR, Graff A, Shute D, et al. Valsartan, a new angiotensin II antagonist for the treatment of essential hypertension: Efficacy, tolerability and safety compared to an angiotensin-converting enzyme inhibitor, lisinopril. *J Human Hypertension* 1997;11: 483-489.
29. Data on file. Novartis Pharmaceuticals.
30. Valsartan (Diovan) package insert.
31. Data on file. Bristol-Myers Squibb Company, 1997.
32. Kochar M, Zablocki CJ, Guthrie R, et al. Irbesartan in combination with hydrochlorothiazide in mild-to-moderate hypertension. *Am J Hypertens* 1997;10:106A.Abstract D5.
33. Tikkanen I, Omvik P, Jensen HJ. Comparison of the angiotensin II antagonist losartan with the angiotensin converting enzyme inhibitor enalapril in patients with essential hypertension. *J Hypertens* 1995;13:1343-1351.
34. Larochelle P, Flack JM, Hannah S, et al. Irbesartan versus enalapril in severe hypertension. *Am J Hypertens* 1997;10:131A. Abstract D103.
35. Data on file. Bristol-Myers Squibb Company.

36. Goldberg A, Sweet C. Efficacy and safety of losartan. *Can J Cardiol* 1995;11 (Suppl F):27F-32F.
37. Kassler-Taub K, Littlejohn T, Elliott W, et al. Comparative efficacy of two angiotensin II receptor antagonists, irbesartan and losartan, in mild-to-moderate hypertension. *Am J Hypertens* In press.
38. Corea L, Cardoni O, Fogari R, et al. Valsartan, a new angiotensin II antagonist for the treatment of essential hypertension: A comparative study of the efficacy and safety against amlodipine. *Clin Pharmacol Ther* 1996;60:341-346.
39. Mimran A, Ruilope L, Kerwin L, et al. Comparison of the angiotensin II receptor antagonist, irbesartan, with the full dose range of enalapril for the treatment of hypertension. Abstract presented at the Eighth European Meeting on Hypertension, June 13-16, 1997; Milan, Italy.
40. Stumpe KO, Haworth D, Hoglund C, et al. Comparison of the angiotensin II receptor antagonist, irbesartan, and atenolol for the treatment of hypertension. *J Hyperten* 1997;15(suppl 4):S115.
41. Schocken DD, Arrieta ME, Leaverton PE, et al. Prevalence and mortality rate of congestive heart failure in the United States. *J Am Coll Cardiol* 1992;20:301-306.
42. The SOLVD Investigators. Effect of enalapril on mortality and the development of heart failure in asymptomatic patients with reduced left ventricular ejection fractions. *N Engl J Med* 1992;327:685-691.
43. Pfeffer MA, Braunwals E, Moye LA, et al. Effect of captopril on mortality and morbidity in patients with left ventricular dysfunction after myocardial infarction: Results of the Survival and Ventricular Enlargement Trial. *N Engl J Med* 1992;327:669-677.
44. Curzen NP, Fox KM. Do ACE inhibitors modulate atherosclerosis? *Eur Heart J* 1997;18:1530-1535.
45. Nolly H, Miatello R, Damiani MT, et al. Possible protective effects of kinins and converting enzyme inhibitors in cardiovascular tissues. *Immunopharmacol* 1997;36:185-191.
46. Dickstein K, Chang P, Willenheimer R, et al. Comparison of the effects of losartan and enalapril on clinical status and exercise performance in patients with moderate or severe chronic heart failure. *J Am Coll Cardiol* 1995;26:438-445.
47. Gottlieb SS, Dickstein K, Fleck E, et al. Hemodynamic and neurohormonal effects of the angiotensin II antagonist losartan in patients with congestive heart failure. *Circulation* 1993;88: 1602-1609.
48. Pitt B, Segal R, Martinez FA, et al. Randomized trial of losartan versus captopril in patients over 65 with heart failure (Evaluation of Losartan in the Elderly Study, ELITE). *Lancet* 1997;349: 747-752.
49. Pitt B, Chang P, Grossman W, et al. Rationale, background, and design of the Randomized Angiotensin receptor antagonist-Angiotensin-converting enzyme enhibitor Study (RAAS). *Am J Cardiol* 1996;78:1129-1131.
50. Diely DG, Cargill RI, Wheeldon NM, et al. Haemodynamic and endocrine effects of type 1 angiotensin II receptor blockade in patients with hypoxaemic cor pulmonale. *Cardiovascular Research* 1997;33:201-208.
51. Parving HH, Tarnow L, Rossing P. Renal protection in diabetes: An emerging role for calcium antagonists. *J Hypertens* 1996; 14(Suppl):S21-S25.
52. Teuscher AU, Weidman PU. Requirements for antihypertensive therapy in diabetic patients: Metabolic aspects. *J Hypertens* 1997;15(Suppl):S67-S75.
53. Kastrup EW, ed. *Facts and Comparisons.* St. Louis, MO: JB Lippincott Co.; 1998:165R-165X.
54. Ibrahim HN, Rosenberg ME, Hostetter TH. Role of the renin-angiotensin-aldosterone system in the progression of renal disease: A critical review. *Semin Nephrol* 1997;17:431-440.
55. Rumuzzi A, Mohamed El. Impact of renin-angiotensin system blockade on structure and function of glomerular membrane components in animal models of kidney disease. *Exper Nephrol* 1996;4(Suppl 1):27-33.
56. Border WA, Noble NA. Interactions of transforming growth factor-b and angiotensin II in renal fibrosis. *Hypertension* 1998;31(part 2):181-188.
57. Toto RD, Adams-Huet B, Fenves AZ, et al. Effect of ramipril on blood pressure and protein excretion rate in normotensive nondiabetic patients with proteinuria. *Am J Kidney Dis* 1996;28: 832-840.
58. De'Oliveira JM, Price DA, Fisher ND, et al. Autonomy of the renin system in type 2 diabetes mellitus: Dietary sodium and renal hemodynamic responses to ACE inhibition. *Kidney International* 1997;52:771-777.
59. Kohzuki M, Yasujima M, Kanazawa M, et al. Do kinins mediate cardioprotective and renoprotective effects of cilazapril in spontaneously hypertensive rats with renal ablation? *Clin Exper Pharmacol Physiol* 1995;1(Suppl):S357-S359.
60. Allen TJ, Cao Z, Youssef S, et al. Role of angiotensin II and bradykinin in experimental diabetic nephropathy. *Diabetes* 1997;46:1612-1618.
61. de Zeeuw D, Gansevoort RT, de Jong PE. Losartan in patients with renal insufficiency. *Can J Cardiol* 1995;11(Suppl F): 41F-44F.
62. Remuzzi A, Perico N, Amuchastegui CS, et al. Short and long-term effect of angiotensin II receptor blockade in rats with experimental disease. *J Am Soc Nephrol* 1993;4:40-49.
63. Kohzuki,M, Yasujima M, Kanazawa M, et al. Antihypertensive and renal-protective effects of losartan in streptozotocin diabetic rats. *J Hypertens* 1995;13:97-103.
64. Chan JC, Critchley JA, Tomlinson B, et al. Antihypertensive and anti-albuminuric effects of losartan potassium and felodipine in Chinese elderly hypertensive patients with or without non-insulin-dependent diabetes mellitus. *Am J Nephrol* 1997; 17:72-80.
65. Kasiske BL, Ma JZ, Kalil RSN, Lousi TA. Effects of antihypertensive therapy on serum lipids. *Ann Intern Med* 1995;122: 133-141.
66. Product information. *Physician's Desk Reference,* 52nd edition. Montvale, NJ: Medical Economics Company; 1998.
67. Sibai BM. Treatment of hypertension in pregnant women. *N Engl J Med* 1996;335:257-265.
68. Textor SC. Renal failure related to angiotensin-converting enzyme inhibitors. *Semin Nephrol* 1997:67-76.
69. Hilleman De, Mohiuddin SM, Lucas BD, et al. Cost-minimization analysis of initial antihypertensive therapy in patients with mild-to-moderate essential diastolic hypertension. *Clin Therapeutics* 1994;16:88-102.
70. McCombs JS, Nichol MB, Newman CM, et al. The costs of interrupting antihypertensive drug therapy in a Medicaid population. *Medical Care* 1994;32:214-226.

Exercise Stress Testing for Coronary Artery Disease

Kevin Berman, MD

Patients with coronary artery disease (CAD) frequently present with intermittent chest discomfort. Unless the description of these events is classic, in terms of precipitating factors, time course, quality, location, and alleviating factors for angina, further evaluation should be undertaken. First-hand observation of the event by the physician is most helpful in diagnosing angina. Determining the threshold for provocation of symptoms and correlating it with an electrocardiogram is useful. This rationale provided the basis for the creation of exercise stress testing to determine the presence or absence of coronary disease by Goldhammer and Scherf in 1933.[1] Their protocols were patient specific. Master, who devised a "two step fitness test," generalized this technique. Unfortunately, the latter was not vigorous, and more vigorous testing to detect disease at an earlier stage was devised.[2] Treadmills and bicycles subsequently became the standard techniques for inducing strenuous exercise and have led to the rise of "maximal stress testing."

Indications for Noninvasive Stress Testing

There are five basic indications for exercise stress testing. The first and most common is to aid in diagnosing the etiology of chest pain in adults, where the story is consistent for, but not necessarily diagnostic of, coronary disease. There should be a reasonable risk of finding disease in the patient; however, the story may not clearly suggest angina. As a subset of this indication, in patients with known disease, stress testing may help to delineate the severity of the disease and may help guide therapy. Those at low risk may continue with observation and medical therapy. Those at high risk should undergo definite revascularization (if possible).

The next common use for stress tests is evaluation of the efficacy of therapy, be it medical or postrevascularization (percutaneous transluminel coronary angioplasty [PTCA], stent, coronary artery bypass graft [CABG], rotoblator, transluminal extraction catheter, directional coronary atherectomy). Drug therapy includes vasodilators, beta blockers, antiarrhythmics, nitrates, calcium channel blockers, aspirin, or a combination of therapies. Again, as a subgroup, some myocardial infarction stress testing can help stratify which patients can proceed to vigorous rehabilitation and which must move more slowly due to angina, arrhythmias, or impaired myocardial reserve. Additionally, patients who wish to undertake an exercise program who clinically demonstrate poor cardiac conditioning may be stratified regarding risk using stress testing.

Stress testing also helps delineate the efficacy of noncoronary cardiac surgery (repair of congenital malformations, valve repair/replacement) and peripheral revascularization. Controversy still remains as to the use of routine testing in patients with high-risk jobs (i.e., jobs in which a sudden cardiac event could lead to major loss of life and injury to others—airline pilots, truck drivers, bus drivers). Unfortunately, there is a significant false-positive rate

Table 1. Indications for Noninvasive Exercise Stress Testing

- Diagnosis of chest pain—pain that is suggestive but not diagnostic of ischemia
- Assess patient with known disease for suitability for rehabilitation
- Evaluate severity of known coronary disease
- Guide rehabilitation in post-infarct patients
- Assess the efficacy of therapy
- Medical therapy
- Invasive/interventional procedures: PTCA/stent/rotoblator/transluminal extractor/directional atherectomy/post
- Post coronary bypass grafting
- Post valve repair/replacement
- Post repair of congenital defects
- Post peripheral revascularization
- Provide screening in high-risk professional or those clinically deconditioned who wish to undertake an exercise program
- Risk factor management
- Assessment of exercise-induced arrhythmias
- Assessment (objective) of exercise tolerance
- Detect early ischemia
- Evaluate for timing of valve repair/replacement

in asymptomatic individuals. Advocates of testing say that it is better to overtest to disprove a false-positive than to risk the general public welfare. The even larger controversy is whether there is any use in "blindly" screening the general public, in whom most are asymptomatic, the evidence of disease is low, and many false-positives will be seen. Applying Bayes' Theorem, which indicates that the prevalence of a disease is directly related to the incidence of disease in a population, seeking out occult disease in the asymptomatic public should not be undertaken. Again, if risk factors exist in an asymptomatic patient, such as strong family history for coronary disease, tobacco abuse, diabetes, hypertension, dyslipidemias, age, or gender, then stress testing in conjunction with these can be judiciously used to predict the risk of developing coronary disease. Naturally, an abnormal test in this setting offers a golden opportunity to modify risk factors to prevent or retard the development of disease.

A third and important indication for stress testing is unmasking exercise-induced arrhythmias. Finally, stress tests are useful in objectively assessing exercise tolerance. It is well known that diminished exercise tolerance may well be an early indicator of ischemia. Exercise testing also may help to objectively determine when a patient's diseased heart valve needs to be replaced. *(Please see Table 1.)*

Issues and Concerns

Unfortunately, the ability to correlate stress tests with coronary angiograms has been poorer than anticipated. There is agreement, however, regarding stress testing and clinical follow-up. There are good epidemiological data to explain why "blindly" screening asymptomatic patients is not as accurate as when the test is used to screen chest pain. Clearly, monitoring heart rate, blood pressure, and exercise tolerance is paramount in accurately using the results of stress testing.

Physiology

Stress testing provides an invaluable assessment of cardiovascular physiology and provides invaluable information regarding a host of cardiac parameters.

Coronary Arterial Reserve

Every organ in the human body has built-in reserve potential. This allows shifting of function from a resting state to a much higher level of function at any given time or to allow continued normal function even in the face of various disease states. In other words, even if the disease state has significantly impaired a large volume of the organ, continued normal function, even at moderately increased demand levels, is maintained.

The cardiovascular system, including the heart, arterial tree, and venous tree, is no exception. Resting states are a poor predictor of functional capacity with vigorous exercise. With exercise, there may be reversal of shunts, changes in pulmonary pressures, and changes in transvalve gradients that are missed at rest but become critical with exercise. Induction of wall motion abnormalities and left ventricular dysfunction with exercise may lead to increased shearing forces and aneurysm formation. Also important is the fact that even with diffuse, advanced coronary disease, there may be no ischemia due to redistribution of flow as well as the intrinsic properties of the blood created by coronary vasodilatation and constriction. Exercise stimulates the myocardium to demand maximal or close to maximal flow safely. To date, it is the only known way of increasing O_2 demand, allowing the unmasking of even moderate impaired coronary flow.

Cardiac Output

With exercise, adult cardiac output may rise to five times as high as its basal state (5 L/min to 25 L/min). This is accomplished through skeletal muscle vasculature vasodilatation. Mean arterial pressure also rises. A 50% increase in pressure is common, resulting in increased myofibril contractility (a prime determinant of O_2 consumption). Mild increases in stroke volume are seen as well. There is limited adaptation of stroke volume in the face of increased cardiac output. Thus, the burden falls to the increased heart rate. Increasing heart rate shortens the systolic ejection phase. With the shortened ejection time, increasing the rate of myofibril tension preserves normal emptying. This adaptation, unfortunately, comes at the expense of increased O_2 consumption.

Myocardial O_2 Consumption

Myocardial O_2 consumption is directly related to myofibril tension, borderline contractile state, and rate of change of the tension. Exercise increases the rapidity of the development of the tension and the degrees of shortening in the myofibrils. Thus, O_2 consumption per contraction increases with exercise. O_2 consumption is dependent on heart rate, which is dependent on the degree of exercise. In non-hypertensive individuals, heart rate is the largest determinant of coronary flow with exercise. Direct measures of wall contractility cannot be practically measured, but the O_2 consumption correlates well with the heart rate/pressure product (heart rate times systolic blood pressure). This index correlates with coronary perfusion in both normal and diseased states. To wit, patients with stable angina develop chest pain at a reproducible rate pressure product. Coronary flow increase is impeded with moderate-to-severe obstruction of the principal coronary arteries and, thus, exercise-induced ischemia is seen. The cornerstone of stress testing is the premise that objective and subjective evidence of exercise-induced ischemia allows the diagnostic presumption of coronary disease.

The most common etiology of exercised-induced ischemia is coronary atherosclerosis. Another cause includes pulmonary disease (failure to obtain proper oxygenation). Because of the remarkable vasodilatory capacity of the coronaries, this etiology is rare. Coronary capillaries dilate and myocardial O_2 extraction, which is extremely efficient, compensates for the pulmonary desaturation. Anemia and carbon monoxide poisoning, which affect O_2 transport, can also cause ischemia. Left ventricular strain and hypertrophy due to aortic stenosis may cause a consumption perfusion mismatch (even if coronaries are normal). Naturally, any of these in the face of coronary disease acts synergistically to produce a mismatch.

It is important to realize that coronary vascular supply is not the limiting factor in assessing cardiac performance. Thus, by using high-performance exercise testing and correlating it with angiography, it was proven that maximal exercise in the face of normal coronaries does not result in ischemia. Again, if the heart, the coronary arteries, and the oxygen transport are normal, standard exercise testing does not result in ischemia. It is important to understand that these "standard" exercise stress tests are based on successively higher levels of exercise. Physiologically, each level serves as a "warm-up" for the next level. If the protocol is changed and sprint-type exercising is performed (i.e., warm-up levels are eliminated) even those with normal coronaries may manifest ischemia. The explanation for this lies in progressive "recruitment" of coronary reserve. This recruitment occurs with normal coronaries. It is vital in patients with mild-to-moderate atherosclerosis to prevent ischemia at levels of less than peak exercise. Angiography done in those with exertional ischemia invariably reveals moderate-to-severe disease.[4-7]

Myocardial Ischemia Secondary to Diminished Coronary Flow

Just how much coronary flow must be reduced to produce ischemia is not known. Minor changes would be virtually impossible to detect in "standardized" stress tests. Often the time exercised does not unmask ischemia. With longer exercise, other factors mitigating maximal exercise (i.e., pulmonary, orthopedic, peripheral, and vascular may prevent unmasking ischemia).

Rough thresholds for ischemia can be determined. In the standard treadmill test, the change from nonischemic to ischemic occurs from one stage to the next. Each stage correlates roughly with a 40% increase in the rate-pressure product.

Coronary Atherosclerosis/ Restriction to Flow

As angiography continues to improve, the ability to discern what level of stenosis correlates with clinical ischemia becomes vital as an offshoot. The degree of stenosis, below which normal health and the ability to remain symptom free, must be defined.

Gould and colleagues studied the degree of occlusion necessary to diminish coronary flow and induce "reactive hyperemia." In the resting state, at least 80% occlusion was needed to decrease coronary flow. A definable drop in inducible hyperemia occurred with 50-70% stenosis. It took at least 70% stenosis to have inducible hyperemia. Logan verified these results with post-mortem study of atherosclerotic arteries.[9]

The geometry of the stenosis obviously affects the degree of disruption to flow. Normal coronaries generally have an amazing degree of reserve. Even though a 50% stenosis implies disease processes at work, a potential for failure of these processes occurs, particularly with progression of decrease. These lesions rarely cause symptoms with "normal" levels of exertion.

The tests available are relatively insensitive to moderate atherosclerosis. Therefore, to enhance accuracy, maximal or near maximal exertion should be the goal of stress testing. Multiple modalities using high-quality leads are vital to detect ischemia.

Despite its insensitivity in predicting pressure coronary anatomy, stress testing is useful for unmasking ischemia. Ellestad and associates found a low level of events in "normal responders" as compared to a significantly higher level in those with a positive stress test (7% of normals had a future event in 4 years vs 46% of positives).[20] Events were defined as angina, MI, and death.

Using ST segments, exercise tolerance, and maximum heart rate, McNeer verified these results.

Clinical Correlates

Chest pain, long held to be a marker of ischemia, unfortunately is not as sensitive as we would like. Chest pain is only 50% as common as ST segment depression in the face of ischemia. The presence of classic angina is presumptive evidence of coronary disease although other conditions, such as critical aortic stenosis, may also result in "non-coronary" chest pain.

One of the problems is in nomenclature. Many patients deny chest pain but will report pressure, burning, and palpitations among other symptoms. Avoidance of the term "pain" may obviate this pitfall.

Discerning the location and radiation pattern of the pain often helps to exclude or include the etiology as coronary disease. Again, there are many variations of the classic anginal pattern and if a high

Table 2. Use of Exercise Testing

Noninvasive Lab
- Assess for ischemia based on ECG
- Assess for ischemia by wall monitor studies
- Assess for ischemia by nuclear tracers (Thallium, Sestambi, etc.)
- Evaluate exercise tolerance
- Occult ischemic disease
- Timing of valvular surgery
- Assess efficacy of treatment
- Congenital disease
- Valvular surgery
- Revascularization

Invasive Lab
- Assess valvular gradients
- Evaluate shunts
- Assess left ventricular function
- Assess coronary reserve metabolism

index of suspicion for coronary disease exists, the diagnosis of coronary disease should not be excluded.

Time of onset and time of disappearance of the pain should be noted and clearly delineated.

ST Segment Changes. The classic positive test occurs when horizontal ST depression in two anatomically contiguous leads is seen. Unfortunately, ST segment changes occur with hypertension, drugs, body habitus, and bundle branch blocks, to name a few.

Arrhythmias. Ventricular and atrial ectopy is not uncommon. Their presence in the absence of structural disease is of no consequence. Generally, an increase in ectopy with exercise, particularly if the history is compatible, is suggestive but not diagnostic for ischemia. Arrhythmias that extinguish with exercise are virtually always benign. In addition, ectopy with ST-T wave changes carry a more significant effect when trying to unmask occult ischemia.

Reduction in Exercise Tolerance. In patients with no valvular disease, no evidence of cardiomyopathy, and no evidence of myocarditis, loss of exercise tolerance is often an early sign of significant coronary disease. A drop in blood pressure (i.e., pump failure in the face of exercise), is an ominous finding strongly suggestive of severe disease. Thus, global ischemia can be unmasked. Unfortunately, regional ischemia can sometimes be missed if the normal myocardium overcompensates for the decreased myocardium and prevents an objective change in exercise tolerance. Thus, exercise tolerance must be used in conjunction with other aspects of stress testing.

Types of Exercise Testing

Exercise testing may be done in the noninvasive lab or in the cardiac catherization lab. Testing in the noninvasive lab hinges on monitoring ECG data. High-intensity exercise as described above is paramount in unmasking coronary disease.

Testing in the cath lab can be achieved by leg ergometry or hand ergometry. The former is often preclusive in the cath lab.

Isometric exercise has gained some interest. The premise is that isometric exercise increases heart rate and systemic vascular resistance and, thus, unmasking ischemia. *(Please see Table 2.)*

Exercise Mode

There are two broad categories defining the method by which exercise testing occurs: physiologic/physical exercise and "chemical" exercise.

The most basic form of exercise stress testing is the treadmill test. The patients are prepared by removing hair, wax, and skin secretions from the chest wall using liquid sandpaper. The electrodes are then applied in a prescribed pattern (which will be discussed later). The patients are then able to stand on the treadmill, which is a mechanically powered machine that automatically changes the speed and angle of incline at predetermined intervals. The goal is to have the patients exercised to at least submaximal levels (85% of predicted heart rate for age), (i.e., 220-age $\times$ 0.85) or maximal predicted heart if possible. Serial ECGs are performed monitoring for ST-T wave changes and ectopy. The patients are frequently questioned regarding whether they feel any symptoms. Heart rate and blood pressure are serially monitored. Once the patients achieve the target heart rate (ideally at least the submaximal rate) or if they cannot go further, the test is terminated. Blood pressure, heart rate, and ECGs are monitored for six minutes into recovery—again looking for ectopy, new ECG changes, resolution of ST-T wave changes, and changes (abnormal) in heart rate and blood pressure. At any point during the test, if significant ischemic symptoms or changes in blood pressure or heart rate suggesting ischemia or incipient pump failure, or ECG changes consistent with ischemia occur, the test should be terminated. The caveat to the final condition is that the baseline ECG should have been normal and no other factors to explain ECG shifts present.

Various protocols (standardized) can be used for exercise testing. In addition, manual changes can be programmed, if needed, to allow the patients to continue and ultimately achieve their target heart rate. *(Please see Table 3.)*

To do an exercise stress test, the patients must be awake and alert. They must also be able to follow instructions. There should be a reasonable expectation that the patients can walk a suitable period to be able to achieve target heart rate. Those with unsteady gaits, neurological defects (making walking restricted), orthopedic problems (ruptured discs, osteoarthritis), or claudication (bad peripheral vascular disease) would not be suitable candidates for exercise stress testing. Encumbrances such as an immobile chest (bandages, rib fractions, recent thorax surgery) or travascular catheters (Swan-Ganz catheter, femoral arterial/venous lines, temporary transvenous pacemakers) would also not be suitable. Foley catheters, orthopedic appliances, and, in some cases, 0_2 may also preclude exercise testing. Patients with severe lung disease would also be poor candidates for exercise testing.

Table 3. Most Common Treadmill Exercise Protocols

	STAGE (MPH)	SPEED (TO GRADE)	ELEVATION (MINUTES)	DURATION (ME)	VO_2/KG/MN
Bruce	1	1.7	10	3	18
	2	2.5	12	3	25
	3	3.4	14	3	34
	4	4.2	16	3	46
	5	5.0	18	3	55
	6	5.5	20	3	—
	7	6.0	22	3	—
	1	3	0	2	10
Naughton	2	3	2.5	2	14
Blake	3	3	5	2	18
	4	3	7.5	2	21
	5	3	10	2	24
	6	3	12.5	2	28
	7	3	15	2	32
	8	3	17.5	2	35
	9	3	20	2	38
	10	3	22.5	2	42
Steffield	0	1.7	0	3	8
Note:	½	1.7	5	3	12
Stage 2-7	1	1.7	10	3	18
See Bruce					

For pure ECG exercise stress testing, the baseline ECG should be normal or have no ST changes that would lead to a false-positive or false-negative test. Absolute contraindications to exercise stress tests are listed in Table 4.

Clinically, a positive test is defined as 1 mm horizontal ST depression in two anatomically contiguous leads or a fall of systolic or diastolic blood pressure more than 15 mmHg upsloping ST depression, symptoms, ST elevation, arrhythmias, and rate-related conduction changes suggestive but not diagnostic for ischemia.

Other forms of exercise testing (other than treadmills) include bicycle riding and variable step. Bicycle riding has the advantage of eliminating thorax problems and can be done with upper extremity indwelling catheters. Their disadvantage is the lack of familiarity that most have with this technique and the higher level of patient cooperation required. Variable step is a useful alternative for elderly or sedentary patients.

Time Course

The length and pattern of exercise is naturally determined by the purpose of the test. Different levels of intensity are required for participation in sports vs. industrial screening vs. risk stratification for high-risk professionals vs. screening for coronary disease.

The test may be fixed or varied both in terms of intensity and duration. If a homogenous population is being tested, then a single level of exercise is suitable. For heterogenous groups or stratification of a group, multiple-level testing is more appropriate.

Termination of the test occurs when either of two conditions is met: 1) further testing would be harmful to the subject, or 2) the goals desired have been obtained. If the patients, prior to achieving the target heart rate/target goals, terminate the test, this is deemed a submaximal or nondiagnostic test.

Open-ended testing refers to testing when the subjects or their reactions determine the end point. Closed-ended testing is milder and of less intense duration.

End points for open-ended testing are heart rate (fixed), heart rate variable (i.e., 90% of maximal heart rate), exercise to symptom leveled maximal endurance, or physiologically proven maximal aerobic capabilities.

Exercise to a Fixed Heart Rate

The underlying premise here is that 10 poorly conditioned individuals or those with cardiac disease (be it coronary, valvular, cardiomyopathy) will achieve the prescribed rate faster than healthy individuals. The disadvantage to the test is it treats all age groups

Table 4. Contraindications to Stress Testing

- Myocardial infarction (incipient/acute/healing)
- Unstable angina
- Critical aortic stenosis
- Acute congestive heart failure
- Uncontrolled hypertension
- Uncontrolled arrhythmias
- High degree AV block
- Acute intercurrent systemic illness
- Refusal of patient to give informed consent

equally. Clearly, older individuals will achieve the prescribed heart rate at a much higher percentage of their maximal capacity. This test optimally tests within the same age range. *(Please see Table 5.)*

Variable Heart Rate Targets

The prime advantage here is that the individual does not exercise to all-out maximal capacity. The sensitivity of the test remains intact. With age, the highest maximal heart rate attainable decreases. Also, among younger subjects, the maximal heart rate attainable varies with athletic (cardiac) conditioning. There is also an intergender variation in the fall in heart rate with age. The test is adjusted for age, sex, and physical training. As an example, one may choose 90% of predicted heart rate as target.

Subjective Maximal Exercise

Patients exercise to their maximum subjective capacity. End points include pain, fatigue, and dyspnea. The disadvantage here lies in what the subjects perceive as their maximal level of exercise.

Maximum Aerobic Activity

Oxygen uptake and use are monitored throughout the test. Maximal aerobic capacity determines the end of the test. This is a cumbersome test suited for the physiological lab but poorly suited for general use.

Determining the Protocol

All protocols share some common threads. An appropriate history and physical should precede all testing. A fasting state or semifasting state is required. At the very least, a light meal should be eaten no later than two hours prior to testing. This prevents the possibility of stomach upset and nausea. More important, blood flow to the heart is not factitiously lower by increasing flow to abdominal organs. Informed consent is obtained. A baseline ECG and relevant laboratory studies should be reviewed to rule out a contraindication to testing.

Age, body habitus, orthopedic and vascular factors, lung disease, and cardiac conditioning help determine the most suitable protocol.

Exercise Electrocardiography

Eithoven performed the first exercise stress test by recording an ECG on a patient after the patient ran up a flight of stairs.[12] Since that time, significant refinement of the technique has occurred. Masters created a step-wise protocol for stress testing by standardizing the test. Improvisation and interpolation of the data were eliminated.

ST Depression/Myocardial Ischemia

It was Feel who first demonstrated the relationship between angina and ST depression. The ST depression was of new onset with the beginning of chest pain and lasted throughout the episode. Three basic forms of ST depression are of clinical significance. *(Please see Table 6.)*

Practical Aspects in Exercise Stress Testing

It is of vital importance that the electrode skin interface be maximized to eliminate motion artifact and allow maximal accuracy in recording the ECG to allow maximal accuracy in interpreting the changes seen.

There is some controversy as to the number of leads required. Some use a single bipolar lead using three electrodes. Mason and

Table 5. Target Heart Rate for Graded Exercise Heart Rate

Age (years)	30	35	40	45	50	55	60	65
Pred. Max HR:								
Men	193	191	189	187	184	182	180	178
Women	190	185	181	177	172	168	163	159
Target HR:								
(90% Max)								
Men	173	172	170	168	166	164	162	160
Women	171	167	163	159	155	151	147	143

colleagues all feel a single lead may miss ischemic changes.[15] At present, the best accepted and most used is the Mason-Likar 12-lead set using the torso and limbs.

Etiology of Falsely Abnormal ECG Tracing

It is beyond the scope of this article to discuss all the causes of false-positive stress testing but some of the more common and clinically relevant will be discussed here.

Elevated Left Ventricular Diastolic Pressure. Pressure overload of the ventricle most commonly occurs with systemic arterial hypertension or with outflow tract obstruction (idiopathic hypertrophic subaortic stenosis [IHSS], aortic stenosis, etc.). Even if atherosclerosis is absent, subendocardial ischemia may be seen. Lepeschkin and colleagues, while studying college students with hypertension, demonstrated exercise-induced ST depression.[16-17]

One of the other caveats in patients with hypertension is that they are frequently treated with diuretics. Hypokalemia is common and this in and of itself causes ST-T wave abnormalities.

Barlow's Syndrome (murmur, chest pain, ventricular ectopy) shows chronic ST-T wave changes even in the absence of coronary disease.

Bundle branch blocks and paradoxical septal activation (Pacemaker, prior cardiac surgery) or any deviation from the normal activation sequence of the ventricles can lead to ST-T wave changes. Such deviation precludes accurate interpretation of the ECG changes seen with exercise. Left bundle branch block, right bundle branch block, interventricular conduction delay, and Wolff-Parkinson-White can all lead to false-positive stress tests.

Drug Effects. Digitalis, a common cardiac drug, frequently leads to false-positive testing even if the baseline ECG does not show "classic" digitalis effect. In addition, adequate levels of digitalis may preclude patients from obtaining their target heart rate. Lastly, digitalis may mask the forme fruste of certain arrhythmias.

Tricyclic antidepressants as well as many other CNS active drugs can lead to false-positive tests, particularly in women.[18] Certain antihypertensives are known to cause false-positive exercise stress tests. Most notably are methyldopa and the potassium "wasting" diuretics. Nitrates, as well as other vasodilatory drugs, allow higher thresholds before ischemia occurs. Beta blockers, a cornerstone in treating ischemic heart disease, often obfuscate the results of stress testing. Beta blockers are more likely to produce false-negative test-blunting of heart rate and antihypertensive effects would have negative test results although significant CAD is present. By recoupling the oxygen supply ratio and by their very properties (antihypertensive and antiarrhythmic), they may lead to a false-positive test.

Mitral Valve Prolapse. Mitral valve prolapse (MVP) is a not uncommon cause of chest pain and arrhythmias, particularly in younger women. Whether due to exercise-induced changes in the mitral apparatus causing a change in electric vectors or basic hormonal changes or a combination, MVP frequently causes ST-T wave changes compatible with ischemia even in the absence of coronary disease.

Interpretation of Study

Clinically, a positive stress test occurs when 1 mm of horizontal ST depression in two anatomically contiguous leads is seen. The deeper the depression and the longer it lasts, the more likely it is that the subject has coronary disease. This assumes none of the aforementioned etiologies for false-positives is present.

Table 6. Types of ST Segment Depression

- Transient ST depression that resolves within one minute of termination of exercise
- Depression occurring with exercise, worsening with exercise, and requiring several minutes of recovery to resolve
- ST elevation compatible with Prinzmetal's angina
- Modest ST elevation secondary to dyskinesia or prior ventricular scarring

ECG responses in men are more likely to correlate with true coronary disease than in women. The most likely explanation for this lies in the increased prevalence of coronary disease in men. With increases in smoking, women in the workforce being exposed to environmental toxins, and the aging of the population (loss of protective effect of female hormones), there has been some decline in the gender gap and stress testing in women often correlates with coronary disease.

Aside from assessing the electrocardiograph data, other parameters must be assessed and evaluated. Blood pressure response, heart rate response, development of arrhythmias, and development or worsening of murmurs are all important in assessing the patient as discussed above. Evaluation of exercise tolerance is also vitally important.

As an interesting note, ST-T wave change correlated with coronary disease in 64% of patients with coronary disease in Cole and Ellestad's study. If exertional angina accompanied these changes, the true positivity of the test exceeded 85%.[19]

A common physiologic variant on ECGs is J point depression as long as the "depression" does not last more than 0.08 seconds after the initial deflection. This is of no clinical relevance. Similarly, in the absence of other clinical or electrocardiographic evidence of ischemia, minor (i.e., less than 1 mm) or upsloping ST depression do not imply ischemia. If any doubt remains after stress testing, imaging with a nuclear agent in conjunction with stress testing should be performed.

Mathematical Evaluation of Stress Testing

Bayes' Theorem states that the predictive value of a test is influenced by its sensitivity and the prevalence of a disease in the population tested. Thus, testing asymptomatic individuals with a low risk factor profile often leads to false-positive tests. Patients with ST depression with mild exercise have a greater than 50% chance of having or developing coronary disease. Those with ischemia at moderate exercise levels have a less than 50% chance. Ischemia only with strenuous exercise confers a less than 20% chance of having or developing disease.[20] *(Please see Table 7.)*

Other Forms of Stress Testing

All of the preceding discussion regarding stress testing by exercise is relevant to the following discussion. Sometimes it is not possible to simply perform an exercise stress test and be able to rely on its results. In addition, sometimes the patient simply can't exercise. In the latter case, other forms of inducing "myocardial stress" must be used.

Nuclear Imaging as an Adjunct to Stress Testing (Thallium, Sestambi, Cardiolyte, etc.). If the patients are otherwise able to exercise but have baseline ECG abnormalities that preclude accurate assessment of the ST-T wave changes, nuclear imaging will help to clarify the picture. Nuclear imaging can be done in one of two ways. In the first case, the patients do a "routine" stress test. At the peak of exercise, thallium or the chosen material is injected. One more minute of exercise is performed and the test is terminated. The patients are previously advised that they must give the observer one minute of warning before they must "terminate" the test. That final minute is important for circulating the tracer. Stress and rest images are obtained. Alternatively, the resting part may be done first and the stress images done later if the appropriate nuclear material is chosen. Nuclear tracers are inert and go where blood supply goes. A defect at stress levels that persist at rest usually connotes a scar. A defect that "fills" in at rest connotes ischemia.

With any test, some disadvantages are present. A fixed lesion may not reperfuse or balance ischemia (e.g., triple vessel disease may be missed). Motion artifact, breast artifact, patient cooperation, and inability to exactly reproduce the same "angle" of examination with rest and stress images may cause false-positive or false-negative tests. Nonetheless, thallium and other nuclear materials distinctively enhance the accuracy of stress tests.

Chemically Induced Stress. If the patients are unable to exercise, chemically induced myocardial stress may be used. Two basic forms are used: 1) cyclic AMP blockers; and 2) dobutamine.

Table 7. Common Statistical Definitions

1.	Sensitivity	=	$\frac{\text{True positives}}{\text{Total positives}}$
2.	Specificity	=	$\frac{\text{True normals}}{\text{Total normals}}$
3.	Accuracy	=	$\frac{\text{True positives + true negatives}}{\text{Total number of tests}}$
4.	True-positive	=	Patient actually has disease predicted by test
5.	True-negative	=	Patient is normal when test predicted normalcy
6.	False-positive	=	Patient disease predicted by test
7.	False-negative	=	Test fails to document disease in patient who actually has the disease
8.	Predictive value	=	$\frac{\text{True positive}}{\text{True + false positives}}$
9.	Relative risk (risk ratio)	=	$\frac{\text{Disease rate in patients with positive test}}{\text{Disease rate in patients with negative test}}$

Drugs, such as persantine and adenosine, block cyclic adenosine monophosphate (C-AMP). C-AMP is responsible for vasomotor tone. If this is blocked, vascular beds dilate (arterial bed). Normally, arteries dilate whereas abnormal ones dilate not as well or not at all. A "steal" phenomenon is created and "ischemia" is seen. The drug is infused over 4-6 minutes. At three minutes, thallium is injected. "Stress" and "rest" pictures are taken and interpreted as above. Serial ECG and BP recordings are made. Since heart rate and BP rarely increase, it is rare to see significant ECG changes.

This form of testing is not physiologic since the heart rate and BPs rarely increase to a significant degree. Exercise tolerance cannot be assessed. Many drugs such as caffeine, xanthines, etc., must be stopped 24-48 hours prior to the test. This may not be practical in patients admitted for 23-hour observation with atypical chest pain. The most significant contraindication is in patients who are dependent on xanthines or with bronchospastic disease. Blocking C-AMP blocks its smooth muscle relaxant effect in bronchioles and may precipitate an attack. C-AMP blockers induce a plethora of effects, not the least of which is chest pain. They correlate poorly with true disease.

The effects of C-AMP blockers can be reversed by administration of theophylline. Despite its drawbacks, C-AMP blockers to induce myocardial stress are important in the clinician's armamentarium. It is particularly useful in patients whose significant increase in heart rate and blood pressure is not desired and in those with significant baseline arrhythmias.

Adenosine may induce high-degree AV block and should be used cautiously in those with baseline AV nodal disease.

The second important drug used for chemical stress testing is dobutamine, a beta agonist. Dobutamine is infused sequentially to a maximum of 40 mcg/kg/mn to achieve the target heart rate. One to two mg of atropine may also be administered. Sequential blood pressure and ECG recordings are performed. At the maximum infusion or when the target heart rate is achieved, nuclear imaging is performed and standard interpretation is undertaken. The ECG changes are just as valid with dobutamine as with exercise. Thus, ST-T wave changes can be construed to mean ischemia if they meet the heretofore described criteria. This is a much more physiologic test than C-AMP blockers since heart rate and blood pressure rise, as does O^2 demand. Arrhythmias induced by dobutamine, however, lose a lot of significance since dobutamine itself induces arrhythmias.

Patients with significant borderline hypertension or baseline arrhythmias may not be suitable for dobutamine. This is, however, an excellent drug in patients who can't exercise or where C-AMP blockers can't be used (particularly COPD patients who have bronchospasm and are xanthine-dependent).

Stress Echocardiography. In patients where the baseline ECG is abnormal and where nuclear imaging is equivocal, stress echocardiography may be invaluable. A baseline echocardiogram is performed. The patient is then exercised on the treadmill. As above, if the patient cannot walk, a chemically induced myocardial stress using dobutamine can be used. Serial ECGs, BP, and HR recordings are made. An echocardiogram is obtained at each stage.

If the patients develop a "regional wall motion abnormality," there is excellent evidence of ischemia. In addition, exercised-induced exacerbation of baseline "minor" valvular abnormalities can be seen. Often, this helps to unmask a chemically induced valvular lesion (mitral stenosis) or an otherwise hard-to-diagnose dynamic valvular lesion that is causing the patient's symptoms.

Table 8. Indications for Stopping Stress Test

- Attainment and maintenance of target heart rate for 1 minute
- Attainment of top stage in protocol used
- Heart rate is ≥ 8 beats more than target heart rate
- End of present stage
- Angina that progresses with exercise
- ST-T wave changes diagnostic of ischemia
- Superventricular tachyarrhythmias
- Ventricular ectopy exacerbated by exercise/precipitated by exercise (> 25% of beats are ectopic)
- Ventricular tachycardia
- Exercise-induced conduction delay
- Signs of impending circulatory collapse (pallor, hypotension, moist clammy skin, profound fatigue)
- Drop in systolic or diastolic blood pressure greater than 15 mmHg
- Profound fatigue/dyspnea
- Subjective desire or need of patient to terminate

The downside to stress echocardiography is that it is labor intensive. Also, the interpreter has to be practiced in assessing wall motion changes—some of which are subtle. The test also assumes that adequate echo images are obtainable. Poor echo windows due to body habitus, among other factors, may preclude use of this modality.

Other Modalities. Stress multigated angiogram (MUGA) scans (exercise, chemical), stress PET scanning, and any combination of the above modalities may be used to unmask ischemic heart disease. Stress MUGA is performed with exercise or chemically induced stress. Baseline and stress MUGA scans are obtained looking for acquired wall motion abnormalities at the peak of "exercise." Stress PET scanning involves chemically induced stress looking for metabolic abnormalities. The goal is to discern scar from hibernating myocardium from ischemic myocardium.

Safety of Stress Testing

The goal of any test is to obtain accurate, clinically useful information in the safest setting possible. We have previously discussed the contraindications to stress testing. (*See Table 4.*)

The stress test should be terminated when either the patient subjectively wishes to terminate the test or the desired goals have been achieved. (*Please see Table 8.*)

As with any test, awareness of, anticipation of, and the ability to treat complications is paramount. The appropriate equipment, including airway management materials, defibrillators, drugs, and a staff well versed in resuscitation must be available. Complications include:

- Arrhythmias (supraventricular, atrial fibrillation/flutter, and atrial tachycardia) and ventricular (PVCs, couplets, ventricular tachycardia)
- AV nodal block
- Vasovagal reactions
- Circulatory failure
- Syncope
- Refractory chest pain, ischemia, and cardiac arrest.

With appropriate vigilance, the more ominous complications as well as the more minor ones can be avoided or, when they occur, can be appropriately treated.

The incidence of complications remains rare. In a large study, Rodimes and Blackburn[21] documented 16 deaths and 40 patients requiring hospitalization. The calculated mortality was 0.01% and morbidity was 0.024%.

Stress Testing vs. Other Measures of Cardiac Ischemia

Previous noninvasive testing sought to reproduce the conditions that precipitated angina. Patients were subjected to stress, heavy meals, cold air, and cold water. Reduced ambient O^2 and ergonovine were also used to induce symptoms. The latter two were used to assess coronary spasm. Unfortunately, these two methods can in and of themselves cause spasms and were not clinically useful. Hand grip testing has been used. All of the above have a low sensitivity and specificity when compared to standard stress testing.

Several invasive tests are used for assessing the patient for coronary disease. All have the drawback of being invasive tests.

Atrial pacing has been used in those who can't perform treadmill tests. The advantage of pacing is that it obviates the need for drugs. The disadvantage is that blood pressure is not raised and even the maximal heart rate response is blunted (even if the absolute number is achieved) since exercise-induced catacholamine discharge does not occur. The aforementioned factors diminish the sensitivity of the test.

Coronary Angiography. These tests definitively document the extent and nature of the stenosis. Unfortunately, the assessment of the degree of stenosis is subjective. In addition, the geometry seen on angiograms may not accurately correlate with the true intravascular geometry (inadequate visualization of arteries distal to stenosis, eccentric lesions, etc.). In addition, what angiographically correlates with a clinically relevant lesion is not always well defined. Many patients with a noncritical lesion (< 50%) suffer an event, whereas those with "tight" lesions do not suffer an event.

Contrast Ventriculography. Injection of contrast in the ventricle during angiography may help define valvular lesions as well as segmental abnormalities. Again, this is an invasive test and interpretation is subjective.

Ambulatory (Holter) Monitoring. ECG monitoring looking for ST segment changes (particularly in patients with presumed silent ischemia) may unmask coronary disease. The advantage is that the patients are "stressed" in their typical environment. The disadvantages include the cost and the time involved in interpretation. This test does seem to be useful in unmasking Prinzmetal's angina, which is often missed on routine stress testing.

Exercise scintigraphy with thallium appears to be a promising technique. One study quoted a 93% sensitivity compared with a 40% sensitivity for ECG stress testing. The relative specificity compared to angiography was 86%, which, if used in the appropriate subpopulation, will be a valuable addition to the clinician's armory.

Conclusion

Stress testing in all its various forms, if applied and appropriately interpreted, is a safe, effective method for assessing the appropriate population for coronary disease. As the techniques continue to evolve, the sensitivity and specificity will improve, making this an invaluable clinical tool.

References

1. Goldhammer S, Scherf D. *Ascher Kim Med* 1933;122:134.
2. Rowell LB, et al. *Am Heart J* 1965;80:461.
3. Borer JS, et al. *N Engl J Med* 1975;292:367.
4. Mason RE, et al. *Circulation* 1967;36:517.
5. Roctman D, et al. *Ann Intern Med* 1970;72:641.
6. Ascoop CA, et al. *Am Heart J* 1971;82:609.
7. Bartel AG, et al. *Circulation* 1974;49:348.
8. Sheffield LT, Roctman D. *Chest* 1973;63:327.
9. Logan SE. *IEEE Trans Biomed Eng* 1975;22:327.
10. Eclestad MH. Stress testing: Principles and practice. Philadelphia: FA Davis Co., 1975, p. 175.
11. Wrener DA, et al. *Circulation* 1976;54/(Suppl II) II-10.
12. Einthoven W. *Arch Ges Physical* 1908;122:517.
13. Master AM, et al. *Am Heart J* 1942;24:777.
14. Fecl H, Siegel ML. *Am J Med Sc* 1928;175:255.
15. Mason RE, Likar I. *Trans Am Clin Clematol Assoc* 1964;76:40.
16. Roitman D, et al. *Ann Intern Med* 1970;72:641.
17. Lepeschkin E, Surawizc B. *N Engl J Med* 1958;258:511.
18. Linhart JW, et al. *Circulation* 1974;50:1173.
19. Cole JP, Ellestad MH. *Am J Cardiol* 1978;41:227.
20. Ellestad MH, Wan MK. *Circulation* 1975;51:363.
21. Rodimes P, Blackburn H. *JAMA* 1971;217:1061.

Supraventricular Tachycardia

Ken Grauer, MD

The emergency department physician often treats patients complaining of palpitations. Most commonly, the cause is trivial and treatment is supportive. Supraventricular tachycardia, however, can represent an annoying, worrisome, and potentially serious arrhythmia that requires accurate diagnosis and management. This chapter deals with the appropriate recognition and differentiation of various types of SVT from ventricular tachycardias and outlines practical guidelines for treatment. Catheter-directed ablation is rarely necessary for the treatment of SVT but is an extremely effective and safe option for the refractory patient.

Definition of SVT

The term supraventricular tachycardia (SVT) is defined as a cardiac rhythm that originates at or above the level of the AV node (i.e., a "supra"- ventricular rhythm) and which manifests a heart rate of 100 beats/min or more. SVTs are commonly encountered in primary care both in the office as well as in the hospital. Practically speaking, the principles involved in evaluation and management of these rhythms are similar in both settings. The key to management lies with accurate diagnosis of the mechanism of the arrhythmia. Once the type of SVT has been established, deciding on optimal treatment becomes far simpler.

Diagnosis of SVT Type

Five key issues should be addressed in assessing any patient who presents with an SVT:

1. Is the patient hemodynamically stable?
2. Is the rhythm truly supraventricular?
3. Is the rhythm regular? If so, what is the rate?
4. Is there evidence of atrial activity?
5. Should a vagal maneuver be used?

Is the Patient Hemodynamically Stable?

This question is by far the most important clinical parameter to assess in any patient who presents with a tachycardia. The importance of addressing this issue first is that if the patient is hemodynamically unstable as a *direct* result of the rapid rate, immediate intervention (i.e., synchronized cardioversion) is essential.

Hemodynamic status is assessed by evaluating the patient's level of consciousness during the tachycardia, the presence or absence of symptoms, and specific hemodynamic parameters such as heart rate and blood pressure. Signs of concern include hypotension, shock, heart failure/pulmonary edema, and/or acute myocardial infarction. Symptoms of concern include chest pain, shortness of breath, and decreased mental status.

Two points should be emphasized. First, the definition of hemodynamic stability is equally applicable to rhythms that are

Figure 1. Lead V_1 Rhythm Strip

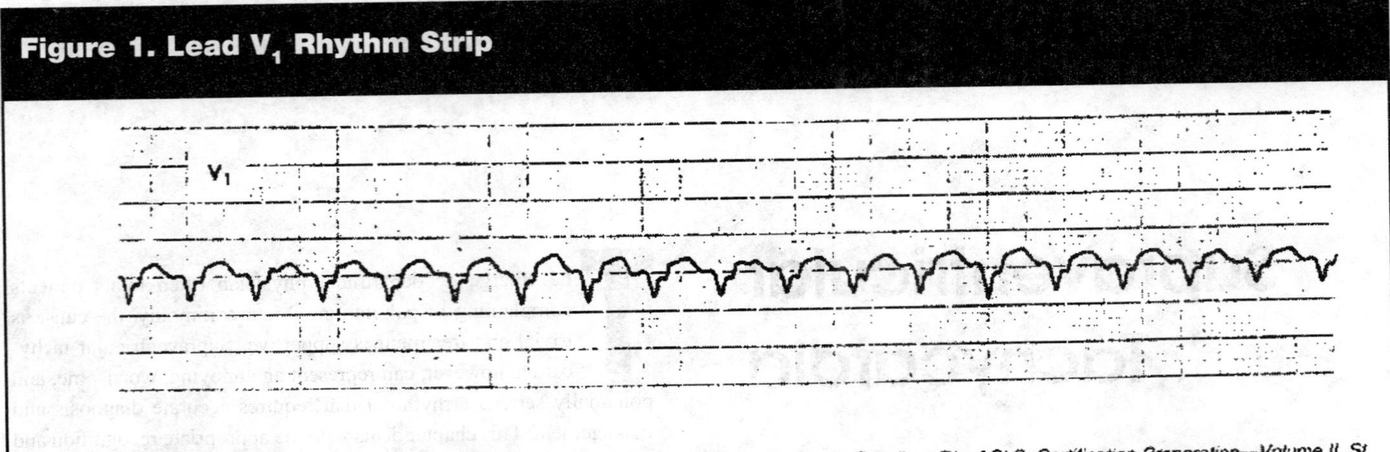

The QRS complex appears to be narrow in this single monitoring lead. Reproduced from Grauer K, Cavallaro DL. *ACLS: Certification Preparation—Volume II.* St. Louis: Mosby-Lifeline, 1993.

supraventricular as it is for ventricular tachycardia (VT). Thus, a patient with tachycardia who is hypotensive, having chest pain, and mentally confused is probably in need of immediate synchronized cardioversion regardless of what the rhythm happens to be. On the other hand, if the patient with tachycardia is asymptomatic (i.e., normotensive and without chest pain, shortness of breath, or mental confusion) then there is probably time for more careful evaluation and a trial of medical treatment, even if the rhythm turns out to be VT.

The second point to emphasize regarding assessment of hemodynamic stability is that sometimes, "You simply have to be there." Although a blood pressure reading of 90 systolic is typically cited as the minimal acceptable level for defining "stability," some patients do tolerate lower readings surprisingly well. Synchronized cardioversion will, therefore, not necessarily be needed for the patient with tachycardia who, despite a systolic blood pressure reading in the 70-80 mmHg range, has no signs or symptoms of hemodynamic decompensation. Clearly, clinical judgment is needed at the bedside for determining the most appropriate course of action.

Is the Rhythm Truly Supraventricular?

Although the focus of this article relates to evaluation and management of patients with supraventricular tachyarrhythmias, it is essential not to assume a supraventricular etiology for a tachycardia until this premise has been firmly established. It is all too easy to get fooled. For example, the tachycardia shown in Figure 1 was interpreted as an SVT on the basis of a narrow-appearing QRS complex in this V_1 monitoring lead. The patient was alert, normotensive, and tolerating the tachycardia without any indication of hemodynamic compromise. Assumption of a supraventricular etiology led to administration of verapamil in an attempt to convert the rhythm. This promptly precipitated ventricular fibrillation, and the patient died.

A 12-lead ECG was obtained on this patient just prior to administration of verapamil. *(Please see Figure 2.)* Unfortunately, the decision to use verapamil in this case was based on the diagnosis of SVT that had been made from the single monitoring lead shown in Figure 1. Retrospective analysis poi nts out several errors in management.

A presumptive diagnosis of SVT should never be made on the basis of patient appearance or hemodynamic status. The clinical reality is that not all patients in sustained VT will immediately decompensate as a result of this rhythm. On the contrary, some patients with sustained VT may tolerate this tachycardia for surprisingly long periods that may last for hours or even days at a time.[1] Compensatory vasoconstriction in such individuals may be sufficient to maintain adequate perfusion and a normal (or near normal) blood pressure. This is especially true for patients who otherwise have good ventricular function and a tachycardia rate that is not excessively fast. On occasion, sustained VT may persist with even hypertensive blood pressure readings and/or heart rates in excess of 200 beats/min. Assessment of clinical parameters (i.e., level of consciousness, rate of the tachycardia, and associated blood pressure) is, therefore, unreliable as a means for distinguishing between those tachycardias that are supraventricular and those that are due to ventricular tachycardia.[2]

In contrast, use of a 12-lead ECG obtained during the tachycardia will often provide invaluable assistance for making this critical distinction.[2,3] Regarding the case just discussed, no more than brief inspection of the 12-lead tracing shown in Figure 2 is needed to implicate a ventricular etiology for this tachycardia. QRS widening that had not been apparent in the V^1 lead shown in Figure 1 is readily seen in virtually all other leads. Awareness of the fact that QRS duration may appear deceptively short in a rhythm strip recording (if a portion of the QRS complex in that lead happens to lie on the baseline) is essential for accurate diagnosis. Final judgment for determining QRS width during a tachycardia should, therefore, be reserved until more than a single monitoring lead has been inspected.

Detailed discussion of electrocardiographic criteria used to distinguish between VT and SVT clearly extends beyond the scope of this article. Nevertheless, several important points can be made. Statistically, the cause of a wide-complex tachycardia (WCT) of uncertain etiology is far more likely to be VT than SVT with either aberrant conduction or preexisting bundle branch block.[2-5] This is particularly true when the patient is an older adult with a history of underlying heart disease (i.e., coronary artery disease, heart failure, or cardiomyopathy) in whom up to 90% of all WCTs are ventricular in etiology.[2,6,7] Two easy-to-remember criteria that are evident on this tracing strongly favor the diagnosis of VT: 1) the bizarre (markedly rightward) mean QRS axis during the tachycardia; and 2) complete negativity (in the form of a QS complex) in left-sided lead V_6.[3,8] Practically speaking then, VT should always be assumed until proven

Figure 2. 12-lead ECG

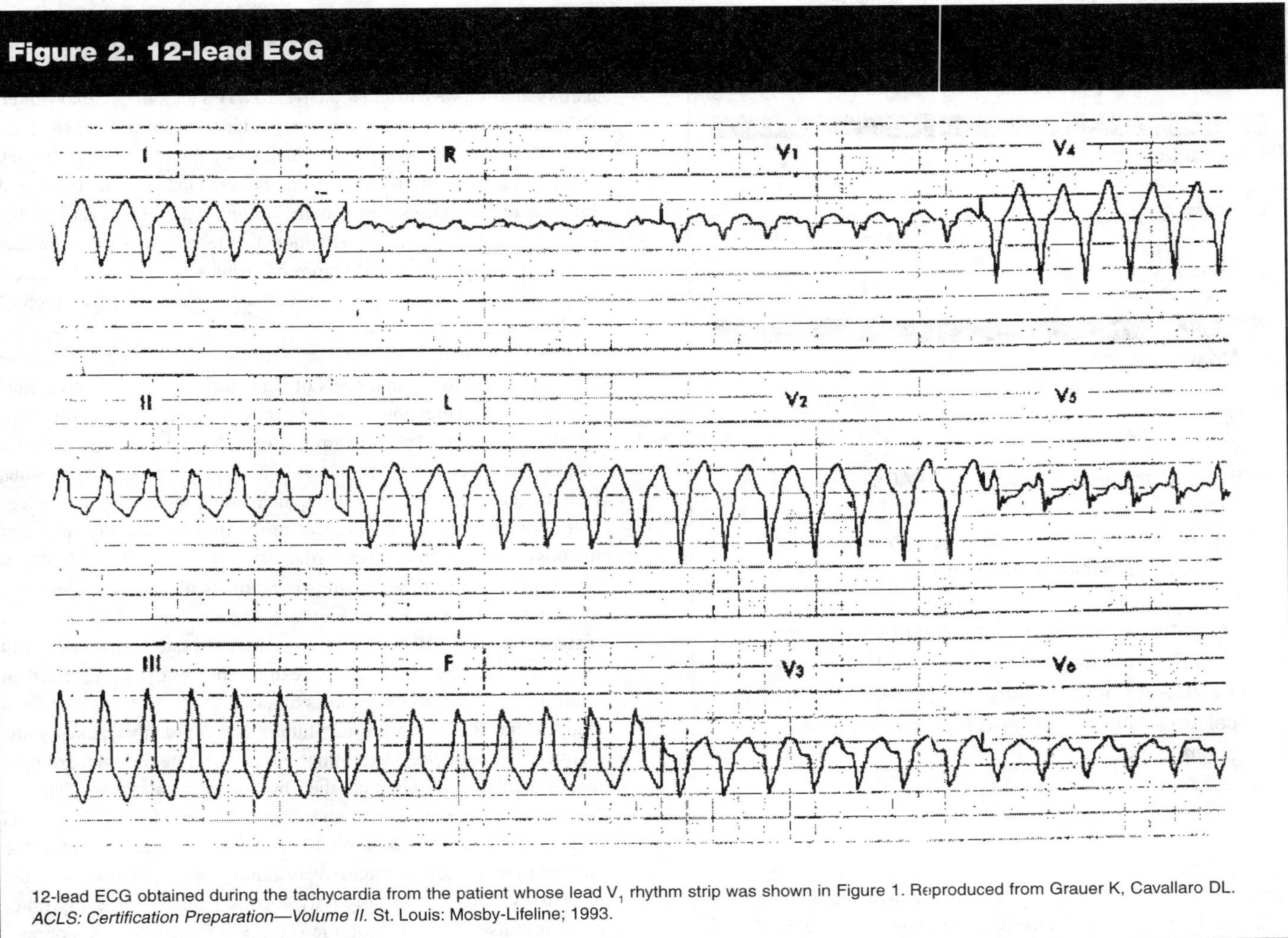

12-lead ECG obtained during the tachycardia from the patient whose lead V_1 rhythm strip was shown in Figure 1. Reproduced from Grauer K, Cavallaro DL. *ACLS: Certification Preparation—Volume II*. St. Louis: Mosby-Lifeline; 1993.

other-wise whenever confronted with a regular, WCT of uncertain etiology. Treat the patient accordingly (i.e., as if the rhythm is VT) until there is evidence to the contrary. If the patient is hemo-dynamically stable, obtaining a 12-lead ECG during the tachycardia may greatly assist in determining the true diagnosis.

Use of verapamil (or diltiazem) is not advised unless one is *certain* that the tachycardia in question is not VT. This potentially lethal mistake was made in the case just discussed. The reason for avoiding IV administration of these calcium-channel blockers when treating a WCT of uncertain etiology is that their negatively inotropic and vasodilatory properties are likely to precipitate deterioration of the rhythm to ventricular fibrillation if the WCT turns out to be VT.[9] As will be discussed shortly, use of either adenosine or procainamide is preferred when *empirically* treating a WCT of uncertain etiology. Adenosine is likely to convert the rhythm if the WCT turns out to be a *reentry* type of SVT. Unlike verapamil and diltiazem, administration of IV adenosine will usually *not* precipitate deterioration of the rhythm (i.e., to ventricular fibrillation) if the WCT turns out to be ventricular tachycardia. As helpful as adenosine may be when a supraventricular etiology is strongly suspected, this drug is unlikely to be of benefit when ventricular tachycardia is the probable etiology. In this situation, we favor consideration of IV procainamide, since this drug may be effective *regardless* of what the etiology of the SVT turns out to be. Procainamide may convert ventricular tachycardia—or at least slow the rate of ventricular tachycardia (i.e., VT at a rate of 140 beats/min is likely to be much better tolerated than VT at a rate of 180 beats/min). Procainamide may also be effective if the rhythm turns out to be PSVT, since it may alter conduction properties in one or both of the reentry pathways. Finally, IV procainamide is a drug of choice for supraventricular tachyarrhythmias associated with the Wolff-Parkinson-White (WPW) syndrome, since this drug slow conduction in the *anterograde* direction down the accessory pathway.

Lidocaine is an effective drug and the agent of choice for the treatment of sustained ventricular tachycardia. However, indiscriminate use of this drug is not recommended when the etiology of a tachycardia is uncertain because lidocaine administration may sometimes paradoxically accelerate the rate of a supraventricular tachycardia.8 As a result, we favor limiting use of this drug to the treatment of those tachycardias that are strongly suspected of being ventricular in etiology.

Determining the Type of SVT: Attention to Rate and Regularity

Our reason for emphasizing the importance of ensuring that the patient is hemodynamically stable and that the rhythm is *truly*

Table 1. Commonly Encountered SVTs

REGULAR SVTS

- Sinus tachycardia
- PSVT (or AVNRT)
- Atrial flutter*

IRREGULAR SVTS

- Atrial fibrillation
- MAT
- Sinus tachycardia with frequent PACs

***Note-** Atrial flutter may occasionally present with an irregular (variable) ventricular response. (See text.)

Abbreviations: SVT-supraventricular tachycardia; PSVT- paroxysmal supraventricular tachycardia; AVNRT- AV nodal reentry tachycardia; MAT- multifocal atrial tachycardia; PACs- premature atrial contractions.

supraventricular is that the approach to management is dramatically different when this is not the case. Attention can now be directed at addressing the remaining key issues which will usually allow determination of the specific type of SVT. Treatment decisions become far simpler once the correct diagnosis is known.

Practically speaking, the number of different types of supraventricular tachyarrhythmias that are commonly encountered in primary care is limited. Differentiation into those that are regular and those that are not is an important step in the diagnostic process. *(Please see Table 1.)* As can be seen from the table, determination that the ventricular response of the SVT is regular essentially limits diagnostic possibilities to three principal entities: 1) sinus tachycardia; 2) paroxysmal supraventricular tachycardia (PSVT); or 3) atrial flutter. Other causes of a regular supraventricular tachycardia do exist (i.e., ectopic atrial tachycardia, SVT with SA nodal reentry, etc.), but they are much less common than the three causes listed in the table, and for practical purposes can usually be ignored. With regard to the entities listed in the table, attention to the rate of the ventricular response, the presence and nature of atrial activity, and, if needed, response to a vagal maneuver will almost always suggest which of the three entities is present.

The points to remember about the rate of the ventricular response relate to the diagnosis of sinus tachycardia and atrial flutter. In a non-exercising adult, the rate of sinus tachycardia will usually not exceed 160 beats/min (or rarely 170 beats/min). Faster rates (of 200 beats/ min or more) may at times be seen with sinus tachycardia in children. However, in an adult, the presence of a regular SVT at a rate exceeding this range limit essentially rules out the possibility of sinus tachycardia.

Application of these diagnostic points is illustrated by analysis of the tachycardia shown in Figure 3. The rhythm in this figure is a regular, narrow QRS complex tachycardia at a rate of just under 200 beats/min. Atrial activity is not readily apparent. As suggested in Table 1, the differential diagnosis of a regular SVT consists of sinus tachycardia, PSVT, and atrial flutter. The rapid rate makes sinus tachycardia unlikely. Determination of the rate in this example makes it also unlikely that the rhythm is atrial flutter. This is because the atrial rate of flutter in an untreated adult patient is almost always close to 300/min (250-350/min range). To protect the patient from having an excessively rapid ventricular response, the normal AV node will usually only allow conduction of every other atrial impulse. This physiologic (i.e., protective) 2:1 AV conduction ratio most commonly results in a ventricular response to flutter that is close to 150 beats/min (300 ÷ 2 = 150/min). Thus, the ventricular rate of the regular SVT seen in Figure 3 is clearly faster than what one would normally expect for a patient in atrial flutter with the usual 2:1 AV conduction ratio. By the process of elimination, this leaves PSVT as the most probable diagnosis of the tachycardia.

In contrast to the diagnostic process just described for differen-

Figure 3. Regular SVT at a Rate of Just Under 200 Beats/Minute

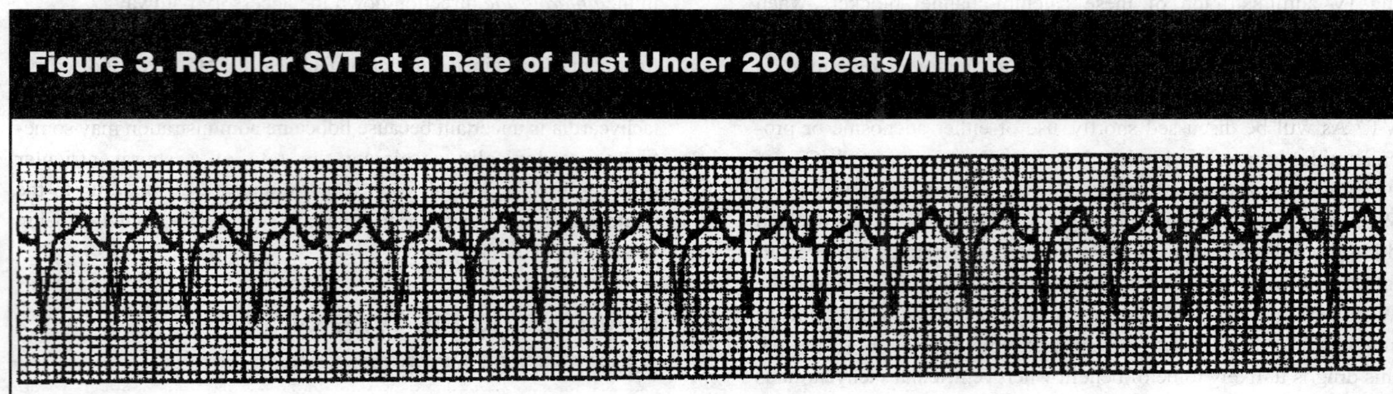

Atrial activity is not readily apparent. Calculation of the rate in this example makes it unlikely that the rhythm is either sinus tachycardia or atrial flutter. *(See text.)* PSVT is therefore the most probable diagnosis. Reproduced from Grauer K. *A Practical Guide to ECG Interpretation.* St. Louis: Mosby-Lifeline; 1993.

Figure 4. Sinus Tachycardia

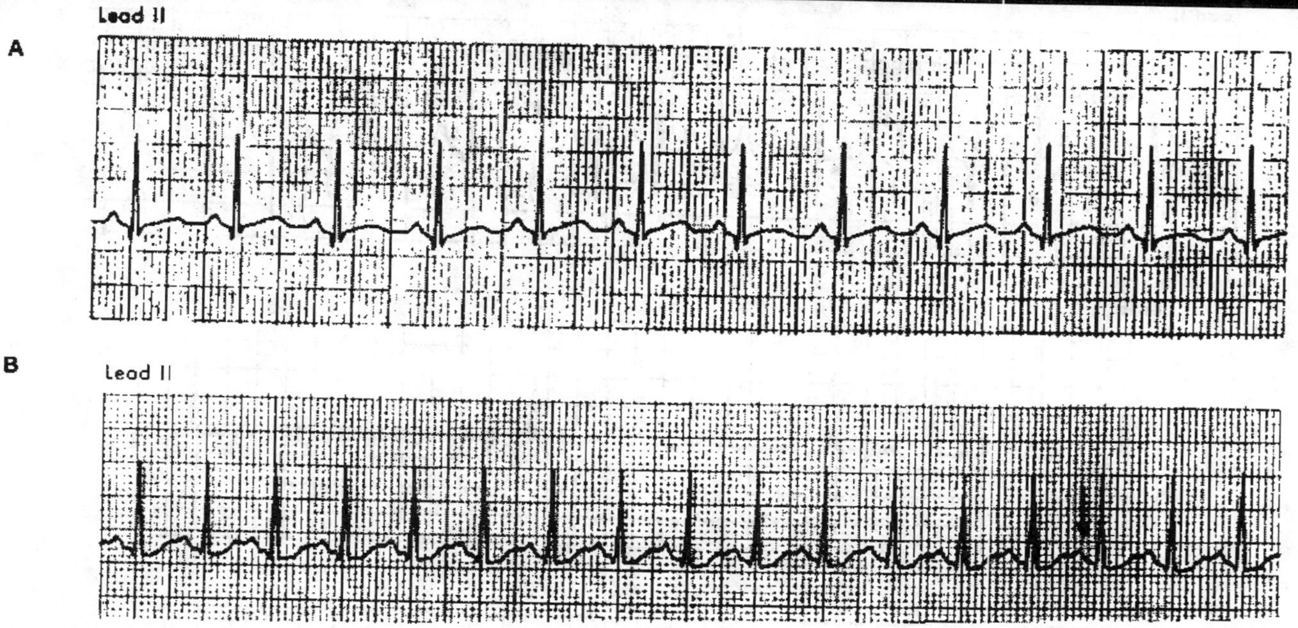

A Lead II

B Lead II

A) Sinus tachycardia. Sinus mechanism is readily recognized by the presence of an upright P wave in lead II and the constant PR interval preceding each QRS complex. B) Sinus tachycardia at a more rapid rate. Because of the fast heart rate, it is much more difficult to recognize a distinct P wave preceding each QRS complex (arrow). Reproduced from Grauer K, Cavallaro DL. *ACLS: A Comprehensive Review—Volume II.* St. Louis: Mosby-Lifeline; 1993.

tiation between the principal types of regular SVTs, recognition of a clearly irregular ventricular response strongly suggests one specific diagnosis: atrial fibrillation. Statistically, this is by far the most common cause of a rapid, irregularly irregular SVT. That said, Table 1 indicates two other entities that may also result in an irregular SVT, which are multifocal atrial tachycardia (MAT) and sinus tachycardia with frequent premature atrial contractions (PACs). Added to this list is the possibility of atrial flutter, which occasionally manifests a variable (irregular) ventricular response. Attention to the presence and nature of atrial activity should facilitate distinction between these entities.

The Presence and Nature of Atrial Activity

Sinus mechanism rhythms are defined by the presence of an upright P wave in standard lead II. This finding is well seen in the example of sinus tachycardia shown in Figure 4A, in which a regular, narrow QRS complex tachycardia (at a rate of 115 beats/min) manifests upright P waves that occur at a constant and normal PR interval before each QRS. The problem arises if the rate of sinus tachycardia is faster, in which case it may be much more difficult to discern a definite P wave preceding each QRS complex. *(Please see Figure 4B.)*

Figure 5. Atrial Flutter with 2:1 AV Conduction

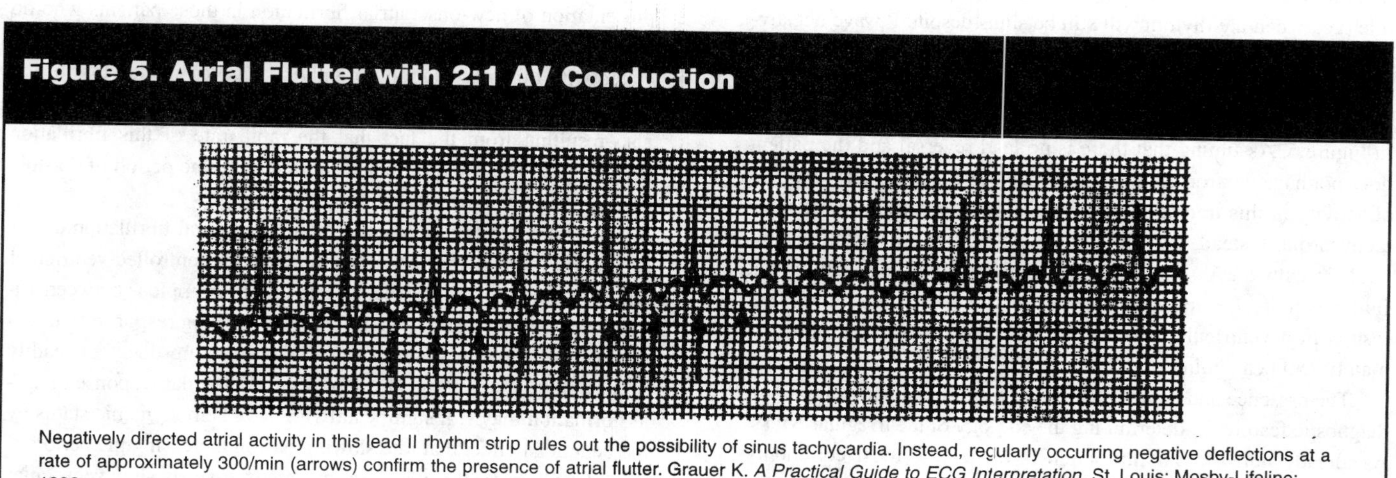

Negatively directed atrial activity in this lead II rhythm strip rules out the possibility of sinus tachycardia. Instead, regularly occurring negative deflections at a rate of approximately 300/min (arrows) confirm the presence of atrial flutter. Grauer K. *A Practical Guide to ECG Interpretation.* St. Louis: Mosby-Lifeline; 1992.

Figure 6. Atrial Fibrillation

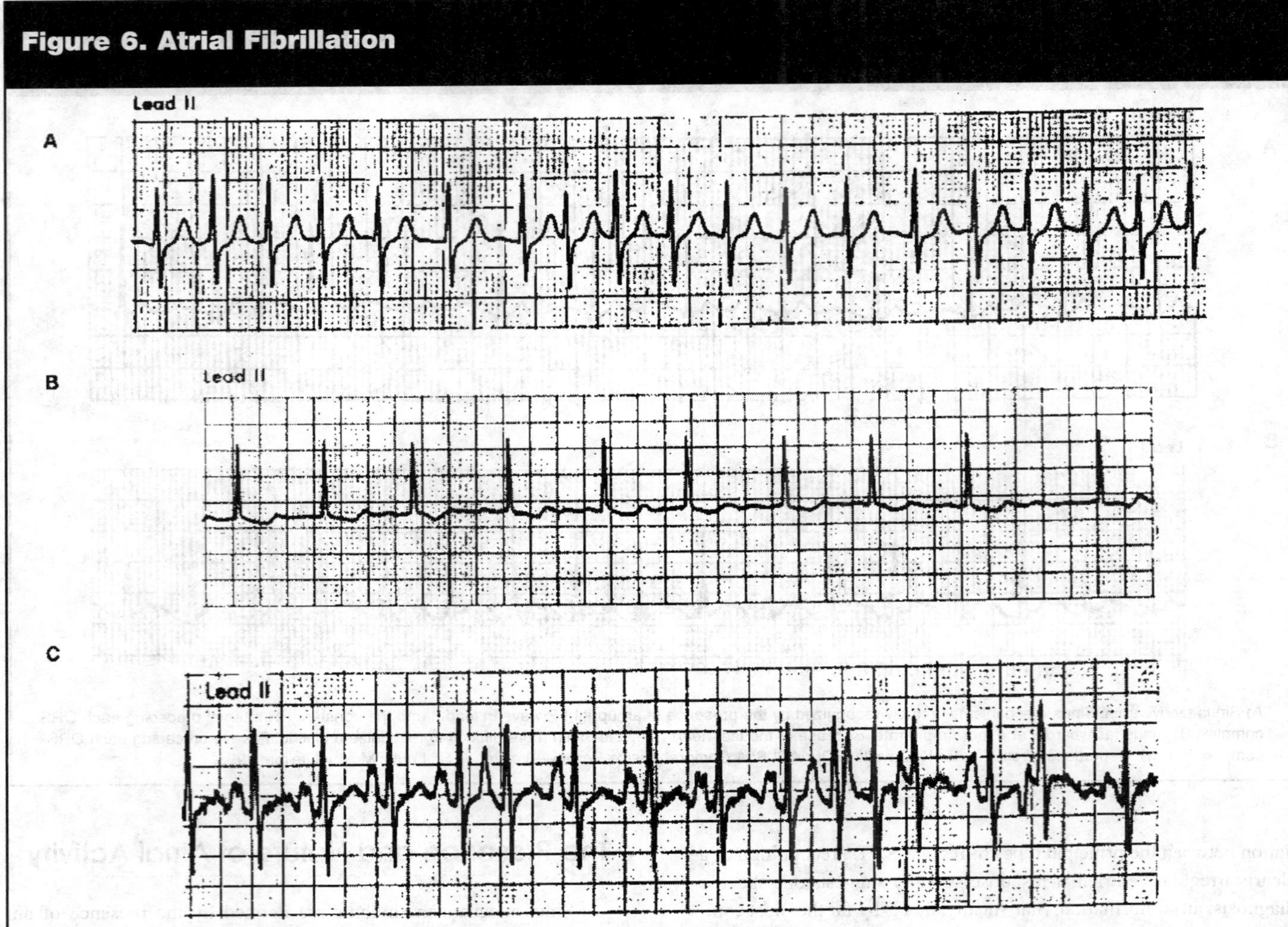

Figure 6. A) Atrial fibrillation with a rapid ventricular response (i.e., with an average heart rate of more than 120 beats/ min). Atrial activity is completely absent in this example. B) Atrial fibrillation with a controlled ventricular response (i.e., with an average heart rate of between 70-110 beats/ min). Fine fib waves are present in this tracing in the form of low amplitude undulations that deform the baseline. C) MAT. Recognition of definite P waves of varying morphology distinguishes this irregular SVT from atrial fibrillation. Reproduced from Grauer K, Cavallaro DL. *ACLS: A Comprehensive Review—Volume I.* St. Louis: Mosby-Lifeline; 1993.

An extremely helpful diagnostic point to consider is that if the P wave is not upright in standard lead II, then the mechanism of the rhythm is unlikely to be sinus. The only exceptions to this general rule (i.e., when the rhythm will still be sinus despite P wave negativity in lead II) are lead reversal and dextrocardia. Both of these conditions are uncommon (if not rare).

Application of the rule regarding P wave polarity is illustrated in Figure 5. Assuming that there is no lead reversal and the patient does not have dextrocardia, the presence of negatively directed atrial activity in this tracing (arrows) rules out the possibility of sinus tachycardia. Instead, the etiology of this regular SVT is atrial flutter, here with 2:1 AV conduction. As expected with this arrhythmia, flutter activity occurs at a rate that is close to 300/minute. This results in a ventricular response of half that amount, or approximately 150 beats/minute.

The presence and nature of atrial activity is an equally important diagnostic feature for determining the etiology of the irregular SVTs. As already noted, atrial fibrillation is by far the most commonly occurring irregular SVT in clinical practice. Identification of this arrhythmia is made by recognizing an irregularly irregular pattern of QRS complexes that occurs in the absence of P waves. This situation is illustrated in Figure 6A, in which the ventricular response to atrial fibrillation is rapid. This rapid response is the most common clinical presentation of new-onset atrial fibrillation in those patients who do not have conduction system disease. Heart failure is frequently associated with this presentation not only because of sudden loss of the atrial "kick" (which accounts for up to 30% of cardiac output), but also resulting from the fact that the rapid rate of this fibrillation rhythm leads to disproportionate shortening of the period of diastole (during which the heart fills).

In contrast to Figure 6A, the example of atrial fibrillation that is shown in Figure 6B occurs with a moderate or controlled ventricular response. The average ventricular rate in this example is between 70-110 beats/ min, reflecting an optimal rate-slowing response to initial treatment. Even when conversion to sinus rhythm does not readily occur in the acute setting, slowing of the ventricular response to atrial fibrillation may still significantly improve hemodynamic status by the beneficial effect that rate slowing has on increasing the period of diastolic filling. At the other extreme, an excessively slow ventricular response to atrial fibrillation (i.e., to an average ventricular rate of

Table 2. Expected Clinical Responses of Various SVTs to Vagal Maneuvers

- **PSVT**—abrupt termination of the tachyarrhythmia with conversion to sinus rhythm- or, no response at all to the vagal maneuver.
- **Sinus tachycardia**—gradual slowing during application of the maneuver- with resumption of the tachycardia after cessation.
- **Atrial fibrillation/flutter**—increased degree of AV block with resultant slowing of the ventricular response. Hopefully this will allow recognition of "telltale" flutter activity (as in figure 7) or underlying fib waves.
- **MAT**—no response.
- **Ventricular tachycardia**—no response.

less than 50-60 beats/minute) is to be avoided, and most often reflects either overuse of rate-slowing medication (i.e., digitalis toxicity) or sick sinus syndrome and the need for pacing.

Note in Figure 6A that evidence of atrial activity is completely lacking in this example of atrial fibrillation. Electrical activity of the fibrillating atria will often be seen, taking the form of low amplitude undulations in the ECG baseline that are usually described as either fine or coarse "fib waves," depending on their size. Fine fib waves are present and distort the otherwise isoelectric ECG baseline in Figure 6B. The important clinical point is not to misinterpret this fibrillatory activity as indication that P waves are present.

To emphasize this point, contrast the appearance of Figure 6C with that of 6A and 6B. All three rhythms are irregularly irregular. Yet the irregular SVT shown in Figure 6C is clearly not the result of atrial fibrillation because definite P waves are seen throughout this rhythm strip. These P waves constantly vary in size, shape, and polarity, suggesting involvement of multiple atrial foci in the genesis of this chaotic rhythm—thus its name, multifocal atrial tachycardia (MAT). Because atrial activity with MAT is often more subtle than its appearance in Figure 6C, diagnosis of this arrhythmia could be easy to overlook unless careful attention is routinely directed at searching for P waves in more than one lead.

Use of a Vagal Maneuver

Recognition of the specific type of SVT will usually be readily apparent from analysis of the ECG parameters of heart rate, regularity, and the presence and nature of atrial activity. At times, however, identification of the type of SVT may not be forthcoming from this initial assessment. In such cases, cautious application of a vagal maneuver may prove invaluable, both as a diagnostic and therapeutic intervention. For example, identification of the flutter activity that we highlighted with arrows in Figure 5 is admittedly a subtle finding. Application of carotid sinus massage (CSM) to this patient at the point marked by the heavy arrow in Figure 7 greatly facilitates recognition of underlying flutter activity by the temporary slowing it produces in the rate of the ventricular response (small arrows in Figure 7).

Vagal maneuvers act by transiently increasing parasympathetic tone while the maneuver is applied. This results in a slowing of conduction through supraventricular and AV nodal tissues. With re-entry tachyarrhythmias such as PSVT that depend on the AV node for their perpetuation, application of a vagal maneuver may serve a therapeutic effect and convert the rhythm to sinus. Termination of the arrhythmia occurs with PSVT if conduction through the AV node is delayed just long enough to interrupt at least a portion of the reentry circuit. With most other types of SVT that are not dependent on the AV node for their perpetuation, use of a vagal maneuver primarily serves a diagnostic purpose. The goal of the procedure in this situation is to produce transient slowing of the ventricular response in the

Figure 7. Application of Carotid Sinus Massage to a Patient in Atrial Flutter

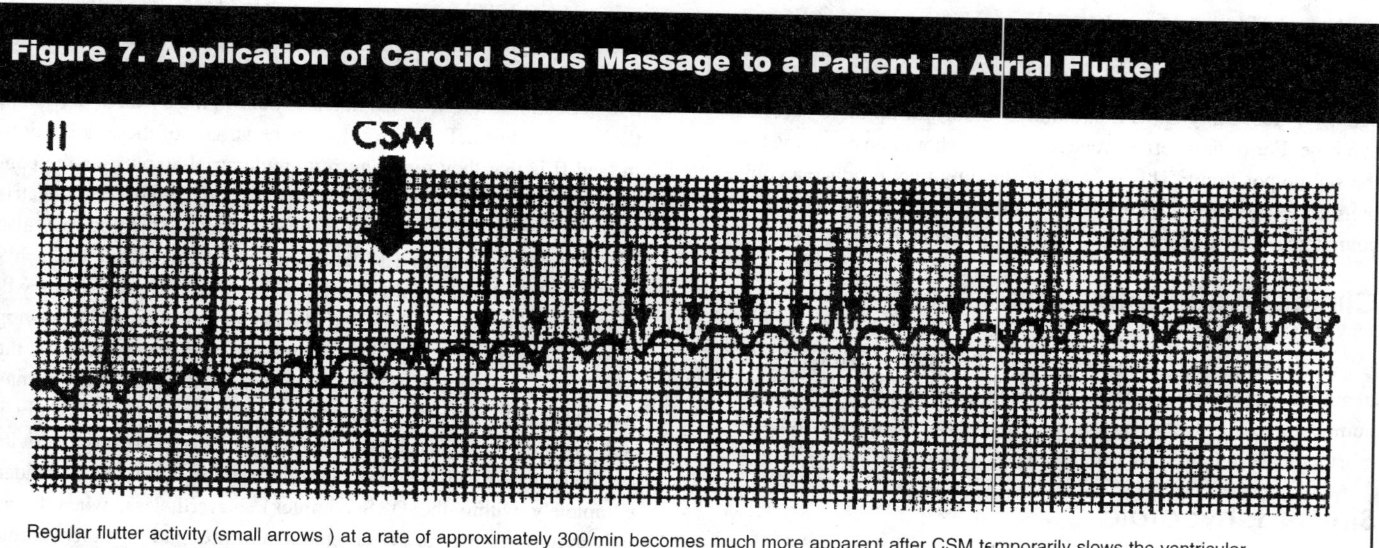

Regular flutter activity (small arrows) at a rate of approximately 300/min becomes much more apparent after CSM temporarily slows the ventricular response. Reproduced from Grauer K. *A Practical Guide to ECG Interpretation.* St. Louis: Mosby-Lifeline; 1992.

hope that this will allow recognition of the presence and nature of underlying atrial activity. *(Please see Figure 7.)* Expected clinical responses of the various cardiac arrhythmias to application of vagal maneuvers are noted in Table 2.

Types of vagal maneuvers include carotid sinus massage, Valsalva, activation of the gag reflex, facial submersion in ice water, eyeball pressure (which is no longer recommended because of the risk of retinal detachment), digital rectal massage, and squatting. Patients with recurrent episodes of PSVT often instinctively learn to perform one or more of these maneuvers on their own to terminate their arrhythmia.

In an emergency care setting, carotid sinus massage is the vagal maneuver performed most often for treatment. Under constant ECG monitoring, the patient's head is turned to the left and the area of the right carotid bifurcation (near the angle of the jaw) is gently but firmly massaged for 3-5 seconds at a time (but no longer!). If right carotid massage is ineffective, the left side may be tried. Never massage both sides simul-taneously. Sufficient pressure must be applied with massage for the procedure to work—so much so that the conscious patient should be alerted that massage will be uncomfortable (and may even be a little painful). Augmentation of the therapeutic effect of CSM can be obtained by performing the procedure a second time in Trendelenburg position (at a decline of about -10°).[10] Massage must be applied in the correct location. All too often, pressure is applied too low (i.e., to the mid-portion of the neck). The carotid sinus (bifurcation) lies high in the neck—just below the angle of the jaw. If PSVT persists despite attention to these details, remember that CSM may still work if reapplied after administration of antiarrhythmic drugs.

It is important to emphasize that CSM is not a totally benign procedure—especially when applied to older individuals.[11] Complications that have been associated with use of CSM include syncope, stroke (from dislodgement of a carotid plaque), sinus arrest, high-grade AV block, prolonged asystole, and ventricular tachyarrhythmias in patients with digitalis toxicity. As a result, the maneuver should probably not be attempted in patients with a history of sick sinus syndrome, cervical bruits (listen to the neck before application!), cerebrovascular disease, or when the possibility of digitalis toxicity exists.

Use of Valsalva is an alternative vagal maneuver that, if performed correctly, may produce an even more potent vagotonic effect than CSM.[12] The patient is asked to forcibly exhale (bear down) against a closed glottis (as if straining at stool) for up to 15 seconds at a time. For optimal effectiveness, Valsalva should be performed in the supine position.[12] This is because standing may produce a compensatory increase in sympathetic tone that at least partially counteracts the vagotonic (parasympathomimetic) effect of Valsalva.

Clinical Approach to Treatment

Once diagnosis of the specific type of SVT has been made, the treatment approach is greatly facilitated. Practically speaking, the number of clinical options needed for successful management of most patients in a primary care setting is limited.

Sinus Tachycardia

The treatment of choice for sinus tachycardia is to identify and correct its underlying cause. With rare exceptions, the rhythm itself should never be treated. For example, if the reason for sinus tachycardia is hypotension from shock, then the treatment of choice is intravascular volume repletion with IV fluid infusion (and not administration of rate-slowing drugs!).

Paroxysmal Supraventricular Tachycardia

Paroxysmal supraventricular tachycardia (PSVT) is an extremely common tachyarrhythmia that occurs in both ambulatory and inpatient settings. Although a majority of patients with PSVT are symptomatic with this arrhythmia (most often in the form of palpitations or the sensation of rapid heart beat), in most cases clinical implications of the rhythm are benign.[13] This is especially true when PSVT occurs in an otherwise healthy young adult. On the other hand, sudden development of this rhythm is likely to be more consequential when it arises in certain other subsets of patients such as the elderly, infants or very young children, and adults with significant underlying cardiac disorders. Hemo-dynamic decompensation is particularly prone to occur in such individuals when the rate of the tachycardia is very rapid and/or the rhythm persists for long periods of time.

Electrocardiographically, the diagnosis of PSVT is suggested by the finding of a regular SVT in which normal atrial activity is lacking. The rhythm most often begins abruptly—which is why it is termed "paroxysmal". Once it begins, the ventricular response tends to be exceedingly regular, most often at a rate of between 140 and 240 beats/minute. *(Please see Figure 3.)* The mechanism of PSVT is almost always one of "re-entry"—in which a portion of the reentry circuit almost invariably involves the AV node. This accounts for the "all-or-none" phenomenon seen with treatment, in which the arrhythmia is likely to either be resistant to vagal maneuvers and AV nodal rate-slowing drugs—or respond dramatically to treatment (with abrupt conversion to sinus rhythm). It also accounts for the increasing tendency in recent years to refer to this rhythm as AVNRT (AV nodal reentry tachycardia) instead of PSVT—reflecting our enhanced understanding of the underlying mechanism.

As noted above, normal (i.e., upright in lead II) P waves will not be seen when the rhythm is PSVT. However, careful attention to the surface ECG will sometimes reveal other evidence of atrial activity—and thereby provide a clue to the mechanism of the arrhythmia. When present, such atrial activity most often takes the form of subtle negative deflections in lead II that notch or deform the terminal portion of the QRS complex. The reason for the negativity of these deflections in lead II is that they represent retrograde atrial activity, as the continuously circulating electrical impulse is conducted back to the atria over the retrograde limb of the reentry pathway. Notching may also be seen in other leads of a 12-lead tracing obtained during the tachycardia, although the polarity of deflections in these other leads will not necessarily be negative. The clinical significance of identifying this atrial activity is that its recognition confirms reentry as the responsible mechanism for the tachycardia—a finding which may have potentially important therapeutic implications. Unfortunately, it will not always be possible to demonstrate retrograde atrial activity on the surface ECG (because these deflections will often be hidden completely within the QRS complex). Nevertheless, when found (which may require careful comparison of pre- and post-tachycardia tracings), less commonly implicated mechanisms of SVT rhythms (such as increased automaticity) are essentially ruled out.

Table 3. Drugs and Doses of AV Nodal Rate-Slowing Agents

DRUG INDICATIONS	DOSING INFORMATION	SIDE EFFECTS
Adenosine PSVT (and other reentry tachyarrhythmias) As a *diagnostic maneuver* (i.e., "chemical Valsalva") in patients with SVT of *uncertain* etiology	**IV Bolus**—initially give 6 mg push. If no response after 1-2 minutes, give 12 mg by IV push, which may be repeated a final time 1-2 minutes later (for a *total* dose of 6 + 12 + 12 = 30 mg). Be sure to give adenosine by IV push (injecting the drug as fast as possible over 1-3 seconds) and follow each dose with a saline flush. Higher than usual doses may be needed for patients receiving theophylline. Lower than usual doses may be needed for patients receiving carbamazepine or dipyridamole.	Adverse effect that may be seen include facial flushing, cough/dyspnea (the drug is a mild bronchoconstictor), chest pain, and bradycardia (which may be marked). Fortunately, these side effects are usually short-lived. The drug should *not* be given to patients with frank bronchospasm or asthma, or to those with a history of sick sinus syndrome or severe conduction syndrome.
Verapamil PSVT Atrial fibrillation/flutter (to control the ventricular response) MAT	**IV Dosing**—Begin with a dose of 2.5-5 mg IV (to be given over a 1-2 minute period). Give the drug *slower* (over 3-4 minutes) to the elderly or to those with borderline blood pressure readings. May give up to 5-10 mg in a dose (and repeat several times in 15-30 minutes needed)—up to total dose of ~30 mg. **Oral Dosing**—120-480 mg/d, divided into three equal doses (or given less often if sustained release preparations are used). May increase the serum digoxin level by up to 50%.	May cause hypotension (give the drug *slowly* by the IV route). Use with caution in patients with impaired left ventricular function. Avoid when treating a wide-complex tachycardia of uncertain etiology. Do not use for rapid atrial fibrillation with WPW (anterograde conduction down the accessory pathway may be accelerated). Should not be given IV within 30 minutes of using an IV beta-blocker. Calcium chloride (500-1000 mg given IV over 5-10 minutes) may be used to treat calcium toxicity. (The effect of diltiazem on the serum digoxin level is minimal.)
Diltiazem Indications are the same as for verapamil	**IV Bolus**—For the average-size adult, begin with an *initial* IV bolus of 0.25 mg/kg (~ 20 mg for an *averaged-size* adult) given over a two-minute period. Use smaller doses (of ~ 10-15 mg) for lighter patients and the elderly. **IV Infusion**—Begin IV infusion at ~ 10 mg/h. Most patients will be controlled at infusion rates of between 10-15 mg/h, although some patients only need 5 mg/h. **Oral Dosing**—90-360 mg daily, divided into three or four equal doses (or given less often if sustained release preparations are used).	Adverse effects and cautions are the same as for verapamil (with the exception that the hypotensive and negatively inotropic effect may be somewhat less for diltiazem).
Digoxin Atrial fibrillation/flutter (to control the ventricular response) PSVT	**IV Dosing**—If the patient has *not* previously been digitalized, consider IV loading with an *initial* dose of 0.25-0.5 mg. This may be followed with 0.125-0.25 mg IV increments given every 2-6 hours (until a *total* loading dose of ~0.75-1.5 mg has been administered over the first 24 hours). The next day, the daily *maintenance* dose may be started. **Oral Dosing**—The daily *oral* maintenance for *most* adults under 60 years old (who have normal function) is 0.25 mg/d. Lower doses (0.125 mg daily—or every other day) are recommended for older patients and/or those with impaired renal function.	Digitalis toxicity may present with nausea, vomiting, changes in color vision, and/or with virtually any cardiac arrhythmia. To minimize the chance of developing digitalis toxicity, lower doses of drug should be used in the elderly, with renal failure, in patients with ischemia or hypokalemia/hypomagnesemia, and/or when drugs that are prone to increase the serum digoxin level are used (such as quinidine and verapamil).
Esmolol PSVT Atrial fibrillation/flutter (to control the ventricular response) Treatment of ventricular tachycardia (especially when underlying ischemia is present)	**IV Dosing**—Administer an *initial* IV loading dose (of 250-500 mcg/kg) over a one-minute period. Follow this with a four-minute infusion at 25-50 mcg/kg/min. If desired response is not obtained, titrate the rate of infusion *upward* by 25-50 mcg/kg/min at 5-10 minute intervals. Although a dose of up to 300 mcg/kg/min may be used, it is generally best *not* to exceed 200 mcg/min (as doing so greatly increases the incidence of hypotension). May thereafter begin use of a longer-acting oral antiarrhythmic agent (and taper esmolol).	Avoid use of esmolol (and other IV beta-blockers) in patients with frank bronchospasm or left ventricular dysfunction. Hypotension is the most common adverse effect from IV infusion of the drug. Should not be given IV within 30 minutes of using IV verapamil or diltiazem.

Table 4. Underlying or Precipitating Conditions to Consider in Association with Atrial Fibrillation

- Heart failure
- Ischemic heart disease (including acute myocardial infarction)
- Hypertensive heart disease
- Rheumatic heart disease (especially mitral stenosis)
- Hyperthyroidism
- Alcohol abuse
- Acute medical illness (i.e., pneumonia, sepsis, shock)
- Acute pulmonary embolism
- Acute sympathetic "trigger" (i.e., use of cocaine, amphetamines)
- Sick sinus syndrome
- Atrial myxoma (a rare but correctable cause)
- "Lone" atrial fibrillation (accounting for 10% of cases of atrial fibrillation in which no precipitating cause is found)

Regarding the treatment of PSVT, use of a vagal maneuver should be considered first. *(Please see Table 2.)* If this is not successful, any of the antiarrhythmic drugs shown in Table 3 may then be tried either alone or in combination. In recent years, the drug that has become the agent of choice for treatment of PSVT in the acute care setting is adenosine. Obvious advantages of adenosine relate to its rapid onset of action and exceedingly short half-life (which is less than 10 seconds in duration). As a result, the clinician will know within a very few minutes if the drug will work or not. Adverse effects can occur with the use of adenosine and most commonly include facial flushing, dyspnea, chest pain, and bradycardia. However, because of the drug's short duration of action, any side effects that do occur will generally be short-lived. Adenosine is therefore well tolerated by most patients, although caution is advised (if the drug is used at all) in patients with sick sinus syndrome or other evidence of conduction system disease, and in those with a history of bronchospasm.

Several key aspects of adenosine dosing should be emphasized. The dose recommended for initial use in adults is 6 mg given by IV push. The drug should be injected IV as rapidly as possible (ideally within 1-3 seconds) and followed immediately with a saline flush to facilitate absorption and prevent deterioration of medication while the drug is still in the IV tubing. If there is no response to this initial dose within 1-2 minutes, a second dose (of 12 mg) may be given by IV push followed 1-2 minutes later by a final 12 mg bolus (for a total dose of 30 mg). If the patient fails to respond to this total dose, adenosine is unlikely to work and another agent should be selected. Higher than usual doses of adenosine are likely to be needed for patients who are also receiving theophylline products (because of competitive antagonism between these two agents). In contrast, lower than usual doses (i.e., 3 mg) should be used for patients who also are taking dipyridamole or carbamazepine.

Drawbacks associated with the use of adenosine are that the drug will generally only be effective for treatment of tachy-arrhythmias that have a reentry mechanism (such as PSVT), and that the ultra-short half-life of this drug may predispose to development of arrhythmia recurrence after the effect of adenosine has worn off. Adenosine may be readministered to patients in the acute care setting; however, recurrence of the arrhythmia suggests that continued control may require the addition of drugs with a longer duration of action.

Another advantage of the rapid onset and short duration of action of adenosine is that even when the drug fails to convert the rhythm, it may still serve a diagnostic purpose in evaluation. This clinical application of adenosine has been referred to as "chemical Valsalva," in which the immediate action of the drug exerts a similar effect as occurs with a vagal maneuver (i.e., it induces transient slowing of the ventricular response that may facilitate detection of subtle underlying atrial activity that was not readily apparent on the initial tracing). Unlike verapamil and diltiazem, IV administration of adenosine is unlikely to precipitate deterioration of a wide-complex tachycardia if inadvertently given to a patient in ventricular tachycardia.[14]

Clinically, adenosine will be successful in converting PSVT to sinus rhythm more than 90% of the time. In those cases when repeated dosing of the drug fails, other rate-slowing agents may still be effective. *(Please see Table 3.)* Verapamil and diltiazem both demonstrate comparable efficacy to adenosine for converting PSVT to sinus rhythm, and these drugs may work when adenosine does not. Alternatively, use of an IV beta-blocker (such as esmolol) could also be tried, although IV beta-blocker administration should be avoided within 30 minutes of giving IV verapamil or diltiazem (because of the potential for this combination to produce excessive rate slowing). Digoxin is another medication that may effectively reduce the long-term recurrence rate of PSVT. However, the relatively delayed onset of action of digoxin (usually 30-60 minutes following IV administration) makes it a far less than optimal agent for acute treatment than IV preparations of the other drugs listed in Table 3.

Several "pearls" should be noted regarding the management of PSVT. First, IV administration of magnesium sulfate may find a place in the treatment approach for acute conversion of PSVT that had been refractory to other measures.[15,16] Use of magnesium might best be considered for selected patients who fail to respond to standard therapy—especially when serum magnesium levels are either known or suspected to be low.[17] Dosing is empiric, and might safely entail IV administration of 1-2 g over a 5-30 minute period—repeating this amount later if needed. Much larger doses of IV magnesium have been used for treatment of cardiac conditions with only a minimal incidence of adverse effects (mainly flushing, mild hypotension, and bradycardia).[18] Temporarily stopping or slowing the rate of infusion usually results in rapid resolution of these problems.

In addition to application of a vagal maneuver, other non-pharmacological interventions also play an important role in the long-term management of many patients with frequent episodes of PSVT. Specifically, careful attention should be directed at identifying and correcting other factors that may be precipitating or exacerbating the arrhythmia. These may include untreated medical conditions (i.e., ischemia, heart failure, hypoxemia, acidosis); serum electrolyte disorders (especially hypokalemia or hypomagnesemia); severe stress (causing unopposed activation of sympathetic tone); and many all too easily overlooked pharmacological interactions (i.e., excessive use of caffeine, alcohol, nicotine effect from smoking, over-the-counter sympathomimetics, diet pills, and/or recreational drugs such as cocaine or amphetamines).

Finally, consideration should be given to the use of intermittent therapy for those patients with recurrent PSVT that only occurs at infrequent intervals.[19,20] Daily treatment with an antiarrhythmic agent is simply not needed when episodes of the arrhythmia only occur a handful of times (or less) in a given year—especially in view of the fact that such episodes are almost uniformly associated with a benign outcome. Prescrip-tion of a carefully designed "antiarrhythmic cocktail" to be taken at home on a prn basis is likely to be far more preferable to such patients (in terms of cost-efficacy and minimization of long-term side effects) to daily prescription of a drug for prevention of an infrequently occurring benign condition.

The contents of an antiarrhythmic cocktail can be individualized to suit patient needs.[20] Combined use of a single dose of an oral rate-slowing agent (most commonly verapamil, diltiazem, or a beta-blocker)—together with a dose of a benzodiazepine will often result in surprisingly rapid conversion of the rhythm (within 30-90 minutes) while the patient remains at home. Non-coated benzodiazepines (i.e., lorazepam, alprazolam) may be administered sublingually for even more rapid effect. In addition to their sedative and calming action, the anxiolytic effect of these drugs may help to convert PSVT by a physiologic mechanism—in that they attenuate sympathetic tone, and may therefore alter conduction properties in one or both limbs of the reentry pathway.

Atrial Fibrillation

Atrial fibrillation is the most commonly occurring sustained cardiac arrhythmia. The rhythm is present in more than 2 million Americans, with a frequency that progressively increases with advancing age. As a result, as many as 7-14% of elderly individuals may develop atrial fibrillation in either intermittent or sustained form at some point during their lifetime.[21]

Electrocardiographically, the diagnosis of atrial fibrillation is suggested by the finding of an irregularly irregular rhythm without the presence of P waves. The ventricular response may be rapid, moderate, or slow. *(Please see Figures 6A and 6B.)* If the ventricular response is rapid and results in the patient becoming hemodynamically unstable, synchronized cardioversion should be immediately performed. Fortunately, this situation is relatively uncommon, so that medical treatment can be attempted first in the vast majority of patients. Sequential goals of management in the hemodynamically stable patient with atrial fibrillation are to identify the underlying (or precipitating) cause of the rhythm *(Please see Table 4)*, to correct the underlying condition if at all possible, to slow the rate if the ventricular response is rapid, to convert the rhythm to sinus, and to prevent thromboembolism.[22] Listing goals in this sequence emphasizes the importance of trying to find an underlying cause that can be corrected since, if accomplished, achieving the remaining therapeutic goals (i.e., slowing the rate, converting the rhythm, and preventing thromboembolism) will all be much easier to attain.

To a large extent, the appropriate work-up of a patient with newly diagnosed atrial fibrillation is based on attempting to identify a potentially correctable cause. In addition to standard laboratory tests (i.e., complete blood count, chemistry profile with serum electrolytes including magnesium), we suggest obtaining a 12-lead ECG (to confirm diagnosis of atrial fibrillation and rule out acute infarction), chest x-ray (looking for evidence of heart failure and/or pulmonary disease), and thyroid function studies (to rule out hyperthyroidism) and eliciting a careful history for assessment of alcohol or stimulant abuse (with drug screening as deemed appropriate). Despite its cost, we strongly favor routinely performing M-mode and 2-D echocardiography on all patients in atrial fibrillation at the earliest opportunity for three important reasons: 1) it is the most helpful noninvasive test for determining the precipitating cause of atrial fibrillation; 2) it provides a measure of left atrial size, which gives some objective indication of the likelihood of being able to convert the arrhythmia and maintain sinus rhythm if conversion is successful; and 3) it assesses left ventricular function, which, together with left atrial size, provides insight regarding the risk of thromboembolic complications and the relative need for long-term anticoagulation.[22,23]

The spectrum of potential clinical presentations of atrial fibrillation is diverse. As already emphasized, the ventricular response associated with new-onset atrial fibrillation is most often rapid, a finding that accounts for the frequent association of heart failure with this rhythm. Palpitations and the sensation of rapid or irregular heart beat may or may not be present. Surprisingly, many patients with atrial fibrillation are either relatively asymptomatic or completely unaware that they are experiencing this rhythm.[13] Others present with a cerebrovascular accident (stroke or transient ischemic attack) as their first manifestation. Any of the medical conditions listed in Table 4 may be seen.

From a clinical perspective, when symptoms are directly attributed to the rhythm itself they are most often the result of the rapid ventricular response. Initial treatment measures should, therefore, be aimed at controlling the ventricular rate. Doing so not only helps to relieve symptoms, but may also reduce ischemia and improve hemodynamic status. This is because decreasing the ventricular rate will most often lead to an increase in coronary flow and cardiac output as a result of the longer period now available for diastolic filling.

Traditionally, digoxin has been the drug selected most often for the purpose of slowing the rapid ventricular response to atrial fibrillation. While still an appropriate indication for this medication, it now appears that other drugs will often be preferable to digoxin in this situation.[24,25] By itself, digoxin does not facilitate conversion of atrial fibrillation to sinus rhythm.[26] As many as 50% of patients with new-onset atrial fibrillation will spontaneously convert to sinus rhythm over the ensuing 12-24 hours regardless of whether they are given digoxin or are simply treated with supportive measures alone.[26,27] The physiological mechanism by which digoxin works to slow the rate of rapid atrial fibrillation is primarily through an increase in vagal (i.e., parasympathetic) tone. As a result, even high doses of the drug will not necessarily be optimally effective in controlling the heart rate of acutely ill patients for whom tachycardia is at least partially mediated by an increase in sympathetic tone (from endogenous secretion of catecholamines, as so commonly occurs with acute stress states).[24] Not generally appreciated is the fact that the vagotonic action of digoxin may produce the opposite effect on atrial tissue as it does on the AV node—leading to shortening of the atrial refractory period and an even greater tendency toward perpetuation of the fibrillatory rhythm.[24,28] For these reasons, an increasing number of clinicians now favor selection of AV nodal slowing agents that exert a more direct action on the AV node (such as IV verapamil or diltiazem) for initial treatment of rapid atrial fibrillation- rather than depending on the indirect vagotonic effect of digoxin. In addition, the onset of action of digoxin is significantly slower than it is for these other agents.

Compared to verapamil, a decided advantage of IV diltiazem is the availability of a formulation for continuous IV infusion. In addition to allowing moment-to-moment dose titration of the drug, use of a continuous IV infusion prolongs the rate-slowing effect of diltiazem compared to a regimen of intermittent bolus dosing (as is used with verapamil).

Direct catecholamine inhibition with beta-blockade (using IV esmolol, or other beta-blocking agents) offers an alternative to IV verapamil or diltiazem that may also be more effective than digoxin for initial slowing of the ventricular response to rapid atrial fibrillation. Combination therapy (i.e., concomitant administration of IV digoxin and either verapamil, diltiazem, or a beta-blocker) may enhance the rate-slowing effect even more by a synergistic action that allows lower doses of each agent to be used.[25,29,30] As previously noted, IV beta-blocker administration should be avoided within 30 minutes of giving IV verapamil or diltiazem. The clinician will, therefore, need to select either an IV calcium channel blocking agent or a beta-blocker for treatment—but not both. Dosing recommendations for IV administration of these rate-slowing drugs are detailed in Table 3.

Added to the list of agents that appear in Table 3 may soon be magnesium sulfate. Recent data suggest that IV magnesium may exert a beneficial rate-slowing effect that may be additive to the effect of other drugs.[31,32] Although more studies clearly are needed before widespread adoption of this drug, consideration might be given at this time to empiric use of magnesium sulfate (in a dose of 1-4 g, infused IV over a period of several hours) for those patients with rapid atrial fibrillation that fails to respond to standard measures—especially when serum magnesium levels are either known or suspected to be low.

Pharmacological considerations for long-term rate control of chronic atrial fibrillation are similar to those suggested for acute management, with the obvious exception that oral medications are used. Despite continued common use of digoxin, oral verapamil, diltiazem, and/or beta-blockers have all been shown to be superior to digoxin for controlling the ventricular response to atrial fibrillation in ambulatory patients—especially in younger and more active adults.[25,33,34] This is because with activity, vagal tone tends to be withdrawn while sympathetic tone is enhanced. In contrast, the indirect vagotonic effect of digoxin is more likely to be effective when used to treat elderly and more sedentary individuals.[24,35]

Conversion of atrial fibrillation to sinus rhythm is a separate facet of management that, in the hemodynamically stable patient, is most often addressed after attending to rate control. This is because drugs used for facilitating conversion to sinus rhythm are different than the drugs that are used for initial rate control. The point to emphasize is that antiarrhythmic agents are not benign. Their use is best limited to those situations in which they are truly needed—and for which they are most likely to exert a beneficial effect.[25,27] As already noted, a substantial percentage of patients with new-onset atrial fibrillation convert spontaneously to sinus rhythm within the first 24 hours of seeking medical attention—simply with supportive measures and efforts aimed at correcting underlying medical conditions that may have precipitated the arrhythmia (i.e., diuresis of patients in heart failure, treatment of ischemia, correction of electrolyte and acid-base disorders, oxygenation of patients with bronchospasm or pneumonia, etc.). Should atrial fibrillation persist despite these measures, consideration might then be directed to the merits of attempting medical or electrical cardioversion for the specific case at hand.

Potential benefits accruing from restoration of sinus rhythm are obvious. Symptoms (i.e., palpitations, dizziness, shortness of breath) are relieved; cardiac hemodynamics are improved (restoration of the "atrial kick" with resultant enhancement of cardiac output); and the long-term risk of thromboembolism will be eliminated. Unfortunately, the process of cardioversion is not without risk. This is especially true for patients who have been in atrial fibrillation for more than 48 hours, in whom there presumably has been time for thrombus formation to occur within the fibrillating (i.e., non-contractile) atrial chambers.[21] Anticoagulation for a period of at least three weeks prior to attempts at elective cardioversion (to allow adequate time for thrombus to organize and become firmly adherent to the atrial wall) will significantly reduce the incidence of postconversion embolization in such patients. However, it will not eliminate this risk entirely; an estimated 1% of patients still develop thromboembolic complications in association with cardioversion even when anticoagulated beforehand.[21] The clinical reality is simply that not all patients with atrial fibrillation are suitable candidates for attempting either medical or electrical cardioversion.

Practically speaking, the chance of converting a patient in atrial fibrillation to sinus rhythm—and maintaining a normal rhythm after conversion—depends on three principal factors. Most important among these is the duration of time that the arrhythmia has been present prior to attempted cardioversion, with the chance of successful conversion decreasing significantly when atrial fibrillation has persisted for longer than six months. The other two factors are left atrial size (conversion to sinus rhythm is less likely when echocardiographic left atrial diameter exceeds 45-50 mm) and identifying and correcting the underlying cause of the rhythm. Given that some risk of stroke remains in association with cardio-version (even among patients who are anticoagulated), this process should probably not be considered for patients who do not have a realistic chance of achieving and maintaining a normal rhythm.

For those patients in whom an attempt at medical cardioversion is felt to be appropriate, any of a number of drugs may be used for this purpose. Traditionally, class IA antiarrhythmic agents (i.e., quinidine, procainamide, or disopyramide) have been selected first. While moderately effective and still frequently used, newer drugs have become available in recent years. These include class IC agents (flecainide and propafenone) and class III drugs (amiodarone and sotalol). Which agent to select in a given situation depends on multiple factors including the expected efficacy and side effect profile of the particular drug, patient specific variables in the case at hand, and individual preferences of the treating clinician.

Table 5. ACCP Consensus Conference Recommendations for Antithrombotic Therapy in Atrial Fibrillation (A Fib)[21]

PATIENTS WITH A FIB AT *HIGHEST* RISK OF STROKE

- Strongly consider long-term oral anticoagulation with **warfarin** for *all* patients with A Fib who are older than age 65. Aim to maintain the INR between 2.0 and 3.0 if at all possible—although a lower level of anticoagulation (i.e., to an INR value that is closer to 2.0) might be preferable for older patients (> 75 years of age) to reduce the risk of age-related bleeding. Clearly, a balance must be reached in elderly patients between the perceived risk of stroke and the increased risk of bleeding with warfarin.
- Strongly consider long-term oral anticoagulation with **warfarin** (to maintain the INR between 2.0 and 3.0) for patients with A Fib who are younger than age 65 if they have one or more of the following risk factors:

mitral stenosis	diabetes
prosthetic heart valves	clinical coronary artery disease
hypertension	thyrotoxicosis
heart failure	

- If, for any reason, anticoagulation is not used in any of these high risk groups (i.e., patient refusal, poor compliance, frequent falling, and/or other factors that might predispose to an increased risk of bleeding), treat with **aspirin** (325 mg/d) unless contraindicated.

PATIENTS WITH A FIB AT LOWER RISK OF STROKE

- Patients with A Fib who are younger than age 65 and do not have any of the risk factors noted above are at relatively low risk of stroke—especially if they have normal left atrial size and no evidence of left ventricular dysfunction on echocardiography. Treatment with *either* **aspirin** *or* **warfarin** is appropriate in such individuals.

Despite its potential for adverse effects, quinidine remains the most commonly chosen drug for initial attempts at medical cardioversion. Successful conversion in the acute setting can be achieved in up to 30% of patients who remain in atrial fibrillation after rate-slowing drugs have been used to control the ventricular response.[25] Continued administration of quinidine following conversion results in maintenance of sinus rhythm at one year in about half of this group, compared to a much smaller number who remain in sinus rhythm when quinidine is stopped.[36] Unfortunately, long-term maintenance therapy with quinidine is associated with an almost three-fold increase in cardiac-related mortality—a finding that raises serious questions about the advisability of continuing this medication for more than a few months following successful conversion.[36] Clearly, long-term treatment with quinidine should not be continued in those patients who despite therapeutic levels of the drug revert to atrial fibrillation in follow-up visits. For those in whom the drug works, the decision must be made as to whether the benefits of maintaining sinus rhythm outweigh the drawbacks associated with long-term use.

Alternative approaches are available. These include selection of another class IA drug (i.e., procainamide or disopyramide), selection instead of a newer antiarrhythmic agent for acute and/or long-term therapy, or acceptance of atrial fibrillation as the patient's chronic rhythm, with commitment to long-term anticoagulation in an attempt to minimize the risk of systemic embolization.

With regard to the other two class IA agents, both procainamide and disopyramide are of almost comparable efficacy to quinidine for converting atrial fibrillation and maintaining sinus rhythm with long-term therapy.[35] Procainamide offers the additional advantage of availability of an IV formulation for more rapid effect. Although data are somewhat limited on the use of these two drugs for treatment of atrial fibrillation, obvious concern exists for the potential of any class IA agent to prolong the QT interval and predispose to development of torsade de pointes and/or sudden death. Other concerns include the significant negative inotropic and anticholinergic effects of disopyramide, and the risk of agranulocytosis and high incidence of drug-induced lupus associated with long-term use of procainamide.

Of the newer antiarrhythmic agents, flecainide may be the most effective for facilitating acute conversion of atrial fibrillation to sinus rhythm. The drug may be given either orally or intravenously, with successful conversion occurring within 4-12 hours in 60-90% of patients.[25,27,37,38,39] Somewhat lower conversion rates are achieved with the other new drugs. Caution is advised when administering any of the newer agents, as they all may depress left ventricular function and/or induce proarrhythmia. Equally important clinically as their potential for facilitating acute conversion of atrial fibrillation is the efficacy of class IC and class III drugs for maintaining sinus rhythm with long-term therapy. Not only are these drugs superior to quinidine (and other class IA agents) for this purpose, but their overall toxicity is also significantly less.[40,41] In particular, use of low dose amiodarone (100-300 mg daily) has been shown to maintain sinus rhythm in up to 70% of patients with long-term therapy—even when left atrial size is large and/or other drugs have been ineffective.[25,42] Adverse effects are noticeably less when these low doses are used. It can be anticipated that future years will see a continued trend toward increased use of these newer agents in appropriate clinical situations.

The final issue to address regarding the management of atrial fibrillation relates to the need for anticoagulation. In patients with chronic nonvalvular atrial fibrillation who are not anticoagulated, the estimated overall risk of embolic stroke is about 5% per year (3-8% range in most studies).[21,22,25] This represents a more than five-fold increased incidence of stroke compared to control subjects who are in normal sinus rhythm. If in addition to atrial fibrillation the patient also has mitral stenosis due to rheumatic heart disease, then the relative risk of stroke is increased more than 15-fold.[43] Thus, the risk of stroke clearly will vary in different subsets of patients with atrial fibrillation. Principal determinants of the magnitude of this risk are the age of the patient (stroke risk progressively increases with advancing age) and the presence and nature of coexisting cardiovascular disease.

Long-term anticoagulation with warfarin significantly decreases the risk of stroke in patients with chronic nonvalvular atrial fibrillation. Combined results from the six major primary prevention trials assessing the benefit of antithrombotic therapy suggest a 68% reduction in risk among warfarin-treated patients.[21] In view of the fact that a majority of strokes in the treated groups from these studies occurred in patients who were not adequately anticoagulated at the time of their event, it is likely that improved compliance with therapeutic objectives might lower the risk of stroke even more.[44] Aspirin is also effective in reducing the risk of stroke in patients with chronic nonvalvular atrial fibrillation. However, the benefit obtained from aspirin is no more than half as effective as full anticoagulation for prevention of stroke.[21] Whether this increased degree of protection conveyed by warfarin is enough to override the inconvenience and greater risk of bleeding associated with long-term use of this treatment is an issue that must be individually decided for each particular case. To facilitate the decision-making process, we summarize the recommendations put forth by the most recent American College of Chest Physicians (ACCP) Consensus Conference on Antithrombotic Therapy. *(Please see Table 5.)*[21]

Atrial Flutter

In our experience, atrial flutter is by far the most commonly overlooked cardiac arrhythmia. Although easy to diagnose when flutter activity is obvious (as it is following carotid sinus massage in Figure 7), recognition of this arrhythmia may be much more difficult when the lead being monitored fails to provide any indication of underlying atrial activity. Use of additional leads (ideally obtaining a 12-lead ECG), maintaining a high index of suspicion (always think flutter whenever the rate of a regular SVT is close to 150 beats/min), and selective use of vagal maneuvers are ways to prevent a missed diagnosis.

Clinically, the overall approach to evaluation and treatment of atrial flutter is surprisingly similar to that for atrial fibrillation. That is, the drugs that are used to achieve rate control and/or convert the rhythm are the same—and synchronized cardioversion is the treatment of choice if the patient becomes acutely unstable. Some important differences do exist, however, between these two arrhythmias. Atrial fibrillation is far more common. Because of the chaotic (and therefore asynchronous) nature of atrial activity with fibrillation, the risk of embolization appears to be much greater than it is with atrial flutter (in which atrial activity is clearly more organized). Unfortunately in recent years, there have been a number of case reports of embolization occurring following cardioversion of patients with pure atrial flutter. This suggests that even though the overall risk of embolization is less with atrial flutter, it may still be prudent to consider anticoagulation in patients with both atrial fibrillation and atrial flutter prior to elective attempts at cardioversion.[21]

Another important difference between these two arrhythmias is in the way they respond to the same therapy. Thus, although digoxin, verapamil, diltiazem, and/or beta-blockers are all used to achieve rate control in each case, it will often be much more difficult to effectively slow the ventricular response to atrial flutter—even when high doses of one or more of these rate-slowing agents are used. In contrast, atrial flutter is the rhythm that generally responds best to synchronized cardioversion (probably reflecting the fact that atrial flutter is a more organized rhythm). As a result, much lower initial energy levels (usually 50 joules) are typically selected for cardioversion of atrial flutter, whereas significantly higher energies (of 200 joules) are likely to be needed for successful cardioversion of atrial fibrillation.

Multifocal Atrial Tachycardia

Next to atrial flutter, MAT may be the most problematic SVT from a diagnostic standpoint. This is because unlike the situation in Figure 6C where multiple P wave forms are easy to identify, the ectopic atrial activity of MAT will not always be evident in the lead being monitored. In such cases, irregularity of the ventricular response may simulate atrial fibrillation. Thus, the key to recognizing MAT is maintaining a high index of suspicion for the rhythm, and obtaining a 12-lead ECG to facilitate the search for P waves in more than a single lead.

MAT occurs primarily in two clinical settings: chronic obstructive pulmonary disease (COPD), and extremely ill patients with multisystem problems that usually require intensive care treatment.[45] The reason why distinction between atrial fibrillation and MAT is so important clinically is that prognosis and management of these two conditions differs dramatically. Digitalization is a treatment of choice for achieving rate control of rapid atrial fibrillation. In contrast, treatment of MAT must be directed at correcting the underlying cause of the arrhythmia. This usually entails correction of hypoxemia for patients with COPD and correction of acidosis, electrolyte abnormalities, sepsis, and shock (in addition to other underlying conditions) for patients with MAT and multisystem disease. Because MAT is notoriously resistant to the rate-slowing effect of digoxin, the tendency is great to develop digitalis toxicity if MAT is mistakenly diagnosed as atrial fibrillation and treated with repeated doses of this medication. Practically speaking, the ventricular response in most cases of MAT is not so rapid as to require specific antiarrhythmic therapy. For those occasional instances when rate control will be needed, verapamil or diltiazem constitute the treatment of choice. Administration of IV magnesium may also be helpful in some cases, even when serum magnesium levels are normal.[45]

References

1. Symanski BJ, Marriott HJL. Ventricular tachycardia—Diagnosis and misdiagnosis: A case report. *Heart Lung* 1995;24:121-123.
2. Grauer K, Cavallaro D. ACLS: Pocket Reference, St. Louis; Mosby Lifeline:1993:106-109.
3. Grauer K. When 12 leads are better than one. In: *A Practical Guide to ECG Interpretation*. St. Louis: Mosby-Year Book; 1992:217-256.
4. Grauer K, Cavallaro D. *ACLS: Certification Preparation—Volume I*. St. Louis: Mosby Lifeline;1993:104.
5. Steinman RT, et al. Wide QRS tachycardia in the conscious adult: Ventricular tachycardia is the most frequent cause. *JAMA* 1989;261:1013-1016.

6. Baerman JM, et al. Differentiation of ventricular tachycardia from supraventricular tachycardia with aberration: Value of the clinical history. *Ann Emerg Med* 1987;16:40-43.
7. Akhtar M, et al. Wide QRS complex tachycardia: Reappraisal of a common clinical problem. *Ann Intern Med* 1988;109: 905-912.
8. Grauer K, Cavallaro D: Differentiation of PVCs from aberrancy. In: *ACLS: A Compre-hensive Review—Volume II*. St. Louis: Mosby Lifeline; 1993:489-546.
9. Stewart RB, et al. Wide complex tachycardia: Misdiagnosis and outcome after emergent therapy. *Ann Intern Med* 1996; 104:766-771.
10. Pomeroy PR. Augmented carotid massage. *Ann Emerg Med* 1992;21:1169-1170.
11. Schweitzer P, Teichholz LE. Carotid sinus massage: Its diagnostic and therapeutic value in arrhythmias. *Am J Med* 1985;78:645-654.
12. Mehta D, et al. Relative efficacy of various physical manoeuvres in the termination of junctional tachycardia. *Lancet* 1988;1:1181-1185.
13. Page RL, et al. Asymptomatic arrhythmias in patients with symptomatic paroxysmal atrial fibrillation and paroxysmal supraventricular tachycardia. *Circulation* 1994;89:224-227.
14. Emergency Cardiac Care Committee and Subcommittees, American Heart Association: Guidelines for cardiopulmonary resuscitation and emergency cardiac care. *JAMA* 1992;268: 2223-2225.
15. LeDuc TJ, Carr JD. Magnesium sulfate for conversion of supraventricular tachycardia refractory to intravenous adenosine. *Ann Emerg Med* 199;:27:375-378.
16. Wesley RC, et al. Effect of magnesium sulfate on supraventricular tachycardia. *Am J Cardiol* 1989;63:1129-1131.
17. Grauer K, et al. New developments in cardiopulmonary resuscitation. *Am Fam Phys* 1991;43:832-844.
18. Woods KL, et al. Intravenous magnesium sulphate in suspected acute myocardial infarction: Results of the second Leicester Intravenous Magnesium Intervention Trial (LIMIT-2). *Lancet* 1992;339:1553-1558.
19. Margolis B, et al. Episodic drug treatment in the management of paroxysmal arrhythmia. *Am J Cardiol* 1980;45:621-626.
20. Rose JSet al. Effective termination of reentrant supraventricular tachycardia by single dose oral combination therapy with pindolol and verapamil. *Am Heart J* 1986;112:759-765.
21. Laupacis A, et al. Antithrombotic therapy in atrial fibrillation. *Chest* 1995;108(Suppl):352S-359S.
22. Ezekowitz MD, Grauer K. Management of chronic atrial fibrillation. *American Family Physician* (Monograph)- Fall, 1993.
23. The Stroke Prevention in Atrial Fibrillation Investigators. Predictors of thrombo-embolism in atrial fibrillation: Echocardiographic features of patients at risk. *Ann Int Med* 1992;116:6-12.
24. Falk RH, Leavitt JI. Digoxin for atrial fibrillation: A drug whose time has gone? *Ann Int Med* 1991;114:573-575.
25. Podrid PJ. Chapter 32, Atrial Fibrillation. In: Parmley WW and Chatterjee K, eds. *Cardiology.* Philadelphia; 1995:1-30.
26. Falk RH, et al. Digoxin for converting recent-onset atrial fibrillation to sinus rhythm: A randomized, double-blind trial. *Ann Int Med* 1987;106:503-506.
27. Donovan KD, et al. Intavenous flecainide versus amiodarone for recent-onset atrial fibrillation. *Am J Cardiol* 1995;75: 693-697.
28. Rawles JM, et al. Time of occurrence, duration and ventricular rate of paroxysmal atrial fibrillation: The effect of digoxin. *Br Heart J* 1990;63:225-227.
29. Roth A, et al. Efficacy and safety of medium- and high-dose diltiazem alone and in combination with digoxin for control of heart rate at rest and during exercise in patients with chronic atrial fibrillation. *Circulation* 1986;73:316-324.
30. Steinberg JS, et al. Efficacy of oral diltiazem to control ventricular response in chronic atrial fibrillation at rest and during exercise. *J Am Coll Cardiol* 1987;9:405-411.
31. Hays JV, et al. Effect of magnesium sulfate on ventricular rate control in atrial fibrillation. *Ann Emerg Med* 1994;24:61-64.
32. Brodsky MA, et al. Magnesium therapy in new-onset atrial fibrillation. *Am J Cardiol* 1994;73:1227-1229.
33. Lang R, et al. Superiority of oral verapamil therapy to digoxin in treatment of chronic atrial fibrillation. *Chest* 1983;83: 491-499.
34. Singh BN, Nademanee K. Use of calcium antagonists for cardiac arrhythmias. *Am J Cardiol* 1987;59:153B-162B.
35. Klein HO, Kaplinsky E. Digitalis and verapamil in atrial fibrillation and flutter: Is verapamil now the preferred agent? *Drugs* 1986;31:185-197.
36. Coplen SE, et al. Efficacy and safety of quinidine therapy for maintenance of sinus rhythm after cardioversion: A meta-analysis of randomized controlled trials. *Circulation* 1990;82: 1106-1116.
37. Kingma JH, Suttorp MJ. Acute pharmacologic conversion of atrial fibrillation and flutter: The role of flecainide, propafenone, and verapamil. *Am J Cardiol* 1992;70:56A-61A.
38. Capucci A, et al. Effectiveness of loading oral flecainide for converting recent-onset atrial fibrillation to sinus rhythm in patients without organic heart disease or with only systemic hypertension. *Am J Cardiol* 1992;70:69-72.
39. Hohnloser SH, Zabel M. Short- and long-term efficacy and safety of flecainide acetate for supraventricular arrhythmias. *Am J Cardiol* 1992;70:3A-10A.
40. Naccarelli GV, et al. Prospective comparison of flecainide versus quinidine for the treatment of paroxysmal atrial fibrillation/flutter. *Am J Cardiol* 1996;77:53A-59A.
41. Reimold SCet al. Propafenone versus sotalol for suppression of recurrent symptomatic atrial fibrillation. *Am J Cardiol* 1993;71:558-563.
42. Chun SH, et al. Long-term efficacy of amiodarone for the maintenance of normal sinus rhythm in patients with refractory atrial fibrillation or rlutter. *Am J Cardiol* 1995;76:47-50.
43. Wolf PA, et al. Atrial fibrillation as an independent risk factor for stroke: The Framingham Study. *Stroke* 1991;22:983-988.
44. Albers GW. Atrial fibrillation and stroke: Three new studies, three remaining questions. *Arch Int Med* 1994;154: 1443-1448.
45. Kastor JA. Multifocal atrial tachycardia. *N Engl J Med* 1990; 322:713-1717.

Deep Venous Thrombosis: Risk Factor Assessment and Diagnosis

Stephen A. Colucciello, MD, FACEP

The management of deep venous thrombosis (DVT) has changed dramatically over the past several years. Advances in both technology and pharmacology have placed the emergency physician in a pivotal role for managing veno-occlusive disease.

DVT is a cause of significant morbidity and mortality.[1-3] Acutely, it causes pain and limits physical activity. A dramatic presentation of DVT known as phlegmasia dolens leads to gangrene, shock, and death. If clots embolize, subsequent pulmonary embolism (PE) can be fatal. Despite resolution of the acute event, destruction of venous valves can lead to recurrent swelling, stasis ulcers, and persistent edema.[1]

Although DVT is a significant cause of mortality in the elderly, even children are not immune. Most patients with venous thrombosis have risk factors, among them: stasis, hypercoagulability, trauma, and/or endothelial injury.

Although the physical examination usually provides clues to the diagnosis, the emergency physician must remember that the clinical examination is neither sensitive nor specific for DVT. Failure to detect a deep venous thrombosis can lead to catastrophic results. A clinical scoring system aids in the diagnosis of patients with leg pain or swelling, and new assays for D-dimer play a growing role. In the past decade, venography has declined, and Duplex ultrasound has become the diagnostic modality of choice.

The emergency physician must aggressively recognize and treat life threats, such as pulmonary embolism and phlegmasia dolens. Heparin is often underdosed, and the use of a weight-based nomogram assists the emergency physician to rapidly achieve a targeted PTT. Low-molecular weight heparin (LMWH) will change practice standards by allowing home treatment of venous thrombosis at lower total cost. The use of thrombolytics remains controversial.

This chapter outlines an outcome-effective clinical approach for DVT management. It will help emergency departments (EDs) design critical pathways for developing a safe and effective treatment program for this common condition.

Epidemiology

Approximately 2 million Americans suffer from DVT each year,[4] but, because most DVT is occult, the true incidence is unknown. Approximately 250,000 patients per year require hospitalization for 5-10 days of intravenous heparin therapy.[5] In addition to those with acute thrombosis, millions more suffer from sequelae such as stasis dermatitis and venous ulcers. While the degree of morbidity is significant, mortality rates are equally problematic. Thromboembolic disease is annually responsible for 200,000 deaths in the United States.[6] The elderly are in greatest jeopardy; DVT is associated with a 21% one-year mortality in this age group.[7] Many in this subgroup die from associated PE, while others succumb from comorbid disease, especially cancer. Even children are at risk for venous thrombosis. Pediatric patients at risk include those with spinal cord injuries, hypercoagulable states, and those with a recent history of central lines.[8]

Etiology and Risk Factors for DVT

Virchow first elucidated the causes of deep venous thrombosis with a description of a classical triad: stasis, hypercoagulability, and endothelial injury. While at least 50% of patients with DVT have risk factors,[9] the strongest risk factor for venous thrombosis is prior thromboembolic disease.[10] *(Please see Table 1.)* Moreover, risk factors are additive in nature.[11]

Stasis. Stasis may arise from prolonged bed rest (4 days or more) or extended travel in a vehicle such as an airplane or automobile. The principal cause of death related to transatlantic flights is not airplane lasagna, but pulmonary embolism. This is known, among other things, as the "economy class syndrome," in which venous thrombosis is induced by cramped quarters in an airplane, usually during transoceanic flights.[12] A cast on the leg also increases venous stasis and impairs the "muscle pump" mechanism that propels blood into the central circulation. Stasis plays a role in thrombosis encountered in the morbidly obese and in individuals with cardiac disease. Limb paralysis from stroke or spinal cord injury is associated with a difficult-to-evaluate syndrome of painless or occult thrombosis.[13]

Hypercoagulability. Surgery and trauma are responsible for up to 40% of all thromboembolic disease, which results from both a hypercoagulable state and immobility. These insults activate the clotting cascade, and indices of thrombosis and fibrinolysis rise rapidly.[14]

Malignancy also accelerates the coagulation cascade and is responsible for up to 4% of all episodes of DVT.[15,16] Activation of the extrinsic pathway via tissue factor plays an important role in clot generation;[17] breast and prostate cancer are common precipitants. Up to 10% of patients with new onset DVT develop cancer within six months after the diagnosis of DVT.[18,19] Recurrent migratory superficial thrombophlebitis caused by malignancy (usually solid tumors) is called Trousseau's syndrome. This condition is resistant to warfarin therapy and may require long-term heparin prophylaxis.[20]

Increased estrogen predisposes to thrombosis due to a fall in protein 'S,' and cigarette smoking significantly enhances this tendency.[19] Increased estrogen occurs during all stages of pregnancy—the first three months postpartum, after elective abortion, and during treatment with oral contraceptive pills (OCPs). Low-dose estrogen OCPs are not associated with an increased risk of DVT. Women with congenital resistance to activated protein C (factor V Leiden mutation) are especially susceptible to thrombosis due to OCPs.[22] Progesterone-only pills and Norplant may slightly increase the risk of thrombosis.

Ten percent of thromboembolic disease is due to acquired or inherited disorders of coagulation. Three of the most common disorders include deficiencies of protein 'S,' protein 'C,' and antithrombin III. While most patients inherit these conditions, they may also be acquired. Because the nephrotic syndrome results in urinary loss of antithrombin III, this diagnosis should be considered in children presenting with thromboembolic disease.[23] Antiphospholipid antibodies accelerate coagulation and include the lupus anticoagulant and anticardiolipin antibodies.[24] Paradoxically, nearly half of these patients have a prolonged PTT on laboratory testing despite being hypercoaguable.[25] Suspect antiphospholipid antibodies when thrombosis occurs in young patients with no other risk factors. This syndrome is especially likely if the patient has arterial thrombosis or venous clot in unusual locations, such as the mesentery or solid organs.[26] Inflammatory processes, such as systemic lupus erythematosus (SLE), sickle cell disease, and inflammatory bowel disease (IBD), also predispose to thrombosis, presumably due to hypercoagulability.

Endothelial Injury. The third aspect of Virchow's triad is endothelial injury. Trauma, surgery, and invasive procedure may dis-

Table 1. Risk Factors for Thromboembolic Disease

Table 1. Risk Factors for Thromboembolic Disease
STASIS
Immobility
Four days bed rest
Long plane ride (economy class syndrome)
Long train or car ride (many hours)
Paralysis: stroke, spinal cord injury
Cast on leg
HYPERCOAGULABILITY (UNDERLYING DISEASE)
Previous thromboembolic disease
Malignancy
Inflammatory conditions (SLE, IBD, PVD)
Nephrotic syndrome (loss of antithrombin III)
Sepsis
COAGULATION DISORDERS—INHERITABLE VS. ACQUIRED
Resistance to activated Protein C
Protein S deficiency
Protein C deficiency
Antithrombin deficiency
Disorders of fibrinogen or plasminogen
Antiphospholipid antibodies (lupus anticoagulant and anticardiolipin)
INCREASED ESTROGEN (CAUSES URINARY LOSS OF PROTEINS AND ANTITHROMBIN III)
Pregnancy
Post-partum < 3 months
Elective abortion or miscarriage
Oral contraceptive pills, other exogenous estrogens
INTIMAL DAMAGE
Intravenous drug abuse
Trauma
Recent surgery
Central lines
MULTIFACTORIAL
Trauma
Recent surgery
Age > 60
Cardiac disease
Obesity
Heart failure
Lower limb arteriopathy

rupt venous integrity.[27,28] In particular, orthopedic surgery of the hip and lower extremities can incite thrombosis. Iatrogenic causes of venous thrombosis are increasing due to the widespread use of central venous catheters, particularly subclavian and internal jugular lines. These lines are an important cause of upper extremity DVT, particularly in children.[29] Femoral lines also generate thrombus in 14% of patients cannulated.[30]

Clinical Pathophysiology

Anatomists describe the venous drainage of the lower extremity in relationship to the muscle fascia. The superficial veins include the greater and lesser saphenous veins, which drain into the deep system via the perforating or communicating veins. A series of valves direct blood flow toward the heart. The pump action of the thigh and calf muscles powers this flow.[31] While some view anatomists as humorless, they have perpetuated a dangerous joke on emergency physicians. The have named a major vessel of the lower extremity the "superficial" femoral vein. However, this structure is a *deep* vein! Three quarters of primary care physicians do not realize this fact and may neglect to anticoagulate the patient when this vein is involved.[32]

The nidus for a clot is often an intimal defect. For example, intravenous catheters, irritating medications, or illicit drugs precipitate superficial thrombophlebitis.[33-35] When a clot forms on an intimal defect, the coagulation cascade promotes clot growth proximally. Thrombus can extend from the superficial veins into the deep system from which it can embolize to the lungs. Nearly 25% of all patients with superficial phlebitis have involvement of the deep system.[36] Males older than age 60, patients with systemic infection, and patients on prolonged bed rest are most likely to develop DVT.[37]

While the vast majority of pulmonary emboli arise from the iliofemoral system, patients with calf vein involvement are also at risk. While *isolated* calf thrombi are unlikely to produce significant pulmonary emboli, up to 15-20% can later propagate and then embolize.[38-40] Once a clot develops, whether proximal or distal, venous hypertension frequently leads to pain and/or swelling. Extensive deep venous thrombosis can even result in compartment syndrome of the thigh and leg.[41] However, many cases of DVT remain asymptomatic until embolization occurs. Anticoagulation of superficial vein thrombosis remains controversial.

Opposing the coagulation cascade is the endogenous fibrinolytic system. After the clot organizes or dissolves, most veins will recanalize in several weeks.[42] Residual clots retract as fibroblasts and capillary development lead to intimal thickening.[43] Venous hypertension and residual clot may destroy valves, leading to the postphlebitic syndrome, which develops within 5-10 years.[44] Edema, sclerosis, and ulceration characterize this syndrome, which develops in 40-80% of patients with DVT.[45,46] In addition to the chronic changes of the postphlebitic syndrome, patients also can suffer exacerbations of swelling and pain, probably as a result of venous dilatation and hypertension. These exacerbations are clinically indistinguishable from recurrent DVT.[47] Accordingly, episodes of acute swelling and pain should be attributed to the postphlebitic syndrome *only after* objective tests confirm no recurrence of DVT.

Pulmonary embolism (PE) is a serious complication of DVT. Many episodes of pulmonary embolism go unrecognized, and at least 40% of patients with DVT have clinically silent PE on VQ scanning,[48] which is not the gold standard for diagnosis of PE. Most cases of PE arise from the iliofemoral system. Massive occlusion of the iliofemoral system can be life- and limb-threatening. Patients who have malignancy, congestive heart failure, massive obesity, or prior DVT are most susceptible to this complication.

Table 2. Important Historical Questions

1. Have you or anyone in your family ever had a blood clot in the leg or lung?
2. Have you been on a long trip (e.g., car, plane, etc.)?
3. Have you recently been bedridden for more than three days?
4. Have you had surgery or trauma in the last 2-3 months?
5. Have you been pregnant in the last three months (therapeutic abortion, miscarriage, current pregnancy)?
6. Are you on birth control pills and do you smoke?
7. Do you have any medical problems (e.g., malignancy, SLE, CHF)?
8. Have you had chest pain or shortness of breath?

Presentation and Physical Examination

Symptomatic patients typically complain of lower extremity pain or swelling. They may report a sense of fullness, which increases with standing or walking.[49] Some individuals may complain of pain in the lower extremity when coughing or sneezing, which is different from electric type pain with cough or sneeze that is associated with sciatica. Venous involvement is usually unilateral unless the vena cava occludes, a rare and catastrophic event. In one study, DVT never occurred in the patients with bilateral symptoms.[50] However, bilateral involvement can occur.

It is important to determine the time course of symptoms and to elicit a history of recent trauma. As a rule, venous thrombosis occurs over several days, and sudden, severe pain is more compatible with muscle rupture or injury. Associated symptoms are also important, especially the presence of chest pain or shortness of breath, which may suggest PE. The medical history should be used to assess risk factors for thromboembolic disease. A history of prior DVT is important, as up to 26% of patients with DVT have had a previous episode.[10] *(Please see Table 2.)*

Physical Examination. A caveat that is nearly 20 years old remains valid today. "A combination of clinical signs and symptoms that included tenderness, swelling, redness, and the assessment of Homans' sign [can] not adequately differentiate patients with or without DVT."[51]

This is not to imply that physical examination is useless, but that a number of physical findings in combination with risk factors assist in the diagnosis of a patient with leg complaints.

Occasionally, a rectal temperature can help distinguish cellulitis from DVT. While patients with DVT may have a low grade fever due to a systemic inflammatory response, this fever rarely exceeds 102°F. To help make this differentiation, it is essential to completely undress

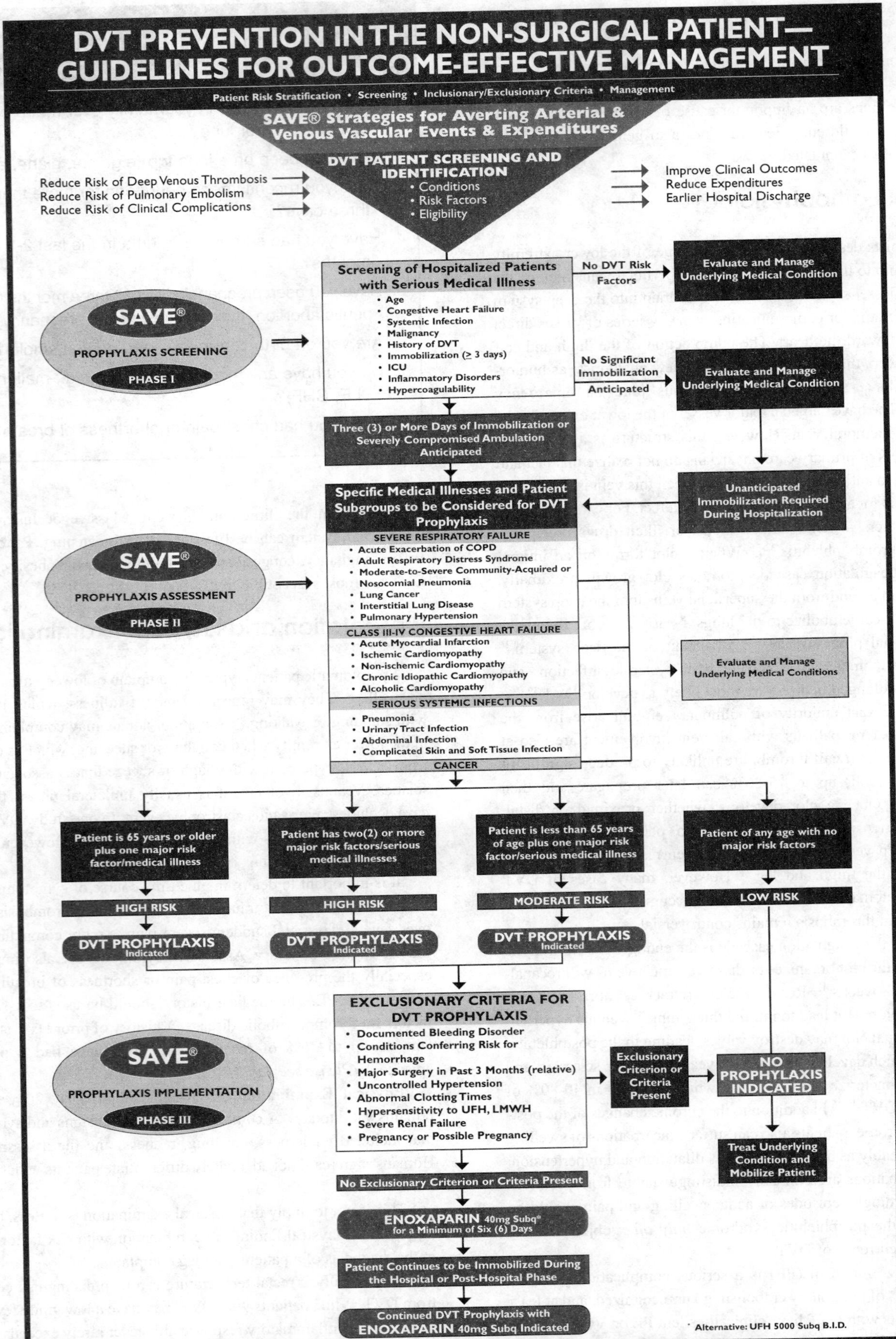
DVT PREVENTION IN THE NON-SURGICAL PATIENT—
GUIDELINES FOR OUTCOME-EFFECTIVE MANAGEMENT
Patient Risk Stratification • Screening • Inclusionary/Exclusionary Criteria • Management
SAVE® Strategies for Averting Arterial & Venous Vascular Events & Expenditures
DVT PATIENT SCREENING AND IDENTIFICATION
• Conditions
• Risk Factors
• Eligibility
Reduce Risk of Deep Venous Thrombosis
Reduce Risk of Pulmonary Embolism
Reduce Risk of Clinical Complications
Improve Clinical Outcomes
Reduce Expenditures
Earlier Hospital Discharge
SAVE® PROPHYLAXIS SCREENING PHASE I
Screening of Hospitalized Patients with Serious Medical Illness
• Age
• Congestive Heart Failure
• Systemic Infection
• Malignancy
• History of DVT
• Immobilization (≥ 3 days)
• ICU
• Inflammatory Disorders
• Hypercoagulability
No DVT Risk Factors
Evaluate and Manage Underlying Medical Condition
No Significant Immobilization Anticipated
Evaluate and Manage Underlying Medical Condition
Three (3) or More Days of Immobilization or Severely Compromised Ambulation Anticipated
Unanticipated Immobilization Required During Hospitalization
SAVE® PROPHYLAXIS ASSESSMENT PHASE II
Specific Medical Illnesses and Patient Subgroups to be Considered for DVT Prophylaxis
SEVERE RESPIRATORY FAILURE
• Acute Exacerbation of COPD
• Adult Respiratory Distress Syndrome
• Moderate-to-Severe Community-Acquired or Nosocomial Pneumonia
• Lung Cancer
• Interstitial Lung Disease
• Pulmonary Hypertension
CLASS III-IV CONGESTIVE HEART FAILURE
• Acute Myocardial Infarction
• Ischemic Cardiomyopathy
• Non-ischemic Cardiomyopathy
• Chronic Idiopathic Cardiomyopathy
• Alcoholic Cardiomyopathy
SERIOUS SYSTEMIC INFECTIONS
• Pneumonia
• Urinary Tract Infection
• Abdominal Infection
• Complicated Skin and Soft Tissue Infection
CANCER
Evaluate and Manage Underlying Medical Conditions
Patient is 65 years or older plus one major risk factor/medical illness
HIGH RISK
DVT PROPHYLAXIS Indicated
Patient has two(2) or more major risk factors/serious medical illnesses
HIGH RISK
DVT PROPHYLAXIS Indicated
Patient is less than 65 years of age plus one major risk factor/serious medical illness
MODERATE RISK
DVT PROPHYLAXIS Indicated
Patient of any age with no major risk factors
LOW RISK
SAVE® PROPHYLAXIS IMPLEMENTATION PHASE III
EXCLUSIONARY CRITERIA FOR DVT PROPHYLAXIS
• Documented Bleeding Disorder
• Conditions Conferring Risk for Hemorrhage
• Major Surgery in Past 3 Months (relative)
• Uncontrolled Hypertension
• Abnormal Clotting Times
• Hypersensitivity to UFH, LMWH
• Severe Renal Failure
• Pregnancy or Possible Pregnancy
Exclusionary Criterion or Criteria Present
NO PROPHYLAXIS INDICATED
Treat Underlying Condition and Mobilize Patient
No Exclusionary Criterion or Criteria Present
ENOXAPARIN 40mg Subq* for a Minimum of Six (6) Days
Patient Continues to be Immobilized During the Hospital or Post-Hospital Phase
Continued DVT Prophylaxis with ENOXAPARIN 40mg Subq Indicated
* Alternative: UFH 5000 Subq B.I.D.

Figure 1. Clinical Suspicion for DVT

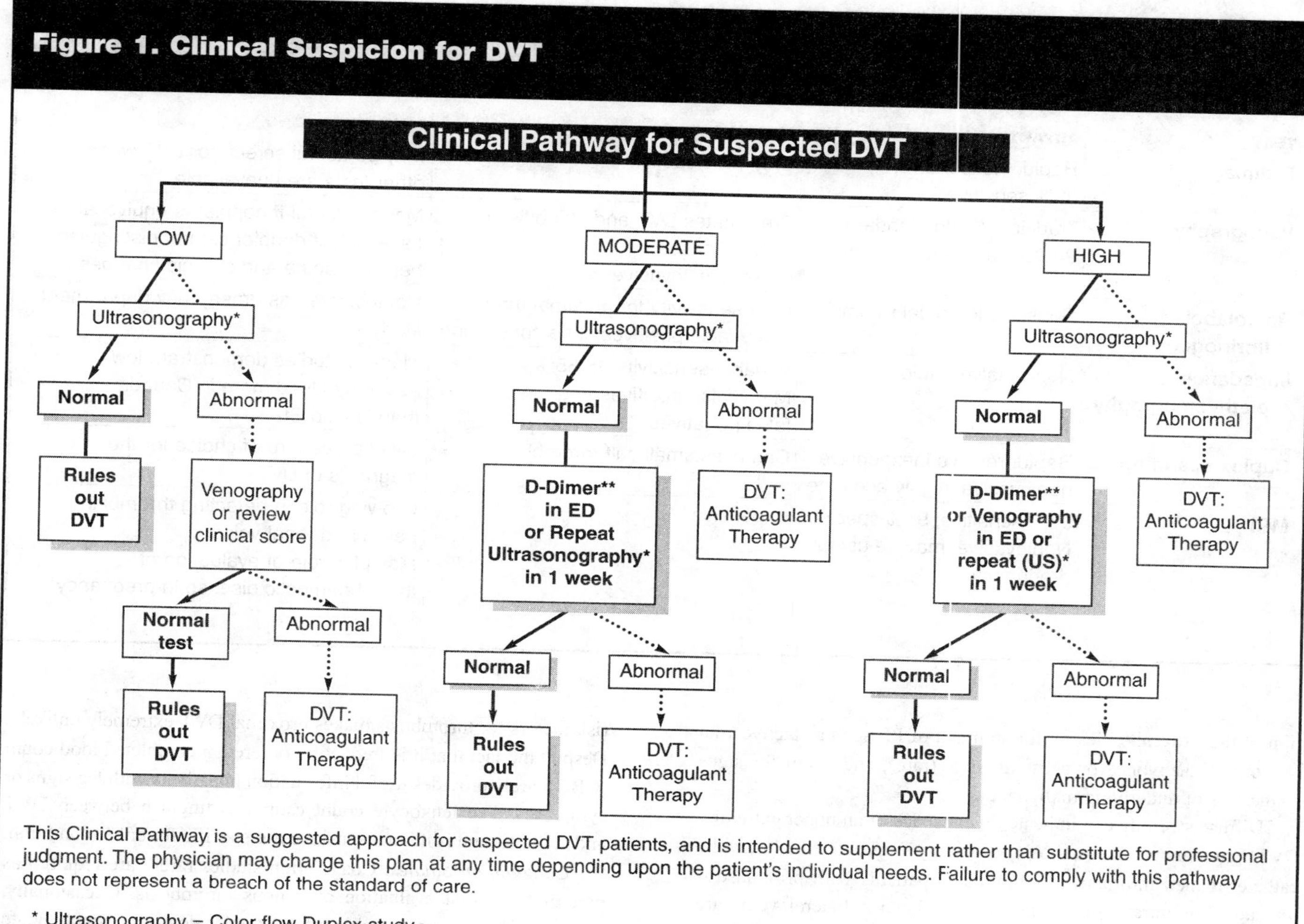

This Clinical Pathway is a suggested approach for suspected DVT patients, and is intended to supplement rather than substitute for professional judgment. The physician may change this plan at any time depending upon the patient's individual needs. Failure to comply with this pathway does not represent a breach of the standard of care.

* Ultrasonography = Color flow Duplex study
** D-Dimer red cell agglutination study

Source: Adapted from Anand. *JAMA* 1998;279:1094-1099.

the patient with leg symptoms and inspect for lymphangitis, erythema, and ulcerations. Clots may become infected, especially in patients with intravenous drug abuse. Remember to examine the entire limb for abnormalities, as lymphangitis may have large "skip" areas. Be alert for psychiatric patients or prisoners who may tie a tourniquet around their thigh to produce factitious DVT.

Lack of discrepancy in calf size does not rule out DVT. Some researches have standardized calf measurements at 10 cm below the tibial tuberosity. While asymmetry of the calves of 1 cm or more is abnormal, such asymmetry does not definitively distinguish between patients with thromboembolic disease and those without.[52] However, asymmetric calf swelling of greater than 3 cm is almost always a significant finding.[53]

Examine the legs for pitting edema; extremities affected by acute thrombosis are frequently warmer than the opposite limb. Palpation includes a search for "cords," which are very specific, although insensitive for thrombosis. Cords are most often detected in the popliteal fossa. Palpate distal pulses and evaluate capillary refill to assess limb perfusion. Pulses may also be diminished in long-standing arterial disease. The presence of pain with passive range of motion of the toes or ankle is an important clue to compartment syndrome. Move and palpate all joints to detect acute arthritis or other joint pathology. Neurologic evaluation may detect nerve root irritation; sensory, motor, and reflex deficits should be noted. Search for a thrill or bruit which is associated with arteriovenous (AV) fistulas. Patients with large fistulas have abnormally high cardiac output, and manual compression of the fistula reflexively slows the heart by reducing the shunt (Branham's sign).[54] Patients with a remote history of a gunshot wound to the extremity are most likely to present with a fistula. Bony tenderness does not rule out DVT. Indeed, up to 65% of patients with DVT will have pain with percussion of the medial tibia.[49] Bancroft or Moses' sign is pain with compression of the calf against the tibia. Some patients with DVT will have more pain with this maneuver than with transverse compression of the gastrocnemius.[55]

A review of venous thrombosis would not be complete without mention of Homans'' sign: pain in the posterior calf or knee with forced dorsiflexion of the foot. It is often present in patients with sciatica. Despite numerous references to Homans'' sign in the medical literature, this finding is inaccurate and unreliable.[56]

Examination of the patient with DVT does not end with evalua-

Table 3. Diagnostic Modalities

TEST	ADVANTAGES	DISADVANTAGES	COMMENTS
D-dimer	Rapid, inexpensive, 93% sensitive	Only 77% specific	May be useful screen for DVT when other tests are unavailable
Venography	Traditional gold standard 90-95% accurate	Precipitates DVT and phlebitis in 1-3% of cases expensive; invasive	May be useful if doppler is equivocal especially if doppler cannot distinguish between acute and chronic changes
Radiolabeled fibrinogen	Sensitive for distal thrombi	Poor sensitivity for proximal thrombi; many false positives; time consuming	Not indicated as emergency department study
Impedance plethysmography	Noninvasive, rapid	Variable sensitivity 65-85% Many false positives and false negatives	Modern studies demonstrate low accuracy. Used more in Canada than United States
Duplex scanning	Rapid, relative inexpensive, noninvasive; highly accurate	Can miss small calf thrombi	Initial procedure of choice for the diagnosis of DVT
MRI	97% sensitive; 95% specific Noninvasive; may be useful pregnancy	Expensive	Growing role in detecting thrombi in pelvic and renal veins. May play role of evaluation of thromboembolic disease in pregnancy

tion of the extremity. Search for stigmata of PE such as tachycardia (common), tachypnea or chest findings (rare), and exam for signs suggestive of underlying malignancy.[18]

Diffuse swelling can indicate the presence of an upper extremity DVT. Effort-induced thrombosis occurs in young, active males, while catheter-related thrombosis is limited to patients with prior instrumentation or intravenous drug abuse. Dilated collateral veins are frequent, but these are more easily seen in Caucasians. Look for arm discoloration and palpable axillary veins.[57]

Diagnostic Studies

Clinical examination alone is able to confirm only 20-30% of cases of DVT.[58] *(Please see Figure 1.)* Because of the limitations associated with the physical examination and history, the diagnosis of DVT must be pursued in any patient who presents with unexplained extremity pain or swelling. A patient who presents with symptoms in both arms or both legs, usually will not be suffering from bilateral thrombosis. Patients with risk factors for bilateral thrombosis, however, who present with bilateral findings, need careful examination. Patients with unilateral complaints and no clear explanation, such as a direct blow to the extremity, twisted ankle, etc., require further evaluation. The presence of risk factors for DVT must decrease the threshold for obtaining imaging studies. Accordingly, nearly all patients with complaints compatible with venous thrombosis, and who have no typical alternative diagnosis, require an imaging study.[59] Patients with suspected DVT who complain of chest pain or shortness of breath should have a VQ CT scan to expedite the diagnosis.

Blood Tests. Two blood tests are valuable in the management of thromboembolic disease: the D-dimer and the INR. Current D-dimer assays have predictive value for DVT, and the INR is useful for guiding the management of patients with known DVT who are on warfarin (Coumadin). While no blood test can conclusively rule in or rule out venous thrombosis, a normal D-dimer in a patient with no risk factors for thrombosis makes proximal DVT extremely unlikely. Despite the fact that it is frequently ordered, a complete blood count (CBC) rarely provides useful information in patients with leg signs or symptoms. The leukocyte count cannot distinguish between DVT and cellulitis and is neither sensitive nor specific for either condition.

Coagulation Studies. Coagulation studies rarely are required as part of the initial evaluation of venous thrombosis. Occasionally, these studies may be valuable after Doppler demonstrates an acute clot, and in patients who develop a clot while on warfarin.

Although most physicians order a PTT *before* starting heparin for DVT, interestingly, this practice is not justified by the literature. For patients not on warfarin, assessment of the PTT will almost never affect management.[60] Obviously, a PTT should be obtained six hours after standard heparin in begun.

PT and INR. If a patient with acute DVT is currently on warfarin, an International Normalized Ratio (INR) is essential for management. It is now well documented that the prothrombin time (PT) is both antiquated and inaccurate, primarily because the sensitivity of thromboplastin reagents differs from batch to batch. Fortunately, the INR adjusts for this lack of standardization by comparing each batch with an International Sensitivity Index.[61,62] Measurement of the PT could be eliminated from clinical practice if replaced by the INR. Adequate anticoagulation for DVT is reflected by an INR between two and three.[61] If a patient with a *sub-therapeutic* INR develops a DVT, they will require more aggressive anticoagulation—first with heparin, and then an increased dose of warfarin. However, a patient who is on warfarin, but sustains an acute clot and has a *therapeutic* INR, requires a Greenfield filter.

Up to 10% of patients with DVT have an underlying coagulation disorder such as antiphospholipid syndrome or protein 'S,' protein 'C,' or antithrombin III deficiency.[1-3] However, measurements of these levels usually are not necessary for emergency management. On occasion, the admitting internist may screen young adults with unexplained thrombosis for more common coagulation disorders.[63]

D-dimer. If an emergency physician wishes to use a single blood test in order to exclude the diagnosis of DVT, the D-dimer assay would be that test. Only 2% of patients with a negative D-dimer (measured by the whole blood agglutination assay) will have DVT. In patients with a low pretest probability, the negative predictive value is 99.4%.[64]

D-dimer is a specific degradation product of cross-linked fibrin. Because concurrent production and breakdown of clot characterize thrombosis, patients with thromboembolic disease have elevated levels of D-dimer. There are three major approaches for measuring D-dimer. The two older tests include the sensitive, but time consuming, enzyme-linked immunoabsorbent assay (ELISA) and a rapid, but less sensitive, latex agglutination.[65] These tests suffered from a specificity of as low as 15-38% in DVT and PE.[66-68] Currently, the most useful assay is the whole blood agglutination test (SimpliRED). This five minute, bedside test is both rapid and sensitive.[69] In one study, this technique had a sensitivity of 93% for proximal DVT, 70% for calf DVT, and an overall specificity of 77%.[69] All D-dimer tests, regardless of the process, are more sensitive for proximal than distal clot, and may miss as many as 30% of calf DVTs.[70,71] False-positive D-dimers occur in patients with recent (within 10 days) surgery or trauma, recent myocardial infarction or stroke, acute infection, disseminated intravascular coagulation, pregnancy or recent delivery, active collagen vascular disease, or metastatic cancer.[69]

In a patient with no risk factors for DVT, a negative D-dimer measured by the whole-blood agglutination assay almost rules out the diagnosis (i.e., there will be less than a 1% chance of proximal DVT).[64] While some physicians may opt to forgo imaging studies in patients with a negative D-dimer, others may be reluctant to rely entirely upon a blood test. It seems reasonable that a negative D-dimer may obviate the need for off-hour Doppler studies in low-risk patients. If a patient presents at night with a swollen leg and a negative red cell agglutination test, imaging usually can be safely postponed until the morning.

Imaging Studies

Imaging studies include both invasive (venography, radiolabeled fibrinogen) and noninvasive (ultrasound, plethysmography, MRI) techniques. *(Please see Table 3.)* Current options are discussed in the next sections.

Venography. While venography aspires to be the "gold standard" modality for the diagnosis of DVT, it is a "gold-plated" standard at best.[72] First, radiologists disagree on interpretation in at least 10% of cases, and 5-15% of all studies are technically inadequate.[72,73] Moreover, side effects are significant and 2-5% of patients develop phlebitis from this painful procedure. The rare case of anaphylaxis remains a significant clinical concern. For the most part, ultrasound has supplanted venography for the initial evaluation of the patient with suspected DVT. If the ultrasound is equivocal or unavailable, venography may be useful. Venography is also useful if the patient has a high clinical probability of thrombosis and a negative ultrasound, and it is also valuable in symptomatic patients with a history of prior thrombosis in whom the ultrasound is non-diagnostic. In these patients, it usually can distinguish between acute events and chronic changes seen on ultrasound. A contrast study can delineate occlusion, recanalization, and collateral channels. Since neither ultrasound nor impedance plethysmography (IPG) is accurate for clot in asymptomatic postoperative patients, venography is the only test that is reliable for the diagnosis of DVT in this population.[74] Fortunately, the emergency physician is rarely faced with this dilemma.

Table 4. Scoring System for Risk of DVT

CLINICAL FEATURE	SCORE
Active Cancer (treatment ongoing or within previous 6 months or palliative)	1
Paralysis, paresis, or recent plaster immobilization of the lower extremeties	1
Recently bedridden for more than 3 days or major surgery, within 4 weeks	1
Localized tenderness along the distribution of the deep venous system	1
Entire leg swollen	1
Calf swelling by more than 3 cm when compared to the asymptomatic leg (measured 10 cm below tibial tuberosity)	1
Pitting edema (greater in the asymptomatic leg)	1
Collateral superficial veins (non-varicose)	1
Alternative diagnosis as likely or greater than that of deep-vein thrombosis	-2

Low probability ≤ 0
Moderate probability 1 or 2
High probability ≥ 3

Source: Anand SS, et al. Does this patient have deep vein thrombosis? *JAMA* 1998;279:1094-1099.

Nuclear Medicine Studies. Because the radioactive isotope incorporates into a growing thrombus, this test can distinguish new clot from an old clot.[75] Despite this fact, I-125 labeled fibrinogen is not a valuable ED study. It is insensitive for detection of proximal thrombi, it takes 24 hours to perform, and is plagued by a high, false-positive rate.[76] For these reasons, nuclear medicine studies should be reserved for the admitting physician.

Plethysmography. Plethysmography measures change in lower extremity volume in response to certain stimuli. By using a tourniquet and respiratory variation, the operator can detect changes in leg volume as a function of venous outflow.[77] Changes in such objective variables as calf circumference, cutaneous blood flow, or electrical resistance occur when there is obstruction of venous return. IPG is based upon changes in electrical resistance, and is the most widely used and accurate form of plethysmography.

IPG is very operator dependent, and early literature displayed a 95% correlation with venography for proximal DVT.[76] However, recent literature shows that the sensitivity of IPG is generally around 65-70%.[78-80] Because any impairment of venous outflow affects plethysmography results, many false positives occur. Postphlebitic syndrome, abdominal tumors, pregnancy, and congestive heart failure (CHF) can produce inaccurate results.[78-80]

Ultrasonography. From an emergency medicine perspective, in most clinical encounters, color-flow Duplex scanning is the imaging test of choice for patients with suspected DVT.[81,82] This test is inexpensive, noninvasive, and widely available. Its name

Table 5. Differential Diagnosis of a Swollen Leg

- DVT
- Post-phlebitic syndrome
- Cellulitis—most important
- Muscle injury/hematoma
- Popliteal cyst (Baker's cyst)
- Superficial phlebitis
- Capillary leak syndrome
- Fracture
- Compartment syndrome
- Nerve root irritation
- Abscess
- Hypoproteinemia
- Congestive heart failure
- Lymphedema
- Malignancy
- Factitious
- AV fistula
- Acute arthritis
- Myositis

derives from the dual use of Doppler flow with two-dimensional scanning. The Doppler component evaluates blood flow for proximal obstruction, and the addition of color flow technology provides the most accurate images. Changes in flow that occur with respiration and from calf compression (phasicity and augmentation) differentiate obstructing from non-obstructing thrombi.[83] The B-mode, or 2-D echo, provides a two-dimensional image of the vein and surrounding structures. The sonographer detects thrombus in the vein by directly visualizing and then compressing the vein with a transducer. Veins filled with clot do not collapse like a normal vein. In addition, the sonographer can distinguish fresh clot from an old clot based upon echogenicity, homogeneity, and collateral flow.[84] The color-flow duplex scan can detect 95-99% of acute thrombi above the knee.[85,86] Ultrasound can also distinguish other causes of leg swelling, such as tumor, popliteal cyst, abscess, aneurysm, or hematoma.[87] Pain, edema, dyspnea, and a history of DVT are most predictive of positive scans.[88]

It should be stressed that ultrasound does have its clinical limitations. High sensitivity testing requires sophisticated, (i.e., expensive) diagnostic equipment. Moreover, scans are very reader dependent and some institutions do not achieve optimal accuracy because of a lack of radiographic expertise. Duplex scanning is less sensitive for clots below the knee and detects only 80% of distal thrombi.[83,89] Supra-inguinal veins are also hard to visualize. In addition, Duplex scans are less likely to detect non-occluding thrombi. During the second half of pregnancy, ultrasound becomes less specific, because the gravid uterus compresses the inferior vena cava, thereby changing Doppler flow in the lower extremities.[90] However, an experienced sonographer may still detect a clot in a pregnant patient by demonstrating a non-compressible vein.

Outcome-Effective Evaluation: A Multi-Modal Approach

Studies suggest that a limited examination of only the common femoral and popliteal veins may be as sensitive as the traditional venous survey and may be performed in half the time.[91] Another approach to saving cost is to limit use of the ultrasound to the symptomatic extremity. This also cuts scanning time by half while maintaining acceptable accuracy.[92]

When the emergency physician suspects DVT and the ultrasound is positive, subsequent treatment is automatic. But what about the patient with a suspected thrombosis who has a negative Doppler? Two to three percent of such patients later prove to have DVT, and some suffer fatal pulmonary embolism.[93,94] For this reason, many authorities recommend at least one additional ultrasound or IPG within the first week of presentation, in all patients with a negative study.[95] In this regard, two normal ultrasounds one week apart essentially exclude the diagnosis of DVT.[96] Serial testing, however, is costly; many patients are lost to follow-up, and the vast majority of patients who do undergo serial studies are disease free. As a result, if a definitive diagnosis can be made in the ED without serial studies, it would save time, money, and perhaps lives. One such strategy is the use of pretest probabilities, a strategy that relies on the patient's risk factors

Risk Factor Analysis and Pretest Probability. Patients with suspected DVT may be divided into those with low, moderate, and high pretest probability. The scoring is based on risk factors, symptoms, and physical signs. *(Please see Table 4.)* In a prospective study, the prevalence of DVT was 85% in the high pretest probability category, 33% in the moderate, and 5% in the low category.[97] If the pretest probability was high and the ultrasound was positive, or if the pretest probability was low and the ultrasound was negative, the results were deemed *concordant*. Patients with ultrasounds concordant with the pretest probability were treated according to the ultrasound results. A patient with a high pretest probability and a positive ultrasound required anticoagulation, while a patient with a low pretest probability and a negative ultrasound required no further treatment. The authors demonstrated that "only 0.6% (3) of 481 (95%; CI, 0.1-1.8) patients with low or moderate pretest probability with a negative initial or serial ultrasound, respectively, developed DVT or PE in the three months of follow-up."[97]

Patients with *discordant* results (i.e., high pretest probability and negative Doppler, or low pretest probability and positive Doppler) were subject to immediate venography. This strategy resulted in the highest diagnostic accuracy rate. Since only 6% of patients with high pretest probability and negative ultrasounds had DVT on venography, the authors suggested such patients might be safely managed with a repeat ultrasound in one week instead of immediate venography. However, they did not test this hypothesis. This study also demonstrated that patients with a low pretest probability and a negative ultrasound did not require serial studies.

Combination D-dimer and Impedance Plethysmography. While using pretest probabilities is one way to eliminate the need for serial studies, the addition of the D-dimer test may be another. One study examined the utility of combining the D-dimer test with IPG. The combination of a negative D-dimer and a negative IPG had a negative predictive value of 98.5% for DVT over the subsequent three months.[64] There is no reason why such results should not apply to patients imaged with Doppler as well. Using this logic, the combination of a negative D-dimer and negative ultrasound may obviate serial studies.

Magnetic Resonance Imaging. Magnetic Resonance Imaging (MRI) represents a significant advance in the diagnosis of DVT. It detects leg, pelvis, and pulmonary thrombi and is 97% sensitive and 95% specific for DVT.[98,99] It distinguishes a mature from an immature clot.[100] Because it is expensive and requires significant patient cooperation, it should not replace ultrasound as the primary screening tool. It is most useful in the second and third trimester of pregnancy when ultrasound becomes less accurate. MRI is safe in all stages of pregnancy.[101]

Differential Diagnosis

The differential diagnosis of the swollen or painful leg is broad. *(Please see Table 5.)* Many conditions can cause bilateral leg edema, secondary to either hypoproteinemia or an increase in venous or lymphatic pressure. Pregnancy, CHF, nephrotic syndrome, liver disease, or capillary leak syndrome can all produce bilateral leg swelling.[47] If prior DVT has unilaterally damaged venous valves, asymmetric swelling will occur with all of these conditions. Abdominal masses such as gravid uterus, hematoma, malignancy, or abscess, can compress a single iliac vein leading to ipsilateral venous stasis.[56]

Patients with the postphlebitic syndrome develop recurrent unilateral pain and swelling that is clinically indistinguishable from acute DVT. Such patients require objective testing for diagnosis. Recognize that ultrasound, IPG, and even venography will be abnormal and difficult to interpret in the presence of chronic changes.

Cellulitis is an important consideration and may be clinically difficult to distinguish from DVT.[102] While fever, chills, and leukocytosis are more common with cellulitis, these findings can occur with DVT. Duplex scanning is the best method to differentiate cellulitis from DVT. One study suggests that a needle aspirate of the edema fluid can identify cellulitis. A protein level greater than 10 g/L of edema fluid denotes infection.[103]

Lymphedema may also produce unilateral leg swelling. In the United States, malignancy is the most likely cause of lymphedema, while in third world countries filariasis is a common cause. Unlike DVT, septic arthritis and other causes of monoarticular arthritis are characterized by joint pain on range of motion. A Baker's cyst is a popliteal cyst filled with synovial fluid that may present as a mass behind the knee.[104] It usually occurs in association with chronic arthritis. Rupture of a popliteal this cyst may produce pseudothrombophlebitis clinically indistinguishable from acute DVT.[105] A ruptured Baker's cyst is best diagnosed by MRI, knee arthrogram, or duplex sonography.[106-108] A tear of the Achilles tendon or a calf muscle (usually soleus) causes acute pain and may be associated with a hematoma or ecchymosis.[109] Arterio-venous (AV) fistula also produces unilateral pain and swelling. A positive straight leg raise sign signals nerve root irritation, while elevations of creatinine kinase characterize significant myositis.

References

1. Milne AA, Stonebridge PA, Bradbury AW, et al. Venous function and clinical outcome following deep vein thrombosis. *Br J Surg* 1994;81:847-849.
2. Zamorski MA, Opdycke RA. Advances in the prevention, diagnosis, and treatment of deep venous thrombosis. *Am Fam Physician* 1993;47:457-469.
3. Carter CJ. The natural history and epidemiology of venous thrombosis. *Prog Cardiovasc Dis* 1994;36:423-438.
4. Hirsh J, Hoak J. Management of deep vein thrombosis and pulmonary embolism. A statement for healthcare professionals. Council on Thrombosis (in constitution with the Council on Cardiovascular Radiology), American Heart Association. *Circulation* 1996;93:2212-2245.
5. Lensing AWA, Hirsh J, Buller HR. Diagnosis of venous thrombosis. In: Colman RW, Hirsh J, Marder VJ, et al, eds. *Hemostasis and thrombosis: Basic principles and clinical practice*. 3rd ed. Philadelphia, PA: J.B. Lippincott; 1994:1297-1321.
6. Ferris EJ. Deep venous thrombosis and pulmonary embolism: Correlative evaluation and therapeutic implications. *Am J Roentgenol* 1992;159:1149-1155.
7. Kniffin WD, Jr., Baron JA, Barrett J, et al. The epidemiology of diagnosed pulmonary embolism and deep venous thrombosis in the elderly. *Arch Intern Med* 1994;154:861-866.
8. Radecki RT, Gaebler-Spira D. Deep vein thrombosis in the disabled pediatric population. *Arch Phys Med Rehabil* 1994;75:248-250.
9. Cogo A, Bernardi E, Prandoni P, et al. Acquired risk factors for deep-vein thrombosis in symptomatic outpatients. *Arch Intern Med* 1994;151:164-168.
10. Coon WW, Willis PWI, Keller JB. Venous thromboembolism and other venous disease in the Tecumseh: Community health study. *Circulation* 1973;48:839.
11. Dunmire SM. Pulmonary embolism. *Emerg Med Clin N Am* 1989;7:339-354.
12. Sahiar F, Mohler SR. Economy class syndrome. *Aviat Space Environ Med* 1994;65:957-960.
13. Weingarden SI. Deep venous thrombosis in spinal cord injury. Overview of the problem. *Chest* 1992;102:63, 6S-9S.
14. Sharrok NE, Go G, Sculco TP, et al. Changes in circulatory indices of thrombosis and fibrinolysis during total knee arthroplasty performed under tourniquet. *J Arthroplasty* 1995;10:523-528.
15. Prins MH, Lensing AW, Hirsh J. Idiopathic deep venous thrombosis. Is a search for malignant disease justified? *Arch Intern Med* 1994;154:1310-1312.
16. Dhami MS, Bona RD. Thrombosis in patients with cancer. *Postgrad Med* 1993;92:131-133, 137-140.
17. Kakkar AK, DeRuvo N, Chinswangwatanakul V, et al. Extrinsic pathway activation in cancer with high factor VIIa and tissue factor. *Lancet* 1995;346:1004-1005.
18. Nordstrom M, Lindblad B, Anderson H, et al. Deep venous thrombosis and occult malignancy: An epidemiological study. *BMJ* 1994;308:891-894.
19. Prandoni P, Lensing AWA, Buller HR, et al. Deep-vein thrombosis and the incidence of subsequent symptomatic cancer. *N Engl J Med* 1992;327:1128-1133.
20. Callander N, Rapaport SI. Trousseau's syndrome. *West J Med* 1993;158:364-371.
21. Alving BM, Comp PC. Recent advances in understanding clotting and evaluating patients with recurrent thrombosis. *Am J Obstet-Gyncol* 1992;167:1184-1191.

22. Vandenbroucke JP, Koster T, Briet E, et al. Increased risk of venous thrombosis in oral contraceptive users who are carriers of factor V Leiden mutation. *Lancet* 1994;344: 1453-1457.
23. DeMattia D, Penza R, Giordano P, et al. Thromboembolic risk in children with nephrotic syndrome. *Haemostasis* 1991; 21:300-304.
24. Ginsberg KS, Liang MH, Newcomer L, et al. Anticardiolipin antibodies and the risk for ischemic stroke and venous thrombosis [see comments]. *Ann Intern Med* 1992;117: 997-1002.
25. Bick RL, Baker WF, Jr. The antiphospholipid and thrombosis syndromes. *Med Clin North Am* 1994;78:667-684.
26. Provenzale JM, Ortel TL. Anatomic distribution of venous thrombosis in patients with antiphospholipid antibody: Imaging findings. *Am J Roentgenology* 1995;165:365-368.
27. Geerts WH, Code KI, Jay RM, et al. A prospective study of venous thromboembolism after major trauma [see comments]. *N Engl J Med* 1994;331:1601-1606.
28. Schmidt U, Enderson BL, Chen Jp, et al. D-dimer levels correlate with pathologic thrombosis in trauma patients. *J Trauma* 1992;33:312-319.
29. Andrew M, David M, Adams M, et al. Venous thromboembolic complications (VTE) in children: First analyses of the Canadian Registry of VTE. *Blood* 1994;83: 1251-1257.
30. Meredith JW, Young JS, O'Neil EA, et al. Femoral catheters and deep venous thrombosis: A prospective evaluation with venous duplex sonography. *J Trauma* 1993;35:187-190.
31. Menzoian JO, Doyle JE. Venous insufficiency of the leg. *Hosp Pract* 1989;24:109.
32. Bundens WP, Bergan JJ, Halasz NA, et al. The superficial femoral vein. A potentially lethal misnomer. *JAMA* 1995; 274:1296-1298.
33. Lisse JR, Davis CP, Thormond-Anderle M. Cocaine abuse in deep venous thrombosis. *Ann Intern Med* 1989;110:571.
34. Samlaska CP, James WD, Simel DL. Superficial migratory thrombophlebitis and factor XII deficiency. *J Am Acad Dermatol* 1990;22:939.
35. Villavicencio JL, Gonzalez-Cerna JL. Acute vascular problems of children. *Curr Probl Surg* 1985;22:1.
36. Jorgensen JO, Hanel KC, Morgan AM, et al. The incidence of deep venous thrombosis in patients with superficial thrombophlebitis of the lower limbs. *J Vasc Surg* 1993;18: 70-73.
37. Lutter KS, Kerr TM, Roedersheimer LR, et al. Superficial thrombophlebitis diagnosed by duplex scanning. *Surgery* 1991; 110:42-46.
38. Philbrick JT, Becker DM. Calf deep venous thrombosis. A wolf in sheep's clothing? *Arch Intern Med* 1988;148: 2131-2138.
39. Saeger W, Genzkow M. Venous thromboses and pulmonary embolisms in post-mortem series: Probable causes by correlations of clinical data and basic diseases. *Pathol Res Pract* 1994;190:394-399.
40. Giachino A. Relationship between deep-vein thrombosis in the calf and fatal pulmonary embolism. *Can J Surg* 1988;31: 129-130.
41. Rahm M, Probe R. Extensive deep venous thrombosis resulting in compartment syndrome of the thigh and leg. A case report. *J Bone Joint Surg—American volume*. 1994;76: 1854-1857.
42. van Ramshorst B, van Bemmelen PS, Hoeneveld H, et al. Thrombus regression in deep venous thrombosis. Quantification of spontaneous thrombolysis with duplex scanning. *Circulation* 1992;86:414-419.
43. Lipchik EO, DeWeese JA, Rogoff SM. Serial long-term phlebography after documented lower leg thrombosis. *Radiology* 1976;120:563.
44. Hopkins NFG, Wolfe JHN. Deep venous insufficiency and occlusion. *Med J* 1992;304:107.
45. Cronan JJ, Leen V. Recurrent deep venous thrombosis: Limitations of ultrasound. *Radiology* 1989;170:739.
46. Colucciello SA, Plotka M. The Patient with Chronic Venous Insufficiency. In: Herr R, Cydulka R, eds. *Emergency Care of the Compromised Patient*. Philadelphia, PA: JB Lippincott; 1994:370-382.
47. Barnes RW, Wu KK, Hoak JC. Fallibility of the clinical diagnosis of venous thrombosis. *JAMA* 1975;234:605.
48. Moser KM, Fedullo PF, LitteJohn JK, et al. Frequent asymptomatic pulmonary embolism in patients with deep venous thrombosis [published erratum appears in *JAMA* 1994;271:1908] [see comments]. *JAMA* 1994;271:223-225.
49. DeGowin RL. *DeGowin and DeGowin's Diagnostic Examination* 6th Ed. New York: McGraw Hill, Health Professionals Division; 1994.
50. Sheiman RG, Weintraub JL, McArdle CR. Bilateral lower extremity US in the patient with bilateral symptoms of deep venous thrombosis: Assessment of need. *Radiology* 1995; 196:379-811.
51. O'Donnell T, Abbott W, Athanasoulis C, et al. Diagnosis of deep venous thrombosis in the outpatient by venography. *Surg Gynecol Obstet* 1980;150:69-74.
52. Stein PD, Henry JW, Gopalakrishnann D, et al. Asymmetry of the calves in the assessment of patients with suspected acute pulmonary embolism. *Chest* 1995;107:936-939.
53. Anand SS, Wells PS, Hunt D, et al. Does this patient have deep vein thrombosis? *JAMA* 1998;279:1094-1099.
54. Anonymous. *Cecil Textbook of Medicine.* Philadelphia, PA: W.B. Saunders; 1988.
55. Sapira JD. *The Art and Science of Bedside Diagnosis.* Baltimore, MD: Urban & Schwarzenberg; 1990.
56. Hirsh J, Hull RD, Raskob GE. Clinical features and diagnosis of venous thrombosis. *J Am Coll Cardiol* 1986;8: 114B.
57. Prescott SM, Tikoff G. Deep venous thrombosis of the upper extremity: A reappraisal. *Circulation* 1979;59:350-355.
58. Huisman MV, Buller HR, ten Cate JW. Utility of impedance

plethysmography in the diagnosis of recurrent deep-vein thrombosis. *Arch Intern Med* 1988;148:681.

59. Cronan JJ. Venous thromboembolic disease: The role of US. [Review]. *Radiology* 1993;186:619-630.
60. McKinley L, Wrenn. Are baseline prothrombin time/partial thromboplastin time values necessary before instituting anticoagulation? *Ann Emerg Med* 1993;22:697-702.
61. Hirsh J, Poller L. The International Normalized Ratio. A guide to understanding and correcting its problems. *Arch Intern Med* 1994;154:282-288.
62. Greenspan RH. Pulmonary angiography and the diagnosis of pulmonary embolism. [Review]. *Prog Cardiovasc Dis* 1994; 37:93-105.
63. Levi PJ, Gonzalez FM, Rush DS, et al. Hypercoagulable states as an evolving risk for spontaneous venous and arterial thrombosis. *J Am Coll Surg* 1994;178:266-270.
64. Ginsburg JS, Kearon C, Douketis J, et al. The use of D-dimer testing and impedance plethysmographic examination in patients with clinical indications of deep vein thrombosis [see comments]. *Arch Intern Med* 1997;157:1077-1081.
65. de Moerloose P, Minazio P, Reber G, et al. D-dimer determination to exclude pulmonary embolism: A two-step approach using latex assay as a screening tool. *Thromb Haemost* 1994;72:89-91.
66. van Beek EJ, van den Ende B, Berkmans RJ, et al. A comparative analysis of D-dimer assays in patients with clinically suspected pulmonary embolism. *Thromb Haemost* 1993;70:408-413.
67. Bounameaux H, Cirafici P, de Moerloose P, et al. Measurement of D-dimer in plasma as diagnostic aid in suspected pulmonary embolism. *Lancet* 1991;337:196-200.
68. Ginsberg JS, Brill-Edwards PA, Demers C, et al. D-dimer in patients with clinically suspected pulmonary embolism. *Chest* 1993;104:1679-1684.
69. Wells PS, Brill-Edwards P, Stevens P, et al. A novel and rapid whole-blood assay for D-dimer in patients wit clinically suspected deep vein thrombosis. *Circulation* 1995; 91:2184-2187.
70. Wells PS, Brill-Edwards P, Stevens P, et al. A novel and rapid whole-blood assay for D-dimer in patients with clinically suspected deep vein thrombosis. *Circulation* 1995; 91:2184-2187.
71. Bounameaux H, Cirafici P, de Moerloose P, et al. Measurement of D-dimer in plasma as a diagnostic aid in suspected pulmonary embolism. *Lancet* 1991;337:196-200.
72. Redman HC. Deep venous thrombosis: Is contrast venography still the diagnostic "gold standard?" *Radiology* 1988;168:277.
73. Hirsh J. Clinical utility of impedance plethysmography in the diagnosis of recurrent deep-vein thrombosis. *Arch Intern Med* 1988;148:519.
74. Kearon C, Julian JA, Newman TE, et al. Noninvasive diagnosis of deep venous thrombosis. McMaster Diagnostic Imaging Practice Guidelines Initiative. *Ann Intern Med* 1998;128:663-677.
75. Wu KK, Hoak JC, Barnes RW. A prospective comparison of four methods for the diagnosis of deep vein thrombosis. *Thromb Diath Haemorrh* 1974;32:260.
76. White GH. Chronic venous insufficiency. In: Wilson SE, ed. *Vascular surgery principles and practice.* New York: McGraw-Hill; 1987:736.
77. Warwick DJ, Thornton MJ, Freeman S, et al. Computerized strain-gauge plethysmography in the diagnosis of symptomatic and asymptomatic venous thrombosis. *Br J Radiol* 1994;67:938-940.
78. Ginsberg JS, Wells PS, Hirsh J, et al. Reevaluation of the sensitivity of impedance plethysmography for the detection of proximal deep vein thrombosis [see comments]. *Arch Intern Med* 1994;154:1930-1933.
79. Anderson DR, Lensing AW, Wells PS, et al. Limitations of impedance plethysmography in the diagnosis of clinically suspected deep-vein thrombosis. *Ann Intern Med* 1993;118: 25-30.
80. Heijboer H, Buller HR, Lensing AWA, et al. A comparison of real-time compression ultrasonography with impedance plethysmography for the diagnosis of deep-vein thrombosis in symptomatic outpatients. *N Engl J Med* 1993;329: 1365-1369.
81. Vogel P, Laing FC, Jeffrey RB, et al. Deep venous thrombosis of the lower extremity: US evaluation. *Radiology* 1987;163:747.
82. Kristo DA, Perry ME, Kollef MH. Comparison of venography, duplex imaging, and bilateral impedance plethysmography for diagnosis of lower extremity deep vein thrombosis. *South Med J* 1994;87:55-60.
83. Polak JF. Doppler ultrasound of the deep leg veins: A revolution in the diagnosis of deep vein thrombosis in monitoring of thrombolysis. *Chest* 1991;99:165S.
84. Abu Rahma RF, Kennard W, Robinson PA, et al. The judicial use of venous duplex imaging and strain gauge plethysmography (single or combined) in the diagnosis of acute and chronic deep venous thrombosis. *Surg Gynecol Obstet* 1992;174:52.
85. Rose SC, Zwiebel WJ, Nelson BD, et al. Symptomatic lower extremity deep venous thrombosis: Accuracy, limitations, and role of colored duplex flow imaging in diagnosis. *Radiology* 1990;175:639.
86. Lewis BD, James EM, Welch TJ, et al. Diagnosis of acute deep venous thrombosis of the lower extremities: Prospective evaluation of color Doppler flow imaging versus venography. *Radiology* 1994;192:651-655.
87. Buchbinder D, McCullough GM, Melick CF. Patients evaluated for venous disease may have other pathologic conditions contributing to symptomatology. *Am J Surg* 1993;166:211-215.
88. Hill SL, Holtzman GI, Martin D, et al. Selective use of the duplex scan in the diagnosis of deep venous thrombosis. *Surg* 1995;170:201-205.

89. Messina LM, Sarpa MS, Smith MA, et al. Clinical significance of routine imaging of iliac and calf veins by color flow duplex scanning in patients suspected of having acute lower extremity deep venous thrombosis. *Surgery* 1993;114:921-927.
90. Douketis JD, Ginsberg JS. Diagnostic problems with venous thromboembolic disease in pregnancy. [Review]. *Haemostasis* 1995;25:58-71.
91. Pezzullo JA, Perkins AB, Cronan JJ. Symptomatic deep vein thrombosis: Diagnosis with limited compression US. *Radiology* 1996;198:67-70.
92. Sheiman RG, Weintraub JL, McArdle CR. Bilateral lower extremity US in the patient with bilateral symptoms of deep venous thrombosis: Assessment of need. *Radiology* 1995; 196:379-381.
93. Cogo A, Lensing AW, Koopman MM, et al. Compression ultrasonography for diagnostic management of patients with clinically suspected deep vein thrombosis: Prospective cohort study. *BMJ* 1998;316:17-20.
94. Ginsberg JS. Management of venous thromboembolism. *N Engl J Med* 1996;335:1816-1828.
95. Koopman MM, van Beek EJ, ten Cate JW. Diagnosis of deep vein thrombosis. *Prog Cardiovasc Dis* 1994;37:1-12.
96. Birdwell BG, Raskob GE, Whitsett TL, et al. The clinical validity of normal compression ultrasonography in outpatients suspected of having deep vein thrombosis. *Ann Intern Med* 1998;128:1-7.
97. Wells PS, Hirsh J, Anderson DR, et al. Accuracy of clinical assessment of deep vein thrombosis. *Lancet* 1995;345: 1326-1330.
98. Spritzer CE, Norconk JJ, Jr., Sostman HD, et al Detection of deep venous thrombosis by magnetic resonance imaging. *Chest* 1993;104:54-60.
99. Evans AJ, Sostman HD, Knelson MH, et al. 1992 ARRS Executive Council Award. Detection of deep venous thrombosis: Prospective comparison of MR imaging with contrast venography. *Am J Roentgenol* 1993;161:131-139.
100. Erdman WA, Jayson HT, Redman HC, et al. Deep venous thrombosis of extremities: Role of MR imaging in the diagnosis. *Radiology* 1990;174:425.
101. Spritzer CE, Evans AC, Kay HH. Magnetic resonance imaging of deep venous thrombosis in pregnant women with lower extremity edema. *Obstet-Gynecol* 1995;85:603-607.
102. Nordestgaard AG, Williams RA. Varicose veins. In: Wilson SE, ed. *Vascular surgery: Principles and practice*. New York; McGraw-Hill: 1987:711.
103. Berlyne GM, Kwan T, Li J, et al. Oedema protein concentrations for differentiation of cellulitis and deep vein thrombosis. *Lancet* 1989;2:728-729.
104. Rosian R, Mandell BF. A 47-year-old woman with a swollen leg. *Cleve Clin J Med* 1995;62:281-284.
105. Gomez J, Kattamis A, Scheneck Jr. Pseudothrombophlebitis in an adolescent without rheumatic disease. A case report. *Clin Ortho Rel Res* 1994;3308:250-253.
106. Lazarus ML, Ray CE Jr, Maniquis CG. MRI findings of concurrent acute DVT and dissecting popliteal cyst. *Magn Reson Imaging* 1994;12:155-158.
107. Soriano ER, Catoggio LJ. Baker's cysts, pseudothrombophlebitis, pseudo-pseudothrombophlebitis: Where do we stand? *Clin Exp Rheumatol* 1990;8:107-112.
108. Brady HR, Quigley C, Stafford FJ, et al. Popliteal cyst rupture and the pseudothrombophlebitis syndrome. *Ann Emerg Med* 1987;16:1151-1154.
109. Thompson JS, Kaufman RL, Beardmore TD. Pseudothrombophlebitis in neuropathic arthropathy. *J Rheumatol* 1989;16:1606.

Deep Venous Thrombosis: Patient Management and Anticoagulation

Stephen A. Colucciello, MD, FACEP

The treatment landscape for managing patients with deep venous thrombosis (DVT) is evolving at a rapid pace. The most important studies affecting current approaches to therapy are those comparing and evaluating the efficacy of unfractionated heparin (UH) vs. low molecular weight heparin (LMWH) for management of patients with DVT, both in and out of the hospital.

These trials, which are impressive in their support of the saftey, suitability, and efficacy of LMWHs, have presented new challenges for the emergency medicine community. In particular, new developments in the management of DVT require emergency physicians to risk stratify patients into those who require hospitalization and those who are amenable to outpatient treatment. In this regard, recent approval of the LMWH, enoxaparin, for out-of-hospital treatment of DVT has positive pharmacoeconomic consequences that must be considered in the equation for DVT management.

Risk stratification of these patients will include a detailed history and evaluation that considers the presence of underlying co-morbid conditions, hemodynamic stability of the patient, exclusion of pulmonary embolism, location of the thrombosis, ability of patient to self-administer LWMH such as enoxaparin on a home basis, and adequate follow-up and support.

This chapter examines the pharmacotherapeutic options available for DVT management. The roles of heparin, LMWHs, and warfarin are examined in detail, and indications for procedural interventions also are discussed. Finally, a management algorithm outlining an outcome-effective approach to managing DVT with LMWH is presented.

Management Principles

The patient with deep venous thrombosis (DVT) rarely requires immediate life-saving interventions. Nevertheless, management protocols must be systematic and precise. *(Please see Table 1.)* Two life-threatening conditions are pulmonary embolism (PE) and phlegmasia dolens. If either diagnosis is clinically obvious, heparin should be started prior to imaging studies. Hypotensive patients with these conditions require rapid crystalloid infusion and thrombolytics.

Patients with suspected DVT require objective testing, preferably with duplex scanning. If venous thrombosis is confirmed, contraindications to anticoagulation should be identified. Patients with absolute contraindications to heparin require vena cava interruption.[1] The filter is 95% effective in preventing PE and has a 10% complication rate on insertion. Since these outcomes are similar to those seen with anticoagulation, some authorities recommend that the filter be the primary intervention for recurrent DVT.[2] In particular, patients with malignancies benefit from this procedure.[3] It should be stressed that filter insertion, itself, is associated with a 22% incidence of DVT at the puncture site.[4] Anticoagulation is the mainstay of treatment. Specific therapeutic agents are discussed below.

Table 1. Management

SUPERFICIAL VENOUS THROMBOSIS
- Use duplex scan to screen for involvement of deep system
- Elevation, non-steroidal anti-inflammatory drugs

DEEP VENOUS THROMBOSIS
- Begin warfarin on the first hospital day or in the ED
- Low-molecular-weight heparin—more effective and safer than standard heparin
- Enoxaparin, approved in the United States for inpatient and outpatient treatment of DVT
- Heparin 80 U/kg load, 18 U/kg/hr drip
- ? Thrombolysis for severe disease in young adults
- Vena cava filter if thrombosis in presence of adequate anticoagulation

PHLEGMASIA DOLENS
- Fluid resuscitation
- Heparinization before imaging studies
- Thrombolysis for patients who do not respond rapidly to heparin
- Thrombectomy for patients unresponsive to thrombolysis

UPPER EXTREMITY THROMBOSIS
- Diagnose with duplex scan
- Catheter directed thrombolysis

CALF THROMBI
- Anticoagulate or perform serial studies to detect propagation

Table 2. Heparin Weight-based Nomogram

Initial dose = 80 U/kg bolus, 18 U/kg/h

ON REPEAT PTT IN 6 HOURS:

PTT less than 40 s—rebolus with 80 U/kg, increase drip by 4 U/kg/h
PTT 40-60 s—rebolus with 40 U/kg, increase drip by U/kg/h
PTT 60-80 s—no change
PTT 80-100 s—decrease drip by 2 U/kg/h
PTT greater than 100—hold drip for 1 hour, then decrease drip by 3 U/kg/h

Source: Pearson SD. A critical pathway to treat proximal lower-extremity deep vein thrombosis. *Am J Med* 1996;100:283-289.

Heparin

Heparin activates antithrombin III to prevent conversion of fibrinogen to fibrin; it accelerates inhibition of factors XII-a, XI-a, IX-a, and X-a.[5] From a pathophysiological perspective, heparin blocks extension of thrombus and reduces the risk of emboli. The drug has a narrow therapeutic window and, in one study, was cited as the most common cause of drug-related deaths in the hospital.[6] Significant bleeding occurs in about 7-30% of patients, and complications occur at the rate of 1-2% per day.[6] The elderly patient and those taking aspirin are at greatest risk for hemorrhagic complications. Fortunately, for the patient and the emergency physician, complications rarely occur with the loading dose or during the first few hours. Thrombocytopenia develops in approximately 3% (reported range, 0.8-26.0%), usually, after 3-5 days.[7] Heparin-induced thrombocytopenia usually is defined as a decrease in the platelet count below 150,000 per cubic millimeter that begins five or more days after the start of heparin therapy, in conjunction with a positive test for heparin-dependent IgG antibodies.[8]

Dosing. Dosing is important. Some studies suggest that, on occasion, clinicians may not give enough heparin, and, consequently, many patients are sub-therapeutic at 24 hours. This can be a serious concern, as delays in anticoagulation may lead to progressive or recurrent thromboembolism.[9] In one study, more than 80% of patients who received heparin according to a weight-based nomogram had therapeutic heparin levels within 12 hours, compared with only 45% of standard (fixed) dose patients.[10] A weight-based nomogram is most likely to achieve a rapid therapeutic response and may reduce the time required to achieve a therapeutic partial thromboplastin time (PTT) by half, as compared to fixed dosing.[11] *(Please see Table 2.)* Measurement of the PTT is not necessary before beginning heparin.[12]

The heparin drip must be continued for 4-5 days, possibly longer for patients with significant iliofemoral thrombosis. When IV heparin is used, the patient should be admitted to the hospital and the consultant should check the activated PTT in six hours. An adequate response is 1.5-2.5 times control.[13,14] Absolute contraindications to heparin include active internal bleeding, malignant hypertension, CNS neoplasm, recent and significant trauma or surgery, and/or a history of heparin-induced thrombocytopenia. Relative contraindications include recent GI bleed or hemorrhagic stroke. Because heparin acts on antithrombin III, patients with antithrombin III deficiency are resistant to the drug. In this case, pretreat with antithrombin III concentrate or fresh frozen plasma to replenish this factor, and then begin standard heparin infusion.[15]

Warfarin (Coumadin)

After starting heparin or another anticoagulation agent (i.e., Low Molecular Weight Heparin [LMWH]) approved for DVT treatment, the emergency physician may order warfarin (Coumadin) 10 mg by mouth. By initiating warfarin on the first hospital day, the patient may be discharged in 4-5 days, by which time the INR will usually be in the 2.0-3.0 range.[16] After discharge, most patients will require three months of anticoagulant therapy.[17] Historically, there has been some controversy regarding the timing of warfarin therapy. The argument against starting warfarin in the emergency department (ED) is largely theoretical. If a patient has a protein C or S deficiency, if warfarin is given without heparin, it may have a procoagulant effect (accelerating pathological thrombosis). However, when heparin is started before warfarin, the patient will be therapeutically anticoagulated before the onset of any procoagulant effect from warfarin. Several authors have documented the safety of early warfarin administration.[18-20] Most tellingly, the American College of Chest Physicians states that "the currently accepted approach is to begin heparin and oral anticoagulant therapy together at the time of diagnosis . . ."[21]

Hospital Therapy. Because of the cost associated with in-hospital treatment of DVT, critical pathways now emphasize outpatient management with enoxaparin when appropriate. There is considerable variation in the management of DVT, even within a single hospital, and clinical pathways may serve to decrease cost and length of stay.[22]

Clinical goals that can affect length of stay include the following:
1.) Heparin bolus in ED using a weight based nomogram;
2.) PTT > 60 within 12 hours of admission;
3.) Oral dose of warfarin within 12 hours of therapeutic PTT (Many experts suggest warfarin be started orally at the same time heparin is given.);
4.) Heparin for > 96 hours before DC;
5.) INR of 2-3 no later than 120 hours after first dose of warfarin; and
6.) Hospital DC within 12 hours of therapeutic INR.[22]

Low Molecular Weight Heparins (LMWHs)

LMWH represents a major advance in the treatment of DVT, especially with the availability of the LMWH, enoxaparin, for treatment of DVT.[23] Some studies that have compared standard intravenous unfractionated heparin (UH) to subcutaneous LMWH show that LMWH has improved antithrombotic effects and has fewer adverse consequences.[24-26] In this regard, a meta-analysis study demonstrated that LMWH reduced thromboembolic complications, clinically important bleeding, and mortality when compared to unfractionated heparin.[27] In addition, because LMWH can be given subcutaneously once or twice a day without need for coagulation tests, home treatment with enoxaparin for DVT has become a clinical reality.

The LMWHs were first synthesized in the 1970s, and comprise a heterogeneous family of refined heparins with a molecular weight that ranges between 4000 and 9000 Daltons.[28] This compares to the 12,000-15,000 Dalton molecular weight of unfractionated heparin. Because LMWH primarily inhibits factor X-a and has little effect on thrombin or platelet aggregation, there are fewer hemorrhagic complications.[29] LMWH usually does not elevate the PTT. For this reason, LMWH is valued for its antithrombotic effect and lack of anticoagulant effect. There is evidence that suggests LMWHs administered subcutaneously in fixed doses adjusted for body weight and without laboratory monitoring may be more effective and safer than adjusted-dose standard heparin. In a major meta-analysis, LMWH reduced symptomatic thromboembolic complications by 53%, clinically important bleeding by 68%, and mortality by 47% when compared to standard heparin.[30] A separate meta-analysis, including more than 2000 patients and 16 controlled trials, found that LMWH significantly reduced thrombus extension (odds ratio, 0.51) and demonstrated a trend toward decreased PE, fewer major bleeds, and lowered morality.[26] Of particular concern to the internist, heparin-induced thrombocytopenia is less common with LMWH than with unfractionated heparin.[31]

The only LMWH currently approved for outpatient and inpatient treatment of DVT in the United States is enoxaparin. The approved dose of enoxaparin for inpatient treatment of DVT, with or without PE is 1 mg/kg q 12 hours SQ or 1.5 mg/kg SQ qd. The dose of enoxaparin for *outpatient* therapy of deep venous thrombosis *without* pulmonary embolism is 1 mg/kg q 12 hours SQ.[32,33]

The safety and use of home treatment of DVT has undergone rigorous investigation. In two recent studies, authors compared adjusted-dose intravenous standard heparin administered in the hospital to fixed-dose subcutaneous LMWH administered twice daily at home.[33,34] *(Pelase see Table 3.)* In both studies, home treatment with LMWH compared favorably with standard in-hospital therapy. Patients treated at home—or with a short hospitalization with early discharge to home—spent 67% less time in the hospital and had greater physical activity and social functioning than their standard heparin cohorts.[34] Some patients had professional home health care assistance with their injectionsp; all had careful follow-up.

Pharmacoeconomic Considerations. With recent approval for DVT treatment, enoxaparin represents a breakthrough in out-of-hospital management of venous thromboembolic disease. It should be stressed that this approach is part of a larger movement to reduce total outcome costs. In a healthcare environment that puts a premium on effective therapy implemented in a cost-optimizing manner, outpatient DVT treatment with enoxaparin requires close examination.

The safety and efficacy of taking low molecular weight heparin at home was previously demonstrated in a clinical trial in which patients with acute proximal deep vein thrombosis were randomized to receive either intravenous standard heparin in the hospital or subcutaneous low molecular weight heparin administered primarily at home. Treatment in the home has the potential to substantially reduce the cost to the health care system.

An economic evaluation was conducted by prospectively collecting data on resource use and health-related quality of life (Medical Outcomes Study Short-Form 36) on the 300 patients who formed the trial stratum presenting with proximal vein thrombosis as outpatients, of whom 151 received standard heparin and 149 received low molecular weight heparin. The primary viewpoint of the analysis was societal, and costs included health care costs, patient travel costs, and productivity costs as a result of time off work. Costs were assessed over a period of three months from randomization. Quality of life was assessed as the change in Short-Form 36 domain scores from baseline to day 7 for each treatment group (all costs are in 1997 Canadian dollars).

There were 11 recurrent thromboembolic events and 1 bleed in the 151 patients who received standard heparin; the corresponding data for the 149 patients receiving low molecular weight heparin were 10 and 4, respectively. The mean cost per patient who received standard heparin was Can $5323 compared with Can $2278 for low molecular weight heparin, a total societal cost savings per patient using low molecular weight heparin of Can $3045 (95% confidence interval, Can $2012-$4050). There was no difference in quality of life between the two groups except for the domain of social functioning, where a greater improvement from baseline to day 7 was observed for the low molecular weight heparin group vs the standard heparin group ($P = 0.005$).

For patients with acute proximal deep vein thrombosis, treatment at home with low molecular weight heparin is less costly than hospital-based treatment with standard heparin. The economic evidence in

Table 3. Considerations in Home Treatment for DVT

MEDICAL EXCLUSIONS
- Concurrent pulmonary embolism (PE)
- Serious co-morbid condition
- Cancer, infection, stroke
- Prior DVT or PE
- Contraindications to anticoagulation
- Familial bleeding disorder
- Known deficiency of Antithrombin III, Protein C, Protein S
- Pregnancy

SOCIAL EXCLUSIONS
- No phone
- Lives far from hospital
- Unable to understand instructions or comply with follow-up
- Family or patient resistance to home therapy

MECHANICS AND PROTOCOLS
- Subcutaneous enoxaparin 1 mg/kg q 12 hours for a minimum of five days and achieving INR of 2-3 (from warfarin therapy)
- Warfarin to be started on first day of therapy
- Need a mechanism to monitor INR during outpatient treatment

CLOSE FOLLOW-UP
- Warn patients to return immediately for shortness of breath, hemorrhage, or clinical decomposition

Adapted from: Levine MN, et al. Ardeparin (low-molecular-weight heparin) vs graduated compression stockings for the prevention of venous thromboembolism. A randomized trial in patients undergoing knee surgery. *Arch Intern Med* 1996;156:851-856; Koopman MM, et al. Treatment of venous thrombosis with intravenous unfractionated heparin administered in the hospital as compared with subcutaneous low-molecular-weight heparin administered at home. The Tasman Study Group. *N Engl J Med* 1996;334:682-687.

favor of outpatient treatment with low molecular weight heparin exhibits dominance; a situation of reduced cost is created with no compromise in clinical outcomes or patients' quality of life.

Outcome Analysis and Implementation Strategies. Among the potential pharmacoeconomic advantages of out-of-hospital treatment with enoxaparin would be fewer admissions, increased patient comfort, and decreased overall costs. A disadvantage is that patients would have to be carefully evaluated to identify those who would be more safely treated in the hospital. In addition, much of the responsibility for treatment would be shifted from medical personnel to the patient and family, requiring self-administration of anticoagulants, self-monitoring for safety and efficacy, and compliance with clinic appointments for dosage adjustments of oral anticoagulants.

Home-Based Treatment of DVT: Maximixing Outcomes. As discussed, paradigm shifts in medication usage should be conservatively undertaken, as clinical experience helps to refine the management program. Initial treatment of DVT at home should follow a protocol in which all aspects of the treatment are clearly defined for the family and follow-up physician. Ideally, each ED should develop a treatment protocol that is written in advance by a team of medical professionals experienced in the treatment of DVT. The protocol should include criteria for patient selection, enoxaparin and warfarin therapy, patient and caregiver education, and monitoring. Each medical facility will need to develop a protocol that fits its own practice patterns.

One of the most important goals is developing criteria to identify patients who qualify for home-based treatment of DVT. As mentioned, most studies evaluating LMWH for outpatient therapy have excluded patients with a high risk of bleeding (malignant hypertension, peptic ulcer disease, recent surgery, known bleeding disorders, thrombocytopenia, high risk of falling), a high risk of recurrent thrombosis (previous CVT, pregnancy), and suspected PE. In addition, patients who resided a long distance from follow-up medical care, who were unable to care for themselves or did not have a competent caregiver in residence, and who were simply too ill to stay at home were not considered candidates from home-based treatment of DVT. Patients had to be willing to participate in their care, including self-administration of medications and follow-up for warfarin dosage adjustment when necessary. With these strict guidelines for patient selection, about 22-58% of patients screened in various studies were considered eligible for home-based treatment of DVT with a LMWH such as enoxaprin.[32,35,36]

Patient Instructions. Detailed instructions must be provided by the emergency medicine team. The patient or caregiver must be taught to administer the medication, monitor for adverse reactions and efficacy, and perform any other self-care deemed necessary (such as bed rest, leg elevation, and use of compression stockings). The patient or caregiver also must know what steps to take in the event of a complication. Instruction should begin immediately after diagnosis and can be provided by a nurse, a pharmacist, or both. Written instructions should also be provided.

Monitoring home-based treatment of DVT with enoxaparin should include compliance, subcutaneous injection technique, local adverse effects from the injections, signs of bleeding, signs of recurrent thrombosis, and initiation and monitoring of warfarin therapy. Much of this monitoring can be done by the visiting nurse, who should see the patient daily during the initial treatment period of 5-9 days.

It may also be useful for a nurse, a pharmacist, or a physician from the treatment team to periodically telephone the patient or caregiver to ensure that treatment is going as planned and that there are no complications. For patients selected to undergo home-based treatment with enoxaparin, the LMWH should be administered for at least five days, and warfarin can be started on the same day as the LMWH or the day after. Blood should be drawn daily to monitor the prothrombin time for the first few days; the International Normalized Ration (INR) should be between 2.0 and 3.0 for two consecutive days before the LMWH is stopped.

Thrombolytic Agents

Thrombolytics are infrequently used for the treatment of DVT in the United States. In a survey of pulmonologists, only 28% had used thrombolytics for DVT.[37] Streptokinase, given as a 24-72-hour continuous infusion, is the only FDA approved thrombolytic regimen for DVT.[38] When compared to heparin, streptokinase produces more rapid resolution of symptoms and preserves venous valve integrity.[39,40] There is weak evidence that thrombolytics may decrease the incidence of the postphlebitic syndrome.[41] Despite these advantages, physicians are reluctant to use streptokinase for treatment of DVT because there is a three-fold risk of significant bleeding compared to heparin.[37] Bleeding complications include major GI hemorrhage, as well as fatal and nonfatal CNS bleeds.[42-44] There is a higher incidence of bleeding with the use of thrombolysis in DVT than in myocardial infarction. This may be related to the prolonged duration of therapy, as well as the higher incidence of comorbid illness with venous thrombosis.[45] Urokinase, which had a small role in the treatment of DVT, has been removed from the market. Informed patients may not accept the increased risk of bleeding from streptokinase, despite a decreased risk of the postphlebitic syndrome.[46] Patients given the choice would rather receive heparin, accepting the risk of postphlebitic syndrome over that of major bleed. In general, the emergency physician should consider thrombolysis in cases of upper extremity DVT, and, perhaps, massive iliofemoral thrombosis. The best candidates are young, otherwise healthy patients with acute onset of severe symptoms and no contraindications to thrombolysis. Inform the patient of the increased risk of bleeding and potentially life-threatening complications associated with thrombolytics.

Special Management Issues

Phlegmasia Dolens. Phlegmasia alba dolens, the painful "milky white" leg occurs when a thrombosis obstructs venous outflow so completely that subcutaneous edema and blanching occur. As the condition worsens and obstruction becomes complete, capillary perfusion ceases and the limb becomes cyanotic; this condition is known as phlegmasia cerulean dolens (PCD). These patients may develop shock, gangrene, a pulmonary embolism, and go on to die.[47] Such massive iliofemoral occlusion is a medical emergency that requires prompt intervention.[48] Resuscitate the hypotensive patient with fluids, and if unresponsive to crystalloid infusions, begin vasopressor therapy with dopamine or norepinephrine. Anticoagulate such patients immediately, based on clinical presentation. Heparin or LMWH may prove sufficient in non-gangrenous forms, but the patient with PCD may require thrombolysis or surgical thrombectomy.[49-51]

Calf Thrombi. The management of venous thrombosis below the knee is controversial.[52] Because many calf thrombi will propagate (32%) and subsequently embolize, some authorities suggest heparin or LMWH, admission, and initiation of warfarin.[53] Others argue that because most calf thrombi will spontaneously resolve, anticoagulation is not necessary.[54] However, patients who are not anticoagulated must undergo serial noninvasive studies to document clot regression.[55] If serial plethysmography or ultrasound show progression, the patient should be anticoagulated. Because noninvasive studies such as ultrasound are less sensitive for distal than proximal thrombi, the emergency physician should schedule serial studies if they still suspect DVT despite a normal initial ultrasound.[56] Alternatively, a negative, sensitive D-dimer study may obviate the need for serial studies, especially if the patient has few risk factors.[57] The optimal number and timing of serial studies has not been clarified, but a negative study at one week generally is adequate to rule out clot progression.[58]

Upper Extremity DVT. Effort thrombosis usually occurs in physically active young males, and may lead to DVT of the upper extremity.[59] Occasionally, a predisposing anatomic cause exists, such as cervical rib or thoracic outlet obstruction.[60] Upper extremity DVT from central lines is observed in children. While it was once thought that upper extremity DVT was benign, clots from the upper extremities can cause significant or even fatal PE.[61] Order duplex scanning to confirm the diagnosis.[62] While heparin may be used, catheter-directed thrombolysis with urokinase was generally accepted as the treatment of choice for upper extremity DVT.[59,60,63] However, no well-designed, controlled, randomized trials demonstrate the superiority of thrombolysis in this condition. Presumably, aggressive therapy will prevent the significant morbidity of recurrent hand and arm swelling. If patients have contraindications to thrombolysis or anticoagulation, placement of a Greenfield filter in the superior vena cava is recommended.

Pregnancy. Women are at increased risk of thrombosis throughout all stages of pregnancy. Prior to 20 weeks of gestation, duplex scanning is safe and accurate, but after 20 weeks, the gravid uterus presses on the inferior vena cava and confounds Doppler flow. An experienced sonographer can still detect clot within the vein by B-mode technology. In general, an indeterminate or non-diagnostic duplex scan in late pregnancy requires an additional study. MRI is an excellent choice, being both accurate and safe.[64] Heparin, which does not cross the placenta, remains the treatment of choice for DVT in pregnancy. LMWH is generally considered safe in pregnancy and is rated category B. After initial intravenous anticoagulation, women with DVT should remain on daily subcutaneous heparin until delivery. Warfarin is *contraindicated* during pregnancy due to its teratogenic effects,[65] but it should be started postpartum if the patient does *not* breast-feed.

Suspected Acute vs. Chronic DVT. Some patients with prior DVT who have recurrent symptoms require a specialized workup.[66,67] However, even in these patients, Duplex scanning remains the initial imaging study of choice.[68] If the study is normal, DVT is unlikely. A scan that clearly demonstrates fresh clot, based on homogeneity and echogenicity, is confirmatory of acute DVT; however, many studies will be equivocal. Patients with DVT can demonstrate persistent abnormalities on ultrasonography months to years after the acute event; in fact, 80% of ultrasounds are abnormal at three months and 50% abnormal at one year.[69] Comparison with a prior duplex scan will differentiate new vs. old changes, but access to a previous scan is oftentimes impossible. A combination of clinical suspicion, D-dimer testing, serial venous ultrasonography, lung scanning, fibrinogen leg scanning, or nuclear magnetic imaging may differentiate between old and new deep venous thrombosis.[68]

Patients with DVT while on Warfarin. If a patient on warfarin develops DVT, the emergency physician must decide if the patient is adequately anticoagulated, which is defined as an INR between 2.0 and 3.0. If the INR is below 2.0, start heparin and increase the daily dose of warfarin. If the INR is greater than 2.0, begin heparin and obtain consultation regarding vena cava filter placement. Most authorities believe that these patients require a filter to prevent PE.[70] A minority opinion recommends heparin and the addition of antiplatelet drug, such as dipyridamole 75 mg by mouth three times a day in addition to the warfarin regimen.[71,72]

Superficial Thrombophlebitis. Superficial thrombophlebitis may propagate into the deep system. Simple, localized phlebitis,

Outpatient Treatment of Deep Venous Thrombosis

Legend

Rx DRUG TREATMENT | Tx THERAPY | Px PROGNOSIS | Dx DIAGNOSIS

Establish a Hospital-Approved Protocol (having undergone multi-speciality review) that provides:

- Standardized therapy
- ED nursing education before D/C
- Close nurse/physician follow-up
- Coordinated warfarin clinic
- In selected cases, ability to admit to ED observation unit

↓

Diagnosis Confirmed by:

- Duplex ultrasonography
- Venography
- Other accepted modalities

↓

Inclusion Criteria: → Does Not Qualify → Inpatient Management

- 18 years old or older
- Not pregnant
- Otherwise healthy, reliable patient who can comply with protocols

↓

None of these Exclusionary Criteria is Present → Exclusionary Criteria Present (Px) → Inpatient Management

- Suspicion of pulmonary embolism
- Geographic inaccessibility
- Already on heparin for > 24 hours
- History of venous thromboembolic disease
- Significant comorbidities
- More than a minimal risk for bleeding
- Known inherited or acquired clotting abnormalities
- No recent spinal anesthesia or catheter insertion
- Morbid obesity
- Renal insufficiency
- Extensive iliofemoral involvement

↓

Consider LMWH agents (Rx)

- Enoxaparin, SQ: 1 mg/kg BID (currently, the only LMWH approved for outpatient treatment of DVT) Agent of choice

↓

Good Education and Follow-up: (2, Px)

- Have patient undergo nursing or pharmacist education with disease awareness, self-injection technique, warning signs and symptoms prompting return, and understanding of possible risks and complications.
- Outpatient follow-up with warfarin clinic, treatment nurse, and physician coordinated prior to discharge.

which develops at the site of a recent IV catheter, is generally benign. The emergency physician should order a duplex scan if the patient has involvement of the saphenous vein or significant risk factors for DVT.[73,74] Treat isolated superficial involvement with compression bandages and nonsteroidal anti-inflammatory drugs.[75] While some authorities recommend venous excision and local thrombectomy,[76]

Table 4. Pitfalls in the Management of Deep Venous Thrombosis

1. Relying on calf measurements and negative Homans signs to rule out DVT
2. Failure to perform objective testings on patients with presumed cullulitis of the leg
3. Failure to evaluate deep system in patients with superficial thrombophlebitis
4. Failure to consider the clinical likellihood of DVT when interpreting Doppler studies
5. Failure to use a weight-based nomogram to dose heparin
6. Failure to either anticoagulate or perform serial studies on patients with isolated calf vein thrombosis
7. Failure to perform a simple screen for malignancy in patients with unexplained deep venous thrombosis

less drastic measures usually suffice. If the patient is an intravenous drug user or is toxic appearing, consider septic thrombophlebitis, and admit for broad-spectrum antibiotics.

Summary

The patient with a painful or swollen leg presents a diagnostic challenge for the emergency physician. *(Please see Table 4 and Figure 1.)* Because of the limitations of physical examination, objective imaging studies are necessary for the majority of patients with unexplained limb complaints. Duplex scanning remains the diagnostic study of choice to evaluate for DVT. The red cell agglutination test of D-dimer is very sensitive for thrombosis, and a negative test makes proximal clot unlikely. Recognition of alternative conditions, such as compartment syndrome, septic arthritis, and cellulitis, is essential for optimal care. A weight-based nomogram is the best means to administer heparin, and ED use of warfarin can decrease hospital stay. Recognize atypical presentations of PE and phlegmasia dolens to institute lifesaving interventions. The use of subcutaneous LMWH is safe and effective and permits home treatment of DVT. Enoxaparin has approval for treatment of DVT, and outpatient management of carefully selected patients will become the standard of care.

References

1. Greenfield LJ, Michna BA. Twelve-year clinical experience with the Greenfield vena caval filter. *Surgery* 1988;104:706.
2. Fink JA, Jones BT. The Greenfield filter as the primary means of therapy in venous thromboembolic disease. *Surg Gynecol Obstet* 1991;172:253.
3. Cohen JR, Grella L, Citron M. Greenfield filter instead of heparin as primary treatment for deep venous thrombosis or pulmonary embolism in patients with cancer. *Cancer* 1992; 70:1993-1996.
4. Ferris EJ, McCowan TC, Carver DK, et al. Percutaneous inferior vena caval filters: Follow-up of seven designs in 320 patients. *Radiology* 1993;188:851-856.
5. Olson ST, Bjork I. Regulation of thrombin activity by antithrombin and heparin. *Sem Thromb Hemostasis* 1994;120: 373-409.
6. Hirsh J, Dalen JE, Deyken D, et al. Heparin: Mechanism of action, pharmacokinetics, dosing considerations, monitoring, efficacy and safety. *Chest* 1992;104:337S-351S.
7. Chong. Heparin induced thrombocytopenia. *Br J Hematol* 1995;89:431-439.
8. Warkentin TE, Levine MN, Hirsh J, et al. Heparin-induced thrombocytopenia in patients treated with low-molecular-weight heparin or unfractionated heparin. *N Engl J Med* 1995;332:1330-1335.
9. Hull RD, Raskob GE, Hirsh J, et al. Continuous intravenous heparin compared with intermittent subcutaneous heparin in the initial treatment of proximal-vein thrombosis. *N Engl J Med* 1986;315:1109-1114.
10. Elliott CG, Hiltunen SJ, Suchyta M, et al. Physician-guided treatment compared with a heparin protocol for deep vein thrombosis. *Arch Int Med* 1994;154:999-1004.
11. Hollingsworth JA, Rowe BH, Brisebois FJ, et al. The successful application of a heparin nomogram in a community hospital. *Arch Int Med* 1995;155:2095-2100.
12. McKinley L, Wrenn. Are baseline prothrombin time/partial thromboplastin time values necesesary before instituting anticoagulation? *Ann Emerg Med* 1993;22:697-702.
13. Hirsh J, Poller L, Deykin D, et al. Optimal therapeutic range for oral anticoagulants. *Chest* 1989;95(sup 2):5S.
14. Bolan CD, Alving BM. Recurrent venous thrombosis in hypercoagulable states. *Am Fam Physician* 1991;44:1741.
15. Humphries JE. Acquired antithrombin-3 deficiency replacement with antithrombin-3 concentrates in a patient with protein S deficiency accelerates response to therapy. *Acta Hematologica* 1993;90:151-154.
16. Zamorski MA, Opdycke RA. Advances in the prevention, diagnosis, and treatment of deep venous thrombosis.. *Am Fam Physician* 1993;47:457-469.
17. Anon. Optimum duration of anticoagulation for deep-vein thrombosis and pulmonary embolism. Research Committee of the British Thoracic Society. *Lancet* 1992;340:873-876.
18. Mohiuddin SM, Hilleman DE, Destache CJ, et al. Efficacy and safety of early versus late initiation of warfarin during heparin therapy in acute thromboembolism. *Am Heart J* 1992;123:729-732.
19. Hull RD, Raskob GE, Rosenbloom D, et al. Heparin for five days as compared with 10 days in the initial treatment of proximal venous thrombosis. *N Engl J Med* 1990;322: 1260-1264.
20. Ansell JE. Oral anticoagulant therapy—50 years later. *Arch Int Med* 1993;153:586-596.
21. Hyers TM, Hull RD, Weg JG. Antithrombotic therapy for venous thromboembolic disease. *Chest* 1992;102:408S-425S.
22. Schoenenberger RA, Pearson SD, Goldhaber SZ, et al. Variation in the management of deep vein thrombosis: Implications for the potential impact of a critical pathway. *Amer J Med* 1996;100:278-282.
23. Ebell MH. Low molecular weight heparins for DVT. *J Fam Pract* 1994;39:501-502.

24. Hull RD, Raskob GE, Pineo GF, et al. Subcutaneous low-molecular-weight heparin compared with continuous intravenous heparin in the treatment of proximal-vein thrombosis. *N Engl J Med* 1992;326:975.
25. de Valk HW, Banga JD, Wester JW, et al. Comparing subcutaneous danaparoid with intravenous unfractionated heparin for the treatment of venous thromboembolism. A randomized controlled trial. *Ann Int Med* 1995;123:1-9.
26. Leizorovicz A, Simonneau G, Decousus H, et al. Comparison of efficacy and safety of low molecular weight heparins and unfractionated heparin in initial treatment of deep venous thrombosis: A meta-analysis. *BMJ* 1994;309:299-304.
27. Lensing AW, Prins MH, Davidson BL, et al. Treatment of deep venous thrombosis with low-molecular-weight heparins. A meta-analysis. *Arch Intern Med.* 1995;155:601-607.
28. Wolf H. Low-molecular-weight heparin. *Med Clin North Am* 1994;78:733-743.
29. Nurmohamed MT, Verhaeghe R, Haas S, et al. A comparative trial of a low molecular weight heparin (enoxaparin) versus standard heparin for the prophylaxis of postoperative deep vein thrombosis in general surgery. *Am J Surg* 1995;169: 567-571.
30. Lensing AW, Prins MH, Davidson BL, et al. Treatment of deep venous thrombosis with low-molecular-weight heparins. A meta-analysis. *Arch Int Med* 1995;155:601-607.
31. Warkentin TE, Levine MN, Hirsh J, et al. Heparin-induced thrombocytopenia in patients treated with low-molecular-weight heparin or unfractionated heparin. *N Engl J Med* 1995;332:1330-1335.
32. Simonneau G, Charbonnier B, Decousus H, et al. Subcutaneous low-molecular-weight heparing compared with continuous intravenous unfractionated heparin in the treatment of proximal deep vein thrombosis. *Arch Intern Med* 1993;153:1541-1546.
33. Levine M, Gent M, Hirsh J, et al. A comparison of low-molecular-weight heparin administered primarily at home with unfractionated heparin administered in the hospital for proximal deep-vein thrombosis. *N Engl J Med* 1996;334:677-681.
34. Koopman MM, Prandoni P, Piovella F, et al. Treatment of venous thrombosis with intravenous unfractionated heparin administered in the hospital as compared with subcutaneous low-molecular-weight heparin administered at home. The Tasman Study Group. *N Engl J Med* 1996;334:682-687.
35. Schafer AI. Low-molecular-weight heparin—An opportunity for home treatment of venous thrombosis (Editorial). *N Engl J Med* 1996;334:724-725.
36. Gibaldi M, Wittkowsky AK. Contemporary use of and future roles for heparin in antithrombotic therapy. *J Clin Pharmacol* 1995;35:1031-1045.
37. Witty LA, Krichman A, Tapson VF. Thrombolytic therapy for venous thromboembolism. Utilization by practicing pulmonologists. *Arch Intern Med* 1994;154:1601-1604.
38. Thomas L, Reichl M. Pulmonary embolism in patients attending the accident and emergency department with pleuritic chest pain. *Arch Emerg Med* 1991;8:48-51.
39. Sherry S. Thrombolytic therapy for deep vein thrombosis. *Semin Intervent Radiol* 1985;2:331-337.
40. Rogers L, Lutcher C. Streptokinase therapy for deep vein thrombosis: A comprehensive review of the English literature. *Am J Med* 1990;88:389-395.
41. Francis CW, Marder VJ. Fibrinolytic therapy for venous thrombosis. *Prog Cardiovasc Dis* 1991;34:193-204.
42. Goldhaber SZ, Buring JE, Lipnick RJ, et al. Pooled analyses of randomized trials of streptokinase and heparin in phlebographically documented acute deep venous thrombosis. *Am J Med* 1984;76:393-397.
43. Bounameaux H, Banga JD, Bluhmki, et al. Double-blind, randomized comparison of systemic continuous infusion of 0.25 versus 0.50 mg/kg/24 h of alteplase over 3 to 7 days for treatment of deep venous thrombosis in heparinized patients: Results of the European Thrombolysis with rt-PA in Venous Thrombosis (ETTT) Trial. *Thromb Haemost* 1992;67: 306-309.
44. Turpie AG, Levine MN, Hirsh J, et al. Tissue plasminogen activator (rt-PA) vs heparin in deep vein thrombosis. Results of a randomized trial. *Chest* 1990;97:172S-175S.
45. Levine MN, Goldhaber SZ, Gore JM, et al. Hemorrhagic complications of thrombolytic therapy in the treatment of myocardial infarction and venous thromboembolism. *Chest* 1995;108:291S-301S.
46. O'Meara JJI, McNutt RA, Evans AT, et al. A decision analysis of streptokinase plus heparin as compared with heparin alone for deep-vein thrombosis. *N Eng J Med* 1994;330: 1864-1869.
47. Baethge BA, Payne DK. Phlegmasia cerulea dolens associated with a lupus anticoagulant. *West J Med* 1991;154:211.
48. Hood DB, Weaver FA, Modrall JG, et al. Advances in the treatment of phlegmasia cerulea dolens. *Am J Surg* 1993;166: 206-210.
49. Hirsh J, Hull RD, Raskob GE. Clinical features and diagnosis of venous thrombosis. *J Am Coll Cardiol* 1986;8:114B.
50. Greenfield LJ. Deep vein thrombosis, prevention and management. In: Wilson SE, ed. *Vascular surgery principles and practice.* New York: McGraw-Hill; 1987:736-757.
51. Smith BM, Shield GW, Riddell DH. Venous gangrene of the upper extremity. *Ann Surg* 1985;201:511.
52. Chapman WHH, Foley KT. Pulmonary embolism from a venous thrombosis distal to the popliteal vein. *Military Med.* 1991;156:252-254.
53. Lohr JM, Kerr TM, Lutter KS, et al. Lower extremity calf thrombosis: To treat or not to treat? *J Vasc Surg* 1991;14: 618-623.
54. Moser KM, LeMoine JR. Is embolic risk conditioned by location of deep venous thrombosis? *Ann Int Med* 1981;94: 439-444.
55. Huisman MV, Vuller HR, et al. Serial impedance plethysmography for suspected deep venous thrombosis in outpatients. *N Engl J Med* 1986;314:823-828.
56. Koopman MM, van Beek EJ, ten Cate JW. Diagnosis of deep vein thrombosis. *Prog Cardiovasc Dis* 1994;37:1-12.
57. Ginsburg JS, Kearon C, Douketis J, et al. The use of D-dimer testing and impedance plethysmographic examination in patients with clinical indications of deep vein thrombosis. *Arch Intern Med* 1997;157:1077-1081.
58. Cogo A, Lensing AW, Koopman MM, et al. Compression ultrasonography for diagnostic management of patients with

clinically suspected deep vein thrombosis: Prospective cohort study. *BMJ* 1998;316:17-20.

59. Hughes MJ, D'Agostino JC. Upper extremity deep venous thrombosis: a case report and review of current diagnostic/therapeutic modalities. *Am J Emerg Med* 1994;12: 631-635.
60. Horattas MC, Wright DJ, Fenton AH, et al. Changing concepts of deep venous thrombosis of the upper extremity: Report of a series and review of the literature. *Surgery* 1988; 104:561-567.
61. Black MD, French GJ, Rasuli P, Bouchard AC. Upper extremity deep venous thrombosis. Underdiagnosed and potentially lethal. *Chest* 1993;103:1887-1890.
62. Cronan JJ. Venous thromboembolic disease: The role of US. [Review]. *Radiology* 1993;186:619-630.
63. Pires LA, Jay G. Upper-extremity deep-vein thrombosis: Thrombolytic therapy with anistrepalase. *Ann Emerg Med* 1993;22:748-750.
64. Spritzer CE, Evans AC, Kay HH. Magnetic resonance imaging of deep venous thrombosis in pregnant women with lower extremity edema. *Obstet-Gynecol* 1995;85:603-607.
65. Hirsh J, Fuster V. Guide to anticoagulant therapy, Part II: Oral anticoagulants. *American Heart Assoc, Circ*. 1994;89: 1469-1480.
66. Colucciello SA, Plotka M. The Patient with Chronic Venous Insufficiency. In: Herr R, Cydulka R, eds. *Emergency Care of the Compromised Patient.* Philadelphia: JB Lippincott; 1994: 370-382.
67. Wells PS, Ginsberg JS. DVT and pulmonary embolism: Choosing the right diagnostic tests for patients at risk. *Geriatrics* 1995;50:29-32, 35-36.
68. Kearon C, Julian JA, Newman TE, et al. Noninvasive diagnosis of deep venous thrombosis. McMaster diagnostic imaging practice guidelines initiative. *Ann Intern Med* 1998;128: 663-677.
69. Heijboer H, Cogo A, Buller HR, et al. Detection of deep vein thrombosis with impedance plethysmography and real-time compression ultrasonography in hospitalized patients. *Arch Intern Med* 1992;152:1901-1903.
70. Stephen JM, Feied CF. Venous thrombosis. Lifting the clouds of misunderstanding. *Postgrad Med* 1995;97:36-42, 45-47.
71. Shattil SJ. Diagnosis and treatment of recurrent venous thromboembolism. *Med Clin North Am* 1984;68:577.
72. Anon. Collaborative overview of randomized trials of antiplatelet therapy-3: Reduction in venous thrombosis and pulmonary embolism by antiplatelet prophylaxis among surgical and medical patients. *BMJ* 1994;308:235-246.
73. Lutter KS, Kerr TM, Roedersheimer LR, et al. Superficial thrombophlebitis diagnosed by duplex scanning. *Surgery* 1991;110:42-46.
74. Yucel EK, Egglin TK, Waltman AC. Extension of saphenous thrombophlebitis into the femoral vein: Demonstration by color flow compression sonography. *J Ultrasound Med* 1992;11:285-287.
75. Messmore HL, Bishop M, Wehrmacher WH. Acute venous thrombosis. Therapeutic choices for superficial and deep veins. *Postgrad Med* 1991;89:73-77.
76. Pulliam CW, Barr SL, Ewing AB. Venous duplex scanning in the diagnosis and treatment of progressive superficial thrombophlebitis. *Ann Vasc Surgery* 1991;5:190-195.

Anticoagulation and Antiplatelet Therapy: Aspirin, Glycoprotein IIb/IIIa Inhibitors, and ADP Platelet Receptor Antagonists

Susan B. Promes, MD
Tammie Quest, MD
Gideon Bosker, MD, FACEP

Anticoagulation. Antiplatelet therapy. Vascular death risk reduction. These are some of the most critical, yet complex, rapidly evolving, controversial, and difficult-to-manage areas in the field of emergency medicine. In fact, from an emergency medicine perspective, a comprehensive understanding of the clinical role that antiplatelet agents and anticoagulants play in mortality reduction and disease prevention has become an area of intense investigation. New therapeutic agents—among them, aspirin, glycoprotein IIb/IIIa inhibitors, enoxaprin, warfarin, and others—represent powerful, proven additions to the arsenal for management of patients at risk for vascular-related disorders. As a result, the increasing role these agents have come to play in managing life-threatening ischemic, arterial, and veno-occlusive syndromes presents new challenges for emergency medicine specialists.

Of special importance is the understanding that these new agents have been investigated in a wide and diverse range of patient subsets. Moreover, all drugs that belong to the same class are not created equal. And, certain classes of drugs, as well as agents within those classes, appear useful only for specific clinical indications, among them: percutaneous coronary intervention (PCI) procedures (angioplasty, stenting, etc.), prevention and treatment of venous thromboembolism, prevention of MI and stroke, atrial fibrillation, unstable angina, non-ST-segment elevation MI, non-Q wave myocardial infarction, or classical MI with ST-segment elevation.

For example, in some cases, a drug may show risk reduction of recurrent ischemic events only in patients who undergo PCI, but not in those treated with only pharmacologic therapy. Not surprisingly, linking agents, or antiplatelet/anticoagulant "cocktails," to specific conditions has become a formidable clinical challenge that requires interpretation of sometimes imperfect, and, sometimes, even conflicting clinical trials. Moreover, when pharmacoeconomic, safety, and efficacy considerations enter into the equation, selecting an outcome-effective anticoagulant or antiplatelet drug can tax even the most analytical mind.

One of the most important priorities for the emergency physician is to recognize indications (DVT, unstable angina, acute MI) that justify acute intervention with these agents in the emergency department (ED). Although general indications for antiplatelet and anticoagulation therapies are widespread, ranging from cardioprevention and unstable angina to non-Q-wave MI and stroke reduction, the optimal agent or class, and its overall effectiveness for specific subgroups and combinations of drugs are still a matter of debate and a subject of ongoing investigation. Interestingly, existing antiplatelet agents, when used alone, have not been found to be clinically effective in the area of veno-occlusive disease, although this may change as future studies report outcomes with newer agents and trials designed to evaluate combined therapy.

In addition, ED physicians also must be able to identify—and in some cases, it may be argued, even screen ED patients for—those individuals (i.e., high-risk patients with chronic atrial fibrillation, patients with recent MI and left ventricular failure, and individuals with coronary artery disease risk factors) who can benefit from the addition of a prevention-oriented antiplatelet agent or anticoagulant on an outpatient basis in order to reduce their risk for such conditions as embolic infarction, stroke, or MI. When patients present to the ED with problems unrelated to arterial or venous occlusive disease, but who, nevertheless, require and may benefit from prevention-oriented drug intervention, physicians should be prepared to refer such individuals for antiplatelet or anticoagulation therapy. Finally, important paradigm shifts also are occurring in the area of DVT treatment. With trials showing the efficacy of low molecular-weight heparins (LMWHs), such as enoxaprin, for treatment of selected patients with DVT, consideration of outpatient treatment for this condition may soon become standard practice in emergency medicine.

To achieve these goals and maximize outcomes associated with anticoagulant and antiplatelet therapy, this chapter will examine indications and clinical effectiveness of three classes of antiplatelet agents currently approved by the FDA, the cyclooxygenase inhibitor (aspirin), the ADP platelet inhibitors, ticlopidine, and clopidogrel, as well as a new class of agents, the GP IIb/IIIa receptor antagonists (abciximab, tirofiban, eptifibatide). Because there are clinically significant differences among these drug classes, and among the drugs within each class, the authors provide detailed analysis of mechanism of actions, indications, drug toxicity, and cost. In addition, considerations related to use of these agents during pregnancy and lactation will be examined.

In the next chapter, the authors turn to the venous side of the thrombosis equation, and examine anti-fibrin drugs, including unfractionated heparin and the exciting new opportunities associated with low molecular heparin preparations (dalteparin and enoxaparin). A review of indications for warfarin and a brief synopsis of newer, direct thrombin inhibitors also will be presented.

Table 1. Vascular and Ischemic Disorders: Therapeutic Options

Condition	Therapeutic Options
ACUTE MYOCARDIAL INFARCTION	Aspirin, enoxaparin (non-Q wave MI), heparin (with certain thrombolytics) eptifibatide, tirofiban
ACUTE PULMONARY EMBOLISM	Heparin, enoxaparin, coumadin
ATRIAL FIBRILLATION	Aspirin, clopidogrel, ticlopidine, heparin, warfarin
DEEP VENOUS THROMBOSIS	Heparin, enoxaparin, ardeparin, dalteparin
DOCUMENTED DEEP VENOUS THROMBOSIS	Heparin, enoxaparin, coumadin
UNSTABLE ANGINA	Aspirin, clopidogrel, ticlopidine, enoxaparin, heparin, abciximab (with planned PCI), eptifibatide, tirofiban
PERCUTANEOUS CORONARY INTERVENTION (PCI)	Heparin, abciximab, eptifibatide, tirofiban
TIA/ISCHEMIC STROKE	Aspirin, clopidogrel, ticlopidine, heparin

Introduction: Role and Significance of Coagulation Disorders in Emergency Medicine

Under normal physiologic conditions, blood components do not interact with an intact vascular endothelium. However, exposure of circulating blood to disrupted or dysfunctional endovascular surfaces initiates a series of complex biochemical events that give rise to the rapid deposition of platelets, erythrocytes, leukocytes, and insoluble fibrin, producing an initial hemostatic plug. Not surprisingly, platelet aggregation is believed to play a major role in the pathogenesis of arterial thrombosis and its associated clinical conditions, including myocardial infarction (MI), stroke, and other ischemia-related diseases. From a therapeutic perspective, evidentiary-based trials have documented that inhibition of platelet aggregation reduces the incidence of both primary and secondary ischemic complications of atherothrombotic disease.

The importance of platelet function, aggregation, and inhibition is related to its central role in normal hemostasis, which can be characterized as a balance between thrombus formation and dissolution. Vascular thrombosis is a dynamic process, in which clot formation and dissolution occur almost spontaneously. The overall extent of thrombosis and the associated circulatory compromise, therefore, is determined by forces that shift the "balance" in one direction or another. In particular, platelets both mediate and participate as cellular components in "white thrombus" formation; these thrombi develop in high-pressure arteries, where circulating platelets adhere to areas of abnormal epithelium. In contrast, venous thrombi consist of a loosely packed network of erythrocytes and fibrin with islands of aggregated platelets (red thrombus). As would be expected, clinical strategies for prevention and/or treatment of arterial thrombotic disease varies considerably from agents used for managing patients with venous thrombosis.

Broadly speaking, these pathophysiological differences explain the clinical observation that anti-fibrin drugs, such as heparin, low molecular weight heparin (LMWH), and warfarin, are effective in syndromes (DVT and PE) associated with venous thrombosis, whereas aspirin and antiplatelet therapies are the mainstay of treatment and prevention for arterial thrombotic syndromes. Moreover, it should be emphasized that, in addition to these well-known medications, there are newer antithrombotics that appear to potentiate the effectiveness of existing treatments for both arterial and venous thrombotic disease. Accordingly, combination or cocktail therapies using multiple agents are likely to hold significant promise. *(Please see Table 1.)*

Inhibition of platelet aggregation, coagulation, clot formation, and thrombus reactivity have become the most important and effective prevention-oriented strategies in patients at risk for cardiovascular disease and stroke. From a pathophysiological perspective, a growing thrombus of aggregated platelet causes reduced arterial blood flow and leads to end-organ ischemic and/or occlusive

Table 2. Antiplatelet Agents: Indications and Cost of Therapy

Agent	Indications	Cost/month or IV course*
CYCLOOXYGENASE INHIBITOR		
Aspirin	2° prevention of MI/ Stroke; Acute coronary and cerebral ischemia syndromes	< $
	Low risk patient subgroups or lone atrial fibrillation	
ADP PLATELET RECEPTOR INHIBITOR		
Ticlopidine	Aspirin failures;	$$
Clopidogrel	Peripheral vascular disease	$$
GP IIb/IIa INHIBITOR		
Abciximab	Unstable angina only when PCI planned within 24 hrs	$$$*
Eptifibatide	Unstable angina, non-Q wave MI,	$$$*
Tirofiban	adjuvant of PCI	$$$*

Drug only cost, does not include monitoring and administration costs
< $ = < $5.00 *$$ = $80-100* *$$$ = ~$1300*[44]

clinical syndromes. Overall, the site, size, and composition of thrombi forming within the arterial circulatory systems is determined by: 1) alterations in blood flow; 2) the thrombogenicity of endovascular surfaces; and 3) the concentration and reactivity of hemostatic proteins and cellular elements.

It should be emphasized that an extremely complex series of events—precipitated by a number of biochemical mediators and physical stressors—is responsible for transforming an atheroma into a highly thrombogenic surface that fosters platelet aggregation and subsequent in situ thrombosis. In this regard, collagen from the exposed subendothelium, tissue factor on the surface of macrophages, adenosine diphosphate (ADP) from red blood cells that are lysed as they pass through stenotic arteries that produce turbulent flow, and the action of shear stress (disruption of laminar flow) all activate platelets and lead to the expression of the active form of the glycoprotein (GP) IIb/IIIa receptor on their surface. These receptors permit platelets to aggregate by attaching to one of several macromolecular ligands. As thrombosis evolves, local thrombin generation acts as an ongoing stimulant for platelet activation and subsequent aggregation.

Aspirin: Cyclooxygenase Inhibitor Par Excellence

Aspirin has become the standard antiplatelet agent for prevention of a wide range of ischemic syndromes. It is used for secondary prevention of MI (both acutely in combination with thrombolytic agents and for long-term oral prophylaxis), for prevention of thromboembolic disease in low-risk patients with chronic atrial fibrillation, as adjunctive therapy with heparin for unstable angina, for TIA prophylaxis, and for many other conditions. Specifically, long-term aspirin therapy reduces the risk of critical cardiovascular and cerebrovascular events (death, stroke, MI, unstable angina) by an average of about 25% compared to placebo.[1-3] Furthermore, it has been shown that aspirin reduces the risk of abrupt vessel closure during percutaneous revascularization. The reasons for aspirin's widespread use are well known. It is simple to administer, it is safe at low doses, and it is cost effective. In fact, to date, no other antiplatelet agent has demonstrated the risk-benefit ratio and low cost that aspirin affords. *(Please see Table 2.)* And yet, despite the benefits of aspirin therapy, experts still do not universally agree as to whether different doses of aspirin have varying magnitudes of clinical benefit, or what the ideal dose of aspirin should be for a particular clinical condition.

Mechanism of Action and Onset of Action. The antiplatelet effect of low-dose aspirin therapy (30-325 mg/d) is due to acetylation of platelet cyclooxygenase. This reaction is irreversible, and studies have shown that aspirin can induce inhibition of this enzyme at doses as low as 30 mg/d.[1,2] Without cyclooxygenase, platelets are unable to make thromboxanes, which are pro-aggregatory and cause vasoconstriction, but cyclooxygenase inhibition also prevents platelets from generating prostacyclins, which cause vasodilation and help maintain GI mucosal integrity. While the inhibition of platelet-derived thromboxanes is the principal antithrombotic mechanism of aspirin, the concomitant reduction of prostacyclins is thought to limit aspirin's value in arterial occlusive disease. At low doses, however, it is thought that inhibition of thromboxanes can occur without inhibiting prostacyclins, therefore allowing the beneficial effects of aspirin to predominate, while minimizing GI side effects.

One of the principal pharmacokinetic advantages of aspirin is its rapid onset of action, which explains its usefulness in acute coronary occlusive syndromes. One-dose therapy with aspirin produces acute inhibition of platelet function within 60 minutes of administration, an effect that lasts about nine days, which represents the approximate half-life of a platelet. Enteric coating will delay onset of inhibition by about 3-4 hours.[3] Currently, there is no oral antiplatelet preparation available that has an onset of action as rapid as "plain" aspirin. This quick onset of action represents a major advantage over other agents for treatment of acute ischemic vascular syndromes. Aspirin is rapidly absorbed by both oral and rectal routes.

As far as monitoring, in patients on chronic aspirin therapy, a routine CBC should be ordered periodically to rule out occult bleeding, and a stool guiac test should be performed. Bleeding time will be prolonged in patients taking aspirin.

Dosing. Aspirin dosing is controversial, with various studies or editorials confirming, recommending, or reporting that aspirin doses from 30 to 1400 mg/d are effective for specific clinical conditions.[4]

Most studies and consensus panels, however, recommend aspirin dosages between 81 and 325 mg/d.[5] *(Please see Table 3.)*

There is also conflicting information with respect to the relationship between aspirin dose and side effects, although lower doses appear to be associated with a lower risk of hemorrhagic complications. Moreover, women seem to be at higher risk for aspirin-related complications. When the the objective is secondary prevention of MI, the goal is to use the lowest dose of aspirin required to inhibit thromboxane, yet spare prostacyclin production. Although the mechanism of gastrointestinal side-effects is not well understood, these complications are thought to be related, at least in part, to inhibition of prostacyclin, which is thought to occur at higher aspirin doses.[6] There have been intriguing reports of "booster" dosing of aspirin, in which patients taking 81 mg/d of aspirin for long-term prevention, take one 325 mg aspirin tablet every 15 days, in order to enhance cardioprotection. Although one study suggests enhanced outcomes with this dosing pattern, additional trials are required to establish the efficacy of this approach.

Table 3. Minimum Recommended Dose of Aspirin for Common Indications

THROMBOTIC DISORDER	MINIMUM EFFECTIVE DAILY DOSE
Stable angina	81 mg
Unstable angina	81 mg
Acute myocardial infarction	160-325 mg
Transient ischemic attack	81 mg
Atrial fibrillation (warfarin contraindicated or young/lone atrial fibrillation)	325 mg
Atrial fibrillation (in addition to warfarin in case of failure)	325 mg
Secondary prevention of MI	81-162 mg

Toxicity. Although aspirin-related side effects are rarely seen within the context of acute administration within the ED setting, physicians must be aware of possible complications of chronic therapy. Aspirin, which has a Class D pregnancy rating, is unsafe in pregnancy; its safety in lactating women is unknown or controversial.

The side effects of aspirin are primarily related to dose but may also be related to length of use.[7] Pooled data from 21 clinical trials suggest that patients on long-term aspirin therapy have 1.5-2.0 times the risk of hematemesis or melena.[8] Both short- and long-term aspirin use may produce gastric erosions and hemorrhage, but long-term use increases the frequency and severity of disease. Aspirin-induced gastric injury, as detected by endoscopy, has been found to be greatest in the first week and tapers off within 2-8 weeks of continuous ingestion.

Aspirin is primarily associated with gastric rather than duodenal ulceration. Antacids, buffering agents, H-2 blockers, proton pump blockers, misiprostol, and enteric coating may reduce gastrointestinal injury, although these agents generally do not need to be administered when aspirin is given in the acute setting.[9] Aspirin, alone, usually does cause generalized, systemic bleeding except in cases of concomitant anticoagulant use, hemophilia, and uremic states.[10-12] The incidence of severe neutropenia with aspirin is approximately 0.02%. If a patient on aspirin develops severe bleeding, packed red blood cells and platelets should be administered. Aspirin-related antiplatelet clinical effects last about nine days, which is the average life of a platelet.

Indications for Aspirin Therapy. The primary indications for acute administration of aspirin in the ED setting include acute myocardial infarction (AMI), unstable angina in low-risk patients with atrial fibrillation, and ischemic cerebrovascular syndromes that have failed warfarin therapy or in patients who are poor candidates for warfarin. However, emergency physicians should also be prepared to counsel other individuals with coronary heart disease (CHD) risk factors who access the ED for non-cardiac problems, but who may benefit from the prevention-oriented benefits of aspirin therapy.

Primary vs. Secondary Prevention. In this regard, aspirin has been evaluated for its effectiveness in both primary and secondary prevention of MI. There have been only a few major trials published to explore the issue of primary prevention. In men, aspirin reduces the incidence of MI, but the net effect on stroke and cardiovascular death remains inconclusive. It should be stressed that the U.S. Physicians Health Study (USPHS)[11] and the British Doctors Trial (BDT)[13] give conflicting results. The USPHS revealed about an 18% reduction of all vascular events (nonfatal MI, nonfatal stroke, or cardiovascular death) among those on aspirin (325 mg qod), with a 33% reduction in non-fatal MI. The BDT noted no significant difference in combined end points of important cardiovascular events, thereby casting the role of aspirin for primary prevention into serious doubt. With regard to primary prevention of stroke, aspirin affords no benefit and may, in fact, be harmful. There was a small increase in hemorrhagic stroke rate in healthy individuals.

An important ingredient in many cocktails for cardioprevention, aspirin is still under-used for secondary prevention against *recurrent* MI. ED physicians should attempt to identify these individuals in the process of taking a drug history in patients with known cardiovascular disease. As emphasized, the use of aspirin for primary prevention in healthy individuals is still somewhat controversial, although most experts recommend its inclusion in cardioprotective regimens in high-risk subgroups. The 1988 American Physicians Health Study was prematurely stopped because of a 40% reduction in first, non-fatal MIs. The British Male Doctors study, however, did not show a reduction in first MIs, thus generating a controversy about the use of aspirin in primary prevention. The Thrombosis Prevention Trial (TPT) also does not support the widespread use of aspirin for primary prevention, because, even in high-risk men, the overall reduction in ischemic heart disease (IHD) events was a modest 20%, and aspirin had no effect on total mortality. Moreover, there are few data on women, at least one-half of the target population.

Low-intensity warfarin was also evaluated in TPT, and its cardioprotective effects for primary prevention were similar to aspirin. However, because warfarin was associated with an excess of dissecting and ruptured aortas, it cannot be recommended for primary prevention, especially in combination with aspirin. However, the case for using aspirin to prevent recurrent MI and coronary events in men at high risk is very strong. The appropriate dose is 81 mg of aspirin per day, with some experts recommending 162 mg/d. So who is eligible for aspirin therapy? Probably, most individuals older than age 50 with no contraindications, diabetics, those with a history of coronary heart disease, stable or unstable angina, history of MI, coronary angioplasty, or coronary bypass graft. The use of aspirin for primary prevention in women at low risk for CAD is not settled because the risk of causing hypertensive hemorrhage is slightly greater in patients on aspirin than those off of aspirin.[14,15]

In general, then, routine aspirin use for primary prevention in healthy individuals may afford no benefit, while placing patients at mild-to-moderate risk for hemorrhagic events. Primary preventive measures, such as lowering cholesterol, blood pressure, estrogen replacement therapy in women, and cessation of smoking, may have more of an effect on prevention of CHD than aspirin alone. However, low-dose aspirin therapy (81 mg/d) is indicated in all individuals who can tolerate the drug with a history of stroke/TIA, MI, angina, documented CHD, and probably, in other risk groups, such as diabetics and individuals with peripheral vascular disease.

Because emergency services are increasingly being integrated into comprehensive health management plans, emergency physicians should identify such high-risk subgroups requiring cardioprevention and ask about aspirin use as part of a drug history. Meta-analysis data suggest that total morbidity and mortality is significantly reduced when aspirin is used for secondary prevention in these subgroups.[16] In patients with a history of cardiovascular or cerebrovascular ischemic events, a meta-analysis of 25 trials, suggest vascular event rates are reduced by about 25%, with the most significant reduction observed in non-fatal MI (32%). In addition, a 20% reduction in risk of stroke has been observed with aspirin.[16]

Acute Coronary Syndromes. The primary indication for acute aspirin administration in the ED is acute coronary artery syndromes. In general, aspirin should be administered to all individuals with known or suspected ischemic coronary syndromes as first-line therapy.[17] If it is unclear whether the patient took their daily aspirin dose, just give it. The side effects are minimal, and the benefit may be substantial.

The Second International Study of Infarct Survival (ISIS-2) demonstrated that 160 mg of aspirin daily, given up to 24 hours after the onset of suspected AMI and continued for one month afterward reduced mortality by 23%.This benefit was maintained for two years and equaled that produced by IV streptokinase.[18] Other agents, such as thrombolytics and anticoagulants may be combined with aspirin, but aspirin must never be forgotten and should be part of any mortality-reducing pathway for managing patients with acute coronary syndromes.

Non-Valvular Atrial Fibrillation (AF). The overall risk of stroke in non-valvular AF is estimated to be about 4.5% per year.[19] Older individuals and those with hypertension, diabetes, previous stroke, heart failure, and coronary heart disease are at greater risk for thromboembolic events than those without these risk factors.

It should be stressed that warfarin, not aspirin, represents first-line therapy for chronic AF in *high-risk patients* (advanced age, prior TIA/stroke, hypertension or diabetes, left ventricular dysfunction, congestive heart failure, left atrial enlargement). However, summary data demonstrates that aspirin alone may be appropriate first-line therapy in those at *low* risk.[20] Persons younger than 75 years, with no high-risk factors ("low-risk"), benefit from aspirin alone, with an acceptable 0.5% primary event-per-year rate of thromboembolic events. Although less effective than warfarin, aspirin has been shown to reduce the risk of stroke by 18-44%.[21] Nevertheless, because high-risk individuals have a much higher primary event rate with aspirin alone vs. warfarin (4.8% vs 3.6%, respectively), aspirin therapy alone is recommended in high-risk patients only if they are intolerant of, or poor candidates for warfarin therapy.

In summary, the Stroke Prevention in Atrial Fibrillation (SPAF) III study has shown that aspirin is effective for preventing cerebrovascular events in low-risk AF patients. On the other hand, patients with chronic AF who are at high risk for embolic events (i.e., those with two or more risk factors from among the following: hypertension, valvular heart disease, elderly, women > 75 years, hypertension, prior stroke, and CHF or LV dysfunction) should be treated with warfarin to achieve an INR in the range of 2.0 to 3.0. Those at low risk (i.e., they do not have any of the risk factors cited above) can be treated with aspirin alone.

The value of antithrombotic therapy in patients with LV dysfunction was evaluated in the Studies of Left Ventricular Dysfunction (SOLVD) trial. The purpose of this investigation was to analyze the SOLVD database to assess the effects of antithrombotic therapy on risk for sudden cardiac death. A multivariate analysis revealed that antiplatelet therapy (primarily aspirin) was associated with a 24% reduction in sudden cardiac death risk, and anticoagulant (warfarin) therapy was associated with a 32% reduction in risk. Interestingly, antiplatelet therapy was not associated with a decreased risk in sudden death in a subset of 923 patients thought to have nonischemic heart failure, but anticoagulant therapy was still associated with a reduced risk in this group. Eligible candidates who have sustained an MI accompanied by an ejection fraction less than 35% will benefit most from warfarin-based anticoagulant therapy.[22]

Valvular Heart Disease. Aspirin alone is not sufficient to prevent thromboembolic complications of valvular heart disease.[23] However, In combination with full-dose warfarin, aspirin has been shown to improve the efficacy above warfarin alone. Unfortunately, the additional benefit is associated with a significant increase in bleeding. In patients who have failed warfarin (i.e., have experienced a thromboembolic event while on warfarin), it is reasonable to add aspirin, even though there is an increased risk of hemorrhagic complications. Patients intolerant of warfarin also may take aspirin.

Peripheral Vascular Disease/Intermittent Claudication. Generally speaking, aspirin should be recommended in all patients with claudication symptoms. Aspirin decreased morbidity and mortality associated with peripheral vascular disease. Patients with claudication have as high as 60% mortality over 10 years, which is due mostly to MI and stroke. Additionally, antiplatelet therapy has been shown to demonstrate a reduced need for surgery.[24]

Venous Thromboembolism. The efficacy of aspirin for prevention of venous thromboembolic disease is uncertain. Currently, there is no conclusive data to date to support the use of aspirin for this indication. The Pulmonary Embolism Prevention Trial is currently in progress.[5]

ADP-Platelet Receptor Inhibitors: Ticlopidine (Ticlid®) and Clopidogrel (Plavix®)

Ticlopidine (Ticlid®) and clopidogrel (Plavix®) are two agents that affect platelet activity (including aggregation) through inhibition of ADP platelet activation. Although these agents usually are not used for *acute* intervention in the ED, they are becoming widely accepted as a "second-line" antiplatelet therapy, especially in patients who cannot tolerate aspirin or who have failures on aspirin therapy.[25]

Table 4. Antiplatelet Agents: Complications, Monitoring, and Pregnancy Profile

Agent	Major Complications	Monitoring	Pregnancy
CYCLOOXYGENASE INHIBITOR			
Aspirin	GI bleeding	None	Class D
ADP PLATELET RECEPTOR INHIBITOR			
Ticlopidine	Neutropenia, ITP, TTP	CBC w/diff q 2 weeks for first 90 days; thereafter, with s/s of infection	Class B
Clopidogrel	Rash, diarrhea, abdominal pain	None	Class B
GPIIb/IIa INHIBITOR			
Abciximab	Generalized bleeding	None	Class C
Eptifibatide	*Note: required concomitant heparin therapy must be closely monitored to prevent excess bleeding*		Class B
Tirofiban			Class B

Moreover, because these medications can cause side effects, ED physicians must be aware of their indications and potential problems.

Compared to aspirin, these agents have been shown to offer convincing, clinically significant benefits with respect to reduction of ischemic events related to certain end points. However, whether these drugs offer outcome-effective advantages over aspirin is more difficult to evaluate when one considers cost of therapy and possible toxicity, especially in the case of ticlodipine. In this regard, ticlopidine should be used cautiously, based on recent reports that individuals taking this drug are at risk for acquiring thrombotic thrombocytopenic purpura (TTP), as well as neutropenia and agranulocytosis. The new antiplatelet agent clopidogrel is similar to ticlopidine and provides protection against recurrent MI that is similar or slightly better than aspirin, but it is not associated with the hematological risks seen with ticlopidine.

Reversal agents are available. Methylprednisolone normalizes bleeding time in patients taking ticlopidine. If significant bleeding develops, a platelet transfusion may be used, except in cases of ticlopidine-induced TTP. Ticlopidine carries a Pregnancy Class B rating, based on animal studies. No adequate and well controlled studies are available in women. The drug is excreted in human breast milk. *(Please see Table 4.)*

From an emergency medicine perspective, use of ADP platelet receptor inhibitors is limited by the rapidity of onset of action, which is slower than it is for aspirin. Because both agents require several days to achieve maximal therapeutic effects, their use is limited in acute ischemic syndromes.[26] The onset of action of ticlopidine increases gradually over a period of four days, with a total duration of activity of about 14 days. Clopidogrel has an onset of action within about two hours and a total duration of activity of about five days. *(See Table 5.)* Nevertheless, emergency physicians will encounter an increasing number of patients who present on these agents or who may require, on a selected basis, initiation of these agents on discharge from the ED.

Mechanism of Action and Dosing. Ticlopidine and clopidogrel are thienopyridine derivatives structurally unrelated to other platelet inhibitors. Structurally, ticlopidine and clopidogrel are nearly identical; specifically, clopidogrel is the (S) active enantiomer of ticlopidine. This structural alteration seems to account for clinically significant differences in potency and toxicity.[25]

Both agents block platelet-platelet adhesion. This action is mediated by selective and irreversible inhibition of ADP to its platelet receptor, thereby affecting the ADP-dependent activation of the GPIIb/IIIa complex. The GPIIb/IIIa complex is required for subsequent fibrinogen binding and, ultimately, thrombus formation. Both agents may take several days to reach maximum effect and both undergo hepatic metabolism.[26,27] From a compliance perspective, clopidogrel, which is dosed at 75 mg/d has potential advantages over ticlopidine, which is dosed 250 mg po bid with food.[28]

Toxicity. As emphasized, the side-effect profile of ticlopidine has been the major factor limiting its use. Ticlopidine has a number of toxic, even potentially life-threatening, effects with which the ED physician should be familiar. Diarrhea, which is encountered in 20-22% of patients, and transaminitis, observed in up to 8% of patients, are the most frequently noted drug-related toxicities. Agranulocytosis, although rare, is one of the most dreaded drug-related complications. In clinical trials with ticlopidine, the overall incidence of neutropenia (ANC < 1200) was 2.4%. Severe neutropenia (ANC < 450) occurred in 0.8% of patients. Mild to moderate neutropenia (ANC 451-1200) occurred in 1.6%. The onset of neutropenia may be sudden, and usually occurs between three weeks and three months after initiation of therapy. Unfortunately, some cases have been detected after three months or longer of drug therapy.

In addition, thrombocytopenia (< 80,000) may be induced in the form of immune thrombocytopenia (ITP) or thrombotic thrombocytopenia purpura (TTP); neutropenia may also complicate these clinical presentations. Fatalities have been reported. Because ticlopidine is metabolized by the liver, it is contraindicated in patients with severe liver impairment. Other contraindications include: active bleeding, hemostatic disorder, and baseline hematopoietic disorder.[28]

In contrast to ticlopidine, clopidogrel has relatively few side effects and is similar to aspirin in its safety profile. The most common

Table 5. Antiplatelet Drugs: Pharmacokinetics

Agent	Onset	Duration
CYCLOOXYGENASE INHIBITOR		
Aspirin	30-60 minutes 9 ± 2 days	75-325 mg
ADP PLATELET RECEPTOR INHIBITOR		
Ticlopidine	< 4 days	14 days
Clopidogrel	2 hours	5 days
GP IIb/IIa INHIBITOR		
Abciximab	< 2 hours	*48 hours*
Eptifibatide	< 1 hour	*2-4 hours*
Tirofiban	5 min.	3-8 hours

adverse reactions associated with clopidogrel include rash, abdominal pain, or dyspepsia; each are reported in about 4-5% of patients. Severe neutropenia may occur but is exceedingly rare. The incidence of severe neutropenia with clopidogrel is similar to that with aspirin (0.04% vs 0.02%), and it is much lower than the 0.8% incidence seen with ticlopidine. No cases of TTP have been reported.[29]

Monitoring. When considering the cost-benefit ratio of ticlopidine, the costs of vigilant monitoring of drug therapy must be included in the equation for drug selection. In this regard, monitoring the complete blood count (CBC), including a differential (neutrophil and platelet counts) is essential in all patients taking ticlopidine. Blood monitoring should be performed once every two weeks for the first three months of therapy. After 90 days, complete blood counts are recommended only when the patient has signs or symptoms of infection. Patients who have a 30% or greater drop in neutrophil count, must be monitored more closely, and considered for alternative therapy (i.e., clopidogrel). Patients who stop therapy for any reason must continue to have their blood monitored for at least two weeks, given the long half-life of the drug.[28] Clopidogrel, in contrast, does not require blood monitoring. Both agents prolong bleeding time.

Indications: Cerebral Ischemia/Stroke. Both ticlopidine and clopidogrel have demonstrated efficacy in reducing risk of recurrent cerebral ischemia and stroke. Although there may be indications for using these agents as initial therapy, their primary role is in patients who have experienced thromboembolic events while on aspirin therapy (i.e., "aspirin failures") and in individuals who require MI or stroke prophylaxis but are intolerant of aspirin. A recent worldwide survey of 185 neurologists in North America and Western Europe who are field leaders in the area of stroke prevention found significant differences in management styles for aspirin failures.[30] More than two-thirds responded that in the setting of aspirin failure, they would stop aspirin and begin another agent such as ticlopidine or some other anticoagulant. The literature supports the position that as an alternative to aspirin, ADP platelet receptor inhibitors are the most effective oral agents, although there are important differences in the relative efficacy and indications for ticlopidine and clopidogrel in stroke and MI prevention.

The clinical data for both clopidogrel and ticlopidine show that both agents are effective in the secondary prevention of cerebral ischemia and stroke.[31] The ticlopidine-based TASS Trial (3069 patients) evaluated patients for a 2-5 year period, and demonstrated a 48% reduction in fatal and non-fatal stroke the first year and about a 24% overall reduction per 100 patients followed for five years (ticlopidine vs aspirin). When composite outcomes of stroke, MI, and vascular death are considered vs. placebo in a meta-analysis trial, risk reductions are 25% for aspirin and 33% with ticlopidine.[32]

In the clopidogrel vs. aspirin CAPRIE Trial (19,185 patients), clopidogrel showed an overall (i.e., when all patient subgroups were combined) relative-risk reduction of 8.7% above the accepted 25% reduction using aspirin therapy, for the combined end points of ischemic stroke, MI, or vascular death.[33] Because of the results of the CAPRIE Trial, clopidogrel carries an expanded indication for prevention of recurrent MI. Interestingly, however, the CAPRIE efficacy data for clopidogrel are not as impressive as the TASS data, especially for stroke prevention.

At least one other aspect of the CAPRIE trial requires special mention. Of special note is the fact that in the *MI subgroup* in the CAPRIE study, there was actually a slightly *higher* incidence of *all end point* (fatal/non-fatal MI or stroke, or other vascular deaths) vascular events observed in the clopidogrel treated patients vs. those on aspirin. Inclusion into the MI group required clinical signs, symptoms, EKG, and laboratory confirmation of MI within 35 days prior to randomization to either aspirin or clopidogrel. Although there was a slight reduction in fatal/non-fatal recurrent MI and fatal stroke in the qualifying MI subgroup (11,630 patients), the increase in "other vascular deaths" was significantly greater in the clopidogrel vs. aspirin group. Other vascular deaths, according to the CAPRIE protocol, were defined as "any deaths that were clearly non-vascular and did not meet the criteria for fatal stroke, fatal myocardial infarction, or hemorrhage. Deaths considered by the Central Validation Committee to be directly related to the qualifying event were classified as other vascular."[33] Accordingly, it would be difficult to justify, at present, to use clopidogrel as the sole agent of choice for overall vascular event/death in patients with recent MI, unless they are unable to tolerate or have failed aspirin therapy.

While these agents appear to offer significant advantage over aspirin in selected patient populations, the cost:benefit ratio should be considered. Cost decision-analysis modeling indicates with respect to cerebral ischemia/infarction, five-year treatment with ticlopidine would reduce the number of lifetime strokes in 100 high-risk patients by two stroke events at an incremental cost compared to aspirin of $31,200-55,000 per quality-adjusted life-year gained.[34] In summary, while the use of the ADP receptor inhibitors can, with qualifications, be recommended for targeted patient subgroups, these agents are expensive when compared to aspirin. The cost per month for aspirin is $3.14 (Bayer), $113.93 for ticlopidine, and $86.76 for clopidogrel.[35]

Acute Coronary Syndromes. Clopidogrel and ticlopidine are less effective than aspirin, but they may be considered as second-line

Table 6. Dosing and Indications for Antiplatelet Agents and Anticoagulation Therapy

Drug or Drug Class*	Clinical Indications	Comments and Warnings
CYCLOOXYGENASE INHIBITOR		
Aspirin	**Atrial fibrillation:** 325 mg q day PO **Angina:** 81 mg q day PO/PR **Acute Myocardial Infarction:** 160-325 mg q day PO/PR **Cerebral Ischemia:** 81 mg q day PO/PR	Thrombocytopenia
ADP RECEPTOR INHIBITORS		
Clopidogrel	Use in the case of "aspirin failures" **Coronary or Cerebral Ischemia:** 75 mg q day PO	Rash GI Upset
Ticlopidine	Use in the case of "aspirin failures" **Coronary or Cerebral Ischemia:** 250 mg bid PO	Neutropenia GI upset Thrombocytopenia
GP IIb/IIIa RECEPTOR INHIBITOR		
Abciximab	**Acute Coronary Syndromes with planned PCI within 24 hours:** 0.25 mg/kg IV bolus (10-60 minutes prior to procedure) then 0.125 mcg/kg/min IV drip for 12 hrs **PCI only:** 0.25 mg/kg IV bolus then 10 mcg/min IV drip for 18-24 hours or until 1 hour after PCI	Must use with heparin. Lasts 1-2 days. Readministration may cause hypersensitivity reaction. GP IIb/IIIa inhibitor of choice
Eptifibatide	**Acute Coronary Syndrome:** 180 mcg/kg IV bolus then 2 mcg/kg/min IV drip up to 72 hours **PCI:** 135 mcg/kg IV bolus then 0.5 mcg/kg/min IV drip for 20-24 hours	Lasts approximately 21/2 hours
Tirofiban	**Acute Coronary Syndrome or PCI:** 0.4 mcg/kg/min IV for 30 min. then 0.1 mcg/kg/min IV	
UFH		
Heparin	**Prophylaxis for DVT:** 5,000 units q 8-12 hrs SQ **Deep Venous Thrombosis, Pulmonary Embolism** **Unstable Angina or PCI:** Bolus 5000-7500 units IV followed by IV drip 1000-2000 units per hour, titrate to therapeutic effect	Thrombocytopenia
LMWH		
Ardeparin	**Prophylaxis for DVT (knee replacement):** 50 units/kg bid SQ	Do not use in patients who have received an LP or spinal anesthesia.
Dalteparin	**Prophylaxis for DVT (abdominal surgery):** 2500 anti Factor Xa units q day SQ-low risk pts 5000 anti Factor Xa units q day SQ-high risk pts	Use caution in renal or liver failure patients. Do not use in patients who have received an LP or spinal anesthesia.
Enoxaparin	**Prophylaxis for DVT (hip/knee replacement):** 30 mg bid SQ **Extended Prophylaxis for DVT (hip replacement) or general surgery:** 40 mg q day SQ **Unstable angina or Non-Q wave MI:** 1 mg/kg q 12 hours SQ **Inpatient therapy for Deep Venous Thrombosis with or w/o Pulmonary Embolism:** 1 mg/kg q 12 hours SQ or 1.5 mg/kg SQ qd **Outpatient therapy of Deep Venous Thrombosis without Pulmonary Embolism:** 1 mg/kg q 12 hours SQ	Use caution in renal failure patients and elderly. Do not use in patients who have received an LP or spinal anesthesia.
Warfarin	**Atrial Fibrillation, Deep Venous Thrombosis, or Pulmonary Embolism:** 5-10 mg PO in ED then titrate dose to therapeutic effect	Monitor PT/INR Multiple drug interactions

** It is important to remember that a complication of all these agents is hemorrhage.*

or alternative therapy when aspirin cannot be tolerated. The delayed onset of action may account, in part, for the inferior results compared to aspirin for management of acute coronary syndromes. Studies, however, do suggest that some antiplatelet therapy is better than none at all.[36]

Peripheral Vascular Disease. Both agents can be considered reasonable alternatives to aspirin in patients with intermittent claudication.[23] Improved morbidity and mortality has been observed in patients on ticlopidine for the indication of intermittent claudication compared to placebo. Although not well quantified, improvement in clinical outcomes with ticlopidine is primarily observed in the area of cardiovascular and neurovascular events, which is consistent with the data in the area of TIA and stroke reduction reported in the TASS trial.[36] Clopidogrel also has been shown to have a relative-risk reduction of vascular events compared to aspirin of 23.8%.

GP IIb/IIIa Receptor Antagonists: Abciximab (ReoPro®), Eptifibatide (Integrilin®), and Tirofiban (Aggrastat®)

Platelet aggregation and thrombus formation may occur despite aspirin use. The glycoprotein (GP) IIb/IIIa receptor antagonists represent the latest generation of powerful platelet inhibitors. With 40,000-80,000 GP IIb/IIIa receptors per platelet, it is not surprising that antagonists to this receptor have demonstrated clinical success in acute coronary syndrome trials.[37-39] Accordingly, incorporation of GP IIb/IIIa receptor blockers into medical stabilization and mortality-reducing regimens for unstable angina has enhanced the safety and reduce the number of invasive procedures. At present, there are multiple trials investigating the adjunctive role of GP IIb/IIIa receptor inhibitors in combination with enoxaparin and fibrinolytic therapies, including tPA. It has also been suggested that platelet aggregation around residual thrombus—a phenomenon that is not resolved by current therapies—may contribute to fibrinolytic therapy failures.

Preliminary results with GP IIb/IIIa receptor antagonists are generally favorable when combined with thrombolytics. As a result, these antiplatelet drugs may offer some additional benefits by permitting lower doses of thrombolytic agents such as tPA to be used in MI (with or without heparin) and, ultimately, by permitting fewer patients to undergo invasive therapy. Although preliminary economic considerations suggest GIIb/IIIa antagonists may be cost-effective by reducing the need for emergent revascularization procedures and the length of hospital stay, a definitive pharmacoeconomic analysis is still awaited.

Unfortunately, drawing definitive conclusions about the current role of GP IIb/IIIa inhibitors for emergency practice is exceptionally difficult, because many of the studies used to support these agents show conflicting or inconsistent results—sometimes related to gender and geographical differences with respect to clinical trial outcomes. In addition, the studies were performed using different treatment regimens in slightly different patient subgroups. Among the trials used to identify the role of GP IIb/IIIa inhibitors are the CAPTURE,[38] EPISTENT,[39] EPIC,[40] and EPILOG[41] trials. Development of oral agents in the GP IIa/IIIb drug class—among them, xemilofiban, orbofiban, sabrafiban—is currently in progress.

Mechanism and Dosing. In the presence of platelet activation by fibrinogen or von Willebrand factor, the GP IIb/IIIa receptors on platelets undergo structural modification, which facilitates platelet aggregation and subsequent thrombus formation. There are currently three GP IIb/IIIa agents available for clinical use, and they differ considerably in indications, dosing, and outcomes. In the case of abciximab and tirofiban, heparin should accompany infusion, with strict attention to dosing per manufacturer recommendations to avoid excess bleeding events.

Abciximab (ReoPro®). Abciximab is the Fab fragment of the chimeric human-murine monoclonal antibody 7E3, which is produced by continuous perfusion in mammalian cell culture. The Fab fragment is extracted and, when given to human subjects, it blocks the GP IIb/IIIa receptor and, therefore, platelet aggregation. Abciximab is administered by intravenous infusion and has a half-life of 10 minutes. Continuous infusion must be maintained for antiplatelet effect. Although abciximab remains in the circulation for two weeks, platelet function returns within 48 hours. It is a non-competitive inhibitor, accounting for a longer half-life than is observed with other agents in its class.

Abciximab is intended for use in combination with aspirin and heparin.[42,43] According to the package insert, it is dosed as a 0.25 mg/kg IV bolus administered 10-60 minutes prior to cardiac catheterization, which is then followed by continuous infusion of 0.125 mcg/kg/min (to a maximum of 10 mcg/min) for 12 hours.

Eptifibatide (Integrilin®). Eptifibatide is derived from the venom of the southeastern pygmy rattlesnake. This cyclic heptapeptide reversibly binds to platelets in a dose- and concentration-dependent manner.

A competitive inhibitor, eptifibatide (in contrast to abciximab) does not maintain inhibition after infusion. Available only as an infusion, 84% platelet inhibition has been observed after a 15 minute infusion. Plasma elimination half-life is approximately 2.5 hours after bolus plus infusion. In clinical trials that have shown eptifibatide to be effective, most patients also received both heparin and aspirin. However, the manufacturer's package insert does not require heparin or aspirin for eptifibatide use.

The dose for managing patients with acute coronary syndromes is 180 mcg/kg bolus with an infusion of 2 mcg/kg/min until discharge or CABG for up to 72 hours. When used for patients undergoing a percutaneous coronary intervention (PCI), the infusion should be decreased to 0.5 mcg/kg/min at the time of procedure, followed by continued infusion for 20-24 hours after PCI, for up to a maximum of 96 hours.

Tirofiban (Aggrastat®). Tirofiban is a non-peptide extraction from the venom of an African snake, the saw-scaled viper. Platelet inhibition occurs within five minutes, and bleeding time returns to normal within 3-4 hours after discontinuation of infusion. The elimination half-life is two hours. The recommended dose is 0.4 mcg/kg/min for a 30 min infusion, then 0.1 mcg/kg/min (one-half the dose for severe renal insufficiency).

Toxicity. Bleeding is the major complication with all agents in this class. The incidence of major bleeding end points (intracranial hemorrhage, a > 5 mg/dL decrease in hemoglobin, or > 15 mg/dL drop in hematocrit) for all three agents ranges between 2.0% and 5.2%. (CP10-14) Minor bleeding episodes are reported to be between 4% and 11%.[37-41] In patients on warfarin in whom PCI is imminent, it is recommended that warfarin be discontinued (and reversed with fresh frozen plasma [FFP] and Vitamin K), and titratable heparin be started. In all cases, in order to reduce the incidence of bleeding complications, heparin should be carefully dosed and monitored, precisely as recommended by the manufacturer of each agent.

Thrombocytopenia is a potentially life-threatening side effect. Mild to severe thrombocytopenia may occur with all three drugs and ranges between 0.5% and 3.2%. It must be stressed that the data may be confounded by the mandatory use of heparin with these agents, and that some reports may reflect heparin-induced thrombocytopenia. Data are limited regarding readministration of agents for subsequent ischemic episodes, but readministration may lead to hypersensitivity, anaphylaxis, thrombocytopenia, or diminished effectiveness.[44-46] Data for use of GIIb/IIIa inhibitors with thrombolytic agents are under investigation (GUSTO-IV). Preliminary results suggest that alteplase may be safer with respect to bleeding than streptokinase when given with eptifibatide.

Abciximab is designated Pregnancy Class C; animal studies have not been conducted. It is not known whether abciximab is excreted into human milk or absorbed systemically after ingestion. Eptifibatide and tirofiban are designated Class B. It is not known if these drugs are excreted into human milk or absorbed systemically after ingestion. Use with caution.

Indications: Acute Coronary Syndromes and Percutaneous Coronary Intervention. Based on results from a number of clinical trials,[37-41] GP IIb/IIIa inhibitors have been approved for treatment of diverse patient populations with ischemic syndromes. Eptifibatide is approved for patients with unstable angina (UA)/non-Q-wave MI (NQMI), regardless of the mode of patient management. It is also indicated for treatment of patients undergoing elective, urgent, or emergency PCI. Abciximab is approved for treatment of patients scheduled to undergo PCI (including those with refractory unstable angina awaiting PCI), while tirofiban HCl is approved for treatment of patients with UA/NQMI (who may be managed either medically or with PCI).

Abciximab, which is approved only as adjunctive therapy for unstable angina when percutaneous coronary intervention is planned within 24 hours, has been studied in three trials. A key inclusionary criterion was that the decision for percutaneous coronary intervention was made prior to starting the drug infusion.[44-46] In addition, all patients enrolled had previous angiographic studies that demonstrated a potential "culprit" lesion. Progression to MI or death after intervention was less than 5% with abciximab compared to 9% with placebo, when evaluated at a 30-day end point.[38]

It should be stressed that when abciximab was evaluated in the CAPTURE Trial (1265 patients) the primary efficacy end point was a composite of death from any cause, nonfatal MI, or urgent repeat intervention or CABG for recurrent ischemia (11.3% for abciximab and 15.9% for placebo) at 30 days. However, at six months in the CAPTURE Trial, there appeared to be minimal, statistically borderline differences between those treated with abciximab and those in the placebo arm.

The finding of only borderline benefit with abciximab at six months is not in agreement with the EPIC Trial (1400 patients) or EPISTENT Trial (2399 patients) results presented at the European Society of Cardiology Meeting in August 1998;[39] these studies, in fact, did demonstrate significant reductions in death/MI/recurrent revascularization end points at six months in specific patient subgroups.[39-41] For example, in the EPISTENT Trial, the improved end points with abciximab were observed primarily in the group of patients who had received the drug and had PCI/stent therapy; in contrast, in those who received abciximab plus PCI (PTCA) treatment, the differences between drug and placebo had only borderline significance.

Overall, abciximab administration to patients undergoing stent implantation reduced the composite end point at 30 days by 51% and by 47% at six months compared to stenting alone. From a practical, emergency intervention perspective, it appears as if abciximab is most advisable in patients who undergo PCI and stent implantation or PTCA. In the EPIC Trial, the reduction in MI/death/revascularization was significant only in abciximab patients who received a bolus of the drug *plus* infusion. Improved end points, including reduction in restenosis, persisted for three years. Other studies have failed to confirm such protracted benefits. The different outcomes among the studies has been explained by the variations in study design. In CAPTURE, patients received abciximab for only one hour after PCTA compared with 12 hours in EPIC and EPILOG. These findings suggest that the infusion of abciximab for 12 hours after PCTA may be critically important in producing a benefit that is sustained over the long term. Currently, abciximab is the GP IIb/IIIa receptor antagonist of choice.

Unfortunately, the data for eptifibatide (Integrilin®) are even more ambiguous, and in some ways problematic, from a cautionary perspective.[47] In U.S. and Canadian studies (3827 patients), the combined death/MI rate at 30 days was 15% for placebo and 11.7% for eptifibatide (22% reduction). However, in Western European studies (3697 patients), there was only a 7% relative reduction (14.8% combined adverse end point in placebo, 13.8% with eptifibatide). More disturbing, however, is the finding that in Latin American (396 patients) and Eastern European (1541 patients) trials, there was a net increase in adverse, combined end points with eptifibatide.[47] In overall worldwide outcome data, in *male* patients there was a 16.9% negative end point rate in those on placebo, and in only 13.9% in the eptifibatide treatment arm.

However, in *worldwide* outcomes evaluating *women*, negative combined end points were observed in 13.7% of females on placebo, and in 14.9% on the eptifibatide arm (i.e., a net increase of 8% in adverse events in the treatment arm). Once again, the Western and Eastern European study groups, as well as the Latin American trials, showed a marked adverse effect of the drug in women. Moreover, the PURSUIT Trial suggests that the greatest benefits with eptifibatide were observed in patients undergoing PCI, not in those managed pharmacologically. Given the gender-specific efficacy, the differences in responsiveness to PCI and non-PCI subgroups, and some of the discrepancies between regional outcomes with eptifibatide, it is probably prudent at the present to limit use of this agent in favor of other modalities (i.e., abciximab or enoxaparin) until additional studies provide clarification.

The tirofiban data are also sufficiently ambiguous to demand further investigation before this agent can be recommended for routine use. In the RESTORE Trial (2141 patients) at 30 days, there were no statistically significant difference in the incidence if the composite end point (death/MI or any repeat intervention) between the groups receiving tirofiban HCl and placebo (12.2% in the placebo group vs. 10.3% in the tirofiban group, P = 0.16). The PRISM study (3200 patients) also failed to demonstrate significant benefit of tirofiban over heparin. In contrast, the PRISM-PLUS Trial (1550) patients showed a 19% (P = 0.024) risk reduction at six months for tirofiban plus heparin vs. heparin alone (for death/MI/repeat revascularization).[48]

In summary, the jury is still out on exactly how prominent a role tirofiban and and eptifibatide should play in ED-based antiplatelet management. There may be a place for these agents, but additional clarification is required. Clearly, among the GP IIa/IIIb receptor antagonists per se, the overall data are more compelling for abciximab, especially in certain subgroups (i.e., those undergoing stent-related procedures as part of PCI). However, when this class is compared to the wide range of end point benefits demonstrated for enoxaprin at the one-year end point (ESSENCE), enoxaprin (Lovenox®) seems to be emerging as the initial agent for consideration in patients with acute coronary syndromes (UA/NQMI). The ED role of the GIIb/IIIa receptor antagonists has yet to be defined.

References

1. The Dutch Study Trial Group. A comparison of two doses of aspirin (30 mg vs 283 mg a day) in patients after a transient ischemic attack or minor stroke. *N Engl J Med* 1991;325: 1261-1266.
2. Antiplatelet Trialists' Collaboration. Collaborative overview of randomized trials of antiplatelet therapy, I: Prevention of death, myocardial infarction, and stroke by prolonged antiplatelet therapy in various categories of patients. *BMJ* 1994;308:81-106.
3. McEvoy (ed). *American Hospital Formulary Service 98 Drug Information.* Bethesda, Maryland: American Society of Health System Pharmacists; 1998.
4. Hart RG, Harrison JG. Aspirin Wars: The optimal dose of aspirin to prevent stroke. *Stroke* 1996;4:585-587.
5. Hirsch J, Dalen JE, Fuster V, et al. Aspirin and other platelet active drugs: The relationship among dose, effectiveness, and side effects. *Chest* 1995;108:247S-257S.
6. Rees WD, Turnberg LA. Reappraisal of the effects of aspirin on the stomach. *Lancet* 1980;2:410-413.
7. Farrel B, Godwin J, Richars S, et al. The United Kingdom transient ischemic attack (UK-TIA) aspirin trial: Final results. *J Neurol Neurosurg Psychi* 1991;54:1044-1054.
8. Roderick PJ, Wilkes HC, Meade TW. The gastrointestinal toxicity of aspirin: An overview of randomized controlled trials. *Br J Clin Pharmacol* 1993;35:219-226.
9. Graham DY, Smith JL. Aspirin and the stomach. *Ann Intern Med* 1986;104:390-398.
10. Chesebro JH, Fuster V, Elveback, et al. Trial of combined warfarin plus dipyridamole or aspirin therapy in prosthetic heart valve replacement: Danger of aspirin compared to dipyridamole. *Am J Cardiol* 1983;51:1537-1541.
11. The Steering Committee of Physicians Health Study Research Group. Preliminary report: Findings from the aspirin component of the ongoing physician's health study. *N Engl J Med* 1988;318:262-264.
12. Goldman S, Copeland J, Moritz T, et al. Improvement in early saphenous vein graft patency after coronary artery bypass surgery with antiplatelet therapy: Results of a Veterans Administration Cooperative Study. *Circulation* 1988;77: 124-321.
13. Peto R, Gray R, Collins R, et al. Randomized trial of prophylactic daily aspirin in British male doctors. *BMJ* 1988;296:313-316.
14. SPAF Investigators. Aspirin for Atrial Fibrillation Stroke Prevention. *JAMA* 1998;279:1273-1277.
15. SPAF. Stroke Prevention in Atrial Fibrillation Investigators warfarin and aspirin. *Lancet* 1996;348:633-638.
16. Acheson J, Archibald D, Barnett H, et al. Antiplatelet trialists collaboration: Secondary prevention of vascular disease by prolonged antiplatelet therapy. *BMJ* 1988;296:320-331.
17. Collins R, Peto R, Baignet C, et al. Aspirin, heparin and fibrinolytic therapy in suspected acute myocardial infarction. *N Engl J Med* 1997;336:847-859.
18. Second International Study of Infarct Survival Collaborative Group. Randomized controlled trial of intravenous streptokinase, oral aspirin, both or neither among 17,187 cases of suspected acute myocardial infarction. *Lancet* 1988;2: 349-360.
19. Kopecky SL, Gersh BJ, McGoon MD, et al. The natural history of lone atrial fibrillation: A population study over three decades. *N Engl J Med* 1987;317:669-674.
20. Stroke Prevention in Atrial Fibrillation Investigators. Warfarin versus aspirin for prevention of thromboembolism in atrial fibrillation: Stroke Prevention in Atrial Fibrillation II Study. *Lancet* 1994;343:687-691.
21. Matchar DB, McCrory DC, Barnett HJM. Medical treatment for stroke prevention. *Ann Intern Med* 1994;121:41-53.
22. SOLVD Investigators. Effect of enalapril on mortality and the development of heart failure in asymptomatic patients with reduced LV ejection fraction. *N Engl J Med* 1992;327: 685-692.
23. Coulshed DS, Fitzpatrick MA. Drug treatment associated with heart valve replacement. *Drugs* 1995;46:897-911.
24. Hiatt WR. Current and future drug therapies for claudication. *Vasc Med* 1997;2:257-262.
25. CAPRIE Steering Committee. A randomized, blinded trial of clopidogrel versus aspirin in patients at risk of ischemic events (CAPRIE). *Lancet* 1996;348:1329-1339.
26. Verstraete M, Zoldhelyi. Novel antithrombotic drugs in development. *Drugs* 1995;49:856-884.
27. Noble S, Goa KL. Ticlopidine: A review of its pharmacology, clinical efficacy and tolerability in the prevention of cerebral ischemia and stroke. *Drugs Aging* 1996;8:214-232.
28. Mosby. Complete Drug Reference 1997. Physician GenRx-Drug Information. *Ticlopidine Hydrochlorinde.* p II-2001-2003.
29. Clopidogrel for reduction of athersclerotic events. In: *The Medical Letter* 1998;40:59-60.
30. Masuhr F, Busch M, Einhaupl. Differences in medical and surgical therapy for stroke prevention between leading experts in North America and Western Europe. *Stroke* 1998;29: 339-345.
31. Gent M, Blakely, JA, Easton JD, et al. The Canadian American Ticlopidine Study (CATS) in thromboembolic stroke. *Lancet* 1989;1:1215-1220.
32. Hass W, Easton J, Adams HJ, et al. A randomized trial comparing ticlopidine hydrochloride with aspirin for the prevention of stroke in high-risk patients. *N Engl J Med* 1989;321:501-507.
33. CAPRIE Steering Committee. A randomized, blinded trial of clopidogrel versus aspirin in patients at risk for ischemic

events (CAPRIE). *Lancet* 1996;348:1329-1339.

34. Oster G, Huse DM, Lacey MJ. Cost-effectiveness of ticlopidine in preventing stroke in high-risk patients. *Stroke* 1994; 25:1149-1156.
35. Cardinale V (ed). 1998 Drug Topics *Red Book.* New Jersey: Medical Economics, Co; 1998.
36. Balsano F, Rizzon V, Scrutinio D. Antiplatelet treatment with ticlopidine in unstable angina. *Circulation* 1990;82:17-26.
37. Mark, DB, Cowper, PA, Berkowitz SC, et al. Economic Assessment of Low-Molecular Weight Heparin (Enoxaprin) Versus Unfractionated Heparin in Acute Coronary Syndrome Patients: Results from the ESSENCE Randomized Trial. *Circulation* 1998;97:1702-1707.
38. The CAPTURE Investigators. Randomized placebo-controlled trial of abciximab before and during percutaneous coronary revascularization. *N Engl J Med* 1997;336: 1689-1696.
39. The EPISTENT Investigators. Randomized placebo-controlled and balloon-angioplasty-controlled trial to assess safety of coronary stenting with use of platelet glycoprotein-IIb/IIIa blockade. *Lancet* 1998;352:87-89.
40. The EPIC Investigators. Use of monoclonal antibody directed against the platelet glycoprotein IIb/IIIa receptor in high-risk coronary angioplasty. *N Engl J Med* 1994;333:956-961.
41. The EPILOG Investigators. Platelet glycoprotein IIn/IIIa receptor blockade and low-dose heparin during percutaneous coronary vascularization. *N Eng J Med* 1997;336:1689-1696.
42. Tcheng J, Ellis SG, George BS. Pharmacodynamics of chimeric glycoprotein IIb/IIIa integrin antiplatelet antibody Fab 7E3 in high risk coronary angioplasty. *Circulation* 1994; 90:1757-1764.
43. Simoons ML, DeBoer MJ, Van der Brand MJBM, et al. Randomized trial of a GPIIb/IIIa platelet receptor blocker in refractory unstable angina. *Circulation* 1994;89:596-603.
44. EPILOG Investigators. Platelet glycoprotein IIb/IIIA receptor blockage and low dose heparin during percutaneous coronary revascularization. *N Engl J Med* 1997;336:1689-1696.
45. CAPTURE Investigators. Randomized placebo-controlled trial of abciximab before, during and after coronary intervention in refractory unstable angina: the CAPTURE study. *Lancet* 1997;349:1429-1435.
46. EPIC Investigators. Use of a monoclonal antibody directed against the platelet glycoprotein IIb/IIIa receptor in high-risk coronary angioplasty. *N Engl J Med* 1997;336:1689-1696.
47. Integrilin, Product Monograph. Cor Key Pharmaceuticals. 1998.
48. Tirofiban (Aggrastat) package insert. Merck Pharmaceuticals. 1998.

Low Molecular Weight Heparin: An Evolving Therapeutic Landscape

Gideon Bosker, MD, FACEP

Since the introduction of low-molecular-weight heparins (LMWHs) to the U.S. market in 1993, their indications have continued to expand. Of most significance to primary care physicians is the recent Food and Drug Administration (FDA) approval of enoxaparin for the outpatient treatment of deep vein thrombosis (DVT). With the ever-increasing emphasis on cost-effective health care, primary care physicians need to be conversant with the role of LMWHs in shortening or even eliminating hospitalization for patients with uncomplicated DVT. This chapter outlines the rationale and indications for outpatient therapy and provides an example of a clinical care pathway for ease of establishing treatment guidelines at local hospitals.

Introduction

Despite the recognition of risk factors and the availability of effective means for prophylaxis, DVT and pulmonary embolism (PE) remain common causes of morbidity and mortality. It is estimated that approximately 600,000 patients per year are hospitalized for DVT in North America.[1] In the United States, symptomatic pulmonary embolism occurs in more than 600,000 patients and causes or contributes to death in up to 200,000 patients annually.[2]

PE is the most common cause of death in patients following total hip replacement, which is one of the top 10 diagnosis-related groups (DRGs) for almost every hospital in this country. PE has been touted as the most common cause of preventable hospital mortality. The postphlebitic syndrome with persistent leg pain, swelling, and ulcerations affects 15 million Americans and may be prevented if thrombosis prophylaxis were routinely used and DVT treated effectively.[3] A recently published cohort analysis indicates that the mortality associated with venous thromboembolism (VTE) may be higher than previously thought.[4]

The treatment landscape for managing patients with DVT is evolving at a rapid pace. The most important studies affecting current approaches to therapy are those comparing and evaluating the efficacy of unfractionated heparin (UFH) vs. LMWH for management of patients with DVT, both in and out of the hospital. These trials, which are impressive in their support of the safety, suitability, and efficacy of LMWHs, have presented new challenges for the emergency medicine community. In particular, new developments in the management of DVT require emergency physicians to risk stratify patients into those who require hospitalization and those who are amenable to outpatient treatment.

Since the clinical introduction of warfarin in the 1950s, the management of VTE in the United States has changed little. Patients with proximal and symptomatic distal DVT are customarily hospitalized and placed on bed rest. They are given a bolus of intravenous UFH with subsequent continuous IV infusion of UFH for 5-6 days until therapeutic anticoagulation with warfarin is achieved, which is defined as an International Normalized Ratio (INR) of 2.0-3.0. The

Table 1. Advantages of LMWH Over UFH

- Less binding to heparin-binding proteins, endothelial cells, and matrix proteins
- More predictable antithrombotic dose response
- Better bioavailability at lower doses
- Less bleeding (possibly)
- Lower risk of heparin-induced thrombocytopenia
- Longer half-life
- No need for APTT monitoring
- Less risk of osteoporosis

heparin dose is adjusted to achieve an activated partial thromboplastin time (APTT) ratio of 1.5-2.5, which commonly correlates with a therapeutic heparin level of 0.2-0.4 IU/mL by protamine titration or an anti-Xa level of 0.3-0.6 IU/mL by a chromogenic assay.[5] The concept of dosing UFH by body weight was introduced by Raschke et al in 1993. This approach resulted in a more rapid achievement of a therapeutic APTT.[6]

Although the complication rate during the hospitalization period for most patients is extremely low, only recently has the possibility of treating DVT on an outpatient or short-stay basis been explored. The need to give UFH by constant IV infusion guided by frequent APTT measurements precluded outpatient therapy or early discharge. The opportunity to initiate outpatient or short-stay programs for DVT treatment has been made possible by the introduction of LMWHs. These LMWHs have significant pharmocokinetic advantages over UFH due to their differences in size and structure.

In this regard, use of LMWH, enoxaparin, for out-of-hospital treatment of DVT has positive pharmacoeconomic consequences that must be considered in the equation for DVT management. Risk stratification of these patients will include a detailed history and evaluation that considers the presence of underlying co-morbid conditions, hemodynamic stability of the patient, exclusion of pulmonary embolism, location of the thrombosis, ability of patient to self-administer an LMWH such as enoxaparin at home, and adequate follow-up and support.

Finally, recent approval of enoxaparin for use in seriously ill medical patients will provide opportunities for reducing complications associated with deep venous thromboembolism in hospitalized patients with respiratory failure, congestive heart failure, and other risk factors that predispose to VTE with or without pulmonary embolism.

Structure of Heparins

LMWH and UFH are glycosaminoglycans made of chains of alternating residues of D-glucosamine and a uronic acid, which may be either glucoronic or iduronic acid.[7] Heparins are commercially prepared most commonly from porcine intestinal mucosa. UFHs are treated by chemical or enzymatic depolymerization to form LMWHs. The mean molecular weight distribution of LMWH is 4000-6000 Daltons compared to about 12,000 Daltons for UFH.[8] The majority of UFH molecules are greater than 18 saccharide units long; however, this is true in less than half of LMWH molecules. These differences in size and structure account for the distinct pharmacological actions of LMWHs.

Mechanism of Action. Heparins exhibit most of their antithrombotic effects by inactivating two important factors in the coagulation cascade: factor Xa and factor IIa (thrombin). Heparin acts as a template to which both antithrombin III and coagulation enzymes bind. The main difference between UFH and LMWH is that LMWH has greater activity against factor Xa than factor IIa (4:1 to 2:1), whereas UFH has similar effects against both. Approximately one-third of UFH and LMWH molecules have a unique pentasaccharide enabling them to bind to antithrombin III and subsequently inhibit factors IIa and Xa. However, only those heparin molecules with at least 18 saccharide units are capable of forming a ternary complex with antithrombin III and factor IIa.[7] Since only about a third of LMWH molecules are large enough to form this ternary structure, they have less effect on factor IIa but retain their antifactor Xa activity.[9] In addition, both UFH and LMWH stimulate the release of tissue factor pathway inhibitor (TFPI) from the endothelium. TFPI complexes with and inactivates factor Xa and factor VIIa and works independently of pentasaccharide binding. Yet another mechanism of action is that heparin inactivates factor IIa by heparin cofactor II.

Pharmacokinetics. The substantial pharmacokinetic advantage of LMWHs is their increased bioavailability resulting from their decreased affinity for circulating plasma proteins. UFHs bind readily to histidine-rich glycoprotein, polymeric vitronectin, platelet factor IV, multimers of von Willebrand factor, fibronectin, macrophages, and endothelial cells.[10] In addition, UFHs exhibit unpredictable anticoagulant activity due to the wide patient variability in plasma concentrations of these heparin-binding proteins. Some of these proteins are acute phase reactants while others are released during the clotting process. To compensate for this binding, higher doses of UFH are required. Frequent laboratory monitoring is also required for UFHs; however, lab monitoring is usually not required for LMWHs due to their superior bioavailability, more predictable dose response effect, and minimal effect on IIa. Exceptions would include patients with renal insufficiency (since both UFHs and LMWHs are eliminated renally) and patients who are markedly obese or underweight.

Because LMWHs do not prolong the APTT, monitoring of the anticoagulant response in these patients can be achieved by following anti-Xa levels. Variation in plasma protein concentrations results in unpredictable renal and hepatic clearance. Because LMWHs bind less to macrophages and endothelium, the renal and hepatic clearance is slower and results in a longer plasma half-life. The improved bioavailability and longer half-life of LMWHs allow them to be dosed conveniently once or twice daily. *(Please see Table 1.)*

Indications for LMWH. LMWHs have been used in Europe and Canada for more than 10 years, during which a great deal of clinical experience has been gained. Enoxaparin was introduced in the United States in 1993. Currently, three LMWHs and one heparinoid are approved by the FDA in the United States. These agents are widely used in the prophylaxis of DVT, particularly in high-risk abdominal surgery patients and in those patients undergoing total hip and knee replacement. The value of extended DVT prophylaxis is supported by the results of a prospective, randomized, double-blind study demonstrating a 63% risk reduction with enoxaparin for 21 days post-discharge after total hip replacement for DVT prophylaxis compared to placebo.[11] There was no significant difference in incidence of adverse events, including bleeding. Enoxaparin is the only LMWH approved by the FDA for extended prophylaxis after hospital discharge in patients with total hip replacement. In addition, enoxaparin is the only LMWH currently indicated for prophylaxis of seriously ill medical patients who meet appropriate inclusionary criteria *(see part II of this series)*. Even though LMWHs are more expensive than UFHs, they are more cost-effective for DVT prophylaxis after major orthopedic surgery.[12] Non-FDA-approved uses include DVT prophylaxis following hip fracture and multiple trauma.

The Fifth American College of Chest Physicians' Consensus Conference on Antithrombotic Therapy has published recommendations for DVT prophylaxis and has identified LMWH as an acceptable pharmacological agent for most at-risk patients.[13] *(See Table 2.)* In addition to VTE prophylaxis and treatment, two LMWHs (enoxaparin and dalteparin) are approved by the FDA for the prevention of thrombotic complications in acute non-Q-wave infarction and unstable angina. A recent study in patients with acute ischemic stroke showed a statistically significant improvement in favor of LMWH compared to placebo in terms of mortality and dependency in daily activities. Hemorrhagic complications during 10 days of treatment were similar between the groups.[14] The use of LMWH has expanded to other clinical settings including pregnancy, vascular surgery grafts, trauma, and spinal cord injury.

Evidence-Based Support for LMWH in VTE. More than 20 published studies have evaluated the safety and efficacy of various LMWHs in the treatment of VTE. Leizorovicz performed a meta-analysis of the literature and found LMWHs to be at least as effective and safe as UFH.[15] In a study of 500 patients, Levine et al compared outpatient enoxaparin at 1 mg/kg subcutaneously bid vs. inpatient UFH administered by IV infusion with APTT monitoring in the treatment of DVT.[16] All patients received warfarin. Patients randomized to enoxaparin spent an average of only 1.1 days in the hospital compared to 6.5 days for UFH. One hundred twenty patients receiving enoxaparin were not hospitalized at all. There was no significant difference in major bleeds between the two groups.

Similarly, Koopman et al randomized 400 patients to nadroparin (a LMWH not available in the U.S.) vs. UFH.[17] Rates of recurrent VTE between the two groups were not significantly different but nearly 40% of the patients assigned to nadroparin did not require hospitalization. Bleeding complications were less frequent in the LMWH-treated patients. In their European multicenter trial, Fiessinger et al showed that 253 patients randomized to dalteparin administered once daily vs. UFH did not have statistical differences in progression of DVTs distal to the inguinal ligament.[18] Hull et al compared the LMWH logiparin to intravenous UFH and demonstrated at least equal effectiveness and safety in the treatment of proximal DVT.[19] In a review of the literature, Brewer concluded that LMWHs are clearly superior to UFH in the treatment of DVT based on efficacy, safety, convenience, and cost.[20]

Enoxaparin was found to be as safe and effective as UFH in a study of 900 patients in the treatment of DVT with or without PE.[21] These results, combined with the study of Levine et al,[16] led the FDA to approve enoxaparin for the inpatient treatment of DVT with or without PE and for outpatient treatment of patients with DVT. Yeager

Table 2. Recommendations for DVT Prophylaxis[13]

Medical patients	
• General medical patients:	Low-dose unfractionated heparin (LDUH) or LMWH (grade A1*)
• Myocardial infarction:	LDUH or full-dose anticoagulation (grade A1); intermittent pneumatic compression (IPC), and elastic stockings (ES) may be useful if anticoagulation contraindicated (grade C1).
• Ischemic stroke:	LDUH or LMWH (grade A1)
• Long-term central lines:	warfarin 1 mg daily or LMWH (grade A1)
Surgery patients	
• General surgery patients:	Low risk: early ambulation Moderate risk: LDUH 2 h preop and q 12 h, ES, IPC, LMWH (grade A1) High risk: LDUH q 8 h or LMWH (grade A1) High risk prone to hematomas and infection: IPC (grade A1) Very high risk: LDUH or LMWH combined with IPC (grade B1) Selected very high risk: warfarin (grade A2) Aspirin *not* to be used in general surgery patients
• Intracranial neurosurgery:	IPC with or without ES. LDUH or LMWH may be acceptable alternatives (grade A1).
• Acute spinal cord injury:	LWMW (grade B1)
• Multiple trauma:	LMWH should be started ASAP (grade A1)
Orthopedic patients	
• Total hip replacement:	LMWH* or warfarin or adjusted dose UFH (grade A1) Adjuvant ES or IPC may provide additional efficacy.
• Total knee replacement:	LMWH,† warfarin, or IPC
• Hip fracture:	LMWH or warfarin (grade A2) Adjuvant IPC may provide additional benefit IVC filters indicated only in high-risk patients in whom anticoagulant-based prophylaxis not feasible due to active bleeding

* Grade A recommendations are more strongly supported by the literature than grade B and grade C recommendations. See reference for complete definitions.

† Emerging level I data suggest 29-31 day duration of LMWH prophylaxis may provide additional protection (grade A2).

Table 3. Comparison of LMWH for DVT Treatment[22]

GENERIC AGENT	TRADE NAME	TREATMENT DOSE	AVERAGE MW (DALTON)	ANTI XA/IIA RATIO	HALF-LIFE (MIN)
Ardeparin	Normiflo	Not evaluated	6000	2:1	200
Dalteparin	Fragmin	100 u/kg bid	5000	2:1	119-139
Danaparoid	Orgaran	750 u bid	5500	28:1	24 hrs
Enoxaparin	Lovenox	100 u/kg bid	4500	4:1	129-180
Nadroparin	Fraxiparine	225 u/kg bid	4500	3.2:1	132-162
Reviparin	Clivarine	100 u/kg bid	4300		NA
Tinzaparin	Logiparin, Innohep	175 u/kg qd	4900	2:1	111

and Matheny have concisely summarized information on various LMWHs that have been successfully used in the treatment of DVT.[22] This information is summarized *in Table 3. Table 4* lists the results of four studies using various LMWHs.

Outpatient or Short-Stay Treatment of VTE. The first step in treatment is accurate diagnosis. No patient should be subjected to the risk, expense, and inconvenience of anticoagulation therapy without an objective, diagnostic confirmation of VTE. With good technique, duplex ultrasonography is adequate to made the diagnosis of DVT. If the results of duplex ultrasonography are unclear, venography remains the gold standard for diagnosis. For PE, diagnostic tests include ventilation/perfusion scan, pulmonary angiography, spiral computerized tomography, and gadolinium magnetic resonance. D-dimer (a fibrin split product) testing is considered a sensitive but not specific test for the diagnosis of VTE. Therefore, normal plasma levels (< 500 μg/L by enzyme-linked immunosorbent assay) provide excellent negative predictive value in patients suspected of having PE and particularly in those with low clinical suspicion.

Baseline laboratory testing should include a complete blood count with platelet count, APTT, and PT/INR. The physician should evaluate the patient's candidacy for thrombolytic therapy, especially in younger patients with acute symptomatic iliofemoral thrombosis. Patients should be considered for a work-up for a hypercoagulable state (e.g., protein C, protein S, anti-thrombin III deficiency, factor V Leiden, antiphospholipid antibodies). Patients who might benefit from a hypercoagulability work-up include those with family history of VTE, development of DVT in the upper extremities, or DVT occurring without obvious provoking factors such as immobility, trauma, or surgery. Treatment with heparin and/or warfarin may make the work-up difficult due to these agents' interference with test results. For example, warfarin lowers protein C and S levels. Similarly, an acute VTE with comorbid conditions may falsely alter the levels due to the increase in acute phase reactants that accompany stress. Because the cost of testing for hypercoagulable states can be substantial and the results do not normally affect the acute treatment decision, it is suggested that the hypercoagulable work-up be done 2-3 weeks after the cessation of therapy.

Consultation with the laboratory director or hematologist may be helpful in determining the scope and timing of any anticipated work-up. Because cancer is a common cause of the hypercoagulable state, patients presenting with unprovoked VTE should be considered for a work-up for occult malignancy. At the very least, these patients should have a thorough history and physical examination and subsequent clinically appropriate cancer screening such as mammography and fecal occult blood testing.

Estrogen replacement therapy or oral contraceptives must be discontinued as they are absolutely contraindicated during the course of therapy for VTE. The dilemma is whether these agents can be safely reintroduced upon completion of therapy in patients who have no major continuing risk factors for DVT. If reintroduced, they should be done so at the lowest possible clinically effective dose.

Only those patients with uncomplicated DVT are eligible for outpatient treatment. *(Please see Table 5.)*

The physician must confirm the diagnosis of DVT and determine that the patient is a candidate for LMWH treatment. Although several LMWHs have been successfully used in the treatment of DVT, currently only enoxaparin has gained FDA approval for the treatment indication. For in-hospital treatment of DVT with or without pulmonary embolism, the approved dose of enoxaparin is either 1 mg/kg SC q 12 hours or 1.5 mg/kg SC q day. For outpatient treatment, the only FDA-approved dosage is 1 mg/kg b.i.d. Enoxaparin is available in 30, 40, 60, 80, and 100 mg prefilled disposable syringes. Multi-dose vials that will make more precise weight-based dosing easier to achieve should be available shortly.

Warfarin may be given 2-4 hours after the initial subcutaneous dose of enoxaparin. Warfarin can temporarily cause a hypercoagulable state due to its effect on depleting protein C and protein S, which both have short half-lives. A commonly used approach is to begin with a dose estimated to be the patient's eventual maintenance dose. For most patients, this will be 5 mg daily with subsequent doses adjusted based on the results of the INR in order to achieve a goal INR of 2.0-3.0. Higher loading doses have not resulted in faster achievement of targeted INR and run the risk of increased bleeding and warfarin skin necrosis. Although not universally agreed upon, patients known to have a hypercoagulable state caused by the antiphospholipid antibody syndrome may require an INR of 3.0-3.5.[23]

The multiple drug-drug and drug-food interactions associated with warfarin warrant an attempt to keep the patient's vitamin K intake and

Table 4. Results of Randomized Clinical Trials of LMWH vs. UFH for DVT Treatment

STUDY REFERENCE	NUMBER OF PATIENTS	AGENTS	RECURRENCE, LMWH/UFH	BLEEDING, LMWH/UFH	MORTALITY, LMWH/UFH
Fiessenger[18]	253	Dalteparin	3.3/1.5	0/1.5	0.8/2.9
Levine[16]	500	Enoxaparin	5.3/6.7	2/1.2	4.5/6.7
Koopman[17]	400	Nadroparin	6.9/8.6	0.5/2.0	6.9/8.1
Hull[19]	432	Tinzaporin	2.8/6.9	0.5/5.0	4.7/9.6

concomitant drug usage stable. Warfarin should be administered in the afternoon or evening to allow for morning INR results to return so that dosing can be appropriately adjusted.

There is no good supporting evidence for the value of routine bed rest, but bed rest with leg elevation would be appropriate for those patients with significant leg pain and swelling until such symptoms resolve.[24]

Patient Education and Follow-Up. Patient education forms the cornerstone of outpatient anticoagulation management. The patient needs to be instructed on signs and symptoms of PE, bleeding, or extension of DVT. Also, the patient needs instruction on proper technique of LMWH administration as well as drug-drug and drug-food interactions with warfarin. Case managers are helpful in securing third-party reimbursement and arranging for home health agency visits if required. Many home health agencies are equipped today with portable finger-stick monitoring devices so that the PT/INR can be obtained immediately and the results called in to the pharmacist or physician for warfarin dosing changes. Platelet counts do not need to be routinely performed if the total course of LMWH administration is expected to be less than seven days. Once the INR is greater than 2.0 for two consecutive days, LMWH can be stopped and the patient continued on warfarin.

Although there is some debate regarding the length of warfarin therapy, it is generally recommended that the minimum duration is three months—although recurrence rates are less when treatment is extended to at least six months for patients with idiopathic VTE.[25] Patients who develop worsening signs and symptoms of DVT extension such as increasing swelling and pain, and those patients who show evidence of PE should be considered for hospital admission. The mortality rate of patients with DVT who are promptly and effectively anticoagulated is extremely low. A meta-analysis indicates the rate of fatal PE during 5-10 days of heparin and three months of oral anticoagulants is around 0.4%.[26] The enclosed supplement provides a sample short-stay DVT clinical pathway that can be readily adapted to an outpatient protocol.

Clinical Considerations with LMWHs

Bleeding. Hemorrhage is the most frequent and significant side effect of heparin. Animal studies have shown hemorrhage is more frequent with UFH than LMWH when given in equipotent doses.[8] LMWHs have less inhibition of platelet function less interaction between platelets and endothelial walls than UFH. Animal studies have shown reduced bleeding in those LMWHs with higher anti-Xa:anti-IIa ratios. Although LMWHs theoretically might cause less bleeding than UFH, recent clinical experience suggests similar bleeding rates. Patients at risk of bleeding include those with peptic ulcer disease and those who have had recent surgery. All patients should be screened at the time of VTE diagnosis and patients at excessive risk for bleeding should be excluded from consideration for outpatient management. Although the package insert for enoxaparin suggests urine analysis and fecal occult blood tests during the course of therapy, the need for such testing is uncertain.

Patients should be educated to promptly report any symptoms of bleeding, such as tarry stools, coffee-ground emesis, weakness, pallor, and fatigue. If bleeding is minor, holding LMWH is usually adequate. If bleeding is major, LMWH's effect can be at least partially reversed with protamine sulfate, a basic protein that neutralizes heparin's anti-IIa activity. It should be administered mg for mg and given slowly over 10 minutes as it may cause hypotension. The total dose should not exceed 50 mg. One study comparing the effects of protamine on UFH and LMWH showed near complete reversal of anti-Xa activity and APTT.[27] However, in patients with prolonged APTT on LMWH, protamine had a minimal effect on anti-Xa.

Heparin-Induced Thrombocytopenia (HIT). There are two forms of thrombocytopenia associated with heparin use. The early

Table 5. Contraindications to Outpatient Treatment

- Hypersensitivity to heparin or pork products
- Pulmonary embolism
- Significant comorbid conditions (e.g., congestive heart failure, chronic obstructive lung disease)
- Pediatric patients (safety and efficacy not established)
- Nursing mothers (not known if drug excreted in human milk and caution should be used in this patient population)
- Known hypercoagulable state and recurrent thromboembolism (relative contraindication)
- Active major bleeding
- History of heparin-induced thrombocytopenia
- Expected noncompliance

form is benign and reverses despite continued heparin use. The severe form is called HIT. This typically does not occur until day 5 of heparin therapy and is an autoimmune reaction. The body forms heparin platelet factor 4-dependent IgG antibodies that bind with platelet antigens.[7] This immune complex results in thrombocytopenia and/or paradoxical thrombosis. If a patient has been exposed to heparin within the last three months, HIT can occur within 24 hours.

There is evidence that the risk of HIT is less with LMWHs than with UFHs. In one large study, the incidence of HIT, defined as a platelet count (< 150 X 10^9/L) at more than four days post-initiation of therapy, was higher in the UFH group than the LMWH group (2.7% vs 0%). When thrombocytopenia is defined as a drop in platelets of greater than 50% in more than four days, the incidence was 5.7% and 0.9%, respectively.[28] HIT is a clinicopathological diagnosis. Platelet activation assays using washed platelets have a sensitivity and specificity of 90% for detection of HIT antibodies. Antigen assays using enzyme-linked immunosorbent antibodies (ELISA) to detect antibodies against heparin/PF4 complexes yield sensitivities and specificities of 80% and 90%, respectively.

HIT rarely presents within five days of heparin administration and platelet counts are not routinely recommended if the duration of heparin administration is expected to be seven days or less and the patient has had no heparin exposure within the previous three months. If the platelet count falls more than 50% from baseline or if the absolute platelet count falls below 100,000 d/L, LMWH should be held pending laboratory confirmation of HIT. If the patient develops HIT and requires continuing anticoagulation, recombinant hirudin should be considered.

Lipid Effects. Heparins exert lipolytic activity and lipase enzymes including lipoprotein lipase. In one study, total cholesterol increased by about 20% in groups given UFH or LMWH for 3-6 months.[29] HDL levels increased more in the UFH group, and LDL increased more than twice that in the LMWH group although this difference was not statistically significant. Since the duration of UFH or LMWH therapy for VTE is typically a few days, these lipid effects are not clinically important.

Osteoporosis. Heparins augment PTH-stimulated bone resorption and stimulate osteoclasts. Generally, increased molecular size and the degree of sulfation are major determinants of heparin's ability to promote bone resorption. Animal studies have shown decreased calcium loss in fetal rat calvaria with LMWH compared to UFH.[30] Also, spinal fractures occur less frequently in humans on long-term LMWH compared to UFH.[31] From these data, it would be expected that LMWHs would result in lower risk of heparin-induced osteoporosis.

Other Side Effects. Skin lesions associated with heparin use include erythematous papules, skin necrosis, and urticaria. Reactions such as asthma, tachycardia, tachypnea, conjunctivitis, rhinitis, angioedema, and shock are less common. Long-term administration of heparin may rarely cause hypoaldosteronism due to the inhibition of aldosterone synthesis.[7]

Renal Insufficiency. LMWHs, like UFHs, are eliminated through the kidneys. It is prudent in patients with renal insufficiency to adjust the dosage accordingly. Data are scarce regarding dose modifications in patients with serum creatinine of greater than 2 mg/dL. LMWHs might be best administered at reduced doses or increased intervals and monitored with anti-Xa levels. If anti-Xa levels are not readily available, reduced doses of UFH should be given and the APTT monitored accordingly.

Obese Patients. In most studies, LMWH has been dosed on the basis of actual body weight. Data on pharmacokinetics and dosing guidelines in obese patients are scarce. In patients weighing more than 130 kg, consider using a modification toward ideal body weight (IBW). A commonly used formula to adjust for ideal body weight is found below:

IBW for men = 50 kg + (2.3 kg X [inches > 5 feet])
IBW for women = 45 kg + (2.3 kg X [inches > 5 feet])
If Actual Body Weight (ABW) < IBW, enoxaparin dosing weight = ABW
If ABW > IBW, enoxaparin dosing weight = IBW + 0.3 (ABW-IBW)

Outcome Analysis and Implementation Strategies. Among the potential pharmacoeconomic advantages of out-of-hospital treatment with enoxaparin would be fewer admissions, increased patient comfort, and decreased overall costs. A disadvantage is that patients would have to be carefully evaluated to identify those who would be more safely treated in the hospital. In addition, much of the responsibility for treatment would be shifted from medical personnel to the patient and family, requiring self-administration of anticoagulants, self-monitoring for safety and efficacy, and compliance with clinic appointments for dosage adjustments of oral anticoagulants.

Home-Based Treatment of DVT

Maximizing Outcomes. As discussed, paradigm shifts in medication usage should be conservatively undertaken, as clinical experience helps to refine the management program. Initial treatment of DVT at home should follow a protocol in which all aspects of the treatment are clearly defined for the family and follow-up physician. Ideally, each ED should develop a treatment protocol that is written in advance by a team of medical professionals experienced in the treatment of DVT. The protocol should include criteria for patient selection, enoxaparin and warfarin therapy, patient and caregiver education, and monitoring. Each medical facility will need to develop a protocol that fits its own practice patterns.

One of the most important goals is developing criteria to identify patients who qualify for home-based treatment of DVT.

As mentioned, most studies evaluating LMWH for outpatient therapy have excluded patients with a high risk of bleeding (malignant hypertension, peptic ulcer disease, recent surgery, known bleeding disorders, thrombocytopenia, high risk of falling), a high risk of recurrent thrombosis (previous CVT, pregnancy), and suspected PE. In addition, patients who resided a long distance from follow-up medical care, who were unable to care for themselves or did not have a competent caregiver in residence, and who were simply too ill to stay at home were not considered candidates from home-based treatment of DVT. Patients had to be willing to participate in their care, including self-administration of medications and follow-up for warfarin dosage adjustment when necessary. With these strict guidelines for patient selection, about 22-58% of patients screened in various studies were considered eligible for home-based treatment of DVT with a LMWH such as enoxaparin.[32,35,36]

Patient Instructions. Detailed instructions must be provided by the emergency medicine team. The patient or caregiver must be taught to administer the medication, monitor for adverse reactions and efficacy, and perform any other self-care deemed necessary (such as bed rest, leg elevation, and use of compression stockings). The patient or caregiver also must know what steps to take in the event of a complication. Instruction should begin immediately after diagnosis and can be provided by a nurse, a pharmacist, or both. Written instructions should also be provided.

Monitoring home-based treatment of DVT with enoxaparin should include compliance, subcutaneous injection technique, local adverse effects from the injections, signs of bleeding, signs of recurrent thrombosis, and initiation and monitoring of warfarin therapy. Much of this monitoring can be done by the visiting nurse, who should see the patient daily during the initial treatment period of 5-9 days.

It may also be useful for a nurse, a pharmacist, or a physician from the treatment team to periodically telephone the patient or caregiver to ensure that treatment is going as planned and that there are no complications. For patients selected to undergo home-based treatment with enoxaparin, the LMWH should be administered for at least five days, and warfarin can be started on the same day as the LMWH or the day after. Blood should be drawn daily to monitor the prothrombin time for the first few days; the International Normalized Ratio should be between 2.0 and 3.0 for two consecutive days before the LMWH is stopped.

Economic Considerations. One of the major impediments to more widespread use of LMWH in the outpatient treatment of DVT is economics. Although LMWHs are more expensive than UFH, the total cost of care is reduced for each event. Currently, financial incentives are misaligned in many U.S. health care facilities. Physicians are commonly reimbursed by patient day, whereas hospitals are typically reimbursed by case rates or DRGs for Medicare patients. Thus, hospitals do not benefit from avoiding hospitalization because they do not receive DRG payment. Physicians do not have any financial incentive to discharge early as their daily revenues will decline. Shortening the hospital stay, however, would result in considerable reduction in cost for the hospital while maintaining the same DRG reimbursement.

Hospitals should, therefore, be motivated to provide the necessary resources of infrastructure and personnel if overall cost savings can be achieved through a shortened hospital stay. If hospitalization can be completely avoided, Medicare patients avoid the substantial out-of-pocket cost of the Part A deductible, which currently is $768 per hospitalization. As Medicare does not cover outpatient prescription medications, these savings would be reduced to a degree by the costs of LMWH. The clinician should keep these financial implications in mind and recognize that elderly patients without supplemental insurance may be at risk for noncompliance. The pharmaceutical company that manufactures enoxaparin has a mechanism to provide enoxaparin for indigent patients and can assist in facilitating home care coverage for eligible patients. Case managers, social workers, and HHAs play crucial roles in the coordinated management of these patients.

In areas of the country with highly penetrated managed care such as California, outpatient protocols have been in place for years with high success.[32] In these settings, capitation payment arrangements often align incentives among physicians, hospitals, and health plans. A recent analysis has demonstrated that LMWHs are highly cost-effective for management of VTE when even a relatively small percentage of patients are eligible for outpatient treatment.[33]

Patient Acceptance. Some patients may be hesitant to have an abbreviated hospitalization or outpatient treatment for a potentially life-threatening condition such as DVT. At least one clinical study investigated patient compliance, acceptance, and satisfaction with such a protocol. In a prospective cohort of 113 consecutive patients presenting with acute DVT, 89 were treated at home with LMWH.[34] During the study, one patient died from a combination of PE and major bleeding. No other patient died during the three-month follow-up. One patient developed bleeding that required readmission to the hospital and five patients developed recurrent DVT. All had active malignant disease and developed their recurrence 2-12 weeks into their course of oral anticoagulation. Of the subjects who completed the satisfaction questionnaire, 75 of 82 (91%) were pleased with home treatment; 44 of 63 (70%) felt comfortable with the self-injection of LMWH; and 71 of 77 (92%) were satisfied with the support and instructions they received during their outpatient management.

Table 6. FDA-Approved Indications for LMWHs and Heparinoids

Ardeparin (Normiflo)

- DVT prophylaxis in total knee replacement

Dalteparin (Fragmin)

- DVT prophylaxis in abdominal surgery
- DVT prophylaxis in total hip replacement
- Unstable angina and non-Q- ave infarctions

Enoxaparin (Lovenox)

- DVT prophylaxis in total hip and total knee replacement and in patients at risk in abdominal surgery
- Unstable angina and non-Q wave infarctions
- Treatment of inpatient DVT with or without PE
- Outpatient treatment of DVT

Danaparoid (Orgaran)

- DVT prophylaxis in total knee replacement

Are LMWHs Interchangeable?

With the increasing introduction of LMWHs in the U.S. marketplace, there is interest as to whether these LMWHs are truly clinically distinct or whether they can be used interchangeably. Fareed et al have demonstrated distinct pharmacologic and biochemical profiles among LMWHs.[35] The Fifth American College of Chest Physicians' Consensus Conference on Antithrombotic Therapy states that although the various LMWHs have similar profiles, they may not be interchangeable clinically.[7] Each is produced through a distinct depolymerization process resulting in products with varying molecular weights, anti Xa:anti IIa activity ratios, release of tissue factor pathway inhibitor, bioavailability, and plasma half-lives.

For these reasons, the FDA has stated that LMWHs cannot be used interchangeably.[36] It is recognized that other LMWHs, including ardeparin and dalteparin, have been used in abbreviated hospitalization and outpatient studies and are currently being used in DVT treatment, particularly in other countries.[34,37] However, due to the ever-present threat of litigation and until more trials comparing LMWHs with each other are available, it would seem prudent to limit the use of LMWHs to those agents that are FDA-approved for their respective indications. (*Please see Table 6*). Nevertheless, the market must be sensitive to the enormous pressure placed on third-party payers, physicians, hospitals, and patients to continually seek cost-effective alternatives.

References

1. Turpie AGG. Management of venous thromboembolism: Optimization by clinical trials. *Haemostasis* 1996;26:220-226.
2. Dalen JE, Albert JS. Natural history of pulmonary embolism. *Prog Cardiovasc Dis* 1975;17:257-270.
3. Prevention of venous thromboembolism. International Consensus Statement. *Int Angiol* 1997;16:3-38.
4. Heit JA, et al. Predictors of survival after deep vein thrombosis and pulmonary embolism. *Arch Intern Med* 1999;159:445-453.
5. Hyers TM, et al. Antithrombotic therapy for venous thromboembolic disease. *Chest* 1998;114:561S-578S.
6. Raschke RA, et al. The weight-based heparin dosing nomogram compared with a "standard care" nomogram. A randomized controlled trial. *Ann Intern Med* 1993;119:874-881.
7. Hirsh J, et al. Heparin and low-molecular-weight heparin. *Chest* 1998;114:489S-510S.
8. Samama MM, et al. New data on the pharmacology of heparin and low molecular weight heparins. *Drugs* 1996;52(Suppl 7):8-15.
9. Thompson-Ford JK. Low-molecular-weight heparin for the treatment of deep vein thrombosis. *Pharmacotherapy* 1998;18: 748-758.
10. Weitz JI. Low-molecular-weight heparins. *N Engl J Med* 1997; 337:688-698.
11. Planes A, et al. Efficacy and safety of postdischarge administration of enoxaparin in the prevention of deep venous thrombosis after total hip replacement: A prospective randomised double-blind placebo-controlled trial. *Drugs* 1996;52(Suppl 7):47-54.
12. Borris LC, Lassen MR. Thromboprophylaxis with low molecular weight heparin after major orthopaedic surgery is cost effective. *Drugs* 1996; 52(Suppl 7):42-46.
13. Clagett GP, et al. Prevention of venous thromboembolism. *Chest* 1998;114:531S-560S.
14. Kay R, et al. Low-molecular-weight heparin for the treatment of acute ischemic stroke. *N Engl J Med* 1995;333:1588-1593.
15. Leizorovicz A. Comparison of the efficacy and safety of low molecular weight heparins and unfractionated heparin in the initial treatment of deep venous thrombosis: An updated meta-analysis. *Drugs* 1996;52(Suppl 7):30-37.
16. Levine M, et al. A comparison of low molecular weight heparin administered primarily at home with unfractionated heparin administered in the hospital for proximal deep-vein thrombosis. *N Engl J Med* 1996; 334:677-681.
17. Koopman MMW, et al. Treatment of venous thromboembolism with intravenous unfractionated heparin administered in the hospital as compared with subcutaneous low molecular weight heparin administered at home. *N Engl J Med* 1996;334:682-687.
18. Fiessinger JN, et al. Once-daily subcutaneous dalteparin, a low molecular weight heparin, for the initial treatment of acute deep vein thrombosis. *Thromb Haemost* 1996;76:195-199.
19. Hull RD, et al. Subcutaneous low-molecular-weight heparin compared with continuous intravenous heparin in the treatment of proximal-vein thrombosis. *N Engl J Med* 1992;326:975-982.
20. Brewer D. Should low-molecular-weight heparins replace unfractionated heparin as the agent of choice for adults with deep venous thrombosis? *J Fam Pract* 1998;47:185-192.
21. Spiro TE. A multicenter clinical trial comparing once and twice-daily subcutaneous enoxaparin and intravenous heparin the treatment of acute deep vein thrombosis. *Blood* 1997; 90(Suppl 1):295A.
22. Yeager BF, Matheny SC. Low-molecular-weight heparin in outpatient treatment of DVT. *Am Fam Physician* 1999;59:945-952.
23. Khamashta MA, et al. The management of thrombosis in the antiphospholipid-antibody syndrome. *N Engl J Med* 1995;332: 993-997.
24. Opinions regarding the diagnosis and management of venous thromboembolic disease. *Chest* 1996;109:233-237.
25. Kearon C, et al. A comparison of three months of anticoagulation with extended anticoagulation for a first episode of idiopathic venous thromboembolism. *N Engl J Med* 1999;340: 901-907.
26. Douketis JD, et al. Risk of fatal pulmonary embolism in patients with treated venous thromboembolism. *JAMA* 1998; 279:458-462.
27. Wolz M, et al. Studies on neutralizing effects of protamine on unfractionated and low molecular weight heparin (Fragmin) at the site of activation of the coagulation system in man. *Thromb Haemost* 1993;73:439-445.
28. Warkentin TE, et al. Heparin-induced thrombocytopenia in patients treated with low molecular weight heparin or unfractionated heparin. *N Engl J Med* 1995;332:1330-1335.
29. Monreal M, et al. Effects of long-term therapy with either heparin or low molecular weight heparin on serum lipid levels. A prospective study. *Haemostasis* 1995;25:283-287.
30. Shaughnessy SG, et al. The effects of low molecular weight heparin and standard heparin on calcium loss from fetal rat calvaria. *Blood* 1995;86:1368-1373.
31. Monreal M, et al. Comparison of subcutaneous unfractionated heparin with a low molecular weight heparin (Fragmin) in patients with venous thromboembolism and contraindications to coumarin. *Thromb Haemost* 1994;71:7.
32. Dedden P, et al. Pharmacy-managed program for home treatment of deep vein thrombosis with enoxaparin. *Am J Health Syst Pharm* 1997;54:1968-1972.
33. Gould MK, et al. Low-molecular-weight heparins compared with unfractionated heparin for treatment of acute deep vein thrombosis. *Ann Intern Med* 1999;130:789-799.
34. Harrison L, et al. Assessment of outpatient treatment of deep-vein thrombosis with low-molecular-weight heparin. *Arch Intern Med* 1998;158:2001-2003.
35. Fareed J, et al. Are the available low-molecular-weight heparin preparations the same? *Semin Thromb Hemost* 1996;22(Suppl 1):77-91.
36. Nightingale SL. Appropriate use of low-molecular-weight heparins. *JAMA* 1993;270:1672.
37. Goldhaber SZ, et al. Abbreviated hospitalization for deep venous thrombosis with the use of ardeparin. *Arch Intern Med* 1998;158:2325-2328.

Venous Thromboembolic Disease

Gideon Bosker, MD, FACEP

In the late 1970s, it was recognized that it might be possible to dissociate the beneficial antithrombotic effects of heparin from its hemorrhagic anticoagulant effects. This insight provided the impetus to fractionate heparin and isolate the antithrombotic effects in the form of low molecular weight heparins (LMWHs). Compared with unfractionated heparin (UFH), LMWHs have superior absorption and pharmacokinetic profiles, similar antithrombotic activities, and potentially fewer hemorrhagic complications. Moreover, LMWHs are proving to be at least as effective as heparin in a number of clinical settings, and they are revolutionizing the management of acute deep venous thrombosis by permitting home-based therapy. Finally, recent landmark studies (MEDENOX) have confirmed the effectiveness of at least one LMWH (enoxaparin) in preventing VTED in seriously ill medical patients. Risk-stratification strategies that identify those subgroups most suitable for prophylaxis are currently being established.

A number of LMWHs have been developed and approved for human use over the past decade. Interestingly, clinical use of LMWHs in the United States is relatively new, with four agents having received FDA approval: ardeparin (Normiflo®; Wyeth-Ayerst Laboratories), dalteparin (Fragmin®; Pharmacia & Upjohn), tinzaparin (Innohep®; Dupont); and enoxaparin (Lovenox®; Aventis Pharmaceuticals, Inc.). All four agents have been approved for management—prophylaxis and/or treatment—of venous thromboembolism (VTE). However, it should be stressed that enoxaparin is the only LMWH approved for VTED prophylaxis, inpatient and outpatient treatment of VTED, and acute management of ACS.

Although head-to-head trials are lacking, several observations and conclusions can be made about the current status of LMWHs in the treatment of venous and arterial thromboembolic disease. The first point is that all of the LMWH trials in ACS involved very high-risk patients, virtually all of whom had either ECG changes or NSTEMI. Nadroparin was superior to placebo in one trial and dalteparin was superior to placebo in both FRISC and FRISC II. This data, in addition to the finding that heparin was superior to placebo, reflects the second point: that high-risk patients should receive some heparin product, and the preferred agent (see below) is enoxaparin.

Of the four large randomized clinical trials, that compared a LMWH with heparin (FRIC, ESSENCE, TIMI-11B, and FRAXIS trials), only two trials, both using enoxaparin (ESSENCE and TIMI-11B), reflected superiority over heparin. Therefore, the third point is that only enoxaparin has been shown to be superior to heparin in the management of patients with unstable angina/NSTEMI. The fourth point is that there is not enough data to support the administration of any LMWH beyond the acute hospital phase and that chronic administration is associated with increased major hemorrhage.

Many factors will affect the future use of LMWHs for ACS. Some cardiologists are concerned about using the long-acting LMWHs at the time of PCI. Another factor is the increased use of antiplatelet agents including the glycoprotein IIb/IIIa inhibitors,

Table 1. The Burden of VTE in Medical Patients: Frequency of DVT in the Absence of Prophylaxis

General medical patients	10-26%	(Cade 1982; Belch et al, 1981)
Stroke	11-75%	(Nicolaides et al, 1997)
Myocardial infarction	17-34%	(Nicolaides et al, 1997)
Spinal cord injury	6-100%	(Nicolaides et al, 1997)
Congestive heart failure	20-40%	(Anderson et al, 1950)
Medical intensive care	25-42%	(Cade, 1982; Dekker et al, 1991; Hirsh et al, 1995)

thromboxane synthetase inhibitors (ridogrel), and ADP binding inhibitors (ticlopidine and clopidogrel). The interaction between these agents is unclear. Even with the rapidly expanding uses of the GP IIb/IIIa inhibitors, anticoagulation with an anti-thrombin agent remains is mandatory in the current management of ACS. Multimodal approaches will be elucidated with new clinical trials. A current algorithm for managing patients with ACS is provided in Figure 1.

With these new developments in clear focus, the purpose of this issue is to update clinicians on recent developments in the use of LMWH for ACS, VTED, and medical prophylaxis for seriously ill patients.

Table 2. Why is Prophylaxis Under-used?

- Clinicians are unaware of the level of VTE risk
- Heterogeneous population
- Perceived difficulties in risk assessment
- Few studies of prophylaxis
  - — poorly defined patient populations
  - — different methods of DVT diagnosis/outcome definition

Acute Coronary Syndromes (ACS): The Role of Heparins

Atherosclerotic plaque disruption associated with endothelial shearing results in thrombin generation and platelet activation. Heparin facilitates the action of circulating antithrombin III, an enzyme that inhibits thrombin and several other activated factors essential for the clotting cascade. Heparin's advantage over aspirin in unstable angina (USA) results from its direct antithrombin action. Although this action prevents new clot formation, it does not dissolve existing thrombus.

Five trials have evaluated the effectiveness of UFH in the management of USA.[1-3] A 1989 double-blind trial randomized 479 patients with USA into groups receiving aspirin, UFH, both, or neither.[3] All treatment arms experienced significantly fewer AMIs than the placebo group. There were no significant differences between treatment groups, but the combination of aspirin and UFH was associated with more episodes of serious bleeding (3.3 vs. 1.7 percent). A similarly designed investigation enrolling 796 men, the RISC trials of 1990 reported that aspirin reduced the risk of AMI and death while heparin had no significant influence on the event rate.[2] It was noted, however, that the group treated with heparin and aspirin had the lowest event rate during the first 5 days following onset of ischemic symptoms.

The latest study to address the use of heparin compared UFH with aspirin in 484 USA patients using a randomized, double-blind design.[4] Patients were followed 5.7 ± 3.3 days. AMI occurred in 0.8% of those treated with heparin and 3.7% of those receiving aspirin. A follow-up of a 1989 study of 479 patients reported reactivation of angina following discontinuation of therapy in significantly more patients who had received heparin than in those treated with aspirin or heparin and aspirin.[5] From this data, while it is not clear which is the better agent, or what the precise advantage combination confers, it is clear that both heparin and aspirin are beneficial in unstable angina.

There are no clear data to support continuous infusion of UFH over intermittent injection for USA, but the ACC/AHA guidelines recommend continuous infusion since it may reduce bleeding complications. The current recommended dosing is a bolus of 80 units/kg followed by a continuous infusion of 18 units/kg/hr to maintain an aPTT of 1.5 to 2.5 times control.[6]

It should be stressed that UFH has several disadvantages as an antithrombotic agent. For example, at therapeutic levels, it can lead to thrombin formation by activating platelets. Also, thrombin generation has been reported after discontinuation of UFH. UFH is difficult to administer, requiring continuous intravenous infusions and frequent monitoring of aPTT. The incidence of heparin-induced thrombocytopenia (HIT) is significant, and is greater in patients receiving GIIB/IIIA antiplatelet receptor inhibitors.

Low Molecular Weight Heparins (LMWHs). To circumvent these limitations and pitfalls of UFH—and also, to evaluate the possibility of improving patient outcomes in ACS—LMWHs such as enoxaparin have been intensively studied as a possible replacement for UFH in patients with USA and other acute coronary ischemic syndromes, including MQMI. From a pathophysiological perspective, LMWHs are more potent inhibitors of thrombin generation than UFH and are resistant to inhibition by activated platelets. The antithrombotic activity provided by LMWHs stabilizes the plaque, allowing the healing plaque to develop a smooth muscle layer with less disruption and diminished plaque propagation rates. This process is referred to as passification. Other benefits that LMWHs possess as compared to UFH include relatively simple dosing, ease of administration, limited requirements for further blood monitoring, and a more predictable anticoagulant effect.[7-9]

The rationale for use of LMWHs in acute coronary ischemic syndromes is supported by a number of evidentiary trials; in fact, the use of LMWHs in unstable angina has been evaluated in five large trials.[10]

Figure 1. Guidelines for Outcome-Effective Treatment of Acute Coronary Syndromes

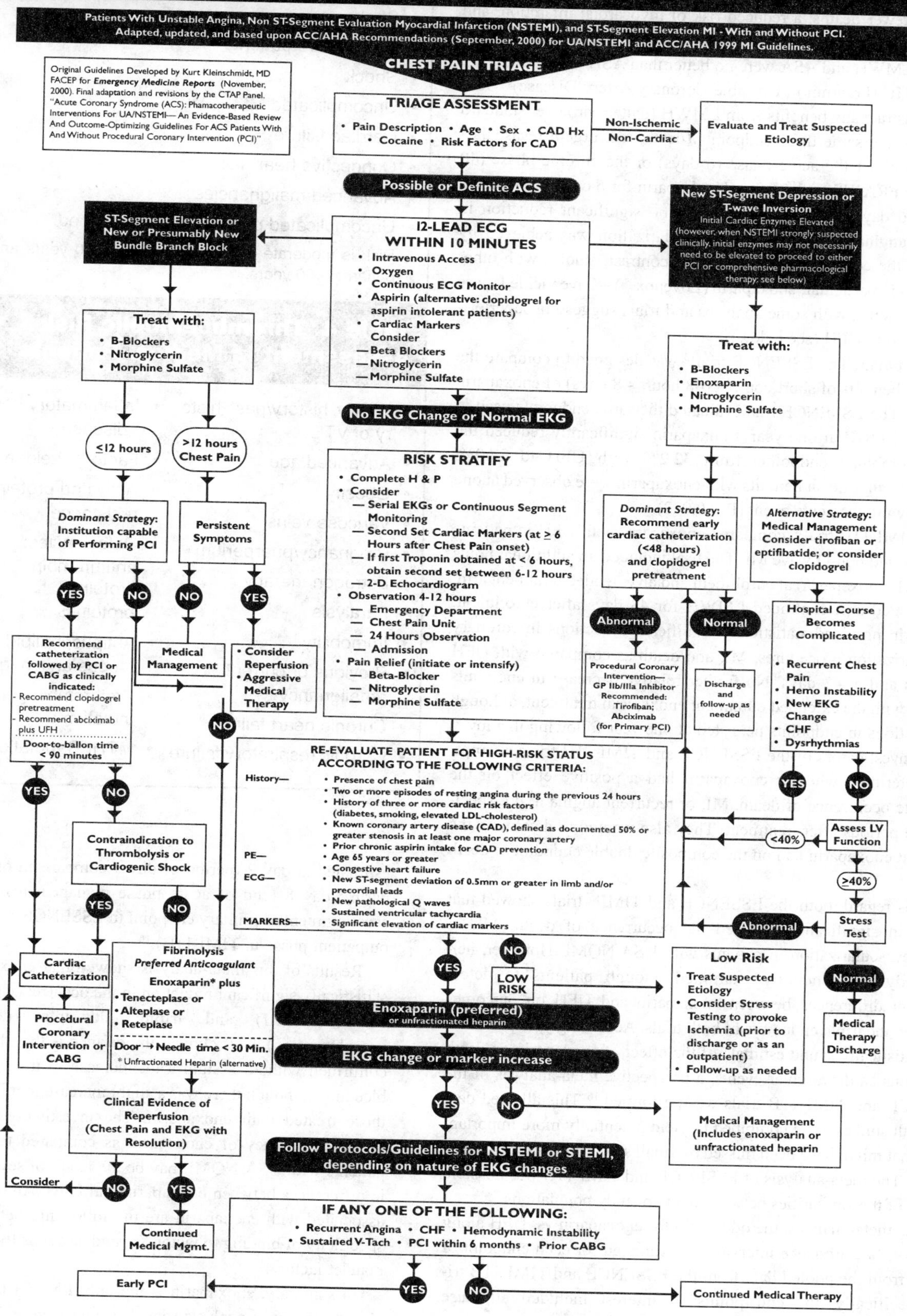

The FRISC (Fragmin® during Instability in Coronary Artery Disease) compared ASA and placebo versus ASA and dalteparin.[11] The addition of LMWH within 72 hours of presentation with ACS resulted in significantly fewer deaths, a reduced risk of myocardial infarction, and fewer urgent revascularization procedures than placebo. By 150 days, however, LMWH and ASA were no better than ASA alone.

The FRIC (Fragmin in Unstable Coronary Artery Disease)[60A] did not demonstrate any benefits from LMWH (dalteparin) over standard UFH using the same three endpoints (death, MI, urgent revascularization) in either the acute phase (6 days) or the chronic phase (40 days). The FRAXIS trial[12] infused nadroparin for 6 or 14 days versus UFH for 6 days. At 90-day follow-up, no significant reduction in recurrent angina, MI, or urgent revascularization was achieved by extending the course of the LMWH. In contrast, studies with other LMWHs—in particular, enoxaparin (Lovenox®)—have yielded more favorable results, with some analyses and trials suggesting superiority compared to UFH (see below).

Enoxaparin. The ESSENCE trial[13] was designed to compare the long-term benefits of short courses (48 hours - 8 days) of enoxaparin and UFH. The ESSENCE trial evaluated the same endpoints used in FRISC and FRIC at one year. Enoxaparin significantly reduced the 30-day combined endpoints from 32.2% with UFH to 27.0%. Statistically significant benefits with enoxaparin were observed at one year following the acute event (P = 0.022).

The TIMI 11B trial[14] compared enoxaparin with UFH in patients with USA and non-Q wave MI. The trial included an additional bolus of LMWH (enoxaparin) at enrollment and an extended treatment arm. The extended arm continued LMWH for 43 days after enrollment. Enoxaparin provided statistically significant reductions in coronary revascularization procedures, MI, and death as compared with UFH at 8 days and at 43 days. No further relative decrease in endpoints occurred with the extended outpatient enoxaparin treatment, although the reductions in endpoints persisted at one year following therapy.

The investigators of the ESSENCE and TIMI 11B trials attempted to determine whether enoxaparin had a positive effect on the composite occurrence of death, MI, or recurrent angina at pre-specified time periods after treatment. They also wanted to determine the effect that enoxaparin had on the composite double endpoint of death and MI.

In this regard, both the ESSENCE and TIMI[15] trials showed that enoxaparin significantly reduced the occurrence of death, MI, or urgent revascularization in patients with USA/NQMI. However, neither study independently examined enough patients to detect significant differences between enoxaparin and UFH on outcomes other than the triple endpoints of both trials. Accordingly, to provide a more statistically sound estimate of the effect of enoxaparin on death and serious cardiovascular events, a prospective meta-analysis of the ESSENCE and TIMI 11B trials was performed.[16] This allowed data from both studies to be combined to yield potentially more important results that might have been missed by small studies due to small sample size. The meta-analysis of ESSENCE and TIMI 11B was possible because of the similarities between the two study populations.

In the meta-analysis, the odds ratio for enoxaparin vs. UFH along with its 95% confidence interval was estimated for each endpoint of interest from the pooled data from the ESSENCE and TIMI 11B trials. Specifically, the end points of interest included all-cause mortality, recurrent myocardial infarction, urgent revascularization, and major hemorrhage. The odds ratio and confidence interval were estimated at day 2 (period of direct comparison of UFH vs. enoxaparin); day 8 (end of acute phase management); day 14 (time of ascertainment of primary endpoint in ESSENCE); and day 43 (end of outpatient phase in TIMI 11B).[16]

Results of this meta-analysis showed that enoxaparin provided a statistically significant reduction in the occurrence of composite double (death/MI) and triple endpoints (death/MI/recurrent vascularization).[16] Of clinical importance is that these benefits were confirmed without a significant increase in the incidence of major bleeding, although there was a slight increase in minor hemorrhage in those treated with enoxaparin. The investigators suggest that the increased efficacy of enoxaparin as compared to UFH in treating patients with USA/NQMI may be the result of several pharmacologic differences between enoxaparin and UFH. Among the advantages associated with enoxaparin are the following: better bioavailability; specificity of binding to factor Xa; and less sensitivity to inhibition of platelet factor 4.

In summary, enoxaparin is the only LMWH that in prospective, clinical and meta-analysis trials has consistently demonstrated superiority over UFH in the management of UA and NQMI. Although

Table 3. Medical Conditions Associated With Increased Risk of VTE

- Stroke
- Critical care patients
- Shock
- Uncomplicated MI
- Cardiac failure
- Congestive heart failure
- Advanced malignancies
- Uncomplicated patients confined to bed*

* Risk is moderate for patients ages 40-60 years and high for patients > 60 years.

Table 4. Thromboembolic Risk Assessment in Medical Patients

- Family history/past history of VTE
- Advanced age
- Obesity
- Varicose veins
- Pregnancy/puerperium
- Estrogen therapy
- Paralysis
- Immobility
- Previous or current malignancy
- Chronic heart failure
- Chronic respiratory failure
- Inflammatory bowel disease
- Factor V Leiden mutation
- Activated protein C resistance
- Defeciencies:
  antithrombin
  protein C
  protein S
- Antiphspholipid antibody/lupus anticoagulant
- Prothrombin gene mutation
- MTHFR mutation*

Table 5. Is Prophylaxis Beneficial in Medical Patients?

Reduction in DVT Frequency

PATIENT GROUP	STUDY	DVT FREQUENCY RISK (%): PLACEBO/UNTREATED	UFH PROPHYLAXIS
General medical patients	Cade, 1982	10	2 (NS)
	Belch et al, 1981	26	4 (P = 0.01 vs. control)
MI	Pooled data#	24	7
Ischemic stroke	Pooled data#	63	23
Intensive care	Cae, 1982	29	13 (P < 0.05 vs. control)
			LMWH PROPHYLAXIS
Elderly patients (> 85 years)	Dahan et al, 1986	9	3 (P < 0.05 vs. control)
Ischemic stroke	Pooled data#	63	16

#Reported in Clagett et al, 1998.
NS = not significant

large trials comparing the LMWHs to each other are lacking, in all studies LMWHs were at least as beneficial as UFH. However, only enoxaparin has demonstrated benefit over UFH in two trials, which enrolled more than 7,000 patients, perhaps because of its higher Xa to antifactor IIa activity.[8] Consequently, LMWHs, especially enoxaparin, should be considered for all patients presenting with ACS without ST segment elevations. Based on these studies, a number of authorities, consensus guidelines, and clinical reviews have encouraged clinicians to use enoxaparin as the preferred agent (rather than UFH) for managing patients with USA and non-Q-wave MI.

Prophylaxis in Seriously Ill Medical Patients

Venous thromboembolism (VTE) remains a major cause of mortality and morbidity in hospital patients, despite the availability of effective prophylactic agents.[17] Interestingly, studies demonstrate that the majority of patients who suffer a fatal pulmonary embolism (PE) have not undergone recent surgery,[18] but PE is rarely suspected as a cause of death in non-surgical patients[19] and prophylaxis is infrequently used,[20] despite consensus statement recommendations.[21-23] The burden of venous thromboembolic disease in non-surgical populations is significant[24,25] with certain medical conditions, among them congestive heart failure, respiratory failure, and systemic infection associated with elevated risk for thromboembolic disease (*See Table 1*). A review of recent studies evaluating risk factors in individual patients will help clarify the need for and value of thromboprophylaxis in clearly defined groups of medical patients.

Burden of Thromboembolic Disease. Compared with surgical populations, far fewer studies have reported on the frequency of VTE in medical patients. However, those figures that are available suggest a moderate risk of deep vein thrombosis (DVT) in general medical patients in the absence of prophylaxis[24,25] according to the risk categories (low, moderate, high) defined for surgical patients.[26] It should be noted that much higher rates of VTE have been observed in specific groups which, accordingly, should be risk-stratified to receive thromboembolic prophylaxis when indicated.[15,23-25,27-29] In this regard, a recent study reported that up to one in 20 hospitalized medical patients with multiple problems and severe immobility may suffer a fatal pulmonary embolism.[30] It should be noted, however, that current management practices emphasizing extensive use of thrombolytics, UFH, GIIB/IIIA inhibitors, LMWH, and antiplatelet agents, may contribute to a reduction in the incidence of VTE, including PE.

In light of the substantial burden of VTE in medical populations, current consensus statements on the prevention of VTE recommend assessment of all hospitalized patients, both medical and surgical, for thromboembolic risk, and use of appropriate prophylaxis. Specific prophylaxis recommendations have been made for patients with stroke and MI by the American College of Chest Physicians (ACCP)[21] and the International Consensus Conference.[23] Prophylaxis is also recommended for other groups of medical patients with clinical risk factors for VTE. However, recommendations are for poorly defined patient groups and vary among consensus documents. For example, recommendations by the UK-based second Thromboembolic Risk Factors (THRIFT II) Consensus Group[22] are based on the individual level of thromboembolic risk assessed for each patient.

Patient Risk Stratification and Prophylaxis. Despite current consensus statement recommendations, surveys show that prophylaxis is still underused in medical settings.[20] Several reasons explain these practice patterns *(Please see Table 2)*. First, despite epidemiological data demonstrating the prevalence of VTE, many clinicians remain unaware of the level of thromboembolic risk in medical settings. The diversity of medical patients, lack of reliable evidence demonstrating risk levels and perceived difficulty in assessing individual thromboembolic risk in the presence of multiple risk factors may contribute to the problem. The paucity of data from well-designed trials demonstrating the efficacy of prophylaxis in medical patients provides a further barrier to widespread use. Finally, even those studies that have been published to date are mostly small, involve poorly defined populations and vary in their endpoints, undermining confidence in their findings and preventing cross-trial comparisons.

From a clinical, need-to-prophylax perspective, a broad range of medical conditions are associated with an increased risk of VTE *(Please See Table 3)*. Some of these have been stratified according to the level of risk they confer,[31] although classifications may vary depending on concomitant risk factors. In particular, stroke, critical care patients, MI, and malignant disease are strongly linked to thromboembolic events. Other medical conditions known to increase the risk of VTE include inflammatory conditions such as systemic lupus erythematosus[32] and inflammatory bowel disease,[33] diabetic ketoacidosis, coma, and the nephrotic syndrome.[31] Recently, patients with severe cardiopulmonary diseases, including congestive heart failure and/or pulmonary infection or respiratory failure, have been identified as a moderate risk group.[21,31,35]

Although the current clinical condition is an important contributor to overall thromboembolic risk, underlying long-term risk factors appear to be at least as important in determining thromboembolic risk in medical patients.[16B] *(Please See Table 4)* Risk factors are similar to those cited for surgical patients, but unlike surgical patients, in medical settings underlying factors may be even more important than the current medical condition in determining overall risk.[31] The THRIFT II report, on which this slide is based, recommends clinical assessment and a series of blood tests to detect congenital and acquired molecular risk factors.[22] The International Consensus Statement suggests a similar series of blood tests for patients with a personal or family history of VTE.[23]

A number of clinical trials have demonstrated a reduction in the frequency of asymptomatic DVT in several medical populations through the use of pharmacological prophylaxis *(Please see Table 5)*. Some of these studies[21,24,25,35] illustrate a substantial reduction in the rate of DVT in medical patients as detected by the fibrinogen uptake test, suggesting that prophylaxis with either UFH or LMWH may be of value in these groups. The validity of these findings is questionable, however, because the fibrinogen uptake test has been shown to be a weak predictor of clinically important VTE.[38] Furthermore, while the benefit in high-risk stroke and MI patients appears significant, the evidence in general medical patients is less conclusive. Given the diversity of general medical patients, there is an urgent need for further investigations to assess the potential benefit of anticoagulant treatment in more clearly defined medical populations.

Nevertheless, three large studies, summarized on the slide, have assessed the impact of thromboprophylaxis on mortality in general medical patients.[37-39] However, all of these have methodological limitations, undermining the reliability of their findings. In one study, Halkin and colleagues[39] treated medical patients with open-label UFH 5000 IU b.i.d. or no treatment until discharge or mobilization. Although only 61% of eligible patients were treated, mortality in the treated group was significantly reduced from the first day of therapy. This effect appeared too early to be explained by a reduction in fatal PE, suggesting that the mortality reduction with UFH may have arisen via multiple mechanisms. In another study by Bergman and colleagues,[39] acute medical patients were randomized to nadroparin 7500 IU o.d. or placebo for 21 days. Mortality was similar in both groups, but the nadroparin group exhibited non-significant reductions in the rate of PE found at autopsy (15.9% vs. 28.3%, P=0.13) and clinical VTE (2.9% vs. 3.9%, P=0.18).

In the third study,[39] Gardlund and colleagues randomized infectious disease patients aged over 55 years to UFH 5000 IU b.i.d. or placebo for three weeks. Autopsy was available in 60% of patients who died. Deaths from PE were significantly delayed in the UFH group, but the six-week mortality rate was similar in both groups. Non-fatal VTE was reduced by UFH. The findings of previous trials of prophylaxis in medical patients have been controversial, as the patient populations and methods used to detect thromboembolism, and the dose regimens vary. Comparative studies with clearly defined populations and reliable end points are therefore required, and if there is a need for antithrombotic therapy, the optimal dosing should be confirmed.

MEDENOX Trial. In response to the need for evidence to clarify the role of prophylaxis in specific non-surgical patient subgroups, the

Table 6. MEDENOX Study

Prophylaxis of VTE in MEDical patients with ENOXaparin

AIMS

- Identify need for prophylaxis in clearly defined group
- Determine optimal dose

STUDY DESIGN

- Phase III, multicenter, randomized, double-blind, placebo-controlled, three parallel group
- Well-defined population: patients hospitalized with an acute medical disorder
- Enoxaparin 20 or 40 mg once daily vs. placebo, administered subcutaneously for 6-14 days
- DVT detected by routine bilateral ascending venography
- Follow-up at 3 months

Table 7. MEDENOX Inclusion Criteria

- Age > 40 years
- Recent immobilization (< 3 days) — autonomous walking distance < 10 meters
- Hospitalization due to one of:
  - heart failure (NYHA class III or IV)
  - acute respiratory failure
  - acute infectious disease/acute rheumatic disorder/active episode of inflammatory bowel disease PLUS pre-defined risk factor for VTE

Table 8. Pre-defined Risk Factors for VTE

- Age > 75 years
- Cancer: Previous or evolving
- History of VTE
- Obesity (BMI ≥ 30 kg/m^2 in males; 28.6 kg/m^2 in females)
- Varicose veins
- Estrogen/antiandrogen therapy (except replacement therapy for menopause)
- Chronic heart failure
- Chronic respiratory failure

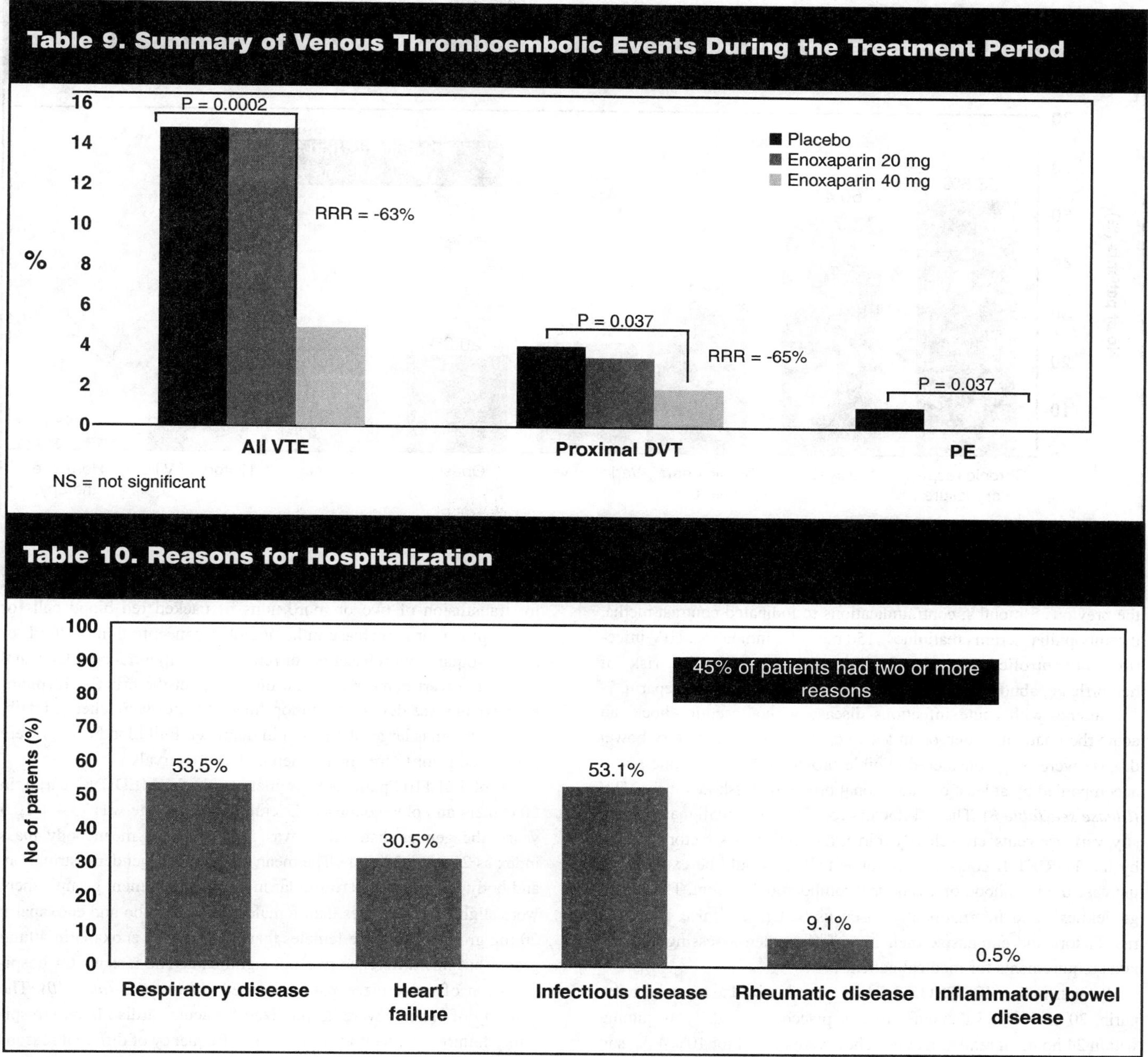

MEDENOX trial was conducted using the LMWH enoxaparin in clearly identified risk groups. In contrast to previous investigations, the MEDENOX trial included a clearly defined patient population—patients immobilized with severe chest (cardiopulmonary) disease—and was designed to answer questions about the need for prophylaxis in this group of medical patients and to determine the optimal dose of LMWH.

The design of the MEDENOX trial included a placebo arm, allowing determination of the thromboembolic risk and the need for prophylaxis in the clearly defined patient group. *(Please see Table 6.)*. According to the THRIFT II classification, the population would be expected to be at moderate risk of VTE, since low-risk patients and those with high-risk conditions (e.g., stroke or MI) were excluded.[22] However, the actual risk level for the defined population has not been confirmed in any previous trial. The use of systematic venography to detect DVT provided a reliable and accurate means of assessing prophylactic efficacy.

Inclusionary criteria for MEDENOX were intended to clearly define risk groups within the general medical population *(See Table 7)*. Patients were considered eligible if they were 40 years of age or older, had been immobilized for less than 3 days, and were hospitalized due to a specific, acute medical condition—in particular, heart failure, respiratory failure, an infectious disease, or a rheumatic disorder. In this regard, it should be stressed that patients with congestive heart failure and/or pulmonary infections have been highlighted in the most recent ACCP consensus statement as a specific target group requiring thromboprophylaxis.[21] Patients randomized in the MEDENOX Trial had a projected hospital stay of at least 6 days. Patients with respiratory failure were considered eligible provided they did not require respiratory support. The primary exclusion criteria were: preg-

Table 11. Risk Factors for VTE

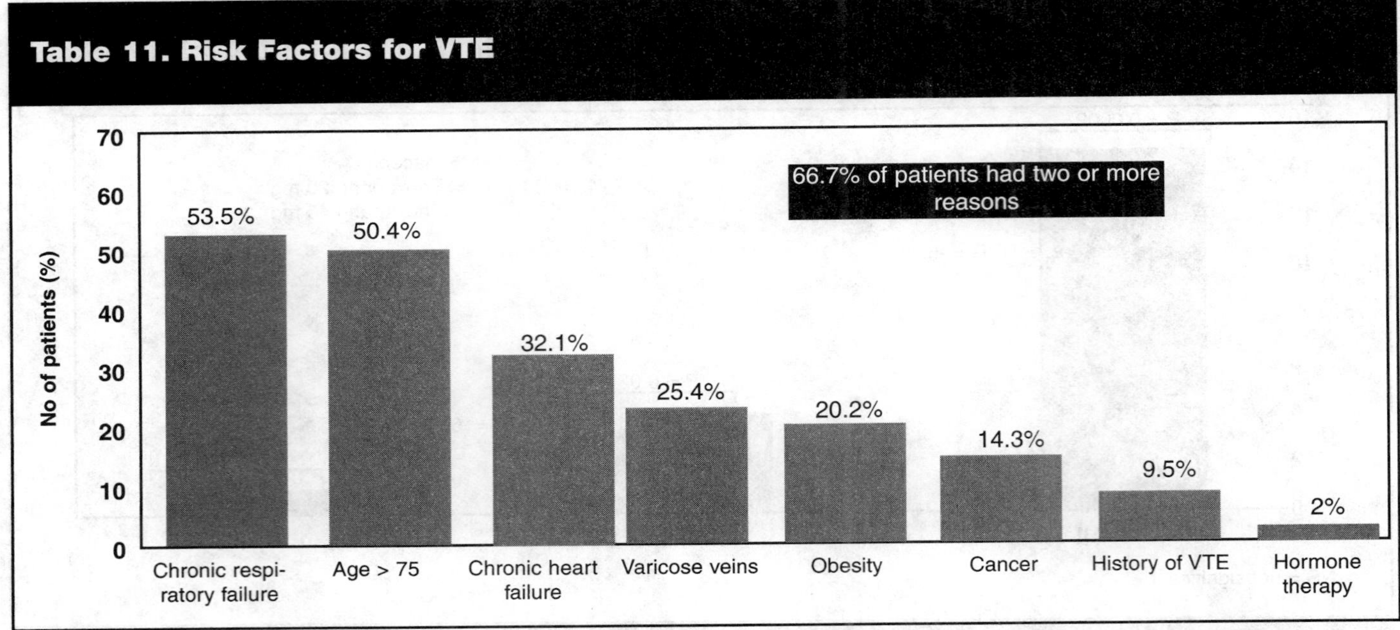

nancy or possible pregnancy, breastfeeding, stroke, major surgery in the previous 3 months; contraindications to iodinated contrast media, thrombophilia, serum creatinine > 150 mmol/L, intubation, HIV infection, uncontrolled hypertension, conditions conferring risk of hemorrhage, abnormal clotting tests, or hypersensitivity to heparin.

Patients with acute infectious disease without septic shock, an acute rheumatic disorder, or an active episode of inflammatory bowel disease were only considered eligible provided the acute illness was accompanied by at least one additional predefined risk factor for VTE *(Please see Table 8)*. The risk factors for VTE (age, malignancy, obesity, varicose veins, etc.) closely mirror the clinical risk factors defined by the THRIFT II consensus document,[22] and would be expected to increase the likelihood of a venous thromboembolic event. The ACCP guidelines[21] and International Consensus Statement[23] also cite these risk factors and emphasize their importance when assessing prophylaxis requirements for medical patients.

Patients in the MEDENOX Trial were randomized to receive enoxaparin, 20 or 40 mg subcutaneously, or placebo once daily, beginning within 24 hours of randomization. They were treated for 10 ± 4 days in the hospital and followed up in person or by telephone contact on day 90 (days 83-110). During follow-up, patients were instructed to report any symptoms or signs of VTE or any other clinical event *(Please see Table 9)*. The primary and secondary efficacy endpoints for MEDENOX were chosen to allow an objective assessment of the risk of VTE in the study population and extent of any benefit of prophylaxis. The primary endpoint was any venous thromboembolic event between day 1 and day 14. All patients underwent systematic bilateral venography at day 10 ± 4, or earlier if clinical signs of DVT were observed. Venous ultrasonography was performed if venography was not possible. Suspected PE was confirmed by high-probability lung scan, pulmonary angiography, helical computerized tomography, or at autopsy.

The primary safety endpoints were hemorrhagic events, death, thrombocytopenia, or other adverse event or laboratory abnormalities. As the principal adverse event associated with anticoagulant therapy, hemorrhage was a key safety outcome. Major and minor hemorrhagic events occurring during treatment were recorded. Major hemorrhage was defined as overt hemorrhage associated with a need for transfusion of two or more units of packed red blood cells or whole blood, or a decrease in hemoglobin concentration of 20g/L or more compared with baseline, or retroperitoneal, intracranial, or fatal bleeding. Overt hemorrhage that did not meet the criteria for major hemorrhage was defined as minor. Injection sites were checked daily for haematomas larger than 5 cm in diameter. Full blood counts were performed prior to treatment, then at 3-day intervals.

A total of 1102 patients were included in the MEDENOX trial, in 60 centers and nine countries. Overall, the mean age was 73.4 ± 10.5 years, the gender distribution was 50:50 and the mean body mass index as 25.0 ± 6.2 kg/m^2. The mean patient ages, gender distribution, and body mass index were similar in all three treatment groups; there were slightly more males than females in the placebo and enoxaparin 20 mg groups, and more females than males in the enoxaparin 40 mg group, but this difference was not significant. The reasons for hospitalization of randomized patients varied *(Please see Table 10)*. The majority of patients were hospitalized for acute cardiac failure, respiratory failure, or infectious disease. The frequency of different reasons for hospitalization was similar across all treatment groups. The number of patients in each hospitalization group suggests that a high proportion of acutely ill medical patients have two or more concomitant conditions, each contributing to the overall thromboembolic risk.

For the study population as a whole, the most prevalent risk factor in addition to the underlying illness was advanced age (50.4%), followed by varicose veins (25.4%), and obesity (20.2%) *(Please see Table 11)*. A similar number and proportion of patients in the three treatment groups exhibited each of the separate risk factors. Just over one-third of patients in each group had chronic cardiac failure, and about half suffered from chronic respiratory insufficiency.

Many of the patients in all three treatment groups had multiple risk factors. Overall, 96.9% of the study population (1068 patients) had at least one additional risk factor for VTE, in addition to their qualifying medical condition (heart failure or acute respiratory failure). Only 31 patients (2.8%) had no additional risk factors, 335 (30.2%) had one risk factor, and 733 (66.7%) had two or more risk factors. This pattern

Table 12. MEDENOX Conclusions

- Patients immobilized with severe cardiopulmonary, infectious, or rheumatic disease are at significant (moderate) risk of VTE.
- Enoxaparin 40 mg once daily given subcutaneously during 6 to 14 days is effective in reducing the risk of VTE by 63% in these patients.
- This is achieved without an increase in adverse events, in particular hemorrhage or thrombocytopenia, as compared to placebo.
- There is a trend toward mortality reduction with enoxaparin 40 mg once daily.

was similar in all treatment groups. The mean number of risk factors per patient was 2.1 ± 1.1, 2.0 ± 1.1 and 2.1 ± 1.1 in the placebo, enoxaparin 20 mg, and enoxaparin 40 mg groups, respectively. Multiple risk factors therefore appear to affect a high proportion of patients with acute cardiopulmonary or infectious disease. Risk factors for VTE have a cumulative effect on total risk.

The mean duration of treatment in MEDENOX was approximately 7 days with a standard deviation of 3 days. Duration of treatment did not differ significantly among the groups. Overall, 16% of patients had less than 6 days treatment (i.e., less than the planned minimum period) and 26% had more than 8 days. No patients were treated for longer than 14 days as per protocol specifications. The use of the continuation of any anticoagulant therapy after the end of the treatment period was left to the individual investigator's judgment. Of the 1102 patients included in the study, 1073 received at least one dose of the study drug and were included in the safety analysis.

Of the 1102 patients enrolled, a total of 866 patients were assessed for primary efficacy at day 14. The incidence of total, proximal, and distal DVT was significantly reduced with enoxaparin 40 mg compared with placebo. By day 14, the incidence of VTE was 14.9% in the placebo group and 5.5% in the enoxaparin 40 mg group, representing a significant 63% relative risk reduction (97% CI: 37-78%; P = 0.0002). Outcomes in the enoxaparin 20 mg group were not significantly different from placebo. A total of four symptomatic non-fatal PEs occurred, three in the placebo group and one in the enoxaparin 20 mg group. Finally, there was a trend toward mortality reduction with enoxaparin. By day 110, death had occurred in 50 (13.9%), 51 (14.7%) and 41 (11.4%) patients in the placebo, enoxaparin 20 mg, and enoxaparin 40 mg group, respectively. The 2.5% reduction in overall mortality in the enoxaparin 40 mg group was clinically meaningful but did not reach statistical significance.

By day 110,798 patients had been assessed for secondary efficacy. The significant reduction in total VTE and proximal and distal DVT observed in the enoxaparin 40 mg group was maintained at the 3-month follow-up. Relative risk reduction at 3-month follow-up: all VTE 59% and proximal DVT 66%. Four additional fatal PEs occurred during follow-up, one in the placebo group (3 weeks after the treatment period ended) and one and two in the enoxaparin 20 mg and 40 mg groups, respectively (2 months after the treatment period ended).

From a clinical safety perspective, there were no significant differences among the groups in the frequency of major or minor hemorrhage, thrombocytopenia, or any other adverse events. Major hemorrhage occurred in 11 patients during the treatment period; the fatal haemorrhage in the enoxaparin 40 mg group was considered unrelated to the study treatment by the investigators. Two additional fatal hemorrhages occurred during follow-up, one in the enoxaparin 20 mg group and one in the enoxaparin 40 mg group, 8 and 3 weeks after discontinuation of the study medication, respectively.

A total of 31 cases of thrombocytopenia occurred during the treatment period (13 cases in the placebo group, 10 in the enoxaparin 20 mg group and 8 in the enoxaparin 40 mg group). Fourteen of them were judged to be probably related to study medication, eight in the placebo group, four in the enoxaparin 20 mg group, and two in the enoxaparin 40 mg group. Remarkably, the three patients who experienced severe thrombocytopenia were all in the placebo group.

Clinical Implications and Analysis. The reason for the efficacy difference between the 20 and 40 mg doses of enoxaparin requires analysis. It may be that the prophylaxis requirements in medical patients differ from those in surgical patients with the "same" risk level. MEDENOX suggests that the 20 mg enoxaparin dose, approved for moderate-risk surgical patients, was insufficient to overcome the prothrombotic state in the population included this trial, which comprised elderly medical patients with multiple risk factors for VTE. Dose recommendations for surgical patients based on risk level clearly cannot be extrapolated to medical patients. The MEDENOX population responded well to the 40 mg dose, which is recommended in high-risk surgical patients. It is possible that the 20 mg dose may be effective in less severely ill medical patients and further studies are required to investigate this question.

The primary conclusions of the MEDENOX trial can be applied directly to clinical practice (*See Table 12*). First, acutely ill medical patients with cardiopulmonary or infectious disease are at significant risk of VTE. Second, enoxaparin, given once daily at a dose of 40 mg for 6 to 14 days reduces the risk of VTE by 63%; and third, the reduction in thromboembolic risk is achieved without increasing the frequency of hemorrhage, thrombocytopenia, or any other adverse event compared with placebo. An additional—and important—conclusion is that enoxaparin 20 mg once daily is not effective in preventing VTE in this patient group, and that these patients require the same dose of prophylaxis as that used in high-risk surgery. It might have been expected to be sufficient, since the frequency of VTE without prophylaxis (15%) falls within the "moderate-risk" category, according to the Salzman and Hirsh classification,[26] and the 20 mg dosage is effective in moderate-risk surgical patients.

Accordingly, the outcomes of the study demonstrate a qualitative difference in the nature of thromboembolic risk in medical and surgical patients. The medical patients randomized in MEDENOX were elderly, severely ill and had multiple underlying risk factors. By contrast, many moderate-risk surgical patients have only the single thrombogenic stimulus of wound healing following surgery. Clearly, medical and surgical patients should be considered separately for prophylaxis purposes, although it is possible that less severely ill medical patients may respond to a 20 mg dose of enoxaparin.

Summary

The introduction of LMWHs has provided a unique opportunity to improve outcomes and reduce cost in the management of selected patients with DVT. The FDA has approved enoxaparin for inpatient treatment of DVT with or without PE and for outpatient treatment of DVT. Managed care organizations and hospitals will embrace the use of LMWHs in short-stay or outpatient treatment protocols as a more cost-effective approach to the traditional but expensive inpatient management with UFH. Primary care physicians need to be familiar with outpatient protocols so that patients are selected appropriately and continuity of care is not jeopardized.

References

1. Lewis HD, Davis JW, Archibald DG, et al. Protective effects of aspirin against acute myocardial infarction and death among men with unstable angina. Results of a Veteran Administration Cooperative Study. *N Engl J Med* 1983;309:396-403.
2. Olatidoye AG, Wu AH, Feng Y, et al. Prognostic role of troponin T versus troponin I in unstable angina pectoris for cardiac events with meta-analysis comparing published studies. *Am J* Cardiol 1998;81:1405-1410.
3. Theroux P, Quimet H, McCans J, et al. Aspirin, heparin, or both to treat acute unstable angina. *N Engl J Med* 1988;319:1105-1111.
4. Theroux P, Waters D, Qui S, et al. Aspirin versus heparin to prevent myocardial infarction during the acute phase of unstable angina. *Circulation* 1993;88:2045-2048.
5. Theroux P, Waters D, Lam J, et al. Reactivation of unstable angina after the discontinuation of heparin. *N Engl J Med* 1992;327: 141-145.
6. ISIS-2 Collaborative Group. Randomized trial of intravenous streptokinase, oral aspirin, both or neither among 17,187 cases of suspected myocardial infarction: ISIS-2. *Lancet* 1988;2:349-360.
7. Hirsch J, Levine MN. Low molecular weight heparin. *Blood* 1992;79:1-17.
8. Hirsh J. Low molecular weight heparin: A review of the results of recent studies of the treatment of venous thromboembolism and unstable angina. *Circulation* 1998;98:1575-1582.
9. Melandri G, Semprini F, Cervi V, et al. Comparison of efficacy of low molecular weight heparin (parnaparin) with that of unfractionated heparin in the presence of activated platelets in healthy subjects. *Am J Cardiol* 1993;72:450-454.
10. Cohen M, Demers C, Gurfinkel EP, et al. A comparison of Low-molecular weight heparin with unfractionated heparin for unstable coronary disease. *N Engl J* Med 1997;337:447-452.
11. FRISC study group. Low molecular weight heparin during instability in coronary artery disease. Fragmin during Instability in Coronary Artery Disease (FRISC) study group. *Lancet* 1996;347: 561-568.
12. Klein W, Buchwald A, Hillis WS, et al. Fragmin in unstable angina pectoris or in non-Q-wave acute myocardial infarction (the FRIC study). Fragmin in Unstable Coronary Artery Disease. *Amer J* Cardiol 1997;80:30E-34E.
13. Cohen M, Demers C, Gurfinkel EP, et al. Low molecular weight heparins in non-ST-segment elevation ischemia: the ESSENCE trial. Efficacy and Safety of Subcutaneous Enoxaparin versus intravenous unfractionated heparin, in non-Q-wave Coronary Events. *Am J Cardiol* 1998;82:19L-24L.
14. Antman EM, McCabe CH, Gurfinkel EP, et al. Enaxaparin prevents death and cardiac ischemic events in unstable angina/non-Q-wave myocardial infarction. Results of the thrombolysis in myocardial infarction (TIMI) 11B trial. *Circulation* 1999;100:1593-1601.
15. Salzman EW, Hirsh J. Prevention of venous thromboembolism. In: Coleman RW, Hirsh J, Marder VJ, et al, Eds. *Hemostasis and Thrombosis: Basic Principles and Clinical Practice.* New York: Lippincott, 1982:986.
16. Antman EM, Cohen M, Radley D, et al. Assessment of the treatment effects of enoxaparins for unstable angina/non-Q-Wave myocardial infarction. TIMI 11B ESSENCE Meta Analysis. *Circulation* 1999;100:1602-1608.
17. Anderson FA, Wheeler HB, Goldberg RJ, et al. A population-based perspective of the hospital incidence and case-fatality rates of deep vein thrombosis and pulmonary embolism. The Worcester DVT study. *Arch Intern Med* 1991;151:933-938.
18. Sandler DA, Martin JF. Autopsy proven pulmonary embolism in hospital patients: Are we detecting enough deep vein thrombosis? *J Royal Soc Med* 1989;82:203-205.
19. Goldhaber SZ, Savage DD, Garrison RI, et al. Risk factors for pulmonary embolism — the Framingham study. *JAMA* 1983; 74:1023-1028.
20. Anderson FA, Wheeler HB, Goldbert R, et al. Physician practices in the prevention of venous thromboembolism. *Ann Intern Med* 1991;115:591-595.
21. Clagett GP, Andersen FA, Heit JA, et al. Prevention of venous thromboembolism. *Chest* 1998;114(5 suppl):531S-560S.
22. Second Thromboembolic Risk Factors (THRIFT II) Consensus Group. Risk of and prophylaxis for venous thromboembolism in hospital patients. *Phlebology* 1998;13:87-97.
23. Nicolaides AN, Bergquist D, Hull R, et al. Consensus statement. Prevention of venous thromboembolism. *Int Angiol* 1997:16: 3-38.
24. Belch JJ, Lowe GDO, Ward AG, et al. Prevention of deep vein thrombosis in medical patients by low-dose heparin. *Scott Med J* 1981;26:115-117.
25. Cade JF. High risk of the critically ill for venous thromboembolism. *Crit Care Med* 1982;10:448-450.
26. Anderson GM, Hull E. The effect of dicoumarol upon the mortality and incidence of thromboembolic complication of congestive heart failure. *Am Heart* J 1950;39:697-702.
27. Hirsh DR, Ingenito EP, Goldhaber SZ. Prevalence of deep venous thrombosis among patients in medical intensive care. *JAMA* 1995;274:335-337.
28. Dekker E, Nurmohamed MT, Heijboer H, et al. Incidence of deep venous thrombosis (deep vein thrombosis) in high-risk intensive care patients. *Thromb Haemost* 1991;65:1348.
29. Diebold J, LÆhrs U. Venous thrombosis and pulmonary embolism. A study of 5039 autopsies. *Path Res Pract* 1991;187:260-266.
30. Baglin TP, White K, Charles A. Fatal pulmonary embolism in hospitalized medical patients. *J Clin Pathol* 1997;50:609-610.
31. Gensini GF, Prisco D, Falciani M, et al. Identification of candidates for prevention of venous thromboembolism. *Semin Thromb Hemost* 1997;23:55-67.
32. Gladman DD, Urowitz. Venous syndromes and pulmonary embolism in systemic lupus erythematosus. *Ann Rheum Dis* 1980;39:340-343.
33. Talbot RW, Heppel J, Dozois RR, et al. Vascular complications of inflammatory bowel disease. *Mayo Clin Proc* 1986;1:140-145.
34. Gallus AS. Anticoagulants in the prevention of venous thromboembolism. In: Hirsh J, Ed. *Antithrombotic Therapy.* London : Bailliere Tindall; 1990:675-677.
35. Dahan R, Houlbery D, Caulin C, et al. Prevention of deep vein thrombosis in elderly medical in-patients by a low molecular weight

heparin: a randomized double-blind trial. *Haemostasis* 1986; 16:159-164.

36. Ledlle FA. Heparin prophylaxis for medical patients? (editorial). *Ann Intern Med* 1998;128:768-770.
37. Halkin H, Goldberg J, Modan M, et al. Reduction of mortality in general medical n-patients by low-dose heparin prophylaxis. *Ann Intern Med* 1982;96:561-565.
38. Bergmann J-F, Caulin C. Heparin prophylaxis in bedridden patients. *Lancet* 1996;348:205-206 (letter).
39. Gardund B for the Heparin Prophylaxis Study Group. Randomized, controlled trial of low-dose heparin for prevention of fatal pulmonary embolism in patients with infectious diseases. *Lancet* 1996;347:1357-1361.

Bradycardia

Richard A. Harrigan, MD
William J. Brady, MD

Bradycardic patients present unique challenges for the emergency department (ED) physician. First, the clinician must determine the stability of the patient and promptly institute any necessary resuscitation measures before proceeding with further evaluation and work-up of the dysrhythmia. Naturally, consideration always should be given to age-related and/or situational parameters associated with bradycardic syndromes. For example, the athletic, 24-year-old female with an ankle sprain, a heart rate of 44, and a blood pressure of 90/60 mmHg requires a much different approach than the 74 year-old presenting with chest pain and the same vital signs. After hemodynamic stability is achieved, the etiology of the bradydysrhythmia can be investigated in more detail.

Defining a bradycardic rhythm requires a working knowledge of the cardiac conduction system and an understanding of the various electrocardiographic manifestations of bradycardia. Moreover, bradycardia is associated with an extensive differential diagnosis. In this regard, after such critical entities as acute myocardial infarction, sepsis, hypoxia, hypoglycemia, and hypothermia have been considered, the differential expands to include a wide variety of other cardiac and systemic conditions. Finally, evaluation and treatment options should be revisited to ensure the underlying condition was addressed in the therapeutic plan.

The following review of the emergency evaluation and treatment of bradycardia includes a practically oriented discussion of the relevant anatomy, followed by a discussion of the electrocardiographic spectrum of bradydysrhythmias. The etiology and pathophysiology of bradycardia will be discussed, considering both cardiac and extracardiac causes. Finally, a review of pharmacologic and non-pharmacologic treatment modalities will be presented.

Cardiac Conduction System: Anatomy and Electrophysiology

A basic understanding of the cardiac conduction system requires a knowledge of relevant structures and their connections, as well as the blood supply to these structures. *(Please see Table 1.)* Normally, impulse conduction commences at the sinoatrial (SA) node, which is located at the junction of the superior vena cava and the right atrium. The SA node is generously innervated by both branches of the autonomic nervous system. The cardiac impulse next traverses intra-atrial fibers to reach the atrioventricular (AV) node, which is located above the ostium of the coronary sinus at the base of the interatrial septum on the posteromedial portion of the right atrial wall.

Emerging from the AV node is the bundle of His, which enters the fibrous skeleton of the heart and runs anteriorly across the membranous interventricular septum. The His bundle then subdivides into right and left bundle branches. The right bundle branch cours-

Table 1. Vascular Supply of the Cardiac Conduction System[1,2]

STRUCTURE	IMMEDIATE BLOOD SUPPLY	CORONARY VASCULAR SUPPLY
SA node	Sinus nodal artery	RCA 60% LCX 40%
AV node	AV nodal artery	PDA (of RCA) 90% LCX 10%
Bundle of His	AV nodal artery	PDA (of RCA) 90% LCX 10%
	Septal perforating arteries	LAD
Right bundle branch	AV nodal artery	PDA (of RCA) 90% LCX 10%
	Septal perforating arteries	LAD
Left bundle branch		
Anterior fascicle	Septal perforating arteries	LAD
Posterior fascicle		LAD PDA (of RCA)

Key:
RCA = right coronary artery
LCX = left circumflex artery
PDA = posterior descending artery
LAD = left anterior descending artery
Percentages refer to inter-, rather than intra-individual variations in blood supply.

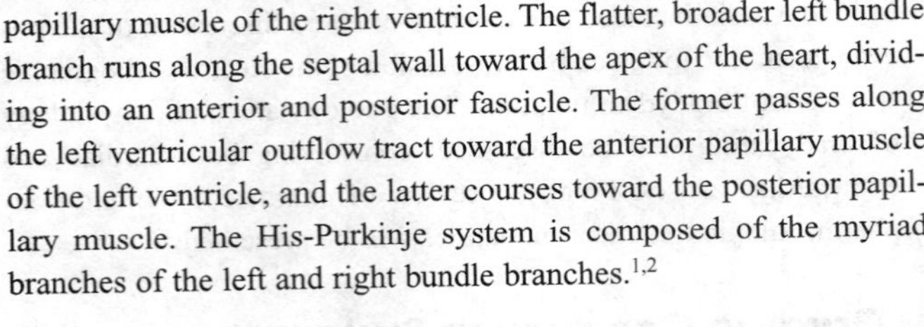

es along the interventricular septum toward the base of the anterior papillary muscle of the right ventricle. The flatter, broader left bundle branch runs along the septal wall toward the apex of the heart, dividing into an anterior and posterior fascicle. The former passes along the left ventricular outflow tract toward the anterior papillary muscle of the left ventricle, and the latter courses toward the posterior papillary muscle. The His-Purkinje system is composed of the myriad branches of the left and right bundle branches.[1,2]

The electrophysiologic manifestations of the anatomical configuration of the conduction system are observed on the electrocardiogram. The duration of the P wave reflects the duration of atrial activation, which proceeds from right atrium to left. The PR interval represents the time interval between the onset of atrial depolarization and the beginning of ventricular depolarization. During this time, the impulse travels from the atria (not including the time it took to move from the SA node itself to the right atrium), through the AV node, the bundle of His, the bundle branches, and the Purkinje fibers, until the ventricular myocardium begins to depolarize.

Ventricular activation is reflected in the duration of the QRS complex.[3] The frequency of P waves, the relationship between P waves and other activation sites, or the absence of the P waves, analyzed along with length of the PR interval, are the most important parameters for assessing bradydysrhythmias. Stated differently, bradydysrhythmias are the result of sinus node dysfunction or AV conduction disorders; these, in turn, are affected by diseases (e.g., myocardial ischemia), conditions (e.g., hypothermia), or drugs (e.g., digoxin) that affect the automaticity and refractoriness of cardiac cells, and conduction of impulses within the system.[1]

Electrocardiographic Analysis

Regular Bradycardia. Sinus bradycardia (SB) is defined as the presence of sinus rhythm with a rate less than 60 beats per minute (bpm); that is, the P wave morphology, the PR interval, and the P-P intervals are all uniform and normal.[1] *(Please see Figure 1.)* The parameters of so-called "normality" must be flexible, however, inasmuch as rates less than 60 bpm may be normal for some individuals. For example, highly trained endurance athletes may exhibit a resting sinus bradycardia of 30 to 40 bpm, due to increased vagal tone.[1,3]

In some cases, lower pacemakers may assume control of rhythm in the absence of sinus node activity. A junctional rhythm is by definition bradycardic, and is characterized by a regular, narrow QRS

Figure 1. Sinus Bradycardia

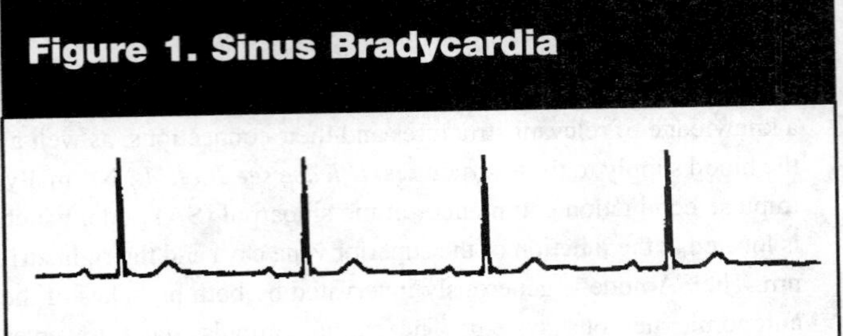

Sinus bradycardia is noted when the ventricular rate is less than 60 bpm, the QRS complex is narrow, the rhythm is regular, and each P wave is associated with a QRS complex.

Reprinted with permission from: Brady WJ, Harrigan RA. Evaluation and management of bradyarrhythmias in the emergency department. *Emerg Med Clin North Am* 1998;16:361-388.

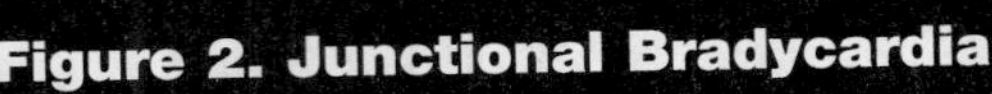

Figure 2. Junctional Bradycardia

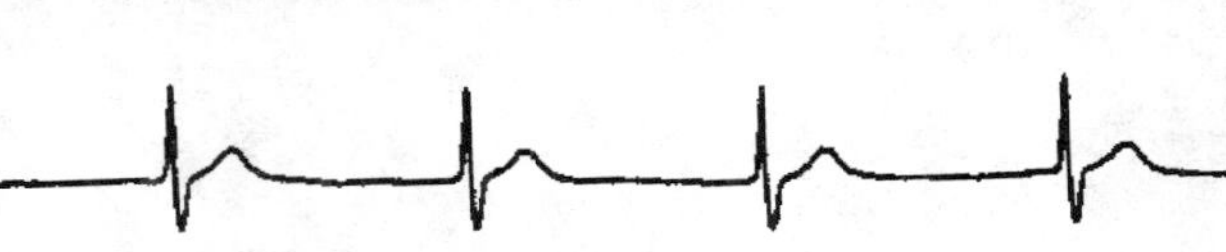

A junctional rhythm is noted with a narrow-QRS complex and ventricular rates of 45-60 bpm.

Reprinted with permission from: Brady WJ, Harrigan RA. Evaluation and management of bradyarrhythmias in the emergency department. *Emerg Med Clin North Am* 1998;16:361-388.

Figure 3. Idioventricular Bradycardia

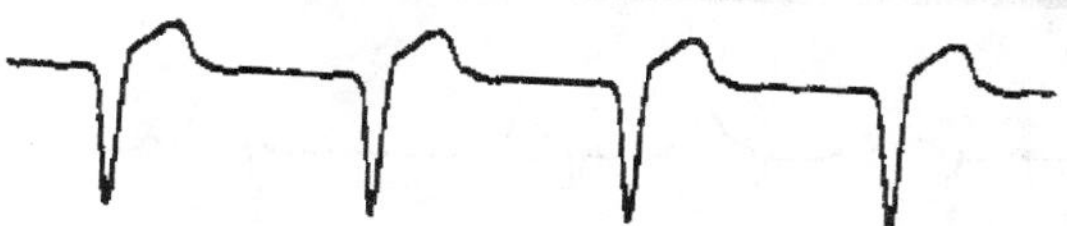

An idioventricular rhythm is noted if the focus of the escape rhythm is found in the His-bundle branch block system; the QRS complex is wide with a rate of 30-45 bpm.

Reprinted with permission from: Brady WJ, Harrigan RA. Evaluation and management of bradyarrhythmias in the emergency department. *Emerg Med Clin North Am* 1998;16: 361-388.

complex rhythm at a rate between 40 to 60 bpm *(Please see Figure 2.)* There may be no evidence of P waves, or retrograde P waves may be seen. Retrograde refers to conduction from, rather than to, the AV node, and the retrograde P may come before, after, or during the QRS complex on the ECG.[3] Junctional rhythms may emanate from the AV node, in which case the rate is higher (45 to 60 bpm). In contrast, slower, narrow complex junctional rhythms (35 to 45 bpm) have been found to originate in the His bundle.[3] An idioventricular rhythm *(please see Figure 3)* usually is between 30 and 40 bpm, but may be as slow as 20 or as rapid as 50 bpm. The QRS complexes are widened abnormally. If the new pacemaker site is located in the ventricular septum, however, the complexes may be close to the upper limits of normal in width. Preexisting intraventricular conduction delays can make a slow junctional escape rhythm indistinguishable from a fast idioventricular rhythm.[3]

Traditionally, the various degrees of AV block (first-, second-, and third-degree) are considered together in a discussion of AV conduction defects. It may be useful to consider bradycardias as regular vs. irregular, as we do the tachycardias. Accordingly, first- and third-degree AV block can be considered here. First-degree AV block *(please see Figure 4)* is a regular rhythm; the P-P and R-R intervals are uniform. The PR interval is prolonged, by definition, to greater than 0.20 seconds; this may be uniform on a tracing or there may be some variability in the degree of prolongation, which may be linked to changes in heart rate and vagal tone.[3] Electrophysiologically, the delay in first-degree AV *block* may be in the atrial fibers, the AV node, or the His-Purkinje system.

Third-degree AV block (complete heart block) also is a regular rhythm. *(Please see Figure 5.)* The P-P and R-R intervals are constant (unless there is sinus arrhythmia, with some variability then being seen in the P-P intervals), but the PR intervals are variable. This is considered by some to be a type of AV dissociation, as the two chambers are functioning independently of each other. Others state that true AV dissociation exists only when increased automaticity of a lower pacemaker renders its rate faster than that of the atria, leaving the ventricle refractory to activation from the slower atrial impulses, as in the case of ventricular tachycardia.[3] In complete heart block, the atrial pacemaker can be either sinus or ectopic, and may be tachycardic or bradycardic, but it is faster than the lower pacemaker, which can be

Figure 4. First-Degree Atrioventricular Block

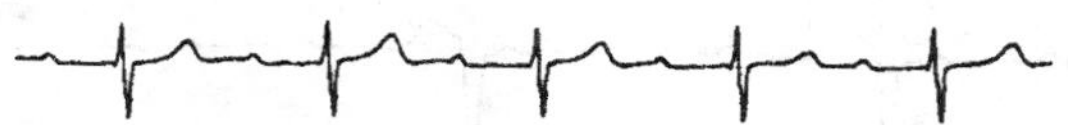

The PR interval is prolonged with a duration greater than 0.20 sec and is constant without progressive change with both a normal P wave and QRS complex. Every atrial impulse is conducted to the ventricles.

Reprinted with permission from: Brady WJ, Harrigan RA. Evaluation and management of bradyarrhythmias in the emergency department. *Emerg Med Clin North Am* 1998;16:361-388.

either junctional or ventricular. *(please see Figure 6.)* The location of that lower pacemaker determines the width of the QRS complexes and the rate of ventricular contraction, as previously discussed.[1,3]

Irregular Bradycardias. Sinus arrhythmia is defined as normal, consistent P wave morphology with variation in the P-P interval of greater than 0.16 seconds. This arrhythmia is seen more commonly in the context of slow rates, so it deserves discussion within the context of sinus bradyarrhythmias. Two types exist: respiratory sinus arrhythmia is the more common variant, in which the rate slows with expiration and speeds up with inspiration. This phasic change results from pulmonary reflex-mediated changes in vagal tone. The less common, non-respiratory sinus arrhythmia has an unknown mechanism, and is more often seen in patients with heart disease.[3] It should be noted that sinus arrhythmia also can present with non-bradycardic rhythms.

Sinus pause and sinus arrest are related entities, primarily differing in the degree rate slowing. Sinus pause is characterized by a transient cessation of impulse generation from the SA node; if this is prolonged, it is classified as sinus arrest. The pathophysiological dis-

Figure 5. Third-Degree Atrioventricular Block with Narrow QRS Complex

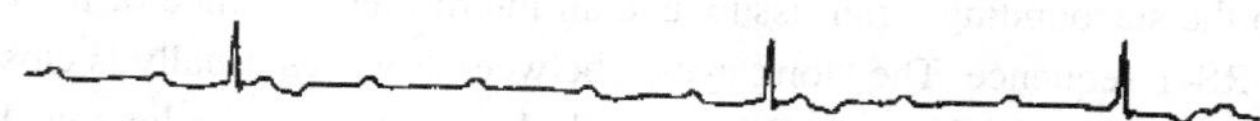

No meaningful relationship is noted between the P waves and the QRS complex. The P waves will appear in a regular rhythm and will "match" through the rhythm strip at a specific atrial rate. The QRS complexes should appear in a regular fashion and also will "march" through the rhythm strip. The duration of the QRS complex and the ventricular escape rhythm is located near the His bundle, the rate is greater than 40 bpm, and the QRS complexes tend to be narrow.

Reprinted with permission from: Brady WJ, Harrigan RA. Evaluation and management of bradyarrhythmias in the emergency department. *Emerg Med Clin North Am* 1998;16:361-388.

Figure 6. Third-Degree AVB with Widened QRS Complex

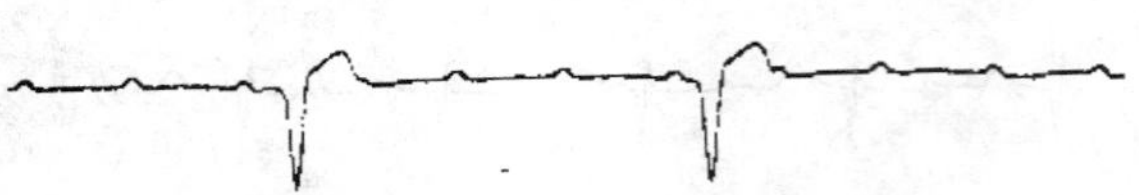

When the site of escape is distal to the His bundle, the rate tends to be less than 40 bpm and the QRS complexes tend to be wide.

Reprinted with permission from: Brady WJ, Harrigan RA. Evaluation and management of bradyarrhythmias in the emergency department. *Emerg Med Clin North Am* 1998;16:361-388.

tinction is not always clear.[3] The sinus pause may be terminated by a sinus beat, an AV junctional complex, or a ventricular escape beat, depending on the length of the pause. Thus, the rhythm is irregular, and bradycardic during the period of pause. There may be periods of other rhythms on a prolonged rhythm strip (e.g., normal sinus rhythm), which are punctuated by bradycardic interludes.

Sinoatrial block (SA block, or SA exit block) is a somewhat confusing entity. The confusion probably stems from the fact that it is difficult to detect on the normal 12-lead surface ECG; in fact, it can only be inferred from the P wave activity.[3] As with AV block, there are three degrees of SA block. Only one variant (second-degree SA block; see next section) can be detected in the ED using 12-lead ECG. First-degree SA block cannot be distinguished on a standard ECG; this entity reflects prolonged conduction time from the SA node to the surrounding atrial tissue, but the P-P, R-R, and PR intervals are uniform. There is a gap in time between SA node impulse formation and P wave occurrence, but the emergency physician cannot detect this by evaluating the ECG at the bedside. Similarly, third-degree SA block cannot be distinguished from sinus arrest at the bedside.

The only SA block that can be distinguished on a standard 12-lead ECG is an irregular rhythm, second-degree SA block. In this conduction disturbance, there is intermittent failure to conduct sinus impulses to the surrounding atrial tissue, and an intermittent absence of the P-QRS-T sequence. The "long cycle" between P waves usually is close to a multiple of the basic P-P interval, the duration of the long cycle being just short of the exact multiple of the P-P interval. As such, it may be difficult to distinguish from marked sinus arrhythmia, blocked premature atrial contractions, and periods of sinus pause.[1,3]

Second-degree AV block is usually, but not always, manifested by an irregular rhythm. There are two types of second-degree AV block: Mobitz Type I and Mobitz Type II. Both feature intermittent failure of atrial impulses to reach the ventricles (i.e., some of the P waves are not followed by QRS complexes). Mobitz Type I features "grouped beating," meaning the QRS complexes appear in groups, separated by a pause, which produces the irregularity. *(See Figure 7.)* The morphology of the P waves and the QRS complexes generally are normal. However, the PR interval progressively lengthens until an atrial impulse cannot reach the ventricle, in which case a "dropped beat" occurs; this represents a nonconducted P wave. An additional feature

Figure 7. Second-Degree, Type I Atrioventricular Block (Wenkebach Block)

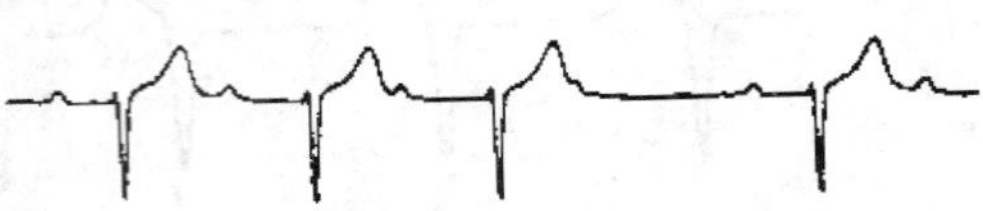

The PR interval is often normal in the first beat of the series. Progressive PR interval lengthening with subsequent beats is observed until an impulse is unable to reach the ventricles, resulting in a nonconducted P wave. After the dropped beat, the PR interval returns to normal and the cycle repeats. P-waves and QRS complexes are usually normal in terms of morphology and total duration. A pattern to the RR interval also is seen with RR interval becoming increasingly shorter. Following the dropped beat, the RR interval in the subsequent beats tend to shorten. One also will notice on the rhythm strip a grouping of beats, referred to as grouped beating of Wenkebach.

Reprinted with permission from: Brady WJ, Harrigan RA. Evaluation and management of bradyarrhythmias in the emergency department. *Emerg Med Clin North Am* 1998;16: 361-388.

is a progressive shortening of the RR interval as the PR interval gets progressively longer.

Taken together, these characteristics are known as the Wenkebach phenomenon. In some cases, there is Type I second-degree AV block without the typical Wenkebach phenomenon, i.e. there is no progressive lengthening of the PR intervals before the dropped QRS. The PR interval may be variable and the RR interval may not progressively shorten. However, in this variety of Mobitz Type I, the biggest increase in the PR interval may be seen just before the nonconducted P, and the shortest PR interval occurs after the nonconducted P.[3] The less commonly encountered Mobitz type II AV block also features intermittently blocked P waves, but in contrast to Type I, the PR intervals are constant in the conducted beats; whether normal or prolonged, they are uniform. *(Please see Figure 8.)* Most patients with Type II AV

Figure 8. Second-Degree, Type II Atrioventricular Block with 3:2 Conduction

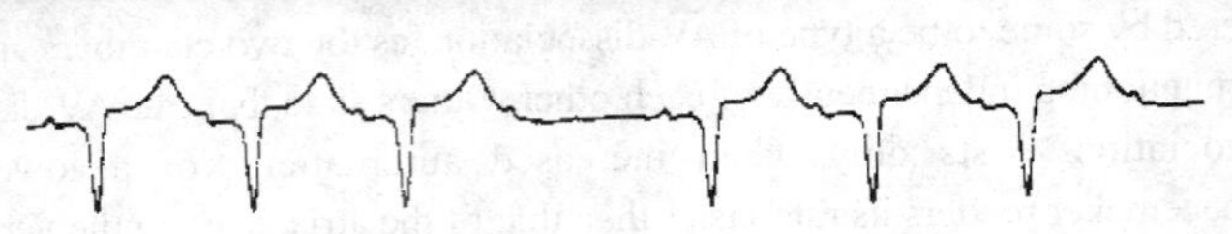

Reprinted with permission from: Brady WJ, Harrigan RA. Evaluation and management of bradyarrhythmias in the emergency department. *Emerg Med Clin North Am* 1998;16:361-388.

Figure 9. Second-Degree, Type II Atrioventricular Block with 2:1 Conduction

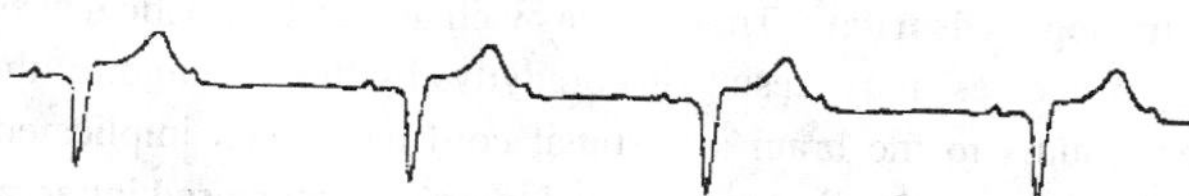

The PR interval is constant without progressive lengthening and may be either normal or prolonged. The QRS complex is widened in most instances. The magnitude of the AVB is expressed as a ration of P waves to QRS complexes. For example, if there are two P waves for every QRS complex, then it is a 2:1 block as seen here. Distinguishing type I from type II block is relatively straightforward unless there is 2:1 conduction as seen in this example. In this situation, there is no way to compare the PR intervals for the conducted beats and hence make the distinction between Mobitz Type I and type II AVBs. The width of the QRS complex in Mobitz Type II block, however, may give the clinician information as to the level of block; Type II AVB is usually characterized by an escape rhythm with a widened QRS complex. Nonetheless, in situations of 2:1 conduction the physician should initially assume the block is a Mobitz II unless proven otherwise, owing to the relatively malignant course of type II AVB.

Reprinted with permission from: Brady WJ, Harrigan RA. Evaluation and management of bradyarrhythmias in the emergency department. *Emerg Med Clin North Am* 1998;16: 361-388.

block have an associated bundle branch block, meaning the block is distal to the His bundle; rarely (approximately one-third of the time) the block is in the bundle of His or in the AV node, rendering a narrow complex QRS.[3] The occasional dropped beats lead to interludes of intermittent bradydysrhythmia.

The magnitude of AV block is expressed as a ratio of P waves to QRS complexes, termed the conduction ratio. When the conduction ratio is 2:1, it is impossible to differentiate the two types of second-degree AV block, since the conduction of every other P wave is blocked; thus, the PR interval cannot be assessed for lengthening. *(Please see Figure 9.)* This may simulate SB, especially if the nonconducted P waves are buried in the preceding T waves.[3] Moreover, like SB, 2:1 AV block is a generally regular rhythm; if there is variability of the conduction ratio over time (on a long rhythm strip), irregularity will become evident, and the differentiation between Mobitz I and II may be clearer.

Differential Diagnosis: Cardiac and Non-Cardiac Causes of Bradycardia

The differential diagnosis of bradycardia is extensive, and can be considered in a number of ways. The following discussion will examine cardiac causes (ischemic and nonischemic), which will be followed by a section on extracardiac causes.

Ischemia. A variety of bradydysrhythmias (bradycardia and conduction block) may complicate acute myocardial infarction (AMI). SB occurs in about 40% of patients with AMI; junctional (20%) and idioventricular (15%) dysrhythmias occur far less frequently. First-, second- (Mobitz Type I), and third-degree AV blocks occur in approximately 15%, 12%, and 8% of AMIs, respectively; Mobitz Type II AV block is very unusual.[4,5] When considering only the unstable bradydysrhythmias, third-degree AV block is the most frequently encountered in this setting (40%). SB (25%) and junctional rhythm (20%) follow complete heart block in frequency of unstable rhythms in AMI.[4,5]

The pathophysiology of bradydysrhythmia in AMI can be multifactorial. In most cases, ischemia or infarction of cardiac tissue is the underlying cause. Other mechanisms that may be associated with the AMI include: hyperkalemia, hypoxia, acidosis, local increase in adenosine concentration, variations in autonomic control, and pharmacotherapy (especially calcium channel antagonists and beta adrenergic blockers). Occurrence of bradydysrhythmia in AMI also varies depending upon the location of the coronary vascular lesion. Inferior AMI is more frequently complicated by bradydysrhythmias; in most cases, this results from occlusion of the right coronary artery (RCA).[3] During the first six hours post-AMI, patients also may abruptly develop compromising bradydysrhythmias due to increased parasympathetic tone; this is characterized by a slow ventricular escape rate, which usually responds well to atropine. After six hours, bradydysrhythmias tend to develop slowly, and may consist of slow ventricular escape rates, but with a poorer response to pharmacotherapy.[6]

Bradycardic conduction disturbances, such as the various AV blocks, also may develop in anterior and anteroseptal infarction, which typically are due to occlusion of the left main coronary artery, the left anterior descending artery (LAD), or its branches. These cases are associated with a poorer response to pharmacotherapy and a worse prognosis.[3] The risk of developing complete heart block, regardless of infarct site, has been found to directly correlate with the degree of conduction disease evidenced by the 12-lead ECG in AMI; the more conduction defects (first- or second-degree AV blocks, bundle branch, or fascicular blocks) occurring on the tracing, the higher the risk of progression to complete heart block.[7] This can have implications for the use of prophylactic ventricular pacing in the setting of AMI.

Nonischemic Cardiac Causes. These disorders are not necessarily directly related to acute cardiac ischemia, injury, or infarct. Sick sinus syndrome (SSS) is a disorder of sinus node impulse formation, or transmission to the atria. It has a variety of electrocardiographic manifestations, including: 1) severe bradycardia; 2) periods of sinus pause or arrest; 3) periods of sinus exit block (SA block); 4) alternating bursts of varying atrial tachycardias and bradycardia (the tachy-brady syndrome); and 5) AV junctional escape rhythms.[3,8,9] These manifestations may occur alone or in combination and are often intermittent, making ambulatory electrocardiographic monitoring a more sensitive tool than a single 12-lead ECG for detection of SSS.[3] SSS is more common in the elderly population, but can be seen in younger patients.

Commonly, there is histopathological evidence of fibrous destruction of nodal and internodal tissue, which is often independent of coronary artery disease.[3,4,5,8-10] Causes of SSS include primary, idiopathic disease as well as ischemic cardiac disease and a multitude of other factors (e.g., rheumatologic, oncologic, metabolic, infectious, structural, and iatrogenic) discussed below.[3] Lenegre's disease is an idiopathic degenerative condition featuring fibrotic changes of the conduction system that may advance to calcification; bradycardia and varying degrees of AV block may be found on the ECG, along with other conduction disease manifestations, such as right bundle branch block and left anterior fascicular block.

Due to similar presentations, Lenegre's disease is often lumped with Lev's disease, another fibrosclerotic process. In this condition, normal sclerotic changes of the cardiac skeletal structures seen with advanced aging also involve the adjacent conduction system.[3,10,11] Although rare (approximately 1 in 22,000 live births), congenital complete AV block has been described, and has been associated with maternal rheumatologic disease, especially systemic lupus erythematosus.[12]

Pharmacologic/Toxicologic. Several medications, most of which are used for treatment of cardiovascular disease, can cause bradycardia when taken in therapeutic amounts. These include some calcium channel antagonists, beta-adrenergic blockers, digoxin, alpha$_2$-adrenergic agonists (e.g., clonidine, methyldopa), and cholinergic agents. It follows that these same agents have the propensity to cause profound bradydysrhythmias when ingested in toxic amounts; indeed, pharmacotoxicity, together with ischemic disease and degenerative processes, account for the majority of cases of AV block.[9]

Virtually all calcium antagonists and beta-adrenergic blockers can cause severe bradycardia and advanced heart block in overdose;[13] among the former group, verapamil has been found to more frequently and profoundly cause these bradydysrhythmias when compared to diltiazem and nifedipine in overdose situations.[14] Amlodipine also has been reported to cause bradycardia in a poisoning scenario.[15]

Digoxin has been reported to cause bradycardia, sinus arrest, SA block, and all degrees of AV block in the setting of overdose; conversely, it also may cause supraventricular or ventricular tachydysrhythmias. Early in acute digoxin toxicity, the depression of SA node function or impairment of AV nodal conduction may respond to atropine; later this response may be lost. One indication for administration of digoxin-specific antibody fragments is progressive bradydysrhythmia unresponsive to atropine.[16] A variety of botanicals with cardiac glycoside activity also have been reported to cause bradydysrhythmias, among them: foxglove, lily-of-the-valley, yew berry, dogbane, Siberian ginseng, and squill.[16-18] Although classically linked with wide-complex tachydysrhythmias, the Type Ia antiarrhythmics (quinidine, disopyramide, and procainamide) and drugs that may behave like them in overdose (e.g., Type Ic antiarrhythmics, tricyclic antidepressants, carbamazepine, quinine, chloroquine, propoxyphene, amantadine, cyclobenzaprine, and thioridazine) may produce heart block.[19]

Opioids, sedative-hypnotics, and alpha$_2$-adrenergic agonists act via central nervous system-mediated mechanisms to produce bradycardia.[19] Methyldopa has been postulated to cause both direct cardiac and central nervous system-mediated bradycardia and first-and second-degree AV block.[19,20] Other pharmacologic agents linked with bradycardia include the following: organophosphates, cholinesterase inhibitors, lithium, phenothiazines, and cocaine.[10,19,21] The latter drug, although classically associated with a hyperadrenergic state and tachycardia, also has been found to cause bradycardia at low doses, and may behave like a type Ia antiarrhythmic in toxic situations.[22] Cardiac conduction abnormalities are not a feature of oral phenytoin overdose;[23] however, the propylene glycol carrier it is mixed with for intravenous delivery has been implicated for concentration- and infusion-rate related bradycardia and heart block.[24]

Neurologic Disorders. Traumatic as well as non-traumatic neurological processes may result in bradydysrhythmias; among the former, trauma to the brain and spinal cord have been implicated. Severe head trauma leading to profound injury and increased intracranial pressure may be accompanied by systemic hypertension and bradycardia (i.e., the Cushing's reflex, which carries a poor prognosis).[10] Severe bradycardia also can be seen after acute injury to the cervical cord; the bradycardia is mediated by disruption of the autonomic nervous system. Specifically, disruption of the sympathetic fibers in this region can cause unopposed parasympathetic effects, leading to slowing of the heart rate.[10] Studies have shown that patients with profound injury to the cervical cord display bradycardia for up to 2-6 weeks post-trauma; vagal stimulatory maneuvers (e.g., suctioning) may exacerbate this bradycardia, resulting in sinus pauses.[25]

Other neurologic diseases associated with bradydysrhythmias include cerebrovascular accident, subarachnoid hemorrhage, seizure (ictal bradycardia syndrome), and Guillain Barré syndrome.[10,26,27] In the first two entities, increased intracranial pressure must be suspected when hypertension also is present. This also should be suspected if vital signs consistent with the Cushing's reflex are seen after seizure and there is a possibility of occult head trauma. Most cases of ictal bradycardia syndrome are seen with temporal lobe seizures; the conduction pauses that may occur can make it difficult to discern whether loss of consciousness was due to a primary cardiac event or the ictal bradycardia syndrome.[26] Autonomic nervous system dysfunction is felt to be responsible for the brady- or tachydysrhythmias, which are associated with severe cases of Guillain Barré syndrome; sinus bradycardia and AV block are both potential cardiac manifestations of the disease.[27]

Infectious Etiologies. Myocarditis can produce a variety of electrocardiographic manifestations, including ST segment and T wave changes, and less commonly, AV block of varying degrees.[3,21,28] A variety of infectious agents cause these changes via differing mechanisms, including direct tissue involvement, immune-mediated toxicity, and toxin-mediated effects. Myriad infectious agents have been linked to myocarditis. *(Please see Table 2.)* Chagas disease can cause both a congestive cardiomyopathy and dysrhythmias, including ventricular dysrhythmias and conduction disease such as AV block.[29] Lyme disease deserves special attention. Up to 10% of patients will develop clinically evident, usually transient, cardiac involvement, and the most common cardiac pathology is AV block. Degrees of heart block may fluctuate within a given patient, including the development of third-degree AV block.[21,30-32]

Rheumatologic Conditions. Most connective tissue disorders can feature involvement of the heart (please see Table 3), and although pericarditis is the most common rheumatologic manifestation in some (e.g., rheumatoid arthritis, systemic lupus erythematosus, and scleroderma), varying degrees of conduction system disease may occur, including AV block.[33-35] Heart block may be seen in up to 25% of patients with Reiter's syndrome, and up to 10% of those with rheumatoid arthritis.[33]

Miscellaneous. Due to its multisystem, infiltrative course, the granulomatous disease sarcoidosis has a propensity to cause heart

Table 2. Infectious Causes of Myocarditis with Potential for Bradydysrhythmia[10,21,28-32]

VIRAL		
Coxsackie B virus	Influenza	Mononucleosis
Hepatitis	Mumps	Rubella
Rubeola	Varicella virus	Respiratory syncytial
BACTERIAL		
Streptococcus	Meningococcus	Mycoplasma
Staphylococcus	Diphtheria	
OTHER		
Trypanosomiasis (Chagus disease)	Syphilis	Lyme disease

Table 3. Rheumatologic Diseases Affecting the Heart with Potential for Bradydysrhythmia[33-35]

- Rheumatoid arthritis
- Scleroderma
- Systemic lupus erythematosus
- Polymyositis
- Reiter's syndrome
- Ankylosing spondylitis
- Sjögren's syndrome
- Behcet's disease
- Wegener's granulomatosis

block. Twenty-five percent of sarcoid patients have histologic evidence of cardiac involvement, with only about one-fifth of those showing clinical cardiac manifestations.[28,36] Although a variety of cardiac pathologies can be seen with sarcoidosis (e.g., conduction system disease—congestive and restrictive cardiomyopathy, supraventricular and ventricular dysrhythmias—the most common presenting cardiac manifestation is complete heart block. The disease has a predilection for involving the interventricular septum.[36] Amyloidosis, a rare systemic infiltrative disease, usually affects the heart by causing a restrictive cardiomyopathy, and the vascular system by inducing orthostatic hypotension. However, it also can cause bradycardia, SSS, and AV block.[28]

Hypothyroidism and hypothermia may produce bradycardia. Hypoadrenalism, hyperparathyroidism, and acromegaly all have been described with bradycardia. Marked electrolytes elevations, including hyperkalemia, hypermagnesemia, and hypercalcemia, also can cause bradydysrhythmias.[10] Hypoglycemia is an unusual cause of compromising bradycardia; neurologic and endocrinologic mediation has been postulated.[37] Among iatrogenic causes, radiation therapy has induced conduction system disease, including heart block, but more commonly damages the pericardium.[38,39] Rejection and ischemia are felt to be responsible for bradydysrhythmias occasionally seen after orthotopic heart transplant.[40]

Reflex-Mediated Causes. Finally, a number of neuroreflexive processes should be considered in the differential diagnosis of bradydysrhythmias; these are not disease processes, but rather cardiac responses to stimuli via neurologic pathways. Most commonly encountered is the vasovagal event. Here, transient bradycardia sometimes leading to syncope occurs, and usually is associated with a painful, stressful, or emetic event.[9,41]

There are two types of hypersensitive carotid sinus syndrome: cardioinhibitory and vasodepressor. The former is manifested by more than three seconds of ventricular asystole during stimulation of the carotid sinus, and results from an oversensitivity of the afferent carotid sinus nerves leading to the efferent vagal response. Cardioinhibitory and vasodepressor responses can occur independently or concomitantly.[9,10] Less commonly seen reflex-mediated bradydysrhythmias sharing a common afferent (fifth cranial nerve) and efferent (10th cranial nerve) pathway include the diving reflex (cold water to the upper face); oculocardiac reflex (trauma or pressure applied to the globe); and maxillofacial reflex (surgical manipulation of the maxillofacial or temperomandibular regions).[10,42,43] Other reflexive mechanisms known to cause bradycardia include rectoprostatic massage; deglutition, micturition, and defecation syncope; and glossopharyngeal neuralgia.[10]

Pharmacotherapy of Bradycardia

Atropine. Generally the first-line therapy for symptomatic bradydysrhythmia, atropine enhances the automaticity of the SA node and AV nodal conduction via a vagolytic mechanism. Indications for atropine include seriously symptomatic sinus bradycardia or AV block, and asystolic cardiac arrest. In adults, the initial dose is 0.5 mg to 1.0 mg intravenously, repeated every five minutes if needed to a maximum vagolytic dose of 0.04 mg/kg (3 mg in a 75 kg patient).[44] The pediatric dose is 0.01 mg/kg. Generally, patients are more likely to respond to the first dose than to subsequent doses, and bradycardia responds more readily than does AV block.[4,5]

There are two major concerns when considering administration of atropine to a patient with symptomatic bradydysrhythmia. One concern is the potential exacerbation of underlying coronary ischemia and precipitation of malignant ventricular dysrhythmias, and the other is the possibility of paradoxical slowing of the rhythm after atropine is given. Regarding the first issue, although atropine may worsen ischemia if given during an acute coronary event,[44,45] so too might hypoperfusion from an unstable bradydysrhythmia adversely affect outcome. Recent data did not reveal evidence of intensification of cardiac ischemia in patients receiving atropine for compromising bradydysrhythmias.[4,5] Development of malignant ventricular dysrhythmias has been found infrequently after administration of atropine for unstable bradydysrhythmia in the prehospital setting, and has a reported incidence of 2-4%.[4,5,46] Knowing the minimal risk associated with this therapy, the emergency physician should nevertheless be prepared and use the agent cautiously.[47-50]

Paradoxical slowing of the heart rate after administration of atropine for unstable bradydysrhythmia has been found rarely in patients with infranodal AV block—Mobitz Type II second-degree AV block and third-degree AV block with a wide QRS complex. The majority of patients with these rhythms do not manifest this paradoxical reaction, however; an awareness of this possible adverse effect in this subgroup of bradydysrhythmias is advisable.[4,5,46,49,51-54]

Isoproterenol. A non-specific beta-adrenergic agonist, isoproterenol causes an increase in chronotropy, inotropy, and conduction

Table 4. Electrocardiographic Waveforms Seen During Transvenous Pacemaker Placement[65-67]

LOCATION	WAVEFORM	
	P wave	*QRS complex*
Superior vena cava	negative	negative
High right atrium	larger/negative	smaller/negative
Mid-right atrium	larger/biphasic	smaller/negative
Low right atrium	smaller/positive	larger/negative
Right ventricle, free	smaller/positive	larger/negative
Right ventricle, against wall		ST segment elevation
Inferior vena cava	smaller/positive	smaller again/negative

velocity via beta-$_1$ receptor stimulation, and smooth muscle relaxation and bronchodilation via beta-$_2$ stimulation. Physiologically, the result is an increase in cardiac output, systolic blood pressure, and myocardial contractility, with a decrease in diastolic blood pressure, systemic vascular resistance, and pulmonary vascular resistance. Although the mean arterial pressure should not be significantly affected, myocardial oxygen demand is increased (due to beta$_1$ effects), and coronary perfusion pressure is decreased (due to beta$_2$ effects). Therefore, isoproterenol is not the drug of choice in situations of acute coronary ischemia, and is relegated to a reserve role—as a bridge, only if needed, between atropine failure or maximization, and pacing, which is actually preferred.

Isoproterenol does have a role in the patient with symptomatic bradydysrhythmia and a denervated, transplanted heart.[44] It should be avoided in digoxin-toxic patients, as increased ventricular ectopy may result.[16] The dose is 2.0 mcg/min, with titration to hemodynamic effect, to a maximum infusion of 10 mcg/min. The half life and duration of effect are short; side effects are predictable from the pharmacology of the drug: tachydysrhythmias, palpitations, ischemia, flushing, dizziness, tremor, and nausea.[44]

Glucagon. This naturally occurring hormone has positive inotropic and chronotropic effects, actions that are not mediated by adrenergic receptors. Inotropic effects exceed chronotropic effects in the failing heart; the reverse is true under normal conditions (in both cases with limited expense of myocardial oxygen consumption).[55] Glucagon has a demonstrated beneficial effect in bradydysrhythmias resulting from calcium channel blocker and beta adrenergic antagonist toxicity;[13,14,56,57] many consider it first-line therapy in these cases, yet reports of its success have been mixed.[55] Recommended dose ranges in the setting of toxicity from these drugs are variable; generally, an initial bolus of 2-10 mg intravenously is suggested, with continuous infusion if necessary at 2-5 mg/hr. In cases requiring large doses, the phenol diluent that accompanies the preparation should be replaced by sterile water, saline, or D_5W to avoid phenol toxicity. In infants, the bolus dose is 50 mcg/kg. Adverse effects include nausea, emesis, hypokalemia, and inconsequential hyperglycemia.[55]

Aminophylline. Because adenosine has been postulated to contribute to some conduction abnormalities seen during acute myocardial infarction, aminophylline—its competitive inhibitor—may play a role in the management of some bradydysrhythmias in this setting.[58] Adenosine appears to be released from ischemic myocardial cells, resulting in prolongation of AV nodal conduction time. The dose is 5-15 mg/kg infused over five minutes. As with isoproterenol, it functions as a medical bridge to more definitive therapy of atropine-resistant bradydysrhythmias—namely, cardiac pacing.

Emergency Cardiac Pacing

Transcutaneous Cardiac Pacing. This technique has evolved in both simplicity and efficacy over time. Indications are stratified into those for prophylactic placement without active pacing, and those for active pacing. Prophylactic placement of transcutaneous pacing apparatus is indicated for stable bradydysrhythmias or conduction disturbances with potential for progression to instability, such as those occurring during acute myocardial infarction. Examples include significant sinus node dysfunction, Mobitz Type II second-degree AV block, third-degree AV block, and new conduction delays (e.g., bundle branch blocks or bifascicular block). Active pacing is indicated for bradydysrhythmias with instability (e.g., hypotension/shock, anginal chest pain or dyspnea, altered sensorium, pulmonary edema) that are unresponsive to medical therapy, and for bradyasystolic arrest.[44]

Pacing of asystolic cardiac arrest is often futile, however, and if instituted, should be employed early to optimize chances of a better outcome.[59,60] Prehospital transcutaneous pacing by emergency medical technicians for asystolic patients (before intubation and/or drug administration by later-arriving paramedics) has not been found to be effective.[61] It has been used in the prehospital arena with success, however, in patients with hemodynamically significant bradycardia.[62] Transcutaneous cardiac pacing is an interim therapy, and should serve only as a bridge to definitive transvenous pacing. Dog studies with pacing for up to 60 minutes have not shown enzyme, electrocardiographic, or histologic evidence of myocardial damage.[63]

Transcutaneous pacemakers generally require two connections to the patient: a set of pads for delivering the pacing current, and leads for monitoring the patient; some units allow both defibrillation and pacing through the same pads. The placement of the pads is generally anterior/posterior, with the anterior pad being as close as possible to the point of maximum cardiac impulse, and the posterior pad being directly opposite the anterior, in the left parathoracic region. When pacing an awake patient, current should be slowly increased until capture is attained—a palpable pulse that correlates with the waveform seen on the unit. In cardiac arrest, the maximum current should be applied initially to assure rapid capture; this can be titrated down to the minimal current that guarantees capture if the patient regains consciousness. Conscious patients may need intravenous medication for pain and anxiety management, as the current necessary may cause significant discomfort. Complications include pain, failure to detect underlying ventricular dysrhythmias (due to technical difficulties in systems without adequate dampening capability for pacing artifact), and theoretically, induction of dysrhythmias. Minor local tissue damage is possible; the magnitude of electrical shock delivered to health care personnel, even during CPR, is trivial.[64]

Transvenous Cardiac Pacing. This procedure yields more definitive control of bradydysrhythmias unresponsive to medical therapy or accompanied by serious signs and symptoms as discussed above. Although it is invasive, the actual delivery of current to pace the heart is better tolerated in most patients than with the transcutaneous method. Central venous access is the first step, and is optimally accomplished via the right internal jugular approach (leaving the left side clear for possible future permanent pacemaker placement). The right subclavian approach may be technically more difficult; the right femoral approach is another possibility, especially in coagulopathic patients in whom a compressible vessel is more desirable.

The transvenous wire optimally is placed with fluoroscopic guidance, which, as a rule, is often not available to the emergency physician who must perform the procedure emergently. Alternatively, the wire can be passed either blindly or semi-blindly with electrocardiographic guidance. The blind approach should be reserved for situations where electrocardiographic guidance is not readily available and the patient is in extremis. The operator should advance the balloon-tipped catheter approximately 10 cm into the venous port, and then turn the pulse generator to the "sense" mode, advancing into the ventricle until cardiac activity is sensed. At this time, the balloon is deflated, the generator is switched to the "pace" mode, and the current is advanced from a minimal setting, used during the first phase (e.g., < 0.2 mA), to a current that is likely to capture the ventricle (e.g., 4 to 5 mA). The monitor is then watched for electrical capture as the wire is advanced up to 10 cm further. If capture does not occur, the wire should be withdrawn the 10 cm distance, and readvanced. If the patient is asystolic, there is no reason to advance the wire in the "sense" mode; the pacing generator should be in the "pace" mode, asynchronous, at maximum output, and advanced looking for evidence of ventricular capture.[65-67]

In a patient with a heart beat, semi-blind placement of the pacing wire with electrocardiographic guidance is a better alternative when fluoroscopy is not available. In this case, the patient should be connected to the limb leads of the ECG machine. A precordial "V" lead from the ECG machine is then connected to the distal, negative terminal of the pacer wire, and serves as an intracardiac electrocardiographic monitor to ascertain location. Table 4 describes the waveforms seen at different points as the wire advances. The general concept is that wave forms grow larger as the chamber they correspond to is entered, and vector cardiographic rules are in place. The balloon should be deflated once in the right ventricle to avoid straying into the right ventricular outflow tract. The wire should then be advanced while monitoring the V lead, with the goal of engaging the wall of the right ventricular apex. Once the operator is satisfied that the right ventricular wall is engaged, the V lead should be disconnected and the pacing generator attached to both pacing wire leads, and the patient can be paced. Chest radiography is used to verify positioning and exclude iatrogenic pneumothorax. On the anteroposterior film, the tip of the wire should be seen in the right ventricle, crossing the midline to the left. If a lateral film can be obtained, the tip of the catheter should be seen curling toward the distal aspect of the sternum. Complications include inappropriate positioning of the wire, induction of dysrhythmias, infection, thrombosis, phlebitis, and perforation of cardiovascular structures traversed en route. The complications related to central venous access also must be anticipated.[65-67]

Finally, pacemaker function should be assessed in terms of both pacing threshold and sensitivity. Pacing threshold is the smallest amount of current necessary to cause ventricular contraction. It is determined by setting the rate at least 10 bpm above the intrinsic heart rate, and then dialing the amperage down until capture is lost. With a properly positioned wire, this should be < 1.0 mA. This process should be repeated two or three times for reliability assessment. Once the threshold has been determined, the output should be set at approximately 2.5 times the threshold to assure capture. If the patient has an underlying rhythm, pacing sensitivity should be assessed. This is defined as the pacemaker's ability to sense adequate cardiac activity, and thus be inhibited. To test this, the pacemaker rate (in demand mode) should be dialed down to 10 to 20 bpm below the intrinsic heart rate; if sensing adequately, paced impulses should disappear from the monitor. Like pacing threshold, this too should be determined two or three times, looking for equivalent results. A post-procedure 12-lead ECG tracing should reveal a left bundle branch block pattern during paced beats if the wire is in the right ventricle.[65-67]

Summary

Bradydysrhythmias are frequently encountered in the ED, and at times require emergent therapy for stabilization. There are a wide variety of bradycardic rhythms, which are best assessed with a 12-lead EKG, and can be stratified into regular and irregular rhythms. While stabilizing the patient and defining the rhythm, the EP must consider a vast differential diagnosis of causality that includes much more than ischemia and infarction, although these are a paramount consideration. Treatment options include observing the rhythm, pharmacotherapy, and cardiac pacing, both transcutaneous and transvenous. Disposition decisions are best made when the nature of the rhythm and its etiology are determined, with consideration of the extent of therapy given to that point, and an assessment of the potential for instability in the immediate future.

References

1. Josephson ME, Zimetbaum P, Marchinski FE, et al. The bradyarrhythmias: Disorders of sinus node function and AV conduction disturbances. In: Fauci AS, Braunwald E, Isselbacher KJ, et al, eds. *Harrison's Principles of Internal Medicine.* 14th ed. New York: McGraw Hill; 1998:1253-1261.
2. Woodburne RT. *Essentials of Human Anatomy.* 7th ed. New York: Oxford University Press; 1983.
3. Chou T, Knilans TK. *Electrocardiography in Clinical Practice: Adult and Pediatric.* 4th ed. Philadelphia: WB Saunders; 1996.
4. Brady WJ, Swart G, DeBehnke DJ, et al. The efficacy of atropine in the treatment of hemodynamically unstable bradycardia and atrioventricular block: Prehospital and emergency department considerations. *Resuscitation* 1999;41:47-55.
5. Swart GS, Brady WJ, DeBehnke DJ, et al. Acute myocardial infarction complicated by hemodynamically unstable bradyarrhythmia: Prehospital and emergency department treatment with atropine. *Am J Emerg Med* 1999;17:647-652.
6. Feigl D, Ashkenazy J, Kishon Y. Early and late atrioventricular block in acute inferior myocardial infarction. *J Am Coll Cardiol* 1984;4:35-38.
7. Lamas GA, Muller JE, Turi ZG, et al. A simplified method to predict occurrence of complete heart block during acute myocardial infarction. *Am J Cardiol* 1986;57:1213-1219.
8. Kerr CR, Grant AO, Wenger TL, et al. Sinus node dysfunction. *Cardiol Clin* 1983;1:187-202.

9. Zipes DP. Specific arrhythmias: Diagnosis and treatment. In: Braunwald E, ed. *Heart Disease: A Textbook of Cardiovascular Medicine.* 5th ed. Philadelphia: WB Saunders; 1997:640-704.
10. Ornato JP, Peberdy MA. The mystery of bradyasystole during cardiac arrest. *Ann Emerg Med* 1996;27:576-587.
11. Myerburg RJ, Castellanos A. Cardiac arrest and sudden cardiac death. In: Braunwald E, ed. *Heart Disease: A Textbook of Cardiovascular Medicine.* 5th ed. Philadelphia: WB Saunders; 1997:742-779.
12. Ross BA. Congenital complete atrioventricular block. *Pediatr Clin North Am* 1990;37:69-78.
13. Cox J, Wang RY. Critical consequences of common drugs: Calcium channel blocker and beta-adrenergic antagonist overdose. *Emerg Med Rep* 1994;15:83-90.
14. Ramoska EA, Spiller HA, Winter M, et al. A one-year evaluation of calcium channel blocker overdoses: Toxicity and treatment. *Ann Emerg Med* 1993;196-200.
15. Koch AR, Vogelaers DP, Decruyenaere JM, et al. Fatal intoxication with amlodipine. *J Toxicol Clin Toxicol* 1995;33:253-256.
16. Lewin NA. Cardiac glycosides. In: Goldfrank LR, Flomenbaum NE, Lewin NA, et al, eds. *Goldfrank's Toxicologic Emergencies.* 6th ed. Stamford CT: Appleton and Lange; 1998:791-808.
17. Cummins RO, Haulman J, Quan L, et al. Near-fatal yew berry intoxication treated with external cardiac pacing and digoxin-specific FAB antibody fragments. *Ann Emerg Med* 1990;19:38-43.
18. Tuncok Y, Kozan O, Cavadar C, et al. Urginea maritima (squill) toxicity. *J Toxicol Clin Toxicol* 1995;22:83-86.
19. Hessler R. Cardiovascular principles. In: Goldfrank LR, Flomenbaum NE, Lewin NA, et al, eds. *Goldfrank's Toxicologic Emergencies.* 6th ed. Stamford CT: Appleton and Lange; 1998: 353-378.
20. Sadjadi SA, Leghari RU, Berger AR. Prolongation of the PR interval induced by methyldopa. *Am J Cardiol* 1984;54:675-676.
21. Huff JS, Syverud SA, Tucci MA. Case conference: Complete heart block in a young man. *Acad Emerg Med* 1995;2:751-756.
22. Goldfrank LR, Hoffman RS. The cardiovascular effects of cocaine. *Ann Emerg Med* 1991;20:165-175.
23. Wyte CD, Berk WA. Severe oral phenytoin overdose does not cause cardiovascular morbidity. *Ann Emerg Med* 1991;20:508-512.
24. York RC, Coleridge ST. Cardiopulmonary arrest following intravenous phenytoin loading. *Am J Emerg Med* 1988;6:255-259.
25. Lehman KG, Lane JG, Piepmeier JM, et al. Cardiovascular abnormalities accompanying acute spinal cord injury in humans: Incidence, time course and severity. *J Am Coll Cardiol* 1987;10: 46-52.
26. Reeves AL, Nollet KE, Klass DW, et al. The ictal bradycardia syndrome. *Epilepsia* 1996;37:983-987.
27. Greenland P, Griggs RC. Arrhythmic complications in the Guillain Barré syndrome. *Arch Intern Med* 1980;140:1053-1055.
28. Wynne J, Braunwald E. The cardiomyopathies and myocarditides. In: Braunwald E, ed. *Heart Disease: A Textbook of Cardiovascular Medicine.* 5th ed. Philadelphia: WB Saunders; 1997:1404-1463.
29. Pimenta, Mirand M, Pereira CB. Electrophysiologic findings in long-term asymptomatic chagasic individuals. *Am Heart J* 1983; 106:374-380.
30. Cox J, Krajden M. Cardiovascular manifestations of Lyme disease. *Am Heart J* 1991;122:1449-1455.
31. Steere AC, Batsford WP, Weinberg M, et al. Lyme carditis: Cardiac abnormalities of Lyme disease. *Ann Intern Med* 1980;93:8-16.
32. Vidaillet HJ, Broste SK, Marx JJ, et al. The 12-lead electrocardiogram of "healthy" ambulatory subjects with positive Lyme serology. *Am J Cardiol* 1993;71:1249-1251.
33. Coblyn JS, Weinblatt ME. Rheumatic diseases and the heart. In: Braunwald E, ed. *Heart Disease: A Textbook of Cardiovascular Medicine.* 5th ed. Philadelphia: WB Saunders; 1997:1776-1785.
34. Lee LA, Pickrell MB, Reichlin M. Development of complete heart block in an adult patient with Sjögren's syndrome and anti-Rho/SS autoantibodies. *Arthritis Rheum* 1996;39:1427-1429.
35. Handa R, Wali JP, Aggarwal P, et al. Wegener's granulomatosis with complete heart block. *Clin Exp Rheumatol* 1997;15:97-99.
36. Sharma OP, Maheshwari A, Thakur K. Myocardial sarcoidosis. *Chest* 1993;103:253-258.
37. Pollock G, Brady WJ, Hargarten S, et al. Hypoglycemia manifested by sinus bradycardia: A report of three cases. *Acad Emerg Med* 1996;3:700-707.
38. Knight CJ, Sutton GC. Complete heart block and severe tricuspid regurgitation after radiotherapy. *Chest* 1995;108:1748-1751.
39. Orzan F, Brusca A, Gaita F, et al. Associated cardiac lesions in patients with radiation-induced complete heart block. *Int J Cardiol* 1993;39:151-156.
40. Weinfeld MS, Kartashov A, Piana R, et al. Bradycardia: A late complication following heart transplantation. *Am J Cardiol* 1996;78: 969-971.
41. Marco CA, Marco AP. Profound bradycardia related to long bone fracture manipulation. *J Emerg Med* 1996;14:305-308.
42. Hirjak D, Zajko J, Satko I. Bradycardia after orbital injury. Case report. *Int J Oral Maxillofac Surg* 1993;22:26-27.
43. Precious DS, Skulsky G. Cardiac dysrhythmia complicating maxillofacial surgery. *Int J Oral Maxillofac Surg* 1990;19:279-282.
44. Cummins RO, ed. *Textbook of Advanced Cardiac Life Support.* American Heart Association; 1997-1999.
45. Richman S. Adverse effect of atropine during myocardial infarction. *JAMA* 1974;228:1414-1416.
46. Warren JV, Lewis RP. Beneficial effects of atropine in the prehospital phase of coronary care. *Am J Cardiol* 1976;37:68-72.
47. Cooper MJ, Abinader EG. Atropine-induced ventricular fibrillation: Case report and review of the literature. *Am Heart J* 1979;97: 225-228.
48. Lazzari JO, Benchuga EG, Elizari MV, et al. Ventricular fibrillation after intravenous atropine in a patient with atrioventricular block. *Pace* 1982;5:196-200.
49. Lunde P. Ventricular fibrillation after intravenous atropine for treatment of sinus bradycardia. *Acta Med Scand* 1976;199:369-371.
50. Massumi RA, Mason DT, Amsterdam EA, et al. Ventricular fibrillation and tachycardia after intravenous atropine for the treatment of bradycardias. *N Engl J Med* 1972;287:336-338.
51. Ng L, Nikolic G. Atropine bradycardia. *Heart Lung* 1991:20: 414-415.
52. Grauer LE, Gershen BJ, Orlando MM, et al. Bradycardia and its complications in the prehospital phase of acute myocardial infarction. *Am J Cardiol* 1973;32:607-611.
53. Stock E. Cardiac slowing, not cardiac irritability, the major problem in the prehospital phase of myocardial infarction. *Med J Austrail* 1971:2:747-750.
54. Stuckey JG. Arrhythmias in the prehospital phase of acute myocardial infarction. *Med J Austrail* 1973:2:29-32.

55. Pollack CV. Utility of glucagon in the emergency department. *J Emerg Med* 1993;11:195-205.
56. Doyon S, Roberts JR. The use of glucagon in a case of calcium channel blocker overdose. *Ann Emerg Med* 1993;22:1229-1233.
57. Love JN, Howell JM. Glucagon therapy in the treatment of symptomatic bradycardia. *Ann Emerg Med* 1997;29:181-183.
58. Goodfellow J, Walker PR. Reversal of atropine-resistant atrioventricular block with intravenous aminophylline in the early phase of inferior wall acute myocardial infarction following treatment with streptokinase. *Eur Heart J* 1995;16:862-865.
59. Falk RH, Jacobs L, Sinclair A, Madigan-McNeil C. External noninvasive cardiac pacing in out-of-hospital cardiac arrest. *Crit Care Med* 1983:11:779-782.
60. Syverud SA, Dalsey WC, Hedges JR. Transcutaneous and transvenous cardiac pacing for early bradyasystolic cardiac arrest. *Ann Emerg Med* 1986:15:121-124.
61. Cummins RO, Graves JR, Larsen MP, et al. Out-of-hospital transcutaneous pacing by emergency medical technicians in patients with asystolic cardiac arrest. *N Engl J Med* 1993;328:1377-1382.
62. Barthell E, Troiano P, Olson D, et al. Prehospital external cardiac pacing: a prospective, controlled clinical trial. *Ann Emerg Med* 1988;17:1221-1226.
63. Syverud SA, Dalsey WC, Hedges JR, et al. Transcutaneous cardiac pacing: Determination of myocardial injury in a canine model. *Ann Emerg Med* 1983:745-748.
64. Syverud S, Hedges JR. Emergency transcutaneous cardiac pacing. In: Roberts JR, Hedges JR, eds. *Clinical Procedures in Emergency Medicine.* 3rd ed. Philadelphia:WB Saunders;1998:225-231.
65. Benjamin GC. Emergency transvenous cardiac pacing. In: Roberts JR, Hedges JR, eds. *Clinical Procedures in Emergency Medicine.* 3rd ed. Philadelphia:WB Saunders;1998:210-225.
66. Vukmir RB. Emergency cardiac pacing. *Am J Emerg Med* 1993;11:166-176.
67. Jafri SM, Kruse JA. Temporary transvenous cardiac pacing. *Crit Care Clin* 1992;8:713-725.

Atrial Fibrillation

Frank Ruiz, MD

Emergency department (ED) physicians encounter atrial fibrillation (AF) in a variety of presentations, ranging from chronic, well-managed, asymptomatic disease to acute hemodynamic compromise associated with a rapid ventricular rate. The ED physician must investigate not only the underlying causes and precipitants of AF, but must also perform a risk assessment concerning the possibility of acute ischemia and determine the need for admission. Furthermore, issues concerning anticoagulation and prevention of thromboembolism must be addressed.

To make matters more complicated, a variety of new strategies and drugs have appeared for rapid rate control and immediate chemical cardioversion. For the patient with AF who is unstable due to decompensated heart failure, acute ischemia, or hypotension, a number of management options are available, and decisions concerning electrical cardioversion are not as straightforward as they are in supraventricular tachycardia (SVT), ventricular tachycardia, or ventricular fibrillation. This review presents targeted strategies for ED evaluation and management of AF. New therapies for acute rate control, chemical cardioversion, and other approaches for the unstable patient are highlighted.

Background

AF is the most common sustained cardiac arrhythmia, with a prevalence of about 0.5-1.0% in the population at large.[1-3] With advancing age the prevalence increases, with 5% of patients older than age 65 having AF.[1-4] Chronic AF is a major risk factor for stroke, carrying a risk of about 3-7% per year in older patients with associated coronary heart disease or CHF who are not receiving coumadin.[5]

The presence of AF indicates a high likelihood of coexisting cardiovascular or systemic disease. Underlying conditions capable of producing AF include hypertensive heart disease, coronary artery disease, valvular heart disease, cardiomyopathies, pericarditis, congenital heart disease, cardiac contusion, Wolff-Parkinson-White syndrome (or other accessory pathways), and cardiac surgery.[5] Systemic conditions associated with atrial fibrillation include thyroid disease, malignancy, ethanol intoxication and withdrawal, severe electrolyte disturbance, sarcoidosis, amyloidosis, pheochromocytoma, and pulmonary embolism.[5,6] About 10% of patients with AF have no associated disease, and are referred to as having lone AF.[7]

The duration of new onset AF varies considerably, with about 30-60% of patients converting spontaneously to sinus rhythm within 24 hours.[8-10] The duration is important, in part, because persistence of the arrhythmia produces electrophysiologic changes in the atria, or "remodeling," that increases the likelihood that the arrhythmia will continue.[11] More importantly, the duration of the arrhythmia is related to the risk of thrombus formation. Patients with AF lasting longer than 48 hours are at risk for developing an atrial thrombus and should not undergo elective attempts at chemical or electrical cardioversion unless they have received adequate anticoagulation.[12] In contrast, patients with brief intermittent episodes of AF in the absence of structural heart disease carry a much lower risk of cardioembolic stroke.[12]

Clinical Features

Patients with new onset AF typically present with symptoms of rapid heart rate, palpitations, and/or shortness of breath. In the absence of underlying conduction system disease, the ventricular response is rapid—usually in the range of 100-160 beats per minute. A pulse deficit is usually present; in other words, the radial pulse is slower than the auscultated apical rate because some of the ventricular contractions, due to inadequate filling times, are not strong enough to transmit a pressure wave to the radial artery.[13]

It should be stressed that patients with slow rates that are not attributable to medications inhibiting AV node conduction may have underlying conduction system disease that will increase the risk of severe bradycardia upon cardioversion. On the other hand, a very rapid (> 160) ventricular rate, accompanied by a wide QRS suggests the presence of an accessory pathway. Normalization of the rate in patients with preexisting AF suggests the possibility of atrial tachycardia, junctional or idioventricular rhythms, or ventricular tachycardia, all of which may result from digoxin toxicity.

Clinical evaluation of patients with AF should include a search for underlying structural heart disease (especially cardiac ischemia) and for systemic conditions that may precipitate the arrhythmia. The history should note the presence of alcohol or illicit drug use, risk factors for coronary artery disease, and symptoms of angina and congestive heart failure. A history of syncope is important because it may be a clue to the presence of sick sinus syndrome or nonsustained ventricular tachycardia. Detection of noncardiac illnesses also are important and may affect management decisions. Evidence of congestive heart failure, valvular heart disease, pericarditis, or thyrotoxicosis should be sought.

Diagnostic Studies

The electrocardiogram is valuable for a number of reasons. First, it will confirm the diagnosis by the presence of irregularly irregular supraventricular beats without discernible P waves. Fibrillatory waves (F waves) may be present and appear as fine, irregular undulations of the baseline, which are sometimes mistaken for flutter waves. Ashman's phenomenon is a transient bundle branch block that produces a wide QRS complex when a long R to R interval is followed by one that is short. Look for electrocardiographic evidence of acute ischemia, new or old infarction, pericarditis, and ventricular hypertrophy. Patients taking digoxin may have characteristic ST depression. Patients taking quinidine or other class IA antiarrhythmic drugs may have QT prolongation.

Additional studies that may be helpful in the ED include a chest x-ray, which may reveal cardiomegaly, congestive heart failure, pneumonia, chronic obstructive pulmonary disease (COPD), tumors of the lung and mediastinum, or evidence of pulmonary embolism as causative or complicating factors. Look for and correct serum electrolyte abnormalities. An elevated creatinine is important to note because digoxin is, in part, renally cleared. If the patient is taking warfarin, check the prothrombin time to make sure the INR is in the range from 2 to 3.

Transthoracic echocardiography, although extremely valuable in the work-up of patients with AF, is deferred to the outpatient setting, or may be performed later in the course of the patient's hospitalization, if admitted. Similarly, a screening thyroid study can be done as an outpatient since results would not be available in the ED.

Slowing the Ventricular Response in AF: Rate Control in the ED

Digoxin. A number of agents are available for rate control in the ED setting. *(Please see Tables 1 and 2.)* Digoxin, the most commonly prescribed cardiac glycoside, is the oldest drug in use for control of the ventricular response in AF. Digoxin inhibits the active transport of sodium and potassium across cell membranes. Inhibition of the sarcolemma ATPase results in an increase in cytoslic calcium, thus increasing the force of myocardial contraction. In specialized conduction cells, including those of the AV node, digoxin causes a *decrease* in automaticity and increases the maximal resting diastolic membrane potential, primarily due to digoxin's vagotonic effects. The effective refractory period in the AV node is increased, and conduction velocity is decreased.[14,15] The clinical result is a decrease in ventricular rate.

Patients with congestive heart failure have chronically elevated sympathetic tone and decreased baroreceptor responsiveness. The infusion of digoxin in the setting of heart failure decreases sympathetic tone by increasing carotid barocептor responsiveness and by increasing cardiac inotropy. The result is a lower blood presssure with a higher cardiac output. Although the use of digoxin does not prolong life in patients with congestive heart failure, its use has been clearly shown to lessen symptoms and to decrease the likelihood of hospitalization.[16] As a result, digoxin is one drug of choice for rate control in AF patients with moderate to severe heart failure.

However, there are two principal drawbacks to the use of digoxin in the ED. The first has to do with its slow onset of action.[17] Of the various protocols for intravenous loading of digoxin, none demonstrates significant slowing of the ventricular response until about four hours or more have passed. Second, digoxin does not prevent adrenergic increases in heart rate.[18] As a result, many ED patients who have a high degree of sympathetic tone (due to pain, respiratory distress, anxiety, alcohol withdrawal, etc.) will not achieve adequate rate control with digoxin. And those ED patients who are sent home on digoxin may be aware of a rapid heart rate upon mild to moderate physical exertion.

Other potential problems with digoxin result from its narrow therapeutic range, toxic effects, and potential drug interactions. Digoxin also has a long elimination half-life (approximately 36-48 hours), and high levels will accumulate in patients with impaired renal function unless dosage and dosing interval are adjusted accordingly. In general, clinical benefit from digoxin in heart failure is seen with serum levels about 1 ng/mL, with an optimal effect at 1.3 ng/mL, although the dose reponse is nonlinear. Unfortunately, in AF, the relationship between dose and response is not as predictable. Clinical signs of toxicity are typically seen with levels of 2-3 ng/mL or higher, although there are some patients who may have evidence of mild toxicity at lower levels. Symptoms of toxicity include confusion, malaise, visual disturbance (intense yellow colors, halos), nausea, vomiting, abdominal pain (which in some cases is due to mesenteric ischemia caused by digoxin-mediated reduction in

Table 1. Targeted Strategies for Rate Control in Atrial Fibrillation

Drug	Comment
PATIENTS WITH MILD OR MODERATE HEART FAILURE AND NORMAL TO HIGH BLOOD PRESSURE	
Diltiazem IV	Expensive, bolus wears off quickly, needs to be followed with a continous infusion
Digoxin IV	Inexpensive, does not cause hypotension, onset of action > 4 hours
PATIENTS WITH SEVERE HEART FAILURE (WHO HAVE FAILED CARDIOVERSION)	
Digoxin	Slow in onset, > 4 hrs
Amiodarone	Slight risk of extreme bradycardia
PATIENTS WITH SEVERE CHF, VOLUME OVERLOAD, AND SIGNIFICANT HYPOTENSION (WHO HAVE FAILED CARDIOVERSION)	
Digoxin	With pressor support (phenylephrine or norepinephrine)
Amiodarone	With pressor support
PATIENTS WITH ISCHEMIC CHEST PAIN OR ACUTE MI (IN PRESENCE OF ONGOING ISCHEMIC PAIN, EMERGENCY DC CARDIOVERSION SHOULD BE PERFORMED)	
Metoprolol IV	Has advantage of decreasing mortality in acute MI
Diltiazem IV	Fairly easy to titrate, some protection against ischemia
WPW AND RAPID AF	
Procainamide	Slows rate through the bypass tract while converting to sinus. (Do not give digoxin, calcium blockers, or beta blockers! They may increase conduction through the bypass tract.)
THYROTOXICOSIS	
β blocker IV	If the patient has concurrent high output CHF, choose esmolol because of its short half-life; otherwise may give propranolol
PATIENTS WITH RAPID RATES AND HYPERTENSION	
Verapamil IV	Less expensive than diltiazem, but with more negative inotropy
Metoprolol IV	Also a potent negative inotrope

splanchnic blood flow), cardiac arrhythmias, especially exccessive slowing of the ventricular response, and accelerated junctional rhythms. Important drug interactions include decreased digoxin clearance with concurrent administration of quinidine, amiodarone, captopril, diltiazem, nifedipine, or verapamil.[14,15]

Hypomagnesemia is known to attenuate the cardiac response to digoxin. Clinical trials have examined the effects of ventricular rate control when intravenous digoxin is given concurrently with intravenous magnesium.[14-16] The results of these clinical trials indicate that the combination of magnesium and digoxin is superior to digoxin alone in achieving rate control.[19,20] Whereas intravenous loading protocols for digoxin may take more than four hours to slow the ventricular response, the *combination* of digoxin and magnesium can achieve a 25% reduction in heart rate in 2-4 hours. Accordingly, if one chooses intravenous digoxin for rate control, magnesium should be added in all patients with known or suspected magnesium deficiency, such as alcoholics, or individuals receiving potent doses of loop diuretics. Do not give magnesium in the the setting of renal insuficiency or renal failure, since toxic doses of magnesium will accumulate rapidly. Even in patients with normal renal function, extremely high doses of magnesium (e.g., 10 gm given intravenously over 6 hours) can cause dangerous pauses.[20]

Table 2. Dosages of Drugs for Rate Control in Atrial Fibrillation

DIGOXIN

0.5 mg IV, then 0.250 mg in one hour (max 1-1.5 mg/24hr)

DIGOXIN AND MAGNESIUM

0.5 mg digoxin IV, 2 gm $MgSO_4$ bolus, then 1 gm $MgSO_4$/hr X 4 hours

DILTIAZEM

0.25 mg/kg IV bolus, 15 min later if needed give second bolus 0.35 mg/kg, then 5-15 mg/hr maintenance

PROPRANOLOL

1 mg IV, repeat in 5 minutes if needed

METOPROLOL

5 mg IV, repeat in 5 minutes if needed

ESMOLOL AND DIGOXIN

0.25-0.5 mg digoxin, repeated in 2 hours

Esmolol dose titration:

Time (min)	*IV Bolus (mg)*	*IV Infusion (mg/min)*
0	10	2
5	10	4
10	20	8
15	20	12
20	20	16

VERAPAMIL

2.5-5 mg IV, repeat in 30 minutes if needed

Beta-Blockers. Beta-1 adrenergic receptor *stimulation* of the heart causes increases in rate, myocardial contractility, conduction velocity, and automaticity. *Blockade* of the beta-1 receptor produces slowing of AV conduction and increased AV node refractoriness which, in AF, results in slowing of the ventricular response. Concommitant decreases in cardiac contractility can result in hypotension or congestive heart failure. Beta-2 receptor blockade may lead to bronchial smooth muscle constriction, and, in diabetic patients, may delay recovery from hypoglycemia because of catecholamine effects on glycogenolysis.[21]

Intravenous beta blockers can produce rapid control of the ventricular response in AF. The beta blockers, metoprolol, propranolol,

Table 3. Transition from Intravenous to Oral Diltiazem

INFUSION RATE	ORAL DILTIAZEM CD DOSE
5 mg/hr	180 mg
10 mg/hr	300 mg
15 mg/hr	360 mg

The infusion is continued for 4 hours after the oral dose is given. Alternatively, one may use short-acting diltiazem at doses of 30, 60, and 90 mg, respectively, with discontinuation of the infusion 2-4 hours later.

and esmolol, are available for intravenous administration.[18] Esmolol, which is metabolized by red cell esterases, has the shortest elimination half-life (9 minutes) and selectively blocks B1 receptors. Esmolol is metabolized to methanol; however, the amount of methanol produced is not significant, and methanol toxicity does not occur. Esmolol's extremely short half-life makes it desirable when there is a risk of hypotension or heart failure. Propranolol blocks both beta-1 and beta-2 receptors and has a plasma half-life of about 3-5 hours. Metoprolol has beta-1 selectivity and has a plasma half-life of about 3-4 hours. Intravenous beta blockers usually are contraindicated in the settings of congestive heart failure, reactive airway disease, and hypotension.

Early studies of esmolol for rate control in AF and atrial flutter reported a 12-48% incidence of hypotension.[18] A subsequent study used esmolol in combination with digoxin in an attempt to minimize the hypotensive and negative inotropic effects of esmolol.[22] Of 21 patients studied, no episode of symptomatic hypotension occurred, and there were only two cases of dyspnea or congestive heart failure. Because no comparison treatment arm was used, it is not known whether the combination of esmolol and digoxin is superior to esmolol alone, either in terms of efficacy or in terms of complication rates. If esmolol is used in AF, a less aggressive dosing protocol should be used than that recommended, in order to minimize the risk of hypotension. When contraindications are absent, intravenous beta blockers are the drugs of choice for rate control in patients with thyrotoxicosis, alcohol withdrawal, hypertension, and in those with a history of angina pectoris or prior myocardial infarction.

Calcium Channel Blockers. The introduction of calcium channel blockers has dramatically improved management of AF. Excitation-contraction coupling in the heart depends on the activation of fast sodium and slow calcium channels. Calcium entering myocytes binds to troponin, freeing actin and myosin to contract. As a result, all calcium channel blockers have the potential to cause negative inotropy. In vascular tissue, increases in cytosolic calcium lead to contraction of smooth muscle. All classes of calcium channel blockers cause a decrease in arterial smooth muscle tone. They do not have significant effects on venous beds and do not increase venous capacitance or diminish preload.

AV node conduction depends, in part, on the rate of recovery of the calcium slow channel. The dihydropyridine calcium channel blockers (e.g., nifedipine) do not block the rate of recovery of the slow channel and consequently do not slow AV conduction. Verapamil (a phenylalkylamine calcium channel blocker) and diltiazem (a benzothiazepine) both decrease the rate of recovery of the slow channel, slowing conduction through the AV node. Verapamil and diltiazem may be associated with negative inotropic effects.[15,23]

When given intravenously, verapamil produces lowering of arterial blood pressure due to direct vasodilatation. There is also a blunting of the reflex tachycardia due to verapamil's negative chronotropic effects. The negative inotropic effects of verapamil are partly compensated by reduction in afterload. In patients with congestive heart failure, verapamil may cause profound hypotension due to diminished cardiac contractility and peripheral vasodilitation. However, in patients *without* preexisting left ventricular dysfunction, verapamil is generally safe and effective in controlling rate; symptomatic hypotension is rare even in otherwise healthy individuals.[24] Diltiazem has a similar effect on the AV node, but it is associated with less negative inotropy, making it a safer drug in patients with borderline low blood pressure or mild-to-moderate congestive heart failure.[25] As a general rule, verapamil is appropriate for rate control in the patient with hypertension and rapid AF, but who has no history of congestive heart failure. Diltiazem is ideal in the normotensive patient, and in the patient with mild-to-moderate heart failure who requires rapid rate control.

The use of diltiazem in the setting of heart failure is not entirely without risk, because there is a small incidence of hypotension.[25] Consequently, diltiazem should not be used in patients with preexisting hypotension or severe heart failure because of the risk of producing shock. One should also bear in mind the financial considerations related to the use of intravenous diltiazem. It is more costly than verapamil. And because of its short duration of action, an initial bolus must be followed by a continuous infusion, requiring nursing monitoring in the ED or, subsequently, in the CCU.

The transition from intravenous to oral diltiazem may take hours to achieve.[26] One protocol for the transition from intravenous to oral diltiazem has been described in the literature. *(Please see Table 3.)* Patients who were stable for two hours on an intravenous infusion of diltiazem were given a dose of long-acting oral diltiazem (diltiazem CD) based on the IV infusion rate. The infusion was stopped four hours after administration of the oral dose. Seventy-seven percent of patients maintained heart rate control during the transition period.

Unstable Patients with Rapid AF

The Patient With Acute Myocardial Infarction (AMI). The patient with AF in the setting of an acute myocardial infarction (AMI) frequently presents a management problem. The incidence of new onset AF in CCU patients with acute infarction is roughly 11-19%.[27,28] In anterior infarction, the arrhythmia may result from diminished left ventricular contractility with subsequent rise in left atrial pressure. In inferior infarction, AF is frequently associated with right ventricular infarction. In selected cases of transmural infarction, AF results from acute pericarditis.[29] Some patients with acute infarction have chronic or paroxysmal AF or comorbidities that predispose to AF such as hypertension or pulmonary disease.

ACLS guidelines recommend immediate electrical cardioversion for patients with serious signs or symptoms; however, these recommendations bear some consideration in the patient with AMI. In some patients with AMI, AF is *chronic*, and there will be a substantial risk of thromboembolism with DC cardioversion if adequate anticoagulation has not been maintained. These patients require immediate rate control with a beta blocker or calcium channel blocker. In patients with *new onset* AF, the arrhythmia frequently converts spontaneously within a short period of time.[27,30] The ventricular response is not always rapid, especially in the setting of inferior infarction, and may not require specific intervention.[31]

For those patients with acute infarction and rapid ventricular rates, success has been reported with the use of intravenous propranolol.[32] Propranolol and metoprolol both have long half-lives, posing a slight risk of prolonged bradycardia. However, early intravenous beta blocker therapy has been shown to decrease mortality in AMI. Esmolol, because of its short half-life, would, in theory, be slightly safer than propranolol or metoprolol. Because of the paucity of published data, however, the routine use of intravenous beta blockade over direct current cardioversion in the acutely infarcting patient cannot be recommended. Intravenous beta blockers would be appropriate in the patient who has failed cardioversion, or in the patient who has a rapid rate without ongoing ischemic chest pain.

Intravenous amiodarone has also been studied in patients with acute atrial fibrillation complicating myocardial infarction, and has the advantage of both achieving rapid slowing of the ventricular response, as well as restoring sinus rhythm in the majority of patients.[33,34] Although complications are rare, amiodarone can cause worsening of congestive heart failure and excessive slowing of the ventricular response.

DC cardioversion is clearly justified in patients with persistent ischemic chest pain and a rapid ventricular response. The risks of DC cardioversion are low; however, cardioversion can result in atrial or ventricular stunning (causing or exacerbating heart failure), inappropriate bradycardia, ventricular tachycardia, and, in rare cases, asystole.[35-40] Failure to synchronize the shock to the R wave may result in ventricular fibrillation.[36,41] Electrical cardioversion generally carries a high success rate (approaching 90%), but, in patients with AMI, there is a substantial risk that the arrhythmia will recur shortly after sinus rhythm is achieved.[33]

AF with Congestive Heart Failure. Patients with congestive heart failure and rapid AF also pose a management dilemma. A rapid ventricular response decreases ventricular filling and compromises cardiac output. The irregularity of the arrhythmia further decreases ventricular contractility and cardiac output.[42] If the degree of congestive heart failure is mild to moderate, then rate control with digoxin or diltiazem may suffice. In patients with severe congestive heart failure, there is a risk of symptomatic hypotension with diltiazem,[25] and digoxin is not capable of rapidly slowing the ventricular response. In these high-risk patients, DC cardioversion carries the slight danger of exacerbating heart failure through ventricular stunning, hypotension, or bradyarrhythmias.[43] There is also the problem of recurrence of the arrhythmia after an initially successful cardioversion.[33]

Some newer studies have addressed the use of intravenous amiodarone in hemodynamically destabilizing AF with severely depressed left ventricular function. Amiodarone has relatively little negative inotropy, and, even if sinus rhythm is not restored, control of the ventricular rate may confer substantial hemodynamic improvement.[33,44-47] In these high risk patients, many of whom require vasopressor support, the conversion rate to sinus rhythm is high, and amiodarone is well tolerated. However, there is a small risk of severe bradycardia, exacerbation of heart failure, and death. No consensus has yet emerged concerning the use of amiodarone in this difficult setting. For the time being, physicians should still attempt emergency DC cardioversion for severely compromised patients with heart failure and rapid ventricular rates. Intravenous amiodarone should be reserved for those patients who fail cardioversion.

AF with Hypotension. In general, a rapid ventricular rate does not lead to hypotension, although this tacharrhythmia will cause decreased cardiac output from impaired ventricular filling. Patients with rapid AF and significant hypotension usually have comorbidities that, combined with a rapid ventricular rate, produce hypotension. One should consider the possibility of intravascular volume depletion (from dehydration or blood loss), drug induced arterial dilatation, pulmonary embolism, cardiac tamponade, septic shock, and cardiogenic shock. Patients with rapid rates and symptomatic hypotension who are not volume overloaded should receive a fluid challenge. Failure to respond to a fluid challenge mandates emergency cardioversion. Patients who fail to respond to emergency cardioversion, or who revert to AF, will require pressor support and rate control with intravenous amiodarone and digoxin.[47] Calcium channel blockers and beta blockers are strictly contraindicated in the setting of hypotension.

The AF Patient with Preexcitation Syndrome. Wolff-Parkinson-White (WPW) and other accessory pathway syndromes can predispose to AF. When AF occurs in this subgroup of patients, activation of the ventricles may occur via the AV node, the accessory pathway, or, simultaneously, by both pathways. It should be stressed that the accessory pathway may be capable of conduction so as to produce ventricular rates faster than those seen with AV node conduction. Drugs used to slow the ventricular rate, by selectively blocking the AV node, may accelerate conduction through the bypass tract, leading to dramatic increases in rate and hemodynamic compromise. Rapidly conducted AF can degenerate into ventricular fibrillation in WPW patients (especially in those who have multiple accessory pathways).[48] Hence, there is some urgency in managing AF in patients with WPW. Intravenous procainamide slows conduction through the bypass tract and may chemically convert the rhythm to sinus. Stable patients should receive intravenous procainamide. Digoxin, beta blockers, or calcium channel blockers should not be used, since they can lead to preferential conduction through the bypass tract. Hemodynamically unstable patients should be shocked immediately, as should patients who fail to respond to procainamide, and patients with rates above 250 (they are at the highest risk of degeneration to VF).[49]

Thyrotoxicosis and AF. Thyroid disease may have a profound effect on cardiac performance. Thyrotoxicosis is characterized by a hyperdynamic circulatory state, in part due to increased total blood volume, decreased systemic vascular resistance, and a shortened circulation time. Thyroid hormone also acts as a positive chronotrope. In addition, left ventricular contractility is enhanced in thyrotoxicosis, as is left ventricular diastolic relaxation. Stroke volume and cardiac output are increased. One typically encounters a sinus tachycardia with a wide pulse pressure. AF is also common, occurring in 9-22% of patients with thyrotoxicosis.[49] The rapid ventricular response is usually refractory to standard doses of digoxin, but responds well to beta blocker therapy. Stable patients with thyrotoxicosis may be treated with oral beta blockers. The nonselective beta blocker propranolol is the drug of choice. Intravenous beta blocker therapy should be given in the ED for patients who require rapid rate control.

Severe thyrotoxicosis may result in a state of high output congestive heart failure. Although beta blockers are generally contraindicated in heart failure, in this setting beta blockade therapy

Table 4. Vaughn Williams Classification of Drugs Used in Atrial Fibrillation

IA	Quinidine, procainamide, disopyramide
IC	Flecainide, propafenone
II	Propranolol, metoprolol, esmolol
III	Sotolol, amiodarone, ibutilide
IV	Diltiazem, verapamil

may lead to rapid and dramatic improvement. Intravenous esmolol is the drug of choice in high-output failure due to thyrotoxicosis. Some patients, however—those who have progressed to an irreversible dilated cardiomyopathy, or may have underlying structural heart disease—will require conventional therapy with diuretics and traditional pre- and afterload reducing agents.

The Young Patient with AF. Although there is some heterogeneity in young (< 35 years) patients with AF, many will have "lone AF." These patients may present with new onset AF, with no apparent cardiac or systemic illnesses to account for the arrhythmia, or they may give a history of recurrent bouts of AF with a prior workup that has revealed no significant pathology. The dilemma is management to determine whether to pursue a rate control strategy or whether to cardiovert. One should base this decision in part upon the patient's history. For example, a patient who has had multiple prior bouts of AF is unlikely to remain in sinus rhythm if cardioverted in the ED, and should be treated with diltiazem to control the ventricular response. Diltiazem is superior to other agents in this setting. Verapamil has a greater potential to lower blood pressure and decrease contractility than diltiazem. Warfarin should not be given if the patient has lone AF since the risk of thromboembolism is extremely low in the absence of anticoagulation. In patients younger than 60 years with lone AF, the risk of thromboembolism is no greater than that of the general population.[50]

A young patient with a first episode of AF should be offered chemical cardioversion with intravenous ibutilide or electrical cardioversion under deep sedation. One should keep in mind that many patients who decline intervention will convert to sinus rhythm spontaneously. In addition, many patients successfully converted to a sinus mechanism (using either ibutilide or electricity) will eventually revert to AF.

Chemical Cardioversion of AF in the ED

Chemical cardioversion of acute AF in the ED has not yet gained widespread use, in part, because of a number of logistic factors. Patients must be carefully selected to minimize the risk of stroke and cardiac complications. Class IA and IC antiarrhythmics have shown moderate efficacy, but have some proarrhythmic and negative inotropic effects, requiring close inpatient monitoring.[51-53] The class III agents, amiodarone and sotolol, have been studied, but conversion rates in some studies have been disappointing, and both drugs require inpatient monitoring. Traditional drugs used to control the ventricular response (digoxin, diltiazem, verapamil, and pure beta blockers) do not reliably convert AF to sinus rhythm.[54] *(See Table 4.)*

Ibutilide is the first practical agent for ED use for chemical cardioversion of patients with new onset AF (< 48 hours). Ibutilide falls into the class III category of antiarrhythmic drugs and has the advantage of intravenous administration and a short half-life, so that within four hours of administration, the drug's electrophysiologic effects (prolongation of repolarization) are completely resolved.[55,56] Unfortunately, conversion rates for patients with AF treated with ibutilide are less than complete, with a reported success rate of about 30-50%.[57]

Ibutilide's effects on repolarization increase the risk of polymorphic ventricular tachycardia. Most of these cases terminate spontaneously; however, about 2% of patients treated with ibutilide will have sustained VT that requires electrical cardioversion.[58] Hence, patients should not be treated with ibutilide unless they are also suitable candidates for electrical cardioversion. Prior to giving ibutilide, patients should be in a fasting state; they must have normal electrolytes (incuding serum magnesium); and there should be no prior history of torsade de pointes, ventricular tachycardia, or sick sinus syndrome. Patients should also be excluded from ibutilide therapy if they have slow heart rates not caused by AV node blocking drugs, or if there is congestive heart failure or hypotension.

The greatest impediment to the practice of chemical cardioversion in the ED has to do with disappointing long-term outcomes. Only a small percentage of patients remain in sinus rhythm in the absence of chronic antiarrhythmic therapy. In general, drugs used to maintain sinus rhythm must be started days prior to chemical or electrical cardioversion. *(See Table 5.)* Ongoing clinical trials including Atrial Fibrillation Follow-Up Investigation of Rhythm Management (AFFIRM) and others will eventually determine which is superior: A strategy of rate control or pharmacological maintainance of sinus rhythm.

Prevention of Thromboembolism

The risk of stroke from cardiac emboli in chronic AF is significant; therefore, ED physicians must address the issue of anticoagulation. The Framingham Heart Study showed an overall risk of stroke of 5% per year in patients with nonvalvular AF.[59] The Stoke Prevention in Atrial Fibrillation (SPAF) study showed a stroke risk of 6.2% per year in non-anticoagulated patients.[60] There are important risk factors for stroke in the setting of AF. The presence of structural heart disease (i.e., left ventricular dysfunction, congestive heart failure, valvular heart disease, coronary artery disease, and left atrial enlargement) identifies a high-risk group for thromboembolism.[61,62] Patients with global left ventricular dysfunction have a stroke risk of 12% per year. Systemic factors that increase the risk of stroke are hypertension (5-6%/year), diabetes (8-9%/year), and prior stroke or TIA (12%/year).[61,62]

A number of clinical trials have prospectively evaluated these risk factors to determine which patients benefit from aspirin therapy alone and which require warfarin to achieve a meaningful reduction in stroke risk without an untoward increase in major bleeding complications. Aspirin, when compared with placebo, reduces the risk of stroke by 22%.[63] Warfarin, in contrast, is associated with a 64% reduction in stroke;[63] however, major bleeding can be expected in 2-3% of patients per year who are treated with warfarin.[63]

SPAF III prospectively identified a low-risk group for stroke in nonvalvular AF.[64] Low-risk patients are those with none of the following risk factors: hypertension or history of hypertension, recent congestive heart failure or left ventricular fractional shortening of 25% or less, previous thromboembolism, and female sex at age older than

Table 5. Emergency Electrical Cardioversion

- Choose a short-acting, intravenous anesthetic, or amnestic agent: Propofol, methohexitol, and midazolam are ideal
- Paddle placement: Hand held-right parasternal 2nd, 3d ICS and left lateral at cardiac apexor defibrillator pad-left parasternal and left posterior chest
- Energy: 200 joules initially, if unsuccessful wait 3 minutes, then 300 joules (if still unsuccessful, 360 joules). Synchronization on the R wave will prevent ventricular fibrillation

Table 6. Anticoagulation Guidelines in Atrial Fibrillation

- Recent congestive heart failure, or fractional shortening less than 25%*
- Rheumatic heart disease*
- Prior thromboembolism*
- Female sex, older than 75 years*
- Hypertension: Treat with warfarin or aspirin depending on patient preference and individual risk of complications
- None of the above risk factors: Treat with aspirin, 325 mg/day

* These risk factors require treatment with warfarin

75 years. Patients with no risk factors may be treated with aspirin (325 mg/day). Patients with hypertension have a moderate risk of stroke. Those patients should receive either aspirin or warfarin depending on the patient's preferences and individual risk of complications from warfarin. Patients with recent congestive heart failure, left ventricular fractional shortening of 25% or less, prior thromboembolism, or female sex older than 75 years have a high (8% per year) risk of stroke and should receive warfarin if there are no contraindications. Care should be taken to keep the INR between 2 and 3, since major bleeding generally occurs when the INR is above 3-3.5.

Numerous studies have demonstrated that 3-4 weeks of anticoagulation prior to attempts at cardioversion decreases the risk of stroke in those patients whose AF has lasted more than 48 hours.[65] *(Please see Table 6.)* In the absence of anticoagulation, there is a 5-7% risk of stroke. The 3-4 week period of anticoagulation prior to cardioversion reduces the risk of stroke to about 1.2%.[66] An alternative strategy is to perform transesophageal echocardiography in patients with AF of greater than 48 hours duration. In the absence of left atrial thrombus, patients may be safely cardioverted with a risk of stroke equivalent to that in patients receiving four weeks of warfarin prior to cardioversion.[66] Following cardioversion, patients should continue on warfarin for one month because return of atrial contractility may be delayed for several weeks in spite of the presence of p waves on the electrocardiogram.[65,67]

Recognition and Treatment of Thromboemboli in AF

Not all strokes that occur in patients with AF are the result of cardiac emboli. AF patients are a heterogeneous group, many of whom have hypertension, diabetes, atherosclerotic disease, and other conditions that predispose to stroke in the absence of a left atrial thrombus. The use of transesophageal echocardiography in AF has led to the recognition that some patients have complex plaque in the aortic arch that predisposes to embolic stroke.[68] The diagnosis of a cardioembolic stroke in a patient with AF is presumptive. In general, a cardioembolic etiology is suggested by the following: a) an infarct involving the cerebral surface territory of a single vessel, b) multiple infarcts occurring in different vascular territories, c) evidence of embolization to the extremities or other organs, and d) hemorrhagic infarction.[69]

The emergency physician evaluating a patient with AF and an acute stroke syndrome should perform a noncontrast head CT to exclude the possibility of a hemorrhage. The prothrombin time and INR should be checked. One should not begin immediate anticoagulation with heparin because of the risk of hemorrhagic transformation of the stroke.[70,71] The purpose of later heparinization is not to treat the acute stroke, but rather to prevent further embolic events. The optimal time to initiating anticoagulation following cardioembolic stroke is controversial. Numerous studies have shown a significant incidence in bleeding complications, without improvement in stroke outcome, when heparin is given immediately. There is no need for the emergency physician to immediately begin a heparin infusion. If heparin is started at the time of admission to the hospital, a continuous infusion is given, without a loading dose, in an attempt to minimize the risk of hemorrhagic transformation.

Cardiac emboli may result in acute limb ischemia, presenting with dramatic severe pain, pallor, coldness of the extremity, and a pulse deficit, in which case immediate anticoagulation with heparin (bolus, then continuous infusion) is indicated. Prompt surgical consultation should be obtained. Catheter or operative embolectomy, or infusion of a fibrinolytic agent is performed to restore perfusion to the ischemic limb. Similarly, sudden thromboembolism to a mesenteric artery will produce bowel ischemia and rapid subsequent infarction requiring immediate operative exploration, thrombectomy, and resection of nonviable bowel with primary anastamosis or a diversion.

Disposition

Because AF, is oftentimes not an ischemia-mediated arrhythmia, not all patients with new onset AF require hospitalization to rule out myocardial infarction.[72] Physicians should base the decision to rule out MI based on the presence of angina or anginal equivalents, features of the electrocardiogram, as well as the patient's general risk for having underlying coronary artery disease. In addition to the possibility of ischemia, there are other compelling reasons to admit patients with new onset AF to the hospital. The presence of decompensated heart failure, myocardial contusion, infective endocarditis, hypotension, syncope, renal failure, pneumonia, stroke, or sepsis are all reasonable indications for admission. Many patients with AF are elderly and have substantial comorbidities, including unsuspected conduction system disease that may lead to excessive bradycardia when drugs are given for rate control.

Some patients with new onset AF will spontaneously convert to sinus rhythm in the ED and may be safely discharged home with appropriate follow-up. Of those patients in whom AF persists, it is usually desirable to achieve restoration of sinus rhythm as soon as possible in order to relieve symptoms, prevent electrical remodeling, and to avoid the need for long-term anticoagulation.[73,74] Hence, one can also justify hospitalization of stable patients with new onset AF if they are likely to undergo attempts at chemical or electrical cardioversion.

Summary

ED evaluation and management of patients with AF is not always straightforward. A number of key points should be kept in mind. Drug therapy to control rate can result in significant side effects, including excessive bradycardia, hypotension, and exacerbation of left ventricular dysfunction. The selection of an agent to control rate should be based upon its side effect profile and the urgency surrounding the patient's symptoms and hemodynamic status. Patients who remain in AF are at significant risk for embolic stroke and will require initiation of appropriate anticoagulation. Finally, the decision to admit to the hospital will depend on the degree of cardiovascular instability, the presence of comorbidities, and the patient's suitability for chemical or electrical cardioversion.

References

1. Krahn AD, Manfreda J, Tate RB, et al. The natural history of atrial fibrillation: Incidence, risk factors, and prognosis in the Manitoba follow-up study. *Am J Med* 1995;98:476-484.
2. Kannel WB, Abbott RD, Savage DD, et al. Epidemiologic features of atrial fibrillation: The Framingham study. *N Engl J Med* 1982;306:1018-1022.
3. Camm AJ, Obel OA. Epidemiology and mechanism of atrial fibrillation and atrial flutter. *Am J Cardiol* 1996;78:3-11.
4. Prytkowsky EN, Benson DW, Fuster V, et al. Management of patients with atrial fibrillation. *Circulation* 1996;93: 1262-1277.
5. Gilligan DM, Ellenbogen KA. The management of atrial fibrillation. *Am J Med* 1996;101:413-421.
6. Ettinger PO, Wu CF, De La Cruz C, et al. Arrhythmias and the "holiday heart": Alcohol associated cardiac rhythm disorders. *Am Heart J* 1978;95:555-562.
7. Baer M, Goldschlager N. Atrial fibrillation: An update on new management strategies. *Geriatrics* 1995;50:22-29.
8. Bellandi F, Dabizzi RP, Di Natale M, et al. Intravenous propafenone: Efficacy and safety in the conversion to sinus rhythm of recent onset atrial fibrillation—A single blind placebo controlled study. *Cardiovasc Drugs Ther* 1996:10: 153-157.
9. Donovan KD, Dobb GJ, Coombs LJ, et al. Reversion of recent onset atrial fibrillation to sinus rhythm by intravenous flecainide. *Am J Cardiol* 1991;67:137-141.
10. Galve E, Rius T, Ballester RB, et al. Intravenous amiodarone in treatment of recent onset atrial fibrillation: Results of a randomized, controlled study. *J Am Coll Cardiol* 1996;27: 1079-1082.
11. Wijffels MC, Kirchhof CJ, Dorland R, at al. Atrial fibrillation begets atrial fibrillation. A study in awake chronically instrumented goats. *Circulation* 1995;92:1954-1968.
12. Laupacis A, Albers G, Dunn M, et al. Antithrombotic therapy in atrial fibrillation. *Chest* 1992;102:4265-4335.
13. Allessie M. Atrial fibrillation. In: Braunwald E et al, eds. *Cardiovascular Disease* p. 654-699.
14. Kelley RA, Smith TW. Pharmocolgic treatment of heart failure. In: Hardman JG, Limbird LE, eds. *The Pharmocologic Basis of Therapeutics*, 9th ed, p. 809-838.
15. Roden DM. Antiarrhythmic drugs. In Hardman JG, Limbird LE, eds. *The Pharmocologic Basis of Therapeutics*, 9th ed, 839-874.
16. The Digitalis Investigation Group. The effect of digoxin on mortality and morbidity in patients with heart failure. *N Engl J Med* 1997;336:525-533.
17. Falk RH, Knowlton AA, Bernard S, et al. Digoxin for conversion of recent onset atrial fibrillation: A randomized, double-blind trial. *Ann Int Med* 1987;106:503-506.
18. Shettigar UR. Management of rapid ventricular rate in acute atrial fibrillation. *Int J Clin Pharmacol Ther* 1994;32: 240-245.
19. Hays JV, Gilman JK, Rubal BJ. Effect of magnesium sulfate on ventricular rate control in atrial fibrillation. *Ann Emerg Med* 1994;24:64-64.
20. Brodsky MA, Orlov MV, Capareli EV, et al. Magnesium therapy in new onset atrial fibrillation. *Am J Cardiol* 1994;73: 1227-1229.
21. Hoffman BB, Lefkowitz RJ. Catecholamines, sympathomimetic drugs, and adrenergic receptor antagonists. In: Hardman JG, Limbird LE, eds. *The Pharmocologic Basis of Therapeutics*, 9th ed, p. 249-264.
22. Shettigar UR, Toole JG, Appunn DO. Combined use of esmolol and digoxin in the acute treatment of atrial fibrillation or flutter. *American Heart J* 1993;126:368-374.
23. Oates JA. Antihypertensive agents and the drug therapy of hypertension. In: Hardman JG, Limbird LE, eds. *The Pharmocologic Basis of Therapeutics*, 9th ed, 781-808.
24. Phillips BG, Gandhi AJ, Sanoski CA, et al. Comparison of intravenous diltiazem and verapamil for the acute treatment of atrial fibrillation and atrial flutter. *Pharmacother* 1997;17: 1238-1245.
25. Goldenberg IF, lewis WR, Dias VC, et al. Intravenous diltiazem in the treatment of patients with atrial fibrillation or flutter and moderate to severe congestive heart failure. *Am J Cardiol* 1994;74:884-889.
26. Blackshear JL, Stambler BS, Strauss WE, et al. Control of heart rate during transition from intravenous to oral diltizem in atrial fibrillation or flutter. *Am J Cardiol* 1996;78: 1246-1250.
27. Madias JE, Patel DC, Singh D. Atrial fibrillation in acute myocardial infarction: A prospective study based on data from a consecutive series of patients admitted to the coronary care unit. *Clin Cardiol* 1996;19:180-186.
28. Hildebrandt P, Jenson G, Kober L, et al. Myocardial infarction 1979-1988 in Denmark: Secular trends in age-related

incidence, in-hospital mortality and complications. *European Heart J* 1994;15:877-881.
29. Nagahama Y, Sugiura T, Takehana K, et al. The role of infarction-associated pericarditis on the occurrence of atrial fibrillation. *European Heart J* 1998;19:287-292.
30. Bertolet BD, Hill JA, Kerensky RA, et al. Myocardial infarction related atrial fibrillation: Role of endogenous adenosine. *Heart* 1997;78:88-90.
31. Madias JE.Atrial fibrillation in acute myocardial infarction: A prospective study based on data from a consecutive series of patients admitted to the coronary care unit (letter to the editor). *Clin Cardiol* 1996;19:618-619.
32. Lemberg L, Castellanos A, Arcebal AG. The use of propranolol in arrhythmias complicating acute myocardial infarction. *Am Heart J* 1970;80:479-487.
33. Cowan JC, Gardiner P, Reid DS, et al. A comparison of amiodarone and digoxin in the treatment of atrial fibrillation complicating suspected acute myocardial infarction. *J Cardiovasc Pharmacol* 1986;8:252-256.
34. Blandford RL, Crampton J, Kudlac H. Intravenous amiodarone in atrial fibrillation complicating myocardial infarction. *BMJ* 1982;284:16-17.
35. Ewey GA. Optimal technique for electrical cardioversion of atrial fibrillation. *Circulation* 1992;86:1645-1647.
36. Lip GY. Cardioversion of atrial fibrilllation. *Postgrad Med J* 1995;71:457-465.
37. Mehta PM, Reddy BR, Lesser J, et al. Severe bradycardia following electrical cardioversion for atrial tachyarrhythmias in patients with acute myocardial infarction. *Chest* 1990;97: 241-242.
38. Garcia-Rubira JC, Romero D, Garcia JT, et al. Transient myocardial injury after elective electrical cardioversion. *Int J Cardiol* 1994;46:283-285.
39. Xiong C, Sonnhag C, Nylander E, et al. Atrial and ventricular function after cardioversion of atrial fibrillation. *Brit Heart J* 1995;74:254-260.
40. Manning WJ, Silverman DI, Katz SE, et al. Impaired left atrial mechanical function after cardioversion: relation to the duration of atrial fibrillation. *J Am Coll Cardiol* 1994;23: 1535-1540.
41. Kerber RE. Transthoracic cardioversion of atrial fibrillation and flutter: Standard techniques and new advances. *Am J Cardiol* 1996;78:22-26.
42. Daoud EG, Weiss R, Bahu M, et al. Effect of an irregular ventricular rhythm on cardiac output. *Am J Cardiol* 1996;78: 1433-1436.
43. Upshaw CB. Hemodynamic changes after cardioversion of chronic atrial fibrillation. *Arch Internal Med* 1997;157: 1070-1076.
44. Hou Z-Y, Chang M-S, Chen C-Y, et al. Acute treatment of recent-onset atrial fibrillation and flutter with a tailored dosing regimen of intravemous amiodarone: a randomized, digoxin controlled study. *Eur Heart J* 1995;16:521-528.
45. Kumar A. Intravenous amiodarone for therapy of atrial fibrillation and flutter in critically ill patients with severely depressed left ventricular function. *South Med J* 1996;89: 779-785.
46. Lie KI, Van Gelder IC. Therapy of recent onset atrial fibrillation and flutter in haemodynamically compromised patients: Chemical cardioversion or control of the ventricular rate? *Eur Heart J* 1995;16:433-434.
47. Clemo HF, Wood MA, Gilligan DM, et al. Intravenous amiodarone for acute heart rate control in the critically ill patient with atrial tachyarrhythmias. *Am J Cardiology* 1998;81: 594-598.
48. Klein GJ, Bashore TM, Sellers TD, et al. Ventricular fibrillation in the Wolff-Parkinson-White syndrome. *N Engl J Med* 1979;301:1080-1085.
49. Woeber KA. Thyrotoxicosis and the heart. *N Engl J Med* 1992;327:94-98.
50. Kopecky SL, Gersh BJ, McGoon MD, et al. The natural history of lone atrial fibrillation: A population-based study over three decades. *N Engl J Med* 1987;317:669-674.
51. Blitzer M, Costeas C, Kassotis J, et al. Rhythm management in atrial fibrillation-with a primary emphasis on pharmocologic therapy: Part 1. *PACE* 1998;21:590-602.
52. Costeas C, Kassotis J, Blitzer M, et al. Rhythm management in atrial fibrillation-with a primary emphasis on pharmocologic therapy: Part 2. *PACE* 1998;21:742-749.
53. Kassotis J, Costeas C, Blitzer M, et al. Rhythm management in atrial fibrillation-with a primary emphasis on pharmocologic therapy: Part 3. *PACE* 1998;21:1133-1142.
54. Jordaens L, Trouerbach J, Calle P, et al. Conversion of atrial fibrillation to sinus rhythm and rate control by digoxin in comparison to placebo. *European Heart J* 1997;18:643-648.
55. Naccarelli GV, Lee KS, Gibson JK, et al. Electrophysiology and pharmacology of ibutilide. *Am J Cardiol* 1996;78:12-16.
56. Roden DM. Ibutilide and the treatment of atrial tachyarrhythmias: A new drug—almost unheralded—is now available to US physicians. *Circulation* 1996;94:1499-1502.
57. Ellenbogen KA, Clemo HF, Stambler BS, et al. Efficacy of ibutilide for termination of atrial fibrillation and flutter. *Am J Cardiol* 1996;78:42-45.
58. Kowey PR, VanderLugt JT, Luderer JR. Safety and risk/benefit analysis of ibutilide for acute conversion of atrial fibrillation/flutter. *Am J Cardiol* 1996;78:46-52.
59. Wolf PA, Dawber TR, Thomas HE, et al. Epidemiologic assessment of chronic atrial fibrillation and risk of stroke: The framingham study. *Neurology* 1978;28:973-977.
60. Stroke prevention in atrial fibrillation investigators. Predictors of thromboembolism in atrial fibrillation: I. Clinical features of patients at risk. *Ann Int Med* 1992;116:1-5.
61. Asinger RW, Hart RG, Helgason CM, et al. Predictors of thromboembolism in atrial fibrillation: I. Clinical features of patients at risk. *Ann Int Med* 1992;116:1-5.
62. Cleland JG, Cowburn PJ, Falk RH. Should all patients with atrial fibrillation receive warfarin? Evidence from randomized clinical trials. *European Heart J* 1996;17:674-681.
63. Flacker GC. Anticoagulation issues in atrial fibrillation. *Cardiol Review* 1998;6:199-202.
64. SPAF III writing committee for the stroke prevention in atrial fibrillation investigators. Patients with nonvalvular atrial fibrillation at low risk of stroke during treatment with aspirin: Stroke prevention in atrial fibrillation III study. *JAMA* 1998; 279:1273-1277.
65. Laupacis A, Albers G, Dunn M, et al. Antithrombotic therapy

in atrial fibrillation. *Chest* 1992;102:426S-433S.

66. Silverman DI, Manning WJ. Role of echocardiography in patients undergoing elective cardioversion of atrial fibrillation. *Circulation* 1998;98:479-486.
67. Harjai KJ, Mobarek SK, Cherif J, et al. Clinical variables affecting recovery of left atrial mechanical function after cardioversion from atrial fibrillation. *J Am Coll Cardiol* 1997; 30:481-486.
68. Stroke prevention in atrial fibrillation investigators committee on electrocardiography. Transesophageal echocardiography corrolates of thromboembolism in high risk patients with nonvalvular atrial fibrillation. *Ann Int Med* 1998;128:639-647.
69. Adams HP, Biller J. Ischemic cerebrovascular disease. in Bradley WG, Daroff RB, Fuichel GM, eds. *Neurology in Clinical Practice,* 2nd ed.
70. Albers GW, Bittar N, Young L, et al. Clinical characteristics and management of acute stroke in patients with atrial fibrillation admitted to U.S. university hospitals. *Neurology* 1997; 48:1598-1604.
71. Sherman DG, Dyken ML, Gent M, et al. Antithrombotic therapy for cerebrovascular disorders: An update. *Chest* 1995; 108:444S-456S.
72. Mulcahy B, Coates WC, Heneman PL, et al. New-onset atrial fibrillation: When is admission medically justified? *Acad Emerg Med* 1996;3:114-119.
73. Mandel WJ. Should every patient with atrial fibrillation have the rhythm converted to sinus rhythm? *Clin Cardiol* 1994;17: 16-20.
74. Phibbs BP. Atrial fibrillation and hospital admission (letter to the editor). *Acad Emerg Med* 1996;3:820.

Syncope

Arthur M. Pancioli, MD
Patsy M. McNeil, MD

Syncope is defined as a sudden, transient loss of consciousness with an accompanying loss of postural tone.[1,2] As every emergency physician knows, this common symptom is oftentimes the first manifestation of a potentially life-threatening disorder that is difficult to evaluate in a comprehensive fashion within the emergency department (ED) setting.

Not infrequently, however, the ED evaluation of syncope will press into service significant technical and physician resources, requiring substantial financial expenditures, that fail to produce a diagnosis. Moreover, a lack of consensus regarding the optimal approach for assessment of patients with syncope further emphasizes the need for a standardized, evidence-based framework to guide ED physicians in these clinical encounters.

The following review emphasizes the importance of the history, physical examination, and electrocardiogram for distinguishing between serious and benign causes of syncope. In addition, an expeditious approach for pinpointing the etiology of syncopal episodes is presented. Finally, this issue is intended to help the emergency physician differentiate high-risk patients with potentially lethal conditions that require admission from low-risk patients who may be safely discharged home with outpatient follow-up.

Epidemiology

Syncope is a common presenting complaint among patients presenting to the ED and accounts for about 1-6% of all ED visits.[3,4] The Framingham study found a 3.3% incidence of syncope in a cohort of patients followed over a 26-year period. Other reports indicate that the lifetime incidence of syncope may be as high as 48%, with a significant percentage of individuals choosing not to seek medical attention.[5,6]

From a practical and statistical perspective, the majority of all patients who have a documented syncopal episode have a benign etiology, they sustain minimal injury, and they have no long-term increase in mortality. Nevertheless, evaluation of syncope is critical, first because it is a common presenting complaint in the ED and second, because patients in whom syncope is the manifestation of a cardiac etiology have a high risk of mortality and sudden death in the absence of appropriate intervention.

In fact, among all patients with syncope, 5-28% present with a cardiac cause, the group with the poorest prognosis. Specifically, syncope of confirmed cardiac origin is associated with a one-year mortality rate of about 18-33%[7-11] as compared to a 6% one-year mortality in patients with syncope of unknown etiology, and 12% one-year mortality in those patients with syncope from other causes.[6,12] The increased mortality is associated with such cardiac precipitants as bradyarrhythmias, ventricular rhythm disturbances, and myocardial infarctions, and are the principal reason that the ED evaluation of syncope attempts to identify and triage patients with syncope of cardiac origin.

In addition, syncope occurs across a broad age range with an estimated 15-20% of all children experiencing at least one episode of syncope before the end of adolescence.[13-15] The incidence of syncope in the elderly is approximately 6% per year, with an overall recurrence rate of 30%.[16] Not surprisingly, syncope is a significant cause of morbidity and mortality in the elderly, in which the trauma resulting from falls is more often associated with major injury than it is in other age groups.[17]

Clinical Pathophysiology. Syncope, from the Greek word *synkope* or "pause," usually is caused by events that result in a transient decrease in cerebral blood flow, glucose metabolism, or oxygen supply. Although individual variation exists, a reduction in cerebral blood flow of greater than 35% will produce syncope, and a disruption of cerebral perfusion for 5-10 seconds results in loss of consciousness.[5] Cerebral blood flow is directly related to maintenance of vascular tone and systemic blood pressure that, in turn, is directly related to heart rate (HR), stroke volume (SV), and cardiac output (CO), as well as systemic vascular resistance (SVR). Four general mechanisms best describe the different types of syncope.[6]

- Vasomotor instability and sudden reduction in SVR (vasodepressor syncope);
- Decreased CO caused by mechanical obstruction (aortic stenosis, atrial myxoma);
- Decreased CO caused by hemodynamically significant arrhythmias (VT, VFIB);
- Decreased perfusion due to cerebrovascular disease (SAH, ischemic stroke, basilar artery migraine, etc.).

General Principles. Patients admitted to the ED who have had transient unconsciousness or presyncopal episodes should be treated as presenting with a major symptom with potentially serious sequelae. They should not be kept waiting in the waiting room and should immediately be admitted into the department and onto a bed. A cardiac monitor should be placed, an intravenous line started, and, in the absence of other contraindications, at least low-flow oxygen administered.

A history should then be taken from the patient with the intention of interviewing appropriate witnesses, especially if the patient does not have knowledge of the events surrounding his or her loss of consciousness. A careful history and physical examination will reveal the cause of the syncope or dizziness in up to 70% of cases.

In the history, careful differentiation of the several conditions causing diminished cerebral blood flow must be made. When faintness is related to primary cardiac pathology, there is usually a combination of dermal pallor and cyanosis. On the other hand, when peripheral circulation is at fault, pallor is usually a striking manifestation and is not accompanied by cyanosis or respiratory disturbances. When the primary disturbance is in the cerebral circulation, the face is likely to be florid and the breathing to be slow and stertorous.

During the attack, a heart rate faster than 150 beats per minute indicates an ectopic cardiac rhythm, while a bradycardia of less than 40 beats per minute suggests complete heart block. In a patient experiencing faintness or syncope attended by bradycardia, one must distinguish between a reflex vasovagal attack and cardiogenic or a Stokes-Adams type of bradycardia. Of course, the electrocardiogram (ECG) is decisive and must be taken in any elderly patient who presents with syncope.

Careful delineation of symptoms before the patient's loss of consciousness (premonitory symptoms), during the event, and after the event will allow the practitioner to place the patient in diagnostic categories that will aid in the diagnosis.

With regard to premonitory symptoms, attention should be given to the period of time during which the attack develops. If the attack begins over a period of seconds, carotid sinus syncope, postural hypotension, sudden AV block, ventricular standstill, or fibrillation is likely. When the symptoms develop gradually during a period of several minutes, hyperventilation or hypoglycemia should be considered. The occurrence of syncope during or after exertion would, of course, suggest aortic outflow obstruction.

The position of the patient at the onset of the attack is important. Epilepsy and syncopal attacks due to hypoglycemia, hyperventilation, or heart block are likely to be independent of posture. Faintness associated with a decline in blood pressure and with tachycardia usually occurs only in the sitting position, whereas faintness associated with orthostatic hypotension is likely to occur shortly after the change from the recumbent to the standing position.

Associated symptoms must also be noted. These include palpitations and numbness and tingling of the hands and face, which are frequent accompaniments of hyperventilation. Genuine convulsions during the attack will also prove diagnostic.

Careful query should be made about the duration of the attack. When the duration is brief (i.e., a few seconds to a few minutes), carotid sinus syncope or one of the syncopal forms of postural hypotension is most likely. A duration of a few minutes but less than an hour suggests hypoglycemia or hyperventilation.

In the physical examination, certain procedures should always be carried out in the patient with syncope. Orthostatic blood pressures with the patient lying, sitting with legs dangling, and standing should be performed, taking careful note of both blood pressure and pulse. A drop in blood pressure without a pulse rise, as indicated before, should indicate a primary autonomic disturbance causing the orthostatic hypotension. As with any patient, note carefully any abnormal vital signs. The thrust of the physical examination should be toward the detection of localizing neurologic signs, with a careful cardiopulmonary examination with specific attention toward suspicious murmurs, abnormal pulse or pulse formation, and bruits.

Etiology

Syncope can result from a variety of causes, ranging from minimal morbidity to severe life-threatening illnesses. These etiologies include: cardiac, vasomotor/neurally mediated, toxic/metabolic, and psychogenic. *(Please see Table 1.)* In addition, syncope also may be of unknown cause.

It should be stressed that the diagnostic yield of confirmed causes in the work-up of syncope is low and, in fact, the specific etiology of syncope is unknown in up to 50% of patients, regardless of how extensive the evaluation.[2,6,18]

Several causes of syncope listed in Figure 1 have presentations that are suggestive of the diagnosis. Unfortunately, few population-based studies have, in sufficient detail, compared the presentations of various types of syncope to permit clear differentiation among different etiologies, according to symptoms or the clinical features. Nevertheless, Figure 2 identifies characteristics of various causes of

Table 1. Differential Diagnosis of Syncope

Cardiovascular Causes	Vasomotor or Neurally Mediated Causes
ARRHYTHMIAS	
Tachycardic arrhythmias	Vasodepressor/vasovagal
Supraventricular tachycardia	Subarachnoid hemorrhage
Ventricular tachycardia	Subdural hemorrhage
Ventricular fibrillation	Ischemic stroke
Wolfe-Parkinson-White	Vertebrobasilar Insufficiency
Bradycardic arrhythmias	Transient ischemic attack
Sick sinus syndrome	Basilar artery migraine
Atrial fibrillation with slow conduction	Glasopharyngeal or Trigeminal neuralgia
2nd and 3rd degree heart block	Situation/Reflex syncope
Pacemaker malfunction	Micturation
Carotid sinus sensitivity	Defecation
Long Q-T syndrome	Post-tussive
Structural	Weightlifters
Aortic stenosis	Post-prandial
Mitral stenosis	Swallow
Pulmonic stenosis	Emotional
Hypertrophic cardiomyopathy	Orthostatic disorder
Restrictive cardiomyopathy	Anemia
Dilated cardiomyopathy	Dehydration
Atrial myxoma	**TOXIC/METABOLIC**
Cardiac tamponade	Drugs
Congenital heart disease	Hypoglycemia
Vascular Disease	Hypoxemia
Aortic dissection	Carbon monoxide poisoning
Myocardial infarction	Other chemicals/ natural gases
Pulmonary embolus	
Pulmonary hypertension	**PSYCHOGENIC**
Air embolism	Anxiety disorder
Subclavian steal	Conversion disorder
Anomalous origin of left coronary artery from the right sinus of Valsalva	Somatization disorder
	Panic disorder
	Breath-holding
	Hyperventilation

syncope that may aid in pinpointing a specific syncopal syndrome or precipitating factor. *(Please see Table 2.)*

Vasodepressor Syncope. The most common cause of syncope, vasodepressor syncope, results from a transient failure of autonomic cardiovascular control mechanisms. Vasodepressor syncope begins with an increase in sympathetic tone accompanied by an increase in blood pressure, heart rate, and systemic vascular resistance. This is followed by an abrupt and inappropriate reversal as vagal tone increases, causing sudden hypotension with or without bradycardia and negative inotropy. A rapid and pronounced loss of consciousness with an accompanying loss of postural tone results. Normally, the neurovascular system is controlled via reflex arcs of autoregulation involving feedback loops within the carotid sinus, aortic arch, and cardiac mechanoreceptors. *(Please see Table 3.)* When these reflex arcs fail, vasomotor instability and sudden reduction in SVR result in vasodepressor syncope or the "common faint." The net result is venous pooling in the lower extremities, withdrawal of sympathetic tone, and increased parasympathetic activity. This, along with decreased venous return to the heart, produces a decrease in cerebral perfusion. Because of the increase in parasympathetic- and, especially, vagal-tone, the patient's symptoms often include feelings of weakness, pallor, sweating, nausea, and abdominal cramping, all of which frequently accompany the common fainting spell.[1,6,17,19]

Vasodepressor or vasovagal syncope accounts for approximately 40% of syncopal episodes. Vasodepressor syncope carries a worse prognosis in the elderly than with younger patients. Approximately 16% of elderly patients experiencing vasodepressor syncope have major morbidity or mortality in the intervening six months, whereas less than 1% of patients younger than age 30 who present with this type of syncope are at such risk.

This is the common faint experienced by most people. Regardless of the precise mechanism, all of these patients experience hypotension accompanied by an inappropriate slowing of the heart rate. The setting is very important in the diagnosis of vasovagal syncope. Typically, these spells occur after an emotional upset, in crowded warm rooms, or during prolonged standing, as seen in children during school assemblies or in soldiers during parades or inspections. They also occur after injurious shocking events or prolonged bed rest, and during pain and fasting. Mild blood loss, poor physical condition, anemia, fever, and organic heart disease also will predispose a person to vasovagal syncope. Such fainting spells occur in approximately 5% of normal blood donors. Full meals and warm baths, which cause diversion of blood away from the brain to the viscera and extremities, also predispose people to these spells.

Patients are always standing or sitting in the premonitory phase before these spells. Very characteristically, there is a spectrum of premonitory symptoms that lasts for at least a few seconds and usually for a few minutes or longer.

Recovery comes after the patient assumes the recumbent position, although pallor and weakness often persist. Episodes may recur within a half-hour if the patient attempts to stand again. Usually, no specific therapy is needed, although pretreatment with atropine in predisposed individuals can reduce this type of syncope. In the ED, an IV infusion of dextrose and normal saline is usually all that is required, along with monitoring. Adrenergic agents are rarely necessary.

Orthostatic Syncope. This type of syncope affects elderly patients who have a disproportion between blood volume and vascular capacitance or a chronic defect or instability of vasomotor reflexes. The character of the syncopal attack is similar to that of the vasovagal or vasodepressor type of syncope. However, the effect of posture is the cardinal feature here. Sudden rising from the recumbent or sitting position is the circumstance in which it is most likely to happen. Elderly patients are particularly predisposed to this type of syncope. They frequently lack physical conditioning and undergo prolonged illness and recumbency. Their flabby muscles allow more pooling of blood in their legs, and they frequently have venous insufficiency, which increases the capacity for the pooling of blood in the legs.

Table 2. Characteristics of Syncope Diagnoses

DIAGNOSIS	ONSET WITH	QUALITIES	NOTE
Arrhythmias[14,30,48]	Unpredictable triggers, although electrolyte imbalance may increase arrhythmic potential	Often sudden in onset. Often in patients with history of organic heart disease or strong family history of sudden death, arrhythmias. Quick post-event recovery of mentation	Increased risk of VT or AV block in males, the elderly, < 3 episodes syncope, < 6 sec warning. Presence of mechanical pacers often deceptively reassuring
Structural Cardiac Disease[11]	Exertion	Rapidly progressive symptoms to syncopal event. Murmurs characteristic. Positional symptoms common with myxoma	Patients with mechanical valves warrant close evaluation if no admittance
Pulmonary embolus[31,32]	Hypercoaguable state, known DVT	Sudden onset. Dyspnea, tachypnea, chest pain	Incidence of syncope associated with PE = 14%. Dx of syncope missed in 70% of patients who survive the first hour
Carotid Sinus Hypersensitivity[6,11]	Carotid sinus stimulation. Tight collars, sudden neck movement, shaving	Rapid onset. Rapid post-event mental clearing. Relatively common disorder, but uncommonly a cause of syncope.	More common in older age range. Must differentiate with VB insufficiency. More often elicited with R-sided carotid massage.
Aortic Dissection[34,48]	—	Ripping pain. Progressive clinical deterioration	Marfan's, syphilis, Cystic medial necrosis
Vasovagal[33,48]	Upright posture. Often triggered with emotion or pain	Brief prodrome of lightheadedness, visual blurring common but not unique. Rapid resolution of symptoms when patient supine	Potentially high morbidity in the elderly. Patients often otherwise healthy. Symptoms alone do not replace rule out of arrhythmic cause
CVA/TIA[6,7,22]	Unpredictable	Focal neurologic findings. Vertigo, ataxia, paresthesia, diplopia	Patient may have history of TIA, atherosclerosis, or hypercoagulable state. 1.5-7.7% of TIAs have syncope
Subarachnoid Hemorrhage[34]	Unpredictable. Sentinel bleeding possible warning	Severe headache of sudden onset with or w/o focal neurologic signs. Nausea and meningeal signs common	Family history contributive. Systolic hypertension > 200 occurs in up to 35% of patients. Cardiac dysrhythmias and ECG changes not uncommon
Vertebrobasilar Insufficiency[35]	Onset with posture change or movement of neck—especially hyperextension	Accompanying symptoms may include visual blurring, blindness, nausea, dysarthria, dysphagia. Symptoms transient	History and exam suggestive, while MRI aids in more definitive diagnosis
Hypoglycemia[3,7]	Increased insulin administration or inadequate p.o. intake	Symptoms of being jittery, diaphoresis,increasing mental status change often precede any loss of consciousness	Any associated syncopal symptoms not usually transient in nature unless hypoglycemia corrected
Hyperventilation[34]	Emotional upset or pain	Gradual onset. Gradual progression to full mental clearance with control of ventilation	Vertigo common. Association with perioral and extremity numbness, carpo pedal spasms
Basilar Artery Migraine[35]	Unpredictable. Triggers may occur, but visual prodrome often absent	Vertigo common and accompanied by vomiting, dysarthria, and commonly unilateral occipital or suboccipital headache	Usually found in younger women. Family history of migraines common

Table 2. Characteristics of Syncope Diagnoses *(continued)*

DIAGNOSIS	ONSET WITH	QUALITIES	NOTE
Glossopharyngeal or Trigeminal Neuralgia[36]	Swallowing is common trigger w/ glossopharyngeal neuralgia. Onset of syncope sudden and usually associated with paroxysmal pain	Pain a more prominent complaint. Syncope rare.	—
Reflex syncope[34]	Urination, defecation, cough, eating, swallowing, emotional upset, or weight lifting	Morbidity more significant than mortality	Cough—Often COPD and male. Seen in pediatric population. Almost never seen in women. Micturation—Often with male nocturia. Esp with ETOH. Swallow—May occur in patients with esophageal or cardiac conduction disorder
Subclavian Steal[4,11]	Exercise of arm on affected side	Global ischemia and syncope rare. Neurologic defects typically only contralateral to side of effected subclavian	—
Pulmonary Hypertension[34]	May have inciting event such as PE or MI	Functional acute obstruction to pulmonary flow decreasing preload and CO	—
Hypovolemia[43]	Prolonged bleeding, emesis, or diarrhea	Orthostatic hypotension often evident. Historical clues usually foundation of diagnosis	Finding source of hypovolemia key in managing disorder
Drug syncope[13,28,40]	Medication administration or without clear association to particular medicine	More prevalent in the elderly. Multiple medications may contribute. Characteristics of syncope vary widely	Note that the elderly overall tolerate antihtn agents well, and agents such as antiparkinson, antidepressants, and neuroleptics should be suspect as well.
Hypoxemia[35]	Any asphyxiating circumstance	Pulmonary source more common but CO, natural gas, chemical source such as bleach/ammonia mix not rare	Source of hypoxemia must be defined
Myocardial Infarction[15,20]	Unpredictable syncope onset	May be caused by multiple causes, including decreased EF, tamponade, arrhythmia	ECHO and angiogram key to management decision making
Anomalous origin of left coronary artery from the Right Sinus of Valsalva[37,38]	Exercise frequently insisting event	Usually an etiology of the pediatric population	Angiogram key to management decision making
Subdural Hematoma[35]	Unpredictable syncope onset	Preceding findings possibly subtle with forgetfulness, persistent headache	May occur at time of head trauma but most typically occurs at prolonged period afterwards
Air embolus	Large intravascular air bolus from iatrogenic or diving source	Symptoms often consistent with pulmonary embolism due to similar mechanism	Hyperbaric oxygen dive may be essential

Table 3. Causes of Drug Syncope

• Vasodilators	• Adrenergic antagonists (a & B)
• Diuretics	• Phenothiazines
• Antidepressants	• Calcium channel blockers
• CNS depressants	• Neuropathic drugs
• Drugs prolonging QT	• Central acting hypertensives
• EtOH, marijuana, cocaine	• Viagra

Furthermore, elderly patients are subject to neuropathies, which are more frequent in their age group. The elderly diabetic patient who gets diabetic neuropathy, which may affect the autonomic nervous system, is particularly at risk. Diabetic neuropathy is very rare in juvenile diabetics. In addition, there is a higher incidence of the chronic complications of alcoholism (including peripheral neuropathy and other degenerative neuronal processes) that occur in geriatric patients.

Furthermore, there are more geriatric patients receiving antihypertensive, vasodilator, and antiparkinsonism drugs—all of which may predispose them to orthostatic hypotension.

Loss of vasoconstrictor reflexes in the resistance and capacitance vessels of the lower extremities, as mentioned above, leads to orthostatic hypotension and syncope. Elderly patients are particularly predisposed to specific abnormalities known as primary autonomic insufficiency or dysautonomias. These defects may occur either in peripheral (postganglionic) or central (preganglionic) neurons.

Cardiac Syncope. Although cardiac syncope has several causes, the principal underlying mechanism is decreased cardiac output due to either decreased stroke volume or heart rate. *(See Table 1.)* Causes of decreased stroke volume include mechanical obstructions (aortic stenosis, atrial myxoma), conditions with decreased ejection fraction (myocardial infarction, cardiomyopathies), and conditions with decreased filling time (tachyarrhythmias). Bradyarrhythmias also may lead directly to decreased cardiac output.[6,20]

Approximately 30-35% of syncopal episodes in the elderly patient result from some type of cardiac dysfunction. The morbidity and mortality of cardiac syncope is significantly higher than with other types of syncope, with a mortality rate of 19% in patients admitted to a medical intensive care unit.

Cardiac syncope results from transient reduction in cerebral perfusion from a primary decrease in cardiac output. It is the one specific cause of syncope that may occur while the patient is in the recumbent or supine position. Loss of consciousness in an elderly patient, especially when sitting or supine, must always suggest cardiac syncope until proven otherwise. The cardinal manifestation of cardiac syncope is loss of consciousness, which can occur in any position. The patient may experience a brief premonitory weakness, palpitations, or chest pain, depending on the cause of the cardiac syncope. It is estimated that 4-7 seconds of asystole are required for the patient to lose consciousness in the upright position, and that as long as 20-30 seconds are required if the patient is recumbent so that such brief premonition is not consistent with cardiac syncope. There are multiple types of cardiac syncope, including bradyarrhythmias, tachyarrhythmias, and mechanical obstruction to cardiac output.

Cardiac syncope, resulting from atrioventricular block, is perhaps the most common type of bradyarrhythmic syncope; syncopal episodes associated with this arrhythmia are known as the Morgagni-Adams-Stokes syndrome. When patients develop heart block, there is a sudden interruption of intraventricular conduction, and asystole will exist (the warm-up period) for 10-90 seconds before any ventricular rhythm begins. During this period of asystole, a dizzy spell of syncope may be experienced by the patient. Often, the clinical picture is that of an elderly individual who complains of brief episodes of dizziness and presyncope that occur without warning, often 2-3 times per day. These episodes frequently occur over a period of several weeks. If the diagnosis is not made and a pacemaker not implanted, 50% of these patients will be dead within one year.

Patients who develop complete heart block from coronary artery disease (CAD) usually have prior evidence of conduction disease if, in fact, previous ECGs are available.

There are, of course, other causes of chronic progressive heart block. Calcific encroachment into the atrioventricular (AV) node and His-Purkinje system, usually in association with aortic valve calcification, is also a relatively frequent cause. Iatrogenic heart block may result from cardiac surgery or valve replacement.

Previous ECGs may help the ED physician suspect the occurrence of complete heart block. Variable patterns that may have been present in these patients include right bundle branch block and left anterior hemiblock—perhaps the most frequent pattern in patients subsequently developing complete heart block, right bundle branch alone, left anterior hemiblock alone, or left bundle branch block alone. A chief problem is the prediction of or the likelihood of progression to complete heart block in patients with bundle branch block on a baseline ECG. Prospective follow-up studies suggest that documented or suspected heart block develops in only 4-6% of cases observed for three and one-half years. However, patients with chronic bifascicular and trifascicular conduction abnormalities show a higher incidence of subsequent heart block when they have histories of syncope (17%) than when they do not (2%).

Neurologic Syncope. Neurologic syncope results from cerebrovascular disease associated with decreased global perfusion or focal involvement of the brainstem. Neurologic syncope may also occur in the setting of such systemic metabolic derangements as hypoglycemia, hypoxemia, or secondary to toxins or drugs.

Syncope in the elderly patient is frequently attributed to transient ischemic attacks (TIAs). Loss of consciousness must involve nonperfusion of the reticular activating system, and as such, TIAs in the carotid distribution usually do not involve loss of consciousness. Vertebrobasilar system TIAs, however, may involve loss of consciousness; however, syncope alone is the exception rather than the rule. Other symptoms associated with vertebrobasilar insufficiency (including diplopia, dysarthria, bilateral weakness, bilateral visual loss, and vertigo) usually accompany loss of consciousness. One specific manifestation of vertebrobasilar TIA that both signals its origin and is relatively pathognomonic of vertebrobasilar insufficiency is the so-called "drop" attack or akinetic collapse. In this type of episode, patients usually do not lose consciousness but experience sudden inescapable paralysis of their extremities, especially the legs, falling to the floor helplessly. This usually signifies TIA of the brainstem, and these attacks are characterized by "tunnel vision," speechlessness, or ptosis.

It must be noted that although the possibility of transient cerebral ischemic attacks must always be considered in older patients who complain of spells of dizziness, virtually all symptoms commonly associated with the usual TIAs are focal in nature, whereas patients with a complete loss of consciousness generally fall into a different diagnostic category. Thus, if a careful description of the patient's symptoms indicated that the event was focal in nature, cerebrovascular disease should be the primary consideration. It should be noted, however, that a combination of extracranial occlusive disease and hypotension from another cause, even if only moderate in severity, may lead to syncope in the geriatric patient. Syncope in elderly patients also occurs during relatively brief runs of supraventricular tachycardia. Bilateral tight carotid stenosis or unilateral stenosis with occlusion of the contralateral carotid is particularly likely to predispose such patients to syncope.

Mechanisms protecting against syncope in the general population may be altered in the elderly due to age-related physiologic changes. The elderly may have a decreased baroreceptor sensitivity, as well as a blunted plasma renin and aldosterone response causing adverse alterations in extra cellular fluid balance.[21,22] Thus, any emotional or physiologic stressor applied to the elderly population results in a lower threshold for syncope.

Syncope and Seizures

Seizure disorders must be in the differential diagnosis of transient loss of consciousness in the elderly patient. Seizures are usually marked by an abrupt loss of consciousness. Unlike syncope, seizures usually occur without warning in more than 50% of cases. As with Stokes-Adams attacks, an abrupt loss of consciousness may occur in the supine position, independent of the patient's activity level or posture and without warning. A careful interview of the patient and witnesses may help distinguish the occurrence of the seizure from syncope. Although 50% of seizures occur without warning, the remainder present with a brief, momentary, premonitory syndrome or aura. This aura usually does not include weakness, dizziness, or graying of vision but, rather, does include discrete neurologic symptoms such as an auditory phenomenon, a queasy stomach, complex visual experiences, or unpleasant olfactory sensations. The seizure can occur even during sleep and may be induced by monotonous music or loud noise. It may begin with a cry as air is emitted and forced through the closed glottis. Characteristically, the eyes turn either to one side or upward, although this sign is of little value in localizing the side of the neurologic deficit. There is usually stertorous breathing and cyanosis rather than pallor. Frequently, tachycardia rather than a slow thready pulse is present.

Perhaps the most characteristic and distinguishing feature between seizures and syncope is the postictal phenomenon. Frequently, patients have been injured during their seizure episode—an occurrence most unlikely in syncope where patients have premonitory warnings to allow them to protect themselves. The period of unconsciousness does tend to be longer in epilepsy than in syncope; urinary and fecal incontinence are frequent in epilepsy and rare in syncope. The return of consciousness, as mentioned, is prompt in syncope and slow in epilepsy. Mental confusion, headache, and drowsiness are common sequelae in epilepsy, while these are rare in the postsyncopal period. Physical weakness with clear sensorium usually characterizes the postsyncopal sensorium. Of course, the occurrence of frequent tonic-clonic movements is much more characteristic of a seizure disorder.

The patient with apparent loss of consciousness may present to the ED with myriad complaints, including "falling out," "passing out," or simply "feeling dizzy." The distinction between syncope and near-syncope frequently depends upon a detailed history or eyewitness recollection. Near-syncope is just as important a symptom and, potentially, carries as significant a risk as syncope. Multiple studies have attempted to pinpoint the etiology of syncope through standardized historical, laboratory, or physical findings.[7,23-26] Unfortunately, there is no simple recipe for determining the cause of syncope in a large percentage of patients. Nevertheless, there are aspects of the history and physical exam that may simplify the diagnosis and help the investigator to focus his/her evaluation. *(Please see Table 2.)*

The Red Flags of Syncope and the ESP Mnemonic

Bosker and Sequeria have encapsulated all of the dangerous aspects of syncope into an appropriate mnemonic device. They term this the ESP approach to syncope. This approach divides the diagnostic assessment of syncope into three distinct phases, the Early premonitory phase, the Syncopal phase, and the Postsyncopal phase. Each of these phases has a mnemonic to signify the respective red flags or situations in which syncope could be potentially dangerous.

The Premonitory Phase. In the early premonitory phase, the appropriate mnemonic for the dangerous situations is summarized by SCENT:

- Supine posture when syncope occurs;
- Cardiac symptoms occur just before the syncope (chest pain, shortness of breath, palpitations);
- Elderly patients should always be considered to have a serious cause of their syncope;
- No warning to the syncope should always imply cardiac or neurologic disease;
- Trauma associated with the syncope is important because the patient with benign syncope usually can protect himself or herself from the fall.

The Syncopal Phase. Red flags can be organized under the mnemonic TIPS.

- Tongue biting;
- Incontinence of urine but especially of stool;
- Prolonged duration of loss of consciousness;
- Seizure activity.

The Postsyncopal Phase. The postsyncopal red flags are organized under the mnemonic CHAN.

- Confusion;
- Headaches;
- Abnormal vital signs;
- Neurologic dysfunction (especially focal dysfunction).

The goals of the evaluation of syncope in the ED are to 1) stabilize any acute clinical needs of the patient; 2) rule out illnesses of immediate potential danger; 3) thoroughly investigate the possibility of syncope of cardiac origin; and 4) determine the appropriate disposition for each patient whether it be an admission to the hospital, referral for outpatient care, or discharge with reassurance. It is impor-

Table 4. Differentiation Among Syncope, Stokes-Adams Syndrome, and Seizures

HISTORY	SYNCOPE	STOKES-ADAMS SYNDROME	SEIZURE
Position	Usually upright	Upright/ supine	Upright/ supine
Skin color	Pale	Pallor/ cyanosis	No change
Injury	Rare	Frequent	Frequent
Episode length	Short	Variable	Long
Tonic/ Clonic jerks	Few	Few	Frequent
Tongue Biting	Rare	Rare	Frequent
Incontinence	Rarely urinary	Rarely urinary	Frequent urinary or fecal
Postictal	Promptly lucid	Promptly lucid	Return to consciousness slow; headache; confusion; weakness prolonged

tant to remember that it is not always necessary or possible to diagnose the cause of each case.

Symptom Categories. The physician must be able to identify and help the patient identify the significant differences between syncope, faintness or presyncope, lightheadedness, vertigo, and seizure disorders. Syncope primarily comprises a generalized weakness of muscles and an inability to stand and is associated with a transient loss of consciousness. Presyncope or faintness contrasts with syncope in that there is no loss of consciousness, but there is a sense of giddiness and lack of strength with a sensation of impending loss of consciousness.

Patients who have syncope usually experience it in an upright position, either sitting or standing, and have ample warning of the impending faint through a sense of "not feeling good." A sense of giddiness is accompanied by the sensation of swaying of surrounding objects. Patients yawn or gape, see spots before their eyes, and hear ringing in their ears. Nausea may accompany these symptoms, sometimes with vomiting. There is a notable pallor or ashen-gray complexion to the skin. The patient is usually profusely diaphoretic. The deliberate onset frequently allows patients to protect themselves from injury, and a hurtful fall from syncope is rare. Loss of consciousness may occasionally be averted if the patient assumes a recumbent position before he or she passes out. Patients usually remain unconscious for a period of seconds to minutes but may be unconscious for as long as 20-30 minutes. They usually lie motionless, but a few clonic jerks of the limbs and face may occur. Generalized tonic-clonic movements do not occur, although occasional urinary incontinence (but not fecal incontinence) may be noted. Once patients awaken, their color returns. They may experience sensations of being weak and may actually lose consciousness again if arising too quickly. Headache, drowsiness, and mental confusion are unusual after a syncopal episode; if these occur, they usually imply the presence of a convulsion.

It is important for the physician to help patients specify whether the complaint of dizziness represents lightheadedness or vertigo. Lightheadedness usually refers to a sensation of giddiness or faintness, while vertigo refers to a feeling of whirling rotation. Patients with vertigo have no alteration of consciousness or no sensation of an impending faint. The key symptom of vertigo is the sensation of motion, which the patient may perceive as veering, staggering, imbalance, or momentary disequilibrium, although many with vertigo may describe the classic sensation of spinning rotation.

The patient may often describe the sensation of being pulled to one side or to the ground as if drawn by a magnet—the phenomenon of impulsion. The feeling of impulsion is particularly characteristic of vertigo. All but the mildest forms of vertigo are accompanied by diaphoresis, pallor, nausea, and vomiting. As a rule, the patient can walk only with difficulty or not at all if the vertigo is intense. Most patients have previously experienced a sensation of vertigo after normal activities, such as riding a merry-go-round. When queried specifically, they often readily recognize the similarity between their symptoms and those previous experiences. If they cannot be specific in distinguishing their "dizziness," provocative maneuvers may be indicated to attempt to reproduce symptoms they have experienced.

History

A targeted evaluation of syncope requires assembling an accurate and detailed history of the sequence of events involved in the syncopal episode. *(Please see Table 4.)* When a cause can be found, studies suggest that the physical exam will lead to the diagnosis in 45-85% of cases.[10,11,15,28,29]

When formulating a history in the patient with syncope, it is essential to obtain an accurate account from all available witnesses. No amount of diagnostic testing can compensate for an incomplete or inadequate initial history. Details of the events preceding loss of consciousness are essential, as well as the play-by-play of events following the syncopal episode. Circumstances surrounding the episode should be ascertained, including the time, place, and duration of the episode, relationships to posture, fasting, eating, exercise, illness, sleep, medications, and patterns of recurrence. *(Please see Table 4.)*

Age-Related Factors. Age is a key element in the approach to syncope, inasmuch as younger and older populations each have special considerations that affect diagnostic and triage strategies. For example, it may be particularly difficult to identify the cause of syncope in the elderly (> 60 years old) because syncope in this age group is more likely to be multifactorial.[6,21,22] In particular, with advanced age, it is more likely that complex pharmacologic regimens and coexisting disease contribute to the event. The elderly may also have age-related physiologic changes that alter the syncopal response. These patients are more likely to have a cardiovascular cause of syncope, exhibiting a two-fold higher incidence than younger patients.[21] Moreover, the incidence of sudden death is three times greater in elderly patients who present with syncope.[21,25,39]

Older patients, on average, take approximately three times as many medications as the general population.[21,40] The potential for drug interactions places the older patient at increased risk for drug-induced syncope. *(Please see Table 3.)* In fact, a recent study identifies neuroleptics, antiparkinsonian medications, and non-tricyclic antidepressants as particularly problematic in patients 65 years and older.[40]

Syncope in the pediatric and adolescent population, in general, is a benign event. Special care should be taken, however, to inquire about syncope during exercise or a strong family history of sudden death, since this may suggest hypertrophic cardiomyopathy, anomalous origin of left coronary artery from the sinus of Valsalva, congenital aortic stenosis, long Q-T syndrome, or catecholamine-sensitive ventricular tachycardia.[14,41]

Adult patients presenting to the ED with syncope will often have cardiac risk factors. Organic heart disease (coronary artery disease, congestive heart failure, valvular heart disease, cardiomyopathy, bundle branch block, bifascicular block, or congenital heart disease) that accompanies syncope is a predictor of arrhythmia or death within one year.[25] These individuals are at a higher risk for arrhythmia and should be examined carefully to exclude potential cardiac causes for the syncopal event. In particular, the presence of three out of four of the following—abnormal ECG, age greater than 45, history of congestive heart failure, or history of ventricular arrhythmia—carries an approximately 10-fold increase in the incidence of serious arrhythmia and or death within one year.[25] Patients who have dilated cardiomyopathy and syncope carry a very high risk for sudden death; 83% of these individuals experience sudden death at 30 months (vs 32% in patients with cardiomyopathy and no syncope).[42] Finally, patients with mechanical pacemakers should undergo careful pacemaker interrogation, since intrinsic pacemaker abnormalities may not be evident on ECG alone.[29]

Physical Examination

Physical examination of the patient with syncope should be performed with special attention to the cardiovascular and neurological organ systems. Vital signs should be assessed for signs of hypovolemia. Tachycardia or hypotension should be noted. Orthostatic vital sign changes may suggest hypovolemia, but are limited by their lack of sensitivity, particularly in the young patient.[43] The patient's heart rate should be correlated with the pulse to ensure perfusion and to assess its regularity. Differential blood pressures in both arms may indicate subclavian steal or aortic dissection. Although obtaining a temperature is often neglected or delayed in busy EDs, it is particularly important in elderly patients, since hypothermia can suggest sepsis or hypoglycemia; hyperthermia also may indicate infection.

The cardiovascular examination should be particularly thorough. The auscultatory exam may be difficult in a noisy ED, but clues to hypertrophic cardiomyopathy, valvular heart disease, and congenital cardiac malformations should be sought. For example, the murmurs of mitral regurgitation and atrial stenosis become less pronounced with the Valsalva maneuver, while the murmurs of hypertrophic cardiomyopathy or mitral valve prolapse become louder and more prolonged.

Although the nonauscultatory exam has become a lost art, it remains useful, particularly in noisy EDs. The chest should be palpated for signs of a ventricular heave or a laterally displaced PMI, suggesting ventricular enlargement. It should also be felt for irregularities of its rhythm, which are frequently found in disorders of enlarged ventricles. Parasternal palpation may reveal a heave suggesting right ventricular pressure or volume overload. A palpable thrill may accompany severe pulmonic or aortic stenosis. Finally, the neck should be evaluated for the presence and character of jugular venous distension. Cann A-waves suggest AVE block due to atrial contraction against a closed mitral valve. In addition, the upstroke of the carotid pulse may be delayed due to aortic stenosis.

Carotid massage may be useful for investigating the possibility of carotid sinus hypersensitivity, although it also carries some risk of ventricular fibrillation, prolonged asystole, and ischemic stroke.[10,11,23] It should never be performed in the presence of carotid bruits, a history of ventricular tachycardia, recent stroke, or myocardial infarction. If indicated, the procedure is performed with the patient in a supine position. If negative, then it may be repeated with the patient standing.

Every patient with syncope deserves a thorough neurologic exam, including the pupils and retina, which should be examined for signs of cerebral edema. The abdomen should be examined for signs of a ruptured abdominal aortic aneurysm. Skin examination may reveal evidence of a thrombotic, embolic, or hemorrhagic process.

Modalities: Uses and Abuses

A number of clinical studies have shown that laboratory tests are of low yield in the evaluation of syncope, unless indicated by history or physical exam.[2,3,7,26] In this regard, laboratory tests frequently contribute to the high cost of syncope evaluations, while contributing little to the diagnosis.[1] One possible exception is the acquisition of a B-HCG when evaluating a female patient of reproductive age with syncope, since the history and physical exam may be unreliable for ruling out pregnancy.

Perhaps the greatest controversy in the evaluation of syncope involves the use of costly diagnostic modalities. The primary value of these ancillary tests lies in their ability to assist the emergency physician in making appropriate referrals and disposition decisions, including admission to the hospital. Although some tests are not routinely available in the ED, the emergency physician can often arrange for them on an outpatient basis.

ECG. Many experts advocate obtaining an ECG on all patients presenting to the ED with syncope, primarily because of the risk of sudden death associated with cardiac syncope. Although the diagnostic yield of mandatory ECG is low, ECGs are inexpensive, readily available, and may lead to a life-saving intervention when a significant diagnostic abnormality is found (e.g., complete heart block). A normal ECG is associated with a low likelihood that syncope is caused by an arrhythmia and carries a low risk of sudden death (providing important prognostic information as well).[20,25] Although the ECG in patients with syncope shows some abnormality in up to 50% of patients, significant abnormalities occur in only 2-11% of patients.[20,23,24]

Holter Monitor/Prolonged ECG Monitoring. Approximately 4% of patients with syncopal symptoms have documented arrhythmias on prolonged ECG monitoring.[29] Holter or prolonged ECG monitoring is useful because syncope often has an unpredictable onset with little reproducibility. Moreover, a static ECG may fail to diagnose transient arrhythmias. Because brief arrhythmias commonly occur in asymptomatic individuals, syncope can only be attributed to an arrhythmia when it is associated with symptoms.

How long should patients be monitored? A 24-hour period has been shown to be the optimal length of time for the initial evaluation, since monitoring beyond 24 hours fails to increase the number of clinically significant arrhythmias detected.[44] The decision to admit patients for monitoring should be driven by clinical indicators of serious illness and, especially, a strong suspicion of a cardiac cause for the syncopal episode. Specifically, when a patient reports syncope without a prodrome and has a history of organic heart disease or an abnormal ECG, then 24 hours of inpatient monitoring is indicated. In patients with non-life threatening recurrent syncope, 24-hour Holter monitoring as an outpatient is a reasonable option. Electrocardiographic loop recording or event monitoring (for periods up to 30 days or longer) may be considered for certain patients with recurrent syncope.

CT Scan, MRI, and EEG. CT scan, MRI, and EEG are indicated in the work-up of syncope only when history or physical exam elicits evidence of neurologic abnormality. Studies investigating the value of EEG have shown that it has negligible use in the absence of history of seizure activity.[23,45] Large-scale studies have not been completed evaluating the role of CT or MRI in the syncope work-up. Still, studies have shown that CT or MRI do not lead to significant findings except when patients have focal neurologic deficits or a history of witnessed seizures.

Echocardiography. Fewer than 5% of all patients with syncope will have echocardiographic manifestations of dilated cardiomyopathy, atrial myxoma, or hypertrophic cardiomyopathy.[4,46] Consequently, the history, physical exam, and ECG are essential for identifying which patients will benefit from echocardiography. In general, however, echocardiography provides no useful additional information in syncope patients in the absence of clinical evidence of heart disease elicited by history, physical examination, or ECG.[46]

Evaluation of Cardiac Ischemia. The prevalence of acute cardiac ischemia among adult syncope patients ranges from 0.5% to 7.0%.[2,8,20] While patients with syncope are often admitted to a telemetry bed to rule out myocardial infarction, patients without chest pain or an ischemic abnormality on initial ECG have a low incidence of acute ischemia as the cause of their syncopal episode.[47] Most experts recommend that further evaluation or cardiac ischemia be reserved for those syncope patients whose history, physical exam, or ECG suggest cardiac ischemia.

Electrophysiologic Studies. Electrophysiologic studies (EPS) involve electrical stimulation of cardiac ventricles to uncover disturbances that predispose to brady or tachyarrhythmias. Although EPS has played an important role in the study of ventricular tachycardia, supraventricular tachycardias, and bradyarrhythmias, it is invasive, expensive, and has a low yield when applied to the wrong patient population. EPS is best used in patients with organic heart disease.[24,46,48] Similarly, EPS for the evaluation of the syncope patient should be guided by several clinical predictors that are associated with an increased sensitivity of finding clinically significant arrhythmias. Organic heart disease and nonsustained ventricular tachycardia detected by Holter monitor increases the likelihood of diagnosing ventricular tachyarrhythmias by EPS. In addition, the presence of organic heart disease with nonsustained ventricular tachycardia by Holter monitor increases the sensitivity of EPS to 100% for detecting clinically significant arrhythmias. Sinus bradycardia,[11] heart block, or bundle branch block by ECG are associated with a 79% sensitivity for bradyarrhythmias at EPS.[44] Without these predictors, clinically significant findings detected through EPS are rare.[24]

Management and Disposition

Hemodynamically, patients with syncope require acute stabilization in the ED, with basic attention to airway, breathing, and circulation. Patients with suspected etiologies such as aortic dissection, ruptured aortic aneurysm, dissecting aneurysm, complete heart block, cardiac tamponade, and subarachnoid hemorrhage require rapid diagnosis and immediate intervention. In unstable syncope patients with an undefined diagnosis, consideration of these entities should be entertained and ruled out as rapidly as possible.

In stable patients, the evaluation should begin with a history, physical exam, and ECG, and proceed to other diagnostic modalities as indicated. If a tentative diagnosis can be made, patients should be categorized into three groups: 1) patients with suspected cardiac syncope who carry a high risk of mortality or sudden death; 2) patients with other life- or limb-threatening conditions, such as subarachnoid hemorrhage, requiring admission; 3) patients sustaining significant injury from a syncopal fall (e.g., hip fractures, subdural hematoma); and 4) elderly patients with an unclear diagnosis, but who have risk factors for cardiac or cerebrovascular disease. Patients who do not fall into these categories can generally be discharged from the ED. Some will require outpatient diagnostic testing or consultation, and others will require simple reassurance and discharge home.

Summary

Because syncope is a symptom suggesting potentially lethal underlying disease, it requires a careful and conscientious approach to patient evaluation. History, physical exam, and ECG form the cornerstone of the ED evaluation, which should focus on ruling out syncope of cardiac etiology with its associated risk of sudden death. Multiple diagnostic tools are currently available, although not all are used in the ED. Each has a potential role in the diagnostic evaluation of syncope, but should be used judiciously.

Although substantial research into syncope has been undertaken in the past 15 years, at this time, no suitable standardized approach to evaluation exists. Because the potential causes of syncope are multiple and wide-ranging, the approach to the evaluation of the patient with syncope must still be individualized. Guidelines will continue to evolve as new modalities of evaluation are created and further study clarifies the boundaries of the syncope evaluation.

References

1. Engel GL. Psychologic stress, Vasodepressor (vasovagal) syncope, and sudden death. *Ann Int Med* 1978;89:403-411.
2. Kapoor WN, Karpf M, Wieand S, et al. A prospective evaluation and followup of patients with syncope. *N Engl J Med* 1983;309:197-204.
3. Day SC, Cook EF, Funkenstein H, et al. Evaluation and

outcome of emergency room patients with transient loss of consciousness. *Am J Med* 1982;73:15-23.

4. Gendelman HE, Linzer M, Gabelman M, et al. Syncope in a general hospital patient population. *NY State J Med* 1983;83: 1161-1165.
5. Dermksian G, Lamb LE. Syncope in a population of healthy young adults. *JAMA* 1958;168:1200-1207.
6. Henderson MC, Prabhu SD. Syncope: Current diagnosis and treatment. *Curr Probl Cardiol* 1997;22:237-296.
7. Junaid A, Dubinsy IL. Establishing an approach to syncope in the emergency department. *J Emer Med* 1997;15:593-599.
8. Eagle KA, Black HR, Cook EF, et al. Evaluation of prognostic classifications for patients with syncope. *Am J Med* 1985;79:455-460.
9. Lempert T. Recognizing syncope: Pitfalls and surprises. *J Royal Soc Med* 1996;89:372-375.
10. Kapoor WN. Diagnostic evaluation of syncope. *Am J Med* 1991;90:91-106.
11. Gilman JK. Syncope in the emergency department. *Emer Med Clin North Am* 1995;13:955-971.
12. Rehm CG, Ross SE. Syncope as etiology of road crashes involving elderly drivers. *Amer Surg* 1995;61:1006-1008.
13. Maniolis AS. Evaluation of patients with syncope: Focus of age-related differences. *Amer Coll Cardiol Current J Rev* 1994;3:13-18.
14. Driscoll DJ, Jacobsen SJ, Porter CJ, et al. Syncope in children and adolescents. *J Amer Coll Cardiol* 1997;29:1039-1045.
15. Ruckman RN. Cardiac causes of syncope. *Ped Rev* 1989;9: 101-108.
16. Lipsitz LA, Wei JY, Rowe JW. Syncope in an elderly institutionalized population: Prevalence, incidence, and associated risk. *Q J Med* 1985;55:45-55.
17. Braden DS, Gaymes CH. The diagnosis and management of syncope in children and adolescents. *Ped Ann* 1997;26: 422-426.
18. Kapoor WN, Hanusa BH. Is syncope a risk factor for poor outcomes? Comparison of patients with and without syncope. *Am J Med* 1996;100:646-655.
19. Kosinski DJ, Wolfe DA, Grubb BP. Neurocardiogenic syncope: A review of pathophysiology, diagnosis, and treatment. *Cardiovasc Reports and Rev* 1993;42:22-29.
20. Geogeson S, Linzer M, Griffith JL, et al. Acute cardiac ischemia in patients with syncope: Importance of the initial electrocardiogram. *J Gen Int Med* 1992;7:379-386.
21. Kapoor WN, Snustad D, Peterson J. Syncope in the elderly. *Am J Med* 1986;80:419-428.
22. Davidson E, Rotenberg Z, Fuchs J, et al. Transient ischemic attack-related syncope. *Clin Cardiol* 1991;14:141-144.
23. Linzer M, Yang EG, Estes NA, et al. Diagnosing syncope. Part 1: Value of history, physical examination, and electrocardiography. *Ann Int Med* 1997;126:989-996.
24. Linzer M, Yang EG, Estes NA, et al. Diagnosing syncope. Part 2: Unexplained syncope. *Ann Int Med* 1997;127:76-78.
25. Martin TP, Hanusa BH, Kapoor WN. Risk stratification of patients with syncope. *Ann Emer Med* 1997;29:459-466.
26. Kapoor WN. Back to basics for the workup of syncope. *J Gen Int Med* 1995;10:695-696.
28. Davidson E, Fuchs J, Rotenberg Z, et al. Drug-related syncope. *Clin Cardiol* 1989;12:577-580.
29. Leung FW, Oill PA. Ticket for admission: Unexplained syncopal attacks in patients with cardiac pacemaker. *Ann Emer Med* 1980;9:527-528.
30. Calkins J, Byrne M, El-Atassi R, et al. The economic burden of unrecognized vasodepressor syncope. *Am J Med* 1993;95: 473-479.
31. Wolfe TR, Allen TL. Syncope as an emergency department presentation of pulmonary embolism. *J Emer Med* 1998;16: 27-31.
32. Cayenne S, Marzo K, Larzar J, et al. Syncope—An under-recognized manifestation of pulmonary embolism. *Resident and Staff Physician* 1998:44-49.
33. Ruiz GA, Peralta A, Gonzalez-Zuelgaray J, et al. Evolution of patients with clinical neurocardiogenic (vasovagal) syncope not subjected to specific treatment. *Am Heart J* 1995;130:345-350.
34. Goldman JM. Syncope In: *The Clinical Practice of Emergency Medicine.* 2nd ed. Philadelphia: AL Harwood-Nuss; 1996:627-630.
35. Wilterdink JL. Sentinel headaches and aneurysmal subarachnoid hemorrhage. *Current Diag in Neurology.* St. Louis: CV Mosby; 1994.
36. Adams RD, Victor M. *Principles of Neurology.* New York, NY; McGraw Hill: 1993.
37. McHarg MS, Shinnar S, Rascoff H, et al. Syncope in childhood. *Ped Cardiol* 1997;18:367-371.
38. Pratt JL, Fleisher GR. Syncope in children and adolescents. *Ped Emer Care* 1980;5:80-82.
39. Olsky M, Murray J. Dizziness and fainting in the elderly. *Emer Med Clin N Am* 1990;8:295-307.
40. Cherin P, Colves A, de Periere CD, et al. Risk of syncope in the elderly and consumption of drugs: A case-control study. *J Clin Epidemiol* 1997;50:313-320.
41. Maron BJ, Roberts WL, McAllister HA, et al. Sudden death in young athletes. *Circulation* 1980;62:218-229.
42. Fruhwald FM, Eber B, Schumacher M. Syncope in dilated cardiomyopathy is a predictor of sudden cardiac death. *Cardiology* 1996;87:177-180.
43. Levitt MA, Lopez B, Liberman ME, et al. Evaluation of the tilt test in an adult emergency medicine population. *Ann Emer Med* 1992;21:713-718.
44. Bass EB, Curtiss EL, Arena VC, et al. The duration of holter monitoring in patients with syncope. Is twenty-four hours enough? *Arch Int Med* 1990;150:1073-1078.
45. Davis TL, Freemon FR. Electroencephalography should not be routine in the evaluation of syncope in adults. *Arch Int Med* 1990;73:593-598.
46. Bachinsky WB, Linzer M, Weld L, et al. Usefulness of clinical characteristics in predicting the outcome of electrophysiologic studies in unexplained syncope. *Am J Cardiol* 1992;69: 1044-1049.
47. Denes P, Uretz E, Erzi MD, et al. Clinical predictions of EP findings in patients with syncope of unknown origin. *Arch Int Med* 1988;148:1922-1928.
48. Calkins J, Shyr Y, Frumin H. The value of the clinical history in the differentiation of syncope due to ventricular tachycardia, atrioventricular block, and neurocardiogenic syncope. *Am J Med* 1995;98:365-373.

tation of emergency department patients with [illegible] of [illegible]. [illegible]

[illegible] M, [illegible] et al. [illegible] syncope in a general hospital patient population. [illegible] 1999;[illegible]

5. Dermksian G, Lamb LE. Syncope in a population of healthy young adults. JAMA 1958;168:1200–1207.
6. Henderson MC, Prabhu SD. Syncope: current diagnosis and treatment. Curr Probl Cardiol 1997;22:237–296.
7. [illegible] A, [illegible]. [illegible] syncope in the emergency department. [illegible]
8. Eagle KA, Black HR, Cook EF, et al. Evaluation of prognostic classifications for patients with syncope. Am J Med 1985;79:455–460.
9. Lempert T. Recognizing syncope: pitfalls and surprises. J R Soc Med 1997;90:[illegible]
10. Kapoor WN. Diagnostic evaluation of syncope. Am J Med 1991;90:91–106.
11. Gilman JK. [illegible] in the emergency department. [illegible]
12. [illegible] SA. Syncope as a cause of road crashes involving elderly drivers. [illegible]
13. [illegible] AS. Evaluation of patients with syncope [illegible]. [illegible]
14. Driscoll DJ, Jacobsen SJ, Porter CJ, et al. Syncope in children and adolescents. J Am Coll Cardiol 1997;29:1039–1045.
15. Ruckman RN. Cardiac causes of syncope. Pediatr Rev 1987;9:101–108.
16. Lipsitz LA, Wei JY, Rowe JW. Syncope in an elderly, institutionalised population: Prevalence, incidence, and associated risk. Q J Med 1985;55:45–54.
17. Benditt DG, [illegible]. The diagnosis and management of syncope in children and adolescents. [illegible]
18. Kapoor WN, Hanusa BH. Is syncope a risk factor for poor outcomes? Comparison of patients with and without syncope. Am J Med 1996;100:646–655.
19. Kosinski D, [illegible]. Neurocardiogenic syncope: [illegible] diagnosis and treatment. [illegible]
20. [illegible] et al. [illegible] in patients with syncope: importance of the signal-averaged electrocardiogram. [illegible]
21. [illegible] Syncope in the elderly. [illegible]
22. [illegible] et al. [illegible] syncope [illegible]
23. Linzer M, Yang EH, Estes NA, et al. Diagnosing syncope. Part 1: Value of history, physical examination, and electrocardiography. [illegible]
24. Linzer M, Yang EH, Estes NA, et al. Diagnosing syncope. Part 2: Unexplained syncope. [illegible]
25. Martin GJ, Adams SL, [illegible]. Prospective evaluation of syncope. [illegible]
26. Kapoor WN. [illegible] of syncope. [illegible]
28. Davidson E, Rotenberg Z, Fuchs J, [illegible]

syncope. Am J Cardiol 1997;79:[illegible]

29. [illegible] et al. [illegible] in patients with [illegible]
30. Calkins H, Byrne M, el-Atassi R, et al. The economic burden of unrecognized vasodepressor syncope. Am J Med 1993;95:473–479.
31. Wolfe TR, Allen TL. Syncope as an emergency department presentation of pulmonary embolism. J Emerg Med 1998;16:27–31.
32. [illegible], Marzo K, [illegible] et al. Syncope: An under-recognized manifestation of pulmonary embolism. [illegible] 1998;[illegible]
33. Raviele A, Proclemer A, [illegible] et al. Evaluation of patients with [illegible] subjected to [illegible]
34. [illegible] Syncope. In: [illegible] Pulmonary Embolism. 2nd ed. [illegible] 1996;[illegible]
35. [illegible] Subclavian [illegible]
36. Adams RD, Victor M. Principles of Neurology. [illegible] New York: McGraw-Hill, [illegible]
37. McHarg ML, Shinnar S, [illegible] H, et al. Syncope in childhood. Pediatr Cardiol 1997;18:367–371.
38. Pratt JL, Fleisher GR. Syncope in children and adolescents. Pediatr Emerg Care 1989;5:80–82.
39. [illegible] Dizziness and fainting in the elderly. [illegible]
40. [illegible] et al. [illegible] of syncope in the elderly and [illegible]: A case-control study. [illegible]
41. Maron BJ, Roberts WC, McAllister HA, et al. Sudden death in young athletes. Circulation 1980;62:218–229.
42. [illegible] Syncope in dilated cardiomyopathy: [illegible] predictor of sudden cardiac death. [illegible]
43. [illegible] Evaluation of [illegible] tachycardia [illegible]
44. Bass EB, Curtiss EI, Arena VC, et al. The duration of Holter monitoring in patients with syncope. Is 24 hours enough? Arch Intern Med 1990;150:1073–1078.
45. Davis TL, Freemon FR. Electroencephalography should not be routine in the evaluation of syncope in adults. Arch Intern Med 1990;150:2027–2029.
46. [illegible] et al. Usefulness of clinical [illegible] in predicting the outcome of electrophysiologic studies in unexplained syncope. [illegible]
47. [illegible] in patients with [illegible]
48. [illegible] The value of the clinical history in the differentiation of syncope due to ventricular tachycardia, atrioventricular block, and neurocardiogenic syncope. Am J Med 1995;98:365–373.

Diagnosis of Abdominal Aortic Aneurysm

Gary Hals, MD, PhD
Michael Pallaci, DO

The clinical scenario is familiar to the experienced emergency physician. An elderly man with a history of hypertension and cigarette smoking arrives to the emergency department (ED) by ambulance complaining of back pain; he is diaphoretic and hypotensive. The diagnosis of abdominal aortic aneurysm (AAA) rupture should be considered at the outset, with confirmation of the diagnosis and prompt surgical intervention being the principal management objectives.

A leaking or ruptured AAA is one of the most dramatic and life-threatening conditions encountered in the ED, and patients with this condition are presenting in ever-increasing numbers to EDs across the country.[1] The increase in the incidence of AAA is due not only to a growing number of elderly, but also to an increase in the absolute frequency of this disease.[1] The fact that many patients have no prior symptoms until their AAAs rupture also adds to the difficulty of management. Even more auspicious is that the natural history of AAA is progressive growth, which culminates in rupture. It should be stressed that while AAA rupture is by far the most frequent complication, infection of aneurysm, aortoenteric fistula, and atheroembolism are additional clinical manifestations of AAA that can complicate both the diagnosis and prognosis of this disease.

Given the natural history of this condition and a mortality rate ranging between 50% and 80%, emergency physicians must be aware of both classic and more insidious presentations of AAA.[2,3] Unfortunately, even when patients present with "classic" signs and symptoms, misdiagnosis is still common and is reported to be as high as 30-60% in some studies.[4,5] Explanation for the unacceptably high misdiagnosis rate have centered on the possible confusion between signs of AAA and more common conditions. In this regard, two common presentations for a leaking AAA include: 1) back pain with hematuria; and 2) left lower quadrant (LLQ) pain with GI bleeding. Inasmuch as renal colic and acute diverticulitis are much more common causes of these symptom complexes, respectively, it is easy to understand why the diagnosis of symptomatic AAA can be difficult even for the experienced ED clinician. Delaying the correct diagnosis of patients with leaking AAA has been reported to double the mortality rate of these patients.[6]

With these issues in clear focus, this chapter will address the diagnostic and clinical challenges faced by the ED physician caring for patients with AAA. The authors also address current thinking about the pathogenesis of AAA, typical and atypical presentations, ED evaluation and stabilization, and late complications following AAA repair.

Introduction

Abdominal aortic aneurysms (AAAs) account for approximately 15,000 deaths each year in the United States and rank as the 13th leading cause of death.[7,8] From an incidence perspective, AAA is found in 2% of the elderly population (age > 65 years), with a higher incidence in males vs. females (9:1). Rupture of an AAA usually is a lethal event, carrying an overall mortality rate of 80-90%;[9,10] a significant percentage of these patients die before arrival to the hospital. Among those who reach the operating room, the mortality rate is still 50%.[11,12] Fortunately, prompt diagnosis and surgical repair before rupture can reduce the mortality rate; the operative survival rate of patients undergoing elective repair is reported to be about 95%.[12]

Definitions. An aneurysm is defined as an irreversible, localized dilatation of an artery to at least 1.5 times of its normal diameter.[13] Nevertheless, there has been some controversy surrounding the exact definition of what constitutes an AAA and its precise anatomical characteristics. Although up to six different definitions have been proposed, the most accepted description is that an aortic aneurysm is an aorta that is dilated 1.5 times that of the adjacent intact aorta.[14] Since the normal diameter of the abdominal aorta is around 2 cm, with some variation in men vs. women (aorta in men > 55 years averages 2.1 cm, and 1.8 cm in women), an aorta measuring 3 cm commonly is used as a defining criterion for an AAA.[15]

Figure 1. Different Types of Aortic Aneurysms[75]

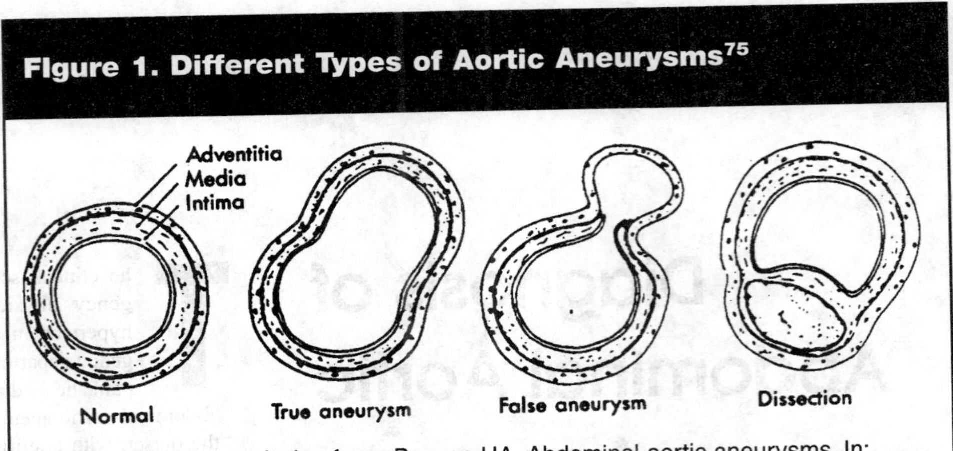

Reproduced with permission from: Bessen HA. Abdominal aortic aneurysms. In: Rosen P, et al, eds. *Emergency Medicine: Concepts and Clinical Practice.* 4th Ed. St. Louis: Mosby-Year Book, Inc; 1998:1374.

A true aneurysm is characterized by involvement of all three layers of the vessel (intima, media, and adventitia), as opposed to a pseudoaneurysm, which involves only the adventitia and/or surrounding tissue. *(Please see Figure 1.)* In other words, a pseudoaneurysm is actually a disruption in the intima and media of the aorta, and only the adventitia/surrounding tissue retains blood within the aortic cavity.

Most AAAs are true aneurysms, whereas pseudoaneurysms of the aorta are primarily seen as late complications of repair. An AAA frequently is confused with an aortic dissection, which can occur in (or involve) an AAA, but which more typically begins in the thoracic aorta. An AAA and acute aortic dissection are separate processes precipitated by different etiologies, clinical findings, diagnostic tests, and treatment strategies. An inflammatory aneurysm is characterized by extensive perianeurysmal and retroperitoneal fibrosis, and dense adhesions of adjacent abdominal organs.[16]

Clinical Anatomy. The aorta is a retroperitoneal structure that lies immediately anterior to the lumbar spine. It enters the abdomen after passing through the aortic hiatus of the diaphragm at T12 along with the thoracic duct and azygous vein. The aorta yields five main vascular branches between the diaphragm and its bifurcation. Almost immediately below the diaphragm it bifurcates into the celiac trunk and superior mesenteric artery (SMA). The renal arteries branch off the aorta about 1 cm inferior to the SMA at approximately the L1-L2 interspace. Note that the L1-L2 level is an important landmark, as greater than 90% of AAAs arise inferior to the renal arteries, and extend from this location to involve the iliac arteries.[17] *(Please see Figure 2a.)*

The next branch is the smaller inferior mesenteric artery (IMA), and the last are the two iliac arteries. The aorta splits into the right and left common iliac arteries about 2-3 cm inferior to the IMA at the level of the umbilicus. The vascular branches arising distal to the renal arteries are often involved in the aneurysm and may require grafting at surgery. There are two main types of aortic aneurysms classified according to their shape. Most AAAs are fusiform with tapering at both ends, while the other type is saccular, with the aneurysm joined to the aorta by a smaller entrance. *(Please see Figure 2b.)*

Clinical Pathogenesis and Risk Factors

Over the course of a lifetime, the aorta is exposed to cumulative physical stress caused by arterial blood pressure. Why then do some individuals develop an AAA, whereas others do not? The precise mechanisms leading to the development of an AAA remain unclear, although it is likely to be the result of a combination of events. In general, the factors leading to aortic aneurysm include those that weaken and increase stress on the aortic wall. Those factors most often identified in this pathophysiological process include: atherosclerosis, hypertension, breakdown of elastin and collagen, inflammation, genetic factors, tobacco smoking, and age. For those interested in more detailed analysis of AAA pathogenesis, an excellent review of the literature is available.[18]

Atherosclerosis. Atherosclerosis was once thought to be the leading cause of AAA, but atherosclerosis generally leads to occlusive arterial disease. Despite this basic difference, there appears to be an etiologic relationship between the two disorders. These conditions share multiple risk factors and there is a clear association between AAA and peripheral artery disease. However, several recent studies have shown that the two diseases have clear epidemiological differences. For example, elevated serum lipid levels have not been found in patient populations with AAA using case-control studies.[19] Furthermore, the makeup of patients with AAA shows a higher proportion of males.[20,21]

Some researchers have suggested that atherosclerosis may be a response to aneurysmal dilatation rather than its cause.[22,23] Others think, based on animal studies, that regression of atherosclerotic plaques can weaken the wall of the aorta and lead to aneurysm formation.[24] The human abdominal aorta has few vasa vasorum to provide nutrients for the media, and it relies on diffusion from surrounding areas. Plaques in the aorta may also impair nutrient diffusion to the media, which can lead to further weakening. Investigations show that atheromatous plaques form preferentially in areas of low shear stress, and the lateral aortic wall just superior to the bifurcation is a region of low shear stress. It seems unlikely that coincidence is the reason that this is a common site for aortic aneurysms to form.[24] Obviously a relationship exists between AAAs and atherosclerosis. However, the details of this association are still being elucidated.

Elastin and Collagen. Another area of recent research has focused on defining the role elastin and collagen, the two principle biochemical components of the aortic wall, play in aneurysm formation. The two proteins are arranged with smooth muscle cells in concentric lamellae in the aortic media. Elastin, as the name suggests, is a very flexible protein. It can expand to double its original length

Figure 2a. Normal Anatomy of the Aorta[105]

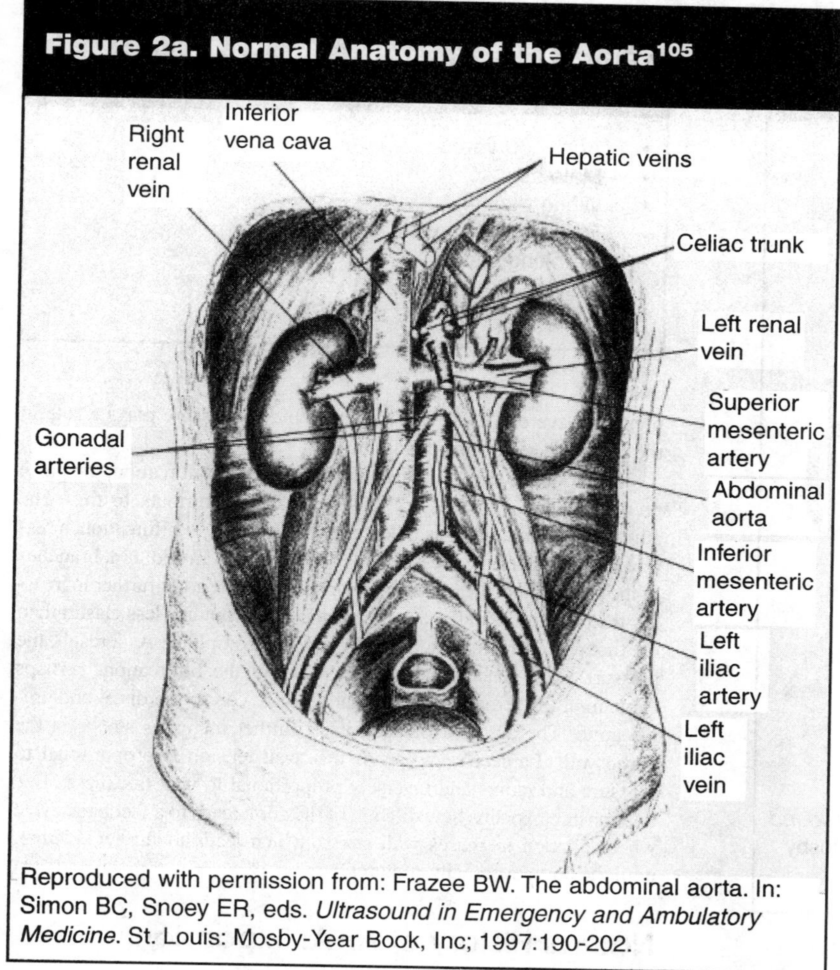

Reproduced with permission from: Frazee BW. The abdominal aorta. In: Simon BC, Snoey ER, eds. *Ultrasound in Emergency and Ambulatory Medicine*. St. Louis: Mosby-Year Book, Inc; 1997:190-202.

and yet still recoil, without damage, to original size. The properties of elastin provide the aorta with the ability to stretch and recoil to original caliber as blood pressure fluctuates with the cardiac cycle. This cyclic stretch and rebound are responsible for the continuous augmentation large arteries provide to cardiac output during diastole.[25]

Collagen, on the other hand, has opposite properties. It is a strong protein that is very resistant to stretching; tests show it has a tensile strength 20 times that of elastin.[26] In fact, if it is stretched to just slightly beyond its original length, structural damage occurs.[27] Collagen in the aorta is coiled when the aorta is at rest. Therefore, as the aorta expands, elastin acts first as the main load-bearing element and stretches easily. As the elastin reaches its maximal length, the collagen is uncoiled so that it now provides support for the aorta. With collagen being very strong and resistant to stretch, the aorta now assumes these properties. Collagen has been likened to a "safety net" for the aorta.[18]

There is mounting evidence that destruction of elastin is a key element in the formation of aortic aneurysms. The abdominal aorta normally contains much less elastin than the thoracic aorta, and aneurysms are more common in the abdomen.[28] The amount of elastin found in the wall of an AAA is considerably reduced (35% to 8%) when compared to a normal abdominal aorta.[29] Moreover, elastin is not synthesized in the adult aorta, and has an impressive half-life of 70 years.[30] This time span correlates with the age of disease onset in many patients, and suggests that aneurysmal formation may be dependent on the amount of total elastin present. (Additional evidence demonstrates that aneurysms can be produced in vivo in animal models by giving intra-arterial elastase, a naturally occurring enzyme that destroys elastin.)[31]

Finally, elevated elastase levels can be found in human AAAs, an activity that persists after aneurysm repair, suggesting that this is likely to be a primary event and not a response to aneurysm formation.[32] However, loss of elastin alone will produce only a slight dilatation of the aorta.[33] As collagen is produced throughout life, the next step is thought to be replacement of the lost elastin by collagen fibers. Indeed, collagen comprises a larger proportion in diseased aortas.[34] Since collagen cannot stretch without damage, significant fragmentation of collagen occurs with time, leading to increasing diameter of the aorta. Although elastin and collagen are important components in the pathogenesis of aneurysm formation, other microfibrillar proteins may also play a role. This is most clearly established in the case of Marfan's syndrome, in which a genetic mutation leads to changes in fibrillin, which can lead to aneurysms and dissection.[35]

Genetic Factors. It is well established that genetics play a role in the development of aneurysms, and that a positive family history is a risk factor for AAA. *(Please see Table 1 for risk factors.)* Approximately 15-20% of first-degree relatives of patients with AAA will also have the disease, and a surprising 20-25% of brothers of patients with AAAs will develop an aneurysm.[36,37] Reminiscent of sickle cell disease, gene mutations causing only a single amino acid substitution on the collagen molecule have been identified as predictive of AAA in one family studied.[38] In contrast to sickle cell, however, this mutation is actually rare in the general population of AAA patients. Other researchers are looking for genetic causes of increased proteolytic enzyme activity, such as elastase and collagenase, since these enzymes are known to be present in increased concentration in the media of AAA.[39] Despite intensive investigation, there is no clear consensus about the role of genetics in the average patient with AAA.

Tobacco Use. The link between smoking and AAA prevalence has been established for more than 20 years.[40] Furthermore, in one study, AAA rupture was four times more common in smokers and 14 times more common in smokers who hand-rolled their cigarettes.[41] The exact mechanism by which this risk is incurred remains unclear. Even as the tar content of cigarettes has decreased by 50% over past two decades, age-adjusted AAA rupture has increased.[41] Hence, attention has focused on other toxic components of smoke.

Chronic obstructive pulmonary disease (COPD) recently has been shown to be a risk factor for rupture of aneurysms less than 5 cm;[42,43] consequently, alpha-1 antitrypsin has been suggested as a link between the two diseases. Alpha-1 antitrypsin is a major inhibitor of proteolytic enzymes, including elastase. Since deficiency of this enzyme is associated with emphysema and rapid destruction of elastin in the lungs, it has been suggested that a similar process could occur in the aorta.[42] At this time, however, clear support for this hypothesis has not been established.

Aortic Inflammation. Inflammatory aneurysms are identified at surgery as those that have thickened walls and dense adhesions to surrounding structures. Interestingly, approximately 4-15% of patients will be found to have an inflammatory AAA at time of surgery.[44,45] These patients also typically have the clinical triad of weight loss, abdominal pain, and elevated erythrocyte sedimentation rate.[44]

At one time, this type of aneurysm was thought to be a separate and distinct disease process from non-inflammatory aneurysms. However, recent research has found that some degree of inflammato-

Figure 2b. Illustration of Fusiform and Saccular Aortic Aneurysms[105]

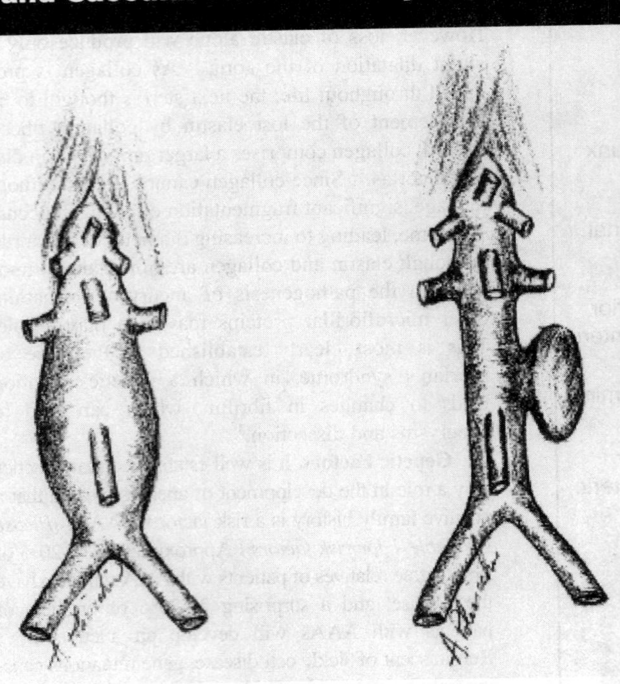

Reproduced with permission from: Frazee BW. The abdominal aorta. In: Simon BC, Snoey ER, eds. *Ultrasound in Emergency and Ambulatory Medicine*. St. Louis: Mosby-Year Book, Inc; 1997:190-202.

Table 1. Risk Factors for AAAs

- Age > 60 years
- Male sex
- White race
- Family history of AAA
- Smoking history
- History of hypertension
- History of coronary artery disease

ry infiltration is present in most AAAs, and the current hypothesis is that an "inflammatory aneurysm" is an extreme example within a continuous spectrum of AAA disease.[46-48] Furthermore, it has been suggested that increased infiltration of the aneurysm by lymphocytes and histiocytes is associated with clinical findings of increased tenderness and increased diameter of the aneurysm.[18] Therefore, the inflammatory process could be an important factor in the equation of aneurysmal dilatation. The fact that inflammatory infiltration does correlate with aneurysm expansion in a rat model supports this hypothesis.[49]

Age. AAAs are uncommon in patients younger than 50 years of age, although they are encountered with increasing frequency as a patient's age increases; overall, 2-4% of patients older than age 50 will have an AAA.[50] The average age at time of diagnosis is between 65 and 70 years.[51]

Interestingly, even the "normal" aorta dilates and develops a thicker wall with age.[52] As discussed in the section on elastin and collagen, loss of elastin and replacement of collagen in the wall of the aorta leads to damage of collagen fibers as they are forced to support wall stresses in the aorta at lower distending pressures. As elastin is not replaced as we age, this process occurs in all individuals. In this regard, the aorta of a 20-year-old patient is nearly three times more elastic than that of a 70-year-old patient.[52,53]

Hypertension. Hypertension has long been known to be a risk factor for AAA. Patients with hypertension and AAA are also at an increased risk for rupture.[54,55] As with other risk factors associated with AAA, it remains unclear whether hypertension is a direct cause of AAA or exacerbates a pre-existing flaw in the aortic wall. It seems clear, however, from the observed effects that normal changes in blood pressure have on AAA, that increased blood pressure plays a role in the pathogenesis of this condition.[54]

As blood travels down the aorta from root to bifurcation, the pulse pressure actually increases.[56] Several factors contribute to this. The aorta tapers in diameter as it descends from thorax to bifurcation, a feature that increases the pressure wave amplitude.[56] In addition, branches of the aorta reflect the pressure wave back into the aorta further increasing the pressure. Finally, the abdominal aorta contains less elastin than the thoracic aorta, making it stiffer and less compliant. As a result, the pressure wave reaches its peak just before the bifurcation, perhaps explaining the remarkable localization of AAAs to the distal abdominal aorta. The act of expansion itself further increases stress on the aortic wall. Laplace's law states that wall tension is proportional to pressure and radius and inversely proportional to wall thickness. This relationship explains how dilation of the aorta leads to a feedback cycle where dilation increases wall stress, which leads to further dilation, until the aorta eventually ruptures.

Natural History of AAA: Expansion and Rupture

Left untreated, most AAAs inexorably enlarge over time until they eventually rupture. Patients die from internal hemorrhage.[57] While other outcomes and complications of AAAs are possible (i.e., embolism or dissection), aortic rupture remains the most common and most dangerous complication for the majority of patients with evolving AAA.

The most significant risk factor for rupture is size of the aneurysm, but interestingly, length or expansion rate have not been shown to correlate with risk of rupture.[57-59] While the average growth rate is quoted at between 2 mm and 5mm per year, individual aneurysms will grow at different rates.[22] One study found that 20% of aneurysms grew more than 4 mm per year, while the remaining 80% grew at a reduced rate, with 15% having no detected growth.[60] What this means is that some aneurysms remain stable for years whereas others grow rapidly without pause; it is impossible to predict with accuracy which aneurysms will follow which time course.

Perhaps, in part due to the forces of Laplace's law, larger aneurysms (> 5 cm) typically grow faster and carry a higher risk for rupture than do smaller ones.[61] Interestingly, many of the studies have been performed exclusively on male patients. A recent review noted that women with AAAs represent 34% of deaths from AAA rupture in 1988, but only around 20% of all surgical cases.[62] The investigators suggested that since women naturally have smaller aortic diameters, a 5 cm aneurysm in a woman represents more advanced disease than a similar size AAA in a male patient. Further study is needed to more accurately define this correlation.

In addition, there is disagreement in the literature about the risk of rupture of intermediate size aneurysms (4-6 cm). Autopsy data from

1977 show a rate of rupture of 60% for those at 10 cm or greater, 23% for those between 4 cm and 5 cm, and 9.5% for those less than 4 cm.[63] However, aneurysm size at autopsy may not be as accurate as it is in a living patient.[60] Furthermore, the data are not consistent and actually vary widely from study to study. Risks of rupture of 1-3% for aneurysms 4-5 cm have been published as recently as 1998.[64] Population-based studies from many areas of the world quote numbers as low as a surprising 0% risk of rupture for aneurysms less than 5 cm.[65-67] Finally, the United Kingdom small aneurysm trial data on 1090 patients with aneurysms less than 5.5 cm in diameter had an overall risk of rupture of only 1% per year for those less than 4.0 cm.[68] Of note is that this is a much larger study than any of the previously mentioned reviews.

Not surprisingly, this controversy has fueled considerable debate about which patients with which size aneurysm truly are at risk of rupture. A recent investigation found that in a population of 161 patients with AAA rupture, the mortality was the same (70% for < 5 cm and 66% for > 5 cm), regardless of size.[42] They found that 10% of aneurysms in their series ruptured at less than 5.0 cm, with 1.2% rupturing at less than 4 cm. COPD and diabetes were associated with a higher rupture risk of smaller aneurysms.

Another study also found COPD and diastolic hypertension to be associated with a higher risk of rupture.[54] This review reported that the highest risk of rupture was associated with aneurysm size greater than 5.0 cm, presence of COPD, and diastolic blood pressure higher than 105 mmHg. The risk of rupture in these patients was 100%, while it was only 2% in patents with aneurysmal size less than 3 cm, no COPD, and diastolic blood pressure lower than 75 mmHg for the same time period (mean, 37 months).[54] A study of 514 patients with aneurysms found advanced age, severe cardiac disease, previous stroke, and cigarette smoking were associated with more rapid growth of smaller aneurysms.[69]

Using a different approach, one author polled members of the Society for Vascular Surgeons on their estimate of risk of rupture in a patient with an AAA varying from 6.5 cm to larger than 7.5 cm in diameter. Remarkably, with 267 surgeons responding, the median estimate of rupture risk was more than twice as high as published estimates, with some guessing the risk even four times higher than published data.[70] As the author points out, other physicians cannot expect consistent recommendations for their patients until better data become available. These data are expected in the next year at the end of a large VA-based study currently in progress.

The variability of data concerning risk of AAA rupture creates a fierce debate about recommendations for elective repair of AAA. While it is true that ED physicians typically are not making decisions concerning when to perform elective repair of AAA, the fact remains that ED physicians may be asked to offer consultation to patients who present to the ED with asymptomatic AAA. In addition, the frequent use of abdominal computed tomography (CT) and ultrasound (US) in the ED has led to an increase in the incidental finding of small AAAs while a patient is being evaluated for other pathology.[71] In fact, small aneurysms now account for 50% of clinically recognized aneurysms.[59] Taken together, these facts imply that the ED physician should at least be aware of the current standard of care regarding elective repair of AAA. *(Please see Table 2.)*

Little debate exists regarding repair of aneurysms larger than 5-6 cm; if the patient is without prohibitive co-morbid conditions, then elective repair is recommended to avoid the high risk of rupture. Mortality from rupture is greater than 90%, while it is less than 5% for elective repair, including data on less-than-perfect operative candidates.[59] Likewise, most surgeons would recommend frequent observation of patients with aneurysms of less than 4 cm rather than immediate repair.

Table 2. Surgical Indications for AAA[44]

- All symptomatic aneurysms
- All saccular aneurysms
- Poor risk patient: size > 6 cm
- Good risk patient: size > 5 cm
- Young, good risk patient: size 4-5 cm

Currently, three trials are under way in Canada, England, and the United States to answer the question of elective repair of aneurysms between 4 cm and 5 cm in diameter. Initial data from the British study of 1090 patients ages 60-76 years with aneurysms of 4-5 cm in diameter suggest that the risk of repair is higher than expected. The operative mortality of 5.8% in this study is higher than the 3% rate in previously published studies.[68,72] In addition, there was no survival advantage for early intervention; the six-year mortality was the same (64%) for operation vs. following with serial US until aneurysm size was larger than 5.5 cm.[72] This trial, then, suggests that elective repair of smaller aneurysms (< 5 cm) is not warranted as a general recommendation. The authors of an accompanying editorial point out that with a lower elective operative mortality, resulting from more judicious patient selection, prophylactic repair of smaller aneurysms might be more compelling.[73] *(Please see Table 2.)*

Finally, a new endovascular stent-grafting technique for treatment of AAA is being evaluated for eventual replacement of the traditional surgical approach.[74] This procedure allows the surgeon to place a stent inside the aneurysm under fluoroscopic guidance from a remote femoral artery puncture, thereby removing the aneurysm from circulation and preventing rupture. Still in an experimental stage, this technique is being used more frequently outside the United States. Complications range from migration or thrombosis of the stent, to embolization, continued dilation of the aneurysm, and leakage of blood into the aneurysm from either end of the stent. Controlled clinical trials are now under way in the United States, and the technique is expected to meet with approval.[74]

Clinical Presentation

Although the clinician may tend to lump the presentation of AAA into those patients who come to the ED with an incidental finding vs. those who have a catastrophic presentation, myriad signs of symptomatic AAA have been described.

Unruptured. The majority of AAAs are detected when they produce symptoms in their "host;" unfortunately, rupture of an AAA is often responsible for the first symptoms the patient experiences. While a significant number of patients do present for evaluation of vague symptoms that ultimately can be linked to the presence of an AAA, the exact incidence of symptoms in patients without AAA rupture remains unknown.[75] Such symptoms may include vague abdominal or back pain, the cause of which may not be clear. These symptoms may be related to erosion into surrounding structures (i.e., vertebral bodies) as the aneurysm expands; this is thought to be a rare occurrence. Some patients complain of an abdominal fullness or notice pulsations.

A high index of suspicion is required in patients with known AAA who complain of pain or tenderness. It should be stressed that most intact aneurysms are not tender, and that new tenderness is highly suggestive of rapid expansion or early rupture. Less frequently, patients with AAA will present with embolic complications or a fistula between the aorta and GI tract or venous structures (see section on

"Atypical Presentations"). Compression of the adjacent duodenum can lead to gradual narrowing. Accompanying symptoms include weight loss and vomiting, a constellation that has been termed the SMA syndrome.[76] Compression of the ureters can cause true renal colic, and compression of nerves and nerve roots can lead to radicular symptoms.

Physical findings of AAA primarily consist of palpating a pulsatile abdominal mass. Other physical findings are of little diagnostic value as they are too nonspecific or insensitive. Bruits are detected in only 5-10% of patients with AAA, and they may result from other sources (i.e., renal or mesenteric artery stenosis).[77] Femoral pulses are typically normal in patients with AAA, unless hypotension from rupture is present. A recent meta-analysis evaluating the diagnostic accuracy of palpation found that results depended on the size of the aneurysm. For aneurysms 3.0-3.9 cm, accuracy was only 29%; for those with aneurysms 5.0 cm or greater, it increased only to 76%.[78] Obesity in the patient was an obvious factor complicating palpation for AAA presence.

The presence of aortic pulsations alone is not predictive of AAA, as the aorta in thin elderly people can be felt easily. Moreover, a torturous aorta in a thin person can mislead the examiner into believing the aortic diameter is bigger than it really is. The accurate way to exam a patient for the presence of an AAA is to palpate on each side of the aorta to determine its width; a value larger than 2.5 cm should prompt further work-up. Concerns that one will cause a rupture if an AAA is present by simple palpation are unfounded. The authors of the meta-analysis found a positive predictive value of only 43% in screening patients for AAA by abdominal exam without other adjunctive modalities. Hence, the bottom line appears to be to palpate patients in whom the diagnosis is in question without fear of inducing rupture, and if an AAA is not detected, a more accurate confirmatory test (i.e., US or CT) is certainly indicated.

Ruptured AAA. Rupture of an AAA usually is a catastrophic event, and patients often present in extremis. The triad of abdominal pain, pulsatile abdominal mass, and hypotension are reported as the "classic" presentation for ruptured AAA. Unfortunately, as with so many diseases, the classic presentation is not the most common one. Indeed, only 30-50% of patients with AAA rupture will present with this triad.[79] The majority of AAA ruptures cause retroperitoneal bleeding as opposed to bleeding into the abdominal cavity itself. The so-called free rupture is more likely to cause rapid exsanguination and death before the patient can reach the ED.[73] Retroperitoneal bleeding is seen in 76-90% of cases, and as a rule the bleeding is to the left.[80] Therefore, back pain is a more common presenting complaint, and should trigger the ED physician to consider and rule out AAA as the diagnosis.

The pain produced by retroperitoneal bleeding is often the initial trigger for the patient's presentation to the ED. Specifically, most patients complain of back, flank, or abdominal pain that is sudden in onset, severe, and constant in nature. It may radiate into the inguinal region, scrotum, or thigh, or even into the chest if the retroperitoneal hematoma spreads superiorly. Severe, sudden pain in a patient with AAA does not always indicate rupture or that bleeding has occurred. Rapidly expanding aneurysms can produce a similar clinical presentation.[81] However, because rapidly expanding aneurysms are at a high risk for impending rupture, all patients with severe pain and a documented AAA should be considered to have a ruptured AAA until proven otherwise. The sudden and intense nature of the pain can cause nausea, vomiting, and/or vasovagal syncope; transient hypotension from blood loss can produce brief syncope in these patients as well.

Initially, most patients can be stabilized in the ED if significant blood loss is not ongoing; in fact, persistent hypotension is usually a late and ominous finding. The duration of symptoms in patients with proven AAA rupture is variable. Some patients with small, contained bleeding in the retroperitoneum may have waited days or even weeks to present for care.[82] Therefore, prolonged duration of pain does not rule out the diagnosis of rupture, and a seemingly stable patient with AAA and a subacute history of back pain still requires evaluation for possible rupture.

Because larger aneurysms are frequently associated with rupture, physical findings in these patients often include a palpable abdominal mass.[83] For example, a retroperitoneal hematoma can sometimes be detected as a non-pulsing mass in the left lower quadrant. However, if the aneurysm is small and the patient is obese, or if abdominal guarding or distension are present, one is much less likely to palpate a mass. In addition, reduced blood pressure can dampen aortic pulsations produced by the aneurysm. Ecchymosis can develop from significant bleeding, and can be seen in the abdominal wall, flank, scrotum, penis, inguinal region, perineum, or perianal area.[84] A hematoma can even present as a mass in the scrotum, simulating an incarcerated hernia.[85] Finally, although not common, the hematoma can compress the femoral nerve, resulting in femoral neuropathy. This produces hip and thigh pain, quadricep muscle weakness, reduced sensation over the anteromedial thigh, and weakened patellar reflex.[75]

Misdiagnosis: Avoiding the Pitfalls

Unfortunately, misdiagnosis of symptomatic AAA is common. In fact, some series report misdiagnosis rates as high as 30-60%.[5,86] In particular, patients with a ruptured AAA are often "missed" if they present in atypical fashion, while the patient with "classical" symptoms may be misdiagnosed as renal colic or diverticulitis.

Several features of symptomatic AAA act in concert to increase risk of ED misdiagnosis. For example, the majority of these patients (> 80%) have no idea that an aneurysm is present at time of rupture, giving the ED physician no historical clues to suggest the diagnosis.[87] Furthermore, AAA rupture is much less common in elderly patients than other diseases that can mimic this condition. That is, when an elderly patient presents with LLQ pain and guaiac positive stools, the likelihood of diverticulitis is much greater than AAA rupture. Complicating the clinical diagnosis is that the "classical triad" of back/abdominal pain, hypotension, and pulsatile mass is actually the exception rather than the rule. One study found only 9% of patients with AAA rupture presented with this triad.[86]

A number of studies have reported the final diagnoses in patients thought to have ruptured AAA but who were found to have other conditions discovered during surgery.[88] One group of researchers found a misdiagnosis rate of 10% over a 10-year time period at their institution.[89] Figure 3 summarizes the final diagnoses in these patients. It should be stressed that almost 75% of these patients still would have required emergency surgery based on their final diagnosis. In addition, 10 of the 16 patients in this series did indeed have AAAs found at surgery; CT scan was done in three of these patients and the results were "misleading" and not helpful in ruling out rupture of AAA. These data provide additional support for the prudent practice of taking unstable patients with a suspected diagnosis of ruptured AAA directly to the OR with limited diagnostic studies.

Many of the conditions that can be confused with AAA rupture are listed in Figure 4.[86] Renal colic is the most frequent misdiagnosis. The fact that AAA can be misdiagnosed as ureteral colic can be explained on the basis of anatomical and clinical pathophysiology. Compression of a ureter by an expanding aneurysm or hematoma can produce renal colic through ureteral obstruction.[86] Consequently, the physician may recognize the renal colic, but fail to ascribe it to an underlying process, such as expanding or ruptured AAA. Pursuit of the underlying etiology is imperative, since most patients with renal colic usually are sent home, where AAA rupture is likely to prove fatal. In the following section, features of AAA linked to misdiagnosis in patients with both typical and atypical presentations will be emphasized.

Classical Presentation. The so-called "classic patient" with AAA rupture can be difficult to recognize. A number of findings and clinical features can complicate the diagnosis. First, the presenting symptoms of rupture are not specific for this entity. Acute abdominal pain has myriad causes in elderly patients, most of which are more common than AAA rupture. Likewise, back pain is often present for other reasons in ED patients, the majority of which are not life threatening. As a result, patients may be inappropriately triaged from the start, putting them at even greater risk.

Elderly patients with back pain and hematuria must be evaluated for AAA. If AAA is present, they should be considered to have acute rupture until proven otherwise. The same can be said for patients with LLQ pain and lower GI bleeding. In addition, any elderly patient with abdominal pain and a mass, especially in the LLQ, should be considered to have a symptomatic AAA unless CT or US shows a normal aorta. In addition, any elderly patient presenting with shock and presumed sepsis needs to be evaluated for presence of an aneurysm. These patients often have mental status changes that preclude them from providing a history of pain which might lead the physician to the correct diagnosis.

Finally, acute myocardial infarction (AMI) can occur as a result of AAA rupture. Patients with AAA often have other arterial disease, and the associated hypotension and cardiovascular stress can precipitate an AMI. Fortunately, most of these patients can give a history of abdominal or back pain in addition to chest pain. Complaints of abdominal or back pain should not be ignored in these patients, especially if they precede the onset of chest discomfort. As will be reiterated later, the best advice is to "think" aneurysm and look for it early to avoid misdiagnosis.

Atypical Presentations. There are several atypical presentations that AAA, with or without rupture, can produce. These atypical presentations include the following: chronic contained rupture, aneurysm dissection, inflammatory aneurysm, aortovenous (AV) or aortoenteric (AE) fistula, and embolic complications. AE fistulas primarily are found as a late complication of AAA repair, and will be discussed in a later section. These complications of AAAs are by no means common, but they do happen and only will be "picked up" by a physician who is looking for them.

Although most patients with AAA rupture present acutely, some have been known to wait for weeks or months prior to detection.[90] In these cases, the rupture occurs in the retroperitoneal space, where it may be contained without further leakage.

Characteristically, these patients have continuous, chronic back pain and a number of complications caused by the retroperitoneal hematoma, such as femoral neuropathy.[91] Even though they may have survived with a "stable" rupture for long periods, they still are at risk for progression to hemorrhage at any time.[92]

Dissection of the abdominal aorta can occur, but this is the rare exception; fewer than 4% of aortic dissections begin in the abdominal aorta.[93] These can occur without the presence of AAA. Fortunately, the symptom complex produced by abdominal aortic dissection is similar to AAA rupture, and the distinction may be recognized during the workup for AAA rupture or detected at surgery.

Inflammatory AAAs are defined by a thickened aneurysmal wall, extensive perianeurysmal and retroperitoneal fibrosis, and dense adhesions of adjacent abdominal organs.[16] Clinically, these patients may present with abdominal or back pain, but also have signs of chronic, smoldering infection such as weight loss, low-grade fevers, and elevated erythrocyte sedimentation rate.[94] Although initially thought to be the result of a completely separate pathological process, most clinical investigators recognize that all AAAs exhibit some degree of inflammatory change; as a result, inflammatory AAAs are thought to be an extreme example of the continuum of AAA disease.[44,95] They are identified in 4-12% of patients with AAAs.[96]

A recent study of 274 patients with AAAs found no ruptures in those patients with inflammatory aneurysms.[94] Despite this report, it is known that inflammatory AAAs can rupture, but it is not known if they are less prone to this complication or if chronic contained rupture

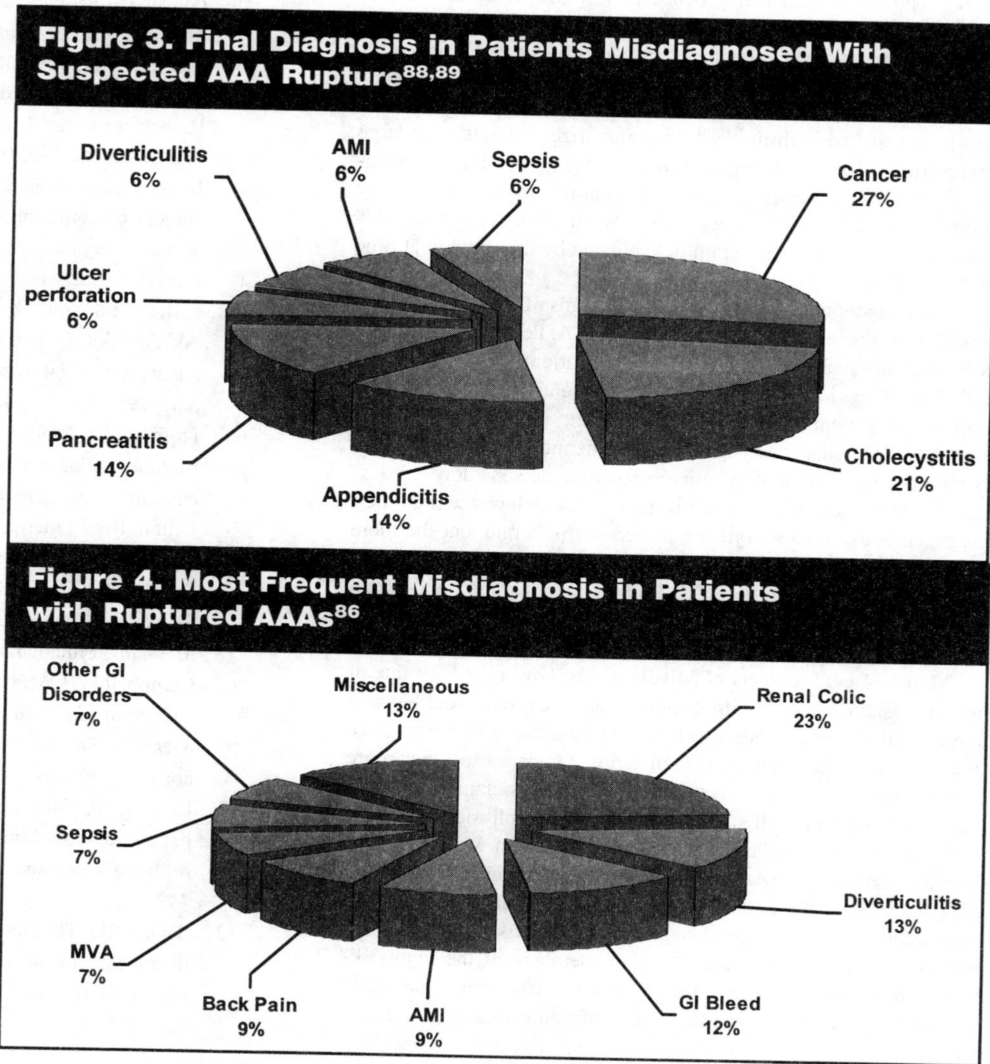
Figure 3. Final Diagnosis in Patients Misdiagnosed With Suspected AAA Rupture[88,89]

Figure 4. Most Frequent Misdiagnosis in Patients with Ruptured AAAs[86]

leads to inflammatory changes in the beginning. Advanced cases on CT and US show a characteristic "mantle core sign" where the lumen of the aorta is compressed into a dumbbell shape by the inflammatory reaction. Ureteral compression (sometimes leading to acute renal failure) is seen in about 10-25% of patients in association with these aneurysms, and often results when the aneurysm extends into the iliac arteries.[97,98] Treatment is the same as for other symptomatic AAAs—expeditious removal—although it may be technically more demanding because of the dense adhesions surrounding the aneurysm.

AV fistulas also can be seen in patients with AAA, but are found in only 1% of elective AAA repairs and in 4% of patients with AAA rupture.[99] AV fistulas occur when the AAA erodes into an adjacent vein. Most commonly, the inferior vena cava or left renal vein is involved.[14] Although an AV fistula can open simultaneously with AAA rupture, the majority of patients with AV fistula have no other sites of aneurysm leakage. The fistula results in shunting of blood from the arterial to venous system and increased venous return. Increased venous pressure can lead to distension of veins in the legs or abdominal wall. It can also produce hematuria through distension and leakage of veins in the bladder wall, or by increased venous pressure in the kidneys. Renal insufficiency can develop from the combination of increased pressure in renal veins, high-output heart failure, and decreased renal blood flow caused by the shunt.

Patients with AV fistula can present with symptoms of high-output failure, including: dilated heart, tachycardia, wide pulse pressure, dyspnea, pulmonary edema, and eventual hemodynamic decompensation. The shunt also can produce a decrease in blood flow in structures distal to the shunt. Patients can present with cool lower extremities and diminished pulses. Since aneurysms that produce AV fistulas usually are large, nearly 90% are palpable in the abdomen.[75] An abdominal bruit can be heard in 75% of patients, and 25% also will have a palpable thrill.[100,101] To summarize, patients with large aneurysms (> 10 cm) and signs of high-output cardiac failure, hematuria, renal insufficiency, signs of venous distension or any combination of the above, need to be evaluated for AV fistula. This can be done with an arteriogram or evaluated by the surgeon at time of AAA repair.

Any patient presenting to the ED with signs of peripheral emboli should be evaluated for the presence of an AAA. Peripheral embolism is another unusual but documented complication of AAA. Overall, embolism to the lower extremities is the presenting symptom in less than 5% of patients with AAA.[14] Rarely, the entire aneurysm will thrombose, simultaneously producing ischemic symptoms in both extremities; more commonly, microemboli are passed "downstream" and generate ischemic symptoms in the distal lower extremities. Larger emboli can cause one leg to become ischemic, but the more common situation is ischemia in one or two toes caused by microemboli (the "blue toe syndrome").[2] Emboli to other intra-abdominal vessels can produce intestinal ischemia, renal ischemia and failure, and neurological deficits (via the spinal artery of Adamkiewicz).

Medico-Legal Aspects of Misdiagnosis. Given the high rate of misdiagnosis of patients with symptomatic AAA, one would expect failure or delay of diagnosis to be a common cause of malpractice suits. While not frequent in overall terms compared to other more common causes of lawsuits (i.e., missed MI), AAA claims are represented in most studies of suits against emergency physicians. In one study of malpractice claims from 1980 to 1987 in Massachusetts, failure to diagnose AAA accounted for 2% of claims (6 of the total 262), and 3% of the dollars paid ($384,000 of $11,800,000).[102] A more recent article also classified AAAs as "high risk" for cases paid against emergency physicians.[103] Other members of the high risk-class included: chest pain, wounds, fractures, pediatric fever/meningitis, central nervous system bleeding, and epiglottitis.[103]

One would expect the data to back up these claims; in other words, patients with misdiagnosis should have a higher mortality rate. One group reported a 50% increase in mortality (35% to 75%, respectively) when studying patients with misdiagnosis from 1975 to 1979.[6] Interestingly, more recent studies have not found the same results. Delay to diagnosis of AAA rupture was not found to be associated with an increased mortality in these patients.[5,86] Several facts are likely to be responsible for this. These include the high baseline mortality (up to 80%) associated with AAA rupture, even when it is rapidly diagnosed.[3] Patients with or without delay of diagnosis in one series had similar mortality rates of 44% and 58%, respectively.[86]

Especially important is that misdiagnosis may be more likely in the subgroup of hemodynamically stable patients. They survive long enough to make it to the ED and appear less critical than those with hypotension on presentation. Perhaps, they survive their protracted course because they have more subtle symptoms and a better prognosis from the onset than those with unrestricted rupture. This suspicion was confirmed in a recent study on the effect of length of ED stay on mortality of patients with ruptured AAA.[104] These investigators reported that prolonged presurgical time was associated with more hemodynamically stable patients, and these patients did have a lower mortality rate. Even so, every effort should be made to avoid delays to diagnosis and treatment.

References

1. Glover JL. Thoracic and abdominal aneurysms. In: *Emergency Medicine—A Comprehensive Study Guide*. 3rd Ed. New York: McGraw Hill; 1992:382-386.
2. Gloviczki P. Ruptured abdominal aortic aneurysms. In: Rutherford RB, ed. *Vascular Surgery*. 4th Ed. Philadelphia: WB Saunders; 1995:1060-1068.
3. Ingolby CJH, Wujanto R, Mitchell JE. Impact of vascular surgery on community mortality from ruptured abdominal aortic aneurysms. *Br J Surg* 1986;73:551-553.
4. Banerjee A. Atypical manifestations of ruptured abdominal aortic aneurysms. *Postgrad Med* 1993;69:6-11.
5. Akkersdijk GJ, Hajo van Bockel J. Ruptured abdominal aortic aneurysm: Initial misdiagnosis and effect on treatment. *Eur J Surg* 1988;164:29-34.
6. Hoffman M, Avellone JC, Plecha FR, et al. Operations for ruptured abdominal aortic aneurysm: A community-wide experience. *Surgery* 1982;91:597-602.
7. Gillum RF. Epidemiology of aortic aneurysm in the United States. *J Clin Epidemiol* 1995;48:1289-1298.
8. Balsano N, Cayten CG. Abdominal aortic aneurysms. In: Schwartz GR, et al, eds. *Principles and Practice of Emergency Medicine*. Philadelphia: Lea & Febiger; 1992:1370-1375.
9. Campbell WB. Mortality statistics for elective aortic aneurysm. *Eur J Vasc Surg* 1991;5:111-113.
10. Mealy K, Salman A. The true incidence of ruptured abdominal aortic aneurysms. *Eur J Vasc Surg* 1988;2:405-408.
11. Rutledge R, Oller DW, Meyer AA, et al. A statewide, population-based time-series analysis of the outcome of ruptured abdominal aortic aneurysm. *Ann Surg* 1996;223: 492-502.
12. Sayers RD, Thompson MM, Nasim A, et al. Surgical management of 671 abdominal aortic aneurysms: A 13-year review from a single center. *Eur J Vasc Endovasc Surg* 1997; 13:322-327.

13. Johnston KW, Rutherford RB, Tilson MD, et al. Suggested standards for reporting on arterial aneurysms. *J Vasc Surg* 1991;13:452-458.
14. Rothrock SG, Green SM. Abdominal aortic aneurysms: Current clinical strategies for avoiding disaster. *Emerg Med Reports* 1994;15:126-136.
15. Goldstone J. Aneurysms of the aorta and iliac arteries. In: Moore W, ed. *Vascular Surgery: A Comprehensive Review*. 4th Ed. Philadelphia: WB Saunders; 1993:401-421.
16. Rasmussen TE, Hallett JW Jr. Inflammatory abdominal aortic aneurysms: A review with new perspectives in etiology. *Ann Surg* 1997;225:1-10.
17. Vowden P, Wilkinson D, Ausobsky JR, et al. A comparison of three imaging techniques in the assessment of an abdominal aortic aneurysm. *J Cardiovasc Surg* 1989;30:891-896.
18. MacSweeney STR, Powell JT, Greenhalgh RM. Pathogenesis of abdominal aortic aneurysm. *Brit J Surg* 1994;81:935-941.
19. Louwrens HD, Adamson J, Powell JT, et al. Risk factors for atherosclerosis in men with stenosing or aneurysmal disease of the abdominal aorta. *Int Angiol* 1993;12:21-24.
20. Norrgard O, Angquist KA, Dahlen G. High concentrations of Lp(a) lipoprotein in serum are common among patients with abdominal aortic aneurysms. *Int Angiol* 1988;7:46-49.
21. Norrgard O, Angquist KA, Johnson O. Familial aortic aneurysms: Serum concentrations of triglyceride, cholesterol, HDL-cholesterol and (VLDL + LDL)-cholesterol. *Br J Surg* 1985;72:113-116.
22. Ernst CB. Abdominal aortic aneurysm. *N Eng J Med* 1993; 328:1167-1172.
23. Tilson M. Aortic aneurysms and atherosclerosis. *Circulation* 1995;92:491-510.
24. Zarins CK, Glagov S, Vesselinovitch D, et al. Aneurysm formation in experimental atherosclerosis: Relationship to plaque evolution. *J Vasc Surg* 1990;12:246-256.
25. Shealy CB, Elliott BM. Abdominal aortic aneurysms, what's changing? *J South Carolina Med Assoc* 1997;93:13-16.
26. Caro CG, Pedley TJ, Schroter RC, et al. Solid mechanics and the properties of blood vessel walls. In: *The Mechanics of the Circulation*. Oxford: Oxford University Press; 1978:86-105.
27. Dobrin PB. Mechanics of normal and diseased blood vessels. *Ann Vasc Surg* 1988;2:283-294.
28. Zatina MA, Zarins CK, Gewertz BL, et al. Role of median lamellar architecture in the pathogenesis of aortic aneurysms. *J Vasc Surg* 1984;1:442-428.
29. Campa JS, Greenhalgh RM, Powell JT. Elastin degradation in abdominal aortic aneurysms. *Atherosclerosis* 1987;65:13-21.
30. Powell JT, Vine N, Crossman M. On the accumulation of D-aspartate in elastin and other proteins of the ageing aorta. *Atherosclerosis* 1992;97:201-208.
31. Anidjar S, Saltzmann J-L, Gentrie D, et al. Elastase-induced experimental aneurysms in rats. *Circulation* 1990;82:973-981.
32. Cohen JR, Faust G, Tenebaum N, et al. The calcium messenger system and the kinetics of elastase release from human neutrophils in patients with abdominal aortic aneurysms. *Ann Vasc Surg* 1990;4:570-574.
33. Anidjar S, Kieffer E. Pathogenesis of acquired aneurysm of the abdominal aorta. *Ann Vasc Surg* 1992;6:298-305.
34. Rizzo RJ, McCarthy WJ, Dixit SN, et al. Collagen types and matrix protein content in human abdominal aortic aneurysms. *J Vasc Surg* 1989;10:265-373.
35. Ramierz F, Periera L, Zhang H, et al. The fibrillin-Marfan syndrome connection. *Bioessays* 1993;15:589-594.
36. Verloes A, Sakalihasan N, Koulischer, L et al. Aneurysms of the abdominal aorta: Familial and genetic aspects in three hundred thirteen pedigrees. *J Vasc Surg* 1995;21:646-655.
37. Majumder PP, St. Jean PL, Ferrell RE, et al. On the inheritance of abdominal aortic aneurysm. *Am J Hum Genet* 1991;48:164-170.
38. Kontusaari S, Kuivaniemi H, Tromp G, et al. A single base mutation in type III procollagen that converts the codon for glycine 619 to arginine in a family with familial aneurysms and mild bleeding tendencies. *Ann N Y Acad Sci* 1990;580: 556-557.
39. Brophy CM, Marks WH, Reily JM, et al. Decreased tissue inhibitor of metalloproteinases (TIMP) in abdominal aortic aneurysm tissue: A preliminary report. *J Surg Res* 1991;50: 653-657.
40. Doll R, Peto R, Wheatley K, et al. Mortality in relation to smoking: 40 years' observations on male British doctors. *BMJ* 1994;309:901-911.
41. Strachan DP. Predictors of death from aortic aneurysm among middle-aged men: The Whitehall study. *Br J Surg* 1991;78: 401-404.
42. Nicholls SC, Gardner JB, Meissner MH, et al. Rupture in small abdominal aortic aneurysms. *J Vasc Surg* 1998;28: 884-888.
43. Cronenwett JL, Murphy TF, Zelencock GB, et al. Actuarial analysis of variables associated with rupture of small aortic aneurysms. *Surgery* 1985;98:472-483.
44. Sterpetti AV, Hunter WJ, Feldhaus RJ, et al. Inflammatory aneurysms of the abdominal aorta: Incidence, pathologic, and etiologic considerations. *J Vasc Surg* 1989;9:643-650.
45. Sternbergh WC III, Gonze MD, Garrard CL, et al. Abdominal and thoracoabdominal aortic aneurysm. *Surg Clin North Am* 1998;78:827-843.
46. Stella A, Gargiulo M, Pasquinelli G, et al. The cellular component in the parietal infiltrate of inflammatory abdominal aortic aneurysms (IAAA). *Eur J Vasc Surg* 1991;5:65-70.
47. Lieberman J, Scheib JS, Googe PB, et al. Inflammatory abdominal aortic aneurysm and the associated T-cell reaction: A case study. *J Vasc Surg* 1992;15:569-572.
48. Koch AE, Haines GK, Rizzo RJ, et al. Human abdominal aortic aneurysms. Immunophenotypic analysis suggesting an immune-mediated response. *Am J Pathol* 1990;137: 1199-1213.
49. Anidjar S, Dobrin PB, Eichorst M, et al. Correlation of inflammatory infiltrate with the enlargement of experimental aortic aneurysms. *J Vasc Surg* 1992;16:139-147.
50. Bengtsson H, Bergqvist D, Sternby NH. Increasing prevalence of abdominal aortic aneurysms: A necropsy study. *Eur J Surg* 1992;158:19-23.
51. Reily JM, Tilson MD. Incidence and etiology of abdominal aortic aneurysms. *Surg Clin North Am* 1989;69:705-711.
52. Spina M, Garbisa S, Hinnie J, et al. Age-related changes in composition and mechanical properties of the tunica media of the upper thoracic human aorta. *Ateriosclerosis* 1983;3:64-76.

53. Imura T, Yamamoto K, Kanamori K, et al. Non-invasive ultrasonic measurements of the elastic properties of the human abdominal aorta. *Cardiovasc Res* 1986;20:208-214.
54. Cronenwett JL, Sargent SK, Wall MH, et al. Variables that affect the expansion rate and outcome of small abdominal aortic aneurysms. *J Vasc Surg* 1990;11:260-269.
55. Spittell JA Jr. Hypertension and arterial aneurysm. *J Am Coll Cardiol* 1983;1:533-540.
56. Dorbin PB. Pathophysiology and pathogenesis of aortic aneurysms: Current concepts. *Surg Clin North Am* 1989;69: 687-703.
57. Glimaker H, Holmberg L, Elvin A, et al. Natural history of patients with abdominal aortic aneurysm. *Eur J Vasc Surg* 1991;5:125-130.
58. Sterpetti AV, Cavallaro A, Cavallari N, et al. Factors influencing the rupture of abdominal aortic aneurysms. *Surg Gynecol Obstet* 1991;173:175-178.
59. Hallet JW Jr. Abdominal aortic aneurysm: Natural history and treatment. *Heart Dis Stroke* 1992;1:303-308.
60. Nevitt MP, Ballard DJ, Hallett JW Jr. Prognosis of abdominal aortic aneurysms: A population-based study. *N Engl J Med* 1989;321:1009-1014.
61. Vardulaki KA, Prevost TC, Walker NM, et al. Growth rates and risk of rupture of abdominal aortic aneurysms. *Br J Surg* 1998;85:1674-1680.
62. Katz DJ, Stanely JC, Zelenock GB. Gender differences in abdominal aortic aneurysm prevalence, treatment and outcome. *J Vasc Surg* 1997;59:235-242.
63. Fielding JWL, Black J, Ashton F, et al. Diagnosis and management of 528 abdominal aortic aneurysms. *BMJ* 1981; 283:355-359.
64. Sternbergh WC, Gonze MD, Garrard CL, et al. Abdominal and thoracoabdominal aortic aneurysm. *Surg Clin North Am* 1988;78:827-834.
65. Johansson G, Swedenborg L. Ruptured abdominal aortic aneurysms: A study of incidence and mortality. *Br J Surg* 1986;73:101-103.
66. Johansson G, Nydahl S, Olofsson P, et al. Survival in patients with abdominal aortic aneurysms. Comparison between operative and nonoperative management. *Eur J Vasc Surg* 1990;4:497-502.
67. Brown PM, Pattenden R, Gutelius JR. The selective management of small abdominal aortic aneurysms: The Kingston study. *J Vasc Surg* 1992;15:21-27.
68. Mortality results for randomized controlled trial of early elective surgery or ultrasonographic surveillance for small abdominal aortic aneurysms. The UK Small Aneurysm Trial participants. *Lancet* 1998;352:1649-1655.
69. Chang JB, Stein TA, Liu JP, et al. Risk factors associated with rapid growth of small abdominal aortic aneurysms. *Surgery* 1997;121:117-122.
70. Lederle FA. Risk of rupture of large abdominal aortic aneurysms. Disagreement among vascular surgeons. *Arch Intern Med* 1996;156:1007-1009.
71. Johnston KW, Scobie TK. Multicenter prospective study of nonruptured abdominal aortic aneurysms. Population and operative management. *J Vasc Surg* 1988;7:69-81.
72. Finlayson S, Birkmeyer J, Fillinger M, et al. Should endovascular surgery lower the threshold for repair of abdominal aortic aneurysms? *J Vasc Surg* 1999;29:973-985.
73. Cronenwett JL, Johnston KW. The United Kingdom small aneurysm trial: Implications for surgical treatment of abdominal aortic aneurysms. *J Vasc Surg* 1999;29:191-194.
74. Ouriel K, Green RM. Arterial disease. In: Schwartz SI, et al, eds. *Principles of Surgery.* 7th Ed. New York: McGraw-Hill; 1999: 931-1005.
75. Bessen HA. Abdominal aortic aneurysms. In: Rosen P, et al, eds. *Emergency Medicine: Concepts and Clinical Practice*, 4th Ed. St. Louis: Mosby-Year Book, Inc; 1998:1806-1819.
76. Sostek M, Fine SN, Harris TL. Duodenal obstruction by abdominal aortic aneurysm. *Am J Med* 1993;94:220-221.
77. Lederle FA, Walker JM, Reinke DB. Selective screening for abdominal aortic aneurysm with physical examination and ultrasound. *Arch Intern Med* 1988;148:1753-1756.
78. Lederle FA, Simel DL. Does this patient have abdominal aortic aneurysm? *JAMA* 1999;281:77-82.
79. Banerjee A. Atypical manifestations of ruptured abdominal aortic aneurysms. *Postgrad Med* 1993;69:6-11.
80. Kiell CS, Ernst CB. Advances in management of abdominal aortic aneurysm. *Adv Surg* 1993;26:73-98.
81. Goldstone J. Aneurysms of the aorta and iliac arteries. In: Moore WS, ed. *Vascular Surgery: A Comprehensive Review.* 4th Ed. Philadelphia: WB Saunders; 1993:401-421.
82. Harris LM, Faggiloi GL, Fiedler R, et al. Ruptured abdominal aortic aneurysms: Factors affecting mortality rates. *J Vasc Surg* 1991;14:812-818.
83. Gaylis H, Kessler E. Ruptured abdominal aortic aneurysms. *Surgery* 1980;87:300-304.
84. Ratzan RM, Donaldson MC, Foster JH, et al. The blue scrotum sign of Bryant: A diagnostic clue to ruptured abdominal aortic aneurysm. *J Emerg Med* 1987;5:323-329.
85. Khaw H, Sottiurai VS, Craighead CC, et al. Ruptured abdominal aortic aneurysm presenting as symptomatic inguinal mass: A report of six cases. *J Vasc Surg* 1986;4: 384-389.
86. Marston WA, Alhquist R, Johnson G, et al. Misdiagnosis of ruptured abdominal aortic aneurysms. *J Vasc Surg* 1992;16: 17-22.
87. Vohra R, Reid D, Groome J, et al. Long-term survival in patients undergoing resection of abdominal aortic aneurysm. *Ann Vasc Surg* 1990;4:460-465.
88. Porcellini M, Benardo B, Del Viscovo L, et al. Intra-abdominal acute diseases simulating rupture of abdominal aortic aneurysms. *J Cardiovasc Surg* 1997;38:653-659.
89. Valentine RJ, Barth MJ, Myers SI, et al. Nonvascular emergencies presenting as ruptured abdominal aortic aneurysms. *Surgery* 1993;113:286-289.
90. Sterpetti AV, Blair EA, Schultz RD, et al. Sealed rupture of abdominal aortic aneurysms. *J Vasc Surg* 1990;11:430-435.
91. Bower TC, Cherry KJ, Pairolero PC. Unusual manifestations of abdominal aortic aneurysms. *Surg Clin North Am* 1989;69:745-754.
92. Jones CS, Reily MK, Dalsing MC, et al. Chronic contained rupture of abdominal aortic aneurysms. *Arch Surg* 1986;121: 542-546.
93. VanMaele RG, DeBock L, Van Schil PE, et al. Limited acute

dissections of the abdominal aorta. Report of 5 cases. *J Cardiovasc Surg* 1992;33:298-304.

94. Sasaki S, Keishu Y, Takigami MD, et al. Inflammatory abdominal aortic aneurysms and atherosclerotic abdominal aortic aneurysms: Comparison of clinical features and long-term results. *Jpn Circ J* 1997;61:231-235.
95. Pennell RC, Hollier LH, Lie JT, et al. Inflammatory abdominal aortic aneurysms: A thirty year review. *J Vasc Surg* 1985;2:859-869.
96. Boontje AH, Van den Dungen JJ, Blanksma C. Inflammatory abdominal aortic aneurysms. *J Cardiovasc Surg* 1990;31: 611-616.
97. Latifi HR, Heiken JP. CT of inflammatory abdominal aortic aneurysm: Development from an uncomplicated atherosclerotic aneurysm. *J Comput Assist Tomogr* 1992;16: 484-486.
98. Nevelsteen A, Lacroix H, Stockx L, et al. Inflammatory abdominal aortic aneurysm and bilateral complete ureteral obstruction: Treatment by endovascular graft and bilateral ureteric stenting. *Ann Vasc Surg* 1999;13:222-224.
99. Lanne T, Bergqvist D. Aortocaval fistulas associated with ruptured abdominal aortic aneurysms. *Eur J Surg* 1992;158: 457-465.
100. Potyk DK, Guthrie CR. Spontaneous aortocaval fistula. *Ann Emerg Med* 1995;25:424-427.
101. Gilling-Smith GL, Mansfield AO. Spontaneous abdominal arterio-venous fistulae: Report of eight cases and a review of the literature. *Br J Surg* 1991;78:421-425.
102. Karcz A, Holbrook J, Auerbach BS, et al. Preventability of malpractice claims in emergency medicine: A closed claims study. *Ann Emerg Med* 1990;19:865-873.
103. Karcz A, Korn R, Burke MC, et al. Malpractice claims against emergency physicians in Massachusetts: 1975-1993. *Am J Emerg Med* 1996;14:341-345.
104. Farooq MM, Freischlag JA, Seabrook GR, et al. Effect of the duration of symptoms, transport time, and length of emergency room stay on morbidity and mortality in patients with ruptured abdominal aortic aneurysms. *Surgery* 1996; 119:9-14.
105. Frazee BW. The abdominal aorta. In: Simon BC, Snoey ER, eds. *Ultrasound in Emergency and Ambulatory Medicine*. St. Louis: Mosby-Year Book, Inc; 1997:190-202.

Management of Abdominal Aortic Aneurysm

Gary Hals, MD, PhD
Michael Pallaci, DO

Even with the current arsenal of ultrasonic and computerized tomographic modalities, all the diagnostic tools available to the emergency department (ED) physician have limitations. For example, bedside ultrasound (US) is an excellent screening tool to identify patients with an abdominal aortic aneurysm (AAA), but is less reliable for detection of vascular rupture. Because of its rapidity of execution, however, US is the better tool for rapid identification of an AAA in an unstable patient.

On the other hand, strong suspicion that an unstable patient has an AAA may be all that is required to transport the patient to the OR for definitive treatment. In contrast, computed tomography (CT) is accurate for both detection of an AAA and identifying leak or rupture; its diagnostic advantages must be weighed against that fact, but the scanning suite often is the last place one wants to put an unstable patient. Accordingly, CT is most useful in evaluation of symptomatic but stable patients.

The alert physician will be aware of post-surgical complications, which are associated with an increased risk of rupture and arteriovenous complications.

With these diagnostic and management issues in mind, this concluding part of our two-part series outlines the diagnostic and management strategies for patients with AAA. The sequencing of diagnostic testing is highlighted, and the role of stabilization prior to surgical intervention is emphasized.

Diagnostic Pathways for AAA: Sequencing, Strategy, and Execution

The appropriate test and sequencing for ED evaluation of patients with a suspected AAA depends on several factors: 1) the stability of the patient; 2) the time delay in performance of the test; and 3) the disposition options available to the ED physician. In the small ED, where limited surgical back up is available, transfer of the patient to more appropriate facilities should take precedence over completing the work-up or even making the diagnosis. When high-risk patients need to be evaluated for a symptomatic AAA, they should be taken to the nearest ED where they can be rapidly taken to the OR if the diagnosis is confirmed.

As a rule, time should not be wasted ordering an evaluation if the patient will be transferred for surgery anyway. In those EDs where adequate surgical consultation is readily available, the question is: "Which test do I order first?" More often than not, the answer is: Order whichever test (US or CT) can be obtained most rapidly.

Overview. Given equal availability of US and CT, bedside US is the test to obtain in order to answer the question of whether there is an aneurysm. It is nearly 100% sensitive for diagnosing the presence of an AAA, it can be executed in a matter of minutes, and it does not require unstable patients to leave the department.[1] While much less accurate than CT in detecting actual rupture, if the patient has the symptoms of rupture and presence of an AAA, this usually is all the information required for the consultant to take the patient to the OR.

CT scanning, on the other hand, is much more accurate for defining the anatomy of the aneurysm; moreover, it can detect involvement of other major arteries (i.e., renal or mesenteric), the

Figure 1. Ultrasound Image of an Abdominal Aortic Aneurysm

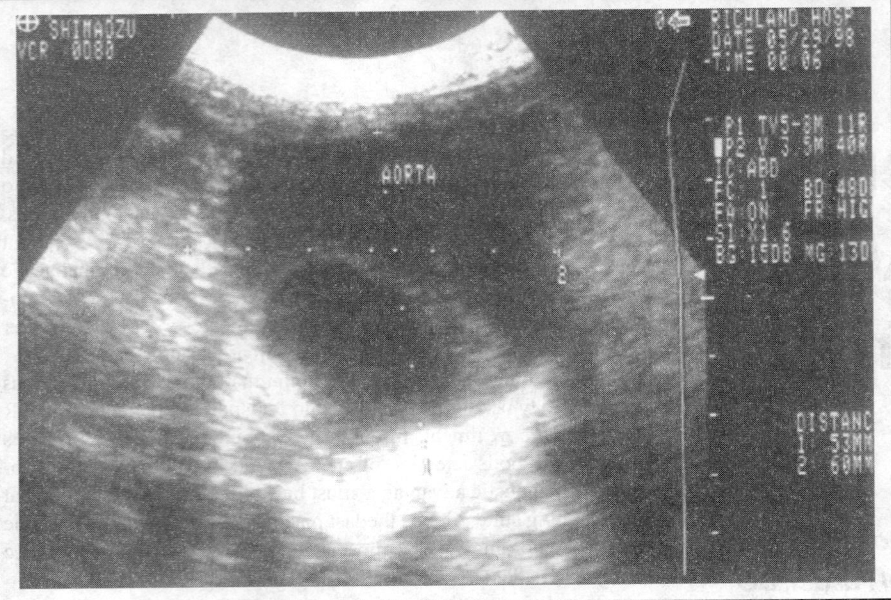

presence of hematoma or thrombus, and involvement of retroperitoneal structures. As an overarching approach to modality selection, the following is true: If it is simply a matter of determining whether the patient has an AAA, then bedside US (if available without delay) will give the best response. If the questions to be answered are, "How does this patient's AAA need to be managed, is there a rupture, and what will be required in the OR?" then CT will provide the best characterization of the management plan.

Plain Films. Unlike the case for most causes of acute abdominal pain, plain radiographs do represent a reasonable initial screening test for the ED physician who is evaluating a patient with suspected AAA. In this case, evidence of AAA is seen in about 60-75% of abdominal films.[2,3] The clinician should attempt to identify a calcified aortic wall, which can be seen on cross-table lateral films in up to 68% of patients.[4] Cautious interpretation is required since the outer rim of the aneurysm may not be calcified, leading the physician to assume the aortic diameter is much smaller than it is in reality.

Other signs that are suggestive of AAA include: paravertebral soft tissue mass, loss of psoas or renal outlines, and rarely, erosion of vertebral bodies from long-standing AAAs.[5] Advantages of plain films for evaluation of these patients primarily are rapid availability of the test and results. Radiographs can be performed at the bedside, preventing the unstable patient from leaving the department. The major disadvantage of plain films is that a negative study cannot exclude the diagnosis. In patients for whom there is a high suspicion for AAA, one should not use plain films unless other options (US or CT) are not rapidly available. If the physician is forced to wait for US or CT, a plain x-ray should certainly be obtained during the waiting period, since confirmation of AAA on plain film may obviate the need for further radiographic evaluation.

Ultrasound. As previously mentioned, US has been shown to be nearly 100% accurate for detecting the presence of AAA.[6] The appearance of an AAA as seen on US is shown in Figure 1. The primary advantages of US is its rapidity, non-invasiveness, and that it can be used in nearly all patients who present with suggestive symptoms. Perhaps the most useful aspect of US is that unstable patients can be evaluated in the ED without interruption of resuscitation and stabilization efforts. Although the study is still in abstract form, one current study demonstrates potential advantages of US over CT. When comparing bedside US to CT scan, the average time to diagnosis was 5.4 minutes for US and 83 minutes for CT. The average time to OR was similarly reduced: 12 minutes in US patients and 90 minutes in those diagnosed by CT scan.[7] Another author found that use of bedside US in the ED was 95% accurate in identifying patients who needed emergency surgery.[6] These patients were hemodynamically unstable and had abdominal pain; the US was used to confirm presence of an aneurysm.

Drawbacks of the US also should be noted. First, US cannot accurately identify rupture in an aneurysm; one study evaluating only 60 patients yielded a sensitivity for extraluminal blood of only 4%.[6] Although failure to identify rupture is a disadvantage, oftentimes identification of the presence of an aneurysm is sufficient to refer the patient for urgent consultation. US can be used to recognize relatively small volumes of intraperitoneal fluid (several hundred ccs), and it has recently been reported that this modality can diagnose AAA rupture in an ED patient.[8]

The fact that most AAAs rupture into the retroperitoneal space—an area that is less accessible to the US—compromises the usefulness of this modality. Abdominal cavity hemorrhage, which is associated with AAA, carries a much higher mortality rate, presumably from unrestricted hemorrhage. Secondly, it is technically difficult to visualize the aorta with US in obese patients, or in those with excessive, overlying bowel gas. Finally, US does not provide the complex data that CT scan can show concerning the relationship of the aneurysm to other vascular structures.

These disadvantages notwithstanding, immediate bedside US is an appropriate modality for rapid and safe identification of AAA in ED patients suspected of having an AAA. One team of investigators has identified three specific situations where limited bedside US should be used in evaluation of the aorta in ED patients: 1) in the presence of abdominal pain and hypotension, where demonstration of normal aorta excludes AAA as the diagnosis early in the work-up; 2) in the stable patient with unexplained abdominal or back pain, in which AAA is one of the few life-threatening diagnoses that needs to be ruled-out early in the patient's course; and 3) every elderly patient with abdominal or back pain with risk factors such as peripheral vascular disease, hypertension, tobacco use, etc.[1]

Computed Tomography (CT). As with US, CT is virtually 100% accurate in detection and measurement of an AAA.[9] Visualization of an AAA as seen by CT is shown in Figure 2. Unlike US, it can also provide accurate characterization of the entire aorta and identify involvement of surrounding vascular or intestinal structures. Obesity or presence of bowel gas does not limit the ability to perform the study. It is also much more accurate than US in identifying rupture.[10] As little as 10 mL of blood can be identified outside the aortic lumen.[11]

CT has even been reported to identify signs of impending rupture in patients with symptomatic AAA. A "high-attenuating crescent" in the aneurysm wall was shown to be indicative of imminent AAA rupture in one recent study.[12] Newer helical CTs can produce three-dimensional reconstructions of an AAA. Typically, IV contrast is given for elective studies, but these are not absolute requirements for emergency scans. IV contrast will help the radiologist identify mural thrombus and periaortic fibrosis, but acute hemorrhage and aneurysm size can still be measured without IV contrast. Withholding IV contrast also will be of benefit to patients with baseline renal insufficiency, as many patients experience renal dysfunction after AAA repair. Oral contrast will aid precise identification of bowel loops, but the time delay required for its use can be a liability for some patients.[13]

While CT provides a wealth of information in the patient being evaluated for symptomatic AAA, it does have several distinct disadvantages. The most important is that the patient must leave the ED to obtain the study, or if the scanner is in the department, the patient must still enter a room where he or she is not accessible for continued resuscitation or treatment. Therefore, use of CT should be reserved only for evaluation of stable patients.

Even though the CT scan is extremely accurate, it still can produce false-negative results. In other words, in some cases, an AAA will be identified but the CT will be negative for acute rupture. Patients have been reported to have a negative CT scan for rupture, but then soon decompensate and a ruptured AAA is found at surgery.[14] These cases emphasize that one should not be lead into thinking a patient's symptoms are not from impending rupture if the CT shows an AAA but no hemorrhage. From a practical, sequencing perspective, if the patient has an AAA and symptoms consistent with possible rupture, the patient should have emergent consultation by a vascular surgeon regardless of whether the CT scan shows the presence of hemorrhage.

In one four-year study, only 8% of patients taken to the OR for an AAA rupture had evidence of hemorrhagic leakage upon surgical evaluation in the OR.[15] Nevertheless, 75% of these patients required surgical repair for AAA or another nonvascular surgical procedure at the time of their laparotomy. Consequently, it is beyond the purview of the emergency physician alone to "make the final call" on whether the AAA is leaking and what kind of surgical procedure is required. This assessment should always be undertaken in collaboration with a surgical consultant. One recent article by a vascular surgeon suggested "that CT has little additional diagnostic value" in the work-up of patients with suspected AAA rupture.[16] He suggested that "if the patient has no medical contraindications to AAA repair, the patient should be taken directly to the OR."

Angiography. Angiography represents another option for evaluation of patients with symptomatic AAA, but this modality should *not* be used by emergency physicians to screen patients for AAA. It often underestimates aortic diameter, as the presence of mural thrombus is common in AAAs and this can produce a normal sized aortic lumen in the presence of a larger aneurysm. Its primary function is for consulting surgeons who may obtain anatomic information that will aid in the surgical plan.

Many vascular surgeons still routinely order arteriography before aneurysm resection, although there is considerable debate in the surgical literature as to whether the information obtained justifies the cost, discomfort, and potential risk to the patient.[11] Currently, the reported indications for arteriography as articulated in the surgical literature include: 1) symptoms of mesenteric ischemia; 2) hypertension or renal dysfunction (i.e., suspicion of renal artery stenosis which could also be repaired at time of surgery); 3) horseshoe kidney; and 4) claudication or other signs/symptoms of coexistent lower extremity occlusive disease.[11] Newer helical CTs with the ability to produce three-dimensional reconstructions have been evaluated for replacement of conventional arteriography. One study found that CT angiography can provide all the necessary imaging for elective aneurysm repair, but it requires twice the radiation dose and three times the amount of contrast dose.[17]

Figure 2. CT Scan of a Ruptured Abdominal Aortic Aneurysm

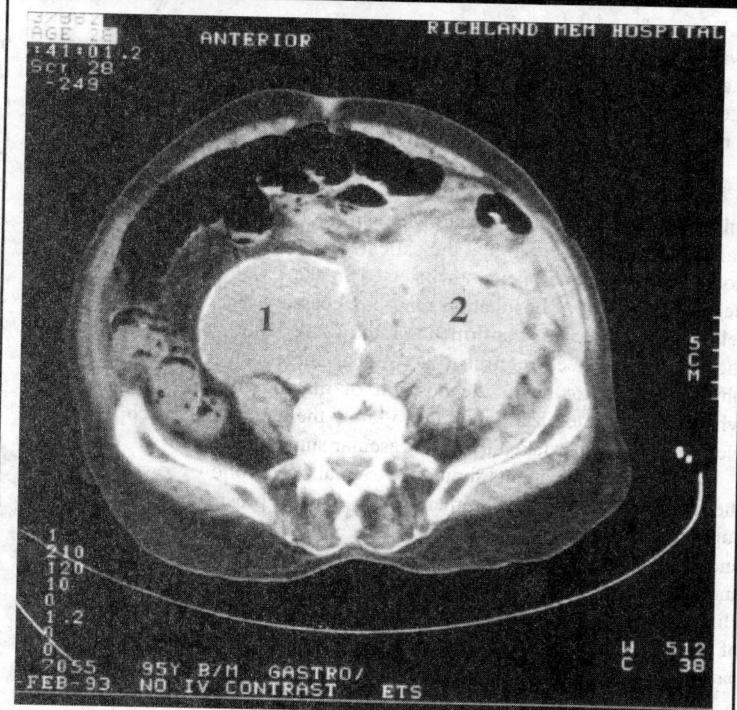

1 = Large abdominal aortic aneurysm
2 = Free blood in the abdominal cavity

Magnetic Resonance Imaging. Magnetic resonance imaging (MRI) offers the advantages of US and CT in that it is accurate for detecting the presence of an AAA. It is even better than CT for defining three-dimensional views of the aorta and surrounding vascular structures. At present, though, the disadvantages prevent its routine use in the ED for evaluation of patients for symptomatic AAA. Most importantly, MRI does not accurately identify acute hemorrhage.[18] Furthermore, the limitations placed by the inability to scan patients with metallic foreign objects (i.e., pacemakers, surgical clips), the lack of accessible monitoring equipment in the MRI room, and the high cost all relegate the use of MRI scans in the setting of AAA to primarily for elective pre-operative evaluation.

Management

The emergency management of patients with AAA requires a systematic and methodical approach, which will be determined by various factors, including the patient's symptoms, co-morbid conditions, and aneurysm size. The resources of each institution (surgical back-up, access to US/CT) also need to be taken into consideration. As mentioned previously, if a patient presents with symptoms strongly suggestive of AAA rupture and with a physical exam consistent with this condition (i.e., palpable pulsatile abdominal mass), the clinician does not need additional information to justify transfer of the patient to the nearest appropriate center if adequate surgical back-up is not available.

Management strategies are identified for three categories of patients: 1) Those with an incidental AAA; 2) patients with a ruptured AAA who are stable; and 3) patients with an AAA who are unstable.

Incidental AAA. With the frequent use of US and CT scans, AAAs are found in increasing numbers in ED patients who are being evaluated for other disease processes. Furthermore, it is estimated that 50% of these "new," previously undetected aneurysms are small (i.e., < 5 cm), and therefore, the approach to the treatment of asymptomatic aneurysms in this size range is controversial.[19]

What is not a matter of debate, however, is that symptomatic AAA requires surgical intervention. Therefore, the burden of proof falls on the emergency physician when an AAA is detected; specifically, one must be certain that the patient's presenting symptoms are not the result of the aneurysm detected in the ED. As mentioned before, appropriate consultation may be necessary to establish this relationship. Once it is confirmed that the AAA is not symptomatic, the patient will need referral to a vascular surgeon. While the ED physician will not be in the position of making the decision of whether to operate, it is important to know the general approach to elective AAA repair taken by most vascular surgeons.

Asymptomatic patients should have serial US to follow growth of the aneurysm. Recent recommendations from a prospective study suggest an interval of one year between US for patients with aneurysms less than 4 cm in size, and every six months for those with aneurysms 4 cm or greater.[20] Since coronary artery disease (CAD) is clinically evident in at least 50% of patients with AAAs,[19] AMI is one of the most common cause of death during or after surgery for these patients.

To provide clinical guidance for managing these patients, one author has suggested three preoperative classes, or risk categories, for patients that are based on their CAD status. Class 1 patients are those at lowest risk, i.e., without evidence of CAD and normal exercise tolerance. These patients may have elective repair without further cardiac evaluation. Class 2 patients represent individuals with known CAD or those with significant risk factors (diabetes, hypertension, etc.). It is recommended that these patients have a preoperative cardiac evaluation with subsequent catheterization and angioplasty if needed. Class 3 patients have significant CAD and are acutely symptomatic or unstable. He suggests these patients undergo cardiac catheterization for evaluation and treatment prior to elective surgery. Relative contraindications to AAA, as recommended by the Joint Council of the Society for Vascular Surgery, include patients with life expectancy of less than two years, recent MI, severe angina, severe pulmonary insufficiency with dyspnea at rest, severe renal dysfunction, intractable congestive heart failure, and advanced dementia.[21] Finally, patients should be given clear discharge instructions concerning who to follow up with and when, as well as specific symptoms that should prompt them to seek immediate medical treatment (abdominal/back pain, GI bleeding, etc).

Ruptured AAA in the Stable Patient. Patients with symptomatic AAA who are able to maintain their cardiovascular status should be treated aggressively. They can decompensate at any time and are likely to give the physician little warning before doing so. Once the diagnosis of ruptured AAA has been established, they should be taken to the operating room as quickly as possible. However, as the mortality for emergency surgery on intact aneurysms is 20-25% compared to 5% for elective repair (primarily from lack of time to address co-morbid conditions), it is not unreasonable for the surgeon to request verification of rupture prior to surgery.[21,22]

In other words, if a bedside US demonstrates the presence of an AAA in a stable patient, the surgeon may appropriately request CT scan for proof of rupture and delineation of anatomy prior to surgery. Although this maneuver is associated with some risk for the patient, as it does delay time to definitive treatment and the patient has a significant risk for sudden, catastrophic collapse at any point, many surgeons will obtain a CT prior to surgery. The decision must weigh the potential benefits of decreased surgical mortality from improved definition of the case vs. increased mortality from delay of surgery. Accordingly, the ED physician should contact the consulting surgeon as soon as the presence of an AAA is established (even from physical exam) and he or she should be closely involved in decisions from that point on. After the presence of an AAA is established, the ED physician should never send the patient for additional studies (such as CT scan) without surgical consultation.

In addition, the patient should have someone at his or her bedside at all times who is capable of resuscitation while the patient is being transported to the OR should he or she suddenly decompensate. Two large bore IVs should be placed as soon as possible and laboratory tests, such as type and crossmatch (for at least 10 units of blood), hemoglobin and hematocrit, chemistry panel for renal function, coagulation studies, urinalysis (UA), and electrocardiogram (ECG), are all indicated. However, no laboratory test should delay transport of the patient.

Finally, the patient may be hypertensive on presentation to the ED. One may be tempted to treat the blood pressure as in patients with thoracic aortic dissection, and reduce it with beta-blockers and nitroprusside. While it "makes sense" that reducing stress on the aortic wall would help slow or prevent further rupture, this approach has not been shown to improve outcomes in any studies. Furthermore, development of hypotension is a risk and this may confuse the clinical picture. Therefore, antihypertensive treatment is not generally recommended, and should not be initiated without discussion with the consultant.

Ruptured AAA in the Unstable Patient. Patients with ruptured AAA are not considered "stable" until the aorta is cross-clamped in the OR. Consequently, these patients should have a rapid ED course and all delays should be avoided prior to transport to the OR. Emergency surgical intervention is the procedure providing definitive benefits in this patient subgroup. At least one study evaluating patients who were taken to emergency surgery who did not have an AAA rupture found that 75% of these patients still required emergency surgical intervention.[23] Use of the MAST (military antishock trousers) suit has been suggested for ED patients with ruptured AAA, but it has not been shown to be beneficial.[5] Therefore, general use in the ED is not recommended, but the suit may be helpful while transporting patients to another facility. These patients should have two large bore IVs and/or central IV access initiated as soon as they arrive. At least 10 units of blood should be ordered, as these patients often require a large volume of blood.[24] Preoperative hypotension is strongly correlated with risk of death in these patients.[25]

Patients with ruptured AAA may develop hypotension and tachycardia secondary to blood loss, or from a combination of hypovolemia and depressed cardiac function. Accordingly, the appropriate degree of volume resuscitation in these critically ill patients is debatable. Some argue that preoperative hypotension slows bloods loss and allows clot formation, much as has been suggested in trauma patients with penetrating injuries.[26] Giving the patient a large volume of crystalloid can promote a dilutional coagulopathy as well.[27] On the other hand, prolonged hypotension in these elderly patients can contribute to end organ problems, such as renal failure and cardiac ischemia. Indeed, most patients who undergo emergent repair of ruptured AAAs die in the early postoperative stage from MI or respiratory or renal failure, which may represent complications of inadequate organ perfusion.[24,25]

As no studies on varying resuscitation strategies in these patients have been published, there is no blood pressure "number" to aim for when caring for a patient with a ruptured AAA. Adequate blood pressure should be maintained to preserve mental status and prevent cardiac ischemia, and the blood pressure required will vary from patient to patient. Blood products should be used early in the resuscitation efforts in order to reduce dilutional coagulopathy.

Few diagnostic studies are necessary in unstable patients with ruptured AAA. One author reported a significantly increased mortality rate in patients with symptomatic aneurysms who underwent more extensive preoperative evaluation.[28] If the physical exam reveals a pulsatile abdominal mass, the patient should be taken to the OR directly. If the physical exam is not diagnostic, bedside US will often demonstrate the presence of an AAA. Documentation of the aneurysm and symptoms consistent with rupture are usually all that is required to take unstable patients to the OR. These patients should not be taken out of the department for any other reason; tests such as CT scan are too risky and time consuming in hypotensive patients. Baseline labs, including chemistry panel, CBC, coagulation studies, UA, and ECG, are all indicated, but none of these values is likely to impact the treatment of the ED patient. Although these patients can be in considerable pain, their low blood pressure usually precludes use of narcotics for pain relief.

At this time, surgery is the only definitive treatment for AAA rupture; endovascular repair currently is being used only in elective repairs. Although the risk of emergent repair remains high (around 50%), without surgery the process is almost certainly fatal.[21,29] Even so, debate is under way in the literature as to whether emergent repair should be withheld from certain patients based on risk factors. Several retrospective studies have attempted to identify prognostic indicators for mortality in patients undergoing emergent AAA repair.[25,30-34]

The following factors have been suggested as preoperative factors that characterize the patient as being in a "higher risk" category: hypotension or shock on admission; age older than 76 years; creatinine greater than 0.19 mmol/L; loss of consciousness after arrival to the ED; hemoglobin less than 9 g/dL; evidence of cardiac ischemia on ECG; history of COPD; and history of transient ischemic attack (TIA) or stroke.[30,34] Intraoperative factors affecting survival include increased cross-clamp time, need for a bifurcated graft, presence of saccular aneurysm, and persistent hypotension in the OR.[31-33] Postoperative events associated with increased risk include renal failure requiring dialysis, mesenteric infarction, and respiratory failure. The results of these studies vary. One group found that patients with three or more of five selected risks (age > 76, creatinine > 0.19 mmol/L, loss of consciousness after arrival, hemoglobin less than 9 g/dL, or ECG ischemia) had 100% mortality.[30] With two factors, the mortality was 72%, and with one it was 37%. This compared to a mortality of 16% with zero risk factors. Based on these results, they suggest that one should consider withholding surgery from the highest risk groups.

On the other hand, another study found that while increased age was indeed a risk factor for death, there was a survival rate of 44% in patients older than 80 years of age operated on in a 10-year period.[25] Furthermore, they also reported that 28% of patients who experienced cardiac arrest before surgery still survived repair.[25] Therefore, no clear criteria have yet been established for withholding surgery from patients with acute rupture. Currently, the only absolute contraindication to surgery is a competent patient who refuses the procedure, which is not a common occurrence. All patients presenting with AAA rupture should be referred to a vascular surgeon for evaluation; even if he or she initially refuses surgery, the patient may change his or her mind after speaking with the surgeon.

Late Complications of AAA Repair

AAA repair, whether elective or emergent, improves the life expectancy of those who survive the surgery. The five-year survival rate after repair is reported to be 76%.[35] However, the presence of CAD or cerebral vascular disease in these patients is correlated with a much lower survival rate of 30-40% over eight years, compared to 60% survival in those without CAD.[19] In one series, 60% of patients had either sustained a MI in the eight years since repair or died from complications of their MI.[19]

Connective tissue disorders associated with aneurysmal disease makes recurrence of a new aneurysm possible. Up to 5% of patients with one aortic aneurysm will eventually develop a new one requiring surgery.[19] The most common sites for new aneurysm after repair are above the original graft or in the thoracic aorta. These patients are also at risk for femoropopliteal aneurysms; 5-15% will develop an aneurysm in this location.[19] Two other significant complications that the ED physician needs to be aware of are graft infection and aortoenteric fistula. These two complications can occur together, with infection leading to fistula. In one recent series, 38% of patients with aortic graft infection also had a graft-enteric fistula.[36] Approximately 3-5% of patients surviving aneurysm repair will experience one of these problems.[19]

Graft Infection. Symptoms of graft infection can occur soon after repair, resulting from contamination during surgery, or they can occur years later, when they are caused by spread of contiguous infection or hematogenous spread. The infected portion may be localized (most commonly the inguinal section), or it may involve the entire graft.[37] As with AAA rupture, the mortality of graft infection is also high. Mortality rates range from 33% in one series of infected grafts without intestinal fistula formation, to 50% in a British series.[38,39] Another recent series found that 100% of 24 patients with graft infection alone presented with symptoms of sepsis.[40] Infection was suspected in an additional 31% of patients diagnosed with aortoenteric fistula (AEF).

Staphylococcus epidermidis is the most common organism isolated from graft cultures, and is thought to enter as a result of contamination during the healing process or later seeding from skin ulcers at distant sites.[39] Presenting symptoms can be divided into two groups of patients: those with sepsis and perigraft infection, and those with graft infection leading to aortoenteric fistula (AEF). Those patients found to be infected with *S. epidermidis* presented with more subtle symptoms of low grade fever, malaise, elevated erythrocyte sedimentation rate, and elevated white blood cell (WBC) count. Signs of graft infection seen on CT scan include perigraft fluid, gas and soft tissue swelling, or false aneurysm formation.[39] A small prospective series comparing CT with indium-labeled WBCs found CT to be more sensitive as a marker for infection.[41]

Unfortunately, the treatment for aortic graft infection requires not only antibiotic therapy, but also graft excision and extra-anatomic bypass. The bypass is typically performed by the axillofemoral route, and leads to a high risk for lower extremity amputation (5-year limb loss rate of 33%) as some bypasses fail or the patient is not a candidate for this surgery at all.[42] Consequently, all patients with a post AAA repair status that includes systemic infections of unknown etiology or those with GI bleeding will need to be evaluated for possibility of graft infection. As will be stressed below, it is wise to assume that the cause of GI bleeding in patients with AAA repair is graft-enteric fistula until proven otherwise. In one series, 75% of patients with GI bleeds were found to have a cause other than an AEF.[39] The converse means that 25% of patients being evaluated for GI bleed after AAA repair did have an AEF.

Aortoenteric Fistula. While fistulae can form between an AAA and intestine prior to repair, these are much more commonly seen after aneurysm repair. The most common site of development is between the proximal aortic anastomosis and the distal duodenum, as this is the nearest intestinal structure and it is fixed in the retroperitoneum. However, fistulas can be formed at any site in the GI tract and may cause upper or lower GI tract bleeding.[43]

Although one could expect the patient to present with massive GI bleeding, the blood loss from an AEF can be acute or chronic, minimal or extensive. As mentioned above, graft infection is thought to be a significant cause of AEF formation. One series of 22 patients with AEF found blood cultures were positive for enteric organisms in 85% of cases.[44] The mean interval in their series from surgery to presentation with AEF was 36 months, but AEF has been reported in patients as long as 14 years after surgery.[44] A significant minority of these patients (22%) presented with a "herald hemorrhage;"[44] i.e., a sudden, brisk bleeding episode leading to hypotension, that ceases spontaneously and is followed by rebleeding hours to days later.

Accordingly, all patients with previous AAA repair and GI bleeding require evaluation for possible AEF. The precise approach depends on the patient's hemodynamic condition. Unstable patients with limited response to resuscitation should be taken to the OR for exploratory surgery to stop bleeding and identify its source. In stable patients, upper GI endoscopy is the recommended initial test, but it is not 100% accurate and its main value may lie in identifying another cause of bleeding.[45] CT scan is also useful, not because it will identify the fistula, but because it can recognize evidence of graft infection. Unfortunately, graft fistulas are only recognized with certainty, at best, 50% of the time, and exploratory surgery is often required in patients with suspected AEF and major GI bleeding to rule-out the diagnosis.[45]

When identified, an AEF requires high-risk, graft replacement surgery. A recent review suggests that surgery for AEF carries a higher mortality than for graft infection alone; only 25% of patients were alive at 18 months after surgery, compared to 60% surviving graft infection alone.[40] Therefore, when a patient with an aortic graft presents to the ED with GI bleeding, consultation with a GI specialist or vascular surgeon is essential to rule-out AEF.

Summary

Patients with AAA are presenting in ever increasing numbers in EDs across the country, due to both an increase in incidence and an increase in the number of elderly patients in the population. Ruptured AAAs account for at least 15,000 deaths per year and represent the 10th leading cause of death in men older than 55 years of age.[46] With these increasing numbers, ED physicians will encounter more patients with symptomatic aneurysms, as well as patients with complications of AAA repair.

Patients with AAA have always been a challenge for emergency physicians because these individuals are often unaware of their disease until the sudden, catastrophic presentation of acute rupture. When patients present with AAA rupture, diagnosis of this condition is often difficult. Any patient older than 50 years of age who presents to the ED complaining of back or abdominal pain and has any of the risk factors (family history, hypertension, vascular disease, tobacco use) should be evaluated with either US or CT for the possibility of AAA.

If an AAA is confirmed, consultation with a vascular surgeon will be required to rule-out acute rupture as the cause of the complaints. Ultimately, the take-home message is: 1) remember to look for an aneurysm in patients with risk factors; 2) keep in mind the best approach for care of patients in the three general conditions encountered (incidental finding, stable rupture, and unstable rupture; and 3) do not assume the patient's complaints are not related to the AAA until proven otherwise. With these points in mind, the ED physician can improve the patient's chances of survival.

References

1. Frazee BW. The abdominal aorta. In: Simon BC, Snoey ER, eds. *Ultrasound in Emergency and Ambulatory Medicine*. St. Louis: Mosby-Year Book, Inc; 1997:190-202.
2. Loughran CF. A review of the plain abdominal radiograph in acute rupture of abdominal aortic aneurysms. *Clin Radiol* 1986;37:383-387.
3. Brewster DC, Darling RC, Raines JK, et al. Assessment of abdominal aortic aneurysm size. *Circulation* 1977;56(Supp 2):164-169.
4. LaRoy LL, Cormier RJ, Matalon TA, et al. Imaging of abdominal aortic aneurysms. *Am J Roentgenol* 1989;152:785-792.
5. Bessen HA. Abdominal aortic aneurysms. In: Rosen P, et al, eds. *Emergency Medicine: Concepts and Clinical Practice*, 4th Ed. Mosby-Year Book, Inc; 1998:1806-1819.
6. Shuman WP, Hastrup W. Suspected leaking abdominal aortic aneurysm: Use of sonography in the emergency room. *Radiology* 1988;168:117-119.
7. Plummer D, Clinton J, Matthew B. Emergency department ultrasound improves time to diagnosis and survival in ruptured abdominal aortic aneurysm. *Acad Emerg Med* 1998;5:417.
8. Miller J, Grimes P, Miller J. Case report of intraperitoneal ruptured abdominal aortic aneurysm diagnosed with bedside ultrasonography. *Acad Emerg Med* 1999;6:661-664.
9. Bernstein EF. Computed tomography, ultrasound and magnetic resonance imaging in the management of aortic aneurysm. In: Hobson RW, Williams RA, et al, eds. *Vascular Surgery: Principles and Practice,* 2nd Ed. New York: McGraw-Hill; 1994.
10. Zarnke MD, Gould HR, Goldman MH. Computed tomography in the evaluation of the patient with symptomatic abdominal aortic aneurysm. *Surgery* 1988;103:638-642.
11. Ouriel K, Green RM. Arterial disease. In: Schwartz SI, et al, eds. *Principles of Surgery,* 7th Ed. New York: McGraw-Hill; 1999:931-1005.
12. Mehard WB, Heiken JP, Sicard GA. High-attenuating crescent in abdominal aortic aneurysm wall at CT: A sign of acute or impending rupture. *Radiology* 1994;192:359-362.
13. Siegel CL, Cohan RH. CT of abdominal aortic aneurysms. *Amer J Roentgenol* 1994;163:17-29.
14. Greatorex RA, Dixon AK, Flower CDR, et al. Limitations of computed tomography in leaking abdominal aortic aneurysms. *BMJ* 1988;297:284-285.
15. Porcellini M, Benardo B, Del Viscovo L, et al. Intra-abdominal acute diseases simulating rupture of abdominal aortic aneurysms. *J Cardiovasc Surg* 1997;38:653-659.
16. Adam DJ, Bradbury AW, Stuart WP, et al. The value of computed tomography in the assessment of suspected ruptured abdominal aortic aneurysm. *J Vasc Surg* 1998;27:431-437.
17. Errington ML, Ferguson JM, Gillesie IN, et al. Complete pre-operative imaging assessment of abdominal aortic aneurysm

with spiral CT angiography. *Clin Radiol* 1997;52:369-377.

18. Durham JR, Hackworth CA, Tober JC, et al. Magnetic resonance angiography in the preoperative evaluation of abdominal aortic aneurysms. *Am J Surg* 1993;166:173-177.
19. Hallet JW Jr. Abdominal Aortic Aneurysm: Natural history and treatment. *Heart Dis Stroke* 1992;1:303-308.
20. Cook TA, Galland RB. A prospective study to define the optimum rescreening interval for small abdominal aortic aneurysm. *Cardiovasc Surg* 1996;4:441-444.
21. Hollier LH, Taylor LM, Ochsner J. Recommended indications for operative treatment of abdominal aortic aneurysms: Report of a subcommittee of the Joint Council of the Society for Vascular Surgery and the North American Chapter of the International Society for Cardiovascular Surgery. *J Vasc Surg* 1992;15:1046-1056.
22. Sullivan CA, Rohrer MJ, Cutler BS. Clinical management of the symptomatic but unruptured abdominal aortic aneurysm. *J Vasc Surg* 1990;11:799-803.
23. Valentine RJ, Barth MJ, Myers SI, et al. Nonvascular emergencies presenting as ruptured abdominal aortic aneurysms. *Surgery* 1993;113:286-289.
24. Johansen K, Kohler TR, Nicholls SC, et al. Ruptured abdominal aortic aneurysm: The Harborview experience. *J Vasc Surg* 1991;13:240-245.
25. Gloviczki P, Pairolero PC, Mucha P, et al. Ruptured abdominal aortic aneurysms: Repair should not be denied. *J Vasc Surg* 1992;15:851-857.
26. Bickell WH, Wall MJ, Pepe PE, et al. Immediate versus delayed fluid resuscitation for hypotensive patients with penetrating torso injuries. *N Engl J Med* 1994;331:1105-1109.
27. Crawford ES. Ruptured abdominal aortic aneurysm: An editorial. *J Vasc Surg* 1991;13:348-350.
28. Donaldson MC, Rosenberg JM, Bucknam CA. Factors affecting survival after ruptured abdominal aortic aneurysm. *J Vasc Surg* 1985;2:564-570.
29. Seeger JM, Kieffer RW. Preoperative CT in symptomatic abdominal aortic aneurysms: Accuracy and efficacy. *Am Surg* 1986;52:87-90.
30. Hardman DT, Fisher CM, Patel MI, et al. Ruptured abdominal aortic aneurysms: Who should be offered surgery? *J Vasc Surg* 1996;23:123-129.
31. Bauer EP, Redaelli C, von Segesser LK, et al. Ruptured abdominal aortic aneurysms: Predictors for early complications and death. *Surgery* 1993;114:31-35.
32. Koskas F, Kieffer E. Surgery for ruptured abdominal aortic aneurysm: Early and late results of a prospective study by the AURC in 1989. *Ann Vasc Surg* 1997;11:90-99.
33. Sasaki S, Yasuda K, Yamauchi H, et al. Determinants of postoperative and long-term survival of patients with ruptured abdominal aortic aneurysms. *Surg Today* 1998;28:30-35.
34. Prance SE, Wilson YG, Cosgrove CM, et al. Ruptured abdominal aortic aneurysms: Selecting patients for surgery. *Eur J Vasc Endovasc Surg* 1999;17:129-132.
35. Moriyama Y, Toyohira H, Saigenji H, et al. A review of 103 cases with elective repair of abdominal aortic aneurysm: An analysis of the risk factors based on post-operative complications and long-term follow up. *Surg Today* 1994;24: 591-595.
36. Goldstone J, Cunningham D. Diagnosis, treatment, and prevention of aorto-enteric fistulas. *Arch Chir Scand Suppl* 1990;555:165-172.
37. Goldstone J. The infected infra-renal aortic graft. *Acta Chir Scand* 1987;538:72-86.
38. Plate G, Hollier LA, O'Brien P, et al. Recurrent aneurysms and late vascular complications following repair of abdominal aortic aneurysms. *Arch Surg* 1985;120:590-594.
39. O'Brien T, Collin J. Prosthetic vascular graft infection. *Br J Surg* 1992;79:1262-1267.
40. McCann RL, Schwartz LB, Georgiade GS. Management of abdominal aortic graft complications. *Ann of Surg* 1993;217: 729-734.
41. Mark AS, McCarthy SM, Moss, AA, et al. Detection of abdominal aortic graft infection: Comparison of CT and in-labeled white blood cell scans. *AJR Am J Roentgenol* 1985; 144:315-318.
42. Quinones-Baldrich WJ, Hernandez JJ, Moore WS. Long-term results following surgical management of aortic graft infection. *Arch Surg* 1991;126:507-511.
43. Peck JJ, Eidemiller LR. Aortoenteric fistulas. *Arch Surg* 1992; 127:1191-1193.
44. Champion MC, Sullivan SN, Coles JC, et al. Aortoenteric fistula. Incidence, presentation, recognition, and management. *Ann Surg* 1982;195:314-317.
45. Calligaro KD, Veith FJ. Diagnosis and management of infected prosthetic aortic grafts. *Surgery* 1991;110:805-813.
46. U.S. Public Health Service. *Vital Statistics of the United States, Vol. II, Mortality, Part A*. Dept. of Health and Human Service, Publ. No. (PHS) 87-1101. Washington, DC: US Government Printing Office; 1987.

Part VI

Gastrointestinal Disease

Acute Appendicitis

Gary Hals MD, PhD

Patients with abdominal pain present some of the most challenging cases encountered in the emergency department (ED). Furthermore, "belly pain" also is one of the most common chief complaints. These patients are seen on every shift, can vary from the infant to the elderly nursing home patient, and often take much more time than the average patient to see and evaluate. Some patients with acute processes that require surgical intervention actually appear quite well early in their course, making it easy to miss the severity of their problem. Likewise, other patients initially appear ill with an "acute abdomen" only to improve dramatically during their ED stay and ultimately be discharged with gastritis or constipation as the cause. Even after a careful and thorough work-up by the best physicians, the end result of these patient encounters is frequently "abdominal pain of uncertain etiology." This diagnosis is applied to 40% of ED patients evaluated and discharged for abdominal pain.[1,2] While this ultimately is the correct diagnosis in many patients, the task of the emergency physician is to identify the subset of patients who require further intervention. The case of acute appendicitis is an important diagnosis to find, and a dangerous one to miss in these patients.

Appendicitis is a relatively common entity encountered in the ED, with one case per 1000 people per year.[3,4] Every person has a 6% lifetime risk of developing appendicitis.[5] It is the most common surgical emergency reported in children and pregnant patients.[6,7] While common, acute appendicitis often is difficult for both ED physicians and surgeons to diagnose accurately. Up to as many as 30% of patients with proven appendicitis are misdiagnosed and discharged by a physician before being correctly identified.[8] The negative laparotomy rate remains in the 20-25% range.[9] The rates are even higher for the elderly, women, and children, a testimony to the difficulty of making this diagnosis in these subgroups. Although morbidity and mortality have been reduced over time, the acceptable rate of perforation remains at about 20%.[10,11] However, the rate approaches a staggering 70% in patients younger than 9 years and older than 60 years of age.[12,13] The mortality rate of simple appendicitis is 0.1%, but increases 20- to 60-fold with perforation.[3,14-16] The rate of wound infection in all patients increases to 35% with perforation.[17,18] It is easy to understand why misdiagnosis of appendicitis is the fifth leading cause of successful litigation against emergency physicians and accounts for 15% of all dollars paid in ED malpractice claims.[8,19]

Atypical presentations and appendicitis in high-risk populations, such as children, the elderly, and pregnant patients, are difficult to detect. The rate of complications, including death, is directly correlated with delay of diagnosis and surgery. The fact that no single laboratory test is 100% accurate for diagnosing appendicitis exacerbates the problem. With all these factors combined, it is not surprising that attempts to diagnose patients with appendicitis can lead to frustration and confusion for both the patient and doctor. Unfortunately, when a case of appendicitis is "missed," it can produce unsatisfactory outcomes for both as well. The following review of acute appendicitis will help to update our perspective on this troublesome disease. A thorough overview of the pathophysiology of acute appendicitis and its clinical features in high-risk patients can help improve outcomes and reduce medico-legal risk.

Introduction

When evaluating a patient in whom the diagnosis of appendicitis is being considered, several key points should be emphasized. Appendicitis is most commonly seen in 10-30-year olds, but can be seen in patients of any age. Although rare in infants, it has been reported.[20] It should be included in the differential of *any* patient seen in the ED with abdominal pain. While most patients will present with right lower quadrant (RLQ) pain, the appendix can be found *anywhere* in the abdomen. One study of more than 10,000 cases revealed that the appendix was retrocecal in 65% of cases and in the pelvis in 31%.[21] Another landmark 40-year review of more than 70,000 cases found the appendix in the right upper quadrant in 4% of the subjects, the left upper quadrant in 0.06% and the left lower quadrant in 0.04%.[22] Undiagnosed congenital malrotation can explain some of these more bizarre locations.

Although not typical, recurrent episodes and even chronic appendicitis are recognized clinical entities.[9,23,24] There are even case reports of patients with ultrasound and clinical findings of acute appendicitis who are followed without surgery, and whose appendix on ultrasound returned to normal.[25,26] One author estimates recurrent appendicitis affects 6% of those individuals ultimately diagnosed with acute appendicitis.[27] Acute appendicitis should be considered even if a patient has had similar episodes of pain before, or if the pain has persisted for longer than 1-2 weeks.

Finally, it is useful to keep in mind the myriad diseases that can be confused with acute appendicitis. At the top of the list are acute gastroenteritis (AGE) and pelvic inflammatory disease (PID). The striking point here is that each of these is more common than acute appendicitis in the ED. Do not neglect to consider the diagnosis of appendicitis in these patients. (Strategies for differentiating these entities from appendicitis will be discussed in later sections). Other conditions less commonly confused with appendicitis, but still important to remember, include: Crohn's disease, mittleschmerz, pancreatitis, testicular torsion, Meckel's diverticulum, diverticulitis, cholelithiasis, bowel obstruction, endometriosis, ovarian cyst, tubo-ovarian abscess, ectopic pregnancy, urinary tract infection, and pyelonephritis. The bottom line is, many patients seen daily with abdominal pain in the ED do not have appendicitis, but, unless the appendix has been taken out, any of them *could* have this condition.

Pathophysiology of Acute Appendicitis

Some of the difficulties in recognizing acute appendicitis can be diminished by an understanding of how this condition develops. Attention to the sequence of events and the body's reaction to them can help the physician identify appendicitis whether the patient presents 12 hours or two days into the disease. The appendix is a blind pouch that arises from the inferior border of the cecum. It contains lymphoid tissue, but the function of the appendix remains a mystery. No detectable loss is noted by its surgical absence; however, even a negative laparotomy *does* carry risks of wound infection, fetal loss, and myocardial infarction, among others.[28-30] While the appendix contains little lymphoid tissue at birth, more develops as we age. This continues, peaking in adolescent years and followed by atrophy of this tissue as we age. This parallels the risk and peak incidence of appendicitis, and might explain why 69% of cases are seen in patients 10-30 years old.[31] Obstruction of the appendix lumen is thought to be the first event in development of appendicitis.[32] Lymph tissue hypertrophy may play a role in luminal obstruction, especially in children. This may explain why acute appendicitis can follow gastroenteritis, upper respiratory infections, measles, or infectious mononucleosis.[33] Unfortunately, when appendicitis develops late in the course of a viral illness, distinguishing between these two entities may be difficult. The theory of lymphatic hyperplasia is also consistent with the fact that the majority of cases occur between October and May, correlating with a higher frequency of enteric infections during this same time.[34]

Obstruction of the appendix lumen is also thought to occur from other factors as well. Some causes of obstruction include fecaliths, strictures, barium, tumors, pinworms, and foreign bodies. Examples of the more unusual foreign bodies include bones, seeds, wood, metal, plastic, and even chewing gum.[34] Obstruction of the lumen triggers a cascade of events culminating in acute appendicitis. First, the epithelial cells lining the appendix continue to secrete mucus after the lumen is blocked. Accumulation of this fluid results in distension of the appendix, which reduces venous

Table 1. Signs and Symptoms Seen in Presentation of Acute Appendicitis[1,4,14,31,37,96,144]

SYMPTOMS	FREQUENCY (%)
Abdominal pain	97-100
Migration of pain to RLQ	49-61
Nausea	67-78
Vomiting	49-74
Anorexia	70-92
Fever	10-20
Diarrhea	4 -16
Constipation	4 -16
SIGNS	
Abdominal tenderness	95-100
RLQ tenderness	90-95
Rebound tenderness	33-68
Rectal tenderness	30-40
Cervical motion tenderness	30
Rigidity	12
Psoas sign	5-3
Obturator sign	5-8
Rovsing's sign	5
Palpable mass	< 5
Mean temperature	37.9°C

Figure 1. Variations in Normal Position of the Appendix

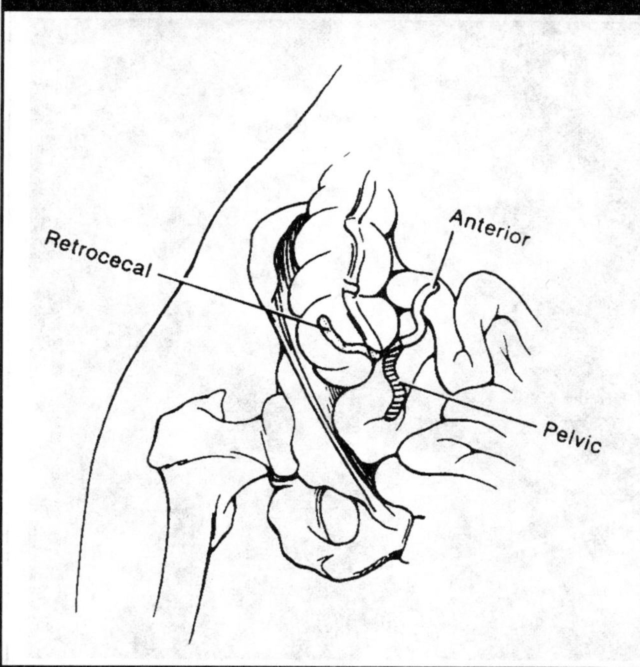

and lymphatic drainage of the appendix. Bacteria multiply in the lumen, and rapidly invade the wall of the appendix. This creates further edema of the appendix and additional stretching of its muscular wall. The sensation of stretch of the appendix wall is transmitted by visceral autonomic nerves entering the spinal cord along T8 to T10. As visceral pain is poorly localized, this explains why the patient feels only vague periumbilical pain. At this stage, the patient has simple appendicitis. It takes an average of 17 hours for patients to present at this stage.[35] Consequently, it is important to realize that patients with only "a few hours" of vague abdominal pain can be well into their course of appendicitis. Identifying patients at this stage of their disease can reduce the risk of subsequent perforation.

If obstruction of the lumen is not relieved, increased intraluminal pressure compromises venous arterial blood supply to the appendix. Subsequent ischemia of the appendix wall leads to necrosis, perforation, and abscess formation. When inflammation indirectly reaches the parietal peritoneum through the inflamed appendix wall or directly through perforation, somatic pain develops. Interestingly, classical rebound RLQ tenderness is actually a sign of probable or impending *perforation*. Stimulation of somatic pain receptors produces stronger, localized RLQ pain. This is the basis of pain migration from the periumbilical area to the RLQ and can be a key feature for differentiating appendicitis from other diseases. Average time from onset of disease to perforation is 34 hours; 72 hours is required for abscess formation.[35] When perforation occurs, the luminal pressure of the appendix decreases, and this may explain why some patients experience a brief period of pain relief. In adults, the abscess is often contained by the omentum. However, young children have a lesser-developed omentum, and rupture of the appendix leads more quickly to diffuse peritonitis.

Atypical Presentations Aren't Rare

Classical presentations aren't really that classical. The patient who presents looking healthy and complains of indigestion can be just as likely to have an acute myocardial infarction as the one that appears ill and complains of "an elephant sitting on my chest." The ED physician quickly learns to be especially vigilant for "atypical" presentations of angina, and to treat these patients conservatively with admission if one cannot safely exclude the diagnosis of unstable angina. While acute appendicitis may not be as common as unstable angina, the ED physician needs to remain suspicious of patients presenting with abdominal pain and sometimes approach them in a similar fashion. In other words, if you cannot safely exclude appendicitis as the diagnosis, it may be prudent to obtain a consult or admit the patient for your protection and theirs. The following discussion will illustrate just how variable the signs and symptoms of acute appendicitis can be.

While no ED physician would miss a patient presenting with the classic symptoms of pain beginning periumbilically and moving to the RLQ and associated with vomiting, anorexia, rebound, and fever, it is essential to realize how many patients present *without* classic features. "Classical" presentations of appendicitis are reported in only 50-60% of patients.[14,19,36,37] Table 1 summarizes the frequency of signs and symptoms seen in patients with proven appendicitis. While most patients present with abdominal pain, only about half (49-61%) give the history of migration of the pain to the RLQ. Only about two-thirds complain of nausea, vomiting, or anorexia. The number with RLQ tenderness is near 100%, but only one-third to two-thirds have rebound tenderness. Worse still, 30% of females can have cervical motion tenderness (CMT) on exam![14,19,36,37] The classic psoas and obturator signs are absent in 85-90% of exams. It is imperative to remember that peritoneal signs are reliably present after perforation has occurred. The mean temperature on presentation does not even reach the classic cut-off of 38°C to define the presence of a fever. The take-home message from these numbers is that one should not discount appendicitis in a patient with abdominal pain just because the "classic" features are not present.

The fact that the appendix can be found in a variety of anatomic locations helps explain some of this variability. *(Please see Figure 1.)* Only when the appendix lies anteriorly can it make contact with the anterior peritoneum and produce a classical presentation. If the appendix tip lies retrocecally, less inflammation will reach the bowel to produce anorexia, nausea, or vomiting. These patients may even present with flank pain instead of abdominal pain. The extreme example of this problem is encountered when the appendix lies in an extraperitoneal position; fortunately, this is an infrequent occurrence. When the appendix is retroileal, inflammation of the ureter occurs, causing testicular pain or lab findings consistent with urinary tract infection. *(See Urinalysis section.)* When the tip reaches the right upper quadrant, as in pregnancy, the findings can be more consistent with acute cholecystitis than appendicitis. *(See section on High-Risk Patient Populations for more information on diagnosis of appendicitis in pregnancy.)*

Diagnostic Tests

No laboratory test can establish the diagnosis of acute appendicitis with 100% accuracy. With this in mind, a patient with a

Figure 2. Examples of CT Findings in Acute Appendicitis

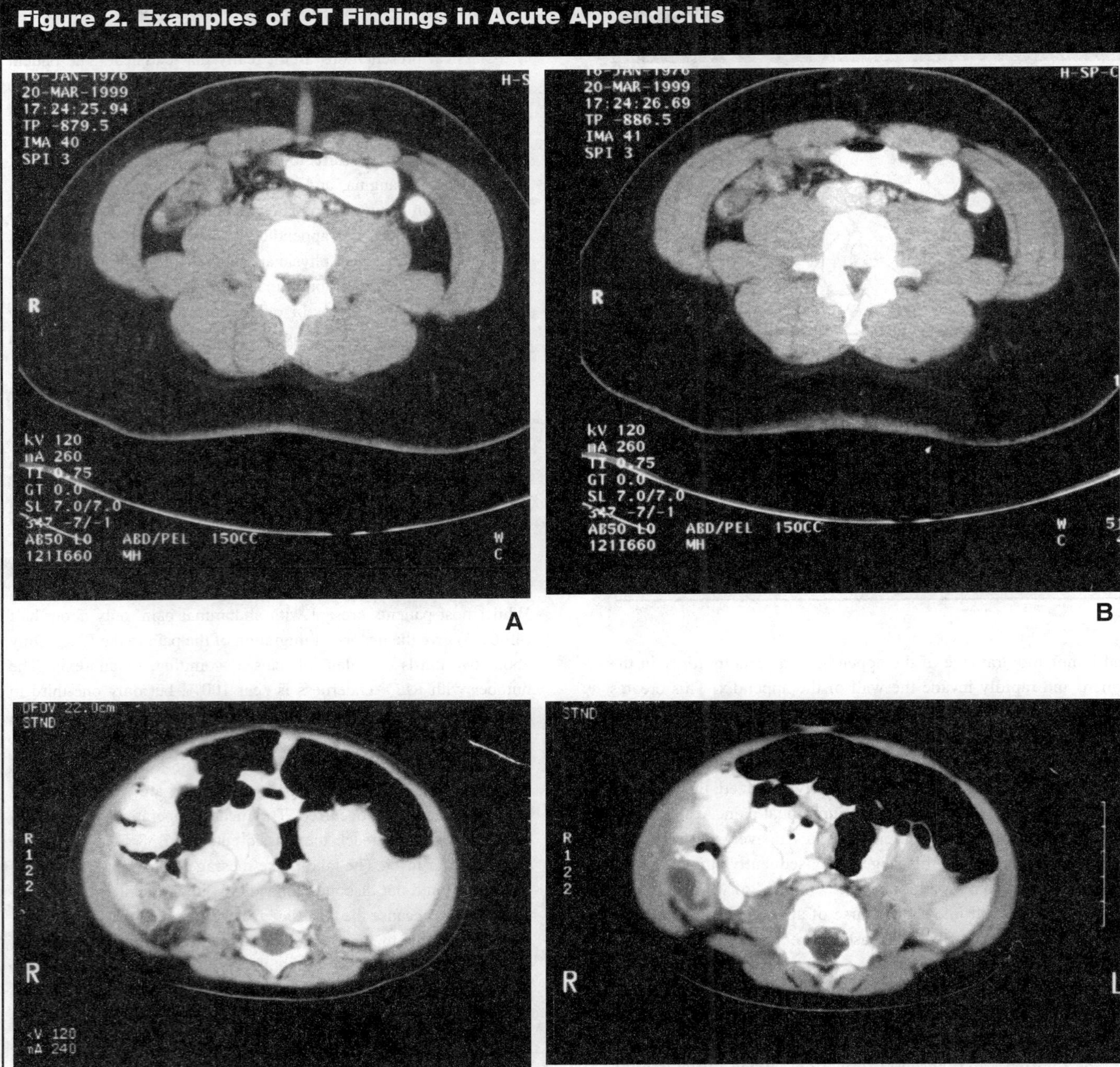

Figure 2 A shows an example of the early findings of simple appendicitis. An enlarged appendix (approximately 1.5 cm) is seen, and in the same patient inflammatory changes are seen in place of the appendix 2 centimeters distal to the first image. The next two figures show an example of CT findings in a more-advanced case of appendicitis. In figure 2 C, a fecalith can be seen just medial to a loculate fluid collection. Figure 2 D shows a well-developed abscess in the same patient, several centimeters distal to the first image.

"classical" presentation should not have any laboratory tests done that will *delay* their transition to surgery. As stated above, however, most patients do not have such a clearcut presentation. In these patients, ancillary tests will be used in combination with observation and repeated exam to help support the diagnosis of appendicitis, or to rule out another diagnosis. The following section will discuss the strengths and weaknesses of commonly used lab tests, as well as recent studies evaluating imaging by computed tomography (CT) and ultrasound. Remember that while some of these tests can be helpful, the most useful "tests" are the history and physical, followed by surgical consultation, and observation when the diagnosis is in doubt.

White Blood Cell Count. The usefulness of the white blood cell count (WBC) for diagnosing acute appendicitis in the ED has long been controversial. The conversation is familiar: The general surgeon/resident asks "What's the white count?" and the ED physician/resident states to the consultant "What difference will it make?" Then, the general surgeon/resident responds with "I'll see the patient after the WBC, films, etc. are done." Fortunately, the issue is slowly being resolved; even the surgical literature is reporting that the WBC is not essential and does not affect the decision to operate.[38] In general, ED physicians still get a WBC count when considering appendicitis, and surgeons will sometimes take the patient to the OR without labs. The best advice is to know the preferences of the consultants with whom you regularly interact, and do as they prefer, or provide them with papers to inform them of the opposing view.

The facts are that leukocytosis is seen in 75-80% of patients with acute appendicitis,[5] and a similar number have an increased number of immature band forms or "left shift."[39] Both of these values alone have been shown not to be useful in ruling out appendicitis, as they are too nonspecific; they can be seen in many of the diseases (AGE, PID) that are confused with appendicitis as well.[40,41] However, several authors report only 4-11% of patients with appendicitis will have *both* a WBC count less than 10,000 and normal differential of less than 75% neutrophils.[5,32,42,43] While the combination of a normal WBC and differential apparently makes appendicitis less likely in these patients, again, it will not rule it out in all patients. It may also take time for this elevation to occur; one study noted that while the WBC count did eventually show elevation, it was still normal in 80% of patients during the first 24 hours.[44,45] Furthermore, some high-risk populations are less likely to present with an increased WBC count. Elderly patients have normal WBC counts in up to 45% of patients on presentation.[46]

Figure 3. Examples of Ultrasound Findings in Acute Appendicitis

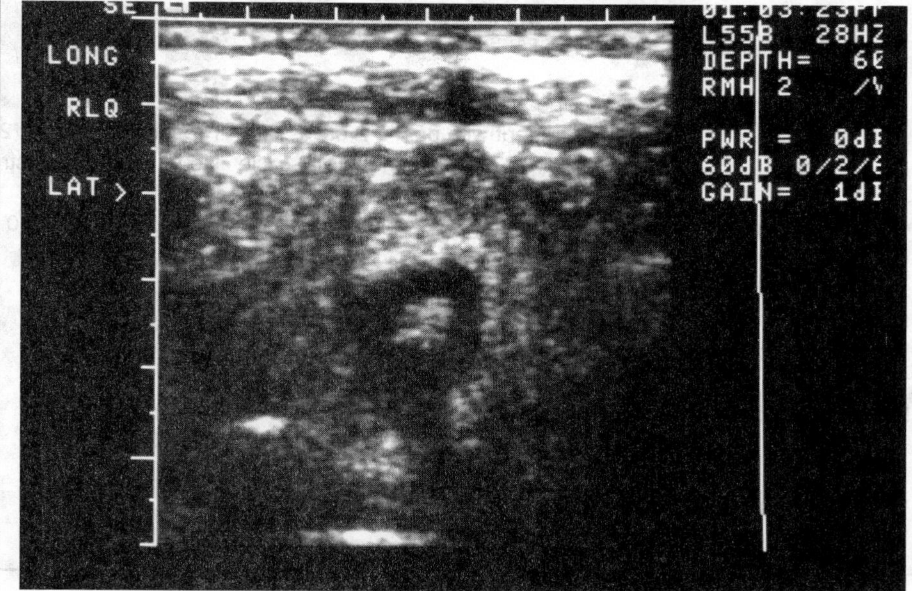

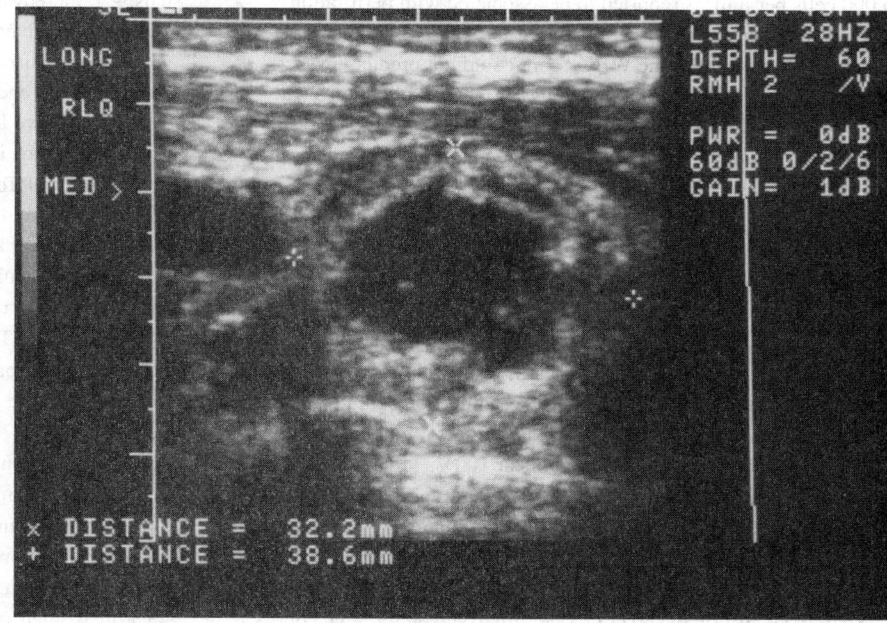

These figures show close-up images of two patients with US findings consistent with appendicitis. Figure 3 A shows an enlarged appendix (approximately 2 cm), with a "bulls eye" finding of central solid matter in the appendix lumen surrounded by free fluid. Figure 3 B shows an example of appendiceal abscess as seen by US.

The typical WBC range for simple appendicitis is between 12,000 and 18,000 cells per mm^3. Unfortunately, many of the diseases that can simulate acute appendicitis (i.e., PID, ovarian cyst rupture, AGE, ectopic pregnancy, etc.) can also produce a WBC in this range. Furthermore, progressive increase of the WBC with time has been shown to be unreliable in differentiating appendicitis from other diseases.[47,48] As mentioned above, a recent article showed that the WBC itself did not affect the decision by surgeons to operate on patients with RLQ pain.[39] In addition, a WBC count of 15,000 to

Table 2. Features that Aid in Differentiation of PID and Appendicitis*

FEATURE:	PELVIC INFLAMMATORY DISEASE	ACUTE APPENDICITIS
Abdominal pain:		
Location	Variable, may radiate to back	Migration to RLQ
Duration	Present with pain > 2 days	Present with pain < 2 days
Onset	Within 7 days of menstrual cycle	No relation to menstruation
Cervical motion tenderness:	Common—82 %**	Less common 28-30 %
Bilateral adnexal tenderness:	More common—58 %	Unusual—8 %
History of prior PID:	More common—44 %	Unusual—8 %
Presence of nausea/ vomiting:	Less common	More common

* No one feature can distinguish reliably between PID and appendicitis.[4]
** All data from reference[4]

25,000 cells per mm^3 is reported to be associated with perforation.[49] However, another recent article reviewing 1919 cases challenges this by showing the height of the WBC count could not predict the presence of perforation. This study found the proportion of patients with an elevated WBC count and perforation at surgery was equal to the proportion perforated with a normal WBC count.[50] This is consistent with other studies.[51,52]

Other serum markers, such as C-reactive protein levels alone,[53] leukocyte elastase,[54] and even technetium leukocyte scans[61] have also been investigated for possible use in diagnosis of appendicitis. However, they have not yet been shown to be consistently reliable to recommend general use.[56,57] Lastly, the combination of C-reactive protein levels with WBC and differential, the "triple test," has also been prospectively evaluated.[58] While the ability to accurately predict appendicitis was again low (37%), the authors did find that there was a high negative predictive value of near 100%.[58] In other words, if all three tests are negative (WBC < 9000, neutrophil differential < 75%, C-reactive protein < 0.6 mg/dL), the likelihood of appendicitis is very small. This may prove useful after further verification with larger numbers of patients.

Urinalysis. A urinalysis (UA) is helpful to screen for renal colic, as appendicitis will not normally produce hematuria alone. But do not be led astray if the UA shows WBCs and bacteriuria. Though most authors state that greater than 30 WBCs is indicative of a urinary tract infection (UTI), if the appendix makes contact with the ureter, the UA in appendicitis can mimic a UTI. In documented appendicitis, up to 30% of UAs will show more than 5 WBC per high power field,[59] and bacteriuria can be present in up to 15%.[60] Finally, do not forget that a urine pregnancy test should be run on all women of childbearing age to rule out ectopic pregnancy.

Plain Radiography. Flat and upright abdominal films have long been used in the ED work-up of patients with suspected appendicitis. Physicians have noted that these tests are of little use in helping make the diagnosis of appendicitis.[61] The infamous fecalith is the only finding specific for appendicitis, but is rarely seen on plain films. The 2% incidence does not justify the expense of obtaining the study.[14,62,63] Other findings reported to be helpful in diagnosing appendicitis (local air-fluid levels, soft tissue mass, psoas obliteration, gas in the appendix, etc.) have also been shown to be present in other diseases[39,64] and in normal individuals.[62,65,66] Ultimately, plain films can help identify other diseases (i.e., bowel obstruction), but they are of little use in patients being evaluated for acute appendicitis.[39]

A similar consensus has been reached concerning the use of a barium enema to diagnose appendicitis. While the obstructed appendix is not supposed to fill with barium, the normal appendix will not fill in 10-12% of individuals,[67-69] thereby generalizing an unacceptable false-positive rate. Other studies have shown the converse as well; the "obstructed" appendix can also completely fill with barium.[67,70] To make matters worse, barium enema is also suspected as a cause of appendicitis.[71] These facts have led most authors to recommend discontinuing use of barium enema in work-up of appendicitis.[72,73]

Computed Tomography. Early studies with computed tomography (CT) found that while this modality is extremely helpful in diagnosing many kinds of abdominal pathology in the ED setting, it was not as helpful in the diagnosis of appendicitis.[74-76] Perhaps the small size and variable location of the appendix caused the initial low yield with CT in appendicitis. However, more recent investigations, including one prospective study,[77] have suggested helical CT to be much more accurate in appendicitis than previously reported. Sensitivities of 97-100%, a specificity of 95%, and an accuracy rate of 98% have been reported.[77,78] Even if appendicitis was not identified using this modality, an alternative diagnosis was found in 54-80% of patients.[77,78] Another retrospective study found that CT negative laparotomy rates decreased to 4% in adult males and 8% in ovulating women,[79] compared to typical rates of 20% in men and 45% in women of childbearing age. Interestingly, the perforation rates were not lower in these same cases, and remained in the 19-22% range.[79] The encouraging sensitivity and specificity rates have led one author to proclaim that "the great mimicker, acute appendicitis, has met its match."[80] However, at least one expert has pointed out that a negative scan will not definitively rule out appendicitis,[74] and a recent review of the subject in the surgical literature emphasizes that improvements in outcome have not been demonstrated with routine use of new technology.[81] Clearly, further studies on larger numbers of patients are needed to settle this controversy. CT scans can be helpful in identification of a phlegmon or appendiceal abscess, but the clinical exam in these patients typically is sufficient for surgical intervention. Finally, CT will not always rule out ovarian pathology, PID, gastroenteritis, or other diseases in the differential, but it does have the advantage over ultrasound in that no pain is produced by the exam and obesity does not impair the study. Figure 2 illustrates typical CT findings of acute appendicitis in both early and advanced cases.

Ultrasound. Ultrasound (US) evaluation of patients with abdominal pain is rapidly expanding in the ED. The US findings in adults include visualization of a non-compressible appendix more than 6-7 mm in outer-wall-to-outer-wall diameter, single-wall diameter greater than 2 mm, dilated lumen, or presence of periappendiceal fluid. One expert team has identified three criteria for the diagnosis of appendicitis by US: 1) a tender, not-compressible appendix; 2) no peristalsis of the appendix; and 3) overall diameter greater than 6 mm.[83] Figure 3 shows an example of a non-compressible, dilated appendix on US and an example of appendiceal abscess. In adults, the sensitivity is reported to be 75-89%[84,85] and the specificity is 95%, yielding an overall accuracy of 87-96%.[84-86] A similar number range has recently been established using US in children with appendicitis,[87-89] although at least two published studies suggest the outcome is not improved by using US in children.[90,91]

The advantages of US are well known. The study is quick, readily available in most EDs, is non-invasive, has low-risk, and has been shown to be accurate.[84,85,92,93] Despite its usefulness, the diagnosis may be difficult if the appendix is not visualized on US. This is especially common in obese patients and patients with perforation and/or abscess.[83] The test may also be problematic if the patient's pain does not allow him or her to tolerate the pressure that must be applied with the probe in the RLQ to permit visualization of the appendix. In this regard, all of the diagnostic criteria depend upon visualization of the appendix, and, if it is not seen on US, the diagnosis of appendicitis is still possible. Indeed, one reason for lack of visualization is perforation, in which case sensitivity is reported to be as low as 29%.[94] Consequently, as good as US can be, it still lacks the ability to rule out the diagnosis 100% of the time. US appears to be most useful in the early stages of disease when the diagnosis is unclear. As in other situations we routinely encounter (i.e., chest pain and negative ECGs), positive findings are helpful, but negative studies mean "keep looking." Repeat exam, consultation, and admission for observation may be required to ensure safety of the patient. Observation in the ED or as an inpatient has been shown to be beneficial in patients with possible appendicitis[14,95] without increasing risk of complications.[96,97]

High-Risk Patient Populations

Unfortunately, healthy, adult men are the only group of patients in which an evaluation for possible appendicitis can be considered "routine." The "atypical" presentation is more likely to be encountered. The following sections review strategies for detecting acute appendicitis in other patient subgroups: ovulating women, pregnant women, children, the elderly, and immunosuppressed patients.

Ovulating Women. The principal reason that diagnosis of appendicitis in women can be difficult is because other, more common conditions, such as pelvic inflammatory disease (PID) and ovarian cyst rupture, may be confused with appendicitis. PID deserves special attention since it can be especially difficult to distinguish from appendicitis. The inflammatory process associated with PID can masquerade as appendicitis, producing RLQ tenderness, elevated WBC, fever, and a history consistent with appendicitis. The

Figure 4. Changes in Normal Position of the Appendix During Pregnancy

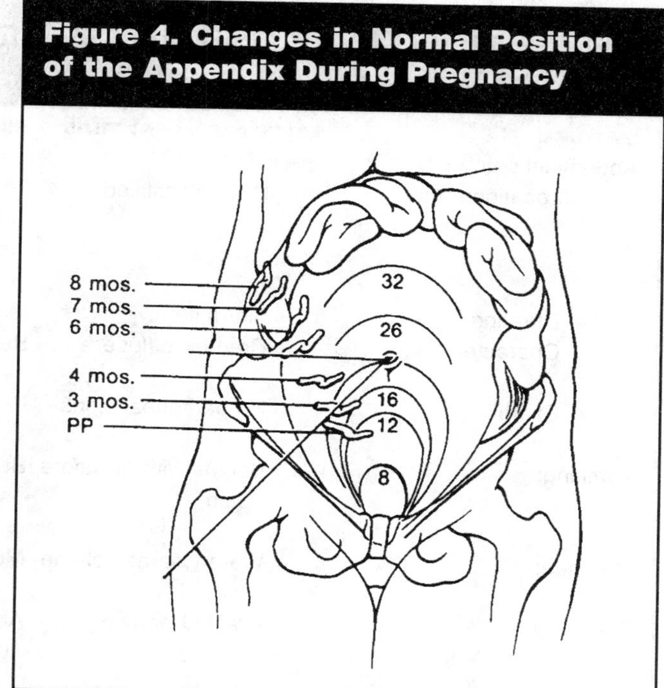

negative laparotomy rate of 30-50% in adult women is testimony to the difficulty of diagnosing appendicitis in this population.[14,98,99] A recent study of 174 non-pregnant women found that 33% had been misdiagnosed before being correctly identified as having appendicitis.[100] The majority of misdiagnosed women had atypical features in their presentations, including diffuse bilateral lower quadrant pain, CMT, and right adnexal tenderness.[100]

Many authors have tried to identify features that would differentiate these two diseases, and have suggested the following. *(See Table 2.)* The presence of anorexia/nausea/vomiting and onset of pain less than one day before presentation make appendicitis more likely in a retrospective review of 1000 cases of appendicitis.[14] Other features identified that made PID more likely were: pain greater than two days before presentation and onset of symptoms within seven days of last menstrual cycle. However, one study specifically looking at the usefulness of the timing of pain and stage of menstrual cycle found no difference between the onset of pain in PID or appendicitis and the stage of the patient's menstrual cycle.[101] Another prospective study suggested four additional criteria: history of sexually transmitted disease, abdominal tenderness other than RLQ, CMT, and bilateral adnexal tenderness.[4] A more recent retrospective review supports these criteria, and adds history of vaginal discharge, urinary symptoms, and discharge at the os as additional features to support a diagnosis of PID.[102]

Although these criteria may aid clinical judgement, they are *not* 100% reliable.[103] For example, CMT can occur with an appendix lying in the pelvis, and, therefore, cannot be used alone to make the diagnosis of PID.[104] Vaginal probe ultrasound may be a useful modality to help reduce the rate of complications and unnecessary surgery in adult women. Another approach recently evaluated is diagnostic laparoscopy, a strategy that reduced the negative appendectomy rate to 5%.[105]

Pregnancy. Although the two conditions may coexist, pregnancy has no influence on the frequency of acute appendicitis;[106] in fact,

Table 3. Features that Aid in Differentiating Between AGE and Appendicitis

FEATURE:	ACUTE GASTROENTERITIS	ACUTE APPENDICITIS
Abdominal pain:		
Location	Poorly localized	Poorly localized early in course, later localized to RLQ
Duration	Intermittent	More constant
Character	Crampy, diffuse	Becomes more severe with time
Exam	No peritoneal signs	Peritoneal signs present
Vomiting:	Begins with or before pain	Begins after pain, sometimes hours later
Diarrhea:	Watery, large volume	Mucoid, small volume
Fever:	Present early on in course	Absent initially, or low grade only

appendicitis occurs equally in each trimester[107] at a rate of about one per 1,500-2,200 pregnancies.[20,108] The risk for both mother and fetus is significant if appendicitis is not diagnosed early in its course, with mortality rates of about 2% for the mother and up to 35% for the baby having been reported.[109] One difficult aspect of diagnosis results from the shifting location of the appendix as pregnancy progresses. *(Please see Figure 4.)* The shifting position of the appendix in pregnancy may lead the physician to confuse appendicitis with cholecystitis or pyelonephritis, both of which are common in later pregnancy. Another problem is the similarity between symptoms encountered in early pregnancy and acute appendicitis; these include anorexia, nausea, vomiting, and mild abdominal pain. In addition, the natural elevation of WBC in pregnancy can further confuse the clinical picture. As a result, US may be the most useful test for confirming the diagnosis of appendicitis in pregnant patients. With US, there is no risk to the patient or fetus, and renal disease or gallstones can easily be identified in most patients. Use of US may lead to early surgical consultation. Ultimately, the best counsel is to be aware that appendicitis can occur in pregnant patients and to document other diagnoses before discharging or admitting the patient. Finally, consultation is mandatory when the clinical picture is not straightforward.

Children

While acute appendicitis is the most common surgical disorder in children, only 5% of visits for abdominal pain in children are due to appendicitis.[1] Seeing so many children with varied causes of abdominal pain, the majority of which are from a benign process, can lull the physician into a sense of false security and can increase the risk of missing the diagnosis. Indeed, up to 50% of children with documented appendicitis who are initially seen by a physician are misdiagnosed.[55,110] Furthermore, the younger the child, the more likely a delay in diagnosis will occur leading to perforation. Children younger than 2 years of age have rates of perforation that approach 100%; the perforation rate is about 71% in the 3-5 year age group, and 40% in the 6 to 10-year-old age group.[110,111] Some of the features associated with perforation include: younger age, home observation after initial visit, pain duration of more than two days, atypical clinical features, and temperature higher than 39°C.[112-114] The incidence of complications, including wound infection and even death, is correlated with perforation which is caused by delay to treatment.

One of the most common misdiagnoses for appendicitis in children is AGE. This is not surprising, since many signs, symptoms, and findings of the two diseases can overlap. Moreover, AGE is very common, and lymphoid hyperplasia secondary to viral illnesses is thought to trigger appendicitis as a result of luminal obstruction. It is impossible, however, to say how many of these "missed" cases of appendicitis actually represent appendicitis following AGE. In either case, several strategies can help reduce the chance of missing appendicitis in the setting of possible AGE. *(Please see Table 3.)* If the child has abdominal pain and vomiting but does not have diarrhea, then AGE should not be listed as a diagnosis and appendicitis should be more strongly considered. Furthermore, the presence of diarrhea does not exclude appendicitis from the differential. One study evaluated the presence of diarrhea in children younger than 3 years with appendicitis and found that diarrhea was present in 33% of cases.[115] Another investigator has pointed out that diarrhea from AGE is usually watery and abundant, whereas the diarrhea associated with appendicitis tends to be less voluminous and may have mucoid stools.[41] Constipation is often cited as a source of abdominal pain in children and is present in 8% of children with appendicitis.[41]

Accordingly, the history of constipation should not "rule out" appendicitis. In one study, constipation predisposed patients to a high misdiagnosis rate.[116]

Fever is often absent early in appendicitis, but much less so with AGE.[41] The temporal relation of vomiting and pain are repeatedly given significance. In AGE, vomiting is said to occur before or concurrent with pain and in appendicitis; vomiting is to begin after pain is noted.[41] Finally, localizing tenderness should never be ignored or interpreted as a feature of AGE. Repeated exams may be necessary to establish localized tenderness, since abdominal exams in children can be difficult to assess within the framework of one attempt. The pain of AGE is more diffuse and crampy, where appendicitis should produce a consistently tender area that is localized. This area may not be localized in the classic "McBurney's point," as barium enema studies have shown that the actual location of the appendix is normally inferior and medial to McBurney's point.[117] One investigation stressed that 15% of appendiceal bases are more than 10 cm from McBurney's point! Therefore, reproducible point tenderness anywhere near the RLQ in a child should raise a strong suspicion for the presence of appendicitis.

Table 4. Suggested ED Management Pathway for Acute Appendicitis*

HIGH CLINICAL PROBABILITY

History and physical examination (including pelvic and rectal)
NPO
Saline lock and fluid resuscitation
Urinalysis
Urine pregnancy test, if applicable
Surgical consultation
Antibiotic (cefotetan or cefoxitin)
Appendectomy

MODERATE CLINICAL PROBABILITY

History and physical examination (including pelvic and rectal)
NPO
Saline lock and rehydration if needed
CBC
Urinalysis
Urine pregnancy test, if applicable
Surgical consultation
Ultrasound or CT
- If positive, appendectomy
- If negative, observation and serial examinations

LOW CLINICAL PROBABILITY

History and physical examination (including pelvic and rectal)
CBC
Urinalysis
Urine pregnancy test, if applicable
Ultrasound or CT if symptoms persist at time of follow-up
Surgical consultation for follow-up
- If follow-up in ED, see in 12-24 hours for repeat examination, with earlier return for increased symptoms

* Adapted from reference [82]

The Elderly

Older patients with abdominal pain can be difficult to evaluate in the ED. Geriatric patients are more likely to have serious pathology, and their vital signs and exam do not always reflect the severity of their underlying illness. Diagnostic problems with appendicitis in the elderly are well-documented. Only 5-10% of cases of appendicitis are diagnosed without delay in patients older than 60 years, but more than 50% of the overall mortality is in this age group.[9,18] Delays to presentation contribute to mortality in the following manner: most patients older than 60 years waited 24-48 hours before presenting to a physician.[118-120] One study noted 17% of patients older than 60 years had been seen and misdiagnosed with a non-surgical problem before being correctly diagnosed with appendicitis.[121] Common surgical misdiagnoses include bowel obstruction, cholecystitis, and peptic ulcer disease.[122] In addition, only 51% of patients were correctly identified as having appendici-

Table 5. Tips to Reduce Malpractice Risk in Suspected Appendicitis[9]

- All patients with RLQ tenderness have appendicitis until proven otherwise.
- Be aware that the "atypical" presentation is the common one.
- Beware of high-risk groups: children, ovulating or pregnant women, the elderly, and the immunocompromised.
- 50% of deaths from appendicitis occur in the elderly. Be especially vigilant for appendicitis presenting in atypical fashion in older patients.
- Vomiting following onset of abdominal pain is more consistent with appendicitis than other diagnoses.
- Document all physical exams well, including rectal/pelvic exams.
- Perform serial abdominal exams and document them. Diagnosing appendicitis is difficult enough without limiting data through incomplete exams.
- Never use a normal WBC to determine that the patient does not have appendicitis.
- Remember *no* test will rule out appendicitis with 100% accuracy.
- Do not give IV narcotics to patients with vague abdominal pain and unclear diagnoses. Always obtain surgical consultation and do *not* discharge patients with abdominal pain requiring narcotic pain relief when there is not a clear non-surgical diagnosis (i.e., mild pancreatitis).
- Use the diagnosis of "abdominal pain of uncertain etiology" for all patients with unclear presentations and explain to the patient that you "do not know yet what is causing their symptoms."
- Never write a discharge diagnosis of acute gastroenteritis if there is no history of diarrhea.
- Consult liberally in cases in which the diagnosis of appendicitis is in question.
- Give complete and clear discharge/follow-up instructions, and document these well.
- Do not send patients home when the diagnosis is in question and there is reasonable doubt that the patient can or will return as directed (i.e., alcoholics, homeless, those without transportation, unreliable parents, etc.)
- Tell every patient discharged from the ED for abdominal pain that "appendicitis can develop in anyone in *only* 24 hours" so they understand the importance of a return visit for continued or worsening pain.

tis before surgery,[18,123] and 50% of patients older than 60 years who died from appendicitis were admitted for three days or more before surgery was performed.[124]

While their perforation rate is similar to that of small children (46-83%),[18,125] this may not be due only to delayed presentations and misdiagnosis. One study noted that in patients presenting within 24 hours of symptom onset, patients older than 50 years of age were twice as likely to have perforation (24% rate) compared to patients in their 30s.[118]

It is speculated that the appendix wall in elderly patients is weaker and perforates more quickly; in addition, older patients may not be able to mount as vigorous a defense. The presence of comorbid conditions in elderly patients also complicates assessment. Finally, physical exam can be misleading. RLQ pain and tenderness were noted to be absent in 23% of older patients,[126,127] and classical pain migration was not present in 60-80% of elderly individuals with appendicitis.[18,128,119] Nausea, vomiting, and anorexia were also noted to occur less often compared to younger adults.[18,118] A more recent review covering a 10-year period highlights the diagnostic challenges: only 20% of patients older than 60 years presented with "classic" anorexia, fever, RLQ pain, and an elevated WBC.[18] As with other high-risk groups, it should be stressed that atypical presentations are common, and, therefore, considering appendicitis in every elderly patient with abdominal pain is essential for improving outcomes.

Immunocompromised Patients

Although patients with HIV come to mind when considering immunocompromised individuals, patients on chronic steroids, sickle cell patients, those taking chemotherapy, diabetics, dialysis patients, and others with depressed immune systems are also at higher risk of complications and misdiagnosis of appendicitis. HIV-positive patients may have other causes of abdominal pain that can confuse the diagnosis (i.e., cryptosporidiosis, lymphoma, and cytomegaloviris [CMV] colitis). While there have been reports of mycobacterial infections mimicking appendicitis,[128] AIDS patients can also have appendicitis due to complications associated with their HIV. Appendicitis arising from Kaposi's sarcoma,[129,130] cytomegalovirus,[131] and mycobacterial infection[132] also have been reported. Patients with immune system dysfunction are at higher risk because their inflammatory response to infection and perforation is diminished, which leads to delayed presentation and masked signs and/or symptoms.[133] The perforation rate is reported to be as high as 50% in one series of HIV patients.[134] The WBC is not helpful in these patients, as bone marrow suppression prevents elevation. The early use of diagnostic laparoscopy has been recommended as an alternative to exploratory surgery in these patients to aid in early diagnosis and reduce complications as well as unnecessary surgery.[135]

Acute Appendicitis Pathway

Management of patients with suspected appendicitis in the ED can be divided into three patient risk groups: those with high, moderate, or low clinical probability of the diagnosis. Table 4 presents a summary of a suggested approach for these three patient groups. Those with a low clinical suspicion after evaluation can be safely sent home from the ED provided good follow-up precautions have been provided and the patient can return after 12-24 hours. From a risk management perspective, it is extremely important to stress to the patient and/or their family the risks of not following up as directed. Those with a moderate clinical suspicion and a negative US should either be observed in the ED for 4-6 hours, or, preferably, admitted to an observation unit for serial exams every 2-4 hours. It is always in everyone's best interest to obtain a surgical consult in patients in whom the diagnosis is unclear after an ED evaluation. Those with high clinical suspicion should not be subjected to any unnecessary delays in the ED before surgery. Intravenous (IV) fluid resuscitation should be initiated, all patients should be NPO, and antiemetics should be given to decrease discomfort from nausea and vomiting. Antibiotics should be initiated in the ED and should provide broad-spectrum anaerobic and gram-negative coverage. Cefotetan or cefoxitin (adult dose 2 grams IV) can both be given as single agents in appendicitis. In children, a triple antibiotic approach is often recommended; ampicillin (100-200 mg/kg/24 hr q 4 hr IV), clindamycin (30-40 mg/kg/24 hr q 6 hr IV), and gentamycin (5.0-7.5 mg/kg/24 hr q 8 hr IV).[136,137] Remember that gentamycin is a "category C" drug in pregnancy (safety has not been established), whereas the cephalosporins are "category B" (usually safe). Preoperative antibiotic use has been shown to reduce complication rates,[138] but should be given in consultation with the admitting physician.

Medication for pain relief in ED patients with severe abdominal pain deserves special attention. In general, every patient who has a high suspicion of appendicitis should be given something for pain relief. Although there is controversy regarding the timing of pain relief in ED patients with significant abdominal pain, prospective studies have shown that appropriate use of IV narcotics does not lead to misdiagnosis of patients with acute abdominal pain; it may actually increase the accuracy of diagnosis by making the exam more fruitful. This concept has support in both the surgical literature,[139,140] and emergency medicine literature.[141,142] In most patients, IV analgesia should be administered after speaking with the consultant, but this should not become a source of a "turf battle" between the ED physician and the surgeon. Simply state that the patient is very uncomfortable, is requesting some relief, and you feel that a small dose of your drug of choice will not alter the patient's diagnosis. By calling the consultant before any pain relief is given, he or she can be given the choice between coming to the ED to examine the patient before IV pain relief, or he or she can be actively involved in which drugs to give and in what doses. If the consultant is opposed to use of analgesia, a good alternative is use of droperidol (Inapsine®). Although this drug is an antiemetic related to haldol, it can reduce anxiety associated with severe pain, as well as alleviate nausea. The patient's perception that the physician cares about their pain enough to give them some relief without delay will help them to endure the wait until more adequate pain relief can be provided. If a surgeon is not immediately available, IV analgesia should be administered.

Risk Management Strategies

The diagnosis of acute appendicitis remains a clinical challenge. As many as 30% of patients with pathologically proven appendicitis have been seen and misdiagnosed by another physician before being correctly identified.[8] One study characterizing the features of misdiagnosis of appendicitis involving litigation against ED physicians found that only 55% of non-pregnant patients presented "classically."[143] Since misdiagnosis of appendicitis is among the top five leading causes of successful malpractice suits against ED physicians in the United States,[8,19] strategies for reducing this risk should be used. Table 5 summarizes several useful points to aid ED physicians in reducing risks when evaluating patients with possible appendicitis.

A recent review of litigation against ED physicians for missed appendicitis identified several features commonly encountered in these cases.[143] Seven statistically significant features of misdiagnosed cases include: lack of distress on presentation, no nausea or vomiting, absence of rebound on exam, lack of guarding on exam, lack of performance of rectal exam, giving narcotic pain medication in the ED, and ED diagnosis of gastroenteritis. In general, the diagnosis was more likely to be missed in patients who presented with atypical features, including lack of severe distress, lack of nausea and vomiting, and absence of rebound and guarding on exam. They suggested that perhaps patients were presenting in the interval after initial perforation and before signs of peritonitis could develop. The fact that the misdiagnosed patients had pain on average for 50% longer than control cases lends support to this interpretation. Patients whose appendicitis was missed also had poor documentation of the history and physical exam in their charts. Location, duration, quality, radiation, and increasing/decreasing features of pain were consistently missing. Physical exams were not complete in that rectal exams were not documented and/or not performed. Almost 50% of patients misdiagnosed were labeled as "gastroenteritis." Interestingly, no patient in this study whose appendicitis was missed had nausea, vomiting, and diarrhea documented as present in their charts. As mentioned before, discharging a patient with the diagnosis of gastroenteritis who does not have diarrhea is not advisable. It may be preferable to characterize the illness as "abdominal pain of uncertain etiology," and share this uncertainty with the patients and their relatives. This will underscore the importance of returning for repeat evaluation.

Although the use of pain medication in appendicitis has been discussed at length, this study makes an important distinction. Narcotic pain relief is appropriate in consultation with an admitting physician for a patient with probable appendicitis. This should not be construed to mean that narcotics should be given to patients in whom the pain is not severe if they are not admitted or have consultation in the ED. This study found that use of narcotic pain relief was more likely to be associated with misdiagnosis in patients labeled as having gastroenteritis. These patients were given the narcotics for vague abdominal symptoms only, and then sent home without consultation. Their control group of patients who were *not* misdiagnosed also had narcotic medications administered, but only after the diagnosis of appendicitis was written in the chart and surgical consultation was obtained. It is estimated that 50% of the missed cases might have been prevented if the patients requiring narcotics for their abdominal pain had been given surgical consultation or admission for observation instead of discharge home. Finally, the important point is that 3% of patients with missed appendicitis *died*, while none of the control group expired. This figure is consistent with a study noting deaths only in misdiagnosed patients.[116]

In a study focusing on children, a misdiagnosis rate of 28% in 181 cases was noted. In these 50 cases of misdiagnosis in children under the age of 13 years, Rothrock et al[116] found the most common misdiagnosis to be AGE. As with the study above, they found misdiagnosed patients presented "atypically" with a mean younger age (5.3 yrs vs 7.9 yrs) and had more complaints of constipation, diarrhea, dysuria, irritability, lethargy, and signs of upper respiratory infections. On physical exam, misdiagnosed patients also were less likely to have abdominal tenderness. Of note, though, is that 48% of the misdiagnosed patients did have maximal tenderness in the RLQ and were *still* not thought to have a surgical problem. This underscores the point that RLQ tenderness in a child should never be considered insignificant until proven otherwise. Finally, physical exams were poorly documented, especially rectal exams. While many physicians may feel the rectal exam is of little use in adults, and at least one study verified this,[144] the results in children are markedly different. Several authors report up to 50-80% of children with appendicitis have localized tenderness on rectal exam and that 25% will have a rectal mass.[145,146]

Summary

Ultimately, the accurate diagnosis of acute appendicitis is difficult even for experienced emergency physicians and surgeons. As discussed in this article, atypical presentations are actually more common. Healthy adult males make up the only group of patients considered to be at low risk for misdiagnosis. The only patient in the ED who is safe from appendicitis is the patient who has already had his or her appendix removed! Only by recognizing the limitations of the diagnostic tests available and by maintaining a high suspicion for appendicitis in the high-risk groups, can the ED physician reduce the risk of misdiagnosis.

In the final analysis, there are three groups of patients—those who have it, those who don't, and those who might. The first group is comprised of those patients who present with exams and histories highly suspicious for appendicitis; they are easily recognized. Second, there are patients with a very low likelihood of appendicitis. These patients are also easily dispositioned, but should not go out the door without "the talk." At the end of the encounter, the ED physician should review the findings and his or her interpretation of the patient's complaint. The patient needs to be sent home with clear, written precautions indicating what to look for (worse belly pain, fever, vomiting, or concern about getting better) and when to return (within 8-12 hours). The patient and his or her relatives need to hear the risks if they do not return as directed (i.e., bad infection that can kill him or her). One version that accomplishes all of these goals in a very brief time is as follows: "Mr./Ms. X, I don't believe you have appendicitis now. However, you still have your appendix, and anyone with one can develop problems in only 24 hours and need surgery. If you feel worse, with more pain, fever, or vomiting you must return to be rechecked or else you can become very sick and even die from this." By keeping information clear, simple, and to the point, the patients are more likely to retain important information. This also gives the patients time to ask questions concerning their evaluation and diagnosis before they leave. While not every patient in a busy ED needs a lengthy discussion before being discharged, spending a few extra minutes with higher-risk patients is time well spent.

The last group is everyone in between; these patients that can be difficult to triage. Until an accurate diagnostic test is available, the patient in whom the diagnosis remains in question after ED evaluation should have surgical consultation and admission for observation. One pediatric series found that adherence to this recommendation reduced the negative laparotomy rate to 1.5%, with a perforation rate of 30%.[147] Both of these are dramatically lower than the typical rates for children.[4] Another recent study of 252 patients found short-term observation of 10 hours significantly improved diagnostic accuracy.[95] The surgeon's adage of "when in doubt, take it out" can be modified for the ED physician to "when in doubt, don't send them out!"

References

1. Brewer RJ, Golden GT, Hitch DC, et al. Abdominal pain: An analysis of 1,000 consecutive cases in a university hospital emergency room. *Am J Surg* 1976;131:219-223.
2. Staniland JR, Ditchburn J, de Dombal FT. Clinical presentation of acute abdomen: Study of 600 patients. *BMJ* 1972;3:393-398.
3. Pieper R, Kager L. The incidence of acute appendicitis and appendectomy: An epidemiological study of 971 cases. *Acta Chir Scand* 1982;148:45-49.
4. Bongard F, Landers DV, Lewis F. Differential diagnosis of appendicitis and pelvic inflammatory disease: A prospective analysis. *Am J Surg* 1985;150:90-96.
5. Catto J. Acute appendicitis. In: Tintinalli JE, et al, eds. *Emergency Medicine—A Comprehensive Study Guide.* 3rd ed. New York: McGraw Hill; 1992:461-463.
6. Janik JS, Firor HV. Pediatric appendicitis: A twenty year study of 1640 children at Cook County (Illinois) Hospital. *Arch Surg* 1979;114:717-719.
7. Babaknia A, Parsa H, Woodruff JD. Appendicitis during pregnancy. *Obstet Gynecol* 1977;50:40-44.
8. Rogers J. Abdominal pain: Foresight. Dallas: American College of Emergency Physicians; Dec 1986, Issue 3.
9. Salkin MS. Appendicitis: Avoiding failure to diagnose. *ED Legal Letter* 1996;7:113-124.
10. Williams GR. Presidential address: A history of appendicitis. With anecdotes illustrating its importance. *Ann Surg* 1983; 197:495-506.
11. Berry J, Malt RA. Appendicitis near its centenary. *Ann Surg* 1984;200:567-575.
12. Stone HH, Sanders JL, Martin JD. Perforated appendicitis in children. *Surgery* 1971;69:673-678.
13. Owens BJ, Hamit HF. Appendicitis in the elderly. *Ann Surg* 1978;187:392-396.
14. Lewis FR, Holcroft JW, Boey J, et al. Appendicitis: A critical review of diagnosis and treatment in 1,000 cases. *Arch Surg* 1975;110:677-684.
15. Mittlepunckt A, Nora PF. Current features in the treatment of acute appendicitis: An analysis of 1,000 consecutive cases. *Surgery* 1966;60:971.
16. Jess P. Acute appendicitis: Epidemiology, diagnostic accuracy, and complication. *Scand J Gastroenterol* 1983;18:161-163.
17. Scher KS, Coil JA. The continuing challenge of perforated appendicitis. *Surg Gynecol Obstet* 1980;150:535-538.
18. Horattas MC, Guyton DP, Wu D. A reappraisal of appendicitis in the elderly. *Am J Surg* 1990;160:291-293.
19. Trautlein JJ, Lambert RL, Miller J. Malpractice in the emergency department—Review of 200 cases. *Ann Emerg Med* 1984;13:709-711.
20. Doherty GM, Lewis FR. Appendicitis: Continuing diagnostic challenge. *Emerg Med Clin North Am* 1989;7:537-553.
21. Wakely CPG. The position of the vermiform appendix as ascertained by an analysis of 10,000 cases. *J Anat* 1933; 67:277.
22. Collins DC. 71,000 human appendix specimens: A final report summarizing forty-year study. *Am J Proctol* 1963; 14:365-381.
23. Mattei P, Sola JE, Yeo CJ. Chronic and recurrent appendicitis are uncommon entities often misdiagnosed. *J Am Coll Surg* 1994;178:385-389.
24. Savrin RA, Clausen K, Martin EW, et al. Chronic and recurrent appendicitis. *Am J Surg* 1979;137:355-357.
25. Heller MB, Skolnick ML. Ultrasound documentation of spontaneously resolving appendicitis. *Am J Emerg Med* 1993; 11:51-53.
26. Migraine S, Atri M, Bret PM, et al. Spontaneously resolving acute appendicitis: Clinical and sonographic documentation. *Radiology* 1997;205:55-58.
27. Barber MD, McLaren J, Rainey JB. Recurrent appendicitis. *Br J Surg* 1997;84:110-112.
28. Chang FC, Hogle HH, Welling DR. The fate of the negative appendix. *Am J Surg* 1973;126:752-756.
29. Hobson T, Rosenman LD. Acute appendicitis—When is it right to be wrong? *Am J Surg* 1964;108:306-312.
30. Law D, Law R, Eiseman B. The continuing challenge of acute and perforated appendicitis. *Am J Surg* 1976;131: 533-535.
31. Rothrock SG. Overcoming limitations and pitfalls in the diagnosis of appendicitis. *Emerg Med Rep* 1992;13:41-52.
32. Arnbjornsson E, Bengmank S. Obstruction of the appendix lumen in relation to pathogenesis of acute appendicitis. *Acta Chir Scand* 1983;149:789-791.
33. Hart LS. Conditions requiring surgery: appendicitis. In: Barkin RM, et al, eds. *Pediatric Emergency Medicine: Concepts and Clinical Practice.* 1st ed. Mosby-Year Book, Inc: 1997:847-850.
34. Brumer M. Appendicitis: Seasonal incidence and postoperative wound infections. *Br J Surg* 1970;57:93-99.
35. Misra SP, Dwivedi M, Misra V, et al. Preoperative sonographic diagnosis of acute appendicitis caused by *Acsaris lumbricoides. J Clin Ultrasound* 1999;27:96-97.
36. Linz DN, Hrabovsky EE, Franceschi D, et al. Does the current health care environment contribute to increased morbidity and mortality of acute appendicitis in children? *J Ped Surg* 1993;28:321-328.
37. Pieper R, Kager L, Nasman P. Acute appendicitis: A clinical study of 1,018 cases of emergency appendectomy. *Acta Chir Scand* 1982;148:51-62.
38. Clarke JR, Schoffstall JM. Appendicitis. In: Schwartz GR, et al, eds. *Principles and Practice of Emergency Medicine.* Philadelphia, Lea & Febiger; 1992:1687-1897.
39. English CD, Allen W, Coppola ED, et al. Excessive dependence of the leukocytosis cue in diagnosing appendicitis. *Am Surg* 1977;43:339-402.
40. McLario D, Rothrock SG. Understanding the varied presentation and management of children with acute abdominal disorders. *Ped Emerg Med Reports* 1997;2: 111-122.

42. Sasso RD, Hanna EA, Moore DL. Leukocytic and neutrophil counts in acute appendicitis. *Am J Surg* 1970;120:563-566.
43. Raftery AT. The value of the leukocyte count in the diagnosis of acute appendicitis. *Br J Surg* 1976;63:143-144.
44. Hoffman J, Rasmussen OO. Aids in the diagnosis of acute appendicitis. *Br J Surg* 1989;76:774-779.
45. Doraiswamy NV. The neutrophil count in childhood acute appendicitis. *Br J Surg* 1977;64:342-344.
46. Freund HR, Rubinstien E. Appendicitis in the aged: Is it really different? *Ann Surg* 1984;50:573-576.
47. Thimsen DA, Tong GK, Gruenberg JC. Prospective evaluation of C-reactive protein in patients suspected to have acute appendicitis. *Surg Gynecol Obstet* 1989;55:466-468.
48. Scott JH III, Amin M, Harty JI. Abnormal urinalysis in appendicitis. *J Urol* 1983;129:1015.
49. Stringel G. Appendicitis in children: A symptomatic approach for a low incidence of complications. *Am J Surg* 1987;154: 631-635.
50. Coleman C, Thompson JE, Bennion RS, et al. WBC count is a poor predictor of severity of disease in the diagnosis of appendicitis. *Am Surg* 1998;64:983-985.
51. Young DV. Results of urgent appendectomy for right lower quadrant tenderness. *Am J Surg* 1989;157:428-430.
52. Graham JM, Pokorny WJ, Harberg FJ. Acute appendicitis in preschool age children. *Am J Surg* 1980;139:247-250.
53. Paajanen H, Maniskka A, Laato M, et al. Are serum inflammatory markers age dependent in acute appendicitis? *J Am Coll Surg* 1997; 184:303-308.
54. Eriksson S, Granstrom L, Olander B, et al. Leucocyte elastase as a marker in the diagnosis of acute appendicitis. *Eur J Surg* 1995;161:901-905.
55. Henneman PL, Marcus CS, Inkiles SH, et al. Evaluation of children with possible appendicitis using technetium 99m leukocyte scan. *Pediatrics* 1990;85:838-843.
56. Hallen S, Asberg A. The accuracy of C-reactive protein in diagnosing acute appendicitis—A meta-analysis. *Scand J Clin Lab Invest* 1997;57:373-380.
57. van Dieijen-Visser MP, Go PM, Brombacher PJ. The value of laboratory tests in patients suspected of acute appendicitis. *Eur J Clin Chem Clin Biochem* 1991;29:749-752.
58. Dueholm S, Bagi P, Bud M. Laboratory aid in the diagnosis of acute appendicitis. A blinded, prospective trial concerning the diagnostic value of leukocyte count, neutrophil differential count, and C-reactive protein. *Dis Colon Rectum* 1989;32: 855-859.
59. Scott JH, Amin M, Harty JI. Abnormal urinalysis in appendicitis. *Urology* 1983;129:1015.
60. Arnbjornsson E. Bacteriuria in appendicitis. *Am J Surg* 1988; 155:356-358.
61. Campbell JPM, Gunn AA. Plain abdominal radiographs and acute abdominal pain. *Br J Surg* 1988;75:554-556.
62. Bakha RK, McNair MM. Useful radiologic signs in acute appendicitis in children. *Clin Rad* 1977;28:193-196.
63. Field S, Guy PJ, Upsdell SM, et al. The erect abdominal radiograph in the acute abdomen: Should its routine use be abandoned? *Br Med J* 1985;290:1934-1936.
64. Shimkin PM. Radiology of acute appendicitis. *AJR Am J Roentgenol* 1978;130:1001-1004.
65. Rothrock SG, Green SM, Harding M, et al. Plain abdominal radiography in the detection of acute medical and surgical disease in children. *Pediatr Emerg Care* 1991;7:281-285.
66. Schnaufer L, Soroosh M. Abdominal Emergencies. In: Fleisher GR and Ludwig S, eds. *Textbook of Pediatric Emergency Medicine.* 3rd ed. Baltimore: Williams and Wilkins; 1993: 1309-1313.
67. Sakover RP, Del Fava RL. Frequency of visualization of the normal appendix with barium enema examination. *Am J Roentgenol Radium Ther Nucl Med* 1974;121:312-317.
68. Hatch Ei, Naffis D, Chanlder NW. Pitfalls in the use of barium enema in early appendicitis in children. *J Pediatr Surg* 1981; 16:309-312.
69. Schey WL. Use of barium in the diagnosis of appendicitis in children. *Am J Roentgenol Radium Ther Nucl Med* 1973; 118:95-103.
70. Dietz WW. Fallacy of the roentgenologically negative appendix. *JAMA* 1969;208:1495.
71. Palder SB, Dalessandri KM. Barium appendicitis. *West J Med* 1988;148:462-464.
72. Preston CA, Karch SB. The influence of gender and use of barium enema on morbidity in acute appendicitis. *Am J Emerg Med* 1989;7:253-255.
73. Smith DE, Kirchmer NA, Stewart DR. Use of the barium enema in the diagnosis of acute appendicitis and its complications. *Am J Surg* 1979;38:829-834.
74. Balthazar EJ, Megibow AJ, Hulnick O, et al. CT of appendicitis. *Am J Roentgenol* 1986;147:705-710.
75. Balthazar EJ, Birnbaum BA, Yee J, et al. Acute appendicitis: CT verses US correlation in 100 patients. *Radiology* 1994; 190:31-35.
76. Balthazar EJ, Megibow AJ, Siegel SE, et al. Appendicitis: Prospective evaluation with high-resolution CT. *Radiology* 1991;180:21-24.
77. Rao PM, Rhea JT, Novelline RA, et al. Helical CT technique for the diagnosis of appendicitis: Prospective evaluation of a focused appendix CT examination. *Radiology* 1997;202: 139-144.
78. Funaki B, Grosskreutz SR, Funaki CN. Using unenhanced helical CT with enteric contrast material for suspected appendicitis in patients treated at a community hospital. *Am J Roentgenol* 1998;171:997-1001.
79. Balthazar EJ, Rofsky NM, Zucker R. Appendicitis: The impact of computed tomography imaging on negative appendectomy and perforation rates. *Am J Gastroenterol* 1998;93:786-771.
80. Malone AJ, Shetty MR. Diagnosis of appendicitis. *Lancet* 1997;14:349.
81. Wilcox RT, Traverso LW. Have the evaluation and treatment of acute appendicitis changed with new technology? *Surg Clin North Am* 1997;77:1355-1370.
82. Greenfield RH, Henneman PL. Disorders of the small intestine. In: Rosen P, et al, eds. *Emergency Medicine: Concepts and Clinical Practice.* 4th ed. Mosby-Year Book, Inc; 1998:2005-2021.
83. Promes SB. Miscellaneous applications: Appendicitis. In: Simon BC, Snoey ER, eds. *Ultrasound in Emergency and Ambulatory Medicine* 1st ed. Mosby-Year Book, Inc; 1997:252-256.

84. Puylaert JB, Rutgers PH, Lalisang RI, et al. A prospective study of ultrasonography in the diagnosis of appendicitis. *N Engl J Med* 1987;317:666-669.
85. Jeffrey RB, Laing FC, Lewis FR. Acute appendicitis: Sonographic criteria based on 250 cases. *Radiology* 1988;167:327-329.
86. Yacoe ME, Jeffry RB. Sonography of appendicitis and diverticulitis. *Radiol Clin North Am* 1994;32:899-912.
87. Crady SK, Jones JS, Wyn T, et al. Clinical validity of ultrasound in children with suspected appendicitis. *Ann Emerg Med* 1993;22:1125-1129.
88. Schulte B, Beyer D, Kaiser C, et al. Ultrasonography in suspected acute appendicitis in childhood—Report of 1285 cases. *Em J Ultrasound* 1998;8:177-182.
89. Ramachandran P, Sivit CJ, Newman KD, et al. Ultrasonography as an adjunct in the diagnosis of acute appendicitis: A four-year experience. *J Pediatr Surg* 1996; 31:164-167.
90. Ford RD, Passinault WJ, Morse ME. Diagnostic ultrasound for suspected appendicitis: Does the added cost produce a better outcome? *Am Surg* 1994;60:895-898.
91. Roosevelt GE, Reynolds SL. Does the use of ultrasonography improve the outcome of children with appendicitis? *Acad Emerg Med* 1998;5:1071-1075.
92. Schwerk WB, Wichtrup B, Rothmund M, et al. Ultrasonography in the diagnosis of acute appendicitis: a prospective study. *Gastroenterol* 1989;97:630-639.
93. John H, Neff, Kelemen M. Appendicitis diagnosis today: Clinical and ultrasonic deductions. *World J Surg* 1993;17: 243-249.
94. Abu-Youseff MM, Phillips ME, Franken EA, et al. Sonography of acute appendicitis. A critical review. *Crit Rev Diagn Imaging* 1989;29:381-408.
95. Graff L, Radford MJ, Werne C. Probability of appendicitis before and after observation. *Ann Emerg Med* 1991;20: 503-507.
96. Jones PF. Active observation in management of acute abdominal pain in children. *BMJ* 1976;2:531-533.
97. White JJ, Santillana M, Haller JA. Intensive in-hospital observation: A safe way to decrease unnecessary appendectomy. *Ann Surg* 1975;41:793-798.
98. Hoffman J, Rasmussen AB. Aids in the diagnosis of acute appendicitis. *Br J Surg* 1989;76:774-779.
99. Pieper R, Kager L. The incidence of acute appendicitis an appendectomy: An epidemiological study of 971 cases. *Acta Chir Scand* 1982;148:51-62.
100. Rothrock SG, et al. Misdiagnosis of appendicitis in nonpregnant women of childbearing age. *J Emerg Med* 1995;13:1-8.
101. Robinson JA, Burch BH. An assessment of the value of menstrual history in differentiating acute appendicitis from PID. *Surg Gynecol Obstet* 1984;159:149-152.
102. Webster DP, Schneider CN, Cheche S, et al. Differentiating acute appendicitis from PID in women of childbearing age. *Am J Emerg Med* 1993;11:569-572.
103. Najem AZ, Barillo DJ, Spillert CR, et al. Diagnosing pelvic inflammatory disease. *JAMA* 1991;266:2594-2604.
104. Henneman PL, Marcus CS, Butler JA, et al. Evaluation of women with possible appendicitis using technetium-99m leukocyte scan. *Am J Emerg Med* 1990;8:373-378.
105. Borgstein PJ, Gordijn RV, Eijsbouts QA, et al. Acute appendicitis—A clear-cut case in men, a guessing game in young women. A prospective study on the role of laparoscopy. *Surg Endosc* 1997;11:923-927.
106. Tamir IL, Bongrad FS, Klein SR. Acute appendicitis in the pregnant patient. *Am J Surg* 1990;160:571-575.
107. Cunningham FG, McCubbin JG. Appendicitis complicating pregnancy. *Obstet Gynecol* 1975;45:415-420.
108. Babaknia A, Parsa H, Woodruff JD. Appendicitis during pregnancy. *Obstet Gynecol* 1977;50:40-44.
109. Kammerer WA. Non-obstetric surgery during pregnancy. *Med Clin North Am* 1979;63:1157-1164.
110. Savrin RA, Clatworthy HW. Appendiceal rupture: A continuing diagnostic challenge. *Pediatrics* 1979;63:36-43.
111. Schorlemmer GR, Herbst CA. Perforated neonatal appendicitis. *South Med J* 1983;76:536-537.
112. Samuels GA. Appendicitis in children. *West Indian Med J* 1971;20:105.
113. Brickman ID, Leon W. Acute appendicitis in childhood. *Surgery* 1966;60:1083.
114. Foster JH, Edwards WH. Acute appendicitis in infancy and childhood: A twenty year study in a general hospital. *Ann Surg* 1957;146:70.
115. Horwitz JR, Gursoy M, Jaksic T, et al. Importance of diarrhea as a presenting symptom of appendicitis in very young children. *Am J Surg* 1997;173:80-82.
116. Rothrock SG, Skeoch G, Rush JJ, et al. Clinical features of misdiagnosed appendicitis in children. *Ann Emerg Med* 1991;20:45-50.
117. Ramsden WH, Mannion RA, Simpkins KC, et al. Is the appendix where you think it is, and if not, does it matter? *Clin Radiol* 1993;47:100-103.
118. Hirsch SB, Wilder JR. Acute appendicitis in hospital patients aged over 60 years. 1974-1984. *Mt Sinai J Med* 1987;54:29-33.
119. Hall A, Wright TM. Acute appendicitis in the geriatric patient. *Ann Surg* 1978;44:147-150.
120. Andersson A, Bergdahi L. Acute appendicitis in patients over 60. *Ann Surg* 1978;44:445-447.
121. Burns RP, Cochran JL, Russell WL, et al. Appendicitis in mature patients. *Ann Surg* 1985;201:695-704.
122. Reiss R, Deutsch AA. Emergency abdominal procedures in patients above 70. *J Gerontol* 1985;40:154-158.
123. Telfer S, Fenyo G, Holt PR, et al. Acute abdominal pain in patients over 50 years of age. *Scand J Gastroenterol* 1988;144(supp):47-50.
124. Albano WA, Zielinski CM, Organ CH. Is appendicitis in the aged really different? *Geriatrics* 1975;30:81-88.
125. Thorbjarson B, Loehr WJ. Acute appendicitis in patients over the age of 60. *Surg Gynecol Obstet* 1967;125:1277-1280.
126. Hubbell DS, Barton WK, Solomon OD. Appendicitis in older people. *Surg Gynecol Obstet* 1960;110:289-292.
127. Hall A, Wright TM. Acute appendicitis in the geriatric patient. *Am Surg* 1978;44:147-150.
128. Visvanathan K, Jones PD, Truskett P. Abdominal mycobacterial infection mimicking acute appendicitis in an AIDS patient. *Aust N Z J Surg* 1993;63:558-560.

129. Chetty R, Slavin JL, Miller RA. Kaposi's sarcoma presenting as acute appendicitis in an HIV-1 positive patient. *Histopath* 1993;23:590-591.

130. Zebrowska G, Walsh NM. Human immunodeficiency virus-related Kaposi's sarcoma of the appendix and acute appendicitis. Report of a case and review of the literature. *Arch Pathol Lab Med* 1991;115:1157-1160.

131. Neumayer LA, Maker R, Ampel NM, et al. Cytomegalovirus appendicitis in a patient with HIV infection. *Arch Surg* 1993;128:467-468.

132. Livingston RA, Siberry GK, Paidas CN, et al. Appendicitis due to *Mycobacterium avium* complex in an adolescent infected with HIV. *Clin Infect Dis* 1995;20:1579-1580.

133. Stellato TA, Shank RR. Gastrointestinal emergencies in the oncology patient. *Semin Oncol* 1989;16:521-531.

134. Savioz D, Lironi A, Zurbuchen P, et al. Acute right iliac fossa pain in acquired immunodeficiency: A comparison between patients with and without acquired immune deficiency syndrome. *Br J Surg* 1996;83:644-666.

135. Binderow SR, Shaked AA. Acute appendicitis in patients with AIDS/HIV infection. *Am J Surg* 1991;162:9-12.

136. Rosser SB, Nazem A. Appendicitis in the pediatric age group. *J Natl Med Assoc* 1988;80:401-403.

137. Bauer T, Vennits B, Holm B, et al. Antibiotic prophylaxis in acute non-perforated appendicitis. The Danish multicenter study group III. *Ann Surg* 1989;209:307-311.

138. Antimicrobial prophylaxis in surgery. *Med Lett Drugs Ther* 1993;35:91-94.

139. Zoltie N, Cust MP. Analgesia in the acute abdomen. *Ann R Coll Surg Engl* 1986;68:209-210.

140. Attard AR, Corlett MJ, Kinder NJ, et al. Safety of early pain relief for acute abdominal pain. *BMJ* 1992;305:554-556.

141. Pace S, Burke TF. Intravenous morphine for early pain relief in patients with acute abdominal pain. *Acad Emerg Med* 1996;3:1086-1092.

142. LoVecchio F, Oster N, Sturmenn K, et al. The use of analgesics in patients with acute abdominal pain. *J Emerg Med* 1997;15:775-779.

143. Rusnak RA, Borer JM, Fastow JS. Misdiagnosis of acute appendicitis: Common features discovered in cases after litigation. *Am J of Emerg Med* 1994;12:397-402.

144. Alvarado A. A practical score for the early diagnosis of acute appendicitis. *Ann Emerg Med* 1986;15:557-565.

145. Bartlett RH, Eraklis AT, Wilkinson RH. Appendicitis in infancy. *Surg Gynecol Obstet* 1970;130:99-105.

146. Brickman ID, Leon W. Acute appendicitis in childhood. *Pediatr Surg* 1960;5:1083-1089.

147. Putnam TC, Emmens RW. Appendicitis in children. *Surg Gyn Obstet* 1990;170:527-532.

[illegible] Bilbao [illegible], Miller [illegible]. Kaposi's sarcoma presenting as [illegible] appendicitis in an HIV-1 positive patient. Histopath[illegible]

130. [illegible] Human immunodeficiency virus-related Kaposi's sarcoma of the appendix and acute appendicitis. Report of a case and review of the literature. [illegible]

131. [illegible] Keller K, Ampel NM, et al. Cytomegalovirus appendicitis in a patient with HIV infection. Arch Surg [illegible]

132. [illegible] RA, Snapper [illegible] [illegible] appendicitis due to [illegible] complex in an adolescent infected with HIV. Clin Infect Dis [illegible]

133. [illegible] Gastrointestinal emergencies in the oncology patient. [illegible]

134. [illegible] Acute right lower quadrant pain [illegible]: A comparison between [illegible] with and without acquired immunodeficiency syndrome. Br J Surg [illegible]

135. [illegible] appendicitis in patients with HIV infection. Am J Surg [illegible]

136. [illegible] appendicitis in the pediatric age group. [illegible]

137. [illegible] Antibiotic prophylaxis in [illegible] appendicitis. The Danish multicenter study [illegible]

138. [illegible]

139. [illegible] acute abdomen [illegible]

140. [illegible] Safety of early pain relief for acute abdominal pain. BMJ 1992;305:554.

141. [illegible] for early pain relief in patients with acute abdominal pain. [illegible]

142. [illegible] The use of analgesics in patients with acute abdominal pain. J Emerg Med [illegible]

143. [illegible] Misdiagnosis of acute appendicitis: Common features discovered in cases after litigation. Am J Emerg Med 1994;[illegible]

144. [illegible] in the diagnosis of acute appendicitis [illegible]

145. [illegible] Appendicitis in infants. [illegible]

146. [illegible] appendicitis in children. [illegible]

147. [illegible] appendicitis in children. [illegible]

Infectious Diarrhea

Earl J. Reisdorff, MD, FACEP
Vincent J. Pflug, DO

Diarrhea is a common complaint among patients seen by emergency department (ED) physicians and is the second most common cause of days missed from school or work.[1] Infectious diarrhea is a special concern in the pediatric population, accounting for the third most common cause for the hospitalization of children in the United States, and responsible for 10% of all pediatric visits to the ED.[2,3] More than 400 deaths per year in the United States are attributed to diarrheal illness.[4]

Though subjectively defined, diarrhea is generally regarded as an increase in stool frequency or content, as well as the production of fecal material of a looser, more watery consistency. In addition, diarrhea may be associated with an increased urgency to defecate, tenesmus, and perianal discomfort. Since no strict definition exists, diarrhea should be characterized in the context of a patient's normal stool pattern. For example, a child that is breast-fed may have more stools than a child who receives an iron-containing formula.

Diarrhea may be noninfectious or infectious in etiology. Noninfectious etiologies are delineated in Table 1. This chapter focuses on infectious causes of diarrheal illness. An understanding of specific terminology is germane to this discussion. Dysentery refers to diarrheal illness associated with abdominal pain, tenesmus, and stool containing blood or mucus. Bacillary dysentery is dysentery caused by Shigella. Enteric fever suggests an acute infectious enteritis associated with bacteremia and systemic symptoms. Typhoid fever is an acute, generalized febrile illness caused by *Salmonella typhi* characterized by fever, a rash (rose spots), splenomegaly, bradycardia, delirium, and leukopenia.

Pathophysiology

Diarrhea results from either an imbalance in the absorptive-secretory processes of the bowel or from intestinal hypermotility. Usually, the intestinal tract is a site of absorption for water and electrolytes. In the case of diarrhea, this physiological process is reversed, and the gut becomes the site of water and electrolyte loss. Most of the morbidity from diarrheal illness is due to dehydration and electrolyte imbalances.

The infectious dose for microorganisms varies from 10^1 to 10^2 organisms for *Shigella* and *Giardia lamblia* up to 10^8 for *Vibrio cholerae* and *Escherichia coli*. Factors that predispose one to acquiring diarrheal illness include H_2-blocker use, broad-spectrum antibiotic use, abnormal intestinal motility, and interruption of the gastric mucosa. Diarrheal disease is caused by pathogens that are typically categorized as *inflammatory* and *noninflammatory. (Please see Table 2.)* Inflammatory pathogens (e.g., *Shigella*) invade the bowel mucosa. Noninflammatory or "secretory" pathogens (e.g., *E. coli*) elaborate enterotoxins. Some bacteria that cause "food poisoning" elaborate toxins even prior to ingestion (e.g., *Staphylococcus aureus, Bacillus cereus*).

Table 1. Differential Diagnosis of Acute Infectious Diarrhea

- Ulcerative colitis
- Crohn's disease
- Mesenteric ischemia
- Appendicitis
- Diverticulitis
- Anal fissures
- Gastritis
- Peptic ulcer disease
- Hemorrhoids
- Juvenile polyps
- Irritable bowel syndrome
- Milk allergy (other food allergies)
- Malrotation with midgut volvulus
- Meckel's diverticulum
- Intussusception
- Henoch-Schönlein vasculitis
- Drugs and toxins: mannitol, phenolphthalein, sorbitol, magnesium-containing antacids, quinidine, colchicine, mushrooms, mercury poisoning

Table 2. Common Infectious Organisms Associated with Diarrheal Syndromes

INFLAMMATORY	
Shigella	*Campylobacter*
E. coli—invasive	*Salmonella*
Clostridium difficile	*Yersinia enterocolitica*
Aeromonas (certain sp.)	*Entamoeba histolytica*
NONINFLAMMATORY	
Vibrio cholerae	*Vibrio vulnificus*
Vibrio parahaemolyticus	*Aeromonas* (certain sp.)
E. coli—enterotoxigenic	Rotavirus
Norwalk agent	Calicivirus
Astrovirus	

Enterotoxin-induced diarrheal stool is watery and contains few fecal leukocytes. The prototypic form of secretory diarrhea (cholera) is caused by *V. cholerae*. In cholera, large amounts of isotonic solution are passed into the bowel, making the patient prone to dehydration. A similar pattern of diarrhea is seen with viruses and enterotoxic *E. coli*. Inflammatory bacteria enter the endothelium of the distal small bowel and colon, producing fever and abdominal pain. The stool may contain blood, mucus, and abundant fecal leukocytes. Common invasive organisms are *Shigella, Campylobacter jejuni*, and *Salmonella*. *Yersinia enterocolitica* and some forms of *E. coli* also are invasive.

Viruses cause most cases of acute infectious enteritis. Common viral pathogens include rotavirus, calicivirus, astrovirus, enteroviruses, Norwalk agent, and enteric adenoviruses (serotype 40 and 41). Viral diarrhea is watery and self-limiting. The peak incidence of most viral diarrhea occurs in the winter and spring months, though enterovirus infections occur in the late summer and early autumn.

Clinical Diagnosis

History. A symptom-specific history must be taken. The history should explore: 1) the mode of onset of the diarrhea (sudden or gradual); 2) the duration of the diarrhea (and associated symptoms); 3) the frequency of stools; 4) the character of the stool (e.g., soft, brown liquid); 5) the presence of mucus or blood; 6) the progression or course of symptoms; 7) the location of any abdominal pain, presence of cramps, or tenesmus; and 8) any significant change in stool odor. Further items for consideration should include the month of occurrence, patient age, day care center participation, recent antibiotic use, travel (rustic and foreign), and exposure to infected persons.

Try to identify foods that may have been contaminated. Patients frequently relate their diarrheal illness to the last thing they ate. Though there is always a "last meal" prior to the onset of symptoms, many organisms have incubation periods from 1-3 days. Therefore, to identify a dietary etiology, a meal history must be taken for the past three days. High-risk foods include chicken, seafood, and undercooked ground beef.

Inquire about the consistency, frequency, and odor of the stool. All stool is foul-smelling. Therefore, one should not ask if a patient's stool smells "bad," but rather if there is a *change* in the stool odor. The presence of mucus or blood suggests an invasive or protozoal process.

Diarrheal illness is more common in children attending day care centers. As many as 50% of day care centers experience diarrhea epidemics during a given year.[5,6] This may be a function of wearing diapers, frequent hand-to-mouth motor activity, and inadequate handwashing practices by staff.

Family pets can be reservoirs for *Campylobacter, Yersinia*, and *Salmonella*. Reptiles have high carriage rates for *Salmonella*.[7] A rare *Salmonella* serotype, *Salmonella tilene,* has recently been described in the United States among children with pet African pygmy hedgehogs.[8]

Among patients with AIDS, organisms causing infectious diarrhea are frequently recovered from the stool, including *Mycobacterium avium intracellulare*, cytomegalovirus, *Cryptosporidium, Salmonella, Campylobacter, Shigella*, herpes simplex, *Isospora belli, Candida, Clostridium difficile, Giardia lamblia, Entamoeba histolytica, Blastocystis hominis, Aeromonas hydrophila,* and adenovirus.[9] Among patients with AIDS, diarrhea tends to be more common in homosexual males (80%) compared to heterosexual men with a history of intravenous drug abuse (58%).[10]

Rotavirus and Norwalk agent infections are most common in the winter months. Enteroviral infections are most prominent in summer and early autumn months. *C. jejuni, Salmonella*, and *E. coli* occur predominantly in the summer months. *Y. enterocolitica* diarrhea is most frequent during the winter.

Gastroenteritis symptoms from 1-7 hours after ingestion suggest the ingestion of *S. aureus* or *B. cereus* preformed enterotoxins. Gastrointestinal symptoms starting 8-14 hours after ingestion suggest *C. perfringens* toxins. Gastrointestinal symptoms beyond 48 hours suggest disease from other infectious agents.

Physical Examination. The physical examination should first focus on the constitutional appearance of the patient, vital signs, and

Table 3. Clinical Characteristics of Inflammatory vs. Noninflammatory Causes of Diarrhea

CHARACTERISTIC	INFLAMMATORY	NONINFLAMMATORY
Onset	Gradual	Sudden
Fever	Present	Absent
Abdominal pain	Common, severe	Less common, mild
Systemic symptoms:		
Nausea, vomiting, headache, myalgias	Common	Uncommon
Abdominal tenderness	Prominent	Minimal
Fecal leukocytes	Present	Absent

Adapted from: Bitterman R. Acute gastroenteritis and constipation. In: Rosen P, Barkin RM, et al, eds. *Emergency Medicine: Concepts and Clinical Practice.* (3rd ed). St. Louis: Mosby Year Book; 1992:1537.

the clinical signs of dehydration. Lethargy or stupor may reflect severe dehydration, bacteremia, or infection with *Campylobacter* or *Shigella.* Fever with relative bradycardia may indicate typhoid fever. The patient may have low blood pressure and orthostatic changes as a consequence of profuse diarrhea.

Examination of the patient's skin may reveal cutaneous icterus, which can occur in patients with gay bowel syndrome (as a consequence of associated viral hepatitis) and in some patients with *Campylobacter* or *Salmonella typhi* enteritis. Icterus is occasionally seen with cytomegalovirus, herpes simplex, or *E. histolytica* infections, which may involve the liver. A rash consisting of rose spots (faint salmon-colored maculopapular lesions on the trunk) is a sign of typhoid fever during the second week of illness. Patients with diarrhea secondary to celiac sprue may develop dermatitis herpetiformis (extensive, itching eruption of vesicles and papules that occur in groups).

Generalized lymphadenopathy may indicate AIDS. Inguinal adenopathy should arouse suspicion of *Chlamydia trachomatis* proctitis (lymphogranuloma venereum) or of associated syphilis or gonorrhea. Examine the throat, since gonorrheal proctitis may be accompanied by a prominent, sometimes symptomatic, exudative pharyngitis. Arthritis, uveitis, or both suggest idiopathic inflammatory bowel disease rather than infectious enteritis. Photophobia, mild conjunctivitis, and arthralgias may, however, be apparent in infectious enteric fevers.

During the abdominal exam, be attentive for palpable tenderness or masses. Patients with acute diarrheal disease may have abdominal wall tenderness from vomiting as well as abdominal cramps from bowel hypermotility. Enteroinvasive organisms such as *Yersinia* and *Campylobacter* can cause pain that mimics appendicitis (pseudoappendicitis). *(Please see Table 3.)* Diffuse tenderness may indicate underlying proctocolitis. Biliary pain or gallbladder tenderness may accompany *Salmonella* or *Campylobacter* infections. Splenomegaly is typically associated with typhoid fever. A mass may point to diverticular disease, colonic carcinoma, or Crohn's colitis.

Rectal examination is imperative. Careful inspection of the perineum and perianal area may reveal hemorrhoids, anal fissures, or fistulous tracts. These perianal problems occur commonly in homosexual males with gay bowel syndrome and in patients with Crohn's disease. A digital rectal examination can detect a carcinoma of the colon or the raised plaques characteristic of pseudomembranous enterocolitis. Obtain a stool sample for occult blood testing.

Laboratory Studies

In the acute setting, laboratory studies are best used to define the degree of dehydration and electrolyte loss. If estimated fluid losses exceed 5% of the total body weight, the serum pH, potassium, sodium, and glucose should be measured. One may further consider ordering a urine specific gravity, serum blood urea nitrogen, and serum creatinine. The complete blood cell count is of limited use, though a high white blood cell count with a left shift (bandemia) more strongly suggests bacterial disease. In typhoid fever, a low white blood cell count is sometimes seen.

If a stool sample is available, a wet prep can be made by mixing a small amount with either normal saline or methylene blue. A routine Gram's stain can also be prepared. One should look for white or red blood cells, mucus strands, and the trophozoites or cysts of parasites. The presence of numerous white cells in clumps and clusters is evidence of a significant inflammatory component in the stool. Blood is often an admixture and may not appear bright red in the diarrheal effluvium. When indicated, stool should be transported promptly to the laboratory for culture. When delays occur, the stool should be refrigerated at 4°C.[10] Most stool cultures check only for *Salmonella, Shigella,* and *Campylobacter*. If *Yersinia*, *Vibrio*, or enterohemorrhagic *E. coli* (0157:H7) is a consideration, the physician should notify the laboratory and request recovery techniques for these pathogens. Likewise, if a parasitic infection is suspected, stool should be specifically studied for ova and parasites. Acid-fast stains help detect *Cryptosporidium* and *Cyclospora*. The latex agglutination assay for *C. difficile* toxin is also requested separately. A rapid slide test has been developed to identify *Campylobacter.* The Rotazyme test is an enzyme-linked immunoadsorbent assay for rotavirus detection. *Giardia* can be diagnosed by using a weighted string and a gelatin capsule (the Enterotest). DNA probes have been developed that rapidly detect *Salmonella, Y. enterocolitica, C. jejuni, Vibrio, C. perfringens,* and a variety of types of *E. coli*.[11] Probes for viruses (rotavirus and enteric adenovirus) and protozoa (*E. histolytica, G. lamblia*) have also been developed. Confirmation of Norwalk disease requires immunoelectronmicroscopy. *S. aureus* food poisoning can be confirmed by culturing *S. aureus* from the vomit of the ill patient.

The primary decision for the physician is when to obtain a stool culture or other stool studies. Microbiologic testing is expensive and unnecessary for most cases of a condition that is typically self-limited. When there is no fever, pain, blood in the stool, mucus in the stool, significant epidemiologic considerations, or special exposures, laboratory tests are unnecessary. However, if the patient has a high fever, tenesmus, bloody diarrhea, severe abdominal pain, weight loss,

Table 4. Grading Clinical Hydration Status

PARAMETER	5%	5-10%	10%
Skin turgor	Slightly decreased	Decreased	Very decreased
Skin color	Pale	Sallow	Ashen
Oral mucosa	Dry	Very dry	Parched
Tears	± Decreased	Absent	Absent
Fontanelle	Normal	Depressed	Sunken
Heart rate	± Increased	Increased	Marked tachycardia
Blood pressure	Normal	± Decreased	Decreased
Urine output	Mild oliguria	Oliguria	Anuria
Level of consciousness	Irritable	Lethargic	Unresponsive

Used with permission: Bonadio WA. Acute infectious enteritis in children. *Emerg Med Clin North Am* 1995;13:68.

day care center participation, rustic or foreign travel, seafood ingestion, or recent antibiotic use, a stool specimen should be examined for fecal leukocytes. If fecal leukocytes are seen, a stool culture for enteric pathogens should be considered. A high fever (≥ 39°C) in the child younger than 1 year with diarrhea is another indication for stool culture.

In addition to the presence of fecal leukocytes, other factors that increase the culture yield for invasive organisms include the abrupt onset of fever, blood in the stools, greater than four stools per day, and no vomiting.[12] Other risk factors that also reflect an increased probability of bacterial enteritis are the abrupt onset of symptoms (< 24 hours), fever higher than 39°C (102.2°F), toxic clinical appearance, diarrhea preceding vomiting at disease onset, more than 10 stools in 24 hours, tenesmus, hematochezia, mucoid stool, severe cramping, abdominal pain, and hypoalbuminemia. In one study, bacterial pathogens were isolated in 40% of diarrheal stools when two of three parameters (hematochezia, temperature ≥ 39°C, > 10 stools/day) were present.[13] Even when fecal leukocytes are present, more than 80% of fecal specimens can still yield a negative culture.[14]

As with stool cultures, not all patients require stool to be sent for ova and parasite smears. Proposed indications for the evaluation of stool for ova and parasites include: parasitic infection suspected by history, immunocompromise, appropriate travel history, homosexual history, public health concerns (food handler, day care worker, etc.), persistent diarrhea, and diarrhea not responsive to appropriate antibiotics.[15]

Bacterial Pathogens

Shigella. *Shigella* isolation rates have been increasing in recent years. Spread by the fecal-oral route, *Shigella* outbreaks have been associated with contaminated food, water, and swimming pools, as well as with day care center participation. Outbreaks are more common in the summer and fall. Shigellosis (infection by *Shigella*) is characterized by fever, abdominal pain, and diarrhea. The stool may be watery and contain blood and mucus (50-75% of cases). Temperatures can reach 40-41°C (104.0-105.8°F) in children. The duration of illness is usually less than five days.

Shigella is highly infectious; ingestion of only 10-100 organisms may cause disease. Patients become symptomatic 36-72 hours after exposure. Though usually a self-limited disease, shigellosis can be fulminating, resulting in dehydration and death. Cultures are negative in about one-third of cases of *Shigella* infection.

Treatment is usually supportive; however, antibiotics do shorten the duration of illness, improve patient nutrition during illness, and limit shedding of bacteria. Antibiotics are recommended in cases in which a patient's symptoms persist to the time of diagnosis.[16] However, resistance to trimethoprim-sulfamethoxazole and ampicillin is an increasing problem. Drugs of choice include third-generation cephalosporins and fluoroquinolones. *(Please see Table 5.)* Children with documented *Shigella* should be excluded from day care participation until negative stool cultures are obtained.[17] Complications of shigellosis include dehydration, Reiter's syndrome, arthralgia, and hemolytic uremic syndrome.

Salmonella. *Salmonella* is the most common bacterial cause of gastroenteritis in the United States, with an estimated two million cases each year.[18] More than half of the outbreaks of *Salmonella* infection are related to the consumption of contaminated water, eggs, poultry, or dairy products.[19,20] Salmonellosis (infection by *Salmonella*) is also spread through fecal-oral contamination. Pets (e.g., turtles, snakes, ducklings, hedgehogs) have also been known to carry the organism. *Salmonella* causes a variety of syndromes, including gastroenteritis, enteric fever, and an asymptomatic carrier state. Nausea and vomiting are frequently followed by diarrhea, abdominal pain, and fever. Diarrheal stool from *Salmonella* is described as having a foul, "rotten-egg" odor. With enteric fever, a prolonged fever is present with bacteremia, reticuloendothelial activation, and multiorgan involvement. The most common sites of bacterial "metastases" include the bones, meninges, endocardium, and kidneys. In the asymptomatic carrier state, the organism can be present for longer than one year.

Typhoid fever is characterized by an unremitting fever with abdominal pain, cramps, and, occasionally, rose spots. In 10-20% of patients, meningismus is present. Oddly, diarrhea may be absent and a cough may be present. Patients may have splenomegaly and bradycardia. People who are immunocompromised (e.g., sickle cell disease, AIDS, asplenia) are particularly susceptible to *Salmonella* infection. The diagnosis is made by the recovery of the organism in the blood, urine, or stool.

Bowel hypermotility should not be inhibited. Antibiotics can prolong the carrier state of *Salmonella*. Nonetheless, antibiotics should be considered in newborns and the elderly as well as in patients with lymphoproliferative disorders, cardiovascular disease, bone or joint disease, joint prostheses, sickle-cell disease, organ transplants, and

Table 5. Drugs of Choice for Bacterial Infections

CAUSE	TREATMENT	PEDIATRIC DOSE	ADULT DOSE
Salmonella (treatment depends on severity)	chloramphenicol	20 mg/kg qid × 2 wks (max, 1 g)	500 mg qid × 7-14 d
	TMP-SMX	TMP 5 mg/kg and SMX 25 mg/kg bid × 2 wks	160/800 mg bid × 14 d
	ampicillin	35 mg/kg (max, 1g) IV q4h for 2 wks	500 mg qid × 7-14 d
	ciprofloxacin	not recommended <17 yrs	750 mg bid x 28 d (fecal carriage)
	norfloxacin	not recommended < 17 yrs	400 mg bid × 28 d (fecal carriage)
Shigella	TMP-SMX	TMP 5 mg/kg and SMX 25 mg/kg bid × 5 d	160/800 mg po bid × 7-14 d
	ampicillin	20 mg/kg IV or po q6h for 5 d	500 mg po qid × 7-14 d
	ciprofloxacin	not recommended < 17 yrs	500 mg bid × 3-5 d
	norfloxacin	not recommended < 17 yrs	400 mg bid × 3-5 d
	ceftriaxone	50-100 mg/kg qd IVPB	1-2 g qd × 7-14 d
Campylobacter (severe or persistent cases)	erythromycin	40-50 mg/kg/d divided qid × 5-7 d	500 mg qid × 5-7 d
	tetracycline	10 mg/kg qid × 7-10 d*	250 mg qid × 7-10 d
	ciprofloxacin	not recommended < 17 yrs	500 mg bid × 3-5 d
	norfloxacin	not recommended < 17 yrs	400 mg bid × 3-5 d
Clostridium difficile	vancomycin	5 mg/kg po qid × 7 d	125-400 mg po qid × 7-10 d
	metronidazole	7 mg/kg po tid × 7 d	500 mg po tid × 7-10 d
Vibrio cholerae	tetracycline	10 mg/kg qid × 7-10 d*	250 mg qid × 7-10 d
	furazolidone	1.25-1.5 mg/kg qid × 7 d	100mg qid × 7 d
	TMP-SMX	TMP 5 mg/kg and SMX 25 mg/kg bid × 5-7 d	160/800 mg bid × 5-7 d
Escherichia coli (severe or persistent cases)	TMP-SMX	TMP 5 mg/kg and SMX 25 mg/kg bid × 5-7 d	160/800 mg bid × 5-7 d
Giardia lamblia	metronidazole	5 mg/kg tid × 7 d	250 mg tid × 7 d
	quinacrine	2 mg/kg tid × 7 d	(> 8yrs) 100 mg tid × 7 d
	furazolidone	1.25-1.50 mg/kg qid × 7 d	100 mg qid × 7 d
Entamoeba histolytica (treatment depends on severity)	metronidazole	5 mg/kg tid × 7 d	250 mg tid × 7 d
	followed by:		
	diiodohydroxyquin	40 mg/kg/d tid × 20 d	650 mg tid × 20 d
	or diloxanide furoate	20 mg/kg/d tid × 10 d	500 mg tid × 10 d; then bid × 3 wks

* Not recommended in children younger than 10 years
TMP-SMX = trimethoprim-sulfamethoxazole

AIDS. Treatment of enteric fever consists of chloramphenicol (50-100 mg/kg/d q6h) for 2-4 weeks. Other antibiotic choices include ampicillin, amoxicillin, or trimethoprim-sulfamethoxazole.

Campylobacter. *Campylobacter* is an enteroinvasive bacteria. Among young adults, *Campylobacter* enteritis is 4-10 times more frequent than *Salmonella* enteritis and 9.5-46.0 times more frequent than *Shigella* enteritis.[14,21] A seasonal predilection occurs from May to October with a peak in July. The ingestion of poultry, beef, and milk, as well as contact with domestic animals, is implicated in disease outbreaks. Infection is characterized by diarrhea (watery with blood and mucus) and mild fever. Two-thirds of patients have abdominal pain that can mimic appendicitis. Treatment is usually supportive, but erythromycin, tetracycline, fluoroquinolones, and aminoglycosides are used if complications or bacteremia are present.

Aeromonas. *Aeromonas* is isolated from aquatic sources, such as fresh water, sewage, marine environments, and drinking water. It is also found in meat and produce. The peak incidence of *Aeromonas* gastroenteritis occurs in the summer through early autumn.[22] Isolation rates have approached 7%, making *Aeromonas* the fourth most common cause of bacterial diarrhea in the United States.[23] The symptoms of *Aeromonas* gastroenteritis include vomiting, fever, and diarrhea that is sometimes bloody. *Aeromonas* primarily affects children younger than 3 years, and the illness usually lasts less than 10 days. Fecal leukocytes are generally absent, and spread to close contacts is rare. The organism is not sought on routine culture in the laboratory. The role of antibiotics in its treatment is uncertain.

Yersinia. Human infection from *Yersinia* usually results by ingesting contaminated food (especially pork), water, or milk. Domestic animals such as household pets are also implicated in the transmission of *Y. enterocolitica*. Water- and food-borne disease as well as fecal-oral transmission have been implicated. Symptoms last 5-14 days and include acute enteritis, dysentery, mild fever, and abdominal pain. Blood is present in the stools of 26% of cases.[24] *Yersinia* enteritis may present as mesenteric adenitis or even mimic appendicitis.[25] The laboratory should be contacted when the physician suspects *Yersinia* as the etiologic agent. Antibiotics are ineffective in altering the course of illness.[26,27] Erythema nodosum, which appears as painful red nodules in the anterior leg, may be present, particularly in women. *Yersinia* is also implicated as a cause of transient synovitis.

Vibrio. *Vibrio cholerae* infections occur only sporadically in the United States, most often in the Gulf Coast states (e.g., Texas and Louisiana). Cholera is most common in the summer and early fall and is associated with drinking contaminated water or the consumption of raw or undercooked shellfish. Cholera can cause profuse watery stools with mucus, giving the classic appearance of "rice-water" stools. Volume losses require aggressive rehydration. Metabolic acidosis and hypokalemia can ensue due to the loss of bicarbonate and potassium in the stool. Though rehydration is the primary treatment, antimicrobial therapy (tetracycline, trimethoprim-sulfamethoxazole, furazolidone) decreases the severity of the diarrhea and hastens the clearance of the organism from the gut.[28]

Vibrio parahaemolyticus and *Vibrio vulnificus* are present in raw and undercooked seafood (particularly oysters, clams, and crabs) taken from the Gulf of Mexico. Diarrhea can be explosive and associated with cramps, vomiting, and dysentery. The average incubation period is 12 hours. Illness usually lasts about three days and the disease is self-limited. Antibiotics do not significantly alter the disease course.[29]

Escherichia coli. Different strains of *E. coli* produce varied patterns of diarrheal illness. Enterotoxic *E. coli* (ETEC) is acquired through the ingestion of food or water contaminated by feces. It is a common cause of traveler's diarrhea. Abdominal cramps, bloating, watery diarrhea, and the urgent need to defecate are characteristic of ETEC. Enteropathogenic *E. coli* (EPEC) causes epidemics of fever, diarrhea, and vomiting in infants (usually those younger than 6 months). It may be severe, lasting 7-14 days. Rehydration is the primary treatment. Antibiotics are used in severe cases. Enteroinvasive *E. coli* (EIEC) causes fever, severe cramps, and watery diarrhea. EIEC is another common cause of traveler's diarrhea. Later in the disease course, there is scant stool tinged with blood and mucus. Enterohemorrhagic *E. coli* (EHEC) is the serotype 0157:H7. EHEC is normally found in cattle bowel flora and contaminates beef during the slaughter process.[30] Humans are infected by ingesting partially cooked contaminated beef. Patients are afebrile with copious watery diarrhea that contains few to no leukocytes. The disease can progress to produce bloody diarrhea, hemolytic uremic syndrome, and death.

Clostridium difficile. *C. difficile* becomes a major pathogen when the endogenous bacterial flora in the gut is altered by an antibiotic. Almost any antibiotic can predispose one to *C. difficile* infections, but ampicillin, clindamycin, and cephalosporins are the most commonly implicated agents.[31] Hospitalized and nursing home patients are at increased risk. Fewer than 10% of patients who have *C. difficile* isolated from the gastrointestinal tract will develop pseudomembranous colitis.[32] Patients with pseudomembranous colitis have watery diarrhea and crampy lower abdominal pain 1-3 weeks after starting antibiotic therapy. Tenesmus, nausea, vomiting, and anorexia may also be present. The treatment of pseudomembranous colitis begins with discontinuing the offending antibiotic. This can be sufficient for mild cases; oral vancomycin or oral metronidazole is required for more severe cases.[33] Antidiarrheal agents should be avoided. Untreated, the disease has a high mortality.

Food Poisoning. *S. aureus* is the most common cause of toxin-related disease, accounting for hundreds to thousands of cases of food poisoning each year.[34] Symptoms usually occur 1-6 hours after ingestion of a food high in salt, protein, or sugar such as ham, potato salad, or similar foods. Meats and dairy products also carry *S. aureus*. Symptoms appear 2-24 hours (most commonly 6-12 hours) after ingestion of the toxin. Symptoms of nausea, vomiting, diarrhea, abdominal pain, and, rarely, fever are usually self-limited, with resolution occurring within 24 hours in most cases.[35]

B. cereus causes clinical disease from both a preformed enterotoxin and another enterotoxin produced in vivo. The preformed toxin causes illness (predominantly vomiting) approximately 1-6 hours after ingestion. This has been described in people eating fried rice. A less common diarrheal illness occurs 6-18 hours after ingestion of poorly refrigerated foods. The watery diarrhea and abdominal cramps usually resolve within 36 hours. Vomiting and fever are rare in the diarrheal form of the disease, but patients can be affected by both.[36]

C. perfringens enteritis can develop 24 hours after ingestion. *C. perfringens* causes abdominal cramps and watery diarrhea. The diarrheal illness occurs when food (especially meat) is allowed to stand at room temperatures. Symptoms start 6-24 hours after ingestion of infected food, with an average of 12 hours to the onset of symptoms. Abdominal cramps and diarrhea are sometimes accompanied by headache, chills, and fever. Vomiting is uncommon.

Viral Pathogens

Rotavirus. Rotavirus is the most common cause of infectious diarrhea in children, with an estimated one million cases each year in the United States.[37] Although the peak incidence is between 6 months and 2 years of age, it can be present at any age. However, clinical disease is less likely in older children and adults. Spread is person-to-person and also fecal-oral. As few as 10 viral particles can cause disease.[38] The virus can survive for days on toys and countertops. The disease occurs in all months, with a seasonal increase during the winter months. Vomiting, watery diarrhea, fever, and abdominal pain usually last 3-8 days. Diarrheal stool from rotavirus has a sour-fruity odor due to carbohydrate malabsorption. The disease is self-limited, and fluid and electrolyte replacement is the primary therapy. Some studies support the use of bismuth subsalicylate to shorten the duration of symptomatic infection. Antimotility agents such as loperamide, diphenoxylate, or codeine are to be avoided.

Enteric Adenovirus. Adenoviruses are best known for causing upper respiratory infections. Serotypes 40 and 41 cause acute gastroenteritis. Transmission is person-to-person by the fecal-oral route. Children younger than 2 years are usually affected. Diarrhea, fever, respiratory symptoms, and, sometimes, vomiting usually last one week.[39]

Other Viruses. Viral etiologies account for 70-80% of all cases of acute infectious enteritis. *(Please see Table 6.)* Calicivirus, astrovirus, enteroviruses, and Norwalk agent all cause infectious enteritis. Transmission, symptoms, and treatment are similar to that of other enteric viruses. There is usually a watery diarrhea void of leukocytes.

Table 6. Viral Causes of Acute Diarrhea

AGENT	CLINICAL SYNDROME	DIARRHEA	VOMITING	FEVER	URI
Rotavirus	Infantile gastroenteritis, winter months, sour-fruity stool	+++	++	++	+
Norwalk agent	Adult gastroenteritis, family outbreaks	+++	+++	+	-
Enteric-type adenovirus	Intestinal "flu"	++	++	+	+
Enterovirus	Mild GI upset, summer months	+	±	+	++
Calicivirus	"Flu" in children < 2 years	++	+	±	-

Protozoal Pathogens

Giardia lamblia. *Giardia* is the most common cause of parasitic gastroenteritis in the United States. Transmission is person-to-person, fecal-oral, or from drinking water contaminated by feces. High-risk groups for giardiasis include travelers, children in day care centers, institutionalized people, and homosexual men. Campers and skiers who drink untreated mountain water are also at risk.[40] Beavers have been a reservoir for the protozoan in Colorado mountain streams. Giardiasis can exist as an acute, chronic, or asymptomatic infection. Giardiasis produces frequent stools, excessive flatulence, and abdominal pain. The "classic" stool of the patient with a *Giardia* infection is foul-smelling, floating, and frothy. Normal stools may occur intermittently during the disease course. Patients complain of abdominal pain, distention, a postprandial urge to defecate, feeling bloated, and feeling gaseous. Weight loss, steatorrhea, vomiting, and fever may also occur. Stools should be submitted for examination for the protozoan. If giardiasis is still suspected after a negative microscopic examination of stool, an Enterotest (string test) or duodenal aspiration can be performed. An antigen test (ELISA) of the stool is another cost-effective method of diagnosis. Antibiotic treatment is accomplished with quinacrine, metronidazole, or furazolidone.[41] An empiric course of metronidazole may be a reasonable, cost-effective intervention. A course of metronidazole is far less expensive than a complete battery of laboratory tests.

Entamoeba histolytica. *E. histolytica* rarely causes diarrhea in the United States. Most infected patients are asymptomatic. Infection results from the ingestion of *Entamoeba* cysts or through anal intercourse. Groups at high risk for amebiasis are those traveling to endemic areas, institutionalized individuals, and homosexual men. Infection is often asymptomatic, but can produce colitis, abdominal tenderness, bloody stools, fever, and weight loss. Of patients with clinical amebiasis, 5-10% will develop extraintestinal manifestations such as an amebic abscess of the liver.[42] Treatment depends on the severity of the clinical disease. Diiodohydroxyquin, metronidazole, and diloxanide furoate are antiprotozoal agents used for amebiasis.[43] Steroids must be strictly avoided in the treatment of *E. histolytica*, mandating its differentiation from inflammatory bowel disease.

Cryptosporidium parvum. *C. parvum* is an intestinal protozoan that commonly causes diarrhea in animals. In the spring of 1993, there were over 400,000 cases caused by a contaminated water supply in Milwaukee. It is a significant pathogen in immunocompromised patients, children in day care settings, and travelers. However, many patients are asymptomatic or experience a transient self-limited diarrheal illness. In the immunocompromised, *Cryptosporidium* causes a profuse, nonbloody, watery diarrhea that produces large volume losses. *Cryptosporidium* may be chronically carried in patients with AIDS. Mild epigastric cramping, nausea, vomiting, anorexia, and even fever may be present. The organism is seen in the stool when prepared with an acid-fast stain. The efficacy of antiprotozoal agents has not been established.[44]

Isospora belli. *I. belli* is similar to *Cryptosporidium,* but no known animal reservoir exists. In immunocompromised patients, *Isospora* infection may be indistinguishable from cryptosporidiosis.[45] Trimethoprim-sulfamethoxazole, metronidazole, and pyrimethamine-sulfadiazine have been used successfully to treat *I. belli*.

Toxin-Mediated Illness. Ciguatera poisoning is a diarrheal illness caused by ingesting fish infected by a dinoflagellate (*Gambierdiscus toxicus*). The disease is more commonly seen in spring and summer. Fish that are commonly affected include sea bass, snapper, grouper, barracuda, mahi-mahi, and skipjack. Ciguatera toxicity is characterized by diarrhea, vomiting, limb paresthesias, hypotension, peripheral muscle weakness, abdominal cramps, and itching. There is usually no fever. Symptoms begin five minutes to 30 hours after ingestion, with an average of about six hours. The disease lasts days to months; fatalities are rare.[46] Treatment involves fluid replacement and the administration of antiemetics and antihistamines. Amitriptyline may also be therapeutic.[47]

Scromboid poisoning causes flushing, diarrhea, headache, erythema, palpitations, nausea, dizziness, chills, thirst, itching, blurred vision, abdominal cramps, and conjunctival injection. It usually lasts less than six hours after ingestion, but weakness and fatigue can persist for prolonged periods. Scromboid poisoning is a form of saurine and histamine toxicity. The fish types that are commonly affected are known as "blood fish" and include tuna, mackerel, bonito, and mahi-mahi. The incubation period is minutes to hours, with complete recovery in 2-10 hours. Treatment involves antihistamines (e.g., diphenhydramine 25-50 mg IV).

Treatment

Rehydration. In treating all diarrheal illness, rehydration and electrolyte replacement is axiomatic. Many commercial preparations (e.g., sports drinks) and "clear liquids" found in the home are often hypertonic or insufficient in sodium and potassium content. *(See Table 7.)* Once initial fluid deficits have been replaced, oral rehydration solutions should be diluted or alternated with free water in order to prevent hypertonic conditions. Indications for intravenous rehydration may include hypotension, persistent vomiting, obtundation,

Table 7. Oral Rehydration Solutions

SOLUTION	NA+	K+	CL-	HCO3-	OSM
WHO	90	20	80	30	330
Hydrate	84	10	59	70	305
Rehydration	75	20	65	30	310
Pedialyte	45	20	35	30	250
Lytren	50	25	45	30	290
Infalyte	50	20	40	30	270
Resol	50	20	50	34	270
Ricelyte	50	25	-	-	200
Gatorade	23	3	-	-	330
Bouillon	72	12	-	-	-
Jell-O	45	18	-	-	-
Cola	2	0	-	13	550
Apple juice	3	20	2.5	0	700
Chicken broth	250	5	250	0	450
Ginger ale	3	1	2	-	540
Tena	0	0	-	0	5

Key: WHO = World Health Organization solution; Na = sodium (mEq/L); K = potassium (mEq/L); HCO_3^- = bicarbonate (mEq/L); Osm = osmolarity (osmoles/L).

paralytic ileus, weight loss of greater than 5% total body weight, moderate to severe metabolic acidosis (serum bicarbonate < 15 mEq/L), symptomatic hypoglycemia, and significant hypernatremia or hyponatremia.

In the past, "resting the gut" had been advocated in treating diarrhea. Gut rest can be tolerated by adults, but children can lose up to 1-2% of their body weight each day from inadequate nutrition. One strategy recommends that instant formula be diluted to half-strength and given along with the oral rehydration solution. Once rehydrated, the infant can be returned to normal feedings. Older children should be encouraged to eat as tolerated. Foods to avoid include fruits and vegetables, due to their high bulk content. Soups have little nutritional value and a high sodium content. High-sugar foods have a high osmotic gradient and can lead to increased diarrhea.

Antimicrobials. Antimicrobials should be used in cases of diarrheal illness when they will shorten the length of the symptomatic infection, reduce shedding of the causative organism, and prevent life-threatening complications. *(Please see Table 5.)* Patients presenting to the ED rarely have a known organism on which to focus treatment. The ideal antibiotic for empiric therapy would be effective against most causative organisms, decrease the symptoms and duration of disease while preventing the development of a carrier state, and decrease organism spread via fecal excretion. Antibiotics such as ampicillin, tetracycline, erythromycin, and trimethoprim/sulfamethoxazole do not provide a wide enough spectrum of coverage, and have been met with increasing resistance of likely causative organisms.[45] Empiric treatment of acute infectious diarrhea with a fluoroquinolone has frequently been shown to shorten the duration of the diarrheal illness.[48] This benefit of shortening the diarrheal illness is of limited value. In addition, due to concerns about toxicity to growing cartilage, the quinolones are not to be used in children or during pregnancy. However, the quinolones have a broad spectrum of coverage for the usual infectious causes of diarrhea, and successfully eradicate the carrier state.[15]

Most causes of acute diarrheal illness are viral in nature and therefore are not responsive to antibiotic therapy. Laboratory studies are often not useful in the acute setting and empiric therapy is of questionable benefit, as described above. For these reasons, antibiotics should be reserved for those cases of acute diarrheal illness where a strong suspicion of a treatable bacterial cause arises from history, epidemiology, and laboratory findings. In addition, the adverse effects of antibiotic use must be considered.[49]

Other Therapy. Additional therapy includes the use of silicates (e.g., kaolin). Silicates are clay suspensions that increase stool consistency but do not significantly alter the amount of water lost in the stool. Bulk-forming fibers (e.g., methylcellulose) may be therapeutic with mild diarrhea. Cholestyramine, an agent used to treat hypercholesterolemia, binds the *C. difficile* toxin as well as other bacterial toxins in the gut. Cholestyramine is constipating in healthy patients.

Anticholinergic and antimuscarinic agents include atropine, hyoscyamine, scopolamine, and dicyclomine. These agents are avoided in diarrheal illness because of the antimotility effects. Although atropine is used in combination with diphenoxylate, the atropine is present only to reduce the abuse potential of the diphenoxylate.

Antisecretory agents include the alpha-agonists, such as clonidine. The exact mechanism is uncertain, but gut motility is slowed. Clonidine can improve diarrhea from diabetes mellitus, vasoactive intestinal polypeptide secreting tumors, and opiate withdrawal.[50,51] However, clonidine has limited efficacy in treating infectious diarrhea.[52] Opiates have antisecretory and antimotility activity. Opiates should generally be avoided in cases of infectious diarrhea.[53]

Loperamide inhibits gut peristalsis and reduces the amount of diarrhea experienced by infected individuals.[54] It also shortens the course of diarrheal illness. Use in children is done cautiously, since complications such as an adynamic ileus, severe vomiting, and respiratory depression from overdose can occur. In adults, since serious adverse reactions are rare, loperamide may be useful.[55]

The therapeutic mechanism of bismuth subsalicylate is uncertain. Theories include the prevention of microbe attachment, decreased enterotoxin production, and limiting the secretory activity. Bismuth subsalicylate is effective in treating traveler's diarrhea and acute diarrhea in children.[56] Salicylate toxicity from bismuth subsalicylate use has been reported.[57,58]

Summary

A careful history and physical examination will guide the physician in developing appropriate management strategies for patients presenting with acute diarrhea. Though laboratory studies often do not allow for an organism-specific diagnosis to be made in the acute setting, they can assist in narrowing the differential diagnosis and assisting the physician in deciding specific management plans. Treatment is often symptomatic with selective use of antimicrobial agents. The guidelines presented here should provide the practicing physician with a practical working approach to the patient with infectious diarrhea.

References

1. Gorbach SL. Gastrointestinal infections. *Curr Opinion Gastroenterol* 1989;6:69. Editorial overview.
2. Seidel JS. Diarrhea and food poisoning. In: Tintinalli JE, Ruiz E, Krome RL, eds. *Emergency Medicine: A Comprehensive Study Guide.* 4th ed. New York: McGraw Hill; 1996:488.
3. DeWitt TG, Humphrey KF, McCarthy P. Clinical predictors of acute bacterial diarrhea in young children. *Pediatrics* 1985; 76:551-556.
4. Marks MI. Infectious diarrhea: Introduction and commentary. *Pediatr Ann* 1994;23:526-527.
5. Keswick BH, Pickering LK, DuPont HL. Prevalence of rotavirus in children in day care centers. *J Pediatr* 1983;103: 85-86.
6. Pickering LK, Evans DG, DuPont HL, et al. Diarrhea caused by *Shigella,* rotavirus, and *Giardia* in day-care centers: Prospective study. *J Pediatr* 1981;99:51-56.
7. Reptile-associated salmonellosis—selected states, 1994-1995. *MMWR Morb Mortal Wkly Rep* 1995;44:347-350.
8. African pygmy hedgehog-associated salmonellosis — Washington, 1994. *Morb Mortal Wkly Rep* 1995;44:462-463.
9. Antony MA, Brandt LJ, Klein RS, et al. Infectious diarrhea in patients with AIDS. *Dig Dis Sci* 1988;33:1141-1146.
10. Hoshiko M. Laboratory diagnosis of infections diarrhea. *Pediatr Ann* 1994;23:570-574.
11. Echeverria P, Sethabutr O, Serichantalergs O. Modern diagnosis (with molecular tests) of acute infectious diarrhea. *Gastroenterol Clin North Am* 1993;22:661-682.
12. Williams EK, Lohr JA, Guerrant RL. Acute infectious diarrhea. II. Diagnosis, treatment and prevention. *Pediatr Infect Dis* 1986;5:458-465.
13. Finkelstein JA, Schwartz JS, Torrey S, et al. Common clinical features as predictors of bacterial diarrhea in infants. *Am J Emerg Med* 1989;7:469-473.
14. Blaser MJ, Wells JG, Feldman RA, et al. Campylobacter enteritis in the United States. *Ann Intern Med* 1983;98: 360-365.
15. Bitterman R. Acute gastroenteritis and constipation. In: Rosen P, Barkin RM, et al, eds. *Emergency Medicine: Concepts and Clinical Practice.* 3rd ed. St. Louis: Mosby Year Book; 1992:1533-1577.
16. Molla AM, Molla AM. Effect of antibiotics on food intake and absorption of nutrients for children with diarrhea due to *Shigella. Rev Infect Dis* 1991;13(suppl 4):S347-S350.
17. Revised guidelines for the control of Shigella sonnei infection and other infective diarrheas. PHLS Working Group. *Commun Dis Rep CDR Wkly* 1993;3:r69-r70.
18. Cohen MB. Etiology and mechanisms of acute infectious diarrhea in infants in the United States. *J Pediatr* 1991;118: S34-S39.
19. Wilder AN, MacCready RA. Isolation of *Salmonella* from poultry. *N Engl J Med* 1966;274:1453-1460.
20. Fry RD. Infectious enteritis. A collective review. *Dis Colon Rectum* 1990;33:520-527.
21. Tauxe RV, Deming MS, Blake PA. *Campylobacter jejuni* infections on college campuses: A national survey. *Am J Pub Health* 1985;75:659-660.
22. Mathewson JJ, Dupont HL. *Aeromonas* species: Role as human pathogens. *Curr Clin Top Infect Dis* 1992;12:26-36.
23. San Joaquin VH, Pickett DA. *Aeromonas*-associated gastroenteritis in children. *Pediatr Infect Dis J* 1988;7:53-57.
24. Marks M, Pai C, Lafleur L. *Yersinia enterocolitica:* A prospective study of clinical, bacteriologic, and epidemiologic features. *J Pediatr* 1980;96:26-31.
25. Olinde AJ, Lucas JF, Miller RC. Acute yersiniosis and its surgical significance. *South Med J* 1984;77:1539-1540.
26. Pai CH, Gillis F, Tuomanen E, et al. Placebo-controlled double-blind evaluation of trimethoprim-sulfamethoxazole treatment of *Yersinia enterocolitica* gastroenteritis. *J Pediatr* 1984;104:308-311.
27. Hoogkamp-Korstanje JA. Antibiotics in *Yersinia enterocolitica* infections. *J Antimicrob Chemother* 1987;20:123-131.
28. Morris JG, Black RE. Cholera and other vibrioses in the United States. *N Engl J Med* 1985;312:343-350.
29. Janda JM, Powers C, Bryant RG, et al. Current perspectives on the epidemiology and pathogenesis of clinically significant *Vibrio* spp. *Clin Microbiol Rev* 1988;1:245-267.
30. Wells JG, Shipman LD, Greene KD, et al. Isolation of the *Escherichia coli* serotype 0157:H7 and other Shiga-like-toxin-producing *E. coli* from dairy cattle. *J Clin Microbiol* 1991;29: 985-989.
31. Bartlett JG. Antibiotic-associated colitis. *Clin Gastroenterol* 1979;8:783-801.
32. Knoop FC, Owens M, Crocker IC. *Clostridium difficile:* Clinical disease and diagnosis. *Clin Microbiol Rev* 1993;6: 251-265.
33. Dinh HT, Kernbaum S, Frottier J. Treatment of antibiotic-induced colitis by metronidazole. *Lancet* 1978;1:338-339. Letter.
34. Bean NH, Griffin PM, Goulding JS, et al. Foodborne disease outbreaks, 5-year summary, 1983-1987. *MMWR Morb Mortal Wkly Rep* 1990;39(SS-1):5.
35. Tranter HS. Food-borne staphylococcal illness. *Lancet* 1990; 336:1044-1046.
36. Terranova W, Blake PA. *Bacillus cereus* food poisoning. *N Engl J Med* 1978;298:143.
37. Ho MS, Glass RI, Pinsky PF, et al. Rotavirus as a cause of diarrheal morbidity and mortality in the United States. *J Infect Dis* 1988;158:1112-1116.
38. Ward RL, Bernstein DI, Young EC, et al. Human rotavirus studies in volunteers: Determination of infectious dose and serological response to infection. *J Infect Dis* 1986;154: 871-880.
39. Uhnoo I, Wadell G, Svensson L, et al. Importance of enteric adenoviruses 40 and 41 in acute gastroenteritis in infants and young children. *J Clin Microbiol* 1984;20:365-372.
40. Wright RA, Spencer HC, Brodsky RE, et al. Giardiasis in Colorado: An epidemiologic study. *Am J Epidemiol* 1977;105: 330-336.
41. Dupont HL, Sullivan PS. Giardiasis: The clinical spectrum, diagnosis and therapy. *Pediatr Infect Dis* 1986;5:S131-S138.
42. Adams EB, McLeod IN. Invasive amebiasis. *Medicine* 1977; 56:325-334.
43. Wolfe MS. The treatment of intestinal protozoan infections. *Med Clin North Am* 1982;66:707-720.

44. Navin TR, Juranek DD. Cryptosporidiosis: Clinical, epidemiologic, and parasitologic review. *Rev Infect Dis* 1984;6:313-327.
45. DeHovitz JA, Pape JW, Boncy M, et al. Clinical manifestations and therapy of *Isospora belli* infection in patients with acquired immunodeficiency syndrome. *N Engl J Med* 1986;315:87-90.
46. Sanders WE Jr. Intoxications from the seas: Ciguatera, scombroid, and paralytic shellfish poisoning. *Infect Dis Clin North Am* 1987;1:665-676.
47. Davis RT, Villar LA. Symptomatic improvement with amitriptyline in ciguatera fish poisoning. *N Engl J Med* 1986; 315:65. Letter.
48. Goodman LJ, Trenholme GM, Kaplan RL, et al. Empiric antimicrobial therapy in domestically acquired diarrhea in urban adults. *Arch Intern Med* 1990;150:541-546.
49. Wiström J, Jertborn M, Ekwall E, et al. Empiric treatment of diarrheal disease with norfloxacin. *Ann Intern Med* 1992;117: 202-208.
50. Fedorak RN, Field M, Chang EB. Treatment of diabetic diarrhea with clonidine. *Ann Intern Med* 1985;102:197-199.
51. Sandgren JE, McPhee MS, Greenberger NJ. Narcotic bowel syndrome treated with clonidine. *Ann Intern Med* 1984;101: 331-334.
52. Rabbani GH, Butler T, Patte D, et al. Clinical trial of clonidine hydrochloride as an antisecretory agent in cholera. *Gastroenterology* 1989;97:321-325.
53. DuPont HL, Hornick RB. Adverse effect of lomotil therapy in shigellosis. *JAMA* 1973;226:1525-1528.
54. Heel RC, Brogden RN, Speight TM, et al. Loperamide: A review of its pharmacological properties and therapeutic efficacy in diarrhoea. *Drugs* 1978;15:33-52.
55. Ericsson CD, Johnson PC. Safety and efficacy of loperamide. *Am J Med* 1990;88(suppl 6a):10s-14s.
56. Gorbach SL. Bismuth therapy in gastrointestinal diseases. *Gastroenterology* 1990;99:863-875.
57. Levy G. Aspirin and bismuth subsalicylate. *Am J Dis Child* 1993;147:1281. Letter.
58. Sainsbury SJ. Fatal salicylate toxicity from bismuth subsalicylate. *West J Med* 1991;155:637-639.

Ischemic Bowel Syndromes

James A. Castellone, MD
Robert D. Powers, MD, FACP, FACEP

The presentation of ischemic bowel disease is frequently subtle, especially in the elderly, and can be confused with many other life-threatening conditions. The fact is, few diseases result in such a high mortality rate as acute mesenteric ischemia; mortality rates range from 50-100% in most series.[1,2] The clinical course is frequently complicated by the fact that these patients have other comorbid conditions, including congestive heart failure (CHF), cardiac arrhythmias, or chronic dehydration.

The emergency physician's primary role in evaluating patients with acute abdominal pain is to distinguish benign abdominal disorders from ischemia-related syndromes. Prompt recognition is essential. If patients with acute mesenteric ischemia are not detected rapidly, the risk of bowel infarction increases dramatically, and the probability of survival is low. A high index of suspicion is required, and, once the diagnosis is strongly supported, invasive evaluation and definitive surgical intervention are mandatory.[2]

With these issues in mind, the purpose of this chapter is to review the relevant anatomy, pathophysiology, and clinical presentations in the emergency department (ED), to improve outcomes in this high-risk population.

Clinical Classification and Anatomy

Generally speaking, mesenteric ischemia can be separated into two distinct classes: acute mesenteric ischemia (AMI) and chronic mesenteric ischemia (CMI). Moreover, AMI can be further subdivided into occlusive (OMI) and nonocclusive (NOMI) mesenteric ischemia. Typically, OMI is the result of either thrombotic or embolic—acute or subacute—arterial or venous occlusion. Approximately 80% of cases of AMI are occlusive in etiology, with arterial emboli or thromboses predominating in 65% of cases and venous thrombosis in 15%.[2-4] Arterial occlusions are the result of emboli in 75% of patients and are caused by in situ thrombosis in the remaining 25%. NOMI, which is associated with low perfusion states with or without microvascular pathology, is responsible for about 20% of patients who present with AMI.[3-6]

Arterial Anatomy. A fundamental understanding of the arterial anatomy of the gastrointestinal tract will aid the clinician in patient evaluation and management. Blood supply to the abdominal organs derives from three major vessels: the celiac trunk, the superior mesenteric artery (SMA), and the inferior mesenteric artery (IMA). Abdominal organs receive their blood supply based upon their embryological development. The pharynx, esophagus, stomach, proximal sections, parts of the duodenum, liver, gallbladder, pancreas and spleen are supplied by the celiac trunk. The distal duodenum, jejunum, ileum, cecum, ascending colon, and two-thirds of the transverse colon receive their blood supply from the SMA. The distal one-third transverse colon, descending and sigmoid colon, and rectum are supplied by the IMA. There is an abundant supply of collateral vessels and thus significant territorial overlap of blood flow that can be clinically significant.[4]

From a clinical perspective, the extensive collateral vasculature of the gastrointestinal tract protects the bowel from massive ischemia. As a rule, if there is occlusion of a mesenteric vessel, collateral vessels, if they are sufficiently patent, provide the needed blood supply. The main anastomotic regions include the pancreaticoduodenal arteries (celiac artery with the SMA), the marginal artery of Drummond (SMA and IMA), and the arc of Riolan (SMA and IMA). If the celiac artery is occluded, then the SMA can provide collateral flow via the pancreaticoduodenal arteries, and the same is true in reverse should the SMA occlude. Should the IMA occlude, then collateral flow via the arc of Riolan and marginal artery can provide anterograde flow. However, the acuity of the occlusion—whether the occlusion is secondary to an embolus or thrombus—and its location will determine whether collateral flow is successful or intestinal necrosis develops.

Venous Vasculature. The general anatomy of the venous circulation parallels the arterial architecture. The inferior mesenteric vein (IMV) facilitates venous return from the IMA distribution to join the splenic vein. Likewise, the superior mesenteric vein (SMV) facilitates blood return from the SMA distribution to meet the splenic vein and form the portal vein that then drains into the liver. In cases of mesenteric venous thrombosis (MVT), portal vein thrombosis, or portal hypertension, the mesenteric venous collateral circulation and portacaval anastamoses become clinically significant.

The major portacaval anastomotic regions are the esophageal veins via the left gastric vein, paraumbilical veins, middle and inferior rectal veins with the IMV, and various retroperitoneal veins. As a result, patients can present clinically with either hematemesis secondary to portal hypertension or portal vein thrombosis or with hematochezia secondary to mesenteric vein thrombosis and venous engorgement.

Abdominal Pain Perception and Neural Innervation. A brief review of the innervation of abdominal viscera is helpful for understanding the progression and presentation of clinical disease in patients with mesenteric ischemia. As might be expected, abdominal pain is the most common presenting chief complaint of patients with AMI. Early in the presentation, pain is nonspecific and out of proportion to the physical findings, which can confound the correct diagnosis.

Visceral nerves that supply the intra-abdominal organs also supply the peritoneum, and are carried in the low thoracic and lumbar splanchnic nerves (T5-L2). Somatic nerves that supply the abdominal wall structures and skin also supply the parietal peritoneum.

One way to evaluate abdominal pain is by differentiating visceral from somatic pain. Visceral pain is derived from receptors located in the visceral peritoneum and is triggered by such stimuli as smooth-muscle contraction or spasm, distension or stretching, and ischemia, but not to physical palpation or temperature. Typically, there is no exacerbation or change in pain quality or quantity with movement. In contrast, somatic pain is derived from receptors located in the parietal peritoneum and is triggered by such stimuli as touch, cutting, ischemia, pressure, heat, or inflammation. Pain is exacerbated by movement because of the change in the relationship between the parietal peritoneum with the inflamed visceral peritoneum. This produces guarding, a phenomenon in which abdominal muscles contract in an attempt to prevent movement. Symptoms associated with visceral pain include salivation, nausea, vomiting, and sweating.

The processing of somatic pain occurs in the cortex and, as a result, has specific localization that is perceived at the respective dermatomal distribution. Somatic pain usually is described as sharp or knife-like and focal, but it can be diffuse as a result of widespread inflammation associated with a ruptured viscus. As is well-known, patients do present in atypical fashion, and significant overlap within the sympathetic nervous system can refer pain to an atypical location.[7-10]

Clinical Pathophysiology: The Mesenteric Ischemic Cascade

Approximately 20-25% of cardiac output is delivered to the small and large intestine, with a 2:1 distribution of SMA to IMA. Eighty percent of this flow is for perfusion of the mucosa and 20% for the muscularis because of the high metabolic requirements of the mucosa. Accordingly, the visceral mucosa is very sensitive to the decreased perfusion and compromised oxygen delivery characterized by ischemic states.

Mesenteric Ischemia. Mesenteric ischemia can result from prolonged periods of vasoconstriction.[11,12] Other precipitating factors include activation of the renin-angiotensin axis; angiotensin II is a potent mesenteric and peripheral vasoconstrictor. Vasopressin, which is released in significant quantities in low-flow states, affects splanchnic vascular resistance to a much greater degree than the systemic circulation and is useful for treating GI hemorrhage.[11-13]

Another significant factor in mesenteric ischemia is the countercurrent exchange mechanism that occurs in the small intestinal villi. In this regard, villi subjected to ischemia result in epithelial cell necrosis that stimulates release of endothelial factors, and leads to the attraction and activation of neutrophils and macrophages into the ischemic tissue. These cells release substances such as protease enzymes, TNF, platelet activating factor, arachadonic acid byproducts (prostaglandins and leukotrienes), and toxic oxygen radicals that produce further endothelial damage, increased vascular permeability, vasoconstriction, inflammation, and necrosis. Digestive enzymes in the intestinal lumen are then able to invade the injured cells, resulting in the leakage of fluid and net movement of fluid into the bowel lumen.[11-13]

From a metabolic perspective, cellular hypoxia results in decreased production of ATP and cellular acidosis. The clinical manifestations of metabolic acidosis are an increased respiratory rate and associated secondary respiratory alkalosis. Reperfusion injury can occur after reestablishment of blood flow. The anaerobic environment leads to the proliferation of anaerobic organisms in the intestinal lumen, absorption into the circulation, and translocation into the peritoneum, resulting in an increased risk for secondary sepsis.[11-14]

Animal models of mesenteric ischemia show that mild ischemia of short duration results in no permanent damage and intestinal mucosal repair. However, moderate to severe ischemia of longer duration does result in significant injury. The earliest injury is at the villus tips resulting in necrotic enterocytes being sloughed into the intestinal lumen. Edema develops within the bowel wall in the lamina propria and mucosal protection decreases. Cellular activation as described previously occurs and transmucosal necrosis ensues.[11-13]

Bowel Injury Patterns: Clinical Correlations. The severity of ischemic injury to the bowel depends upon the duration of ischemia,

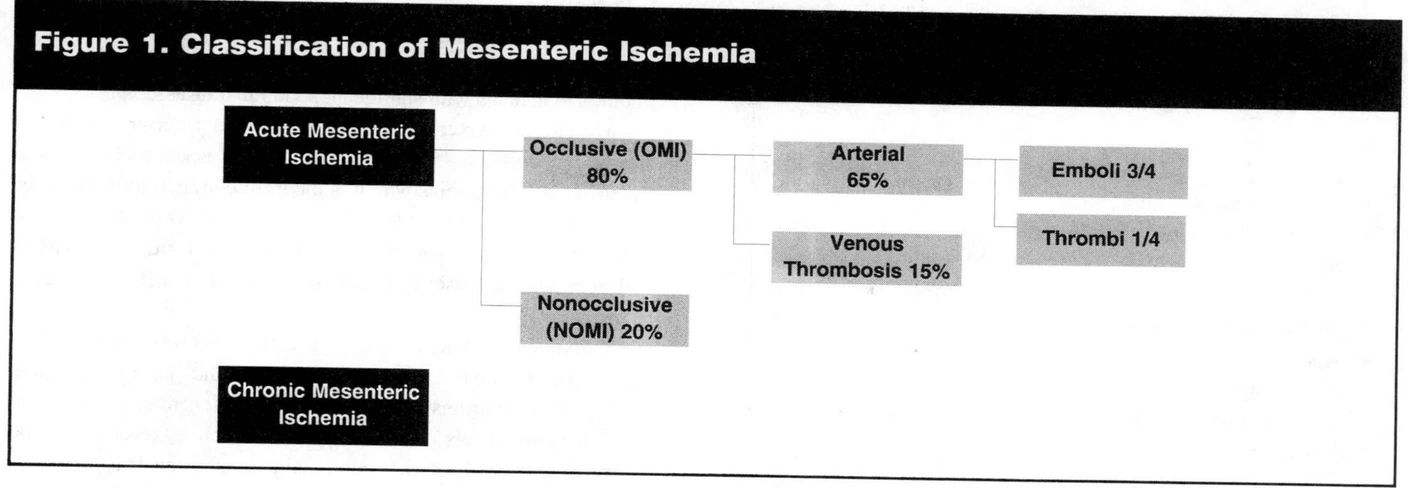

the etiology of the ischemia (embolus, thrombus, or low-flow state), and the integrity of the collateral circulation. As emphasized, collateral circulation protects the gut from developing ischemia. Moreover, it has been shown that, as a rule, at least two of the three major mesenteric vessels (celiac, SMA, and IMA) must be diseased in order to produce ischemia. However, acute occlusion of the SMA alone can result in acute mesenteric insufficiency. When a major mesenteric vessel is occluded, collateral vessels open immediately in response to the decreased arterial pressure distal to the occlusion. However, if the occlusion is prolonged, vasoconstriction develops regardless of whether the occlusion was secondary to an arterial embolus, thrombus, or low-flow state. It has been shown that even after an obstructed vessel is opened, vasoconstriction may persist.

Precise patterns and the extent of bowel injury secondary to ischemic insult depend upon etiologic factors, underlying anatomy, and compensatory mechanisms of the patient. Generally speaking, major emboli to the SMA do not lodge proximally, as is seen with thrombi, but they tend to occlude the vessel distally to branches of the middle colic and jejunal arteries. Consequently, the injury pattern usually involves the distal jejunum, the ileum, and the ascending colon, whereas the proximal jejunum, and transverse and distal colon are spared. Minor emboli to the SMA may involve distal branches, resulting in a focal segmental injury pattern. Arterial thromboses lodge at the origin of the vessel, and they occur much more commonly in the SMA due to the angle of take-off from the aorta—45° vs. the celiac axis which is 90°. As a result, the entire small bowel from proximal jejunum to distal colon is affected by proximal thrombosis of the SMA.

Nonocclusive Mesenteric Ischemia. In NOMI, most of the small intestine and portions of the large intestine are affected in a patchy injury pattern. The splenic flexure is commonly affected because its perfusion is dependent on distal SMA and IMA branches. The descending and sigmoid colon are also commonly affected. In mesenteric venous thrombosis, the injury pattern usually involves short segments of the proximal and middle small intestine. Venous engorgement and extravasation of blood into the tissues is a common finding. *(Please see Figure 1.)*

Mechanical Causes of Ischemia. Mechanical causes that result in external compression of the bowel wall (incarcerated hernia, intussusception, volvulus, adhesions), and, therefore, the major vessels, are more common than primary vascular occlusions. The resulting injury pattern will be determined by the anatomic site of bowel compression. Ischemic injury also occurs proximally to obstructive lesions of the colon. Ischemic colitis is the most common form of intestinal ischemia secondary to obstructing or partially obstructing lesions of the colon (e.g., cancer), and ulcerative colitis. The spectrum of injury ranges from superficial ulcers to gangrenous necrosis and perforation. [11-13,15]

Ischemic Bowel Syndromes: Clinical Presentations and Diagnostic Pitfalls

Patients suffering from ischemic bowel disease can present with a wide range of signs and symptoms, ranging from vague abdominal discomfort to frank peritonitis and septic shock. Morbidity and mortality caused by mesenteric ischemia are linked to the time delay in making the diagnosis and underlying host factors.

Diagnostic Challenges. AMI remains a challenging diagnosis, primarily because of the lack of physical findings in these patients who complain of pain early in the ischemic process. At the other end of the spectrum are those patients with advanced ischemia who present with obvious surgical abdominal disease with significant physical findings. However, once peritonitis has occurred, the ischemic process is well-advanced and the mortality is greater than 70% in most published reports.

Overall, using an aggressive diagnostic approach has been shown to reduce mortality to approximately 45%. Lack of peritoneal signs is a positive predictive factor, with 90% of patients surviving who present without peritoneal signs and have AMI diagnosed at angiography.[1] Accordingly, the challenge lies in making the diagnosis when a patient presents early in the course of their ischemia.

Mesenteric Arterial Embolism. The median age of patients presenting with mesenteric arterial embolism is 70 years, with approximately two-thirds of patients with arterial embolism being women.[2] The overwhelming majority of emboli lodge in the SMA, although thrombotic emboli to the celiac trunk have been reported; emboli consisting of tumor and cholesterol have also been documented.[2]

SMA embolism has a more favorable prognosis than bowel ischemia secondary to thrombosis of the SMA. This is because

Table 1. Risk Factors Associated with AMI Embolism

- Advanced age
- Coronary artery disease
- Cardiac valvular disease
- History of dysrrhythmias
- Atrial fibrillation
- Post-myocardial infarction mural thrombi
- History of thromboembolic events
- Aortic surgery
- Aortography
- Coronary angiography
- Aortic dissection
- Congestive heart failure

emboli lodge distally to the middle colic and jejunal branches, sparing the proximal jejunum and distal colon. Emboli originating in the left atrium or ventricle are the most common cause of SMA embolism. Risk factors include advanced age, coronary artery disease, cardiac valvular disease, history of dysrrhythmias, atrial fibrillation, post-myocardial infarction mural thrombi, history of thromboembolic events, aortic surgery, aortography, coronary angiography, aortic dissection; one case has been reported following colonoscopy.[3-6,16] *(Please see Table 1.)*

Approximately 20% of patients have a previous history of peripheral emboli. Patients recently converted to sinus rhythm from atrial fibrillation are particularly susceptible to thromboembolism. Reports have shown that there is a delay in normal mechanical contractility in the atrium after the conversion to normal sinus rhythm in atrial fibrillation, and, consequently, emboli have occurred days after conversion in patients without atrial thrombi at the time of conversion.[5]

Patients typically complain of the sudden onset of severe periumbilical pain, which is consistent with the innervation and vascular supply to the SMA distribution. Associated symptoms such as nausea, vomiting, and frequent bowel movements are more likely if the ischemia is secondary to an acute vascular occlusion.[4,12,17] Pain may be the only presenting symptom, and it is typically intense but poorly localized. In a report of 82 patients with SMA embolus over 22 years, one study reported typical abdominal pain in only 74.5% of patients while finding it absent or atypical in 23%.[18]

Clearly, the most consistent finding is pain that is out of proportion to the physical findings. This is explained by the fact that only the visceral structures are ischemic early on, and the parietal peritoneum (which would affect physical findings) has not been irritated yet because transmural necrosis with its associated inflammatory process adjacent to the parietal peritoneum has not occurred. Accordingly, the abdomen may be soft with only mild tenderness. One review reported that more than than two-thirds of patients presented without typical signs, such as absent bowel sounds, abdominal distension or guarding, that are indicative of a significant abdominal process. Additionally, blood in the rectum was present in only 16% of patients.[13] The presence of occult blood has also been reported as being present in 25% of patients.[2,13]

When the ischemic process becomes transmural, peritoneal signs become evident. Caution must be taken when a patient is on corticosteroids, since this may blunt an appropriate inflammatory response and, therefore, suppress pain and fever and mask typical findings in patients with significant abdominal disease.[8]

Mesenteric Arterial Thrombosis. The superior mesenteric artery originates at a 45° angle off the ventral aspect of the abdominal aorta, which explains why it is the most common location in the mesenteric circulation for thrombotic occlusion. Thrombotic occlusion portends a less favorable prognosis than occlusion secondary to embolization because a larger segment of intestine becomes ischemic.

Thrombosis usually occurs in the area of atherosclerotic narrowing in the proximal SMA. In most cases, the proximal jejunum through the distal transverse colon becomes ischemic. SMA thrombosis usually occurs in patients with chronic, severe, visceral atherosclerosis; a history of abdominal pain after meals is present in 20-50% of these patients.[2,6,19] Patients are often elderly, have associated coronary artery disease, severe peripheral vascular disease, or hypertension.

One large trial reported on a series of autopsies, in which coronary, cerebral, and mesenteric arteries were examined to evaluate the frequency of atherosclerosis in the visceral arteries.[19] They found that the percentage of cases with visceral atherosclerosis increased with increasing age. Five percent of patients younger than 40 years old had moderate mesenteric arterial stenosis, 14% in 40-59 year olds, 33% in the 60-79 age group, and 67% in those older than 80 years. Atherosclerotic changes were rare in distal mesenteric arteries with no luminal narrowing. Fifteen percent of autopsy cases had at least two significant mesenteric arterial stenoses; none of these patients had reported symptoms of chronic mesenteric ischemia. The celiac artery was the most common site of mesenteric arterial stenosis, followed in decreasing frequency by the SMA and IMA. They also found a strong association between mesenteric artery and coronary artery atherosclerosis.[19]

Patients with SMA thrombosis present with the gradual onset of abdominal pain and distension. A history of postprandial abdominal pain and weight loss in those with symptoms of chronic mesenteric ischemia can be elicited in fewer than half of cases. Finding subjective complaints that are well out of proportion to the physical findings is characteristic. Nausea and vomiting found in mesenteric arterial occlusion has been attributed to ischemic gastroparesis. As a result, patients with severe nausea and vomiting may have decreased-to-no bowel sounds secondary to this process, without peritoneal findings. These patients usually present later than patients with acute mesenteric insufficiency secondary to embolization, and they may well have had pain for 12-24 hours. Patients frequently will have physical findings consistent with peripheral vascular disease, such as carotid, femoral, or abdominal bruits, or decreased-to-absent peripheral pulses. Again, massive abdominal distension, absent bowel sounds, muscular guarding, rebound and localized tenderness, and rigidity indicate advanced necrosis of bowel.[6,15,20]

Mesenteric Venous Thrombosis. The mean age of presentation ranges from 48-60, but intestinal ischemia secondary to MVT can occur at any age.[21-23] AMI itself is rare and ischemia secondary to MVT accounts for only 5-15% of cases. A few significant clinical factors should be emphasized. MVT occurs in a younger patient population, and the mortality rate is lower than the other causes of AMI, ranging from 20-50%.[6,24] MVT has been traditionally classified as either primary (unknown etiology) or secondary to a predisposing

Table 2. Risk Factors Associated with Mesenteric Venous Thrombosis

Hypercoagualable or Hematologic Disorders
Polycythemia vera
Myeloproliferative disorders
Sickle cell disease
Antithrombin III deficiency
Protein C deficiency
Protein S deficiency
Hyperfibrinogenemia
Thrombocytosis
Deep venous thrombosis
Malignancy
Estrogen therapy/OCP
Pregnancy
Postoperative
Inflammatory Conditions
Pancreatitis
Diverticulitis
Appendicitis
Cholangitis
Peritonitis
Intra-abdominal abscess
Ileocolitis/IBD
Sepsis
Trauma
Operative venous injury
Post-splenectomy
Blunt or penetrating abdominal injury
Sclerotherapy of esophageal varices
Other
Congestive heart failure
Renal failure
Decompression sickness
Portal hypertension

condition. *(Please see Table 2.)* Primary MVT accounts for approximately 20% and secondary thrombosis for approximately 80% of cases. Hypercoagulable states associated with MVT include polycythemia vera, myeloproliferative disorders, antithrombin III deficiency, protein C and S deficiencies, DVT, malignancy, estrogen therapy, and pregnancy. One study of 30 patients with MVT secondary to hypercoagulable states noted polycythemia vera as the most common etiology, comprising 35% of the cases.[21] Portomesenteric venous thrombosis occurs in patients with portal hypertension, cirrhosis, and following sclerotherapy for esophageal varices. Intra-abdominal inflammatory conditions such as pancreatitis, diverticulitis, appendicitis, peritonitis, abscesses and ileocolitis have all been shown to cause MVT. Additionally, up to 60% of patients with MVT have a history of peripheral deep venous thrombosis.[6,21-29]

Inadequate venous drainage results in massive vascular congestion and fluid sequestration, which can lead to hypovolemia, hemoconcentration, and, eventually, if untreated, cardiovascular collapse. Mesenteric arterial vasospasm uniformly coexists with venous occlusion and persists despite resolution of the occlusion. Portal vein thrombosis can produce esophageal varices and splenomegaly and can present as hematemesis or an upper gastrointestinal bleed. Splenic vein thrombosis, as seen after splenectomy or in pancreatic inflammatory conditions, may present as an upper GI bleed with varices within the stomach but without intestinal ischemia. Superior mesenteric vein thrombosis will result in small intestinal ischemia, and inferior mesenteric vein thrombosis is usually of no consequence.[22,23,29]

The clinical presentation of MVT depends upon the acuity of the venous occlusion and covers the spectrum from acute onset to insidious evolution of abdominal pain. In general, symptoms tend to develop less rapidly than with acute arterial insufficiency. It should be stressed that MVT may have an acute, subacute, or chronic onset.

A number of studies have helped characterize this ischemic syndrome.[21,22] The symptoms of acute MVT include abdominal pain in 83-100% of patients, which, typically, is described as being out of proportion to the physical findings. The abdominal pain has a mean duration of 5-14 days, but 25% of patients present within 48 hours. Anorexia has been noted in 53-54%, vomiting in 41-77%, diarrhea in 36%, constipation in 13-34%, and hematemesis in 9-42% of patients. Physical findings include abdominal tenderness in 95-97%, distension in 51-84%, decreased bowel sounds in 42-77%, stool positive for occult blood in 26-54%, guarding in 42-53%, shock in 6-32%, and fever (> 38° C) in 24-47% of patients.[21,22,25]

The abdominal pain in MVT is described as being diffuse and nonspecific initially, but it later becomes constant in nature. Gastrointestinal bleeding, whether upper or lower, signifies bowel infarction and necrosis. The abdominal distension may not be accompanied with tympany to percussion due to massive venous congestion within the bowel wall, lumen, and peritoneal cavity. A significant number of patients present with fever and shock, indicative of cardiovascular collapse from hypovolemia, sepsis, and advanced disease.

Subacute MVT occurs in patients with venous thrombi and abdominal pain for several weeks to months but, even without evidence of intestinal infarction, some patients also complain of associated nausea or diarrhea. There are usually no physical findings. Chronic MVT is defined as patients without abdominal pain with thrombosis. These patients typically present with gastrointestinal bleeding from esophageal varices associated with thrombosis of the portal or splenic veins.[22-24]

Nonocclusive Mesenteric Ischemia. Acute mesenteric insufficiency due to NOMI occurs in approximately 20% of all cases with bowel ischemia.[30] One study conducted over a 13-year period reported a mean age of 59. The study emphasized the presence of precipitating illnesses, which result in low-flow states and can occur in younger patients.[30]

The pathogenesis of NOMI appears to be multifactorial. Mesenteric vasoconstriction can result from the shunting of blood flow to the vital organs (heart and brain) during periods of hypotension or shock. Whether the hypotensive state is due to a primary cardiac event such as cardiogenic shock, an arrhythmia, or in a patient with sepsis, the end result is the shunting of blood away from the splanchnic circulation to the central circulation. The main mediators of this process appear to be angiotensin II and vasopressin.[31]

Ergot alkaloid poisoning, cocaine abuse, and calcium-channel blocking agent use and overdose have also been shown to result in

Table 3. Risk Factors and Conditions Associated with Nonocclusive Mesenteric Ischemia

Advanced age
Cardiovascular disease
Congestive heart failure
Cardiac arrhythmias
Cardiogenic shock
Post myocardial infarction
Post cardiopulmonary bypass
Peripheral vascular disease
Preceding hypotensive episode
Sepsis
Dehydration
Diuretic therapy
Drug-induced splanchnic vasoconstriction
digoxin
catecholamines/vasopressors/alpha agonists
ergot alkaloid poisoning
cocaine abuse
calcium channel blocker use and overdose
Endogenously mediated splanchnic vasoconstriction
angiotensin II
vasopressin
catecholamines
Diabetes
Exercise

nonocclusive ischemia secondary to severe mesenteric vasoconstriction.[2,32,33] NOMI occurs in exacerbations of CHF, cardiogenic shock, and after cardiopulmonary bypass.[15,36,38] In 3066 patients who underwent cardiopulmonary bypass over a five-year period, the incidence of postoperative NOMI was .36% (11 patients). A significant number of patients with NOMI have had long-term treatment with digitalis. Studies suggest that patients with CHF and increased portal venous pressure who are on digitalis may be susceptible to mesenteric vasoconstriction and NOMI.[2,34]

Clinically, patients who present with NOMI are often critically ill, usually as a result of the precipitating event that has led to the splanchnic vasoconstriction. Precipitating conditions include: cardiogenic shock with a myocardial infarction, congestive heart failure, or, in the intensive care unit, placement on vasopressors for the treatment of septic shock. Accordingly, abdominal pain in any patient with the risk factors described previously must raise the clinical suspicion of NOMI. *(Please see Table 3.)* If delays in diagnosis result, then the condition will progress and, if peritoneal findings appear, the patient may not be salvageable.

In general, the signs and symptoms of NOMI are similar to those of acute mesenteric ischemia. One retrospective review of NOMI over a 13-year period found abdominal pain to be present in 77% of patients, nausea and vomiting in 38%, diarrhea in 23%, and anorexia in 23%. In 54% of patients, abdominal tenderness and distension were present, and 46% had decreased bowel sounds. In 38% of patients, the presenting complaint of abdominal pain was diffuse and without signs of peritonitis, whereas the other 62% presented with peritonitis. Patients who presented early had a mortality of 40% and those who presented late had a mortality rate of 100%. The overall mortality rate in this study was 77%.[30]

Chronic Mesenteric Ischemia. CMI, also known as "intestinal angina," is a rare form of intestinal ischemia. Chronic mesenteric ischemia occurs in a 3:1 ratio of women to men and patients are generally older than 60 years of age. CMI is usually the result of severe stenosis of the proximal ostial portion of the main mesenteric arteries. *(Please see Table 4.)* Intestinal ischemia secondary to CMI is rare because of the rich collateral circulation previously described between the three main mesenteric arterial pathways. Those patients that do go on to develop CMI usually do not develop symptoms until at least two of the three major mesenteric arteries (CA, SMA, IMA) are occluded or significantly stenosed.

The severe pain that occurs in these patients appears to be the result of blood flow changes between the stomach and small intestine during a meal ingestion. After atherosclerosis, the second most likely cause of CMI is the celiac axis compression syndrome. In this syndrome, the median arcuate ligament of the diaphragm may compress the celiac axis during expiration and can result in CMI. However, only one-third of patients with celiac axis compression syndrome have postprandial abdominal pain, and weight loss is often absent. Celiac axis compression remains a diagnosis of exclusion.[2,35]

Several case reports have noted young patients with a history of cocaine abuse with postprandial abdominal pain, weight loss, and food aversion with diagnostic occlusion of the celiac and SMA. Cocaine is thought to cause intimal injury and platelet aggregation leading to thrombosis in addition to the vasospasm at the time of it's use. The results of studies show that cocaine potentiates arterial thrombosis not only of the mesenteric vasculature but also of the coronary circulation, which results in mesenteric and coronary ischemia.[36]

Clinically, patients complain of epigastric or periumbilical pain which is dull, deep, crampy, or aching in character. The pain characteristically begins 15-30 minutes after eating, increases in severity, and then slowly diminishes over the subsequent 1-4 hours. The pain intensity depends upon the size of the meal, and, as the occlusive process progresses, patients develop symptoms with smaller and smaller meals, ultimately leading to the avoidance of food. As a result, patients develop significant weight loss. Physical examination usually reveals a patient who is cachectic (depending on the duration of the symptoms), has a soft and nontender abdomen with bowel sounds, and no signs of peritonitis.[2,35,36]

Patient Evaluation and Use of Diagnostic Modalities

Laboratory Testing. Patients older than 50 years of age who present with abdominal pain need a thorough investigation to determine the etiology of their pain. Unfortunately, laboratory investigations in acute mesenteric ischemia are neither sensitive nor specific.

Putative markers for intestinal ischemia include: creatine phosphokinase (CPK), alkaline phosphatase, diamine oxidase, hexosaminidase, lactate dehydrogenase (LDH), aspartate transferase (AST/SGOT), leukocyte counts, electrolytes, hemoglobin/hemat-

Table 4. Risk Factors and Conditions Associated with Chronic Mesenteric Ischemia

Arteriosclerosis (95%)
Peripheral vascular disease
Diabetes mellitus
SMA intimal dissection
Celiac axis compression syndrome
Fibromuscular dysplasia
Cocaine abuse
Ergot alkaloid poisoning
Vasculitis/arteritis
radiation therapy
autoimmune mediated (SLE, RA, scleroderma)
polyarteritis nodosa

ocrit, amylase, inorganic phosphate, serum lactate levels, and intestinal fatty acid binding protein. Unfortunately, none of these tests have been proven to be beneficial prior to the onset of intestinal necrosis.

One study has shown that the seromuscular enzyme CPK was elevated earlier and to a greater extent than the other seromuscular enzymes (LDH, AST) and mucosal enzymes (diamine oxidase and alkaline phosphatase). This investigation reported a sensitivity of 54% at two hours after experimentally induced ischemia secondary to SMA ligation and 75% at four hours with a specificity of 83% at both two and four hours. CPK levels were shown to rise in 3-4 hours and reach a peak at about eight hours.[38]

Studies examining the leukocyte count show it to be elevated in most cases of mesenteric ischemia. Leukocyte counts of 10-15,000/mm^3 are present in approximately 25% of cases, 15-30,000 in 50%, and 25% of patients have values greater than 30,000.[17] However, in early mesenteric ischemia, the leukocyte count may not be elevated, and the diagnosis of mesenteric ischemia can not be ruled out by a normal white blood cell count, but it probably makes the diagnosis less likely.[38]

Analysis of electrolytes also lacks sensitivity and specificity in early mesenteric ischemia. The finding of a metabolic acidosis would signify a significant pathologic process, but other abdominal surgical emergencies also have an associated metabolic acidosis. One study reported that in patients with SMA emboli, only 42% had a metabolic acidosis and it was shown not to be statistically significant.[39] The serum amylase has been shown to be elevated in half of patients up to twice the normal values.[17]

Serum inorganic phosphate levels have been shown to be an indicator for intestinal ischemia in several retrospective studies. Up to 80% of patients with intestinal infarction have been shown to have increased levels, and, in cases where blood was obtained early (4-12 hours) after the onset of symptoms, 94% of patients had elevated levels vs. control patients with non-ischemic surgical abdominal emergencies.[39] One group examined the lactate level in patients with acute abdominal disease. They reported a sensitivity of 100% and a specificity of 42% for mesenteric ischemia.[40]

Further clinical trials are needed in order to evaluate serum markers in diagnosing acute mesenteric ischemia.

Plain Radiography. The first radiological evaluation that should be performed on patients suspected of having acute mesenteric ischemia are abdominal and chest x-rays to exclude the presence of free air or bowel obstruction. In rare instances, plain films of the abdomen reveal findings consistent with ischemic bowel such as pneumatosis intestinalis, portal venous gas, or a thickened bowel wall with thumbprinting.[13,41] However, in the majority of cases, plain films will be normal, and in early mesenteric ischemia, normal x-rays are the rule.[42]

Abnormal findings on plain films that are nonspecific for mesenteric ischemia include an ileus, gasless abdomen, small bowel pseudo-obstruction, splenic flexure cut-off sign, and free air. Findings highly suggestive of ischemia include a thickened bowel wall with thumbprinting, intramural air (pneumatosis intestinalis), and portal venous gas. Pneumatosis intestinalis results from mucosal ischemia and damage followed by dissection of intraluminal gas into the submucosa.[42,43] In one study on diagnostic imaging in mesenteric infarction of patients with proven AMI, 67% had air fluid levels, 18% had dilated bowel loops, 10% had a gasless abdomen, 2% had pneumatosis, and portal venous gas was present in 2%.[44]

Computed Tomography. Due to the availability, improved quality, and speed of computed tomography (CT), it is commonly used for assessing undiagnosed abdominal pain in the ED. Findings in AMI include normal studies, nonspecific findings such as focal or diffuse bowel wall thickening, focal dilated fluid filled bowel loops, mesenteric edema, engorgement of mesenteric veins, peritoneal fluid, and intra-abdominal air. Specific findings include pneumatosis intestinalis, portal venous gas, mesenteric vessel occlusion, and enlargement of a thrombosed vein.

The sensitivity of CT in AMI has been reported to be from 64-82%.[42,44,45] CT has been shown to be the most sensitive test for detecting thrombosis in the mesenteric venous bed and, therefore, is useful for confirming the diagnosis of MVT.[21] One group relies upon contrast-enhanced CT as their first imaging study, especially when there is a strong suspicion for MVT.[22] However, as will be discussed for patients with suspected AMI of unknown etiology, CT is not the first study of choice.

Ultrasonography. Ultrasound is used with increased frequency for the initial evaluation of patients with abdominal pain in the ED. Duplex ultrasound can identify major arterial or venous occlusions and additional findings suggestive of AMI. However, the usual shortcomings of abdominal ultrasound, such as respiratory motion, intra-abdominal gas, obesity, and the inability to satisfactorily visualize mesenteric vessels at all times prevent its use as an initial modality for diagnosing AMI.

Findings in patients with AMI include small intestinal bowel wall thickening (> 5 mm), decreased or absent peristalsis, MVT, and intraperitoneal fluid.[42] In a study on Doppler sonography for detection of AMI due to SMA occlusion, bowel wall abnormalities were detected in only 50% of patients (3 of 6), and the correct diagnosis of SMA occlusion was noted in five of six patients. Duplex ultrasound has been reported to be reliable for CMI and MVT, but very few studies have evaluated its use in AMI.[42,46]

Magnetic Resonance Imaging (MRI). MRI is useful for delineating the mesenteric vessels and bowel wall and has been shown to be better than nonenhanced CT but equal to contrast-enhanced CT for evaluating the mesenteric venous system. However, no studies

Figure 2. An Aggressive Diagnostic Approach to Acute Mesenteric Ischemia

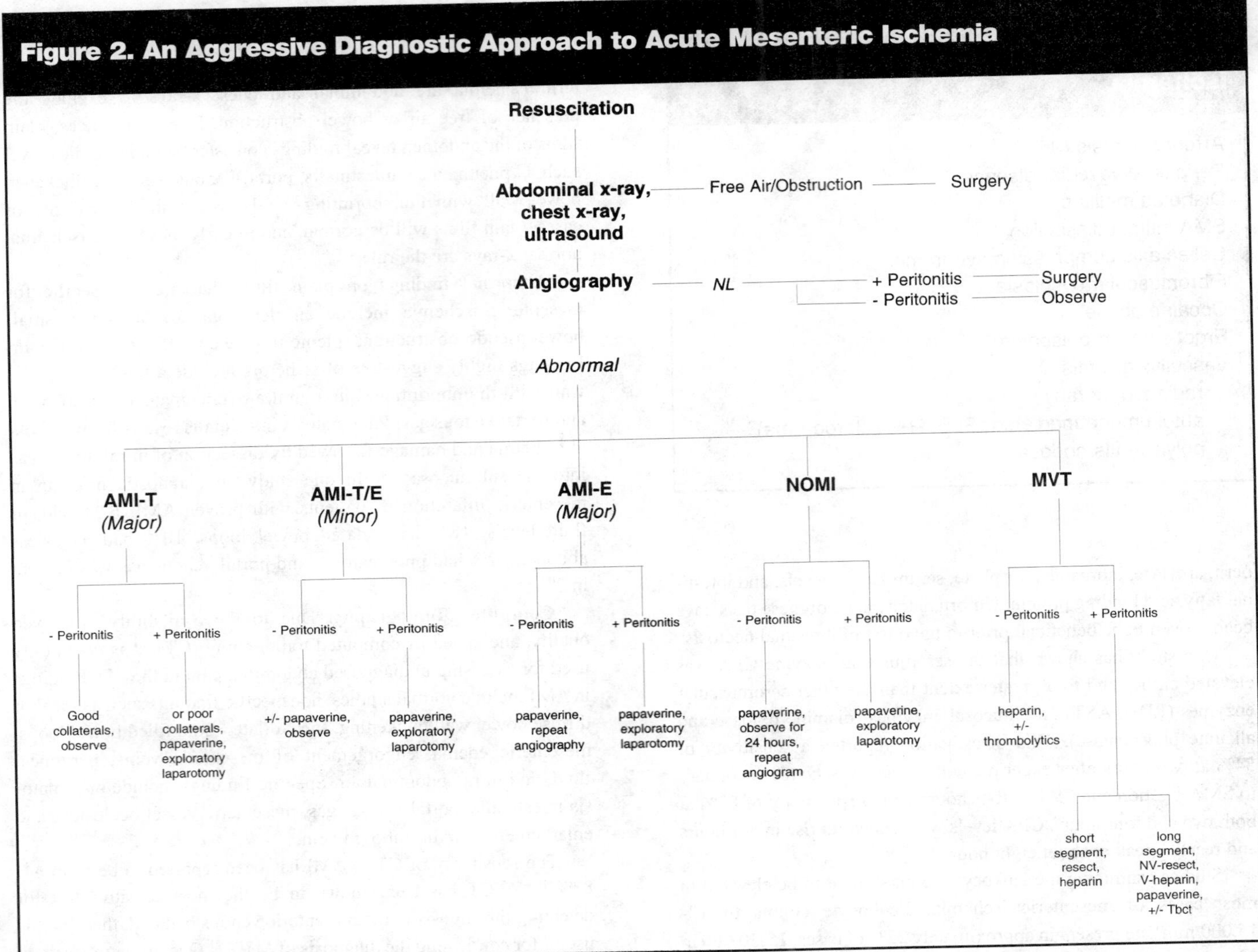

have been reported for its use in AMI. An advantage of MRI is the avoidance of ionizing radiation, but the disadvantages, which include the duration of the exam and the lack of 24 hour availability, are significant.[24,42]

Laparoscopy. Laparoscopy demonstrates intra-abdominal fluid and transmural necrosis but does not evaluate the mucosa. Additionally, increased intraperitoneal pressures can decrease mesenteric arterial flow if greater than 20 mmHg. Therefore, a patient can experience an acute mesenteric ischemic event that may not be detected with laparoscopy.[3]

Endoscopy. Endoscopy can visualize mucosal injury at the site of injury but will give no information regarding the serosa, and a transmural infarct can go undetected. Additionally, there is a risk of perforation with a friable ischemic bowel wall.[3]

Angiography. Angiography is the gold standard for the diagnosis of AMI and is also used for therapeutic infusion of the vasodilator papaverine.[2,15,47,48] However, the use of angiography to diagnose AMI remains controversial. Most clinical monographs on AMI recommend that after obtaining plain abdominal films to rule out the presence of free air or obstruction, angiography must be obtained early, especially in those patients in whom there is a strong clinical suspicion for AMI.

Many of the controversies and intervention bifurcation points surrounding timing and indications for angiography are highlighted in a landmark study by Moneta and Lee.[2] In this study, the authors conclude that in patients without peritoneal signs, the use of angiography may avoid surgical intervention and may identify patients with NOMI who can be treated with an infusion of papaverine via a catheter secured in the superior mesenteric artery. In addition, these investigators recommend that patients suspected of having AMI secondary to emboli or thrombi—as opposed to NOMI—should undergo surgery, and patients with a delayed onset suspected of having NOMI should undergo angiography prior to laparotomy.[2] However, other reports strongly suggest that patients diagnosed with either emboli or thrombi who do not have peritonitis can also be started on papaverine and have repeat angiography in 24 hours and avoid surgery.[3-5]

The majority of the clinical literature favors angiography if no peritoneal findings are present. *(Please see Figure 2.)* Should peritoneal findings be present then preoperative angiography may be performed. One problem with obtaining angiography is that it may delay surgical intervention, and that patients with peritoneal signs cannot afford such a delay in the face of ongoing ischemia. One group advocates that patients with physical findings that necessitate immediate surgical intervention should undergo angiography and that intra-arterial vasodilator therapy can be started intra- or postoperatively.[32]

Another group identifies mesenteric angiography as "the key to diagnosing mesenteric ischemia before bowel infarction and prior to laparotomy, as a definitive diagnosis cannot be made clinically." Furthermore, it is essential to obtain angiography and a diagnosis prior to infarction in order to decrease morbidity and mortality. An operative strategy regarding treatment can be made with information obtained from angiography. The following procedures may be considered: thrombectomy, embolectomy, endarterectomy, revascularization, and angioplasty, depending upon the etiology.[48]

Patients who are hypotensive, or on vasopressor support are not suitable for angiography because the severe mesenteric vasoconstriction may prevent differentiation of NOMI from OMI and intra-arterial vasodilators are also contraindicated.[48]

An Aggressive Diagnostic Approach. Because of the high mortality associated with AMI, especially when peritoneal findings are present and patients have an infarcted bowel, it is essential that those patients with possible mesenteric ischemia be detected early in the course of their illness to decrease the mortality. Studies have been done using an aggressive diagnostic approach in establishing the presence of mesenteric ischemia and providing treatment options. These studies suggest that mortality can be decreased from 70-90% to 45-50%; if the diagnosis is established prior to the development of peritonitis, it can be decreased to 10%.[1,24,41]

To identify all cases of AMI, the clinician must accept a significant percentage of patients with negative angiograms. As a general rule, therefore, patients who are older than 50 years of age, complaining of the sudden onset of abdominal pain for more than two hours' duration, and have significant risk factors for AMI (thrombosis, embolus, NOMI, MVT), should be considered eligible for the management scheme outlined in the algorithm outlined in *Figure 2*.[1]

ED Management

Stabilization and Initial Management. Initial treatment in the ED requires appropriate resuscitation, which includes intravenous fluid replacement, correction of predisposing or precipitating causes of ischemia, maintaining adequate oxygenation, and the institution of antibiotic coverage.[1,13,17,49]

After initial resuscitative efforts have been started, correction of any predisposing or precipitating causes of ischemia must be addressed. The main pathophysiological insult is a lack of mesenteric blood flow so cardiac output must be maintained. Patients presenting with CHF, dysrrhythmias, or in cardiogenic shock need immediate therapy. In patients with significant hypotension that is unresponsive to fluid resuscitation, vasopressors may be used, but the lowest possible dose should be infused, and alpha agonists should be avoided, with ionotropes being the preferred agents.[1,13]

In patients in shock, there is a lack of adequate end-organ perfusion; it is essential to maintain adequate oxygenation. If there is a lack of oxygen content due to decreased hemoglobin, then blood should be given. Endotracheal intubation and mechanical ventilation should be instituted when indicated. Patients suspected of having mesenteric ischemia who appear acutely ill should have parenteral antibiotic therapy started as soon as possible to cover for gram-negative enteric bacteria as well as anaerobes after blood cultures are drawn.[13]

An important factor in hypotensive patients is the increased renin-angiotensin-aldosterone axis and antidiuretic hormone (ADH) secretion. Since angiotensin is a potent mesenteric vasoconstrictor, it has been proposed that angiotensin converting enzyme (ACE) inhibitors may be beneficial in blunting the severe mesenteric vasoconstriction, but no studies have been done to examine this therapy in AMI.[13]

Papaverine. Since mesenteric vasoconstriction is present in patients with occlusive as well as nonocclusive etiologies, intra-arterial infusion into the superior mesenteric artery of papaverine is an important method for increasing mesenteric perfusion, and is considered definitive therapy in patients with NOMI. Papaverine is a potent inhibitor of phosphodiesterase, which degrades cyclic adenosine monophosphate (cAMP). Therefore increased cAMP results in vascular smooth-muscle relaxation. Infusion into the SMA is the most effective way of relieving mesenteric vasoconstriction.

Papaverine is started at angiography and continued postoperatively if laparotomy is performed. The dosing is 60 mg IV bolus followed by a 30-60 mg/h continuous infusion at a concentration of 1 mg/mL. Since 90% of papaverine is metabolized by the liver with each pass, there are no systemic effects noted as a result.[5,14,58,60] It has been reported that papaverine improves survival 20-50%.[12] Tolazoline is another vasodilator that has been used in patients with mesenteric vasoconstriction.[1]

Medical and Surgical Interventions: The Overview. Surgical consultation should be obtained early for all patients with suspected AMI. Immediate surgery is necessary for patients with peritonitis, for those requiring restoration of arterial or venous flow, and for the resection of necrotic bowel. In patients found to have massive small and large intestinal necrotic bowel who are not expected to survive, resection may not be indicated.

AMI With Embolism. There are many treatment options for AMI secondary to embolism. Once embolism is confirmed as the etiologic factor at angiography, and papaverine infusion is started, then laparotomy should be performed to evaluate bowel viability. Surgical intervention may involve arteriotomy with embolectomy and bowel resection if nonviable necrotic bowel is found. If bowel viability is equivocal, then the surgeon may perform a second look procedure 12-24 hours postoperatively to avoid extensive bowel resection at initial laparotomy.[15]

Patients without peritoneal signs with minor emboli, who achieve pain relief with vasodilator infusion, may be managed nonoperatively with repeated angiograms.[1] *(Please see Figure 2.)* Intra-arterial infusion into the superior mesenteric artery (SMA) with thrombolytic agents has been used successfully in patients with confirmed embolism without evidence of peritonitis, normal abdominal films, and no evidence of an ileus.[50] One report suggests that thrombolytics may take 36 hours to dissolve the embolus, thus exposing the bowel to a prolonged ischemia. Therefore, the authors do not recommend their use in AMI.[1] In contrast, there have been several case reports supporting the use of urokinase and streptokinase in SMA emboli in patients without peritonitis with a duration of abdominal pain less than eight hours from the onset.[51-53] Postoperative anticoagulation is recommended for all patients, but determining the proper time to start heparin remains controversial.[18]

AMI With Thrombosis. Acute mesenteric ischemia secondary to thrombosis also is treated initially with a papaverine infusion started at angiography. Several interventions are available to the surgeon.

Patients without peritoneal signs with minor thrombi may be treated with papaverine only. Patients with major thrombi with good collateral vasculature, also without peritoneal signs, may be observed in the hospital without a papaverine infusion. *(Please see Figure 2.)* Patients with peritoneal signs and documented thrombosis require laparotomy as do patients with major thrombi and poor collateral flow even in the absence of peritoneal findings.

Preoperative angiography enhances the decision-making process regarding surgical revascularization. Endarterectomy, thrombectomy, and mesenteric revascularization with aortomesenteric bypass grafting have been the traditional methods of treatment with better long-term results using thrombectomy and bypass grafting.[1,6,12,15]

A retrospective review evaluated 16 patients who underwent percutaneous transluminal angioplasty (PTA) of the celiac, SMA, and IMA.[54] The study included patients with chronic mesenteric ischemia and acute mesenteric ischemia secondary to thrombosis, which made interpretation difficult. Two of the 16 with an obvious acute presentation had unsuccessful primary PTA, with one resulting in death and the other requiring surgical revascularization. Recurrence rates after surgical revascularization have been reported at 7-50%, whereas recurrence rates for PTA have been from 17-63% requiring repeat PTA.[54,55] Because of the danger of recurrence and extensive potential bowel loss, in addition to lack of methods to monitor bowel injury, PTA is not recommended for acute SMA thrombosis.[1]

AMI With MVT. AMI secondary to MVT mandates treatment with anticoagulation, as soon as the diagnosis is made. The aim is to limit the extent of thrombosis and to prevent recurrent thromboses.[6,12] Numerous studies have shown that patients not treated with anticoagulation postoperatively had a significant increased incidence of recurrence with higher mortality rates.[23] Therefore, heparin is the initial treatment of choice, followed by long term warfarin therapy.[6] In patients without peritonitis, anticoagulation may be the only form of treatment instituted, but scattered studies on thrombolytic therapy have been performed.[56] Necrotic nonviable bowel requires resection and revascularization should precede resection. Patients with equivocal bowel may require a second-look operation at 12-24 hours.[6,57] There are also some reports of success with portomesenteric venous thrombectomy, but most patients with acute MVT have diffuse vein thrombosis not amenable to such therapy.[21,23]

NOMI. Patients diagnosed angiographically with NOMI are immediately started on intra-arterial papaverine for severe mesenteric vasoconstriction. *(Please see Figure 2.)* In patients without peritoneal signs, papaverine is the treatment of choice followed by repeat angiography at 12-24 hours. In patients with peritonitis, exploratory laparotomy is indicated immediately, with necrotic or nonviable bowel being resected and papaverine infusion continued postoperatively with repeat angiography in 24 hours. Therapy for NOMI remains nonsurgical unless there is evidence of peritonitis and necrotic bowel. Nonsurgical treatment includes correcting any underlying conditions that resulted in the diffuse mesenteric vasoconstriction, such as CHF, arrhythmias, or hypotension, in an effort to increase mesenteric blood flow. Additional therapy includes aggressive fluid resuscitation, antibiotics, and papaverine as has been previously addressed.[1,6,12,15,30,32] Captopril has been recommended because of the significant increase in angiotensin and its potent mesenteric vasoconstrictive effects, but clinical reports in humans are lacking.[32]

CMI. CMI does not require emergent intervention unless there is AMI in a patient with underlying CMI. Patients with CMI can develop low-flow states, making them susceptible to NOMI in addition to OMI secondary to thromboembolism. Typically, patients with CMI are severely malnourished and require preoperative parenteral nutrition. Resolution of symptoms in patients with CMI requires mesenteric revascularization with the goal of therapy being the restoration of blood flow and alleviating abdominal pain. Successful interventions have included endarterectomy, PTA, and bypass grafting.[6,35]

Angioplasty is considered a reasonable alternative to surgery in patients who are high surgical risks, because the location of the lesion occurs at the origin of the artery making success with angioplasty less likely. Additionally, patients with initial successful PTA have a high recurrence rate requiring repeat PTA or surgical intervention.[12,58] Vascular bypass grafting is the procedure of choice for patients with CMI. Studies have revealed that multiple vessel bypass decreases the recurrence rate from 50% to 11% vs. single vessel bypass.[12] Thus, the vast majority of patients with CMI who present to the ED with abdominal pain will require vascular surgery consultation for definitive intervention.

Summary

AMI is a potentially lethal disease that requires early diagnosis. Due to the lack of physical findings in patients with early mesenteric insufficiency, an aggressive diagnostic approach is recommended in the appropriate clinical setting in order to avoid delays in diagnosis, which have been shown to have a significant impact on mortality. NOMI is a disease that continues to be unrecognized until the clinical picture is far advanced. Only clinicians with a high index of suspicion in those patients with the appropriate risk factors will suspect NOMI, which will facilitate an early diagnosis prior to the onset of intestinal necrosis, gangrene, peritonitis, and cardiovascular collapse.

Patients suspected of having AMI require early surgical consultation, and elderly patients with undiagnosed abdominal pain also need surgical consultation. A major pitfall is the failure of emergency physicians to obtain angiography in patients older than 50 with more than two hours of abdominal pain who have risk factors for AMI. Failing to obtain angiography results in failing to diagnose patients while they are still salvageable. Clinical judgement must prevail, and evaluation should be individualized.

References

1. Kaleya R, Sammartano R, Boley S. Aggressive approach to acute mesenteric ischemia. *Surg Clin North Am* 1992;72: 157-184.
2. Moneta G, Lee R. Diagnosis of intestinal ischemia. In: Rutherford R. *Vascular Surgery Vol. 2.* Philadelphia: WB Saunders; 1995:1267-1278.
3. McGovern R, Franco R. Acute mesenteric ischemia after colonoscopy. *Am J Gastroenterol* 1995;90:170.
4. Taylor L, Porter J. Treatment of acute intestinal ischemia caused by arterial occlusions. In: Rutherford R. *Vascular Surgery Vol 2.* Philadelphia: WB Saunders; 1995:1278-1285.
5. Halkin A, Leibowitz, D. Management of acute mesenteric ischemia. *New Engl J Med* 1996;335:594.

6. Flinn W, Bergan J. Visceral ischemic syndromes: Obstruction of the superior mesenteric artery, celiac axis, and inferior mesenteric artery. In: Sabiston D, et al. eds. *Textbook of Surgery: The Biological Basis of Modern Surgical Practice.* Philadelphia: WB Saunders; 1997:1750-1759.
7. Stern J. Arteries to the gut and to its associated structures. In: *Essentials of Gross Anatomy.* Philadelphia: FA Davis Company; 1988:214-223.
8. Sterns E. Acute abdominal pain. In: *Clinical Thinking in Surgery.* Norwalk: Appleton and Lange; 1988:359-374.
9. Silen W. The principles of diagnosis in acute abdominal disease. In: *Cope's Early Diagnosis of the Acute Abdomen.* 18th ed. Oxford: Oxford University Press; 1991:3-19.
10. Sinanan M. Acute abdomen and appendix. In: Greenfield L, Mulholland M, Oldham K, et al. *Surgery: Scientific Principles and Practice.* Philadelphia: JB Lippincott; 1993:1120-1130.
11. Patel A, Kaleya R, Sammartano R. Pathophysiology of mesenteric ischemia. *Surg Clin North Am* 1992;72:31-41.
12. Levine J, Jacobson E. Intestinal ischemic disorders. *Dig Dis* 1995;13:3-24.
13. Unknown. Acute mesenteric ischemia: Pathophysiology, diagnosis, and treatment. *Disease-a-Month* 1993;39:131-210.
14. Zimmerman B, Granger D. Reperfusion injury. *Surg Clin North Am* 1992;72:65-83.
15. Schneider T, Longo W, Ure T, et al. Mesenteric ischemia: Acute arterial syndromes. *Dis Colon Rectum* 1994;37:1163-1174.
16. Scully R, Mark E, McKneely F, et al. Case records of the Massachusetts General Hospital: Weekly clinicopthological exercises. *N Engl J Med* 1995;332:804-810.
17. Walls R, Ho K. Mesenteric ischemia and infarction. In: Harwood-Nuss A, et al. eds. *The Clinical Practice of Emergency Medicine.* Philadelphia: Lippincott-Raven; 1996; 181-184.
18. Batellier J, Kieny R. Superior mesenteric artery embolism: Eighty-two cases. *Ann Vasc Surg* 1990;4:112-116.
19. Jarvinen O, Laurika J, Sisto T et al. Arteriosclerosis of the visceral arteries. *VASA* 1995;24:9-14.
20. Glover J, Blossom G. Mesenteric ischemia. In: Tintinalli J, Ruiz E, Krome R, et al. *Emergency Medicine: A Comprehensive Study Guide.* 4th ed. New York: McGraw-Hill; 1996:387-389.
21. Rhee R, Gloviczki P, Mendonca CT, et al. Mesenteric venous thrombosis: Still a lethal disease in the 1990s. *J Vasc Surg* 1994;20:688-697.
22. Boley S, Kaleya RN, Brandt LJ, et al. Mesenteric venous thrombosis. *Surg Clin North Am* 1992;72:183-202.
23. Kazmers A. Intestinal ischemia caused by venous thrombosis. In: Rutherford R. *Vascular Surgery Vol 2.* Philadelphia: WB Saunders; 1995:1288-1300.
24. Cecil B, Brandt L. Vascular disorders of the intestine. In: Bennett J, Plumb F. *Cecil Text book of Medicine.* 20th ed. Philadelphia: WB Saunders; 1997:20.
25. Hilaly M, Abu-Zidan F. Mesenteric vein thrombosis: Is it one disease? *Eur J Vasc Endovasc Surg* 1995;9:103-106.
26. Zigrossi P, Campanini M, Borden G, et al. Portal and mesenteric thrombosis in protein s deficiency. *Am J Gastroenterol* 1996;91:163-165.
27. Krummen D, Cannova J, Screiber H. Conservative management strategy for pancreatitis-associated mesenteric venous thrombosis. *Am Surg* 1996;62:432-434.
28. Coralnick J, Budin J, Sedarat A. Inferior mesenteric vein thrombosis in Crohn's Disease: CT diagnosis. *J Comput Assist Tomogr* 1996;20:168-169.
29. Reinus J, Brandt L, Boley S. Ischemic diseases of the bowel. *Gastroenterol Clin North Am* 1990;19:319-343.
30. Howard T, Plaskon L, Wiebke EA, et al. Nonocclusive mesenteric ischemia remains a diagnostic dilemma. *Am J Surg* 1996; 171:405-408.
31. Wilcox, M, Howard T, Plaskon L, et al. Current theories of pathogenesis and treatment of nonocclusive mesenteric ischemia. *Dig Dis Sci* 1995;40:709-716.
32. Rivers S, Veith F. Nonocclusive mesenteric ischemia. In: Rutherford R. *Vascular Surgery Vol 2.* Philadelphia: WB Saunders 1995;1284-1289.
33. Gennaro M, Ascer E, Matano R, et al. Acute mesenteric ischemia after cardiopulmonary bypass. *Am J Surg* 1993;166: 231-235.
34. Kim E, Gewertz B. Chronic digitalis administration alters mesenteric vascular reactivity. *J Vasc Surg* 1987; 5:382.
35. Cunningham C, Reilly L, Stoney R. Chronic visceral ischemia. *Surg Clin North Am* 1992;72:231-245.
36. Myers S, et al. Chronic intestinal ischemia caused by intravenous cocaine use: Report of two cases and review of the literature. *J Vasc Surg* 1996;23:724-729.
37. Cipolla D, Boley S, Luchs S, et al. Chronic mesenteric ischemia presenting as chronic diarrhea and weight loss with pneumatosis intestinalis. *Gastroenterologist* 1996;4:134-141.
38. Thompson J, Bragg L, West W. Serum enzyme levels during intestinal ischemia. *Ann Surg* 1990;211:369-373.
39. Kurland B, Brandt L, Delany H. Diagnostic tests for intestinal ischemia. *Surg Clin North Am* 1992;72:85-104.
40. Lange H, Jackel R. Usefulness of plasma lactate concentration in the diagnosis of acute abdominal disease. *Eur J Surg* 1994; 160:381-384.
41. Hockberger R, Henneman P, Boniface K. Mesenteric vascular occlusion. In: Rosen P, et al. *Emergency Medicine: Concepts and Clinical Practice* Vol 2. St. Louis: Mosby; 1992: 1638-1642.
42. Wolf E, Sprayregen S, Bakal C. Radiology in intestinal ischemia. *Surg Clin North Am* 1992;72:107-124.
43. Scholz F. Ischemia bowel disease. *Radio Clin North Am* 1993;31:1197-1218.
44. Klein H, Lensing R, Kosterhalfen B, et al. Diagnostic imaging of mesenteric infarction. *Radiology* 1995;197:79-82.
45. Taourel P, Deneuville M, Praden J, et al. Acute mesenteric ischemia: Diagnosis with contrast-enhanced CT. *Radiology* 1996;199:632-636.
46. Danse E, et al. Acute intestinal ischemia due to occlusion of the superior mesenteric artery: Detection with Doppler sonography. *J Ultrasound Med* 1996;15:323-326.
47. Walker J, Dire D. Vascular abdominal emergencies. *Emerg Med Clin North Am* 1996;14:571-592.
48. Bakal C, Sprayregen S, Wolf E. Radiology in intestinal ischemia: Angiographic diagnosis and management. *Surg Clin North Am* 1992;72:125-141.

49. Jamieson W, et al. Myocardial and circulatory performance during ischemic phase of superior mesenteric artery occlusion. *Can J Surg* 1993;36:435-439.
50. Turegano-Fuentes F, de Tomas-Palacios J, Perez-Diaz D, et al. Acute arterial syndromes in mesenteric ischemia. *Dis Colon Rectum* 1995;38:778-779.
51. Turegano-Fuentes F, Simo Muerza G, Echenaguisa Belda A, et al. Successful intra-arterial fragmentation and urokinase therapy in superior mesenteric artery embolisms. *Surgery* 1995;117:712-714.
52. Gallego A, Ramirez P, Rodriguez JM, et al. Role of urokinase in the superior mesenteric artery embolism. *Surgery* 1996;120:111-113.
53. McBride K, Gaines P. Thrombolysis of a partially occluding superior mesenteric artery thromboembolus by infusion of streptokinase. *Cardiovasc Intervent Radiol* 1994;17:164-166.
54. Hallisey M, et al. Angioplasty for the treatment of visceral ischemia. *J Vasc Intervent Radiol* 1995;6:785-791.
55. Bocchini T, Hoffman J, Zuckerman D. Mesenteric ischemia due to an occluded superior mesenteric artery treated by percutaneous transluminal angioplasty. *J Clin Gastroenterol* 1995; 20:86-88.
56. Rivitz SM, Geller SC, Hahn C, et al. Treatment of acute mesenteric venous thrombosis with transjugular intramesenteric urokinase infusion. *J Vasc Intervent Radiol* 1995;6:219-228.
57. Babu S, Shah P. Celiac territory ischemic syndrome in visceral artery occlusion. *Am J Surg* 1993;166:227-230.
58. Taylor L, Porter J. Treatment of chronic visceral ischemia. In: Rutherford R, et al. *Vascular Surgery Vol 2.* Philadelphia: WB Saunders; 1995;1301-1311.

Peptic Ulcer Disease

Russell Yang, MD, PhD

It seems today that more and more in medicine can be explained by the germ theory. Add to that list peptic ulcer disease. Physicians had become rather dogmatic in assigning the cause of ulcer disease as having "too much acid." Due to very original and exciting research first starting in Australia, we have now established the bacterial etiology of peptic ulcer disease. With this new knowledge comes more precise therapy. Those of us who are seasoned veterans have witnessed the remarkable advances in medicine over the past several decades in regard to ulcer disease. Some remember the bland diet regimens, antiacids, and the development of H_2 blockers, sucralfate, and proton-pump inhibitors—all of which have made ulcer surgery almost an anachronism. It is indeed somewhat curious and ironic that we now return to the relatively simple modality of antibiotics.

This chapter highlights the appropriate diagnosis and management of patients suffering the ravages of *Helicobacter pylori* infection and highlights the new FDA guidelines. Perhaps we were right after all in the "old days" when we told patients they had gastritis. The "itis" is more true now than ever.

Introduction

Helicobacter pylori (H. pylori) is a gram-negative organism named for its spiral shape and predilection for gastric tissue.[1] *H. pylori* infects more than 90% of duodenal ulcer patients and 70% of patients with gastric ulcers.[38] As such, eradication of *H. pylori* represents a major advancement in the treatment of peptic ulcer disease. The exact mechanism by which *H. pylori* causes ulcers is not known, but its eradication reduces the risk of ulcer recurrence from 60-90% to less than 10%.[38] Thus, careful selection of individuals for eradication is cost-effective and can improve the quality of life for those individuals.

With the widespread penetration of managed care, physicians will be increasing their roles in the treatment and management of peptic ulcer disease. Understanding the risk factors and epidemiology as well as the diagnostic methods available for *H. pylori* is important. Furthermore, knowledge of the current treatment regimens is crucial to render effective eradication of *H. pylori.*

Who Gets *H. pylori*?

The epidemiology of *H. pylori* is well-established.[1] *(Please see Table 1.)* Individuals from crowded urban living conditions and poor socioeconomic status have a high prevalence of *H. pylori* infection. Indeed, the *H. pylori* prevalence is twice as high in persons whose incomes are less than $5000 per year as compared to those who earn more than $25,000 per year.[2]

H. pylori is an acquired infection, and the mode of transmission is not clear. In developing countries, infection occurs early so that most individuals are infected in their childhood (approaching

Table 1. Factors Influencing the Risk for *Helicobacter pylori* Infection

Age
Living/lived in a developing country
Crowded urban living conditions
Poor socioeconomic status
Low income
Lower education level
Minority population
Familial infection with *Helicobacter pylori*

Table 2. Possible Mechanisms of Ulcer Pathogenesis by *Helicobacter pylori*

A. Production of locally toxic products, including ammonia, vacuolating cytotoxin, proteases, and lipases
B. Stimulation of a mucosal immune response with release of inflammatory mediators, generation of an antibody response, and production of cytokines (e.g., interleukin-8)
C. Alteration of gastrin secretion and elevated acid secretion

80%).[39] In developed countries, the infection occurs later, with approximately 50% of individuals becoming infected by the time they reach 60 years of age.[3] In the United States, minority populations (black and Hispanic) have an increased rate of *H. pylori* as compared to whites.[4] Furthermore, an individual who has parents or siblings infected with *H. pylori* is much more likely to harbor *H. pylori*.[5] Although the mode of transmission in these studies has not been established, fecal-oral or person-to-person transmission is suspected.[6]

The precise mechanisms by which *H. pylori* causes peptic ulcer disease is not known.[7] *(Please see Table 2.)* Ammonia production by the bacterial urease may cause injury to gastric tissue. *H. pylori* also produces a vacuolating cytotoxin which disrupts gastric epithelial cells. In addition, the protective gastric mucous layer may also be destroyed by proteases and lipases elaborated by *H. pylori.* Stimulation of a mucosal immune response may also cause damage. Furthermore, *H. pylori* does increase gastrin levels, resulting in enhanced acid production, which eventually leads to ulcer formation.[8] Indeed, elevated gastrin levels return to normal following eradication of *H. pylori* in duodenal ulcer patients.[9]

Infection with *H. pylori* is associated with antral gastritis. As noted earlier, a high proportion of duodenal and gastric ulcers in patients not taking nonsteroidal anti-inflammatory drugs (NSAIDs) have *H. pylori* infection. Conversely, only 15-20% of *H. pylori*-infected people develop ulcer disease.[10] Thus, it is probably a culmination of factors, such as age of acquisition, host's health status, and the virulence of the *H. pylori* strain, that leads to ulcer disease.

How Do You Test for *H. pylori* Infection?

Both invasive and non-invasive methods for confirming the presence of *H. pylori* are available.[11-13] *(Please see Table 3.)* Overall, false-negative results occur in about 5-15% of cases using any of these methods.

In patients for whom esophagogastroduodenoscopy (EGD) is indicated, gastric mucosal biopsy specimens can be easily obtained. The specimen can then be tested for the presence of bacterial urease by histological examination or culture. Histologic examination is considered to be the gold standard for the diagnosis of *H. pylori*.[14] Generally, sampling more than one area of the stomach can increase the yield of detection.[11,40] Rapid urease testing is quick and inexpensive when compared to histology, and false-positive results are uncommon (90% sensitivity and nearly 100% specificity). Results are usually available within five hours and yield a sensitivity of 85-90% and a specificity of 95-100%.[13] Urease testing is performed by placing a gastric biopsy specimen in a well with urea and a pH indicator, which signals the change in pH. Thus, if the biopsy specimen contains *H. pylori,* then the enzyme urease degrades the urea to ammonia resulting in a color change. Therefore, given the inexpensive cost of rapid urease testing, histologic examination should be performed when *H. pylori* infection is suspected and the urease test is negative (i.e., when a false-negative rapid urease test is suspected or when histology may yield additional information (e.g., malignancy).[11] Cultures for *H. pylori* are the least sensitive of the invasive testing methods and are primarily a research tool to test for antimicrobial sensitivity.[13]

The nonendoscopic methods for determining the presence of *H. pylori* include serologic/whole blood testing and the recently FDA-approved urea breath test. Qualitative serologic/whole blood testing for antibodies (IgG) to *H. pylori* is inexpensive and about as sensitive (90%) as invasive methods.[37] In a comparison of four commercially available serology tests, the sensitivity ranges from 84% to 97%.[37] Serologic/whole blood testing is used most commonly since it is simple and can be easily performed. However, this methodology is not reliable in confirming *H. pylori* status after eradication since antibody levels fall slowly (over months). In addition, serologic tests do *not* distinguish which patients with dyspepsia actually have ulcer disease.

Urea breath tests offering a 95% sensitivity and specificity are now available and take advantage of urease production by *H. pylori.* Patients drink a liquid containing a non-radioactive (13C) or radioactive (14C) labelled urea. In the presence of *H. pylori,* the bacterial urease hydrolyzes the urea, releasing labelled CO_2, which is absorbed into the blood and then released though expired air.[15] A sample of expired air is sent to the laboratory for examination. The urea breath test is useful to document eradication of *H. pylori* after antibiotic therapy. Recent treatment with bismuth compounds, antibiotics, or proton pump inhibitors (omeprazole or lanzoprazole) can lead to false negative results. Therefore, it is generally recommended that the urea breath test be performed at least four weeks after therapy has been discontinued.[15]

In summary, it not always necessary to perform endoscopy to diagnose *H. pylori.* For the initial diagnosis without endoscopy, serologic testing is the test of choice. When performing endoscopy, the rapid urease assay is less expensive, although histologic examination

Table 3. Diagnostic Testing for *Helicobacter pylori*

Test	Approximate Cost	Sensitivity/ Specificity
Endoscopic biopsy (performed in endoscopy unit)		
— Rapid urease testing	$15	85-90%/95-100%
— Histology	$125	90-100%/90-100%
— Culture/Sensitivity	$250	90%/100%
Non-endoscopic Tests (performed in office)		
— Serum (qualitative)	$10	70-100%/50-100%
— Serum (quantitative)	$75	90-95%/90%
— Whole blood (fingerstick) (qualitative)	$10	80%/90%
— Urea breath test (13C)	$250	95%/95-100%
— Urea breath test (14C)		95%/95-100%

remains the gold standard. For evaluation after eradication therapy, the urea breath test is preferred. *(Please see Table 4.)*

Who Should be Tested for *H. pylori*?

Primary care physicians should test for *H. pylori* in all patients with known ulcer disease including current disease, prior history, or those on maintenance therapy. Furthermore, patients with a history of complicated ulcer diseases (bleeding, penetration, etc.) should also be tested.[38]

H. pylori is associated with gastric adenocarcinoma, and individuals infected with *H. pylori* do have an increased chance of developing cancer (3-6 fold).[16] Furthermore, some gastric non-Hodgkin lymphomas and mucosa-associated lymphoid tissue (MALT) lymphomas are also linked to *H. pylori* infection. In fact, cure of some MALT lymphomas has been reported simply by bacterial eradication.[17] Thus, these individuals should be tested for the presence of *H. pylori*.

It is not known at present if prophylactic eradication of *H. pylori* will prevent the development of gastric cancer in high-risk individuals (i.e., first-degree relatives).

Dyspepsia without demonstrable ulcer disease is very common and is probably secondary to several etiologies. The role of *H. pylori* in these patients has not been established; therefore, routine testing of these individuals is not warranted.[18]

How to Treat for *H. pylori*

Following the above guidelines, the primary care physician should only treat those individuals who test positive for *H. pylori*. NSAID-related ulcers should be treated with antibiotics only if *H. pylori* is present; approximately 50% of patients with NSAID-related ulcers are infected with *H. pylori*.[35]

Table 4. Application of Diagnostic Tests for *Helicobacter pylori*

Test of choice when endoscopy is not indicated
- serology or whole blood testing

Test of choice when endoscopy is performed
- rapid urease assay

Test of choice to confirm eradication
- urea breath test

Conventional anti-ulcer therapy is important for symptomatic relief and to enhance ulcer healing. Most studies have examined the role of H_2 receptor antagonists and proton pump inhibitors in the treatment of *H. pylori.* The four H_2 blockers (ranitidine, cimetidine, nizatidine, famotidine) are equally effective and are generally well-tolerated.[19] Cimetidine has more drug-drug interactions (particularly with warfarin, phenytoin, and theophylline) because of its inhibition of cytochrome p450. The H_2 blockers have no intrinsic anti-*Helicobacter* activity.

The proton pump inhibitors (omeprazole and lanzoprazole) relieve pain and heal ulcers more rapidly than the H_2 receptor antagonists.[20] These agents are well tolerated and may have some intrinsic anti-microbial activity against *H. pylori,* but they are more expensive than the other available agents. The role of other anti-ulcer agents such as antacids and sucralfate is not clear.[21] Misoprostol, a prostaglandin analogue, is indicated only for ulcer prevention in patients on chronic NSAID therapy.[22]

At present, no single antibiotic can reliably eradicate *H. pylori* infection.[23] Because *H. pylori* is a non-invasive organism residing in the mucous layer overlying gastric mucosa, many antibiotics cannot achieve high enough levels of penetration to be effective. Thus, single agent therapy should not be used and can lead to bacterial resistance.

Multiple drug regimens have been studied, and several regimens have received FDA approval. *(Please see Table 5.)* Successful eradication of *H. pylori* is influenced by local resistance patterns and compliance with awkward regimens. In general, high eradication rates are achieved when at least two antimicrobials are combined with either a bismuth compound (e.g., Pepto Bismol), which has topical antimicrobial activity, or an antisecretory agent, such as a proton pump inhibitor or an H_2-receptor antagonist (> 80%).[25] Regimens containing only one antimicrobial agent are not recommended because of cure rates of less than 70%.[23,24]

Two dual drug regimens to eradicate *H. pylori* have been approved by the FDA.[24] Initially, omeprazole plus amoxicillin was shown to be effective against *H. pylori,* but subsequent studies did not confirm its efficacy. More recently, omeprazole plus clarithromycin has resulted in eradication rates of approximately 80%, and this regimen appears to be well-tolerated.[25] Combination therapy with ranitidine bismuth subcitrate and clarithromycin may give slightly higher rates of eradication, but this therapy has been less well studied.[26] At present, it is recommended to add another antibiotic (e.g., tetracycline or amoxicillin) to achieve acceptable eradication rates.[18,24]

Standard triple therapy (bismuth, metronidazole, and tetracycline) for 14 days is the original regimen first reported to successfully

Table 5. Selected *Helicobacter pylori* Treatment Regimens

Dual Therapy

1. Omeprazole (40 mg q D or 20 mg bid)
   or lanzoprazole (30 mg bid)
   + clarithromycin (500 mg bid)
   followed by omeprazole 20 mg qd
   or lanzoprazole (30 mg qd)
   for an additional two weeks

Duration: 14 days

Eradication: 80%

Relative: +++

2. Rantidine bismuth subcitrate (RBC)
   (400 mg bid) +
   clarithromycin (500 mg bid)
   followed by RBC for an additional two weeks

Duration: 14 days

Eradication: 80%

Relative: +++

Triple Therapy

1. Bismuth based
   bismuth subsalicylate (2 tab qid)
   + metronidazole (250 mg qid)
   (or clarithromycin 500 mg tid may be substituted but not yet FDA approved)
   + tetracycline (500 mg qid)
   followed by H_2RA or PPI for two additional weeks

Duration: 14 days

Eradication: > 90%

Relative: +

2. Proton Pump Inhibitor based
   Lanzoprazole (30 mg bid)
   (omeprazole 20 mg bid may be substituted but not yet FDA approved)
   + clarithromycin 500 mg bid
   + metronidazole 500 mg bid
   (or amoxicillin 1000 mg bid)

Duration: 14 days (may be given for 7 or 10 days with slightly less efficacy)

Eradication: > 90%

Relative: ++

eradicate *H. pylori*.[27] This regimen is usually given with an H_2 receptor antagonist or a proton pump inhibitor and results in greater than 90% eradication rates in compliant patients (i.e., adherence to at least 60% of the treatment regimen).[28] Clarithromycin (500 mg bid) can be substituted for metronidazole if nitroimidazole resistance is problematic. Substitution of amoxicillin (500 mg qid) for tetracycline reduces eradication rates to 80%.[23] Similarly, doxycycline could not be substituted for tetracycline.[23] Thus, standard triple therapy is relatively inexpensive, but taking 15-17 pills per day and a relatively high rate of side effects (> 30%) limit its effectiveness.[28] Usually, an H_2 receptor antagonist or proton pump inhibitor is added to the treatment regimen to reduce ulcer pain and to ensure ulcer healing.[18]

Newer triple therapies comprised of a proton pump inhibitor (omeprazole or lanzoprazole) and two antimicrobial agents also provide excellent eradication rates of *H. pylori* (> 90%). These therapies are better tolerated, leading to greater compliance. *(See Table 5.)* These regimens are better accepted because they can be given for only one week, do not contain bismuth, and can be administered twice a day. Usually, one of the antibiotics is clarithromycin since it is able to eradicate *H. pylori* in up to 40% of cases as a monotherapy and because its levels are enhanced in the mucous layer when given with a proton pump inhibitor (omeprazole).[29,30]

The duration of therapy of these regimens can be varied. Per protocol eradication rates for treatment lengths of seven, 10, and 14 days range from 86%, 91%, and 95%, respectively.[31] Thus, patients should be encouraged to adhere to treatment regimens for as long as prescribed, since decreased compliance can render an otherwise acceptable regimen ineffective. The mnemonic "3-2-1" for three drugs given twice a day for one week may be useful in remembering the various drug regimens.

Resistance may occur to metronidazole and to clarithromycin, particularly if either agent is given alone.[25] Bacterial resistance occurs rarely to tetracycline and and amoxicillin but not at all to bismuth.[32,41] Prior antibiotic exposure predicts individual and regional variation and should be considered in selecting an appropriate regimen. Non-compliance is a problem due to the side effects and complexity of the available regimens. To minimize compliance problems, shorter courses of therapy are desired (e.g., 1 week). Additionally, two products are available to help patients adhere to their complex regimens. Helidac therapy is supplied as 14 blister cards, each containing eight bismuth salicylate tablets, four metronidazole tablets (250 mg each), and four tetracycline tablets (500 mg each). Tritec is a combination product of ranitidine and bismuth subcitrate. Although convenient, this combination is more expensive than if each agent were purchased separately.

Thus, selection of the appropriate eradication regimen should be done on an individual basis. Penetration of managed care into the practice of medicine has made decision-making more complicated due to restricted formularies. However, if a regimen is not well-tolerated, even if it is less expensive, it may end up costing more because of more returned office visits, further testing (including repeated endoscopy), or additional eradication regimens and decreased customer satisfaction.

Follow-up After *H. pylori* Eradication

Confirming eradication of *H. pylori* after completing treatment is not routinely required in uncomplicated and symptom-free patients.[33] Confirmation is recommend in patients with a history of refractory or complicated ulcers. Serologic testing is not recommend since slowly declining antibody titers may result in false-positive results. The urea breath test is the test of choice because it is reliable, non-invasive, and should only be performed more than four weeks after the last dose of antibiotics to prevent false-negative results. Endoscopy with biopsy is the most expensive method to confirm eradication.

Management of patients once *H. pylori* has been eradicated is controversial and should be determined on a case-by-case basis. In general, once the antibiotic regimen has been administered, antisecretory treatment with an H_2 blocker or proton pump inhibitor can be given for a patient with complicated ulcer disease. In these patients, confirmation of *H. pylori* eradication is useful. Reinfection rates with *H. pylori* are considered to be low[34] and depend upon the prevalence of *H. pylori* infection, socioeconomic status, age, geographical location, developing vs. developed countries, and timing of follow-up period.[42]

In patients taking NSAIDs who are also *H. pylori*-infected, treatment of their ulcer should involve both eradication of the *H. pylori* and cessation of the NSAID (if possible) since both are independent risk factors for ulcer disease.[35,36]

Conclusions

The discovery of H. pylori has revolutionized the care of the peptic ulcer disease patient. Eradication of *H. pylori* greatly reduces the risk of ulcer recurrence and can eliminate the need for chronic antiulcer therapy. Current regimens have proven effective but are often complex and associated with many adverse effects. In the future, more effective regimens requiring shorter treatment courses and with more favorable side effect profiles will be developed.

References

1. Graham DY, et al. Epidemiology of *Helicobacter pylori* in an asymptomatic population in the United States. *Gastroenterol* 1991;100:1495-1501.
2. Fierdorek SC, Malaty HM, Devans DL, et al. Factors influencing the epidemiology of *Helicobacter pylori* infection in children. *Pediatrics* 1991;88:578-582.
3. EUROGAST Study Group. Epidemiology of and risk factors for *Helicobacter pylori* infection among 3194 asymptomatic subjects in 17 populations. *Gut* 1993;34:1672-1676.
4. Veldhuyzen van Zanten SJO, Pollak PT, Best LM, et al. Increasing prevalence of *Helicobacter pylori* infection with age: Continuous risk of infection in adults rather than a cohort effect. *J Infect Dis* 1994;169:434-437.
5. Drumm B, Perez-Perez GI, Blaser MJ, et al. Intrafamilial clustering of *Helicobacter pylori* infection. *N Engl J Med* 1990;322:359-363.
6. Mitchell HM, Lee A, Carrick J. Increased incidence of *Campylobacter pylori* infection in gastroenterologists: Further evidence to support person-to-person transmission of *H. pylori. Scand J Gastroenterol* 1989;24:396-400.
7. Dunn BE. Pathogenic mechanisms of *Helicobacter pylori. Gastroenterol Clin North Am* 1993;22:43-57.
8. El-Omar EM, Penman ID, Ardill JES, et al. *Helicobacter pylori* infection and abnormalities of acid secretion in patients with duodenal ulcer disease. *Gastroenterol* 1995;109: 681-691.
9. Moss SF, Calam J. Acid secretion and sensitivity to gastrin in patients with duodenal ulcer: Effect of eradication of *Helicobacter pylori. Gut* 1993;34:888-892.
10. Hunt RH. The role of *Helicobacter pylori* in pathogenesis: The spectrum of clinical outcomes. *Scand J Gastroenterol* 1996;31(Suppl 220):3-9.
11. Cohen H, Laine L. Endoscopic methods for the diagnosis of *Helicobacter pylori. Aliment Pharmacol Ther* 1997;11(Suppl 1):3-9.
12. Cutler AF, Harstad S, Ma CK, et al. Accuracy of invasive and noninvasive tests to diagnose *Helicobacter pylori. Gastroenterol* 1995;109:136-141.
13. Loffeld RJLF, Stobberingh E, Arends JW. A review of diagnostic techniques for *Helicobacter pylori* infection. *Dig Dis Sci* 1993;11:173-180.
14. Genta RM, Robason GO, Graham DY. Simultaneous visualization of *Helicobacter pylori* and gastric morphology: A new stain. *Hum Pathol* 1994;25:221-226.
15. Brown KE, Peura DA. Diagnosis of *Helicobacter pylori* infection. *Gastroenterol Clinics of North Am* 1993;22: 105-116.
16. Howden CW. Clinical expressions of *Helicobacter pylori* infection. *Am J Med* 1996;100:27S-34S.
17. Rogerrero E, Zucca E, Pinotti G, et al. Eradication of *Helicobacter pylori* infection in primary low-grade gastric lymphoma or mucosa-associated lymphoid tissue. *Ann Intern Med* 1995;122:767-769.
18. Soll AH for the Practice Parameters Committee of the American College of Gastroenterology. Consensus statement: Medical treatment of peptic ulcer disease. Practice guidelines. *JAMA* 1996;275:622-629.
19. Jones DB, Howden CW, Bruget DW, et al. Acid suppression in duodenal ulcer: A meta-analysis to define optimal dosing with antisecretory drugs. *Gut* 1987;28:1120-1127.
20. Valenzuela JE, Berlin RG, Snape WJ, et. al. U.S. experience with omeprazole in duodenal ulcer. Multicenter double-blind comparative study with ranitidine. *Dig Dis Sci* 1991;36: 761-768.
21. Korman MG. *Helicobacter pylori* eradication: Therapy other than with bismuth or proton-pump inhibitors. *Scan J Gastroenterol* 1996;31 Suppl 220:41-43.
22. Cryer B, Feldman M. Strategies for preventing NSAID-induced ulcers. *Drug Ther* 1994;July:26-32.
23. Chiba N, Rao BV, Rademaker JW, et al. Meta-analysis of the efficacy of antibiotic therapy in eradicating *Helicobacter pylori. Am J Gastroenterol* 1992;87:1716-1727.
24. Unge P, Berstad A. Pooled analysis of anti-*Helicobacter pylori* treatment regimens. *Scand J Gastroenterol* 1996:31(Suppl 22):27-40.
25. Hunt RH. Eradication of *Helicobacter pylori* infection. *Am J Med* 1996;100:42S-51S.
26. Ciociola AA, Webb DD, Turner K. Dual and triple therapy regimens of antisecretory agents and antibiotics for the eradication of *Helicobacter pylori:* An overview. *Scan J Gastroenterol* 1996;31 (Suppl 218):3-9.
27. Graham DY, Law GO, Klein PD, et al. Effect of treatment of

Helicobacter pylori infection on the long-term recurrence of gastric or duodenal ulcer: A randomized, controlled study. *Ann Intern Med* 1992;116:705-708.

28. Graham DY, Law GO, Malaty HM, et al. Factors influencing the eradication of *Helicobacter pylori* with triple therapy. *Gastroenterol* 1992;102:493-496.
29. Goddard AF, Spiller RC. The effect of omeprazole on gastric juice viscosity, pH and bacterial counts. *Aliment Pharmacol Ther* 1996;10:105-109.
30. Gustavson LE, Kaiser JF, Edmonds AL, et al. Effect of omeprazole on the concentrations of clarithromycin in plasma and gastric tissue at steady state. *Antimicrob Agents Chemother* 1995;39:2078-2083.
31. Laine L, Estrada R, Trujillo E, et al. Randomized comparison of differing periods of twice-a-day triple therapy for the eradication of *Helicobacter pylori. Aliment Pharmacol Ther* 1996;10:1029-1033.
32. Olson C, Edmonds A. Primary susceptibility of *C. pylori* to clarithromycin compared to metronidazole in patient with duodenal ulcers associated with *H. pylori* infection. *Gut* 1995;37(Suppl 2):A814.
33. Penston JG. Review article: Clinical aspects of *Helicobacter pylori* eradication therapy in peptic ulcer disease. *Aliment Pharmacol Ther* 1996;10:469-486.
34. Penston JG. *Helicobacter pylori* eradication—Understandable caution but no excuse for inertia. *Aliment Pharmacol Ther* 1994;8:369-389.
35. Laine LA. *Helicobacter pylori* and complicated ulcer disease. *Am J Med* 1996;100:52S-59S.
36. Laine I, Comineli F, Sloane R, et al. Interactions of NSAIDs and *Helicobacter pylori* on gastrointestinal injury and prostaglandin production: A controlled double-blind trial. *Aliment Pharmacol Ther* 1995;9:127-135.
37. Chey WD, Murthy UK, Linscheer WG, et al. A comparison between four different commercially available serology tests for *Helicobacter pylori. Gastroenterol* 1996;110:A80 (abstract).
38. NIH Consensus Development Panel on *Helicobacter pylori* in Peptic Ulcer Disease. *JAMA* 1994;272:65-69.
39. Malaty HM, Evans DG, Evans DJ, et al. *Helicobacter pylori* in Hispanics: Comparison with blacks and whites of similar age and socioeconomic class. *Gastroenterol* 1992;103:813-816.
40. Genta RM, Graham DY. Comparison of biopsy sites for the histopathologic diagnosis of *Helicobacter pylori:* A topographic study of H. pylori density and distribution. *Gastrointest Endoscopy* 1994;40:342-345.
41. Adamek RJ, et al. Primary and acquired *H. pylori* resistance to clarithromycin, metronidazole, and amoxicillin. *Gastroenterol* 1996;110:A48.
42. Van der Ende A, Van Der Hulst RWM, Dankert J, et al. Reinfection versus recrudescence in *Helicobacter pylori* infection. *Aliment Pharmacol Ther* 1997;11(Suppl 1):55-61.

Food-borne Illness

Charles M. Seamens, MD, FACEP
Gary Schwartz, MD, FAAP

The emergency department (ED) physician is often presented with complaints that patients attribute to items that they happened to eat that day. When patients seek advice about whether their complaint might be the result of a food-borne illness, it is important that the ED physician is able to determine what is and is not a foodborne illness, treat the problem, and counsel the patient appropriately. When the index of suspicion for a food-borne illness is high, this information should be reported to the local health department authorities for definitive diagnosis and epidemiological management.

More than 250 different diseases and syndromes have been associated with contaminated food or drink.[1] Estimates of the number of cases of food-borne disease in the United States range from 6.5 to 81 million cases per year, with from 525 to more than 7000 associated deaths.[1] More precise estimates are lacking for two reasons: 1) Patients with food-borne disease often do not seek medical care because the symptoms are mild and self-limited; and 2) oftentimes, the patient or clinician does not recognize the link between food and the illness.[1] In fact, it is estimated that fewer than 5% of food poisoning cases are recognized and reported.[2]

The risk of food-borne illness depends on the type of food, its source of production, how it is prepared and handled, and the consuming host's resistance to the infectious agent.[1] The great majority of food items that cause these diseases are raw or undercooked foods of animal origin, such as meat, milk, eggs, cheese, fish, or shellfish.[3]

Background

The number of food poisoning cases in the United States are increasing, in large part because the eating habits of many Americans have changed over the years. In this regard, Americans have increased consumption of food prepared by commercial service establishments, where food service workers and handlers may be hired with inadequate training or attention to proper sanitation and hygiene. In addition, fresh fruit, vegetables, and other cold food items are now mass produced and sold through large and complex distribution networks, where sanitation quality assurance standards are suboptimal. Imported foods comprise an increasing proportion of the diet and, oftentimes, are shipped from developing countries where food hygiene and basic sanitation measures and protocols are poorly monitored.[3] The size and complexity of these operations can magnify the public health significance of food-borne contamination.[1]

The most common foodborne diseases are infections caused by such bacteria as *Salmonella* and *Campylobacter*, or by viruses, such as Norwalk or hepatitis A.[3] Food poisoning caused by bacteria comprises about two-thirds of U.S. poisoning outbreaks linked to a known etiology.[4] Specifically, about 75% of reported cases of bacterial food poisoning in the United States can be traced to *Campylobacter*, *Salmonella*, *Staphylococcus*, and *Clostridium per-*

Table 1. Food-Borne Syndromes[5,43]

ORGANISM	INCUBATION	DURATION	FEVER	VOMITING	DIARRHEA
S. aureus	1-6 hr	< 24 hr	-	+	+
B. cereus (emetic)	1-6 hr	< 24 hr	-	+	-
B. cereus (diarrheal)	6-24 hr	< 24 hr	-	-	+
C. perfringens	6-24 hr	< 24 hr	±	±	+
Heavy metal	5-120 min	< 24 hr	-	+	-
Norwalk virus	24-48 hr	24-48 hr	+	+	+
ETEC	16-72 hr	5-10 d	±	-	+
EIEC	16-48 hr		+		+
EHEC	1-8 d	5-10 d	-	+	+
Nontyphoidal *Salmonella*	6-48 hr	< 7 d	+	±	+
Typhoidal *Salmonella*	1-3 wk	3-4 wk	+	+	+
Shigella	16-72 hr	1 d-1 mo	+	+	+
Campylobacter	16-48 hr	3-5 d	+	+	+
V. parahemolyticus	5-24 hr	1-3 d	+	+	+
Ciguatera	1-30 hr	wks-mos	-	+	+
Scombroid	10-180 min	4-6 hr	-	-	+
Paralytic shellfish	5 min-4 hr	hrs-days	-	±	±
C. botulinum	12-36 hr	wks-mos	-	-	-
MSG	< 1 hr	1-6 hr	-	-	-

fringens. The pathogenesis of diarrhea associated with foodborne illness involves either a) the production of enterotoxin causing secretory diarrhea; b) inflammation from a cytotoxin; or c) direct invasion of intestinal mucosa by the organism.[5] Toxin-mediated gastroenteritis is caused by ingestion of performed toxin or by toxin produced after ingestion and is characterized by watery diarrhea and the absence of fever, vomiting, or bloody diarrhea.[5] Syndromes caused by ingestion of performed toxins are characterized by a shorter incubation period of 1-6 hours and a shorter duration of illness, usually less than 12 hours.[5] In contrast, syndromes caused by *in vivo* production of toxin or by direct mucosal invasion are characterized by a longer incubation period (6-72 h) and a longer duration of illness (1-10 d).[5] *(Please see Table 1.)* One clinical feature that suggests a toxin or chemical etiology rather than an infectious cause is the simultaneous occurrence of gastrointestinal and neurologic signs and symptoms.[6]

Spectrum of Food-Borne Syndromes

Campylobacter. *Campylobacter* has surpassed salmonella to become the most common cause of bacterial food poisoning.[7] This is somewhat surprising since the organism was not considered a human pathogen until the 1970s; currently more than 2 million cases of human *Campylobacter* infections are reported in the United States each year.[8] Interestingly, one factor that has been cited to explain the increased incidence of *Campylobacter* infections, is the change in food consumption, away from red meat in favor of poultry in a cholesterol-conscious socitey.

Campylobacter, which infects more than half of the chickens in the United States,[9] requires a body temperature of approximately 40°C for incubation, making poultry an ideal source host.[10] Also contributing to the high rate of infection are the methods by which chickens are raised. Most chickens sold in the United States are produced by the broiler method, which involves raising large number of chickens in enclosed areas with unlimited food and water. These chickens frequently become infected within the first two or three weeks of life and remain infected until they are harvested at 6-7 weeks of life. In addition to becoming infected in the chicken houses, chicken meat also can be cross-contaminated when infected chicken meat is mixed with non-infected meat at the processing plant. Water, unpasteurized milk, and red meat are less common sources of *Campylobacter* infection. Sick pets, such as dogs and cats, may also be a source of infection.[11] *Campylobacter* rarely is spread person-to-person. If this does occur, it is usually spread among young children.

Campylobacter is derived from a greek word meaning "curved rod." There are multiple species of *Campylobacter*, but only four that are pathogenic in humans, *C. jejuni, C. coli, C. lari,* and *C. upsaliensis*. Most important of these species is *C. jejuni,* which causes 90% of human infections.[12] From an epidemiological perspective, infections tend to occur in children younger than 4 years and in adults 15-44 years of age. The peak time of the year for *Campylobacter* infections is May-June, although, most cases of food poisoning caused by campylobacter are sporadic, making it more difficult to identify the exact source.

Campylobacter has an incubation period of 1-7 days, with most patients developing symptoms within 24-72 hours. The organism can cause a range of symptoms from mild diarrhea of brief duration to severe diarrhea, cramps, and gastrointestinal bleeding. In most cases the disease is self limiting, lasting 3-5 days. Malaise may follow for a period of 1-2 weeks. In addition to the gastrointestinal complaints, patients may present with influenza-like symptoms and may have a fever as high as 39-40°C.

Complications from *Campylobacter* are rare and include bacteremia, which is seen in approximately 1% of infected patients and, for the most part, is generally limited to neonates, the elderly, and immunocompromised patients.[13] Of special note is the fact that bacteremic patients are at risk for developing meningitis, cholecystitis, and urinary tract infections. Late complications include Guillain Barré Syndrome (GBS) and reactive arthritis.[14] In fact, it is estimated that up to 40% of GBS may be caused by *Campylobacter* infection; this complication typically occurs anywhere from one to three weeks after the initial infection.[14] Fortunately, death from *Campylobacter* is a rare complication.

Treatment measures beyond supportive care are required only for high-risk patients, such as neonates, the elderly, and immunocompromised patients. Treatment for neonates consists of erythromycin and, for adults, is either erythromycin (500 mg twice a day for 5 days) or a fluoroquinolone. Local resistance patterns should also be considered since there is increasing resistance to fluoroquinolones. Although the disease is self limited, about 10% of infected patients will require hospitalization.[7] Patients may return to work at any time, unless they are involved in catering or health care-related activities, in which case they should return to work only after symptoms have resolved. There is no need to reculture infected patients who have improved clinically.

Salmonella. *Salmonella* is the second most common cause of food poisoning.[7] Although *Salmonella* is ubiquitous, its primary reservoir is in the intestinal tracts of infected or colonized animals, such as chicken, cattle, and pigs, which are sources that commonly infect humans. While fresh fruit and vegetables are less likely to carry *Salmonella*, *Salmonella* can be spread though consumption of eggs. In the past, fecal contamination through small cracks in the egg shell lead to infected eggs. This method of contamination is much less likely due to improved sanitary conditions. Presently, most eggs become contaminated through transovarian spread with an intact shell. Still, it is estimated that each year one in every 50 egg consumers will be exposed to *Salmonella*-contaminated eggs; overall, about three-quarters of all *Salmonella enteritis* outbreaks being traced back to infected eggs.[15] In the past, pet turtles spread *Salmonella* to children, but these turtles have been banned from sale since 1975.

Interestingly, *Salmonella* food poisoning is more common in industrialized countries than it is in less developed, emerging countries where good sanitation is less common. It has been suggested that less developed countries tend to grow food locally and process it on a smaller scale, which minimizes cross contamination. Additional reasons for higher infection rates among industrialized countries include the practice of feeding animals meat packing byproducts, which may be infected, and overcrowding on farms and in slaughter houses.

Salmonella is a gram-negative rod that causes infection though ingestion of the organism. There are several thousand subtypes of *Salmonella*, but fewer than 200 of these infect humans. Approximately one-half of *Salmonella* infections are caused by *S. typhimurium* and *S. enteriditis*.[16] *Salmonella* species are sensitive to heat and acid and, therefore, are frequently killed by cooking or by gastric acids in the stomach. For this reason, a large inoculum is typically required to cause infection. Organisms that survive passage through the stomach will attempt to invade the intestinal mucosa of the distal ileum or proximal colon and replicate. Although the precise manner by which salmonella causes symptoms is not yet known, it is thought to be due to inflammatory mediators.

Infections most commonly occur in the warmer months, with a peak incidence in August and September. Most infections occur in children younger than 5 years, with a higher incidence in children younger then 1 year, and in adults older than 60 years. Patients at highest risk for infection include those who are immunocompromised, have low gastric pH (patients on H2 blockers, post gastrectomy, etc.), have altered gastrointestinal motility, have altered intestinal flora (on antibiotics), or have diabetes.

Gastroenteritis is the most common presentation of *Salmonella* infection. Typically, symptoms occur 6-48 hours after ingestion, but can have a shorter onset with larger inoculum sizes.[17] The illness usually begins with nausea, vomiting, myalgias, headache, and diarrhea. The diarrhea may be mild or severe and may present with gross blood per rectum. Abdominal cramps are present in three-quarters of patients.[18] Temperature elevation to 38-39°C is common and usually lasts less than two days, unless the patient is infected with *S. typhi*, in which case the fever can persist for weeks. Unfortunately, the presentation in the elderly, who are at high risk of complications, may be varied. Laboratory testing is nonspecific and usually includes a normal peripheral white blood cell count and moderate number of white cells and red cells on microscopic examination of stool.

Most patients with *Salmonella enteritis* will have a self limiting disease and should do well with supportive care measures such as good fluid intake. More aggressive treatment, including antibiotics, is warranted in neonates, the elderly, and in other immunocompromised patients who are at risk for systemic illness. The systemic complications of *Salmonella* infection typically begin with bacteremia, which is observed in 5-10% of high-risk patients.[18] The antibiotic of choice for adults is a fluoroquinolone.[19] For neonates, the preferred agents are ampicillin, trimethoprim-sulfamethoxazole, and ceftriaxone.[20] Treatment should begin within 48 hours from the onset of illness in order to be maximally effective.[21] Immunocompetent patients usually are not treated since the disease is self limited and antibiotics may prolong the excretion of the organism.[23-25] Furthermore, resistance to the antibiotic can occur with unnecessary treatment.[18]

In addition to bacteremia, reactive arthritis occurs in approximately 5% of infected patients and can last for years.[25] This disability has been correlated with radiographic evidence of joint damage. A clinical risk factor for arthritis is prolonged diarrhea during the acute illness. Another complication is prolonged excretion of the organism because of a chronic carrier state. Osteomyelitis, which can result from *Salmonella* bacteremia, is a complication most often encountered in patients with sickle cell anemia.

Prevention primarily involves limiting cross contamination in processing plants and food preparation areas. This should include preventing cross contamination by kitchen utensils and thorough hand washing. Fortunately, the organism can be killed from thorough cooking. Eggs cooked at 140°F and maintained at this temperature for 26 seconds, or at 160° for only 10 seconds, should be free of *salmonella*.[26] Food heated to the appropriate temperature in a microwave oven may not be free of contamination because of uneven heating.[27]

***Escherichia coli* O157:47.** This cause of food poisoning has received much attention in the past several years due to a number of outbreaks in fast food restaurants and meat packing plants. First isolated only 16 years ago in Michigan and Oregon, *E. coli* O157:47 is now known to be present throughout the world.[28] Most cases are reported in the United States and Canada. Ground beef is the primary source of *E. coli* infections in humans. Infection can result either directly from infected cattle or from cross contamination when large amounts of ground beef are mixed together. Infected meat can cause significant numbers of ill people since only a small number of bacteria are needed to cause illness. *E. coli* is not known to cause disease in cattle. Therefore, even healthy animals may transmit the organism. Other possible sources include unchlorinated water supplies, swimming in fecally contaminated lakes, or person-to-person transmission. The latter is a significant problem affecting young children in daycare and the elderly in nursing homes.[29,30]

E.coli O157:H7 is a gram-negative, noninvasive pathogen that attaches to the gastrointestinal mucosa. It is the third leading cause of diarrhea in regions of the United States. In patients with *bloody* diarrhea, *E. coli* can be isolated in much higher percentage of stool cultures. The disease caused by this pathogen is thought to be mediated by two cytoxins. These cytoxins are similar to those produced by shigella, and are called shigella-like toxins (SLT) 1 and 2.

Infections most commonly occur during the warm months—June through September—with an incidence as high as 6.1 infections per 100,000 per year in children younger than 5 years old.[31] The incubation period is as short as one day, or as long as eight, and averages between three and four days. After the incubation period, infected patients can present with a spectrum of clinical manifestations that may include bloody diarrhea, hemolytic uremic syndrome (HUS), or death. The illness typically begins with severe cramps and non-bloody diarrhea that turns bloody by the second or third day of illness. The cramps can be severe enough to mimic an acute abdomen. Bloody diarrhea is present in 90% of patients and can be of variable severity.[32] Diarrhea typically lasts 3-7 days, with 10-11 stools on the worst day. Nausea and vomiting are common complaints, affecting one-half of these patients.[32] An elevated temperature may or may not be present.

Typically, the disease lasts about one week without treatment, although approximately one-fourth of infected patients will require hospitalization.[7] Most hospitalized patients will require only supportive therapy such as intravenous fluids, but some patients will develop HUS (6% of infected patients) and a small percentage (5%) of these patients will die.[33-35]

HUS is the most worrisome complication of *E. coli* O157:47 infection and is a common cause of acute renal failure in children. It usually occurs 5-10 days after the onset of diarrhea and is characterized by microangiopathic hemolytic anemia, thrombocytopenia, and renal failure. Of patients who develop HUS, the mortality is about 5%, with one-third of survivors sustaining a persistent disability.[31] Exactly how the pathogen causes HUS is unknown, but is thought to be mediated by the shigella-like toxins. Central nervous system complications such as irritability, lethargy, seizure, or coma are seen in approximately 30% of patients with HUS.[35] Risk factors for the development of HUS include age younger than 2 years, severe gastrointestinal prodrome, fever, and a leukocytosis (> 12,000 WBCs/mm^3).[34-36] HUS is rarely seen in the absence of bloody diarrhea.

There is controversy as to how this disease is best treated. There is some consensus for a treatment plan that includes supportive care measures *without* antibiotics, since there is speculation that antibiotics may increase toxin release as bacteria are lysed. However, there are no good studies to support this approach, and some authorities use antibiotics at the outset. Antimotility agents are also thought to potentially worsen the condition, and, therefore, are not recommended.[36] Treatment is primarily supportive, with attention to fluid and electrolyte balance and monitoring for the development of complications.

Ciguatera. Ciguatera fish poisoning is the most commonly reported food-borne disease associated with eating fish in the United States; this condition is even more common in the tropics and subtropics.[37,38] The Pacific Islands and Caribbean region are considered endemic areas.[39] In the United States, 90% of cases occur in Hawaii and southern Florida, but even fish caught in North Carolina waters have been implicated in ciguatera poisonings.[37] Due to travel and importation of ciguatoxic fish, outbreaks have the potential to occur anywhere.[37] Disease may occur in nonendemic areas in individuals who have consumed fish caught in endemic areas that have been transported into nonendemic areas, and in individuals consuming infected fish in endemic areas and then flying home to nonendemic areas shortly thereafter.[37,38,40] Hence, cases of ciguatera poisoning have been diagnosed in nonendemic states, among them Texas, Louisiana, New York, Massachusetts, and Maryland. The incidence is probably underestimated because the disease is not always recognized, it is misdiagnosed, or it goes unreported.[37,41]

Ciguatera outbreaks have been reported in association with the ingestion of more than 400 species of fish.[6] Grouper, red snapper, amberjack, and barracuda are the most common species of fish implicated.[6,41] Species known to be toxic in a significant percentage of cases are often barred from sale because of the fear of ciguatera poisoning (e.g., barracuda in southern Florida). Interestingly, ciguatoxic fish look, smell, and taste normal.[42,43]

Ciguatoxin is a naturally occurring toxin found in algae-associated microorganisms that live in coral reefs.[37,41] The ciguatoxins become concentrated in larger fish, making them more toxic.[37,40] Ciguatera does not appear to harm the sea creatures and produces toxicity only in birds and mammals that feed upon them.[42] Fish merely transport the toxin up the food chain.[41] Becaue the toxin appears to be concentrated in the head, viscera, and roe, these parts of the fish should never be eaten.[41]

The ciguatera syndrome may actually be caused by eight or nine ciguatoxins.[44] The toxins, which act as sodium channel agonists in nerve, muscle, and cardiac cells, are odorless, colorless, tasteless, and both heat and acid stable.[37] Moreover, these toxins are unaffected by normal cooking procedures and they cannot be eliminated by salting, drying, smoking, or marinating.[37,38]

People of all ages can be affected. Symptoms are highly variable and frequently subjective.[44] The same fish may produce mild symptoms in some patients, while other persons may exhibit a more severe illness.[40] Geographic and seasonal differences in the number of ciguatoxic fish, the mixture of toxins, and patient susceptibility account for variability in clinical symptomatology of symptoms.[44] Not surprisingly, children seem to be more sensitive. A history of multiple ciguatoxin exposures has been linked to progressively more severe symptoms with each exposure.[38] Death may occur in patients who have eaten parts of the fish that contain higher levels of the toxin.[38]

Clinical manifestations appear 2-30 hours (mean, 5 hours) after eating a toxic fish.[6,40] Duration, severity, order, and occurrence of symptoms may vary considerably. Gastrointestinal symptoms lasting 1-2 days are often the first manifestations of poisoning and include abdominal pain, nausea, vomiting, painful defecation, and diarrhea.[37,40]

Neurologic symptoms are the most bothersome and persistent complaints.[37] Paresthesias and sensory reversal of hot and cold sensation has been considered the symptomatic hallmark of ciguatera poisoning; these symptoms may occur within three hours of ingestion of contaminated fish.[43,44] Pruritis and paresthesias, described as uncomfortable tingling sensations, most often develop in the extremities, oral cavity, and pharynx.[37,40] Perceptions of loose teeth and ataxia can occur.[38,42] Pupillary size, reflexes, and body temperature are normal.[37] Neurological symptoms usually resolve after 1-2 weeks.[38] Pain, paresthesias, pruritis, and weakness may persist for several weeks, followed by an increase in symptoms following ingestion of animal proteins.[40] Chronic symptoms have been reported and may be the result of permanent nerve damage.[44]

Cardiovascular symptoms often occur within 2-5 days after ingestion.[37] Bradycardia, hypotension, and T wave abnormalities have been reported.[37,40,41] Bradycardia has been associated with the amount of fish eaten and the size of the fish and is more common in older victims.[41] Ciguatoxin causes an increase in parasympathetic tone and impairs sympathetic reflexes.[38] Pulmonary edema also has been reported.[44] Cardiovascular symptoms usually resolve within five days after onset.[38] Other symptoms include dysuria, chills, sweating, vertigo, neck stiffness, rash, a metallic taste, and polymyositis.[40]

Breast-fed infants also may be at risk because mothers with ciguatera poisoning who breast feed have reported excessive nipple pain and diarrhea in their infants.[37,38,40] It also may be possible to transmit ciguatera through sexual intercourse. Because ciguatoxin is concentrated in the gonads of fish, the same has been suggested of humans.[38]

Symptoms, which may vary in severity, tend to disappear in a few days, however, they may become chronic and last for months or even years.[40,41,44] Patients may become sensitized to the toxin, with symptoms initially disappearing, only to return at a later date following ingestion of alcohol or animal protein.[37,44]

Treatment of ciguatera remains symptomatic and supportive.[38,40] Successful management of neurologic symptoms has been accomplished with IV mannitol (1 g/kg),[44] which is most effective if given within the first 48 hours of symptoms, but may still be moderately effective if administered after that time. Mannitol may provide some relief even after several months.[37,44] Mannitol does not seem to affect cardiovascular or gastrointestinal symptoms, but it does reduce the severity and duration of neurological symptoms.[38] The mechanism of mannitol's effect is obscure.[40] It should be used with caution in patients with severe dehydration caused by vomiting.[38] Amitriptyline, tocainide, and mexilitene have been shown to be of some symptomatic benefit.[37,41,43] Some experts recommend that steroids, opiates, and barbiturates be avoided in this disease.[37]

Ciguatera is rarely fatal, but morbidity is high and symptoms may be debilitating and prolonged.[37,40] It is difficult to diagnose ciguatera with any degree of confidence because reliable methods for detecting ciguatoxins in humans are not widely available.[40,43,44] However, ciguatoxin can be detected by commercially available test kits, using a stick-enzyme immunoassay.[42] Rapid immunoassays for identification of ciguatoxic fish are currently being developed.[37]

Scombroid. In contrast to ciguatera, in which the fish are toxic when caught, fish responsible for causing scombroid become toxic *after* they are caught.[6] Scombroid is caused by improper refrigeration of fish, which encourages bacterial growth and degradation of the fish flesh, resulting in the conversion of histidine to histamine.[42] Bacterial growth also produces a histamine-like toxin, saurine.[6] Both of these substances are unaffected by normal cooking temperatures.[37] Fish of the scombroid family, including bluefin and yellowfin tuna, skipjack, and mackeral, are usually responsible for this condition. Such non-scombroid fish as dolphin fish (mahimahi) or marlin may also produce this syndrome.[6,42,44] These fish often have a bitter, peppery, or metallic taste. Unfortunely, they also may taste, smell, and appear perfectly normal.[6,42,43]

Symptoms consist of an histamine-like reaction, which occurrs 10-30 minutes after ingestion. These include flushing, rash, hot sensations of the skin (especially of the head and face), headache, dizziness, burning sensation on the mouth and throat, diarrhea, and, rarely, bronchospasm.[37,42,44,63] Symptoms are usually self limited and resolve after 3-6 hours. Antihistamines such as diphenhydramine are effective.[44]

Paralytic Shellfish Poisoning. The symptoms of paralytic shellfish poisoning begin shortly after ingestion. A gastrointestinal prodrome is seen during the first 30 minutes to several hours, followed by sensory disturbances of the face and limbs.[6,42,43] Saxitoxin, the principal offender, blocks sodium channels and inhibits peripheral nerve conduction.[42,43,45] Disturbances include paresthesias of the mouth, lips, face, and fingertips. This is followed by dysphagia, dysphoria, and weakness.[45] Paralytic features predominate during the next few hours.[42] Most deaths associated with paralytic shellfish poisoning are caused by saxitoxins and occur within the first 12 hours of ingestion; the deaths result from diaphragmatic paralysis and respiratory depression.[43,45,46]

The diagnosis is suggested by a recent history of mussel or scallop consumption, appearance of typical symptoms, and detection of toxin in the uneaten shellfish.[44,45,46] There are no antitoxins available and treatment is supportive. Ingestion of alcohol increases absorption of the toxin.[46] Lavage may help remove unabsorbed toxin.[46] Cooking does not destroy the toxin.[45]

Other Seafood Toxins and Syndromes. Poisonous seafood produces a number of different toxins that are capable of producing a variety of syndromes. Diarrhetic shellfish poisons, such as okadic acid, pectenotoxins, and dinophysistoxins, produce gastrointestinal disorders such as diarrhea.[44] Domoic acid, which is found in mussels and dungeness crab, causes the syndrome of amnesic shellfish poisoning.[42-44]

Neurologic shellfish poisoning is caused by the brevitoxins, a heat stable neurotoxin that can be aerosolized by the surf and produces transient respiratory and mucous membrane irritation.[43,44] Brevitoxins also cause neurological dysfunction, such as paresthesias, reversal of hot and cold sensations, ataxia, depression of cardiovascular and respiratory function, and such GI symptoms as nausea, vomiting, and diarrhea.[44-45] Palytoxin-induced symptoms consist of severe headache and paresthesia followed by paralysis.[44] Palytoxin is a coronary vasoconstrictor. Ischemia is widespread, causing anoxia in major organs.[44] Palytoxin may cause symptoms similar to ciguatera, as well as intense muscle contractions and rhabdomyolysis.[37]

Puffer fish poisoning from tetrodotoxin causes symptoms within 30 minutes of ingestion and begins with parasthesias, usually tingling of the tongue and mouth; this progresses to vomiting, diarrhea, abdominal pain, and ultimately, ascending motor paralysis, hypotension, respiratory failure, and death.[47-49]

Nonparalytic shellfish poisoning is a relatively mild form of seafood poisoning.[42] Symptoms typically occur within three hours of ingestion and consists of a syndrome of gastrointestinal and sensory disturbances of face and limbs, including paradoxical sensory disturbances with reversal of hot and cold sensation.[42] Motor, respiratory, and bulbar musculature are not affected.[42] *(See Table 2.)*

Staphylococcus aureus **Intoxication.** *S. aureus* is the most common cause of toxin-related food poisoning in the United States.[5] Because its symptoms are frequently self-limited, the true incidence of this syndrome is likely much higher.[43] Intoxication occurs from preformed toxins, which accumulate in foods that have been inadequately refrigerated.[43] Food that typically causes *S. aureus* poisoning has previously been cooked and contains a large proportion of protein, salt, and sugar.[43,51,52] Staphylococci thrive in high concentrations of salt and sugar that other organisms cannot tolerate.[53] Meat and meat products, especially ham and chicken, are most commonly implicated. Other implicated foods include fish and shellfish, milk and milk products, cream filled cakes, and potato and macaroni salads.[43,52,54] Since toxigenic staph are ubiquitous, most foods are contaminated with small numbers of viable organisms at some point before consumption.[51] Even foods from cans and jars have been implicated.[53]

Improper storage of previously cooked food is most often implicated as a cause, but contaminated equipment and poor personal hygiene may also account for transmission of disease.[52] In most instances, it is the food handler who contaminates the food.[54] However, only about one-third of implicated food handlers had lesions on their hands or nose indicative of staphyloccal infection (e.g., furuncles).[52] Between 30% and 50% of the general population carry *S.aureus* and one-third to one-half of these carry enterotoxigenic strains.[54]

Five Staphylococcal enterotoxins have been identified: A, B, C, D, and E.[55] Staphylococci that produce A or A and D together account for the majority of cases of food poisoning.[52,55] Temperatures normally used for cooking will not destroy these heat-resistant toxins. Since staphylococci enterotoxin are colorless, odorless, and tasteless, foods containing the toxins usually look and taste normal.[42,51,53,55]

Staphylococcal food poisoning occurs rapidly after ingestion of the contaminated food.[43] The incubation period may vary in relation to individual susceptibility, the amount of toxin in the food, and the amount of food ingested.[53] Sudden onset of nausea, vomiting, abdominal pain, and watery diarrhea usually occurs 30 minutes to eight hours after eating contaminated food.[5,52,53] Fever is rare, and symptoms usually last less than 12-24 hours.[5,43,52]

Treatment is supportive; attempts to eradicate staphylococcus with antibiotics are not recommended since this disease is toxin-mediated.[43] Definitive diagnosis can be made by culturing the implicated food, the vomitus, or the stools of the patient.[43] Because the illness is mediated by toxins and not infection, secondary transmission does not occur.[43] Although the duration of illness is short and almost always self-limited, the hospitalization rate may be as high as 14% and a few deaths have occurred.[52,53]

Bacillus cereus **Intoxication.** *Bacillus cereus* is a ubiquitous aerobic, spore forming, gram-positive rod that produces gastrointestinal illness. As with other food-borne illnesses, the incidence is under-reported because the illness is self-limiting and, usually, is not severe.[56] If the illness is reported, it still may go undetected because not all state public health laboratories make *B. cereus* testing routinely available.[56]

Although the spore is not particularly heat stable, spores of some strains are able to withstand relatively high temperatures, particularly if the food has a high fat content, which seems to have a protective effect.[57] Meat has been identified as a vehicle of transmission in multiple outbreaks of *B.cereus*, but the illness is most commonly associated with fried rice.[58] *B.cereus* is frequently present in uncooked rice.[56] If the cooked rice is maintained at room temperature while it drains, spores can germinate and a heat stable enterotoxin is produced that can survive brief heating such as stir frying.[5,43,56,57] Toxin production is enhanced by the addition of protein in the form of egg or meat.[57] Consequently, the enterotoxin may be preformed in the food or it may be produced within the small intestine.[57]

B. cereus not only produces gastrointestinal illness, but it is also responsible for nongastrointestinal infections including wound infections, infections of lines and shunts, ocular infections, primary cutaneous infections, endocarditis, CNS infections, and respiratory infections.

B. cereus causes two distinct gastrointestinal syndromes: an acute emetic syndrome within 1-6 hours of consumption and a diarrheal syndrome 8-16 hours after ingestion.[43] In the emetic syndrome, low numbers of contaminating organisms produce a heat stable enterotoxin that is consumed.[43] The preformed toxin is stable to trypsin, pepsin, and pH extremes.[43,56,58] The clinical presentation of the emetic syndrome caused by *B. cereus* food poisoning is characterized by the acute onset of nausea, vomiting, and abdominal pain, which usually resolve within about 10 hours.[5,43] Diarrhea occurs in one-third of patients.[57] In particular, the emetic syndrome is strongly associated with ingestion of fried rice obtained from

Table 2. Toxins and Syndromes

TOXIN	SYNDROME
Ciguatoxin	Ciguatera
Histamine, saurine	Scombroid
Saxitoxin	Paralytic shellfish poisoning
Domoic acid	Amnesic shellfish poisoning
Tetrodotoxin	Pufferfish poisoning
Brevitoxin	Neurologic shellfish poisoning
Okadaic acid	Diarrhetic shellfish poisoning

Chinese restaurants.[43,57] The emetic syndrome is more common than the diarrheal syndrome, which is associated with ingestion of a variety of prepared foods that have been inadequately refrigerated.[43] The diarrheal syndrome is mediated by a heat-labile enterotoxin that is produced in vivo after ingestion of the organism.[5]

This enterotoxin is sensitive to heating, proteolytic enzymes, and acids.[56,58] Abdominal cramps and profuse watery diarrhea develop 6-24 hours after ingestion and lasts 24 hours.[5,56,57] Vomiting is unusual and fever is uncommon.[12,25,56,58] The diarrheal syndrome resembles *C. perfringens* food poisoning.[25]

Supportive therapy is usually not needed, and the patient recovers within 24 hours.[57] There is no role for antimicrobial therapy.[57] Diagnosis is complicated by natural contamination of many foodstuffs with spores, and the detection of *B.cereus* in the absence of clinical symptoms may not always signify food-borne disease.[57] Stool cultures are not generally useful in *B.cereus* intoxication.[58] In most cases, expensive reference laboratory biological tests are needed to conclusively prove the presence of toxigenic strains and to establish an association between foodstuffs and symptoms.[57]

Clostridium perfringens. *Clostridium perfringens* is an anaerobic, spore-forming, gram-positive bacillus.[43] It is present in human (95% of normal adults harbor *C. perfringens* in their stool) and animal feces, soil, water, and air, and is a contaminant of most commercially available meat and poultry products.[51,52] Five types of *C.perfringens* are recognized, and most cases of self-limited diarrheal disease are caused by Type A strains.[55] The 24-hour illness caused by type A organisms is found almost exclusively in meat and poultry products when there has been a delay between cooking and consumption of the meat products.[43] Type C strains can cause severe hemorrhagic necrotizing jejunitis accompanied by bloody diarrhea, severe abdominal pain, and shock; these strains are uncommon in developed countries.[55]

Clostridial spores germinate and multiply rapidly after cooking in foods that have been allowed to sit for 2-3 hours or longer.[43,55] The contaminated food is ingested and a heat sensitive enterotoxin is produced.[43] Ingestion of spores does not produce the illness; the toxin must be produced within the GI tract to cause the illness.[43] The attack rate is approximately 50% in individuals who are exposed to contaminated food.[43]

After an incubation period of 6-24 hours, patients experience epigastric pain, abdominal cramps, and watery diarrhea.[5] Fever, nausea, and vomiting occur less commonly.[5] Symptoms resolve within 12-24 hours.[5,43]

The diagnosis is confirmed by a) identifying the organism in suspected food; b) a high spore count in the patients stool; or c) by isolating organisms with the same serotype from stool and suspected food.[43] The CDC criteria for diagnosis rely on organism and spore counts in food and feces. Serotyping of the isolates can be helpful.[52]

Listeria. The identification of food as the major vector for human listeriosis was made in the early 1980s in an outbreak caused by coleslaw contaminated with *Listeria* from vegetables that had been fertilized with sheep manure.[59] An estimated 1850 persons become seriously ill with listeriosis in the United States each year.[60]

Listeria monocytogenes is a motile, gram-positive rod.[12] It is found in the stools and the female genital tract of 1% of normal individuals.[43,59] *Listeria* has also been found in dish cloths, kitchen and bathroom drains, refrigerator vegetable compartments, and toothbrushes.[61] The bacterium also has been found in a variety of raw foods, such as uncooked meats and vegetables.[59,60] Vegetables can become contaminated from soil or manure.[60] Chicken seems particularly susceptible to listeria contamination.[62] Foodborne outbreaks of listeriosis associated with lettuce, cabbage, milk, cheese, shellfish, raw vegetables, and turkey frankfurters have been identified.[1,43] When *Listeria* is isolated from processed foods, it is usually not the result of inadequate heating or refrigeration. Rather, food is usually contaminated after processing.[60] *Listeria* is killed by pasteurization, but is unique in its ability to grow at refrigerated temperatures.[4,61] Little is known of the pathogenesis of adult listeriosis. Despite its widespread occurrence, only a minority of people acquire the disease after ingesting contaminated food. Its virulence may depend on the immune status of the individual and the particular strain ingested.[59,62]

Diagnosis is made difficult by a prolonged incubation period. The time between eating the food and the onset of symptoms varies from several days to five weeks. *Listeria* produces a self-limited febrile gastroenteritis, as well as myalgias, arthralgias, and headache.[4] It is not detected by routine stool cultures.[4,59]

Two major types of human listeriosis occur: materno-fetal and adult. Pregnant women are about 20 times more likely than other healthy adults to get listeriosis.[60] Pregnant women develop a self-limiting flu-like illness that may lead to birth complications. The infant may become infected either by transplacental passage of listeria following maternal bacteremia or by contact with infected maternal vaginal secretions. In adults, as well as neonates, listeriosis may present as a meningitis and, sometimes, as a septicemic illness. The adult disease is thought to occur predominately in immunocompromised individuals. Healthy adults and children can occasionally get infected with *Listeria*, but they rarely become seriously ill.[60] The mortality rate of immunocompromised individuals with listeriosis is about 25-30%.[59]

***Vibrio* Infections.** *Vibrio* are curved, gram-negative, flagellated rods so named because they are so motile that they appear to vibrate.[51] In the United States, *Vibrio* infections are most common in states bordering the Gulf of Mexico.[63] Most food-borne illness in the United States caused by *Vibrio* is caused by two species, *V. vulnificus* and *V. parahemolyticus*. *Vibrio* bacteria are natural inhabitants of marine environments and can cause gastroenteritis, wound infections, and septicemia.[63] *V. vulnificus* is commonly found in U.S. coastal waters and, presumably, in all species of coastal shellfish.[64]

V. vulnificus infection more often follows eating raw or undercooked oysters, and *V. parahemolyticus* infection is more likely to be associated with eating shrimp or crabs.[45] *Vibrio* infections may occur in persons who live some distance from the Gulf Coast, but have recently consumed raw shellfish while visiting the Gulf of Mexico.[63] Outbreaks typically occur during the summer and fall when the water is warmer and the *Vibrio* can multiply quickly.[41] The majority of patients with *Vibrio gastroenteritis* have ingested seafood, especially raw oysters, within 37 days before the onset of illness.[63] Consumption of raw clams and other seafood is a less common cause.[63] *Vibrio* contamination does not alter the appearance, taste, or odor of oysters.[65]

V. vulnificus may both invade the mucosa *and* produce a enterotoxin.[55] Therefore, not unexpectedly, fever, chills, and headache in addition to gastrointestinal symptoms, are common manifestations of this infection.[55] GI symptoms include watery or bloody diarrhea, abdominal cramping, nausea, and vomiting.[55,63] The mean duration of illness is about eight days.[63] In the case of *V. parahaemolyticus*, a similar syndrome occurs after an incubation period of 12-24 hours. The duration of illness is about 1-3 days.[45] No treatment is required for *V. parahaemolyticus* as the disease does not seem to be altered by antibiotics.[66,67] Treatment of *V. vulnificus* consists of doxycycline, a third generation cephalosporin, and an aminoglycoside.[68] Patients with liver disease, impaired immune systems, and diabetes should be warned against eating raw or partially cooked molluscan shellfish because of the increased risk of fulminant infections.[64,65]

Hepatitis A Shellfish Infections. Unlike bacteria, viruses do not multiply or produce toxins in food; food items merely act as vehicles for their transfer.[69] Most infections associated with consumption of oysters, clams, cockles, and mussels are viral in origin.[69] Clams, oysters, and mussels harvested from waters contaminated by raw sewage are the most frequent cause of food-borne viral hepatitis A.[43] Soft fruits, such as strawberries and raspberries, have also been implicated.[69] Other foods also have been implicated, but the true source is usually contaminated water.[43] It is difficult to associate a specific food item with the illness because of the long incubation period, which may be as long as 2-8 weeks.[64] Cases of gastroenteritis reported 24 hours after eating shellfish, which is then followed by hepatitis A 3-4 weeks later have been recorded.[69] Symptoms include fever, malaise, jaundice, nausea, and abdominal pain.[43] Diarrhea is rare.[43] There is no carrier state and no chronic state associated with HAV infection.[70] Treatment is supportive.[43] Infection with hepatitis A in chronic carriers of hepatitis B and C is associated with high morbidity and mortality.[71]

Norwalk Virus Infection. Foods most commonly associated with the Norwalk virus include poorly cooked or raw shellfish, especially oysters and clams. Contamination often occurs when these shellfish filter untreated infectious sewage.[72] Contaminated drinking water also has been implicated.[43,73] Steaming shellfish until the shells open does not adequately destroy the virus.[45,74] Outbreaks occur year round and affect older children and adults, but not infants or young children.[75] The infectious virus may be excreted in the feces of food handlers for at least 48 hours after they recover from infections.[75]

Symptoms typically appear 24-48 hours after ingestion of contaminated food products,[43,64] and include the rapid onset of nausea, vomiting, nonbloody diarrhea, cramps, headache, and malaise. These symptoms resolve over a 24-48 hour period.[43] The abdominal symptoms are frequently associated with fever and leukocytosis.[76] Gastroenteritis caused by Norwalk virus is unusual in young children.[39] Older children and adolescents are likely to experience vomiting more frequently than diarrhea, while adults experience diarrhea more than vomiting.[39] Complications are rare and patients usually recover fully.[45]

Treatment with bismuth subsalicylate has been shown to decrease the duration of symptoms.[43] The diagnosis is made by documenting a rise in antibody titer or by identifying the virus in the stool. These tests are not widely available.[43]

Heavy Metal Poisoning. Heavy metal poisoning is a rare cause of gastroenteritis and results from gastric irritation caused by copper, zinc, iron, tin, or cadmium.[6,43,77] These illnesses are uaually associated with acidic or carbonated beverages that have been stored in, or allowed to come in contact with, metal containers or tubing, such as soft drink dispensers or metal containers.[6,43,78,79] Common symptoms of acute heavy metal ingestion caused by copper and tin include bloating, nausea, vomiting, cramps, diarrhea, and a metallic taste that usually occur 5-60 minutes after ingestion.[6,43,79,80] Copper poisoning is suggested by vomitus that is blue or green in color.[81] Cadmium may be found in seafoods such as oysters, clams, and lobsters, as well as grains and peanuts. Cadmium and zinc cause myalgias, nausea, vomiting, abdominal pain, diarrhea, and weakness. Cadmium is also associated with increased salivation.[43,81] Symptoms are usually self limited and abate gradually over hours.[43] The best, although expensive, method to make the diagnosis is to assay for individual heavy metals in the beverage fluid.[43]

Infant Botulism. Botulism is caused by ingestion of *C. botulinum*, an anaerobic, gram-positive, spore producing organism that is both heat and cold tolerant. The organism is found in contaminated foods and is ubuiquitous in the environment. Home-canned asparagus, green beans, peppers, and other vegetables are frequent sources of infection. Jams and jellies are rarely a cause of botulism because their high sugar content prevents growth of *C. botulinum*.[82] In other parts of the world, garlic, fish, and meats are leading causes, but these foods rarely cause botulism in the United States.[83,84] Infants may contract the disease through ingestion of *Clostridial* spores. Contaminated honey is a classic but uncommon source of spores.[85] More frequently, spores are contracted from some other environmental source.[86] After ingestion of spores, the *Clostrdial* toxin must be produced *in vivo* for symptoms to occur. Most environmental exposures of infant botulism have been described in California, Utah, and Pennsylvania where the levels of spores are high.

Infant botulism is the most common form of botulism, and affects children between 2 and 6 months of age.[86] The incubation period can range from three to 30 days. Infant botulism frequently presents as nonspecific symptoms that may include lethargy, weakness, poor feeding, and constipation. On exam, the child will have poor head control and hypotonia, as well as cranial nerve abnormalities such as ptosis and impaired gag and suck reflexes. These symptoms can be difficult to distinguish from those seen in a septic child.

Whereas infants usually ingest the spores, adults typically become infected after ingesting the preformed neurotoxin.The *Clostridial* neurotoxin binds to peripheral nerve endings, where it interferes with the release of neurotransmitters and causes a flaccid paralysis. There are seven different neurotoxin subtypes labelled A-G, but only A, B, and E cause illness in humans.[87]

The presentation of botulism in adults is different than in children. Typically, the incubation period is 12-36 hours, but may take up to 10 days for symptoms to develop.[88] Adults also present with impaired cranial nerve function, which is more easily detected than it is in infants. Other common complaints include difficulty with speech and swallowing, and visual complaints such as blurrred vision and diplopia. As the disease progresses, a descending weakness develops; this is associated with autonomic dysfunction, including dry mouth, urinary retention, and hypotension. Sensation usually remains intact; there is no CNS involvement and sensorium is unaffected.

Triavalent botulism antitoxin is the treatment of choice for botulism and must be administered as soon as possible after symptoms develop. The antitoxin neutralizes only unbound toxin, so patients may not improve immediately after administration, although they should not worsen either. The antitoxin is derived from an equine source, and up to 9% of patients may develop a hypersensitivity reaction or serum sickness.[89] Antibiotic use is controversial, but if antimicrobials are used, penicillin is the drug of choice. Treatment, otherwise, is supportive. Mechanical ventilation may be necessary until the neurotoxin's effects diminish. In adults and children who do not require immediate intubation, respiratory status should still be observed in an intensive care setting. Approximately 80% of affected children will have some degree of respiratory compromise.[90]

Monosodium Glutamate. Monosodium glutamate is a powdered food additive used as a flavor enhancer.[43] Symptoms include a burning sensation, facial pain, chest tightness, headache, nausea, abdominal pain, diaphoresis, and palpitations.[91,92] The association between monosodium glutamate and the classic symptoms of the Chinese Restaurant Syndrome is tenuous. These symptoms may be due to monosodium glutamate or they may be due to a variety of other ingredients such as allergenic proteins (nuts, seafood), preservatives (sulfites, nitrites, etc.), food dyes, or histamine.[92,93] The symptoms are self-limited.

Another, yet uncommon, cause of food-borne illness are parasitic infections. These include Cryptosporidium, Entamoeba histolytica, and Giardia lamblia. Each of these organisms is spread via the fecal/oral route, but can contaminate food and water. The contaminated water can be from a lake, stream, or municipal water supply, since chemical decontamination of drinking water may not kill cryptosporium. Filtration will remove the parasite, but it is not used by all communities treating their water supply. The presenting complaints of a symptomatic patient with parasitic intestinal infection are non-specific, including diarrhea, abdominal cramping, and low-grade fever. To diagnose these types of infection, evidence of parasites should be found on microscopic examination of a fresh stool specimen. Often, multiple stool specimens (3 or more) are needed to make a diagnosis. Mucosa biopsy can also be helpful in making the diagnosis. Treatment for Giardia is metronidazole, while E. histolytica is treated with a combination of metronidazole followed by iodoquinol. Cryposporidium has no effective treatment, but is a self limited disease in immunocompetent patients. Unfortunately, immunocompromised patients can have a prolonged problem if they become infected, and, therefore, should be knowledgeable on how Cryptosporidium is spread in order to avoid possible exposure.

Evaluation of Diarrhea

Most diarrheal disease is mild and self-limited, does not require hospitalization, and does not require laboratory evaluation, unless there is evidence of significant dehydration or systemic toxicity.[94,95] Routine bacteriologic testing is not cost effective and usually does not alter treatment.[96] However, patients who are sick enough to require hospitalization should have a complete blood count with differential and electrolyte studies performed.[95] Enterocolitis with fever, cramping abdominal pain, and blood and mucus in the stools also requires laboratory evaluation.[94]

The practice of dividing diarrheal infections into inflammatory vs. noninflammatory presentations is based on the supposition that a patient with bloody stools, tenesmus, fever, persistent abdominal cramping, and the presence of fecal leukocytes is infected with an invasive bacterial pathogen such as *Shigella* and will require antimicrobial therapy.[96] However, because there is significant overlap among the syndromes caused by bacterial pathogens (i.e., some invasive bacteria cause watery diarrhea without fever, blood, or abdominal pain, as would be typical in cases of noninflammatory diarrhea) the utility of this classification is somewhat limited.[96]

To avoid the unecessary cost associated with culturing every patient with diarrhea, stool cultures should be reserved for patients with blood, mucus, and WBCs in the stool, for those with significant toxicity or dehydration, or for patients with an underlying immunocompromising illness.[95] The most simple and helpful test for identifying patients who may need antibiotics is the stool WBC examination.[94] Fecal leukocytes usually are not present in diarrhea caused by viruses and toxins.[75,97] The yield of positive cultures increases for patients in whom fecal leukocytes are detected.[96] One study found that bloody and watery diarrhea with leukocytes resulted from *Shigella, Salmonellae*, or *Campylobacter* in about 83% of cases.[98] The positive and negative predictive values of the fecal leukocyte test are approximately 45% and 93%, respectively.[96] The absolute fecal leukocyte count is not predictive of a specific infection and their absence does not preclude bacterial diarrhea.[98] For diarrheal disease caused by *Shigella*, the sensitivity of the fecal leukocyte test is about 73%. For other pathogens, the sensitivity is about 50%.[96] It has yet to be proven that patients with fecal leukocytes benefit more from antimicrobial therapy than those without fecal leukocytes.[96]

Stool cultures are indicated to help identify cases in which antimicrobial therapy should be given in order to shorten the course of illness and to prevent spread to contacts.[94] The clinician should be familiar with the capabilities of their hospital's laboratory. Most laboratories are able to test for *Salmonella*, *Shigella,* and *Campylobacter*. The laboratory should be notified of suspicion of less common organisms such as *V. parahemolyticus* or *E. coli* O157:H7.[96]

Collection of stool is optimally performed within 30 minutes of passage.[98] Consequently, although the practice of giving a specimen kit to the patient to take home may be more convenient for the clinician, this approach will likely decrease diagnostic yields. Refrigeration of specimens also may decrease yields inasmuch as cold temperatures decrease viability of *Shigella* and *Salmonella* to some extent.[98] Stool cultures should not be taken with a swab.[98] Two stool cultures will yield a detection rate of 99%, and this appears to be the standard for routine workups.[96]

Salmonella is easily isolated and serotyped.[66] *Campylobacter* must be cultured on selective media and usually must be requested specifically because it is not cultured routinely. Enteropathic *E. coli* (EPEC) testing is complex and expensive.[98] The rate of recovery of *E. coli* O157:H7 is highest during the first few days after the onset of diarrhea and drops off significantly after seven days.[96] A latex agglutination test is available to identify *E. coli* O157:H7.[66] There is no specific culture medium that differentiates Enterohemorrhagic *E. coli* (EHEC) from other pathogenic types of *E. coli,* but sorbitol-MacConkey agar is a good screening media in combination with serotyping.[67] Serologic tests are available, but are not routinely useful.[66] *V. parahaemolyticus* is easily identified by culture.[66] Diagnosis of *V. vulfinicus* infections is made by stool, wound, or blood cultures on special media.[68] *(Please see Table 3.)*

Because many different microorganisms may cause diarrhea, a variety of tests, in addition to bacterial cultures may be needed to

Table 3. Diagnosis of Food-Borne Illness[100]

ORGANISM	DIAGNOSIS
S. aureus	Culture organism in vomitus or food
B. cereus	Culture organism in stool and food
C. perfringens	Culture organism in stool and food
C. botulinum	Demonstrate toxin in stool or food, culture organism in stool
S. enteritidis	Culture organism in stool
C. jejuni	Culture organism in stool
Viral gastroenteritides	Demonstrate virus in stool and antibody in blood
E. coli	Culture organism in stool

establish an etiology.[94] The gram stain can easily demonstrate *C. jejuni*, a gram-negative rod, with sensitivities as high as 94%, and specificities greater than 99%. Unfortunately, the gram stain has no value for detecting any other common pathogen, since these cannot be differentiated from normal stool flora.[96,98]

Laboratory confirmation of the cause of viral food-borne gastroenteritis requires either detection of the virus in the stool or a rise in virus-specific antibody.[39] Identification of viruses that cause gastroenteritis depends largely upon examination of stool specimens by electron microscopy.[69,70] Specimens should be stored without freezing, and should be examined within 48-72 hours after onset of symptoms, after which the virus concentration in stool declines below levels detectable by electron microscopy.[4] Antibody to Norwalk virus begins to develop within five days after onset of illness, peaks within three weeks, and begins to decline by week 6.[39] Enzyme-linked immunosorbent assay (ELISA) and radioimmunoassay tests may be used to detect the Norwalk virus, but they are not widely used.[39,75,95] Polymerase chain reaction (PCR) has shown promise in detection of Norwalk viruses not only in feces and vomitus but also the shellfish itself.[73] Unless PCR is available, it is not practical to examine food remnants because the number of virus particles will be much too low for other currently available detection methods.[69]

Since HAV is excreted mainly before infection is apparent, stool specimens are inappropriate. Laboratory diagnosis of infection depends on detection of specific anti-HAV IgM in serum.[69]

The diagnosis of botulism can be made by detection of the toxin in the serum or stool, or by culturing the organism from stool or gastric samples. Obtaining a stool specimen for analysis may be problematic since constipation is often a problem with botulism. Enema fluid can be cultured as an alternative. Toxin isolation is best done within three days of ingestion, but is positive in only 50% of cases. To distinguish botulism from other paralytic disorders, electromyography may be necessary.

For some cases, antibiotic therapy may be required to minimize the duration of illness, reduce morbidity, or reduce the contagiousness.[95] Several studies have shown that empirical therapy for acute diarrheal disease with fluoroquinolones, regardless of the infecting organism, reduces the number of stools, as well as other signs and symptoms.[96,99] However, ciprofloxacin is no more effective than placebo in reducing the duration of diarrhea in patients with positive bacteriology.[99] Consequently, it seems the precise role of fluoroquinolones in gastroenteritis needs to be further delineated.

Summary

The use of new technologies, such as irradiation of food stuffs, may play a critical role in ensuring the microbial safety of the food supply in the future.[1] In the meantime, people should be counseled to cook their meat thoroughly, and to be sure that juices or drippings from raw meat or poultry do not contaminate other foods.[3]

As the safety of foodstuffs receives more media scrutiny, more patients with concerns about food-borne illness will present to the ED. Emergency physicians will be called upon to make these diagnoses and provide treatment. In this regard, the ED physician must recognize these syndromes, be aware the difficulty in making the diagnosis, but not be tempted to waste resources trying to confirm the precise etiology of all patients who present with food-borne illness. Surveillance summaries on foodborne illnesses can be obtained by writing:

Public Inquiries, Office of Public Affairs, Centers for Disease Control, 1600 Clifton Road, Atlanta, Georgia, 30333.[71]

The authors greatly appreciate the assistance of Keith Wrenn, MD, in the preparation of this manuscript.

References

1. Hedberg CW, MacDonald KL, Osterholm MT. Changing Epidemiology of Food-Borne Disease: A Minnesota Perspective. *Clin Infect Dis* 1994;18:671-678.
2. Chicken: What you don't know can hurt you. *Consumer Reports* 1998;63:12-18.
3. Food and Water Borne Bacterial Diseases @http://www.cdc.gov/ncidod/disease/bacter/foodborn.htm
4. Food poisoning, listeriosis, and febrile gastroenteritis. *Nutr Rev* 55:57-60.
5. Afghani B, Stutman HR. Toxin-related diarrheas. *Ped Ann* 1994;3:549-555.
6. Hughes JM, Horwitz MA, Merson MH, et al. Foodborne disease outbreaks of chemical etiology in the United States, 1970-1974. *Am J Epidem* 1977;105:233-244.
7. Foodborne Diseases Active Surveillance Network. 1996. *Morb Mortal Wkly Rep MMWR* 1997;46:258-261.
8. Allos BM, Blaser MJ. *Campylobacter jejuni* and the expanding spectrum of related infections. *Clin Infect Dis* 1995;20:1092-2101.
9. Humphrey TJ, Henley A, Lanning DG. The colonization of broiler chickens with *Campylobacter jejuni*: Some epidemiological investigations. *Epidemiol Infect* 1993;110: 601-607.
10. Wood RC, MacDonald KL, Osterholm MT. *Campylobacter Enteritis* outbreaks associated with drinking raw milk during youth activities. *JAMA* 1992;268:3228-3230.
11. Blaser MJ, Laforce FM, Wang WL. Reservoirs for Human Campylobacteriosis. *Clinic Res* 1979;27:40A.

12. Tauxe RV, Gargrett-Bean N, Patton CM, et al. *Campylobacter* isolates in the United States, 1982-1986. *Morb Mortal Wkly Rep MMWR* 1988;37:1-12.
13. Skirrow MB, Sutcliffe E, Benjamin J. *Campylobacter bacteremia* in England and Wales, 1981-91. *Epidemiol Infect* 1993;110:567-573.
14. Allos BM. Association between *Campylobacter* infection and Guillain-Barré Syndrome. *J Infect Dis* 1997;176:(S)125-128.
15. *Salmonella enteiditidis* infection. CDC website at http:/www.cdc.gov/ncidod/publications/brochures/salmon.htm
16. Hargrett-Bean NT, Pavia AT, Tauxe RV. *Salmonella* isolates from humans in the United States, 1984-1986. *Morb Mortal Wkly Rep MMWR* 37;(SS-2)25-31.
17. Mintz ED, Cartter ML, Hadler JL, et al. Dose response effects in an outbreak of *Salmonella enteritidis*. *Epidemiol Infect* 1994;112:13-23.
18. Lee LA, Puhr ND, Maloney EK, et al. Increase in antimicrobial resistant *Salmonella* infections in the United States, 1989-1990. *J Infect Dis* 1994;170;128-134.
19. Stanford JP, Gibert DN, Moellering RC, et al. *The Sanford Guide to Antimicrobiol Therapy, 27 Ed.* 1997.
20. Report of the Committee on Infectious Diseases 1997. American Academy of Pediatrics. Elk Grove, IL.
21. Wistrom J, Norrby SR. Fluoroquinolones and bacterial enteritis, when and for whom? *J Antimicrob Chemother* 1995;36:23-39.
22. Smith ER, Badley WD. Treatment of *Salmonella enteritis* and its effect on the carrier state. *CMA Journal* 1971;104:1004-1006.
23. Antibiotics prolong *Salmonella* excretion. *BMJ* 1969: 699-700.
24. Aserroff B, Bennett JV. Effect of antibiotic therapy in acute salmonellosis on the fecal excretion of *salmonella*. *N Engl J Med* 1969;281:636-640.
25. Thompson GT, DeRubeis DA, Hodge MA, et al. Post *Salmonella* reactive arthritis: Late clinical sequelae in a point source cohort. *Am J Med* 1995;98:13-21.
26. Doyle MP. Questions and answers. *JAMA* 1994;272:895.
27. Evans MR, Parry SM, Ribeiro CD. *Salmonella* outbreak from microwave cooked food. *Epidemiol Infect* 1995;115:227-230.
28. Riley LE, Remis RS, Helgerson SD, et al. Hemorrhagic colitis associated with a rare *Escherichia Coli* serotype. *N Engl J Med* 1983;308:681-685.
29. Carter AO, Borczyk AA, Carlson JAK, et al. A severe outbreak of *Escherichia coli* O157:47 associated hemorrhagic colitis in a nursing home. *N Engl J Med* 1987;317:1496-1500.
30. Spika JSA, Parsons JE, Nordenberg D, et al. Hemolytic uremic syndrome and diarrhea associated with *Escherichia coli* O157:47 in a day care center. *J Pediatr* 1986;109:287-291.
31. Ostroff SM, Kobayashi JM, Lweis JH. Infections with *Escherichia coli* O157:47 in Washington State. *JAMA* 1989;262:355-359
32. Bell BP, Goldoft M, Griffin PM, et al. A Multistate outbreak of *Escherichia coli* O157:47 associated bloody diarrhea and hemolytic uremic syndrome from hamburgers. *JAMA* 1994;272:1349-1353.
33. *Escherichia coli* O157:47 outbreak at a summer camp—Virginia 1994. *MMWR Morb Mortal Wkly Rep* 1995;44:419-421.
34. Martin DL, MacDonald KL, White K, et al. The epidemiology and clinical aspects of the Hemolytic Uremic Syndrome in Minnesota. *N Eng J Med* 1990;323:1161-1167.
35. Siegler RL, Pavia AT, Christofferson RD, et al. A 20-year population based study of postdiarrheal hemolytic uremic syndrome in Utah. *Pediatrics* 1994;94:35-40.
36. Cimolai N, Carter JE, Morrison BJ, et al. Risk factors for the progression of *Escherichia coli* 1057:H7 enteritis to hemolytic uremic syndrome. *J Peds* 1990;116:589-592.
37. Swift AEB, Swift TR. Ciguetera. *Clin Tox* 1993;31:1-29.
38. Beadle A. Ciguatera Fish Poisoning. *Military Med* 1997;162:319-322.
39. Hedberg CA, Osterholm MT. Outbreaks of food-borne and waterborne viral gastroenteritis. *Clin Micro Rev* 1993;6:199-210.
40. Glaziou P, Legrand A. The epidemiology of *Ciguatera* fish poisoning. *Toxicon* 1994;8:863-873.
41. Noone J. A case of *Ciguatera* fish poisoning. *J Emerg Nurs* 1996; 22:101-104.
42. Watters MR. Organic neurotoxins in seafoods. *Clin Neuro Neurosurg* 1995;97:119-124.
43 Bishai WR, Sears CL. Food poisoning syndromes. *Gastroenterol Clin NA* 1993;22:579-608.
44. Tosteson TR. The diversity and origins of toxins in *Ciguetera* fish poisoning. *PRHSJ* 1995;14:117-129.
45. Noble RC. Death on the half-shell: The health hazards of eating shellfish. *Perspect Bio Med* 1990;33:313-322.
46. Food and Water Borne Bacterial Diseases@ http://www.cdc.gov/ncidod/disease/bacter/shelfish.htm
47. Sun K, Wat J, So P. Puffer Fish Poisoning. *Anaesth Intens Care* 1994;22:307-308.
48. LangeWR. Puffer fish poisoning. *Am Fam Phys* 1990;42:1029-1033.
49. Tetrodotoxin poisoning associated with eating puffer fish transported from Japan-California, 1996. *JAMA* 1996;275:163.
50. Sun KO. Management of puffer fish poisoning. *Br J Anaesth* 1995; 75:500.
51. Grady GF, Keusch GT. Pathogenesis of bacterial diarrheas. *N Eng J Med* 1971;285:831-841.
52. Holmberg SD, Blake PA. Staphylococcal food poisoning, New facts and old misconceptions. *JAMA* 1984;251:487-489.
53. Outbreak of staphyloccal food poisoning associated with precooked ham-Florida, 1997. *Morb Mortal Wkly Rep MMWR* 1997;46:1189-1191.
54. Wieneke AA, Roberts D, Gilbert RJ. Staphylococcal food poisoning in the United Kingdom, 1969-90. *Epidemiol Infect* 1993;110: 519-531.
55. Plotkin GR, Kluge RM, Waldman RH. Gastroenteritis: Etiology, pathophysiology and clinical manifestations. *Medicine* 1979;58: 95-114.

56. *Bacillus cereus* food poisoning associated with fried rice at two child day care centers-Virginia, 1993. *Morb Mortal Wkly Rep MMWR* 1994;43:177-178.
57. Drobniewski FA. *Bacillus cereus* and related species. *Clin Microbiol Rev* 1993;6:324-338.
58. Luby S, Jones J, Dowda H, et al. A large outbreak of gastroenteritis caused by diarrheal toxin-producing *Bacillus cereus*. *JID* 1993;167:1452-1455.
59. Lacey RW. Food-borne bacterial infections. *Parasitology* 1993;107(S):S75-S93.
60. Preventing Foodborne Illness: Listeriosis@ http://www.cdc.gov/ncidod/disease/bacter/foodborn/lister.htm
61. Brumer RR, Giffel MC, Spoorenberg E, et al. *Listeria* species in domestic environments. *Epidemiol Infect* 1996;117:437-442.
62. Wilson IG. Occurrence of *Listeria* species in ready to eat foods. *Epidemiol Infect* 1995;115:519-526.
63. Hlady WG, Klontz KC. The epidemiology of *Vibrio* infections in Florida, 1981-1993. *J Infect Dis* 1996;173: 1176-1183.
64. Rippey SR. Infectious diseases associated with *Molluscan* shellfish consumption. *Clin Microbiol Rev.* 1994;7: 419-425.
65. Warning about *Vibrio* infections and raw *Molluscan* shellfish consumption. *JAMA* 1993;269:1361.
66. Qadri SMH. Infectious diarrhea. *Postgrad Med* 1990;88: 169-184.
67. Cheney CP, Wong RKH. Acute infectious diarrhea. *Med Clin NA* 1993;77:1169-1196.
68. Questions and answers about Vibrio vulnificus@http://www.cdc.gov/ncidod/disease/bacter/foodborn/vibriovu.htm
69. Appleton H. Foodborne viruses. *Lancet* 1990;336: 1362-1364.
70. Alcoff J. Viral hepatitis. *J Fam Pract* 1982;15:141-162.
71. Morse DL, Guzewich JJ, Hanrahan JP, et al. Widespread outbreak of clam and oyster gastroenteritis: Role of Norwalk virus. *N Engl J Med* 1986;314:678-681.
72. Kohn MA, Farley TA, Ando T, et al. An outbreak of Norwalk virus gastroenteritis associated with eating raw oysters. *JAMA* 1995;272: 466-471.
73. Sugieda M, Nakajima K, Nakajima S. Outbreaks of Norwalk-like virus-associated gastroenteritis traced to shellfish: Coexistence of two genotypes in one specimen. *Epidemiol Infect* 1996;116: 339-346.
74. Kirkland KB, Meriwether RA, Leiss JK, et al. Steaming oysters does not prevent Norwalk-like gastroenteritis. *Pub Health Rep* 1996;111:527-530.
75. Blacklow NR, Greenberg HB. Viral gastroenteritis. *N Engl J Med* 1991;325:252-264.
76. Taterka JA, Cuff CF, Rubin DH. Viral gastrointestinal infections. *GI Clin NA* 1992;21:303-330.
77. Benoy CJ, Hooper PA, Schneider R. The toxicity of tin in canned fruit juices and solid foods. *Fd Cosmet Toxicol* 1971;9:645-656.
78. Spitalny KC, Brondum J, Vogt RL, et al. Drinking-water-induced copper intoxication in a Vermont family. *Pediatrics* 1984;74:1103-1106.
79. Barker WH, Runte V. Tomato juice-associated gastroenteritis, Washington and Oregon, 1969. *Am J Epidemiol* 1972;96:219-226.
80. Taylor A. Detection and monitoring of disorders of essential trace elements. *Ann Clin Biochem* 1996;33: 486-510.
81. Louria DB, Joselow MM, Browder AA. The human toxicity of certain trace elements. *Ann Int Med* 1972;76:307-319.
82. CDC. Foodborne Botulism-Oklahoma, 1994. *Morb Mortal Wkly Rep MMWR* 1995;44:200-202.
83. St. Louis ME, Peck Sh, Bowering D, et al. Botulism from chopped garlic: Delayed recognition of a major outbreak. *Ann Int Med* 1988; 108:363-368.
84. Centers for Disease Control. Fish Botulism-Hawaii, 1990. *Morb Mortal Wkly Rep MMWR* 1991;40:412-414.
85. Arnon SS, Midura TF, Damus K, et al. Honey and other environmental risk factors for infant botulism. *J Pediatr* 1979;94;331-336.
86. Long SS. Botulism in infancy. *Pediatr Infect Dis* 1984;84: 266-271.
87. Woodruff BA, Grufflin JF, McCroskey LM, et al. Clinical and laboratory comparison of botulism from toxin types A, B, and E in the United States, 1975-1988. *J Infect Dis* 1992;166:1281-1286.
88. Shapiro BE, Soto O, Shafqat S, et al. Adult botulism. *Muscle Nerve* 1997;20:100-102.
89. Black RD, Gunn RA. Hypersensitivity reactions associated with botulinum antitoxin. *Am J Med* 1980;69:567-570.
90. Schreiner MS, Firel EM, Ruddy R. Infant botulism: A review of 12 years' experience at The Children's Hospital of Philadelphia. *Pediatrics* 1991;87:159-165.
91. Zautcke JL, Schwartz JA, Mueller EJ. Chinese restaurant syndrome: A review. *Ann Emerg Med* 1986;15:1210-1213.
92. Pulce C, Vial T, Verdier F, et al. The Chinese restaurant syndrome: A reappraisal of monosodium glutamate's causative role. *Adv Drug Tox Rev* 1992;11:19-39.
93. Tarasoff L, Kelly MF. Monosodium L-Glutamate: A double-blind study and review. *Fd Chem Tox* 1993;31: 1019-1035.
94. Overall JC. Is it bacterial or viral? Laboratory differentiation. *Ped Rev* 1993;14:251-261.
95. Leung AKC, Robeson WLM. Acute diarrhea in children. *Postgrad Med* 1989;86:161-173.
96. Hines J, Nachamkin I. Effective use of the clinical microbiology laboratory for diagnosing diarrheal diseases. *Clin Infect Dis* 1996;23:1292-1301.
97. Sabol VK, Diarrhea. *AACN Clin* 1997;8:425-436.
98. Adler PM. Stool examination: Culture versus gram stain. *Ann Emerg Med* 1986;15:337-340.
99. Welsby PD. Infectious diseases. *Postgrad Med J* 1994;70: 74-85.
100. Katelaris PH, Farthing MJG. Traveler's diarrhea: Clinical presentation and prognosis. *Chemother* 1995;41:40-47.

Acute Geriatric Abdomen

Richard Caesar, MD, FACEP

The acute geriatric abdomen poses what is arguably one of the most puzzling, treacherous, and challenging diagnostic dilemmas facing the emergency department (ED) physician. Compared to other organ systems, the gastrointestinal tract is frequently the source of nebulous complaints and neglected symptomatology.

Sudden onset of abdominal discomfort in an elderly patient almost always generates a complex and extensive differential diagnosis. Consider the case of the 80-year-old man who presents to the ED with severe epigastric pain, fever, and vomiting. He has a history of gallstones—which are present in up to one-half of individuals 80 years or older—that could be responsible for his symptoms. But this may not tell the whole story. For example, the stone might be causing acute cholecystitis at the cystic duct, or it may have already made its descent to the ampulla of Vater and precipitated biliary pancreatitis. Management will depend on which of these events is responsible for his symptoms. Even a serum amylase may not pinpoint the precise etiology.

Without question, an abdominal ultrasound examination should be performed. But even if this procedure confirms the presence of stones, perhaps they have been present for 30 years, and are only a "red herring." It may be that this patient, who also has been on prednisone and ibuprofen for his osteoarthritis, is declaring his first episode of peptic disease with a penetrating ulcer, as do 50% of patients in this age group as their initial presentation. We know gastrointestinal hemorrhage cannot be ruled out merely because there is no blood in the emesis. And without a definitive diagnosis, immediate decisions must still be made regarding additional studies, surgical consultation, and pain relief. This patient, who also is in rapid atrial fibrillation and is not on thromboembolic prophylaxis, cannot recall whether he has ever had an irregular pulse; consequently, his presentation demands that we consider impending small bowel infarction, secondary to embolization of a left aerial thrombus to the superior mesenteric artery.

Each of these disorders can present with the original constellation of complaints that includes epigastric pain, fever, and vomiting, and each condition also can progress to mental obtundation and shock. But the same presentation can also be seen with gastroenteritis in the 80-year-old patient, in whom a diagnostic laparotomy and/or costly noninvasive procedures will be decidedly unhelpful and unnecessary.

Without the luxury of time, the ED physician must consider multiple simultaneous conditions in an unstable elderly patient and decide which, if any, are responsible for the patient's acute symptomatology. Given the complexities and contradictions encountered with the acute geriatric abdomen, this is a difficult and frustrating exercise at best. To improve the diagnostic accuracy and clinical management of older patients who present with acute abdominal complaints, this article presents a systematic approach—one that combines laboratory, radiographic, and clinical parameters—that will help decipher the causes of gastrointestinal symptoms in the acutely ill geriatric patient.

Table 1. Causes of Abdominal Pain in the Elderly

Causes
Abdominal pain of unknown etiology
Constipation
Cholelithiasis
Acute cholecystitis
Intestinal obstruction
Acute pancreatitis
Gastroenteritis
Duodenal ulcer
Abdominal aortic aneurysm
Appendicitis
Mesenteric ischemia
Obstructive uropathy
Gastroenteritis
Volvulus

Table 2. Common Anatomic Pain Sites for Specific Caues of Acute Abdominal Disorders in the Elderly

RIGHT UPPER QUADRANT AND FLANK	
Cholecystitis	Intestinal obstruction
Pyelonephritis	Retrocecal appendicitis
Penetrating ulcer	Pancreatitis
Choledocholithiasis	Gastric ulcer
EPIGASTRIUM	
Pancreatitis	Gastritis
Duodenal ulcer	Early appendicitis
Penetrating ulcer	Mesenteric ischemia
Colon carcinoma	Abdominal aortic aneurysm
LEFT UPPER QUADRANT AND FLANK	
Splenic enlargement	Diverticulitis
Pyelonephritis	Bowel obstruction
RIGHT LOWER QUADRANT	
Appendicitis	Bowel obstruction
Hernia	Pyelonephritis
Cholecystitis	Diverticulitis
Psoas abscess	Leaking aneurysm
LEFT LOWER QUADRANT	
Diverticulitis	Bowel obstruction
Hernia	Leaking aneurysm
Pyelonephritis	Abdominal wall hematoma
HYPOGASTRIUM	
Diverticulitis	Cystitis
Bladder obstruction	Appendicitis
Prostatism	Hernia
Bowel obstruction	Colon carcinoma

Diagnostic Pitfalls

Emergency physicians with experience in clinical geriatrics readily acknowledge the bewildering array of obstacles to evaluating the acute abdomen in this patient population. First, many older patients are poor historians. Dementia, in particular, can obscure time-honored symptoms, putting the clinician at a considerable disadvantage. The older patient also is far more likely to have undergone previous laparotomy. The resulting adhesions and other forms of scarring not only increase the likelihood of intestinal obstruction but alter the three-dimensional relationships of intra-abdominal structures. Consequently, signs and symptoms in these patients can deviate from classical patterns.

Given that elderly patients are often poor and misleading historians, and that their acute abdominal complaints can suggest an intimidating variety of both trivial and life-threatening pathology, it is not surprising that older patients with abdominal pain consume a disproportionate amount of time and resources in the ED. *(Please see Tables 1 and 2.)* Comparing lengths of stay in the ED of elderly (> 65 years) vs. younger patients, and categorizing major complaints into shortness of breath, chest pain, and abdominal pain, one study observed that the discharged geriatric patient with abdominal pain was the single most time consuming of all ED visitors, with almost two and a half hours spent, on average, in the department.[1] Furthermore, despite well-documented higher admission rates for elderly (47%) vs. the nonelderly (18), when patients with abdominal complaints were discharged from the ED, their recidivism rate was nearly twice as high (29% vs 15%) as younger patients with similar complaints.

Laboratory Database and Radiographic Evaluation

Evaluation of the older patient with abdominal symptomatology must be systematic and comprehensive. Although no single laboratory or radiographic test is absolutely required for initial evaluation of these patients, an extended database consisting of a CBC, amylase, liver function studies, alkaline phosphatase, and urinalysis is appropriate. When dehydration or electrolyte disturbances are suspected, measurement of serum electrolytes, blood urea nitrogen (BUN), and creatinine levels may help guide therapy. Unfortunately, laboratory results will usually not be diagnostic, and further evaluation with radiographic studies is an inevitable part of the evaluation of acute abdominal pain in the older age group.

The cost-effectiveness and utility of the abdominal plain film depends on the clinical context. Most studies suggest that plain film examination is a relatively low-yield procedure when used as a screening tool in patients presenting with diffuse or nonspecific findings, particularly in patients with acute gastrointestinal bleeding or in acute disease of the biliary or genitourinary system.[2,3] Nevertheless, in those patients thought to have large or small bowel obstruction, volvulus, perforation, ischemia, infarction, or peritoneal signs suggestive of peritonitis, plain film evaluation is clinically useful.

Careful inspection of the abdominal series—which may consist of a posterior-anterior (PA) chest film, supine and upright films of the abdomen, and, in some centers, decubitus or cross-table supine films of the abdomen—may yield clues that point to a specific diagnosis. For example, pleural effusions are commonly found in association with disease of the pancreas, such as pancreatic carcinoma, hepatic disease, or subphrenic abscess, which may be accompanied by elevation of the hemidiaphragm, with or without mottled gas in the subphrenic space. Esophageal perforation secondary to protracted vomiting, esophageal foreign body, or esophageal carcinoma will demonstrate pleural effusion in about 60% of cases.

Abnormal Gas Patterns. When evaluating abnormal gas patterns, a systematic approach that addresses the following questions may be useful: Is the air inside or outside the bowel? If the air is intraluminal, the emergency physician should consider ileus, bowel obstruction, or gas outline in a mucosal lesion. On the other hand, of the air is extraluminal, it is helpful to distinguish between peritoneal free air, loculated air collections (i.e., abscess), and retroperitoneal air. On occasion, air may follow a distinct anatomic structure such as intramural air, biliary air (emphysematous cholecystitis), or portal venous air.

Pneumoperitoneum. True pneumoperitoneum in an older, nontraumatized patient is most often caused by bowel perforation, usually a perforated duodenal or gastric ulcer. Approximately 70% of such perforations demonstrate pneumoperitoneum.[4] Less commonly, pneumoperitoneum is the result of severe inflammatory disease of the bowel as in severe colitis or toxic megacolon, bowel ischemia, bowel obstruction, or prolonged ileus. The clinician should always look for associated bowel dilatation in the presence of pneumoperitoneum and correlate this finding with the duration of symptoms. Immediate onset of bowel distension usually indicates a bacterial peritonitis due to a large perforation, whereas chemical peritonitis will have a delay in onset of bowel dilatation.

Obstruction and Hens. Classically, mechanical obstruction results in bowel dilatation due to the accumulation of air and fluid proximal to the point of obstruction, but diminished bowel caliber occurs distal to the point of obstruction with little or no air or fluid present because peristalsis moves the bowel contents rectally. Consequently, in patients with mechanical obstruction, differential air fluid levels are identified proximal to the obstruction and usually appear as short segments at varying heights through the abdomen. Occasionally, gas is resorbed from the distended fluid-filled loops and the abdomen may appear totally gasless.

Progressive thickening of the bowel wall (> 3 mm in diameter), so-called "thumbprinting" secondary to submucosal edema, hemorrhage, or infiltration of bowel suggest vascular compromise. The presence of crescenteric or curvilinear air lucency within the intramural portion of the bowel in the face of increasing obstruction or ileus indicates vascular compromise or infarction which, in the elderly, can occur in the setting of mesenteric ischemia or arterial embolism.

Diverticulitis. The initial plain films in the patient with diverticulitis may be normal or may demonstrate localized ileus or distal bowel obstruction. The presence of extraluminal gas or mottled air suggests the presence of sinus tracts, fistulas, or abscesses.

Pinpointing the Diagnosis

Mechanical Obstruction. Mechanical obstruction in the gastrointestinal tract has a number of causes. For example, in the esophagus, it frequently results from foreign body impaction at a web, a benign stricture, and, less often, from carcinoma. In the stomach, gastric outlet obstruction is often secondary to severe inflammatory changes of peptic ulcer disease or is caused by a malignancy, whereas in the small bowel, adhesions from prior surgery, inflammatory bowel disease, tumors, and acute appendicitis must be considered in the differential diagnosis. Although uncommon, internal hernias are an important—and, frequently, misdiagnosed—cause of mechanical large bowel obstruction in the geriatric patient.

Small Bowel Obstruction. Signs and symptoms of small bowel obstruction are not distinctive or unique in the geriatric population. If the obstruction is complete, diffuse colicky abdominal pain, distention, nausea, vomiting, and eventual obstipation are usually present. "Rushes" and "tinkles" may be auscultated during resistance to peristalsis.

The elderly individual is statistically more likely to have undergone a laparotomy than his younger counterpart and, consequently, is more likely to develop postoperative adhesive scarring. Adhesions may become a problem relatively soon after surgery (weeks or months) or, in a more insidious fashion, with symptoms manifesting themselves many years after the offending surgery. As with all age groups, adhesions are the most common etiology for small bowel obstruction in the elderly. The majority can be treated conservatively, with bowel rest, nasogastric suction, and hydration. However, a significant percentage will not resolve spontaneously and must undergo surgical lysis of adhesions, thus contributing to a vicious cycle of adhesion formation-obstruction-laparotomy with surgical "takedown" of adhesions, and renewed scarring.

Hernias. With the exception of adhesive scarring in men, inguinal hernias are the most common etiology for bowel obstruction in the geriatric population. Indirect inguinal hernia occurs when intestinal structures pass through the internal inguinal ring and through the inguinal canal. Among elderly men, direct inguinal hernia is a more frequent cause for obstruction. This results from protrusion and occasional incarceration of intestinal contents with Hesselbach's area, owing to gradual weakening of the transversalis fascia. Direct inguinal hernias are uncommon in older women, in whom the femoral variety accounts for up to one-third of hernias. Femoral hernias descend through the femoral canal, beneath the inguinal ligament, and present as a palpable mass at or above the inguinal ligament itself.

Large Bowel Obstruction. Obstruction of the large intestine is more likely to be partial and intermittent and to be associated with feculent emesis and heme-positive stools. Unlike small bowel obstruction, the most common cause of large bowel obstruction in the elderly is malignancy. Indeed, colonic cancer is the single most common cancer among the entire geriatric population. Colonic cancer represents 30% of all malignancies among men and 40% among women in the older age group. The left colon is by far the most common site with up to two-thirds of all lesions within reach of the sigmoidoscope.

Volvulus. Volvulus accounts for up to 10% of all cases of large bowel obstruction in those younger than age 60 and about 15% in the elderly.[5] The condition is characterized by rotation of a segment of bowel around the axis of its mesentery, a topologic derangement that compromises vascular supply and obstructs and causes distention of the involved lumen. Eighty-five percent of these cases involve the sigmoid colon, where elongation of the affected region (so-called

Table 3. Biliary Tract Ultrasound

MAJOR DIAGNOSTIC CRITERIA
Stone present
Nonvisualization of the gallbladder
MINOR DIAGNOSTIC CRITERIA
Wall thickening
Sonographic Murphy's sign
Gallbladder enlargement
Round gallbladder shape
Pericholecystic fluid
ADVANTAGES
Accuracy
Rapidity of performance
Minimal preparation
No ionizing radiation
Other structures "screened"
COST
Average: $230

"redundancy") in the elderly predisposes them to this form of bowel obstruction. Fifteen percent of cases are cecal in origin and are characterized by a twisted, dilated cecum that is transposed or "flipped" over into the right upper quadrant on the plain film. A so-called "bird's beak" narrowing at one end of the dilated segment of bowel identifies the proximal portion of obstruction.

Treatment of cecal and sigmoid volvulus are markedly different. When volvulus involves the sigmoid, the distended lumen can usually be decompressed with the passage of a soft rectal tube (through a sigmoidoscope) with detorsion of the mesenteric axis. When the likelihood of peritoneal contamination is low, barium enema is often therapeutic. With recurrent episodes of sigmoid volvulus (which is seen in more than 50% of patients), partial colonic resection with anastomosis is generally preferred over detorsion and fixation. Cecal volvulus, on the other hand, invariably requires laparotomy, often with right hemicolectomy and ileocolonic anastomosis. Mortality rates, which vary from 24-40% in all first episodes of volvulus, are ascribed to a delay in diagnosis and underlying illness.

Biliary Tract Emergencies. Biliary tract emergencies arise as a result of obstruction caused by calculi in the gallbladder and the biliary tree or neoplasms of and around the biliary tree. The three most common biliary tract emergencies in the elderly include acute cholecystitis, acute cholangitis, and acute pancreatitis, all of which are potentially lethal conditions, especially in the elderly. The incidence of stones within the gallbladder (cholelithiasis) and common bile duct (choledocholithiasis)—as well as inflammation of the gallbladder (cholecystitis)—increases significantly with each decade of life.[6] Various studies report that after age 50, there is approximately a 5% increase in the incidence of cholecystitis with each decade of life, ranging from a 25% incidence during the sixth decade to greater than 55% during the eighth decade. In one large Swedish study, one-fourth of all patients older than 70 who presented with an acute abdomen were found to have cholecystitis.[7] The incidence of common bile duct stones roughly doubles during the same period. With age, the level of biliary cholesterol increases, raising the lithogenic index of bile and making the development of stones more likely.

Signs and symptoms of cholecystitis in the elderly are variable. Older patients with acute disease will most often complain of epigastric or right subcostal pain radiating to the back or right shoulder. If the pain subsides after several hours, the diagnosis of biliary colic without cholecystitis may be entertained. However, pain, fever, and vomiting that persist usually indicate the presence of acute cholecystitis. In the elderly, fever and leukocytosis may be delayed, although signs of peritoneal irritation (percussion tenderness, rebound and/or involuntary guarding over the epigastrium or right upper quadrant) may actually occur earlier in the natural history of the disease. If complications such as a gangrene or perforation develop, the patient may present with hypotension and frank septic shock.

At the more benign end of the spectrum of presentation are recurrent episodes of transient, uncomplicated cystic duct obstruction—usually the result of multiple smaller calculi—which present with vague and less specific symptomatology. As a rule, the history is characterized by little more than subjective complaints of eructation, flatulence, relative anorexia, or mild fatty food intolerance; these symptoms may be accompanied by poorly localized upper abdominal or flank discomfort. Peptic disease, occult malignancy, right lower lobe pneumonia, variant angina, and upper urinary tract disease must also be ruled out while the biliary tree is targeted for examination.

If asymptomatic biliary tract stones are documented with abdominal ultrasound, the clinician must determine the best approach to an elderly patient with so-called, "silent" gallstones. Several factors should be kept in mind. First, the presence of a single large gallstone is associated with a substantially higher risk of complications than is so-called "biliary gravel," or multiple small stones. Second, complications such as gangrene and/or perforation occur much more rapidly after the onset of initial symptoms in the geriatric population, which means that surgery is usually the more prudent course in this age group.

In this regard, it should be emphasized that in the case of elective cholecystectomy, age alone is associated with only a negligibly increased mortality rate. However, in the emergent surgical setting, advanced age becomes a significant risk factor. One large study reviewed 137 cases of patients older than 70 undergoing cholecystectomy and divided them into elective and emergent surgical groups.[8] There was a 60% greater rate of complications among the emergent cholecystectomies, and an almost fourfold greater mortality rate in the elderly (12.5% vs 3.8%).

Ultrasonography. During the past few years, ultrasonic evaluation of the biliary system has emerged as an integral part of the emergency evaluation of patients with acute abdominal complaints. The most important change has been the development of real-time (as opposed to static) imaging, which can now organize hundreds of thousands of ultrasonic tomograms on several planes into detailed and coherent images. In evaluating patients with possible cholelithiasis or cholecystitis, a number of major and minor diagnostic criteria are defined sonographically. Complete non-visualization of the gallbladder or the sonographic presence of gallstones are both considered major criteria, along with evidence of dilated ducts. The sensitivity of

Table 4. Empiric Antibiotic Therapy for Management of Acute Abdominal Conditions in the Elderly

ABDOMINAL AORTIC ANEURYSM

Cefazolin 1 g IV or
Vancomycin 1 g IV (for hospitals where methicillin-resistant *S. aureus* or *S. epidermidis* causes infections)

APPENDICITIS (NON-PERFORATED)

Cefoxitin 1 g IV or
Cefotetan 1 g IV

APPENDICITIS (PERFORATED)

Ampicillin-sulbactam 1.5-3.0 g IV q6h plus
Tobramycin 100-120 mg IV loading, then 80-100 mg IV q8h or
Tobramycin 100-120 mg IV loading, then 80-100 mg IV q8h plus
Clindamycin 600-900 mg IV q8h

BACTERIAL CHOLANGITIS/BILIARY SEPSIS

Mezloxicillin, azlocillin, or piperacillin 3 g IV q4-6h IV plus
Metronidazole 1 g IV over 1 h, then 500 mg IV q6h or
Ampicillin-sulbactam 3 g IV q6h plus
Tobramycin 80-100 mg IV q8h

BACTERIAL PERITONITIS

Ampicillin-sulbactam 3 g IV q6h plus
Tobramycin 80-100 mg IV q8h or
Imipenem/cilastin 0.5-1.0 g IV q6-8h or
Ticarcillin/clavulanate 3.1 g IV q4-6h plus
Tobramycin 80-100 mg IV q8h

CHOLECYSTITIS

Mezloxicillin, azlocillin, or piperacillin 3 g IV q4-6h or
Ampicillin-sulbactam 3 g IV q6h plus
Tobramycin 80-100 mg IV q8h or
Ticarcillin/clavulanate 3.1 g IV q4-6h

DIVERTICULITIS (MILD)

Trimethoprim-sulfa DS 1 po bid or
Ciprofloxacin 250-500 mg po bid plus
Metronidazole 250 mg po tid 10 days

DIVERTICULITIS (MODERATE TO SEVERE)

Ampicillin-sulbactam 1.5-3.0 g IV q6h plus
Tobramycin 100-120 mg IV loading, then 80-100 mg IV q8h or
Tobramycin 100-120 mg loading, then 80-100 mg IV q8h plus
Clindamycin 600-900 mg IV q8h

INTRA-ABDOMINAL ABSCESS

Ampicillin-sulbactam 1.5-3.0 g IV q6h plus
Tobramycin 100-120 mg loading, then 80-100 mg IV q8h or
Tobramycin 100-120 mg loading, then 80-100 mg IV q8h plus
Clindamycin 600-900 mg IV q8h

PREOPERATIVE PROPHYLAXIS (LAPAROTOMY FOR RUPTURED VISCOUS)

Cefoxitin 1 g IV q6h or
Cefotetan 1 g IV q1 2h plus
Tobramycin 100-120 mg loading, then 80-100 mg IV q8h or
Clindamycin 600 mg IV q6h plus
Tobramycin 100-120 mg IV loading, then 80-100 mg IV q8h

these major criteria is about 85%, while their specificity is greater than 95%. Minor diagnostic criteria include gallbladder wall thickening(> 4-5 mm), tenderness of the gallbladder when palpated during examination (sonographic Murphy's sign), gallbladder enlargement (> 5 cm in any dimension), round gallbladder shape, and evidence of pericholecystic fluid. Of these, wall thickening appears to be the most statistically reliable. More to the point, one study has demonstrated that the combination of a sonographic Murphy's sign in the presence of gallbladder enlargement on ultrasound was 99% predictive of "patients needing a cholecystectomy" regardless of the specific diagnosis.[9] The so-called screening abdominal ultrasound has been shown to detect nonbiliary causes of pain in the upper abdomen in 24-35% of patients without gallbladder disease.[9] *(Please see Table 3.)*

Management. Initial management of acute cholecystitis is conservative, consisting of IV fluids, nothing by mouth, parenteral analgesics, and broad-spectrum antibiotics. *(Please see Table 4.)* If the patient is vomiting or has evidence of gastric distension or ileus on plain radiographs of the abdomen, a nasogastric tube should be inserted. Surgical cholecystectomy remains the treatment of choice in patients with acute cholecystitis. Indications for prompt surgery in the asymptomatic geriatric patient with documented gallstones include the following: 1) single large stone; 2) diabetes mellitus; 3) obesity; 4) immuno-suppressive illness; 5) history of pancreatitis; 6) possible common bile duct involvement; and 7) absence of significant concomitant disease.

These recommendations represent a general reversal of attitudes toward gallbladder surgery in the elderly. Rather than viewing the elderly as too fragile for surgery or as a group for whom laparotomy should be postponed until a near-terminal precarious moment, it has been shown that the older population fares just as well as their younger counterparts under controlled (i.e., elective) conditions.[10] When definitive surgical treatment is delayed in an otherwise appropriate operative candidate, complications become increasingly likely. The increasing use of laparoscopic cholecystectomy, which obviates the need for general anaesthesia and minimizes blood loss, scarring, and overall operative stress, makes delays in surgical intervention even less acceptable.[11-13]

Perforation of the Gallbladder. Because elderly patients are more prone to atherosclerotic vascular disease, they are also more susceptible to perforation secondary to ischemic changes within the gallbladder wall. Whereas the gallbladder may take weeks to rupture after the onset of obstructive symptoms in the younger patient, perforation in the elderly may occur as early as 3-4 hours after the onset of symptoms. Generally, perforation is a condition limited to elderly men, in which mortality rates between 15% and 25% are reported.[14] Sequelae of perforation include bile peritonitis, cholecystenteric fistula with or without gallstone ileus, and generalized abscess formation. Surgical intervention in this condition is mandatory.

Gallstone Hens. Gallstone ileus is a dramatic but relatively uncommon complication of perforation in which a large stone erodes through the gallbladder wall and migrates into the adjacent small bowel. The stone, which is usually at least 2.5 cm in size, moves distally and eventually causes mechanical small bowel obstruction at the ileocecal valve or at a more proximal narrowed site. The condition can be diagnosed on plain film of the abdomen if the characteristic triad of air in the biliary tree, gallstone in the intestine, and evidence of small intestinal obstruction is present. For reasons that are unclear, gallstone ileus is more common among women and, in one study, was the etiology for 20% of intestinal obstructions in female patients older than age 65.[15]

Emphysematous Cholecystitis. Emphysematous cholecystitis is believed to be secondary to severe vascular insufficiency within the gallbladder wall, where compromised tissue permits growth of *Clostridium perfringens* or other gas-producing anaerobic organisms. Radiographically, the gallbladder appears as a distended radiolucent cavity on the abdominal plain film, which is often the only diagnostic procedure necessary to confirm the diagnosis. Gas may also be visible and will appear in the gallbladder lumen, wall, or pericholecystic soft tissue and ducts. Emphysematous cholecystitis occurs in only 1% of all patients with cholecystitis and is five times more common in males. This condition should be suspected in any diabetic male with symptoms referable to the biliary tree.

Acalculous Cholecystitis. Any condition that predisposes to stagnation or concentration of bile predisposes to acalculous cholecystitis,[16] including prolonged narcotic use, dehydration, or low-flow hemodynamic states, such as congestive heart failure. Common in men older than age 65, acalculous cholecystitis frequently presents as a complication of an unrelated insult, such as a major trauma, burns, or septicemia. Because of its association with other serious pathology and its predilection for older patients, acalculous cholecystitis has a higher mortality rate (6.5%) than the more common calculous variety (4%). Surgical treatment is mandatory unless otherwise contraindicated.[17]

Cholangitis. Usually associated with gram-negative bacteria such as *Escherichia coli* and *Klebsiella* species, as well as anaerobes, acute cholangitis is a serious and potentially lethal disorder requiring prompt recognition and treatment. The most common cause of acute cholangitis in the United States is choledocholithiasis, which is present in about 10-20% of patients with cholelithiasis. The surgical literature describes the physical findings of ascending cholangitis with the so called Charcot's triad: right upper-quadrant pain, spiking fever, and jaundice. By definition, ascending cholangitis arises retrograde from the intestinal tract, producing infection of the common, cystic, and hepatic ducts. Back pressure from obstructed, infected bile introduces bacteria into capillaries and lymphatics, generating quick onset of systemic symptoms. A separate and far less common entity, suppurative cholangitis, results when the gallbladder obstructs secondary to stone, stricture, or neoplasm, and then fills with frank pus. These patients will usually rapidly go on to septic shock.[18]

Antibiotic coverage must be broad spectrum, because the microbiology of biliary infections includes both aerobes and anaerobes. Among aerobes, *E. coli, Klebsiella* species, *Enterobacter* species, and enterococcus predominate. The major anaerobes are *Bacteroides fragilis* and *Clostridium* species. Pure aerobic and mixed aerobic-anaerobic infections occur in about equal frequencies, while purely anaerobic infections are rarely seen.

When cholangitis is suspected in the ED, fluid support and antibiotic therapy (see previous section) should be initiated promptly. Particular attention must be paid to coagulation studies since a significant percentage of patients with either suppurative or nonsuppurative cholangitis develop disseminated intravascular coagulopathy. Definitive treatment may include endoscopic papillotomy to decompress and drain the duct prior to cholecystectomy. In skilled hands, papillotomy is quick and may be performed without the risks of general anesthesia, allowing time for hemodynamic stabilization prior to surgery in the emergent setting.

Peptic Ulcer Disease

Among all age groups, 10% of patients with peptic ulcer disease will present with an acute surgical abdomen as their initial manifestation of this condition. In the elderly, 50% of patients will present in this manner, of which 35-40% will present with a rigid, board-like, quiet abdomen (with or without signs of shock) as their first and only manifestation of peptic disease. Consequently, peptic ulcer disease and its complications should never be far from the top of the differential diagnosis in elderly patients who present with upper or midabdominal pain,[19] with or without evidence of gastrointestinal bleeding.

Complication rates are high, with one series reporting a bleeding or perforation rate of 31 % in patients between the ages of 60 and 64 and 76% in patients 75-79 years of age.[19] Frank hemorrhage accounts for up to two-thirds of the complications of peptic ulcer disease, with perforation and outlet obstruction comprising the remainder of cases. In the general population, the ratio of duodenal to gastric ulcer approaches 10 to 1. Among the elderly, however, it declines to 2 to 1. This relative increase in gastric ulceration has significant consequences. While accounting for only one-third of all ulcers documented in this age group, gastric ulceration accounts for over two-thirds of ulcer-related mortality in this same group.

Elderly patients with peptic ulcer disease are more likely to be on steroids or nonsteroidal anti-inflammatory agents, which compromise the gastrointestinal mucosa. One large study of elderly patients who expired in the hospital revealed a fourfold greater death rate from peptic ulcer/upper gastrointestinal hemorrhage in patients taking nonsteroidal anti-inflammatory drugs (NSAIDs) than those who did not.[20] Additional investigations have demonstrated that NSAIDs can mask symptoms of preexistent peptic disease, thus delaying diagnosis and increasing morbidity and mortality.

Pancreatitis. Pancreatitis is the most common nonsurgical etiology for abdominal pain requiring hospitalization in the geriatric population.[21,22] Though not widely appreciated, its incidence increases with age, because the elderly are statistically (with exposure through time), pharmacologically, and pathophysiologically more vulnerable to all the following predisposing factors leading to pancreatitis: 1) alcoholism; 2) biliary tract disease; 3) penetrating ulcer; 4) infection (usually viral, but occasionally *E. coli* or *Pseudomonas*, *Staphylococcus*, or *Klebsiella* species); 5) hypertriglyceridemia; 6) drug reactions (thiazides, furosemide, NSAIDs, sulfonamides, erythromycin, tetracycline, corticosteroids, acetaminophen, estrogens); 7) hypercalcemia; 8) carbon monoxide exposure; and 9) hypothermia. Distinguishing among these etiologies is important for prevention of recurrence.

Acute pancreatitis can be divided into clinical categories that reflect the underlying processes. In the elderly, as in the younger age group, interstitial (edematous) pancreatitis comprises 80-95% of cases, with hemorrhagic (necrotizing) pancreatitis comprising 5-15%. Presentation includes epigastric pain, penetrating in nature, accompanied by low-grade fever, nausea, vomiting, and signs of volume depletion. But even in the presence of extensive inflammation, the elderly (as they do with cholecystitis) present at one end or the other of the clinical spectrum. Signs and symptoms of the geriatric patient with acute pancreatitis may be nonspecific, poorly localized, with the patient ill but not in acute distress. There may be anorexia for 1-2 days, upper or midabdominal pain, mild nausea, and little else. At the other extreme, some patients will present with agonizing epigastric or chest pain, hypotension, and shock. Cullen's sign (periumbilical ecchymosis) or Grey Turner's sign (flank ecehymosis) may be present with hemorrhagic pancreatitis. A certain subpopulation, estimated at 10%, arrives without complaint of pain or emesis but simply with unexplained hypotension and altered mental status. The relatively early onset of hemodynamic collapse in acute pancreatitis, which may even be associated with transient ST- and T-wave changes on electrocardiogram, may be related to so-called myocardial depressant factor (MDF) elaborated by the inflamed or ischemic pancreas. Interestingly, geriatric women are affected significantly more frequently than men.

Diagnostically, hyperamylasemia has been the cornerstone of clinical evaluation, but the nonspecificity of this enzyme elevation in the setting of a fragile, elderly patient limits its diagnostic usefulness.[23] For example, hyperamylasemia can be seen in pneumonia, renal insufficiency, peptic disease, mesenteric vascular compromise, and other disorders. However, on occasion, the magnitude of hyperamylasemia is more specific and quite helpful, as in biliary pancreatitis, where enzyme elevation may be five- to tenfold greater than normal, well above the range of elevation seen in the other disorders just mentioned. The ratio of amylase-to-creatinine clearance is also helpful. A value of greater than 5% (in the absence of diabetic ketoacidosis) is diagnostic of pancreatitis. While seen in a variety of other gastrointestinal disorders, the so-called sentinel loop (essentially a localized region of paralytic ileus) is also frequently associated with pancreatitis.

An area of mystery and relative controversy concerns the pulmonary complications of pancreatitis in all age groups.[24] Simple hypoxemia is the most common complication. In the elderly, however, the incidence of objective findings on chest x-ray (ranging from small areas of basilar atelectasis to effusions, infiltrates, and frank pulmonary edema) is significantly increased and the severity of radiographic changes is directly related to the degree of pancreatic inflammation. The pulmonary edema of acute pancreatitis in the geriatric population usually begins 2-3 days after the initial presentation and appears to be associated with serum triglyceride elevation. Mortality rates for the initial presentation of acute pancreatitis are 15% in patients younger than age 50, 30% in the 50- to 70-year-old group, and 40% in patients older than age 70.[21-24] Interestingly, however, one study of 268 patients in Britain demonstrated that while mortality from pancreatitis was increased in the elderly, these deaths were generally secondary to associated illnesses that were prevalent in this age group.[24] When only deaths due to complications of acute pancreatitis were analyzed, the mortality rate was not significantly different between young and older patients.

Appendicitis. Unlike its relatively straightforward presentation in the young adult, acute appendicitis in the older patient often presents with minimal symptomatology. For this and other reasons, clinicians have traditionally maintained an insufficient index of suspicion for appendicitis in the geriatric patient.[25] Reasons for this are clear. In the normal course of aging, the appendix typically involutes, and appendectomies in patients older than age 60 account for only 8% of all those performed. (This figure is partially misleading, as a significant number of patients may have had incidental appendectomies as part of previous laparotomies in their younger years.) Geriatric patients with acute appendicitis still account for 5-7% of all acute abdominal emergencies in this age group.[26] Because of a low index of suspicion, however, significant delays in diagnosis have been found to be four times as common in patients in their seventh decade as compared to those patients in the fourth decade of life. Moreover, appendiceal perforation is more common in the elderly as compared to the general population.

Approximately 40-50% of geriatric patients going to laparotomy with acute appendicitis are incorrectly diagnosed preoperatively.[25,27] These diagnostic errors, which lead to perforation of the inflamed appendix, are due primarily to the relative lack of both magnitude and specificity of the signs and symptoms in this subgroup.

Not infrequently, the older patient may ascribe his or her discomfort to ongoing problems such as constipation and may have treated himself or herself with enemas for hours or even days prior to presentation. In addition, anatomical changes caused by previous surgery may produce unusual patterns of symptomatology; for example, the appendix may rupture into an inguinal or femoral hernial sac or be anatomically relocated due to adhesive scarring from previous surgeries. A landmark study of 94 elderly patients with appendicitis reflects the problematic aspects of this condition both to the patient, who must decide to obtain treatment, and to the physician, who must make the diagnosis and arrange prompt surgery. In 83% of patients, more than 24 hours elapsed between the onset of symptoms and initiation of surgery, while in 53%, more than 48 hours had elapsed. As expected, the incidence of complications (perforation, gangrene, abscess) increased dramatically with delayed treatment. All four deaths were in patients older than age 80 who had perforated after a surgical delay of greater than 24 hours.[27]

Errors in diagnosis ranged from metastatic colon cancer and intestinal obstruction to incarcerated inguinal hernia and PID. For the clinician who, in the elderly, expects the 8-24 hours of epigastric or periumbilical pain followed by localization to the right lower quadrant with fever and leukocytosis, lifesaving laparotomy will be dangerously delayed. This disease is frequently missed in the elderly because it is not uncommon for the pain to remain poorly localized in these patients. Rebound and involuntary guarding on abdominal exam are seen in only 50% of cases. Such symptoms as constipation (rather than 1-2 episodes of diarrhea frequently found in younger patients) and abdominal distention are not uncommon; rigors and/or hypothermia signify progression to perforation. As in most cases of sepsis among the elderly, a white blood cell count differential characterized by increased bands without leukocytosis is a poor prognostic sign.

A number of studies undertaken since 1992 demonstrate the superiority of urgent diagnostic laparotomy over temporization in these patients.[11,28,29] Graham and colleagues found that of 79 likely candidates for appendectomy, 52 were ruled out laparoscopically, sparing these patients considerable mortality.[12] Interestingly, the presence of hypochromic microcytic anemia with heme-positive stools in the setting of acute appendicitis is highly suggestive of appendicitis secondary to neoplastic obstruction.

Diverticular Disease. Diverticulosis, defined as simple herniation of the bowel wall that does not violate the serosa, occurs in 2% of Americans younger than age 30, in 50% of Americans older than age 60, and increases thereafter.[30] Most patients are asymptomatic, but they may experience constipation (as both a cause and effect of diverticular disease) and bloating with mild discomfort. Among the elderly, simple diverticulosis is an important cause of lower gastrointestinal bleeding, second only to vascular ectasia and other arteriovenous malformations. The sigmoid colon is the area most commonly affected and is the only colonic segment involved in 65% of patients. Fifteen percent of patients with documented diverticulosis will have at least one episode of significant hemorrhage that is generally not associated with pain and usually resolves spontaneously. In most cases, a single diverticulum is responsible and up to 25% of patients will suffer a recurrence.[30] Bleeding that fails to subside may be treated with vasoconstrictor agents (e.g., vasopressin) instilled via selective mesenteric angiography. This method has been reported to be successful in greater than 90% of patients.

Although diverticulosis can remain asymptomatic for years, with inflammation and/or violation of the outer (serosal) bowel surface, complications ensue. In this regard, perforation may result in peritonitis or the contaminated area may be walled off by omentum, small bowel, or bladder, resulting in a pericolic abscess or chronic fistula formation. The abscess itself is not only a source of infection but may also cause bowel obstruction. In the early phase of diverticulitis, the presentation often consists of well-localized left lower quadrant pain exacerbated by defecation. Guarding on abdominal examination and, at times, a palpable mass (in the nonobese subject) will also be evident. Distal lesions may be palpable as a mass on rectal exam. Fever and leukocytosis of some degree are the rule, with the caveat, as in all potential abdominal catastrophes herein discussed, that the elderly patient may be unable to mount an elevated white blood cell count or fever, particularly in the face of overwhelming sepsis. On occasion, if the involved area is adjacent to the urinary bladder, pyuria and hematuria may result. Any suspicion of an inflammatory lesion in this setting rules out the use of barium enema, as contents under pressure may initiate or extend bowel rupture.[31]

Clinical decisions regarding inpatient vs. outpatient therapy for diverticulitis depend on the severity of the disease process. Stable patients without peritoneal findings at the younger end of the geriatric age spectrum can usually be sent home with enterically active wide-spectrum antibiotics (e.g., sulfamethoxazole and trimethoprim, amoxicillin, ciprofloxacin), bed rest, liquid diet with stool softeners, and pain medication as necessary. Older patients who are more toxic and/or unable to take oral medications and fluids must be admitted for intravenous hydration while the bowel is placed completely at rest (i.e., npo with continuous nasogastric suction). They should receive parenteral antibiotic therapy (e.g., ampicillin-sulbactam [Unasyn] 1.5-3.0 g/q6h IV or another antibiotic providing coverage against anaerobes and gram-negative aerobic enteric organisms). As a rule, most cases subside with conservative measures, but in the significantly ill patient who fails to respond within 24-36 hours, or in whom abscess or fistula formation is suspected, temporary diverting colostomy with partial resection of the involved segment and eventual re-anastomosis is generally recommended.

Acute Lower Gastrointestinal Hemorrhage. Defined as bleeding distal to the ligament of Treitz, lower gastrointestinal hemorrhage is most closely associated with a patient's age, the average being 65.[32] In this age group, diverticulosis and angiodysplasia are the most common etiologies, while in roughly 10% of patients no source can be found.[33] In many cases the astute clinician can correlate signs and symptoms with likely bleeding sites and pathophysiology. A history of bright red blood noted on the toilet paper suggests hemorrhoids or anal fissure. Formed stool streaked with blood implies the presence of malignancy or benign polyp. Hematochezia or melena (maroon or black in color) denotes ascending colon or small bowel hemorrhage, or rapid bleeding from a more proximal site.

Like diverticulosis, angiodysplasia is a directly age-related phenomenon. Over time, normal intermittent distention of the cecum and right colon causes recurrent obstruction to venous outflow where veins penetrate the muscularis layer. This increases the back pressure, resulting in the formation of arteriovenous shunts.[34] Also like diverticulosis, bleeding will stop spontaneously in 80% of cases, while the recurrence rate is higher (up to 50%).[34] For the emergency physician, recognition of the actual or potentially unstable patient, prompt fluid resuscitation/transfusion, and coordination of specialty care are paramount. Definitive treatment includes laser photocoagulation, electrocoagulation, or surgical resection.

Mesenteric Vascular Occlusion

Among the most age-specific gastrointestinal catastrophes is the acutely ischemic bowel secondary to mesenteric vascular occlusion or insufficiency. While this condition occasionally occurs in younger patients at risk for atherosclerotic cardiovascular disease, this is primarily a disease of the elderly, in whom risk increases with advancing age.[35]

When faced with the patient complaining of abdominal pain, there is a natural tendency to think diagnostically in terms of primary alimentary endorgan dysfunction. In this setting, the differential diagnosis will include hepatic, biliary, or primary gastrointestinal disease. Although this is appropriate, it should be stressed that when dealing with the elderly patient, a primary vascular etiology for abdominal pain (e.g., abdominal aortic aneurysm) must always be entertained, both because of a greater statistical likelihood of occurrence in this age group and because of the dire consequences associated with a delay in diagnosis. While not within the scope of this review, the diagnosis of abdominal aortic aneurysm must be considered in any at-risk patient with abdominal pain, particularly the elderly hypertensive/vasculopathic male. Naturally the presence of a pulsatile abdominal mass, asymmetric lower extremity pulses, or pain radiating to the back or flank raises further suspicion.[36,37]

Etiologies for acute mesenteric ischemia include superior mesenteric artery embolus in about 30-35% of cases, superior mesenteric artery thrombosis in 10-15% of cases, and the syndrome of "nonocclusive mesenteric ischemia" (NOMI) in 40-50% of patients. These etiologies will be discussed separately, but it is useful to think of them collectively, since many features of their diagnoses and treatment are identical.

The patient with acute mesenteric ischemia usually is an elderly male who complains of diffuse abdominal pain, the severity of which is disproportionate to objective findings (i.e., severe discomfort with minimal objective findings). Often, there is a history of cardiovascular disease, such as recent myocardial infarction, congestive heart failure (or other "low-flow states"), or atrial fibrillation. The abdominal pain is deep and visceral in nature; the patient may be doubled over and is usually very still. The difficulty in diagnosis stems from the fact that early in the ischemic process, often including the early stages of infarction, the clinician is presented with few objective physical manifestations of concern. Besides the pain, abdominal distention and gastrointestinal bleeding may be the only findings until widespread bowel necrosis is well under way. Even these signs may be unreliable. In many patients fever, rigors, nausea and vomiting, leukocytosis, and vascular collapse occur in varied but rapid succession. Laparoscopy, although useful for diagnosing transmural infarction, is not reliable for evaluating earlier stages of mucosal ischemia in which blood is shunted to the serosa and the normal intestinal appearance is preserved for the eye of the direct observer. Because of these diagnostic pitfalls, mortality figures for combined causes exceed 70%.

Acute Superior Mesenteric Artery (SMA) Thrombosis. Preexisting atherosclerosis is usually the setting for acute thrombotic obstruction in the mesenteric vasculature. The lesion typically forms within the first 2 cm of the artery's branch point from the aorta, where chronic turbulence of flow results in maximal plaque formation. Patients with thrombotic etiology for their vascular occlusion may report a history of postprandial "intestinal angina," usually upper abdominal in location, crampy in nature, and occurring 30-60 minutes after a meal.

SMA Embolus. Embolic occlusion, approximately twice as common as thrombotic occlusion, is most often seen in the elderly man with cardiovascular disease. Because of its acute angle as it takes off from the aorta, the superior mesenteric artery is well designed for harboring emboli, which most often originate from a mural thrombus in the left heart. Atrial fibrillation is an important risk factor. While these patients do not generally report a history of prior intestinal angina, they often have a history of previous embolic disease involving cerebral, iliofemoral, or other major arteries. It has been noted in one study that 20% of those patients presenting with SMA occlusion have been shown to have synchronous emboli in other arteries.

Syndrome of Nonocclusive Mesenteric Ischemia. In this condition, which probably accounts for as many as one-half of all cases of mesenteric infarction, no specific obstructive lesion is discovered, but one or more of a variety of factors ultimately results in greatly reduced blood flow to the splanchnic bed. Hemorrhagic shock or hypovolemia from any cause can reduce flow to the mesentery, where, in this setting, splanchnic vasoconstriction (to divert blood to the heart and brain) compounds the problem. Similarly, patients with low output states from chronic congestive heart failure, recent myocardial infarction with reduced left ventricular function, and other primary cardiac causes are also at risk. Interestingly, because of more aggressive and sophisticated fluid resuscitation and monitoring of volume status along with more liberal usage of systemic vasodilators to unload the failing heart, this "low-flow" etiology appears to be declining in frequency.

Treatment. Elderly patients with mesenteric infarction, hemodynamic instability, and metabolic derangements are very poor operative candidates. Angiography, however, is a far less invasive maneuver and is being used with relative success both diagnostically and therapeutically in conditions associated with mesenteric ischemia. In a patient suspected of mesenteric occlusion, angiography will usually demonstrate the presence or absence of an obstructing lesion, and define the lesion as an embolus, thrombus, or low-flow splanchnic constrictive state. It will demonstrate the presence or absence of adequate collateral vessels around an obstruction and provide the basis for a rational decision regarding eventual laparotomy with intestinal resection and/or arterial dilatation or reconstruction. Occasionally a potent local vasodilator such as papaverine is selectively infused angiographically, often as a temporizing measure while surgical decisions are being made. The value of angiographic thrombolysis has not been determined so far.

Empiric Antibiotic Therapy

Because the risk of postoperative complications associated with acute abdominal disorders in the elderly is almost twice as great as in younger patients, antibiotic management must be aggressive and, in general, provide a spectrum of coverage that is broad enough to address polymicrobial infections associated with organisms of the gastrointestinal tract. As a rule most acute abdominal conditions in the elderly will require a combination of two agents-one to cover anaerobic and non-*Pseudomonas* gram-negative organisms and one to cover Pseudomonas species, if indicated. *(See Table 4.)* However, when perforation of a viscus has not occurred, a single agent may suffice.

Technologic Issues

Technology is making increasingly sophisticated procedures more available for diagnosis of acute abdominal pain.[38-43] While we recognize that in 1994, the ED physician is not likely to order an endoscopic retrograde cholangiopancreatogram (ERCP) or to schedule lithotripsy, the rationale for such procedures and their role in the diagnosis and treatment of various conditions should be understood by an informed primary care physician. The emergency physician will often be consulted by patient and family on any of a variety of issues and may indeed decide, for example, in the setting of the acute abdomen, whether a surgeon or radiologist is the next clinician to be contacted. We have seen that for the geriatric patient with abdominal pain, diagnostic delay is not an uncommon source of increased morbidity and mortality. Thus, a potent argument can be made for earlier and more complete evaluation (including one or more imaging studies) within the ED setting. Merely admitting the elderly patient for "expectant observation" while waiting for his or her lab values or physical examination to drastically change is no longer acceptable.

Until recent years, imaging studies of the acute abdomen, particularly in the ED, were largely limited to the standard abdominal plain film series. While this is a useful confirmatory tool when obstruction or perforation is strongly suspected, it is otherwise minimally useful. A total of 1780 patients reviewed by Eisenberg and associates demonstrated significant abnormality in only 10% of plain films, while a prospective study by McCook showed only a 2% incidence of clinically useful positive findings from this examination.[44] And while the abdominal plain film has been a reliable tool in the setting of bowel obstruction, Megibow and coworkers have shown the superiority of the abdominal CT scan, which was not only 95% accurate in diagnosing bowel obstruction, but could specifically identify hernias, neoplasms and adhesions, which together combined to account for 80% of obstructions in this series.[45]

Ultrasound and Appendicitis. Until recent years, the emergency clinician evaluating appendicitis has had little support from diagnostic imaging. Plain films of the abdomen might show an appendicolith in a small minority of cases, indicating appendicitis in the appropriately symptomatic patient. But the sensitivity of plain films was unacceptably poor. Beginning in 1981 with initial case reports, this decade has generated improved technology and increasingly discriminating sonographic criteria for the diagnosis of appendicitis. These criteria include: 1) visualization of a noncompressible appendix (an noninflamed appendix will not visualize on ultra sound); 2) the presence of fecaliths; and 3) maximal appendiceal diameter exceeding a certain length (6 mm is a figure currently used). Additionally, periappendiceal fluid and inflammatory changes in the periappendiceal fat can sometimes be identified. With these kind of criteria, one study found the technique was 90% sensitive and greater than 96% specific with 94% accuracy.[21]

An important study prospectively evaluated 100 patients with right upper-quadrant pain but without nausea, fever, or leukocytosis-a clinical setting common in the geriatric population. Here the CT scan was 98% sensitive, 83% specific, and 93% accurate in making the diagnosis of appendicitis. It also picked up other causes of pain in 17% of those original 100 patients, including ileocolitis, diverticulitis, pyelonephritis and pancreatitis. Thus, in the geriatric patient in whom appendicitis remains a possibility but where diverticulitis, neoplasm, or bowel ischemia are also likely, the abdominal CT scan may be the procedure of choice. It should be noted, however, that a CT scan in this setting will require administration of oral contrast material to completely opacify the gastrointestinal tract-a potential liability in the imminently presurgical candidate. Furthermore, Taourel and colleagues looked at 40 "difficult" cases in which diagnosis was unclear despite routine lab work, plain films, and surgical consultation.[47] Diagnoses prior to CT scan were compared to post-CT diagnoses, and both were compared with discharge diagnoses. CT scans were able to correctly diagnose 38 of 40 patients, while the pre-CT clinical diagnoses were accurate in only 50% of patients.

Ultrasonic Evaluation of the Pancreas. Diagnostic specificity in ruling in (or out) pancreatic disease in the elderly is a less critical matter than specificity in assessing the appendix or biliary tree. The decision whether to hospitalize the patient is based largely on the clinical presentation (e.g., hemodynamic status, degree of pain, tolerance of fluids and medications) rather than narrowly on the presence or absence of pancreatitis. Nonetheless, in the geriatric patient with abdominal pain, the process of ruling in pancreatitis as the etiology for abdominal symptomatology is valuable; once ruled in, surgery is rarely a consideration and further diagnostic procedures may be delayed pending clinical assessment and treatment of the patient's immediate condition.

The ED physician should not hesitate to consult with the radiologist to help explain abdominal pain or elevated enzyme levels. The advantages of ultrasound in the acute setting are its rapidity of performance, multidirectional imaging capacity, relative low cost, and accuracy in detailing the full length of the common bile duct. In this setting, the radiologist will describe a gland that is focally or diffusely enlarged (with edema) with more irregular margins and increased echogenicity. Biliary pancreatitis will reveal the presence of stones, while chronic disease may disclose pseudocyst formation.

While providing more extensive detail of pancreatic anatomy, there would appear to be little justification for "screening CT scans" in the setting just described. As a follow-up, either for inpatient or outpatient studies, CT is invaluable. However, in the evaluation of the patient with negative or equivocal ultrasonic findings, who has as-yet-undiagnosed abdominal pain, the decision whether to obtain immediate surgical consult, to admit, or to discharge the patient must be made on clinical grounds.

Summary

Elderly patients with acute abdominal catastrophes frequently present with atypical symptoms of prolonged duration. Cholecystitis, intestinal obstruction, and appendicitis remain the most common etiologies for the surgical abdomen in the elderly; acute pancreatitis is the most common nonsurgical abdominal etiology for hospital admission. Moreover, a high index of suspicion should be maintained for vascular etiologies causing abdominal complaints in the elderly.

Because the rate of misdiagnosis is high in this population, evaluation must be systematic and will include plain radiography of the abdomen when indicated, and if a diagnosis cannot be made with this modality, ultrasonic evaluation is mandatory in almost all cases prior to discharge from the ED. In addition, there is a need for an aggressive approach to elective surgery in selected cases where prognosis is often comparable to that in younger subjects but significantly worse under emergent conditions.

Finally, with the regular use of ultrasonographic assessment and enhanced clinical skills on the part of emergency physicians, it is possible to reduce the number of elderly patients discharged from EDs departments who are suffering from mild or nebulous symptoms that are actually harbingers of impending abdominal catastrophe.

References

1. Baum SA, Rubenstein Z. Old people in the emergency room: Age related differences in emergency department use and care. *J Am Geriatr Soc* 1987;35:398-404.
2. Eisenberg RL, Heineken P, et al. Evaluation of abdominal radiography in the diagnosis of abdominal pain. *Ann Surg* 1984;197:464469.
3. McCook TA, Ravin CE, Rice RP. Abdominal radiographs in the emergency department: A prospective analysis. *Ann Emerg Med* 1982;1:7-8.
4. Rice RP, Thompson WL, et al. The diagnosis and significance of intraluminal gas in the abdomen. *Radial Clin North Am* 1982;20:819.
5. Wertkin MG, Aufses AH. Management of volvulus of the colon. *Dis Colon Rectum* 1978;21:40-45.
6. Crump C. The incidence of gallstones and gall bladder diseases. *Surg Gynecol Obstet*1979;53;447-455.
7. Fenjo G. Acute abdominal disease in the elderly: Experience from two series in Stockholm. *Am J Surg* 1982;143:751-754.
8. Margiotta DZ, et al. Fragmentation of gallstones by extracorporeal shock waves. *N Engl J Med* 1986;314: 751-754.
9. Carroll BA. Preferred imaging techniques for the diagnosis of cholecystitis and cholelilithiasis. *Ann Surg* 1989;210:1-12.
10. Glenn F. Surgical management of acute cholecystitis in patients 65 years of age and older. *Ann Surg* 1981;193:56-59.

11. Graham A, Henley C. Laparoscopic evaluation of acute abdominal pain. *J Laparoendosc Surg* 1991;1:165-168.
12. Custer GG, Gilroy SB. The role of laparoscopy in the diagnosis of acute appendicitis. *Am Surg* 1992;58:627-629.
13. Meador JH, et al. Laparoscopic cholecystectomy: Report of 82 cases. *South Med J* 1991;84:186-189.
14. Blake R, Lynn J. Emergency abdominal surgery in the aged. *Br J Surg* 1976;63:956-960.
15. Day EA, Marks C. Gallstone ileus. *Am J Surg* 1975;128: 552-558.
16. Long RN, Heimbach DM. Acalculous cholecystitis in critically ill patients. *Am J Surg* 1978;136:31-36.
17. Long RN, et al. Acalculous cholecystitis in critically ill patients. *Am J Surg* 1978;136:31-36.
18. Pollock EW, Ring ER. Percutaneous decompression of benign and malignant biliary obstruction. *Arch Surg* 1979; 114:148-151.
19. Leverat M, et al. Peptic ulcer in patients over 60: Experience in 287 cases. *Am J Dig Dis* 1966;11:279-285.
20. Griffin ML, et al. Non-steroidal anti-inflammatory use and death from peptic ulcer in elderly persons. *Ann Intern Med* 1988;109:359-363.
21. Hoffman E, Perez E. Acute pancreatitis in the upper age groups. *Gastroenterology* 1959;36:675-685.
22. Mallory A, Kern F. Drug induced pancreatitis: A critical review. *Gastroenterology* 1980;78:813-820.
23. Jam I, et al. Elevated serum amylase activity in the absence of clinical pancreatic or salivary gland disease. *Am J Gastroenterol* 1978;70:480-488.
24. Warshaw AL, et al. The pathogenesis of pulmonary edema in acute pancreatitis. *Ann Surg* 1975;82:505-510.
25. Wolfe W, et al. Acute appendicitis in the aged. *Surg Gynecol Obstet* 1952;94:239-247.
26. Kauvar DR. The geriatric acute abdomen. *Clin Geriatr Med* 1993;9:547-558.
27. Hirsch SB, Wilder JR. Acute appendicitis in hospital patients over 60 (1974-84). *Mt. Sinai J Med* 1987;54::29-33.
28. Forde KA. The role of laparoscopy in the evaluation of the acute abdomen in critically ill patients. *Surg Endosc* 1992;6: 219-221.
29. Koruda MJ. Appendicitis: Laparoscopic strategy in diagnosis and treatment. *N Carol Med J* 1992;53:196-198.
30. Lichtiiger S, Kombluth A, et al. Lower gastrointestinal bleeding. In: Taylor MB, Gollan LL, et al, eds. *Gastrointestinal Emergencies.* 1st ed. Baltimore: Williams and Wilkins; 1992:358.
31. Deckman RC, Cheskin LJ. Diverticular disease in the elderly. *J Am Geriatr Soc* 1993;41:986-993.
32. Browder W, Cerise EJ. Impact of emergency angiography in massive lower gastrointestinal bleeding. *Ann Surg* 1986;204:530.
33. Boley SJ, DiBiase A. Lower intestinal bleeding in the elderly. *Am J Surg* 1979;137:57.
34. DeMarkles MP, Murphy JR. Acute lower Gastrointestinal Bleeding. *Med Clin North Am* 1993;77:1095-1096.
35. Boley SJ, et al. An aggressive roentgenologic and surgical approach to acute mesenteric ischemia. In: Hyus L. *Surgery Annual.* New York: Appleton-Century-Crofts; 1973.
36. Chalmers RT, et al. Abdominal aortic aneurysms in the elderly. *Br J Surg* 1993;80:1122-1123.
37. Paty PS, et al. Aortic replacement for abdominal aortic aneurysm in elderly patients. *Am J Surg* 1993;166-193.
38. Takada T, et al. Ultrasound diagnosis of acute appendicitis. *Int Surg* 1986;71:9-13.
39. Reid MH, Phillips HE. The role of CT and ultrasound imaging inbiliary tract disease. *Surg Clin North Am* 1981;61: 787-825.
40. Martin K, Doubilet P. How to image the gall bladder in suspected cholecystitis. *Ann Intern Med* 1988;722-729.
41. Jeffrey RB, Laing FC. Acute appendicitis: Sonographic criteria based on 250 cases. *Radiology* 1988;167:327-329.
42. Clark LR, et al. Pancreatic imaging. *Radial Imag North Am* 1985;26:489-501.
43. Ungar JA. Acute care imaging techniques:a clinical approach. In: Schwartz et al, eds. Emergency Medicine: The Essential Update. Philadelphia: W.B. Saunders Co; 1989.
44. Brazaitis MP, Dachman AH. Radiologic evaluation of acute abdominal pain of intestinal origin. *Med Clin N Am* 1993; 77:941.
45. Megibow AJ, Balthazar EJ, et al. Bowel obstruction: Evaluation with CT. *Radiology* 1991;180:313-318.
46. Balthazar EJ, Megibow AJ, Siegel SE, et al. Appendicitis: Prospective evaluation with high resolution CT. *Radiology* 1991;180:21-24.
47. Taourel P, Baron MP, Prade J, et al. Acute abdomen of unknown origin: Impact of CT in diagnosis and management. *Gastrointest Radial* 17:287294.

Intestinal Gas Complaints

Fabrizis L. Suarez, MD, PhD
Michael D. Levitt, MD

Patients frequently attribute a variety of symptoms to the presence of excessive gastrointestinal gas. These symptoms may take the form of excessive eructation, bloating and abdominal distention, or abnormal volume, or malodor of flatus. Unfortunately, objective verification of the existence of these problems is difficult, if not impossible. Thus, the physician must commonly rely upon the patient's self-perception that there is an abnormality. This unfortunate situation is further complicated by the lack of scientific information concerning the appropriate diagnostic and therapeutic approach to gaseous complaints. As a result, the physician usually treats gaseous problems without clear-cut evidence that a problem actually exists and with treatments of highly questionable efficacy.

In this chapter, the authors review what is known about the origin, diagnosis, and treatment of gaseous complaints. Although many of these problems may not be susceptible to therapy, it is hoped that this review will allow the physician to respond to the complaint of "too much gas" in a cost-effective, rational fashion.

Physiology of Bowel Gas

An understanding of the factors that deliver gas to and remove gas from the gut facilitates a rational response to gaseous complaints. Five gases are present in quantitatively important volumes in the human gut: N_2, O_2, H_2, CO_2, and CH_4 (methane).[1,2] None of these gases has an odor. The characteristic unpleasant odor of intestinal gas, as will be discussed, appears to result primarily from the presence of trace quantities of sulfur-containing compounds such as H_2S.[3]

Figure 1 summarizes the mechanisms by which gas enters and leaves the human gut. The four mechanisms that deliver gas to the lumen and the specific gases delivered by these mechanism are: 1) air swallowing → O_2 and N_2; 2) interaction of bicarbonate and acid → CO_2; 3) diffusion from the blood → CO_2, N_2, and O_2; and 4) bacterial fermentation reactions → CO_2, H_2, CH_4, and a wide variety of trace gases including gases containing sulfur such as H_2S. Gases can be removed from the gut via: 1) eructation and passage per anus; 2) diffusion into the blood; and 3) consumption of gas by bacteria. The net of these processes proximal to a given site in the gut determines the volume and composition of gas passing that site; the net of these processes throughout the entire gut determines the volume and composition excreted per rectum.

It is apparent from the above that diffusion can contribute to or reduce the volume of gut gas. The direction of net diffusion of gas (i.e., into or out of the lumen) is determined by the partial pressurue difference of the gas in the lumen and the blood. Gases whose sole source in the body is intraluminal production such as H_2 and CH_4 always diffuse from lumen to blood.[4] Following absorption, these gases are carried by the blood to the lungs, where they are efficiently cleared in expired air. To determine the fractions of these gases that are absorbed and passed per rectum, subjects have been housed in airtight rooms for several-day periods.[5] The total excretion rate of H_2 and CH_4 (via lungs and anus) was determined from the difference in concentration of the gas in the air entering and leaving the room. Measurements of the gases in expired air permitted determination of the rates that the gas was absorbed and excreted by the lungs. Usually, about 50% of each gas was absorbed and excreted on the breath, although when gas passage was very rapid, a smaller fraction was absorbed. Measurements of the excretion rate of H_2 and CH_4 on the breath provide a simple, noninvasive means of assessing the gut production of these gases.

Nitrogen and CO_2 are normally present in the blood; thus, these gases have the potential to diffuse from the blood into the lumen as well as from lumen to blood. For example, air contains very little CO_2; therefore, when air is swallowed, CO_2 diffuses from the blood perfusing the stomach into the lumen. However, in the duodenum, acid reacts with duodenal bicarbonate producing very high concentrations of CO_2, and this gas now diffuses from lumen to blood.[6] Because CO_2 diffuses very rapidly, virtually all this CO_2 is probably absorbed in the small bowel. In the colon, the bacteria often produce large amounts of CO_2 that is not totally absorbed, and flatus often contains sizable quantities of CO_2.[2,3]

Figure 1. Mechanisms and Sites of Gas Delivery and Removal from the Gastrointestinal System

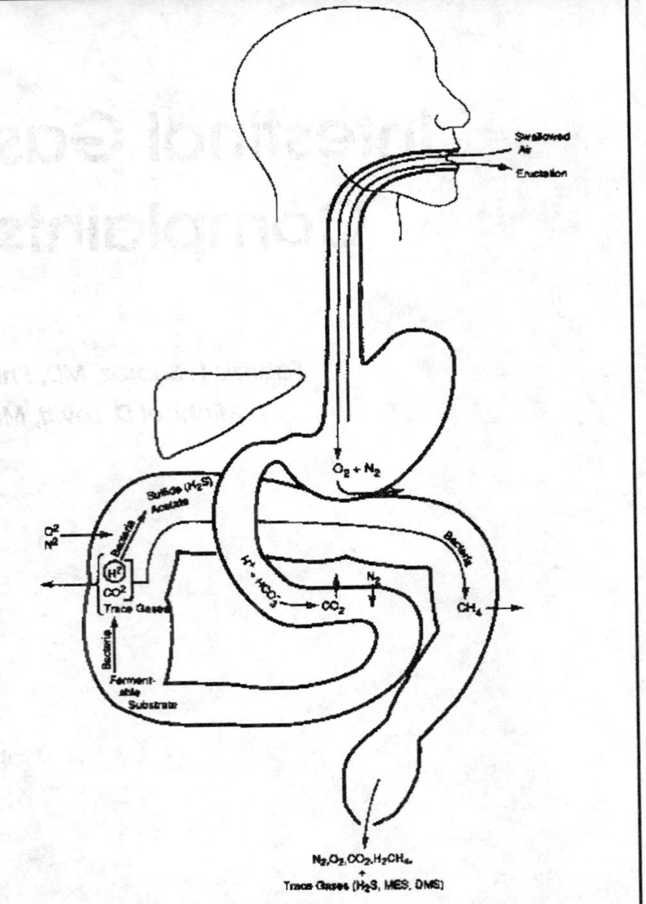

Clinical Complaints of Gas

The patient uses the terminology "gas" to refer to a variety of complaints including excessive eructation, abdominal discomfort and bloating, or passage of excessively voluminous or malodorous gas per rectum. A crucial aspect of the patient's history is to determine exactly which of these complaints is the problem since they have different origins and different treatments.

Excessive Eructation

Several centuries ago, postprandial belching indicated appreciation for the meal; today, however, eructation is generally socially unacceptable. One socially acceptable form of eructation is esophageal speech, which allows laryngectomized patients to form words via controlled belching.[7]

The mechanism of belching has been studied using radiological and manometric techniques.[8-10] McNally et al demonstrated that the pressure in the human stomach plateaued at 4-7 mmHg during distention of the stomach with air.[8] This finding suggests relaxation of both the gastric and abdominal musculature in response to increasing intragastric volume. At intermittent intervals, the lower esophageal sphincter (LES) opened, a common gastroesophageal cavity was established, and the subject belched. The requirement for relaxation of LES in belching is supported by the frequently observed inability of subjects to belch following fundoplication.[11] A belch also requires relaxation of the upper esophageal sphincter (UES). Kahrilas et al proposed that gaseous distention of the esophageal body induces relaxation of the UES.[10] Interestingly, UES pressure increases in response to fluid distention of the esophagus,[10] suggesting that the characteristics of esophageal contents may influence UES function.

Virtually every analysis of gas aspirated from the stomach has demonstrated that the predominant components are N_2 and O_2, the atmospheric gases.[12] Gases produced in the gut—CO_2, H_2, and CH_4—usually represent a minor fraction of this gas, although with gastric outlet obstruction, bacterial overgrowth in the stomach can lead to appreciable bacterial gas production. Thus, ordinarily, a belch is derived from swallowed air rather than gas produced in the stomach.

Using ultrafast computerized tomography, it was recently demonstrated that a mean of 17 mL of air accompanied each swallow of a 10 mL bolus of liquid.[13] Thus, 1700 mL of air

Figure 2. Algorithm for the Evaluation of the Patient Complaining of Excessive Flatus

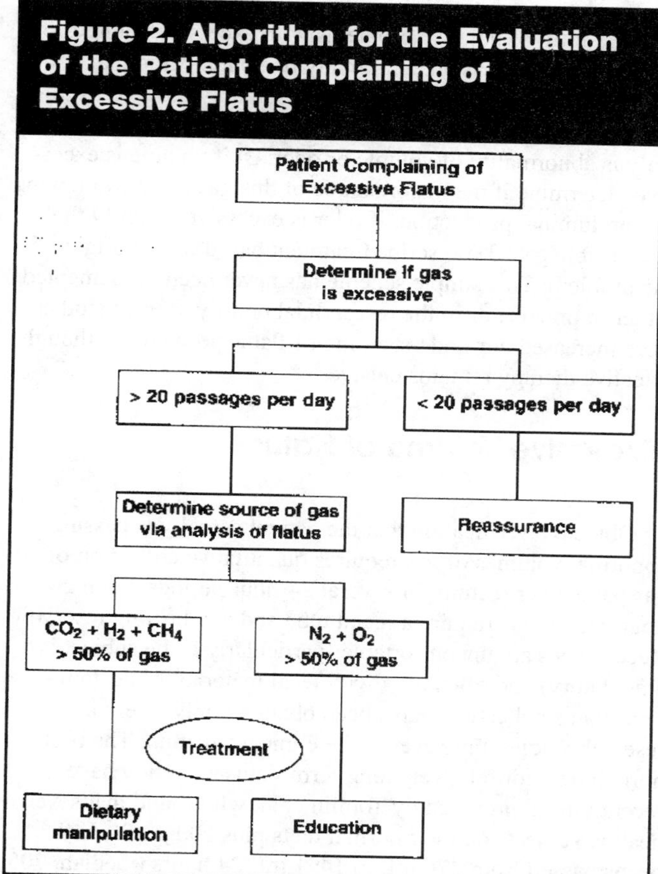

Table 1. Foods Containing Non-Absorbable Carbohydrates

TYPICAL FOOD SOURCES	NON-ABSORBABLE CARBOHYDRATES
Dietetic candies, sugarless gum	Sugar alcohols: mannitol, sorbitol, xylitol
Soft drinks, honey	Fructose
Legumes: soybeans, baked beans	Oligosaccharides: raffinose, stachyose
Complex carbohydrates: wheat, corn, potatoes	Resistant starch, retrograde starch
Grains, fruits, and vegetables	Fiber: cellulose, hemicellulose
Citrus fruits, beans, oat products	Pectins, gums, mucilages
Lactose*	Dairy products

* Only in lactose maldigester individuals.

(1350 mL of N_2) will be swallowed each day with the roughly one liter of liquid ingested per 24 hours. The swallowing of saliva and food will deposit additional N_2 in the stomach, and it seems likely that over 2000 mL of N_2 is swallowed each day. However, healthy subjects were found to excrete a mean of only about 250 mL of N_2 per 24 hours in flatus.[14] It is not possible to establish an appreciable positive N_2 gradient between lumen and blood; therefore, N_2 absorption from the gut is negligible. It follows that the vast majority of swallowed N_2 must be eliminated via recognized or unrecognized eructation.

In addition to the air swallowing that accompanies food and liquid ingestion, some subjects unconsciously aspirate air into the esophagus, often in an attempt to initiate an eructation. All or most of this air is immediately eructed from the esophagus, although the patient believes that the gas is emanating from the stomach. This maneuver results in a what might be termed a "pseudo" belch (i.e., a belch that clears gas from the esophagus, as opposed to the "true" belch that removes gas from the stomach).

Occasional belching is a normal phenomenon usually observed postprandial. Excessive and uncontrollable belching reflects excessive air swallowing or aspiration. The belching patient virtually never recognizes that excessive air swallowing is occurring, and conscious efforts to stifle air swallowing are seldom effective.

Hypersalivation from gum chewing, smoking, oral irritation, a chronic postnasal drip, nervousness, and tension are alleged to be associated with aerophagia, and treatment of these conditions should presumably be beneficial. Repeated "pseudo" eructation may result from attempts to alleviate discomfort in the stomach or esophagus (most commonly reflux esophagitis), and, for some reason, this maneuver seems to temporarily alleviate the discomfort. Treatment designed to eliminate the cause of the discomfort often leads to a decrease in eructation. While it has been claimed that it is difficult to swallow air if a tongue blade or some other object is held between the teeth, the effectiveness of this treatment has not been objectively evaluated. There is little scientific evidence that drugs such as simethicone, antispasmodics, or sedatives are useful in the treatment of excessive eructation. Of interest is a recent report by Spiegel of a 71-year-old subject with incessant eructation of four months' duration who was successfully treated with hypnosis.[15]

Abdominal Bloating and Distention

Frequently, the patient complaining of too much "gas" is referring to sensations of abdominal bloating or distention. In general, patients and health providers believe that excessive intestinal gas is the cause of such symptoms. However, using a washout technique, we found normal volumes of gas (< 200 mL) in the intestines of bloating subjects.[2] In addition, a study using computerized tomography found no evidence of increased intestinal gas in patients complaining of bloating,[16] and abdominal roentgenographs in patients complaining of bloating seldom demonstrate abnormal volumes of gas. Lastly, periods of high breath hydrogen excretion do not correlate with symptoms of discomfort in bloating patients.[17] Thus, it appears that complaints of bloating and distention are usually indicative of an "irritable" bowel that causes the patient to perceive that the intestine is over-distended when no such distention actually exists. This concept is supported by the observation that bloating patients have an enhanced pain response to balloon-induced

Figure 3. Volume of the Main Sulfur-Containing Gases in 16 Subjects

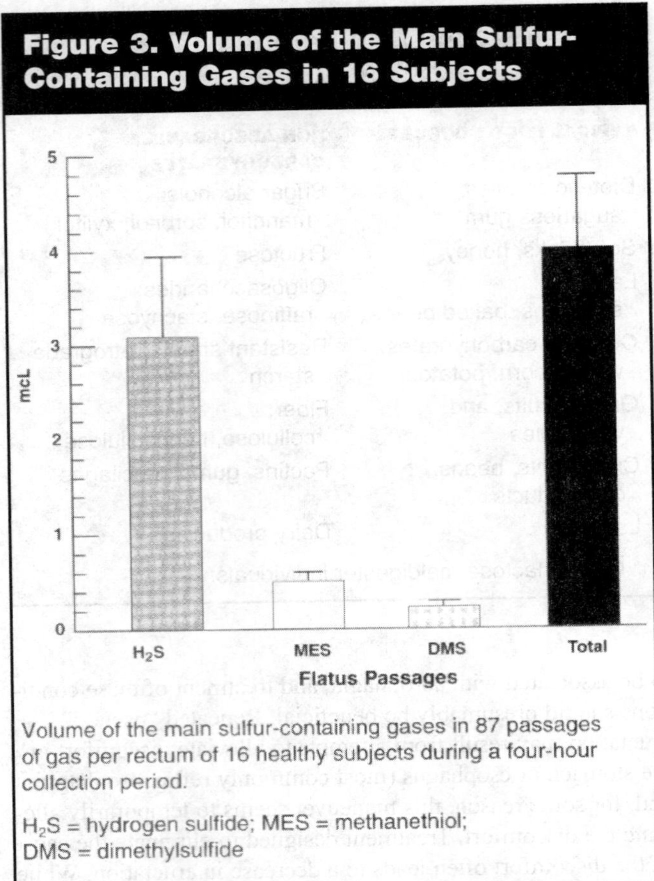

Volume of the main sulfur-containing gases in 87 passages of gas per rectum of 16 healthy subjects during a four-hour collection period.

H_2S = hydrogen sulfide; MES = methanethiol; DMS = dimethylsulfide

bowel distention.[18] It also is possible that feelings of distention reflect increased volume of solid or liquid luminal contents. For example, we found that healthy subjects complained of mild distention and "gas" following ingestion of fiber.[19] These subjects had no increase of flatus or breath H_2 excretion, and it appeared that the fiber-induced increase in luminal bulk was responsible for the sensation of distention.

It should be stressed that partial bowel obstruction also presents with bloating and distention. Thus, the work-up required for these complaints depends upon the age of the patient, duration of the problem, and associated symptoms. The subject younger than 40 years of age with a multiple-year history and no systemic symptoms is unlikely to have an obstructing lesion, and a minimal workup is indicated. In contrast, an elderly patient with a brief history of symptoms requires a more thorough evaluation.

We are aware of no data to indicate that treatments designed to reduce bowel gas benefit patients with functional bloating and distention. Therapy should generally be directed toward treatment of the underlying irritable bowel.

Rectal Gas Complaints

Patients not infrequently complain that their passage of rectal gas represents a major social problem. This complaint can take the form of putative problems with excessive volumes of flatus or gas that has an abnormally bad odor. A rational approach to this complaint would presumably proceed as follows *(please see Figure 2)*: 1) objectively determine if there truly is abnormality of volume or odor; 2) if volume is excessive, determine if the major source of this gas is air swallowing or intraluminal production; if odor is excessive, identify the responsible gas; 3) prescribe treatment based on the origin of the problem. This simple scheme has never been implemented either in practice or in the research laboratory. Recent studies have increased our understanding of flatus problems, although effective therapy remains elusive.[3,14]

Excessive Volume of Flatus

Objective verification that the patient actually is passing abnormal volumes of gas requires quantitative collection of all gas passed per rectum for several 24-hour periods. Such 24-hour collections require a rectal tube and a collecting reservoir. Rectal tubes are uncomfortable (particularly if the subject is ambulatory) and often plug with fecal material. Thus, long-term flatus collections have been obtained only rarely in research studies and never in the clinical situation. The best normal data for relatively long-term flatus excretion have recently been provided by Tomlin et al, who found that seven healthy subjects on their normal diets plus 200 g of baked beans passed from 476 mL to 1491 mL/24 hours (median, 705 mL/24 hours).[14]

Quantitative collections of rectal gas are only possible with highly motivated patients. A much simpler measure of flatus normality is a count of flatus passages, a technique we have used extensively in research studies designed to assess gas excretion after ingestion of lactose, lactulose, beans, and fiber.[20-22] A study involving 20 healthy subjects ingesting their ad lib diets indicated that healthy controls pass gas an average of 10 times per day, with an upper limit of normal (mean ± SD) of 20 times per day.[19] No statistically significant difference in the frequency of gas passage was observed with gender or age. The finding of statistically significant increases in gas passages when the diet was supplemented with lactulose or pinto beans, two stimuli known to increase gas production in the colon, supports the ability of this technique to identify a real increase in flatulence. However, since an individual passage of gas can vary in volume from 17 mL to 375 mL,[4] flatulence frequency obviously is not a perfect quantitative indicator of gas passage.

In practice, patients generally complain of excessive frequency rather than excessive volume of gas passage. As the initial step in the evaluation of such a patient, we recommend that the subject maintain a meticulous recording of each flatus passage for a one-week period. There is a good deal of misunderstanding as to what constitutes normal for flatus frequency, and these recordings frequently show a normal frequency (i.e., < 20 passages per day). In this situation, no further diagnostic tests are indicated, and reassurance should be provided to the subject as to his or her "normality." While patients may not be

Table 2. Correlation Between the Concentration of Sulfur-Containing Gases and Odor Intensity of Flatus Passages*

Odor Intensity§	H_2S‡	MES‡	DMS‡	Total Sulfur-Containing Gases
Judge 1	r = 0.644	r = 0.248	r = 0.333	r = 0.628
	P < 0.001	P = 0.071	P = 0.014	P = < 0.001
Judge 2	r = 0.437	r = 0.304	r = 0.227	r = 0.444
	P = 0.001	P = 0.026	P = 0.099	P = 0.001

* Data were analyzed by the Pearson correlation coefficient. N = 54 flatus passages.

§ Odor intensity was rated on a linear scale ranging from 0 (no odor) to 8 (very offensive).

‡ H_2S = Hydrogen sulfide; MES = Methanethiol; DMS = Dimethylsulfide

completely satisfied by this reassurance, further evaluation is not indicated when no abnormality exists.

If flatus frequency is appreciably greater than 20 times per day, the assumption is that the patient is passing excessive gas, and the next step should be to determine the origin of the gas. There are two possible sources of excessive bowel gas: intraluminal production and swallowed air. The quantitatively important gases produced in the lumen are CO_2, H_2, and CH_4, whereas air swallowing delivers N_2 and O_2 to the gut. Thus, the analysis of a carefully collected flatus sample provides a quick means of determining the source of the gas.

The collection of a rectal gas sample is most easily achieved using a rectal tube attached to a syringe via a three-way stopcock.[4] It should be stressed that the initial gas sample collected contains large amounts of air from the dead space of the tube. Thus, several gas samples must be collected and discarded via the free arm of the three-way stopcock before collecting the sample for analysis. The O_2 content of the sample provides a simple internal control with regard to atmospheric contamination of the sample. Rectal gas always contains low levels of O_2 (< 5%), whereas atmosphere contains 21% O_2. Samples containing greater than 5% O_2 are not a reliable indicator of flatus composition

While our laboratory is one of the few in the country capable of routinely carrying out a complete analysis of rectal gas, detectors used for analysis of breath H_2, CH_4, and CO_2 are widely available. With appropriate dilution (H_2 and CH_4 may require dilutions of 5000-fold), the contribution of gases produced in the lumen can be measured with these detectors. If the analysis shows that H_2, CO_2, and CH_4 represent the majority of flatus, the gas is being produced in the gut. If these gases comprise the minority of the flatus sample, it can be assumed that N_2 must be the major component, and that air swallowing is the major source of the gas.

Excessive rectal gas is commonly assumed, both by physicians and the lay public, to result from intraluminal production as opposed to swallowed air. In reality, there have been too few studies of flatulent subjects to determine if this assumption is correct.[23] We have recently studied a very flatulent patient (up to 120 passages of gas per day) who had been subjected to innumerable expensive diagnostic tests in the belief that the patient must have an abnormality of the gut that caused excessive gas production.[24] Analysis of flatus samples on three occasions showed that virtually all the rectal gas was N_2 (i.e., excessive air swallowing was the source of the flatus). In this situation, therapy should be directed toward the reduction of air swallowing (see eructation section). Given that eructation appears to be an important determinant of the quantity of swallowed air that enters the intestine, treatment with carminotives that enhance belching (i.e., peppermint water) theoretically could reduce rectal gas excretion.

When flatus consists of non-atmospheric gases, H_2, CO_2, and CH_4, fermentation reactions carried out by the intestinal flora are the source of the rectal gas. The quantity of gas produced is a function of the availability of fermentable substrates (primarily carbohydrates) to the colonic flora and the gas-releasing ability of the flora.[25]

The colon contains bacteria that produce gas and other organisms that efficiently consume gas. The net of these two competing processes determines the amount of gas available for excretion. For example, fermentation of 10 g of carbohydrate can liberate 3400 mL of H_2.[26] Since healthy subjects are thought to malabsorb about 30 g of carbohydrate each day, more than 10,000 mL of H_2 should be produced in the colon per 24 hours. This volume of H_2 would obviously produce very severe flatulence. However, only about 5% of the H_2 that is produced in the colon is actually excreted;[27] the other 95% is consumed by bacteria that use this gas for methane production or sulfate reduction.[28-30]

The substrate used by the colonic flora for gas production may be of endogenous or exogenous (dietary) origin. Mucin is a carbohydrate-rich compound that is produced endogenously. For a dietary carbohydrate to serve as substrate for fermentation reactions in the colon, the carbohydrate must be incompletely absorbed in the small bowel. In patients with diffuse intestinal disease (celiac disease, for example), all dietary carbohydrates may be malabsorbed. Healthy subjects also may incompletely absorb a variety of carbohydrates.

Since absorption of carbohydrates requires that these compounds be digested to the monosaccharide form, malabsorption may reflect the inability to digest a carbohydrate or the inability to absorb certain monosaccharides (i.e., sorbitol). Table 1 lists various foods that contain non-absorbable carbohydrates. Examples of foods that are malabsorbed due to incomplete digestion include lactose, in lactase-deficient subjects, and legumes, which contain oligosaccharides such as raffinose that are totally indigestible by humans. Of particular interest is the demonstration that the commonly ingested sources of starch, such as wheat, potatoes, corn, and oats, increase breath H_2 excretion, indicating incomplete absorption.[31] The resistance to digestion of these foodstuffs appears to result from the inability of amylase to gain access to the starch as opposed to an inherent indigestibility of the starch molecule. Refrigeration of cooked wheat products such as pasta aggravates this maldigestion by causing the starch to crystallize in a process called retrogradation.[32]

The vast majority of subjects complaining of excessive flatus have no recognizable disorder of the intestinal tract. Thus, extensive diagnostic studies are generally not indicated unless there is some other evidence of a malabsorptive disorder. In particular, there is no gross anatomical lesion that could cause excessive flatulence, and expensive endoscopic and radiological studies are not useful.

Theoretically treatment of excessive flatus due to gas production in the gut may involve: 1) enhancement of digestion of carbohydrates using exogenous enzymes; 2) removal of the offending foodstuff(s) from the diet; or 3) alteration of the colonic flora.

The most common situation in which exogenous enzymes are recommended for increased gas is when lactose is ingested by lactase-deficient subjects. However, our controlled studies showed that flatus frequency was only mildly but not statistically significantly increased when lactase-deficient subjects ingested one or two cups of milk with breakfast and dinner.[33] Thus, the use of lactase preparations should be limited to the situation in which lactose is ingested in very appreciable quantities (i.e., > 2 cups per day). Lactase preparations can be added to milk, which is then incubated overnight, or taken as tablets with milk or milk products. A preparation that contains the enzyme required for digestion of the oligosaccharides in legumes (Beano) is available over-the-counter. Unfortunately, our studies have suggested that when this enzyme is used in accordance to the product insert, flatus frequency is not diminished.

Dietary alterations to reduce gas require elimination of most of the foods listed in Table 1. This is extremely difficult because of the multiple complex carbohydrates, such as wheat and potatoes, that are malabsorbed. Rice is the only complex carbohydrate that is completely absorbed.[34] A diet that contains no complex carbohydrates markedly reduces gas production.[14] Unfortunately, such a diet is found to be relatively unpalatable by the average American.

Lastly, induction of a flora that tends either to produce little gas or that efficiently consumes gas would be a useful therapeutic tool. There is some evidence that feeding subjects large quantities of nonabsorbable carbohydrates (such as lactose to lactose malabsorbers) induces a flora rich in lactobacilli, organisms that ferment carbohydrate via a non-gaseous pathway.[35,36] As a result, less gas is produced following lactose ingestion.

There is no evidence that any known manipulation can induce a flora that more effectively consumes gas. Antibiotic therapy does not appear to be a useful means of reducing colonic gas production due either to a failure of antibiotics to reduce gas producing organisms or, more likely, to a reduction of gas-consuming organisms.

Malodorous Flatus

Despite the enormous amount of discussion devoted to the topic of flatus odor, there has been minimal study of the factors responsible for this odor.[3] It was taught for many years that the offensive odor of flatus resulted from its content of aromatic breakdown products of proteins such as indole and skatole. However, Moore et al, in an elegant study of human feces, concluded that these aromatic compounds were present in very low concentration and that these compounds had an odor distinctly different from human feces.[37] These workers concluded that three sulfur-containing gases—methanethiol, dimethyldisulfide, and trimethylsulfide—were the major offensive gases elaborated by human feces.

We recently carried out the first systematic study designed to identify the odoriferous components of human flatus.[3] In this study, 87 individual flatus passages obtained from healthy subjects were collected via rectal tube and analyzed for sulfur containing gases. In contrast to the findings of Moore et al with human feces, we found the predominant sulfur gases in flatus to be H_2S, methanethiol, and dimethylsulfide *(please see Figure 3),* with H_2S being the predominant gas. The discrepancy between our findings and those of Moore et al appears to reflect the fact that the compounds we observed in flatus are all highly volatile and thus would rapidly leave the feces for the gas space. In contrast, two of the compounds observed by Moore and co-workers in feces, dimethyldisulfide and trimethylsulfide, have very low volatility. Thus, it is not surprising that these compounds are found in feces but not the surrounding gas phase (i.e., flatus).

While sulfur-containing gases are present in very low concentrations (< 0.01%) in flatus, these compounds have a very powerful, offensive odor. To actually determine if these gases were responsible for flatus malodor, it was necessary to employ the only instrument capable of judging the offensiveness of an odor—the human nose. In what is known as the "sniff test,"[38] two judges, previously shown to have excellent olfactory discrimination, blindly ejected a small amount of flatus contained in a syringe at a distance of about 5 cm from the nose. The offensiveness of the odor was rated on a linear scale. As shown in Table 2, a highly significant correlation was observed between the intensity of malodor and the concentrations of the sulfur gases. Such a correlation could indicate that the gases were associated with the presence of other odoriferous compounds as opposed to being cause of the odor. Thus, further experiments were carried out in which flatus samples were treated with zinc, which avidly binds the sulfhydryl components of H2S and methanethiol. This treatment markedly reduced the odor, indicating that the two sulfur-containing gases were very likely responsible for much of the offensive smell of flatus. Lastly, artificial flatus samples comprised of the three sulfur containing gases in concentrations typical of flatus were blindly presented to our judges.

These mixture were rated to be offensive and to have a fecal-like odor.

On the basis of the above evidence, we concluded that the sulfur gases were the predominant, but probably not the only offensive malodorous component of flatus. This knowledge simplifies studies of flatus odor in that the objective measurement of the concentration of gases can be employed in place of the time-consuming subjective evaluation of odor. Studies of the sulfur gases showed, somewhat contrary to expectation, that flatus from males had a lower concentration of sulfur gases than did gas collected from females.[3] However, the stimulation of the nose that results from flatus passage is a function of the amount of offensive gas released per passage as opposed simply to the concentration of these gases. When the larger volume of flatus passages in males vs. females (119 ± 11.9 mL vs 88 ± 8.9 mL) was taken into account, the actual volume of sulfur gas released per passage showed no gender difference.

We also indirectly investigated the "silent but deadly" concept, which proposes that quiet flatus passages are more offensive than noisy passages. While we did not employ an audiometer to measure the sound of the passages, it seems likely that large volume passages are more noisy than small passages. Thus, if the "silent but deadly" concept were correct, the quantity of sulfur gases should have been inversely correlated with the size of the passages. This was not the case, and, in fact, there was a strong positive correlation between the volume of sulfur gases and the volume of the passage.

The only treatment presently that has been claimed to reduce flatus odor is a fabric-covered, charcoal-lined cushion sold under tradename of "Toot Trapper" (UltraTech Products. Inc., Houston, TX). The manufacturer of this cushion claims that the cushion absorbs odoriferous gases in flatus, hence limiting the odor that escapes into the environment. Objective testing of the efficacy of this cushion requires a means of accurately determining the quantity of sulfur gases that escapes the cushion. To this end, we fabricated gas-tight mylar pantaloons that were sealed at the waist and the thighs with duct tape. The cushion was tested by inserting the active cushion, an identical appearing placebo cushion (charcoal encased in mylar), or no cushion into the pantaloons. The subjects sat on a wooden chair, and a small tube was situated at the anus. A mixture of the sulfur-containing gases was infused at the anus, and the quantity of gases escaping into the environment of the pants was determined. The cushion clearly was effective as evidenced by the more than 90% reduction in sulfur gases that occurred with the active cushion. The placebo cushion produced about a 50% reduction in sulfur gases, apparently due to reactivity of these gases with the fabric of the cushion. We conclude that the cushion is effective but unwieldy. Present experiments are being directed to miniaturizing the cushion and searching for compounds that bind sulfur gases in the colon.

References

1. Kirk E. The quantity and composition of human colonic flatus. *Gastroenterol* 1949;12:782-794.
2. Levitt MD. Volume and composition of human intestinal gas determined by means of an intestinal washout technique. *N Engl J Med* 1971;284:1394-1398.
3. Suarez FL, Furne JK, Springfield JR, Levitt MD. Identification of gases responsible for the odor of human flatus and evaluation of a device purported to reduce this odor. *Gastroenterol* 1997;112:A45.
4. Suarez FL, Furne JK, Springfield JR, Levitt MD. Insights into human colonic physiology obtained from study of flatus composition. *Am J Physiol* 1997;272:G1028-G33.
5. Christl SU, Murgatroyd PR, Gibson GR, Cummings JH. Quantitative measurement of hydrogen and methane from fermentation using a whole body calorimeter. *Gastroenterol* 1992;102: 1269-1277.
6. Fordtran JS, Walsh JH. Gastric acid secretion rate and buffer content of the stomach after eating. Results in normal subjects and in patients with duodenal ulcer. *J Clin Invest* 1973;52:645-657.
7. Pope CE. II. Heartburn, dysphagia and other esophageal symptoms. In Sleisinger MH, Fordtran JS, (eds). *Gastrointestinal diseases: Pathophysiology, diagnostic and management,* 4th ed. Philadelphia, PA: WB Saunders Company 1989:200-203.
8. McNally FE, Kelly JE, Ingelfinger FJ. Mechanism of belching: effects of gastric distention with air. *Gastroenterol* 1964;46: 254-259.
9. Castell CD. The lower esophageal sphincter: physiology and clinical aspects. *Ann Intern Med* 1975;83:390-401.
10. Kahrilas PJ, Dodds WJ, Dent J, Wyman JB, Hogan WJ, Arndorfer RC. Upper esophageal sphincter function during belching. *Gastroenterol* 1986;91:133-40.
11. DeMeester TR, Bonavina L, Albertucci M. Nissen fundoplication for gastroesophageal reflux disease. Evaluation of primary repair in 100 consecutive patients. *Ann Surg* 1986;204:9-20.
12. Maddock WG, Bell JL, Tremaine MJ. Gastrointestinal gas. Observation of belching during anesthesia, operations an pyelography and rapid passage of gas. *Ann Surg* 1949;130:512.
13. Pouderoux P, Gulchin AE, Shezhang L, Kahrilas PJ. Esophageal bolus transit imaged by ultrafast computerized tomography. *Gastroenterol* 1996;110:1422-1428.
14. Tomlin J, Lowis C, Read NW. Investigation of normal flatus production in healthy volunteers. *Gut* 1991;32:665-669.
15. Spiegel SB. Uses of hypnosis in the treatment of uncontrollable belching: A case report. *Am J Clin Hypnosis* 1996;38:263-270.
16. Maxton DG, Martin DF, Whorwell PJ, Godfrey M. Abdominal distention in female patients with irritable bowel syndrome: Exploration of possible mechanisms. *Gut* 1991;32:662-664.
17. Haderstorfer B, Psycholgin D, Whitehead WE, Schuster MM. Intestinal gas production from bacterial fermentation of undigested carbohydrate in irritable bowel syndrome. *Am J Gastroenterol* 1989;84:375-378.
18. Ritchie J. Pain from distention of pelvic colon by inflating a balloon, in the irritable bowel syndrome. *Gut* 1973;14:125-132.
19. Levitt MD, Furne J, Olsson S. The relation of passage of gas and abdominal bloating to colonic gas production. *Ann Intern Med* 1996;124:422-424.
20. Suarez FL, Savaiano DA, Levitt MD. A comparison of symptoms in people with self- reported severe lactose intolerance after drinking milk or lactose-hydrolyzed milk. *N Engl J Med* 1995;333:1-4.
21. Zumarraga LM, Levitt MD, Suarez FL. Absence of Gaseous Symptoms During Ingestion of Commercial Fiber Preparations. Aliment Pharmacol Therapeutics 1997 (in press).

22. Strocchi A, Corazza G, Ellis CJ, et al. Detection of malabsorption of low doses of carbohydrate: accuracy of various breath H_2 criteria. *Gastroenterol* 1993;105:1404-1410.
23. Levitt MD, Lasser R, Schwartz J, Bond JH. Studies of a flatulent patient. *N Engl J Med* 1976;295:260-262.
24. Levitt MD, Furne J, Aeolus MR, Suarez FL. Evaluation of an extremely flatulent patient: Case report and proposed diagnostic and therapeutic approach. 1997. Submitted for publication.
25. Strocchi A, Levitt MD. Intestinal Gas. In: Sleisenger MH, Fordtran JS, eds. *Gastrointestinal and Liver Diseases.* 6th ed. Philadelphia, PA: W.B. Saunders Company 1998:153-160.
26. Wolin MJ. Interaction between H_2-producing species. In: Schlegel HG, Pfenning N, eds. Microbial formation and utilization of gases. Gottingen, Germany: Goltze Press; 1976:141-147.
27. Christl SU, Murgatroyd PR, Gibson GR, Cummings JH. Production, metabolism, and excretion of hydrogen in the large intestine. *Gastroenterol* 1992;102:1269-1277.
28. Levitt MD, Gibson GR, Christl SU. Gas metabolism in the large intestine. In: Gibson GR, Macfarlane GT, eds. *Human colonic bacteria: Role in nutrition, physiology, and disease.* Boca Raton, FL: CRC Press, Inc. 1995:131-154.
29. Gibson GR, Cummings JH, Macfarlane GT, et al. Alternative pathways for hydrogen disposal during fermentation in the human colon. *Gut* 1990;31:679-683.
30. Levitt MD, Berggren T, Hastings J, Bond JH. Hydrogen (H_2) catabolism in the colon of the rat. *J Lab Clin Med* 1974;84:163-167.
31. Anderson IH, Levine AS, Levitt MD. Incomplete absorption of the carbohydrate in all-purpose wheat flour. *N Engl J Med* 1981;304:891-892.
32. Englyst HN, Wiggins HS, Cummings JH. Determination of the non-starch polysaccharides in plant foods by gas-liquid chromatography of constituent sugars as alditol acetates. *Analyst* 1982;107:307-318.
33. Suarez FL, Savaiano DA, Arbisi P, Levitt MD. Tolerance to the daily ingestion of two cups of milk by individuals claiming lactose intolerance. *Am J Clin Nutr* 1997;65:1502-1506.
34. Kerlin P, Wong L, Harris B, Capra S. Rice flour, breath hydrogen and malabsorption. *Gastroenterol* 1984;87:578-585.
35. Hertzler SR, Levitt MD, Savaiano DA. Colonic adaptation to the daily lactose feeding in lactose maldigesters reduces lactose intolerance. *Am J Clin Nutr* 1996;64:1232-1236.
36. Price KR, Lewis J, Wyatt GM, Fenwick GR. Flatulence-causes, relation to diet and remedies. *Nahrung* 1988;32:609-626.
37. Moore JG, Jessop LD, Osborne DN. Gas-chromatographic and mass-spectrometric analysis of the odor of human feces. *Gastroenterol* 1987;93:1321-1329.
38. Schimidt NF, Missan SR, Tarbet WJ, Cooper AD. The correlation between organoleptic mouth-odor rating and levels of volatile sulfur compounds. *Oral Surg* 1978;45:560-567.

Chronic Hepatitis C

Robert A. Levine, MD

Chronic hepatitis C virus (HCV) infection is the liver disease of this era. Predictions for the 21st century are that liver-related deaths from HCV will increase fourfold and orthotoptic liver transplantation sixfold, respectively. This is related to the fact that the currently infected pool of patients with HCV will peak in the next 10-20 years. Patients with chronic HCV are burdened with both the fear of dying of this disease and the stigma of living with it.

The recent National Institutes of Health Consensus Conferences on chronic HCV solidified the justification for a selective approach to treatment. Nevertheless, the high profile of chronic HCV has led to a sense of urgency about treating all newly recognized patients. This approach has caused the variable natural history of this disease to be overlooked. The debate about whom to treat has failed to focus attention on the alternate approach of waiting for better emerging therapies for the subset of patients with histologically minimal or mild chronic HCV. Practitioners may be more confident about postponing treatment in patients with minimal hepatitis on liver biopsy since they are less likely than patients with more moderate or severe necroinflammatory activity or fibrosis to progress to cirrhosis.

Background

Infection with the hepatitis C virus is a global health problem. An estimated 170 million people are chronically infected worldwide. In the United States, the prevalence of antibody to hepatitis C is estimated to be 1.8% and approximately 4 million persons in the United States currently have chronic HCV.[1,2]

Like acute hepatitis A or B, it is usually subclinical and less than 25% of patients develop jaundice. Fulminant hepatitis is rare, if it occurs at all. The number of acute cases of hepatitis C has decreased during the past decade from more than 150,000 to 30,000. Eighty-five percent of patients with HCV develop chronic infection. HCV contributes to the deaths of 10-12,000 Americans per year and is the principal cause of chronic liver disease, cirrhosis, and hepatocellular cancer (HCC). Among patients with chronic HCV, 20% progress to cirrhosis after 20-50 years and, thereafter, 1-5% develop HCC in 10-20 years.[3] Most patients remain asymptomatic for many decades and may never develop progressive or symptomatic liver disease. Approximately 20% of patients at the first time they are evaluated with liver biopsy already have cirrhosis. Alcohol abuse has a deleterious effect on the natural history of chronic HCV.

There remains disagreement as to the prognosis of patients with chronic HCV. In our experience, there is a large subpopulation of chronic HCV in which there is less progression to cirrhosis, if it occurs at all, when patients initially have histologically minimal or mild chronic HCV.[4] Those with more moderate or severe hepatitis and/or significant fibrosis are much more likely to develop cirrhosis.

Epidemiology

From a demographic point of view, HCV infection has its highest incidence among persons aged 20-39 years and males predominate slightly.[5] African Americans have substantially higher prevalence of HCV infection than do caucasians and probably a lesser response to treatment, although the latter has not been yet established.

Identifying Patients at Risk

One of the problems is to identify individuals at risk for disease progression. Three independent factors have been noted with an increased rate of fibrosis progression: age of infection older than 40 years, daily alcohol ingestion more than 50 g, and male sex. In addition, the histological picture of a liver biopsy is extremely important in prognosticating progression. As shown in Table 1, patients with no significant fibrosis and minimal or mild necroinflammation are at much lower risk of progression than those with moderate or severe necroinflammation and septal fibrosis or nodularity. The liver biopsy remains the cornerstone of risk identification. Strong predictors of progression to cirrhosis in 10 years are patients with a high grade of necroinflammation, septal fibrosis, or incomplete nodularity. The liver biopsy is more likely to identify the risk of progression than is the genotype or viral load. There is no correlation between HCV-RNA level and histology.[6] In many ways, a liver biopsy may be cost-effective since current therapy is expensive, is ineffective in the majority of patients, and has side effects that may be significant. It is critical to use the liver biopsy to recommend which patients have a better or worse prognosis. Conceivably, the role of liver biopsy may decrease in the future if emergent therapies become more cost-effective than the current therapies.[7] Some have argued that treatment of all patients with chronic HCV is cost-effective and would cut the lifetime incidence of cirrhosis from 66% to 60%.[8-9]

Alcohol is probably the most important high-risk factor as evidenced by the fact that moderate alcohol consumption is associated with a two- to three-fold greater risk of cirrhosis and decompensated liver disease.[10,11] In alcoholic users, 58% develop cirrhosis by the second decade, whereas only 10% of individuals who do not use alcohol develop cirrhosis in that same period.[11] Since alcohol is the most important factor to enhance disease progression and more than 10 g/d is addictive, in our center we recommend that patients not have any alcohol intake if they have chronic HCV.

As shown in Table 1, it is questionable whether genotype or viral levels show a correlation with disease activity and outcome strong enough to justify their use in assessing prognosis in individual patients. In general, patients with genotypes HCV-2 and HCV-3 have the best response in contrast with those with HCV-1, who have the worst. Unfortunately, these parameters have a low predictive value compared to the liver biopsy, which is the gold standard for prognostication.

Since chronic HCV is usually asymptomatic until irreversible liver damage has occurred, it is critical for the primary care providers to make a timely diagnosis and have a high index of suspicion for this disease. In order to obtain proper screening tests to detect asymptomatic infection during routine examinations, the practicing physicians should be familiar with the risk factors for acquiring chronic HCV, which include the patients with elevated alanine aminotransferase (ALT), intravenous drug abuse, hemophiliacs, hemodialysis patients, health care workers with exposure to blood-blood products,[12] persons with needle-stick injury, transplant recipients, transfusion/blood product recipients prior to 1990, persons with a tattoo or body piercing, HIV-positive individuals, persons who inhale cocaine, employment in patient care or clinical laboratory work, persons who are sexually active with multiple partners, exposure to a sex partner or a household member who has a history of hepatitis, and a low socioeconomic level. Although hepatitis C is associated with a history of tattoos, it has not been demonstrated that the transmission occurs also from ear piercing, acupuncture, or medical, surgical, or dental procedures.[13]

Transfusions

Currently, the transfusion rate is extremely rare, being less than 1.5% per recipient or approximately 0.02% per unit transfused.[13] Prior to 1990, however, before the advent of a screening test for HCV, there was a high prevalence rate. Persons with hemophilia have extremely high prevalence rates of HCV infection up to 90% because effective procedures to inactivate viruses in patients receiving clotting factor concentrate prepared from plasma pools was lacking.[13] Since December 1994, all immune globulin transfusion products are inactivated for HCV RNA.

Injecting and Other Illegal Use

Sharing syringes and needles is associated with high prevalence of HCV. After five years of injecting, as many as 90% of drug users are infected with HCV. The history of intranasal cocaine is one of the more recently recognized modes of transmission through probably epistaxis or contaminated straws. Studies suggest that as many as 14% of the general population have used cocaine at least once.[13]

Nosocomial and Occupational Exposure

Nosocomial transmission of HCV is possible if infection-controlled techniques of disinfection are inadequate and con-taminated equipment is shared among patients. Reports are rare of such a transmission, other than in chronic hemodialysis units. The latter prevalence ranges from as low as 10% to as high as 60%.[13]

Health care, emergency medical, and public safety workers who have exposure to blood in the workplace are at risk for being infected with HCV. However, the prevalence of HCV infection among health care workers, including surgeons, is no greater than the general population and averages 1-2%, and is 10 times lower than that for chronic hepatitis B infection.[13]

The average incidence of antibody seroconversion after unintentional needle sticks for sharp exposures from an HCV-positive source is 1.8% (range, 0-7%).[13]

Other Exposures

Percutaneous HCV transfusion has been associated with unusual folk medicine practices, tattooing, body piercing, and commercial barbering. High-risk sexual practices have a 6% prevalence of anti-HCV.[13] The prevalence among nonsexual household contacts of persons with chronic HCV infection is unknown.

Table 1. Risk of HCV Disease Progression

Low Risk	High Risk
Female	*Male*
Age < 35 years at acquisition	Age > 40 years at acquisition
No alcohol use	Alcohol use > 50 g daily
Mild necroinflammation (grades 1-2)	Moderate/severe necroinflammation (grades 3-4)
No/minimal fibrosis (stages 0/1)	Septal fibrosis/nodularity (stages 2-4)

The average rate of perinatal HCV infection among infants born to HCV-positive, HIV-negative women is 5-6%.[13-15] These findings are based solely on detection of anti-HCV and HCV RNA, respectively. HCV RNA can be detected in infected infants as early as 1-2 months. The rate of passage of HCV antibodies from mother to child is less than 1%, and the rate of HCV viremia in infants after perinatal transmission is uncommon.[13-15]

Although injecting-drug use accounts for 60% of HCV transmission, other exposures such as occupational, hemodialysis, household, and perinatal together account for approximately 10% of HCV infections. Thus, potential risk factors can usually be identified if a proper history is asked. Ideally, less than 10% of patients should have no recognized source of infection if the physician pursues with an intensive history, but in practice about 40% remain without a likely source of their disease.

Pathogenesis

The host immune response is activated in chronic HCV, particulary T-cell-mediated activity. The latter contributes to hepatic damage. Unfortunately, humoral, cellular immune, and cytokine responses are not apparently sufficient to eradicate HCV in most patients. Direct viral cytopathicity does not appear to account for the liver damage in this disease.[16]

HCV demonstrates heterogeneity within the viral genome so that most patients infected have evidence of multiple quasispecies that differ somewhat in nucleotide sequence. Because of the quasispecies phenomenon and the high rate of mutation of the genome, chronic HCV is the ultimate outcome and not the exception. Host factors, in particular the immune system, play a role in the development of chronic infection. A better understanding of the immune system's contribution to this disease will provide insight into better future therapy.

Clinical Features and Natural History

Approximately 15-20% of persons resolve their infection without sequellae, as shown by the persistent absence of HCV RNA in the serum and normalization of ALT levels. In the remaining 80-85% chronic HCV infection develops, with persistent or fluctuating ALT elevations indicating active liver disease in two-thirds of these patients and in one-third of the remaining patients of chronically infected persons, ALT levels remain normal.

It is critical to recognize that a single ALT determination cannot be used to exclude ongoing hepatic injury or subclinical hepatitis since there is fluctuation in ALT levels in this infection. It is recommended by most experts that patients have at least three separate abnormal ALT determinations over a 6-12 month period at least one month apart to increase the likelihood of the presence of chronic infection.

The cause of this disease is insidious and progressive without physical signs and symptoms in most patients during the first two or more decades after infection. Asymptomatic persons are recognized during blood donor screening by HCV-positive virology or by elevated ALT levels that may be detected during routine physical examinations.

Cirrhosis develops in approximately 20-25% of persons with chronic HCV over 20-50 years and HCC in 1-5%. However, once cirrhosis is established, the rate of HCC may be as high as 1-4% annually.

Many of these patients are associated with various factors that have a synergistic effect on the severity of their liver disease. As cited in Table 1, these factors include alcoholic intake,[10-11] male gender, being older than 40 years at infection, and having more necroinflammatory histologic activity on liver biopsy. In contrast, when patients are carefully avoiding certain risk factors, the prognosis seems much improved without progression to cirrhosis. A notable example of this is more than 200 Irish women in Dublin who have been followed two decades after they received HCV-contaminated Rh factor immune globulin in the maternity hospital. Eventually, only 2.4% had evidence of cirrhosis and none died from the disease.[17] Thus, longer term follow-up studies are needed to assess the ultimate consequences of chronic HCV.

Extrahepatic manifestations of chronic HCV include cryoglobulinemia, membranoproliferative glomerulonephritis, and porphyria cutanea tarda. There are other suggested extrahepatic conditions, but these have not been established. Recognized extrahepatic manifestations of the disease are probably of immunologic origin.

Diagnosis and Monitoring

A variety of tests are available for diagnosing patients with chronic hepatitis C and monitoring their response to treatment. These include ALT for biochemical determination; enzyme immunoassays (EIAs) and recombinant immunoblot assays (RIBA)

Table 2. Serologic Assays for Hepatitis C Virus (HCV) Infection

Test/Type	Application	Comments
• **Hepatitis C virus antibody (anti-HCV)** EIA (enzyme immunoassay) Supplemental assay (i.e., recombinant immunoblot assay [RIBA])	Indicates past or present infection, but does not differentiate between acute, chronic, or resolved infection All positive EIA results should be verified with a supplemental assay	Sensitivity ≥ 97% EIA alone has low-positive predictive value in low-prevalence populations
• **HCV RNA (hepatitis C virus ribonucleic acid) Qualitative tests** Reverse transcriptase polymerase chain reaction (RT-PCR) amplification of HCV RNA by in-house or commercial assays (e.g., Amplicor HCV)	Detect presence of circulating HCV RNA Monitor patients on antiviral therapy	Detect virus as early as 1-2 weeks after exposure Detection of HCV RNA during course of infection might be intermittent; a single negative RT-PCR is not conclusive False-positive and false-negative results might occur
• **Quantitative tests** RT-PCR amplification of HCV RNA by in-house or commercial assays (e.g., Amplicor HCV Monitor) Branched chain DNA (bDNA) assays (e.g., Quantiplex HCV RNA assay)	Determine concentration of HCV RNA useful for assessing the likelihood of response to antiviral therapy	Less sensitive than qualitative RT-PCR Should not be used to exclude the diagnosis of HCV infection or to determine treatment end point
• **Genotype** Several methodologies available (e.g., hybridization, sequencing)	Group isolates of HCV based on genetic differences, into six genotypes and > 90 subtypes With new therapies, length of treatment might vary based on genotype	Genotype 1 (subtypes 1a and 1b) most common in United States and associated with lower response to antiviral therapy

Source: Adapted from CDC. U.S. Department of Health and Human Services. Recommendations for prevention and control of hepatitis C virus (HCV) infection and HCV-related chronic disease. *MMWR Morb Mort Wkly Rep* 1998;47(no. RR-19):1039.

for serologic detection of anti-HCV; polymerase chain reaction (PCR) assay and signal amplification assay (branched DNA) for direct detection of HCV RNA in serum; and liver biopsy for assessing histologic activity and stage of disease. (*See Tables 2-4 and Figure.*)

Serological Tests for Hepatitis C

Enzyme immunoassay (EIA). A second-generation enzyme immunoassay (EIA-2) for detecting antibody against HCV (anti-HCV) is the key test to suggest chronic HCV. Its antibody is not detected in the serum until months after exposure and may take as long as 6-12 months to appear. The sensitivity of this assay is approximately 92-95% and usually a positive EIA-2 in a patient with elevated ALT and risk factors for HCV is diagnostic. At this point, the patients should be referred to a gastroenterologist or hepatologist for further evaluation. *(Please see Table 2.)*

Recombinant immunoblot Assay (RIBA). The RIBA assay is positive when at least two antigens are present and implies that a previous positive anti-HCV test was a true-positive. One positive antigen is considered indeterminate and none negative. If the RIBA is indeterminate or negative, hepatitis C is unlikely. This supplemental test with RIBA is probably not cost-effective. However, if the diagnosis of HCV is in question, a RIBA could be obtained in an individual who is anti-HCV-positive by EIA-2. Specifically, if the patient has hypergammaglobulinemia, the possibility of autoimmune hepatitis, or when liver enzymes are normal and no risk factors are present, then the RIBA may be helpful for confirmation and to exclude the rare false-positive tests from an anti-HCV-negative individual.

HCV RNA Detection. This test detects the presence of the virus itself and, therefore, can be used to differentiate patients who

Table 3. Persons who Should be Tested for Hepatitis C Virus (HCV) Infection Based on Their Risk for Infection or a Recognized Exposure

- Persons who injected illegal drugs, including those who injected once or a few times many years ago and do not consider themselves as drug users, who received clotting factor concentrates produced before 1987, who were ever on chronic (long-term) hemodialysis, or have persistently abnormal alanine aminotransferase levels
- Prior recipients of transfusions or organ transplants, including:
  persons who were notified that they received blood from a donor who later tested positive for HCV infection
  persons who received a transfusion of blood or blood components before July 1992
  persons who received an organ transplant before July 1992
- Healthcare, emergency medical, and public safety workers after needle sticks, sharps, or mucosal exposures to HCV-positive blood
- Children born to HCV-positive women
- Recipients of transplanted tissue (e.g., corneal, musculoskeletal, skin, ova, sperm)
- Intranasal cocaine and other noninjecting illegal drug users
- Persons with a history of tattooing or body piercing
- Persons with a history of multiple sex partners or sexually transmitted diseases
- Long-term steady sex partners of HCV-positive persons

Source: Adapted from CDC. U.S. Department of Health and Human Services. Recommendations for prevention and control of hepatitis C virus (HCV) infection and HCV-related chronic disease. *MMWR Morb Mort Wkly Rep* 1998;47(no. RR-19):1039.

have ongoing infection and those who have cleared the virus from the circulation. Qualitative HCV RNA detection uses reverse transcription polymerase chain reaction (RT-PCR), which is the most sensitive technique for the presence of HCV RNA. Quantitative HCV-RNA is especially important when viral counts are low. Thus, measurement of HCV RNA levels can confirm the diagnosis of HCV when it is in doubt.

Currently, the RT-PCR is the most sensitive assay available for serum HCV RNA with detection limits ranging from 100 to 2000 copies/mL. Signal amplification assays, such as branched chain quantitation of HCV, are less sensitive (e.g., 200,000 virus equivalents/mL) but appear to be reproducible from one laboratory to another. HCV RNA measurements may be useful to monitor treatment. HCV RNA should be the primary test for confirming the diagnosis of hepatitis C infection and determining treatment response. No hepatitis C test predicts the severity of the liver disease.

Because there is a lack of standardization between the various PCR assays available, values from different assays cannot be compared. It is critical to use the same laboratory while monitoring viral load during treatment.

Liver Biopsy. Biopsy confirms an early diagnosis of chronic HCV and excludes any other alternative or coexisting diseases such as hemochromatosis or alcohol-related illness. It is the only accurate way to determine hepatitis activity, stage of fibrosis and severity, thereby providing important prognostic information by determining the baseline extent of liver damage. As previously mentioned, patients with minimal hepatitis and no significant fibrosis may not be chosen for treatment, while those most likely to have progressive liver damage have at least moderate- to-severe inflammation and necrosis and/or portal bridging fibrosis.[4,18,19]

Diagnostic Algorithm

All patients with elevated ALT levels, with or without associated risk factors for hepatitis C, should be tested for anti-HCV by enzyme immunoassay (EIA). For those patients without risk factors who are anti-HCV positive, serum HCV RNA should be determined by PCR. If HCV RNA results are positive, a liver biopsy should be performed. If HCV RNA results are negative, retesting should be performed within several months. If again negative, results should be dismissed as a false-positive EIA and other causes of elevated ALT should be evaluated. For those patients with no associated risk factors and with normal ALT levels, confirmation of HCV exposure should be obtained with either the RIBA test for anti-HCV or the PCR assay for HCV RNA. The former is approximately as expensive as the latter test; thus, in our center we prefer PCR. This test is also more reliable than branched chain quantitation of viral load. Patients with HCV risk factors and elevated ALT levels should then, in preparation for treatment, have a liver biopsy performed followed by quantitation of HCV RNA. *(Please see Figure.)*

ALT

ALT levels fluctuate greatly and do not necessarily reflect the presence of infection, severity of disease, or degree of disease progression. Most studies have shown only a weak correlation between serum ALT and histologic severity.[6] Approximately 10% of patients who lose HCV RNA during treatment continue to have elevated ALT. About 10% of patients who normalize ALT during treatment continue to have HCV RNA in serum.

Treatment

Despite a decade of experience with treatment for chronic HCV, only in the past 2-3 years has significant progress in treating this disease become evident. An expanding armamentarium of treatment options and new insights about the virus and disease progression has led clinicians to be more aggressive in treatment of certain populations of patients with HCV. Although there may be a subgroup of patients wherein the prognosis is relatively good with virtually no progression to cirrhosis (those patients with minimal hepatitis and no significant fibrosis on liver biopsy),[4] in others the progress is insidious leading to severe fibrosis, cirrhosis, and HCC. Despite the fact that monotherapy with interferon has been present for the last decade, 6-12 months of such therapy is less than ideal because of its limited effectiveness with less than 15% of patients showing sustained virological responses. A multidrug approach, as in HIV infection, may prove to be useful for patients with more aggressive hepatitis C. Currently, combination interferon/ribavirin therapy has produced sustained virological responses in about 40-50% of patients who either relapse after an initial response to interferon alone or are treatment-naive patients being administered this combination treatment for 6-12 months.[4,20-22] Both types of therapy appear to be cost-effective. Patients who experience sustained virological, biochemical, and/or histological responses represent the minority of those treated today. In the future, emerging therapies hopefully will provide better improvement in these parameters.

There is evidence that longer treatment of 18-24 months might lead to better results, although also to more adverse side effects.[23-24] New research with other treatment approaches suggests that higher starting doses (induction dosing),[25] longer treatment at a given dose, maintenance therapy, and the use of a prolonged form of interferon may augment the current treatment and possibly increase the sustained response.

Successful treatment, whether defined as sustained eradication of the virus from the blood or sustained normalization of serum ALT, improves the patient's quality of life.[26] Moreover, histological improvement can be measured in patients who have initial liver biopsies before treatment and subsequent follow-up biopsies.[26,27] The latter may be the best correlate of good prognosis in patients who respond to therapy and are followed for many years. Even in nonresponders to interferon treatment, liver biopsy usually shows some improvement.[27]

Interferons

Type 1 interferons (alpha, beta, omega, and consensus) share common biologic activity. Three type 1 interferons are currently licensed for the treatment of chronic HCV in the United States. Interferon alfa-2b and interferon alfa-2a are human recombinant interferons, and interferon alfacon-1 (consensus interferon) is a synthetic interferon derived by scanning the sequences of several natural interferon subtypes and assigning the most frequently observed amino acid in each corresponding position. This latter drug shows promising treatment results for achieving sustained virus eradication in relapsed patients treated with more intensive high-dose regimens.[28]

Interferon therapy for chronic HCV has been shown to normalize ALT levels, reduce HCV RNA to undetectable levels, reduce hepatic inflammation, and improve liver histology. A secondary goal is to improve the long-term outlook by delaying progression to cirrhosis, reducing the risk of liver failure and HCC, and decreasing the need for liver transplantation.

Table 4. Persons for Whom Routine Hepatitis C Virus (HCV) Testing is not Recommended

- Health care, emergency medical, and public safety workers
- Pregnant women
- Household (nonsexual) contacts of HCV-positive persons
- The general population

Source: Adapted from CDC. U.S. Department of Health and Human Services. Recommendations for prevention and control of hepatitis C virus (HCV) infection and HCV-related chronic disease. *MMWR Morb Mort Wkly Rep* 1998;47(no. RR-19):1039.

Interferon and Ribavirin Combination Therapy

Ribavirin appears to work synergistically with interferon to produce superior antiviral effects. The main side effect of ribavirin alone or in combination with IFN has been hemolytic anemia. However, this resolves and hemoglobin baseline levels return upon stopping treatment.

Recent studies report that the combination of interferon and ribavirin for initial treatment of patients with chronic HCV and for treatment in patients with relapsed hepatitis C who previously responded to interferon alone demonstrates success rates, as defined by prolonged (6 months) clearance of plasma viral RNA with presumptive eradication of the virus and concomitant improvement in histopathology.[10,20,21,27] The percentages for combination therapy are in the range of 31% for 24 weeks and 38% for 48 weeks, respectively. Such results compare with 6% and 13% for control groups receiving interferon alone, at 24 and 48 weeks, respectively. Sustained rates appear to be maintained for many years if HCV-RNA is found to be undetectable after six months of cessation of therapy.[29]

It appears that interferon in combination with ribavirin is the treatment of choice for patients with previous responses to interferon and subsequent relapse. Clinical studies are being undertaken to determine whether nonresponders should be treated with combination therapy.

Who Should be Treated?

In general, patients with chronic HCV who are at greatest risk for progression to cirrhosis are those patients with persistently elevated ALTs, positive HCV RNA levels, and a liver biopsy with moderate necroinflammatory changes or fibrosis. On the other hand, for patients with elevated ALT levels but minimal inflammatory changes on the liver biopsy and no significant fibrosis, they may be monitored with repeated measurements of ALT and an occasional liver biopsy every 3-5 years since their progression to cirrhosis is minimal and slow.[4,26]

Patients with risk of decompensated cirrhosis should not undergo treatment and those with decompensation should be recommended for liver transplantation. Compensated cirrhosis was previously thought to be a negative variable for response, but newer treatments may prove to be as effective in cirrhotic as in noncirrhotic patients. (*Please see Table 5.*)

It is not clear which factors increase the likelihood of response to therapy for chronic HCV.[30,31] Previously, it was thought that low pretreatment HCV RNA levels, viral genotype other than 1, and mild histologic disease were important. While viral genotype 1a or 1b may carry a lower response to therapy, the level of HCV RNA is controversial. On the other hand, in our center, we believe that minimal hepatitis among patients with mild histologic disease separates a subset population may never need subsequent treatment with monotherapy or combination therapy.[4]

Patients who are drinking excessive amounts of alcohol, who are injecting illegal drugs, and who are noncompliant should not be entered into treatment programs. Other contraindications for treatment with interferon include major depressive illness, cytopenias, hyperthyroidism, renal transplantation, and evidence of autoimmune disease. The best results with interferon monotherapy are 15-25% achievement of a sustained response as measured by normalization of HCV RNA and ALT at least one year after therapy is stopped.[23,26] Many of these have histological improvement.[23,26,27] The treatment with a standard dose of interferon is rarely effective in those who do not respond at the end of therapy.

The Patient with Normal ALT Levels

Patients with persistently normal ALT values are currently not treated with interferon outside of clinical trials.[26,32-36] Patients who have documented persistently normal ALT have a spectrum of his-

Figure. Hepatitis C Virus (HCV)-Infection-Testing Algorithm for Asymptomatic Persons

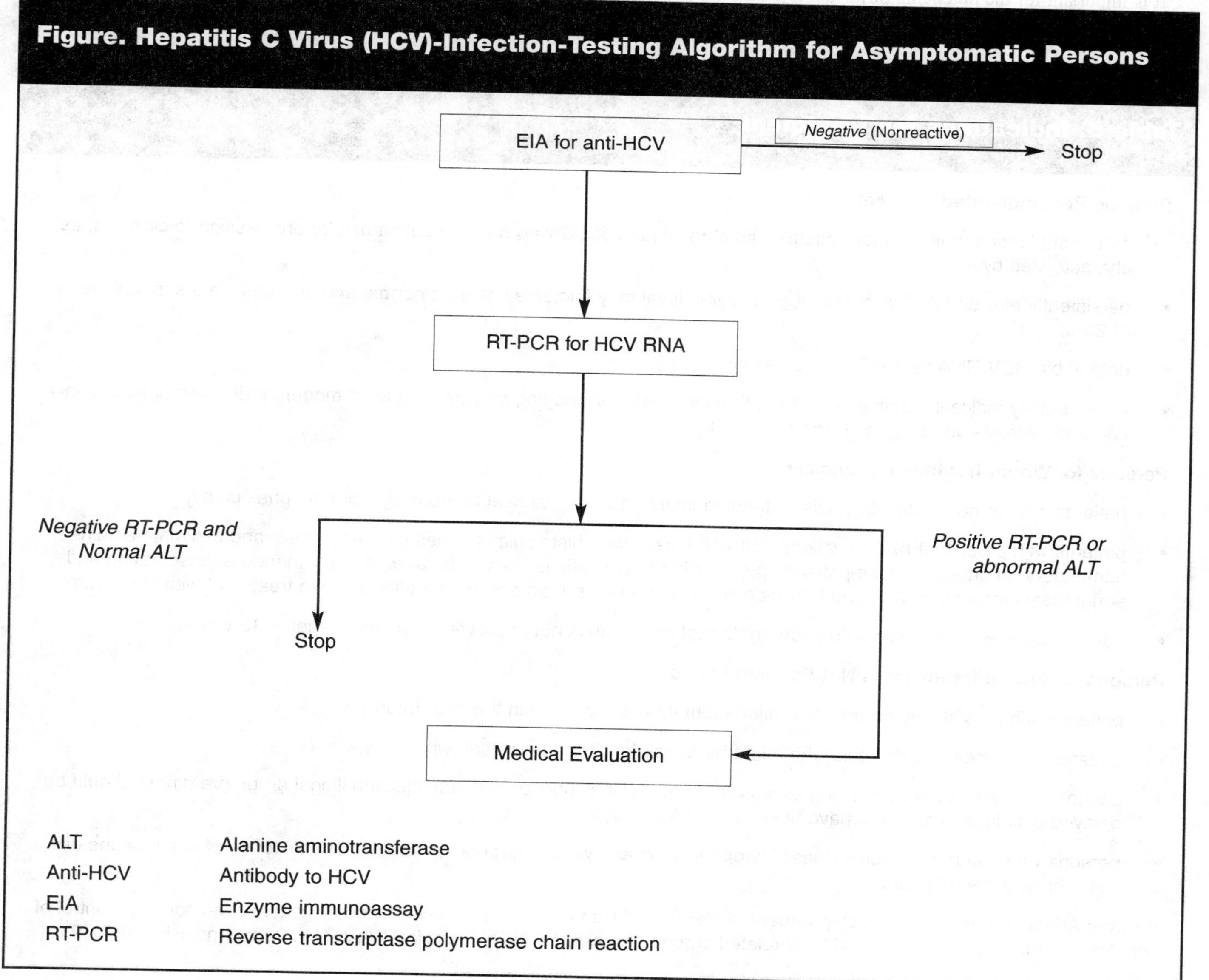

ALT — Alanine aminotransferase
Anti-HCV — Antibody to HCV
EIA — Enzyme immunoassay
RT-PCR — Reverse transcriptase polymerase chain reaction

tological abnormalities, most of which are associated with minimal or very mild hepatitis.[4] Progression of this disease with normal ALT is extremely slow, with the median time to cirrhosis being estimated as long as 80 years and therapeutic response uncertain.[4,35] Large, prospective, randomized control trials are needed to assess the effects of various treatments in this group of patients. Currently, most patients are not being treated for HCV if they have normal ALT values.[4]

With the relative success of combination therapy, there are many hepatologists who do treat this type of patient with combination drugs. The sustained response rate in patients with normal ALT may be shown in the future to be similar to patients with elevated enzymes. At present, in our center, we believe that patients with normal ALT and minimal hepatitis demonstrated on liver biopsy should not be treated because they have a good prognosis.[35] In rare instances, treatment could be indicated for this group in a mother-to-be or an active surgeon.

Side Effects of Treatment

It is important for the practicing physician to be aware of the side effects that patients will have after receiving interferon and/or combination therapy. Five to 15% of patients discontinue treatment and 10-40% must take reduced doses because of side effects. The most common of these, which occur in more than 10% of patients, are flulike symptoms (fevers, headaches, fatigue, myalgia, ascenia, rigors, arthralgias, and dizziness), and in 5-10% of patients gastrointestinal symptoms (nausea, anorexia, diarrhea), alopecia, irritability, and depression occur. Severe side effects have been observed in less than 2% of patients but include autoimmune disease, among which most commonly is thyroid dysfunction, including hypo- and hyperthyroidism, seizure disorder, acute cardiac and renal failure, retinopathy, and sepsis. The only irreversible side effect of interferon is hypothyroidism or hyperthyroidism, which occurs frequently but in a ratio of 5:1, respectively.

Bedtime administration and prophylactic acetaminophen may minimize or prevent the flulike symptoms, which generally decrease with continued treatment.

Ribavirin used in combination therapy can produce hemolytic anemia that may be problematic for patients with a pre-existing anemia, bone marrow suppression, or renal failure. Ribavirin is also teratogenic and female patients should avoid becoming pregnant during therapy.

Table 5. Indications for Treatment

Persons Recommended for Treatment

Treatment is recommended for patients with chronic hepatitis C who are at greatest risk for progression to cirrhosis, as characterized by:

- persistently elevated ALT level (although enzyme level may fluctuate between normal and abnormal in a subpopulation of 20%)
- detectable HCV RNA by a PCR-based assay
- a liver biopsy indicating active hepatitis with either portal or bridging fibrosis or at least moderate degrees of inflammation and necrosis and stage > 1 and grade > 1

Persons for Whom Treatment Is Unclear

- patients with compensated cirrhosis (without jaundice, ascites, variceal hemorrhage, or encephalopathy)
- patients with persistent ALT elevations, but with less severe histologic changes (i.e., no fibrosis and minimal necroinflammatory) changes in these patients, progression to cirrhosis is likely to be slow, if at all; therefore, observation and serial measurements of ALT and liver biopsy every 3-5 years is an acceptable alternative to treatment with interferon
- patients ages < 18 years or > 60 years (note that interferon is not approved for patients ages < 18 years).

Persons for Whom Treatment Is Not Recommended

- patients with persistently normal ALT values (but this may change in the near future)
- patients with advanced cirrhosis who might be at risk for decompensation with therapy
- patients who are currently drinking excessive amounts of alcohol or who are injecting illegal drugs (treatment should be delayed until these behaviors have been discontinued for ≥ 6 months)
- persons with major depressive illness, cytopenias, hyperthyroidism, renal transplantation, evidence of autoimmune disease, or who are pregnant

Source: Adapted from CDC. U.S. Department of Health and Human Services. Recommendations for prevention and control of hepatitis C virus (HCV) infection and HCV-related chronic disease. *MMWR Morb Mort Wkly Rep* 1998;47(no. RR-19):1039.

Table 6. Preventive Measures for Patients with Chronic HCV

- Do not drink alcohol
- Do not start any new medicines, including over-the-counter and herbal medicines, without checking with their doctor
- Do get vaccinated against hepatitis A, and, for those at risk for hepatitis B, also with B vaccine
- Do not donate blood, body organs, other tissue, or semen
- Do not share toothbrushes, dental appliances, razors, or other personal-care articles that might have blood on them
- Do cover cuts and sores on the skin to keep from spreading infectious blood or secretions
- HCV-positive persons with one long-term steady sex partner do not need to change their sexual practices. They should discuss the risk, which is low but not absent, with their sex partner. If they want to lower the limited chance of spreading HCV to their partner, they might decide to use barrier precautions (e.g., latex condoms). They discuss with their partner the need for counseling and testing

Source: Adapted from CDC. U.S. Department of Health and Human Services. Recommendations for prevention and control of hepatitis C virus (HCV) infection and HCV-related chronic disease. *MMWR Morb Mort Wkly Rep* 1998;47(no. RR-19):1039.

Certain contraindications require cessation or reduction in the dosage of interferon. These include laboratory tests in which reversible reductions are observed during therapy in more than 10% of patients, including hemoglobin, white blood cell counts, and granulocyte counts. In the presence of ribavirin, a hemolytic anemia is expected in virtually all patients but is modest in nature and the drug can be continued in more than 95% of patients without cessation or reduction in dose.

A Minority Cure for HCV

Since interferon is successful in only a minority of patients and there is breakthrough during therapy and relapse after therapy, patients should be treated only if there are clear indications. These indications include elevated ALT enzyme, no contraindications to therapy, compliance, absence of alcohol for at least six months, and the willingness to commit to 6-12 months of therapy. Unfortunately, even in these treated patients, a sustained response is often not obtained in the majority. Nevertheless, for those who do respond it appears that sustained response can be maintained for subsequent years and at least for 3-5 years.[23,27,29] In such patients, it is possible that they may be cured of their infection and their risk of further disease progression will be minimal, if at all.

The "cure" for chronic HCV remains elusive. However, the outlook for new and more effective therapies is promising and current treatments have been more effective than earlier therapies. The end point of treatment depends on achievement of sustained clearance of serum HCV RNA that is influenced, in turn, by the patient's viral replication and immune balance.

New Treatments

New formulations of interferon include pegylated interferon that are conjugated with polyethylene glycol (PEG) molecules and have a much longer half-life than conventional interferon. Current trials are under way regarding their ability and effectiveness. Such treatment may make long-term interferon therapy more tolerable. It appears that there may be a four-fold higher rate of viral clearance after 12 weeks of PEG therapy compared to those with nonpegylated monotherapy. Combination therapies like that approved recently for interferon and ribavirin may involve combining PEG interferon with ribavirin and/or other nucleosides in the years to come.

Long-acting interferons are produced by attaching a long "tail" of PEG to interferon. This increases the half-life of interferon from six hours to nearly five days and allows PEG-interferons to be administered once weekly. These agents are currently in Phase 3 clinical trials and, in some of these trials, it appears that the loss of HCV RNA can be achieved in nearly two-thirds of the treated patients (Mitchell L. Shiffman, MD, personal communication). The rate of long-term sustained response has yet to be defined.

The limited success of vaccine strategies has stimulated the search for adjunct therapies and antiviral medications that inhibit viral entry, replication, and assembly. Inhibition of serine protease, helicase, or RNA polymerase activity may be the most promising approach for antiviral treatment of HCV infection. The nonstructural 3/4A serine protease of HCV RNA genome is especially well characterized.[37] It is required for viral replication and is the first molecular target for which new antiviral agents are being developed. A protease inhibitor would be likely to block both the establishment of viral infection and viral production in chronically infected cells. Several candidate protease inhibitors are currently under intense preclinical study.

Preventive Measures

Tables 6 and 7 illustrate preventive measures for patients with chronic HCV, for high-risk persons, and procedures for post-exposure of health-care personnel.

Summary of Treatment Response

Response to therapy is monitored by complete eradication of HCV RNA from the serum. A negative serum HCV-RNA six months after cessation of therapy (sustained response) is the most useful predictor of long-term virologic response. After 3-6 months of treatment if patients have detectable viral load, then there is a low likelihood of achieving a sustained response with either monotherapy or combination therapy. All of these patients should probably discontinue treatment, since less than 1% will subsequently achieve long-term sustained viral eradication. Patients with

Table 7. Preventive Measures for Persons with High-Risk Drug or Sexual Practices

Persons who use or inject illegal drugs should be advised to:

- Stop using and injecting drugs
- Enter and complete substance-abuse treatment, including relapse-prevention programs
- Use latex condoms correctly and every time to protect themselves and their partners from diseases spread through sexual activity or to have sex with only one uninfected partner or not to have sex at all
- Get vaccinated against hepatitis B and, if appropriate, hepatitis A

biochemical and virological normalization at the end of treatment still have more than a 40% virologic relapse.

Retreatment of relapsers and nonresponders with the same dose of interferon is associated with a low rate of sustained response. In contrast, it is possible that retreatment with higher doses of interferon for a prolonged duration may increase the sustained response in such relapsed patients, even possibly in previous nonresponders. The latter observations need to be confirmed in larger clinical trials.

Combination therapy has been approved currently for patients with a history of relapse, that is in patients who previously responded to treatment but relapsed following discontinuation of therapy. Sustained response is achieved in 40-50% of naive patients and patients following retreatment. Nonresponders are difficult to treat. It is conceivable that as many as 20% of nonresponders may lose their HCV RNA during treatment, but it is yet unclear how many of these will achieve long-term sustained response.

Studies have shown that a six-month sustained clearance of viral load from serum after stopping treatment indicates a long-term favorable outcome.[27] More than 90% of these patients remain HCV-RNA negative for 5-10 years, associated with histologic improvement in all patients.[29] Patients studied for HCV-RNA in liver tissue specimens were concomitantly found to be nonreactive.[29]

Treatment strategies for chronic HCV under evaluation involve increasing the duration of therapy, modifying interferons, induction followed by maintenance therapy, and new antiviral drugs. Some of the latter agents may have an even better therapeutic response than currently approved drugs. There is increasing evidence that treatment may decrease subsequent development of complications, such as decompensated cirrhosis and HCC. Future studies may confirm whether the expected incidence of cirrhosis and HCC may be reduced in treated compared to untreated patients.

References

1. Alter MJ, Mast EE. The epidemiology of viral hepatitis in the United States. *Gastroenterol Clin North Am* 1994;23: 437-455.
2. Alter MG. Epidemiology of hepatitis C. *Hepatology* 1997; 26(suppl):62S-65S.
3. Tong MJ, et al. Clinical outcomes after transfusion-associated hepatitis C. *N Engl J Med* 1995;332:1463-1466.
4. Levine RA. Treating histologically mild chronic hepatitis C: Monotherapy, combination therapy, or tincture of time? *Ann Intern Med* 1998;129:323-326.
5. Alter MJ, et al. Risk factors for acute non-A, non-B hepatitis in the United States and association with hepatitis C virus infection. *JAMA* 1990;264:2231-2235.
6. Reedy DW, et al. AST/ALT ratio ≥ 1 is not diagnostic of cirrhosis in patients with chronic hepatitis C. *Dig Dis Sci* 1998;43:2156-2159.
7. Carroll L. Interferon suggested for all hepatitis C cases. Selecting patients who would benefit long term may not be cost effective. *JAMA* 1998;280:2088-2093.
8. Wong JB. Interferon treatment for chronic hepatitis B or C infection: Costs and effectiveness. *Acta Gastroenterol Belgica* 1998; 61:238-242.
9. Wong JB, et al. Pretreatment evaluation of chronic hepatitis C risks, benefits, and costs. *JAMA* 1998;280:2088-2093.
10. Pessione F, et al. Effect of alcohol consumption on serum hepatitis C virus RNA and histologic lesions in chronic hepatitis C. *Hepatology* 1998;27:1717-1722.
11. Wiley TE, et al. Impact of alcohol on the histological and clinical progression of hepatitis C infection. *Hepatology* 1998;28:805-809.
12. Conry-Cantilena C, et al. Routes of infection, viremia, and liver disease in blood donors found to have hepatitis C virus infection. *N Engl J Med* 1996;334:1691-1696.
13. CDC. U.S. Department of Health and Human Services. Recommendations for prevention and control of hepatitis C virus (HCV) infection and HCV-related chronic disease. *MMWR Morb Mort Wkly Rep* 1998;47:1-39.
14. Granovsky MO, et al. Hepatitis C virus infection in the mothers and infants cohort study. *Pediatrics* 1998;102: 355-359.
15. Ohto H, et al. Transmission of hepatitis C virus from mothers to infants. *N Engl J Med* 1994;330:744-750.
16. Lau DT-Y. Mechanisms of hepatic toxicity. IV. Pathogenetic mechanisms involved in hepatitis C virus-induced liver diseases. *Am J Physiol (Gastrointest Liver Physiol)* 1998;38: G1217-G1220.
17. Crowe J, et al. Presentation of hepatitis C in a unique uniform cohort 17 years from inoculaton [Abstract]. *Gastroenterology* 1995;108:A1054.
18. Poynard T, et al. Natural history of liver fibrosis progression in patients with chronic hepatitis C. The OBSVIRC, METAVIR, CLINIVIR, and DOSVIRC groups. *Lancet* 1997;349:825-832.
19. Yano M, et al. The long-term pathological evolution of chronic hepatitis C. *Hepatology* 1996;23:1334-1340.
20. McHutchison JG, et al. Interferon alfa-2b alone or in combination with ribavirin as initial treatment for chronic hepatitis C. *N Engl J Med* 1998;339:1485-1492.
21. Davis GL, et al. Interferon alfa-2b alone or in combination with ribavirin for the treatment of relapse of chronic hepatitis C.*N Engl J Med* 1998;339:1493-1499.

22. Reichard O, et al. Randomised, double-blind, placebo-controlled trial of interferon a-2b with and without ribavirin for chronic hepatitis C. The Swedish Study Group. *Lancet* 1998;351:83-87.
23. Marcellin P, et al. Long-term histologic improvement and loss of detectable intrahepatic HCV RNA in patients with chronic hepatitis C and sustained response to interferon-a therapy. *Ann Intern Med* 1997;127:875-881.
24. Poynard T, et al. Randomised trial of interferon a2b plus ribavirin for 48 weeks or for 24 weeks versus interferon a2b plus placebo for 48 weeks for treatment of chronic infection with hepatitis C virus. *Lancet* 1998;352:1426-1432.
25. Lee WM, and the Roferon Study Group. Response to 6 or 12 months of treatment using an induction regimen of interferon alfa-2a in non-cirrhotic patients with chronic hepatitis C. *Hepatology* Submitted, 1999.
26. National Institutes of Health Consensus Development Conference Panel statement: Management of hepatitis C. *Hepatology* 1997;26(Suppl 1):2S-10S.
27. Sobesky R, et al. Modeling the impact of interferon alfa treatment on liver fibrosis progression in chronic hepatitis C: A dynamic view. *Gastroenterology* 1999;116:378-386.
28. Heathcote EJ, et al. Re-treatment of chronic hepatitis C with consensus interferon. *Hepatology* 1998;27:1136-1143.
29. Lau DT-Y, Leiner DE, Ghany MG, et al. 10-Year follow-up after interferon-alpha therapy for chronic hepatitis C. *Hepatology* 1998;28:1121-1127.
30. Shiratori Y, et al. Predictors of the efficacy of interferon therapy in chronic hepatitis C virus infection. Tokyo-Chiba Hepatitis Research Group. *Gastroenterology* 1997;113: 558-566.
31. Pagliaro L, et al. Interferon-a for chronic hepatitis C: An analysis of pretreatment clinical predictors of response. *Hepatology* 1994;19:820-828.
32. Serfaty L, et al. Interferon alfa therapy in patients with chronic hepatitis C and persistently normal aminotransferase activity. *Gastroenterology* 1996;110:291-298.
33. Silverman AL, et al. Alfa interferon treatment of hepatitis C virus RNA-positive patients with normal or near-normal alanine aminotransferase levels. *Am J Gastroenterol* 1997; 92:1793-1795.
34. Van Thiel DH, et al. Chronic hepatitis C in patients with normal or near-normal alanine aminotransferase levels. The role of interferon a2b therapy. *J Hepatol* 1995;23:503-508.
35. Mathurin P, et al. Slow progression rate of fibrosis in hepatitis C virus patients with persistently normal alanine transaminase activity. *Hepatology* 1998;27:868-872.
36. Naito M, et al. Serum hepatitis C virus RNA quantity and histological features of hepatitis C virus carriers with persistently normal ALT levels. *Hepatology* 1994;19: 871-875.
37. Major ME, Feinstone SM. The molecular virology of hepatitis C. *Hepatology* 1997;25:1527-1538.

Nonulcer Dyspepsia

Nicholas J. Talley, MD

The term dyspepsia is currently considered to encompass patients with epigastric pain or discomfort.[1,2] Those patients who have predominant heartburn or acid regurgitation, the classic symptoms of gastroesophageal reflux disease (GERD), should not be considered to have dyspepsia even if they also suffer from epigastric pain or discomfort; these patients have GERD until proven otherwise. Only a minority of patients with dyspepsia are found to have a definite structural explanation for the symptoms, such as peptic ulcer disease, after appropriate testing. Hence, most patients with dyspepsia end up with a label of nonulcer (or functional) dyspepsia following investigations.[1,2] There is increasing evidence that nonulcer dyspepsia is a heterogeneous condition, but conceptually two broad clinical subsets exist: one group has predominant pain (referred to now as ulcer-like dyspepsia) while another group has predominant bloating, fullness, nausea or early satiety rather than pain (and are referred to as dysmotility-like dyspepsia).[2]

Epidemiology

Dyspepsia is remarkably common in the general population. Studies from the United States suggest that one in four persons experience recurrent upper abdominal pain or discomfort each year.[3] Only a minority of subjects with dyspepsia seek medical care, or in other words become patients.[3] While dyspepsia and nonulcer dyspepsia are common conditions, the natural history remains relatively poorly defined. There is a turnover of symptoms; approximately one-third of patients with dyspepsia lose their symptoms over a 12- month period, which is balanced by a similar number of other subjects who experience the symptoms in the population, leading to a stable prevalence from year to year.[3] However, most patients reporting the onset of symptoms are relapsers rather than new cases. The incidence of nonulcer dyspepsia is probably less than 1% per year. Factors that explain the onset and disappearance of symptoms in the general population remain undefined. The relatively high disappearance rate presumably explains in part the placebo response in this condition, which in clinical trials has been observed to be approximately 20-40%.[4]

Nonulcer dyspepsia does not cause any known mortality. Older studies suggested that the risk of peptic ulcer disease was not increased in nonulcer dyspepsia.[5] However, recent randomized, controlled trials of *Helicobacter pylori* eradication therapy in the condition have reported the incidence of peptic ulcer disease to be approximately 5% over 12 months of follow-up.[6,7] This is not confined to patients who remain *H. pylori* positive and presumably in part reflects the background use of nonsteroidal anti-inflammatory drugs including low-dose aspirin. However, this rate of peptic ulcer disease has implications for management, as discussed later.

Etiology and Pathophysiology

The cause and pathophysiology of nonulcer dyspepsia remains inadequately defined. It is likely to be a multi-factorial condition. However, new pathophysiological information has come to light in recent years that has provoked changes in patient management.

Gastric Acid

It has been confirmed that acid secretion overall is not increased in patients with nonulcer dyspepsia compared with healthy controls.[8] However, in a Scottish study, *H. pylori*-positive infected nonulcer dyspepsia patients who received gastrin releasing peptide, which simulates the postprandial state, had an abnormally increased acid secretion compared with controls.[8] Unfortunately, *H. pylori*-negative nonulcer dyspeptic patients were not assessed in this study and the results remain to be confirmed.

There are conflicting data on whether acid infusion into the stomach or duodenum can induce symptoms. Overall, it appears unlikely that acid infusion into the stomach induces dyspepsia, but increased acid exposure in the duodenum may be of more relevance. A recent study showed that nausea could be induced by duodenal acid infusion in those patients who had duodenal dysmotility (presumably increasing acid exposure time because of reduced clearance). These results suggest that both abnormal acid exposure and abnormal neuromuscular function may together be a mechanism capable of causing symptoms.[9]

Abnormal Gastric Sensation

Mechanosensory stimulation by inflation of balloons in the gastric fundus has shown that patients with nonulcer dyspepsia as a group have abnormal sensory thresholds; they sense the balloon at lower pressures and/or volumes compared with healthy controls.[10-12] Although only small numbers of patients have been studied, approximately 50% appear to have this abnormality. It remains less certain whether the abnormality is localized to the gastric mucosa or reflects sensitisation of the spinal cord or even higher up in the central nervous system. A number of new drugs are currently in development that aim to block abnormal gut sensation, although these are not yet available.

Disturbed Gastric Emptying

It has been observed that one-quarter to one-half of patients with nonulcer dyspepsia have a delay in gastric emptying, although usually this abnormality is relatively modest.[13,14] Typically, these patients have underlying antral hypomotility that accounts for the delay in emptying. Drugs are available that will accelerate gastric emptying but a correlation between symptom relief and increased gastric emptying per se is, at best, weak. Hence, this abnormality alone is unlikely to account for symptoms in those affected.

Figure 1. Seroprevalence of *H. pylori* in Dyspepsia Subgroups Among Blood Donors

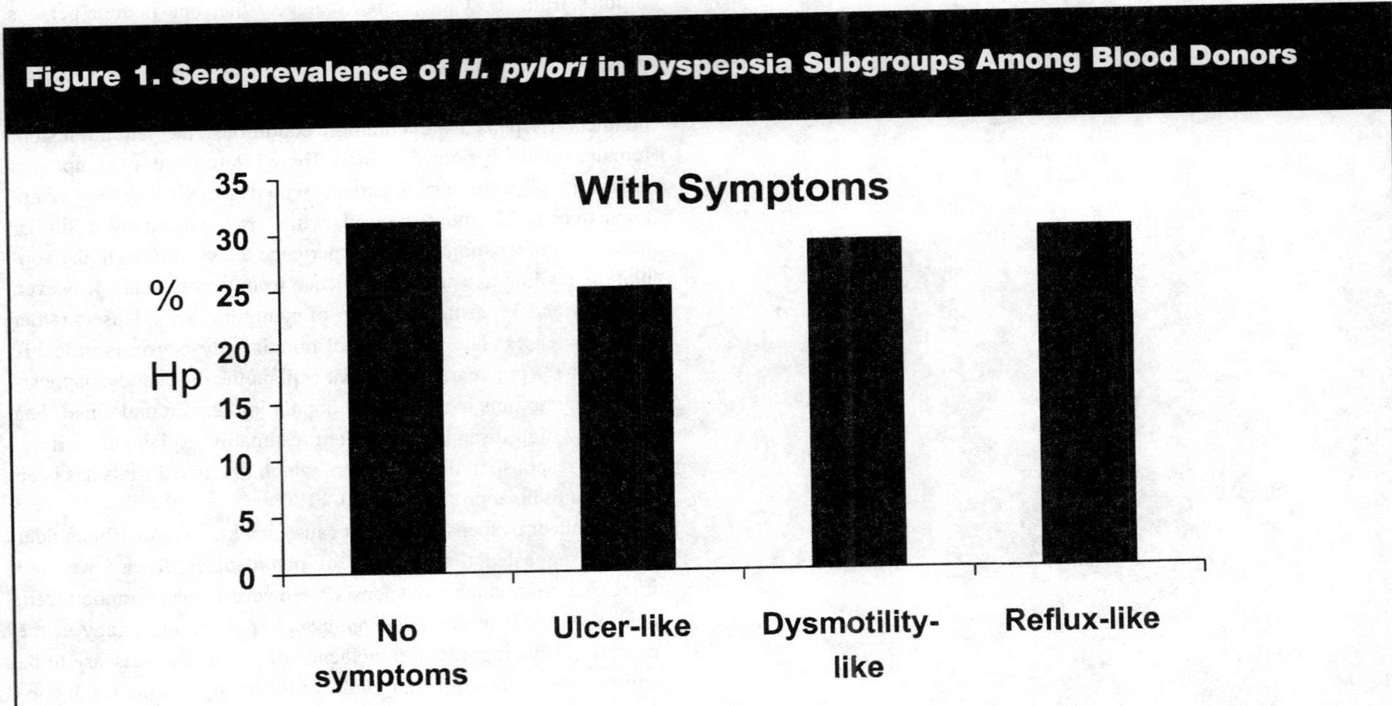

Note the similar prevalence of infection among all groups.

Source: Holtman G, et al. Dyspepsia in healthy blood donors. Pattern of symptoms and association with *Helicobacter pylori*. *Dig Dis Sci* 1994;39:1090-1098.

Abnormal Relaxation of the Gastric Fundus

In health, the gastric fundus relaxes on ingestion of a meal, allowing normal distribution of food in the stomach and promoting controlled emptying of chyme into the small intestine. Recently, it has been observed that this mechanism is impaired in about 40% of patients with nonulcer dyspepsia.[15-17] Lack of relaxation of the fundus is associated in particular with the inability to finish a normal sized meal (early satiety).[15] Drugs inducing fundic relaxation can result in symptom improvement, and this is an exciting new development as described below.

Psychological Distress

The relationship between anxiety and depression as well as life event stress and nonulcer dyspepsia continues to be of interest.[18] Overall, there is reasonable evidence that patients with nonulcer dyspepsia are more anxious and depressed than controls although it has also been suggested that this may reflect selection bias (those who present for medical care with nonulcer dyspepsia may have more psychological distress than nonpatients; psychological factors may, therefore, drive health care seeking and this may explain the apparent association). There is some limited evidence that centrally acting drugs (e.g., the tricyclic antidepressants) are of value in nonulcer dyspepsia, but this observation could be just as well explained by peripheral rather than central mechanisms of action.[19]

Helicobacter pylori

H. pylori infection (and the associated histological gastritis) occurs in up to 50% of patients with nonulcer dyspepsia, although the prevalence depends on age, socioeconomic status, and ethnic background. It has been controversial whether *H. pylori* is causally linked to nonulcer dyspepsia.[20] Clinical studies have suggested that *H. pylori* infection may be more prevalent in nonulcer dyspepsia than age-matched controls, although the data have not been particularly convincing.[20] There is no evidence that specific symptoms are linked to *H. pylori* infection in nonulcer dyspepsia.[21] *(Please see Figure 1.)* It has been postulated that the infection may set the scene for dyspepsia later in life because of the neuromodulatory influences of inflammatory mediators released in response to the infection.[20] However, the benefit of eradication of the infection in adults has been relatively disappointing, as described below.

Diet

While many patients relate symptoms of dyspepsia to food ingestion, the influence of dietary components has been a neglected field. There is evidence that a high fat intake can induce symptoms.[22] The role of food intolerance and food allergy is likely to be small but remains relatively undefined.

Clinical Features

Patients with nonulcer dyspepsia have, by definition, chronic or recurrent epigastric pain or discomfort. Most patients have multiple symptoms, although they can usually identify the most bothersome (or predominant) complaint. Symptoms are not always related to meals. A small proportion of patients are woken by pain at night, contrary to classical teaching. Peptic ulcer cannot be distinguished from nonulcer dyspepsia by symptom patterns alone.[23]

Pain that is severe or very severe, lasts for hours and episodically needs to be carefully evaluated; this classical pattern suggests biliary pain rather than nonulcer dyspepsia and may be due to gallstones or, rarely, biliary dyskinesia.[1] Patients who present with epigastric pain or discomfort relieved by defecation, or associated with an increase or decrease in stool consistency or stool frequency, are likely to have irritable bowel syndrome rather than nonulcer dyspepsia, and these patients should be managed accordingly.[2] Weight loss can occur in nonulcer dyspepsia although this is then usually associated with a significant underlying gastric motility disturbance; other causes of weight loss also need to be considered in this clinical setting (e.g., pancreatic disease and eating disorders).

Physical examination is essentially normal in nonulcer dyspepsia. There may be mild epigastric tenderness that is of no diagnostic value. Abdominal wall pain needs to be distinguished; these patients characteristically have pain that is increased by tensing the abdominal wall muscles.

Diagnosis

To make a firm diagnosis, an esophagogastroduodenoscopy is required.[1] This test should be conducted when patients are off antisecretory therapy; recent use of antisecretory drugs may mask current peptic ulcer disease or reflux esophagitis and lead to misdiagnosis. An upper GI x-ray is less satisfactory but remains a common substitute. Any patient with alarm (red flag) features (e.g., age > 45 years at onset, weight loss, dysphagia, vomiting, anemia or bleeding) deserves prompt endoscopy.[1]

The clinical features alone are unfortunately insufficient to allow a firm diagnosis of nonulcer dyspepsia. However, in the patient who has a typical history, the provisional diagnosis can be considerably strengthened by noninvasively testing for *H. pylori* (for example, by ordering a locally validated serology test). *H. pylori*-negative patients are extremely unlikely to have peptic ulcer disease (or gastric cancer). Similarly, patients not ingesting traditional nonsteroidal anti-inflammatory drugs (NSAIDs) are at low risk for ulcer disease. Thus, younger patients who have no alarm features, a typical history, and who are *H. pylori* negative and not ingesting NSAIDs can be given a provisional diagnosis of nonulcer dyspepsia with reasonable certainty, and treated accordingly. Furthermore, if the patient fits the other criteria above but is infected with *H. pylori*, then currently the American Gastroenterological Association recommends a strategy of treating the infection empirically; this abolishes most active ulcers and the ulcer diathesis, and is safe and costeffective compared with endoscopy (unless endoscopy is very inexpensive).[1,23,24]

Differential Diagnosis

There are three key structural conditions that need to be considered in the patient who presents with nonulcer dyspepsia. Peptic ulceration is an important cause of episodic dyspepsia. However, the vast majority of patients with an ulcer are either *H.*

pylori positive or ingest NSAIDs, or have both risk factors.[1] The new COX-2 specific NSAIDs do not cause ulceration.[25] An increasing number of peptic ulcers are being identified that are *H. pylori* negative and NSAID negative, but overall the prevalence of this condition is very low and the clinical importance of these ulcers remains undefined.

The second condition that can be confused with nonulcer dyspepsia is gastroesophageal reflux disease. Upper GI x-ray is inadequate for documenting GERD; a hiatal hernia (unless very large or a rolling type) is of little relevance.[1] Esophagogastroduodenoscopy will only identify one-third to one-half of cases of true gastroesophageal reflux disease, although if esophagitis is present (based on the finding of mucosal breaks) this is unequivocal evidence of GERD. Most of the remaining endoscopy negative patients can be identified by taking an adequate history (they suffer with predominant heartburn), although some misclassification with nonulcer dyspepsia is inevitable.[26] Routinely, 24-hour esophageal pH testing should not be considered but, in difficult cases, this test can be helpful.

The third condition that is of concern to both patients and physicians is gastric cancer. This is relatively rare in the United States but in older patients always requires exclusion. For this reason, endoscopy is recommended for all patients older than 45 years of age presenting with dyspepsia initially.[1] Unfortunately, most patients with gastric cancer have advanced incurable disease; they also typically have alarm features such as weight loss, dysphagia, recurrent vomiting, bleeding, or anaemia, and so can often be reasonably readily identified in practice.[27]

Management

Once a diagnosis of nonulcer dyspepsia has been made, reassurance and explanation are key initial steps in management.[28] Many patients have presented to see their physician because of anxiety or a fear of serious disease, and will continue to consult unless this fear is allayed.[29] Patients appreciate being given a firm diagnostic label, and no patient with nonulcer dyspepsia should be denied this type of reassurance.[2]

It is useful to next carefully review the patients symptomatology and try to ascertain what symptom is most bothersome or predominant.[2] If epigastric pain is predominant (ulcer-like dyspepsia), there is increasing evidence that potent acid suppression (preferably with a full dose proton pump inhibitor) is of value in this subset of cases.[30,31] On the other hand, if the predominant symptom is bloating, nausea, early satiety or fullness, then patients do not respond to acid suppression any better than placebo.[30] This group of patients should be considered for a prokinetic initially.[32] Cisapride is the current drug of choice because unlike metoclopramide it does not have central nervous system side effects. However, cisapride has been associated with prolongation of the QT interval and rarely sudden death, usually in patients receiving other drugs that increase the blood levels of cisapride (e.g., erythromycin, clarithromycin, antifungals, nefazodone, anti-retrovirals), or in patients with severe underlying cardiac disease or electrolyte disturbances.

If treatment fails with one of these first-line pharmacological approaches after 4-8 weeks, it may be worthwhile switching between antisecretory and prokinetic therapy for a period as some-

Figure 2. Relief of Dyspepsia in the Final Week of the Trial, 12 Months After Eradication Therapy for *H. pylori* or Placebo

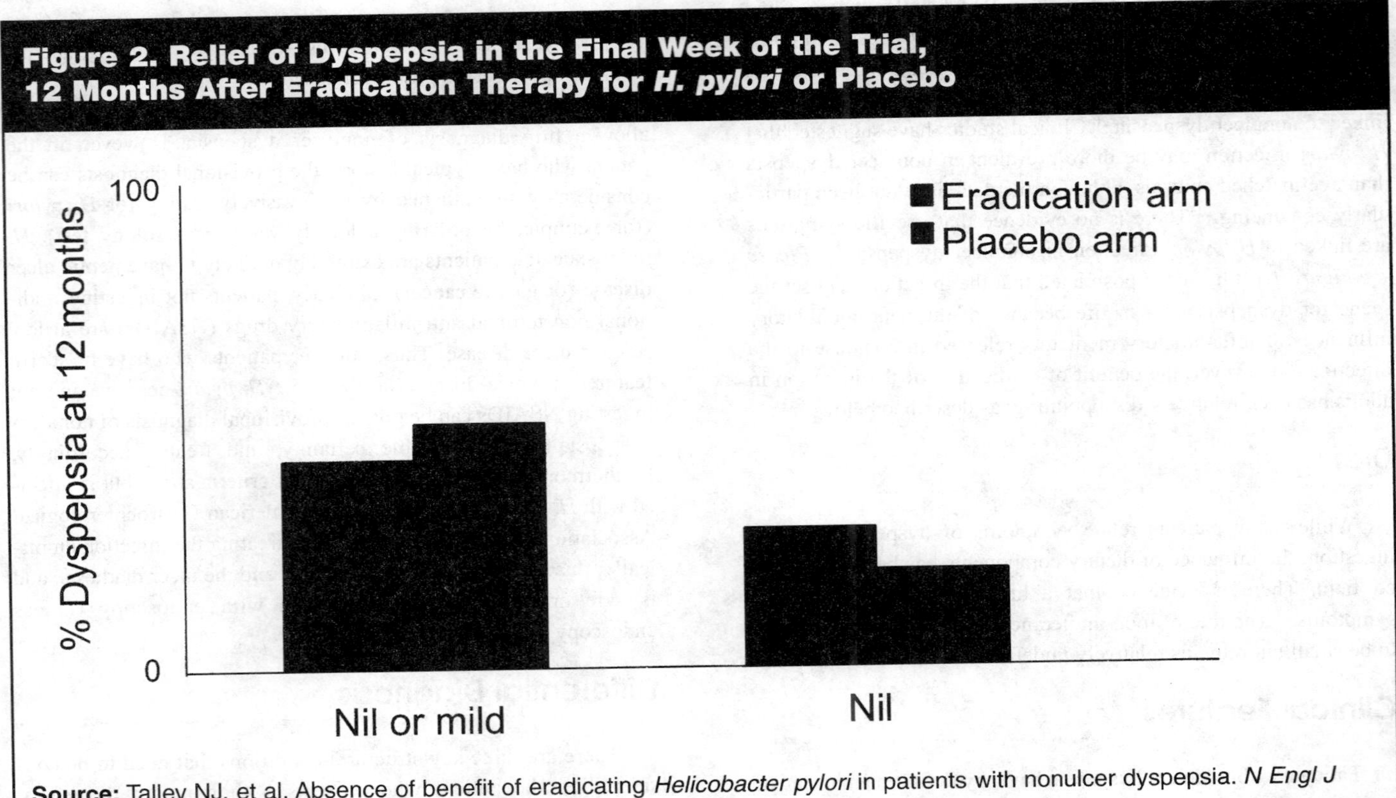

Source: Talley NJ, et al. Absence of benefit of eradicating *Helicobacter pylori* in patients with nonulcer dyspepsia. *N Engl J Med* 1999;341:1106-1111.

times patients will respond to this change.[1,2] If treatment is successful, it should be stopped after 4-8 weeks and the patients clinical course observed. Many patients will only require short intermittent courses of therapy to adequately control their chronic symptomatology.[33]

Some patients will fail to respond to this approach. Recent evidence suggest that a subset of these patients with postprandial distress have a failure of fundic relaxation. Cisapride does relax the fundus.[34] Another class of drugs that appears to relax the fundus are the serotonin type 1A receptor agonists. The antimigraine drug sumitriptan and the anxiolytic buspirone in small studies both appear to be useful for inducing fundic relaxation and reducing postprandial symptoms in some patients.[35,36] Clonidine may also be of value in this group of patients anecdotally. However, none of these new treatments is currently firmly established to be of benefit.

In patients with resistant symptoms, the diagnosis needs to be reconsidered. Atypical GERD, depression and rare causes of dyspepsia (e.g., pancreatic cancer, celiac disease, metabolic conditions) should be excluded. Next, consideration should be given to a trial of antidepressant therapy. There is some evidence that a low-dose tricyclic antidepressant can be of value for some patients with nonulcer dyspepsia, although adequate controlled trials are as yet unavailable.[19] For example, amitryptiline can be started at the dose of 10-20 mg before bed and if necessary slowly titrated up. If successful, therapy should be continued for a period of approximately six months and then tapered off.

The value of therapy to eradicate *H. pylori* in nonulcer dyspepsia has recently been carefully evaluated in large, randomized, double-blind, placebo-controlled clinical trials.[6,7,37,39] Most of the high-quality trials have been negative *(please see Figure 2)*. However, it remains conceivable that perhaps 5% of patients with nonulcer dyspepsia do respond to *H. pylori* eradication therapy (the trials have not been large enough to detect this effect size). Furthermore, *H. pylori* eradication does prevent the development of peptic ulceration in at least some patients with nonulcer dyspepsia, and, therefore, may have other value. Overall, however, eradication therapy appears to induce symptom relief that is similar to placebo, and if this treatment is considered patients need to be appropriately informed.

The value of behavioral therapy and psychotherapy in nonulcer dyspepsia remains inadequately tested. However, some patients will benefit from psychological interventions[2] and the strategy should be considered for patients with recalcitrant symptoms.

References

1. Talley NJ, et al. AGA technical review: Evaluation of dyspepsia. American Gastroenterological Association. *Gastroenterology* 1998;114:582-595.
2. Talley NJ, et al. Functional gastroduodenal disorders. *Gut* 1999;45(Suppl 2):37-42.
3. Talley NJ, et al. Onset and disappearance of gastrointestinal symptoms and functional gastrointestinal disorders. *Am J Epidemiol* 1992;136:165-177.
4. Veldhuyzen van Zanten SJO, et al. Drug treatment of functional dyspepsia: A systematic analysis of trial methodology with recommendations for the design of future trials. Report of an international working party. *Am J Gastroenterol* 1996;91:660-673.
5. Janssen HA, et al. The clinical course and prognostic determinants of non-ulcer dyspepsia: A literature review. *Scand J Gastroenterol* 1999;34:546-550.
6. Talley NJ, et al. Absence of benefit of eradicating *Helicobacter pylori* in patients with nonulcer dyspepsia. *N Engl J Med* 1999;341:1106-1111.
7. Blum AL, et al. Lack of effect of treating Helicobacter pylori infection in patients with nonulcer dyspepsia. *N Engl J Med* 1998;339:1875-1881.
8. McColl KE. Role of gastric acid in the aetiology of dyspeptic disease and dyspepsia. *Baillieres Clin Gastroenterol* 1998;12:489-502.
9. Samsom M, et al. Abnormal clearance of exogenous acid and increased acid sensitivity of the proximal duodenum in dyspeptic patients. *Gastroenterology* 1999;116:515-520.
10. Schmulson MJ, Mayer EA. Gastrointestinal sensory abnormalities in functional dyspepsia. *Baillieres Clin Gastroenterol* 1998;12:545-556.
11. Marzio L, et al. Proximal and distal gastric distension in normal subjects and *H. pylori*-positive and -negative dyspeptic patients and correlation with symptoms. *Dig Dis Sci* 1998;43:2757-2763.
12. Salet GA, et al. Responses to gastric distension in functional dyspepsia. *Gut* 1998;42:823-829.
13. Perri F, et al. Patterns of symptoms in functional dyspepsia: role of *Helicobacter pylori* infection and delayed gastric emptying. *Am J Gastroenterol* 1998;93:2082-2088.
14. Stanghellini V, et al. Predominant symptoms identify different subgroups in functional dyspepsia. *Am J Gastroenterol* 1999;94:2080-2085.
15. Tack J, et al. Role of impaired gastric accommodation to a meal in functional dyspepsia. *Gastroenterology* 1998;115: 1346-1352.
16. Thumshirn M, et al. Gastric accommodation in non-ulcer dyspepsia and the roles of *Helicobacter pylori* infection and vagal function. *Gut* 1999;44:55-64.
17. Berstad A, et al. Gastric accommodation in functional dyspepsia. *Scand J Gastroenterol* 1997;32:193-197.
18. Olden KW. Are psychosocial factors of aetiological importance in functional dyspepsia? *Baillieres Clin Gastroenterol* 1998;12:557-571.
19. Mertz H, et al. Effect of amitriptyline on symptoms, sleep, and visceral perception in patients with functional dyspepsia. *Am J Gastroenterol* 1998;93:160-165.
20. Talley NJ, Hunt RH. What role does *Helicobacter pylori* play in dyspepsia and nonulcer dyspepsia? Arguments for and against *H. pylori* being associated with dyspeptic symptoms. *Gastroenterology* 1997;113(Suppl 6):S67-77.
21. Holtmann G, et al. Dyspepsia in healthy blood donors. Pattern of symptoms and association with *Helicobacter pylori. Dig Dis Sci* 1994;39:1090-1098.
22. Feinle C, et al. Effects of duodenal nutrients on sensory and motor responses of the human stomach to distension. *Am J Physiol* 1997;273(3 Pt 1):G721-726.
23. Agreus L, Talley NJ. Challenges in managing dyspepsia in general practice. *BMJ* 1997;315:1284-1288.

24. Heaney A, et al. A prospective randomised trial of a "test and treat" policy versus endoscopy based management in young *Helicobacter pylori* positive patients with ulcer-like dyspepsia, referred to a hospital clinic. *Gut* 1999;45:186-190.
25. Laine L, et al. A randomized trial comparing the effect of Rofecoxib, a cyclooxygenase 2-specific inhibitor, with that of ibuprofen on the gastroduodenal mucosa of patients with osteoarthritis. *Gastroenterology* 1999;117:776-783.
26. Dent J, et al. An evidence-based appraisal of reflux disease management—the Genval Workshop Report. *Gut* 1999; 44(Suppl 2):S1-S16.
27. Christie J, et al. Gastric cancer below the age of 55: Implications for screening patients with uncomplicated dyspepsia. *Gut* 1997;41:513-517.
28. Fisher RS, Parkman HP. Management of nonulcer dyspepsia. *N Engl J Med* 1998;339:1376-1381.
29. Quartero AO, et al. What makes the dyspeptic patient feel ill? A crosssectional survey of functional health status, *Helicobacter pylori* infection, and psychological distress in dyspeptic patients in general practice. Gut 1999;45:15-19.
30. Talley NJ, et al. Efficacy of omeprazole in functional dyspepsia: double-blind, randomized, placebo-controlled trials (the Bond and Opera studies). *Aliment Pharmacol Ther* 1998;12:1055-1065.
31. Jones R, Crouch SL. Low-dose lansoprazole provides greater relief of heartburn and epigastric pain than low-dose omeprazole in patients with acid-related dyspepsia. *Aliment Pharmacol Ther* 1999;13:413-419.
32. Finney JS, et al. Meta-analysis of antisecretory and gastrokinetic compunds in functional dyspepsia. *J Clin Gastroenterol* 1998;26:312-320.
33. Meineche-Schmidt V, et al. Impact of functional dyspepsia on quality of life and health care consumption after cessation of antisecretory treatment. A multicentre 3 month follow-up study. *Scand J Gastroenterol* 1999;34:566-574.
34. Tack J, et al. The influence of cisapride on gastric tone and the perception of gastric distension. *Aliment Pharmacol Ther* 1998;12:761-766.
35. Tack J, et al. Influence of fundus-relaxing drug on meal-related symptosm in dyspeptic patients with hypersensitivity ot gastric distention. *Gastroenterology* 1999;116:(G1419) A324.
36. Tack J, et al. A placebo-controlled trial of busiprone, a fundus-relaxing drug, in functional dyspepsia: Effect on symptoms and gastric sensory and motor function. *Gastroenterology* 1999;116:(G1423)A325.
37. McColl K, et al. Symptomatic benefit from eradicating *Helicobacter pylori* infection in patients with nonulcer dyspepsia. *N Engl J Med* 1998;339:1869-1874.
38. Talley NJ, et al. Eradication of *Helicobacter pylori* in functional dyspepesia: randomised double blind placebo controlled trial with 12 months' follow up. The Optimal Regimen Cures Helicobacter Induced Dyspepsia (ORCHID) Study Group. *BMJ* 1999;318:833-837.
39. Greenberg PD, Cello JP. Lack of effect of treatment for *Helicobacter pylori* on symptoms of nonulcer dyspepsia. *Arch Intern Med* 1999;159:2283-2288.

Obesity

John P. Foreyt, PhD
Victor R. Pendleton, PhD

We are witnessing an epidemic of obeseity in our society. More than half the adult population of the United States is affected. This increase in prevalence is having a deleterious effect on the health of our population. Overweight and obesity are strongly associated with morbidity and mortality. Although genetic predisposition may play a minor role in the increasing prevalence, the environmental factors that affect food intake, eating behavior, and physical activity are the primary determinants. There is a strong need for a structured approach to obesity management. The basic principles include a comprehensive clinical assessment, achievable weight loss goals, and realistic lifestyle changes in dietary behavior and activity levels. Imparting the lifestyle strategies for achieving long-term eating and physical activity habits is essential for successful management. Self-monitoring is the most critical one for maximizing chances of success. Many primary care physicians (PCPs) are reluctant to prescribe drugs to treat obesity even though there are efficacious agents available to help patients manage their diet. Antiobesity drugs can serve as important adjuncts for patients who struggle with dietary change. Surgical approaches also can be effective treatments for obesity and help some severely obese patients achieve medically significant sustained weight losses. The recognition that obesity is a chronic disease for which there is no cure has increased concerns about future generations. More effective methods of prevention are needed if we are ever to stem this major public health problem.

Introduction

Obesity is among the most pervasive public health problems in the United States.[1] It is a deceptively complex, multifactorial chronic disease of appetite regulation and energy metabolism involving the integration of metabolic, physiological, biochemical, genetic, behavioral, social, and cultural factors.[2,3] While our understanding of how obesity develops is incomplete, there is agreement about the health risks of being obese. Obesity is associated with increased morbidity and mortality. It is related to type 2 diabetes, hypertension, dyslipidemia, coronary heart disease, stroke, gallbladder disease, osteoarthritis, sleep apnea, respiratory problems, and some cancers.[4-6]

Obesity is seen by many in the general public as the result of gluttony and sloth. It would disappear if only obese individuals would "eat less and exercise more." Unfortunately, obesity is a striking disease with respect to the amount of effort needed and the vigilance required for its management.[7] Published studies suggest that although individuals who complete weight loss programs lose about 10% of their weight, virtually all of them gain it back within five years.

The purpose of this chapter is to briefly review for the PCP what is known about the disease of obesity and to describe currently used strategies for its management.

Definition

Obesity is an excess of body fat. It has been defined as the point at which health risks are believed to accelerate. This point is defined as more than 25% body fat in men and more than 33% in women.[8] Assessment strategies for estimating body fat include hydrodensitometry (underwater weighing), air displacement plethysmography, dual x-ray absorptiometry (DXA), isotope dilution, total body potassium, skinfold measurements, bioelectrical impedance, ultrasound, total body conductivity (TOBEC), computed tomography (CT), magnetic resonance imaging (MRI), and neutron activation.

In hydrodensitometry, the person is weighed using a specialized scale while completely submerged under water. The principle behind the technique is that fat floats and nonfat components sink. This technique was the gold standard until the advent of DXA. The DXA method requires the person to lie on a table while low-energy x-rays are beamed through the body. Estimates of lean body mass, body fat, and bone content are possible. The cost of the DXA equipment ranges from $40,000-$100,000. People weighing in excess of 300 lbs may not be testable because of the structural limitations of the equipment. The skinfold technique involves the measurement of subcutaneous fat at predefined points on the body using a special pincher-type device known as a skin caliper.

The skinfold technique is a common method of estimating body fat because it involves the use of inexpensive equipment and is easy to administer. The technique may be less reliable than previously mentioned methods because of variation in measurement instrumentation and problems with inter-rater reliability. Because the jaws of the caliper open only so far, extremely large fat deposits may preclude the use of this technique. In bioelectrical impedance, a weak electric current is passed through the body. The principle behind this technique is that current flow is facilitated through hydrated, fatfree tissue and is impeded by dense adipose tissue. Therefore, the more body fat, the higher the impedance. Though this technique is modern in its use of technology, it may be less accurate than previously mentioned methods due to its sensitivity to the person's level of hydration. For example, women who are menstruating or individuals who have recently consumed alcoholic beverages may produce inaccurate results.

Body fat can be estimated using a portable ultrasound meter. This device measures subcutaneous fat using sound reflectance. This technique has good reliability and does not limit the size of the person to be evaluated. TOBEC is a technique that relies on the changes in electromagnetic characteristics as a function of fat and water. Like the DXA, the equipment is expensive but may be useful in specialized research settings.

Though accurate, the imaging techniques, CT and MRI, are also expensive. In a clinical setting for the treatment of obesity, the cost/benefit ratio of this high-end equipment may be prohibitive. Less expensive techniques, such as skinfold measurement and ultrasound, performed according to established protocols, can produce results with 95-97% accuracy.[9] This level of accuracy is probably enough for the PCP. However, even these techniques require time and equipment.

In order to reduce the time and effort necessary to capture a useful measure of body composition, quicker ways are used to define obesity. Body mass index (BMI), expressed as weight in kilograms divided by height in meters squared (kg/m^2), has emerged as the favored measure among researchers and is increasingly being used clinically by PCPs. The BMI is significantly correlated with total body fat. *(Please see Table 1.)* The cutoffs defining adult underweight, normal weight, and obesity in terms of BMI are given in Table 2. The advantages of using the BMI for PCPs are its ease of use and its accuracy in measuring both weight and height. It allows the same criteria to be applied independent of gender. It is a good estimation of excess body fat in BMIs greater than 25, and works especially well in BMIs greater than 30. The BMI does not work well with highly muscled athletes who have abnormally high levels of lean muscle mass. At this time, the BMI categories are restricted to men and women who are past puberty. Categorizing growing children by BMI could result in erroneous estimates of body composition.[9] BMI categories for use with children are not presently available. The BMI also can be determined using inches and pounds: (weight in pounds divided by height in inches squared × 703 [i.e., $lbs/in^2 \times 703$]).

Prevalence

Currently, 55% of the adult U.S. population is overweight or obese.[1,6] As indicated in Table 2, the definition of overweight is a BMI of 25 or greater, and obesity is a BMI of 30 or greater. A total of 32.6% of the adult population is overweight and 22.3% is obese. Table 3 illustrates the rise in the percentage of the U.S. population from 1960-1994[6] that is obese. The highest prevalence of obesity is in the minority population, with 36.5% of black women and 33.3% of Mexican-American women having BMIs greater than 30. The lowest prevalences of obesity are white men (20.0%) and black men (20.6%). Obesity increases with age through age 59 then declines. Men in their 50s have an obesity prevalence of 28.9%; women, 35.6%.

The prevalence of childhood obesity also is increasing, with estimates ranging from 20-30%.[10,11] Childhood obesity predicts adult obesity. One-third of all obese adults were obese as children.[12] The Bogalusa heart study suggests that there has been a 50% increase in obesity of 6- to 11-year-olds since 1973 and that the trend is continuing.[13] Another study reported an 80% increase in the incidence of obese children becoming obese adults.[14] Adults with the onset of obesity in childhood have more severe obesity and earlier onset of comorbidities. The likelihood of an obese child becoming an obese adult increases as children age and remain obese.

Etiology and Pathogenesis

The epidemic of obesity that we are currently experiencing is the result of an imbalance between energy expenditure and caloric intake. The causes of this imbalance are related to genetic predisposition and changes in the human environment and lifestyle.[15,16] The ability to store fat during periods of ample food availability is an environmentally selected trait that increases the individual's chances of survival during periods of famine.[16,17] Researchers have theorized that the human genome is characterized by susceptibilities that interact with environmental factors to produce obese phenotypes.[17] Ironically, the major environmental factors that interact to produce the harmful and ever-increasing levels of adiposity in modern society are the high availability of calorie-dense foods and the absence of a physically demanding environment.[18-20]

Assessment

Assessment is useful in the design and optimization of treatment approaches. Assessment helps the provider target specific problem areas for change. Typical areas of assessment are degree of obesity, diet/eating patterns, physical activity patterns, emotional state, and readiness to change. Degree of obesity can be useful in selecting the most appropriate treatment modality. For example, cognitive-behavioral strategies have been used most often with individuals who are overweight to moderately obese (BMI from 25-40).[6] Other approaches, such as surgery, may be indicated for patients with severe obesity (BMI > 40).[6]

Dietary Assessment. Considering the major role of diet in the pathogenesis of obesity, evaluation of dietary patterns is often an important component of treatment planning. On the other hand, the labor-intensive nature of traditional assessment methods, such as 24-hour recall and food-frequency questionnaires, challenges the primary care provider's ability to deliver quality service in a time-efficient manner. In response to this dilemma, brief dietary assessment questionnaires have been developed. Some of these questionnaires are targeted to the dietary management of specific medical conditions. Examples of such instruments are the MEDFICTS Dietary Assessment Questionnaire[21] and the Rate Your Plate[22] dietary assessment questionnaire, which target management of cholesterol, and the Eating Pattern Assessment Tool,[23] which is aimed at patients interested in maintaining a heart-healthy diet. These tools assess the frequency at which certain food groups are eaten per week, as well as typical serving sizes. These results, though targeted for the management of specific medical conditions, are generalizable to obesity management because they provide a description of the patient's daily eating patterns. One advantage of these brief assessment tools is that the primary care provider is able to capture reliable data about the general eating patterns of the patient with a minimum of time expended. Another advantage is that the patient gains self-awareness of eating behavior. Many of these instruments are self-scored and guide the patient through a process of goal setting to achieve a healthier diet. If more detailed records of eating behavior are desired, it is best acquired with the assistance of, or referral to, a registered dietitian.

Physical Activity Assessment. The issues related to the assessment of physical activity are similar to those of eating behavior. Treatment planning can be enhanced by knowledge of physical activity patterns but the cost in time of traditional assessment methods is often prohibitive. General patterns of physical activity may be efficiently determined using the Self-Administered 7-Day Physical Activity Recall Questionnaire.[24] This simple, two-question instrument provides a means of capturing general information regarding the patient's level of moderate to vigorous physical activity during the most recent seven-day period. Although this instrument does not provide detailed information at the kcal level, it may provide enough data to guide the provider in treatment planning and recommendations.

Emotional Assessment. A 24% prevalence of depression was reported in a recent study of outpatients in a primary care setting.[25] The prevalence among obese patients who also binge eat is high.[26] Assessment of emotional status is important in the treatment of obesity.[27] Many patients suffering from depression will have difficulty adhering to a weight management program. Depressed patients may

Table 1. Body Mass Index (BMI) Table

HEIGHT / BMI	19	20	21	22	23	24	25	26	27	28	29	30	35	40
	WEIGHT (In Pounds)													
4'10"	91	96	100	105	110	115	119	124	129	134	138	143	167	191
4'11"	94	99	104	109	114	119	124	128	133	138	143	148	173	198
5'	97	102	107	112	118	123	128	133	138	143	148	153	179	204
5'1"	100	106	111	116	122	127	132	137	143	148	153	158	185	211
5'2"	104	109	115	120	126	131	136	142	147	153	158	164	191	218
5'3"	107	113	118	124	130	135	141	146	152	158	163	169	197	225
5'4"	110	116	122	128	134	140	145	151	157	163	169	174	204	232
5'5"	114	120	126	132	138	144	150	156	162	168	174	180	210	240
5'6"	118	124	130	136	142	148	155	161	167	173	179	186	216	247
5'7"	121	127	134	140	146	153	159	166	172	178	185	191	223	255
5'8"	125	131	138	144	151	158	164	171	177	184	190	197	230	262
5'9"	128	135	142	149	155	162	169	176	182	189	196	203	236	270
5'10"	132	139	146	153	160	167	174	181	188	195	202	207	243	278
5'11"	136	143	150	157	165	172	179	186	193	200	208	215	250	286
6'	140	147	154	162	169	177	184	191	199	206	213	221	258	294
6'1"	144	151	159	166	174	182	189	197	204	212	219	227	265	302
6'2"	148	155	163	171	179	186	194	202	210	218	225	233	272	311
6'3"	152	160	168	176	184	192	200	208	216	224	232	240	279	319
6'4"	156	164	172	180	189	197	205	213	221	230	238	246	287	328

Source: Adapted from NIH/NHLBI Clinical Guidelines.[6]

Table 2. Adult Obesity Classification Using BMI

	BMI
Underweight	< 18.5
Normal weight	18.5-24.9
Overweight	25-29.9
Mild obesity	30-34.9
Moderate obesity	35-39.9
Severe obesity	> 40

ultimately experience more success if the depression is treated before a weight loss program is begun.[28,29] A number of well-documented instruments helpful in identifying depression are available, including the Beck Depression Inventory for Primary Care (BDI-PC) and the Center for Epidemiologic Studies Depression Scale (CES-D).[30] The BDI-PC is a self-administered seven-item questionnaire that reliably identifies depression in a primary care setting.[25] The CES-D is a 20-item self-administered scale that has good psychometric properties, is brief, easy to use, and is a public document.

Stage of Change Assessment. Obese patients will present at different levels of readiness to change. Understanding where the patient is in this regard may help the therapeutic process by guiding the selection of treatments that are congruent with the patient's desire to change. The Stages of Change model was proposed to facilitate this process.[31] It categorizes people with problem conditions into one of five stages: precontemplation, contemplation, preparation, action, and maintenance. Precontemplators may not be at all concerned with their condition. Contemplators may be concerned but not yet decided on taking action. If the patient is not ready to begin a weight management program, suggestions to take action will probably fall on deaf ears. A different approach, involving education and personalization of risk factors, may be the most appropriate intervention for these individuals. Patients in the preparation stage may have decided to do something about their condition but have not yet begun. Such patients may need encouragement to take action and to make a commitment to their health and well-being. Patients who are ready to take action, or who have recently begun taking action, would benefit most from behavioral interventions such as goal setting and self-monitoring. They may use information describing community resources and group activities available to help them meet their goals. People in the maintenance stage would benefit from moral support and recognition of the good things they are doing for themselves. Table 4 describes some diagnostic questions that are useful in determining the patient's current stage of change.

Lifestyle Change Strategies

In the management of obesity, the primary focus should be to increase physical activity, normalize caloric consumption, and create realistic expectations of success. There are seven basic lifestyle change strategies to help patients make the necessary adjustments in eating and physical activity to lose and maintain body weight.

Table 3. Obesity Trends (%) in the United States (BMI > 30; ages 20-80+)[6]

	Men (%)	Women (%)
1960-1962	10.4	15.1
1971-1974	11.8	16.1
1976-1980	12.2	16.3
1988-1994	19.5	25.0

Set Realistic Goals. Goals for losing weight frequently differ between patient and physician. Unrealistic goals need to be addressed early. The average weight a patient will lose in a treatment program is about 8-10%;[6] many patients want to lose much more than that. One strategy is to help the patient set moderate short-term goals and focus on the health benefits of even modest amounts of weight loss. The patient is encouraged to re-evaluate periodically and to reset goals if necessary. This method has the dual benefit of providing the patient with feelings of success for having met short-term goals, while approaching the long-term goal at a moderate pace that is conducive to long-term maintenance. Patients may benefit from being reminded that setting unrealistic goals is setting oneself up for failure.

Self-Monitoring. The most important lifestyle change strategy is self-monitoring. Self-monitoring involves the observation and recording of specific personal behaviors, related feelings, and environmental cues.[32] For the patient working to manage obesity, the purpose of self-monitoring is to raise the awareness of eating and physical activity behavior and the factors contributing to it. The patient is asked to record foods eaten and aspects of the environmental situation in which the eating occurred. Feedback—in the form of calories, food groups, or fat grams—can help the patient see what changes need to be made. Also, consistent recording symbolizes compliance, which may be reinforcing in and of itself.

Although it is desirable for patients to be accurate in the records they keep, absolute accuracy is not necessary. Less accurate recording may still lead to improvement because of the patient's increased awareness of diet and activity patterns, and the factors that influence them.[33,34] Self-awareness enables the patient to target areas for change that will have the greatest effect. Studies have shown self-monitoring to be consistently related to improved treatment outcomes, and patients report that it is one of their most helpful tools.

We find that physicians often do not like to ask their patients to keep food diaries, and patients do not like to fill them out. Yet, diaries are the single most useful tool for raising patients' awareness of their eating and physical activity patterns. The food diary is the most helpful behavioral strategy we have. Encourage patients to keep one.

Stimulus Control. Stimulus control involves the identification and modification of the environmental factors contributing to overeating or underexercising.[33] After environmental factors to overeating and/or sedentary behavior have been identified using a diary, stimulus control techniques may be used to weaken or eliminate the influence of the cues. For example, if food availability is found to be a cue for overeating, then eliminating tempting foods from the house might result in reduced caloric consumption. Another

Table 4. Sample Questions for Determining Exercise Behavior Stage of Change

Which statement most accurately describes you?

Precontemplation—I do not exercise and have no plans to start.

Contemplation—I plan to begin exercising in the next six months.

Preparation—I plan to begin exercising in the next month.

Action—I have begun exercising on a consistent basis during the past six months.*

Maintenance—I have been exercising on a consistent basis for more than six months.

* Consistent exercise = 3 or more times per week for 20 minutes or more.

example is when patients identify a lack of motivation as the reason for missing scheduled exercise sessions. In such cases, telephone reminders or participation in an exercise group may be useful in motivating patients to stay on track. Laying out exercise clothes and walking shoes before going to bed may make it easier for patients to exercise when waking up the next morning.

Cognitive Restructuring. Cognitive restructuring involves changing inaccurate beliefs.[35] This procedure encourages patients to examine their inner dialogues (i.e., their thoughts and feelings about themselves and their obesity). It challenges them to change those who are determined to be inaccurate or counterproductive. For example, some patients believe that losing weight will result in happiness in many other aspects of their lives. If such patients lose weight but do not achieve happiness in the other areas, they may become discouraged and return to old behavior patterns. Patients who have endured a lifetime of obesity may have problems seeing themselves as new leaner persons. Failure or relapse may be expected because of these distorted self-images. The purpose of cognitive restructuring is to identify self-defeating cognitions and to help patients replace them with more productive ones. Having patients write down and repeat positive self-affirmations, such as "I will walk at least 30 minutes today," can often serve as helpful reminders for behavior change.

Stress Management and Inoculation Training. Stress is a strong predictor of overeating and relapse.[36] Therefore, it is not surprising that stress management and inoculation training are useful in the management of obesity because they teach the patient techniques for identifying, handling, and reducing stress. Some of these techniques include diaphragmatic breathing, progressive muscle relaxation, and meditation. Inoculation seeks to develop in the patient the ability to resist environmental stimuli that might ordinarily lead to relapse. Inoculation is done by exposing the patient to the stimulus and practicing successful negotiation of it.[37] Exposure may be done in vivo or through guided imagery. For example, the stimulus may be the offer of a piece of cake at a birthday party or the feelings of anger toward a coworker. Successful negotiation may be practiced by selecting from options such as walking away, declining the offer, or taking a time-out to reduce the state of arousal.

Relapse Prevention Training. Relapse prevention training normalizes relapse as part of the weight-loss process.[33,37] It teaches patients to accept relapse as a possible eventuality and prepares them to manage the relapse by minimizing the damage and getting back on track as soon as possible. By anticipating relapse and having coping strategies in place, a full relapse may be avoided.

Social Support. Studies consistently show the value of support systems in improving compliance with obesity management programs.[33,38,39] Incorporating social support consists of including others in the patient's management program. This may be done by encouraging the participation of family members and friends, or by referring the patient to a group of like-minded people with similar goals. Social support may also be achieved by encouraging the patient to seek out group exercise and recreation programs. Social support facilitates the obesity management process and benefits the patient by providing positive social influence to adopt new behaviors, by developing self-acceptance, and by providing an outlet for the frustrations often experienced by obese people trying to make lifestyle changes.

Pharmacotherapy

According to the recommendations of the NIH/NHLBI clinical guidelines, drugs may be a useful adjunct to modifications in behavior, including diet and physical activity. The recommendation of the guidelines is that "weight loss drugs may only be used as part of a comprehensive weight loss program including diet and physical activity for patients with a BMI of 30 or greater with no concomitant obesity-related risk factors or diseases, or for patients with a BMI of 27 or greater with concomitant obesity-related risk factors or disease."[6,40] Currently, there are two drugs for obesity that are approved by the Food and Drug Administration (FDA) for long-term use: sibutramine (Meridia) and orlistat (Xenical).

Sibutramine. Sibutramine was initially developed as an antidepressant. Weight loss was noticed in depressed patients who took the drug who were not actively attempting to lose weight. Sibutramine is a serotonin and noradreneline reuptake inhibitor.[41] It has been studied in randomized, double-blind, placebo-controlled trials lasting 6-12 months. More than 20 trials involving obese subjects have been reported. Subjects have included those with uncomplicated obesity and those with dyslipidemia and type 2 diabetes. Dose-response relationships were observed. Weight losses were significantly greater in the sibutramine-treated subjects than in those receiving placebo. Sibutramine-treated subjects typically lost about 6-10% of body weight over 6-12 months.

Adverse events are predictable based on its pharmacology. There is a mean increase in blood pressure of 1-2 mm Hg and a mean increase in heart rate of four beats per minute. In some patients, sibutramine may substantially increase blood pressure. Potentially clinically significant increases in blood pressure have been reported with an incidence of 2% relative to placebo in uncomplicated obesity. Sibutramine should be used with caution in patients with a history of hypertension and should not be given to patients with uncontrolled or poorly controlled hypertension. The physician should monitor blood pressure in all patients.

There has been no reported increase in ischemic coronary events, arrhythmias, or cerebrovascular events with use of sibutramine. There have been no cases of primary pulmonary hypertension attributable to sibutramine reported and no increase in valvular heart disease compared with placebo subjects. No neurotoxicity has been seen. Drug interactions include monoamine oxidase inhibitors (MAOIs), selective serotonin reuptake inhibitors (SSRIs), erythromycin, and ketoconazole.

Orlistat. Orlistat is a lipase inhibitor that works by reducing the body's absorption of dietary fat.[42,43] It is a nonsystemic drug that blocks 30% of dietary fat. It works in the gastrointestinal tract. To date, there have been seven one- and two-year randomized, double-blind, placebo-controlled trials involving more than 4000 patients. In all studies, patients who took orlistat lost significantly more weight than those receiving a placebo. Almost three times as many patients taking orlistat achieved weight loss of more than 10% compared to placebo. Twice as many lost at least 5%. Orlistat-treated patients showed improvements in total and low-density lipoprotein (LDL) cholesterol, blood pressure, and fasting insulin and glucose.

Orlistat is contraindicated in patients with chronic malabsorption syndrome or cholestasis, and in patients taking cyclosporine or with a known sensitivity to any component of orlistat. Orlistat treatment effects include changes in bowel habits such as oily or loose stools, the need to have a bowel movement quickly, bloating, or oily spotting. They tend to occur when patients consume more than 30% of calories from fat. These effects may be minimized once the patient lowers the fat in the diet to less than 30%. Because orlistat blocks dietary fat, it reduces absorption of fat-soluble vitamins A, D, E, and K, and beta carotine. Patients on orlistat require a multivitamin supplement containing fat-soluble vitamins.

Surgery

The NIH/NHLBI clinical guidelines recommend that "surgical intervention is an option for carefully selected patients with clinically severe obesity (a BMI of ≥ 40 or ≥ 35 with comorbid conditions) when less intensive methods of weight loss have failed and the patient is at high risk for obesity-associated morbidity and mortality."[6]

Severely obese patients are often not helped by more conservative weight loss approaches, including lifestyle change strategies. The NIH consensus conference on surgical approaches for weight loss concluded that this aggressive approach is reasonable for severely obese persons who are at increased risk for premature death and that the potential benefits are greater than the risks.[44] Weight losses following surgery may be as much as 100 lbs or more over 12 months. The ongoing Swedish Obesity Study (SOS) reported that gastric bypass resulted in greater weight losses than gastroplasty at 12 months (93 lbs vs 67 lbs, respectively).[45] Comorbidities also show significant improvements following surgery.

Diet

There are numerous randomized controlled trials that demonstrate the efficacy of adhering to a balanced, reduced calorie diet.[6,46] Reduced calorie diets based on USDA guidelines, which create a deficit of 500-1000 calories per day, are indicated for any program aimed at achieving weight loss of 1-2 pounds per week.[6] The USDA guidelines describe food choices that promote good health. These are presented in the form of recommended numbers of servings from the five major food groups *(please see Figure 1)*.

Figure 1. The Food Guide Pyramid

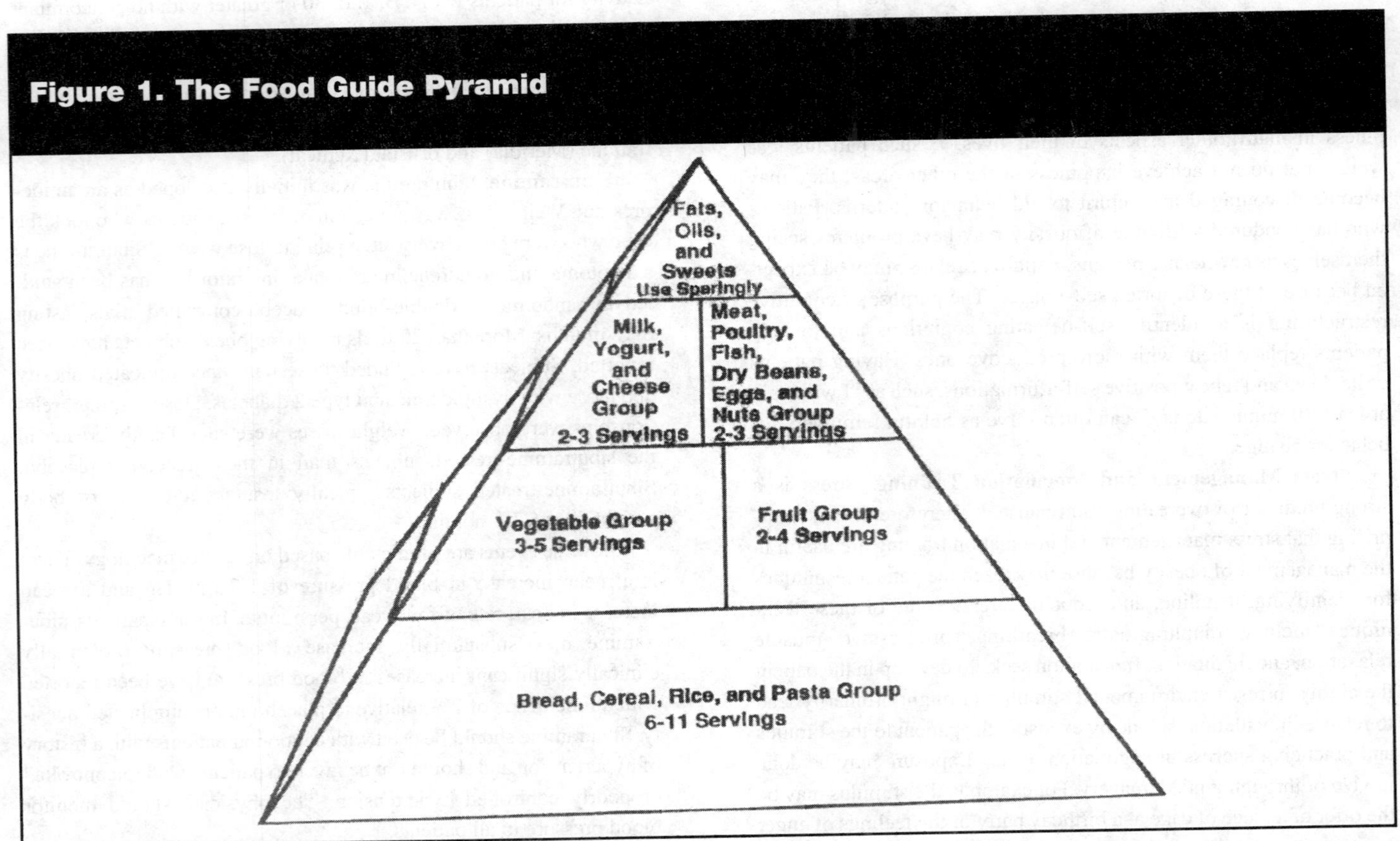

Reduced Caloric Consumption. The USDA standard serving for meat is 3 oz. Serving sizes in restaurants today frequently exceed 8 oz. The standard serving size for popped popcorn is 3 cups. At the movies, 16-cup servings are common. In fast-food lines, the offer of "super-sizing" is standard. These trends make reduced caloric consumption difficult. Many patients do not understand standard portion sizes. Descriptions of typical serving sizes are useful in helping patients conceptualize the amount of food that makes up a recommended serving. The USDA provides useful pamphlets to assist in patient education.[47]

Normalized eating refers to eating in accordance with a person's daily caloric requirements. Daily caloric requirements represent the intake necessary to maintain current body weight. Patients need to know their requirements. Daily caloric requirements can be estimated using the following age- and gender-specific formulas[48]:

Men:

18-30 y: RMR = 15.4 × weight (kg)-27 × height (m) + 717
30-60 y: RMR = 11.3 × weight (kg) + 16 × height (m) + 901
> 60 y: RMR = 8.8 × weight (kg) + 1128 × height (m)-1071

Women:

18-30 y: RMR = 13.3 × weight (kg) + 334 × height (m)-35
30-60 y: RMR = 8.7 × weight (kg-25 × height (m) + 865
> 60 y: RMR = 9.2 × weight (kg) + 637 × height (m)-302

Estimates of daily caloric requirements can be calculated by multiplying the RMR by an activity factor of 1.3 for women and men. This factor assumes a predominantly sedentary lifestyle, which is common for obese patients. For example, a 49-year-old man who is 6 feet tall and weighs 230 lbs:

RMR = 11.3 × 104.3 + 16 × 1.84 + 901 = 2109
Daily caloric requirement = 2109 × 1.3 = 2742

A daily deficit of 500 calories will result in a weight reduction of 1 lb per week, which is in accordance with current obesity management guidelines. The caloric content of many foods is given on the packaging. Pocket handbooks are also available that contain the energy value of unpackaged foods such as fruits and vegetables. Applying the self-monitoring techniques mentioned above, patients could use this information to select meals based on caloric content and thereby achieve better control toward maintaining their intake goals. The self-awareness produced by the self-monitoring effort keeps patients focused on intake and interested in the caloric content of the food they plan to eat.

In practice, it is not always possible to determine the caloric content of food choices. This is especially true when eating in restaurants and with friends. In such cases, self-monitoring is still helpful and should be continued, but the focus should shift from calories to portion sizes and fat content. It is helpful to conceptualize servings in three sizes: small, medium, and large. By selecting food in small portion sizes, especially foods that are high in percentage of calories from fat, patients can eat out with a minimum of deviation from their weight-loss trajectory.

The evidence is strong that balanced, reduced-calorie diets, with choices made according to the USDA guidelines, are effective in facilitating weight loss. Balance, variety, and moderation are still the secrets of a diet conducive to successful weight management.

Physical Activity

When designing the physical activity component of an intervention, the type, frequency, intensity, and duration of the activities should be considered. Moderate aerobic activity is well suited for weight reduction. The types of activities selected should be matched to the patient's physical and psychological attributes and limitations. For example, many obese people do not like bicycle riding because of the discomfort caused by narrow seats. Others avoid swimming because of the embarrassment they experience when their bodies are exposed. Compliance may be facilitated if patients can identify modes of physical activity that they find suitable.[49,50]

Physical activity should be worked into the patient's lifestyle to ensure consistency. Accepted guidelines suggest that physical activity be performed at least five days per week.[49,50] A gradual approach that builds up to this recommended level of activity will allow time for physical and psychological adaptations to occur and will lower the chance of injury. For obese patients beginning a program of increased physical activity, moderate intensity is indicated. During aerobic exercise, a simple test known as the "Talk Test" can be useful in assessing activity intensity. Patients are at the appropriate level of intensity if they are just barely breathing hard and are still able to carry on a conversation. This level also corresponds to a perceived level of exertion equal to 7, on a scale from 1 to 10. Duration of exercise should begin slowly, perhaps at about 10 minutes, and gradually increase to 30 minutes or more per day.[49,50]

Patients should keep in mind that the focus of physical activity is weight loss. Maximum physical exertion is not required. Moderate intensity can be as effective as higher intensity exertion in achieving caloric expenditure. For example, the number of calories expended to walk a mile in 15 minutes is roughly the same as required to walk a mile in 20 minutes. No doubt that walking at the more rapid pace burns calories at a faster rate per minute, but the slower walker will eventually make up the difference by walking for a longer time. Explaining the benefit of moderate intensity exercise in this way may lead the patient to value modest efforts and contribute to overall program adherence. General increases in physical activity should also be encouraged. Simple modifications, such as taking the stairs and parking a bit further out in the parking lot, can add up over the course of weeks and months.

Weight loss will be directly related to frequency, intensity, type, and duration of physical activity, as well as to caloric intake. Table 5 illustrates the amount of exercise necessary to burn off the calories from several different types of foods while walking at a normal pace (approximately 3 mph). Relating information in this way may help the patient put that extra piece of candy into perspective.

Problems Frequently Encountered by Primary Care Providers

Successful management of patient obesity is not a simple process. This section discusses some of the specific problems often faced by the primary care provider working with obese patients.

Side Effects of Medications. Some medications have weight gain as a side effect. These medications are obviously counterproductive to any weight loss effort. Some medications bring about feelings of drowsiness and lethargy. Patients taking these medications may find increased levels of physical activity exceedingly hard to maintain. Some of these medications are given in Table 6.

Physicians should consider the tradeoffs of these medications when treating obese patients.

Lack of Patient Motivation. Patients present at different levels of motivation. Meeting patients where they are and moving them through the change continuum can increase motivation. Patients should be screened for readiness to change before beginning an obesity management program, and treatment modalities should be selected accordingly. For example, the questions in Table 4 may be used to assess the patient's readiness to change exercise behavior. If patients are in the precontemplation stage, efforts to raise their consciousness may be most helpful. Precontemplators may be defending against embarrassment, shame, or feelings of hopelessness. Providers may help precontemplators to become aware of their defenses. Providers may also help precontemplators by normalizing their feelings and expanding their options. Providers may solicit the aid of family members in this effort.

When working with patients in the contemplation stage, a provider may seek to arouse them emotionally by encouraging them to take a good hard look at themselves and asking if they are really satisfied with themselves, or if they have enough self-love to try to help themselves. If patients are in the preparation stage, the provider could encourage them to make a commitment. A written and signed agreement between the provider and the patient is a powerful technique because it personalizes the commitment and fortifies the provider-patient alliance. If patients are in the action or maintenance stage, the provider can provide kudos and suggestions regarding specific problems they may be having with the program. Using this screening technique and meeting patients where they are is an effective way of increasing motivation in patients who lack it.[31]

Risk of Injury During Exercise. Sedentary individuals are vulnerable to injury when activity levels are increased. These types of injuries may be dermatologic, orthopedic overuse, or the result of falls. The provider should warn patients about these potential problems and encourage them to take the necessary precautions. In general, sedentary patients should begin the program slowly to allow time for gradual physical adaptations to occur. The benefits of consistent moderate physical activity should be emphasized.

Patient Discomfort. Obese patients are likely to experience discomfort during physical activity that may negatively affect exercise adherence. For example, a recent study reported that severely obese women who were tested using walking and cycle ergometry experienced more distress than normal controls.[51] These results suggest that walking, which is generally considered to be a moderate-intensity activity, may be more intense for obese individuals. Patients should be advised to select activities in a manner that anticipates and minimizes discomfort.

Patient Feelings of Hopelessness. Some patients may feel powerless to lose weight because of previous failures and/or a belief in their genetic destiny to be obese. Effective treatment planning includes resources to identify and restructure these types of distorted and counterproductive cognitions. Continuous provider reinforcement is useful as well as patient participation in supportive group activities with members that model the desired behavior and results.

Provider Bias. Patient-provider alliance building is an effective method of improving program compliance.[41] Provider preconceptions and bias regarding obese people may prevent the development of a strong alliance.[52] There is considerable research showing that discrimination against the obese exists in our society. Providers should be aware of the possibility that they may carry negative feelings toward obese patients that might come out during patient visits. Obese patients may be more sensitive to interpersonal cues because of the discrimination they experience.

Strategies to Promote Adherence

Table 7 lists some important strategies that help patients adhere to obesity management programs. These strategies include suitable selection of treatment modalities, self-awareness, frequent follow-up, access to a support system, access to information and education, realistic goals, anticipation, and commitment.

Selection of suitable treatment modalities should be done in conjunction with the patient. Screening for depression and readiness to begin a change program are appropriate first steps. Understanding the patient's likes, dislikes, motivations, and time and resource constraints can facilitate constructive problem-solving and lead to feasible program plans. If the patient has chosen unrealistic goals, the provider might try changing the terminology to remove the emotion from the situation. For example, if an obese person is ashamed of the amount of weight gained and is adamant about losing 100 lbs in six months, the provider might try changing the terminology from pounds to BMI units. Focusing on the reduction of BMI units might eliminate some of the shame-based pressure felt by the patient to "lose weight."

Obesity is notoriously refractory, so it is likely that some form of continuous or intermittent long-term care model will be needed for most obese patients. Patients will benefit from frequent clinical and weigh-in visits. The more weigh-in visits, the better the results. Organizing weight management groups that meet weekly and are facilitated by members of the primary care team is an effective way of getting patients in for frequent weigh-ins.

Social support can motivate patients to persevere when they might otherwise falter. Frequent exposure to like-minded individuals may encourage the patient to want to emulate the behavior of dedicated people in the group. When patients have a support group, they have somewhere to go with their problems, where people care and will listen to them and offer suggestions and comfort. Peer support is useful in promoting adherence. Providers can help patients reach their goals by encouraging them to create a plan that involves social support and by organizing weight management groups facilitated by members of the primary care team.

Primary care providers can help patients stay on track by providing education about obesity and strategies to deal with barriers to adherence. Education might consist of pamphlets describing healthy eating or exercise guidelines. Even information about the illnesses associated with obesity might be helpful in motivating some patients to stay the course. Strategies to address exercise boredom or eating out are useful to patients adhering to a weight loss program. For example, if patients are bored with their exercise program, the provider might help them identify options or emphasize decreasing sedentary activity (e.g., cut down on the time watching television), rather than increasing physical activity. If patients are having difficulty sticking to the dietary guidelines because they eat out frequently, the provider might suggest that they focus on portion sizes when the options are limited.

Providers should focus on developing collaborative relationships with patients and seek their full support for the success of the program. This can be facilitated by contracting with patients in writing to formalize their agreement to participate fully in the obesity management effort.

Finally, providers would do well to model the behaviors that they request of their patients. Patients are more likely to accept advice from providers whom they feel are practicing what they preach.

Summary

Obesity is a chronic disease for which there is no cure. Its management requires eternal vigilance. Currently available management strategies can help obese patients improve their health and well-being. We need to increasingly turn our attention to general preventive approaches to reduce continued weight gain in our patients and to target intervention approaches in a manner that will result in the greatest benefit.

References

1. Mokdad AH, et al. The spread of the obesity epidemic in the United States, 1991-1998. *JAMA* 1999;282:1519-1522.
2. Howard BV, et al. Studies of the etiology of obesity in Pima Indians. *Am J Clin Nutr* 1991;53(6 Suppl):1577S-1585S.
3. Weinsier RL, et al. The etiology of obesity: Relative contribution of metabolic factors, diet, and physical activity. *Am J Med* 1998; 105:145-150.
4. Pi-Sunyer FX. Comorbidities of overweight and obesity: Current evidence and research issues. *Med Sci Sports Exerc* 1999;31(11 Suppl):S602-608.
5. Calle EE, et al. Body-mass index and mortality in a prospective cohort of U.S. adults [see comments]. *N Engl J Med* 1999; 341:1097-105.
6. National Institutes of Health (NIH) and National Heart Lung and Blood Institute (NHLBI), Clinical Guidelines on the Identification, Evaluation, and Treatment of Overweight and Obesity: The Evidence Report. 1998, Washington, D.C.: Government Press.
7. Brownell KD, Wadden TA. Etiology and treatment of obesity: Understanding a serious, prevalent, and refractory disorder. *J Consult Clin Psychol* 1992;60:505-517.
8. Bray GA. *Contemporary Diagnosis and Management of Obesity*. Newton, Pa.: Handbooks in Health Care Co.; 1998.
9. McArdle WD, et al. *Exercise Physiology: Energy, Nutrition, and Human Performance*. 3rd ed. Philadelphia: Lea & Febiger; 1991.
10. Troiano RP, Flegal FM. Overweight children and adolescents: Description, epidemiology, and demographics. *Pediatrics* 1998;101(Suppl):497-504.
11. Gortmaker SL, et al. Increasing pediatric obesity in the United States. *Am J Dis Child* 1987;141:535-540.
12. Dietz WH. Childhood weight affects adult morbidity and mortality. *J Nutr* 1998;128(2 Suppl):411S-414S.
13. Freedman DS, et al. Secular increases in relative weight and adiposity among children over two decades: The Bogalusa Heart Study. *Pediatrics* 1997;99:420-426.
14. Schonfeld-Warden N, Warden CH. Pediatric obesity. An overview of etiology and treatment. *Pediatr Clin North Am* 1997;44:339-361.
15. AACE/ACE Obesity Task Force, AACE/ACE position statement on the prevention, diagnosis, and treatment of obesity. 1998, The American Association of Endocrinologists and the American College of Endocrinology.
16. Poston WS, 2d, Foreyt JP. Obesity is an environmental issue. *Atherosclerosis* 1999;146:201-209.
17. Skinner BF. *Science and Human Behavior*. New York: Free Press; 1965.
18. Eaton SB, et al. Stone agers in the fast lane: Chronic degenerative diseases in evolutionary perspective. *Am J Med* 1988;84:739-749.
19. Eaton SB, et al. *The Paleolithic Prescription*. New York: Harper & Row; 1988.
20. Brown PJ, Bentley-Condit VK. Culture, evolution, and obesity. In: Bray GA, Bouchard C, James WPT, eds. *Handbook of Obesity*. New York: Marcel Dekker; 1998: 143-155.
21. National Cholesteral Education Program. Short dietary questionnaire to assess adherence to a step I and step II diet. In: *Second Report of the Expert Panel on Detection, Evaluation, and Treatment of High Blood Cholesterol in Adults*. 1993, National Institutes of Health. National Heart, Lung, and Blood Institute: Bethesda, MD. p. IIA-1.
22. SCORE, Rate Your Plate. 1988, Memorial Hospital: Rhode Island.
23. Physician Based Nutrition Program and Department of Medicine and Division of Epidemiology, Eating pattern assessment tool. 1990, University of Minnesota: Minneapolis, Minn.
24. Blair SN. How to assess exercise habits and physical fitness. In: Matarazzo JD, et al, eds. *Behavioral Health*. New York: Wiley; 1984:424-447.
25. Steer RA, et al. Use of the Beck depression inventory for primary care to screen for major depression disorders. *Gen Hosp Psychiatry* 1999;21:106-111.
26. Marcus MD. Binge eating in obesity. In: Fairburn C, Wilson GT, eds. *Binge Eating: Nature, Assessment, and Treatment*. New York: Guilford Press; 1993:77-96.
27. Webber EM. Psychological characteristics of binging and nonbinging obese women. *J Psychology* 1994;128:339-351.
28. Clark MM, et al. Depression, smoking, activity level, and health status: Pretreatment predictors of attrition in obesity treatment. *Addict Behav* 1996;21:509-513.
29. Tanco S, et al. Well-being and morbid obesity in women: A controlled therapy evaluation. *Int J Eat Disord* 1998;23: 325-339.
30. Miller GD, Harrington ME. Center for epidemiologic studies depression scale. In: St. Jeor ST, ed. *Obesity Assessment: Tools, Methods, Interpretations*. New York: Chapman & Hall; 1997:457-464.
31. Prochaska JO, et al. *Changing for Good: The Revolutionary Program that Explains the Six Stages of Change and Teaches you how to Free Yourself from Bad Habits*. New York: W. Morrow; 1994.
32. Baker RC, Kirschenbaum DS. Self-monitoring may be

necessary for successful weight control. *Behavior Therapy* 1993;24:377-394.

33. Foreyt JP, Goodrick GK. Factors common to successful therapy for the obese patient. *Med Sci Sports Exerc* 1991;23:292-297.
34. Foreyt JP, Poston WSC. Building better compliance: Factors and methods common to achieving a healthy lifestyle. In: Gotto AM, et al, eds. *Drugs Affecting Lipid Metabolism: Risk Factors and Future Directions*. Dordrecht, The Netherlands: Kluwer Academic Publishers; 1996:489-496.
35. Foreyt JP, Goodrick GK. Evidence for success of behavior modification in weight loss and control. *Ann Intern Med* 1993;119:698-701.
36. Pendleton VR, et al. Stress and the outcome of treatment for binge eating. In press.
37. Foreyt JP, Goodrick GK. Attributes of successful approaches to weight loss and control. *Appl Prev Psychiatr* 1994;3: 209-215.
38. Kayman S, et al. Maintenance and relapse after weight loss in women: Behavioral aspects. *Am J Clin Nutr* 1990;52: 800-807.
39. Klem ML, et al. The psychological consequences of weight gain prevention in healthy, premenopausal women. *Int J Eat Disord* 1997;21:167-174.
40. Niego SH, et al. Subjective or objective binge: Is the distinction valid? *Int J Eat Disord* 1997;22:291-298.
41. Luque CA, Rey JA. Sibutramine: A serotonin-norepinephrine reuptake-inhibitor for the treatment of obesity. *Ann Pharmacother* 1999;33:968-978.
42. Hvizdos KM, Markham A. Orlistat: A review of its use in the management of obesity. *Drugs* 1999;58:743-760.
43. Davidson MH, et al. Weight control and risk factor reduction in obese subjects treated for 2 years with orlistat: A randomized controlled trial [see comments] [published erratum appears in *JAMA* 1999;281(13):1174]. *JAMA* 1999;281:235-242.
44. National Institutes of Health Consensus Development Conference Statement, Gastrointestinal surgery for severe obesity. *Am J Clin Nutrition* 1992;55:615S-619S.
45. Naslund I. The size of the gastric outlet and the outcome of surgery for obesity. *Acta Chir Scand* 1986;152:205-210.
46. Hyman FN, et al. Evidence for success of caloric restriction in weight loss and control. Summary of data from industry. *Ann Intern Med* 1993;119(7 Pt 2):681-687.
47. United States Department of Agriculture, The Food Guide Pyramid. Home and Garden Bulletin Number 252. 1992, Washington, D.C.: U.S. Government Printing Office.
48. *Report of a Joint FAO/WHO/UNU Expert Consultation, Energy and Protein Requirements*. 1985, World Health Organization: Geneva.
49. U.S. Preventive Services Task Force, Counseling to promote physical activity. In: *Guide to Clinical Preventive Services: Report of the U.S. Preventive Services Task Force*, 2nd ed. Baltimore, Md.: Williams & Wilkins; 1996:chap. 55.
50. U.S. Department of Health and Human Services, physical activity. In: Dickey LL, ed. *Clinician's Handbook of Preventive Services: Put Prevention into Practice*. Waldorf, Md.: American Nurses Pub.; 1994:311-317.
51. Mattsson E, et al. Is walking for exercise too exhausting for obese women? *Int J Obes Relat Metab Disord* 1997;21: 380-386.
52. Maddox GL, Liederman V. Overweight as a social disability with medical implications. *J Med Educ* 1969;44:214-220.

Part VII

Obstetrics and Gynecology

Preconceptional Care

Elmar P. Sakala, MD, MA, MPH

Most physicians providing obstetric care can recall seeing a patient on the first prenatal visit with a maternal complication or fetal abnormality that might have been prevented by appropriate counseling and intervention prior to the pregnancy. Some patients are ignorant of the following effects on the developing embryo: 1) medical conditions they are suffering from; 2) medications they are taking; 3) occupational hazards they are exposed to; or 4) social practices they are engaging in. With organogenesis beginning as early as 17 days after conception, it is easy to understand why waiting until the onset of prenatal care may have little effect on providing the ideal environment for the developing conceptus.

Preconceptional counseling seeks to optimize pregnancy outcome by identifying individuals with risk factors, then providing interventions to prevent the development of a condition or disease that could jeopardize the mother, fetus, or neonate. Preconceptional care should be an integrated component of all primary care services, particularly as part of initial and annual visits for family planning services. Preconceptional care and counseling should be offered by primary care physicians to all women in their reproductive years as well as to their partners.

Primary care physicians provide the first contact between the patient and the health-care system. The majority of health-care visits of patients in their reproductive years are through primary care providers. The bulk of preventive care services occurs within the framework of the primary care health system. It is understandable then that the partnership between primary care doctors and their patients holds the key to optimal health-care outcomes, including pregnancy.

The Value of Prenatal Care

The achievement of optimal outcomes of pregnancy has been attributed, to a great degree, to the early enrollment of pregnant women into prenatal care. Prenatal care is traditionally initiated once pregnancy has been detected and seeks the following basic aims: 1) to identify known risks to either the mother or the fetus (e.g., women with Rh negative blood types); 2) to prevent the actualization of risks identified (e.g., administering prophylactic Rh immune globulin to Rh negative women); 3) to diagnose latent problems early enough to treat and thereby prevent any morbidity or mortality (e.g., obtain cultures and treat promptly if positive: cervical [for gonorrhea and chlamydia]; vaginal [for bacterial vaginosis and group B -hemolytic strep]; urine [for asymptomatic bacteriuria]); 4) to limit the adverse sequelae of problems that cannot

Table 1. The Focus of Preconceptional Care

1. **Discontinue Harmful and Addictive Habits**
   a. Alcohol
   b. Smoking
   c. Cocaine
2. **Discontinue Teratogenic Prescription Medications**
   a. Lithium
   b. Phenytoin
   c. Valproic acid
   d. Isotretinoin
   e. Warfarin
3. **Adopt Healthy Dietary Habits**
   a. Folic acid supplementation
   b. Normalization of body weight
   c. Avoid anorexia and bulemia
4. **Identify Risk of Preventable Perinatal Infections**
   a. Hepatitis B virus
   b. Rubella
   c. Toxoplasmosis
   d. HIV
5. **Normalize Blood Nutrient Substrates**
   a. Glucose
   b. Phenylalanine
   c. Iron
6. **Modify Psychosocial Risk Factors**
   a. Lack of social support
   b. Conditions of high stress and anxiety
7. **Provide Genetic Counseling**
   a. Tay-Sachs disease
   b. Sickle-cell anemia
   c. Cystic fibrosis

be detected and treated early (e.g., prompt delivery of a patient with severe preeclampsia or timely administration of maternal corticosteroids to induce surfactant production in preterm fetuses).

These aims parallel the three tiers of preventive care in the health care system. Aims 1 and 2 above illustrate the most basic tier, which is primary prevention—identification of risk factors and provision of interventions so that the condition or disease never develops. Aim 3 illustrates secondary prevention, the next tier of preventive care—early identification of a problem and prompt treatment to prevent disability. Aim 4 is the third tier, which is tertiary prevention—the treatment of a major problem after it has developed to prevent disability.

Many studies support the premise that the interventions involved in such an organized prenatal care sequence contribute to decreasing maternal and perinatal morbidity and mortality. Maternal mortality rates in the United States have indeed fallen precipitously over the last 50 years. Perinatal mortality rates have similarly fallen significantly, even though U.S. perinatal mortality lags behind those of other industrialized countries in the Western world.

Limitations of Prenatal Care

Some perinatal mortalities and morbidities occur unpredictably. For these cases, no risk factors were present to suggest a problem would develop prior to the adverse event. Accordingly, corrective action was not possible. Examples include pre-eclampsia, umbilical cord accidents, and fetal anomalies arising from new mutations.

However, other adverse pregnancy outcomes potentially could have been prevented. Examples include intrauterine fetal death from abruptio placenta in a cocaine user and fetal macrosomia in a woman with poorly controlled adult-onset diabetes mellitus. The relevant risk factors were clearly present, but they were either not identified or appropriate intervention was not provided in a timely fashion.

But even if the sequence of risk identification and preventive intervention is initiated after pregnancy has occurred, optimal maternal and perinatal outcomes may still not be realized. Reasons for this inadequacy of prenatal care may be any of the following:

1. Many of the risks identified during prenatal care may already have had their destructive effect on the fetus by the time prenatal care starts. Waiting to address the existing pregnancy risks until after conception may be like closing the barn door after the horse is already out. An example is the development of neural tube and cardiac anomalies in the fetus of a woman with juvenile-onset diabetes mellitus whose blood glucose values were out of control during early embryogenesis.

2. The process of modification of maternal lifestyle behaviors that are harmful to the fetus may be of such an intensity and lengthy duration that their adverse effect will have already occurred by the time the behaviors are finally changed. Examples include the development of fetal alcohol syndrome in heavy-drinking women and the growth-restricted newborns of tobacco-smoking women.

3. Counseling for genetic risks after conception has occurred precludes avoiding pregnancy by seeking permanent sterilization and the consideration of artificial insemination by donor. An example is informing a woman who is already pregnant that she is a carrier for hemophilia and that 50% of her sons will be affected and 50% of her daughters will be carriers.

Thus, it makes intuitive sense to advance the preventive aspects of prepregnancy planning far enough before conception that the risks identified can be eliminated or at least modified as much as possible before pregnancy occurs. This lays the theoretical basis for the focus of preconceptional counseling.

Preconceptional Care is Primary Prevention

While prenatal care focuses on all three tiers of prevention (primary, secondary, and tertiary), preconceptional care is uniquely and distinctively primary prevention in nature. Its singular focus is on identification of risks to mother and baby, followed by health promotion to eradicate those risks. The focus of the following specific aspects of comprehensive preconcep-

Table 2. Key Elements in Preconceptional Counceling

1. Who initiated the preconceptional counseling? Patient or physician?
2. How many decisions by the patient are required? A single decision, or multiple repetitive decisions?
3. What is the duration of behavior change required by the patient?
4. What is the nature of the targeted behavior change? Restricted or complex?
5. Does the target of the recommendation involve addictive substances?
6. Is the adverse behavior the consequence of psychiatric conditions?
7. Does the recommended behavior change have the support of the patient's family, cultural, and social group?
8. Is the rationale behind the recommendation understood by the patient?
9. How extensive is the economic cost of the recomendation to the patient?

tional care is fundamentally on the adoption of behaviors that enhance the health of the mother and baby along with the discontinuance of behaviors hazardous to them.

The Focus of Preconceptional Care

Discontinue Harmful and Addictive Habits. Alcohol use among pregnant women is common in the United States. It is the most commonly abused psychoactive drug during pregnancy, with use rates of 6-20% depending on the population studied. Women in the childbearing age group are the most likely to use alcohol. Fetal exposure to alcohol is associated with major perinatal problems. Severe birth defects, facial malformations, growth retardation, central nervous system dysfunction, as well as learning and behavioral problems are noted. In heavy drinkers (2-3 drinks per day), the incidence of miscarriage doubles to 30%, and the rate of low birth weight doubles to 25%. Fetal alcohol syndrome is the primary cause of mental retardation in children.[1] The risk of some abnormality in the fetus exposed to heavy alcohol use is approximately 50%. Since no safe level of alcohol consumption has been established, advise your patients to avoid all alcohol prior to conception and throughout pregnancy.

Smoking in pregnancy is associated with infertility, preterm labor, low birthweight babies, and higher perinatal morbidity and mortality. A dose-response relationship has been shown between the number of cigarettes smoked during pregnancy and newborn birthweight reduction. Long-term adverse neonatal physical, emotional, and intellectual effects from prenatal nicotine exposure have been documented.[2,3] The U.S. Office of Smoking and Health states that smoking is an important preventable cause of adverse pregnancy outcomes.[4,5] It is essential to advise women to modify smoking habits and to aim at quitting smoking prior to pregnancy.[6-8]

Cocaine use in pregnancy is widespread. This habit, even if limited to only the first trimester, can result in spontaneous abortion, placental abruption, premature birth, intrauterine growth restriction (IUGR), and fetal anomalies. These anomalies are thought to have a vasospastic etiology resulting from cocaine constriction of fetal blood vessels that leads to decreased regional circulation. Neonatal central nervous system dysfunction has been well described as a consequence of maternal cocaine use. Women who stop cocaine use by the second trimester have a normal incidence of premature delivery and IUGR.[9] Inform your patients that stopping cocaine use prior to pregnancy has major perinatal benefits.

Discontinue Teratogenic Prescription Medications. The following section details a number of commonly used systemic pharmacological preparations that have been associated with serious teratogenic effects on the developing embryo.

Lithium. The use of this antidepressant drug during the first trimester may be related to an increased incidence of congenital defects, particularly of the cardiovascular system. One-third of the heart defects noted are that of the rare Ebstein's anomaly.[10] Consider using antidepressants other than lithium for your depressed female patients prior to conception and during the first trimester.

Phenytoin. Epileptic women taking phenytoin, either alone or in combination with other anticonvulsants, have a 2-3 times greater risk over the general population for delivering a child with congenital defects. Fetal hydantoin syndrome, first described in 1968 by Meadow, is found in 10% of infants exposed to phenytoin in utero.[11] Findings noted include craniofacial dysmorphism, prenatal and postnatal growth delay, mental retardation, congenital heart defects, cleft lip and palate, and distal digital hypoplasia.[12] If possible, prescribe anticonvulsants other than phenytoin to epileptic women prior to them attempting pregnancy.

Valproic Acid. This is another anticonvulsant with significant teratogenic potential. The prevalence of meningomyelocele related to valproic acid monotherapy in pregnancy is estimated to be 2.5% when used between day 17-20 after conception.[13] A characteristic pattern of minor facial defects has also been described, along with defects involving digits, urogenital tract, and mental and physical growth. Since valproic acid readily crosses the placenta, avoid prescribing it to epileptic women considering pregnancy.[14]

Isotretinoin. This vitamin A isomer is used for the treatment of severe, recalcitrant cystic acne. A high percentage of isotretinoin users are women in their childbearing years; up to 40% are women aged 13-19 years. This agent is a potent teratogen when taken orally but not topically. It has a characteristic anomaly pattern involving the central nervous, craniofacial, and cardiovascular systems.[15] Current recommendations are that you advise patients that systemic isotretinoin should be stopped at least one month prior to conception.[16]

Warfarin. This oral anticonvulsant was first described in 1966 as causing fetal embryopathy.[17] The critical period of exposure

Table 3. Predictors of Success in Preconceptional Counseling

1. **Highest success**
   a. Counseling is initiated by patient
   b. Intervention requires only a single decision by the patient
2. **Moderate success**
   a. The duration of the behavior change is short
   b. The nature of the targeted behavior change requires limited but multiple patient decisions
   c. The economic cost to the patient is limited
3. **Limited success**
   a. The targeted behavior involves addictive substances
   b. The recommended behavior change is not endorsed by the patient's family, cultural, or social group
   c. The nature of the behavior change is extensive and pervasive

appears to be between the 6th and 9th weeks of gestation, with 30% of exposed fetuses developing fetal warfarin syndrome.[18] Common characteristic findings include nasal hypoplasia (due to failure of nasal septum development) and stippled epiphyses. Exposure after the first trimester carries the risk of central nervous system defects, probably from fetal hemorrhage.[19] Change women on warfarin anticoagulation therapy to subcutaneous heparin prior to conception.

Adoption of Healthy Dietary Habits. Neural tube defects (NTD) may be more frequent in lower socioeconomic groups and in women with diets lacking in certain vitamins. Incidence is higher in subsequent pregnancies of women who had a previous fetus with a NTD. Folic acid supplementation initiated at least 28 days prior to conception appears to reduce the rate of recurrent NTDs in subsequent pregnancies.[20] Recent studies suggest that if you prescribe 4 mg/d of folate preconceptionally to your at-risk patients, their serious anomaly rate can be reduced by 70%.[21] Low maternal prepregnancy weight, especially when combined with low pregnancy weight gain, is associated with increased perinatal mortality and morbidity.[22,23] High maternal prepregnancy weight is associated with hypertension, fetal macrosomia, glucose intolerance, and difficult labor and delivery.[24] Encourage your preconception patients to normalize their body weight, thereby improving their pregnancy outcome.

Anorexia and bulimia are psychiatric conditions with major nutritional consequences, particularly for the pregnant woman and her fetus. Therapy is complex, prolonged, and unpredictable in outcome.[25,26]

Identification of Risk for Preventable Perinatal Infectious Diseases. Hepatitis B virus (HBV) is a significant perinatal problem due to the risk of vertical transmission from mother to baby. The prevalence of surface antigen carriers in the United States is less than 1% but approaches 20% in individuals from the Far East as well as in the Alaskan Eskimo.[27] Up to 10% of these infected individuals will develop a chronic carrier state with long-term risks including liver failure, cirrhoses, and liver cancer. Neonates born to women who are hepatitis B "c" antigen positive have a 90% chance of becoming chronic carriers. If your preconception female patients do not know their HBV status, order a simple blood screening test to identify whether they have the HBV antigen. For patients who are negative but at risk for HBV, recommend the series of preconception vaccinations thereby protecting not only themselves but also their future newborns.[28]

Rubella infection in pregnancy, although mostly benign for the mother, may cause spontaneous first trimester loss, fetal demise, or congenital rubella syndrome in the newborn. The widespread use of attenuated live rubella virus vaccine has almost abolished congenital rubella syndrome. Recommend immunization to your non-pregnant rubella-susceptible preconception patients to protect their future offspring.

Primary maternal toxoplasmosis infection in pregnancy can result in IUGR, stillbirth, and severe neonatal central nervous system sequelae including mental retardation and deafness. The earlier in gestation the infection, the more severe the fetal effects. It is transmitted to humans by ingestion of the sporozoa oocytes contained in raw meat or in infected cat feces. Currently, no immunization against toxoplasmosis is available, but you can identify seronegative women prior to pregnancy. Then, counsel them about appropriate preparation of meat and handling of cat litter.

Human immunodeficiency virus (HIV) infection is increasing most rapidly in heterosexual women of childbearing age. Acquired immunodeficiency syndrome (AIDS) is the fifth leading killer of American women between the ages of 15 and 45.[28a] Vertical transmission of HIV from an infected mother to her fetus and neonate occurs at a rate of 30%, with an extremely rapid progression in the newborn to AIDS. Immunization against HIV is nor currently available. All women should be offered HIV testing and should be asked regarding sexual partners and sexual practices. All primary physicians should be actively educating their patients regarding safer sex practices and the hazards of HIVto the newborn.

Normalization of Blood Nutrient Substrates. Glucose. Congenital malformations are the most frequent cause of neonatal death in infants of overt diabetic mothers. Anomalies are seen at a rate up to three times that of the general population. These anomalies, occurring with an incidence of 6-9%, involve skeletal, cardiovascular, genitourinary, and central nervous system defects.[29] The mechanism of anomaly establishment has been shown to be substantially due to elevated plasma glucose levels. The critical gestation age for development of these malformations is before the seventh week of gestation, when most women have not even enrolled for prenatal care. Encourage overt diabetic women to achieve euglycemia before and during early pregnancy because repetitive studies show their congenital anomaly rates can be reduced to the same level as the general population.[30-32]

Phenylalanine. Phenylketonuria (PKU) is an autosomal recessive inborn error of metabolism in which blood levels of the amino acid phenylalanine are markedly elevated due to pheny-

Table 4. Ideal Opportunities for Preconceptional Care

1. Initial family planning visits
2. Annual family planning visits
3. Premarital examinations
4. Discontinuance of contraceptive methods
5. Finding of negative pregnancy test
6. Infertility evaluation

lalanine hydroxylase deficiency. Untreated PKU in infants and developing children results in mental retardation. The affected fetus of a woman who is only a carrier is not at risk in utero. However, the affected fetus of a pregnant woman with overt PKU is at high risk for mental retardation, microcephaly, and IUGR if the mother eats a phenylalanine unrestricted diet. If you place your PKU patients on a low-phenylalanine diet prior to conception and continue it throughout the pregnancy, fetal damage from high phenylalanine levels can be significantly reduced.[33]

Iron. Iron deficiency anemia is eight times more common in women than in men, mostly due to menstrual blood losses and pregnancy demands. The reduction in circulating red blood cell hemoglobin does not occur until the bone marrow stores are completely depleted. If a woman's iron stores are marginal prior to conception, even though she may not be manifestly anemic, the increased iron demands of pregnancy may drain whatever bone marrow stores remain, making her overtly anemic. While maternal iron deficiency does not affect the fetus, due to active transport of iron across the placenta to meet fetal requirements, it clearly adversely affects the oxygen-carrying capacity of the woman leaving her tired and weak. Assess women planning pregnancy for evidence of iron deficiency anemia, then place them on iron supplementation to restore bone marrow stores before pregnancy occurs.

Modification of Psychosocial Risk Factors. Epidemiologic studies have identified psychosocial conditions associated with increased perinatal mortality as well as morbidities such as preterm birth.[34] Preconception risk assessment by a sensitive interviewer provides an opportunity to identify such adverse conditions. Examples of psychosocial risk factors under the general category of lack of social support include: living in an abusive relationship, living alone, single marital status, and being a single parent. Examples of conditions with high stress and anxiety include: psychiatric condition, lack of employment, low income, inadequate housing, and limited formal education. Any efforts on your behalf that can successfully modify or correct the psychosocial condition prior to conception would appear to enhance the outcome of pregnancy once it occurs.[35]

Genetic Counseling. Genetic counseling involves advising a family regarding the risk of adverse consequences from the occurrence or risk of occurrence of a genetic disorder within the family. The family at risk is advised of what is known; the severity, anticipated course, prognosis, and management of the disorder; the risk of occurrence; and the choices available for avoiding recurrence.[36] Much genetic counseling occurs retrospectively, after the birth of an affected infant.

The increased risk of aneuoploidy associated with advanced maternal age is the most common indication for invasive perinatal testing. While the risk is progressive throughout adult life, the curve begins to accelerate at about 35 years of age. The primary reason for this increased risk is a higher incidence of nondisjunction events, resulting in trisomies (-21, -18, -13) and 47,XXX and 47,XXY.[36a]

Set up your initial patient history forms to ask screening questions to identify risk for the most common disorders, then provide counseling to detected carriers. Examples are screening for Tay-Sachs disease in Ashkenazy Jews or French Canadians, and for sickle-cell anemia in people of African, Mediterranean, Middle Eastern, or Caribbean descent. Screening for cystic fibrosis may be offered to patients with a family history of the disease.

Provide preconceptional identification of carrier status, and it will allow women and their partners to understand autosomal recessive risks outside of the emotional context of pregnancy. This allows both informed decision-making about conception and planning for further desired testing should pregnancy occur.

Although genetic counseling can often provide a quantifiable risk of occurrence or recurrence, it is limited in actual primary prevention. Most often, the options available are: 1) get pregnant and take a chance followed by early prenatal diagnosis with possible pregnancy termination if the fetus is affected; 2) avoid pregnancy by male and/or female sterilization; 3) achieve pregnancy through artificial and/or assisted reproduction with donor sperm and/or donor ovum; or 4) adopt a child. For an overview of the focus of preconceptional care, see Table 1.

Predictors of Success in Preconceptional Counseling

While it is relatively easy to distinguish which risk factors are associated with perinatal mortality and morbidity, the likelihood of successfully changing or modifying those risk factors prior to conception is variable. The following considerations will heavily affect the probability of successful preconception behavior change.[37] *(Please see Tables 2 and 3.)*

1. Who initiated the preconception counseling? The patient or the clinician?

2. How many decisions by the patient are required? A single decision, or multiple and repetitive decisions?

3. What is the duration of behavior change required by the patient? Short or prolonged?

4. What is the nature of the targeted behavior change? Restricted or complex?

5. Does the target of the recommendation involve addictive substances?

6. Is the adverse behavior the consequence of psychiatric conditions?

7. Does the recommended behavior change have the support of the patient's family, cultural, and social group?

8. Is the rationale behind the recommendation understood by the patient?

9. How extensive is the economic cost of the recommendations to the patient?

Highest Success Counseling Scenarios. The following characteristics identify situations that have the highest chance for successful preconception primary prevention. Unfortunately, they represent a relatively small fraction of the total opportunities that exist for preconceptional interventions. All health-care professionals, regardless of their interest or training, whether nursing aides or subspecialist physicians, need to ensure that the following opportunities for preconceptional counseling are not missed.

a. Counseling is initiated by the patient. Most often this occurs if the patient has experienced an unfavorable outcome with a previous pregnancy. Examples include: an overt diabetic woman delivers a baby with caudal regression syndrome; a child is born with a previously undiagnosed spina bifida. The motivation for behavior change by the patient is maximal; thus, the likelihood of following through with recommendations for preconception glycemic control or folate supplementation is greatest. The main causes of failure in patient-initiated encounters are default on the part of the clinician to either provide the needed information and management or failure to refer the patient to a professional who does have the required interest and expertise.

b. Intervention requires only a single decision by the patient. The best example is immunization against serious perinatal infectious diseases, such as rubella and hepatitis B. The practice of administering rubella immunization immediately postpartum to susceptible women prior to discharging them from the maternity unit has been an extremely effective preconception intervention. Equally efficacious has been the identification of hepatitis B surface-antigen positive gravidas and the administration to their newborn of active vaccination as well as passive immunization with hepatitis B immunoglobulin. The limiting steps in such cases are: 1) failure to identify the risk status of the patient by not performing an appropriate prenatal screening test; or 2) failure to set up or implement protocols, thereby not administering immunizations when they are indicated.

Moderate Success Counseling Scenarios. The following characteristics identify the situations that have a significant chance for successful preconception primary prevention. These represent a somewhat larger fraction of the total opportunities that exist for preconceptional interventions. Even though these cases call for a greater degree of time spent in health education and promotion with the patient, the likelihood of seeing a successful outcome is good. With the increasing emphasis placed on primary care by changes in the health-care system, a strong case can be made for primary care physicians of all disciplines to pursue the following preconceptional counseling scenarios.

a. The duration of the behavior change is short. If an adverse intrauterine environment can be modified during a relatively short but critical period of embryogenesis, major congenital anomalies could potentially be prevented. An example is the achievement of euglycemia by an overt diabetic woman at the time of conception and for the first eight post-conceptional weeks. The interval of time required to obtain the benefit is only a few months, which makes the possibility of patient compliance reasonable. The limitations in implementing this intervention are both patient and clinician related.

Patient-related limitations include failing to take the initiative to control blood glucoses early enough to achieve eu-glycemia prior to conception. The initial motivation may be present, but, since conception seldom occurs when planned or desired, the level of drive may dwindle over time. Glucose control, even though of relatively short duration, does involve complex behaviors including: frequent monitoring of blood glucose levels, selection of appropriate food-mix, timing of eating, timing and regularity of exercise, as well as adjustment of insulin dosages. The more complex the behavior change, the more challenging the implementation.

Clinician-related limitations may be related to primary prevention not being as exciting to many specialists as acute care. The physician's focus is often on the pressing chief complaint rather than the less urgent, but just as important, preventive activity. Additionally, preventive activities are often not well reimbursed by third-party payers.

b. The nature of the targeted behavior requires limited but multiple patient decisions. Taking pharmacologic preparations at critical periods of the pregnancy can potentially prevent congenital anomalies. An example is folate supplementation preconceptionally and in the early post-conceptional weeks. The target behavior is restricted in scope, limited to a single daily tablet of folic acid. However, the behavior must be repeated daily over a period of months. The same patient and physician limitations apply here as in the previous section.

c. The economic cost to the patient is limited. Changes that have no cost to the patient have the highest probability of successful implementation. If additional cash outlay is required, the lower the dollar amount required, the more likely the recommended change will take place. An example is the recognition of an epileptic woman considering pregnancy of the need to substitute a non-teratogenic (more expensive) anticonvulsant medication for a teratogenic (less expensive) anticonvulsant.

Limited Success Counseling Scenarios. The following situations have limited probability for successful preconception primary prevention. However, they have the greatest potential for improving maternal and perinatal outcomes since they represent the greatest proportion of total challenges that exist for preconceptional interventions. Because of the inherent nature of these circumstances, these patient encounters can be exceptionally challenging, demanding, and frustrating. Special skills in communication, motivation, and education are called into play in these situations. Not all primary care physicians have the time, the interest, or the training to deal with these challenging cases. However, all physicians should be familiar with other health-care professionals, specialists, or community resources that are able to assist the patient in behavior change.

a. The targeted behavior involves addictive substances. Smoking during pregnancy has numerous adverse perinatal consequences. Yet, efforts to enhance smoking cessation are complicated by the addictive properties of nicotine. Successful intervention will often require the skills of professionals specially trained in addiction medicine. In spite of the limited response rate, your effort to decrease preconception use of addictive substances is well justified.

b. The recommended behavior change is not endorsed by the patient's family, cultural, or social group. This is a key limitation of many approaches to treatment of dependency conditions such as cocaine use. The patient may, within an isolated rehabilitation setting, stay "clean" for a prolonged period of time. However, when she returns to her previous social and cultural milieu, where cocaine use is part of the accepted and promoted lifestyle, the old habit may well be resumed.

c. The nature of behavior change is extensive and pervasive. Many of the hazards to the developing embryo and fetus are the consequence of lifestyle habits that are deeply ingrained into the everyday life of the woman. The limited success in motivating a change in such aspects of lifestyle is because change requires an extensive alteration in the woman's behavior and how she experiences her life. Examples of such behaviors include: smoking cigarettes, consuming alcohol, ingesting an unhealthy diet, and experiencing excessive physical or emotional stress. Changes in each of these behaviors have the potential to improve the outcome of pregnancy.

Although such behaviors are recognized to be statistically associated with less than optimal pregnancy outcomes, the majority of babies born to women practicing these behaviors have no grossly identifiable abnormalities. The hope that such anecdotal "satisfactory" outcomes will somehow repeat often underlies the half-hearted efforts by both patients and health-care providers in modifying these harmful behaviors. Don't wait until after pregnancy to encourage patients to start changing extensive and pervasive behavior. Begin addressing them now, before conception takes place.

Who Should Perform Preconceptional Counseling?

One would expect physicians providing pregnancy care would be tuned in to the importance of providing this service. Since many OB/GYN physicians and some family practitioners provide the major part of obstetrical care, it would seem appropriate to expect them to be in the forefront of preconceptional counseling. However, all primary care practitioners who provide family planning information or services have a significant role to play, whether they be internists, family doctors, pediatricians, nurse practitioners, nurse midwives, or physician assistants. Preconceptional care should be made available to all women and their partners as an integrated part of primary care services, particularly as part of initial and annual family planning service visits.[8] Ideal opportunities for discussing pregnancy planning are visits when patients: 1) present for premarital examinations, 2) come for discontinuance of contraceptive methods, 3) are found to have a negative pregnancy test, or 4) seek infertility care. *(Please see Table 4.)* Patients receiving such services indicate an overwhelmingly positive response to the counseling. These avenues may serve to meet most of the high success scenarios and many of the moderate success ones.

However, broad changes in lifestyle habits and patterns (such as smoking tobacco, drinking alcohol, and poor nutritional habits) will not come about by health-care professionals waiting for patients to come to them. Such lifestyle changes include the challenging and difficult issues involved in the limited success scenarios. And yet, the greatest benefit of preconceptional change can arise from these, since women participating in these adverse behaviors number in the millions.

Helping professionals from all aspects of society should participate in preconceptional counseling in its broadest sense. School health personnel need to work with the teaching staff. Clergy need to be educated to discuss these principles in premarital counseling. The broadcast and print media need to be employed through public service messages on a wider scale to alert families at risk regarding the significance of making healthy choices.

Summary

1. Prenatal care often starts too late to interrupt injurious events and harmful influences to the developing embryo, many of which may antedate the pregnancy or be present at the time of conception.

2. Preconceptional care is mostly primary prevention in that it identifies women with risk factors and provides interventions so the adverse condition is removed and the harmful effect is never actualized.

3. Health education and motivation of behavior change are crucial to preconceptional counseling.

4. The focus of preconceptional care includes: discontinuing harmful and addictive habits, discontinuing teratogenic prescription medications, adopting healthy dietary habits, identifying risk for preventable perinatal infectious diseases, normalizing blood nutrient substrates, modifying psychosocial risk factors, and providing genetic counseling.

5. Characteristics can be identified that distinguish high vs. low likelihood of success in behavior change. Physicians are more likely to participate in preventive scenarios initiated by the patient or those involving a single decision by the patient. Physicians may not always be adequately trained or interested in dealing with the low success scenarios that involve addictive substances or require extensive and pervasive lifestyle change.

6. Preconceptional care should be part of all initial and annual primary care encounters.

7. Helping professionals from all aspects of society should participate in preconceptional counseling in its broadest sense.

References

1. Warren KR, Bast RJ. Alcohol related birth defects: An update. Public Health Rep 1988;188:638-642.
2. Institute of Medicine: Preventing Low Birthweight. Washington D.C., National Academy Press; 1985:119.
3. U.S. Public Health Service Expert Panel on the Content of Prenatal Care: Caring for our Future. Washington, D.C. Public Health Service, Department of Health and Human Services; October

1989:25-30.

4. Office of Smoking and Health: The health consequences of smoking for women: A report of the Surgeon General. Rockville, Maryland: U.S. Department of Health and Human Services, Public Health Service; 1980.
5. Office of Smoking and Health: The health consequences of smoking for women: A report of the Surgeon General. Rockville, Maryland: U.S. Department of Health and Human Services, Public Health Service; 1990.
6. Aaronson NK, Ershoff DH. Smoking cessation in pregnancy: A self-help approach. *Addic Behav* 1985;10:103-108.
7. Chasnoff IJ, et al. Cocaine use in pregnancy. *N Engl J Med* 1985;313:666-669.
8. Pettiti B, Coleman C. Cocaine and the risk of low birthweight. *Am J Pub Health* 1990;80:25-28.
9. Chasnoff IJ, Griffith DR, MacGregor SN, et al. Temporal patterns of cocaine use in pregnancy: Perinatal outcome. *JAMA* 1989;261:1741-1743.
10. Nora JJ, Nora AH, Toews WH. Lithium, Ebstein's anomaly, and other congenital heart defects. *Lancet* 1974;2:594-595.
11. Meadow SR. Anticonvulsant drugs and congenital abnormalities. *Lancet* 1968;2:1296-1297.
12. Hanson JW, Smith DW. The fetal hydantoin syndrome. *J Pediatr* 1975;87:285-287.
13. Lindhout D, Schmidt D. In utero exposure to valproate and neural tube defects. *Lancet* 1986;1:1392- 1393.
14. Lammer EJ, Sever LE, Oakley GP. Teratogen update: Valproic acid. *Teratology* 1987;35:465-473.
15. Lammer EJ, Chen DT, Hoar RM, et al. Retinoic acid embryopathy. *N Engl J Med* 1985;313:827-828.
16. Anonymous. Adverse effects with isotretinoin. *FDA Drug Bull* 1983;13:21-23.
17. DiSaia PJ. Pregnancy and delivery of a patient with a Starr-Edwards mitral value prosthesis. *Obstet Gynecol* 1966;28:469-471.
18. Hall JG, Pauli RM, Wilson KM. Maternal and fetal sequelae of anticoagulation during pregnancy. *Am J Med* 1980;68:122-124.
19. Chong MKB, Harvey D, DeSwiet M. Follow-up study of children whose mothers were treated with warfarin during pregnancy. *Br J Obstet Gynaecol* 1984;91:1070-1074.
20. Laurence KM, James N, Miller MH, et al. Double-blind randomized controlled trial of folate treatment before conception to prevent recurrence of neural tube defects. *BMJ* 1981;282:1509-1511.
21. MRC Vitamin Study Research Group. Prevention of neural tube defects: Results of the Medical Research Council Vitamin Study. *Lancet* 1991;338:131.
22. Naeye RL. Weight gain and the outcomes of pregnancy. *Am J Obstet Gynecol* 1979;135:3-9.
23. Abrams BF, Laros RK. Prepregnancy weight, weight gain, and birth weight. *Am J Obstet Gynecol* 1986;154:503.
24. Johnson SR, Kolberg BH, Varner MW, et al. Maternal obesity and pregnancy. *Surg Gynecol Obstet* 1987;164:431-437.
25. Fairburn CG, Stein A, Jones R. Eating habits and eating disorders in pregnancy. *Psychosomatic Med* 1992;54:665-672.
26. Stewart DE. Reproductive functions in eating disorders. *Ann Med* 1992;24:287-291.
27. Arevalo JA. Hepatitis B in pregnancy. *West J Med* 1989;150: 668-670.
28. Cohen M, Cohen H. Current recommendations for viral hepatitis. *Contemp Obstet Gynecol* 1990;35:56-60.
28a. International Trade Administration. U.S. Industrial Outlook. U.S. Department of Commerce, Washington. 1991;44:1.
29. Kalter M, Warkany J. Congenital malformations. *N Engl J Med* 1983;308:424-431; 491-497.
30. Goldman JA, Dicker D, Feldberg D, et al. Pregnancy outcome in patients with insulin-dependent diabetes mellitus with preconceptional diabetic control: a comparative study. *Am J Obstet Gynecol* 1987;155:293-297.
31. Kitzmiller JL, Gavin LA, Gin GD, et al. Preconception care of diabetes: glycemic control prevents congenital anomalies. *JAMA* 1991;265:731-736.
32. Scheffler RM, Feuchtbaum LB, Phibbs CS. Prevention: The cost-effectiveness of the California Diabetes and Pregnancy Program (CDPP). *Am J Pub Health* 1992;82:168-175.
33. Rohr FJ, Doherty LB, Waisbren SE, et al. New England Maternal PKU Project: Prospective study of untreated and treated pregnancies and their outcomes. *J Pediatr* 1987;110:391-398.
34. Thompson JE. Maternal stress, anxiety, and social support during pregnancy: Possible directions for prenatal intervention. In: Merkatz IR, Thompson JE, Mullen PD, Goldberg RL, ed. New Perspectives on Prenatal Care. New York: Elsevier Science Publishing Co, Inc; 1990.
35. Jack BW, Culpepper L. Preconception care. *J Fam Pract* 1991;32: 306-314.
36. Taysi K. Preconceptional counseling. *Ob Gyn Clins North Am* 1988;15:167-178.
36a. Ferguson-Smith MA, Yates JRW. Maternal age-specific rates for chromosome aberrations and factors influencing them: Report of a collaborative European study on 52965 amniocentesis. *Prenatial Diag* 1984;4:5-7.
37. Sakala EP, Ho E. Preconception counseling: Improving pregnancy outcomes by starting before prenatal care. *Clin Consult Obstet Gynecol* 1994;6:244-251.

Ectopic Pregnancy: Part I

Gary Hals, MD, PhD
Antoinette Tolbert, MD

Women frequently present to the emergency department (ED) for complications relating to pregnancy. In particular, vaginal bleeding is one of the most common presenting complaints of women during the first 20 weeks (or first half) of pregnancy. In fact, nearly 40% of women experience vaginal bleeding during the course of their pregnancy, and up to 15% of clinically recognized pregnancies terminate in miscarriage.

Pregnant patients presenting with bleeding complications require special attention because hemorrhage may represent life- or fetus-threatening complications. In this regard, the incidence of ectopic pregnancy (EP) has increased steadily over the past three decades, with ectopic pregnancies now accounting for about 2% of total identified pregnancies in the United States.[1]

The serious consequences of EP are well-known to emergency practitioners. It is the leading cause of death in the first trimester, and accounts for 9-13% of all pregnancy-related deaths.[2,3] Although EP is the second leading cause of maternal mortality among all races, it is the leading cause in African-American women.[4] Approximately 90% of these deaths are the result of uncontrolled maternal hemorrhage.[5]

To make matters worse, EP can be difficult to diagnose. One study suggests that up to 50% of patients with EP are misdiagnosed on their first ED visit.[6] Another recent study of misdiagnosed ectopic pregnancies found the correct diagnosis was not made until an average of eight days after initial presentation.[7] Once an EP has progressed to rupture, the only treatment option is surgery—either laparoscopically or by full laparotomy.

An important challenge in these patients is timely identification of those women with complicated ectopic pregnancies from the larger group of individuals with self-limiting, spontaneous miscarriage. In this regard, however, it should be emphasized that even among patients with spontaneous miscarriage, a significant subset will advance to serious complications such as uterine infection or prolonged bleeding, both of which may require aggressive management. Finally, a few patients with vaginal bleeding early in their pregnancies will suffer from such unusual conditions, among them, trophoblastic disorders such as hydatidaform mole and choriocarcinoma.

Of special significance is that medical management of EP has dramatically altered treatment of these patients, but use of noninvasive management options requires early diagnosis to be successful. Accordingly, ED physicians are now under increasing pressure to diagnose EP very early in its course—and prior to complications—to take advantage of new medical advances in the management of this condition.

In the obstetrical literature, bleeding complications of pregnancy traditionally have been divided into those manifesting during the first half pregnancy, and those occurring in the second half of pregnancy. Generally speaking, vaginal bleeding in patients presenting before 20 weeks of gestation is associated with specific etiologies and treatments, whereas bleeding that occurs beyond 20 weeks is linked to an alternate differential diagnosis and management scheme.

From a clinical perspective, the work-up of patients in the first 20 weeks consists primarily of evaluation for EP or spontaneous miscarriage, whereas after 20 weeks, the most common serious causes of bleeding are placenta previa or abruption. Furthermore, it should

Table 1. Risk Factors for Ectopic Pregnancy

LESSER RISK
Previous pelvic or abdominal surgery
Cigarette smoking
Vaginal douching
Age of 1st intercourse < 18 years
GREATER RISK
Previous genital infections (e.g., PID)
Infertility (In vitro fertilization)
Multiple sexual partners
GREATEST RISK
Previous ectopic pregnancy
Previous tubal surgery or sterilization
Diethystilbestrol exposure in utero
Documented tubal pathology (scarring)
Use of intrauterine contraceptive device

Adapted from: Pisa MD, Carson SA. Ectopic pregnancy. In: Scott JR, et al, eds. *Danforth's Obstetrics and Gynecology.* 8th ed. Philadelphia: Lippincott Williams & Wilkins; 1999:155-172; and Mallett VT. Ectopic pregnancy. In: Pearlman MD, Tintinalli JE, eds. *Emergency Care of the Woman.* New York: McGraw Hill; 1998:21-28.

be stressed that the fetus is considered viable after about 24 weeks gestation, which means the ED physician actually has two patients in most patients who present with bleeding during the second half of pregnancy.

With these issues in clear focus, the authors review the ED evaluation and management of vaginal bleeding encountered during the first 20 weeks of gestation.

Current diagnostic and management strategies recommended in these patients are presented so they can be applied in the ED setting, treatment tables are provided to streamline access to clinical information, and new advances in therapy are highlighted.

Ectopic Pregnancy: Overview and Epidemiology

Any pregnancy in which the embryo implants outside the uterine cavity is defined as an EP. With the extremely rare exception of an abdominal pregnancy that successfully reaches term, the presence of an EP presents the ED physician with the following dilemma: 1) a fetus located in an ectopic location cannot reach maturity; and 2) its continued presence in that location represents a potentially life-threatening condition for the mother. Stated simply, hemorrhagic shock secondary to EP accounts for 6-7% of all maternal deaths.[8]

Unfortunately, the incidence of EP in the United States has increased steadily over time. In 1983, 70,000 ectopic pregnancies were reported in the United States, with an incidence of 4.5 per 1000 pregnancies.[9] Since then, the incidence has continued to increase, with 19.7 ectopics reported per 1000 pregnancies in 1992.[10] The two principal explanations for this rise include the following: 1) an increase in the prevalence of risk factors for EP (especially pelvic inflammatory disease [PID]); and 2) an increase in the sensitivity for detecting the condition in its early stages (i.e., transvaginal ultrasound [TVU] and more sensitive serum pregnancy testing).

Confirmation of EP also has important implications for future fertility of the patient. Specifically, the chances for successful subsequent pregnancies are lowered; one study suggests that only 33% of patients with a history of EP will have a subsequent pregnancy progress to live birth.[11] A history of an EP is also a strong risk factor for occurrence of future ectopic pregnancies.

Risk Factors. Risk factors for development of EP are listed in Table 1. As many as 50% of patients with an EP will give history of one of more of these risk factors.[12] A common theme among all risk factors is scarring of the fallopian tubes. Damage to the tubes often results from previous pelvic infection, especially from chlamydia and/or gonorrhea. In one study, the EP rate was 4% in women with salpingitis proven by laparoscopy, compared to 0.7% in women with healthy fallopian tubes.[13] In another study, 38% of tubes in women with EP had microscopic evidence of PID.[14]

The risk of repeated infection proportionally increases the likelihood of EP. For example, after two infections the risk for EP is about 35%, and after three or more prior infections the risk rose to about 75%.[13] It follows that pelvic surgery and previous sterilization procedures can lead to tubal scarring and, accordingly, increase in risk for EP. It should be stressed that a history of tubal ligation does not rule out the possibility of an EP. Reports of patients having EP after tubal ligation are not rare, and these patients are also at higher risk of rupture as EP is not always included in the differential of these patients.[15,16]

In the case of non-infectious risk factors, the link with an increased risk for EP is less clear. Cigarette smoking slightly increases the risk for ectopic implantation, but it is believed to be an association rather than a direct cause. It is theorized that impaired immune function found in smokers may predispose them to PID, alterations in tubal motility, or that it is associated with a lifestyle that is associated with acquisition of key risk factors.[17,18] Interestingly, use of vaginal douches is associated with increased an risk of EP, although the precise mechanism is not understood. Clearly, use of intrauterine devices (IUDs) for contraception increases risk of EP; interference with intrauterine implantation appears to be the mechanism. Finally, the use of diethylstilbestrol (DES) by a pregnant woman will produce fallopian tube deformities in her female offspring. Therefore, if a patient's mother used DES, she will be at higher risk for developing an EP.

Clinical Pathophysiology. Interestingly, the condition of EP appears to a uniquely human malady. No animal model is has been identified in which this condition has been documented. Consequently, much of what is known about the pathophysiology of EP is based on direct observation rather than animal testing.

After fertilization, the trophoblast (pre-embryo) implants in an abnormal site, usually in the fallopian tube. When the trophoblast implants, it invades blood vessels in the tubal wall, thereby accessing a blood supply necessary for further growth. Although the embryo is growing, it does so at a slower rate than normal, since the tissue in which it has implanted is not designed to support its growth. Consequently, human chorionic gonadotropin (beta-hCG) levels may not rise at the normally predicted rate, a feature that is useful for diagnosis. However, once the embryo attains a certain size, three outcomes are possible: 1) The embryo may be aborted into the abdominal cavity where it will be reabsorbed or continue as an abdominal pregnancy (very rare); 2) the embryo may be spontaneously absorbed in the fallopian tube; or 3) the tubal wall may rupture and result in significant blood loss that may be life threatening.

Although researchers have tried to identify specific risk factors for rupture in EP, these have been very difficult to determine. In one series of 236 ectopic pregnancies, about 26% of ectopic pregnancies terminated in in rupture.[21] Interestingly, rupture occurred in some patients with beta-hCG levels as low as 100 mIU/mL.[21] In another series of 693 ectopic pregnancies, the mean gestational age for rupture was 7.2 ± 2 weeks.[22] No differences were detected in beta-hCG levels among women who did and did not have rupture. However, the rate of rupture in patients with beta-hCG levels lower than 100 mIU/mL was 11%.[22] Moreover, rupture was more common in patients with their first EP than in those with repeat cases, perhaps indicating that previous experience with the disease shortened the time to diagnosis.

Figure 1. Frequency and Sites of Ectopic Pregnancy Implantation

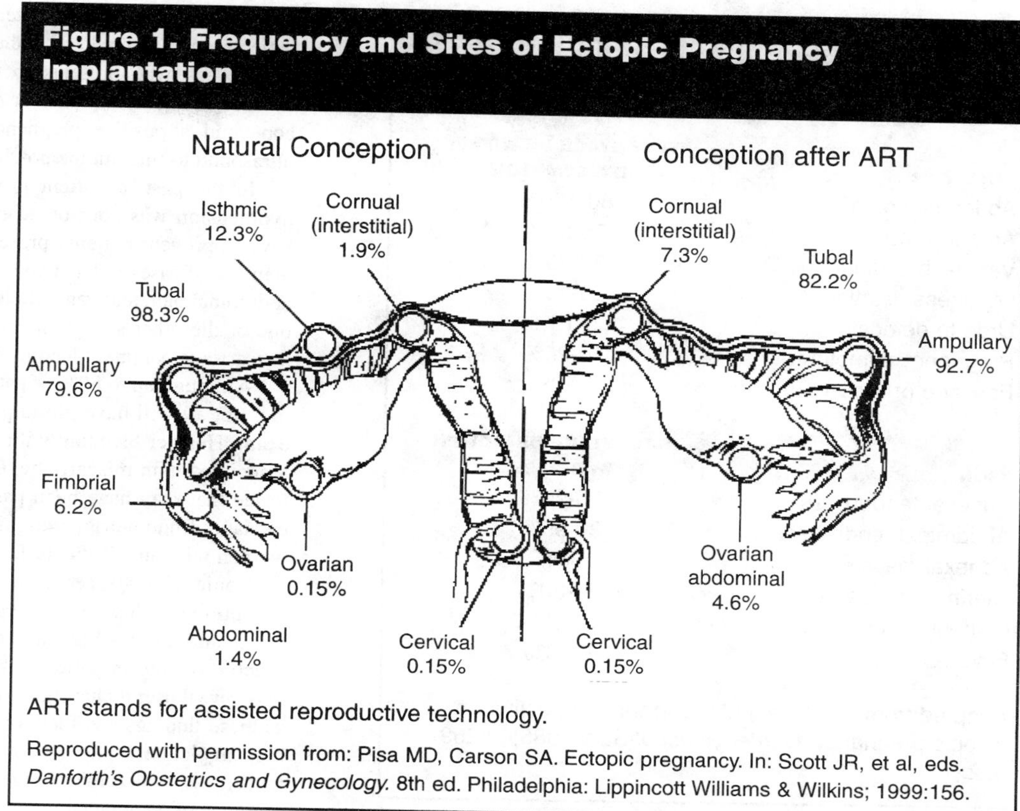

ART stands for assisted reproductive technology.

Reproduced with permission from: Pisa MD, Carson SA. Ectopic pregnancy. In: Scott JR, et al, eds. *Danforth's Obstetrics and Gynecology.* 8th ed. Philadelphia: Lippincott Williams & Wilkins; 1999:156.

It is suspected that abnormalities in the fallopian tube (i.e., scarring) slow migration of the trophoblast through the tube and increase risk for ectopic implantation. While this may explain the majority of ectopic pregnancies, this does not explain those that implant in the cervix. Figure 1 illustrates various sites in which ectopic pregnancies are known to occur and the frequency of their occurrence. Note that in the case of natural reproduction, 98% of ectopic implantations occur in the fallopian tubes. With assisted reproduction, tubal pregnancies still account for 82% of all ectopic pregnancies.

Of clinical significance is the observation that two specific implantation sites are associated with a significantly higher maternal mortality rate (i.e., cornual and interstitial ectopic gestations). Because the myometrium is more distensible than the fallopian tube, these locations permit the embryo to grow to a much larger size before rupture. As a result, rupture may occur as late as 10-14 weeks during gestation, which produces more bleeding from the relatively vascular uterus.[23] Although cornual locations account for only 4.7% of ectopic pregnancies, they carry a 2.2% overall maternal mortality rate.[24]

Associated with the highest relative maternal risk, abdominal pregnancy carries a mortality rate that is about 7.7 times greater than all other forms of EP combined.[25] As Figure 1 indicates, abdominal pregnancies are diagnosed in only 1.4% of all ectopics produced through natural reproduction. If the fetus survives such a pregnancy, malformations are present in up to 40% of infants.

An especially problematic and high risk variation of EP is the heterotopic pregnancy. In this case, a normal uterine pregnancy coexists with an EP. In 1948, this was a very rare condition and was reported in only 1 in 30,000 pregnancies.[26] However, the ED physician should be aware that the heterotopic pregnancy is becoming increasingly common. In this regard, data from the 1980s show a rate of 1 in 10,000 pregnancies, and the most recent estimates vary from 1 in 3889 to 1 in 6778 pregnancies.[27-29] However, in the case of assisted reproduction, the heterotopic pregnancy rate soars to a staggering 1-8 per 100 pregnancies.[27]

As with isolated EP, the most common implantation site for the ectopic fetus is the fallopian tube (94%).[27] As one would expect, the presence of heterotopic pregnancy confounds the work-up and diagnostic evaluation of these patients. First, beta-hCG levels are not helpful since the concomitant intrauterine pregnancy will produce normal levels of beta-hCG. In addition, the pelvic ultrasound detects only about 50% of tubal heterotopic pregnancies.[30] As might be expected, few patients are diagnosed before the EP becomes symptomatic or ruptures, and almost 50% are admitted for emergency surgery after rupture occurs as the presenting symptom.[30]

Although case reports exist of normal delivery of the intrauterine pregnancy after rupture of the ectopic in a few patients, the most frequent outcome is loss of both fetuses when rupture occurs.[31] Finally, it is also important to know that there have been a few case reports of bilateral ectopic pregnancies. The essential clinical point concerning heterotopic pregnancies is that during a work-up for an EP, if the patient is found to have an intrauterine pregnancy, there is still a risk for presence of a coexisting ectopic.

Clinical Presentation

Although they may not compel the patient to seek medical attention, the first symptoms a woman with EP experiences are those associated with early pregnancy. As expected, these include nausea with or without vomiting, breast tenderness, and amenorrhea. However, because the vascularly compromised embryo is producing lower amounts of beta-hCG than if it were normally implanted, symptoms of pregnancy may not be as pronounced in some patients; in fact, no more than 25% of patients report pregnancy-related symptoms before diagnosis of their EPs.[33]

Symptoms precipitated by structural changes or hormonal perturbations are more typical, and frequently provide the first clue to diagnosis. In particular, as the embryo grows, myriad symptoms can be produced by distension of the fallopian tube. *(Please see Table 2,*

Table 2. Presenting Signs and Symptoms of Ectopic Pregnancy

SYMPTOM	PERCENTAGE OF WOMEN WITH SYMPTOM
Abdominal pain	80-100%
Amenorrhea	75-95%
Vaginal bleeding	50-80%
Dizziness, fainting	20-35%
Urge to defecate	5-15%
Pregnancy symptoms	10-25%
Passage of tissue	5-10%

SIGN	PERCENTAGE OF WOMEN WITH SIGN
Adnexal tenderness	75-90%
Abdominal tenderness	80-95%
Adnexal mass	50%
Uterine enlargement	20-30%
Orthostatic changes	10-15%
Fever	5-10%

Adapted from Weckstein LN. Current perspective on ectopic pregnancy. *Obstet Gynecol Surv* 1985;40:259-272.

which summarizes presenting signs and symptoms of EP.) Note that nonspecific abdominal pain or pelvic pain has been reported in 80% of patients with EP at 4-6 weeks gestation.[33] Patients may also report having "normal" periods, light periods, or spotting. This bleeding can occur at the time of an expected period, further confusing the patient about her pregnancy status. Up to 20% of patients do not report missing a period, and 15% of patients rupture prior to "missing" their first period.[20,34] Bleeding can sometimes be linked to insufficient beta-hCG levels, which cannot support the integrity of the uterine lining at these lower hormone levels. Furthermore, patients with cornual ectopics can progress to a later stage of pregnancy and may present with more severe symptoms as late as 12-14 weeks of gestation.

As an EP progresses, the greatest danger to the patient is risk of fallopian tube rupture. The symptoms of rupture produce the "classical" presentation of an EP. These symptoms include sudden, severe unilateral abdominal pain, vaginal bleeding, and a history of amenorrhea. As one might expect, "classical" symptoms are uncommon and this particular history is neither sensitive nor specific.

Loss of blood into the peritoneal cavity usually will produce symptoms of peritoneal irritation, but the quantity and location of the blood will greatly influence the symptom complex. For example, smaller amounts of bleeding may only produce tenderness, rebound, and guarding in the pelvic area, and the patient's abdominal exam may not yield any significant findings. At least one study suggests that absence of pain and tenderness is not an absolutely reliable negative predictor for rupture, since about 4% of women with hemoperitoneum secondary to a ruptured ectopic are pain free.[8,20]

Another recent study of an inner city population found almost 10% of EP patients with rupture had no pain and 36% had no adnexal tenderness on pelvic exam.[6] Therefore, absence of pain and tenderness will not always alert the clincian to patients with a life-threatening rupture. However, with larger amounts of blood loss, the patient will exhibit signs of hypovolemia, including orthostasis, syncope, tachycardia, and hypotension. Syncope is common in these patients, and EP should be in the differential for any woman of reproductive age who presents to the ED with syncope. Even in the absence of significant pain or other symptoms, a woman with syncope and a positive pregnancy test in the ED should have an ultrasound to rule out the possibility of ectopic rupture.

In the past, a patient presenting with an adnexal mass and hypotension was considered typical of EP. As detection methods have improved, patients presenting in shock now make up fewer than 5% of cases.[20] The two most common complaints are of lower abdominal pain and vaginal bleeding, but the patient may have only one or the other symptom. In contrast to the case of spontaneous miscarriage, vaginal bleeding in EP is often mild.

Although up to 80% of patients will complain of vaginal bleeding, not all will have blood present in the vaginal vault on pelvic exam. Heavier bleeding with passage of clots is more likely to be associated with miscarriage. One should take care to examine any tissue that may have been passed and assumed to be from a miscarriage. Endometrial sloughing can also cause heavy bleeding in women with an EP, due to falling beta-hCG levels. If fetal parts or chorionic villi are seen, an ectopic is highly unlikely, with the exception of a heterotopic pregnancy.

In addition to abdominal tenderness, which frequently is a nonspecific finding in patients of child-bearing years, the pelvic exam may reveal useful clues that suggest the presence of an EP. As useful as these findings are, they too can be nonspecific and obfusacte the clinical picture. Up to 66% of women with EP have cervical motion tenderness, which may suggest the diagnosis of PID. Although the presence of an adnexal mass is an important sign of EP, this finding is present in only up to 60% of cases, even in those patients who are under general anesthesia.[37] Moreover, up to 20% of patients will have adnexal masses on the opposite side, presumably from a corpus luteum cyst on the uninvolved ovary.[38]

The uterus in a patient with suspected EP should be softened and normal size, or slightly enlarged but smaller than expected by gestational dates. This finding is reported in up to 70% of cases, although one study found that 26% of patients were thought to have a 6-8 week uterus.[20,39] Because the uterus will be enlarged consistent with the gestational period in the case of heterotopic pregnancy, finding a normal sized uterus will not rule out presence of an ectopic.

The authors of one review went so far as to suggest that a pelvic digital and speculum exam should not be performed in these patients.[36] In a series of 382 patients with EP, they found that these exams did not yield any information that changed management of these patients. While this may be the case in women who ultimately are found to have EP, the pelvic exam is still useful in diagnosing conditions that can be confused with EP. And it is especially helpful to identify patients who have an open os, as this subgroup is much more likely to have a spontaneous miscarriage than EP.

Diagnostic Strategy: Multi-Modal Synthesis

The ED evaluation of a patient with suspected EP primarily relies on the determination of serum hormone levels and the use of ultrasound imaging. Culdocentesis and diagnostic laparoscopy are still indicated in certain situations, and also will be discussed. However, these techniques are adjuncts to the primary modalities and are indicated in difficult-to-diagnose subgroups. It should be emphasized that Rh status must be verified in every patient with vaginal bleeding to avoid the failure to treat Rh-negative mothers with Rhogam.

Human Chorionic Gonadotropin. Beta-hCG is a glycoprotein hormone produced by both ectopic and normally implanted trophoblastic cells. Currently available monoclonal antibody assays can detect the presence of beta-hCG as soon as 2-3 days postimplantation. In a normal pregnancy, the level of this protein doubles about every two days up to a value of 10,000 mIU/mL. After this level, doubling no longer occurs, and serial beta-hCG measurements are not clinically helpful.

Specifically, the beta-hCG level should increase by 66% every 1.8-3 days for the first 6-7 weeks beginning 8-9 days after ovulation.[49] After 9-10 weeks gestation, the levels decline. This is an important clinical distinction. In the majority of ectopic pregnancies (or conditions associated with an abnormally developing fetus), beta-hCG levels will not consistently rise at the expected rate. The trophoblastic tissue does not obtain an adequate blood supply when implanted ectopically, and therefore, it does not grow at the expected rate. Abnormal beta-hCG levels are defined as those that fall, plateau, or fail to reach the predicted slope before 9-10 weeks gestation.

One should keep in mind that there are exceptions to this rule, that is, 10% of normal pregnancies can manifest abnormal doubling times, and similarly, up to 15% of ectopic pregnancies can have a normal doubling time.[44] Even accounting for such variations, most obstetrical texts take the position that documented failure of beta-hCG levels to double in 48 hours is diagnostic of a nonviable pregnancy and permits uterine curettage to empty the uterus.[19]

Typically, a urine pregnancy test is ordered to verify the presence of beta-hCG in the urine and, if positive, a serum quantitative level may then be obtained in order to verify if the level is above the discriminatory level for ultrasound. Alternatively, one may proceed directly to ultrasound, and if an intrauterine pregnancy is seen, a quantitative level may not be required. However, if no intrauterine pregnancy is identified, the quantitative level will be needed to interpret the ultrasound results. *(Please see section on Ultrasound.)* Even though normally rising levels can be seen early in ectopic pregnancies, nearly 90% of patients with documented EP will have low, plateauing, or declining levels on their initial visit.[50]

As outlined, the quantitative level of beta-hCG is useful in management decisions and for interpreting results of the ultrasound. With current ultrasound technology, most series state that early evidence of intrauterine pregnancy should be seen by transabdominal ultrasound with beta-hCG levels of 6500 mIU/mL, or at 1500 to 2000 mIU/mL using TVU.[9,23] Consequently, absence of a gestational sac in a patient whose beta-hCG indicates that a pregnancy should be detectable by these ultrasonographic modalities increases the likelihood for EP. Clinically, the beta-hCG level can be followed in stable patients in whom the level is too low to expect ultrasound visualization of a normal intrauterine pregnancy. The level should be rechecked in 48 hours; the importance of this repeat test should be communicated to the patient, and it should documented that this was stressed to the patient.

Although beta-hCG levels are a cornerstone in the diagnosis of EP, caution is advised when interpreting the results in specific patients, inasmuch as some patients with EP never attain beta-hCG levels greater than 1500 mIU/mL. Low levels, however, do not predict a benign course in every patient. A recent study of 1263 patients with suspected EP found that 60% of women with EP never had beta-hCG levels rise to greater than 1500 mIU/mL.[51] Another study found a four-fold increase in risk of EP in women with beta-hCG levels less than 1000 mIU/mL, with rupture occurring in 29% of these patients.[6]

In conjunction with these results, the ED physician should be aware that ectopic rupture requiring surgery is well documented in patients with low (< 100 mIU/mL) or even absent beta-hCG levels (rupture at < 10 mIU/mL), and that it is imprudent to believe that there is no danger of rupture at levels below 1500 mIU/mL.[21,52,53] In other words, if a patient has a beta-hCG below 1500 mIU/mL and is in shock without other obvious cause, ruptured EP has not been ruled out and the patient should be treated accordingly.

Progesterone. As early as the mid 1980s, use of a single, quantitative serum progesterone level has been reported in the literature to be of use in the diagnosis of EP.[40] Progesterone is produced by the corpus luteum in response to the presence of a pregnancy. In contrast to beta-hCG levels, progesterone levels change little in the first 8-10 weeks of gestation. An important point is that progesterone levels normally fall after 10 weeks gestation. When dates are unclear, a low level can be misleading if the patient has a normal pregnancy advanced beyond 10 weeks.[41] Otherwise, when a pregnancy fails during the first 8-10 weeks, progesterone levels fall.

Current data suggest that a single progesterone level higher than 25 ng/mL is consistent with a viable intrauterine pregnancy, and that this level was found to exclude EP with a 97.5% sensitivity.[19,20] Moreover, 25% of viable intrauterine pregnancies have levels below 25 ng/mL.[12] Many authors report that a level below 5 ng/mL is 100% diagnostic of a non-viable pregnancy.[19] However, a low level does not correlate with the location of the pregnancy.[42]

The American College of Obstetrics and Gynecology (ACOG) currently recommends that "no single progesterone value will definitively confirm the viability or nonviability of an intrauterine pregnancy or the presence of an EP."[43] Most authors still suggest that when beta-hCG levels fail to rise as predicted, a progesterone value below 5 ng/mL permits diagnostic evacuation of the uterus in cases in which an EP cannot be distinguished from a spontaneous miscarriage.[44,45] It is important to realize that variation can be present; the lowest progesterone level associated with an EP reported thus far is 5.1 ng/mL.[46] Furthermore, 2% of ectopic pregnancies have been reported to have levels higher than 25 ng/mL.[47]

Because of these inconsistencies and imperfect sensitivities for detection of EP, use of progesterone levels to diagnose EP is currently controversial. A recent meta-analysis of 26 studies found that serum progesterone levels are not sensitive enough to distinguish between EP and non-EP.[45] This study, however, did confirm that low serum levels are sufficiently accurate to distinguish between pregnancy failure and a viable pregnancy. Although current ACOG guidelines state that no single level can identify a failed pregnancy, current recommendations from the literature are as follows: A single progesterone level greater than 25 ng/mL is highly suggestive of a viable intrauterine pregnancy, but is not considered sufficient evidence by ACOG to discontinue a work-up for EP.[20]

One recent study found use of a progesterone level in patients with beta-hCG less than 1000 mIU/mL increased the accuracy of diagnosis.[48] When the progesterone level was less than 5 ng/mL in patients with a beta-hCG less than 1000 mIU/mL, abnormal pregnancy was diagnosed with a specificity of 94% and sensitivity of 100%.[48] When the level is less than 5 ng/mL, a patient may undergo uterine curettage if chorionic villi are found and EP is ruled out. However, if no villi are found, laparoscopy is indicated to exclude EP.[44] Levels between 5 ng/mL and 25 ng/mL are indeterminate. Although serum progesterone levels are inexpensive, they are not always available in every ED within a useful time frame. If and when the value of progesterone levels are clarified, they may add utility to the other modalities used for evaluation of EP.

Ultrasound. From a clinical, patient assessment perspective, TVU has become the single most valuable modality for the work-up of patients suspected of having an EP. It is the only technique available, other than laparoscopy, that permits the physician to identify the specific location of the pregnancy.

The beta-hCG level at which signs of pregnancy can first be seen ultrasonographically is called the discriminatory threshold. Although

Figures 2a and 2b. Ultrasound Images of a Normal Gestational Sac and Pseudogestational Sac

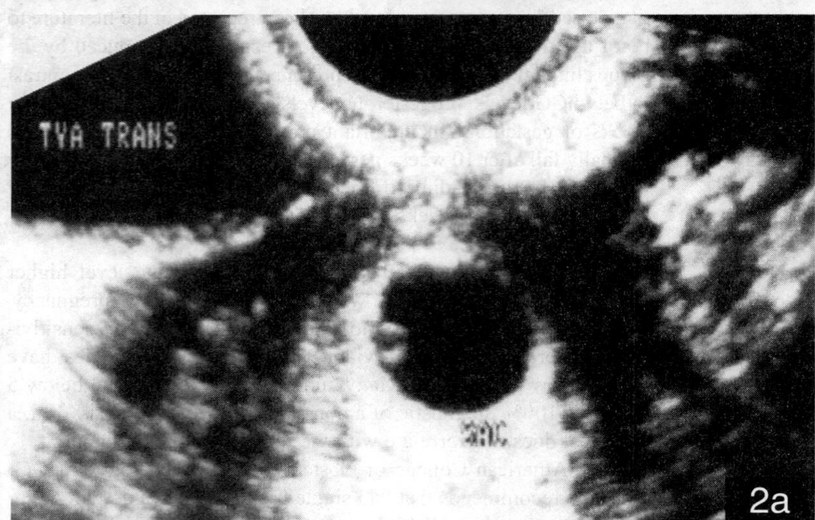

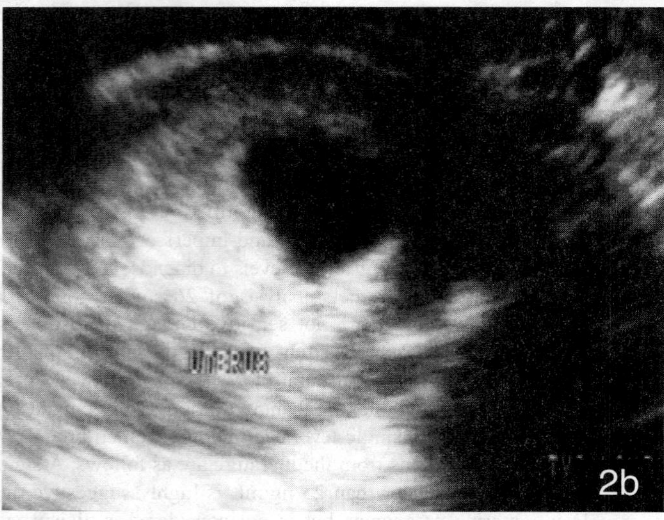

In Figure 2a, the yolk sac is seen an a small hyperechogenic circle on the left margin of the gestational sac. **In contrast, Figure 2b** shows a pseudogestational sac where the sac is irregular in shape, has no yolk sac, and represents fluid in the endometrial cavity. One can see how a early gestational sac without yolk sac development can be confused with a pseudogestational sac.

the precise beta-hCG value varies among institutions, a recent study reported that with TVU, a gestational sac was visible with beta-hCG levels of 1398 ± 155 mIU/mL.[54] Another study found that a level greater than 1500 mIU/mL was associated with 94% EP diagnosis rate on TVU.[55] However, in another study, only 33% of patients with EP were identified when the levels were less than 1000 mIU/mL.[56]

Consistent with these data is the fact that most authors report a discriminatory beta-hCG threshold of between 1000 mIU/mL and 2000 mIU/mL. These levels corresponded with beta-hCG determinations made only 34.8 ± 2.2 days from the patient's last menstrual period.[56] Accordingly, TVU has the capability, assuming sufficiently high and "discrminatory" beta-HCG levels are detected, to identify a pregnancy location as soon as one week after missing a menstrual period.

An important exception to the discriminatory level is the case of multiple gestations. With twins, the beta-hCG level can be greater than 2000 mIU/mL and there may be no ultrasonogrpahic findings of intrauterine pregnancy as would be expected in a single gestation.[57] Transabdominal ultrasound is less sensitive and is reported to identify a gestational sac in patients with beta-hCG values of 6500 mIU/mL. Clearly, transabdominal ultrasound is less accurate, and it should be no surprise that up to 50% of cases of EP have indeterminate transabdominal ultrasound results.[58] In addition, a level of 6000 mIU/mL level is attained in only 25% of ectopic pregnancies, further reducing the usefulness of transabdominal ultrasound.[58]

Departmental Ultrasonography. Increasingly, ED physicians are performing their own ultrasonographic studies in the ED, with recent studies confirming the safety and effectiveness of this practice. One investigator found that when properly trained, ED physicians performing an ultrasound had a 90% sensitivity and 88% specificity in their diagnosis of EP.[59] A second study found that readings by gynecologists agreed with 93% of ultrasonographic studies performed by ED physicians.[60] In addition, the waiting time for ED patients was reduced by an average of 70 minutes when the ED physician performed the ultrasound as compared to those seen in consultation by Ob/Gyn residents.[61] The number of patients requiring consultation was reduced 85%.[61]

Because an increasing percentage of ED physicians are learning to use ultrasonographic techniques for evaluation of EP as well as other conditions, the ultrasonographic findings in early pregnancy will be discussed in this review. The first sign of pregnancy with TVU is a gestational sac, which appears as a round hypoechogenic collection of fluid surrounded by a hyperechogenic rim representing the trophoblast. A gestational sac can be seen as early as 2-3 weeks after implantation in a normal pregnancy. *(Please see Figure 2a.)* It is important to note that a pseudogestational sac also can be seen, and may be confused with a normal pregnancy.

A pseudogestational sac is actually a fluid collection inside the endometrial cavity. *(Please see Figure 2b.)* This is the result of bleeding of the endometrium caused by the extrauterine pregnancy, and it will conform to and fill the endometrial cavity. A gestational sac is eccentrically placed within the uterine wall, as it is implanted in the endometrium. A normal gestational sac has (or will develop) a yolk sac within it (please see Figure 2a), whereas a pseudogestational sac will not. Because the yolk sac may not always be visible at the time of first ultrasound, care must be taken in interpreting these early findings of pregnancy on ultrasound.

Misinterpretation of the pseudogestational sac as a sign of intrauterine pregnancy is one of the most common causes of misdiagnosis of EP by TVU.[62] To complicate matters, in a study on misdiagnosis of EP, pseudogestational sacs were seen in 20% of patients initially misdiagnosed on their first ED visit.[63] The next finding after development of the yolk sac is visualization of the embryonic pole followed by actual cardiac motion. Caution is urged in interpretation of these ultrasound images because interstitial pregnancies can be very hard to distinguish from normal implantations. In addition, implantation of the embryo in the horn of a bicornuate uterus can be difficult to interpret with discriminating accuracy on ultrasound, as can cervical implantation. Furthermore, abnormally developing pregnancies or spontaneously reabsorbing pregnancies may also present problems in interpretation. In the case of interstitial, cervical, or bicornuate uterus, additional diagnostic information may be obtained with magnetic resonance imaging (MRI), provided that the patient is stable enough to undergo this type of testing.

Ultrasonograhic evidence of EP requires observation of a definite pregnancy outside the uterine boundary (most often in the fallopian tubes), or finding a complex adnexal mass that represents an EP. When a gestational sac is seen in the tube, one will be able to visualize a hypoechogenic fluid collection surrounded by a hyperechogenic ring. The ring consists of a decidual reaction of the fallopian tube, and is termed the "tubal ring" sign or "ring of fire." This finding is common and is seen in 60-70% of ectopic pregnancies.[64] In one series, the presence of a tubal ring correlated with a mean beta-hCG of 4300 mIU/mL.[65]

Inasmuch as the fallopian tube is an inhospitable location for pregnancy development, many tubal pregnancies do not develop normally. For example, in the largest series to date (380 surgically confirmed ectopic pregnancies) cardiac motion was only seen in 4% of patients with EP, and this finding correlated with an average beta-hCG level of 10,744 mIU/mL.[66] Bleeding into the gestational sac is common, however, and can lead to thrombus formation inside the sac. This may produce a confusing ultrasound picture, with visualization only of a complex adnexal mass. Presence of such a mass is, however, still suggestive of EP and should heighten suspicion of the diagnosis in the appropriate clinical setting. Additional caution is urged in the case of ovarian pregnancies because the EP can be very difficult to distinguish from a normal ovarian cyst. Serial ultrasonographic studies may be necessary to identify an enlarging gestational sac.

The ED physician must be familiar with the limitations of ultrasonographic technology. First, the usefulness and predictive value of the ultrasound generally depends as much on the skill level and experience of the operator. For ED physicians performing their own ultrasound, the primary utility of TVU is to identify an empty uterus (or a normal intrauterine pregnancy) in a patient whose beta-hCG level is above the discriminatory threshold. Indeed, a recent study found patients suspected of EP whose first ultrasound study showed an empty uterus were at highest risk compared to other patients whose ultrasound showed intrauterine fluid or debris.[67] In other words, if the level is between 1000 mIU/mL and 2000 mIU/mL and no signs of intrauterine pregnancy are seen, the patient is assumed to have an EP.

Therefore, definitive failure to identify an intrauterine pregnancy and absent ultrasound findings of an EP are sufficient to maintain a high suspicion of an ectopic when the beta-hCG is above the discriminatory threshold. If ultrasound findings indicate definitive evidence of an EP (an identified ectopic fetus), the diagnosis is certain. If suspicious but indeterminate findings (fluid in the cul-de-sac without intrauterine pregnancy [IUP], adnexal mass without IUP), then the diagnosis is strengthened but not certain.

Numerous studies have shown that use of TVU does reduce indeterminate ultrasound findings compared to transabdominal ultrasound, but it is not 100% accurate in every case. Even with a definitive adnexal mass or cul-de-sac fluid, the positive predictive value for EP is reported to be about 94%.[68] Other studies show that adnexal masses are seen in only 15-35% of patients with an EP.[69,70] Another recent study found that among patients with beta-hCG greater than 1500 mIU/mL, about 24% of those who had indeterminate TVU findings eventually had an EP confirmed.[71] A novel suggestion by one author was to subdivide indeterminate ultrasound findings into high-, medium-, and low-risk patients. High-risk patients were defined as those having an empty uterus, medium-risk patients had non-specific intrauterine fluid collections, and low-risk patients had intrauterine echogenic debris (blood clots).[72] One study of 132 patients with EP found there were no definitive ultrasound findings for the presence of rupture.[73]

Recently, there has been debate in the literature about the usefulness of the thickness of the endometrial stripe as seen on TVU. Some authors suggest that the thickness of the stripe in the uterine cavity alone can be predictive the location of the pregnancy. In a 1996 retrospective study of 47 women with ectopic pregnancies, one author found that the endometrial stripe was always less than 6 mm.[74] In comparison, 37 women who ultimately were proven to have normal intrauterine pregnancies had stripe thickness greater than 6 mm.[74] However, a more recent study of 676 patients (42 with EP) found that a thin endometrial stripe alone was not predictive of EP.[75] Another study found that there was predictive value of the endometrial stripe, but that it was limited to patients with beta-hCG levels less than 1000 mIU/mL.[76] Finally, one author found that gestation age and endometrial stripe thickness could not distinguish between patients with and without EP.[77] Larger studies will likely be needed to clarify this issue.

Other Diagnostic Tests: Uterine Curettage, Culdocentesis, and Laparoscopy. Three other diagnostic tests may be useful in the diagnosis of EP: 1) uterine curettage; 2) culdocentesis; and 3) laparoscopy. While these procedures are beyond the purview of the ED physician (with the exception of culdocentesis), it is important to understand when these tests are indicated and what their limitations are.

Uterine curettage involves physically scraping the uterine cavity in an effort to obtain evidence of a intrauterine pregnancy. This is performed only when serum hormones indicate a non-viable pregnancy (progesterone < 5 ng/mL or falling/plateauing beta-hCG). Typically, chorionic villi are identified (by floating tissue obtained in saline) when a failed intrauterine pregnancy is present. When villi are not seen, diagnosis of completed miscarriage can still be made if the beta-hCG level falls 15% or more 8-12 hours after the procedure.[44] When no villi are seen and beta-hCG levels do not fall, EP is highly suspected. Ectopic pregnancy is diagnosed in this situation if the beta-hCG plateaus or continues to rise after the procedure.[44] Curettage is most useful in patients with an indeterminate ultrasound. In one study of patients with indeterminate scans, the incidence of EP was 40% when no villi were seen on curettage.[78]

Culdocentesis was used much more often before widespread availability of TVU. It is still indicated in situations where ultrasound is unavailable and EP is highly suspected, or in an unstable patient where time is critical. It can be accurate in the case of ruptured ectopic. Up to 90% of patients with a ruptured ectopic will have a positive culdocentesis result.[34] As one might expect, the results are not as good with unruptured ectopics. Only 65% of these patients will have a positive culdocentesis result.[79] In culdocentesis, a tenaculum is used to elevate the cervix anteriorly and a 20-gauge spinal needle is inserted below the cervix to obtain fluid from the cul-de-sac.

Caution is urged in interpreting indeterminate results, as they can be difficult to decipher. A positive result is determined when nonclotted blood (> 0.5 cc) is obtained.[79] Indeterminate results are when a dry tap, clotting blood (> 0.5 cc), or serous fluid (> 5 cc) is obtained. Presumably, clotting blood is from pelvic veins, as defibrinators in the peritoneum should prevent clotting of free peritoneal blood. One needs to remember, though, that rapid bleeding into the peritoneum can produce clotting blood on a culdocentesis, but that the patient's condition should clue one to the severity of the blood loss. Bloody culdocentesis fluid can also be obtained from a hemorrhagic corpus luteum cyst, but the fluid normally has a hematocrit of less than 12%.[80]

Dry taps are seen in 10-20% of culdocentesis procedures, and can be obtained in patients who actually have peritoneal blood from a ruptured ectopic.[34] Thus, a dry tap should not be confused with a negative result. Aspiration of only small amounts of serous fluid (0.3-5.0 cc) is a negative culdocentesis result. These can be seen in the case of a non-hemorrhagic corpus luteum cyst rupture, but are found in up to 5% of women with EP as well.[34] As culdocentesis is not a technically difficult procedure, the key is to know how to interpret the results correctly if one is forced to rely on this in patient work-up for EP.

Finally, laparoscopy can be both diagnostic and therapeutic for EP. Use of laparoscopy is indicated in patients with peritoneal signs and equivocal results from previous testing with ultrasound, culdocentesis, or uterine curettage. It can also used alone for treatment when the diagnosis has been made by other means, although many patients are now managed medically.

References

1. Ectopic pregnancy: United States: 1990-1992. *MMWR Morb Mortal Wkly Rep* 1995;44:46-48.
2. Goldner TE, Lawson HW, Xia Z, et al. Surveillance of ectopic pregnancy—United States, 1970-1989. *MMWR Morb Mortal Wkly Rep* 1993;42:73-85.
3. NCHS. Advanced report of final mortality statistics, 1992. Hyattsville, MD: US Department of Health and Human Services, Public Health Services, CDC; 1994. (Monthly vital statistics report; vol 43, no. 6, Suppl).
4. Bernstein J. Ectopic pregnancy: A nursing approach to excess risk among minority women. *J Obstet Gynecol Neonatal Nurs* 1995;24:803-810.
5. Grimes DA. The morbidity and mortality of pregnancy: Still risky business. *Am J Obstet Gynecol* 1995;170:1489-1494.
6. Kaplan BC, Dart RG, Moskos M, et al. Ectopic pregnancy: Prospective study with improved diagnostic accuracy. *Ann Emerg Med* 1996;28:10-17.
7. Robson SJ, O'Shea RT. Undiagnosed ectopic pregnancy: A retrospective analysis of 31 "missed" ectopic pregnancies at a teaching hospital. *Aust N Z Obstet Gynaecol* 1996;36:182-185.
8. Jehle D, Krause R, Braen GR. Ectopic Pregnancy. *Emerg Med Clin North Am* 1994;12:55-71.
9. Ory SJ. New options for diagnosis and treatment of ectopic pregnancy. *JAMA* 1992;267:534-537.
10. Ectopic Pregnancy—United States, 1990-1992. *JAMA* 1995; 273:533.
11. Fylstra DL. Tubal pregnancy: A review of current diagnosis and treatment. *Obstet Gynecol Surv* 1998;53:320-328.
12. Stovall TG, Kellerman AL, Ling FW, et al. Emergency department diagnosis of ectopic pregnancy. *Ann Emerg Med* 1990;19:1098-1102.
13. Westrom L. Effect of acute pelvic inflammatory disease on fertility. *Am J Obstet Gynecol* 1975;121:707-713.
14. Bone NL, Greene RR. Histological study of uterine tube with tubal pregnancy: A search for evidence of previous injection. *Am J Obstet Gynecol* 1961;82:1166.
15. Peterson HB, Xia Z, Hughes JM, et al. The risk of ectopic pregnancy after tubal sterilization. U.S. Collaborative Review of Sterilization Working Group. *N Engl J Med* 1997;336: 762-767.
16. Hendrix NW, Chauhan SP, Maier RC. Ectopic pregnancy in sterilized and nonsterilized women. A comparison. *J Reprod Med* 1998;43:515-520.
17. Chow W, Daling JR, Cates W, et al. Epidemilogy of ectopic pregnancy. *Epdemiol Rev* 1987;9:70-94.
18. Ankum WM, Mol BWJ, Van der Veen F, et al. Risk factors for ectopic pregnancy: A meta-analysis. *JAMA* 1996;65: 1093-1099.
19. Pisa MD, Carson SA. Ectopic pregnancy. In: Scott JR, et al, eds. *Danforth's Obstetrics and Gynecology.* 8th ed. Philadelphia: Lippincott Williams & Wilkins; 1999:155-172.
20. Mallett VT. Ectopic pregnancy. In: Pearlman MD, Tintinalli JE, eds. *Emergency Care of the Woman*. New York: McGraw Hill; 1998:21-28.
21. Falcone T, Mascha EJ, Goldberg JM, et al. A study of risk factors for ruptured tubal ectopic pregnancy. *J Women's Health* 1998;7:459-463.
22. Saxon D, Falcone T, Mascha EJ, et al. A study of ruptured tubal ectopic pregnancy. *Obstet Gynecol* 1997;90:46-49.
23. Dorfman SF, Grimes DA, Cates W Jr, et al. Ectopic pregnancy mortality, United States, 1979-1980: Clinical aspects. *Obstet Gynecol* 1984;64:386-390.
24. Felmus LB, Pedowitz P. Interstitial pregnancy: A survey of 45 cases. *Am J Obstet Gynecol* 1953;66:1271-1279.
25. Attapattu JAF, Menon S. Abdominal pregnancy. *Int J Gynaecol Obstet* 1993;43:51-55.
26. DeVoe R, Pratt J. Simultaneous intrauterine and extrauterine pregnancy. *Am J Obstet Gynecol* 1948;56:1119-1126.
27. Reece EA, Petrie RH, Sirmans MF, et al. Combined intrauterine and extrauterine gestations: A review. *Am J Obstet Gynecol* 1983;146:323-330.
28. Bello GV, Schonolz D, Mashirpur J, et al. Combined pregnancy: The Mount Sinai experience. *Obstet Gynecol Surv* 1986;41:603-613.
29. Hann LE, Bachmann DM, McArdle C. Coexistent intrauterine and ectopic pregnancy: A reevaluation. *Radiology* 1984;152: 151-154.
30. Rojansky N, Schenker JG. Heterotopic pregnancy and assisted reproduction: An update. *J Assist Reprod Genet* 1996;13: 594-601.
31. Chandra PC, Schiavello HJ, Briggs SL, et al. Heterotopic pregnancy with term delivery after rupture of a first-trimester tubal pregnancy. A case report. *J Reprod Med* 1999;44: 556-558.
32. DeGraaf FL, Demetroulis C. Bilateral tubal ectopic pregnancy: Diagnostic pitfalls. *Br J Clin Pract* 1997;51:56-58.
33. Hockberger RS. Ectopic pregnancy. *Emerg Med Clin North Am* 1987;5:481-493.
34. Abbott JT. Acute complications related to pregnancy. In: Rosen P, et al, eds. *Emergency Medicine: Concepts and Clinical Practice*. 4th edition. Mosby-Year Book, Inc; 1998: 2342-2364.
35. Weckstein LN. Current perspective on ectopic pregnancy.

Obstet Gynecol Surv 1985;40:259-272.
36. Mol BW, Hajenius PJ, Engelsbel S, et al. Should patients who are suspected of having an ectopic pregnancy undergo physical examination? *Fertil Steril* 1999;71:155-157.
37. Pagano R. Ectopic pregnancy: A seven year survey. *Med J Aust* 1981;2:586-588.
38. Weckstein LN, Boucher AR, Tucher H, et al. Accurate diagnosis of early ectopic pregnancy. *Obstet Gynecol* 1985;65: 393-397.
39. Brenner PF, Ray S, Mishell DR. Ectopic pregnancy: A study of 300 consecutive surgically treated cases. *JAMA* 1980;243: 673-676.
40. Matthews CP, Coulson PB, Wild RA. Serum progesterone levels as an aid in the diagnosis of ectopic pregnancy. *Obstet Gynecol* 1986;68:390-394.
41. Stern JJ, Voss, F, Coulam CB. Early diagnosis of ectopic pregnancy using receiver-operator characteristic curves of serum progesterone concentrations. *Hum Reprod* 1993;8: 775-779.
42. Valley VT, Mateer JR, Aiman EJ, et al. Serum progesterone and endovaginal sonography by emergency physicians in evaluation of ectopic pregnancy. *Acad Emerg Med* 1998;5: 309-313.
43. ACOG practice bulletin. Medical management of tubal pregnancy. *Int J Gynecol Obstet* 1999;65:97-103.
44. Stovall TG, Ling FW, Carson SA, et al. Serum progesterone and uterine curettage in differential diagnosis of ectopic pregnancy. *Fertil Steril* 1992;57:456-458.
45. Mol BW, Limjer JG, Ankum WM, et al. The accuracy of a single serum progesterone measurement in the diagnosis of ectopic pregnancy: A meta analysis. *Human Reprod* 1998;13: 3220-3227.
46. Stovall TG, Ling FW, Cope BJ, et al. Preventing ruptured ectopic pregnancy with a single serum progesterone. *Am J Obstet Gynecol* 1989;160:1425-1428.
47. McCord ML, Muram D, Buster JE, et al. Single serum progesterone as a screen for ectopic pregnancy: Exchanging specificity and sensitivity to obtain optimal test performance. *Fertil Steril* 1996;66:513-516.
48. Dart R, Dart L, Segal M, et al. The ability of a single serum progesterone value to identify abnormal pregnancies in patients with beta-human chorionic gonadotropin values less than 1,000 mIU/mL. *Acad Emerg Med* 1998;5:304-309.
49. Cunningham FG, MacDonald PC, Gant NT, et al. *Williams Obstetrics,* 19th ed. Norwalk, CN: Appleton & Lange; 1993.
50. Romero R, Kadar N, Copel JA, et al. The value of serial human chorionic gonadotropin testing as a diagnostic tool in ectopic pregnancy. *Am J Obstet Gynecol* 1986;155:392-394.
51. Barnhart K, Mennuti MT, Benjamin I, et al. Prompt diagnosis of ectopic pregnancy in an emergency department setting. *Obstet Gynecol* 1994;84:1010-1015.
52. Hochner-Celnikier D, Ron M, Goshen R, et al. Ruptured ectopic pregnancy following disappearance of serum beta subunit of hCG. *Obstet Gynecol* 1992;79:826-827.
53. Taylor RN, Padula C, Goldsmith PC. Pitfall in the diagnosis of ectopic pregnancy: Immunocytochemical evaluation in a patient with false-negative serum beta-hCG levels. *Obstet Gynecol* 1988;71:1035-1038.
54. Leach RE, Ory SJ. Modern management of ectopic pregnancy. *J Reprod Med* 1989;34:324-338.
55. Barnhart KT, Simhan H, Kamelle SA. Diagnostic accuracy of ultrasound above and below the beta-hCG discriminatory zone. *Obstet Gynecol* 1999;94:583-587.
56. Dart RG, Kaplan B, Cox C. Transvaginal ultrasound in patients with low beta-human chorionic gonadotropin values: How often is the study diagnostic? *Ann Emerg Med* 1997;30: 135-140.
57. Kadar N, Bohrer M, Kemmann E, et al. The discriminatory human chorionic gonadotropin zone for endovaginal sonography: A prospective, randomized study. *Fertil Steril* 1994;61:1016-1020.
58. Romero R, Kadar N, Castro D, et al. The value of adnexal sonographic findings in the diagnosis of ectopic pregnancy. *Am J Obstet Gynecol* 1988;158:52-55.
59. Durham B, Lane B, Burbridge, L, et al. Pelvic ultrasound performed by emergency physicians for the detection of ectopic pregnancy in complicated first-trimester pregnancies. *Ann Emerg Med* 1997;29:338-347.
60. Mateer JR, Aiman EJ, Brown MH, et al. Ultrasonographic examination by emergency physicians of patients at risk for ectopic pregnancy. *Acad Emerg Med* 1995;2:867-873.
61. Burgher SW, Tandy TK, Dawdy MR. Transvaginal ultrasonography by emergency physicians decreases patient time in the emergency department. *Acad Emerg Med* 1998;5: 802-807.
62. Rumack C, Wilson S, Charboneau JW. *Diagnostic Ultrasound.* St Louis: Mosby; 1991.
63. Abbott J, Emmans LS, Lowenstein SR. Ectopic pregnancy: Ten common pitfalls in diagnosis. *Am J Emerg Med* 1990;8: 515-522.
64. Shalev E, Yarom I, Bustan M, et al. Transvaginal sonography as the ultimate diagnostic tool for the management of ectopic pregnancy: Experience with 840 cases. *Fertil Steril* 1998;69: 62-65.
65. Atri M, Bret PM, Tulandi T, et al. Ectopic pregnancy: Evolution after treatment with transvaginal methotrexate. *Radiology* 1990;176:359-364.
66. Brown DL, Doubilet PM. Transvaginal ultrasound for diagnosing ectopic pregnancy: Positive criteria and performance characteristics. *J Ultrasound Med* 1994;13: 259-266.
67. Dart R, Dart L, Mitchell P. Normal intrauterine pregnancy is unlikely in patients who have echogenic material identified within the endometrial cavity at transvaginal ultrasound. *Acad Emerg Med* 1999;6:116-120.
68. Cattanach S. Ectopic pregnancy: We can still miss the diagnosis. *Austral Fam Physician* 1994;23:190-196.
69. Russell SA, Filly RA, Damato N. Sonographic diagnosis of ectopic pregnancy with endovaginal probes: What really has changed? *J Ultrasound Med* 1993;3:145-151.
70. Frates MC, Laing FC. Sonographic evaluation of ectopic pregnancy: An update. *AJR* 1995;165:251-259.
71. Braffman BH, Coleman BG, Ramchandani P, et al. Emergency department screening for ectopic pregnancy in an emergency department setting. *Radiology* 1994;190:797-802.
72. Dart R, Howard K. Subclassification of indeterminate pelvic

ultrasonograms: Stratifying the risk of ectopic pregnancy. *Acad Emerg Med* 1998;5:313-319.

73. Frates MC, Brown DL, Doubilet PM, et al. Tubal rupture in patients with ectopic pregnancy: Diagnosis with transvaginal US. *Radiology* 1994;191:769-772.
74. Spandorfer SD, Barnhart KT. Endometrial stripe thickness as a predictor of ectopic pregnancy. *Fertil Steril* 1996;66:474-477.
75. Mehta TS, Levine D, McArdle CR. Lack of sensitivity of endometrial thickness in predicting the presence of an ectopic pregnancy. *J Ultrasound Med* 1999;18:117-122.
76. Dart R, Dart L, Mitchell P, et al. The predictive value of endometrial stripe thickness in patients with suspected ectopic pregnancy who have an empty uterus at ultrasonography. *Acad Emerg Med* 1999;6:602-608.
77. Mol BW, Hajenius PJ, Engelsbel S, et al. Are gestational age and endometrial thickness alternatives for serum human chorionic gonadotropin as criteria for the diagnosis of ectopic pregnancy? *Fertil Steril* 1999;72:643-645.
78. Dart R, Dart L, Mitchell P, et al. The utility of dilatation and evacuation procedure in patients with symptoms suggestive of ectopic pregnancy and indeterminate transvaginal ultrasonography. *Acad Emerg Med* 1999;6:1024-1029.
79. Elliot M, Riccio J, Abbott J. Serous culdocentesis in ectopic pregnancy: A report of two cases caused by coexistent corpus luteum cysts. *Ann Emerg Med* 1990;19:407-410.
80. Hallatt JG, Steele CH, Snyder M. Ruptured corpus luteum with hemoperitoneum: A study of 173 surgical cases. *Am J Obstet Gynecol* 1984;149:5-9.

Ectopic Pregnancy: Part II

Gary Hals, MD, PhD
Antoinette Tolbert, MD

Because both noninvasive pharmacotherapeutic options, as well as myriad surgical approaches, are available for managing patients with ectopic pregnancy (EP), emergency physicians are faced with the challenge of risk-stratifying patients into subgroups that are eligible for a specific therapeutic program. More than anything, this means confirming the diagnosis of EP as early as possible in the natural history of the condition, thereby permitting consideration of a wider range of management approaches.

These clinical obstacles to making a precise diagnosis are well known, and consequently, a systemic approach to patient evaluation is recommended. During the first 20 weeks of gestation, the differential diagnosis of EP includes spontaneous miscarriage and other trophoblastic disorders. Fortunately, with the availability of serum hormone analysis, transvaginal ultrasonography, and more invasive strategies, the diagnosis of EP can be confirmed early in pregnancy, thereby permitting a greater percentage of patients to be treated with noninvasive, medical approaches such as methotrexate.

Spontaneous miscarriage also requires a systematic approach to diagnosis to identify patients who can be treated expectantly vs. those who require dilatation and curettage.

Trophoblastic disorders, although not common, also may confuse the diagnosis, and must be excluded in the majority of cases.

This chapter presents an algorithmic approach to the differential diagnosis of vaginal bleeding during the first 20 weeks of pregnancy. Finally, risk-stratification strategies are discussed in detail that permit the physician to select the least invasive treatment strategy for individual patients with EP and other disorders during early pregnancy.

Differential Diagnosis of Ectopic Pregnancy: Improving Accuracy of Detection

The incidence of EP increased nearly five-fold between 1980 and 1992, a period during which the diagnosis of this condition also became more accurate.[1] In the 1970s, for example, establishing an accurate diagnosis of pregnancy in these patients was a significant problem; in fact, the false-negative rate for pregnancy tests in patients with EP was reported to be as high as 50%.[2] Fortunately, the diagnostic challenge in patients with EP has been minimized by the availability of increasing sensitive laboratory tests.

Presently, the pregnancy tests most commonly used in the emergency department (ED) are based on the enzyme-linked immunosorbent assay (ELISA), and are highly sensitive and specific. Beta-hCG urine concentrations of approximately 20 mIU/mL and 10 mIU/mL in serum can be detected in the most sensitive ELISA tests. False negatives are reported to be as low as 1% for urine testing and 0.5% for serum testing. False negatives may occur in the presence of renal failure and dilute urine and very early in pregnancy.[3,4] Current transvaginal ultrasonographic technology can identify intrauterine pregnancies at around 35 days gestation or beginning during the first week after a missed period.

Table 1. Differential Diagnosis of Ectopic Pregnancy

• Normal intrauterine pregnancy	Threatened or incomplete miscarriage
• Ovarian cysts (rupture, unruptured)	Appendicitis
• Acute salpingitis	Tubo-ovarian abscess
• Gastroenteritis	Torsion of ovary or fibroid
• Diverticulitis	Renal calculi
• Pyelonephritis	Endometriosis

Adapted from: Mallett VT. Ectopic pregnancy. In: Pearlman MD, Tintinalli JE, eds. *Emergency Care of the Woman*. New York: McGraw Hill; 1998:21-28; and Lewis FR, Holcroft JW, Boey J, et al. Appendicitis: A critical review of diagnosis and treatment in 1,000 cases. *Arch Surg* 1975;110:677-684.

Preventing Misdiagnosis. Despite quantifiable improvements in diagnostic technology, the misdiagnosis of EP is not an infrequent occurrence. In one older review of 86 fatal ectopic pregnancies, almost 50% of these patients had seen a physician and were given an alternate diagnosis prior to their death.[5]

A more recent review published in 1990 still reported that up to 40% of patients later confirmed as having an EP were misdiagnosed on their first ED visit.[6] The authors examined 28 patients with misdiagnosis and compared them to 37 patients in whom the diagnosis was successfully made during their first visit to the ED. They found that misdiagnosed patients had fewer complaints of severe pain and had less tenderness on exam than the control group. A significant percentage of misdiagnosed patients had no complaints of pain whatsoever on their first visits. About 56% of ultrasonographic exams in the missed patients were considered nondiagnostic, but these were transabdominal studies. Nine of the 28 patients had culdocentesis on the first visit, and all of the taps were nondiagnostic. The beta-hCG levels in patients with missed ED varied widely, ranging from 100 mIU/mL to greater than 10,000 mIU/mL.

The time required to make an accurate diagnosis of EP in patients who were initially misdiagnosed varied from 24 hours to 15 days. Several conclusions and recommendations aimed at preventing misdiagnosis of EP were presented. First, the most common misdiagnosis was spontaneous miscarriage. Many of these patients presented with crampy abdominal pain during the initial presentation, and in some cases, the pain decreased with time. In several cases, the passage of tissue was interpreted as a sign of miscarriage, although this diagnosis was not subsequently confirmed by examination of the tissue for villi. (Note: In EP, endometrial tissue may slough off and give the appearance of products of conception but no chorionic villi will be found under close examination.)

Of special concern was the finding that almost 32% of patients in whom the diagnosis was originally missed had signs of hypovolemia during their first visit, a finding that was attributed to causes other than blood loss. Some patients had orthostatic changes of greater than 30 mmHg in blood pressure, and others had a 14% decrease in their hematocrit. These changes were inappropriately explained as being a result of dehydration or hemodilution from saline administration, or they were simply overlooked. Finally, all of the women in whom EP was missed had a history of at least one risk factor for EP.

Differential Diagnosis. The differential diagnosis of EP is summarized in Table 1. Among the list of diseases that may be confused with EP, threatened or incomplete miscarriage is the most common misdiagnosis. These patients can present in a very similar fashion; they may have have falling beta-hCG levels, and occasionally, ultrasonographic findings may be similar. From a diagnostic perspective, an os that is open to a fingertip is indicative of a spontaneous miscarriage, and can be a useful physical finding. When the clinician is in doubt of the diagnosis, the patient should undergo uterine curettage to examine for chorionic villi. If none are seen, the patient is at very high risk for EP and should proceed to diagnostic laparoscopy. Finally, heterotopic pregnancy is much more common in patients using assisted reproduction techniques. Consequently, identification of an intrauterine pregnancy or confirmation of miscarriage may not be enough to rule out ectopic in this subgroup of patients.

Ovarian cysts are common in early pregnancy, and they also have a propensity to rupture. When a ruptured cyst produces hemoperitoneum, this condition may be difficult to distinguish from the rupture of an EP.[7] Although a culdocentesis can be helpful in some cases, clinical evidence of hemoperitoneum in these patients will usually require surgical intervention to confirm the correct diagnosis and establish an appropriate treatment plan.

Patients with pelvic inflammatory disease (PID) also may be confused with women suspected of having an EP. Although PID is rare in pregnancy because presence of the cervical mucus plug should prevent ascending infection, in rare cases PID may still be seen in the earlier stages. One possible explanation is that the infection was present prior to the pregnancy. In addition, patients with EP can present with fever, further confusing the picture. However, presence of a positive pregnancy test obligates the physician to rule out EP first, even if the working diagnosis is PID or tubo-ovarian abscess. A transvaginal ultrasound study can sometimes confirm a diagnosis, but in some patients only a laparoscopic examination will be confirmatory. *(Please see Figures 1-3.)*

Appendicitis is easily misdiagnosed in women of childbearing age, with reported negative laparotomy rates approaching 50% in pregnant patients.[8] Pregnant women can be even more confusing. Right lower quadrant pain/tenderness, elevated white blood cell counts, and fever are overlapping findings in both diseases. In some cases, a laparoscopic study is required for final diagnosis. Complications of endometriosis, ovarian torsion, or torsion of a uterine fibroid can also be confused with EP, but in these patients ultrasound studies can often identify the problem. In summary, when faced with a pregnant patient, laparoscopy may be required to differentiate between EP and other diagnoses with similar presentations.

Diagnostic Algorithms. A number of diagnostic algorithms have been proposed to assist in rapid and efficient identification of patients with EP. The objective of these algorithms is to reduce the rate of misdiagnosis. Many diagnostic algorithms for stable patients have been developed, an example of which is presented in Figure 4.[9-11]

Up to 20% of patients with EP will have signs of hemodynamic instability or significant peritonitis; clearly, these patients should be resuscitated with ABCs in mind and they should have urgent surgical consultation. For the remaining 80% of patients, algorithms can be useful. Proposed algorithms of EP detection vary, but in general, they rely on a combination of serum markers and transvaginal ultrasound.

Without exception, a single (or serial) beta-hCGs or progesterone level is required as part of the systematic evaluation of all patients suspected of having EP. These levels are interpreted in conjunction with transvaginal ultrasonographic studies. If there is ultrasonographic evidence of EP, the patient should receive either medical or surgical treatment for EP. However, if the beta-hCG is above the discriminatory threshold (around 1500 mIU/mL) and the ultrasound is indeterminate or shows no intrauterine pregnancy, the patient is still considered to be high risk for an EP, and appropriate consultation is required.

One large series found a 25% incidence of EP in patients with beta-hCG greater than 1500 mIU/mL and nondiagnostic ultrasound.[12] If the beta-hCG is less than the discriminatory threshold, the patient may still have EP, but the diagnosis will typically be unclear until serial beta-hCG levels can be taken. It may be possible to follow these patients in the outpatient setting, with the consultant monitoring the serial enzyme levels and repeating ultrasound studies to confirm the diagnosis. All discharged patients should be given appropriate instructions for EP and threatened miscarriage.

Outpatient follow-up consists of repeat beta-hCG in 48 hours and ultrasound if the level rises above the discriminatory threshold. Ultrasound has been shown in a large series to be diagnostic in 80% of patients with beta-hCG above 1500 mIU/mL.[13] Although using serial beta-hCG levels has been shown to be 97% sensitive and 95% specific, a potential disadvantage of this approach is delay of diagnosis.[14]

Figure 1. Ultrasound Image of Ectopic Pregnancy

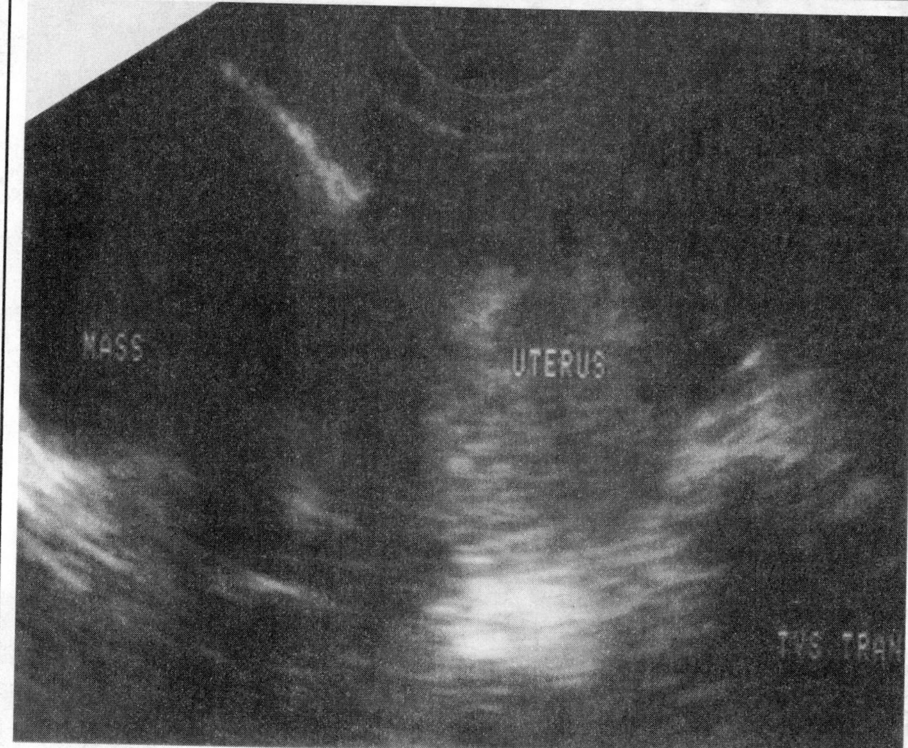

In Figure 1, a large hyperechogenic mass is noted adjacent to the uterus, representing an ectopic pregnancy.

Algorithms that rely on a single progesterone level have been shown to be 100% accurate in one series, and have the advantage of not requiring serial levels.[10] If the ultrasound is not diagnostic, and the progesterone is higher than 25 ng/mL, the pregnancy is likely to be normal. Uterine curettage for diagnosis is performed in cases where the progesterone level is less than 5 ng/mL, or when serial beta-hCG levels plateau or fall. It should be stressed that even when beta-hCG levels never rise above the discriminatory threshold, the patient is still at considerable risk of EP. Uterine curettage is again recommended to distinguish between failed intrauterine pregnancy and EP.

Several precautions are advised when managing patients in the outpatient setting. First, the ED physician should note that the rupture has been reported in individuals with very low beta-hCG levels—in some cases in patients with a level as low as less than 10 mIU/mL.[15] The patient should not be discharged to stay at home alone. If sudden hypotension develops, she may not be able to call for help. Finally, any patient who is being evaluated for possible EP and is to be discharged should not be sent out without a phone call to the OB/GYN consultant who will be performing the follow-up visit.

Ensuring appropriate and timely follow-up for these patients is essential. Making their obstetrician aware of the situation gives them the chance to call the patient and remind them to follow-up if the patient does not choose to do so on her own. Patients in whom follow-up cannot be reasonably assured, for whatever reason, should be referred for inpatient evaluation or observation.

Management of Ectopic Pregnancy

Overview. Fortunately, the care of patients with suspected EP has greatly improved over the years. The first successful surgery for EP was performed in 1883, and until recently, surgical intervention was the mainstay of treatment.[16] In decades past, the diagnosis of EP usually was not made until the operation was performed, and one needed high suspicion of the diagnosis to commit to laparotomy. As a result, most patients were not treated until symptoms of rupture had become clear, making early intervention all but impossible.

The introduction of laparoscopic surgical techniques further improved management of patients with EP. The performance of a salpingotomy (removal of the involved section of the fallopian tube) or linear salpingostomy (removal of products of conception via an incision in the tube) also marked improvements in management by increasing the chance for future fertility in these patients. However, the most dramatic change in therapy was the introduction in 1982 of medical treatment, the mainstay of which is methotrexate, in a select subset of eligible patients.[17]

When indicated and appropriate, methotrexate is now commonly used for medical management of EP and has shown success rates equivalent to those of surgical intervention.[17] As a result, early diagnosis of EP is now more important than ever because it permits consideration of different treatment options, decreases morbidity and mortality, and may help reduce the incidence of future ectopic pregnancies. The following section will review and summarize cur-

Figure 2. Ultrasound Image of Free Fluid in Cul-de-sac

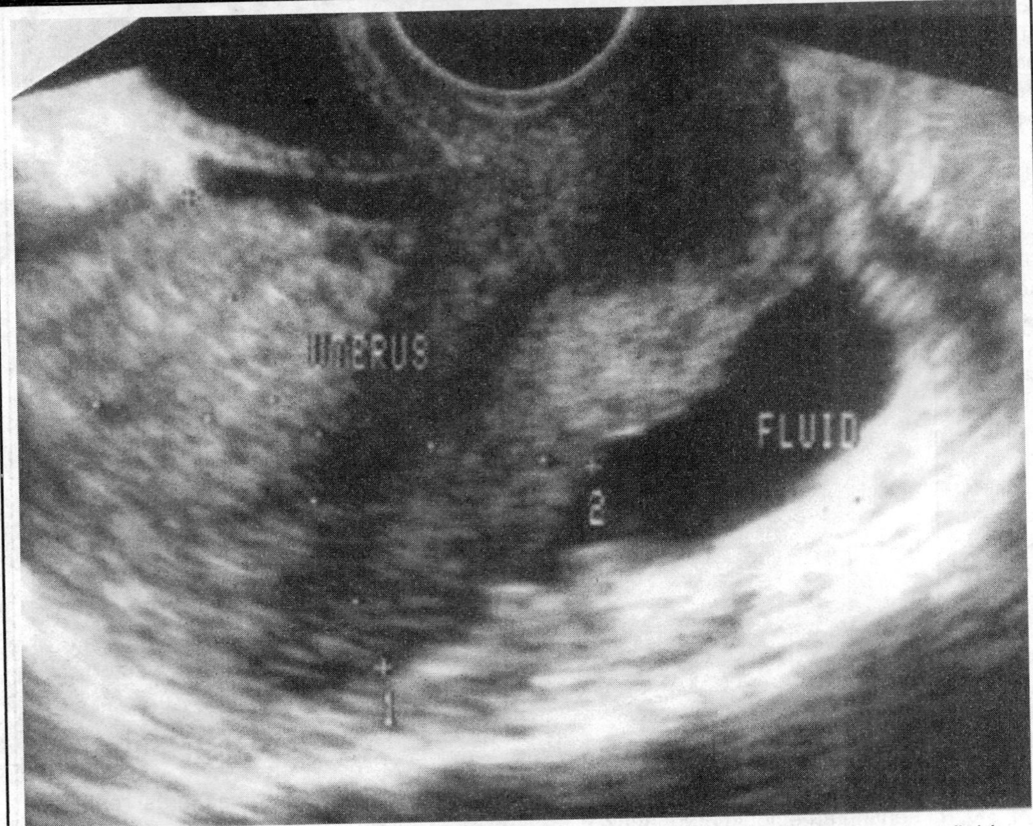

In Figure 2, the ectopic pregnancy is not seen, but evidence of rupture is seen as free fluid in the cul-de-sac.

rently recommended medical and surgical management strategies in patients with confirmed EP.

Medical Management. In many medical centers, medical management of EP is now considered to be the treatment of choice for EP. The reasons for this include lack of surgical complications and lower cost of treatment.

In the United States in 1990, it was estimated that the total cost of care for EP was $1.1 billion. In one study conducted at a university-based teaching hospital, average total cost was $1563 for medical treatment, $6626 for laparoscopic treatment, and $8001 for laparotomy.[18]

Mean length of hospital stay also varied-2.5 days for laparoscopic care vs. 5.2 days for laparotomy.[18]

After the initial report of successful medical management in 1982, many clinical trials followed and all found that outcome with medical treatment for unruptured EP was similar to that for laparoscopic salpingostomy.[18] So far, however, only one randomized comparison comparing the two treatments has been performed. In 1997, one group presented data demonstrating that in patients without signs of rupture, methotrexate was as effective as laparoscopic salpingostomy.[17] Furthermore, they found that subsequent rates of successful pregnancies were also the same in both treatment groups.[20] Methotrexate has also been used successfully to treat more unusual ectopic locations, such as cornual pregnancies, that previously were only managed with surgery.

To maximize the usefulness, safety, and efficacy of medical management, certain inclusionary and exclusionary patient criteria must be met. In particular, contraindications are designed to avoid treating more advanced cases in which the risk of rupture is significant. Contraindications to medical treatment of EP include: obvious signs of rupture (hemoperitoneum, severe pain), diameter of adnexal mass (> 3-4 cm on ultrasound), beta-hCG greater than 2000 mIU/mL, evidence of cardiac activity, and/or suspected heterotopic pregnancy.[21] Accordingly, early diagnosis of EP is essential for optimizing patient outcomes and enabling the consultant to use this approach.

Methotrexate is currently the drug of choice for medical management of EP. This agent inhibits synthesis of purines and pyrimidines and, therefore, prevents DNA synthesis and cell division. Clearly, methotrexate is not specific for ectopic tissue, and its side effects include bone marrow suppression, hepatotoxicity, stomatitis, pulmonary fibrosis, and photosensitivity.[21] Side effects can be treated and minimized with leucorvorin.[22]

Two methotrexate regimens currently are used: single dose and "variable" dose treatment. Single dose is used more often and, although it is more convenient, it is slightly less successful than the variable dose method. Single-dose methotrexate therapy has been reported to have an overall success rate of 82%, with 4% of the total treated group requiring a second dose for rising beta-hCG levels and 14% eventually requiring surgical intervention for bleeding or rupture.[19] In contrast, variable dose regimens were successful in 93% of patients; both regimens have similar rates of success for subsequent pregnancy (58% variable, 61% single dose).[23]

Methotrexate treatment may administered as inpatient treatment, but single-dose therapy given intramuscularly can also be performed in the outpatient setting, thereby avoiding hospitalization. If a patient is being discharged from the ED with an injection of methotrexate, the importance of follow-up with their OB to obtain serial beta-hCG levels must be stressed, as well as educating the patient about warning signs of rupture. Lastly, one is reminded to always check the Rh status in these patients, and treat Rh-negative mothers with Rhogam. *(Please see section on Rhesus Factor.)*

Surgical Treatment. When the first successful surgical treatment of EP was performed in 1883, four patients survived the procedure—an amazing outcome at the time.[16] In 1973, the first laparoscopic surgery was performed, and it soon became the surgical treatment of choice for EP.[24] As with medical management, early diagnosis of EP is essential to avoid open laparotomy.

The laparoscopic approach has been shown superior to laparotomy in three different prospective randomized trials.[25] In this regard, use of the laparoscope leads to lower cost, shorter hospital stays, less blood loss, less analgesia, shorter operating room times, and more rapid return to work. The ability to carry a successful subsequent pregnancy is similar with either method. The laparoscope has been used with good results in treatment of less common ectopic locations as well, including ovarian, interstitial, and early abdominal pregnancies. For traditional tubal pregnancies, linear salpingostomy (removal of products of conception via an incision in the tube) instead of traditional salpingectomy (removal of the entire tube) produced better future fertility rates, but has a higher risk of recurrent EP.

Persistent EP is one of the main complications of surgery, and occurs in 8% of linear salpingostomy patients vs. 4% of laparotomy patients.[25] This complication results from the presence of retained trophoblastic tissue, and is diagnosed by following beta-hCG levels after surgery. If the beta-hCG level has not fallen to less than 50% of the preoperative value on the first postoperative day, there is an 85% chance of persistent EP.[26] Persistent EP can be treated successfully by single-dose methotrexate.

Figure 3. Ultrasound Image of Tubal Ring

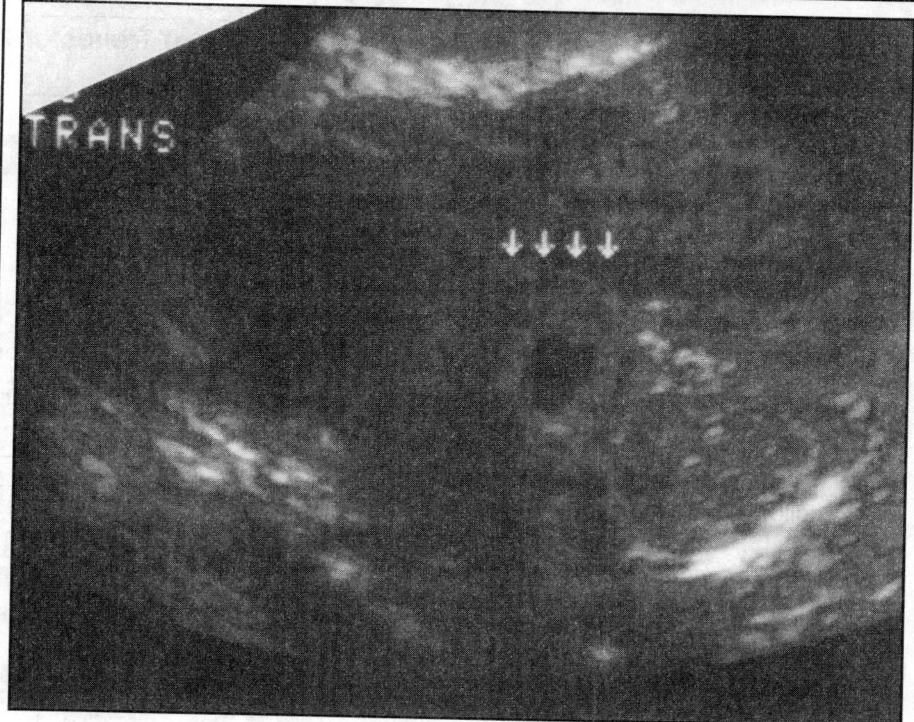

In Figure 3, a tubal ring or "ring of fire" sign is seen. A small, hypoechogenic mass is seen surrounded by a hyperechogenic area representing an ectopic gestational sac and surrounding decidual reaction.

New Treatment Advances. Two new treatment approaches have recently been developed for EP. The first is direct injection of ectopic tissue with methotrexate using ultrasonographic guidance. This approach was first described in 1987, and to date 12 studies totaling 406 patients have been published.[25] Substances other than methotrexate have also been used (i.e., hyperosmolar glucose) in attempts to avoid the potential toxicity of methotrexate.[27] In fact, this approach is associated with fewer side effects, yet produces higher local concentrations of methotrexate.

The direct injection technique can be used in patients with baseline hepatic or renal abnormalities, in whom systemic methotrexate may be contraindicated. The biggest disadvantage is that the technique requires an experienced operator to reduce risk of infection, bleeding, and tubal damage at the injection site. At present, direct injection is only being performed at a few centers and lacks general acceptance. Success rates are similar to single-dose systemic methotrexate, with an 81% overall success rate among the 406 patients included.[28] A 47% rate of successful subsequent pregnancy was reported.[28]

Ironically, the second "new approach" replicates a strategy that was used before surgical intervention was developed (i.e., "expectant management"). Before the advent of surgery, EP was not a uniformly fatal disease, with some patients having spontaneous regression or tubal abortion without deleterious effects. The "watchful waiting" approach was again attempted in an effort to preserve fertility when salpingectomy was the only surgical option, and it is currently begin explored again in an effort to reduce risks and costs of treatment.

The first study reporting on the outcomes of expectant management was in 1955, and the results were problematic.[29] Only 57% of patients resolved, 20% needed surgery for persistent symptoms, and another 23% needed surgery for catastrophic bleeding.[102] Given these results, it is not surprising that no additional attempts using this technique were reported again until 1982. In fact, strict selection criteria for patients has led to a total of 363 patients being reported in 12 studies world-wide since 1982.[30]

Current studies select for patients at very low risk for rupture. The range of beta-hCG levels in these studies is between 250 mIU/mL up to 2,500 mIU/mL.[31,32] Other studies simply select patients with falling beta-hCG levels or the following: a tubal mass of less than 2-3 cm diagnosed by laparoscope, empty uterus on ultrasound, and lack of fetal cardiac motion.[30] Interestingly, when these inclusionary and exclusionary criteria are used, studies have reported an overall success rate of 67%, with rupture in only 2.5% of patients.[30]

It is important to note that some of the ruptures have occurred in patients with very low beta-hCG levels (i.e., between 41 mIU/mL and 212 mIU/mL).[30] Subsequent successful pregnancy rates of 68% were reported for the 363 patients.[30] Overall, the authors suggest that up to 15-20% of patients with a diagnosis of EP may be appropriate candidates for expectant management. They suggest the following criteria to identify eligible patients: minimal pain, minimal vaginal bleeding, no rupture (free fluid), falling beta-hCG levels with initial levels less than 1,000 mIU/mL, no ectopic cardiac motion, and ectopic mass less than 3 cm.[30] Current American College of Obstetrics and Gynecology (ACOG) recommendations suggest this approach can be used in patients with a decreasing beta-hCG less than 200 mIU/mL. Patients must understand the associated risk of

Figure 4. Algorithm for ED Evaluation of Vaginal Bleeding or Pain in the First Twenty Weeks of Pregnancy

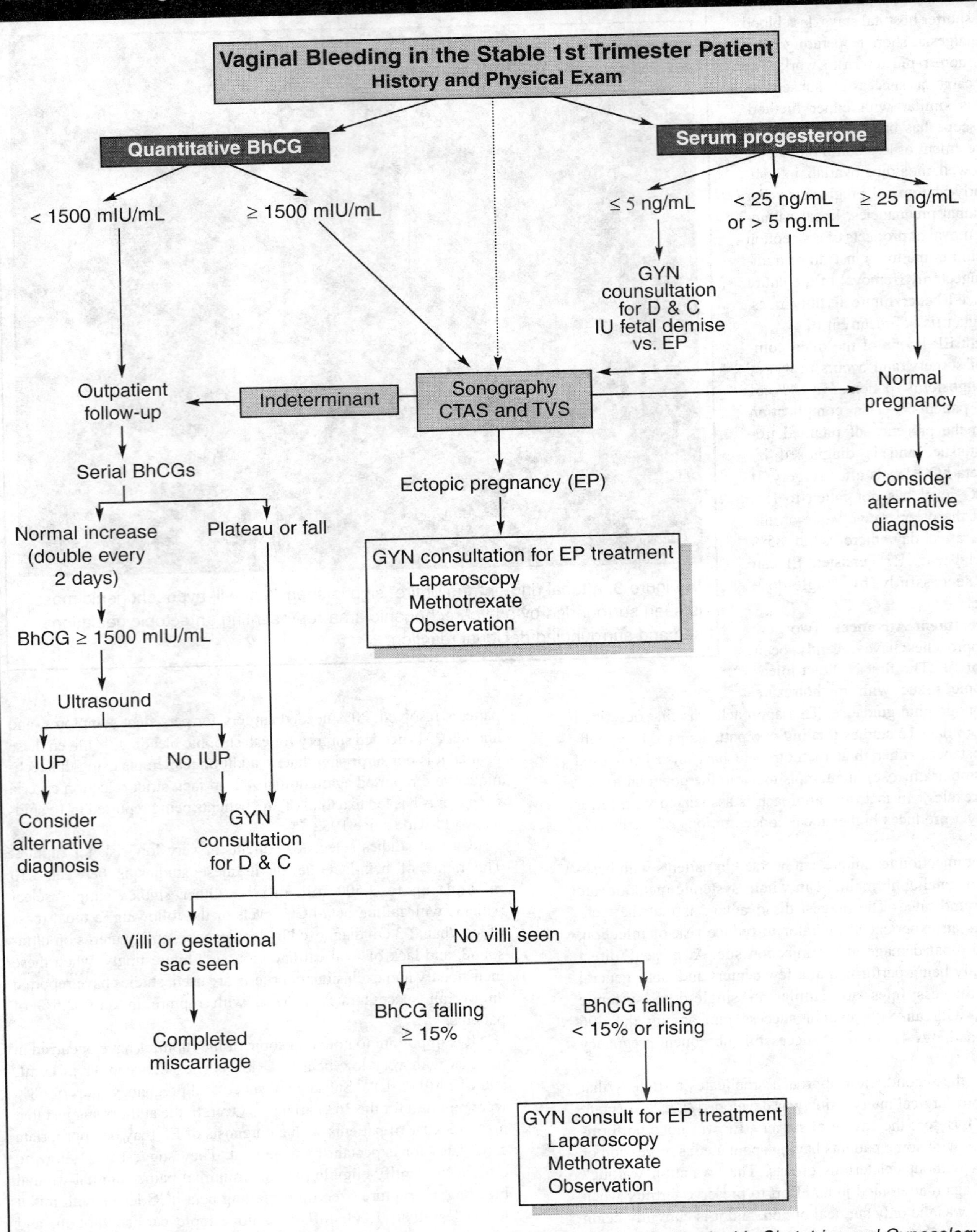

Adapted from Pisa MD, Carson SA. Ectopic pregnancy. In: Scott JR, et al, eds. *Danforth's Obstetrics and Gynecology*. 8th ed. Philadelphia: Lippincott Williams & Wilkins; 1999:155-172; and Abbott JT. Acute complications related to pregnancy. In: Rosen P, et al, eds. *Emergency Medicine: Concepts and Clinical Practice*. 4th edition. Mosby-Year Book, Inc; 1998:2342-2364.

rupture, bleeding, and that a need for further treatment may be required.[33]

Spontaneous Miscarriage

Spontaneous miscarriage is a common diagnosis in patients with vaginal bleeding that occurs during the first half of pregnancy. It is estimated that 15% of clinically proven pregnancies end in miscarriage, with the majority occurring before 12 weeks gestation.[34] Moreover, because some patients may miscarry before they are known to be pregnant, the actual miscarriage rate may be as much as 2-3 times higher than reported.

Up to 20% of pregnant women will experience vaginal bleeding during the first weeks of pregnancy, and as many as 50% of them will progress to miscarriage.[35] The risk of miscarriage varies greatly with age. For patients younger than 20 years, the risk averages only 12%, whereas in patients older than 45 years it approaches 50%.[36] As the term "abortion" has a negative connotation to many patients, it is gradually being replaced in the literature with "miscarriage." This section will review causes and risk factors for spontaneous miscarriage, and discuss in detail the ED evaluation and management of various presentations of miscarriage.

When evaluating pregnant patients with vaginal bleeding, ED physicians must recognize that maternal trauma from domestic abuse is common and, at times, may be occult in its presentation. Hence, all pregnant women should routinely be screened for abuse. A history of substance abuse, depression, or multiple ED visits should alert the physician to the possibility of abuse. The abuser is usually confrontational toward the staff and overprotective of the patient. Abuse is more likely to be identified if the patient is questioned in a private setting and in a non-judgmental and direct manner.[37] Emotional status and safety must be addressed before the patient is discharged from the ED.[38]

Pathophysiology. Spontaneous miscarriage may result from abnormal embryo development or from maternal factors. Up to 50% of women with spotting or cramping early in pregnancy will have an abnormal intrauterine pregnancy on initial ultrasound, with many of these embryos being morphologically abnormal.[39] Approximately 33% of miscarried specimens lost before 9 weeks are due to anembryonic development, termed a "blighted ovum."[40] In this case, only an empty gestational sac is seen on ultrasound.

The significant percentage of embryonic abnormalities represents a natural process that eliminates almost 95% of cytogenetic defects before birth. The rate of identified chromosome defects in miscarried embryos from the first trimester approaches 60%, and falls to 7% by the end of the 24th week.[34] In most cases, the parents have normal karyotypes, and the abnormal conceptus is the result of a random genetic error. However, a small number of parents may carry balanced translocations and they will give rise to recurrent miscarriages. Patients with recurrent miscarriage require obstetric evaluation to identify the cause when possible, as some will be due to treatable conditions such as cervical incompetence.

Much attention in the lay press has been given to chemical and infectious agents as a potential cause of spontaneous miscarriage, including tobacco use, coffee, alcohol, illicit drugs, Salmonella, shingles, Mycoplasma, and various sexually transmitted diseases. While many of these agents can increase the risk of miscarriage, it is felt that such extrinsic factors account for a small percentage of spontaneous miscarriage.[41] An important point is that birth control pills, video display terminals, minor abdominal trauma in the first trimester, and diagnostic x-rays less than 10 rads have been shown *not* to increase pregnancy loss.[42]

ED Evaluation and Management. Patients who present to the ED early in pregnancy with abdominal pain and/or vaginal bleeding are at risk for spontaneous miscarriage. As mentioned previously, any patient with complaints that may be related to pregnancy (nausea, vomiting, abdominal pain, syncope, etc.) needs to have a pregnancy test in the ED. Similarly, any patient in the early stages of pregnancy with abdominal pain or vaginal bleeding should be evaluated for EP before the diagnosis of miscarriage can be made (Please see previous sections on EP).

When evaluating patients with suspected miscarriage, pertinent historical facts include dates and features of last menstrual period, drug use, obstetric and gynecologic history, as well as general medical and surgical histories. The physical exam should always include a pelvic exam, but this may be deferred to the obstetric consultant if the patient is nearing the end of the first half of pregnancy. In general, when the uterus is at the umbilicus by palpation, the patient is roughly 20 weeks pregnant. Vaginal exams are contraindicated in the second half of pregnancy when the patient presents with vaginal bleeding until placenta previa has been ruled out by ultrasound. Even minor trauma caused by a vaginal exam can result in catastrophic maternal hemorrhage in these patients.

In patients who are clearly in the early stages of pregnancy-(i.e., they have low beta-hCG levels and no significant uterine enlargement), the pelvic exam can be useful to verify that bleeding is coming from the os and not from a non-obstetrical cause such as hemorrhoids. Cultures for chlamydia and gonorrhea should be obtained. If there is bleeding from the os, one may determine if the os is open by gently attempting to pass a fingertip into the os, but one should never force the fingertip into the os. Probing with foreign objects (i.e., cotton swabs) is not recommended.

One should feel for adnexal masses or tenderness, and any tissue that is obtained should be sent for pathological verification of the presence of chorionic villi. Before sending the tissue to the lab, it can be examined in saline suspension using a low power microscope. Organized blood clots will appear firm with shredded edges, whereas chorionic villi appear with feathery edges. Up to 50% of specimens can be accurately identified by this means.[43] Diagnostic testing consists of quantitative beta-hCG and/or progesterone levels followed by transvaginal ultrasound (refer to previous discussion of diagnostic evaluation and diagnostic algorithms for EP).

The differential diagnosis of vaginal bleeding in the first half of pregnancy has been discussed. It is important to realize that spontaneous miscarriage is the most common misdiagnosis associated with EP. Several other disorders can easily be confused with spontaneous miscarriage. Hemorrhagic urinary tract infections (UTIs) can cause "vaginal bleeding" and can be differentiated using a catheterized urine specimen. An important point to remember is that all UTIs are treated in pregnancy to reduce the risk of miscarriage.

Non-obstetrical bleeding, such as hemorrhoids, also can occur. Cervical lesions are often friable and bleed easily. When a cervical lesion is found on exam, cervical carcinoma is always a concern. However, one should not biopsy these lesions in the ED as biopsy may lead to significant bleeding. Implantation bleeding is relatively common, and is more likely when it occurs around the time of an expected period. Bleeding can also be caused as the embryo invades the highly vascular endometrial tissue. The bleeding can vary from spotting to that associated with a normal period, and therefore, it can be a source of confusion for the patient when dates are calculated. Once EP has been ruled out, there are several types of spontaneous miscarriage that may be encountered. These are discussed in the sections below.

Threatened Miscarriage. A threatened miscarriage is defined as any amount of uterine bleeding in the first 20 weeks of pregnancy without passage of tissue or cervical dilation. The bleeding associated with threatened miscarriage can vary from a brownish discharge to bright red vaginal bleeding. The bleeding can start and stop repeatedly over the course of many days, and is often associated with uterine cramping or low backache.

On physical exam the cervix will be closed and uneffaced, and no tissue will be passed. Ultrasound can diagnose intrauterine pregnancy after as little as 5.5 weeks of gestation, but the ultrasound at 3-4 weeks gestation usually will be indeterminate.[44] Very early in pregnancy, an ultrasound finding of an empty uterus can still represent a normally developing pregnancy, an abnormal pregnancy destined to miscarry, or an ectopic. As mentioned above, ectopic must be ruled out using serial beta-hCG levels (or another diagnostic approach).

Ultrasonographic findings consistent with miscarriage include: abnormal gestational sac size or small embryo for dates, slow fetal heart rates, or large (> 20 mm) empty gestational sacs. In a recent ultrasound study of 78 women with intrauterine echogenic material (blood clots) with no gestational sac, all underwent spontaneous miscarriage.[45] Up to 95% of pregnancies will continue to live birth if a normal fetal heart rate is found at 8 weeks gestation.[46] The rate of pregnancy loss is only 1% when a live fetus is present at 14-16 weeks gestation.[44] To date there is no convincing evidence that any treatment will change the outcome in patients diagnosed with threatened miscarriage.

Patients with threatened abortion may be discharged with mandatory obstetrical follow-up and good return instructions (i.e., return for increased bleeding, passage of tissue, fever, worse pain, etc). Serial beta-hCG levels are typically followed as an outpatient and falling levels or decreasing gestational size on repeat ultrasound indicate a poor prognosis for the embryo. Alternatively, a single progesterone level may be predictive of fetal outcome. A single progesterone level over 25 ng/mL has been shown to be useful in predicting the presence of a viable pregnancy prognosis.[42,47] In a study of 358 women with threatened miscarriage, 148 had live births, 175 patients continued to spontaneous miscarriage, and there were 35 ectopic pregnancies. A single progesterone level over 25 ng/mL had a 90% sensitivity in discriminating between failing and non-failing pregnancies.[48]

Once fetal demise has occurred, the options for treatment include expectant management or uterine curettage. There has been debate in the literature as to whether expectant management or curettage is the better treatment. A pooled literature review found no difference between expectant management and surgical treatment; each was 93% successful.[49] Furthermore, expectant management has the advantage of a lower incidence of uterine perforation and infection compared to surgery. Another author found similar results, and suggested women with minimal intrauterine tissue, minimal bleeding or pain, and no signs of infection were good candidates for expectant management.[50] Medical management can be added in the form of prostaglandin (misoprostol) or antiprogesterone (mifepristone). However, a recent randomized trial found additional medical treatment was not superior to expectant management alone, and another author proposed larger trials to compare the two options.[51,52]

Inevitable/Incomplete Miscarriage. Although previously classified as separate entities, these two categorizations represent the same process of early pregnancy loss. They present in a similar fashion and are treated in a similar manner. Inevitable miscarriage is defined as vaginal bleeding or passage of tissue in conjunction with cervical dilation. An open cervix, defined as one through which a fingertip can easily pass into the os, is an important physical finding used to identify a spontaneous miscarriage.

Incomplete miscarriage occurs when products of conception have incompletely passed, a condition that usually is associated with vaginal bleeding and cramping. Retained tissue is more common in the second trimester and can result in profuse bleeding. Other than the occasional passage of only one twin, there is no fetal survival with inevitable or incomplete miscarriage. Complete evacuation of the uterus is advised to reduce maternal complications of bleeding and infection. Again, tissue obtained should be sent for pathological confirmation of villi to rule out the possibility of EP.

Uterine curettage can be performed as an outpatient, but the procedure should be executed by the consultant unless the ED physician is specifically trained in the procedure. Complications include blood loss, uterine perforation, and infection. After completion, the patient should be observed for several hours for signs of significant blood loss, and then followed-up with in 24-48 hours for re-examination and verification of falling beta-hCG levels.

Complete Miscarriage. A complete miscarriage occurs when all the products of conception have passed and vaginal bleeding has stopped. If the diagnosis is certain, no further treatment is required. If it is in question, ultrasound may be performed to evaluate for retained products. If these are detected, uterine curettage is the recommended treatment.

Missed Miscarriage. A missed miscarriage is defined by retention of products of conception for a prolonged period of time after documented fetal demise. The reason that some embryos do not spontaneously abort is unknown. Beta-hCG levels may fall to zero without passage of tissue, and the patient may no longer report symptoms of pregnancy. Most patients do eventually abort the fetus; coagulation defects from retained products of conception are rare in the first half of pregnancy. As expectant management may be emotionally difficult for the patient once diagnosed, most prefer uterine curettage for first trimester and dilation and curettage for second trimester cases.

Septic Miscarriage. Fortunately, the incidence of sepsis as a complication of miscarriage has dramatically decreased and is an uncommon cause of maternal mortality. Any type of spontaneous or elective miscarriage may lead to uterine infection and sepsis. The patient will typically present with fever, abdominal pain/tenderness, and uterine pain. The patient may be unaware of the preceding pregnancy and miscarriage, or she may not be forthcoming with this history for multiple reasons.

The ED physician needs to maintain a high suspicion for this possibility when contemplating PID as an alternative diagnosis. In most cases, the beta-hCG will still be positive and should provide a clue to the diagnosis. In advanced cases, the patient may present in septic shock. When the diagnosis of uterine infection from miscarriage is considered, the patient needs to be treated for potential sepsis and receive fluid resuscitation.

Cervical cultures and gram stains, a tetanus booster when indicated, and flat/upright x-ray studies should be included to rule out free air or foreign bodies. The infections tend to be polymicrobial, and the following antibiotic regimens are recommended: Triple antibiotic coverage is used, with one choice from each category below. Coverage for gram-positive anaerobic or aerobic organisms can be provided with penicillin G, ampicillin, or any cephalosporin.[34] Gram-negative aerobic organisms are treated with aminoglycosides or aztreonam, and gram-negative anaerobic bacteria with clindamycin or metronidazole. Monotherapy with ampicillin/sulbactam, ticarcillin clavulanate, or piperacillin tazobactam is also acceptable.

Regardless of the choice, antibiotic coverage should be promptly administered. It is important to remember that early evacuation of the uterus is required for treatment of these patients and should be performed within several hours of presentation. Thus, prompt diagnosis and consultation are essential. Patients should be admitted to an ICU setting, as some will experience complications of sepsis syndrome (respiratory distress syndrome, coagulopathies, etc).

Rhesus Factor. When managing patients with EP or miscarriage, it can be easy to forget the Rh factor status. However, all pregnant patients with vaginal bleeding need a Rh factor test regardless of the cause. Almost 15% of patients are Rh negative and are at risk for carrying an Rh positive fetus. As Rh positive fathers greatly outnumber negative ones, and verification of the father's Rh status is problematic and impractical, any Rh negative mother is treated.

The maternal immune system will view the fetal blood as foreign and make antibodies against the Rh factor. As antibodies readily cross the placenta, any subsequent pregnancy will be at increased risk for hemolytic disease. This is often fatal for subsequent fetuses, so prevention is paramount. Sensitization can occur as early as eight weeks gestation, and the risk is estimated at 9% at 12 weeks gestation.[42] Recommendations are a 50 microgram IM injection of Rhogam (Rh immune globulin) for patients less than 12 weeks and 300 micrograms IM for patients greater than 12 weeks. As gestational dates can be notoriously inaccurate and there is no additional risk with the higher dose, many physicians opt for the 300 microgram dose in all patients. While Rhogam is ideally given at the time of ED presentation, it can be given up to 72 hours after bleeding and still be equally effective. Usefulness may be found even as late as 2-4 weeks after bleeding.[42]

Trophoblastic Disorders

Trophoblastic disorders represent abnormal proliferation of trophoblastic tissue. These disorders include complete mole (no recognizable fetal tissue), partial mole (fetal tissue with trophoblastic tissue), invasive hydatidiform mole, and choriocarcinoma.

Molar pregnancies can arise from a normal pregnancy, an EP, spontaneous miscarriage or an elective abortion. They occur in approximately 1 in 1000 pregnancies overall, with patients younger than 20 years or older than 40 years and women with a history of miscarriages being at increased risk.[53] The risk increases by at least fivefold in women who are older than 40 years of age. The risk increases tenfold if the patient has had a prior molar pregnancy. The risk of choriocarcinoma increases 5- to 24-fold for women older than 40 years of age. However, the most important risk factor of choriocarcinoma is a history of a hydatidiform mole. The risk of choriocarcinoma in these patients has been estimated to be 1000 times that of the general population.[54]

Patients with trophoblastic disorder most commonly present with vaginal bleeding, severe or persistent hyperemesis, and early development of preeclampsia. As the trophoblastic tissue expands at a much faster rate than a normal pregnancy, a large uterus for dates is often found on exam. Quantitative beta-hCG levels are also much higher than those found in normal pregnancy. Ultrasound will show a "snow storm" pattern secondary to the molar vesicles.[4] Fifteen percent of molar pregnancies can progress to choriocarcinoma, which can metastasize to the lungs, vagina, brain, liver, bowel, spleen, or kidney.[52]

A patient who presents to the ED and is found to have trophoblastic disease should have a chest x-ray to rule out pulmonary metastases. Obstetric consultation is mandatory in all cases. Depending on the age of the patient and the desire for fertility, treatment consists of dilation and curettage or hysterectomy. A beta-hCG level should be obtained each week following treatment until levels have normalized for three weeks. Levels should then be drawn monthly for 6-12 months. The patient should use contraception for at least one year following the molar pregnancy.[52] Chemotherapy is utilized in choriocarcinoma and in molar pregnancies that have stable or rising beta-hCG levels. Fortunately, trophoblastic disease is highly responsive to chemotherapy.

Summary

The diagnosis of pregnancy can be easily overlooked in the ED. Bleeding complications during the first half of pregnancy are common, and any patient with vaginal bleeding, abdominal pain, or other symptoms of pregnancy should have pregnancy ruled out. If the patient is found to be pregnant, EP should be ruled out. EP is still a leading cause of maternal death. The ED physician needs to maintain a high index of suspicion for these patients to reduce potential morbidity and mortality. Patients should also be evaluated for spontaneous miscarriage or its complications, as well as trophoblastic disease. Rhogam should be given to all Rh-negative patients.

Obstetrical consultation will be required for most patients while in the ED, and certainly all will require further follow up visits with an obstetrician. Finally, as the grief reaction of early pregnancy loss can be severe in some patients, referral to psychiatric counseling or social worker consultation before discharge should be considered. These reactions are common in the ED, as a recent study of 44 ED patients with spontaneous miscarriage found that 80% experienced a significant grief reaction.[55]

References

1. Ectopic Pregnancy—United States, 1990-1992. *JAMA* 1995; 273:533.
2. Schwartz RO, DiPietro DL. Beta-hCG as a diagnostic aid for suspected ectopic pregnancy. *Obstet Gynecol* 1980;56: 197-203.
3. Jehle D, Krause R, Braen GR. Ectopic Pregnancy. *Emerg Med Clin North Am* 1994;12:55-71.
4. McKennett M, Fullerton JT. Vaginal bleeding in pregnancy. *Am Family Phys* 1995;53:639-646.
5. Dorfman SF, Grimes DA, Cates W Jr, et al. Ectopic pregnancy mortality, United States, 1979-1980: Clinical aspects. *Obstet Gynecol* 1984;64:386-390.
6. Abbott J, Emmans LS, Lowenstein SR. Ectopic pregnancy: Ten common pitfalls in diagnosis. *Am J Emerg Med* 1990;8: 515-522.
7. Hertzberg BS, Kliewer MA, Paulson EK. Ovarian cyst rupture causing hemoperitoneum: Imaging features and the potential for misdiagnosis. *Abdom Imaging* 1999;24:304-308.
8. Lewis FR, Holcroft JW, Boey J, et al. Appendicitis: A critical review of diagnosis and treatment in 1,000 cases. *Arch Surg* 1975;110:677-684.
9. Kaplan BC, Dart RG, Moskos M, et al. Ectopic pregnancy: Prospective study with improved diagnostic accuracy. *Ann Emerg Med* 1996;28:10-17.
10. Stovall TG, Kellerman AL, Ling FW, et al. Emergency department diagnosis of ectopic pregnancy. *Ann Emerg Med* 1990;19:1098-1102.
11. Mol BW, van der Veen F, Bossuyt PM. Implementation of probabilistic decision rules improves the predictive value of algorithms in the diagnostic management of ectopic pregnancy. *Hum Reprod* 1999;14:2855-2862.
12. Barnhart KT, Simhan H, Kamelle SA. Diagnostic accuracy of ultrasound above and below the beta-hCG discriminatory zone. *Obstet Gynecol* 1999;94:583-587.

13. Destefano F, Peterson HB, Layde PM, et al. Risk of ectopic pregnancy following tubal sterilization. *Obstet Gynecol* 1982; 60:326-330.
14. Ankum WM, Mol BWJ, Van der Veen F, et al. Risk factors for ectopic pregnancy: A meta-analysis. *JAMA* 1996;65: 1093-1099.
15. Hochner-Celnikier D, Ron M, Goshen R, et al. Ruptured ectopic pregnancy following disappearance of serum beta subunit of hCG. *Obstet Gynecol* 1992;79:826-827.
16. Tait RL. Classic pages in obstetrics and gynecology by Lawson Tait: Five cases of extra-uterine pregnancy operated upon at the time of rupture. *Am J Obstet* 1972;113:129.
17. Tenaka T, Hayashi H, Kutsuzawa T, et al. Treatment of interstitial ectopic pregnancy with methotrexate: Report of a successful case. *Fertil Steril* 1982;37:851-852.
18. Stovall TG, Bradham DD, Ling FW, et al. Cost of treatment of ectopic pregnancy: Single-dose methotrexate versus surgical treatment. *J Women's Health* 1994;3:445-450.
19. Hajenius PJ, Engelsbel S, Mol BW, et al. Randomized trial of systemic methotrexate versus laparoscopic salpingostomy in tubal pregnancy. *Lancet* 1997;350:774-779.
20. Lau S, Tulandi T. Conservative medical and surgical management of interstitial ectopic pregnancy. *Fertil Steril* 1999;72:207-215.
21. Buster JE, Pisarska MD. Medical management of ectopic pregnancy. *Clin Obstet Gynecol* 1999;42:23-30.
22. Stovall TG, Ling FW, Carson SA, et al. Nonsurgical diagnosis and treatment of tubal pregnancy. *Fertil Steril* 1990;54: 537-548.
23. Pisarska MD, Carson SA, Buster JE. Ectopic pregnancy. *Lancet* 1998;351:1115-1120.
24. Shapiro HI, Adler DH. Excision of an ectopic pregnancy through the laparoscope. *Am J Obstet Gynecol* 1973;117: 290-291.
25. Yao M, Tulandi T. Current status of surgical and nonsurgical management of ectopic pregnancy. *Fertil Steril* 1997;67: 421-433.
26. Spandorfer SD, Sawin SW, Benjamin I, et al. Postoperative day 1 serum human chorionic gonadotropin level as a predictor of persistent ectopic pregnancy after conservative surgical management. *Fertil Steril* 1997;68:430-434.
27. Gjelland K, Hordnes K, Tjugum J, et al. Treatment of ectopic pregnancy by local injection of hypertonic glucose: A randomized trial comparing administration guided by transvaginal ultrasound or laparoscopy. *Acta Obstet Gynecol Scand* 1995;74:629-634.
28. Natofsky JG, Jorge L, Mayer JC, et al. Ultrasound-guided injection of ectopic pregnancy. *Clin Obstet Gynecol* 1999;42: 39-47.
29. Lund J. Early ectopic pregnancy. *J Obstet Gynaecol Br Emp* 1955;62:70-76.
30. Cohen MA, Sauer MV. Expectant management of ectopic pregnancy. *Clin Obstet Gynecol* 1999;42:48-54.
31. Carp HJA, Oelsner G, Serr DM, et al. Fertility after nonsurgical treatment of ectopic pregnancy. *J Reprod Med* 1986;31:119-122.
32. Madinen JI, Kivijarvi AK, Irjala KMA. Success of nonsurgical management of ectopic pregnancy. *Lancet* 1990;335:1099.
33. ACOG practice bulletin. Medical management of tubal pregnancy. *Int J Gynecol Obstet* 1999;65:97-103.
34. Scott JR. Early pregnancy loss. In: Scott JR, et al, eds. *Danforth's Obstetrics and Gynecology.* 8th ed. Philadelphia: Lippincott Williams & Wilkins; 1999:143-153.
35. Turner LM. Vaginal bleeding during pregnancy. *Emerg Med Clin North Am* 1994;12:45-54.
36. Warburtin D, Kline J, Stein Z, et al. Cytogenetic abnormalities in spontaneous abortions of recognized conceptions. In: Porter IH, ed. *Perinatal Genetics: Diagnosis and Treatment.* New York: Academic Press; 1986:133.
37. Greenberg EM, McFarlane J, Watson MG. Vaginal bleeding and abuse: Assessing the pregnancy women in the emergency department. *MCN Am J Matern Child Nurs* 1997;22:182-186.
38. Poole GV, Martin JN Jr, Perry KG Jr, et al. Trauma in pregnancy: The role of interpersonal violence. *Am J Obstet Gynecol* 1996;174:1873-1877.
39. Goldstein SR. Sonography in early pregnancy. *Clin Obstet Gynceol* 1994;37:681-692.
40. Byrne JBL, Ward K. Genetic factors in recurrent abortion. *Clin Obstet Gynecol* 1994;37:693-704.
41. Brent RL, Beckman DA. The contribution of environmental teratogens to embryonic and fetal loss. *Clin Obstet Gynecol* 1994;37:646-670.
42. Mallett VT. Ectopic pregnancy. In: Pearlman MD, Tintinalli JE, eds. *Emergency Care of the Woman.* New York: McGraw Hill; 1998:21-28.
43. Lindahl B, Ahlgren M. Identification of chorionic villi in abortion specimens. *Obstet Gynecol* 1986;67:79-81.
44. Goldstein SR. Embryonic death in early pregnancy: A new look at the first trimester. *Obstet Gynecol* 1994;84:294-297.
45. Dart R, Dart L, Mitchell P. Normal intrauterine pregnancy is unlikely in patients who have echogenic material identified within the endometrial cavity at transvaginal ultrasound. *Acad Emerg Med* 1999;6:116-120.
46. Simpson JL, Mills JL, Holmes LB, et al. Low fetal loss rates after ultrasound-proved viability in early pregnancy. *JAMA* 1987;258:2555-2557.
47. Pisa MD, Carson SA. Ectopic pregnancy. In: Scott JR, et al, eds. *Danforth's Obstetrics and Gynecology.* 8th ed. Philadelphia: Lippincott Williams & Wilkins; 1999:155-172.
48. Al-Sebai MA, Kingsland CR, Diver M, et al. The role of a single progesterone measurement in the diagnosis of early pregnancy failure and the prognosis of fetal viability. *Br J Obstet Gynaecol* 1999;102:364-369.
49. Geyman JP, Oliver LM, Sullivan SD. Expectant, medical, or surgical treatment of spontaneous abortion in first trimester of pregnancy? A pooled quantitative literature evaluation. *J Am Board Fam Pract* 1999;12:55-64.
50. Hurd WW, Whitfield RR, Randolph JF Jr., et al. Expectant management versus elective curettage for the treatment of spontaneous abortion. *Fertil Steril* 1997;68:601-606.
51. Nielsen S, Hahin M, Platz-Christensen J. Randomized trial comparing expectant with medical management for first trimester miscarriages. *Br J Obstet Gynaecol* 1999;106:804-807.
52. Ballagh SA, Harris HA, Demasio K. Is curettage needed for uncomplicated incomplete spontaneous abortion? *Am J*

Obstet Gynecol 1998;179:1279-1282.

53. Viera AJ, Clenny TL, Shenenberger DW. Vaginal Bleeding at 16 Weeks. *Am Family Phys* 1999;59:649-651.
54. Freedman RS, Tortolero-Luna G, Pandey DK, et al. Gestational trophoblastic disease. *Obstet Gynecol Clin North Am* 1996;23:545-571.
55. Zaccardi R, Abbott J, Koziol-MaLain J. Loss and grief reactions after spontaneous miscarriage in the emergency department. *Ann Emerg Med* 1993;22:799-804.

Medical Disorders in the Pregnant Patient

Gary Hals, MD, PhD
Todd Crump, MD

While an emergency department (ED) physician is completing the chart of a young woman treated for community-acquired pneumonia, the nurse presents the clinician the results of the patient's pregnancy test. The nurse says,"It turns out she's pregnant after all. Do we need to do anything different now?" For many patients treated in the ED for common medical disorders who also happen to be pregnant, this is a challenging question. And the answer is "Yes." In many cases, the patient's pregnancy will significantly alter levels of baseline labs, the approach to diagnosis, and selection of therapeutic agents.

In 1999, the world population is projected to reach 6 billion people. According to the U.S. Census, about 8% of women from ages 14 to 44 years were pregnant during 1994, resulting in 3.9 million live births.[1] One study evaluating pregnancy rates of ED patients found that female patients presenting to this clinical environment have a pregnancy rate of around 10%.[2] As an experienced physician knows, diagnosing a patient with an "unexpected" pregnancy is hardly a rare event. Pregnant patients often present to the ED for complications relating to their pregnancy, among them vaginal bleeding, miscarriage, and early labor. But these patients also are at risk for—and suffer from—common diseases that affect non-pregnant individuals. To further complicate ED care of these patients, pregnancy may affect many aspects of a women's physiology, including changes in baseline cardiovascular and respiratory status. Accordingly, ED physicians need to be aware of the impact pregnancy will make on day-to-day diagnostic and management decisions in this patient population.

With these issues in focus, this chapter reviews the basic alterations of physiology associated with normal pregnancy. Most importantly, the authors present a comprehensive review of ED treatment of a variety of common medical disorders in the context of pregnancy. Disorders discussed in detail include asthma, diabetes, hypertension, pneumonia, deep venous thrombosis (DVT), pulmonary embolism (PE), urinary tract infection (UTI), pyelonephritis, and human immunodeficiency virus (HIV) infection. The authors also summarize approaches to drug therapy in pregnancy and include a discussion of drugs that are and are not safe for use in pregnancy.

Physiologic Changes Associated with Pregnancy

Pregnancy affects virtually every organ system. These changes are designed to accommodate the developing fetus, and adapt the mother's body to withstand the "growing" metabolic demands of pregnancy as it progresses. These changes also can modify the approach to pregnant women's medical care, inasmuch as baseline "normal" laboratory test levels change throughout gestation. For example, physicians should be aware that alterations occur in arterial blood gas measurements. This may affect care of the pregnant patient with asthma. For example, a woman's ability to tolerate an asthma attack in late pregnancy may be compromised as compared to her response when not pregnant. The following section will review clinically important alterations in a pregnant women's physiology and their effects on baseline laboratory tests. *(Please see Table 1.)*

Table 1. Summary of Laboratory Changes in Pregnancy

LAB TEST	NORMAL RANGE	PREGNANCY EFFECT	GESTATIONAL TIMING
Sodium	135-145 mEq/L	lower 2-4 mEq/L	By midpregnancy
Potassium	3.5-4.5 mEq/L	lower 0.2-0.3 mEq/L	By midpregnancy
Creatinine	0.6-1.1 mg/dL	lower 0.3 mg/dL	By midpregnancy
Creatinine phosphokinase	26-140 U/L	raise 2-4 fold	After labor (mb bands also)
Glucose (fasting)	65-105 mg/dL	lower 10%	Gradual fall
Fibrinogen	200-400 mg/dL	raise 600 mg/dL	By term
Urea nitrogen	12-30 mg/dL	lower 50%	First trimester
Hematocrit	36-46%	lower 4-7%	Nadir at 30-34 weeks
Hemoglobin	12-16 g/dL	lower 1.4-2.0 g/dL	Nadir at 30-34 weeks
Leukocyte count	4000-10,000/mm^3	raise 3500/mm^3	Gradual increase to term (up to 25,000/mm^3 in labor)
Platelets	150,000	400,000/mm^3	Slight decrease

Adapted from: Barclay ML. Critical physiologic alterations in pregnancy. In: Pearlman MD, Tintinalli JE, eds. *Emergency Care of the Woman*. New York: McGraw Hill; 1998:303-312.

Hematology. During pregnancy, plasma volume increases by approximately 33% (450 mL). Benefits associated with this increase include compensation for blood loss associated with delivery and minimizing the effects of gravity and maternal position on fetal circulation. This increase occurs gradually and mirrors the growth of the fetus. However, red cell mass expands at a slightly slower rate, which in turn, produces a dilutional anemia early in pregnancy that can be mistaken for a pathologic process. Survey studies suggest that the mean hemoglobin level in pregnancy is between 10.2 g/dL and 11.6 g/dL.[3] Similarly, serum proteins are also diluted, and the resulting lower colloid osmotic pressure may be responsible for dependent edema. By term, total blood volume increases by an average of 45% above pre-pregnancy levels. The clinical consequences of expanded blood volume may require dosing changes in some medications, inasmuch as an expanded intravascular space can dilute the concentration of such drugs as anticonvulsants and antihypertensive agents.

The white blood cell (WBC) count typically ranges from 5,000/mL to 12,000/mL during pregnancy. This is accompanied by a small left shift, which may confuse the clinical picture when evaluating pregnant women for signs of infection. Some authors also report decreased leukocyte function characterized by decreased chemotaxis and adherence.[4] Whether these changes induce compromised immune function in pregnancy is not conclusively established. It is established, however, that pregnancy affects the coagulation pathway. Although the clotting time of whole blood is unchanged, certain coagulation factors (VII, VIII, IX, and X) are produced at increased levels, thereby shortening prothrombin and partial prothromboplastin times. As a consequence, the risk of thromboembolism in pregnancy is 1.8 fold greater than in the non-pregnant state, and further 5.5 fold in the postpartum period.[3] Finally, the platelet count decreases slightly during pregnancy, and the blood sedimentation rate is markedly elevated from increased fibrinogen levels, which is rendered almost useless as a screening test in pregnancy.

Cardiovascular Alterations. A number of fundamental cardiovascular parameters are altered by pregnancy. These changes help accommodate anatomic alterations and metabolic demands produced by uterine growth and fetal development. In this regard, heart rate, heart size, and stroke volume are increased during pregnancy, especially in its later stages; cardiac output increases by 30-50% to 6.2 L/min.[5] The increase in cardiac work is frequently accompanied by the characteristic systolic murmur of pregnancy. Arterial blood pressure and vascular resistance also decrease during normal pregnancy; the systolic blood pressure decreases 5-10 mmHg, while diastolic pressure decreases 10-15 mmHg as compared to pre-pregnancy levels.[3] A 12% increase in heart size, combined with upward displacement of the diaphragm by an enlarging uterus, produce a larger cardiac silhouette on chest x-ray. The electrocardiogram (ECG) is also affected by a shift in the heart's position, with left-axis deviation being a common finding. Finally, ST-segment and T-wave changes have been reported in 14% of normal pregnant women.[6]

Changes in a woman's posture, especially later in pregnancy, can make a significant impact on her circulatory status. Compression of the inferior vena cava and aorta by an enlarged uterus is exacerbated when the mother is supine and can produce a 25-30% decrease in cardiac output.[7] Placing the patient in the left lateral decubitus will dramatically reduce this effect. This manipulation should be considered when caring for pregnant patients, especially those restrained by cervical spine immobilization. Venous pressures below the diaphragm are normally increased during pregnancy, a finding that is exacerbated in the supine position. Increased venous pressure can cause dependent edema, venous stasis, varicose veins, and hemorrhoids.

Pulmonary. As pregnancy progresses and the uterus occupies a greater percentage of the abdominal cavity, the diaphragms are progressively elevated. A woman's thorax increases in circumference to compensate, and several baseline respiratory values are changed relative to the non-pregnant state. Tidal volume, alveolar, and minute ventilation are all increased in pregnancy. These changes are perceived by the mother, with 70% of normal, healthy women reporting symptoms of dyspnea in pregnancy.[5] Interestingly, respiratory rate and vital capacity are unchanged. Peak flow rates do not differ between pregnant and non-pregnant healthy women of matched build, even during the third trimester.[8] In general, the pregnant woman is in a state of partially compensated respiratory alkalosis during pregnancy. The PCO_2 is decreased by 10 mmHg to a "normal" pregnant range of about 30 mmHg.[9] Serum bicarbonate is decreased to the range of 18-22 mEq/L, and the "normal" pH in pregnancy is increased to 7.40-7.45.

Knowledge of these alterations in baseline values is important when evaluating blood gas measurements in pregnant women being treated for pneumonia, asthma, or diabetic ketoacidosis (DKA). As a rule, changes in respiratory status can help the mother perform more efficient gas exchange and compensate for additional fetal oxygen consumption. However, the increased gas exchange can lead to problems as well. Hypoxia, hypercarbia, or hypocarbia all occur more rapidly, especially with assisted ventilation. The added fetal oxygen demand and higher affinity of fetal hemoglobin for oxygen can also lead to significant maternal hypoxia, especially when the mother suffers from hypoventilation, regardless of the etiology.

Renal Effects. Pregnancy affects renal anatomy and kidney function in several ways. The expanding uterus compresses ureters in the second and third trimesters of pregnancy, putting the women at increased risk for hydronephrosis. The glomerular filtration rate (GFR) increases by 50% by the second trimester.[10] The increased GFR leads to a decreased level of "normal" creatinine. The normal serum creatinine level in pregnancy is 0.5-0.75 mg/dL. Accordingly, a serum creatinine higher than 1.0 mg/dL is considered abnormal in pregnancy. Drugs excreted primarily by the kidneys (i.e., aminoglycosides and magnesium sulfate) require special attention to dosing in pregnant patients. Impaired tubular reabsorption of glucose and increased GFR lead to glycosuria, which increases risk for urinary tract infection (UTI), including pyelonephritis.

Table 2. Common Asthma Triggers and How to Avoid Them

TRIGGER	AVOIDANCE
Allergy	Common allergans include dust and mold in the home. Air filtration may be helpful.
Exercise	Get plenty of exercise, but warm up before. Swimming may be preferred to other sports.
Respiratory Infections	Avoid people with colds and flu by avoiding crowded indoor areas in winter when risk of infection is high. Consider influenza and pneumococcal vaccines.
Emotional Stress	Learn to relax and breath properly during an attack. Learn coping skills and stress management techniques.
Lung Irritants	Avoid known irritants. Stay indoors when air pollution is bad. Never smoke and avoid being near smokers.
Weather	Cover mouth with a scarf on cold days.
Drugs	Avoid aspirin, NSAIDs, drugs that contain them.

Adapted from: Mawhinney H, Spector SL. Optimum management of asthma in pregnancy. *Drugs* 1986;32:178-87.

Gastrointestinal Effects. Heartburn is frequent in pregnancy. This symptom is due, in part, to hormonally induced relaxation of the esophageal sphincter and decreased gastric tone, and from higher gastric pressures caused by uterine expansion. Moreover, depressed motility of the small bowel and increased colonic absorption of water can lead to increased complaints of constipation. Cholestasis is increased in pregnancy, and this may be due to reduced contractility of the gallbladder caused by elevated progesterone. The prevalence of symptomatic cholesterol stones is increased in pregnancy, which leads to an increased incidence of cholecystitis in pregnancy. To make matters worse, common surgical disorders such as cholecystitis or appendicitis are more difficult to diagnose in the pregnant patient. In the past, the majority (about 70%) of pregnant patients with cholecystitis were successfully managed medically,[11] in large part because pregnancy was considered a contraindication to laparoscopic treatment. However, at least one recent series suggests laparoscopic intervention is safe and effective in the pregnant patient.[12] Serum albumin decreases to 3.0 g/dL and serum alkaline phosphatase increases up to 400% compared to nonpregnant levels. These changes, along with clinical findings of spider angiomata and palmar erythema caused by increased estrogen levels, may suggest the presence of liver disease, but as a rule they are normal findings in pregnancy.

Asthma

Asthma is a chronic inflammatory disorder of the airways involving many cell types. Susceptible individuals will suffer from wheezing, dyspnea, chest tightness, and coughing.[13] The overall prevalence of asthma in the United States is nearly 5% of the population.[14] Asthma affects about one of every 100 pregnant women,[15] making it the most common respiratory disorder and potentially the most serious disease complicating pregnancy.[16] The precise etiology of asthma is unknown, although genetic and environmental factors seem to be involved. *(Please see Table 2.)*[14] Extrinsic asthma is thought to be triggered by inhalation of an allergen, and is IgE-mediated. A person is labeled as having intrinsic asthma when no specific allergen can be identified.

Pregnancy alters the course of asthma in the gravid woman in the following way: One-third of pregnant patients experience improvement, one-third remain the same, and one-third experience worsening of their symptoms.[17] There is significant risk to both the mother and child with worsening of asthma symptoms. Asthma was associated with an increased perinatal mortality two times that of controls in one recent study.[18] Moreover, another study noted an increase in complications such as hyperemesis, preeclampsia, and hemorrhage in patients with asthma, as well as an increase in neonatal mortality and premature birth.[19] Encouragingly, another study found no differences in mortality when comparing pregnant asthmatic women who were treated with steroids to those without asthma.[20] These data underscore the importance of aggressive medical management of pregnant patients who present to the ED with acute exacerbations of bronchial asthma.

Pathophysiology. As mentioned previously, numerous physiologic and structural changes alter pulmonary function during pregnancy. Hyperemia, hypersecretion, and mucosal edema of the respiratory tract result from increases in circulating estrogen levels. The gravid uterus increases abdominal girth, elevates the diaphragm, and widens the costal angle.[21] Pregnant women experience an increase in tidal volume, a decrease in expiratory reserve volume, residual volume, and functional residual capacity, while vital capacity is unchanged.[22] Alveolar hyperventilation results in a decreased PCO_2 from 34-40 to 27-34 mmHg, which is typically seen by 12 weeks of gestation.[9] As might be expected, the frequency of asthma exacerbations peaks around the sixth month of gestation;[23] the most severe symptoms occur between the 24th and 36th weeks.[24]

Briefly, the pathophysiology of asthma includes the following: 1) contraction of airway smooth muscle resulting in increased airway resistance; 2) increased mucus secretion with small airway obstruction; 3) hyperinflation of the lungs with increased residual volume; and 3) bronchial hyperreactivity caused by histamine, prostaglandins, and leukotrienes. Mast cell degranulation appears to trigger the asthma cascade and results in the release of chemical mediators, which lead to increased airway resistance and bronchospasm. In the case of pregnancy, respiratory alkalosis cannot be maintained in the face of reduced ventilation, and acidosis develops. Because of the baseline changes in arterial blood gas values in pregnancy (decreased PCO_2 and increased pH), it is important to realize that a PCO_2 of 38- 40 mmHg and pH of 7.38-7.4 in a symptomatic pregnant patient is evidence that normally expected alveolar hyperventilation is no longer being maintained. A patient with these arterial blood gas values is at significant risk for maternal hypoxemia, subsequent fetal hypoxia, and respiratory failure.

Presentation. The pregnant patient presenting with an exacerbation of asthma may complain of dyspnea, productive or non-productive cough, and/or a tight chest. Symptoms tend to be worse at night and may be preceded by allergic rhinitis or a viral illness. On physical exam, the patient typically has an increased respiratory rate, a rapid pulse, and elevated blood pressure. Auscultation of the chest reveals diminished breath sounds, wheezing, rhonchi, and a prolonged expiratory phase. In addition, the patient may be utilizing accessory muscles. Recalling that "all that wheezes is not asthma," the differential diagnosis should include acute bronchitis, vocal cord dysfunction, pulmonary embolism, and congestive heart failure.[14] Although rare, peripartum cardiomyopathy can produce new onset congestive failure that is accompanied by wheezing and dyspnea. These patients often have no history of previous symptoms of heart failure and the diagnosis can be missed if not considered.

Management. Leukocyte count with differential may show eosinophilia, and pulmonary function tests consistent with an obstructive pattern may be seen. A hand-held peak flow meter may be used in place of spirometry. The chest x-ray may be normal, it may demonstrate hyperinflation, or reveal complications such as pneumonia, pneumothorax, or pneumomediastinum.[14] Clearly, the possible deleterious effects to the fetus are a concern when ordering roentgenograms in the pregnant woman. However, recent data indicate that x-ray doses used in clinical radiography (30-100 millirads for a single film) are below the level at which statistically significant increases in fetal anomalies arise (> 5 rad). Nevertheless, abdominal shielding is recommended as it reduces external scatter of radiation.[25]

Management of the pregnant asthmatic in the ED includes administration of oxygen to maintain a PaO_2 a level greater than 60 mmHg or 95% O_2 saturation. Inability to maintain PO_2 higher than 60 mmHg is an indication for intubation and for possible emergency delivery if the fetus has developed to a viable stage.[26] In all patients with significant symptoms, baseline arterial blood gases and pulse oximetry should be performed. In patients with significant symptoms and potentially viable pregnancies (gestational age > 24 weeks), fetal monitoring (ideally in the form of a continuous heart monitor) is mandatory. The presence of abnormal fetal heart patterns (heart rate > 160 bpm or < 120 bpm) require emergent obstetrical consultation. Because formal pulmonary function tests are impractical or unavailable in the ED, peak expiratory flow rates should be measured and followed for improvement. Beta-agonists such as albuterol should be administered via a nebulizer up to every 20 minutes for up to three doses. Alternatively, for patients who experience difficulty with inhaled medications, terbutaline 0.25 mg may be injected subcutaneously every 20-30 minutes as needed for a total of three doses. Epinephrine may be injected subcutaneously 0.1 mg to 0.3 mg of a 1:1,000 solution in patients who are failing initial therapy.

If the patient's peak expiratory flow rate returns to 70% of normal, she may be discharged to home. Patients with severe disease may be given a short course of oral corticosteroids (40 mg q day or 20 mg po bid for 5 days) in consultation with their obstetrician. If the peak flow is less than 70%, the patient should be hospitalized, continued on beta agonists, and methylprednisolone should be initiated at a dose of 80 mg every six hours. A peak flow rate below 25% or a PCO_2 greater than 35 mmHg is indicative of respiratory failure and warrants intensive care unit admission, and if indicated, intubation.[27] Other signs indicating the need for hospitalization include persistent tachycardia (> 120 bpm), respiratory rate higher than 30 /min, or if the patient is unable to walk unaided for short distances in the ED.

Fortunately, most pregnancies complicated by asthma are uneventful. However, poorly controlled asthma requiring inpatient admission carries an increased risk of prematurity and low birth weight.[28] Other fetal complications of uncontrolled asthma include increased risk of perinatal death, intrauterine growth retardation, preterm birth, and low birth weight.[16] In addition, uncontrolled asthma and maternal hypoxia may result in fetal hypoxia. Conditions associated with uncontrolled asthma such as hypertension, hypocapnia, alkalosis, and dehydration may reduce uteroplacental blood flow, thereby further reducing fetal oxygenation.[29]

Management of asthma during pregnancy with the possible exception of oral steroid therapy, does not differ significantly from that of the nonpregnant population.[14] The mainstay of prophylaxis is inhaled corticosteroids. In one study, inhaled steroids resulted in a 75% reduction of asthma exacerbations compared to the control group.[30] Rescue therapy still requires a beta-agonist. Additional therapies, among them, cromolyn, nedocromil, long-active beta-2 agonists, theophylline, leukotriene antagonists, and ipratropium bromide, have been used without evidence of adverse outcomes on pregnancy.[14] Although steroids may be used in severe cases, one study found these agents may increase the risk of preeclampsia.[31] While routinely used for outpatient treatment of non-pregnant patients, use of oral steroids should not be initiated for outpatient management without discussing this treatment plan with the patient's obstetrician. ED physicians must be cautious when prescribing medications in the pregnant patient. As a rule, pregnant patients are concerned about potential, drug-related effects on their baby and look to their obstetrician for approval before taking medications. Accordingly, the ED physician should not hesitate to contact the patient's obstetrician for advice on medications. Disposition from the ED should include educating the patient about avoiding potential asthma triggers such as allergens, exercise, infection, emotional stress, lung irritants, weather changes, and certain medications.[15]

Hypertension

Hypertension is one of the most common complications of gestation, affecting almost 10% of all pregnancies in the United States.[32] Fetal complications include intrauterine growth retardation, fetal death in utero, and premature delivery. Adverse maternal outcomes, which are similar to those in the non-gravid population, include stroke, heart disease, and renal failure.[33] Worldwide, hypertensive disorders are responsible for 15-20% of maternal deaths.[33]

Although pregnancy is characterized by an increase in cardiac output and expanded blood volume,[34] the gravid woman undergoes such marked vasodilatation that the mean arterial pressure typically falls by approximately 10 mmHg.[35] As seen in Table 1, the definition of hypertension in pregnancy is a blood pressure higher than 140/90 mmHg. The American College of Obstetricians and Gynecologists (ACOG) has classified hypertensive disorders into four broad categories: preeclampsia-eclampsia; chronic hypertension; chronic hypertension with superimposed preeclampsia; and transient hypertension.[36] Table 3 lists precise definitions of each of these four types of hypertension encountered in pregnancy.

Preeclampsia. The clinical hallmark of preeclampsia includes the classic triad of hypertension, edema, and proteinuria.[32] In preeclampsia, elevated blood pressure is defined as a systolic blood pressure increase of 30 or more mmHg over average readings which were obtained before 20 weeks gestation, or an increase of 15 mmHg or greater in diastolic blood pressure compared to early or pregestation measurements. If baseline pressures are not known, a systolic blood pressure of 140 mmHg or a diastolic blood pressure of 90 mmHg is sufficient to meet the criteria for preeclampsia. This classification scheme defines proteinuria as 30 mg per dL, ("1+") on a dipstick urine, or greater than 300 mg in a 24-hour urine collection. Edema is defined as 1+ pedal edema that fails to resolve with rest; facial or hand edema; or weight gain exceeding 2 kg in a one-week period.[32]

Risk factors associated with preeclampsia include nulliparity, extremes of reproductive age, a family or personal history of preeclampsia, a previous diagnosis of hypertension, renal disease, diabetes mellitus, multiple gestations, hydatidiform mole, and hydrops fetalis.[32,37]

The etiology of preeclampsia is currently debated. One theory proposes that preeclampsia is related to defective implantation of the placenta with subsequent placental hypoperfusion.[38] The placenta releases substances that, in turn, induce the vascular endothelium to produce procoagulants, vasoconstrictors, and mitogens.[38] Pathologic changes seen in the brain, heart, and liver of patients with preeclampsia mimic the changes seen in hypovolemia, indicating that hypoperfusion rather than hypertensive vascular injury may be responsible for the clinical finding in preeclampsia.[37,39] Other theories include imbalances of prostacyclin and thrombaxane, immunologic abnormalities, increased vascular reactivity to vasoactive agents, and genetic variations of the angiotensinogen gene. To date, no one theory has been proven conclusively.[38]

Maternal complications of preeclampsia include convulsions, cerebral hemorrhage, placental abruption with disseminated intravascular coagulopathy, pulmonary edema, renal failure, liver hemorrhage, and death.[40] The HELLP Syndrome (hemolysis, elevated liver enzymes, and low platelet count) may occur with hepatic ischemia and intravascular coagulation.[41] Complications of preeclampsia are the second leading cause of maternal death in pregnancies beyond 20 weeks.[42] In the fetus, pre-eclampsia may cause growth retardation, hypoxemia, acidosis, prematurity, and death.[40]

In addition to the classic triad of hypertension, edema, and proteinuria, the preeclamptic patient may present with a multitude of constitutional signs and symptoms. She may have visual changes, tinnitus, headache, tachycardia, nausea, vomiting, hematemesis, and oliguria.[41] On physical exam, the blood pressure should be noted and compared to pregestational or early gestation measurements. The blood pressure should also be measured in the sitting position after five minutes of rest.[43] In addition to maternal vital signs, the fetus should be monitored for signs of distress. Other findings on physical exam may include hyperreflexia, diplopia, hepatomegaly, and edema.[41]

Table 3. Classification of Hypertension During Pregnancy

Chronic Hypertension: Hypertension (BP > 140/90 mmHg) that is present and observable before pregnancy or that is diagnosed before the 20th week of gestation. Hypertension diagnosed for the first time during pregnancy and persisting beyond the 42nd day postpartum.

Preeclampsia-eclampsia: Increased blood pressure accompanied by proteinuria, edema, or both, which usually occur after 20 weeks gestation (or earlier with trophoblastic diseases such as hydatidiform mole or hydrops).

PREECLAMPSIA SUPERIMPOSED

On Chronic Hypertension: Chronic hypertension (defined above) with increase in blood pressure (30 mmHg systolic, 15 mmHg diastolic, or 20 mmHg mean arterial pressure) together with the appearance of proteinuria or generalized edema.

Transient Hypertension: The development of elevated blood pressure during pregnancy or in the first 24 hours postpartum without other signs of preeclampsia or preexisting hypertension (a retrospective diagnosis).

Adapted from: National High Blood Pressure Education Program Working Group Report on High Blood Pressure in Pregnancy. *Am J Obstet Gynecol* 1990:163(5 Pt 1):1691-1712.

Multiple laboratory findings are associated with preeclampsia, although there is no single test that serves as a reliable early indicator. Uric acid levels are typically elevated (greater than or equal to 5 mg per dL). A complete blood count (CBC) may be useful for detecting thrombocytopenia. The hematocrit increases with preeclampsia, but may actually decline if hemolysis develops. A peripheral smear may demonstrate schistocytes. Other supporting labs include an elevated lactate dehydrogenase level, an elevated transaminase level, a rising serum creatinine, hypoalbuminemia, and prolonged prothrombin and activated partial thromboplastin time.[44]

When possible and appropriate, definitive and curative therapy for preeclampsia is delivery of the fetus.[37] Consequently, any ED patient in whom preeclampsia is considered a possible diagnosis will require urgent obstetrical consultation. Specific indications for delivery include imminent eclampsia, multiorgan dysfunction, fetal distress, or gestational age beyond 34 weeks.[45] Some researchers have described protocols for expectant management of the preeclamptic patient at less than 34 weeks of gestation.[40]

Other therapies that should be initiated in the ED include blood pressure control and careful monitoring of fluid status. Parenteral hydralazine has traditionally been used in pregnancy and is considered safe and effective for management of preeclampsia.[46] A 5 mg bolus of hydralazine is initiated followed by 5-10 mg every 20-30 minutes to achieve a goal systolic pressure of 130-150 mmHg and a diastolic pressure of 90-100 mmHg.[32, 47] If hydralazine is ineffective, a second agent may be required. Labetalol or nitroprusside may be used. Angiotensin-converting enzyme (ACE) inhibitors should not be used in pregnancy because serious fetal side effects (i.e., renal damage) are possible. Fluid intake should be limited to 100 cc per hour.

If pulmonary edema or oliguria develops, a pulmonary artery catheter may be placed to monitor hemodynamic status.[32]

Although a comprehensive discussion outlining management of eclampsia is beyond the scope of this review, seizure prophylaxis is an integral part of preeclampsia management.[48] Magnesium sulfate is the drug of choice, a loading regimen consisting of a 6 gram bolus given over 30 minutes, followed by 2 grams per hour continuous infusion is recommended.[40] The serum target range for magnesium is a level of 4-7 mEq/L (from a baseline of around 2 mEq/L).

Exceeding this target range will put the woman at serious risk for magnesium toxicity so levels should be monitored closely. Clinical findings of toxicity include loss of deep tendon reflexes (around 10 mEq/L) and, ultimately, respiratory depression and cardiac arrest (> 13 mEq/L). Because the magnesium ion functions as a weak calcium channel blocker, the treatment for magnesium "overdose" is 1 gram of calcium gluconate IV over 2 minutes. Because delivery of the fetus is frequently the definitive treatment for the preeclamptic woman, consultation with an obstetrician is critical and should be initiated early in the patient's care.

Chronic Hypertension. Chronic hypertension in pregnancy may be diagnosed if the patient has a history of hypertension before pregnancy, has persistently elevated blood pressures greater than or equal to 140/90 mmHg before 20 weeks gestation, or persistent hypertension beyond 42 days postpartum.[37] Chronic hypertension complicates approximately 2-5% of all pregnancies.[31] The cardiovascular changes of pregnancy have been described earlier. Peripheral vasodilatation may lead to a drop in blood pressure during pregnancy, thus masking hypertension in a patient previously diagnosed with this condition. Between 15% and 20% of chronic hypertensives will develop superimposed preeclampsia, which is diagnosed by quantitative urine protein measurement, assessing for edema, and monitoring previously mentioned labs. Patients with chronic hypertension carry a three-fold increased risk for placental abruption and subsequent maternal hemorrhage.[49] In patients with superimposed renal insufficiency, there is a higher incidence of preeclampsia, preterm delivery, and fetal growth retardation.[50] Fetal complications include fetal growth restriction, as well as higher mortality rates, primarily due to the increased incidence of superimposed preeclampsia.[33, 51]

Chronic hypertension usually is detected from routine vital signs, although the patient with severe hypertension may present with signs and symptoms attributable to end organ damage. The differential diagnosis includes preeclampsia, superimposed preeclampsia, and secondary hypertension. The most common forms of secondary hypertension are the result of renal disease, renovascular disease, hyperaldosteronism, Cushing's syndrome, and pheochromocytoma.[33]

When evaluating a pregnant patient with chronic hypertension, several physical findings and laboratory tests may direct the course of therapy. The physical exam should include appropriate blood pressure measurements as previously described, a fundoscopic examination, chest auscultation, and a survey for renal artery bruits. Coarctation of the aorta is a rare but potentially serious problem that needs to be considered in this patient population.[52] Laboratory tests should include a metabolic panel to assess renal function and glucose. Persistently elevated serum glucose with fluctuating blood pressure warrants an assay for urine vanillylmandelic acid and metanephrines to rule out pheochromocytoma. Urinalysis should be performed to assess for proteinuria. A 24-hour urine collection may be necessary to measure creatinine clearance. A chest x-ray and electrocardiogram may be necessary if heart failure is suspected.[52]

When deciding whether to treat elevated blood pressure, the emergency physician must evaluate and weigh the maternal risks vs. fetal risks of drug exposure. Consultation with the patient's obstetrician is advised to assist in making this decision. Current guidelines recommend treatment if the diastolic blood pressure exceeds or equals 100 mmHg. If renal disease or other end organ damage is present, then treatment should be initiated if the diastolic pressure is 90 mmHg.[32] The most widely used antihypertensive drugs for pregnant patients are methyldopa and hydralazine. Once the maximum dose of methyldopa (4 grams per day) and hydralazine (400 mg per day) have been reached, a third agent may be added. Labetalol, atenolol, and nifedipine are recommended options.[52] Propranolol, thiazide diuretics, and angiotensin converting enzyme inhibitors should not be used due to potential adverse maternal and fetal side-effect profiles.[53]

Pneumonia

Pneumonia is the most common non-obstetric infectious cause of death during pregnancy and the puerperium.[54] In the pre-antibiotic era, maternal mortality due to pneumonia was as high as 32%,[55] but use of antibiotics has reduced this rate to as low as 3.5%.[56] However, immunocompromised states associated with HIV, the increased incidence of drug use, and postponed childbearing may be contributing to the recent increase in the number of cases of pneumonia complicating pregnancy.[57]

While the frequency of pneumonia in the pregnant patient is similar to that in the nongravid population, multiple respiratory, physiological, and mechanical changes, along with alterations in cellular immunity, make the gravid woman more susceptible to pulmonary insults.[57] As discussed previously, the gravid uterus elevates the diaphragm and widens the costal angle. An increase in the transverse diameter of the chest makes clearing respiratory secretions more difficult and further aggravates airway obstruction from pulmonary infections.[58] Diminished functional residual capacity associated with pregnancy is accompanied by a 20% increase in oxygen consumption that makes brief periods of hypoxia difficult to tolerate.[59] Immunologically, there is a diminished lymphocyte proliferation response, decreased natural killer cell activity, and decreased numbers of helper T-cells.[60] While these changes in immunity do not necessarily place the pregnant woman at greater risk for infection, they may make viral and fungal pneumonias more virulent.[61]

Pathophysiology. Pathogens causing pneumonia in pregnant women are similar to those encountered in the general population. Two-thirds are bacterial in nature, with *Streptococcus pneumoniae* being the most common organism.[61] Patients typically present with complaints of fever, chills, pleuritic chest pain, cough productive of purulent or blood-tinged sputum, and dyspnea. [57] On physical exam, the patient may have dullness to percussion, tactile fremitus, and egophany. [61] Adjunctive tests include a complete blood count with differential, a chest x-ray, sputum gram stain with culture, and blood cultures. [57] The second most common bacterial pathogen is *Haemophilus influenza*. This gram-negative bacillus is more likely to occur in patients with chronic illness, smokers, and in patients with influenza infection.

Klebsiella pneumoniae may develop in immunocompromised patients and cause abscess formation. *Staphylococcus aureus* is a potential pathogen when the patient is recovering from influenza.[61]. Atypical organisms, such as *Mycoplasma, Legionella*, and *Chlamydia* cause pneumonias which have a gradual onset with antecedent myalgias, headaches, and low grade fevers. The cough is more non-productive, but sputum produced may be more mucoid than purulent. Chest x-ray demonstrates interstitial patchy infiltrates rather than lobar consolidation. Adjunctive tests include complete blood count, serum cold agglutinins, and titers for suspected pathogens.[57]

The most common viral pneumonia is influenza, typically type A.[61] The patient may complain of malaise, headache, fever, chills, cough, and other upper respiratory symptoms.[61] The physical examination may not elicit typical findings of pneumonia. Adjunctive tests include a chest x-ray, which may show a unilateral patchy infiltrate.[61] Of potential concern is the development of bacterial superinfection with *Staphylococcus aureus, Haemophilus influenzae, pneumococcus*, or gram-negative organisms.[61] In addition to influenza, *varicella* is a potential etiologic agent in pneumonia in the gravid patient. In fact, pneumonia more often complicates *varicella* infection in pregnant patients as compared to the general population.[62] It occurs most frequently during the third trimester and develops approximately five days after the appearance of the typical rash of varicella. In addition to the skin lesions, the patient may present with oral lesions, dyspnea, cough, pleurisy, and malaise. The chest x-ray may demonstrate patchy infiltrates.[61]

Other potential pathogens include *Pneumocystis carinii, Mycobacterium, Cryptococcus, Coccidioides immitis,* and *Blastomycoses. Pneumocystis carinii* pneumonia (PCP) is the principal cause of pregnancy-associated AIDS death in the United States.[61] Patients with PCP may present with fever, tachypnea, dyspnea, and nonproductive cough. Adjunctive tests include an arterial blood gas which shows a decrease in PO_2 and respiratory alkalosis, and a chest x-ray which demonstrates bilateral alveolar disease. Sputum silver stains are diagnostic.[61] While uncommon, varicella pneumonia carries grave risk for both mother and child, with a maternal mortality reported to be as high as 35%.[3] The key to the diagnosis is appearance of pneumonia symptoms 2-5 days after the onset of varicella fever and rash. Because of the high potential for mortality, any pregnant woman with varicella pneumonia requires hospitalization and treatment with acyclovir.[57]

Management. Pregnant patients presenting to the ED with respiratory complaints should have a thorough history, including immunization history and documentation of previous immunity to *varicella*. The social history should address habits such as smoking, alcohol abuse, drug abuse, high-risk sexual behaviors, occupational history, and travel history.[57] The medical history should address chronic medical conditions, including heart disease, asthma, bronchitis/pneumonia, anemia, and immunocompromising conditions such as HIV, hemoglobinopathies, renal disease, and advanced age. The practitioner should also ascertain whether the patient is undergoing chemotherapy or taking other immunosuppressive agents.[57]

The differential diagnosis of upper respiratory complaints in the gravid female includes dyspnea of pregnancy, pneumonia, bronchitis, asthma, pulmonary embolism, pneumothorax, pulmonary edema, congestive heart failure, and hyperventilation. Management of the patient includes antimicrobials as indicated, as well as supportive care and careful monitoring of maternal and fetal health. Obstetrical consultation is advised for each of these steps. Pre-term labor has been reported in women with pneumonia. While disagreement continues to persist regarding the need for hospitalization, some authors would recommend inpatient admission for all pregnant women with a radiographically confirmed pneumonia.[63] Given the fact that leading researchers recommend parenteral antibiotics, hospitalization becomes a logical choice for patient care.[57] Other factors to guide one's decision to admit include severity of illness and comorbid factors. Certainly, no pregnant women with pneumonia should be sent home without consulting her obstetrician.

Bacterial pneumonia, as well as viral pneumonia complicated by bacterial superinfection, should be treated with correct spectrum antibiotics. A second- or third-generation cephalosporin, combined with erythromycin or intravenous azithromycin, will cover most anticipated pathogens as well as atypical organisms. Gram-negative and anaerobic coverage using an aminoglycoside or clindamycin, respectively, may be added as clinically indicated.[57] Penicillins, cephalosporins, erythromycin, azithromycin, and clindamycin have no known harmful effects on the fetus. However, gentamicin poses a risk of ototoxicity and nephrotoxicity to both the mother and the fetus.[64] A beta-lactam with a beta-lactamase inhibitor, third-generation cephalosporin, or an anti-pseudomonal antimicrobial may be added for nosocomial pneumonias.[64]

Published reports have described use of amantadine and ribavirin for treatment of influenza pneumonia, with successful outcomes and no evidence of teratogeny.[65] Pregnant patients with PCP should be treated with trimethoprim-sulfamethoxazole, a category "C" drug. (See section on drugs in pregnancy on page 69).

Because trimethoprim is a folic acid antagonist, folate supplementation should be given. Sulfamethoxazole has the potential to cause kernicterus if given near the time of delivery.[61]

Supportive measures include supplemental oxygen, chest physiotherapy, and beta agonist breathing treatments if reactive airway disease is also present. The head of the bed should be elevated, and positional changes should be encouraged. Adequate control of fever is also recommended. Beyond 24 weeks gestation, the fetus should be continuously monitored. Maternal fluid status and electrolytes should be followed closely, and intubation should be performed as clinically indicated. Delivery should occur for obstetric purposes only.[57]

Maternal outcomes have improved dramatically since the aggressive use of antibiotics. Complications in the gravid female are similar to those of the general population, including respiratory distress necessitating intubation, empyema, and pneumothorax. Comorbid illness and underlying risk factors may dictate severity of disease and subsequent complications.[61] Similarly, poor fetal outcomes are associated with comorbid medical illness in the mother. Premature labor and fetal death have been documented as complications of maternal pneumonia with a frequency ranging from 4% to 44%.[61] These data do not account for the unknown effects of specific microorganisms, medications, fever, and hypoxia.

Deep Venous Thrombosis

Venous thromboembolism (VTE) is another leading cause of maternal morbidity and mortality in pregnancy, accounting for 14% of all maternal deaths from 1980-1985.[66] VTE is five times more likely to occur during pregnancy when compared to a nonpregnant woman of similar age,[67] with some authors suggesting VTE occurs in 1 in 1000 to 1 in 2000 pregnancies.[67] Evidence suggests that VTE is more likely to occur postpartum than in the antepartum period, and that the risk is higher in patients who have undergone cesarean section vs. vaginal delivery.[68] Other risk factors for VTE include history of VTE, instrumentation during delivery, bedrest, obesity, advanced maternal age, multiparity, and blood abnormalities. These include presence of antiphospholipid antibody, activated protein C resistance, antithrombin III deficiency, myeloproliferative disorders, paroxysmal nocturnal hemoglobinemia, deficiency of protein C or protein S, homocystinemia, hyperprothrombinemia, and dysfibrinogenemia.[69]

Pregnancy is a risk factor for venous thrombosis, as each element of Virchow's triad (stasis, endothelial damage, and hypercoagulability) is present.[67] Physiologic increases in venous distensibility and capacitance lead to increased stasis, which is exacerbated by compression of pelvic vessels. Endothelial damage occurs during delivery, as the placenta separates, or during surgery. Hypercoaguability in pregnancy is caused by an increased concentration of coagulation factors, especially factors II, VII, X, and fibrin. *(Please see Table 4.)* Concomitantly, there is a decrease in protein S, a coagulation inhibitor. This is accompanied by inhibition of the fibrinolytic system, which is greatest during the third trimester.[67]

Pregnant patients who present to the ED with suspected DVT may complain of leg discomfort and ankle swelling, which are also encountered as part of pregnancy. Accordingly, one should inquire about risk factors. On physical exam, the affected lower extremity may be tender and swollen with a 2 cm increased circumference relative to the unaffected limb.[70] DVT usually begins in the deep proximal veins and has a predilection for the left leg during pregnancy.[71] Homan's sign is present in less than one-third of patients with DVT.[67] Other signs suggestive of DVT include a palpable cord, change in limb color, or cool extremities.[70]

Diagnosis. The differential diagnosis for DVT includes a number of musculoskeletal disorders, as well as superficial thrombophlebitis, impaired venous or lymphatic flow, and Baker's cyst. [67] Because pregnant patients are at increased risk for DVT and because this diagnosis is virtually impossible to confirm from a history and physical alone, any pregnant patient with complaints suggestive of a DVT should have an imaging study performed. Noninvasive imaging such as duplex Doppler scanning is the preferred initial test for the diagnosis of DVT. When performed by an experienced practitioner, sensitivity approaches 98% for detecting symptomatic calf or proximal DVT with a 95% specificity.[72] Iliac vessels may be difficult to visualize in the presence of a gravid uterus, so comparison with the unaffected leg is useful. Repeating the Doppler exam in 2-3 days has also proven useful for detecting thrombi not previously visualized.[70] Impedance plethysmography (IPG) has a sensitivity of 95% and specificity of 98% for detecting proximal vein thrombi.[73] IPG records changes in electrical resistance caused by venous volume changes in the involved limb.[70]

Venography has been the standard against which other imaging studies are evaluated for their usefulness in detecting DVT. Nevertheless, the majority of physicians prefer duplex Doppler scanning for obvious reasons. Venography is a technically difficult, invasive exam associated with potential side effects from the contrast dye, such as pain, swelling, tenderness, and erythema;[70] these symptoms can simulate the presence of a DVT. In addition, DVT may be a complication of venography. And while duplex Doppler scanning and IPG are considered safe to maternal and fetal health, venography carries small, but potential risks associated with radiation exposure to both the mother and the fetus.[70] However, it should be stressed that the amount of radiation required for routine venography has not been associated with adverse fetal outcomes.[67]

From a practical, radiation exposure perspective, venogram of one extremity exposes the fetus to 0.3 rad; exposure to the fetus of less than 5 rad has not been associated with fetal abnormalities. Advantages of venography include the ability to detect calf and proximal iliac clots, which may be missed by Doppler study. Most experts recommend either serial Doppler study or venography in a woman with an initially negative Doppler and a high clinical suspicion of DVT.[67-70] Serial Doppler studies are typically performed 2-7 days following the initial exam. Proponents of this approach argue that this will prevent pregnant women from getting potentially unnecessary antigcoagulation; the disadvantage is that a patient with a DVT may have treatment withheld until a second study yields the diagnosis.

Table 4. Guidelines for Anticoagulation in Pregnancy

PREGNANT:

1. Baseline lab values: CBC, PT, PTT.
2. Heparin loading dose: 80 U/kg (or 5000 U) IV bolus.
3. Continuous heparin infusion of 1300 U/hr for DVT and 1500 U/hr for PE.
4. Check PTT every 6 hours and adjust infusion to maintain PTT between 1.5 and 2.5 times the patient's baseline.
5. Rebolus with 5000 U heparin if PTT is not prolonged and increase rate of infusion.
6. Repeat PTT every 6 hours for first 24 hours, then check daily unless outside of therapeutic range.
7. Check platelets every day or every other day for first 10 days of heparin to monitor for heparin-induced thrombocytopenia.

POSTPARTUM:

Heparin therapy as above including:

1. Begin warfarin (Coumadin) therapy on the first day of heparin treatment at 5 mg to 10 mg daily.
2. Check the PT daily and adjust dose to maintain INR between 2.0 and 3.0.
3. Stop heparin after INR of 2.0 to 3.0 is reached for 4 to 7 consecutive days.
4. Continue oral anticoagulation for 3 months to maintain INR of 2.0 to 3.0.

Adapted from: Rutherford SE, Phelan JP. Deep venous thrombosis and pulmonary embolism in pregnancy. *Obstet Gynecol Clin North Am* 1991;18:345-370.

Pulmonary Embolism

When evaluating a pregnant patient for DVT, the diagnosis of PE should also be considered. The classic symptoms of PE include shortness of breath and pleuritic chest pain. Additional symptoms include cough and hemoptysis. On physical exam, the patient may appear tachypneic and apprehensive. Chest auscultation may reveal crackles, an increased pulmonic second heart sound, and a pleural friction rub. The differential diagnosis includes asthma, dyspnea of pregnancy, pneumonia, bronchitis, pulmonary edema, congestive heart failure, and pneumothorax. Although a discussion of diagnostic testing for PE follows, some clinicians argue that in some situations treatment without a confirmed diagnosis of PE may be acceptable. In other words, a patient with chest pain who has newly diagnosed DVT may be assumed to have a pulmonary embolism and managed clinically without additional testing.

Usually, however, adjunctive testing will be necessary to make the diagnosis of PE, as well as to rule out other causes of dyspnea. The arterial blood gas (ABG) may reveal a diminished PO_2 of more than 85 mmHg, or widened alveolar-arterial gradient (> 20 mmHg). While up to 20% of patients with PE will have normal ABG readings (20% have a PO_2 > 80 mmHg), a much smaller percentage will have a normal A-a gradient.[74] During the third trimester, the ABG should be obtained in the sitting position, as the PO_2 may be lowered by as much as 15 mmHg when obtained from the patient in the supine position.[67] As pregnancy changes the baseline pulmonary physiology, ABG testing may be even more important in "sicker" patients to obtain data on their oxygenation and carbon dioxide retention. In contrast, ABG screening may not be necessary in healthy appearing patients in whom PE simply needs to be "ruled out"; these patients can proceed directly to VQ scan.

The most common abnormality noted on electrocardiogram is tachycardia; however, right axis shift, T-wave inversion, and the classic $S_1Q_3T_3$ pattern, though rare, may be present.[70] A shielded chest x-ray is necessary to rule out pneumonia and pulmonary edema, and can also be used to interpret ventilation-perfusion (VQ) scans if performed. Nonspecific abnormalities such as atelectasis, pleural effusion, and elevation of the hemidiaphragm may be present in up to 80% of patients.[67] Lastly, although D-dimer levels may be sensitive for diagnosis of PE in non-pregnant patients, their use in pregnant patients has not been evaluated.

The most important screening test for PE in the pregnant patient is the VQ scan. A high probability scan is sufficient to warrant treatment.[69] A normal or near normal scan excludes the diagnosis of PE. Unfortunately, most patients with a PE have a VQ scan interpreted as low or intermediate probability for PE. These patients must then undergo the more invasive pulmonary angiography. Patients should be reassured that the amount of radiation exposure from the combined chest x-ray, VQ scan, and angiography is less than the amount of exposure associated with adverse fetal outcomes.[67] Disadvantages of VQ scan include the time required for the test (2-3 hours) and the potential difficulty of obtaining the test in a timely manner during the middle of the night. Chest CT scan is another alternative to the VQ scan, but specific data in pregnant patients are lacking compared to non-pregnant populations.

The issue of additional radiation exposure from chest CT is also of concern. Advantages however, include the fact that CT is usually easier to obtain than a VQ scan and takes much less time to perform. Newer technology of helical CT, and CT angiography are even more accurate that standard CT scan but still may miss more distal (smaller) emboli. The accuracy of CT angiography also depends on the quality of the bolus contrast injection. More information about the use of CT scanning for the diagnosis of PE can be found in a recent review.[75] Radiation exposure can be of concern to expectant mothers undergoing testing in the ED, and one can reassure the patient that VQ scans are considered safe in pregnancy.[76] Exposure to less than 5 rad per year is considered safe in humans, and a chest CT will expose the patient to between 2 and 5 rad. For reference, an abdominal film will expose the patient to between 0.9 rad and 2.2 rad, depending on the size of the patient. New generation CT scans have very focused beams with minimal scatter, and shielding of the abdomen during the study will protect the fetus from nearly all radiation exposure.

Management. A pregnant patient with suspected pulmonary embolism or a clinically evident DVT warrants hospitalization, anticoagulation, and supportive care in consultation with the patient's obstetrician.[67] Supplemental oxygen should be provided to reverse hypoxia and maintain a PO_2 of more than 60 mmHg. Intubation criteria are similar to those given for asthma, with intubation indicated for inability to maintain adequate fetal oxygenation (i.e., PO_2 of < 60 mmHg) or for uncontrolled rising maternal PCO_2. Patients with hypercapnia and obtundation may require intubation with mechanical ventilation. Fluid resuscitation and pressors such as dopamine may be required to maintain adequate blood pressure (systolic pressure > 80 mmHg), with the realization that uterine blood flow may be compromised. Narcotic analgesics should not be withheld.[67]

Only pregnant patients with life-threatening manifestations of PE (i.e., a large PE with hypoxia and hypotension) should be treated with a fibrinolytic agent such as tissue plasminogen activator.[68,77] There are currently no data on the risk of placental abruption or potential injury to the fetus. These agents are contraindicated post partum secondary to bleeding complications. Other contraindications include recent surgery, bleeding disorders, and marked hypertension.[69] Emergency thoracotomy and embolectomy may be beneficial as a last-ditch effort for critically ill patients, but this procedure is beyond the purview of most ED physicians. It should be stressed, however, that when a pregnant patient near term (> 34-36 weeks) does arrest, emergency C-section offers the only chance of survival for the fetus and greatly increases the effectiveness of CPR in the mother.

Anticoagulation for DVT and/or PE should be initiated with heparin, generally adhering to the same recommendations as for non-pregnant patients. Heparin is relatively safe during pregnancy as it does not cross the placenta. Some studies have been done evaluating heparin in pregnancy that support its safety.[68,70] An initial bolus of 80 units/kg is followed by a continuous infusion of 18 units/kg of heparin per hour intravenously. The activated partial thromboplastin time (aPTT) is measured every six hours for the first two days of therapy, and adjustments in heparin infusion are made to keep the aPTT between 1.5 and 2.5 times the patient's baseline.

After 5-7 days of intravenous heparin, therapy throughout the remainder of pregnancy consists of 2-3 subcutaneous injections of heparin daily, with dosing being adjusted based on the aPTT. Subcutaneous heparin should be discontinued with the onset of regular uterine contractions. Protamine sulfate may be administered if the aPTT is greater than 2.7 times the control. Thrombocytopenia is a well-known side effect of heparin administration, and therefore a baseline platelet count is necessary. Platelet counts should be monitored daily or every other day during the first 10 days of therapy.[79] Up to one-third of women on long-term heparin therapy suffer from reduction in bone density.[68]

Low molecular weight heparin (LMWH) has proven to be effective in preventing and treating DVT, and has been used in at least one small study of six women; no complications were reported and effective DVT prevention was confirmed in these patients.[80] A more extensive study is required to establish safety of LMWH use in pregnant patients. However, in support of LMWH use, data indicate that it does not cross the placenta; LMWH has less heparin-induced thrombocytopenia, and in the case of enoxaparin, can be given as a once-daily injection. Oral warfarin therapy may be initiated safely in the postpartum period, but not during pregnancy.[67] Warfarin is a known teratogen, causing nasal hypoplasia, stippled epiphyses, and central nervous system abnormalities. In addition, because warfarin crosses the placenta, the fetus is at increased risk of neonatal hemorrhage during delivery.[68] A final option for treatment is a Greenfield filter. Use of this filter has been reported in pregnant patients to prevent PE.[81] Newer, removable filters are being tested currently in non-pregnant patients and may provide treatment alternatives in the future.[82]

Urinary Tract Infection

Pathophysiology. The three most common forms of urinary tract infections in pregnant women can be characterized as asymptomatic bacteriuria, cystitis, and pyelonephritis. While most urinary tract infections in pregnancy are asymptomatic, it should be stressed that maternal and fetal complications can occur in the absence of symptoms. Furthermore, normal physiologic changes of pregnancy increase the maternal risk for development of pyelonephritis and its associated complications. As early as the seventh week of gestation, dilation of the renal pelvis and ureters occurs, resulting in hydroureter, which progresses until term.[83] The right collecting system is affected more than the left because of to the drop of the right ureter into the pelvic cavity.[84]

Throughout gestation, the kidneys increase in length by one centimeter, and the bladder changes position, becoming an abdominal rather than a pelvic organ.[85] Elevated progesterone levels facilitate smooth muscle relaxation, resulting in bladder expansion and diminished ureteral peristalsis.[86] There are also data to suggest that the physiologic and anatomic effects of estrogens in pregnancy may increase the virulence of *E. coli*.[87] Diminished renal concentrating ability may decrease the natural antibacterial properties of urine.[83] Other risk factors for urinary tract infections in pregnancy include a history of recurrent urinary tract infections, an anatomic abnormality in the urinary tract, neurogenic bladder, diabetes mellitus, lower socioeconomic status, multiparity, sexual intercourse, and sickle cell trait.[88]

Organisms causing urinary tract infection are derived from normal perineal flora and affect both pregnant and nonpregnant patients. Most organisms grown in culture are coliforms, with *E. coli* being the most common, followed by *Klebsiella* and *Enterobacter* species, as well as *Proteus mirabilis*.[89] Occasional gram-positive organisms have been isolated.[88] Recent data demonstrate uropathogenic strains of *E. coli* which predominate in pregnant women.[90]

Asymptomatic Bacteriuria. Asymptomatic bacteriuria is defined as persistent bacterial colonization of the urinary tract without urinary tract symptomatology.[86] The prevalence of asymptomatic bacteriuria is 5-10%, which is the same for pregnant and nonpregnant women.[91] The gravid woman with bacteriuria, however, is at increased risk for developing pyelonephritis. This complication occurs in up to 20-30% of untreated gravid women.[86] In addition, asymptomatic bacteriuria has been associated with preterm delivery and low birth weight.[86] Diagnosis is typically confirmed by detection of greater than 100,000 colony-forming units of a single organism per milliliter of urine on culture, although some authors also recommend treatment with lower colony counts (20,000-50,000).[92] Gram staining is reported to be the best, most rapid screening test available with a 90% sensitivity and 88% specificity rate, but it can be technician dependent.[93] In many obstetric offices, urine cultures are typically the diagnostic test of choice, inasmuch as a routine urinalysis is inadequate to diagnose infection of the urinary tract during pregnancy.[94] Newer, rapid-culture techniques have been advocated, but none have become widely accepted as good screening tests.[86] In the ED, it is recommended that physicians use a catheterized specimen to help guide treatment. Cultures can be sent, but only they are of practical value if follow-up on culture results is obtained. Many EDs have personnel dedicated to this task, but another option is to communicate with the patient's obstetrician that tests have been sent to assure follow-up. Treatment of asymptomatic bacteriuria is essentially the same as that for cystitis.

Cystitis. Cystitis presents as dysuria, hematuria, urinary frequency, urgency, and suprapubic discomfort; a positive urine culture with absence of pyelonephritis symptoms is characteristic.[86] Cystitis complicates 0.3-1.3% of pregnancies.[95] Because many of the symptoms of cystitis can be encountered in pregnancy without the presence of infection, the urine culture remains the gold standard for diagnosis.[86] As mentioned above, ED physicians should rely on a urinalysis by catheterization in combination with clinical symptoms to diagnose cystitis in these patients. Pathogens isolated in cystitis are similar to those recovered in asymptomatic bacteriuria.[95] However, a patient with symptoms of cystitis and a "sterile" urine culture should be evaluated and/or treated for *Chlamydia trachomatis* infection. A single dose of 1 gram of azithromycin has been shown to be effective for uncomplicated *Chlamydia* infection in pregnancy.

Much effort has been focused on evaluating single dose therapy vs. three-day and 7- to 10-day courses of antibiotics for asymptomatic bacteriuria and cystitis. Approximately 70-80% of patients have elimination of bacteriuria after 7-10 days of antibiotics. The efficacy rates are similar for three-day courses of antimicrobials[88] or single-dose treatment. Although single dose therapy has showed promising results, some authors recommend further study to evaluate this treatment duration.[86,96] Regardless of length of therapy, appropriate follow up to document eradication of bacteriuria is essential.[88]

Historically, ampicillin and amoxicillin have been used because they have proven safe in pregnancy and achieve high urinary concentrations. However, ampicillin resistance to *Escherichia coli* has approached 30% in the United States.[97] Cephalexin 250 mg to 500 mg four times daily for 3-7 days has been advocated. Cephalexin costs around $0.60 per 250 mg, but resistance to *Enterococcus* can be up to 90%.[98] Cephalosporins along with penicillin have a well-documented risk of anaphylaxis. Nitrofurantoin 100 mg four times daily has extensive use during pregnancy but poses a risk of hemolytic anemia in patients with glucose-6-phospate dehydrogenase deficiency. In addition, nitrofurantoin costs around $1.50 per 100 mg and resistance of up to 20% by organisms causing cystitis has been reported.[99] Sulfisoxazole 500 mg, four times daily is another option but should be avoided near term secondary to risks of hyperbilirubinemia. Trimethoprim is relatively contraindicated in the first trimester due to its antifolate properties.[86,88] Trimethoprim/sulfisoxazole costs roughly $0.40 per tablet and resistance has been reported to be in the 30% range.[99] As bacterial resistance can vary by geographic region, becoming educated about resistance rates reported in one's area of practice is advised.

A follow-up urine culture should be performed one week following therapy for asymptomatic bacteriuria or cystitis. Approximately 20-30% of pregnant patients will have another positive urine culture requiring an additional 7-10 days of therapy with a different antibiotic. A second treatment failure would require adjunctive testing for a structural abnormality.[88] Eradication of a persistent or recurrent infection may require suppressive dosing throughout the remainder of pregnancy.[88] Unlike asymptomatic bacteriuria, there are no data to suggest cystitis increases the risk of preterm delivery and low birth weight.[86]

Pyelonephritis. Acute pyelonephritis complicates 1-2% of all pregnancies. It is more common after midpregnancy and occurs unilaterally in more than 50% of cases; the right side is affected more than the left. The infectious agent usually ascends from the lower urinary tract and contains p-fimbriae adhesins in 75-90% of cases.[100] Widespread screening and treatment of asymptomatic bacteriuria has led to a dramatic decline in the incidence of pyelonephritis from 4% to approximately 1%.[95] In addition to cystitis-like symptoms, patients with pyelonephritis may present with fever, chills, flank pain, nausea, and vomiting.

On physical examination, there is often costovertebral angle tenderness. A striking aspect of fever in these patients is its labile nature, with fevers as high as 107°F, rapidly followed by hypothermia (down to 93°F).[101] These findings are thought to result from bacterial endotoxins. Adjunctive tests include urinalysis and urine culture. Presumptive diagnosis must be made, however, without the urine culture as results take 24 hours and emergent treatment is indicated. One to two bacteria per high power field in an unspun urine specimen, or 20 bacteria per high power field in a spun urine specimen correlates with 100,000 colony-forming units per milliliter on urine culture. White cell casts confirm the diagnosis but are not always present. Blood cultures are not always indicated, as isolated organisms are typically the same as in the urine culture.[86]

Nearly all pregnant patients with pyelonephritis are dehydrated because of fever and emesis; therefore, fluid resuscitation should be initiated. A subset of patients will develop sepsis syndrome with diminished cardiac output despite adequate fluid resuscitation, and vasopressors may be required. Endotoxins, which alter the alveolar-capillary permeability membrane, may lead to pulmonary edema and respiratory insufficiency in 2-8% of pregnant patients with pyelonephritis.[102] Patients with this complication are typically tachypneic, tachycardiac, and febrile. Arterial blood gas will reveal hypoxemia, and the chest x-ray will show pulmonary edema and, possibly, adult respiratory distress syndrome. Fluid overload and the use of tocolytics worsen this clinical scenario. Careful monitoring of fluid balance and supplemental oxygen should be instituted. Respiratory distress requires intubation and mechanical ventilation to prevent fetal hypoxia.[86]

Another complication of antepartum pyelonephritis is renal dysfunction. It is usually transient, occurs in 25% of cases, and resolves over several days.[86] Serum creatinine levels should be monitored and nephrotoxic antibiotics should be avoided or adjusted appropriately.[86] Pyelonephritis may be associated with preterm delivery and low birth weight, but the strength of such an association is not confirmed.[86] Most clinical symptoms resolve after the first two days of therapy. Urine cultures typically become sterile within 24 hours of initiating antibiotics. Nevertheless, 30-40% of patients suffer relapse or reinfection. Monthly urine cultures may be indicated to prevent recurrence of pyelonephritis. In addition, suppressive therapy with nitrofurantoin, 100 mg each night, may prevent recurrent disease.[92]

Traditionally, the gravid woman with pyelonephritis has been admitted to the hospital for parenteral antibiotics, supportive care, and monitoring. This practice has been called into question over the last several years, with some studies advocating outpatient treatment for selected patients.[103] A randomized, controlled trial demonstrated that outpatients receiving intramuscular ceftriaxone and inpatients receiving intravenous cefazolin had similar rates of persistent or recurrent bacteriuria and recurrent pyelonephritis.[86] Nevertheless, currently established therapy consists of intravenous antibiotics continued 1-2 days after the patient is afebrile, followed by a one- to two-week course of oral antibiotics. As with ampicillin, first-generation cephalosporins are compromised by an increasing antimicrobial resistance rate. Consequently, the addition of an aminoglycoside to ampicillin or a third-generation cephalosporin has been advocated. Many physicians question the role of aminoglycoside therapy due to concerns of maternal nephrotoxicity and fetal ototoxicity.[86] Clinical trials have demonstrated the efficacy of ceftriaxone, which is preferable due to its once-daily dosing, monotherapeutic efficacy, and safety profile.[104]

Diabetes Mellitus

Approximately 3-5% of all pregnancies are complicated by diabetes mellitus (DM). Most of these cases are attributed to gestational diabetes, while a half percent are secondary to previously diagnosed Type I and Type II diabetes mellitus.[105] Type I diabetes (insulin dependent) is usually diagnosed before the age of 30 and is characterized by a deficiency of insulin. Type II diabetics are typically older than 40 years old and overweight. Their disease process involves peripheral resistance to insulin, increased hepatic production of glucose, and a relative pancreatic insufficiency of insulin production.[106] Even though these patients typically do not require insulin, all diabetics are "brittle" during pregnancy and therefore, Type II diabetics should be converted to an insulin regimen during pregnancy. Another form of diabetes occurs secondary to various medical disorders.[107] Most obstetricians follow the White Classification of diabetes in pregnancy. This classification describes the severity of diabetes and its manifestations.[108] *(Please see Table 5.)*

The increased insulin resistance in pregnancy is due, in part, to secretion of human placental lactogen and placental growth hormone.[107] Patients using insulin before pregnancy may note a doubling of their insulin requirements during pregnancy. In addition, elevated levels of circulating estrogen, progesterone, and prolactin may diminish peripheral sensitivity to insulin during pregnancy.[109] Other complicating factors include increased body weight, increased fat deposition, higher caloric intake, and diminished physical activity, all of which decrease insulin sensitivity during a "normal" pregnancy.[107] However, in patients with Type I diabetes, hypoglycemic reactions are common during the first trimester.

Table 5. White Classification of Diabetes in Pregnancy

CLASS	DESCRIPTION
A	Abnormal glucose tolerance test, but asymptomatic or normal glucose achieved with diet control
B	Adult-onset diabetes (> age 20 yr) and short disease duration
C	Youth-onset diabetes (age 1-19 yr) or relatively long disease duration (10 to 19 years)
D	Childhood onset (< age 10 yr), very long disease duration (> 20 yr), or evidence of background retinopathy
E	Any diabetes with evidence of vascular disease in the pelvis (diagnosed by plain films)
F	Any diabetes with the presence of renal disease
R	Any diabetes with the presence of proliferative retinopathy
RF	Any diabetes with both renal disease and proliferative retinopathy
G	Any diabetes with a previous history of multiple pregnancy losses
H	Any diabetes with atherosclerotic heart disease
T	Any diabetes postrenal transplantation

Adapted from: Hare JW. Gestational diabetes and the White Classification. *Diabetes Care* 1980;3:394.

In gestational diabetes, the increased demand for insulin cannot be met by endogenous production. The onset of gestational diabetes (or at least its recognition) occurs during pregnancy in patients without previous diagnosis of Type I or Type II diabetes.[110] Overall, gestational diabetes is 10 times more common than Type I and Type II diabetes combined.[107] Risk factors for gestational diabetes include history of a previous pregnancy complicated by gestational diabetes, a history of large-for-gestational-age infant, obesity, age older than 30 years, and a family history of Type II diabetes. In addition, certain ethnic groups, including Native Americans, African Americans, and Hispanic Americans, are at increased risk for developing gestational diabetes.[107] Furthermore, up to half of all patients with gestational diabetes will develop Type II diabetes later in life.[105] The American College of Obstetrics and Gynecology recommends that all pregnant women between 24 and 28 weeks gestational age be screened for diabetes.

Fetal Effects

Poor glycemic control during pregnancy is linked to fetal complications, as well as to poor maternal outcomes. Perhaps the most well known complication is fetal macrosomia. Maternal hyperglycemia leads to fetal hyperglycemia secondary to passive diffusion of nutrients across the placenta. Excessive fetal insulin production then causes increased fetal fat deposition.[111] Macrosomia increases the risk of birth asphyxia, shoulder dystocia, brachial plexus injury, fracture of the clavicles and humerus, and increases the need for forceps delivery and cesarean section.[107] Between 30% and 50% of neonates born to diabetic mothers will go on to develop neonatal hypoglycemia (serum glucose less than 40 mg/dL) secondary to elevated endogenous insulin levels and abrupt discontinuation of maternal nutrient supply.[112] Other neonatal complications include respiratory distress syndrome, neonatal hypocalcemia, and hyperbilirubinemia, all of which are linked to poor glycemic control.[107]

Congenital malformations occur at 2-4 times the expected frequency in diabetic mothers, especially in those with poor glycemic control at conception and throughout the first trimester.[113] Consequently, most of these birth defects are seen in Type I and Type II diabetics rather than in patients with gestational diabetes. The most common anomalies are ventricular and atrial septal defects, transposition of the great vessels, neural tube defects, gastrointestinal atresias, and urinary tract malformations.[107] In addition, there is an association between first trimester spontaneous abortion and diabetic pregnancies.[104] The mechanism for these complications is unclear, but may be related to hyperosmolality, ketosis, disruption of glycolysis, DNA glycosylation, oxygen free radicals, cell membrane lipid peroxidation, and inhibition of growth factors.[107]

Maternal Effect

Other medical complications of pregnancy appear to be more common in diabetics. Pre-term labor may be seen in up to 30% of diabetic pregnancies.[115] Hypertensive disorders, including preeclampsia and eclampsia also are more common in diabetes, especially in pregestational diabetics who may already have vasculopathies and renal insufficiency.[107] ED physicians are frequently the first clinicians to diagnose diabetes, and a high-risk obstetric team should be consulted when this occurs. Unfortunately, many of the birth defects described occur so early in pregnancy that complications may have already developed by the time pregnancy is diagnosed. Nevertheless, encouraging strict glycemic control can improve long-term outcomes.

Regardless of the presenting symptom, a careful history should be obtained, including last menstrual period, obstetric history, gynecologic history, medical history, medications and diet. Glucometer readings should be assessed, and the review of systems should identify any illness which may worsen glycemic control. On physical examination, vital signs must be reviewed, and the patient's mental status addressed, since fluctuations in serum glucose may alter sensorium. Fetal heart tones should be assessed, and careful documentation of the fundal height and uterine size recorded, given the propensity for macrosomia. Laboratory studies should include a serum glucose and other appropriate tests depending on the presenting complaint. If DKA is suspected, serum ketones should be drawn, and an arterial blood gas performed to evaluate acid-base status.[105]

Diabetic Ketoacidosis

As might be expected, insulin-dependent pregnant patients are at higher risk for DKA, which complicates about 2% of pregnancies in insulin-dependent patients.[116] Although maternal mortality is low, fetal mortality ranges from 50% to 90% in DKA.[117] Patients without diabetes often become ketotic during early pregnancy as a result of hyperemesis gravidarum, and hyperemesis is often a trigger for DKA. It should be stressed that the "normal" pH of pregnancy is mild alkatosis, so the patient in DKA may have a pH of near 7.40 but still be in DKA. Also, a pregnant patient is defined as hyperglycemic with a serum glucose reading of only 200 mg/dL. Thus, the criteria for diagnosis of DKA in pregnancy are much more strict than in a non-pregnant patient. In general, DKA is treated with ICU admission, insulin, fluids, and volume monitoring. However, fetal heart rate monitoring is recommended starting at gestational age of 12 weeks, and beyond 24 weeks continuous fetal and uterine monitoring are advised. Although uterine contractions are commonly seen in DKA, they ordinarily do not result in delivery if the pregnancy is not near term. Therefore, tocolytic drugs should not be used without evidence of significant cervical dilation.

Disposition

The criteria for admission of pregnant patients with complications of diabetes should be emphasized. Hyperemesis gravidarum predisposes pregnant patients with diabetes to DKA and significant risk of fetal death. If a patient is unable to eat and drink adequately, the possibility of hypoglycemia should be considered. Consequently, any pregnant diabetic with hyperemesis should be admitted. As in non-diabetics, significant ketosis increases the risk of neurologic defects in the fetus. Any pregnant diabetic who cannot clear their ketosis with IV fluids in the ED should also be admitted. As many of the congenital defects seen in the children of diabetics arise from derangements in organogenesis (first trimester), diagnosis of pregnancy in a diabetic patient who is not under adequate glycemic control (abnormal serum glucose is > 200 mg/dL) should also be considered for admission. As diabetic pregnancies are, by definition, high-risk pregnancies, the ED physician should consult obstetric colleagues when caring for these patients. Many centers have a high-risk team to care for pregnant diabetics, which includes primary providers, endocrinologists, nutritionists, and social workers. Contact with consultants should be done to assure follow-up any time pregnant diabetics present to the ED and are discharged. Finally, educating diabetic patients about their disease process, including preconception counseling, is critical to improving both maternal and fetal outcomes.

Human Immunodeficiency Virus

An unfortunate reality of the HIV epidemic is infection in the pregnant woman. Nearly 25% of cases of acquired immunodeficiency syndrome (AIDS) occur in women, of which 85% are in their childbearing years.[118,119] To make matters worse, many HIV-infected women are unaware of their serostatus.[120] Vertical transmission of the virus occurs in 25-59% of deliveries if the mother is untreated.[111] This type of transmission of the HIV virus accounts for around 1800 HIV-infected babies born each year in the United States.[121] Accordingly, perinatal transmission accounts for the majority of HIV-1 infections among U.S. children.[122]

One of the relevant questions concerning vertical transmission is: How is the virus passed from mother to child? The bottom line is that although all of the risk factors are not thoroughly understood, a lower CD4 count and higher viral load in the mother increase the risk of viral transmission.

Several aspects of precipitous deliveries in HIV-positive mothers are relevant to emergency practice. For example, episiotomies and use of scalp electrodes in routine deliveries should be avoided in the ED setting unless clinically indicated, as they may play a role in transmission of the virus. Likewise, breast feeding in known HIV-positive mothers also should be avoided. Zidovudine (AZT)

Table 6. Recommended Prophylactic Regimens for Pregnancy in HIV Patients

ALL PATIENTS:
- Pneumococcal vaccine (0.5 mL IM as a one time dose)
- Yearly influenza vaccine (0.5 mL IM)
- Isoniazid for patients with positive TB test, TB history, or chest x-ray evidence of previous TB (300 mg po daily for 12 months)

PATIENTS WITH CD4 COUNT < 200 MM³:
- Trimethoprim/sulfamethoxazole for *pneumocystis carinii* pneumonia (1 single strength po daily)

PATIENTS WITH CD4 COUNT < 50 MM³:
- Azithromycin for *Mycobacterium avium* complex (1200 mg po weekly)

treatment in pregnancy has been shown to reduce rates of vertical transmission from 25% to only 8%.[123] Although relatively little data are available, use of AZT in pregnancy has not been associated with any specific congenital abnormalities. Therefore, all pregnant women seen in the ED with HIV infection not already taking AZT should be encouraged to discuss AZT use with their OB-GYN.

Often a patient will be seen in the ED, and their HIV status will be in question. There are several clinical presentations that should alert the ED physician to consider HIV infection. Recurrent sinusitis, bronchitis, or pneumonia in an otherwise young, healthy patient is one presentation. Unexplained weight loss or fever, herpes zoster, nonhealing genital ulcers, oral thrush, and chronic vaginal candidiasis are all known to be associated with HIV infection as well. Abnormal blood cell counts such as neutropenia or thrombocytopenia also raise the possibility of HIV infection. HIV screening tests should be offered to all pregnant women, although the test need not necessarily be ordered in the ED. When an HIV test is ordered in the ED, it is useful to notify the OB consultant who will be following the patient. The ED physician also should be aware that in 1993, the CDC expanded the definition of AIDS to include the following: CD4 count higher than 200/mm³ (or < 14% total lymphocytes), pulmonary tuberculosis, recurrent bacterial pneumonia (> 1 episode in 1 year), and invasive cervical cancer. Pregnant patients presenting with any of the above scenarios should also be evaluated for HIV infection.

When a pregnancy is confirmed in an HIV-positive woman in the ED, or in a patient strongly suspected of having HIV, the following maternal screening tests should be ordered: CD4 count, assay for viral load, CBC, liver function tests, tuberculin skin testing, chest x-ray, serology for toxoplasmosis and cytomegalovirus, as well as testing for other sexually transmitted diseases. Pap smears should also be done as there is an increased incidence of cervical dysplasia in HIV-positive patients. The ED physician should also be aware of the currently recommended prophylactic regimens for pregnant HIV-positive patients. *(Please see Table 6.)*

As mentioned above, it is recommended that all HIV-positive, pregnant patients take AZT for prophylaxis against transmission of the virus to their child. When a pregnant patient presents to the ED in labor, and is known to be HIV infected, the following additional steps are recommended. If the patient is in active labor or has had spontaneous rupture of membranes, and the patient is not enrolled in a clinical trial, the patient should be given AZT in a 2 mg/kg bolus dose followed with a 1 mg/kg/hr continuous infusion. Amniotomy, episiotomy, and scalp electrodes should not be routinely used unless clinically indicated to limit the exposure of the baby to maternal secretions. Obviously, urgent consultation with obstetric colleagues is mandatory. Lastly, infection with HIV also predisposes the mother to greater morbidity and mortality from common bacterial infections associated with childbirth and the postpartum period. Many authors recommend routine use of prophylactic antibiotics for childbirth in HIV-positive patients; as HIV treatments change frequently, the obstetric consultant should be asked for guidelines in this area.

Table 7. Disorders that May Present as Hyperemesis Gravidarum

CAUSES OF INCREASED VOMITING ASSOCIATED WITH PREGNANCY
- Hydatidaform mole
- Multiple gestations
- Pregnancy-induced hypertension
- Placental abruption

CAUSES OF VOMITING NOT ASSOCIATED WITH PREGNANCY
- Appendicitis
- Cholelithiasis
- Pancreatitis
- Hepatitis
- Thyrotoxicosis
- Bowel obstruction
- Peptic ulcers
- Diabetic ketoacidosis
- Increased intracranial pressure
- Pyelonephritis
- Medications

Adapted from: Hod M, Orvieto R, Kaplan B, et al. Hyperemesis gravidarum: A review. *J Reprod Med* 1994;39:605-612; Cosmas JM. Nausea and vomiting in early pregnancy. In: Pearlman MD, Tintinalli JE, (eds). *Emergency Care of the Woman.* New York: McGraw Hill; 1998:49-56.

Hyperemesis Gravidarum

While not a condition of non-pregnant women, nausea and vomiting of pregnancy and hyperemesis gravidarum affect a large number of pregnant women and generate many ED visits. Nausea and vomiting of pregnancy is characterized by the typical "morning sickness" seen early in pregnancy, but also affects some women more in the afternoon or evening than the morning. It complicates 50-90% of all pregnancies.[124] Although reoccurring daily in many cases, this type of vomiting is normally self-limited. Less commonly, intermittent vomiting will persist throughout a pregnancy.

Nausea and vomiting of pregnancy begins around the 4th to 6th week of gestation, peaks around week 8 to 12, and usually ends around the 20th week. In contrast, vomiting of hyperemesis is pro-

Table 8. Drugs Considered Safe in Pregnancy[151]

PAIN MEDICATIONS
- Acetaminophen
- Propoxyphene (Darvocet)
- Codeine—can lead to addiction and newborn withdrawal if used excessively

ASTHMA MEDICATIONS
- Theophylline
- Terbutaline
- Cromolyn Sodium
- Beta-adrenergic agonists (albuterol, isoproterenol, metaproterenol)
- Corticosteroids—do cross the placenta, inhaled to a much lesser degree

ANTIBIOTICS
- Penicillins
- Cephalosporins (except cefaclor, cephalexin and cephradine)[152]
- Sulfonamides (except in 3rd trimester)
- Sulfamethoxazole/trimethoprim (controversial in 1st trimester)
- Nitrofurantoin (Macrodantin—will not treat bacteremia)
- Antituberculosis drugs
- Erythromycin (except erythromycin esto- late Ilosone)
- Clindamycin

ANTIVIRALS
- Acyclovir
- Zidovudine (AZT)

ANTIFUNGALS
- Imidazoles (clotrimazole or miconazole — except in 1st trimester)

ANTICOAGULANTS
- Heparin (data with low molecular weight heparin are limited)

ANTICONVULSANTS
- Phenytoin, valproic acid, and carbamazepine are all associated with defined malformation syndromes but many physicians feel benefits for the mother outweigh risks to the fetus. Do not prescribe without OB or neurologist recommendation.

ANTIEMETICS*
- Promethazine (Phenegran)
- Proclorperazine (Compazine)
  *Stress other remedies first (crackers in a.m., frequent small meals, etc.)
- Ginger (shown better than placebo)
- Metoclopramide (Reglan)

DECONGESTANTS*
- Diphenhydramine (Benadryl)
  *Nasal sprays absorbed less than po medications

ANTIHYPERTENSIVES
- Methyldopa (Aldomet)
- Hydralazine (Apresoline)
- Atenolol (Tenormin)

GASTROINTESTINAL DRUGS
- H2 blockers:
  - Ranitidine (Zantac)
  - Famotidine (Pepcid)
- Sucralfate (Carafate)

ANTIDEPRESSANTS
- Amitriptyline (Elavil)
- Fluoxetine (Prozac)

WOUND CARE
- Lidocaine

longed and intractable, and is associated with dehydration, ketonemia, electrolyte abnormalities, metabolic alkalosis, and weight loss of 5-10% of the patient's pre-pregnancy weight. Compared to nausea and vomiting of pregnancy, hyperemesis affects only 2% of pregnancies.[125] Even though not as many patients are affected, the majority of them require multiple ED visits and admissions during the course of the pregnancy. One study found a readmission rate of 27% in 140 women with diagnosis of hyperemesis.[126]

Risk factors reported for hyperemesis include multiple gestations, previous spontaneous miscarriage, and history of hyperemesis.[127] Hyperemesis also occurs more frequently in first pregnancies. Because nausea and vomiting of pregnancy are self-limiting and rarely require intervention other than rehydration, reassurance, and advice on avoiding nausea, this section will focus on a discussion of hyperemesis gravidarum.

Etiology. Many factors have been suggested and investigated as a cause of hyperemesis, but to date no clear mechanism has been elucidated. Beta-hCG levels and other hormonal factors, as well as metabolic, toxic, and psychosocial factors have all been proposed as contributing factors in many cases. Beta-hCG levels have been suggested as a cause of hyperemesis, as the incidence is higher in patients with multiple gestations and molar pregnancies. One author found 26% of patients with molar pregnancies also had hyperemesis.[128] In addition, the peak of nausea and vomiting roughly coincides with peak levels of beta-hCG in the 6th to 12th week of pregnancy. Despite these facts, comparisons of measured beta-hCG levels in patients with and without hyperemesis yield conflicting results. Some authors report a correlation,[129] while others do not.[130]

Levels of other hormones, including cortisol, estrogens, progesterone, prolactin, growth hormone, and follicle stimulating hormone, have been evaluated and do not show any abnormal levels in patients with hyperemesis.[127] Up to 66% of patients with hyperemesis will have evidence of increased thyroid function,[131] with some exhibiting transient clinical thyrotoxicosis. It appears that beta-hCG itself causes the increase in T4 in these patients,[132] although the significance of this finding is not yet clear. In addition, many women with hyperemesis also have an acquired vitamin B6 deficiency.[133] Again the significance of this fact in the cause and effect relationship of hyperemesis remains unclear. One recent article suggested a possible link between presence of *H. pylori* infection and hyperemesis; treatment of the infection resulted in resolution of symptoms.[134] Lastly, psychological factors including immaturity, chemical dependency, depression, and hysteria have all been suggested as causative factors. As with other theories, the disagreement in the literature on the relationship of psychological factors and hyperemesis remains today. The most recent articles suggest they play a role, but are not causative.[135]

Diagnosis. Patients with hyperemesis will have clinical signs of dehydration. Dry mucus membranes, poor skin turgor, and orthostatic signs and symptoms are often present. Along with these findings, they often have a variety of electrolyte and laboratory abnormalities. These include elevated hematocrit, elevated blood urea nitrogen (BUN), hyponatremia, hypokalemia, ketonuria or ketonemia, and metabolic alkalosis with paradoxical aciduria. Accordingly, appropriate lab tests in patients suspected of hyperemesis include a CBC, serum electrolytes, BUN, creatinine, urinalysis, and serum ketones. Mild changes in liver enzymes and bilirubin may also be found in some patients.

There are many disease states which, initially, can present in a similar fashion to hyperemesis, and therefore, can lead to misdiagnosis. Hence, diagnosis of hyperemesis in the ED can be considered one of exclusion. Table 7 provides a list of conditions that should be considered in the differential diagnosis of hyperemesis. Although the association with twins, molar pregnancies, and hyperemesis is well known, it is easy to overlook these as an underlying cause. The presence of a molar pregnancy carries a risk for the mother and making the diagnosis early can reduce this risk. An abnormally high beta-hCG for a particular stage of pregnancy can be a clue that one of these conditions is present, but an ultrasound will be needed to rule them out.

Many gastrointestinal disorders also can be confused with hyperemesis. As pain is not often a part of hyperemesis, any right upper or lower quadrant pain should prompt an evaluation for cholecystitis or appendicitis. Additional laboratory tests should be ordered in patients in whom pancreatitis or hepatitis is considered. As stated above, hyperemesis can produce mild elevations in liver enzymes but not the dramatic elevations as typically seen in acute hepatitis. Likewise, amylase and lipase may be slightly elevated in hyperemesis but not to the degree typically seen in acute pancreatitis. Although transient thyrotoxicosis may be seen in hyperemesis, any patient with these findings will require admission to ensure it is indeed transient. Any diabetic patient with symptoms of hyperemesis needs admission as DKA and hypoglycemia are common complications. Lastly, many medications are associated with vomiting and the patient should be asked about use of such medications, including non-prescription use.

Management. When treating ED patients with hyperemesis, the focus should be on rehydration, correcting electrolyte imbalances, and if possible, diminishing vomiting. Unless the patient has only minimal electrolyte changes, urinary ketones that can be cleared while in the ED, can hold down po liquids, and has good OB follow-up, she will likely be admitted. General admission criteria include: weight loss of more than 10% of pre-pregnancy level, persistent vomiting when NPO, inability to correct elec-

Table 9. Drugs to Avoid in Pregnancy[151]

DRUG	UNTOWARD EFFECTS
Asprin	Increases bleeding risk at delivery, decreased uterine contractility, no teratogenic effects
NSAIDs	Chronic use may lead to oligohydramnios or neonatal pulmonary hypertension, best to avoid use
Selected Cephalosporins:	
Cefaclor, Cephalexin, Cephradine	Associated with possible teratogenic effects[152]
Tetracyclines	Discolor teeth
Aminoglycosides	Ototoxicity when taken in first trimester
Quinolones	Bind to cartilage and bone, consequences are debated
Metronidazole (Flagyl)	Effects in humans at normal doses are debated
Lindane	A neurotoxin with toxicity noted primarily in overexposure
Antiseizure Drugs:	
Phenytoin, valproic acid Carbamazepine	All associated with defined malformation syndromes—do not prescribe without OB or neurologist recommendation
ACE inhibitors	Renal failure, oligohydramnios, limb and craniofacial deformities
Lithium	Congenital heart disease (Ebstein anomaly)
Warfarin (Coumadin)	Congenital fetal defects
Propranolol (Inderal)	Generally considered safe, may be associated with low birth weight
Terfenadine (Seldane)	Polydactyly
Phenylpropanolamine (Entex LA)	Increased risk of birth defects
Pseudoephedrine (Sudafed)	Increased risk of gastroschisis
Cimetidine (Tagamet)	Possible antiandorgenic effects in fetus
Benzodiazipines	Possible fetal syndrome similar to fetal alcohol syndrome
Oral Contraceptives	Possible cardiac defects in fetus when used in 1st trimester
Isotrentinoin (Accuatane)	Associated with multiple birth defects, spontaneous abortion
Propylthiouracil (PTU)	Induces fetal goiter
Oral hypoglycemics	Cross placenta and induce fetal hypoglycemia
Recreational Drugs:	
Tobacco	Increased prematurity, fetal growth retardation
Alcohol	Fetal alcohol syndrome
Cocaine	Increased spontaneous abortions, placental abruption, preterm labor and microcephaly

trolyte abnormalities, and uncertainty of the diagnosis of hyperemesis.[136]

Regardless of whether the patient is admitted or not, initial rehydration with IV fluids should be started early. At least one author suggests that rehydration and correction of electrolytes is more important and more helpful in controlling a patient's vomiting than use of medications for nausea.[127] An initial bolus of up to 40 mL/kg of 5% dextrose in either lactated Ringer's or normal saline should be started. These patients often require up to 5 liters of fluid for initial rehydration.[136] Nothing should be given by mouth until dehydration and electrolyte disturbances have been corrected. If this can be done without admission, then small amounts of clear liquids can be initiated.

Many antiemetics can be safely used in pregnancy, and these can be helpful as adjunctive therapy for intractable vomiting. *(Please see Table 8)*. Promethazine (Phenergan), prochlorperazine (Compazine), metoclopramide (Reglan), trimethobenzamide (Tigan), diphenhydramine (Benadryl), and dimenhydrinate (Dramamine) in standard doses have all been used to treat either nausea and vomiting of pregnancy or hyperemesis without any known side effects or fetal risk.[136,137] One recent study found intravenous ondansetron was not effective in treatment of hyperemesis.[138] Several others have reported success using oral methyprednisolone, and one found it more effective than Phenergan.[139,140]

Because many patients are at risk for reoccurrence of vomiting, the following suggestions may be helpful. Patients should eat smaller, more frequent meals and avoiding strong odors, high-fat content foods, and sweet drinks. Patients can also be reassured that the presence of nausea and vomiting early in pregnancy is generally associated with improved pregnancy outcome. Lower incidence of spontaneous miscarriage and perinatal mortality is reported for women who suffer from increased nausea and vomiting early in pregnancy.[141,142] However, there are reports of a higher proportion of low birth weight infants born to women with the diagnosis of hyperemesis.[143] Another study found that intrauterine growth restriction correlated with a weight loss of more than 5% of the mother's pre-pregnancy weight.[144]

Rare and unusual complications of hyperemesis have been reported, and can require emergency intervention. These complications include Wernike's encephalopathy from thiamine deficiency, upper GI bleeding from ulcers or Mallory-Weiss tears, retinal hemorrhage, coagulopathies from vitamin K deficiency, aspiration pneumonia, rhabdomyolysis, and renal or hepatic damage.[145-147] Similarly, some patients will require more aggressive treatment due to continued inability to tolerate po intake. Use of Dobhoff feeding tubes, total parenteral nutrition, percutaneous feeding tubes, and elective termination of the pregnancy have all been reported.[148-150]

Drugs in Pregnancy

Treating pregnant patients in the ED can be stressful if the ED physician is not aware of which drugs can and cannot be safely used in pregnant patients. Although specific drug therapies have been discussed under the appropriate disease states above, this section will provide a brief overview of drug treatment in pregnancy and concentrate on drugs that are recommended for specific conditions, as well as drugs that are known to be associated with fetal or maternal complications. Before discussing specific drugs, a review of the Food and Drug Administration categories of drug labeling for use in pregnancy is helpful.

It should be stressed that the majority of data concerning drug use in human pregnancy is anecdotal, as actual drug testing cannot be ethically performed on pregnant women. Therefore, many drugs that are considered "safe" are so because they have been used for many years without apparent effect. Pregnant patients should always be informed that, as a rule, it is best to avoid drug use in pregnancy, since long-term side effects may not be apparent for many years to come. However, they should not be deterred from using drugs that are needed to treat potentially dangerous conditions (i.e., antibiotics in cystitis), and patients should be reassured that many drugs (i.e., acetomenophen) have been used for years without any known side effects.

Category A. Controlled studies in women fail to demonstrate a risk to the fetus, and the possibility of fetal harm appears remote.

Category B. No evidence exists of risk for humans. Animal studies do not indicate a risk to the fetus, there are no controlled human studies, or animal studies do shown an adverse effect on the fetus, but well-controlled studies in pregnant women have failed to demonstrate a risk to the fetus.

Category C. Use may cause risk to the fetus. Studies have shown the drug to have animal teratogenic or embryocidal effects, but no controlled studies in women are available. Potential benefit of use may outweigh potential harm.

Category D. Positive evidence of human fetal risk exists, but in certain situations (e.g., life-threatening situations or serious diseases for which safer drugs cannot be used or are ineffective) use of the drug may outweigh potential risks.

Category X. Studies in animals or humans have demonstrated fetal abnormalities, or evidence demonstrates fetal risk based on human experience, or both, and the risk clearly outweighs any possible benefit.

Table 9 summarizes commonly used drugs and emphasizes their recommendations for use in pregnant patients.

References

1. Fertility of American Women. Washington, DC: Fertility Statistics Branch, Bureau of the Census, U.S. Gov. Printing Office, 1994;20-482.
2. Ramoska E, Sacchetti A, Nepp M. Reliability of patient history in determining the possibility of pregnancy. *Ann Emerg Med* 1989;18:48-50.
3. Hansen WF, Hansen AR. Problems in pregnancy. In: Tintinalli JE, Ruiz E, Krome RL, eds: *Emergency Medicine: A Comprehensive Study Guide*, 4th Ed. New York, McGraw-Hill; 1996:564-575.
4. Krause PJ, Ingardia CJ, Pontius LT, et al. Host defense during pregnancy: Neutrophil chemotaxis and adherence. *Am J Obstet Gynecol* 1987;157:274-280.
5. Barclay ML. Critical physiologic alterations in pregnancy. In: Burrow GN & Duffy TP, eds: Pearlman MD, Tintinalli JE, eds. *Emergency Care of the Woman*. New York: McGraw Hill; 1998:303-312.
6. Oram S, Holt M. Innocent depression of the ST segment and flattening of the T-wave during pregnancy. *J Obstet Gynecol Br Commonw* 1961;68:765-770.
7. Ueland K, Novy MJ, Petersen EN, et al. Maternal cardiovascular dynamics: IV. The influence of gestational age on the maternal cardiovascular response to posture and exercise. *Am J Obstet Gynecol* 1969;104:856-864.
8. Brancazio LR, Laifer SA, Schwartz T. Peak expiratory flow rate in normal pregnancy. *Obstet Gynecol* 1997;89:383-386.

9. Martinez FG. Pulmonary disorders during pregnancy. In: Pearlman MD, Tintinalli JE, eds. *Emergency Care of the Woman*. New York: McGraw Hill; 1998:191-227.
10. Dunlop W. Serial changes in renal haemodynamics during normal human pregnancy. *Br J Obstet Gynaecol* 1981;88: 1-9.
11. Landers D, Carmona R, Crombleholme W, et al. Acute cholecystitis in pregnancy. *Obstet Gynecol* 1987;69:131-133.
12. Elderin SC. Laparoscopic cholecystectomy in pregnancy. *Am J Surg* 1993;165:625-627.
13. National Heart, Lung, and Blood Institute. National Institutes of Health International Consensus report on diagnosis and management of asthma. Bethesda:1992.
14. Terr AI. Asthma and reproductive medicine. *Obstet Gynecol Surg* 1998;53:699-707.
15. Mawhinney H, Spector SL. Optimum management of asthma in pregnancy. *Drugs* 1986;32:178-187.
16. Luskin AT. An overview of the recommendations of the Working Group on Asthma and Pregnancy. *J Allergy Clin Immunol* 1999;103:S350-S353.
17. Juniper EF, Newhouse MT. Effect of pregnancy on asthma: A systematic review and meta-analysis. In: Schatz M, Zeiger RS, Claman HC, eds. *Asthma and Immunological Diseases in Pregnancy and Early Infancy*. New York: Marcel Dekker; 1993:401-427.
18. Greenberger PA, Patterson R. Beclomethasone diproprionate for severe asthma during pregnancy. *Ann Intern Med* 1983; 98:478-480.
19. Bahna SL, Bjerkedal T. The course and outcome of pregnancy in women with bronchial asthma. *Act Allergol* 1972;27:397-406.
20. Schatz M, Patterson R, Zeitz S, et al. Corticosteroid therapy for the pregnant asthmatic patient. *JAMA* 1975;233:804-807.
21. Elkus R, Popovich J. Respiratory physiology in pregnancy. *Clin Chest Med* 1992;13:555-565.
22. Cugell D, Frank N, Gaensler E, et al. Pulmonary function in pregnancy: Serial observations in normal women. *Am Rev Tuberc* 1953;67:568-597.
23. Gluck JC, Gluck PA. The effects of pregnancy on asthma: A prospective study. *Ann Allergy* 1976;37:164-168.
24. Schatz M, Harden K, Forsythe A, et al. The course of asthma during pregnancy, postpartum and with successive pregnancies: A prospective analysis. *J Allergy Clin Immunol* 1988;81:509-517.
25. Brent RL. The effect of embryonic and fetal exposure to x-ray, microwaves, and ultrasound: Counseling the pregnant and nonpregnant patient about these risks. *Semin Oncol* 1989;16:347-368.
26. Gordon M, Niswander KR, Berendes H, et al. Fetal morbidity following potentially anoxigenic obstetric conditions. VII. Bronchial asthma. *Am J Obstet Gynecol* 1970;106:421-429.
27. Clark SL. Asthma in pregnancy. *Obstet Gynecol* 1993;82: 1036-1040.
28. Jana N, Khunnu B, Saha, et al. Effect of bronchial asthma on the course of pregnancy, labor, and perinatal outcome. *J Obstet Gynaecol* 1995;21:227-232.
29. Cousins L, Catanzarite VA. Fetal oxygenation, acid-base balance, and assessment of well-being in the pregnancy complicated by asthma or anaphylaxis. In: Schatz M, Zeiger RS, Claman HN, eds. *Asthma and Immunologic Diseases in Pregnancy and Early Infancy*. New York: Marcel Dekker; 1998:27.
30. Stenius-Aarniala BS, Teramo KA, Hedman J. Acute asthma during pregnancy. *Thorax* 1996;51:411-414.
31. Schatz M, Petitti D, Chilingar L, et al. The safety of asthma and allergy medications during pregnancy. *J Allergy Clin Immunol* 1997;100:301-306.
32. National High Blood Pressure Education Program Working Group Report on High Blood Pressure in Pregnancy. *Am J Obstet Gynecol* 1990:163(5 Pt 1):1691-1712.
33. August, P. Hypertensive disorders in pregnancy. In: Burrow GN & Duffy TP, eds. *Medical Complications During Pregnancy*. 5th ed. Philadelphia: W.B. Saunders; 1999:53-77.
34. Poppas A, Shroff SG, Korcarz CE, et al. Serial assessment of the cardiovascular system in normal pregnancy: Role of arterial compliance and pulsatile arterial load. *Circulation* 1997;95:2407-2415.
35. Bader ME, Bader RA. Cardiovascular hemodynamics in pregnancy and labor. *Clin Obstet Gynecol* 1968;1:924-939.
36. Hughes EC, ed. Obstetric-Gynecologic Terminology. Philadelphia, 1972:422-423.
37. Roberts JM, Redman CW. Preeclampsia: More than pregnancy induced hypertension. *Lancet* 1993;341: 447-1451.
38. Roberts JM, Taylor RN, Musci TJ, et al. Preeclampsia: An endothelial cell disorder. *Am J Obstet Gynecol* 1989;161: 1200-1204.
39. Zamorski MA, Green LA. Preeclampsia and hypertensive disorders of pregnancy. *Am Fam Physician* 1996;53: 1595-1604.
40. Witlin AG, Sibai BM. Hypertension in pregnancy. *Ann Rev Med* 1997;48:115-127.
41. Roberts JM. Pregnancy-related hypertension. In: Creasy RK, Resnik R, eds. *Maternal-fetal Medicine: Principles and Practice.* 3rd ed. Philadelphia: Saunders; 1994:804-843.
42. Kaunitz AM, Hughes JM, Grimes DA, et al. Causes of maternal mortality in the United States. *Obstet Gynecol* 1985;65:605-612.
43. The 1988 Report of the Joint National Committee on Detection and Treatment of High Blood Pressure. *Arch Intern Med* 1988;148:1023-1038.
44. Dekker GA, Sibai BM. Early detection of preeclampsia. *Am J Obstet Gynecol* 1991;165:160-172.
45. Schiff E, Friedman SA, Sibai SM. Conservative management of severe preeclampsia remote from term. *Obstet Gyncol* 1994;84:626-630.
46. Paterson-Brown S, Robson SC, Redfern N, et al. Hydralazine boluses for the treatment of severe hypertension in preeclampsia. *Br J Obstet Gynaecol* 1994;101:409-413.
47. Joint National Committee on Detection, Evaluation and Treatment of High Blood Pressure. *The Fifth Report of the Joint National Committee on Detection, Evaluation, and Treatment of High Blood Pressure*. Bethesda: National Institutes of Health, 1993.
48. Pritchard JA, Cunningham FG, Pritchard SA. The Parkland

Memorial Hospital protocol for the treatment of eclampsia: Evaluation of 245 cases. *Am J Obstet Gynecol* 1984;148:951-963.

49. Ananth CV, Savitz DA, Williams MA. Placental abruption and its association with hypertension and prolonged rupture of membranes: A methodologic review and meta-analysis. *Obstet Gynecol* 1996;88:309-318.
50. Cunningham FG, Cox SM, Harstad TW, et al. Chronic renal disease and pregnancy outcome. *Am J Obstet Gynecol* 1990;163:453-459.
51. Rey E, Couturier A. The prognosis of pregnancy in women with chronic hypertension. *Am J Obstet Gynecol* 1994;171: 410-416.
52. Sibai, BM. Diagnosis and management of chronic hypertension in pregnancy. *Obstet Gynecol* 1991;78:451-461.
53. Schoenfeld A, Segal J, Friedman S, et al. Adverse reactions to antihypertensive drugs in pregnancy. *Obstet Gynecol Surv* 1986;41:67- 73.
54. Kaunitz AM, Hughes JM, Grimes DA, et al. Causes of maternal mortality in the United States. *Obstet Gynecol* 1985;65:605-612.
55. Findland M, Dublin TD. Pneumococcic pneumonias complicating pregnancy and the puerperium. *JAMA* 1939; 112:1027-1032.
56. Oxorn H. The changing aspects of pneumonia complicating pregnancy. *Am J Obstet Gynecol* 1955;70:1057-1063.
57. Goodrum LA. Pneumonia in pregnancy. *Semin Perinatol* 1997;21:276-283.
58. Nyhan D, Bredin C, Quigley C. Acute respiratory failure in pregnancy due to staphylococcal pneumonia. *Ir Med J* 1983;76:320-321.
59. Leontic E. Respiratory disease in pregnancy. *Med Clin North Am* 1977;61:111-128.
60. Sargent IL, Redman C. Immunologic adaptations of pregnancy. In: Reece EA, Hobbins JC, Mahoney MJ, et al, eds. *Medicine of the Fetus and Mother*. Philadelphia: JB Lippincott Co., 1992:317-327.
61. Rigby FB, Pastorek JG II. Pneumonia during pregnancy. *Clin Obstet Gynecol* 1996;39:107-119.
62. Rodrigues J, Niederman MS. Pneumonia complicating pregnancy. *Clin Chest Med* 1992;13:679-691.
63. Cunningham F. Pulmonary disorders. In: Paterson L, ed. *Williams Obstetrics*. Norwalk, CT: Appleton and Lange; 1994:1-14.
64. Hornby P, Abrahams T. Pulmonary pharmacology. *Clin Obstet Gynecol* 1996;39:17-35.
65. Kirshon B, Faro S, Zurawin RK, et al. Favorable outcome after treatment with amantadine and ribavirin in a pregnancy complicated by influenza pneumonia: A case report. *J Reprod Med* 1988;33:390-401.
66. Rochat RW, Koonin LM, Atrash HK, et al. Maternal mortality in the United States: Report from the Maternal Mortality Collaborative. *Obstet Gynecol* 1988;72:91-97.
67. Toglia MR. Management of venous thromboembolism during pregnancy. In: Pearlman MD, Tintinalli JE, eds. *Emergency Care of the Woman*. New York: McGraw Hill; 1998:183-190.
68. Ginsberg JS, Hirsh J. Use of antithrombotic agents during pregnancy. *Chest* 1998;114:524S-530S.
69. McPhedran P. Venous thromboembolism during pregnancy. In: Burrow GN & Duffy TP, eds. *Medical Complications During Pregnancy*. 5th ed. Philadelphia: W.B. Saunders; 1999:97-109.
70. Rutherford SE, Phelan JP. Deep venous thrombosis and pulmonary embolism in pregnancy. *Obstet Gynecol Clin North Am* 1991;18:345-370.
71. Bergqvist A, Bergqvist D, Hallbook T. Deep vein thrombosis during pregnancy: A prospective study. *Acta Obstet Gynecol Scand* 1983;62:443-448.
72. Elias P, LeCorff G, Bouvier JL, et al. Value of real time B mode ultrasound imaging in the diagnosis of deep vein thrombosis of the lower limbs. *Int Angiol* 1987;6:175-182.
73. Markisz JA. Radiographic and nuclear medicine diagnosis. In: Goldhaber SZ, ed. *Pulmonary Embolism and Deep Vein Thrombosis*. Philadelphia: WB Saunders; 1985:41-75.
74. McFarlane MJ, Imperiale TF. Use of the alveolar-arterial oxygen gradient in the diagnosis of pulmonary embolism. *Am J Med* 1994;96:57-62.
75. Remy-Jardin M, Jardin J. Spiral CT angiography of the pulmonary circulation. *Radiology* 1999;212:615-636.
76. Balan KK, Critchley M, Vedavathy KK, et al. The value of ventilation-perfusion imaging in pregnancy. *Br J Radiol* 1997;70:338-340.
77. Ramin SM, Ramin KD, Gilstrap LC. Anticoagulants and thrombolytics during pregnancy. *Semin Perinatol* 1997;21: 149-153.
78. Howie PW. Anticoagulants in pregnancy. *Clin Obstet Gynaecol* 1986;13:349-363.
79. Toglia MR, Nolan TE. Venous thromboembolism during pregnancy: A current review of diagnosis and management. *Obstet Gynecol Surv* 1997;52:60-72.
80. Gillis S, Shushan A, Eldor A. Use of low molecular weight heparin for prophylaxis and treatment of thromboembolism in pregnancy. *Int J Gynaecol Obstet* 1992;39:297-301.
81. Thomas LA, Summer RR, Cardwell MS. Use of Greenfield filters in pregnant women at risk for pulmonary embolism. *South Med J* 1997;90:215-217.
82. Ponchon M, Goffette P, Hainaut P. Temporary vena caval filtration. Preliminary clinical experience with removable vena caval filters. *Acta Clin Belg* 1999;54:223-228.
83. Lindheimer MD, Katz AL. The kidney in pregnancy. *N Eng J Med* 1970;283:1095-1097.
84. Patterson TF, Andriole VT. Bacteriuria in pregnancy. *Infect Disease Clin North Am* 1987;1:807-822.
85. Krieger JN. Complications and treatments of urinary tract infections during pregnancy. *Urol Clin North Am* 1986;13: 685-693.
86. Millar LK, Cox SM. Urinary tract infections complicating pregnancy. *Infect Disease Clin North Am* 1997;11:13-26.
87. Sandberg T, Stenqvist K, Svanberg-Eden C, et al. Host-parasite relationship in urinary tract infections during pregnancy. *Prog Allergy* 1983;33:228-235.
88. Patterson TF, Andriole VT. Detection, significance and therapy of bacteriuria in pregnancy. *Infect Dis Clin North Am* 1997;11:593-608.
89. MacDonald P. Alexandar D, Catz C, et al. Summary of a

workshop on maternal genitourinary infections and the outcome of pregnancy. *J Infect Dis* 1983;147:596-605.

90. Hart AH, Pham T, Nowicki S, et al. Gestational pyelonephritis associated *Escherichia coli* isolates representing a nonrandom closely related population. *Am J Obstet Gynecol* 1996;174:983-989.
91. Whalley P. Bacteriuria of pregnancy. *Am J Obstet Gynecol* 1967;97:723-738.
92. Cunningham FG. Urinary tract infections during pregnancy. In: Pearlman MD, Tintinalli JE, eds. *Emergency Care of the Woman*. New York: McGraw Hill; 1998: 303 - 312.
93. Bachman JW, Heise RH, Naessens JM, et al. A study of various tests to detect asymptomatic urinary tract infections in an obstetric population. *JAMA* 1993;270:1971-1974.
94. Lenke RR, VanDorsten JPV. The efficacy of the nitrite test and microscopic urinalysis in predicting urine culture results. *Am J Obstet Gynecol* 1981;140:427-429.
95. Harris RE, Gilstrap LC. Cystitis during pregnancy: A distinct clinical entity. *Obstet Gynecol* 1981;57:578-580.
96. Andriole VT, Patterson TF. Epidemiology, natural history, and management of urinary tract infections in pregnancy. *Med Clin North Am* 1991;75:359-373.
97. Duff P. Pyelonephritis in pregnancy. *Clin Obstet Gynecol* 1984;27:17-31.
98. Jones RN, Kugler KC, Pfaller MA, et al. Characteristics of pathogens causing urinary tract infections in hospitals in North America: Results from the SENTRY Antimicrobial Surveillance Program, 1997. *Diag Microbiol Infect Dis* 1999;35:55-63.
99. Cormican M, Morris D, Corbett-Feeney G, et al. Extended spectrum beta-lactamase production and fluoroquinolone resistance in pathogens associated with community acquired urinary tract infection. *Diagn Microbiol Infect Dis* 1998;32:317-319.
100. Stenqvist K, Sandberg T, Lidin-Janson G, et al. Virulence factors of *Escherchia coli* in urinary isolates from pregnant women. *J Infect Dis* 1987;156:870-877.
101. Lucas MJ, Cunningham FG. Urinary infection in pregnancy. *Clin Obstet Gynecol* 1993;36:855-868.
102. Cunningham FG, Lucas MJ, Hankins GD. Pulmonary injury complicating antepartum pyelonephritis. *Am J Obstet Gynecol* 1987;156:797-807.
103. Millar LK, Wing DA, Paul RH, et al. Outpatient treatment of pyelonephritis in pregnancy: A randomized controlled trial. *Obstet Gynecol* 1995;173:597-602.
104. Sanchez-Ramos L, McAlpin KJ, Adair D, et al. Pyelonephritis in pregnancy: Once-a-day ceftriaxone versus multiple doses of cefazolin. *Am J Obstet Gynecol* 1995;172: 129-133.
105. Lorenz RP. Diabetes during pregnancy. In: Pearlman MD, Tintinalli JE, eds. *Emergency Care of the Woman*. New York: McGraw Hill; 1998:239-246.
106. DeFronzo R. Lilly Lecture 1987. The triumvarate: Beta cell, muscle, liver: A collusion responsible for NIDDM. *Diabetes* 1988;37:667-687.
107. Inzucchi SE. Diabetes in pregnancy. In: Burrow GN & Duffy TP, eds. *Medical Complications During Pregnancy*. 5th ed. Philadelphia: W.B. Saunders Co.; 1999:25-51.
108. Hare JW. Gestational diabetes and the White Classification. *Diabetes Care* 1980;3:394.
109. Ryan E, Ennis L. Role of gestational hormones in the induction of insulin resistance. *J Clin Endocrinol Metab* 1988:67:341-347.
110. National Diabetes Group: Classification and diagnosis of diabetes mellitus and other categories of glucose intolerance. *Diabetes* 1979;28:1039-1057.
111. Pedersen J. Weight and length at birth of infants of diabetic mothers. *Acta Endocrinol* 1954;16:330-347.
112. Ogata E. Perinatal morbidity in offspring of diabetic mothers. *Diabetes Rev* 1995;3:652.
113. Kucera J. Rate and type of congenital anomalies among offspring of diabetic women. *J Reprod Med* 1971;7:73-82.
114. Miodovnik M, Lavin J, Knowles H, et al. Spontaneous abortion among insulin dependent diabetic women. *Am J Obstet Gynecol* 1984;150:372-376.
115. Mimouni F, Miodovnik M, Siddiqi T. High spontaneous premature labor rates in insulin dependent pregnant women: An association with poor glycemic control and urogenital infection. *Obstet Gynecol* 1988;14:175-180.
116. Montoaro MN, Myers VP, Mestman JH, et al. Outcome of pregnancy in diabetic ketoacidosis. *Am J Perinatol* 1983; 10:17-20.
117. Reece EA, Homko C. Diabetes-related complications of pregnancy. *J Nat Med Asssoc* 1993;85:537-545.
118. Espanol T, Caragol I, Bertran JM. Evolution of immunologic abnormalities in HIV infection by vertical transmission. *Acta Pediatr* 1994;400(suppl):35-38.
119. Ellerbrock TV, Bush TH, Chamberland ME, et al. Epidemiology of women with AIDS in the United States, 1981 through 1990: A comparison with heterosexual men with AIDS. *JAMA* 1991;265:2971-2975.
120. Centers for Disease Control and Prevention: World AIDS Day. *MMWR Morb Mortal Wkly Rep* 1996:45:1005.
121. Viscarello RR, Copperman AB, DeGennaro NJ. Is the risk of perinatal transmission of HIV increased by intrapartum use of spiral electrodes or fetal scalp pH sampling? *Am J Obstet Gynecol* 1994;170:740-743.
122. Sperling RS. Human immunodeficiency virus infection in pregnancy. In: Pearlman MD, Tintinalli JE, eds. *Emergency Care of the Woman*. New York: McGraw Hill; 1998:273-279.
123. Boyer PJ, Dillon M, Navaie M, et al. Factors predictive of maternal-fetal transmission of HIV-1: Preliminary analysis of zidovudine given during pregnancy and/or delivery. *JAMA* 1994;271:1925-1930.
124. Broussard CN, Richter JE. Nausea and vomiting of pregnancy. *Gastroenterol Clin North Am* 1998;27:123-151.
125. Klebanoff M, Koslowe P, Kaslow R, et al. Epidemiology of vomiting in early pregnancy. *Obstet Gynecol* 1985;66: 612-616.
126. Godsey RK, Newman RB. Hyperemesis gravidarum: A comparison of single and multiple admissions. *J Reprod Med* 1991;36:287-290.
127. Hod M, Orvieto R, Kaplan B, et al. Hyperemesis gravidarum: A review. *J Reprod Med* 1994;39:605-612.
128. Glick MM, Dick EL. Molar pregnancy presenting with hyperemesis gravidarum. *J Am Osteopath Assoc* 1999;99:

162-164.

129. Kauppila A, Huhtaniemi I, Ylikorkala O. Serum chorionic gonadotropin and pregnancy-specific beta-1-glycoprotein in predicting pregnancy outcome and in association with early pregnancy vomiting. *Gynecol Obstet Invest* 1984;18:49-53.
130. Soules MR, Hughes CL, Garcia JA, et al. Nausea and vomiting of Role of human chorionic gonadotropin and 17-hydroxyprogesterone. *Obstet Gynecol* 1980;55:696-700.
131. Reinken L, Gant H. Vitamin B6 nutrition in women with hyperemesis gravidarum during the first trimester of pregnancy. *Clin Chim Acta* 1974;55:101-102.
132. Hershman JM. Human chorionic gonadotropin and the thyroid: Hyperemesis gravidarum and trophoblastic tumors. *Thyroid* 1999;9:653-657.
133. Kimura A, Amino N, Tamaki H, et al. Gestational thyrotoxicosis and hyperemesis gravidarum: Possible role of hCG with higher stimulating activity. *Clin Endocrinol* 1993;38:345-350.
134. Jacoby EB, Porter KB. *Helicobacter pylori* infection and persistent hyperemesis gravidarum. *Am J Perinatol* 1999;16: 85-88.
135. Deuchar N. Nausea and vomiting in pregnancy: A review of the problem with particular regard to psychosocial and social aspects. *Br J Obstet Gynecol* 1995;102:6-8.
136. Cosmas JM. Nausea and vomiting in early pregnancy. In: Pearlman MD, Tintinalli JE, eds. *Emergency Care of the Woman*. New York: McGraw Hill; 1998:49-56.
137. Nelson-Piercy C. Treatment of nausea and vomiting in pregnancy. When should it be treated and what can be safely taken? *Drug Saf* 1998;19:155-164.
138. Sullivan CA, Johnson CA, Roach H, et al. A pilot study of intravenous ondansetron for hyperemesis gravidarum. *Am J Obstet Gynecol* 1996;174:1565-1568.
139. Safari HR, Fassett MJ, Souter IC, et al. The efficacy of methyprednisolone in the treatment of hyperemesis gravidarum: A randomized, double-blind, controlled study. *Am J Obstet Gynecol* 1998;179:921-924.
140. Safari HR, Alsulyman OM, Gherman RB, et al. Experience with oral methyprednisolone in the treatment of refractory hyperemesis gravidarum. *Am J Obstet Gynecol* 1998;178: 1054-1058.
141. Weigel MM, Weigel RM. Nausea and vomiting of early pregnancy and pregnancy outcome: An epidemiological study. *Br J Obstet Gynecol* 1989;96:1312-1318.
142. Tierson F, Olson C, Hook EB. Nausea and vomiting of pregnancy and association with pregnancy outcome. *J Obstet Gynecol* 1986;155:1017-1022.
143. Chin RKH, Lao TT. Low birth weight and hyperemesis gravidarum. *Eur J Obstet Gynecol* 1988;28:179-183.
144. Gross S, Librach C, Cecutti A. Maternal weight loss associated with hyperemesis gravidarum: A predictor of fetal outcome. *Am J Obstet Gynecol* 1989;160:906-909.
145. Gardian G, Voros E, Jardanhazy T, et al. Wernicke's encephaolopathy induced by hyperemesis gravidarum. *Acta Neurol Scand* 1999;99:196-198.
146. Robinson JN, Banerjee R, Thiet MP. Coagulopathy secondary to vitamin K deficiency in hyperemesis gravidarum. *Obstet Gynecol* 1998;92:673-675.
147. Fudaka Y, Ohta S, Mizuno K, et al. Rhabdomyolysis secondary to hyperemesis gravidarum. *Acta Obstet Gynecol Scand* 1999;78:71.
148. Hsu JJ, Clark-Glena R, Nelson DK, et al. Nasogastric enteral feeding in the management of hyperemesis gravidarum. *Obstet Gynecol* 1996;88:343-346.
149. Levine MG, Esser D. Total parenteral nutrition for the treatment of severe hyperemesis gravidarum; marginal nutritional effects and fetal outcome. *Obstet Gynecol* 1988;72:102-107.
150. Serrano P, Velloso A, Garcia-Luna PP, et al. Enteral nutrition by percutaneous endoscopic gastrojejunostomy in severe hyperemesis gravidarum: A report of two cases. *Clin Nutr* 1998;17:135-139.
151. Niebyl JR. Drug use in pregnancy and lactation. In: Pearlman MD, Tintinalli JE, eds. *Emergency Care of the Woman*. New York: McGraw Hill; 1998: 165-178.
152. Briggs GG, Freeman RK, Yaffe SJ. *Drugs in pregnancy and lactation. 4th Ed.* Baltimore: Williams & Wilkins; 1994: 148-149.

Vaginal Bleeding in Pregnancy

Gary Hals, MD, PhD

We have all been there, and the clinical decision-making process can be daunting: "Doctor," the nurse informs us, "the new patient in the OB-GYN room is having severe vaginal bleeding. She's 26 weeks pregnant." This is a presentation that will quicken the pulse and raise the anxiety level of most emergency department (ED) physicians, even the most seasoned clinicians who fully appreciate the differential diagnosis and possible complications. Pregnant women with this chief complaint are especially stressful for the ED physician for a number of reasons. First, the clinician will be concerned that the mother may deliver a premature, but potentially viable child. Once a pregnancy has reached about 24 weeks, the fetus is potentially viable, but it may require critical, invasive interventions. In such cases, survival of the fetus may depend on appropriate, life-supporting interventions administered by the ED physician and/or neonatologist caring for the child during the first few minutes, or hours, of life.

Even in the absence of fetal delivery, the ED physician will usually simultaneously have to manage the care of two "patients," one of which (the fetus) primarily can be assessed only by data obtained from the fetal monitor or ultrasonographic evaluation. Another complicating factor is that although most ED physicians have adequate "book knowledge" about such cases, they often lack sufficient hands-on clinical experience. In this regard, most ED physicians are comfortable with precipitous term deliveries, but emergency resuscitation of a preterm infant presents an unfamiliar challenge. Most emergency medicine residency programs are based at medical centers with active obstetrical residencies; as a result, these patients oftentimes bypass the ED, entirely depriving the ED physician of first hand experience with these patients.

Although pregnancy is classically divided into 13-week trimesters, the approach to vaginal bleeding in pregnancy is to divide the pregnancy into the first half (< 20 weeks) and second half (> 20 weeks) of gestation. One factor justifying such a division is that conditions associated with late second-trimester bleeding are similar to that are produced during the third trimester. First-trimester bleeding is common, occurring in about 40% of pregnancies. In contrast, bleeding during the last half of gestation occurs in only 3-4% of all pregnancies, and is associated with a perinatal mortality rate of 23-32%.[1]

The purpose of this chapter is to review the current evidence-based recommendations related to the diagnosis and management of vaginal bleeding that occurs during the second half of pregnancy. Finally, the relative lack of experience and high risk nature of these patients—and their associated conditions—demand that the ED physician keep abreast of clinical advances in this area to provide state-of-the-art care for these ED patients.

Introduction

From a practical, clinical perspective, causes of vaginal bleeding during the second half of pregnancy can be divided into obstetrical and non-obstetrical causes. Obstetrical causes of vaginal bleeding during this period include the following: 1) placental abruption; 2) placenta previa; 3) uterine rupture; 4) vasa previa (or

Figure 1. Illustration of the Different Types of Placental Abruption

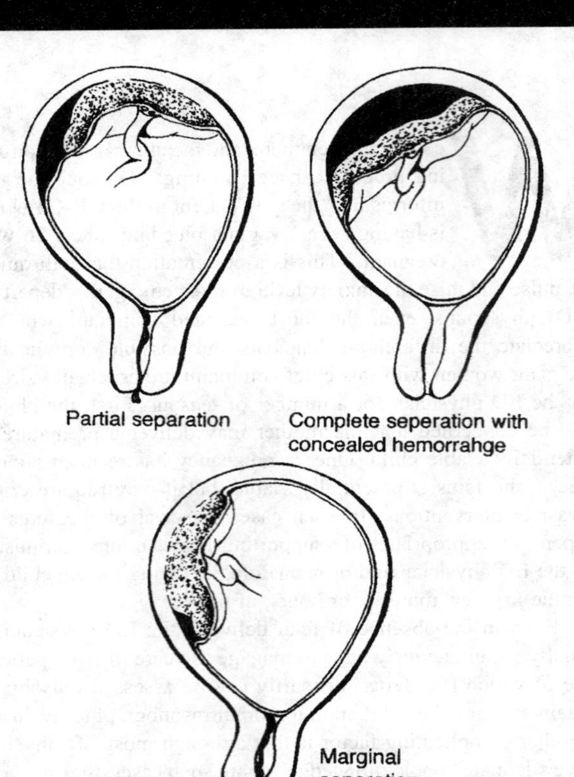

Grade 1 abruption is shown in the bottom diagram as marginal separation. **Grade 2** abruption is shown in the upper left as partial separation. **Grade 3** abruption is shown in the upper right as complete separation with concealed hemorrhage.

Reproduced with permission from: Scott JR. Placenta previa and abruption. In: Scott JR, et al, eds. *Danforth's Obstetrics and Gynecology.* 8th ed. Philadelphia: Lippincott Williams & Wilkins; 1999:412.

Table 1. Clinical Findings in Placental Abruption: Grade-Dependent Maternal and Fetal Profiles

GRADE 1:

Slight or minimal vaginal bleeding (spotting) and limited uterine irritability (no organized contractions) are typically present. Maternal blood pressure is unchanged, and maternal serum fibrinogen level is normal (normal maternal fibrinogen concentration is 450 mg/percent). Fetal heart rate is normal, between 120 bpm and 160 bpm.

GRADE 2:

External uterine bleeding is mild to moderate, similar to that of a heavy period. Uterine irritability is evident, with tetanic contractions at times. Maternal hypotension is absent in supine position, but orthostatic symptoms may be present. Resting maternal pulse rate may be elevated. Fibrinogen levels are lowered to the range of 150 mg/percent to 250 mg/percent. Fetal distress is evident as manifested by compromised fetal heart rate patterns.

GRADE 3:

Bleeding is moderate to severe but may be underestimated by external losses. Painful uterine contractions are present and they are often tetanic in nature. Hemodynamic instability is evident by maternal hypotension and tachycardia. Fibrinogen levels often are reduced to less than 150 mg/percent, representing a blood loss of approximately 2000 mL. Maternal coagulopathies (thrombocytopenia, clotting factor, and fibrinogen depletion) are often present. Fetal death is

isolated fetal hemorrhage); and 5) the "bloody show" associated with onset of labor. Each of these conditions will be discussed, highlighting risk factors, diagnosis, and ED management.

Nonobstetrical causes of bleeding during the last 20 weeks of pregnancy rarely cause significant bleeding. Nevertheless they may occur, and entities that should be considered include lesions of the vagina, cervical polyps or cancer, friable condyloma acuminata, hemorrhoids, and postcoital trauma. It should be emphasized that because the cervix is much more vascular during the later phases of pregnancy, there may be more bleeding than is typically associated with these cervical lesions. As a result, biopsies of cervical lesions should be performed only by an experienced obstetrician. If bleeding is minor (simple spotting), if there is a verifiable history of recent trauma (speculum exam or intercourse), and if a bleeding site is identified on exam that does not originate from the os, then the patient can be reassured that the bleeding is not serious. Nevertheless, any patient with a diagnosis of non-obstetrical vaginal bleeding should be cautioned about warning signs that indicate more serious bleeding, and these women should be referred directly to their obstetrician for urgent follow-up in the event of more serious hemorrhage.

Finally, it is important to stress that basic physiological changes occur in pregnancy that protect the mother from natural blood loss associated with delivery. For example, by 40 weeks gestation, plasma volume dramatically increases by 33% (450 mL), and total blood volume increases by an average of 45% above pre-pregnancy levels. This augmentation of blood volume occurs gradually and mirrors the growth of the fetus. However, the red cell mass expands at a slightly slower rate, producing a dilutional anemia that is most pronounced in early pregnancy. Consequently, the mean hemoglobin level during pregnancy is 10.2 g/dL to 11.6 g/dL.[2] As a result, from a physiological perspective, the mother may tolerate blood loss slightly better than a non-pregnant patient with the same degree of hemorrhage, but on the other hand, the resulting anemia may be more profound as a result of fluid shifts and resuscitation with saline. Fibrinogen levels are also increased in pregnancy, rising up to three times the pre-pregnancy level by term.

Placental Abruption

Placental abruption (or abruptio placenta) is defined as premature separation of a normally implanted placenta from its attachment to the uterus before birth of the fetus. Abruption occurs most frequently during the third trimester; about 80% of all cases will occur shortly before the onset of labor, although this complication may occur at any time after 20 weeks of gestation.[3] Placental separation during the first 20 weeks is considered part of the process of spontaneous abortion.[4] The incidence of abruption is between 1 in 86 and 1 in 200 live births, and therefore, complicates approximately 1% of all pregnancies.[3] Even so, abruption is the most common cause of intrapartum fetal death, with an associated mortality rate of 25-50%. The majority of these deaths are due to complications of premature birth (respiratory distress syndrome, intraventricular hemorrhage, and necrotizing enterocolitis). As a result, placental abruption accounts for up to 15% of all perinatal deaths.[5] Morbidity also is significant, with permanent neurological deficits reported in up to 14% of surviving infants.[6] Abruption can also produce significant complications in the mother, among them, life-threatening maternal hemorrhage, severe coagulopathies, and the need for emergency Cesarean section (C-section); these complications account for significant maternal morbidity and mortality.

Placental separation occurs in varying degrees of severity, and is generally classified according to the following schemata: 1) complete or Grade 3; 2) partial or Grade 2; and 3) mild or Grade 1, in which case separation involves only the placental margin. *(Please see Figure 1.)* These classes of placental abruption correlate reasonably well with clinical findings and prognostic outcomes for both mother and fetus. Fortunately, Grade 3 (severe) abruptions are the least common, occurring in only 15-24% of clinically recognized cases of abruption.[1,7] Grade 2 (moderate) abruptions account for about 27-45% of cases, and Grade 1 (mild) abruptions are seen in 40-48% of cases.[1,7] A key point to remember is that the amount of external bleeding associated with abruption may not correlate with the extent or severity of the abruption and this may create a sense of false security. In this regard, for example, concealed hemorrhage occurs when the bleeding is contained inside the uterus, and these abruptions may be as dangerous to the mother and fetus as those characterized by severe external bleeding. Important and characteristic clinical findings for each class of abruption are summarized in Table 1.

Clinical Pathophysiology. In placental abruption, bleeding is thought to initiate from abnormal small vessels in the basal layer of the decidua or from fetoplacental vessels. As bleeding progresses, a hematoma enlarges beneath the placenta, sheering it from the uterus. Bleeding may be seen vaginally, or it may be concealed entirely inside the uterus. *(Please see Figure 1.)* As a result, the amount of visible or external bleeding may not necessarily correlate with maternal blood loss or grade of abruption.

Fetal compromise in abruption results from fetal hypoxia associated with the placenta's decreased ability to perform gas exchange. Additional risks include fetal blood loss through the disrupted placenta, maternal Rh sensitization, amniotic fluid embolism, and maternal disseminated intravascular coagulation (DIC). In severe abruption, microvascular coagulation is thought to stimulate the maternal fibrinolytic system, resulting in critical depletion of platelets and clotting factors, a serious clinical event that places the mother at risk for additional bleeding.

When a concealed abruption occurs, intrauterine pressures rise and, as a result, uterine muscles are unable to contract sufficiently around fractured vessels in order to inhibit further bleeding. Blood may also dissect into the fetal membranes or into the wall of the uterus. The clinical, disruptive effects of abruption on the fetus depend almost entirely upon the degree of separation of the placenta. Marginal separation from the uterus may produce no notable effects, whereas in complete abruption, fetal death is almost unavoidable. In almost 50% of cases characterized by severe abruption, the fetus is dead by the time the mother is admitted to the hospital.[8] As would be expected, varying degrees of separation between marginal and complete separation will have variable effects on the fetus.

Table 2. Risk Factors for Placental Abruption

- Maternal hypertension
- Eclampsia and preeclampsia
- History of previous abruption
- Uterine distension (multiple gestations, hydramnios, or tumors)
- Vascular disease (collagen vascular disorders, diabetes)
- Tobacco smoking
- Cocaine use
- Microangiopathic hemolytic anemia
- Premature rupture of membranes
- Uterine blunt trauma (domestic abuse, automobile collisions)
- Short umbilical cord

The precise etiology of placental abruption currently remains unclear, but several risk factors have been identified. The most important risk factor appears to be maternal hypertension. Hypertension in pregnancy is defined as a blood pressure 140/90 mmHg, an increase in systolic pressure of greater than 30 mmHg, or an increase in diastolic pressure of greater than 15 mmHg as compared to pre-pregnancy values. Although hypertension is a risk factor for all types of abruption, the correlation is most striking with Grade 3 abruption where 50% of cases are associated with either pregnancy-induced or chronic maternal hypertension.[4] Transient rises in blood pressure precipitated by cocaine use also can increase risk of abruption.[9] Furthermore, any condition that predisposes the mother to vascular disease (i.e., preeclampsia, diabetes, collagen vascular diseases, and chronic renal disease) is associated with increased risk for abruption. Finally, a variety of other conditions also are associated with increased risk for abruption. *(Please see Table 2.)*

It should be stressed that a previous placental abruption greatly increases the risk for abruption in subsequent pregnancies by more than 10-fold.[10] Because blunt abdominal trauma is also a risk factor for abruption, this etiology should be considered in any trauma evaluated during the second half of pregnancy. A history of trauma, especially from domestic abuse, also should be elicited in any pregnant woman presenting with abdominal pain or bleeding. Data now confirms that physical trauma currently complicates one out of every 12 pregnancies, and that spousal abuse is a leading cause in these cases.[1] Several, newer studies have identified maternal cigarette use, advanced maternal age, and male fetal gender as additional risk factors for abruption.[11] A link between intrauterine growth retardation and increased risk for abruption also has been proposed.[12]

Clinical Presentation. The classical presentation of placental abruption is characterized by sudden onset of abdominal pain, uterine contractions, and vaginal bleeding. In clinical practice, however, the presentation of abruption is highly variable. This variability results from the various degrees of placental separation. Typically, patients with more severe placental separation will present with more severe and "classical" symptoms. For example, in

Figure 2. Ultrasound Image of Placental Abruption

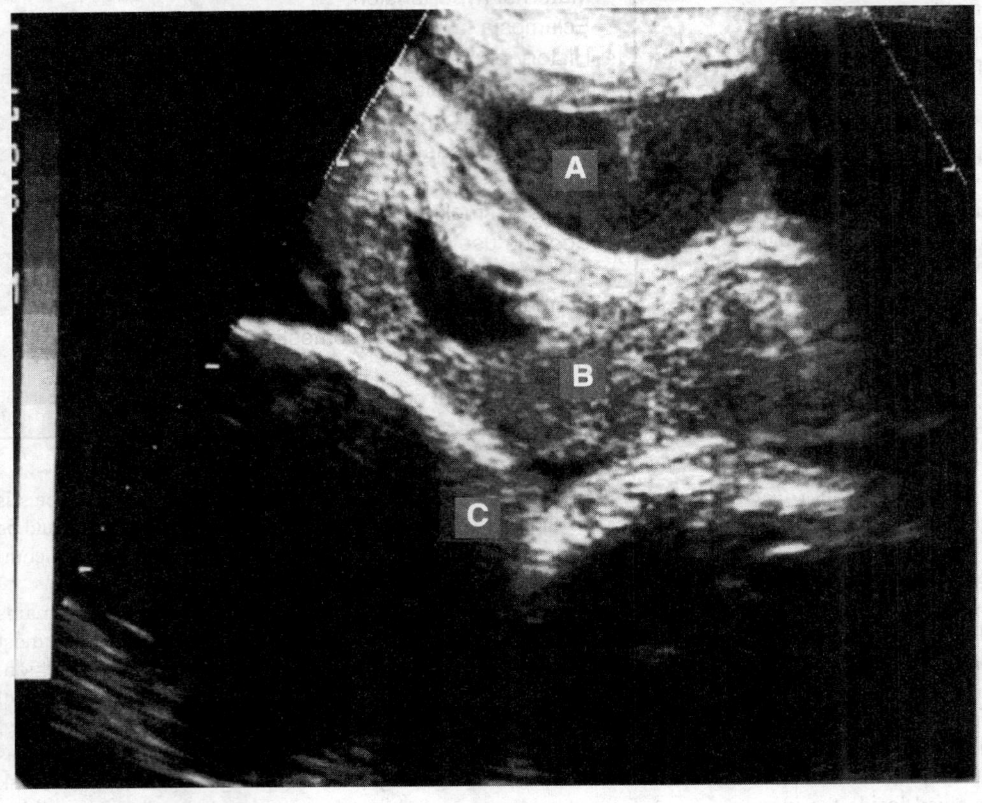

A = Retroplacental Clot
B = Placenta
C = Fetus
Ultrasound image provided by E. Horger, MD, University of South Carolina School of Medicine, University Specialty Clinics, Department of OB/GYN, Columbia, SC 29203.

Grade 3 abruption, severe and abrupt abdominal and/or back pain is common. Although the pain is constant, painful uterine contractions will be superimposed. When uterine tetany occurs, there will be no cyclical nature to the patient's pain. Frequently, by the time an exam is performed, the fetus will be in severe distress (bradycardic) or even dead.

Severe abruptions also can cause maternal cardiovascular shock that is accompanied by hypotension and tachycardia. Complications of shock (adult respiratory distress syndrome and acute tubular necrosis) may be apparent at the time of ED presentation. Hematuria, easy bruising, and continued bleeding at puncture sites are signs of DIC that may be seen early in the clinical course. Patients with severe abruption are suffering from hypovolemic shock and should be viewed as hypotensive multi-trauma patients in terms of their complications. Accordingly, aggressive fluid resuscitation and early transfusion should be instituted. *(Please see Patient Management section.)* Finally, any patient presenting with vaginal bleeding during the second half of pregnancy should never have a vaginal or rectal exam done until the possibility of placenta previa has been ruled out by ultrasonographic studies.

Patients with Grade 1 abruption usually will present with more subtle findings and may be difficult to diagnose. In this regard, pain may not be present with smaller separations, although in most cases uterine irritability (mild contractions) is present. Vaginal bleeding is seen in only 80% of cases because bleeding is concealed in the intrauterine space in the remaining 20% of patients.[1] Patients with concealed hemorrhage have a higher maternal mortality rate, perhaps because of failure to recognize the severity of maternal blood loss during the initial patient encounter. As smaller abruptions will not affect the fetal heart rate, a common misdiagnosis in these patients is early onset labor. Although these patients may not require any intervention if their abruption remains small, they should be carefully monitored for signs of worsening separation. A significant number of patients with mild abruption will have no signs or symptoms. Almost 30% will be diagnosed at the time of delivery when a small retroplacental clot is identified.[1]

Patients with Grade 2 abruptions typically present with more classic symptoms, but may not manifest symptoms of hypovolemic shock as early as patients with severe abruptions. However, the onset of symptoms may be gradual or sudden. Several significant findings can alert the ED physician that this is not simply a case of early onset labor. The uterus is often tender and fails to relax between contractions. Vaginal bleeding, when not concealed, is moderate by abruption standards but is much more pronounced than the typical "bloody show" of labor. Once again, it should be emphasized that the amount of vaginal bleeding is often misleading, and that if the patient presents with symptoms of more extensive blood loss, appropriate intervention is required. Fetal distress is common in Grade 2 abruptions, a finding that should prompt urgent obstetric consultation.

Laboratory Studies. From a practical, clinical perspective, the take-home message is that placental abruption, for the most part, is a clinical diagnosis. There are no pathognomonic laboratory studies that accurately establish the diagnosis. Given that premise, research is being conducted to identify serum markers for abruption. Thrombomodulin (a marker of endothelial cell damage) has been reported to be a sensitive marker for abruption, and may prove to be clinically useful in the future.[13] Currently, useful laboratory markers center are associated with the appearance of complications, most notably DIC.

DIC can be triggered by massive hemorrhage, which in turn stimulates production of tissue thromboplastin, resulting in extensive microvascular clotting (hence the name disseminated intravascular coagulation). These clots stimulate the fibrinolytic cascade, which leads to extensive consumption of platelets, fibrinogen, and other clotting factors. Maternal fibrinogen levels are normally in the range of 450 mg/percent, and the volume of blood

Figure 3. Illustration of the Different Types of Placenta Previa

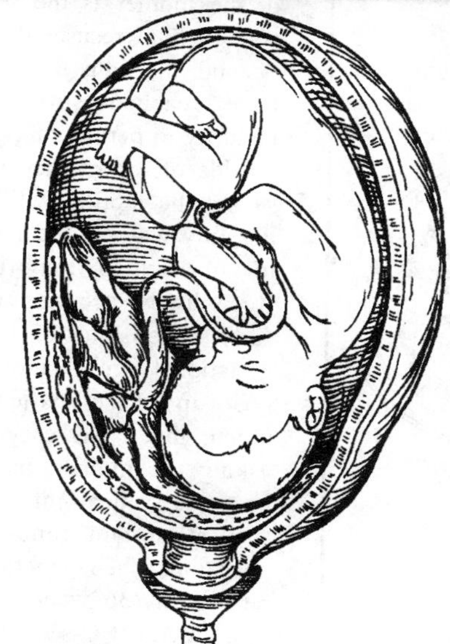
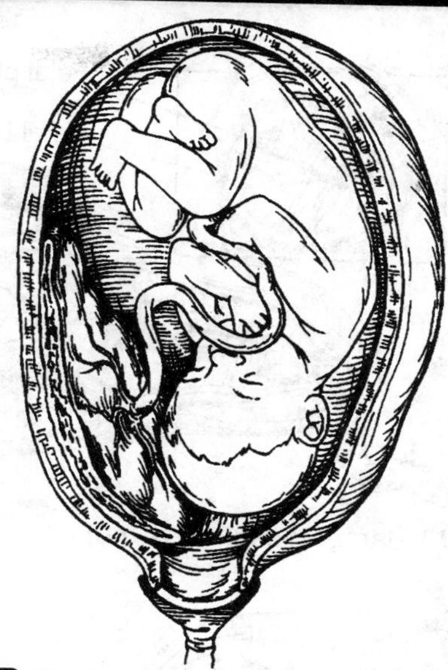
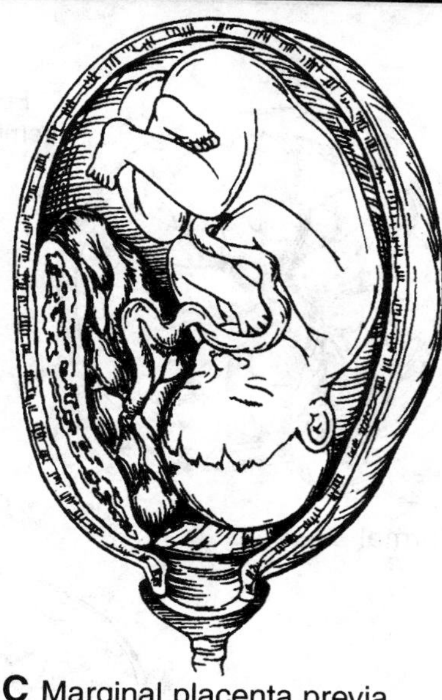

A Total placenta previa **B** Partial placenta previa **C** Marginal placenta previa

Reproduced with permission from: VanDeKerkhove KM, Johnson TRB. Bleeding in the second half of pregnancy: Maternal and fetal assessment. In: Pearlman MD, Tintinalli JE. eds. *Emergency Care of the Woman*. New York: McGraw Hill; 1998:79.

lost roughly correlates with the decrease in fibrinogen levels. The majority of patients experiencing a significant drop in fibrinogen level will ultimately require transfusion of blood products. At levels of 300 mg/percent, maternal coagulation abnormalities begin to manifest themselves with spontaneous bleeding at puncture sites. A fibrinogen level of 150 mg/percent correlates with a maternal hemorrhage of more than 2 liters. As the average blood loss in a Grade 3 abruption is 2.5 liters or more, the fibrinogen level may provide a rough estimate of the severity of placental separation, as well as fetal prognosis.

As there may be a delay in obtaining a fibrinogen level in some centers, another "crude" alternative may be used.[14] In the "poor man's fibrinogen assay," a red top tube of blood is allowed to sit at room temperature. If a clot does not form within 6 minutes or forms and lyses within 30 minutes, a coagulation defect is probably present and the fibrinogen level is less than 150 mg/percent.[14] Other lab values related to DIC include low platelets, prolonged PT or PTT, and raised D-dimer levels (released in fibrin degradation).

Finally, placental separation may introduce fetal blood into the maternal circulation, which can be detected by the Kleihauer-Betke test. While this test also can be used to dose Rhogam in these patients, a major disadvantage of this test is the long processing time. Clinical decisions, therefore, should be based on other data and this test should be limited to use as a screening tool for identifying patients with minimal or Grade 1 abruption, especially in cases where there is no other evidence for abruption except clinical suspicion.

Imaging Studies. During the first 20 weeks of pregnancy, imaging studies provide a reliable modality for clinical diagnosis. Unfortunately, this is not the case for placental abruption. Initial studies evaluating the usefulness of this technique found that ultrasound missed a surprising 98% of placental separations.[14] More advanced ultrasound technology, however, has greatly reduced the false-negative diagnosis rate, but ultrasonographic evaluation will still fail to detect up to 50% of abruptions.[14]

When present, a number of ultrasonographic findings are consistent with the diagnosis of placental abruption. Hematomas may be seen either in the subchorionic (between the placenta and the membranes), retroplacental (between placenta and uterine wall), or preplacental (between the placenta and amniotic fluid) compartments. *(Please see Figure 2.)* Interestingly, the precise location of the hematoma can affect the prognosis of the fetus. In particular, large retroplacental hematomas (> 60 mLs or greater than 50% of placental surface affected) will produce fetal death in about 50% of cases, whereas an equivalent subchorionic hemorrhage will cause fetal death in only 10% of cases.[15] Therefore, the primary purpose of ultrasound in diagnosis of abruption is to rule out other causes of vaginal bleeding in late pregnancy, most notably placenta previa. In these cases, ultrasound also can be used to assess for the fetal heartbeat.

Magnetic resonance imaging (MRI) is the only other diagnostic modality currently used to identify abruption. It has the advantage of high sensitivity. However, the lack of access to the test, as well as time and expense involved, do not make MRI a viable option in most emergency departments. At present, its use is relegated to clinically stable patients in whom the diagnosis is suspected, but in whom the diagnosis cannot be established by other means.

Patient Management. Treatment of patients with placental abruption depends, in part, on the degree of placental separation and the hemodynamic stability of mother and fetus. Stable patients with suspected or proven Grade 1 abruption (mild) should be admitted for observation and, in some cases, elective delivery. Patients with a higher grade abruption will manifest, or will unpredictably manifest, signs of hemorrhagic shock. The fetus may show signs of distress, or in the most severe cases, they will already have lost a heartbeat by the time of presentation to the ED.

Hence, all patients should have a fetal monitor placed, regardless of their initial presentation. They should be treated with close moni-

Figure 4. Illustration of Placental Abnormalities Leading to Placenta Previa

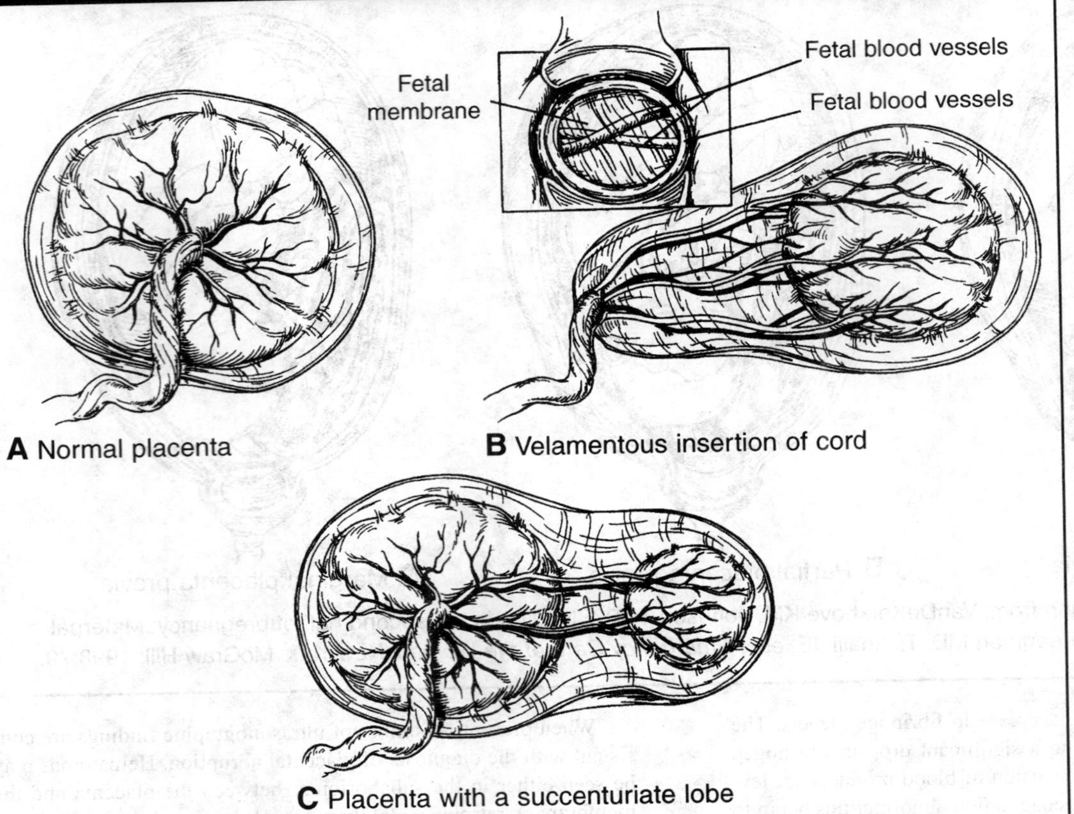

A Normal placenta

B Velamentous insertion of cord

C Placenta with a succenturiate lobe

The inset at the top shows the view of a dilated cervix with fetal blood vessels visible just inside the uterus.
Reproduced with permission from: VanDeKerkhove KM, Johnson TRB. Bleeding in the second half of pregnancy: Maternal and fetal assessment. In: Pearlman MD, Tintinalli JE. eds. *Emergency Care of the Woman*. New York: McGraw Hill; 1998:84.

toring, two large-bore IV lines, and a type and cross for 2-4 units of blood should be obtained. Coagulation studies (CBC, PT/PTT, fibrinogen level, D-dimer) should be ordered STAT and repeated if the patient's condition deteriorates. Blood products should be utilized for anemia or as the patient's condition dictates. Correction of coagulopathy caused by DIC also is recommended. Immediate consultation with an obstetrician is mandatory, as no patient with a suspected abruption should ever be discharged to home.

Patients with large, concealed hemorrhages are at risk for uterine rupture, and decompression of the uterine cavity may be done by amniotomy (rupture of membranes). As a rule, ED physicians should not perform this procedure, but if consultation is unavailable, remember that it may improve the mother's condition. A small incision is made in the membranes bulging through the os, but should only be performed in patients with suspected concealed hemorrhage when all other resuscitative measures are failing.

Resuscitation of the mother takes priority over all clinical contingencies, and when required, type O negative blood may be used for resuscitation if time does not permit type and crossmatch. Transfusion of platelets and fresh frozen plasma can also be used to treat coagulopathies associated with DIC. While it is true that there are two patients involved in patient management, the mother's hemodynamic stability takes precedence. Improvement of the mother's circulation will often improve that of the fetus if distress is present, and therefore, resuscitation of the mother is the first step in fetal resuscitation. Second, the fetus may not have reached sufficient maturity to permit survival outside of the mother and saving the mother will be the only way for the fetus to survive to maturity. Accordingly, accurate and early establishing of fetal gestational age is another goal in these patients. Often, this is as easy as asking the mother, but it becomes critical information at certain times in gestation. When the fetus is near term (36 weeks and up), emergent C-section is a more likely option than in patients in whom fetal viability is in question.

A fetus younger than 23-24 weeks is considered non-viable for survival outside the mother. Consequently, from a practical clinical perspective, it is of paramount importance to establish the age of the fetus. If the mother is unsure of dates, an urgent ultrasound will help clarify gestational age. If the fetus is clearly preterm, most obstetricians use magnesium sulfate or subcutaneous terbutaline to control uterine contractions and prevent actual labor. When the fetus is potentially viable, fetal monitoring and urgent consultation with a neonatal team or pediatrician also should be performed early. Although considerable controversy exists about the management of patients with abruption and a preterm fetus, most authors recommend trying to prevent labor until the fetus is clearly viable. When delivery is indicated, the method of choice is also debated in the obstetric literature. C-section may be the fastest method of delivery, but it also will increase blood loss and the risk of complications, especially when DIC is present. Alternatively, vaginal delivery may be associated with decreased blood loss, but can take a prolonged course with additional stress on the fetus.

Likewise, management of patients with fetal demise and coagulopathy is also controversial, since emergent C-section will considerably increase maternal blood loss and risk. Therefore, C-section should only be performed as a last resort in those patients in whom maternal hemorrhage is uncontrollable by any other means. With so much debate on the most outcome-effective approach, the primary goal of the ED physician should be to stabilize the patient(s) and deliver them to the care of obstetricians and pediatricians who can make these controversial decisions.

Once the patient is stabilized, she may need to be transferred to an appropriate center for further evaluation and treatment. However, transfer should not be attempted until the patient is sufficiently stabilized to undergo transport without additional risk. Finally, Rh-negative mothers should be treated with Rhogam. Recommendations are for 50 microgram IM injection in patients less than 12 weeks and 300 micrograms IM for those 12 weeks or more. Alternatively, one may simply use 300 micrograms for all Rh-negative patients, as gestational dates can be inaccurate and there is no additional risk with the higher dose.

Figure 5. Ultrasound Image of Placenta Previa

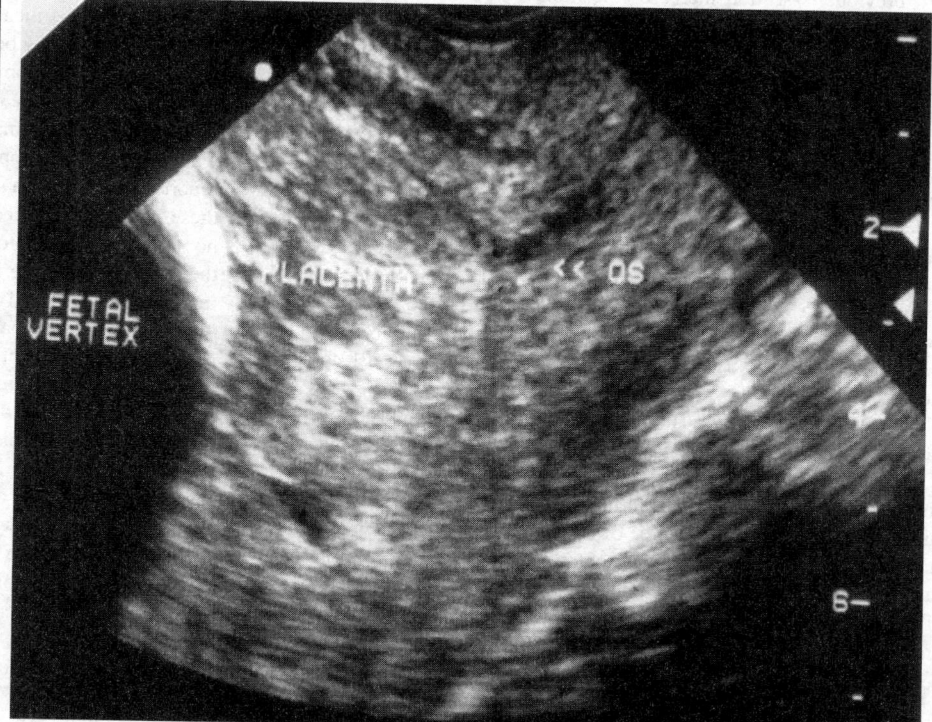

The fetal vertex is shown on the left. The cervical os is identified on the right, with the placenta labeled between the fetus and os.

Ultrasound image provided by E. Horger, MD, University of South Carolina School of Medicine, University Specialty Clinics, Department of OB/GYN, Columbia, SC 29203.

Placenta Previa

Placenta previa is another important cause of bleeding during the later half of pregnancy. This condition is defined as the improper implantation of the placenta over the cervical os; in other words, the placenta is inappropriately positioned between the cervix and the presenting fetal part, thereby impairing unencumbered descent of the fetus. The incidence of previa is similar to abruption, occurring in approximately one in 200 live births.[4]

Three different types of previa have been identified and are characterized as follows: marginal, partial, and total. *(Please see Figure 3.)* They are defined according to the extent to which the placenta encroaches on the cervix. Marginal previa occurs when the placenta extends up to the os, but does not cover it. Partial previa is defined by partial occlusion of the os by the placenta, with an incidence reported to be as high as 3% of all cases of previa.[14] Total previa, as the name suggests, occurs when the placenta completely covers the os. The incidence of total previa is estimated to occur in 20-43% of all cases of previa.[16] In contrast to abruption, the classification of previa neither predicts mortality of mother or fetus nor forecasts management approaches. Any patient with any type of previa can develop life-threatening hemorrhage during labor. The preferred method of management for all patients with previa is delivery by C-section.

Pathophysiology. The mechanism by which placenta previa causes serious—and potentially life-threatening—vaginal bleeding during the later half of pregnancy is relatively clear. Hemorrhage results from early separation of the placenta from the uterus. *(Please see Figure 4.)* This typically occurs from gradual thinning of the cervix in anticipation of delivery. Bleeding can also be induced from physical exertion, labor, local trauma (intercourse or digital examination by a physician), or it may have no apparent trigger.

Regardless of the cause, the comparative lack of muscle tissue in the lower uterine segment is predisposed to bleeding from the placenta as it separates from the uterine wall. The lower the attachment of the placenta, and the earlier in pregnancy that the lower uterus begins to change, the earlier bleeding occurs. The first bleeding episode typically ceases on a self-limited basis, but recurs as cervical changes become more pronounced. Nearly 33% of patients are diagnosed before 30 weeks gestation, but up to another 33% are not diagnosed until after 36 weeks gestation.[1] In one study, 5-15% of patients were diagnosed at 17 weeks.[16] However, almost 90% of these patients had resolution of the previa by term.[17] In contrast to abruption, the fetus is generally compromised from the bleeding unless a larger portion of the placenta detaches or maternal blood loss is extensive. The primary danger to the fetus is from preterm delivery precipitated by the bleeding episodes. As one would expect, the earlier in pregnancy that bleeding begins, the worse the perinatal risk. Interestingly, there is an association between fetal growth retardation and congenital abnormalities and children born to mothers with placenta previa.[18,19]

Although the mechanism of bleeding is clear, the reasons for improper placental implantation in these patients are not well characterized. Most authors agree that a host of factors are involved and some may be more important in the individual patient. Risk factors most commonly cited are multiparity (large number of previous pregnancies), prior C-section, prior placenta previa, multiple gestation (twins, etc.), and prior abortion with curettage.[4] A common theme among the risk factors is the scarring of the uterus. Uterine scars are formed by surgical procedures, such as C-section or elective abortion, or they may result from previous placental implantation.

Some authors suggest the placenta implants in the lower uterine segment to "avoid" previously damaged uterine muscle, where implantation may be more difficult or may impair subsequent placental function. Whatever the explanation, the presence of a scar from previous C-section increases the mother's risk for previa by about six-fold, yielding a 1-4% risk for previa in any pregnancy after C-section.[20] The risk increases in direct correlation to the number of uterine surgeries. In patients with a history of four or more C-sections, there is nearly a 10% risk of placenta previa.[21] This risk is not affected by the orientation of the C-section incision (transverse vs vertical), and appears to be a result of the presence of previous uterine trauma alone. The evidence for multiparity as a risk factor for previa also is strong. Placenta previa is seen in 1 out of 20 grand multiparas and only 1 in 1500 nulliparas.[1] In the uncommon case of multiple gestations, the larger surface area of the placenta (or placentas) gives rise to an increased risk of previa simply by the relatively decreased surface area of the uterus. As with abruption, male fetal sex and maternal cigarette use also have been found to increase risk for placenta previa.[12,22]

Clinical Presentation. In contrast with placental abruption, patients with previa typically present with painless vaginal bleeding; in fact, almost 70% of patients with previa will present in this fashion.[14] Another 20% will have uterine contractions associated with pain. Clearly, this can be a source of confusion for the physician as painful bleeding is the classical presentation of placental abruption. It is important to note that the pain associated with previa is usually milder than pain in patients with significant placental abruption. The remaining 10% of patients will be incidentally diagnosed at time of C-section or during the course of a routine ultrasound.[14]

Even though the majority of patients with previa present with painless vaginal bleeding, less than 50% of patients who present with these signs and symptoms are ultimately diagnosed with previa.[1] In previa, the blood noted usually is bright red in color. It will be necessary to verify that blood is coming from the os and not from another vaginal source, and a speculum exam is required to verify this. However, it is very important for the ED physician to be clear about the risks of performing a vaginal exam in any patient with bleeding in the second half of pregnancy. While placenta previa does not often cause life-threatening hemorrhage on its own (in the absence of labor), iatrogenic trauma of the cervix can produce bleeding that is dangerous both to mother and child. Therefore, any patient with vaginal bleeding in the later half of pregnancy where previa is in question should not undergo any invasive exam of the vagina until previa is ruled out.

When an exam is performed by the obstetrician, it is performed as a "double set-up" exam. The patient undergoes vaginal exam in the OR with all the necessary equipment and personnel to proceed immediately with an emergency C-section in the event dangerous bleeding is induced by the exam. Obviously, the exam is performed in this fashion if the fetus is considered viable for delivery. In the absence of these conditions, it is never "safe" to perform any invasive vaginal exam (speculum or digital) in a patient with previa. The only possible exception to this may be in an ED where there is no access to an obstetrician or ultrasound. A very gentle and limited speculum exam may be indicated to verify the bleeding is coming from the os and not from another, less worrisome source. Even in this setting, it can be argued that if no consultant is available, the patient should be transferred to an ED where appropriate consultation exists before attempting a potentially dangerous maneuver.

Imaging Studies. Apart from standard laboratory tests used to guide resuscitative efforts in a mother with significant hemorrhage, ultrasound is virtually the only test required for evaluation of a patient suspected of having placenta previa. *(Please see Figure 5.)* As with abruption, MRI is being investigated as a tool for diagnosis, but currently is not recommended for ED use.[23] As mentioned above, ultrasound should be done to rule out previa as a diagnosis before any invasive vaginal exams are performed. Therefore, in stable patients with bleeding during the second half of pregnancy, ultrasound should be performed as rapidly as possible to clarify the patient's diagnosis. With a hemodynamically unstable patient, resuscitation and emergency C-section may be the only treatment indicated.

Because it is completely non-invasive, transabdominal ultrasound is the technique of choice to rule out previa. This is not to say that transvaginal exams are not potentially safe and more accurate when performed by appropriately trained individuals. Several authors report that transvaginal exams are safe and provide better data in these patients.[24-26] Recommendations are that the probe be inserted no more than 3 cm into the vagina, and that no contact is made with the cervix or lower uterine segment in order to avoid iatrogenic bleeding. Images obtained by transvaginal ultrasound are of superior quality, and this approach avoids poor images that frequently are produced in obese patients and those with full urinary bladders. When using the transabdominal approach, it is recommended that a second scan be obtained with an empty bladder to increase accuracy. Likewise, when the placenta is implanted posteriorly or laterally in the uterus, diagnostic transabdominal images are difficult to obtain. Overall, the accuracy of transabdominal ultrasound is reported to be in the 93-97% range, with 2-6% false-positive and 2% false-negative rates.[25,27] Comparison to previous ultrasound studies is very useful, but not always available when the patient presents to the ED.

It should be stressed that up to 90% of patients diagnosed with placenta previa before 20 weeks gestation will resolve by term delivery.[17] The term "placental migration" has been used to explain this fact. The term is somewhat of a misnomer, as it is improbable that the placenta actually separates and re-implants to account for this observation. A more likely explanation is that the lower uterine segment structure changes with time and grows disproportionately. Another possibility is that the placenta may also undergo relatively more growth away from the cervix. Whatever the exact mechanism, it is surprising to find that 73% of patients with total previa diagnosed in the second trimester will regress to a lesser degree of previa.[28] Marginal previa will be found at term in only 2.5% of cases diagnosed in the second trimester.[28] Another author reports that up to 5% of all pregnant women will have evidence of some type of placenta previa on ultrasound in the second trimester.[1] Furthermore, 95% of these patients will have no symptoms, no previa at term, and a normal ultrasound by 28 weeks.[1] Therefore, a history of previa diagnosed early in the patient's pregnancy does not mean that the condition will still present at the time of their ED visits.

Finally, it should be noted that the other important function of ultrasound in these patients is to establish fetal gestational age and potential fetal viability outside the mother. As will be seen in the next section, management of patients with placenta previa is greatly influenced by whether a viable or near-term fetus exists at time of the mother's presentation.

Patient Management. Care of the patient with documented or suspected placenta previa and late term vaginal bleeding can be complex. As with abruption, management is determined by the severity of maternal hemorrhage and fetal viability as judged by gestational age and current vital signs. Patients who present with bleeding complications of previa often do so late in their pregnancy. As maternal blood volume has increased by 20-40% by term, the mother may tolerate substantial blood loss (500 mLs) without affecting vital signs. Therefore, when the vital signs show evidence of hypovolemia, one should assume that blood loss has been catastrophic and treat the patient accordingly. Consequently, any "sick" patient with bleeding and previa requires full efforts at maternal volume resuscitation, including large bore IVs (or central access) and early transfusion of appropriate blood products. Urgent consultation in these cases is required inasmuch as emergency C-section may be life-saving for the mother and the fetus.

The general approach to a stable patient with vaginal bleeding in the second 20 weeks of gestation requires an accurate, relevant history of the event, including history of complications during the current as well as during previous pregnancies, an overview of general medical conditions, and a history of potential trauma (intercourse, recent medical exams, etc.). A physical exam—excluding a vaginal or rectal exams—should be performed. Reportedly, placenta previa is more likely when a "high presenting part" of the fetus is palpated on abdominal exam. The physician is reminded not to forget a "5th vital sign" in these patients (i.e., fetal heart monitoring, which is the standard of care in any patient with late trimester bleeding).

A transabdominal ultrasound exam should be obtained early in the work-up of any patient in whom placenta previa is suspected. If evidence of previa is obtained on ultrasound, the obstetrician will proceed with a C-section or expectant management, depending on the condition of mother and fetus, fetal gestational age, and the severity of maternal bleeding. When the fetus is clearly viable, significant improvements in perinatal mortality have been noted with early use of C-section.[1] A recent evaluation of C-section in previa, however, found that regional anesthesia is associated with lower blood loss and may be a safer alternative than general anesthesia for delivery in these patients.[29] In patients in whom the fetus is clearly not viable outside the mother, the pregnancy is supported in the hospital until fetal maturity can be established. Use of tocolytics in this setting remain controversial, and up to 33% of patients will fail expectant management.[30] Such complications as DIC and renal failure less frequently are seen in cases of previa as compared to abruption. Maternal mortality is now less than 1%, and perinatal mortality is less than 5% with current therapies.[1]

Vasa Previa

Although rare, vasa previa is a potentially important cause of painless late trimester bleeding. The condition is distinguished by the fact the vaginal bleeding in vasa previa is completely of fetal origin. Consequently, in contrast to other causes of obstetrical hemorrhage, the mother, for all practical purposes, is not physically endangered by this type of hemorrhage. This condition results from a defect in placental formation. Typically, the umbilical cord is inserted in a lateral (velamentous) position on the placenta. The umbilical vessels travel through the placental membranes unsupported by other placental tissue. As these vessels travel across the cervix, in advance of the presenting fetal anatomy, they are at risk of rupture and isolated, fetal hemorrhage.

Vasa previa can also be caused by presence of an extra lobe on the placenta. Most often, the umbilical vessels are torn at time of labor or during artificial rupture of the membranes, but bleeding also may occur spontaneously late in pregnancy. As the fetal blood volume is quite small (up to 500 mLs), seemingly insignificant amounts of vaginal bleeding can result in fetal exsanguination. While vasa previa complicates only 1 in 2000-5000 pregnancies, perinatal fetal mortality from rupture of these vessels approaches 75%.[31]

As might be expected, diagnosis of this condition can be difficult in the ED setting. If the condition is not detected prior to ED presentation, the fetus may expire before the diagnosis is confirmed. Ultrasound findings of a bi-lobed placenta will certainly heighten suspicion, but are not diagnostic._Transvaginal color-flow Doppler has been used to diagnose vasa previa, but the technique is still being developed and transvaginal ultrasound is not yet the standard of care to rule out placenta previa.[32] Most authors still recommend first ruling out placenta previa before pursuing other diagnoses. Vaginal instrumentation (the best way to diagnose vasa previa) in patients with potential placenta previa is currently contraindicated.

Laboratory tests are available that will detect the presence of fetal hemoglobin or nucleated red blood cells in the expelled blood. However, the lack of availability of these tests when needed, the length of time required to perform them, and their inaccuracy render them less useful clinically. The ED physician, however, should be aware, though, of the "Apt" test.[33] The "Apt" test is used to distinguish fetal from maternal red blood cells in vaginal blood, based on the higher resistance of fetal hemoglobin to alkaline conditions.

Clinical suspicion for this condition should be heightened when the mother presents with a small volume, bleeding episode, and absence of other maternal symptoms (significant uterine pain, signs of large volume blood loss), but the fetal monitor shows significant fetal distress. Specifically, one should search for fetal tachycardia, sinusoidal fetal heart rate pattern, or variable decelerations that coincide with membrane rupture. The presence of any of these fetal distress patterns combined with "minor" vaginal bleeding and lack of maternal symptoms suggest vasa previa. Emergency C-section is virtually the only method of fetal salvage in these cases, and delays in obtaining an emergent obstetrical consultation will increase an already high fetal mortality.

Uterine Rupture

Uterine rupture is a devastating event. Maternal mortality approaches 40% in the worst cases, and the fetal mortality is even higher.[4] Risk factors for this condition have two themes in common: weakness of the uterine wall (typically associated with surgical scars), and increased intrauterine pressures. The most common causes of uterine scarring are previous C-section, fibroid removal, or other procedures that divide the uterine wall. Increased intrauterine pressures can be seen with concealed placental abruption, blunt abdominal trauma, and other placental abnormalities. Placenta acreta/increta/percreta are conditions where the placenta invades the uterine wall from just below the surface (acreta) to completely through it (percreta). Invasive moles and chroiocarcinoma are also risk factors for uterine rupture.

Clinical signs of uterine rupture include a sudden increase in uterine pain or irritability, loss of previously normal contraction patterns, and fetal heart rate abnormalities. At times, the physician may be able to palpate fetal parts on abdominal exam. As expected, intra-abdominal bleeding can vary from small to clinically significant volumes, depending on the extent of the uterine tear. True maternal blood loss is often much greater than the amount of vaginal bleeding. Both mother and fetus often suddenly decompensate during "normal" labor and emergent action is required. The severity of the patient's condition will usually preclude any attempt at imaging or other diagnostic maneuvers. In the worst case scenario, it also may mean that definitive treatment is needed before consultants arrive. Obviously, this is a disastrous situation, and only an emergent C-section will possibly salvage the fetus (or just to control maternal hemorrhage).

Summary

Pregnancy is an important but potentially stressful time in a woman's life. When an unexpected, potentially dangerous event such as vaginal bleeding occurs, it is extremely upsetting for the expectant mother and father. While the ED physician may not always be able to bring good news to these patients, in many cases early intervention can make the difference between life and death for the fetus, and at times the mother as well.

Placental abruption and placenta previa are the two most common causes of vaginal bleeding in the second half of pregnancy. Therefore, any patient presenting to the ED with bleeding in later pregnancy may be suffering from one of these conditions until proven otherwise. The ED physician must first recognize the potential danger, and realize that patients may be more ill than they first appear. Resuscitation of the mother, fetal monitoring, fetal gestational age estimates, an ultrasound to rule out previa as a cause, and obstetrical consultation should be performed in all cases. Early pediatric consultation is also essential when dealing with a viable fetus. The ED physician must recognize that early delivery is essential in cases of severe bleeding.

References

1. Scott JR. Placenta previa and abruption. In: Scott JR, et al, eds. *Danforth's Obstetrics and Gynecology.* 8th ed. Philadelphia: Lippincott Williams & Wilkins; 1999:407-418.
2. Hansen WF, Hansen AR. Problems in pregnancy. In: Tintinalli JE, Ruiz E, Krome RL, eds. *Emergency Medicine: A Comprehensive Study Guide,* 4th Ed. New York: McGraw-Hill; 1996:564-575.
3. Pritchard J. Obstetric hemorrhage. In: Pritchard J, MacDonald P, eds. *Williams Obstetrics*. New York: Appleton-Century-Crofts; 1980:485.
4. VanDeKerkhove KM, Johnson TRB. Bleeding in the second half of pregnancy: Maternal and fetal assessment. In: Pearlman MD, Tintinalli JE. eds. *Emergency Care of the Woman.* New York: McGraw Hill; 1998:303-312.
5. Pritchard JA, Cunningham G, Pritchard SA, et al. A prospective controlled study of outcome after trauma during pregnancy. *Am J Obstet Gynecol* 1990;162:1502-1505.
6. Abdella TN, Sibai BM, Harp JM, et al. Perinatal outcome in abruptio placentae. *Obstet Gynecol* 1984;63:365-370.
7. Hurd W, Miodovnik M, Hertzberg V, et al. Selective management of abruptio placentae: A prospective study. *Obstet Gynecol* 1983;61:467-473.
8. Knab DR. Abruptio placentae. An assessment of the time and method of delivery. *Obstet Gynecol* 1978;52:625-629.
9. Landy HJ, Hinson J. Placental abruption associated with cocaine use: A case report. *Repro Toxicol* 1987;1:203-205.
10. Ananth CV, Savitz DA, Williams MA. Placental abruption and its association with hypertension and prolonged rupture of membranes: A methodologic review and meta-analysis. *Obstet Gynecol* 1996;88:309-318.
11. Kramer MS, Usher RH, Pollack R, et al. Etiologic determinants of abruption placentae. *Obstet Gynecol* 1997;89:221-226.
12. Andres RL. The association of cigarette smoking with placenta previa and abruptio placentae. *Semin Perinatol* 1996; 20:154-159.
13. Magriples U, Chan DW, Bruzek D, et al. Thrombomodulin: A new marker for placental abruption. *Thromb Haemost* 1999; 81:32-34.
14. Benedetti TJ. Obstetric hemorrhage. In: Gabbe SG, Niebyl JR, Simpson JL, eds. *Obstetrics: Normal and Problem Pregnancies,* 3rd Ed. New York: Churchill Livingstone; 1996: 499-532.
15. Nyberg DA, Mack LA, Benedetti TJ, et al. Placental abruption and placental hemorrhage: Correlation of sonographic findings with fetal outcome. *Radiology* 1987;358:357-361.
16. Cotton D, Ead J, Paul R, et al. The conservative aggressive management of placenta previa. *Am J Obstet Gynecol* 1987; 168:1424-1429.
17. Rizos N, Doran T, Miskin M, et al. Natural history of placenta previa ascertained by diagnostic ultrasound. *Am J Obstet Gynecol* 1979;133:287-291.
18. Brar HS, Platt LD, DeVore GR et al. Fetal umbilical velocemetry for the surveillance of pregnancies complicated by placenta previa. *J Reprod Med* 1988;33:741-744.
19. McShane PM, Heyl PS, Epstein MF. Maternal and perinatal morbidity resulting from placenta previa. *Obstet Gynecol* 1985;65:176-182.
20. Chattopadhyay S, Kharif H, Sherbeeni J. Placenta previa and accreta after previous cesarean section. *Eur J Obstet Gynecol Reprod Biol* 1993;52:151-156.
21. Clark S, Koonings P, Phelan J. Placenta previa/accreta and prior cesarean section. *Obstet Gynecol* 1985;66:89-92.
22. Demissie K, Breckenridge MB, Joesph L, et al. Placenta previa: A preponderance of male sex at birth. *Am J Epidemiol* 1999;149: 824-830.
23. Thorp JM Jr, Wells SR, Wiest HH, et al. First trimester diagnosis of placenta previa by magnetic resonance imaging. *Am J Obstet Gynecol* 1998;178:616-618.
24. Thorp JM, Councell RB, Sandridge DA, et al. Antepartum diagnosis of placenta previa percreta by magnetic resonance imaging. *Obstet Gynecol* 1992;80:506-508.
25. Tan NH, Abu M, Woo JLS, et al. The role of transvaginal ultrasonography in the diagnosis of placenta previa. *Aust NZ J Obstet Gynecol* 1995;35:42-45.
26. Farine D, Fox, HE, Jakobson S, et al. Vaginal ultrasound for the diagnosis of placenta previa. *Am J Obstet Gynaecol* 1988; 159:566-569.
27. Leerentveld, RA, Gilberts EC, Arnold M, et al. Accuracy and safety of transvaginal sonographic placental localization. *Obstet Gynecol* 1990;76:759-762.
28. Zelop C, Bromley B, Frigoletto FJ, et al. Second trimester sonographically diagnosed placenta previa: Prediction of persistent previa at birth. *Int J Gynaecol Obstet* 1994;44: 207-210.
29. Fredericksen MC, Glassenberg R, Stika CS. Placenta previa: A 22-year analysis. *Am J Obstet Gynecol* 1999;180:1432-1437.
30. Watson WJ, Defalo RC. Magnesium sulfate tocolysis in selected patients with placenta previa. *Am J Perinatol* 1990;7: 251-253.
31. Kouyoumkjian A. Velamentous insertion of the umbilical cord. *Obstet Gynecol* 1980;56:737.
32. Harding JA, Lewis DF, Major CA, et al. Color flow Doppler—A useful instrument in the diagnosis of vasa previa. *Am J Obstet Gynecol* 1990;163:1566-1568.
33. Odunski K, Bullough CH, Henzel J, et al. Evaluation of chemical tests for fetal bleeding from vasa previa. *Int J Gynaecol Obstet* 1996;55:207-212.

Abnormal Vaginal Bleeding

Charles Seamens, MD
Corey M. Slovis, MD, FACP, FACEP

Vaginal bleeding is one of the most common complaints of women presenting to the emergency department (ED). Therefore, it is very important for the ED physician to have expertise in the initial evaluation and treatment of vaginal bleeding. Pregnancy-related causes of abnormal uterine bleeding must always be considered early in the differential diagnosis of any reproductive-age woman. Because the diagnosis of pregnancy always alters the approach to the patient with vaginal bleeding, a pregnancy test is imperative before proceeding to treatment.

The causes of abnormal vaginal bleeding that are nonpregnancy-related fall into two categories: 1) hormonal imbalance of estrogen and/or progesterone, or 2) an anatomic lesion. Derangement of estrogen-progesterone balance is most commonly due to anovulatory states and occurs at the extremes of a woman's reproductive life.[1] Anatomic lesions can cause severe bleeding and usually require histological identification.

Although most episodes of abnormal vaginal bleeding do not cause acute medical complications, diagnosis and treatment are essential because menses is the main source of iron loss in the menstruating woman. Increased vaginal blood loss is the most common cause of iron-deficiency anemia in women of reproductive age.[2]

This chapter focuses on causes of vaginal bleeding unrelated to pregnancy with an emphasis on etiology, diagnosis, and treatment.

Terminology

There are a number of terms used to describe vaginal bleeding that describe the quantity, frequency, or cause of the bleeding. Because a woman's perception of blood loss is highly subjective, objective evaluation of these patients is difficult. Some of the terms used to describe these pathological states require definition. *Menorrhagia* is derived from the Greek word men, meaning month, and rhegynai, meaning to burst forth.[2] Menorrhagia is defined as menstrual cycles in which bleeding is either excessive or prolonged. Menstrual blood loss is considered excessive if it exceeds 80 mL per period cycle. While menorrhagia affects women of all ages, half of all patients presenting with the problem are younger than age 40, and about 20% are adolescents.[3] Menorrhagia is very common in women during their reproductive years and is seen in 9-14% of all women in this age group.[4] *Metromenorrhagia* refers to prolonged or excessive uterine bleeding that occurs at irregular intervals. *Oligomenorrhea* is defined as uterine bleeding episodes that occur from intervals of 35 days to six months.[3] Women with this pattern may have ovulatory, anovulatory, or mixed ovulatory-anovulatory bleeding. Most commonly, oligomenorrhea is due to a hypothalamic cause.[5] *Polymenorrhea* is regular bleeding that occurs at intervals shorter than 21 days. *Amenorrhea* refers to the absence of uterine bleeding for at least six months.[6] *Intermenstrual bleeding* is defined as bleeding that occurs between regular men-

Figure 1. Hormonal Variation During the Menstrual Cycle

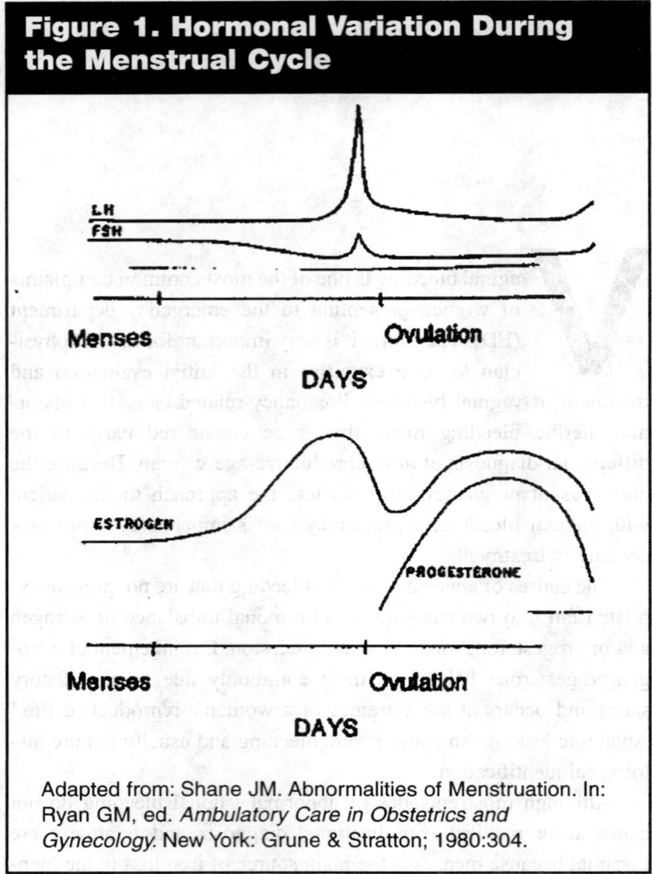

Adapted from: Shane JM. Abnormalities of Menstruation. In: Ryan GM, ed. *Ambulatory Care in Obstetrics and Gynecology.* New York: Grune & Stratton; 1980:304.

strual cycles. The amount of bleeding is variable and typically les s frequent than metrorrhagia. Intermenstrual bleeding may also be referred to as breakthrough bleeding. Probably the most common cause of intermenstrual bleeding is that caused by oral contraceptive pills (OCPs).

Normal Menstruation

To understand vaginal bleeding in the disease state, it is essential to have a detailed understanding of normal menstruation and the hormonal influences that are crucial to this process.

The normal menstrual cycle depends on a complex interaction of hormonal events that have profound anatomical and physiological consequences. Normal menses is based on the relative amounts of estrogen and progesterone, which, in turn, are regulated by the hypothalamus' secretion of two releasing factors: luteinizing hormone (LH) and follicle-stimulating hormone (FSH). Estrogen stimulation approximately six months prior to menarche initiates endocervical mucus production and desquamation of vaginal epithelial cells. Thus, prior to beginning true menstrual flow, peripubescent girls will begin to experience physiological leukorrhea.[7]

Each menstrual cycle is divided into three phases: *proliferative* (follicular), *secretory* (luteal), and *menstrual*. By convention, the first day of the menstrual bleeding cycle is considered day 1, and subsequent days are numbered serially until the next menstrual bleeding.[8]

Proliferative Phase. The first phase of menses is called the proliferative phase because of the dramatic proliferation and growth of the endometrial wall of the uterus. FSH and LH stimulate the uterus to increase its wall thickness. This phase of the menstrual cycle varies the most in duration. It usually lasts about 10 days.[9]

At the beginning of the menstrual cycle (approximately days 4 and 5), the hypothalamus synthesizes and secretes gonadotropin-releasing hormone, which stimulates the secretion of the gonadotropins LH and FSH from the pituitary gland.[5] FSH stimulates the formation of about 1000 ovarian follicles in the ovaries during each menstrual cycle. FSH and LH cause the maturing follicles to produce and secrete three classes of sex steroids: estrogens, androgens, and progestins.

Estrogen, the most important sex steroid at the early stage of follicular development, provides the primary feedback inhibition to the pituitary gland and its secretion of FSH.[9] A positive feedback mechanism also develops with the leading follicle—the graafian follicle. This follicle secretes the majority of estradiol. This estrogen is the most potent, develops the most FSH and LH receptors, and secretes even more estradiol. Estradiol secretion peaks around the 14th day.[5,10] The estrogen levels also exert positive feedback on LH. Approximately 24-36 hours before ovulation, estrogen levels rise sharply, causing a further decline of FSH and an LH peak. This LH surge in turn triggers ovulation.[9] *(Please see Figure 1.)*

The high estrogen levels of the proliferative phase stimulate the growth of the endometrium from 1 mm at the time of menstruation to 5 mm at the time of ovulation.[10] Another action of estrogen during the proliferative phase is the synthesis of progesterone receptors.[5]

The endometrial threshold is a theoretical representation of the amount of estrogen stimulation required to prime the endometrium so that bleeding can occur.[11] In other words, a certain amount of estrogen must be present for a certain amount of time to sufficiently thicken the wall of endometrium. The amount of endometrial tissue produced during this phase is directly proportional to the levels of circulating estrogen.[9] Only estrogen priming of the endometrium can produce bleeding; progesterone administration without estrogen priming will not cause bleeding.[8] After ovulation, progesterone production increases, and the secretory phase begins.[3]

Secretory Phase. The LH surge and subsequent ovulation caused by increased estradiol heralds the beginning of the secretory phase. The LH surge also causes production of progesterone in the dominant follicle 12-24 hours before ovulation.[5,9] The increasing progesterone secretion plays a major role in both successful ovulation and development of the corpus luteum following ovulation.

A smaller FSH surge also occurs and causes: 1) increased androgen production in the degenerating follicles; 2) progesterone production in the dominant follicle; 3) the remaining follicles to become atretic; and 4) an ovulatory stimulus. This ovulatory stimulus is accomplished by stimulating prostaglandin production essential for follicle rupture. Birth control pills inhibit FSH and LH secretion, thus neither the LH surge nor ovulation take place.[9]

After ovulation, the graafian follicle develops and becomes the corpus luteum. It produces progesterone, which antagonizes the action of estrogen by inducing enzymatic conversion of estradiol to estrone, a less potent estrogen. Remember, estrogen's action is to stimulate growth. Progesterone, therefore, indirectly halts the growth of the endometrium since it inhibits estrogen.[9,11] Progesterone causes the endometrial stroma to become compact, and secretory changes occur within the glands.[3]

The secretory phase begins on the day after ovulation, continues for 14 days, and is much more constant in duration than the more

Table 1. Common Causes of Abnormal Uterine Bleeding at Different Ages

ADOLESCENCE
Anovulatory uterine bleeding, coagulation disorders, pregnancy-related causes, functional ovarian cysts, breakthrough bleeding, withdrawal bleeding
REPRODUCTIVE AGE
Pregnancy related causes, dysfunctional uterine bleeding, anatomic lesions, anticoagulant therapy, thyroid disease
PERIMENOPAUSAL AGE
Anatomic lesions, anovulatory dysfunctional uterine bleeding, bleeding disorders, liver disease, anticoagulant therapy
POSTMENOPAUSAL AGE
Anatomic lesions, bleeding disorders, liver disease, anticoagulant therapy, trauma

variable proliferative phase.[5] The corpus luteum functions for approximately 14 days under LH stimulation, during which it gradually involutes if pregnancy has not occurred. Both estrogen and progesterone levels then return to basal levels, initiating a cascade of events that culminates in menstruation.[3,5,10] If fertilization and implantation occur, the trophoblast will begin to secrete β-hCG and maintain the function of the corpus luteum.

Menstruation. Menstruation is due to estrogen and progesterone withdrawal. The bleeding is self-limited because the endometrium responds in an orderly and progressive fashion in shedding down to the basal layers.[3,8]

During menstruation, blood flow is facilitated by local fibrinolytic activity in the endometrial blood vessels.[5] Cessation of menstrual bleeding, on the other hand, depends on clotting occurring at the disrupted end of the spiral endometrial arteries, prolonged vasoconstriction, and the active proliferation and regeneration of the endometrium.[5]

If ovulation does not occur, an abnormal pattern of uterine bleeding results. This is because estrogen's effects are not balanced by those of progesterone and, thus, unopposed estrogenic stimulation occurs. Bleeding then proceeds in a disordered fashion. Periods can be excessive in frequency and amount, or they may be infrequent and lighter at irregular intervals.[5]

Normal Menstrual Cycles. The normal menstrual cycle is 21-35 days. Variability in the cycle occurs in the proliferative (follicular) phase; the secretory (luteal) phase is more consistent, lasting 12-14 days. Normal menstrual flow usually occurs over 2-6 days. Flow is usually heaviest for the first 1-3 days and then tapers off.[3,10,12] The average blood loss per cycle is 20-60 mL, with median expected blood loss approximately 30-40 mL.[3,5,13] Menstrual blood loss of 80 mL or more is considered excessive and results in a greater risk of iron-deficiency anemia.[10,13,14] Although there is patient-to-patient variability in the length, duration, and amount of menstrual blood loss, these parameters remain relatively constant for individuals from cycle to cycle. Usually, the only time a woman seeks medical advice for this problem is when she perceives a deviation from her norm.[10]

Etiologies of Abnormal Vaginal Bleeding

Abnormal vaginal bleeding takes place for a variety of reasons. Increased menstrual blood loss may be due to anovulatory or ovulatory disorders, chronic systemic illnesses, organic reproductive pathology, blood dyscrasias, anatomic lesions, or trauma. *(Please see Table 1.)*

Dysfunctional Uterine Bleeding. Dysfunctional uterine bleeding (DUB) refers to abnormal vaginal bleeding that is usually hormonal in etiology. This entity remains a common cause of abnormal vaginal bleeding. The hormonal abnormalities can be the result of endogenous abnormal hormone production or the result of exogenously given sex steroids (i.e., OCPs).

As stated previously, the endometrial threshold is the amount of estrogen stimulation required to prime the endometrium so that bleeding can occur. The pattern and magnitude of the abnormal bleeding is thought to depend on not only the level of circulating estrogen, but also on the fluctuations that occur at that level. Women with low estrogen levels are likely to have intermittent spotting and light bleeding. Women with higher levels of estrogens often have a prolonged interval of amenorrhea followed by excessive episodes of bleeding.[5] If, for some reason, estrogen levels are insufficient to reach the endometrial threshold, bleeding will not occur.[8,11]

There are two variations of estrogen breakthrough bleeding. The first is associated with estrogen levels that are well above the endometrial threshold required to prime the endometrium. Estrogen stimulates the growth of the endometrium, while progesterone matures the endometrium and inhibits the endometrial growth effects of estrogen. In anovulatory states, with no progesterone inhibition, unopposed estrogenic stimulation causes the endometrial lining to become quite thick and vascular. Since ovulation has not occurred, and, thus, no progesterone is being produced, the bleeding usually seen in normal menstruation does not occur. Areas of endometrium outgrow their hormonal support and degenerate, causing irregular and prolonged bleeding.[8] Rather than an orderly shedding of the endometrium, the thick endometrium becomes friable and intermittently breaks down to bleed. The resultant bleeding due to inefficient endometrial shedding may be prolonged, profuse, and irregular. This type of anovulatory bleed is a very common cause of abnormal uterine bleeding in young women.[11]

The other type of estrogen breakthrough bleeding is associated with relatively low, but constant, levels of estrogen that tend to hover at levels around the bleeding threshold. Portions of the endometrium degenerate and spotting occurs.

Progesterone withdrawal bleeding occurs only after the endometrium has been primed with estrogenic stimulation. Progesterone alone cannot induce bleeding because it does not cause proliferation of the endometrium. When estrogen therapy is continued as progesterone is withdrawn, progesterone withdrawal bleeding occurs. This type of bleeding is relatively uncommon.[12]

When exogenous synthetic sex steroid hormones are administered, most commonly OCPs, abnormal vaginal bleeding can be seen due to a variety of mechanisms resulting in breakthrough bleeding or withdrawal.

Breakthrough bleeding occurs more frequently on progestin-only pills or pills with low doses of estrogen and progestin and is annoying enough that the OCPs are often discontinued.[5] Replacing them with a different pill formulation, usually one with a higher dose of estrogen, may reduce breakthrough bleeding. Breakthrough bleeding can indicate reduced birth-control efficacy, so additional contraception (if birth control is desired), such as a barrier method, should be advised until the bleeding resolves.[14]

Intermenstrual bleeding is common when patients first begin OCPs but usually resolves within three months of starting the drug. Intermenstrual bleeding while on OCPs is usually due to missed pills or variable ingestion times. Patients should be carefully counseled about the importance of taking the OCP every day. Taking the pill at the same time each day decreases the frequency of breakthrough bleeding.[14]

Drug interactions have also been implicated in breakthrough bleeding in patients on OCPs. The most common drugs causing breakthrough bleeding are anticonvulsants, such as phenytoin, phenobarbital, carbamazepine and, primidone, and some antibiotics, like penicillins, tetracylines and trimethoprim-sulfamethoxazole.

Anatomic Pelvic Disease. *Cervical Lesions.* The vulva, vagina, and cervix may have abnormalities, such as tumors, infections, or lacerations.[10] Lesions of the cervix can cause abnormal vaginal bleeding that must be differentiated from intrauterine sources. If present, cervical polyps will usually be visible within the cervical os and are usually erythematous, friable and painless. Their presenting symptom is commonly postcoital or intermenstrual bleeding.[3] Cervical or vaginal condyloma can also be a source of bleeding. In addition, trauma to the cervix or vagina, especially with atrophic, postmenopausal mucosa, can be the source of vaginal bleeding.[5]

Uterine Lesions. Benign lesions of the uterus are a much more common cause of abnormal uterine bleeding than malignancies.[5] Perimenopausal women frequently become metromenorrhagic because of anovulation, but in many cases this occurs in combination with anatomic lesions such as uterine fibroids, polyps, and neoplasia.[5,14] Uterine leiomyomas or fibroids occur in 20-25% of women by age 40 and in up to 50% of women overall.[14,15] The majority of leiomyomas are asymptomatic. About 30% of patients with leiomyomas complain of abnormal uterine bleeding. Fibroids are a common incidental finding, and the presence of fibroids does not indicate that they are the cause of the excessive bleeding until other causes have been ruled out.[14] Large, intramural uterine leiomyomas can cause menorrhagia by enlarging the surface area of the endometrial cavity or by altering the uterine and endometrial vasculature.[15] Submucosal and intraluminal polypoidal leiomyomas disrupt the endometrial vessels and are more likely to cause abnormal uterine bleeding.[5,16] The bleeding associated with leiomyomas is cyclic and can be profuse.[3]

As with fibroids, adenomyosis is another cause of an enlarged uterus. Uterine adenomyosis occurs when endometrial tissue is imbedded in the myometrium and can contribute to abnormal uterine bleeding.[5,16]

Endometriosis is a variable condition that undoubtedly may be accompanied by normal bleeding, but clinical evidence suggests that it is also associated with menorrhagia, though not frequently.[16,17]

Endometrial polyps are most frequently encountered in women between the ages of 40 and 55 and may be found solitary or multiple, pedunculated or sessile.[3]

Malignant tumors of the uterus become more common as age progresses. Endometrial carcinoma occurs most commonly between the ages of 50 and 75 years, although 20-25% of cases occur before menopause.[5] Leiomyosarcoma must be suspected when menorrhagia does not respond to treatment and is associated with progressive uterine growth.[18] One % of women, between ages 40 and 60 years, with presumed uterine leiomyomas with symptoms significant enough to warrant hysterectomy had a diagnosis of leiomyosarcoma postoperatively.[5] Anatomical lesions are probably better diagnosed by hysteroscopy and ultrasound than by the traditional D&C. [1,17,19-30]

The presence of an IUD can produce intermenstrual bleeding. The IUD creates a foreign body reaction in the uterus that results in a local inflammatory reaction in the endometrium and shows potent fibrinolytic activity.[18,31] This bleeding is generally well-tolerated by the patient with proper reassurances. Other causes of abnormal uterine bleeding can coexist with the IUD. These should be considered if there is significant deviation from an established bleeding pattern from month to month.[5] The duration and the amount of menstrual blood loss are increased by inert or copper-containing IUDs. On the other hand, progesterone-containing IUDs diminish menstrual blood loss.[15] Bleeding directly due to the IUD is relieved when the device is removed, often with the next cycle.[5]

Clinical Approach

Vaginal Bleeding in Adolescence. Adolescents often present with abnormal uterine bleeding, which is usually due to anovulatory cycles. There is a delay in the maturation of the positive feedback mechanism that is necessary for the LH surge and subsequent ovulation. For this reason, the initial cycles after menarche are usually anovulatory.[10] The slowly maturing hypothalamic-pituitary axis is quite vulnerable to various physiological and pathological processes.[5,12,13] This is not in itself a pathological condition but a part of normal maturation that occurs at varying rates in individual girls.[12] In the first year of menarche, around 55% of menses are anovulatory. It takes an average of 15 months to complete the first 10 menstrual cycles.[7] The adolescent tends to have cycles of variable lengths, anovulation being associated with both short and long cycles.[7] Most adolescents who experience dysfunctional bleeding eventually begin ovulating regularly.[14] Although it is sometimes difficult to decide when to do a pelvic exam in girls age 10-16 years, those who are sexually active with hemodynamic compromise, significant anemia, or pain should have a pelvic examination. Cultures for sexually transmitted diseases should also be obtained.

A neoplastic cause of dysfunctional uterine bleeding is highly unlikely during adolescence. Provided that pregnancy has been excluded, therapy can be commenced without further investigations. Treatment can be stopped after 3-6 months and the patient observed to see whether a normal menstrual pattern develops.

Keep in mind that excessive uterine bleeding in adolescence may be the initial manifestation of an underlying coagulopathy.[5] In one population of hospitalized adolescents with excessive menstrual bleeding, only 74% were diagnosed with DUB—close to 20% had a coagulation disorder and 7% had other pathology.[12,33]

Vaginal Bleeding in Reproductive-Age Women. As in all patients, it is essential to obtain a complete history, including a menstrual history and reproductive history.[3] In the active reproductive years, anovulatory bleeding is a less frequent cause of menstrual irregularity.[5] Pregnancy must always be excluded as an etiology.

The clinician must try to estimate the amount of blood loss the patient is experiencing. Menstrual bleeding that is associated with clotting or that lasts longer than seven days is very suggestive of substantial blood loss.[10] The presence of iron-deficiency anemia is most often the only practical way to determine whether bleeding has been excessive.

If the clinician determines that the frequency and amount of blood loss is excessive, then further evaluation is indicated. Initial laboratory tests should include hemoglobin, platelet count, a pregnancy test, and, as based on history, coagulation studies.

Vaginal Bleeding in Perimenopausal and Postmenopausal Women. Dysfunctional uterine bleeding occurs most often at the extremes of the reproductive years. Perimenopausal women also have an increased rate of dysfunctional uterine bleeding.[3] A detailed menstrual history is of utmost importance in guiding use of other diagnostic studies, especially in the older woman. A complete obstetrical history should also be taken, including previous gynecological surgeries as well as past and current use of medications. Coexistent diseases may be the etiology of present uterine bleeding.[5]

Anovulatory cycles often occur during the perimenopausal years. As the ovary ages, it becomes less sensitive to FSH and LH and produces less estrogen despite normal to elevated levels of gonadotropins. Although sufficient estrogen is present to stimulate proliferation of the endometrium, the high level of estrogen needed to induce the midcycle surge of LH is not reached, resulting in continuous estrogen stimulation of the endometrium. Just as in the adolescent, the continuous estrogen stimulation leads to a vascular, friable endometrium that may bleed intermittently or slough at irregular intervals.[10,14]

In this age group, the diagnosis of anovulatory bleeding is one of exclusion, as any uterine bleeding in the postmenopausal years, particularly intermenstrual bleeding, is categorically abnormal and requires further investigation. In one study, there was a 30% incidence of significant pathology on a cohort of perimenopausal bleeders, of which two-thirds had malignant or premalignant potential.[5] It is a mistake to assume that abnormal uterine bleeding in this age group is a self-limited, benign process.

Menorrhagia

The definition of menorrhagia requires objective measurement of the amount of menstrual blood loss. The patient's own reports and perception of excessive blood loss may not always be a true reflection of measured menstrual loss.[5,18]

Subjective assessments of the amount of menstrual blood loss and clinical parameters, such as duration of menses or number of napkins and tampons used, have not been accurate.[15,18,34] Evaluating women with this common subjective complaint can be very difficult because there is no practical method to quantify menstrual blood loss, especially in the ED.

Women complaining of menorrhagia can only base their assessment on their own menstrual history and on their perception of what the norm is for other women.[35] It is possible for a woman who has been menstruating excessively over many months or years to classify her menses as light if the heavy loss is reduced. Similarly, a woman who normally loses 20 mL with each period may classify her period as heavy when it doubles to 40 mL, which is within a normal range.[34]

Many women are unable to judge the severity of their vaginal bleeding. In a study by Hallberg and associates, 40% of women with excessive uterine bleeding (> 80 mL) considered their periods normal or even light. Some women with light periods viewed their bleeding as severe.[13] Some authors consider 60 mL to be a more realistic upper limit of normal. Even if this amount is used as the upper limit of normal, another study indicated 40% of women whose bleeding fell below this level perceived their menstrual periods to be heavy.[18,36] The age of the patient appears to affect her perception of blood loss. Younger women perceived their daily menstrual loss as being excessively heavy, while the older women perceived a similar loss as light or moderate.[36]

Physicians often feel they can assess menstrual blood loss by inquiring about the number of sanitary pads or tampons used each period. Many women who mistakenly perceive their menstrual periods as heavy use a large numbers of pads or tampons per period, although some of these pads are barely discolored after use.[36] Objectively measured menstrual blood loss does not always correlate with pad or tampon count. In general, however, sanitary napkins absorb more blood than tampons.

The most accurate method to quantify the amount of menstrual blood loss is the alkaline hematin method. Blood loss can be accurately measured by collecting all tampons and pads used during the menses, blended with a known amount of sodium hydroxide, extracting the hemoglobin, and quantifying it by spectrophotometry.[14] Although this is an easy laboratory method to perform in research circumstances, it is far too laborious in general practice, let alone the ED.[10,15,37,38] Clinically, a very helpful objective measure for ED evaluation is the assessment of blood hemoglobin or serum ferritin concentrations, because two-thirds of women with objective menorrhagia develop iron-deficiency anemia.[39]

History. Menorrhagia may be due to systemic, local, or iatrogenic disorders. Initial assessment begins with a complete medical and gynecological history. The length and interval of the patient's normal menstrual cycles should be ascertained. Then, the amount, including duration and timing of excessive blood flow, should be assessed as accurately as possible.[40] The history should specifically determine the presence of clots and flooding. Associated symptoms of pain, nausea, bruising, or petechiae and any history of abnormal nongynecological bleeding should be sought. A history of medication use, especially use of aspirin or coumadin, should be obtained. Sexual activity, method of contraception, the presence of an IUD, and the possibility of pregnancy are historically important.

The possibility of a threatened abortion, complete or incomplete abortion, and ectopic pregnancy must be ruled out by pregnancy testing. History alone may be unreliable because the patient may have irregular menses, may not know she is pregnant, or may be too frightened or embarrassed to admit to the possibility of pregnancy.[7]

Any history of systemic diseases, particularly thyroid, renal, or hepatic diseases, should be noted, as should any history suggestive of coagulopathies.[3] Coagulopathies may initially present as menorrhagia that is directly proportional to the severity of the underlying coagulopathy.[5] Menorrhagia occurs in the majority of women with bleeding disorders.[41] Patients often give a history of excessive bleeding after dental extractions or other procedures. However, this history may be missed if not specifically asked for. For example, in women, the most common manifestations of von Willebrand's disease is menorrhagia, as well as postoperative and postpartum bleeding. Similarly,

Table 2. Combination Monophasic OCPs

DRUG	ESTROGEN	PROGESTIN	COST*
Loestrin 1/20	ethinyl estradiol	norethindrone	$25.24
Loestrin 1.5/30	ethinyl estradiol	norethindrone	$25.24
Brevicon 21,28	ethinyl estradiol	norethindrone	$22.08
Modicon 21	ethinyl estradiol	norethindrone	$24.17
Norinyl 1/35 21,28	ethinyl estradiol	norethindrone	$21.41
Ortho-Novum 1/35	ethinyl estradiol	norethindrone	$22.06
Levlen 21,28	ethinyl estradiol	levonorgestrel	$20.58
Nordette 21	ethinyl estradiol	levonorgestrel	$25.29
Lo/Ovral	ethinyl estradiol	norgestrel	$26.21
Ovral	ethinyl estradiol	norgestrel	$35.79
Demulen 1/30	ethinyl estradiol	ethynodiol diacetate	$23.32
Demulen 1/50	ethinyl estradiol	ethynodiol diacetate	$26.00
Norinyl 1/50 21,28	mestranol	norethindrone	$21.41
Ortho-Novum 1/50	mestranol	norethindrone	$22.06
Desogen	ethinyl estradiol	desogestrel	$19.55
Ortho-Cept 21	ethinyl estradiol	desogestrel	$22.20

*cost to pharmacy of one month's supply

Adapted from: Choice of contraceptives. *Med Lett* 1995;37:9-12.

von Willebrand's disease is said to be the most common hereditary disorder associated with menorrhagia.[42]

Since the liver is the major site of synthesis of coagulation factors, both acute and chronic liver disease can affect menstrual function. The use of warfarin or aspirin can lead to increased menstrual bleeding as well.[14,15]

Subclinical hypothyroidism has long been implicated as a cause of menorrhagia. Generally, the severely hypothyroid patient eventually becomes amenorrheic, but she may experience anovulatory bleeding before this. The excessive bleeding generally resolves with thyroid replacement therapy.[5,14,43]

The relationship between hemodialysis and menorrhagia remains confusing.[15] While most patients on chronic hemodialysis develop frank amenorrhea, hypermenorrhea has also been described.[44]

The polycystic ovary syndrome is most often characterized by infrequent menses, yet heavy uterine bleeding also may occur, especially after a long period of amenorrhea. This syndrome should be considered in the hirsute, overweight, relatively infertile teenager.[40]

In order to treat appropriately, it is usually important to determine whether the bleeding is ovulatory or anovulatory in nature. Bleeding that occurs at regular cyclic intervals and is preceded by premenstrual symptoms such as breast tenderness or fullness, water weight gain, mood swings, variable libido, abdominal bloating or cramping, nausea, edema, and headache is likely ovulatory.[3,7] Bleeding abnormalities associated with ovulatory cycles include menorrhagia and intermenstrual bleeding.[14]

Anovulatory uterine bleeding normally occurs at the beginning and end of a woman's reproductive years. At both ends of menstrual life, this expected phenomenon may produce enough symptoms to require specific diagnosis and treatment. These anovulatory states are due to a change in the hypothalamic-pituitary influence on the ovaries, not the inability of the uterus to respond properly.[5] The perimenopausal woman has a less responsive ovary but mature hypothalamic mechanism while the adolescent has a more responsive ovary and an immature hypothalamic axis.[5]

Physical Examination. As with any other patient who is bleeding, vital signs should be carefully evaluated, and any abnormalities should be addressed. A complete physical examination is important, specifically looking for pallor, petechiae, or bruising.

All women of reproductive age should have a pelvic examination. The pelvic exam may uncover adnexal, uterine, and lower genital tract abnormalities, and the bimanual vaginal exam is the time-honored method of assessment of pelvic masses.[8,19] On bimanual exam, an enlarged uterus raises the suspicion of pregnancy, and this possibility needs to be excluded.[10] Unfortunately, not all masses are able to be detected by palpation. Factors that may reduce the accuracy of the bimanual exam include the examiner's experience, the patient's weight, and degree of relaxation. Transvaginal sonography is more accurate for detecting adnexal and uterine masses than the bimanual exam, but it should be used in a complementary fashion instead of replacing the pelvic exam.[8,19] Any woman with disturbing symptomatology and a normal pelvic exam should undergo transvaginal ultrasound to confirm the absence of cysts or neoplasms.[19,20]

Treatment. The lack of objective evidence of increased blood loss in many patients complaining of menorrhagia must be seriously considered when justifying the appropriateness of any therapy. The choice of medical therapy for abnormal uterine bleeding depends primarily on the etiology and is affected by the patient's age, coexisting medical disorders, coexisting reproductive tract disorders, and, most importantly, the severity of blood loss. The drug of choice depends on whether the bleeding is associated with anovulatory or ovulatory cycles and the age and contraceptive needs of the patient.[35]

If a careful history and physical examination do not reveal a systemic or structural illness, certain patients can be treated for dysfunctional uterine bleeding without further studies. Adolescents and women under the age of 35 with short-term ovulatory dysfunction can be treated with OCPs.[14] *(Please see Table 2.)* Probably the best options for treatment of menorrhagia are OCPs or NSAIDs. OCPs decrease menstrual bleeding by 50% and reduce dysmenorrhea. OCPs may be effective in the management of bleeding caused by fibroids.[14]

Progestational Agents. Progestins have an anti-estrogen effect that is mediated by the conversion of estradiol to the less potent estrone.[5,45] Progesterone therapy can be used to suppress a heavy episode of bleeding and on a regular maintenance basis. Two regimens may be used, either a higher dose and taper down, or a lower dose and increase, as needed to arrest the bleeding.

Medroxyprogesterone acetate or norethisterone may be given in a dosage of 30-40 mg/d initially for one week, decreasing by 10 mg/d each week until a daily dosage of 10 mg is reached. The bleeding should stop in the first week, but if it does not, the dosage can be increased to 40-50 mg/d. Once the patient has been free of bleeding for 3-4 weeks, the progesterone can be stopped and a withdrawal bleed should occur.

The other regimen is to give progesterone 10 mg/d initially and increase the dosage each day until the bleeding stops. Once the bleeding has been controlled, the dosage can then be maintained for a total of 3-4 weeks. Norethindrone 5 mg taken twice daily can be used in a similar fashion.[10]

Patients on cyclic progesterone should be counseled to use a barrier method of contraception if they are sexually active because this regimen is not effective for birth control.[14] Occasional ovulation does occur. The side effects of medroxyprogesterone are weight gain, abdominal bloating, mood changes, anxiety, nausea, edema, headaches, acne, and exacerbation of epilepsy and migraines.[3,35,46]

Depot medroxyprogesterone acetate is also available and is administered by intramuscular injection. A major disadvantage of this drug is that after a single injection a sustained progestational effect can last up to six months. However, this agent may have a role in the treatment of dysfunctional uterine bleeding for the poorly compliant or mentally incompetent patient. An effective dose is 150 mg every three months.[10]

Medicated IUDs that release levonorgestrel in a controlled manner have been shown to substantially reduce menstrual blood loss.[46] The levonorgestrel has local effects on the endometrium and limited systemic absorption. Up to half of the women who use them will become amenorrheic.[1,35]

In the perimenopausal patient who has had structural lesions excluded, treatment with monthly progesterone can be started. This treatment may be continued until no further withdrawal bleeding occurs, which signifies ovarian failure. At this time estrogen replacement can be added to the regimen. The estrogen should not contain more than 35 mcg.

Estrogens. The healing effect of estradiol may be the result of the induced growth of the endometrium. It also promotes coagulation by increasing fibrinogen levels, clotting factors, platelet aggregation, and by decreasing capillary permeability.[10]

Chronic bleeding and long-term treatment with oral contraceptives or progestational therapy can result in atrophic changes in the endometrium that make it prone to bleeding. Thus, estrogen therapy may be effective in the anovulatory patient who presents with persistent bleeding despite a D&C with evidence of minimal endometrial tissue.

For these patients, intravenous conjugated estrogens can be used effectively at a dose of 25 mg every four hours, with a maximum of three doses. Immediately after the bleeding has stopped, progestational therapy should be started.[10]

NSAIDs. NSAIDs inhibit the enzyme cyclooxygenase in the arachidonic acid cascade, decreasing the production of prostaglandins.[4,18] Menorrhagia may be associated with an excess of PGE_2 (vasodilator) function in the endometrium over PGF_2 (vasoconstrictor) function.[35] NSAIDs, therefore, may be useful in treating menorrhagia by decreasing PGE_2 concentrations. For patients with menorrhagia, NSAIDs will reduce blood from menses by 30-50%.[15,47,48]

Patients with menorrhagia caused by structural lesions, such as fibroids, may not respond to NSAIDs.[14,15] Patients should be instructed to begin the NSAIDs on the first day of the menstrual period and to continue them on a scheduled basis until menstrual bleeding stops.[14,15] NSAIDs reduce menstrual flow, have the advantage of also reducing dysmenorrhea, and may be used in combination of with OCPs.[18] The advantages of NSAIDs include their relative paucity of side effects, low cost, and need for use only at the time of bleeding. They are particularly suitable as first-line therapy for the large group of women with ovulatory menorrhagia.[35] After cessation of therapy, patients can be expected to revert to their original pattern of bleeding. Although it is also a prostaglandin inhibitor, aspirin is not effective for menorrhagia, and, even at doses of 1500 mg or 3000 mg, does not diminish menstrual blood loss. The higher dose may even increase menstrual blood loss. Little is known about the effect that low dosages of aspirin have on blood loss.[15]

Danazol. Danazol (Danocrine), a 2,3-isoxazol derivative of 17 ethinyl-testerone, has undesirable androgenic side effects but has been used successfully in some patients for reduction of menstrual flow.[5,49] Danocrine 200-400 mg every day for 25 days a month has been helpful with menorrhagia.[47,50,51] The most acceptable dosage appears to be 200 mg/d.[51] At this dosage, most women will still experience regular menstruation (higher doses cause amenorrhea) and relief from dysmenorrhea.[35]

Uterine Contracting Agents. Uterine contracting agents, such as ergotamine, do not diminish the amount of menstrual blood loss and are therefore useless and even dangerous having precipitated myocardial infarction.[15,52,53]

Others. Tamoxifen, vitamin E, and subcutaneous desmopressin have been tried in special cases with apparent success.[39] Effective treatments for menorrhagia in patients with bleeding disorders are combination OCPs, oral or intramuscular progesterone, or progesterone-containing IUDs. If contraception is not desired, prostaglandin inhibitors are the drugs of choice.[41] Combination OCPs and antifibrinolytics are relatively contraindicated in women receiving oral anticoagulant therapy. Since combination OCPs are relatively contraindicated, and inert or copper-containing IUDs increase menstrual blood loss, continuous administration of progesterone is the contraceptive of choice in women receiving oral anticoagulant therapy.[41]

The use of synthetic gonadotropin-releasing hormone agonists (GnRH-a) have also been used to control abnormal uterine bleeding. The mechanisms of menstrual blood loss reduction is probably related to the low-circulating estrogen levels.[54,55]

Dysfunctional Uterine Bleeding

The following therapeutic approach has been described by Gupey and Ahlstrom after pregnancy states and anatomic lesions have been excluded:[40]

Mild DUB. Women who are not anemic or have very mild anemia with a hematocrit of 35% or greater or a hemoglobin of 10-11 g/dL or higher have mild DUB. Management consists of reassurance, iron supplementation, and follow-up with a gynecologist.[7,40]

Moderate DUB. Moderate DUB is usually associated with significant but not life-threatening anemia. Hematocrits typically run in the 25-35 % range, corresponding to a hemoglobin of 9-10 g/dL. The goals of treatment for dysfunctional uterine bleeding are to control the acute bleeding as well as avert future episodes of bleeding.[10] Pharmacological treatment should be started for patients who find their bleeding patterns intolerable or who have iron-deficiency anemia.[14]

Hormonal therapy is required to regulate the bleeding and thereby limit blood loss. Therapy tides the patient over until her own endocrine system matures or readjusts itself. Many regimens have been recommended and used successfully, including estrogen alone, estrogen and synthetic progestin, and synthetic progestin alone.[33,40] For the patient who is acutely bleeding, a low-dose oral contraceptive can be administered at a dose of 1-4 pills a day. This regimen should be continued for one week and then decreased to one pill a day.[10] Combined estrogen and progestin in the form of an oral contraceptive pill is used most frequently to treat moderate DUB, but many other treatment regimens exist and work well. A low-dose combined OCP is given orally for 21 days, followed by a short withdrawal bleed during seven days of placebo pills. Hormonal therapy should not be stopped before the hemoglobin level has returned to normal and iron stores replenished. If hormonal therapy is started when the patient is actively bleeding, a higher dose of estrogen and synthetic progestin is often needed to stop flow. The patient is instructed to take up to four OCP tablets per day initially until bleeding stops, and then to gradually taper down to one tablet per day over a period of a week or so. Extra hormonally active (not placebo) pills from a different package of OCPs should be used for this purpose.[40] *(Please see Table 2.)*

Possible side effects of hormonal use are nausea and breast tenderness. Patients should be warned about breakthrough bleeding or spotting. It is especially important to warn girls and their mothers that stopping the medication abruptly will result in resumption of bleeding and worsening of anemia. Iron supplementation may be given as ferrous gluconate 325 mg tid. There is no evidence that hormonal medication is harmful to the maturing hypothalamic-pituitary-ovarian axis or that it stunts growth.[7,40]

Severe DUB. Patients with severe bleeding over a short period of time may show hemodynamic compromise with hypotension and tachycardia. These patients require immediate hospitalization along with prompt and aggressive therapy. There are two goals to acute therapy: first and foremost, the restoration of hemodynamic stability; the next, the cessation of uterine bleeding.[40]

Estrogen can be administered intravenously as Premarin, the water-soluble conjugated equine estrogen, to control uterine bleeding acutely. A dose of 25 mg of Premarin can be given every 4-6 hours until bleeding slows considerably (up to a maximum of four doses).[56] Premarin is associated with: 1) increased fibrinogen levels within six hours of administration; 2) increased factors V and IX; 3) platelet aggregation; and 4) decreased capillary permeability.[55] Concurrently (because bleeding will soon recur), a high-dose combination estrogen and synthetic progestin tablet can also be given. Enovid 5 mg (mestranol 75 mg and norethynodrel 5 mg) can be given orally every six hours, or ethinyl estradiol in a dose of 500 mcg (0.5 mg) and medroxyprogesterone (Provera) 20 mg can be used instead.[7,40]

For those patients placed on hormonal therapy, an antiemetic is often required during the first few days of this hormonal regimen, as nausea and vomiting frequently accompany the high estrogen doses. One Enovid 5 mg can be continued daily for a total of 21 days and then stopped to allow a withdrawal bleed. Menstrual flow should then be controlled using a low-dose combination OCP beginning within one week of stopping the Enovid 5 mg and continuing for at least three cycles. Iron replacement therapy should be encouraged. In most patients, the menses become regular and DUB does not recur.[33,40]

For those patients with intractable severe bleeding or life-threatening vaginal bleeding, an emergent D&C may be necessary. The evacuation of blood clots from the cavity and the removal of hypertrophic endometrial tissue will cause a temporary cessation of bleeding. The reduction of bleeding can be short-lived, and without further treatment, many patients resume a pattern of menorrhagia.[1,5,27,57] D&C may remedy bleeding from polyps, submucous leiomyomas, or retained products of conception.[27]

Other Means to Control Uterine Hemorrhage. Uterine tamponade using a Foley catheter has been used successfully to control uterine hemorrhage. The procedure consists of inserting the largest caliber of Foley catheter that can be inserted through the cervix with ease. Anesthesia is not typically required. The balloon is distended with saline until the bleeding stops. Occasionally, patients who have been bleeding excessively have large uteri, and balloon sizes up to 15-30 mL have been used. Patients with fibroids may need 30-40 mL of saline instilled. Blood will sometimes drip through a large caliber Foley catheter, so further tamponade is required by clamping the Foley catheter. The balloon is usually left in place for 12-24 hours to control bleeding.[58]

Summary

As a frequent complaint of women presenting to the ED, vaginal bleeding represents an important clinical problem for the emergency physician. A working understanding of the normal menstrual cycle is helpful when organizing a differential diagnosis and evaluation and treatment plan. In the absence of ectopic pregnancy, vaginal bleeding generally is not immediately life-threatening. A thorough evaluation of the potential etiologies, however, must be initiated in the ED, along with simultaneous treatment of the bleeding and associated clinical effects when appropriate. As with many ED patients, proper follow-up is necessary once evaluation and treatment have been initiated in the ED setting.

References

1. Brill AI. What is the role of hysteroscopy in the management of abnormal uterine bleeding? *Clin Obstet Gynecol* 1995;38:319-345.
2. Rees M. Menorrhagia. *BM J* 1987;294:759-762.
3. Galle PC, McRae MA. Abnormal uterine bleeding. *Postgrad Med* 1993;93:73-76, 80-81.
4. Duncan KM. Nonsteroidal anti-inflammatory drugs in menorrhagia. *Ann Pharmacother* 1993;27:1353-1354.
5. Jennings JC. Abnormal uterine bleeding. *Med Clin North Am* 1995;79:1357-1376.
6. Kempers RD. Dysfunctional uterine bleeding. In: Speroff L, et al, eds. *Obstetrics and Gynecology.* Philadelphia: J.B. Lippencott Co.; 1990:1-11.

7. Altchek A. Dysfunctional uterine bleeding in adolescence. *Clin Obstet Gynecol* 1977:20:633-650.
8. Carter J, Fowler J, Carson L, et al. How accurate is the pelvic examination as compared to transvaginal sonography? *J Reprod Med* 1994;39:32-34.
9. Hochbaum SR. Vaginal bleeding. *Emerg Med Clin North Am* 1982;5:429-442.
10. Bayer S, De Cherney AH. Clinical manifestations and treatment of dysfunctional uterine bleeding. *JAMA* 1993;269:1823-1828.
11. Strickler RC. Dysfunctional uterine bleeding. *Postgrad Med* 1979;66:135-146.
12. Carlson KJ, Nichols DH, Schiff I. Indications for hysterectomy. *N Engl J Med* 1993;328:856-860.
13. Hallberg L, Hogdahl A, Nilsson L, et al. Menstrual blood loss—A population study. *Acta Scand Obstet Gynecol* 1966;45:321-351.
14. Walthen PI, Henderson MC, Witz CA. Abnormal uterine bleeding. *Med Clin North Am* 1995;79:329-342.
15. van Eijkeren MA, Christiaens GCML, Scholten PC, et al. Menorrhagia: Current drug treatment concepts. *Drugs* 1992;43:201-209.
16. Fraser IS. Hysteroscopy and laparoscopy in women with menorrhagia. *Am J Obstet Gynecol* 1990;162:1264-1269.
17. Fraser, IS. Hysteroscopy and laparoscopy in women with menorrhagia. *Am J Obstet Gynecol* 1991;164: 47-52.
18. Fraser IS. Efficacy of mefenamic acid in patients with a complaint of menorrhagia. *Obstet Gynecol,* 1981;58:543-551.
19. Dodson M. Use of transvaginal ultrasound in diagnosing the etiology of menometrorrhagia. *J Reprod Med* 1994;39:362-372.
20. Emanuel MH, Verdel MJ, Wamsteker K, et al. A prospective comparison of transvaginal ultrasonography and diagnostic hysteroscopy in the evaluation of patients with abnormal uterine bleeding: Clinical implications. *Am J Obstet Gynecol* 1995;172: 547-552.
21. Motashaw ND, Dave S. Diagnostic and therapeutic hysteroscopy in the management of abnormal uterine bleeding. *J Reprod Med* 1990:35:616-620.
22. Nasri MN, Shepherd JH, Setchell ME, et al. The role of vaginal scan in measurement of endometrial thickness in postmenopausal women. *Br J Obstet Gynecol* 1991;98:470-475.
23. Goldstein SR, Nachtigall M, Snyder JR, et al. Endometrial assessment by vaginal ultrasonography before endometrial sampling in patients with postmenopausal bleeding. *Am J Obstet Gynecol,* 1990;163:119-123.
24. Valle RF, et al. Hysteroscopic evaluation of patients with abnormal uterine bleeding. *Surg Obstet Gynecol* 1981;153: 521-526.
25. Varner RE, Sparks JM, Cameron CD, et al. Transvaginal sonography of the endometrium in postmenopausal women. *Obstet Gynecol* 1991;78: 195-199.
26. Townsend DE, Fields G, McCausland A, et al. Diagnostic and operative hysteroscopy in the management of persistent postmenopausal hemorrhage. *Obstet Gynecol* 1993;82:419-421.
27. Grimes DA. Diagnostic dilation and curettage: A reappraisal. *Am J Obstet Gynecol* 1982;142:1-6.
28. Brooks PG, Serden S. Hysteroscopic findings after unsuccessful dilatation and curettage for abnormal uterine bleeding. *Am J Obstet Gynecol* 1988;158:1354-1356.
29. Smith JJ, Schulman H. Current dilatation and curettage practice: A need for revision. *Obstet Gynecol,* 1985; 65:516-518.
30. Stode RJ, Kanbour A. Prehysterodomy curettage. *Obstet Gynecol* 1975;45:537-541.
31. Sheppard BL, Bonnar J. The effects of intrauterine contraceptive devices on the ultrastructure of the endometrium in relation to bleeding complication. *Am J Obstet Gynecol* 1983;146;829-839.
32. Mansfield MJ, Eman SJ. Adolescent menstrual irregularity. *J Reprod Med* 1984; 29:399-410.
33. Claessen EA, Cowell CA. Acute adolescent menorrhagia. *Am J Obstet Gynecol* 1981;139:277-280.
34. Chimbira TH, Anderson ABM, Turnbull AC. Relationship between measured menstrual blood loss and patient's subjective assessment of loss, duration of bleeding, number of sanitary towels used, uterine weight, and endometrial surface area. *Br J Obstet Gynaecol* 1980; 87:603-609.
35. Liddell H. Menorrhagia. *N Z Med J* 1993;106:255-257.
36. Fraser IS, McCarron G, Markum R, et al. A preliminary study of factors influencing perception of menstrual blood loss volume. *Am J Obstet Gynecol* 1990;149:788-793.
37. New T, Barnard G, Collins W. A rapid method for measuring menstrual blood loss using automatic extraction. *Conception* 1977;16:269-281.
38. Shaw ST. On qualifying menstrual blood loss. *Contraception* 1977;16:283-284.
39. Magos AL. Management of menorrhagia. *BMJ* 1990;300:1537-1538.
40. Gupey SM, Ahlstrom P. Common menstrual disorders. *Pediatr Clin North Am* 1989;36:551-571.
41. van Eijkeren MA, Christians GCML, Haspels AA, et al. Measured menstrual blood loss in women with a bleeding disorder or using oral anticoagulant therapy. *Am J Obstet Gynecol* 1990;162:1261-1263.
42. Fraser IS, McCarren G, Markum R, et al. Measured menstrual blood loss in women with menorrhagia associated with pelvic disease or coagulation disorder. *Obstet Gynecol* 1986;68:630-633.
43. Wilansky DL, Greisman B. Early hypothyroidism in patients with menorrhagia. *Am J Obstet Gynecol* 1989;673-677.
44. Perez RJ, Lipner H, Abdulla N, Cicotto S, et al. Menstrual dysfunction of patients undergoing chronic hemodialysis. *Obstet Gynecol* 1979;51:552-555.
45. Crosignani PG, Rubin B. Dysfunctional uterine bleeding. *Human Reprod* 1990; 5:637- 638.
46. Farquhaw C. Management of dysfunctional uterine bleeding. *Drugs* 1992; 44: 578-584.
47. Thorneycroft IH. Medical management of abnormal uterine bleeding in the patient in her 40s. *Obstet Gynecol Clin North Am* 1993;20:333- 336.
48. Nygren KG, Rybo G. Prostaglandins and menorrhagia. *Acta Obstet Gynecol Scand Suppl.* 1983;113:101-103.
49. Dockeray CJ, Sheppard BL, Bonnar J. Comparison between mefenamic acid and danazol in the treatment of established menorrhagia. *Br J Obstet Gynaecol* 1989; 96:840-844.

50. Bonduella M, Walker JJ, Calder AA. A comparative study of danazol and norethisterone in dysfunctional uterine bleeding presenting as menorrhagia. *Postgrad Med J* 1991:67: 833-836.
51. Cameron IT, Leask R, Kelly RW, et al. The effects of danazol, mefenamic acid, norethisterone and a progesterone —Impregnated coil on endometrial prostaglandin concentrations in women with menorrhagia. *Prostaglandins* 1987;34: 99-109.
52. Higham JM, O'Brien PMS, Shaw RW. Assessment of menstrual blood loss using a pictorial chart. *Br J Obstet Gynaecol* 1990;97:734-739.
53. Chimbura, TH, Anderson ABM, Naish C, Cope E, et al. Reduction of menstrual blood loss by danazol in unexplained menorrhagia: Lack of effect of placebo. *Br J Obstet Gynaecol,* 1980;87:1152-1158.
54. Shaw RW, Faxer HM. Use of superactive luteinizing hormone releasing hormone (LHRH) against in the treatment of menorrhagia. *Br J Obstet Gynaecol* 1984; 91:913-916.
55. Petrucco OM, Fraser IS. The potential for the use of GnRH agonists for treatment of dysfunctional uterine bleeding. *Br J Obstet Gynaecol* 1992;Suppl 7:34-36.
56. DeVore GB, Owens O, Kase N. Use of intravenous premarin in the treatment of dysfunctional uterine bleeding—A double-blind randomized control study. *Obstet Gynecol,* 1982; 59:285-291.
57. Haynes PJ, Hodgson H, Anderson ABM, et al. Measurement of menstrual blood loss in patients complaining of menorrhagia. *Br J Obstet Gynaecol* 1977;84:763-768.
58. Goldrath MH. Uterine tamponade for control of acute uterine bleeding. *Am J Obstet Gynecol* 1983;147:869-872.

Preeclampsia/ Eclampsia

Robert Schwab, MD

Preeclampsia/eclampsia has been called the "disease of theories."[1] Although it is a relatively common entity and has been the subject of a large body of research, the search for an inciting agent and a unifying pathophysiological mechanism has generated more questions than answers. Even the definition of the disease has been a source of controversy. Nevertheless, research has yielded a great deal of information that has markedly improved maternal and fetal outcomes, and work continues to enhance efforts at prevention of this often devastating condition.

Ideally, diagnosis and treatment of preeclampsia is the domain of the obstetrician. However, emergency physicians must be prepared to correctly diagnose subtle presentations and manage acute emergencies associated with this disease. Emergency physicians serving lower socioeconomic patient populations with limited access to prenatal care can expect to see acute, life-threatening manifestations of this condition. But, subtle presentations mimic common illnesses for which any patient may present to the ED. Thus, all emergency physicians should be familiar with common presentations and emergency management.

This chapter will summarize current information regarding the epidemiology, etiology, pathophysiology, and clinical sequelae of preeclampsia/eclampsia. Common ED presentations and an approach to diagnosis and treatment of emergent manifestations will be discussed. The information contained in this chapter will assist the emergency physician in restoring and preserving fetal and maternal well-being until definitive care can be undertaken by an obstetrician.

Introduction

Preeclampsia (PE) is the term used to describe a disorder of pregnancy characterized by hypertension, proteinuria, and often edema, usually manifesting after the 20th week of gestation. A diagnosis of eclampsia is made when a patient demonstrates seizure activity or coma in addition to signs and symptoms of PE.

Discussions and definitions of PE have emphasized the hypertensive aspects of the syndrome. A reasonable working definition of hypertension in pregnancy is a systolic pressure above 140 mmHg or 30 mmHg above pre-pregnancy levels, or a diastolic pressure above 90 mmHg or 15 mmHg above pre-pregnancy levels.[2] Ideally, the diagnosis should be made based on two measurements at least six hours apart, but the emergency physician often must act based on a single reading.[3]

Hypertension in pregnancy does not, by itself, define PE. There are four categories of hypertension in pregnancy currently recognized by the American College of Obstetricians and Gynecologists.[2] Only when hypertension is accompanied by proteinuria (300 mg or more excreted over a 24-hour period) can the diagnosis of PE be established; additional supportive findings include the presence of diffuse pitting edema or a weight gain of five or more pounds in one week.[4]

Epidemiology

Incidence and Risk Factors. Until relatively recently, PE was estimated to occur in 7% of all deliveries, but this figure was based on study samples that were not necessarily representative of the national population. A more comprehensive epidemiological study suggests that the true incidence of PE is closer to 3%, and that eclampsia occurs in roughly 0.05% of all deliveries.[5]

Risk factors for *preeclampsia* have been described in a number of large studies.[6-13] Although awareness of these risk factors is important for targeted screening efforts, such screening is impractical and unnecessary in the ED. However, review of risk factors aids the understanding of theories regarding mode of transmission. Daughters and sisters of preeclamptic women have more than a fourfold relative risk for the development of PE, while young maternal age, nulliparity, and twin pregnancies are associated with a threefold relative risk.[5,9,10] Eighty-five percent of all cases of PE occur in primigravidas. Other risk factors associated with a relative risk between 1 and 2 include multiparous women conceiving by a new partner, unmarried women, women with a history of barrier contraceptive use, and black women, although the rate of PE among blacks and other minorities appears to be declining.[5,9-11] A previous history of PE conveys increased risk, as does a history of diabetes, hypertension, or renal disease.[12,13] For unknown reasons, pregnant smokers have a decreased incidence of PE.[12]

Etiology. The precise etiology of PE remains unknown, but epidemiological studies have suggested that genetic and immunological factors are involved. Statistical analysis of Mendelian models of inheritance applied to observed incidences of PE support the hypothesis that homozygosity for a single recessive gene shared by mother and fetus leads to development of this disorder.[15]

Evidence supporting an immunological etiology is provided by the association with nulliparity, barrier contraception, and multiparous women conceiving by a new partner. This theory proposes that the immunological response to an unknown antigen is protective. Studies have demonstrated altered immunological activity of various types in women with pregnancy-induced hypertension.[16-20]

The hypothesis that accounts for nearly all the observed associations postulates genetic transmission of a gene that modulates the immune response. Human leukocyte antigen (HLA) sharing between mother and fetus has been observed with greater frequency in women with pregnancy-induced hypertension; attention has been focused on the HLA-DR4 antigen, but the relative importance of maternal, paternal, and fetal alloantigens has not yet been defined.[21-24]

Pathophysiology

Site of Origin. The clinical course of the disease suggests a primary role for the placenta, since it is delivery of the placenta that is essential in reversing the signs and symptoms of PE.[9] Association of the disease with hydatidiform molar and twin pregnancies, conditions in which the amount of trophoblastic tissue is increased, also implicates the placenta as an essential component of the disease process.[25]

Microscopic examination of trophoblastic tissue from women with PE has revealed a consistent finding that appears to validate the clinical observations. In normal pregnancies, the uterine spiral arteries are invaded by trophoblast at 14-16 weeks' gestation, converting these arteries to low-resistance, high-volume vessels that do not respond to vasoconstrictors.[1] Uteroplacental perfusion is thus maximized. In PE, invasion of the trophoblast is incomplete, and the spiral arteries retain responsiveness to vasoconstrictors.[26] The resulting uteroplacental hypoperfusion and ischemia is thought to elaborate toxins that lead to the pathophysiological derangements found in women with this disorder.[9]

Hyperdynamic Model. This model proposes that increased cardiac output is the fundamental derangement in PE.[13,27] Elevated cardiac output, which also occurs in normal pregnancies, has been demonstrated in preeclamptic women long before the development of hypertension, proteinuria, and edema, and earlier than the expected trophoblastic invasion of the spiral arteries.[27] It is postulated that hyperperfusion leads to maximal compensatory vasodilation, after which capillary beds are damaged by exposure to elevated pressures and flow.

Endothelial Cells. Vascular endothelial cells play an integral role in regulating vascular tone, hemostasis, and vascular permeability. During normal pregnancy, these cells adapt to the altered physiological state to produce vasodilation, a blunted response to vasopressors, and hypercoagulability.[9] In PE, endothelial cells lose their normal response to physiological changes and demonstrate new responses, leading ultimately to diffuse vasospasm, alteration in coagulability, and increased permeability.

Mediators. Blood concentrations of a number of substances manufactured or regulated by endothelial cells have been found to be altered in PE, suggesting that these substances may mediate the observed pathophysiological changes. Vasospasm and increased responsiveness to angiotensin II are partly attributed to increased angiotensin II binding-site density on platelets, and may also be due to increased levels of endothelin, a potent vasoconstrictor that increases pressor effects as well.[1,28-31] Imbalance occurs between vasodilatory prostaglandins (prostacyclin) and vasoconstrictive prostaglandins (thromboxane), with the ratio in preeclamptic women favoring thromboxane.[32] Other vasodilatory substances secreted by endothelial cells have been shown to be present in lower concentrations in preeclamptic women. The net effect of these observed alterations is unopposed vasoconstriction and diminished perfusion.[33]

Endothelial cells also regulate intravascular coagulation. In normal pregnancy, levels of fibrinogen and several clotting factors increase, while plasminogen levels decrease.[34] This hypercoagulability of pregnancy is altered in PE. Thrombocytopenia is common and is thought to be due to increased consumption by adherence to injured vessels.[9] The elevated thromboxane/prostacyclin ratio favors platelet adherence. Although there is controversy regarding the contribution of coagulopathy to the pathophysiology of PE, it is clear that a subset of patients experience significant consumptive coagulopathy and bleeding problems.[34]

Finally, dysfunction of the endothelial cell alters its ability to regulate vascular permeability. This has been demonstrated experimentally in patients with PE, and is manifest clinically as proteinuria and edema.[35]

Clinical Sequelae of Preeclampsia/Eclampsia

In women with PE, diffuse endothelial dysfunction leads to multisystem disease and diffuse organ dysfunction. Some of these derangements in organ function occur quite early and may serve as markers for later complications. Others manifest much later and occur only in severe disease.

Cardiovascular. Hemodynamic data from women with PE have produced nonuniform conclusions. Many believe that elevated systemic vascular resistance is a fundamental abnormality of the disorder, but Easterling and associates have demonstrated that elevated cardiac output is a fundamental abnormality in women who develop PE, and that this abnormality occurs long before the development of clinical disease.[13,27] It appears that vasospasm and elevated vascular resistance occur much later and only in a subset of women who develop more severe manifestations of the illness.

Plasma volume in normal pregnancy increases by 40-50%.[1] In women with PE, the plasma volume does not increase as much.[35] Renal losses, loss of intravascular oncotic pressure, and increased capillary permeability all play a role in diminishing plasma volume.

Renal. Renal blood flow is increased in patients with PE.[36] Glomerular filtration rate and creatinine clearance decrease by approximately 25% compared with normal pregnancy, but often remain above prepregnancy levels.[34] Uric acid clearance decreases markedly; elevated uric acid may be an early indicator of the disease.[34]

Hepatic. Liver involvement in PE is usually mild and clinically insignificant.[34] In a subset of patients with severe disease, however, the liver appears to be a primary target organ, and liver dysfunction can be severe.[37] Areas of focal parenchymal necrosis containing microthrombin and fibrinogen can bleed to form subcapsular hematomas.[37,38] Hepatocellular necrosis leads to elevations in transaminases that range from mild elevations to values up to 4000 IU/L.[37,38] Bilirubin can be elevated as well, but prothrombin time is usually normal, suggesting that hepatic function is generally preserved.

Hematologic. The most common hematologic abnormality found is thrombocytopenia, the etiology of which is thought to be enhanced consumption through adherence to damaged endothelium.[39] The altered prostacyclin/thromboxane ratio favors platelet adherence as well. The combination of platelet activation and damage to endothelial cells, which secrete prostaglandins, procoagulants, heparin, and tissue plasminogen-activating factor, enhances consumption of clotting factors, reversing the hypercoagulability of normal pregnancy. Most of these changes remain subclinical, however; thrombocytopenia is typically mild, and clinical diffuse intravascular coagulation (DIC) is uncommon.[9]

Placental. Two abnormalities are observed in women with PE. The first involves failure of trophoblastic invasion of uterine spiral arteries. The second abnormality has been termed atherosis, which describes placental vessels that are occluded by aggregates of platelets, fibrin, and lipophages.[9] The net effect is placental ischemia and areas of infarction.

Neurologic. Severe neurologic dysfunction in conjunction with other signs and symptoms of PE defines eclampsia. Seizures are the primary manifestation of central nervous system involvement, but coma and focal findings can be seen as well.[3,40] Cerebral hemorrhage, edema, vasospasm, and thrombosis all can occur.[34] Microscopically, the pathological changes resemble those of patients with hypertension and hypertensive encephalopathy. Cerebral hemorrhage is the leading cause of maternal death from eclampsia.

Presenting Signs and Symptoms

Mild Preeclampsia. Most commonly, PE will be diagnosed based on the asymptomatic development of hypertension, proteinuria, or edema discovered during routine prenatal care. However, be alert to the possibility of detecting asymptomatic PE in any pregnant patient presenting to the ED. Blood pressure measurement is routinely performed during triage. Ask the patient what her baseline blood pressure has been, or check the medical record. Look for edema during the physical examination. Do not be misled by isolated lower-extremity edema, which is common and not indicative of a pathological process. Since edema may be absent, and relative hypertension can be difficult to ascertain, the finding of proteinuria may be the only clue to mild PE. Anything more than trace protein on a urine dipstick is cause for concern. EDs seeing a large number of patients who neglect routine prenatal care should consider urine dipstick screening of all pregnant patients presenting after the 20th week of gestation.

Consider admitting patients found to have hypertension, proteinuria, or generalized edema after the 20th week of gestation. Urgent referral to an obstetrician is adequate for patients less than 20 weeks who have hypertension and/or proteinuria to assess the need for therapy and to rule out hydatidiform disease.

Severe Preeclampsia. Suspect severe disease in patients with PE who have any symptoms other than swelling. Indeed, the presence of headache, altered mental status, visual changes, abdominal pain, or seizures defines severe disease. *(Please see Table 1.)* Oliguric patients may complain of diminished urine output, although isolated acute renal failure in PE is rare.[41] Complaints of abnormal bleeding and bruising are uncommon but suggestive of severe disease as well. In general, symptomatic patients will have higher blood pressure and 3+ to 4+ proteinuria on urine dipstick testing. Other physical findings, such as cyanosis, jugular venous distension, and pulmonary rales are sometimes found in patients with severe disease. Look carefully for signs of coagulopathy, such as petechiae and bruising, and for papilledema and hyperreflexia, which indicate central nervous system involvement. Be alert, however, to the patient with vague, nonspecific symptoms, such as headache, blurred vision, nausea, or abdominal pain, particularly in the epigastrium or right upper quadrant. In the absence of obvious hypertension or other dramatic physical findings, these patients present a diagnostic challenge. Initiate a complete diagnostic workup on any patient in the second or third trimester of pregnancy who presents with neurological or gastrointestinal symptoms.

HELLP Syndrome. It is unclear whether patients with PE who are found to have Hemolysis, Elevated Liver function tests, and Low Platelets (HELLP) represent a subset of severe disease or a manifestation of underlying medical illness in pregnancy.[42,43] However, this entity, which affects up to 10% of severe preeclamptics and 30-50% of eclamptics, results in hepatocellular necrosis and liver dysfunction, has a higher complication rate (one-third develop DIC), and higher mortality.[42,44] Despite the seriousness of this disease entity, many patients with the HELLP syndrome present without hypertension or marked proteinuria. Presenting symptoms are typically vague and nonspecific, including nausea, malaise, and mild abdominal pain.[42] Although these symptoms relate to the underlying hepatic dysfunction, jaundice, hypoglycemia, and signs of coagulopathy are uncommon.[38] Thus, this

Table 1. Definition of Severe Preeclampsia

TWO OR MORE OF THE FOLLOWING SIGNS:

- Systolic blood pressure of 160 mmHg or diastolic pressure of 110 mmHg recorded six hours apart with the patient at bed rest
- Proteinuria, 5g/24 hours or 3+ to 4+ protein on dipstick
- Oliguria, urine output less than 400 mL/24 hours, or less than 30 mL/hour for two consecutive hours
- Cerebral or visual disturbances, including eye changes
- Pulmonary edema
- Epigastric pain
- Evidence of hemolysis, abnormal results from liver function tests, and/or thrombocytopenia
- Generalized convulsions and no history of seizure disorder

Adapted from: Stone JL, Lockwood CJ, Berkowitz GS, et al. Risk factors for severe preeclampsia. *Obstet Gynecol* 1994;83:357-361.

Table 2. Differential Diagnosis of Preeclampsia

Thrombotic microangiopathies (MHA): TTP, HUS, Sepsis, Drugs

Fibrinogen consumptive disorders (DIC): Hypovolemia, Hemorrhage, Sepsis, Acute fatty liver

Connective tissue disorders: SLE, Scleroderma, Primary renal disease

Adapted from: Martin JN, Stedman CM. Imitators of preeclampsia and HELLP syndrome. *Obstet Gynecol Clin North Am* 1991;18:181-198.

life-threatening entity often presents a significant diagnostic challenge. Exercise caution in examining the liver of patients with HELLP syndrome, since overly vigorous palpation may precipitate the rare but catastrophic complication of hepatic subcapsular hematoma rupture.

Differential Diagnosis. Table 2 lists the major diagnoses to be considered in patients thought to have PE. Knowledge of the differential diagnosis is critical to appropriate emergency management of the patient with suspected PE because, in addition to resuscitation and provision of supportive care, the emergency physician must initiate a complete diagnostic evaluation and recognize those entities that require immediate, adjunctive therapy. Failure to consider and then identify sepsis or the need for immediate surgical intervention will lead to unnecessary morbidity and mortality. When a diagnosis of PE is made based on history and physical findings alone, consider the possibility of cocaine intoxication, which has been a common misdiagnosis.[45] Most diagnostic confusion, however, occurs in patients thought to have the HELLP syndrome.

Diagnostic Evaluation. A detailed laboratory evaluation is essential for any patient suspected of having PE, because significant abnormalities often cannot be detected clinically. Order a complete blood count, platelet count, and peripheral blood smear. Mild thrombocytopenia is common, and, in severe cases, anemia plus the presence of fragmented red blood cells on peripheral smear provides evidence of microangiopathic hemolysis. Obtain a coagulation profile, including prothrombin time, partial thromboplastin time, fibrinogen, and fibrin degradation products. These are usually normal, except in severe disease. Assess renal and hepatic function: order electrolytes, glucose, BUN, creatinine, uric acid, LDH, AST, ALT, and bilirubin (direct and indirect). Mild elevations of BUN and creatinine are consistent with HELLP syndrome but can also be seen in thrombotic thrombocytopenic purpura. Marked renal dysfunction is suggestive of hemolytic-uremic syndrome. Extremely high levels of transaminases and hypoglycemia are seen in acute fatty liver of pregnancy. Any significant abnormality in these studies mandates admission.

Initiate a 24-hour urine collection to assess proteinuria and creatinine clearance as well as a drug screen in patients who are admitted. Obtain urine, blood, and cervical specimens for culture and sensitivity in women with fever or other signs of sepsis.

Tests such as anti-nuclear antibodies, rheumatoid factor, and Coomb's test can be deferred to the consultant. However, do not delay important imaging studies. Obtain a chest x-ray in patients with dyspnea, chest pain, or clinical signs of cardiopulmonary dysfunction. Order a CT scan of the head in any patient with headache, hyperreflexia, focal neurological findings, seizure, or altered mental status. Finally, consider performing or ordering pelvic ultrasonography to assess fetal well-being, and to rule out abruptio placentae or hydatidiform disease in consultation with the patient's OB/GYN. Also, consider ultrasonography of the liver and gallbladder when clinical findings are suggestive.

Treatment

General Principles. Although delivery of the fetus and placenta is the only definitive treatment, expectant management of women remote from term improves fetal outcome without undue risk to the mother.[44] Women with mild PE who are able to comply with home therapy recommendations and return for frequent reassessment may be managed as outpatients, although hospitalization for initial assessment of maternal/fetal well-being may be recommended. Patients with severe PE should be transferred to a tertiary care center for intensive monitoring and management.

Hypertension. There is controversy regarding the level at which treatment for hypertension is required. Prior to the 20th week of gestation, only hypertension with evidence of end-organ dysfunction requires emergent therapy. After 20 weeks, evidence of end-organ dysfunction defines a hypertensive emergency requiring immediate therapy. A blood smear consistent with microangiopathic hemolytic anemia indicates severe microvascular damage and the need for emergent therapy as well. Initiate therapy immediately in patients with severe PE, including otherwise asymptomatic patients with blood pressure readings of 160/110 mmHg or higher. Untreated, the

Table 3. Pharmacologic Management of Hypertension and Seizures

Drug	Dose/Route	Indications
ANTIHYPERTENSIVE THERAPY		
Hydralazine	5-10 mg IV repeat q20min to 60 mg maximum	First-line therapy for blood pressure >160/110 mmHg, severe preeclampsia, HELLP, or end-organ dysfunction
Labetalol	50-100 mg IV;	Alternative first-line therapy repeat q30min to 300 mg max
Nitroprusside	0.2 mcg/kg/min IV; increase as needed	Use when hydralazine or labetalol are ineffective or contraindicated to desired response
ANTICONVULSANT THERAPY		
Magnesium sulfate	4-6 g IV over 20 min then 1-2 g/h	Severe preeclampsia, eclampsia, preeclampsia near term
Phenytoin	20 mg/kg IV at 12.5 mg/min to 1500 mg maximum	Eclampsia
Diazepam	5-10 mg IV; repeat as necessary to 30 mg total	Status epilepticus

generalized vasospasm that causes these significant elevations in blood pressure can lead to cerebral hemorrhage, congestive heart failure, acute renal failure, and abruptio placentae. Women whose baseline blood pressure is low may be at high risk with readings far below 160/110 mmHg. Good clinical judgment and close consultation with the obstetrician are needed to decide when to initiate emergent therapy in these patients.

Use caution when initiating anti-hypertensive therapy. For asymptomatic patients, the goal should be to lower the pressure to around 120/80 mmHg.[46] Patients demonstrating end-organ dysfunction or a microangiopathic process should have their diastolic pressure lowered to their usual baseline or 90 mmHg, preferably within one hour.[41,47] However, overly aggressive therapy can lead to hypotension, which may exacerbate uteroplacental ischemia.[47] Since the use of antihypertensive agents in asymptomatic patients with mild elevations of blood pressure is controversial, leave these therapeutic decisions to the consultant.[47] For hypertensive emergencies, familiarity with a few agents is sufficient to effectively manage these potentially life-threatening situations.

Treatment should be rapid and controlled. Oral agents are inappropriate choices, since absorption is slow and often unpredictable. Intramuscular absorption is similarly unpredictable in these patients due to systemic vasospasm.[47] Three intravenous agents are available that should provide effective control of hypertension in nearly all patients with PE.[41] *(Please see Table 3.)*

Hydralazine has traditionally been the drug of choice for treatment of severe hypertension in pregnancy. Its arteriolar vasodilatory effects produce a reflex tachycardia and increase in cardiac output which is theoretically helpful in maintaining uterine perfusion.[47] Give 5-10 mg intravenously every 20 minutes to a maximum dose of 60 mg.[46] Side effects include overshoot hypotension, headache, and flushing.

An alternative first-line agent for treatment of hypertensive emergencies in PE is labetalol, which possesses both alpha- and beta-antagonist effects as well as beta-2-agonist properties.[41] These effects combine to produce vasodilatation and a lowering of systemic vascular resistance. Advantages of labetalol over hydralazine include more rapid onset of action and less overshoot hypotension.[41] The effective dose and duration of action of labetalol are more variable, however. Begin with a dose of 50 mg intravenously, and repeat it every 30 minutes to a total dose of 300 mg. Once effective blood-pressure control is achieved, give repeat doses every three hours.[48] Side effects include tremulousness and flushing.

Adverse effects on the fetus are uncommon with hydralazine or labetalol, making the risk-benefit ratio quite low. Should these agents prove ineffective, use sodium nitroprusside.

Unlike the first-line agents, sodium nitroprusside has an extremely short duration of action and must be administered as a continuous infusion. It is a powerful arteriolar and venous smooth-muscle relaxant that is quite effective in lowering blood pressure rapidly. Nitroprusside has the further advantage of allowing minute-by-minute titration for very precise control of blood pressure. Its main disadvantage relates to its metabolic products—cyanide and thiocyanate. Both can be dangerous to mother and fetus, although the safety profile of nitroprusside in PE is good.[41,49]

Nevertheless, begin nitroprusside infusions at a lower-than-usual dose in patients with PE; start at 0.2 mcg/kg/min, rather than the usual 0.5 mcg/kg/min. Monitor closely for thiocyanate toxicity, which manifests as blurred vision, tinnitus, or altered mental status.

These three agents should provide an adequate formulary for treating hypertensive emergencies in PE. Other agents, such as methyldopa and nifedipine, have been used to control blood pressure but are not suitable for managing emergent conditions. Do not use diuretics except to treat pulmonary edema, since they will further reduce the already diminished plasma volume. ACE inhibitors have been associated with harmful fetal effects and are contraindicated in pregnancy.[47] Good communication with the consultant will guide nonemergent therapy.

Seizures. Prevention of seizures is of paramount importance, since eclampsia has a significantly higher maternal and perinatal mortality than does preeclampsia.[4] Although the precise pathophysiological mechanism underlying eclamptic seizures is unclear, cerebral vasospasm, edema, ischemia, and ionic shifts between intra- and extracellular compartments are thought to contribute.[50,51] Whatever the cause, appropriate prophylaxis and treatment of seizures can usually be achieved with magnesium sulfate, phenytoin, and diazepam. *(Please see Table 3.)*

Magnesium sulfate has been used in the management of PE for many years, and a recent large trial confirms its efficacy in preventing eclamptic seizures.[52] Since magnesium blocks calcium channels in smooth muscle and has been shown to prevent and reverse vasospasm experimentally, its efficacy in preventing seizures has a theoretical mechanistic basis.[51] There is much less controlled evidence in support of magnesium's utility in terminating seizures. In experimental settings, magnesium sulfate does not dampen neuronal firing, and so cannot be classified as an anticonvulsant.[50] Still, the widespread acceptance of magnesium sulfate as the drug of choice for the prevention and treatment of eclampsia renders these theoretical discussions clinically irrelevant.[47] Empiric data confirm that seizures occur uncommonly in patients receiving magnesium sulfate, and that magnesium prevents recurrence in 85-90% of eclamptic patients who receive the drug after an initial seizure.[53] Indications for initiating magnesium therapy include severe PE, eclampsia, and preeclampsia near term.

Give magnesium sulfate intravenously; the loading dose is 4-6 g, diluted in normal saline or 5% dextrose infused over 5-20 minutes. Follow this with a maintenance infusion of 1-2 g/hr controlled by an infusion pump. Monitor the patients closely for side effects. Magnesium toxicity can lead to respiratory paralysis and cardiac arrest, but hyporeflexia generally precedes more serious adverse effects.[54] Check patellar reflexes at least every hour, and monitor urine output and respiratory rate as well. In addition, check a serum magnesium level approximately one hour after initiating therapy; the therapeutic serum magnesium concentration is 4-7 mEq/L.[47]

Phenytoin is a commonly used anticonvulsant that can also be used for seizure prophylaxis. Although the incidence of seizures in patients receiving phenytoin prophylaxis is low, magnesium sulfate remains the drug of choice for prophylaxis of seizures in preeclamptic patients.[50,52] For termination of seizures, phenytoin possesses proven anticonvulsant properties, making it a logical therapeutic option. Opinions differ as to whether magnesium or phenytoin is more effective in terminating eclamptic seizures.[47,50] If the patient is already receiving magnesium, adding phenytoin seems logical. When patients are not being treated, magnesium is the best first choice, since it can be given more rapidly than phenytoin and is safer than diazepam.

Give 20 mg/kg (to a maximum dose of 1500 mg) of phenytoin intravenously by infusion at a rate not to exceed 50 mg/min.[50] Since serum protein levels tend to be lower in patients with PE, free phenytoin levels are higher, increasing the potential for toxicity.[50] Consider reducing the rate of infusion to 12.5 mg/min, and monitor the patient continuously for hypotension and cardiac arrhythmias. Other signs of phenytoin toxicity include lethargy and nystagmus. Check a phenytoin level one hour after the infusion is completed. Therapeutic levels are 10-20 mcg/mL. Neonatal toxicity has not been reported in patients treated for brief periods near term.[47,50]

Diazepam is effective in terminating seizures in eclamptic patients.[47,50] Its use in the United States has been limited by reports of fetal respiratory depression, hypotonia, heart beat variability, and maternal respiratory depression.[47,53] However, the risks of continued seizures and potential toxicity must be weighed against the benefit of terminating seizure activity. Diazepam can be given quite rapidly, which is advantageous for the termination of seizures. Consider using it when patients on magnesium manifest prolonged seizures or status epilepticus requiring immediate termination.

Give 5-10 mg intravenously over one minute, repeated as necessary up to a total dose of 30 mg.[47] Monitor the patient's respiratory status closely, and be prepared to provide ventilatory support. Avoid diazepam if possible when delivery is imminent, since the drug may depress neonatal respiration and cause hypotonicity.[50]

Other Emergent Manifestations. Patients with PE may present with other potentially life-threatening manifestations of the disease.[41] Central nervous system involvement may produce coma secondary to hemorrhage or cerebral edema with increased intracranial pressure. Cardiogenic and noncardiogenic pulmonary edema can occur. Patients with HELLP syndrome are at risk for rupture of hepatic subcapsular hematoma, which leads to massive intraperitoneal hemorrhage, and for other hemorrhagic complications secondary to DIC. Management of these life-threatening presentations involves standard therapy of the underlying problem along with good supportive care, prompt consultation, and delivery of the fetus and placenta as soon as possible.

Cardiopulmonary Arrest. Cardiopulmonary arrest is an uncommon complication of PE. Causes include massive hemorrhage, hypoxia secondary to pulmonary edema, or central nervous system dysfunction. Hypermagnesemia due to inadvertent overdose or secondary to alterations in renal function may also cause rapid decline in cardiopulmonary function. Be prepared to treat with intravenous calcium. Once cardiopulmonary arrest occurs, initiate CPR and resuscitate according to established protocols. Although resuscitation of the mother always is the first priority, outcome of cardiopulmonary arrest in women near term is improved by emergent perimortem cesarean section.[55,56] Removal of the fetus, a mechanical impediment to effective CPR, improves chances for maternal survival. Furthermore, fetal outcome improves, as time from cardiac arrest to delivery is decreased. If delivery can be accomplished within 15 minutes of cardiac arrest, the risk of neurological sequelae for the surviving infant is substantially lowered.

Summary

PE is a disorder that can present with very subtle, nonspecific symptomatology, or with dramatic, life-threatening complications. An understanding of the underlying pathophysiological derangements will assist in anticipating complications and initiating a diagnostic evaluation. Familiarity with a limited number of drugs will allow appropriate treatment until definitive care can be undertaken by the obstetrical consultant.

References

1. Pipkin FB, Rubin PC. Preeclampsia—the "disease of theories." *Br Med Bull* 1994;50:381-396.
2. National High Blood Pressure Education Program Working Group. Report on high blood pressure in pregnancy. *Am J Obstet Gynecol* 1990;163:691-712.
3. Smith MA. Preeclampsia. *Prim Care* 1993;20:655-664.
4. Fadigan AB, Sealy DP, Schneider EF. Preeclampsia: Progress

and puzzle. *Am Fam Physician* 1994;49:849-856.
5. Saftlas AF, Olson DR, Franks AL, et al. Epidemiology of preeclampsia and eclampsia in the United States 1979-1986. *Am J Obstet Gynecol* 1990;163:460-465.
6. Zlatnik FJ, Burmeister LF. Dietary protein and preeclampsia. *Am J Obstet Gynecol* 1983;147:345-346.
7. Eskenazi B, Fenster L, Sidney S. A multivariate analysis of risk factors for preeclampsia. *JAMA* 1991;266:237-241.
8. Chesley LC. History and epidemiology of preeclampsia/eclampsia. *Clin Obstet Gynecol* 1984;27: 801-820.
9. de Groot CJM, Taylor RN. New insights into the etiology of preeclampsia. *Ann Med* 1993;25:243-249.
10. Coonrod DV, Hickok DE, Zhu K, et al. Risk factors for preeclampsia in twin pregnancies: A population-based cohort study. *Obstet Gynecol* 1995;85:645-650.
11. Klonoff-Cohen MS, Savitz DA, Cetalo RC, et al. An epidemiologic study of contraception and preeclampsia. *JAMA* 1989; 262:3143-3147.
12. Stone JL, Lockwood CJ, Berkowitz GS, et al. Risk factors for severe preeclampsia. *Obstet Gynecol* 1994;83:357-361.
13. Easterling TR, Benedetti TJ. Preeclampsia: A hyperdynamic disease model. *Am J Obstet Gynecol* 1989;160:1447-1453.
14. Kilpatrick DC, Liston WA, Gibson F, et al. Association between susceptibility to preeclampsia within families and HLA-DR4. *Lancet* 1989;ii:1063-1065.
15. Liston WA, Kilpatrick DC. Is genetic susceptibility to preeclampsia conferred by homozygosity for the same single recessive gene in mother and fetus? *Br J Obstet Gynaecol* 1991;98:1079-1086.
16. Jenkins DM, Need J, Rajah SM. Deficiency of specific HLA antibodies in severe pregnancy preeclampsia/eclampsia. *Clin Exp Immunol* 1977;27:485-486.
17. Scott JS, Jenkins DM, Need JA. Immunology of preeclampsia. *Lancet* 1978;i:704-706.
18. Sridama V, Yang S-L, Moawad A, et al. T-cell subsets in patients with preeclampsia. *Am J Obstet Gynecol* 1983;147: 566-569.
19. Massobrio M, Benedetto C, Bertini E, et al. Immune complexes in preeclampsia and normal pregnancy. *Am J Obstet Gynecol* 1985;152:578-583.
20. Vasquez-Escobosda C, Perez-Medina R, Gomez-Estrada H. Circulating immune complexes in hypertensive disease of pregnancy. *Obstet Gynecol* 1983;62:45-48.
21. Jenkins DM, Need JA, Scott JS, et al. Human leukocyte antigens and mixed lymphocyte reaction in severe preeclampsia. *BMJ* 1978;i:542-544.
22. Bolis PF, Bianchi MM, La Fianza A, et al. Immunogenetic aspects of preeclampsia. *Biol Res Preg* 1987;8:42-45.
23. Kilpatrick DC, Gibson F, Livingston J, et al. Preeclampsia is associated with HLA-DR4 sharing between mother and fetus. *Tissue Antigens* 1991;35:178-181.
24. Hoff C, Peevy K, Giattina K, et al. Maternal-fetal HLA-DR relationships and pregnancy-induced hypertension. *Obstet Gynecol* 1992;80:1007-1012.
25. Page EW. The relation between hydatid moles, relative ischemia of the gravid uterus, and placental origin of eclampsia. *Am J Obstet Gynecol* 1939;37:291-293.
26. Pijnenborg R, Anthony J, Davey DA, et al. Placental bed spiral arteries in the hypertensive disorders of pregnancy. *Br J Obstet Gynaecol* 1991;98:648-655.
27. Easterling TR, Benedetti TJ, Schmucker BC, et al. Maternal hemodynamics in normal and preeclamptic pregnancies: A longitudinal study. *Obstet Gynecol* 1990;76:1061-1069.
28. Taylor RN, Varma M, Teng NNH, et al. Women with preeclampsia have higher plasma endothelin levels than women with normal pregnancies. *J Clin Endocrinol Metab* 1990;71:1675-1677.
29. Dekker GA, Kraayenbrink AA, Zeeman GG, et al. Increased plasma levels of the novel vasoconstrictor peptide endothelin in severe preeclampsia. *Eur J Obstet Gynecol Reprod Biol* 1991;40:215-220.
30. Mastrogiannis DS, O'Brien WF, Krammer J, et al. Potential role of endothelin-1 in normal and hypertensive pregnancies. *Am J Obstet Gynecol* 1991;165:1711-1716.
31. Nova A, Shibal BM, Barton JR, et al. Maternal plasma level of endothelin is increased in pre-eclampsia. *Am J Obstet Gynecol* 1991;165:724-727.
32. Friedman SA. Preeclampsia: A review of the role of prostaglandins. *Obstet Gynecol* 1988;71:122-137.
33. Pinto A, Sorrentino R, Sorrentino P, et al. Endothelial-derived relaxing factor released by endothelial cells of human umbilical vessels and its impairment in pregnancy-induced hypertension. *Am J Obstet Gynecol* 1991;164:507-513.
34. Davison JM. Preeclampsia as a multisystem disease. *Adv Exper Med Biol* 1989;252:119-131.
35. Gallery EDM, Brown MA. Volume homeostasis in normal and hypertensive human pregnancy. *Clin Obstet Gynecol* 1987;1:835-851.
36. Gallery EDM, Gyory AZ. Glomerular and proximal renal tubular function in pregnancy-associated hypertension: A prospective study. *Eur J Obstet Gynecol Reprod Biol* 1979; 9:3-12.
37. Martin JM, Stedman CM. Imitators of preeclampsia and HELLP syndrome. *Obstet Gynecol Clin North Am* 1991;18: 181-198.
38. Sibai BM. The HELLP syndrome (hemolysis, elevated liver enzymes, and low platelets): Much ado about nothing? *Am J Obstet Gynecol* 1990;162:311-314.
39. Gibson B, Hunter D, Neame PB, et al. Thrombocytopenia in preeclampsia and eclampsia. *Semin Thromb Hemost* 1992;8: 234-245.
40. Royburt M, Seidman DS, Serr DM, et al. Neurologic involvement in hypertensive disease of pregnancy. *Obstet Gynecol Surv* 1991;46:656-664.
41. Barton JR, Sabai BM. Acute life-threatening emergencies in preeclampsia-eclampsia. *Clin Obstet Gynecol* 1992;35: 402-413.
42. Martin JN, Stedman CM. Imitators of preeclampsia and HELLP syndrome. *Obstet Gynecol Clin North Am* 1991;18: 181-198.
43. Goodlin RC. Preeclampsia as the great impostor. *Am J Obstet Gynecol* 1991;164:1577-1581.
44. Magann EF, Martin JN. Complicated postpartum preeclampsia-eclampsia. *Obstet Gynecol Clin North Am* 1995;22: 337-356.

45. Towers CV, Pircon RA, Nageotte MP, et al. Cocaine intoxication presenting as preeclampsia and eclampsia. *Obstet Gynecol* 1993;81:545-547.
46. Gallery EDM. Hypertension in pregnancy: Practical management recommendations. *Drugs* 1995;49:555-562.
47. McCombs J. Treatment of preeclampsia and eclampsia. *Clin Pharmacother* 1992;11:236-245.
48. Naden RP, Redman CWG. Antihypertensive drugs in pregnancy. *Clin Perinatol* 1985;12:521-538.
49. Shoemaker CT, Meyers M. Sodium nitroprusside for control of severe hypertensive disease of pregnancy: A case report and discussion of potential toxicity. *Am J Obstet Gynecol* 1984;149:171-173.
50. Repke JT, Friedman SA, Kaplan PW. Prophylaxis of eclamptic seizures: Current controversies. *Clin Obstet Gynecol* 1992;35:365-374.
51. Sadeh M. Action of magnesium sulfate in the treatment of preeclampsia-eclampsia. *Stroke* 1989;20:1273-1275.
52. Lucas MJ. A comparison of magnesium sulfate with phenytoin for the prevention of eclampsia. *N Engl J Med* 1995;333:201-205.
53. Sibai BM. Magnesium sulfate is the ideal anticonvulsant in preeclampsia-eclampsia. *Am J Obstet Gynecol* 1990;162: 1141-1145.
54. Chao A. The patellar reflex in preeclamptic women with subtherapeutic and therapeutic serum magnesium levels. *J Reprod Med* 990;97:110-117.
55. Marx GF. Cardiopulmonary resuscitation of late-pregnant women. *Anesthesiology* 1982;56:156.
56. Katz VL, Dotters DJ, Droegemueller W. Perimortem cesarean delivery. *Obstet Gynecol* 1986;68:571-576.

Pelvic Inflammatory Disease

Charles Stewart, MD, FACEP
Gideon Bosker, MD, FACEP

Pelvic inflammatory disease (PID): Dangerous, deceptive, and debilitating. As practitioners know, the diagnosis of PID frequently is difficult to confirm and, typically, the patients are young and tend to be non-compliant with their treatment regimens. Moreover, the sequelae of inadequate treatment can have devastating consequences, and the number of antibiotic options, combinations, and treatment protocols is nothing less than daunting. Frequently managed in the ED setting, PID is a term that is most commonly used to describe infection of the uterus, fallopian tubes, and adjacent pelvic structures that is not associated with surgery or pregnancy. An estimated 1 million women per year are diagnosed with PID—a condition that is particularly common and problematic among lower socioeconomic groups in urban areas.[1,2]

In addition to the acute manifestations of the infection, long-term sequelae such as ectopic pregnancy and infertility occur in 25% of cases.[1-3] In 1998, the direct and indirect costs of the disease and its complications were estimated to be greater than $5 billion. In view of the effect of this infection, a systematic approach to diagnosis and therapy is mandatory for all emergency and primary care practitioners who encounter patients with this condition and its related complications.

In virtually all cases, PID results from ascending spread of organisms from the cervix and vagina to the upper genital tract. Sexual transmission of *Neisseria gonorrhea* and/or *Chlamydia trachomatis* accounts for more than half of all cases of PID, but *H. hominis* and other organisms have also been implicated.[1,2,6] *N. gonorrhea* is the major cause of PID in urban areas, where gonococcal infection is prevalent, whereas *C. trachomatis* is responsible for a greater proportion of cases among college students, in whom gonococcal infection is less common.

Organisms such as *E. coli* and other enteric pathogens, especially anaerobes, also may cause PID, especially when the normal vaginal flora (lactobacilli) are supplanted with other organisms. However, infection in the upper genital tract does not always result in clinically recognizable disease; indeed, many women with adverse sequelae associated with PID, such as infertility, have no known history of the disease.[4,5]

Accordingly, a high index of suspicion and a low threshold for initiating treatment in PID are essential for facilitating detection and optimizing patient outcomes. Clinical vigilance should be applied to all women of child-bearing age with pelvic pain. Lower abdominal tenderness, adnexal tenderness, and pain on manipulation of the cervix are present in physical examination in up to 90% of women.[1,6,7] Other manifestations, such as elevated erythrocyte sedimentation rate or C-reactive protein and abnormal vaginal discharge vary widely in frequency. At present, there are no effective ways to detect clinically silent disease.

Although laparoscopic visualization of inflamed fallopian tubes and pelvic structures is possible and, according to some experts, represents a "gold standard" for the diagnosis, it is seldom practical in the acute setting. As a rule, therefore, the emergency physician must initiate empiric antibiotic therapy for PID based on clinical criteria, regional resistance patterns, patient history, and patient compliance patterns rather than on the basis of culture results.

Because new and highly effective treatment regimens have been introduced for PID, emergency physicians now have a number of therapeutic options available for managing problematic and, frequently, poorly compliant patients with this condition.[8-10] Many of the regimens are published in the Centers for Disease Control and Prevention (CDC) guidelines, and other drugs have not yet become part of the most current guidelines, but have indications for PID.

Overview

Pelvic inflammatory disease (PID) represents a spectrum of infections and inflammatory disorders of the uterus, fallopian tubes, and adjacent pelvic structures. Variable in presentation and caused by myriad bacterial and atypical organisms, PID may include any combination of endometritis, salpingitis, tubo-ovarian abscess, oophoritis, and in its more extreme manifestation, pelvic peritonitis. Since the infection most often involves the fallopian tubes, salpingitis is commonly used as a synonym for PID, although this is not strictly correct.

Because reporting rates for PID probably do not reflect the estimated prevalence of the disease in the community, most experts agree that the true incidence of PID is not known and may never be confirmed with any degree of accuracy. Moreover, many episodes of PID are not recognized by the patient or the clinician. And although sexually transmissible diseases (STDs) are reportable entities, there is no mandatory reporting for PID, even though the etiologic organisms associated with PID are similar to those encountered with STDs. Finally, clinical diagnosis of this disease can be difficult, and definitive confirmation of pelvic inflammation and/or infection by laparoscopy and/or culture usually are lacking. As a result, estimating the prevalence of PID from chart reviews may not yield an accurate accounting of how many cases occur annually in the United States.

Despite the aforementioned difficulties with reporting, diagnosing, and confirming PID, the CDC estimates that one out of every 10 women will have at least one episode of PID during her reproductive years.[11] During each of the past five years, at least 1 million women have been diagnosed with PID annually and more than 200,000 women have been hospitalized annually as a result of this condition. At least one-quarter of women with PID will have major complications, including infertility, ectopic pregnancy, chronic pelvic pain, tubo-ovarian abscesses, and/or pelvic adhesions. Overall, the annual estimated cost of treating PID and its complications is estimated to be more than $5 billion annually in the United States alone.[12,13]

Etiology and Clinical Pathogenesis

PID is thought to arise from an ascending infection of the female genital tract. As a rule, the upper female genital tract is sterile. Presumably, PID results when pathogenic microorganisms spread from the cervix and vagina to the upper portions of the genital tract to such structures as the salpinx, ovaries, and adjacent structures. Predicting exactly which pathogens are responsible for individual cases of PID can be difficult, and consequently, expert panels recommend broad spectrum antibiotics (usually, but not always, two- or multiple-drug combinations) that are active against sexually transmissible agents such as *Neisseria gonorrhoeae* and *Chlamydia trachomatis,* as well as against anaerobes and gram-negative organisms.

Clearly, in some patients, pelvic infection is not transmitted sexually but is the consequence of a trans-cervical procedure such as dilation and curettage, suction abortion, or insertion of an intrauterine device (IUD). As a result, more often than not, decisions regarding initial antibiotic therapy, spectrum of coverage, and patient disposition in PID will have to be made on the basis of clinical judgment (empiric treatment is the rule) rather than culture-driven parameters.

Treatment recommendations for PID are constantly under review, updated, and published regularly STDs by the CDC (usually, every two years). Empiric regimens recommended by this organization are designed to reflect etiologic patterns, changes in antimicrobial drug resistance, compliance issues, cost, and efficacy data generated by well-designed clinical trials. Because the CDC analyzes a broad range of clinical, epidemiological, and pharmacological data to generate its recommendations, CDC treatment pathways for PID commonly are incorporated into emergency department, hospital, and public health clinic protocols for disease management.

Not uncommonly, however, certain agents shown to be highly effective for management of PID or STDs will have been approved for these clinical indications by the Food and Drug Administration (FDA), but because of timing considerations related to review and publication of the CDC Guidelines, these antibiotics may not appear in the most current CDC recommendations. Many of these FDA-approved antibiotics eventually do go on to become part of the CDC guidelines, albeit after a "lag" period between gaining formal FDA indication and formal publication in the CDC Guidelines. Emergency physicians, as well as other clinicians, including OB-GYN specialists, should be aware of the possible discrepancies between antibiotics approved by the FDA for PID and those agents recommended in current CDC publications.

Finally, it should be stressed that there are wide regional and international variations in etiologic agents involved in PID.[13] Reports of quinolone resistance among gonococcal species in Asia is just one example requiring clinical consideration. Because of these geographical variations, a therapeutic regimen that is highly effective in one area may be suboptimal in another. In particular, antibiotics that can be used successfully in North America and Europe may be inappropriate for treating patients with PID or STDs in Asia and Africa.

Specific Etiologic Organisms. In North America, the etiology of PID, to a great degree, has been characterized by the use of cervical cultures and/or immunofluorescent tests for gonorrhea and chlamydia. Using these diagnostic techniques, chlamydia has been shown to be responsible for 25-50% of all cases of PID. In addition, 10-20% of female patients who are infected with gonorrhea will progress to PID.

Although PID caused by gonorrhea generally requires *parenteral* therapy, uncomplicated gonococcal urthethris can be treated with single-dose therapy. There are a variety of effective regimens based on quinolones, cephalosporins, and the macrolide azithromycin that vary considerably in cost. It should be stressed that because up to

30% of patients with gonorrhea may also have coexisting chlamydial infection, chlamydia must always be empirically treated along with gonorrhea. The importance of effective communication in enhancing compliance with medication regimens cannot be overemphasized.[5] Because significant noncompliance has been reported with seven-day doxycycline regimens for treatment of uncomplicated chlamydia cervicitis or urethritis, one-dose therapeutic modalities (these would include azithromycin 1 gm po once for uncomplicated chlamydial infection and a choice of several once-dose options for uncomplicated gonococcal infection) are generally preferred.

Infection with chlamydia is problematic because up to 70% of cases are asymptomatic, which predisposes to chronic, subclinical inflammation and tubal scarring. Recent data suggest that one-third of women 15-19 years of age and up to half of those younger than 15 years become reinfected with *Chlamydia* within six years of initial diagnosis.[14] A latent chlamydial infection with prolonged inflammatory response may further predispose to ascending infection or to direct effects of the chlamydial infection. Studies confirm that chlamydial infection causes more severe tubal scarring than gonorrhea and is more likely to be associated with chronic PID.[15]

Polymicrobial Infection. The natural history of PID is not fully elucidated, although one current hypothesis suggests that the infection begins with *Chlamydia* and/or gonorrhea.[16] The vaginal and cervical environment becomes altered as these organisms proliferate; changes in pH, availability of oxygen and nutrients, and the presence of microbiologic waste products encourage the overgrowth of endogenous and anaerobic flora, causing a co-existent bacterial vaginosis. If host defenses ebb or are compromised, organisms ascend along contiguous mucosal surfaces into the endometrium and then into the fallopian tubes.

Culture-based studies that evaluated culdocentesis specimens obtained from hospitalized patients with the clinical diagnosis of PID suggest that mixed infections are responsible for up to 70% of cases with PID.[17] These polymicrobial infections typically include both anaerobic and aerobic microorganisms. When samples are obtained by laparoscopy alone, a polymicrobial etiology is confirmed in only about 30-40% of cases.

From an etiologic perspective, anaerobes such as *Bacteroides*, *Peptostreptococcus,* and *Peptococcus* may have been reported, as have facultative bacteria, including *Gardnerella vaginalis, Streptococcus, E. coli,* and *Haemophilus influenzae.* Organisms associated with bacterial vaginosis have been confirmed by endometrial biopsy. These organisms include *Prevotella bivia, Peptostreptococcus, Ureaplasma urealyticum,* and *Mycoplasma hominis.*[18] The broad range of organisms known to cause PID generally requires empiric treatment with a combination of antimicrobial agents with activity against chlamydia and gonococcus, and in the majority of cases, against anaerobic organisms as well.

Risk Factors

A disease of younger women, PID occurs almost exclusively in sexually active women and is most common in adolescents. Risk factors include sexual activity, particularly with multiple sexual partners, young age, and certain types of mechanical contraception. There is considerable overlap between the risks of acquiring a STD and the risk for contracting PID.

Age. Women younger than 25 years of age comprise more than 75% of all cases of PID and have a 10-fold increase in incidence as compared to older women.[19] Sexually active teenagers are more than three times more likely to have PID than women with similar activity who are 25-29 years of age.[20] Physiologically, the risk of infection with PID is enhanced by the greater permeability of the cervical mucous plug in adolescents and by greater exposure of columnar epithelium in the cervix during adolescence. In addition, teenagers are more likely to have multiple sexual partners, whether in parallel or serially. Teenagers frequently are sexual "risk-takers" and indulge in unprotected sex and inconsistent use of barrier contraception.

Women with multiple sexual partners are at increased risk of acquiring diseases such as gonorrhea and chlamydia, which predispose PID. Other sexual behaviors that have been associated with increased risk of PID include multiple new partners within the past 30 days and an increased frequency of sexual intercourse.

Method of Contraception. A number of studies have implicated intrauterine devices as a predisposing factor for PID.[21] The intrauterine device may increase susceptibility by altering the microbiologic milieu in the cervix and uterus, by impairing local host defenses with a "foreign body" effect, or by dragging vaginal flora into the uterus during insertion. Recent studies, including data from users of the current copper "T" device with progesterone show that most of the increased risk occurs within the first four months after the insertion of the device. Again, women without other significant risk factors for STDs have less risk of developing PID after insertion of an IUD.[22,23]

Barrier contraception appears to reduce the risk for PID, presumably because it may protect against some cervical infections. A number of studies demonstrate that there is *increased detection* rate of lower genital tract infection caused by chlamydia in patients who use oral contraceptives.[24] On the other hand, oral contraceptive users also seem to have a *lower* risk for developing PID. This paradox may be explained by the fact that there is a higher detection rate associated with oral contraceptive users—and therefore, earlier treatment—or it may be explained by the existence of some protective factor produced by oral contraceptives.

Other Factors. Menses may increase the risk of PID. Retrograde flow may spread infection from the uterus out to the fallopian tubes. This has been shown to occur in 25% of healthy women.[25] Classically, gonococcal PID occurs within a week of the onset of menses. In contrast, chlamydial PID does not appear to be temporally associated with menses. Recent studies have shown that vaginal douching may also predispose to the development of PID. Mechanical pressure causes upward spread of lower genital tract infection. Alteration of the pH creates a hospitable environment for infection. Abnormal bacterial flora of the vagina or "bacterial vaginosis" may also be a risk factor for PID.[18] In this disease, there is a predominance of anaerobic flora, an alkaline pH, and a significant reduction in lactobacilli. A purulent discharge is often present.

Complications and Adverse Sequelae

Long-term sequelae occur in about 25% of patients who have had PID. The most common, and dreaded, complications include infertility and ectopic pregnancy, both of which result from scarring of the fallopian tubes. Additional complications include recurrent infections, chronic pelvic pain, and dyspareunia.

Fitz-Hugh-Curtis Syndrome. Fitz-Hugh-Curtis syndrome is an extra-pelvic manifestation of PID. The presenting complaint is right upper quadrant abdominal pain which is secondary to to peri-hepatic inflammation.[26,27] This complication is seen in about 5-20% of all women with PID.[28] The syndrome includes pain (radiation to the right shoulder or back is common) and tenderness in the hepatic region and may be associated with abnormal liver function tests. String adhesions in the area of the liver may be seen on laparoscopy. The etiology may be due to spillage of purulent material from the fimbriated end of the fallopian tube.

Tubo-ovarian Abscess. Tubo-ovarian abscess (TOA) occurs as a complication in 7-16% of all cases of acute PID.[18] The process begins when salpingitis results in spillage of infected exudate onto the ovary. The ovary then adheres to the tube as the exudate covers its surface. The site of last ovulation may be particularly vulnerable and may become the focus for infection to spread within the body of the ovary.[18] As many as 15% of tubo-ovarian abscesses will rupture and soil the peritoneum, creating an acute surgical abdomen. Although chlamydia and gonorrhea may be isolated from the cervix of patients with TOA, only rarely are these organisms found within the abscess itself. Rather, the organisms most often cultured from the abscess are facultative anaerobes and strict anaerobes.[29] Ultrasound is the most useful technique for confirming the diagnosis of a tubo-ovarian abscess. Transvaginal ultrasound has a sensitivity of 85% and a specificity of almost 100% in the diagnosis of a tubo-ovarian abscess.[30]

Chronic Pelvic Pain. Extratubal scarring can produce pelvic adhesions that may result in chronic pain. The rate of hospital admission for conditions associated with abdominal pain is much higher in individuals with proven PID than in those without a history of this disease. Specifically, women with PID have 10 times as many subsequent admissions for nonspecific abdominal pain as controls.[31] Admission diagnoses include chronic pelvic pain, gynecological pain, and non-specific abdominal pain.

Ectopic Pregnancy and Infertility. Scarring and structural changes in the fallopian tubes are well-documented consequences of PID and increase the risk for tubal pregnancy. Specifically, the rate of ectopic pregnancy is increased four-fold in women who have had documented cases of PID.[32] The greater the number of recurrences of the original infection, the more scar tissue that is built up in the tubes. Gradual accretion of scar tissue from recurrent episodes of inflammation hampers ciliary function and may partially or completely occlude the fallopian tubes. It also is well documented that tubal changes are responsible for the increased risk of infertility that is associated with PID infections.[33] In one large study of more than 1800 women, infertility was correlated with the severity of salpingitis and the number of episodes of PID, with each episode of PID almost doubling the rate of infertility.[33] In one prospective study, infertility due to tubal occlusion occurred in 8% of women after one episode of PID, in 19.5% after two episodes, and in 40% after three or more episodes.[34] Furthermore, as previously mentioned, many cases of PID are clinically silent, but as many as 70% of women who are infertile due to tubal obstruction have serum antibodies against chlamydia vs. only about 25% of women who are infertile for other reasons.[2,3,7]

Interestingly, more than one-half of patients with tubal factor infertility give no history of PID.[33] In most of these patients, however, antibodies to *Chlamydia* or gonorrhea are found, indicating prior infection. Nevertheless, both gross and microscopic examination of the fallopian tubes of women with tubal factor infertility fails to differentiate between patients with and without a history of PID.

Diagnosis and Evaluation

The definitive diagnosis of PID requires invasive testing. This can include an endometrial biopsy showing evidence of endometritis, laparoscopy with abnormalities consistent with PID, or transvaginal sonography showing thickened, fluid-filled tubes with or without free pelvic fluid or a tubo-ovarian abscess.[35]

Laparoscopy. Most experts agree that laparoscopy is still the "gold standard" for establishing the definitive diagnosis of PID. Despite the usefulness of this technique, the majority of patients managed in the emergency department receive a presumptive diagnosis on the basis of clinical criteria alone, in large part because laparoscopy simply requires more technical skill, surgical risk, and cost than clinical pathways and protocols have been willing to support. Moreover, it is unlikely that laparoscopy will ever become practical as a screening procedure. Despite these limitations, laparoscopy is an important technique when the diagnosis of PID is in question or during situations in which the patient fails to improve. In a substantial number of patients, an alternate diagnosis such as appendicitis, ovarian tumor, ectopic pregnancy, or ovarian cyst may be identified.[36] Finally, although laparoscopy is considered the cornerstone of diagnosis in PID, there are limitations to this technique; since the laparoscope examines only the external surfaces of the tube and adjacent structures, early disease localized to the intra-tubal wall may be missed.[37]

Pelvic Ultrasound. Pelvic ultrasound has been well studied in PID and is useful for identifying tubal and ovarian pathology, with a reported sensitivity rate of up to 93%.[38] Although it is not necessary to obtain an ultrasound in every case of suspected PID, this modality is useful for making the diagnosis of tubo-ovarian abscess, for detecting other complications of PID, and for eliminating other entities in the differential diagnosis, such as ectopic pregnancy. As a general rule, ultrasound should be performed if a pelvic or a tubal mass is suspected. Moreover, an ultrasound is mandatory in a pregnant patient with abdominal pain. In addition, any patient who is treated with appropriate antibiotics and does not improve after 48 hours of therapy should have a pelvic ultrasound to exclude structural disease.[39] Transvaginal ultrasound is not only better for image quality and anatomic detail, but is more comfortable for most patients.

CT Scanning. Although CT scanning is not specifically mentioned in the CDC guidelines, this imaging technique can identify pelvi pathology consistent with PID and may be helpful for distinguishing among conditions with a similar presentation.

Major and Minor Determinants. Despite the advantages of these techniques, most women suspected of having PID in the ED are treated on the basis of a presumptive diagnosis generated by clinical signs and symptoms. Unfortunately, culture or other isolation of a sexually transmitted organism usually will not be available, rarely is an endometrial biopsy obtained, and direct visualization of the pelvic organs is the exception rather than the rule.

Typically, then, the presumptive diagnosis of PID is made in women who are sexually active who present with lower abdominal pain and are found to have cervical, uterine, or adnexal tenderness on pelvic examination. Not surprisingly, these criteria for clinical diagnosis have low sensitivity and specificity. PID, which is one of many conditions producing such symptoms, probably accounts for less than one-half of cases associated with this presentation.

Because clinical contingencies usually require that antibiotic treatment be initiated on the basis of noninvasive evaluation, the CDC has recommended minimum criteria required for empiric treatment of PID. These major determinants include lower abdominal tenderness, adnexal tenderness, and cervical motion tenderness.[39] Other authors have used these same major criteria but have also added the requirement that at least one minor determinant also be present. Unfortunately, these criteria have not been evaluated systematically in studies that correlate clinical examination with findings at laparoscopy.[40] Minor determinants (i.e., signs that may increase the suspicion of PID) include:

- Fever (oral temperature > 101°F; > 38.3°C);
- Vaginal discharge. One study notes that an increased WBC in the vaginal discharge was the laboratory test with the highest sensitivity in diagnosing PID.[41]
- Documented STD. Laboratory documentation of cervical infection with either gonorrhea or Chlamydia establishes presence of a milieu of PID. If a patient with a documented STD presents with abdominal pain, PID should be strongly suspected.
- Erythrocyte sedimentation rate (ESR). This test may be used to assist in the diagnosis of PID. It is nonspecific and can be elevated in a number of inflammatory conditions.
- C-reactive protein. C-reactive protein is an acute phase protein synthesized in the liver. The serum concentration increases a few hours after injury or inflammation and reaches a peak 24-48 hours later. Elevated C-reactive protein is seen in PID, and may be useful in early diagnosis of this disease.[42] Unfortunately, it is not specific and seen with a number of inflammatory conditions or injuries.
- Systemic signs. Nausea and vomiting may be found in patients with PID, but these symptoms are more common in other diseases such as appendicitis.
- Dyspareunia. Dyspareunia may be the first symptom that brings a patient to the emergency department. *(Please see Table 1.)*

Limitations of Diagnostic Criteria. One large study has demonstrated that no single historical, clinical, or laboratory finding, nor any combination of these, is both perfectly sensitive and specific for establishing the diagnosis of PID.[43] In large part, this is because the disease presents with a wide range of symptoms, depending on the severity of the disease. Moreover, the evolution of symptoms in PID is oftentimes gradual and the early complaints are mild, especially when *Chlamydia* is the offending organism.[44] PID due to *Chlamydia* tends to be associated with sexual activity at a very young age, and these patients are less likely to present for medical care during the early stages of disease. Minimum diagnostic criteria for PID include the presence of lower abdominal tenderness, adnexal tenderness, and cervical motion tenderness, although the entire triad may not be noted in early cases of PID. Instead, the patient may only complain of dyspareunia, spotting, fever, and/or abnormal vaginal or cervical discharge.

In summary, it should be stressed that the clinical diagnostic criteria are insensitive and nonspecific; false-positive and false-negative diagnoses are common. Unfortunately, the only alternative is to examine the pelvic anatomy directly with laparoscopy, but this invasive approach is not always feasible, as it requires general anesthesia, and is costly.[45] It is mandatory that other causes for the complex of symptoms should be identified. Specific diagnoses that should be considered include ectopic pregnancy, a ruptured ovarian cyst, endometriosis, and appendicitis.

Table 1. Laboratory Evaluation for Pelvic Inflammatory Disease

- Complete blood count with differential
- Pregnancy test of choice (unless patient is already known to be pregnant)
- Tests for chlamydia and gonorrhea
- RPR or VDRL tests for syphilis
- Pelvic sonogram
- C-reactive protein or erythrocyte sedimentation rates may be helpful.

Atypical Pelvic Inflammatory Disease. As noted earlier, there is a large reservoir of atypical PID. Attempts to find demographic, clinical, or behavioral predictors of atypical PID are disappointing, to say the least. In one study of 283 women with tubal occlusion or adhesion, 84% reported no history of PID.[46] The patient with atypical disease was more likely to be married, educated, and have a higher income than those with overt PID. They were less likely to report a history of gonococcal or herpes infections, and were more likely to report multiple partners.

Authors of one study felt that atypical PID was a sexually transmitted disease, but that it was caused by organisms other than *Chlamydia trachomatis, Neisseria gonorrhoeae*, trichomoniasis, or *Mycoplasma* species.[47] These clinical patterns suggest that identification of patients with atypical disease is difficult. Future efforts to identify women with atypical PID will have to rely on metabolic or immunological markers. Perhaps urine screening for chlamydia, gonorrhea, or some as yet unidentified pathogen will prove fruitful in the future.

Management: Antibiotic Guidelines and Patient Disposition

As emphasized, a high index of suspicion and a low threshold for initiating treatment are important for facilitating detection and appropriate management of PID. This approach should be applied to all women of child-bearing age with pelvic pain. Although laparoscopic visualization of inflamed fallopian tubes and pelvic structures is possible and, according to some experts, serves as a "gold standard" for the diagnosis, it is seldom practical. As a rule, the emergency physician must initiate antibiotic therapy on clinical grounds, despite the limitations of this approach. From a clinical perspective, however, lower abdominal tenderness, adnexal tenderness, and pain on manipulation of the cervix are present in physical examination in up to 90% of women, and the presence of this triad will mandate treatment in nearly all cases.[1,6,7] Other manifestations, such as elevated erythrocyte sedimentation rate or C-reactive protein and abnormal vaginal discharge vary widely in frequency. At present, there are no effective ways to detect clinically silent disease.

Because new and highly effective treatment regimens have been introduced for PID, emergency physicians now have a number of therapeutic options available for managing problematic and, frequently, poorly compliant patients with PID.[8-10] In this regard, the CDC recommends a number of possible regimens, most of which mandate the use of a broad-spectrum cephalosporin administered parenterally (initially) along with an oral agent effective against chlamydia, such as doxycycline. Commonly used regimens for inpatient treatment of PID include the combination of cefoxitin, ceftriaxone, or cefotetan plus doxycycline; plus intravenous metronidazole followed by oral therapy with metronidazole plus doxycycline; gentamicin plus clindamycin; and intravenous ampicillin-sulbactam plus doxycycline. Although not included as part of the current CDC recommendation guidelines, intravenous azithromycin therapy followed by oral azithromycin (preferably in combination with an anti-anaerobic agent such asmetronidazole) for the treatment of PID has been shown to be safe and effective. Because azithromycin is FDA-approved for this indication, it will be included in treatment tables in conjunction with CDC-recommended regimens when applicable.

CDC Guidelines for Inpatient Therapy.[51] The CDC has established treatment guidelines for PID, identifying specific patient subgroups that have a higher risk for severe or fertility-compromising disease and, therefore, require hospitalization and inpatient therapy. Most of these recommendations are based on clinical common sense. For example, the ED physician should admit patients in whom the diagnosis is uncertain or who may have surgical diseases such as appendicitis or ectopic pregnancy. Likewise, if the patient with suspected PID fails to respond to outpatient therapy, the next appropriate step is to admit the patient and treat with intravenous antibiotics.

Nearly all patients with severely symptomatic PID should be hospitalized for an initial course of parenteral antibiotic therapy and pain management. In addition, those with potentially complicating disease should also be admitted. Hospitalization should also be considered when the patient is a substance abuser or a young adolescent, and in patients who are unreliable for clinical follow-up, are pregnant, have a possibility of surgical pathology, or are unable to tolerate outpatient therapy.

Antibiotic Therapy: Polymicrobial Vs. Monotherapeutic Approaches. The ideal drug for treatment of PID would be one that has a short course of therapy, is associated with few side effects, could be taken orally, and is inexpensive. It should also induce resistance only infrequently and should be effective against all important PID pathogens. Unfortunately, there is no single drug that satisfies all of these requirements in all patients.

Consequently, the majority of recommended or approved drug regimens for treatment of PID require two or more agents. *(Please see Table 2.)* Although azithromycin is FDA-approved as a single drug agent for PID, most clinicians add an additional agent to cover anaerobic pathogens. In general, treatment plans requiring more than one drug are associated with decreased compliance unless all drugs can be given simultaneously under the supervision of a clinician to confirm compliance. Increasing the number of drugs also increases the potential for side effects and interactions. Clearly, use of more than one drug increases cost.

Single-drug therapy may not be either appropriate or possible because of the possibility of infection with multiple organisms including anaerobes, facultative anaerobes, and aerobic organisms. Since specific microbiologic diagnoses are rarely made, treatment should be directed against a wide range of suspected organisms. The therapeutic agents should include agents that are active against both *N. gonorrhea* and *C. trachomatis*, as well as facultative gram-negative rods and anaerobes.

The CDC has recommended multiple drug therapy for treatment of PID since 1982.[49] These regimens are perhaps the oldest among all current CDC recommendations.[50] In a recent analysis of multiple drug regimens for the treatment of PID, the CDC recommendations were among the six best in clinical response.[18] They have pooled clinical cure rates ranging from 92% to 94%.[51,52] Changing patterns of drug resistance may provoke the next substantial change in recommendations.

Out-of-Hospital Antimicrobial Management for PID

Approaches to managing patients in the ED/outpatient environment requires additional discussion, since there are now other approved regimens in addition to those recommended by the CDC. Most of the CDC-endorsed regimens for outpatient management use a cephalosporin as an important component of the treatment plan. *(Please see Table 3.)* In this regard, the optimum choice of cephalosporin for outpatient regimens is still unclear, although ceftriaxone is widely used. Cefoxitin has better anaerobic coverage, but ceftriaxone is more effective against gonorrhea. Other cephalosporins have been proposed, including ceftizoxime and cefotaxime. These are less well studied.

Azithromycin. The evolving and increasingly important role of azithromycin requires special attention, since it offers dosing advantages that make it attractive to emergency practice. One study evaluated results in a total of 221 women with PID treated with the following regimens: 1) azithromycin monotherapy (administered as 500 mg IV as the initial dose on day 1, followed by 250 mg daily for 6 additional days); 2) azithromycin in combination with metronidazole; and 3) metronidazole (either intravenous metronidazole 500 mg bid on day 1 followed by oral administration of 500 mg bid for 11 days or oral administration of 500 mg bid for 12 days), plus doxycycline (100 mg po bid 14 days), plus cefoxitin (2 gm IV or IM) with probenecid 1 g on the first day of treatment.[53,63]

In an intent-to-treat analysis conducted 15 days after therapy with these regimens, 93% of the patients receiving azithromycin alone, 94% of patients receiving azithromycin plus metronidazole, and 93% of those receiving the triad of cefoxitin, doxycycline, and metronidazole were either cured or improved. The bacteriologic eradication rates for all three regimens were in the 93-95% range. Azithromycin was well-tolerated in patients with PID. The most common side effects were diarrhea (8.5%) and nausea (6.6%). The addition of metronidazole to azithromycin increased slightly the incidence of gastrointestinal side effects, with 10.3% reporting nausea, 3.7% abdominal pain, and 2.8% vomiting.[53]

Based on these data, azithromycin IV (500 mg qd for 1 or 2 days) followed by oral azithromycin 250 mg po qd to complete a total of seven days of therapy should be considered a primary treatment modality for managing patients who require initial intravenous therapy for PID caused by *C. trachomatis, N. gonorrhoeae*, or *M. hominis*. The timing of the switch from intravenous to oral therapy should be made by the physician, who should make this decision based on clinical parameters. Moreover, it should be stressed that when anaerobic infection is strongly suspected to play an etiologic role in any individual patient with PID, the ED physician should combine an antimicrobial agent such as metronidazole that provides anaerobic coverage along with azithromycin.

Although many patients with PID, especially those who appear to be systemically toxic, have abdominal rebound tenderness, have WBC counts greater than 15,000, have a unilateral mass suggestive of tubo-ovarian abscess, have a history or profile indicating risk for poor medication compliance, are in the adolescent age group, and those in whom preservation of fertility is a high priority will require hospitalization, a significant percentage can be treated with initial IV or IM therapy in the ED, followed by oral therapy out of the hospital to complete the antimicrobial course.

As outlined, current options for out-of-hospital management of mild PID include the well-established regimen of ceftriaxone 500 mg IM, followed by doxycycline 100 mg po bid for 14 days with or without metronidazole 500 mg po tid for 10-14 days. These CDC-endorsed regimens have an excellent track record for efficacy and safety. With approval of the azithromycin IV/oral sequenced combination regimen outlined above, it is now possible to streamline therapy for PID into a seven-day course, and substantially reduce the number of oral doses required to complete the treatment course.

The practical implications for the ED physician are as follows: If, on the basis of the clinical findings, the ED physician deems that a patient with mild PID can be managed out of the hospital, and that a single intravenous dose of azithromycin in the ED is sufficient prior to oral therapy, then azithromycin should be administered as an infusion at a rate of 2 mg/mL over 1 hour, or 1 mg/mL over three hours. Azithromycin IV should always be infused over a period of not less than one hour, and should never be administered by bolus or intramuscular injection. If patients with PID have signs and symptoms that suggest the need for more than one intravenous dose, hospitalization will usually be necessary.

The one-hour minimum infusion time required for this antibiotic is not as convenient as the IM route of administration required for the ceftriaxone (plus oral doxycycline) regimen. However, the post-parenteral therapy phase of the azithromycin treatment regimen (which requires only an additional 6 days of oral therapy following the IV dose) is considerably more convenient and compliance-enhancing (both with respect to daily dose frequency and duration of therapy) than the ceftriaxone regimen, which requires consolidation with 28 oral doses of doxycycline over a 14-day period. In a patient population at high risk for noncompliance, the azithromycin regimen offers a potential window of opportunity that should be considered in this difficult patient population.

Other Antibiotics. It should be stated that there is a diversity of opinion regarding newer antibiotics for the treatment of PID, and to some extent, there is a paucity of

Table 2. Antibiotic Treatment Regimens of Choice for Inpatient/Hospitalized Management of PID

INPATIENT PARENTERAL REGIMEN OPTION ONE*

Azithromycin IV (500 mg qd for 1 or 2 days) followed by oral azithromycin 250 mg po once daily to complete a total of 7 days

Plus (as clinically indicated for suspicion for anaerobic infection) Metronidazole 500 mg IV every 8 hours

*This is an FDA-approved regimen that does not currently appear in the CDC Guidelines for PID management.

INPATIENT PARENTERAL REGIMEN OPTION TWO

Cefotetan 2 g IV every 12 hours

Plus

Doxycycline 100 mg IV or po every 12 hours*

or

Cefoxitin 2g IV every 6 hours

Plus

Doxycycline 100 mg IV or po every 12 hours*

*Parenteral therapy can be discontinued 24 hours after the patient improves. Oral therapy should be started with doxycycline 100 mg bid and continued for 14 days total therapy. If a tubo-ovarian abscess is present, many providers will use clindamycin or metronidazole to provide better coverage of anaerobic bacteria.

INPATIENT PARENTERAL REGIMEN OPTION THREE

Clindamycin 900 mg IV every 8 hours

Plus

Gentamicin 2mg/kg loading dose IV or IM (with 1.5 mg/kg maintenance dose every 8 hours)

Parenteral therapy can be discontinued 24 hours after the patient improves clinically. Oral therapy should then be started and continued for a total of 14 days of therapy. Oral therapy should consist of doxycycline 100 mg bid and clindamycin 450 mg qid. Clindamycin continues to have better coverage of *Bacteroides* species than the cephalosporins. This makes regimen option 2 particularly effective when there is a tubo-ovarian abscess or advanced disease where anaerobic organisms are more probable. A major disadvantage of the clindamycin plus aminoglycoside regimen is the ototoxicity of the aminoglycoside. This may be decreased with therapeutic serum level monitoring.

ALTERNATIVE PARENTERAL REGIMEN OPTIONS

Ofloxacin 400 mg IV every 12 hours

Plus

Metronidazole 500 mg IV every 8 hours

or

Ampicillin/sulbactam 3 g IV every 6 hours

Plus

Doxycycline 100 mg PO or IV every 12 hours

or

Ciprofloxacin 200 mg IV every 12 hours

Plus

Doxycycline 100 mg PO or IV every 12 hours

Plus

Metronidazole 500 mg IV every 8 hours

Table 3. Antibiotic Treatment Regimens of Choice for ED/Outpatient Management of PID

OUTPATIENT/ED TREATMENT REGIMEN OPTION ONE

Azithromycin 500 mg as a single dose *intravenously* given in the emergency department *followed by* oral azithromycin 250 mg once daily orally to complete a total of seven days of therapy.*

Plus/Minus

Metronidazole 500 mg orally twice daily for 14 days (as clinically indicated for suspicion of anaerobic infection—usually recommended)

*The FDA-approved regimen for azithromycin treatment of PID specifies 1 to 2 days of intravenous azithromycin therapy (500 mg) followed by oral azithromycin (250 mg) to complete a seven-day course of therapy. Because it is possible to give a single intravenous dose in the emergency department (this dose would constitute day 1 of IV therapy), this would satisfy the minimal FDA criteria of 1 to 2 days of intravenous therapy. Patients, who on the basis of clinical signs and symptoms, require in-hospital management may be more suitable for 2 days of intravenous therapy in the inpatient setting.

ED/OUTPATIENT ORAL TREATMENT REGIMEN OPTION TWO

Ceftriaxone 250 mg IM once

Plus

Doxycycline 100 mg orally twice daily for 14 days

Plus/Minus

Metronidazole 500 mg orally twice daily for 14 days (as clinically indicated for suspicion of anaerobic infection—usually recommended)

ED/OUTPATIENT ORAL TREATMENT REGIMEN OPTION THREE

Cefoxitin 2 g IM plus probenecid 1 gram orally concurrently

Plus

Doxycycline 100 mg orally twice daily for 14 days

Plus/Minus

Metronidazole 500 mg orally twice daily for 14 days (as clinically indicated for suspicion of anaerobic infection—usually recommended)

ED/OUTPATIENT ORAL TREATMENT REGIMEN OPTION FOUR

Ofloxacin 400 mg orally twice daily for 14 days

Plus

Metronidazole 500 mg orally twice daily for 14 days

good data. Multiple authors recommend diverse antibiotic regimens with both new single drugs and various combinations of antibiotics.[54] Clinical judgment, experience, and local resistance patterns should help direct the clinician toward the optimal regimen in any given patient. Multiple, small studies exist to support these diverse antibiotic regimens, but statistically significant studies are not common.

A number of practical aspects of antimicrobial treatment for this disease should be pointed out, so that clinical outcomes can be optimized. For example, many clinicians add metronidazole to outpatient regimens to ensure adequate anaerobic coverage. This view is endorsed in both the 1993 and the 1998 CDC recommendations. Metronidazole lacks activity against both gram-positive and gram-negative aerobic organisms. As mentioned, azithromycin has no significant activity against many anaerobic organisms encountered in PID, so it should usually be used with an additional agent such as metronidazole.

The quinolone story also is changing rapidly and requires special scrutiny. The lack of reliable activity of the older quinolones such as ciprofloxacin against *Chlamydia* means that these agents should not be used to treat PID. Moreover, growing quinolone resistance among *N. gonorrhoeae* infections may make a significant impact on the utility of these agents in the near future.[55] Ofloxacin has established efficacy against *Chlamydia* when given for at least seven days.[56,57] It has shown good results in well-controlled, published studies, hence its inclusion in the CDC outpatient protocols and alternative inpatient protocols. Of concern, however, is the growing resistance rates to the quinolones in general (especially in Asia) and ofloxacin in particular. Disturbingly, increasing resistance among *E. coli* species also has been reported.[58]

While several new combination regimens have been proposed for treatment of PID, none of these have been adequately evaluated for clinical efficacy in the treatment of PID. In small studies, there is a statistically higher cure rate using "newer" antibiotics. In one small study of 100, patients treated with clindamycin and aztreonam had a clinical response rate of 98%.[59] Other small studies with piperacillin had response rates of 95%, but only 60 patients were involved. Imipenem is a broad spectrum antimicrobial with good anaerobic coverage. When combined with cilastatin to decrease renal excretion, imipenem may be a potential antibiotic for the treatment of PID. In three studies with this drug, there was a 94.7% clinical response rate in PID patients.[60] However, imipenem does not adequately cover Chlamydia, so another agent would be required.

Disposition, Adjunctive Therapy, and Follow-up

All women seen in the ED with suspected or confirmed PID require a pregnancy test to determine appropriate management. If present, intrauterine devices should be removed once antibiotic therapy is initiated. Close follow-up of outpatients within 24-48 hours after treatment is started is important. Failure to improve indicates the need for reassessment of the diagnosis (using laparoscopy, ultrasonography, or hospitalization) rather than a change in antibiotic therapy.

Male sexual partners of patients with PID need to be evaluated; this should include examination for sexually transmitted infections other than chlamydial and gonococcal disease, although, as a minimum, they must be treated for these two infections. Women who have had PID should be advised against the use of intrauterine devices and to protect themselves as much as possible against subsequent sexually transmitted infection to reduce their likelihood of infertility and other long-term sequelae. In women with concomitant HIV infection, hospitalization and intravenous therapy are indicated.

In addition to antibiotics, there are adjunctive therapies that may mitigate damage to the reproductive system. Non-steroidal anti-inflammatory agents may mitigate the damage caused in the tubes.[61]

There are no significant human data available and animal studies show inconclusive results.[62] Certainly, ibuprofen and similar agents are inexpensive and well tolerated. They may give substantial relief when pain is a significant symptom. Bed rest is advocated in other countries for treatment of PID and more patients are hospitalized in these countries. There is no data to support or refute a benefit from this practice.

If the patient is HIV positive, inpatient therapy and IV antibiotics using one of the two recommended regimens is the most prudent course. Recommendations do not otherwise differ for the HIV-positive or immunocompromised patient.

Finally, the ED physician should ensure that the sexual partner(s) are treated. This may not only decrease the likelihood of recurrent disease, but may decrease the chance of spreading the disease to others. No woman should be considered adequately treated until her partner(s) are also treated. Screen target groups regularly for STDs. This would include sexually active teenagers, inmates of jails, illicit drug users, and those with multiple sexual partners. Women who report a new sexual partner should always be offered screening for sexually transmitted diseases.

References

1. Therapy for Sexually Transmitted Diseases. *Med Lett* 1994; 913:1-4.
2. Ambulatory PID Research Group. Multicenter randomized trial of ofloxacin versus cefoxitin and doxycycline in outpatient treatment of pelvic inflammatory disease. *South Med J* 1993;6:604-610.
3. McCormack WM. Pelvic inflammatory disease. *N Engl J Med* 1994;330:115-119.
4. Friedland IR, McCracken GH. Management of infections caused by antibiotic-resistant Streptococcus pneumoniae. *N Engl J Med* 1994;331:377-382.
5. Raz R. Stamm WE. A controlled trial of intravaginal estriol in postmenopausal women with recurrent urinary tract infections. *N Engl J Med* 1993;329:753-756.
6. Soper DE, Brockwell NJ, Dalton HP. Microbial etiology of urban emergency department acute salpingitis: Treatment with ofloxacin. *Am J Obstet Gynecol* 1992;3:653-660.
7. Sweet RL. Pelvic inflammatory disease. *Hosp Pract* 1993; 28(suppl 2):25-30.
8. Rolle C. (Tuscon Medical Center, personal communication).
9. Evaluation of new anti-infective agents for the treatment of acute pelvic inflammatory disease. *Clin Infect Dis* 1992;15(suppl): S33-S42.
10. Witkin SS, Ledger WJ. New directions in diagnosis and treatment of pelvic inflammatory disease. *J Antimicrob Chemother* 1994;2:197-199.
11. CDC 1993 sexually transmitted diseases treatment guidelines. *MMWR Morb Mortal Wkly Rep* 1993;42(RR14):75.
12. Newkirk GR. Pelvic inflammatory disease: A contemporary approach. *Am Fam Physician* 1996;53:1127-1135.
13. Washington AE, Katz P. Cost of and payment source for pelvic inflammatory disease. Trends and projections, 1983 through 2000. *JAMA* 1991;266:2565-2569.
14. Dan M, Samra Z, Katz A, et al. Etiology of acute pelvic inflammatory disease proven by laparoscopy. *Sex Trans Dis* 1993;20:158-163.
15. Hillis SD. PID prevention: Clinical and societal stakes. *Hosp Prac* 1994;29:121-130.
16. Braverman PK, Strasburger VC. Sexually transmitted diseases. *Clin Ped* 1994;33:26-37.
17. Sopor DE, Brockewee NJ, Dalton HP. Microbial etiology of urban emergency department acute salpingitis: Treatment with ofloxacin. *Am J Obstet Gynecol* 1992;167:653-660.
18. Rome ES. Pelvic inflammatory disease: The importance of aggressive treatment in adolescents. *Cleveland Clin J Med* 1998; 65:369-376.
19. Hillis SD. PID prevention: Clinical and societal stakes. *Hosp Prac* 1994;29:121-130.
20. Westrom L. Incidence, prevalence, and trends of acute pelvic inflammatory disease and its consequences in industrialized countries. *Am J Obstet Gynecol* 1980;138(7 Pt 2):880-892.
21. Aral SO, Mosher WD, Cates W Jr. Self-reported pelvic inflammatory disease in the United States, 1988. *JAMA* 1991; 266:2570-2573.
22. Rice Pa, Schacter J. Pathogenesis of pelvic inflammatory disease. *JAMA* 1991;266:2587-2593.
23. Farley TM, Rosenberg MJ, Rowe PJ, et al. Intrauterine devices and pelvic inflammatory disease: An international perspective. *Lancet* 1992;339:785-788.
24. Chi IC. A bill of health for the IUD: Where do we go from here? *Adv Contracep* 1994;10:121-131.
25. Cates W Jr. Wasserheit JN, Marchbanks PA. Pelvic inflammatory disease and tubal infertility: the preventable conditions. *Ann N Y Acad Sci* 1994;709:179-195.
26. Faro S, Martens M, Maccato M, et al. Vaginal flora and pelvic inflammatory disease. *Am J Obstet Gynecol* 1993;169: 470-474.
27. Fitz-Hugh T. Acute gonoccocic peritonitis of the right upper quadrant in women. *JAMA* 1934;102:2094-2096.
28. Curtis AH. A cause of adhesions in the right upper quadrant. *JAMA* 1930;94:1221-1222.
29. Wald ER. Pelvic inflammatory disease in adolescents. *Curr Probl Pediatr* 1996;26:86-97.
30. Landers DV, Sweet RL. Tubo-ovarian abscess: Contemporary approach to management. *Rev Infect Dis* 1983;5:876-884.
31. Cacciatore B, Leminen A, Ingman-Friberg S, et al. Transvaginal sonographic findings in ambulatory patients with suspected pelvic inflammatory disease. *Obstet Gynecol* 1992; 80:912-916.
32. Buchan H, Vessey M, Goldacre M, et al. Morbidity following pelvic inflammatory disease. *Br. J Obstet Gynecol* 1993;100: 558-562.
33. Soper DE. Pelvic inflammatory disease. *Infect Dis Clin N Am* 1994;8:821-840.
34. Hooton TM, et al.Randomized comparative trial and cost analysis of 3-day antimicrobial regimens for treatment of acute cystitis in women. JAMA 1995;273:41-5.
35. Westrom L. Incidence, prevalence, and trends of acute PID and its consequences in industrialized countries. *Am J Obstet Gynecol* 1980:138:880-892.
36. Westrom L, Joesoef R, Reynolds B, et al. Pelvic inflammatory disease and fertility. A cohort study of 1844 women with

laparoscopically verified disease and 657 control women with normal laparoscopic results. *Sex Transm Dis* 1992;19:185-192.

37. Soper DE. Pelvic inflammatory disease. *Infect Dis Clin N Am* 1994;8:821-840.
38. Dan M, Samra Z, Katz A, et al. Etiology of acute pelvic inflammatory disease proven by laparoscopy. *Sex Trans Dis* 1993;20:158-163.
39. CDC 1998 sexually transmitted diseases treatment guidelines. *MMWR Morb Mortal Wkly Rep* 1998;47(RR1):80.
40. Wald ER. Pelvic inflammatory disease in adolescents. *Curr Probl Pediatr* 1996;26:86-97.
41. Peipert JF, Boardman L, Hogan JW, et al. Laboratory evaluation of acute upper genital tract infection. *Obstet Gynecol* 1996;87:730-736.
42. Reljic M, Gorisek B. C-reactive protein and the treatment of pelvic inflammatory disease. *Int J Gynecol Obstet* 1998;60: 143-150.
43. Kahn JG, Walker CK, Washington AE, et al. Diagnosing pelvic inflammatory disease: A comprehensive analysis and considerations for developing a new model. *JAMA* 1991;266: 2594-2604.
44. Miller KE. Sexually transmitted diseases. *Primary Care* 1997;24:179-193.
45. Paavonen J. Pelvic inflammatory disease. From diagnosis to prevention. *Dermatol Clin* 1998;4:747-756.
46. Gates W Jr., Joesoef MR, Goldman MB. Atypical pelvic inflammatory disease: Can we identify clinical predictors? *Am J Obstet Gynecol* 1993;169:341-346.
47. Grodstein F, Goldman MB, Cramer DW. Relation of tubal infertility to history of sexually transmitted diseases. *Am J Epidemiol* 1993;137:577-584.
48. Wald ER. Pelvic inflammatory disease in adolescents. *Curr Probl Pediatr* 1996;26:86-97.
49. Abbott M. New directions in the diagnosis and treatment of pelvic inflammatory disease. *J Antimicrob Chemother* 1994; 33:352-353.
50. Wald ER. Pelvic inflammatory disease in adolescents. *Curr Probl Pediatr* 1996;26:86-97.
51. CDC 1998 sexually transmitted diseases treatment guidelines. *MMWR Morb Mortal Wkly Rep* 1998;47(RR1).
52. Landers DV, Wolner-Hanssen P, Paavonen J. Combination antimicrobial therapy in the treatment of acute pelvic inflammatory disease. *Am J Obstet Gynecol* 1991;164: 849-858.
53. Data on file, Pfizer, Inc. New York, NY
54. CDC Sexually transmitted diseases treatment guidelines. 1993. *MMWR Morb Mortal Wkly Rep* 1993;42(RR-14):78-80.
55. Dodson MG. Antibiotic regimens for treating acute pelvic inflammatory disease. *J Reprod Med* 1994;39:285-296.
56. Washington E, Burg AO. Preventing and managing pelvic inflammatory disease: Key questions, practices, and evidence. *J Fam Pract* 1996;43:283-293.
57. Walker CK, Workowski KA, Washington AE, et al. Anaerobes in pelvic inflammatory disease: Implications for the Centers for Disease Control and Prevention's guidelines for treatment of sexually transmitted diseases. *Clin Infect Dis* 1999;28(Supp 1):S29-S36.
58. Hemsell DL, Wendel GD Jr., Hemsell PG, et al. Inpatient treatment for uncomplicated and complicated acute pelvic inflammatory disease: Ampicillin/sulbactam vs. cefoxitan. *Inf Dis Obset Gynecol* 1993;1:123-129.
59. Walker CK, Kahn JG, Washington AE, et al. Pelvic inflammatory disease: Meta-analysis of antimicrobial regimen efficacy. *J Inf Dis* 1993;168:969-978.
60. Erbelding E, Quinn TC. The impact of antimicrobial resistance on the treatment of sexually transmitted diseases. *Infec Dis Clin N Am* 1997;11:889-903.
61. Ridgeway GL. Quinolones in sexually transmitted diseases. *Drugs* 1995;49(Suppl 2):115-122.
62. Tartaglione TA, Hooton TM. The role of fluoroquinolones in sexually transmitted diseases. *Pharmacol* 1993;13:189-201.
63. Pfizer product mongraph. Azithromycin for IV injection.

Sexually Transmissible Diseases

Charles Stewart, MD, FACEP
Gideon Bosker, MD, FACEP

Despite aggressive public education programs and a well-documented association between infection with common sexually transmissible diseases (STDs) and facilitation of HIV transmission, STDs are on the rise, and are frequently encountered in the emergency department (ED) setting. *(Please see Table 1.)* Prompt diagnosis and outcome-effective management of common STDs will reduce the incidence of complications (i.e., pelvic inflammatory disease [PID]) associated with gonococcal and chlamydial infections. The Centers for Disease Control and Prevention (CDC) publishes treatment recommendations for these conditions, and emergency physicians must be familiar with the range of treatment options and the precise indications for initiating therapy.

As a rule, uncomplicated gonorrhea is treated with single-dose therapy. There are a variety of effective drug regimens based on quinolones, cephalosporins, and the macrolides; treatment options vary considerably in cost—a factor that may dictate usage patterns in specific hospital environments. Although only one infectious agent may be involved, empiric treatment of chlamydia is required when gonococcal disease is suspected, and conversely, antimicrobial coverage of *Neisseria gonorrhoeae* is required when chlamydial infection is the most likely etiology.

The importance of effective communication for the purpose of enhancing compliance with medication regimens cannot be overemphasized. Because significant noncompliance has been reported with doxycycline, one-dose therapeutic modalities (e.g., azithromycin 1 g po once for uncomplicated chlamydial infection and a choice of several agents for uncomplicated gonococcal infection [GC]) are generally preferred.

With an estimated annual cost of up to $5 billion to treat primary chlamydial infection and related complications (PID, infertility, chronic pelvic pain), it has become abundantly clear that the chlamydia problem deserves special attention. From an emergency therapeutics perspective, it should be stressed that, to a significant degree, the chlamydia epidemic has grown significantly because of poor patient compliance with the traditional, seven-day course of bid doxycycline. Although this regimen is highly effective for uncomplicated chlamydia when it is taken in its entirety, noncompliance with the drug regimen has been identified as a potential weak link between the emergency physician's prescription pad and optimal clinical outcomes.[1]

For example, in one real world study that followed patients from the time of diagnosis to prescription generation to antibiotic pill consumption, only 65% of all patients prescribed a seven-day course of doxycycline therapy reported sufficient intake of the antimicrobial to achieve expected clinical cure of their chlamydial infection.[1-3] When this degree of noncompliance occurs, a significant percentage of patients will return for retreatment because of therapeutic failures. In addition, these patients increase the chances of infecting their present and future sexual partners, who will then have to access the healthcare system for treatment.

Table 1. Some Sexually Transmissible Diseases

DISEASE	IMPLICATED ORGANISM
Gonorrhea	*Neisseria gonorrhea*
Chlamydia	*Chlamydia trachomatis*
Syphilis	*Treponema pallidum*
Chancroid	*Haemophilus ducreyi*
Lymphogranuloma venereum	*Calymmatobacterium granulomatis*
Gardnerella	*Gardnerella vaginalis*
Genital herpes	Herpes simplex virus
Cytomegalovirus	
Hepatitis virus A and B	
AIDS	HIV
Genital condylomata	Human papilloma virus
Trichomonas	*Trichomonas vaginalis*
Giardia	*Giardia lamblia*
Scabies	*Sarcoptes scabiei*
Pediculosis	*Pedicululs pubis*

Table 2. Clinical Manifestations of Gonorrhea

50% of men and women may be asymptomatic

PATIENT	SYNDROME	FREQUENCY
Men	Conjunctivitis	Rare
	Gonococcal urethritis	85-90% of cases
	Epididymitis	Most common cause
	Prostatitis	Common
	Proctitis (anal intercourse)	Uncommon
	Pharyngitis	Uncommon
	Disseminated disease	Rare
Women	Conjunctivitis	Rare
	Cervicitis	Common, 10-20%
	Acute urethral syndrome	Up to 50% of cases
	Salpingitis	20-25% of cases
	Perihepatitis	Uncommon
	Proctitis	Common
	Pharyngitis	Common
	Disseminated disease	Rare
Neonates	Conjunctivitis (May also develop disease in any exposed mucous membrane surface)	25-50% of exposed infants

The end result of noncompliance-mediated therapeutic failures, as well as failure to diagnose these conditions, is "turnstile STDs," a phenomenon in which pharmacologic reservicing for STDs is required because of therapeutic failures associated with inadequate adherence to medication regimens. These observations strongly support the use of single-dose therapy that is administered under clinical supervision, on site, in the ED or clinic for treatment of uncomplicated chlamydial infections. Finally, it should be stressed that emerging resistance to quinolones among certain gonococcal species may affect decisions regarding antimicrobial treatment.

The purpose of this chapter is to update the emergency physician on current advances in the diagnosis and management of common, uncomplicated STDs (complications of STDs, such as PID, were covered in the previous issue). New diagnostic modalities are highlighted and outcome-effective treatment options are provided.

Gonococcal Infection

Life Cycle. *Neisseria gonorrhoeae* is a facultative, intracellular parasite that contains a typical, gram-negative cell wall. It is characteristic of gonococcal infection that these microbes are able to invade and divide inside epithelial cells. Interestingly, some strains of gonorrhea are "auxotrophs," infectious variants which, because they are unable to synthesize certain amino acids, must acquire these nutrients from the host organism to permit propagation. *N. gonorrhoeae* divides by binary fission every 20-30 minutes. To a great degree, intracellular replication allows the organism to evade host immune defenses. Local tissue damage is the result of a toxin produced by the gonococcal organisms. Although it is speculated that the majority of tissue damage is toxin-mediated, immune response mechanisms may also play a role.

Spectrum of Disease. Transmission of gonorrhea requires physical contact with the infected tissue. It is estimated that about 50% of patients harboring *N. gonorrhoeae* are asymptomatic (i.e., they are colonized with the organism and potentially infectious). The remaining 50% of patients will have characteristic symptoms, 20% of which will have local complications. Overall, about 1-2% of patients will have disseminated gonococcal infection (DGI), which may be symptomatic. Variations in presentation, from asymptomatic to severely symptomatic, reinforce the importance of definitive treatment in all patients suspected of having infection, as well as treatment of their sexual partners.

The vectors for transmission have been well studied. Male to female transmission of *N. gonorrhoeae* is the most efficient transport vector, although there is strong evidence that receptive anal intercourse is also an efficient vector. It should stressed that although oral transmission occurs, this vector is less efficient in transmitting infection than sexual intercourse. *(Please see Table 2.)*

Urethritis. Urethritis is the most common manifestation of *N. gonorrhoeae* infection in men. The incubation period ranges from 3-7 days, and the disease usually manifests symptoms within 10-14 days after the exposure. Characteristic symptoms include a purulent urethral discharge and dysuria. The urethral discharge ranges in color from clear to yellow and, therefore, although not diagnostic, all urethral discharges in men should be presumed to be gonococcal in origin unless culture results suggest otherwise. The majority of cases of gonococcal urethritis in men are symptomatic, with 85-90% of men developing symptoms of an acute infection. Moreover, the more pronounced the discharge, the more likely it is that gonorrhea is present.

From an emergency management perspective, it must be emphasized that chlamydial and gonococcal infections frequently coexist, a clinical finding that explains why treatment protocols including antimicrobial agents directed at both organisms have become standard. For example, if a patient has documented chlamydial infection, the chance of co-infection with gonorrhea is between 25-50%. Overall, the ratio of men with non-gonococcal urethritis (NGU) to men with gonococcal urethritis in most geographical areas is about 4:1. Although the diagnosis of gonococcal urethritis is usually straightforward in men, in women gonococcal urethritis may mimic a urinary tract infection (UTI). As might be expected, dysuria and frequency of urination are common symptoms of gonococcal urethritis in women. Consequently, the presence of pyuria in the absence of bacteriuria in a sexually active female should direct the physician toward evaluation of gonococcal disease.

In young women, acute cystitis and urethritis occur in the absence of classical criteria for bacteriuria (10^5 bacteria per mL of urine) in as many as 50% of cases.[4-6] The constellation of dysuria, frequency of urination, and pyuria in the absence of "significant" bacteriuria has been termed the acute urethral syndrome. In many cases, this syndrome is caused by low-level infections with *Escherichia coli* (10^2-10^4 organisms per mL) or with a sexually transmitted pathogen such as *Chlamydia trachomatis.*

The modern standard for a positive urine culture in a patient with dysuria is now widely accepted to be 10^2 rather than 10^5 organisms per mL. Sexually transmitted pathogens can cause urethritis, vaginitis, and prostatitis, conditions that can clinically mimic the infections of classic uropathogens such as *E. coli.* Microorganisms, including *Trichomonas vaginalis, N. gonorrhoeae, C. trachomatis,* and *Ureaplasma urealyticum,* are common offenders. Urethritis and epididymitis caused by sexually transmitted pathogens are increasingly common among promiscuous males, and UTI may be associated with HIV or herpes virus infection.

Cervicitis. Approximately 10-20% of women who are infected with *N. gonorrhoeae* will present with acute cervicitis. Nevertheless, clinicians should be aware that about 50% of patients with clinical cervicitis will have no complaints, even though they harbor the infection and can transmit the organism. The presence of a purulent cervical exudate in conjunction with cervical friability characterizes the clinical presentation of gonococcal cervicitis. As many as 50% of women infected with gonorrhea will have gonococcal urethritis, although this diagnosis frequently is missed in the female population.[7] In addition, women who have had a hysterectomy can still become infected with gonorrhea; in these individuals, urethral cultures may be necessary to confirm the diagnosis. Although the classical literature on the subject suggests that clinical symptoms tend to follow menstruation, the precise incubation period is not well established for this disease. Typically, however, symptoms generally occur within 10 days of exposure and typically may include the following: 1) vaginal discharge; 2) dysuria; 3) increased frequency of urination; 4) abnormal uterine bleeding; and 5) lower abdominal pain with or without PID.

Epididymitis. Epididymitis is probably the most common and severe complication of gonococcal infection encountered in men. Symptoms include swelling of the epididymal gland next to the testis and accompanying pain in the epididymis. Chlamydia and gonorrhea are the most common causes of acute epididymitis in men younger than age 35. Unfortunately, this disease may be easily confused with acute testicular torsion. A differential point that may aid in diagnosis is that gonococcal epididymitis most often presents with concurrent urethritis. Evaluation of men older than 35 years is sometimes considered problematic, since the classical teaching states that epididymitis is infrequently caused by a STD (either GC or Chlamydia) in men older than age 35. Although this is true on a statistical and epidemiological basis, a STD cannot be ruled out by age of the patient alone. The most common causes for epididymitis are insertive anal intercourse or iatrogenic instrumentation of the urethra.

Proctitis. In the male population, this disease is associated with receptive anorectal sex. Interestingly, about 33-50% of women who have cervical gonorrhea may acquire anorectal infection; in this population, gonococcal proctitis is not related to anorectal intercourse.[7] Of special clinical importance is the fact that 80% of patients who have gonococcal proctitis will have no symptoms, which means the physician must have a high index of suspicion and perform anal cultures when the diagnosis is entertained. As is the case with urethritis, this condition may be due to either gonorrhea or Chlamydia. The most common symptoms include the following: 1) anal irritation; 2) rectal bleeding; 3) rectal discharge; 4) rectal itching (pruritus ani); 5) painful defecation; 6) constipation; and 7) tenesmus. Treatment must include screening for repeat and recurrent infection. The initial treatment course fails in up to 35% of cases.[8]

Pharyngitis. Gonorrheal pharyngitis is transmitted by oral sex. As many as 10-20% of women who have cervical gonorrhea have positive pharyngeal cultures.[9] From a detection point of view, ED physicians should be aware that 90-95% of patients with oral gonorrhea are asymptomatic. When present, symptoms may include oropharyngeal erythema, uvular erythema, and tonsillitis. Chlamydia also may cause occasional cases of pharyngitis; clinical symptoms are mild if present. Because GC pharyngitis is often resistant to usual therapy, close follow-up is mandatory.

Conjunctivitis. Gonococcal ophthalmia used to be a problem affecting newborns in the United States. In the current environment, it is occurring with increasing frequency among sexually active adults. The most common cause is autoinoculation. The condition is characterized by a rapidly developing purulent exudate, and ulceration that may cause perforation of the globe. It usually appears 2-3 days after delivery and can be prevented by instillation of silver nitrate, tetracycline, or erythromycin eye drops after delivery. Although gonococcal conjunctivitis has a more acute onset and produces a more purulent exudate than Chlamydia, these findings are not specific enough to be useful for clinical differentiation.

Pregnancy. Pregnancy does not provide protection from gonococcal infection. In fact, clinically apparent gonococcal infection occurs in pregnant women as frequently as it does in non-pregnant women. From the standpoint of evaluating the pregnant patient, it should be pointed out that there is an increased rate of oropharyngeal gonorrhea in pregnant women. The higher rate of oropharyngeal infection is partially offset by a decreased rate of PID in pregnancy.

Septic abortion, premature delivery, and disseminated gonococcal infection (DGI) all occur in pregnancy. Perinatal GC can also produce pharyngeal, vaginal, or rectal infections in the newborn. Ophthalmia neonatorum is a serious systemic disease, which is now more common in Third World countries.

Disseminated Gonococcal Infection. DGI is the most common systemic complication of acute gonorrhea and occurs in 0.5-3.0% of patients with untreated mucosal infection.[7] For reasons that are not entirely clear, DGI is more common in women than in men. Disseminated gonococcal infection is a complex syndrome characterized by a pustular rash and joint findings; it may also be called arthritis-dermatitis syndrome. Specifically, the following manifestations are encountered in the accompanying percentage of cases: 1) joint and skin findings (69%); 2) joints only (23%); 3) skin only (7%); and 4) endocarditis (1%).

The incubation period for DGI ranges from about 7-30 days and the rash typically is detectable about seven days after menses. Gonorrhea still is the most common cause of septic arthritis in patients younger than 45 years.[10] The usual sites of involvement include the distal joints and the extremities. Rarely, endocarditis can result from hematogenous dissemination of the gonococcal organism.

Diagnosis of Gonorrhea

Although patients usually are treated empirically with antibiotics for suspected gonococcal infection, it is important to establish the diagnosis and report confirmed cases to public health authorities. Diagnostic confirmation of disease will also guide treatment of sexual partners and permit follow-up in patients with resistant strains, complications, or difficult-to-treat clinical subgroups.

Culture. Culture of the organism remains the "gold standard" for diagnosis of gonorrhea. Routine culture for the organism is mandatory even when the diagnosis is evident, since culture results permit evaluation of the strain of *N. gonorrhoeae,* monitoring of antimicrobial susceptibility, and epidemiological surveillance. The full complement of information required to characterize epidemiological patterns and generate organism- and region-specific treatment recommendations can be obtained only from culture results.

The culture technique that is selective for gonorrhea is modified Thayer-Martin medium. The sensitivity rate of bacterial culture using Thayer-Martin medium is about 96-98%, with a turnaround time of about 48 hours. Specimens should be obtained with a Dacron swab, because cotton swabs inhibit growth. Various transport systems containing CO_2 releasing devices are available and are especially useful if the laboratory is either slow to respond or is located a significant distance from the emergency department.

The usual sites of culture are urethral for males and cervical for females. It is important to do a rectal culture if the patient has engaged in receptive rectal intercourse. It is equally important to check and, when indicated, perform a culture of, the pharynx if there are symptoms or if it is a known or suspected site of exposure.

Gram Stain. Although not definitive and limited in sensitivity (especially in females), gram stain of a urethral discharge is an excellent screening and diagnostic test for males. When interpreted by an experienced individual, the test is both sensitive and specific.[11] Unfortunately, there is a high false-positive rate in specimens obtained from cervical smears, so a positive test is only suggestive of GC infection in females. Although not usually performed, gram stain and culture of a female's urethra is as sensitive as it is in males. Likewise, discharge from a Bartholin's gland yields a high sensitivity for gonorrhea. Overall, the sensitivity rates for gram stain specimens obtained from various anatomical sites are reported to be as follows: 1) urethral (96%, either sex); 2) cervical (50%); 3) conjunctiva (95%); 4) rectal (< 50%); and 5) pharyngeal (< 50%).[11]

DNA Techniques. Of special diagnostic significance is the finding that DNA testing is more accurate and reliable in females than are culture results. In contrast, the opposite appeared to be true for males infected with gonorrhea (i.e., culture results appear to be more specific and sensitive).[12] The extreme sensitivity of DNA-based tests in women makes it possible to detect the presence of a single gonococcal organism in samples of freshly voided urine, tampons, and distal vaginal secretions.[13]

Both polymerase chain reaction (PCR) and ligase chain reaction (LCR) techniques have been used for the diagnosis of gonorrhea. Commercially available DNA probe (Gen-Probe-Pace II) and LCR tests (Abbott LCR) can detect *N. gonorrhoeae* directly from cervical or urethral specimens. These assay systems will detect both gonorrhea and Chlamydia infections from a single swab sample.

Similar technology (the AMPLICOR *N. gonorrhoeae* PCR test) has been shown to detect gonorrhea in urine specimens with better accuracy than current urethral swabs (90-95% sensitivity with 98-100% specificity).[14,15] When the cost of preventing a case of PID caused by GC or Chlamydia is computed, urine-based LCR screening appears to be the most cost-effective diagnostic and clinical screening strategy.[16] In asymptomatic, sexually active adolescent females, using a urine-based LCR assay will prevent the greatest number of cases of PID.

Based on these findings, DNA probes are likely to become the standard test for diagnosing Chlamydia and gonorrhea in the near future. Because the tubes used for collection of specimens cause lysis of the organism, the specimen obtained cannot be used for subsequent culture.[17] Moreover, bacterial culture is more expensive and may not necessarily be a more useful clinical test.

Other Diagnostic Modalities. Other confirmatory methods for culture have been used, but are not as well studied. These include antigen detection techniques such as enzyme immunoassay (EIA), nucleic acid probes, and direct fluroscein antigen (DFA). They offer rapid turnaround and office-based performance; they are inexpensive. Unfortunately, these tests are compromised by relatively poor sensitivity and specificity (60-90% sensitivity).

Treatment of Gonococcal Infection

Antimicrobial therapy for gonococcal infection has undergone a dramatic change over the past two decades. In particular, changes in therapy over time have had to account for developing resistance patterns and geographical variations related to antimicrobial resistance. When penicillin was first used for treatment of gonorrhea, the minimum inhibitory concentration was 0.003 to 0.03 mg/L. Since that time, there has been a slow but inexorable increase in the upper range of the minimum inhibitory concentration (MIC). By the 1960s, many strains of *N. gonorrhoeae* had developed intermediate to complete resistance to penicillin, a resistance trend that has continued until the present day.

The evolution of gonococcal resistance has challenged infectious disease experts and epidemiologists at the CDC to identify an "ideal" agent for the treatment of gonorrhea. In the best of all worlds, such a drug would be effective against all types of gonococcal resistance patterns, and all bacterial strains, regardless of geographic location and would produce clinical cure at all sites of infection. Because empiric treatment of the patient with gonorrhea also includes coverage of chlamydia, it would be advantageous for the therapeutic agent to have activity against *Chlamydia*, as well as incubating syphilis. If the drug could be given orally as a single dose, if its cost was sufficiently attractive, and if the the drug had minimal side effects, it

Table 3. Treatment of Uncomplicated Gonorrhea

URETHRAL, RECTAL, OR CERVICAL SITE

Cefixime [a] 400 mg po once
  or
Ceftriaxone [a] 125 mg IM once
  or
Ciprofloxacin [bc] 500 mg po once
  or
Oxyfloxacin [bc] 400 mg po once
  Plus
Azithromycin 1 g orally once [d] (to cover possible or presumed uncomplicated, coexisting chlamydial infection)
  or
Doxycycline [c] 100 mg po twice a day for 7 days [d]

Alternative parenteral medication
Spectinomycin 2 g IM [e]
Ceftizoxime 500 mg IM one time
Cefotaxime 500 mg IM one time
Cefotetan 1 g IM once
Cefoxitin 2 g IM once with probenecid 1 g orally

Alternative quinolones
Enoxacin 400 mg po once [f]
Lomefloxacin 400 mg po once [f]
Norfloxacin 800 mg po once [f]

PHARYNGEAL SITE

GC of the pharynx is more difficult to eradicate. Few antigonococcal drugs can reliably cure pharyngeal GC infections more than 90% of the time.[20]
Ceftriaxone [a] 125 mg IM once
  or
Ciprofloxacin [bc] 500 mg po once
  or
Oxyfloxacin [bc] 400 mg po once
  Plus
Azithromycin 1 g orally once [d] (to cover possible or presumed uncomplicated, coexisting chlamydial infection)
  or
Doxycycline [c] 100 mg po twice a day for 7 days [d]

GONOCOCCAL CONJUNCTIVITIS

Ceftriaxone [a] 1 g IM once
  or
Spectinomycin 2 g IM [g]

[a] Contraindicated if penicillin allergy
[b] Contraindicated during pregnancy
[c] Contraindicated in growing children
[d] Used for treatment of presumed coexisting Chlamydia infection
[e] Useful in treatment of patient who cannot tolerate cephalosporins and quinolones
[f] There is no advantage in use of these drugs over ciprofloxacin.
[g] Spectinomycin is unreliable for GC pharyngitis. Patients should be reevaluated 3-5 days after treatment with this drug. It should be reserved only for those with a known allergy to ceftriaxone.

Table 4. Treatment of Gonococcal Disease in Pregnancy

TREATMENT OF CHOICE

One of the recommended cephalosporins or spectinomycin
  Plus
Erythromycin base 500 mg po qid for 7 days [d]

Patient Follow-up. It is essential to treat all contacts of the index case who have had sexual relations with the index case within 60 days. Testing and retreatment is indicated only if there is persistence of symptoms. Only ceftriaxone is effective against incubating syphilis, and therefore, testing for coexistence of syphilis is more important when other agents are used for therapy. Gonorrhea is reportable in all states. Such cases should be reported either to the local public health authorities or to the designated authority.

Patients should be instructed to avoid sexual intercourse until:

1) the entire course of therapy is completed; 2) their sexual partners are treated; and 3) they and their sexual partners no longer have symptoms. As noted earlier, spectinomycin is an unreliable drug for the treatment of GC pharyngitis. It should be reserved only for those patients with a known allergy to ceftriaxone.[20] Patients who are treated with this drug must be re-evaluated 3-5 days after therapy.

[d] Used for treatment of presumed coexisting Chlamydia infection

would satisfy all the criteria for the perfect anti-gonococcal agent. Unfortunately, such a drug does not yet exist.

Nevertheless, a variety of newer (post-penicillin era) antibiotics are available that are effective against otherwise resistant strains of gonorrhea. These agents are reliable when administered orally, and some are reliable when given by injection. Among the classes/agents approved for treatment of gonorrhea are the cephalosporins, quinolones, and the macrolide azithromycin.

Plasmid-Mediated Resistance. There are two forms of drug resistance: plasmid-mediated and chromosome-mediated resistance. The mechanism of plasmid-mediated penicillin resistance is linked to a bacterial enzyme that breaks down the beta-lactam ring of penicillin, rendering it ineffective. This form of resistance was first described in 1976, and since that time many strains of gonorrhea have been identified that exhibit this kind of resistance. It is also a very effective mechanism of resistance to tetracycline. The abbreviation, PPNG, is used to indicate penicillinase-producing *N. gonorrhoeae*, whereas the abbreviation TRNG is used to indicate tetracycline resistant *N. gonorrhoeae.*

Chromosomal-Mediated Resistance. In this mechanism of drug resistance, there is a genetic mutation in the gonococcus strain that results in altered cell wall permeability to antibiotics. Chromosome-mediated resistant *N. gonorrhoeae* (CMRNG) strains are usually resistant to both tetracycline and penicillin. They may also be resistant to cefoxitin and spectinomycin. Unlike beta-lactamase-mediated antibiotic resistance, chromosomal-mediated resistance cannot be easily detected in the laboratory.[18]

Resistance Patterns. Nationwide, about 20-30% of gonococcal isolates in the United States exhibit some resistance to penicillin and tetracycline. About 8-10% exhibit PPNG resistance; 3-5% are TRNG; 3-5% are both PPNG and TRNG, and 10-20% demonstrate CMRNG to both penicillin and tetracycline. In addition, it should be stressed that resistance to quinolones is being encountered with increasing frequency in the Far East.[19]

Current Treatment Recommendations. Oral therapy consisting of a single dose of the drug, administered under supervision, with medication intake observed by medical providers, is considered to be the best available approach to therapy of uncomplicated gonococcal infection.[20] This approach is associated with the lowest cost for both the patient and the institution and minimizes the possibility of noncompliance. *(Please see Table 3 for treatment recommendations.)*

It should be emphasized that concurrent treatment for *Chlamydia* is still considered to be essential. It is felt that the cost of therapy is less than the cost of testing. Although this contention may no longer be valid with newer DNA probes for Chlamydia, current standard of care mandates antimicrobial coverage for chlamydia. It is also felt that dual therapy may decrease the incidence of antimicrobial-resistant GC in the United States.

Ceftriaxone is the currently recommended intramuscular drug of choice for treatment of gonococcal infection. It has a long history of excellent results and few ceftriaxone-resistant strains of gonorrhea have been reported. Ceftriaxone has the highest cure rate of all currently recommended GC drugs.[20] Using lidocaine or sterile saline solution will reduce the discomfort associated with the injection.

There is still some debate and confusion about the appropriate dose of intramuscular ceftriaxone. The former recommendation for treatment of gonorrhea was 250 mg of ceftriaxone. Many authorities still feel that the currently recommended lower dose of 125 mg will lead to resistant microbes and, therefore, continue to use 250 mg IM.[21] Because ceftriaxone is not presently available in a 125 mg vial, smaller facilities must either use 250 mg of the drug or discard the excess medication. This is not a problem for facilities that have a significant chance of treating more than one patient with a STD in a 24-hour period. If the patient's sexual partner is present in the ED, then treatment using the other half of a 250 mg vial solves several problems simultaneously. Another approach is to use a recommended single-dose oral cephalosporin such as cefixime 400 mg po. Although these agents have a slightly lower cure rate than IM ceftriaxone, the cure rate with cefixime is still a very acceptable 98%.

Although CDC recommendations include quinolones as first-line agents for treatment of uncomplicated GC, this class appears to have several major drawbacks. Currently, the CDC recommendations include a single dose of either ofloxacin or ciprofloxacin. Because of reports of strains that have become increasingly resistant to quinolones, some authorities are becoming less enthusiastic about recommending quinolones for treatment of GC unless the patient has a significant allergy to cephalosporins.

In this regard, a number of factors should be considered. First, quinolones have no significant activity against syphilis, whereas the cephalosporins have substantial efficacy. Quinolones cannot be used in the pregnant patient or in patients younger than 16 years. *(Please see Table 4.)* In addition, gonorrhea can develop resistance to the quinolones relatively rapidly. This has been shown in both the laboratory and in the clinical environment. Although quinolones are currently recommended by the CDC, the reports includes a caveat about multiple reports of quinolone-resistant GC throughout the world.[20]

Table 5. Clinical Manifestations of Chlamydia

50-75% of men and women may be asymptomatic

PATIENT	SYNDROME	FREQUENCY
Men	Conjunctivitis	Rare
	Nongonococcal urethritis	30-50% of cases; Most common
	Postgonococcal urethritis	cause
	Epididymitis	Common
	Prostatitis	Very rare
	Proctitis (anal intercourse)	Uncommon
Women	Conjunctivitis	Rare
	Cervicitis	Very common
	Acute urethral syndrome	20-25% of cases
	Salpingitis	20-25% of cases
	Perihepatitis	Uncommon
Neonates	Conjunctivitis	25-50% of exposed infants
	Pneumonitis	10-20% of exposed infants

Fluoroquinolone-resistant strains account for approximately 10% of all gonococcal strains in Hong Kong and the Republic of the Philippines.[22] If the patient has acquired GC in Asia, then quinolones are definitely not recommended due to the increasing incidence of quinolone-resistant gonorrhea in this geographic region. Strains of gonococci with decreased susceptibility to ciprofloxacin appear to have become endemic in Cleveland, Ohio.[23] This resistance may limit the future use of the quinolones for treatment of gonorrhea in the United States.

None of the quinolones are effective as single-dose therapy against Chlamydia.[24,25] This means that dual therapy for Chlamydia and gonorrhea will require either extended administration of quinolones or dual drug therapy. Of these, the dual drug therapy is both cheaper and more certain when a single-dose antibiotic such as azithromycin is employed.

Chlamydial Infection

The major problems associated with uncomplicated chlamydial infection are difficulty of detection and diagnosis and, on the treatment side, noncompliance with medications. Definitive diagnosis is not possible using any one or more clinical criteria in either the female or male.[26] In women, a presentation spectrum ranges from one that is asymptomatic to one characterized by pain associated with a severely eroded, hypertrophic cervix with a mucopurulent discharge. *(Please see Table 5.)* In males, the patient may be normal or present with any of the symptoms described above for gonococcal disease.

Culture. Chlamydia cannot be identified on a gram stain. Either the Chlamydia organisms must be cultured (a difficult proposition) or the organism must be identified by other means. Culture of the organism by a competent laboratory is 100% specific, but is far from perfectly sensitive.[27] Confirming the diagnosis of chlamydia by culture is currently the legal standard for sexual assault and child abuse cases. Interestingly, although culture is the "gold" standard of diagnosis, Chlamydia culture is problematic. Naturally, a positive Chlamydia culture is 100% specific, but because of problems that are inherent with live culture techniques, this test is only about 80% sensitive. Since the organism is intracellular, culture techniques must use live media; the lab requires special expertise with this culture. Smaller hospitals may simply not have the ability to adequately culture this organism well. Moreover, cultures are expensive ($50 or more each), and it takes about three days to get results.

Direct Fluroscein Antigen (DFA) Detection. In this technique, samples from swab or scrapings are incubated with fluorescein-stained, monoclonal antibody. Slides are evaluated for presence of fluorescein stain. These tests are less sensitive than tissue culture, but non-culture antigen detection methods are easier to handle than cultures and less expensive, costing about $6-12 per test. Performance depends upon the skill of the laboratory staff. Based on product literature and studies, greater than 90% sensitivity and 95% specificity is associated with Microtrak, and greater than 90% sensitivity and specificity is associated with Chlamydiazyme.

Enzyme Immunoassay. The enzyme immunoassay (EIA) test detects the presence of antigen to Chlamydia from anatomic specimens. An antibody-coated solid phase (either polystyrene beads or welled plates of membranes) are used to capture Chlamydia lipopolysaccharide antigen. The antigen is then detected by a second antibody labeled with enzymes that produce a color reaction. The change in color is read by a spectrophotometer. EIA and DFA are equally sensitive and specific when used in women for screening tests. The EIA is a rapid test that takes from 20 minutes to two hours to perform. A one-day turnaround time from most labs is not unusual. There is an office-based kit available that costs about $5-10 per test.

Nucleic Acid Probes. This technique uses DNA or RNA amplification probes to detect Chlamydia in clinical specimens, including urine, tampons, and self -collected distal vaginal secretions (AMPLICOR Chlamydia trachomatis Test; Roche Diagnostic Systems, Inc., Branchburg, N.J.).[16,28] This technique has far better sensitivity and specificity than culture.[29] A major advantage is that the sample can be split and tested for GC at the same time.

As noted in the section on GC, these tests are extremely sensitive and may be able to detect as little as a single organism. Indeed, they may be able to quickly monitor patients for both diagnosis and effectiveness of therapy with simply a urine specimen or a self-collected vaginal swab.[30,31] The authors believe that nucleic acid probes will soon replace cultures as both the standard and the legal test in the foreseeable future. Although there are abundant papers detailing the specificity and sensitivity of cultures in infants and children, there is not a wealth of experience with the nucleic

Table 6. Treatment of Uncomplicated Chlamydia

TREATMENTS OF CHOICE

Azithromycin 1 g po, once given under supervision in the clinic or emergency department or practitioner's office, if possible. *Note:This is the only single-dose therapy for Chlamydia.*

or

Alternative Treatment of Choice

Doxycycline 100 mg bid po for 7-10 days.[a]

ALTERNATIVE TREATMENTS FOR CHLAMYDIA

Erythromycin base 500 milligrams orally four times daily for 7 days. [a]

or

Erythromycin ethylsuccinate 800 mg orally four times daily for 7 days. [a]

or

Ofloxacin 300 mg twice a day for 7 days (contraindicated in patients who are pregnant and/or < 16 years) [a]

RECOMMENDED TREATMENTS FOR CHLAMYDIA IN THE PREGNANT PATIENT

Erythromycin base 500 milligrams orally four times daily for 7 days

or

Amoxicillin 500 mg orally three times a day for 7 days.

ALTERNATIVE TREATMENTS FOR CHLAMYDIA IN THE PREGNANT PATIENT

Erythromycin base 250 mg orally four times daily for 14 days. [a]

or

Erythromycin ethylsuccinate 800 mg orally four times daily for 7 days. [a]

or

Erythromycin ethylsuccinate 400 mg orally four times daily for 14 days. [a]

or

Azithromycin 1 g po, once (Many authorities feel that this drug should completely replace erythromycin even in the pregnant patient, although it does not yet carry formal approval for use in the pregnant patient. Azithromycin carries a class B pregnancy rating).[32]

[a] When an extended duration medication such as doxycycline is employed, the patient should be given the entire course of medication when discharged. Compliance is often unreliable with these medications and any measure possible to improve compliance is appropriate. In one study, even when the doxycycline is given to the patient, only 25% of the patients will complete the full course of doxycycline as directed.

acid amplification techniques. They are not currently recommended as a legal test for rape or in child abuse cases. As more information is collected, this is likely to change.

Cytology. Although cytology is sometimes recommended, it is generally not helpful; it has poor sensitivity and specificity. Cytologic examination looks for inclusion bodies of Chlamydia on scraping smears stained with Giemsa stain. It is a technique that works better with conjunctival scrapings than with pap smears.

Treatment of Uncomplicated Chlamydial Infection

Presumed chlamydial infection should be treated in the following circumstances and patient subgroups: 1) individuals suspected of having non-gonococcal urethritis; 2) individuals suspected of having gonococcal infection; 3) women who present with mucopurulent cervicitis; 4) women who present with a clinical picture consistent with PID; and 5) sexually active men with epididymitis. A follow-up appointment for test of cure should be considered for pregnant women, in patients in whom an "alternative" (i.e., non first-line) agent has been employed, and when there is suspected non-compliance with medications. HIV and immunosuppressed patients may be refractory to an initial treatment course and may therefore require and extended duration of treatment.

Antibiotic Regimens. In populations where noncompliance with medication is likely and when follow-up is unlikely or nonexistent, a single dose of azithromycin (1 gram), consumed by the patient under supervision on site may be more cost-effective approach to the treatment of uncomplicated chlamydial infection. *(See Table 6.)* In fact, when the cost of complications associated with doxycycline noncompliance and the overall outcome cost of azithromycin are compared, the total outcome costs associated with azithromycin are less than with doxycycline.[33] This is despite the higher drug acquisition cost of azithromycin. Unfortunately, azithromycin is not yet approved for use in the pregnant patient and further studies are probably indicated before routine use is advisable. Rifampin and sulfonamides also have good activity against Chlamydia but these agents are not recommended by the CDC.

As a general rule, two factors will influence choice of therapy. Treatment with most agents requires an extended treatment duration (greater than 5 days.) Although resistance to any of the customarily used antibiotics has not been clinically significant, there are some Chlamydial species that have started to exhibit increasing tolerance for tetracycline and derivatives. All of the major antimicrobial agents can cause gastrointestinal side effects. Many patients will not complete the full course of therapy because of this discomfort.

Tetracyclines are contraindicated in pregnancy and in growing children. If the patient is pregnant, an erythromycin regimen should be used. There is some evidence that if the pregnant patient has severe gastrointestinal side effects while taking erythromycin, there will be subtherapeutic levels of erythromycin.[34] This would mean that another regimen would be appropriate in these pregnant patients.

All sexual contacts within the last 60 days should be treated. Timely treatment of sexual partners is essential for decreasing the risk of reinfecting the index patient and stopping the spread of infection. In most patients, a "test of cure" is not needed, unless symptoms persist. There are groups in which recurrence or reinfection is more likely. In one study, a two- to three-fold increased risk of chlamydial persistence or recurrence was observed among women who were younger than 25 years and white or who reported: 1) a recent, new partner; 2) multiple partners; 3) a partner who may have had multiple partners at the time of enrollment; or 4) that not all partners were treated during the one-month follow-up period after initiation of treatment.[35] In these patients, a "test of cure" may be appropriate one month after treatment.

Finally, *Chlamydia* infection increases the chance of HIV transmission. In addition, HIV infection probably causes altered manifestations of *Chlamydia* infection. Since the two diseases are related at least in the manner in which they are transmitted, if the patient has *Chlamydia* or a high risk for Chlamydia, HIV testing is appropriate.

References

1. Katz BP, Zwickl BW. Compliance with antibiotic therapy for *Chlamydia trachomatis* and *Neisseria gonorrhoeae. Sex Trans Dis* 1992;6:351-354.
2. McCormack WM. Pelvic inflammatory disease. *N Engl J Med* 1994;330:115-119.
3. Therapy for sexually transmitted diseases. *Med Lett Drugs Ther* 1994;913:1-4.
4. Faro S. New considerations in treatment of urinary tract infections in adults. *Urology* 1992;39:1-11.
5. Raz R, Stamm WE. A controlled trial of intravaginal estriol in postmenopausal women with recurrent urinary tract infections. *N Engl J Med* 1993;329:753-756.
6. Arav-Boger R, et al. Urinary tract infections with low and high colony counts in young women. Spontaneous remission and single-dose vs. multiple-day treatment. *Arch Int Med* 1994;154:300-304.
7. Zenilman JM. Update on bacterial sexually transmitted disease. *Urol Clin N Am* 1992;19:25-34.
8. Wexner SD. Sexually transmitted diseases of the colon, rectum, and anus. *Dis Col and Rect* 1990;33:1048-1062.
9. Martien K, Emans SJ. Treatment of common genital infections in adolescents. *J Adoles Health Care* 1987;8:129-136.
10. Cucurull E, Espinoza LR. Gonococcal arthritis. *Rheum Dis Clin North Am* 1998;;24:305-322.
11. Bowie WR. Approach to men with urethritis and urologic complications of sexually transmitted diseases. *Med Clin N Am* 1990;74:1543-1557.
12. Carroll KC, Aldeen WE, Morrison M, et al. Evaluation of the Abbott LCx ligase chain reaction assay for detection of *Chlamydia trachomatis* and *Neisseria gonorrhoeae* in urine and genital swab specimens from a sexually transmitted disease clinic population. *J Clin Microbiol* 1998;36: 1630-1633.
13. Gray RH, Wawer MJ, Girdner J, et al. Use of self-collected vaginal swabs for detection of *Chlamydia trachomatis* infection [letter]. *Sex Transm Dis* 1998;25:450.
14. Chapin-Robertson K. Use of molecular diagnostics in sexually transmitted diseases. *Diag Microbiol Infec Dis* 1993;16: 173-184.
15. Koumans EH, Johnson RE, Knapp JS, et al. Laboratory testing

for Neisseria gonorrhoeae by recently introduced nonculture tests: A performance review with clinical and public health considerations. *Clin Infect Dis* 1998;27:1171-1180.

16. Shafer MA, Pantell RH, Schachter J. Is the routine pelvic examination needed with the advent of urine-based screening for sexually transmitted diseases? *Arch Pediatr Adolesc Med* 1999;153:119-125.
17. Hall GS. Probe technology for the clinical microbiology laboratory. *Arch Path Lab Med* 1993;117:578-583.
18. Stamm WE. Problems in the treatment of bacterial sexually transmitted diseases. *Am J Med* 1987;82(suppl 4A):307-310.
19. Denver STD/HIV Prevention Training Center. Sexually transmitted disease clinician's update. Feb. 4-5, 1999.
20. Centers for Disease Control and Prevention. 1998 Guidelines for treatment of sexually transmitted diseases. *Morb Mortal Wkly Rep MMWR* 1998;(No. RR-1).
21. Villarino ME, Shulte JM. Diagnosis and therapy for common sexually transmitted diseases. *Derm Clin* 1992;10:459-468.
22. Knapp JS, Fox KK, Trees DL, et al. Fluoroquinolone resistance in *Neisseria gonorrhoeae. Emerg Infect Dis* 1997;3: 33-39.
23. Gordon SM, Carlyn CJ, Doyle LJ, et al. The emergence of *Neisseria gonorrhoeae* with decreased susceptibility to ciprofloxacin in Cleveland, Ohio: Epidemiology and risk factors. *Ann Intern Med* 1996;125:465-470.
24. Ridgway GL. Quinolones in sexually transmitted diseases. *Drugs* 1993;45:134-138.
25. Corrado ML. The clinical experience with ofloxacin in the treatment of sexually transmitted diseases. *Am J Obstet Gynecol* 1991;5:1396-1399.
26. Stewart CE. Male urinary tract infections. *Emerg Med Clin North Am* 1988;6:617-630.
27. Bell TA. Chlamydia infections in adolescents. *Med Clin North Am* 1990;74:1225-1233.
28. Stary A. Urethritis: Diagnosis of nongonococcal urethritis. *Dermatol Clin* 1998;16:723-726.
29. Smith IW, Morrison CL, Patrizio C, et al. Use of a commercial PCR kit for detecting *Chlamydia trachomatis. J Clin Pathol* 1993;46:822-285.
30. Morre SA, Sillekens PT, Jacobs MV, et al. Monitoring of *Chlamydia trachomatis* infections after antibiotic treatment using RNA detection by nucleic acid sequence based amplification. *Mol Pathol* 1998;51:149-154.
31. Polaneczky M, Quigley C, Pollock L, et al. Use of self-collected vaginal specimens for detection of *Chlamydia trachomatis* infection. *Obstet Gynecol* 1998;91:375-378.
32. Adair CD, Gunter M, Stovall TG, et al. Chlamydia in pregnancy: A randomized trial of azithromycin and erythromycin. *Obstet Gynecol* 1998;91:165-168.
33. Magid D, Douglas JM Jr, Schwartz JS. Doxycycline compared with azithromycin for treating women with genital *Chlamydia trachomatis* infections: An incremental cost-effectiveness analysis. *Ann Intern Med* 1996;124:389-399.
34. Larsen B, Glover DD. Serum erythromycin levels in pregnancy. *Clin Ther* 1998;20:971-977.
35. Hillis SD, Coles FB, Litchfield B, et al. Doxycycline and azithromycin for prevention of chlamydial persistence or recurrence one month after treatment in women. A use-effectiveness study in public health settings. *Sex Transm Dis* 1998;25:5-11.

Sexually Related Trauma

Charles Stewart, MD, FACEP

Although most of the attention directed toward conditions associated with adult sexual activity has focused on life-threatening infectious complications such as AIDS, many hazardous consequences of sexual activity fall into the category of sexual trauma. In this regard, it is important to distinguish between injuries caused by violent, non-consensual acts and those associated with a wide range of behaviors practiced by consenting adults. In most emergency departments (EDs), systematic protocols have been established for the assessment and management of sexual trauma in both adult and pediatric patients who are victims of sexual assault or abuse. Few resources, however, are available for guiding the approach to history-taking, physical examination, and therapeutic intervention in patients with traumatic injuries caused by voluntary sexual practices.

In an age characterized by increasing experimentation with novel sexual aids, unusual erotic practices, mechanical devices, and aggressive masturbatory techniques, it is not surprising that the medical literature is replete with recent reports on traumatic injuries associated with sexual behavior.[1-4] While many of these conditions reflect superficial injuries—abrasions, minor lacerations, contact dermatitis, etc.—caused by vigorous foreplay, masturbation, or intercourse,[5-7] other practices such as fisting, foreign body insertions, and vaginal insufflation are sometimes associated with life-threatening complications ranging from colonic perforation to air embolism.[3,8-10]

Given the range and potential hazards associated with sexual activity by consenting adults, this timely report is designed to highlight and discuss both common and unusual complications resulting from contemporary erotic practices. Injuries or diseases related to child sexual abuse, sexual violence (i.e., rape), and unprotected intercourse or sexual activity in patients known to be HIV-positive, are not covered in this review, which stresses the spectrum of injuries resulting from voluntary sexual practices.

Injuries to the Penis

Because of its capacity for rolling and escaping most injuries except for direct penetration by knife or bullet, the penis is not easily traumatized in the flaccid state. When erect, however, it is more easily damaged, with one review noting that 50% of penile injuries occurred during sexual intercourse, while an additional 21% were characterized as sequelae of other erotic practices.[11] Most traumatic injuries involving the penis are minor and usually are not reported to health care providers. For example, minor trauma to the meatus or shaft of the penis can result from allergens, mechanical trauma, intercourse, oral sex, or chemical irritants. These mechanically induced lesions—as well as those mediated by chemical substances—are often seen in young men who have recently started to masturbate. Penile edema associated with topical aphrodisiacs, irritants, or trauma may involve the prepuce or distal shaft of the penis and can occur as a result of pre-coital or coital activity. Contact allergies to latex, such as that contained in condoms, also can be problematic. Localized meatitis and, occasionally, urethritis can be seen in patients who have had prolonged or vigorous intercourse. Uncircumcised patients are at higher risk for sustaining such injuries, which are sometimes accompanied by local infections. Small lacerations to the frenulum, which are not uncommon, usually can be managed simply by suture repair and dressing.

Although not a sex-related injury in the strict sense, zipper injuries to the penis deserve special mention. Many physicians approach these injuries with a scalpel, which can produce significant anxiety in the patient. In general, however, disassembly of the zipper is a better solution than excision of the foreskin.[12,13] Local anesthetic is a priority both for patient comfort and as a prelude to definitive therapy. Disengagement of the zipper mechanism is most easily accomplished by cutting the transverse bar with appropriate wire cutters. When this is not possible, excision of the entrapped skin, which usually incorporates the prepuce, is a minor procedure using a suture repair that can be performed quickly under local anesthesia.

Human bites causing serious injury to the penis, though uncommon do occur in the setting of sexual activity. The associated wounds tend to be superficial and should be managed with copious irrigation, debridement, and antibiotics (ampicillin clavulanate, 500 mg po tid x 10 days) directed at anaerobic organisms and other mouth flora.

Larger lacerations may be self-inflicted, and can result accidentally from unusual masturbatory techniques or aids (i.e., a vacuum cleaner) or from deliberate attempts at self-mutilation. Sex magazines have promoted vacuum cleaners as masturbatory aids, but neglect to tell their readers that in some models the fan blades are extremely close to the intake and can cause extensive injuries to the inserted penis.[1,2] Lovers' quarrels also may result in severe injuries, which may range from degloving lesions and deep lacerations to avulsions of the glans, shaft, corpora cavernosa, and urethra. These patients require urological consultation and definitive surgical repair.

Although rare, penile amputations have been reported.[1,2] Most result from self-mutilatory practices in psychologically disturbed patients, but occasionally, a wrathful lover may wreak this kind of havoc. The amputated penis requires re-anastomosis of the urethra, both corpus cavernosa, the two dorsal arteries, the two dorsal penile nerves, and the dorsal vein of the penis. Successful penile replantation requires methodology unique to centers and surgeons specializing in microsurgical techniques. When such facilities are not available, and the patient must await transfer, bleeding should be controlled, and the severed member should be refrigerated until the procedure is performed. The success rate of penile replantation is variable, with better results observed in cases involving more distal penile amputations.

Traumatic Penile Lymphangitis. Following mechanical injuries, the next most common sexually related lesion of the penis is traumatic penile lymphangitis. There are several synonyms for this condition, including Hoffman's lymphangitis and non-venereal sclerosing lymphangitis.[14] Traumatic penile lymphangitis is characterized by a palpable cord-like structure along the shaft of the penis or about the dorsal corona.[15] Although the etiology is uncertain, it is thought to occur from repetitive or prolonged penile stimulation in individuals with a variant in lymphatic drainage to the penis.

Patients with traumatic lymphangitis of the penis usually present with a significant other who is worried about the look or feel of the penis. The lesion is usually asymptomatic and the patient should be reassured that the disorder is completely benign. With sexual abstinence, the lesion usually resolves rapidly, although sometimes many weeks are required for complete resolution. The usefulness of nonsteroidal anti-inflammatory drugs, antiviral agents and surgical excision has not been proved.[16,17]

Inserted Foreign Bodies

Foreign objects have been introduced into the urethra for a variety of autoerotic, psychiatric, therapeutic (dilation or cleansing) or, sometimes, very obscure reasons. Objects used for these purposes have included wire, cords, pens, crayons, pencils, nails, thermometers, rods of various materials, candles, and paper clips.[18] Some patients may conceal a history of foreign body insertion and present with complications such as cystitis, urethritis, urinary retention, or weak urinary stream. Additional trauma may occur when the patient attempts to remove the article with household tools.

Diagnosis and therapy is guided by radiographic demonstration of the object. Plain abdominal x-rays, ultrasonography, xerography,[18] and retrograde urethrograms may aid in assessment and localization. The patient should not be catheterized until diagnostic studies have been obtained, inasmuch as blind catheterization may exacerbate the problem.

Urological referral for surgical removal of these objects is required for nearly all patients. Objects distal to the urogenital diaphragm can often be removed by endoscopy, whereas those proximal to this site will likely require surgical removal. Following removal, patients should be re-examined to ensure that no retained fragments, lacerations, perforations, or additional foreign bodies are present. Complications include abscess, urinary infection, stricture, urinary incontinence, hemorrhage, retained foreign body, and anatomical deformity.[3]

Rarely, foreign bodies are implanted intentionally in penile subcutaneous tissue in an attempt to enhance the partner's sexual pleasure.[19] These objects can cause characteristic foreign body reactions and soft tissue infections, and are managed by removal and debridement, and, when necessary, antibiotic therapy.

External Foreign Bodies

A number of stimulatory practices have been associated with penile trauma, one of which involves placement of a snug, so-called, "cock ring" around the penis or penis and scrotum. Cock rings may be made of makeshift materials, or elaborately designed, in which case they are usually fashioned from leather, polished wood, steel, plastic or rubber. Cords, laces, and sections of metal tubing also have been used, as well as at least one commercial device that has been marketed for the treatment of impotence.

Complications occur when the ring fits too tightly around the erect penis, which can result in significant penile edema, thus preventing removal of the ring by the patient. Sequelae include ischemia, swelling, skin ulceration, extensive skin loss, and occasionally, deep tissue loss or amputation.[15] Thrombosis of blood within the penis has occurred in patients with sickle cell disease. Penile numbness, coldness, discoloration, and ecchymosis also have been reported with cock rings and therapeutic devices.

Local anesthesia is almost always required to remove external objects such as cock rings, which can be disengaged with a standard ring cutter. Removal of rings made of tempered steel and thicker objects may require more specialized equipment.[4] Cutting the object in two places will often facilitate removal.[4]

Alternatively, a compression technique in which the portion of the penis distal to the ring is wrapped in silk sutures or umbilical tape may be attempted, although the author has not found this approach to be particularly successful. If the edema formation has not progressed too far, the corpus cavernosum can be irrigated with heparinized saline, facilitating removal of trapped blood from the penis. In extremely severe cases, it may be necessary to remove the entire penile skin to reduce the entrapped tissue volume. Skin grafting will be required later.

Children may present with hair, rubber bands, or thread wrapped around the penis, causing a tourniquet-like effect.[4,20] This was first described by Guillimeau in 1612.[21,22] This traumatic lesion also can be seen in the setting of sexual abuse.[23]

"Fractured" Penis

Penile fracture, though uncommon, was first described by Malis in 1925. Since then about 200 cases have been reported in the literature.[24,25,26] The true incidence is not known because the injury is probably underreported.[27]

Fractured penis is a misnomer inasmuch as humans do not have an osseous structure in the penis. Anatomically, the injury represents a tear in the tunica albuginea of one or both corpora cavernosa. Rents, however, have also been observed in patients who give a history of an erect penis that has been bent double or struck with an object or fist. The patient frequently hears and feels a loud "crack or pop" and then loses the erection.[28-30] This injury occurs in the erect penis only.[31] The most common causes are bending or striking the penis during masturbation or as an attempt to reduce an erection. Cases have been reported in which the patient falls during standing intercourse, is kicked, or attempts to reduce an erection.[32]

Because the history and physical findings are characteristic, the diagnosis of fracture of the penis rarely presents difficulty.[33] Following the fracture, extravasation of blood from the tunica results in deformity, discoloration, and a hematoma of the middle of the penis. The penis will often deviate to the side opposite the site of the tear.[34] Urethral bleeding can occur when laceration of the tunica extends into the urethral mucosa.[35] Generally, patients who have hematuria associated with penile fracture will have a urethral laceration rather than complete avulsion; therefore, most will be unable to void. Although blood at the meatus and inability to void have been reported as classic symptoms of penile fracture, it should be stressed that absence of these findings does not rule out urethral injury.[36] If the lesion includes Buck's fascia, the hematoma will extend into the scrotum and the perineum.[28] In lesions that are confined by Buck's fascia, the hematoma will be limited to the penile shaft.[37]

Variations of penile fracture have been seen. In one case report, the deformity was caused by rupture of the deep dorsal vein rather than the tunica albuginea.[38] The clinical findings were identical to rupture of the tunica.

Blunt trauma to the penis also may cause impotence without fracture of the penis.[39] This may occur during masturbation or from accidents. The etiology appears to be a leak in the tunica albuginea that communicates with the dorsal vein, caused by an axial load on or an acute angulation of the erect penis. In these cases, penile swelling and ecchymosis may be absent.

The usual recommendations for emergency management include ice packs, splinting with tongue blades, and analgesics, although there is no evidence that the first two measures are of any significant benefit. Relief of pain, however, is always appropriate.

Suspicion of a urethral injury should be investigated with retrograde urethrogram. Catheterization of the patient is somewhat controversial and should be performed, if possible, by a urological consultant.[40] Most injuries will resolve promptly without stricture with either urethral or suprapubic catheterization, which is necessary if the patient experiences difficulty voiding. Occasionally, complications can occur. The tip of the catheter may convert a mucosal contusion or minimal laceration into a full thickness tear. If blood is found in the meatus, suprapubic cystostomy may be more appropriate.

Emergent urological referral is indicated in all of these cases, because prompt surgical repair has a far better outcome than conservative therapy.[41-44] Repair includes evacuation of the hematoma and surgical repair oflhe defect in the tunical albuginea.[45-48]

Flail Penis. A variant of the fractured penis is a flail penis resulting from rupture of the suspensory liganlent of the penis. This injury most often results from a fall during standing intercourse. Diagnosis is made by palpation of a gap between the base of the shaft of the penis and the symphysis pubis. An abnormal angle is noted during erection. Urological referral is indicated.

Penile Implant Fractures and Failures. Penile prostheses are occasionally used to allow individuals who can't achieve an erection the opportunity to participate in sexual activities. These prostheses can either be malleable or inflatable and each has its own set of complications. Infections, aneurysms, and erosions associated with insertion of foreign bodies occur, although infrequently.[49] In addition, fractures, cylinder rupture, leaks, and pump defects have been described.[50-51] These problems require urological consultation.

Urethral Tear

Bleeding from the meatus and urethral injury also has been described in reverse coitus insertion of the penis into the shaft of another penis.[52] In these rare cases, the patient does not feel or hear the "snap, crack, or pop," and a fracture of the corpus cavernosum is not found. These unusual lesions appear to heal without repair or sequelae. In all such cases, the patient should be evaluated as if a penile fracture has occurred.

Priapism

Although not strictly a sexually related injury, priapism may follow excessive sexual arousal or, in some cases, may be associated with drug therapy (i.e, trazodone, etc.). Painful sustained erection also can be associated with sickle cell disease, leukemia, paraplegia, iatrogenic causes, and tumors.[53] Priapism occurs in a bimodal distribution with one peak in the 5-10 year age group and another in the 20-25 year age group.

Priapism in younger patients is most frequently associated with either neoplasm or sickle cell disease, whereas in older men the cause is most frequently idiopathic. *(Please see Table 1.)* Many "conservative" treatments for priapism have been tried over the years, including cold showers, ice packs, pressure dressings, ice water enemas, hot water enemas, sedatives, analgesics, estrogens, anticoagulants, amyl nitrate, hypotensive drugs, and anesthesia—both spinal and general.[54]

Table 1. Causes of Priapism[51]

Sickle cell disease	Leukemia, lymphoma
Iatrogenic—papaverine injection	Trauma
Medications	Perineal
Antipsychotics	Spinal
Antihypertensives	Systemic diseases
Anticoagulants	Coagulopathy
Adrenal steroids	Hypertension
Marijuana	Vasculitis
Psychedelic drugs	Nephrotic syndrome
Cocaine	Rheumatoid arthritis
Sexual activity	Toxins
Neoplasms	Scorpion venom
Pelvic tumors	Idiopathic

Early treatment should be directed toward correction of the underlying disease, if one is present. In African American patients, early treatment should include hydration and oxygenation.

Initial attempts at definitive therapy include the use of analgesics and intracavernous adrenergic agents such as epinephrine or ephedrine. Epinephrine (and other adrenergic agents such as ephedrine) constrict inflow channels while relaxing the outflow channels. Epinephrine (1 mg/L of normal saline solution) may be administered as several bolus injections (at 10 minute intervals) or, alternatively, the drug can be infused as a slow drip into the corpus over a 30-60 minute period. After this procedure, it may be necessary for the patient to intermittently squeeze the penis to aid venous outflow.

If pharmacologic therapy is not successful, either a surgical shunt or an attempt at needle drainage is indicated. Although shunting with a large-bore needle may be successful, it is less reliable than a scalpel incision extending from the glans into one corporal compartment, with rongeur of the intervening septum to assure patency of the shunt. A second shunt between the spongiosum and cavernosum at the base of the penis is the next recommended procedure. If this also is unsuccessful, the physician should use blood gas studies to direct subsequent therapy.

Needle drainage is accomplished using a large-bore needle to remove sludged blood and to create a temporary shunt between the corpus cavernosum and the glans. This procedure requires local anesthesia. Following aspiration of the sludged blood, gentle irrigation with about 10 cc of saline should be performed to remove any residual thrombi. It may be necessary to repeat this irrigation 8-10 times.

Blood gas results on the aspirated blood will separate patients into two categories—those with ischemic priapism and non-ischemic priapism. If penile blood gases demonstrate a low pH, low pO_2, and a high CO_2, the priapism is ischemic.[55] In ischemic priapism, aspiration and irrigation are unlikely to be successful in reducing the erection. These patients will often need surgery to restore venous drainage. If the blood gases are compatible with arterial blood, there is no ischemic component, in which case aspiration and irrigation may be sufficient for clinical resolution.

Compressive dressings may cause ischemic skin necrosis and, if employed, should be relatively loose, and examined frequently for evidence of compression ischemia. Patients with prolonged priapism may not respond to aspiration or irrigation because the blood has already clotted. This may result in massive tissue ischemia and, rarely, loss of penile tissue.[56] Protracted, untreated priapism may cause corpus cavernosum fibrosis and result in impotence in as many as 50% of victims.[57]

Scrotal Inflation. For unknown reasons, some men may inject saline or water into the scrotum to enlarge it.[118] Scrotal inflation may cause severe infections similar to Fournier's gangrene of the scrotum. Participants will often use intravenous fluid, tubing, and needles to perform the "inflation." It is uncertain if this technique is done because of exhibitionism or to enhance autoerotic sexual pleasure. It is clearly dangerous and should be discouraged.

Vaginal Injuries

The normal vagina in the unaroused adult female is H-shaped when viewed head-on. During sexual arousal, the lower third of the vagina becomes vasocongested, as the upper vagina expands in length and diameter as the cervix is pulled up and away from the perineum. The internal diameter increases as much as three times and lengthens by as much as 10-20%.[5] During the arousal and plateau phase of sexual response, the outer third of the vagina becomes congested and swells to "hug" the penis.

Although sexual arousal may permit some accommodation, anatomically significant mismatches between the size of the penis and vagina can produce traumatic injuries in the female. Even with so-called "normal intercourse," vaginal injuries in women are more common than penile injuries in men. In this regard, minor mucosal trauma can be confirmed with vital stains even after normal intercourse. This "normal" vaginal trauma is confined to an area near the introitus and the lower part of the hymen. Posterior fourchette tears may be identified with staining methods in 10% of sexually active, post-adolescent women and in 28% of sexually active adolescents.[58,59] Fortunately, true impalement injuries due to sexual activity are unusual.[60] If the object that caused the impalement is no longer in place, assessment of the injury can be difficult.

Every patient who presents to the ED with vaginal bleeding after intercourse should have a pelvic examination, including speculum inspection of the entire vaginal vault. This should be followed by a rectal and abdominal examination. A flat plate and upright film of the abdomen may show free air or a foreign body. As in other patients with abnormal vaginal bleeding, a pregnancy test is mandatory. A sonogram of the pelvis may be helpful in delineating the extent of injury or identifying fluid in the cul-de-sac.

Lower-third Vaginal Lacerations. Lower vaginal lacerations are more common in virginal women. The classic lower laceration is, of course, the hymenal tear. These are usually minor and are seen in the inferior borders of the introitus. Violent defloration can cause extension of these tears into the surrounding anterior introital tissues. Rarely, female genital injury may result from human bites.[61] Cleansing with betadine and antibiotics are usually required for management.

Deep or Upper Two-thirds Vaginal Lacerations. Deep or upper lacerations account for 75% of repairs required following sexual intercourse or sexual insertion of foreign bodies into the vagina.[1] Most patients present with significant vaginal bleeding or pain. In about 3-10% of these cases, bleeding is serious enough to produce hypovolemic shock.[1] Extension into the peritoneum occurs in about

1% of these lacerations, which may be caused by deep penile penetration and impact, or foreign body insertions. Most lesions are about 3-5 cm long and are located posteriorly and on the right side of the vaginal wall.

Foreign objects are suspected as etiologic agents in 5-60% of cases.[1] Despite the range of important traumatic vaginal injuries that can result from sexual trauma, foreign body insertion into the vagina is safer and less likely to result in hospitalization than insertion of similar objects into the rectum.[62,63] Other factors cited as possible precipitants of vaginal injuries include a lapse in sexual activity, disproportionately large penile size of partners, brutality or violence, unestrogenized post-menopausal tissues, and variant positions of intercourse.[64]

Hemorrhage is almost universal in these patients and can be severe to life-threatening. Deaths from exsanguination have been reported.[8] Ruptures that extend into the abdomen may be complicated by rectal tears or intraperitoneal perforation. Following intra-abdominal perforation, evisceration may occur.

All vaginal wounds should be considered contaminated and the patient should receive a broad-spectrum antibiotic that is active against both aerobic and anaerobic organisms, as well as a tetanus booster. This is particularly true if there is a foreign body involved.[9] Therapy consists of control of hemorrhage with vaginal packing, and volume replacement followed by definitive repair. Prompt recognition and treatment of vaginal lacerations are essential for reducing morbidity and mortality.

Vaginal Insufflation Syndrome. Cunnilingus, oral stimulation of the female's genitalia, is a common sexual practice. A variation of this consists of blowing air into the vagina. Although this is not strictly a vaginal lesion, it is otherwise difficult to classify. In these patients, air enters the vagina, continues through the cervix, uterine cavity, Fallopian tubes and then into the peritoneal cavity. In rare patients, an anatomic abnormality such as a vaginal-peritoneal fistula may facilitate air passage into the peritoneum.[65] Other related causes of insufflation include douching with a bulb syringe and with effervescent fluid.[66] *(Please see Table 2.)*

In the non-pregnant patient, vaginal insufflation may lead to either asymptomatic or symptomatic pneumoperitoneum. Symptomatic patients may complain of sudden onset of abdominal pain or sharp, pleuritic chest pain with dyspnea.[67,68] There may be radiation to one or both shoulders. Abdominal examination is most often unremarkable, and the patients do not appear to be toxic.

The upright abdominal x-ray may demonstrate air under the diaphragm, a worrisome finding that may suggest catastrophic abdominal disease. Exploratory laparotomy may be required, but in many cases, serial observation demonstrates resolution of the pneumoperitoneum over 24-48 hours.

Vaginal Insufflation During Pregnancy. In the pregnant patient, vaginal insufflation can cause lethal venous air embolism to the heart, and in the setting of a septal defect, can disseminate emboli to other organs as well.[69] The pathophysiology of this condition is fairly well defined. During pregnancy, the vagina becomes highly distensible and can expand to hold 1-2 liters of air. During insufflation, the air may pass through the cervix, dissect the amniotic membrane and uterine wall, and pass into the uterine veins enroute to the heart.[69] Other reported causes of air embolism during pregnancy include douching, powder insufflation, manual foreplay, vigorous vaginal intercourse, and abortion attempts.[70-72]

Table 2. Sources of Free Air in the Abdomen[6,66,70]
Perforated viscus
Recent surgical procedures
Peritonitis with gas-forming organisms
Pneumomediastinum
Pneumatosis cystoides intestinalis
Gynecological procedures
Pyosalpinx with gas-forming organisms
Douching
Vaginal cuff dehiscence
Orogenital insufflation

The clinical presentation is characterized by abrupt onset of dyspnea, chest pain, seizures (occasionally), tachypnea, tachycardia, hypotension, vaginal bleeding, wheezing, pulmonary edema, transient loud murmurs, cardiovascular collapse, and focal neurological deficits. Air embolism may also cause bronchospasm and coagulopathy. In severe cases, seizures, and collapse can progress rapidly to death. The history is often misleading or unobtainable, which can delay diagnosis and therapy. Most case reports are postmortem.

Hypoxemia, acidosis, and coagulopathies are quite common. Rarely, a chest x-ray may demonstrate right-heart or pulmonary artery air. Pulmonary edema after air embolism has also been noted.[73]

Emergency therapy consists of placing the patient into Trendelenburg position and administering 100% oxygen. If available, hyperbaric therapy will decrease the size of the embolus. If the patient has cardiovascular collapse, a central venous catheter may be placed in an attempt to remove the air.

Vaginal insufflation-induced air embolus has a fetal and maternal mortality rate of about 90%. Although vaginal insufflation is considered to be an unsafe sexual practice, coitus and routine cunnilingus can be practiced safely during pregnancy. It should be stressed, however, that coitus should not be practiced by patients with threatened abortion, prior abortions due to uterine abnormalities, incompetence of the cervix, premature dilation of the cervix, or rupture of the amniotic membranes.

Alternative Orifices

According to anecdotal reports, sexual intercourse has been attempted in every natural and artificial orifice, from colostomies to urethral sex.[6] Consequently, the examiner should ensure that no further trauma is visible at other orifices.

Gender-Independent Lesions in Men and Women

Oral Lesions. The incidence of oral sex has been steadily increasing, with one survey reporting that 90% of married couples in their 30s have practiced this form of sexual behavior in one form or another.[74] The practice is popular among heterosexuals as well as the male and female homosexual populations.[75,76]

Lesions associated with oral sex are usually not serious and, in most cases, resolve spontaneously. Nevertheless, recognition of syndromes associated with oral sex requires a high index of suspicion and persistent questioning by the physician to determine the source of these lesions. In general, oral lesions can be subdivided into categories: those caused by fellatio, and those associated with cunnilingus. Anilinctus— stimulation of the anus with the tongue—produces lesions similar to those encountered with cunnilingus.[1]

Fellatio. Oral trauma caused by fellatio can be caused either by negative pressure or by impact of the penis against the soft tissues of the oropharynx. Physical findings are subtle and include submucosal hemorrhages or ecchymosis on the posterior oral pharynx. The uvula is usually spared. These purplish lesions are typically painless and flat and, not uncommonly, they are incidental findings uncovered during examination of the oral pharynx. In other cases, patients may notice the lesions during self-examination and present to the physicians with anxiety about AIDS, oral candidiasis, herpes, or some other sexually transmitted disease. Rarely, the suction activity associated with fellatio can produce large coalescent bands in the oral cavity that resemble lesions seen in Kaposi's sarcoma.

The diagnosis is confirmed by the presence of characteristic lesions and a history of fellatio. To exclude other possible causes, a VDRL or RPR should be drawn to ensure that these are not lesions of secondary syphilis. In general, oral lesions associated with fellatio resolve in 7-10 days, as long as the patient abstains from this sexual practice. If the lesions do not resolve within this time frame, additional diagnostic studies may be required.

Cunnilingus Syndrome. The cunnilingus syndrome consists of pain on the surface of the tongue and throat, and especially around the lingular frenulum. Frequently, a small ulcer or abrasion will develop in this area. The lesion is caused by repetitive thrusting motion of the tongue used for cunnilingus, and, specifically, by the trauma associated with the tongue scraping against the sharp surfaces of the lower incisors.

Because oral ulcers are associated with many conditions and have many etiologies, persistence of these lesions for more than 10 days is an indication for biopsy in most cases. A VDRL should be ordered in these patients. The examiner should also inspect for ill-fitting dentures. Aggressive toothbrushing and hard foods also can produce this clinical picture.

Treatment consists of abstinence from cunnilingus for 7-10 days. A topical anesthetic may be applied with a cotton-tipped applicator for pain control if necessary. In severe, recurrent cases, the patient may require a dentist to smooth or polish the lower incisors to decrease the chance of recurrence. The patient also should be instructed to choose a different position of his/her partner to change the angle of impact on the incisors.

Anorectal Injuries. Although anorectal stimulation and trauma is more common among male homosexuals, a significant percentage of heterosexuals as well as homosexual females also engage in some form of anal stimulation. In fact, a study in the mid-1970s reported that 8% of women included some form of anal intercourse as a regular part of their sexual repertoire, a finding that was reconfirmed in 1988.[71,78] Erotic anal activities include anal intercourse, enemas, insertion of foreign bodies into the anus, and anilinctus. Among these, only anilinctus is relatively safe for the recipient.

It should be stressed that the use of anal orifices for sexual gratification may be dangerous and is a documented behavioral vector for many serious—even, life-threatening—conditions, including venereal warts, syphilis, gonorrhea, AIDS, hepatitis, and other sexually transmitted organisms.

Anal Masturbation and Foreplay. Anal masturbation usually is performed as part of genital masturbation, and is characterized by manipulation of the anal orifice or insertion of small objects into the anus. The most common method is to simply insert a finger into the rectum or to stimulate the outer anal rim. When practiced in the setting of heterosexual intercourse, manipulation of the anus is most used for arousal as part of sexual foreplay.[79]

Insertion of knotted cords or small beads on a string into the anus are a common sexual theme.[80] During both foreplay and masturbation, however, it is easy to lose control of small objects, especially if they are well-lubricated and the individual is sexually aroused.

Enemas. An enema may be used to cleanse the rectum prior to anal intercourse or manipulation, or, on the other hand, it can be a direct source of erotic stimulation. Arousal may be shared by both the individual giving the enema as well as the person receiving it.

The most important complication of enemas is laceration or perforation of the anus or rectum by the enema nozzle. This complication is more common when a hard nozzle is used instead of a soft rubber rectal tube, when the injection pressure is too great, or when insertion of the enema nozzle is accomplished while the recipient is in the sitting position.[7] The participant also may use an excessive volume of enema solution, a practice that can lead to colonic rupture and, rarely, to water intoxication. People participating in sadomasochistic behavior—as well as inexperienced individuals—have also been known to inject irritating substances into the rectum that can produce a diffuse colitis.

Finally, intoxicating substances such as cocaine, alcohol, or hallucinogens can be inserted into the rectum during sexual activity. These substances are rapidly absorbed through the rectal mucosa and produce psychological and behavioral effects similar to those observed with intravenous injection of these drugs.

Anal Tears. Anal instrumentation or intercourse can produce minor trauma to local structures. Complications include anal fissures, hemorrhoidal tears, mucosal abrasions, ulcerations, contusions, and cryptitis. In one series, 45% of these injuries were caused by penile anal intercourse, 30% by fist intercourse, and 16% by foreign bodies.[81] The remaining 9% were not characterized.

The evaluation of patients suspected of having traumatic injuries associated with anal manipulation or foreign body insertion should be thorough and systematic. In all cases, an upright abdominal and chest x-ray should be obtained to ensure that the patient does not have a pneumoperitoneum. Depending upon the radiographic findings, the patient should then be proctoscoped. This aggressive approach to diagnosis is important because incomplete examination accounts for a false negative examination in up to 30% of patients.

Treatment of uncomplicated lacerations, abrasions, and tears includes abstinence, warm-water sitz baths, stool softeners, and topical analgesic preparations. The patient also should be counseled about the use of more gentle stimulatory practices to prevent recurrences.

In general, non-perforating mucosal lacerations seldom cause major problems. Most patients with these lesions will show no signs of peritoneal irritation or bleeding. However, patients who demonstrate persistent bleeding, or who have deep mucosal lacerations may require surgical repair. These patients should be admitted. Operative repair is generally indicated for torn sphincter muscles, extensive lacerations of the mucosa, and submucosal lacerations.

Retained Rectal Foreign Bodies

Foreign bodies may be inserted into the anus for erotic stimulation, smuggling contraband substances, or cleansing of the rectum. It appears that the only limit on the size of the object inserted is the size of the rectum.[82] Common and uncommon objects inserted into the rectum include dildoes and vibrators, fruits, vegetables, bottles, baseballs, and broomsticks.[83] What may be characterized as bizarre items that are occasionally inserted into the anus include, but are not limited to: gerbils and hamsters, cement, and anal plugs used for bondage and sadomasochistic practices.[84] For additional examples, the reader is referred to a comprehensive review of the world literature on this subject.[85]

Because the use of rectal foreign bodies for sexual arousal is common among gay men, it is not surprising that men outnumber women in reported cases of retained foreign bodies by more than 25 to 1.[86] In addition, it should be noted that males have a higher angle between rectum and anus, which increases the tendency for an object to become impacted. Females may have rectal lesions from forced sexual activities.[87] Foreign body insertion in females is most often performed by the vaginal route, which appears to offer advantages over the rectum, in sensation, control, lubrication, and distensibility.[85]

Removal. Before definitive removal of a retained object(s) is attempted, the emergency physician should confirm that insertion or subsequent manipulation of the object(s) has not caused rectal or colonic perforation.[88] This possibility can usually be excluded by performing a thorough examination of the rectum and a careful abdominal exam. In addition, a flat and upright radiograph of the abdomen should be obtained in all patients prior to removal. This study can be helpful for excluding or confirming the presence of free air. Moreover, it can also demonstrate the configuration of single or multiple objects, and it may help characterize the position of unusually shaped or sharply pointed foreign bodies.

Once perforation is excluded, therapy should be directed toward expeditious removal of the object. Successful removal is enhanced by achieving relaxation of the anal sphincter and obtaining a secure grip on the object. *(Please see Table 3.)*

Following a successful removal, the patient's rectum and colon should be examined thoroughly with a proctoscope to ensure that all foreign objects have been removed and that there is no sign of bowel wall injury. Repeat radiographs may be necessary. If there is any suspicion of bowel perforation either before or during the procedure, surgical consultation should be obtained. In addition, the patient should be admitted for observation and surgical exploration or repair, if indicated.

Use of cathartics is controversial and some authors feel that this will cause hemorrhage, further impaction, or lead to perforation.[89] A high-fiber diet may decrease the incidence of perforation. Preoperative antibiotics will decrease the risk of bacteremia and peritonitis in the event of subclinical perforation.

Perforations. Perforation of the colon or rectum represents a potentially lethal complication of anal erotic activities. Rectal perforations are usually produced by foreign bodies in an attempt for stimulation. Only rarely are perforations the result of rectal intercourse. Sadistic assaults on homosexuals—gay bashing—may include packing the victim's rectum with foreign objects.[73]

Higher perforations can present with usual signs of intraperitoneal contamination, rapid development of abdominal pain, tachycardia, tachypnea, fever, and a rigid abdomen. These patients need intravenous antibiotics, fluid resuscitation, and rapid surgical intervention. Lower perforations may be extraperitoneal and will require antibiotics and presacral drainage.

"Fisting." A special note should be made of a behavior known as "fisting," "handballing," brachiopractic eroticism, or fist fornication.[90] In this practice, the hand and forearm are inserted into the rectum for erotic stimulation. Although this technique is well-known in the homosexual community, it is infrequently practiced—i.e., less than 5% of homosexuals admit to participation in these activities.[1] Willing participants tend to use drugs or alcohol to help them relax. Because intoxicating substances can cloud the appropriate response to pain, they increase the potential for life-threatening injuries.

Table 3. Caveats for the Removal of Retained Rectal Foreign Bodies

- In general, surgical procedures are required for objects that are either impossible to grasp or are located out of the clinician's reach. These patients should be admitted and placed at bed rest. After 24 hours, the foreign body will often be close to the rectum and can then be extracted under spinal anesthesia.
- If the retained object is fragile (e.g., a light bulb), and there is significant risk of bowel damage if the foreign body breaks during removal, the procedure should be performed by a surgeon in the operating room.
- Blind instrumentation is discouraged, since this markedly increases the chance of an iatrogenic perforation.
- When removal is attempted in the ED, it is preferable to grasp the object directly, dislodge it from the sacral hollow, and then guide it out of the rectum.
- If the object is difficult to grasp, lateral vaginal wall retractors or smooth malleable retractors can be inserted and the object grasped with an instrument under direct visualization.[91]
- Snares and piercing tenaculums may afford a better grip.[92] Hollow objects that have the hollow portion facing the examiner may be filled with casting plaster and a small loop or ring inserted into the plaster before it hardens.[93] Once the plaster has set, the cord attached to the ring is gently pulled to permit removal.
- Foley catheters, Blakemore tubes, and suction catheters have all been used to expedite removal through air insufflation, which decreases the suction effects of objects that occupy the entire lumen of the bowel.[94,95]
- Spinal anesthesia, local anal blocks, or intravenous sedation may help relax the anal sphincter.

Note: About 30% of foreign bodies cannot be successfully removed in the ED and, therefore, will require surgical intervention.

Injuries resulting from this activity range from simple anal tears to life-threatening perforation of the colon. The threat to the patient is increased by delay in seeking treatment; management of mucosal tears, erosions, and lacerations is similar to that described for retained foreign bodies in the previous section.

Counseling May Be Needed

Accurate diagnosis of traumatic conditions associated with sexual activity usually requires not only a high index of suspicion, but a streetwise approach to identifying a specific etiologic behavior from a wide range of eccentric practices that have infiltrated the contemporary sexual landscape. Whereas some injuries related to sexual trauma are relatively easy to identify (i.e., penile fracture), others (i.e., vaginal insufflation syndrome, rectal foreign body insertion, etc.) may be much more difficult to evaluate and manage.

Regardless of the condition—or, for that matter, the sexual proclivities and orientations of patients who have sustained trauma—one of the principal obstacles complicating assessment of sexually related injuries is the absence of an adequate, reliable, and thorough history from the patient. Because the mechanism of injury, characterization of sexual aids, and descriptions of pre-injury sexual practices are essential for making a prompt, precise diagnosis, emergency physicians should attempt to establish patient trust, provide reassurance, minimize embarrassment, and feel skilled to undertake a direct, no-holds-barred line of questioning during the history-taking process.

Once the diagnosis is established, patient counseling is frequently required to prevent recurrence of similar injuries. These medical advice sessions should be conducted in a gentle, but persuasive manner, and with the understanding by the physician that sexual practices perceived as unusual or deviant by one person may be routine for another.

References

1. Geist RF. Sexually related trauma. *Emerg Med Clin North Am* 1988;6:439-466.
2. Benson RC. Vacuum cleaner injury to penis. A common urologic problem? *Urology* 1985;25:41-44.
3. Aliabadi H, Cass AS, Gleich, et al. Self-inflicted foreign bodies involving lower urinary tract and male genitals. *Urology* 1985;26:12-16.
4. Bhat AL, Kumar A, Mathur SC, Gangwal KC. Penile strangulation. *Br J Urol* 1991;68:618-621.
5. Metsala P, Nienen H. Traumatic lesions of the vagina. *Acta OB Gyn* 1968;47:82-488.
6. Elam AL, Ray VG. Sexually related trauma: A review. *Ann Emerg Med* 1986;15:576-584.
7. Agnew J. Hazards associated with anal erotic activity. *Arch Sex Behav* 1986;15:307-314.
8. Fain DB, McCormick GM. Vaginal fisting as a cause of death. *Am J Forensic Med Pathol* 1989;10:73-75.
9. Horowitz MD, Dove DB, Eismont FG, et al. Impalement injuries. *J Trauma* 1985;25:914-916.
10. Fatteh A, Leach WB, Wilkinson CA. Fatal air embolism in pregnancy resulting from orogenital sex play. *Forensic Sci Int* 1973;2:247.
11. Pryor JP, Hill JT, Packham DA, et al. Penile injuries with particular reference to injury to the erectile tissue. *Br J Urol* 1981;53;42-46.
12. Griffin GC. Ouch, my zipper's stuck. *Postgrad Med* 1987; 82:324.
13. Nolan JF, Stillwell TJ, Sands JP. Acute management of the zipper entrapped penis. *J Emerg Med* 1990;8:305-307.
14. Aragona P, Piazza R, Artibani W, Dante S. The so-called Hoffman's lymphangitis of the penis: Is it a lymphangitis or a phlebitis. *Int Urol Nephr* 1988;20:139-15.
15. Sieunarine K. Non-venereal sclerosing lymphangitis of the penis associated with masturbation. *Br J Urol* 1987;194-195.
16. Gharpuray MB, Tolat SN. Nonvenereal sclerosing lymphangitis of the penis. *Cutis* 1991;47:421-422.
17. Broaddus SB, Leadbetter GW. Surgical management of persistent, symptomatic non-venereal lymphangitis of the penis. *J Urol* 1982;127:987-988.
18. Oesterling JE, Bromberg WD, Albertson PC. Xeroradiography and ultrasonography in the evaluation of a penile injury. *J Urol* 1986;135:791-793.
19. Lim KB, Seow CS, Tulip T, et al. Artificial penile nodules. Case reports. *Genitourin Med* 1986;62:123-125.
20. Haddad FS. Penile strangulation by human hair: Report of three cases and review of the literature. *Urol Int* 1982;37: 375-388.
21. Haddad FS, Re: Penile tourniquet injury due to a coil of hair. *J Urol* 1985;134:1220. Letter.
22. Mariani PJ, Wagner DK. Topical cocaine prior to treatment of penile tourniquet syndrome. *J Emerg Med* 1986;4: 205-207.
23. Garty BZ, Mimouni M, Varsano I. Penile tourniquet syndrome. *Cutis* 1983;31:431-432
24. Godec CJ, Reiser R, Logush AZ. The erect penis—Injury prone organ. *J Trauma* 1988;28:124-126.
25. Malis J. Penile Fracture. *Arch F Klin Chir* 1925;129:651.
26. Tsang T, Demby AM. Penile fracture with urethral injury. *J Urol* 1992;147:466-468.
27. Brotzman GL. Penile fracture. *J Am Brd Fam Phy* 1991;4: 351-353.
28. Klein FA, Smith MJ, Vernon-Miller N. Penile fracture: Diagnosis and management. *J Trauma* 1985;25:1090-1092.
29. Agrawal SK, Morgan BE, Shafique M, et al. Experience with penile fractures in Saudi Arabia. *Br J Urol* 1991;67:644-646.
30. Kuymcuoglu U, Erol D, Baltaci L, et al. Traumatic rupture of the corpus cavernosum. *Int Urol Neph* 1990;22:363-366.
31. Creecy AA, Beazlie FS Jr. Fracture of the penis: Traumatic rupture of corpora cavernosa. *J Urol* 1957:78:620.
32. Ruckle HC, Hadley HR, Lui PD. Fracture of the penis: Diagnosis and management. *Urology* 1992;40:33-35.
33. Tiong JTK, Taylor A, England E, et al. Fracture of the penis—Review with case report. *Aust NZ J Surg* 1988;58: 428-431.
34. Lehman E, Kremer S. Fracture of the penis. *Surgery, Gyn and Obst* 1991;171;148-150.
35. Cumming J, Jenkins JD. Fracture of the corpora cavernosa and urethral rupture during sexual intercourse. *Br J Urol* 1991;67:327-332.

36. Tsang T, Demby AM. Penile fracture with urethral injury. *J Urol* 1992;17:466-468.
37. Cockrell SN, Quick G. Lower urinary tract trauma. *Resident and Staff Physician* 1990;36:47-64.
38. Nicely ER, Costabile RA, Moul JW. Rupture of the deep dorsal vein of the penis during sexual intercourse. *J Urol* 1992;147:150-152.
39. Penson DF, Seftel AD, Krane RJ, et al. The hemodynamic pathophysiology of impotence following blunt trauma to the erect penis. *J Urol* 1992;148:1171-1180.
40. El-Sherif AE, Dauleh M, Allowneh N, et al. Management of fracture of the penis in Qatar. *Br J Urol 1991*;68:622-625.
41. Oesterwitz H, Bick C, Braun E. Fracture of the penis. Report of 6 cases and review of the literature. *Int Urol Nephrol* 1984;16:123.
42. Ozen HA, Erkan I, Alkibay T, et al. Fracture of the penis and long-term results of surgical treatment. *Br J Urol* 1986;58: 551-552.
43. Anselmo G, Fandella A, Faggiano L, et al. Fractures of the penis: Therapeutic approach and long-term results. *Br J Urol* 1991;67:509-511.
44. Wespes E, Libert M, Simon J, et al. Fracture of the penis: Conservative vs. surgical treatment. *Eur Urol* 1987;13: 166-168.
45. Geiderman JM, Paris PM. Fracture of the penis. *Ann Emerg Med* 1980;9:435-437.
46. Meares EM Jr. Traumatic rupture of the corpus cavernosum. *J Urol* 1971;105:407.
47. Mellinger BC, Douenias R. New surgical approach for operative management of penile fracture and penetrating trauma. *Urology* 1992;34:429-432.
48. Taha SA, Sharayah A, Kamal BA, et al. Fracture of the penis: Surgical management. *Int Surg* 1988;73:63-64.
49. Kessler R. Complications of inflatable penile prostheses. *Urology* 1981;18:470.
50. Goulding FJ. Fracture of the Hydroflex penile implant. *Urology* 1987;30:490-491.
51. Huisman TK, Macintyre RC. Mechanical failure of Omniphase penile prosthesis. *Urology* 1988;31:515-516.
52. Mohapatra TP, Kumar S. Reverse coitus: Mechanism of urethral injury in male partner. *J Urol* 1990;144:1467-1468.
53. Fernandez JA, Basha MA, Wilson GC. Emergency treatment of papaverine priapism. *J Emerg Med* 1987;5:289-291.
54. O'Brien WM, O'Connor KP, Lynch JH. Priapism: Current concepts. *Ann Emerg Med* 1989;18:980-983.
55. Winter CC, McDowell G. Experience with 105 patients with priapism:Update review of all aspects. *J Urol* 1988;140: 980-983.
56. Yealy DM, Hogya PT. Priapism. *Emerg Med Clin North Am* 1988;6:509-520.
57. Jackson SC, Walker JS. Self-administered intraurethral chlorpromazine: An unusual cause of priapism. *Am J Emerg Med* 1991;9:171-175.
58. McCauley J, Gorman RL, Guzinski G. Toluidine blue in the detection of perineal lacerations in pediatric and adolescent sexual abuse victims. *Pediatrics* 1986;78:1039-1043.
59. McCauley J, Guzinski G, Welch R, et al. Toluidine blue in the corroboration of rape in the adult victim. *Am J Emerg Med* 1987;5:105-108.
60. Kennedy D, Becher R, Laferte R, et al. Transvaginal intra-abdominal impalement injury. *South Med J* 1992;32: 618-619.
61. Mathelier AC. Vulvar hematoma secondary to a human bite: A case report. *J Reprod Med* 1987;32:618-619.
62. Benjamin HB, Klamecki B, Haft JS. Removal of exotic foreign objects from the abdominal orifices. *Am J Proctol* 1969;20:413-417.
63. Haft JS, Benjamin HB, Zeit W. Foreign bodies in the female genitourinary tract. Some psychosexual aspects. *Med Asp Hum Sexual* 1974;8:54-78.
64. Haney AF. Vaginal evisceration after forcible coitus with intra-abdominal ejaculation. *J Reprod Med.* 1978;21: 254-256.
65. Varon J, Laufer MD, Sternbach GL. Recurrent pneumoperitoneum following vaginal insufflation. *Am J Emerg Med* 1991;9:447-448.
66. Wright FW, Lumsden K. Recurrent pneumoperitoneum due to jejunal diverticulosis. With a review of the cases of spontaneous pneumoperitoneum. *Clin Radiol* 1975;26: 327-331.
67. MacGregor JS, Wu AW, Rubin HR. Pleuritic chest pain in a postpartum woman. *Arch Emerg Med* 1991;8:271-273.
68. Smally AJ. Referred shoulder pain in a sexually active woman. *Hosp Practice* 1989;62-64.
69. Bernhardt TL, Goldmann RW, Thombs PA, et al. Hyperbaric oxygen treatment of cerebral air embolism from orogenital sex during pregnancy. *Crit Care Med* 1988;16:729-730.
70. Eckert WG, Katchis S, Dotson P. The unusual accidental death of a pregnant woman by sexual foreplay. *Am J Forensic Med Pathol* 1991;12:247-249.
71. Lifshultz D, Donoghue EP. Air embolus during intercourse in pregnancy. *J Forensic Sci* 1983;28:1021-1022.
72. Ragan WD. Antepartum air embolism. *J Indian Med Assoc* 1981;74:30.
73. Kaufman BS, Kaminsky SJ, Rackow EC, et al. Adult respiratory distress syndrome following orogenital sex during pregnancy. *Crit Care Med* 1987;15:703-704.
74. Shope DR. *Interpersonal Sexuality*. Philadelphia: WB Saunders; 1975:71.
75. Gagnon JH, Simon W. The sexual scripting of oral genital contacts. *Arch Sex Behav* 1987;16:1-25.
76. Califia P. Lesbian sexuality. *J Homosex* 1979;4:255-266.
77. Bolling DR. Prevalence, goals and complications of heterosexual anal intercourse in a gynecologic population. *J Reprod Med* 1977;19:120-124.
78. Evans BA, Bond RA, Macrae KD. Sexual behavior in women attending a genitourinary medicine clinic. *Genitourin Med* 1988;64:43-48.
79. Hite S. *The Hite Report*. New York: Macmillan;1976.
80. Comfort A. *The Joy of Sex*. New York: Simon and Shuster; 1972.
81. Barone JE, Yee J, Nealon TF Jr. Management of foreign bodies and trauma of the rectum. *Surg Gynecol Obstet* 198;156:453-457.
82. Bush RA, Owen WF. Trauma and other noninfectious problems in homosexual men. *Emerg Med Clin North Am*

1986;70:59-566.

83. Stokes M, Jones DJ. Colorectal trauma. *Br Med J* 1992;305: 302-305.
84. Eckert WG, Katchis S. Anorectal trauma: Medicolegal and forensic aspects. *Am J Forensic Med Pathol* 1989;10:3-9.
85. Busch DB, Starling JR. Rectal foreign bodies: Case reports and a comprehensive review of the world's literature. *Surgery* 1986;100:512-519.
86. Busch DB, Starling JR. Rectal foreign bodies: Case reports and comprehensive review of the world's literature. *Surgery* 1986;100:512-519.
87. Brunner RG, Shatney CH. Diagnostic and therapeutic aspects of rectal trauma. *Am Surg* 1987;53:215-219.
88. Bloom RR, Nakano PH, Gray SW, et al. Foreign bodies of the gastrointestinal tract. *Am Surg* 1986;52:618-621.
89. Rocklin MS, Apelgren KN. Colonoscopic extraction of foreign bodies from above the rectum. *Am Surg* 1989;56: 119-123.
90. Shook LL, Whittle R, Rose EF. Rectal fist insertion: An unusual form of sexual behavior. *Am J Forensic Med Pathol* 1985;6:319-324.
91. Aquino MM, Turner JW. A simple technique for removing an impacted aerosol-can cap from the rectum. *Dis Colon* Rectum 1986;29:675.
92. Kantarian JC, Riether RD, Sheets JA, et al. Endoscopic retrieval of foreign bodies from the rectum. *Dis Colon Rectum* 1987;30:902-904.
93. Bakaleinik M. Foreign bodies of the gastrointestinal tract, surgical considerations. *Mil Med* 1989;154:11-14.
94. Crass RA, Tranbough RF, Kudsk KA, et al. Colorectal foreign bodies and perforation. *Am J Surg* 1981;142:85-88.
95. Wigle RL. Emergency department management of retained rectal foreign bodies. *Am J Emerg Med* 1988;6:385-389.

Prevention of Cervical Cancer

Allan Hubbell, MD, MSPH

Primary care physicians are on the front lines of efforts to improve cervical cancer control in the United States. Despite advances in screening, diagnosis, and treatment, cervical cancer remains one of the most common cancers among women in this country. Nearly 5000 women died of the disease in 1996. This figure is particularly disturbing because cervical cancer is almost entirely preventable. Even more disturbing are data suggesting that the decline in cervical cancer rates that have occurred over the last 40 years are leveling off, and it appears that incidence rates are actually rising in some groups of women. Therefore, it is important for primary care physicians to be knowledgeable about current recommendations for the prevention of this disease and about the factors that limit the effectiveness of preventive efforts.

Some of the recent developments related to cervical cancer prevention include the growing consensus that the human papillomavirus (HPV) is causally related to this disease and that infection with specific types of HPV put women at high risk. Ongoing studies are evaluating vaccines for this virus and determining whether HPV testing should be a routine part of cervical cancer screening programs. In the meantime, regular screening with the Papanicolaou (Pap) smear is the best preventive measure. Widespread adoption of the Bethesda System for interpreting Pap smears has provided more uniformity to the reporting of results. Moreover, new guidelines regarding the frequency of performing Pap smears from the U.S. Preventive Services Task Force provide a valuable reference for primary care physicians who are developing or revising plans for cervical cancer prevention in their offices.

Barriers to cervical cancer screening and follow-up continue to exist particularly among women who are elderly, socioeconomically disadvantaged, or ethnic minority members. Unfortunately, these are the very women who are at increased risk for developing cervical cancer. A number of studies have suggested approaches for improving screening for these women, but much more work is necessary. Another problem concerns follow-up of women who have abnormal Pap smears. Some studies have shown that up to 60% of women with abnormal smears do not return for additional care. Recommendations for triaging women with abnormal smears who do follow-up are in a state of evolution, but some reasonable guidelines are available. Primary care physicians can play major roles in assuring that their own patients receive appropriate preventive care and in helping community-based screening programs increase the number of women who participate.

This chapter will review these issues in some detail including current information about cervical cancer epidemiology, risk factors, etiology, screening techniques, screening frequency, and follow-up recommendations.

Epidemiology and Risk Factors

Cervical cancer remains an important public health problem, ranking second only to breast cancer as the most common malignancy among women in the world.[1] In the United States, there were approximately 15,700 new cases of cervical cancer and 4900 deaths from this disease in 1996.[2] The disease ranked ninth in incidence and accounted for 6% of all cancers among women. Invasive cervical cancer occurs across a broad age range but is most frequent in the fifth and sixth decades of life. Incidence rates for carcinoma in situ (CIS) are highest among the 25-29 age group.[3] In the last 40 years, the incidence and mortality rates for cervical cancer have declined in the United States and in most other developed countries, largely due to the introduction of screening with the Pap smear. Unfortunately, these declining trends have recently leveled off, and the rates of cervical cancer are actually increasing among young white women.[4]

Many of the risk factors for cervical cancer are related to sexual activity. They include having multiple sexual partners (four or more), early age at first sexual intercourse (before age 18), and history of sexually transmitted diseases.[5] Characteristics of males whose partners develop cervical cancer include history of genital warts, poor hygiene, number of sexual partners, and practice of unsafe sexual behaviors.[6] Other factors such as low socio-economic status, cigarette smoking, dietary factors, and immunosuppression have also been linked to cervical cancer.[7-10]

With the availability of effective screening, cervical cancer has become a disease of the economically disadvantaged. For example, higher risk for cervical cancer has been associated with Hispanic and black populations.[11-14] Women in these ethnic groups may be more likely to experience factors contributing to development of the disease, such as having male partners who have multiple sex partners and using barrier methods of birth control less frequently.[12,15] In addition, numerous studies have found that screening, treatment, and follow-up practices for Hispanics and black women are not as thorough as they are for other groups.[16-18]

Etiology and Pathophysiology

A sexually transmitted agent has long been suspected in the etiology of cervical cancer. Such an agent would explain why most of the risk factors are associated with sexual activity. There is strong evidence that HPV is causally related to cervical cancer.[19] Indeed, HPV DNA has been detected in more than 90% of invasive cervical cancer tumors.[20,21] However, infection with HPV is also very prevalent in the general population, and not all women with HPV develop cervical cancer. Therefore, recent attention has focused on viral types of HPV which have been consistently associated with cervical tumors. Several types, principally 16, 18, 31, 33, and 36, have been implicated with development of cervical cancer[21,22-24] and its precursors.[21,24-26]

HPV infection in itself is not sufficient for development of cervical cancer. Many investigations have suggested the joint contribution of other factors such as Epstein-Barr virus,[27] cytomegalovirus,[28] polyamines and their oxidases,[29] cigarette smoking,[30,31] host genetic factors,[32] and patient age.[33] A proposed etiologic model suggests that HPV plays an initiating role, possibly in conjunction with some of these co-factors. According to the model, the development of dysplasia of cervix and progression to invasive cancer is affected by a complex interaction of host and environmental factors.[34-36] In particular, the viral proteins E6 and E7 produced by high-risk types of HPV appear to be critical for malignant transformation because of their ability to inactivate certain tumor-suppressor proteins.[37]

Screening

Because cervical cancer is usually asymptomatic until late stages, prevention of the disease through regular Pap smear screening is of critical importance. The natural history of the disease is such that there is a well-defined progression from pre-malignant disease to cancer, and this process can occur over a long period of time.[38,39] These characteristics make cervical cancer ideally suited for preventive efforts.[40]

Effectiveness of Screening. The effectiveness of the Pap smear as a screening test has never been tested in a randomized controlled trial but has been suggested by a number of other types of investigations. Case control studies have shown a strong negative association between screening and invasive disease.[41,42] Moreover, most countries that have instituted mass Pap screening programs have noted a corresponding drop in invasive cervical cancer and mortality.[43-45] While these observational studies do not constitute direct evidence that screening was responsible for the findings, the large body of supportive evidence has prompted the adoption of routine cervical cancer screening in many countries.

Unfortunately, not all women receive regular Pap smear screening. The unscreened populations include older women, the uninsured, ethnic minorities, especially Hispanics and elderly blacks, and poor women, particularly those in rural areas.[7,8] The barriers to cervical cancer screening have been well described. They include poverty, lack of health insurance, limited transportation, language difficulties, lack of child care, lack of telephone access, and certain cultural-based attitudes and health behaviors.[7,8,18]

A number of studies have evaluated interventions aimed at improving the use of Pap smears. The interventions have included reminder systems[46] and educational materials about cervical cancer.[47,48] In addition, several projects have evaluated culturally specific programs to improve cervical cancer screening in different ethnic groups, including church-based education[49] and consejeras[50] for Hispanic women and talking circles for American Indian women.[51] Most of the studies indicate that the methods improve the rates of Pap smear use, at least in the short term. To improve the effectiveness of cervical cancer screening, it is important for primary care physicians to assure that their own patients receive appropriate screening. They may also wish to participate in community-based programs that reach out to the medically indigent.

Frequency of Screening. The recommended frequency of cervical cancer screening is based largely on expert opinion. In 1988, the American Cancer Society, the National Cancer Institute, the American College of Obstetricians and

Gynecologists, the American Medical Association, the American Academy of Family Physicians, and others recommended that all women who were sexually active or who had reached age 18 should have annual Pap smears.[52] The recommendation allowed for less frequent testing after three or more annual smears had been negative. The groups differed somewhat in their recommendations regarding other issues such as the age that Pap smear testing should be discontinued.

The U.S. Preventive Services Task Force, the gold standard for evidence-based clinical prevention recommendations, recently issued an updated set of guidelines that differed slightly from those above.[53] *(Please see Table 1.)* The group recommended that testing should begin at the age when a woman first engages in sexual intercourse, that Pap smears should be performed at least every three years, and that the interval between screening should be based upon risk factors (i.e., multiple sexual partners). In addition, the Task Force found insufficient evidence to recommend for or against an upper age limit for Pap smear testing, but stated that it would be reasonable to discontinue testing in women older than the age of 65 years who had regular screening in which the smears were consistently negative. Finally, the group recommended that women who had undergone a hysterectomy in which the cervix was removed did not require Pap smear testing unless the hysterectomy was performed for treatment of cervical cancer.

Cost-Effectiveness of Screening. While there is little debate about the benefits of cervical cancer screening, there have been few formal analyses of its cost-effectiveness. The supportive evidence for Pap smears has been derived from many studies indicating reductions in the incidence of invasive disease. Cervical cancer screening may contribute to reductions in the incidence of disease, a shift in stage of diagnosis, improved survival rates, and, ultimately, reductions in avoidable mortality. Therefore, there is a general consensus that the use of the Pap smear as a screening technique is cost-effective if standardized protocols are followed.[54]

Performance and Interpretation of Pap Smears. Methods of specimen acquisition, preparation, and evaluation of the Pap smear have changed little since its introduction in the 1940s. Although it is highly effective in screening for preinvasive lesions of the cervix, a single test has a false-negative rate estimated to be 20% (usual estimates range from 10% to 45%) or a sensitivity of 80%.[55] Approximately one-half of the false negatives are due to inadequate specimen sampling, and the other half are attributed to a failure to identify the abnormal cells or to interpret them accurately. Although reliable data are lacking, the specificity of the single Pap smear is probably at least 90%.[56] To improve the adequacy of the cervical smear specimen, a variety of sampling devices is available (e.g., spatula, endocervical brush, broom, and cotton swab). Controlled studies have shown that using an endocervical brush in combination with a spatula is more likely to collect endocervical cells than using a spatula or a cotton swab.[57] There is conflicting evidence, however, that the endocervical brush increases the detection rate for abnormal smears or affects clinical outcomes.[58,59]

Pap smears are not read as simply positive or negative but rather as a continuum of findings. Traditionally, Pap smear abnormalities were classified as mild dysplasia at one end of the spectrum and invasive carcinoma at the other end. In the 1960s, the term cervical intraepithelial neoplasia (CIN) was coined to describe histological findings.[60] CIN refers to a spectrum of intraepithelial changes beginning with those traditionally classified as mild dysplasia and ending with CIS. A grading system for CIN classifies lesions from 1 to 3 based upon the percentage of cells from the basement membrane to the surface that are undifferentiated. When one-third or less of the distance from the basement membrane to the surface is involved, the lesions are called CIN 1; when more than one-third but less than two-thirds is involved, they are called CIN 2; and, when more than two-thirds is involved, they are called CIN 3. When malignant cells penetrate the underlying basement membrane of the epithelium and infiltrate the stroma, the lesion is called invasive cervical cancer. Invasive cervical cancer is also classified into three grades: grade 1, or well differentiated carcinoma; grade 2, or moderately differentiated carcinoma; and grade 3, or poorly differentiated carcinoma.[61]

In 1988, the National Cancer Institute convened a panel to address the issue of classification of Pap smears.[62,63] The resulting Bethesda System (as modified in 1991) is now used by most laboratories in this country; therefore, primary care providers should be familiar it. The Bethesda System evaluates the specimen for adequacy, uses diagnostic terminology, and makes recommendations pertaining to the smear when necessary. *(Please see Table 2.)* Among the diagnostic terminologies are low-grade squamous intraepithelial lesions (LSIL) and high-grade squamous intraepithelial lesions (HSIL). LSIL are consistent with HPV and mild dysplasia, whereas HSIL include moderate and severe dysplasia and CIS. Another category of abnormal squamous cells is atypical squamous cells of undetermined significance (ASCUS). The glandular cell abnormalities are divided into two categories: atypical glandular cells of unde-

Table 1. Pap Smear Screening Recommendations by the U.S. Preventive Services Task Force, 1996

- Regular pap smears are recommended for all women who are or who have been sexually active and who have a cervix.
- Testing should begin at the age when women first engage in sexual intercourse. Adolescents whose sexual history is thought to be unreliable should be presumed to be sexually active at age 18.
- Pap smears should be performed at least every three years. The testing interval should be recommended by the physician based upon risk factors.
- There is insufficient evidence to recommend for or against an upper age limit for pap testing but recommendations can be made on other grounds to discontinue regular testing after age 65 in women who have had regular normal screening tests.
- Women who have had a hysterectomy, including removal of the cervix, for reasons other than cervical cancer or its precursors do not require pap testing.

termined significance (AGUS) and adenocarcinoma. Many laboratories now report lesions using both the histological and the cytological classifications (i.e., CIN I/LSIL or CIN III/HSIL).

Management of Patients with Abnormal Pap Smears

Performing the screening Pap smear is only the first step in the process of cervical cancer control. It is important for patients with abnormal Pap smears to return for follow-up and to receive appropriate treatment for the abnormalities. Failure to return for follow-up results in fewer women diagnosed with CIN and higher rates of invasive disease.

Patient Follow-Up. Rates of failure to return for follow-up and treatment after abnormal Pap test results vary, but typical estimates in mostly socioeconomically disadvantaged groups range from 30% to 40%.[64] Many of the factors affecting Pap screening behavior, such as language, knowledge, culture and barriers to health care, also affect failure to return for follow-up.

A few studies have evaluated interventions aimed at improving rates of follow-up for abnormal Pap smears. The programs have included educational pamphlets, personalized follow-up letters, educational slide-tape programs, providing transportation, and structured telephone counseling.[64-68] Like programs aimed at improving Pap smear screening, most of these programs improved follow-up rates somewhat. However, much more work is needed in this important area.

Management Options. Guidelines for the management of women with abnormal Pap smears are in a state of evolution as the value of HPV testing as a screening procedure is being evaluated. Because of the strong association of high-risk HPV types with cervical cancer, HPV testing may be included in future screening recommendations.[37] In the meantime, reasonable guidelines are available that take into consideration the type of Pap smear abnormality and the likelihood that the abnormality will progress to invasive cervical cancer.[37] Lesions consistent with ASCUS and LSIL are relatively unlikely to progress, whereas those consistent with HSIL are relatively likely to progress. In a multicenter study of LSIL, approximately two-thirds of the lesions regressed during long-term follow-up.[69] On the other hand, HSIL lesions were clearly preinvasive and often progressed to invasive cervical cancer if untreated.[70]

Based on these considerations, patients with ASCUS or LSIL may be triaged according to whether their lesions are at low or high risk for becoming clinically significant.[37] *(Please see Table 3.)* Women with ASCUS or LSIL who are at high risk include those over the age of 26, unreliable for follow-up, with a past history of abnormal cytology, unknown to the physician, with multiple sexual partners. In this scheme, patients with ASCUS or LSIL and a normal-appearing cervix should have a repeat Pap smear in six months. Those whose repeat smear suggests minor-grade cytologic atypia but are considered at low risk for developing higher grade lesions are followed at six-month intervals for up to two years and receive colposcopy only if the low-grade abnormality persists. Those women considered at high risk for progression would receive colposcopy as the

Table 2. The 1991 Bethesda System

ADEQUACY OF SPECIMEN

Satisfactory for evaluation
Satisfactory for evaluation but limited by (specific reason)
Unsatisfactory for evaluation (specify reason)

GENERAL CATEGORIZATION (OPTIONAL)

Within normal limits
Benign cellular changes; see descriptive diagnosis
Epithelial cell abnormality; see descriptive diagnosis

DESCRIPTIVE DIAGNOSES

Benign cellular changes
- Infection
  - *Trichomonas vaginalis*
  - Fungal organisms morphologically consistent with *Candida sp.*
  - Predominance of coccobacilli consistent with shift in vaginal flora
  - Bacteria morphologically consistent with *Actinomyces sp.*
  - Cellular changes associated with herpes simplex virus
  - Other
- Reactive changes
- Reactive cellular changes associated with:
- Inflammation (includes typical repair)
- Atrophy with inflammation ("atrophic vaginitis")
- Radiation
- Intrauterine contraceptive device (IUD)
- Other

Epithelial cell abnormalities
- Squamous cells
- Atypical squamous cells of undetermined significance (ASCUS)*
- Low-grade squamous intraepithelial lesion (LSIL) encompassing HPV ** mild dysplasia/CIN I
- High-grade squamous intraepithelial lesion (HSIL) encompassing moderate and severe dysplasia, CIS/CIN II, and CIN II
- Squamous cell carcinoma
- Glandular cell
  - Endometrial cells, cytologically benign, in a postmenopausal woman
  - Atypical glandular cells of undetermined significance (AGUS)*
  - Endocervical adenocarcinoma
  - Endometrial adenocarcinoma
  - Extrauterine adenocarcinoma
  - Adenocarcinoma, not otherwise specified

Other malignant neoplasams: specify

Hormonal evaluation (applies to vaginal smears only)
- Hormonal pattern compatible with age and history
- Hormonal pattern incompatible with age and history; specify
- Hormonal evaluation not possible due to . . . (specify)

* Atypical squamous or glandular cells of undetermined significance should be further qualified as to whether a reactive or a premalignant/malignant process is favored.

** Cellular changes of HPV (previously termed "koilocytotic atypia" or "condylomatous atypia") are included in the category of low-grade squamous intraepithelial lesion.

next step. Generally, it is recommended that all patients with a lesion suspicious for cervical cancer on pelvic exam should receive a biopsy. Those patients with an unequivocally abnormal smear suggestive of HSIL should receive colposcopy. *(Please see Table 3.)*

Patients requiring colposcopy should be evaluated by a physician who is skilled with this procedure. The colposcopist uses a magnifying lens to view the cervix after an application of a dilute solution of acetic acid. Colposcopy enables the physician to evaluate the location and size of the lesion and to direct biopsies that will determine the definitive diagnosis made by histology. In a large review of articles by expert colposcopists, the sensitivity of colposcopy was 94% and the specificity was 51%. A colposcopic examination may also be either satisfactory or unsatisfactory. A satisfactory exam is one in which both the lesion and the squamocolumnar junction can be seen in entirety.

In general, management of abnormal Pap smears is a two-step process: biopsy and then treat. Classic teaching of colposcopy suggests obtaining biopsies of the colposcopically "worse" areas. Generally, acetowhite epithelium is considered abnormal, and as vascular atypias appear and become increasingly irregular, the suspicion for invasion increases. However, what seems to be the worst area may not necessarily be the area of occult invasion. Therefore, some experts recommend curettage in all non-pregnant patients with documented SIL (particularly during the learning curve of colposcopy) to establish a disease-free endocervical canal.[37] They also recommend taking multiple biopsies including the squamocolumnar junction of the abnormal transformation zone.

Combined cytology, colposcopy, and histology will usually allow the physician to distinguish between patients with invasive cancer and those with SIL. Women with invasive disease should be treated according to the clinical stage of the lesion. Women with SIL should be treated on the basis of the histological biopsy diagnosis.[10] Patients with CIN I require no further treatment because the majority of these lesions resolve spontaneously. On the other hand, patients with CIN II or CIN III require treatment to prevent development of invasive disease. There are two approaches to treating these lesions. The first approach uses conservative outpatient techniques including cryotherapy, laser vaporization, and the loop electric excision procedure (LEEP). These procedures may be used when the entire lesion and the entire transformation zone can be seen by colposcopy, there is no evidence of endocervical involvement, there is no discrepancy between the Pap smear results and the biopsy results, there is no evidence of an adenomatous lesion, and there is no evidence of invasive disease. The second approach is a surgical procedure called cervical conization or cone biopsy. This procedure involves resection of a conical area of cervical tissue that includes part of the endocervical canal. Patients who do not meet criteria for conservative management should undergo cone biopsy. *(Please see Table 4.)*

An alternative to the biopsy first, treat afterward approach is one that uses LEEP as a diagnostic and treatment (see and treat) method.[37] This approach is less expensive than a cone biopsy because it is an office procedure. However, LEEP is appropriate only when colposcopy confirms the presence of an unequivocally abnormal transformation zone. Otherwise, the two-step approach should be used.

Table 3. Management Options for Patients with Abnormal Pap Smears

Pap smear consistent with ASCUS and LSIL.

- Repeat pap smear
- If repeat pap smear is negative, follow with annual pap smear
- If repeat pap smear continues to show abnormalities, determine risk of patient
  - —Low-risk patients may be followed every six months for up to two years. If the abnormality continues to exist, perform colposcopy and biopsy.
  - —High-risk patients should receive colposcopy and biopsy.

Papsmear consistent with HSIL (or persistent or high-risk LSIL—see above)

- Perform colposcopy and biopsy
  - —If biopsy results are consistent with CIN I, provide careful observation and follow-up
  - —If biopsy results are consistent with CIN II or III, perform cryotherapy, laser vaporization, LEEP, or cone biopsy
  - —If biopsy results are consistent with invasive disease, perform staging procedures

Future Directions

There are a number of exciting new developments that may help to improve the prevention of cervical cancer. Some of them include educational efforts that encourage behavioral changes to prevent infection; development of a vaccine against HPV; and testing for HPV during screening efforts.

Based upon strong evidence that HPV infection is causative in cervical cancer, a recent NIH Consensus Conference on Cervical Cancer recommended several approaches to prevention.[19] Among other things, the group recommended more educational efforts directed toward adolescents and health care providers regarding the strong causal link between acquisition of HPV as a sexually transmitted disease and development of cervical cancer and its precursors. They also recommended the delay of the onset of sexual intercourse and the use of barrier methods of contraception in the sexually active.

The group also looked forward to the development of an effective prophylactic vaccine against HPV. However, although experimental animal studies have demonstrated that vaccination against HPV is possible,[71] many conceptual issues must be addressed before the vaccines are available for clinical trials. In addition to the construction of the vaccine, issues such as the immune response following vaccination and the selection of target populations will be complex to resolve. Some clinical trials

Table 4. Indications for Cone Biopsies

- Unsafisfactory coloscopy (the entire lesion and the entire transformation zone could not be visualized)
- Evidence of endocervical involvement
- Discrepancy between pap smear and biopsy results (pap smear results are worse)
- Evidence of adenomatous lesion (adenocarcinoma in situ or adenocarcinoma)
- Evidence of invasive cancer on pap smear, cervical biopsy, or colposcopy

have used vaccines as part of a therapeutic regimen,[72] but none have used it as primary prevention.

Finally, the group noted the advantages of developing better predictive markers for progression of SIL to cervical cancer. While the Pap smear remains the best screening test for cervical cancer, much uncertainty still exists regarding which patients with LSIL will progress to HSIL or invasive cancer. Identifying HPV types could provide important information about which patients should undergo colposcopy and which patients could be followed safely with Pap smears. For example, patients with high-risk HPV types (i.e., 16 and 18) might benefit from more aggressive management. Several large clinical trials are currently under way to determine whether HPV testing can effectively triage patients, to develop clinical management guidelines and provide prognostic information, and to identify areas for cost reduction in screening and treatment.[37]

References

1. Parkin DM, Muir CS, Whelan S, et al. Cancer Incidence in Five Continents, vol. VI. IARC Scientific Publications No. 120. World Health Organization, International Agency for Research on Cancer, Lyon, 1992.
2. Parker SL, Tong T, Bolden S, et al. Cancer statistics, 1996. *Ca-A Cancer J Clinicians* 1996;46:5-27.
3. Cramer DW, Cutler SJ. Incidence and histopathology of malignancies of the female genital organs in the United States. *Am J Obstet Gynecol* 1974;118:443-460.
4. Devesa S, Young J, Brinton L, et al. Recent trends in cervix uteri cancer. *Cancer* 1989;62:2184-2190.
5. de Vet HC, Sturmans F. Risk factors for cervical dysplaia: implications for prevention. *Public Health* 1994;108:241-249.
6. Agarwal SS, Sehgal A, Sardana S, et al. Role of male behavior in cervical carcinogenesis among women with one lifetime sexual partner. *Cancer* 1993;72:1666-1669.
7. Calle EE, Flanders WD, Thun MJ, et al. Demographic predictors of mammography and Pap smears screening in U.S. women. *Am J Public Health* 1994;83:53-60.
8. Hayward RA, Shapiro MF, Freeman HE, et al. Who gets screened for cervical and breast cancer: Results from a new national survey. *Arch Intern Med* 1988;148:1177-1181.
9. Phillips AN, Smith GD. Cigarette smoking as a potential cause of cervical cancer: Has confounding been controlled? *Int J Epidemiol* 1994;23:42-49.
10. Cannistra SA, Niloff JM. Cancer of the uterine cervix. *N Engl J Med* 1996;334:1030-1038.
11. Morrison EAB, Ho G, Vermund ST, Goldberg GL, et al. Human papillomavirus infection and other risk factors for cervical neoplasia: A case-control study. *Intl J Cancer* 1991;49:6-13.
12. Peters RK, Thomas D, Hagan DG, et al. Risk factors for invasive cervical cancer among Latinas and non-Latinas in Los Angeles County. *J Nat Cancer Inst* 1986;77:1063-1077.
13. Becker T, Wheeler CM, Key CR, et al. Cervical cancer incidence and mortality in New Mexico's Hispanics, American Indians, and Non-Hispanic Whites. *Western J Med* 1992;156: 376-379.
14. Snipes KP, Perkins CI, Wright WE, Young JL. Cancer incidence and mortality by race/ethnicity in California, 1988-1991. Sacramento: California Department of Health Services, Cancer Surveillance Section, 1994.
15. Zunzunegui MV, King MC, Coria CF, et al. Male influences on cervical cancer risk. *Am J Epidemiol* 1986;123:302-307.
16. Elder JP, Castro FG, de Moor C, et al. Differences in cancer-risk-related behaviors in Latino and Anglo adults. *Preventive Medicine* 1991;20:751-763.
17. Harlan LC, Bernstein AB, Kessler LG. Cervical cancer screening: Who is screened and why? *Am J Public Health* 1991;81: 885-891.
18. Hubbell FA, Chavez LR, Mishra SI, et al. Beliefs about sexual behavior and other predictors of Papanicolau smear screening among Latinas and Anglo women. *Arch Intern Med* 1996; 156:2353-2358.
19. National Institutes of Health Consensus Development Conference Statement: cervical cancer, April 1-3, 1996. National Institutes of Health Consensus Development Panel. *Monogr Natl Cancer Inst* 1996;21:1-26.
20. Bosch FX, Manos MM, Munoz N, et al. Prevalence of human papillomavirus in cervical cancer: a worldwide perspective. International biological study on cervical cancer (IBSCC) Study Group. *J Natl Cancer Inst* 1995;87:796-802.
21. Liaw KL, Hsing AW, Chen CJ, et al. Human papillomavirus and cervical neoplasia: A case-control study in Taiwan. *Int J Cancer* 1995;62:565-571.
22. Cox JT. Epidemiology of cervical intraepithelial neoplasia: The role of human papillomavirus. *Baillieres Clin Obstet Gynaecol* 1995;9: 1-37.
23. Kjaer SK, van den Brule AJ, Bock JE, et al. Human papillomavirus—the most significant risk determinant of cervical intraepithelial neoplasia. *Int J Cancer* 1996;65:601-606.
24. Munoz N, Bosch FX, de Sanjose S, et al. The role of HPV in the etiology of cervical cancer. *Mutat Res* 1994;305:293-301.
25. Eluf-Neto J, Booth M, Munoz N, et al. Human papillomavirus and invasive cervical cancer in Brazil. *Br J Cancer* 1994;69:114-119.
26. Bosch FX, Munoz N, de Sanjose S, et al. Human papillomavirus and cervical intraepithelial neoplasia grade III/carcinoma in situ: A case-control study in Spain and Columbia. *Cancer Epidemiol Biomarkers Prev* 1993;2:415-422.
27. Dillner J, Lenner P, Lehtinen M, et al. A population-based seroepidemiological study of cervical cancer. *Cancer Res* 1994;54: 134-141.
28. Shen CY, Ho MS, Chang SF, et al. High rate of concurrent genital

infections with human cytomegalovirus and human papillomaviruses in cervical cancer patients. *J Infect Dis* 1993;168:449-452.

29. Fernandez C, Sharrard RM, Talbot M, et al. Evaluation of the significance of polyamines and their oxidases in the aetiology of human cervical carcinoma. *Br J Cancer* 1995;72:1194-1199.
30. Fairley CK, Tabrizi SN, Gourlay SG, et al. A cohort study comparing the detection of HPV DNA from women who stop and continue to smoke. *Aust N Z J Obstet Gynaecol* 1995;35:181-185.
31. Simons AM, Mugica van Herckenrode C, Rodriguez JA, et al. Demonstration of smoking-related DNA damage in cervical epithelium and correlation with human papillomavirus tyupe 16, using exfoliated cervical cells. *Br J Cancer* 1995;71:246-249.
32. Gregoire L, Lawrence WD, Kukuruga D, et al. Association between HLA-DQB1 alleles and risk for cervical cancer in African-American women. *Int J Cancer* 1994;57:504-507.
33. Marrero M, Valdes O, Alvarez M, et al. Detection of human papillomavirus by nonradioactive hybridization. *Diagn Microbiol Infect Dis* 1994;18:95-100.
34. Munoz N, Bosch FX, Shah KV, et al. (Eds). The Epidemiology of Cervical Cancer and Human Papillomavirus. Lyon, France; IARC, 1992.
35. Schiffman MH. Recent progress in defining the epidemiology of human papillomavirus infection and cervical neoplasia. *J Nat Cancer Inst* 1992;84:394-398.
36. Schiffman MH, Bauer HM, Hoover RN, et al. Epidemiologic evidence showing that human papillomavirus infection causes most cervical intraepithelial neoplasia. *J Natl Cancer Inst* 1993;85: 958-964.
37. Ferenczy MD, Jenson AB. Tissue effects and host response: The key to the rational triage of cervical neoplasia. *Ob Gyn Clins North Am* 1996;23:759-783.
38. Barron BA, Richart RM. Statistical model of the natural history of cervical carcinoma. II. Estimates of the transition time from dysplasia to carcinoma in situ. *J Nat Cancer Inst* 1970;45:1025-1030.
39. Kashigarian M, Dunn JE. The duration of intraepithelial and preclinical squamous cell carcinoma of the uterine cervix. *Am J Epidemiol* 1970;92:221-222.
40. Perez CA, Kurman RJ, Stehman FB, et al. Uterine Cervix. In: Principles and Practice of Gynecologic Oncology, 1st ed. Hoskins WJ, Perez CA, Young RC (eds.) Philadelphia: JB Lippincott Company; 1992.
41. La Vecchia C, Decarli A, Gentile A, et al. Pap smear and the risk of cervical neoplasia: Quantitative estimates from a case-control study. *Lancet* 1984;2:779-782.
42. Herrero R, Brinton La, Reeves WC, et al. Screening for cervical cancer in Latin America: A case-control study. *Int J Epidemiol* 1992;1050-1056.
43. Cramer DW. The role of cervical cancer in the declining morbidity and mortality of cervical cancer. *Cancer* 1974;34:2018-2027.
44. Miller AB, Lindsay J, Hill GB. Mortality from cancer of the uterus in Canada and its relationship to screening for cancer of the cervix. *Int J Cancer* 1976;17:602-612.
45. Benedet JL, Anderson GH, Matisic JP. A comprehensive program for cervical cancer detection and management. *Am J Obstet Gynecol* 1992;166:1254-1259.
46. McPhee SJ, Bird JA, Fordham D, et al. Promoting cancer prevention activities by primary care physicians. Results of a randomized controlled trial. *JAMA* 1991;266:538-544.
47. McPhee SJ, Bird JA, Jenkins NH, et al. Promoting cancer screening. A randomized controlled trial of three interventions. *Arch Intern Med* 1989;149:1866-1872.
48. Yancey A, Tanjasiri SP, Ryan M, et al. Increased cancer screening behavior in women of color by culturally sensitive video exposure. *Prev Med* 1995;24:142-148.
49. Castro FG, Elder J, Coe K, et al. Mobilizing churches for health promotion in Latino communities: Companeros en al Salud. *Monogr Natl Cancer Inst* 1995;18:127-135.
50. Navarro AM, Senn KL, Kaplan RM, et al. Por La Vida Intervention model for cancer prevention in Latinas. *Monogr Natl Cancer Inst* 1995;18:137-145.
51. Hodge FS, Frederick L, Rodrigues B, et al. American Indian women talking circle. *Cancer* 1996;78:1592-1597.
52. American Cancer Society. Guidelines for the cancer-related checkup: an update. Atlanta: American Cancer Society; 1993.
53. U.S. Preventive Services Task Force. Guide to clinical preventive services: Report of the U S Preventive Services Task Force. 2nd ed. Baltimore: Wilkins and Wilkins; 1996.
54. Eddy DM. Screening for cervical cancer. *Ann Intern Med* 1990; 113:214-226.
55. Soost HJ, Lange HJ, Lehmacher W, et al. The validation of cervical cytology: Sensitivity, specificity, and predictive values. *Acta Cyto* 1991;35:8-14.
56. Tawa K, Forsythe A, Cove JK, et al. A comparison of the Papanicolaou smear and the cervigram: sensitivity, specificity, and cost analysis. *Obstet Gynecol* 1988;71:229-235.
57. Koonings PP, Dickinson K, d'Ablaing G, et al. A randomized clinical trial comparing the Cytobrush and cotton swab for Papanicolaou smears. *Obstet Gynecol* 1992;80:241-245.
58. Cauthen DB, Cullison M, Symm B, et al. Use and effectiveness of the Cytobrush in the primary care setting. *J Am Board Fam Pract* 1991;5:365-368.
59. Alons-van Kordelaar JM, Boon ME. Diagnostic accuracy of squamous cervical lesions studied in spatula-cytobrush smears. *Acta Cytol* 1988;32:801-804.
60. Richart RM. Cervical intrepithelial neoplasia. *Pathol Annu* 1973;8:301-328.
61. Regan JW, Fu YS. The uterine cervix. In Silverberg SG (ed). Principals and Practice of Surgical Pathology, vol 2. New York: Wiley; 1983.
62. National Cancer Institute Workshop. The 1988 Bethesda System for reporting cervical/vaginal cytological diagnoses. *JAMA* 1989;262: 931-934.
63. Broder S. The Bethesda System for reporting cervical/vaginal cytologic diagnoses: report of the 1991 Bethesda Workshop. *JAMA* 1992;267:1982.
64. Marcus AC, Crane LA, Kaplan CP, et al. Improving adherence to screening follow-up among women with abnormal Pap smears: Results from a large clinic-based trail of three intervention strategies. *Medical Care* 1992;30:216-229.
65. Carey P, Gjerdingen DK. Follow-up of abnormal Papanicoulaou smears among women of different races. *J Fam Pract* 1993;37: 583-587.
66. Michielutte R, Diseker RA, Young LD, et al. Noncompliance in screening follow-up among family planning clinic patients with cervical dysplasia. *Preventive Med* 1985;14:248-258.
67. Lacey L, Whitefield J, DeWhite W, et al. Referral adherence in an

inner city breast and cervical cancer screening program. *Cancer* 1993;72:950-955.

68. Paskett ED, White E, Carter WB, et al. Improving follow-up after an abnormal Pap smear: A randomized controlled trial. *Prev Med* 1990;19:630-641.
69. Montz FJ, Monk BJ, Fowler JM, et al. Natural history of the minimally abnormal Papanicolaou smear. *Obstet Gynecol* 1992;80: 385-388.
70. McIndoe WA, McLean MR, Jones RW, et al. The invasive potential of carcinoma in situ of the cervix. *Obstet Gynecol* 1984;64: 451-458.
71. Campo MS. Human papilloma viruses and cervical cancer. Stern P, Stanley M (eds). Oxford University Press; 1993.
72. Chen L, Ashe S, Brady WA, et al. Costimulation of antitumor immunity by the B7 counterreceptor for the T lymphocyte molecules CD28 and CTLA. *Cell* 1992;71:1093-1102.

Premenstrual Syndromes

Meir Steiner, MD, PhD, FRCPC

Women with troublesome premenstrual symptoms are often seen by primary care physicians. Most women of reproductive age experience physical or psychological symptoms premenstrually; however, for some women these symptoms are so severe as to seriously disrupt their social and occupational functioning. These women may meet criteria for premenstrual dysphoric disorder, which is diagnosed through prospective symptom charting. In addition, there is a subgroup of women who experience premenstrual magnification of a concurrent psychiatric or medical illness. All women presenting with premenstrual complaints should be instructed to chart their symptoms prospectively for at least two menstrual cycles to facilitate diagnosis. Lifestyle and low-risk therapies have demonstrated efficacy for women with mild-to-moderate symptoms. Women who fail conservative therapies may benefit from treatment with low-dose serotonin reuptake inhibitors. Suppression of ovulation with hormonal agents is the last line of therapy and should be used only in severe, refractory cases.

Introduction

Epidemiologic surveys have estimated that as many as 75% of women of reproductive age experience some symptoms attributed to the premenstrual phase of the menstrual cycle.[1] More than 100 physical and psychological symptoms have been reported;[2] however, most women are able to manage these symptoms through lifestyle changes and conservative therapies. This phenomenon is often classified by the generic term of Premenstrual Syndrome (PMS) and most often refers to any combination of symptoms that appear during the week prior to menstruation which resolve within a week of onset of menses.[3] Conversely, 3-8% of women in this age group report premenstrual symptoms of irritability, tension, dysphoria, and lability of mood which seriously interfere with their lifestyle and relationships.[4] So disruptive is the latter that a series of research diagnostic criteria for what is now labelled Premenstrual Dysphoric Disorder (PMDD) have been developed and published in the 3rd revised and 4th editions of the Diagnostic and Statistical Manual of Mental Disorders.[5,6] *(Please see Table 1.)* Women who are found to meet the diagnostic criteria of PMDD do not usually respond to conservative and conventional interventions, and they often seek out the expertise of their primary care physician.[6a-c]

Table 1. Summary of PMDD Criteria*

A. Symptoms must occur during the week before menses and remit a few days after onset of menses.

Five of the following symptoms must be present, with at least one being 1, 2, 3, or 4.

1. Depressed mood or dysphoria
2. Anxiety or tension
3. Affective lability
4. Irritability
5. Decreased interest in usual activities
6. Concentration difficulties
7. Marked lack of energy
8. Marked change in appetite, overeating, or food cravings
9. Hypersomnia or insomnia
10. Feeling overwhelmed
11. Other symptoms (i.e., breast tenderness, bloating)

B. Symptoms must interfere with work, school, usual activities, or relationships

C. Symptoms must not merely be an exacerbation of another disorder

D. Criteria A, B, and C must be confirmed by prospective daily ratings for at least two cycles

* Adapted from the *DSM-IV*.[6]

Etiology

The etiology of PMS, and specifically PMDD, is still largely unknown. Attempts have been made to explain the phenomena in terms of biology, psychology, or psychosocial factors, but most of these explanations have failed to be confirmed by laboratory and treatment-based studies.

As is true for all female-specific mood disorders, the role of female sex hormones in PMDD has been considered of central importance. To date, however, studies attempting to attribute the disorder to an excess of estrogen, a deficit of progesterone, a withdrawal of estrogen, or changes in estrogen-to-progesterone ratio have been unable to find specific differences between women with PMDD and those without the disorder.[7] Some investigators have suggested that progesterone and progestogens may actually provoke rather than ameliorate the cyclical symptom changes of PMDD.[8] The hypothesis that ovarian cyclicity is important in the etiology of PMDD is, nevertheless, supported by some but not all studies in which the medical suppression of ovulation resulted in the disappearance of premenstrual mood disturbances and physical symptoms.[9-18]

The current consensus seems to be that normal ovarian function (rather than hormone imbalance) is the cyclical trigger for PMDD-related biochemical events within the central nervous system and other target tissues. A psychoneuroendocrine mechanism triggered by the normal endocrine events of the ovarian cycle seems the most plausible explanation.[19] This viewpoint is attractive in that it encourages investigation of the neuroendocrine-modulated central neurotransmitters and the role of hypothalamic-pituitary-gonadal (HPG) axis in PMDD.

Of all the neurotransmitters studied to date, increasing evidence suggests that serotonin (5-HT) may be important in the pathogenesis of PMDD.[20-24] PMDD also shares many of the features of other mood and anxiety disorders that have been linked to serotonergic dysfunction.[25-27] In addition, reduction in brain 5-HT neurotransmission is thought to lead to poor impulse control, depressed mood, irritability, and increased carbohydrate craving—all mood and behavioral symptoms associated with PMDD.[28] Reciprocity between fluctuations in ovarian steroids and serotonergic function has been established in animals showing that estrogen and progesterone influence central serotonergic neuronal activity. In the hypothalamus, estrogen induces a diurnal fluctuation in 5-HT,[29] whereas progesterone increases the turnover rate of 5-HT.[30] More recently, several studies concluded that 5-HT function also may be altered in women with PMDD.

The current consensus is that women with PMDD may be behaviorally or biochemically sub- or supersensitive to biological challenges of the serotonergic system. It is not yet clear whether these women present with a trait or state marker of PMDD.

Risk Factors

Epidemiologic surveys from around the world continue to demonstrate convincingly that, for adult women, the lifetime prevalence of mood disorders is substantially higher than it is among men. Most of these studies confirm that the ratio of affected women to men is approximately 2:1, and this ratio is maintained across ethnic groups.[31] The higher incidence of depression among women is primarily seen from puberty on and is less marked in the years after menopause.[32] The relationship between PMDD and other psychiatric disorders is complicated by the observation that a high proportion of women presenting with PMDD have a history of previous episodes of mood disorders and that women with an ongoing mood disorder report premenstrual magnification of symptoms as well as an emergence of new symptoms. Likewise, several family studies have identified a concordance in rates of premenstrual tension between first degree female family members.[32a-b]

Presentation and Diagnosis

To aid in the study of menstrual cycle disorders, each menstrual cycle is characterized as containing two prominent phases; the follicular phase occurs after the onset of menses, and the luteal phase refers to the premenstrual interval. The temporal relationship between fluctuations in psychopathology and different phases of the menstrual cycle is well documented. It is therefore essential to ascertain whether the presenting premenstrual symptomatology is unique to the luteal phase or whether it is a worsening of an ongoing, persisting physical or psychiatric disorder. A definition of the follicular phase as days 7-11 and the luteal phase as days -2 through -6 is appropriate in clinical settings.

Women presenting with premenstrual complaints should be instructed to chart their symptoms daily for at least two, preferably three, menstrual cycles in order to measure within cycle symptom changes. The current emphasis is on prospective, self-report instruments that are easy to administer and score without jeopardizing validity. The Daily Record of Severity of Problems (DRSP) assesses 20 symptoms associated with PMDD and specifically measures functional impairment in work and social realms.[33] The Premenstrual Record of Impact and Severity of Menstruation (PRISM)[34] and the Calendar of Premenstrual Experiences (COPE)[35] are more detailed one-page calendars that have also been validated and used in clinical trials. These calendars allow respondents to rate a variety of physical and psychological symptoms, indicate negative and positive life events, record concurrent medications, as well as track menstrual bleeding and cycle length.

As a result of the lack of objective diagnostic tests for PMS or PMDD, a complete history must be collected in these women. In addition to a retrospective history of the premenstrual symptomatology, this interview should also include a complete review of physical systems (including gynecological, endocrinological, allergies, etc.) and medical disorders, as well as a psychiatric history and a detailed review of family loading for mental illness. As the symptoms of anemia and thyroid disease often mirror those of PMS or PMDD, the patient should undergo laboratory investigations if there are any hints of an underlying medical cause for the symptoms. In addition, women who are suspected to meet criteria for PMDD should be assessed at least once during each cycle phase to ensure that the patient subjectively endorses phase-appropriate mood symptoms which supports their daily charting (none or minimal during follicular phase; lifestyle impairing during the luteal phase).

The Diagnostic and Statistical Manual of Mental Disorders, 4th edition (*DSM-IV*)[6] multiaxial classification system includes five axes, each of a different domain of information that may help the clinician in the comprehensive and systematic evaluation of the patient. It draws attention to the various major mental disorders (Axis I) and personality disorders (Axis II); to general medical conditions (Axis III); to psychosocial and environmental factors (Axis IV); and provides a global assessment of functioning (Axis V). In using the *DSM-IV* criteria for PMDD (please see Table 1), a certain familiarity with the multiaxial system is assumed. Thus, for PMDD, criterion C is crucial in excluding any current Axis I, II, or III illness or episode. The other essential features of the *DSM-IV* PMDD criteria are the "on-offness" of symptoms and the emphasis on core mood symptoms (criterion A), the requirement that the symptoms must interfere markedly with lifestyle (criterion B), and, most importantly, that the disorder must be confirmed prospectively by daily ratings for at least two menstrual cycles. Prospective daily rating of symptoms is now the only acceptable means of confirming a provisional *DSM-IV* diagnosis of PMDD. The DRSP, PRISM, and COPE daily calendars contain the core symptoms and most of the additional symptoms considered for the *DSM-IV* diagnosis of PMDD. In using one of the daily calendars, the clinician must identify a priori the patient's chief complaints and the symptoms to be followed throughout treatment. Daily symptoms are rated by the patient using scales which range from none (for a score of 0) to severe (for a score of 7 on the PRISM, 3 on the COPE). Scores for the symptoms of interest are added for the five follicular days and the five luteal days, and these total phase scores are then compared.

Investigators have typically followed a diagnostic severity criterion which is applied in addition to the criteria listed for PMDD in the *DSM-IV*. Conventionally, a within-cycle increase in symptom scores (worsening) of at least 30% from follicular to luteal phase scores is required in order to meet PMDD diagnostic criteria.[36] More recently, it has been suggested that within-cycle worsening of at least 50% is necessary to confirm diagnosis and merit psychopharmacologic intervention.[37] The within-cycle percent change is calculated by subtracting the follicular score from the luteal score, dividing by the luteal score and multiplying by 100 ([luteal-follicular/ luteal] × 100). Thus, a patient presenting with a mean follicular score of 20 and luteal score of 50 would demonstrate a within-cycle symptom increase of 60%. A change in score of this proportion demonstrates the "on-offness" of this symptomatology and is typical of women who meet criteria for PMDD.

Upon completion of the two-cycle prospective diagnostic assessment phase, women may qualify for one of the following diagnostic categories:

A. PMDD: Women who receive this diagnosis meet criteria for PMDD only. They have no other concurrent psychiatric disorder or unstable medical condition but may have a history of a past psychiatric disorder. They have charted symptoms daily for at least two cycles, and their chief complaints include one of the four core symptoms and at least five of the 11 total symptoms (please see Table 1). The symptoms have occurred with most menstrual cycles during the past year and have interfered with social or occupational roles. Their symptoms demonstrate clear worsening premenstrually and remit within a few days after the onset of the follicular phase. In addition, worsening between the follicular and luteal phases must be at least 30%.

B. PMS: Women who receive this diagnosis do not meet all *DSM-IV* criteria for PMDD but do demonstrate symptom exacerbation premenstrually. Only one troublesome symptom is required for this diagnosis, although the symptom must be restricted to the luteal phase of the menstrual cycle, reach a peak shortly before menstruation, and cease with the menstrual flow or soon after.

C. Premenstrual Magnification: Women who receive this diagnosis may meet most of the diagnostic criteria for PMS or PMDD but, in the process of being assessed, have also been identified to have a current major psychiatric disorder or an unstable medical condition. Medical disorders that are commonly exacerbated during the luteal phase include migraine headaches, allergies, asthma, seizures, and genital herpes. Psychiatric conditions that can be magnified include depression, anxiety, panic, bulimia, substance abuse, mania, and psychosis.

D. Other Psychiatric Diagnosis Only: These women do not demonstrate premenstrual symptoms that meet criteria for PMDD but do meet *DSM-IV* criteria for another psychiatric disorder. Women meeting criteria for Intermittent Depressive Disorder or Cyclothymia may also fall into this category, where the cyclical nature of their symptoms does not necessarily match the phases of their menstrual cycle.

E. No Diagnosis: In these women, the diagnosis of PMS or PMDD cannot be made, and medical, gynecological, and psychiatric screening is negative. These women experience disruptive symptoms that tend to occur throughout the cycle. It is often difficult to delineate the exact problem. Careful examination of the entire diary, especially the follicular phase, and discussion with the patient may show low-grade psychiatric or medical problems such as situational, vocational, or marital stress, irritable bowel syndrome, chronic fatigue syndrome, headache, fibromyalgia or other pain syndromes, as well as sleep disorders.

Applying these criteria to women who seek help for premenstrual complaints will facilitate the primary care physician in planning management interventions.

Treatment

Women who present with an Axis I, II, or III disorder and premenstrual magnification should be treated for the primary disorder at the discretion of the supervising clinician. Referral to an appropriate specialist is often indicated for newly diagnosed disorders.

A wide range of therapeutic interventions has been tested in the treatment of premenstrual symptoms. For women who do not meet criteria for PMS, PMDD, or other physical and psychological disorders, conservative treatments are appropriate, and management without pharmacologic interventions should be encouraged. Unfortunately, there have been few randomized controlled trials (RCT) to determine the efficacy of these more conservative interventions (please see Table 2); however, there is some evidence that these patients may best respond to individual or group psychotherapy in combination with lifestyle changes. Recommended dietary changes (especially during the luteal phase) should include the reduction or limitation of tobacco, chocolate, caffeine, and alcohol. Some women report improvement with small, frequent complex carbohydrate meals and vitamins and minerals when taken in moderation. Patients should be encouraged to decrease excess sodium in the diet when edema or fluid retention occurs and, if possible, to reduce weight to within 20% of their ideal weight. Regular exercise is important and particularly effective when combined with the regular practice of stress management techniques. Patients should also be taught to review their own monthly diaries and identify triggers to symptom exacerbation.

PMS

Women who meet criteria for PMS should also be encouraged to practice lifestyle changes and may respond to some of the tested low-risk therapies (please see Table 3):

a. *Vitamin B6* has demonstrated mixed efficacy in clinical trials, with most trials demonstrating ambiguous or negative results using a wide range of dosing strategies from 50 mg daily to 500 mg daily.[38] Because of reports of peripheral sensory neuropathy, dosing in clinical practice should not exceed 150 mg daily to be given during the last two weeks of each cycle.

b. *Calcium* 1000 mg daily demonstrated significant improvement in one clinical trial.[39] No untoward side effects were reported with this dose.

c. *Oral magnesium* 360 mg daily from the fifteenth day of the menstrual cycle to the onset of menstrual flow significantly improved premenstrual pain and negative affect in one RCT.[40]

d. *Optivite* is a vitamin/mineral supplement that was superior to placebo in one RCT.[41] Clinically, up to six Optivite tablets daily during the luteal phase of the menstrual cycle may relieve symptoms.

e. *Vitamin E* (alpha tocopherol) was superior to placebo in women with benign breast disease who scored the severity of their premenstrual symptoms before and after two months of Vitamin E therapy.[42] Vitamin E therapy can safely be used at 400 IU daily.

f. *Evening Primrose Oil* (gamma linolenic acid) has not demonstrated efficacy superior to placebo in several RCTs and should not be recommended as treatment for PMS or PMDD.[43]

g. *Naproxen sodium* improved pain and behavior in one RCT when taken seven days premenstrually[44] and menstrual migraine specifically in another RCT when it was taken daily.[45]

h. *Mefenamic acid* was superior to placebo for improving physical and mood symptoms in one RCT;[46] however, the use of this medication should be limited (7-10 days) because of gastric side effects.

i. *Spironolactone* 100 mg daily from day 12 of the menstrual cycle until the first day of the next menstrual cycle significantly reduced bloating compared to placebo in one RCT.[47] The potential for diuretic abuse and serious contraindication of potassium supplements necessitates the use of this drug for severe symptoms only.

j. *Bromocriptine* of at least 5 mg daily has demonstrated significant improvement in premenstrual mastodynia[48] but has not demonstrated efficacy with the mood symptoms associated to the premenstruum. RCT evidence suggests that a dosing range of 1.25-7.5 mg daily during the luteal phase of the menstrual cycle is appropriate for clinical use.

Women who continue to experience severe premenstrual symptoms after the commencement of low-risk therapies may be considered for the pharmacotherapies indicated for PMDD.

PMDD

Therapeutic interventions for women who meet criteria for PMDD who fail conservative therapies range from treatment of

Table 2. Conservative Therapies

Charting	Daily charting of symptoms
Diet	Reduce or eliminated, especially in the luteal phase: Salt, chocolate, caffeine, and alcohol. Small, frequent complex carbohydrate meals. Vitamins and minerals in moderation.
Exercise	Moderate, regular, aerobic
Stress reduction	Stress management course and/or counselling if necessary
Relaxation	Relaxation course or audio tape
Relationship	Assertiveness course and/or marital counselling if necessary
Self-help groups	If available
Education	Self-help books

the most troublesome symptoms with psychotropic medications to hormonal therapy to eliminate ovulation.

Listed below is a summary of the RCT evidence for the most common therapies used to treat PMDD. It is important to note that only studies that used prospective diagnostic criteria that could meet the *DSM-IV* PMDD classification[6] have been cited.

I. Psychotropic Medications *(Please See Table 4)*

a. *Serotonin Reuptake Inhibitors (SRIs).* SRIs have proven to be very successful in the treatment of PMDD symptoms. Of the selective serotonin reuptake inhibitors (SSRIs), fluoxetine 20 mg daily has been proven superior to placebo in several RCTs.[37,49-52] Sertraline 50-150 mg daily[53] and paroxetine 10-30 mg daily[54] have also demonstrated efficacy in single RCTs. Pilot studies have demonstrated the efficacy of intermittent SRI dosing during the last two weeks of the menstrual cycle;[55-56] however, these finding have yet to be confirmed by a larger RCT. The SRI clomipramine has also been proven superior to placebo in two RCTs, using 25-75 mg daily[57] or during the luteal phase of each menstrual cycle only.[58] Thus, the SRIs to date have demonstrated their effectiveness in significantly improving the psychological and physical symptoms of PMDD as compared to placebo, with only mild, mostly tolerable side effects. The side effects profile is similar between SRIs, and the most troublesome include headache, nausea/gastrointestinal upset, sleep disturbance/insomnia, tremulousness, sweating, dry mouth, and anorgasmia. These side effects can usually be managed through dosing changes, the use of intermittent vs. daily dosing schedules, or by switching to other SRI compounds.

b. *Benzodiazepines (Anxiolytics).* Because of the mood disorder component of PMDD, benzodiazepines, particularly anxiolytics, have also been tested for the treatment of this disorder. Alprazolam has successfully alleviated the symptoms of PMDD in several[59-62] but not all[63] RCTs. The risk of dependence and concerns regarding withdrawal prompted investigators to test the efficacy of alprazolam vs. placebo

Table 3. Low-Risk Therapies (not symptom-specific), Evidence Based

Vitamin B6	100 mg daily
Calcium	1000 mg daily
Magnesium ion	360 mg daily (14 days before menses)
Optivite	up to 6 tablets daily
Vitamin E	400 IU daily
Evening primrose oil	Demonstrated lack of efficacy

when administered in the luteal phase only. Patient-modified dosing was allowed, and efficacious dosing ranged from 0.25 to 5 mg daily for 6-14 days prior to menstruation.[59-62] Sedation and drowsiness were the two most frequently identified side effects of this treatment. Significant improvements in mood and physical symptoms were reported for the positive studies.[56-62] The 5-HT1A partial antagonist busiprone has also demonstrated efficacy in one RCT when administered with a mean daily dose of 25 mg, for the 12 days prior to menstruation.[64]

II. Hormonal Therapy *(Please See Table 5)*

a. *GnRH Agonists.* GnRH agonists can reversibly suppress the menstrual cycle, and this is often called "medical ovariectomy" or "medical menopause." GnRH agonists have proven to be very successful in most but not all clinical trials. Unfortunately, the long-term use of GnRH agonists has been inhibited by the occurrence of side effects which mimic menopause and the potential for hypoestrogenism and osteoporosis. Preliminary evidence suggests that "add-back" therapy with low-dose estrogen and progesterone replacement therapy may prevent some of these side effects.[15] The suggested dosing for the various agonists include: buserelin (400-900 mcg daily, intranasally),[12,13] subcutaneous D-Trp6-Pro9-NEt-GnRH (50 mcg daily),[16] subcutaneous Histrelin (100 mcg daily),[15] and monthly subcutaneous goserelin (3.6 mg).[66] Intramuscular depot leuprolide (3.75 mg per month) was significantly superior to saline placebo in one RCT,[9] whereas at the dose of 7.5 mg per month, it was not.[65] Intramuscular leuoprolide at 3.75-7.5 mg monthly or intranasal buserelin 400-900 mcg daily are the most appropriate GnRHa treatments for clinical use. Addback therapy should consist of conjugated estrogen 0.625 mg daily (Monday-Saturday) and 10 mg of medroxyprogesterone acetate daily for 10 days during every fourth menstrual cycle.

b. *Estradiol.* Estradiol treatment can suppress ovulation and thus has been proven effective in reducing the symptoms of PMDD, although adjunct progestogen therapy is necessary to prevent endometrial hyperplasia. Luteal phase only administration of Premarin was ineffective in one RCT;[67] however, transdermal estradiol or estradiol implants combined with luteal phase noresthisterone, medroxyprogesterone, or dydrogesterone improved physical and mood symptoms in three RCTs.[18,68,69] Transdermal estradiol (100-200 mcg patches) applied twice weekly with low-dose progestogen addback daily from day 17 to 26 of each cycle is appropriate for clinical use.

Table 4. Psychotropic Medications, Evidence Based

Fluoxetine	20 mg daily
Sertraline	50-150 mg daily
Paroxetine	10-30 mg daily
Clomipramine	25-75 mg daily (14 days before menses)
Alprazolam	0.25-5 mg daily (6-14 days before menses)
Busiprone	25 mg daily (12 days before menses)

c. *Danazol.* Danazol is a synthetic androgen, capable of suppressing the HPG axis. While danazol has been proven to be superior to placebo in several RCTs,[70-73] the adverse effect profile of this treatment is considerable and is the result of both its androgenic activity and anti-estrogen properties. The most prominent adverse events are amenorrhea, acne, and weight gain. Tested doses include 100-400 mg daily, and both mood and physical symptoms improved significantly when compared to placebo. The most prominent side effect at this dosing range was altered menstrual cycle length. One study of women with PMS found that danazol 200 mg daily from the onset of symptoms to the onset of menses significantly improved mood symptoms and bloating compared to placebo.[74] Clinical dosing at 200-400 mg daily is appropriate.

d. *Progesterone.* Progesterone has been shown to be no more effective than placebo in treating PMS or PMDD symptoms in the majority of trials and should not be used as a primary treatment for these disorders.[62,75]

e. *Oral contraceptives.* Oral contraceptives suppress ovulation while maintaining menstruation due to periodic steroid withdrawal. Oral contraceptives have their own side effects, which are often similar to the symptoms of PMS or PMDD. The one RCT testing oral contraceptives in this population was a negative study that supported the conclusions of other less rigorous research.[76] Until additional studies ahve been done, oral contraceptives should not be used to treat PMS or PMDD.

To date, no one intervention has proven to be effective for all women with PMDD. SSRIs, as well as clomipramine, continue to be proven as efficacious in women with PMDD who have failed conservative treatment, and they are currently the first treatment of choice. Alprazolam and buspirone have demonstrated efficacy in the reduction of psychological symptoms in RCTs; however, side effects and possible dependence inhibit maximum efficacy.

The last line of treatment for women with PMDD who do not report efficacy with the symptom-modifying drugs are the GnRH agonists. Due to the potential long-term side effects of this treatment, low-dose estrogen-progesterone addback should be considered over the short-term. Estradiol and danazol may also be effective, and gynecological interventions, such as surgery, may need to be considered.[10,11]

Table 5. Hormonal Therapies, Evidence Based

GnRH agonists	
Buserelin	400-900 mcg daily intranasal
Leuoprolide	3.75-7.5 mg monthly, intramuscular injection
PLUS addback	conjugated estrogen 0.625 mg daily (Monday-Saturday) and 10 mg medroxyprogesterone acetate daily for 10 days during every fourth menstrual cycle
Estradiol	100-200 mg patches (2 per week)
PLUS addback	progestrogen day 17-26 each cycle
Danazol	200-400 mg daily
Progesterone	demonstrated lack of efficacy
Oral contraceptives	Insufficient data; 1 negative RCT

Assessment of Efficacy

Patients should be assessed every two weeks (i.e., during the follicular and luteal phases, respectively) within the first month of commencing therapy, and they should be instructed to continue to chart symptoms daily. Dosing strategies vary; however, most recent investigations have demonstrated the efficacy of most therapeutic drugs at low doses. If efficacy has not been attained after several dosing increases, other treatment options should be considered. There is also increasing evidence that response will be relatively immediate in this population; therefore, if there is no change in symptomatology an alternate therapy should be considered within 2-3 menstrual cycles. Continued symptom charting will help to track efficacy, symptom response to dosing changes, symptoms upon termination of therapy, and real vs. perceived side effects. For example, women who report headaches or nausea as side effects are often surprised to see that they rated these symptoms just as severe prior to commencing therapy.

Investigators have yet to reach a consensus on how to define efficacy. Clinically, the easiest way to define efficacy is by the reduction of luteal symptoms so that the luteal symptoms remit significantly or the follicular to luteal difference is less than 30%. What has become obvious is that the intervention alone cannot predict efficacy, and more consideration is now being given to past psychiatric history as well as to family psychiatric history, especially of mood disorders in the families of women with PMDD.

Summary

The recent inclusion of research diagnostic criteria for PMDD in the *DSM-IV* validates the findings that some women in their reproductive years have extremely distressing emotional and behavioral symptoms premenstrually and should help clinicians recognize these women. PMDD can be differentiated from PMS, which is primarily reserved for milder physical symptoms and minor mood changes, as well as premenstrual magnification, which occurs when physical and/or psychological symptoms of a concurrent psychiatric and/or medical disorder are magnified during the premenstruum.

The etiology of PMS and PMDD is still largely unknown. The current consensus seems to be that normal ovarian function (rather than hormone imbalance) is the cyclical trigger for PMDD-related biochemical events within the central nervous system and other target tissues.

Increasing evidence suggests that 5-HT may be important in the pathogenesis of PMDD. The serotonergic system is in close reciprocal relationship with gonadal hormones. Women with PMDD may be behaviorally or biochemically sub- or supersensitive to biological challenges of the serotonergic system. It is not yet clear whether these women present with a trait or state marker of PMDD.

To apply the *DSM-IV* criteria for PMDD, women must chart symptoms daily for at least two cycles, and their chief complaints must include one of the four core symptoms (irritability, tension, dysphoria, and lability of mood) and at least five of the 11 total symptoms. The symptoms should have occurred with most menstrual cycles during the past year and have interfered with social or occupational roles. In addition, the charting of troublesome symptoms should demonstrate clear worsening premenstrually and remit within a few days after the onset of menstruation. Changes in symptoms from the follicular to luteal phase should be at least 30% to make a diagnosis of PMDD.

Treatment options range from the conservative lifestyle and stress management to treatment with psychotropic medications and hormonal or surgical interventions to eliminate ovulation for the more extreme cases.

SSRIs, as well as clomipramine, continue to be proven as efficacious in women with PMDD who have failed conservative treatment. These interventions have demonstrated excellent efficacy with almost immediate relief and minimal side effects. Recent investigations of SRIs have also demonstrated success at low doses. Most investigators now suggest that if efficacy has not been attained after several dosing increases, other treatment options should be considered. There is also evidence of success with GnRH agonists, estradiol, and danazol. Unfortunately, many women are unable to tolerate the side effects of these interventions.

Taken together, these data indicate that treatment may be accomplished by either eliminating the hormonal trigger or by reversing the sensitivity of the serotonergic system.

References

1. American College of Obstetrics and Gynecology Committee. Premenstrual syndrome. *Int J Gynecol Obstet* 1995;50:80-84.
2. Budeiri DJ, et al. Clinical trials of treatment of premenstrual syndrome: Entry criteria and scales for measuring treatment outcomes. *Br J Obstet Gynaecol* 1994;101:689-695.
3. World Health Organization. Mental, Behavioral and Developmental Disorders. Tenth Revision of the International Classification of Diseases (ICD-10). Geneva: World Health Organization, 1992.
4. Johnson SR. The epidemiology and social impact of premenstrual symptoms. *Clin Obstet Gynecol* 1987;30: 367-376.
5. American Psychiatric Association. *Diagnostic and Statistical Manual of Mental Disorders,* Third Edition. Washington, DC, American Psychiatric Association, 1987:367-369.
6. American Psychiatric Association. *Diagnostic and Statistical Manual of Mental Disorders,* Fourth Edition. Washington, DC, American Psychiatric Association, 1994:717-718.

6a. Klein TA. Office gynecology for the primary care physician, part II: Pelvic pain, vulvar disease, disorders of menstruation, premenstrual syndrome, and breast disease. [Review]. *Med Clin N Am* 1996;80: 321-336.

6b. Szewczyk M, Chennault SA. Women's health. Depression and related disorders. [Review]. *Primary Care Clin Office Pract* 1997;24:83-101.

6c. Allan TR, Goldstein L. Selective serotonin reuptake inhibitors in the treatment of mood disorders in primary care: Depression and premenstrual syndrome. *Connecticut Med* 1996;60:215-219.

7. Roca CA, et al. Implications of endocrine studies of premenstrual syndrome. *Psychiatr Ann* 1996;26:576-580.
8. Hammarback S, et al. Cyclical mood changes as in the premenstrual tension syndrome during sequential estrogen-progestogen postmenopausal replacement therapy. *Acta Obstet Gynecol Scand* 1985;64:393-397.
9. Brown CS, et al. Efficacy of depot leuprolide in premenstrual syndrome: Effect of symptom severity and type in a controlled trial. *Obstet Gynecol* 1994;84:779-786.
10. Casper RF, Hearn MT. The effect of hysterectomy and bilateral oophorectomy in women with severe premenstrual syndrome. *Am J Obstet Gynecol* 1990;162:105-109.
11. Casson P, et al. Lasting response to ovariectomy in severe intractable premenstrual syndrome. *Am J Obstet Gynecol* 1990;162: 99-105.
12. Hammarback S, Backstrom T. Induced anovulation as treatment of premenstrual tension syndrome. A double-blind cross-over study with GnRH-agonist versus placebo. *Acta Obstet Gynecol Scand* 1988;67:159-166.
13. Hussain SY, et al. Buserelin in premenstrual syndrome. *Gynecol Endocrinol* 1992;6:57-64.
14. Mezrow G, et al. Depot leuprolide acetate with estrogen and progestin add-back for long-term treatment of premenstrual syndrome. *Fertil Steril* 1994;62:932-937.
15. Mortola JF, et al. Successful treatment of severe premenstrual syndrome by combined use of gonadotrophin-releasing hormone agonist and estrogen/progestin. *J Clin Endocrinol Metab* 1991;72: 252A-252F.
16. Muse KN, et al. The premenstrual syndrome. Effects of a 'medical ovariectomy.' *N Engl J Med* 1984;311:1345-1349.
17. Smith RN, Studd JW. Estrogens and depression in women. In: Lobo RA, ed. *Treatment of the Postmenopausal Woman: Basic and Clinical Aspects.* New York: Raven Press; 1993:129-135.
18. Watson NR, et al. Treatment of severe premenstrual syndrome with estradiol patches and cyclical oral norethisterone. *Lancet* 1989;2: 730-732.
19. Rubinow DR, Schmidt PJ. The treatment of premenstrual syndrome—forward into the past. *N Engl J Med* 1995;332:1574-1575.

20. Steiner M, et al. Serotonin and gender specific psychiatric disorders. *Int J Psychiatry Clin Pract* 1997;1:3-13.
21. Rapkin A. The role of serotonin in premenstrual syndrome. *Clin Obstet Gynecol* 1992;35:629-636.
22. Rojansky N, et al. Imipramine receptor binding and serotonin uptake in platelets of women with premenstrual changes. *Gynecol Obstet Invest* 1991;31:146-152.
23. Steiner M. Female-specific mood disorders. *Clin Obstet Gynecol* 1992;35:599-611.
24. Yatham LN. Is 5-HT1A receptor subsensitivity a trait marker for late luteal phase dysphoric disorder? A pilot study. *Can J Psychiatry* 1993;38:662-664.
25. Endicott J. The menstrual cycle and mood disorders. *J Affective Disord* 1993;29:193-200.
26. Pearlstein TB, et al. Prevalence of axis I and axis II disorders in women with late luteal phase dysphoric disorder. *J Affective Disord* 1990;20:129-134.
27. Wurtman JJ. Depression and weight gain: The serotonin connection. *J Affective Disord* 1993;29:183- 192.
28. Meltzer HY. Serotonergic dysfunction in depression. *Br J Psychiatry* 1989;155:25-31.
29. Cohen IR, Wise PM. Effects of estradiol on the diurnal rhythm of serotonin activity in microdissected brain areas of ovariectomized rats. *Endocrinology* 1988;122:2619-2625.
30. Ladisich W. Influence of progesterone on serotonin metabolism: A possible causal factor for mood changes. *Psychoneuroendocrinology* 1977;2:257-266.
31. Weissman MM, Olfson M. Depression in women: Implications for health care research. *Science* 1995;269:799-801.
32. Weissman MM, et al. Affective disorders. In: Robins LN, Regiers DA, eds. Psychiatric Disorders in America. New York: Free Press; 1991:53-80.
32a. Kendler, et al. Genetic and environmental factors in the etiology of menstrual, premenstrual, and neurotic symptoms; a population-based twin study. *Psychol Med* 1992;22:85-100.
32b. Freeman, et al. Effects of medical history factors on symptom severity in women meeting criteria for premenstrual syndrome. *Obstet Gynecol* 1988;72:236-239.
33. Endicott J, Harrison W. The daily record of severity of problems. Available from Dr. Endicott, New York State Psychiatric Institute, Biometrics Unit, 722 West 168th Street, New York, NY 10032.
34. Reid RL. Premenstrual syndrome. *Curr Probl Obstet Gynecol Fertil* 1985;8:1-57.
35. Mortola JF, et al. Diagnosis of premenstrual syndrome by a simple, prospective, and reliable instrument: The calendar of premenstrual experiences. *Obstet Gynecol* 1990;76:302-307.
36. National Institute of Mental Health. NIMH Premenstrual Syndrome Workshop Guidelines; April 14-15, 1983; Rockville, MD: National Institute of Mental Health.
37. Steiner M, et al. Fluoxetine in the treatment of premenstrual dysphoria. *N Engl J Med* 1995;332:1529- 1534.
38. Kleijnen J, et al. Vitamin B6 in the treatment of premenstrual syndrome—A review. *Br J Obstet Gynaecol* 1990;97:847-852.
39. Thys-Jacobs S, et al. Calcium supplementation in premenstrual syndrome: a randomized crossover trial. *J Gen Intern Med* 1989;4: 183-189.
40. Facchinetti F, et al. Oral magnesium successfully relieves premenstrual mood changes. *Obstet Gynecol* 1991;78:177-181.
41. London RS, et al. Effect of a nutritional supplement on premenstrual symptomatology in women with premenstrual syndrome: A double-blind longitudinal study. *J Am Coll Nutrition* 1991;10: 494-499.
42. London RS, et al. Efficacy of alpha-tocopherol in the treatment of premenstrual syndrome. *J Reprod Med* 1987;32:400-404.
43. Budeiri DJ, et al. Is evening primrose oil of value in the treatment of premenstrual syndrome. *Controlled Clin Trials* 1996;17:60-68.
44. Facchinetti F, et al. Naproxen sodium in the treatment of premenstrual syndromes: A placebo controlled study. *Gynecol Obstet Invest* 1989;28:205-208.
45. Sances G, et al. Naproxen sodium in menstrual migraine prophylaxis: a double-blind placebo controlled study. *Headache* 1990;30: 705-709.
46. Mira M, et al. Mefenamic acid in the treatment of premenstrual syndrome. *Obstet Gynecol* 1986;68:395-398.
47. Vellacott ID, et al. A double blind, placebo controlled evaluation of spironolactone in the premenstrual syndrome. *Curr Med Res Opin* 1987;10:450-456.
48. Andersch B. Bromocriptine and premenstrual symptoms: A survey of double blind trials. *Obstet Gynecol Surv* 1983;38:643-646.
49. Stone AB, et al. Fluoxetine in the treatment of late luteal phase dysphoric disorder. *J Clin Psychiatry* 1991;52:290-293.
50. Menkes DB, et al. Fluoxetine's spectrum of action in premenstrual syndrome. *Int Clin Psychopharmacol* 1993;8:95-102.
51. Wood SH, et al. Treatment of premenstrual syndrome with fluoxetine: A double-blind, placebo- controlled crossover study. *Obstet Gynecol* 1992;80:339-344.
52. Su TP, et al. Fluoxetine in the treatment of premenstrual disorder. *Neuropsychopharmacology* 1997;16:346-356.
53. Yonkers KA, et al. Sertraline in the treatment of premenstrual dysphoric disorder. *Psychopharmacol Bull* 1996;32:41-46.
54. Eriksson E, et al. The serotonin reuptake inhibitor paroxetine is superior to the noradrenaline reuptake inhibitor maprotiline in the treatment of premenstrual syndrome. *Neuropsychopharmacology* 1995;12:167-176.
55. Smoller JW, Halbreich U. Intermittent luteal phase sertraline treatment of dysphoric premenstrual syndrome. Abstract. *Biol Psychiatry* 1997;41:120S.
56. Steiner M, et al. Intermittent fluoxetine dosing in the treatment of women with premenstrual dysphoria. Abstract. *Psychopharmacol Bull* 1997 (in press).
57. Sundblad C, et al. Clomipramine effectively reduces premenstrual irritability and dysphoria: a placebo controlled trial. *Acta Psychiatr Scand* 1992;85:39-47.
58. Sundblad C, et al. Clomipramine administered during the luteal phase reduces the symptoms of premenstrual syndrome. *Neuropsychopharmacology* 1993;9:133-145.
59. Smith S, et al. Treatment of premenstrual syndrome with alprazolam: Results of a double-blind, placebo-controlled, randomized crossover clinical trial. *Obstet Gynecol* 1987;70:37-43.
60. Harrison W, et al. Treatment of premenstrual dysphoria with alprazolam. *Arch Gen Psychiatry* 1990;47:270-275.
61. Berger CP, Presser B. Alprazolam in the treatment of two subsamples of patients with late luteal phase dysphoric disorder: A double-blind, placebo-controlled crossover study. *Obstet Gynecol* 1994;84:379- 385.
62. Freeman EW, et al. A double-blind trial of oral progesterone, alpra-

zolam, and placebo in the treatment of severe premenstrual syndrome. *JAMA* 1995;274:51-57.

63. Schmidt PJ, et al. Alprazolam in the treatment of premenstrual syndrome: A double-blind, placebo- controlled trial. *Arch Gen Psychiatry* 1993;50:467-473.
64. Rickels K, et al. Buspirone in the treatment of premenstrual syndrome [Letter]. *Lancet* 1989;i:777.
65. Helvacioglu A, et al. Premenstrual syndrome and related hormonal changes. *J Reprod Med* 1993;38:864-870.
66. West CP, Hillier H. Ovarian suppression with the gonadotrophin-releasing hormone agonist goserelin (Zoladex) in management of the premenstrual tension syndrome. *Hum Reprod* 1994;9: 1058-1063.
67. Dhar V, Murphy BE. Double-blind randomized crossover trial of luteal phase estrogens (Premarin) in the premenstrual syndrome (PMS). *Psychoneuroendocrinology* 1990;15:489-493.
68. Magos AL, et al. Treatment of the premenstrual syndrome by subcutaneous oestradiol implants and cyclical oral norestisterone: Placebo controlled study. *BMJ* 1986; 292:1629-1633.
69. Smith RN, et al. A randomized comparison over 8 months of 100 micrograms and 200 micrograms twice weekly doses of transdermal oestradiol in the treatment of severe premenstrual syndrome. *Br J Obstet Gynecol* 1995;102: 475-484.
70. Hahn PM, et al. A randomized, placebo-controlled crossover trial of danazol for the treatment of premen-strual syndrome. *Psychoneuroendocrinology* 1995;20:193-209.
71. Gilmore DH, et al. Danazol for premenstrual syndrome: A preliminary report of a placebo-controlled double-blind study. *J Int Med Res* 1985;13:129-130.
72. Deeny M, et al. Low dose danazol in the treatment of premenstrual syndrome. *Postgrad Med J* 1991;67:450-454.
73. Watts JF, et al. A clinical trial using danazol for the treatment of premenstrual tension. *Br J Obstet Gynaecol* 1987;94:30-34.
74. Sarno AP, et al. Premenstrual syndrome: Beneficial effects of periodic, low-dose danazol. *Obstet Gynecol* 1987;70:33-36.
75. Altshuler LL, et al. Pharmacological management of premenstrual disorder. *Harvard Rev Psychiatry* 1995;2: 233-245.
76. Graham CA, Sherwin BB. A prospective treatment study of premenstrual symptoms using a triphasic oral contraceptive. *J Psychosom Res* 1992;36:257-266.

Menstrual Abnormalities

Edward Onusko, MD
Rancie Hannah, MD

Abnormal uterine bleeding is a common complaint in most primary care practices. An average human female will have as many as 400 menstrual cycles during her reproductive years. As many as 31 per 1000 consults annually to a practice[1] or 20% of women at some time in their lives[2] will present to their physicians with the complaint of abnormal periods. The prevalence of numerous possible etiologies that can give rise to abnormal uterine bleeding varies based on the age and reproductive status of the patient. Anovulatory menstrual cycles and hormonal imbalances are common, especially at the extremes of a woman's reproductive life cycle (< 20 and > 40 years old). The term dysfunctional uterine bleeding (DUB) is used to describe the syndrome of abnormal menstrual patterns caused by a variety of hormonal imbalances. In approximately one-quarter of cases of menstrual abnormalities, an organic or pathologic etiology such as pregnancy (or complications thereof), neoplasm (either benign or malignant), infection, or secondary disease conditions (such as a coagulation disorder) can account for the abnormality.[3] Accurate diagnosis of abnormal uterine bleeding can be challenging. A careful history and physical exam are indispensable in the evaluation, since many cases provide no sensitive physical abnormalities or useful laboratory findings to complement the clinician's diagnostic acumen. Evaluation of amenorrhea will not be included in the scope of this chapter.

Normal Menstrual Physiology

The physiologic mechanisms of the normal menstrual cycle are not completely understood, but a basic comprehension of the cyclic hormonal variations and end organ responses is important for understanding the pathologic processes that result in abnormal conditions *(please see Figure 1)*.

Menstruation is the physiologic shedding of the inner lining of the uterus, or endometrium, which occurs on average once per month. Cycles are considered normal if they occur at 28-day intervals, give or take seven days. Pubertal females tend to have a greater variability of cycle length secondary to immaturity of neuroendocrine controls. Uterine bleeding usually lasts from two to seven days, resulting in a blood loss averaging 35 mL (range, 15-50 mL). Blood loss greater than 80 mL per cycle is considered to be abnormal and can with time result in considerable iron deficiency. Subjective estimations by patients of the volume of vaginal blood lost or number of sanitary pads used are notoriously insensitive markers for actual uterine blood loss but may allow for a rough approximation of flow. Ten to fifteen pads or tampons would be consistent with a uterine blood loss of around 60 mL.

Menarche occurs when the hypothalamus signals the pituitary gland to begin manufacturing the gonadotropic hormones FSH (follicle-stimulating hormone) and LH (luteinizing hormone). This

Table 1. Defining Abnormal Bleeding

Menorrhagia	Regularly occurring menses with excessive or prolonged flow
Metrorrhagia	Irregularly occurring menses
Menometrorrhagia	Irregularly occurring menses with excessive or prolonged flow
Polymenorrhea	Regular menses at intervals less than 21 days
Oligomenorrhea	Regular menses at intervals greater than 35 days

is accomplished by the action of hypothalamic GnRH (gonadotropin-releasing hormone), which is released in pulsatile fashion through the hypothalamic-pituitary portal system. FSH action at the ovaries allows the maturation of a cohort of primordial follicles. This period of the cycle is known as the follicular phase. The largest follicle that contains the most FSH receptors is responsible for production of increasing amounts of estradiol, the most physiologically potent estrogenic compound, from androgen precursors. Estradiol along with inhibin, a glycoprotein also produced by the developing follicle, serve as both positive and negative feedback mechanisms at the level of the pituitary.

First, in response to increasing amounts of estradiol and inhibin, FSH levels begin to fall and the remaining follicles in the cohort undergo atresia. With the dominant follicle remaining and estradiol concentrations greater than a critical level for 2-3 days, the pituitary is triggered to release a surge of LH, leading to rupture of the dominant follicle and ovulation. Following ovulation, the follicle proceeds into the luteal phase with production of progesterone by the granulosa cells that remain. If not supported by rising concentrations of BHCG from a fertilized ovum, the corpus luteum regresses and progesterone levels fall.

During follicular development, the endometrial tissue, responding to increasing levels of estrogens, begins to grow during what is termed the proliferative phase of the uterine cycle. Estrogen serves to stimulate the production of endometrial growth factors that permit replication of both endometrial glandular and supportive stromal elements. The endometrial thickness increases to approximately 8-9 mm (post-menses thickness is approximately 1-2 mm). High estrogen concentrations also allow for an up-regulation of additional estrogen receptors and progesterone receptors on endometrial cells. With unopposed and continuous estrogen available, the endometrium will continue to proliferate.

The secretory phase of the endometrial cycle begins with ovulation and the development of the corpus luteum from the remaining elements of the dominant follicle. The rising concentration of progesterone from the corpus luteum exerts an anti-estrogenic effect on the endometrium that causes an arrest of the proliferative phase by down-regulation of both estrogen and progesterone receptors. Progesterone serves to induce endometrial glandular cell differentiation and to organize stromal elements in preparation for possible implantation of a fertilized ovum. Endometrial prostaglandins are also altered by the concentration of progesterone. PGF2a and thromboxane are the major vasoconstrictive agents and PGE exerts a vasodilatory effect. Progesterone withdrawal causes an increase in the ratio of PGF2a to PGE, with a resultant constriction of the spiral arteries of the uterus and local ischemia of the endometrium with the onset of menses. Completion of menses requires clot formation at the spiral arteries secondary to the action of thromboxane and regeneration of the basal layer of the endometrium through the effect of estrogen.

Etiologies

There are a wide variety of causes of abnormal vaginal bleeding *(please see Table 2)*. It is useful to view this subject from the perspective of what phase of the female reproductive life cycle the patient is in. For example, the usual causes of abnormal vaginal bleeding in a postmenopausal female are much different from the usual causes in an adolescent.

Causes of Abnormal Bleeding—Preadolescent

Although urogenital bleeding in prepubertal females is uncommon, some causes are worth mentioning. Hormonal causes may be the result of exogenous estrogens in the form of prescription medications such as oral contraceptives that may be ingested or topically applied by unsuspecting children. If a sufficient dosage is taken, the endometrium may be stimulated to proliferate and withdrawal of the estrogen source may cause bleeding. Newborn females may have a sanguineous discharge or frank bleeding secondary to withdrawal of maternal estrogens transferred in utero.[4] No specific therapy is necessary and bleeding usually stops within 10 days. More likely causes of bleeding in children are localized disorders of the urogenital tract secondary to trauma, abuse, foreign bodies, urethral prolapse, or infection.

Causes of Abnormal Bleeding—Adolescents

Abnormal uterine bleeding becomes a significant and common presenting complaint once a female reaches the pubertal age. Approximately 90% of cases in nonpregnant adolescents are secondary to DUB.[5] True DUB is defined as excessive, prolonged, unpatterned bleeding from the endometrium that is unrelated to secondary disease states or anatomic abnormality. On a physiologic level, DUB in adolescents is caused by immaturity of the hypothalamic-pituitary-ovarian endocrine axis; therefore, ovulatory cycles do not always occur. FSH from the pituitary acts on the ovarian cells, producing estrogen. However, critical estradiol concentrations are not achieved for positive feedback stimulation of LH release (or hypothalamic-pituitary controls fail to initiate the LH surge). The net result is failure of adequate LH to induce ovulation in a developing follicle, absence of ovarian luteal-phase progesterone, and a prolonged proliferative phase of the endometrium. Without the presence of regularly cycling progesterone concentrations, the endometrium grows to excessive and unstable thickness.

Eventually, secondary to either abrupt estrogen withdrawal or insufficient blood supply for the excessive endometrial tissue, patchy sloughing of the endometrium occurs. Bleeding is usually prolonged due to the lack of coordination of the shedding process and lack of appropriate local control of the event by chemical mediators (prostaglandins and thromboxane). Establishment of regular ovulatory cycles usually occurs with time. On average, the younger the age at menarche, the less time is required to establish a majority of ovulatory cycles.[6]

Despite the absence of ovulation, most postmenarchal cycles do not differ significantly in length from normal limits due to an intact negative feedback system, whereby rising estrogen concentrations inhibit further FSH release, which, in turn, inhibits estrogen production by ovarian follicles. This cyclical pattern is responsible for maintaining the rather regular pattern of menses, as the resultant estrogen withdrawal bleeding prevents excessive endometrial thickening between cycles.[7]

DUB may also occur with ovulatory cycles as a result of insufficiency of the corpus luteum ("luteal phase defect"). Periods are usually regular in timing but duration of menses is increased. Resultant blood loss may be excessive.[8] This is less common in adolescents than in older women.

Disorders of hemostasis should be considered as a cause of abnormal or excessive uterine bleeding. These include diseases that affect platelet number or function (such as idiopathic thrombocytopenic purpura, von Willebrand's disease, or leukemia), as well as disruption of intrinsic coagulation factors (hereditary coagulopathies, hepatic or renal failure). Medications such as aspirin or warfarin may also contribute to problem bleeding. In one retrospective case series, 3% of adolescents presenting with abnormal uterine bleeding were diagnosed with a new hematologic disorder. Several others were known to have pre-existing coagulopathies.[9]

Polycystic Ovary Syndrome (PCOS)

The classic syndrome complex of oligomenorrhea, hirsutism, obesity, and polycystic ovaries was first described in 1935 by Stein and Leventhal. It is now appreciated that there is a clinical spectrum of related androgen excess syndromes in many women with anovulatory cycles, in which any of these four signs may be minimal or absent.[10] Although these syndromes are still incompletely understood, a possible underlying mechanism may be hypersecretion of LH. The consequences of high baseline LH levels include:

- stimulation of ovarian theca cell conversion of cholesterol to androgens (i.e., hyperthecosis);
- suppression of FSH, which a) limits ovarian granulosa cell aromatization of androgens to estrogens, and b) prevents normal development of ovarian follicles;
- subsequent systemic androgenic effects of hirsutism, acne, unfavorable lipid profiles, male-pattern adipose distribution;
- conversion of excess androgens to estrogens by adipose tissue, which stimulates the endometrium; and
- chronic anovulation, which prevents the protective effect of cyclic progesterone on the endometrium.[2]

Chronic anovulation from many different etiologies can cause negative effects from both androgen and estrogen excess. Associated pathologies include insulin resistance syndromes, cardiovascular disease, and structural abnormalities of the ovaries. Which of these are the primary disorders and which are secondary results is often unclear.

Causes of Abnormal Bleeding—Reproductive Age

Pregnancy-related complications must always be an initial consideration in this population. These can often be easily ruled out with measurement of urine or serum B-HCG levels. Ectopic pregnancy, spontaneous or threatened abortion, and gestational trophoblastic disease are all considerations.

Hormonal abnormalities (DUB) are still the most common causes of abnormal bleeding in this age group. Low levels of estrogen provide inadequate support to the endometrium and cause irregular, prolonged, but usually light bleeding patterns (estrogen withdrawal bleeding). Sustained levels of excess estrogen, which may result from anovulation, cause periods of amenorrhea followed by acute, heavy bleeding (estrogen breakthrough bleeding).

Other endocrine disorders include hypothyroidism (menorrhagia), hyperthyroidism (oligo- or amenorrhea and elevated estrogen

Figure 1. Menstrual Physiology

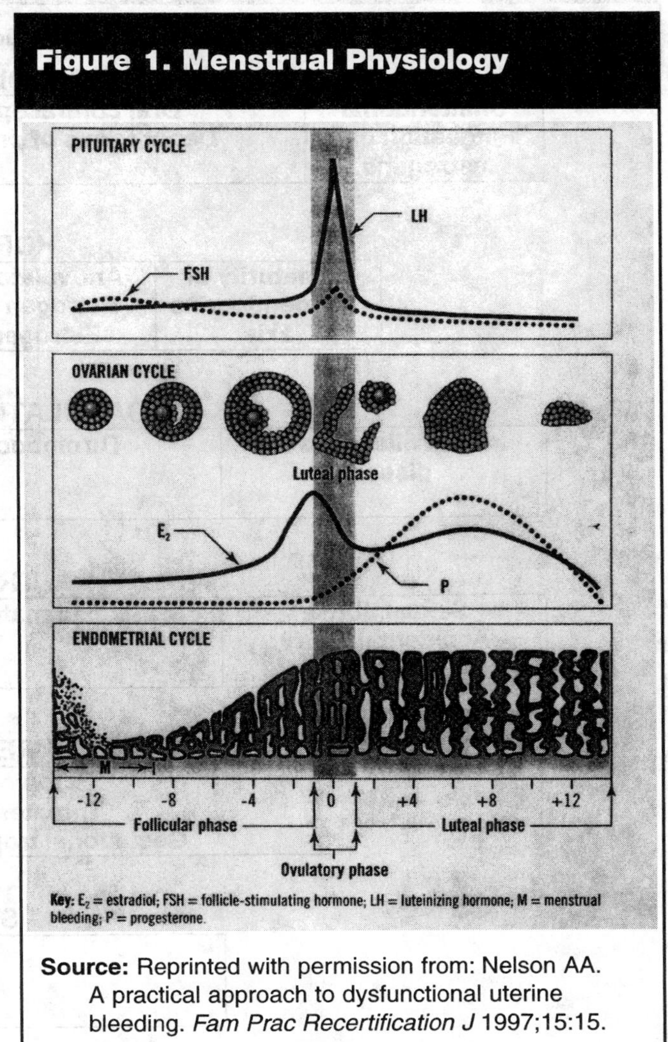

Key: E_2 = estradiol; FSH = follicle-stimulating hormone; LH = luteinizing hormone; M = menstrual bleeding; P = progesterone.

Source: Reprinted with permission from: Nelson AA. A practical approach to dysfunctional uterine bleeding. *Fam Prac Recertification J* 1997;15:15.

levels), diabetes mellitus (anovulation, obesity, insulin resistance, androgen excess), and androgen excess disorders.

Exogenous hormones (oral contraceptives) are a common cause of abnormal vaginal bleeding. Because of the relatively low-dose pills currently in use, missing a single day's dose, or even taking the day's dose later than usual, may result in intermenstrual bleeding. Even though oral contraceptive pills are often prescribed to correct anovulatory bleeding patterns, the balance of estrogenic and progestational effects of combination pills prescribed for contraception may not be right for an individual patient and may result in bleeding irregularities. Long acting hormone preparations such as depo-medroxyprogesterone acetate (Depo-Provera) may cause abnormal vaginal bleeding.

Certain medications have also been associated with abnormal uterine bleeding. Obviously, any anticoagulant (coumadin, heparin, aspirin) has the potential to alter platelet function or clotting factors. Phenytoin, phenothiazines, steroids, tricyclic antidepressants, and lithium may also contribute to abnormal menses by interfering with normal hormonal balance.

Anatomic (structural) lesions are much more common in this age group vs. adolescents. Endometrial (or cervical) polyps and submucosal leiomyomata (fibroids) are treatable causes of vaginal blood loss.[11]

Endometrial hyperplasia and endometrial carcinoma are significant concerns that must be considered in any adult woman with a vaginal bleeding disorder. Age older than 35-40 years is typically used as an indicator of risk, since only 2-5% of cases of endometrial cancer occur in women younger than 40 years.[12] Other risk factors for significant endometrial pathology include hypertension, obesity, impaired carbohydrate metabolism, late onset of menopause, nulliparity, irregular menses, and unopposed exogenous estrogen. Ash et al suggest that patients with a pattern of predominantly irregular menstrual cycles in the preceding 12 months are at highest risk of abnormal endometrial histology, regardless of age.[12]

Smoking more than 16 cigarettes per day is associated with a threefold greater risk of abnormal bleeding patterns, probably due to the anti-estrogenic effects of nicotine.

Table 2. Selected Causes of Menstrual Abnormalities in the Life Cycle

Preadolescence → Adolescence → ReproductiveYears → Perimenopausal → Postmenopausal

EXOGENOUS HORMONES

Unintentional ingestion of estrogens	Oral contraceptive pills Depot forms of progesterone	Hormone replacement therapy

HORMONAL

Immaturity of neuroendocrine axis	Anovulatory syndromes Estrogen breakthrough Estrogen withdrawal	Ovarian failure

COAGULATION DISORDERS

von Willebrand's disease	Thrombocytopenia	Coagulopathies, medical conditions such as hepatic failure, warfarin therapy

TRAUMA

Sexual abuse Accidental injury	Inflammation from STDs	Vaginal atrophy

PREGNANCY-RELATED DISORDERS

Ectopic pregnancy Threatened abortion Gestational trophoblastic disease

STRUCTURAL PATHOLOGY

Fibroids Endometrial dysplasia Carcinoma

Sexually transmitted diseases are a common cause of vaginal bleeding. For example, chlamydia is a common cause of cervicitis, which may result in intermenstrual vaginal spotting.

Causes of Abnormal Vaginal Bleeding—Perimenopausal

As women near the end of their reproductive years, the hypothalamic-pituitary axis tends to remain intact, but the aging ovary is less responsive to gonadotropins and produces less active follicles. Decreased production of estrogen from these follicles fails to trigger the LH surge required for ovulation and corpus luteum formation, resulting in more anovulatory cycles. Menopause may be defined clinically as the absence of menses for one year.[13] Cycles tend to shorten (due to a shortened follicular phase) or become intermittently anovulatory. One study found the median age for the beginning of menopause to be 47.5 years, age at menopause 51.3 years, with a perimenopausal duration of 4-5 years.[14] Eight percent of women become menopausal before age 40.

In this relatively older population of women, endometrial carcinoma must be carefully considered as a cause of abnormal bleeding patterns. However, loss of ovarian function with a resultant change in menstrual patterns is an inevitable result of normal aging, and every woman does not need to necessarily undergo diagnostic intervention at the time of menopause. Each patient needs to have individualized counseling and risk factor assessment.

Structural lesions (such as fibroids) and medical conditions that result in abnormal bleeding patterns (such as hepatic or renal failure) occur more frequently with aging.

Causes of Abnormal Bleeding—Postmenopausal

In the absence of hormone therapy, any vaginal bleeding after menopause should undergo evaluation for a neoplastic lesion.[15] Other common causes of postmenopausal bleeding include exogenous estrogens, atrophic vaginitis/endometritis, endometrial or cervical polyps, and endometrial hyperplasia.

Despite the fact that in the majority of postmenopausal patients the benefits of hormone replacement therapy (osteoporosis reduction and favorable effect on the lipid profile) probably outweigh the adverse risks (thrombotic events and carcinoma of the breast), 1) less than 20-30% of eligible women take it long term,[16] and 2) about 70% of women who are started on replacement therapy stop it within a year, most often secondary to unwanted vaginal bleeding.[17] There is no clear definition of "abnormal bleeding" in postmenopausal women who are taking hormone replacement therapy.

Diagnostic Evaluation

A careful history and physical examination should allow the practitioner to formulate a focused diagnostic plan based on age, risk factors for neoplastic disease, fertility vs. contraceptive concerns, etc. Age of menarche, detailed description of the pattern of bleeding (menstrual diaries may be useful), current medications, previous OB/GYN history, family history, desire for contraception, review of systems to screen for associated medical problems, risk factors for sexually transmitted diseases, and tobacco use are all important aspects of the patient's history. A complete physical exam including breast and pelvic exams should be done. Signs of androgen excess (hirsutism, acne, etc.), structural pelvic lesions (e.g., fibroids), thyromegaly, and many other physical findings may suggest an etiology for the bleeding abnormalities. Acanthosis nigricans (hyperpigmentation of the neck, axillae, and inguinal region) suggests a state of hyperinsulinemia.[18]

Pregnancy should be ruled out as the cause of abnormal vaginal bleeding in any woman of reproductive age. Bleeding disorders may be screened by coagulation studies (PT/PTT) and platelet count. Von Willebrand's disease should be suspected with excessive bleeding at menarche. It may be diagnosed by an abnormal bleeding time and abnormal quantitative or functional assays for von Willebrand's factor. Diagnostic studies for systemic diseases such as hypothyroidism, hyperthyroidism, renal disease, hepatic injury, malnutrition, etc., may be used as clinically indicated.[19] Testing for sexually transmitted diseases may be indicated in sexually active women.

The traditional method for evaluation of women at risk for endometrial carcinoma is endometrial biopsy. Endovaginal ultrasound may be useful in selecting out a low-risk subpopulation of peri- or postmenopausal women (endometrial thickness less than 5 mm) who do not require further diagnostic intervention.[20-22] Infusion of saline into the uterine cavity may improve diagnostic accuracy of ultrasound.[23] Although the high negative predictive value of transvaginal ultrasonography makes it a useful test to screen for low-risk patients, the positive predictive value is poor.[24] Office hysteroscopy (direct visualization of the endometrium via saline infusion and insertion of a flexible scope) is useful for diagnosing endometrial polyps and directing biopsy of suspicious-appearing lesions.[25] A Pap test should always be considered as well, although it will be diagnostic in only about 50% of cases of endometrial carcinoma.

The diagnosis of anovulatory disorders is usually made by putting together the overall clinical picture rather than by a single diagnostic test. In PCOS, a properly timed LH:FSH ratio (> 2:1) is usually present, along with clinical and/or laboratory findings of hyperandrogenism (elevated free testosterone levels) and chronic anovulation (in the absence of secondary causes such as hyperprolactinemia, adult-onset congenital adrenal hyperplasia, and neoplasm). The ovaries may be structurally normal; therefore, the diagnosis cannot be excluded on the basis of imaging or direct observation of them. DUB is primarily a diagnosis of exclusion, implying an imbalance in the hypothalamic-pituitary-ovarian endocrine axis.[26]

Therapeutic Interventions

Abnormal vaginal bleeding found to be secondary to a specific etiology should be treated by correction of the underlying abnormality. Examples would be thyroid hormone replacement in hypothyroidism, or hysterectomy for endometrial carcinoma.

Women taking exogenous female hormones (either oral contraceptives or postmenopausal hormone replacement therapy) may benefit from a change in their regimen. There are a large number of hormone preparations (including all the oral contraceptive pills [OCPs]) available, with varying estrogen and progestin potency, in multiple combinations. If there is a clear pattern of hormonal abnormality, such as estrogen breakthrough bleeding (i.e., bleeding early in the cycle), a specific change in the content of the hormone prescription may be indicated (e.g., increase the pill's estrogenic potency early in the cycle). There are few definitive, evidence-based data on therapeutic manipulation of estrogen/progestin preparations, however, and the patient's bleeding does not often follow a specific pattern. Therefore, a trial of simply changing to a different estrogenic or progestational preparation may result in a more satisfactory menstrual pattern. A complete discussion of the use of OCPs and postmenopausal hormone replacement therapy is beyond the scope of this article.

Management of DUB may be based on age and other factors. In the adolescent population, anovulatory cycles may simply be observed while awaiting maturation of the endocrine axis. Regular cycling with a progestational agent, or combination oral contraceptives (particularly if contraception is desired), may be used to regulate the menses. The adult, reproductive-age patients with DUB are more at risk for adverse effects of chronic anovulation such as development of abnormal endometrial histology. Cycling with 5-10 days of progestin each month should prevent these complications. Estrogen/progestin oral contraceptive combinations may also be used, though the thromboembolic risks of estrogen supplementation increase with advancing age. Perimenopausal women may be cycled with progestin until they complete menopause, at which time chronic hormone replacement therapy may be initiated.[14]

Acute, heavy bleeding episodes of some urgency should be treated with high-dose estrogen therapy.[11] The estrogen may be given either orally (conjugated equine estrogens 10 mg every 6 hours) or intravenously (25 mg every 2-4 hours). Usually, the bleeding is controlled within 24 hours and the patient is switched to oral maintenance estrogen of 10 mg per day for 21-25 days, with oral medroxyprogesterone acetate 10 mg per day given with the last 7-10 days of estrogen. Normal menses should then follow the withdrawal of both hormones. An alternative is to start treatment with combination estrogen/progestin preparations (i.e., birth control pills) 3-4 tablets per day with eventual tapering of the dose over 3-4 weeks. Urgency of treatment is suggested by hemodynamic instability (postural hypotension), marked anemia (hemoglobin < 7 g/dL), or prominent symptomatology (lightheadedness). Visual evaluation of blood loss by the patient is often not a reliable indicator of the objective severity of blood loss.

Nonsteroidal anti-inflammatory drugs (NSAIDs) have been shown to reduce vaginal bleeding via antiprostaglandin effects.[11] They may be used alone or in combination with hormonal manipulation, particularly for the treatment of DUB. Use may be throughout the period of menses or limited to the first three days. Ibuprofen, mefamanic acid, meclofenamate sodium, and naproxen have all been successfully used for this indication. NSAIDs have the additional benefit of relieving other symptoms of dysmenorrhea, such as cramps.

Danazol is a synthetic agent with antiestrogenic and weak androgenic actvities.[27] It has been useful for the treatment of endometriosis, as well as in reducing the severity of unexplained menorrhagia.[28] It has a high incidence of unpleasant side effects and results in infertility secondary to suppression of ovulation, which limits its clinical usefulness.

Gonadotropin-releasing hormone agonists work by disrupting the pulsatile, physiologic release of hypothalamic GnRH. These agents include leuprolide (Lupron), nafarelin (Synarel), goserelin (Zoladex), and histrelin (Supprelion). Their antigonadotropin action results in induction of amenorrhea or reduction of menorrhagia. Unpleasant side effects (nausea, etc.), expense, and loss of bone density with long-term use also limit the usage of these agents as treatments for abnormal vaginal bleeding. Their endocrine effects (anti-gonadotropin) make them useful agents in the treatment of endometriosis, prostate cancer, breast cancer, induction of endometrial thinning prior to endometrial ablation, uterine leiomyomas, and precocious puberty.[29]

If the primary goal of treatment of an anovulatory syndrome is the restoration of fertility, ovulatory agents such as clomiphene (Clomid, Serophene) may be used. This drug appears to act on the hypothalamic-pituitary axis in anovulatory women via modification of intracellular estrogen receptors, with resultant induction of ovulation.

Surgical options include hysterectomy or hysteroscopic endometrial ablation (using laser, "rollerball" electrocoagulation, etc.).[27] Dilatation and curettage may be necessary to achieve control of a single serious bleeding episode unresponsive to hormonal treatment but does not particularly result in long-term improvement in patterns of abnormal bleeding.

Weight loss in cases of PCOS may be effective in reducing insulin resistance, decreasing free testosterone, and restoring ovulation.[30]

Summary

A review of the basic hormonal mechanisms behind normal and abnormal menstrual cycles has led us to explore the various diagnostic and treatment options available for women at various stages in the life cycle. Thoughtful review of an individual patient's clinical presentation and risk factor profile is necessary to direct appropriate management decisions.

The authors wish to thank Marsha Tomlin and her staff for their assistance in the preparation of this manuscript.

References

1. Chen BH, Giudice LC. Dysfunctional uterine bleeding. *West J Med* 1998;169:280-284.
2. Nelson AL. A practical approach to dysfunctional uterine bleeding. *Fam Pract Recertification* 1997;19:14-40.
3. Smith CB. Pinpointing the cause of abnorma l uterine bleeding. *Womens Health Prim Care* 1998;1:835-844.
4. Hoekelman RA, et al. *Primary Pediatric Care*. 3rd ed. St. Louis, MO: Mosby; 1997:1140-1143.
5. Dealy MF. DUB in adolescents. *Nurse Pract* 1998;23:12-25.
6. Apter D, Vihko R. Early menarche, a risk factor for breast cancer, indicates early onset of ovulatory cycles. *J Clin Endocrinol Metab* 1983;57:82-86.
7. Goldfarb AF. *Clinical Problems in Pediatric and Adolescent Gynecology*. New York, NY: Chapman and Hall; 1996:61-68.
8. Lavin C. DUB in Adolescents. *Curr Opin Pediatr* 1996;8: 328-332.
9. Falcone T, et al. DUB in adolescents. *J Reprod Med* 1994;39:761-764.

10. Dawood MY, et al. *Menstrual Disorders*. Patient Care—Supplement Medical Economics Publishing. May 15, 1992:1-21.
11. Chuong CJ, Bronner PF. Management of Abnormal Uterine Bleeding. *Am J Obstet Gynecol* 1998;175(3 part 2):787-792.
12. Ash SJ, et al. Endometrial biopsy in DUB. *J Reprod Med* 1996;41:892-896.
13. Oriel KA, Schrager S. Abnormal uterine bleeding. *Am Fam Physician* 1999;60:1371-1380.
14. Pinkerton JV, et al. Individualized care for the perimenopausal woman. *Patient Care* 1999;3:47-73.
15. Hillard PA. Benign diseases of the female reproductive tract: Symptoms and signs. In Novak's Gynecology. 12th ed. 331-354.
16. Notelovitz M. How to adjust estrogen therapy to patient response. *Patient Care* 2000;34:99-115.
17. Spencer CP, et al. Management of abnormal bleeding in women receiving hormone replacement therapy. *BMJ* 1997; 315:37-42.
18. Patel SR, et al. Polycystic ovary syndrome: How best to establish the diagnosis. *Womens Health Prim Care* 2000; 3:55-69.
19. Galle PC, McRae MA. Abnormal uterine bleeding. Finding and treating the cause. *Postgrad Med* 1993;93:73-81.
20. Smith-Bindman R, et al. Endovaginal ultrasound to exclude endometrial cancer and other endometrial abnormalities. *JAMA* 1998;280:1510-1517.
21. Weber AM, et al. Vaginal ultrasonography versus endometrial biopsy in women with postmenopausal bleeding. *Am J Obstet Gynecol* 1997;177:924-929.
22. Holbert TR. Transvaginal ultrasonographic measurement of endometrial thickness in postmenopausal women receiving estrogen replacement therapy. *Am J Obstet Gynecol* 1997; 176:1334-1339.
23. Goldstein SR, et al. Ultrasonography-based triage for perimenopausal patients with abnormal uterine bleeding. *Am J Obstet Gynecol* 1997;177:102-108.
24. Langer RD, et al. Transvaginal ultrasonography compared with endometrial biopsy for the detection of endometrial disease. *N Engl J Med* 1997;337:1792-1798.
25. Widrich T, et al. Comparison of saline infusion sonography with office hysteroscopy for the evaluation of the endometrium. *Am J Obstet Gynecol* 1996;174:1327-1334.
26. Baughan DM. Challenges in the management of the patient with dysfunctional uterine bleeding. *Fam Pract Recertification* 1993;15:68-78.
27. Rosenfeld JA. Treatment of menorrhagia due to dysfunctional uterine bleeding. *Am Fam Physician* 1996;53: 165-172.
28. Higham JM, Shaw RW. A comparative study of danazol, a regimen of decreasing doses of danazol, and norethindrone in the treatment of objectively proven unexplained menorrhagia. *Am J Obstet Gynecol* 1993;169:1134-1139.
29 Speroff L, et al. *Clinical Gynecologic Endocrinology and Infertility*. 5th ed. Baltimore, MD:Williams and Wilkins; 1994:145-161.
30. Patel SR, et al. Polycystic ovary syndrome: Today's approach. *Womens Health Prim Care* 2000;3:109-113.

Management of the Menopausal Patient: Part I

Redonda Miller, MD
Katherine K. Chang, MD

While health care maintenance, prevention, and management of common medical conditions are often thought of as the "bread and butter" of primary care medicine, a significant portion of most physicians' practices also involves attention to the normal physiologic changes associated with aging. Menopause falls into this realm, and its effects on women are numerous. The hormonal changes that are the hallmark of menopause result in the physical and psychological symptoms that may prompt a visit to the doctor.

Vasomotor symptoms, often referred to as "hot flashes," are one of the most common problems of perimenopausal women. Up to 75% of women may experience these sensations. Less recognized (and reported) are urogenital symptoms, including pruritis, dyspareunia, and urinary incontinence. Psychological manifestations, including depression, decreased libido, and cognitive changes, are some of the most distressing symptoms for women. A familiarity with the various options for treatment of each of these problems, including appropriate use of hormone replacement therapy (HRT), is crucial for effective patient management.

Beyond the self-reported symptoms are systemic changes that are not immediately apparent to patients. Physicians must counsel women on the effect of menopause on the development of osteoporosis and cardiovascular disease. Again, there are varied approaches to treatment, ranging from dietary modification to HRT to exciting new drugs that are revolutionizing women's health, including newer generation bisphosphonates and selective estrogen-receptor modulators (SERMs).

This chapter and the next will take a comprehensive clinical approach to menopause. In this chapter, Drs. Miller and Chang focus on the physiologic changes of menopause, many of the resultant clinical manifestations, and options for treatment. The next chapter will discuss the cardiovascular effects of menopause, the special case of premature ovarian failure, and the general approach to use of HRT, including the controversy over its advantages and disadvantages.

Background

Menopause affects every woman at some point in her life. The average age of menopause is 51, but it commonly occurs anytime between the ages of 45 and 55. As the lifespan of women continues to increase into the 80s, they can expect to live more than a third of their lives after menopause. Women experience the symptoms and sequelae of menopause in varying degrees of severity, and they pose a significant source of morbidity (*see Table 1*). Many of these consequences can be alleviated by HRT. While not every woman is a candidate for HRT, many eligible women remain reluctant to use it. Recent data suggest that, in the United States, only 20% of postmenopausal women with an intact uterus and 38% who have undergone hysterectomy are current users of HRT.[1]

Physiology

"The menopause" is technically defined as the last menses and cannot be dated with certainty until periods have been absent for 12 months. Menopause is often used more colloquially to refer to the time period between the initial prolongation and irregularity of a woman's menstrual cycle and the complete cessation of menses with its consequent symptoms. Hormone levels may fluctuate for 2-5 years prior to the last menses. This antecedent period, together with the first 12 months after the menopause, is better termed "the perimenopause."

Menopause results from the fall in estradiol (the main form of estrogen produced by the ovaries) that accompanies the progressive atresia of ovarian follicles. This atresia also results in decreased levels of inhibin, a glycoprotein produced by the ovaries. The loss of negative feedback of inhibin on the pituitary gland causes an elevation in the pituitary gonadotropin, follicle-stimulating hormone (FSH). The level of the other pituitary gonadotropin, luteinizing hormone (LH), also increases, but FSH levels rise more quickly and to a higher level. An FSH level greater than 30 mIU/mL is supportive of menopause in a nonmenstruating woman, but clinicians should be aware that FSH can intermittently fluctuate to high levels in the perimenopause as well. Measurement of the FSH can be helpful in certain clinical situations when the diagnosis is unclear, such as in an amenorrheic woman who lacks other symptoms or in a woman with premature menopause. Most often, however, menopause remains a clinical diagnosis.

Clinical Manifestations: Vasomotor Symptoms

Vasomotor symptoms are the most common reasons women seek medical attention during menopause.[2] Symptoms are most frequent during the first 2-3 postmenopausal years.[3] Among postmenopausal women, the reported prevalence of vasomotor symptoms varies widely across cultures, ranging from 70-75% in the United States and Europe to 20% in Asian cultures.[4-6] In addition, marked variability exists in the frequency, duration, and intensity of vasomotor symptoms. The majority of affected women experience mild symptoms that do not significantly interfere with daily activities,[7] while about 20-45% seek medical help for more troubling symptoms.[4,8] Studies have found that women who have undergone surgical menopause have an increased number, duration, and severity of vasomotor complaints compared with those who have undergone natural menopause.[3,5] Vasomotor symptoms typically last 0.5-5 years after natural menopause, although in some women they may persist for more than 15 years.[3]

Etiology. While the cause of vasomotor disturbances is likely multifactorial, involving hormonal, psychogenic, and metabolic components, estrogen withdrawal has been shown to be the precipitating factor, acting directly or indirectly to alter the body's thermoregulatory center in the hypothalamus. It is hypothesized that a sudden downward shift of the body's setpoint temperature triggers vasomotor symptoms. Evidence suggests that β-endorphin, an endogenous opioid, and calcitonin gene-related peptide (CGRP), a potent vasodilator, may be key mediators.[9,10]

Table 1. Symptoms and Sequelae of Menopause

Vasomotor Symptoms
- hot flashes

Breast Changes

Urogenital Symptoms
- vaginal dryness
- incontinence
- frequent UTIs

Cognitive Effects
- irritability
- depression
- decreased libido

Loss in Bone Density

Cardiovascular Effects
- decrease in HDL
- increase in LDL
- loss of vasodilation

Vasomotor Signs and Symptoms. The hot flash is a subjective sensation of intense warmth, beginning in the head and neck and spreading downward into the upper arms and torso. A prodromal syndrome of nausea, headache, lightheadedness, vertigo, or palpitations may precede the episode. It is often accompanied by sweating, which may be drenching, as well as visible flushing over the affected areas. Finally, chills or shakes may occur, with the entire episode lasting 30 seconds to five minutes.[8] The term "hot flush" refers to the objective events that occur during the hot flash. These events include an increase in skin conductance, rise in peripheral temperature, and subsequent decrease in central temperature.[11] Women who have hot flashes are more than twice as likely to report insomnia,[12] possibly reflecting the fact that hot flashes occur most commonly at night. Indeed, secondary effects of sleeplessness and early morning awakenings are particularly troubling for many, contributing to the fatigue, irritability, and forgetfulness associated with sleep deprivation. Caffeine, alcohol, spicy foods, sexual activity, a hot and humid environment, and psychological stress have been identified as potential trigger factors for hot flashes.[7]

Treatment Options. Short-term conventional HRT has been shown to be effective in treating both vasomotor symptoms and secondary insomnia in most postmenopausal women *(please see Table 2)*.[11,13] Various oral preparations of estrogen may be used, with a linear relationship between dose and symptom reduction.[14] In a woman who still has her uterus, progestin (synthetic progesterone) can be given sequentially or continuously. Recently, low-dose (0.025 mg) transdermal estrogens have also been shown to be effective in ameliorating vasomotor complaints.[15] Vasomotor symptoms are usually relieved during the first cycle of treatment, and up to four weeks may be needed to evaluate maximal therapeutic efficacy.[16,17] Estrogen replacement therapy also significantly improves self-reported sleep measures in both symptomatic and asymptomatic postmenopausal women.[13]

Besides HRT, several other therapies have shown success in relieving vasomotor symptoms *(please see Table 2)*. Clonidine (0.1, 0.2, or 0.4 mg p.o. b.i.d.) is one such option, although its efficacy is not as high as HRT, and its usage may be limited by side effects such as dizziness, fatigue, headaches, and irritability.[18] For those with persistent, severe symptoms, combination estrogen-androgen therapies may benefit those women who have failed estrogen-alone therapy.[19] Veralipride (100 mg po qd), a dopamine antagonist, is another alternative. Side effects include mild breast discharge and an increased serum prolactin level, and seems to be safe for short-term use.[20] A relatively new drug, tibolone (2.5 mg po qd), has shown promising results in relieving hot flashes in European studies but is currently not available in the United States. A synthetic steroid analogue with mixed estrogenic, progestogenic, and androgenic effects, tibolone has the advantage of a low rate of vaginal bleeding (7% in one study), but it also has rare side effects of venous and leg problems.[21] Progestins alone, in oral (medroxyprogesterone acetate 10 mg qd),[22] long-acting injectable (depomedroxyprogesterone acetate 50, 100, or 150 mg q month),[23] or transdermal (20 mg qd)[24] forms, is also effective. Other alternative medicine approaches, such as soy supplementation (20 g/d), have been promoted, but more studies will be needed to prove their efficacy.[25]

Breast Changes

With the loss of estrogen at menopause, glandular tissue of the breast undergoes involution. Replacement of supporting collagen by adipose tissue leads to sagging and drooping. Both breast density and fibrocystic changes decrease, making mammography easier to interpret. Most women report a loss in breast size. HRT can increase epithelial call proliferation and density of the postmenopausal breast[26] but can also cause significant breast pain and tenderness, particularly in breasts that have not been exposed to estrogen in years. Likewise, an increase in breast density from HRT can be detected mammographically, which can hamper early breast cancer diagnosis.[27]

Urogenital Symptoms

Urogenital Changes. In postmenopausal women, urogenital atrophy is often underreported, underdiagnosed, and undertreated. Women may not bring up urogenital issues with their physicians due to embarrassment, or they may believe that symptoms are simply inevitable products of aging. Yet, urogenital symptoms are prevalent in postmenopausal women and contribute significantly to lower quality of life. In a study of 1200 postmenopausal women, nearly half experienced some form of lower genital tract disorder (vaginal dryness, difficulty with intercourse, itching, discharge, or smarting pain), and nearly 30% reported some degree of urinary incontinence.[28] Symptom onset can be varied, occurring during the perimenopause or developing insidiously, up to 10 or more years after the cessation of menses. Early recognition and treatment of these problems in women can provide a great deal of comfort, as well as preclude the development of more serious consequences in the future.

Pathophysiology. While urogenital aging is attributed to both estrogen deficiency and the aging process, the exact role of estrogen in the pathogenesis of symptoms is incompletely understood. Estrogen is known to help maintain the health and integrity of genital and urinary structures[29]; estrogen receptors are found throughout the female genital tract and the lower urinary tract,[30] reflecting their common embryonic origin, the urogenital sinus. These receptors are not only limited to the urogenital tract but are also found in supporting pelvic muscles and ligaments.[31] Thus, urogenital structures may deteriorate in part because of the loss of estrogen's stimulation during menopause.

Estrogen also promotes relatively more acidic conditions in the vagina through colonization with lactic-acid-producing lactobacilli.

Table 2. Therapies for Vasomotor Symptoms

	Agents	Side Effects
Estrogen-based preparations	• Estrogen compounds (oral, transdermal) • Estrogen/progestin combinations (oral, transdermal)	Nausea, headaches, breast tenderness, bleeding
Progestin-only preparations	• Oral medroxyprogesterone acetate • Depomedroxyprogesterone acetate (depot injectable) • Transdermal cream	Breast tenderness, irritability, depression, headaches
α-adrenergics	• Clonidine	Dizziness, fatigue, headaches, irritability
Dopamine antagonists	• Veralipride	Breast discharge, increased prolactin levels
Synthetic steroids	• Tibolone	Venous and leg disorders
Phytoestrogens	• Soy protein	Unknown

This environment is more resistant to infection.[32] Without estrogen, women have a drier, less acidic vaginal environment and, subsequently, more frequent infections. The vaginal flora shifts toward a predominance of *Escherichia coli* and other fecal gram-negative bacteria that can serve as a potential reservoir for urinary tract infections (UTIs).

Signs and Symptoms of Urogenital Aging. With the withdrawal of estrogen during menopause, atrophic changes occur. In the vagina, this leads to itching, burning, and dryness, which occurs most frequently 4-6 years after menopause.[3] Dyspareunia and secondary loss of interest in sexual activity may follow. Since both the thickness and vascularity of the vaginal wall are estrogen dependent,[32] postmenopausal women have thinner vaginal walls that are more susceptible to trauma and have less ability to heal. Vaginitis occurs with greater frequency, and weakened support muscles may lead to prolapse.

In the urinary tract, atrophic changes lead to dysuria and urinary incontinence. Recurrent UTIs also occur.

Treatment. Estrogen replacement therapy is effective in improving the signs and symptoms of urogenital atrophy. While estrogen has been known to improve vaginal dryness, itching, atrophic vaginitis, and dyspareunia, its effects on urinary symptoms have only recently been investigated. Estrogen subjectively improves urinary incontinence in postmenopausal women.[33,34] Combining estrogen therapy with α-adrenergic drugs may provide significantly more benefit than estrogen alone.[33] Estrogen also prolongs the time to recurrence among postmenopausal women with recurrent UTIs.[35] (Interestingly, cranberry juice was found to reduce the incidence of bacteriuria and pyuria in elderly women, although clinical correlation with symptoms of UTI in this study was lacking.)[36]

Local vaginal estrogen therapy results in higher tissue levels in the urogenital tract compared to oral administration, and thus may be an important mode of delivery for treatment of associated conditions *(please see Table 3)*. In general, much lower doses of estrogen are needed to relieve urogenital atrophy than are needed to treat vasomotor symptoms,[37] opening the door to treatment with unopposed estrogen without eliciting a proliferative endometrium. Local estrogen treatment is available in a variety of forms, including vaginal creams (containing conjugated equine estrogen, micronized estradiol, or diethylstilbestrol), vaginal estriol pessaries, estradiol vaginal rings, and intravaginal estradiol tablets. Since all forms have good safety profiles and are comparably effective in relieving symptoms, individual preferences may dictate choice of administration. The estradiol vaginal ring has been shown to be a well-tolerated option,[38] with the most frequent side effect of leukorrhea (whitish discharge).[39] Patients seem to prefer the ring over both the vaginal pessary, which can be messy to administer and may cause increased vaginal discharge,[38] and estriol vaginal cream.[40] The intravaginal tablet, an easy and hygienic alternative, is effective at relieving symptoms at a dose as low as 25 mg without systemic effects or stimulation of the endometrium.[41]

Unfortunately, none of the low-dose estrogens used in vaginal delivery systems confers benefit on bone mineral metabolism or cardiovascular disease when used alone. Postmenopausal women who are receiving systemic HRT and continue to have urogenital symptoms may benefit from the addition of local treatment. However, the primary care physician must keep in mind that local estrogen preparations may have systemic effects as well.

Table 3. Vaginal Estrogen Preparations

Vaginal Preparation	Comments
Cream	Messy administration
Estriol pessary	Increased vaginal discharge Messy administration Discomfort
Estradiol ring	Leukorrhea
Intravaginal estradiol tablet	Disposable applicator Applied once or twice weekly

As for nonhormonal therapies, vaginal dryness can also be addressed through over-the-counter vaginal lubricants or a moisturizing vaginal gel. The gel, while superior in efficacy to other lubricants,[42] is not as effective as estrogen in treating vaginal dryness.[43] It remains an alternative to local estrogen therapy or as an adjunct to systemic HRT.

Cognitive Effects

Psychological Symptoms. Many women report psychological symptoms at the time of menopause, including irritability, inability to concentrate, memory loss, anxiety, and depression. Whether these symptoms are direct consequences of menopause or are simply secondary effects of sleep deprivation (from nocturnal hot flashes), other physical symptoms, or changing life roles remains controversial. HRT can have a placebo effect that makes the issue even murkier. A recent longitudinal analysis of more than 2500 women did not find an association between depression and natural menopause unless the women had a long perimenopausal period with increased symptoms or had a prior history of depression.[44] While efficacy data are inconclusive, most experts would recommend a trial of HRT for amelioration of minor psychological symptoms, such as irritability and difficulty with concentration, particularly if other indications for HRT are present. A supportive familial environment is probably most helpful. Physicians should ensure that the patient is not suffering from major depression, as this is more serious and usually warrants other therapies, such as selective serotonin reuptake inhibitors.

Libido. A decrease in libido is a common symptom reported by perimenopausal women. Lack of sexual interest is often multifactorial in nature and may be related to psychological factors, such as depression and low self-image, and physical effects, such as dyspareunia secondary to vaginal dryness. A decline in the ovarian androgens, androstenedione and testosterone, may also play a role. Many authors have suggested that the supplementation of standard HRT with androgens has beneficial effects on sexual functioning, although large, well-controlled studies are lacking. One study involving 34 postmenopausal women with low libido found significantly improved sexual activity and satisfaction when testosterone was added.[45] Other benefits of estrogen-androgen therapy have been touted, including improvement in vasomotor symptoms, cognition, and bone density. The long-term safety of testosterone in women is unknown, but further research is ongoing in this area.

Dementia. Recently, there has been interest in the possibility that estrogen use may prevent or delay the development of dementia, particularly Alzheimer's disease. Several epidemiological studies have suggested a preventive role for HRT, and a recent meta-analysis estimated a 29% decline in the risk of dementia among estrogen users.[46] Proposed mechanisms include the abilities of estrogen to serve as an antioxidant, inhibit neuronal apoptosis, and possibly affect metabolism of β-amyloid. Estrogen's effect, however, appears to be mainly preventive, as a large, randomized, controlled trial resulted in no benefit to women with already established disease.[47] Definite conclusions regarding HRT and the prevention of dementia are difficult to draw at this time, and prevention of dementia should not be the sole indication for HRT in a postmenopausal woman.

Bone Loss

Background. Osteoporosis is a huge health problem that is frequently underrecognized by physicians. It is estimated to affect more than 25 million people and cost roughly $13.8 billion annually in the United States.[48] Much of this cost is due to the significant morbidity and mortality from the most serious complication of osteoporosis, hip fractures. Patients who suffer a hip fracture have a 20% chance of dying within one year, a 50% chance of requiring assistance to ambulate, and a 25% chance of requiring permanent nursing home placement.[49] Postmenopausal women are particularly susceptible to osteoporosis, as bone loss occurs most rapidly in the first five years after menopause. During this time, up to 15% of bone density may be lost. In addition to menopause, other risk factors include white or Asian race, low body weight, family history, and smoking.

Osteoporosis is the result of an imbalance between bone formation and bone resorption. Estrogen plays an antiresorptive role, the exact mechanism of which is unknown. Estrogen receptors have been localized on both osteoblasts and osteoclasts. Postmenopausal bone loss is thus related to the decline in estrogen, with an ensuing increase in bone resorption. This bone loss may occur at a rate of 2-5% per year for up to five years and then decreases to about 1% per year.[50] Cancellous bone found in the spine and wrist is predominantly affected.

Screening. Screening for osteoporosis should begin at the first office visit in a perimenopausal woman. A thorough history of all risk factors should be obtained. The physician should also measure height on an annual basis, as loss of height is often an early sign of osteoporosis. A loss of a half inch or more is an indication for concern.

Measurement of bone mineral density (BMD) is an important tool for assessing the risk of future fracture for a woman. Dual-energy X-ray absorptiometry (DEXA) scanning is the most common method used for this measurement. The test is easy to perform, uses little radiation, is cheap (on the order of $200), and takes approximately 10 minutes. According to World Health Organization criteria, BMD is classified according to the DEXA T-score as normal (T-score > -1), osteopenic (T-score between -1 and -2.5), or osteoporotic (T-score ≤ -2.5).[51] While appealing in thought, DEXA scanning has not yet been proven to be cost-effective for the universal screening of women. Most experts recommend measuring BMD in women at menopause if they have one or more risk factors for osteoporosis, if they are undecided about HRT, if incidental osteopenia is found by x-ray, or if they present with a fracture *(please see Table 4)*. A study looking at the influence of bone densitometry on women's decisions about HRT found that women who were diagnosed with low BMD were more likely than normal women to begin some measure to prevent fractures (94% vs 56%; $P < 0.01$) and more likely to start HRT (38% vs 8%; $P < 0.01$).[52]

Table 4. Indications for Bone Density Measurement in Perimenopausal Women

- One or more risk factors for osteoporosis
- Aid in decision about hormone replacement therapy
- Osteopenia found incidentally by x-ray
- Presentation with fracture

Management. Perimenopausal women should be counseled about the rapid bone loss associated with menopause. Since osteoporosis is a clinically silent disease until fracture occurs, most women do not pay enough attention to its prevention. Physicians should advise women about the bone-preserving effects of exercise. Weight-bearing exercises, such as jogging or stair-climbing, are most beneficial. Other modifiable risk factors, such as smoking or heavy alcohol use, should also be addressed.

Ensuring that perimenopausal women are receiving enough calcium is critical. According to National Osteoporosis Foundation (NOF) guidelines, all women (pre- and postmenopausal) should consume 1000 mg of elemental calcium a day. Postmenopausal women not taking estrogen, women older than 65 years, and women with a diagnosis of osteoporosis should receive 1500 mg of calcium per day. Foods rich in calcium include dairy products, dark green vegetables, sardines, salmon, and nuts. If a woman's diet is inadequate, calcium supplements should be prescribed. Calcium carbonate is least expensive, but for women who have chronic gastrointestinal illnesses or who are taking antacids, calcium citrate is better absorbed.

Recommendations regarding dietary intake of vitamin D suggest perimenopausal women should receive at least 400 IU per day. Supplementation is generally not necessary in most women but should be considered in patients with malabsorption syndromes or who lack adequate exposure to sunlight (housebound or nursing home residents). Women with diagnosed osteoporosis should have 800 IU of vitamin D per day.

Further management of perimenopausal bone loss must take into account other risk factors, including the BMD if measured. Preventive therapy should be administered in any woman at significant risk. A T-score of -1.5 or less on DEXA scanning is no longer an indication for prevention, but for active treatment (NOF guidelines). This discussion will focus primarily on prevention.

For prevention in a high-risk woman, strong consideration should be given to estrogen replacement, as it prevents bone loss and may even increase bone mass by a few percentage points when started at menopause. Long-term use (at least 7-10 years) results in a decrease in the osteoporotic fracture rate by 50%.[53] All forms of estrogen seem to be effective. For women who cannot tolerate usual doses of esterified estrogens (0.625 mg), smaller doses (0.3 mg) were recently shown to be effective in preserving BMD.[54] Unfortunately, if estrogen is discontinued, its protective effect on bone slowly wanes.

For women unable to take HRT but at significantly high risk of osteoporosis, other preventive therapies are available. Raloxifene, a selective estrogen-receptor modulator, is a promising alternative. When given at 60 mg per day, it has been shown to result in a 2.5% greater BMD compared to placebo at two years.[55] Other useful agents are the bisphosphonates, which act by inhibiting bone resorption. These medications are effective and are usually considered second-line therapies in women who cannot tolerate estrogens. A 5 mg daily dose of alendronate was shown to prevent bone loss and actually increase BMD by up to 3.5% at two years.[56] In osteoporotic patients, a 10 mg dose of alendronate will increase bone density up to 9% at three years with a concomitant decrease in vertebral fractures by 44%.[57] Risedronate is a newer bisphosphonate that appears to be equally efficacious, but FDA approval is pending at the time of this writing. Finally, calcitonin administered nasally at a dose of 200 IU q.d. is a safe and well-tolerated alternative. Although considered somewhat weaker than the other agents discussed above, postmenopausal women experienced an increase in BMD of 2% at two years.[58] It is reasonable to combine HRT with bisphosphonates or calcitonin in patients at significant risk, but definitive data have not yet been published documenting additive benefits.

Additional Information

Patients frequently request additional sources of information for further reading. The following are several resources particularly helpful to patients:

1. *Menopause Guidebook*. Obtained through: The North American Menopause Society, P.O. Box 94527, Cleveland, OH 44101-4527.
2. www.menopause.org
3. www.discoveryhealth.com
4. www.drkoop.com
5. www.nof.com
6. www.mediconsult.com

References

1. Keating NL, et al. Use of hormone replacement therapy by postmenopausal women in the United States. *Ann Intern Med* 1999;130:545-553.
2. Anderson E, et al. Characteristics of menopausal women seeking assistance. *Am J Obstet Gynecol* 1987;156:428-433.
3. Berg G, et al. Climacteric symptoms among women aged 60-62 in Linkoping, Sweden, in 1986. *Maturitas* 1988;10:193-199.
4. McKinlay SM, Jefferys M. The menopausal syndrome. *Br J Prev Soc Med* 1974;28:108-115.
5. Thompson B, et al. Menopausal age and symptomatology in a general practice. *J Biosoc Sci* 1973;5:71-82.
6. Tang GW. The climacteric of Chinese factory workers. *Maturitas* 1994;19:177-182.
7. Barbo DM. Menopause. In: Wallis LA, et al, eds. *Textbook of Women's Health*. Philadelphia, PA: Lippincott-Raven Publishers; 1998:721-729.
8. Fox SC, Wallis LA. Transition at menopause. In: Wallis LA, et al, eds. *Textbook of Women's Health*. Philadelphia, PA: Lippincott-Raven Publishers; 1998:117-123.
9. Wardlaw SL, et al. β-Endorphin in hypophyseal portal blood: Variations throughout the menstrual cycle. *Endocrinology* 1982;111:879-882.
10. Wyon Y, et al. Postmenopausal women with vasomotor symptoms have increased urinary excretion of calcitonin gene-related peptide. *Maturitas* 1998;30:289-294.
11. Tataryn IV, et al. Objective techniques for the assessment of postmenopausal hot flashes. *Obstet Gynecol* 1981;57:340-344.
12. Clayden JR, et al. Menopausal flushing: Double-blind trial of a nonhormonal medication. *BMJ* 1974;1:409-412.
13. Polo-Kantola P, et al. When does estrogen replacement therapy improve sleep quality? *Am J Obstet Gynecol* 1998;178:1002-1009.
14. Steingold KA, et al. Treatment of hot flashes with transdermal estradiol administration. *J Clin Endocrinol Metab* 1985;61:627-632.
15. Utian WH, et al. Efficacy and safety of low, standard, and high dosages of an estradiol transdermal system (Esclim) compared with placebo on vasomotor symptoms in highly symptomatic menopausal patients. *Am J Obstet Gynecol* 1999;181:71-79.
16. Haas S, et al. The effect of transdermal estradiol on hormone and metabolic dynamics over a six-week period. *Obstet Gynecol* 1995;85:529-537.
17. Belchetz PE. Hormonal treatment of postmenopausal women. *N Engl J Med* 1994;330:1062-1070.
18. Laufer LR, et al. Effect of clonidine on hot flashes in postmenopausal women. *Obstet Gynecol* 1982;60:583-586.
19. Simon J, et al. Differential effects of estrogen-androgen and estrogen-only therapy on vasomotor symptoms, gonadotropin secretion, and endogenous androgen bioavailability in postmenopausal women. *Menopause* 1999;6:138-146.
20. Melis GB, et al. Effects of the dopamine antagonist veralipride on hot flushes and luteinizing hormone secretion in postmenopausal women. *Obstet Gynecol* 1988;72:688-692.
21. Egarter C, et al. Efficacy, tolerability, and rare side effects of tibolone treatment in postmenopausal women. *Int J Gynecol Obstet* 1999;64:281-286.
22. Albrecht BH, et al. Objective evidence that placebo and oral medroxyprogesterone acetate therapy diminish menopausal vasomotor flushes. *Am J Obset Gynecol* 1981;139:631-635.
23. Morrison JC, et al. The use of medroxyprogesterone acetate for relief of climacteric symptoms. *Obset Gynecol* 1980;138:99-104.
24. Leonetti HB, et al. Transdermal progesterone cream for vasomotor symptoms and postmenopausal bone loss. *Obstet*

Gynecol 1999;94:225-228.
25. Washburn S, et al. Effect of soy protein supplementation on serum lipoproteins, blood pressure, and menopausal symptoms in perimenopausal women. *Menopause* 1999;6:7-13.
26. Hofseth LJ, et al. Hormone replacement therapy with estrogen or estrogen plus medroxyprogesterone acetate is associated with increased epithelial proliferation in the normal postmenopausal breast. *J Clin Endocrinol Metab* 1999;84:4559-4565.
27. Leung W, et al. Mammographic density in women on postmenopausal hormone replacement therapy. *Surgery* 1997;122:669-673.
28. Iosif CS, Becassy Z. Prevalence of genitourinary symptoms in the late menopause. *Acta Obstet Gynecol Scand* 1984;63: 257-260.
29. Semmens JP, Wagner G. Estrogen deprivation and vaginal function in postmenopausal women. *JAMA* 1982;248:445-448.
30. Iosif CS, et al. Estrogen receptors in the female urinary tract. *Am J Obstet Gynecol* 1981;141:817-820.
31. Smith P, et al. Steroid hormone receptors in pelvic muscles and ligaments in women. *Gynecol Obstet Invest* 1990;30: 27-30.
32. Sarrel PM. Sexuality and menopause. *Obstet Gynecol* 1990; 75:26S-32S.
33. Elia G, Bergman A. Estrogen effects on the urethra: Beneficial effects in women with genuine stress incontinence. *Obstet Gynecol Survey* 1993;48:509-517.
34. Fantl JA, et al, and The Hormones and Urogenital Therapy Committee. Estrogen therapy in the management of urinary incontinence in postmenopausal women: A meta-analysis. First report of the Hormones and Urogenital Therapy Committee. *Obstet Gynecol* 1994;83:12-18.
35. Bjaren E. A randomized, open, parallel-group study on the preventive effect of an estradiol vaginal ring (Estring) on recurrent urinary tract infections in postmenopausal women. *Am J Obstet Gynecol* 1999;180:1072-1079.
36. Avorn J, et al. Reduction of bacteriuria and pyuria after ingestion of cranberry juice. *JAMA* 1994;271:751-754.
37. Heimer G, Samsioe G. Effects of vaginally delivered estrogens. *Acta Obstet Gynecol Scand* 1996;(S163)75:1-2.
38. Henriksson L, et al. A comparative multicenter study of the effects of continuous low-dose estradiol released from a new vaginal ring versus estriol vaginal pessaries in postmenopausal women with symptoms and signs of urogenital atrophy. *Am J Obstet Gynecol* 1994;171:624-632.
39. Bachmann G. The estradiol vaginal ring—A study of existing clinical data. *Maturitas* 1995;S22:S21-S29.
40. Barentsen R, et al. Continuous low dose estradiol released from a vaginal ring versus estriol vaginal cream for urogenital atrophy. *Eur J Obstet Gynecol Reprod Biol* 1997; 71:73-80.
41. Eriksen PS, Rasmussen H. Low dose 17b-estradiol vaginal tablets in the treatment of atrophic vaginitis: A double-blind placebo controlled study. *Eur J Obstet Gynecol Reprod Biol* 1992;44:137-144.
42. Bachmann GA, et al. Vaginal dryness in menopausal women: Clinical characteristics and non-hormonal treatment. *Clin Pract Sexuality* 1991;7:25-32.
43. Bygdeman M, Swahn ML. Replens versus dienoestrol cream in the symptomatic treatment of vaginal atrophy in postmenopausal women. *Maturitas* 1996;23:259-263.
44. Avis NE, et al. A longitudinal analysis of the association between menopause and depression. Results from the Massachusetts Women's Health Study. *Ann Epidemiol* 1994; 4:214-220.
45. Davis SR, et al. Testosterone enhances estradiol's effects on postmenopausal bone density and sexuality. *Maturitas* 1995;21:227-236.
46. Yaffe K, et al. Estrogen therapy in postmenopausal women: Effects on cognitive function and dementia. *JAMA* 1998; 279:688-695.
47. Mulnard RA, et al. Estrogen replacement therapy for treatment of mild to moderate Alzheimer disease. A randomized controlled trial. *JAMA* 2000;283:1007-1015.
48. Ray NF, et al. Medical expenditures for the treatment of osteoporotic fractures in the United States in 1995: Report from the National Osteoporosis Foundation. *J Bone Miner Res* 1997;12:24-35.
49. Barrett-Connor E. The economic and human costs of osteoporotic fracture. *Am J Med* 1995;98:3S-8S.
50. Riggs BL, et al. Differential changes in bone mineral density of the appendicular and axial skeleton with aging: Relationship to spinal osteoporosis. *J Clin Invest* 1981;67: 328-335.
51. WHO Study Group. Assessment of fracture risk and its application to screening for postmenopausal osteoporosis: Report of a WHO Study Group. WHO Technical Report Series 843, Geneva, Switzerland: World Health Organization. 1994;1-129.
52. Rubin SM, Cummings SR. Results of bone densitometry affect women's decisions about taking measures to prevent fractures. *Ann Intern Med* 1992;166:990-995.
53. Weiss NS, et al. Decreased risk of fractures of the hip and lower forearm with postmenopausal use of estrogen. *N Engl J Med* 1980;303:1195-1198.
54. Genant HK, et al. Low-dose esterified estrogen therapy: Effects on bone, plasma estradiol concentrations, endometrium, and lipid levels. *Arch Intern Med* 1997;157: 2609-2615.
55. Delmas PD, et al. Effects of raloxifene on bone mineral density, serum cholesterol concentrations, and uterine endometrium in postmenopausal women. *N Engl J Med* 1997;337:1641-1647.
56. Hosking D, et al. Prevention of bone loss with alendronate in postmenopausal women under 60 years of age. *N Engl J Med* 1998;338:485-492.
57. Cummings SR, et al. Effect of alendronate on risk of fracture in women with low bone density but without vertebral fractures: Results from the Fracture Intervention Trial. *JAMA* 1998;280:2077-2082.
58. Reginster JY, et al. A double-blind, placebo-controlled, dose-finding trial of intermittent nasal salmon calcitonin for prevention of postmenopausal lumbar spine bone loss. *Am J Med* 1995;98:452-458.

Obstet Gynecol 1996;[illegible]

26. [illegible] S, et al. Effect of soy protein supplementation on [illegible] lipoproteins, blood pressures, and menopausal symptoms in perimenopausal women. Menopause [illegible]
27. [illegible] L, et al. Hormone replacement therapy with estrogen or estrogen plus medroxyprogesterone acetate associated with increased epithelial proliferation in the [illegible] postmenopausal breast. J Clin Endocrinol Metab 1999;84:[illegible]
27. [illegible] W, et al. [illegible] density in women on [illegible] postmenopausal hormone replacement therapy. [illegible] 1997;[illegible]
28. [illegible] C, et al. Prevalence of genitourinary symptoms in the late menopause. Acta Obstet Gynecol Scand 19[illegible]
29. [illegible] R, Wexler [illegible]. Estrogen deprivation and vaginal function in postmenopausal women. JAMA 1982;248:445-[illegible]
30. [illegible] C, et al. Estrogen receptors in the female urinary tract. J Urol Clin [illegible] 1981;[illegible]
31. [illegible] P, et al. [illegible] hormone receptors in pelvic muscles and ligaments in women. [illegible] 1990;[illegible]
32. [illegible] PM. [illegible] and menopause. Obstet Gynecol 1990;75:[illegible]
33. [illegible] O, Bergman A. Estrogen effects on the urethra: beneficial effects in women with genuine stress incontinence. Obstet Gynecol [illegible]
34. [illegible] P, et al. The [illegible] Therapy Committee. Estrogen therapy in the management of urinary incontinence in postmenopausal women: a meta-analysis. First report of the Hormones and Urogenital Therapy Committee. Obstet Gynecol 1994;83:[illegible]
35. [illegible] P. A randomized, open, parallel-group study on the preventive effect of an estradiol-releasing vaginal ring (Estring) on recurrent urinary tract infections in postmenopausal women. Am J Obstet Gynecol 1999;180:1072-1079.
36. [illegible] L, et al. [illegible] of bacteriuria and pyuria after ingestion of cranberry juice. JAMA 1994;271:[illegible]
37. Henriksson L, [illegible]. Effects of a vaginally delivered estrogen [illegible]. [illegible] 1996;[illegible]
38. Henriksson L, et al. A comparative multicenter study of the effects of continuous low-dose estradiol released from a new vaginal ring versus estriol vaginal pessaries in postmenopausal women with symptoms and signs of urogenital atrophy. Am J Obstet Gynecol [illegible]
39. [illegible] The estradiol vaginal ring: a study of existing clinical data. Maturitas 1995;22:[illegible]
40. [illegible] Low dose estradiol releasing vaginal ring versus estriol [illegible] in the treatment of urogenital atrophy. [illegible]
41. [illegible] PS, [illegible]. [illegible] treatment of vaginal [illegible] [illegible] vaginitis: A double-blind placebo-controlled study. [illegible]
42. Bachmann [illegible] vaginal [illegible] in menopausal women: [illegible] characteristics and [illegible] hormonal [illegible]. [illegible]
43. Bachmann G, Notelovitz M, Kelly S, et al. Long-term non-hormonal treatment of the symptomatic treatment of vaginal atrophy in postmenopausal women. Maturitas 1996;23:[illegible]
44. Avis NE, et al. A universal menopausal syndrome? [illegible] association between menopause and depression. Results from the Massachusetts Women's Health Study. Ann Epidemiol 1994;4:214-220.
45. Davis SR, et al. Testosterone enhances estradiol's effects on postmenopausal bone density and sexuality. Maturitas 1995;21:[illegible]
46. [illegible] K, et al. Estrogen therapy in postmenopausal women. Effects on cognitive function and dementia. JAMA 1998;279:[illegible]
47. Mulnard RA, et al. Estrogen replacement therapy for treatment of mild to moderate Alzheimer disease: a randomized controlled trial. JAMA 2000;283:1007-1015.
48. Ray NF, et al. Medical expenditures for the treatment of osteoporotic fractures in the United States in 1995: Report from the National Osteoporosis Foundation. J Bone Miner Res 1997;12:24-35.
49. Barrett-Connor E. The economic and human costs of osteoporotic fracture. Am J Med 1995;98:3-8S.
50. Riggs BL, et al. Differential changes in bone mineral density of the appendicular and axial skeleton with aging: Relationship to spinal osteoporosis. J Clin Invest 1981;67:328-335.
51. WHO Study Group. Assessment of fracture risk and its application to screening for postmenopausal osteoporosis: Report of a WHO Study Group. WHO Technical Report Series 843. Geneva, Switzerland: World Health Organization, 1994:1-129.
52. Rubin SM, Cummings SR. Results of bone densitometry affect women's decisions about taking measures to prevent fractures. Ann Intern Med 1992;116:990-995.
53. Weiss NS, et al. Decreased risk of fractures of the hip and lower forearm with postmenopausal use of estrogen. N Engl J Med 1980;303:1195-1198.
54. Genant HK, et al. Low-dose esterified estrogen therapy: Effects on bone, plasma estradiol concentrations, endometrium, and lipid levels. Arch Intern Med 1997;157:2609-2615.
55. Delmas PD, et al. Effects of raloxifene on bone mineral density, serum cholesterol concentrations, and uterine endometrium in postmenopausal women. N Engl J Med 1997;337:1641-1647.
56. Hosking D, et al. Prevention of bone loss with alendronate in postmenopausal women under 60 years of age. N Engl J Med 1998;338:485-492.
57. Cummings SR, et al. Effect of alendronate on risk of fracture in women with low bone density but without vertebral fractures: Results from the Fracture Intervention Trial. JAMA 1998;280:2077-2082.
58. Reginster JY, et al. A double-blind, placebo-controlled, dose-finding trial of intermittent nasal salmon calcitonin for prevention of postmenopausal lumbar spine bone loss. Am J Med 1995;98:452-458.

Management of the Menopausal Patient: Part II

Redonda Miller, MD
Katherine K. Chang, MD

The menopause presents a unique set of challenges to both patient and physician alike. Patients must adjust to the physical and psychological changes in their bodies brought on by the fall in estradiol levels, while physicians must go beyond simple reassurance and advise patients on the pros and cons of various forms of treatment.

Many women are aware of the potential beneficial effects of hormone replacement therapy (HRT) on bone density, but fewer recognize its cardioprotective role in addressing the increased risk of coronary heart disease that accompanies menopause. Any discussion of HRT must take into account these and other advantages but must also not ignore potential disadvantages. With the advent of the Internet, patients' access to many sources of information (and misinformation) has grown tremendously; it is the duty of the primary care physician to provide accurate and reliable recommendations to help women decide whether HRT is right for them. The decision also must factor in the newer agents available to women, including the selective estrogen receptor modulators (SERMs) and phytoestrogens.

In the last chapter, an introduction to the physiology and clinical manifestations of menopause was given. Part II continues that discussion with a review of the cardiovascular changes during menopause and the importance of recognizing premature ovarian failure. The authors conclude with an overview of the various options for treatment and a decision-making approach for the primary care physician.

Cardiovascular Effects

Coronary heart disease (CHD) is the leading cause of mortality for women in America; menopause, both natural and surgical, is associated with an increase in the risk for CHD. In fact, the relative risk for CHD in postmenopausal women compared to age-matched premenopausal women is 2.7[1]; estrogen replacement therapy lowers the risk of developing and dying from CHD by 50%.[2]

Cardiovascular Changes with Menopause

With the decline of estrogen levels during menopause, several changes occur that serve to increase cardiovascular risk. One easily recognizable effect is the conversion to a more atherogenic lipid profile. Within six months of the cessation of menses, total cholesterol, LDL cholesterol, and triglycerides increase significantly. Conversely, HDL cholesterol shows a gradual decline over the two years preceding cessation of menses.[3] HDL has been shown to be particularly protective in women, and low serum HDL levels are strong predictors of CHD death in women, more so than elevated LDL and total cholesterol levels.[4] After adjusting for other cardiac risk factors, women with HDL levels of less than 50 mg/dL have a relative risk of 1.74 for death from CHD.[4]

In addition, a higher level of plasminogen-activator inhibitor type 1 (PAI-1), an essential inhibitor of fibrinolysis, is found in postmenopausal women compared to premenopausal women.[5] Studies have shown that increased plasma levels of PAI-1 are associated with a higher risk of atherosclerosis and subsequent myocardial infarction and stroke.[6]

Finally, both lipoprotein (a) and homocysteine levels are increased in the plasma of postmenopausal women.[7] Each is believed to be an independent risk factor for atherosclerotic disease. Increased plasma homocysteine confers a risk for CHD similar to smoking or hyperlipidemia and powerfully increases the risks associated with smoking and hypertension.[8]

While blood pressure and weight also have an effect on cardiovascular health, these do not change appreciably during the menopause.[9]

Hormone Replacement Therapy and Cardioprotection

Numerous epidemiological studies have found that, in primary prevention settings, a reduced risk of CHD exists in postmenopausal women who use HRT. In patients with existing CHD, the issue is murkier. Estrogen does not seem to have any significant influence on stroke incidence.[10]

One mechanism of cardioprotection is through alterations in the lipid profile. Oral estrogen replacement therapy in standard doses reverses the adverse lipid effects of menopause, increasing HDL levels by 13-18% and decreasing LDL levels by 11-19%.[11] Higher daily doses of estrogen do not substantially enhance these effects,[12] which generally occur within six months of beginning therapy. The increase in HDL may account for up to 50% of the CHD risk reduction afforded by estrogen therapy.[13] Transdermal estradiol produces similar, but more moderate lipid profile changes, as would be expected by a route of administration that lacks hepatic first-pass metabolism and its direct effects on cholesterol synthesis. Of note, oral conjugated estrogen therapy does increase serum triglycerides in a dose-dependent manner, which may be of concern in treating women who already have high levels.[11]

Oral conjugated estrogen, either alone or combined with progestin therapy, reduces plasma PAI-1, lipoprotein (a), and total homocysteine levels.[13-15] Estrogen may also have other lipid-independent cardioprotective effects, including vasodilation, alteration of cholesterol metabolism and deposition, and calcium antagonism.

Progestins, as a class, increase LDL and decrease HDL. Accordingly, estrogen's beneficial effect on LDL and HDL is attenuated with the addition of progestins to HRT.[10] Micronized progesterone may be less detrimental than other forms of progestins.[9] Despite the consequences on the lipid profile, observational studies suggest that the cardioprotective effects of postmenopausal estrogen combined with progestins in primary prevention remain.[16]

The role of estrogen in secondary prevention of CHD is more controversial. Observational data have suggested a positive effect of estrogen on survival in established CHD patients.[17] However, the only randomized trial to date looking at combination HRT as secondary prevention for CHD—the recent Heart and Estrogen/Progestin Replacement Study (HERS)—did not show a positive effect.[18] After an average follow-up of four years, researchers found an early increase in cardiovascular events and no overall cardiovascular benefit, leading to a recommendation of not starting HRT for secondary prevention of CHD. Yet, after the initial increase in risk during the first year of therapy, possibly due to an immediate prothrombotic effect, risk decreased in subsequent years, suggesting a possible long-term benefit. This study has tempered enthusiasm for estrogen use in secondary prevention, and it will be important to follow further reports from the HERS group and additional randomized trials to better assess true cardiovascular benefit from HRT.

Premature Ovarian Failure

Premature ovarian failure is defined as loss of ovarian function before the age of 40 and is more common than most physicians realize. Up to 1% of women may be affected.[19] There are many causes of premature ovarian failure, including Turner's syndrome; autoimmune disorders such as rheumatoid arthritis, systemic lupus erythematosis, and myasthenia gravis; and physical insults such as surgery, chemotherapy, or radiation therapy. Some cases remain idiopathic. Women who undergo premature menopause have more severe vasomotor symptoms and more significant impairment of sexual functioning. Because these women will spend a significantly larger proportion of their lives without estrogen, they are at markedly increased risk for osteoporosis and heart disease. These women should universally be started on HRT and continued at least until the natural age of menopause (50 years of age) to prevent long-term health consequences.

Hormone Replacement Therapy Considerations: Advantages of HRT

There are many advantages of HRT *(please see Table 1)*. The most obvious to the patient is the relief of vasomotor symptoms and vaginal dryness. Perhaps even more important is the role estrogen plays in the prevention of chronic diseases. It is well documented that the use of estrogen at menopause prevents bone loss. In osteoporotic patients, bone density may even increase up to 5% per year for several years, and the hip fracture rate may decline by 50%. Estrogen also affords a 50% reduction in cardiac events, the leading cause of death among women. Each of these is discussed in the earlier sections.

Disadvantages of HRT

Despite the many positive effects of HRT, physicians must also be aware of the disadvantages *(please see Table 1)*. When confronted with the choice of using HRT, most women claim that their biggest fear is the possible increased risk of breast cancer. Numerous epidemiological studies have tried to address this issue with conflicting results, and no one study is definitive. The Nurses' Health Study[20] suggested that the relative risk of breast cancer for women currently using estrogen is 1.3, which translates into a 30%

Table 1. Advantages and Disadvantages of HRT

Advantages of HRT

- relief of vasomotor symptoms
- decrease in vaginal dryness
- stabilization ± increase in bone density
- improved lipid profile
- decrease in cardiovascular risk

Disadvantages of HRT

- breast tenderness
- vaginal spotting
- increased risk of gallstones
- increased risk of thromboembolic disease
- questionable increased risk of breast cancer

increase in risk. Risk was related to the duration of use, with use over 5-10 years being more significant. No increased risk was found in past users. On the other hand, the Iowa study found that women with a family history of breast cancer who used HRT did not have a significantly increased incidence of breast cancer, even with use of more than five years.[21] Despite the questionable increased risk, all studies (except one)[20] examining mortality from breast cancer in hormone users have documented lower mortality for women on HRT. This may reflect earlier diagnosis in HRT users who are more likely to have regular mammograms, or that estrogen exposure results in better differentiated tumors that are less aggressive.[21,22]

In women with a uterus, more than two decades of evidence have linked the use of unopposed estrogen with adenocarcinoma of the endometrium. A recent meta-analysis estimated this risk to be 2.3 times that of nonusers. With 10 or more years of exposure, the relative risk climbed to 9.5 and remained elevated five years after discontinuation.[23] Adding a progestin negates this risk to that of placebo[24] and should be considered standard in nonhysterectomized women. While some irregular bleeding is anticipated with initiation of continuous HRT, any woman who continues to have irregular bleeding at 6-8 months should undergo further work-up, including possible transvaginal ultrasound and endometrial biopsy. Likewise, any late-onset uterine bleeding warrants evaluation.

Unlike oral contraceptives, HRT is associated with only a small increase in the risk of venous thromboembolism, predominantly in current users. The risk is estimated to be 2.5-3.5 times that of nonusers.[18,25] This is usually not considered to be a deterrent to HRT use.

Women who use HRT are at a modestly increased risk of gallbladder disease.[18] This is presumed to be related to estrogen's ability to enhance uptake and turnover of cholesterol in the liver. Cholesterol concentration is then increased in the bile, leading to a

Table 2. Contraindications to Hormone Replacement Therapy

Absolute

- Personal history of breast cancer
- Acute thromboembolic disease

Relative

- Strong family history of breast cancer
- Unexplained vaginal bleeding
- Past history of thromboembolic disease
- Chronic hepatitis

greater chance of stone formation. Mortality from gallbladder disease is not increased in HRT users.

Minor side effects include breast tenderness and breakthrough vaginal bleeding, which are often short-lived. Less well-substantiated are reports of weight gain, nausea, and headaches.

Despite these disadvantages, the absolute contraindications to HRT are relatively few *(please see Table 2)*. Most experts would agree that a personal history of breast cancer or acute thromboembolic disease falls into this category. Other conditions formerly thought to be contraindications, however, are being re-evaluated in light of the increasingly documented benefits of estrogen.

Methods of Delivery

There are several methods of delivery of hormone replacement for postmenopausal women *(please see Table 3)*. Each has unique features that may make one method more attractive than another for the individual patient. In women who have undergone hysterectomy, estrogen may be administered alone without a progestin. Currently available preparations provide oral, transdermal, or vaginal delivery. Orally, conjugated estrogens are the most widely used and studied. These are less potent than the ethinyl estradiol found in oral contraceptives but are adequate to restore physiologic status. Transdermal estrogen provides a convenient option for women since it may be applied only one or two times per week. The drawback of the transdermal route is the less beneficial effect on the lipid profile since first-pass metabolism through the liver is lost. However, this may be desirable in women with chronic liver disease or high triglyceride levels. Vaginally applied estrogens are useful to ameliorate vaginal dryness, but they lack systemic effects and, therefore, do not prevent bone density loss or provide cardioprotection.

In a patient with an intact uterus, estrogen must be administered with a progestin (synthetic progesterone) to prevent endometrial hyperplasia and possible adenocarcinoma.[24] Medroxyprogesterone acetate is commonly used because its androgenic activity is weaker than other progesterone derivatives. The progestin may be added in one of several ways. It may be given in a cyclical fashion, resulting in periodic sloughing of the endometrium. If done in this fashion, it is usually given on days 16-25 of a woman's cycle. In 70-90% of cases, women find the continued monthly menses associated with cycling to be inconvenient. Alternatively, progestin may be delivered on a continuous basis as medroxyprogesterone acetate 2.5 mg q.d. Regardless of method, the addition of a progestin to estrogen counteracts some of the positive effects on the lipid profile. In particular, HDL cholesterol is not increased as much, but significant benefit remains compared to placebo.[9] Micronized progesterone, a newer and less widely available preparation, can be delivered continuously or cyclically, and seems to result in less detrimental changes in the lipid profile. It is well tolerated and still maintains its protective effects on the uterus.[9]

Some physicians have advocated adding androgens to HRT for menopausal women, particularly if they experience diminished libido, cognitive difficulties, or low mood. Small studies have suggested some effect,[26] but large randomized clinical trials are lacking. Adding an androgen does not diminish the ability of estrogen to relieve vasomotor symptoms or increase bone density.[27] In contrast to standard HRT, however, HDL cholesterol decreases with the addition of testosterone, which may have a bearing on long-term cardioprotection in women. Other potential side effects include acne, hirsutism, weight gain, and aggressiveness, although these have mainly been reported with higher doses. An oral combination preparation of esterified estrogens and methyltestosterone is now available (Estratest). Progestin must still be given in a woman with a uterus.

Selective Estrogen Receptor Modulators

Selective estrogen receptor modulators (SERMs) are a relatively new class of drugs being used for HRT. These drugs bind to the estrogen receptor and have both agonist and antagonist effects, depending on the target organ.[28] Tamoxifen is a first-generation SERM that was approved by the FDA in 1969. Because it blocks the effect of estrogen on the breast, it has been used extensively as adjuvant therapy for prevention of receptor-positive breast cancer recurrence. Drawbacks include the onset or worsening of hot flashes, endometrial hyperplasia with the attendant risk of neoplasia, and increased risk of thrombosis. Other SERMs under development include droloxifene and toremifene, each with varying levels of

Table 3. Forms of Hormone Replacement Therapy

FORM OF HRT	DOSE	COMMENTS
Estrogens	conjugated: 0.625 mg po qd esterified: 0.625 mg po qd estradiol: 1 mg po qd estropipate: 0.625 mg po qd	• use only in hysterectomized women • initial breast tenderness • benefits: improvement in vasomotor sxs; relief of vaginal dryness; cardio protection; osteoporosis prevention
Cyclical estrogens and progestin combination alone	estrogen: one of the above preparations on days 1-25 AND medroxyprogesterone: 10 mg po qd on days 16-25 OR miconized progesterone: 200 mg po qd on days 16-25	• monthly withdrawal bleeding • benefits comparable to estrogen
Continuous conjugated estrogens and progestin alone **combination**	estrogen: one of the above po qd AND medroxyprogesterone: 2.5-5 mg po qd OR miconized progesterone: 100 mg po qd	• vaginal spotting • benefits comparable to estrogen
Transdermal estrogen	estradiol: 0.05-0.1 mg topically 1-2 × per week	• use only in hysterectomized women or must add a progestin • easier for compliance • less benefit on lipid profile • less risk in patients with liver disease
Estrogen and androgen combination	esterified estrogens and methyltestosterone: 0.625/1.25 mg po qd	• ? benefit on libido • must add a progestin in women with a uterus

Table 4. Estrogen vs. Raloxifene for HRT

	Estrogen	Raloxifene
Hot flashes	↓	0 or ↑
Breast tenderness	↑	0
Uterine hyperplasia and bleeding	↑	0
Cholesterol:		
HDL	↑	0
LDL	↓	↓
Bone mineral density	↑↑	↑
Venous thromboembolism	↑	↑

estrogen agonist and antagonist properties.

Raloxifene is a newer generation SERM that has received a lot of attention for use as HRT in postmenopausal women. At a dose of 60 mg q.d., raloxifene provides estrogenic effects on the bone and lipid profile, and antiestrogenic effects on the breast and endometrium. Similar to estrogen, raloxifene inhibits bone resorption primarily in cancellous bone. On average, at two years women gain 2-3% in bone mineral density over placebo[29,30] and have a relative risk of vertebral fracture of 0.7 compared with controls.[30] In addition, raloxifene decreases total and LDL cholesterol but has no effect on HDL and triglycerides. No studies have yet documented the vasodilatory effects that estrogen has or whether a long-term benefit on cardiovascular outcomes exists.

Regarding its antiestrogenic properties, raloxifene has no effect on endometrial thickness as measured by transvaginal ultrasound,[29] and the incidence of uterine bleeding appears to be less with raloxifene than with estrogen. Recent data demonstrated the protective effect of raloxifene on breast tissue in postmenopausal women. In a randomized, placebo-controlled trial, the risk of invasive breast cancer was reduced by 76% over three years in women on raloxifene.[31] Trials are currently under way comparing tamoxifen and raloxifene for prevention of breast cancer recurrence. Not surprisingly, raloxifene's antiestrogenic effect on the breast leads to less breast tenderness than estrogen.

Drawbacks of raloxifene include the lack of relief of vasomotor symptoms, with persistent (and possible worsening of) hot flashes in menopausal women, and the failure to raise HDL cholesterol. The risk of venous thromboembolic disease is also increased threefold, similar to estrogen.[28]

Overall, raloxifene provides many benefits to postmenopausal women, but, at this time, estrogen remains the first choice for most women in the perimenopause *(please see Table 4)*. Increases in bone density are significant but do not appear to be as great as with estrogen, and long-term cardiac benefits are not yet known. A direct comparison between raloxifene and estrogen has not been published. Thus, raloxifene should serve as a useful alternative for women who cannot tolerate or prefer not to take estrogen.

Phytoestrogens

Phytoestrogens are naturally occurring plant-based substances with weak estrogenic effects. The most common forms are isoflavones, found in soybeans and soy products, and lignans, found in flaxseed, vegetables, legumes, and cereals. The clinical importance of the estrogenic effects of these compounds is debated, although more data suggesting some efficacy are accumulating. A recent study found that perimenopausal women given a daily dietary soy supplement had a 45% reduction in daily hot flushes at 12 weeks compared to a 30% reduction in the placebo arm.[32] Regarding potential benefits on the lipid profile, a meta-analysis of 38 controlled clinical trials found that the consumption of soy protein rather than animal protein resulted in significantly decreased levels of total cholesterol, LDL cholesterol, and triglycerides.[33] One concern with these compounds is whether high intake may result in endometrial hyperplasia in women with a uterus, similar to the effect of unopposed estrogen. More data are needed before these compounds can be recommended as a replacement for long-term HRT.

Deciding with Individual Patients

For each menopausal woman, the choice of whether to pursue HRT is a personal one. They should be aware that, despite the many benefits of HRT, up to 20% of women prescribed estrogen for the first time discontinue it during the first year, 10% use it intermittently, and up to 30% never have the prescription filled.[34] Common reasons for discontinuation include intolerance of side effects such as breast tenderness and vaginal spotting, as well as fear of breast cancer.

HRT should not be a universal recommendation. The benefits and risks associated with HRT are different for each woman, and they must be weighed on an individual basis. A distinction must also be made as to whether the woman is interested in short-term use for relief of vasomotor symptoms or long-term use to prevent chronic conditions such as osteoporosis and CHD. Short-term use is fairly riskfree and requires less discussion.

Regarding long-term use, a woman with significant risk factors for osteoporosis or CHD may benefit from long-term HRT. A woman with a personal or strong family history of breast cancer may not. Many attempts have been made to quantify the risk associated with each condition to aid clinicians in their counseling endeavors. The Nurses' Health Study provided information regarding the use of HRT and all-cause mortality. Current hormone users were found to have a lower risk of death (relative risk, 0.63) than nonusers. This reduction was largest in women with cardiac risk factors. The benefit decreased with use of more than 10 years (due to breast cancer deaths) but still remained significant.[35]

Another study used decision analysis to examine the effect of long-term HRT on life expectancy, taking into account the risk of CHD, breast cancer, and hip fracture.[36] The results indicated that HRT should increase life expectancy for nearly all women. Women with at least one cardiac risk factor would benefit, even if a first-degree relative had breast cancer. In this model, the risk of HRT outweighed the benefit only in women without risk factors for CHD or hip fracture, but who had two first-degree relatives with breast cancer.

Clearly, each woman will have her own risk/benefit profile regarding HRT, as well as personal preferences about methods of delivery and tolerance of side effects. Discussion of these factors and close communication between physician and patient are essential in order for the menopausal woman to make an informed decision.

Additional Information

Patients frequently request additional sources of information for further reading. Listed below are several resources particularly helpful to patients.

- *Menopause Guidebook*. Obtained through: The North American Menopause Society, P.O. Box 94527, Cleveland, OH 44101-4527.
- www.menopause.org
- www.discoveryhealth.com
- www.nof.com
- www.mediconsult.com

References

1. Gordon T, et al. Menopause and coronary heart disease. *Ann Intern Med* 1978;89:157-161.
2. Stampfer MJ, Colditz GA. Estrogen replacement therapy and coronary heart disease: A quantitative assessment of the epidemiologic evidence. *Prev Med* 1991;20:47-63.
3. Jensen J, et al. Influence of menopause on serum lipids and lipoproteins. *Maturitas* 1990;12:321-331.
4. Bass KM, et al. Plasma lipoprotein levels as predictors of cardiovascular death in women. *Arch Intern Med* 1993; 153:2209-2216.
5. Gebara OC, et al. Association between increased estrogen status and increased fibrinolytic potential in the Framingham Offspring Study. *Circulation* 1995;91: 1952-1958.
6. Juhan-Vague I, et al. Fibrinolytic factors and the risk of myocardial infarction or sudden death in patients with angina pectoris. *Circulation* 1996;94:2057-2063.
7. Wouters MG, et al. Plasma homocysteine and menopausal status. *Eur J Clin Invest* 1995;25:801-805.
8. Graham IM, et al. Plasma homocysteine as a risk factor for vascular disease: The European Concerted Action Project. *JAMA* 1997;277:1775-1781.
9. The Writing Group for the PEPI Trial. Effects of estrogen or estrogen/progestin regimens on heart disease risk factors in postmenopausal women: The Postmenopausal Estrogen/ Progestin Interventions (PEPI) Trial. *JAMA* 1995;273: 199-208.
10. Stampfer MJ, et al. Postmenopausal estrogen therapy and cardiovascular disease: Ten-year follow-up from the Nurses' Health Study. *N Engl J Med* 1991;325:756-762.
11. Walsh BW, et al. Effects of postmenopausal estrogen replacement on the concentrations and metabolism of plasma lipoproteins. *N Engl J Med* 1991;325:1196-1204.
12. Bush TL, et al. Cardiovascular mortality in noncontraceptive use of estrogen in women: Results from the Lipid Research Clinics Program Follow-up Study. *Circulation* 1987;75: 1102-1109.
13. Koh KK, et al. Effects of hormone-replacement therapy on fibrinolysis in postmenopausal women. *N Engl J Med* 1997;336:683-690.
14. Espeland MA, et al. Effect of postmenopausal hormone therapy on lipoprotein(a) concentration. *Circulation* 1998;97:979-986.
15. Mijatovic V, et al. Postmenopausal oral 17ß-estradiol continuously combined with dydrogesterone reduces fasting serum homocysteine levels. *Fertil Steril* 1998;69:876-882.
16. Grodstein F, et al. Postmenopausal estrogen and progestin use and the risk of cardiovascular disease. *N Engl J Med* 1996;335:453-461.
17. Sullivan JM, et al. Estrogen replacement and coronary artery disease. Effect on survival in postmenopausal women. *Arch Intern Med* 1990;150:2557-2562.
18. Hulley S, et al. Randomized trial of estrogen plus progestin for secondary prevention of coronary heart disease in postmenopausal women. *JAMA* 1998;280:605-613.
19. Davis SR. Premature ovarian failure. *Maturitas* 1996; 23: 1-8.
20. Colditz GA, et al. The use of estrogens and progestins and the risk of breast cancer in postmenopausal women. *N Engl J Med* 1995;332:1589-1593.
21. Sellers TA, et al. The role of hormone replacement therapy in the risk for breast cancer and total mortality in women with a family history of breast cancer. *Ann Intern Med* 1997;127:973-980.
22. Bonnier P, et al. Clinical and biologic prognostic factors in breast cancer diagnosed during postmenopausal hormone replacement therapy. *Obstet Gynecol* 1995;85:11-17.
23. Grady D, et al. Hormone replacement therapy and endometrial cancer risk: A meta-analysis. *Obstet Gynecol* 1995;85:304-313.
24. The Writing Group for the PEPI trial. Effects of hormone replacement therapy on endometrial histology in postmenopausal women: The Postmenopausal Estrogen/ Progestin Interventions (PEPI) trial. *JAMA* 1996;275: 370-375.

25. Daly E, et al. Risk of venous thromboembolism in users of hormone replacement therapy. *Lancet* 1996; 348:977-980.
26. Davis SR, et al. Testosterone enhances estradiol's effects on postmenopausal bone density and sexuality. *Maturitas* 1995;21:227-236.
27. Watts NB, et al. Comparison of oral estrogens and estrogens plus androgen on bone mineral density, menopausal symptoms, and lipid-lipoprotein profiles in surgical menopause. *Obstet Gynecol* 1995;85:529-537.
28. Khovidhunkit W, Shoback DM. Clinical effects of raloxifene hydrochloride in women. *Ann Intern Med* 1999; 130:431-439.
29. Delmas PD, et al. Effects of raloxifene on bone mineral density, serum cholesterol concentrations, and uterine endometrium in postmenopausal women. *N Engl J Med* 1997;337:1641-1647.
30. Ettinger B, et al. Reduction of vertebral fracture risk in postmenopausal women with osteoporosis treated with raloxifene: Results from a 3-year randomized clinical trial. Multiple Outcomes of Raloxifene Evaluation (MORE) investigators. *JAMA* 1999;282:637-645.
31. Cummings SR, et al. The effect of raloxifene on risk of breast cancer in postmenopausal women: Results from the MORE randomized trial. *JAMA* 1999;281:2189-2197.
32. Albertazzi P, et al. The effect of dietary soy supplementation on hot flushes. *Obstet Gynecol* 1998;91:6-11.
33. Anderson JW, et al. Meta-analysis of the effects of soy protein intake on serum lipids. *N Engl J Med* 1995;333: 276-282.
34. Cauley JA, et al. Prevalence and determinants of estrogen replacement therapy in elderly women. *Am J Obstet Gynecol* 1990;163:1438-1444.
35. Grodstein F, et al. Postmenopausal hormone therapy and mortality. *N Engl J Med* 1997;336:1769-1775.
36. Col NF, et al. Patient-specific decisions about hormone replacement therapy in postmenopausal women. *JAMA* 1997;277:1140-1147.

Part VIII

Eye, Ear, Nose, and Throat

Glaucoma

Izak F. Wessels, MD, FRCSE, FRCOphth, FACS

Glaucoma describes a family of different disease entities associated with progressive visual field loss and atrophy of the retinal ganglion cells and nerve fiber layer, with excavation of the optic disc. On average, one in 25 persons ages 50 or older will have glaucoma; less than one half of those will have been diagnosed or received treatment. In African Americans glaucoma occurs 2-4 times more commonly, and the disease also progresses more rapidly. Tragically, the diagnosis is too often made only after extensive damage has occurred and there is no possibility of restoring what has been lost. The primary care physician (PCP) is likely to encounter patients with glaucoma, since the indolent nature of this disease does not result in self-referral. Therefore, a high index of suspicion, basic understanding of mechanism of the disease and awareness of the more obvious signs will facilitate appropriate management.

This chapter attempts to improve glaucoma awareness, as well as provide such important practical points as are relevant to the PCP. The first point includes being able to assess an anterior chamber for depth and performing palpation to detect severely elevated pressure in acute angle closure. The next two include evaluating the optic nerve and awareness of the pattern of visual field loss in glaucoma. Visual field loss is often on the side toward the opposite eye. PCPs should be aware that a pressure measurement can be normal in glaucomatous eyes. Medication effectiveness can be improved by nasolacrimal occlusion. Awareness of the categories of medications, their side effects, and the important interactions with other conditions particularly emphasizes the common side effects that must be recognized and monitored by the PCP. PCPs should be aware of the different surgical options for glaucoma. Some of the common surgical procedures are briefly listed, noting those elements important to the PCP.

Introduction

Glaucoma is not defined by a specific intraocular pressure but rather as an optic neuropathy that can occur at any intraocular pressure depending on the optic nerve susceptibility of the individual person. Treatment effectively prevents progression, if the appropriate medication has been selected, the patient complies well, and where necessary, judicious surgical intervention is performed in a timely manner.

Glaucoma is a leading cause of blindness worldwide, and is estimated to result in more than 6 million bilateral blind people in the year 2000.[1] This paper will review three clinically important types of glaucoma. The first is closed angle glaucoma. Although uncommon, it may present as a medical emergency. Every PCP should be able to use simple evaluations to exclude this condition. The next is congenital glaucoma. While this condition is extremely rare, it must not be overlooked, since early diagnosis and treatment are critically important for visual function. Finally, most emphasis will be placed on the prevalent chronic open angle glaucoma.[2,3]

The practical points presented (anterior chamber depth, palpating for grossly elevated pressure, and recognizing the classic optic disc changes with a direct ophthalmoscope) lie well within the scope of physicians and nurse practitioners.[4,5] Traditionally, ophthalmologists have diagnosed and treated glaucoma both medically and surgically. More recently, the scope of practice of optometrists has expanded in most (but not all) states to include the diagnosis and medical treatment of glaucoma. They can be a valuable resource to the PCP for evaluating, selecting, and implementing therapy, as well as follow-up and appropriate referral for surgery.

Acute Angle Closure Glaucoma. This is a distinctly uncommon disease, except in specific ethnic groups.[6,7] Nevertheless, patients with an acute attack may present first to a PCP. The usual complaint is that of one eye spontaneously becoming excruciatingly painful, with blurred vision and haloes around lights.[8] There is a mid-dilated, poorly responsive pupil, hazy cornea, and diffused corneal light reflex (due to the corneal edema scattering the reflection, as if the cornea is covered with fine dewdrops), all due to the markedly elevated pressure.[9]

Useful confirmatory tests include noting the depth of the anterior chamber (the distance between the cornea and iris) and whether the iris is bowed forward. By shining a light across the eye from the side, the normally flat iris is uniformly illuminated; any forward bowing will result in illumination only on the side of the iris closest to the light. The iris lying on the other side of the pupil will appear to be in a shadow (*see Figure 1*). Furthermore, by gently palpating the eye through the closed upper lid (*see Figure 1*), the markedly elevated pressure will be quite obvious.

Certain individuals are at higher risk: females 3:1 compared to males, those older than 55, those with autosomal dominant inheritance, those with Eskimo or Asian ancestry, those with farsighted eyes (hyperopia), and patients with a smaller than normal cornea.[6] Because a markedly elevated intraocular pressure stimulates the oculocardiac reflex (via the vagus nerve) other findings include bradycardia, dizziness, nausea, and frequently, vomiting. These findings might mislead the PCP to consider an acute intra-abdominal problem, while the ocular symptoms may be overlooked.[10] It is common to treat acute angle closure glaucoma with virtually all pressure lowering medications, including beta blockers and alpha agonists. Ignoring the problem can result in irreversible blindness after just a few hours. Immediate, urgent referral is necessary, and treatment includes systemic (IV or PO) acetazolamide (diamox); aqueous suppressants and miotic drops (≤ 2% pilocarpine); and placing the patient in a supine position to allow the iris to fall back from the anterior chamber angle and permit the fluid to drain. Parenteral (mannitol) and oral (glycerol) hyperosmotic agents also may be required.[11] Certainly, the definitive treatment is a peripheral iridotomy, and the sooner it can be performed the better.

Figure 1. Anterior Chamber Depth

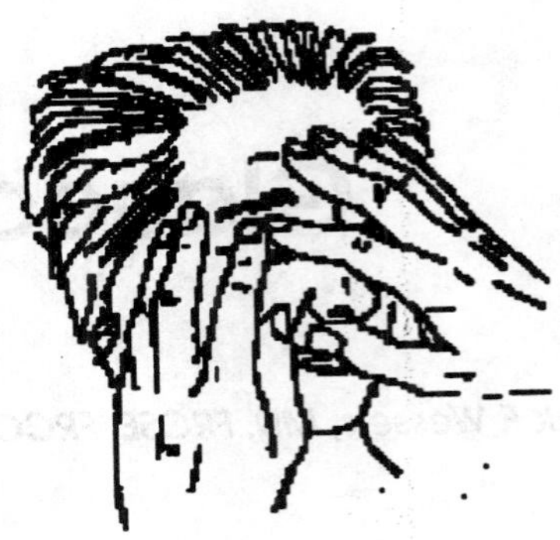

Tactile tension relies on gently palpating the eye through the closed lid. While this cannot provide sufficient accuracy for managing open angle glaucoma, it will reveal marked differences in the intraocular pressures between the two eyes. A normal eye tension feels just slightly firmer than palpating the tip of the nose.

Note that the common labeling on medications as "not for use in glaucoma" applies only to angle closure cases, in which anticholinergic side effects can provoke pupil dilation and result in angle occlusion. Patients with the far more common open angle glaucoma need not be concerned. Primary open angle glaucoma and acute glaucoma are totally different in pathogenesis, symptoms, and treatment.

The symptoms and signs of acute glaucoma are so characteristic that recognition usually is easy and treatment can be begun early enough to prevent permanent angle damage and secondary glaucoma. Secondary angle closure may occur after vascular insult to retina, also as a complication of severe diabetic retinopathy.

Pediatric Glaucoma. Pediatric glaucoma, although exceedingly rare, should be readily apparent due to markedly enlarged corneal diameters: the immature infant eye stretches when there is elevated intraocular pressure, but this may be overlooked if the disease is bilateral. If detected early, the optic nerve may recover.[11] Parents may notice the light sensitivity due to swelling of the cornea, as well as persistent tearing; the latter symptom should not be mistaken for the far more common cause of a congenitally obstructed nasolacrimal duct.

Open Angle Glaucoma. Previously known as chronic simple glaucoma, primary open angle glaucoma is asymptomatic until late in its course, and appropriate screening by PCPs can greatly help reduce the incidence of irreversible

Figure 2. Angle Closure Glaucoma

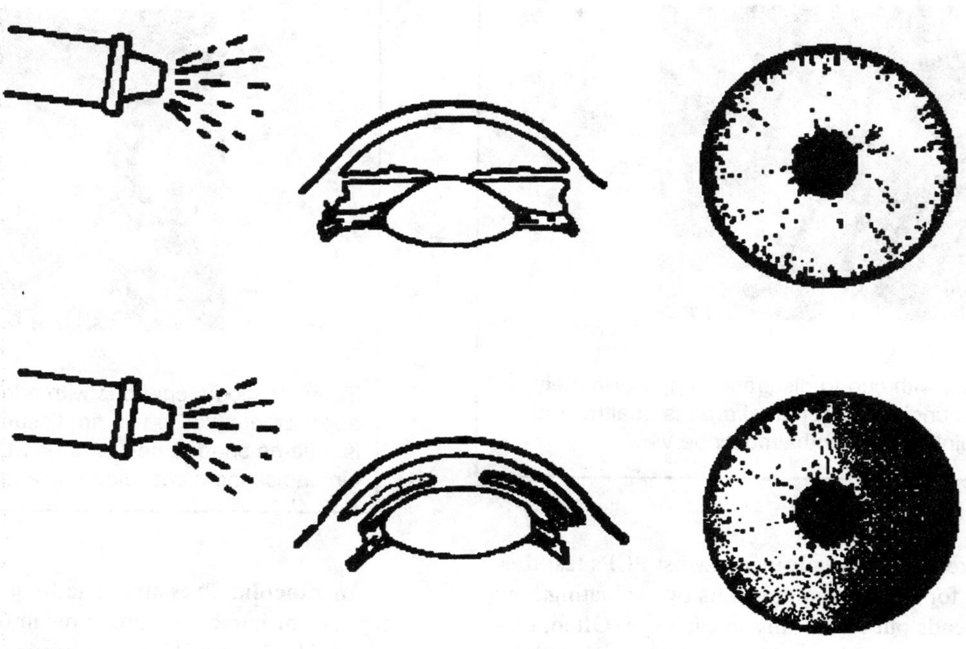

In angle closure glaucoma, the anterior chamber is shallow because the iris is bowed forward (bottom illustration). A light source held to the side and shining across the eye will show uniform illumination of the anterior surface of the iris (upper illustration). A significant convexity of the iris will result in uneven illumination, with a shadow on the iris on the side away from the light.

visual loss.[13-15] Glaucoma is common, even more so in African Americans.[3] Not every patient needs to be treated: the life expectancy, functional ability, and ocular health in general can guide therapy.[16,17] The progression is exceedingly slow; simply by being under treatment seems to result in fewer problems. Glaucoma case finding is feasible in general practice.[18-21] Direct ophthalmoscopy proved to be the most valuable single test in diagnosing glaucoma, and the combination of measurement of intraocular pressure and direct ophthalmoscopy was shown to be the most likely method of diagnosing glaucoma or identifying glaucoma suspects.[9,19,20]

Other methods of identifying the disease include a questionnaire-based algorithm for detection of overall eye disease, with a relative sensitivity/specificity of 90%/44%; determining decreased distance visual acuity (≤ 20/40), 61%/72%; dilated fundus examination, 79%/82%; tonometry, 27%/96%; and supra-threshold visual field testing, 70%/67%.[20] This indicates that fundus examination has the highest sensitivity and specificity.

The intraocular pressure plays an important role, despite the absence of a specific number distinguishing between disease and health.[4,16,22] A severely elevated pressure can result in vascular occlusion, but even mild elevation can, over years, be associated with progressive damage. While there is not an absolute level above which glaucoma can be diagnosed, lowering the pressure can delay or prevent visual loss. This finding has facilitated treatment that varies from close observation to topical and systemic medications. Attempts to improve the fluid flow and drainage include: openings to bypass obstructions (e.g., peripheral iridotomy that can be curative for narrow angle glaucoma) and improve fluid drainage (goniotomy for congenital glaucoma, laser trabeculoplasty, and trabeculectomy for open angle glaucoma); implanting a device to improve drainage; and laser or cryoablation of the secretory structures.[11]

Diagnosis

Four parameters together help make the diagnosis vision, evidence of typical glaucomatous field loss, optic nerve cupping, and intraocular pressure.[20,23]

Visual Field Loss. Modern, computerized test devices permit measuring the visual field more quickly and consistently than is possible with manual methods. Unfortunately, the field loss is not that specific or sensitive and usually only detects

Figure 3. Normal Disc

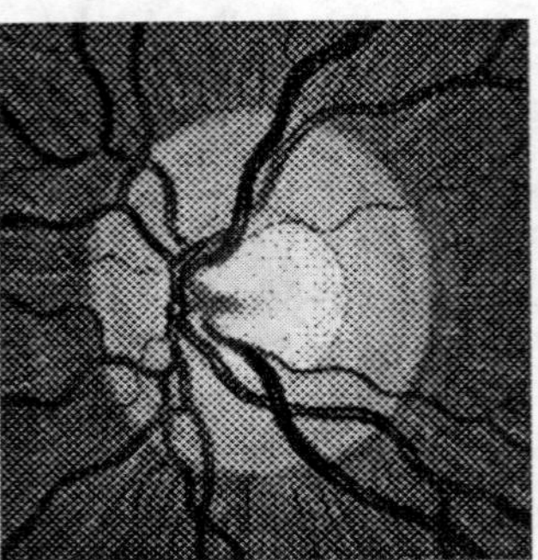

A normal disc, with cup to disc ratio of approximately 0:3. The surrounding neuroretinal area is healthy and will appear pink in the ophthalmoscope view.

Figure 4. Early Glaucoma Changes

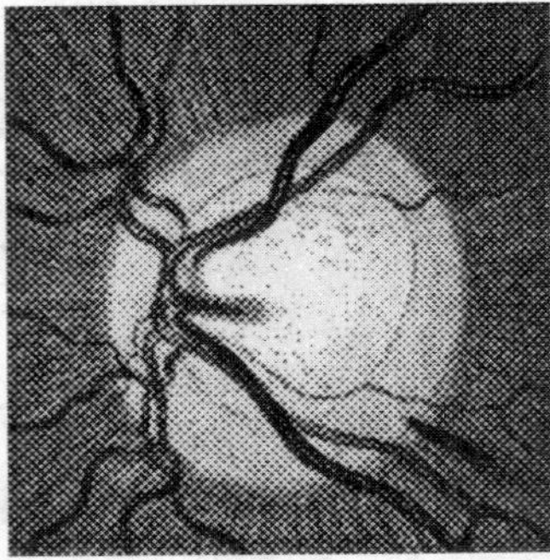

Early glaucoma changes with a larger cup (ratio of approximately 0:7). The rim tissue is narrower, and there is a flame shaped hemorrhage at the 5 o'clock disc margin, indicating a vasculopathy and potential for field loss.

damage that is relatively far advanced. Most PCPs test the peripheral field for driving requirements by evaluating how far the field extends out temporally in each eye. Often, the first area of the visual field to suffer loss lies on the nasal side, while the other eye (usually with asymmetric and nonoverlapping field loss) will have good function. Moreover, the onset and progression is so gradual as to be imperceptible until it is extremely advanced.[24]

The Optic Disc Contour. Practitioners routinely use the direct ophthalmoscope to evaluate the optic nerve (for papilledema, optic atrophy, as well as for glaucoma). It helps to be familiar with the appearance of a normal disc *(please see Figure 1)*. This recognition can best be achieved by routine use of the ophthalmoscope on all patients, including normals.[25] Several specific findings should be noted.

The optic nerve head shows an increase in the area occupied by the optic cup. *(Please see Figure 2.)* The extreme case is obvious *(please see figure 3)*, but obviously it is best to suspect the disease before irreversible visual field loss has occurred. Early signs include vertical enlargement of the cup, a focal area of thinning of the rim. Ultimately, the vessels become displaced nasally, and "bayonet" as they dip under the rim after crossing.

Flame shaped hemorrhages on the disc margin are markers for more rapid visual field loss. *(Please see Figure 2.)*

The astute observer may notice a loss of the normal nerve fiber layer sheen adjacent to the disc. The nerve fiber layer is more noticeable when using the green filter on the ophthalmoscope. *(Please see Figures 2 and 3.)*

Specific findings indicating a greater risk for damage include large nerves, peripapillary atrophy, and prominent laminar dots.[22,26] While the appearance of the disc alone is not sufficient to make the diagnosis, its evaluation is critically important. The ability to appropriately evaluate an optic disc is greatly facilitated by a brief training course.[12,13,19]

Intraocular Pressure. The frequency of distribution (histogram) of intraocular pressures in the general public is a skewed bell curve.[11] Normal pressure is considered as 17 mmHg, with two standard deviations (i.e., 95% of the sample included), including 12-22 mmHg. Only 10% of patients with pressures above 24 will develop glaucoma; but with higher pressures, the risk increases (50% will develop damage if the pressure is > 27 and almost all will have damage if the pressure remains > 30 after 15 years). In eyes with glaucoma the mean pressure is only 23, while one-third will have pressures in the "normal" range. The intraocular pressure varies during the day (usually highest in the morning), and requires relatively expensive delicate instruments as well as meticulous technique to measure the pressure.

There is, indeed, no single diagnostic procedure to give a "yes" or "no" answer. The intraocular pressure is nothing more than a significant risk factor.[2] While pressure measurements are important for follow up and management, the PCP should not rely on pressure measurements alone for diagnosis. The PCP has a special role in encouraging those on glaucoma medications to comply with their medication use. Since there are no obvious signs of benefit, compliance is a major problem, more so since medication does not cure but only preserves what remains.[27]

Medical Treatment

The goal of therapy is not simply to lower the pressure in the eye.[28] The patient in whom the disease does not appear to be rapidly progressing, and who is without much functional disability and has a relatively short remaining lifespan, should not receive drastic treatment. Consideration must be given to not worsen the overall well being of the patient, especially

Figure 5. Advanced Glaucoma

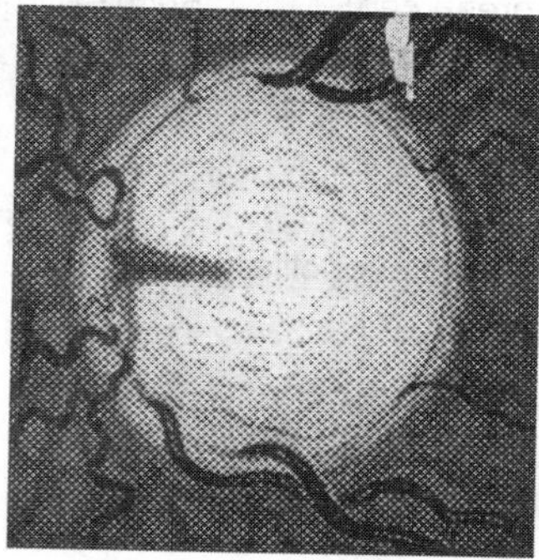

There is hardly any disc substance around the large cup, with the ratio approaching 1. At this point, the disc itself is not able to withstand much further insult.

because glaucoma medications have numerous side effects.[27-29] However, noncompliance remains a major problem, and surgical intervention may be required to prevent visual loss.

The newer agents are extremely potent, with many potential interactions as well as serious systemic side effects.[29] It is not commonly realized that eye drops are extremely concentrated.[30] Timolol 0.5% in each mL contains the same dose as a 5 mg tablet. Each milliliter usually produces an average of 20 drops; therefore, a daily dose of one drop in each eye will deliver 0.5 mg, which can result in toxic systemic levels in the case of a child. In susceptible adults, this drug may cause bronchospasm, reduced exercise tolerance, fatigue, impotence, and even congestive heart failure.

Nasolacrimal punctal occlusion is a beneficial technique to reduce side effects by minimizing systemic absorption of the drops.[27] The patient puts a clean finger over the nose where the upper and lower lids meet and pushes directly onto the bone. Then they instill the drop (usually an assistant is needed) and gently close the lids, without forcible blinking. To achieve a good effect, they should remain thus for 3 minutes or longer. By this simple maneuver, the amount of drug entering the nose is drastically reduced. The nasal mucosa would otherwise allow immediate absorption directly into the systemic circulation. Lacrimal occlusion also markedly increases the contact time with the eye and a higher dose can be delivered, allowing a reduction in the frequency of instillation without noticeable loss of effect.

Categories of Medications

Parasympathomimetics. Pilocarpine, carbachol, and others all act directly on the muscarinic receptors to cause contraction of the muscles of the ciliary body, which may open the drainage meshwork to increase outflow. They also cause pupil constriction (and headache), while other cholinergic side effects (diarrhea and gastrointestinal upset) may occur. A subclass of indirect parasympathomimetics acts by inhibiting acetylcholine esterase. While only rarely used now, the PCP should be aware of their potentiation of the effects of succinyl choline (scoline) muscle relaxants. Furthermore, all parasympathomimetics can worsen inflammation (uveitis) and may increase retinal detachment risk.

Adrenergic Sympathomimetics. Epinephrine was at one time used frequently, but has been replaced by a prodrug dipivefrin (Propine) that only becomes activated within the eye. Known side effects include aggravation of hypertension, thyrotoxicosis, and interactions with MAO inhibitors. More specific alpha agonists have become available, including apraclonidine (Iopidine) and brimonidine (Alphagan). These agents may cause side effects due to interaction with MAO inhibitors, or in patients with liver or kidney impairment. The sympathomimetic effect can obviously provoke or worsen problems such as Raynaud's phenomenon, thromboangiitis obliterans, or symptoms due to coronary or cerebral artery disease.

Beta-blockers. These drops are used more frequently than almost all the other drugs put together.[31] There are numerous agents available, both selective and nonselective.[32] They often have systemic side effects (loss of exercise tolerance, impotence, elevation of blood lipids, bradycardia, cardiac arrhythmias, bronchospasm, depression, etc.) that may be overlooked as due to other factors. Other signs include worsening of chronic obstructive pulmonary disease; reactive airway disease; bradycardia; heart block; heart failure; myasthenia gravis; depression; and interaction with digitalis, quinidine, and reserpine.

Carbonic Anhydrase Inhibitors. These can also cause significant side effects, ranging from a metallic taste to lethargy, weight loss, poor appetite, nausea, and GI upset. Other, more serious problems include renal impairment, calcium kidney stones, and hypokalemia that obviously will potentiate digitalis toxicity. Patients who are allergic to sulfonamides can suffer from catastrophic Stevens Johnson syndrome and aplastic anemia. Even those without sulfa allergies may develop aplastic anemia. These agents can increase the effect of aspirin.

Prostaglandins. Latanoprost (xalatan) is extremely potent; therefore, the medication is dilute, but the cost is high. It functions by increasing uveoscleral absorption and thus increases aqueous absorption through a different pathway than the trabecular meshwork. Frequent side effects range from an allergic conjunctivitis to permanent darkening of light brown/green colored irides. Being a prostaglandin analog, it may aggravate ocular inflammation (uveitis, cystoid macular edema, etc.).

Since each drug has a particular benefit as well as relative contraindications, the selection and prescription is beyond the scope of this brief review. While it is important for the PCP to have some knowledge of the potential interactions, the choice and prescription would best be left to those practitioners familiar with these agents.

Table 1. Details of Complaints Reported During Treatment (Glucosamine)

Category	Effect	Side Effects	Interactions
Parasympathomimetics	Increase outflow (note: these drops usually have a green cap)		Succinyl choline
Pilocarpine		pupil constriction, GI upset	
Carbachol		inflammation (uveitis), retinal detachment	
Phospholine Iodide		brow ache (due to spasm of ciliary muscle)	
Adrenergic Drugs	Increase aqueous outflow		MAO inhibitors
Epinephrine		aggravation of hypertension,	
Dipivefrin (Propine)		thyrotoxicosis	
Alpha Agonists	Decrease aqueous production		
Apraclonidine (Iopidine)		liver kidney impairment	
Brimonidine (Alphagan)		Raynaud's phenomenon,	
		thromboangiitis obliterans, and	
		coronary or cerebral artery disease	
Beta-blockers	Decrease aqueous production		Quinidine, reserpine, digitalis
Timolol (Timoptic)		impotence	
Betaxolol (Betoptic)		elevation of blood lipids	
Levobunolol (Betagan)		bronchospasm COPD reactive airway disease	
Metipranolol (Optipranolol)		myasthenia gravis	
Carteolol (Ocupress)		bradycardia, heart block, heart failure depression, and loss of exercise tolerance	
Carbonic Anhydrase Inhibitors	Decrease aqueous production		
Oral			
Methazolamide (Neptazane)		renal impairment	sulfa allergy
Acetazolamide (Diamox)		calcium kidney stones, hypokalemia	aspirin digitalis
Topical			
Dorzolamide (Trusopt)			
Brinzolamide (Azopt)			
Prostaglandins	Increase outflow through uveoscleral pathway		
Latanoprost (Xalatan)		allergic conjunctivitis; permanently darken a light iris, cystoid macular edema, uveitis	

Surgery

There is a range of different surgical options, the precise indications and techniques of which are less important to the PCP than an awareness of potential complications.

Laser Trabeculoplasty. A blue-green laser is used to place mild burns just in front of the filtration area on the inside of the cornea peripherally. The burns decrease the resistance to outflow and consequently the pressure decreases. While usually only effective for a few years, it can minimize or avoid totally the need for medications temporarily.[33]

Trabeculectomy. This surgery is the most often performed glaucoma surgery, and is used to create an alternative pathway with reduced resistance to flow. After lifting the conjunctiva, a partial thickness flap of sclera is dissected, followed by removing the remaining tissue holding the aqueous back. When the partial thickness outer flap is repositioned, the aqueous fluid now only has to traverse the thinner flap, and it usually more easily percolates through to collect under the conjunctiva and be absorbed. Currently, anti-fibrotic agents (e.g., mitomycin C, 5 Fluoro uracil) are used to prevent the flap from scarring down and blocking the outflow. Often, a thin-walled bleb develops at the site of a successful trabeculectomy surgery. This thin area (obviously visible as an avascular fluid filled vesicle) can sometimes permit infectious organisms to easily penetrate the eye and produce a severe infection. PCPs should be able to recognize the presence of the bleb under the eyelid, and more aggressively manage even minor conjunctivitis in these high-risk patients.

Drainage Tubes. In cases with marked scarring, or in whom trabeculectomies have failed, a permanent plastic tube can be implanted into the anterior chamber to help the aqueous fluid leak out. Various devices are commercially available, each named after its inventor, e.g., Ahmed, Molteno, Baerveldt, etc.

Ciliary Ablation. The aqueous fluid is produced by the ciliary body, and glaucoma results from production exceeding absorption. As a corollary to increasing the absorption of the fluid, it is logical to attempt to surgically reduce the production. Any damage to the ciliary body will result in a reduction in inflow and intraocular pressure. Cryotherapy or laser surgery can ablate the ciliary body and effectively reduce the pressure, although the magnitude of effect is difficult to control.

Summary

There are several points of importance for the PCP.

Acute closed angle glaucoma often presents as an emergency (frequently with symptoms apparently originating elsewhere). The shallow anterior chamber and palpably elevated intraocular pressure is very helpful. Peripheral iridotomy is curative.

Glaucoma can occur in children.

Open angle glaucoma is a common disease that lacks a specific diagnostic test. There is no red line for the intraocular pressure. Measuring the pressure accurately is not simple, and the reading must be interpreted in the light of the visual field test and the contour of the optic nerve head.[34]

Changes of the optic nerve (increased cupping, bleeding on the margin, and loss of thickness of the rim) will frequently present to the PCP. Like most other skills, it becomes easier to recognize abnormalities with practice. Screening for glaucoma ought to be part of every general medical practice.[35,36]

Glaucoma medicines are potent, and frequently cause patients to present to the PCP with side effects. Furthermore, other medications can interact with glaucoma: e.g., systemic corticosteroids may elevate the intraocular pressures and cause glaucomatous damage in the 5% of genetically predisposed individuals.

Early referral to a qualified optometrist or ophthalmologist is strongly recommended to facilitate timely treatment.[37,38] Consultation with suitably qualified optometrists (certain states) may facilitate management.

Surgical treatment can be successful. However, the eye may be at significant risk for endophthalmitis due to a thin (conjunctiva only) and often avascular layer separating the organisms on the conjunctiva from the inside of the eye.

References

1. Thylefors B, Negrel AD. The global impact of glaucoma. *Bull World Health Organ* 1994;72:323-326.
2. Leske MC, Warheit-Roberts L, Wu SY. Open-angle glaucoma and ocular hypertension: The Long Island glaucoma case-control study. *Ophthalmic Epidemiol* 1996;3:85-96.
3. Sommer A, et al. Relationship between intraocular pressure and primary open angle glaucoma among white and black Americans. The Baltimore Eye Survey. *Arch Ophthalmol* 1991;109:1090-1095.
4. Higginbotham EJ. Glaucoma: A preventable cause of blindness. *Md Med J* 1997;46:412-414.
5. Hanson CM, Hodnicki DR. Glaucoma screening: An important role for NPs. *Nurse Pract* 1987;12:14, 18, 21.
6. Drance SM. Angle closure glaucoma among Canadian Eskimos. *Can J Ophthalmol* 1973;8:251-254.
7. Anderson DR, et al. The physiologic characteristics of relative pupillary block. *Am J Ophthalmol* 1991;111:344-350.
8. Hodes BL, Choromokos EA. Glaucoma. Some practical considerations on a common disease. *Postgrad Med* 1978;64:111-120.
9. Faigen M. The early detection of glaucoma in general practice. *Aust Fam Physician* 2000;29:282-285.
10. Cullom RD, Chang B. *The Wills Eye Manual: Office and Emergency Room Diagnosis of Eye Disease*. 3rd ed. Philadelphia: JB Lippincott; 1994.
11. Shields MB. Textbook of Glaucoma, 4th ed. Baltimore, Md: Lippincott Williams & Wilkins; 1998.
12. Podolsky MM. Exposing glaucoma. Primary care physicians are instrumental in early detection. *Postgrad Med* 1998;103:131-136, 142-143, 147-148.
13. Pass M, Chaudhry I, Wong S. Recognizing glaucoma. A guide for the primary care physician. *Postgrad Med* 1996;99:247-248, 251-252, 257-259.
14. Wormald RP, Rauf A. Glaucoma screening. *J Med Screen* 1995; 2:109-114.
15. Sommer A. Glaucoma screening: Too little, too late? *J Gen Intern Med* 1990;5(5 Suppl):S33-37.
16. Georgopouls G, et al. Risk factors in ocular hypertension. *Eur J Ophthalmol* 1997;7:357-363.
17. Spaeth GL. Proper outcome measurements regarding glaucoma: the inadequacy of using intraocular pressure alone. *Eur J Ophthalmol* 1996;6:101-106.
18. Margolis KL, Rich EC. Open-angle glaucoma. *Prim Care* 1989; 16:197-209.
19. Margolis KL, et al. Physician recognition of ophthalmoscopic signs of open-angle glaucoma: effect of an educational program. *J Gen Intern Med* 1989;4:296-299.

20. Wang F, et al. Evaluation of screening schemes for eye disease in a primary care setting. *Ophthalmic Epidemiol* 1998;5:69-82.
21. Strahlman E, et al. Vision screening in a primary care setting. A missed opportunity? *Arch Intern Med* 1990;150:2159-2164.
22. Haefliger IO. Risk factors associated with glaucoma. *Klin Monatsbl Augenheilkd* 1997;210:265-268.
23. Davies P. Health promotion in general practice. *Aust Fam Physician* 1991;20:23-29.
24. David R. Changing therapeutic paradigms in glaucoma management. *Exp Opin Invest Drugs* 1998;7:1063-1086.
25. Garway-Heath DF, Hitchings RA. Quantitative evaluation of the optic nerve head in early glaucoma. *Br J Ophthalmol* 1998;82: 352-361.
26. Anderson DA. The management of elevated intraocular pressure with normal discs and visual fields. Therapeutic approaches based on high risk factors. *Surv Ophthalmol* 1977;21:479-489.
27. Zimmerman TJ, Zalta AH. Facilitating patient compliance in glaucoma therapy. *Surv Ophthalmol* 1983;28:S252-258.
28. Lewis PR, Phillips TG, Sassani JW. Topical therapies for glaucoma: What family physicians need to know. *Am Fam Physician* 1999;59:1871-1879, 1882.
29. Skorin L Jr. New medical therapies in glaucoma management. *J Am Osteopath Assoc* 1997;97:582-583.
30. Diamon JP. Systemic adverse effects of topical ophthalmic agents. Implications for older patients. *Drugs Aging* 1997;11: 352-360.
31. Van Buskirk EM, Fraunfelder FT. Ocular beta-blockers and systemic effects. *Am J Ophthalmol* 1994;98:623-624.
32. Frishman WH, Fuskbrumer MS, Tannenbaum M. Topical ophthalmic beta-adrenergic blockade for the treatment of glaucoma and hypertension. *J Clin Pharmacol* 1994;34:795-803.
33. Pederson JE. Glaucoma. A primer for primary care physicians. *Postgrad Med* 1991;90:41-45, 48.
34. Liesegang TJ. Glaucoma: Changing concepts and future directions. *Mayo Clin Proc* 1996;71:689-694.
35. Wun YT, Lam CC, Shum WK. Impaired vision in the elderly: A preventable condition. *Fam Pract* 1997;14:289-292.
36. Sweet EH, Tark E. Eye care by primary care physicians. A survey of internists and family practitioners in the Sacramento, California, area. *Ophthalmology* 1991;98:1454-1460.
37. Ettinger ER, Schwartz MD, Kalet AL. Referral patterns of primary care physicians for eye care. *J Am Optom Assoc* 1993; 64:468-470.
38. Shields T, Sloane PD. A comparison of eye problems in primary care and ophthalmology practices. *Fam Med* 1991;23: 544-546.

Inflammatory Conditions of the Head and Neck

Madeleine Ponder, MD, DVM
Rita K. Cydulka, MD, FACEP

Inflammatory diseases of the head and neck can result in significant morbidity to the patient if the diagnosis is missed and appropriate therapy delayed. This chapter presents the most common infectious inflammatory conditions of the head and neck, offers guidelines for diagnosis, differentials that should be considered, and the latest recommendations for therapy.

Otitis Media

Definition. Otitis media is an inflammation of the middle ear. Otitis media with effusion is an inflammation of the middle ear with a collection of fluid in the middle ear. Acute otitis media is an inflammatory process of the middle ear of less than three weeks' duration. Chronic otitis media implies inflammation beyond three months with a perforation in the tympanic membrane.[1]

Otitis media is one of the most common infections of childhood. It is the most common reason for a visit to a pediatrician's office after well-baby care. By age 3, children may be categorized into three groups of approximately equal size relative to acute infection of the middle ear. One group is free of ear infections, a second group may have occasional episodes of otitis, and a third group is otitis prone and subject to repeated episodes of acute otitis media. The peak incidence occurs between the ages of 6 and 13 months. Boys are affected more frequently than girls. There is a higher incidence and an increased severity of otitis media among caucasians, Native Americans, and Eskimos. Poor socioeconomic status and living in households with many members increases the frequency of otitis media. Other factors associated with an increased incidence of otitis media include day-care attendance, parental smoking, inhalant or food allergies, and craniofacial deformities such as those associated with cleft palate, Down, Crouzon, Apert, or Turner syndromes.[2] The incidence of otitis media increases in the winter and early spring.[3] Children who are breast fed have significantly fewer episodes of otitis media.[2,4]

Pathophysiology. Eustachian tube dysfunction is the single most important factor in the development of otitis media. In children, eustachian tube function is not as good as in adults. Dysfunction may be caused by viral infections or by anatomic abnormalities. Viral infections are responsible for up to 25% of cases of otitis media. Viruses that affect the middle ear include influenza A virus, respiratory synctial virus, coxsackievirus, adenovirus, and parainfluenza virus. The most common bacterial pathogen is *Streptococcus pneumoniae,* accounting for 29% of otitis media cases. *Haemophilus influenzae* and *Moraxella catarrhalis* also are common pathogens. Less frequently, *Streptococcus pyogenes* and *Staphylococcus aureus* are found. In neonates, gram-negative bacteria play an important role.[5] Other uncommon etiologies include *Mycobacterium tuberculosis, Mycoplasma pneumoniae, Pneumocystis carinii, Pseudomonas aeruginosa,* and *Chlamydia trachomatis*.[5,6]

Diagnosis. The signs and symptoms of otitis media in children include fever, dizziness, irritability, decreased appetite, nausea,

Table 1. Antimicrobial Therapy for Acute Otitis Media[9,10]

ANTIBIOTIC	PEDIATRIC DOSE	ADULT DOSE	ADVANTAGES	DISADVANTAGES
Amoxicillin	less than 20 kg: 40 mg/kg/d PO divided q8h × 10 d	250 mg PO TID × 10 d	Inexpensive	Resistance
Erythromycin/Sulfisoxazole	30-50 mg/kg/d PO divided q6h × 10 d	250-500 mg PO q6h × 10 d		Compliance
Amoxicillin/Clavulanate	< 40 kg: 40 mg/kg/d PO divided q8h × 10 d	250 mg PO q8h × 10 d		GI upset
Ceftriaxone	50 mg/kg IM single dose		Compliance	Pain at injection site
Cefuroxime	30 mg/kg/d PO divided BID ×10 d; max, 1000 mg/d	250 mg PO BID × 10 d	Store liquid at room temp	Adjust dose in renal failure
Cefprozil	6 mos-12yrs: 15 mg/kg PO q12h ×10 d	500mg PO q24h × 10 d	Flavor, compliance	Must refrigerate liquid
Cefaclor	40 mg/kg/d PO divided q8h ×10 d; max, 1000 mg/d	250mg PO q8h × 10 d		Must refrigerate liquid
Loracarbef	< 13 yrs: 30 mg/kg/d PO divided q12h × 10 d	200mg PO q12h × 10 d	Compliance, store at room temp	Adjust dose in renal failure
Cefpodoxime	10 mg/kg/d PO (max, 400 mg/d) or 5 mg/kg/d PO q12h × 10 d	100 mg PO Q12h × 10 d	Compliance	*C. difficile* colitis, must refrigerate liquid
Cefixime	< 50 kg: 8 mg/kg/d or 4 mg/kg BID PO × 10 d	400 mg Qd or 200 mg BID PO × 10 d	Compliance, store at room temp	Adjust dose in renal failure
TMP-SMX	8 mg/kg (TMP) PO divided BID × 10 d	1 DS PO BID × 10 d	Compliance	Adjust dose in renal failure

vomiting, and diarrhea. Otoscopy may reveal a thickened, inflamed tympanic membrane (TM). There may be a loss of the light reflex, bullae on the TM, or air-fluid levels within the middle ear. Pneumatic otoscopy is helpful in determining whether fluid is present in the middle ear. Tympanometry is useful as an adjunctive test.[7] However, tympanometry results may be misleading in patients with cerumen impactions as well as small or angulated external auditory canals. Tympanocentesis is indicated for patients who are seriously ill with toxic signs or symptoms, who have an unsatisfactory response to therapy, who have suppurative complications, and in newborns or immunocompromised patients in whom an unusual organism is suspected.[8]

Treatment. Medical management of acute otitis media involves the use of antimicrobials. *(Please see Table 1.)* Nasal decongestants may be of some benefit in correcting eustachian tube obstruction.

Pressure-equalizing tubes are the mainstay of surgical therapy. Current recommendations for tympanostomy tube placement are for children with three or more infections in six months, four episodes in 12 months, or recurrent otitis media despite a one-month trial of prophylactic antibiotics.[11] Adenoidectomy is of benefit in children who develop recurrent otitis media after extrusion of tympanostomy tubes or for children with persistent middle ear effusion for longer than three months in spite of antibiotic therapy.[12,13]

Complications. The most common medical complication of otitis media is TM perforation. The most common developmental complication of otitis media is hearing loss. A middle ear effusion produces a 25-35 dB conductive hearing loss that can be significant and produce delays in language development. Other serious complications include cholesteatoma, acute mastoiditis, hearing loss, facial nerve paralysis, otitic hydrocephalus, epidural abscess, subdural empyema, and lateral venous sinus thrombosis.[1] It is important to maintain a high index of suspicion for complications in patients who present with severe pain, sensorineural hearing loss, facial paralysis, or severe vertigo.

Emergency Situations. Any patient with a suspected intracranial complication must be treated emergently. Computed tomographic scanning can aid in the diagnosis of intracranial and intratemporal complications.

Otitis Externa

Definition. Otitis externa is an infection of the external auditory canal (EAC). Necrotizing external otitis (formerly known as malignant otitis externa) is a potentially life-threatening infection that begins in the external auditory canal and can extend to the skull base.

Epidemiology. Otitis externa is a common disease. It accounts for up to 30% of patient visits to otolaryngologists.[14] The primary groups affected are children and diabetics.

Etiology. Otitis externa has multiple etiologies. Anatomic factors, such as the congenitally narrow EACs seen in Downs syndrome, play a large role in the development of otitis externa. An acquired EAC stenosis secondary to inflammation also can predispose to the development of otitis externa. Other factors include exposure to heat, humidity, swimming, and trauma to the EAC from fingernails and cotton swabs.[14] Immunocompromised and diabetic individuals are more likely to develop otitis externa.[15] *Staphylococcus aureus* is the most common bacteria isolated from acute otitis externa.[16] Less common are *Staphylococcus epidermidis,* hemolytic *Streptococci, Escherichia coli, Proteus mirabilis, Enterococcus,* and *Pseudomonas aeruginosa*.[14] *Pseudomonas aeruginosa* is predominantly responsible for necrotizing otitis externa.[17] Fungal infections can occur and are often misdiagnosed. The most common fungal etiologies are *Aspergillus, Candida, Penicillium,* and *Alternaria*.[18]

Pathophysiology. Acute otitis externa (commonly called swimmer's ear) is caused by a breakdown in the auditory canal's protective barriers: the skin and cerumen. Warmth and humidity destroy the protective cerumen layer in the external auditory canal. As the cerumen is destroyed the canal becomes pruritic. Fingernails and cotton swabs then injure the skin, allowing a route of entry for bacteria. Once the protective layers have been destroyed, bacteria penetrate and establish an infection. Infection and inflammation lead to edema, purulent discharge, and pain. The infection may spread from the auditory canal to the auricle and periauricular tissues.

Clinical Features. Pruritis is the earliest symptom of otitis externa. Scratching leads to trauma of the skin, which favors secondary bacterial infection. As the infection worsens, the canal becomes edematous and erythematous. Initially, the otorrhea is clear but may become seropurulent. Pain is a prominent feature of acute bacterial otitis externa. Pain may occur at rest, when chewing, or when manipulating the ear.[16] Fungal otitis externa may present with pruritis, a sensation of something in the ear, otorrhea, tinnitis, or otalgia.[18]

Diagnosis. Acute otitis externa is best diagnosed by looking for the clinical findings of the disease, observation of otorrhea, edema and erythema of the EAC, and pain on manipulation of the tragus. Fungal otitis externa may also have visible fungal hyphae in the EAC. Cultures identify specific pathogens.

Treatment. The treatment regimen requires pain control and thorough cleaning of the EAC and removal of debris. Antibiotic therapy (usually topical) and education about the prevention of recurrent disease are axiomatic. Cortisporin otic suspension is the first-line topical therapy for uncomplicated acute bacterial otitis externa. If the canal is severely edematous, it may be necessary to place a wick in the canal for delivery of topical antibiotics. Patients with wicks in place need to be followed on a daily basis to suction debris from the canal and to ensure that the infection is improving. Patients not requiring a wick should be able to clean and irrigate their ears 2-3 times daily (prior to the instillation of antibiotic drops) with an acidifying solution such as aluminum sulfate-calcium sulfate (Domboro). This will help remove debris so that the antibiotic can get to the site of infection. The acidic pH also decreases bacterial and fungal growth. Topical antibiotics should be continued for 2-3 days after the cessation of symptoms. Oral antibiotics are indicated for severe infections with erythema of the auricle or any soft-tissue involvement. The treatment of fungal otitis externa involves thorough cleaning of the external canal, frequent irrigation with Domboro solution, and drying with boric acid powder and a topical antifungal agent. Current recommendations for topical therapy include clotrimazole, nystatin, or tolnaftate.[18] Patients should be instructed to keep ear canals dry, which means the use of ear plugs during swimming and showering. Other than ear plugs, foreign objects (fingernails and cotton swabs) must be kept out of the ear canals.

Complications. Acute otitis externa usually clears with therapy and has few lasting effects. Recurrent episodes of otitis externa and chronic otitis externa may lead to EAC stenosis, perichondritis, or chondritis. Erysipelas, cellulitis, and necrotizing otitis externa are rare complications of otitis externa.[20]

Emergency Situations. Necrotizing otitis externa is the most serious potential complication of otitis externa. It is most commonly seen in diabetic patients but has also been reported in immunocompromised patients. Poor tissue microcirculation is felt to be the underlying defect that allows the infection to spread. The infection usually begins in the external auditory canal and can extend to the base of the skull. It can lead to cranial nerve deficits, jugular vein thrombosis, cavernous sinus thrombosis, intracranial abscess, and meningitis.[21] *P. aeruginosa* is the bacteria felt to be responsible for the infection. The clinical features of the disease include a long-standing infection of the EAC that does not resolve with appropriate therapy. The patient may have had persistent otalgia for longer than one month and prolonged purulent otorrhea for several weeks with granulation tissue in the canal. As the infection spreads to the skull base, the cranial neuropathies can develop. Diagnosis is based on clinical features, culture of *Pseudomonas,* and imaging studies. Mastoid radiographs may demonstrate bone destruction, but a CT scan is the imaging modality of choice. CT scan with contrast will demonstrate soft-tissue thickening and bony erosion.[17] The therapy for necrotizing otitis externa includes thorough cleaning of EAC including removal of granulation tissue. Anti-*Pseudomonas* intravenous antibiotics are required for 3-6 weeks. Oral ciprofloxacin use has been reported; however, up to 20% of *Pseudomonas* become resistant to ciprofloxacin in the six-week treatment period. Rarely, surgical debridement of osteomyelitic tissue is required to clear the infection.[21]

Pharyngitis

Definition. Pharyngitis is a mucosal and submucosal inflammation of the throat that can include the oropharynx, nasopharynx, hypopharynx, adenoids, and tonsils.

Epidemiology. Pharyngitis is a common disease in all age groups. Sore throat is the third most common reason for office visits in the United States.[22] While most attention is focused on Group A beta-hemolytic streptococcal pharyngitis, there are many other causes of pharyngitis.

Etiology. Pharyngitis can be due to bacterial, viral, mycobacterial, or fungal infectious agents, connective tissue disorders, and neoplasms. Bacterial pathogens that produce pharyngitis include: Group A beta-hemolytic *Streptococci, staphylococcus aureus, Haemophilus influenzae* type B, *Bordetella pertussis, Corynebacterium* species, *Treponema pallidum, Neisseria gonor-*

rhoeae, and *Klebsiella rhinoscleromatis*.[23,24] Of these organisms, Group A beta-hemolytic *Streptococcus* is the most frequently implicated cause.[25] Viral pharyngitis may be secondary to infections with adenovirus, rubeola (measles), Epstein-Barr virus, (infectious mononucleosis), cytomegalovirus, human papillomavirus, and herpes simplex virus.[25] Mycobacterial pharyngitis is rare but must be considered in the differential diagnosis. *Mycobacterium tuberculosis* and *Mycobacterium leprae* may both affect the pharynx and nasopharynx. *M. bovis* and *M. avium intracellulare* must be included in the differential of pharyngitis in immunocompromised patients.[26] Fungal infections also should be considered in immunocompromised individuals. The most common fungal infection is *Candida albicans*. Others include cryptococcus, rhinosporidium, histoplasma, blastomyces, and aracoccidioidomycosis.[27]

Noninfectious causes of pharyngitis that must be differentiated from infectious causes include sarcoidosis, Wegener's granulomatosis, Crohn's disease, lymphoma, squamous cell carcinoma, and metastatic tumors.[28-30]

Pathophysiology. Many pharyngeal infections actually begin in the nose and paranasal sinuses. The pharynx can become secondarily infected via postnasal drainage. Lymphatic drainage of the pharynx is to the retropharyngeal, deep cervical, jugular, and lateral pharyngeal lymph nodes. Therefore, any infection of the pharynx can lead to infection of the draining lymph nodes and result in abscess formation in the retropharyngeal and parapharyngeal spaces.[31]

Clinical Features. Group A beta-hemolytic *Streptococcus* is the most frequently identified agent responsible for pharyngitis. It has a seasonal predilection for late fall through early spring. Up to 30% of sore throats in children and 10% of sore throats in adults are caused by Group A beta-hemolytic *Streptococcus* during that time of year. Patients may present with a mild sore throat followed by fever, difficulty swallowing, cervical adenopathy, abdominal pain, and myalgias. The pharyngitis may be exudative with a white plaque on the tonsils or may appear as mild pharyngeal erythema. Streptococci may produce an erythrogenic toxin that results in the characteristic sand paper rash of scarlet fever. The rash can begin on the second day of the illness. It appears first on the trunk and spreads over the entire body. Desquamation may occur one week later.[22]

Staphylococcus aureus and *Haemophilus influenzae* pharyngitis may be indistinguishable in appearance from streptococcal infection. One may see exudates or pustules on the tonsils. *Haemophilus* infection may lead to significant airway compromise from local inflammation and edema of the epiglottitis, supraglottitis, and vocal cords.

Bordetella pertussis is a disease of primarily the trachea and bronchi, but the pharynx and larynx may also be affected. The characteristic pharyngeal finding is a mucopurulent exudate secondary to epithelial necrosis. Common clinical manifestations in children include characteristic spasms of coughing, an inspiratory whoop, conjunctival injection, coryza, fever, and sneezing.[32] Neurologic findings can include dysphagia, hoarseness, palatal paralysis, proximal limb weakness, and paresthesias.[33]

Corynebacterium diphtheriae produces an exotoxin that leads to epithelial necrosis and diptheritic membrane formation. The membrane is gray to black in appearance and is firmly adherent to the underlying tissue. The membrane may extend to the glottis, subglottis, and trachea, resulting in airway obstruction. The exotoxin may also produce respiratory and circulatory collapse, cranial nerve palsies, and more weakness.[34] It is important to recognize this disease and institute therapy.

Treponema pallidum and *Neisseria gonorrhoeae* are sexually transmitted diseases that can affect the pharynx. Syphilis manifestations in the pharynx include chancre formation (painless ulceration) and lymphadenopathy.[23] Gonococcal pharyngitis presents as sore throat, tonsillar hypertrophy, and lymphadenopathy.[35]

Adenovirus is a common cause of upper respiratory infections and pharyngitis. Characteristic findings in viral pharyngitis are lymphoid proliferation in the pharyngeal mucosa along with conjunctivitis.

Rubeola (measles) is characterized by fever, coryza, conjunctivitis, cutaneous rash, pharyngitis, and Koplik's spots, which are small gray spots on the buccal mucosa surrounded by erythema and inflammation. These spots are considered pathognomonic for measles.

Epstein-Barr virus (EBV infectious mononucleosis) is a herpesvirus that produces pharyngitis and is characterized by fever, myalgias, fatigue, exudates on the tonsils, lymphadenopathy, hepatosplenomegaly, atypical lymphocytes, and heterophile antibodies. Symptoms last 1-3 weeks; however, fatigue may persist for several months.[36]

Cytomegalovirus (CMV) is also in the herpesvirus family. CMV infection results in signs and symptoms similar to those found in EBV infection except that heterophile antibodies are absent.[37]

Primary infection with the herpes simplex virus may produce a pharyngitis characterized by vesicular lesions that are clustered. More commonly, HSV produces gingivostomatitis and cervical lymphadenopathy.[38]

Human papillomavirus infection rarely affects the pharynx, but it can infect any squamous epithelial cells in the body. It may present as multiple papules in the pharynx. It is associated with mucosal neoplasms.[39]

Mycobacterial infections of the pharynx may present as inflammation or ulcerations. They are more common in the immunocompromised patient. A pharyngeal infection may spread to the eustachian tube and the middle ear. Tuberculous otitis media may be the only manifestation of the disease.[26]

Fungal infections are also rare in immunocompetent individuals. *Candida albicans* is the most common fungal pharyngeal infection in the immunocompromised patient. *Candida* infection may present as painful ulcerative lesions or as mucosal plaques. Other fungal infections lead to granuloma formation that may be difficult to distinguish clinically from systemic granulomatous diseases such as Wegener's granulomatosis, sarcoidosis, and Crohn's disease. Lymphoma and cutaneous malignancies may be difficult to differentiate from granulomatous diseases.

Diagnosis. Much has been written on the cost-effective diagnosis of Group A beta-hemolytic streptococcal (GAS) pharyngitis. Breese developed a nine-part scoring system to determine the probability of infection with GAS. The patients with the highest likelihood of having GAS were those who presented in February, March, or April, age 5-10 years, a white blood cell (WBC) count between 13,500 and 20,400 cells/mm^3, a fever to 100.5° F, a sore throat, a cough, a headache, an abnormal pharynx, and abnormal cervical glands. However, this only identifies 70% of children and 30% of adults with GAS pharyngitis.[40] When properly performed, a rapid GAS antigen detection test has a sensitivity of 76-87% and a speci-

Table 2. Antimicrobial Therapy of Strep Pharyngitis

ANTIBIOTIC	DOSE	ROUTE	DURATION	ADVANTAGES	DISADVANTAGES
Penicillin	Children: 40 mg/kg/d divided TID; max daily dose, 750 mg. Adults: 500 mg BID or TID	PO	10 days	Inexpensive	Frequency of dosing and duration of therapy
Benzathine penicillin	Wt < 27 kg: 600,000 U Wt > 27 kg: 1,200,000 U	IM IM	One-time dose	Compliance	Pain at injection site
Erythromycin estolate	20-40 mg/kg/d divided BID-QID	PO	10 days	Use in penicillin-allergic patients	GI side effects, compliance
Erythromycin ethyl succinate	40 mg/kg/d divided BID-QID	PO	10 days	Use in penicillin-allergic patients	GI side effects, compliance
Azithromycin	Children: 10 mg/kg on day 1 then 5 mg/kg/d for four more days. Adults: 500 mg on day 1, then 250 mg/d for four days	PO	5 days	Compliance	

Adapted from: Dajani A, Taubert K, Ferrieri P, et al. Treatment of acute streptococcal pharyngitis and prevention of rheumatic fever: A statement for health professionals. *Pediatrics* 1995;96:758-764.

ficity of 90-96%. Confirmatory culture should be performed on all patients with a negative rapid antigen test.[22,40]

Culture of the pharynx for other bacterial pathogens is rarely indicated since cultures may take up to 3-4 days to complete. Diagnosis must be made based on clinical picture and therapy instituted prior to having culture results. Cultures should be used to confirm the diagnosis, but therapy should not be delayed while awaiting culture results.

Viral cultures are rarely indicated in the immunocompetent patient. A presumptive diagnosis of viral pharyngitis is made based on negative bacterial cultures. In the immunocompromised patient, other etiologies need to be considered and cultures, biopsies, and serologies may be indicated. If infectious mononucleosis is suspected, then a latex agglutination test or heterophile antibody test can be performed.

Treatment. The primary goal of therapy in GAS pharyngitis is the prevention of rheumatic fever. The antibiotic of choice is oral penicillin. Intramuscular benzathine penicillin may be used in patients who are unlikely to complete a 10-day course of oral antibiotics. In the penicillin-allergic patient, erythromycin estolate or erythromycin ethyl succinate is effective. Azithromycin may also be used in the penicillin-allergic patient. Oral cephalosporins are also effective but not recommended for patients with anaphylactic reactions to penicillin.[41] Steroids also may serve as an adjunct to antibiotics in relieving the pain of pharyngitis. The current recommendations for recurrent streptococcal pharyngitis are to educate the patient about the importance of compliance with antibiotic therapy, consider cultures of family members, try other antibiotics, and to consider long-term antibiotic therapy or tonsillectomy. Low-dose penicillin therapy (125-250 mg BID) for weeks to months has been suggested for treatment of the carrier state.[25] *(Please see Table 2.)*

The indications for tonsillectomy are controversial. Current recommendations are for recurrent tonsillitis (4 or more episodes per year), recurrent peritonsillar abscess, or suspicion of malignancy. Some authors recommend tonsillectomy for patients with fewer episodes of recurrent tonsillitis in the face of valvular heart disease, poorly controlled diabetes mellitus, ventriculoperitoneal shunt, a history of febrile seizures, or suspicion of malignancy.[42]

Complications. Several serious potential complications should be considered when evaluating the patient with pharyngitis. The early recognition of impending airway obstruction is critical in order to prevent lethal consequences. The potential for airway obstruction should be considered in patients unable to swallow their own secretions, who have noisy or stridorous respirations, and who have an alteration in their voice. The airway obstruction can be secondary to inflammatory changes of the mucosa resulting in acute narrowing of the airway or it may be from abscess or phlegmon formation with extrinsic compression of the airway. Patients with a peritonsillar abscess may also have inflammation of the surrounding structures, including the epiglottis, resulting in airway obstruction.

Peritonsillar abscess and deep neck infections can also be complications of pharyngitis. Pharyngeal hemorrhage is a rare complication resulting from erosion into a vascular structure. If erosion of an artery occurs, rapid exsanguination can occur.

Rheumatic fever is an immune disease caused by Group A beta-hemolytic *Streptococcus*. The bacteria elicit an immune response, causing immune complexes to form. Symptoms include carditis, polyarthritis, chorea, erythema marginatum, subcutaneous nodules, and fever.[43] During epidemics of streptococcal pharyngitis, up to 3% of untreated patients may develop rheumatic fever.[43]

Splenic rupture is a rare complication of infectious mononucleosis that must be considered in patients with left upper quadrant pain and falling hematocrit.[44]

Lemierre's syndrome (septic thrombophlebitis of the internal jugular vein) is a serious complication of an infection of the lateral pharyngeal space that can result from pharyngitis. The organisms most commonly associated with this complication are *Fusobacterium necrophorum, Bacteroides* sp., *Streptococcus* sp., *Peptostreptococcus* sp., and *Eikenella corrodens*.[45] Septicemia can develop several days after a tonsillar or peritonsillar infection. Signs and symptoms include pain in the submandibular area and distant metastatic abscesses from septic emboli.[46,47]

Epiglottitis/Supraglottitis

Definition. Epiglottitis (more appropriately termed supraglottitis) is an infectious process that produces inflammation and edema of the supraglottic structures. The supraglottic structures involved include the epiglottis, uvula, base of the tongue, aryepiglottic folds, arytenoids, false vocal cords, and adjacent pharyngeal walls. Airway obstruction can occur secondary to edema of any of the supraglottic structures.[48]

Epidemiology. Epiglottitis is an uncommon disease most frequently caused by *Haemophilus influenzae* type b (Hib).[49] It occurs more frequently in males, with a 3:2 male-to-female ratio in children and a 1.8:1 male-to-female ratio in adults.[48,50] There is a seasonal predilection for spring and fall, with peak incidences in March and November.[50] Prior to 1990, the average age of children affected with epiglottitis was 36 months. With the development of the Hib vaccine in 1990 for use in children beginning at age 2 months, the incidence of epiglottitis in children has decreased dramatically. Since 1990, the average age affected has increased to 55 months.[50] The annual incidence in children has decreased from 10.9 per 10,000 hospital admissions to 1.8 per 10,000 hospital admissions since 1990.[51] The annual incidence in adults remains stable at 1.8 cases per 100,000.[48,52]

Etiology. Prior to the Hib vaccine, acute infectious epiglottitis was caused by Hib in approximately 76% of cases. Studies of epiglottitis since the development of the Hib vaccine have demonstrated Hib in approximately 23% of patients younger than 2 years.[51] The most common organism isolated in blood cultures is Hib. Other etiological agents for epiglottitis include *Pneumococcus, S. aureus*, Group A *Streptococci*, other *Haemophilus* species, *C. albicans, Neisseria, E. coli, Enterobacter cloacae*, and viruses.[48,51,53]

Pathophysiology. Infection of the supraglottic structures leads to inflammation and edema that can produce sudden total airway obstruction, leading to hypoxia and death.

Clinical Features. In children, the duration of symptoms is about 12 hours prior to presentation. There is usually a history of prior upper respiratory infection. The most common presenting complaints are fever, sore throat, and dysphagia. Signs most commonly seen include respiratory distress, stridor, drooling, toxic appearance, cyanosis, shock, average fever of 38.8° C (101.8° F) and a mean WBC count of 19.2 x 10^9/L.[51] In one study, 92% of children with epiglottitis presented with respiratory distress; stridor was observed in 82% of children.[51] Children tend to sit with a characteristic upright posture with their neck extended and arms providing support of the trunk. This position maximizes the size of the supraglottic airway.

Adults with epiglottitis usually have a different presentation. The duration of symptoms prior to presentation is 36 hours to four days. The most common presenting symptoms are odynophagia and a change in voice. In one study, 100% of patients with epiglottitis presented with odynophagia as their primary complaint, while 75% of these same patients presented with a change in voice.[54] Less commonly seen are dyspnea, drooling, stridor, pharyngitis, fever, cervical adenopathy, cough, and hemoptysis.[48]

Diagnosis. In children, epiglottitis is suspected from the clinical presentation. Children with epiglottitis are at extreme risk of acute airway obstruction. Therefore, it is important to avoid any manipulation of the child that might result in worsening distress. Once the diagnosis of epiglottitis is suspected, examination of the airway should be attempted in the operating room or in the ED, provided all necessary arrangements are made for appropriate control of the airway.

In adults, the disease course is usually more indolent. Endoscopy or indirect laryngoscopy should be performed to assess the supraglottic structures for evidence of supraglottitis and to aid in the treatment plan.

Adjunctive diagnostic tests may be indicated in both children and adults. Lateral soft tissue radiograph of the neck may reveal a thickened epiglottis known as the "thumb sign." Another key radiographic finding is thickening of the aryepiglottic folds. False thickening of the epiglottis can occur from rotational artifact and edema from noninfectious causes (e.g., allergies). Although not diagnostic, the WBC count may be elevated and demonstrate a left shift. Blood cultures and throat cultures can be performed, but therapy should be initiated prior to culture results. In patients taken to the operating room, laryngeal cultures can also be obtained.[48] Latex particle agglutination tests are available for the rapid diagnosis of Hib.[49]

Differential Diagnosis. Epiglottitis must be differentiated from laryngotracheobronchitis (croup). Croup is a disease of younger children (6 months to 3 years). It produces narrowing of the airway and similar signs and symptoms as seen in epiglottitis. Children with croup tend to have a longer course of illness, worsening at night, a "barky" cough, and lack the characteristic posture of children with epiglottitis. However, in children younger than 6 months, croup and epiglottitis can appear identical. An anteroposterior soft-tissue radiograph reveals subglottic narrowing or the "steeple sign."[49,55]

Treatment. When considering treatment options for epiglottitis, it is important to remember that acute airway obstruction is a significant risk. In children, this risk is greater and can occur with more rapidity than in adults. It is imperative when treating children with epiglottitis to keep the child as calm as possible until the airway is secure. The child who appears stable and in no acute distress should be manipulated as little as possible until medical personnel are prepared to control the airway. Attempts to place IV catheters and draw blood should only be attempted if the child is very cooperative. The child should not be separated from his or her parent or guardian. Otolaryngology consult should be placed emergently. The child should be transported to the operating room for controlled evaluation of the airway. With all necessary equipment available for tracheotomy and intubation, an attempt should be made to evaluate the supraglottic structures. Indirect laryngoscopy, flexible fiberoptic endoscopy, or rigid endoscopy can be performed. Intubation can be extremely difficult in children with epiglottitis. The tissue at the tracheal opening is very edematous, and the only indication of the opening may be small air bubbles formed while breathing.

Neuromuscular blocking agents can obscure this finding and should be avoided if possible. Based on the appearance of the supraglottic structures, an artificial airway (intubation or tracheostomy) may be required. The length of intubation required in children varies from 1-7 days.[50] The decision to extubate is based on the presence of an air leak around the endotracheal tube, or when direct laryngoscopy shows a significant reduction in supraglottic edema.[53] Patients who do not require an artificial airway should be observed closely in the intensive care unit setting.

Adult epiglottitis is often not as fulminant, and the evaluation of the supraglottic airway can be safely performed in the ED. Once the diagnosis of epiglottitis is established, the patient should have an intravenous catheter placed for prompt administration of antibiotics. For patients with evidence of impending airway obstruction, endotracheal or nasotracheal intubation should be performed. Tracheostomy is required if intubation is unsuccessful.[56] Adult patients with no respiratory symptoms may be safely observed in the intensive care unit setting.[48] All nonintubated patients should be placed on warm, humidified air.

In both children and adults, antibiotic therapy is initiated as early as possible. Second- or third-generation cephalosporins as well as ampicillin/sulbactam can be used.[10,48] For penicillin- and cephalosporin-allergic patients, aztreonam and chloramphenicol are also effective.[10]

The use of corticosteroids in the management of epiglottitis is controversial. Steroids have not been proven to reduce the need for airway intervention or hasten the recovery in acute adult epiglottitis.[48]

Complications. In addition to the potential for acute airway obstruction, there are other complications of epiglottitis. The most frequent complication in children after respiratory arrest is premature extubation. Infrequently seen are pulmonary edema, pericardial effusion, acidemia, seizures, and bradycardia. Children may also have concomitant *H. influenzae* meningitis.[51] The mortality rate of children with epiglottitis is approximately 1.6%.[50]

The most frequent complications in adults include pneumothorax, congestive heart failure, retropharyngeal abscess, and deep vein thrombosis.[48] Acute airway obstruction has been reported in adults even when closely observed in the ICU setting.[57]

Sinusitis

Definition. Sinusitis is an inflammatory condition of the paranasal sinuses, which include the frontal, ethmoid, sphenoid, and maxillary sinuses. Acute sinusitis is an infectious sinusitis that resolves completely with medical therapy with no permanent mucosal damage. In children, chronic sinusitis is defined as 12 weeks of persistent symptoms and signs or six episodes per year of recurrent acute sinusitis (each lasting at least 10 days) in association with persistent changes on CT scan four weeks after medical therapy. In adults, chronic sinusitis is defined as eight weeks of persistent symptoms and signs or four episodes per year of recurrent acute sinusitis (each lasting at least 10 days) in association with persistent changes on CT scan four weeks after medical therapy.[60]

Epidemiology. Sinusitis is the United States' most common health care complaint and is a tremendously important disease in terms of the cost to the American health care system.[61] Sinusitis accounts for nearly 12 million annual visits to physicians. Its prevalence is increasing in all age groups.[62]

Etiology. Sinusitis is caused by bacterial, viral, and fungal infections. Over half of community-acquired sinusitis is caused by *H. influenzae* and *S. pneumoniae*.[63] Other bacterial pathogens include *S. aureus*, *S. pyogenes*, *M. catarrhalis*, alpha hemolytic *Streptococci*, *Peptostreptococcus*, *Fusobacterium*, and *Bacteroides*.[64] *Pseudomonas*, *Klebsiella*, and other gram-negative species are commonly associated with hospital-acquired sinusitis.[63] Viruses associated with sinusitis include rhinovirus, influenza virus, parainfluenza virus, and adenovirus.[63] Mycobacteria and fungi should be considered in the differential for chronic sinusitis that does not respond to standard therapy.[27,62]

Pathophysiology. The ethmoid and maxillary sinuses are present at birth. The ethmoid sinuses are fully developed by age 14. The maxillary sinuses reach adult size during adolescence. The sphenoid sinus develops after age 2. The frontal sinus begins to develop around age 6.[64] The paranasal sinuses are connected to the nasal passages by ostia. Sinuses are lined with ciliated epithelium that moves mucous in the direction of the ostia. This system clears inhaled particles from the sinuses. Obstruction of the ostia can occur from chronic inflammation, hypertrophy of the mucosa, nasal polyps, and anatomic variants such as septal deviation.[65] Ostia obstruction favors bacterial growth and the development of acute sinusitis.

Clinical Features. Facial tenderness and pain, nasal congestion, and purulent nasal discharge are the hallmarks of acute sinusitis. Other common signs and symptoms include headache, cough, anosmia, pain when chewing, halitosis, fever, epiphora, and edema of the eyelids.[59] Patients often report a recent history of URI. Signs and symptoms vary depending on the sinus involved. *(Please see Table 3.)*

Diagnosis. Pain on palpation over the sinuses and purulent nasal discharge are highly suggestive of sinusitis. Transillumination of the maxillary and frontal sinuses can be helpful in the diagnosis of a non-aerated sinus. Nasal endoscopy is becoming more available and may obviate the need for radiographs in the diagnosis of sinusitis.[65] The utility of plain sinus radiographs is controversial. Plain sinus radiographs are inadequate in the evaluation of the ethmoid sinuses, the source of the majority of sinusitis.[62] Waters, Caldwell, and lateral radiographic views can occasionally yield diagnostic information.[62] However, studies have demonstrated only a 44% correlation between plain maxillary sinus radiographs and subsequent findings of sinusitis on endoscopy.[65] CT scan of the sinuses is the gold standard for the diagnosis of sinus disease. MRI has limited usefulness in the diagnosis of sinusitis. MRI is more sensitive than CT scan for the detection of fungal sinusitis and in the differentiation of inflammatory processes from neoplasms.[66] Sinus cultures assist in the therapy of nosocomial, fungal, and chronic sinusitis or sinusitis in the immunocompromised patient.[67,68]

Differential Diagnosis. The differential diagnosis of sinusitis includes allergic rhinitis, vasomotor rhinitis, nasal obstruction, rhinorrhea, and post-nasal discharge.[65] A good history and endoscopic examination are useful in differentiating between these disorders.

Treatment. The therapy of acute sinusitis is directed at re-establishing patency of the sinus ostia, reducing inflammation of the sinus and nasal mucosa, promoting removal of mucous from the sinuses, and treating the infection with antibiotics.

Table 3. Clinical Findings in Sinusitis[61]

SITE OF SINUSITIS	PRESENTING COMPLAINTS	PAIN WORSENED WITH:	PAIN IMPROVED WITH:	OTHER FACTORS
Ethmoid	Nasal congestion Purulent rhinorrhea Periorbital or Temporal headache	Coughing Straining Supine position	Head upright	Tender at medial canthus
Maxillary	Pain over cheekbone Toothache Temporal headache Periorbital pain	Head upright	Supine position	Tender over maxillary sinus
Frontal	Severe headache	Supine position	Head upright	Tender over frontal sinus
Sphenoid	Diffuse headache Fever	Supine position Bending forward Valsalva	Head upright	Visualized best on CT scan

Complications. There are several potential serious complications of sinusitis. The most common complication involves the orbital structures, since the eye is surrounded on three sides with sinuses. Orbital and periorbital cellulitis, orbital abscess, and blindness have all been observed.[58] Other complications include osteomyelitis of the frontal and maxillary bones and intracranial extension of disease.[69] Potential intracranial complications of sinusitis include brain abscess, subdural empyema, meningitis, cavernous sinus thrombosis, and epidural abscess.[70] Exacerbation of asthma is another potential complication of sinusitis.[71]

Special Situations. Cystic fibrosis also leads to an alteration in the function of the paranasal sinuses and is associated with nasal polyposis. Sinusitis in patients with cystic fibrosis is usually due to *P. aeruginosa* infection. Evaluation of the child with recurrent sinusitis or nasal polyposis should include a sweat chloride test.[58]

Kartagener's syndrome or immotile cilia syndrome tremendously impairs the mucociliary function of the paranasal sinuses. As a result, bacteria and mucous are not cleared from the sinuses, enhancing the risk for recurrent bacterial sinusitis. Medical therapy is the same as for community-acquired sinusitis.[72]

Nasal manipulation in the seriously ill hospitalized patient is common. Nasal oxygen, nasogastric tubes, and nasotracheal tubes all cause intranasal injury and interference with the normal sinus function. This can lead to impairment of the ostia and result in sinusitis. The bacterial agents most commonly seen in the nosocomial setting include *P. aeruginosa* and *Klebsiella pneumoniae.* Nosocomial sinusitis is usually polymicrobial, and 60% of organisms are enteric.[73] In addition, fungi must be considered. The removal of any nasal tubes is an important part of the therapy in addition to the standard therapy for acute sinusitis.[67]

In HIV-infected patients, chronic sinusitis is most often due to *P. aeruginosa, S. aureus,* or anaerobic bacteria.[68] Other bacteria associated with sinusitis in HIV patients include *S. viridans*, *S. pneumoniae, Propionibacterium acnes*, and *Legionella pneumophillia.*[68] Cytomegalovirus has been implicated as well.[68] Fungal infections are more common in HIV patients. Fungi associated with sinusitis in these patients include *Aspergillus, Zygomycosis,* and *Candida.*[68] Early culture is imperative to direct therapy. Sinusitis has been implicated as a potential trigger for the severe weight loss seen in patients with AIDS wasting syndrome.[68]

Deep Neck Abscesses

Definition. There are several potential spaces in the head and neck where abscesses can form. The spaces that can be involved include the subcutaneous tissue, the canine space, the buccal space, the masticator space, the parotid space, the submandibular space, the lateral pharyngeal space, the peritonsillar space, and the retropharyngeal space. The term "deep neck space" refers to a potential space enclosed by the deep cervical fascia. Deep neck spaces include the masticator space, the parotid space, the submandibular space, the lateral pharyngeal space, the peritonsillar space, and the retropharyngeal space. This discussion primarily focuses on the two most common abscess sites: the peritonsillar and retropharyngeal spaces. A peritonsillar abscess is also known as a quinsy. Cellulitis of the submandibular space is also known as Ludwig's angina.[74]

Epidemiology. In children, 49% of head and neck space infections are peritonsillar, 22% retropharyngeal, 14% submandibular, 11% buccal, 2% lateral pharyngeal, and 2% canine space infections.[74] The incidence of peritonsillar abscess in patients age 5 to 59 years is 30.1 per 100,000 person-years. There are approximately 45,000 cases per year of peritonsillar abscess.[75] Although retropharyngeal abscess formation was formerly felt to be exclusively a disease of children, a recent small study demonstrated 70% of patients with retropharyngeal abscesses were adults.[76]

Diabetes mellitus and HIV infection are associated with an increased risk for the development of deep neck abscesses.[76,77] There is also an increased incidence of retropharyngeal abscesses in patients with low socioeconomic status and poor living conditions.[76]

Etiology. Deep neck abscesses are commonly polymicrobial and usually contain oral flora. The bacteria most commonly associated with deep neck abscesses include beta-hemolytic *Streptococci*, *S.*

aureus, Bacteroides sp., *S. viridans,* and *K. pneumoniae.*[76,78] Overall, there is a relatively high incidence of beta-lactamase producing organisms and gram negative organisms.[74]

Pathophysiology. Pharyngotonsillitis is the most common condition associated with the development of a deep neck infection. Other less common conditions leading to deep neck infections include dental infection, viral upper respiratory infection, pharyngitis, foreign body ingestion, trauma (including intubation, adenoidectomy, and esophagoscopy), congenital cysts, and bacteremia.[74]

Abscesses involving the subcutaneous tissue, the canine space, the buccal space, the masticator space, the submandibular space, and the retropharyngeal space are most commonly of dental origin. Periodontal infections can spread to the local facial planes, producing abscesses, or can spread via the deep fascia or lymphatics to the deep neck spaces. Suppuration of the retropharyngeal lymph nodes can lead to abscess formation.[79]

Peritonsillar abscesses usually originate from tonsillitis. Infection spreads to the space between the tonsillar capsule and the lateral pharyngeal wall and the supratonsillar space. When purulent material remains in this space, a peritonsillar abscess ensues. If untreated, the purulent material can rupture and drain into the pharynx or spread to the lateral pharyngeal space where it can track along the carotid sheath.[80]

Clinical Features. Abscesses of the subcutaneous tissue, the canine space, and the buccal space usually present with localized swelling and inflammation. Patients may complain of pain, toothache, odynophagia, sore throat, or fever. Trismus may develop if the infection spreads to the masticator space.[79]

Peritonsillar abscess usually presents as prolonged unilateral tonsillitis or sore throat. Patients may have dysphagia, odynophagia, a muffled or "hot potato" voice, otalgia, and inability to swallow. Patients usually have tender cervical lymph nodes. The examination of the pharynx reveals a unilateral erythematous bulging soft palate, tender to palpation. This soft tissue mass may displace the uvula to the contralateral side. There may also be significant localized edema of the soft palate, uvula, and lateral pharyngeal walls. If the abscess has spread to the lateral pharyngeal space, the patient can present with suppurative jugular thrombophlebitis, 11th and 12th cranial neuropathies, or with hemorrhage associated with erosion into the carotid artery.[80]

Retropharyngeal abscesses usually present with fever, lethargy, poor oral intake, pain, swollen neck, odynophagia, difficulty breathing, difficulty swallowing, cervical lordosis, or hyperextension of the neck. Intraoral examination may be unremarkable or a bulging posterior pharyngeal wall. Stridor or airway obstruction may be present in severe cases.[81]

Diagnosis. The diagnosis of deep neck abscesses is based primarily on history and physical examination. Confirmation of a peritonsillar abscess can be made with needle aspiration of purulent material. A lateral soft tissue radiograph of the neck taken on inspiration with the neck extended may reveal thickening of the prevertebral tissue. Normal thickness of the prevertebral tissue at the second cervical vertebrae is 7 mm. Normal thickness of the prevertebral tissue at the sixth cervical vertebrae is 22 mm. The thickness of the prevertebral tissue should be less than 50% of the width of the adjacent vertebral body.[81] A lateral soft tissue radiograph may also demonstrate displacement of the airway anteriorly.[82]

A CT scan is useful in the evaluation of the patient with suspected deep neck abscess. CT scan can aid in diagnosis, the differentiation between cellulitis and abscess, determining the extent of the disease, and planning operative intervention.[83,84]

Differential Diagnosis. The differential diagnosis of deep neck space infections must include cellulitis. Often this differentiation can only be made intraoperatively. It is also important to differentiate a retropharyngeal abscess from Kawasaki disease. Several reports of retropharyngeal cellulitis from Kawasaki disease exist in the literature. The differentiation is based on identification of other characteristic findings of Kawasaki disease, including nonexudative conjunctivitis, oral cavity changes, polymorphous exanthem, peripheral edema, erythema of the palm and soles, and nonsuppurative cervical adenopathy.[85,86]

Treatment. Incision and drainage is the therapy of choice for any abscess of the head and neck. Studies have demonstrated a 90% efficacy of needle aspiration of a peritonsillar abscess vs. a 100% efficacy of incision and drainage.[87] Tonsillectomy has been recommended based on a recurrence rate of peritonsillar abscesses of 10-15%.[75]

Tracheostomy may be indicated for evidence of impending airway obstruction. Tracheostomy is more commonly used in the management of retropharyngeal abscesses and in Ludwig's angina where airway obstruction can develop rapidly.[77]

Antibiotics should be instituted at the earliest opportunity. Cultures should be sent and antibiotic coverage adjusted to the culture results. Studies have demonstrated that about 10-50% of organisms isolated from peritonsillar abscesses are resistant to penicillin.[75] Clindamycin is the antibiotic currently recommended for the treatment of deep neck abscesses. Other antibiotic alternatives include amoxicillin/clavulanate, ampicillin/sulbactam, or imipenem. Combination therapy includes the use of cefoxitin with gentamicin, ampicillin/sulbactam or clindamycin with gentamicin, ceftazidime, or aztreonam.[10]

Complications. The most common complication of deep neck abscesses is reacummulation of purulent material requiring repeated incision and drainage. Other potential complications include necrotizing cervical fasciitis, aspiration of purulent material and the development of pneumonia, erosion into a great vessel resulting in hemorrhage, and cranial neuropathies from dissection along fascial planes and sepsis.[77]

Parotitis

Definition. Parotitis is an infection and inflammation of the parotid gland. Parotitis can be divided into two categories: acute and chronic.

Epidemiology. The parotid gland is the most common salivary gland affected by infection. Bacterial parotitis is uncommon and is more commonly seen in the postoperative patient.[89] Viral parotitis secondary to mumps is more common in the winter and spring. The incidence of mumps has declined significantly with the widespread use of the mumps vaccine.[90]

Etiology. Bacterial parotitis is more common in the postoperative patient. Poor intraoral hygiene may also be a factor in the development of parotitis. The bacteria most commonly associated with parotitis include: *S. aureus, S. pneumoniae, E. coli, H. influenzae,* and *Bacteroides* sp. *Actinomycosis* and *M. tuberculosis* are rare causes of parotitis. Mumps virus is the most common viral etiology of parotitis.[27,91,92]

Pathophysiology. Stasis of saliva is felt to be the major precipitating factor in the postoperative patient. Stasis can occur from obstruction of the parotid duct (secondary to sialoliths or stenosis) or from a decreased production of saliva. Infection can develop with salivary stasis as saliva is a good medium for bacterial growth.

Clinical Features. Patients with bacterial or viral parotitis can present with unilateral or bilateral parotid enlargement, pain in the gland, trismus, fever, and overlying induration. Patients with mumps parotitis may also present with epididymitis, orchitis, or meningitis. Purulent material may be expressed from the parotid duct.

Diagnosis. The diagnosis is based on the physical examination and is confirmed by expressing purulent material from the parotid duct. Antibody titers to mumps virus are confirmatory. CT scan or ultrasound are indicated in the evaluation of the parotid gland if abscess formation is suspected or if there is evidence of extension of infection into deep neck spaces.

Differential Diagnosis. The differential diagnosis of parotid swelling is extensive. Cat scratch disease can cause chronic periparotid lymph node inflammation that mimics parotitis.[93] Many inflammatory conditions can affect the parotid gland, including sarcoidosis and Sjögren's syndrome. HIV infection is associated with a lymphoproliferative disorder of the parotid glands that can produce bilateral parotid swelling. Parotid and parotid duct neoplasms can also produce inflammation and swelling of the parotid glands.

Treatment. The goals of therapy are to reopen the parotid duct (if it is blocked), increase the production of saliva to flush out the infection, and antibiotics. The patient should be adequately hydrated. Intraoral hygiene must be addressed and improved. Massage of the parotid gland is helpful in the removal of inspirated secretion. Cultures should be taken of any purulent material expressed from the duct to aid in antibiotic therapy. Techniques to increase the flow of saliva include the use of sour lozenges such as lemon drops.

Current recommendations for antibiotic coverage for bacterial parotitis include amoxicillin/clavulanate, ampicillin/sulbactam, clindamycin, cefoxitin, or vancomycin in combination with metronidazole.[10]

Incision and drainage is the recommended therapy for patients with an abscess. Canulation of the parotid duct may be required to bypass a stenotic area or to assist in the removal of a sialolith. Chronic recurrent parotitis unresponsive to medical management may necessitate parotidectomy.

Complications. Potential complications of parotitis include abscess formation, extension of infection into deep fascial planes, destruction of the parotid gland, and septicemia. Chronic recurrent parotitis can lead to parotid atrophy and xerostomia.

Summary

The wide range of potential inflammatory conditions that can affect the head and neck present a challenge to the emergency physician. Disabling and life-threatening complications occur rarely but must be considered. Squamous cell carcinoma and other neoplasms must be considered in the differential for any inflammatory condition of the head and neck in any patient with worsening, persistent, or recurrent symptoms that fail to improve with appropriate therapy.

References

1. Bluestone CD, Klein JO, Paradise JL, et al. Workshop on effects of otitis media on the child. *Pediatrics* 1983;71: 639-652.
2. Giebink GS. Preventing otitis media. *Ann Otol Rhinol Laryngol* 1994;103:20-23.
3. Bluestone CD. Special series: Management of pediatric infectious disease in office practice: Chronic otitis media with effusion. *Pediatr Infect Dis J* 1982;1:180-187.
4. Daly K. Risk factors for otitis media sequelae and chronicity. *Ann Otol Rhinol Laryngol* 1994;103:39-42.
5. Klingman EW. Treatment of otitis media. *Am Fam Phys* 1992;45:242-250.
6. Kirsch CM, Wehner JH, Jensen W, et al. Tuberculous otitis media. *South Med J* 1995;88:363-366.
7. Margolis RH, Hunter LL, Giebink GS. Tympanometric evaluation of middle ear function in children with otitis media. *Ann Otol Rhinol Laryngol* 1994;103:34-38.
8. Paradise JL. Treatment guidelines for otitis media: The need for breadth and flexibility. *Pediatr Infect Dis J* 1995;14: 429-435.
9. Green SM, Rothrock SG. Single-dose intramuscular ceftriaxone for acute otitis media in children. *Pediatrics* 1993;91: 23-29.
10. Fairbanks DNF. *Antimicrobial Therapy in Otolaryngology Head and Neck Surgery.* 8th ed. Alexandria, VA: AAO-HNS; 1996.
11. Kleinman LC, Kosecoff J, Dubois RW, et al. The medical appropriateness of tympanostomy tubes proposed for children younger than 16 years in the United States. *JAMA* 1994;271: 1250-1255.
12. Gates GA. Adenoidectomy for otitis media with effusion. *Ann Otol Rhinol Laryngol* 1994;103:54-58.
13. Paradise JL, Bluestone CD, Rogers KD. Efficacy of adenoidectomy for recurrent otitis media in children previously treated with tympanostomy-tube placement. *JAMA* 1990;263: 2066-2073.
14. Russell JD, Donnelly M, McShane DP, et al. What causes acute otitis externa? *J Laryngol Otol* 1993;107:898-901.
15. Tierney MR, Baker AS. Infections of the head and neck in diabetes mellitus. *Infect Dis Clin North Am* 1995;9:195-216.
16. Cantor RM. Otitis externa and otitis media. *Emerg Med Clin North Am* 1995;13:445-455.
17. Grandis JR, Curtin HD, Yu VL. Necrotizing (malignant) external otitis: Prospective comparison of CT and MR imaging in diagnosis and follow-up. *Radiol* 1995;196:499-504.
18. Lucente F. Fungal infections of the external ear. *Otolaryngol Clin North Am* 1993;26:995-1006.
19. Bressler K, Shelton C. Ear foreign-body removal: A review of 98 consecutive cases. *Laryngoscope* 1993;103:367-370.
20. Linstrom CJ, Lucente FE. Infections of the external ear. In: Bailey BJ ed. *Head and Neck Surgery—Otolaryngology.* Philadelphia: Lippincott Co.; 1993:1549.
21. Evans P, Hofmann L. Malignant external otitis: A case report and review. *Am Fam Physician* 1994;49:427-431.
22. Pichichero ME. Culture and antigen detection tests for strep-

tococcal tonsillopharyngitis. *Am Fam Physician* 1992;45: 199-205.
23. Fiumara NJ, Walker EA. Primary syphilis of the tonsil. *Arch Otolaryngol* 1982;108:43.
24. Goldberg SN, Canalis RF. Rhinoscleroma as a cause of airway obstruction. *Ear Nose Throat J* 1980;59:6.
25. Pichichero ME. Controversies in the treatment of streptococcal pharyngitis. *Am Fam Physician* 1990;42:1567-1576.
26. Manolidis S, Frenkiel S, Yoskovitch A, et al. Mycobacterial infections of the head and neck. *Otolaryngol Head Neck Surg* 1993;109:427-433.
27. Emmanuelli JL. Infectious granulomatous diseases of the head and neck. *Am J Otolaryngol* 1993;14:155-167.
28. Lazarus AA. Sarcoidosis. *Otolaryngol Clin North Am* 1982;15:621.
29. Kihiczak D, Nychay S, Schwartz R, et al. Protracted superficial Wegener's granulomatosis. *J Am Acad Dermatol* 1994; 30:863-866.
30. Taylor CE, Smith CJ. Oral manifestations of Crohn's disease without demonstrable gastrointestinal lesions. *Oral Surg Oral Med Oral Pathol* 1975;39:58.
31. Wenig BM, Kornblut AD. Pharyngitis. In: Bailey BJ, ed. *Head and Neck Surgery—Otolaryngology.* Philadelphia: Lippincott Co.; 1993:553.
32. Klein JO. Pertussis. In: Reece RM. *Manual of Emergency Pediatrics.* Philadelphia: WB Saunders Co.; 1992:472.
33. Holmes RK. Diphtheria. In: Wilson JD, et al. *Harrison's Principles of Internal Medicine.* New York: McGraw-Hill; 1991:571.
34. Feigin RD, Stechenberg BW. Diphtheria. In: Feigin RD, Cherry JD, eds. *Textbook of Pediatric Infectious Diseases.* Philadelphia: WB Saunders; 1987.
35. Tice AW, Rodriquez VL. Pharyngeal gonorrhea. *JAMA* 1981; 246:2717.
36. Pelton SI. Infectious mononucleosis (Epstein-Barr syndrome). In: Reece RM. *Manual of Emergency Pediatrics.* Philadelphia: WB Saunders Co.; 1992:446.
37. Hanshaw JB. Cytomegalovirus infections. In: Feigin RD, Cherry JD, eds. *Textbook of Pediatric Infectious Diseases.* Philadelphia: WB Saunders; 1987.
38. Stewart DC. Sexually transmitted diseases in children and adults. In: Reece RM. *Manual of Emergency Pediatrics.* Philadelphia: WB Saunders Co.; 1992:489.
39. Arends MJ, Wyllie AH, Bird CC. Papillomaviruses and human cancer. *Hum Pathol* 1990;21:686.
40. Pichichero ME. Group A streptococcal tonsillopharyngitis: Cost-effective diagnosis and treatment. *Ann Emerg Med* 1995;25:390-406.
41. Dajani A, Taubert K, Ferrieri P, et al. Treatment of acute streptococcal pharyngitis and prevention of rheumatic fever: A statement for health professionals. *Pediatrics* 1995;96: 758-764.
42. Randall DA, Parker GS, Kennedy KS. Indications for tonsillectomy and adenoidectomy. *Am Fam Physician* 1991;44: 1639-1646.
43. Talbot-Stern JK. Arthritis, tendonitis, and bursitis. In: Rosen P. *Emergency Medicine Concepts and Clinical Practice.* St. Louis: Mosby; 1992:820-821.
44. Polis M. Viral infections. In: Rosen P. *Emergency Medicine Concepts and Clinical Practice.* St. Louis: Mosby; 1992: 2298.
45. Lustig LR, Cusick BC, Cheung SW, et al. Lemierre's syndrome: Two cases of postanginal sepsis. *Otolaryngol Head Neck Surg* 1995;112:767-772.
46. Alvarez A, Schreiber JR. Lemierre's syndrome in adolescent children—Anaerobic sepsis with internal jugular vein thrombophlebitis following pharyngitis. *Pediatrics* 1995;96: 354-359.
47. Ahkee S, Srinath L, Huang A, et al. Lemierre's syndrome: Postanginal sepsis due to anaerobic oropharyngeal infection. *Ann Otol Rhinol Laryngol* 1994;103:208-210.
48. Frantz TD, Rasgon BM, Quesenberry CP. Acute epiglottitis in adults, analysis of 129 cases. *JAMA* 1994;272:1358-1360.
49. Cressman WR, Myer CM. Diagnosis and management of croup and epiglottitis. *Pediatr Clin North Am* 1994;41: 265-276.
50. Senior BA, Radkowski D, MacArthur C, et al. Changing patterns in pediatric supraglottitis: A multi-institutional review, 1980 to 1992. *Laryngoscope* 1994;104:1314-1322.
51. Gorelick MH, Baker D. Epiglottitis in children, 1979 through 1992: Effects of *Haemophilus influenzae* Type b immunization. *Arch Pediatr Adolesc Med* 1994;148:47-50.
52. Frantz TD, Rasgon BM. Acute epiglottitis: Changing epidemiologic patterns. *Otolaryngol Head Neck Surg* 1993;109: 457-460.
53. Valdepena HG, Wald ER, Rose E, et al. Epiglottitis and *Haemophilus influenzae* immunization: The Pittsburgh experience—A five-year review. *Pediatrics* 1995;96:424-427.
54. Barrow HN, Vastola AP, Wang RC. Adult supraglottitis. *Otolaryngol Head Neck Surg* 1993;109:474-477.
55. Newth CJL, Levison H. Diagnosing and managing croup and epiglottitis. *J Resp Dis* 1981:Feb;22-41.
56. Andreassen UK, Baer S, Nielsen TG, et al. Acute epiglottitis—25 years experience with nasotracheal intubation, current management policy and future trends. *J Laryngol Otol* 1992; 106:1072-1075.
57. Mayo-Smith M. Fatal respiratory arrest in adult epiglottitis in the intensive care unit. *Chest* 1993;104:964-965.
58. Wald ER. Sinusitis in children. *N Engl J Med* 1992;326: 319-323.
59. Stafford CT. The clinician's view of sinusitis. *Otolaryngol Head Neck Surg* 1990;103:870-875.
60. Lund VJ, Kennedy DW. Quantification for staging sinusitis. *Ann Otol Rhinol Laryngol* 1995;104:17-21.
61. Kennedy DW. Overview. *Otolaryngol Head Neck Surg* 1990;103:847-854.
62. Kennedy DW, Gwaltney JM, Jones JG, et al. Medical management of sinusitis: Educational goals and management guidelines. *Ann Otol Rhinol Laryngol* 1995;104:22-30.
63. Winther B, Gwaltney JM. Therapeutic approach to sinusitis: Antiinfectious therapy as the baseline of management. *Otolaryngol Head Neck Surg* 1990;103:876-879.
64. Reilly JS. The sinusitis cycle. *Otolaryngol Head Neck Surg* 1990; 103:856-862.
65. Roberts DN, Hampal S, East CA, et al. The diagnosis of inflammatory sinonasal disease. *J Laryngol Otol*

1995;109:27-30.

66. Zinreich SJ. Paranasal sinus imaging. *Otolaryngol Head Neck Surg* 1990;103:863-869.
67. Rouby J-J, Laurent P, Gosnach M, et al. Risk factors and clinical relevance of nosocomial maxillary sinusitis in the critically ill. *Am J Respir Crit Care Med* 1994;150:776-783.
68. Tami TA. The management of sinusitis in patients infected with the human immunodeficiency virus (HIV). *Ear Nose Throat J* 1995;74:360-363.
69. Dolan RW, Chowdhury K. Diagnosis and treatment of intracranial complications of paranasal sinus infections. *J Oral Maxillofac Surg* 1995;53:1080-1087.
70. Lerner DN, Choi SS, Zalzal GH, et al. Intracranial complications of sinusitis in childhood. *Ann Otol Rhinol Laryngol* 1995;104:288-293.
71. Marney SR. Pathophysiology of reactive airway disease and sinusitis. *Ann Otol Rhinol Laryngol* 1996;105:98-100.
72. Kinney TB, Deluca SA. Kartagener's syndrome. *Am Fam Prac* 1991;44:133-134.
73. Borman KR, Brown PM, Mezera KK, et al. Occult fever in surgical intensive care unit patients is seldom caused by sinusitis. *Am J Surg* 1992;164:412-416.
74. Ungkanont K, Yellon RF, Weissman JL, et al. Head and neck space infections in infants and children. *Otolaryngol Head Neck Surg* 1995;112:375-382.
75. Herzon FS. Peritonsillar abscess: Incidence, current management practices, and a proposal for treatment guidelines. *Laryngoscope* 1995;105:1-17.
76. Pontell J, Har-El G, Lucente FE. Retropharyngeal abscess: Clinical review. *Ear Nose Throat J* 1995;74:701-704.
77. Sethi DS, Stanley RE. Deep neck abscesses—Changing trends. *J Laryngol Otol* 1994;108:138-143.
78. Har-El G, Aroesty JH, Shaha A, et al. Changing trends in deep neck abscess: A retrospective study of 110 patients. *Oral Surg Oral Med Oral Pathol* 1994;77:446-450.
79. Herr RD, Murdock RT, Davis RK. Serious soft tissue infections of the head and neck. *Am Fam Prac* 1991;44:878-888.
80. Passy V. Pathogenesis of Peritonsillar abscess. *Laryngoscope* 1994;104:185-190.
81. Hartmann RW. Recognition of retropharyngeal abscess in children. *Am Fam Physician* 1992;46:193-196.
82. DeClercq LD, Chole RA. Retropharyngeal abscess in the adult. *Otolaryngol Head Neck Surg* 1980;88:684.
83. Sakaguchi M, Sato S, Asawa S, et al. Computed tomographic findings in peritonsillar abscess and cellulitis. *J Laryngol Otol* 1995;109:449-451.
84. Lazor JB, Cunningham MJ, Eavey RD, et al. Comparison of computed tomography and surgical findings in deep neck infections. *Otolaryngol Head Neck Surg* 1994;111:746-750.
85. Pontell J, Rosenfeld RM, Kohn B. Kawasaki disease mimicking retropharyngeal abscess. *Otolaryngol Head Neck Surg* 1994;110:428-430.
86. Hester TO, Harris JP, Kenny JF, et al. Retropharyngeal cellulitis: A manifestation of Kawasaki disease in children. *Otolaryngol Head Neck Surg* 1993;109:1030-1033.
87. Wolf M, Even-Chen I, Kronenberg J. Peritonsillar abscess: Repeated needle aspiration vs. incision and drainage. *Ann Otol Rhinol Laryngol* 1994;103:554-557.
88. Pripp CM, Blomstrom P. Epiglottitis and torsades de pointes tachycardia. *Br Heart J* 1994;72:205-208.
89. Lary B. Postoperative suppurative parotitis. *Arch Surg* 1964;89:653.
90. Wagenvoort JH, Hansen M, Bentahar-Grouw BJ, et al. Epidemiology of mumps in the Netherlands. *J Hyg* 1980;85:313.
91. Rice DH. Diseases of the salivary glands—Non-neoplastic. In: Bailey BJ, ed. *Head and Neck Surgery—Otolaryngology*. Philadelphia: Lippincott Co.; 1993:476.
92. Bennhoff DF. Actinomycosis: Diagnostic and therapeutic considerations and a review of 32 cases. *Laryngoscope* 1984;94:1198-1217.
93. Margileth A, Zawadsky PM. Chronic lymphadenopathy in children and adolescents. *Am Fam Prac* 1985;31:166-180.

Sinusitis

Karl Lorenz, LT, MC, USNR

The ubiquitous nature of upper respiratory complaints in primary care requires the practitioner to be facile in the diagnosis of diseases of the respiratory tract and to be cost-effective in providing treatment. The National Ambulatory Medical Care Survey of office-based physicians documented that over the period 1980-1992, fever, cough, and nasal congestion were among the five most common complaints noted in visits that led to the prescription of antibiotics, and sinusitis was the fifth most common diagnosis rendered to patients receiving antibiotics in 1992.[1]

Sinusitis is typically divided into acute, subacute, and chronic sinusitis. Acute sinusitis is defined by symptoms of less than one month's duration, and chronic sinusitis is defined by symptoms of more than three months' duration. Developments in understanding the pathophysiology of sinusitis, trends in the imaging of sinusitis, the marketing of many new drugs for the treatment of sinusitis, and new surgical therapies mandate that practitioners reacquaint themselves with this common condition. This review will discuss the approach to acute and chronic bacterial sinusitis as encountered in the primary care setting.

Anatomy

Understanding contemporary diagnosis and treatment of sinus disease requires an appreciation for the anatomic relationship of the sinuses. The eight sinuses are bilateral pneumatized spaces located within the maxillary, ethmoid, sphenoid, and frontal bones that are developmentally complete by the age of 18.[2] The ethmoid sinuses are composed of a group of smaller air spaces or cells along the lateral nasal wall that are separated by thin bony walls and are divided into anterior and posterior groups.

The sinuses are lined with ciliated columnar epithelium and communicate with the nasal cavity via openings or ostia. The sinuses are coated with a bilayered mucous blanket that contains antibacterial factors and undergoes constant renewal as the top layer is circulated by ciliary action toward the ostia.[3]

The work of Messerklinger[4] and Stammberger[5] elucidated the crucial role of the osteomeatal complex (OMC) in the pathogenesis of sinusitis. This complex anatomic area includes the uncinate process, infundibulum, hiatus semilunaris, the cells of the anterior ethmoid, and the ostia of the maxillary and frontal sinuses. Any inflammatory process affecting the OMC can secondarily result in obstruction and inflammation of the maxillary and frontal sinuses. Medical or surgical therapy that alleviates this obstruction will allow resolution of infection and restoration of mucociliary clearance of the involved sinuses.

Pathophysiology

A number of factors contribute to the development of sinusitis by causing anatomic obstruction, impairing mucociliary function,

Table 1. Factors Associated with Sinusitis

Allergy
Anatomic factors (septal deviation, choanal atresia)
Apical dental infections
Barotrauma (swimming/diving)
Ciliary dyskinesia
Diabetes
Foreign body
HIV infection
Immunodeficiency states
Malignancy (especially hematologic)
Nasal polyps
Nasogastric tubes
Nasotracheal/orotracheal intubation
Trauma/surgery of the head and neck
Upper respiratory infection
Yellow nail syndrome

or degrading the immunologic integrity of the sinuses. Additionally, trauma or direct extension of infection are responsible for some cases of sinusitis. *(Please see Table 1.)* Bacteria are thought to enter the ostia under normal conditions and are readily cleared, but may be introduced under conditions that are favorable for infection. As demonstrated in animal models, neither bacterial inoculation nor ostial closure is sufficient to result in infection of the sinuses, but when both are present, bacterial sinusitis results.[6]

Upper respiratory infection is one of the most common antecedents of sinusitis in the primary care setting. A recent computed tomographic (CT) study of the common cold demonstrated radiographic sinusitis in a majority of patients with symptoms of an acute upper respiratory infection and nasal congestion. Most of these abnormalities resolved in patients restudied within 1-2 weeks.[7] Only a small minority of patients affected by common colds go on to develop bacterial sinusitis in community surveys.[8]

Presumably, viral infection sets the stage for bacterial superinfection of the sinuses through a number of mechanisms. Both viral and bacterial infection of the sinuses cause the development of local edema, decreased mucociliary transport, epithelial desquamation, and increased goblet cell numbers.[9] After bacterial infection is introduced in the closed space of the sinus, relative hypoxia and leukocyte products, including lactate and other organic acids, provide an environment that is favorable for the growth of gram-negative and anaerobic organisms, which are prominent species in chronic infections.[6] Irreversible damage to respiratory mucosa then supervenes, and chronic bacterial sinusitis results.

Allergic rhinitis is another factor commonly implicated in the development of sinusitis in primary care. It has been demonstrated that acute challenge with nasal allergen induces radiographic changes of sinusitis and increased blood flow in affected sinuses. The relationship of these acute changes to bacterial sinusitis in primary care has been debated since studies have not consistently demonstrated a relationship between seasonal allergy and the occurrence of acute sinusitis. The association between allergy and sinusitis is most apparent in patients with chronic sinus disease.[10]

Bacteriology

The bacteriology of sinusitis differs between acute and chronic phases. In acute sinusitis, single organisms predominate and include *S. pneumoniae* and *H. influenzae,* which are present in 60-70% of isolates obtained by antral puncture. Other isolates less frequently obtained include other streptococcal species, *S. aureus, M. catarrhalis, Neisseria* species, anaerobes, and gram negative organisms.[11-14]

Chronic sinusitis is characterized by mixed infections consisting of multiple aerobes and anaerobic organisms. In studies of sinus aspirates or biopsies of chronically infected sinus mucosa, gram-negative and anaerobic species predominate.[15-16] Important organisms include constituents of normal oropharyngeal flora, and many of the isolates are notable for their beta-lactamase production. The same pathogens have been identified in the complications that ensue from chronic sinusitis, and beta-lactamase resistance is an important factor to consider in treatment.[17]

Patients with recent hospitalization or HIV infection may present with sinusitis. Gram-negative organisms and anaerobes in mixed infections are primary concerns in patients presenting after hospitalization involving instrumentation of the oropharyngeal tract.[18] The limited microbiologic data available suggest that *S. aureus* and resistant gram-negative infections, particularly pseudomonas, as well as other typical opportunistic organisms, cause sinusitis in patients with HIV infection.[19]

Differential Diagnosis

Sinusitis must be considered in any patient presenting with upper respiratory complaints. Patients with sinusitis commonly complain of rhinorrhea and nasal congestion, which can be symptoms of several diseases. *(Please see Table 2.)* Seasonal and perennial allergic rhinitis are notable for prominent sneezing, pruritis, watery rhinorrhea, and congestion and may demonstrate pale, edematous nasal mucosa on exam of the anterior nares. Patients with allergy are often notable for the geographic or seasonal nature of their symptoms.

Patients with nonallergic rhinitis often have symptoms provoked by similar nonspecific stimuli, although the diagnosis may be difficult to distinguish apart from negative testing for specific allergens, and a subset of these patients exhibit nasal eosinophilia. Vasomotor rhinitis presents in a subset of patients with perennial rhinitis symptoms. It is often worse in winter and notable for negative tests for allergens and a failure to respond to antiinflammatory therapy. All patients with rhinorrhea and nasal congestion should be interviewed for the use of topical decongestants, since rebound effects from their use can result in recalcitrant unrelieved nasal congestion known as rhinitis medicamentosa.[20]

Table 2. Differential Diagnosis of Rhinorrhea/Nasal Congestion

Seasonal allergic rhinitis
Perennial allergic rhinitis
Non-allergic rhinitis with eosinophilia
Rhinitis medicamentosa
Drugs/medication (prazosin, guanethidine, reserpine, cocaine)
Mechanical/anatomic obstruction
Cerebrospinal fluid rhinorrhea
Pregnancy
Hypothyroidism
Wegener's granulomatosis
Sinusitis (viral, bacterial, fungal)

A number of drugs are notable for their effects on nasal vasculature and can produce nasal congestion. Although guanethidine and reserpine are rarely prescribed, prazosin is an antihypertensive that has been reported to cause nasal congestion in 1-4% of recipients.[21] A number of mechanical factors should be considered in patients presenting with sinonasal complaints; these include nasal polyps, which can be associated with aspirin hypersensitivity and septal deviation. Pregnancy and hyperthyroidism both produce nasal congestion and rhinorrhea through their effects on vascular tone. Wegener's granulomatosis is an uncommon hemmorrhagic vasculitis affecting the upper and lower respiratory tract in which exacerbations have been associated with respiratory infections.

Signs and Symptoms of Sinusitis

The rhinorrhea of sinusitis is typically purulent and accompanied by other symptoms as outlined in Table 3. A number of investigators have examined the relationship of symptoms and signs of sinusitis and sinus radiography by ultrasound or plain radiography.[22-24] A study of ultrasound of the maxillary and frontal sinuses in patients whose physicians clinically suspected sinusitis identified a history of the common cold, pain with forward bending, purulent nasal secretion, pain in teeth, and unilateral maxillary pain as independent predictors of sinusitis.[23] A primary care study of male veterans compared the history and physical exam for sinusitis to plain radiographs and identified maxillary toothache, abnormal transillumination, poor response to decongestants, purulent secretion, and history of colored nasal discharge as predictors of sinusitis.[24] Headache has been clearly associated with sinusitis in case reports of headache relieved by the treatment of sinusitis.[25] The clinicians' overall impression has been validated as the best predictor of sinusitis in primary care.[24]

Table 3. Symptoms and Signs of Sinusitis

Abnormal transillumination
Cough
Dental pain
Facial pain (maxillary, frontal)
Fever
Headache
Hyposmia/anosmia
Nasal obstruction
Nasal polyps
Nasal speech
Pain induced by forward bending
Preceeding upper respiratory infection
Purulent nasal discharge

Diagnosis of Sinusitis: Radiography

A number of methods are available to the primary care practitioner to confirm a diagnosis of sinusitis. Often imaging is not necessary, especially when a high clinical suspicion for sinusitis exists and the patient has not previously been treated. Radiographic confirmation may be desirable when: 1) the patient is very ill; 2) the patient is immunocompromised (malignancy, HIV infection); 3) potential complications of sinusitis are present; 4) the patient has failed to respond to prior treatment; or 5) surgical therapy is anticipated.

Plain radiographs are commonly available for imaging the paranasal sinuses. The Water's view optimizes the projection of the maxillary sinuses in a posterior/anterior view along the occipitomental plane with the chin elevated. The Caldwell view allows for examination of the frontal and ethmoid sinuses by using an occipitofrontal beam while the nose and forehead are in contact with the film. The lateral film is best for visualizing the sphenoid and frontal sinuses. The submental vertex also allows visualization of the sphenoid and ethmoid sinuses.

Plain radiographs can evaluate the presence or absence of sinusitis, which is suggested by mucosal thickening, air-fluid levels, or complete opacification; however, plain radiography is unable to define detailed anatomy and cannot visualize the osteomeatal complex. A number of studies have correlated the findings of mucosal thickening, air-fluid levels, or opacification with the finding of fluid on aspiration of the sinuses in symptomatic patients. Fluid is found in a percentage of patients proportional to the degree of mucous membrane thickening visible on plain radiographs with the highest yield of aspiration in patients with complete opacification.[26] Only 5% of an asymptomatic population will have mucosal abnormalities consisting of thickening greater than 5 mm if examined by standard sinus radiography, although as many as 10% will exhibit polypoid mucosal changes.[27]

Computed tomography (CT) of the sinuses can be performed using either a complete series or a limited coronal series. A number of factors affect CT interpretation and can be minimized by ordering clinicians. Acute upper respiratory infection causes mucosal and sinus changes as noted and obscures relevant chronic changes that have bearing on surgical therapy. CT scans performed for chronic disease should be performed in the patient's most asymptomatic phase. Additionally, patients with polyposis may benefit from steroid nasal sprays for 4-6 weeks prior to scanning, although polyposis still makes interpretation of changes difficult.[28]

CT provides a detailed assessment of sinus anatomy including resolution of bony detail and the osteomeatal unit that is critical to surgical planning. Anatomic variations that may narrow the osteomeatal complex and contribute to sinusitis are identified including, in order of frequency, concha bullosa (aerated middle turbinate), nasal septal deformity, paradoxical middle turbinate (a middle turbinate with its curvature concave to the nasal septum), Haller cells (ethmoid cells extending along the medial roof of the maxillary sinus), prominent ethmoid bulla, and deviations of the uncinate process. Sixty-two percent of one studied population with chronic sinusitis had at least one of these anatomic variations compared to 11% of a normal control group.[29] Results of computed tomography must be correlated with the clinical presentation and endoscopic findings. CT should not be used alone to determine surgical intervention, since a high percentage of the asymptomatic population demonstrate mucosal disease.[30]

In addition to its use in presurgical planning for chronic sinusitis, CT may be selectively useful as a diagnostic study in ill patients with acute sinusitis. CT is much more sensitive at detecting the radiographic changes of sinusitis, and its specificity is not hampered by overlying bone and soft tissue that can make interpretation of plain films difficult.

Although CT scanning is very sensitive for detecting sinusitis, mucosal thickening must be interpreted with caution. Patients without clinical sinusitis demonstrate a high prevalence of abnormal findings on CT examination of the sinuses; thus, CTs in patients with a low clinical suspicion for sinusitis must be interpreted cautiously. Studies of patients referred for CT scan of the head for conditions other than sinusitis report sinus abnormalities in 15-40% of patients scanned. Notably, complete sinus opacification is a rare abnormality even in an asymptomatic population, occurring in only approximately 1% of sinuses studied, and thus should always be regarded as a sign of potentially significant sinus disease.[30,31]

A recent comparison of plain radiography of the sinuses with CT demonstrated the potential diagnostic superiority of CT in ill patients with possible sinusitis. In a small study of emergency room patients with acute sinusitis, although plain films demonstrated air-fluid levels or complete opacification of the maxillary sinus in most cases detected by CT, they failed to demonstrate ethmoidal, frontal, or sphenoidal air-fluid levels or opacification.[32]

Magnetic resonance imaging (MRI) has proven useful in distinguishing fungal infection of the sinuses and in distinguishing benign inflammatory from neoplastic conditions. MRI does not provide information about bony anatomy, and its role in restricted to the evaluation of potential fungal or neoplastic disease in chronic sinusitis.

Medical Treatment

The ancillary treatment of sinusitis is largely empirical, and strategies are similar for acute and chronic bacterial disease. Ancillary treatments for sinusitis include decongestants, mucolytics, and nasal steroid preparations. Alpha-adrenergic decongestants include both topical and systemic preparations. Although many preparations are effective in restoring nasal patency, topical preparations must be used cautiously because of their potential for rebound and overuse, and systemic preparations may have the advantage of promoting patency in tissue not directly accessible to topical decongestants.[33]

Ancillary treatments that may promote mucociliary clearance include nasal saline irrigation and medications such as guaifenesin. Topical saline sprays may be given several times daily to promote liquefaction and clearance of secretions and for symptom relief.

A number of additional therapies may be considered in patients with allergic rhinitis. Topical steroid preparations have not been shown to be definitely helpful in treating sinusitis in the setting of allergic rhinitis, but their use is reasonable and relatively inexpensive. Aqueous preparations may be helpful in a subset of patients who find other preparations irritating. Additionally, antihistamines are useful adjunctive treatment for allergic rhinitis. In acute sinusitis, antihistamines should be avoided because of their drying effect on nasal secretions, which may impair mucocilliary clearance, but they are useful in long-term therapy.

The importance of antibiotic therapy in acute and chronic sinusitis has not been well tested. First, it is not clear when viral or allergic sinusitis is superseded by bacterial infection. As demonstrated in CT study of the common cold and in the few placebo-controlled trials of antibiotic therapy in sinusitis, many patients with acute sinusitis will have spontaneous resolution of their symptoms without treatment.[7,34]

Additionally, the superiority of beta-lactamase drugs has not been proven in acute treatment of sinusitis, although patients in whom initial therapy fails will often be infected with resistant species.[34] Thus, reasonable choices for initial therapy include drugs like trimethoprim-sulfamethoxazole or amoxicillin. In the event of clinical failure, secondary therapy should include a drug active against beta-lactamase-resistant species such as amoxicillin-clavulanate, an oral cephalosporin, a macrolide or azolide, or a quinolone in combination with a drug active against gram-positive species, such as clindamycin.[35]

In addition to beta-lactamase production, the presence of penicillin-resistant pneumococci must be considered in treatment failure after initial therapy with a penicillin because these organisms have also been identified with increasing frequency in sinusitis, particularly in children.[36] The cost of a 10-day course of therapy with selected antimicrobials for the treatment of sinusitis is shown in Table 4.

The efficacy of an initial 10-day course of therapy has been demonstrated in studies employing repeated sinus puncture, and recently the efficacy of a three-day course has been suggested in a randomized trial employing empirical therapy in patients with sinusitis defined by symptoms and compatible findings on plain radiography.[37]

Table 4. Costs of Selected Antimicrobials for the Treatment of Sinusitis*

ANTIMICROBIAL	DOSAGE	AVERAGE WHOLESALE PRICE
Trimethoprim-sulfamethoxazole	800/160 mg TAB bid	$7.63
Ampicillin	500 mg CAP qid	$10.23
Amoxicillin	500 mg CAP tid	$3.68
Amoxicillin-clavulanate	500 mg CAP tid	$86.45
Cefaclor	500 mg CAP tid	$115.44
Cefuroxime axetil	500 mg TAB bid	$131.98
Loracarbef	400 mg PULVULE bid	$80.97
Cefixime	400 mg TAB bid	$131.34
Azithromycin	250 mg CAP (6 doses)	$36.22
Clarithromycin	500 mg TAB ID	$65.20
Ciprofloxacin	500 mg TAB bid	$68.37
Clindamycin	150 mg CAP qid	$48.31

* Based upon a 10-day course of therapy, average wholesale cost to the pharmacist

Another important patient category to consider for treatment is patients with symptoms and normal plain radiographs. Recently, the outcomes of patients with symptoms but normal radiography were evaluated. These patients had a profile of symptoms similar to patients with radiographic sinusitis, but with a lower prevalence of physical exam findings, and were given diagnoses of allergic rhinitis, sinusitis, viral infection, bronchitis, or other diagnoses. The symptoms of cough and itchy eyes tended to predict treatment success or failure. Patients having only cough responded better to conservative treatment, possibly because of true viral infection. Patients with itchy eyes tended to have a more protracted course, possibly associated with allergic rhinosinusitis, which tends to be more difficult to treat over the short term.[38]

Complications of Sinusitis

Orbital complications most frequently result from acute ethmoiditis. They are classified into four categories: periorbital (preseptal) edema, subperiosteal abscess, orbital cellulitis, and orbital abscess. Periorbital edema is the least serious of these complications. The orbital septum acts as an anatomic barrier to posterior spread of the infection from the eyelids into the true orbit. Patients will present with eyelid edema but will not have orbital abnormalities such as visual loss, chemosis, proptosis, or limitation of extraocular motion. These signs will be present with the more severe and threatening subperiosteal abscess, orbital cellulitis, or orbital abscess. CT scan confirms the presence of orbital involvement and allows exact assessment of the sinus disease. Consultation with an ophthalmologist is imperative. Visual acuity must be monitored closely since optic nerve inflammation and compression may occur as the infection progresses. Intravenous antibiotics are the mainstay of treatment. Surgical decompression of the orbit and drainage of involved sinuses is indicated when the CT demonstrates an abscess, for deteriorating visual acuity, or if there is no improvement in the symptoms in 48-72 hours.

Intracranial complications of sinusitis include meningitis, epidural abscess, subdural abscess, venous sinus thrombosis, and brain abscess. Meningitis is the most common intracranial complication of sinusitis. The sphenoid sinus is the most frequent source, followed by the ethmoid, frontal, and maxillary sinuses. Meningeal signs and symptoms are the same as for other sources of meningitis. Treatment of meningitis consists of intravenous antibiotics and the surgical drainage of the involved sinus.

Most cases of intracranial abscesses are secondary to frontal sinusitis. The symptoms of epidural abscesses may consist only of a mild increase in headache, so the index of suspicion must be high. Subdural abscesses and brain abscesses generally present with more headache, fever, and meningeal signs. The clinical course may be rapid with progression to seizures, neurologic deficits, and a reduction in the level of consciousness. CT scan with contrast is the preferred method to confirm the presence of the intracranial complications of sinusitis. Neurosurgical consultation is imperative. Treatment consists of intravenous antibiotics, drainage of sinus disease, and craniotomy with drainage of the intracranial abscess.

The frontal bone is the most frequent site of osteomyelitis that results as a complication of sinusitis. Signs include a soft doughy edema over the frontal bone (Pott's puffy tumor) associated with lid edema, fever, and headache. A CT scan confirms the diagnosis and evaluates the possibility of a concurrent intracranial abscess. Treatment consists of intravenous antibiotics combined with surgery tailored to the presence of abscess and sinus disease.

Nasal Endoscopy

Nasal endoscopic examination is necessary in the evaluation of refractory sinonasal disease. Examination with a nasal speculum and headlight alone will not allow a sufficient view of the osteomeatal complex. Endoscopy allows the clinician to more accurately delineate the character of the sinonasal mucosa and to observe the presence of abnormal secretions or polyps. It allows more detailed study of those anatomic variations which may contribute to osteomeatal complex obstruction. Finally, it allows the effect of treatment to be followed more accurately and may preclude repeated radiographic evaluations.[39]

Nasal endoscopy is an office procedure within the capability of the primary care provider. Flexible or rigid endoscopes may be used. 25-degree or 30-degree angled rigid scopes are generally preferred by otolaryngologists for sinonasal examination because of their superior optical quality and because they can more easily be used to move the anesthetized middle turbinate medially in order to allow complete inspection of the middle meatus. Flexible endoscopes are easier on the patient. They may also be a more versatile and cost-effective instrument for the primary care provider since they can be advanced past the nasopharynx and allow examination of the hypopharynx and larynx.

Prior to endoscopic examination, the nasal cavity is sprayed with a decongestant and a topical anesthetic (4% lidocaine or 2% pontocaine). The nasal septum, floor of the nose, inferior turbinate, sphenoethmoidal recess, middle turbinate, and middle meatus are inspected in turn. The nature of the sinonasal mucosa is studied, and the presence of abnormal secretions, polyps, or anatomic variations is noted.[39]

The Role of the Otolaryngologist

Most patients with acute sinusitis and many with chronic sinusitis will improve when placed on appropriate medical therapy. Cases of sinusitis that are refractory to medical management, including treatment of associated conditions such as allergy, should be referred to an otolaryngologist for evaluation. Indications for referral to an otolaryngologist are listed in Table 5.

Table 5. Indications for Referral to an Otolaryngologist

- Complication of sinusitis
- Severe acute sinusitis
- Failure of medical therapy
- Frequent recurrent sinusitis
- Immunocompromised patient (AIDS, hematologic malignancy)
- Associated with anatomic nasal obstruction (nasal polyps, septal deviation)

The concept that most cases of sinusitis originate in the anterior ethmoid sinuses and are due to obstruction of the relatively small anatomic area of the osteomeatal complex has drastically altered the surgical approach to refractory sinusitis. The basic aim of functional endoscopic sinus surgery is to remove diseased mucosa and correct anatomic abnormalities in the area of the osteomeatal complex (OMC).[40] Success in relieving obstruction of the OMC restores drainage of adjacent sinuses. Return of efficient mucociliary clearance allows the mucosa of chronically infected sinuses to resume a normal character in the weeks and months following surgery. Because virtually all of the diseased mucosa is removed from the anterior ethmoid cells, destructive surgical intervention in the frontal and maxillary sinuses is unnecessary. Hence, the morbidity of previously favored procedures such as the Caldwell-Luc approach and external ethmoidectomy is avoided.

Patients with recurrent acute or chronic sinusitis refractory to medical management and allergy intervention are candidates for functional endoscopic sinus surgery.[41] The surgery may be performed on an outpatient basis in the majority of cases and can be performed under general anesthesia or local anesthesia with sedation. Several techniques are available for the performance of the surgery.[40] Rigid 0-degree, 30-degree, and 70-degree telescopes are used. The uncinate process is removed along with the ethmoid bulla. This procedure uncovers the ostium of the maxillary sinus, which is enlarged with biting forceps if necessary. If only the maxillary sinus is involved, then the surgery can be concluded. More typically, diseased mucosa must be cleared from other anterior ethmoid cells and the frontal recess and frontal sinus ostium cleared. Anatomic abnormalities such as a concha bullosa or deviated nasal septum are corrected if present. The posterior ethmoid and sphenoid sinuses are addressed only if involved. If indicated, the posterior ethmoid is reached endoscopically through the basal lamella and the dissection carried back to the sphenoid. On conclusion of the surgery, the nose is packed or not at the discretion of the surgeon. Postoperative care is crucial and includes frequent saline irrigation to clear mucus and blood clots. Meticulous periodic cleaning of the surgical site promotes healing, reduces scarring, and prevents recurrence of osteomeatal complex obstruction. After surgery, it may take months for the mucosal changes associated with long-standing chronic sinusitis to heal. Antibiotics and adjuvant medical therapy may be necessary during this period.[42]

Outcome studies of endoscopic sinus surgery have shown a high favorable response rate; however, there are no randomized trials comparing surgery with aggressive medical management. In a retrospective study of 155 patients who underwent endoscopic surgery, Matthews and colleagues reported that 90% of patients believed surgery was beneficial. Patients with facial pain showed the greatest improvement. All patients having simultaneous septoplasty had successful outcomes. Opacification of the sphenoid sinus correlated with a poor outcome.[43]

Symptomatic improvement does not entirely correlate with endoscopic resolution of disease. A combined prospective and retrospective study by Kennedy measured outcomes in 120 endoscopic surgery patients. After a mean follow-up of 18 months, 85% of patients reported marked improvements in symptoms; 45% of the operative sites had some evidence of residual disease as determined by the presence of drainage, scarring, inflammation, or mucosal hypertrophy.[44]

Functional endoscopic sinus surgery is a relatively safe procedure, but it is not without major risks. These include orbital injury, nasolacrimal duct injury, and cerebrospinal fluid leak. In a residency training program, a study of 337 patients on whom surgery was performed showed a 1.5% incidence of major complications.[45]

Summary

Sinusitis commonly presents in the primary care setting. It often occurs in association with viral upper respiratory infection, and most cases of acute sinusitis will resolve spontaneously without antibiotic treatment. Osteomeatal complex obstruction promotes an environment favorable to bacterial infection and is often found in association with maxillary or frontal sinusitis. If underlying infection and obstruction is treated early, obstruction may resolve and allow return of normal sinus function; however, persistent obstruction can result in irreversible damage to mucosa and chronic bacterial sinusitis. Medical therapy for acute sinusitis should include coverage of *H. influenzae* and *S. pneumoniae,* and polymicrobial infections by beta-lactamase-resistant organisms must be considered in treatment of chronic sinusitis. Medical therapy should also include treatment of associated conditions such as allergy that may contribute to chronic sinusitis. When sinusitis persists despite adequate medical therapy, nasal endoscopy should be considered to evaluate anatomic factors. Surgical consultation for aspiration and functional endoscopic surgery should be considered.

References

1. McCaig LF, Hughes JM. Trends in antimicrobial drug prescribing among office-based physicians in the United States. *JAMA* 1995;273:214-219.
2. Facer GW, Kern EB. Sinusitis: Current concepts and management In: Baily BJ, Johnson JT, Kohut RI, Pillsbury HC, Tardy ME (eds). *Head and Neck Surgery—Otolaryngology.* Philadelphia: Lippincott; 1993:342-349.
3. Kaliner MA. Human nasal host defense and sinusitis. *J Allergy Clin Immunol* 1992;90:424-430.
4. Messerklinger W. *Endoscopy of the Nose.* Baltimore: Urban and Schwarzenberg; 1978.
5. Stammberger H. *Functional Endoscopic Sinus Surgery.* Philadelphia: BC Decker; 1991.
6. Stierna P, Kumlien J, Carlsöö B. Experimental sinusitis in rabbits induced by aerobic and anaerobic bacteria: Models for reasearch in sinusitis. *J Otolaryngol* 1991;20:376-378.
7. Gwaltney JM, et al. Computed tomographic study of the common cold. *N Engl J Med* 1994;330:25-30.
8. Gwaltney JM. Sinusitis. In: Mandell GL, Bennett JE, Dolin R (eds). *Principles and Practice of Infectious Diseases.* New York: Churchill Livingstone; 1995:585-590.
9. Norlander T, Westrin KM, Stierna P. The inflammatory response of the sinus and nasal mucosa during sinusitis: implications for research and therapy. *Acta Otolaryngol Stockh* 1994;Suppl 515:38-44.
10. Karlsson G, Holmberg K. Does allergic rhinitis predispose to sinusitis? *Acta Otolaryngol Stockh* 1994:Suppl 515:26-29.
11. Evans FO, et al. Sinusitis of the maxillary antrum. *N Engl J Med* 1975;293:735-739.
12. Hamory BH, et al. Etiology and antimicrobial therapy of acute maxillary sinusitis. *J Infect Dis* 1979;139:197-202.
13. Savolainen S, Ylikoski J, Jousimies-Somer H. Differential diagnosis of purulent and non-purulent acute maxillary sinusitis in young adults. *Rhinology* 1989;27:53-61.
14. Gwaltney JM, et al. The microbial etiology and antimicrobial therapy of adults with acute community-acquired sinusitis: A fifteen-year experience at the University of Virginia and review of other selected studies. *J Allergy Clin Immunol* 1992;90:457-462.
15. Brook I, Thompson DH, Frazier EH. Microbiology and management of chronic maxillary sinusitis. *Arch Otolaryngol Head Neck Surg* 1994;120:1317-1320.
16. Ito K, et al. Bacteriology of chronic otitis media, chronic sinusitis, and paranasal mucopyocele in Japan. *Clin Infect Dis* 1995;(Suppl 2)20:S214-S219.
17. Brook I, Frazier EH. Microbiology of subperiosteal orbital abscess and associated maxillary sinusitis. *Laryngoscope* 1996;106:1010-1013.
18. Rouby JJ, et al. Risk factors and clinical relevance of nosocomial maxillary sinusitis in the critically ill. *Am J Respir Crit Care Med* 1994;150:776-783.
19. Grant A, et al. Paranasal sinus disease in HIV antibody positive patients. *Genitourinary Med* 1993;69:208-212.
20. Knight A. The differential diagnosis of rhinorrhea. *J Allergy Clin Immunol* 1995;95:1080-1083.
21. *Physicians' Desk Reference;* 1996:1938.
22. Axelsson A, Runze U. Symptoms and signs of acute maxillary sinusitis. *J Otolaryngol Relat Spec* 1976;38:298-308.
23. Van Dujin NP, Brouwer HJ, Lamberts H. Use of symptoms and signs to diagnose maxillary sinusitis in general practice: Comparison with ultrasonography. *BMJ* 1992;305:684-687.
24. Williams JW, et al. Clinical evaluation for sinusitis: Making the diagnosis by history and physical examination. *Ann Intern Med* 1992;117:705-710.
25. Clerico DM. Sinus headaches reconsidered: Referred cephalgia of rhinologic origin masquerading as refractory primary headaches. *Headache* 1995;35:185-192.
26. Axelsson A, et al. The correlation between the radiological examination and the irrigation findings in maxillary sinusitis. *Acta Otolaryng* 1970;69:302-306.
27. Fascenelli FW. Maxillary sinus abnormalities: Radiographic evidence in an asymptomatic population. *Arch Otolaryng* 1969;90:190-193.
28. Bingham B, Shankar L, Hawke M. Pitfalls in computed tomography of the paranasal sinuses. *J Otolaryngology* 1991;20:414-418.
29. Zinreich J. Imaging of inflammatory sinus disease. *Otolaryngologic Clin N Am* 1993;26:535.
30. Havas TE, Motbey JA, Gullane PJ. Prevalence of incidental abnormalities on computed tomographic scans of the paranasal sinuses. *Arch Otolaryngol Head Neck Surg* 1988;114:856-859.
31. Calhoun KH, et al. CT evaluation of the paranasal sinuses in symptomatic and asymptomatic populations. *Otolaryngol Head Neck Surg* 1991;104:480-483.
32. Burke TF, Guertler AT, Timmons JH. Comparison of sinus x-rays with computed tomography scans in acute sinusitis.

Academic Emerg Med 1994;1:235-239.

33. Zeiger RS. Prospects for ancillary treatment of sinusitis in the 1990s. *J Allergy Clin Immunol* 1992;90:478-495.
34. Wald ER, Chiponis D, Ledesma-Medina J. Comparative effectiveness of amoxicillin and amoxicillin-clavulanate potassium in acute paranasal sinus infections in children: A double-blind, placebo-controlled trial. *Pediatrics* 1986;77: 795-800.
35. Bartlett JG. Antiobiotic selection in sinusitis. *Arch Otolaryngol Head Neck Surg* 1996;122:422-423.
36. Nelson CT, et al. Activity of oral antibiotics in middle ear and sinus infections caused by penicillin-resistant *Streptococcus pneumoniae:* Implications for treatment. *Pediatr Infect Dis J* 1994;13:585-589.
37. Williams JW, et al. Randomized controlled trial of 3 vs. 10 days of trimethoprim/sulfamethoxazole for acute maxillary sinusitis. *JAMA* 1995;273:1015-1021.
38. Holleman DR, Williams JW, Simel DL. Usual care and outcomes in patients with sinus complaints and normal results of sinus roentgenography. *Arch Fam Med* 1995;4:246-251.
39. Kennedy DW, et al. Medical management of sinusitis: Educational goals and management guidelines. *Ann Otol Rhinol Laryngol* 1995;104 Suppl. 167:22.
40. Rice DH. Endoscopic sinus surgery. *Otolaryngol Clin N Am* 1993;26:613.
41. Reuler JB, et al. Sinusitis: A review for generalists. *Western J Med* 1995;163:40.
42. Evans KL. Diagnosis and management of sinusitis. *BMJ* 1994;309:1415.
43. Matthews BL, et al. Endoscopic sinus surgery: Outcome in 155 cases. *Otolaryngol Head Neck Surg* 1991;104:244.
44. Kennedy DW. Prognostic Factors, outcomes and staging in ethmoid sinus surgery. *Laryngoscope* 1992;102(Suppl 57):1.
45. Ramadan HH, Allen GC. Complications of endoscopic sinus surgery in a residency training program. *Laryngoscope* 1995; 105:376.

Ophthalmologic Emergencies

David D. Markoff, MD, FACS
David Chacko, MD, PhD

The presentations of eye-threatening problems may be subtle or dramatic. Pain may or may not be present. Loss of vision is not always a prominent initial complaint, although subsequent visual testing may reveal significant field or perceptual deficits. But regardless of the initial impression, the clinical and medico-legal consequences of inappropriately managed emergencies of the eye can be devastating. Consequently, patient evaluation must always be systematic, precise, and meticulously documented.

The fact is, perhaps more than many other conditions, eye-related emergencies require accurate diagnosis, thorough evaluation, and targeted management to optimize clinical outcomes. Moreover, the range of ocular and retinal pathology requiring emergency treatment is broad, and most patients with unusual conditions or acute onset of blindness will require opthalmologic consultation as part of their management plan.

"Red eye" is one of the most common symptoms triggering a visit to the emergency department for evaluation of an opthalmologic problem. Some causes are relatively benign—allergic reaction, subconjunctival hemorrhage, bacterial conjunctivitis—whereas other etiologies such as angle closure glaucoma or endopthalmitis can be sight-threatening and will require emergent treatment, including surgery to preserve vision.

Trauma to the eye requires not only a thorough physical examination with a slit lamp, but additional modalities such as plain radiography or CT scanning may be necessary to detect orbital penetration delineate the location of an intraorbital foreign body. In the case of blunt trauma to the globe, it is imperative to evaluate the likelihood of orbital rupture. Chemical trauma/burns to the globe requires toxin-specific management,with targeted therapy depending on the nature of the offending agent. Prompt ocular lavage is a mainstay of treatment for these injuries.

Deciphering the cause of non-traumatic visual loss is an essential component of emergency opthalmologic management. The most common causes include optic nerve dysfunction, retinal pathology, or retinal vascular occlusion, all of which can be suspected during the initial encounter and require immediate treatment to preserve vision. Diplopia, another common presentation, may suggest an acute neurologic deficit, which can be either vascular (i.e., a third CN palsy precipitated by a posterior communicating artery aneurysm) or degenerative (multiple sclerosis) in etiology.

The purpose of this chapter is to provide a concise and focused review of common eye emergencies managed in the ED setting. Stressing those conditions that require immediate treatment for preservation of vision, this review outlines a systematic approach to the opthalmologic examination, presents guidelines for testing, indications for referral, and outcome-effective management pathways.

Table 1. The Ocular Examination

- Visual Acuity
- External-lids, lashes, lacrimal, periorbital
- Pupils
- Extraocular motility
- Visual fields
- Biomicroscopy
- Intraocular pressure
- Fundoscopy

Ocular Examination

The eye examination can be broken down into the eight parts listed in Table 1.

For both medical and legal reasons, visual acuity should be checked on every patient who presents with an eye problem. This is usually done for distance vision with a standard acuity chart (Snellen) and recorded for first the right eye and then the left eye. A near card can also be used and is especially helpful for bedridden patients. Acuity can be checked both with and without correction, although the most important piece of information is usually the "best corrected" acuity. If the patient did not bring or does not have glasses, a pinhole occluder can give a good approximation of corrected acuity. The external examination should look for signs of trauma, lid disease, proptosis, etc.

Pupillary examination is important, especially in patients with significant loss of vision. The swinging flashlight test is used to check for a relative afferent pupillary defect.[1]

Extraocular movements (EOMs) are checked by having the patient follow an object while holding their head still. Look especially for any evidence of muscle palsy or restriction. Defer EOM testing if an open globe injury is suspected.

A confrontation visual field is performed by presenting two objects (usually both hands of the examiner) in front of each eye separately and having the patient state whether they can count the fingers on each hand. This is especially helpful for picking up hemianopic field defects.

Biomicroscopy of the anterior segment of the eye is best performed using a slit lamp. A direct ophthalmoscope with the +10 lens in place also works well. Look especially for abnormalities of the cornea, anterior chamber (i.e., hyphema), and iris.

Intraocular pressure is tested unless an open globe is suspected. A Goldmann type applanation tonometer is best. The portable Tonopen (Mentor) also works well in the emergency setting.

Fundoscopic examination is best performed through dilated pupils (use 1% tropicamide and 2.5% phenylephrine). Carefully document any dilating drops given in patients with head trauma.[2] A direct ophthalmoscope gives a good view of the optic nerve, macula, and vessels. Indirect ophthalmoscopy is needed for the peripheral retinal exam.

Table 2. Red Eye Findings

Discharge

Clear or watery discharge with allergic processes, superficial abrasions, and viral infections. Yellowish or purulent discharge most common with bacterial conjunctivitis.

Preauricular adenopathy

Seen with most viral infections, including herpes simplex. Gonococcus only bacterial conjunctivitis with a preauricular node.

Membrane

Fibrinous membrane over palpebral conjunctiva most commonly seem with adenoviral or herpetic viral infections, streptococcus or gonococcus bacterial infections, and with chemical burns.

Red Eye

A red eye can signify a sight-threatening process or a benign self-limited disease. Examination findings which help to separate various etiologies are listed in Table 2.

Common non-traumatic causes of red eye, along with recommended treatments, are listed below. (Traumatic causes are given in a later section.)

Subconjunctival Hemorrhage. Usually spontaneous onset with no pain or decreased vision. Exam shows solid, bright red patch on bulbar conjunctiva with sharp borders. If the patient has any history of trauma, look for further injury. Treat by observation. If there are multiple recurrences or other signs of excessive bleeding, check clotting parameters.[3]

Allergic Reactions. The patient has symptoms of itching, burning, and watering. There is often a history of systemic allergic problems. Exam shows injected conjunctiva, possibly chemosis, and watery discharge. Treat by cool compresses, removal of offending allergen, and medications if necessary. Naphazoline and others are available over the counter. Histamine blockers, such as levocarbastine, help acute symptoms. Mast cell inhibitors (lodoxamide tromethamine, cromolyn) help prevent future attacks. Olopatadine hydrochloride combines both histamine blockade and mast cell inhibition.

Viral Infections (Non-herpetic). Patients often have a history of exposure to "pink eye" or concurrent upper respiratory infection. Exam shows preauricular adenopathy, watery discharge, possible conjunctival membrane. The cornea may have grayish round subepithelial lesions. The patient may have eyelid edema, especially with adenovirus. Treatment for most viral conjunctivitis is cool compresses and observation (adenoviral infections can take 2-3 weeks to clear and are highly contagious). An antibiotic, such as erythromycin ointment 1-2 times/day, can be used as prophylaxis against secondary bacterial infection. Topical steroids can help the acute symptoms but tend to prolong the course, especially of corneal infiltrates.[4]

Herpes Simplex. This usually presents with pain or foreign body sensation and decreased vision. Exam may show a tender preauricular node, corneal dendrite that stains with fluorescein (acute HSV) or hazy, edematous patch in cornea (disciform HSV). Treatment is topical trifluridine eight times/day for 5-7 days until dendrite heals. Debridement of the dendrite with a cotton-applicator at the slit lamp may also help hasten healing.[5] The ability to differentiate between HSV keratitis and conjunctivitis is important. Prompt referral to an ophthalmologist is recommended.

Bacterial Conjunctivitis. This presents with a history of yellowish discharge and eyelids mattered together upon awakening. It can be mild to severe. Hyperacute or extremely severe cases of purulent conjunctivitis are often due to gonococcus, which is also the only bacterial conjunctivitis to have preauricular adenopathy. Examination shows mild-to-severe conjunctival injection and purulent discharge. Most cases of bacterial conjunctivitis are mild and self limited. Treatment should be with an earlier generation antibiotic such as 10% sodium sulfacetamide qid for 5-7 days.[6] Overuse of later generation broad spectrum antibiotics (such as the topical flouroquinolones) should be avoided because of the emerging problems of resistance.[7] Non-responding infections should be cultured and treatment adjusted based on culture results. Gonococcal infection requires systemic treatment (ceftriaxone),[8] ocular lavage, and topical erythromycin, along with appropriate reporting and treatment of partners.

Bacterial Keratitis. Patients have a history of photophobia, pain, and decreased vision. It is more common in soft contact lens wearers, especially if lenses are worn overnight. The patient may have had a predisposing insult to corneal epithelium, such as an abrasion from mild trauma or misdirected eyelashes. Examination shows marked conjunctival injection, whitish ulcer in the superficial cornea, anterior chamber reaction, and occasionally hypopyon. Get ophthalmology consultation for culture and scraping of cornea and possible admission to the hospital. Treatment is usually started with hourly, around-the-clock, broad spectrum topical antibiotics. One of the flouroquinolones (oflaxacin or ciprofloxacin) is usually used initially with adjustment of medications based on culture results.[9] Homatropine 5% bid will help to reduce ciliary spasm and pain.

Fungal Keratitis. The symptoms are similar to bacterial keratitis. The exam shows a more lacy appearance to the corneal infiltrate and needs to be referred to an ophthalmologist. There is often a history of superficial corneal trauma from plant material. Treat patients with natamycin drops after obtaining cultures. Fungal ulcers may require surgical debridement.

Endophthalmitis. History of recent (usually within 48-72 hours) intraocular surgery or trauma. There is usually a sudden decrease in vision to hand motions or light perception levels. Exam shows marked conjunctival injection, discharge, possible eyelid edema, hazy cornea, and marked anterior chamber cellular reaction with hypopyon. The fundus is often not visible secondary to vitreous inflammation. Endophthalmitis is a true ophthalmic emergency and requires immediate evaluation and treatment by an ophthalmologist. Treatment consists of vitreous tap or vitrectomy, intravitreal antibiotics and possibly steroids, and intensive topical antibiotics. Prognosis depends on the causative organism and the length of time to treatment.[10]

Eyelid Infections (Preseptal Cellulitis). There is a history of spontaneous onset or recent minor lid trauma. Exam shows an erythematous and edematous eyelid. The globe is normal to mildly injected. Vision, extraocular motility, pupils, and optic nerve head are usually normal. Look for a hordeolum (infection around base of eyelash) or chalazion (enlarged meibomian gland) as the inciting event. Use warm compresses qid if evidence of chalazion. If there is early infection and no material for Gram's stain, treat empirically with amoxicillin/clavulanate 250-500 mg po tid in adults and appropriate adjusted dose in children.[11] More severe cases may require incision and drainage of eyelid and treatment with appropriate IV antibiotics based on Gram's stain and culture. Careful differentiation must be made between preseptal and orbital cellulitis.

Orbital Cellulitis. Patients give a history of pain, decreased vision, and possible diplopia. They may have sinusitis (especially ethmoiditis), recent orbital trauma, or recent dental surgery. Examination shows swollen, erythematous lids, mild to severe proptosis, limitation of EOMs, decreased vision, and possible afferent pupillary defect. Workup includes a CT scan (look for signs of sinusitis, subperiosteal abscess, and orbital abscess) and appropriate cultures. Patients are admitted and given broad spectrum coverage with IV antibiotics (clindamycin and ceftazidime). ENT consultation should be obtained.[12] In diabetics with ketoacidosis and immunocompromized patients, consider fungal infection (mucormycosis), which is life threatening and requires immediate treatment with IV, Amphotericin B, surgical debridement, and possibly hyperbaric oxygen.[13]

Dacryocyctitis. Patients give a history of purulent discharge and pain over the medial canthal region. Exam shows edema and erythema over region of the lacrimal sac and often reflux discharge through the puncta with pressure over the lacrimal sac. Treat by taking cultures and starting oral antibiotics (amoxicillin/clauvulanate 250-500 mg po tid or cephalexin 500 mg po q 6 h). Definitive treatment is surgical dacryocystorhinostomy.[14]

Uveitis or Inflammation of the Uveal tissue (Iris and Choroid). The most common emergent presentation is as iritis. A history of pain, photophobia, and decreased vision is given. Exam shows ocular injection, especially at the corneal scleral limbus and whitish deposits on the posterior cornea (keratic precipitates). Flare and cells are seen in the anterior chamber with a tangential slit beam. A hypopyon may be present and there may be dilated vessels on the iris. Funduscopic exam is needed to rule out posterior uveitis. Intraocular pressure may be elevated from inflammatory cells or decreased from ciliary body inflammation. Often no laboratory workup needed acutely for isolated, primary iritis. Treat with intensive topical steroids (Prednisolone acetate 1% every hour) and cycloplegics (atropine 1% or homatropine 5% bid).[15] Ophthalmologic follow-up is required for steroid taper and further diagnostic work-up, especially if any evidence of posterior (choroidal) involvement.

Acute Angle-Closure Glaucoma. Patients usually present with sudden onset of redness, decreased vision, intense pain, possibly nausea, and emesis. This is more common in farsighted patients. Examination shows marked ocular injection, especially at the limbus. The cornea is edematous. The pupil may be mid-dilated and non-reactive. The intraocular pressure is elevated, often markedly to 60 or 70 mmHg. The fellow eye is also at significant risk for angle closure and can be examined for narrow angles at the slit lamp. Angle closure is a true ophthalmologic emergency that requires immediate treatment. Ocular massage should be done immediately

Table 3. Common Chemicals Involved in Eye Injuries

Common Substances	Compound	Class
Battery acid	Sulfuric acid (H_2SO_4)	Acid
Bleach	Sulfurous acid (H_2SO_3)	Acid
Cement and mortar	Lime ($Ca(OH)_2$	Alkali
Chrome plating solution	Chromic acid (Cr_2O_3)	Acid
Drain cleaner	Lye (NaOH)	Alkali
Glacial acetic acid	Acetic acid (CH_3COOH)	Acid
Glass and tile cleaners	Ammonia (NH_3)	Alkali
Glass frosting acid	Hydrofluoric acid	Acid
Fertilizers	Ammonia (NH_3)	Alkali
Hydrochloric acid	Hydrochloric acid	Acid
Industrial cleaners	Sulfuric acid	Acid
Plaster	Lime ($Ca(OH)_2$)	Alkali
Sparklers and firecrackers	Magnesium hydroxide	Alkali
Vinegar	Acetic acid (Ch_3COOH)	Acid
Whitewash	Lime ($Ca(OH)_2$)	Alkali

as this can sometimes break the attack. Topical aqueous suppressants (timolol, brominidine, dorzolamide) are placed in the eye. Miotics, such as pilocarpine 2%, are given. Oral osmotics like 50% glycerin are given to help decrease intraocular pressure. As soon as possible, a surgical peripheral iridectomy (laser or incisional) is performed. Prophylactic peripheral iridectomy is usually placed in the fellow eye within 1-2 weeks.[16]

Carotid Cavernous Fistula. There are two main types, low flow and high flow. The low flow type is usually found in elderly, hypertensive patients without a history of trauma. They present with a red eye secondary to dilated episcleral vessels, elevated intraocular pressure, and may have proptosis. Treatment is by control of blood pressure and observation or, in more severe cases, interventional radiology. High flow types are usually found in younger patients following blunt or penetrating head trauma. The vision may be decreased. There is marked ocular vascular engorgement externally and internally, and usually marked exophthalmos. This requires emergent treatment. Interventional radiologic treatment methods are usually used with attempted embolic closure of the fistula.[17]

Traumatic Visual Loss

Chemical Burns. Exposure of the eye to chemicals is a true ocular emergency. Prompt and vigorous lavage is crucial to successful management. IV solutions, such as Ringers or normal saline attached to a large bore IV tubing, can be used to irrigate the eye at a rate of 500 cc/30 minutes. The eye should be kept open and the topical anesthesia using proparacaine or tetracaine is recommended to facilitate the irrigation. Sometimes, special irrigating contact lenses are used but this is not necessary. Great care must be taken to have the patient move the eye in all directions and careful inspection of the fornices must be undertaken during irrigation. Five minutes after cessation of irrigation, the pH of the eye should be checked and the range should be from pH 6.8-7.4. If pH is outside of this range, further irrigation is necessary.

A complete history of the incident with identification of the chemical and duration of exposure prior to irrigation is crucial. *(Please see Table 3.)* Acids cause surface proteins to precipitate and coagulate, confining the chemical to the surface of the eye and limiting the damage. The most common causes of acid injury are sulfuric, sulfurous, hydrofluoric, acetic, chromic, and hydrochloric acid.[18] Alkalis saponify and solubilize cell membranes, allowing penetration into the eye and resulting in significant deep damage to the eye. The most common causes of alkali injury are ammonia, lye, potassium hydroxide, magnesium hydroxide, and lime.[18] For all chemical injuries, a thorough examination of the lids with eversion of the lids to examine the fornices for particular matter is important. Calcium hydroxide particles may be more easily removed with a cotton tip applicator soaked in EDTA. Slit lamp exam of the cornea and conjunctiva with fluorescein is necessary to check for staining defects in the cornea. The intraocular pressure should be checked using the tonopen or Goldmann applanation tonometer. Prompt referral to an ophthalmologist is recommended at this point. If the IOP is elevated, Diamox 250 mg tablet and one drop of a topical beta blocker such as timoptic 0.5% will help decrease pressure. One drop of cycloplegic agent (scopolamine 0.25%) and topical antibiotic ointment (erythromycin) must be given with oral medications for pain control.

Eyelid Lacerations

Trauma to the eyelids and orbit can pose a severe threat to eyesight. The history must include relevant information about blunt vs. sharp objects, type of object, and velocity of the object. Thorough examination of the eyelids, globe, motility, and palpation of the orbital rim is important. Presence of lid lacerations requires careful cleaning of the wound and determination of tissue loss. Unless the patient comes with tissue in a plastic bag, tissue loss is rare, even in a complex lid laceration with multiple full thickness laceration with significant exposure of the globe. Great care must be taken not to discard any tissue or excise what appears to be macerated tissue from the surface of the lid. If the laceration is lateral to the puncta, chances of canalicular laceration are remote. If the laceration is medial to the puncta and includes the lid margins, there is a possibility of canalicular laceration. For all lacerations involving the lid margins and/or medial lid, either an ophthalmologist or skilled facial plastics specialist should close the wound, taking care to maintain the integrity of the canalicular system with stents. The repair of lid lacerations should be considered urgent and, in most cases, a delay of 12-36 hours does not alter the surgical result.[19] Lid lacerations lateral to the puncta can be closed easily with 6.0 silk or nylon suture superficially and 6.0 vicryl for deeper structures such as the tarsal plate. Care should be taken to horizontally close lacerations as often as possible, because vertical closure can result in cicatricial ectropion with exposure and drying of the eyes. Prophylactic antibiotics are indicated if given within three hours of injury, but since the lids are highly vascular, the chances of infection are reduced and the majority of lids do well.[20]

Orbital Fractures

If examination of the orbital walls with gentle palpation reveals crepitus, subcutaneous air, or a severe restriction to ocular motility, further evaluation with a CT scan of the orbit is indicated to rule out orbital fractures.[21] Orbital fractures are commonly seen with blunt trauma to the orbit. Careful evaluation of the eye by an ophthalmologist prior to surgery is important and presence of diplopia with restriction of motility needs to be determined. Differentiating between a paretic muscle and an entrapped muscle that is restricting motility (leash effect) is important. Timing of repair is controversial, with some experts suggesting initial aggressive surgical repair[22,23] and others suggesting delay of repair until the orbit has been re-evaluated in 10-14 days.[24] Inferior orbital fractures need only be repaired if there is diplopia within the central 20° of gaze, significant enophthalmos, or recession of the globe into the maxillary sinus. Too often, surgery is performed immediately, not allowing time for orbital edema to subside so that a better evaluation of motility can be performed.

Intraorbital Foreign Body

If an orbital foreign body is noted on CT scan or on x-ray, proper history to determine type of foreign body is extremely important. If the foreign body is composed of organic matter, such as wood or vegetable matter, it must be removed to prevent orbital cellulitis. Foreign bodies made from copper are not well tolerated and also should be removed. Copper alloys from brass and bronze are fairly well tolerated and inert substances, such as glass, plastic, iron, lead, steel, and aluminum, are well tolerated and can be left in the orbit. BBs and shotgun pellets are typically made of 80-90% lead and 10-20% iron.

Corneal Foreign Bodies

Corneal foreign bodies are the most common workplace injury, accounting for nearly 35% of all eye injuries at the workplace.[25] There is usually a history of grinding wheel work or metal upon metal contact. Thorough examination of the cornea and the anterior chamber with a slit lamp is imperative to rule out intraocular foreign bodies. Careful examination of the conjunctiva under the upper and lower lids up to the fornix is necessary to remove particles trapped in the lid conjunctiva. Superficial foreign bodies may be removed by irrigation but foreign bodies embedded in the cornea need to be removed at the slit lamp using a 25-gauge needle or foreign body spud. Residual rust and material must be removed with a foreign body bur. If the foreign body is in the visual axis, it would be prudent to refer to an ophthalmologist and have them remove the foreign body to limit size of the scar and, thus, decrease risk of vision loss. After removal, a cycloplegic agent (Cyclogyl 1%) and a broad spectrum antibiotic ointment is given to prevent corneal infection until the defect is healed.

Intraocular Foreign Bodies

Patients with a history of trauma with a sharp object or high-speed missile are at high risk for corneoscleral laceration and possible intraocular foreign body. Signs, such as a shallow anterior chamber, subconjunctival hemorrhage, hypotony, hyphema, cataract, and decreased vision can all point to a ruptured globe. Orbital CT scans with thin slices are the gold standard for detection of intraocular foreign bodies. Presence of an intraocular foreign body on CT scan requires an emergent referral to an ophthalmologist. The globe should not be manipulated excessively and an eye shield should be placed. Substances, such as copper, iron, steel, and organic material, need to be removed immediately because of the risk of toxicity to the retina or endophthalmitis. *(Please see Table 4.)* Patients should undergo a pars plana vitrectomy and removal of the foreign body.[26] Prognosis for vision is poor—especially if the foreign body has imbedded in the retina because of the risk of proliferative vitreoretinopathy (PVR).[27] In patients with PVR, significant scar tissue develops on the retinal surface and can result in a tractional retinal detachment with poor visual outcomes. All patients with an intraocular foreign body will have a corneal or scleral laceration and will need surgical repair of the laceration. (*See section on Corneal and Scleral Lacerations.*)

Corneal Abrasions and Erosions

In patients complaining of severe pain, erythema with edema of the eyelids, and photophobia, one must strongly consider corneal abrasion in the differential diagnosis. The patient may indicate a history of trauma, contact lens wear, herpes infection, or acute onset of pain upon awakening. Patients should be evaluated with the slit lamp

Table 4. Commonly Encountered Intraocular Foreign Bodies

Class of Foreign Body	Activity	Management
Copper	Severe inflammatory	Remove immediately
Glass	Inert	Remove
Iron	Severe inflammatory response	Remove immediately
Lead	Mild inflammatory	Remove
Nickel	Mild inflammatory	Remove
Organic—wood, plants, and cilia	Severe inflammatory	Remove immediately
Plastic	Inert	Remove
Steel	Severe inflammatory	Remove immediately
Stone	Inert	Remove

using both regular light and cobalt blue light with fluorescein dye in a topical anesthetic. If an epithelial defect exists, it will take up the dye and fluoresce yellow against the blue background illumination. The examiner should have the patient blink his eyelid. If there is pooling of the dye without an abrasion, the yellow fluorescein will be displaced. With an abrasion, the region of yellow fluorescein will remain fixed on the cornea. Care must be taken to differentiate between a corneal abrasion and the dendrite seen in *Herpes keratitis*. Treatment with broad spectrum antibiotic drops (sulfacetamide 10% or polytrim) and cycloplegic drops (Cyclogyl 1%) are recommended. Currently, there are significant questions as to the benefits of a pressure patch over no patch.[28,29] If patients are not patched, topical nonsteroidal agents, such as diclofenac or ketorolac, are recommended for pain control.[30,31] Contact lens-associated abrasions need gram negative coverage with an aminoglycoside and a cycloplegic without patching. These abrasions need to be carefully monitored to ensure that a corneal ulcer does not occur.

Patients with a history of acute onset of pain and redness upon awakening frequently have a history of a previous large corneal abrasion. In these patients, the adhesion complexes between the epithelium and the basement membrane have been damaged, resulting in recurrent corneal erosions. Slit lamp exam reveals either a full thickness epithelial defect or an epithelial irregularity with mobile epithelium. The epithelium needs to be debrided and treatment is the same as for a corneal abrasion. After the epithelium is healed, copious lubrication is necessary for 6-8 weeks—especially lubricating ointment at night. If erosions recur, than surgical intervention to increase adhesion complexes is necessary.

Conjunctival Lacerations

Sometimes, patients with mild pain, red eye, foreign-body sensation, and a history of trauma will only have conjunctival laceration on careful examination of the globe. Exploration of the site and possible CT scan of the orbit may be indicated to rule out rupture of the globe. The laceration limited to the conjunctiva will rapidly heal and may need antibiotic ointment for 4-7 days. Large laceration (> 1.5 cm) may be sutured but most need no surgical repair. These patients should be re-examined within one week if the laceration is large.

Corneal and Scleral Lacerations

Lacerations of the globe can occur due to blunt trauma, missiles, or sharp objects. The sclera and cornea are usually resistant to blunt trauma but, with sufficient force, scleral rupture can occur. Compressive forces rarely cause rupture at the impact site, but ruptures actually occur at a remote site where the sclera is the thinnest. The sclera is the thinnest at the junction of the cornea and the sclera (limbus) and posterior to the insertion of the rectus muscles. Usually, scleral ruptures occur in the superonasal and superotemporal quadrants, are solitary, and extend from the limbus to the equator of the globe. Laceration due to missiles and sharp objects occur mostly in the front of the eye and can involve both the cornea and sclera. Signs of rupture include hyphema, cataract, vitreous hemorrhage, visual acuity of light perception or no light perception, ocular hypotony, and subconjunctival hemorrhage. If a laceration of the cornea and sclera is suspected, place a shield over the eye and, if one is not available, fashion one with the bottom of a styrofoam cup and obtain an ophthalmology consult immediately. Do not attempt to finish the exam as this may cause further extrusion of ocular contents. An orbital CT scan to rule out intraocular foreign bodies is highly advisable, and prompt surgical repair with proper ophthalmic follow-up is needed. Injuries greater than 20 mm in length and injuries caused by blunt trauma or missiles generally have a poor visual prognosis.[32] After primary repair of the lacerations, vitreoretinal surgery to re-attach the retina or remove retinal traction has greatly improved visual outcomes.[33]

Traumatic Iritis and Hyphema

The four phases of blunt injury are compression, decompression, overshooting, and oscillations.[34] Anterior-posterior compression results in equatorial expansion, shortening of the visual axis, and posterior displacement of the lens and iris. Extreme stretching of the ocular tissue results in specific types of injury to iris, trabecular meshwork, ciliary body, lens, retina vitreous, choroid, sclera, and optic nerve. The net result can be a breakdown in the blood-aqueous barrier and the blood-retinal barrier. Depending on the extent of the damage, it can result either in traumatic uveitis or in traumatic hyphema.

If the patient complains of pain, photophobia, and tearing, a careful slit lamp examination must be done to check for anterior flare (protein) and cells (white blood cells). Since the signs for uveitis can be subtle, referral to an experienced eyecare provider is preferred.

Flare and cell in the anterior chamber indicates traumatic uveitis, which runs a brief and benign course.[35] Cycloplegics drops (Cyclogyl 1% qid) and prednisone drops (Prednisolone acetate 1% qid) for one week will reduce the inflammation and recheck of the eye in one week is recommended.

Patients with blood in the anterior chamber or on slit lamp exam have a hyphema. These patients deserve a thorough examination by an ophthalmologist to rule out possibility of a ruptured globe. There is a high risk of rebleed within five days of the initial trauma and elevated intraocular pressures. Historically, patients were hospitalized for hyphema, but there appears to be no significant difference in rebleeding rates and clinical outcomes between hospitalized patients and those treated at home.[36,37] Close outpatient follow-up and strict bedrest is necessary to prevent rebleeds.[38] Cycloplegia with Atropine 1% bid and topical steroids (prednisolone acetate 1% qid) are given to enhance patient comfort but have not been shown to prevent rebleed or improve outcome. Antifibrinolytic agents, such as aminocaproic acid, can be used both systemically or topically to stabilize the clot for five days and decrease the rate of rebleed.[39-41] Patients with hyphema should be examined every day for five days post-trauma and then two days after cessation of aminocaproic acid to check for rebleed and elevated intraocular pressures. Approximately 5% of patients with hyphema will develop uncontrollable intraocular pressures, prolonged clot duration, and corneal blood staining. These patients will need surgical intervention to remove clot mass from the anterior chamber. Great care must be taken to avoid vision loss from uncontrolled glaucoma or corneal bloodstaining and pressure control is vital.

Retinal Edema, Retinal Tears, and Vitreous Hemorrhage

Traumatic forces can cause violent movement of the vitreous away from the retina, resulting in a coup or contrecoup lesion in the retina. Types of injuries most often encountered are retinal tears and nontearing retinal injury resulting in retinal edema or retinal hemorrhages.[42] Retinal edema, called Berlin's edema or commotio retinae, can be seen in the retinal periphery or the posterior pole. If it involves the macula or fovea, the patient will usually complain of decreased vision because of photoreceptor disruption.[43] Direct ophthalmoscopy may reveal a whitish gray central retinal lesion that may be difficult to note without a dilated exam. Patients that have sustained blunt trauma to the retina do not need emergent surgical intervention but need to be monitored by an ophthalmologist because they may develop sequelae, such as retinal pigment epithelium atrophy or macular hole.[44] If a macular hole develops, surgical intervention to repair the hole should be considered. Retinal hemorrhages should be observed and will be reabsorbed with time. They usually do not cause chronic vision loss.

Occasionally, patients will complain of decreased vision and there is a poor view of the retinal. If the vitreous is detached from the retina and a retinal vessel is broken, bleeding can occur in the vitreous cavity making it impossible to evaluate the retina with ophthalmoscopy. If there is no rupture of the globe, vitreous hemorrhages need to be monitored carefully with diagnostic ultrasound called B-scan to rule out retinal tears or retinal detachment. Patients should be monitored monthly until the hemorrhage resolves. Some retina specialists would perform a vitrectomy to improve vision and avoid other complications sooner than six months if the vitreous hemorrhage persists.

Traumatic retinal tears most commonly occur at the anterior edge of the retina, at its junction with the ciliary body, and are called retinal dialysis.[45] Often, the retinal dialysis is not visible at the time of injury due to its location and it may be overlooked on subsequent exams. Many retinal detachments associated with retinal dialysis are first diagnosed more than one year after the injury. The inferotemporal and superonasal quadrants are most frequently involved.[46] Careful history and follow-up examination might prevent progression to a retinal detachment. If a retinal tear is seen, laser photocoagulation or freezing therapy will stabilize the retina. Patients who have a history of previous trauma, flashing lights, and a grey curtain over the eye are at high risk for a retinal detachment. Prompt referral to an ophthalmologist for an indirect ophthalmoscopic examination might prevent further delay in diagnosis and surgical repair. Visual prognosis is good when retinal breaks or detachments are diagnosed and repaired within six weeks of surgery.[47] The patient may undergo placement of air in the globe, scleral buckle, or pars plana vitrectomy for repair of retinal detachment.

Lens Subluxation/Dislocation

Compressive forces from trauma can cause dehiscence of zonules supporting the lens. Decentration of the lens with some partial zonular dehiscence is called subluxation. Total zonular disruption can lead to lens dislocation into the vitreous cavity or into the anterior chamber. Usually, the lens capsule is intact and there is minimal inflammation. In the majority of cases, observation and a thorough eye exam with refraction for visual rehabilitation is sufficient. However, in cases of subluxed lenses with the edge of the lens in visual axis or dislocated lenses with angle closure glaucoma, surgical intervention is necessary. Although many ophthalmologists still use intracapsular lens extraction, pars plana lens removal has had promising results.[48]

Optic Nerve Trauma

Patients with an injury to the optic nerve may have decreased visual acuity, visual field deficits, or a relative afferent pupillary defect. Examination of the pupils with the swinging flashlight test must be performed, but sometimes because of corneal opacities, hyphema, or lid edema, it is difficult to assess the injured eye. In this instance, checking the consensual response in the other eye will help the examiner determine the status of the nerve. Trauma to the nerve may be direct, such as in penetrating injuries due to projectiles or objects that lacerate the nerve. Orbital fractures and high velocity

Table 5. Retinal Causes of Acute Non-Traumatic Visual Loss

	Age-related Macular Degeneration	Central retinal Artery Occlusion	Central Retinal Vein Occusion	Retinal Detachment
History	metamorphopsia to sudden loss of central vision, usually elderly	amaurosis fugax episodes, sudden loss of vision, middle age to elderly	rapid (over several days) to sudden loss of vision, usually elderly but can be seen in young adults	dark shadow over vision, often preceded by flashes and floaters
Visual Acuity	small decrease to loss of central vision	usually severe loss to count fingers or no light perception	moderate to severe loss	normal to severe loss depending on macular status
Pupils	no afferent defect	large afferent defect on affected side	often have afferent defect	afferent defect in relation to size of detachment
Retina	drusen (yellow spots), pigment clumping, hemorrhage	milky, swollen retina with cherry red spot over fovea, may see hollenhorst plaque	widely scattered retinal hemorrhage and whitish retinal infarcts	elevated, whitish, billowy retinal tissue—may see tear in retina
Optic Nerve	not affected	usually pale, may be swollen	swollen, congested vessels with hemorrhage	usually normal—may be obscured by detachment
Emergency Treatment	referral for fluoroscein angiogram within 24-48 hours	immediate ocular massage, IOP anterior chamber paracentesis	treat any IOP elevation	referral to ophthalmologist for repair
Long-Term Treatment	laser treatment for eligible lesions, long-term prognosis poor[18]	if not reversed acutely prognosis very poor; watch for neovascularization[19]	close observation for neovascular complications, possible laser tx[20]	pneumatic retinopexy or scleral buckling or vitrectomy used to repair[21]

projectiles can also cause severe contusion of the nerve. The first due to compression by bone fragments and the latter due to dissipation of significant energy in close proximity to the nerve. Increased tissue pressure from orbital air or retrobulbar hemorrhage can cause optic nerve compression and tractional forces on the globe can completely avulse the optic nerve from the eye.[49,50] Usually, disc edema, hemorrhage, or avulsion can be seen with ophthalmoscopy.

Indirect trauma can occur when there is no initial ophthalmoscopic evidence of injury to the eye. Many times, the severity of injury is not proportional to the amount of vision loss and it can occur immediately or is delayed. Concussive forces shear axons at the lamina cribrosa at the entry of the nerve into the eye. Optic atrophy with pale optic nerve is then seen 3-6 weeks later. Generally, the prognosis for recovery of vision is poor in traumatic optic nerve injuries, but IV corticosteroids given for 3-5 days have been shown to be beneficial. Treatment should be immediately initiated.

Non-Traumatic Visual Loss

Acute, non-traumatic visual loss presents special diagnostic challenges. Important historical points include time of onset, quality and severity of visual loss, mono- or binocularity, duration of loss, and associated ocular and systemic diseases. It is helpful to think through the globe structure from anterior to posterior to sort out the various etiologies of acute non-traumatic visual loss. Corneal causes include corneal erosions (can be spontaneous or associated with corneal epithelial dystrophy's or bullous kerotapathy), infectious keratitis, or toxic reactions to chemicals or medications. Anterior chamber causes include acute iritis and spontaneous hyphema. Lenticular causes include cataract (usually posterior subcapsular type that can progress fairly rapidly and be "suddenly" noted by patient). Vitreous causes include spontaneous vitreous hemorrhage (often in diabetics with proliferative retinopathy) or pars planitis (idiopathic inflammation of vitreous usually found in young adults).

Retinal and optic nerve diseases are probably the most common causes of acute non-traumatic visual loss. *(Please see Table 5.)* Central retinal artery occlusion requires immediate ophthalmologic treatment to attempt to preserve vision.

Optic Nerve Disorders

Optic nerve dysfunction causes decreased visual acuity, color vision, and almost always presents with an afferent pupillary defect. The optic nerve can appear swollen, congested, and possibly pale, or

Figure 1. Anisocoria Flowchart

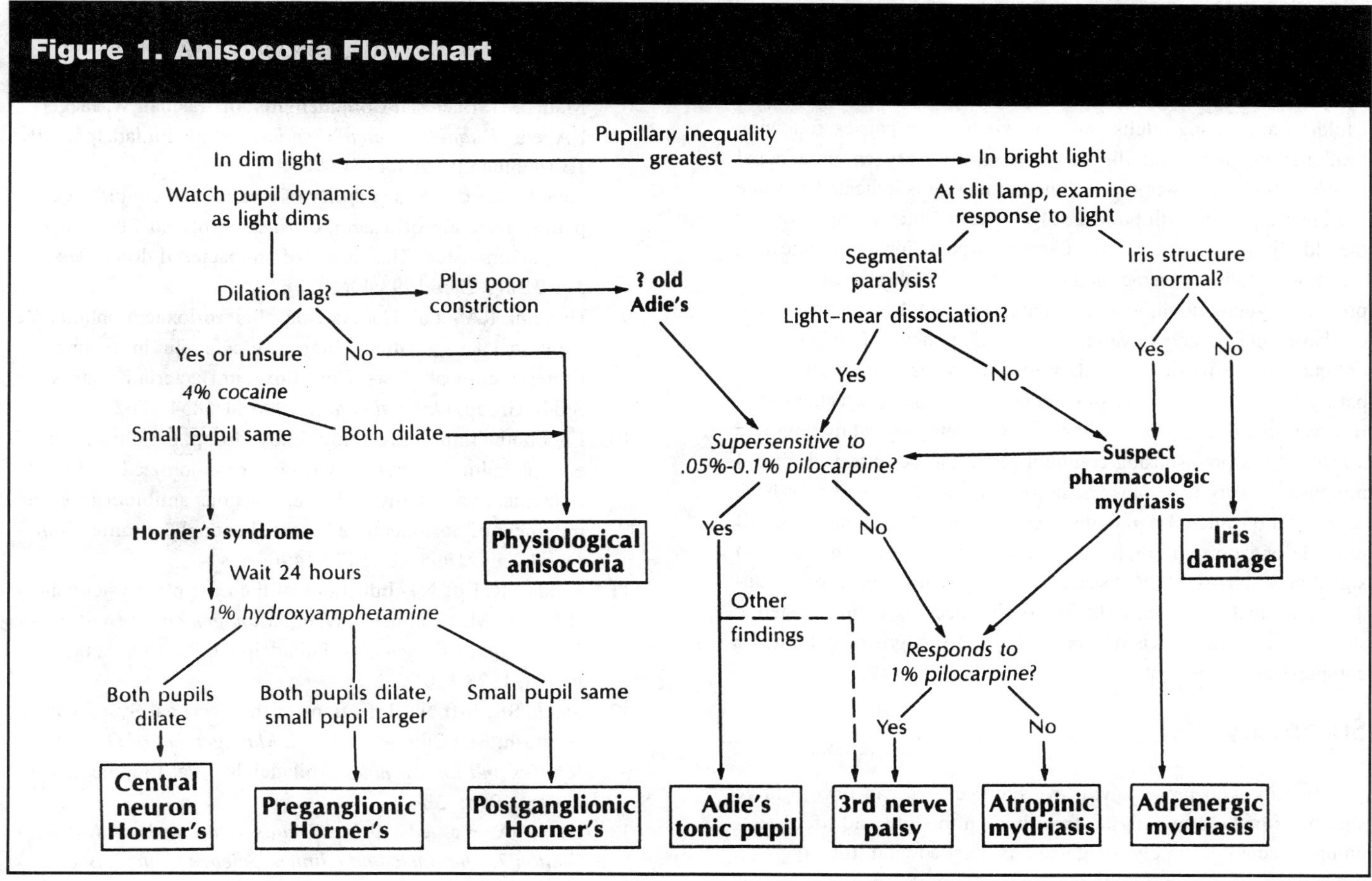

it can look normal if the insult is retrobulbar. Optic neuritis is seen in younger patients (15-45 age group). Examination will show the above findings and there may be pain with extraocular movements. Vision can fall to low levels and then usually recovers, although often not completely. Treatment is based on results of the optic neuritis treatment trial. Oral steroids should not be used. High dose IV steroids may help hasten recovery in severe cases.[55] Anterior ischemic optic neuropathy (AION) is more common in older patients. It is found in both arteritic (age > 55) and non-arteritic (age 45-65) forms. The arteritic form is associated with giant cell arteritis. Patients may have profound loss of vision in one eye and may have an associated central retinal artery occlusion. If untreated, the second eye has a significant chance of also losing vision. Patients usually have temporal artery tenderness and systemic symptoms, such as jaw claudication, weight loss, and fever. Westergren sedimentation rate (> 47) and c-reactive protein level (> 2.45 mg/dL) can help with the diagnosis.[56] If a patient has a clinical presentation consistent with giant cell arteritis, high-dose systemic steroids should be started immediately and a temporal artery biopsy should be arranged. The non-arteritic form of anterior ischemic optic neuropathy is often found in patients with underlying systemic hypertension or diabetes mellitus. There is no proven treatment for non-arteritic AION.

Anisocoria

Anisocoria, or a difference in pupil size, can be a benign physiological state or a sign of a serious, life-threatening intracranial disease. Important historical points are any recent trauma, any previously noted anisocoria, any foreign material in eyes, and any headache, diplopia, or other neurological symptoms. An efficient, accurate decision tree is shown in Figure 1. Obtain ophthalmologic consultation if any doubt exists as to the cause of the anisocoria. Any anisocoria in conjunction with a third nerve palsy ("blown pupil" on the ipsilateral side) requires emergent neuroradiologic workup and possible emergent neurosurgical intervention if an intracranial aneurysm is found.[57]

Diplopia

Diplopia, or double vision, can be separated into binocular diplopia (present only with both eyes open) or monocular diplopia (still present with one of the eyes closed). Other important historical points are time of onset, whether the diplopia is intermittent or constant, directions of gaze in which diplopia worsens, antecedent trauma, and any previous ocular surgeries, especially strabismus surgeries. During the examination, pay special attention to the pupils and extraocular motility exam. Occlude first the right eye, then the left eye to determine if any shifts or correcting movements occur. Alternating the occluder between the eyes rapidly can also help to elicit any abnormalities. Categorize the ocular alignment as normal, esotropic, exotropic, or vertical misalignment. Carefully check the full range of extraocular movements to determine if any visible muscle palsy is present. If the patient notes diplopia is worse or only present in certain directions of gaze, this can be a good clue of what muscles are malfunctioning. True monocular diplopia is usually caused by an abnormality of the cornea, lens, or central retina. A complete dilated examination is usually required to find the cause. Children and young adults can have sixth nerve palsies following head trauma or a viral illness, or it may signify an intracranial process. Aggressive workup with neuroimaging is indicated.[58] Acute third nerve palsies with pupil involvement in either young adults or the elderly may represent the effects of a posterior communicating artery aneurysm. Neuroradiologic workup and multiple sclerosis can present in young adults with any pattern of EOM involvement that can have a high degree of variability. Elderly patients often have sixth or fourth nerve palsies secondary to a microvascular insult. These patients often have hypertension, diabetes, or generalized atherosclerotic vascular disease. If they have no other neurological findings and a history of a predisposing condition, they can be observed for 3-4 months.[59] If they have other neurological findings, worsen, or have no resolution after 3-4 months, perform an MRI. Acute onset of diplopia or worsening diplopia in patients with Graves disease can signal new activity of the disease. This may require emergent evaluation and treatment (i.e., radiation, orbital decompression, systemic steroids) if decreased vision, increased IOP, or signs of optic nerve compression are present.

Summary

Patients who present with eye emergencies can have a large variety of pathology, ranging from benign to sight and life threatening. Accurate, timely diagnosis is needed and this requires careful slit lamp and ophthalmoscopic examination by the physician to determine whether an emergency eye consult is necessary. In patients with red eye, the physician must be able to rule out conditions that are site threatening prior to treating a patient for conjunctivitis. In a traumatic vision loss after an initial evaluation, the patient should be promptly referred to an ophthalmologist. In patients with suspected rupture of the globe or intraocular foreign body, one must obtain an orbital CT scan, place an eye shield, and let the ophthalmologist determine the extent of the injury. Sight threatening mistakes are usually made only when physicians attempt to manage ocular emergencies without the benefit of an experienced eye care specialist.

References

1. Mead MD. Evaluation and Initial Management of Patients with Ocular and Adnexal Trauma. In: Albert DM, Jakobiec FA, eds. *Principles and Practice of Ophthalmology*. WB Saunders; 1994: 3367.
2. Congdon NG, MacCumber MW. Ocular Evaluation In: MacCumber MW, ed. *Management of Ocular Injuries and Emergencies*. Philadelphia, Pa: Lippincott-Raven; 1998:36.
3. Cullom RD, Chang B, eds. *The Wills Eye Manual*. 2nd ed. Philadelphia, Pa: Lippincott-Raven; 1994:119-120.
4. Berlin MW, et al, eds. *External Disease and Cornea, Section 8, The Basic and Clinical Science Course*. San Francisco, Ca: American Academy of Ophthalmology; 1993:97.
5. Harris LL, O'Brien TP. Infectious Conjunctivitis and Keratitis. In: MacCumber MW, ed. *Management of Ocular Injuries and Emergencies*. Philadelphia, Pa: Lippincott-Raven; 1998:200.
6. Manis MJ. Bacterial Conjunctivitis. In: Tasman W, Jaeger EA, eds. *Duane's Clinical Ophthalmology*. Philadelphia, Pa: JB Lippincott; 1994:4.
7. Knauf HP, et al. Suseptibility of corneal and conjunctival pathogens to ciprofloxacin. *Cornea* 1996;1:66-71.
8. No authors listed. The choice of antibacterial drugs. *Med Lett Drugs Ther* 1998;40(1023):38.
9. Hunduik RA, et al. Comparison of ciprofloxacin ophthalmic solution 3% to fortified tobramycin-cefazolin in treating bacterial corneal ulcers. Ciprofloxacin Bacteria Keratitis Study Group. *Ophthalmology* 1996;11:1854-1862.
10. Endophthalmitis Vitrectomy Study Group. Results of the endophthalmitis vitrectomy study: A randomized trial of immediate vitrectomy and of intravenous antibiotics for the treatment of postoperative bacterial endophthalmitis. *Arch Ophthalmol* 1995;113:1479-1496.
11. Sadda SR, Iliff NT. Infections of the Lacrimal System and Orbit. In: MacCumber MW, ed. *Management of Ocular Injuries and Emergencies*, Philadelphia, Pa: Lippincott-Raven; 1998:130.
12. Sadda SR, Iliff NT. Infections of the Lacrimal System and Orbit. In: MacCumber MW, ed. *Management of Ocular Injuries and Emergencies*, Philadelphia, Pa: Lippincott-Raven; 1998:132.
13. Nerad JA, et al, eds. *Orbit, Eyelids, and Lacrimal System, Section 7, The Basic and Clinical Science Course*. San Francisco, Ca: American Academy of Ophthalmology; 1995:63.
14. Cullom RD, Chang B, eds. *The Wills Eye Manual*. 2nd ed. Philadelphia, PA: Lippincott-Raven; 1994:143.
15. Rao NA, et al, eds. *Intraocular Inflammation and Uveitis, Section 9, The Basic and Clinical Science Course*. San Francisco, CA: American Academy of Ophthalmology; 1995:81-82.
16. Simmons RJ, et al. Primary Angle Closure Glaucoma. In: Tasman W, Jaeger EA, eds. *Duane's Clinical Ophthalmology, vol 3 Chapter 53*. Philadelphia, PA: JB Lippincott; 1994:13-14.
17. Troost BT, Glaser JS. Aneurysms, Arteriovenous Communications, and Related Vascular Malformations. In: Tasman W, Jaeger EA, eds. *Duane's Clinical Ophthalmology, vol 2 Chapter 17*. Philadelphia, PA: JB Lippincott; 1994:20-21.
18. Wagoner, MD. Chemical injuries of the eye: Current concepts in the pathophysiology and therapy. *Surv Ophthalmol* 1997;41:275-313.
19. Rubin PA, Shore JW. Penetrating Eyelid and Orbital Trauma. In: Albert DM, Jakobiec FA, eds. *Principles and Practice of Ophthalmology*. WB Saunders; 1994:3432.
20. Westfall CT, Shore JW. Isolated fractures of the orbital floor: Risk of infection and the role of antibiotic prophylaxis. *Ophthalmic Surg* 1991;22:409-411.
21. Mucci B. A new perspective on blow-out fracture of the orbit. *Injury* 1997;28:555-556.
22. Levin LM, Kademani D. Clinical considerations in the

management of orbital blow-out fractures. *Compend Contin Educ Dent* 1997;18:596-598.

23. Sires BS, et al. Oculocardiac reflex caused by orbital floor trapdoor fracture: An indication for urgent repair. *Arch Ophthalmol* 1998;116:955-956.
24. Seiff SR, Good WV. Hypertropia and the posterior blowout fracture: Mechanism and management. *Ophthalmology* 1996;103: 152-156.
25. Nicaeus T, et al. An analysis of 148 outpatient treated occupational accidents. *Klin Monatsbl Augenheilkd* 1996; 209:7-11.
26. Kazokoglu H, Saatci O. Intraocular foreign bodies: Results of 27 cases. *Ann Ophthalmol* 1990;22:373-376.
27. Cardillo JA, et al. Post-traumatic proliferative vitreoretinopathy. The epidemiologic profile, onset, risk factors, and visual outcome. *Ophthalmology* 1997;104: 1166-1173.
28. Hart A, et al. The management of corneal abrasions in accident and emergency. *Injury* 1997;28:527-529.
29. Patterson J, et al. Eye patch treatment for the pain of corneal abrasion. *South Med J* 1996;89:227-229.
30. Jayamanne DG, et al. The effectiveness of topical diclofenac in relieving discomfort following traumatic corneal abrasions. *Eye* 1997;11:79-83.
31. Kaiser PK, Pineda R. A study of topical nonsteroidal anti-inflammatory drops and no pressure patching in the treatment of corneal abrasions. Corneal Abrasion Patching Study Group. *Ophthalmology* 1997;104:1353-1359.
32. Esmaeli B, et al. Visual outcome and ocular survival after penetrating trauma. A clinicopathologic study. *Ophthalmology* 1995;102:393-400.
33. Pieramici DJ, et al. Open-globe injury. Update on types of injuries and visual results. *Ophthalmology* 1996;103: 1798-1803.
34. Hersh PS, et al. Anterior Segment Trauma. In: Albert DM, Jakobiec FA, eds. *Principles and Practice of Ophthalmology*. WB Saunders; 1994:3385-3390.
35. Seymour R, Ramsey MS. Unusually severe traumatic uveitis associated with occult ankylosing spondylitis. *Can J Ophthalmol* 1991;26:156-158.
36. Kennedy RH, Brubaker RF. Traumatic hyphema in a defined population. *Am J Ophthalmol* 1988;106:123-130.
37. Clever VG. Home care of hyphemas. *Ann Ophthalmol* 1982; 14:25-27.
38. Shiuey Y, Lucarelli MJ. Traumatic hyphema: outcomes of outpatient management. *Ophthalmology* 1998;105:851-855.
39. Crouch ER, Frenkel M. Aminocaproic acid in the treatment of traumatic hyphema. *Am J Ophthalmol* 1976;81:355-360.
40. Fourman S. Topical aminocarpoic acid in the treatment of patients with traumatic hyphema. *Arch Ophthalmol* 1998; 116:395-396.
41. Crouch ER Jr, et al. Topical aminocaproic acid in the treatment of traumatic hyphema. *Arch Ophthalmol* 1997; 115:1106-1112.
42. Williams DF, et al. Posterior segment manifestations of ocular trauma. *Retina* 1990;10:35-44.
43. Liem AT, et al. Reversible cone photoreceptor injury in commotio retinae of the macula. *Retina* 1995;15:58-61.
44. Yanagiya N, et al. Clinical characteristics of traumatic macular holes. *Jpn J Ophthalmol* 1996;40:544-547.
45. Ross WH. Traumatic retinal dialyses. *Arch Ophthalmol* 1981;99:1371-1374.
46. Zion VM, Burton TC. Retinal dialysis. *Arch Ophthalmol* 1980;98:1971-1974.
47. Johnston PB. Traumatic retinal detachment. *Br J Ophthalmol* 1991;75:18-21.
48. Omulecki W, et al. Pars plana vitrectomy, lensectomy, or extraction in transscleral intraocular lens fixation for the management of dislocated lenses in a family with Marfan's syndrome. *Ophthalmic Surg Lasers* 1998;29:375-379.
49. Espaillat A, To K. Optic nerve avulsion. *Arch Ophthalmol* 1998;116:540-541.
50. Tsopelas NV, Arvanitis PG. Avulsion of the optic nerve head after orbital trauma. *Arch Ophthalmol* 1998;116:394.
51. Macular Photocoagulation Study Group. Argon laser photocoagulation for neovascular maculopathy. Five-year results from randomized clinical trials. *Arch Ophthalmol* 1991;109:1109-1114.
52. Heckenlively JR, et al, eds. *Retinal and Vitreous, Section 12, The Basic and Clinical Science Course*. San Francisco, CA: American Academy of Ophthalmology; 1995:185-188.
53. Central Vein Occlusion Study Group. A randomized clinical trial of early panretinal photocoagulation for ischemic central vein occlusion. The Central Vein Occlusion Study N Report. *Ophthalmology* 1995;102:1434-1444.
54. Cullom RD, Chang B, eds. *The Wills Eye Manual*. 2nd ed. Philadelphia, PA: Lippincott-Raven; 1994:250.
55. Beck RW, et al. A randomized, controlled trial of corticosteroids in the treatment of acute optic neuritis. *N Engl J Med* 1992; 326:581-588.
56. Hayreh SS, et al. Giant cell arteritis: Validity and reliability of various diagnostic criteria. *Am J Ophthalmol* 1997;123: 285-296.
57. Kerrison JB, Miller NR. Traumatic and Other Acute Disorders of Eye Movements and Pupils. In: MacCumber MW, ed. *Management of Ocular Injuries and Emergencies*. Philadelphia, PA: Lippincott-Raven; 1998:370-371.
58. Bajandas FJ, Kline LB. Neuro-ophthalmology Review Manual. 3rd ed. Thorofare, NJ: Slack; 1988:83.
59. Bajandas FJ, Kline LB. Neuro-ophthalmology Review Manual. 3rd ed. Thorofare, NJ: Slack; 1988:84.

The Red Eye

Kenneth H. Butler, DO
Earl J Reisdorff, MD, FACEP

A frequently encountered manifestation of infectious, chemically mediated, or idiopathic inflammatory processes, the acutely painful "red eye" is an important, and diagnostically challenging, ophthalmologic problem managed in the emergency department (ED) setting. Afflicting both young and old individuals—and variable in the severity and acuteness of its presentation—red eye can be caused by a wide spectrum of conditions that range in morbidity from minor to life-threatening disorders. *(Please see Table 1.)*

Generally speaking, less serious causes of red eye include such conditions as viral and bacterial conjunctivitis, hordeolum, and blepharitis, whereas more worrisome, vision-compromising disorders consist of narrow-angle glaucoma, uveitis, and orbital cellulitis. Not surprisingly, diagnostic accuracy is enhanced by the recognition that many disorders producing red eye are age-specific. For example, whereas pediatric patients are at risk for developing *Haemophilus influenzae* periorbital cellulitis and *Chlamydia*- or gonococcal-induced ophthalmia neonatorum, adults are more likely to present with traumatic hyphemea, subconctival hemorrhage, and glaucoma.

Even though many patients with red eye have garden-variety bacterial conjunctivitis that is easily managed with topical antibiotics, not infrequently differential diagnosis of this complaint is difficult. Consequently, nearly all evaluations of this condition should include—at the very least—a visual acuity exam, a qualitative assessment of pain, a description of pupillary function, a slit lamp exam, and when indicated, tonometric measurement of intraocular pressure. Frequently, however, further assessment of the eye will be necessary, requiring additional diagnostic techniques that include, but are not limited to, funduscopic examination, blood cultures, gram stain and culture, fluoroscein staining of the cornea, and, occasionally, CT or MRI scanning.

The etiology of red eye usually can be rapidly identified using simple examination techniques and historical information. For example, the extent of inflammation in periorbital tissues helps distinguish periorbital cellulitis from disorders confined to the eyelids and the lacrimal apparatus. Photophobia suggests a disorder involving the anterior chamber, whereas pain exacerbated by the consensual light reflex strongly suggests uveitis. When orbital discomfort is completely relieved by a topical anesthetic, the condition is usually confined to the cornea and conjunctivae. A firm globe suggests glaucoma.

This chapter presents a systematic approach to the differential diagnosis of red eye, and provides a detailed discussion of therapeutic options ranging from antimicrobial therapy to methods for lowering intraocular pressure. Practical, hands-on techniques for performing a thorough ophthalmologic examination are also reviewed. Finally, detailed illustrations and rapid-access management tables have been incorporated in order to facilitate emergency diagnosis and management of these conditions.

Figures 1-4. Anatomical Structures of the Eye

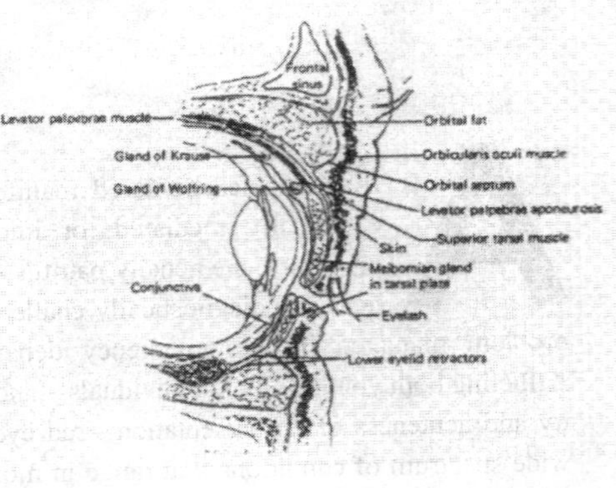

Figure 1. Cross section anatomy of the eyelids. Used with permission: Vaughan DG, Asbury T, Riordan-Eva P, eds. *General Ophthalmology.* 13th ed. Norwalk: Appleton & Lange, 1992, pg 19.

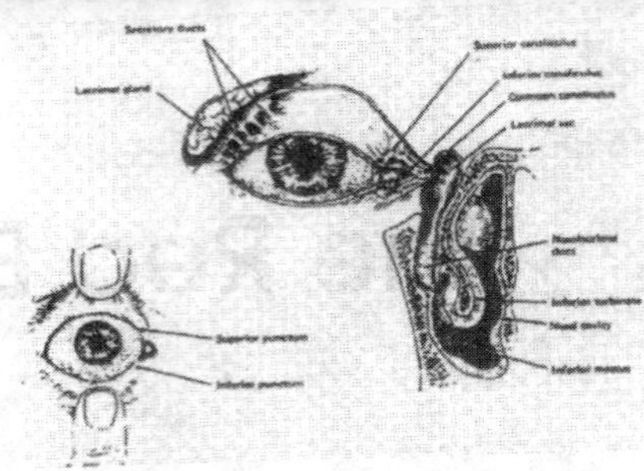

Figure 2. The lacrimal system. Used with permission: Vaughan DG, Asbury T, Riordan-Eva P, eds. *General Ophthalmology* 13th ed. Norwalk: Appleton & Lange, 1992, pg 21 as modified from Thompson J, Elstrom ER. Radiology of the nasolacrimal passageways. *Med Radiogr Photogr* 1949;25:66.

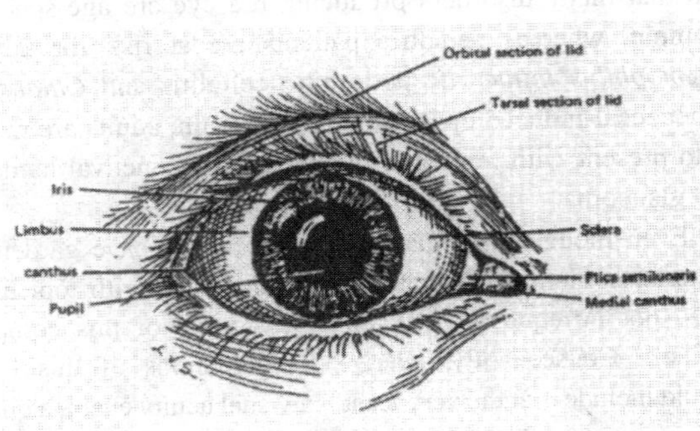

Figure 3. External landmarks of the eye. Used with permission: Linder HH, ed. *Clinical Anatomy.* Norwalk: Appleton & Lange, 1989, pg 83.

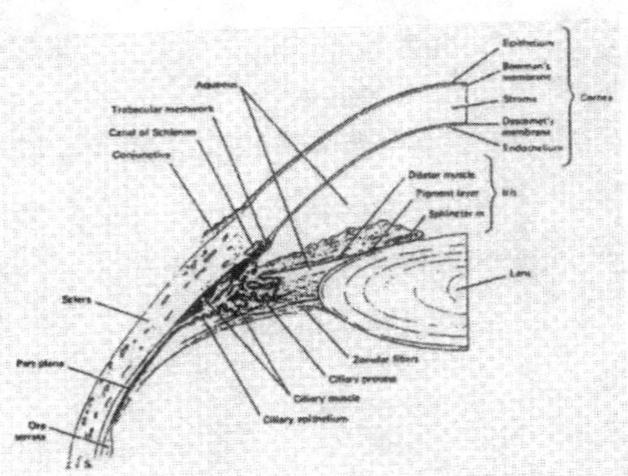

Figure 4. Anterior chamber and surrounding structures. Used with permission: Vaughan DG, Asbury T, Riordan-Eva P, eds. *General Ophthalmology* 13th ed. Norwalk: Appleton & Lange, 1992, pg 12.

Visual Acuity: Vital Sign for the Eye

Evaluation of visual acuity provides important information regarding clarity of the cornea, lens, and vitreous humor as well as the integrity of the visual pathway from the retina to the occipital cortex. In most cases, the visual acuity should be measured prior to any physical manipulation of the eye or local instillation of ophthalmic medications. Typically, acuity is measured at 20 feet and written as a ratio in which the patient's results are compared to those of a visually "normal" person.

This portion of the exam should be performed using the patient's corrective lenses (this should be noted on the chart). If the patient does not have his or her corrective lenses, a pin-hole test should be performed. This is done by having the patient look through a pinhole that is made by placing several holes close together in a piece of paper and using an 18-gauge needle. Refractory errors will improve when looking through a pinhole, but decreased vision due to organic lesions will not improve. If patients are unable to read letters, the vision should be recorded using one of the following: finger counting (e.g., "FC at 4 ft"); hand movement (HM); light perception (LP); and no light perception (NLP).

Physical Examination

A systematic examination will direct the physician to almost all causes of the red eye. After the visual acuity is determined, two drops of a topical ophthalmologic anesthetic is usually applied to the affected eye. The eye is inspected, starting with the periorbital tissues, followed by evaluation of the conjunctivae, cornea, and sclera. The pupillary response is determined; the extraocular muscles are assessed with respect to range of motion and funduscopy is performed. The lacrimal apparatus is palpated and the eyelids are completely everted, inspecting for follicle formation and retained foreign bodies. The globe is then palpated (avoiding the anterior chamber) for firmness. Fluorescein stain is applied, and the cornea is examined using a cobalt blue light source. Finally, a slit lamp examination is performed in order to identify foreign bodies or corneal erosions, and to detect abnormalities in the anterior chamber—i.e, flare, keratic bodies, and blood (hyphema).

Differential Diagnosis of Red Eye: Lid Disorders

Blepharitis. Blepharitis is an inflammatory disorder of the eyelid margins, in a process that may be associated with conjunctivitis. Anterior blepharitis is generally divided into staphylococcal (ulcerative) and seborrheic (non-ulcerative) categories.[1] The seborrheic form is characterized by hyperemia of the lid margins and greasy scales surrounding the eyelashes. Therapy for this variant of anterior blepharitis consists of meticulous lid hygiene and scale removal with gentle washing, usually with baby shampoo. Neonates may develop this condition along with seborrheic dermatitis of the scalp (cradle cap).

The ulcerative (staphylococcal) form of blepharitis produces inflammation of the follicles and lashes which, if inadequately treated, can lead to local abscess formation. Patients most commonly present with erythematous eyelid margins that are stippled with multiple, crusting, suppurative lesions. These crust-laden lesions can be extracted only with difficulty, and attempts at removal often cause dislodgement of eyelashes. *Staphylococcal blepharitis* may be further complicated by formation of a hordeolum (sty), chalazion, or keratitis (inflammation of the cornea).[2] Mild cases of anterior staphylococcal blepharitis are treated with a topical antistaphylococcal agent; oral, systemic therapy is frequently added for severe cases.

Posterior blepharitis results when the meibomian gland becomes plugged, producing a caseous secretion. *(Please see Figure 1.)* In this disorder, the lids may eventually roll inward, causing injury to the tarsal conjunctiva and cornea. Treatment usually consists of oral antistaphylococcal antibiotics.

Hordeolum. A hordeolum (or sty) is an acute suppurative, nodular inflammatory process—sometimes accompanied by frank abscess formation—involving the meibomian glands of the eyelids. *Staphylococcus aureus* is the most common infectious agent. The patient will present with an acutely tender erythematous and edematous lid margin, where abscess pointing can often be visualized at the eyelash follicle. Not uncommonly, a hordeolum will point to the conjunctival surface or to the skin, where spontaneous rupture is possible. Treatment consists of warm compresses[3] 3-4 times daily and application of ophthalmic ointment with antistaphylococcal coverage (i.e., gentamicin ophthalmic ointment) to the conjunctival sac every three hours. If there is no resolution of symptoms in 48 hours, surgical drainage may be necessary.

Chalazion. Sometimes evolving from a hordeolum, a chalazion represents granulomatous inflammation that develops around a sebaceous gland in the eyelid. The acute process frequently produces marked lid edema and may spontaneously drain through the skin or subconjunctival surface. Initial treatment during the early stages consists of warm compresses, which are used to localize the process and achieve spontaneous drainage.[3] Although topical antibiotics probably do not directly affect the inflammation, they are sometimes used empirically as adjunctive therapy to decrease local bacterial flora. Surgical drainage of a chalazion may be necessary if the inflammatory process becomes chronic.[4]

Table 1. Conditions Causing Red Eye

Eyelid	**Iris**
Blepharitis	Uveitis
Hordeolum (sty)	Glaucoma—acute narrow angle
Chalazion	
Lacrimal	**Conjunctiva**
Dacryadenitis	Ophthalmia neonatorum
Dacryocystitis	Bacterial
	Viral
Orbit	Allergic
Periorbital cellulitis	
Orbital cellulitis	**Trauma**
	Burns (chemical and thermal)
Sclera	Corneal abrasions
Episcleritis	Intraorbital foreign body
Scleritis	Ruptured globe
Cornea	Penetrating ocular injury
Corneal abrasions	
Keratitis	
Neurologic	
Cavernous sinus thrombosis	

Lacrimal Disorders

Dacryoadenitis. Most often encountered in children, dacryoadenitis is an acute inflammation of the lacrimal gland, which is located in the superior temporal quadrant of the orbit. *(Please see Figure 2.)* In children, dacryoadenitis is frequently associated with a viral infection, whereas in adults it is often a manifestation of gonococcal infection.[5] Dacryoadenitis may be caused by contiguous extension from bacterial conjunctivitis or lid cellulitis. The clinical presentation is characterized by pain, swelling, and erythema of the temporal aspect of the upper lid. Treat with warm compresses and oral antibiotics.

Dacryocystitis. Precipitated by obstruction of the nasolacrimal duct, dacryocystitis is a suppurative infection of the lacrimal sac, which is located in the inferonasal quadrant of the orbit. Dacryocystitis is most often encountered in infants and postmenopausal women, and is rare in other patient sub-groups, unless caused by trauma or a dacryolith.[6] Patients usually present with swelling, redness, and tenderness surrounding the medial canthus, and often, mucoid material may be expressed from the lacrimal sac. *(Please see Figure 3.)* Acute dacryocystitis in children is usually caused by Haemophilus influenzae. Prompt antimicrobial treatment with amoxicillin-clavulanate will minimize the risk of orbital cellulitis. *(Please see Table 2.) S. aureus* and beta-hemolytic streptococcus are the most common pathogens in adults.

Management of the afebrile pediatric patient consists of outpatient antibiotic therapy with amoxicillin-clavulanate, whereas severely ill

Table 2. Drug Therapy for Conditions Causing Red Eye

Dacryocystitis
- **Amoxicillin-Clavulanate**
  - Child 20-40 mg/kg/24 hr ÷ q 8 hr po
  - Adult 250-500 mg q 8 hr po
- **Dicloxacillin**
  - Child 12-25 mg/kg/24 hr ÷ q 6 hr po
  - Adult 125-500 mg/dose q 6 hr po
- **Cephalexin**
  - Child 25-50 mg/kg/24 hr ÷ q 6-12 hr po
  - Adult 250-1000 mg/dose q 6-12 hr po
- **Cefuroxime**
  - Child 50-100 mg/kg/24 hr ÷ q 6-8 hr IM or IV
  - Adult 0.75-3 mg/dose q 6-8 hr IM or IV

Periorbital Cellulitis
- **Cefaclor**
  - Child 40 mg/kg/24 hr ÷ q 8 hr po
  - Adult 250-500 mg/dose q 8 hr po
- **Cefuroxime**
  - Child 100-150 mg/kg/24 hr ÷ q 6-8 hr IV
  - Adult 0.75-3 g/dose q 6-8 hr IV (max dose 9 g/24 hr)
- **Nafcillin**
  - Child 100-200 mg/kg/24 hr ÷ q 6 hr IV
  - Adult 500-2000 mg/dose q 4-6 hr IV (max dose 12 g/24 hr)

Orbital Cellulitis
- **Cefuroxime**
  - Child (<6 yr) 100-150 mg/kg/24 hr ÷ q 8 hr IV
- **Nafcillin**
  - Child 150-200 mg/kg/24 hr ÷ q 6 hr IV
  - Adult 500-2000 mg/dose q 4-6 hr IV (max dose 12 g/24 hr)
- **Chloramphenicol**
  - Child 50-100 mg/kg/24 hr ÷ q 6 hr IV
  - Adult 50-100 mg/kg/24 hr IV (max dose 4 g/24 hr)
- **Vancomycin**
  - Child 30-50- mg/kg/24 hr ÷ q 8 hr IV
  - Adult 2 g/24 hr ÷ q 6-12 hr IV

Conjunctivitis
- **Sulfonamide Ophthalmic Solution (10, 15, 30% solutions)**
  - Dose: 1-3 drops in lower conjunctival sac q 2-3 hr/day
- **Sulfonamide Ophthalmic Ointment**
  - Dose: Apply small amount to lower conjunctival sac 1-4 times daily and at bedtime
- **Gentamicin Ophthalmic Solution**
  - Dose: 1-2 drops 4-6 times daily
- **Gentamicin Ophthalmic Ointment**
  - Dose: Apply small amount to lower conjunctival sac 2-3 times daily
- **Tobramycin Ophthalmic Solution**
  - Dose: 1-2 drops 4-6 times daily
- **Bacitracin Ophthalmic Ointment**
  - Dose: 1-2 drops 4-6 times daily
- **Erythromycin Ophthalmic Ointment**
  - Dose: Apply small amount to lower conjunctival sac 2-3 times daily
- **Ciprofloxacin Ophthalmic Solution**
  - Dose: 1-2 drops 4-6 times daily

Glaucoma
- **Pilocarpine (2-4% solution)**
  - Dose: 1-2 drops q 15 min until pupil constricts, then 1-2 drops qid
- **Timolol (0.5% solution)**
  - Dose: 1-2 drops bid
- **Acetazolamide**
  - Dose: 500 mg po, IM, or IV

Iritis
- **Homatropine (2-5% solution)**
  - Dose: 1-2 drops q 3-4 hr
- **Prednisolone (1% solution)**
  - Dose: 1-2 drops q 2 hr while awake, q 4 hr at night

children should be hospitalized and treated with intravenous cefuroxime. *(Please see Table 2.)* Adults with mild cases should be treated with oral dicloxacillin (500 mg po qid) or oral cephalexin (500 mg po qid). Febrile adults who appear acutely ill require hospitalization and treatment with intravenous nafcillin or cefazolin. Acute dacryocystitis usually responds to antibiotics, warm compresses, and relief of the obstruction, which may require surgery.

Periorbital (Preseptal) Cellulitis

Localized in the soft tissues anterior to the orbital septum, periorbital cellulitis usually presents with fever, erythema and edema of the eyelids, chemosis, orbital pain, and conjunctivitis. *(Please see Figure 1.)* With respect to differential diagnosis, extraocular muscle use is unrestricted with periorbital cellulitis, but usually is restricted with orbital cellulitis. The physician should search for violaceous discoloration of the eyelids and surrounding tissues, which is characteristic of *H. influenzae* infection. Common predisposing factors include: a recent history of respiratory tract infection; sinusitis; acute or chronic otitis media; eyelid or facial trauma; and infection of adjacent structures.[7,8]

Periorbital cellulitis, which occurs more frequently than orbital infections, is most commonly seen in patients 5 years old and younger,[8] with a peak incidence between 6 months and 2 years. The most common pathogens in children are *H. influenzae* and *Streptococcus pneumoniae*, whereas in adults *S. aureus* and beta-hemolytic streptococcus are the most common etiologic agents. Periorbital cellulitis caused by human bites are associated with an increased risk of infection with anaerobic organisms.[9]

Laboratory evaluation should include a complete blood cell count (CBC), which usually demonstrates an elevated white blood cell count in the 10,000-15,000 cells/mm^3 range; severe cases can produce WBC counts of more than 20,000 cells/mm.[3] Blood cultures should be obtained in pediatric patients, although most will not yield a pathogen. Because *H. influenzae* type B infection can lead to meningitis, routine lumbar puncture is recommended by some authors. In most cases, however, lumbar puncture is of limited help unless signs of meningeal irritation are present.[10,11] Percutaneous aspirates for gram stain and culture, however, are recommended.

Oral penicillinase-resistant penicillins or a cephalosporin (cefaclor) are appropriate antimicrobial choices for mild cases in which outpatient therapy is deemed suitable. Intravenous nafcillin or a third-generation cephalosporin, combined with chloramphenicol or ampicillin-sulbactam for anaerobic organisms, are reasonable choices for more severe infections requiring hospitalization. When a single agent is preferred, intravenous (IV) cefuroxime is frequently used because of its efficacy against both *H. influenzae* and *S. pneumoniae*. A CT or MRI scan is indicated if orbital cellulitis is suspected.[12] Because of the possibility of central nervous system (CNS) complications, hospitalization is strongly recommended in moderate to severe infections.

Table 3. Differential Diagnosis of Common Causes of Inflamed Eye

	Acute Conjunctivitis	Acute Iritis	Acute Glaucoma	Corneal Trauma or Infecction
Incidence	Extremely common	Common	Uncommon	Common
Discharge	Moderate to copious	None	None	Watery or purulent
Vision	No effect on vision	Slightly blurred	Markedly blurred	Usually blurred
Pain	None	Moderate	Severe	Moderate to severe
Conjunctival injection	Diffuse; more toward fornices	Mainly circum-corneal	Diffuse	Diffuse
Cornea	Clear	Usually clear	Steamy	Change in clarity related to cause
Pupil size	Normal	Small	Moderately dilated and fixed	Normal
Pupillary light response	Normal	Poor	None	Normal
Intraocular pressure	Normal	Normal	Elevated	Normal
Gram stain	Causative organisms	No organisms	No organisms	Organisms found in corneal ulcers due to infection

Used with permission from Vaughan DG, Asbury T, Riordan-Eva P. *General Ophthalmology* 13th ed. Norwalk, Appleton & Lange, 1992.

Orbital Cellulitis

Orbital cellulitis is a potentially serious infection which can be complicated by CNS involvement, visual loss, cavernous sinus thrombosis, osteomyelitis, and, on rare occasions, death. Early signs and symptoms include proptosis, orbital discomfort, and ophthalmoplegia, which is caused by edema of orbital adipose and soft tissues.

Pediatric patients with orbital cellulitis are usually older than 6 years of age, febrile, and appear acutely ill.[13] Most cases result from a sinus infection.[14] Physical findings include localized pain, redness, edema of the eyelids, chemosis, and conjunctival injection. These findings are similar to those found in periorbital cellulitis. However, with orbital cellulitis, diffuse soft tissue inflammation may be severe enough to cause axial displacement of the eye. Non-axial (lateral) displacement of the eye suggests a focal subperiosteal or orbital abscess.

The most common etiologic agents include bacteria associated with sinusitis. These agents include: *S. aureus, Streptococcus pyogenes, S. pneumoniae*, and *H. influenzae*. When orbital cellulitis occurs in the setting of trauma, infections caused by *S. aureus, Clostridium sp.*, and anaerobes as well as polymicrobial infections predominate. Orbital cellulitis is rare in infancy, but, when present, is usually caused by *H. influenzae*. The assessment of visual acuity may be difficult in infants. Nevertheless, the presence of an ipsilateral afferent pupillary defect (Marcus-Gunn pupil) should be considered a sign of significant visual impairment in this age group.[9]

With respect to diagnostic confirmation, a CT scan or MRI of the orbital apex is mandatory. Axial and coronal cuts through the orbit will help define preseptal and orbital inflammation.[15-17] Other conditions, such as orbital abscess, sinusitis, periosteal mass, foreign body, and globe displacement can be distinguished by CT or MRI scan.

All patients suspected of having orbital cellulitis should have blood cultures drawn. In children, blood cultures are more likely to be positive when *H. influenzae* is the etiologic agent.[18] Nevertheless, in older children and adults, blood cultures are rarely positive.[19] Aspirates from abscesses and infected sinuses are generally more helpful in making a diagnosis.

Patients with orbital cellulitis should be admitted for IV antibiotics. In patients younger than 6 years of age, cefurox-ime is recommended. Older patients are treated with cloxacillin or nafcillin in combination with chloramphenicol. In penicillin-allergic patients, vancomycin can be substituted for a penicillinase-resistant penicillin.[20] Patients should be reassessed frequently while in the ED, where overall clinical condition, changes in temperature, mental status, visual acuity, proptosis, ophthalmoplegia, pupillary findings, and funduscopic changes should be noted and documented.

Conjunctivitis

Conjunctivitis is a common ophthalmologic problem, in large part because the conjunctivae are exposed to many environmental irritants, allergens, occupation-related chemicals, and microorganisms. Noxious agents can cause edema, inflammation, hypertrophy, cell death, and exfoliation. There also may be edema of the stromal layer (chemosis), hypertrophy of the lymphoid layer of the stroma (follicle formation), and a conjunctival exudate frequently forms on the lid margins. *(Please see Table 3.)* It should be stressed that most cases of mild conjunctivitis are self-limited (since they are caused by a virus) and respond well to topical antibiotics and ocular hygiene. Although topical antibiotics do not enhance resolution of viral conjunctivitis, they are used empirically in almost all cases of conjunctival inflammation because it is difficult to distinguish clinically between bacterial and viral causes of this condition.

The differential diagnosis of conjunctivitis includes several conditions.and, distinguishing among them can be difficult. For example, patients with allergic conjunctivitis complain of ocular "itching" and tearing associated with sneezing and nasal congestion. The conjunctivae are usually mildly injected and there may be dramatic chemosis. Topical antihistamines and vasoconstrictors may provide relief.

Bacterial Conjunctivitis. Bacterial infection of the conjunctiva usually produces a purulent or mucopurulent conjunctivitis. A wide range of bacteria can infect the conjunctiva and there is considerable variation with the age of the patient, location, and season. *S. aureus* is the most common etiologic agent in bacterial conjunctivitis. *S. pneumoniae* and *H. influenzae* are prominent pathogens in children.[21] Usually, patients complain of irritation, a "gritty" sensation, and tearing in one or both eyes. A mucopurulent discharge is common, but visual acuity is seldom affected. The conjunctiva will be diffusely injected without involvement of the perilimbic area. *(Please see Figure 3.)* There may also be subconjunctival petechial hemorrhages that are most characteristic of *H. influenzae*. Examination of the superior tarsal conjunctiva may reveal follicles which are suggestive of Chlamydia trachomatis infection.

Purulent, hyperacute bacterial conjunctivitis is most often caused by *Neisseria gonorrhoeae*, which characteristically produces an intense, inflammatory response accompanied by a copious purulent discharge, and edema of the eyelids and conjunctiva. The exudate will demonstrate gram-negative intracellular diplococci. Neisseria conjunctivitis is a reportable disease and sexual partners should be evaluated.

Viral Conjunctivitis. Viral conjunctivitis, which is usually associated with adenovirus infection, can range in severity from a mild self-limited infection to a serious, disabling disease. There may be bilateral involvement with a profuse serous discharge and photosensitivity. Sometimes, the patient will report migration of the infection from one eye to the other. The usual presentation consists of conjunctival injection, chemosis, lid edema, and a marked follicular response, which is best seen on the inner surface of the inferior eyelid. There also may be punctate fluorescein staining of the cornea.

Infection with herpes simplex virus (HSV), which is reported to cause up to 500,000 cases of HSV conjunctivitis in the United States annually, produces discrete epithelial lesions on the cornea that usually form branching (dendritic) ulcers.[22,23] In addition to characteristic corneal lesions, herpetic vesicles are often present on the face or eyelids. HSV infection in the newborn must be treated with intravenous acyclovir. In patients who have HSV infection in this age group, the physician should attempt to exclude concurrent encephalitis, chorioretinitis, and hepatitis.

Acute hemorrhagic conjunctivitis is endemic to most countries and is commonly seen in Florida. The presentation consists of abrupt onset of conjunctivitis, edema, serous drainage, and conjunctival hemorrhage, and it usually resolves spontaneously within 5-7 days.[24]

Neonatal Conjunctivitis (Ophthalmia Neonatorum). Microbial inoculation of the newborn conjunctiva from the maternal genital tract frequently occurs during birth. Inoculation can also complicate cesarean section, especially when amniotic membranes have been ruptured for more than three hours. Bacterial conjunctivitis in the immunologically immature or premature infant can lead to meningitis and sepsis. Bacterial causes of neonatal conjunctivitis include *Escherichia coli*, *S. aureus*, and *H. influenzae*. The most virulent pathogens are *N. gonorrhoeae* and *C. trachomatis* and usually require hospital admission. The diagnosis can usually be made by performing conjunctival smears for gram stain, culture, and a chlamydia assay.[25] Chemical conjunctivitis is common in the newborn and is usually due to the inflammation caused by silver nitrate prophylaxis. The condition is usually mild and resolves within three days.

Treatment of Conjunctivitis. Because most conjunctival infections are viral in nature, the majority will resolve spontaneously. In practice, however, because it is difficult to distinguish between bacterial and viral etiologies, topical antibiotic therapy may hasten resolution and is required for management in nearly all cases. *(Please see Table 2.)* Moreover, since conjunctivitis is extremely contagious, antibiotics usually are applied to both eyes, even when unilateral disease is present; this prevents the spread of infection from one eye to the other.

Sodium sulfacetamide is widely used for topical therapy and is available in a 10% or 30% concentration. Despite the efficacy of this preparation, *S. aureus* has become increasingly resistant to sodium sulfacetamide. When this organism is strongly suspected, gentamicin or tobramycin can be used. These aminoglycosides also are effective against *Pseudomonas aeruginosa* and gram-negative bacilli, but they have less activity against *Neisseria* and *Haemophilus*. Bacitracin is effective against gram-positive organisms (e.g., *Staphylococcus*, *Streptococcus*), whereas erythromycin is effective against N. gonorrhoeae, *N. meningitidis*, and *H. influenzae*, but less so against S. aureus, *S. pneumoniae*, and *S. pyogenes*.[26] Fluoroquinolones (though expensive) are highly effective against a broad spectrum of organisms, including *P. aeruginosa*.[27-29] Specifically, ciprofloxacin is effective in almost 90% of patients without serious side effects.[30] Fluoroquinolones are contraindicated in children and pregnant patients.

Conjunctivitis due to *N. gonorrhoeae* requires systemic and topical treatment. Intravenous penicillin G or intramuscular aqueous procaine penicillin G should be used. Alternative therapy includes ceftriaxone given as a single dose.[31] Topical therapy should include penicillin G or bacitracin ophthalmic ointment. Topical steroids should be avoided.

Uveitis (Iritis)

The uveal tract is composed of the iris, the ciliary body, and the choroid (the middle layer of the globe). Uveitis is inflammation of the uveal tract, which is usually confined to the iris and the anterior chamber. Presentation of acute uveitis usually includes blurred vision, ocular pain, conjunctival injection, a watery discharge, and photophobia, which is caused by inflammation of the anterior uvea and spasm of the ciliary body. A simple bedside test for assessment of uveitis is the consensual light reflex. The affected (red) eye is covered and a bright light is shined into the uncovered, unaffected eye. If pain is induced in the red eye, uveitis should be strongly suspected. Blurred vision usually results from clouding of the aqueous humor, cornea, or lens. Uveitis can be associated with minor trauma, chronic inflammatory conditions (e.g., ulcerative colitis), and systemic infections (e.g., Lyme disease). Uveitis can be difficult to diagnose in the absence of ocular redness; in these cases, patients may have isolated pain that is relieved by ibuprofen.

Conjunctival vascular congestion produces a circumcorneal (ciliary) "flush." The inflamed anterior uveal tract causes protein and cells to extravasate into the aqueous humor, which can be detected by slit-lamp examination. Increased protein circulating within the aqueous is called flare. Fine white deposits (keratic precipitates) on the surface of the cornea may occur. Accumulation of fibrin in the anterior chamber can result in adhesions between the pupillary margin of the iris and the lens called synechiae, which may produce miosis and pupillary irregularities. The intraocular pressure (IOP) may elevate due to decreased flow of aqueous humor out of the anterior chamber. Anticholinergic preparations (e.g., Homatropine 1-5%, soptoatropine 1%) dilate the pupil to help prevent synechiae formation. However, atropine is contraindicated if acute narrow-angle glaucoma is suspected. Topical steroids (prednisolone acetate 1% solution [Econopred Plus, Pred Forte]) that decrease the inflammatory response should be used cautiously because they can result in secondary glaucoma and cataract formation as well as exacerbate herpes simplex keratitis. Oral non-steroidal anti-inflammatory agents (NSAIDS) are also used. Patients with uveitis should be referred for ophthalmologic evaluation.

Episcleritis and Scleritis

Episcleritis is characterized by inflammation of the thin layer of vascular elastic tissue overlying the sclera just beneath the conjunctiva. Resembling a localized conjunctivitis, it usually involves a single quadrant of the globe and is usually self-limited and benign. Unlike conjunctivitis, the inflammation in episcleritis is deeper, salmon-colored, and the dilated vessels do not always blanch with topical phenylephrine.

Scleritis, which is often bilateral, is a destructive process involving the sclera, and is usually associated with systemic disease or infection. It is characterized by the destruction of collagen, cellular infiltration, and a vasculitis. It is often bilateral. Patients present with severe orbital pain, scleral edema, and diffuse nodular patches of deeply injected scleral tissue that may have a violaceous hue. Lacrimation and photophobia are common. Systemic NSAIDs are used, although a short-term, high-dose course with systemic corticosteroids is recommended by some authors.[7] Ophthalmologic referral is imperative.

Glaucoma

Glaucoma is characterized by an elevated intraocular pressure (IOP). Because the optic nerve can be damaged, emergent ophthalmologic consultation is mandatory. Three major types of glaucoma have been identified: open-angle, narrow-angle (angle-closure), and congenital. Congenital and open-angle glaucoma rarely cause acute symptoms. Acute narrow-angle glaucoma, however, is an urgent, painful condition, requiring immediate treatment.

The IOP is regulated by the flow of the aqueous humor out of the anterior chamber. Acute narrow-angle glaucoma usually occurs where there is a preexisting narrowing of the anterior chamber angle. A tight contact forms between the iris and lens, blocking the outflow of aqueous humor from the posterior chamber. *(Please see Figure 4.)* When the pupil dilates, the iris bulges anteriorly, thus obliterating the anterior angle between the cornea and the iris. This process blocks reabsorption of aqueous humor, producing an acute rise in the IOP.

Acute episodes of narrow-angle glaucoma are characterized by ocular redness, visual blurring, perception of halos forming around objects due to corneal edema, mild to severe pain, nausea and vomiting, and a poorly reactive, mid-dilated pupil. Triggering phenomena include stress, a darkened environment, and pharmacologic agents (e.g., anticholinergic agents).

When the IOP rises rapidly, fluid is forced into the cornea, causing edema. As corneal edema increases, the visual acuity diminishes. The patient develops impaired vision, perilimbal injection, conjunctival edema, a "steamy" cornea, and flare cells in the anterior chamber. A simple test to confirm narrow-angle glaucoma is to shine a penlight across the eye from the temporal side. In the normal eye, the entire iris will illuminate. In the eye with narrow-angle glaucoma, a shadow will appear on the nasal side due to the bulging of the iris (iris bombé).[31] A slit lamp examination must be performed to estimate the anterior chamber depth.

The diagnosis of acute narrow-angle glaucoma is made by documenting an elevated IOP with the use of a Schiötz tonometer, which measures the amount of corneal indentation produced by the direct application of a preset weight. The "softer" the eye, the more a given force will indent the cornea. Schiötz tonometry is performed with the patient resting in the supine position; a topical anesthetic is instilled. The patient looks forward at a fixed point and the tonometer is lowered until the concave end balances completely upon the cornea. The corneal resistance will displace the plunge upward; the higher the IOP, the greater the corneal resistance. A number is read off the tonometer, which is then converted to an IOP using a standard chart. If the scale reads zero, additional weight is placed on the tonometer until a reading is obtained. A pressure of 20 mmHg or less is considered normal. In acute attacks, the pressure may exceed 50 mmHg. If tonometry is unavailable, simple finger ballottement is often helpful. With the patient looking down, the examiner presses each index finger into the globes, alternately applying pressure. The normal eye has some compressibility; the eye with glaucoma feels rock-like.

Acute management of narrow-angle glaucoma requires use of agents that release the iris from the trabecular meshwork. Initial therapy consists of pilocarpine (2-4%), which will open the angle and should be instilled every 15 minutes until pupillar constriction is achieved. It should be noted that when the IOP is high, the iris is ischemic and, in some cases, pilocarpine may not be effective until the IOP is diminished. Prophylactic pilocarpine (1%) is given to the unaffected eye.

When necessary, aqueous humor production can be decreased with timolol (0.5% Timoptic), a topically administered beta-blocker,[33] which will decrease the IOP within one hour, and achieve a peak effect within two hours. Systemic carbonic anhydrase inhibitors, such as acetazolamide (Diamox), also suppress aqueous production.[34] The vitreous volume can be rapidly reduced by the use of hyperosmotic agents (i.e., mannitol), which lower IOP by osmotic diffusion and diuresis as well as by decreasing aqueous humor formation. The effects may be seen within 10 minutes of administration, and have a duration of action of up to five hours. Oral glycerol may be used, but only with caution in the diabetic patient.[35] Definitive treatment of acute narrow-angle glaucoma is with a surgical iridotomy.

Ocular Trauma

Corneal Abrasion. Patients who have sustained a corneal abrasion present to the ED with acute pain, lacrimation, foreign body sensation, photophobia, and blepharospasm, which can usually be relieved with a topical anesthetic. Most often, physical exam reveals ciliary injection and an area of epithelial loss that will stain with fluorescein and is identified with a cobalt blue filter. Careful inspection of the bulbar and tarsal conjunctiva should be performed by everting the eyelids. The examiner should search for a retained foreign body, rust ring, or contact lens. If present, they should be removed. Multiple corneal abrasions caused by a retained foreign body repeatedly grating across the cornea is referred to as the ice rink sign. Some patients with a corneal abrasion will suffer from recurrent corneal erosion, which can occur weeks to months after the initial injury. In this syndrome, pain is frequently experienced during the night or upon awakening.

Treatment includes patching the eye, use of a topical broad-spectrum antibiotic for infection prophylaxis, and tetanus prophylaxis when indicated. A cycloplegic agent (e.g., Cyclogyl 1%) may increase comfort, but is not required in most cases. The pressure patch (using two eye pads together) is applied to provide comfort and to minimize local corneal trauma from lid movement as the epithelium heals. The patch should be left on for at least 24-48 hours. With respect to follow-up, the patient is reexamined in 36-48 hours to monitor healing and exclude any infection. A follow-up examination is essential.

Contact lens-related abrasions are associated with an increased incidence of gram-negative bacterial infection especially from *Pseudomonas*.[36] With lens abrasions, an antibiotic with gram-negative coverage (gentamicin, tobramycin) is used and an eye patch is avoided. Oral analgesics may be given. Topical anesthetics are contraindicated; they delay healing and can promote further injury due to a loss of the protective reflexes. Contact lens wearers should abstain from lens wear for at least one week.

Chemical Injuries. The most serious chemical burns are caused by strong alkaline agents such as ammonia, lye, potassium hydroxide, magnesium hydroxide (found in sparklers), and lime (plaster, cement).[37-38] Alkalis are toxic to ophthalmologic structures because they rapidly penetrate the cornea and can cause damage to the entire anterior segment of the eye. Tissue destruction is mediated by the hydroxyl ion in alkali compounds, which causes liquefaction necrosis. Opacification of the cornea or an extensive avascular segment of the sclera suggests considerable ocular damage.

Acid burns, although severe, are often limited to the ocular surface. Restricted destruction is explained by the fact that most acids coagulate epithelial and stromal proteins, forming a barrier to deep penetration. Of the many acids that can cause injury, sulfuric acid (found in automobile batteries) is most common.

Treatment for serious chemical burns begins at the scene, and consists of copious water irrigation using the nearest available source (hose, shower). Irrigation should be continued during transport to the ED. Treatment should be continued upon arrival and the examination should be started without any interruption of therapy. Topical anesthetic agents are given for pain relief and eyelid retractors are inserted to permit easy visualization. Irrigation should be continued for up to 40 minutes with a physiologic solution (Dacriose, 0.9 normal saline), using a Morgan lens to facilitate irrigation. The eyelids should be everted in the search for retained particles. A litmus paper test should be performed after irrigation to confirm that the pH of the tears is in the 7.3-7.7 range. It should be emphasized that alkali material can continue to leach out of the anterior chamber for several hours. As a result, repeated litmus testing and continued irrigation may be required. All patients with moderate to severe chemical burns should be examined by an ophthalmologist.

Traumatic Hyphema. Hyphema (blood in the anterior chamber) is a common manifestation of blunt trauma. The extent of hyphema should be described by the volume of blood filling the anterior chamber (e.g., one-third, one-half, all of the anterior chamber). Blunt impact to the eye distorts the normal architecture producing a rapid increase in IOP, equatorial stretching of the globe, and posterior displacement of the lens and iris. Hemorrhage originates from the blood vessels of the iris and ciliary body.[39]

A complete eye examination is required to exclude a ruptured globe in all patients with blunt trauma. The visual acuity, IOP, and an illustration of the hyphema must be documented in the chart. Rebleeding is suggested by bright red blood layering over darker, clotted blood and an increase in the size of the hyphema. Traumatic iritis and traumatic mydriasis may accompany a hyphema. The patient should have the head of the bed elevated to 30 degrees, minimize movement, receive analgesics or sedatives, and be referred to an ophthalmologist for follow-up evaluation.

Cavernous Sinus Thrombosis

Although rare, thrombosis of the cavernous sinus may follow infections of the midface, sphenoid sinusitis, or ethmoid sinusitis. *S. aureus* is recovered in two-thirds of cases with *Pneumococcus* and *Streptococcus sp.* identified in the majority of remaining cases. *H. influenzae* should be considered in children younger than 5 years. Cavernous sinus thrombosis (CST) may be difficult to clinically differentiate from orbital cellulitis. Headache, fever, proptosis, chemosis, and ptosis develop in more than 90% of cases of CST. With respect to the differential diagnosis, cranial nerve palsies are characteristic of CST and commonly involve the third and sixth cranial nerves, with a lateral gaze palsy frequently seen as an early neurological finding.

As the disease progresses, the pupil usually becomes fixed and dilated. If the sympathetic plexus is interrupted, the pupil becomes small and fixed, but this is rare. Eventually, cranial nerves III, IV, V, and VI become involved, producing paralysis or paresis of the extraocular muscles. There is often pain and paresthesias along the maxillary and ophthalmic divisions of the trigeminal nerve. Patients develop an altered mental status and may become lethargic or comatose. Meningeal signs and papilledema are common.

A moderate leukocytosis is common and cerebral spinal fluid (CSF) analysis shows a mononuclear and neutrophilic pleocytosis, an elevated protein level, and a normal glucose level. Blood cultures may be positive in the early stages of the disease; *S. aureus* is the most common isolate.[40-42] Orbital venography is the radiologic procedure of choice, but MRI may emerge as the primary diagnostic technique.

Empiric antibiotic treatment should be started until culture results return. A penicillinase-resistant synthetic penicillin and chloramphenicol for anaerobic coverage is recommended. Anticoagulation with intravenous heparin and use of thrombolytic agents have been successful in some cases,[42,43] but their use is controversial.

Summary

Infectious and inflammatory conditions causing red eye can involve a wide variety of ophthalmological compartments and structures. In this regard, treatment is highly variable and diagnosis-specific. Consequently, a thorough understanding of the anatomy of the lacrimal system, the orbit, and periorbital structures is essential for appropriate management. Detailed historical information also is required to make a precise diagnosis and should include: onset and duration of symptoms, nature and location of pain, presence or absence of photophobia, itching, visual changes, recent injuries and occupational exposure, previous eye surgery, and a history of systemic or ocular diseases. Finally, triage personnel must be aware of the urgency of certain ocular complaints (i.e., chemical burns) so that treatment can be initiated promptly.

References

1. McCulley JP, Dougherty JM, Deneau DG. Classification of chronic blepharitis. *Am Acad Ophthalmol 1*982;89: 1173-1180.
2. Thygeson P. Complications of staphylococcic blepharitis. *Am J Ophthalmol* 1969;68:446-449.
3. Judge J. Overview of the red eye. *J Ophthalmic Nursing Technology* 1992;11:197-202.
4. Gaston H. Managing the red eye. *Practitioner* 1989;233: 1566-1572.
5. Sullivan JH. Lids and lacrimal apparatus. In Vaughan DG, Asbury T, Riordan-Eva P, eds. *General Ophthalmology* 13th ed. Norwalk: Appleton & Lange; 1992:88.
6. Sullivan JH. Lids and lacrimal apparatus. in Vaughan DG, Asbury T, Riordan-Eva P, eds. *General Ophthalmology* 13th ed. Norwalk: Appleton & Lange; 1992:89.
7. Yanofsky NN. The acute painful eye. *Emerg Med Clin North Am* 1988;6:21-42.
8. Jackson K, Baker SR. Periorbital cellulitis. *Head Neck Surg* 1987;9:227-234.
9. Lessner A, Stern GA. Preseptal and orbital cellulitis. *Infect Dis Clin North Am* 1992;6:933-952.
10. Antoine GA, Grundfast KM. Periorbital cellulitis. *Int J Pediatr Otohinolaryngol* 1987;13:273-278.
11. Ciarallo LR, Rowe PC. Lumbar puncture in children with periorbital and orbital cellulitis. *J Pediatr* 1993;122:355-359.
12. Goldberg F, Berne AS, Oski FA. Differentiation of orbital cellulitis from preseptal cellulitis by computed tomography. *Pediatrics* 1978;62:1000-1005.
13. Israele V, Nelson JD. Periorbital and orbital cellulitis. *Pediatr Infect Dis J* 1987;6:404-410.
14. Jackson K, Baker SR. Clinical implications of orbital cellulitis. *Laryngoscope* 1986;96:568-574.
15. Jones DB, Steinkuller PG. Strategies for the initial management of acute preseptal and orbital cellulitis. *Trans Am Ophthalm Soc* 1988;LXXXVI:94-112.
16. Hirsch M, Lifshitz T. Computerized tomography in the diagnosis and treatment of orbital cellulitis. *Pediatr Radiol* 1988; 18:302-305.
17. Williams SR, Carruth JAS. Orbital infection secondary to sinusitis in children: diagnosis and management. *Clin Otolaryngol* 1992;17:550-557.
18. Gellady AM, Shulman ST, Ayoub EM. Periorbital and orbital cellulitis. *Pediatrics* 1978;61:272-277.
19. Weiss A, Friendly D, Eglin K, et al. Bacterial periorbital and orbital cellulitis in childhood. Am Acad Ophthalmol 1983; 90:195-203.
20. Noël LP, Clarke WN, MacDonald N. Clinical management of orbital cellulitis in children. *Can J Ophthalmol* 1990;25: 11-16.
21. Groothuis JR, Thompson J, Wright PF. Correlation of nasopharyngeal and conjunctival cultures with middle ear fluid cultures in otitis media. *Clin Pediatr* 1986;25:85-88.
22. External ocular infections and inflammatory disease. In *Vision Research: A National Plan* 1983-1987. Washington D.C.: National Eye Institute, 1983, U.S. Department of Health and Human Services Publication NIH 83-2472. pg113.
23. Howes DS. The red eye. *Semin Ophthalmol* 1990;5:15-23.
24. Asbell PA, de la Pena W, Harms D, et al. Acute hemorrhagic conjunctivitis in Central America: First enterovirus epidemic in the Western Hemisphere. *Ann Ophthalmol* 1985;17: 205-210.
25. Grosskreutz C, Smith LBH. Neonatal conjunctivitis. *Inter Opthalmol Clin* 1992;32:71-79.
26. Steinert RF. Current therapy for bacterial keratitis and bacterial conjunctivitis. *Am J Ophthalmol* 1991;112:10S-14S.
27. Neu HC. Microbiologic aspects of fluoroquinolones. *Am J Ophthalmol* 1991;112:15S-24S.
28. Cokingtin CD, Hyndiuk RA. Insights from experimental data on ciprofloxacin in the treatment of bacterial keratitis and ocular infections. *Am J Ophthalmol* 1991;112:25S-28S.
29. Leibowitz HM. Antibacterial effectiveness of ciprofloxacin 0.3% ophthalmic solution in the treatment of bacterial conjunctivitis. *Am J Ophthalmol* 1991;112:29S-33S.
30. Leibowitz HM. Clinical evaluation of ciprofloxacin 0.3% ophthalmic solution for treatment of bacterial keratitis. *Am J Ophthalmol* 1991;112:34S-47S.
31. Laga M, Naamara W, Brunham RC, et al. Single-dose therapy of gonococcal ophthalmia neonatorum with ceftriaxone. *N Engl J Med* 1986;315:1382-1385.
32. Pederson JE. Glaucoma. A primer for primary care physicians. *Postgrad Med* 1991;90:41-48.
33. Airaksinen PJ, Saari KM, Tiainen TJ, Jaanio E-AT. Management of acute closed-angle glaucoma with miotics and timolol. *Brit J Ophthalmol* 1979;63:822-825.
34. Everitt DE, Avorn J. Systemic effects of medication used to treat glaucoma. *Ann Intern Med* 1990;112:120-125.
35. Oakley DE, Ellis PP. Glycerol and hyperosmolar nonketotic coma. *Am J Ophthalmol* 1976;81:469-472.
36. Catania LJ. Management of corneal abrasions in an extended-wear patient population. *Prim Care Update* 1988;1: 123-133.
37. Harris LS, Cohn K, Galin MA. Alkali injury from fireworks. *Ann Ophthalmol* 1971;August:849-851.

38. Wagoner MD, Kenyon KR. Chemical Injuries. In: Shingleton BJ, Hersh PS, Kenyon KR, eds. *Eye Trauma*. St. Louis: Mosby Yearbook, 1991:79-94.
39. Wilson FM. Traumatic hyphema. pathogenesis and management. *Ophthalmology* 1980;87:910-919.
40. Ali SM, Ahmed SH. Cavernous sinus thrombosis in children. *J Trop Pediatr* 1992;38:194-195.
41. Thatai D, Chandy L. Dhar KL. Septic cavernous sinus thrombo-phlebitis: a review of 35 cases. *J Ind Med Assoc* 1992;90;290-292.
42. DiNubile MJ. Septic thrombosis of the cavernous sinuses. *Arch Neurol* 1988;45:567-572.
43. Karlin RJ, Robinson WA. Septic cavernous sinus thrombosis. *Ann Emerg Med* 1984;13:449-455.

Part IX

Geriatric Medicine

Depression in the Elderly

David Bienenfeld, MD

When the losses, threats, and stresses of late life give rise to depression, older people are likely to turn first to their primary care physicians (PCPs) for help. Coming to the office with complaints of fatigue or generalized somatic discomfort, they may quickly be found to display emotional disturbances. The physician can easily be confused by the many displays of depressive conditions in the elderly and might be tempted to regard such distress as an inevitable consequence of aging in contemporary society. Treatment of geriatric depression in a frail population often seems like a daunting task.

Depression in the elderly, however, can be recognized and characterized with some clarity. Secondary depression due to medical illness or treatment must be identified. Treatment options include antidepressants, psychotherapy, and electroconvulsive therapy.

Epidemiology

Among community-dwelling Americans older than age 65, the point prevalence of major depression is 1-4%, compared with 3-5% across all age groups. But when combined with minor depressive syndromes, the prevalence among elderly in the community is about 15%. In primary care settings, depressive syndromes have been detected in about 20% of patients; in nursing homes, up to 30%.[1-4] Risk factors for depression regardless of age, include:

- female sex;
- unmarried status;
- poverty;
- social isolation;
- prior history of depressive illness.

Additional risk factors in older individuals include:

- loss or grief;
- caretaking responsibilities;
- medical illness in self or spouse.[5]

The relative decrease in detection of major depression in older adults may be a function of cohort effect, prevalence of dementia, losses to suicide, or age-biased diagnostic criteria.[3] In any event, fully 50-70% of cases of major depression go undetected by PCPs. Since 15% of elderly depressives will die of suicide and more than three quarters of those who commit suicide have seen the PCP within the prior month, it is essential for the PCP to recognize depression in the aging patient.[6,7]

Stress and Strain

At first blush, it seems easy to understand why depression is so common in latter years. Aging is hard. The body becomes more vulnerable to disease and disability. Friends and relatives become ill and die. The elderly are at risk for the loss of financial security and their familiar living environments. And, in a youth-centered culture such as ours, older people are threatened with an even greater loss: the loss of respect of others. As one wag put it: "Old age ain't for sissies." So it is tempting to conclude that because life is stressful, people get depressed. But this formulation is suspect.

First, concluding that depression is a "normal" reaction to age-related difficulties is analogous to thinking that it is "normal" for someone with a gunshot wound to the abdomen to lose a liter of blood every few minutes. Just because a response may be normative doesn't mean it is not pathological. Depression is suffering, and it demands attention.

Second, the relationship between stressors and depressive outcome has always proven to be empirically tenuous. Even though most people undergo the same stressors, the majority are not depressed. One person may become suicidally depressed at the death of a spouse, while another sees it as relief for both parties from longstanding suffering. Some people are devastated by retirement—others experience it as a rebirth. Perhaps the more fitting question is, with all the hard things about getting old, why are most old people not depressed?[8]

These losses and threats constitute stressors. Stress is something external to individual and results in symptoms only when it produces strain. The vulnerability to strain is a characteristic of the host, just as different individuals have different susceptibility to the same exposure to a viral infection. Psychological resistance is a product of defense mechanisms, perceptual prejudices, and behavioral responses that are gathered under the rubric of coping. Because the range of stressors in late life is so broad, it is the person with the widest range of coping skills who will be most able to adapt; the person with a limited range of coping skills will be more vulnerable to experiencing strain, which is often manifest as depression.[9]

Recognition

Older patients in particular are often not accustomed to putting feelings into words and may instead describe, "bad nerves," or "funny feelings all over." The clinician can help by offering mood statements, such as, "You sound sad," or, "Are you feeling blue?" It is useful to pay as much attention to facial expression and tone of voice as to the content of speech.[10]

Most clinicians are familiar with the classic "neurovegetative" signs of depression: insomnia, anorexia, constipation, and diminished libido. These features become less discriminatory as people age. Sleep problems are commonplace in late life, appetite normally diminishes with age, constipation is endemic among the elderly, and few practitioners would comfortably define what constitutes abnormal libido in a 75 year-old person.

More useful than these traditional features are the melancholic symptoms listed in the DSM-IV:[11]

- Loss of pleasure (anhedonia) or loss of reactivity of mood to environmental events
- Psychomotor agitation or retardation
- Early morning wakening or midnight wakening
- Pathological guilt
- Diurnal variation (typically feeling worst in the morning and better in the afternoon or evening)
- Weight loss (> 5% over a few months or less)

These signs and symptoms may be indicative of neurotransmitter dysfunction and tend to correlate with the likelihood of antidepressant response.

Patterns of Depression

Depression is not a homogenous entity. People bring to their physicians different patterns that may be organized as depression the symptom, depression the syndrome, and depression the disease. One person may have elements of two or three patterns simultaneously.

As a *symptom*, depression may represent simple sadness, grief, mourning, or an adjustment disorder with depressed mood. Patients with this pattern come to the physician describing a subjective sense of psychological distress, linked by the patient to an identifiable loss or threat. They will typically complain of tearfulness, nervousness, pessimism, guilt, or diminished interest or energy, and they may have some melancholic features. Past history or family history of affective disorders is not remarkable in this group.

These are patients for whom the major thrust of therapy will be overcoming or adapting to loss. It helps the patient first to see the sense in a frightening situation and to know that he/she is not crazy. Such patients will often need permission to mourn, as family and others may discourage it. Education to families on this count is important, and elders need a context in which to mourn at their own pace without guilt. Such patients may also benefit from temporary symptomatic treatment with antianxiety agents or hypnotics. They typically do not need antidepressant treatment.

Patients with a depressive *syndrome* experience a general sense of dysphoria resulting from a particular characteristic vulnerability to environmental stressors. They come to clinical attention with a more chronic and pervasive disturbance of mood, affect, and behavior than those with grief or sadness; the relationship of mood to precipitant is more tenuous. The subjective sense of sadness is often lost in a cloud of negativism, anxiety, and worry. Affective disturbances may be overshadowed by fatigue, accident-proneness, or forgetfulness. Melancholic signs are not uncommon. If these signs are present, antidepressants are likely to be of help.

But these people often suffer from chronic depression because they have deficient coping capacities. Medication may relieve some of the symptoms, but leaves much of the distress. Thus, formal psychotherapy is generally necessary for optimal treatment outcome. At the least, psychiatric referral can tell the

Table 1. Risk Factors for Suicide

Sex
Age
Depression
Previous attempt(s)
Ethanol abuse
Rational thinking impairment
Social supports lacking
Organized plan
No job
Sick

PCP if medication is likely to be helpful and if psychotherapy is indicated.

Depression may present itself as a *disease*, in the form of major depression or the depressed phase of bipolar disorder. These patients come to attention with a profound sense of sadness, hopelessness, guilt, or despair, or sometimes just nameless fear or agitation. They may well be psychotic at the time of first presentation. Melancholic features are almost invariably present and are more severe than in a depressive syndrome. A credible link to any environmental precipitant is rare.

These people have a disease of the brain. They need somatic treatment for their depression. Paradoxically, they may be easier to treat in the primary care or long-term care setting than those with less severe depressions because the vulnerability of their coping mechanisms is not an issue. Consultation from a psychiatrist may help the PCP choose the best antidepressant or decide if hospitalization or electroconvulsive therapy (ECT) would be better choices. But most can be managed if recognized properly and treated aggressively.

Suicide

The assessment of geriatric depression is not complete without an evaluation of suicide risk. Rates of suicide are alarmingly high and about one in seven people with serious depression will die at his/her own hand. It is most notable that older people make relatively fewer unsuccessful suicide attempts than younger ones; thus, the clinician has fewer chances to intervene and prevent such deaths.[12]

Risk factors for suicide can be recalled with the mnemonic "SAD PERSONS" *(please see Table 1)*. Sex and age are interactive; women's risk peaks between 55 and 65 years of age, men's risk continues to rise after age 60. Rational thinking can be impaired by late-life cognitive disorders. Physical illness, social isolation, unemployment, and alcohol use are particularly strong correlates of suicide risk.[13,14]

PCPs are advised to recall the "Rules of Sevens":[12-14]

- One in **seven** recurrent depressions ends in suicide.
- **70%** of suicides suffer from major depression.
- **70%** of suicides have seen a physician (usually a PCP) within the prior six weeks.
- Suicide is the **seventh** leading cause of death in the United States.

Depression Secondary to Medical Conditions and Treatments

Particularly in the primary care setting, it is vital to consider medical conditions that may lie behind depressive symptoms. Some medical illnesses have features that resemble depression, such as the weakness and fatigue of anemia or diabetes. Other diseases, like Parkinson's disease or stroke, can alter brain chemistry in ways similar to primary depression.

Table 2 lists some of the more important medical causes of secondary depressions. Major depression occurs in 40-50% of patients with Parkinson's disease and is associated with poorer motor and cognitive function than in non-depressed Parkinson's patients.[15] At least one in four stroke victims will suffer an episode of depression.[16] Similarly, the risk of major depression in cancer patients is about 25%, particularly with metastatic visceral malignancies; an additional 25% will suffer from dysthymic disorder or adjustment disorder.[17]

Notably absent from the list of medical conditions associated with depression is menopause. The common wisdom that menopause carries with it a vulnerability to affective illness is not substantiated by empirical study. Except in the case of surgical menopause or in women with a prior history of depression, depressive illness is no more common in menopausal women than in nonmenopausal peers. When depression does appear in such women, it should be evaluated and treated as a condition warranting its own attention.[18-21]

Not only medical disorders, but also the treatments commonly prescribed to aging patients can produce depressive features *(please see Table 3)*. Since depressed elders frequently exhibit anxiety, prescription of benzodiazepines is tempting. However, these agents do not treat depression, they can exaggerate the apathy and withdrawal of depression, and their use can lead the clinician to postpone initiation of definitive antidepressant treatment. Antipsychotic medications, given to people without frank hallucinations or delusions, can produce dysphoria and other depressive features. They are often prescribed for people with dementia who do not have formal psychoses. Among the antihypertensive agents, only those with central nervous mechanisms of action are worrisome; calcium channel blockers and ACE inhibitors are not likely to harm mood or affect.[23]

Table 2. Medical Conditions Associated with Depression[22]

Central Nervous System Disorders
- Parkinson's disease
- Stroke
- Tumors

Endocrine Disorders
- Diabetes
- Thyroid

Cancer

Infections
- Common flu
- Pneumonia

Anemia

Autoimmune disorders
- Polymyalgia rheumatica
- Temporal arteritis

* Adapted from Conn DK[22]

Antidepressant Therapy

When melancholic features are present, antidepressant therapy is generally indicated. Of the major classes of antidepressants—tricyclics (TCAs), selective serotonin reuptake inhibitors (SSRIs), and newer mixed-action agents—all are approximately equally effective. About two-thirds of elders who complete a course of treatment will experience significant symptom relief from major depression. Thus, the selection of agents is generally based on tolerability and safety.[24]

Desipramine and nortriptyline cause limited pharmacodynamic or pharmacokinetic interactions with other drugs; however, they can be the target of such interactions. For example, SSRIs will increase serum levels of the TCAs.[26]

Selective Serotonin Reuptake Inhibitors. These agents are, appropriately, the mainstay of antidepressant therapy in aging individuals. They have no α-1 adrenergic affinity; except for paroxetine, they have negligible muscarinic or histaminic blockade. Notably, they do not impair cognition. Their major side effects are the products of their therapeutic mode of action (i.e., enhancement of serotonin transmission). These effects are gastrointestinal (nausea, anorexia, diarrhea), central nervous (insomnia or sedation, nervousness, dizziness, tremor, headache), and sexual (diminished libido, anorgasmia, delayed ejaculation, impotence). All these effects are dose-related. Since SSRIs have a fairly flat dose-response curve, increasing drug dose generally increases adverse effects without substantially enhancing therapeutic effects.[25,27]

Table 3. Medications Associated with Depression[23]

Psychotropic
- Benzodiazepines
- Antipsychotics

Antiparkinsonian
- L-Dopa
- Amantadine

Antihypertensive
- Propranolol
- Methyldopa
- Clonidine
- Reserpine
- Hydralazine

Other
- Steroids

Drug interactions with SSRIs are complex because of their influence on the cytochrome P450 system. Fluoxetine is the widest and most potent inhibitor of P450 isoenzymes, paroxetine is moderately problematic, and sertraline and citalopram are the narrowest and least potent P450 inhibitors.

Other Agents. Nefazodone is a weak inhibitor of serotonin reuptake but a potent antagonist at the 5-HT2 receptor. As a result, it does not produce sexual dysfunction, but often produces drowsiness—sometimes to a prohibitive extent. Other side effects may include nausea and dizziness. Nefazodone inhibits the CYP 450 3A isoenzyme, which is responsible for 50% of known oxidative drug metabolism, including its own metabolism.[25,26]

Venlafaxine is a mixed action, noradrenergic and serotonergic, antidepressant. It has no affinity for muscarinic, histaminic or α-1 adrenergic receptors. It may cause transient nausea, dizziness, nervousness, sexual dysfunction, and anorexia. Its drug interaction profile is similar to that of sertaline and citalopram.[24,26,27]

Mirtazapine has a novel mode of action, primarily blocking histamine-1 receptors (with some activity at 5HT2A, 5HT2C, 5HT3, and α-2 sites). The histamine-1 blockade produces a secondary increase in both noradrenergic and serotonergic transmission. It does not produce nausea or sexual side effects and does not alter sleep physiology. It is moderately sedating and usually causes increased appetite and weight gain. Because of its multiple loci of action, it can produce pharmacodynamic interactions with a variety of histaminergic, serotonergic, and α-adrenergic drugs. It has few pharmacokinetic (cytochrome P450) interactions.[26,28]

Bupropion is an antidepressant with mild dopaminergic activity. It is generally well tolerated, it has little anticholiner-

Table 4. Comparison of Major Antidepressants[25-29]

Drug	Significant active metabolites	Plasma half-life parent plus active	Muscarinic anticholinergic effects	Sedation	Agitation, nervousness, insomnia	Geriatric dose initial/ maximum (mg/d)
TCAs						
Desipramine	Yes	24-96 h	Moderate	Moderate	Rare	10/150
Nortriptyline	Yes	36-48 h	Moderate	Moderate	Rare	10/100
SSRIs						
Citalopram	Yes	36-90 h	None	Little/none	Rare	10/40
Fluoxetine	Yes	8-18 d	None	Little/none	Common	10/80
Paroxetine	No	30 h	Moderate	Moderate	Rare	10/40
Sertraline	No	36 h	None	Mild	Rare	25/200
Other						
Mirtazapine	No	40-60 h	None	Moderate	Rare	15/45
Nefazodone	Yes	24 h	None	Severe	None	200/600
Venlafaxine	Yes	12 h	None	Mild	Common	37.5/300

gic activity, and it causes almost no sexual dysfunction. It does have a tendency to cause seizures at doses not far above the therapeutic range and must be given in multiple doses daily. Dosing is highly variable from patient to patient. Bupropion's efficacy relative to the TCAs and SSRIs has been questioned. It may potentiate the action of co-administered dopaminergic and noradrenergic drugs, and bupropion levels can rise with concurrent administration of fluoxetine.[25,26]

Trazodone was a transitional drug between the TCAs and SSRIs. It is a weak serotonin-2A receptor antagonist. While it has a wide therapeutic index, it causes dose-dependent drowsiness, dizziness, and confusion. Its adrenergic blocking properties cause constipation and postural hypertension. The efficacy of trazodone in geriatric populations has not been widely studied. Its drug interaction profile is similar to that of nefazodone.[26]

Table 4 provides a comparison of the major antidepressants useful in older patients in primary care.

Some depressive symptoms may begin to resolve within a short while, but most will take several weeks. In the elderly, the time course of response may be even further prolonged, and full antidepressant response may not occur for as long as two months, even at full antidepressant dose. Once remission is achieved, the full dose of antidepressant should be continued for a minimum of two years (compared with 6-9 months in younger patients). While conventional wisdom may lead the practitioner to reduce the acute antidepressant dose for maintenance therapy, this practice is not generally successful and is not supported by research. At all ages, "the dose that gets you better is the dose that keeps you better."[30,31] Since the risk of relapse increases with age, and since severity of depression increases with recurrent episodes, lifetime maintenance therapy is recommended by many experts *(please see Table 5)*.[30-32]

Tricyclic Antidepressants. Most TCAs have both adrenergic and serotonergic therapeutic actions. Unfortunately, they also act at other neurotransmitter sites that contribute to their many side effects. Muscarinic anticholinergic effects include dry mouth, urinary retention, diminished visual accommodation, cognitive impairment, and tachycardia. Histaminic effects include sedation, increased appetite, and weight gain. Alpha-adrenergic blockade causes orthostatic hypotension. Additionally, all TCAs have Type I antiarrhythmic effects, which may adversely affect cardiac conduction. Most worrisome, TCAs are potentially lethal in overdose and have a much narrower ratio of toxic to therapeutic dose than most other treatment options.[24,25]

Tertiary amine TCAs (e.g., amitriptyline, imipramine) have more numerous and more intense side effects than secondary amine agents, and should rarely, if ever, be prescribed for elderly patients. Secondary amines, such as nortriptyline and desipramine, are somewhat safer and better tolerated.[25]

Electroconvulsive Therapy (ECT)

While ECT is certainly not in the armamentarium of the PCP, it remains an invaluable intervention for treatment-refrac-

Table 5. Indications for Lifetime Maintenance Antidepressant Therapy

Age 50 or older at first episode
Three or more episodes at any age
Two episodes and: • Age 40 or older • Family history of recurrent major depression • Family history of bipolar disorder • First episode before age 20 • Both episodes severe or life threatening within the prior three years

tory depression at all ages and remarkably safe and effective in late life. In primary major depression, ECT induces remission in 80-90% of patients, and its efficacy does not decrease with age. It is particularly indicated in patients who have failed to respond to, or who have been unable to tolerate, multiple antidepressants; and in those whose depression represents an imminent threat to health or survival. There is some indication that patients with delusional depression respond better to ECT than to antidepressants.[33]

Contemporary techniques of anesthesia and ECT stimulus have drastically reduced the adverse effects of cognitive impairment and damage to teeth and bones that were common several decades ago. Unilateral electrode placement is significantly less injurious to memory than bilateral placement. Adequate paralysis makes fractures and dislocations rare even in patients with severe osteoporosis.[34]

Psychotherapies

In those patients whose vulnerability to depression is based on inadequate coping mechanisms or maladaptive personality style, and in those who experience depressive symptoms in the face of major life stressors, psychotherapy is no less valuable in late life than it is in earlier adulthood. A number of modalities have proven useful in elderly patients.[35]

Psychodynamic Psychotherapy. This examines the patient's interpretation of life events and his/her defense mechanisms. Unconscious feelings or conflicts are brought to light, and more adaptive interpretations are adopted.

Cognitive Therapy. This sees depression as a result of self-defeating thinking patterns. The therapist helps the patient identify automatic thoughts that lead to feelings of hopelessness and futility. Patient and therapist test the veracity of these beliefs and undertake experimental adoption of more adaptive cognitions. Behavioral homework is a vital feature.

Interpersonal Therapy. This focuses on losses and role transitions as stressors underlying depression. The therapy helps the patient identify these effects and reformulate his/her role in the social environment.

Group Therapy. This can provide an opportunity for depressed elders to break the shell of depressive isolation. Identification with others and confrontation of self-defeating beliefs and behaviors, help the patient overcome depressive ideation and behaviors.

Family Therapy. This may be a useful adjunct to individual treatment. Families may discourage the expression of depressed feelings and may distance themselves from the depressed elder. Family stressors may be the precipitant for the depression. With identification and clarification, the family can become allies of the treating physician.

Summary

While most people negotiate the currents of late life without emotional disturbance, a large number experience the pain of depression. The PCP is often the first source of contact for them. Depression may present as a reaction to stressful developments, a pattern of maladaptive coping, or an episode of severe emotional illness. Depression can also be a secondary effect of the diseases to which the elderly are subject and to the medications they may be prescribed.

With proper recognition, the PCP can implement safe and effective treatment. The SSRIs are generally efficacious and well tolerated, and there is a range of other pharmacologic agents available. After consultation, psychotherapy may be recommended in addition to, or instead of, medication.

Usually, therapeutic outcome in older adults with depression is encouraging. By identifying the condition and implementing treatment, the physician can restore pleasure and meaning to his/her depressed patients' lives.

References

1. Banazak DA, Wills C, Collins C. Late-life depression in primary care: Where do we go from here? *J Am Osteopathic Assn* 1998;98:489-497.
2. Lepine JP, Bouchez S. Epidemiology of depression in the elderly. *Intl Clin Psychopharm* 1998;13(suppl5):7-12.
3. Beekman AT, Copeland JR, Prince MJ. Review of community prevalence of depression in later life. *Br J Psychiatry* 1999;174:307-311.
4. Birrer RB. Depression and aging too often do mix. *Postgrad Med* 1998;104:143-149.
5. Unutzer J, Katon W, Sullivan M, Miranda J. Treating depressed older adults in primary care: Narrowing the gap between efficacy and effectiveness. *Milbank Quarterly* 1999;77:225-256.
6. Ruggles DJ. Depression in the elderly: A review. *J Am Acad Nurse Practitioners* 1998;10:503-507.
7. Schwenck TL, Klinkman MS, Coyne JC. Depression in the family physician's office: What the psychiatrist needs to know—the Michigan depression project. *J Clin Psychiatry* 1998;59(suppl20):94-100.
8. Bienenfeld D. Psychology of aging. In: Bienenfeld D, ed. *Verwoerdt's Clinical Geropsychiatry*. 3rd ed. Baltimore, Md: Williams and Wilkins; 1990:26-44.
9. Vaillant GE, Vaillant CO. Natural history of male psychological

health, XII: A 45-year study of predictors of successful aging at age 65. *Am J Psychiatry* 1990;147:31-37.

10. Silver IL, Herrmann N. Comprehensive psychiatric evaluation. In: Sadavoy J, Lazarus LW, Jarvik LF, Grossberg GT, eds. *Comprehensive Review of Geriatric Psychiatry—II*. Washington, London: American Psychiatric Press; 1996: 223-250.
11. American Psychiatric Association. *Diagnostic and Statistical Manual of Mental Disorders*. 4th ed. Washington, DC: American Psychiatric Association; 1994:383-384.
12. Merrill J, Owens J. Age and attempted suicide. *Acta Psychiatrica Scand* 1990;82:385-388.
13. Hawton K, Fagg J. Deliberate self-poisoning and self-injury in older people. *Int J Ger Psychiatry* 1990;5:367-373.
14. Nowers M. Deliberate self-harm in the elderly: A survey of one London borough. *Int J Ger Psychiatry* 1993;8:609-614.
15. Evans DL, Staab JP, Petit JM, et al. Depression in the medical setting: Biopsychological interactions and treatment considerations. *J Clin Psychiatry* 1999;60(suppl 4):40-55.
16. Robinson RG, Starr LB, Price TR. A two-year longitudinal study of mood disorders following stroke: Prevalence and duration at six-month follow-up. *Br J Psychiatry* 1984;144:256-262.
17. McDaniel JS, Musselman DL, Porter MR, et al. Depression in patients with cancer: Diagnosis, biology, and treatment. *Arch Gen Psychiatry* 1995;52:89-99.
18. Nicol-Smith L. Causality, menopause and depression: A critical review of the literature. *BMJ* 1996;313:1229-1232.
19. Pearce MJ, Hawton K. Psychological and sexual aspects of the menopause and HRT. *Baillieres Clin Obstet Gynaecol* 1996;10: 385-399.
20. Dennerstein L. Well-being, symptoms and the menopausal transition. *Maturitas* 1996;23:147-157.
21. Depressive symptoms in the perimenopause: Prevalence, assessment, and guidelines for treatment. *Harvard Rev Psychiatry* 1998;6:121-132.
22. Conn DK. Other dementias and mental disorders due to general medical conditions. In: Sadavoy J, Lazarus LW, Jarvik LF, Grossberg GT, eds. *Comprehensive Review of Geriatric Psychiatry—II*. Washington, London: American Psychiatric Press; 1996:497-528.
23. Depression Guideline Panel. *Depression in Primary Care: Vol. 1. Detection and Diagnosis*. Rockville Md: U.S. Department of Health and Human Services, Public Health Service, Agency for Health Care Policy and Research; 1993:67-71.
24. Roose SP, Suthers KM. Antidepressant response in late-life depression. *J Clin Psychiatry* 1998;59(suppl 10):4-8.
25. Flint AJ. Choosing appropriate antidepressant therapy in the elderly. *Drugs Aging* 1998;13:269-280.
26. Preskorn SH. Outpatient Management of Depression: A Guide for the Primary-Care Practitioner. 2nd ed. Caddo Okla: Professional Communications; 1999.
27. Montgomery SA. Efficacy and safety of the selective serotonin reuptake inhibitors in treating depression in elderly patients. *Internat Clin Psychopharmacol* 1998;13(suppl 5):49-54.
28. Baumann P. Care of depression in the elderly: Comparative pharmacokinetics of SSRIs. *Internat Clin Psychopharmacol* 1998;13(suppl 5):35-43.
29. Davis KM, Mathew E. Pharmacologic management of depression in the elderly. *Nurse Pract* 1998;23:16-28.
30. Montano CB. Primary care issues related to the treatment of depression in elderly patients. *J Clin Psychiatry* 1999;60 (suppl 20):45-51.
31. Greden JF. Antidepressant medication: When to discontinue and how to stop. *J Clin Psychiatry* 1993;54 (suppl):39-45.
32. Depression Guideline Panel. *Depression in Primary Care: Vol. 2. Treatment of Major Depression*. Rockville Md: U.S. Department of Health and Human Services, Public Health Service, Agency for Health Care Policy and Research; 1993:110-112.
33. Fink M. Who should get ECT? In: Coffey EC, ed. *The Clinical Science of Electroconvulsive Therapy*. Washington, London: American Psychiatric Press; 1993:3-16.
34. Beyer JL, Weiner RD, Glenn MD. *Electroconvulsive Therapy: A Programmed Text*. 2nd ed. Washington, London: American Psychiatric Press; 1993:17-24.
35. Wheeler BG, Bienenfeld D. Principles of individual psychotherapy. In: Bienenfeld D, ed. *Verwoerdt's Clinical Geropsychiatry*. 3rd ed. Baltimore, Md: Williams and Wilkins; 1990:204-222.

Hypertension in the Elderly

Norman M. Kaplan, MD

Hypertension is present in more than 50% of people older than age 65. Almost two-thirds of the hypertension in those older than age 65 is purely or predominantly systolic in nature, reflecting the progressive atherosclerosis of large capacitance vessels, which amplify the pulse wave velocity and produce an early return of pulse wave reflection in systole. Care is needed in making the diagnosis, preferably with multiple out-of-the-office blood pressure (BP) measurements. In addition, postural hypotension frequently accompanies systolic hypertension and, if present, must be managed before treatment of the hypertension.

Treatment of isolated systolic hypertension (ISH) in the elderly provides, in the short term, even greater protection against the various hypertension-induced morbidities and mortalities than does treatment of younger hypertensives. Six major randomized controlled trials have documented the benefits of therapy of the elderly. All but the most recent were diuretic-based, and it should be noted that β–blocker-based therapy has not been shown to benefit the elderly. On the basis of these trials, JNC-6 recommends a diuretic as the preferred treatment of ISH but adds a long-acting dihydropyridine as an appropriate alternative. Other drugs may be useful, including α-blockers for those elderly men with prostatism. In the Swedish Trial in Old Patients-2 study, small doses of an ACE inhibitor provided equal benefit against cardiovascular mortality as did conventional therapy (diuretic, β-blockers or both) or low doses of a calcium channel blocker.

In the enthusiasm to apply these major benefits of therapy to the large population of vulnerable elderly hypertensives, sight should not be lost of the well-described antihypertensive efficacy of multiple lifestyle modifications and of the multiple potential hazards of indiscriminate therapy.

By appropriate use of non-drug and drug therapies, the elderly hypertensive can be protected, sometimes against death but to an even greater degree against debilitating morbidities, surely justifying their therapy.

The Scope of the Problem

The most rapidly expanding part of the population in the United States and other developed societies is the elderly, defined as age 65 or older. Projections estimate that more than 20% of the U.S. population will be older than 65 by the year 2030 with almost 1 million being older than age 100.[1] The provision of health care for this large group of elderly people will cost a great amount. From the age of 65 until

Figure 1. Mean Systolic and Diastolic Blood Pressures by Age and Race or Ethnicity for Men and Women 18 Years of Age and Older in the U.S. Population

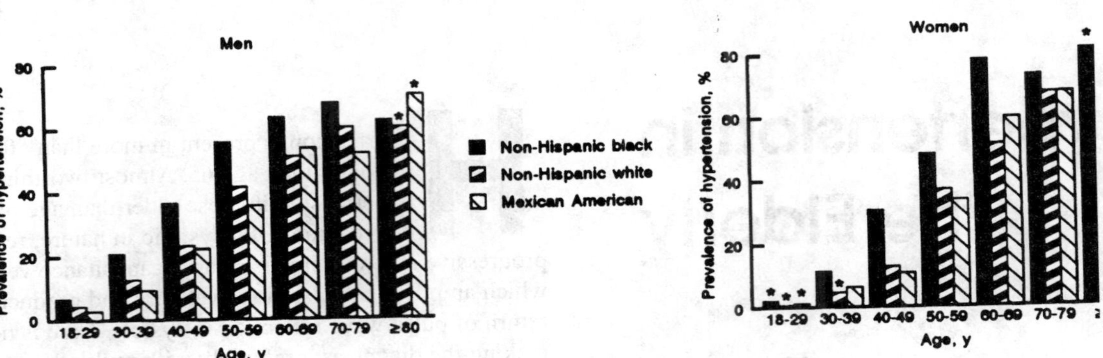

Thick solid line, non-Hispanic whites; thin solid line, Mexican-Americans. Data from the NHANES III Survey. (Reprinted with permission from Burt VL, Whelton P, Roccella EJ, et al. Prevalence of hypertension in the U.S. adult population. Results from the Third National Health and Nutrition Examination Survey, 1988-1991. *Hypertension* 1995;25:303-313.)

death, the cumulative cost of health care is estimated to average $150,000 per person who dies at age 75; $250,000 per person dying at age 90; and $400,000 per person dying at age 100.[1] Much of the increased costs will be consumed by nursing home care, which as will be noted, could be reduced by effective treatment of hypertension.

The Burden of Hypertension. As the population ages, the incidence of hypertension progressively rises *(please see Figure 1)*. By age 65, the majority of people will be hypertensive—the prevalence reaching almost 80% among African-American women. Most of this hypertension is predominantly or purely systolic in nature, reflecting the progressive rise in systolic pressure with age, accompanied by the usual fall in diastolic pressure with age, accompanied by the usual fall in diastolic pressure *(please see Figure 2)*. In the Framingham cohort, almost two-thirds of the hypertension seen among those older than age 65 was ISH.[2]

The Changing Pattern of Blood Pressure

The progressive rise in systolic blood pressure and the usual fall in diastolic pressure noted in Figure 2 is a reflection of the arteriosclerotic and atherosclerotic rigidity of the large capacitance arteries (aorta and major branches) that is almost invariable in people living in developed societies. Thereby the difference between the systolic and diastolic levels, the pulse pressure, progressively widens and, as will be noted, becomes the best prognostic indicator for cardiovascular risk.

As Izzo and colleagues describe:[3] "Age-related changes in BP are manifestations of a generalized process of increasing arterial stiffness (or decreasing compliance) that results from the progressive replacement of elastin by collagen in the walls of large arteries. This process of diffuse arteriosclerosis leads to dilation and lengthening of the aorta and its immediate branches through fibrosis and hypertrophy of the arterial muscularis. Arteriosclerosis inevitably accompanies aging in Western societies, but its development is clearly accelerated by the presence of hypertension and the age at which it is expressed varies with the degree of BP elevation.

"Arteriosclerosis can be differentiated pathophysiologically from atherosclerosis, which is primarily related to the effects of abnormal cholesterol oxidation and deposition in the inner layers of large arteries. Atherosclerosis begins as endothelial dysfunction and macrophage uptake of oxidized lipids into the vessel walls and is accelerated by the coexistence of hypertension."

In addition to the higher pressure developing within marrowed capacitance arteries, the arterial rigidity adds another mechanism that Weisfeldt has nicely described:[4]

"As aging stiffens the central aorta, the left ventricle continues to eject the same amount of blood at the same rate into the aorta. As a result, the velocity of movement of blood down the arterial system accelerates with age. This acceleration in pulse wave velocity extends down the entire arterial tree. When the pulse wave reaches the iliac bifurcation, it is reflected and transmitted back toward the aorta. Moreover, like the forward transmission, the backward transmission wave is also accelerated.

"In the young (20-year-old) aorta, the rate of transmission forward and backward is slow enough so that systole has been completed by the time the reflected wave returns to the heart. This has the effect of raising aortic diastolic pressure after the aortic valve has closed. This does not increase cardiac work and tends to maintain aortic blood pressure during diastole…In the elderly (80-year-old), the reflected wave returns well before the aortic valve shuts. This elevates systolic left ventricular and arterial blood pressure increasing the

Table 1. Nonpharmacological and Pharmacological Measures in the Management of Postural Hypotension Due to Neurogenic Failure

Nonpharmacological Measures

To Be Avoided

- Sudden head-up postural change (especially on walking)
- Prolonged recumbency
- Straining during micturition and defecation
- High environmental temperature (including hot baths)
- Large meals (especially with refined carbohydrates)
- Alcohol
- Drugs with vasodepressor properties

To Be Introduced

- Arise slowly
- Head-up tilt during sleep
- Small, frequent meals
- 16 oz of water before arising
- Isometric exercise before arising

To Be Considered

- Elastic stockings
- Abdominal binders

Pharmacological Measures

- Starter drug—Fludrocortisone
- Sympathomimetics—Ephedrine, Midodrine
- Specific targeting—Octreotide, Desmopressin, Erythropoietin

Adapted from: Mathias C, Kimber J. *Annu Rev Med* 1999;50:317-336.

work of the left ventricle in ejecting blood. This reflected wave has the additional effect in the elderly of decreasing the diastolic aortic pressure that supports coronary flow. Clearly, this is a potentially important hemodynamic change and may have significant implications for the choice of antihypertensive strategy."

The Implications of Blood Pressure

Since the widening pulse pressure typically seen with aging reflects the arterio- and atherosclerotic changes occurring within the vasculature, it comes as no surprise that this measure is the best predictor of the risk for vascular diseases that are mainly induced by arterio- and atherosclerosis. As Kannel notes, for many years, until the 1970s, most attention was directed to the diastolic blood pressure, both to diagnose hypertension and to monitor therapy.[2] Starting in the 1970s and accelerating through the 1980s, there was increasing awareness of the even greater influence of systolic levels. More recently, particularly as more data involved the elderly population, the pulse pressure, reflecting the separate contributions of both the rising systolic and the falling diastolic levels, has been clearly found to be even more accurately predictive of future cardiovascular diseases including coronary, cerebrovascular, and renal diseases as well as congestive heart failure.[5] However, as Izzo et al note:[3]

"Pulse pressure, although slightly more robust than systolic BP as a risk indicator, is considerably less straightforward to use clinically than systolic BP, and it has not yet been validated as a surrogate end point for morbidity or mortality in a prospective randomized clinical trial."

Therefore, systolic BP will remain the major focus of concern in the elderly with the caveat that too low a diastolic pressure may also deserve attention, as will be described.

Postural Hypotension

Often accompanying the vascular rigidity that leads to a rising systolic and falling diastolic pressure, there is with age a progressive loss of sensitivity of the baroreceptor reflexes that are largely responsible for the maintenance of a normal BP despite changes in posture and activity.[6] As many as 30% of elderly people with systolic hypertension will have a fall of 20 mmHg or more in systolic pressure when they stand (i.e., postural hypotension).[7] As a consequence, symptoms of cerebral hyperfusion may occur leading to falls and subsequent trauma. The falls in pressure when standing are usually most pronounced upon arising in the morning when syspurthelic nervous activity must immediately rise from the low levels induced by supine sleeping. In some, sylanchnic pooling of blood after meals may also lead to hypotension.

Recognition of the Problem. All elderly and diabetic patients should be asked about symptoms that could connote postural and post-proudial hypotension. Their examination should always include careful measurement of, first, BP after five minutes supine and then repeated measurements immediately and after two minutes of standing. If necessary, the patient can hold on to the table but must bear their weight on their upright body. If a reading is not taken immediately upon standing, a rapid and significant postural fall may be missed since the reflex may still be active but slow.[8]

Management. If the systolic falls more than 20 mmHg, corrective measures should be taken before treatment of the seated/supine hypertension is attempted; otherwise, the postural symptoms will likely be aggravated by whatever antihypertensive therapy that is used. The helpful maneuvers are listed in Table 1. Since the greatest fall in BP usually occurs upon arising, it is helpful to raise the head of the bed by 12-15°, maintaining sympathetic nervous system activity through the night so the change upon arising is not so abrupt. Before standing, the patient should do 3-5 isometric exercises such as tightly squeezing a tennis ball—raising the BP by 30-40 mmHg. If these maneuvers aren't enough, drinking 16 oz of water before

Figure 2. Prevalence of High Blood Pressure by Age and Race or Ethnicity for Men and Women 18 Years of Age and Older in the U.S. Population

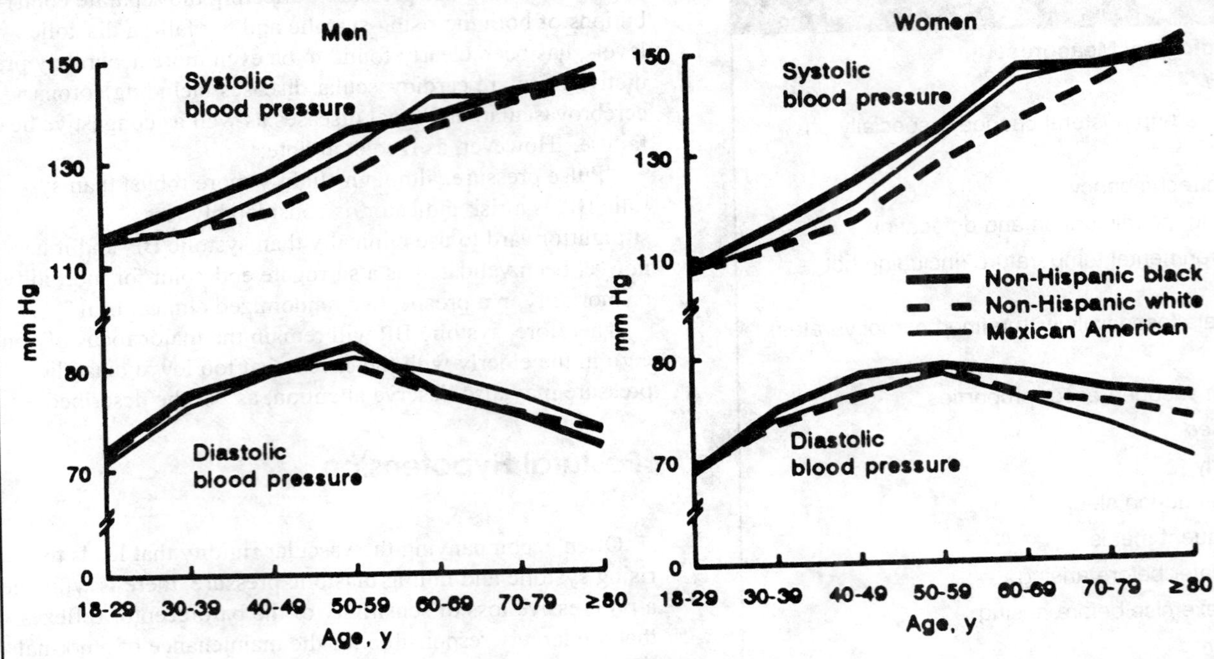

Solid bars, non-Hispanic black; heavy cross-hatching, non-Hispanic white; light cross-hatching, Mexican-American; estimate based on a sample size that did not meet the minimum requirements of the NHANES III design or relative systolic ejection murmur of more than 30%. Data from NHANES III. (Reprinted with permission from: Burt VL, Whelton P, Roccella EJ, et al. Prevalence of hypertension in the U.S. adult population. Results from the Third National Health and Nutrition Examination Survey, 1988-1991. *Hypertension* 1995;25:303-313.)

standing has been found to raise systolic BP by 30-40 mmHg in patients with significant autonomic insufficiency.[9]

Lifestyle Modifications

Once postural hypotension, if present, is managed, the systolic hypertension should be treated, first with lifestyle changes and then, if needed, with one or more antihypertensive drugs.

The lifestyle changes universally recommended are listed in Table 2. Some of these are even more useful in the elderly: The response to sodium reduction is greater, and the effect of smoking cessation may be profound with an immediate decrease in BP and improvement to cerebral blood flow.

The best documentation of the benefits of both sodium reduction and weight loss in the elderly comes from the large and long Trial of Nonpharmacologic Interventions in the Elderly (TONE).[10] In this trial, 975 elderly hypertensives who were being well controlled on medication had their medications stopped. They were then randomly placed on one of four regimens: sodium reduced diet; weight loss by caloric restriction and exercise; both sodium reduction and weight loss; or no change in either (i.e., usual care). They were then carefully monitored for the return of hypertension while remaining on no antihypertensive medication for 30 months.

As seen in Figure 3, the results were impressive. Even though the average amount of sodium reduction (40 mm/d) and weight loss (10 lbs) was relatively small, their effect was significant. Whereas only 16% of those on usual care

Table 2. Lifestyle Modifications for Hypertension Prevention and Management

- Lose weight if overweight
- Limit alcohol intake
- Increase aerobic physical activity (30-45 minutes most days of the week)
- Reduce sodium intake to no more than 100 mmoL/d (2.4 g of sodium or 6 g of sodium chloride)
- Maintain adequate intake of dietary calcium and magnesium
- Stop smoking and reduce intake of dietary saturated fat and cholesterol

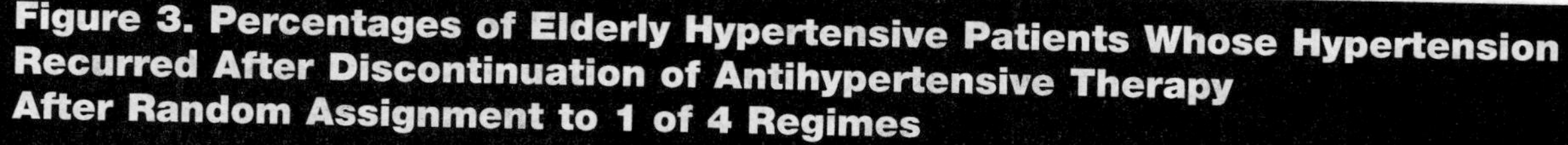

Figure 3. Percentages of Elderly Hypertensive Patients Whose Hypertension Recurred After Discontinuation of Antihypertensive Therapy After Random Assignment to 1 of 4 Regimes

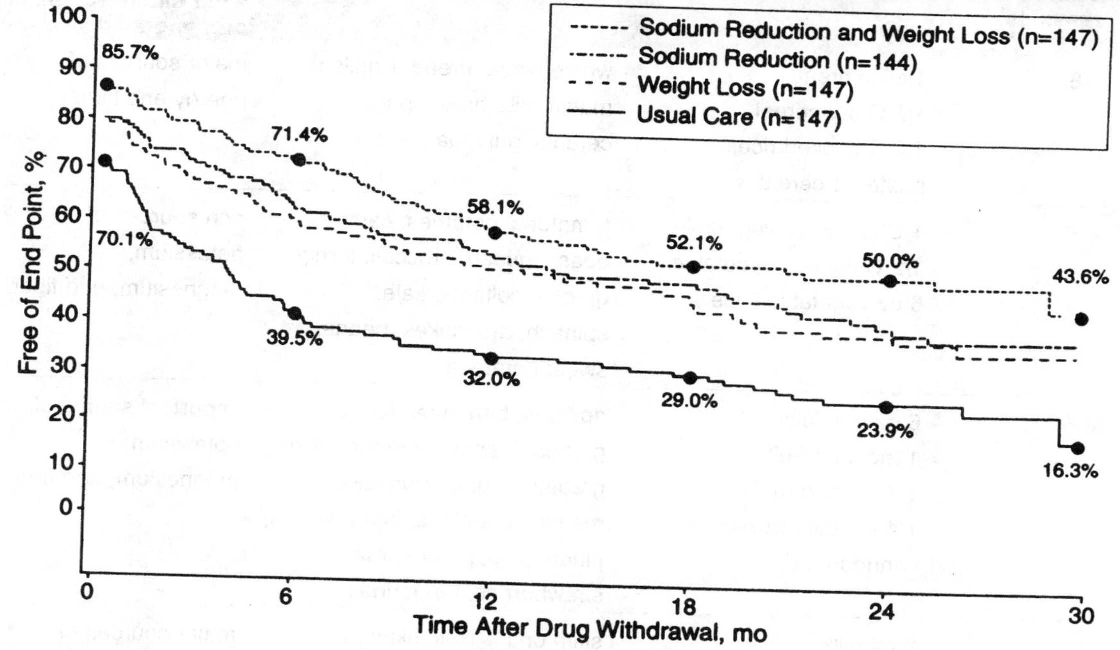

Reprinted with permission from: Whelton P, Appel L, Espeland M, et al. Sodium reduction and weight loss in the treatment of hypertension in older persons. *JAMA* 1998;279:839-846.

remained normotensive on no drugs over 30 months, twice as many of those on either lifestyle regimen and three times as many on both remained normotensive.

These data are strong affirmations of the major benefits to be derived from even relatively small degrees of sodium reduction and weight loss. Though not separately evaluated, regular aerobic and resistance exercise can be equally effective, not only in lowering BP but also in reducing glucose intolerance and dyslipidemia.[11]

Moderation of alcohol consumption is also important. Those who drink more than two portions per day (a portion equals 1.5 oz of spirits, 4 oz of wine, or 12 oz of beer) should be strongly advised to cut back to no more than two per day both to reduce BP and to remove other dangers of excess alcohol. However, regular daily drinking of as little as one-half to two portions per day clearly provides protection against myocardial infarction, stroke, and overall mortality.[12]

Consumption of a diet rich in fresh fruits and vegetables and low in saturated fat can also lower BP while reducing other cardiovascular risks.[13] The DASH diet is also relatively low in sodium (130 mm/d), and further benefit has been noted when additional sodium reduction is added to this diet (*see Table 3*).

Antihypertensive Drug Therapy

If lifestyle changes are not enough to lower systolic BP to below 160 mmHg, antihypertensive drug therapy should be given. Whether to give drugs to the large group of elderly people with "borderline" systolic hypertension (i.e., levels between 140 and 160 mmHg), remains an open issue. Most recent guidelines from expert committees recommend drug therapy for those with systolic levels above 140 mmHg if they are at high risk because of the coexistence of diabetes, renal insufficiency, or congestive heart failure.[14-17] However, absent data from randomized controlled trials (RCTs) in relatively low-risk elderly patients with systolic levels below 160 mmHg, there is generally hesitation in treating such patients. Trials now in progress should soon provide evidence of the wisdom of treating such patients.

Selection of Initial Therapy. All of these expert committee guidelines agree on the choices of initial drug therapy for elderly patients with ISH: a low dose of a long reacting diuretic or dihydropyridine calcium channel blocker (DHP-CCB) (*please see Table 4*). The "compelling" indications shown in the World Health Organization-International Society of Hypertension (WHO-ISH) guideline[15] shown in Table 4 are in agreement with those from the U.S. Joint National Committee[14] and other recent guidelines.[16,17]

The choice of a low-dose diuretic or a DHP-CCB is based on data from the RCTs that have been nicely summarized by Staessen et al[18] (*please see Figure 4*). In this meta-analysis of all eight published outcome trials in the elderly with ISH, involving 15,693 patients who were followed up for an aver-

Table 3. The DASH Diet

FOOD GROUP	DAILY SERVINGS	SERVING SIZES	EXAMPLES AND NOTES	SIGNIFICANCE OF EACH FOOD GROUP TO THE DASH DIET PROGRAM
Grains and grain potatoes	7-8	1 slice bread 1/2 C dry cereal 1/2 C cooked rice, pasta, or cereal	whole wheat bread, English muffin, pita bread, bagel, cereals, grits, oatmeal	major sources of energy and fiber
Vegetables	4-5	1 C raw leafy vegetable 1/2 C cooked vegetable 6 oz vegetable juice	tomatoes, potatoes, carrots, peas, squash, broccoli, turnip greens, collards, kale, spinach, artichokes, beans, sweet potatoes	rich sources of potassium, magnesium, and fiber
Fruits	4-5	6 oz fruit juice 1 medium fruit 1/4 C dried fruit 1/4 C fresh, frozen, or canned fruit	apricots, bananas, dates, grapes, oranges, orange juice, grapefruit, grapefruit juice, mangoes, melons, peaches, pineapples, prunes, raisins, strawberries, tangerines	important source of potassium, magnesium, and fiber
Low-fat or nonfat dairy foods	2-3	8 oz milk 1 C yogurt 1.5 oz cheese	skim or 1% milk, skim or lowfat buttermilk, nonfat or lowfat yogurt, part-skim mozzarella cheese, nonfat cheese	major sources of protein
Meats, poultry, and fish	2 or less	3 oz cooked meats, poultry, or fish	select only lean; trim away visible fats; broil, roast, or boil, instead of frying; remove skin from poultry	rich sources of protein and magnesium
Nuts, seeds, and legumes	4-5 per week	1/5 oz or 1/3 C nuts 1/2 oz or 2 Tbsp seeds 1/2 C cooked legumes	almonds, filbers, mixed nuts, peanuts, walnuts, sunflower seeds, kidney beans, lentils	rich sources of energy, magnesium, potassium, protein, and fiber

age of 3.8 years, active treatment (either diuretic-based or DHP-CCB based) reduced total mortality by 13%, cardiovascular mortality by 18%, all cardiovascular events by 26%, stroke by 30%, and coronary events by 23%. Staessen et al calculated the number of elderly ISH patients who would need to be treated for five years to prevent a fatal or nonfatal event: 26 for any cardiovascular event, 48 for a stroke, and 64 for a heart attack. The number needed to treat was lower in men older than age 70 and in those who had survived a previous cardiovascular complication.

Patients Older Than Age 80. The benefits of antihypertensive drug therapy have been shown to extend to those older than age 80. In a subgroup meta-analysis of the 1670 participants in the RCTs who were 80 years or older, treatment was shown to prevent 34% of strokes, 22% of major cardiovascular events, and 39% of heart failure.[19] As noted in Figure 4, in all RCTs of patients older than age 60 with ISH, total mortality was reduced much less than was morbidity—not surprising since it is likely that no medical intervention can prolong the duration of life to a significant degree in older people. However, the reduction of morbidity that makes life so difficult for the elderly provides more than enough rationale for the use of appropriate antihypertensive therapy.

In the Syst-Eur trial involving active treatment with the DHP-CCB nitrendipine, the incidence of dementia was reduced by 50%, from 7.7 in those on placebo to 3.8 cases

Table 4. Guidelines for Selecting Drug Treatment of Hypertension

CLASS OF DRUG	COMPELLING INDICATIONS	POSSIBLE INDICATIONS	COMPELLING CONTRAINDICATIONS	POSSIBLE CONTRAINDICATIONS
Diuretics	Heart failure Elderly patients Systolic hypertension	Diabetes	Gout	Dyslipidemia Sexually active males
β-blockers	Angina After myocardial infarct Tachyarrhythmias	Heart failure Pregnancy Diabetes	Asthma, COPD Heart block*	Dyslipidemia Athletes and physically active patients Peripheral vascular disease
ACE inhibitors	Heart failure Left venticular dysfunction After myocardial infarct Diabetic nephropathy		Pregnancy Hyperkalaemia Bilateral renal artery stenosis	
Calcium antagonists	Angina Elderly patients Systolic hypertension	Peripheral vascular disease	Heart block†	Congestive heart failure‡
α-blockers	Prostatic hypertrophy	Glucose intolerance Dyslipidemia		Orthostatic hypotension
Angiotensin II antagonists	ACE inhibitor cough	Heart failure	Pregnancy Bilateral renal artery stenosis Hyperkalemia	

* Grade 2 or 3 atrioventricular block

† Grade 2 or 3 atrioventricular block with verapamil or diltiazem

‡ Verapamil or diltiazem. Angiotensin converting enzyme (ACE)

per 1000 patient-years in those on treatment.[20] Whether such protection can accompany other forms of antihypertensive therapy is not known since no other published data on the incidence of dementia have appeared.

Other Drugs. As noted in Table 4, elderly patients with other coexisting diseases should be provided appropriate therapy. Examples include: β-blockers for those with coronary disease, particularly if they have survived a myocardial infarction; ACE inhibitors for those with heart failure or diabetic nephropathy; α-blockers for those with prostatism.

On the other hand, β-blockers alone have not provided primary protection against coronary disease in the elderly.[21] Moreover, in the patients enrolled in the Antihypertensive and Lipid Lowering (ALLHAT) trial, the α-blocker doxazosin did not protect against the development of heart failure as well as did the diuretic chlorthalidone, leading to discontinuation of that portion of the ALLHAT trial.[22] Nonetheless, both β-blockers and α-blockers should be used if they are otherwise indicated, but not as primary choices for the broader range of ISH patients.

The Place for ACE Inhibitors. ACE inhibitors may turn out to be an appropriate choice for more elderly patients than those shown in Table 4. In a large, nonplacebo RCT of three different drug therapies in 6614 patients aged 70-84 years with combined systolic and diastolic hypertension (BP > 180/105 mmHg), those on an ACE inhibitor did as well as those on conventional therapy (diuretic + beta-blocker or a DHP-CCB).[23] The ACE inhibitor-treated third had fewer heart attacks and episodes of heart failure than the CCB-treated third.

Moreover, half of the 9297 high-risk patients older than age 55 with vascular disease or diabetes plus one other cardiovascular risk factor who were enrolled in the Heart Outcomes Prevention Evaluation (HOPE) study and received the ACE inhibitor ramipril did significantly better than the half who did not receive the ACE inhibitor.[24] These patients, most with hypertension, many with diabetes, had little additional fall in BP (2-3 mmHg) beyond that provided by their other therapies to which the ACE inhibitor was added.

Figure 4. Summarized Results in 15,693 Older Patients with Isolated Systolic Hypertension Enrolled in Eight Trials of Antihypertensive Therapy

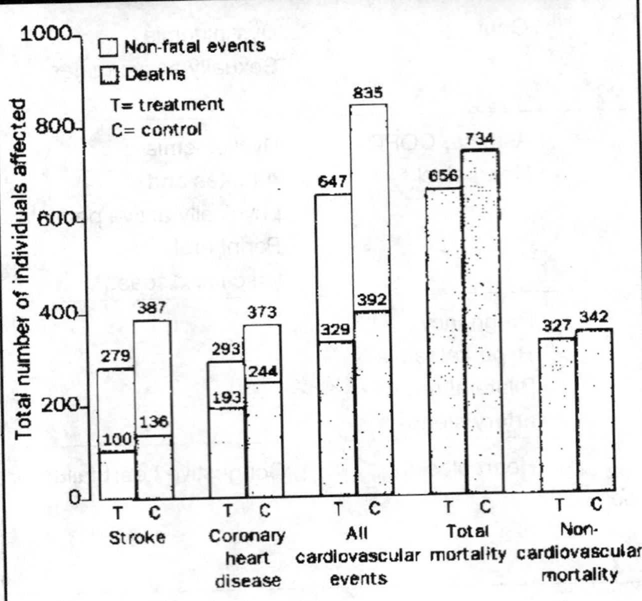

T = treated; C= control.

Reprinted with permission from: Staessen JA, Gasowski J, Wang JG, et al. Risks of untreated and treated isolated systolic hypertension in the elderly: Meta-analysis of outcome trials. Lancet 2000;355:865-872.

Table 5. Guidelines in Treating Hypertension in the Elderly

- Check for postural and postprandial hypotension before starting
- Choose drugs that will help other concomitant conditions
- Start with small doses, titrating gradually
- Use longer acting, once-daily formulations
- Avoid drug interactions, particularly from over-the-counter medications (e.g., NSAIDs)
- Look for subtle drug-induced adverse effects (e.g., weakness, dizziness, depression, confusion)
- Monitor home BPs to avoid over and under treatment
- Aim for the goal of SBP = 140-145, DBP = 80-85

Therefore, the significant additional benefits of the ACE inhibitor have been attributed to additional effects beyond the antihypertensive effect.

These additional benefits of ACE inhibitors may or may not apply to the rapidly expanding group of angiotensen II—receptor blockers (ARBs). All of the expert committee guidelines[14-17] recommend that they be used only in those in whom an ACE inhibitor is needed but who cannot tolerate that drug, usually because of cough, since there are no outcome data on their use in hypertension. The only currently available head-to-head comparison of an ACE inhibitor (captopril) against an ARB (losartan), performed in 3152 patients aged 60 years or older with class II-IV heart failure, confirms the wisdom of this recommendation: Those on the ACE inhibitor did better than did those on the ARB.[25]

Effects on Pulse Pressure. As previously noted, cardiovascular risk in the elderly reflects both the rise in systolic pressure and the fall in diastolic pressure—both reflections of atherosclerotic rigidity of large arteries. Therefore, not surprisingly, the wide pulse pressure that combines the two altered levels of BP adds even more prognostic certainty than either BP level alone.[26] In the last few years, as the importance of wide pulse pressure has been recognized, interest has risen on the effects of various antihypertensive therapies on pulse pressure in addition to their effects on systolic hypertension alone.

In all of the studies of elderly patients with ISH, a greater antihypertensive effect has been noted on the elevated systolic levels than on the already low diastolic levels. For example, in the Systolic Hypertension in the Elderly Program (SHEP) trial, the average reductions provided by the diuretic-based therapy were 25 mmHg and 9 mmHg, respectively: 170 mmHg systolic reduced to 145, 77 mmHg diastolic reduced to 68.[27] In the Syst-Eur trial wherein the average pretreatment BPs were 174/85 mmHg, the effects of CCB-based therapy were on average a 23 mmHg fall in systolic and a 7 mmHg fall in diastolic levels.[28]

In the only currently completed comparative trial of representative drug from each major class, the VA Cooperative Study involving 1292 men with an average pretreatment BP of 152/99, only those given a diuretic had a reduction in pulse pressure after one year of therapy, whereas the pulse pressure rose in those on the other classes of antihypertensive agents.[29] These data, though suggestive, are not definitive and may not even apply to the elderly with ISH.

On the other hand, limited experience with nitrate therapy, specifically isosobide mononitrate, has shown a somewhat more selective fall in systolic levels than in diastolic levels, presumably reflecting a greater reduction in arterial rigidity than that provided by other drugs.[30] No large-scale trials are currently available but one or another agent that reduces vascular rigidity by providing nitric oxide may turn out to be particularly useful in the elderly.

The Potential Danger of Reductions in Diastolic Pressure. The desire to reduce only the elevated systolic pressures and not to reduce the already low diastolic pressures further comes both from observational data on the additional risks seen with naturally low diastolics[3,4] and from data in patients whose diastolics were lowered by antihypertensive therapy.[27,31] Among the patients enrolled in the SHEP trial who received diuretic-based therapy, a higher rate of cardiovascular events (mainly strokes) was seen in those whose diastolics were lowered by 5 mmHg or more than in those whose diastolics were lowered less.[27] In a prospective population cohort study of 2351 elderly hypertensives (average BP of 157/80 mmHg), there was a significant increase in the risk of stroke in those whose diastolic pressure was reduced to below 65 mmHg by antihypertensive therapy.[31]

Therefore, caution is advised in the treatment of ISH in the elderly: If the already low diastolic pressures are inadvertently reduced to below 65 mmHg, therapy should be slowed or reduced. It should be noted that even with the apparent added risk of those whose diastolics fell in the SHEP trial, those treated did better than did those whose systolic hypertension was not treated (i.e., left on placebo). The need for treatment of ISH remains unequivocal. However, caution is advised not to lower diastolic levels too much to avoid the "J-curve" seen with significant reductions in pressure.

The Special Needs of Diabetic Hypertensives. At any age, the coexistence of diabetes with hypertension markedly increases cardiovascular risk. The elderly, including those with ISH, share this increased risk. Therefore, there is a need to treat them more intensively to levels of BP considerably lower (i.e., to below 130/80), than recommended for nondiabetic patients.[14] The need for this more intensive therapy was shown in the massive Hypertension Optimal Treatment (HOT) trial.[32] Among the 1501 diabetic hypertensives, those whose diastolic pressures were reduced the most (average, 81 mmHg) had half as many major cardiovascular events as did those whose pressures were reduced the least (average, 85 mmHg).

The HOT trial used the DHP-CCB felodipine as baseline therapy, but many patients also needed additional therapies of an ACE inhibitor (41%), β-blocker (28%), or diuretic (22%). On the basis of considerable data documenting the special benefits of ACE inhibitors in diabetics along with the strong evidence of the benefits of ramapril in the 3577 diabetics enrolled in the HOPE trial,[33] an ACE inhibitor ought to almost always be the initial drug used in a diabetic hypertensive. If, as is likely, more therapy is needed, a diuretic and then a DHP-CCB would be logical additions since they provided excellent protection in the SHEP and Syst-Eur trials.[34] Beta-blockers may also be considered since in the United Kingdom Prospective Diabetes Study (UKPDS), atenolol did somewhat better than did captopril in reducing cardiovascular events in 1200 diabetic hypertensives over a nine-year follow-up.[35]

However the BP is lowered, a goal of well below 140/90 mmHg should be sought in diabetic hypertensives, particularly if diabetic nephropathy is present. When more intensive antihypertensive therapy, along with more intensive control of diabetes and dyslipidemia, was provided to such patients, the incidences of progressive renal, neurological, and retinal disease were markedly reduced.[36] Therefore, as difficult and costly as it may be, intensive management of these high-risk patients is clearly needed.

Summary

Table 5 lists appropriate guidelines for the treatment of hypertension in the elderly. Such patients may pose multiple barriers to effective control but, with caution and persistence, they should benefit from currently available management.

References

1. Spillman B, Lubitz J. The effect of longevity on spending for acute and long-term care. *N Engl J Med* 2000;342:1409-1415.
2. Kannel W. Elevated systolic blood pressure as a cardiovascular risk factor. *Am J Cardiol* 2000;85:251-255.
3. Izzo J, Levy D, Black H. Importance of systolic blood pressure in older Americans. *Hypertension* 2000;35:1021-1024.
4. Weisfeldt Myron. Aging, changes in the cardiovascular system, and responses to stress. *Am J Hypertens* 1988;11:41S-45S.
5. Franklin S. Is there a preferred antihypertensive therapy for isolated systolic hypertension and reduced arterial compliance? *Curr Hypertens Reports* 2000;2:253-259.
6. Mathias C, Kimber J. Postural hypotension: Causes, clinical features, investigation, and management. *Annu Rev Med* 1999; 50:317-336.
7. Kaplan NM. Primary hypertension: Natural history, special populations, and evaluation. In: *Clinical Hypertension*. 7th ed. Baltimore, Md: Williams & Wilkins; 1998.
8. Caine S, Alsop K, Mahon M. Overlooking orthostatic hypotension with routine blood-pressure equipment. *Lancet* 1998;352: 458.
9. Jordan J, Shannon J, Black B, et al. The pressor response to water drinking in humans: A sympathetic reflex? *Circulation* 2000;101:504-509.
10. Whelton P, Appel L, Espeland M, et al. Sodium reduction and weight loss in the treatment of hypertension in older persons. *JAMA* 1998;279:839-846.
11. Kelley G, Kelley K. Progressive resistance exercise and resting blood pressure: A meta-analysis of randomized controlled trials. *Hypertension* 2000;35:838-843.
12. Gaziano J, Gaziano T, Glynn R, et al. Light-to-moderate alcohol consumption and mortality in the physicians' health study enrollment cohort. *J Am Coll Cardiol* 2000;35:96-105.
13. Appel L, Moore T, Obarzanek E, et al. A clinical trial of the effects of dietary patterns on blood pressure. *N Engl J Med* 1997;336:1117-1124.
14. Joint National Committee. The sixth report of the Joint National Committee on Detection, Evaluation, and Treatment of High Blood Pressure. *Arch Intern Med* 1997;360:757-764.
15. Guidelines Subcommittee. 1999 World Health Organization-international society of hypertension guidelines for the management of hypertension. *J Hypertension* 1999;17:151-183.
16. Ramsay LE, Williams B, Johnston GD, et al. Guidelines for management of hypertension: Report of the third working party of the British hypertension Society. *J Hum Hypertens* 1999;13: 569-592.
17. Feldman R, Campbell N, Larochelle P, et al. 1999 Canadian recommendations for the management of hypertension. *CMAJ* 1999;161:S1-S22.

18. Staessen JA, Gasowski J, Wang JG, et al. Risks of untreated and treated isolated systolic hypertension in the elderly: Meta-analysis of outcome trials. *Lancet* 2000;355:865-872.
19. Gueyffier F, Bulpitt C, Boissel J-P, et al. Antihypertensive drugs in very old people: A subgroup meta-analysis of randomised controlled trials. *Lancet* 1999;353:793-796.
20. Forette F, Seux M-L, Staessen JA, et al. Prevention of dementia in randomised double-blind placebo-controlled Sys-Eur trial. *Lancet* 1998;352:1347-1351.
21. Messerli F, Grodzicki T. Antihypertensive therapy in the elderly: Evidence-based guidelines and reality. *Arch Intern Med* 1999;159:1621-1622.
22. The ALLHAT Officers and Coordinators for the ALLHAT Collaborative Research Group. Major cardiovascular events in hypertensive patients randomized to doxazosin vs chlorthalidone. *JAMA* 2000;283:1967-1975.
23. Hansson L, Lindholm LH, Ekbom T, et al. Randomised trial of old and new antihypertensive drugs in elderly patients: Cardiovascular morbidity and mortality in the Swedish Trial in Old Patients with hypertension-2 study. *Lancet* 1999;354: 1751-1756.
24. The Heart Outcomes Prevention Evaluation Study Investigators. Effects of an angiotensin-converting-enzyme inhibitor, ramipril, on cardiovascular events in high-risk patients. *N Engl J Med* 2000;342:145-153.
25. Pitt B, Poole-Wilson P, Segal R, et al. Effect of losartan compared with captopril on mortality in patients with symptomatic heart failure: Randomised trial—The Losartan Heart Failure Survival Study ELITE II. *Lancet* 2000;355:1582-1587.
26. Blacher J, Staessen J, Girerd X. Pulse pressure not mean pressure determines cardiovascular risk in older hypertensive patients. *Arch Intern Med* 2000;160:1085-1089.
27. Somes G, Pahor M, Shorr R, et al. The role of diastolic blood pressure when treating isolated systolic hypertension. *Arch Intern Med* 1999;159:2004-2009.
28. Staessen J, Fagard R, Thijs L, et al. Randomised double-blind comparison of placebo and active treatment for older patients with isolated systolic hypertension. *Lancet* 1997;350:757-764.
29. Cushman W, Materson B, Reda D, et al. Pulse pressure changes with six classes of antihypertensive agents and placebo. *Am J Hypertens* 2000;13:22A.
30. Stokes G, Ryan M, Brnabic A. A controlled study of the effects of isosorbide mononitrate on arterial blood pressure and pulse wave form in systolic hypertension. *J Hypertens* 1999;17: 1767-1773.
31. Voko Z, Bots M, Hofman A, et al. J-shaped relation between blood pressure and stroke in treated hypertensives. *Hypertension* 1999;34:1181-1185.
32. Hansson L, Zanchetti A, Carruthers G, et al. Effects of intensive blood-pressure lowering and low-dose aspirin in patients with hypertension: Principal results of the hypertension optimal treatment (HOT) randomised trial. *Lancet* 1998;351:1755-1762.
33. Heart Outcomes Prevention Evaluation (HOPE) Study Investigators. Effects of ramipril on cardiovascular and microvascular outcomes in people with diabetes mellitus: Results of the HOPE study and MICRO-HOPE substudy. *Lancet* 2000;355:253-259.
34. Tuomilehto J, Rastenyte D, Birkenhager W, et al. Effects of calcium-channel blockade in older patients with diabetes and systolic hypertension. *N Engl J Med* 1999;340:677-684.
35. UK Prospective Diabetes Study Group. Efficacy of atenolol and captopril in reducing risk of macrovascular and microvascular complications in type 2 diabetes: UKPDS 39. *BMJ* 1998;317: 713-720.
36. Gaede P, Vedel P, Parving H-H, et al. Intensified multifactorial intervention in patients with type 2 diabetes mellitus and microalbuminuria: The Steno type 2 randomised study. *Lancet* 1999;353:617-622.

Osteoporosis: Prevention and Treatment

Cesar Libanati, MD

Recent improvements in diagnostic testing coupled with the rapidly expanding number of therapeutic options for the prevention and treatment of osteoporosis have resulted in growing recognition of this disease as a silent epidemic of major proportion. Primary care physicians are uniquely positioned to help prevent the occurrence of osteoporotic fractures in the aging population. This chapter summarizes recent developments in osteoporosis prevention and treatment. It is intended to assist primary care physicians in keeping up with this rapidly evolving field.

The clinical consequence of osteoporosis is the development of skeletal fractures after minimal or no trauma (i.e., after a fall from a standing height or less). Osteoporotic fractures occur primarily at the wrist, the spine, or the hip. Hip fractures, the most morbid complication of osteoporosis, occur at a rate of approximately 250,000 per year in the United States.[1] Although we lack up-to-date estimates, based on 1995 data, the annual costs associated with the care of osteoporotic fractures likely exceed $10 billion in the United States.[2] These expenditures are expected to escalate to $40 billion by the year 2025.

Generally speaking, osteoporotic fractures are the result of reduced bone strength due to bone loss leading to low bone mass and microarchitectural deterioration of trabecular bone.[3] Clinically speaking, that definition translates to a decrease in bone density (mass/unit volume of bone) that can now be measured with excellent precision and accuracy in the office setting. Thus, bone density testing provides the basis for the identification of patients with low bone density and for the implementation of therapeutic recommendations much like blood pressure measurements or cholesterol testing enable physicians and patients to recognize the need for intervention and tailor treatment for hypertension and hypercholesterolemia, respectively.

Osteoporosis Causes

The risk of developing an osteoporotic fracture primarily relates to the amount of bone present at any given moment. This, in turn, is the result of the maximum amount of bone achieved during early adulthood (peak bone mass) minus the accumulated bone loss. Two pathogenic mechanisms, alone or in combination, can result in osteoporosis: 1) conditions that result in reduced peak bone mass; and 2) accelerated or prolonged bone loss.

Osteoporosis is more prevalent in whites than in blacks, and in women than in men, reflecting the fact that blacks and males achieve higher peak bone mass than whites and females, respectively. Genetics appear to play a major role in the determination of peak bone mass as suggested by the fact that almost 98% of peak bone mass is achieved by the end of the second decade of life.[4] The booming identification of candidate genes associated with bone density underscores the polygenic regulatory mechanisms of peak bone density.[5-8] Undoubtedly, environmental factors such as calcium intake and weight bearing may also play a role in the attainment of peak bone density. Research into the mechanisms responsible for maximizing peak bone density is a logical approach to attempt to prevent osteoporosis. Unfortunately, while it is clear that reduced calcium intake or suboptimal exercise early in life can result in a deficit in peak bone mass and should be avoided. The opposite (i.e., supplemental calcium intake or increased exercise during adolescence) does not necessarily result in a sustained improvement in peak bone mass.

After peak bone mass has been attained, age-related bone loss occurs. This bone loss is universal but it accelerates in females during menopause due to the decrease in estrogen production.[9,10] While menopause is the most common cause responsible for estrogen deficiency, other conditions associated with a diminished estrogen production, such as exercise-associated amenorrhea, surgical oophorectomy, anorexia nervosa, or hyperprolactinemia, will result in bone loss. Recent evidence also points to estrogen deficiency as a significant factor responsible for senile male osteoporosis.[11] Later in life, in addition to estrogen deficiency, other physiological changes may contribute to bone loss: calcium malabsorption, leading to secondary hyperparathyroidism and a decline in growth factors at both the endocrine and the local tissue levels, further leads to a negative bone balance and a reduction in bone mass in both sexes.[12] Accordingly, the incidence of osteoporosis increases with age; approximately 20% of women in their seventh decade of life, 30% of women in their eighth decade of life, and 70% of women older than 80 years suffer osteoporosis.[1]

Accelerated bone loss is common in conditions such as immobilization, malabsorption, hyperparathyroidism, hypo-gonadism, multiple myeloma, and glucocorticoid therapy. Patients suffering from those conditions may benefit from bone density determination. In general, a good history, a physical examination, and few appropriate laboratory evaluations enable physicians to rule out these secondary causes of osteoporosis.

Diagnosis

A number of clinical risk factors have historically been associated with the risk of developing osteoporosis. Among these we recognize: female gender, increasing age, family history, Caucasian or Asian race, estrogen deficient state, nulliparity, sedentarism, lifelong history of low calcium intake, smoking, excessive alcohol or caffeine consumption, and long term use of glucocorticoid drugs. However, these risk factors, used alone or in combination, have only a limited predictive value in clinical practice and cannot be relied upon to always identify patients with low bone density and increased risk for fracture. The presence of an osteoporotic fracture is a noteworthy exception and patients who have already sustained a fragility fracture have a markedly increased risk of sustaining further fractures independent of their bone density level or other risk factors.[13,14] This observation can help identify osteoporotic patients in daily clinical practice. It also underscores the need to identify and treat patients before their first osteoporotic fracture has occurred. In this regard, it is well accepted that bone density is the strongest predictor of fracture risk (with roughly a doubling in the fracture risk for each unit of standard deviation decrease in bone density).[15] Other factors such as propensity to fall[14] and greater height[16] increase fracture risk, while thiazide diuretics appear to reduce hip fracture risk in elderly subjects.[17]

Because bone density is such a strong predictor of fracture risk, bone density testing has become the cornerstone for osteoporosis diagnosis and also provides guidelines for pharmacologic intervention.

Bone Density Testing

With the advent and availability of bone density testing, we can now determine the risk for fracture in an individual patient much like we can determine the risk for stroke or heart disease from blood pressure or cholesterol measurements. In fact, the relationship between bone density and fracture risk is stronger than the widely accepted relationship between cholesterol and coronary artery disease. Bone density can be assessed by a number of different techniques such as dual X-ray absorptiometry (DXA), quantitative computed tomography (QCT), and quantitative ultrasound (QUS). DXA and QCT allow bone density measurements at a central or peripheral skeletal location; QUS determinations are limited to peripheral skeletal sites. Evidence indicates that bone density measurements obtained with any of the available methods are intercorrelated and that bone density measured by any of those methods indicates fracture risk. Peripheral measurements rely on density evaluations at the forearm, calcaneus, phalanges, or tibia. Central measurements are those performed at the spine and hip, the two areas of clinical relevance in osteoporosis.[18] Peripheral density measurements offer the advantage of being lower cost and portable, thus, potentially enabling the screening of a large number of patients. Their disadvantage is that a normal peripheral density measurement does not necessarily rule out osteoporosis or osteopenia in the hip or spine. Patients with risk factors for osteoporosis may benefit more from a central than a peripheral bone density measurement since a normal peripheral bone density test in those patients does not exclude osteopenia or osteoporosis at a central site. Recommendations are being developed to ensure the most cost-effective use of peripheral and central bone density technologies.[18] *(Please see Table 1.)*

Central DXA measurements are preferred and have become the standard for clinical testing[20,21] largely due to the fact that this technique is highly reproducible and that adequate reference databases are available for spine and hip DXA measurements in clinical practice. This latter point is of major relevance since the diagnosis of normal, osteopenic, and osteoporotic densities relies on the comparison of the density of the individual studied, expressed in units of T-Score, to that of a normal young reference population. Although less than ideal, the standardization of bone density reporting in terms of T-Scores has facilitated interpretation of bone density. The World Health Organization's proposed definition of normal, osteopenia and osteoporosis based on T-Score analysis is now widespread and has been incorporated into diagnostic and treatment algorithms. Simply stated, a T-Score is simply the absolute density level of the patient being measured expressed in terms of units of standard deviation from the "ideal" or peak bone density achieved during young adulthood (the T-Score is calculated using the following formula: T-score = [density of the individual - young normal bone density]/standard deviation of young normal). Although the cutoff points for the classification of osteopenic (a bone density resulting in a T-Score between –1 and –2.5) and osteoporotic (a bone density resulting in a T-Score inferior to –2.5) densities is somewhat arbitrary since the

Table 1. Indications for Bone Density Testing

- Estrogen-deficient women at clinical risk for osteoporosis
- Individuals with vertebral abnormalities
- Individuals receiving, or planning to receive, long-term glucocorticoid (steroid) therapy
- Individuals with primary hyperparathyroidism
- Individuals being monitored to assess the response of an approved osteoporosis drug therapy

relationship between fracture risk and bone density is continuous, it provides a useful framework for test interpretation and patient evaluation and management.[22] The lower the density in the osteopenic or osteoporotic range, the more negative the T-Score. Since the calculation of the T-Score involves density comparison to that of a normal young population, it is ideal that a young reference database common to all manufacturers and techniques be used for standardization.[23,24] Such a common reference database is available for hip measurements with central densitometers (NHANES III database[25]). A Z-Score is also included in most density reports. The Z-Score is the absolute density level of the patient expressed in terms of units of standard deviation from the "expected" density for an age-, sex-, and race-matched individual. Although the use of the Z-Score is less well defined than that of the T-Score, a low Z-Score (i.e., inferior to –2.0) helps the ordering physician by alerting that the patient may have lost greater amount of bone than expected.

Another advantage of DXA over the other available techniques is that expected changes in density in response to different therapies are well documented both at the spine and hip and, thus, enable educated decisions regarding treatment response during follow-up of individual patients.

Both hip and spine need to be measured. The spine allows for precise follow-up of response to therapy and the hip density is necessary, in the elderly, to avoid false-negative diagnoses due to the presence of degenerative changes that may artifactually increase the bone density determination in the spine.

Patients with normal spine and hip densities may not need to worry about osteoporotic fractures and may not require any form of pharmacological intervention (estrogen replacement therapy [ERT] after menopause may still be advisable based on cardiovascular risk profile and menopausal symptoms). Subjects with osteopenia should be carefully counseled, treated, and followed such that, at least, no further bone loss develops. Finally, patients with osteoporosis require active intervention aimed at fall prevention and pharmacologic therapy to increase bone density and decrease fracture risk.

Biochemical Markers of Bone Formation and Bone Resorption

Bone balance is the result of bone formation minus bone resorption. Both bone formation and bone resorption may be assessed by means of chemical measurements of skeletal-specific proteins or byproducts of collagen breakdown in serum and urine. Bone formation markers (i.e., alkaline phosphatase, osteocalcin) are available but their use outside of research studies is hampered by poor precision, daily or seasonal variance, and the lack of FDA-approved therapeutic agents to increase bone formation. Bone resorption markers (urinary hydroxyproline and the newer collagen cross links such as pyridinoline, deoxypyridinoline, N-telopeptides, and C-telopeptides) have been proposed to assist in the identification of patients likely to sustain fractures (independent of bone density) in the identification of individuals with rapid bone loss and in the monitoring of antiresorptive therapeutic responses. The rationale behind these applications is simple: if bone resorption and bone loss are correlated and if antiresorptive therapies (such as estrogen, alendronate, raloxifene, and calcitonin) are effective at decreasing bone resorption and reducing fracture risk, then a marker of bone resorption could be used to identify patients more likely to benefit from therapeutic intervention and monitor the efficacy of the treatment.[26-29] Although these strategies prove correct when applied to large number of study patients, the use of these markers for the identification or follow-up of individual subjects in clinical practice may be limited. The limitations arise, in part, from the large variance (15-30%) in marker measurements. While duplicate measurements would improve the variance, they would also result in greater expenditure. Recent reports further question the usefulness of these markers in day-to-day practice.[30,31] To date, we cannot provide evidence-based guidelines for the use of these biochemical markers in the diagnosis or monitoring of osteoporotic patients with the possible exception of bone resorption marker decrease after three months of alendronate therapy—enabling some prediction of the bone density to increase later.[32]

Prevention and Treatment Strategies

The main objective in the prevention and treatment of osteoporosis is the maintenance of skeletal integrity by 1) achieving the highest possible peak bone density; 2) arresting bone loss; and 3) preventing falls.

More studies are needed to enable recommendations that will undeniably contribute to a higher peak bone density. Until then, it is important to encourage a balanced diet including at least 1300 mg of calcium during the adolescent years and 1000-1500 mg afterward, to promote weight bearing exercise, and to recommend avoidance of alcohol and tobacco products. Detailed information about calcium content in food products is widely available in food labels. As a rule of thumb, a cup of milk or 2 oz of cheese provide approximately 300 mg of calcium.

Daily calcium supplementation (1000-1500 mg) along with 400-800 IU vitamin D have been shown to reduce the rate of bone loss in women greater than five years postmenopause and should be given concomitantly with all other pharmacological interventions. While adequate calcium intake via food or supplementation may help achieve maximum peak bone density, slow bone loss and decrease (particularly when combined with vitamin D) fracture risk[33] in some patients, it is now well accepted that calcium and vitamin D alone may not prevent the development of osteoporosis in large number of patients.

As previously mentioned, bone loss may begin after peak bone density is achieved and accelerates during menopause with the great-

Table 2. Available FDA Approved Drugs for the Management of Osteoporosis

Drug	Dosage	Indication	Comments
Estrogen	See text	Prevention and Treatment	Ongoing Women Health Initiative Study will hopefully allow evidence-based recommendations regarding ideal onset, dosage and length of therapy
Raloxifene	60mg PO QD	Prevention	No breast or uterine tissue stimulation; Decrease in cholesterol similar to estrogen
Alendronate	5 mg PO QD 10 mg PO QD	Prevention Treatment	Adherence to strict instructions on how to take the medicine essential. Well-documented reduction in spine and hip fracture risk.
Calcitonin	200 IU QD (nasal) 50-100 IU QD SQ	Treatment	Modest analgesic effect. Not indicated in the early post-menopausal years.
Calcium	See text	Prevention/Treatment	Calcium alone may not prevent the development of osteoporosis
Vitamin D	400-800 IU QD	Prevention/Treatment	May help reduce hip fracture incidence in the elderly

est bone loss occurring in the first 5-7 menopausal years.[34,35] The perimenopausal years, therefore, constitute a unique window when primary care providers could have a major effect by discussing and instituting therapeutic plans to prevent bone loss. Bone density testing at this time of life can assist the female patient and her doctor to make a well-informed decision about the need to institute measures to prevent osteoporosis. Another advantage of bone density testing is that it increases acceptance of ERT.[36] Females who are not willing or incapable of receiving ERT and have osteopenic densities may consider alternative agents such as alendronate and raloxifene, which are now FDA approved to prevent bone loss. After the age of 65, a bone density test should be performed, if not previously done, in that individual to decide if pharmacologic therapy should be considered to prevent or treat osteoporosis. *(Please see Table 2.)*

Estrogen Replacement Therapy

Estrogen deficiency after menopause predictably leads to bone loss and osteoporosis. Accordingly, ERT is the accepted standard of practice for the prevention and for the treatment of osteoporosis. All postmenopausal women without contraindications should consider ERT. Contraindications to estrogen administration include family or individual history of breast cancer; estrogen dependent neoplasia; undiagnosed genital bleeding; and a history of or active thromboembolic disorder.

Because the greatest rate of bone loss occurs in the first years after cessation of ovarian function, ERT should be initiated at the onset of menopause to prevent bone loss accumulation. Recent placebo-controlled studies to evaluate the effect on alendronate[37] or raloxifene[38] in the prevention of osteoporosis in postmenopausal women included an estrogen-treated arm. Conjugated estrogens, at a dose of 0.625 mg per day, resulted in approximate increases in bone density at the spine and the hip of 5% and 3%, respectively, at 24 months.

Unfortunately, we lack well-controlled prospective studies to evaluate the ideal dose and the optimal duration of estrogen therapy to prevent osteoporosis. Accordingly, there are no clear recommendations regarding the optimal duration of ERT. From a skeletal standpoint, bone density assessment at regular intervals (possibly every 3-5 years) provides density data to help determine if continuation of ERT may be further recommended. Baseline and repeat bone density testing remains the sole test that allows documenting maintenance. The importance of repeat bone density testing is stressed by reports of development of osteoporosis despite compliance with ERT[39] and of bone loss occurring in patients followed longitudinally while receiving ERT.[40] If ERT is discontinued and no other therapies are instituted, serial bone density measurements should be continued to monitor for accelerated bone loss known to occur after ERT is stopped.[41] Although ERT may be most beneficial if started early after cessation of menses, elderly patients also increase bone density and decrease fracture incidence if receiving ERT.[42]

Different estrogen preparations are currently available for the prevention and treatment of osteoporosis. The route of administration (oral or transdermal) does not seem to affect the efficacy of estrogen. Conjugated estrogens and transdermal estradiol are commonly prescribed at a dose of 0.625 mg and 0.05 mg, respectively, for the prevention of postmenopausal osteoporosis. For the treatment of postmenopausal osteoporosis conjugated estrogens doses of 0.625-1.25 mg daily are most commonly used.

Although we also lack good studies of estrogen's effect on fracture, several small studies and epidemiological observations reveal a lower incidence of fractures in osteoporotic women treated with estrogen.[41,43-45] Estimates of fracture risk reduction from ERT vary between 20% and 60% and the greatest fracture benefit from estrogen therapy may occur if estrogen is used for 10 years or longer.

The benefits of ERT are not limited to bone. Estrogens decrease total cholesterol and low-density lipoprotein levels and increase high-density lipoprotein (HDL) levels.[46] Estrogens also cause vasodilatation and other direct benefits on the endothelium. Based on these actions and few well-controlled studies, we have widely accepted that estrogens reduce cardiovascular morbidity and mortality.[47] While most beneficial effects of estrogen on the lipid profile are maintained if a progestin is added, this therapy tends to reduce the increase on HDL characteristic of estrogen's action. The cardiovascular benefit of estrogen supplementation was recently questioned by the publication of the results of the Heart and Estrogen/Progestin Replacement Study.[48] This research reported that treatment with oral conjugated estrogen and medroxyprogesterone, during a follow-up period of approximately four years, did not reduce the overall rate of coronary events in postmenopausal women with established atherosclerotic heart disease. Far from settling the issue, this study stresses the notion that estrogen therapeutic recommendations regarding dosage and length of therapy need to be individualized rather than generalized. The results of the ongoing Women's Health Initiative Study will hopefully provide data to allow evidence-based recommendations regarding the ideal onset, dosage, and recommended length of ERT. Other major potential beneficial effects of ERT such as colon cancer and Alzheimer's disease incidence reductions while exciting also remain to be formally studied.

Unfortunately, ERT has side effects. ERT results in endometrial hyperplasia and doubles the risk of endometrial cancer in women with an intact uterus. This increased risk can be easily eliminated by the addition of medroxyprogesterone acetate either cyclically (12-14 days/month) at a dose of 5-10 mg or continuously at a dose of 2.5-5 mg daily. Other adverse events related to ERT are breast tenderness, weight gain, headaches, and libido changes. Unfortunately, most women who receive prescriptions for ERT stop therapy within a few months. The side effects, together with concerns about increased breast cancer risk, account for the poor compliance observed with ERT. The breast cancer risk, if present, is likely related to the cumulative time on estrogen supplementation. Evidence suggests a small increase in breast cancer risk after 10-15 years of estrogen supplementation.[49,50] Again, the Women's Health Initiative Study may help clarify the relationship between ERT and breast cancer risk. Until that study is completed, the availability of selective estrogen receptors modulators, which result in positive effects on bone and lipid profile while avoiding breast or uterine tissue stimulation, offer an alternative to females concerned about the possible increase in breast cancer risk or those who have been on continuous ERT for more than a decade. Finally, ERT results in a small increase in thromboembolic events.[51]

Selective Estrogen Receptor Modulators

With the discovery and molecular understanding of the function and tissue distribution of two distinct estrogen receptors, a new group of drugs has emerged to potentially improve estrogen's beneficial actions while reducing or avoiding altogether estrogen's known side effects. These drugs have been termed selective estrogen receptor modulators (SERMs). SERMs act as either estrogen analogs or estrogen antagonists depending on the tissue and on the presence or absence of endogenous estrogen. The oldest of all SERMs is tamoxifen, which was recently approved for the prevention of breast cancer in selected populations. Tamoxifen prevented bone loss at the spine but not at the wrist in postmenopausal women.[52]

Raloxifene, a new SERM, was recently approved by the FDA for the prevention of osteoporosis based on the results of large, randomized, placebo-controlled, double-blind studies.[38] When used at a dose of 60 mg per day, raloxifene demonstrated modest but statistically significant increases (1.5%-2% in 24 months) in bone density at the hip and spine compared to calcium supplemented groups. This increase in density was approximately half of that seen in those patients receiving ERT but raloxifene therapy was not associated with uterine stimulation. Raloxifene therapy was recently shown to be associated with a significant decrease in vertebral fracture risk compared to placebo[53] and, thus, may also prove beneficial in the treatment of established osteoporosis in addition to the already approved use for osteoporosis prevention.

Raloxifene also results in a beneficial effect on the lipid profile similar to that seen with estrogen (raloxifene does not improve total HDL cholesterol but does not increase triglycerides either). It remains to be proven if this effect on lipids will positively affect cardiovascular morbidity and mortality. The results of a double-blind, placebo-controlled, five-year study initiated in 1998, the Raloxifene Use for the Heart, will in time hopefully address this important question.

Possibly, the most exciting aspect of raloxifene therapy is the lack of breast stimulation and the possibility that, like tamoxifen, it may provide a protective effect against certain types of breast cancer. Preliminary reports indicate that raloxifene therapy results in a 50-70% reduction in breast cancer risk.[54] Again, ongoing studies will provide a more definite answer to the reduction in breast cancer risk reportedly associated with raloxifene administration.

Raloxifene may be taken at any time during the day and without regard to foods or medicines with the exception of cholestiramine, which prevents intestinal absorption of raloxifene. Raloxifene may be better tolerated than ERT and raloxifene administration resulted in fewer dropout rates than ERT as a result of side effects.[55] Minor common side effects associated with raloxifene therapy include hot flashes and leg cramps. Serious side effects include an increased risk of venous thromboembolism (deep venous thrombosis, pulmonary embolism, and retinal vein thrombosis).[38] Although rare and similar in incidence to patients receiving ERT, thromboembolic adverse events are serious enough to recommend stopping raloxifene and prompt evaluation in patients complaining of leg pain or swelling, unexplained shortness of breath or hemoptisis, or changes in vision while receiving raloxifene therapy. Raloxifene should not be used before menopause and should be discontinued in patients who become immobilized.

Bisphosphonates

Alendronate is an oral bisphosphonate approved for the treatment and prevention of osteoporosis in women. Alendronate exerts its effect on bone by inhibiting osteoclasts and thereby reducing bone resorption without negatively affecting mineralization. Large-scale, randomized, placebo-controlled, double-blind studies have demonstrated that alendronate, given at a dose of 5 mg and 10 mg per day, is effective at maintaining and increasing bone density, respectively.[37,56]

The recommended dose for prevention of osteoporosis is 5 mg per day. This dose resulted in significant increases in lumbar (3.5%) and hip (2%) densities when compared to placebo. These increases were slightly but not significantly different from those observed in the ERT arm of the trial. The recommended dose for the treatment of osteoporosis is 10 mg per day. With this dosing, bone density significantly increased at the spine and the hip by about 7% and 4%, respectively at 36 months. These increases in density were associated with an approximate 50% reduction in fracture risk at both skeletal sites. Subgroup analysis revealed similar reductions in fracture risk regardless of age, degree of baseline bone resorption, or absolute pretreatment bone density level.

Alendronate has also been documented to prevent and improve osteoporosis associated with prednisone therapy.[57]

The effect of combination therapy such as alendronate and estrogen is currently under evaluation. Preliminary reports indicate that an additive effect on bone density occurs when these two agents are used in combination.[58]

Regardless of the dosage used, patients should be instructed to take the alendronate pill in the morning with 2-3 glasses of water, at least 30 minutes before any food or beverages. Because bisphosphonates are poorly absorbed and because these groups of drugs bind tightly to other compounds, it is important that no other medication be taken at the same time, particularly calcium preparations. Patients should also be instructed against lying down after taking alendronate to avoid gastro-esophageal reflux. Esophagitis, a side effect rarely observed in the research trials but reported after the drug was approved and released for general use by the FDA, emphasizes the importance to adhering to the recommendations on how to take the drug. Alendronate is not recommended for use in patients with severe renal insufficiency or hypocalcemia.

Because alendronate exclusively exerts its effect on the skeletal system, follow-up bone density is a logical tool to monitor therapy. In the controlled trials, the majority of patients responded to therapy with maintenance or improvement in bone density. If this is proven the case in real practice, a follow-up of bone density may not be routinely required with this form of therapy, particularly in those patients who demonstrate a decrease in their bone resorption marker. As with any test, bone density testing while on alendronate should only be performed if the result will influence therapeutic recommendations.

Calcitonin

Calcitonin, a naturally occurring hormone, has long been used for the treatment of osteoporosis. Until recently, the only calcitonin available was an injectable form. Recently, a nasal spray form was approved for the treatment of postmenopausal osteoporosis. Presently available calcitonins include salmon calcitonin (injectable and nasal spray) and human calcitonin (injectable only). In the treatment of osteoporosis, calcitonin may be given as either 50 IU or 100 IU intramuscularly or subcutaneously daily or every other day[59] or as 200 IU intranasally every day.[60] The nasal spray, at a dose of 200 IU/d, alternating nares, results in a modest but not significant increase in bone density at the spine (2%) compared to placebo-treated subjects. For reasons still poorly understood, the increase in bone density associated with calcitonin administration may be transient. Although recent abstract reports regarding a reduction in fracture occurrence with nasal calcitonin therapy are encouraging, the effect of this therapy on hip fracture remains to be demonstrated. Patients who have suffered an acute osteoporotic fracture[61] may benefit from the analgesic effect of calcitonin, a unique characteristic of this agent.

Calcitonin is an alternative to estrogen and alendronate therapy in women who cannot tolerate or refuse these therapies and may be useful in the management of painful acute osteoporotic fractures. It is generally well tolerated with minimal adverse effects. Because of the possible, albeit rare, allergic reaction to salmon, calcitonin skin testing should be done before initiation of parenteral therapy in patients with suspected allergy to calcitonin. Adverse effects occurring with parenteral therapy include nausea or vomiting and transient vasomotor symptoms. These side effects are self-limited and can be managed with a reduction in the administered dose. Nasal calcitonin side effects are primarily limited to rhinitis.

The Immediate Future

While the past decade resulted in major diagnostic and therapeutic developments leading to 1) improved recognition of patients at risk for fracture before fractures occur by means of bone density testing; and 2) an increased availability of agents to halt bone loss and reduce future fracture occurrence, the medical community is still lagging in the use of both the diagnostic tools and the therapeutic agents. As a result, many unrecognized patients with osteopenia continue to lose bone and many patients with osteoporosis continue to fracture. The immediate future calls for the recognition that osteopenia and osteoporosis need to be considered in the differential diagnosis in all women after the menopause. This goal can only be accomplished if primary care providers recognize the importance of this disease.

The More Distant Future

All currently approved therapeutic agents for the prevention and treatment of osteoporosis share one common mechanism of action: they inhibit or decrease bone resorption. While this group of agents is effective at maintaining or mildly increasing bone density, we now need agents that would result in ample gains in bone density to correct the large bone density deficits characteristic of severe osteoporosis. This can only be accomplished by agents that stimulate bone formation. Parathyroid hormone peptides, growth hormone, and growth factors are anabolic agents currently under different phases of development to treat osteoporosis. It is likely that one such agent will become available in the next 5-10 years.

Conclusion

The increasing availability of bone density testing to identify patients at risk for osteoporotic fractures, coupled with the FDA approval of alternatives to ERT for the prevention and treatment of osteoporosis, signals a turning point in our battle against this morbid condition. Calcium with or without vitamin D supplementation is encouraged but may not prevent osteoporosis. Bone density testing allows the accurate and rapid identification of patients at risk for osteoporotic fractures and provides the basis for pharmacologic intervention. ERT should be considered in all postmenopausal women without contraindications. Alternatives to estrogen for osteoporosis prevention include the new SERM raloxifene (60 mg/d) or the bisphosphonate alendronate (5 mg/d). For the treatment of osteoporosis, estrogen and alendronate (10 mg/d) result in significant increases in bone density. Alendronate therapy has been associated with proven reductions in fracture risk at both the spine and hip. Calcitonin offers a safe alternative although the effect on density is modest and the effect on fracture, particularly at the hip, is less well documented.

References

1. Prestwood K, Weksler ME. Osteoporosis: Up-to-date strategies for prevention and treatment. *Geriatrics* 1997; 52:92-98.
2. Ray NF, et al. Medical expeditures for the treatment of esteoporotic fractures in the USA in 1995: Report from the National Osteoporosis Foundation. *J Bone Miner Res* 1997;12:24-35.
3. Consensus Development Conference, Prophylaxis and treatment of osteoporosis. *Am J Med* 1991;90:107-110.
4. Bonjour JP, et al. Critical years and stages of puberty for spinal and femoral bone mass accumulation during adolescence. *J Clin Endocrinol Metab* 1991;73:555-563.
5. Garnero P, et al. Collagen I a 1 Sp1 polymorphysm, bone mass, and bone turnover in healthy French premenopausal women: The OFELY study. *J Bone Miner Res* 1998;13: 813-817.
6. Zmuda JM, et al. Genetic variation in a2hs-glycoprotein is related to calcaneal broadband ultrasound attenuation in older women. *Calcif Tissue Int* 1998;63:5-8.
7. Greenfield EM, Goldberg VM. Genetic determination of bone density. *Lancet* 1997;350:1263-1264.
8. Rosen CJ, et al. Association between serum insulin growth factor-I (IGF-I) and a simple sequence repeat in IGF-I gene: Implications for genetic studies of bone mineral density. *J Clin Endocrinol Metab* 1998; 83(7):2286-2290.
9. Hui SL, et al. Effects of age and menopause on vertebral bone density. *Bone Miner* 1987;2:141-146.
10. Richelson LS, et al. Relative Contributions of aging and estrogen deficiency to postmenopausal bone loss. *N Engl J Med* 1984;311:1273-1275.
11. Khosla S, et al. Relationship of serum sex steroids levels and bone turnover markers with bone mineral density in men and women: A key role for bioavailable estrogen. *J Clin Endocrinol Metab* 1998; 83(7):2266-2274.
12. Hilliker S, et al. The pathogenesis of primary osteoporosis. In: H Slavkin H and P Price (eds.) *Chemistry and Biology of Mineralized Tissues.* Elsevier Science Publishers, 1992: 455-463.
13. Kotowicz MA, et al. Risk of hip fracture in women with vertebral fracture. *J Bone Miner Res* 1994;9:559-605.
14. Cummings SR, et al. Risk factors for hip fracture in white women: Study of Osteoporotic Fractures Research Group. *N Engl J Med* 1995; 332767-773.
15. Marshall D, et al. Meta-analysis of how well measures of bone density predict occurrence of osteoporotic fractures. *BMJ* 1996;312(7041):1254-1259.
16. Hemenway D, et al. Body height and hip fracture: A cohort study of 90,000 women. *Int J Epidemiol* 1995;24:783-786.
17. Jones G, et al. Thiazide diuretics and fractures: can meta-analysis help? *J Bone Miner Res* 1995;10:106-111.
18. Wahner HW. Use of densitometry in the management of osteoporosis. In: Marcus R, Feldman D, Kelsey J, eds. *Osteoporosis.* Academic Press 1996;1055-1074.
19. Miller PD, et al. The challenges of peripheral bone density testing. Which patients need additional central density skeletal measurements? *Journal of Clinical Densitometry* 1998;1:211-217.
20. Grampp S, et al. Comparisons of noninvasive bone mineral measurements in assessing age-related loss, fracture discrimination, and diagnostic classification. *J Bone Miner Res* 1997;12:697-711.
21. Genant HK, et al. Noninvasive assessment of bone mineral and structure: State of the art. *J Bone Miner Res* 1996;11: 707-730.
22. Kanis JA. Assessment of fracture risk and its application to screening for postmenopausal osteoporosis: Synopsis of a WHO report. *Osteoporosis Int* 1994;4:368-381.
23. Faulkner KG, et al. Discrepancies in normative data between Lunar and Hologic DXA systems. *Osteoporos Int* 1996;6: 432-436.
24. Greenspan SL, et al. Precision and discriminatory ability of calcaneal bone assessment technologies. *J Bone Miner Res* 1997;12:1303-1313. Published erratum appears in *J Bone Miner Res* 1997;12:1957.
25. Looker AC, et al. Updated data on proximal femur bone mineral levels of US adults. *Osteoporos Int* 1998;8:468-489.
26. Garnero P, et al. Increased bone turnover in late postmenopausal women is a major determinant of osteoporosis. *J Bone Miner Res* 1996;11:337-349.
27. Rosen CJ, et al. The predictive value of biochemical markers of bone turnover for bone mineral density in early postmenopausal women treated with hormone replacement or calcium supplementation. *J Clin Endo Metab* 1997;82: 1904-1910.
28. Slemenda C, et al. Sex steroids and bone mass: A study of changes about the time of menopause. *J Clin Invest* 1987; 80:1261-1269.
29. Garnero P, et al. Comparison of new biochemical markers of bone turnover in late postmenopausal osteoporotic women in response to alendronate treatment. *J Clin Endocrinol Metab* 1994;79:1693-1700.
30. Ott SM, et al. Ability of bone biochemical markers to predict 4-year changes in bone density in postmenopausal women. *J Bone Mineral Res* 1998;23(5S):1044.
31. Hannon RA, et al. Long-term variability of biochemical markers of bone turnover in postmenopausal women. *J Bone Mineral Res* 1998; 23(5S):1045.
32. Greenspan SL, et al. Early changes in biochemical markers of bone turnover predict the long-term response to alendronate therapy in representative elderly women: A randomized clinical trial. *J Bone Miner Res* 1998;13:1431-1438.
33. Cumming RG, Nevitt MC. Calcium for prevention of osteoporotic fractures in postmenopausal women. *J Bone Mineral Res* 1997;12:1321-1329.
34. Lindsay R, et al. Prevention of spinal osteoporosis in oophorectomized women. *Lancet* 1980;2:1151-1153.
35. Nachtigall LE, et al. Estrogen replacement therapy. I. A 10-year prospective study in the relationship to osteoporosis.

Obstet Gynecol 1979;53:277-281.

36. Silverman SL, et al. Effect of bone density information on decisions about hormone replacement therapy: A randomized trial. *Obstet Gynecol* 1997;89:321-325.
37. Hosking D, et al. For the Early Postmenopausal Intervention Cohort Study Group. Prevention of bone loss with alendronate in postmenopausal women under 60 years of age. *N Engl J Med* 1998; 338:485-492.
38. Delmas P, et al. Effects of raloxifene on bone mineral density, serum cholesterol concentrations and uterine endometrium in postmenopausal women. *N Engl J Med* 1997;337:1641-1647.
39. Nelson H, et al. Osteoporosis and fractures are common in older postmenopausal women using estrogen. *J Bone Mineral Res* 1998; 23(5S):1013.
40. Ensrud KE, et al. Hip and calcaneal bone loss increase with advancing age: longitudinal results from the study of osteoporotic fractures. *J Bone Miner Res* 1995;10: 1778-1787.
41. Quigley ME, et al. Estrogen therapy arrests bone loss in elderly women. *Am J Obstet Gynecol* 1987;156:1516-1523.
42. Cauley JA, et al. Estrogen replacement therapy and fractures in older women. Study of Osteoporotic Fractures Research Group. *Ann Intern Med* 1995;122:9-16.
43. Weiss NS, et al. Decreased risk of fractures of the hip and lower forearm with postmenopausal use of estrogens. *N Engl J Med* 1980; 303:1195-1198.
44. Williams AR, et al. Effect of weight, smoking, and estrogen use on the risk of hip and forearm fractures in postmenopausal women. *Obstet Gynecol* 1982;60:695-699.
45. Ettinger B, et al. Long-term estrogen replacement therapy prevents bone loss and fractures. *Ann Intern Med* 1985;102: 319-324.
46. The Postmenopausal Estrogen/Progestins Interventions (PEPI) Trial. Effects of estrogen or estrogen/progestin regimens on heart disease risk factors in postmenopausal women. *JAMA* 1995;273:199-208.
47. Grodstein F, et al. Postmenopausal hormone therapy and mortality. *N Engl J Med* 1997;336:1769-1775.
48. Hulley S, et al. The Heart and Estrogen/progestin Replacement Study (HERS) Research Group. Randomized Trial of Estrogen Plus Progestin for Secondary Prevention of Coronary Heart Disease in Postmenopausal Women. *JAMA* 1998;280:605-613.
49. Hulka BS. Hormone-replacement therapy and the risk of breast cancer. *Cancer* 1990;40:289-296.
50. Speroff L. Postmenopausal hormone therapy and mortality. *Obstet Gynecol* 1996;87:44S-54S.
51. Daly E, et al. Risk of venous thromboembolism in users of hormone replacement therapy. *Lancet* 1996;348:977-980.
52. Love RR, et al. Effects of tamoxifen on bone mineral density in postmenopausal women with breast cancer. *N Engl J Med* 1992;326:852-856.
53. Ensrud K, et al. The effect of 2 and 3 years of raloxifene on vertebral and non-vertebral fractures in postmenopausal women with osteoporosis. *J Bone Mineral Res* 1998;23(5S): 1013.
54. Goldhirsch A, et al. New treatments for breast cancer: breakthroughs for patient care or just steps in the right direction? *Ann Oncol* 1998;9:973-976.
55. Walsh BW, et al. Effects of raloxifene on serum lipids and coagulation factors in healthy postmenopausal women. *JAMA* 1998;279:1445-1451.
56. Liberman UA, et al. For the alendronate Phase III osteoporosis treatment study group. Effect of oral alendronate on bone mineral density and the incidence of fractures in postmenopausal osteoporosis. *N Engl J Med* 1996;333:1437-1443.
57. Saag KG, et al. Alendronate for the prevention and treatment of glucocorticoid-induced osteoporosis. *N Engl J Med* 1998; 339:292-299.
58. Greenspan S, et al. Effect of alendronate and estrogen, alone or in combination, on bone mass and turnover in postmenopausal osteoporosis. *J Bone Mineral Res* 1998; 23(5S):1107.
59. Civitelli R, et al. Bone turnover in postmenopausal osteoporosis: Effect of calcitonin treatment. *J Clin Invest* 1988;82:1268-1274.
60. Overgaard K, et al. Effect of salmon calcitonin given intranasally on bone mass and fracture rates in established osteoporosis. A dose-response study. *Br Med J* 1992;305: 556-561.
61. Lyritis GP, et al. Analgesic effect of salmon calcitonin in osteoporotic vertebral fractures: A double-blind placebo-controlled clinical study. *Calcif Tissue Int* 1991;49:369-372.

Management of Geriatric Patients in Skilled Nursing Facilities

Keith Doram, MD, FACP, MBA, CMD

There is a real need for efficient and efficacious medical management of geriatric patients in skilled nursing facilities (SNFs). The number of geriatric patients in SNFs is increasing primarily due to the overall increase in the population of the aged in our society. These patients consume the largest and most disproportionate amount of our healthcare dollars and resources. The government is concerned about the future solvency of Medicare as it is projected that the geriatric population (those > 65 years) will increase from 13% to 20% of the U.S. population by the year 2020.[1] The U.S. Bureau of the Census estimates that the geriatric population 80 years of age and older is expected to increase to 6.1 million by 2010 and more than double to 12.3 million by 2040 (a rate 2.5 times that of the rest of the U.S. population). The Census data also show that 90% of all SNF patients are older than age 65 and of those, 45% are older than 85.[2] Currently, almost 2 million people live in the nation's 20,000 SNFs, and this is expected to reach 3.4 million by the year 2030.[3]

More and more practitioners find themselves caring for the frail, elderly, and often high-risk complicated patients in the unique and challenging environment of the SNF.[4] These practitioners are under increasing pressures to deliver cost-effective quality medical care. This chapter is intended to provide the SNF healthcare provider with relevant and practical clinical information and practice guidelines that will better enable the medical staff to provide for the special needs of the geriatric patient. Physicians will be encouraged to develop their assessment/ plans being mindful of the useful information contained in the nationally standardized and mandated minimum data set (MDS) and resident assessment protocols (RAPs).

Across the continuum of acute care hospitals (ACHs), transitional/subacute care facilities, and nursing homes (NHs), all use skilled nursing personnel. Functionally, the main differences between the types of SNFs have related to the severity of illness and intensity of service(s) required. Subacute care facilities generally are capable of providing more intensive services than traditional SNFs or NHs but less than ACHs. Subacute care units are often found within ACHs and the typical patient is elderly (> 75% older than 65), less likely to be cognitively impaired, on more medications, and more likely to be rehospitalized.[5] The focus will primarily be on traditional SNFs (i.e., NHs). Table 1 displays some of the major differences between ACHs and SNFs.

Key issues in the management of geriatric patients in SNFs:

- Governmental regulations
- Functional status
- Medication usage
- Agitation and dementia
- Nutrition
- Preventive measures
- Special treatment considerations

Table 1. Differences Between Acute Care Hospitals and Skilled Nursing Facilities

Characteristic	Acute Care Hospital	Skilled Nursing Facility
Patient care	Physician-driven	Nurse-driven
Progress notes	Daily	Every 30-60 days and PRN
Patient length of stay	Days	Weeks to years
Severity of illness	Acute and unstable	Chronic and stable
Facility surveys	Every three years using JCAHO standards	Every year using government regulation standards
Patient care updates	Done daily at bedside	Done mostly over the telephone PRN

SNF Regulations

Prior to the institution of Medicare and Medicaid legislation in 1965, each state had oversight of SNFs. However, most states had few, if any, mechanisms in place to ensure that a minimally acceptable quality of care was being provided to the patients admitted to SNFs. The resultant public health concerns led to the development of federal-government-issued regulations for SNFs involved in Medicare and Medicaid in 1974.[6]

These regulations, however, did little to improve the quality of care for SNF patients. The regulations were not well received and the states often knowingly allowed their SNFs to remain out of compliance with the regulations. Therefore, in 1983, the Health Care Financing Administration (HCFA) contracted with the Institute of Medicine (IOM) to make recommendations that would "serve as a basis for adjusting federal (and state) policies and regulation governing the certification of nursing homes to make those policies and regulations as appropriate and effective as possible."[7] Congress used the recommendations resulting from the HCFA-IOM alliance report as a basis for the regulatory changes incorporated into the Omnibus Budget Reconciliation Act of 1987 (OBRA 1987), Public law 100-203. Federal and state surveyors use interpretive guidelines based on OBRA 1987 for their inspection surveys of SNFs. States may also have other specific requirements (e.g., California's Title 22 Regulations), that directly affect SNFs.

OBRA Regulations for Medical Director (Section 483.75)

Prior to OBRA 87, most SNF medical directors were just clinicians who cared for the majority of patients in the SNF and were in essence the "de facto physicians" for any and all clinical questions or issues that would arise. OBRA 87 stipulates that all SNFs have a medical director. However, there are more reported medical directors positively associated with hospital-based SNFs and with having a high proportion of Medicare residents.[8] The physician who serves as the medical director must assume specific interactive and proactive administrative responsibilities for the design, measurement, assessment, and improvement of the quality of care. The medical director should meet regularly with the administrator and the director of nursing (DON) and should organize and monitor the medical staff.

OBRA Regulations for Attending Physicians (Section 483.40)

The attending physician should personally approve of the patient's admission and admission orders. A complete history, physical, assessment, and plan should be completed by the attending physician within 72 hours of each patient's admission. Generally, each patient requires a progress note every 30 days, although more or less frequent evaluations are allowed (and are billable). The physician should review the patient's total program, including the minimum data set (MDS) and resident assessment protocols (RAPs).

Patient Rights (Section 483.10) and Physical Restraints (483.13(a))

The patient has the right to choose and contact his/her own personal physician, receive medical care in privacy, be informed of his/her medical condition, and refuse treatment.

There are many potential harms associated with the use of physical restraints (e.g., strangulation, skin and musculoskeletal injury, loss of personal dignity, etc.). Therefore, OBRA 87 requires that there should not be any undue use of chemical or physical restraints unless they are medically indicated to treat the resident's symptoms. Restraints are not to be used for "discipline or convenience." After one year of implementation of this regulation, the use of restraints in the United States decreased by approximately 33%.[9]

Medication Usage (Section 483.25(1))

One of the main objectives of the Nursing Home Reform Amendments (included in OBRA 87) was the reduction of antipsychotic drug use in SNFs.[10] The IOM committee stated in 1986 that excessive use of psychoactive medication is an indicator of poor-quality care.[11] The regulations make the SNF directly responsible for physician prescribing patterns regarding psychoactive medication. SNFs are subject to potential financial penalties if physicians fail to comply with the OBRA interpretive usage guidelines.[12] Essentially, physicians need to have clear and documented medical indications for use of psychoactive medications in SNF residents. Psychoactive drugs with shorter half-lives and fewer associated side effects are preferred.

Patient Assessment (Section 483.20)—Minimum Data Set and Resident Assessment Protocols

The MDS/RAPs are a comprehensive, standardized, and reproducible nursing generated functional assessment instrument

Table 2. Resident Assessment Protocols (RAPs)

1. Delirium
2. Cognitive loss/dementia
3. Visual function
4. Communication
5. Activities of daily living function/rehabilitative potential
6. Urinary incontinence and in-dwelling catheter
7. Psychosocial well being
8. Mood state
9. Behavior problem
10. Activities
11. Falls
12. Nutritional status
13. Feeding tubes
14. Dehydration/fluid maintenance
15. Dental care
16. Pressure ulcer
17. Antipsychotic drug use
18. Physical restraints

mandated by OBRA in 1991 to be used by all SNFs certified by Medicare and Medicaid (or Medical).[13] The MDS must be completed no later than 14 days after admission, annually, quarterly, and after any significant change in the patient's physical or mental condition. All SNFs are required to send the MDS/RAPs report via modem to HCFA. (It is anticipated that in the future HCFA will correlate physicians' billings with the MDS report and any significant discrepancies found may result in Medicare audits.)

Most physicians who manage patients in SNFs are still unfamiliar with the MDS and RAPs. The MDS assessment includes the medical history, medical status, physical and mental functional status, sensory and physical impairments, nutritional status and requirements, special treatments or procedures, psychosocial status, discharge potential, dental condition, activities, potential, rehabilitation potential, cognitive status, and drug therapy. The scored responses on the MDS trigger the use of RAPs, which involve 18 common clinical syndromes that occur in SNFs, especially the geriatric patients *(please see Table 2.)*

The medical staff should make greater use of the information contained in the MDS and RAPs algorithms. The nurses are responsible for completing the MDS/RAPs and they rely on the physicians' comprehensive assessment of the patient—especially diagnoses and conditions that affect function. Primary examples of these types of diagnoses and health conditions are contained in various sections of the MDS *(please see Table 3)*.[14]

SNFs are nurse-orientated and the physician or practitioner must rely on timely telephone (or other) communication with the SNF nurses in order to adequately care for their elderly patients. The nurses are required to notify the physician to verify admission orders and to notify him/her of any significant changes in the patient's status. The number and complexity of patients a physician has will determine the frequency of communication required. Ouslander and colleagues published useful guidelines for notification of physicians or mid-level practitioners concerning changes in the patient's status.[15] The symptoms, signs, laboratory, and other prompters of immediate versus nonimmediate notification as outlined in these guidelines are summarized in Table 4. These guidelines are not meant to be all inclusive.

Functional Status

Geriatric patients will usually have two or more chronic illnesses that can affect function (e.g., osteoarthritis, ASHD, etc.). Elderly patients admitted to SNFs are usually higher risk (higher acuity) patients who have significant impairment of function due to more advanced chronic illnesses (e.g., moderate to severe dementia, stroke, osteoporosis-related hip fractures, etc.). However, often a lower acuity patient has to be admitted to a SNF simply because there are insufficient family and/or social support persons available at home.

Healthcare outcomes are better predicted by functional status than medical diagnoses.[16] Two reliable and validated standardized tests of functional status are the instrumental activities of daily living (IADL) and activities for daily living (ADL)—these are also found in the MDS.[17,18] Inability to perform one or more ADL is more likely to cause an elderly person to be admitted to a SNF than one or more losses of IADL functions *(please see Table 5)*.

Podsiadio and Richardson have shown that geriatric patients were independent for basic transfers if they could complete "up & go" tasks (such as chair transfers, toilet transfers, walk 50 yards, etc.) in time scores of less than 20 seconds.[19] In addition to assessing IADL and ADL, the physician should focus on aspects of the history and physical exam that can affect function *(please see Table 6)*.

Whenever possible, every effort should be aimed at bringing the entire multidisciplinary team (social services, physical and occupational therapy, nursing, physician, etc.) together to maintain and improve the functional status of each elderly SNF resident. Doing this will help ensure their best possible healthcare outcome.

Medication Usage

The elderly consume more than 33% of our nation's prescription medications, even though they currently represent only about 13% of the U.S. population.[24] The reason for this statistic is obvious—the geriatric patients have more chronic symptomatic illnesses. Unfortunately, adverse drug reactions are more likely to occur in the elderly. This is due to several age-related pharmacokinetic changes that affect drug bioavailability, half-life, and the volume of distribution *(please see Table 7)*.[25] For example, acidic drugs, such as salicylates, warfarin, phenytoin, and valproate, are bound primarily by albumin. Basic drugs, such as lidocaine, meperidine, propranolol, and carbamazepine, are mostly bound by alpha1-acid glycoprotein.[26] Additional factors that can affect drug

Table 3. Diagnoses and Health Conditions of the MDS

Disease Diagnoses

Heart/Circulation

a. Arteriosclerotic heart disease (ASHD)
b. Cardiac dysrhythmias
c. Congestive heart failure (CHF)
d. Hypertension (HTN)
e. Hypotension
f. Peripheral vascular disease
g. Other cardiovascular disease

Neurological

h. Alzheimer's disease
i. Dementia other than Alzheimer's
j. Aphasia
k. Cerebrovascular accident (stroke)
l. Multiple sclerosis
m. Parkinson's disease

Pulmonary

n. Emphysema/asthma/COPD
o. Pneumonia

Psychiatric/Mood

p. Anxiety disorder
q. Depression
r. Manic depressive (bipolar disease)

Sensory

s. Cataracts
t. Glaucoma

Other

u. Allergies
v. Anemia
w. Arthritis
x. Cancer
y. Diabetes mellitus
z. Explicit terminal prognosis
aa. Hypothyroidism
bb. Osteoporosis
cc. Seizure disorder
dd. Septicemia
ee. Urinary tract infection in last 30 days
ff. None of the above

Health Conditions

Problem Conditions

a. Constipation
b. Diarrhea
c. Dizziness/vertigo
d. Edema
e. Fecal impaction
f. Fever
g. Hallucination/delusions
h. Internal bleeding
i. Joint pain
j. Pain—resident complains or shows evidence of pain daily or almost daily
k. Recurrent lung aspirations in last 90 days
l. Shortness of breath
m. Syncope (fainting)
n. Vomiting
o. None of the above

Accidents

a. Fell in the past 30 days
b. Fell in the past 31-180 days
c. Hip fracture in the last 180 days
d. None of the above

levels, such as inflammatory disorders, renal or hepatic diseases, and drug-drug interactions, are more likely to be present in the geriatric patient.

The goals of drug therapy in the elderly must always be assessed and reassessed. For example, the therapeutic goals for a highly functional 68-year-old female diabetic will undoubtedly be different than for a bed-bound, severely demented 88-year-old female diabetic patient. Also, in Wallace and Verbeeck's opinion, the use of insulin sliding scales or other more aggressive glucose-lowering therapies is strongly discouraged in the geriatric Type II diabetic SNF patient. Wallace and Verbeeck have found that writing the following standing orders for Type II diabetics is acceptable and helps prevent unnecessary telephone calls and the more acutely dangerous symptomatic hypoglycemia: capillary blood glucose (CBG) checks PRN (but usually not more than once per day) and the nurse is to call the physician for any CBG less than 55 mg/dL or for two or more CBG levels that are greater than 250 mg/dL. The guidelines recommended by the American Diabetic Association should be modified according to what is reasonable.

As a general rule, when antipsychotic and anxiolytic medications (e.g., haloperidol, resperidone, lorazepam, etc.) are indicated, they should be started at one-third to one-half the dose of that normally used in the younger adult patient.

The safest tricyclic antidepressents (TCAs) to use are nortriptyline or desipramine—and they should primarily be given (in low doses) to patients for pain syndromes (e.g., peripheral neuropathy, etc.).

The other TCAs should not be prescribed in the older SNF patient for either depression or pain syndromes given the many other safer therapeutic options that are now available (e.g., selective serotonin reuptake inhibitors).

We now know that the elderly can benefit from the same medical interventions of the younger or middle-age adult. Increasingly, based on landmark clinical trial data that included many elderly patients (e.g., West of Scotland Study—pravastatin; Scandinavian Simvastatin Survival Study; and the Cholesterol and Recurrent Events trial—pravastatin), expert consensus panels are recommending a more aggressive stance in the treatment of various acute and chronic disorders in the elderly (e.g., the National Cholesterol Expert Panel [NCEP] guidelines).[27] For example, following these NCEP treatment guidelines in the appropriate patient can result in a significant reduction in heart attacks and strokes—leading causes of death and disability in the elderly patient.

The main questions to ask regarding drug therapy in the SNF geriatric patient are:

1. What medications have been proven to best improve and/or maintain function?
2. What medications can be stopped?
3. What are the safest drugs and what are their lowest effective doses?

Agitation and Dementia

The most common psychiatric disorder in the elderly is dementia, especially in those older than 85 years (wherein an estimated 40-50% may have dementia—two-thirds of which are secondary to probable Alzheimer's disease [AD]).[28] In the SNF setting, 70-90% of residents have one or more of the psychiatric diagnoses found in the American Psychiatric Association's *Diagnostic and Statistical Manual of Mental Disorders*, the majority being AD.[29]

All patients with dementia should be evaluated for possible reversible causes such as hypothyroidism, vitamin B_{12} deficiency, pseudodementia (depression), and neurosyphilis. A history of stroke should raise suspicion for multiinfarct dementia—the second leading cause of dementia in the elderly. Aggressive implementation of proven stroke prevention measures should be done in all appropriate geriatric patients (e.g., treatment of hypertension, use of warfarin in patients with atrial fibrillation, reduction of LDL-

Table 4. Immediate and Nonimmediate Notification Problems

Immediate Notification (Acute) Problems—Physician is notified directly or by beeper right away

Nursing staff should call 911 (for full code status patients) in situations requiring immediate action (e.g., respiratory/cardiac arrest or rapid deterioration of signs and symptoms prior to physician response)

Symptoms that are sudden in onset, represent a marked change from baseline, or are unrelieved by the already prescribed therapy (e.g., chest pain, new or worsening confusion, shortness of breath, slurred speech, weakness, dizziness/vertigo, musculoskeletal pain, severe headache, cough, nausea/vomiting/diarrhea, suicidal ideations, etc.)

Signs such as temperature > 101°F rectally, respiratory rate > 28/min, resting pulse > 110 or < 55/min, systolic blood pressure > 200 or < 90 torr, syncope, seizure, severe bleeding, laceration requiring sutures, fall with suspected serious injury, abnormal drainage, acute confusion or agitation, or new focal neurologic deficit

Laboratory results that are requested as "stat" or "same day," any "panic level" as reported by the laboratory, hematocrit < 30, WBC > 12,000, sodium (Na) < 125 or > 155, potassium (K) < 3.0 or > 5.5 (in nonhemolyzed specimen), glucose > 250 or < 60 in anyone and < 90 in a diabetic on hypoglycemic agents, BUN > 40, symptomatic UTI with positive UA, positive radiograph report that may require immediate intervention (e.g., pneumonia, fracture)

Medication errors of import (overdose or underdose) of cardiac, psychotropic, or hypoglycemic drugs

Nonimmediate Notification (Subacute) Problems

Persistent symptoms or complaints by patient or family member (e.g., constipation, anorexia, urinary incontinence, recurrent falls, weakness, ataxia, itching, etc.)

Persistent signs such as progressive weakness, significant weight loss, incontinence of stool or urine, skin rashes, chronic agitation or confusion, etc.

Other issues could include poorly controlled blood pressure or diabetes, medication issues, annual H & P lab and diagnostic study results

Table 5. Functional Assessment Tests

Activities of Daily Living (ADL)*	
1. Continence	4. Bathing
2. Transferring	5. Dressing
3. Toileting	6. Feeding
* Arranged in logical order patterned after the usual functions a person would perform after arising from bed in the morning.	
Instrumental Activities of Daily Living (IADL)	
Managing finances	Housekeeping
Taking medications	Food preparation
Using transportation	Shopping
Laundry	Telephone

cholesterol in patients with coronary artery disease, use of aspirin, etc.).

Although memory loss, decreasing ability to perform IADLs and ADLs, and progressive loss of higher cognitive function have a major effect on a person's quality of life, it is often the behavioral problems that arise in patients with dementia that present the greatest challenges to caregivers and attending physicians.

There are many nonpharmacologic approaches to management of behavioral disturbances in dementia, including: behavioral ("time outs," distraction, choice, conditioning); environmental modification (feeding, increasing or decreasing stimulation, signs/pictures); group programs (music, exercise, planned activities); touch (reassuring and caring); routines (familiar possessions and clothing); use of family members for feeding and to be in their SNF environment; and improving communication between patients and caregivers.[30]

Cholinergic agents (e.g., tacrine and donepezil) are the first class of drugs that have been approved by the FDA for the treatment of AD, although other agents such as estrogen replacement therapy may also be beneficial.[31] Tacrine and donepezil have approximately equal efficacy as shown by the Alzheimer's Disease Assessment Scale-Cognitive Subscale (ADAS-Cog), which measures memory, language, and praxis-heavily weighted toward memory.[32] Donepezil has the best tolerability and safety profile of the two and 82% of patients either improved or had no further cognitive decline after 24 weeks of therapy—it is the preferred agent.[33] The clinical trials were performed in mild to moderately severe AD as defined by the National Institute of Neurological and Communicative Disorders and Stroke-Alzheimer's Disease and Related Disorders Association (NINCDS-ADRADA),[34] as well as the *Diagnositic and Statistical Manual of Mental Disorders*, 3rd edition revised (DSM-III-R)[35] criteria for the diagnosis of probable Alzheimer's disease. The MMSE score of the individuals studied was between 10 and 26.

Donepezil has also been used in the treatment of advanced (severe) Alzheimer's (i.e., those with MMSE scores of 0). These anecdotal case studies have shown improvements in the ADL functional abilities but not in the IADL.[36] Family and caregiver satisfaction is especially related to improvement in ADLs. Although prospective clinical trial studies need to be performed in advanced AD patients, Shua-Haim and colleagues recommend that consideration for donepezil therapy be given to all AD patients.

Agitation and other behavioral problems encountered in patients with dementia are often difficult to manage in SNFs. Antipsychotic drugs can effectively reduce acute agitation and can have a role in the management of chronic behavioral disorders. However, many considerations have to be addressed, including OBRA 87 regulations on the use of antipsychotics, and the frequent and severe side effects associated with these medications.

There has been a significant decline in the short- and long-term use of antipsychotic drug usage in SNFs in the post-OBRA 87 era. This decrease in antipsychotic drug usage has resulted in an improvement in the quality of SNF care, but additional research is needed to determine the effects on patient outcomes.[37] Table 8 displays preferred treatment guidelines as adapted from an Expert Consensus Panel for Agitation in Dementia.[38]

Guiding principle: Always seek to know why the patient is agitated and initially try environmental (nondrug) interventions in the mildly agitated patient. The cause for delirium should always be determined and managed expeditiously.

Nutrition

Nutritional problems are extremely common in the geriatric patient. The adequate assessment and treatment of nutritional deficiencies in SNF patients is a key quality-of-care issue and affects healthcare outcomes. There is a decline in food intake as one gets older in spite of the increase in weight that occurs during middle age.[39] This finding suggests a change in the resting metabolic rate and physical activity that is associated with aging. Other factors that foster anorexia and the increased likelihood of nutritional deficiencies developing in the geriatric patient include: declines in olfaction and taste,[40] increased levels of cholecystokinin (a gastrointestinal satiety hormone),[41] gender differences in leptin (fat cell hormone that decreases food intake and increases metabolism) levels,[42] and circulating cytokines (e.g., cachectin).[43]

A body mass index less than 19, the unintentional loss of 5% body weight in less than 30 days (or a loss of 10% in < 6 months), and an albumin less than 3.5 mg/dL all suggest the presence of malnutrition. Table 9 shows one instrument, "SCALE," that has been shown to aid in the identification of malnutrition[44] and correlates well with the well-validated Mini Nutritional Assessment (MNA).[45]

Once malnutrition is diagnosed it is important to attempt to correct the underlying problem and facilitate adequate nutritional intake. Review all medications closely; many drugs can cause gastrointestinal problems and anorexia (e.g., most SSRIs, antibiotics, digitalis, nonsteroidal anti-inflammatory agents, etc.). Delirium, dementia, depression, and other illnesses (e.g., febrile illnesses, infections, congestive heart failure, pain syndromes, neuromuscular disorders, terminal cancers, renal failure, etc.) can adversely affect nutritional update.[46]

Dietary supplements can be helpful in malnourished patients. Carbohydrate-rich liquid supplementation is less likely to cause satiation than more fat-rich liquid supplements.[47] Frequent feeds, encouraging family to bring favorite snacks or meals, avoidance of

Table 6. Important Factors of Geriatric History and Physical Exam that can Affect Functional Status

- General—weight, height, body mass index (key indicator of nutritional status)
- Eyes—check visual acuity; r/o presbyopia, cataracts, glaucoma, macular degeneration
- Ears—check for presbycusis (high-frequency acuity loss)—use finger rub or whispered voice
- Mouth—oral hygiene, dentition (loose dentures, missing teeth, malocclusion)
- Lungs—quantify dyspnea or any chronic lung disorders
- Cardiovascular—check for bruits, heart gallops, congestive heart failure, atrial fibrillation; check pulses and orthostatic changes
- Gastrointestinal—rectal exam for occult blood, masses, or fecal impaction
- Genitourinary—r/o atrophic vaginitis, urinary incontinence, prostate hypertrophy
- Musculoskeletal—r/o osteoporosis, arthritis; check muscle strength
- Neurological—check gait and balance by direct observation (consider using Tinnetti exam);[20] r/o focal neurological deficits or peripheral neuropathy
- Mental status—r/o cognitive impairment (mental status testing); can do quick short-term memory testing by asking patient to recall 3 unrelated words/objects after spelling "WORLD" backward—if patient is not completely accurate do a full Mini-Mental State Exam (MMSE);[21] check for depression using the Geriatric Depression Scale,[22,23] agitation, or thought disorders
- Endocrine—r/o diabetes, hypothyroidism, or hyperlipidemia
- Skin—check for decubitae (if present, is highly suggestive of impaired mobility)

restricted diets, and a supportive eating environment are all important measures that can be taken. If long-term enteral feeding tubes are required, gastrostomy tubes are preferred over nasogastric enteral feeding tubes, and continuous enteral feeding techniques are preferred over bolus feeding in the nonambulatory patient (due to an increased risk of aspiration associated with bolus feeding). It is important to note that there is no difference in survival between tube-fed and those who were not. Generally, most patients require 25-30 kcal/kg ideal body weight (IBW) per day for maintenance (20 kcal/kg/d to lose weight and 40 kcal/kg/d to gain weight).

Prevention

The U.S. Preventive Services task force has published preventive recommendations to be used in the asymptomatic elderly patient.[48] However, evidence-based preventive measures with directly proven benefit in the asymptomatic elderly person include: tobacco use history, blood pressure measurements, blood glucose and cholesterol testing, evaluating vision and hearing, initiating estrogen replacement for women, and ensuring current tetanus, influenza, and pneumococcal immunizations.[49] Mammography, pelvic exams, hemoccult stool testing, and prostate-specific antigen testing can also be useful in the appropriate SNF patient.

Approximately 25% of the tuberculosis (TB) cases in the United States occur in elderly persons and SNF patients are at an even higher risk.[50] All SNF patients/residents should receive a two-step tuberculin skin test on admission or a screening chest radiograph. The established recommendations by the Centers for Disease Control should be followed regarding the surveillance, containment, assessment, and reporting of TB infection and TB disease.[51]

Prevention and treatment of decubitus ulcers primarily relate to increasing a patient's functional status and mobility. Otherwise, frequent turning (at least every 2 hours) and a red-uction in skin moisture and friction are fundamental therapies.

More aggressive use of proven medical therapies that can help prevent stroke—the leading cause of chronic disability in the United States—should be considered in the appropriate patient. These therapies include: warfarin use in atrial fibrillation,[52] HMG-Coenzyme A reductase inhibitor use in coronary artery disease,[53] antihyperten-

Table 7. Age-Related Changes Affecting Medications

- Decrease in total body water weight (plasma volume remains essentially unchanged)
- Decrease in glomerular filtration rate and renal clearance
- Decrease in hepatic blood flow and hepatic clearance
- Decrease in cell membrane receptors and sensitivity
- Increase in relative body fat content
- Albumin concentration decreases and alpha1-acid glycoprotein concentration increases

sive treatment,[54] and other alternative treatments in patients with known atherosclerosis (e.g., aspirin, ticlodipine, clopidogrel).[55]

Special Treatment Considerations

Physical Restraints and Falls. Try to avoid their use if at all possible. The more functional SNF geriatric patients may be more likely to fall. However, if they are restrained they may be even more susceptible to serious injury.[56] Look closely at reasons for repeat falls in any SNF geriatric resident.

Urinary Incontinence. Look for treatable causes (e.g., delirium/dementia, urinary tract infections, atrophic vaginitis, medications, diabetes, restricted mobility, and stool impaction) and categorize the incontinence as stress, urge, or overflow and treat accordingly. Avoid using indwelling or external catheters unless the patient has severe pressure sores, is in hospice care, or has expressed a preference for catheter use.

Pressure Ulcers. Good SNFs should be able to keep the incidence of pressure ulcers less than 5%. Adequate nursing protocols and SNF policies are essential. Try not to use topical agents containing povidone or hydrogen peroxide because they may delay the healing process. If wet-to-dry dressings are ordered, make sure they are changed frequently enough. The aim is to keep the inside of the wound/ulcer moist but the surrounding skin dry. Shallow stage II-III decubitae can often be managed conservatively and respond well to hydrocolloid, 1% silver sulfadiazine, transparent adhesive dressing, bacitracin zinc, and similar topical dressings.[57] In Alvarez and associates' opinion the single most important risk factor for pressure ulcer development is immobility.

Hospice. Judicious use of this valuable service is warranted. However, all patients who have less than six months to live do not have to be enrolled in a hospice program—even though they may technically qualify. Hospice is a healthcare resource that should be used appropriately. Hospice can be helpful especially in terminal patients with significant pain and suffering and in aiding families who are having difficulty coping with the death and dying process.

Diagnostic Testing/Hospitalization/Advanced Directives. Each SNF geriatric patient is different. Although many may carry

Table 8. Agitation in Patients with Dementia: Expert Panel Treatment Guidelines

Environmental Intervention Options

- Mild and severe agitation—education and support for family and caregivers
- Mild agitation—structured routines, reassurance, socialization
- Severe agitation—supervision and environmental safety

Medications and Specific Presentations of Agitation

- Psychosis—(acute) conventional high potency antipsychotic = CHAP; (long-term) risperidone, CHAP
- Depression—(without psychosis) antidepressant alone: sertraline or paroxetine; (with psychosis) antidepressant + antipsychotic (consider electroconvulsive therapy)
- Anxiety—(acute) benzodiazepine: lorazepam, consider oxazepam; (long-term) buspirone
- Insomnia—(acute) trazodone, consider lorazepam or zolpidem; (long-term) trazadone
- "Sundowning"—(acute) trazodone; consider CHAP, resperidone, olanzapine; (long-term) trazodone; consider resperidone, olanzapine, or CHAP
- Aggression or anger—(mild, acute) trazodone; (mild, long-term) divalproex, selective serotonin reuptake inhibitor = SSRI, trazodone, buspirone; (severe, acute) CHAP, risperidone; (severe, long-term) divalproex, resperidone, or CHAP
- Osteoarthritic pain—despiramine or nortryptiline, SSRIs, trazodone

IM Medication for Acute Interventions—haloperidol alone, consider lorazepam alone

Safest Medications for Long-Term Use—SSRIs, buspirone

Safest Medication Choices for Patients with High Medical Comorbidity

- Antipsychotics—risperidone
- Anxiolytics—buspirone
- Anticonvulsants—divalproex
- Antidepressants—SSRIs
- For sleep—trazodone

Medication Least Likely to Cause Drug Interactions—buspirone

Table 9. SCALE: A Malnutrition Detection Instrument

S	Sadness (Geriatric Depression Scale)
C	Cholesterol less than 160 mg/dL
A	Albumin less than 3.5 mg/dL
L	Loss of 5% of body weight
E	Eating problems (physical or cognitive)

the same diagnoses, the decision to do more advanced testing, hospitalize, etc., will depend on several factors particular for each individual. The primary guiding questions are: 1) "Will this test or treatment significantly improve this patient's quality of life?" 2) "What is the patient's (or surrogate decision-maker's) informed decision as stated in his/her advanced directives?"

The attending physician should provide the patient (and family) with the treatment options accompanied with his/her recommendations. The physician can be helpful in providing guidance to the patient and their family. Most patients want to be assured of no undue pain or suffering and to maintain their personal dignity. Physicians and practitioners can be of great assistance in helping families cope with death and dying.

Summary

The number of geriatric patients in SNFs will continue to grow substantially. It is therefore essential that physicians become more knowledgeable about the aging process and maintain a sensitivity to the particular needs of the geriatric SNF resident. The attending physician should always seek to appropriately maximize the elderly SNF resident's functional status and to prescribe proven therapies that improve outcomes and quality of life. In most patients, but especially in the elderly, concerns about the quality of life supercede longevity issues.

The attending physician should be aware of the unique environment of the SNF and the governing OBRA regulations. He/she should make use of the MDS and RAPs in developing the specific treatment goals of each patient and should communicate effectively with the nursing staff.

Physicians caring for geriatric patients in SNFs should also consider subscribing to relevant publications by the American Geriatrics Society and the American Medical Directors Association (AMDA).

References

1. Calkins E, Davis PJ, Ford AB: *The Practice of Geriatrics*. Philadelphia: W.B. Saunders;1986.
2. FIND/SVP: *The Long Term Care Market: A Market Intelligence Report*. New York; FIND/SVP, 1993.
3. Ouslander J, Osterweil D, Morley J. *Medical Care in the Nursing Home*. 2nd ed. New York, New York: McGraw-Hill; 1997.
4. Shaughnessy PW, Dramer AM. *N Engl J Med* 1990;332: 1-27.
5. Smith RL, Osterweil D. The medical director in hospital-based transitional care units. *Clinics in Geriatric Medicine (Medical Direction in Long-term Care)*. Philadelphia: W.B. Saunders Co., Vol. 11(3), August 1995:375.
6. Institute of Medicine, Committee on Nursing Home Regulation. *Improving the Quality of Care of Nursing Homes*. Washington, DC: National Academy Press 1986.
7. Feldman J, Boulter C, eds. *Minimum Data Set Plus: Multistate Nursing Home case Mix and Quality Demonstration Training Manual*. Natick, MA: Eliot Press, 1991.
8. McCarthy JF, et al. *Annals of Long-Term Care* 1999;7: 35-43.
9. Kane RI, et al. *Annual Review of Public Health* 1993;14: 545-584.
10. Elon R, Pawlson LG. *J Am Geriatr Soc* 1992;2:394-398.
11. Institute of Medicine, Committee on Nursing Home Regulation. *Improving the Quality of Care of Nursing Homes*. Washington, DC: National Academy Press, 1986.
12. Elon RD. Omnibus Budget Reconciliation Act of 1987 and its implications for the medical director. *Clinics in Geriatric Medicine (Medical Direction in Long-Term Care)*. Philadelphia: W.B. Saunders Co., Vol. 11(3), August 1995: 426.
13. Zisselman MH, et al. *Annals of Long-Term Care* 1998;6: 200.
14. State Operations Manual. Minimum Data Set 2.0. US Department of Health and Human Services. Health Care Finance Administration (HCFA). Washington, DC: 1997
15. Ouslander J, et al. *J Am Geriatr Soc* 1990;38:490-492.
16. Norain P, et al. *J Am Geriatr Soc* 1988;36:775-783.
17. Lawton MP, Brody EM. *Gerontologist* 1969;9:179-186.
18. Katz S. *J Am Geriatr Soc* 1983;31:721-727.
19. Podsiado D, Richardson S. *J Am Geriatr Soc* 1991;39:142.
20. Tinetti ME. *J Am Geriatr Soc* 1986;34:119.
21. Folstein MF, et al. *J Psychiatr Res* 1975;12:189-198.
22. Yesavage JA, et al. *J Psychiatr Res* 1983;17:37-49.
23. Burke WJ, et al. *J Am Geriatr Soc* 1992:40:922-935.
24. Stason WB, et al. *J Am Coll Cardiol* 1987;10:18A-22A.
25. Yuen GJ. *Clin Geriatr Med* 1990;6:257-267.
26. Wallace SM, Verbeeck RK. *Clin Pharmacokinet* 1987;12: 41-72.
27. Summary of the Second Report of the National Cholesterol Education Program Expert Panel on Detection, Evaluation, and Treatment of High Blood Cholesterol in Adults. *JAMA* 1993;269:3015.
28. Evans DA, et al. *JAMA* 1989;262:2551-2556.
29. Rovner BW, et al. *Am J Psychiatry* 1986;143:1446-1449.
30. Grossberg GT. *Alzheimer's Disease—Management Today* 1998;1:4-7.
31. Yaffe K, et al. *JAMA* 1998;279:688-695.
32. Olin JT, Schneider LS. *Int J Geriatr Psychiatry* 1995;10: 753-756.
33. Rogers SL, et al. *Dementia* 1996;7:293-303.
34. Mckhann G, et al. *Neurology* 1984;34:939-944.
35. American Psychiatric Association. Committee on Nomenclature and Statistics. *Diagnostic and Statistical*

Manual of Mental Disorders. 3rd ed rev. Washington, DC: APA;1987:121.

36. Shua-Haim JR, et al. *Annals of Long-Term Care* 1999;7: 67-71.
37. Shorr RI, et al. *JAMA* 1994;271:358-362.
38. Alexopoulos GS, et al. The Expert Consensus Guideline Series: Treatment of agitation in older persons with dementia. Postgraduate Medicine Special Report; April 1998.
39. *MMWR Morb Mortal Wkly Rep* 1994;43:116-125.
40. Morley JE. *Am J Clin Nutr* 1997;66:760-773.
41. Bertelemy P, et al. *J Am Geriatr Soc* 1992;40:R755-R761.
42. Sih R, et al. *J Clin Endocrinol Metab* 1997;82:1661-1667.
43. Merguid MM, et al. *Nutrition* 1996;12:557-562.
44. Morley JE, et al. *Annals of Long-Term Care* 1998; 6(Supp E:1-12.
45. Guigoz Y, et al. *Nutr Rev* 1996;54:S59-S65.
46. Morley JE, Silver AJ. *Ann Intern Med* 1995;123:850.
47. Shafer RB, et al. *Am J Physiol* 1985;248:R479-R483.
48. U.S. Preventive Services Task Force. *Guide to preventive services*. 2nd ed. Baltimore: Williams Wilkins, 1996.
49. Frame PS. *Am Fam Physician* 1999;59:1747-1750.
50. Yoshikawa TT. *Nursing Home Medicine* 1995;3:207.
51. *MMWR Morb Mortal Wkly Rep* 1990;39(No. RR-10):1.
52. Atrial Fibrillation Investigators. *Arch Intern Med* 1994;154: 1449-1457.
53. Hebert PR, et al. *JAMA* 1997;278:313-321.
54. SHEP Coorperative Research Group. *JAMA* 1991;265:3255-3264.
55. Matchar DB, et al. *Ann Intern Med* 1994;121:41-53.
56. Capezuti E, et al. *J Gerontol A Biol Sci Med Sci* 1998;53: M47-M52.
57. Alvarez O, et al. *Wounds*. Wayne, PA: Health Management Publications Inc., 1989:35-51.

Community-Acquired Pneumonia in the Elderly

Gideon Bosker, MD, FACEP

A common cause for admission of elderly patients from the emergency department (ED) to the hospital, community-acquired pneumonia (CAP) is a serious, growing health problem in the United States. It has an incidence estimated at 4 million cases annually.[1,2] Approximately 600,000 hospitalizations for CAP are reported each year at an annual cost of about $23 billion.[1,3] Mortality rates among the most seriously affected patients (the majority of whom are in the geriatric age group) approaches 40%, and causative pathogens are identified in fewer than 50% of patients.[4-6] Accordingly, empiric antibiotic regimens frequently are chosen in the elderly population on the basis of results of clinical trials.

Despite a general consensus that empiric treatment of CAP in elderly patients requires, at the least, mandatory coverage of such organisms as *Streptococcus pneumoniae, Haemophilus influenzae,* and *Moraxella catarrhalis,* as well as atypical organisms (*Mycoplasma pneumoniae, Chlamydia pneumoniae,* and *Legionella pneumophila),* antibiotic selection strategies for achieving this spectrum of coverage vary widely. New treatment guidelines for CAP have been issued by some national associations (Infectious Disease Society of America [IDSA]) and the Centers for Disease Control and Prevention (CDC) Drug-Resistant Streptococcus pneumoniae Therapeutic Working Group. These newer strategies are in addition to those contained in the guidelines published by the American Thoracic Society (ATS).

Deciphering the strengths, subtleties, and weaknesses of recommendations issued by different authoritative sources can be problematic and confusing. Because patient disposition practices and treatment pathways vary among institutions and from region to region, management guidelines for CAP in the geriatric patient must be "customized" for the local practice environment. Unfortunately, no single set of guidelines is applicable to every patient or practice environment; therefore, clinical judgment must prevail. This means taking into account local antibiotic resistance patterns, epidemiological and infection incidence data, and patient demographic features.

It also is becoming clear that the outcomes for CAP in the elderly can be maximized by using risk-stratification criteria that predict mortality associated with CAP. Associated clinical findings such as hypotension, tachypnea, impaired oxygen saturation, multi-lobar involvement, elevated blood urea nitrogen, and altered level of consciousness are predictive of more serious disease, as are age and acquisition of CAP in a nursing home environment. These factors may assist clinicians in initial selection of intravenous antibiotic therapy for hospitalized patients.

Because of important advances, changes, and refinements that have occurred in the area of CAP treatment over the past year, this landmark review presents a comprehensive, state-of-the-art assessment of guidelines for management of the geriatric patient with CAP. Special emphasis has been given to both epidemiological data demonstrating the importance of correct spectrum coverage with specific macrolides or fluoroquinolones and the selection of initial intravenous antibiotics for in-hospital management of CAP. The need to provide prophylaxis against venous thromboembolic disease (VTED) in elderly patients with pneumonia and/or congestive heart failure (CHF) or respiratory failure also is addressed.

In addition, a detailed analysis and comparison of monotherapeutic (azithromycin or levofloxacin) vs. two-drug (cephalosporin plus a macrolide) approaches for initial therapy is provided. To ensure our readers are current with and can apply the latest evidence-based strategies for CAP treatment to their elderly population, detailed antibiotic selection guidelines are provided. Drawing upon consensus panels and association guidelines, these antimicrobial protocols are linked to risk-stratification criteria and specific clinical profiles of elderly patients presenting to the hospital or acute ambulatory setting with CAP.

Diagnosis and Evaluation

The annual incidence of pneumonia in patients older than 65 years is about 1%.[7] The typical presentation of pneumococcal pneumonia with fever, rigors, shortness of breath, chest pain, sputum production, and abnormal lung sounds is easy to recognize. Unfortunately, the changing epidemiology of pneumonia presents a greater diagnostic challenge. Atypical agents or opportunistic infections in immunocompromised patients have a much more subtle presentation. Pneumonia in older patients frequently has an insidious presentation with fewer characteristic features of pneumonia, which may be confused with CHF or respiratory compromise associated with chronic long disease.

The definitive, etiologic diagnosis of pneumonia is verified by the recovery of a pathogenic organism(s) from either the blood, sputum, or pleural fluid in the setting of a patient with a radiographic abnormality suggestive of pneumonia. In the case of atypical organisms, the diagnosis is made by the comparison of acute and convalescent sera demonstrating a rise in appropriate titers, or by other sophisticated techniques such as direct florescent antibody testing. The Gram's stain is occasionally helpful in establishing the diagnosis, but requires practitioners or technicians who are highly skilled in this diagnostic methodology. An adequate Gram's stain must have fewer than 25 epithelial cells per low-powered field. The finding of more than 10 gram-positive, lancet shaped diplococci in a high-powered field is a sensitive and specific predictor of pneumococcal pneumonia. Unfortunately, the Gram's stain will rarely be helpful in determining other causes of pneumonia.

Transtracheal aspiration or bronchial washings are a more accurate means of obtaining specimens for Gram's stains and culture, although this procedure is rarely indicated in the outpatient setting. Overall, fewer than 50% of patients with CAP will be able to produce sputum. Of these, one-half of the sputum specimens obtained will be inadequate. When an adequate Gram's stain is obtained, however, it has a negative predictive value of 80% when compared to a sputum culture. The blood culture is helpful in about 15% of patients, while serology will establish the diagnosis in 25% of patients.[7,8] About 40% of sputum cultures will identify a pathologic organism. Bronchoscopy and thoracentesis may occasionally be necessary, but these procedures generally are reserved for seriously ill patients, particularly those who require management in the ICU setting.[3,5,8]

Signs and Symptoms. Especially in the elderly patient, the signs and symptoms of pneumonia may be mimicked by many disorders, including pulmonary embolism (PE), CHF, lung cancer, hypersensitivity pneumonitis, tuberculosis, chronic obstructive pulmonary disease (COPD), granulomatosis disease, and fungal infections. A variety of drugs also can induce pulmonary disease. Cytotoxic agents, non-steroidal anti-inflammatory drugs (NSAIDs), and some antibiotics, including sulfonamides and certain antiarrhythmics, such as amiodarone or tocainide, can mimic pulmonary infection. In addition, common analgesics, including salicylates, propoxyphene, and methadone, also may precipitate acute respiratory symptoms. Such collagen vascular diseases as systemic lupus erythematosus, polymyositis, and polyarteritis nodosa may cause fever, cough, dyspnea, and pulmonary infiltrates, thereby mimicking symptoms of pneumonia. Rheumatoid arthritis can cause an interstitial lung disease, although it does not usually cause fever or alveolar infiltrates.

Initial Stabilization and Adjunctive Measures

Prompt, aggressive, and adequate supportive care must be provided to geriatric patients who present to the hospital with pneumonia. As is the case with other serious conditions, supportive care frequently must be performed in conjunction with the history, physical examination, and diagnostic testing. Among initial stabilization measures, managing the airway and ensuring adequate breathing, oxygenation, ventilation, and perfusion are of paramount importance.

Upon arrival to the hospital, oxygenation status should be assessed immediately using pulse-oximetry. Patients with an arterial oxygen saturation of less than 90% should receive supplemental oxygen. Arterial blood gases are especially helpful in patients suspected of hypercarbia and respiratory failure. This laboratory modality may be useful in patients with COPD, decreased mental status, and fatigue. Patients with hypoxia who do not respond to supplemental oxygen, as well as those with hypercarbia accompanied by respiratory acidosis, may be candidates for mechanical ventilation. This may be accomplished with either intubation and mechanical ventilation or non-invasive ventilation (bilevel positive pressure ventilation [BiPAP]). Recent studies have shown BiPAP to be successful in treating patients with respiratory failure due to pneumonia.[9] When this technique is available to the emergency physician, it may avert the need for endotracheal intubation and its potential complications.

Patients with evidence of bronchospasm on physical exam, as well as those with a history of obstructive airways disease (asthma or COPD), may benefit from inhaled bronchodilator therapy.

Evidence of inadequate perfusion may range from mild dehydration with tachycardia to life-threatening hypotension due to septic shock. Patients with septic shock usually will show evidence of decreased tissue perfusion, such as confusion and oliguria in association with a hyperdynamic circulation. In either case, initial therapy consists of intravenous fluids (normal saline or lactated Ringer's solution) administered through a large bore IV. In elderly patients, fluid overload is a potential complication, and it is wise to administer IV fluids in bolus doses with frequent assessment of response.

Risk Stratification and Patient Disposition: Outpatient Vs. Inpatient Management

Overview. Determining whether to admit or discharge an elderly patient with pneumonia is one of the most important, and potentially, cost-incurring decisions an emergency physician, pulmonologist, or internist can make. For this reason, there have been increasing efforts to identify patients with CAP who can appropriately be treated as outpatients.[10-13] The disposition decision for geriatric patients with pneumonia should take into account the severity of the pneumonia, as well as other medical and psychosocial factors that may affect the treatment plan and clinical outcome.[14-16]

In the absence of respiratory distress or other complicating factors, many young adults can be adequately treated with appropriate oral antibiotic therapy. This is less often the case for the elderly patient with CAP, because comorbid conditions and other risk factors may complicate the course of the illness. Even when following appropriate treatment and dispositon, patients may have symptoms, including cough, fatigue, dyspnea, sputum production, and chest pain that can last for several months. To address this issue of patient disposition and treatment setting, a variety of investigators have proposed criteria to identify patients requiring hospitalization. Patients felt to be at low risk have a median length of stay of seven days, while those at medium risk have a median length of stay of 12-13 days.

Among the factors most physicians use to make admission decisions for pneumonia are the presence of hypoxemia, overall clinical status, the ability to maintain oral intake, hemodynamic status, and the patient's home environment. Using clinical judgment, however, physicians tend to overestimate the likelihood of death from pneumonia.[14] These findings have led some investigators to employ more stringent prediction rules. For example, the chest radiograph may help identify patients who are at high risk for mortality. The presence of bilateral effusions, moderate-size pleural effusions, multi-lobar involvement, and bilateral infiltrates are associated with a higher risk of mortality.

A recent landmark study outlined below presented a prediction rule (Pneumonia Severity Index [PSI]) to identify low-risk patients with CAP.[11] Using such objective criteria as patient age, coexistent medical conditions, and vital signs, patients are assigned either to a low-risk class, which has a mortality rate of about 0.1% in outpatients, or to higher risk categories. Patients with any risk factors are then evaluated with a second scoring system that assigns individuals to one of three higher risk categories, which have mortality rates ranging from 0.7% to 31%.[14] In addition to the factors noted in this prediction rule, patients who are immunocompromised as a result of AIDS or chronic alcohol use frequently require hospitalization.

Once the clinician has determined hospitalization is required, the need for intensive care unit (ICU) admission also must be evaluated. A variety of factors are associated with an increased risk for mortality, including increasing age (> 65 years), alcoholism, chronic lung disease, immunodeficiency, and specific laboratory abnormalities, including azotemia and hypoxemia. These patients may require admission to the ICU.

Prognostic Scoring. There have been many efforts to assess severity and risk of death in patients with pneumonia.[15,17-20] The study by Fine and colleagues has received considerable attention and is used as a benchmark by many clinicians.[14] This study developed a prediction rule, the PSI, to assess 30-day mortality in patients with CAP. The rule was derived and validated with data from more than 52,000 inpatients, and then validated with a second cohort of 2287 inpatients and outpatients as part of the Pneumonia PORT study. Subsequent evaluation and validation has been performed with other cohorts, including geriatric patients and nursing home residents.[21,22]

In this risk-stratification scheme, patients are assigned to one of five risk classes (1 is lowest risk, 5 is highest risk) based upon a point system that considers age, co-existing disease, abnormal physical findings, and abnormal laboratory findings. Elderly patients cannot be assigned to Class 1, as a requirement is age younger than 50 years.[14]

In older patients, age contributes the most points to the overall score. For example, it should be noted that males ages older than 70 years and females ages older than 80 years would be assigned to Class 3 on the basis of age alone, without any other risk factor. In the Fine study, patients assigned to Class 1 and 2 were typically younger patients (median age, 35-59 years) and patients in Class 3-5 were older (median age, 72-75 years).

Outpatient management is recommended for Classes 1 and 2, brief inpatient observation for Class 3, and traditional hospitalization for Classes 4 and 5.[15,15,23] For a geriatric patient to qualify for outpatient treatment based on these recommendations, he or she would have to be younger than 70 years of age if male or younger than 80 years of age if female, and have no additional risk factors. Inpatient observation or traditional hospitalization would be recommended for all other patients based on this rule. Other studies have suggested outpatient management for Class 3 patients.[11,24]

Geriatric patients considered eligible for management as outpatients must be able to take oral fluids and antibiotics, comply with outpatient care, and must be able to carry out activities of daily living (ADLs) or have adequate home support to assist with ADLs.[14-16] Other factors cited in previous studies but not included in the PSI also have been found to increase the risk of morbidity or mortality from pneumonia. These include: other comorbid illnesses (diabetes mellitus, COPD, post-splenectomy state), altered mental status, suspicion of aspiration, chronic alcohol abuse or malnutrition, and evidence of extrapulmonary disease.[8] Additional laboratory studies that may suggest increased severity of illness include white blood cell count less than 4 or greater than 30, absolute neutrophil count less than 1, elevated protime or partial thromboplastin time, decreased platelet count, or radiographic evidence of multilobar involvement, cavitation, and rapid speeding.[8]

Severe pneumonia may require ICU admission. In the Fine study, 6% of patients in Class 3, 11% of patients in Class 4, and 17% of patients in Class 5 required ICU admission.[14] The ATS guidelines define severe pneumonia as the presence of at least one of the following: respiratory rate greater than 30, severe respiratory failure ($PaO_2/FIO_2 < 250$), mechanical ventilation, bilateral infiltrates or multilobar infiltrates, shock, vasopressor requirement, or oliguria (urine output < 20 cc per hour). The presence of at least one of these is highly sensitive (98%) but only 32% specific for the need for ICU management.[25] It is emphasized that the above guidelines for admission should not supersede clinical judgment when assessing the need to hospitalize patients.[8,14,15,23]

Antibiotic Selection for the Elderly Patient with Pneumonia

Introduction. Antibiotic therapy is the mainstay of management for geriatric patients with CAP. It should be stated at the outset that antibiotic therapy should be initiated promptly, as soon as the diagnosis is strongly suspected or confirmed, and after appropriate microbiological studies or samples have been obtained. Because the elderly are at high risk for acquiring pneumonia, many of the guidelines issued by consensus panels, clinical experts, and scientific associations, including those of the IDSA, the ATS, and the CDC Drug-Resistant Streptococcus pneumoniae Therapeutic Working Group, apply directly to this patient population. Therefore, these recommendations should be studied in detail to arrive at sensible, empiric pharmacotherapeutic interventions for the elderly patient with pneumonia. Although the CDC group makes no specific recommendations for geriatric patients, their guidelines apply to all adult patients; hence, their conclusions are applicable to the geriatric patient with CAP.

Consensus Panels. It should be stressed that there is no absolute or consistent consensus on precisely which drug, or combination of drugs, constitutes the most outcome-effective choice for pneumonia in the geriatric patient. Most panels and guideline documents agree that antimicrobial coverage must include sufficient activity against the bacterial pathogens *S. pneumoniae, H. influenzae*, and *M. catarrhalis*, as well as against the atypical pathogens *Mycoplasma, Legionella*, and *C. pneumoniae*. Therefore, such agents as azithromycin and levofloxacin which, because of their activity against both bacterial and atypical pathogens commonly encountered in CAP, have supplanted cephalosporins as preferred monotherapeutic options for treatment of appropriate patients with pneumonia.

Beyond this non-negotiable caveat mandating coverage for the six aforementioned pathogens, there are important differences among recommendations and expert panels for empiric treatment of pneumonia. Variations among the guidelines usually depend upon: 1) their emphasis or focus on the need to empirically cover drug-resistant *Streptococcus pneumoniae* (DRSP) species as part of the initial antimicrobial regimen; 2) their concern about using antimicrobials (fluoroquinolones) with an over-extended (too broad) spectrum of coverage; 3) their concern about the potential of growing resistance to a class (fluoroquinolones) which has agents that currently are active against DRSP species; 4) their preference for monotherapeutic vs. combination therapy; 5) when the guidelines were released (recent vs several years old); and 6) their emphasis on drug costs, patient convenience, and options for step-down (IV to oral) therapeutic approaches. Clearly, these factors and the relative emphasis placed on each of them will influence antimicrobial selection for the geriatric patient with pneumonia.

With these issues and drug selection factors in mind, the most recent guidelines issued by the CDC Drug-Resistant Streptococcus pneumoniae Therapeutic Working Group attempts to both risk-stratify and "drug-stratify" patients according to their eligibility for receiving agents as initial empiric therapy that have activity against DRSP. Before presenting a detailed discussion of the current treatment landscape for CAP, the following points from this expert panel should be emphasized. First, the relative importance of *S. pneumoniae* as a cause of outpatient CAP in the elderly patient is difficult to determine. Nevertheless, a review of the literature suggests that *S. pneumoniae* accounts for 2-27% of all cases of CAP treated on an outpatient basis.[7,26,27] In addition, surveillance studies have suggested that about 7% of invasive *S. pneumoniae* species in the United States showed a significant degree of penicillin resistance.[28] Hence, this group estimates that only 0.14% (7% of 2%) to 1.9% (7% 0f 27%) of outpatients with bacterial pneumonia have pneumococcal infections with levels of resistance high enough to warrant consideration of alternative treatment.

This analysis has made the CDC panel conclude that because outpatient CAP in patients who are appropriately triaged and risk-stratified is generally not immediately life-threatening and because *S. pneumoniae* isolates with penicillin MICs of no less than 4 mcg/mL are uncommon, antibiotics with predictable activity against highly penicillin-resistance pneuomococci are not necessary as part of the initial regimen. From a practical, drug-selection perspective, the working group, therefore, suggests that oral fluoroquinolones are not first-line treatment in elderly outpatients with CAP because of concerns about emerging resistance. Consequently, oral macrolide or beta-lactam monotherapy is recommended by the CDC working group as initial therapy in patients with pneumonia considered to be amenable to outpatient management.

It should be noted, however, that even for hospitalized (non-ICU) patients, the panel, while noting the effectiveness of monotherapy with selected fluoroquinolones, recommends the combination of a parenteral beta-lactam (cefotaxime, ceftriaxone, etc.) plus a macrolide (azithromycin, erythromycin, etc.) for initial therapy.[2] Regardless of the panel or critical pathway, one of the important consistent changes among recent recommendations for initial, empiric management of patients with CAP is mandatory inclusion of a macrolide (which covers atypical pathogens) when a cephalosporin (which has poor activity against atypical pathogens) is selected as part of the regimen.

For critically ill patients, first-line therapy should include an intravenous beta-lactam, such as ceftriaxone or cefotaxime, and an intravenous macrolide, such as azithromycin or erythromycin (see discussion below). The option of using a combination of a parenteral beta-lactam (cefotaxime, ceftriaxone, etc.) plus a fluoroquinolone with improved activity against DRSP also is presented. Once again, however, this committee issues clarifying, and sometimes cautionary, statements about the role of fluoroquinolone monotherapy in the critically ill patient, stating that caution should be exercised because the efficacy of the new fluoroquinolones as monotherapy for critically ill patients has not been determined.[2]

Clearly, however, fluoroquinolones are an important part of the antimicrobial arsenal in the elderly, and The CDC Drug-Resistant Streptococcus pneumoniae Therapeutic Working Group has issued specific guidelines governing their use in the setting of outpatient and inpatient CAP. In general, this panel has recommended that fluoroquinolones be reserved for selected patients with CAP, and these experts have identified specific patient subgroups that are eligible for initial treatment with extended-spectrum fluoroquinolones. For hospitalized patients, these include adults for whom one of the first-line regimens (e.g., cephalosporin plus a macrolide) has failed, those who are allergic to the first-line agents, or those who have a documented infection with highly drug-resistant pneumococci (i.e., penicillin MIC ≥ 4 mcg/mL).[2] The rationale for this approach is discussed in subsequent sections below.

With these considerations in focus, the purpose of this antimicrobial treatment section is to review the various recommendations, consensus panel statements, clinical trials, and published guidelines. A rational analysis of this information also will be performed, in order to generate a set of guidelines and protocols for specific populations as these issues relate to the geriatric patient.

Antibiotic Overview. A brief overview of agents that have been used for treatment of CAP will help set the stage for outcome-effective drug selection. *(Please see Table 1.)* The first-generation cephalosporins have significant coverage against gram-positive organisms. By comparison, third-generation cephalosporins have less gram-positive coverage and increased coverage against aerobic gram-negative rods.[29] Ceftazidime has coverage against *Pseudomonas*, while cefoperazone has a somewhat higher MIC. Some of the second-generation cephalosporins, such as cefoxitin, cefotetan, and cefmetazole, provide coverage against *Bacteroides* species. Imipenem has broad coverage against aerobic and anaerobic organisms. Aztreonam provides significant coverage for gram-negative bacilli such as *Pseudomonas*.

Among the beta-lactams, the CDC Drug-Resistant Streptococcus pneumoniae Therapeutic Working Group identifies cefuroxime axetil, cefotaxime sodium, ceftriaxone sodium, or ampicillin-sulbactam as recommended empiric agents. The group notes, however, that among these agents, cefotaxime and ceftriaxone have superior activity against resistant pneumonococci when compared with cefuroxime and ampicillin-sulbactam.[2]

The aminoglycosides are active against gram-negative aerobic organisms. These agents are generally used for elderly patients with severe CAP, particularly when it involves *Pseudomonas*. As a rule, they are combined with a third-generation cephalosporin or an extended spectrum quinolone antibiotic, monobactam, or an extended spectrum penicillin when used in these circumstances.[30]

The tetracyclines are active against *Streptococcus pneumoniae, H. influenza, Mycoplasma, Chlamydia*, and *Legionella*. There is, however, a growing incidence of *S. pneumoniae* resistance to tetracyclines.[31] These agents are alternatives to the macrolide antibiotics for empiric therapy for CAP in young, healthy adults.[32] Convenience and coverage advantages of the new macrolides, however, have thrust the tetracyclines into a secondary role for managing CAP. Clindamycin has activity against the anaerobes, such as *B. fragilis, S. pneumoniae,* and *S. aureus*.[33,34] Its anaerobic coverage makes it a consideration for the treatment of pneumonia in nursing home patients suspected of aspiration. Metronidazole also has activity against anaerobic bacteria such as *B. fragilis*. It is used in combination with other antibiotics for the treatment of lung abscesses, aspiration pneumonia, or anaerobic infections.

Appropriate and Adequate Intensity of Antimicrobial Coverage. Because macrolides and extended spectrum quinolones are effective, appropriate agents for treatment of CAP, they frequently get equal billing as initial choice agents for management of CAP. Despite their excellent track record and proven efficacy, however, the macrolides and extended spectrum quinolones have clinically significant differences that should be considered in the antibiotic treatment equation for CAP. Accordingly, a careful analysis of the benefits and potential pitfalls of these agents should include a full accounting of the relevant similarities and differences. It will help emergency physicians and intensivists develop criteria that suggest the appropriateness and suitability that each of these classes may have in specific patient subgroups.

Although the previously cited six organisms (*S. pneumoniae, H. influenzae,* and *M. catarrhalis*, and atypical pathogens *Mycoplasma, Legionella,* and *C. pneumoniae*) are the most commonly implicated pathogens in elderly patients with CAP, the patients also are susceptible to infection with gram-negative enteric organisms such as *Klebsiella, Escherichia coli,* and *Pseudomonas*. In other cases, the likelihood of infection with DRSP is high. When infection with these pathogens is likely, intensification of empiric coverage should include antibiotics with activity against these gram-negative species and/or DRSP.

Table 1. Cost of IV Antibiotics for CAP in the Elderly

DRUG AND DOSAGE	DAILY DRUG COST (WAC)* COST/DAY
Azithromycin IV 500 mg	$18.96
Ceftriaxone 1 gm IV qd	36.06
Levofloxacin 500 mg IV qd	33.00
Erythromycin 500 mg IV qid	5.20
Ciprofloxacin 400 mg IV bid	48.00
Cefotaxime 1 g IV tid	25.00
Tricarcillin-clavulanate 3.1 g qid	48.32

* WAC = Wholesale acquisition cost.
Hospital formulary pricing guide, August 1999. WAC may not necessarily reflect actual pharmacy costs or costs associated with drug administration cost comparisons.

Clinical features or risk factors that may suggest the need for intensification and expansion of bacterial and/or atypical pathogen coverage include the following: 1) increasing fragility (> 85 years of age, comorbid conditions, previous infection, etc.) of the patient; 2) acquisition of the pneumonia in a skilled nursing facility; 3) the presence of an aspiration pneumonia, suggesting involvement with gram-negative or anaerobic organisms; 4) chronic alcoholism, increasing the likelihood of infection with *Klebsiella pneumoniae*; 5) pneumococcal pneumonia in underlying disease-compromised individual who has not been vaccinated with pneumococcal polysaccharide antigen (Pneumovax); 6) history of infection with gram-negative, anaerobic, or resistant species of *S. pneumoniae*; 7) history of treatment failure; 8) previous hospitalizations for pneumonia; 9) patient requires or has had previous ICU hospitalization for pneumonia; 10) acquisition of pneumonia in a community with high and increasing resistance among *S. pneumoniae* species; and 11) immunodeficiency and/or severe underlying disease. Many of the aforementioned risk groups also can be treated with the combination of a third-generation cephalosporin plus a macrolide, in combination with an aminoglycoside when indicated.

As emphasized earlier in this review, most consensus panels, infectious disease experts, textbooks, and peer-reviewed antimicrobial prescribing guides recommend, as the initial or preferred choice, those antibiotics that, within the framework of monotherapy or combination therapy, address current etiologic and mortality trends in CAP. As a general rule, for empiric initial therapy in patients without modifying host factors that predispose to enteric gram-negative or pseudomonal infection they recommend those antibiotics that provide coverage against the bacterial pathogens *S. pneumoniae, H. influenzae,* and *M. catarrhalis,* as well as against atypical pathogens *Mycoplasma, Legionella,* and *C. pneumoniae*.[35]

Correct Spectrum Coverage. When antimicrobial monotherapy is desirable, cost-effective, and/or clinically indicated, extended spectrum quinolones and advanced generation macrolides best satisfy the empiric coverage requirements for patients with CAP. These antimicrobial agents are among the therapeutic classes of choice for management of CAP in the outpatient setting. *(Please see Tables 2 and 3.)*

Although third-generation cephalosporins, beta-lactam antibiotics, and TMP/SMX (trimethoprim-sulfamethoxazole) are still deemed valuable by many authorities and practitioners (in particular, in combination with other agents for in-hospital management of CAP), these agents have been allocated for the most part to secondary or alternative status for oral therapy. This is because they are not, as a rule, clinically indicated for treatment of atypical organisms, including *Mycoplasma, Legionella,* and *C. pneumoniae*, whose increasing importance now demand initial, out-of-the-gate coverage.

Because advanced generation macrolides and extended spectrum quinolones constitute the principal oral and intravenous treatment options for CAP, the following sections will discuss indications, clinical trials, side effects, and strategies for their use in CAP. The focus of the discussion will be on newer antibiotics that: 1) provide coverage of bacterial and atypical organisms causing CAP; 2) are available for both outpatient (oral) and in-hospital (IV) management; and; 3) are able, when indicated, to provide compliance-enhancing and cost-effective treatment within the context of antimicrobial monotherapy. It should be stressed that these agents also may be used as part of combination therapy for CAP. Antibiotics satisfying these criteria are azithromycin and levofloxacin.

Advanced Generation Macrolides: Correct Spectrum First-Line Coverage

The established new generation macrolide antibiotics include the erythromycin analogues azithromycin and clarithromycin.[36,37] Compared to erythromycin, which is the least expensive macrolide, the major advantages of these newer antibiotics are significantly decreased gastrointestinal side effects, which produce enhanced tolerance, improved bioavailability, higher tissue levels, and pharmacokinetic features that permit less frequent dosing and better compliance, as well as enhanced activity against *H. influenzae*.[38,39] In particular, the long tissue half-life of azithromycin allows this antibiotic to be prescribed for a shorter duration (5 days) than comparable antibiotics given for the same indications.

Macrolides in CAP Therapy: An Overview. Given the cost differences between azithromycin and clarithromycin, as well as the improved compliance patterns associated with short-duration therapy, any rational approach to distinguishing between these agents must consider prescription, patient, and drug resistance barriers. *(Please see Table 4.)*

From the outset, it is fair to say that these macrolides, to a great degree, have supplanted the use of erythromycin (as well as cephalosporins and tetrayclines) in community-acquired infections of the lower respiratory tract. In some institutions, this is not the case. Although erythromycin, in particular, has been considered by some to be the antibiotic of choice for CAP, its lack of efficacy against *H. influenzae*, as well as its adverse gastrointestinal side effects, potential for drug-drug interactions, and poor compliance profile, are now recognized as clinically important liabilities in emergency practice.[40,41] It is, however, effective against pneumococcal pneumonia, Mycoplasma pneumonia, and many atypical infections, including Legionella. *(Please see Table 4.)* Food decreases the absorption of erythromycin, which interferes with drug metabolism; therefore, many experts caution this drug should not be considered for use in elderly patients on theophylline or warfarin.[22,35]

From the perspective of providing definitive, cost-effective, and compliance-promoting therapy, the newer macrolide antibiotics, which include both azithromycin and clarithromycin, have recently emerged as some of the drugs of choice-along with the new, extended spectrum quinolones-for outpatient management of CAP.[42] When used as oral agents, they play a central role in management of pneumonia in otherwise healthy elderly individuals who do not require hospitalization.

From an emergency medicine and in-hospital management perspective, the value and desirability of macrolide therapy has been significantly enhanced by availability of the intravenous formulation of azithromycin, which has been approved for hospitalized patients with CAP. Unlike penicillins, cephalosporins, and sulfa-based agents, azithromycin has the advantage of showing in vitro activity against both atypical and bacterial offenders implicated in CAP.[43,44]

The macrolides also have the advantage of a simplified dosing schedule, especially azithromycin, which is given once daily for only five days (500 mg po on day 1 and 250 mg po qd on days 2-5). *(Please see Table 5.)* Clarithromycin requires a longer course of therapy and is more expensive. Clarithromycin costs approximately $68-72 for a complete, 10-day course of therapy vs. $42-44 for a complete course of therapy with azithromycin. Clarithromycin, however, is another alternative among macrolides for outpatient treatment of CAP. It is now available in once-daily formulation (1000 mg/d for 10 days) for oral use, but an intravenous preparation is not currently available. In general, the decision to use a macrolide such as azithromycin rather than erythromycin is based on weighing the increased cost of a course of therapy with azithromycin against its real-world advantages, which include a more convenient dosing schedule, its broader spectrum of coverage, its favorable drug interaction profile, and its decreased incidence of gastrointestinal side effects, which occur in 3-5% of patients taking a five-day, multiple-dose regimen.[45] The introduction of a tablet formulation permits consumption of the antibiotic without regard to food ingestion.

Azithromycin. From a practical, clinical, and cost perspective, the newest and, perhaps, most important advance in the area of macrolide therapy is the availability of intravenous azithromycin for the management of hospitalized patients with moderate or severe CAP.[46-48] Currently, azithromycin is the only advanced generation macrolide indicated for parenteral therapy in hospitalized patients with CAP due to *C. pneumoniae, H. influenzae, L. pneumophila, M. catarrhalis, M. pneumoniae, S. pneumoniae,* or *Staphylococcus aureus*.[43,44,48,49] This coverage would be considered correct spectrum coverage for empiric therapy of CAP in the elderly patient.

The comparative trials demonstrating clinical success (patients who were cured or improved at 10-14 days post-therapy) rates of about 77% and concomitant bacteriologic response rates of about 96% for frequently isolated pathogens with azithromycin in CAP were conducted in a wide variety of patients with moderate and severe pneumonia. These included a significant percentage of patients who were 65 years of age or older, had an abnormal respiratory rate (> 30 breaths per minute), a PaO_2 of less than 60 mmHg, and/or BUN greater than 20 mg/dL.[43,44,48] Many of these patients had concurrent

Table 2. Empiric Antimicrobial Therapy of Choice for Outpatient‡ and In-Hospital Management of Elderly Patients with Community-Acquired Pneumonia

PATIENT PROFILE/ETIOLOGIC AGENTS	FIRST-LINE ANTIBIOTIC THERAPY†	ALTERNATIVE FIRST-LINE ANTIBIOTIC THERAPY
Otherwise Healthy **> 60 years of age** (Patients deemed to be suitable for outpatient/oral therapy, i.e., no systemic toxicity, high likelihood of compliance, and supportive home environment)*	Azithromycin PO	Levofloxacin PO OR Cefuroxime plus azithromycin PO OR Clarithromycin
In-Hospital (not in intensive care unit) underlying risk factors or comorbid conditions: In-Hospital management (COPD, history of pneumonia, diabetes, etc.)	Azithromycin IV OR Azithromycin IV plus ceftriaxone OR Cefotaxime plus azithromycin IV	Imipenem IV plus azithromycin IV OR Levofloxacin IV
CAP acquired in the nursing home environment (increased likelihood of gram-negative, *E. coli, Klebsiella pneumoniae*)	Ceftriaxone IV plus azithromycin IV OR Levofloxacin IV	Ceftriaxone plus erythromycin IV OR Cefotaxime plus azithromycin IV
CAP in the elderly individual with chronic alcoholism (Increased likelihood of *Klebsiella pneumoniae* infection)	Ceftriaxone IV plus azithromycin IV OR Levofloxacin IV	Ceftriaxone plus erythromycin IV OR Cefepime IV plus azithromycin IV
Severe CAP acquired in an area or institution with significant prevalence (> 20%) of *S. pneumoniae* species showing high-level or complete resistance to macrolides, cephalosporins, and/or penicillin, but maintaining high sensitivity to extended spectrum quinolones)	Levofloxacin IV OR Levofloxacin IV plus Ceftriaxone IV	Vancomycin¶ plus azithromycin IV
Severe CAP complicated by structural disease of the lung (bronchiectasis): Increased likelihood of *Pseudomonas* and polymicrobial infection	Cefepime IV plus levofloxacin IV plus/minus aminoglycoside OR Ciprofloxacin IV plus aminoglycoside IV plus azithromycin IV	Ciprofloxacin IV plus cefepime IV plus azithromycin IV OR Carbapenem IV plus azithromycin IV plus aminoglycoside
CAP in a patient with suspected aspiration (increases the likelihood of gram-negative and anaerobic infection**)	Levofloxacin IV plus clindamycin IV OR Azithromycin IV plus ampicillin-sulbactam IV	Levofloxacin IV plus ampicillin-sulbactam IV
Severe CAP in a compromised host with a previous hospitalization for, or who resides in a community or facility with a high reported incidence of methicillin-resistant *S. aureus* (MRSA)***	Levofloxacin IV plus vancomycin IV OR Ceftriaxone IV plus azithromycin IV plus vancomycin IV	Levofloxacin IV plus vancomycin IV
CAP patient with severe pneumonia requiring ICU hospitalization***	Ceftriaxone IV plus levofloxacin IV plus/minus aminoglycoside (*Pseudomonas* strongly suspected) OR Ceftriaxone IV plus azithromycin IV plus/minus anti-pseudomonal agent	Ciprofloxacin IV plus aminoglycoside IV plus azithromycin IV OR Cefotaxime IV plus azithromycin IV plus/minus aminoglycoside

* Oral therapy/outpatient treatment recommendations are appropriate only for those otherwise healthy patients with CAP of mild enough severity that they are judged to be suitable candidates for outpatient management with oral antibiotics.
§ Quinolones are restricted for use in patients > 18 years of age.
¶ If *S. pneumoniae* demonstrates complete resistance to extended spectrum quinolones (very rare), third-generation cephalosporins, and macrolides, then vancomycin may be required as part of initial therapy, although this would be necessary only in rare circumstances.
† First-line therapy recommendations take into consideration cost of the drug (which may vary from one institution to another), convenience of dosing, daily dose frequency, spectrum of coverage, side effects, and risk of drug-drug interactions.
** When anaerobic organisms are suspected as one of the possible etiologic pathogens in a patient with CAP, clindamycin or a β-lactam/β-lactamase inhibitor (ampicillin/sulbactam, tricarcillin/clavulanate, or ticarcillin/tazobacatam) is recommended.
***High community prevalence of, previous history of hospitalization, or increasing local incidence of methicillin-resistant *S. aureus* (MRSA) in a patient with a clinical presentation consistent with *S. aureus* pneumonia; vancomycin should be considered as component for initial therapy.
‡ Adapted from references 2, 3, 5, 6-8, 11, 35, 41, 43, 44, 46, 47, 54, 64, 66

diseases or syndromes, including emphysema, chronic airway obstruction, asthma, diabetes, and/or were cigarette smokers.[50]

As would be expected, the efficacy of this macrolide was compared to clinical outcomes with a cephalosporin (cefuroxime) used with or without erythromycin. In a randomized, comparative investigation, therapy with intravenous azithromycin alone followed by oral azithromycin was as effective as intravenous treatment with the designated second-generation cephalosporin, cefuroxime followed by oral cefuroxime axetil, with or without the addition of oral or intravenous erythromycin.[50]

Azithromycin dosing and administration schedules for hospitalized patients are different than for the five-day course used exclusively for outpatient management, and these differences should be noted. When this advanced generation macrolide is used for hospitalized patients with CAP, 2-5 days of therapy with azithromycin IV (500 mg once daily) followed by oral azithromycin (500 mg once daily to complete a total of 7-10 days of therapy) is clinically and bacteriologically effective. For patients requiring hospitalization, the initial 500 mg intravenous dose of azithromycin should be given in the ED.

Like the oral formulation, IV azithromycin appears to be well-tolerated, with a low incidence of gastrointestinal adverse events (4.3% diarrhea, 3.9% nausea, 2.7% abdominal pain, 1.4% vomiting), minimal injection-site reactions (less than 12% combined injection-site pain and/or inflammation or infection), and a low incidence of discontinuation (1.2% discontinuation of IV therapy) due to drug-related adverse patient events or laboratory abnormalities.[51]

Initial Intravenous Management: Macrolide Monotherapy (Azithromycin) vs. Combination Therapy

As emphasized earlier, prompt administration of intravenous antibiotics in the ED can improve clinical outcomes in patients with CAP. Consequently, once diagnostic tests, including cultures and radiographs (when appropriate), have been performed, initial antibiotic therapy for hospitalized patients should be administered in the ED, especially if delays in getting the patient admitted are anticipated.

Although antibiotic recommendations based on risk-stratification criteria, historical features, site where the infection was acquired, and other modifying factors are provided in Table 3, institutional protocols, hospital-based critical pathways, resistance features, and other factors will influence antibiotic selection.

Table 3. Infectious Disease Society of America (IDSA) Consensus Report Guidelines

OUTPATIENT MANAGEMENT: PREFERRED ANTIMICROBIALS IN MOST PATIENTS (IN NO SPECIAL ORDER)

- Macrolide*, Extended-spectrum fluoroquinolones**, or doxycycline***
- Alternative options: Amoxicillin/clavulanate and some second-generation cephalosporins (cefuroxime, cefpodoxime, or cefprozil). *Note:* These will not be active vs. atypical agents.

* Macrolide: azithromycin, erythromycin, or clarithromycin; azithromycin or clarithromycin is preferred if *H. influenzae* infection is suspected

** Fluoroquinolone: levofloxacin is preferred.

*** Increasing resistance to *S. pneumoniae* is observed in some geographical regions

IN-HOSPITAL-GENERAL MEDICAL WARD MANAGEMENT: PREFERRED ANTIMICROBIALS IN MOST PATIENTS (IN NO SPECIAL ORDER)

Preferred:
- β-lactam[a] with a macrolide[b] *OR*
- An intravenous fluoroquinolone (levofloxacin) with expanded coverage against *S. pneumoniae*

Alternative:
- Cefuroxime with a macrolide[b] *OR*
- Azithromycin (alone)

IN-HOSPITAL-INTENSIVE CARE UNIT MANAGEMENT: PREFERRED ANTIMICROBIALS IN MOST PATIENTS (IN NO SPECIAL ORDER)

Preferred:
- Azithromycin, erythromycin, or a fluoroquinolone plus cefotaxime, ceftriaxone, or a β-lactam-/β-lactamase inhibitor[d]

MODIFYING FACTORS

- Structural disease of lung (bronchiectasis): Add anti-pseudomonal penicillin, carbapenem, or cefepime plus macrolide[b] or fluoroquinolone[c] *plus* an aminoglycoside
- Likelihood of or previous history of pseudomonal infection: Add antipseudomonal penicillin, carbapenem, or cefepime plus macrolide[b] or fluoroquinolone[c] plus an aminoglycoside.
- High community prevalence or local incidence of methicillin-resistant *Staphylococcus aureus* (MRSA) in a patient with clinical presentation suggestive of *S. aureus* pneumonia: consider adding vancomycin.
- Penicillin allergy: Fluoroquinolone[c] with or without clindamycin
- Suspected aspiration: Fluoroquinolone[c] plus clindamycin or a β-lactam-/β-lactamase inhibitor[d]

[a] β-lactam: Cefotaxime or ceftriaxone
[b] Macrolide: Azithromycin, clarithromycin, or erythromycin
[c] Fluoroquinolone: Levofloxacin or another fluoroquinolone with enhanced activity against *S. pneumoniae*
[d] β-lactam-/β-lactamase inhibitor: Ampicillin/sulbactam, ticarcillin/clavulanate, or piperacillin/tozabactam; for structural disease of the lung; ticarcillin/clavulanate or piperacillin/clavulanate

Adaptation and Summary of Preferred Antimicrobial Recommendations from the Infectious Disease Society of America, IDSA 1998

Despite variations in hospital or departmental protocols, certain requirements regarding drug selection for CAP are relatively consistent. For example, from an empiric antibiotic selection perspective, what appears to be non-negotiable for managing the majority of patients with CAP, is providing mandatory antimicrobial coverage against *S. pneumoniae, H. influenzae, M. catarrhalis, Legionella, M. pneumoniae,* and *C. pneumoniae*. As mentioned earlier, consensus reports and national guidelines support this strategy (see section on Consensus Guidelines for Antibiotic Therapy below). Within the framework of monotherapy, IV azithromycin (500 mg IV for 2-5 days, followed by 500 mg PO to complete a 7-10 day course) is recommended by many institutional protocols for ward (i.e., non-ICU) patients with CAP who do not have modifying factors (i.e., aspiration,

Table 4. Macrolides: Approved Spectrum of Coverage in Community-Acquired Pneumonia

Antibiotic	Indicated* for Treatment of CAP Caused by These Organisms						
	S. pneumoniae	*H. influenzae*	*M. catarrhalis*	*M. pneumoniae*	*C. pneumoniae*	*L. pneumophilia*	*S. aureas*
Azithromycin**	Yes	Yes	Yes	Yes	Yes	Yes	Yes
Clarithromycin	Yes			Yes	Yes		
Erythromycin	Yes			Yes		Yes	

*Indicated, i.e., according to FDA approved indications as specified in the package insert for each agent. The agent may, however, show *in vitro* activity against organisms for which clinical indications have not yet been established.

** Intravenous formulation of azithromycin.

immunosuppression, alcoholism, etc.) that suggest the likelihood of gram-negative pneumonia.[35,49,51,52]

For hospitalized patients, at least two days of intravenous azithromycin therapy is recommended (the first dose of which can be given in the ED), followed by transition to oral therapy at the discretion of the physician based on clinical factors. It should be noted that intravenous azithromycin is currently the only macrolide that carries an indication for in-hospital, intravenous-to-oral step-down, monotherapeutic management of appropriately risk-stratified patients with CAP. When combination cephalosporin/macrolide therapy is the accepted hospital protocol, among the macrolides available, IV azithromycin is recommended by this author as the co-therapeutic agent (i.e., in combination with a cephalosporin) of choice in the elderly for the following reasons: 1) it can be administered on a once-daily basis, thereby minimizing human resource costs associated with drug administration; 2) it is the only macrolide indicated for in-hospital, intravenous-to-oral stepdown, monotherapeutic management of CAP caused by *S. pneumoniae, H. influenzae, M. catarrhalis, Legionella pneumophila, M. pneumoniae, C. pneumoniae*, or *S. aureus*—an important efficacy and spectrum of coverage benchmark; 3) at $19-22 per day for the intravenous dose of 500 mg azithromycin, its cost is reasonable; 4) the intravenous-to-oral step-down dose of 500 mg has been established as effective in clinical trials evaluating hospitalized patients with CAP; and 5) azithromycin has excellent activity against *Legionella pneumophila*, a pathogen commonly implicated in the geriatric patient with CAP. The decision to use azithromycin as a monotherapeutic agent, or in combination with a cephalosporin for initial therapy of CAP, will be determined by intra-institutional pathways and protocols, based on consensus recommendations and association guidelines as presented in this article.

Critical Pathways and Protocols. The decision to employ a monotherapeutic regimen with IV azithromycin for inpatient treatment of CAP usually will be based on intra-hospital infectious disease protocols and local susceptibility patterns, which may risk-stratify patient subgroups appropriate for monotherapy. When patients with CAP are hospitalized in the ICU or there is a significant likelihood of gram-negative infection (i.e., *Klebsiella, E. coli,* or *P. aeruginosa*), monotherapy with a macrolide is not appropriate, and CDC group's recent consensus report stresses the importance of using an IV macrolide in combination with other agents, in particular, third-generation cephalosporins such as ceftriaxone or cefotaxime.[2] In these patients, a macrolide should be used in combination with a cephalosporin (and when anti-pseudomonal coverage is necessary, an anti-pseudomonal cephalosporin and/or an aminoglycoside also may be required) or alternatively, an extended spectrum fluoroquinolone such as levofloxacin should be considered, although combination therapy also has been advocated with this agent in severely ill patients.[2] When anaerobic organisms are suspected, clindamycin or a beta-lactam/beta-lactamase inhibitor is appropriate.

Accordingly, a number of critical pathways for pneumonia therapy recommend use of two-drug therapy for CAP. The therapy typically is the combination of an IV cephalosporin such as ceftriaxone plus a macrolide, which usually is administered, initially, by the intravenous route when the patient's condition so warrants. Perhaps the important change in CAP treatment since publication of the American Thoracic Guidelines in 1993 is the current general consensus that atypical organisms such as *L. pneumophila, C. pneumoniae*, and *M. pneumoniae* must be covered empirically as part of the initial antibiotic regimen. Whereas previous consensus guidelines indicated that macrolides could be added to a cephalosporin on a "plus or minus" basis for initial CAP treatment, it is now felt that coverage of the atypical spectrum, along with coverage of *S. pneumoniae, H. influenzae,* and *M. catarrhalis,* is mandatory.[2] New guidelines from the IDSA and CDC now reflect this strategy which, in practical terms, means that a macrolide such as azithromycin or erythromycin (or a fluoroquinolone with activity against atypical organisms) will be part of almost every empirical antimicrobial regimen used for CAP.

Although virtually all protocols using combination cephalosporin/macrolide therapy specify intravenous administration of the cephalosporin, guidelines specifying whether initial macrolide therapy should be by the intravenous or oral route are less concrete. Recent CDC guidelines recommend intravenous macrolide therapy for patients hospitalized in the ICU, while oral therapy is permissible in conjunction with an IV cephalosporin in the medical ward patient.[2] Because atypical infections such as *L. pneumophila* are associated with high mortality rates, especially in the elderly, and because hospitalized patients with CAP, by definition, represent a sicker cohort, it is prudent and, therefore, advisable that initial macrolide therapy in the hospital be administered by the intravenous route. The author of this review, therefore, recommends IV azithromycin therapy as the preferred initial, empiric agent in the elderly, whether used as monotherapy or in combination with another agent. Step-down to oral therapy can be accomplished when the patient's clinical status so dictates, or when culture results suggest this is appropriate.

It should be pointed out that while some consensus panels (IDSA 1997 CAP Guidelines) support the use of IV azithromycin in hospitalized CAP patients as monotherapy or as the macrolide component of combination therapy, other panels (CDC Therapeutic Working Group) support its use specifically as the macrolide component of combination therapy along with such as agents as ceftriaxone, cefuroxime, or cefotaxime. Although each institution will determine its preferred approach to these options, recent studies lend support to the notion that IV azithromycin monotherapy for hospitalized patients (45% of which were > 64 years of age) with CAP admitted to a general medical ward is equal in efficacy to a 1993 ATS-suggested regimen of cefuroxime with the addition of erythromycin when clinicians believe it is necessary.[43] In one study, which excluded patients with aspiration, as well as those with evidence of gram-negative infection known to be resistant to the study medications, the authors also conclude that gastrointestinal tolerance of the azithromycin regimen was better than the suggested ATS regimen, and that azithromycin therapy was associated with a shorter length of stay as compared with the ATS-suggested regimen.[43]

Another prospective, randomized multicenter trial compared the efficacy and safety of azithromycin monotherapy with those of a combination of cefuroxime plus erythromycin as empirical therapy in hospitalized patients with CAP.[44] Data from 245 patients (67 received azithromycin monotherapy, 78 received combination cefuroxime and erythromycin) were evaluated, and it was found that clinical cure was achieved in 91% (61 of 67) of the patients in the azithromycin group and in 91% (71 of 78) of those in the combination group. *Streptococcus pneumoniae* and *Haemophilus influenzae* were isolated in 19% and 13% of the total patient population, respectively; atypical pathogens accounted for 33% of the etiologic diagnoses, with *Legionella pneumophila, Chlamydia pneumoniae,* and *Mycoplasma pneumoniae* being identified in 14%, 10%, and 9% of patients, respectively. The investigation, which excluded nursing home residents, concluded that treatment with azithromycin was as effective as cefuroxime plus erythromycin in the empirical management of CAP in immunocompetent patients who were hospitalized.[44]

Both the aforementioned studies conclude that, in a selected population of patients with CAP, azithromycin monotherapy is as effective as a combination regimen (i.e., cefuroxime plus erythromycin) that is consistent with guidelines published by the ATS, Canadian Community-Acquired Pneumonia Consensus Group, and the IDSA.

Extended Spectrum Fluoroquinolones, Indication for Initial Empiric Use: Intensifications of Coverage and Patient Selection

The extended spectrum quinolone levofloxacin is indicated for treatment of CAP. Because levofloxacin is used both as an oral agent and intravenously in the hospital setting, has indications for use in suspected DRSP pneumonia, and is the most widely used fluoroquinolone for this indication, the discussion below will focus on levofloxacin.

However, another recently introduced extended spectrum fluoroquinolone, gatifloxacin (Tequin) is also available for both intravenous and oral therapy for the treatment of pneumonia, and has appropriate spectrum of coverage for bacterial and atypical pathogens causing pneumonia. It may play an increasingly important role in the management of these patients. Currently, though, clinicians have had more practical experience with the fluoroquinolone, levofloxacin, and therefore, this review will focus primarily on this fluoroquinolone representative from this antimicrobial class. Among oral agents, the fluoroquinolone moxifloxacin (Avelox) is also available.

Levofloxacin. Levofloxacin, the S-enantiomer of ofloxacin, is a fluoroquinolone antibiotic that, when compared with older quinolones, also has improved activity against gram-positive organisms, including *Streptococcus pneumoniae*. This has important drug selection implications for the management of patients with CAP and exacerbations of COPD. The active stereoisomer of ofloxacin, levofloxacin is available in a parenteral preparation or as a once daily oral preparation that is given for 7-14 days.

Levofloxacin is indicated for the treatment of adults (> 18 years) with mild, moderate, and severe pulmonary infections, including acute bacterial exacerbation of chronic bronchitis and CAP.[53] It is active against many gram-positive organisms that may infect the lower respiratory tract, including *S. pneumoniae* and *Staphylococcus aureus*, and it also covers atypical pathogens, including *Chlamydia pneumoniae, Legionella pneumophila*, and *Mycoplasma pneumoniae*. It is also active against gram-negative organisms, including *E. coli, H. influenzae, H. parainfluenzae, Klebsiella pneumoniae*, and *Moraxella catarrhalis*. Although it is active against *Pseudomonas aeruginosa* in vitro and carries an indication for treatment of complicated UTI caused by *Pseudomonas aeruginosa*, levofloxacin does not have an official indication for CAP caused by this gram-negative organism.

Several studies and surveillance data suggest that some newly available, expanded spectrum fluoroquinolones, including levofloxacin (which is approved for PRSP), are efficacious for the treatment of *S. pneumoniae*, including penicillin-resistant strains.[2,54,55] In one study, microbiologic eradication from sputum was reported among all 300 patients with pneumococcal pneumonia treated with oral levofloxacin.[54] In a study of in vitro susceptibility of *S. pneumoniae* clinical isolates to levofloxacin, none of the 180 isolates (including 60 isolates with intermediate susceptibility to penicillin and 60 penicillin-resistant isolates) was resistant to this agent.[55] In addition, a surveillance study of antimicrobial resistance in respiratory tract pathogens found levofloxacin was active against 97% of 9190 pneumococcal isolates and found no cross-resistance with penicillin, amoxicillin-clavulanate, ceftriaxone, cefuroxime, or clarithromycin.

Despite high level activity against pneumococcal isolates and a formal indication for levofloxacin use in suspected DRSP lower respiratory tract infection, the CDC Drug-Resistant Streptococcus pneumoniae Therapeutic Working Group's recent guidelines do not advocate the use of expanded spectrum fluoroquinolones (among them, levofloxacin, sparfloxacin, or grepafloxacin) for first-line, empiric treatment of pneumonia. This is because: 1) of their broad, perhaps, over-extended spectrum of coverage that includes a wide range of gram-negative organisms; 2) of concern that resistance among pneumococci will emerge if there is widespread use of this class of antibiotics; 3) their activity against pneumococci with high penicillin resistance (MIC ≥ 4 mcg/mL) makes it important that they be reserved for selected patients with CAP; 4) use of fluoroquinolones has been shown to result in increased resistance to *S. pneumoniae* in vitro; and 5) population-based surveillance in the United States has shown a statistically significant increase in ofloxacin resistance among pneumococcal isolates between Jan. 1, 1995, and Dec. 31, 1997 (unpublished data, Active Bacterial Core Surveillance, CDC).[2]

From a practical, drug selection perspective, The CDC Drug-Resistant Streptococcus pneumoniae Therapeutic Working Group has recommended that fluoroquinolones be reserved for selected patients with CAP, and these experts have identified specific patient subgroups that are eligible for initial treatment with extended-spectrum fluoroquinolones such as levofloxacin. For hospitalized patients, these include adults and elderly patients for whom one of the first-line regimens (cephalosporin plus a macrolide) has failed, those who are allergic to the first-line agents, or those who have a documented infection with highly drug-resistant pneumococci (i.e., penicillin MIC ≥ 4 mcg/mL).[29]

When given orally, levofloxacin is dosed once daily, is well absorbed orally, and penetrates well into lung tissue.[56] It is active against a wide range of respiratory pathogens, including atypical pathogens and many species of *S. pneumoniae* resistant to penicillin.[57,58] In general, levofloxacin has greater activity against gram-positive organisms than ofloxacin and is slightly less active than ciprofloxacin against gram-negative organisms.[59,60]

Levofloxacin is available as both an oral and parenteral form, and the oral and IV routes are interchangeable (i.e., same dose). Levofloxacin is generally well tolerated (incidence of adverse reactions, < 7%). Levofloxacin is supplied in a parenteral form for IV use and in 250 mg and 500 mg tablets. The recommended dose is 500 mg IV or orally qd for 7-14 days for lower respiratory tract infections. Food does not affect the absorption of the drug, but levofloxacin should be taken at least two hours before or two hours after antacids containing magnesium or aluminum, as well as sucralfate, metal cations such as iron, and multivitamin preparations with zinc.

Dosage adjustment is recommended in patients with impaired renal function (clearance < 50 mL/min).[53] The drug is well-tolerated, with the most common side effects including nausea, diarrhea, headache, and constipation. All quinolones have been associated with cartilage damage in animal studies, and therefore, they are not recommended for use in children, adolescents, and pregnant and nursing women.

Comparative trials (generally available in abstract form) suggest that levofloxacin is as effective as cefuroxime axetil, cefaclor, and amoxicillin/clavulanate in upper or lower respiratory infections.[61,62] In patients with CAP, IV levofloxacin with step-down-to-oral therapy was superior to ceftriaxone with step-down therapy to cefuroxime axetil.[63] About 22% of patients in the cephalosporin arm required the addition of erythromycin or doxycycline due to the presence of atypical respiratory pathogens. The clinical response rates (cure plus improvement) were 88-97% for levofloxacin. Microbiological eradication was reported to be 94-98% in patients in whom a microbiological pathogen could be identified; however, a large number of patients (32-43%) were not evaluable for this end point.[61-63]

It should be emphasized that, currently, such macrolides as azithromycin also are recommended for pneumonia in ambulatory, otherwise healthy adults. And, for older patients, an oral cephalosporin, such as cefuroxime axetil plus a macrolide to provide coverage of atypical pathogens may be considered.[56]

Empiric Antibiotic Coverage for Community-Acquired Pneumonia: Matching Drugs with Patient Profiles

A variety of antibiotics are available for outpatient management of pneumonia. *(Please see Table 3.)* Although the selection process can be daunting, as mentioned, a sensible approach to antibiotic selection for patients with pneumonia is provided by treatment categories for pneumonia generated by the Medical Section of the American Lung Association and published under the auspices of the ATS.[64] This classification scheme, which is now almost seven years old, not only helps make clinical assessments useful for guiding therapy, but it is also predictive of ultimate prognosis and mortality outcome. New, more recently devised consensus panel recommendations also are available and will be discussed.

The most common pathogens responsible for causing CAP include the typical bacteria: *S. pneumoniae, H. influenzae*, and *M. catarrhalis*, as well as the atypical pathogens: *Mycoplasma, Legionella*, and *Chlamydia pneumoniae*.[65] *H. influenzae* and *M. catarrhalis* are both found more commonly in patients with COPD. Clinically and radiologically, it is difficult to differentiate between the typical and atypical pathogens; therefore, coverage against all these organisms may be necessary. In patients producing sputum containing polymorphonuclear leukocytes, the sputum Gram's stain may contain a predominant organism to aid in the choice of empiric therapy. For most patients, therapy must be entirely empiric and based on the expected pathogens.[66,52] *(Please see Table 3.)*

Therefore, for the vast majority of otherwise healthy patients who have CAP, but who do not have comorbid conditions and who are deemed well enough to be managed as outpatients, therapy directed at *S. pneumoniae, H. influenzae, M. pneumoniae, Chlamydia pneumoniae, Legionella pneumophila,* and *M. catarrhalis* is appropriate. From an intensity and spectrum of coverage perspective, coverage of both the aforementioned bacterial and atypical species has become mandatory.

In these cases, one of the newer macrolides, should be considered one of the initial agents of choice. The other monotherapeutic agents available consist of the extended spectrum quinolones, which provides similar coverage and carries and indication for initial therapy in this patient subgroup.

For the older patient with CAP who is considered stable enough to be managed as an outpatient, but in whom the bacterial pathogen list also may include gram-negative aerobic organisms, the combined use of a second- or third-generation cephalosporin or amoxicillin-clavulanate plus a macrolide has been recommended. Another option may consist of an advanced generation quinolone.

Some experts emphasize that in non-smoking adults without COPD (i.e., patients at a low risk for having *H. influenzae*), therapy with erythromycin should be strongly considered.[66] This is a matter of clinical judgment, but in any event, the newer macrolides, azithromycin and clarithromycin, are recommended in cases of erythromycin intolerance. In patients with COPD, either TMP-SMX or doxycycline usually provides adequate coverage against *S. pneumoniae* and *H. influenzae*, but TMP-SMX will not cover atypical pathogens.

Use of the older quinolones is not recommended for empiric treatment of community-acquired respiratory infections, primarily because of their variable activity against *S. pneumoniae* and atypical organisms. Although the older quinolones (i.e., ciprofloxacin) should generally not be used for the empiric treatment of CAP, they may provide an important option for treatment of bronchiectasis, particularly when gram-negative organisms such as *Pseudomonas* are cultured from respiratory secretions.[67] In these cases, ciprofloxacin should be used in combination with another anti-pseudomonal agent when indicated.

The most important issue for the emergency physician or pulmonary intensivist is to ensure that the appropriate intensity and spectrum of coverage are provided, according to patient and community/epidemiological risk factors. In many cases, especially when infection with gram-negative organisms is suspected or there is structural lung disease, this will require shifting to and intensifying therapy with an extended spectrum quinolone. However, in most cases of non-ICU patients admitted to the hospital, azithromycin IV as monotherapy or a cephalosporin plus azithromycin is recommended, depending on institutional protocols.

In this regard, determining which of these antibiotics (macrolides vs extended spectrum quinolones) should be considered "workhorse" drugs in the ED or hospital setting, for initial CAP treatment requires thoughtful analysis that takes into account cost, convenience, spectrum of coverage, host risk factors, and patient risk stratification.

In the case of azithromycin, its five-day duration of therapy, $39-$42 cost per course of treatment, and targeted coverage of *S. pneumoniae, H. influenzae, M. catarrhalis, Chlamydia*, and *M. pneumoniae*, must be weighed against the longer duration and slightly greater cost per treatment course for the quinolones and the fact that their spectrum of coverage includes not only the appropriately targeted, aforementioned organisms commonly implicated in CAP, but also extensive activity against gram-negative organisms, which may not always be required, especially in otherwise healthy individuals. This over-extended spectrum of coverage may exert resistance pressure on gram-negative organisms frequently encountered in a hospital setting; therefore, quinolone use should be risk-stratified to an appropriate subset.

From a cost-effectiveness perspective, it appears that when gram-negative coverage of *Klebsiella* and other species is not required, the advanced generation macrolide azithromycin represents a sensible choice as initial therapy, especially in individuals without underlying problems. However, in patients in whom gram-negative infection is more of a concern, the extended spectrum quinolone is an important alternative to combination therapy consisting of a third-generation cephalosporin plus a macrolide such as azithromycin.

Finally, there is an increasing problem in the United States concerning the emergence among hospitalized pneumonia patients of *S. pneumoniae* that is relatively resistant to penicillin and, less commonly, to extended-spectrum cephalosporins. These isolates also may be resistant to sulfonamides and tetracyclines.[64,68,69] Except for vancomycin, the most favorable in vitro response rates to *S. pneumoniae* are seen with extended spectrum quinolones. See Table 3 for a summary of current recommendations for initial management of outpatient and in-hospital management of patients with CAP.

Antimicrobial Therapy and Medical Outcomes. A recent study has helped assess the relationship between initial antimicrobial therapy and medical outcomes for elderly patients hospitalized with pneumonia.[70] In this retrospective analysis, hospital records for 12,945 Medicare inpatients (≥ 65years of age) with pneumonia were reviewed. Associations were identified between the choice of the initial antimicrobial regimen and three-day mortality, adjusting for baseline differences in patient profiles, illness severity, and process of care. Comparisons were made between the antimicrobial regimens and a reference group consisting of patients treated with a non-pseudomonal third-generation cephalosporin alone.

Of the 12,945 patients, 9751 (75.3%) were community-dwelling and 3194 (24.7%) were admitted from a long-term care facility (LCF). Study patients had a mean age of 79.4 years ± 8.1 years; 84.4% were white, and 50.7% were female. As would be expected, the majority (58.1%) of patients had at least one comorbid illness; and 68.3% were in the two highest severity risk classes (IV and V) at initial examination. The most frequently coded bacteriologic pathogens were *S. pneumoniae* (6.6%) and *H. influenzae* (4.1%); 10.1% of patients were coded as having aspiration pneumonia, and in 60.5% the etiologic agent for the pneumonia was unknown.

The three most commonly used initial, empiric antimicrobial regimen in the elderly patient with pneumonia consisted of the following: 1) a non-pseudomonal third-generation cephalosporin only (ceftriaxone, cefotaxime, ceftizoxime) in 26.5%; 2) a second-generation cephalosporin only (cefuroxime) in 12.3%; and 3) a non-pseudomonal third-generation cephalosporin (as above) plus a macrolide in 8.8%. The 30-day mortality was 15.3% (95% CI, 14.6%-15.9%) in the entire study population, ranging from 11.2% (95% CI, 10.6%-11.9%) in community-dwelling elderly patients to 27.5% (95% CI, 26%-29.1%) among patients admitted from a LCF.[70]

As might be predicted, this study of elderly patients with hospitalization for pneumonia demonstrated significant differences in patient survival depending upon the choice of the initial antibiotic regimen. In particular, this national study demonstrated that, compared to a reference group receiving a non-pseudomonal third-generation cephalosporin alone, initial therapy with a non-pseudomonal plus a macrolide, a second-generation cephalosporin plus a macrolide, or a fluoroquinolone alone was associated with 26%, 29%, and 36% lower 30-day mortality, respectively. Despite the fact that these regimens are compatible with those recommended by the IDSA and CDC, only 15% of patients received one of the three aforementioned regimens associated with reduced mortality rates.

For reasons that are not entirely clear, patients treated with a beta-lactam/beta-lactamase inhibitor plus a macrolide or an aminoglycoside plus another agent had mortality rates 77% and 21% higher than the reference group, respectively.

Role of Specific Pathogens in CAP. Prospective studies for evaluating the causes of CAP in elderly adults have failed to identify the cause of 40-60% of cases of CAP, and two or more etiologies have been identified in 2-5% of cases. The most common etiologic agent identified in virtually all studies of CAP in the elderly is *Streptococcus pneumoniae,* and this agent accounts for approximately two-thirds of all cases of bacteremic pneumonia.

Other pathogens implicated less frequently include *H. influenzae* (most isolates of which are other than type B), *Mycoplasma pneumo-*

Table 5. Available Macrolides for Monotherapy or Co-Therapy in Elderly, Hospitalized Patients with Community-Acquired Pneumonia

Antibiotic	Spectrum of coverage*	Daily dosing frequency	IV to oral stepdown**	Is agent available for IV monotherapy of CAP?
Azithromycin IV	*S. pneumoniae* *H. influenzae* *M. catarrhalis* *M. pneumoniae* *C. pneumoniae* *L. pneumophila*	once daily	available and indicated	yes
Erythromycin IV	*S. pneumoniae* *M. pneumoniae* *L. pneumophila*	four times daily	available	no
Clarithromycin oral (IV not available)	*S. pneumoniae* *M. pneumoniae* *C. pneumoniae*	twice daily	not available	no

*Spectrum of coverage refers to approved indications as they pertain to in-hospital treatment of CAP for organisms specified.
**Refers to availability of IV to oral step-down using the *same* agent, i.e., IV azithromycin to oral azithromycin, IV erythromycin to oral erythromycin, etc.

niae, C. pneumoniae, S. aureus, Streptococcus pyogenes, Neisseria meningitidis, M. catarrhalis, Klebsiella pneumoniae and other gram-negative rods, *Legionella* species, influenza virus (depending on the time of year), respiratory syncytial virus, adenovirus, parainfluenza virus, and other microbes. The frequency of other etiologies, (e.g., *Chlamydia psittaci* [psittacosis], *Coxiella burnetii* [Q fever], *Francisella tularensis* [tularemia], and endemic fungi [histoplasmosis, blastomycosis, and coccidioidomycosis]), is dependent on specific epidemiological factors.

The selection of antibiotics, in the absence of an etiologic diagnosis (gram stains and culture results are not diagnostic), is based on multiple variables, including severity of the illness, patient age, antimicrobial intolerance or side effects, clinical features, comorbidities, concomitant medications, exposures, and the epidemiological setting.

Consensus Guidelines for Antibiotic Therapy

Consensus Report Guidelines: Infectious Disease Society of America. The IDSA through its Practice Guidelines Committee provides assistance to clinicians in the diagnosis and treatment of CAP. The targeted providers are internists and family practitioners, and the targeted patient groups are immunocompetent adult patients. Criteria are specified for determining whether the inpatient or outpatient setting is appropriate for treatment. Differences from other guidelines written on this topic include use of laboratory criteria for diagnosis and approach to antimicrobial therapy. Panel members and consultants were experts in adult infectious diseases.

The guidelines are evidence based where possible. A standard ranking system is used for the strength of recommendations and the quality of the evidence cited in the literature reviewed. The document has been subjected to external review by peer reviewers as well as by the Practice Guidelines Committee, and was approved by the IDSA Council in September 1998. *(Please see Table 3.)*

Centers for Disease Control Drug-Resistant Streptococcus pneumoniae Therapeutic Working Group Guidelines. One of the important issues in selecting antibiotic therapy for the elderly patient is the emerging problem of DRSP. To address this problem and provide practitioners with specific guidelines for initial antimicrobial selection in these patients, the CDC Drug-Resistant Streptococcus pneumoniae Therapeutic Working convened and published its recommendations in May 2000.[2] Some of the important clinical issues they addressed included the following: 1) what empirical antibiotic combinations (or monotherapeutic options) constituted reasonable initial therapy in outpatients, in hospitalized (non-ICU) patients, and in hospitalized intubated or ICU patients; 2) what clinical criteria, patient risk factors, or regional, epidemiological features constituted sufficient trigger points to include agents with improved activity against DRSP as initial agents of choice; and 3) what antibiotic selection strategies were most appropriate for limiting the emergence of fluoroquinolone-resistant strains.

Their conclusions with respect to antibiotic recommendations overlap significantly with the IDSA recommendations and the existing 1993 ATS guidelines. The specific differences contained in the Drug-Resistant Streptococcus pneumoniae Therapeutic Working Guidelines involve primarily the sequence in which antibiotics should be chosen in order to limit the emergence of fluoroquinolone-resistant strains, a preference for using combination drug therapy, cautionary notes about using fluoroquinolones as monotherapy in critically ill patients, reserving use of fluoroquinolones for specific patient populations, and detailed guidance regarding the comparative advantages among agents in each class.

Oral macrolide (azithromycin, clarithromycin, or erythromycin) or beta-lactam monotherapy is recommended by the CDC working group as initial therapy in patients with pneumonia considered to be amenable to outpatient management. For inpatients not in an ICU, this group recommends for initial therapy the combination of a parenteral beta-lactam (cefotaxime, ceftriaxone, etc.) plus a macrolide (azithromycin, erythromycin, etc.).[2] Hence, one of the most important, consistent changes among recent recommendations for initial, empiric management of patients with CAP is mandatory inclusion of a macrolide (which covers atypical pathogens) when a cephalosporin (which has poor activity against atypical pathogens) is selected as part of the initial combination regimen.

For critically ill patients, first-line therapy should include an intravenous beta-lactam, such as ceftriaxone or cefotaxime, and an intravenous macrolide such as azithromycin or erythromycin. The option of using a combination of a parenteral beta-lactam (cefotaxime, ceftriaxone, etc.) plus a fluoroquinolone with improved activity against DRSP is also presented. Once again, however, this committee issues clarifying, and sometimes cautionary, statements about the role of fluoroquinolone monotherapy in the critically ill patient, stating that caution should be exercised because the efficacy of the new fluoroquinolones as monotherapy for critically ill patients has not been determined.[2]

Clearly, fluoroquinolones are an important part of the antimicrobial arsenal in the elderly, and The CDC Drug-Resistant Streptococcus pneumoniae Therapeutic Working Group has issued specific guidelines governing their use in the setting of outpatient and inpatient CAP. It recommend fluoroquinolones be reserved for selected patients with CAP, among them: 1) adults, including elderly patients, for whom one of the first-line regimens (cephalosporin plus a macrolide) has failed; 2) those who are allergic to the first-line agents; or 3) those patients who have a documented infection with highly drug-resistant pneumococci (i.e., penicillin MIC ≥ 4 mcg/mL).

Prevention of Venous Thromboembolism

Background. Although antibiotic therapy, oxygenation, and maintenance of hemodynamic status are the primary triad of emergency interventions in elderly patients with pneumonia, there has been an increasing recognition of the risk for venous thromboembolic disease (VTED) incurred by immobilized elderly patients with infections such as pneumonia, especially when accompanied by CHF and/or respiratory failure. Emergency physicians, as well as attending physicians admitting such patients to the hospital, should be aware that the risk of VTED is significant enough to require prophylaxis in elderly patients with CAP who are likely to be immobilized for a period of three days or more (i.e. can ambulate less than 10 meters per day), and who have such risk factors as obesity, previous history of VTED, cancer, varicose veins, hormone therapy, chronic heart failure (NYHA Class III-IV), or chronic respiratory failure.[71]

From a practical perspective, this subset of patients should be strongly considered for prophylaxis to reduce the risk of VTED. Based on recent studies, the presence of pneumonia in a patient 75 years or older is, in itself, a criterion for prophylaxis against VTED, and when these factors are accompanied by CHF (Class III-IV) or respiratory failure, prophylaxis should be considered mandatory if there are no significant contraindications.[71] It should be added that The American College of Chest Physicians (ACCP) guidelines[72] and International Consensus Statement[73] also cite risk factors for VTED and emphasize their importance when assessing prophylaxis requirements for medical patients.

Evidence for Prophylaxis. The data to support a prophylactic approach to VTED for serious infections in the elderly is growing. The studies with subcutaneous unfractionated heparin (UFH) are inconclusive, although this agent is used for medical prophylaxis. Despite the recognition of risk factors and the availability of effective means for prophylaxis, DVT and PE remain common causes of morbidity and mortality. It is estimated that approximately 600,000 patients per year are hospitalized for DVT in North America.[74] In the United States, symptomatic PE occurs in more than 600,000 patients and causes or contributes to death in up to 200,000 patients annually.[75]

With respect to the risk of VTED in older patients with infection, one study group randomized infectious disease patients ages older than 55 years to UFH 5000 IU bid or placebo for three weeks. Autopsy was available in 60% of patients who died. Deaths from PE were significantly delayed in the UFH group, but the six-week mortality rate was similar in both groups. Non-fatal VTE was reduced by UFH. The findings of previous trials of prophylaxis in medical patients have been controversial, as the patient populations and methods used to detect thromboembolism, and the dose regimens vary, undermining the value of the findings. Comparative studies with clearly defined populations and reliable end points were therefore required to determine appropriate patient subgroups for antithrombotic therapy.[76]

The MEDENOX Trial. In response to the need for evidence to clarify the role of prophylaxis in specific non-surgical patient sub groups, the MEDENOX trial was conducted using the LMWH enoxaparin in a clearly identified risk groups.[71] In contrast to previous investigations, the MEDENOX trial included a clearly defined patient population (patients immobilized with severe chest [cardiopulmonary] disease) and was designed to answer questions about the need for prophylaxis in this group of medical patients and to determine the optimal dose of LMWH.[71]

Patients in the MEDENOX Trial were randomized to receive enoxaparin, 20 or 40 mg subcutaneously, or placebo once daily, beginning within 24 hours of randomization. They were treated for 10 (4 days in hospital and followed up in person or by telephone contact on day 90 (range, day 83-110). During follow-up patients were instructed to report any symptoms or signs of VTE or any other clinical event. The primary and secondary efficacy end points for MEDENOX were chosen to allow an objective assessment of the risk of VTE in the study population and extent of any benefit of prophylaxis. The primary end point was any venous thromboembolic event between day 1 and day 14. All patients underwent systematic bilateral venography at day 10 or earlier if clinical signs of DVT were observed. Venous ultrasonography was performed if venography was not possible. Suspected PE was confirmed by high probability lung scan, pulmonary angiography, helical computerized tomography, or at autopsy.[71] The primary safety end points were hemorrhagic events, death, thrombocytopenia, or other adverse event or laboratory abnormalities.[71]

A total of 1102 patients were included in the MEDENOX Trial, in 60 centers and nine countries. The study excluded patients who were intubated or in septic shock. Overall, the mean age was 73.4 the gender distribution was 50:50 male/female and the mean body mass index was 25.0. The mean patient ages, gender distribution, and body mass index was similar in all three treatment groups; there were slightly more males than females in the placebo and enoxaparin 20 mg groups, and more females than males in the enoxaparin 40 mg group, but this difference was not significant. The reasons for hospitalization of randomized patients varied.

The majority of patients were hospitalized for acute cardiac failure, respiratory failure, or infectious disease, with pneumonia being the most common infection in those older than age 70. For the study population as a whole, the most prevalent risk factor in addition to the underlying illness was advanced age (50.4%). By day 14, the incidence of VTE was 14.9% in the placebo group and 5.5% in the enoxaparin 40 mg group, representing a significant 63% relative risk reduction (97% CI: 37-78%; P = 0.0002) in VTE.

The primary conclusions of the MEDENOX Trial can be applied directly to clinical practice. First, acutely ill elderly medical patients with cardiopulmonary or infectious disease are at significant risk of VTE. Second, enoxaparin, given once daily at a dose of 40 mg for 6-14 days reduces the risk of VTE by 63%; and third, the reduction in thromboembolic risk is achieved without increasing the frequency of hemorrhage, thrombocytopenia, or any other adverse event compared with placebo. This study strongly suggests that elderly, immobilized patients admitted to the hospital with severe pneumonia, especially if accompanied by respiratory failure or Class III-IV CHF, should, if there are no contraindications to the use of anticoagulants, be considered candidates for prophylaxis with enoxaparin, 40 mg SC qd upon admission to the hospital to prevent VTED.

References

1. Sue DY. Community-acquired pneumonia in Adults. *West J Med* 1994;161:383-389.
2. Heffelfinger JD, Dowell SF, et al. A report from the Drug-resistant Streptococcus pneumoniae Therapeutic Working Group. Management of community-acquired pneumonia in the era of pneumococcal resistance. *Arch Int Med* 2000;160:1399.
3. Bartlett JG, Mundy M. Community-acquired pneuominia. *N Engl J Med* 1995;333:1618-1624.
4. Fine MD, Smith MA, et al. Prognosis and outcomes of patients with community acquired pneumonia. A meta-analysis. *JAMA* 1996;275:134-141.
5. Bates JH, Campbell AL, et al. Microbial etiology of acute pneumonia in hospitalized patients. *Chest* 1992;101:1005-1012.
6. Fang GD, Fine M, Orloff, et al. New and emerging etiologies for community-acquired pneumonia with implications for therapy-prospective multicenter study of 359 cases. *Medicine* 1990;69:307-316.
7. Marrie TJ. Community-acquired pneumonia: Epidemiology, etiology, treatment. *Infect Dis Clinic North Am* 1998;12:723-740.
8. American Thoracic Society: Guidelines for the Initial Management of adults with Community-Acquired Pneumonia: Diagnosis, Assessment of Severity, and Initial Antimicrobial Therapy. *Am Rev Respir Dis* 1993;148:1418-1426.
9. Confalonieri M, Potena A, Carbone G, et al. Acute respiratory failure in patients with severe community-acquired pneumonia. A prospective randomized evaluation of noninvasive ventilation. *Am J Respir Crit Care Med* 1999;160:1585-1591.
10. Hoe LK, Keang LT. Hospitalized low-risk community-acquired pneumonia: Outcome and potential for cost-savings. *Respirology* 1999;4:307-309.
11. Marrie TJ, Lau CY, Wheeler SL, et al. A controlled trial of a critical pathway for treatment of community-acquired pneumonia. *JAMA* 2000;283:749-755.
12. Dean NC, Suchyta MR, Bateman KA. Implementation of admission decision support for community-acquired pneumonia. A pilot study. *Chest* 2000;117:1368-1377.
13. Flanders WD, Tucker G, Krishnadasan A, et al. Validation of the pneumonia severity index: Importance of study-specific recalibration. *J Gen Intern Med* 1999;14:333-340.
14. Fine MJ, Auble TE, Yealy DM, et al. A prediction rule to identify low-risk patients with community-acquired pneumonia. *N Engl J Med* 1997;336:243-250.
15. Auble TE, Yealy DM, Fine MJ. Assessing prognosis and selecting an initial site of care for adults with community-acquired pneumonia. *Infect Dis Clin North Am* 1998;2:741-759.
16. Dean NC. Use of prognostic scoring and outcome assessment tools in the admission decision for community-acquired pneumonia. *Clin Chest Med* 1999;20:521-529.
17. Farr BM, Sloman AJ, Fisch MJ. Predicting death in patients hospitalized for community-acquired pneumonia. *Ann Intern Med* 1991;115:428-436.
18. Fine JM, Smith MA, Carson CA, et al. Prognosis and outcomes of patients with community-acquired pneumonia. *JAMA* 1996;275:134-141.
19. Houston MS, Silverstein MD, Suman VJ. Risk factors for 30-Day mortality in elderly patients with lower respiratory tract infection. *Arch Intern Med* 1997;157:2190-2195.
20. Conte HA, Chen YT, Mehal W, et al. A prognostic rule for elderly patients admitted with community-acquired pneumonia. *Am J Med* 1999;106:20-28.
21. Ewig S, Kleinfeld T, Bauer T, et al. Comparative validation of prognostic rules for community-acquired pneumonia in an elderly population. *Eur Respir J* 1999;14:370-375.
22. Mylotte JM, Naughton B, Saludades C, et al. Validation and application of the pneumonia prognosis index to nursing home residents with pneumonia. *JAGS* 1998;46:1538-1544.
23. Marston BJ, Plouffe JF, et al. Incidence of community-acquired pneumonia requiring hospitalization. Results of a population-based active surveillance study in Ohio. The Community-Based Pneumonia Incidence Study Group. *Arch Int Med* 1997;157:1709-1718.
24. Atlas SJ, Benzer TI, Borowsky LH, et al. Safely increasing the proportion of patients with community-acquired pneumonia treated as outpatients. An interventional trial. *Arch Intern Med* 1998;158:1350-1356.
25. Ewig S, Ruiz M, Mensa J, et al. Severe community-acquired pneumonia. Assessment of severity criteria. *Am J Respir Crit Care Med* 1998;158:1102-1108.
26. Brentsson E, Lagergard T. Etiology of community-acquired pneumonia in outpatients. *Eur J Clin Microbiol* 1986;5:446-447.
27. Langille DB, Yates L, Marrie TJ. Serological investigation of pneumonia as it presents to the physician's office. *Can J Infect Dis* 1993;4:328.
28. Whitney CG, Barrett N, et al. Increasing prevalence of drug-resistant Streptococcus pneumoniae (DRSP): Implications for therapy for pneumonia. In: *Programs and Abstracts of the 36th Annual Meeting of the Infectious Disease Society of America*, Nov. 12-15, 1998. IDSA, Abstract 51.
29. Cleeland R, Squires E. Antimicrobial activity of ceftriaxone: A review. *Am J Med* 1984;77:3.
30. Mandell LA. Antibiotics for pneumonia therapy. *Med Clin N Am* 1994;78:997-1014.
31. Gopalakrishna K, Lerner P. Tetracycline-resistant pneumococci: Increasing incidence and cross resistance to newer tetracyclines. *Am Rev Respir Dis* 1973;108:1007.
32. Mandell L. Community-acquired pneumonia: Etiology, epidemiol-

ogy and treatment. *Chest* 1995;108(sup):35S-42S.
33. Edelstein P. Legionnaires' disease. *Clin Infect Dis* 1993;16:741.
34. Garrison D, DeHaan R, Lawson J. Comparison of in vitro antibacterial activities of 7-chloro-7-deoxylincomycin, lincomycin, and erythromycin. *Antimicrob Agents Chemother* 1968;1967:397.
35. Antibiotic Update 1998: Outcome-effective treatment for bacterial infections managed in the primary care and emergency department setting. *Emerg Med Rep* 1997;18:1-24.
36. Enoxacin-A new fluoroquinolone. *Med Lett Drugs Ther* 1992;34:103-105.
37. Cooper B, Lawer M. Pneumococcal bacteremia during ciprofloxacin therapy for pneumococcal pneumonia. *Am J Med* 1989;87:475.
38. Flynn CM, et al. In vitro efficacy of levofloxacin alone or in combination tested against multi-resistant *Pseudomonas aeruginosa* strains. *J Chemother* 1996;8:411-415.
39. Dholakia N, et al. Susceptibilities of bacterial isolates from patients with cancer to levofloxacin and other quinolones. *Antimicrob Agents Chemother* 1994;38:848-852.
40. Garibaldi RA. Epidemiology of community-acquired respiratory tract infections in adults. Incidence, etiology, and impact. *Am J Med* 1985;78:32-37.
41. Fang GD, Fine M, Orloff J, et al. New and emerging etiologies for community-acquired pneumonia with implications for therapy. *Medicine* 1990;69:307-316.
42. Habib MP, et al. Intersci Conf Antimicrob Agents Chemother 1996;36. Abstract L002. 36th Interscience Conference on Antimicrobial Agents and Chemotherapy. New Orleans, LA. Sept. 15-18, 1996.
43. Plouffe J, Schwartz DB, Kolokathis A, et al. Clinical efficacy of intravenous followed by oral azithromycin monotherapy in hospitalized patients with community-acquired pneumonia. *Antimicrob Agents Chemother* 2000;44:1796-1802.
44. Vergis EN, Indorf A, et al. Azithromycin vs cefuroxime plus erythromycin for empirical treatment of community-acquired pneumonia in hospitalized patients. A prospective, randomized, multicenter trial. *Arch Int Med* 2000;160:1294-1300.
45. File TM, et al. Abstr Intersci Conf Antimicrob Agents Chemother 1996;36. Abstract L001 (LM1). 36th Interscience Conference on Antimicrobial Agents and Chemotherapy. New Orleans, LA. Sept. 15-18, 1996.
46. The choice of antibacterial drugs. *Med Lett Drugs Ther* 1996;38: 25-34.
47. Clarithromycin and azithromycin. *Med Lett Drugs Ther* 1992;34: 45-47.
48. Pfizer, Inc. Azithromycin package insert.
49. Pfizer product monograph. Azithromycin for IV injection.
50. Whitman MS, Tunkel AR. Azithromycin and clarithromycin: Overview and comparison with erythromycin. *Infect Control Hosp Epidemiol* 1992;12:357-368.
51. Data on file, Pfizer, Inc. New York, NY.
52. Zimmerman T, Reidel KD, Laufen H, et al. Intravenous toleration of azithromycin in comparison to clarithromycin and erythromycin. In Abstracts of the 36th Interscience Conference on Antimicrobial Agents and Chemotherapy. Washington, DC: American Society Microbiology; 1996:16 Abstract A82.
53. Mundy LM, et al. Community-acquired pneumonia: Impact of immune status. *Am J Respir Crit Care Med* 1995;152:1309-1315.
54. File TM, Dunbar L, et al. A multicenter, randomized study comparing the efficacy and safety of intravenous and/or oral levofloxacin versus ceftriaxone and/or cefuroxime in treatment of adults with community-acquired pneumonia. *Antimicrob Agents Chemother* 1997:41:1965-1972.
55. Kulgman KP, Capper T, et al In vitro susceptibility of penicillin-resistant *S. pneumoniae* to levofloxacin, selection of resistant mutants, and time-kill synergy studies of levofloxacin combined with vancomycin, telcoplanin, fusidic acid, and rifampin. *Antimicrob Agents Chemother* 1996;40:2802-2804.
56. Levaquin Product Information. Ortho-McNeil Pharmaceuticals. January 1997.
57. Vincent J, et al. Pharmacokinetics and safety of trovafloxacin in healthy male volunteers following administration of single intravenous doses of the prodrug, alatrofloxacin. *J Antimicrob Chemother* 1997;39(supp B):75-80.
58. Spangler SK, et al. Activity of CP 99,219 compared with those of ciprofloxacin, grepafloxacin, metronidazole, cefoxitin, piperacillin, and piperacillin-tazobactam against 489 anaerobes. *Antimicrob Agents Chemother* 1994;38:2471-2476.
59. Child J, et al. The in-vitro activity of CP 99,219, a new naphthyridone antimicrobial agent: A comparison with fluoroquinolone agents. *J Antimicrob Chemother* 1995;35:869-876.
60. Brighty KE, et al. The chemistry and biological profile of trovafloxacin. *J Antimicrob Chemother* 1997;39(supp B):1-14.
61. Hoogkamp-Korstanje JAA. In-vitro activities of ciprofloxacin, levofloxacin, lomefloxacin, ofloxacin, pefloxacin, sparfloxacin, and trovafloxacin against gram-positive and gram-negative pathogens from respiratory tract infections. *J Antimicrob Chemother* 1997;40:427-431.
62. Barry AL, et al. In vitro activities of five fluoroquinolone compounds against strains of *Streptococcus pneumoniae* with resistance to other antimicrobial agents. *Antimicrob Agents Chemother* 1996;40:2431-2333.
63. Visalli MA, et al. Activity of CP 99,219 (trovafloxacin) compared with ciprofloxacin, sparfloxacin, clinafloxacin, lomefloxacin and cefuroxime against ten penicillin-susceptible and penicillin-resistant pneumococci by time-kill methodology. *J Antimicrob Chemother* 1996;37:77-84.
64. American Thoracic Society, Medical Section of the American Lung Association. *Am Rev Respir Dis* 1993;148:1418-1426.
65. Fine MJ, et al. The hospital discharge decision for patients with community-acquired pneumonia. Results from the Pneumonia Patient Outcomes Research Team cohort study. *Arch Intern Med* 1997;157: 47-56.
66. American Thoracic Society. Guidelines for the initial management of adults with community-acquired pneumonia: Diagnosis, assessment of severity, and initial antimicrobial therapy. *Am Rev Respir Dis* 1993;148:1418-1426.
67. Thys JP, Jacobs F, Byl B. Role of quinolones in the treatment of bronchopulmonary infections, particularly pneumococcal and community-acquired pneumonia. *Eur J Clin Microbiol Infect Dis* 1991;10:304-315.
68. Piscitelli SC, Danziger LH, Rodwold KA. Clarithromycin and azithromycin: New macrolide antibiotics. *Clin Pharm* 1992;11: 137-152.
69. Ortquist A, et al. Oral empiric treatment of community-acquired pneumonia. *Chest* 1996;110:1499-1506.
70. Gleason PP, Meehan TP, Fine JM, et al. Associations between initial antimicrobial therapy and medical outcomes for hospitalized elderly patients with pneumonia. *Arch Intern Med* 1999;159: 2562-2572.
71. Samama MM, Cohen AT, Darmon JY, et al. A comparison of enoxaparin with placebo for the prevention of thromboembolism in acutely ill medical patients. Prophylaxis in Medical Patients with Enoxaparin Study Group. *N Engl J Med* 1999:341:793-800.
72. Clagett GP, Andersen FA, Heit JA, et al. Prevention of venous thromboembolism. *Chest* 1998;114(5 suppl):531S-560S.

73. Nicolaides AN, Bergquist D, Hull R, et al. Consensus statement. Prevention of venous thromboembolism. *Int Angiol* 1997:16:3-38.
74. Anderson FA, Wheeler HB, Goldberg RJ, et al. A population-based perspective of the hospital incidence and case-fatality rates of deep vein thrombosis and pulmonary embolism. The Worcester DVT study. *Arch Intern Med* 1991;151:933-938.
75. Sandler DA, Martin JF. Autopsy proven pulmonary embolism in hospital patients: Are we detecting enough deep vein thrombosis? *J Royal Soc Med* 1989;82:203-205.
76. Gardund B for the Heparin Prophylaxis Study Group. Randomized, controlled trial of low-dose heparin for prevention of fatal pulmonary embolism in patients with infectious diseases. *Lancet* 1996; 347:1357-1361.

Dementia

Fredric Hustey, MD

Emergency department (ED) encounters involving older patients with cognitive impairment are common. The incidence of dementia increases dramatically in the very elderly, the fastest growing subset of our geriatric population. Dementia also is prevalent in nursing home patients, who are often transferred to the ED for evaluation. The presence of dementia, which may not be recognized or documented, makes the evaluation of the older patient even more difficult. An accurate history may not be obtainable, which can lead to diagnostic uncertainty and more extensive work-ups. Dementia also has important implications for medical decision making and patient disposition. Furthermore, as the number of older ED patients increases, we can expect to see more patients presenting primarily for evaluation of cognitive impairment. Since some causes, such as depression or hypothyroidism, are potentially reversible, an accurate evaluation becomes even more critical.

This chapter examines the topic of dementia with an emphasis on etiologies, including potentially reversible causes; rapid ED assessment using simple screening tools; and avoiding pitfalls, such as differentiating dementia from delirium. Future issues will examine mental status changes in the elderly and delirium in greater detail.

Introduction

As the proportion of elderly in the population continues to increase, emergency physicians are likely to encounter geriatric issues with increasing frequency. The emergency department (ED) evaluation of these patients often is challenging. In one survey, the majority of emergency physicians indicated that the evaluation of common clinical problems, such as chest pain and altered mental status, was more difficult and time-consuming for older patients. They also reported insufficient training and very few continuing medical education hours on geriatric emergency medicine topics.[1] Because of the emphasis on illnesses of high acuity in the ED, there may be a lack of understanding and recognition for less acute but equally important age-specific disease processes in the geriatric ED patient. One of the most common of these is the syndrome of dementia. There is a high prevalence of dementia in older ED patients. One study found one-third of geriatric ED patients had unrecognized cognitive impairment.[2] This significant finding has important implications for emergency physicians. Obtaining an accurate medical history may be difficult in these patients. In addition, these patients carry a special risk for adverse outcomes after ED evaluation. The presence of dementia in the elderly patient can affect medication and discharge instruction compliance, resulting in an increased morbidity and mortality. Lack of recognition and delay in treatment may also contribute to poor long-term outcome. Emergency physicians are in a unique position to aid these patients. In order to achieve this, an increase in physician education and awareness is needed.

Definition

Dementia is a clinical syndrome described by a chronic, pathologic loss of intellectual function severe enough to interfere with

Table 1. Definition of Dementia[6]

1. Chronic impairment of memory of such severity as to interfere with daily, social, or occupational activities, with at least one of the following additional deficits:
   - aphasia
   - agnosia
   - apraxia
   - impaired executive functioning
2. Dementia cannot be diagnosed in the presence of delirium.

daily social or occupational activities.[3,4] It differs from the mild cognitive impairment associated with normal aging,[5] which does not significantly interfere with daily functioning. The hallmark of dementia is a progressive deterioration of memory. In order to confirm the diagnosis, patients must also exhibit at least one other deficit in cognitive function. *(Please see Table 1.)* This may include a language disturbance (aphasia), agnosia (difficulty recognizing or identifying familiar objects despite intact sensory function), apraxia (difficulty executing learned motor tasks despite intact motor function), or impairment in executive functioning (planning, organizing, abstracting, etc.).[6]

Epidemiology

Although dementia can occur in nearly all age groups, it is primarily a disease of the elderly. Prevalence ranges from 10% to 17% in those older than age 65, but increases dramatically as age progresses.[7-11] Approximately 1% of patients age 60 have dementia, while it affects nearly 50% of those 85 years and older.[12] There is no single cause or pathologic process responsible for dementia. More than 55 different illnesses can bring about the clinical syndrome.[13]

Dementia has a tremendous effect on both society and the health care system. Patients with dementia utilize a larger proportion of health care resources and have a higher morbidity and mortality rate than the general population corrected for age.[9,14] Dementia is also one of the leading contributors to the development of long-term functional dependence in the elderly, exceeding coronary artery disease and stroke.[9] This often results in placement of patients with dementia into extended care facilities, where extensive resources are devoted to the care and assistance of these patients. Family members caring for these patients are also affected. Those surrounding the patient frequently suffer from related depression and social stress.[15] The scope of dementia's effect on the health care system will continue to grow. The prevalence and mortality from dementia are expected to increase exponentially in the United States over the next 20-40 years, along with the rapid expansion of the geriatric population.[16-18]

Etiologies

Etiologies of dementia may be broadly grouped into two categories: those that are potentially curable or reversible, and those that are universally degenerative and progressive. *(Please see Table 2.)* Many cases of dementia are the result of multiple disease processes. The most common single cause of dementia is Alzheimer's disease, which accounts for more than half of all cases.[3,4] Vascular dementia comprises the next largest group, accounting for 10-20% of all dementia. Nearly all of the remaining cases are accounted for by a variety degenerative disorders, leaving fewer than 1% of causes considered potentially curable or reversible.[4,19] Although most causes of dementia are considered irreversible, there are still a variety of treatments available that can improve symptoms and slow functional decline. It is important to recognize these patients and to refer them for further evaluation and treatment.

Alzheimer's disease is perhaps the most widely recognized form of dementia. It accounts for nearly 50-70% of all cases.[3,4] It is characterized by an irreversible decline in cognitive function, primarily involving memory and language capabilities. Short-term memory is notably affected, and is usually one of the earliest findings. Language impairment may initially manifest as difficulty with word finding in spontaneous speech, and can progress to frank aphasia. In addition to memory and language deficits, patients also have difficulty processing visual and spacial information. This can lead to difficulty identifying or recognizing familiar objects or faces (agnosia) and misperceptions (e.g., mistaking shrubs or trees for people).[4] The inability to perform learned motor tasks (apraxia) is also a feature of Alzheimer's disease. As the dementia progresses, patients develop a progressive disorientation to time and place. This is nearly a universal finding in all patients with Alzheimer's disease.[3]

Psychiatric symptoms are frequently a part of Alzheimer's dementia as well. Patients may become withdrawn or increasingly hostile. Psychotic features are not uncommon. Hallucinations (predominantly visual) occur in up to 25% of patients;[4] paranoid delusions may be present in up to 50%.[20] Depression and suicidal ideation are also common findings.[21]

Unlike other dementia, disorders of movement (tremor, rigidity) are uncommon in Alzheimer's disease, and are usually present only in advanced cases. Presence of these features early in the course of the dementia should lead to questioning the diagnosis of Alzheimer's disease.

Research continues to aid us in the understanding of the pathophysiology of Alzheimer's disease. The "cholinergic hypothesis" associates cognitive decline with cholinergic neuronal destruction in the brain.[22] The result is an overall deficit of cholinergic neurotransmitter activity. Pathologic formation of B-amyloid leads to characteristic neuritic plaque formation in the brain.[23] Hyperphosphorylated tau-proteins collect to form neurofibrillary tangles.[24]

These processes appear to be concentrated in specific regions of the brain. Nearly all patients with Alzheimer's disease have progressive atrophy of the hippocampal and parahippocampal regions of the temporal lobe. The general cortical atrophy that follows is less specific. PET and SPECT imaging studies frequently reveal severe metabolic and perfusion deficits in the parietal and temporal lobes of Alzheimer's patients as well.[25,26]

The diagnosis of Alzheimer's disease is still confirmed postmortem, with cerebral tissue revealing characteristic neurofibrillary tangle and amyloid plaque deposition concentrated in the temporal and parietal lobes.[27]

A genetic link to Alzheimer's dementia has been strongly implicated. A gene identified on chromosome 19, the apolipoprotein (APOE) 4 allele, has been shown to both increase risk of development and decrease age of onset.[28] Interestingly, the presence of a different allele (APOE-2) has been shown to have a protective effect.[29] Many cases of Alzheimer's disease however, appear to be sporadic and not genetically linked.

Vascular dementia is second in frequency only to Alzheimer's disease in the elderly, and is responsible for approximately 10-20% of all dementia. Unlike Alzheimer's dementia, extrapyramidal dysfunction is not uncommon. Rigidity, masked facies, gait disturbance, and other parkinsonian features may be evident.[30] Co-existing dementia and focal neurologic deficit from prior cerebrovascular insult should always arouse suspicion of vascular dementia. More subtle motor deficits, such as impaired motor reaction time to external stimuli, are often present as well.[31] The course typically fluctuates but is always progressive.

In multi-infarct dementia, associated risk factors for the development of the disease should be present. Patients often have a history of stroke, poorly controlled hypertension, or peripheral vascular disease. Computed tomography (CT) and magnetic resonance imaging (MRI) findings are non-specific but may include visualization of multiple prior lacunar infarcts, white matter low attenuation,[32] including peri-ventricular white matter disease, and generalized atrophy. There are currently no widely accepted criteria for the diagnosis of vascular dementia.[4]

It is important to recognize there are many causes of vascular dementia other than repetitive small infarcts occurring from cerebrovascular disease (multi-infarct dementia [MID]). These include, but are not limited to autoimmune and infectious vasculitis (as with systemic lupus or neurosyphillis); subdural hematomas; and embolic disease (as in endocarditis). These potentially reversible causes must be entertained in the differential diagnosis of the patient presenting with a vascular dementia.

Occasionally, dementia may present with a predominance of psychiatric symptoms. This is the case with frontotemporal dementia (FTD). FTD occurs at an earlier age than most other degenerative dementia, with a mean onset reported at age 56.[33] Subtle personality changes, disinhibition, psychotic features (hallucinations and delusions), and other psychiatric symptoms often precede frank dementia by several years.[33] This often leads to an initial psychiatric diagnosis early in the course of the disease. There may be impairment of executive functioning, including difficulty with planning, goal setting, and speech. Motor dysfunction and parkinsonian features may also develop.[27] There is a strong familial inheritance of frontotemporal dementia, although many cases still appear to be sporadic.[33-35] Neuropathological findings are nonspecific, and include frontotemporal atrophy, gliosis of gray and white matter, and neutrophil vacuolization.[35]

Another common cause of dementia is that seen in Parkinson's disease. Typical movement disorders associated with Parkinson's accompany symptoms of dementia. Dementia with parkinsonism as an early feature often progresses much more rapidly than Alzheimer's dementia.[4]

Although previous studies have suggested that a significant number, estimated at 11%, of cases of dementia are potentially reversible,[36] more recent literature suggests that only approximately 1% are likely to reverse.[4,19] Common causes of reversible dementia include normal pressure hydrocephalus, vitamin B12 deficiency, hypothyroidism, and subdural hematoma. Early evaluation and detection of these reversible causes of cognitive impairment may lead to earlier treatment and, more importantly, improved outcomes.

Normal pressure hydrocephalus (NPH) is characterized by a classic triad of urinary incontinence, ataxia, and cognitive dysfunction. However, the diagnosis should be entertained in all patients presenting with gait disturbance and dementia. A history of urinary incontinence may be lacking in up to 50% of cases.[36] Gait disturbance may present initially as mild unsteadiness and progress to a shuffling gait as in Parkinson's disease. Cognitive impairment is often difficult to distinguish from Alzheimer's disease, but apraxia and aphasia are extremely uncommon. Head CT will often suggest the diagnosis, demonstrating the classic findings of enlarged ventricles without convolutional atrophy. Radionuclide cisternography will demonstrate reflux of cerebrospinal fluid into ventricles and delayed pericerebral diffusion.[36]

Table 2. Some Common Causes of Dementia

TYPE OF DEMENTIA	
Irreversible	***Reversible***
Alzheimer's disease	Normal pressure hydrocephalus
Multi-infarct dementia	Hypothyroidism
Frontotemporal dementia	Vitamin B_{12} deficiency
Parkinson's disease	Syphilis
Multiple sclerosis	Vasculitis
Huntington's chorea	Adrenal insufficiency
	Cushing's disease
	Chronic subdural hematomas
	Depression (pseudodementia)

Treatment of patients with normal pressure hydrocephalus has varying success. Ventriculoperitoneal shunting occasionally results in a complete reversal of symptoms, although residual deficits or no improvement at all are common outcomes.[19] Overall, only 30-50% of patients show improvement with treatment.[37]

Vitamin B12 deficiency is another common cause of potentially reversible dementia. Patients often have other symptoms typical of B12 deficiency, including a painful red tongue, parasthesias in the extremeties, and megaloblastic anemia. This diagnosis cannot be excluded in the setting of a normal erythrocyte count or morphology, since megaloblastic anemia is often absent. An abnormal cyanocobalamin levels confirm the diagnosis. As the deficiency progresses, there is less chance of reversal. Even with treatment the prognosis remains poor, although recovery does rarely occur.[38,39]

Hypothyroidism is the most common endocrine dysfunction to present with dementia. History may reveal fatigue, cold intolerance, constipation, and weight gain. Evidence of a hypometabolic state, alopecia, or the classic delay in relaxation of deep tendon reflexes on physical exam should also arouse suspicion. With treatment, full recovery can occur; however, reversal is usually incomplete.[40]

In the patient with a history of falls, chronic subdural hematomas may precipitate dementia. The prognosis after surgical intervention is limited, although some patients will have significant improvement.[41]

Depression in the elderly frequently induces symptoms resembling dementia (pseudodementia). Differences may be subtle but may include a shorter duration and a more acute onset of symptoms than in the patient with true dementia.[4] A history of psychiatric disease or emotional stressor may be elicited. Patients with depression may appear disinterested when questioned, and memory deficits may improve with coaxing. Often, a trial of anti-depressant therapy will result in resolution of symptoms.[19]

Dementia and the Emergency Department

The emergency department evaluation of the patient with dementia begins with recognition. The physician should always be on guard for evidence of abnormal cognition, regardless of the chief complaint.

Figure 1. Short, Portable Mental Status Questionnaire

- ❑ 1. What is the date today? (Month? Date? Year?)
- ❑ 2. What day of the week is it?
- ❑ 3. What is the name of this place?
- ❑ 4. What is your telephone number? Phone # from chart: ___ ___ ___/___ ___ ___-___ ___ ___ ___
  OR
  What is your street address? Address from chart:
  ____
- ❑ 5. How old are you?
- ❑ 6. When were you born? Date of birth from chart: ___ ___/___ ___/___ ___ ___ ___
- ❑ 7. Who is president of the United States now?
- ❑ 8. Who was president before him?
- ❑ 9. What was your mother's maiden name?
- ❑ 10. Subtract 3 from 20 and keep subtracting 3 from each new number, all the way down.

Used with permission from: Pfeiffer E. A short portable mental status questionnaire for the assessment of organic brain deficit in elderly patients. *J Am Geriatr Soc* 1975;23:433-441.

A wealth of potential information can be gained from closely observing the patient while gathering the history. The patient may have unusual difficulty relating events. Individuals may also have difficulty recalling medications taken or significant elements of his or her medical history. Trouble with word finding or aphasia may also be uncovered. Individuals in daily contact with the patient (such as family members or caregivers) should always be interviewed as well. They can help clarify the acuity of disease progression, and will often provide further evidence of cognitive dysfunction. They may relate alterations in personality, sleep disturbances, difficulty remembering tasks or medications, and evidence of apraxia. During the remainder of the physical examination, inability with activities of daily living may be evident. Patients may be poorly groomed and inappropriately dressed. During this phase, any evidence of abnormal cognition should compel the physician to further explore the possibility of dementia.

There are a variety of brief screening tools that can be useful to the emergency physician in further assessing cognitive function.[9] These may be useful if the emergency physician suspects undocumented cognitive impairment or has concerns about patient disposition or follow-up, especially in elderly patients who live alone. The Short Portable Mental Status Questionnaire (SPMSQ)[42] (see Figure 1) and the Orientation-Memory-Concentration Test (OMC)[43] (see Figure 2) are the most commonly used. Both of these tests are easy to administer and can be completed quickly in the ED. The SPMSQ consists of 10 items and focuses on orientation. Five or more errors on the SPMSQ provide evidence of cognitive impairment. The OMC consists of six items, and can be easily administered in the ED in less than 2 minutes.[2] It is reliable, valid, and has a better sensitivity for milder levels of impairment than the SPMSQ.[10,44] It is also unique in that scores have been related to neuropathologic findings of dementia at autopsy.[43] A weighted score of more than 10 on the OMC test is indicative of at least moderate cognitive impairment. Despite their ease of use, screening tests such as these are underutilized. For this reason, a group from Yale developed a simple, two-part test for detecting dementia in the outpatient setting. The Time and Change test involves only two tasks: to identify, given two tries and 1 minute, the correct time from an analog clock set at 11:10; and to sort out a dollar in change from three quarters, seven dimes, and seven nickels (given 2 tries in 2 minutes).[45] This test proved to be 63% sensitive and 96% specific for detecting dementia. While some cases of dementia will be missed, any patient who passes the test is unlikely to have even mild dementia. While screening tools such as these will help the physician assess cognition in greater detail, they should not be used to establish a formal diagnosis of dementia. They should, however, arouse suspicion for dementia when the results are abnormal and prompt the physician to refer these patients for further assessment. In the ED setting, physicians may find these screens useful to document possible acute or subacute cognitive impairment and then, based on the history and examination, determine if a significant organic cause might be present.

It is difficult, if not impossible, to do a complete laboratory and radiologic evaluation of the patient with suspected dementia in the ED. Furthermore, there is no "dementia protocol" outlining specific labs and x-rays, as the more than 55 clinical conditions that can precipitate dementia make each patient unique. The National Institutes of Mental Health and the National Institutes of Neurological Communicative Disorders recommend that all patients with dementia have a complete blood count, metabolic panel, set of electrolytes, thyroid function panel, vitamin B12 and folate levels, serology for syphilis, urinalysis, chest radiograph, and electrocardiogram as part of the initial screening evaluation.[3] There is still much debate over the routine use of neuroimaging studies (head CT, MRI) in the evaluation of all patients with dementia.[19,25,26,31,45] While these studies are costly and yields are low, they play an important role in excluding potentially reversible causes of dementia (NPH, subdural hematomas). A lack of classic examination findings is not always reliable in excluding these etiologies from the differential diagnosis. Neuroimaging studies may also be helpful in identifying specific etiologies for "irreversible," or degenerative dementia. For example, MRI studies revealing hippocampal and parahippocampal atrophy may help to confirm a diagnosis of Alzheimer's disease. As treatment options vary with the cause of the dementia, these studies are important in helping to direct further therapy.

It is impractical to carry out a complete work-up for dementia in the ED. Many of these tests are appropriately deferred to the physician to whom the patient is later referred. One approach might be to screen all patients with new suspicion of dementia with a complete blood count, serum glucose, set of electrolytes, and a metabolic panel. Further testing could be selectively obtained based on results of the history and physical examination. For example, the patient with a risk for subdural hematoma, focal neurologic deficit, or evidence of normal pressure hydrocephalus warrants a head CT in the ED. Suspicion of myxedema warrants assessment of thyroid functions. An erythrocyte sedimentation rate should be completed for all patients with suspected vasculitis. Review the differential diagnosis for potentially reversible causes when formulating a care plan for each patient. A relatively recent onset of symptoms may carry a higher risk for morbidity, and should result in a more aggressive search.

Differential Diagnosis

It is important to distinguish dementia from other diseases that may also affect cognition. Delirium should always be considered in the differential diagnosis of the patient with an abnormal mental status. Unlike dementia, delirium is a more acute condition and is usually reversible with treatment. *(Please see Table 3.)* While patients with delirium may exhibit cognitive dysfunction, the primary problem is a clouding of consciousness and a reduced awareness of the surrounding environment. Patients often display abnormal levels of alertness, and may be hypoactive or hypervigilant. There is invariably an attention deficit, with an impaired ability to maintain, focus, and shift concentration. Hallucinations are also more common in the patient with delirium. Symptoms tend to fluctuate in severity over the course of the day. Delirium is often an indication of serious underlying illness, and is associated with high morbidity and mortality. Patients with delirium always warrant an aggressive search for underlying causes and usually require hospitalization. Dementia cannot be diagnosed in the presence of a delirium.

Major depressive disorder is often difficult to distinguish from dementia. Both disorders may present with memory impairment and changes in effect. Patients with depression often seem disinterested and apathetic during memory testing, and deficits often improve with coaxing. This is in contrast to the patient with dementia, who gives incorrect answers despite an adequate effort to remember. Depression is also more likely to exhibit a more discreet onset and shorter duration. Finally, patients with depression may be more likely to complain of a memory deficit, while it is often the family of the patient with dementia who first mentions the complaint.[4]

Finally, it is important to differentiate dementia from the mild cognitive impairment associated with normal aging. These patients exhibit mild impairment in memory, which does not affect daily function.

Disposition

The dementia itself is often not the deciding factor in determining the patient's disposition. Co-existing abnormalities found during the evaluation may necessitate hospitalization (urosepsis, subdural hematoma, etc.). However, there are also special circumstances to consider in the patient with dementia. The effect of cognitive impairment on treatment compliance should be considered. For example, a patient with uncomplicated pneumonia discharged to home may return with sepsis because of antibiotic noncompliance resulting from confusion over medication instructions. Such patients lacking adequate home support to assist with compliance should be hospitalized. Patients incapable of performing necessary self-care functions and with limited home support should also be hospitalized. This may be evidenced by unusually poor hygiene (such as the presence of urine or feces in clothing), dehydration, or poor nutritional status. Family or caregiver frustration may lead to abuse. Other options for disposition include follow-up assessment at home by home-health nurses and use of sub-acute units, including ED-based observation units. All patients with dementia and suspicion of elder abuse should be hospitalized for further evaluation.

Pitfalls

There are several potential pitfalls to avoid when evaluating the ED patient with dementia. These include failing to recognize the presence of dementia, failing to refer patients for further evaluation of cognitive impairment, misperceiving dementia as a medically untreatable and terminal process, and assuming a patient with dementia has been evaluated and managed by a primary care physician.

Emergency physicians may be overlooking the presence of an abnormal mental status in large numbers of geriatric patients.[46] The pace of the ED often results in the urge to focus narrowly on the chief complaint. Subtle evidence of dementia may be ignored. A patient might display problems with word finding while relating a history. Short-term memory impairment may manifest as unusual difficulty in remembering details, or reciting or complying with medications. Failure to interview individuals in close contact with the patient may leave additional evidence uncovered. Often patients are unaware of cognitive difficulties and will deny any problems if asked.

Table 3. Delirium or Dementia?

	DELIRIUM	DEMENTIA
Onset	Acute	Insidious
Progression	Fluctuating	Stable
Attention	Disordered	Normal
Hallucinations	Visual	Absent
Delusions	Fleeting	Absent (unless advanced or FTD)
Cognition	Disordered	Impaired

Even when dementia is recognized, ED management may be sub-optimal. The perception of dementia as an illness of lower acuity may result in an incomplete or superficial evaluation.[47] Attributing senility to the normal process of aging can be more detrimental to the patient. The physician may decide that no further evaluation is necessary, depriving the patient of potential therapies, resources, or cures.

It is important to refer all patients with suspected dementia for further evaluation and treatment. Geriatric assessment units, used in consultation with the patient's primary care physician, can be of assistance in this evaluation. If the cause of dementia is discovered, interventions can be instituted that slow or even reverse disease progression. This is true even with degenerative, or so-called irreversible dementia such as Alzheimer's or MID. Cholinesterase inhibitors such as Tacrine and Donazepil can be used to slow cognitive deterioration and delay institutionalization in many patients with Alzheimer's disease.[48-51] Early psychosocial intervention has also been shown to postpone institutionalization.[22] Dementia-related behavioral symptoms often respond to anti-depressant therapy with selective serotonin re-uptake inhibitors. Psychotic features can be managed with newer and safer neuroleptic agents. In patients with vascular dementia, secondary prevention of cerebral infarcts may be effective in slowing the course.[52] Most of these treatments are appropriately deferred to the patient's primary physician, who after further evaluation may identify a specific cause for the dementia.

Early recognition and referral of all patients with dementia has important prognostic significance. There is a much greater chance of curing a reversible dementia early in the course of the disease. Deficits also become more prominent as the dementia remains untreated. Early treatment of Alzheimer's disease may have a dramatic effect on prognosis as well.[53]

Patients at high risk for failure to refer may be those in which underlying dementia is most readily apparent. Avoid the urge to assume that if the condition is obvious and chronic, it has at some point been addressed by the primary care provider. While family members may recognize there is a significant memory problem, they may not have arranged for further evaluation because of believing that there is nothing medically that can be done. Any assumption that the dementia is currently being treated should be confirmed by asking the patient and family.

Conclusion

Dementia is highly prevalent among elderly patients seen in the ED. It is important for emergency physicians to recognize the special risks that apply to these patients. In the short term, ED outcome can be adversely affected by an inability to understand and comply with discharge instructions. Emergency physicians are also in a position to dramatically alter the long-term outcome of these patients. While most cases of dementia are considered irreversible, all cases are treatable when recognized and accurately diagnosed. Prognosis may be dependent on how early these treatments are initiated in the course of the disease. Early recognition and appropriate referrals initiated in the ED may significantly alter the prognosis and quality of life of patients with dementia.

References

1. McNamara RM, Rousseau E, Sanders AB. Geriatric emergency medicine: A survey of practicing emergency physicians. *Ann Emerg Med* 1992;21:796-801.
2. Gerson LW, Counsell SR, Fontanarosa PB, et al. Case finding of cognitive impairment in elderly emergency department patients. *Ann Emerg Med* 1994;23:813-817.
3. Johnson JC, Sims R, Gottlieb G. Differential diagnosis of dementia, delirium and depression. *Drugs & Aging* 1994;5:431-445.
4. Geldmacher DS, Whitehouse PJ. Current concepts: Evaluation of dementia. *N Engl J Med* 1996;335:330-336.
5. Huppert F, Wilcock G. Ageing, cognition and dementia. *Age & Ageing* 1997;4:20-23.
6. Diagnostic and Statistical Manual of Mental Disorders, 4th Ed. American Psychiatric Association; 1994.
7. Larson EB, Kukall WA, Katzman RL. Cognitive impairment: Dementia and Alzheimer's disease. *Ann Rev Pub Health* 1992;13:431-439.
8. Erkinjuntti T, Ostbye T, Steenhuis R, et al. The effect of different diagnostic criteria on the prevalence of dementia. *N Engl J Med* 1997;337:1667-1674.
9. Aguero-Torres H, Fratiglioni L, Winblad B. Natural history of Alzheimer's disease and other dementias: Review of the literature in the light of the findings from the Kungsholmen Project. *Inter J Geriatr Psych* 1998;13:755-766.
10. Fillenbaum GG, Landerman LR, Simonsick EM. Equivalence of two screens of cognitive functioning: The Short Portable Mental Status Questionnaire and the Orientation-Memory-Concentration test. *J Am Geriatr Soc* 1998;46:1512-1518.
11. Gao S, Henrie HC, Hall KS, et al. The relationship between age, sex, and the incidence of dementia and Alzheimer disease: A meta-analysis. *Arch Gen Psych* 1998;55:809-815.
12. Evans DA, Funkenstein HH, Albert MS, et al. Prevalence of Alzheimer's disease in a community population of older persons: Higher than previously reported. *JAMA* 1989;226: 2551-2556.
13. Mayeux R, Foster NL, Rossor M, et al. The clinical evaluation of patients with dementia. In: Whitehouse PJ, ed. *Dementia*. Vol. 40 of Contemporary neurology series. Philadelphia: F.A. Davis; 1993:92-129.
14. Lanska DJ. Dementia mortality in the United States. Results of the 1986 National Mortality Followback Survey. *Neurol* 1998;50:362-367.
15. Braekhus A, Oksengard AR, Engedal K, et al. Social and depressive stress suffered by spouses of patients with mild dementia. *Scan J Prim Health* 1998;16:242-246.
16. Lanska DJ, Schoenberg BS. The epidemiology of dementia: Methodological issues and approaches. In: Whitehouse PJ, ed. *Dementia.* Vol. 40, Contemporary neurology series. Philadelphia: F.A. Davis, 1993:3-33.
17. Jorm AF. *The epidemiology of Alzheimer's disease and related disorders*. London: Chapman and Hall; 1990:54-76.
18. Jorm AF, Koren AE, Jacomb PA. Projected increases in the number of dementia cases for 29 developed countries: Application of a new method for making projections. *Acta Psych Scan* 1988;78:493-500.
19. Van Crevel H, van Gool WA, Walstra GJ. Early diagnosis of dementia: which tests are indicated? What are their costs? *J Neurol* 1999;246:73-78.
20. Mendez MF, Martin R, Smyth KA, et al. Psychiatric symptoms associated with Alzheimer's disease. *J Neuropsych Clin Neurosci* 1990;2:28-33.
21. Draper B, MacCuspie-Moore C, Brodaty H. Suicidal ideation and the "wish to die" in dementia patients: The role of depression. *Age & Ageing* 1998;27:503-507.
22. Schneider LS. New therapeutic approaches to cognitive impairment. *J Clin Psych* 1998;11:8-13.
23. Murphy GM, Tamminga CA. Amyloid plaques [Images in Neuroscience]. *Am J Psych* 1995;152:1258
24. Trojanowski JQ, Lee VM-Y. Phosphorylation of neuronal cytoskeletal proteins in Alzheimer's disease and Lewy body dementias. *Ann N Y Acad Sci* 1994;747:92-109.
25. Small GW, Leiter F. Neuroimaging for diagnosis of dementia. *J Clin Psych* 1998;11:4-7.
26. Scheltens P. Early diagnosis of dementia: Neuroimaging. *J Neurol* 1999;246:16-20.
27. Drachman DA, Newell KL. Weekly clinicopathological exercises: Case 12-1999: A 67-year-old man with three years of dementia. *N Eng J Med* 1999;340:1269-1276.
28. Corder Eh, Saunders AM, Strittmatter WJ, et al. Gene dose of apolipoprotein E type 4 allele and the risk of Alzheimer's disease in late onset families. *Science* 1993;261:921-923.
29. Corder EH, Saunders AM, Risch MJ, et al. Apolipoprotein E type 2 allele and the risk of late onset Alzheimer's disease. *Nature Genet* 1994;7:180-183.
30. Kotsoris H, Barclay LL, Kheyfets S, et al. Urinary and gait disturbances as markers for early multi-infarct dementia. *Stroke* 1987;18:138-141.
31. George AE, de Leon MJ, Golomb J, et al. Imaging the brain in dementia: Expensive and futile? *Amer J Neuroradiol* 1997;18:1847-1850.
32. Amar K, Lewis T, Wilcock G, et al. The relationship between white matter low attenuation on brain CT and vascular risk factors: A memory clinic study. *Age & Ageing* 1995;24: 411-415.
33. Chow TW, Miller BL, Hayashi VN, et al. Inheritance of frontotemporal dementia. *Arch Neurol* 1999;56:817-822.
34. Lynch T, Sano M, Marder KS, et al. Clinical characteristics of a family with chromosome 17-linked disinhibition-dementia-parkinsonism-amyotrophy complex. *Neurology* 1994;44:1878-1884.
35. Foster NL, Wilhemsen K, Sima AAF, et al. Frontotemporal dementia and parkinsonism linked to chromosome 17: A consensus conference. *Ann Neurol* 1997;41:706-715.

36. Clarfield AM. The reversible dementias: Do they reverse? *Ann Intern Med* 1988;109:476-486.
37. Vanneste J, Augustijn P, Dirven C, et al. Shunting normal-pressure hydrocephalus: Do the benefits outweigh the risks? A multicenter study and literature review. *Neurology* 1992; 42:54-59.
38. Teunisse S, Bollen AE, Gool WA, et al. Dementia and subnormal levels of vitamin B12: Effects of replacement therapy on severity of dementia. *J Neurol* 1996;243:522-529.
39. Chatterjee A, Yapundich R, Palmer CA, et al. Leukencephalopathy associated with cobalamin deficiency. *Neurology* 1996;46:832-834.
40. Haupt M, Kurz A. Reversibility of dementia in hypothyroidism. *J Neurol* 1993;240:333-335.
41. Alexander EM, Wagner EH, Buchner DM, et al. Do surgical brain lesions present as isolated dementia? A population-based study. *J Am Geriatr Soc* 1995;43:138-143.
42. Pfeiffer E. A short portable mental status questionnaire for the assessment of organic brain deficit in elderly patients. *J Am Geriatr Soc* 1975;23:433-441.
43. Katzman R, Brown T, Fuld P, et al. Validation of a short orientation-memory-concentration test of cognitive impairment. *Am J Psychiatry* 1983;140;734-739.
44. Davis PB, Morris JC, Grant E. Brief screening tests versus clinical staging in senile dementia of the Alzheimer type. *J Am Geriatr Soc* 1990;38:129-135.
45. Froelich TE, Robinson JT, Inouye SK. Screening for dementia in the outpatient setting: The time and change test. *J Am Geriatr Soc* 1998;46:1506-1511.
46. Lewis LM, Miller DK, Morley JE, et al. Unrecognized delirium in ED geriatric patients. *Amer J Emer Med* 1995;13: 142-145.
47. Birrer R, Singh U, Kumar DN. Disability and dementia in the emergency department. *Emer Med Clin of North Am* 1999;17:505-517.
48. Shea C, MacKnight C, Rockwood K. Donepezil for treatment of dementia with Lewy bodies: A case series of nine patients. *Inter Psychogeriatrics* 1998;10:229-238.
49. Knopman D, Schneider L, Davis K, et al. Long-term tacrine (Cognex) treatment: Effects on nursing home placement and mortality, Tacrine Study Group. *Neurology* 1996;47:166-177.
50. Minthon L, Gustafson L, Dalfelt G, et al. Oral tetrahydroaminoacridine treatment of Alzheimer's disease evaluated clinically and by regional cerebral blood flow and EEG. *Dementia* 1993;4:32-42.
51. Nordberg A, Lilja A, Lundqvist H, et al. Tacrine restores cholinergic nicotinic receptors and glucose metabolism in Alzheimer patients as visualized by positron emission tomography. *Neurobiol Aging* 1992;13:747-758.
52. Amar K, Wilcock G. Vascular dementia. *BMJ* 1996;312: 227-231.
53. van Reekum R, Simard M, Farcnik K. Diagnosis of dementia and treatment of Alzheimer's disease. Pharmacologic management of disease progression and cognitive impairment. *Can Fam Physician* 1999;45:945-52.

Orthopedic Emergencies in the Elderly

Steven F. Fisher, MD
Selim Sumer, MD, MS, FACEP

The world's aging population is a distinct segment of society with specific medical concerns. While the majority of the orthopedic injuries afflicting the elderly are not immediately life-threatening, these injuries precipitate untimely mortality. Furthermore, orthopedic injuries lead to long-term morbidity and a significant decline in function, which may greatly restrict the independence of some individuals.

This chapter is devoted to addressing the common orthopedic concerns encountered by the elderly. Common fractures, predisposing factors, therapeutic techniques, and preventive measures will be discussed. The value of a thorough evaluation and the prompt initiation of care by emergency physicians will be stressed. Moreover, to be better advocates for their patients, emergency physicians should be well versed in the preventative strategies that may benefit patients who are at risk.

Epidemiology

Fractures in the elderly are of great medical and economic concern. The proportion of the world's elderly population continues to grow rapidly, largely because of an increased life expectancy. Improved health care and heightened health consciousness account for this longevity. By the year 2020, the U.S. Census Bureau predicts that the average life expectancy will be 82.0 years for women and 74.2 years for men.[1] In fact, this segment of the population is now the fastest growing group in the United States and other developed countries.[2] As the elderly population continues to grow, so will their encumbrance upon an already overwhelmed health care system. For this reason, strategies for improved medical care and prevention must be devised. Similarly, the demand for emergency physicians well-versed in the management of fractures in the elderly will increase to counter the challenge of an increasing number of elderly patients presenting with common fractures. As the emergency department is the portal to medical care for many, the emergency physician must be cognizant of current therapies and preventative strategies in order to reduce morbidity, mortality, and the costs of hospitalization. Furthermore, the task of coordinating the multidisciplinary care of patients often befalls the emergency physician.

Predisposing Factors

The etiology of fractures in the elderly may be subdivided into intrinsic and extrinsic factors. Intrinsic factors are those predisposing conditions innate to bone, such as osteoporosis and other disease-related processes. Conversely, extrinsic factors, such as trauma and elder abuse, are those that are not related to the innate properties of bone. Most commonly, traumatic injuries affecting the elderly are the result of falls or motor vehicle accidents. Excepting non-traumatic osteoporotic or pathologic fractures, the elderly are susceptible to the same mechanical forces placed upon younger people in traumatic injury. The elderly, however, cannot tolerate these same mechanical forces and suffer heightened injury.

Osteoporosis. Osteoporosis is the most common metabolic bone disease in the United States and a significant cause of morbidity among the elderly. Affecting the physical and psychological prosperity of nearly 28 million Americans, it is one of the most predominant diseases associated with aging.[3] In addition to aging, osteoporosis is the consequence of genetic, hormonal, and nutritional factors, as well as physical forces.[4] It is characterized by a concomitant reduction in bone mass and deterioration in skeletal microarchitecture, which ultimately compromises bone integrity. Moreover, the link between osteoporosis and the preponderance of fractures in the elderly cannot be disputed.

For Caucasian women, the lifetime risk of suffering a hip fracture is 19%, a distal forearm fracture is 16%, and a vertebral fracture is 15.6%. In fact, a Caucasian woman has a 40% chance of suffering one of these fractures during her lifetime.[5] Furthermore, in the United States, approximately 80% of osteoporotic fractures occur in women, and the age-specific incidence of these fractures is higher in women than men.[6] Although the number of men afflicted with osteoporosis is unknown, estimates of lifetime fracture risk range from 13% to 25%.[7]

Osteoporosis alters the usual balance between formation and resorption of bone during remodeling. Bone is resorbed by osteoclasts at a greater rate than it is formed by osteoblasts, resulting in a loss of both bone mass and density. Due to this unbalanced resorption, the bone becomes so fragile that it cannot withstand the normal mechanical forces placed upon it. Ultimately, a fracture occurs and osteoporosis becomes a clinically evident problem. The most common orthopedic injuries associated with osteoporosis are vertebral compression fractures, distal radius fractures, and proximal femur (hip) fractures. Hip fractures result in considerable morbidity and mortality.[8] Vertebral compression fractures and distal radius fractures also lead to significant morbidity, and in the case of vertebral fractures, also substantial mortality. No matter the specific outcome, few with an osteoporosis-related fracture elude a reduction in quality of life.

Heightened bone resorption commences circa the beginning of menopause in many women (type I), and age-related bone loss (type II) becomes evident in the sixth decade of life in many men and women.[9] In women, bone mass and density peak between menarche and the fourth decade.[10] Thereafter, there is a small premenopausal decline in bone mass, but the onset of menopause propagates a more precipitous loss of bone mineral density. In fact, interruption of the endogenous supply of estrogen during menopause appears to increase the activation of new remodeling sites.[11] An increased number of active remodeling units leads to the complete penetration of trabecular bone. The consequence of which appears to be a loss of the template upon which new bone may be formed and a subsequent permanent deficit in bone mass and structure.[12] The average rate of decline in bone mineral density in untreated women is highest during the initial five years after the onset of menopause or after the discontinuation of estrogen replacement. In fact, an annual loss of approximately 2-4% of bone mineral density can be expected.[13] Although bone loss persists indefinitely, the rate of such loss gradually declines to approximately 1-1.5% per year by 10 years postmenopause. In one study, however, a possible acceleration of bone loss was noted after the age of 70.[14]

In men, the three major causes of osteoporosis are alcohol abuse, glucocorticoid excess, and hypogonadism. These etiologies account for 40-50% of all men with osteoporosis.[7] Nevertheless, it is important to consider occult gastrointestinal (GI) disease when treating a man whose osteoporosis is not readily explained. Interestingly, these men are typically not symptomatic of GI manifestations. The list of other potential causes of osteoporosis in men is extensive. Unfortunately, when all known or likely causes are ruled out, approximately 40-50% of men will not have a known etiology.[15] Therefore, the diagnosis of idiopathic osteoporosis in men is common. An arbitrary upper age limit is imposed for this diagnosis, as eventually age alone can account for bone loss in both men and women.[16]

Measurement of bone mass is used in the diagnosis and monitoring of osteoporosis. The methods for measuring bone mass have improved greatly in recent years. Specifically, dual energy x-ray absorptiometry (DXA), quantitative computed tomography (QCT), and single-photon absorptiometry (SPA) currently are the most commonly used techniques. DXA allows for the rapid and precise determination of the body's bone mineral mass, in addition to lean vs. fat soft-tissue composition. More importantly, the x-ray-based system evaluates bone mineral density at individual anatomic locations such as the spine, hip, and forearm. Conversely, QCT offers the advantage of less radiation while quantifying the absorption of ionizing radiation by calcified tissues. These measurements are then compared to standard reference material in order to calculate bone mineral equivalents. QCT, however, is limited by its high cost. Finally, SPA employs a beam of low-energy photons to assess bone mineral density at peripheral sites such as the radius or calcaneous, where the thickness of surrounding soft-tissue is low and may be controlled. It has the advantages of being radiation-free and having low cost.[17]

DXA, however, has been the most successful technique due to its ability to measure bone mass at virtually all skeletal sites. This is important, as bone mass at one site cannot be predicted from measurements performed at another site, even in the same individual.[18] Therefore, assessment at particular sites is preferable. Nevertheless, all of the aforementioned modalities, as well as prospective techniques currently under development, may be excellent predictors of future fracture risk.

Falls. Falls are a common event in the lives of older persons, and may result in significant morbidity, mortality, and health care utilization. Nearly 20% of elderly adults require the assistance of another person or a device (such as a cane or walker) to ambulate. Furthermore, such assistance is necessary in almost 40% of patients age 85 older.[19] Per annum, falls occur in 32% of individuals between the ages of 65 and 74, in 35% of those between ages 75 and 84, and in 51% of those 85 years or older.[20] Approximately 4-6% of falls in elderly persons result in fractures, one-fourth of which occur at the hip.[21] Additionally, falls account for 12% of all deaths (directly or indirectly) in the aged.[20] More often, falls result in restriction of mobility or activity and can lead to a loss of independence and fear. This fear is validated by the fact that more than two-thirds of those elderly who fall will do so again within six months.[22] Decreased confidence in the ability to safely ambulate can lead to further functional decline, depression, feelings of helplessness, and social isolation. Furthermore, the inability to rise after a fall is distressing and dangerous. Elder persons found on the ground for prolonged periods are at increased risk of subsequent complications, not limited to dehydration, hypothermia, decubitous ulcers, pneumonia, and rhabdomyolysis.

Falls are the result of different etiologies and circumstances. Unearthing the precipitant of a fall is as vital as the identification and treatment of the subsequent injuries. Identified risk factors for falling include age, cognitive impairment, medications, chronic disease, vertigo, and impairments in strength, balance, and gait.[21] The combined number of risk factors is also quite pertinent. One community-based prospective study demonstrated that 8% of elderly persons with no risk factors, as opposed to 78% of those with four or more risk factors, fell within the year.[23] Additionally, the chance of suffering multiple falls directly increased with the number of risk factors.[24]

As individuals age, they are inevitably besieged with multiple medical conditions, which may lead to an increased susceptibility to falls. It is estimated that known syncope accounts for 2-15% of falls in the elderly, but many syncopal episodes go unidentified. Thus, it should be considered a potential precipitant of all unwitnessed falls and, therefore, investigated.[25] The most frequent causes of syncope in elder persons are vasovagal reactions, cardiac arrhythmias, and orthostatic hypotension.

Likewise, delirium is another common antecedent for falls in the elderly. Approximately 10% of elderly patients older than age 65 meet the criteria for delirium. Unfortunately, fewer than 25% of delirious patients are identified.[26] Gait disorders, another precipitant of falls, are present in 20-50% of the elderly population.[27] These disorders may be attributed to multiple factors, including chronic diseases that impair sensory, cognitive, neurologic, or musculoskeletal function. Last, medications also can be a cause of falls. Drugs implicated included sedatives-hypnotics, diuretics, and cardiac medications.

The realization that a fall may be a sentinel event in the life of an aged person should prompt emergency physicians to initiate appropriate interventions for these people. The diagnostic assessment of an elderly person who has suffered a fall should focus on identifying risk factors that can be ameliorated to reduce the likelihood of future falls. (The basic components of the clinical assessment are outlined in Table 1.) The coordination of multi-specialty care through appropriate referrals is paramount. Interventions that improve functional status or curb functional decline may increase a patient's well-being as well as longevity.

Pathological Fractures. Pathological fractures are those that result from a focal disease process, which compromises the integrity of bone. Typically, the fracture occurs during normal activity or with minor trauma. The two most common etiologies of pathological fractures are malignancies and Paget's disease. Metastatic carcinoma remains the most common malignancy of bone.[28] In fact, the most likely primary cancers to invade bone are breast, lung, thyroid, kidney, and prostate. Multiple myeloma is the most common primary malignancy of bone, but other cancers of the hematopoietic system, such as lymphoma and leukemia, may precipitate pathologic fractures.[28] Less commonly, osteosarcoma and chondrosarcoma, cancers of the bone itself, may lead to fractures as well.

Paget's disease (osteitis deformans), a pathological increase in bone turnover, is a common bone disorder in the geriatric population. Second only to osteoporosis, it is characterized by the resorption of normal bone and the excessive deposition of abnormal bone.[29] Although the newly formed bone is dense, it is structurally abnormal and a precursor to pathological fractures. While Paget's disease may involve only one bone, typically multiple sites are implicated in an asymmetrical distribution. In 75% of cases, the affected sites include the pelvis, the lumbar spine, and the femur.[30]

Ninety-five percent of patients with Paget's disease are asymptomatic, making it difficult to diagnose. For those patients who do experience symptoms such as bone pain, skeletal deformity, and fracture; diagnosis is difficult nevertheless because such symptoms may be attributed to concomitant or pre-existing arthritic changes. In fact, up to 30% of patients who experience symptoms do so for at least 10 years prior to diagnosis.[30] While its presentation is insidious, Paget's disease leads to significant morbidity in elder persons.[31] In fact, it may affect up to 3% of adults older than age 40.[32]

Elder Abuse. Elder abuse is a real and significant problem that plagues the elderly population and is an occasional cause of fractures. The House Select Committee on Aging estimates that 1-2 million elder Americans are abused each year.[33] The true prevalence of elder abuse may be much higher, however, as many cases are not reported.[34] In fact, a Boston survey demonstrated that only one in 14 cases of elder abuse is reported, and reporting is rarely done by physicians. One Michigan study demonstrated that only 2% of reported cases in the state were made by physicians.[35]

Emergency physicians may be the only persons to encounter a victim of elder abuse and are, therefore, uniquely positioned to identify and assist them. A random survey in 1992, however, revealed that only 27% of emergency physicians had protocols available for the appropriate management of suspected elder abuse. Interestingly, 75% of these physicians reported having algorithms in place for suspected child abuse.[36] In contrast to cases of suspected child abuse, mandatory reporting of elder abuse may infringe upon the autonomy and privacy of the competent adult. Furthermore, mandatory reporting may discourage abused elderly from seeking medical care because of the fear of embarrassment and institutionalization. For these reasons, elder abuse may necessitate specific laws and management that differ from classic abuse models. Nevertheless, mandatory reporting laws exist in all 50 sates and the District of Columbia.[37]

Elder abuse is typically divided into four categories: physical, emotional, financial, and neglect.[38] Sexual abuse is often included within the category of physical abuse. Similarly, neglect may be divided into "passive neglect" and "active neglect." The active form of neglect implies that the caregiver willfully fails to provide essential care, while passive neglect may result from a caregiver's ignorance or lack of skills.[39]

An elderly patient's chief complaint may be indicative of abuse. Falls, dehydration, and failure to thrive may reflect abusive situations. A thorough physical exam may uncover signs of abuse. These signs

Table 1. Imperatives in Assessment of the Elderly Patient Who Has Sustained a Fall

PERTINENT HISTORY	PHYSICAL EXAMINATION
Precipitants of Fall	General appearance
Loss of balance	Vital signs, including orthostatics
Environmental hazards	Hydration status
Postural change	Nutritional status
Medication alterations	Mental status
Alcohol use	Focal neurologic deficit
Elder abuse	Signs of neurologic disease
Associated Symptoms	Evidence of traumatic injury
Chest pain	Decreased visual acuity
Dyspnea	Carotid bruits
Palpitations	Cardiac bruits
Lightheadedness	Cardiac murmurs or arrhythmias
Vertigo	Abdominal masses or bruits
Weakness	Arthritic changes
Confusion	Motion limitation
Comorbid Conditions	**FUNCTIONAL ASSESSMENT**
Previous CVA	**Gait and balance**
Parkinsonism	Rising from chair
Osteoporosis	Walking
Seizure disorder	Turning
Cardiac disease	Sitting down
Joint dysfunction	**Mobility**
Sensory deficit	Command of assistive devices
Prior fall	Endurance
Alcohol abuse	**Activities of Daily Living**
Pertinent Medications	Bathing
Antihypertensives	Dressing
Diuretics	Continence
Antidepressants	Transferring
Narcotics	
Neuroleptics	
Sedatives	

may include bruises and fractures of various ages, rope and restraint marks, habitual and neurotic disorders, and signs of general neglect. Avoiding confrontation and asking non-judgmental questions regarding a caregiver's difficulties in caring for an elderly patient may uncover signs of an abusive relationship. Victims are likely to withhold information regarding abuse, as they often feel embarrassed or guilty. Additionally, they may fear retaliation by the caregiver or subsequent institutionalization.

Treatment

Although the elderly are subject to the same mechanisms of injury as younger people, their response to injury is unique. Traditional trauma-care protocols, which have been devised for younger patients, should be adapted or augmented for the elderly. The declining health and reduced physiologic reserves of the elderly lead to worsened outcomes after traumatic injury. Additionally, the cause of the patient's traumatic injury must be investigated. Often, acute illness, myocardial events, and syncopal episodes may have precipitated the mechanism that resulted in the patient's injury. The emergency physician should attempt to recreate the injury scene in order to predict potential injuries the patient may have suffered.

Initially, the principles regarding the care of the multiply injured elderly patient remain the same as those of the younger patient. Priority must be placed upon a proper primary survey. The patient's airway must be secured utilizing a manual airway maneuver, oropharyngeal or nasopharyngeal adjuncts, or endotracheal/nasotracheal intubation. Should these techniques fail, a surgical airway via cricothyrotomy should be obtained. Concurrent with airway maintenance, the patient's cervical spine should be immobilized. Cervical immobilization is necessary to prevent spinal cord injury in the presence of an occult vertebral fracture or ligamentous neck injury that may compromise the integrity of the spinal column. Immobilization may be accomplished by manually holding the head in neutral anatomic position. This position must be maintained during all movements, transports, and procedures, including intubation. While this is best accomplished utilizing a hard cervical collar secured to a hard board with rigid lateral support material, the elderly patient may require some modifications. Arthritis or severe thoracic kyphosis may alter the normal anatomic positioning of the neck, which may be held in severe flexion. This altered anatomy poses a significant challenge, and proper immobilization may require additional support under the patient's head.

After the airway is secured and the cervical spine satisfactorily stabilized, proper ventilation must be assured. Should the patient's respiratory status be uncertain or in jeopardy, assistance should be provided with bag-valve-mask ventilation and high flow oxygen. Furthermore, any precipitants of ventilatory compromise must be sought. The presence of pneumothorax and hemothorax should be ruled out and, if present, treated immediately with tube thoracostomy. Subsequently, adequate circulation should be assessed and maintained. Visible hemorrhage should be controlled with appropriate, direct pressure. Concurrently, fluid resuscitation via large-bore peripheral intravenous catheters should be initiated with crystalloid fluid and/or blood products as necessary. The use of pneumatic anti-shock garments (PASG) is controversial, but may stabilize the pelvis and have a role in maintaining circulatory pressure in trauma patients with pelvic fractures. Most importantly, immediately life-threatening causes of circulatory compromise, such as pericardial tamponade, tension pneumothorax, and massive pulmonary embolism, must be detected and alleviated.

Only after the primary survey is complete should the assessment of musculoskeletal trauma begin. Nevertheless, the role of musculoskeletal trauma in precipitating immediate mortality or severe morbidity should not be underestimated. Elderly patients who possess poor physiological reserve may develop shock subsequent to blood loss. In fact, an isolated femur fracture, which may lead to a liter or more of blood loss, can precipitate hemorrhagic shock. Nevertheless, the hypotensive trauma patient with an obvious lower extremity injury necessitates a full traumatic work up to ensure that concomitant cardiac, pulmonary, abdominal, renal, pelvic, or spinal injuries do not exist.

Hip Fractures

Introduction. Sustaining a hip fracture is a devastating event, which leads to hospitalization, surgical correction, increased morbidity and mortality, reduced mobility, and often, the inability to live independently. The long-term morbidity associated with hip fractures is significant. In fact, one study found that only half of the patients who could walk independently prior to a hip fracture regained this capability.[40] Further, one-third of patients with hip fractures became totally dependent upon others to perform the most basic activities of daily living.[41] Elderly patients who suffer a hip fracture experience a 12-20% reduction in survival, with 5-20% excess mortality within the first year, after a hip fracture as compared to patients of the same age, race, and gender who have not suffered the same.[8,42,43]

Epidemiology. Projections estimate that the annual number of hip fractures worldwide will rise to 6.26 million by the year 2050.[44] This projected increase can be attributed to the growth of the world's elderly population, most prominently in Asia, Africa, Latin America, and the Middle East. In fact, these areas of the world are projected to account for more than 70% of the estimated 6.26 million hip fractures in the year 2050.[45] Similarly, in North America the number of hip fractures is increasing with the projected incidence of 650,000 per annum by the year 2050. Currently, more than 350,000 Americans fracture their hips each year and more than 90% are attributed to falls.[46] It is important to note, however, the age-specific incidence rates of hip fractures concurrently are increasing with the expanding elderly population.[47] For this reason, the projected increase in hip fractures cannot be based solely upon an aging population.

The frequency of hip fractures varies markedly between populations and races. Whites of Northern European and North American descent account for the highest incidence of hip fractures worldwide. Minority populations also suffer significant morbidity and mortality from hip fractures. Rates of fractures in both Asian and Hispanic populations are significant, and the incidence of hip fractures increases exponentially with age in every cluster. The lifetime risk of a hip fracture is 5-6% in Caucasian men and 16-18% in Caucasian women.[48] Ninety percent of all hip fracture patients are older than age 65.[49] In fact, by the age of 80, one-fifth of all women have suffered a hip fracture. By the age of 90, almost half of all women will have broken a hip.[50] In 1990, worldwide, the incidence of hip fractures in women was approximately double that of men. The preponderance of fractures in women is explained by a lower bone mass and density, as well as a higher frequency of falling.[45] Thus, while hip fractures may be more prevalent in some populations, they are a significant cause of morbidity and mortality in all groups.

Evaluation. After the initial evaluation and stabilization of the elderly trauma patient, the secondary survey may commence. The clinical presentation of a hip fracture may vary greatly with the type of fracture involved. Non-displaced fractures may be relatively symptom free, while displaced fractures are likely to be accompanied by severe pain and loss of function. Often, patients with displaced fractures will be unable to ambulate and the extremity may be shortened and externally rotated. If a traction device has been placed in the field, it should be removed to facilitate an adequate examination. The extremity should be immediately assessed for sites of external bleeding and obvious deformities.

Figure 1. Femoral Neck Fracture

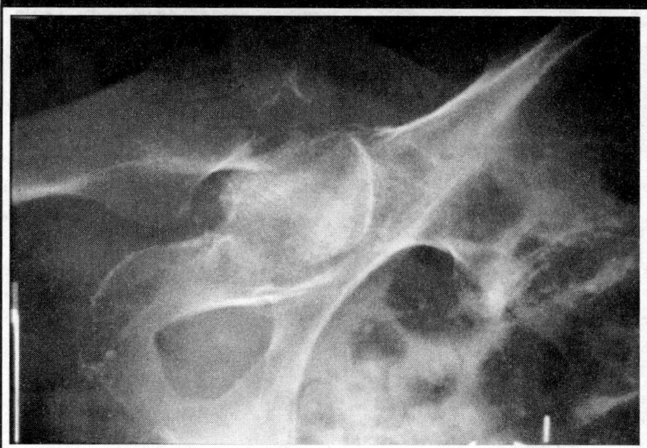

Figure 2. Intertrochanteric Fracture

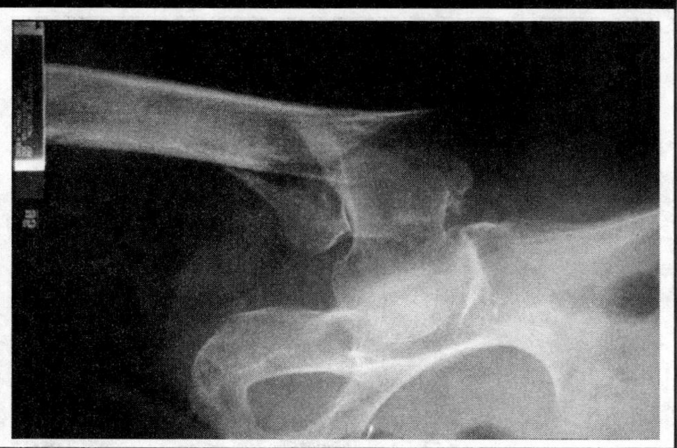

Importantly, any wound near a likely fracture should be considered an open fracture until proven otherwise and wrapped in a sterile dressing. The extremity should be palpated for areas of tenderness, swelling, deformity, or crepitus. Furthermore, an examination of the distal extremity for vascular or neurologic compromise is imperative. Pulse discrepancies, coolness, pallor, paresthesia, and motor abnormalities are suggestive of an arterial injury. Similarly, paresis, paralysis, and paresthesia are indicative of neurologic compromise.

Once identified, an injured extremity may be immobilized and supported. A position of comfort (flexion, abduction, and external rotation at the hip) may be achieved with a pillow beneath the thigh.[51] A Hare traction splint may be applied to reduce the fracture as well as discomfort. Importantly, there are two contraindications to the application of the Hare splint or any other traction device. First, sufficient traction to reduce an open fracture should not be applied. Realigning the contaminated ends before debridement of the wound in the operating room may precipitate or propagate infection. Second, traction should be avoided when injury to the sciatic nerve is suspected. Further force upon an already stretched or partially torn nerve could be devastating.[52]

Initial radiographic assessment of the hip includes an anteroposterior view of the hip and pelvis. If a high index of suspicion for hip fracture exists, a cross-table lateral view may be obtained initially as well. The cross-table lateral view is preferred to the frogleg lateral view, which requires positioning that is difficult for patients with hip fractures and a subsequently reduced range of motion. Furthermore, frogleg positioning may result in increased displacement of the fracture fragments. An internal rotation view of the hip may allow identification of otherwise occult nondisplaced or impacted fractures. Typically, the view is obtained with the lower extremity in 15 degrees of internal rotation, which allows visualization of the entire femoral neck. When a suspected fracture remains unidentified, a technetium bone scan or magnetic resonance imaging (MRI) may be utilized. The sensitivity and specificity of bone scanning, 93% and 95% respectively, are not altered by the patient's age or time after injury.[53] Similarly, MRI has been shown to be equally efficacious in locating occult fractures.[54] Following radiographic studies, the extremity should be re-immobilized for comfort.

The majority of patients with hip fractures are in severe pain and, in addition to immobilization, parenteral analgesia should be provided when not contraindicated by an associated injury. Alternatively, femoral nerve blockade may be attempted. Also, prophylactic antibiotics, when not contraindicated, should be initiated in patients who are likely to undergo immediate internal fixation. Typically, a parenteral bolus of a first-generation cephalosporin should be sufficient.[55] Antibiotics are also recommended for open fractures. Importantly, the size and perceived cleanliness of the wound dictates the antibiotic regimen that should be utilized. In reasonably clean wounds of less than one centimeter, a first-generation cephalosporin should be ample. Conversely, dirty wounds and/or those greater than one centimeter may require increased gram-negative coverage, such as an aminoglycoside.[56] Penicillin may be added to the antibiotic regimen if the wound is grossly contaminated and potentially inoculated with clostridia.[57] Furthermore, the patient's tetanus status must be determined. For those elderly persons whose vaccination history indicates unknown or partial immunization, tetanus immune globulin (TIG) and tetanus vaccine (Td) should be administered concomitantly.

Finally, all fractures of the proximal femur necessitate orthopedic consultation. Unless a specific contraindication to surgical repair exists, surgical intervention is required. In fact, surgical management with early mobilization, to avoid the sequelae of prolonged immobilization, is the generally accepted therapy in the elderly. Surgical correction of the fracture should take place as soon after the injury as possible, but only after stabilization of the patient is ensured. Interestingly, when the factors of age, sex, and number of comorbidities were controlled in one prospective study, delaying the operative management of the fracture by 48 hours doubled the patient's risk of mortality during the first postoperative year.[58] Therefore, it is imperative that an orthopedic surgeon be contacted promptly and encouraged to expeditiously perform operative repair. Also, the emergency physician should obtain appropriate preoperative laboratories such as a complete blood count, type and screen, coagulation studies, and urinalysis, in addition to an ECG and chest x-ray, to facilitate the process.

Femoral Neck Fractures

The femoral neck, which connects the femoral head to the shaft of the femur in the region of the trochanters, is extremely susceptible to fracture in the elderly. *(Please see Figure 1.)* Age-related bone loss or osteoporosis is believed to be the major determinant of the incidence of femoral neck fracture; hence, as previously noted, an increased preponderance of these fractures can be expected as the population ages.[59] The mean age of patients suffering this fracture is 74 to 78 years.[60] Often, because femoral neck fractures are associated with osteoporosis, the inciting traumatic event may be seemingly trivial. In fact, many femoral neck fractures may occur before the

Figure 3. Vertebral Compression Fracture

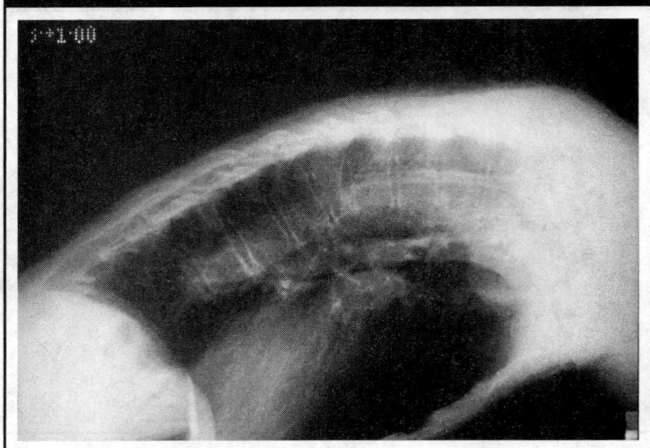

Figures 4a and b. Distal Radius Fracture

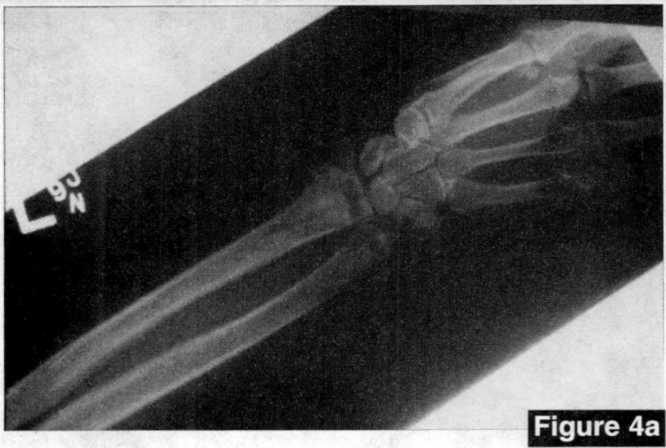

Figure 4a

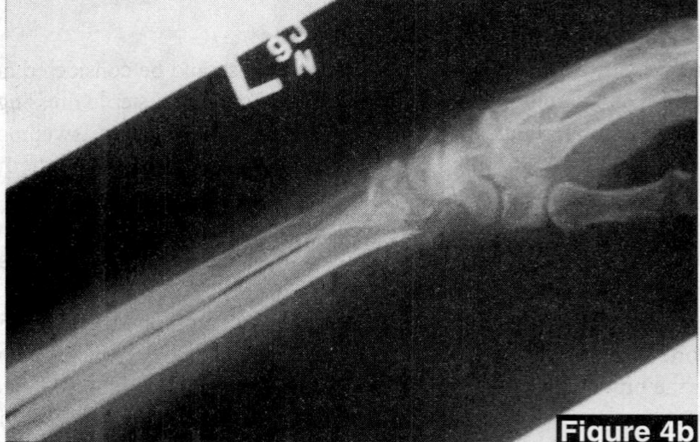

Figure 4b

Figure 4a shows an antero-posterior (AP) x-ray of the fracture.
Figure 4b shows a lateral x-ray of the fracture.

patient hits the ground.[61] In older adults, hip fractures *cause* falls almost as frequently as they *result* from falls.

Classification. The Garden classification system is most commonly used to describe femoral neck fractures. The system is based upon the degree of displacement of the fracture fragments. This potentially complex classification system may be simplified by grouping types I and II (non-displaced) and types III and IV (displaced). This simplification allows femoral neck fractures to be appropriately classified as to treatment and prognosis and, therefore, obviates the need for further differentiation.[62]

Treatment. Surgical management of femoral neck fractures is the therapy of choice, barring relative contraindication because of severe medical or mental problems. Impacted or non-displaced femoral neck fractures should undergo in situ internal fixation with multiple screws or pins. Some authors prefer three cannulated 6.5 mm cancellous lag screws inserted in parallel under fluoroscopy.[63] Interestingly, internal fixation is not advocated for displaced femoral neck fractures in the elderly. A high rate of nonunion and osteonecrosis has led to the implementation of primary prosthetic replacement as the therapy of choice.[63] Nevertheless the treatment decision should be based upon the individual patient. Emphasis should be placed upon the patient's age, associated medical problems, extent or comminution of the fracture, and the quality of bone.

Intertrochanteric Fractures

The intertrochanteric region, which encompasses both the greater and lesser trochanters, is the transitional area between the femoral neck and shaft. Trabecular bone, which effectively transmits and disburses mechanical stress, is prominent in this region. As opposed to the femoral neck, the intertrochanteric region is well vascularized and not at great risk of osteonecrosis or nonunion. *(Please see intertrochanteric fracture in Figure 2.)*

Classification. The Evans classification system is utilized to describe intertrochanteric fractures. The system is based upon fracture stability and the ability to convert an unstable fracture to a stable reduction.[64] This classification system, however, may be difficult to reproduce, and intertrochanteric fractures may be better classified simply as stable or unstable. In general, stability is based upon whether the posteromedial cortex is intact.

Treatment. Operative management is advocated for virtually all intertrochanteric fractures. Instability or comminution of the fracture site, however, may necessitate anatomic fracture alignment, in addition to fixation. Fixation of the fracture may be accomplished with a sliding hip screw or an intramedullary nail and hip screw. In studies comparing these methods, both have been found to have a similar operative management, hospital course, complication rate, and implant failure. The intramedullary nail and hip screw, however, may lead to femoral shaft fractures at the nail tip or distal locking bolts.[65] Therefore, the sliding hip screw is advocated by some authors.[66] Regardless of the management selected, early weight-bearing ambulation should be encouraged following fixation.

Vertebral Fractures

Introduction. Elderly patients sustain a substantial number of spinal fractures because of osteoporotic changes associated with aging. The most clinically relevant of these changes is the demineralization of the vertebral body. Patterns of injury vary considerably, however, suggesting that other factors may contribute to spinal injury as well.[67] Compression fractures of the vertebrae may occur spontaneously or with minimal trauma, such as occurs with coughing or simple household tasks like removing laundry from the washer. Multiple vertebral fractures may precipitate severe impairment, including kyphosis and the loss of the lumbar lordosis. Moreover, the eventual impairment of chest wall function in severe and debilitating kyphosis may reduce vital

Table 2. The Frykman Classification

TYPE I	TYPE II	TYPE III	TYPE IV	TYPE V	TYPE VI	TYPE VII	TYPE VIII
Extra-articular	Extra-articular	Involvement of the radio-carpal joint	Involvement of the radio-carpal joint	Involvement of the radio-ulnar joint	Involvement of the radio-ulnar joint	Involvement of both joints	Involvement of both joints
Intact ulnar styloid	Fractured ulnar styloid	Intact ulnar styloid	Fractured ulnar styloid	Intact ulnar styloid	Fractured ulnar styloid	Intact ulnar styloid	Fractured ulnar styloid

capacity.[68] Therefore, diminished thoracic space may result in decreased exercise tolerance and the ability to perform the activities of daily life. Similarly, the compression of abdominal contents may be disfiguring and extremely painful. Reduced abdominal space may lead to premature satiety and accelerated weight loss.[69]

Epidemiology. Secondary to osteoporosis, more than 500,000 vertebral fractures occur annually in elderly patients in the United States.[4] Vertebral fractures occur more frequently than fractures of the proximal femur or distal radius in women older than age 65. In fact, one-third of women in this age group sustain a vertebral fracture. By age 75, 90% of the population will have had plain radiographs demonstrating vertebral body compression.[70] *(Please see Figure 3.)*

Evaluation. Patients with vertebral fractures usually develop back pain that leads to radiological assessment. Of note, however, pain in the lumbar or sacral regions is less predictive of vertebral compression fractures than is pain in the thoracic area. While height loss of more than 1 inch is a sensitive indicator of compression, it can occur without fractures due to narrowing of vertebral disks and postural changes. Conversely, many patients may be asymptomatic and their vertebral fractures found incidentally. Importantly, the most frequent fractures are in the thoracic vertebrae below T6 and in the lumbar vertebrae.[71]

When evaluating the aged spine, primary or metastatic disease must be considered as a potential etiology in vertebral body collapse. This diagnosis, however, is often difficult to make based solely on radiographic studies. While MRI may facilitate a diagnosis, a definitive diagnosis can only be made through examination of vertebral body fragments recovered during surgery.[67]

Treatment. Multiple vertebral fractures have a considerable impact upon the elderly by reducing their ability to engage in the activities of daily life. Recent findings contradict prior research on patients with vertebral fractures and suggest that the functional impact of these fractures can, in fact, be substantial. In one study, patients with vertebral fractures scored substantially lower on physical performance measures, such as functional reach and mobility skills, and their walking was slower, with reduced endurance.[72] Moreover, patients who have suffered a vertebral fracture are at increased risk of future peripheral and vertebral fractures. Consequently, these patients lose self-esteem and may become depressed.[69,73] The goals of acute management, therefore, are to maximize pain control, to expeditiously mobilize the patient, and to initiate appropriate social services.

Distal Radius Fractures

Introduction. The forearm is a complex structure that provides mechanical stability and enables coordinated movement of the wrist and elbow. Integrity of forearm is essential for intricate movements of the hand; therefore, fractures of the forearm may have a devastating effect upon a patient's ability to perform even simple activities.

Epidemiology. Distal forearm fractures are the most common fractures encountered in orthopedics and account for approximately 15% of all fractures requiring emergency care.[74] Women older than age 50 have been shown to have a significant increase in the incidence of distal radius fractures, while men older than age 70 had only a minimal increase.[74] In fact, one study found that more than 85% of all distal radius fractures occur in women older than age 50.[75] Also of note, prior to age 70, distal forearm fractures occur more frequently than hip fractures.[76]

Evaluation. A detailed understanding of anatomic relationships in the forearm provides the basis for evaluation in the emergency department. Muscles anchored to the dorsum of the forearm enable extension of the wrist and digits. Similarly, muscles attached volarly enable flexion of the same. Importantly, these muscular attachments may precipitate significant displacement of bones upon fracturing the wrist. For this reason, clinical and radiographic evaluations must be systematic and thorough. *(Please see Figures 4a and b.)* Radiographs should include the joints above and below the suspected fracture site.

Classification. Numerous eponyms exist for fractures in this region, resulting in considerable confusion in the literature, as well as in clinical practice. Furthermore, no universally accepted classification system exists. While the literature regarding classification has evolved significantly, eponyms are still frequently used by clinicians to describe fractures. Examples of common eponyms include Colles' fracture and Smith's fracture which, respectively, describe dorsal and volar angulation of the displaced metaphyseal fracture. While eponyms allow for a rapid and simplified description of a fracture, a classification system should provide information as to the type and complexity of a fracture, in addition to a basis for treatment. For example, the Frykman classification system describes a distal radius fracture involving the radiocarpal or radioulnar joints with or without involvement of the ulnar styloid. *(Please see Table 2.)* This classification system categorizes fractures into types I-VIII. The complexity and difficulty of management increases respective to the type.[77] More recent schemes have sought to describe fracture stability and direct reduction techniques and operative indications. Nevertheless, no perfect scheme exists at this time.

Treatment. Nondisplaced fractures of the distal radius are amenable to non-operative treatment. After appropriate radiographic evaluation, the fracture may be immobilized in a short arm cast. Alternatively, the extremity may be immobilized initially with only a volar splint to allow for severe swelling. It should be noted that fiberglass is preferable to plaster in the elderly, as it is much lighter and permits greater mobility.

Displaced fractures, however, necessitate either closed or open reduction. Fracture reduction should be attempted in all closed displaced distal radius fractures. Importantly, due to atrophic skin, the elderly are susceptible to soft-tissue injury during attempted closed reduction. For this reason, the forearm should be pre-wrapped in web roll and the fingers placed carefully in the finger traps. Additionally, excessive traction upon and exaggeration of the fracture should be avoided.[78] After fracture reduction, the forearm should be immobilized in a sugar-tong splint. The fracture, as well as the splint, should then be assessed radiographically.

The criteria for appropriate reduction of distal radius fractures remains controversial. Younger patients will tolerate only minimal post-reduction displacement or deformity at the fracture site. In these patients, a poor reduction may lead to debilitating pain and poor functional outcome. Conversely, elderly patients, particularly those who lead sedentary lifestyles, may tolerate more post-reduction displacement or angulation. Importantly, the patient must be re-assessed in one week. At that time, the sugar-tong splint may be changed to a short-arm cast. Additionally, if the fracture reduction has been compromised, it may be re-attempted. Repeated manipulation of the fracture, however, has been reported to lead to a satisfactory outcome less than half of the time.[79] If signs of fracture instability exist after reduction, surgical intervention may be indicated. Importantly, in the elderly, functional requirements must be reviewed prior to subjecting a patient to surgical repair. Those with multiple medical problems, cognitive deficits, and sedentary lifestyles may be better managed non-operatively.

Figure 6. Hip Fracture Risk Reduction

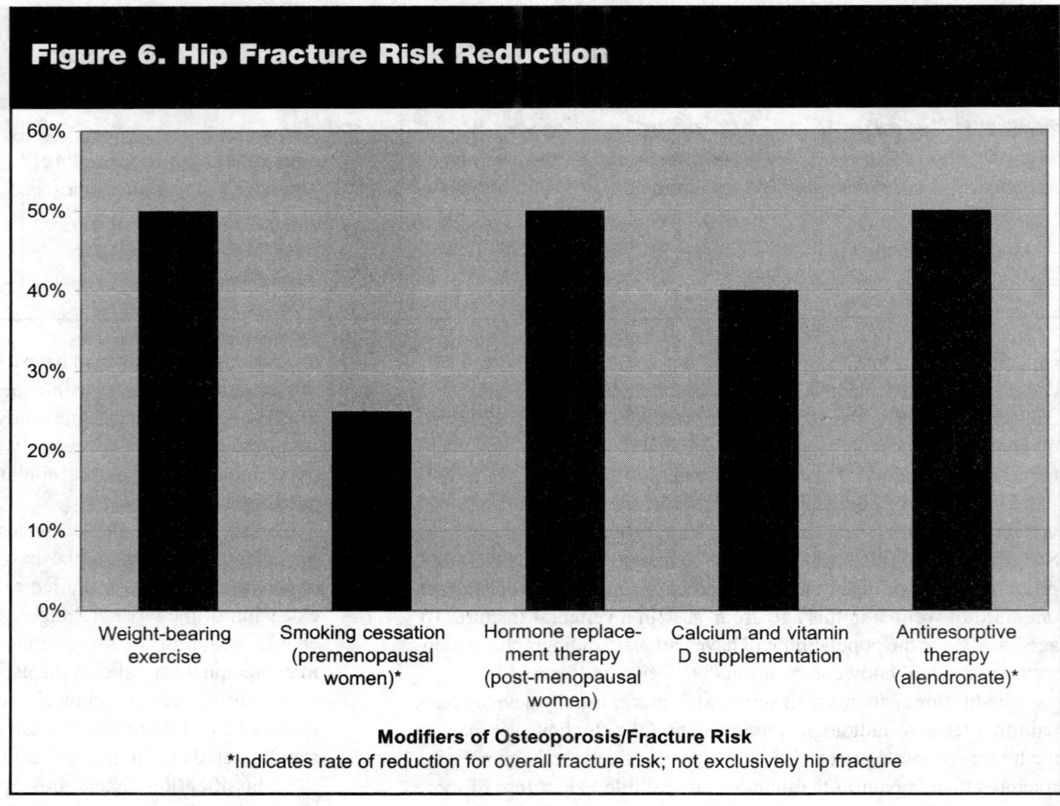

*Indicates rate of reduction for overall fracture risk; not exclusively hip fracture

Fractures with a high degree of displacement, comminution, and soft-tissue injury may necessitate operative management. External fixation is typically the preferred approach in the elderly, because of the high frequency of comminution and osteopenia.[75] Alternatively, open reduction and internal fixation is indicated for complex fractures involving articular surfaces, which are inherently unstable. Open fractures require aggressive management. Antibiotic therapy, tetanus toxoid, and surgical debridement are imperative. Following debridement, external fixation is typically advocated for fracture stabilization. While specific indications exist for either operative technique, they are well beyond the scope of this chapter.

Although in the majority of patients, the long-term functional consequences of sustaining a distal forearm fracture are minimal, some patients do experience restricted activity, chronic pain, and limited function.[80] For these patients, the chronic pain associated with distal forearm fractures can alter their daily routine. These effects, however, can be ameliorated by the immediate initiation of treatment and physical therapy. In fact, the elderly may benefit greatly from a formal physical therapy regimen to maximize rehabilitation. Informal rehabilitation, however, may begin while the patient is still in the emergency room with finger range-of-motion exercises.[81]

Prevention

The prevention of diseases associated with old age should commence in youth. The value of primary prevention (hindering the development of disease processes) or secondary prevention (arresting the progression of disease) dissipate with increasing age; hence, a greater burden is placed upon tertiary prevention (minimizing disability due to disease). Importantly, an accurate assessment of the geriatric patient in the emergency department may identify those at risk for osteoporosis and other age-related conditions.

Osteoporosis. Alterations in lifestyle, such as regular weight-bearing exercise, smoking cessation, and reduced alcohol consumption may significantly reduce an individual's susceptibility to osteoporosis. A sedentary lifestyle may reduce the mechanical forces exerted upon the skeleton and precipitate bone loss through increased resorption. Thus, physical activity is perhaps the most important means to improve bone mass and inhibit bone loss.[48] Regular weight-bearing exercise may reduce the risk of hip fracture by at least 50%.[82] Physical activity is also associated with improved muscle strength, stability, reaction time, balance, and coordination. Additionally, a woman who undergoes smoking cessation prior to menopause will reduce her fracture risk by approximately 25%.[82] Furthermore, alcohol decreases bone density, while simultaneously increasing one's risk of falling.[83] Therefore, avoidance of excessive alcohol consumption is also of great importance.

In postmenopausal women, estrogen replacement therapy reduces the risk of hip fracture by at least 50%.[84] In fact, hormone replacement therapy has been shown to be efficacious in reducing bone loss by approximately 40%.[85] Estrogen appears to be most beneficial during the period of accelerated bone loss that occurs immediately after the onset of menopause. However, the high cost and fleeting benefits of estrogen therapy compromise its utility. Moreover, the merit of initiating estrogen therapy in women well into menopause remains uncertain. Conversely, one group demonstrated in a controlled trial that transdermal estrogen therapy reduced bone loss and fractures in women ages 47-75 who were all newly treated.[86]

Women should take calcium 1500 mg and vitamin D 750 units daily to deter the progressive loss of bone associated with osteoporosis. By doing so, they may reduce the risk of hip fractures by as much as 40%.[22] In fact, the NIH Consensus Conference in 1994 recommended a daily intake of 1500 mg calcium for all persons older than age 65.[87] Furthermore, one report regarding calcium and vitamin D3 found that an intake of 1500 mg/d of calcium and 800 units of vitamin D resulted in 43% fewer hip fractures and a 32% reduction in all non-vertebral fractures in those older than age 68.[88]

Antiresorptive therapy via bisphosphonates, such as alendronate, results in high bone mineral density and reduces fracture incidence by approximately 50% within two years of treatment.[89] Bisphosphonates bind to bone surfaces and interfere with the resorptive actions of mature osteoclasts.[90] They may also inhibit osteoclast activity by causing osteoblasts to release osteoclast-inhibiting substances.[91] Moreover, bisphosphonates may indirectly decrease circulating IL-6 levels which stimulates osteoclasts.[92] According to one study on women with postmenopausal osteoporosis, 10 mg of alendronate, daily, maximized spinal bone mass.[93] *(Please see Figure 6.)*

Unfortunately, the identification and treatment of osteoporosis is not atop the priority list of many primary care health providers; hence, as patient advocates, emergency physicians must be cognitive of the disease and its disastrous effects. Proper recognition and appropriate referral will help those who suffer from osteoporosis and osteoporosis-related fractures tremendously.

Falls. In addition to therapies aimed at preventing or limiting osteoporosis, attention must be focused on other factors that precipitate fractures in the elderly. These include neuromuscular and sensory impairment, medicinal side effects, and environmental hazards. Investigations regarding the treatment of older persons to reduce the number or impact of identifiable risk factors are underway. Treatment of these risk factors could potentially decrease the incidence of falls. Older people who fall often reduce their level of activity secondary to fear of further falls and subsequent injury. However, a reduction in activity level leads to further deterioration and greater risk of falling in the future. A regular exercise regimen should include stretching exercises and activities to strengthen muscles in the arms and legs. For example, walking 3-5 times per week is a simple and effective means to increase life expectancy and functional independence and to reduce the risks of heart disease, osteoporosis, and depression.[22]

Many members of the elderly population are concurrently taking several medications. By doing so, they may be compromising their levels of alertness. Specific medications, dosing alterations, and polypharmacy are closely associated with an increased risk of falling.[94] Multiple studies have implicated sedatives, antidepressants, neuroleptics, and antihypertensives as particularly likely medications to precipitate a fall.[21] As many as 25% of elderly persons 65 years or older ingest at least one of 20 medications considered unsafe in the aged. Approximately 5% of this population are taking two or more of these drugs.[22]

Environmental factors that jeopardize the elderly should be altered. Importantly, 44% of falls occur in the presence of environmental hazards.[23] Precipitants such as stairs, inadequate lighting, slippery or uneven flooring, electrical cords, and perilous transfers from bed to wheelchair or commode could likely be remedied with appropriate environmental evaluations by out-of-hospital providers. For example, the use of nightlights, handrails, stable footware, even flooring, and secured rugs should be encouraged in order to alleviate common household risks. Moreover, many falls are associated with poor vision; hence, ophthalmologic evaluation should be sought regularly.[22]

Alternatively, in one randomized clinical trial conducted among elderly nursing home residents with a high risk of falling, the use of energy absorbing hip pads reduced the risk of fracture by more than 50%.[95] In addition, new assistive technology has introduced seats that give high-risk patients a biomechanical advantage to decrease bone stress. For example, a spring-loaded seat elevator that assists the elderly individual in standing reduces stress upon the hip.[96] These methods of prevention may be beneficial in those who have already progressed beyond earlier preventative strategies.

Elder Abuse. The identification and avoidance of elder abuse are essential to the prevention of fractures in the elderly. According to adult protective services, public and professional awareness is the most significant factor in identifying and preventing elder abuse.[97] Additionally, social and home health care services may be extremely beneficial in assessing patients at risk of being abused. While these services may be helpful, they must be activated by physician reporting. Emergency physicians must be cognizant of patient autonomy, while complying with mandatory reporting laws. Victims should be made aware that reporting is intended to make community services available—not to compromise their independence. Also, it must be stressed that emergency care is accessible at any time. Currently, physicians fail to report elder abuse because they are unfamiliar with the law, wary of offending patients, preoccupied with time limitations, and incognizant of available resources.[39]

Conclusion

While the majority of the orthopedic injuries afflicting the elderly are not immediately life-threatening, these injuries may precipitate untimely mortality, significant morbidity, and reduced independence. As the elderly population continues to grow, so will their encumbrance upon an already overwhelmed health care system. The emergency physician must, therefore, be cognizant of current therapies and preventative strategies in order to reduce morbidity, mortality, and the costs of hospitalization. Furthermore, the task of coordinating the multidisciplinary care of elderly patients often befalls the emergency physician. Most importantly, the elderly are a distinct segment of society and must be treated as such. To this end, it is absolutely imperative for emergency physicians to recognize the unique characteristics of the elderly and tailor their management accordingly.

The authors would like to thank Rachael Fisher, JD, Associate Attorney, Choate, Hall & Stewart, Boston, MA, for help with the preparation of this paper.

References

1. Schneider EL, Guralnik JM. The aging of America: Impact on health care costs. *JAMA* 1990;263:2335-2340.
2. Eliastam M. Elderly patients in the emergency department. *Ann Emerg Med* 1989;18:1222-1229.
3. Lindsay R. *Osteoporosis: A Guide to Diagnosis, Prevention, and Treatment.* New York: Raven Press; 1992.
4. Riggs BL, Melton LJ. Involutional osteoporosis. *N Engl J Med* 1986;314:1676-1686.
5. Melton LJ, Atkinson EJ, O'Fallon WM, et al. Long-term fracture risk prediction with bone mineral measurements made at various skeletal sites. *J Bone Miner Res* 1991;6: S136.
6. Melton, LJ III. Epidemiology of Fractures. In: Riggs BL, Melton LJ III et al, eds. *Osteoporosis: Etiology, Diagnosis and Management.* Philadelphia: Raven Press; 1995:225-248.
7. Looker AC, Orwoll ES, Johnston Jr CC, et al. Prevalence of low femoral bone sensitivity in older US adults from NHANES III. *J Bone Miner Res* 1997;12:1761-1768.
8. Mullen JO, Mullen NL. Hip fracture mortality: A prospective, multifactorial study to predict and minimize death risk. *Clin Orthop* 1992;280:214-222.

9. Prince RL, Smith M, Dick IM, et al. Prevention of postmenopausal osteoporosis: A comparative study of exercise, calcium supplementation, and hormone-replacement therapy. *N Engl J Med* 1991;325:1189-1195.
10. Bonjour JP, Rizzoli R. Bone Acquisition in Adolescence. In: Marcus R, Feldman D et al, eds. *Osteoporosis*. San Diego: Academic Press; 1996:465-476.
11. Eriksen EF. Normal and pathological remodeling of human trabecular bone: Three dimensional reconstruction of the remodeling sequence in normals and in metabolic bone disease. *Endocr Rev* 1986;7:379-408.
12. Parfitt AM. Skeletal Heterogeneity and the Purposes of Bone Remodeling: Implications for the Understanding of Osteoporosis. In: Marcus R, Feldman D et al, eds. *Osteoporosis*. San Diego: Academic Press; 1996:315-329.
13. Ross PD. Risk factors for osteoporotic fracture. *Endocr Metab Clin* 1998;27:289-301.
14. Ensrud KE, Palermo L, Black D, et al. Hip and calcaneal bone loss increase with advancing age: Longitudinal results from the Study of Osteoporotic Fractures. *J Bone Miner Res* 1995;10: 1778-1787.
15. Orwoll ES. Osteoporosis in men. *Endocr Metab Clin* 1998;27: 349-367.
16. Bilezikian JP. Commentary: Osteoporosis in men. *Endocr Metab Clin* 1999;84:3431-3435.
17. Garnero P, Delmas PD. Diagnostic evaluation update. *Endocr Metab Clin* 1997;26:913-936.
18. Duboeuf F, Braillon P, Chapuy MC, et al. Bone mineral density of the hip measured with dual-energy x-ray absorptiometry in normal elderly women and in patients with hip fracture. *Osteoporosis Int* 1991;1:242-249.
19. Close J, Ellis M, Hooper, et al. Prevention of falls in the elderly trial: A randomized controlled trial. *Lancet* 1999;353: 93-97.
20. Nelson RC, Amin MA. Falls in the elderly. *Emerg Med Clin North Am* 1990;8:309-324.
21. King MB, Tinetti ME. Progress in geriatrics: Falls in community-dwelling older persons. *J Am Geriatr Soc* 1995; 43:1146-1154.
22. Baraff LJ, Della Penna R, Williams N, et al. Practice guidelines for the ED management of falls in community-dwelling elderly persons. *Ann Emerg Med* 1997;30:480-492.
23. Tinetti ME, Speechley M, Ginter SF. Risk Factors for falls among elderly persons living in the community. *N Engl J Med* 1988;319:1701-1707.
24. Nevitt MC, Cummings SR, Kidd S, et al. Risk factors for recurrent nonsyncopal falls. *JAMA* 1989;261:2663-2668.
25. Olsky M, Murray J. Dizziness and fainting in the elderly. *Emerg Med Clin North Am* 1990;8:295-307.
26. Lewis LM, Miller DK, Morley JE, et al. Unrecognized delirium in ED geriatric patients. *Am J Emerg Med* 1995;13: 142-145.
27. Sudarsky L. Geriatrics: Gait disorders in the elderly. *N Engl J Med* 1990;322:1441-1446.
28. Higinbotham NL, Marcove RC. The management of pathological fractures. *J Trauma* 1965;5:792-798.
29. Hamdy RC. *Paget's Disease of Bone: Assessment and Management*. London: Praeger Publishers; 1981:2.
30. Kanis JA. Paget's Disease of Bone. In: Goldman L, Bennett JC, eds. *Cecil Textbook of Medicine*. Philadelphia: W.B Saunders Co.; 2000:1414-1416.
31. Lyles KW, Lammers JE, Shipp KM, et al. Functional and mobility impairments associated with Paget's disease of the bone. *J Am Geriatr Soc* 1995; 43:502-506.
32. Siris ES. Extensive personal experience: Paget's disease of bone. *J Clin Endocrinol Metab* 1995;80:335-338.
33. Subcommittee on Health and Long-Term Care of the Select Committee on Aging, House of Representatives. *Elder Abuse: A Decade of Shame and Inaction*. Washington DC: US Government Printing Office; 1990.
34. Pillemer K, Finkelhor D. The prevalence of elder abuse: A random sample survey. *Gerontologist* 1988;28:51-57.
35. Homer AC, Gilleard C. Abuse of elderly people by their carers. *BMJ* 1990;301:1359-1362.
36. McNamara RM, Rousseau E, Sanders AB. Geriatric emergency medicine: A survey of practicing emergency physicians. *Ann Emerg Med* 1992;21:796-801.
37. Subcommittee on Health and Long-Term Care of the Select Committee on Aging, House of Representatives. *Elder Abuse: A Decade of Shame and Inaction*. Washington DC: US Government Printing Office; 1992.
38. Lachs MS, Pillemer K. Abuse and neglect of elderly persons. *N Engl J Med* 1995;332:437-443.
39. Kleinschmidt KC. Elder abuse: A review. *Ann Emerg Med* 1997;30:463-472.
40. Wolinsky FD, Fitzgerald JF, Stump TE. The effect of hip fracture on mortality, hospitalization, and functional status: A prospective study. *Am J Public Health* 1997;87:398-403.
41. Jensen JS, Bagger J. Long-term social prognosis after hip fracture. *Acta Orthop Scand* 1982;53:97-101.
42. Eiskjaer S, Ostgard SE, Jakobsen BW, et al. Years of potential life lost after hip fracture among postmenopausal women. *Acta Orthop Scand* 1992;63:293-296.
43. Aharonoff GB, Koval KJ, Skovron ML. Hip fractures in the elderly: Predictors of one year mortality. *J Orthop Trauma* 1997;11:162-165.
44. Cooper, C. Hip fractures in the elderly: A worldwide projection. *Osteoporosis Int* 1992;2:285-289.
45. Melton, LJ. Hip fractures: A worldwide problem today and tomorrow. *Bone* 1993;14:1s-8s.
46. Grisso JA, Kelsey JL, Strom BL, et al. Risk factors for falls as a cause of hip fracture in women. *N Engl J Med* 1991; 324:1326-1331.
47. Melton LJ, O'Fallon WM, Riggs BL. Secular trends in the incidence of hip fractures. *Calcif Tissue Int* 1987;41:57-64.
48. Kannus P, Parkkari J, Sievanen H, et al. Epidemiology of hip fractures. *Bone* 1996;18:57-63.
49. American Academy of Orthopedic Surgeons. Position Statement on the Prevention of Hip Fractures. 1998.
50. Thorngren KG. Fractures in older persons. *Disabil Rehabil* 1994;16:119-126.
51. Needoff M, Radford P, Langstaff R. Preoperative traction for hip fractures in the elderly: A clinical trial. *Injury* 1993;24: 317-318.
52. Rudman N, McIlmail D. Emergency department evaluation and treatment of hip and thigh injuries. *Emerg Med Clin*

2000;18:29-53.

53. Holder LE, Schwarz C, Wernicke PG, et al. Radionuclide bone imaging in the early detection of fractures of the proximal femur (Hip): Multifactorial analysis. *Radiology* 1990;174:509-515.
54. Rizzo PF, Gould ES, Lyden JP, et al. Diagnosis of occult fractures about the hip: Magnetic resonance imaging compared with bone-scanning. *J Bone Joint Surg Am* 1993;75:395-401.
55. Burnett JW, Gustilo RB, Williams DN, et al. Prophylactic antibiotics in hip fractures. *J Bone Joint Surg* 1980;62: 457-462.
56. Gustilo RB, Merkow RL, Templeman D. The management of open fractures. *J Bone Joint Surg* 1990;72:299-304.
57. Gregory P, Sanders R. The management of severe fractures of the lower extremities. *Clin Orthop* 1995;318:95-105.
58. Zuckerman JD, Skovron ML, Koval KJ, et al. Postoperative complications and mortality associated with operative delay in older patients who have a fracture of the hip. *J Bone Joint Surg* 1995;77:1551-1556.
59. Birge SJ. Osteoporosis and hip fracture. *Clin Geriatr Med* 1993;9:69-86.
60. Lawton JO, Baker MR, Dickson RA. Femoral neck fractures—Two populations. *Lancet* 1983;2:70-72.
61. Nguyen ND, Oesterling BR, McLaughlin RE, et al. Femoral neck fractures in the elderly patient: A preventable injury. *Am J Emerg Med* 1996;14:288-290.
62. Garden RS. Low angle fixation in fractures of the femoral neck. *J Bone Joint Surg* 1961;43:647-663.
63. Koval KJ, Zuckerman JD. Femoral Neck Fractures. In: Koval KJ, Zuckerman JD, eds. *Fractures in the Elderly.* Philadelphia: Lippincott-Raven; 1998:178-181.
64. Evans EM. The treatment of trochanteric fractures of the femur. *J Bone Joint Surg* 1949;31B:190-203.
65. Brible SH, Patel AD, Bircher M, et al. Fixation of intertrochanteric fractures of the femur: A randomized prospective comparison of the gamma nail and the dynamic hip screw. *J Bone Joint Surg* 1991;73B:330-334.
66. Koval KJ, Zuckerman JD. Intertrochanteric Fractures. In: Koval KJ, Zuckerman JD, eds. *Fractures in the Elderly.* Philadelphia: Lippincott-Raven; 1998:178-181.
67. Main WK, Cammisa FP, O'Leary PF, et al. The Spine. In: Koval KJ, Zuckerman JD, eds. *Fractures in the Elderly.* Philadelphia: Lippincott-Raven; 1998:143-158.
68. Culham EG, Jimenez HA, King CE. Thoracic kyphosis, rib mobility, and lung volumes in normal women and women with osteoporosis. *Spine* 1994;19:1250-1255.
69. Silverman SL. The clinical consequences of vertebral compression fracture. *Bone* 1992;13s:27-31.
70. Cohen LD. Fractures of the osteoporotic spine. *Orthop Clin North Am* 1990;21:143-150.
71. Raisz LG, Kream BE, Lorenzo JA. Metabolic Bone Disease. In: Wilson JD, Foster DW, Kronenberg HM, et al, eds. *Wilson: Williams Textbook of Endocrinology*. Philadelphia: W. B. Saunders Co.; 1998:1211-1240.
72. Lyles KW, Gold DT, Shipp KM, et al. Association of osteoporotic vertebral compression fractures with impaired functional status. *Am J Med* 1993;94:595-601.
73. Gold DT, Shipp KM, Lyles KW. Managing patients with complications of osteoporosis. *Endocrinol Metab Clin North Am* 1988;27:485-496.
74. Bengner U, Johnell O. Increasing incidence of forearm fractures: A comparison of epidemiologic patterns 25 years apart. *Acta Orthop Scand* 1985;56:158-160.
75. Dinowitz MI, Koval KJ, Meadows S. Distal Radius. In: Koval KJ, Zuckerman JD, eds. *Fractures in the Elderly*. Philadelphia: Lippincott-Raven; 1998:127-141.
76. Baron JA, Barrett JA, Karagas MR. The epidemiology of peripheral fractures. *Bone* 1996;18:209-213.
77. Frykman G. Fracture of the distal radius including sequelae: Shoulder hand finger syndrome, disturbance in the distal radioulnar joint and impairment of nerve function. A clinical and experimental study. *Acta Orthop Scand* 1967; 108s:1-155.
78. Leung KS, Shen WY, Tsang HK, et al. An effective treatment of comminuted fractures of the distal radius. *J Hand Surg* 1990;15A:11-17.
79. McQueen MM, MacLaren A, Chalmers J. The value of remanipulating Colles' fractures. *J Bone Joint Surg* 1986;68B:232-233.
80. Field J, Atkins RM. Algodystrophy is an early complication of Colles' fracture: What are the implications? *J Hand Surg* 1997;22:178-182.
81. Dias JJ, Wray CC, Jones JM, et al. The value of early mobilization in the treatment of Colles' fractures. *J Bone Joint Surg* 1987;69B:463-467.
82. Law MR, Wald NJ, Meade TW. Strategies for the prevention of osteoporosis and hip fracture. *BMJ* 1991;303:453-459.
83. Smith R. Prevention and treatment of osteoporosis: Common sense and science coincide. *J Bone Joint Surg* 1994;76: 345-347.
84. Felson DT, Zhang Y, Hannan MT, et al. The effect of postmenopausal estrogen therapy on bone density in elderly women. *N Engl J Med* 1993;329:1141-1146.
85. Cauley JA, Seeley DG, Ensrud K, et al. Estrogen replacement therapy and fractures in older women: Study of Osteoporotic Fractures Research Group. *Ann Intern Med* 1995;122:9-16.
86. Lufkin EG, Wahner HW, O'Fallon WM. Treatment of postmenopausal osteoporosis with transdermal estrogen. *Ann Intern Med* 1992;117:1-9.
87. Optimal Calcium Intake. *NIH Consensus Statement* 1994; 12:1-31.
88. Chapuy MC, Arlot ME, Duboeuf F, et al. Vitamin D3 and calcium to prevent hip fractures in elderly women. *N Engl J Med* 1992;327:1637-1642.
89. Black DM, Cummings SR, Karpf DB, et al. Randomized trial of effect of allendronate on risk of fracture in women with existing vertebral fractures. *Lancet* 1996;348: 1535-1541.
90. Rodan GA, Fleisch HA. Bisphosphonates: Mechanisms of action. *J Clin Invest* 1996;97:2692-2696.
91. Vitte C, Fleisch H, Guenther HL. Bisphosphonates induce osteoblasts to secrete an inhibitor of osteoclast-mediated reabsorption. *Endocrinology* 1996;137:2324-2333.
92. Lissoni P, Cazzaniga M, Barni S, et al. Acute effects of

pamidronate administration on srum levels of interleukin-6 in advanced solid tumor patients with bone metastases and their possible implications in the immunotherapy of cancer with interleukin-2. *Eur J Cancer* 1997;33:304-306.

93. Liberman UA, Weiss SR, Broll J, et al. Effect of oral alendronate on bone mineral density and the incidence of fractures in postmenopausal osteoporosis. *N Engl J Med* 1995;333:1437-1443.
94. Cumming RG, Miller JP, Kelsey JL, et al. Medications and multiple falls in elderly people: The St. Louis OASIS Study. *Age Ageing* 1991;20:455-461.
95. Lauritzen JB, Petersen MM, Lund B. Effect of external hip protectors on hip fractures. *Lancet* 1993;314:11-13.
96. Weiner DK, Long R, Hughes MA, et al. When older adults face the chair-rise challenge: A study of chair height availability and height-modified chair-rise performance in the elderly. *J Am Geriatr Soc* 1993;41:6-10.
97. United States General Accounting Office. Elder Abuse: Effective Reporting Laws and Other Factors. Washington DC: Report to the Chairman, Subcommittee on Human Services, Select Committee on Aging, House of Representatives, 1991.

Subdural Hematoma

Stephen W. Meldon, MD
Sarah Delaney-Rowland, MD

Due to advancements in medical technology, better access to health care, and improved living conditions, the geriatric population in the United States is rapidly expanding. This dramatic increase in the number of older persons will put a much larger population at risk for injury. Improving outcomes in this fragile population requires the need for a better understanding in the diagnosis, treatment, and management of geriatric injuries. Elderly trauma patients have an increased mortality rate and worse outcomes despite similar or less injury severity than nonelders.[1,2] The explanation for this difference lies in those factors unique to the older patient. Diminished physiologic reserve associated with aging, atypical clinical presentations, and comorbidities contribute to worse trauma outcomes in this age group. Important comorbidities include preexisting central nervous system (CNS) disease and other concurrent medical illnesses such as cardiovascular disease, lung disease, and coagulopathy. Geriatric trauma, though not completely distinct from nongeriatric trauma, does require an expanded fund of knowledge and specialized skills.

Head trauma is a significant contributor to poor outcomes in the elderly. As a cause of trauma-related deaths, it is second only to shock. Several differences exist when head injuries are compared in elder and nonelder populations. These include mechanism of injury, clinical presentation, operative intervention, and radiographic findings on neuroimaging. The sex ratio of head injuries in the elderly is approximately 1:1, whereas in nonelder head-injured patients there is a much higher incidence with males. The most common mechanism of injury in the elderly is falls, compared with motor vehicle crashes (MVC) in the younger population. [3-6] Alcohol is involved less frequently in older injured patients. The elderly have a higher rate of positive computerized tomography (CT) scans and an increased need for neurosurgical intervention. Clinical presentations also differ, with 12% of older patients having a normal neurological examination and a positive CT scan, compared with 7% in the younger age group.[3] Overall, elderly patients have worse outcomes, with increased hospital admissions, worse functional outcomes, and increased injury-related deaths.[7,8] Elderly patients with head injuries and Glasgow Coma Scale (GCS) score of less than 8 have greater than 80% mortality rate.[9]

With this background in mind, this chapter will focus on subdural hematomas, the most common, significant intracranial injury in elders. Etiologies, diagnosis, and management of acute and chronic subdural hematomas will be discussed. In addition, atypical clinical presentations and CT findings will be emphasized.

Definition

A subdural hematoma (SDH) refers to a collection of blood between the dura and the brain. SDHs are three times more frequent in the elderly population.[10] Most result from bleeding originating from bridging veins, which are prone to injury following acceleration/deceleration movement of the brain. Prognosis depends on several factors: the degree of underlying brain injury; the size and pressure of the expanding hematoma; and the patient's age. Prognosis is especially poor in the elderly.

SDHs are commonly classified into three types, depending on the time of symptom onset following the initial injury. Although these time frames are somewhat arbitrary, the significant differences in CT findings, treatment, and outcome make this classification useful.

Acute subdurals are symptomatic within 24 hours after injury. Usually there is an associated decreased level of consciousness on presentation. CT scan demonstrates a hyperdense, crescent-shaped collection between the calvarium and the cortex. Acute subdurals are more common in younger patients and tend to be associated with major trauma.[11] Approximately one-third of acute subdurals have other associated focal brain injuries. They may occur in association with cortical contusions, subarachnoid hemorrhages, and diffuse axonal injury.[11] Morbidity and mortality are much higher when compared to chronic SDHs.

Subacute SDHs are symptomatic between 24 hours and two weeks after the injury. Presentations include complaints of headache, altered mental status, motor weakness, or hemiparesis. CT scan demonstrates a hypodense or isodense (when compared to brain parenychma) fluid collection.

Chronic subdurals generally become symptomatic more than two weeks after the initial injury. The signs and symptoms may be nonspecific, such as mild mental status changes and difficulty walking, or more dramatic, such as focal weakness, hemiparesis, and altered level of consciousness. Chronic subdurals occur in older individuals, are often associated with trivial trauma, and are seldom associated with injury to underlying brain. One study found that the majority of chronic subdurals occurred in patients older than 50 years of age and none had associated focal brain injuries.[11]

After review of the literature, one study defined chronic SDH by the following criteria: hematomas resulting in urgent neurologic deficits 20 days after trauma, or if no trauma has taken place, hematomas that have existed for at least three weeks; hematomas not accompanied by evidence of fresh cerebral injury or cerebral injury that has failed to heal; or hematomas with pronounced, neomembranous organization.[12]

A subdural hygroma, also referred to as a traumatic subdural effusion, is a collection of blood-tinged fluid in the subdural space. Absolute distinction between chronic SDHs and subdural hygromas is not always possible because the subdural fluid is often a mixture of CSF and blood. Evidence exists to indicate that subdural hygromas may become chronic SDHs.[13-15] The mechanism of formation is not entirely understood. They may result from tears in the subarachnoid space that permit CSF to escape into the subdural space, or from effusions from injured vessels with abnormal permeability. The most common signs and symptoms are headache, nausea, and vomiting; decreased level of consciousness; and focal deficits. CT scan demonstrates a crescent-shaped collection that has the same density as CSF. Subdural hygromas are usually associated with minor or trivial trauma. They occur more frequently in older patients, with the majority of patients in their sixth decade.[16]

Epidemiology

Accurate incidences of acute and chronic SDHs are difficult to assess. The number of elders is rapidly increasing, placing more patients at risk for these injuries. A recent epidemiologic study found that fall-induced severe head injuries in elders was increasing at a rate that was not due simply to demographic changes.[17] In addition, reported incidences of small acute and chronic SDH have clearly increased secondary to widespread use of CT scanning.

One prospective U.S. population-based study found the average annual incidence of clinically important SDH to be 46.7 per 100,000. Using the 65-74 year old group as a reference, the relative risk for SDH was five times higher in 75- to 84-year-olds and 13 times greater in those older than 85.[18]

A retrospective study covering a seven-year period found the overall incidence of chronic SDHs was 1.72 cases/100,000 population/year. The study also reported that the incidence was greatly influenced by increasing age. In patients aged 60 to 69 years, the incidence rose to 8.4 cases/100,000 population/year, and the incidence further doubled for populations older than 70 years of age.[19] Kudo et al assessed the epidemiological trends on Awaji Island in 1992 and found the overall incidence of chronic subdural was 13.1 (per 100,000 population/year); the incidence was 17 times greater in people 65 years or older (58.1 compared to 3.4 in younger persons). If these numbers were extrapolated to all of Japan by the year 2020, the incidence would increase to 16.3/100,000 population/year.[20]

Falls remain the most significant mechanism of injury in this group. An increasing number and incidence of fall-induced severe head injuries exists in the geriatric population.[17] One study found that 59% of their elderly population who required CT scans for evaluation of closed head trauma sustained their trauma from falls.[21] The study found MVCs responsible for closed head injuries in the elderly in only 20% of the population studied. Other investigators have found similar results.[22,23] However, the increasing number of older drivers may have a significant effect on both the prevalence of older patients involved in MVCs and the incidence of head injuries and SDH.

Etiology

Common predisposing conditions for the development of SDHs include coagulopathy, vascular malformations, renal dialysis, CSF shunts, and head trauma. Head trauma is the most frequent causative factor leading to the development of SDHs. Although direct trauma to the dura, brain, or skull or a pre-existing arachnoid cyst can lead to the formation of a SDH, the most common mechanism is traumatic acceleration/deceleration injury.

The trauma required to produce a chronic SDH is often mild and is usually not accompanied by period of unconsciousness.[19,24-26] The interval from time of trauma to presentation is variable, ranging from three weeks to 12 years.[24,26] However, a history of trauma often is not elicited from the patient or the patient's family. In multiple studies, a history of trauma was documented in only 55-65% of patients with chronic SDHs.[27,28]

This is in contrast to acute SDHs in which the trauma required to produce an acute subdural is usually severe. Most patients present within hours of the initial injury.

Anticoagulation plays a significant role in the predisposition for SDH. In one review of 116 anticoagulant-related intracranial hemorrhages, approximately 40% were chronic subdurals and nearly 80% of patients were older than 80 years of age.[29] Since warfarin use has increased steadily during the last decade, consideration of anticoagulant-related SDH in the elderly becomes even more important.[30] The risk of SDH also is increased with other bleeding diatheses such as hemophilia, thrombocytopenia, and hepatogenic coagulopathies.[24]

Uncommon etiologies for subdural bleeding other than trauma include rupture of a cerebral aneurysm or arteriovenous malformation (AVM), brain tumors, meningeal carcinomatosis, and sarcoidosis.[31-34] A rare cause of chronic SDHs is local infection.[35]

Other at-risk populations include renal dialysis patients and alcoholics. Renal dialysis patients' predisposition stems from platelet dysfunction, anticoagulation, and intracranial hypotension.[36] Alcoholic patients are predisposed to the development of SDHs because of frequent trauma (such as falls), cerebral atrophy, and coagulopathies associated with cirrhosis. Alcohol abusers have a significantly higher incidence of acute SDH and have increased postoperative morbidity and mortality compared to non-alcoholics.[37]

Pathophysiology

Acute SDHs usually occur when the brain is subjected to a high-energy, short-duration force from trauma.[38] This mechanism produces shearing forces that not only tear the bridging veins and result in an acute SDH, but also often produce frontal and temporal cerebral contusions. Shear forces also damage the cerebral vasculature and disturb cerebral autoregulation.[38] Cerebral vascular damage may be responsible for the high incidence of associated cerebral edema, which predisposes to secondary ischemic brain damage.[39]

The mechanism responsible for the development of subdural hemorrhage is a traumatic acceleration/deceleration of the head. This results in differential movement of the brain relative to the skull and in tearing or stretching of cortical bridging veins.[40] The elderly are predisposed to bleeding via this mechanism because of generalized cerebral atrophy and an increase in venous fragility. Cortical bridging veins are short, straight trunks that pass directly from the dura to the brain. These bridging veins are placed under stress as the atrophying brain separates from the dura. Since these thin, fragile veins are firmly adherent to both the dura and the mobile cerebral hemisphere, they are intolerant of significant movement and bleed easily when injured.[41] Acute subdurals also may develop from chronic SDHs as a result of recurrent trauma or following surgical evacuation of a chronic subdural hemtoma.[42]

In contrast, the pathophysiology of chronic SDHs is complex and involves slow evolution and development of the hematoma over a prolonged time period.[35] The unique pathophysiology characterizing chronic SDHs was initially described using light microscopy more than half a century ago.[43] On the first day, the outer surface of the developing hematoma is covered with a thin layer of fibrin and fibroblasts begin to migrate from the undersurface of the dura toward the clot. On day four, a membrane forms on the outer surface of the clot and subsequently enlarges. After approximately two weeks, there exists a thin inner membrane covering the liquefied hematoma. Some subdurals will reabsorb spontaneously, while others will create a chronic SDH by gradual increase in the volume of the encapsulated fluid.

Two theories have been proposed to explain the growth of chronic SDHs. Gardner postulated that partial clot liquefaction increased the protein content within the encapsulated space and thus increased the oncotic pressure within the chronic subdural. The resulting osmotic gradient then caused SDH enlargement.[44] Flaws with Gardner's hypothesis include a normal oncotic pressure following breakdown of red blood cells and identical osmolality of surgically removed SDH, venous blood, and CSF.[45,46]

The second hypothesis suggests that recurrent bleedings account for the expansion of chronic SDHs.[24,47] Ito et al administered Cr51-labeled red blood cells intravenously 6-24 hours prior to the evacuation of SDHs and found up to a 28% concentration of fresh blood within the subdural.[48] The recurrent hemorrhage appears to originate from dilated, abnormal vessels contained in the outer membrane of the hematoma.[49] Angiogenesis factor, found in increased quantities in chronic SDH, contributes to the development of the increased vascularity of the outer membrane. A coagulopathic environment exists within chronic SDHs, and abnormal levels of fibrinolytic enzymes and increased fibrinolytic activity increase the likelihood of hemorrhage.[50-52]

Another mechanism to explain the development of a chronic SDH is transformation of a subdural hygroma into chronic SDH. In one study, this was a common occurrence, with one-fourth of patients with traumatic subdural effusion developing a chronic SDH.[16] This may occur as a result of new head trauma, which causes a tear in the bridging veins within or external to the subdural fluid collection. However, most patients with such a transformation deny any recent head trauma.[15,40] Another plausible mechanism involves multiple, recurrent microhemorrhages occurring from the subdural hygroma membrane.[15] It is hypothesized that brain atrophy may predispose patients to this transformation; however, it has been observed in patients as young as 18 years of age.[13,15]

The pathogenesis of subdural hygromas is still unknown but is believed to involve minor trauma that results in the separation of the dura-arachnoid interface, producing a potential subdural space. Proliferation of the dural border cell layer results in a neomembrane with hyper-permeable capillaries.[53,54] A subsequent efflux of CSF or leakage of serous fluid into the subdural space occurs, creating the subdural hygroma.[54,55] Repeated microhemorrhages in the subdural hygroma may occur from either bridging vein trauma or bleeding from the neomembranes, resulting in a chronic SDH.

Clinical Presentations and Differential Diagnosis

SDH has been referred to as the "great neurologic imitator."[56,57] SDHs can mimic stroke, dementia, and other neurological diseases such as Parkinson's. Symptoms may be insidious and nonspecific, and a history of head trauma is often lacking. Subtle presentations include mild headache, subtle mental status change, and gait disturbances. SDH must be considered in any older person with an alteration in mental status, especially in those prone to falls or on anticoagulants. Acute changes in a patient's activities of daily living (ADLs: bathing, dressing, continence, toileting, feeding, and transfers) may be indicative of an acute medical event such as a SDH.

Acute SDHs often present with a clear history of trauma followed by headache and altered level of consciousness. Evidence of direct head trauma such as cephalohematomas or scalp lacerations, however, may be mild or absent. Patients commonly present with a lucid interval and then acutely deteriorate. Acute SDH were present in 17-38% of cases involving "talk and die" patients.[58,59] Focal neurological deficits and new gait disturbances may occur. Signs of increased intracranial pressure (ICP) may be noted, but are less likely to be present initially in the elderly because of preexisting brain atrophy. Pupillary changes and posturing are ominous signs. It should be reemphasized that the precipitating trauma, such as a fall from a standing height, may be mild. Patients with subacute SDH often complain of worsening headaches 7-14 days after trauma.[60] There may be evidence of old injuries including healing lacerations or abrasions.

The presenting symptoms of chronic SDH are highly variable. Symptoms may occur acutely and suggest other cerebrovascular events. The difficulty in diagnosis is compounded in patients with multiple comorbid conditions and in those who are unable to give a detailed history. The most common presenting symptoms are headache, mental status changes, and hemiparesis.[25,27,61] Headache is the presenting complaint in 30-90% of patients.[19,28,57,62] The description of the headache ranges from mild and generalized to severe with sudden onset. Headache severity may increase with coughing, straining, and exercise. Nausea and vomiting may occur. Mental status changes can present as dementia, mild confusion, and various levels of decreased consciousness, including obtundation.[19,57,62]

A recent retrospective analysis found the three most common presentations of chronic subdurals to be symptoms of increased ICP, fluctuating drowsiness, and progressive dementia.[26]

Presenting complaints may mimic stroke or transient ischemic attacks (TIA). Symptoms vary and include aphasia, hemiparesis, and hemisensory defects.[63-66] Possible mechanisms to explain this presentation include decreased regional blood flow from intermittent vessel compression, vascular displacement from parenchymal swelling, and electrophysiologic aberrations such as seizures or cortical depression.[63,65,67] Given that the elderly population has higher rates of atherosclerotic disease, focal deficits resulting from decreased cerebral blood flow are more likely. One study hypothesized that these events are temporally associated with repeated episodes of bleeding into the hematoma.[65]

Patients with chronic SDHs may present with psychiatric symptoms of depression, paranoia, schizophreniform psychosis, manic-depressive psychosis, catatonia, and vague personality and intellectual changes.[35,68,69] Although geriatric depression is becoming increasingly recognized, other acute or new-onset psychiatric illnesses are uncommon in this age group, and organic etiologies such as SDH should be sought.

Chronic SDHs also may mimic Parkinson's disease in their presentation or cause an exacerbation of symptoms in patients who have Parkinson's. Explanations for this finding include dysfunction of the frontopontine pathways or disturbances of basal ganglia function.[70,71]

Seizures are both an initial symptom and a risk factor for the development of a SDH. The incidence of seizures with chronic SDHs is approximately 4-6% and decreases to 2-3% following neurosurgical treatment.[57,62,72]

Although the physical findings of chronic SDH may be varied, the findings tend to correspond to the patient's presenting symptoms. Papilledema is indicative of increased ICP, but is found less commonly in geriatric patients since any underlying brain atrophy can accommodate a large expanding mass before ICP raises significantly. Common neurological signs include aphasia, cranial nerve palsies, hemiparesis, hemisensory deficits, gait disturbances, and hemianopsia.[19,25,28,62]

The majority of subdural hygromas are asymptomatic. However, symptomatic presentations include irritability, drowsiness, headache, confusion, and depressed level of consciousness.[15]

Posterior fossa SDH represent a very rare clinical entity, if newborns are excluded. They occur in less than 2% of all SDHs.[25,73] Posterior fossa SDHs result from occipital trauma that injures bridging vessels or venous sinuses. Clinical presentations include complaints of nausea, vomiting, headache, decreased level of consciousness, cranial nerve palsies, nuchal rigidity, cerebellar signs and symptoms, and papilledema. There are often signs of brainstem compression: miosis, mydriasis, nystagmus, anisocoria, flaccid or hypertonic limbs, and eye deviation. The clinical course is rapid and decline usually occurs within the first nine hours after injury.[73] Prognosis is dismal; less than 5% of patients survive. Negative outcome predictors include: advanced age, rapid clinical deterioration, brainstem compression, associated intracranial lesions, delayed surgery, and completely obliterated posterior fossa cisterns on head CT.[73,74]

Although uncommonly found in the head-injured geriatric patient, a review of head injuries and SDHs in the elderly would be lacking without a brief consideration of epidural hematomas. An epidural hematoma refers to a collection of blood between the inner table of the skull and the dura. It is most commonly caused by a direct contact or impact injury with a forceful deformity of the skull. Eighty percent are associated with a skull fracture crossing the middle meningeal artery or a dural sinus. Most are in the temporal-parietal region. Epidurals are usually unilateral; however, there is a high incidence of other intracranial lesions, including subarachnoid hemorrhage and contusions. Unlike subdurals, epidurals develop rapidly since the bleeding source is usually arterial. Slower progression may occur if the bleeding is from a dural sinus. The classic presentation is a loss of consciousness followed by a "lucid interval" (a brief period of improving mental status). A depressed level or secondary loss of consciousness follows. Common complaints include severe headache, sleepiness, dizziness, nausea, and vomiting. Mortality is much lower compared to acute SDH. CT scan demonstrates a hyperdense, biconvex, ovoid, or lenticular collection with sharply defined margins.

Epidural hematomas are seen much less commonly than subdurals in the elderly. This is thought to be the result of the close attachment of the dura to the periosteum of the inner table, which obliterates the potential space and prevents the hematoma from developing.

Differential diagnosis of SDH includes dementia, stroke, TIA, encephalitis, adverse drug reactions, psychiatric disorders, brain tumors, and subarachnoid hemorrhage. *(See Table 1.)* Careful history and physical examination can help differentiate these conditions.[18] Older patients, however, often have underlying neurological disease and differentiating acute findings; cognitive impairment and changes from the patient's baseline may be difficult. Liberal use of CT scanning is recommended in this population.[41] Antiplatelet and anticoagulant therapy should not be instituted in patients with focal or transient neurological deficits until SDH is excluded.[64,75]

Diagnostic Studies

The diagnosis of acute and chronic SDHs has changed considerably since the advent of CT scanning. Prior to this, the diagnosis was suggested by abnormal skull radiographs and confirmed by cerebral angiography. Plain films were abnormal in up to 50% of cases (demonstrating depression or lateral displacement of the pineal gland); however, this finding was neither sensitive nor specific.[25,57,62] Angiography was the standard means for diagnosing SDHs for many years, with accuracy approaching 99%. Subdurals would appear as an avascular region between the cortical surface of the brain and the inner table of the skull.[25,28,62] Angiography, still in use just two decades ago, was invasive, time consuming, and not without risk. Radioisotope brain scans have also been used in the past to detect SDHs. They were only reliable in well-developed hematomas and had high false-negative rates in patients with scalp trauma, Paget's disease, infection, and tumor.[56,76-78]

Noncontrast head CT scans provide a reliable, noninvasive means for detecting acute and chronic SDHs. A peripheral area of either high or low density, when contrasted with normal brain tissue, is easily identified. As was alluded to above, a SDH is a dynamic entity; therefore, its appearance on CT scans depends upon the phase of its development.[79-81]

In the acute setting, SDHs usually appear as a hyperdense crescentic-shaped mass overlying the cortical surface. *(Please see Figure 1.)* Since the subdural space is continuous around each hemisphere, the hematoma is free to completely surround these structures while respecting the midline and tentorial margins.[81] Occasionally, a hyperacute SDH may appear hypodense if imaged prior to clot formation. Hypodense areas may also appear within an acute SDH (mixed-density SDH) because of active bleeding.[82] Acute SDH can also appear hypodense in patients with significant underlying anemia (hemoglobin concentrations less than 8-10 g/dL).[83] Although usually easily visualized, acute SDH can be difficult to appreciate if the collection occurs under the temporal lobe or along tentorial surfaces. *(Please see Figure 2.)*

Between the first and third weeks after formation, a SDH may become isodense to brain tissue because of lysis of red blood cells and resorption of hemoglobin. *(Please see Figure 3.)* Effacement of sulci, inward displacement of the normal gray-white junction, deformation of normal ventricular anatomy, and obliteration of basal cisterns may indirectly identify these isodense collections.[79,84,85] Medial displacement of cortical sulci away from the inner table of the skull is highly suggestive of isodense SDH. Conversely, good visualization of the cortical sulci extending to the inner table of the skull rules out an isodense SDH.[86] Bilateral isodense subdurals are more difficult to detect but may appear as obliteration of basal cisterns and blunting of the normal gyral and sulcal anatomy.[84] In addition, small compressed ventricles, although not a specific finding, should suggest the possibility of bilateral isodense SDHs.[86] Contrast-enhanced CT scans are useful for visualization of isodense subdurals. Contrast enhancement of the cortical surface and inner membrane of the SDH, which are displaced from the inner table of the skull, allows for easier detection.[85,87,88] A scanning delay of 3-6 hours allows for visualization of the hematoma itself.[89]

In the third week, the clot becomes hypodense relative to brain tissue and is usually readily apparent on CT scan. *(Please see Figures 4 and 5.)* Chronic SDH commonly occur bilaterally, especially in the very elderly (older than 75 years).[90] Acute hemorrhage can occur in a chronic SDH after only minor trauma. Blood tends to layer on the fibrovascular membranes that bridge the subdural space, creating a multilocular appearance.[81] *(Please see Figure 6.)* This should be differentiated from the layering of blood products (hematocrit effect) seen in acute subdurals when patients are left undisturbed for several hours.

Subdural hygromas, which are often frontal, are also hypodense fluid collections. *(Please see Figure 7.)* Differential diagnosis includes chronic SDH or brain atrophy with enlargement of the subarachnoid space.[91] Hygromas usually arise 1-2 weeks after trauma, which helps differentiate them from chronic SDH. As with chronic SDHs, fluid in the subdural space tends to collect anteriorly, especially in elderly patients. The distinction between these two entities is not always possible radiographically, unless a CT scan was performed at the time of the initial trauma.

Although CT remains the imaging modality of choice for detecting SDHs in the acute setting, magnetic resonance imaging (MRI) has better sensitivity.[69] SDHs have shorter T1 and longer T2 values when compared to normal brain. Chronic SDH are often hyperintense on T1 and T2 weighted scans and are rarely isodense on T1 images.[61,92,93] Low intensity T2 images due to recurrent bleeding are common in symptomatic chronic SDH, and MRI findings correlate well with the age of the hematoma and onset of symptoms.[94] MRI also clearly demonstrates isodense SDH better than CT. It is also significantly better at identifying small or transversely oriented SDH collections, interhemispheric SDH, and SDH at the base of the skull and in the posterior fossa, since it eliminates the bone artifact seen on CT.[95,96] Postcontrast MRI can predict progression of acute SDH. Diffuse enhancement, which indicates active bleeding, has been shown to be very sensitive in predicting enlarging hematomas.[97]

Chronic SDHs can also be detected on EEG by diffuse or unilateral voltage suppression, delta activity, or depression of a rhythm; however, the EEG may also be normal or demonstrate nonspecific findings and imaging is still required to make the diagnosis.[43,56,77]

Accurate and rapid diagnosis of SDHs is imperative for successful management. The size (measured in mm) and density of the SDH should be noted. Other important CT findings include the degree of midline shift (also noted in mm), effacement of ventricles and cisterns, and associated intracranial hematomas or subarachnoid hemorrhage.

Management

As with all acutely ill or injured patients, initial management of head injuries begins with rapid assessment and attention to airway, breathing, and circulation (ABCs). Attention to the ABCs will limit secondary insults from hypoxemia and increased ICP. Initial assessment should assess the patient's level of consciousness and responsiveness and pupillary reactivity. The GCS is a rapid, reliable, and reproducible score for head injury patients. It is useful both for predicting prognosis and for frequent reassessment of these patients. *(Please see Table 2.)*

Table 1. Differential Diagnosis for SDH

- ❑ Stroke/TIA
- ❑ Normal pressure hydrocephalus
- ❑ Parkinson's disease
- ❑ Infection (meningitis, brain abscess)
- ❑ Dementia
- ❑ Psychiatric illness
- ❑ CNS tumor
- ❑ Adverse drug reactions

Indications for endotracheal intubation include airway control and hyperventilation. Although a GCS of 8 or less often indicates loss of airway protection, snoring respirations, accumulation of secretions in the oral pharynx, and lack of cough or gag response provide more direct evidence of the need for airway protection. In the setting of normal respiratory function, intubation will also ensure adequate oxygenation. Since critical management decisions are often based on serial neurological examinations and GCS scores, routine use of long acting paralytic agents is not advocated.[98]

The role of hyperventilation in the management of acute head injury is somewhat controversial.[99,100] The benefit of hyperventilation is that it reduces $PC0_2$, causing a subsequent cerebral vasoconstriction, which in turn reduces ICP. The goal is a $PC0_2$ of approximately 30-35 mmHg; levels less than 35 mmHg should be avoided in the first 24 hours post-injury. However, it is now recognized that maintaining cerebral perfusion pressure (CPP) should guide therapy in traumatic brain injuries. CPP is defined as the mean arterial pressure (MAP) minus ICP. Ideally, CPP should be kept at approximately 70 mmHg.[101] The beneficial affects of hyperventilation appear short-lived, and hyperventilation can actually lower cerebral blood volumes and thus reduce CPP. Despite these controversies, hyperventilation remains commonly used in patients with documented or suspected increased ICP.

Osmotic diuresis, another common means of ICP management, is also controversial.[101-103] Mannitol at doses of 0.5-1.0 gm/kg IV is commonly used as a temporizing measure in the setting of acute changes in the neurologic exam (such as posturing or other evidence of herniation), increasing hematoma size, or uncontrollable ICP. Osmotic diuretics, such as mannitol, should be used to maintain CPP greater than or equal to 70 mmHg in the euvolemic or hypervolemic patient. Injudicious use in the hypovolemic patient can result in lowering the MAP with a resulting decrease in CPP. This may be especially critical in the elderly trauma patient, since accurate evaluation of volume status can be difficult.[104] If hypovolemia is present or suspected, volume replacement should be employed, and followed by pressors if necessary to maintain the MAP. The most commonly used pressors include norepinephrine (Levophed; 3-12 micrograms/minute IV) or phenylephrine (Neo-Synephrine; 40-180 micrograms/minute IV). Pressor agents should not be used for neurological resuscitation without ICP and MAP monitoring.[101]

Figure 1. Acute SDH

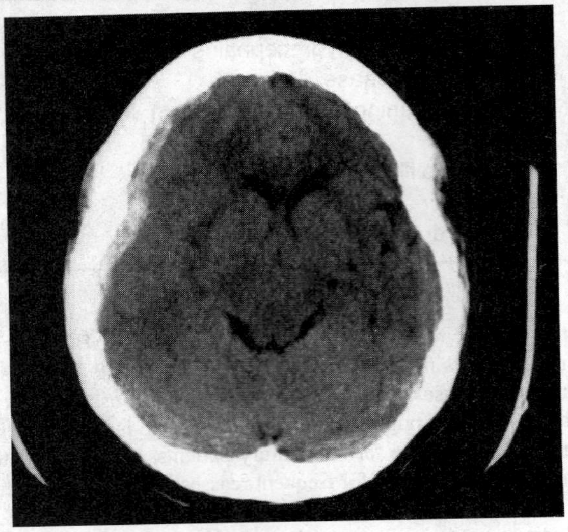

Figure 2. Acute SDH Along Falx

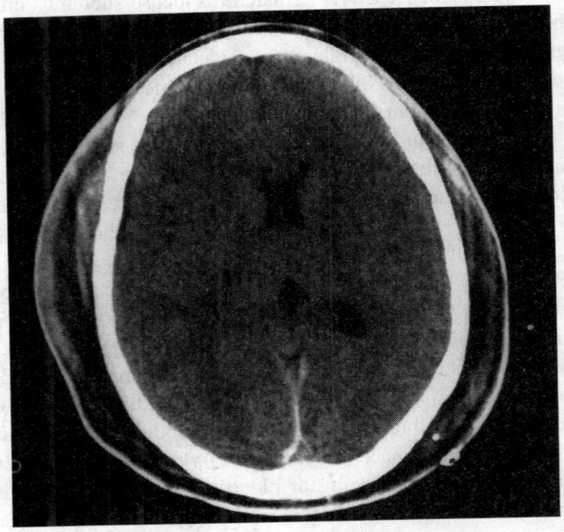

Note asymmetrical appearance of falx.

Specific management of acute and chronic subdurals, including indications for neurosurgical interventions, will be discussed below.

Management of acute SDHs depends on the patient's neurological exam, including GCS and CT findings, with attention to SDH size, midline shift, and cistern effacement. Patients who have an acute SDH with a thickness of 10 mm or less and a shift of the midline structures of 5 mm or less can often be treated nonoperatively.

In one large, retrospective series of patients with acute SDH, 61% were managed nonoperatively.[105] These patients tended to have small SDH (< 10 mm), higher GCS scores (mean of 11), and less evidence of associated brain injury (open paramesencephalic cisterns and less midline shift). For patients with GCS scores of 9-15, craniotomy was not associated with a difference in outcome. The importance of the pre-hospital and admitting GCS scores for determining treatment also has been examined. Patients with stable GCS scores who did not meet CT criteria for surgery were treated conservatively in one prospective study. Fifteen of 65 patients were managed nonoperatively; two required subsequent operations. Functional outcomes were achieved in two-thirds of patients treated with nonoperative management.[98] In another series of acute SDH patients with GCS scores between 11 and 15, 93% achieved a good outcome with nonoperative treatment.[106] As these studies suggest, if

Figure 3. Isodense (Subacute) SDH

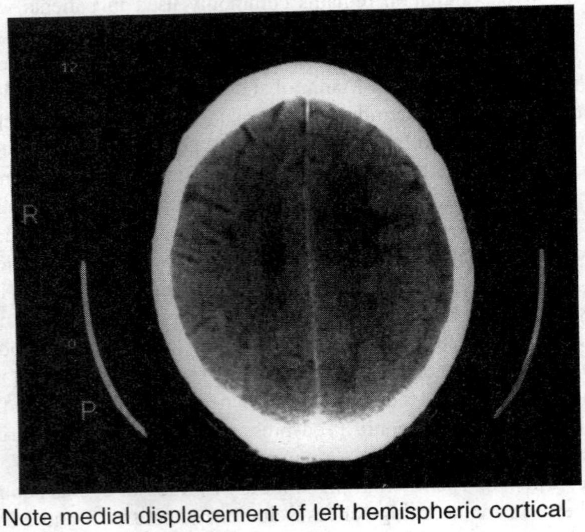

Note medial displacement of left hemispheric cortical sulci.

Figure 4. Chronic SDH with Typical Hypodense Appearance

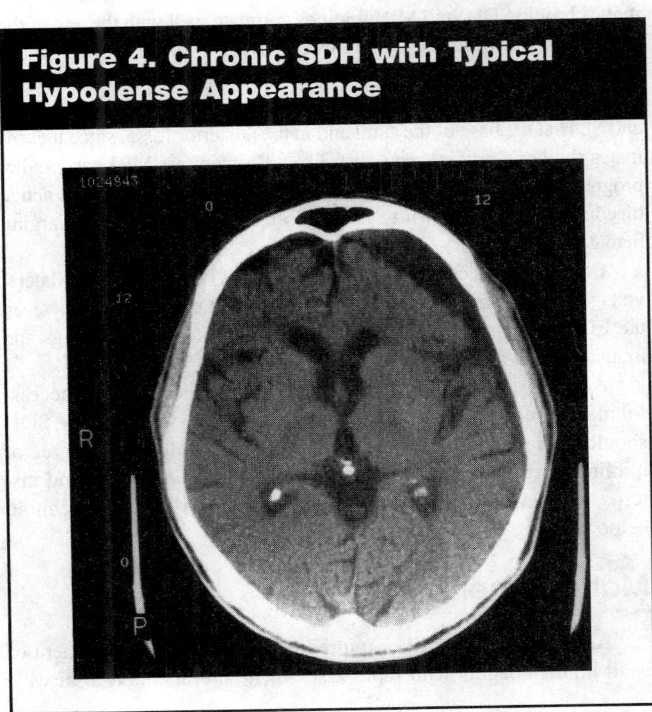

Figure 5. Chronic SDH with Neomembrane

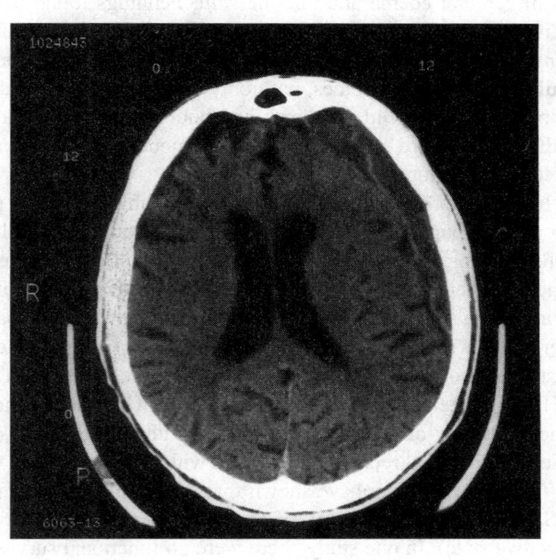

a small hematoma is not a source of intracranial hypertension or significant neurologic dysfunction, then evacuation provides no advantage.

Conversely, large SDH with shift greater than 5 mm are usually associated with an elevated ICP. In these instances, prompt craniotomy and evacuation is necessary and management of the acute SDH generally takes precedence over other injuries. Early surgery is most important for a subset of patients with pure acute SDHs and a lucid interval after injury. In these cases, associated cerebral damage is mild and neurologic deterioration results from increased ICP due to the hematoma itself. Numerous studies have demonstrated lower mortality (approximately 50% survival) in this group of patients with prompt surgical treatment.[107-109]

Figure 7. Subdural Hygroma (Bilateral)

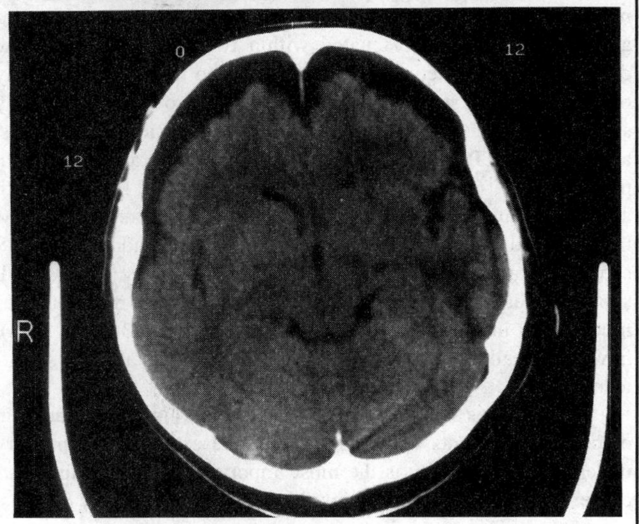

Figure 6. Chronic SDH (Bilateral) with Acute Hemorrhage

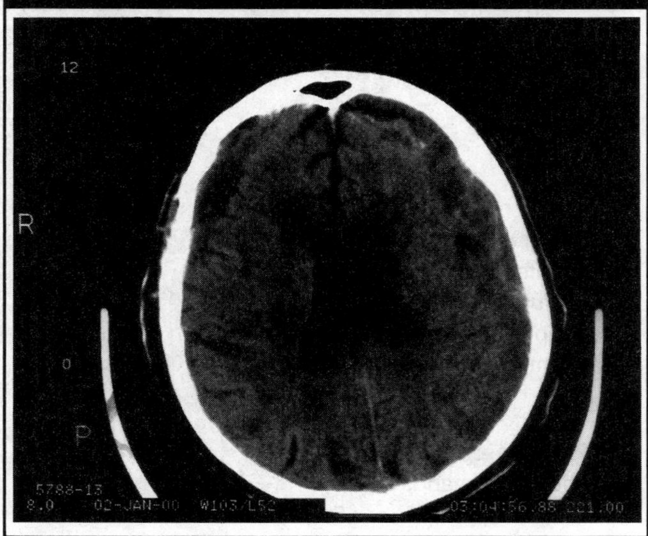

Operative treatment of acute SDHs consists of craniotomy for evacuation of the clot and may include subsequent placement of subdural or intraventricular pressure-monitoring devices. Overall surgical mortality rates range from 33% to 100%.[73,110,111] Emergency department burr holes are not useful for the diagnosis or treatment of acute SDH. The thick, nonliquid nature of the clot often prohibits evacuation through a small burr hole and generally requires a craniotomy in most cases.[112]

If not surgically removed, the SDH may be expected to resolve into liquefied clot within 4-6 weeks and eventually be completely absorbed.[39,113] Resolution of acute SDH is primarily seen in young, healthy adults with relatively small hematomas.

The treatment of chronic SDHs is a matter of debate; however, a simplified approach consists of either conservative or operative management. Since chronic SDH is a primary disease of the elderly, treatment modalities ideally should be minimally invasive, expedient, and have the best therapeutic result. Conservative medical management involves mannitol and glucocorticoid administration.[114] Surgical evacuation involves craniotomies, burr holes, twist drill craniotomies, or small trephine. The method is determined by the amount of hemorrhage and consistency of the hematoma as assessed by CT or MRI. Morbidity and mortality following surgical evacuation ranges from 5% to 11% and is affected by type of surgical procedure.[35]

Burr hole craniotomy is the most accepted surgical treatment of chronic SDHs. It has been shown to be an effective treatment with a low incidence of complications in spite of patients' advanced age and associated comorbid diseases.[24,27,28] Recent technical advances have resulted in lower mortality, reduced re-operative rate, and shorter duration of in-patient stay.[115,116]

Craniotomy with extensive membranectomy is a more invasive surgical technique with a higher rate of complication.[24] The use of this technique as the initial treatment of chronic SDH has declined and it is now reserved as a secondary treatment following unsuccessful initial procedures.[27,28,117]

Re-accumulation of chronic SDH after burr hole craniotomy is a known complication.[24,27,118] Re-accumulation of hematoma with fresh blood is more likely with large excisions of the external membrane and may be related to excessive drainage volume.[118] A recent study involving very elderly patients recommends that re-operation

Table 2. Glasgow Coma Scale (GCS)

Response	Score
EYE OPENING	
Spontaneous	4
To voice	3
To pain	2
None	1
VERBAL RESPONSE	
Oriented	5
Confused	4
Inappropriate words	3
Incomprehensible	2
None	1
MOTOR RESPONSE	
Obeys commands	6
Localizes pain	5
Withdraws (pain)	4
Flexion (pain)	3
Extension (pain)	2
None	1
Total GCS	*3-15*

for persistent fluid collections not be performed if there is clinical improvement in the patient.[115]

Spontaneous resolution of chronic SDHs is rarely observed. CT findings associated with spontaneous resolution include chronic subdurals that are low density or isodense, that are small in size and associated with ventricular dilation, and those that are found in patients with mild or no clinical signs or symptoms.[15,119,120] The mechanism responsible for this spontaneous resolution is hypothesized to involve decreased fibrinolytic activity of the hematoma capsule and of the fluid.[119]

Other complications from surgical evacuations include subdural empyema, brain abscess, cellulitis, bone-flap infection, and meningitis. Seizures are also a postoperative complication so anticonvulsants are begun preoperatively and continued for six months. Further complications include acute intracerebral hematoma after evacuation. This may occur by hemorrhage into previously undetected areas of contusion, a sudden increase in cerebral blood flow coupled with faulty autoregulation, and damage to parenchymal vessels secondary to rapid shift of cranial contents. Complications also include brain stem hemorrhage, cerebral edema, tension pneumocephalus, and SIADH.

Post-op results of chronic SDH evacuation are dependent on neurologic condition of patients at the time of admission.[27]

Prognosis

Acute SDHs generally carry a poor prognosis, especially in the elderly. Mortality rates range from 50% to 80% and have not changed significantly in four decades.[25,121-124] One study found mortality to be four times higher in older patients than in younger ones.[125] Important prognostic factors in addition to age include neurologic presentation, CT scan findings, and delays in craniotomy and hematoma evacuation.

One group examined 315 patients with severe head injuries.[126] Patients with SDH had 66% mortality and worse outcomes as measured by the Glasgow Outcome Scale. Predictors of mortality included older age, low motor score on the GCS, and CT scan findings of cerebral edema and midline shift. Pennings found not only significantly worse survival (79% mortality vs 36% mortality for younger patients) in older patients with severe brain injuries, but also significantly worse outcomes, with only one older patient making a favorable recovery. Older patients had both early and late hospital deaths and one-third were attributed to pulmonary, cardiac, or multisystem organ failure.[127]

Important prognostic factors that are available to the ED physician include pupillary response and GCS. Although bilateral fixed pupils is typically an ominous sign in patients with traumatic intracranial hemorrhage, in one series a full 25% of patients with this finding made a good recovery.[128] In this study, however, no patients older than the age of 65 survived and the most important predictor of negative outcome in these patients was the presence of an acute SDH. One recent series examined the initial GCS score and outcome.[121] Ninety-one percent of patients with a high GCS (9-15) achieved functional recovery, compared with 23% of patients with a low GCS (3-8). Others have shown that the simple combination of GCS and age can be predictive of poor outcomes (death or persistent vegetative state). In one study, there were no functional survivors in patients with an age older than 60 and a GCS score of less than 5.[129] As the authors note, these findings should not be used to decide if treatment is warranted, but instead should be used to guide clinicians and families toward rational treatments and realistic expectations.

CT findings can also help predict outcomes in patients with acute SDH. One report showed that a hematoma thickness less than 10 mm had only a 10% mortality, while mortality rose to 90% with hematomas greater than 30 mm.[123] The authors noted a significant increase in mortality (less than 50% survival) with a hematoma thickness greater than 18 mm and a mid-line shift greater than 20 mm. Just as importantly, evidence of brain swelling (additional midline shift not explained by hematoma size alone) was a significant factor in outcome. Fifty percent mortality was associated with brain swelling displacement of only 3 mm and patients with swelling greater than 5 mm had only a 25% chance of survival.

The timing of acute SDH evacuation has also been evaluated in regard to prognosis. One group reviewed 82 patients with acute SDH and coma and found that time from injury to operation was the most significant factor in reducing mortality.[130] Patients who underwent surgery within four hours had a 30% mortality compared to 90% who had surgery after four hours. Interestingly, patient age did not affect survival. Others have noted improved survival if extra-axial hematomas are evacuated within two hours of neurologic deterioration.[124] Functional outcome was also improved with early operation. Not all studies have shown such improvement with early surgery. Another group found age older than 65, low GCS scores, and elevated ICPs, but not timing of surgery, to be associated with poor outcome.[109] A recent, larger study examined 211 patients with acute SDH and GCS ranging from 3 to 15. Factors found to be independently associated with outcome were age, admission GCS scores, overall injury severity, and pupillary reactivity.[105] In a small subset of patients with large acute SDH and coma, mortality was much lower in those undergoing early craniotomy (30% vs 59%); however, small numbers accounted for the lack of statistical significance.

These studies suggest that although age is an important factor in outcomes in patients with acute SDHs, the extent of the primary underlying brain injury is the most important factor affecting outcome. Functional recovery is possible, even in very elderly patients, if their initial presentation shows only mild impairment in consciousness (i.e., GCS scores of 12 or higher).[131,132]

In contrast to acute SDH, chronic SDH have a much better outcome. Prognosis is often determined by the patient's condition on admission, general health, and comorbid diseases.[15,25,120] Mortality of patients surgically treated for chronic SDH is approximately 10%. Three-fourths of patients return to their baseline functional level postoperatively.[133] The use of burr hole craniotomy and closed-system drainage also limits the surgical risk and can be offered even to very elderly and frail patients. Good outcomes (absent or only mild neurological deficits) have been reported in 76% of older patients treated for chronic SDH by this method.[134] These findings reflect the pathophysiology of this entity and the low incidence of significant underlying brain injury.

Few studies have addressed factors influencing function and independence as a long-term outcome in the geriatric head-injured population. One study found that in geriatric trauma patients with a GCS of less than 8, none returned to independent living.[135] Another study found that 33% of head-injured elderly patients had a change in domicile following their discharge from the hospital.[136]

Older adults sustaining mild and moderate head injury show cognitive and behavioral changes and disturbances in mood persisting for greater than one year post-injury.[137,138] A review examining cognitive performance in geriatric patients following a closed head injury found that 50% had generalized deterioration and dementia thought to be a consequence of their head trauma.[139] Elderly head injured patients perform more poorly at word naming and word fluency, memory testing, and other cognitive abilities than age-matched controls.[137,140] These cognitive disturbances may predispose these patients to more falls and as a consequence increase the risk of subsequent head injuries.

Additional Aspects

Pitfalls. Several pitfalls can occur in the evaluation of elderly patients with SDHs. The most important pitfall is simply not considering the diagnosis. In the elderly, acute SDHs can occur after seemingly minor head trauma or following insignificant injury mechanisms such as a fall. Chronic subdurals may be especially hard to diagnose since there is often no history or seemingly remote history of head trauma. As noted above, presentations can be subtle or can mimic other disease processes such as worsening Parkinson's disease or dementia. Histories should be obtained or confirmed with family members or caregivers. A history of acute changes in mentation, behavior, or ADLs is potentially significant. The possibility of a SDH in these patients should be kept in mind and if suspected, a CT scan should be obtained.

Conversely, the presence of a small chronic SDH or subdural hygroma may be found in older patients who have other causes for acute mental status change, such as severe hyporthyroidism or hyperosmolar coma. Although beyond the scope of this article, other common etiologies for altered mental status or delirium in older patients such as infection, congestive heart failure, or electrolyte abnormalities should be sought. Careful attention to the history, physical examination (such as signs of hypothyroidism), and laboratory evaluation (electrolytes, renal function, and glucose levels) can be very helpful in assessing these complex patients.

As noted above, CT scans are very sensitive at detecting acute and chronic SDHs. Two pitfalls in CT diagnosis can occur, however. The first, as noted previously, is missing a subacute SDH. The other is missing an acute SDH in an unusual location, such as a parafalcine or tentorial SDH. Careful review, along with neuroradiological consultation (using tele-radiology if necessary), should limit these occurrences.

In addition, the possibility of a cervical spine injury (CSI) should be considered in all patients with a history of trauma and SDH. CSI are not uncommon in the older patient. These injuries most often occur following minor trauma, with falls (70%) being the most common mechanism. CSI in the elderly often involve the upper cervical spine (C1 and C2) and spinal cord injury is either absent or incomplete.[141] Radiographic evaluation should include an adequate view of the odontoid. CT scans may be necessary if plain films are not conclusive or suspicious for acute injury.

Disposition

Disposition of older patients with SDH is fairly straightforward. Absolute indications for emergent neurosurgical consultation include GCS score of 8 or less in the setting of trauma, and CT findings of acute SDH with or without mass affect or obliteration of basal cisterns.[101] Patients with acute SDH require admission to an intensive care unit (ICU) setting. If neurosurgical care is not immediately available, patients should be promptly transferred.

Patients with chronic SDH also require neurosurgical consultation, with the urgency of the evaluation depending on the patient presentation, such as the presence of neurologic deficits or an abnormal GCS score. Patients with small chronic SDH and minimal abnormalities on neurologic examination warrant admission for observation and neurosurgical consultation. Patients found to have cystic hygromas are at risk for development of chronic SDH and should followup with their primary care physician who can arrange neurosurgical evaluation as appropriate. Other important factors in disposition include the patient's living arrangements and consideration of elder abuse.

Summary

SDHs are common in elder persons and will increase in incidence as our population grows older. Acute SDHs can occur after varying degrees of trauma and often have devastating outcomes in this age group, especially if diagnosis and treatment are delayed. Initial management of acute head injuries and SDH should be familiar to all emergency physicians. Chronic SDHs are more insidious and can mimic a number of other disease processes in the very elderly. Maintaining a high index of suspicion and liberal use of CT scanning can allow one to make this difficult diagnosis and thus maximize outcomes for this at-risk population.

References

1. Osler T, Hales K, Baack B, et al. Trauma in the elderly. *Am J Surg* 1988;156:537-543.
2. Finelli FC, Jonsson J, Champion HR, et al. A case control study for major trauma in geriatric patients. *J Trauma* 1989; 29:541-548.
3. Nagurney JT, Borczuk P, Thomas SH. Elder patients with closed head trauma: A comparison with nonelder patients. *Acad Emer Med* 1998;5:678-684.
4. Baker SP, O'Neill B, Ginsberg MJ, et al. *The Injury Fact Book,* 2nd ed. New York: Oxford University Press; 1992.
5. Sattin RW, Huber DAL, DeVito CA, et al. The incidence of fall injury events among the elderly in a defined population. *Am J Epidem* 1990;131:1028-1037.
6. Rakier A, Guilburd JN, Soustiel JF, et al. Head injuries in the elderly. *Brain Inj* 1995;9:187-193.

7. Champion HR, Copes WS, Buyer D, et al. Major trauma in geriatric patients. *Am J Pub Health* 1989;79:1278-1282.
8. van der Sluis CK, Timmer HW, Eisma WH, et al. Outcome in elderly injured patients: Injury severity versus host factors. *Injury* 1997;28:588-592.
9. Levy DB, Hanlon DP, Townsend RN. Geriatric trauma. *Clin Geriatr Med* 1993;9:601-620.
10. Evans R. Trauma and Falls. In: Sanders AB, ed. *Emergency Care of the Elder Person*. St. Louis: Beverly Cracon Publications; 1996:150-170.
11. Lee KS, Park YT, Bae HG, et al. Pathogenesis and fate of traumatic subdural hygroma. *Br J Neurosurg* 1994;8:551-558.
12. Yamashima T, Yamamoto S. Clinicopathological classification of chronic subdural hematoma. *Zent bl Fneurochir* 1985;46: 304-314.
13. Lee KS, Doh JW, Bae HG, et al. Relations among traumatic subdural lesions. *J Korean Med Sci* 1996 Feb;11:55-63.
14. Lee KS, Bae WK, Doh JW, et al. Origin of chronic subdural hematoma and relation to traumatic subdural lesions. *Brain Inj* 1998;12:901-910.
15. Park C, Choi KH, Kim MC, et al. Spontaneous evolution of posttraumatic subdural hygroma into chronic subdural hematoma. *Acta Neurochir (Wien)* 1994;127;41-47.
16. Murata K. Chronic subdural hematoma may be preceded by persistent traumatic subdural effusion. *Neurl Med Chir (Tokyo)* 1993;33:691-696.
17. Kannus P, Palvanen M, Niemi S, et al. Increasing number and incidence of fall-induced severe head injuries in older adults: Nationwide statistics in Finland in 1970-1995 and prediction for the future. *Am J Epidemiol* 1999;149:143-150.
18. Alexander EM, Wagner EH, Buchner DM, et al. Do surgical brain lesions present as isolated dementia: A population-based study. *J Am Geriatr Soc* 1995 Feb;43:138-143.
19. Fogelholm R, Heiskanen O, Waltimo O. Chronic subdural hematoma in adults. Influence of patient's age on symptoms, signs and thickness of hematoma. *J Neurosurg* 1975;42:43-46.
20. Kudo H, Kuwamura K, Izawa I, et al. Chronic subdural hematoma in elderly people: Present status on Awaji Island and epidemiological prospect. *Neurol Med Chir (Tokyo)* 1992; 32:207-209.
21. Nagurney JT, Borczuk P, Thomas SH. Elderly patients with closed head trauma after a fall: Mechanisms and outcomes. *J Emer Med* 1998;16:709-713.
22. Oreskovich MR, Howard JD, Copass MK, et al. Geriatric trauma: Injury patterns and outcome. *J Trauma* 1984;24:565.
23. Roy CW, Pentland B, Miller JD. The causes and consequences of minor head injury in the elderly. *Injury* 1986;17:220-223.
24. Markwalder T-M. Chronic subdural hematomas: A review. *J Neurosurg* 1981;54:637-645.
25. McKissock W, Richardson A, Bloom WH. Subdural hematoma: A review of 389 cases. *Lancet* 1960;1:1365-1369.
26. Kotwica Z, Brzezinski J. Clinical pattern of chronic subdural hematoma. *Neurochirurgia* (Stuttg) 1991;34:148-150.
27. Krupp WF, Jans PJ. Treatment of chronic subdural hematoma with Burr-hole craniostomy and closed drainage. *Br J Neurosurg* 1995;9:619-627.
28. Richter HP, Klein HJ, Schafer M. Chronic subdural hematomas treated by enlarged Burr hole craniotomy and closed system drainage retrospective study of 120 patients. *Acta Neurochir* (Wien) 1984;71:179-188.
29. Mattle H, Kohler S, Huber P, et al. Anticoagulation-related intracranial extracerebral hemorrhage. *J Neurol Neurosurg Psychiatry* 1989;52:829-837.
30. Smith NL, Psaty BM, Furgerg CD, et al. Temporal trends in the use of anticoagulants among older adults with atrial fibrillation. *Arch Intern Med* 1999;159:1574-1578.
31. Bassett RC, Lemmen LJ. Subdural hematoma associated with bleeding intracranial aneurysm. *J Neurosurg* 1952;9:443-450.
32. Boop WC Jr, Chou SN, French LA. Ruptured intracranial aneurysm complicated by subdural hematoma. *J Neurosurg* 1961;18:834-836.
33. Russell DS, Cairns H. Subdural false membrane or hematoma (pachymeningitis internal iaemorrhagica) in carcinomatosis and sarcomatosis of the dura mater. *Brain* 1934;57:32-48.
34. Modesti LM, Binet EF, Collins GH. Meningtomas causing spontaneous intracranial hematomas. *J Neurosurg* 1976;45: 437-441.
35. Traynelis VC. Chronic subdural hematoma in the elderly. *Clin Geriatr Med* 1991;7:583-598.
36. Kopitnik TA, deAndrade R Jr, Gold MA, et al. Pressure changes within a chronic subdural hematoma during hemodialysis. *Surg Neurol* 1989;32:289-293.
37. Sonne NM, Tonnesen H. The influence of alcoholism on outcome after evacuation of subdural hematoma. *Br J Neurosurg* 1992;6:125-130.
38. Gennarelli TA, Speilman GM, Langfitt TW, et al. Influence of the type of intracranial lesion on outcome from severe head injury. A multicenter study using a new classification system. *J Neurosurg* 1982;56:26-32.
39. Adams JH. Brain Damage in Fatal Non-missile Head Injury. In: Vinken PJ, Bruyn GW, Klawans HL, eds. *Handbook of Clinical Neurology*, Vol 57. Amsterdam: Elsevier Science Publishers; 1990;43-63.
40. Cooper PR. Post-traumatic Intracranial Mass Lesion. In: Cooper PR, ed. *Head Injury*, 3rd ed. Baltimore: Williams & Wilkins; 1993:275-329.
41. Mandavia D. Newton K. Geriatric trauma. *Emerg Med Clin North Am* 1998;16:257-274.
42. Turgut M, Akalan N, Saglam S. A fatal acute subdural hematoma occurring after evacuation of "contralateral" chronic subdural hematoma. *J Neurosurg Sci* 1998;42:61-63.
43. Munro D, Merritt HH. Surgical pathology of subdural hematomas. Based on a study of one hundred and five cases. *Arch Neurol* 1936;35:64-78.
44. Gardner WJ. Traumatic subdural hematoma with particular reference to the latent interval. *Arch Neurol Psych* 1932;27: 847-858.
45. Rabe EF, Flynn RE, Dodge, PR. A study of subdural effusions in an infant with particular reference to the mechanisms of their persistence. *Neurology* 1962;12:79-92.
46. Weir B. The osmolality of subdural hematoma fluid. *J Neurosurg* 1971;34:528-533.
47. Putnam TJ, Cushing H. Chronic subdural hematoma: Its pathology, its relations to pachymeningitis hemorrhagica and its surgical treatment. *Arch Surg* 1925;11:329-393.
48. Ito H, Yamamoto S, Saito K, et al. Quantitative estimation of

hemorrhage in chronic subdural hematoma using the 51Cr erythrocyte labeling method. *J Neurosurg* 1987;66:862-864.
49. Sato S, Suzuki J. Ultrastructural observations of the capsule of chronic subdural hematoma in various clinical stages. *J Neurosurg* 1975;43:569-578.
50. Ito H, Komai T, Yamamoto S. Fibrinolytic enzyme in the lining walls of chronic subdural hemtoma. *J Neurosurg* 1978;48:197-200.
51. Kawakami Y, Chikama M. Tamiya T, et al. Coagulation and fibrinolysis in chronic subdural hematoma. *Neurosurgery* 1989;25:25-29.
52. Saito K, Ito H, Hasegawa T, et al. Plasmin-0_2-plasmin inhibitor complex and 0_2-plasmin inhibitor in chronic subdural hematoma. *J Neursurg* 1989;70:68-72.
53. Friede RL, Schachenmayr W. The origin of subdural neomembranes: II. Fine structure of neomembranes. *Am J Pathol* 1978;92:69-84.
54. Hasegawa M, Yamashima T, Yamashita J, et al. Traumatic subdural hygroma: Pathology and meningeal enhancement on magnetic resonance imaging. *Neurosurgery* 1992;31:580-585.
55. Fobben ES, Grossman RI, Hackney DB, et al. MR characteristics of subdural hematomas and hygromas at 1.5 T. *AJR* 1989;153:589-595.
56. Potter JF, Fruin AH. Chronic subdural hematoma—The Great Imitator. *Geriatrics* 1977;32:61-66.
57. Luxon LM, Harrison MJ. Chronic subdural hematoma. *Q J Med* 1979;48:43-53.
58. Lobato RD, Rivas JJ, Gomez PA, et al. Head-injured patients who talk and deteriorate into coma. *J Neurosurg* 1991;75:256-261.
59. Marshall LF, Gautile T, Klauber MR, et a.: The outcome of severe closed head injury. *J Neurosurg* 1991;75:S28-S36.
60. Nomura S, Oritz T, Tsurutani T, et al. Subacute subdural hematoma: Report of 3 cases. *Nippon Geka Hokan* 1996;65:30-35.
61. Maggio WW. Chronic Subdural Hematoma in Adults. In: Apuzzo MLJ, ed. *Brain Surgery*, Vol 2. New York: Churchill Livingstone, 1993;1299-1314.
62. Cameron MM. Chronic subdural hematoma: A review of 114 cases. *J Neurol Neurosurg Psychiatry* 1978;41:834-839.
63. Mishriki YY. Subdural hematoma mimicking a transient ischemic attack due to antihypertensive medication. *South Med J* 1999;92:905-906.
64. Cher LM, White OB. Subdural hematoma presenting with transient neurological deficits. *Med J Aust* 1992;156:654-655.
65. Moster ML, Johnston DE, Retnmuth OM. Chronic subdural hematoma with transient neurological deficits: A review of 15 cases. *Ann Neurol* 1983;14:539-542.
66. Russell NA, Goumnerova L, Atack EA, et al. Chronic subdural hematoma mimicking transient ischemic attack. *J Trauma* 1985;25:1113-1114.
67. Ikeda K, Ito H, Yamashita J. Relation of regional cerebral blood flow to hemiparesis in chronic subdural hematoma. *Surg Neurol* 1990;33:87-95.
68. Black DW. Subdural hematoma: A retrospective study of the great neurologic imitator. *Postgrad Med* 1985;78:107-115.
69. Elie M, Primeau F, Cole MG. Chronic subdural hematoma in the elderly: A case report. *J Geriatr Psychiatry Neurol* 1996; 9:100-101.
70. Wiest RG, Burgunder JM, Krauss JK. Chronic subdural haematomas and Parkinsonian syndromes. *Acta Neurochir* (Wien) 1999;141:753-758.
71. Ellis GL. Subdural hematoma in the elderly. *Emerg Med Clin North Am* 1990;8:281-294.
72. Rubin G, Rappaport ZH. Epilepsy in chronic subdural hematoma. *Acta Neurochir* (Wien) 1993;123:39-42.
73. Borzone M, Rivano C, Altomonte M, et al. Acute traumatic posterior fossa subdural hematomas. *Acta Neurochir* (Wien) 1995;135:32-37.
74. Tsai FY, Teal JS, Itabashi HH, et al. Computed tomography of posterior fossa trauma. *J Comput Assist Tomog* 1980;4:291-305.
75. Ferro JM, Pinto AN, Falcao I, et al. Diagnosis of stroke by the noneurologist. A validation study. *Stroke* 1998;29:1106-1109.
76. Cowan RJ, Maynard CD, Lassiter KR. Technetium-99m pertechnetate brain scans in the detection of subdural hematomas: A study of the age of the lesion as related to the development of a positive scan. *J Neurosurg* 1970;32:30-34.
77. Lusins J, Jaffe R, Bender MB. Unoperated subdural hematomas: Long-term follow-up study by brain scan and electroencephalography. *J Neurosurg* 1976;44:601-607.
78. Raskind R, Glover MB, Weiss SR. Chronic subdural hematoma in the elderly: A challenge in diagnosis and treatment. *J Am Geriatr Soc* 1972;20:330-334.
79. Haar Fl, Lott TM, Nicholas P Jr. The usefulness of CT scanning for subdural hematomas. *Neurosurgery* 1977;1:272-275.
80. Scotti G, Terbrugge K, Melancon D, et al. Evaluation of the age of subdural hematomas by computerized tomography. *J Neurosurg* 1977;47:311-315.
81. Klufas RA, Hsu L, Patel MR, et al. Unusual manifestations of head trauma. *AJR* 1996;166:675-681.
82. Reed D, Robertson WD, Graeb DA, et al. Acute subdural hematomas: Atypical CT findings. *AJNR* 1986;7:417-421.
83. Smith WP, Batnitzky S, Rengachary SS. Acute isodense subdural hematomas: A problem in anemic patients. *AJR* 1981;136:543-546.
84. Weisberg LA. The significance of nonvisualization of the cortical sulcal spaces on computed tomography. *Comput Radiol* 1982;6:337-341.
85. Weisberg LA. Analysis of the clinical and computed tomographic findings in isodense subdural hematoma. *Comput Radiol* 1986;10:245-252.
86. Kim KS, Hemmati M, Weinberg PE. Computed tomography in isodense subdural hematoma. *Radiology* 1978;128:71-74.
87. Hayman LA, Evans RA, Hinck VC. Rapid-high-dose contrast computed tomography of isodense subdural hematoma and cerebral swelling. *Radiology* 1979;131:381-383.
88. Marcu H, Becker H. Computed-tomography of bilateral isodense chronic subdural hematomas. *Neuroradiology* 1977;14:81-83.
89. Karasawa H, Tomita S, Suzuki S. Chronic subdural hematomas: Time-density curve and iodine concentration in enhanced CT. *Neruoradiology* 1987;29:36-39.
90. Spallone A, Giuffre R, Gagliardi FM, et al. Chronic subdural hematoma in extremely aged patients. *Eur Neurol* 1989;29:

18-22.

91. Deltour P, Lemmerling M, Bauters W, et al. Posttraumatic subdural hygroma: CT findings and differential diagnosis. *JBR-BTR* 1999;82:155-156.
92. Hosoda K, Tamaki N, Masumura M, et al. Magnetic resonance images of chronic subdural hematomas. *J Neurosurg* 1987;67: 677-683.
93. Sipponen JT, Sepponen RE, Sivula A. Chronic subdural hematoma: Demonstration by magnetic resonance. *Radiology* 1984;150:79-85.
94. Kaminogo M, Moroki J, Ochi A, et al. Characteristics of symptomatic chronic subdural haematomas on high-field MRI. *Neurorad* 1999;41:109-116.
95. Kelly AB, Zimmerman RD, Snow RB, et al. Head trauma: Comparison of MR and CT experience in 100 patients. *AJNR* 1988;9:699-708.
96. Romano VA, Toffol GJ. Confirmation of traumatic interhemispheric subdural hematoma by magnetic resonance imaging. *J Emerg Med* 1994;12:369-373.
97. Tomida M, Muraki M, Uemura K, et al. Post contrast magnetic resonance imaging to predict progression of traumatic epidural and subdural hematomas in the acute stage. *Neurosurgery* 1998;43:66-71.
98. Servadei F, Nasi MT, Cremonini AM, et al. Importance of a reliable admission Glasgow Coma Scale score for determining the need for evacuation of posttraumatic subdural hematomas: A prospective study of 65 patients. *J Trauma* 1998;44: 868-873.
99. Muizelaar JP, Marmarou A, Ward JD, et al. Adverse effects of prolonged hyperventilation in patients with severe head injury: A randomized clinical trial. *J Neurosurg* 1991;75:731-739.
100. Obrist WD, Langfitt TW, Jaggi JL, et al. Cerebral blood flow and metabolism in comatose patients with acute head injury. *J Neurosurg* 1984;61:241-253.
101. Gruen P, Liu C. Current trends in the management of head injury. *Emerg Med Clin North Am* 1998;16:63-83.
102. Cruz J, Miner ME, Allen SJ, et al. Continuous monitoring of cerebral oxygenation in acute brain injury: Injection of mannitol during hyperventilation. *J Neurosurg* 1990;73: 725-730.
103. Mendelow AD, Teasdale GM, Russell T, et al. Effect of mannitol on cerebral blood flow and cerebral perfusion pressure in human head injury. *J Neurosurg* 1985;63:43-48.
104. Scalea TM, Simon HM, Duncan AO, et al. Geriatric blunt multiple trauma: Improved survival with invasive monitoring. *J Trauma* 1990;30:129-136.
105. Dent DL, Croce MA, Menke PG, et al. Prognostic factors after acute subdural hematoma. *J Trauma* 1995;39:36-42.
106. Croce MA, Dent DL, Menke PG, et al. Acute subdural hematoma: Non-surgical management of selected patients. *J Trauma* 1994;36:820.
107. Stone JL, Lowe RJ, Jonasson O, et al. Acute subdural hematoma: Direct admission to a trauma center yields improved results. *J Trauma* 1986;26:445-450.
108. Singounas EG, Sfakianos G, Sourtzis I, et al. "Benign" acute subdural haematomas. *Acta Neurochir* (Wien) 1990;106: 140-144.
109. Wilberger JE, Harris M, Diamond DL. Acute subdural hematoma: Morbidity and mortality related to timing of operative intervention. *J Trauma* 1990;30:733-736.
110. St. John JN, French BN. Traumatic hematomas of the posterior fossa. A clinicopathological spectrum. *Surg Neurol* 1986;25:457-466.
111. Hecimovic I, Blagus G, Kristek B, et al. Successful treatment of traumatic acute posterior fossa subdural hematoma: Report of two cases. *Surg Neurol* 1999;51:247-251.
112. Lowe JG, Northrup BE. Traumatic Intracranial Hemorrhage. In: Evans RW, ed. *Neurology and Trauma.* Philadelphia: WB Saunders; 1996;140-150.
113. McCormick WF. Pathology of Closed Head Injury. In: Wilkins WH, Rengachay SS, ed. *Neurosurgery*. Vol 2. New York: McGraw-Hill; 1965:1544-70.
114. Drapkin AJ. Chronic subdural hematoma: Pathophysiological basis for treatment. *Br J Neursurg* 1991;5:467-473.
115. Zingale A, Albanese V, Romano A, et al. Traumatic chronic subdural hematoma over 80 years. A preliminary prospective study. *J Neurosurg Sci* 1997;41:169-173.
116. Smely C, Madlinger A, Scheremet R. Chronic subdural hematoma - A comparison of two different treatment modalities. *Acta Neurochir* (Wien) 1997;139:818-825.
117. Tyson G, Strachan WE, Newman P, et al. The role of craniectomy in the treatment of chronic subdural hematomas. *J Nuerosurg* 1980;52:776-781.
118. Matsumoto K, Akagi K, Abekura M, et al. Recurrence factors for chronic subdural hematomas after burrhole craniostomy and closed system drainage. *Neurol Res* 1999 Apr;21:277-280.
119. Nakamura H, Ogawa T, Hashimoto T, et al. Reevaluation on resolving subdural hematoma. *Neurol* 1981;21:491-500.
120. Naganuma H, Fukamachi A, Kawakami M, et al. Spontaneous resolution of chronic subdural hematomas. *Neurosurgery* 1986;19:794-798.
121. Koc RK, Akdemir H, Oktem IS, et al. Acute subdural hematoma: Outcome and outcome prediction. *Neurosurg Rev* 1997;20:239-244.
122. Massaro F, Lanotte M, Faccani G, et al. One hundred and twenty-seven cases of acute subdural hematoma operated on. Correlation between CT scan findings and outcome. Acta Neurochir *(Wien)* 1996;138:185-191.
123. Zumkeller M, Behrmann R, Heissler HE, et al. Computed tomographic criteria and survival rate for patients with acute subdural hematoma. *Neurosurgery* 1996;39:708-712.
124. Haselberger K, Pucher R, Auer LM. Prognosis after acute subdural or epidural hemorrhage. *Acta Neurochir* (Wien) 1988;90:111-116.
125. Howard III MA, Gross AS, Dacey RJ, et al. Acute subdural hematomas: An age-dependent clinical entity. *J Neurosurg* 1989;71:858-863.
126. Fearnside MR, Cook RJ, McDougal P, et al. The Westmead Head Injury Project outcome in severe head injury. A comparative analysis of pre-hospital, clinical and CT variables. *Br J Neurosurg* 1993;7:267-279.
127. Pennings JL, Bachulis BL, Simons CT, et al. Survival after severe brain injury in the aged. *Arch Surg* 1993;128:787-794.
128. Sakas DE, Bullock MR, Teasdale GM. One-year outcome following craniotomy for traumatic hematoma in patients with fixed dilated pupils. *J Neurosurg* 1995;82:961-965.

129. Quigley MR, Vidovich D, Cantella D, et al. Defining the limits of survivorship after very severe head injury. *J Trauma* 1997; 42:7-10.
130. Seelig JM, Becker DP, Miller JD, et al. Traumatic acute subdural hematoma. Major mortality reduction in comatose patients treated within four hours. *N Engl J Med* 1981;304: 1511-1518.
131. Caggetti B, Cossu M, Pau A, et al. The outcome from acute subdural and epidural intracranial hematomas in very elderly patients. *Br J Neurosurg* 1992;6:227-232.
132. Jamjoom A. Justification for evacuating acute subdural hematomas in patients above the age of 75 years. *Injury* 1992;23:518-520.
133. Bollmer D, et al. Age and outcome following traumatic coma: Why do older patients fare worse, in report on Traumatic Coma Data Bank. *J Neurosurg* 1991;75(suppl):537-549.
134. Ernestus RI, Beldzinski P, Lanfermann H, et al. Chronic subdural hematoma: Surgical treatment and outcome in 104 patients. *Surg Neurol* 1997 Sep;48:220-225.
135. VanAalst JA, Morris JA, Kendle H, et al. Severely injured geriatric patients return to independent living: A study of factors influencing function and independence. *J Trauma* 1991;31:1096-1102.
136. Wilson JA, Pentland B, Currie CT, et al. The functional effects of head injury in the elderly. *Brain Inj* 1987;1:183-188.
137. Goldstein FC, Levin HS, Goldman WP, et al. Cognitive and behavioral sequelae of closed head injury in older adults according to their significant others. *J Neuropsy Clin Neurosci* 1999;11:38-44.
138. Luukinen H, Viramo P, Koski K, et al. Head injuries and cognitive decline among older adults. *Neurol* 1999;52: 557-562.
139. Mazzucchi A, Cattelani R, Massale G, et al. Head injured subjects aged over 50 years: Correlation between variables of trauma and neuropsychological follow-up. *J Neurology* 1992; 239:256-260.
140. Aharon-Peretz J, Kliot D, Amyel-Zvi E, et al. Neurobehavioral consequences of closed head injury in the elderly. *Brain Injury* 1997;11:871-875.
141. Spivak JM, Weiss MA, Cotler JM, et al. Cervical spine injuries in patients 65 and older. *Spine* 1994;19:2302-2306.

Heart Failure in the Elderly

William Franklin Peacock IV, MD, FACEP

Disproportionally represented in the elderly, heart failure (HF) is the single most economically expensive disease in the United States. Because of the aging of America, and the relative success in treating coronary artery disease, the future impact of HF may be epidemic in proportion. Until recently, there was little improvement in HF outcome, and the diagnosis of HF was a death sentence. Currently, five-year survival for HF is worse than that predicted for most cancers.

Today, therapeutic advances are markedly improving outcomes. To ensure effective treatment, the clinician should have a clear understanding of the divergent pathology in the two main categories of HF and their effects on the aging myocardium. Systolic HF results from pump inadequacy. This is in contradistinction to diastolic HF, where ventricular pumping performance is maintained, but a loss of compliance prevents adequate cardiac filling. The normal aging process increases the overall stiffness of the cardiovascular system, but systolic function is preserved. These distinctions are critical when selecting treatment options.

This chapter reviews the physiologies of the aging myocardium and the pathologic consequences of the two main types of HF. Clinical diagnostic methods, interventions, and confounders appropriate to care of the elderly HF patient are detailed, and there is a focus on the medical treatment of HF in the aged.

Introduction/Epidemiology

HF is one of the greatest challenges facing the United States health care system. It affects nearly 5 million Americans, and many more with asymptomatic dysfunction who are likely to become symptomatic within the next five years.[1,2] *(Please see Table 1.)* It is the only cardiovascular disease increasing in both incidence and prevalence, and its death rate has increased sixfold over the last 40 years.[2,3]

HF disproportionally effects the elderly. Less than 1% of those younger than age 50 are affected, but prevalence doubles each decade, and by age 80 nearly 10% are stricken.[4] Of those older than 65 years, HF is the leading cause of hospitalization and accounts for about 700,000 annual admissions.[3,5] Furthermore, since HF patients are usually older, management is complicated by high rates of coexisting disease. The expectation that the number of Americans older than age 65 will double in the next 30 years is the impetus to develop more effective therapies.[4]

HF is the most expensive diagnosis in the Medicare system. As reported at the Heart Failure Society of America 1999 Annual Meeting, current costs are estimated at \$23.1 and \$14.7 billion for inpatient and outpatient care, respectively. The cost of HF hospitalizations doubles that of all forms of cancer.[6]

Prognosis. The prognosis of HF is poor. Once symptomatic, two-year mortality is about 35%. Over the next six years, it increases to 80% for men and 65% for women. Symptoms do predict outcome. The yearly risk of death with mild to moderate symptoms is 5-10%, vs. 30-40% with severe symptoms. After pulmonary edema, only 50% survive one year, and following cardiogenic shock, 50-85% die within one week. The New York Heart Association (NYHA) HF class is the most commonly used

Table 1. Annual Impact of Heart Failure[1,2]

NUMBER OF PATIENTS	RESULT
43,000	HF is principal cause of death[4]
250,000	Deaths in which HF contributes[2,38]
500,000	New cases
3,500,000	Co-contributor to inpatient hospitalization
11,000,000	Outpatient visits
20,000,000	Asymptomatic cardiac dysfunction

Table 2. New York Heart Association Classifications for Heart Failure

- **I. No limitation:** Asymptomatic during usual daily activities
- **II. Slight limitation:** Mild symptoms during ordinary daily activities
- **III. Moderate limitation:** Symptoms noted with minimal activities
- **IV. Severe limitation:** Symptoms present even at rest

prognostic scale. *(Please see Table 2.)* Despite poor sensitivity and high inter-observer variability, the scale is useful for predicting mortality. Older patients, once rated as class IV, have a one-year mortality of greater than 50%.[7]

Pathophysiology. HF can present precipitously following acute myocardial infarction (AMI), and is due to pump failure. As cardiac output (CO) declines, BP and peripheral perfusion decrease. Vasoconstriction may preserve BP at a cost of increased systemic vascular resistance (SVR), which raises myocardial O_2 demand and may exacerbate ischemia. As the heart fails, increasing intracardiac pressures develop, pulmonary congestion occurs, and death follows if the pathologic cascade is not interrupted. Symptomatically hypotensive HF patients (i.e., cardiogenic shock) require aggressive circulatory support in an ICU environment. Their care is not covered here.

Less acute presentations, with chronic recidivism, are the more common presentation of HF in the ED environment. When myocardial stress or injury result in a reduction of CO, compensatory mechanisms may partially preserve circulatory function. The responses include neurohormonal activation, which results in increasing levels of norepinephrine (NE), vasopressin, and stimulation of the renin-angiotensin system. The combined effects are sodium and water retention and increased vascular tone. The secondary consequences are elevation of intracardiac pressures. At this stage, patients may be asymptomatic, but the mechanisms initiating cardiac remodeling are established. Interruption and attenuation of cardiac neuroendocrine responses to incipient HF form the theoretical basis for beta-blockade and ACE inhibitor therapies.

HF and the Aging Heart

The consequences of aging include extensive functional and structural myocardial changes. Aging is associated with increases in ventricular wall thickness and myocardial interstitial collagen.[7] This significantly impacts diastolic function, resulting in impaired ventricular relaxation and increased LV wall stiffness.[7] However, in the absence of concurrent cardiovascular disease, resting systolic function is well preserved and measures of cardiac function are unaffected by age in healthy patients.[7,8] The summary effect of age on the cardiovascular system is a loss in the ability to respond to stress.[8]

Aging results in events that contribute to an increased risk of developing HF. These effects include increased systemic vascular impedance, impaired ventricular relaxation, decreased ventricular compliance, and impaired myocardial metabolism.[4,7,8] With aging, a decrease in vascular elasticity and increased impedance to ventricular ejection accentuate systolic hypertension.[9]

Diminished cardiac relaxation and increased ventricular stiffness predispose to diastolic HF and have consequences in relation to atrial dynamics. Greater ventricular stiffness impairs early diastolic ventricular filling.[7] Consequently, atrial contraction becomes more important; as much as 30-40% of end diastolic LV volume is because of atrial contraction.[8] Thus, the older patient is more dependent upon atrial kick and will be more symptomatic if atrial fibrillation occurs.[8]

Aging also diminishes β1 and β2 receptor responsiveness. This decreases maximal heart rate and contractility and impairs peripheral vasodilation. Cellular energy handling is affected by aging; specifically, mitochondrial ATP production is decreased in the elderly.[8,9]

All these changes impair the ability of the aging heart to respond to cardiovascular stress (e.g., exercise, infection, etc). Older patients are more sensitive to hypertension, atrial fibrillation, and cardiac ischemia; conditions that are all more common in the elderly.

Etiology. HF may arise from numerous sources. *(Please see Table 3.)* Decompensation of previously established HF is the final common pathway of cardiac stress from numerous sources. *(Please see Table 4.)* Hypertension and coronary artery disease account for more than 70% of HF cases in both the young and elderly. However, in the elderly, the etiology more frequently is multifactorial.[8] In the older adult, ischemic heart disease, with a history of MI, is the most common cause of dilated cardiomyopathy.[8] Valvular heart disease, specifically calcific aortic stenosis and mitral regurgitation, is increasingly common in the elderly.[4] Lastly, hypertensive hypertrophic cardiomyopathy and cardiac amyloidosis more frequently occur in older patients, while alcoholic and dilated idiopathic cardiomyopathies tend to affect younger patients.[4,10]

Congestive HF

HF commonly presents with fluid overload. However, low CO HF syndromes, that are accompanied by dehydration and intravascular depletion, occur without congestion. Therefore, congestive HF refers only to the fluid overloaded state; it does not reflect myocardial contractility. Fluid status is independent of CO. Both diastolic and systolic HF patients may suffer from congestion.

Systolic vs. Diastolic HF. Ventricular wall tension is a product of afterload (systolic BP) and ventricular radius. Elevated wall tension stimulates cardiac remodeling. Myofibers either hypertrophy or die (apoptosis) and form scar tissue. Why apoptosis occurs is unclear. It is this predominate response (hypertrophy vs apoptosis) that determines HF type. While elements of both systolic and diastolic HF can occur together, this distinction is helpful when designing treatment plans.

Systolic HF. A normal ejection fraction (EF) is 60%; an EF of less than 40% is considered systolic dysfunction. Impaired cardiac contractility is the hallmark of systolic HF. In the normal heart, increasing preload results in improved cardiac contractility (i.e., the Frank Starling mechanism). This is lost in systolic HF. With cardio-

Table 3. Major Etiologies of Heart Failure

- Coronary artery disease
- MI complications
  Acute mitral regurgitation, papillary muscle rupture, cardiac free wall rupture
- Sustained arrhythmia
- Uncontrolled hypertension
- Valvular rupture or disease
- Myocarditis
- Acute pulmonary embolus
- Pericardial disease/tamponade
  Effusion, constrictive pericarditis
- Hyperkinetic states
  Anemia, thyrotoxicosis, A-V Fistula (e.g., dialysis)
- Infiltrative disorders
  Amyloidosis, sarcoidosis, hemochromatosis
- Infectious
  Endocarditis
- Toxin
  Alcoholic cardiomyopathy

Table 4. Examples of Common Causes of Heart Failure Decompensation

- **Exacerbation of comorbidities:**
  Acute MI, emphysema, uncontrolled hypertension, atrial fibrillation, hyperthyroidism, anemia, diabetes
- **Superimposed infection:**
  Pneumonia, urinary tract infection
- **Social issues:**
  Medication or dietary non-compliance, excessive alcohol
- **Iatrogenic causes:**
  Negative inotropic medications (e.g., verapamil, nifedipine, etc.)
  Non-steroidal anti-inflammatory medication

vascular stress (e.g., walking, volume expansion) the myocardium cannot improve contractility. Increasing venous return results in elevated intra-cardiac pressures that may lead to pulmonary congestion and edema. The process of systolic HF involves impaired contractility, neurohormonal activation, increased intracardiac volume and pressure, and enhanced afterload sensitivity. The most common etiologies of systolic HF are, in descending frequency, coronary artery disease (in two-thirds), hypertension, idiopathic cardiomyopathy, valvular heart disease, other specific cardiomyopathies, and myocarditis.[2,11]

Diastolic HF. Age-related cardiac changes predispose the older patient to diastolic HF.[12] In those younger than age 60, only 6% of HF patients have diastolic dysfunction, as compared to rates of 21% in 61- to 70-year olds, and 41% in those older than 70.[13] In diastolic HF, LV systolic function is preserved and the EF is normal or increases. Pathologically, impaired ventricular relaxation and ventricular stiffness result in an abnormal diastolic pressure/volume relationship. Common etiologies of diastolic HF are listed in Table 5.

Diastolic HF patients are volume sensitive. Significant preload reduction or afterload increases may cause hypotension. As in systolic HF, circulatory congestion is a common ED presentation. Between 30% and 50% of HF patients have circulatory congestion without LV dysfunction.[14] The majority of the elderly will also have underlying hypertension, coronary artery disease, or valvular heart disease.[12]

HF type is difficult to diagnose at the bedside; consequently, echocardiograms are often obtained.[7] In one small study, a diastolic BP of 105 mmHg or greater and absence of jugular venous distention (JVD) was specific (100%) but insensitive (30%) in indicating preserved LV contractility.[14]

Ultimately, diastolic HF therapy is directed at the underlying etiology. *(Please see Table 5.)* Although diastolic dysfunction is a common cause of HF in the aged, treatment is mainly empiric since there are very few large, controlled trials to guide therapy.

Right vs. Left Heart Failure. Left and right HF are sometimes differentiated. Left HF presents with dyspnea, fatigue, weakness, cough, and orthopnea in the absence of peripheral edema, JVD, or hepatojugular reflux (HJR). Right HF results in peripheral edema, JVD, HJR, and ascites, without marked pulmonary symptoms. Since this a closed system, abnormally elevated cardiac pressures/volumes are quickly reflected into the contralateral system. This distinction better describes valvular dysfunction.

Arrhythmia and Sudden Death. Ventricular arrhythmias are common, and HF carries the greatest risk for sudden death. Non-sustained ventricular tachycardia (NSVT) occurs in 30-40% of patients with dilated cardiomyopathy, and premature ventricular contractions (PVCs) are found in 95% of patients with advanced HF. The sudden death risk is proportional to the EF decrease and HF severity.[15] Although arrhythmia is common, neither Holter nor electrophysiologic studies predict sudden death.[16] Ventricular arrhythmias by Holter monitoring predict all-cause mortality, but are non-specific for sudden death, so therapy is guided by symptoms. Syncope, resuscitation after cardiac arrest, sustained VT, symptomatic NSVT, and ventricular fibrillation (VF), prompt aggressive management.

Atrial fibrillation (AF) is common in the elderly, especially in those with HF.[17] Furthermore, the elderly are more symptomatic when this arrhythmia occurs. If AF is acute or is associated with HF exacerbation, attempts at cardioversion are warranted. Chronic antiarrhythmic therapy for AF is less useful.

Half of HF deaths are caused by pump failure. Sudden death occurs in 10-40%, and is due to VF or VT in half.[15,16,18] The remaining sudden deaths die from unexplained hypotension or bradycardia progressing to pulseless electrical activity.[19] Therapies to decrease sudden death have had little success. Prophylactic antiarrhythmics (e.g., encainide, flecainide) increase mortality by pro-arrhythmic and negative inotropic effects.[20] Amiodarone lacks pro-arrhythmic effects but has many non-cardiac side effects. In trials of amiodarone vs. placebo, overall cardiac mortality was unchanged, but there was a 35% reduction in arrhythmic deaths.[21] Implantable defibrillators may offer hope, but there is insufficient research to currently recommend them.

Clinical Course

HF frequently follows a pattern of worsening symptoms at home, prompting an ED visit, ED stabilization and diagnosis, then hospitalization. While the average hospitalization for HF patients is 3-7 days, it can be considerably longer in patients older than age 75.[10] This

Table 5. Diastolic Heart Failure Etiologies[87]

- Restrictive cardiomyopathy
  - Cardiac amyloidosis
- Constrictive pericarditis
- Ischemic heart disease
  - Post-infarction scarring/remodeling
- Hypertrophic heart disease
  - Hypertrophic cardiomyopathy
  - Chronic hypertension
  - Aortic stenosis
  - Mitral or tricuspid stenosis

cycle repeats, with increasing frequency and worsening disability, until death in five years. Frequent hospitalizations affect the patients' quality of life and consume significant health care resources.

Diagnosis/ED Evaluation. The diagnosis of HF may be difficult since no single finding is pathognomonic. In the elderly, HF is both under- and over-diagnosed because routinely used diagnostic elements are neither sensitive nor specific.[4,7,22] This is because of a high rate of confounding comorbidities and the fact that the elderly frequently have more advanced disease at diagnosis.[17] The greater severity of disease in the older patient at presentation is hypothesized to be caused by a more sedentary lifestyle that does help identify symptoms until physical limitations are severe.[17]

In primary care, the initial diagnosis of HF may be falsely positive in more than half of patients. Symptoms that mimic HF are often caused by occult cardiac ischemia, obesity, and chronic obstructive pulmonary disease (COPD) exacerbations.[23] Gender also may lead to misdiagnosis;[23,24] in one study HF was correctly determined in only 18% of women vs. 36% of men.[24] Diagnostic criteria for HF may aid the clinician. The Framingham criteria require one major and two minor criteria to be met for diagnosis.[25,26] *(Please see Table 6.)* Using the Boston criteria, increasing points confer a higher probability of HF.[27] *(Please see Table 7.)* In the Boston scale, a score of 4 or greater detects a pulmonary artery occlusion pressure (PAOP) of 12 mmHg or higher with a sensitivity of 90% and a specificity of 85%. While validated, these criteria have limited usefulness when patients are asymptomatic.

History. The common complaints of HF are shortness of breath, dyspnea on exertion, orthopnea, peripheral edema, weight gain, paroxysmal nocturnal dyspnea, cough, and fatigue. In the elderly, the classic symptoms of HF (i.e., exertional dyspnea, fatigue, orthopnea) are neither sensitive nor specific.[4,7] Exertional symptoms may not be reported in older sedentary patients. Thus, non-specific complaints of generalized weakness, anorexia, nausea, fatigue, mental disturbances, altered breathing, and dry cough may be the presenting complaints for HF in the elderly.[7,22]

When taking the history, search for signs of AMI. AMI should always be considered diagnostically as a cause of HF. The clinician should keep in mind that the elderly have a higher frequency of silent or occult AMI presentation. He or she should ascertain the patients' CAD risk factors and determine if there are any other events that may worsen or precipitate HF. These include hypertension, anemia, hyperthyroidism, worsening comorbidity, over-the-counter medication use, electrolyte abnormalities, or occult infection. Dietary and medication non-compliance can decompensate HF, so habits are queried. Arrhythmia worsens underlying HF and is suggested by palpitations. Lastly, check for alcohol or drug use, and their withdrawal, since these adversely affect cardiac function.

Table 6. Framingham Criteria for the Diagnosis of Heart Failure

MAJOR CRITERIA

Paroxysmal nocturnal dyspnea
Neck vein distention
Rales
Cardiomegaly
Acute pulmonary edema
S_3 gallop
Increased venous pressure (> 16 cm H_2O)
Positive HJR

MINOR CRITERIA

Extremity edema
Night cough
Dyspnea on exertion
Hepatomegaly
Pleural effusion
Vital capacity reduced by one-third of normal
Tachycardia (≥ 120)

Non-Compliance. Non-compliance with HF treatment is a pernicious problem for many reasons: Diuretics may cause nocturia, dietary restrictions are onerous, fluid restriction is uncomfortable, medication costs can be exorbitant, and complicated multi-drug regimens can be difficult for the elderly. Therapeutic simplification and education are critical for success; their importance cannot be overemphasized.

Physical Examination. Airway is paramount. Once stability is ensured, further evaluation should proceed. Vital signs should be checked. Note that resting tachycardia is uncommon in the elderly.[7] Lung sounds, peripheral edema, JVD, HJR, and extra heart sounds help detect fluid overload. Skin mottling, from poor peripheral perfusion, is associated with markedly increased hospital mortality (odds ratio, 17.5).[28] The cardiac point of maximal impulse (PMI) can help estimate HF chronicity; in longstanding HF, cardiac remodeling may shift the PMI laterally.

In the elderly, physical exam limitations are significant. Edema, rales, and the presence of an S_3 or S_4 are neither sensitive nor specific.[4,7] Finding an S_4 is of little value; it may simply reflect age-related diastolic dysfunction.[4] Ankle edema is common in older patients and probably should not be considered cardiac in origin unless other signs of HF are present.[10] Finally, in chronic HF, the physical signs of congestion have a poor predictive value for identifying high PAOP.[29]

ECG. The ECG is crucial. It is fastest diagnostic test, and screens for arrhythmia, electrolyte imbalance (e.g., hyperkalemia), drug toxicity (e.g., digoxin), and suggests the chronicity and etiology of HF (e.g., LVH). If new ischemic changes are noted, immediate ICU admission is warranted. A diagnosis of systolic HF is unlikely in the presence of a normal 12 lead ECG, which has good sensitivity but poor specificity for detecting systolic dysfunction.[30] ECG also has prognostic value; five-year mortality in dilated cardiomyopathy is worse when abnormal Q waves, QRS duration longer than 0.12 s, or left bundle branch block are present.[14]

Laboratory Tests. Since occult AMI may cause or decompensate HF, cardiac enzymes should be obtained. In the ED setting,

Table 7. Boston Criteria for Diagnosing Congestive Heart Failure

HISTORY	SCORE
Dyspnea at rest, or orthopnea	4
Nocturnal dyspnea	3
Dyspnea while walking	2
Dyspnea on stair climbing	1
CHEST X-RAY	
Alveolar pulmonary edema	4
Interstitial pulmonary edema	3
Bilateral pleural effusions	3
Cardiothoracic ratio > 0.5	3
Kerley A lines	2
PHYSICAL EXAMINATION	
HR 91-110 bpm	1
HR > 110 bpm, or JVD > 6 cm H_2O	2
JVD and edema or hepatomegaly	3
Basilar rales	1
Rales > basilar	2
Wheezing or S_3 gallop	3

cardiac enzymes diagnose but don't exclude AMI.[31] If the enzymes are elevated, ICU admission is needed. Diuresis may cause electrolyte changes, and electrolyte levels are indicated. Serum BUN and creatinine also should be measured, as renal function is commonly affected by HF therapy. A complete blood count (CBC) evaluates for anemia, and if hepatomegaly is present, liver enzymes may differentiate passive congestion from other etiologies.

In the elderly, thyroid function testing is considered, especially if AF is present.[1] Toxicology testing (e.g., digoxin) is guided by presentation, with alcohol and drug screening performed when abuse is suspected. Hypomagnesemia is considered with arrhythmia or severe hypokalemia. Arterial blood gas measurements are performed selectively; they should be obtained in those at risk of CO_2 retention or those who appear severely ill.

Radiology. All elderly patients with suspected HF need a chest radiograph (CXR). A negative CXR does not exclude abnormal LV function. CXRs can exclude some confounding pathologies (e.g., pneumonia), but physicians should remember that co-morbidities are more likely in the aged. CXR findings of HF are cardiomegaly, Kerley lines, increased pulmonary vascularity, and pleural effusion. Symptoms may precede chest x-ray changes by hours, so treatment should not be withheld while waiting for a CXR or if CXR results are normal.

CXRs also have significant limitations. Cardiomegaly is helpful, and a cardiothoracic (CT) ratio higher than 60% predicts increased five-year mortality.[15] But because of intrathoracic cardiac rotation, CXRs are insensitive for its detection.[32] In one study of HF with proven cardiomegaly, 22% of patients had CT ratios of less than 50%.[32] Likewise, pleural effusion can be missed by CXR. The sensitivity, specificity, and accuracy of the supine CXR for pleural effusion is only 67%, 70%, and 67%, respectively.[33]

Use of the portable CXR (pCXR) in the ED is common. HF findings on pCXR are, in descending frequency, dilated upper lobe vessels (cephalization), cardiomegaly, interstitial edema, enlarged pulmonary artery, pleural effusion, alveolar edema, prominent superior vena cava, and Kerley lines.[34] But, pCXR sensitivity for HF is poor. Only dilated upper lobe vessels are detected in more than 60% of HF patients. Increasing HF severity is associated with more positive pCXR findings. With the exception of Kerley lines (11%) and prominent vena cava (44%), all other pCXR findings occur in at least two-thirds of severe HF cases.[34]

In chronic HF, CXRs are unreliable. Pulmonary congestion is undetectable by CXR in 39% of patients with mild to moderate PAOP elevation (16-29 mmHg), and in 53% with severe elevation (> 30 mmHg). PAOP is important; survival and quality of life improve when it is normalized.[29]

The gold standard for thoracic fluid assessment is unclear, although thoracic computed tomography (CT) scan has been proposed. If chest CT scan, PAOP, and CXR are done simultaneously, pulmonary fluid will be seen on the CT scan prior to detection on CXR and before PAOP elevates.[35-37] However, in elderly symptomatic ED patients, CT scan is difficult.

Echocardiography. EF is the most important measurement in HF.[2] This is especially true in the elderly, for whom a high frequency of diastolic HF exists. There is no correlation between symptoms and EF, but measuring EF is diagnostic and determines HF type.[30] Once systolic HF is established, repeat measures are not needed. If systolic HF is not established, or it has been a long time since the last EF measurement, reassessment by echocardiogram can be helpful. Other methods of EF determination are available (e.g., angiogram, cardiac MRI), but are not available or are less useful in the ED setting.

Differential Diagnosis. Many problems mimic acute HF. Breathlessness is common, so conditions causing dyspnea should be included in the differential diagnosis. AMI is also an early consideration. It must always be excluded as the primary cause of presentation, or as the etiology of a HF exacerbation.

An exacerbation of COPD is easily confused with acute HF. Both may present with acute dyspnea and abnormal lung sounds. Worsening of either can precipitate an exacerbation of the other. The history may help differentiate the two diagnoses (e.g., diuretic noncompliance), as well as a careful physical (evaluating for peripheral edema, HJR, S_3, etc). Severe hypertension and peripheral vasoconstriction are suggestive of acute HF, even with marked wheezing. The chest x-ray is helpful, but its limitations have been noted.

Pneumonia, or other pulmonary pathologies, may mimic or exacerbate HF. Fever, productive cough, pleuritic chest pain, focal abnormalities on CXR, and leukocytosis suggests this diagnosis. Acute breathlessness also results from pulmonary embolism (PE). Acute onset, pleuritic pain, and a normal ECG, suggest PE. ABGs may demonstrate increases in the alveolar-arterial (A-a) oxygen gradient, because of ventilation perfusion mismatch; however, this is also seen in HF. The CXR can be misleading because chronic HF findings may be unrelated to the presentation. Ventilation perfusion scan or pulmonary angiography may be considered.

Finally, peripheral edema is seen in HF, but is non-specific as it is found in hypoproteinemia, hepatic or renal failure, and vascular stasis.

Supportive Therapy

Oxygen. Supplemental O_2 should be provided, with therapy guided by pulse oximetry. Supplemental O_2 assists in dyspnea relief and may decrease hypoxic anxiety. Since hypoxia is a greater risk than hypercarbia, O_2 is not withheld because of CO_2 retention concerns.

Cardiac Monitoring. Cardiac monitoring in the ED is needed. It can diagnose arrhythmia contributing to HF and aid in the detection of electrolyte abnormalities from diuresis or ACEI use.

IV Access. HF may cause ventricular arrhythmia, and prompt therapy may be required. Any delays while attempting peripheral IV placement may have adverse consequences. IV access should be obtained early in ED management.

Medications

Diuretics. While diuretics prompt relief of fluid overload, compared to young patients, the elderly are less responsive.[8] Diuretics are used in all patients with congestion, irrespective of HF type, but are not recommended as monotherapy since they do not change mortality rates.[2,38] Loop diuretics promote free water and sodium loss, maintaining efficacy until renal function is severely impaired. This is in contrast to distal tubule diuretics (thiazides, potassium sparing agents, etc.) that are not as effective in patients with renal insufficiency.[2]

Diuretics alter efficacy and toxicity of other HF medications, especially in the older patient.[4] Dosing is best guided by daily body weight measurement. Complications include electrolyte depletion (i.e., Na^+, K^+, Mg^{++}), to which the elderly are more susceptible, as well as hypotension, azotemia, and neurohormonal activation.[4,8] Excessive diuresis is avoided in the elderly because of the built-in volume sensitive diastolic dysfunction of aging. Diuretic resistance may be overcome by IV use, combination diuretic therapy, or a brief course of an agent that augments renal blood flow (e.g., dobutamine).[1,2]

Furosemide is an effective loop diuretic. In ED patients with acute dyspnea and pulmonary congestion, twice the daily oral dose may be given (max: 180 mg) as an IV push, as long as there is adequate BP. If the patient is not on a loop diuretic, 40 mg is a good initial dose. Alternatively, 1 mg bumetadine equals 40 mg furosemide.[39] If urinary output is still poor after three hours, double and repeat the dose. Output goals are 500 cc within two hours. If the creatinine exceeds 2.5 mg/dL, halve output goals. If output remains poor, admission is needed. Diuretic response predicts outcome. In acute pulmonary edema, poor diuresis is associated with higher mortality, and net urine output of less than 1 liter is more common in those failing observation unit therapy.[28,40]

Digoxin. Digoxin improves myocardial contractility at all ages, controls ventricular rate in AF, and is recommended in systolic HF.[2,41] It has no effect on mortality, but decreases HF deaths and hospitalizations, even in those older than 80 years.[42] Aging changes in lean body mass and renal function lower the therapeutic index in the elderly. If the patient is older than 70 years, appropriate serum levels are 0.5 to 0.9 ng/mL.[41,43]

Toxicity causes arrhythmias (e.g., heart block, ectopic or re-entrant rhythms), gastrointestinal symptoms (nausea, vomiting), and neurologic complaints (visual disturbances, disorientation, confusion). Toxicity is suggested with elevated serum levels but occurs at lower levels with hypokalemia or hypomagnesemia. The elderly may be more susceptible to the neurologic and cardiac manifestation of digoxin toxicity. Up to 20% of elderly patients on chronic therapy experience toxicity at least once.[44] Serum digoxin levels are increased by quinidine, verapamil, spironolactone, flecainide, propafenone, and amiodarone. The dose of digoxin should be decreased if these drugs are added. Digoxin dosing in systolic HF is 0.125 to 0.25 mg qd. For rate control of AF, doses higher than 0.25 mg qd are not recommended.

Vasodilators: Angiotensin-Converting Enzyme Inhibitors (ACEIs). Angiotensin II (AII) may cause or worsen HF. It causes vasoconstriction, aldosterone secretion, sympathetic activation, and contributes to vascular hypertrophy.[45] ACEIs prevent the conversion of angiotensin I (AI) to AII, and prevent bradykinin degradation (an anaphylaxis mediator) by ACE.

ACEI use decreases hospitalizations and mortality, improves symptoms, and attenuates cardiac remodeling in systolic HF.[19,46,47] They function as balanced vasodilators in that they provide both arterial and venous dilation.[48] They lower arterial blood pressure, intracardiac end-diastolic pressures, cardiac work, myocardial oxygen consumption, and decrease neurohormonal activation and sodium and water retention and may reduce complex ventricular arrhythmia.[48] All of these effects are beneficial in systolic HF.

Despite that renin-angiotensin system function declines with age, the beneficial effects ACEIs are preserved in the elderly. These effects are most pronounced in older patients. In post-MI patients with EF less than 40%, captopril decreased mortality by 8% in those 55 years or younger, 13% in those 56-64, and 25% in those 65 years or older.[49] Others support these findings.[50] All elderly patients with systolic HF, even if asymptomatic, should have a trial of ACEI.[2,38,48] With congestive symptoms, ACEIs should be combined with diuretics. In the elderly, ACEIs are at least as effective as in the young, but rates of ACEI prescribing are lower.[4,51] Age is not a contraindication for ACEI use.[51]

ACEIs can cause hypotension or worsening renal insufficiency, especially in the setting of volume depletion. With chronic ACEI use, these complications may be due to over-diuresis or HF progression. If congestion is present, suspect HF progression; in its absence, decrease the diuretic dose. Renal deterioration may also occur following NSAID usage.

ACEIs also may cause hyperkalemia. It may result from deteriorating renal function, ongoing K^+ supplementation, or concurrent K^+ sparing diuretics.

Idiosyncratic angioedema occurs in less than 1% of ACEI users, even after chronic use. If this occurs, stop the ACEI and assess for critical anaphylaxis. Therapy is routine, but the patient is barred from future ACEI use.

Within months of ACEI use, a non-productive cough occurs in 5-15%. The cough usually resolves within 1-2 weeks after stopping ACEIs and returns on re-introduction. Due to the benefit of ACEIs, tolerating the cough is encouraged. In the ED, cough should prompt a search for other pathology (e.g., early pulmonary edema or pneumonia) as well.

In the elderly, the initial ACEI dose should be low, and then titrated up. Target doses for ACEIs are: captopril, 50mg tid; enalapril or lisinopril, 20 mg qd; or ramipril, 5 mg bid.[4] But, if titration fails, even low doses may confer some benefit.[4]

Vasodilators: Angiotensin II (AII) Receptor Blockers (ARBs). Stopping AII synthesis by ACEI is desirable, but AI is still converted to AII by other chymases. ARBs block the AII receptor, providing AII inhibition while keeping ACE activity intact. Intact ACE degrades bradykinin, therefore decreasing complications from its accumulation (e.g., cough, anaphylaxis).

ARBs are used if ACEIs cause angioedema or intractable cough. They are as likely as ACEIs to cause hypotension, worsen renal function, and induce hyperkalemia. To date, trials are inconclusive as to whether ARBs prolong life and decrease morbidity like ACEIs.[52,53] Therefore, ARBs are not ACEI substitutes. They are used after failure of a prior ACEI trial or can be added to an ACEI regimen if symptoms persist.[2]

ARBs are well tolerated in the elderly and complication rates are comparable to placebo.[48,54,55] The rate of hyperkalemia is similar to that found with ACEIs, and is associated with the same risk factors.[55] A common ARB is losartan, dosed at 50 mg daily. The initial dose is lowered in those on high-dose diuretics, and potassium and renal function must be monitored.

Vasodilators: Hydralazine and Isosorbide Dinitrate (HISDN). An alternative to ACEI or ARBs, but with less benefit,

HISDN is not used unless marked ACEI/ARB intolerance exists.[1,2,46,56] There is no use of either agent alone for HF.

Beta-Blockers. Sympathetic activation, mediated by norepinephrine, results in many events contributing to HF.[57] *(Please see Table 8.)* Beta-blockers interfere with the neurohormonal effects and lead to a decrease in both mortality and hospital admissions.[58-63] In a large study of 10,000 patients, beta-blockers decreased mortality by 65%, lowered hospitalizations, and improved symptoms.[63] Beta-blockers are recommended in NYHA class II or III systolic HF.[2] They are usually combined with diuretics and ACEIs. Data currently are insufficient to indicate use in class IV HF.[2]

Contraindications include bronchospastic disease, symptomatic bradycardia, or advanced heart block (without pacemaker protection). They should be used cautiously in asymptomatic bradycardia (heart rate < 60). Diabetes is not a contraindication.[62] Beta-blockers should not be initiated in decompensated HF and should be avoided if fluid retention requires IV diuresis, if IV inotropes are anticipated, or if hospitalization is needed. Since ED HF is usually symptomatic, initiating beta-blockers is difficult in this environment.

Carvedilol is the only FDA-approved HF beta-blocker, and should be begun after stabilization of diuretics, ACEI, and digoxin dosing. Starting dose is 3.125 mg bid.[64] It is slowly increased, at two-week intervals, based on tolerance. Common complications are bradycardia, hypotension, dizziness, and diarrhea. Metoprolol also is commonly used. The initial dose is 6.25 mg qd, and gradually should be increased to 50 mg bid.

Decompensated HF patients on beta-blockers are a challenging management problem. Beta-blocker termination may cause deterioration, but further dosing can worsen tenuous hemodynamics. A short course of IV inotrope, while giving a lower beta-blocker dose, may allow stabilization by other measures (e.g., IV diuretics, vasodilators).

Spironolactone. Aldosterone has detrimental cardiac effects, independent of AII. Its antagonism by spironolactone can improve HF. The mortality risk and cardiac hospitalizations of NYHA class IV HF decreases by 32% when spironolactone is added to routine therapy.[65,66] Thus, NYHA class IV HF may be trialed on low-dose spironolactone therapy, 12.5-25 mg/d.[2,65] At this dose, serious hyperkalemia risk is similar to placebo, but gynecomastia is a common adverse event. Spironolactone is not recommend if the creatinine is greater than 2.5 mg/dL or K^+ is greater than 5.0 mEq/L. Serum K^+ is checked one week after initiation of therapy and after dose changes. There is insufficient evidence for spironolactone in NYHA class I or II HF.

Specifics of Systolic HF Therapy. Standard therapy in systolic HF usually consists of the combination of ACEIs, digoxin, and diuretics for the relief of fluid overload. Beta-blockers are added as appropriate, and in NYHA IV HF, spironolactone is prescribed.

Calcium channel blockers (CCBs) are not recommended.[1,2] Short-term use may result in pulmonary edema and cardiogenic shock. Long-term use increases the risk of worsening HF and death.[67-70] These adverse effects may be because of the CCBs' negative inotropicity. Amlodipine, which has not been demonstrated to have a clear adverse mortality effect, may be used for other compelling clinical reasons.

Specifics of Diastolic HF Therapy. Since most large trials focus on the treatment of systolic HF, guidelines for diastolic HF therapy are largely empiric.[4] In diastolic HF, diuretics are appropriate if congestion or edema is present, but one should avoid excessive diuresis. Hypotension, confusion, and azotemia may result if intravascular depletion (decreased preload) causes cardiac output to fall.

Other diastolic HF medications are beta-blockers, CCBs, and ACEIs.[17] Beta-blockers slow heart rate, which prolongs filling time and improves stroke volume, decreases symptoms, and helps prevent ischemia. In one small study of elderly HF patients (mean age, 81), with an EF 40% or lower, beta-blockers improved survival.[71] In contradistinction to systolic HF, CCBs may reduce ischemia and ventricular hypertrophy in diastolic HF. They also have a beneficial effect on diastolic function. Verapamil may improve symptoms and exercise capacity in the elderly diastolic HF patient.[72] ACEIs can improve LV compliance by reducing hypertrophy. In 21 elderly patients, enalapril improved exercise capacity, LV mass, and diastolic function.[44] However, the mortality-reducing benefits of ACEIs in diastolic HF remains unproven in the aged.[10,30]

Table 8. Effects of Norepinephrine Contributing to Heart Failure Development

1. Increases SVR by vasoconstriction; increases ventricular volume/pressure.
2. Impairs renal sodium excretion.
3. Induces cardiac hypertrophy.
4. Increases myocardial cellular automaticity, may provoke arrhythmia.
5. Contributes to hypokalemia.
6. Contributes to apoptosis by stimulating growth and oxidative stress.

Nitrates and digoxin may be of use in diastolic HF when impaired ventricular relaxation is the primary etiologic factor. But, since they decrease preload, and cause a resultant decline in CO, they should be used with caution. Digoxin, often considered contraindicated in diastolic HF, may have similar benefits to those seen in systolic HF.[4] In 988 patients randomized to either placebo or digoxin, digoxin had no overall mortality effect but decreased HF deaths and hospitalizations by 18%.[42]

Appropriate ACEI use in diastolic HF is unclear. However, since hypertension is a common precipitant of diastolic HF, its use may be of benefit in these patients. Some support the use of ACEIs in diastolic HF.[48]

A useful approach in diastolic HF is to use beta-blockers if the resting heart rate exceeds 75, or ACEIs if it is less than 75—provided there are no contraindications to their use.[4] These drugs can be combined with diuretics and nitrates to relieve congestion or edema. In refractory cases, digoxin is considered.

Measures with Limited Risk/ Benefit Analysis

Intermittent Inotropic Therapy. Intuitively, inotropes would seem to be of use to augment contractility and decrease SVR by vasodilation. Short-term use does improve CO, but there is no lasting benefit in symptoms or outcome.[2,6] In fact, chronic IV use increases mortality, and so is not recommended.[2,6,73,74] Appropriate uses are as a bridge to stabilization in decompensated patients on beta-blockers, or while instituting definitive therapy (e.g., heart transplant).

Anticoagulation. The risk of thromboembolism in stable HF patients is 1-3% annually, and is highest in those with lowest EFs.[75,76] Conversely, anticoagulation risk is high in the elderly.[11,18] Many use warfarin in HF, but there are few data to support this prac-

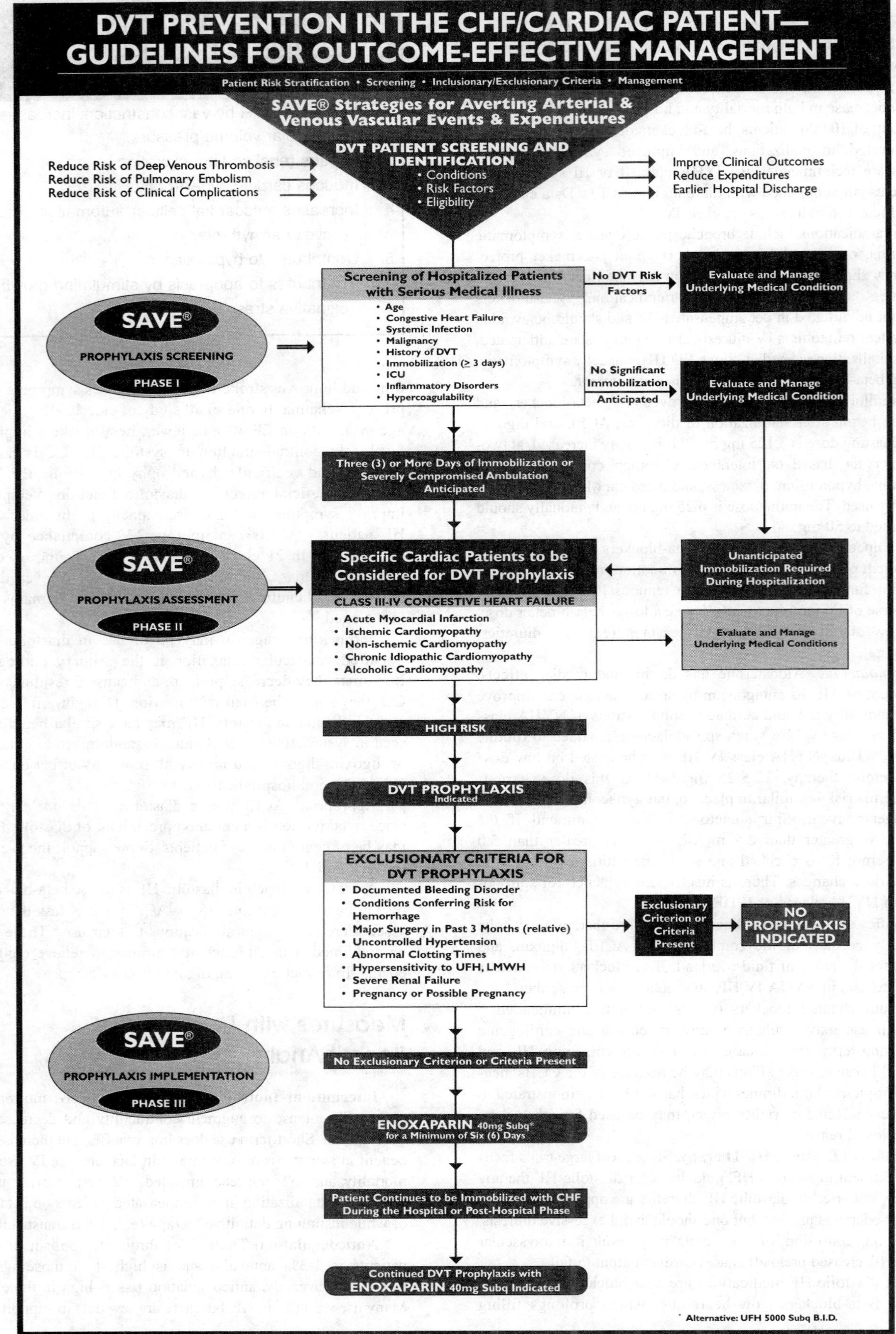
DVT PREVENTION IN THE CHF/CARDIAC PATIENT—
GUIDELINES FOR OUTCOME-EFFECTIVE MANAGEMENT
Patient Risk Stratification • Screening • Inclusionary/Exclusionary Criteria • Management
SAVE® Strategies for Averting Arterial & Venous Vascular Events & Expenditures
DVT PATIENT SCREENING AND IDENTIFICATION
• Conditions
• Risk Factors
• Eligibility
Reduce Risk of Deep Venous Thrombosis
Reduce Risk of Pulmonary Embolism
Reduce Risk of Clinical Complications
Improve Clinical Outcomes
Reduce Expenditures
Earlier Hospital Discharge
SAVE®
PROPHYLAXIS SCREENING
PHASE I
Screening of Hospitalized Patients with Serious Medical Illness
• Age
• Congestive Heart Failure
• Systemic Infection
• Malignancy
• History of DVT
• Immobilization (≥ 3 days)
• ICU
• Inflammatory Disorders
• Hypercoagulability
No DVT Risk Factors
Evaluate and Manage Underlying Medical Condition
No Significant Immobilization Anticipated
Evaluate and Manage Underlying Medical Condition
Three (3) or More Days of Immobilization or Severely Compromised Ambulation Anticipated
SAVE®
PROPHYLAXIS ASSESSMENT
PHASE II
Specific Cardiac Patients to be Considered for DVT Prophylaxis
CLASS III-IV CONGESTIVE HEART FAILURE
• Acute Myocardial Infarction
• Ischemic Cardiomyopathy
• Non-ischemic Cardiomyopathy
• Chronic Idiopathic Cardiomyopathy
• Alcoholic Cardiomyopathy
Unanticipated Immobilization Required During Hospitalization
Evaluate and Manage Underlying Medical Conditions
HIGH RISK
DVT PROPHYLAXIS
Indicated
EXCLUSIONARY CRITERIA FOR DVT PROPHYLAXIS
• Documented Bleeding Disorder
• Conditions Conferring Risk for Hemorrhage
• Major Surgery in Past 3 Months (relative)
• Uncontrolled Hypertension
• Abnormal Clotting Times
• Hypersensitivity to UFH, LMWH
• Severe Renal Failure
• Pregnancy or Possible Pregnancy
Exclusionary Criterion or Criteria Present
NO PROPHYLAXIS INDICATED
SAVE®
PROPHYLAXIS IMPLEMENTATION
PHASE III
No Exclusionary Criterion or Criteria Present
ENOXAPARIN 40mg Subq*
for a Minimum of Six (6) Days
Patient Continues to be Immobilized with CHF During the Hospital or Post-Hospital Phase
Continued DVT Prophylaxis with ENOXAPARIN 40mg Subq Indicated
* Alternative: UFH 5000 Subq B.I.D.

tice.[1,2] Patients with AF should receive warfarin, with dosage adjustments to keep the INR between 2.0 and 3.0.[1] Most elderly patients in sinus rhythm who have no history of a past embolic event probably do not need anticoagulation.[17]

Non-Steroidal Anti-Inflammatory Drugs (NSAIDs). NSAIDs inhibit diuretics and ACEIs, worsen both cardiac and renal function, and should be avoided in HF.[1,2] With few data for guidance, routine use of aspirin for MI prophylaxis in coronary artery disease, in the setting of concurrent ACEI treatment for HF, is controversial; however, current recommendations are to maintain once daily dosing of aspirin (75-325 mg) to diminish the risk of cardiovascular events in patients with CAD.

Antiarrhythmics. HF patients are sensitive to the pro-arrhythmic and cardiodepressant effects of antiarrhythmics, and antiarrhythmics do not decrease sudden death risk.[20,77] Suppression of asymptomatic ventricular arrhythmias is usually unnecessary. However, after resuscitation from sudden death, VF, or sustained VT, electrophysiologic testing and device placement may be considered.[2]

Class I antiarrhythmics are not used in HF except for immediate treatment of life-threatening ventricular arrhythmias.[1,2,77,80] Some class III agents (e.g., amiodarone) do not increase sudden death risk.[78,79] Therefore, they are preferred for atrial arrhythmias.[2] But, due to toxicity, amiodarone is not routinely recommended to prevent sudden death if the patient has already been treated with mortality-reducing drugs (ACEIs, beta-blockers).[2]

Disposition

Inpatient Admission Criteria for ED HF Patients. No published criteria exist. Patients with sustained VT, symptomatic arrhythmia, unstable vital signs, unstable airway, ischemic chest pain, new ECG changes, and AMI enzyme elevations, are admitted to an ICU. Severe electrolyte abnormalities may require a monitored bed. If the patient is congested and unable to attain output goals, or if dyspnea is unrelieved after therapy, admission is warranted. A low admission threshold should be used in the very elderly, in the presence of severe comorbidity, or if the home environment precludes successful outpatient management. Hemodynamically stable patients with fluid overload may be considered for observation unit admission.

Discharge Criteria. Patients with a good diuretic response, dyspnea resolution, and edema improvement, are expected to do well. Ambulation prior to discharge is an effective method to evaluate functional reserve and may help determine the ability to perform activities of daily living. In addition, if ACEI therapy is initiated or up-titrated in the ED, ambulation prior to discharge will assure that the revised therapies do not cause orthostatic hypotension.

Discharge Instructions. Patients should receive instruction on the signs and symptoms of worsening HF, and be educated on when to return to the ED. This should specifically include daily weight monitoring, appropriate responses to weight changes, and when to contact their physician. A written list of their medications and doses should be provided, as well as contact phone numbers for future follow-up. They should be encouraged to stop smoking, to reduce alcohol intake, and to exercise.

Dietary and Social Work Evaluation. An important part of HF management is the home environment. Barriers to obtaining medications, attending outpatient appointments, and adhering to dietary constraints (low sodium diet) need to be determined and eliminated. Failure to address these factors often results in minimal improvement and contributes to frequent readmission.[80] Since dietary non-compliance is a major contributor to multiple hospitalizations, education is important. Dietary consultation should be arranged, and can be accomplished over the phone.

Readmission. In the elderly, multiple simultaneous disease process are common. This complicates management and contributes to the high re-hospitalization rate. HF 90-day readmit rates are 33-47%, and in Medicare patients older than 65 years, nearly 50% are readmitted within 3-6 months.[2,81] Risk factors for re-admission are increasing age, male gender, prior admission within six months, and an initial hospitalization longer than one week.[82] Other contributors are a failed social support system (21%), inadequate follow-up (20%), and non-compliance of diet (18%) or medication (15%). Overall, 90-day readmits are possibly preventable in 38%, and probably preventable in 15%.[80]

A multidisciplinary approach, including physicians, nurses, home care specialists, and pharmacists, decreases 90-day readmission rates, improves quality of life, and lowers costs.[4,80,81,83] This is also true for the ED observation unit, where discharge rates increased by 50%, 90-day ED HF re-visits decreased more than 50%, and HF re-hospitalization decreased by two-thirds after instituting a multidisciplinary approach.[84,85]

Quality Improvement Programs. Like inpatient care, ED management of HF is part of the QI process. Indicators of appropriate levels of care, such as adequate diuretic use and appropriate ACEI treatment, should be documented. Unexpected events, morbidity, and mortality should be reviewed. Patients should be followed for frequency of revisits. Since poor 90-day readmission rates are associated with lower quality inpatient care, this also should be tracked in observation unit HF patients.[86]

Summary

Treatment for HF in the elderly is similar to that of the younger cohort. However, the underlying pathology is significantly different, the confounders more complex, and the diagnosis more difficult. Although the management challenges are greater, and the ultimate prognosis worse when compared to the younger HF patient, our understanding of HF has increased and new therapies offer hope to our elderly patients with heart failure.

References

1. Guidelines for the evaluation and management of heart failure: Report of the American College of Cardiology/American Heart Association task force on practice guidelines (Committee of Evaluation and Management of Heart Failure). *Circ* 1995;92:2764-2784.
2. Packer M, Cohn JN. Consensus recommendations for the management of chronic heart failure. *Am J Cardiol* 1999;83: 2A,1A-38A.
3. Massie BM, Shah NB. Evolving trends in epidemiologic factors of heart failure: Rationale for preventative strategies and comprehensive disease management. *Am Heart J* 1997; 133:703-712.
4. Friesinger GC. Ed. *Cardiology Clinics, Cardiovascular Disease in the Elderly*. Philadelphia: WB Saunders; 1999.
5. O'Connell JB, Bristow MR. Economic impact of heart failure in the United States: Time for a different approach. *J Heart Lung Trans* 1994;13:S107-112.
6. Packer M, Carver JR, Rodeheffer RJ, et al for the PROMISE Study Research Group. Effect of oral milrinone on mortality in severe chronic heart failure. *N Engl J Med* 1991;325:

1468-1475.

7. Tresch DD. The clinical diagnosis of heart failure in older patients. *J Am Geriatr Soc* 1997;45:1128-1133.
8. Rich MW. Epidemiology, pathophysiology, and etiology of congestive heart failure in older adults. *J Am Geriatr Soc* 1997;45:968-974.
9. Wei JY. Age and the cardiovascular system. *N Engl J Med* 1992;327:1735-1739.
10. Doughty R, Andersen V, Sharpe N. Optimal treatment of heart failure in the elderly. *Drugs and Aging* 1997;10: 435-443.
11. Anonymous. Studies of left ventricular dysfunction (SOLVD) Crationale, design and methods: Two trials that evaluate the effect of enalapril in patients with reduced ejection fraction. *Am J Cardiol* 1990;66:315-322.
12. Tresch DD, McGough MF. Heart failure with normal systolic function: A common disorder in older people. *J Am Geriatr Soc* 1995;43:1035-1042.
13. Wong WF, Gold S, Fukuyama O, et al. Diastolic dysfunction in elderly patients with congestive heart failure. *Am J Cardiol* 1990;66:1257-1259.
14. Ghali JK, Kadakia S, Cooper RS, et al. Bedside diagnosis of preserved versus impaired left ventricular systolic function in heart failure. *Am J Cardiol* 1991;67:1002-1006.
15. Batsford WP, Mickleborough LL, Elefteriades JA. Ventricular arrhythmias in heart failure. *Card Clin* 1995;13: 87-91.
16. Hobbs RE, Czerska MD. Congestive heart failure. Current and future strategies to decrease mortality. *Postgrad Med* 1994;96: 167-172.
17. Senni M, Redfield MM. Congestive heart failure in elderly patients. *Mayo Clin Proc* 1997;72:453-460.
18. Stevenson WG, Stevenson LW, Middlekauff HR, et al. Sudden death prevention in patients with advanced ventricular dysfunction. *Circ* 1993;88:2953-2961.
19. The SOLVD Investigators. Effect of enalapril on survival in patients with reduced left ventricular ejection fractions and congestive heart failure. *N Engl J Med* 1991;325:293-302.
20. The Cardiac Arrhythmia Suppression Trial (CAST) investigators. Preliminary report: effect of encainide and flecainide on mortality in a randomized trial of arrhythmia suppression after myocardial infarction. *N Engl J Med* 1989; 321:406-412.
21. Julian DG, Camm AJ, Fangin G, et al. Randomized trial of effect of amiodarone on mortality in patients with left ventricular dysfunction after recent myocardial infarction: EMIAT. *Lancet* 1997;349:667-674.
22. Wenger NK, Franciosa JA, Weber KT. Heart failure. 18th Bethesda conference. Cardiovascular disease in the elderly. *JACC* 1987;10:73A-76A.
23. Remes J, Miettinen H, Reunanen A, et al. Validity of clinical diagnosis of heart failure in primary health care. *Eur Heart J* 1991;12:315-321.
24. Francis CM, Caruana L, Kearney P, et al. Open access echocardiography in management of heart failure in the community. *BMJ* 1995;310:634-636.
25. McKee PA, Castelli WP, McNamara PM, et al. The natural history of congestive heart failure: The Framingham study. *N Engl J Med* 1971;285:1441-1446.
26. Ho KKL, Anderson KM, Kannel WB, et al. Congestive heart failure/myocardial responses/valvular heart disease: Survival after the onset of congestive heart failure in Framingham heart study subjects. *Circ* 1993;88:107-115.
27. Marantz PR, Kaplan MC, Alderman MH. Clinical diagnosis of congestive heart failure in patients with acute dyspnea. *Chest* 1990;97:776-781.
28. Le Conte P, Coutant V, N'Guyen JM, et al. Prognostic factors in acute cardiogenic pulmonary edema. *Am J Emerg Med* 1999;17:329-332.
29. Chakko S, Woska D, Marinez H, et al. Clinical, radiographic, and hemodynamic correlations in chronic congestive heart failure: Conflicting results may lead to inappropriate care. *Am J Med* 1991;90:353-359.
30. Gillespie ND, Darbar D, Struthers AD, et al. Heart Failure: A diagnostic and therapeutic dilemma in elderly patients. *Age Aging* 1998;27:539-543.
31. Peacock WF, Emerman CL, McErlean ES, et al. Troponin T: Insensitive for outcome prediction in low risk suspected acute coronary syndrome ED observation unit patients. *Acad EM* 1998;5:519.
32. Kono T, Suwa M, Hanada H, et al. Clinical significance of normal cardiac silhouette in dilated cardiomyopathy—Evaluation based upon echocardiography and magnetic resonance imaging. *Jpn Cir J* 1992;56:359-365.
33. Ruskin JA, Gurney JW, Thorsen MK, et al. Detection of pleural effusions on supine chest radiographs. *AJR* 1987;148: 681-683.
34. Chait A, Cohen HE, Meltzer LE, et al. The bedside chest radiograph in the evaluation of incipient heart failure. *Radiol* 1972;105:563-566.
35. Shiro K, Takaaki N, Mashiko I. Early diagnosis and estimation of pulmonary congestion and edema in patients with left-sided heart disease from histogram of pulmonary CT number. *Chest* 1996;109:1439-1445.
36. McGredie, M. Measurement of pulmonary edema in valvular heart disease. *Circ* 1967;36:381-386.
37. Luepker R, Liander B, Korsgren M, et al. Pulmonary extravascular and intravascular fluid volume in resting patients. *Am J Cardiol* 1971;28:295-302.
38. Clinical Practice Guideline, Number 11. Heart Failure: Evaluation and care of patients with left-ventricular systolic dysfunction. US Department of Health and Human Services. June, 1994. *AHCPR* publication No. 94-0612.
39. Bumetadine. In: *Physician's Desk Reference*, 2441-43. Montvale, NJ: Medical Economics Co.; 1998.
40. Peacock W, Aponte J, Craig M, et al. Predictors of unsuccessful treatment for congestive heart failure in the emergency department observation unit. *Acad EM* 1997;4: 494.
41. Ware JA, Snow E, Luchi JM, et al. Effect of digoxin on ejection fraction in elderly patients with congestive heart failure. *J Am Geriatri Soc* 1984;32:631-635.
42. The Digitalis Investigation Group. The effect of digoxin on mortality and morbidity in patients with heart failure. *N Engl J Med* 1997;336:525-533.
43. Slatton ML, Irani WN, Hall SA, et al. Does digoxin provide

additional hemodynamic and autonomic benefit at higher doses in patients with mild to moderate heart failure and normal sinus rhythm? *J Am Coll Cardiol* 1997;29: 1206-1213.
44. Aronow WS, Kronzon I. Effect of enalapril on congestive heart failure treated with diuretics in elderly patients with prior myocardial infarction and normal left ventricular ejection fraction. *Am J Cardiol* 1993;71:602-604.
45. Francis G, Cohn J, for the V-HeFT VA Cooperative Studies Group. Plasma norepinephrine, plasma renin activity and congestive heart failure. *Circ* 1993;87:41-48.
46. Cohn JN, Johnson G, Ziesche S, et al. A comparison of enalapril with hydralazine-isosorbide dinitrate in the treatment of chronic congestive heart failure. *N Engl J Med* 1991;325:303-310.
47. The CONSENSUS Trial Study Group. Effects of enalapril on mortality in severe congestive heart failure: Results of the Cooperative North Scandinavian Enalapril Survival Study (CONSENSUS). *N Engl J Med* 1987;315:1429-1435.
48. Aronow WS. The ELITE study. What are its implications for the drug treatment of heart failure? Evaluation of Losartan in the elderly study. *Drugs Aging* 1998;12:423-428.
49. Pfeffer MA, Braunwald E, Moye LA, et al. Effect of captopril on mortality and morbidity in patients with left ventricular dysfunction after myocardial infarction: Results of the survival and ventricular enlargement trial. *N Engl J Med* 1992;327:669-677.
50. Ambrosioni E, Borghi C, Magnani B. Survival of myocardial infarction long-term evaluation (SMILE) investigators. The effect of the angiotensin-converting-enzyme inhibitor zofenopril on mortality and morbidity after anterior myocardial infarction. *N Engl J Med* 1995;332:80-85.
51. Garg R, Yusef S, for the Collaborative Group on ACE Inhibitor Trials: Overview of randomized trials of Angiotensin-converting enzyme inhibitors on mortality and morbidity in patients with heart failure. *JAMA* 1995;273: 1450-1456.
52. McKelvie R, Yusuf S, Pericak D, et al. Comparison of candesartan, enalapril, and their combination in congestive heart failure: Randomized Evaluation of Strategies for Left Ventricular Dysfunction (RESOLVD pilot study). *Eur Heart J* 1998;19(supp):133.
53. Pitt B, Segal R, Martinez FA, et al. On behalf of Elite Study Investigators. Randomized trail of losartan versus captopril in patients over 65 with heart failure (Evaluation of Losartan in the Elderly Study, ELITE). *Lancet* 1997;349:747-752.
54. Burrell LM, Johnston CI. Angiotensin II receptor antagonists. Potential in elderly patients with cardiovascular disease. *Drugs Aging* 1997;10:421-434.
55. Goldberg AI, Dunlay MC, Sweet CS. Safety and tolerability of losartan potassium, an angiotensin II receptor antagonist, compared with hydrochlorothiazide, atenolol, felodipine ER, and angiotensin-converting enzyme inhibitors for the treatment of systemic hypertension. *Am J Cardiol* 1995;75: 793-795.
56. Cohn JN, Archibald DG, Ziesche S, et al. Effect of vasodilator therapy on mortality in chronic congestive heart failure: Results of the Veterans Administration Cooperative Study. *N Engl J Med* 1986;314:1547-1552.
57. Packer M. Adrenergic blockade in chronic heart failure: Principles, progress, and practice. *Prog Cardio Dis* 1998; 41(Supp 1):39-52.
58. Colucci WS, Packer M, Bristow MR, et al. For the US Carvedilol Study Group. Carvedilol inhibits clinical progression in patients with mild symptoms of heart failure. *Circ* 1996;94:2800-2806.
59. Tsuyuki RT, Yusuf S, Rouleau JL, et al. Combination neurohormonal blockade with ACE inhibitors, angiotensin II, antagonists and beta-blockers in patients with congestive heart failure: Design of the Randomized Evaluation of Strategies for Left Ventricular Dysfunction (RESOLVED) pilot study (phase II). *Eur Heart J* 1998;19(Supp):308.
60. The International Steering Committee. Rationale, design, and organization of the Metoprolol CR/XL randomized intervention trial in heart failure (MERIT-HF). *Am J Cardiol* 1997;80(Supp 9B):54J-58J.
61. CIBIS Investigators and Committees. A randomized trial of b-blockade in heart failure: The Cardiac Insufficiency Bisoprolol Study (CIBIS). *Circ* 1994;90:1765-1773.
62. Bristow MR, Gilbert EM, Abraham WT, et al. For the MOCHA Investigators. Carvedilol produces dose-related improvements in left ventricular function and survival in subjects with chronic heart failure. *Circ* 1996;94:2807-2816.
63. Tsuyuki RT, Yusuf S, Rouleau JL, et al. Combination neurohormonal blockade with ACE inhibitors, angiotensin II antagonists and beta-blockers in patients with congestive heart failure: Design of the Randomized Evaluation of Strategies for Left Ventricular Dysfunction (RESOLVD) Pilot Study. *Can J Cardiol* 1997;13:1166-1174.
64. Prescribing Information: Coreg, 1998. SmithKline Beecham Pharmaceuticals, Philadelphia, PA.
65. Pitt B, Zannad F, Remme WJ, et al. The effect of spironolactone on morbidity and mortality in patients with severe heart failure. Randomized Aldactone Evaluation Study Investigators. *N Engl J Med* 1999;341:709-717.
66. The Rales Investigators. Effectiveness of spironolactone added to an angiotensin-converting enzyme inhibitor and a loop diuretic for sever chronic congestive heart failure (The Randomized Aldactone Evaluation Study [RALES]). *Am J Cardiol* 1996;78:902-907.
67. Elkayam U, Weber L, McKay C, et al. S. Spectrum of acute hemodynamic effects of nifedipine in severe congestive heart failure. *Am J Cardiol* 1985;56:560-566.
68. Barjon JN, Rouleau JL, Bichet D, et al. Chronic renal and neurohumoral effects of the calcium entry blocker nisoldipine in patients with congestive heart failure. *J Am Coll Cardiol* 1987;9:622-630.
69. Elkayam U, Amin J, Mehra A, et al. A prospective, randomized, double-blind, crossover study to compare the efficacy and safety of chronic nifedipine therapy with that of isosorbide dinitrate and their combination in the treatment of chronic congestive heart failure. *Circ* 1990;82:1954-1961.
70. Goldstein RE, Boccuzzi SJ, Cruess D, et al. Diltiazem increase late-onset congestive heart failure in post-infarction patients with early reduction in ejection fraction. The Adverse Experience Committee and the Multicenter

Diltiazem Post-infarction Research Group. *Circ* 1991;83: 52-60.

71. Aronow WS, Ahn C, Kronzon I. Effect of propranolol versus no propranolol on total mortality plus nonfatal myocardial infarction in older patients with prior myocardial infarction, congestive heart failure, and left ventricular ejection fraction ³ 40% treated with diuretics plus angiotensin-converting enzyme inhibitors. *Am J Cardiol* 1997;80:207-209.
72. Arrighi JA, Dilsizian V, Perrone-Filardi P, et al. Improvement of the age-related impairment in left ventricular diastolic filling with verapamil in the normal human heart. *Circ* 1994;90:213-219.
73. Lubsen J, Just H, Hjalmarsson AC, et al. Effect of pimobendan on exercise capacity in patients with heart failure: Main results for the Pimobendan in Congestive Heart Failure (PICO) trial. *Heart* 1996;76:223-231.
74. Cohn JN, Goldstein SO, Greenberg BH, et al. A dose-dependent increase in mortality with vesnarinone among patients with severe heart failure. *N Engl J Med* 1998;338: 1810-1816.
75. Cioffi G, Pozzoli M, Forni G, et al. Systemic thromboembolism in chronic heart failure. A prospective study in 406 patients. *Eur Heart J* 1996;17:1381-1389.
76. Baker DW, Wright RF. Management of heart failure. IV. Anticoagulation for patients with heart failure due to left ventricular systolic dysfunction. *JAMA* 1994;272:1614-1618.
77. The Cardiac Arrhythmia Suppression Trail II Investigators. Effect of antiarrhythmic agent moricizine on survival after myocardial infarction. *N Engl J Med* 1992;327:227-233.
78. Doval HC, Nul DR, Grancelli HO, et al, for Grupo de Estudio de la Sobrevida en la Insuficiencia Cardiaca en Argentina (GESICA). Randomized trial of low-dose amiodarone in severe congestive heart failure. *Lancet* 1994; 344:493-498.
79. Singh SN, Fletcher RD, Fisher SG, et al for the Survival Trial of Antiarrhythmic Therapy in Congestive Heart Failure. Amiodarone in patients with congestive heart failure and asymptomatic ventricular arrhythmias. *N Engl J Med* 1995; 333:77-82.
80. Vinson JM, Rich MW, Sperry JC, et al. Early readmission of elderly patients with congestive heart failure. *J Am Geriatr Soc* 1990;38:1290-1295.
81. Rich MW, Vinson JM, Sperry JC, et al. Prevention of readmission in elderly patients with congestive heart failure. *J Gen Int Med* 1993;8:585-590.
82. Krumholz HM, Parent EM, Tu N, et al. Readmission after hospitalization for congestive heart failure among Medicare beneficiaries. *Arch Intern Med* 1997;157:99-104.
83. Rich MW, Beckham V, Wittenberg C, et al. A multidisciplinary intervention to prevent the readmission of elderly patients with congestive heart failure. *N Engl J Med* 1995;333:1190-1195.
84. Albert NM, Peacock WF. Patient outcome and costs after implementation of an acute heart failure management program in an emergency department observation unit. *J Int Soc Heart Lung Trans* 1999;18:92.
85. Peacock WF, Albert NM, Kies P, et al. Emergency department observation unit heart failure protocol decreases adverse outcome rates. *J Card Fail* 1999;5:77.
86. Ashton CM, Kuykendall DH, Johnson ML, et al. The association between the quality of inpatient care and early readmission. *Ann Intern Med* 1995;122:415-421.
87. Grossman W. Diastolic dysfunction in congestive heart failure. *N Engl J Med* 1991;325:1557-1564.

Altered Mental Status

Sandra M. Schneider, MD, FACEP

The chief complaint usually goes something like, "Doctor, my grandmother has been acting strange lately . . . can you tell me what's wrong with her?" When the clinical scenario begins like this, confusion is frequently a part of the evaluation process as well as the patient's presentation. The fact is, altered mental status is a common and, in most cases, rather difficult syndrome to decipher and assess accurately within the diagnostic and temporal constraints of the ED setting. In some cases, however, the causes of delirium and dementia can be identified. For example, the patient with a traumatic head injury, the individual who has ingested an overdose of sedative/hypnotics, or the infant with high fever and signs of meningitis rarely presents a diagnostic dilemma.

The elderly, on the other hand, usually present more of a challenge. Their picture is complicated by the fact that many older patients have a chronic, poorly described dementia, which may make it difficult to distinguish between chronic abnormalities in the patient's baseline mental status and acute clinical deterioration. In addition, the caretaker who accompanies these patients frequently offers little more than, "She's not herself." Finally, the differential diagnosis is extensive and, as a rule, few clues are available from either the history or physical exam.

By necessity, the workup for altered mental status is often "shotgun" in nature and relies upon a battery of expensive tests that includes virtually anything that is available on a stat basis. Frequently, even this database proves to be insufficient for making a definitive diagnosis; therefore, additional radiological modalities are employed early in the evaluation process. In addition, the admission decision often overrides the diagnostic process, and sometimes degenerates into a three-way battle between overstressed family members, hospital or insurance gatekeepers, and emergency physician intermediaries.

This chapter characterizes the multiple etiologies that can cause altered mental status in the elderly. To optimize outcomes in this patient subgroup, a systematic approach to differential diagnosis and an ordered sequence for evaluating these challenging encounters are presented.

Pathophysiological Considerations

Generally speaking, alterations in level of consciousness may be caused by a structural defect in the brain, a lack of adequate substrate necessary for cerebral function, or the presence of exogenous or indigenous toxins. In particular, alertness requires an intact mid-pons, midbrain, thalamus, and cerebral hemisphere. The brain requires an adequate supply of glucose and oxygen to supply energy to the cerebral tissue. Toxins may interfere with oxygen supply (carbon monoxide or cyanide) or neurotransmission. Systemic illness may interfere with substrate supply (hypoglycemia, hypotension), adversely affect neurotransmission, or create false neurotransmitters (uremia, hepatic coma).

Original studies on the pathophysiology of delirium postulated a decrease in cerebral metabolism[1] that may be due to impairment of liberation or conservation of the chemical fuels for the brain, disturbances of the normal ionic passage across membranes, changes in water and electrolyte content, or impaired synthesis of macromolecules required by neurons.[2] When impaired metabolism is accompanied by endogenous or exogenous stress (such as increased demand for neurotransmitters or decrease in oxygen), the reserve capacity of the brain may be insufficient to sustain normal cognitive function.

This theory is consistent with one of the most common etiologies of delirium. Increasing age is accompanied by chronic cholinergic deficiency in the central nervous system. Consequently, when an anticholinergic medication is ingested in vulnerable patients, a substantial decrease in neurotransmitters occurs and delirium develops.[3] Acetylcholine is essential for cognitive functioning, attention, and for maintaining a normal sleep-wake cycle.[2]

In this regard, both hypoxemia and hypoglycemia are known to inhibit acetylcholine synthesis.[4] Other stresses, such as hypercortisolemia, from both endogenous and exogenous sources may lead to delirium.[5] Other authors suggest that delirium is caused by mechanisms involving the dysfunction of beta-endorphinergic neurons and, perhaps, an imbalance of cholinergic, noradrenergic, and serotonergic neuronal networks and neurotransmission.[6,7] Adding support to this theory is the fact that alcohol withdrawal is associated with enhanced central noradrenergic activity, which is the most likely cause of delirium associated with this condition.[8-10]

In contrast, dementia is caused by widespread neuronal degeneration. This is true whether dementia presents in the elderly or in individuals less than 65 years of age. Although aging itself is associated with a gradual loss of neurons, intellectual capacity usually remains intact, unless there is underlying disease. In dementia, excessive cortical neuronal degeneration (such as is seen with Alzheimer's disease) leads to loss of language, perception, and calculation. Huntington's disease causes degeneration in the basal ganglia, thalamus, and deep white matter, changes that appear to slow information processing and produce a flattened affect.

Definitions, Incidence, and Prevalence

Emergency evaluation of elderly patients who present with altered mental status requires distinguishing between two common conditions: delirium and dementia. Organic brain syndrome is defined as a disorder of orientation, memory, intellect, judgment, and affect resulting from diffuse impairment of brain tissue.[11] This syndrome may manifest itself as confusion, abnormal behavior, or an alteration in mental status (either lethargy or hyperactivity). Although there are several specific disorders that produce altered mental status among the elderly, dementia and delirium are of special importance to the emergency practitioner; therefore, these entities will be discussed in detail.

Dementia. Dementia is characterized by chronic loss of intellectual function. Generally speaking, patients will demonstrate significant alterations in both short- and long-term memory. In addition, they also may have impairments in abstract thinking and judgment, gross personality changes, and disturbance of cortical functions such as aphasia, apraxia, agnosia, or constructional difficulty. As might be expected, these abnormalities are significant enough to interfere with daily activity. However, in contrast to delirium, dementia almost always develops over months or years and is usually, but not always, permanent. Moreover, dementia is usually progressive. Mental function may fluctuate over time, but rarely does it return to normal.

Delirium. Delirium is an acute organic dysfunction characterized by global cognitive impairment, attention abnormalities, a decrease in level of consciousness, a change in psychomotor activity (increase or decrease), and a disorder in the sleep/wake cycle. In general, symptoms associated with delirium will have an organic etiology that is either metabolic, infectious, or structural in nature. Almost without exception, the patient's symptoms are global in nature (i.e., cognition, perception, and memory are all affected). From a diagnostic perspective, it should be stressed that the onset of delirium is usually acute and can be measured in hours to days. Once the delirium clears, the patient often returns to baseline mental function.

Delirium and dementia are common disorders in the elderly population.[12,13] Most studies evaluating the incidence and prevalence of this disorder have focused on the hospitalized elderly. Based on these investigations, delirium is present prior to admission in about 15% of hospitalized elderly, whereas an additional 3-12% of patients develop delirium during their hospital stay.[12-16]

In contrast, dementia is present in almost 5% of all individuals over the age of 65, in 20% of patients over the age of 80, and in more than 30% of those over 90.[17,18] Acute delirium is a common associated syndrome in patients with chronic dementia. In one study, 45% of patients with acute delirium had an underlying dementia.[19] Accordingly, establishing baseline cognitive and psychomotor function, or dysfunction, in the setting of an ED is a major challenge for practitioners faced with distinguishing between new-onset delirium and exacerbation of chronic dementia.

Dementia: Precipitants and Prognosis

Alzheimer's Disease. The most common cause of dementia is Alzheimer's disease, accounting for 50-90% of all cases.[20-22] The precise anatomic diagnosis of Alzheimer's disease usually is established only at autopsy, which demonstrates characteristic neurofibrillary tangles and neuritic plaques (previously called senile plaques). Choline acetyltransferase, the enzyme required for synthesis of acetylcholine, is decreased in Alzheimer's disease. Somatostatin, a neurotransmitter for locomotion, sedation, excitation, catatonia, temperature regulation, feeding, learning, and memory, is also reduced in the cerebrospinal fluid (CSF) of Alzheimer's patients and several other forms of dementia.[20-22] Some Alzheimer's patients produce abnormal somatostatin, whereas others have decreased levels.[23-25]

Multi-Infarct Dementia. The next most common cause of dementia is cerebrovascular disease, which accounts for 5-10% of all cases.[20-22] In this context, dementia results from multiple, discrete cerebral infarcts. Multi-infarct dementia occurs most often as a result of embolic disease originating in the carotid arteries; occasionally, the cardiac emboli may be the source. Vasculitis and small-vessel disease associated with chronic hypertension represent other potential causes of multi-infarct dementia.

Infection. Several chronic infections also can produce dementia. Although HIV-associated dementia occurs primarily in younger patients, the elderly can and do participate in high-risk behavior and acquire HIV disease. Nearly 90% of patients with AIDS will show CNS changes at autopsy, and 30-40% will have clinical dementia AIDS dementia is often rapid in onset. CNS lymphomas may cause focal or diffuse abnormalities.[26]

It should be stressed that CNS infection is a potentially reversible cause of dementia and delirium. Such infections as cryptococcal meningitis, toxoplasmosis, progressive multifocal leukoencephalopathy, cytomegalovirus, herpes virus, and viral meningitis are frequently amenable to treatment and should be considered in the differential diagnosis. Creutzfeldt-Jacob disease is a transmittable form of dementia from an as-yet-unidentified virus-like agent.

Alcoholism. Alcoholism is mistakenly thought of as a disease of youth, yet it is estimated that nearly 10% of the elderly have a drinking problem.[27] More than one-third of elderly alcoholics begin abusing alcohol late in life.[27] This often occurs following a life change such as retirement or death of a spouse. Social clues for alcohol abuse, such as driving under the influence, poor performance at work, and observation of increased drinking by a friend or spouse, are often missing in the isolated lives of the elderly. While drinking is common, intoxication is not.[27]

The toxic effects of alcohol on CNS function are exaggerated in patients of advanced age. In this regard, the blood concentration per amount ingested is higher in the elderly due to a lowered volume of distribution. In addition, gastric alcohol dehydrogenase levels may be depleted, especially in patients with coexisting gastric pathology. Alcohol withdrawal is also more severe in the elderly.[27] In particular, withdrawal symptoms last for a longer duration, and such symptoms as disorientation, delirium, and hallucinations are reported more frequently.[28] There is some suggestion that repeated episodes of alcohol withdrawal are associated with more severe withdrawal symptoms in the future (i.e., a "kindling-like" effect[28]). The mortality rate from delirium tremens is higher in the elderly and approaches 40%.[29]

Finally, alcohol may cause permanent structural damage in the brain tissue of elderly consumers. Brain shrinkage, which is observed in alcohol abusers of all ages, is more pronounced and is irreversible in the elderly. Cognitive impairment is reported in 50% of elderly alcoholics.[28]

Dementia: Assessment and Intervention

From the perspective of emergency practice, the practitioner must recognize potentially treatable causes of dementia. In general, these reversible or treatable etiologies fall into three categories: 1) structural lesions of the CNS; 2) metabolic and systemic illness; and 3) neuropsychiatric disorders.

Structural Lesions of the CNS. In elderly patients presenting with dementia of unknown etiology, the physician must maintain a high index of suspicion for space-occupying lesions of the CNS which, in the geriatric patient, may include such conditions as chronic subdural hematoma, meningioma, or glioma. Unfortunately, these entities may be impossible to distinguish from one another on the basis of the physical exam alone. Patients with hydrocephalus may present in a similar manner.

Radiographic imaging with computerized tomography (CT) or magnetic resonance imaging (MRI) can distinguish among these structural abnormalities and will usually help direct treatment in order to prevent further deterioration. It should be noted that if a subdural hematoma has been present for several weeks, absorption of blood from the hematoma may occur, thereby rendering the subdural hematoma isodense. These changes can make it difficult to detect on CT scan, in which case contrast studies or an MRI may be required to confirm the diagnosis.

Metabolic and Systemic Illness. Dementia may be the presenting complaint of myriad metabolic diseases, including chronic liver failure, vitamin B_{12} deficiency, and hypothyroidism. Terminal illness associated with malignancy, cerebrovascular disease, and chronic renal failure may also produce a dementia-like picture.

Neuropsychiatric Disease. Depression is a common condition in the elderly and may occur as the result of progressing dementia. When faced with loss of a loved one, increasing disability, financial insecurity, or emotional isolation, depression in the elderly usually deepens. Classic findings of depression, such as decreased appetite, difficulty sleeping, and general immobility, should not be considered "normal" in the elderly. The Geriatric Depression Scale may be a helpful tool for detecting depression in this patient population.[29]

Delirium: Clinical Presentation and Prognosis

Delirium was one of the earliest mental disorders described by clinical neurologists.[6] It can occur in patients with normal mental function as well as in patients with underlying dementia. Delirium often presents with a prodrome of anxiety, restlessness, disturbed dreams, and transient hallucinations.[2] Patients usually progress to a global disorder characterized by disturbed cognitive abilities, attention deficits, and psychomotor hyper- or hyporeactivity. These patients may have a reduced attention span in response to external stimuli, accompanied by the inability to select and shift to new areas. These disturbances lead to withdrawal, disorganized thinking, and memory deficits.

Patients who are delirious may have difficulty distinguishing hallucinations from reality. Their thinking becomes disordered and fragmented, and often these patients cannot solve problems, anticipate reactions, or grasp abstract meanings. Speech becomes rambling or incoherent. Memory is impaired with respect to registration, retention, and recall. In particular, short-term memory is patchy, although long-term memory may be spared (in contrast to dementia, for which long-term memory is more seriously affected).

Psychomotor disturbances are nearly always present in delirium. In this regard, patients may be hyper- or hypoactive. Although hyperactivity may present a bigger problem for caretakers, hypoactivity is more common. Not uncommonly, there is increased somnolence in the day and excessive wakefulness at night. Dreams may extend into daytime hours and patients may have difficulty telling dreams from reality.

The frail elderly are at increased risk for delirium, especially those individuals with underlying dementia.[2,30] In one study, over 60% of frail elderly patients requiring hospitalization presented with delirium as part of their clinical picture.[17] In hospitalized elderly patients who were not considered frail by screening tests, 37% presented as falls and 32% presented with delirium.[30] Finally, almost one-third of demented patients requiring hospitalization have delirium.[17]

Course and Prognosis. As previously emphasized, delirium is generally a transient event, whereas dementia is usually characterized as a permanent, progressive condition. Temporally speaking, delirium generally lasts less than four weeks, although in the advanced elderly it may persist longer. In one study, delirium lasted less than 24 hours in 20% of patients, 1-3 days in 30%, and more than 30 days in 13% of patients.[1] Most patients will fully recover to their original baseline. From a diagnostic point of view, it should be emphasized that delirium can appear in the terminal phase of cancer and other serious diseases.

The hospital mortality rate in patients with acute delirium is eight times greater than that of age-matched controls.[12] This increased mortality probably reflects morbidity associated with the acute illness that precipitated the delirium. However, the six-month mortality rate in patients who presented with delirium is also higher as compared to controls.[12] More than one-half of patients with acute delirium and no history of dementia will return to independent living.[19] However, when dementia is the precipitating cause of delirium, only 14% of patients will return to an independent living situation.[19]

Delirium: Differential Diagnosis and Acute Management

Poorly understood and inconsistently described in the medical literature, delirium represents a clinical diagnosis that can be caused by a wide range of clinical disorders. From a practical diagnostic perspective, the presence of delirium is no more specific than dyspnea or headache. Frequently, the clinical impression cannot be confirmed by laboratory testing, radiographic modalities, or EEG. Moreover, although there are many specific causes of delirium (see discussions below), many patients will have more than one etiology for their delirium, a feature that further complicates patient evaluation.

Because the elderly are brittle when it comes to cognitive and physiologic function, virtually any disease can precipitate delirium in an elderly person. A small insult can unmask a vulnerable person. The following conditions and etiologies require diligent investigation in patients presenting to the ED with delirium.

Drug Toxicity. In the majority of studies evaluating the etiology of acute delirium, prescription medications were identified as the most common precipitant of this syndrome, having contributed to delirium in 22-39% of cases.[31-33] The drugs discussed in the following sections are of special clinical importance, either because of their frequent association with delirium or because of their capacity for producing CNS changes that precipitate the need for emergency evaluation. In this regard, practitioners should recognize that virtually any medication may cause delirium, including the sedative/hypnotics, narcotics, digitalis, propranolol, penicillin, cephalosporins, sulfonamides, lithium, anticonvulsants, nonsteroidal anti-inflammatory drugs, aspirin, and cimetidine.[33-38]

Anticholinergic Medications. Drug ingestion with an anticholinergic medication should be considered at the top of the differential diagnosis when evaluating a delirious elderly patient, especially one with a previously normal mental status. In particular, anticholinergics contained in over-the-counter (OTC) preparations are, perhaps, the most common and most frequently overlooked causes of acute delirium in the elderly patient.[38]

In young adults, anticholinergic overdose is associated with hallucinations, hyperthermia, diffuse erythema, mydriasis, tachycardia, and hypertension. In the elderly, peripheral signs are limited, whereas confusion and hallucinations are common. These CNS manifestations can occur with therapeutic doses of anticholinergic medications. Addition of an OTC drug with anticholinergic properties (diphenhydramine) to a prescribed medication with anticholinergic side effects can precipitate delirium in the vulnerable patient. Among medications commonly used in the elderly, meperidine, cimetidine, tricyclic antidepressants, antipsychotics, anti-Parkinsonian agents, and ranitidine can produce significant anticholinergic side effects. In addition, lithium can inhibit cyclic guanosine monophosphate (GMP), thereby decreasing serum acetylcholine levels and increasing toxicity of anticholinergic medication. Despite the increased sensitivity of elderly patients to drugs with anticholinergic properties, in one study 60% of nursing home residents and 23% of ambulatory elderly were prescribed medications with anticholinergic effects.[39]

Sedative/Hypnotics. As might be expected, the elderly display increased sensitivity to sedating drugs. Nearly 33% of elderly patients admitted to the hospital use prescription sedative/hypnotics.[17] Long-acting sedative/hypnotics initially used for sleep are often extended to control aberrant daytime behavior. Paradoxically, the residual physiological effects of a sedative taken at night may cause or exacerbate the daytime behavior problems, especially in patients with dementia.

The diagnosis is suggested by a recent history of sedative/hypnotic use. Fortunately, most sedative/hypnotics can be evaluated on a typical drug screen. Levels reported in the therapeutic range do not exclude drug-induced delirium in the elderly patient. Unless significant symptoms such as respiratory depression are present, there is usually no need for aggressive therapy. However, benzodiazepine and narcotic antagonists may be useful when significant symptoms are present and the agent has been identified. These antagonists should be used with caution. Controlling agitated behavior and providing a protective environment is generally all that is needed. Symptoms will resolve spontaneously as serum and tissue drug levels decrease over time.

Aspirin. Aspirin overdose may be difficult to diagnose on the basis of history alone. Although confusion may be prominent in elderly patients suffering from aspirin toxicity, metabolic abnormalities such as a primary respiratory alkalosis are frequently the first indication of impending toxicity. In the majority of cases, aspirin toxicity is the result of unintentional overuse of prescribed and OTC drugs rather than deliberate overdose. The usual scenario is characterized by patients who are prescribed high-dose salicylates and who then unwittingly supplement their prescription with OTC, aspirin-containing preparations.

The toxic effects of these OTC preparations should not be underestimated. For example, 60 mL of Pepto Bismol can produce a salicylate level of 4 mg/dL. Oil of wintergreen, which is sometimes used as an external liniment, contains 7000 mg of salicylate per teaspoon. Consequently, even small ingestions of oil of wintergreen can be fatal. When applied externally to a large surface area of the body, enough salicylate can be absorbed to produce toxic effects.

Although respiratory alkalosis is the most common initial finding in salicylate toxicity, just about any acid-base disturbance can be seen in adults. Mild dehydration, hypoglycemia, and noncardiac pulmonary edema are frequently part of the clinical picture. In chronic ingestions, progressive neurologic deterioration can be seen despite declining serum levels. Salicylates can become trapped in the brain; therefore, CNS levels may be high despite lower serum levels.

Confirmation of salicylate toxicity is made with laboratory measurement of serum aspirin levels. Although salicylate levels greater than 25 mg/dL predictably cause symptoms in most adults, lower levels can produce neuropsychiatric change in the elderly, especially in the presence of fever, dehydration, or renal dysfunction.

Treatment is directed at stabilization of the patient and enhancing elimination of the drug. Drug absorption is decreased by removing the drug with activated charcoal. Drug elimination is increased by urine alkalization or hemodialysis. Hemodialysis is indicated when the serum level is greater than 100 mg/dL for an acute ingestion or over 60 mg/dL in the case of chronic ingestion or when serious symptoms are present, including cardiac or renal failure, intractable acidosis, seizures, or severe fluid imbalance.

Substance Abuse. Stated simply, the elderly are not immune from drug abuse. In fact, many isolated elderly individuals can successfully conceal a severe drug abuse pattern. When social or medical circumstances change precipitously, signs of drug or alcohol withdrawal can present a confusing picture. Family members are often unaware of the abuse, and patients may be embarrassed to disclose a pattern of surreptitious drug consumption. Withdrawal symptoms in which delirium is the primary manifestation can occur when immobility or the presence of family members prevents access to drug sources, or when a companion who provided the patient with an addictive substance dies.

Once the diagnosis is confirmed, treatment is similar to that employed in younger patients. Clonidine can suppress the physiologic signs of withdrawal but may cause severe hypotension in the elderly; hence, it should be used with great caution.

Other Medications. Steroid-induced psychosis can result from the use of exogenous steroids. There is some evidence to suggest that this phenomenon may also occur with high endogenous cortisol levels in the elderly.[33-36] The hypothalamic-pituitary-adrenal axis deteriorates with age, thereby reducing susceptibility to stress in the geriatric patient. Trauma, burns, acute myocardial infarction, or recent surgery may produce enough endogenous cortisol to produce a reversible psychosis. Naturally, a history of prescription steroid medication use should suggest the diagnosis of steroid-induced delirium.

Finally, it should be emphasized that polypharmacy is the rule in the elderly. In this regard, multiple physician prescribing sources (cardiologist, urologist, neurologist, etc.) may lead to drug-drug interactions that can produce delirium.

Infection

Infection is a frequent cause of delirium in the elderly patient, with one study reporting infectious etiologies in 23% of elderly patients presenting with delirium.[16] Encapsulated bacteria such as *Streptococcus pneumoniae*, Group B *Streptococcus*, and *Escherichia coli* are common offending agents in the elderly, in whom they produce considerable mortality and morbidity.[40-41] In addition, the elderly are predisposed to infection (e.g., tuberculosis, listeriosis, legionella, and Herpes zoster) from intracellular organisms.

Urinary Tract Infection. Urinary tract infections (UTIs) are a common precipitant of delirium in the elderly. In men 65-70 years of age, the incidence of bacteriuria is 3%; this rises to 20% in men over 70 years.[39] The incidence in women 65-70 years of age is 20% and may be as high as 50% in those over the age of 80.[42] Elderly patients with a particular predisposition for acquiring UTIs include those with prostatic hypertrophy, cystocele, or neurogenic bladder, where a large post-void residual permits bacterial overgrowth. Among patients with indwelling catheters, urinary tract colonization is nearly universal, and infection is common. The risk of infection in the setting of an indwelling Foley catheter increases with time in a linear fashion, approaching 20% after two weeks and 50% after one month.[43]

Elderly patients with UTIs commonly present with limited urinary symptoms. Malaise, fatigue, fever, and confusion can dominate the clinical picture. Significant fever should suggest the possibility of sepsis, which is more common in chronically debilitated patients. Delirium can occur without fever, although other signs of sepsis, such as tachycardia or leukocytosis, may be present.

The urine usually shows the presence of white blood cells and bacteria. There is usually a leukocytosis, often with a left shift. Although *E. coli* is the most frequent pathogen isolated, *Proteus*, *Klebsiella*, *Enterobacter*, *Serratia* and *Pseudomonas* are frequently isolated in the elderly. Because the majority of the elderly will have complicated infections with organisms that may be resistant to many antimicrobial agents, urinary culture and sensitivity are important. In the patient who presents with delirium or fever, broad coverage with a third-generation cephalosporin, with or without aminoglycoside, is appropriate.

Pulmonary Infection. Pulmonary infections are the fifth leading cause of death in the elderly.[44] Nearly 80% of all deaths due to pneumonia are seen in the elderly population.[45] Not only are immunological defenses compromised with age, but an increase in lung-closing volume makes the lungs more susceptible to atelectasis and pneumonia, especially in patients who are supine for long periods.[46] In part, this accounts for the increased incidence of pneumonia that is observed after hip fracture and the decreased incidence in patients with early ambulation.

Pneumonia is a common infectious cause of delirium in the elderly, and it should be suspected in patients who present with fever, cough, and shortness of breath. Although chronic illness and advanced age can blunt these signs, the incidence of asymptomatic pneumonia is low.[47] Physical examination may be unreliable. Rales and rhonchi may be entirely absent, or they may be present chronically as a result of senile emphysema or chronic obstructive pulmonary disease.

A chest x-ray is mandatory in any elderly patient who presents with delirium, regardless of the pulmonary findings. A chest x-ray will confirm the diagnosis of pneumonia; however, false-negative radiographs occur in up to 15% of cases.[46] Moreover, the pattern of infiltrates may not be helpful in identifying an etiologic organism. For example, pneumococcal pneumonia in the elderly frequently presents as bronchopneumonia rather than in a more characteristic lobar pattern. Sputum is difficult to obtain but may be invaluable for the diagnosis. Up to 20% of pneumonias in the elderly may be due to mixed pathogens.[48] The most common etiologic agents include *Streptococcus pneumoniae*, *Haemophilus influenzae*, *Mycoplasma*, *Moraxella catarrhalis*, and gram-negative species such as *Klebsiella*.

Hospitalization is indicated for most elderly patients with pneumonia and in all patients who present with mental status changes. Prior use of antibiotics will increase gram-negative infections due to altered mouth flora. Beta-lactam therapy within the prior three

Table 1. Mini Mental Status Exam

Points		Max.
Orientation	date	5
	place	5
Registration	recall three objects	3
Attention	serial 7's, 'world' spelled backward, backward counting	5
Recall	three objects recalled later	3
Language	name pencil, wristwatch	2
	repeat "no if, ands, or buts"	1
	follow three-part command	3
	read and obey "close your eyes"	1
	write a sentence	1
	copy a design	1

SCORING

A score of 30 is considered normal. Scores are intended to monitor the patient's progress over time.

months is associated with the appearance of penicillin-resistant pneumococci.[48] Aspiration is associated with pneumonia due to *S. pneumoniae* and anaerobes. As is the case in alcoholics, *Klebsiella* is also common.

When available, sputum and Gram's stain should be used to guide antibiotic coverage. Community-acquired infections should be treated with a macrolide plus a second-generation cephalosporin, such as cefuroxime 1.5 g q 12h, or a third-generation agent, such as ceftriaxone 1-2 g q 12-24h. In hospital- or nursing home-acquired disease, or if the patient has underlying, complicating disease, two-drug coverage should be considered. Parenteral antibiotics are indicated for all patients with pulmonary infiltrates and mental status changes. Treatment should be continued for 14-21 days.

Sepsis. Confusion is one of the earliest signs of sepsis in the elderly patient. The reasons for altered mental status are multifactorial. Bacteremia associated with gram-negative organisms may be accompanied by the release of endotoxin and other chemotactic agents that produce profound physiologic changes, including hypoxia, hypotension, and mental status changes such as delirium. In many cases, the source of sepsis is readily identifiable. In the elderly, UTI, pneumonia, skin infections, and cholecystitis are the most common sources of bacteremia. Initial symptoms may be restricted to the aforementioned organ system, but progression to multi-organ system involvement may be rapid, especially in debilitated patients. In some patients, sepsis occurs in the absence of a primary source.

The diagnosis of sepsis in the setting of delirium may be complicated by the inability to obtain a reliable history that would help guide the clinician toward a source of infection. In addition, fever is inconsistently present in the elderly, in whom hypothermia may be the only sign of underlying infection. In this regard, a fever in excess of 40°C can cause clouding of consciousness and delirium, even in the normal functioning elderly. In individuals with underlying dementia or advanced age, minimal temperature elevations can cause delirium. Occasionally, administering antipyretics may help clear the patient's mental status.

Metabolic Derangements

Fluid and electrolyte imbalances represent the third most common cause of delirium in the elderly.[16] Among those metabolic conditions that can produce profound mental status changes, hyperosmolar non-ketotic coma (HNKC) is of special importance.

Patients with HNKC present with a decrease in mental status, poor skin turgor, and dry mucus membranes. Physical exam may reveal signs of underlying disease or the inciting cause. Laboratory data revealing an osmolality level greater than 350 mmol/L confirms the diagnosis.[49] An osmolality level greater than 400 mmol/L is associated with a poor prognosis. Level of consciousness is usually correlated with the serum and cerebral osmolality. Treatment is directed at fluid restoration.

Risk factors for dehydration are similar to those associated with hyperosmolar non-ketotic coma. Environmental heat exposure is a major risk to the elderly. In order to acclimate to a hot environment, individuals may dehydrate up to 1-2 liters. Moreover, the elderly have a diminished thirst reflex.

Hyponatremia occurs in water overload states, particularly congestive heart failure and conditions associated with excessive secretion of antidiuretic hormone (ADH). Hypoxia may be an important factor, although studies attempting to correlate hypoxia to postoperative delirium have been inconclusive.[50-52]

Hypoxia is an important cause of delirium in the elderly and may result from many conditions, including pneumonia, obstructive pulmonary disease, pulmonary embolism, and congestive heart failure. Therapy is directed at the underlying disorder.

Cardiopulmonary Disease

Except for pneumonia, pulmonary disease is not a common etiology for mental status changes. In patients with long-standing chronic obstructive pulmonary disease (COPD), however, acute retention of CO_2 can cause a depressed level of consciousness. The diagnosis of COPD is generally well-established, and there is usually an inciting event such as pneumonia or an increase in wheezing or mucus production. Deterioration is gradual except when supplemental oxygen is applied, causing the PCO_2 to increase rapidly in patients with hypoxic respiratory drive.

Hypoxia can also cause mental status changes, but when this occurs chronically, it is well-tolerated. Patients with normal baseline function and normal oxygen-carrying capacity should tolerate a PO_2 level as low as 60 mmHg without mental status changes.

Acute Pulmonary Embolism. Acute pulmonary embolism may be extremely difficult to diagnose. Small recurrent pulmonary emboli are particularly difficult to detect and may present with only transient periods of confusion. Tachycardia and dyspnea may be overlooked or dismissed as part of bizarre behavior. Abnormal pulse oximetry or arterial blood gases during an episode of confusion should alert the physician to the possibility of pulmonary embolism. However, some cases of small, recurrent pulmonary emboli may produce little or no change in PO_2 or oximetry. The diagnosis is established by standard ventilation/perfusion scans. When these are indeterminate, pulmonary angiography may be necessary.

Hypotension. Regardless of the etiology, hypotension will decrease delivery of necessary substrates to the brain, producing mental status changes. While significant hypotension may be tolerated in a healthy young person, the elderly have little reserve, and a moderate insult may lead to rapid decrease in blood pressure and loss of consciousness. While hypotension is typically detected at the time of triage into the ED, elderly patients can develop hypotension while in the ED. When a previously oriented person becomes combative, sedated, or confused, a recheck of vital signs and repeat physical exam are indicated. Rapid correction of the hypotension with fluids and pressors, if indicated, will stabilize the patient until the cause(s) of the hypotension can be corrected.

Central Nervous System Disease. Except for dementia, structural abnormalities of the CNS represent an unusual cause of acute delirium. Chronic subdural hematoma can cause delirium in the elderly; however, it is more likely to cause dementia. With age, the brain shrinks, stretching the bridging vessels. Minor trauma causes shearing of the bridging vessels and may produce slow bleeding, resulting in a subdural hematoma. The trauma may be forgotten or not disclosed. Abuse of the elderly should always be considered. Patients with history of a head injury, evidence of abuse, or a history of alcoholism should have a CT scan performed.

Cerebrovascular Disease. Stroke is common in the elderly and may present with profound mental status changes, including delirium, focal neurological deficits, or focal impairments. Thrombotic stroke in the non-dominant hemisphere, particularly in the perisylvian cortex, can cause delirium without focal neurologic impairment.

Psychiatric Disease. Except for depression, new-onset psychiatric disease is unusual in the geriatric patient. Hence, psychiatric conditions should be a diagnosis of last resort when evaluating a confused elderly person. However, psychosocial changes in the environment can exacerbate symptoms of delirium and dementia. Mild-to-moderate delirium can worsen as a result of impaired vision or hearing. Unfamiliar environments (i.e., noisy, crowded EDs), loss of day/night orientation, and an endless stream of new faces and procedures may produce behavioral and cognitive deterioration.

ED Assessment

Transient Delirium. In some cases, delirium may be a transient event caused by hypoglycemia, hypotension, or a seizure disorder. These patients may present with a wide range of symptoms, including decreased level of consciousness, confusion, or agitation. Transient ischemic attacks and postictal states should be considered in the differential diagnosis. Petit mal seizures, although uncommon, can cause periodic episodes of confusion.[53] In fact, up to 12% of the elderly with grand mal seizures will not display active tonic-clonic movements.[53] In these patients, post-ictal confusion is a difficult diagnosis to confirm. The key to the diagnosis is continued improvement of confusion followed by confirmation of a seizure disorder. Patients with dysrhythmias also may experience transient decreases in cerebral blood flow and present with transient confusion.

Table 2. Confusion Assessment Method

ACUTE ONSET AND FLUCTUATING COURSE AND INATTENTION
Evidence of an acute change from baseline
Behavior increasing or decreasing in severity
Difficulty focusing attention
Easily distracted
Difficulty keeping track of what was said
OR
DISORGANIZED THINKING AND ALTERED LEVEL OF CONSCIOUSNESS
Rambling or irrelevant conversation
Unclear or illogical flow of ideas
Unpredictable switching from subject to subject
Hyperalertness or lethargy

Patients whose delirium resolves in the ED should be watched for at least 1-2 hours to ensure this is not a fluctuation in their delirious episode. In general, however, delirium does not completely clear to baseline and then recur. Patients who remain at baseline may be safe for discharge depending on the suspected underlying cause of the episode. A patient with hypoglycemia may be discharged after treatment, whereas patients who experience a new seizure or transient ischemic attack may require hospitalization to initiate workup.

Assessment Tools for ED Evaluation of Altered Mental Status. It should be stressed that delirium represents a constellation of abnormal cognitive signs and symptoms, many that can be considered "soft." In this regard, families may complain that their relative has been confused, or "not themselves." In the ED, however, the clinician may encounter only a passive, compliant patient whose loss in mental faculties may represent chronic deterioration. As a result, the challenge of distinguishing between acute cognitive deterioration and baseline mental status impairments is a priority when evaluating this patient subgroup.

Unfortunately, there are few adequate screening tests that are able to detect mental function abnormalities and, in particular, that will reliably differentiate exacerbation of chronic dementia from acute delirium. Perhaps the best known test is the Mini-Mental Status Exam.[17] *(Please see Table 1.)* Similar to the Glasgow Coma Scale, this screening tool detects problems in cognitive function and can be used over time to detect fluctuations. It is easy to perform and is easily remembered. However, it cannot confirm the cause(s) of the mental function abnormality, nor can it distinguish dementia from delirium.

A second screening tool that may be more helpful in distinguishing delirium from dementia, but is more complex to administer, is called the Confusion Assessment Method.[38] *(Please see Table 2.)* It is based upon a diagnostic algorithm, has a high sensitivity and specificity for the detection of delirium (> 90%), and its interobserver reliability is especially good.[54] However, its usefulness in the ED may be limited.

It appears as if delirium is under-diagnosed in the emergency setting. A recent study reported on a group of 385 patients presenting to an urban ED.[55] All patients were screened for delirium using the

Table 3. Sedating Drugs to Decrease Agitation in the Elderly

DRUG	DOSE	FREQUENCY	SIDE EFFECTS
Haloperidol	0.5-2.0 mg IM IV PO	every 30-60 min	orthostatic hypotension, decrease in seizure threshold, dystonic reaction, neuroleptic malignant syndrome
Droperidol	5 mg IM IV	every 30 min	same as haloperidol
Lorazepam	0.5-1.0 mg IM	every 60 min	respiratory depression, orthostatic hypotension
Phenobarbital	150-100 mg IM IV	every 60 min	cardiovascular and respiratory depression

Confusion Assessment Method as well as the Mini Mental Status Exam and the Geriatric Depression Scale. In this study, 10% of ED patients 65 years of age or older had screening scores consistent with delirium. Yet, the diagnosis of delirium was made in only 17% of patients with these positive screens. Interestingly, 62% of patients with positive screens were admitted, usually with a diagnosis of infection. Of those who were discharged, nearly half were diagnosed as "status post-fall—no significant injury."

Emergency physicians are not the only clinicians demonstrating difficulties recognizing delirium in the elderly patient. Primary care physicians also fail to recognize this condition in a significant percentage of patients.[56] Other studies have shown that 32-67% of cases go unrecognized.[38] In many cases, the cause is apparent but the delirium is overlooked or dismissed as part of the disease process. For example, most experienced emergency physicians have come to expect delirium in a seriously infected elderly patient. At other times, the diagnosis is missed in the hypoactive patient.[38] The hyperactive patient poses a danger to himself and attracts attention, while the quiet one may be overlooked. Perhaps the biggest obstacle to recognizing delirium in the ED is lack of baseline information. Who is delirious, and who is demented? Inadequate information about the baseline may be volitional on the part of the family/caretaker in order to attain a reprieve from care.

When these assessment problems arise, screening tools may be helpful. In this regard, the Confusion Assessment Method appears to be able not only to detect acute delirium in the previously well patient but is also fairly accurate at detecting delirium in the demented patient.[57] It is probably best to employ these methods in cases where the baseline status is in doubt. However, no screening tool is perfect.

Targeted Management Principles

Appropriate treatment measures should be initiated in the elderly patient with altered mental status while the initial evaluation is proceeding. In this regard, supplemental oxygen, antipyretic measures, and fluid replacement if dehydration is detected should be accomplished early in the patient encounter. Initial stabilization of airway, breathing, and circulation always take priority.

As far as therapy for rapidly reversible conditions, hypoglycemia should always be considered in insulin-requiring diabetics. Although rare, insulinoma and aspirin overdose also may present with hypoglycemia. Rapid bedside assessment of serum glucose or, when appropriate, empiric administration of 25 cc of 50% dextrose should be considered in all elderly patients with acute altered mental status. Although empiric glucose administration can increase the osmolality rate in patients with hyperglycemia, this is preferable to prolonged hypoglycemia. Clinical judgment should prevail.

Narcotic abuse is occasionally encountered in the elderly patient. Intentional narcotic overdose can occur in the setting of suicide attempts, especially in elderly, depressed males with terminal conditions.[58] It can also occur when patients ingest the wrong medication and from OTC medications such as dextromethorphan.[59] Consequently, it is prudent to consider a trial of naloxone in all elderly patients with altered mental status.[60,61] Flumazenil can be used to reverse the sedative effects of benzodiazepines. However, this drug should be used with caution since it also reverses any protective effect that benzodiazepines may have on seizure threshold, especially in patients with concomitant tricyclic antidepressant overdose. As a result, use of this agent should be limited to patients with severe benzodiazepine overdose who have not ingested any other substances.

History. Once these initial interventions are completed and the patient is stabilized, the history should be directed at establishing the following: 1) the pre-existing (i.e., baseline) mental status; 2) the pattern and rapidity of the mental status change onset; 3) an assessment of safety measures that may be required in the ED environment (i.e., the need for restraints or sedatives); 4) assessment of rapport with family members; 5) identifying possible precipitating causes of the mental status change; and 6) identifying home needs, if the patient is suitable for discharge.

In particular, the history should be directed at deciphering possible causes of the mental status change. A complete medication history is vital, as is documentation of OTC medication use. Any history of alcohol abuse or use is important. It is also imperative to establish how well the informant knows the patient. During the history, the physician should assess the patient and surroundings to ensure safety precautions are in place. The side rails of the hospital stretcher should be up at all times. Attention to the environment by all caregivers is important.

A thorough physical exam is mandatory and may yield clues that may explain the patient's mental changes. Particular emphasis should be placed on the neurologic exam and the mini mental status exam that is used to document the patient's current level of function. *(Please see Table 1.)*

Restraints. Elderly patients who present with delirium tend to present with hyperactivity or hypoactivity. The hyperactive patient frequently poses an immediate management challenge. When required, both physical and chemical restraints should be available for more aggressive control of patients. Soft restraints such as a posey will remind a patient to remain in bed. For patients with severe delirium, wrist restraints assist in keeping the patient in bed and prevent dismantling of dressings, tubes, and other restraining devices. More aggressive maneuvers, such as leather restraints or four-point restraints, are rarely needed and should be used only for patient safety. In some states, the use of restraints requires a physician order and adequate physician documentation establishing the need for the restraint accompanied by frequent (every 15 minutes) documented visual checks of the patient.

Generally speaking, the use of aggressive restraints suggests the need for chemical sedation. Physical restraints may frighten family members as well as visitors and other patients, especially when accompanied by loud verbal protests from the patient. Explain the reason for the restraints in a loud clear voice that all in close proximity can hear. Although this rarely penetrates the patient's delirium, it may relieve the concerns of others in the ED.

If it is determined that restraints are needed, chemical restraints are usually preferable to physical restraints. The goals of treatment are to inhibit dangerous behavior and calm the patient in order to complete the necessary evaluation. Unfortunately, most sedating drugs (e.g., haloperidol, droperidol) have anticholinergic or extrapyramidal side effects that, on occasion, may exacerbate the delirium. Moreover, many of these agents may cause hypotension or produce undesirable cardiac or respiratory effects. Medications useful for behavorial control of elderly patients with acute delirium are outlined in Table 3.

Laboratory Evaluation. Because the differential diagnosis is extensive, the ED physician is often tempted to take a shotgun approach to laboratory workup of the elderly patient with mental status changes. However, the history and initial physical exam may direct the laboratory workup and permit a more cost-effective, targeted approach. Clearly, if the diagnosis remains in doubt, a tiered approach to laboratory assessment may be the most productive strategy. *(Please see Table 4.)*

In these patients, a screening battery might include a CBC and differential, BUN, creatinine, electrolytes, alcohol level, urinalysis, chest x-ray, and pulse oximetry. An ECG is mandatory since older patients with acute myocardial infarction may present with confusion as part of the initial clinical picture. If these initial tests are normal, urine and serum toxicology screens as well as a CT scan should be considered. The CT scans may be especially helpful if there is a focal neurologic finding or history of head trauma.[62] Although abnormal findings are frequent, they are generally chronic in nature.[34,63]

If the etiology of delirium is still in doubt after the initial database is reviewed, an arterial blood gas, calcium, magnesium, and phosphate levels, as well as thyroid function studies can be sent to the laboratory. In patients with fever or leukocytosis, blood cultures should be drawn and a lumbar puncture considered. In the absence of fever, lumbar puncture is not particularly helpful, although the presence of immune deficiency or HIV infection will improve the yield of this procedure.[64] In the past, EEG has been suggested to assist in the diagnosis of delirium. However, in clinical practice, it has a high false-negative and false-positive rate, and its usefulness in the acute setting is unproven. Newer techniques using serial quantitative EEG may be more promising.[65]

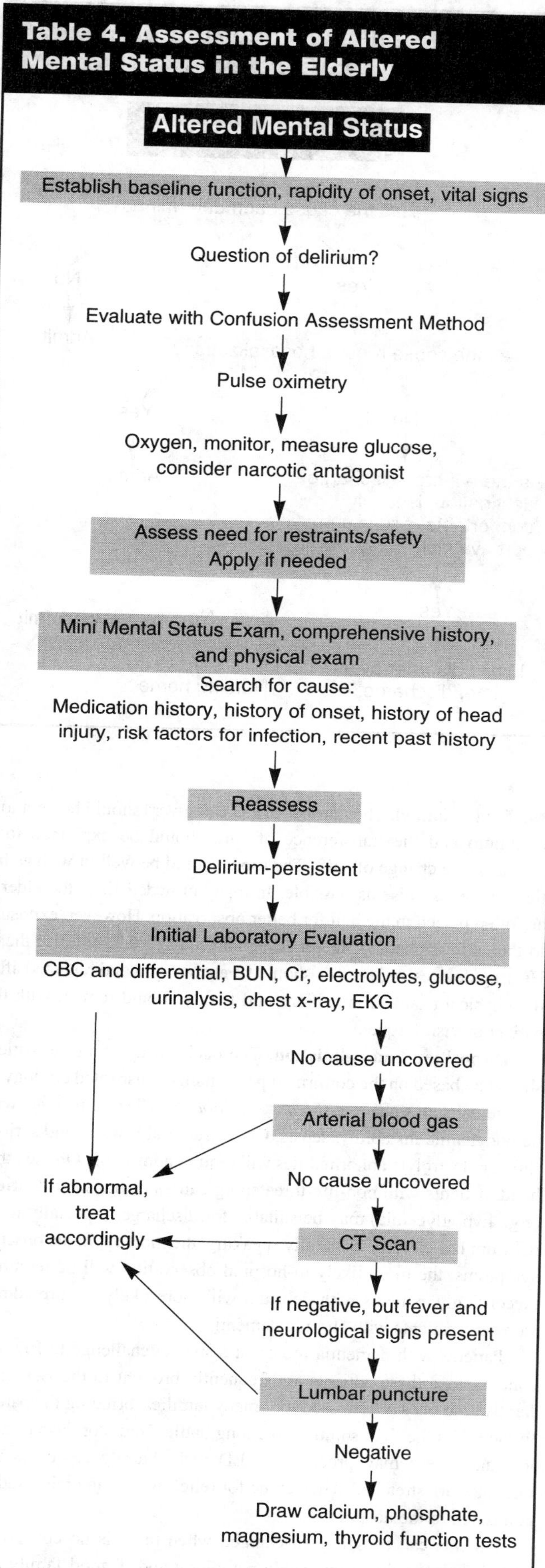

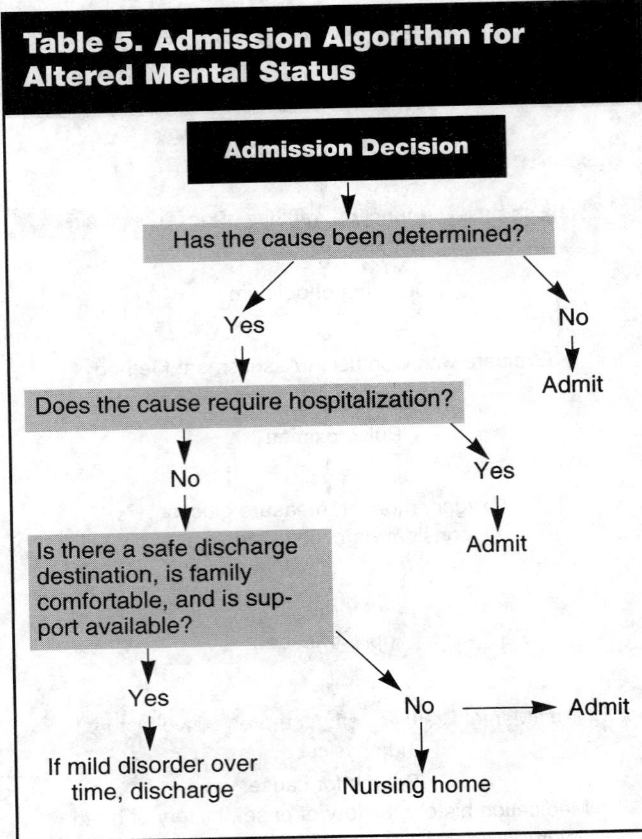

Table 5. Admission Algorithm for Altered Mental Status

ED Personnel. The number of ED caregivers should be kept to a minimum and the transference of care should be explained to a patient at the change of shift. The room should be well lit with as little extraneous noise as possible. In many crowded EDs, the elderly are often placed in the hall for better observation. However, exposure to the endless chaos of the environment may further confuse them. Hearing devices and glasses should be encouraged and replaced after the physical exam. Companions and family should remain with the patient or visit frequently.

Disposition and Admission. The decision to admit the patient should be based on the confirmed precipitant or suspected etiology of the mental status change. *(Please see Table 5.)* Clearly, patients with hemodynamic instability, sepsis, CNS structural lesions, and serious fluid or electrolyte abnormalities will require admission. On the other hand, patients with non-life-threatening causes of transient delirium (e.g., hypoglycemia) may be suitable for discharge, especially if the delirium has cleared. Generally speaking, the more rapid the onset of symptoms, the more likely in-hospital observation will be required. Accordingly, patients with delirium will more likely require admission than patients with chronic dementia.

Patients with dementia represent a special challenge to ED personnel, since these patients are frequently brought to the ED when family resources are stressed. For many families, bringing the patient to the ED is the final solution to a long battle. Hours or days of anxiety and stress may precede the ED visit. Family resources and tolerance are stretched. They come for relief, which, in their mind, is admission to the hospital.

Patients can be safely discharged when there is no concern of underlying significant reversible pathology and if good family and community support services are immediately available. Increasingly, insurance gatekeepers will apply pressure to reduce hospital use in these and other cases.

Summary

The elderly patient with altered mental status represents a clinical challenge for the ED physician. Many social, psychiatric, environmental, and medical problems must be managed simultaneously. The diagnostic evaluation must be systematic and thorough. Attempts to distinguish between acute delirium and exacerbation of chronic dementia are pivotal the the decision-making process. Appropriate laboratory examinations followed by targeted radiographic examination will frequently yield a diagnosis. In addition, it should be stressed that delirium is usually the result of underlying processes such as infection, drug toxicity, or metabolic derangements. Finally, the ED physician is required to make appropriate decisions about who will benefit from acute medical care and who will need respite care—a triage call that is not easy to make based on a brief clinical encounter.

References

1. Sirois F. Delirium: 100 cases. *Can J Psychiatry* 1988;33:375.
2. Lipowski ZJ. Update on delirium. *Psychiatr Clin North Am* 1992;15:335.
3. Itil T, Fink M. Anticholinergic drug-induced delirium: Experimental modification, quantitative EEG, and behavioral correlations. *J Nerv Ment Dis* 1966;143:492.
4. Engel GL, Romano J. Delirium, a syndrome of cerebral insufficiency. *J Chronic Dis* 1959;9:260.
5. Kral VA. Confusional states. In: Howells JG, ed. *Modern Perspectives in the Psychiatry of Old Age.* New York: Brunner/Mazel; 1975:356-362
6. Lipowski AJ. *Delirium: Acute Confusional States.* New York: Oxford University Press; 1990.
7. Koponen H, Stenback U, Mattila E, et al. CSF beta-endorphin immunoreactivity in delirium. *Biol Psychiatry* 1989;25:938.
8. Beresin EV. Delirium in the elderly. *J Geriatr Psychiatry Neurol* 1988;1:127.
9. Gillick MR, Serrell NA, Gillick LS. Adverse consequences of hospitalization in the elderly. *Sci Med* 1982;16:1033.
10. Linnoila M. Alcohol withdrawal and noradrenergic function. *Ann Intern Med* 1987;107:875.
11. *Diagnostic and Statistical Manual of Mental Disorders*, 3rd ed. revised. Washington DC: American Psychiatric Association; 1987.
12. Francis J, Martin D, Kapoor WN. A prospective study of delirium in hospitalized elderly. *JAMA* 1990;263:1097.
13. Rockwood K. Acute confusion in elderly medical patients. *J Am Geriatr Soc* 1989;37:150.
14. Seymour DG, Henschke PJ, Cape RDT, et al. Acute confusional states and dementia in the elderly: The role of dehydration/volume depletion, physical illness and age. *Age Aging* 1980;9:137.
15. Francis J, Kapoor WN. Delirium in hospitalized elderly. *J Gen Intern Med* 1990;5:65.

16. Rockwood K. The occurrence and duration of symptoms in elderly patients with delirium. *J Gerontol* 1993;48:M162.
17. Kolbeinsson H, Jonsson A. Delirium and dementia in acute medical admissions of elderly patients in Iceland. *Acta Psychiatr Scand* 1993;87:123.
18. Inneichen B. Measuring the rising tide. How many dementia cases will there be by 2001? *Br J Psychiatry* 1987;150:193.
19. Purdie FR, Honigman B, Rosen P. Acute organic brain syndrome: A review of 100 cases. *Ann Emerg Med* 1981;10:455.
20. Davies P, Terry RD. Cortical somatostatin-like immunoreactivity in cases of Alzheimer's disease and senile dementia of the Alzheimer type. *Neurobiol Aging* 1981;2:9.
21. Aronin N, Cooper PE, Lorentz LJ, et al. Somatostatin is increased in the basal ganglia in Huntington disease. *Ann Neurol* 1983;13:519.
22. Vecsei L, Widerlov E. Preclinical and clinical studies with somatostatin related to the central nervous system. *Prog Neuropsychopharmacol Biol Psychiatry* 1990;14:473.
23. Koponen HJ, Leinonen E, Lepola U, et al. A long-term follow-up study of cerebrospinal fluid somatostatin in delirium. *Acta Psychiatr Scand* 1994;89:329.
24. Kowall NW, Beal MF. Cortical somatostatin, neuropeptide Y and NADPH diaphorase neurons: Normal anatomy and alterations in Alzheimer's disease. *Ann Neurol* 1988;23:105.
25. Gomez S, Puymirat J, Valade P, et al. Patients with Alzheimer's disease show an increased content of 15 kDalton somatostatin precursor and lowered level of tetradecapeptide in their cerebrospinal fluid. *Life Sci* 1986;39:623.
26. Fauci AS, Lane C. The acquired immunodeficiency Syndrome (AIDS). In: Wilson JD, Braunwal LE, Isselbacher KJ, et al. *Harrison's Principles of Internal Medicine. 12th ed.* New York: McGraw Hill 1991;1406.
27. Liskow BI, Rinck C, Campbell J, et al. Alcohol withdrawal in the elderly. *J Stud Alcohol* 1989;50:414.
28. Bower KJ, Mudd S, Blow FC, et al. Severity and treatment of alcohol withdrawal in elderly versus younger patients. *Alcohol Clin Exp Res* 1994;18:196.
29. Feuerlein W, Reiser E. Parameters affecting the course and results of delirium tremens treatment. *Acta Psychiatr Scand* 1986;73(suppl 329):120.
30. Jarrett PG, Rockwood K, Carver D, et al. Illness presentation in elderly patients. *Arch Intern Med* 1995;155:1060.
31. Francis J, Strong S, Martin D, et al. Delirium in elderly general medical patients: Common but often unrecognized. *Clin Res* 1988;36:771A.
32. Williams MA, Ward SE, Campbell ED. Confusion: Testing versus observation. *J Gerontol Nurs* 1986;14:25.
33. Purdie FR, Honigman B, Rosen P. Acute organic brain syndrome: A review of 100 cases. *Ann Emerg Med* 1981;10:455.
34. Moses H, Van Kaden BA. Neurologic consultations in a general hospital: Spectrum of iatrogenic disease. *Am J Med* 1986; 81:955.
35. The Medical Letter. Drugs that cause psychiatric symptoms. *Med Lett Drugs Ther* 1989;31:113.
36. Larson ME, Kukell WA, Buchner D, et al. Adverse drug reactions associated with global cognitive impairment in elderly persons. *Ann Intern Med* 1987;107:169.
37. Snavely SR, Hodges GR. The neurotoxity of antibacterial medicine. *Ann Intern Med* 1984;101:92.
38. Inouye SK. The dilemma of delirium: Clinical and research controversies regarding diagnosis and evaluation of delirium in hospitalized elderly medical patients. *Am J Med* 1994; 97:278.
39. Blazer DG, Federspiel CF, Ray WA, et al. The risk of anticholinergic toxicity in the elderly: A study of prescribing practices in two populations. *J Gerontol* 1983;38:31.
40. Walford RL. Studies in immunogerontology. Henderson award lecture. *J Am Geriatr Soc* 1982;30:617.
41. Plewa MC. Altered host response and special infections in the elderly. *Emerg Clin North Am* 1990;8:193.
42. Salzman RL, Peterson PK. Immunodeficiency of the elderly. *Rev Infect Dis* 1987;9:1127.
43. Schneider EL. Infectious diseases in the elderly. *Ann Intern Med* 1983;98:395.
44. LaCroiz AZ, Lipson S, Miles TP, et al. Prospective study of pneumonia hospitalizations and mortality of U.S. older people: The role of chronic conditions, health benefits, and nutritional status. *Public Health Rep* 1989;104:350.
45. Centers for Disease Control. (Pneumonia and influenza mortality—United States, 1988-1989 season.*) Morb Mortal Wkly Rep* 1989;38:97.
46. Sims RV. Bacterial pneumonia in the elderly. *Emerg Clin North Am* 1990;8:207.
47. Fedullo AJ, Swinburne AJ. Relationship of patient age to clinical features and outcome for in-hospital treatment of pneumonia. *J Gerontol* 1985;40:29.
48. Verghese A, Berk SL. Bacterial pneumonia in the elderly. *Clin Rep Aging* 1989;3:1.
49. Daugirdas JT, Kronfol NO, Tzamaloukas AH, et al. Hyperosmolar coma: Cellular dehydration and serum sodium concentration. *Ann Intern Med* 1989;110:855.
50. Neilson WR, Gelb AW, Casey JE, et al. Long-term cognitive and social sequelae of general versus regional anesthesia during arthroplasty in the elderly. *Anesthesiology* 1990;73:1103.
51. Moller JT, Svennild I, Johannessen NW. Association between intraoperative pulse oximetry monitoring and postoperative cognitive function. *Br J Anaesth* 1993;71:340.
52. Hornbein TF, Townes BD, Schoene RB, et al. The cost to the central nervous system of climbing to extremely high altitudes. *N Engl J Med* 1989;321:1714.
53. Francis J, Kapoor WN. Delirium in hospitalized elderly. *J Gen Intern Med* 1990;5:65.
54. Inouye SK, van Dyck CH, Alessi CA, et al. Clarifying confusion: The confusion assessment method. *Ann Intern Med* 1990;113:941.
55. Lewis LM, Miler DK, Morley JE, et al. Unrecognized delirium in ED geriatric patients. *Am J Emerg Med* 1995;13:142.
56. Johnson JC, Kerse NM, Gottlieb G, et al. Prospective versus retrospective methods of identifying patients with delirium. *J Am Geriatr Soc* 1992;40:316.
57. Edmonds HL Jr, Griffiths LK, Van der Laken J, et al. Quantitative electroencephalographic monitoring during myocardial revascularization predicts postoperative disorientation and improves outcome. *J Thorac Cardiovasc Surg* 1992;103:555.
58. Ellenhorn MJ, Barceloux DG. Medical Toxicology. New

York: Elsevier 1988; 99-100.

59. Schneider SM, Michelson EA, Boucek CD, et al. Unusual presentation of dextromethorphan poisoning. *Am J Emerg Med* 1991;9:237.
60. Sorensen SC, Matteson K. Naloxone as an antagonist in severe alcohol intoxication. *Lancet* 1978;2:688.
61. Nuotto E, Palva ES, Lahdenranta U. Naloxone fails to counteract heavy alcohol intoxication. *Lancet* 1983;2:167.
62. Francis J, Kapoor WN. Acute mental change: When are head scans needed? *Clin Res* 1991;39:575A.
63. Koponen H, Hurri L, Stenback U, Riekkinen PJ. Acute confusional states in the elderly: A radiological evaluation. *Acta Psychiatr Scand* 1987;76:726.
64. Wolfson L, Katzman R. The neurologic consultation at age 80. In: Katzman R, Rowe JW, eds. *Principles of Geriatric Neurology.* Philadelphia: FA Davis; 1992:339-355
65. Jacobson SA, Leuchter AF, Walter DO, et al. Serial quantitative EEG among elderly subjects with delirium. *Biol Psychiatry* 1993;34:135.

Toxicologic Syndromes in the Elderly

Suzanne K. Elliott, MD
Richard Y. Wang, DO, FACEP, DACMT

Toxicologic syndromes in the elderly can refer to a wide range of specific signs or symptoms that occur in this population as a result of exposure to both toxins and prescribed medications. These syndromes are produced by either direct effects associated with medication intake or from withdrawal symptoms, both of which can lead to potentially dangerous outcomes ranging from confusion and syncope to delirium and seizures.

Generally speaking, these adverse drug reactions (ADRs) tend to occur more frequently and are associated with increased mortality with advancing age.[1,2] The overall incidence of ADRs in geriatric patients varies from 5.6-10.0%.[3] However, the true incidence may be underestimated because patients and physicians may fail to recognize varied and subtle presentations of drug-mediated pathology. It is estimated that 70-80% of ADRs are dose related.[3,4] In fact, the problem is more widespread than is widely appreciated. In one German study, 12% of the elderly had been given at least one prescription that failed to consider either age-related changes in renal function, clinical illness resulting from drug effects, contraindications, or the effects of co-existing diseases.[5]

Interestingly, about 75% of all ADRs in elderly patients are associated with four classes of drugs: cardiovascular, central nervous system (CNS), non-steroidal anti-inflammatory drugs (NSAIDs), and gastrointestinal (GI) agents.[6] An estimated 3-8% of all hospital admissions are associated with ADRs; in the geriatric population, the proportion of admissions associated with drug-related adverse events increases to 10-12%.[3,7] Aspirin, NSAIDs, and cardiovascular drugs comprised 91% of the ADRs necessitating hospital admissions in one study.[7]

Since the majority of these patients present to the emergency department (ED), it is critical for clinicians practicing in this setting to identify and manage toxicologic syndromes related to medication use. This can be difficult in the elderly because the clinical manifestations of ADRs are varied and can easily be attributed to other diseases. *(Please see Table 1.)* This chapter presents a symptom-oriented approach to the management of this challenging patient population.

The Elderly: A Population at Risk

Elderly patients with chronic illnesses are at high risk for drug toxicity. An average of 3-5 chronic medical conditions coexist in ambulatory elderly Americans, while in those institutionalized, this increases to 10.[8] Studies suggest that patients with concurrent illnesses who are in poor health may be more susceptible to ADRs because they lack the necessary physiologic reserve to compensate for drug-induced insults.[4] Other age-related risk factors for drug toxicity include physical impairments such as poor eyesight and diminished dexterity, which can interfere with reading prescription labels and opening containers. Failing memory can be responsible

Table 1. Selected Agents and Their Toxicologic Syndromes in Geriatric Patients

ANTICHOLINERGIC MEDICATIONS

- Tachycardia
- Elevated temperature
- Delirium
- Lethargy
- Mydriasis
- Flushed skin
- Dry mucous membranes
- Diminished bowel sounds
- Urinary retention

ANTIHYPERTENSIVE MEDICATIONS (CENTRAL ALPHA-ADRENERGIC AGONIST)

- Lethargy
- Miosis
- Respiratory depression with periods of apnea
- Bradycardia
- Hypotension (late)

CARDIAC GLYCOSIDES (DIGOXIN)

- Disorientation
- Syncope
- Visual color aberrations
- Nausea
- Vomiting
- Bradycardia
- Hypotension
- Atrioventricular nodal block
- Ventricular dysrhythmia

CHOLINERGIC MEDICATIONS

- Tachypnea
- Tachycardia
- Bradycardia
- Salivation
- Lacrimation
- Urination
- Diarrhea
- Vomiting
- Bronchospasm
- Fasciculations
- Weakness

LITHIUM

- Delirium
- Lethargy
- Diarrhea
- Hyperreflexia
- Tremor
- Myoclonus
- Ataxia
- Methylxanthine:
- Tachycardia
- Hypertension followed by hypotension
- Nausea
- Vomiting
- Abdominal pain
- Delirium
- Leukocytosis
- Lactic acidosis
- Hyperglycemia
- Hypokalemia

OPIOIDS

- Lethargy
- Miosis
- Respiratory depression
- Diminished bowel activity

SALICYLATES

- Tachypnea
- Hyperpnea
- Elevated temperature
- Nausea
- Vomiting
- Tinnitus
- Delirium
- Lethargy
- Respiratory alkalosis
- Anion-gapped metabolic acidosis

SYMPATHOMIMETIC MEDICATIONS

- Tachycardia
- Hypertension
- Elevated temperature
- Delirium
- Diaphoresis
- Hyperactive bowel sounds
- Leukocytosis
- Lactic acidosis
- Hyperglycemia
- Hypokalemia

for either excessive consumption of medications or failure to take them as prescribed.[9,10]

In addition, the elderly are at a greater risk for toxic drug effects because of physiologic changes that occur with the aging process. There is a notable decrease in total body water, muscle mass, plasma proteins, and an increase in body fat. This leads to a smaller volume of distribution and a higher plasma drug concentration for water-soluble drugs.[11-13] Toxic drug effects may also be potentiated as a result of diminished hepatic and renal function. In the liver, these changes are the result of decreased hepatic mass and blood flow, as well as a reduction in some enzymatic processes.[11,13,14] Hepatic blood flow decreases by an estimated 40-45% in the elderly, and this is in part due to diminished cardiac output.[5] The combination of these changes makes the elderly more susceptible to toxic effects of hepatically metabolized drugs such as diazepam, propranolol, and morphine.[14,15]

Generally speaking, glomerular filtration, renal tubular secretion, and renal blood flow naturally decrease with age.[16] Average renal function is reduced by about 50% at the age of 90.[17] Because of decreasing muscle mass with age, a decrease in glomerular filtration usually is not accompanied by an increase in serum creatinine. Consequently, serum creatinine is not an accurate measure of renal function in the elderly.[5,16] Aminoglycoside, digoxin, atenolol, and lithium toxicity can result from reduced renal clearance.[14] Renal function in elderly patients, especially those with decreased effective circulating blood volume (i.e., patients with congestive heart failure) is strongly dependent on prostaglandin-mediated blood flow, which may be inhibited by NSAIDs and can produce further deterioration.[2]

Central Nervous System Syndromes

Assessment and Differential Diagnosis. Assessment and management of altered mental status and confusion in the elderly patient represent important and common clinical problems. The delirious patient is characterized by the acute onset of diffuse impairment of cognitive function, clouding of consciousness, behavioral agitation, or hallucinations. The physician must be able to discern organic from functional causes, because medical processes have a higher rate of mortality than psychiatric disorders.[18] The large spectrum of medical conditions causing agitated delirium include metabolic (e.g., hypoglycemia, hyponatremia), structural, infectious, vascular, traumatic, neurologic, and toxicologic disorders. Drug toxicity was the most commonly identified cause of delirium in one review of patients older than 70 years.[11] Alzheimer's, Parkinson's disease, and cerebrovascular accidents predisposed these patients to delirium and may serve as risk factors.[11]

Delirium. In one important study, delirium, toxic psychosis, and depression accounted for 50% of the ADRs that were admitted to the psychiatric unit.[19] All implicated medications were psychopharmacologic agents (e.g., neuroleptics, antidepressants, benzodiazepines, and anti-Parkinson's), except in two instances in which digoxin and an antiepileptic agent were the causative agents.[19] Medications with anticholinergic effects are more commonly associated with delirium in later life than any other drug class.[20] Some of these agents include the anti-Parkinson's drugs, cycloplegics, Type IA antiarrhythmics, cyclic antidepressants, antihistamines, and neuroleptics.[8] *(Please see Table 2.)*

Given the wide range of drugs producing toxicity in the elderly,the clinician must inquire about over-the-counter (OTC) and ophthalmic drug use during the initial evaluation. In this regard, diphenhydramine, scopolamine, and phenylpropanolamine contained in OTC medications are important causes of delirium.[11] Parasympatholytic ophthalmic agents (e.g., tropicamide [Mydriacyl]) also have been associated with anticholinergic psychosis.[8]

Typical manifestations of anticholinergic toxicity include dry mucocutaneous membranes, mydriasis, diminished bowel sounds, urinary retention, and hallucinations.[21] Central anti-cholinergic findings range from sedation, mild confusion, and inability to concentrate to marked agitated delirium. The relative cholinergic deficit accompanying normal aging may explain the increased sensitivity to drugs blocking central muscarinic receptors in this population.[8]

Among hospitalized patients in one investigation, opioids were found to be the leading cause of drug-induced delirium.[11]

This was followed by benzodiazepines, anticholinergics, NSAIDs, and alcohol or sedative-hypnotic withdrawal.[11] Multiple cases of reversible delirium or cognitive dysfunction have been reported with benzodiazepine use in the elderly, especially at higher doses. Some of these manifestations included hallucinations, bizarre behavior, psychosis, nightmares, amnesia, and impulsive actions.[15,22]

Sedative-hypnotics were noted to be the most common cause of delirium from an ADR in patients older than 60. [23] As a rule, emergency physicians should avoid the use benzodiazepines with long half-lives—and, possibly, those agents metabolized by microsomal oxidation—in the elderly because of diminished liver function in this subgroup and the propensity to accumulate medication. It should be noted that these agents can result in toxicity even at therapeutic dosing. Confusion has been observed with a number of benzodiazepines, including triazolam, flurazepam, diazepam, and chlordiazepoxide.[12,21]

Finally, salicylate intoxication should also be considered in any elderly patient with unexplained confusion and an acid-base disorder. Age-related renal insufficiency and diminished oral intake of fluids can contribute to salicylate toxicity in this population.[16] Confusion, anxiety, and insomnia also have all been associated with NSAID use.[24] These agents include naproxen and ibuprofen, both of which are now available without prescription.

Table 2. Drugs That Can Cause Delerium

ANALGESICS
Opioids
Salicylates
ANTICHOLINERGICS
Antihistamines (diphenhydramine)
Anti-Parkinson's medications
Antispasmodics
Cyclic antidepressants (e.g., amitriptyline, doxepin)
Cycloplegics
Neuroleptics
Antipsychotics (e.g., phenothiazines, haloperidol)
ANTIHYPERTENSIVES
Centrally acting (e.g., clonidine)
Beta-adrenergic blockers
Postganglionic sympathetic blockers (e.g., reserpine)
CORTICOSTEROIDS
HYPOGLYCEMICS
LITHIUM
SEDATIVE-HYPNOTICS
Benzodiazepines
Withdrawal
SYMPATHOMIMETICS
Amphetamines
Ephedrine
Methylxanthines
Phenylpropanolamine
Phenylephrine

Agitation. Sedative-hypnotic agents can also produce states of agitation upon abrupt cessation or significant decrease in use. The time of onset and severity of these withdrawal symptoms are dependent on the half-life of the agent, with more serious withdrawal manifestations generally observed in agents with shorter half-lives. Initial manifestations include minor sympathomimetic findings, such as tachycardia, hypertension, agitation, skin flushing, hyperactive bowel sounds, and diaphoresis. As the syndrome progresses, hallucinations, seizures, fever, and delirium occur,with significant risk for cardiovascular collapse and death.[25] Significant withdrawal symptoms can be managed with diazepam 5-10 mg IV every 5-10 minutes. In the event that diazepam is ineffective after adequate dosing, phenobarbital 120 mg IV every 15-30 minutes can be given until sedation is achieved. Adequate respirations and oxygenation must be assured.

Neuroleptic Malignant Syndrome. Altered consciousness and agitation are also observed in neuroleptic malignant syndrome (NMS), a condition that is characterized by four essential signs: fever, muscle rigidity, autonomic instability, and altered consciousness.[26-28] Rigidity, hyperthermia, and tachycardia represent the most common initial manifestations of NMS.[29] The proposed mechanism for NMS is depletion of central dopamine stores, and the precipitating cause is either an increase in the dose or introduction of an antidopaminergic agent (e.g.,phenothiazine) or the withdrawal of a dopaminergic agent (e.g., levodopa, bromocriptine, amantadine). The latter cause is most notable in Parkinson's patients undergoing a "drug holiday."[26] Identifiable risk factors for the development of NMS include high dosages and frequent administrations, intramuscular depot therapy, and agents with high anti-dopaminergic activity (e.g., haloperidol).

Concurrent medical illnesses are commonly associated with NMS,[29] which is commonly seen in young men and has been reported most frequently with the use of haloperidol (Haldol) and fluphenazine (Prolixin).[26,27] In spite of the tendency of NMS to occur in the younger population, the elderly are still at risk because of their varied and increased medication use. Neuroleptic medications are administered to 25-50% of residents of nursing homes, intermediate care facilities, and rest homes.[27] Moreover, these drugs are frequently used as antiemetics and for control of agitation. If NMS is suspected, the medication list in the elderly must be carefully reviewed for neuroleptics and "hidden" dopamine antagonists, such as metoclopramide (Reglan), prochlorperazine (Compazine), and hydroxyzine (Vistaril).[30]

Management of Delirium. Management of the delirious elderly patient begins with stabilization of airway and vital signs, followed by administration of oxygen, glucose, and thiamine. Naloxone (Narcan) is indicated in cases of unexplained coma and respiratory depression. If intracranial pathology (traumatic, infectious, neoplastic, or vascular) is suspected, a head CT scan should be ordered, and consultation with the appropriate specialist should be obtained. Laboratory tests to assist the clinician in determining the etiology of delirium include a CBC, blood glucose, electrolytes, BUN, serum osmolality, calcium, serum ketones, arterial blood gas analysis, and appropriate serum drug levels. A comprehensive urine toxicology screen may also assist in the diagnosis.

If a specific diagnosis has not been made after initial evaluation, selective pharmacologic management for the agitated delirium should be avoided because many drugs may contribute to the patient's morbidity and mortality. For example, the use of neuroleptic agents can contribute to hypotension, seizures, hyperthermia, and worsening of NMS. Benzodiazepines, however, appear to be safe and effective in most cases, while the diagnostic evaluation is in progress. As the patient's toxicologic syndrome becomes better defined, more specific therapeutic interventions can be considered.

Lethargy. Sedative-hypnotic agents are probably the most common cause of CNS depression in the elderly patient. *(See Table 3.)* The incidence of drowsiness and fatigue with benzodiazepines (e.g., diazepam, chlordiazepoxide, flurazepam, nitrazepam) has been shown to significantly increase with age in hospitalized patients.[15] These effects are most notable at higher doses and in agents with a long elimination half-life (e.g., flurazepam [Dalmane]). Delayed reaction time and impaired psychomotor performance have also been noted with benzodiazepine use.[15] More profound CNS depression, including obtundation, may be noted with either morphine or diazepam use in the elderly with hepatic or renal insufficiency or advanced cardiopulmonary disease.[31] Opioid toxicity is recognized by the clinical triad of miosis, respiratory depression, and coma.

Table 3. Drugs That Can Cause Lethargy

ANALGESICS
Opioids
ANTICHOLINERGICS
Antihistamines
Anti-Parkinson's medications
Antispasmodics
Cyclic antidepressants
Cycloplegics
Neuroleptics
ANTICONVULSANTS
Carbamazepine
ANTIHYPERTENSIVES
Centrally acting (e.g., clonidine)
Beta-adrenergic blockers
HYPOGLYCEMICS
SEDATIVE-HYPNOTICS
Benzodiazepines
Barbiturates
Chloral hydrate
Ethanol
Ethchlorvynol
Glutethimide
Meprobamate

Diuretic therapy may also produce generalized fatigue and muscle weakness, which can result from electrolyte abnormalities or dehydration.[9,21] Cardiovascular agents such as calcium-channel blockers, central alpha-adrenergic agonists (e.g., clonidine), and beta-blockers may induce lethargy from either direct CNS effects or diminished cardiac output with subsequent hypoxia. Coma from hypoglycemia during sulfonylurea therapy tends to occur more commonly in the elderly (especially in patients > 85 years), and in patients with renal and hepatic disease, alcoholism, and erratic eating habits.[32]

Lithium toxicity in the elderly patient with compromised renal function may present with stupor, coma, hyperreflexia, clonus, and tremors. As discussed earlier, anticholinergic medications (e.g., neuroleptics, tricyclic antidepressants) may also produce stuporous states.

It should be stressed that the differential diagnosis in these patients is extensive. The elderly patient presenting in a stuporous or comatose state may be suffering from a drug toxicity (e.g., opioids, sedative-hypnotics, cyclic antidepressants), CNS abnormality (e.g., cerebrovascular insult), or metabolic derangement (e.g., hypoglycemia, hepatic encephalopathy). It is important for the clinician to consider a wide differential and to perform a thorough examination when approaching these patients. Initial treatment involves the stabilization of airway and vital signs and a diagnostic evaluation as discussed above. Use of the benzodiazepine antagonist flumazenil is not recommended because of the likelihood of precipitating withdrawal symptoms, including seizures.

Clinical Depression. The overall prevalence of major depression in the elderly ranges from 2-14%, with an additional 15% experiencing milder forms of depression.[33] Depression in the elderly may be seen with the use of opioids, phenothiazines, centrally acting antihypertensives, sedative-hypnotics and from withdrawal from stimulants and steroids.[21,24,33] Chronic benzodiazepine use may cause a mixed dementia-depression syndrome that presents with behavioral disinhibition, visual-motor incoordination, depression, amnesia, and confusion.[34] Most patients with cognitive impairment from benzodiazepines are chronic users and symptoms develop insidiously.[23]

Headache. Causes of headaches from drug-induced states are cranial vasodilation, sudden increase in blood pressure, and elevated intracranial pressure. Metabolic consequences of certain medications (e.g., hypoglycemia, hypoxia) may result in headaches as well. Nitroglycerin use in elderly patients withangina frequently causes headache, which is mediated by cephalic vasodilation. OTC sympathomimetic agents, such as phenylpropanolamine, pseudoephedrine, and oxymetazoline (Afrin), may cause hypertension with subsequent headache through alpha-adrenergic receptor stimulation.

Indirect sympathomimetic agents such as phenylpropanolamine and tyramine-containing products (e.g., wines, cheeses, pickled herring) can also cause headaches when taken with monoamine oxidase-inhibiting (MAOI) agents. MAOI use is complicated by many potentially life-threatening drug-drug interactions, and clinicians should be aware of their increased use in the treatment of major depressive disorders. These agents block the intracellular metabolism of norepinephrine, serotonin, and other catecholamines, resulting in increased concentrations and sympathomimetic symptoms when released. Abrupt withdrawal from chronic beta-adrenergic blocking agents and clonidine therapy may also lead to uncontrolled hypertension and complaints of headache from unopposed catecholamine stimulation of adrenergic receptors.[35] Resumption of the patient's usual antihypertensive dose should result in reduction of the blood pressure within two hours.

Finally, precipitous decreases in steroid dosage after long-term therapy may result in headaches, elevated intracranial pressure, and papilledema. The mechanism is unclear but may be related to steroid-induced adrenal suppression. Prednisone and triamcinolone are most commonly associated with this occurrence.[36] Treatment is to increase the steroid dose and then to taper it over a prolonged period of time.

Cardiovascular Syndromes

Syncope and Near-Syncope. Syncope and near-syncope appear to be the most common presentations of ADRs in the elderly.[37] Hypotension and dysrhythmias are frequently responsible for these clinical manifestations. In one nursing home study, postural hypotension and supraventricular tachycardia were responsible for 20% and 10%, respectively, of all reported ADRs.[6] The elderly are more susceptible to the effects of lowered blood pressure because of a normally sustained higher mean arterial blood pressure and impaired homeostatic responsiveness. Diminished cardiac reserve and altered sinus node and baroreceptor sensitivity limit the reflex tachycardia necessary to maintain cardiac output and organ perfusion.[21,33,37]

Table 4. Drugs That Can Cause Syncope or Near-Syncope

DYSRHYTHMIAS
Beta-adrenergic blockers
Calcium-channel blockers
Digoxin
Type 1A, 1C antiarrhythmics (e.g., encainide, flecainide, quinidine)
HYPOTENSION/ORTHOSTASIS
Antianginals
Antihypertensives
Anti-Parkinson's medications
Cyclic antidepressants
Diuretics
Lithium (nephrogenic diabetes insipidus)
Neuroleptics
METABOLIC
Hypoglycemics

Antihypertensive and cardiac medications contribute to hypotension by inducing peripheral vasodilation, myocardial depression, or hypovolemia.[37] *(Please see Table 4.)* Diuretics may cause syncope from volume depletion and electrolyte disturbances,[21] whereas calcium-channel and beta-adrenergic blockers may produce similar symptoms from bradycardia, myocardial suppression, and vasodilation.[5] Neuroleptics and cyclic antidepressants contribute to postural hypotension as a result of peripheral alpha-adrenergic blockade, which is most notable in the first two weeks of use.

Antiarrhythmic therapy, particularly with the Type 1A and 1C class"as well as digoxin therapy" can produce syncope as a result of dysrhythmias and heart block. Torsades de pointes has been observed with the use of the Type 1A agents in the setting of QT prolongation.[5] Torsades de pointes has also been noted from drug interactions between second-generation antihistamines (e.g., terfenadine) and enzyme inhibitors such as erythromycin, ciprofloxacin, and ketoconazole. Chronic digoxin toxicity most commonly occurs in the elderly and results from either diminished renal clearance, diuretic-induced hypokalemia, or drug-drug interactions. Common digoxin interactions are observed with erythromycin and quinidine. Treatment of life-threatening dysrhythmias may require digoxin immune antibodies (Digibind).

Abnormalities in blood glucose can also cause syncope or near-syncope, and the clinician should always review the patient's medication list for hypoglycemic agents as well as those medications predisposing to hyperglycemia (e.g., thiazide diuretics).[21]

Pulmonary Manifestations

Dyspnea. Hyperventilation consists of increased alveolar ventilation in response to carbon dioxide production from cellular metabolism. Most processes that increase body oxygen consumption (e.g., fever, agitation, metabolic demands) will also increase respiratory drive in an effort to eliminate carbon dioxide.

Hypoxia-induced cerebral edema produces hyperventilation in an attempt to reduce intracranial pressure. Toxins such as methylxanthines (e.g., theophylline), cocaine, and other sympathomimetics cause direct stimulation of the respiratory center in the brain. *(Please see Table 5.)*

Salicylate-induced prostaglandin inhibition may lead to worsening of age-related renal insufficiency and chronic salicylate intoxication, whose manifestations in the elderly include tachypnea, acid-base disorders, noncardiogenic pulmonary edema, and cerebral edema.[16] NSAID therapy can also diminish renal function and lead to fluid retention, hyperkalemia, and congestive heart failure.[17] Elderly patients with parenchymal lung damage may be at risk for opioid and sedative-hypnotic-induced noncardiogenic pulmonary edema. Treatment is generally directed at removal of the offending agent, diuretic therapy, and respiratory support with positive end-expiratory pressure. Beta-adrenergic blockers have been shown to cause bronchospasm and congestive heart failure in elderly patients without known pulmonary disease or impaired left ventricular function.[21]

Toxins that produce a diminished level of consciousness may suppress the respiratory center and cause hypoventilation. Some of the drugs known to cause respiratory depression include the opioids, sedative-hypnotics, and cyclic antidepressants. In addition to decreased respirations and drowsiness, patients may exhibit restlessness, confusion, tachycardia, and diaphoresis from hypoxia. The initial management for drug-induced hypoventilation is discontinuation of the offending agent, arterial blood gas-directed respiratory support, and evaluation for other causative agents.

Myasthenia Gravis. Patients with myasthenia gravis may present with respiratory failure from muscle paralysis due to overmedication with pyridostigmine. Pyridostigmine is an acetylcholinesterase inhibitor that is commonly used by myasthenics to counteract the weakness of their disease. Too much pyridostigmine can result in cholinergic crisis and produces salivation, lacrimation, urination, defecation, GI cramps, and emesis (SLUDGE). Excessive cholinergic stimulation of nicotinic receptors can lead to muscle fatigue and masquerade as a myasthenic crisis. Patients with severe disease who are on large doses of medications are most likely to overmedicate themselves and present in cholinergic crisis.

Muscle weakness resulting from a myasthenic crisis (inadequate therapy) can be differentiated from cholinergic crisis by lack of cholinergic symptoms and by administration of edrophonium. Edrophonium is an acetylcholinesterase inhibitor that will improve muscle strength within seconds in the patient requiring more drug therapy. The effect is transient but serves as a diagnostic tool. If the patient's condition worsens with edrophonium,the presenting condition is most likely cholinergic crisis, in which case the patient's medications should be stopped until the cholinergic crisis resolves and response to edrophonium once again occurs.

ADRs involving the GI tract are common and account for about 20% of all ADRs in the elderly.[6] These side effects may present as mild GI symptoms, such as nausea and vomiting, or more severe problems, such as GI bleeding. GI bleeding is a significant complication of drug therapy in elderly patients. In particular, NSAIDs are associated with more adverse GI effects than any other drug class.[17,38] Roughly 20% of hospital admissions for bleeding ulcers in patients older than 60 years result from NSAIDs. In this population, death from upper GI bleeding is four times more likely in NSAID users

Table 5. Drugs That Can Cause Tachypnea

BRONCHOSPASM
Beta-adrenergic blockers
Drug-induced anaphylaxis
CENTRAL STIMULATION
Salicylates
Sympathomimetics
METABOLIC ACIDOSIS
Salicylates
PULMONARY EDEMA
Cardiogenic:
Beta-adrenergic blockers
Calcium-channel blockers
Noncardiogenic:
NSAIDs
Salicylates
Thiazide diuretics
Opiates
Sedative-hypnotics
Gastrointestinal presentations

than in non-users.[17] Larger studies demonstrate similar findings, in that the elderly have a higher incidence of GI hemorrhages, perforations, and fatalities as a result of NSAID therapy.[24] Impairment of blood flow and changes in gastric mucosa associated with *Helicobacter pylori* gastritis may predispose to NSAID-induced gastric damage in the elderly.[17]

Corticosteroids and anticoagulants are also routinely associated with GI bleeding.[1] Steroids have been shown to significantly increase the incidence of GI hemorrhage and peptic ulceration.[39] Bleeding disorders secondary to anticoagulation therapy with warfarin are the most common cause of iatrogenic hospital admissions.[21] Age greater than 65 years is an independent risk factor associated with major bleeding disorders from warfarin therapy.[12] The elderly are more susceptible to bleeding diatheses because they exhibit greater inhibition of vitamin K-dependent clotting factor synthesis than younger patients with similar comparable doses.[12]

Nausea and vomiting due to medications are commonly due to either direct gastric mucosa irritation or stimulation of the central chemotactic trigger zone. Common offending agents include salicylates, NSAIDs, colchicine, digoxin, codeine, erythromycin, and theophylline. Potassium supplements and quinidine preparations can become lodged in the esophagus and cause ulcerations, perforations, and resultant strictures.[14] This occurrence appears to be due to the irritating nature of the medication and ingesting the pill in the semi-recumbent position without adequate fluid intake.

Opioid and anticholinergic agents are common causes of constipation, which may require hospitalization in the elderly for paralytic ileus.[21] Diarrhea is quinidine's most common side effect and may be especially problematic in the elderly because of electrolyte disturbances, which can induce dysrhythmias.[5]

Table 6. Extrapyramidal Disorders

TYPE	TIME OF ONSET	THERAPY
Dystonia	Early (2-3 days)	Discontinue agent. Diphenhydramine (1-2 mg/kg IM, 25-50 mg tid-qid po), benztropine (1-2 mg IM, 1-2 mg bid po), or trihexyphenidyl (2-5 mg tid-qid po). A benzodiazepine
Akathisia	Early (5-60 days)	Reduce dose of agent. Diphenhydramine (1-2 mg/kg IM, 25-50 mg tid-qid po), benztropine (1-2 mg IM, 1-2 mg bid po), or trihexyphenidyl (2-5 mg tid-qid po). A benzodiazepine
Parkinsonism	Early to late (usually within 72 days)	Reduce dose of agent. Diphenhydramine (1-2 mg/kg IM, 25-50 mg tid-qid po), benztropine (1-2 mg IM, 1-2 mg bid po), or trihexyphenidyl (2-5 mg tid-qid po).
Tardive dyskinesia	Late (prolonged use)	Avoid long-term and high-dose use of agent. Avoid anticholinergics.

Urological Syndromes

Diminished Urinary Output. A decrease in urine output in an elderly patient should alert the clinician to search for serious problems, including both mechanical obstruction as well as drug toxicity. Although many drugs are associated with urinary retention or renal impairment, none are more common or potentially devastating than the NSAIDs.)[10,14] Normal age-related impairment of renal function may be exacerbated by NSAIDs secondary to inhibition of prostaglandins that promote renal vasodilation.[10] Medullary ischemia can ensue and lead to analgesic nephropathy. Patients at risk for NSAID-induced nephropathy include those with renal vascular disease, congestive heart failure, cirrhosis with ascites, intrinsic renal parenchymal disease, and diuretic use.[17,40]

Diminished urinary output from urinary retention can also be due to anticholinergic agents when these drugs are used in men with enlarged prostates.[21] These medications, which impair contraction of the bladder, include antihistamines, cyclic antidepressants, and Type 1A antiarrhythmic agents (e.g., disopyramide). Nebulized ipratropium bromide (Atrovent), commonly used to treat COPD, also inhibits cholinergic activation of smooth muscle and can cause urinary retention in older men.[5,8]

Polyuria. Polyuria and increased thirst from lithium-induced nephrogenic diabetes insipidus usually occur within the first six weeks of therapy.[41] Lithium inhibits the actions of vasopressin in the kidneys, which results in failure to concentrate urine during water deprivation. These symptoms, combined with a low urine-specific gravity, should suggest this diagnosis. There is no specific therapy for nephrogenic diabetes insipidus aside from discontinuing the lithium.

Movement Disorders

Neuroleptic agents are associated with involuntary movement disorders, termed extrapyramidal symptoms (EPSs). These include acute dystonia, akathisia, drug-induced Parkinsonism (akinesia), and tardive dyskinesia.[27] *(Please see Table 6.)* These agents have inhibitory effects on dopaminergic and cholinergic receptors. When neuroleptic antidopaminergic activity exceeds that of their anticholinergic activity at the level of the basal ganglia, hyperkinesis results. As many as 50% of new cases of Parkinsonism may be drug-related,[14] and severe symptoms often necessitate hospital admission.[19]

Tardive dyskinesia is a chronic debilitating disorder that develops as a late complication of neuroleptic therapy. It is characterized by involuntary lip smacking and other dance-like and writhing movements. Tardive dyskinesia has a higher incidence in the elderly and can be precipitated by a reduction in drug dosage after long-term therapy. Anticholinergic agents can worsen the dyskinesia.[31] Metoclopramide-induced movement disorders were noted during early drug clinical evaluations and included trismus, torticollis, facial spasms, opisthotonos, and oculogyric crisis.[42] Long-term treatment with this medication has been associated with tardive dyskinesia, especially in elderly women.[42] Consequently, metoclopramide should be limited to short-term use, and safer agents should be used.[42]

Skin Manifestations

Adverse skin manifestations to systemic medications are most often morbilliform or exanthematous in appearance and may be accompanied by mucosal involvement, facial edema, fever, or lymphadenopathy. When multiple agents are involved, the most recently prescribed is usually suspect and should be discontinued. The continued use of the offending agent can lead to more serious reactions, including toxic epidermal necrolysis, hypersensitivity syndrome, or serum sickness.[43] As part of the initial assessment, the clinician needs to consider other etiologies (e.g., infection, primary skin disorders, collagen vascular diseases, malignancies) as they may present in a similar fashion.

Table 7. Drugs That Can Cause Tinnitus

Aminoglycosides
Caffeine
Ethacrynic acid
Furosemide
NSAIDs
Salicylates
Quinine
Quinidine

Toxic erythema, or a generalized red macular rash, is one of the most common drug-induced skin manifestations. The penicillin derivatives and sulfonamide antibiotics are frequently involved, as are the barbiturates and NSAIDs. Calamine lotion, systemic antihistamines, and steroids are usually beneficial as treatment.

Toxic epidermal necrolysis (TEN) and the related Stevens-Johnson syndrome are commonly drug induced. Stevens and Johnson initially described the condition with febrile erosive stomatitis, severe ocular involvement, and a disseminated purpuric macular skin eruption, often with necrotic centers.[43] In severe cases, this can include limited areas of epidermal detachment (e.g., body surface area [BSA] < 10%). With more extensive skin involvement (e.g., BSA > 20-30%), sheet-like loss of epidermis is seen and the condition is then called TEN. The process is a Type III immune complex disorder. TEN carries a significant mortality rate and warrants intensive care management, often in a burn unit.

The efficacy of systemic steroids for TEN is unproven and predisposes the patient to secondary infections.[43] TEN primarily occurs in older women (mean age, 63), while Stevens-Johnson syndrome tends to occur in the young (mean age, 25).[44] More than 100 compounds have been implicated with both syndromes, although carbamazepine, trimethoprim-sulfamethoxazole, and sulfa-doxine/pyrimethamine (Fansidar) have the highest incidence.[43]

Urticaria and angioedema are common skin manifestations of hypersensitivity reactions. Medications cause mast cells to release histamines and other vasoactive amines that cause vasodilation and soft-tissue edema. Swelling of the larynx and surrounding airway is life-threatening and requires immediate therapy with antihistamines and epinephrine, as well as urgent airway management. Mast-cell degranulation can occur by direct stimulation, Type I IgE mediation, or Type III complement activation. The penicillin derivatives, anesthetics, and radiocontrast agents are most commonly associated with IgE-mediated immediate hypersensitivity reactions.[43] Opioids can produce direct histamine release from mast cells. Urticaria from salicylate and NSAID use results from inhibition of prostaglandins, which promote mast-cell stabilization. Middle-age and elderly patients are particularly susceptible to aspirin-induced angioedema.[17] Although rare, angiotensin-converting enzyme inhibitors (ACEIs) cause angioedema by allowing the buildup of the vasoactive amine bradykinin. Patients with hereditary angioedema appear to be predisposed to developing this complication.[45]

Anticoagulant-induced skin necrosis is a rare and devastating complication of warfarin therapy that occurs in obese female patients with protein C deficiency. The rash appears on day 7-10 of therapy and manifests as red, painful plaques that evolve to necrosis with hemorrhagic blisters. It is frequently seen on fatty areas of the body, including the breasts, hips, and buttocks. This syndrome results from a transient hypercoagulable state with thrombus formation. Treatment includes stopping warfarin therapy, administering vitamin K1, anticoagulation with heparin, and administration of monoclonal antibody-purified protein C concentrate.[43]

Petechiae and ecchymosis may herald adverse effects such as agranulocytosis, granulocytopenia, thrombocytopenia, and aplastic anemia from NSAID use. Aplastic anemia from pyrazole NSAIDs has been seen mainly in patients older than age 60 and on a minimum of six months of drug therapy.[17] The incidence of drug-induced blood dyscrasias peaks in the 60- to 70-year age group and is associated with a 62% mortality.[1]

Vision and Hearing Impairments

It is estimated that of patients older than 65, 43% are visually impaired and 25-45% are hearing impaired.[40] Any medication with the potential to exacerbate either of these problems may prove devastating to such a compromised population.

Tinnitus is the sensation of sound not originating from either mechanical or electrical signals. It usually results from spontaneous neurologic discharge of damaged sensory hair cells of the cochlear nerve. Impaired hearing in the elderly often prevents detection of tinnitus resulting from salicylate, quinine, or quinidine toxicity.[5,16] These drugs cause a constellation of toxic symptoms called cinchonism, which includes nausea,vomiting, tinnitus, and visual disturbances.[5] Although a variety of drugs can cause tinnitus, only the aforementioned agents consistently cause tinnitus at toxic doses. Other agents that cause tinnitus are loop diuretics, aminoglycosides, NSAIDs, and caffeine. *(Please see Table 7.)*

Medications with anticholinergic effects frequently cause mydriasis and blurred vision. This results from an inability to accommodate and may precipitate narrow- or closed-angle glaucoma.[8,33] Scopolamine transdermal patches used for motion sickness can cause anisocoria when topical cross-contamination occurs with the affected pupil. Amiodarone (Cordarone) can produce corneal microdeposits that may produce rainbow-colored halos around bright lights.[5] Chronic digoxin toxicity may also cause colored visual disturbances.[2]

Summary

Adverse effects from medications represent a serious health care problem in the geriatric population. These patients are at risk for these toxicologic syndromes because of polypharmacy and maturing body physiology. Clinical manifestations of ADRs are varied and can affect any organ system of the body. These features make it very difficult for the emergency physician to identify them. However, a symptom-oriented approach and a careful review of the patient's medications can facilitate management of these cases.

References

1. Castleden CM, Pickles H. Suspected adverse drug reactions in elderly patients reported to the Committee on Safety of Medicines. *Br J Clin Pharmacol* 1988; 26:347-353.
2. Oh VMS. Multiple medications: Problems of the elderly patient. *Intl Dental J* 1991;41:348-358.
3. Nolan L, O'Malley K. Prescribing for the elderly. Part I: Sensitivity of the elderly to adverse drug reactions. *J Am Geriatr Soc* 1988; 36:142-149.
4. Chrischilles EA, et al. Self-reported adverse drug reactions and related resource use. *Ann Intern Med* 1992;117:634-640.
5. Lynch RA, Horowitz LN. Managing geriatric arrhythmias II: Drug selection and use. *Geriatrics* 1991;46:41-54.
6. Gerety MB, et al. Adverse events related to drugs and drug withdrawal in nursing home residents. *J Am Geriatr Soc* 1993;41:1326-1332.
7. Colt HG, Shapiro AP. Drug-induced illness as a cause for admission to a community hospital. *J Am Geriatr Soc* 1989; 37:323-326.
8. Feinberg M. The problems of anticholinergic adverse effects in older patients. *Drugs Aging* 1993;3:335-348.
9. Beard K. Adverse reactions as a cause of hospital admissions in the aged. *Drugs Aging* 1992;2:356-367.
10. Hodinka L. Improving the risk-benefit ratio of NSAID therapy in the elderly. *Scand J Rheum* 1991;91S:3-8.
11. Bowen JD, Larson EB. Drug-induced cognitive impairment. *Drugs Aging* 1993;3:349-357.
12. Gurwitz JH, Avorn J. The ambiguous relation between aging and adverse drug reactions. *Ann Intern Med* 1991;114: 956-966.
13. Menkes CJ. Renal and hepatic effects of NSAIDs in the elderly. *Scand J Rheum* 1989;83S:11-13.
14. Brawn LA, Castleden CM. Adverse drug reactions: An overview of special considerations in the management of the elderly patient. *Drug Safety* 1990;5:421-435.
15. Kruse WHH. Problems and pitfalls in the use of benzodiazepines in the elderly. *Drug Safety* 1990;5:328-344.
16. Karsh J. Adverse reactions and interactions with aspirin. Considerations in the treatment of the elderly patient. *Drug Safety* 1990;5:317-327.
17. Nuki G. Pain control and the use of non-steroidal analgesic anti-inflammatory drugs. *Br Med Bull* 1990;46:262-278.
18. Rabins EA. Psychiatric disorders associated with epilepsy. *Psychiatr Clin North Am* 1978;1:101-115.
19. Hermesh H, et al. Contribution of adverse drug reaction to admission rates in an acute psychiatric ward. *Acta Psychiatr Scand* 1985;72:104-110.
20. Tune L, et al. Anticholinergic effects of drugs commonly pre-scribed for the elderly: Potential means for assessing risk of delirium. *Am J Psychiatry* 1992;149:1393-1394.
21. Fox FJ, Auestad AE. Geriatric emergency clinical pharmacology. *Emerg Med Clin North Am* 1990;8:221-265.
22. Rothschild AJ. Disinhibition, amnestic reactions, and other adverse reactions secondary to triazolam: A review of the literature. *J Clin Psychiatry* 1992;53:12(suppl):69-79.
23. Larson EB, et al. Adverse drug reactions associated with global cognitive impairment in elderly persons. *Ann Intern Med* 1987;107:169-173.
24. Kromann-Anderson H, Pedersen A. Reported adverse reactions to and consumption of nonsteroidal anti-inflammatory drugs in Denmark over a seventeen-year period. *Dan Med Bull* 1988;35:187-192.
25. George CF, Robertson D. Clinical consequences of abrupt drug withdrawal. *Med Toxicol* 1987;2:367-382.
26. Dickey W. The neuroleptic malignant syndrome. *Prog Neurobiol* 1991;36:425-436.
27. Nierenberg D, et al. Facilitating prompt diagnosis and treatment of the neuroleptic malignant syndrome. *Clin Pharmacol Ther* 1991;50:580-585.
28. Parikh AM, Camara EG. Neuroleptic malignant syndrome. *Am Fam Physician* 1988;37:296-398.
29. Rosenberg MR, Green M. Neuroleptic malignant syndrome. *Arch Intern Med* 1989;149:1927-1931.
30. Olmsted TR. Neuroleptic malignant syndrome: Guidelines for treatment and reinstitution of neuroleptics. *South Med J* 1988;81:888-891.
31. Hershey LA. Avoiding adverse drug reactions in the elderly. *Mt. Sinai J Med* 1988;55:244-250.
32. Seltzer HS. Severe drug-induced hypoglycemia: A review. *Comp Ther* 1979; 5:21-29.
33. Bressler R, Katz MD. Drug therapy for geriatric depression. *Drugs Aging* 1993;3:195-219.
34. Kramer SI, Reifler BV. Depression, dementia, and reversible dementia. *Clin Geriatr Med* 1992;8:289-297.
35. Gerber JG, Nies AS. Antihypertensive agents and the drug therapy of hypertension. In: Gilman AG, Rall TW, Nies AS, et al, eds. *The Pharmacological Basis of Therapeutics*. 8th ed. New York: Perga-mon Press Inc; 1990:784-813.
36. Ahlskog JE, O'Neill BP. Pseudotumor cerebri. *Ann Intern Med* 1982;97:249-256.
37. Hanlon JT, et al. Syncope and presyncope associated with probable adverse drug reactions. *Arch Intern Med* 1990; 150:2309-2312.
38. Langman MJS. Ulcer complications and nonsteroidal anti-inflam-matory drugs. *Am J Med* 1988;84(2A):15-19.
39. Messer J, et al. Association of adrenocorticosteroid therapy and peptic-ulcer disease. *N Engl J Med* 1983;309:21-24.
40. Mazanec DJ. Conservative treatment of rheumatic disorders in the elderly. *Geriatrics* 1991;46:41-45.
41. Bucht G, et al. Renal function and morphology in long term lithium and combined lithium-neuroleptic treatment. *Acta Med Scand* 1980;208:381-386.
42. Stewart RB, et al. Metoclopramide: An analysis of inappropriate long-term use in the elderly. *Ann Pharmacother* 1992;26:977-979.
43. Roujeau JC, Stern RS. Severe adverse cutaneous reactions to drugs. *N Engl J Med* 1994;331:1272-1285.
44. Schopf E, et al. The toxic epidermal necrolysis and Stevens-Johnson syndrome. *Arch Dermatol* 1991;127:839-842.
45. Slater EE, et al. Clinical profile of angioedema associated with angiotensin converting enzyme inhibition. *JAMA* 1988; 260:967-970.

Oncologic Emergencies

Murray Flotre, BSc, MD, CCFPM

As recently as 30 years ago, the diagnosis of cancer was essentially a death warrant. Fortunately, that statement is no longer true, as more than 40% of patients with cancer can expect to be cured with aggressive surgery, chemotherapy, and radiation therapy.[1] Moreover, the quality of life of oncology patients has improved markedly, and their five-year survival rate rivals that of patients with congestive heart failure.[2] Despite this improved outlook, malignant diseases remain a major cause of morbidity and mortality. Cancer is the second leading cause of death in the United States, and oncologic patients account for more than 20 million physician visits annually.[3]

Most cancer patients are managed by an oncology team that consists of their primary care physician, oncologist, surgeon, and radiation therapist. However, because patients with problems representing emergency complications of malignancy frequently present to the emergency department, the emergency physician must be able to accurately diagnose oncologic emergencies and rapidly institute appropriate therapy.[1] Moreover, some patients have a de novo diagnosis of malignancy made in the ED, and the emergency physician must be familiar with the presentation of cancer and its early signs and symptoms.[4]

Numerous emergencies occur in patients with cancer. Acute problems can arise from the local effects of the primary tumor, result from local or distant metastases, be the manifestation of a systemic complication of the malignancy, or represent an adverse effect of medical or radiotherapy. In addition, even though the severity of most problems related to malignant disease usually justifies immediate hospitalization, the urgency of the specific oncologic emergency determines the urgency of the therapeutic intervention. For example, imminently life-threatening problems such as cardiac tamponade or severe hypercalcemia mandate immediate, aggressive treatment, whereas with other problems such as spinal cord compression and delays in diagnosis and intervention directly effect the ultimate outcome.

The following chapter highlights some of the major emergency complications of malignancy. The authors begin by discussing one of the most lethal oncologic emergencies, fever and granulocytosis, and describe unique diagnostic and therapeutic considerations. Next, the authors address three major problems related to tumor compression—neoplastic cardiac tamponade, epidural spinal cord compression, and superior vena cava syndrome. After outlining the pathophysiology and treatment of malignant hypercalcemia, the authors describe two relatively uncommon oncologic emergencies, leukostasis and the tumor lysis syndrome, and conclude with an overview of the clinical problems related to cerebral metastases. As the population ages and the lifespan of the cancer patient increases, emergency physicians can expect to encounter more of the problems associated with this disorder. By proper evaluation and management of oncologic emergencies, emergency physicians should be able to help prolong and improve the quality of life for patients with cancer.

Approach to Emergencies in Cancer Patients

Patients with cancer are subject to a unique constellation of medical, surgical, and metabolic emergencies that can arise either directly or indirectly from their primary tumor. There are several important priorities in the evaluation and management of oncologic emergencies: identifying the source of the problem, determining the urgency of the condition, considering the acute problem in its proper perspective, coordinating a multidisciplinary treatment plan, and responding to the psychological needs of patients and their families.

Source of the Problem. Identifying the etiology of an oncologic emergency poses a difficult challenge. Do the acute symptoms and signs exist because of an effect from the primary tumor or metastases or as a complication of therapeutic agents or interventions? Which organ system is involved? Is the problem localizable to the central nervous system, respiratory tract, or cardiovascular system, or is there multisystem dysfunction? Does the emergency represent local tumor compression with vital organ obstruction, such as superior vena cava syndrome or acute airway compression? Or is the presenting problem related to systemic biochemical and metabolic derangements, such as with hypercalcemia?

Determining Urgency. Even more importantly, the emergency physician must rapidly determine the urgency of the acute problem. *(Please see Table 1.)* Does the constellation of presenting signs and symptoms represent a critical, life-threatening illness that mandates immediate intervention? Or is the condition acute or urgent, not requiring life-saving intervention but requiring careful evaluation and aggressive treatment? In these cases, physicians usually have the time to analyze the diagnostic possibilities, weigh various treatment options, and involve appropriate consultants.

Because oncology patients certainly can and do experience more commonplace emergencies, physicians should adhere to the principles of performing a thorough evaluation and considering common differential diagnostic possibilities in order to avoid missing these problems. For example, acute mental status changes in a patient with known lung cancer should call to mind the possibilities of hypoglycemia, hypoxemia, and drug overdose as well as cerebral metastases and hypercalcemia.

Proper Perspective. Considering the presenting problem within the framework of the patient's underlying disease process may provide key information to help place the acute crisis in its proper perspective.[5] Important details include the following: type, stage, and extent of the primary tumor; current chemotherapy or radiotherapy regimens; likelihood of remission with effective therapy; associated medical conditions; treatment plan once the acute emergency has resolved; and probability of cure or symptom control.

In addition, emergency physicians should maintain a positive and empathetic approach. Determinations about quantity and quality of life are difficult to answer in the emergency setting.[6] Physicians should not allow their values to intervene in ethical decisions that impact patients with cancer. Instead, clinicians should obtain pertinent information from the patient and family regarding their wishes and expectations pertaining to heroic or life-saving interventions.'

Table 1. Oncologic Emergencies Grouped by Urgency of Diagnosis and Treatment

Immediate:
Granulocytopenia with fever
Neoplastic cardiac tamponade
Airway obstruction
Cerebral herniation

Acute:
Spinal cord compression
Hypercalcemia
Superior vena cava syndrome
Leukostasis
Tumor lysis syndrome
Cerebral metastasis
Renal failure
Coagulation abnormalities

Urgent:
Hyperuricemia
Pathologic fractures

Adapted from: Schmaier AH. *Oncologic Emergencies. Res Staff Phys 1983;*29:63-76.

Multidisciplinary Approach. Effective management of oncology patients often requires a multidisciplinary approach that combines the knowledge and skills of the emergency physician, oncologist, radiologist, and surgeon. To achieve optimal outcome, emergency physicians should involve these cancer specialists early in the evaluation and treatment of patients with oncologic emergencies.

Response to Psychological Needs. The diagnosis of cancer is frightening for the patient and is usually accompanied by anxiety and uncertainty. Acute emergencies resulting from malignancy often intensify the feelings of helplessness, loss of control, and fear of death that many cancer patients and their families experience. Physicians also may encounter the common responses of anger, denial, withdrawal, and depression.

Emergency physicians should be sensitive to the psychological needs of oncology patients and their families. An effective response to the reactions and mental stresses produced by the various cancer-related problems requires physicians to be empathetic, understanding, and considerate, in addition to providing treatment for the acute oncologic disorder.

Neutropenia, Immunosuppression, and Infection

Infection is one of the most common acute emergencies and is a frequent cause of death in cancer patients. The presence of significant fever in these immunocompromised patients represents bacterial infection in 55% to 70% of cases but also can result from tumor necrosis, chemotherapy, radiation therapy, transfusion, and inflammation.[8,9]

Granulocytopenia and Infection. Serious and often overwhelming infection typically occurs shortly after a course of radiation or chemotherapy, when the already immunodeficient patient's defenses are at their lowest level and susceptibility to infection is the greatest. In addition to the malnutrition, impaired humoral immunity, and altered cellular immunity found in patients with cancer, radiation therapy and chemotherapeutic agents further reduce host defenses by lowering the immune and inflammatory response, producing myelosuppression, and impairing leukocyte mobility and phagocytosis.[8,9] Not surprisingly, overwhelming infection is the most common cause of death in cancer patients receiving active treatment.[10]

Granulocytopenia, described variously as an absolute polymorphonuclear leukocyte count less than 1,000/mm^3 or 500/mm^3, is the single most important factor that predisposes cancer patients to serious infection.[4,9] Patients with severe granulocytopenia (less than 100/mm^3) have an 80% chance that an associated infection will be fatal.[4]

Clinical Considerations. Because many diagnostic investigations used to evaluate infectious diseases rely on a neutrophil response, granulocytopenia also complicates the search for the infective focus. For example, physicians commonly look for white cells in the urine and infiltrates in the lung. But unfortunately, both of these responses may be absent with granulocytopenia. Consequently, clinicians fail to identify a definite cause for significant fever in nearly half of neutropenic patients.[8,9,11]

The most likely sources of serious infection in cancer patients are the respiratory, urinary, and gastrointestinal tracts. Physicians should perform a careful history and physical examination searching for subtle symptoms and signs, while focusing on these three systems.

Routinely obtain a complete blood count; urinalysis; gram stains of sputum and urine; cultures of blood, urine, and sputum; and a chest radiograph. Obtain additional radiographic studies, such as abdominal x-rays, and perform other diagnostic procedures, such as lumbar puncture, based on clinical evaluation. Although routine surveillance cultures of the nose, throat, gingiva, and rectum are indicated for granulocytopenic patients with hematologic malignancies, these studies usually contribute little to the overall management of patients with solid tumors.[12]

Dangerous Pathogens. Bacterial agents are the predominant cause of acute infections in cancer patients, although viruses fungi, and parasites are involved in both primary infections and secondary complications. Gram-negative organisms, especially *E. coli, Proteus, Klebsiella*, and *Pseudomonas*, are commonly isolated and account for 60% of life-threatening infections.[4,8,9] Gram-negative bacteremia carries a mortality of greater than 50% and is the most common cause of death in neutropenic cancer patients.[13] Frequently encountered gram-positive infections include *Streptococcus pneumoniae sepsis* and pneumonia and *Staphylococcus aureus* and *Staphylococcus epidermis* infections, especially when an indwelling catheter or intravenous line is present.

Because of immunosuppression, cancer patients are at risk for viral and opportunistic infections, which further complicate diagnosis and therapy.[14] Localized or disseminated viral infections with herpes simplex, herpes zoster, or cytomegalovirus are common. Fungal pathogens, particularly candida albicans are a major problem in neutropenic patients on broad-spectrum antibiotics. Opportunistic infections, especially with *Pneumocystis carinii*, but also with *Aspergillus*, *Cryptococcus*, and *Histoplasma*, are likewise important pathogenic agents.

Empiric Antibiotic Therapy. After obtaining cultures, emergency physicians should initiate empiric antibiotic therapy while the patient is in the ED. Though physicians have a wide range of effective agents at their disposal (indeed, the choice of empiric antibiotics is an ever-changing subject surrounded by much controversy and debate), a regimen should have a broad enough spectrum to cover likely pathogens and be effective against rapidly progressive infections. Standard therapy for the febrile, neutropenic patient is a bacteriocidal, synergistic two-drug regimen consisting of a semisynthetic penicillin with activity against *Pseudomonas* and an aminoglycoside. Despite the development of newer broad spectrum single agents, the two antibiotic regimen remains the therapy of choice and carries a higher success rates (80% vs 59%) than single agents.[9]

Currently, the combination of ticarcillin and gentamicin has the best efficacy to toxicity ratio.[8,15] If indicated, carbenicillin may be substituted for ticarcillin. A cephalosporin (cefazolin, cefoxitin, ceftriaxone, cefotaxime, or ceftazidime) with an aminoglycoside is another effective regimen. Other useful agents include ticarcillin/clavulanate or imipenem/cilastatin.

Additional Measures. Patients with clinical evidence of gram-negative sepsis—fever, hypotension, acute mental obtundation, and increased respiratory rate—mandate aggressive therapy that includes airway stabilization; vigorous fluid resuscitation; and, when necessary, vasoactive agents. The issue of high-dose corticosteroids is hotly contested, yet their efficacy in septic shock remains unproven.

Neoplastic Cardiac Tamponade

Neoplastic cardiac processes are discovered in approximately 21% of autopsies performed on cancer patients and primarily consist of pericardial involvement, including acute effusive, post-radiation, or constrictive pericarditis and neoplastic cardiac tamponade. Although rarely encountered clinically, malignant pericardial tamponade can occur abruptly and, if unrecognized, may result in the death of an otherwise potentially viable patient.

Etiology and Hemodynamics. Neoplastic pericardial effusion is the most common cause of malignant cardiac tamponade.[16] Other causes include post-irradiation pericarditis with effusion, fibrosis, or both, and rarely, tumor encasement of the entire heart in a thick, constrictive neoplastic hull. Eighty percent of cases of malignant pericardial involvement occur secondary to direct tumor invasion or distant metastases, and most commonly are due to carcinoma of the lung or breast, leukemia, or lymphoma.[16-21] Primary malignant tumors of the pericardium occur less frequently but are characterized by rapid accumulation of large volumes of bloody pericardial fluid.

The hemodynamic consequences of malignant pericardial effusions depend on the volume of fluid, the rapidity of its accumulation, and the distensibility of the pericardium. Patients may tolerate large collections of fluid (up to 500 ml) if the accumulation is gradual.[22] Compensatory mechanisms, including tachycardia, peripheral vasoconstriction, and decreased renal blood flow prompting sodium and water retention, are effective in maintaining cardiac output up to a

Table 2. Signs and Symptoms of Neoplastic Cardiac Tamponade

SYMPTOM/SIGN	% OF CASES
Dyspnea	50
Cough	36
Pleural effusion	29
Hepatomegaly	28
Thoracic pain	26
Orthopnea	21
Cyanosis	19
Venous distension	18
Edema (leg)	17
Cardiac enlargement	16
Pulmonary rales	11
Dysphagia	10
Splenomegaly	9
Systolic murmur	5
Hoarseness	5
Hemoptysis	4
Paradoxic pulse	3
Ascites	3
Syncope	2
Diastolic gallop	2
Distant heart sounds, hiccup, PND, pulsus alternans, palpitation, friction rub, paroxysmal SVT	1 each

Adapted from: Theologides A. Neoplastic cardiac tamponade. *Semin Oncol* 1978;5:181-192.

certain point. However, once a critical mass of fluid in the pericardium is reached, further accumulation interferes with ventricular filling and emptying. In cases in which intrapericardial pressure increases to the point that the compensatory mechanism cannot counterbalance the decreased cardiac stroke volume (as a function of either excess fluid volume or sudden intrapericardial bleeding), the emergency physician may be confronted with a critically ill patient with impaired consciousness, respiratory distress, and cardiovascular collapse.

Clinical Features. Even though the development of neoplastic cardiac tamponade is usually preceded by symptoms and signs of malignant pericardial effusion, the diagnosis of this oncologic emergency is often missed.[17-21] Early in the course, symptoms may be subtle and nonspecific and commonly include dyspnea, cough, atypical chest pain, and weakness. *(Please see Table 2.)*

Clinical findings suggestive of tamponade include the following: diminished heart tones, hypotension with narrow pulse pressure, tachycardia, jugular venous distension, and pulsus paradoxus greater than 10 mm Hg. Some authorities suggest that a 10% decrease in systolic blood pressure with deep inspiration is a better indicator than the classic 10 mm Hg fall in systolic pressure.[23]

The clinical triad of dyspnea, distended neck veins, and hypotension occurring in a patient with known malignancy should always raise the suspicion of malignant pericardial tamponade. Differential diagnostic considerations include superior vena cava obstruction, massive pulmonary embolism, and congestive heart failure.

Diagnostic Studies. The ECG and chest radiography may provide additional supporting evidence for neoplastic tamponade. ECG findings, which may be nonspecific, and can be altered by the pericardial fluid; however, they include low voltage, sinus tachycardia, ST segment elevation, and nonspecific ST-T wave abnormalities.[16-18,10,21] Total electric alternans (involving simultaneous alterations of the configuration of the P waves and QRS complexes) are considered pathognomonic for pericardial effusion with tamponade." Chest x-ray findings of cardiomegaly (classically described as a "water bottle heart"), normal pulmonary vasculature, and absence of pulmonary edema are highly suggestive of pericardial effusion.[16,17] However, a normal chest x-ray does not rule out effusion and tamponade. Up to 200 ml of fluid can accumulate in the pericardium without radiographic evidence of cardiac enlargement.[20] Echocardiography readily confirms the diagnosis of neoplastic cardiac tamponade, is highly sensitive, and can be used to guide pericardiocentesis.

Pericardiocentesis. Emergency percutaneous pericardiocentesis may be necessary and can prove life-saving in patients with decompensated malignant pericardial tamponade. Perform immediate pericardiocentesis in patients with cardiac tamponade and impaired consciousness, vascular collapse with pulsus paradoxus greater than 50% or pulse pressure and pulse pressure less than 20 mm Hg, and severe respiratory distress with cyanosis and dyspnea.[17,24]

Prior to performing the procedure, provide high flow oxygen and intravenous fluids. Avoid positive pressure ventilation because it increases both intrapleural and intrapericardial pressures and reduces venous return. Carefully monitor the ECG and hemodynamic status throughout the procedure. Ideally, and if time permits, use echocardiographic guidance. Risks of pericardiocentesis include myocardial and coronary artery trauma, hemorrhage from an injured vessel, cardiac dysrhythmias, and sudden death.

Patients with neoplastic cardiac tamponade often display dramatic improvement following withdrawal of as little as 50 to 100 ml of pericardial fluid, but physicians should remove the maximal amount of fluid and leave an indwelling pericardial catheter to prevent recurrence.[16,17] Also, send samples of pericardial fluid for cytologic and chemical analysis. Once the patient is stabilized, the oncologist and surgeon can decide on more definitive treatment, such as pericardial window, pericardiectomy, radiotherapy, or intrapericardial pharmacotherapy.

Acute Spinal Cord Compression

Spinal cord compression by metastases is a frequent, serious, and potentially treatable complication of cancer.[25-27] Epidural spinal cord compression is usually a late sign of metastatic disease, but on occasion it can be the initial manifestation of a malignant process, Prompt diagnosis and treatment are required to reverse existing neurologic deficits and restore function.[28]

Etiologic Considerations. Approximately 5% of cancer patients experience spinal cord compression at some time during their disease.[29,30] Most tumors that metastasize to the spinal cord are extradural and reach the epidural space by direct extension from metastasis to the vertebral body or through the intervertebral foramen. Intramedullary metastases are much less common and probably arise from hematogenous spread.[9,31]

Any tumor that metastasizes to bone can cause cord compression. Lung, breast, prostate, and kidney carcinomas and multiple myeloma are most commonly involved. Tumors that invade the paravertebral gutters, such as lymphomas and neuroblastomas, also are frequently implicated.

Level of Spine Involvement. Approximately two-thirds of cases of spinal cord compression occur in the thoracic spine, with the other one-third distributed evenly between the cervical and lumbar regions.[26,31] The level at which the metastatic focus arises depends on the primary site. For example, carcinoma of the breast or lung most commonly metastasizes to thoracic vertebrae, whereas colon carcinoma typically involves the lumbar spine.[26,28,31]

Symptoms and Signs. Regardless of the primary tumor, the presentation of metastatic spinal cord compression is usually the same. Back pain is the presenting complaint in 96% of patients, followed by weakness (75%), autonomic dysfunction (bowel or bladder problems or both, 50%), and sensory loss.[4,28]

Back pain is usually present for weeks or months before the appearance of neurologic symptoms. Patients often describe two types of pain: 1) a steady, dull, aching, midline pain that usually corresponds with the site of bony metastasis and 2) a radicular pain that usually occurs later in the course.

Cord compression in the cervical or lumbosacral region usually produces unilateral radicular pain that may involve only one extremity. Radicular pain originating in the thoracic region is usually bilateral and often is described as a band-like constriction around the chest or abdomen. In patients without a prior diagnosis of cancer, clinicians may have difficulty differentiating radicular pain arising from the thoracic spine from nonmalignant disorders such as pleurisy, pancreatitis, or cholecystitis. Likewise, pain arising from metastatic lumbosacral cord compression must be differentiated from pain resulting from a herniated intervertebral disc.

A suggestive clue to the presence of metastatic spinal cord compression is worsening of pain when the patient is supine. Some patients report that they must sleep sitting upright in order to be comfortable enough to sleep the night through. Moreover, even though patients with widespread cancer often have pain in multiple areas of their bodies, physicians should suspect metastatic spinal involvement when patients complain of any new or progressive pain in the neck or back.

Evidence of neurological dysfunction typically appears weeks or months after the onset of pain. Patients may complain of paraparesis, sensory deficits, urinary incontinence or retention, or difficulty ambulating. Clinicians frequently discover symmetric extremity weakness, gait disturbance, sensory loss, hyporeflexia, or signs of bowel and bladder dysfunction. Prompt intervention is necessary to prevent permanent neurological functional loss. however, once paraplegia is established, patients seldom return to full ambulatory status.[25,28]

Radiographic Studies. Approximately 90% of patients with spinal metastases have abnormal plain x-rays. Radiographic findings include pedicle erosion, lytic or sclerotic lesions, and diminished vertebral body height. However, a normal plain film does not rule out the possibility of metastatic spinal cord compression.[9,26,31] If the neurologic examination is suggestive of spinal cord compression, promptly obtain additional confirmatory studies.

Even if the neurologic examination is normal, all patients with abnormal plain films require urgent evaluation for epidural metastases.[32] Myelography is the traditional diagnostic procedure, although MRI and high resolution CT also reliably demonstrate spinal cord compression.[25,26,30] Radionuclide bone scans are sensitive for documenting bony metastases but are not useful for diagnosing or predicting epidural cord compression.

Treatment. As soon as tine diagnosis of malignant spinal cord compression is suspected, institute treatment immediately. Without prompt treatment, mild weakness may progress very rapidly and result in severe, irreversible weakness.[9,28] The combination of high-dose corticosteroids and rapid radiation therapy is the treatment of choice. High-dose steroids (dexamethasone 100 mg IV in divided doses) reduce cord edema, decrease local inflammation, and appear to have an oncolytic effect.[25,26,28] Following pretreatment with steroids, patients should receive the first dose of radiation, optimally within two hours of diagnosis. Surgery is reserved for the following situations: nature of the primary tumor is unknown; diagnosis of malignancy is in doubt; spinal instability; involved region already has received maximal radiation; progressive symptoms after several doses of radiation.

Outcome. Outcome is most closely related to the type of tumor and its radiosensitivity. Prognosis also depends on the patient's pretreatment status, the level and degree of spinal cord compression, and the rapidity of neurological decompensation.[26,28] Patients with lymphoma and myeloma usually fare the best, with nearly 50% achieving satisfactory outcome (defined as normal sphincter control and ambulaiion for longer than three months), whereas only 10% to 15% of those patients with lung or kidney cancer will have a similar functional outcome.

Superior Vena Cava Syndrome

Obstruction of the superior vena cava (SVC) results from compression, thrombosis, or infiltration and gives rise to characteristic physical findings, termed the SVC syndrome.[33-40] Approximately 3% to 10% of all patients with lymphoma or lung cancer develop the SVC syndrome at some point during their disease process. Seventy-five percent of cases of SVC obstruction arise from bronchogenic carcinoma; 1.5% are caused by lymphomas, predominantly non-Hodgkin's; and 7% are due to mediastinal metastases, especially from breast cancer.[9,33-36] Benign etiologies are uncommon and include aortic aneurysm, retrosternal thyroid, constrictive pericarditis, tuberculous mediastinitis, and thrombosis secondary to central venous catheterization or an implanted cardiac pacemaker.[37,38] In one-third to one-half of cases, SVC thrombosis occurs along with the obstruction."

Anatomic Considerations. The SVC is a thin-walled, low-pressure, compressible vessel. It is bounded anteriorly by the sternum; posteriorly and to the right by the right mainstem bronchus, and is surrounded by chains of lymph nodes that drain the right thoracic cavity and the inferior part of the left thorax. As expected from these anatomic relationships, right-sided lung tumor is the most common cause of SVC compression.[4,33,37] In addition, because of the proximity of the SVC and the spinal cord, the SVC syndrome and acute spinal cord compression occasionally occur simultaneously.[37,39]

Clinical Features. SVC syndrome usually has an insidious onset, and patients often are unaware of an underlying malignancy.

Table 3. Symptoms, Signs, and Complications of Hypercalcemia

Neurologic
Fatigue, muscle weakness, hyporeflexia, lethargy, apathy, disturbance of perception and behavior, stupor, coma

Renal
Polyuria, polydipsia, renal insufficiency

Gastrointestinal
Anorexia, nausea, vomiting, constipation, abdominal pain

Cardiovascular
Hypertension, arrhythmias, digitalis sensitivity

Adapted from: Fields AL, Josse RG, Bergsagel DE. Oncologic Emergencies: Metabolic Emergencies. In: Devita UT, el al, eds. Cower, *Principles and Practice in Oncology*, Philadelphia: JB Lippincott Co.; 1985:1866-1881.

Dyspnea is the most common presenting symptom and is present in over half of patients.[37] Forty percent of patients complain of swelling of the face, trunk, or upper extremities, and 20% present with chest pain, cough, or dyspnea, either alone or in combination.[35,37] Other patients may experience syncope, headache, head or facial congestion, or fullness in the arms, face, or neck. On physical examination, about 60% to 70% of patients have neck vein and upper chest vein distension, nearly 50% have facial edema and plethora, and the majority are tachypneic.[9,37] Patients with the SVC syndrome and associated increased intracranial pressure usually have blurred vision, papilledema, and alterations in mental status ranging from obtundation to coma.

On chest x-ray, the majority of patients have an isolated lung mass and often an enlarged mediastinum, and 25% have a right-sided pleural effusion. Chest CT is useful for demonstrating the location and cause of obstruction. Fiberoptic bronchoscopy with biopsy, mediastinoscopy, scalene node biopsy, or limited thoracotomy are indicated to establish the tissue diagnosis. Contrary to earlier literature concerning the management of the SVC syndrome, current studies stress the importance of promptly obtaining the tissue diagnosis and indicate that these procedures seldom cause significant morbidity or mortality.[41]

Management. Once the clinical diagnosis of SVC syndrome is suspected, promptly institute therapy in attempt to achieve symptomatic relief. Elevate the head of the bed to help decrease cerebral edema, provide supplemental oxygen to correct hypoxia, and administer corticosteroids to patients with respiratory insufficiency in an effort to decrease edema at the site of obstruction. Because of increased venous pressures, avoid venipuncture and venous access in the upper extremities, and use lower extremity veins only when necessary. Diuretics may help to temporarily reduce venous pressures but must be used cautiously. Patients with SVC syndrome have decreased venous return to the right heart, and diuretic-induced hypovolemia may cause shock. Obtain immediate consultation with the oncology team.

Depending on the tissue diagnosis, urgent chemotherapy for If; SVC syndrome and approximately 75% to 80% of patients experience prompt relief of symptoms.[33,34,37]

Hypercalcemia

Hypercalcemia is the most common metabolic complication of cancer and occurs in 10% to 20% of patients with cancer at some point during their disease.[42] If unrecognized or inadequately treated, hypercalcemia can be life-threatening.[43] Roughly 80% of hypercalcemic episodes associated with malignancy are caused by solid tumors, particularly carcinoma of the lung, breast, and prostate.‘” Hematologic malignancies such as multiple myeloma, lymphoma, and leukemia comprise the remaining 20%.[9]

Mechanisms of Hypercalcemia. Hypercalcemia associated with malignant disease results from two primary mechanisms, which may occur alone or in combination. First, hypercalcemia can result when tumor cells directly invade the bone and subsequently cause bone destruction. The second mechanism occurs in the absence of bony destruction and involves stimulation of osteoclasts by a variety of tumor-elaborated polypeptides possessing parathyroid hormone activity. Other chemical mediators implicated in the development of hypercalcemia of malignancy include E-series prostaglandins, parathormone, and osteoclast-activating factor.[45]

In addition, cancer patients are at high risk for hypercalcemia because of two other factors: 1) immobilization due to pain, weakness, or fractures; and, 2) dehydration resulting from vomiting and diarrhea associated both with tumor effect and chemotherapy. Clinical manifestations. Many patients present with the clinical triad of hypercalcemia consisting of back pain, constipation, and decreased alertness. Other common clinical features include anorexia, vomiting, polyuria, and hypertension, although a wide variety of symptoms and signs is possible. *(Please see Table 3.)* The severity of clinical findings correlates with the rate of development of hypercalcemia and the degree of serum calcium elevation. In cases of hypercalcemia of malignancy, calcium elevation generally occurs rapidly, and symptoms are usually prominent at relatively lower levels (12 mg/l to 14 mg/dL). The age of the patient, associated metabolic disturbances, and underlying medical illnesses also are important factors in determining the severity of symptoms.

Therapy. Principles of emergency therapy include correcting dehydration, increasing calcium excretion, and decreasing calcium removal from bone.[46] *(Please see Table 4.)* Administer normal saline to replace volume deficits, increase glomerular filtration, and promote saline diuresis, which results in concomitant increases in calcium excretion. Volume deficits may bc substantial, and some patients require 2 to 3 L of saline intravenously over the first few hours of therapy. In elderly patients or those with cardiac disease, careful monitoring is essential, and Swan-Ganz catheterization may be necessary.

After volume status is adequately restored, administer furosemide (40 to 80 mg) to augment renal sodium and calcium excretion. Carefully follow fluid and electrolyte status to avoid problems with volume depletion, hypokalemia, and hypomagnesemia. Corticosteroids should be administered empericaIly in obtunded or comatose patients with serum calcium levels greater than 14 mg/dl and may be indicated in other patients as part of the chemotherapeutic regimen. Mithramycin effectively lowers serum

Table 4. Acute Management of Hypercalcemia

Calcium < 13 mg%; patient minimally symptomatic
1. Oral hydration if possible
2. Mobilize
3. Monitor serum calcium and creatinine

Calcium 13-15 mg%; patient moderately symptomatic
1. Hydrate with IV normal saline 4-6 L/24 hours
2. Furosemide 40-80 mg every 12-24 hours; start after blood volume is restored
3 Potassium 40-80 mEq/24 hours
4. Monitor serum calcium, creatinine, electrolytes, magnesium, intake and output, and daily weights

Calcium > 15 mg%; patient markedly symptomatic
1. Hydrate with IV normal saline 6-10 L/24 hours; consider monitoring with Swan-Ganz catheter
2. Furosemide 40-80 mg every six hours after volume is restored
3. Potassium 15-20 mEq/L of saline
4. After 24 hours, if calcium not responding satisfactorily, consider:
   A. calcitonin 3-8 MRC units/kg IM every six hours,
   or
   B. mithramycin 25 µg/kg IV
5. Monitor calcium, creatinine, electrolytes, magnesium, intake and output
6. If creatinine remains elevated and urine output poor, consider hemodialysis

Adapted from: Bull FE. Hypercalcemia in cancer. In: Yarbro JW, Bornstein RS, eds. *Oncologic Emergencies.* New York City: Grune & Stratton; 1981:l97-214.

calcium by inhibiting bone resorption' and is most useful for hypercalcemia refractory to saline diuresis, but is not routinely administered in the ED.

Tumor Lysis Syndrome

Tumor lysis syndrome is a product of the extreme sensitivity that certain tumors have to antineoplastic drugs and radiation.[42] Leukemia and lymphoma arc most commonly involved, but some solid tumors, such as small-cell lung carcinoma, also are implicated.

Pathophysiology. Rapidly growing tumors that shrink very quickly when exposed to either chemotherapy or radiation create the risk for precipitating tumor lysis. Rapid destruction of tumor cells results in release of their intracellular contents, notably potassium and phosphorus. The result is profound electrolyte abnormalities, including hyperkalemia, hyper-phosphatemia, hyperuricemia, and hypocalcemia. These electrolyte imbalances may lead to life-threatening complications, particularly cardiac dysrhythmias, neuromuscular symptoms, and acute renal failure.

Risk Factors. Patients at highest risk are those with high white blood cell counts or bulky tumors. Both situations increase the potential number of cells to be broken down and the likelihood of electrolyte imbalance. Renal function prior to the start of antineoplastic therapy is very important in determining whether electrolyte imbalance will occur and how severe it will be. Poor renal function or pre-existing hyperuricemia puts the patient at high risk.[43]

Clinical Features. The clinical presentation depends on which electrolyte abnormality is the most prominent. If hypocalcemia predominates, then muscle cramps, tetany, ventricular dysrhythmias, confusion, and convulsions may be the presenting findings.[42,48] Hyperuricemia can cause nephropathy, oliguria, or hematuria." Hypoephosphatemia leads to hypocalcemia and renal failure by producing high levels of calcium phosphate that precipitate in the kidney. Hyperkalemia is the most worrisome complication because of the potential for producing life-threatening ventricular dysrhythmias or sudden death.[9,42]

Prevention and Therapy. The oncologist must take measures to prevent the development of the tumor lysis syndrome. Anti-neoplastic therapy should be delayed until hyperuricemia is corrected and renal function is optimized. Allopurinol, forced diuresis, high flow intravenous fluids, and urinary alkalinization are useful prophylactic measures.[42,48] If the tumor lysis syndrome occurs, emergency physicians should consider early hemodialysis.[49] *(See Table 5.)* Hemodialysis promptly lowers potassium, uric acid, and phosphate levels and is potentially life-saving in severe cases.

Leukostasis

Myeloblastic crisis (or "blast crisis") is a medical emergency characterized by extreme leukocytosis that occurs in patients with acute lymphocytic, acute non-lymphocytic, and chronic granulocytic leukemias. Hyperleukocytosis (greater than 100,000 leukocytes/mm^3) with a high percentage of blast CELLS carries the potential for microvascular sludging (or leukostasis) of these immature cells.to the less mature the cell, the more "sticky" it is, a phenomenon that partially explains the occurrence of blast crisis in acute myelogenous leukemia, where immature cell types predominate, but not in other

Table 5. Suggested Criteria for Hemodialysis Therapy in Patients With Tumor Lysis Syndrome

Serum potassium ≥ 26 mEq/L (6 mmol/L)
Serum uric acid ≥ 210 mg/dL (590 µmol/L)
Serum creatinine ≥ 110 mg/dL (880 µmol/L) .
Serum phosphorus ≥ 110 mg/dL (phosphate ≥ 3.2 mmol/L) or rapidly rising
Volume overload
Symptomatic hypocalcemia

Adapted from: Fields AL, Josse RG, Bergsagel DE. Oncologic Emergencies: Metabolic Emergencies. In: Devita UT, et al, eds. *Cancer, Principles and Practice of Oncology.* Philadelphia: JB Lippincott Co.; 1985:866-1881.

Table 6. Presenting Signs and Symptoms of Intracerebral Metastases

SYMPTOMS	% OF CASES	SIGNS	% OF CASES
Headache	53	Impaired cognitive function	77
Focal weakness	40	Hemiparesis	66
Behavioral and mental change	31	Unilateral sensory loss	27
Ataxia	20	Papilledema	26
Seizures	15	Ataxia	24
Aphasia	10	Aphasia	19

Adapted from: Posner JB. Neurologic complications of systemic cancer. *Disease a Month* 1978;25:1-60.

leukemias, such as chronic lymphocytic leukemia, where the majority of cells are mature.

Target Organs. Leukostasis most commonly affects the lungs and brain. Once pulmonary leukostasis occurs, leukocytes invade the alveolar epithelium and release vasoactive peptides, generate free oxygen radicals, and cause destruction of the pulmonary parenchyma. Patients with pulmonary leukostasis typically present with dyspnea and tachypnea. Depending on the degree of lung involvement, symptoms can range from relatively mild to quite severe and may mimic the adult respiratory distress syndrome.

Leukostasis in the cerebral microcirculation causes diapedesis of leukemic cells into the perivascular space and results in leukemic cellular deposits with tumor mass formation. Life-threatening cerebral infarction, hemorrhage, or both can occur.[4,9,50]

Management. The goal of therapy is reduction of the number of circulating leukocytes. Keep the patient well hydrated with intravenous and (when possible) oral fluids, promote urinary alkalinization with sodium bicarbonate, and administer allopurinol (600 mg initially followed by 300 mg daily) to prevent hyperuricemia. Hydroxyurea (4 to 8 g/day) is effective for reducing the circulating leukocyte pool.

If neurologic or respiratory symptoms are severe, leukophoresis is indicated to reduce the circulating leukocyte count to below 70,000/mm^3.[26] In cases with severe neurologic symptoms and signs, administer a single dose of cranial radiation to arrest leukostasis, destroy perivascular deposits, and potentially prevent significant cerebral vascular accidents.[9]

Cerebral Metastases

Approximately 20% of cancer patients experience symptoms and signs of central nervous system involvement, and at autopsy, nearly 35% of cancer patients are found to have CNS metastases.[4,26-31,51] The majority of cerebral metastases occur secondary to lung carcinoma and reach the brain by hematogenous spread.[24] Carcinoma of the breast, colon, and thyroid; hypernephromas; and malignant melanomas also commonly metastasize to the brain. In general, except for lung carcinoma, most cancers have pulmonary metastases before CNS spread.[4,52] Some tumors originating in the nasopharynx or middle ear metastasize to the skull, meninges, and brain by direct invasion and affect the cerebral hemispheres more often than the cerebellum or brain stem.[31,53]

Neurologic Features. Symptoms and signs of intracranial metastases may be difficult to differentiate from those caused by primary brain tumors, cerebrovascular accidents, and CNS abscesses. *(Please see Table 6.)*

Patients with cerebral metastases frequently complain of headache. The headache may be focal or diffuse, is characteristically worse on awakening, and often improves somewhat after getting out of bed. As intracranial pressure increases, headaches increase in both frequency and severity, and other neurologic symptoms develop.[29,31]

Neurologic dysfunction depends on the type and size of the lesion and the structure involved. Physicians commonly encounter progressive unilateral motor weakness or sensory loss, speech difficulties, gait disturbances, visual symptoms, behavioral abnormalities, and impaired cognitive function.[30,31] Clinicians often note a discrepancy between the patient's complaint and the physical examination findings. For example, only 31% of patients and families complain of some behavioral or mental change, and yet 77% display significant deficits on mental status testing.[30]

Generalized or focal seizures frequently occur in cancer patients with CNS involvement and may be the initial sign of intracranial metastases.[26,27] Focal seizures may help to determine the site of metastases. By increasing cerebral metabolism and cerebral blood

Table 7. Cerebral Herniation Syndromes

1. Transtententorial Herniation
   A. Uncal Herniation
      - Headache
      - Vomiting
      - Unilateral pupillary dilatation
      - Rapid progression to stupor and coma
      - Decorticate and decerebrate posturing
   B. Central Herniation
      - Headache
      - Progressive drowsiness
      - Small reactive pupils
      - Cheyne-Stokes respiration
      - Paucity of focal motor signs
      - Bilateral extensor plantar responses
2. Tonsillar (Foramen Magnum) Herniation
   - Headache
   - Vomiting
   - Hiccoughs
   - Stiff neck (meningismus)
   - Rapid progression to stupor and coma
   - Skew deviation of the eyes
   - Irregular respirations
   - Hypertension

Adapted from: Bisel HF, Wroblewski F, LaDue JS. Incidence and clinical manifestation of cardiac metastases. *JAMA* 1953;153:712-715.

Table 8. Treatment of Intracranial Metastases

I. Acutely Decompensating Patients
- A. Mannitol I-2 @kg IV stat followed by 20 g every six hours if needed
- B. Dexamethasone 100 mg IV stat, then 25 mg qid
- C. Hyperventilate to lower $PaCO_2$ to 25-30 mm Hg

II. Stable Patients with Multiple Cerebral Metastases or Systemic Disease
- A. Dexamethasone 4 mg q6h po (or more often if needed to control symptoms)
- B. Radiation therapy to entire brain
  1. 500 rads qd x 3 days
  2. Four days rest
  3. 300 rads qd x 8 days
  4. total 3,900 rads in 2 weeks

III. Stable Patients with Single Cerebral Metastasis and No Systemic Disease
- A. Dexamethasone 4 mg q6h po (or more if needed)
- B. Surgical extirpation and/or radiation therapy (to entire brain)
- C. After surgery, taper steroids as tolerated

Adapted from: Posner JB. Neurologic complications of systemic cancer. *Disease a Month* 1978;25:I-60.

flow, and therefore cerebral volume, seizures also cause increased intracranial pressure and may precipitate cerebral herniation in the patient with a previously compensated mass lesion.

As with any seizure, clinicians can reduce the risk of physical injury and aspiration by rapid evaluation and prompt effective treatment.[54] Rule out other causes for the seizure, including metabolic disturbances, such as hypoglycemia or hyponatremia, toxic ingestions, CNS infections, and intracerebral hemorrhage.

As the tumor grows and reaches a critical mass, intracranial pressure increases, the brain substance shifts in the direction of least resistance and ultimately moves caudally through the tentorium or foramen magnum.[26] Which of the cerebral herniation syndromes that results depends on the tumor location, its rate of growth, and the direction of brain tissue displacement. *(See Table 7.)*

Cranial CT scanning is the best single test to diagnose intracranial metastases. Both unenhanced and enhanced scans are necessary to obtain maximum information about the metastatic lesion and, on occasion, will provide information about the probable primary site.[27,30,31] Avoid lumbar puncture in patients with suspected cerebral metastases because of the risk of causing cerebral herniation. If meningitis is suspected, perform CT scan first to rule out cerebral metastases.[30]

Management. Emergency management of patients with acute complications arising from cerebral metastases depends on the clinical status. Sustained or repetitive seizures require aggressive therapy. Clinicians may use diazepam (5 mg IV every five minutes to a total dose of 20 to 30 mg) or lorazepam (2 to 4 mg IV) to abort the acute episode and then administer phenytoin or phenobarbital (15 mg/kg IV infused at 20 mg/min) for sustained anticonvulsant effect.[26,55] Some patients will require active airway control measures and ventilatory support.

Emergency physicians must intervene rapidly upon diagnosing impending cerebral herniation. *(Please see Table 8.)* Mainstays of therapy include endotracheal intubation with hyperventilation, IV mannitol and high-dose corticosteroids, and emergent consultation with The radiotherapist and neurosurgeon.

Effectively Managing Oncologic Emergencies

Patients with cancer can experience a variety of potentially life-threatening events. Major complications of malignancy include those related to myelosuppression and overwhelming infection; those resulting from local tumor compression, such as cardiac tamponade, spinal cord compression, and superior vena cava syndrome; those producing systemic effects, notably hypercalcemia, tumor lysis, and Ieukostasis; and those manifesting with acute neurologic dysfunction caused by cerebral metastases. To respond effectively to the complex challenges created by these problems, physicians must be familiar with the etiology, pathophysiology, clinical presentation, and multidisciplinary treatment of acute oncologic emergencies. Coupling this knowledge with an empathetic approach, emergency physicians can provide substantial improvements in both the quality and quantity of life for patients with cancer.

References

1. *Cancer Facts and Figures* 1986. New York City, American Cancer Society, 1986.
2. Kennedy BJ: Who says it is terminal? (Editorial) *JAMA* 1978;239:138.
3. Johnston HM. Silverstein S. Oncologic emergencies. In: Rosen P, Baker FJ, Barkin RM, et al (eds): *Emergency Medicine: Concepts and Clinical Practice.* St. Louis: CV Mosby; 1988:1665.
4. Schmaier AH: Oncologic Emergencies. *Res Staff Phys* 1983;29:63-76.
5. Yarbro JW, Bornstein RS, eds. *Oncologic Emergencies*. New York City: Grune & Stratton; 1981:VIII.
6. Kalia S, Tintinalli JE. Emergency evaluation of the cancer patient. *Ann Emerg Med* 1984;13:723.
7. Rosen P, Honigman B. Life and death. In: Rosen P, Baker FJ, Barkin RM, et al, eds. *Emergency Medicine: Concepts and Clinical Practice*. St. Louis: CV Mosby; 1988:5.
8. Rodriguez V, Ketchel SJ. Acute infection in patients with malignant disease. In: Yarbro JW, Bornstein RS, eds. *Oncologic Emergencies*. New York City: Grune & Stratton; 1981:273-300.
9. Jar& TG: Managing the cancer-related emergency. *Emergency Medicine* 1990;22:58-82.
10. Inagaki J, Rodriguez V, Bodey GP: Causes of death in cancer patients. *Cancer* 1974;33:568-573.
11. Pizza PA, Robichaud KJ, Wesley R, et al. Fever in the pediatric and young adult patient with cancer. *Medicine*

1982;61:153-165.

12. Kramer BS, Pizz PA, Robichaud KJ, et al. Role of serial microbiologic surveillance and clinical evaluation in the management of cancer patients with fever and granulocytopenia. *Am J Med* 1982;72:561-568.
13. Keichel SJ. Rodriguez V: Acute infections in the cancer patient. *Semin Oncol 1978;*5:167.
14. Pennigton JE: Infection in the compromised host. *Seminars in Infect Dis* I: IX-68, 1978.
15. The EORTC International Antimicrobial Therapy Project Group: Three antibiotic regimens in the treatment of infection in febrile granulocytopenic patients with cancer. *J Infect Dis* 1978;137: 14-29.
16. Theologides A Neoplastic cardiac tamponade. *Semin Oncol* 1978;5:181-192.
17. Theologides A. Neoplastic cardiac tamponade. In: Yarbro JW, Bornstein RS, eds. *Oncologic Emergencies*. New York City: Grune & Stratton; 1981:1-21.
18. Johnson FE, Wolverson MK, Sundaram M, et al. Unsuspected malignant pericardial effusion causing cardiac tamponade. *Chest* 1982;82:501-503.
19. Fraser RS, Viloria JB, Wang N. Cardiac tamponade as a presentation of extracardiac malignancy. *Cancer* 1980;45: 1697-1703.
20. Biran S. Hochman A. Levij IS, Stern S: Clinical diagnosis of secondary tumors of the heart and pericardium. *Dis Chest* 1969;3:202-208.
21. Bisel HF, Wroblewski F, LaDue JS. Incidence and clinical manifestations of cardiac metastases. *JAMA* 1953;153: 712-715.
22. Esposilo D: Emergency complications of malignancy. In: Tintinalli JE, Krome RL, Ruiz E, eds. *Emergency Medicine—A Comprehensive Study Guide*. 2nd ed. New York City: McGraw-Hill; 1988:540.
23. Reddv PS, Curtiss El, O'Toole JD, et al. Cardiac tamponade; Hemodynamic observations in man. *Circulation* 1978;58:265-272.
24. Spodick DH: Acute cardiac tamponade: Pathologic physiology, diagnosis, and management. *Prog Cardio Dis* 1967;10: 64-96.
25. Gilbert RW, Kim JH, Posner JB. Epidural spinal cord compression from metastatic tumor: Diagnosis and treatment. *Ann Neural* 1978;43:40-51.
26. Silverstein SR, Marx JA. Neurologic emergencies in patients with cancer. *Topics In Emerg Med* 1986;8:1-ll.
27. Cairncross JG, Posner JB. Neurologic complications of systemic cancer. In: Yarbro JW. Bornstein RS, eds. *Oncologic Emergencies*. New York City: Grune & Stratton; 1981:73-96.
28. Carabell SC: Oncologic Emergencies; central nervous system emergencies. In: Devita UT, et al, eds. *Cancer, Principles and Practice of Oncology*. Philadelphia: JB Lippincott Co.; 1985:1860-1866.
29. Posner JB. Neurological complications of systemic cancer. *Med Chin Varrlt Am* 1979;63:783-800.
30. Posner JB. Neurologic complications of systemic cancer. *Disease Month* 1978;25:1-60.
31. Arsenault L. Melastatic cancer and the nervous system. *Focus on Crit Care* 1984;l:39-47.
32. Rodichok LD, Harper GR, Ruckdeschel JC. Early diagnosis of spinal epidural metastases. *Am J Med* 1981;70:1181-1187.
33. Simpson JR, Perez CA, Presant CA, et al. Superior vena cava syndrome. In: Yarbro JW. Bornstein RS, eds. *Oncologic Emergencies.*New York City: Grune & Stratton; 1981:43-72.
34. Rubin P, Green J, Holzwasser G, et al. Superior vena cava syndrome: Slow-low dose versus rapid high-dose schedules. *Radiology* 1963;81:388-401.
35. Perez CA, Presant CA. Van Amburg AL: Management of superior vena cava syndrome. *Sem in Oncol* 1978;5:123-134.
36. Ghosh BC, Cliffton EE. Malignant tumors with superior vena cava obstruction. *New York State J Med* 1973;73:283-289.
37. Carabell SC, Goodman RL. Oncologic emergencies; superior vena cava syndrome. In: Devita UT, et al, eds. *Cancer. Principles and Practice of Oncology*. Philadelphia: JR Lippincott Co.; 1985:1855-1860.
38. Silverstein GE, Burke G, Goldberg D, et al. Superior vena caval system obstruction caused by benign endothoracic goiter. *Dis Chest* 1969;565:19-523.
39. Rubin P, Hicks GL. Biassociation of superior vena caval obstruction and spinal cord compression. *New York State J Med* 1973;73:2176-2182.
40. Parish JM, Marschke RF, Dines DE, et al. Etiologic considerations in superior vena cava syndrome. *Mayo Clin Proc* 1981;56:407-413.
41. Ahmann FR. A reassessment of the clinical implications of the SVC syndrome. *J Clin Oncol* 1984;2:961-969.
42. Fields AL, Josse RG, Bergsagel DE. Oncologic emergencies: metabolic emergencies. In: Devita UT, et al, eds. *Cancer, Principles and Practice of Oncology*. Philadelphia: JB Lippincott Co.; 1985:1866-1881.
43. Miach PJ, Dawborn JK, Martin TJ, et al. Management of the hypercalcemia of malignancy by peritoneal dialysis. *Med J Austral* 1975;1:782-784.
44. Mundy GR, Martin TJ. The hypercalcemia of malignancy: pathogenesis and management. *Metabolism* 1982;31:1247-1277.
45. Tashjian AH Jr. Prostaglandins, hypercalcemia, and cancer. *N Engl J Med* 1975;293:1317-1318.
46. Bull FE. Hypercalcemia in cancer. In: Yarbro JW, Bornstein RS, eds. *Oncologic Emergencies*. New York City: Grune & Stratton; 1981:197-214.
47. Mundy GR, Wilkinson R, Heath DA. Comparative study of available medical therapy for hypercalcemia of malignancy. *Am J Med* 1983;74:421-432.
48. Bell R, Forbes TK, Sulivan JR. Complications of tumor overkill when associated with high dose methotrexate therapy. *Clin Exp Pharmacol Physiol* 1979;(Suppl):47-55.
49. Cohen LF, CI al. Acute tumor lysis syndrome: A review of 37 patients with Burkitt's Iymphoma. *Am J Med* 1980;68:486-491.
50. Hoagland HC, Perry MC. Blast cell crisis in acute or chronic leukemia *JAMA* 1976;235:1888-1889.
51. Posner JB, Chemik NT. Intracranial metastases from systemic cancer. *Adv Neurol* 1978;19:575-87.
52. Simionescu M: Metastatic tumors of the brain. *J Neurosurg* 1960;17:361-373.
53. Kindt G: The pattern of location of cerebral metastatic

tumors. *J Neurosurg* 1964;1:54-57.

54. Nealon N. Neurologic complications in the cancer patient. In: Howland WS, Graziano C, eds. *Critical Care of the Cancer Patient*. Chicago; Year Book; 1985.
55. Sacks C. Seizures and status epilepticus in adults. In: Tintinalli JE, Krome RL, Ruiz E, eds. *Emergency Medicine—A Comprehensive Study Guide*, 2nd ed. New York City: McGraw-Hill; 1988:563.

Part X

Dermatologic Disorders

Immunologic and Toxin-Mediated Syndromes

William J. Brady, MD, FACEP

The emergency physician is often faced with acute presentations of dermatological disorders. In this regard, the chief complaint of "rash" is encountered in approximately 5% of emergency department (ED) visits nationwide; in addition, cutaneous findings help the physician make the correct diagnosis and determine appropriate management in another 5% of ED cases. Overall, one in 10 ED visits will require expertise in dermatologic disorders.[1]

The emergency physician is frequently the first, and only, clinician who examines a patient with a "rash." Accordingly, he or she must make the diagnosis, stabilize the patient, select proper therapy, and arrange for a timely disposition with appropriate consultation. The physician's ability to identify the dermatologic disorder not only determines the treatment pathway, but also may influence patient outcomes. Although most patients with dermatological diseases can be adequately managed on an outpatient basis with appropriate follow-up, some conditions are potentially life-threatening and require immediate diagnosis, intensive management, and in-hospital disposition.

The pitfalls of managing dermatological syndromes are well-known. Two studies addressing the management of patients with dermatological disorders are revealing. The first, a study of academic internists, demonstrated that 40% of dermatologic cases were misdiagnosed and appropriate referral was not made.[1] Among 40% who were misdiagnosed, 64% were treated inappropriately. The precise clinical significance of inappropriate treatment was not addressed; however, one case of impetigo was treated with topical steroids, and antifungal agents were prescribed for a case of psoriasis. In this same study, 33% of dermatology referrals were deemed unnecessary.[1] Although there are no data on the appropriateness of diagnosis and treatment of dermatological disorders by emergency physicians, these specialists may have similar diagnostic and disposition difficulties.

The second study stresses the importance of visual diagnosis and pattern recognition in evaluating patients with dermatologic complaints. Several groups of physicians at different levels of training were given 100 color slides of various skin lesions; the accuracy of diagnosis, as well as the time to diagnosis were noted. Second-year medical students made the correct diagnosis in only 21% of cases, while their fourth-year colleagues scored slightly higher—a 31% accuracy rate. Second-year family medicine residents were correct 55% of the time, while primary care physicians made the correct diagnosis in 66% of cases. In contrast, dermatologists were correct in approximately 90% of cases. Interestingly, an accurate diagnosis was inversely associated with response time.[2]

With these issues in mind, the purpose of this chapter is to present a step-by-step approach to the recognition and treatment of common and challenging dermatological conditions encountered in the ED.

Table 1. Etologic Classifications of Urticaria (Acute and Chronic Forms)

FOOD AND FOOD ADDITIVES
• Shellfish, eggs, nuts, strawberries, wheat, yeast, various dyes and preservatives
MEDICATIONS
• Penicillins, NSAIDs, sulfa drugs, morphine, dextran, quinine, ACE inhibitors
INFECTIOUS AGENTS
• Bacteria (URI, UTI, dental, chest), fungus (particularly candidiasis), virus (hepatitis B, mononucleosis), protozoa (giardia, malaria), helminths
HORMONAL
• Pregnancy, premenstrual
INHALANTS
• Pollens, spores, mites, dust, aerosols, and volatile chemical agents
PHYSICAL STIMULI
• Pressure, exertional, solar, extremes of temperature, vibratory
MALIGNANCY
• Lymphomas, various carcinomas
RHEUMATOLOGIC DISEASE
• Serum sickness, rheumatic fever, SLE, rheumatoid arthritis, leukocytoclastic vasculitis
GENETIC

Table 2. Causes of Urticaria and Angioedema

MEDICATIONS
Aspirin, other salicylates, and NSAIDs
Codeine and other narcotic agents
Antibiotics—penicillins and sulfa drugs
ACE inhibitors
INGESTANTS/CONTRACTANTS
Food—shellfish, nuts, and strawberries
Inhalants—pollen, spores, and mites
Volatile chemicals and aerosols
Cosmetics
Animal and plant materials
PHYSICAL STIMULI
Extremes of temperature
Exercise
Pressure
Vibration
INFECTIONS (ACUTE, SUBACUTE, AND CHRONIC)
Viral
Bacterial
Parasitic

Urticaria and Angioedema

Urticaria, also referred to as hives or wheals, is a common and distinctive skin reaction that is encountered at least once in up to 20% of the general population; atopic individuals experience urticarial reactions even more frequently. Urticarial reactions result from vasodilation and transudation of fluid into the superficial skin layers (the epidermis); angioedema, which is produced by a similar process, occurs in deeper skin structures. Urticaria and, to a lesser extent, angioedema are classified as either acute or chronic: A chronic episode is arbitrarily defined as hives persisting for six weeks or longer. Although men and women are affected equally by acute urticaria, women in the fourth decade or older are more likely to experience the chronic form. The emergency physician should be aware that such dermatologic findings may be the initial or an early event that may culminate as a potentially life-threatening, multisystem allergic reaction (i.e., anaphylaxis).

A broad range of etiologies *(Please see Tables 1 and 2)* may be responsible for producing such reactions, including various foods and food additives, medications, infectious agents, inhalants, rheumatologic disease states, physical stimuli, hormones, and genetic predispositions. In any particular case, the precise trigger is not always identified despite extensive investigation and subspecialty consultation; overall, patients with acute urticarial events will have a triggering agent identified in only 50-60% of cases, whereas in chronic cases the precipitating factor is confirmed in only 5-20% of cases.[3,4]

Clinical Pathophysiology. The pathogenesis of urticaria and angioedema is complex and involves a number of triggering events and associated cellular reactions. Once exposed to a triggering mechanism, a cascade of cellular events is set in motion. All such triggers—regardless of the ultimate cellular response—result in the release of histamine and other mediators of allergic phenomena, which produce the clinical manifestations of urticaria and angioedema. Precipitant stimulate production of cyclic-GMP from GTP, which generates activating enzymes. These enzymes cause degranulation of intracellular histamine storage depots and other preformed mediators of allergic reaction. Released from mast cells, eosinophils, and basophils via this process, histamine is the primary mediator of any allergic reaction. A number of stimulatory events can lead to histamine release, including 1) cross linking of cellular antibodies via antigens (i.e., food, medications, inhalants); 2) cholinergic stimulation (i.e., acetylcholine); 3) physical stimuli, including temperature extremes, vibration, pressure, etc.; 4) nonimmunologic stimuli such as morphine, lobster, strawberries, etc.; and 5) anaphylatoxins, including complement fragments C3a and C5a. Upon its release, histamine produces an increase in vascular permeability and leakage of plasma fluids into the tissues.

The location of the reaction within the skin will determine characteristics of dermatologic manifestations. Urticaria results from

Table 3. Lesions of Uticaria and Angioedema

URTICARIA

Erythematous/white nonpitting papules/plaques
Peripheral erythematous ring or a zone of pallor
Localized/well-circumscribed
Coalescent lesions resembling an "orange peel"
Excoriations and other local skin trauma

ANGIOEDEMA

Nonpitting and asymmetric edema
Involving the oral cavity, genitalia, hands, and feet
Scattered urticarial lesions

capillary vasodilation and increased permeability in the epidermis; similar events in the dermis and subcutaneous tissues manifest as angioedema. Other related pathogenic actions include alterations in the arrachidonic acid pathways, complement-mediated responses, IgE-dependent hypersensitivity reaction, the actions of various chemotactic factors, and leukocyte infiltration.

Clinical Presentation and Diagnosis. The presentation of urticaria and angioedema usually are straightforward, and the diagnosis generally does not present difficulty. Patients with urticaria complain of pruritus, which can range range from mild and irritating to severe and disabling; they may also note burning or stinging sensations or superficial pain. The cutaneous reaction of urticaria consists of localized, well-circumscribed, raised, erythematous papules and plaques; the individual lesions vary in size from small, measuring 1-2 mm in diameter, to very large, with involvement of an entire body area. Individual lesions may coalesce, forming one large, confluent plaque that can cover the entire trunk. The skin is said to resemble an "orange peel." The lesions may be surrounded by either an erythematous ring or a zone of pallor; alternatively, normal skin may directly abut the lesion. Excoriations and other local skin trauma may be seen in the patient with the intensely pruritic rash. True urticaria frequently appears abruptly and resolves quickly with appropriate therapy. Individual lesions are transient in nature, usually resolving within 1-3 hours, while new lesions may appear in other body areas. Single lesions rarely persist beyond a 24 hours.[3,4]

Angioedema. Angioedema is a more pronounced form of urticaria. It may involve any area of the body (skin or mucous membrane), especially the face, oral cavity, genitalia, hands, and feet. Some patients may note only mild pruritus or related skin discomfort, whereas others may not complain of any skin irritation but identify only an unusual appearance or bodily dysfunction (i.e., inability to speak with lingual edema, airway compromise with laryngeal or lingual edema, or abdominal pain and emesis with gastrointestinal edema). The edema is usually nonpitting and asymmetric in distribution, and may be accompanied by scattered urticarial lesions. Angioedema usually is characterized by a slow progression to full development yet usually resolves within 24 hours. *(Please see Table 3 for a list of cutaneous lesions encountered in the patients with urticaria and angioedema.)*

Table 4. Differential Diagnosis of Urticaria and Angioedema

Erythema multiforme
Urticarial vasculitis
Kawasaki disease

Table 5. Antihistamines Useful in the Management of Urticaria/Angioedema

Medication	Adult Dose	Pediatric Dose
Diphenhydramine (Benadryl)	25-50 mg po/IV q6h	4-6 mg/kg/24h po/IV q6-8h (max 200 mg/24h)
Hydroxyzine (multiple names)	25-100 mg po/IV q8h	2-4 mg/kg/24h po/IV q8-12h (max 200 mg/24h)
Astemizole* (Hismanal)	10 mg po q24h	10 mg po q24h**
Cetirizine (Zyrtec)	5-10 mg po q24h	5-10 mg po q24h**
Fexofenadine (Allegra)	60 mg po q12h	not recommended***
Loratadine	10 mg po q24h	10 mg po q24h**

* Indication limited to chronic idiopathic urticaria (see package insert for details).

** Pediatric use is only recommended in children 6 years or older (see package insert for details).

*** Pediatric use is not recommended in package insert.

The persistence of individual urticarial or angioedematous lesions beyond 24 hours should prompt consideration of alternative diagnoses, including urticarial vasculitis, Kawasaki syndrome, and erythema multiforme (EM). Allergic-mediated urticaria and angioedema tend to be relatively transient in nature with marked pruritus (urticaria only). Lesions resulting from a vasculitic process, Kawasaki disease, or EM will manifest little to no pruritus and will remain fixed in place for several days to weeks; in addition, other lesion morphologies may also be encountered. Patients with nonallergic hives may also note the presence of fever, malaise, myalgias, arthralgias, and abdominal pain. *(Please see Table 4 for the differential diagnosis of urticaria.)*

Management. Mild cases of acute urticaria can be treated with oral antihistamines (H_1 antagonists), including diphenhydramine (adult: 25-50 mg q6h; children: 4-6 mg/kg/24 hr given q6-8h not to exceed 200 mg in 24 hours) or hydroxyzine (adult: 25-100 mg q8h; children: 2-4 mg/kg/24 hr q8-12h not to exceed 200 mg in 24 hours).

Table 6. Lesions of EM

Erythematous papule/macule
Maculopapule
Iris (or target) lesion
Uritcarial lesion
Vesiculobullous
Mucous membrane involvement

Table 7. Differential Diagnosis of EM

Herpetic infection
Vasculitis
Toxic epidermal necrolysis
Primary blistering disorders
Pemphigus and pemphigoid
Toxic-infectious erythemas

Additional medication-related therapy is probably not indicated in mild cases. In the moderate to severe case of urticaria, without respiratory or cardiovascular compromise, widespread body surface involvement and/or marked pruritus may be disabling due to pronounced pruritus. In these cases, parenteral therapy may be required to achieve a more rapid response to treatment. However, the oral route is recommended in all but extreme cases. H_1-antagonists may be used as noted above via the intramuscular or intravenous routes. Oral or parenteral H_2-antagonists (e.g., ranitidine or famotidine) have also demonstrated some benefit in urticaria, particularly in idiopathic and chronic forms of the disorder. Subcutaneous epinephrine in a 1:1000 concentration may be used in severe cases of pruritus at a dose of 0.3 mL for adults and 0.01 mL/kg for children not to exceed 0.3 mL; the beneficial effects of epinephrine will appear within several moments of administration and last for up to one year. Susphrine, a "sustained effect" version of epinephrine, may be administered subcutaneously at one-half the epinephrine dose; the therapeutic effects of Susphrine are prolonged and may last for 4-6 hours. Systemic steroids—prednisone by mouth or methylprednisolone IV—are used in patients with symptomatically disabling reaction.[5] Both urticarial and angioedematous reactions not accompanied by airway involvement or hemodynamic compromise may be managed on an outpatient basis.

Additional medication options are available for the management of pruritus associated with chronic urticaria. These agents, termed the second-generation antihistamines, include astemizole, cetirizine, fexofenadine, loratadine, and terfenadine; terfenadine has been recently withdrawn from the market due to the risk of potentially fatal medication reactions. In general, these newer antihistamines offer the advantages of reduced dosing frequency and less sedative effect; these agents, however, are more costly than the traditional antihistamines. In general, comparisons of these new medications to hydroxyzine are favorable; comparisons among these second-generation agents do not demonstrate significant differences.[6,7] *(Please see Table 5 for a list of the various antihistamine medications used in the management of urticaria.)*

Angioedema cases associated with potential airway compromise represent medical emergencies. Intravenous antihistamines (H_1- and H_2-antagonists) and steroids, as well as subcutaneous epinephrine (or IV), may be required. Securing the airway via fiberoptic-guided endotracheal intubation or cricothyroidotomy may also be necessary. Admission to permit additional airway observation and/or management is required in patients with oropharyngeal angioedema.

The use of topical antihistamine preparations is discouraged because these topical antihistamine agents are readily absorbed and dosing is difficult to predict. Accidental overdosage may occur in patients who aggressively apply the preparations. Topical steroids have no proven clinical benefit and, therefore, are not recommended. Of course, attention toward identification and elimination of the trigger is warranted in all forms of urticaria and angioedema. Most cases of urticaria and angioedema will resolve in 1-3 days without sequelae. A minority of patients will require additional diagnostic evaluation aimed at trigger identification.

Erythema Multiforme

Erythema multiforme (EM) represents an acute inflammatory skin disease with a broad clinical spectrum that ranges from a localized papular eruption of the skin (EM minor) to a severe, multisystem illness (EM major) with widespread vesiculobullous lesions and erosions of the mucous membranes (Stevens Johnson Syndrome [SJS]). Lyell disease (toxic epidermal necrolysis [TEN]) is also considered a form of EM major in certain classification schemes,[8] though such controversy will not effect management and disposition decisions for the emergency physician. The disorder strikes all age groups, with the highest incidence in young adults (20-40 years of age). It affects males twice as often as females and occurs commonly in the spring and fall. Many factors have been implicated in the etiology of EM, including infection, drugs, and malignancies.[9] Drug reactions (particularly antibiotics and anticonvulsants) and malignancies are important causes of EM in older patients, whereas mycoplasma and herpetic infections are the most common precipitants in children. Approximately 50% of all cases lack an identifiable etiology.

The pathogenesis of EM remains largely unknown. Most likely, it is the result of a hypersensitivity reaction. Immunoglobulin and complement components can be demonstrated in the cutaneous microvasculature via immunofluorescence studies of skin biopsy specimens; in addition, there are circulating immune complexes in the serum, and a mononuclear cell infiltrate on histologic examination.[8]

Clinical Presentation and Diagnosis. Patients with EM frequently report malaise, fever, myalgias, arthralgias, diffuse pruritus, and/or a generalized burning sensation before the development of skin lesions. The morphological configuration of the lesions is quite variable. *(Please see Table 6.)*

Maculopapular and target (iris) lesions are the most characteristic. Erythematous papules appear symmetrically on the dorsum of the hands and feet, as well as the extensor surfaces of the extremities. The maculopapule evolves into the classic target lesion over the next 24-48 hours. As the maculopapule enlarges, the central area becomes cyanotic, and occasionally is accompanied by central purpura and/or a vesicle. Urticarial plaques may also occur with or without the iris lesion in a similar distribution. In contrast to true urticaria, EM lesions are approximately the same size (1-2 cm), nonpruritic, and

Table 8. Lesions of TEN

Warm, tender erythroderma
Vesicle
Bulla
Vesiculobulla
Exfoliation
Muccous membrane involvement

Table 9. Differential Diagnosis of TEN

Erythema multiforme
Toxic shock syndrome (staph and strep)
Staphylococcal scalded skin syndrome
Exfoliative drug reactions
Primary blistering disorders
Pemphigus and pemphigoid
Kawasaki syndrome

persist for 1-2 weeks. Partially formed target lesions may resemble urticaria. Vesiculobullous lesions, which may be pruritic and painful, develop within pre-existing maculopapules or plaques, usually on the extensor surface of the arms and legs and less frequently involving the trunk. Vesiculobullous lesions are most often found on mucosal surfaces, including the mouth, eyes, vagina, urethra, and anus.

Lesions develop in successive crops during a 2-4 week period and heal over a course of 5-7 days. Scarring is rarely a problem except in cases of secondary infection or in heavily pigmented patients in whom hypopigmentation or hyperpigmentation may occur. Recurrence may be noted on repeat exposure to the etiological agent, which is a special concern in cases associated with herpes simplex infection or medication use.[10]

Complications of EM include fluid and electrolyte deficiencies, secondary infection, sepsis, ophthalmological sequelae, and multiorgan failure syndrome. In particular, the ophthalmological sequelae may be severe and disabling in that permanent visual impairment may occur. Occular involvement occurs in approximately 10% of patients with EM minor while the SJS variant experiences ophthalmological lesions in almost three-quarter of cases.[11] The differential diagnosis of EM includes herpetic infection, vasculitis, toxic epidermal necrolysis, various primary blistering disorders (pemphigus and pemphigoid), urticaria, Kawasaki disease, and the toxic-infectious erythemas. *(Please see Table 7.)*

Management. Outpatient treatment of EM minor with topical corticosteroids is sometimes possible. However, steroids should not be applied to eroded areas of the skin. Dermatological consultation and close follow-up are strongly encouraged. Those patients with extensive disease, systemic toxicity, and/or mucous membrane involvement require hospitalization, optimally in the intensive care or burn unit setting in which secondary infections, fluid deficits, electrolyte disorders, and nutritional demands are best managed.

Systemic steroids are commonly used to provide symptomatic relief, but are of unproven benefit as far as duration and outcome of EM.[12-14] Some studies suggest an increased incidence of infection with systemic steroid therapy.[13] Many authorities recommend a short, intensive steroid course, particularly in drug-related cases, with abrupt cessation in 3-5 days if no favorable response is noted. This rapid intensive steroid therapy is felt to offer the patient the possible benefits steroids, while avoiding the complications of corticosteroid use.

Systemic analgesics and antihistamines will provide symptomatic relief. Stomatitis is treated with diphenhydramine and viscous lidocaine mouth rinses. Blisters are treated with cool, wet Burow's solution (aluminum sulfate/calcium acetate in aqueous solution) compresses. Occular involvement should be monitored by an ophthalmologist; unfortunately, burst steroid therapy does not appear to reduce either the chance of development or significant existing ocular lesions.[11] EM, particularly SJS, has significant morbidity and a mortality rate of approximately 10%, despite aggressive therapy. The most common causes of death are sepsis and fluid-electrolyte deficits.

Toxic Epidermal Necrolysis

Toxic epidermal necrolysis (TEN) is an explosive dermatosis characterized by tender erythema, bullae formation, and subsequent exfoliation with associated systemic toxicity. As previously stated, TEN may present as a severe form of EM major.[8] TEN is found in all age groups and shows no predilection to gender. The syndrome has multiple etiologies, with medications most commonly implicated.[8,9,15-18] The most frequently encountered medications include antibiotics, anticonvulsants, and nonsteroidal anti-inflammatory drugs (NSAIDs). In one large series, a drug was identified as the causative agent in 77% of cases, with the following medications implicated: sulfonamide antibiotics (30 cases); NSAID, especially phenylbutazone and oxicam derivatives (29 cases); anticonvulsants (7 cases); allopurinol (3 cases); chlormezanone (3 cases); and miscellaneous medications (7 cases), including aspirin, antipyretics, and non-sulfa antibiotics.[19] Malignancy, however, is another causative factor in TEN.[20,21c] In many cases, an etiology is not found. Patients with HIV are particularly prone to TEN for unknown reasons.[22]

The pathogenesis of TEN is poorly understood, but it is felt to be partly immunological.[23] Human lymphocyte antigen (HLA) typing has suggested a possible genetic predisposition (increased incidence of HLA-B_{12} in many patients).[24]

Clinical Presentation and Diagnosis. Patients with TEN often present with a prodrome suggestive of a viral illness, including malaise, anorexia, arthralgias, fever, and upper respiratory infection symptoms. The prodromal symptoms, if present, occur 1-2 weeks prior to the development of dermatological findings. Skin tenderness, pruritus, tingling, or burning may be reported during this period.[20,21]

The onset of objective skin findings is characterized by warm erythema, which initially involves only the face (in areas around the eyes, nose, and mouth) and genitalia, but later becomes generalized. *(Please see Table 8.)* The erythematous areas become tender and confluent within hours of onset. Tender erythema is especially characteristic of early TEN. Flaccid, ill-defined bullae appear within the areas of erythema. Lateral pressure with a finger on normal skin adjacent to bullous lesion dislodges the epidermis, producing denuded dermis and demonstrating Nikolski's sign. The bullae form along the cleavage plane between the epidermis and the der-

Table 10. TSS Case Definition

MAJOR CRITERIA

- Fever—Temperature > 102°F
- Rash—Erythroderma (localized or diffuse) followed by peripheral desquamation in 5-14 days.
- Mucous membrane—Hyperemia of oral and vaginal mucosa and of conjunctiva
- Hypotension—History of dizziness, orthostatic changes, or hypotension

MULTISYSTEM MANIFESTATIONS

- CNS—Altered mentation without focal neurological signs
- Cardiovascular—Evidence of distributive shock (loss of peripheral vascular resistance, hyperdynamic cardiac state, and increased vascular permeability); heart failure with or without pulmonary congestion; and supraventricular or ventricular dyshrythmias, nonspecific T-wave/ST-segment changes, and atrioventricular blocks
- Pulmonary—Adult respiratory distress syndrome
- Gastrointestinal—Vomiting and diarrhea
- Hepatic—Elevations (at least twice normal) in bilirubin, alkaline phosphatase, and the transaminases
- Renal—Blood urea nitrogen and/or creatinine at least twice normal; abnormal urinary sediment without urinary tract infection oliguria
- Hematological—Thrombocytopenia or thrombocytosis; anemia; leukopenia or leucytosis
- Musculoskeletal—Myalgias; arthralgias, rhabdomyolysis
- Metabolic—Hypocalcemia; hypophosphatemia
- Absence of other etiological agent—Cultures of all body fluids negative (may be positive for *S. aureus*); no serological evidence of leptospirosis, rickettsial disease, or rubeola; no clinical evidence of Kawasaki syndrome

Note: The diagnosis of TSS requires the presence of all four major criteria and three or more indications of multisystem involvement.

mis. The epidermis is then shed in large sheets, leaving raw, denuded areas of exposed dermis.

Stomatitis and conjunctivitis may precede the erythematous rash by 24-48 hours. Mucous membrane involvement is an early, characteristic finding of TEN. Oral lesions, which typically are blistering and are characterized by subsequent erosions, are found in the vast majority of patients. Orolabial lesions are disfiguring and often impair adequate oral intake, which may contribute to the significant fluid deficits present in most cases. The eyes are also commonly affected (approximately 75% of patients),[11,20,21] producing purulent conjunctivitis, painful erosions, and potential blindness. Anogenital lesions are found in about one-half of all TEN patients. In 60-65% of cases, there are simultaneous oral, ocular, and anogenital lesions. Additional mucous membrane involvement may be seen in the respiratory, gastrointestinal, and genitourinary tracts.[25]

The average time of onset of symptoms after exposure to the inciting agent is about two weeks. Cutaneous extension follows an unpredictable time course, ranging from 24 hours to 15 days, with a minority of severe cases demonstrating rapid, extensive involvement within 24 hours. The extent of skin involvement is variable, with an average of approximately 40% of body surface area. Sequelae include cutaneous and mucosal scarring, hypopigmentation/hyperpigmentation, and blindness. The differential diagnosis of TEN includes staphylococcal scalded skin syndrome (SSSS), EM, toxic shock syndrome (staphylococcal and streptococcal), exfoliative drug reactions, primary blistering disorders (pemphigus and pemphigoid), and Kawasaki disease. *(Please see Table 9.)*

The two major complications and leading causes of death in TEN are infection (pneumonia[25] and sepsis) and hypovolemia accompanied by electrolyte disorders. A broad range of pathogens are usually found, with staphylococcal and pseudomonal species predominating. The mortality rate has been reported to be 25-30%.[19,22] The following clinical variables are associated with poor prognosis: advanced age, extensive disease, idiopathic nature, multiple medication use, azotemia, hyperglycemia, leukopenia, and thrombocytopenia.

Management. Management of TEN requires hospitalization, optimally in a critical care setting or burn unit. In most cases, therapy is similar to the approach for the burn patient. Immediate concerns center on protecting and monitoring an adequate airway, as well as restoration and maintenance of circulatory volume. Correction of significant electrolyte disorders should also be addressed. Prompt, aggressive antibiotic administration is necessary in suspected or documented infection; initial prophylactic antibiotics are not recommended by most authorities.[22] Petrolatum gauze dressings applied to denuded areas provide a partial barrier against fluid and electrolyte losses. Elimination and/or treatment of any inciting factor is required. As with EM major, any ocular complaints or findings should be explored early by an ophthalmologist; the response to aggressive steroid therapy does not appear to alter the progression of ocular manifestations of TEN.[11]

Exfoliative Dermatitis

Exfoliative dermatitis, a cutaneous reaction produced in response to a drug or a chemical agent or to an underlying systemic disease, refers to a condition in which most or all of the skin surface is affected by a scaly erythematous dermatitis. Men are afflicted twice as often as women; at least 75% of patients are older than 40 years.[26-28] The mechanisms responsible for exfoliative dermatitis are not known.

Exfoliative dermatitis can have an abrupt onset, especially when it is associated with a drug, contact allergen, or malignancy. In contrast, exacerbations related to an underlying cutaneous disorder usually evolve more slowly. One study demonstrated that exfoliative dermatitis tends to be a chronic condition with a mean duration of five years when related to a chronic illness;[26] a shorter course often follows suppression of the underlying dermatosis, discontinuation of causative drugs, or avoidance of allergen. Both idiopathic and chronic disease-related exfoliative dermatitis can continue for 20 or more years; death is rare solely due to exfoliative dermatitis.

Clinical Presentation and Diagnosis. Generalized erythema and warmth is noted and is similar to that seen in patients with TEN;

the erythema is accompanied by scaling or flaking and patients often complain of pruritus with tightness of the skin. In contrast to the patient with TEN, tenderness of the involved skin is usually not present, in contrast to the TEN patient. The patient usually presents with a low-grade fever. Active erythroderma is complicated by excessive heat loss that may manifest as hypothermia. The widespread and marked cutaneous vasodilation may result in high-output congestive heart failure in patients with little cardiovascular physiologic reserve. Disruption of the epidermis results in increased transepidermal water loss, and continued exfoliation can produce significant protein loss and negative nitrogen balance. Chronic inflammatory exfoliation produces many changes, such as dystrophic nails, thinning scalp and body hair, and patchy or diffuse pigmentation changes.

Various erythrodermas may mimic exfoliative dermatitis; however, the presence of ichthyosis in other family members, the lifelong presence of disease, and the morphologic detail in scale and anatomic distribution make differentiation easy.

Management. Considerable effort must be made to identifiy the underlying etiology. This requires taking a careful history to document previous cutaneous disease and recent drug use, as well as laboratory tests, to establish whether there is a possible association with malignancy. Biopsy of involved skin and lymphadenopathy are indicated. Some patients respond to application of topical corticosteroids and oral antihistamines for their pruritus and low-grade pain. A significant percentage of patients require systemic corticosteroids. When systemic steroids are used, the patient can apply bland lotions or creams rather than topical corticosteroid preparations. Tepid colloidal baths, such as cornstarch or oatmeal powder suspension, are of some benefit as well. A patient with a newly diagnosed case of exfoliative dermatitis or one who is experiencing an acute exacerbation should be hospitalized for aggressive skin care, supportive therapy, and continued evaluation. Caution must be exercised in these patients. Those with widespread erythroderma require conservative management with an inpatient disposition and early dermatologic consultation.

Toxic Shock Syndrome

In 1978, Todd et al described a multisystem illness presenting with fever, shock, and erythroderma followed by desquamation; the authors noted an association between the illness and infection with toxigenic *Staphylococcus aureus*—the syndrome was named toxic shock syndrome (TSS).[29] Initially, the vast majority of cases involved menstruating women using extra-absorbent tampons.[30] With removal of these tampons from the market and increased physician awareness of the illness, a 30-50% increase in nonmenstrual cases has been reported.[31,32] Nonmenstrual cases of TSS involve either colonization with or infection by a *S. aureus* species capable of toxin production; this syndrome has been reported in association with acute infection and the presence of indwelling foreign bodies.

Women experience 85-90% of all cases of TSS.[33,34] The preponderance of cases in women is largely the result of the continued prevalence in menstrual cases. TSS has been reported in all age groups from neonatal to geriatric, but is most commonly encountered in patients 15-34 years of age, with one-third of cases occurring in the 15-19 age group and two-thirds in patients younger than 25 years of age. Patients with a nonmenstrual source of TSS are often older (27 years of age) than those with a menstrual etiology (22 years of age).[35]

Table 11. Differential Diagnosis of Toxic-Infectious Erythemas

Scarlet fever
Rocky Mountain spotted fever
Leptospirosis
Rubeola
Meningococcemia
Streptococcal TSS
Staph scalded skin syndrome
Kawasaki disease
Toxic epidermal necrolysis
Stevens-Johnson syndrome
Gram-negative sepsis
Exfoliative drug eruptions
Localized bullous lesion

Infection with, or colonization by, toxin-producing strains of *S. aureus* is required for the development of TSS. *S. aureus* can be isolated from specific soft tissue sites in the majority of cases, although blood cultures are often sterile. The numerous manifestations of illness are felt to originate from both the actions of a specific staphylococcal toxin and from myriad humoral mediators of acute injury.

Protean clinical manifestations of TSS range from a mild, trivial disease, often misdiagnosed as a viral syndrome, to a rapidly progressive, potentially fatal, multisystem illness. Criteria for the diagnosis of TSS are defined in the case definition. *(Please see Table 10.)* In this regard, the typical patient with TSS will present with erythroderma, fever, hypotension, and other evidence of organ involvement. A prodrome of fever, chills, arthralgias, myalgias, nausea, vomiting, and diarrhea may precede the more dramatic manifestations of the syndrome by 2-4 days. The majority of patients are hospitalized after 1-2 days of active illness. In addition to the characteristics listed in the case definition, TSS also is identified by its sudden onset and rapid progression to multisystem dysfunction.[35]

The dermatological hallmark of TSS is a nonpruritic, blanching macular erythroderma, which is a characteristic feature and an important criterion for the diagnosis. As a result, the erythroderma is diffuse, although it may be confined to the extremities or trunk and frequently resembles a typical sunburn. The rash, however, may be subtle and is often missed altogether in heavily pigmented patients or in patients examined in a poorly illuminated room. By definition, the rash is noted at presentation and may resolve in 3-5 days. If the patient survives, a fine desquamation of the hands and feet follows in 5-14 days. Other dermatological manifestations include conjunctival and mucosal hyperemia, petechiae, alopecia, and fingernail loss.

The differential diagnosis *(please see Table 11)* is broad, and includes scarlet fever, Rocky Mountain spotted fever, leptospirosis, rubeola, meningococcemia, streptococcal TSS, SSSS, Kawasaki disease, toxic epidermal necrolysis, SJS, gram-negative sepsis, and exfoliative drug eruptions.

Management of patients with TSS is dictated by the severity of their illness. As in any patient presenting in extremis, the emergency physician must perform a rapid, thorough assessment of the ABCs, insure a stable airway and ventilatory status, and support hemodynamic status. After stabilizing the patient, subsequent management objectives include identification and removal of any potential source of *S. aureus* and associated toxin (e.g., foreign bodies such as nasal packing or vaginal tampon, infected wound, and abscess). Finally, the patient must be monitored closely for evidence of organ system dysfunction. The vast majority of patients with TSS will require hospital admission and the patient who is critically ill is best managed in the intensive care unit. Vigorous fluid resuscitation, use of vasopressors and inotropic agents, and endotracheal intubation with mechanical ventilation are potential management options.

Antibiotic therapy with an appropriate antistaphylococcal agent is recommended. The use of antibiotics will not alter the course of the disease, but it has been shown to reduce the rate of recurrence, which is more common in menstrual cases. The use of corticosteroids is controversial and, currently, cannot be recommended.[2,10]

Toxic Streptococcal Syndrome

A syndrome similar to TSS, caused by *Streptococcus* organisms, has been described.[36,37] Streptococcal TSS (STSS) is a clinical syndrome involving multiple organ systems and is characterized by fever, hypotension, and skin findings. A retrospective review of hospital records from 1985 to 1990 identified 128 patients, aged 6 months to 96 years, with invasive group A streptococcal infection.[38] The causative agent of this clinical disorder is *Streptococcus pyogenes* (group A *Streptococcus*), a *Streptococcal* species that produces extracellular proteins called streptococcal pyrogenic exotoxins (SPEs). The presence of invasive streptococcal infection seems to be a common etiologic factor in STSS. One review noted that 75% of cases of STSS were associated with soft-tissue infections, among them cellulitis, myositis, and fasciitis.[39]

The clinical presentation of STSS is similar to that of staphylococcal TSS. Virtually all patients present with fever and hypotension. Skin findings, including swelling, erythema, or bullae, are found in up to 80% of patients. Subsequent desquamation is less common than in staphylococcal TSS.[40] From a clinical perspective, the clinician should consider STSS as a diagnostic possibility in any patient with fever, skin findings, and hypotension associated with a soft-tissue infection. The same major and minor criteria used to confirm the diagnosis of staphylococcal TSS are helpful for identifying patients with STSS. *(Please see Table 10.)* According to a consensus document, clinical features must include isolation of group A streptococci (*S. pyogenes*), hypoperfusion of target organs, and evidence of multisystem dysfunction.

Because as many as 75% of cases of STSS have an associated soft-tissue infection, exhaustive search for a site of infection is warranted. In this regard, a thorough skin examination is essential; the emergency physician should look for erythema, bullae, skin discoloration, and cellulitis. Palpation of muscle groups may demonstrate tenderness, indicating possible myositis or fasciitis. In extremity infections (myositis, fasciitis), elevated intracompartmental pressures may produce a compartment syndrome. Muscle compartment pressure monitoring may aid in making the diagnosis. The differential diagnosis of STSS is similar to that for staphylococcal TSS.

Management. Successful management of STSS requires early recognition and aggressive supportive care. As with TSS, prompt attention to ABCs and rapid correction of any derangements in these functions must be performed. The most important aspect of early management is aggressive fluid resuscitation. The clinical examination, chest radiograph, and arterial blood gas analysis should be monitored closely for impending respiratory failure. Because soft-tissue infection plays a large role in STSS, aggressive management of these infections is essential. Whether external or internal, the site of infection should be identified, and, if appropriate, quickly incised, and drained; debridement of nonviable tissue is essential. In severe myositis or fasciitis, limb amputation may be necessary to prevent fatal sepsis.[41] Because STSS is often associated with a focus of infection and bacteremia, parenteral anti-streptococcal antibiotics are required. Initially, this requires a combination of antibiotics to provide broad coverage until the pathogen is identified. Additional coverage is based on final culture and sensitivity results. Because of multisystem involvement and the propensity toward renal failure and ARDS, intensive care unit admission with invasive hemodynamic monitoring is usually necessary. Milder cases with appropriate monitoring may be managed outside of the intensive care unit.

Staphylococcal Scalded Skin Syndrome

Staphylococcal scalded skin syndrome (SSSS), also known as Ritter's disease, staphylococcal epidermal necrolysis, or staphylococcal epidermolytic syndrome, develops in patients with a clinically inapparent staph infection caused by a toxigenic organism. SSSS is one of several staphylococcal epidermolytic toxin syndromes, including bullous impetigo and scarlatiniform (staphylococcal scarlet fever) eruption. SSSS occurs in sporadic cases, as well as in outbreaks in nurseries and similar groupings of infants and toddlers aged 6 months to 6 years.[42] A large case series of SSSS showed that 62% of patients were younger than 2 years of age, with 98% of patients younger than age 6.[43] Children who are afflicted with SSSS usually are healthy and otherwise normal, in contrast to adults who develop this disorder. The rare adult case occurs in individuals with chronic immunosuppression (e.g., steroid therapy) or moderate-to-severe renal insufficiency. The exotoxins involved, collectively known as exfoliatin, are elaborated by the bacteria, released into the circulation, and are responsible for such clinical manifestations as erythroderma followed by desquamation. The patient's immune response to antigenic toxin produces fever and irritability.

The exotoxin produces an antibody-mediated immune response directed against the toxin. Antitoxin antibodies are found in more than 75% of the population older than 10 years of age.[44] This finding explains the rarity of the syndrome in older children and adults. Additionally, the rare adult case results from inadequate renal clearance of the toxin in patients with chronic renal disease and suppressed immunity. Infants and children have creatinine clearances approaching 50% of adult values. In the adult with chronic renal disease or the pediatric patient with normal renal function, this relatively low creatinine clearance theoretically allows accumulation of the toxin with subsequent clinical disease.[45,46]

SSSS frequently begins as a clinically inapparent staphylococcal infection of the conjunctiva, nasopharynx, or umbilicus. The disease course can be divided into three phases: 1) initial/erythroderma; 2) exfoliative; and 3) desquamation and recovery. Initially, the patient (or parent) notes the sudden appearance of a tender diffuse erythroderma; localized disease also has been described. The involved skin may have a sandpaper texture similar to the rash of scarlet fever (which presents with a nontender rash). The tender erythema of SSSS is prominent in the perioral, periorbital, and groin regions, as well as in the skin creases of the neck, axilla, popliteal, and antecubital areas. The mucous membranes are spared.

The exfoliative stage begins on the second day of the illness. Erythematous skin wrinkles and peels off at sites of minor trauma or with minimal lateral pressure with the examiner's fingertip, illustrating the positive Nikolski's sign (also found in TEN). Large, flaccid, fluid-filled bullae and vesicles appear next. These lesions rupture easily and are shed in large sheets; the underlying tissue resembles scalded skin and rapidly desiccates. During the exfoliative phase, the patient is often febrile and irritable. After 3-5 days of illness, the involved skin desquamates, with recovery of normal skin within 7-10 days. The vast majority of patients survive with supportive care. Additionally, cultures of the blood, nasopharynx, conjunctiva, and any obviously infected site are recommended, although the clinical utility is of these cultures is questionable since they are usually sterile due to toxigenic nature of the syndrome. The differential diagnosis of SSSS includes toxic epidermal necrolysis, TSS, exfoliative drug eruptions, staphylococcal scarlet fever, and localized bullous impetigo. *(Please see Table 11.)*

Management of the patient with SSSS includes fluid resuscitation and correction of electrolyte abnormalities, as well as identification and treatment of the source of the toxigenic *Staphylococcus*. Appropriate anti-staphylococcal antibiotics, preferably a penicillinase-resistant penicillin, is recommended. Fluid deficits and associated electrolyte deficiencies can be clinically significant because of loss of the skin as a protective barrier, reduced oral intake, and associated fever. Corticosteroids are contraindicated because of the interference with proper immune system functions. Most patients, with the exception of neonates, do not require topical therapies. The newborn may be treated with topical sulfadiazine or its equivalent. Wet dressings are not recommended. The majority of cases require antibiotics and careful monitoring.

Cutaneous Vasculitis

Vasculitis refers to a series of diseases caused by blood vessel inflammation. These conditions are characterized by perivascular inflammatory cell infiltration, vessel necrosis, and leukocytoclasis. Vasculitis may be a primary disease process or develop secondarily to other systemic abnormalities. The effects of vasculitis may be confined to the skin or may involve multiple organ systems. The pathogenesis of vasculitis is not well understood. This section will deal with cutaneous vasculitis as both a primary skin disorder and as well as a reflection of underlying systemic disease.

In cases in which an etiology for cutaneous vasculitis is identified, the most common causative syndrome was rheumatoid arthritis (13%). Other precipitants include food reactions, medications (penicillin, cephalosporins, cyproheptadine, procainamide, thiazide, aspirin), infections (group A streptococcal upper respiratory tract infections, bacterial otitis media, and viral hepatitis), collagen vascular diseases, and regional enteritis. In one large series, no such agent or syndrome was found in the majority of cases (54%).[33]

Clinical Presentation and Diagnosis. A detailed history is mandatory in patients with cutaneous vasculitis. Drug use (over-the-counter, illegal, and prescription) and infectious exposures should be documented. The history and review of systems may show evidence of systemic involvement. Clinical findings may include arthralgias, myalgias, arthritis, myositis, and renal involvement with hematuria and proteinuria; gastrointestinal involvement may be characterized by abdominal pain, nausea, bloody stools, hematemesis, and pancreatitis. Pulmonary, cardiac, ocular, and neurological symptomatology are less common.

Physical examination will demonstrate the vasculitic skin lesions. Other findings will depend on the presence of associated systemic illness. The most common skin manifestation of vasculitis is palpable purpura.[47,48] Other associated lesions include urticaria, ulcerative lesions, erythematous papules and nodules, vesiculobullous lesions, and livedo reticularis.[47-49] Lesions associated with cutaneous vasculitis commonly are located symmetrically on the lower extremities, usually on the feet and ankles.[47-49] The majority of patients will have a limited disease course without significant discomfort; the lesions, however, with their alarming and disfiguring appearance, usually prompt the ED visit. The disease usually lasts several weeks to months; the rare patient may have a chronic or relapsing course over a several year period.

Laboratory values are nonspecific in the evaluation of cutaneous vasculitis. Most patients will have an elevated erythrocyte sedimentation rate or C-reactive protein, especially if there is an associated connective tissue disease. Patients may have an abnormal complete blood cell count with anemia, leukopenia, or leukocytosis; thrombocytosis may be seen due to the "acute-phase-reactant" nature of the platelet; eosinophilia may be present. Urinalysis and renal function tests may show azotemia, hematuria, pyuria, and proteinuria; the urinalysis is an excellent screening tool for systemic vasculitis. The stool may be positive for gross or occult blood. Definitive confirmation of the diagnosis is made with a skin biopsy.

Management. Antihistamines may be prescribed for symptomatic relief and they may prevent development of new skin lesion. Steroids may be used for severe disease. Prednisone 60 mg/d, in divided doses, usually will control cutaneous manifestations. Because the disease course is usually limited to several weeks, steroids should be tapered after the cutaneous symptoms have been controlled. Painful arthralgias and myalgias can be treated with NSAIDs. If cutaneous involvement is secondary to exogenous agents (drugs, food, or infection), they should be identified and removed. Vasculitis associated with systemic illness should resolve with treatment of the underlying disorder.[47-49] Although most patients will respond to conventional treatment, some will develop recurrent skin disease during steroid taper, which may be refactory to further therapy. Numerous therapeutic approaches have been suggested, with variable success in patients with recalcitrant disease, including chronic corticosteroid use, colchicine, and dapsone.

Patients with isolated cutaneous vasculitis or mild systemic symptomatology can be treated symptomatically and discharged home. Although identification of the etiological factor is recommended, the majority of the cases are idiopathic and identification may not be possible. Early dermatological follow-up is essential. Outpatients with cutaneous vasculitis should be watched closely for development of systemic disease.

References

1. McCarthy GM, Lamb GC, Russell TJ, et al. Primary care-based dermatology practice: Internists need more training.

J Gen Int Med 1991;6:52-56.

2. Norman GR. The development of expertise in dermatology. *Arch Dermatol* 1989;125:1063-1070.
3. Beltrami VS. Urticaria and angioedema. *Dermatol Clin* 1996;14:171-182.
4. Zuberbier T. Acute urticaria: Clinical aspects and therapeutic responsiveness. *Acta Derm Venereol* 1996;76:295-303.
5. Pollack CV, Romano TJ. Outpatient management of acute urticaria: The role of prednisone. *Ann Emerg Med* 1995;26: 547-552.
6. Tharp MD. Cetirizine: A new therapeutic alternative for chronic urticaria. *Cutis* 1996;58:94-98.
7. Goldsmith P, Dowd PM. The new H_1 antihistamines. *Dermatol Clin* 1993;11:87-97.
8. Paquet P, Pierard GE. Erythema multiforme and toxic epidermal necrolysis: A comparative study. *Am J Dermatopathol* 1997;19:127-132.
9. Rzany B, Hering O, Mockenhaupt M, et al. Histopathological and epidemiological characteristics of patients with erythema exudativum multiforme major, Stevens-Johnson syndrome, and toxic epidermal necrolysis. *Brit J Dermatol* 1996;135: 6-11.
10. Nesbit SP, Gobetti JP. Multiple recurrences of oral erythema multiforme after secondary Herpes simplex: Report of a case and review of the literature. *J Am Dermatol Assoc* 1986;112: 348-352.
11. Power WJ, Ghoraishi M, Merayo-Lloves J, et al. Analysis of the acute opthalmic manifestations of the erythema multiforme/Stevens-Johnson syndrome/toxic epidermal necrolysis disease spectrum. *Ophthal* 1995;102:1669-1676.
12. Patterson R, Dykewicz MS, Gonzales A, et al. Erythema multiforme and Stevens-Johnson syndrome: Descriptive and therapeutic controversy. *Chest* 1990;98:331-336.
13. Snook DL, McDonald CJ. Dermatologic manifestations of critical illness. *J Crit Illness* 1988;5:9-16.
14. Kakourou T, Klontza D, Soteropoulou F, et al. Corticosteroid treatment of erythema multiforme major (Stevens-Johnson syndrome) in children. *Eur J Pediatr* 1997;156:90-93.
15. Lyell A. Toxic Epidermal Necrolysis: An eruption resembling scalding of the skin. *Br J Dermatol* 1956;68:355-361.
16. Kauppinen K. Cutaneous reactions to drugs with special reference to severe bullous mucocutaneous eruptions and sulphonamides. *Acta Derm Venerol* 1972;52(suppl 68):1-89.
17. Ruiz-Maldonado R. Acute disseminated epidermal necrosis types 1, 2 and 3: Study of sixty cases. *J Am Acad Dermatol* 1985;13:623-635.
18. Lyell A. Toxic epidermal necrolysis (the scalded skin syndrome): A reappraisal. *Br J Dermatol* 1979;100:69-86.
19. Guillaume JC, Roujeau JC, Revuz J, et al. The culprit drugs in 87 cases of toxic epidermal necrolysis. (Lyell's syndrome). *Arch Dermatol* 1987;123:1166-1170.
20. Criton S, Devi K, Sridevi PK, et al. Toxic epidermal necrolysis—A retrospective study. *Int J Dermatol* 1997;36:923-925.
21. Murphy JT, Purdue GF, Hunt JL. Toxic epidermal necrolysis. *J Burn Care Rehab* 1997;18:417-420.
22. Porteous DM, Berger TG. Severe cutaneous drug reactions (Stevens-Johnson syndrome and toxic epidermal necrolysis) in human immunodeficiency virus infection. *Arch Dermatol* 1991;127:740-741.
23. Synder RA, Elias PM. Toxic epidermal necrolysis and staphylococcal scalded skin syndrome. *Dermatol Clin* 1983;1: 235-248.
24. Revuz J, Penso D, Roujeau JC, et al. Toxic epidermal necrolysis: Clinical findings and prognosis factors in 87 patients. *Arch Dermatol* 1987;123:1160-1165.
25. McIvor RA, Zaidi J, Peters WJ, et al. Acute and chronic respiratory complications of toxic epidermal necrolysis. *J Burn Care Rehab* 1996;17:237-240.
26. Abrahams I, McCarthy J, Sanders S. 101 Cases of exfoliative dermatitis. *Arch Dermatol* 1963;87:96-103.
27. Nicolis GD, Helwig EB. Exfoliative dermatitis: A clinicopathologic study of 135 cases. *Arch Dermatol* 1973;108: 788-796.
28. Wong KS, Wong SM, Tham SM, et al. Generalized exfoliative dermatitis: A clinical study of 108 patients. *Ann Acad Med* 1988;17:520-526.
29. Todd J, Fishaut M. Toxic-shock syndrome associated with phage-group I staphylococci. *Lancet* 1978;2:1116-1118.
30. Tofte RW, Williams DN. Toxic shock syndrome. *Postgrad Med* 1983;73:275-280, 285-288.
31. Centers for Disease Control and Prevention. Annual summary 1984. Reported morbidity and mortality in the United States. *Morb Mortal Wkly Rep MMWR* 1986;33:1-135.
32. Freedman, JD, Beer DJ. Expanding perspectives on the toxic shock syndrome. *Adv Intern Med* 1991;36:363-397.
33. Centers for Disease Control and Prevention. Summary of Notifiable Diseases, United States, 1988. *Morb Mortal Wkly Rep MMWR* 1989;37:1-57.
34. Broome CV. Epidemiology of toxic shock syndrome in the United States: Overview. *Rev Infect Dis* 1989;11:S14-S21.
35. Knudson P, Charney M, Salcido D. Post-traumatic toxic shock syndrome. *J Trauma* 1988;28:121-123.
36. Willoughby R, Greenberg RN. The toxic shock syndrome and streptococcal pyrogenic exotoxins. *Ann Int Med* 1983;98:559.
37. Cone LA, Woodard DR, Schlievert PM, et al. Clinical and bacteriologic observations of a toxic shock-like syndrome due to *Streptococcus pyogenes*. *N Engl J Med* 1987;317:146-149.
38. Hoge CW, Schwartz B, Talkington DF, et al. National Centers for Disease Control and Prevention: The changing epidemiology of invasive group A streptococcal infections and the emergence of streptococcal toxic shock-like syndrome: A retrospective population-based study. *JAMA* 1993;269:384-389.
39. Kohler W. Streptococcal toxic shock syndrome. *Int J Med Microbiol* 1990;272:257-264.
40. Stevens DL, Tanner MH, Winship J, et al. Severe group A streptococcal infections associated with a toxic shock-like syndrome and scarlet fever toxin A. *N Engl J Med* 1989;321:1-7.
41. Aitken DR, Mackett MC, Smith LL. The changing pattern of hemolytic streptococcal gangrene. *Arch Surg* 1982;117: 561-567.
42. Resnick SD. Staphylococcal toxin-mediated syndromes in childhood. *Semin Dermatol* 1992;11:11-18.
43. Melish ME, Glasgow LA. Staphylococcal scalded skin syndrome: The expanded clinical spectrum. *J Pediatr* 1971;78: 958-967.

44. Elias PM, Fritsch P, Epstein EH. Staphylococcal scalded skin syndrome. *Arch Dermatol* 1977;113:207-219.
45. Fritsch P, Elias P, Varga J. The fate of staphylococcal exfoliation in newborn and adult mice. *Br J Dermatol* 1976;95:275-284.
46. Melish ME, Chen FS, Murata MS. Epidermolytic toxin (ET) production in human and experimental staph infection. *Clin Res* 1979;27:114A (abstr).
47. Ekenstam E, Callen JP. Cutaneous leukocytoclastic vasculitis: Clinical and laboratory features of 82 patients seen in private practice. *Arch Dermatol* 1984;120:484-489.
48. Sanchez NP, Van Hale HM, Su WP. Clinical and histopathologic spectrum of necrotizing vasculitis: Report of findings in 101 cases. *Arch Dermatol* 1985;121:220-224.
49. Winkelmann RK, Ditto WB. Cutaneous and visceral syndromes of necrotizing or "allergic" angitis: A study of 38 cases. *Medicine* 1964;43:59-89.

Infectious Syndromes

William J. Brady, MD, FACEP

In this chapter, the author provides detailed clinical strategies for diagnosis and management of common, and, in some cases, life-threatening diseases that present with prominent dermatological manifestations. The review begins with herpes zoster infection and culminates with syndromes characterized by widespread blistering.

Herpes Zoster Infection

Both acute varicella and varicella zoster infections are caused by the same virus—*Herpesvirus varicellae*. The primary infection is acute varicella, which manifests in childhood as chicken pox. In contrast, varicella zoster infections (VZI) represent reactivation of a previously dormant virus in a patient with incomplete or compromised immunity; VZI is also referred to as shingles. In the case of the initial illness (i.e., chicken pox), the virus travels via individual cutaneous nerves to the dorsal root ganglia, where it remains latent until reactivation. At the time of reactivation, which usually occurs as a result of diminished immunologic function, the virus migrates down specific sensory nerves to the skin and produces shingles.

The specific factors leading to VZI are unknown, but likely involve reduced immune function in patients with a significant comorbid illness and/or medications associated with immunosuppressive properties. In particular, patients with lymphoma, leukemia, and diabetes mellitus are at highest risk for development of VZI. In addition, patients with altered immune function due to medication effects, organ transplant recipients, and patients with severe rheumatologic illness are more likely to acquire VZI. In most cases, it is difficult to determine whether the primary illness or medical therapy is responsible for reactivation.

Patients of all ages can be afflicted with VZI, with 10% of the population experiencing at least one episode of VZI in their lifetime.[1] However, children who develop chicken pox before the first 2 months of age are reported to be at increased risk for VZI later in life.[2] In addition, patients with an "unexplained" episode of VZI should be questioned about risk behaviors for HIV infection; appropriate testing should follow inasmuch as VZI may be an early manifestation of the acquired immunodeficiency syndrome in high-risk individuals.[3] Generally speaking, an exhaustive search for an underlying malignancy is probably not warranted in patients with VZI, since patients with VZIs are not more likely to have cancer.[4]

Patients with no documented history of chicken pox also may present with VZI. These cases result from either transplacental exposure to varicella or they have had a mild case of chicken pox that was clinically unrecognized. Contact with a patient with active shingles is unlikely to cause VZI in a patient with past chicken pox; however, the patient without a previous episode of varicella infection can acquire chicken pox from such an exposure.

Clinical Presentation and Diagnosis. The rash associated with shingles is characterized by vesicles and/or papules grouped

Table 1. Lesions of Varicella Zoster (Shingles)

- Close grouping/clustering of lesions
- Arrayed on an erythematous base
- Papulovesicles with clear/purulent fluid
- Ultimate ulcer formation with crusting
- Lesions vary in size

together on an erythematous base. Classical features of this herpes infection include the close grouping or clustering of lesions arrayed in an inflamed area of otherwise normal skin. *(Please see Table 1.)* The lesions initially appear as papulovesicles with clear fluid; over several days, the fluid within the vesicles may become cloudy and may eventually rupture. Eventually, there is blister and ulcer formation. The lesions vary in size in contrast to the vesicles seen in the Herpes simplex infections.

As a rule, the lesions of VZI appear along an individual dermatome. Occasionally, adjacent dermatomes may be involved. About two-thirds of all zoster infections involve the trunk, followed by the head and facial region, extremities, and perineal regions. In the case of VZI involving the truncal area, lesions may appear over a period of several days in centripetal fashion, with the initial cluster often located on the patient's back, just lateral to the midline. Subsequent lesions "move around the dermatome" toward the patient's flank and eventually around to the anterior aspect of the thorax over a 5-10 day period. As a rule, the clusters are discrete and are separated by areas of normal skin; in severe cases, the cluster may become confluent along the dermatome.

Unilateral involvement, which abruptly halts at the midline, is helpful in identifying the rash of VZI; occasionally, a few lesions may erupt just beyond the midline, and this is not inconsistent with the diagnosis. Approximately 50% of cases with VZI, especially patients with AIDS or reticuloendothelial malignancy, will experience viremia. These individuals may exhibit solitary lesions, usually totaling less than 30, which are scattered across the body. This finding, alone, does not indicate disseminatiof the disease. Patients with AIDS, individuals on immunosuppressive medications, and those with active reticuloendothelial malignancy more often demonstrate dissemination. Patients with Hodgkin's disease are especially prone to dissemination, with 15-50% of cases demonstrating involvement of the skin, lungs, and central nervous system. This group has a 10-25% mortality.[5] Death from VZI is rare in patients with other types of malignancy.

Pain, which may precede the skin manifestations by 4-5 days, is a prominent symptom in most patents, especially in the elderly.[6] Interestingly, intense pain is a less often encountered complaint in the young patient.[6] Complaints of pain prior to the presence of skin lesions may make the diagnosis difficult, especially in the older patient. A high index of suspicion is required during the initial prodrome, and the diagnosis should be considered in individuals who report severe head, chest, back, or abdominal pain occurring in a dermatomal distribution.

Other sensations that may be noted include pruritus, paresthesias, hypesthesia, and hyperesthesia. Constitutional symptoms such as fever, myalgias, and headache may also be reported by patients at the onset of illness. These prodromal symptoms, including the segmental pain, usually decrease in severity or resolve with appearance of the skin lesions. As is the case with pre-eruptive dermatomal pain, younger patients are less likely to experience other prodromal symptoms. The emergency physician must also be aware of and direct attention toward the psychosocial issues of the the patient with VZI; many older patients will note a sense of helplessness and depression during this infection.[6] In fact, suicide, with the VZI as the triggering event, has been reported.

Ocular involvement, which is common in patients with VZI, affects the ophthalmic branch of the fifth cranial nerve Corneal involvement is likely if vesicular lesions are observed in the lateral portion of the nose, implicating the nasociliary nerve. Hutchinson's sign is noted with lesions involving the distal portion of the nose. This degree of involvement may range from a keratoconjunctivitis without sequelae to a severe keratitis with vision-threatening corneal ulceration and scarring.

Fluorescein staining in conjunction with a comprehensive slit lamp examination of the cornea is essential in all cases of facial VZI. It should be stressed that a negative examination in a patient who has an obvious vesicular rash in the distribution of the third ophthalmic branch of the trigeminal nerve should not dissuade the EP from considering the possibility of corneal involvement; pain and skin lesions frequently appear before any objective ophthalmological findings are observed. The presence of Hutchinson's sign should alert the EP to the possibility of eventual corneal involvement—whether or not corneal lesions are noted at the time of initial examination. In contrast to ophthalmologic findings, involvement of the maxillary and mandibular branches of the fifth nerve will produce intraoral vesicles.

In addition to sensory complaints, other neurologic findings include paralysis and bladder dysfunction. Motor impairment is not common, although partial paresis of an extremity may be seen; complete return of motor function can be expected. The Ramsey Hunt syndrome is seen in patients with facial VZI. Viral movement along the seventh cranial nerve from the geniculate ganglion produces pain in the auricular and lateral facial areas. In addition, vesicles are seen on the tympanic membrane, in the external auditory canal, and on the concha and pinna. Facial nerve paralysis and hearing deficits are common. Auditory nerve involvement is seen in approximately 40% of cases, and is accompanied by partial hearing loss and vertigo.[7] Sacral VZI may produce bladder dysfunction with S2, S3, and/or S4 dermatomal involvement. Regional lymphadenopathy may also be seen in these patients.

Mild cases of VZI will heal uneventfully in 2-4 weeks, whereas severe infections will produce more extensive skin surface involvement, with ulceration and secondary staphylococcal infection. The following factors are associated with an increased risk for severe, localized VZI: older age, HIV infection, ongoing immunosuppressive therapy, and reticuloendothelial malignancy. Scarring, hypopigmentation, and keloid formation are not uncommon. VZI in the pregnant patient, regardless of stage of pregnancy, does not appear to affect either the mother or the fetus.

Postherpetic Neuralgia. Postherpetic neuralgia may be the most dreaded complication of the disease. This type of pain is the major cause of morbidity in patients with recent or remote zoster infections; the mechanism for postherpectic neuralgia been established. From a clinical perspective, however, the pain is often severe, intractable, and exhausting; elderly patients have committed suicide due to the severe pain and lack of relief. The incidence of pain increases with age as does both the magnitude and the duration of pain. The majority of patients under age 30 years do not experience postherpetic pain. By age 40, however, the risk of prolonged pain increases to approximately 30% and, by age 70 years, to 75%.[6] Interestingly, the severity of subsequent pain is not related to the lesion size or severity of the initial infection.[8] Patients with VZI involving the fifth cranial nerve reportedly experience postherpetic pain more often and for longer periods than do individuals with other VZI in other dermatomal distributions.

The differential diagnosis of herpes zoster infection is broad. *(Please see Table 2.)* Any process involving focal blistering and necrosis can produce similar lesions. Accordingly, the differential diagnosis of herpes zoster infection includes dermatitis herpetiformis, H. simplex virus infection, contact dermatitis (e.g., eczematous dermatitis), primary blistering disorders (pemphigus vulgaris and bullous pemphigoid), fixed drug eruptions, erythema multiforme, pyoderma gangrenosum, focal vasculitis, purpura fulminans, diabetic ulcer, bedsores, thermal/friction blisters, and factitious injection. Neuralgia occurring in an erythematous area and lacking vesicular lesions may also be confused with bacterial cellulitis.

Management. Most cases of VZI should be treated with reassurance, oral and/or parenteral pain medication as required, antihistamines, and topical therapy. Many patients are concerned about the disfiguring nature of the lesions; the physician should provide reassurance that lesions will resolve without such sequelae. As a rule, pain should be managed with oral NSAIDs and/or narcotic agents; parenteral narcotic agents may be helpful in patients with severe pain, which may require multiple administrations; alternatively, pain of less than five weeks duration may be treated with regional nerve block or epidural anesthesia. Antihistamine therapy may help relieve the intense pruritic and/or burning sensations encountered in the elderly patient.

Cool compress (tap water or Burow's solution) and calamine lotion will provide relief for superficial pain and pruritus. Such compresses applied for 15-20 minutes four times daily will macerate vesicles, remove crusts, and suppress bacterial growth. Short periods in a cool shower will also reduce superficial skin complaints. Topical steroids are not of benefit. Patients should also be cautioned about contagion toward contacts without a prior history of varicella infection.

Intravenous and oral high-dose acyclovir, if instituted within 48-72 hours of lesion appearance, may reduce discomfort, duration, and the intensity of the infection. There is also evidence to suggest that acyclovir and valacyclovir will reduce the likelihood of developing postherpetic neuralgia.[9,10] In general, acyclovir should be offered to patients who present early in the disease course (i.e., within 72 hours of eruption). Antiviral therapy is strongly recommended in patients who have large lesions, in those who have significant comorbidity, in patients who are using immunosuppressive medications, or those who have ophthalmic zoster. After 72 hours of symptoms, such therapy is unlikely to be of much benefit in the immunocompetent patient.[11,12] Approximately 50% of patients with VZI will present to the physician within this three-day time period, and therefore, will be candidates for this therapeutic approach.[6]

It should be stressed that other antiviral agents are available for the acute treatment of VZI. In addition to acyclovir, valacyclovir 44c and famciclovir 44d also are acceptable.[13] In general, these agents do not offer significant advantage over acyclovir in the treatment of VZI except for reduced dosing frequency, which may increase compliance and, therefore, improve outcome.

Table 2. Differential Diagnosis of Varicella Zoster (Shingles)

- Dermatitis herpetiformis
- Herpes simplex virus infection
- Contact dermatitis (e.g., eczematous dermatitis)
- Primary blistering disorders (pemphigus vulgaris and bullous pemphigoid)
- Fixed drug eruptions
- Erythema multiforme
- Pyoderma gangrenosum
- Focal vasculitis
- Purpura fulminans
- Diabetic ulcer
- Bedsores
- Thermal/friction blisters
- Factitious injection
- Bacterial cellulitis

Patients and physicians should recognize the importance of initiating antiviral therapy as soon as symptoms are noted and the diagnosis can be confirmed. In this regard, administration of the initial dose of the antiviral agent in the emergency department (ED) represents a sound approach, since reduction of symptoms and minimizing post-herpetic neuralgia are both time-sensitive phenomena. In addition to temporal barriers to the success of antiviral therapy, cost factors also must be considered. Antiherpetic agents are costly. In this regard, a recent survey of patients with VZI demonstrated that the majority were unwilling to use expensive agents if success was not likely.[6] *(Please see Table 3 for a listing of the various antiviral agents available for treatment of the VZI patient.)*

The use of systemic steroids for reducing the incidence of postherpetic neuralgia is controversial. As a rule, it is prudent to discuss this option with a dermatologist or an infectious disease consultant on an individual, case-by-case basis. Several reports suggest that if systemic steroids are used early in the eruptive stage of the illness, they may reduce the likelihood of postherpetic pain. Clearly, however, the use of steroids late in the disease course does not produce benefit. In any event, the risk of precipitant disseminated disease is minimal in patients who do not have a malignancy or immunodeficiency disorder.

Patients with severe VZI may require inpatient therapy and urgent dermatologic consultation, but this is the exception rather than the rule. Such cases are characterized by pain unresponsive to oral agents; large areas of local infection requiring aggressive wound care; secondary bacterial infection of herpetic skin lesions; active immunosuppressive or antineoplastic medication therapy; ophthalmic zoster; focal neurologic deficits; or disseminated disease.

Table 3. Oral Antiviral Therapy Used in the Management of VZI

MEDICATION	DOSE
• Zivorax (acyclovir)	800 mg po 5 times/ 24 hr
• Valtrex (valacyclovir)	1 g po q8h for 7 days
• Famvir (famciclovir)	500 mg po q8h for 7 days

Rocky Mountain Spotted Fever

Rocky Mountain spotted fever (RMSF) is a potentially fatal multisystem illness caused by *Rickettsia rickettsii* that is most often introduced to humans via a tick vector. RMSF has been reported in most regions of the United States, with the exception of Maine, Alaska, and Hawaii.[14] The disease is most frequently encountered in the mid- and south-Atlantic coastal states. RMSF is seasonal, with the majority (95%) of cases occurring in the spring and summer. Five to 700 cases are reportedly annually in the United States. Moreover, the condition is associated with a mortality rate ranging from 3% to 7%, but only in patients who are correctly diagnosed and appropriately treated. In heavily pigmented patients, a much higher mortality rate (16%) is noted, which may reflect difficulty in detecting the characteristic rash, and subsequent delays in initiating therapy. It should be stressed that in the absence of timely management, the mortality rate increases to 30-70%.[15,16]

Rickettsia rickettsii is spread to humans via a tick bite. Although not proven, authorities state that the tick must remain attached to the patient for at least six hours in order to transmit disease. After introduction of the organism into body tissues, it disseminates via the blood stream, invades vascular endothelium, and multiplies, a pathophysiological sequence that accounts for the widespread, multisystem nature of the illness. The histopathology is consistent with a necrotizing vasculitis.

Clinical Presentation and Diagnosis. After exposure to the tick and introduction of the organism into the body, the patient usually will present with the triad of fever (94%), headache (88%), and myalgias (85%). These symptoms become prominent approximately one week (range, 3-21 days) after the tick bite. Additional complaints may include photophobia, nausea, vomiting, abdominal pain, dry cough, malaise, and confusion. Typically, the rash in classic RMSF is evident four days (range, 1-15 days) after the onset of fever and other symptoms.[15] In a minority of patients (usually adults), the rash is not noted at any point of the disease course. This entity, also called Rocky Mountain "spotless" fever, occurs in approximately 15% of cases. In many instances, Rocky Mountain spotless fever may actually be Ehrliciosis.

The rash first appears on the wrists and ankles, and spreads rapidly to the palms and soles. As the rash moves centrally, the proximal extremities, trunk, and face are involved. The skin lesions at onset are described as discrete macules or maculopapules that blanch with pressure from the examiner's finger. The initial lesions evolve into petechiae during a 2-4 day period, fade slowly over 2-3 weeks, and heal, occasionally with resultant hyperpigmentation. Rarely, the petechiae may coalesce into ecchymotic areas with eventual gangrene of the distal extremities, nose, ear lobes, scrotum, and vulva.

The overall severity of the rickettsial infection is proportional to both the magnitude of the rash and the rapidity of its progression. Additional clinical findings include focal pulmonary infiltrates; myocarditis, which can be associated with dysrhythmias and cardiogenic shock; peripheral edema caused by herpatic dysfunction and hypoalbuminemia; prerenal renal failure; various neurological findings, including altered mental status, coma, seizures, focal deficits, and meningismus with cerebral spinal fluid pleocytosis; and disseminated intravascular coagulation. The most common cause of death is irreversible, distributive shock related to visceral and central nervous system dissemination of the rickettsial organism.

Diagnosis is largely clinical, and is based on the triad of headache, fever, and myalgias in a patient who has the potential for tick exposure. Even if there is no rash at presentation, the informed clinician should not rule out the possibility of RMSF, since the dermatological manifestations develop late in the disease course, and a minority of patients have the "spotless" variety. Laboratory values are not helpful in making the initial diagnosis, but increases in antibody titer can confirm RMSF in 10 days to two weeks. Immunofluorescent staining of a skin lesion is a new technique, providing a rapid means for diagnosis that is both highly sensitive and specific. The results, however, can be difficult to interpret in inexperienced hands.

The differential diagnosis includes meningococcemia (less orderly, more rapid rash progression) and endemic typhus (dissimilar rash distribution in a less ill patient). Additional entities deserving consideration include disseminated gonococcemia, secondary syphilis, viral exanthem, and disseminated intravascular coagulation.

Management. As in other entities, attention should be paid to establishing an adequate airway with ventilation and oxygenation, coupled with insuring systemic perfusion. Antibiotic therapy includes tetracycline for nonpregnant patients older than 8 years; children and the pregnant patient are best managed with chloramphenicol. Monitoring and supportive management are best performed in a critical care setting, especially in the case of patients who present with obvious disease and the potential for multiorgan failure. Patients who present with possible RMSF (i.e., they have had possible tick exposure and symptomatology characteristic of "viral syndrome") are best managed with a course of oral antibiotic therapy and close medical follow-up.

If the patient presents with a tick embedded in the skin, it should be removed. Using blunt curved forceps, the examiner grasps the tick as close to the skin surface as possible and pulls upward with a steady even pressure. Twisting and jerking movements of the forceps may cause the tick mouth parts to remain embedded in the skin. Steady even pressure for approximately 3-5 minutes will cause the tick to slowly back out of the skin. After the tick has been removed, the wound is thoroughly cleaned and irrigated and then properly bandaged. Tetanus prophylaxis is considered at this point. During the procedure, the examiner should use rubber gloves to shield himself or herself from potential infectious disease.

An alternative method for field use involves a thread or string. A loop is made in the thread and placed over the tick closest to the skin surface. With similar gentle traction the tick is slowly removed from the skin. Regardless of the method of removal, squeezing or pressure on the tick body should be avoided since this may cause injection of tick body fluids into the patient and increase the likelihood of infection.

Meningococcal Disease

Meningococcemia is a potentially fatal infectious illness caused by the gram-negative diplococcal bacterium *Neisseria meningitidis*. Meningococcal disease presents across a wide clinical spectrum in both acute and chronic forms. The acute entities include pharyngitis, meningitis, sepsis, or a combination of central nervous system and systemic infection; this clinical syndrome is most frequently encountered. The chronic variant (which will not be discussed here) is rare and occurs most often in patients with specific complement deficiencies. The chronic state infrequently progresses to acute disease. Meningococci are present in the nasopharynx of 2-20% of the general population (the carrier state); during epidemics, the organism is found in up to 30% of people without evidence of active disease.[17]

Meningococcal disease is commonly encountered in the pediatric setting. The illness usually strikes patients younger than 20 years, with the vast majority of cases occurring in children and infants younger than 5 years. Epidemic outbreaks occur when a virulent strain of the organism is introduced into a closed, confined population. The highest rates of infection are reported in the winter and spring months, although sporadic cases appear throughout the year.[18]

The organism is transmitted via aerosolized droplets of respiratory secretions from asymptomatic carriers and less frequently from actively infected patients. The mortality rate ranges from 5% to 28%; the majority of patients who are treated appropriately early in the course of the disease will recover.[17,19-22] It should be stressed that patients with acute meningococcal infection who exhibit signs of circulatory insufficiency, a peripheral white blood cell count of less than 10,000 cells/mm^3, or a coagulopathy have a high probability of developing organ system failure followed by death.[23]

Clinical Presentation and Diagnosis. Following exposure to the organism, clinical infection usually develops within 3-4 days (range, 2-10 days) and then progresses rapidly to severe illness. The patient may complain of severe headache, sudden fever, nausea, vomiting, myalgias, arthralgia, and a stiff neck. A rash is frequently noted on presentation and is an invaluable clue to suspecting the diagnosis early in the disease course. The mental status is often altered, ranging from agitated confusion to coma. On rare occasions, the patient with fulminant disease will present in septic shock.

Dermatological manifestations of multisystem meningococcal disease include petechia, urticaria, hemorrhagic vesicles, macules, and/or maculopapules. The classical petechial lesions are found on the extremities and trunk, but also are noted on the palms, soles, head, and mucous membranes. The petechiae evolve into palpable purpura with gray necrotic centers, which is a pathognomic finding for meningococcal infection. Skin findings result from invasion by the organism into the skin and subsequent destruction of the vascular endothelium. Histopathological analysis demonstrates an infectious vasculitis.

Fulminant meningococcal disease, which is encountered in less than 5% of patients, presents with sudden onset of prostration, petechiae with areas of ecchymosis, and distributive shock. This rapidly progressive variant of meningococcemia is complicated by purpura fulminans, which represents an aggressive form of disseminated intravascular coagulation. Large ecchymotic areas—usually, on the extremities, acral portions of the face, and genitalia—become necrotic or gangrenous. Patients who survive this fulminant disease will have gangrenous tissue that will auto-amputate or require surgical removal.

The diagnosis of acute meningococcal disease is suggested by the presence of an ill-appearing patient with an associated petechial rash accompanied by nonspecific symptoms of fever, headache, altered sensorium, and body aches. Additional historical points, physical signs, and laboratory findings supportive of the diagnosis include known exposure to active disease, rapid progression of nonspecific symptoms with the associated petechial rash, gram stain of skin lesions or cerebral spinal fluid demonstrating gram-negative intracellular diplococci, and latex agglutination of the cerebrospinal fluid. The differential diagnosis includes RMSF, TSS, acute gonococcemia, bacterial endocarditis, vasculitis (Henoch-Schonlein prupura or leukocytoclastic vasculitis), enteroviral infections, and bacterial sepsis (gram positive and gram negative) with disseminated intravascular coagulation.

Management. After stabilizing respiratory and hemodynamic parameters, parenteral antibiotics should be administered immediately. Prudent and proactive management suggests antibiotics should be administered as soon as possible in any patient suspected of acute disease. In this regard, an uncertain diagnosis or diagnostic studies such as head computerized tomographic scan should not delay empiric antibiotic administration.

Initial empiric therapy should also provide coverage of *Haemophilus influenzae, Streptococcus pneumoniae*, and *Neisseria meningitidis*. Appropriate agents include third generation cephalosporins such as ceftriaxone; due to the increased prevalence of cephalosporin-resistant pneumococcus, parenteral vancomycin should also be administered on an empirical basis. Once laboratory evidence confirms meningococci, intravenous penicillin should be used; it represents the drug of choice for this infection. Chloramphenicol is an alternative agent. Chemoprophylaxis with rifampin or ciprofloxacin is used for close contacts of the patient and in medical personnel, including prehospital caregivers, who have or may have been exposed to respiratory secretions.

Kawasaki Syndrome

Kawasaki disease (KD), also known as mucocutaneous lymph node syndrome, is an acute febrile illness that occurs primarily in children; the onset occurs from the neonatal period to early adolescence and the mean age at diagnosis is 2.6 years. Rare adult cases have been reported. The diagnosis of adult KD remains a challenge due to the age presentation.[24]

KD was first described in Japan, although cases are commonly encountered both endemically and epidemically in the Americas, Europe, and Asia. The major clinical features include: prolonged fever with a duration greater than five days; conjunctivitis and other mucosal changes; lymphadenopathy; and erythematous exanthem, with subsequent desquamation. The precise cause of KD is not known, but an immune response to an infectious agent or environmental toxin is suspected. Both short- and long-term morbidity and mortality result from cardiac involvement in the form of myocardial infarction, malignant arrhythmias, and acute congestive heart fail-

Table 4. Kawasaki Disease Diagnostic Criteria

Presence of prolonged fever (greater than 5 days) with four of the following features:

- Bilateral conjunctivitis
- Mucous membrane changes (red or fissured labia, erythematous pharynx, "strawberry" tongue)
- Polymorphous, erythematous rash (papules, vesicles, bullae, urticarial plaques)
- Extremity changes (erythema/edema of palms/soles, desquamation)
- Lymphadenopathy (at least one node measuring 1.5 cm in diameter)

ure. Mortality in the United States and Japan, which usually results from cardiac dysfunction, has been reported to be 1-2%.[25]

Clinical Presentation and Diagnosis. As with many disease states encountered in emergency medicine, the diagnosis does not depend upon a specific laboratory test. Rather, the diagnosis should be considered in a young child with unexplained, prolonged fever associated with rash and conjunctivitis. The Centers for Disease Control and Prevention in Atlanta have defined KD according to the following criteria *(please see Table 4)*: The presence of prolonged fever (greater than 5 days) accompanied by four of the following features 1) bilateral conjunctival injection; 2) mucous membrane changes (red or fissured labia, erythematous pharynx, "strawberry" tongue); 3) erythematous rash; 4) extremity changes (erythema and edema of palms and/or soles, desquamation); and 5) lymphadenopathy (at least one node measuring 1.5 cm in diameter). The fever is a constant feature and is usually lacking chills and sweats; it abruptly appears, spiking to 101°F to 104°F, and responds poorly to antipyretic therapy. The mean duration of fever at diagnosis is approximately nine days, with a range of five days to one month.

Mucosal changes in KD are seen in the conjunctivae as well as other areas. Conjunctivitis is an almost constant feature, and is characterized by bilateral involvement. Typically, the bulbar conjunctiva demonstrates congestion; at times, the palpebral portion of the conjunctiva is also affected. Uveitis is frequent, and is reported in up to 70% of cases. In contrast to EM major, the conjunctival process in KD lacks ulceration and significant discharge.

The orolabial mucosal surface also is frequently affected, and it too represents another "almost constant feature," of the disease, which presents within three days of fever onset with erythema of the pharynx and fissuring of the lips. The lips then become desiccated, complicated by further fissuring, while ulcerations may appear in an oropharyngeal distribution. The lingual papillae become hypertrophied, resulting in the "strawberry tongue" appearance similar to that seen in scarlet fever.

The rash, which is always erythematous and, frequently, polymorphous, is noted soon after onset of the fever. It resembles the dermatologic findings of EM with erythematous lesions of multiple form. The most frequently seen forms include a diffuse maculopapular eruption and urticarial lesions. Perineal involvement is common, usually with erythematous maculopapules which then coalesce. Vesiculopapules are seen on the extensor surfaces of the large joints.

Table 5. Differential Diagnosis of Kawasaki Syndrome

- Erythema multiforme
- Urticarial vasculitis
- Kawasaki disease
- Toxic-infectious erythemas
- Exfoliative drug reactions

Desquamation occurs first in the perineal area followed by the distal extremities; diffuse skin loss is uncommon. Extremity changes include edema of the distal structures that may be so painful as to limit ambulation. Lymphadenopathy is seen in three-fourths of patents with KD. Firm, nontender lymph nodes are seen and may be limited to a single node.

Additional organ system involvement can be seen in the the heart, with coronary artery inflammation and aneurysmal formation, pericarditis, and myocarditis complicated by arrhythmias, myocardial infarction, and/or acute CHF. Cardiac involvement is seen in approximately 20% of children with KD, and is the major cause of mortality. KD-related death may also occur many years later due to sudden cardiac death or myocardial infarction, both of which may result from aneurysms. Aseptic meningitis, polyarthritis, urethritis, and hydrops of the gallbladder are also seen in the KD patient; the most frequent laboratory abnormality seen is thrombocytosis, which typically ranges from 600,000 to 1.5 million, and which appears on the 10th day of illness. Other laboratory findings include leukocytosis with left shift, alterations in the hepatic transaminases, sterile pyuria, and CSF pleocytosis. *(Please see Table 5 for the differential diagnosis of KD.)*

Treatment. In addition to resuscitation and stabilization, the patient with suspected or confirmed KD should be admitted to the hospital for further diagnostic evaluation and monitoring of possible cardiac complications. Specific therapy includes aspirin and intravenous gamma globulin.

Bullous Diseases

Pemphigus Vulgaris and Bullous Pemphigoid. Of the autoimmune, "blistering" diseases, two—pemphigus vulgaris (PV) and bullous pemphigoid (BP)—are of importance to the emergency physician because of their severity, potential for rapid progression, and associated comorbidity.

PV is a generalized, mucocutaneous, autoimmune, blistering eruption with a grave prognosis. It is characterized by intraepidermal acantholytic blistering. Before the efficacy of systemic steroids in the treatment of pemphigus was noted in the 1950s, the disease had a one-year mortality rate of more than 90%. Today, only 10% of patients succumb to their disease, with most of these deaths resulting from immunosuppressive medication side-effects.[26]

BP is a generalized, mucocutaneous, blistering disease of the elderly, with an average age of 70 years at the time of initial diagno-

Table 6. Lesions of the Bullous Diseases

- Large, flaccid bulla
- Nikolski's sign
- Ulcers
- Exfoliation
- Mucous membrane involvement

sis.[27] Although the blisters are deeper in the skin than in PV (below the epidermal basement membrane), the prognosis is better. There is usually less associated comorbidity with a more rapid response to therapy.

Pathologically, both PV and BP are characterized by the presence of unique antigen/autoantibody systems. The presence of these autoantibodies may be detected using immunofluorescence techniques. PV is a prototypical autoimmune disease that, like Goodpasture's syndrome and myasthenia gravis, exhibits pathogenic autoantibodies. The autoimmune nature of PV was demonstrated by passive transfer experiments. These studies showed that the intraperitoneal administration of pemphigus IgG into neonatal Balb/c mice lead to blister formation with the histological, ultrastructural, and immunofluorescent features of PV.[28] Although autoantibodies have been detected in BP, they have not been proven to be pathogenic. Recent research has identified the autoantigens in many of the autoimmune bullous diseases, and molecular genetics techniques have been used to clone the genes in BP and PV.[29,30]

Clinical Presentation and Diagnosis. The primary lesions of PV are vesicles or bullae that vary in diameter from less than 1 cm to several centimeters; they commonly first affect the head, trunk, and mucous membranes. The blisters are usually clear and tense, originating from normal skin or atop an erythematous or urticarial plaque. Within 2-3 days, the bullae become turbid and flaccid. Rupture soon follows, producing painful denuded areas. These erosions are slow to heal and are prone to secondary infection. Nikolski's sign is invariably positive in PV and absent in other autoimmune blistering diseases. *(Please see Table 6 for the dermatologic lesions common to PV.)*

Mucous membranes are affected in 95% of PV patients; in as many as 25% of these patients, the mucous membranes are the primary sites of involvement. Blisters on mucous membranes are more transitory than those on the skin in that they are more vulnerable to rupture; this is particularly true in the mouth, where ragged ulcerative lesions readily develop after inadvertent biting of the tissues. A few lesions will produce little discomfort, but extensive involvement of the tongue, cheeks, and oropharynx may be extremely painful—so painful that it interferes with the patient's alimentation and nutrition.

BP is characterized by the presence of tense blisters (up to 10 cm in diameter) that arise from either normal skin or from erythematous or urticarial plaques; ulceration with tissue loss follows. Sites of predilection include the intertriginous and flexural areas. Pruritis, occasionally accompanied by a burning sensation, is noted with the appearance of the blistering. Frank pain in the lesions is rarely present. *(Please see Table 6 for the dermatologic lesions common to BP.)*

Table 7. Differential Diagnosis of Bullous Diseases

- Toxic epidermal necrolysis
- Erythema multiforme
- Autoimmune blistering diseases
- Burns
- Severe contact dermatitis
- Bullous diabeticorum
- Friction blisters

Lesions of the oral cavity occur in BP, but with less consistency and severity than in PV. Because the blisters in the oral cavity rupture very easily and heal without scarring, involvement in the mouth is often overlooked. Oral involvement may occur in as many as 40% of patients.[31] It is unusual for oral mucosal lesions to precede the cutaneous eruption as in PV, reported in only two of 36 patients in one series.[32]

The differential diagnosis of PV and BP *(see Table 7)* include all of those diseases that can present with primary skin blistering, including TEN, EM, other autoimmune blistering diseases, burns, severe contact dermatitis, bullous diabeticorum, and friction blisters. The nature of the clinical presentation, histology, and immunofluorescence testing should yield the correct diagnosis in the patient with generalized blistering.

Management. Limited oral intake and accelerated protein, fluid, and electrolyte losses through the involved skin can rapidly lead to hypoalbuminemia with significant hypovolemia and electrolyte disturbances in both PV and BP. Consequently, initial inpatient dermatological care is warranted in most cases with extensive blistering to initiate high-dose systemic steroid and immunosuppressive therapy.

Dermatological consultation is imperative at the time of the initial patient encounter in the ED. The cutaneous surfaces involved with blisters or eroded areas should be treated as burns with the application of silver sulfadiazine cream or antibiotic ointments with clean dressings. The pain originating from oral lesions may be partially relieved with soothing mouth washes (Cepacol [Marion Merrell Dow, Kansas City, MO] diluted 1:4 or 1:1 mixture of diphenhydramine elixir with Mylanta [Johnson & Johnson-Merck, Fort Washington, PA]) or with viscous lidocaine. Oral hygiene should be maintained via frequent mouth washes with normal saline or chlorhexidine gluconate (Peridex [Proctor and Gamble, Cincinnati, OH]) oral rinse solutions. Close observation and rapid treatment with appropriate antibiotics for superficial infection is imperative because the most frequent site for subsequent sepsis is the denuded cutaneous surface.

Currently, treatment with corticosteroids results in the complete recovery of some patients and control of the disease in others if the therapy is continued. Still, 10% of PV patients die either from the disease or complications of therapy, with adverse prognosis associated with the extent of disease at presentation and delay in treatment past six months from the onset. Ultimately, PV does remit. After a mean of 8.7 years in a cohort of PV patients, 45% were free of disease and off of therapy, and 38% were clinically free of disease on low-dose maintenance steroid therapy.[33]

BP is also managed by systemic steroids, especially when there is widespread disease. Mild disease, arbitrarily defined as less than 20 lesions, usually responds to lower doses of steroids, (e.g., 20-40 mg of prednisone per day). BP had a 25% mortality rate before the introduction of steroid treatment. Today, patients with BP usually recover from the disease, although treatment may be necessary for months and even years. In one series, 16% of patients were still under active treatment for their disease after three years.[33] Complications from systemic therapy with corticosteroids and immunosuppressants have special hazards to be considered in treating elderly patients with concomitant disease, including diabetes, hypertension, and glaucoma.[34]

References

1. Funaki B, Elpern DJ. Herpes zoster incidence in younger age groups. *J Am Acad Dermatol* 1987;16:883-884.
2. Baba K, Yabuuchi H, Takahashi M, Ogra PL. Increased incidence of herpes zoster in normal children infected with varicella zoster virus during infancy: Community-based follow-up study. *J Pediatr* 1986;108:372-377.
3. Friedman-Kein AE. Herpes zoster: A possible early clinical sign for the development of acquired immunodeficiency syndrome in high-risk individuals. *J Am Acad Dermatol* 1986; 14:1023-1028.
4. Ragozzino MW. Risk of cancer after herpes zoster: A population-based study. *N Engl J Med* 1982;307:393-397; Feuyo MA, Lookingbill DP. Herpes zoster and occult malignancy. *J Am Acad Dermatol* 1984;11:480-482.
5. Mazur MH, Dolin R. Herpes zoster at the NIH: A 20 year experience. *Am J Med* 1978;65:738-744.
6. Goh CL, Khoo L. A retrospective study of the clinical presentation and outcome of herpes zoster in a tertiary dermatology outpatient referral clinic. *Int J Dermatol* 1997;36:667-672.
7. Scott MJ, Scott MJ. Ipsilateral deafness and herpes zoster ophthalmicus. *Arch Dermatol* 1983;119:235-236.
8. Watson PN, Evans RJ. Postherpetic neuralgia: A review. *Arch Neurol* 1986;43:836-840.
9. Wood MJ. How to measure and reduce the burden of zoster-associated pain. *Scand J Inf Dis* 1996;100(suppl):55-58.
10. Jackson JL, Gibbons R, Meyer G, et al. The effect of treating herpes zoster with oral acyclovir in preventing postherpetic neuralgia. A meta-analysis. *Arch Int Med* 1997;157:909-912.
11. Acosta EP, Fletcher CV. Valacyclovir. *Ann Pharmacother* 1997; 31:185-191.
12. Crumpacker C. The pharmacological profile of famciclovir. *Semin Dermatol* 1996;15(Suppl):14-26.
13. Stein GE. Pharmacology of new antiherpes agents: Famciclovir and valacyclovir. *J Am Pharm Assoc* 1997;NS37: 157-163.
14. Woodward TE. Rocky Moutain spotted fever: Epidemiological and early clinical signs are keys to treatment and reduced mortality. *J Infect Dis* 1984;150:465-468.
15. Anonymous. Rocky Mountain spotted fever—United States, 1985. *Morb Mortal Wkly Rep MMWR* 1986;35:247-249.
16. Westerman EL. Rocky Mountain spotless fever: A dilemma for the clinician. *Arch Intern Med* 1982;142:1106-1107.
17. Peltola H. Meningococcal disease: Still with us. *Rev Infect Dis* 1983;5:71-91.
18. Walker DH, Burday MS, Folds JD. Laboratory diagnosis of Rocky Mountain Spotted Fever. *South Med J* 1980;73: 1443-1446.
19. Edwards MS, Baker CJ. Complications and sequelae of meningococcal infections in children. *J Pediatr* 1981;99: 540-545.
20. Gardlund B. Prognostic evaluation in meningococcal disease: A retrospective study of 115 cases. *Intensive Care Med* 1986; 12: 302-307.
21. Emparanza JI, Aldamiz-Echevarria L, Perez-Yarza EG, et al. Prognostic score in acute meningococcemia. *Crit Care Med* 1988;16:168-169.
22. Tesoro LJ, Selbst SM. Factors affecting outcome in meningococcal infection. *Am J Dis Child* 1991;145:218-220.
23. Algren JT, Lal S, Cutliff SA, et al. Predictors of outcome in acute meningococcal infection in children. *Crit Care Med* 1993;21: 447-452.
24. Butler DF, Hough DR, Friedman SJ, et al. Adult Kawasaki disease. *Arch Dermatol* 1987;123:1356-1361.
25. Morens DM, Anderson LJ, Hurwitz ES. National surveillance of Kawasaki disease. *Pediatr* 1980;65:21-5.
26. Seidenbaum M, David M, Sandbank M. The course and prognosis of pemphigus: A review of 115 patients. *Int J Dermatol* 1988;27: 580-584.
27. Lever WF. Pemphigus and pemphigoid: A review of the advances made since 1964. *J Am Acad Dermatol* 1979;1: 2-31.
28. Anhalt GJ, Labib RS, Voorhees JJ, et al. Induction of pemphigus in neonatal mice by passive transfer of IgG from patients with the disease. *N Engl J Med* 1982;306:1189-1196.
29. Amagai M, Klaus-Kovtun V, Stanley JR. Autoantibodies against a novel epithelial cadherin in pemphigus vulgaris, a disease of cell adhesion. *Cell* 1991;67:869-877.
30. Diaz LA, Ratrie H III, Saunders WS, et al. Isolation of a human epidermal cDNA corresponding to the 180-kD autoantigen recognized by bullous pemphigoid and herpes gestationis sera. Immunolocalization of this protein to the hemidesmosome. *J Clin Invest* 1990;86:1088-1094.
31. Person JR, Rogers RS. Bullous and cicatricial pemphigoid: Clinical, histopathologic, and immunopathologic correlations. *Mayo Clin Proc* 1977;52:54-66.
32. Venning VA, Frith PA, Bron AJ, et al. Mucosal involvement in bullous and cicatricial pemphigoid. A clinical and immunopathological study. *Br J Dermatol* 1988;118:7-15.
33. Burton JL, Harman RRM, Peachey RDG, et al. Azathioprine plus prednisone in treatment of pemphigoid. *Br Med J* 1978;2: 1190-1191.
34. Gallant C, Kenny P. Oral glucocorticoids and their complications: A review. *J Am Acad Dermatol* 1986;14:161-177.

Part XI

Orthopedic and Rheumatological Disorders

Common Sports Injuries: Part I

Clayton F. Holmes, EdD, PT, ATC

Each year, sports injuries account for approximately 500,000 visits to the doctor.[1] Athletes who present as sports participants may be male or female, preadolescent, adolescent, or older. In the latter group, many of the injuries are musculoskeletal in nature. The joints most commonly involved are shoulder, ankle, and knee. This article, divided into two parts, describes the clinical presentation, examination, and intervention of several of the more common pathologies derived from sports-related injury.

Ankle Injuries

Boney Anatomy. The ankle joint is made up of three bones: the tibia, the fibula, and the talus. In addition, the talus sits on top of the calcaneus forming another joint called the talo-calcaneal or sub-talar joint.[2]

Ligaments. The lateral ligaments include the anterior talofibular ligament (ATFL) and the calcaneofibular ligament (CFL) *(please see Figures 1 & 2)*.[2,3]

The deltoid ligament resides medially. It is a triangular shaped ligament that fans out from the medial malleolus to the navicular, talus, and calcaneus.[2] Other major ligament structures include the interosseus ligaments and the anterior and posterior tibio-fibular ligaments.[3] Each of these ligaments plays major stabilizing roles relative to the ankle and foot.[4] Musculotendinous structures include the tendons of the peroneus longus and brevis on the lateral aspect that traverse the lateral aspect of the ankle while the medial aspect of the ankle includes the tibialis posterior tendon, the flexor digitorum longus, and the flexor hallucis longus tendons.[2]

Biomechanics. Both the ankle joint proper and the subtalar joint contribute to the motions of inversion and eversion. Other motions that occur at the ankle are plantar flexion and dorsiflexion. The distal fibula, or lateral malleolus, extends further distally than the medial malleolus does. In addition, the dome of the talus is wedge-shaped from front to back. The dome of the talus is wider posteriorly than it is anteriorly. This means that when the ankle moves into dorsiflexion, the bones are more congruent; therefore, the ankle is more stable. Converseley, when the ankle is in plantar flexion, it is less stable.

General Considerations: Ankle History and Physical Exam

Ankle injuries are the most common injuries that occur in the athletic arena.[4,5] Common injuries include sprains, fractures, and tendon injuries.[4] When performing a history of the ankle injury, it is critical to determine the mechanism of injury of the ankle.[3-5] In most instances, the athlete will be able to recall this in some detail, but if the athlete cannot recall the mechanism of injury, there may have been an onlooker who could determine the mechanism of injury. This may be a teammate, coach, or athletic trainer.

General physical exam considerations include position of the foot—specifically, both the weight bearing and the non-weight bearing neutral position.[5] A relatively normal gait can occur if the athlete can maintain the neutral position of the foot. In addition, this inspection should include the typical concern regarding swelling and ecchymosis. This swelling may be isolated over the sinus tarsi or it may be general edema. If this is a chronic sprain that has not been well taken care of, there may be pitting edema or general edema that is pitted when pressed. For example, this could occur if the athlete uses heat too soon after an acute injury.

The athlete should also be asked to perform active range of motion. This includes plantar flexion, dorsiflexion, inversion, and eversion. These motions are usually limited by swelling and pain.

A neurovascular exam including strength and sensation should be performed on all acute injuries. This includes evaluation of a distal pulse (tibialis posterior and/or dorsalis pedis) and an evaluation of dermatomes and myotomes. Dermatomes are as follows: L-4 anterior medial lower leg, L-5 anterior lateral lower leg, S-1 lateral border of the foot, and S-2 is posterior leg *(please see Table 1)*.[6] Myotomes should be checked for relative strength and dermatomes should be checked to determine if sensory input is intact to light touch.

Ankle Sprains

Different authors use different classifications of ankle sprains.[4,5,7] In general, sprains are defined as damage to ligaments. Sprains are graded according to a cross-sectional microtrauma that occurs within each ligament. In other words, the anterior talofibular ligament could have a 1st degree (stretch), 2nd degree (partial tear), or a 3rd degree (complete tear) sprain *(please see Table 2)*.[8] However, Nitz has described ankle sprains differently.[8] In fact, he described 1st degree sprains as isolated anterior talofibular ligament sprains, 2nd degree sprains as those sprains involving other ligaments including the deltoid ligament, and 3rd degree sprains as those that involve tearing ATFL, deltoid ligaments, and involvement of ATFL and CFL. Perhaps a more appropriate classification is to modify the Nitz classification to include only the tibiofibular or high ankle sprain as the third degree. Regardless of the categorization scheme that is used, it is clear that anterior talofibular ligament involvement is present in the vast majority of ankle sprains.[3-5,7] In addition, the lateral ligaments are involved 85% of the time.[7]

Figure 1. Lateral View of Tendons and Ligaments Responsible for Maintaining Ankle Articulation

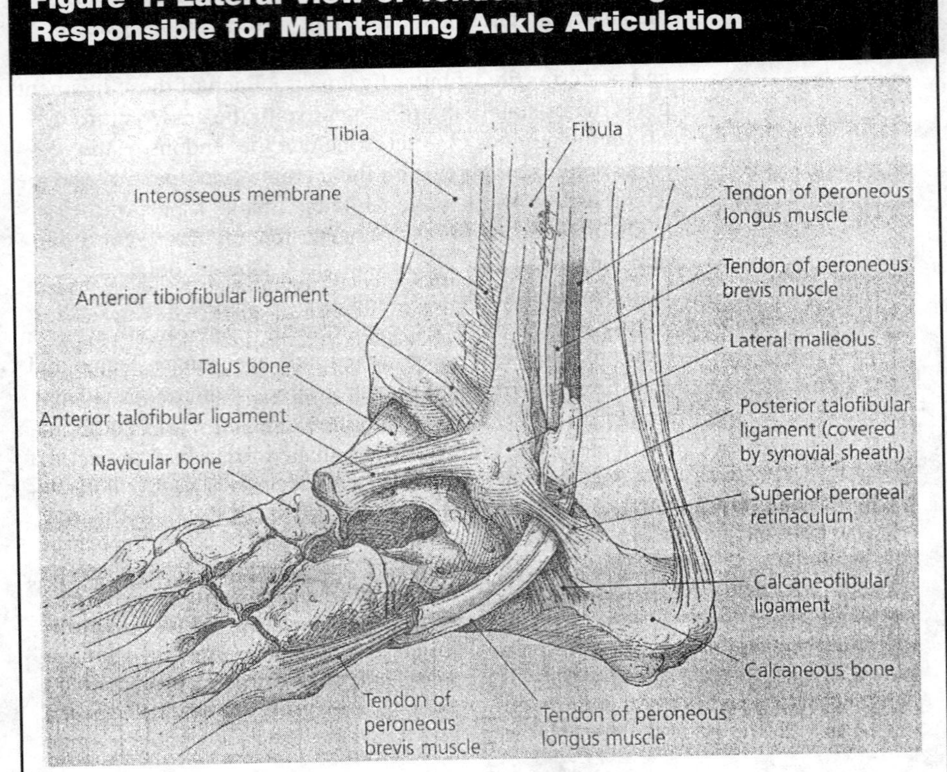

Reprinted with permission from: *Am Fam Physician* 1998;57:475. ©1998 by Floyd E. Hosmer.

Grade I Ankle Sprains: History and Specific Physical Examination. The mechanism of injury of the classic lateral ankle sprain, primarily involving the anterior talofibular ligament, is plantar flexion with inversion.[4,5,7] These sprains, while very common, can also be somewhat debilitating. In fact, if these sprains are not well taken care of, including a full course of rehabilitation, then reoccurrence of an ankle sprain is much more likely to occur.[9]

Inspection may indicate minimal or no swelling, which may be restricted to the sinus tarsi immediately overlying the ATF. The most common special tests used to evaluate the lateral ligaments include the anterior drawer test and the medial talar rock test. The anterior drawer test is performed specifically to evaluate the integrity of the anterior talofibular ligament. One hand stabilizes the distal leg while the other hand grasps the calcaneus and a force in an anterior direction from heel to toe is directed across the foot *(please see Figures 3 & 4)*.[10] The medial talar rock is performed to test the integrity of the calcaneal fibular ligament. While performing this test, the foot is held in neutral with one hand

Table 1. Dermatomes of the Lower Extremity

Nerve Root	Dermatome Description
L1	lower back and groin
L2	anterior thigh
L3	anterior distal thigh and knee
L4	medial lower leg
L5	lateral lower leg
S1	posterior lower leg to mid calf
S2	posterior lower leg from mid calf up

Adapted from: Reese NB. Muscle and Sensory Testing. 1st ed. Philadelphia, Pa: WB Saunders Company; 1999.

while the other hand stabilizes the distal leg. The foot is then rocked into inversion, thus mimicking the mechanism of injury.[5] Both of these tests are highly specific for a grade 1 ankle sprain.

Grade I Ankle Sprain: Treatment/Rehabilitation. Treatment of grade 1 ankle sprains includes ice and rest acutely (mnemonic: R.I.C.E. = rest, ice, compression, elevation). The key to determining whether the athlete needs crutches is this: "Can the athlete ambulate with a normal gait?" If the athlete can ambulate with a normal gait, he or she may not need crutches or may just need one crutch (on the opposite side of the injury). If, however, the athlete has to walk with a limp, he or she needs crutches. However, with a grade 1 sprain, crutches should be only for relative rest. The athlete should practice a heel-toe gait while walking on crutches.[11]

As soon as the athlete can ambulate and has full range of motion without pain, then he or she is ready to begin aggressive rehabilitation. This is usually performed by a physical therapist and entails strengthening of possible structures that were injured including the peroneals with exercises such as resisted eversion using a thera-band. Perhaps, more importantly, this is a program of proprioceptive training. This begins in a static environment and then progresses to a dynamic environment. For example, a static environment could be nothing more than a single leg stance while the dynamic environment may include a BAPST board and/or a slide board, single-leg hops, etc. It is critical to note that the athlete is not prepared to go back to his or her activity until a rehabilitation program is completed. In this way, the athlete is less likely to have a recurrence of injury.[4,5] Other therapeutic interventions that are common to the treatment of ankle sprains include early active range of motion exercises and kryokinetics. At a maximum, return to full activity occurs within 7-10 days.[4]

Ice should continue as the primary physical agent until swelling has stopped. Ice could then be replaced by contrast bath and then progressing to moist heat. This also is commonly followed by manual interventions including mobilization techniques, including low-grade mobilization techniques, to improve the nutritional status of the joint. As with any injury, morbidity is the primary consideration with regard to progression. For example, if pain and swelling increase in the ankle after the rehabilitation session, then obviously the rehabilitation was too aggressive. This rarely happens, particularly with grade 1 ankle sprains.

Finally, the vast majority of grade 1 ankle sprains should be protected for the remainder of the season. Common protections include taping by

Figure 2. Deltoid Ligaments of the Ankle

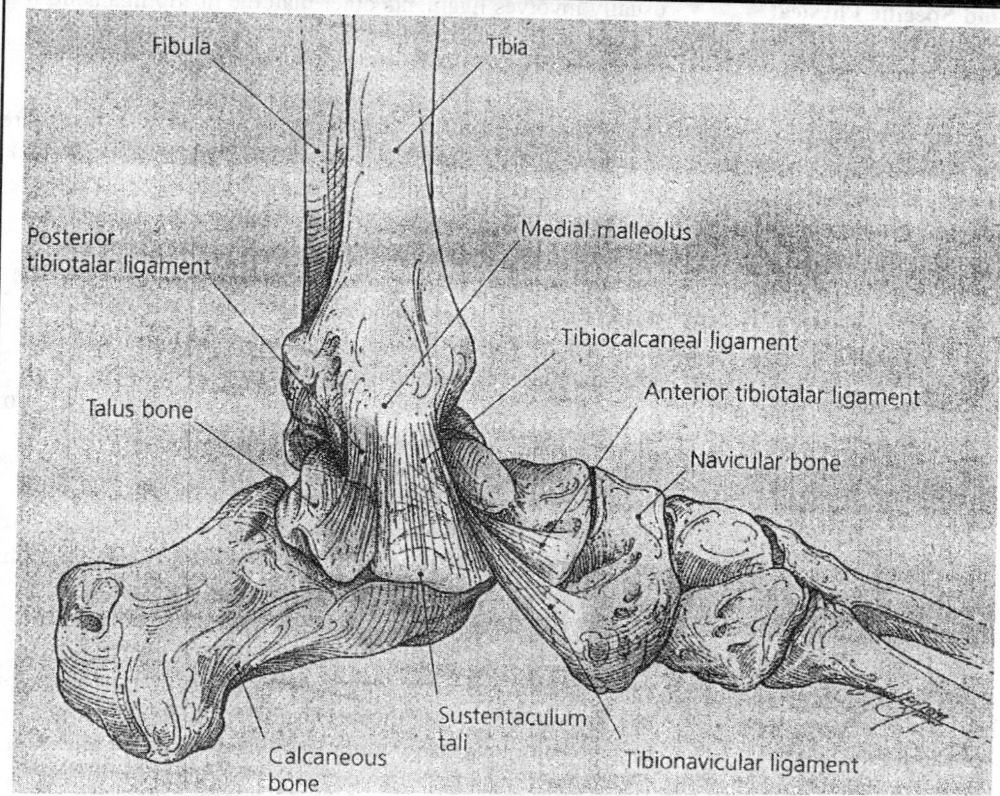

Reprinted with permission from: Am Fam Physician 1998;57:475. ã1998 by Floyd E. Hosmer

Table 2. Nitz Categories of Ankle Sprains

Grade 1	lateral ligament involvement
Grade 2	lateral and medial ligaments involved
Grade 3	lateral, medial, and tibiofibular ligaments involved

Adapted from: Nitz AJ, et al. Nerve injury and grades II and III ankle sprains. Am J Sports Med 1985;13: 177-182.

Figure 3. Medial Talar Rock

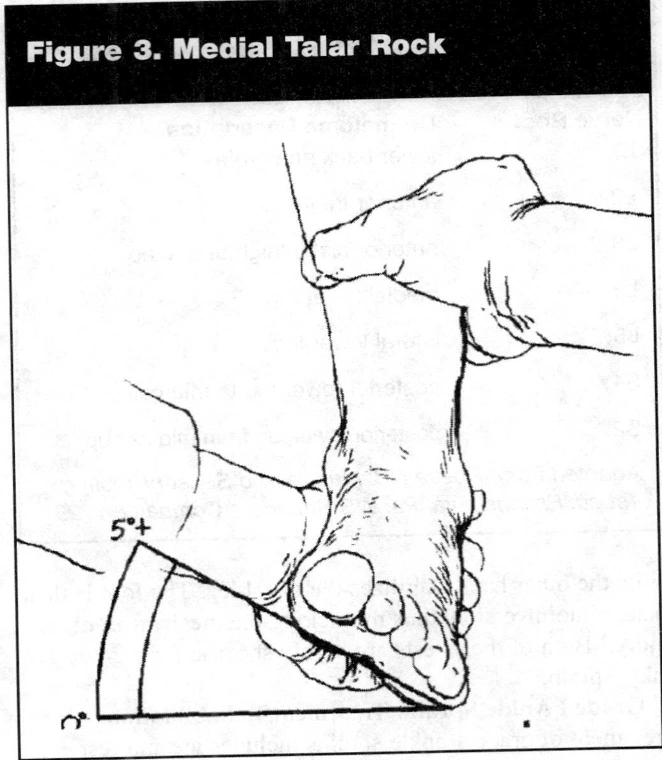

someone who is proficient in athletic taping (e.g., an athletic trainer or physical therapist). It is interesting to note that Wilkerson and Nitz reported that the U-shaped pad was extremely beneficial in decreasing swelling after a grade 1 ankle sprain.[12] This pad should be put under tape.[5] Another possible preventive measure is bracing instead of taping. Bracing has been shown to be as effective as taping in many instances, which may be due to proprioceptive feedback.[13,14] Bracing has also been shown to be more cost-effective than taping when used.[15]

This rehabilitation is followed by a more functional rehabilitation in which the athlete mimics his or her sport and is slowly returned to that sport. This is the last phase of any rehabilitation in athletic injury. This rehabilitation should be directed by a physical therapist or an athletic trainer.[4,7,9]

Grade II Ankle Sprains: History and Specific Physical Exam. Grade 2 ankle sprains are those involving the deltoid ligament and take longer to heal.[8] This is primarily because most feet pronate and the deltoid ligament bears more weight than the lateral ligaments of the ankle.[4] Fortunately, these only constitute about 5% of ankle sprains.[4]

The mechanism of injury here is the opposite of the 1st degree sprain. That is, eversion is involved. When violent eversion occurs at the ankle, the fibula should be evaluated for fracture.

Inspection may reveal a more general swelling and obvious point tenderness over the deltoid ligament to palpation (medial joint line). In addition, a talar rock into eversion is often done to test the integrity of the deltoid ligament. This is performed in the same manner as inversion except the foot is rocked into eversion rather than inversion.[10,16] Ecchymosis will appear much more frequently with grade 2 sprains and will overlie the medial joint.

Grade II Ankle Sprain: Treatment. Treatment is similar to that of the grade 1. The athlete may be out of action somewhere between two to four weeks (for grade 2 sprains).[4]

Grade III Ankle Sprains. Again, according to a modified Nitz classification, grade 3 sprains are syndesmosis sprains usually involving the anterior tib-fib ligament.[8] Since the anterior tib-fib ligament traverses the talocural joint, it is much more difficult to heal. Specifically, every time the athlete bears weight, the talocural space is spread apart and this further traumatizes the tib-fib ligament.

History considerations include the mechanism of injury, which in this case is quite often a torsional stress. In other words, the talus rotates within the talocural joint. This injury usually involves ligaments other than the tib-fib ligament. It can include the interossseous ligament and the ligaments below the medial and lateral ligaments (ATF, CF, and deltoid).[8]

Inspection will be similar to that of a grade 2 sprain. There may be point tenderness over the anterior tib-fib ligament. In the acute phase, weight bearing and active range of motion will be painful. Strength should not be tested secondary to pain. The squeeze test, which is performed by compressing the fibula and the tibia at the mid-portion of the lower leg, is a common special test performed to determine if there is a syndesmosis sprain. Pain in an area of the anterior talocural joint may indicate a syndesmosis sprain.[5]

Radiographs. The Ottawa Ankle Rules have been put into place to determine the need for x-rays when ankle sprain is suspected to rule out fractures *(please see Table 3)*.[3] Their usefulness has been demonstrated.[3,17]

Grade III Ankle Sprains: Treatment. There is some controversy with regard to immobilization of the grade 3 or high ankle sprain.[4,5] Quite often, the use of an air cast in both severe grade 2 and grade sprains 3 is used. The athlete will definitely be nonweight bearing for a time with a grade 3 sprain to allow some healing to occur before weight bearing begins on the tib-fib ligament. Once the athlete gains full range of motion, rehabilitation can begin. This rehabilitation will follow much the same course as the grade 1. Obviously, the rehabilitation will be much slower and the ankle may take 4-8 weeks to heal.[4]

Figure 4. Lateral Talar Rock

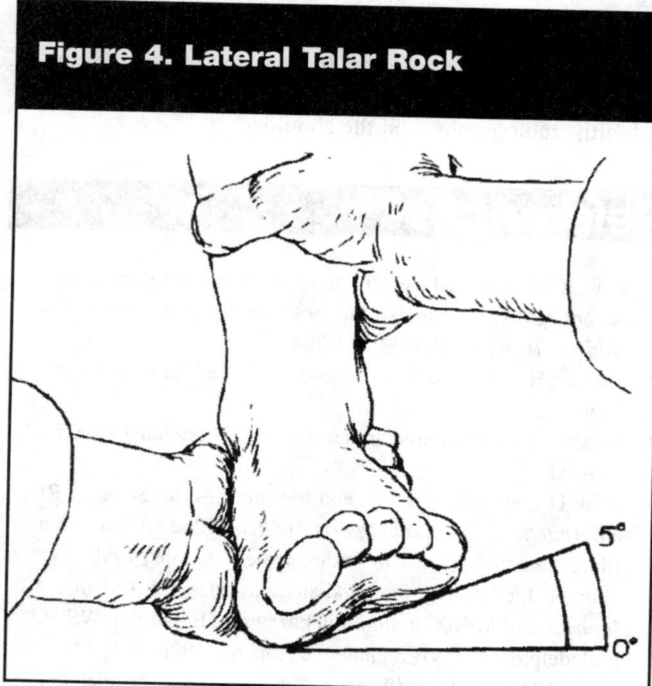

Table 3. Ottowa Ankle Rules for Radiographic Series Following Acute Ankle Injuries

Ankle Radiographs are required only if the patient presents with pain in the malleolar zone and any of the following:

- boney tenderness at tip of lateral malloelus
- boney tenderness at tip of medial malloelus
- presents with inability to bear weight

Foot Radiographs are required only if patient has pain in the midfoot zone and any of the following:

- boney tenderness at the base of the fifth metatarsel
- boney tenderness at the navicular
- presents with inability to bear weight

Adapted from: Wexler RK. The injured ankle. Am Fam Physician 1998;57(3):474-480.

Tendonitis

History/Pathophysiology. Tendonitis about the ankle and foot is also a relatively common condition. Unlike ankle sprains that present with a history of trauma, tendonitis presents with a history of insidious onset. In other words, no specific mechanism of injury is recalled. This is not always true and acute tendonitis can occur. However, many times tendonitis occurs from chronic overuse. Table 4 summarizes common tendonitis sites, common causative factors, and signs and symptoms. The pathophysiology of tendonitis is relatively simple. Most tendons have a diminished blood supply relative to the rest of the contractile mechanism. In other words, poor blood supply can lead to an inability to recover from microtrauma. As that microtrauma accrues, at some point a critical mass of fibers is involved and the pain begins. As mentioned previously, this pain can slowly grow to a point to where many people have had tendonitis for several months before they seek help. Other common sites of tendonitis are the tibialis posterior, the tibialis anterior, and the paroneal tendon, but by far the most common is the achilles tendon.[5]

Specific Physical Examination. Achilles tendonitis is relatively common. Quite often, pain occurs just proximal to the insertion of the calcaneus. This could be due to faulty foot mechanics. Acutely, however, a heel lift should be used. It is also important to evaluate the athlete's footwear. Many times, injuries such as tendonitis occur when shoes are "worn out." A list of training areas that cause tendonitis is included in Table 4. Signs and symptoms include pain with active movement. This pain may or may not be aggravated by weight bearing. There will be pain with passive stretching of the same tendon. Obviously, with palpation there will be localized tenderness. There may be swelling or thickening of the tendon in addition to some possible crepitious around the perry tendon tissues. Tendonitis pain is usually more prevalent in the early morning. As the day wears on, the blood supply of the tendon improves with motion and pain decreases.[5]

Treatment. Treatment for tendonitis about the ankle usually involves some form of orthotic fabrication and usually some form of heel lift. In addition, a course of rehabilitation should be undertaken usually by a physical therapist and/or athletic trainer.[4,5,9] Initially, treatment should be relatively conservative. Obviously, changes in any training errors that have occurred should be a primary consideration. Lower leg alignment should also be evaluated. Typical rehabilitation usually includes some form of heat to improve blood flow, followed by active exercises within the tolerance of pain (exercise should not increase the pain). Common exercises include stretching of the tendon with contract-relax techniques that may include weight bearing on a trampoline progressing to weight bearing on ground. Functional rehabilitation will always include proprioceptive training such as static single-leg stance followed by balance in a dynamic environment (BAPST board, sliding board, etc.). The critical point of rehabilitation is the last phase of rehabilitation, which is the return to play. This should be done very slowly. Stress across the tendon should be increased slowly as activities of the sport should be mimicked in a lower load environment. This may be in water or on a trampoline. The athlete then progresses to a soft flat level surface, such as a grass field, and finally progresses to his or her athletic surface. These injuries generally occur in runners. The last surface that the athlete would return to would be a hard concrete surface. In fact, it is preferable that all athletes train on a softer surface.[4,5,9]

Table 4. Tendonitis in the Lower Leg, Ankle, and Foot

Common Sites

- Achilles tendon just above its insertion into the calcaneous
- Tibialis posterior just behind the medial malleolus
- Tibialis anterior on the dorsum of the foot just under the extensor retinaculum
- Peroneal tendon behind the lateral malleolus and at the insertion into the base of the fifth metatarsal

Common Causative Factors

- Faulty foot mechanics producing friction and compression between the tendon, sheath, and underlying boney structure, or causing compression of the tendon against the shoe
- Poor footwear that creates poor mechanics or is not fit properly
- Training errors that include:
  Intensity too high, with poor work:rest ratio;
  Muscle fatigue leading to mechanical breakdown of foot function
  Poor training surface (dirty gym floor), sudden change from soft to hard or hard to soft (road camber change when running)
  Sudden changes in program such as adding hills, sprints, or distance
  Returning or progressing too quickly following an illness
  Poor flexibility in the gastrocnemius soleus muscle, which increases twist and whipping action of Achilles tendon because foot must increase pronation to increase dorsiflexion of the ankle joint in weight-bearing position; this in turn can produce chronic overstretching of Achilles tendon and result in microtears of tendon
  Trauma (direct blow)
- Infection from an overlying cut or a penetrating wound into the tendon

Signs and Symptoms

- Pain with active movement, aggravated in weight bearing
- Pain on passive stretching
- Localized tenderness
- Possible swelling and/or thickening in the tendon and peritendon tissues
- May have "snowball crepitus"
- Morning stiffness at site of lesion; this also occurs following any period of inactivity during the day when the part is not moved for 15-20 minutes or longer

Adapted from: Athletic Injuries and Rehabilitation. Zachazewski JE, Quillen WS, eds. Philadelphia, Pa: WB Saunders Company; 1996.

Part II of Common Sports Injuries will discuss knee injuries, including the anatomy, history, and physical exam; ACL tears, rehabilitation, the patella femoral joint, patellar tendonitis, radiographs, and the shoulder.

References

1. Powell JW, Barber-Foss KD. Injury patterns in selected high school sports: A review of the 1995-1997 seasons. *Journal of Athletic Training* 1999;34:277-284.
2. Netter FH. *Atlas of Human Anatomy*. 2nd ed. East Hanover, NJ: Novartis; 1997.
3. Wexler RK. The injured ankle. *Am Fam Physician* 1998;57: 474-480.
4. Funk DA, et al. Leg, ankle, and foot injuries. In: Schenck RC, ed. *Athletic Training and Sports Medicine*. 2nd ed. Rosemont, Ill: American Academy of Orthopaedic Surgeons; 1999.
5. Taunton J, et al. Leg, foot, and ankle injuries. In: *Athletic Injuries and Rehabilitation*. Zachazewski JE, Quillen WS, eds. Philadelphia, Pa: WB Saunders Company; 1996.
6. Reese NB. *Muscle and Sensory Testing*. 1st ed. Philadelphia, Pa: WB Saunders Company; 1999.
7. Pfeffer GB. Foot and ankle. In: Snider RK, ed. *Essentials of Musculoskeletal Care*. 1st ed. Rosemont, Ill: American Academy of Orthopaedic Surgeons; 1997.
8. Nitz AJ, et al. Nerve injury and grades II and III ankle sprains. *Am J Sports Med* 1985;13:177-182.
9. Anderson KJ, et al. Recurrent anterior subluxation of the ankle. *J Bone Joint Surg Am* 1952;34A:853-860.
10. Hoppenfeld S, Hutton R. *Physical Examination of the Spine and the Extremities*. New York, NY: Prentice Hall; 1976.
11. Holmes CF, Schenck RC. Applied principles in treatment and rehabilitation. In: *Athletic Training and Sports Medicine*. Schenck RC, ed. Chicago, Ill: American Academy of Orthopedic Surgeons; 1999:852-857.
12. Wilkerson GB, Nitz AJ. Dynamic ankle stability: Mechanical and neuromuscular interrelationships. *J Sports Rehabil* 1994;3: 43-57.
13. Carroll MJ, Rijke AM, Perrin DH. Effect of the Swede-O ankle brace on talar tilt in subjects with unstable ankles. *J Sports Rehabil* 1993;2:261-267.
14. Feuerbach JW, Grabiner MD. Effect of the aircast on unilateral postural control: Amplitude and frequency variables. *J Orthop Sports Phys Ther* 1993;17:149-154.
15. Gross MT, et al. Comparison of support provided by ankle taping and semirigid orthosis. *J Orthop Sports Phys Ther* 1988;9: 33-39.
16. Magee DJ, et al. Shoulder injuries. In: Zachazewski JE, Quillen WS, eds. *Athletic Injuries and Rehabiliation*. 1st ed. Philadelphia, Pa: WB Saunders; 1996.
17. Gilliagn B, et al. Application of the Ottawa Ankle Rules in children: A retrospective analysis. *Pediatrics* 1999;104:688.

Common Sports Injuries, Part II

Clayton F. Holmes, EdD, PT, ATC

Each year, sports injuries account for approximately 500,000 visits to the doctor.[1] Athletes who present as sports participants may be male or female, pre-adolescent, adolescent, or older. In the latter group, many of the injuries are musculoskeletal in nature. The joints most commonly involved are shoulder, ankle, and knee. This chapter, divided into two parts (please see chapter 146), describes the clinical presentation, examination, and intervention of several of the more common pathologies derived from sports-related injuries.

Knee Injuries

Anatomy. The knee proper is made up of the proximal tibia and the distal femur. In addition, the patella femoral joint, which is usually considered part of the knee, is made up of the patella and its articulation with the condyles and the intercondyler notch of the distal femur.[2] The knee and patellofemoral joint will be addressed separately with regard to examination and treatment.

Biomechanics. It should be noted that the knee is not a hinge joint (i.e., it does not move in one single plane). During knee flexion in open chain (the foot is free in space), the tibia slides posteriorly on the condyles of the femur. In closed chain, during knee flexion and extension, the femur slides and rolls on the tibia. In addition, axial rotation occurs as the femur internally rotates during terminal extension, in closed chain, the tibia externally rotates during open chain.[3] Normal walking causes knee joint forces of 2-4 times the body weight, 50-100% of that of which is transmitted through the meniscus.[4] In addition, in the patella femoral joint, the patella acts as a lever for the quadriceps mechanism providing stronger knee extension. The Q angle (quadricep's angle formed by the anterior superior illiac spine, the middle of the patella, and the tibial tubercle) identifies a possible anatomic predisposition for patello-femoral problems. If this angle is greater than 20°, it is considered a predisposition to pathology (< 15-20° is considered a predisposition to pathology).[3]

Evaluation

History and Physical Exam of Knee Injuries. History is the most critical of any knee evaluation. As a matter of fact, some authors indicate that the history alone can be diagnostic 90% of the time. This is only true if the physician understands the typical mechanisms of injury and implications of acuteness vs. chronicity of the injury.[4] As with an acute ankle

Figure 1. Lachman Test

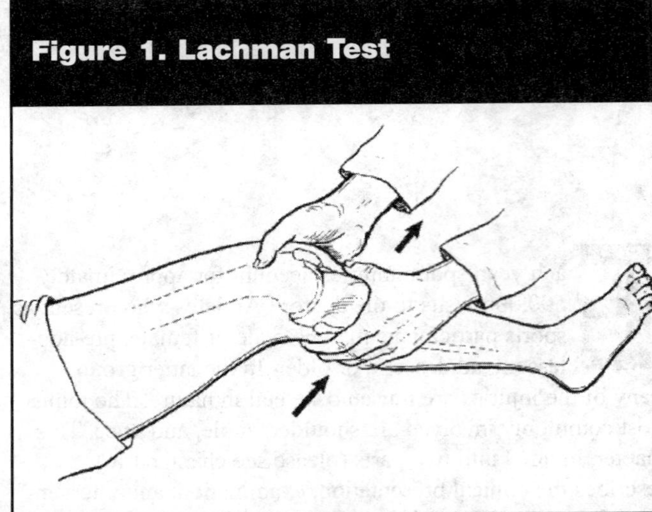

Figure 2. Valgus Stress Test for Medial Collateral Ligament

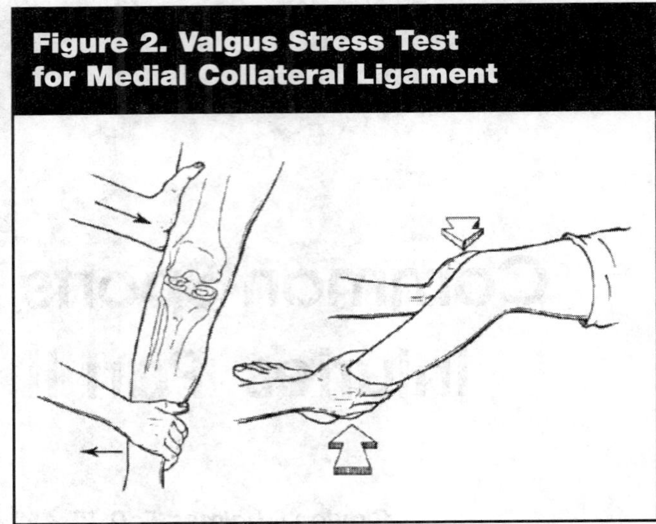

injury, an acute knee injury should include a complete neurovascular exam, specifically including the distal pulse. A major deformity about the knee, a pale foot, or an inability to move the foot and toes may suggest fracture or dislocation of the knee. A dislocation of the knee proper (tibia femoral joint) is an emergent condition and often requires surgery.[5]

Other than obvious deformity, inspection should focus on a specific determination of the type of swelling. Specifically, a distinction should be made between hemarthrosis and soft tissue swelling. A hemarthrosis is an intra-articular accumulation of blood. This is obviously from a highly vascular structure such as the anterior cruciate ligament (ACL). In fact, a hemarthrosis within 12-24 hours after an incident means that there is a 70% chance that there is an ACL tear. The hemarthrosis should be distinguished from soft tissue swelling, which is more likely edema and has a "water balloon" appearance. If the hemarthrosis does occur within 2-3 hours, the physician should first suspect an ACL tear, which occurs most often. Second, the physician should suspect a patellar dislocation, and an osteochondral fracture third.[4]

In the acute knee, palpation to confirm deformity is more common than palpation of specific structures to illicit pain. In fact, the entire knee may be painful, and illiciting pain from palpation is not specific.[4] The same is generally true for range of motion in the acute knee.

Several special tests can also be performed to check the integrity of the major ligaments. Specifically, the Lachman test should be performed to test the integrity of the anterior cruciate ligament.[7,8] (*Please see Figure 1.*[6]) In this test, the examiner stabilizes the tibia with one hand while translating the proximal tibia anteriorally with the other hand. The posterior cruciate ligament is often tested with a posterior drawer test. In this test, the examiner places the hip in approximately 45° of flexion, the knee in approximately 90° of knee flexion, and translates the tibia posteriorly with the thenar imminences of both hands on the proximal tibia and the thumbs on the joint line.[4]

The valgus stress test is performed with the patient in supine position on the table and the examiner stabilizing the lateral thigh with one hand while moving the distal tibia in a valgus direction. This tests the integrity of the medial collateral ligament *(please see Figure 2)*.[6] Conversely, the varus stress test done with the medial thigh stabilized while the distal tibia is forced in a varus direction tests the integrity of the lateral collateral ligament *(please see Figure 3)*.[4,6]

Lastly, the McMurray test tests for meniscus tears. In this test, the patient lies supine and the examiner grasps the heel of the patient's foot. Then the examiner fully flexes the knee while palpating the joint line for clicks and locks. The hip is put into external rotation to test the medial meniscus and internal rotation to test the lateral meniscus as the examiner slowly brings the leg into partial extension while performing a varus stress on the knee. The varus stress on the knee evaluates the medial compartment. To evaluate a lateral meniscus tear, the examiner applies a valgus stress on the knee while internally rotating the foot. Pain over the joint line may be indicative of a tear. Obviously, a click or clunk is also indicative of a meniscus tear.[4,8]

Perhaps the most common test of the integrity of the patella femoral joint is the apprehension test. In this test, the patella, with knee extended but in slight flexion, is displaced laterally. If the athlete becomes apprehensive about this technique, this is usually indicative of patella dislocation.[8]

Specific Injuries

Anterior Cruciate Ligament Tears. ACL tears occur most commonly in contact sports. Contact sports include football, basketball, soccer. (See Holmes CF. The Preparticipation Evaluation. *Primary Care Reports* 2000;6:189-196.)

History and Specific Physical Exam. The mechanism for an ACL tear is most commonly a rotation or pivoting of the knee with the foot planted on the ground. This usually occurs during noncontact (i.e., the most severe injury that can occur to the knee in athletics, the ACL tear is usually a noncontact injury).[4] The foot is usually planted, the knee is flexed, and

Figure 3. Varus Stress Test for Lateral Collateral Ligament

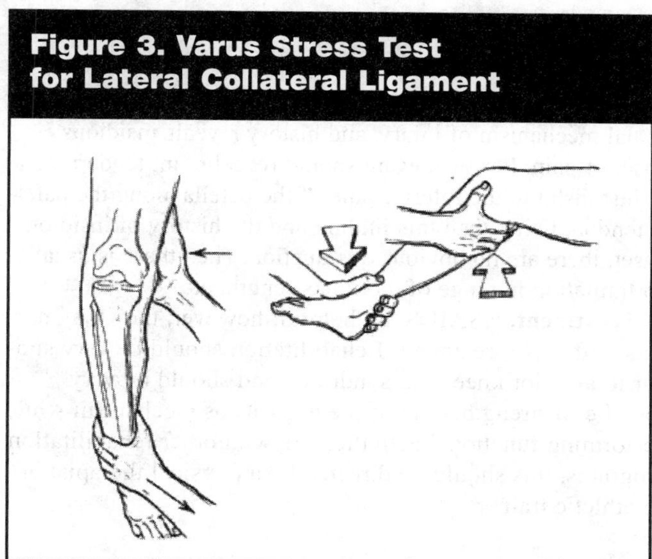

Table 1. Ottawa Knee Rules

- Age 55 years or older; or
- Tenderness at head of fibula; or
- Isolated tenderness of the patella (no bone tenderness of knee other than patella); or
- Inability to flex to 90°; or
- Inability to bear weight both immediately for four steps; or
- Unable to transfer weight twice onto each lower limb regardless of limping.

Adapted from: Wexler RK. The injured ankle. *Am Fam Physician* 1998;57(3)474-480.

the athlete suddenly changes direction, thus applying a rotational force to the knee. The same mechanism of injury can occur during contact. This usually occurs during contact to the leg as in a roll block in football. However, this occurs most commonly in non-contact environments with the foot planted.[4,9]

Physical examination includes an athlete who is limping and who usually cannot straighten his or her knee. This may be due to the ACL stump. As mentioned previously, if the hemarthrosis develops within 2-24 hours, this is also indicative of a possible ACL. All four of the previously mentioned ligaments should be tested (ACL, PCL, MCL, and LCL). There are frequently other ligament injuries with an ACL tear.[4,9]

Treatment. Early immobilization is controversial.[4] Some authors indicate that since this condition will definitely require surgery, the athlete should begin early motion and weight bearing as soon as possible. The feeling is that the athlete should go into surgery with as normal of a knee as possible. Others like to control the forces across the knee with the possible assumption that the ACL may only be partially torn. Whatever the case, the athlete should be referred to an orthopaedist immediately. Most athletes who have this injury and want to return to sports will require surgical reconstruction. Very few athletes can return to sport without an ACL.[10] If an athlete is willing to give up the sport that caused the injury and perform only "straight-line sports," then he or she may get by without surgery.[4]

Rehabilitation. Whether postsurgical or cruciate deficient, initial treatment should focus acutely on symptom reduction, including swelling reduction and the re-establishment of normal gait. In addition, the athlete should attempt to maintain full terminal extension and gain flexion as soon as possible. Functional rehabilitation includes partial squats, stationary bike, and some type of stepper machine. Bracing has not been shown to be successful after ACL reconstruction, but some type of bracing may be necessary for the cruciate deficient knee[11] (i.e., the athlete who chose not to have the surgery). ACL tears in children are problematic. Some suggest that an ACL reconstruction should not be performed on a child until he or she reaches Tanner's developmental stage 3.[12]

Medial Collateral Injuries. Isolated medial collateral ligament injuries (MCL) and/or combination of ACL injuries are frequently seen in contact sports.[4] This is due primarily to the presence of a natural physiologic valgus at the knee. Therefore, when forces cross the knee, the medial collateral ligament is more likely to receive stress than the lateral collateral ligament. The mechanism of injury is usually valgus stress. This valgus stress could occur with a lateral blow to the side of the knee with the foot planted. If the foot is not planted, the lateral blow is not as likely to cause an MCL injury. There are three grades of sprains as defined by the amount of microtrauma that has occurred. A 1st degree is a stretch, a 2nd degree is a partial tear, and a 3rd degree is a complete tear (*please see Table 1*).

The most common physical examination finding is a tender MCL. This may be at the distal insertion (proximal tibia), midsubstance, or proximal insertion of the sprain. There is also pain with forced flexion. This is because the MCL is taut during flexion. Swelling may be localized to the medial side of the knee and ecchymosis is usually obvious. There are two components to the medial collateral ligament, a superficial and a deep layer. The superficial layer is most commonly injured. As with all four ligament stress tests, as well as the McMurray's test, they should be performed to rule out concomitant and/or meniscus injury.[4]

The treatment for the majority of MCL tears is definitely nonsurgical for grades 1 and 2 sprains. A severe grade 3 sprain that is not isolated and includes other, concomitant injuries, may be a surgical candidate. However, the vast majority of MCL tears are nonsurgical.[13] Grade 1 sprains are not immobilized; however, grade 2 and 3 sprains may be immobilized for a period of 1-2 weeks. Severe grade 3 sprains may be immobilized for a short period of time; however, immobilization should be limited due to morbidity secondary to immobilization, such as decreased motion and atrophy of the quadriceps mechanism. As with the cruciate deficient knee, rehabilitation can be functional and include partial squats, a stepper machine, and/or stationary bike. Weight bearing should be performed as tolerated. As with other crutch-type activities, the primary factor in determining weight-bearing status is the normalization of gait. If the athlete does not have a normal gait, some type of ambulation assistance is needed. If the athlete has a normal gait with some verbal cueing then crutches may not be needed. This can be determined by a physical therapist and the functional rehabilitation should be performed by a physical therapist or athletic trainer.[4,14]

Prognosis is very good with isolated MCL sprains. Grade 1 and mild grade 2 MCL sprains generally return 10-14 days after injury, whereas isolated grade 3 sprains may be out for up to five weeks.[15]

The Patella Femoral Joint

Patella femoral pain or anterior knee pain syndrome is perhaps more common than traumatic knee injures. It is more prevalent in the female population due to an increased Q angle.

History and Specific Physical Examination. Patella femoral pain does not migrate beyond the anterior aspect of the knee and is usually chronic in nature with a history of insidious onset. Patella femoral pain is a common presentation in adolescent athletes. Inspection may indicate mild effusion but more often does not. The peri-patella region may be point tender to palpation. Often, a medial plica is also inflamed, thus making the medial aspect of the peri-patella region even more sensitive. While range of motion may not be affected, strength may be affected. Observation and strength testing of the quadriceps muscles should indicate atrophy present when compared side to side. Special tests include the apprehension test, which is positive for possible chronic subluxation events or dislocation. In addition, compression of the patella while the athlete performs flexion and extension may elicit crepitus at the patella femoral joint. This has classically been indicative of patella femoral arthralgia but may also be indicative of general inflammation.[18]

Treatment acutely includes nonsteroidal anti-inflammatory drugs (NSAIDS); however, a specific rehabilitation program is essential to return the athlete to his or her activity. Rehabilitation should focus on quadricep strengthening. This may include exercises, such as partial squats, short arc quads, straight-leg raises, and stationary bike (with the seat high to decrease total knee flexion). In addition, aquatic therapy is often helpful with these patients. While the patient returns to activity, the water creates an environment where the patient can mimic sports activities in a setting with diminished forces. A physical therapist or athletic trainer should direct the rehabilitation program.[16]

Patellar Tendonitis

History and Specific Physical Examination. There is no actual mechanism of injury, and history reveals insidious onset of pain. Physical exam should reveal point tenderness at or just distal to the inferior pole of the patella along the patella tendon. Other than this finding and the history of insidious onset, there are no obvious dysfunctions (i.e., there is usually no limitation in range of motion, strength, etc).[4]

Treatment. NSAIDS are helpful; however, they may not be an effective treatment. Rehabilitation should be very similar to anterior knee pain syndrome and should be very specific to strengthening of the quadriceps mechanism while performing functional activities. As with other rehabilitation programs, this should be directed by a physical therapist or an athletic trainer.[4,16]

Radiographs

As with the ankle for acute injuries, Ottawa Rules can be followed (*see Table 2*).[16]

Decision Rule for Radiography in Acute Knee Injuries. A knee examination is required for acute knee injury in patients with one or more of these findings related to age, tenderness, or function (*please see Table 2*).[16]

Ottawa Rules have been put in place in emergency rooms and have improved specificity related to prescription of radiographs and the presence of fracture. Specifically at the knee, this has been done because approximately 1.3 million patients present annually in ER departments with acute knee trauma; however, only an estimated 6% of those patients have suffered fracture.[17] Ottawa Rules notwithstanding, most athletic injuries to the knee will meet this criteria (i.e., for example an ACL or MCL injury to the knee will many times be painful in weight bearing). The athlete will not have been able to continue to participate in athletics. Therefore, these criteria will have been met and a radiograph will be obtained. These criteria may not be met for chronic knee injuries. For chronic knee pain, radiographs can be used in this instance to assess joint space narrowing, specifically to assist patella femoral alignment or the possibility of malalignment. In addition, osteochondritis, desecans, loose bodies, cysts, and rare tumors can also be ruled out.[4] Three views are commonly taken: a bilateral standing position to assess patella femoral alignment should be done in weight-bearing position at a 45° angle of flexion; second, a lateral view at 60° of flexion; and third, a merchant view of the patella at 30° of flexion. The posterio-anterior view can provide a view of the femoral notch, which should be evaluated when cruciate injury is suspected for a possible cruciate evultion fracture. The lateral view can be used to assess tibia femoral alignment when possible significant knee injuries are suspected to rule out a tibia femoral dislocation. In chronic knee injuries, this can also be used to identify tibia "ossicles and fractures." A merchant view assesses patella femoral joint space and alignment.[4]

Table 2. Shoulder vs. Cervical Region Pathology

Cervical Region	Shoulder
Pain at rest	Pain with use
Pain with neck motion	Pain working overhead
Pain with pressure on neck	Feeling of instability
Aggravated by postural positions	Local palpable tenderness
Pain distal to shoulder	Pain in deltoid region
Reflex changes	Pain mainly on dominant side
Altered peripheral sensation	Relief with local injection
Decreased cervical spine motion	

Adapted from: Zachazewski JE, Quillen WS, eds. *Athletic Injuries and Rehabilitation.* Philadelphia, Pa: WB Saunders Company; 1996.

Shoulder

Anatomy/Biomechanics. The shoulder complex is made up of three bones and four articulations. The bones are the clavicle, scapula, and humerus. The four articulations are the sternoclavicular joint, the scapulothoracic articulation, the acromioclavicular joint, and the glenohumeral joint.[2] It is important to note that during glenohumeral movement, particularly flexion or abduction, moving the hand into an overhead position, that rotation of the clavicle occurs. This motion occurs at the sternoclavicular joint. In addition, there is an arthrokinematic sliding that occurs at the acromioclavicular joint as the scapula raises and rotates on the clavicle. The arthrokinematic motion of the glenohumeral joint is as follows: the head of the humerus rolls upward during abduction or flexion and at the same time slides downward. Suffice it to say that for normal shoulder motion to occur, normal motion is required at all four articulations.[3]

For this motion to occur, two force couples occur that use muscles of both the rotator cuff and the scapula stabilizers. The muscles of the rotator cuff are as follows: supraspinatus, which has a direct pull to abduct at the shoulder, infraspinatus, teres minor, and subscapularis, which all have the ability to pull the humerus down, thus causing the sliding down during abduction. In addition during abduction, the rhomboids, the middle and lower trapezius, and the deltoid rotate the scapula laterally.[3]

One other clinically significant anatomical consideration is the coracoacromial arch, which is made up of the coracoacromial ligament along with the acromion. This arch makes up the roof of the lateral aspect of the shoulder, an area that is "implicated in some acromial impingement."[18] The supraspinatus tendon arises from the head of the humerus and dives toward the scapula in this arch in addition to overlying the supraspinatus tendon.[2] Also, the subaccromial/subdeltoid bursa is under the arch.[2] Both of these structures along with the biceps tendon are commonly "impinged." For this reason, both spurpraspinatus tendonitis and bicep tendonitis fall under the general umbrella of impingement.

History and Physical Examination: General Considerations. Perhaps the most critical factor when performing a history is to rule out concomitant cervical spine dysfunction. In order to do this, a cervical spine exam must be performed. This should include a dermatome and myotome check and also should include active range of motion. For example, painful active range of motion of the cervical spine might indicate a component of cervical spine dysfunction in addition to shoulder pathology. Other findings specific to cervical spine dysfunction would be decreased reflexes, and possibly a positive cervical compression test.[18] In addition, cervical spine pain could radiate along the C-5, C-6 dermatome, a common site of cervical spine dysfunction.[19] Pain above the glenohumeral joint (e.g., in upper trapezius or levator trigger points) could be indicative of either cervical spine or shoulder pathology (*see Table 3*).[19] Table 3 has identified some clinical features of cervical spine pathology vs. shoulder pathology.

General Considerations of Physical Examination. Inspection of the shoulder should include the presence or absence of atrophy of the rotator cuff musculature and an evaluation of cervical spine posture. For example, the classic forward head posture may be indicative of cervical spine as a contributing factor to shoulder pain. Active range of motion should include overhead motion such as flexion and abduction. In addition, extension and external and internal rotation should be performed actively. Both quantity and quality of motion should be evaluated, and a patient's report of pain should be noted during range of motion as well. Strength testing is critical in the shoulder. Quite often, strength is limited secondary to pain. With shoulder conditions, strength testing should be done. A gross strength test should include abduction at 90°, flexion at 90°, and should include isometric testing performed in the following positions: abduction at 90°, flexion at 90°, internal and external rotation with the arm at the side and the elbow at 90°. In addition, test strength in the "plane of the scapula."[3] This is the actual plane in which the the glunohumeral joint functions, and it is as follows: abduction to 90° then horizontal abduction of 30°. Pain in this plane may specifically be indicative of impingement. In addition, a specific, acute neurovascular exam including a dermatome and myotome check of the entire upper extremity should be performed.

Impingement

Impingement is a general term that is inclusive of several distinct clinical entities. Some of these clinical entities include supraspinatus tendonitis, subaccromial/subdeltoid bursitis, and biceps tendonitis. These conditions have been generally labeled impingement because the mechanism of injury (chronic overhead motion) is the same for all three conditions. When considering the general history of the shoulder patient, there should be attention paid to onset. While it is possible to have acute impingement, insidious onset of pain is much more common as a presentation. The specific mechanism of injury for impingement is chronic overhead motion. This is a common condition seen in throwers; specifically, the serve in volleyball, the throw in baseball, or the throw in football have been commonly implicated. Physical exam (PE) findings include point tenderness in the subacromial region and/or over the biceps tendon, a painful arc during active range of motion-abduction. In addition, conservative treatment is similar. Impingement may not present with any abnormal findings under inspection. Palpation may reveal point tenderness in the subacromial region and/or across the biceps tendon. Range of motion again may not present with abnormal findings with regard to quantity of motion (i.e., the athlete will be able to perform range of motion through the full range), but the subtle qualities in motion may be present. For example, during abduction the athlete may have a "hitch" somewhere in the range of 70-100°. This is called a painful arc and is indicative of some form of impingement.[8] Strength, tested as previously described, may be positive. Again, the strength limitation will be subtle if impingement is present, and this may occur during resistive abduction or resisted external rotation, and resistance in the plane of the scapula.[18]

Several special tests have been described for different types of impingement. Perhaps the most common is the Jobe position, or the empty can test.[18] In this test, the athlete places his or her arm in the plane of the scapula, then severe internal rotation occurs (i.e., the athlete is described as emptying a can with his or her hand). Resistance is then applied about the forearm. If this is painful, it is specifically indicative of supraspinatus involvement. Other impingement tests have been described. Two that are very common are the Neer impingement test and the Hawkins-Kennedy impingement test.[18-20] In the Neer impingement test, the athlete goes into full flexion. Then the examiner places one hand behind the shoulder and the other hand at the elbow and forces the arm further into flexion. Pain in the shoulder is indicative of impingement.[19] In the Hawkins-Kennedy impingement test, the athlete again places his or her arm in the plane of the scapula. At this point, severe internal rotation is applied with resistance. Again, pain in the subacromial region in this instance is also indicative of impingement. The most common special test used for biceps tendonitis is the speed test.[19] In this test, the athlete places his or her arm at 90° of shoulder flexion with the elbow fully extended. At this point, resisted flexion occurs. The elbow is fully extended and the arm is externally rotated. At this point, the palm is facing upward and the athlete attempts to push the palm further upward while the examiner forces the arm down. Pain in the anterior aspect of the shoulder is indicative of biceps tendonitis.[19,20]

Special Tests Related to Instability. Instability is much more difficult to evaluate specifically relative to special tests. The most commonly used special test is called the anterior apprehension test. In this test, the athlete lays supine and the examiner places the arm in 90° of abduction and full external rotation. If anterior instability is present, the athlete will usually be apprehensive about putting the arm in this position.[8] In addition, in evaluating general instability, the examiner should again lay the athlete in supine position and then mobilize the humerus by sliding the head of the humerus near the joint line anteriorly and posteriorly, visualizing specific movement and end points. This should be compared to the other side.[19]

Treatment. Treatment, obviously acutely, initially includes NSAIDS—perhaps the most common followed by physical agents. Ice and heat are both used at this time. Since there is possible anatomic predisposition to impingement and if this condition does not resolve initially, it should be referred to an orthopedist. Acutely, the exercise that is most commonly given is the pendulum, or Codman's, exercise. In this exercise, the athlete bends forward and hangs the arm loosely at a 90° angle. At this point, the athlete swings the trunk causing the arm to swing in a pendelum motion or in a circular motion beginning with small circles and progressing to bigger circles. This exercise should be done 3-5 times a day for 2-3 minutes. This exercise allows blood flow to the impinged regions to improve and perhaps allows healing to occur.

Impingement requires a consistent rehabilitation program that should be performed by a physical therapist or athletic trainer. Strengthening exercises acutely should target both the rotator cuff and the scapula stabilizers, which have more recently been implicated as a possible source of abnormal biomechanics leading to impingement.[19] Initially, exercises will be performed isometrically and later performed isotonically. As mentioned previously, exercises such as the Codman's and other range-of-motion exercises are critical in both the prevention and rehabilitation of these conditions. In fact, Codman's should be performed as a warm-up and cool-down exercise in all throwing athletes.

The last phase of rehabilitation is always return to activity. When dealing with a throwing athlete, this should be done in

Figure 4. Shoulder Instability Spectrum

Vague Sense of Shoulder Dysfunction

(**A**traumatic **M**ultidirectional Instability in **B**oth Shoulders that responds to Intensive **R**ehabilitation. If surgery necessary, **I**nferior Capsular Shift Used [**AMBRI**])

Repetitive Microtrauma

Subluxation (Voluntary/Involuntary)

Frank Disclocation
(Trauma)

(**T**raumatic, **U**nidirectional Instability with **B**ankart Lesion Requiring **S**urgery [**TUBS**])

a very gradual manner, again supervised by a physical therapist or athletic trainer.[14]

The last phase of any rehabilitation is return to activity, and should include a functional throwing program for any throwing athlete. For example, a baseball player who wants to get back to the overhead throwing motion after impingement should first start by tossing the ball a few feet with the therapist. This should be followed by tosses of increasing length. Possibly starting as low as 10 ft and progressing out to 100 ft. At some point, the athlete will start to progress in terms of velocity and instead of tossing, begin throwing. All of this is guarded by pain. If, at any point, the athlete begins to experience pain, then he or she should go back to the previous stage and stay there until the pain subsides. Usually the throwing program does not have to be discontinued, but a regression to the previous step will suffice. This progression continues until the athlete is back throwing at the level he or she wants to throw. If the athlete is a pitcher, the last step is obviously to pitch off the mound.[21]

Instability

Instability is a complex condition that many feel occurs along a continuum.[22] For example, it can present as only a general sense of shoulder instability (*please see Figure 4*)[19] all the way to traumatic dislocation. There are three basic classifications of instability. They are traumatic, a-traumatic, and acquired.[23] Traumatic dislocation has a definite mechanism of injury that usually includes abduction and external rotation with applied force to the shoulder, thus resulting in the humeral head dislocating anteriorly. A frank dislocation usually presents at the emergency room and is easily identified. PE findings include dislocation on radiograph and obvious deformity of the glenohumeral joint. An a-traumatic dislocation can occur with athletes with what some would call general hypermobility—those who have instability in multiple directions.[19] The history of the patient with acquired instability may include multiple instances of reported shoulder dislocation quite often with self-reduction.[19]

PE Findings may include atrophy of the deltoid rotator cuff muscles and/or scapula stabilizers. Point tenderness can occur in the anterior or the posterior aspect of the shoulder, and there may or may not be an active range of motion limitation, depending on whether the athlete presents acutely. Acquired instability is a condition in which the history of the athlete usually includes swimming, gymnastics, baseball, and pitching.[19] Theoretically, there is a chronic repetitive microtrauma that occurs, thus causing this acquired instability. The athlete's shoulder becomes extremely mobile and this may be a precursor to a traumatic dislocation. However, this athlete may present with only a vague sense of instability and, more commonly, this athlete will present with a vague sense of instability. PE findings would be similar to those of a-traumatic instability. Again, all instability may occur along a continuum. Both a-traumatic instability and acquired instability may have a positive apprehension test. The most commonly used special test is called the anterior apprehension test. In this test, the athlete lies supine and the examiner places the arm in 90° of abduction and full external rotation. If anterior instability is present, the athlete will usually be apprehensive about putting the arm in this position.[8]

Instability is a very complex clinical entity and should usually be referred to a sports medicine orthopedist for further evaluation. Nonsurgical rehabilitation, however, is often successful in these patients. Rehabilitation is similar to that described under impingement, with a focus on rotator cuff strengthening and scapular stabilizers strengthening. However, when subluxations or dislocations occur more than once, the athlete should be referred to an orthopedist.

Acromioclavicular Joint

Perhaps one of the most common injuries in contact sports, particularly football, is the AC sprain.

History. AC sprains usually occur because of a direct fall on the "point of the shoulder," thus driving the clavicle upward. There are basically three types of AC sprains, although some divide type 3 into three subgroups: grade 1 usually includes minimal damage, usually to the AC ligament. PE will include local tenderness in palpation. The patient may have a loss in range of motion in grade 1 stress and x-rays are usually normal. This is the most common AC sprain. In a grade 2 AC sprain, there is an additional injury to the acromioclavicular capsule, and the acomioclavicular and corococlavicular ligaments. This is evident as the clavicle is raised on inspection and there is a separation at the AC joint on stress x-ray. Grade 3 includes significant injury to the capsule in addition to the acromioclavicular and the corococlavicular ligament. While grade 1 and 2 may be treated conservatively, grade 3 may be treated surgically. There is usually significant deformity with the end of the clavicle displaced superiorly. A grade 1 should cause very little loss of time to athletic participation; however, a grade 2 may include some period of healing—possibly up to six weeks. Both grade 1 and 2 respond well to traditional rehabilitation efforts including physical agents and strengthening exercises.[19]

Summary

Common sports injuries include ankle sprains, knee injuries, impingement, instability, and AC sprains of the shoulder. All of these injuries require a physician who understands that the ultimate goal is usually to go back to the activity that caused the injury in the first place—the chosen sport. Knowledge regarding examination, initial treatment, and rehabilitation will aid the athlete in reaching his or her goal.

References

1. Powell JW, Barber-Foss KD. Injury patterns in selected high school sports: A review of the 1995-1997 seasons. *Journal of Athletic Training* 1999;34:277-284.
2. Netter FH. *Atlas of Human Anatomy*. 2nd ed. East Hanover, NJ: Novartis Medical Education; 1997.
3. Norkin CC, Lavangie PK. *Joint Structure and Function: A Comprehensive Analysis*. 2nd ed. Philadelphia, Pa: FA Davis Company; 1992.
4. Shelbourne DK, et al. Knee injuries. In: Schenck RC, ed. *Athletic Training and Sports Medicine*. Rosemont, Ill: American Academy of Orthopaedic Surgeons; 1999.
5. Schenck RC. Classification and Treatment of Knee Dislocations. *Orthopedic Special Edition* 1998;4:35-38.
6. Irrgang JJ, et al. The knee: Ligamentous and meniscal injuries. In: Zachazewski JE, ed. *Athletic Injuries and Rehabilitation*. Philadelphia, Pa: WB Saunders Company; 1996:623-692.
7. Taunton J, et al. Leg, foot, and ankle injuries. In: Zachazewski JE, Quillen WS, eds. *Athletic Injuries and Rehabilitation*. Philadelphia, Pa: WB Saunders Company; 1996.
8. Hoppenfeld S, Hutton R. *Physical Examination of the Spine and the Extremities*. New York, NY: Appleton-Century-Crofts; 1976.
9. Shelbourne KD, et al. Anterior cruciate ligament injuries. In: Reider B, ed. *Sports Medicine: The School-Age Athlete*. Philadelphia, Pa: WB Saunders Company; 1996:329-347.
10. Kannus P, Jarvinen M. Conservatively treated tears of the anterior cruciate ligament. *J Bone Joint Surg* 1997;69A:1007-1012.
11. Shelbourne KD, Gray T. Anterior cruciate ligament reconstruction with autogenous patellar tendon graft followed by acclerated rehabilitation: A two- to nine-year follow up. *Am J Sports Med* 1997;25:786-795.
12. Shelbourne KD, Patel DV, McCarroll JR. Management of anteriorcruciate ligament injuries in skeletally immature adolescents. *Knee Surg Sports Traumatol Arthrosc* 1996;4: 68-74.
13. Rettig AC, Rubinstein RA. Medial and lateral ligament injuries of the knee. In: Scott W, ed. *The Knee*. St. Louis, Mo: Mosby-Year Book; 1994.
14. Anderson BC. *Office Orthopedics for Primary Care Diagnosis and Treatment*. 2nd ed. Philadelphia, Pa: WB Saunders Company; 1998.
15. Jones RE, Henley MB, Francis P. Nonoperative management of isolated grade III collateral ligament injury tears in high school football players. *Clin Orthop* 1986;213:137-140.
16. Wexler RK. The injured ankle. *Am Fam Physician* 1998;57: 474-480.
17. Stiell IG, et al. Prospective validation of a decision rule for the use of radiography in acute knee injuries. *JAMA* 1996;275: 611-615.
18. Thompson WO, et al. Shoulder injuries. In: Schenck RC, ed. *Athletic Training and Sports Medicine*. Rosemont, Ill: American Academy of Orthopaedic Surgeons; 1999.
19. Magee DJ, et al. Shoulder injuries. In: Zachazewski JE, Quillen WS, eds. *Athletic Injuries and Rehabiliation*. Philadelphia, Pa: WB Saunders Company; 1996.
20. Pfeffer GB. Foot and ankle. In: Snider RK, ed. *Essentials of Musculoskeletal Care*. 1st ed. Rosemont, Ill: American Academy of Orthopaedic Surgeons; 1997.
21. Wilk PT, et al. Interval throwing program for the shoulder. In: Andrews JR, ed. *The Athlete's Shoulder*. New York, NY: Churchill Livingstone; 1994:569-628.
22. Jobe F, et al. The shoulder in sports. In: Rockwood CA, Matsen FA, eds. *The Shoulder*. 2nd ed. Philadelphia, Pa: WB Saunders Company; 1998:1214-1238.
23. Neer CS, Foster CR. Inferior capsular shifts for involuntary inferior and multi-directional instability of the shoulder. *J Bone Joint Surg Am* 1980;62A:897-908.

Serological Tests in Rheumatic Diseases

Keith K. Colburn, MD
Myron E. Chu, DO

After a thorough history and physical examination, a physician normally formulates a differential diagnosis. If the patient has symptoms and signs suggestive of a connective tissue disease, which tests should the doctor order? What do the test results mean? How does one use the information provided by these tests? This chapter discusses how to use laboratory tests in rheumatic diseases. Put in their proper perspective, laboratory tests help rule out, confirm, or sub-classify a disease process. Therefore, it is extremely important to have a clear knowledge of the patient's history and an appropriate physical examination before one can interpret laboratory tests; otherwise, information from these tests is relatively useless. To make sense of test results, it is essential that the doctor know the rheumatic disease process, criteria for the diagnoses of these diseases, and what the test results mean in the context of the disease one is suspecting. In using a test to rule out or confirm a diagnosis, one must understand "sensitivity" (the percent of positive test results in patients with a given disease), "specificity" (the percent of negative test results in patients without the disease in question), and "positive and negative predictive values" in the setting of one's reference laboratory. This chapter reviews the context of ordering clinical laboratory tests on patients with suspected connective tissue diseases.

Introduction

Immunologic tests assist the clinician in the diagnosis and management of patients with rheumatic diseases. Recently the thrust of managed care is to have primary care physicians order and interpret test results that are usually obtained by subspecialists. This chapter will help to illustrate the clinical application and proper interpretation of the more commonly ordered rheumatologic laboratory tests.

Before a test is ordered, the physician must have in mind a course of action to follow in response to the outcome of the test. In general, immunologic tests are usually obtained for disease screening, help in confirming a diagnosis based on the history and clinical findings, assessing specific organ involvement, monitoring disease activity, and/or monitoring drug toxicity.[1] It should be remembered that if a certain test does not have the potential to significantly contribute to or alter the diagnosis or course of therapy, it might be better left undone.

The use of a test to confirm or exclude a diagnosis is determined by its sensitivity, specificity, and positive or negative predictive value.[2] Sensitivity is defined as the percent of positive test results in patients with a given disease. Specificity is defined as the percent of negative test results in

Table 1. Determination of Sensitivity, Specificity, and Predictive Values

	Disease	No Disease	Total
Abnormal Tests	TP*	FP	TP+FP
Normal Tests	FN⁺	TN	FN+TN
Total	TP+FN	FP+TN	

*TP = true positive, TN = true negative

⁺FP = false positive, FN = false negative

Sensitivity = TP/(TP+FN)

Specificity = TN/(TN+FP)

Positive predictive value = TP/(TP+FP)

Negative predictive value = TN/(TN+FN)

Prevalence = (TP+FN)/[(TP+FN)+(FP+TN)]

patients without the disease in question. Tests that are very sensitive are used to exclude a diagnosis. An extremely sensitive test is positive in almost all patients who have a certain disease; therefore, a negative test is strong evidence against the presence of that disease, but it is not necessarily diagnostic. A good example of a highly sensitive test with very little disease specificity is an anti-nuclear antibody (ANA) test, which, if negative, nearly always rules out a diagnosis of systemic lupus erythematosus (SLE).

Tests with high specificity can help confirm a diagnosis. A good example of a very specific test is the anti-Smith antibody test, which, if positive, is almost always associated with the diagnosis of SLE. However, in immunologic tests, high specificity is frequently coupled with low sensitivity; therefore, a negative highly specific test does not exclude the presence of a specific disease. Anti-Smith antibodies, although very specific for SLE, are present in the sera of only 20% of SLE patients. If a test has a low specificity for a disease, a positive test result does little to confirm a diagnosis.

The positive predictive value is the probability that a patient with a positive test result actually has the disease, whereas the negative predictive value is the probability that a person with a negative test result does not have the disease. The positive or negative predictive values of a test will vary with the prevalence of the disease in the particular population tested. As the prevalence of a disease decreases in the population, it becomes less likely that the test represents a false-positive result. Prevalence is simply the fraction of the population who have the disease. Table 1 shows how sensitivity, specificity, and predictive values are calculated.

It is essential for clinicians to remember that a diagnosis of a rheumatologic disease should be made to a large extent based on a knowledgeable history, then on the physical examination, and, to a much lesser extent, on laboratory and other tests. The laboratory tests should be used to help support a clinical judgment. It is important to also know the limits of the tests that are ordered to fully appreciate their value.

The following is a discussion of the use of the laboratory for rheumatic diseases.

The Laboratory Evaluation in Systemic Lupus Erythematosus

Systemic lupus erythematosus (SLE) is an autoimmune disease that can affect most organ systems. Myriad clinical manifestations can result, as well as a variety of autoantibodies to various components of the cell. A few of these antibodies may be pathogenic in certain features of SLE disease processes.

LE Cell Phenomenon. In 1948, Hargraves noticed that the bone marrow smears of patients with SLE had white blood cells containing peculiar intracytoplasmic inclusions.[3] These white blood cells were termed LE cells and were at first considered to be diagnostic of SLE. The LE cell, usually a polymorphonuclear white blood cell, phagocytizes a homogeneously staining globular material called a hematoxylin body. The hematoxylin body consists of modified nuclear material, IgG, and complement. The LE cell phenomenon usually occurs in vitro but occasionally can be seen in vivo, as in SLE pleural, ascitic, pericardial, and synovial fluids. It was initially thought that the LE cell test was exclusively seen in SLE. However, specificity of this test is relatively low, since the LE cell phenomenon can be seen in rheumatoid arthritis, lupoid hepatitis, drug reaction, and in some cases of scleroderma and dermatomyositis. The LE cell test is positive in only 70-80% of patients with active SLE and in fewer patients with SLE in remission.[2] A positive test, because of its limited sensitivity, does not confirm the presence of SLE, and, by the same token, a negative test, because of the limited sensitivity, does not exclude the diagnosis of the disease. The LE cell preparation is now considered to be outdated, insensitive, and nonspecific and is rarely ordered by knowledgeable clinicians. Interest in the LE cell preparation test seems to have taken on more of an historical nature.

Antinuclear Antibody Test. Antinuclear antibodies (ANA) belong to a large family of autoantibodies that react with antigens present in cell nuclei. The method most commonly used in the clinical laboratory for determining ANAs is the indirect immunofluorescent test using human tissue culture cells, such as human epithelial cells (Hep-2 cells), as substrate. By comparison, the ANA test done by enzyme-linked immunoassays (EIA) has an unsatisfactory sensitivity and specificity and is clinically less useful.[4]

The serum ANA is the most sensitive test done on patients with SLE. It is positive in 95-99% of untreated SLE patients.[5] The degree of positivity of the ANA test may also be important, because the positive predictive value of the test increases with higher titers.[6] Although the sensitivity of the ANA test is very high, the specificity is poor. The positive ANA can be found in patients with various rheumatic diseases, including rheumatoid arthritis (RA), scleroderma, juvenile rheumatoid arthritis

Table 2. ANA Patterns, Their Associated Diseases, and Antibody Tests

ANA Test Pattern	Disease Association	More Specific Autoantibody Tests
Homogeneous	Nonspecific Drug-induced SLE	Nonspecific Anti-histone Abs (Test must be chosen based on clinical impression)
Speckled	Sjögren's syndrome La(SS-B)	Ro(SS-A)
	Mixed connective tissue disease	RNP
	SLE	Sm (Smith)
	Scleroderma	Scl-70
	CREST	Centromere
Rim	SLE	dsDNA
Nucleolar	Scleroderma	
None	ANA negative SLE	Ro(SS-A) La(SS-B)

Table 3. Some Drugs that May Induce Lupus-Like Syndrome

Definite	Possible
Procainamide	Phenytoin
Hydralazine	Atenolol
INH	Captopril
Chlorpromazine	Penicillamine
Methyldopa	Quinidine
	Nitrofurantoin
	Propylthiouracil

(JRA), Sjögren's syndrome, and mixed connective tissue disease (MCTD). The positive ANA may also be found in the serum of patients with hepatitis C infection, interstitial pulmonary fibrosis, pneumoconiosis, silicosis, chronic active hepatitis, malaria, leprosy, certain drugs, and neoplasms of various organs. A serum ANA is present in some healthy people, especially the elderly.

Because of its high sensitivity, the ANA is most useful when it is negative. A negative test result nearly excludes the diagnosis of SLE. Although ANA-negative SLE occurs, it is extremely rare, found in only 1% of patients with active disease.[7] Some patients with SLE, however, develop a negative ANA as their disease remits, either spontaneously or from therapy.[8] Disappearance of a positive ANA test occurs in approximately 10-20% of SLE cases, but this percentage can increase to 30-50% for those SLE patients who develop renal failure and are treated with dialysis.[8] It should be noted that some patients with SLE who exhibit clinical remission will maintain high ANA titers. This persistent elevated ANA titer should not be used as an indicator for initiating therapy. ANA titers of less than 1:40 or 7 IU/mL (using the new international units) are considered normal.

When the ANA test is positive, the fluorescent pattern may be somewhat helpful in subclassifying the rheumatic diseases. Four types of patterns of nuclear fluorescence have been described in which the titer is also provided. No single pattern has been found to be diagnostic of any specific disease, but there have been strong associations. Additionally, all or any combination of patterns may appear simultaneously, and any one pattern may somewhat obscure the others.

The four patterns of ANA fluorescent nuclear staining are homogeneous (diffuse), speckled, peripheral (rim), and nucleolar. *(Please see Table 2.)* The most common ANA pattern is the non-specific, homogeneous pattern seen in patients with SLE as well as RA, Sjögren's syndrome, and scleroderma. The speckled pattern is commonly seen in patients with SLE, MCTD, scleroderma, RA, liver disease, ulcerative colitis, and in some healthy people.[2] The peripheral pattern is often detected in SLE patients who have active nephritis. The nucleolar pattern is less frequently seen but is more commonly associated with scleroderma and rheumatologic overlap syndromes with sclerodermatous features.[7]

Anti-Double Stranded DNA. If the clinician suspects a diagnosis of SLE or a disease process with clinical features of SLE in which the ANA result is positive, then further antibody tests are warranted. The ANA includes antibodies to both single- and double-stranded DNA. Anti-single stranded DNA (anti-ssDNA) antibodies are not specific for SLE because they occur in patients with different autoimmune diseases. Anti-double-stranded DNA (dsDNA) antibodies, or anti-native DNA (nDNA) antibodies, are considered to be characteristic of SLE and occur in as many as 70% of patients with active SLE and, especially, with lupus nephritis. The anti-dsDNA antibody test does not predict lupus nephritis nor other particular SLE disease manifestations, but because these antibodies often fluctuate in parallel with disease activity, test results are used as an SLE disease monitor.[7] The specificity for a positive anti-dsDNA test is about 95%.

Anti-Smith Antibody. Anti-Smith antibodies (anti-Sm) were identified in 1966 and named after SLE patient Shirley Smith. Anti-Sm antibodies are 99% specific for SLE. The sensitivity, however, is approximately 20%. The anti-Sm antibody test does not correlate with any particular feature of SLE nor does it vary greatly with time.[9] A word of caution is indicated here, as it is a common clerical error to confuse "anti-Sm" with "anti-smooth muscle" when ordering tests. The anti-smooth muscle antibody test is associated with autoimmune chronic active hepatitis and other liver diseases. Therefore, writing out "anti-Smith" instead of "anti-Sm" may ensure that the correct test is performed.

Table 4. Clinical and Laboratory Features of APS

Clinical	
***Major Features**	**Other (proposed) Clinical Features**
Venous thrombosis (DVT, PE, etc.)	Livedo reticularis
Arterial thrombosis (CVA, MI, gangrene)	Endocardial valvular vegetations
Thrombocytopenia	Positive Coomb's test
Pregnancy loss	Migraine headaches
	Leg ulcers
	? Pulmonary hypertension
	? Chorea
	? Avascular necrosis
Laboratory	
Anti-cardiolipin antibody test medium to high positive IgG >20 GPL units, IgM > 20 MPL units	
Positive lupus anticoagulant test	

** A diagnosis of APS should be based on a history of one major clinical feature (preferably not explainable by any other predisposing condition) and a positive laboratory test (which has remained positive for several weeks to months).*

Table 5. Drugs Associated with Myopathy

alcohol	ipecac	colchicine
cyclosporin	gemfibrozil	penicillin
penicillamine	hydralazine	vincristine
corticosteroids	phenytoin	cimetidine
heroin	lovastatin	hydroxychloroquine
chloroquine	levodopa	
zidovudine	procainamide	

Anti-Ribonucleoprotein Antibody. In 1972, Sharp et al described a group of patients with overlapping clinical features of SLE, polymyositis, and scleroderma and coined the term "mixed connective tissue disease" or MCTD.[10] Serum antibodies to ribonucleoprotein (anti-U1snRNP) are a feature of patients with MCTD. These U1snRNP antibodies were previously referred to as ribonucleoprotein (RNP) or nRNP (nuclear RNP) antibodies. Patients also have high serum titers of speckled ANA. Antibodies to ribosomal RNP most often account for cytoplasmic staining in immunofluorescence. These antibodies are called "extractable nuclear antigens" or ENAs, because they are easily extractable in normal saline solution. There are more than 20 different anti-ENA antibodies described, but the two major ones are anti-U1snRNP, and the anti-Sm, which has been previously discussed above. Anti-U1snRNP is a small nucleoprotein particle containing U1RNA (uridine-rich RNA). Antibodies to U1snRNP are present in 35-45% of patients with SLE and, by definition, virtually all patients with MCTD.[11] When SLE is present, anti-Sm antibodies are usually accompanied by anti-U1snRNP antibodies. The anti-U1snRNP antibody test is not useful in monitoring disease activity or predicting SLE flares. High titers do not seem to be associated with worse disease.

The clinician should suspect MCTD in a patient with overlapping clinical features of SLE, scleroderma, and polymyositis with a high titer speckled ANA. If the patient's serum contains anti-U1snRNP alone, then the diagnosis of MCTD is likely. However, in patients with these overlapping features, if the serum is negative for anti-RNP antibodies, the term "undifferentiated connective tissue disease" is used for the diagnosis.

An ENA panel is often ordered, which usually includes the anti-Sm and the anti-U1snRNP. A laboratory should have a listing of the component tests offered on each panel. However, rather than ordering a panel, it is better to order the necessary tests individually.

Anti-ribosomal P Antibody. Antibodies to ribosomal P proteins (anti-ribosomal P) are detected in 12-16% of patients with non-psychotic SLE and are quite rare in other rheumatic diseases.[12] These antibodies, however, are detected in 45-90% of patients with severe depression associated with psychosis due to SLE.[13] Yet, there has been great controversy regarding the clinical correlation of these antibodies with neuropsychiatric SLE. A positive test for anti-ribosomal P protein antibodies is not diagnostic of lupus psychosis because almost 50% of patients with anti-ribosomal P antibodies have no severe behavioral problems.[13] If CNS lupus is suspected, the history and clinical physical examination ought to be used as the basis for the diagnosis. The clinician considering ordering the anti-ribosomal P antibody test should remember that the results obtained may not help to support or rule out CNS lupus and consequently will not alter the diagnosis nor the planned course of treatment.

Sjögren's Antibodies: Anti-Ro/SSA and anti-La/SSB. Anti-SSA(anti-Ro) and anti-SSB(anti-La) are circulating antibodies that are frequently seen together in patients with primary Sjögren's syndrome and subacute cutaneous lupus. However, they may occur in other connective tissue diseases with or without associated primary Sjögren's syndrome. Anti-SSA antibodies are found in approximately 25-35% and anti-SSB antibodies in about 25% of patients with SLE.[1,14] The serum of less than 1% of normal individuals has the anti-SSA antibody, and those that do have the antibody have low levels. Children born to mothers with a positive serum anti-SSA antibody test run a significant risk of having neonatal heart block, which will be discussed below under "Neonatal Lupus." There is a high frequency of subacute cutaneous lupus with the presence of circulating anti-SSA and anti-SSB antibodies. This subset of SLE patients with a photosensitive, non-scarring skin rash with either annular or psoriasiform morphology tends to

Table 6. Brief Differential Diagnosis of Muscle Weakness

Proximal Muscle Weakness
- polymyositis
- dermatomyositis
- vitamin D deficiency
- adrenal insufficiency
- hypophosphatemia
- hypothyroidism

Glycogen Storage Disease
- McArdle's disease
- adult onset acid maltase deficiency

Lipid Storage Myopathies
- carnitine deficiency
- carnitine palmityltransferase deficiency

Neuromuscular Disorders
- genetic muscular dystrophies (Dechenne's, Becker's, etc.)
- myasthenia gravis
- Eaton-Lambert syndrome
- myotonic dystrophy
- Guillain Barré
- diabetes
- porphyria
- amyotrophic lateral sclerosis

Infections
- viral (influenza, EBV, HIV, coxsackie virus)
- bacterial (staphylococcus, streptococcus, clostridium)
- parasitic (toxoplasmosis, trichinosis, cysticercosis)

Non-neuromuscular Causes of Weakness
- hypotension
- hypoxia
- hypoglycemia
- anemia
- malignancy
- malnutrition
- cerebrovascular insufficiency
- hypercapnia

Table 7. Some Diseases Associated with Rheumatoid Factor

Rheumatic Diseases	Bacterial Infections
rheumatoid arthritis	subacute bacterial endocarditis
SLE	syphilis
scleroderma	tuberculosis
MCTD	Lyme disease
Sjögren's syndrome	leprosy
sarcoid	brucellosis
mixed cryoglobulinemia	
Viral Diseases	**Parasitic Diseases**
AIDS	trypanosomiasis
Rubella	kala-azar
cytomegalovirus	malaria
hepatitis	schistosomiasis
mononucleosis	
influenza	

have less frequent visceral involvement. Patients with the so-called ANA-negative SLE often have subacute cutaneous lupus and may test positive for anti-SSA antibodies and rheumatoid factor (RF).

Neonatal Lupus. Neonatal lupus syndrome present at birth, or shortly thereafter, is characterized by a lupus skin rash, transient or permanent congenital heart block, cytopenias, and liver inflammation. The mother of the infant has SLE or some form of systemic connective tissue disease and tests positive for the anti-SSA antibody. Because of transplacental transfer of maternal IgG, the infant tests positive for anti-SSA antibodies. The risk of having a child with the syndrome is higher if the mother has both antibodies to SSA and SSB, but the risk is lower if the mother has isolated SSA in low titers.[7] The presence of anti-SSA antibodies increases the risk of giving birth to an infant with congenital heart block to about 5%.[14] Since anti-SSA and anti-SSB antibodies readily cross the placenta, they can be used as markers for neonatal lupus. Careful monitoring of the fetus should be done before as well as after delivery. Laboratory tests on the infant should include a CBC and platelets to evaluate cytopenias as well as an ANA, anti-dsDNA, anti-SSA, and anti-SSB antibodies.

Anti-Histone Antibodies in Drug-Induced Lupus. A negative anti-histone antibody test is used to help rule out a clinical diagnosis of drug-induced lupus. The clinical features of drug-induced lupus are often less severe than those of SLE, of which the most commonly reported symptoms are fever, arthritis, and serositis.[15] CNS and renal involvement are rare in drug-induced lupus. Anti-histone antibodies occur in more than than 90% of cases. However, anti-histone antibodies are not specific for drug-induced SLE, since they are also found in 25% of patients with SLE.[16] Antibodies to single-stranded DNA may be present, but antibodies to double-stranded DNA are typically absent.[15] *(Please see Table 3.)*

Complement. The complement system is a group of proteins that functions as a mediator of inflammation. The protein components interact with each other and with other aspects of the immune system. Complement activation is a cascade reaction. Patients with active SLE, especially with nephritis, frequently show evidence in their serum of activitation of the complement pathway by depression of the levels of C3, C4, and CH50. Lowered serum complement levels may indicate both consumption of components and a decrease in complement synthesis as in lupus nephritis. It is not practical and cost-effective to measure most of the complement components because they are unstable. CH50 and C3 are the most useful initial measures of the complement system. The CH50 is a measure of the integrity of the entire classical complement cascade, but not the alternative pathway. C3 is the most stable complement component, and its depression indicates activity in either or both classical and alternative pathways. CH50 and C3 should be assessed together, because low levels of either may indicate an SLE flare. C4 is also a measure of the classic complement pathway and may also be low in active SLE. However, C4 by itself may not be an accurate indication of SLE activity, as it is commonly low in people who have an inherited deficiency of C4. The prevalence of complement deficiency in the general population is estimated at 0.03%, and it appears that C2 deficiency is the most common inherited deficiency in the white population.[17] In rheumatologic disorders such as SLE, the incidence

Table 8. Factors that Influence the Erythrocyte Sedimentation Rate

alcohol	ipecac	colchicine
cyclosporin	gemfibrozil	penicillin
penicillamine	hydralazine	vincristine
corticosteroids	phenytoin	cimetidine
heroin	lovastatin	hydroxychloroquine
chloroquine	levodopa	
zidovudine	procainamide	

of C2 deficiency may be as high as 5.9%.[18] SLE in C2-deficiency individuals tends to be different than the general population in that the age of onset is earlier and there is a higher incidence of males.[17] Milder renal involvement is noted in C2-deficient SLE individuals as well as lower ANA titers, but the prevalence of anti-SSA antibodies is increased.[17]

Anti-Phospholipid Antibodies

Patients with the anti-phospholipid antibody syndrome (APS) may have recurrent vascular thrombosis, pregnancy loss, and thrombocytopenia associated with a persistantly positive lupus anticoagulant (LAC) test and/or moderat-to-high levels of anticardiolipin antibody (ACL) levels. *(Please see Table 4.)* There is a strong correlation of APS and SLE, although APS can be seen alone. Cardiolipin is a phospholipid that was isolated in 1941 from beef heart by Mary Pangborn during investigations of serologic tests for syphilis.[19] Patients with APS but without SLE are often referred as having primary APS (PAPS). These individuals usually do not develop SLE.

Antiphospholipid (APL) antibodies can either be drug induced or autoimmune. Infections such as syphilis, Lyme disease, and HIV-1 (HTLV-1) can induce APL antibodies, while chlorpromazine and other drugs that can cause a drug-induced lupus can also produce APL antibodies. However, clinical APS occurs with autoimmune-, not drug-induced, APL antibodies.[20] Autoimmune-induced APL antibodies are frequently present in sustained high serum titers most often of IgG isotype.[20] Infection-induced APL antibody titers tend to be of IgG and IgM isotypes and of lower, transient titers. Drug-induced APL antibodies are primarily of IgM isotype.[20]

In the presence of the appropriate clinical manifestations, a positive serum LAC, ACL, or both help to confirm a diagnosis of APS. A positive LAC test is suggested by the following clinical findings: 1) A prolonged partial thromboplastin time (PTT); 2) failure to correct the abnormal clotting time by mixing patient serum with normal serum (suggesting the presence of a clotting inhibitor); and 3) normalization of the test with freeze-thawed platelets or phospholipids.[21] Serum ACL antibody tests are usually measured with a standardized EIA for each of the isotypes. IgG results are reported in GPL units, IgM in MPL units, and IgA in APL units. IgG values above 20 GPL units are considered positive and above 40 are most specific for APS.[22]

In the absence of APL antibodies, the differential diagnosis for unexplained arterial or venous thrombosis or pregnancy loss includes, among other conditions, use of birth control pills by a smoker, nephrotic syndrome, vasculitis, accelerated atherosclerosis, factor V Leiden activated protein C resistance, homocystinuria, Buerger's disease, malignancy, protein C and S deficiency, and anti-thrombin III deficiency.[22]

Wegener's Granulomatosis

Antineutrophil Cytoplasmic Antibodies (ANCA). Wegener's granulomatosis (WG) is an uncommon, multisystem disease of unknown etiology that occurs in young or middle-aged adults with a slight preponderance toward men and is almost always fatal if untreated. The major features of WG include a triad of necrotizing granulomatous vasculitis of the upper and lower respiratory tracts and glomerulonephritis. To confirm the diagnosis in patients with suspected WG and rule out other processes, such as systemic infections and malignancies, it is essential to have tissue evidence, preferably from an open lung biopsy.[23]

Antineutrophil cytoplasmic antibodies (ANCA) were first described in 1982 in the serum of patients with systemic vasculitis and glomerulonephritis and were later identified as a marker for WG.[23] On immunofluorescent staining of alcohol-fixed PMNs, two patterns of ANCA can be recognized. C-ANCA is identified by a coarse, granular, centrally-accentuated pattern that decreases in intensity toward the periphery of the cell. The C-ANCA is specific for proteinase 3. Proteinase 3 is a 29-kd serine protease found in the azurophilic granules of the neutrophil and is the major antigen for C-ANCA. The other recognized ANCA pattern is P-ANCA, an artifact of ethanol fixation. Ethanol causes the rearrangement of positively charged granule constituents around and on the negatively charged nuclear membrane, resulting in an artifactual perinuclear pattern. The major antigen for P-ANCA is myeloperoxidase, a lysosomal enzyme found in neutrophils.

C-ANCA is reported in the sera of as many as 90% of patients with active WG.23 In active, limited WG, the sensitivity of C-ANCA tests is 60-67%[24] and can decrease to 41-43% in patients with inactive disease.[25] Thus, although the sensitivity of a positive C-ANCA is high, a negative result does not necessarily exclude the diagnosis of WG, especially in patients with limited or inactive WG. Using the C-ANCA to monitor disease activity was suggested, since C-ANCA titers often parallel WG disease activity,[24] but its usefulness is still not clear.

P-ANCA can be found in the sera of 80% of patients with active pauci-immune necrotizing and crescentic glomerulonephritis.[26] A positive P-ANCA can be a useful marker for vasculitis-associated cresentic glomerulonephritis as well as Churge-Strauss syndrome.[27] In patients with ANCA-associated glomerulonephritis, approximately 90% of the positive P-ANCA results are secondary to anti-myeloperoxidase antibodies.[27] P-ANCA tests that are positive but are myeloperoxidase-negative have poor specificity and are associated with inflammatory bowel disease, chronic active hepatitis, primary sclerosing cholangitis, and normal controls.[28]

WG is a rare disease, and the prevalence in the population may markedly influence the predictive value of a positive C-ANCA test. If used as a screening test, a positive C-ANCA test result may often be falsely positive.[23] The C-ANCA test is most valuable when the clinical situation suggests a diagnosis of vasculitis and the clinician is considering several diagnoses, including WG.[23] However, a positive C-ANCA test does not substitute for a tissue biopsy to make the diagnosis of WG, because one does not want to start a patient on a two- or three-year course of cyclophosphamide without an accurate diagnosis.

Scleroderma Antibodies

Scleroderma or systemic sclerosis (SSc) is a connective tissue disease in which there is fibrosis of the skin and visceral organs. The disease is rare in childhood and peaks at 50-60 years of age. There is a preponderance for females, although the female-to-male ratio varies with age, the highest being 15:1 during childbearing years.[29] Little is known about the etiology of SSc. Isolated cases of SSc may be secondary to exposure to vinyl-chloride, benzene, or the chemotherapeutic agent, bleomycin. Diffuse scleroderma includes the distal and proximal extremities, the internal organs, the face, and the trunk of the body. CREST syndrome (calcinosis, Raynaud's, esophageal dysmotility, sclerodactyly, telangiectasis) is a limited form of scleroderma involving the distal extremities and the face. The ANA is positive in 70-90% of individuals with SSc and 60-90% of those with CREST.

Scl-70 antibodies or anti-DNA-topoisomerase I are almost exclusively seen in SSc, although only 20-40% of patients with SSc have a positive test. Anti-centromere antibodies are present in 60-90% of patients with CREST, but only 10-15% of patients with SSc. Anti-centromere antibodies are occasionally detected in patients with Raynaud's syndrome.[30]

Polymyositis/Dermatomyositis

Polymyositis and dermatomyositis are idiopathic inflammatory myopathies that are characterized by proximal limb weakness, neck flexor weakness, and, occasionally, muscle pain. The laboratory hallmarks of these muscle diseases are elevated serum creatine kinase (CK) and aldolase levels. The LDH and transaminases may also be elevated. There are reported cases of patients with normal CK and serum aldolase levels but with muscle biopsies positive for the presence of an inflammatory myopathy. An electromyelogram (EMG) is a sensitive test for evaluating an inflammatory myopathy. Over 90% of patients with polymyositis/dermatomyositis will have the typical findings of irritability of myofibrils (fibrillation potentials) on needle insertion at rest and short duration, low amplitude, complex (polyphasic) potentials on contraction. However, there is little correlation between the amount of weakness or functional disability and the EMG findings.[31] Reviewing medications of a patient with suspected myopathy may also be rewarding, because several drugs have been associated with a myopathy, including corticosteroids, zidovudine, and cimetidine.[31] *(Please see Table 5.)*

Antibodies to the Jo-1 antigen (histydyl-tRNA synthetase) are present in the sera of 18-31% of adult patients with polymyositis and rarely in dermatomyositis.[30] Anti-Jo-1 antibodies also appear to be a marker for interstitial lung disease in polymyositis.

The anti-Mi-2 antibody is an antinuclear antibody found in the sera of only 5-10% of myositis patients, but it is strongly associated with the rash of dermatomyositis, especially in juvenile dermatomyositis.[31] The anti-PM-Scl (originally anti-PM-1) antibody is only occasionally detected in myositis patients and identifies a small subset of individuals with features of systemic sclerosis with myositis. See Table 6 for a brief differential diagnosis of muscle weakness.

Sjögren's Syndrome

Sjögren's syndrome (sicca syndrome) is a chronic, slowly progressive disease that primarily affects the exocrine glands by lymphocytic infiltration, destroying and replacing functional epithelium. Patients present with characteristic symptoms of dry eyes (xerophthalmia), dry mouth (xerostomia), and, often, parotid gland swelling and vaginal dryness. The Schirmer's tear test and Rose Bengal staining of the corneal epithelium as well as sialometry and sialography can be used to help make the diagnosis of Sjögren's syndrome. A minor salivary gland biopsy may also be useful.

Two antibodies, anti-SSA and anti-SSB, are common in the sera of patients with Sjögren's syndrome. The antibodies are not specific for Sjögren's syndrome, and, as previously mentioned, may be found in other autoimmune diseases, such as SLE. Anti-SSA(Ro) antibodies are present in approximately 40-45% of patients with Sjögren's syndrome and 25-35% with SLE.[14,32] Anti-SSB(La) antibodies are detected in approximately 50% of patients with Sjögren's syndrome and in up to 25% with SLE.[32]

Rheumatoid Arthritis

Rheumatoid Factor. In the 1940s, Waaler and Rose and colleagues discovered that the majority of sera of patients with rheumatoid arthritis (RA) agglutinated sheep red blood cells sensitized with rabbit anti-erythrocyte antibodies.[33,34] They referred to these antibodies as rheumatoid factors (RF). RFs are autoantibodies directed against antigenic determinants on the Fc fragment of IgG. The development of radioimmunoassay (RIA) and enzyme-linked immunosorbent assay (EIA) methods have facilitated the more precise quantification of IgM, IgG, and IgA rheumatoid factors. The most commonly measured RF is IgM antibody to IgG by latex agglutination or, more recently, by nephelometry. IgM RFs are multivalent and are efficient agglutinators of antigen-coated particles. Studies indicate that RFs are present in the serum of 75-80% of patients with RA and at some time during the disease course. Diseases other than RA in which positive RF test results are frequently found include rheumatic diseases (Sjögren's syndrome, SLE, cryoglobulinemia, etc.), viral infections, chronic inflammatory diseases, and neoplasms after chemotherapy or radiotherapy.

RF is found in the sera of 5% of healthy persons in the general population and increases with age to 10-25% of individuals over 65 years old.[35] Therefore, the positive predictive value remains poor at about 6% and must be interpreted in light of other clinical features. RF tests can be performed by nephelometry or agglutination. There is some variation in the sensitivity of RF detection depending on which technique is used. Agglutination using latex particles or bentonite is more sensitive but less specific than tests that employ sheep red cells.[36] The sensitivity of RF for RA patients by nephelometry is between 61-75%.[37] See Table 7 for a more complete list of diseases associated with RF.

The pathologic role of RF in RA remains unclear. The RF titer does not correlate with disease activity, but it is generally considered that high titer RFs are associated with more severe disease, including the presence of rheumatoid nodules and extra-articular features. The RF test sub-classifies RA patients into seropositive and seronegative disease. Patients with "RA" but negative for RF need to be watched more closely for the development of a different diagnosis, such as psoriatic arthritis or one of the spondyloarthropathies.

Other Laboratory Tests

Erythrocyte Sedimentation Rate (ESR). The erythrocyte sedimentation rate (ESR) is a general indicator of inflammation and is a measure of the speed at which red blood cells (RBCs) settle in uncoagulated blood. The ESR is considered to be a sensitive test for chronic inflammation, but it is not very specific. Elevated ESR values can be seen in conditions such as infection, malignancy, oral contraceptive use, pregnancy, hyperthyroidism, hypothyroidism, etc.

The mechanism of the ESR has to do with the reaction of proteins in the presence of inflammation. With the presence of acute phase reactants (the most abundant being fibrinogen), the RBCs tend to aggregate in a stacked coin fashion, which is referred to as "rouleau" formation. Other serum proteins, such as alpha- and gamma-globulins, also influence the ESR but to a lesser extent. The higher the intensity of inflammation with more fibrinogen production and increased rouleau formation, the higher the ESR.

There are two common methods of measuring ESR: Wintrobe and Westergren. The Wintrobe method is limited by a short tube (100 mm) and, consequently, limits the high readings obtained with the Westergren tube (200 mm) in some of the more serious rheumatic diseases. The ESR is a measurement in millimeters (mm) of the distance the RBCs fall in a column of uncoagulated blood in one hour. A Westergren ESR of less than 10 mm in males and 20 mm in females is considered normal. An increased ESR is often seen with aging. Anemia has a profound effect on the Wintrobe and Westergren ESR. The blood of anemic patients will markedly increase the ESR because there are fewer RBCs, leaving relatively more space for the rouleau to rapidly settle to the bottom. A rule of thumb for correcting the increased ESR due to anemia is for every 1% Hct below normal, substract 2 mm from the reported ESR. A less frequently used test, the zeta sedimentation rate, does not need to be corrected for anemia.

The ESR is often helpful in following the course of an inflammatory process and may help in distinguishing inflammatory RA from tendonitis, bursitis, and conditions like non-inflammatory osteoarthritis. The ESR is a cornerstone in the diagnosis of polymyalgia rheumatica and temporal arteritis in which the ESR is often very high. However, the ESR is of limited value in diagnosing joint symptoms. A careful history and joint examination for synovitis is far more important than an ESR value. Additionally, changes in ESR values do not always correlate with clinical disease activity in RA. The ESR should not be used to screen asymptomatic persons for diseases, as fewer than six in 10,000 persons in the general population will benefit from the test even after a history and physical examination is done.[38] Table 8 shows factors that influence the ESR.

The Complete Blood Count (CBC). The CBC is important for monitoring patients with autoimmune diseases and their treatment of those diseases. These patients often have a normochromic, normocytic anemia (anemia of chronic disease). Patients with arthritis often take aspirin and various NSAIDs and may be prone to blood loss from the GI tract. A Coomb's positive hemolytic anemia should be suspected in an SLE patient with a low hemoglobin and hematocrit. Patients taking cytotoxic medications for diseases such as active SLE, RA, or vasculitis need to be screened with a CBC because they may develop bone marrow suppression. Active SLE or Felty's syndrome may cause a very low WBC, whereas treatment of a disorder with corticosteroids or infection may increase the WBC count. The eosinophil count in the differential component of the CBC is useful in certain diseases such as Churg-Strauss, Wegener's granulomatosis, and eosinophilic fasciitis.

A low platelet count may be seen in active SLE, APS, idiopathic thrombocytopenic purpura, or heparin therapy. Platelets are acute phase reactants and may be increased in RA and other chronic connective tissue diseases.

Chemistry Profiles. With advancing technology, the chemistry profiles often replace the selection of appropriate individual tests; however, specific tests in these panels are often needed to monitor features of certain diseases and toxicities of treatment. Regular liver and kidney function tests are mandatory for patients with rheumatic diseases who are being treated with cytotoxic agents such as cytoplasphomide, azathioprine, and methotrexate. The blood urea nitrogen and creatinine (BUN and Cr) are important for detecting and monitoring renal involvement and drug toxicity in diseases such as SLE, scleroderma, and uric acid nephropathy in gout patients. Periodic serum Cr tests are mandatory for patients taking NSAIDs and cytotoxic drugs like cyclosporin. Serum uric acid levels are important in monitoring allopurinol dosage in gout, as the goal of long-term therapy is to achieve and maintain a serum uric acid level of 4.0-4.5 mg/dL. An elevated serum calcium level may signal possible hyperparathyroidism as a cause of pseudogout or of osteoporosis, which can be managed by treating the underlying cause.

Urinalysis. The basic urinalysis is very helpful for monitoring disease activity in many rheumatic diseases. A 24-hour urine collection will quantitate nephrotic range proteinuria in active SLE. A routine UA may help in monitoring the safety of NSAID use and gold therapy. Proteinuria of less than 150 mg in a 24-hour period is considered normal. Less than 500 mg of protein over 24 hours in patients with SLE is often tolerated but must be followed closely. A higher degree of proteinuria may indicate the need for further investigation and treatment. Red and white blood cells and/or casts in the urine may suggest glomerulonephritis, as seen in patients with SLE and vasculitis.

Synovial Fluid. Synovial fluid analysis can be very helpful in establishing a diagnosis of gout, pseudogout, or infection. Immediate synovial fluid analysis is mandatory in active monoarticular arthritis because the differential diagnosis includes diseases with potentially disastrous outcomes (i.e., infection) if undetected and treatment is delayed.

Conclusion

Laboratory tests assist the clinician in confirming or excluding and classifying diagnostic impressions based on a thorough history and examination of a patient. The immunologic laboratory tests are helpful in the connective tissue diseases only if the clinician is aware of the limitations of each test, including their sensitivity and specificity and the reliability of the laboratory that is performing the tests. If the clinician does not take all available information into account, the laboratory test results obtained could be misleading. In today's environment of cost containment and managed care and, more importantly, to practice good medicine, a clinician should know the question that the test ordered is supposed to answer regarding confirming, excluding, or classifying diagnostic impressions.

References

1. Moder KG. Use and interpretation of rheumatologic tests: A guide for clinicians. *Mayo Clin Proc* 1996;71:391-396.
2. Wong LG, Colburn KK. Laboratory tests in rheumatology. In: Spiegel TM, ed. *Practical Rheumatology.* New York: Wiley and Sons; 1983:143-168.
3. Hargraves MM, et al. Presentation of two bone marrow elements: The "tart cell" and the "L.E." cell. *Proc Staff Meet Mayo Clin* 1948;23:25-28.
4. Peter JB, Reyes HR. *Use and interpretation of tests in rheumatology,* First edition. Santa Monica, CA: Specialty Laboratories, Inc.; 1996:11-12.
5. Wernick R. Avoiding laboratory test misinterpretations in geriatric rheumatology. *Geriatrics* 1989;44:61-80.
6. Mills JA. Systemic lupus erythematosus: Review article. *N Engl J Med* 1994;330:1871-1879.
7. von Mühlen CA, Tan EM. Autoantibodies in the diagnosis of systemic rheumatic diseases. *Semin Arth Rheum* 1995;24:323-358.
8. Reichlin M, Harley JB. Antinuclear antibodies: An overview. In: Wallace DJ, Hahn BH, eds. *Dubois' Lupus Erythematosus.* Philadelphia: Williams & Wilkins; 1997:397-405.
9. Peter JB. *Use and Interpretation of Tests in Clinical Immunology.* Eighth edition. Santa Monica, CA: Specialty Laboratories, Inc.; 1991:224-225.
10. Shart GC, et al. Mixed connective tissue disease. An apparently distinct rheumatic disease syndrome associated with a specific antibody to an extractable nuclear antigen (ENA). *Am J Med* 1972;52:148-159.
11. Prockop DJ, et al. Collagen in normal and diseased connective tissue. In: McCarty DJ, Koopman WJ, eds. *Arthritis and Allied Conditions,* Volume I . Philadelphia: Lea and Febiger; 1993: 213-262.
12. Isshi K, Hirohata S. Association of anti-ribosomal P protein antibodies with neuropsychiatric systemic lupus erythematosus. *Arthritis Rheum* 1996;39:1483-1490.
13. Peter JB. *Use and interpretation of tests in clinical immunology.* Eighth Edition. Santa Monica, California: Specialty Laboratories, Inc., 1991:214.
14. Peter JB. *Use and interpretation of tests in clinical immunology.* Eighth Edition. Santa Monica, CA: Specialty Laboratories, Inc., 1991:230-231.
15. Gladman DD, Urowitz MB. Systemic lupus erythematosus. In: *Primer on the rheumatic diseases,* 10th edition. Atlanta: Arthritis Foundation; 1993:106-111.
16. Hannaman RA. Rheumatology. In: *MedStudy a Condensed Review of Internal Medicine.* 6th Edition. Woodland Park, CO: MedStudy Corp.; 1996:7.
17. Frank MM. Complement in disease: Inherited and acquired complement deficiencies. In: *Santer's Immunologic Diseases,* 5th edition, Volume I. New York: Little, Brown & Co.;1995:484-500.
18. Atkinson JP. Complement deficiency: Predisposing factor to autoimmune syndromes. *Clin Exp Rheumatol* 1989;7:95.
19. Roubey RA. Antiphospholipid antibody syndrome. In: McCarty DJ, Koopman WJ, eds. *Arthritis and Allied Conditions,* Volume I. Baltimore: Williams & Wilkins; 1997:1393-1406.
20. Lockshin MD. Antiphospholipid antibody syndrome. *Rheumatic Dis Clin North America* 1994;20:45-59.
21. Harris EN. Antiphospholipid syndrome. In: *Primer on the rheumatic diseases.* 10th Edition. Atlanta: Arthritis Foundation; 1993:116-117.
22. Harris EN. Diagnosis & management of antiphospholipid syndrome. *Hospital Practice* 1994;29:65-76.
23. Rao JK, et al. The role of antineutrophil cytoplasmic antibody (C-ANCA) testing in the diagnosis of Wegener's granulomatosis: A literature review and metaa-analysis. *Ann Intern Med* 1995;123: 925-932.
24. Nolle B, et al. Anticytoplasmic autoantibodies: Their immunodiagnostic value in Wegener's granulomatosis. *Ann Intern Med* 1984; 111:28-110.
25. St. Claire EW. Vasculitis. In: Weisman MH, Weinblatt ME, eds. *Treatment of the Rheumatic diseases: Companion to the Textbook of Rheumatology.* Philadelphia: WB Saunders, 1995:137-159.
26. Falk RJ, Jennette SC. Anti-neutrophil cytoplasmic autoantibodies with specificity for myeloperoxidase in patients with systemic vasculitis and idiopathic necrotizing and crescentic glomerulonephritis. *N Engl J Med* 1988;318:1651-1657.
27. Jennette JC, Falk RJ. Anti-neutrophil cytoplasmic autoantibody-associated glomerulonephritis and vasculitis. *Am J Pathol* 1989; 135:921-930.
28. Hannaman RA. Rheumatology. In: MedStudy a Condensed

Review of Internal Medicine. 6th Edition. Woodland Park, CO: MedStudy Corp.; 1996:13-14.

29. LeRoy EC, Silver RM. Systemic sclerosis and related syndromes. In: *Primer on the rheumatic diseases,* 10th edition. Atlanta: Arthritis Foundation; 1993:118-120.
30. Metzger AL, Morris RI. Rheumatology Diagnostics Laboratory, Inc. Reference Cards. Santa Monica, CA.
31. Medsger TA, Oddis CV. Inflammatory muscle disease. In: Klippel JH, Dieppe PA, eds. *Rheumatology.* St. Louis: Mosby; 1994:6.12.1-6.12.14.
32. Moutsopoulos HM, Tzioufas AG. Sjögren's syndrome. In: Klippel JH, Dieppe PA, eds. *Rheumatology.* St. Louis: Mosby; 1994:6.27.1-6-27-13.
33. Waaler E. On the occurrence of a factor in human serum activating the specific agglutination of sheep blood corpuscles. *Acta Path Microbiol Scand* 1940;17:172-188.
34. Rose HM, et al. Differential agglutination of normal and sensitized sheep erythrocytes by sera of patients with rheumatoid arthritis. *Proc Soc Exper Biol Med* 1948;68:1-6.
35. Lipsky PE. Rheumatoid arthritis. In: Isselbacher KJ, Braunwald E, Wilson JD, Martin JB, Fauci AS, Kasper DL. eds. *Harrison's Principles of Internal Medicine.* San Francisco: McGraw Hill; 1994:1648-1655.
36. Wigley FM. Rheumatoid Arthritis. In: Barker LR, Burton JR, Zieve PD, eds. *Principles of Ambulatory Medicine,* 4th edition. Philadelphia: Williams & Wilkins; 1995:943-974.
37. Leavelle DE. *Mayo Medical Laboratories Interpretive Handbook.* Mayo Medical Laboratories, Rochester, MN; 1988:133-134.
38. Sox HC, Liang MH. The erythrocyte sedimentation rate: Guidelines for rational use. *Ann Intern Med* 1986;104:515-523.

Polymyalgia Rheumatica

JDaryl Miller, MD
Susan H. Allen, MD, PhD
Sara E. Walker, MD

Polymyalgia rheumatica is associated with severe pain and stiffness that involves the proximal muscles of the shoulders and hips. The disorder primarily affects elderly Caucasians of northern European ancestry. Here, the authors provide a primary care physician's guide to polymyalgia rheumatica, including clinical features, laboratory tests, and diagnostic criteria. They also point out common problems associated with this disorder, such as giant cell arteritis and osteoporosis.

Definition

Polymyalgia rheumatica is a clinical syndrome that is characterized by muscle aching and stiffness, without weakness, that involves the neck and shoulder girdle and pelvic girdle. The disorder is largely limited to patients over the age of 50 years. Polymyalgia rheumatica is of great interest to the primary care practitioner. The diagnosis is based upon careful clinical assessment, and the symptoms are controlled rapidly and dramatically with low-dose corticosteroid treatment. Polymyalgia rheumatica can be an important clue to the existence of serious underlying illness. A classic association is giant cell arteritis.[1-3] There is increasing recognition that a polymyalgia rheumatica-like syndrome can be a marker for myelodysplastic disorders[4] and Lyme disease.[5]

History

The term polymyalgia rheumatica was adopted in 1959 by Barber to name a set of troublesome symptoms associated with elevation of the erythrocyte sedimentation rate (ESR).[6] This syndrome had been described earlier under a number of synonyms, including "senile rheumatic gout," "periarthrosis humeroscapularis," "myalgic syndrome of the elderly with systemic reactions," and "pseudo-polyarthrite rhizomelique." Barber differentiated polymyalgia rheumatica from polymyositis and other inflammatory rheumatic diseases.[6] He also noted that patients had immediate response to treatment with corticosteroids, with a good prognosis in uncomplicated disease.

Epidemiology

There are many reports of polymyalgia rheumatica in northern Europe[7,8] and the northern United States.[9] In Goteborg, Sweden, 220 patients were identified in 1985-1987 with well-defined polymyalgia rheumatica and negative biopsies of the temporal artery. The average annual incidence for the entire population was 17 cases/100,000. The predilection for older individuals was illustrated by the finding that the average annual incidence for persons age 50 years and older was 50 cases/100,000.[7] In the northern United States, the incidence of polymyalgia rheumatica resembled the Swedish experience. A study in Olmsted County, Minnesota

(1970-1991) found that the annual age- and sex-adjusted incidence in individuals aged 50 and older was 52/100,000.[9] A study conducted more recently (1987-1994) in Tromso, Norway, used negative temporal artery biopsies to exclude giant cell arteritis in 256 cases. The annual incidence in this population was 113/100,000 residents.[8]

Polymyalgia rheumatica clearly increases as the population ages. After the age of 80 years, the annual incidence was 78/100,000 in Goteborg[7] and 97/100,000 in Olmsted County.[9] Occurrence in women is about twice that in men and may be as high as 79% in women.[7] The syndrome involves white individuals almost exclusively. Persons of northern European ancestry are affected more commonly than southern Europeans, and the syndrome is rare among blacks and Asians (reviewed in reference 10).

Etiology

Genetic predisposition, infection, and immunological abnormalities appear to contribute to the etiology of polymyalgia rheumatica.[11] The increased occurrence of polymyalgia rheumatica in people of northern European heritage, as well as aggregation in some families,[12] point to hereditary factors. Polymyalgia rheumatica, giant cell arteritis, and rheumatoid arthritis are all associated with HLA DR4. Patients with polymyalgia rheumatica and giant cell arteritis share the associated sequence polymorphism encoded by the second hypervariable region of the HLA DRB1 gene. The HLA DRB1*04 allele was found in 76% of patients with polymyalgia rheumatica, and all HLA DRB1*04 alleles were represented in this group.

In contrast, rheumatoid arthritis is linked to a sequence motif in the third hypervariable region of DRB1 alleles. Expression of HLA DR4 in rheumatoid arthritis was restricted to the HLA DRB1*0401 and HLA DRB1*0404/8 alleles.[13] A more recent report from the United Kingdom has, however, emphasized genetic similarity between polymyalgia rheumatica and rheumatoid arthritis. The rheumatoid arthritis shared epitope, QKRAA/QRRAA, was present in 75% of polymyalgia rheumatica patients.[14]

Finding antibodies directed against self antigens in patients with polymyalgia rheumatica suggests that autoimmune responses have a role in the etiology. Anticardiolipin antibodies were present in 17% of patients who presented with the uncomplicated disease.[15] Another group of patients had antibodies to nuclear lamin B2 protein that reacted with the lamin-specific C terminus.[16] IgG anti-endothelial cell antibodies occurred in 53% of polymyalgia rheumatica patients.[17] The means whereby these antibodies might contribute to an inflammatory illness, however, have not been defined.

The theory that polymyalgia rheumatica is mediated by a systemic immune response was supported initially by reports of circulating immune complexes and depleted CD8+ (cytotoxic suppressor) T-cells.[18] T-cell depletion is not found consistently, however, in polymyalgia rheumatica. Recently, numbers of these cells were reported as normal,[19] and some cases had clonal expansion of CD8+ cells with a distinct J beta 2.7 gene segment usage.[20]

The association of fever, leukocytosis, and acute phase reactions with polymyalgia rheumatica suggest that the syndrome may be caused by infection. Enteroviral infection[21] and Lyme disease[5] in the elderly may present with signs and symptoms that mimic polymyalgia rheumatica. In Denmark, two epidemics of Mycoplasma pneumoniae infection were associated with peak incidence of polymyalgia rheumatica and the associated disease, giant cell arteritis. Other peaks were related to epidemics of *Chlamydia pneumoniae* and parvovirus B19.[22] Polymyalgia rheumatica has also occurred after treatment with intravesical Bacillus Calmette-Guerin.[23] The assumption that polymyalgia rheumatica is a result of infection was weakened by the report of a survey of 48 newly diagnosed patients. The prevalence of antibodies to *Chlamydia pneumoniae*, cytomegalovirus, enteroviruses, and respiratory syncytial virus was similar in the patients and in 22 age-matched controls. Two patients did have IgM antibodies to enteroviruses.[24]

Pathophysiology

Epidemiologic data suggest that an appropriate genetic background contributes to development of polymyalgia rheumatica, and an infectious agent may trigger aberrant immune responses in a susceptible individual. The disease is characterized by striking muscle stiffness and pain, and muscles may display electromyographic abnormalities (fibrillation potentials, complex repetitive discharges) that improve after treatment with corticosteroids.[25] The histological appearance of skeletal muscle is relatively normal. Inflammation is not present, but Type II fiber atrophy has been reported,[25] and immunoglobulin deposits were found in the perifascicular area of the perimysium.[26] It is generally accepted that these changes are of little consequence, and diseased skeletal muscle is almost certainly not the cause of the painful symptoms of polymyalgia rheumatica. To underscore this fact, the muscle tissue in polymyalgia rheumatica has normal metabolic function.[27]

Recently, it has been appreciated that inflamed bursae and joints contribute to the striking proximal pain and stiffness that characterize this disease. A patient presenting with polymyalgia rheumatica and bilateral diffuse swelling of the hands had magnetic resonance imaging (MRI) and was shown to have synovitis of the glenohumeral joint, tenosynovitis of the extensor tendons of the hand, and marked inflammation of bursae about the shoulder. Subsequent MRI studies of 13 cases revealed that all had evidence of subacromial and subdeltoid bursitis. Three patients were studied after two months of corticosteroid treatment, and two showed resolution of periarticular disease.[28] Arthroscopic biopsies of the shoulder joint have produced abnormal synovium with vascular proliferation; the tissue was infiltrated by macrophages and T-cells. HLA class II antigens and vascular cell adhesion molecule-1 (VCAM-1) were expressed strongly in cells of the synovial lining layers. Synovial vascularity and expression of HLA class II and VCAM-1 antigens were decreased following corticosteroid therapy.[29,30]

It has been proposed that polymyalgia rheumatica is triggered by an aberrant immune process that originates in arteries. This theory is based partially upon the observation that 10-15% of persons with polymyalgia rheumatica have giant cell arteritis proven by biopsy of the temporal artery.[2] The means whereby vascular lesions could produce the symptoms of polymyalgia rheumatica are not clear. In "pure" polymyalgia rheumatica, the vessels that supply skeletal muscle and synovium do not usually have visible changes of arteritis. It is possible that giant cell arteritis affects these vessels on a subclinical level. This supposition was supported by the finding that temporal artery biopsies in polymyalgia rheumatica, which did not have visible inflammatory changes, were nevertheless abnormal. These segments of artery contained messenger RNA (mRNA) for a number of cytokines, including interleukin (IL)-2 in high levels, IL-1 beta, IL-6, and tumor necrosis factor (TNF)-alpha. Temporal artery biopsies from patients with histological evidence of giant cell arteritis also contained transcripts of these cytokines. In addition, the vessels involved in giant cell arteritis contained interferon (IFN)-gamma mRNA.[31] The presence of this cytokine may be a key factor in the progression to overt arterial inflammation.[2]

Clinical Features

The classic symptoms of polymyalgia rheumatica are muscle pain and stiffness, and these symptoms often form the basis of the chief complaint. The shoulder girdle is commonly the first area to become symptomatic, and pain is also experienced in the neck, upper back, upper arms, lower back, and hip girdle. The pain is typically severe, aching in nature, and bilateral. Pain is accentuated by movement of the joints, but the pain is not localized to the joints. The symptoms appear to arise in muscles, tendinous attachments, and bursae.

Patients have prominent stiffness, resembling that found in rheumatoid arthritis. The stiffness is present in the morning, tends to wear off with movement, and recurs later in the day if the patient is inactive. The pain and stiffness may occur so abruptly that the patient remembers the date and hour of onset, or the onset may be gradual.

Constitutional symptoms that may be associated with polymyalgia rheumatica include malaise, fatigue, weight loss, and depression. Low-grade fever has been reported in polymyalgia rheumatica,[9] but high spiking fever suggests underlying infection or giant cell arteritis.

Patients are limited functionally due to the pain and stiffness and may describe difficulties in acts that require use of the proximal musculature (brushing the hair or teeth, rising from the supine or sitting position). It should be emphasized, however, that the muscles are not truly weak.[2]

On physical examination, the typical patient is an elderly Caucasian with a sad and distressed facial expression. Because giant cell arteritis can occur in patients with polymyalgia rheumatica, it is a good idea to carefully palpate both temporal arteries and the branches of these vessels in the scalp. Finding normal vessels does not eliminate the possibility of arteritis. It is well recognized that involved arteries can pulsate and have no tender areas. Just the same, finding a tender segment of temporal artery can be an important clue to the presence of giant cell arteritis. A tender area is the preferred location for an arterial biopsy.

The musculoskeletal examination usually reveals normal muscle bulk, tone, and strength. Tenderness may be elicited over the paracervical muscles and the glenohumeral joints. Muscle testing is difficult because there is considerable pain with movement. If the patient has not moved the painful shoulders for a period of months, the result will likely be restriction of active and passive abduction, elevation, internal rotation, and external rotation.

Synovitis should be sought on the physical examination, because about one-fourth of patients have evidence of peripheral arthritis at the onset of disease.[32] Careful palpation of the sternoclavicular joints, wrists, metacarpophalangeal joints, and knees may reveal swelling and tenderness.[2]

A newly recognized finding is diffuse swelling with pitting edema that can involve hands or feet.[33] *(Pelase see Figure 1.)* The involved areas are painful, and pain is intensified when joints in the area are moved. The swollen part is occasionally warm but not erythematous. The swelling often extends beyond joint margins and occasionally follows tendons.[33] Distal extremity swelling with pitting edema reflects synovial inflammation in joints and tenosynovial membranes.[27]

Figure 1. Patient with Polymyalgia Rheumatica

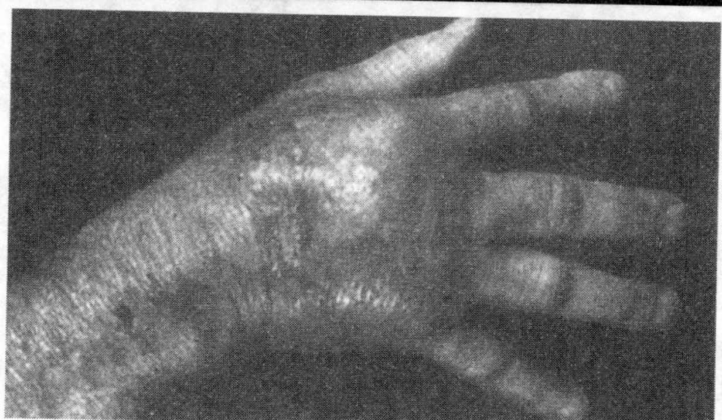

Diffuse swelling of the hand and fingers with pitting edema in a patient with polymyalgia rheumatica. Swelling resolved after the patient was treated with corticosteroids.

Hunder GG. Giant cell arteritis and polymyalgia rheumatica. *Med Clin N Am* 1997;81:195-219. Used with permission from the publishers.

Carpal tunnel syndrome can be a "hidden" manifestation of polymyalgia rheumatica and has been reported as the presenting manifestation.[34] Therefore, patients who are suspected of having this diagnosis should be questioned about nocturnal pain and paresthesias involving the thumb, index finger, and middle finger, and the examiner should note if there is atrophy of the thenar eminence, weakness in abduction or opposition of the thumb, or diminished sensation in the distribution of the median nerve.

Laboratory Tests

The key to diagnosis in polymyalgia rheumatica is an elevated ESR. This test is an indirect means of assessing concentrations of acute phase reactants, which enhance erythrocyte aggregation by binding to the red cell membrane and neutralizing the positive surface charge. In the Westergren ESR test, anticoagulated blood sits in a vertical tube. If acute phase proteins are elevated, the erythrocytes aggregate and fall rapidly. The test value is the number of mm that the red cell column falls in one hour. *(Please see Table 1.[35])*

Most of the published diagnostic criteria for polymyalgia rheumatica require an ESR above 40 mm/hour,[36-38] but values are often as high as 100 mm/hour or greater.[2]

In some instances, the ESR is not increased in patients who otherwise meet established criteria for polymyalgia rheumatica. Helfgott and Kieval found ESR of 30 mm/hour or less in 26 of 117 (22%) of patients.[39] The proportion of men in this group was unusually high (58%), and anemia was less common compared to high-ESR polymyalgia rheumatica patients.[39] Other authors reported that a sedimentation rate lower than 40 mm/hour was associated with a lower

Table 1. Abnormal Laboratory Tests in Polymyalgia Rheumatica

Acute phase reactants	↑↑ ESR
	↑ C-reactive protein
	↑ Alpha 2 globulins
	↑ Fibrinogen
Blood count	Normochromic, normocytic anemia
	↑ Platelet count
Liver enzymes	↑ Alkaline phosphatase
	↑ SGOT/SGPT
Other	↓ Albumin
	↑ Serum IL-6
	↑ Factor VIII/von Willebrand's factor

Adapted from: Dwolatzky T, Sonnenblick M, Nesher G. Giant cell arteritis and polymyalgia rheumatica: Clues to early diagnosis. *Geriatrics* 1997;52:38-44; and from data published in references 41-43.

frequency of constitutional findings such as weight loss.[40] Anemia was absent in the low-ESR patients.

Other laboratory findings are typical of systemic inflammation: increased concentrations of acute phase reactants (C-reactive protein, alpha2 globulins, fibrinogen), mild-to-moderate normocytic normochromic anemia, and elevation of the platelet count. Gamma globulins are increased in one-third of patients.[37] Serum complement, which behaves as an acute phase reactant, is normal or increased.

Tests for both ESR and C-reactive protein are helpful in evaluating the atypical case. Only 1.4% of polymyalgia rheumatica patients present with normal ESR and normal C-reactive protein.[32]

Liver enzymes, especially alkaline phosphatase, are increased in approximately one-quarter of patients, and one-third are hypoalbuminemic.[37] Increased prothrombin has been reported. Enzymes that reflect muscle inflammation, such as creatine kinase and aldolase, are normal. Tests for antinuclear antibodies and rheumatoid factor are negative, and there is no substantial evidence of renal disease.[2]

Elevated serum concentrations of the inflammatory cytokine, IL-6, occurred in 12 of 13 cases,[41] and IL-6 levels were increased when the disease relapsed.[42]

Factor VIII/von Willebrand factor may be elevated in polymyalgia rheumatica. This finding is somewhat nonspecific because the factor is increased in a heterogeneous group of disorders that are associated with endothelial cell damage. The significance of high factor VIII levels in polymyalgia rheumatica is not clear; factor levels did not correlate with disease activity, the ESR value, or levels of acute phase reactants.[43]

Synovial fluid reflects mild inflammation. The leukocyte count is expected to be 1000-20,000 cells/mm^3, with 40-50% neutrophils.

Diagnostic Criteria

In 1979, Bird reported a collaborative study in which 146 patients with polymyalgia rheumatica in Great Britain were compared with 253 other patients whose diseases resembled polymyalgia rheumatica.[36] It was proposed that patients having three of seven criteria had polymyalgia rheumatica with 92% sensitivity and 80% specificity. *(See Table 2.[44])* Other sets of published diagnostic criteria have emphasized the diagnostic importance of pain, recent onset of symptoms, elevated ESR, morning stiffness, older age (over 50 years), systemic symptoms such as weight loss and fever, elevation of acute phase reactants other than the ESR, and muscle tenderness.[38]

An important finding in polymyalgia rheumatica is that treatment with low doses of corticosteroids (10-20 mg prednisone a day) produces prompt relief of symptoms. This response is so predictable and dramatic that some authors consider it a diagnostic criterion.[37,38,45,46]

Differential Diagnosis

The diagnosis of polymyalgia rheumatica is based on clinical findings with supportive data from laboratory tests. It is a diagnosis of exclusion, in that the clinician must rule out a wide variety of diseases that can present with constitutional symptoms, proximal myalgias, and high ESR. Diseases that mimic polymyalgia rheumatica are listed in Table 3.

Elderly-onset rheumatoid arthritis, with onset at 60 years of age or older, can have an abrupt polymyalgia-like onset. The shoulders and hips are involved early, the metacarpophalangeal joints may be spared, and subcutaneous nodules appear to be less common than in younger rheumatoid arthritis patients. The ESR tends to be high with elderly onset. If the test for rheumatoid factor is negative, it may be impossible to differentiate elderly-onset rheumatoid arthritis from polymyalgia rheumatica until the patient has been observed for 6-12 months. Response to low-dose oral prednisone, 5-15 mg daily, is excellent. Some clinicians believe that efficacy of second-line remittive agents is reduced, and these drugs may be more toxic in the elderly rheumatoid arthritis patient.[47]

The elderly patient who presents with bilateral pitting edema of the hands and/or feet, joint pain, and an elevated ESR is a diagnostic puzzle. The possibilities that need to be considered are polymyalgia rheumatica with distal pitting edema and remitting seronegative symmetrical synovitis with pitting edema (RE3PE). Polymyalgia rheumatica can be associated with distal pitting edema that results from synovial inflammation in the joints and about tendons. This finding was reported in 19 (8%) of members of a population cohort of 245 patients with polymyalgia rheumatica.[33] The soft tissue swelling usually developed gradually, involved both sides, and was present in either hands or feet or in all four extremities. Some cases had recurring episodes, but erosions and joint destruction did not occur. Clues to the correct diagnosis are a very high ESR and strongly positive tests for acute phase reactants, such as C-reactive protein. Tests for rheumatoid factor are negative. These patients have poor response to nonsteroidal anti-inflammatory drugs (NSAIDs) but do improve dramatically after treatment with modest doses of corticosteroids. The prognosis is good.[33,48]

RS3PE is a syndrome of elderly Caucasians, primarily men, who have the abrupt onset of proximal myalgias, symmetrical synovitis involving the wrists and small joints of the hands, and pitting edema

Table 2. Diagnostic Criteria for Polymyalgia Rheumatica

- Bilateral shoulder pain and stiffness
- Onset of illness within two weeks
- Initial ESR higher than 40 mm/hour
- Morning stiffness exceeding one hour
- Age older than 65 years
- Depression and/or loss of weight
- Bilateral upper arm tenderness

Any three criteria discriminated between polymyalgia rheumatica and other conditions with sensitivity of 92% and specificity of 80%.[36]

Adapted from: Cimmino MA, Salvarani C. Polymyalgia rheumatica and giant cell arteritis. *Balliere's Clin Rheumatol* 1995;9:515-527 and based upon data in Bird HA, et al. An evaluation of criteria for polymyalgia rheumatica. *Ann Rheum Dis* 1979;38:434-439.

of the hands, feet, and ankles. These patients have elevated ESR and are sero-negative for rheumatoid factor. Most are positive for the HLA-B27 antigen. They show prompt improvement with corticosteroids. The prognosis is very good; the episode occurs only once.[49]

Myopathies (polymyositis, drug-induced) may present with proximal muscle aching but are distinguished from polymyalgia rheumatica by true proximal muscle weakness and elevated creatine kinase. Malaise and muscle and joint pain are common presenting symptoms in systemic lupus erythematosus. Skin rash and renal involvement are two factors that can differentiate lupus from polymyalgia rheumatica. Serum complement levels are expected to be low in many cases of active lupus, whereas high levels are characteristic of polymyalgia rheumatica. The diagnosis of lupus is established by finding positive tests for antinuclear antibodies. Multiple myeloma and Waldenstrom's macroglobulinemia are characterized by paraproteinemia, and lymphomas are suspected if lymph nodes or spleen are enlarged. Very careful attention must be paid to the blood counts and peripheral blood smears in these patients, because myelodysplastic syndromes and leukemias can present with polymyalgia-like symptoms.[4] The diagnosis of paraneoplastic syndrome associated with a solid tumor rests upon a thorough evaluation of the geriatric patient, with the realization that occult malignancies are classic causes of weight loss, anemia, and elevated ESR. Subacute bacterial endocarditis can reproduce many findings of polymyalgia rheumatica, including aching pain in the proximal muscles and weight loss. A patient with a significant heart murmur or peripheral embolization, especially if fever is present, should have blood cultures and an echocardiogram. Infection with enterovirus can produce polylmyalgia-like pain that should be transient.[21] Lyme disease can present with musculoskeletal pain and fatigue and should be considered if the patient has been in an endemic area.[5] The ESR is elevated in about one-half of Lyme disease patients, but it is rare to see elevations to the very high values that are characteristic of polymyalgia rheumatica.[50] Amyloidosis is associated with severe muscle pain but

Table 3. Differential Diagnosis: Diseases that can Mimic Polymyalgia Rheumatica

- Rheumatoid arthritis and RS3PE syndrome
- Myopathies (inflammatory, drug-induced)
- Systemic lupus erythematosus
- Hematopoietic malignancies

  Multiple myeloma, macroglobulinemia of Wandenstrom, myelodysplastic syndromes, lymphoma
- Paraneoplastic syndromes

  Renal cell carcinoma

  Adenocarcinomas (uterus, stomach, pancreas, colon, prostate, unknown origin)
- Infections (subacute bacterial endocarditis, viral infection, Lyme disease)
- Amyloidosis
- Hypothyroidism
- Bone pain (metastatic cancer, metabolic bone disease)
- Fibromyalgia

Adapted from Brooks RC, McGee SR. Diagnostic dilemmas in polymyalgia rheumatica. *Arch Intern Med* 1997;157:162-168 and from data published in references 5, 47, 49, and 50.

can be differentiated from polymyalgia rheumatica by the presence of other findings such as skin lesions, cardiac involvement, and enlarged liver and spleen. The patient with hypothyroidism may not feel well and can present with proximal muscle weakness. In this individual, hoarseness, a slow heart rate, and typical changes in skin, hair, and the deep tendon reflexes are clues to the underlying disorder. Metastatic cancer and Paget's disease typically produce deep, distressing pain that is localized over the affected areas. The pain of metastases is worse at night. Symptomatic osteomalacia can be complicated by painful microfractures. A careful clinical assessment will determine that this pain is skeletal and not in tendons, bursae, muscles, or joints. Fibromyalgia is characterized by pain that is often described as "all over the body," fatigue upon waking, classic tender points, and a normal ESR.

Temporal Artery Biopsy in Polymyalgia Rheumatica. Polymyalgia rheumatica can be a marker for giant cell arteritis (temporal arteritis), which is diagnosed in 10-15% of polymyalgia rheumatica patients.[2] Because it is impractical to obtain a temporal artery biopsy in every patient with polymyalgia rheumatica, Rodriguez-Valverde and associates attempted to select patients who were most at risk for giant cell arteritis.[51] Predictors that suggested the presence of giant cell arteritis were high spiking fevers, new onset of headache, jaw claudication, amaurosis, abnormal temporal arteries, and elevated liver enzymes.[51] These features should guide the physician and the patient in the decision to obtain a biopsy.

The question has been raised that some patients with multiple risk factors almost certainly have arteritis, and a biopsy might not be necessary. Even though the diagnosis of giant cell arteritis seems assured on a clinical basis, it is recommended that a temporal artery be biopsied. A positive biopsy provides a clear basis for undertaking treatment that is potentially hazardous in the aged patient. Patients with giant cell arteritis require initial treatment with 60 mg of prednisone daily. This dose is necessary to control the inflammatory vasculitis and to prevent blindness. In contrast, the polymyalgia rheumatica patient who does not have giant cell arteritis will require a lower dose in the range of 5-20 mg daily. Occasionally, an arterial biopsy will disclose a disease that mimics giant cell arteritis. An example is amyloidosis with involvement of the temporal artery.[52]

In the Rodruguez-Valverde study, patients who were unlikely to have giant cell arteritis as a complication of polymyalgia rheumatica were 70 years of age or younger, without headache, and without cranial features of giant cell arteritis.[51] Cranial features were defined as abnormal temporal arteries (decreased or absent pulses, arterial thickening, swelling, or tenderness), amaurosis (transient or permanent loss of vision), and jaw claudication. The risk of giant cell arteritis was very low, occurring in one of 59 patients without clinical evidence of cranial vessel involvement.[51]

It seems appropriate to avoid biopsy in polymyalgia rheumatica patients without cranial features of arteritis and to treat with low-dose corticosteroids.[51] The patient and doctor should realize, however, that there is a small possibility of giant cell arteritis occurring in a low-risk patient who is receiving low-dose steroid treatment. Close follow-up and good communication is necessary so that fever, headache, or visual symptoms will be reported promptly.

Therapy of Polymyalgia Rheumatica

The original series of patients reported by Barber included two patients who responded to phenylbutazone and three patients who had spontaneous remission.[6] No patients received corticosteroids. Some patients have responded to NSAIDs. Chuang described 96 patients with polymyalgia rheumatica who were identified in a 10-year period in Olmsted County.[37] Thirty were treated with aspirin, and nine received other NSAIDs. Duration of disease was shorter (median, 8 months), and there were fewer relapses compared to patients treated with corticosteroids. The good outcomes were thought to result from milder disease in these patients. They had higher pre-treatment hemoglobin and lower pre-treatment ESR values, compared to the patients who received corticosteroids.[37]

There may be a role for NSAID treatment in selected patients with mild polymyalgia rheumatica, but many clinicians believe that low-dose prednisone is the treatment of choice. NSAID treatment often fails. In about two-thirds of individuals who receive aspirin or other NSAIDs initially, it is necessary to switch to corticosteroids in order to adequately control pain and stiffness.[37] Furthermore, low-dose prednisone provides immediate relief. Within 24-48 hours of starting this treatment, patients experience dramatic improvement in myalgic and constitutional symptoms.

A starting dose of 5-20 mg of prednisone a day is usually effective. Occasionally, a dose of 25 mg is required. Behn examined the prospective course of treated polymyalgia rheumatica.[53] The corticosteroid dose was regulated with a goal of suppressing symptoms and keeping the ESR below 30 mm per hour. Starting treatment with prednisolone, 5-10 mg per day, gave satisfactory control in 94% of the patients with uncomplicated disease. Other investigators reported relapse in 65% of patients treated with the 10 mg dose. Relapses occurred in only 10% of those who received 20 mg daily.[54]

Patients should remain on the starting dose of prednisone for a minimum of four weeks. The rate of dose taper is guided by the clinical response. Resolution of symptoms is more important than reduction in the ESR. For those taking 10 mg or less of prednisone a day, a reduction of the daily dose in 1 mg increments at four-week intervals is acceptable. If the dose is greater than 10 mg, it can be decreased by 2.5 mg every four weeks until the patient is taking 10 mg per day. Subsequent reductions should be in 1 mg increments. The duration of treatment is generally two years, and prednisone can be tapered and discontinued in most patients.

Patients whose disease is not controlled, or who have significant corticosteroid side effects, should be considered for treatment with a steroid-sparing drug. In one series, 65% of polymyalgia rheumatica patients treated with an average daily prednisone dose of 9.5 mg had at least one adverse event. The risks of diabetes mellitus, vertebral fractures, and hip fractures were 2-5 times greater compared to controls.[55] Methotrexate treatment reduced the amount of prednisone taken over a one-year period in one group of patients,[56] but other investigators concluded that it had no steroid-sparing effect.[57] Dapsone is another possible choice for adjunct treatment.[5]

Corticosteroid-Induced Osteoporosis

Glucocorticoids inhibit calcium absorption, increase urinary calcium excretion, decrease bone formation, and increase bone resorption. The greatest loss of bone occurs during the first 6-12 months of therapy and is predominantly due to increased bone resorption. Trabecular bone is affected more than cortical bone, and the trabecular volume may decrease by 20%.[59]

A major challenge facing clinicians prescribing long-term corticosteroid therapy is to monitor and, if possible, minimize the effects on bone density. Most health care providers recognize that post-menopausal women, especially those with preexisting osteoporosis, are at increased risk. It is important to recognize that men are equally at increased risk. Cumulative dose and duration of therapy are the most important risk factors. The incidence of fracture increases with higher cumulative doses and may be as high as 50% in individuals receiving 30 g of prednisone. The most common fracture sites are the vertebrae, ribs, and pelvis.[60] In a cohort of 43 patients with temporal arteritis treated initially with high-dose prednisone, one-third experienced fractures within the first 12 months of therapy.[61] Low-dose prednisone also places patients at risk. A dose of 8 mg per day is associated with an annualized bone loss of 3%.

Table 4 outlines a rational management strategy for glucocorticoid-induced osteoporosis. The American College of Rheumatology has recommended supplementation with high doses of vitamin D (50,000 IU, 3 times per week) or calcitriol (0.5 mcg per day). The potential complication of hypercalcemia with these doses is a major concern. Others have suggested that a weekly dose of 50,000 IU of vitamin D for the first several months of prednisone therapy is an appropriate dose.[62] The 25-hydroxyvitamin D level should be main-

Table 4. Management of Corticosteroid-Induced Osteoporosis

INITIATE LIFESTYLE MODIFICATIONS

- Eliminate adverse health habits—smoking and alcohol excess
- Refer to physical therapist for exercise training including a weight-bearing exercise program, back extension and isometric abdominal exercises, proximal muscle strengthening exercises, and fall prevention strategies
- Dietary intervention: Daily elemental calcium intake of 1500 mg and at least 400-800 IU of vitamin D; 2-3 g sodium restricted diet; caloric restriction; diet high in protein and potassium; American Diabetes Association dietary recommendations for patients with diabetes mellitus

PHARMACOLOGICAL PROPHYLAXIS AND TREATMENT

- Vitamin D, 50,000 IU a week for three months if the 25-hydroxyvitamin D level is below the upper limit of normal. Then re-evaluate with another 25-hydroxyvitamin D level.
- Thiazide diuretic to reduce hypercalciuria
- Hormone replacement therapy in postmenopausal women and testosterone therapy in men, if there are no contraindications
- Anti-resorptive therapy: calcitonin, bisphosphonate

tained within the upper limits of normal. The daily elemental calcium intake should be 1500 mg in divided doses. Thiazide diuretics may be used to decrease hypercalciuria.

Anti-resorptive therapy should be prescribed at the onset of corticosteroid therapy, when the prednisone dose is highest and the greatest bone loss occurs. Hormone replacement therapy should be prescribed in all postmenopausal women, regardless of the bone mineral density result, if there are no contraindications. Hypogonadal men should receive parenteral or transdermal testosterone replacement. Another anti-resorptive therapy such as calcitonin or a bisphosphonate such as etidronate or alendronate should be prescribed if hormone replacement is refused or contraindicated. Parenteral salmon calcitonin (100 IU, 3 times a week) showed no benefit compared to the control group in a two-year intervention trial in 48 patients with newly diagnosed polymyalgia rheumatica, temporal arteritis, and other vasculitides treated with corticosteroids.[63] However, the nasal spray preparation of salmon calcitonin (200 IU per day) did prevent vertebral bone loss after one year in patients with polymyalgia rheumatica.[64]

Intermittent cyclical etidronate (400 mg per day for 2 weeks followed by 11 weeks with no drug) has been shown to prevent glucocorticoid-induced bone loss in patients with polymyalgia rheumatica and giant cell arteritis.[65] Alendronate (10 mg per day) shows potential usefulness in preventing and treating corticosteroid-induced osteoporosis.[66]

Bone mineral density testing should be repeated in six months to assess efficacy of therapy. A change in anti-resorptive treatment or additional anti-resorptive treatment should be considered when the bone loss is greater than 5%.

Summary

Polymyalgia rheumatica is associated with severe pain and stiffness that involves the proximal muscles of the shoulders and hips. Elevated sedimentation rate and elevated acute phase reactions are hallmarks of this disease. It is primarily a disorder of elderly Caucasians of northern European ancestry. The genetic background of affected individuals has similarities to that of patients with giant cell arteritis and rheumatoid arthritis. Recently, anticardiolipin antibodies, antibodies to nuclear lamin B2 protein, and anti-endothelial cell antibodies have been linked to polymyalgia rheumatica. Earlier reports of depleted CD8+ T-cells are now open to question. Skeletal muscle, the apparent site of pain in this disease, is relatively normal, but intense inflammation has been identified in bursae, joints, and tenosynovial areas. Giant cell arteritis is associated with polymyalgia rheumatica. It is noteworthy that the temporal arteries of polymyalgia rheumatica patients contain high levels of IL-2 mRNA, whereas arteries involved in giant cell arteritis express IFN-gamma mRNA. The physical examination in polymyalgia rheumatica is relatively normal, but the clinician should look carefully for evidence of temporal artery involvement, inflamed joints, carpal tunnel syndrome, and diffuse swelling with pitting edema that can involve hands or feet. The differential diagnosis includes rheumatoid arthritis, myopathies, systemic lupus erythematosus, and a number of malignancies. Infections (bacterial endocarditis, enteroviral infection, Lyme disease) and amyloidosis can present with a polymyalgia rheumatica-like picture. Ten to 15% of patients with polymyalgia rheumatica have giant cell arteritis, and temporal artery biopsies should be considered in those with high fever, jaw claudication, amaurosis, and/or abnormal temporal arteries. Most patients with uncomplicated polymyalgia rheumatica respond dramatically to low-dose prednisone. Because steroid-treated patients are at risk for osteoporosis and fractures, anti-osteoporosis measures should be instituted at the beginning of therapy.

References

1. Hunder GG, Disney TF, Ward LE. Polymyalgia rheumatica. *Mayo Clin Proc* 1969;44:849-875.
2. Hunder GG. Giant cell arteritis and polymyalgia rheumatica. *Med Clin N Am* 1997;81:195-219.
3. Swannell AJ. Polymyalgia rheumatica and temporal arteritis: Diagnosis and management. *BMJ* 1997;314:1329-1332.
4. Berthelot JM, et al. Joint manifestations in myelodysplastic syndromes. A report of three cases presenting as polymyalgia rheumatica. *Rev Rhum Engl Ed* 1997;64:95-100.
5. Schwartzberg M, Weber CA, Musico J. Lyme borreliosis presenting as a polymyalgia rheumatica-like syndrome. *Brit J Rheumatol* 1995;34:392-398.
6. Barber HS. Myalgic syndrome with constitutional effects. Polymyalgia rheumatica. *Ann Rheum Dis* 1957;16:230-237.
7. Schaufelberger C, Bengtsson BA, Andersson R. Epidemiology and mortality in 220 patients with polymyalgia rheumatica. *Brit J Rheumatol* 1995;34:261-264.
8. Tore Gran J, Myklebust G. The incidence of polymyalgia rheumat-

ica and temporal arteritis in the county of Aust Agder, south Norway: A prospective study 1987-94. *J Rheumatol* 1997;24:1739-1743.
9. Salvarani C, et al. Epidemiology of polymyalgia rheumatica in Olmsted County, Minnesota, 1970-1991. *Arthritis Rheum* 1995;38:369-373.
10. Hazleman BL. Polymyalgia Rheumatica and Giant Cell Arteritis. In: Klippel JH, Dieppe PA (eds): *Rheumatology.* St. Louis: Mosby, 1994:6.18.1-6.18.8.
11. Cimmino MA. Genetic and environmental factors in polymyalgia rheumatica. *Ann Rheum Dis* 1997;56:576-577.
12. Zauber P, Zhang L, Berman E. Familial occurrence of temporal arteritis. *J Rheumatol* 1997;24:611-612 (letter).
13. Weyand CM, et al. HLA-DRB1 alleles in polymyalgia rheumatica, giant cell arteritis, and rheumatoid arthritis. *Arthritis Rheum* 1994;37:514-520.
14. Haworth S, et al. Polymyalgia rheumatica is associated with both HLA-DRB1*0401 and DRB1*0404. *Brit J Rheumatol* 1996;35:632-635.
15. Chakravarty K, et al. A longitudinal study of anticardiolipin antibody in polymyalgia rheumatica and giant cell arteritis. *J Rheumatol* 1995;22:1694-1697.
16. Brito J, et al. Autoantibodies to human nuclear lamin B2 protein. Epitope specificity in different autoimmune diseases. *J Immunol* 1994;153:2268-2277.
17. Le Tonqueze M, et al. The relationship of anti-endothelial cell antibodies to anti-phospholipid antibodies in patients with giant cell arteritis and/or polymyalgia rheumatica. *Autoimmunity* 1995;20:59-66.
18. Benlahrache C, et al. Decrease of the OKT8 positive T cell subset in polymyalgia rheumatica. Lack of correlation with disease activity. *Arthritis Rheum* 1983;26:1472-1480.
19. Uddhammar A, et al. Peripheral blood lymphocyte subsets in polymyalgia rheumatica. *Clin Rheumatol* 1995;14:62-67.
20. Martinez-Taboada VM, Goronzy JJ, Weyland CM. Clonally expanded CD8 T cells in patients with polymyalgia rheumatica and giant cell arteritis. *Clin Immuno Immunopathol* 1996;79: 263-270.
21. Stevens RJ, Hughes RA. Polymyalgic presentation of enterovirus infection: A cause of diagnostic confusion. *Ann Rheum Dis* 1996;55:147-148 (letter).
22. Olling P, Olsson AT, Elling H. Synchronous variations of the incidence of temporal arteritis and polymyalgia rheumatica in different regions of Denmark; association with epidemics of mycoplasma pneumoniae infection. *J Rheumatol* 1996;23: 112-119.
23. Genereau T, et al. Polymyalgia rheumatica with temporal arteritis following intravesical Calmette-Guerin bacillus immunotherapy for bladder cancer. *Clin Exp Rheumatol* 1996;14:110 (letter).
24. Uddhammar A, et al. Antibodies against *Chlamydia pneumoniae,* cytomegalovirus, enteroviruses and respiratory syncytial virus in patients with polymyalgia rheumatica. *Clin Exp Rheumatol* 1997;15;299-302.
25. Bromberg MB, Donofrio PD, Segal BM. Steroid-responsive electromyographic abnormalities in polymyalgia rheumatica. *Muscle Nerve* 1990;13:138-141.
26. Shintani S, et al. Immunofluorescence study of immune complexes in polymyalgia rheumatica. *J Neurol Sci* 1995;128:103-106.
27. Mattei JP, et al. P-31 magnetic resonance spectroscopy demonstrates unaltered muscle energy utilization in polymyalgia rheumatica. *Arthritis Rheum* 1997;40:1817-1822.
28. Salvarani C, et al. Proximal bursitis in active polymyalgia rheumatica. *Ann Intern Med* 1997;127:27-31.
29. Meliconi R, et al. Leukocyte infiltraiton in synovial tissue from the shoulder of patients with polymyalgia rheumatica. Quantitative analysis and influence of corticosteroid treatment. *Arthritis Rheum* 1996;39:1199-1207.
30. Meliconi R, et al. Synovial expression of cell adhesion molecules in polymyalgia rheumatica. *Clin Exp Immunol* 1997; 107:494-500.
31. Weyand CM, et al. Tissue cytokine patterns in patients with polymyalgia rheumatica and giant cell arteritis. *Ann Intern Med* 1994;121:484-491.
32. Myklebust G, Gran JT. A prospective study of 287 patients with polymyalgia rheumatica and temporal arteritis: Clinical and laboratory manifestations at onset of disease and at the time of diagnosis. *Brit J Rheumatol* 1996;35:1161-1168.
33. Salvarani C, Gabriel S, Hunder GG. Distal extremity swelling with pitting edema in polymyalgia rheumatica. Report of nineteen cases. *Arthritis Rheum* 1996;39:73-80.
34. Herrera B, et al. Carpal tunnel syndrome heralding polymyalgia rheumatica. *Scand J Rheumatol* 1997;26:222-224.
35. Dwolatzky T, Sonnenblick M, Nesher G. Giant cell arteritis and polymyalgia rheumatica: Clues to early diagnosis. *Geriatrics* 1997;52:38-44.
36. Bird HA, et al. An evaluation of criteria for polymyalgia rheumatica. *Ann Rheum Dis* 1979;38:434-439.
37. Chuang T, et al. Polymyalgia rheumatica. A 10 year epidemiologic and clinical study. *Ann Intern Med* 1982;97:672-680.
38. Brooks RC, McGee SR. Diagnostic dilemmas in polymyalgia rheumatica. *Arch Intern Med* 1997;157:162-168.
39. Helfgott Sm, Kieval RI. Polymyalgia rheumatica in patients with a normal erythrocyte sedimentation rate. *Arthritis Rheum* 1996;39:304-307.
40. Gonzalez-Gay MA, et al. Polymyalgia rheumatica without significantly increased erythrocyte sedimentation rate. *Arch Intern Med* 1997;157:317-320.
41. Roche NE, et al. Correlation of interleukin-6 production and disease activity in polymyalgia rheumatica and giant cell arteritis. *Arthritis Rheum* 1993;36:1286-1294.
42. Caplanne D, Le Parc J, Alexandre J. Interleukin-6 in clinical relapses of polymyalgia rheumatica and giant cell arteritis. *Ann Rheum Dis* 1996;55:403-404.
43. Olsson A, Elling P, Elling H. Serological and immunohistochemical determination of von Willebrand factor antigen in serum and biopsy specimens from patients with arteritis temporalis and polymyalgia rheumatica. *Clin Exp Rheumatol* 1990;8:55-58.
44. Cimmino MA, Salvarani C. Polymyalgia rheumatica and giant cell arteritis. *Balliere's Clin Rheumatol* 1995;9:515-527.
45. Jones JG, Hazleman BL. Prognosis and management of polymyalgia rheumatica. *Ann Rheum Dis* 1981;40:1-5.
46. Healey LA. Long-term follow-up of polymyalgia rheumatica: Evidence for synovitis. *Semin Arthritis Rheum* 1984;13:322-328.
47. van Schaardenburg D, Breedveld FC. Elderly-onset rheumatoid

arthritis. *Semin Arthritis Rheum* 1994;23:367-378.

48. Chaoquat D. Peripheral joint involvement in polymyalgia rheumatica. *Rev Rhum* [Engl Ed] 1997;64:184-188.
49. Russell EB, et al. Remitting, seronegative, symmetrical synovitis with pitting edema—13 additional cases. *J Rheumatol* 1990; 17:633-639.
50. Paparone PW. Polymyalgia rheumatica or Lyme disease? How to avoid misdiagnosis in older patients. *Postgrad Med* 1995;97: 161-170.
51. Rodriguez-Valverde V, et al. Risk factors and predictive models of giant cell arteritis in polymyalgia rheumatica. *Am J Med* 1997;102:331-336.
52. Salvarani, et al. Primary systemic amyloidosis presenting as giant cell arteritis and polymyalgia rheumatica. *Arthritis Rheum* 1994;37:1621-1626.
53. Behn AR, Perera T, Myles A. PMR and corticosteroids: How much for how long? *Ann Rheum Dis* 1983;48:658-651.
54. Kyle V, Hazleman BL. Treatment of PMR and GCA: I. Steroid regimens in the first two months. *Ann Rheum Dis* 1989;48: 658-661.
55. Gabriel SE, et al. Adverse outcomes of antiinflammatory therapy among patients with polymyalgia rheumatica. *Arthritis Rheum* 1997;40:1873-1878.
56. Ferraccioli G, et al. Methotrexate in polymyalgia rheumatica: Preliminary results of an open, randomized study. *J Rheumatol* 1996;23:624-628.
57. Feinberg HL, et al. The use of methotrexate in polymyalgia rheumatica. *J Rheumatol* 1996;23:1550-1552.
58. Doury P, et al. The use of dapsone in the treatment of giant cell arteritis and polymyalgia rheumatica. *Arthritis Rheum* 1983; 26,689-690 (letter).
59. Canalis E. Mechanism of glucocorticoid action on bone: Implications of glucocorticoid-induced osteoporosis. *J Clin Endocrinol Metab* 1996;81:3441-3447.
60. Wolinsky-Freidland M. Drug-induced metabolic bone disease. *Endocrinol Metab Clin N Am* 1995;24:395-420.
61. Nesher G, et al. Analysis of steroid related complications and mortality in temporal arteritis: A 15-year survey of 43 patients. *J Rheumatol* 1994;21:1283-1286.
62. Lukert B. Glucocorticoid-induced osteoporosis. In: Marcus R, et al (eds). *Osteoporosis.* San Diego: Academic Press; 1996; 801-802.
63. Healey, et al. A randomized controlled trial of salmon calcitonin to prevent bone loss in corticosteroid-treated temporal arteritis and polymyalgia rheumatica. *Calcif Tissue Int* 1996;58:73-80.
64. Adachi JD, et al. Salmon calcitonin nasal spray in the prevention of corticosteroid-induced bone loss. *Br J Rheumatol* 1994; 33:348-350.
65. Mulder H, Struys A. Intermittent cyclical etidronate in the prevention of corticosteroid-induced bone loss. *Br J Rheumatol* 1994;33:348-350.
66. Saag K, et al. Alendronate for the management of glucocorticoid-induced ostroporosis: Results of the multicenter U.S. Study. *Arthritis Rheum* 1997;40:S134 (abstract).

Systemic Lupus Erythematosus

Keith K. Colburn, MD

Systemic lupus erythematosus (SLE) is a very complicated autoimmune syndrome potentially involving all organ systems. A plethora of autoantibodies are produced in patients with SLE, including some that appear to be pathogenic for certain features of the disease, most notably anti:dsDNA antibodies. The minimum requirement for the diagnosis of SLE is to know and understand the 11 American College of Rheumatology diagnostic criteria. Treatment of patients with SLE is related to the severity of the disease and may be somewhat benign for mild disease or very risky for severe, life-threatening complications, including nephritis, pulmonary hemorrhage, and serious CNS involvement. The leading cause of death in SLE is related to complications of treatment. This article will help guide physicians through the many facets of the diagnosis and treatment of patients with SLE.

Introduction and History

Systemic lupus erythematosus (SLE) is a syndrome with many different presentations and can affect most organ systems. SLE is a prototype of autoimmune diseases in which a wide variety of autoantibodies are produced, some of which may be pathogenic, causing tissue injury. The most characteristic of these antibodies are to double-stranded (ds) or native DNA.[1]

Sir William Osler first described the syndrome of SLE with its systemic manifestations in 1895.[2] Prior to that time, lupus was considered a destructive skin disease. Osler suggested that the pathophysiology of SLE was based on the inflammation of blood vessels, or vasculitis. Soon others described specific pathogenic lesions in multiple organs, including glomerulonephritis, heart valve vegetations, arthritis, pericarditis, and numerous other findings now associated with SLE.[3] The first diagnostic test for SLE, the lupus erythematosus cell prep (LE prep), was described by Hargraves in 1948, followed by an increase in the frequency of detection of this disease.[4] The discovery of the LE prep opened the door to the understanding of the immunologic basis of SLE.

In the early 1950s, with the advent of the use of corticosteroids to treat patients with SLE, a marked improvement in the prognosis of lupus was noted.[5] The subsequent explosion of information using newer immunologic, molecular biologic, and genetic tools has substantially increased the understanding of SLE and improved the treatment of this disease. However, the etiology of lupus still remains a mystery.

The essentials of the diagnosis and management of patients with SLE are in the understanding and recognition of the disease manifestations. It is especially important to be familiar with the American College of Rheumatology (ACR) diagnostic criteria *(please see Table 1)* and know what, when, and how much to treat.[6] The cause of death in SLE patients often has an iatrogenic basis related to the lack of early recognition and the inappropriate treatment of the actual or presumed manifestations of this disease.

Epidemiology

SLE is primarily a disease of young women of childbearing age between 15 and 40 years old. However, the onset of the disease can range from infancy to old age. SLE affects approximately 1 in 2000 individuals in the general population, although the prevalence varies with race, ethnicity, and socioeconomic status.[5] Females make up 80-90% of SLE patients, which affects as many as 1 in 1000 women. In North America and Northern Europe, there are about 40 cases of SLE per 100,000 population, with a higher incidence and tendency to more severe disease in black Americans and Hispanics .[7] The prevalence in children and older adults is approximately 1 per 100,000. An investigation for drug-induced lupus should be considered in older patients with symptoms suspicious of SLE.

Although the precise immunologic events involved in the development of SLE remain poorly understood, a basic model of pathogenesis has emerged. In this model, an environmental trigger acts upon a genetically susceptible individual to create T-cell and B-cell defects that result in increased autoantibody production.[1] The nature of the environmental trigger(s) initiating SLE is one of the least understood features of pathogenesis. Sex hormones, ultraviolet light exposure, drugs, and various infections modify the expression of this disease but may be quite distinct from a more general triggering agent. Many infections are thought to induce flares of activity in lupus, and some may actually predispose an individual to develop SLE. Such infections include parvovirus, CMV, and hepatitis C.[1]

CD4+ (helper) T cells are the driving forces in the pathogenesis of SLE.[10] The specificities of many "self" antigens remain unknown. The evidence suggests, however, that B cells are driven by self antigens in a T-cell-dependent process that involves somatic mutation, affinity maturation, and IgM to IgG class switching.[1]

In population studies of SLE patients, the association of disease with specific class II major histocompatibility complex (MHC) alleles is weak and generally consistent only within a given ethnic group.[1] For example, in Caucasians, there is an association of the human leukocyte antigen (HLA)-DR2 and/or (HLA)-DR3 with an increased incidence of SLE, but the relative risk is less than five times that of the general population.[1] In contrast, class II MHC genes appear to exert a strong influence on the production of specific antinuclear antibodies.[1] The antibody response to several lupus autoantigens is strongly associated with particular MHC class II (HLA-DQ) alleles as well as combinations of class II gene products.

Inherited complement deficiencies, some of which are determined by genes encoded within the MHC, show a powerful effect on disease susceptibility that is demonstrable across racial and ethnic groups. Complement genes for C4 (C4A and C4B) and C2 are encoded within the class III HLA region.[8] A complete lack of the C4A and C4B genes leads to a lupus-like syndrome in most of the patients described. Homozygous C4A deficiency is present in 13-15% of SLE patients compared to less than 1% of healthy controls (relative risk, approximately 15-20 times the general population). Heterozygous C4A deficiency is present in 35-60% of SLE patients compared to 13-20% of healthy controls (relative risk, approximately 2-3). In patients with a homozygous C2 deficiency, nearly 20-30% will develop an autoimmune disease with features resembling SLE.[8] Lupus is also associated with inherited complement deficiencies determined by genes encoded outside the MHC (e.g., Clq or Clrls) that cannot be explained by linked HLA genes. The mechanism by which complement deficiencies may influence the development of lupus is unknown but may involve defects in the clearance of immune complexes or viral particles.

An association of SLE with apoptosis (programmed cell death) was recently proposed.[9] Several genes regulate apoptosis, including genes that inhibit (i.e., *Bcl-2* gene) or promote (i.e., apoptosis-1/*Fas* gene) cell death. The abnormal expression of apoptosis-related genes (e.g., the over-expression of *Bcl-2* or defects in the *Fas* gene) is associated with the development of lupus-like systemic autoimmune disease in animals.[9] A soluble form of the *Fas* protein, an apoptosis-signaling receptor molecule on the surface of lymphocytes, was found in the sera of some patients with SLE.[10] Injection of normal mice with this soluble form of the *Fas* protein resulted in the inhibition of apoptosis and the appearance of autoimmune features.[11]

The major immunologic feature recognized in patients with SLE is autoantibody production. These antibodies are directed to a host of self molecules found in the nucleus, cytoplasm, and the surface of cells. Serum antinuclear antibodies (ANA) directed against components of the cell nucleus are the most characteristic autoantibodies of SLE and are found in more than 95% of patients.[12] Many different autoantibodies are detected in patients with SLE. The types and occurrences of these antibodies are shown in Table 2.

Clinical Manifestations

General or Constitutional Manifestations. Virtually all organ systems can be affected by SLE. Polyarthritis and dermatitis are the most common presenting symptoms and the most frequent clinical manifestations of SLE. *(Please see Table 3.)* Patients diagnosed with SLE may present with one or more disease features, including arthritis, thrombocytopenia, pericarditis, etc. *(Please see Table 4.)* These symptoms may persist or recur for months or years before the diagnosis is confirmed by the appearance of other features. Constitutional manifestations including malaise, overwhelming fatigue, fever, weight loss, and a variety of disturbances of cognition or affect, including anxiety and depression, are frequently described by patients as early symptoms.

Cutaneous and Mucocutaneous Involvement. There are several types of skin involvement in SLE patients. The butterfly rash presents as an erythematous, elevated, pruritic, and sometimes painful lesion across the face in a malar distribution that, on biopsy, shows nonspecific inflammation, although immune deposits at the dermal-epidermal junction are seen by immunofluorescence. Approximately two-thirds of patients with SLE have photosensitivity, defined as a skin rash due to an unusual reaction to sunlight. Solar radiation may also exacerbate systemic disease activity. Reports indicate that up to 70% of patients with photosensitivity are positive for antiSSA (AntiRo) antibodies.[13] Skin lesions on patients with SLE are either acute, subacute, or chronic. Some acute manifestations include bullous lesions and generalized erythema, which may or may not be photosensitive in nature.[14] The clinical feature most characteristic of subacute cutaneous lupus is a superficial, nonindurated, and nonscarring photosensitivity-induced skin rash.[15] In chronic cutaneous SLE, patients may have a discoid rash with scarring. The histologic exam-

Table 1. ACR Diagnostic Criteria for SLE*

CRITERION	DEFINITION
1. Malar rash	Fixed erythema, flat or raised, over the malar eminences, tending to spare the nasolabial folds
2. Discoid rash	Erythematous raised patches with adherent keratotic scaling and follicular plugging; atrophic scarring may occur in older lesions
3. Photosensitivity	Skin rash as a result of unusual reaction to sunlight, by patient history or physician observation
4. Oral ulcers	Oral or nasopharyngeal ulceration, usually painless, observed by physician
5. Arthritis	Nonerosive arthritis involving two or more peripheral joints, characterized by tenderness, swelling, or effusion
6. Serositis	a) Pleuritis—convincing history of pleuritic pain or rub heard by physician or evidence of pleural effusion OR b) Pericarditis—documented by ECG or rub or evidence of pericardial effusion
7. Renal disorder	a) Persistent proteinuria greater than 0.5 grams per day or greater than 3+ if quantitation not performed OR b) Cellular casts—may be red cell, hemoglobin, granular, tubular, or mixed
8. Neurologic disorder	a) Seizures—in the absence of offending drugs or known metabolic derangements (e.g., uremia, ketoacidosis, or electrolyte imbalance)
9. Hematologic disorder	a) Hemolytic anemia—with reticulocytosis OR b) Leukopenia—less than 4000/mm^3 total on two or more occasions OR c) Lymphopenia—less than 1500/mm^3 on two or more occasions OR d) Thrombocytopenia—less than 100,000/mm^3 in the absence of offending drugs
10. Immunologic disorder	a) Positive LE cell preparation OR b) Anti-DNA: antibody to native DNA in abnormal titer OR c) Anti-Sm: presence of antibody to Sm nuclear antigen OR d) False positive serologic test for syphilis known to be positive for at least six months and confirmed by *Treponema pallidum* immobilization or fluorescent treponemal antibody absorption test
11. Antinuclear antibody	An abnormal titer of antinuclear antibody by immunofluorescence or an equivalent assay at any time and in the absence of drugs known to be associated with "drug-induced lupus" syndrome

* The proposed classification is based on 11 criteria. For the purpose of identifying patients in clinical studies, a person shall be said to have systemic lupus erythematosus if any four or more of the 11 criteria are present, serially or simultaneously, during any interval of observation.

Reprinted with permission of the American College of Rheumatology from: Tan EM, Cohen AS, Fries JF, et al. The 1982 revised criteria for the classification of systemic lupus erythematosus (SLE). *Arthritis Rheum* 1982;25:1271-1277.

ination of skin from affected areas in subacute cutaneous lupus erythematosus showed a relatively sparse, superficial inflammatory cell infiltrate. Patients with lupus usually show the classic dermal-epidermal junctional staining by immunofluorescence, or "lupus band," indicating an immune complex mediated process.[16] The lupus band test is often positive in "unaffected" areas of the skin of patients with lupus and in patients with other diseases. According to the opinion of many rheumatologists, including the authors, the lupus band test is not cost-effective and produces little clinically useful information. Therefore, we do not routinely perform this biopsy.[13] Some, however, argue that the lupus band test differentiates discoid lupus from SLE, because discoid lupus has a positive band test in only the skin lesions, whereas SLE will often have a positive test in both a rash and non-affected areas of skin.

The mechanisms for the pathophysiologic effects of ultraviolet light are not fully understood. However, recent studies in patients with SLE showed that ultraviolet light may induce the synthesis of or facilitate translocation to the plasma membrane of antigens such as

Table 2. Major Autoantibodies in SLE

AB	%
ANA	> 95%
Anti-dsDNA	40-60%
Anti-ssDNA	70%
Anti-Smith	25-30%
Anti-ribonuclear protein	35%
AntiSSA (Ro)	35%
AntiSSB (La)	20%
Anticardiolipin Abs	75%
Antihistone Abs	70%
Antiribosomal P Abs	20%

Table 3. The Most Common Presenting Manifestations of SLE

1.	Arthritis/arthralgias	55%
2.	Rash	20%
3.	Nephritis	5%
4.	Fever	5%
5.	Pleuritis/Pericarditis	5%
6.	Seizures	3%
7.	Raynaud's	2%
8.	Others	5%

the SS-A(Ro), SS-B(La), Smith, and ribonucleoprotein. Increased expression of antigens related to SLE at the plasma membrane may provide an initial antigenic stimulus for the development of specific autoantibodies and be involved in an antibody-mediated or cytotoxic cell-mediated immune response.[14] It is very important for patients with SLE to protect themselves from direct sunlight. Oral ulcers are usually painless and occur in up to 35% of patients with SLE.[1] Raynaud's phenomenon occurs in 10-45% of patients with SLE, depending on the series, and is the result of vasospasm and vascular damage, especially apparent with the classical white, blue, and red color changes in the fingers.[1] Alopecia is observed in up to 45% of SLE patients some time during their disease. It can occur also with some of the therapy for SLE. The hair loss may be diffuse or patchy, associated with discoid lesions.[1]

Musculoskeletal Involvement. Arthralgia and arthritis occur in about 95% of patients with SLE. Approximately 75% of lupus patients develop true arthritis.[17] The arthritis may be migratory or persistent and chronic and may include any joint, although typically the small joints of hands, wrists, and knees are symmetrically involved.[10] SLE patients with arthritis usually do not develop joint erosions. Some patients develop metacarpal-phalangeal (MCP) and proximal interphalangeal (PIP) joint subluxations in the late stages of their disease, referred to as Jaccoud's arthritis.

Features of SLE overlap with autoimmune diseases including rheumatoid arthritis, scleroderma, poly/dermatomyositis, and Sjogren's syndrome usually sequentially, although they can also exist concomitantly.[1] The best known of these "overlap" syndromes is mixed connective tissue disease (MCTD). MCTD can have findings of any of the five diseases mentioned above but originally was described with features of SLE, poly/dermatomyositis, and scleroderma and, by definition, has to have circulating antibodies to the ribonucleoprotein, U_1 RNP. Patients with MCTD are less likely to develop nephritis than those with SLE but tend to develop scleroderma changes late in their course. Overlapping features of SLE with rheumatoid arthritis are seen in a few patients. The coexistence of SLE and RA may be determined by having clinical criteria for both diseases including radiological findings.[18]

Patients with SLE commonly complain of muscle pain and weakness. Although true myositis may coexist with SLE, fibromyalgia, drug-induced myopathy secondary to corticosteroids, antimalarials, and other drugs, or coexisting thyroid disease may cause muscular symptoms.[10]

Renal Involvement. The kidney is the most commonly involved internal organ in patients with SLE. Approximately 50-75% of renal biopsies from SLE patients reported in several series show evidence of nephritis.[19] Clinically active renal disease is manifested by the presence of proteinuria (> 500 mg/24 hours), cellular casts, hematuria (> 5 RBCs/hpf), or pyuria (> 5 WBCs/hpf) in the absence of other causes of kidney damage.

The World Health Organization (WHO) classification of SLE *(Table 5)* lists the types of glomerulonephritis found in patients with SLE.[20] According to statistics from WHO, only three out of 148 patients with SLE studied had truly normal kidney biopsies, suggesting that most have varying degrees of renal pathology. Lupus nephritis may also involve the kidney interstitium. The pathogenesis of lupus nephritis includes precipitation of immune complexes with autoantibodies that react with DNA (anti-dsDNA antibodies) and other cellular components in the glomeruli and interstitium of the kidney.[21] Studies correlating the type and severity of nephritis revealed several features that appear to promote pathogenecity, including the quantity of circulating antibodies, charge, class, isotype, idiotype, avidity for DNA, and efficiency of complement fixation.[21] Furthermore, cross-reactivity of anti-DNA autoantibodies with glomerular cell surface antigens, as well as with normal components of basement membrane and mesangial matrix, probably promotes immune complex formation and influences the location of these deposits within the glomerulus.[22]

Neuropsychiatric Involvement. Neuropsychiatric involvement of patients with SLE *(please see Table 6)* ranges from simple headache to CNS vasculitis. Other unusual manifestations of CNS lupus include Parkinsonism, cerebellar ataxia, pseudotumor cerebrae, hypothalamic dysfunction, aseptic meningitis (related to NSAID use), myasthenia-like syndrome, Eaton-Lambert syndrome, and thrombotic thrombocytopenic purpura. Peripheral nervous system involvement of SLE is also noted in approximately 10% of patients and includes sensory or motor myopathies, Guillain Barré-like syndrome, and mononeuritis multiplex.

The pathogenesis of neuropsychiatric SLE includes vasculitic-induced blood vessel occlusion, antibody against brain tissue,

Table 4. Approximate Cumulative Incidence of Clinical Manifestations in SLE Patients

Arthralgia or arthritis	90%
Rash	85%
Fever	75%
Renal involvement	> 50%
Pleuritis	50%
Pericarditis	35%
Alopecia	30%
CNS symptoms	25%
Raynaud's phenomenon	20%
Oral and nasal ulcers	20%
Psychosis	15%

Table 5. World Health Organization Classification of Lupus

	Histology	Prognosis
I	Normal	Excellent
II	Mesangial lupus nephritis	Good
III	Focal proliferative lupus nephritis	Moderate
IV	Diffuse proliferative glomerulonephritis	Poor
V	Membraneous glomerulonephritis	Moderate
VI	Glomerulosclerosis	Poor

hypercoagulable status due to antiphospholipid antibodies, and other secondary causes such as infection, metabolic derangement, and side effects of drugs that are used for treatment of SLE.[10]

Recently, circulating antineuronal and anti-ribosomal P antibodies were found in many patients with CNS lupus.[23] The pathogenic significance of these findings needs further study.

Hematological Manifestation. Anemia, leukopenia, and thrombocytopenia are frequent manifestations of SLE. Patients with SLE often have normocytic normochromic anemia. Coomb's positive hemolytic anemia is frequently present. Circulating antierythropoietin antibodies were recently reported as a possible mechanism of anemia in SLE patients.[24]

Leukopenia with white blood cell counts of less than 4000/mm^3 or lymphopenia with cell counts less than 1500/mm^3 on two or more occasions are part of the diagnostic criteria of SLE. *(See Table 1.)* However, other causes of decreased WBC counts including malignancy, infection, and drug-induced leukopenia should be excluded before attributing the low WBC count to SLE.

Thrombocytopenia with a platelet count of less than 100,000/mm^3 in the absence of other causes is found in up to 25% of SLE patients. Antiplatelet autoantibodies bind to one or more surface glycoproteins (usually the glycoprotein II-IIIa complex). The antibody-coated platelets are ingested in the spleen, liver, lymph nodes, and bone marrow by macrophages with receptors for the Fc region of immunoglobulin. A number of patients with SLE and thrombocytopenia have circulating antiphospholipid antibodies and have a co-existing antiphospholipid syndrome.[25] Spontaneous bleeding is rare in patients with platelet counts of more than 5000/mm^3. However, thrombocytopenia is often a marker of severe disease with poor prognosis.[26] It is important to recognize that a positive antinuclear antibody (ANA) test is also reported in up to 30% of patients with chronic idiopathic thrombocytopenic purpura.[27]

Other Clinical Manifestations of SLE. SLE affects the heart in several ways, including pericarditis, myocarditis, coronary artery disease, and endocarditis. Pericarditis is the most common cardiac manifestation of SLE, occurring in about 20-30% of patients, and usually presents with mid-anterior chest pain. Myocarditis, which is probably vasculitic, is suspected when SLE patients have cardiomegaly, arrhythmias, or conduction defects and usually co-exists with pericarditis during the active phases of SLE. Sterile vegetations of the heart valves, or Liebman Sacks' endocarditis, is a less common cardiac manifestation of SLE. It was recently suggested that Liebman Sacks' endocarditis is often a part of the antiphospholipid syndrome. The prevalence of Liebman Sacks' endocarditis has decreased since treatment with corticosteroids was introduced in the 1950s. It is important to differentiate lupus endocarditis from infective endocarditis. It is also important to prophylactically treat patients with lupus endocarditis with antibiotics when they have any medical or dental procedure. Coronary artery disease is becoming more common in patients with SLE, because they are living longer and because of the effects of high doses of corticosteroids used to treat their disease.[28] Coronary artery vasculitis is not commonly found in SLE patients.

The pulmonary manifestations of systemic lupus include pneumonitis, pulmonary hemorrhage, hypertension, and embolism. Lupus pneumonitis is a clinical dilemma that requires careful diagnosis, because it must be differentiated from an infectious pneumonia. It may at times be necessary to treat patients both with corticosteroids and antibiotics until the etiology is clear. Pulmonary hemorrhage from vasculitis is associated with a 50-60% mortality rate and is a true medical emergency.[29] Pulmonary hypertension is more commonly associated with long-term restrictive lung disease and Raynaud's syndrome.

Gastrointestinal symptoms in patients with SLE are relatively common and present as abdominal pain, anorexia, nausea, and/or vomiting. Peritoneal inflammation is the most likely cause of GI symptoms, but mesenteric vasculitis or pancreatitis are dangerous complications of SLE and need to be considered in the presence of abdominal symptoms.[30] Abdominal pain may be masked in patients being treated with cortico-steroids and may perforate a viscous with very few symptoms to alert the physician of serious complications.

Laboratory Findings

The serum antinuclear antibody test (ANA) is positive in more than 95% of patients with SLE. The ANA is the most sensitive laboratory test for SLE and, therefore, is the most effective for a screening test for lupus. Since the ANA is not very specific, it is most

Table 6. Nervous System Involvement of SLE

Seizure disorder
Psychosis
Depression
Cerebrovascular accident
Movement disorder
Headache
Pseudotumor cerebri
Transverse myelitis
Mononeuritis multiplex
Guillain-Barré syndrome
Organic brain syndrome
Cranial nerve palsy
Peripheral neuropathy
Aseptic meningitis
Hypothalamic dysfunction
Myasthenia
Eaton-Lambert syndrome
Cerebellar ataxia
Thrombotic thrombocytopenic purpura

valuable when it is negative, because its absence almost rules out SLE as a diagnosis.[30] In contrast, antibodies to the Smith antigen (anti-Sm antibodies) and the anti-native or anti-ds DNA antibodies are highly specific for SLE and, therefore, make very good confirmatory tests for the diagnosis of SLE.[30] Table 2 lists a number of the antibodies found in SLE. AntiSSA (Anti-Ro) antibodies are often detected in Sjogren's syndrome, and also in about 30% of patients with SLE. AntiSSA antibodies are very important to detect in pregnant patients with lupus, because these antibodies are frequently associated with neonatal heart block, requiring much closer monitoring of the fetus during pregnancy.[31] Infants of mothers with antiSSA antibodies may also have transient features of SLE, including a rash, hematologic abnormalities of SLE, and/or abnormally elevated liver function tests. Anti-SSB (Anti-La) antibodies, also seen in Sjogren's, are found in patients with SLE in 20-30% of cases.

It is very important to screen patients with SLE for the antiphospholipid syndrome, because of the potentially serious consequences of thromboembolic events associated with this condition. It is important to test the patient for anticardiolipin antibodies (especially the IgG antibodies), as they are most often associated with thromboembolic events. Measuring serum for the presence of the lupus anticoagulant may diagnose other patients with antiphospholipid syndrome not recognized with the anticardiolipin antibody test. In some cases, anticardiolipin antibodies and the lupus anticoagulant may be negative, but the serum anti-β-2 glycoprotein I antibodies may be present and are very significant for a high risk of thromboembolic events.[32] The diagnosis of the antiphospholipid syndrome is not only associated with increased thromboembolic events but also spontaneous abortions and thrombocytopenia.

One index of the activity of SLE that can be monitored is measuring serum complement levels, which may be depressed. A decreased serum level of C3, C4, or CH50, along with a rising titer of anti-double-stranded DNA antibodies, may warn the physician of an impending SLE flare, which should result in more frequent monitoring of the patient and earlier treatment of a potentially serious flare.[33]

Other tests that are important to do in systemic lupus include a CBC, which may detect a depressed white blood cell (WBC) count and evidence of hemolytic anemia or thrombocytopenia. A Coomb's test may help in detecting hemolytic anemia associated with SLE. Anti-histone antibodies are present in the sera of 95% of patients with drug-induced lupus. The most common offending drugs include procainamide, hydralazine, and isoniazide.[34] Many other drugs are also suspected to cause drug-induced lupus. *(Please see Table 7.)* The symptoms of drug-induced lupus are milder but similar to those in patients with SLE, except that the kidney is not usually involved. Stopping the offending drug usually resolves the symptoms. There are other antibodies measured in patients with SLE that have more research value than clinical significance.[1]

Diagnosis of SLE

The diagnosis of SLE should be made on a clinical basis and supported by specific laboratory tests. The key to the diagnosis of SLE in a patient in your office is to know the American College of Rheumatology (ACR) revised 1982 criteria for the diagnosis of systemic lupus.[6] *(Please see Table 1.)* If the patient has four of these criteria confirmed, either on examination or historically, SLE is the most likely diagnosis. Occasionally, however, one can be fooled, and a patient with other diseases, such as hepatitis, subacute bacterial endocarditis (SBE), or other autoimmune diseases may demonstrate four criteria for SLE. In more than 95% of the cases, however, SLE will be the correct diagnosis. In a recent news bulletin, the ACR recommended that the tenth criterion drop the LE prep and add the presence of one of the serum antiphospholipid antibodies.

There are other clinical features also important to recognize in SLE that help with diagnosis. Table 3 outlines the most common presenting features of SLE. The differential diagnosis one must consider on presentation of a patient suspected to have SLE is immense. One can be easily confused, if unable to fit all the multisystem signs and symptoms together into the syndrome of SLE. Recognizing that a patient has a multisystems disease narrows the choices one has to pick from, such as RA, one of the vasculidities, other autoimmune diseases, malignancies, fibromyalgia, and infectious diseases, such as SBE, HIV, hepatitis B or C, etc. If the ANA test is negative, one can almost rule out SLE. However, if the ANA is positive, the rest of the ACR criteria and other clinical findings need to be applied to help select SLE from your differential diagnosis. A patient may not have four criteria but can appear to have SLE. This type of patient is often given the diagnosis of a "lupus-like syndrome." Rarely a patient may be diagnosed with "ANA-negative SLE." Expert opinion is needed to help with this diagnosis.

Table 7. Drugs Known to Cause a Lupus-Like Syndrome

Procainamide
Hydralazine
Isoniazide
Hydantoins
Chlorpromazine
Methyldopa
D-penicillamine
Interferon-r

Table 8. Adverse Effects of Glucocorticoid

Infection
Osteoporosis
Avascular necrosis
Peptic ulceration with combination treatment of NSAIDs
Hypertension
Coronary artery disease
Cataracts
Weight gain
Mood disturbance
Glucose intolerance

Management of SLE

It is sobering to note that the leading cause of death in SLE is from infection, which usually has an iatrogenic component.[35] It is extremely important not to undertreat or overtreat SLE. A rule of thumb in treatment of SLE is that mild disease requires mild treatment, and severe, catastrophic disease requires heroic treatment. This requires a great deal of experience in managing this disease, and even then, there are treatment failures. Complications of treatment, including infections and drug toxicities, or failure to treat adequately in a timely manner, are responsible for most of the morbidity and mortality seen in SLE. The inappropriate use of cortico-steroids often represents the greatest threat to a patient's well being of any of the drugs used in treatment of lupus. The major side effects of corticosteroids are listed in Table 8. When using high doses of corticosteroids for serious complications of SLE, our goal as clinicians should be to get the patient on the lowest effective dose as soon as possible. If one can control SLE adequately, it is often desirable to have the patient on an alternate-day schedule within 4-6 weeks of the initiation of treatment. The use of concurrent drugs, such as hydroxychloroquine, azathioprine, methotrexate, cyclosporine, cyclophosphamide, and others, if indicated, will often help limit the dose of corticosteroids.[36] One must weigh the potential toxicities of each of these drugs in determining the "best" therapeutic regimen for each patient.

Cases of severe nephritis, central nervous system involvement, pulmonary hemorrhage, and other forms of systemic vasculitis require the rapid initiation of high doses of cortico-steroids with cytotoxic medications, especially cyclophosphamide.[33]

Skin and Mucocutaneous Lesions. Protection of the skin from ultraviolet light is very important and includes such measures as applying sunblock to prevent photosensitivity reactions, and using umbrellas, wearing hats and long sleeve shirts, etc. to prevent sunlight from striking the skin. Topical cortico-steroid creams and hydroxychloroquine are effective in treating some of the rashes of systemic lupus. Intralesional injections of corticosteroids can be helpful for discoid lupus. Raynaud's phenomenon is usually relatively mild and seasonal in SLE. The more simple cases can be treated by keeping hands and feet warm with gloves and socks and taking calcium channel blockers, especially nifedipine.[37] Mucocutaneous lesions, if painful, can be treated with topical corticosteroids available in a dental paste.

Musculoskeletal Lupus. Arthritis and arthralgias generally should be treated with nonsteroidal anti-inflammatory drugs (NSAIDs) and hydroxychloroquine, if needed. Corticosteroids for the arthritis treatment alone adds more toxic side effects than are warranted in most cases. If the arthritis is severe, low doses of prednisone (7.5 mg or less) may be necessary and ancillary to steroid-sparing drugs like methotrexate or azathioprine similar to the treatment of rheumatoid arthritis.[36]

Cardiopulmonary Lupus. Pleurisy and/or pericarditis (polyserositis) can often be treated symptomatically with NSAIDs, but one may at times need to use low to moderate doses of corticosteroids in the range of up to 0.5 mg/kg/d of prednisone until symptoms clear.[33] For severe pericarditis or pleurisy with pleural effusion, intravenous pulse methylprednisolone of 1000 mg daily for 2-3 days followed by oral prednisone 1-2 mg/kg/d should be given.[33] The dose of prednisone should be slowly tapered back to the maintenance dose watching closely for exacerbations of the symptoms. Frequent flares of the polyserositis may require steroid-sparing treatment with azathioprine or methotrexate.

SLE-related pulmonary hemorrhage requires heroic intervention because of a 60% mortality rate.[29] Treatment with pulse methylprednisilone 1000 mg/d along with cyclophosphamide, ventilator assistance in an ICU setting, intravenous immunoglobulin, and apheresis are among the modalities that have been tried.

Interstitial lung disease either from the SLE or the drugs used in the treatment of lupus occurs occasionally. An open lung biopsy may be needed to differentiate between an infectious agent and an autoimmune mediated process. The acute process is treated with high doses of corticosteroids often followed by cytotoxic drugs used in other high-risk manifestations of lupus.[29]

Pulmonary hypertension and myocarditis are rare but must be anticipated and treated appropriately similarly to other forms of severe SLE previously mentioned.

Coronary artery disease is becoming more common as lupus patients are living longer.[28] Corticosteroids are thought to be a major contributor to early atherosclerosis and may be a good reason to use cytotoxic drugs to limit the amount of corticosteroids to low doses and alternate-day therapy where the risk of long-term complications outweighs the risks of azathioprine, methotrexate, cyclophosphamide, and similar drugs.

Kidneys. Mesangial lesions (WHO Class II) usually do not cause significant signs or symptoms of nephritis and are not regularly treated. Lupus nephritis with focal glomerulonephritis (WHO Class III) may only require low-dose prednisone in the neighborhood of 10-15 mg every other day. If low-dose, alternate-day corticosteroids are not effective in controlling the nephritis, most studies support the use of azathioprine long term to limit the dose of corticosteroids used and to preserve kidney function. However, patients with severe kidney involvement, especially diffuse, proliferative glomerulonephritis (WHO Class IV), the most aggressive form of lupus nephritis, may need to be started on therapy with 1 g of methylprednisolone IV daily for about 3-5 days to rapidly decrease the inflammatory activity in the glomeruli.[37] These patients should then be treated with approximately 80-120 mg of prednisone daily in divided doses, and I would argue for a goal to get the patient on alternate day therapy (even if it is 120 mg every other day) by 4-6 weeks of treatment. The recognized definitive treatment of lupus nephritis is pulse IV cyclophosphamide in a dose of 0.5-1.0 g/m^2 body surface area (10-20 mg/kg) once monthly for six months and often every three months thereafter indefinitely.[35] This treatment protocol has markedly reduced end-stage renal disease in systemic lupus from 75% of patients in four years on prednisone alone to less than 10% in 10- to 20-year follow-up studies. The IV pulse of cyclophosphamide compared with oral administration markedly decreases the toxicity of this drug, including hemorrhagic cystitis, infection, sterility, etc.[37] The addition of mesna in a dose equal to cyclophosphamide post-cyclophosphamide infusion also limits hemorrhagic cystitis.

Other experimental therapies for diffuse proliferative lupus nephritis include plasmapheresis, which may acutely reduce the antibody load and, consequently, disease activity but results in rapid rebound of anti-DNA antibody levels and disease activity, if not supplemented by corticosteroids and cyclophosphamide.[38] Intravenous immunoglobulin in small series was effective in life-threatening situations.[39] Cyclosporine A (3-5 mg/kg) also appears to be effective, especially in treating the nephrotic syndrome associated with membranous glomerulonephritis (WHO Class V).[40] Cyclosporine may be added to the long-term treatment protocols of lupus nephritis in the future, whereas plasmapheresis and IV immunoglobulin are far too expensive and of questionable long-term value in the treatment of lupus nephritis and are therefore usually saved for life-threatening, catastrophic complications of lupus.

Attention to the treatment of hypertension by the clinician is very important to the long-term outcome of lupus nephritis. However, the nephritis worsens in some patients and they develop end-stage kidney disease with glomerulosclerosis (WHO Class VI) and ultimately start dialysis. These patients become candidates for kidney transplant and do fairly well, even though the newly transplanted kidney may occasionally develop lupus nephritis.[41] Therefore, it is often important to follow the patient's anti-double-stranded DNA antibodies and serum complement levels to help predict whether the patient may have a flare of his lupus nephritis in the near future and treat the patient aggressively.[42]

Nervous System. CNS lupus that is catastrophic in nature can be managed by basically the same treatment as for severe, catastrophic lupus nephritis, with high doses of corticosteroids and with IV cyclophosphamide. The psychosis of CNS lupus responds to corticosteroids. However, high doses of cortico-steroids can also cause a psychosis that is difficult to differentiate in patients treated for SLE. Psychotropic drugs for neuropsychiatric lupus on a long-term basis may be needed, such as haloperidol and/or chlorpromazine for severely agitated patients.[43] Patients with chronic organic brain syndrome from CNS vasculitis respond poorly to aggressive therapy. They would be better managed by early recognition and aggressive treatment when immunologic features are still present. Seizure disorders in lupus can be treated with anticonvulsants, such as phenytoin but also may require corticosteroids in the initial acute phases of CNS lupus.

Strokes occur from several mechanisms in about 5% of patients with lupus at some time during their disease.[44] Strokes are often a result of arterial thrombosis, a thromboembolism due to vegetations breaking loose in Liebman Sacks' endocarditis. In patients with SLE, stroke is most commonly associated with the antiphospholipid syndrome, which will be discussed later. Patients with SLE and antiphospholipid syndrome may also develop chorea, which resolves spontaneously within a few weeks. Transverse myelitis associated with loss of urinary or anal sphincter control and paralysis occurs uncommonly in patients with lupus, most often coexisting with the antiphospholipid syndrome. Treatment of transverse myelitis is with high doses of corticosteroids and cytotoxic agents, especially with cyclophosphamide. The treatment is not very successful at reversing the neurological findings but may help arrest the progress of the disease.

Hematologic Abnormalities in SLE. Anemia occurs often in patients with active SLE. The cause of this anemia may be blood loss (i.e., NSAID-induced GI blood loss), anemia of chronic disease, immunosuppressive treatment, and hemolytic anemia (often Coombs positive). The treatment of the anemia needs to be aimed at the underlying cause, and if obscure, a bone marrow aspiration and biopsy may need to be done. Mild or moderate hemolytic anemia usually responds to cortico-steroids and, if needed, azathioprine to reduce the dose of the corticosteroids to acceptable levels.[33] Danocrine is an alternative drug for hemolytic anemia, but masculinizing effects limit its use. Severe hemolytic anemia is treated similarly to other forms of catastrophic SLE.

Leukopenias caused by SLE usually are not low enough and do not need to be treated, but medication-induced neutropenia may require granulocyte-monocyte-colony stimulating factor (GM-CSF) or similar means to increase WBCs.

Thrombocytopenia below 35,000 counts may need treatment with corticosteroids, and if severe and life-threatening, is treated similarly to severe hemolytic anemia. The hemolysis may also require IV immunoglobulin and ultimately a splenectomy, if other treatments fail.[33]

Pregnancy and Lupus. It is best for patients with SLE to have their disease under good control for several months before contemplating pregnancy. SLE will flare in about 60% of cases during pregnancy, although it is argued by some investigators that this is not substantially different than the flare rate for non-pregnant lupus patients over an equivalent period of time.[45] Oral contraception is controversial for SLE patients, but some feel it is safer than pregnancy. However, all pregnancies in patients with SLE should be considered high risk and followed regularly by a trained high-risk obstetrician. Premature delivery occurs in about 45% of pregnancies in SLE patients, and loss of the fetus occurs in 15%.[45] Of special concern are patients positive for circulating antiSSA antibodies, the antiphospholipid syndrome, and patients with active lupus needing cytotoxic medications. Frequent monitoring of the heart of the fetus with four chamber echocardiogram for the development of heart block is necessary for those positive for antiSSA antibodies. The antiphospholipid syndrome will be discussed below.

Patients should be strongly urged not to get pregnant until discontinuing cyclophosphamide and methotrexate for three months because these medications are potentially severely detrimental to the fetus. NSAIDs should not be used except for a few days at a time in the second and third trimesters and not at all near the time of birth, because of their effect on the fetal ductus arteriosis. Severe flares of SLE should be treated with high doses of corticosteroids during pregnancy and, if necessary, supplemented with azathioprine. Intravenous cyclophosphamide should not be used, especially in the first trimester, except in severe life-threatening situations.

Antiphospholipid Syndrome. The antiphospholipid syndrome, as mentioned above, is frequently associated with the manifestations of CNS lupus, particularly stroke, chorea, and transverse myelitis.[46] The antiphospholipid syndrome is also usually present in other thromboembolic complications of SLE. Patients who are diagnosed with the antiphospholipid syndrome must be anticoagulated and their protime maintained at an INR of between 3 and 4. Even then, some of these patients may continue to thrombose multiple vessels. Spontaneous abortions in female patients with SLE are most frequently associated with the antiphospholipid syndrome. Patients with a history of spontaneous abortions who become pregnant and have antiphospholipid syndrome should be treated with aspirin and heparin, approximately 10,000-20,000 units subcutaneously twice a day, from early pregnancy until the fetus is delivered.[47] Some authors recommend adding corticosteroids (15-20 mg/d), if the serum level of anticardiolipin antibodies rises suddenly. If a pregnant patient with lupus and the antiphospholipid syndrome has not experienced fetal loss in the past, some would argue that corticosteroids in moderate doses and aspirin may improve the fetal outcome.[48] However, in those patients with a history of miscarriages, subcutaneous heparin—preferably low molecular weight heparin to limit osteoporosis, is the drug of choice.

Experimental Treatments for SLE. There are experimental therapies used with varying degrees of success in systemic lupus, especially in patients with rather severe, catastrophic forms of SLE. A number of new potential therapeutic interventions are being tested by research laboratories, including vaccinations, tolerizing procedures, antibodies against surface molecules on B and T cells, and other cytotoxic drugs. IV gammaglobulin is sometimes used in patients with SLE who have rather severe thrombocytopenia, hemolytic anemia, and other major complications of lupus.[33] This treatment appears to have been successful in many cases, but double-blind studies proving its efficacy have not as yet been published. The manipulation of sex hormone levels is used, especially in thrombocytopenia, with the use of danazol. In open trials, dihydroepiandrosterone (DHEA) was used in mild to moderate lupus with some success.[49]

The Prognosis

The prognosis of patients with SLE has improved considerably since the early 1950s, with the five-year survival rate at about 85%, 10-year survival at 75%, and 15-year survival at about 65%.[50] Prior to 1950, the four-year survival rate was at about 50%. Changes in treatment of SLE since the 1950s are largely responsible for this improvement. However, SLE still remains a very dangerous and fatal disease, if not managed appropriately.

Summary

In summary, systemic lupus erythematosus is a disease of the immune system manifested by production of numerous autoantibodies, some of which, including anti-double-stranded DNA antibodies, are pathogenic for disease manifestations of some features of lupus. SLE affects virtually all organ systems and, in its moderate to severe forms, needs very close attention by physicians familiar with the disease and its complications. It is important to know the diagnostic criteria for SLE in order to recognize the disease, especially in its earlier forms when it is much more treatable. SLE remains one of the most fascinating and troubling diseases facing physicians.

References

1. Hahn B. Pathogenesis of SLE. In: Kelley WN, Harris ED, Ruddy S, Sledge CB, eds. *Textbook of Rheumatology.* 5th Ed. Philadelphia: W.B. Saunders; 1997:1015-1027.
2. Rothfield NF. Systemic lupus erythematosus: Clinical aspects and treatment. In: McCarty DJ, ed. *Arthritis and Allied Conditions: A Textbook of Rheumatology.* 11th Ed. Philadelphia: Lea & Febiger; 1989:1022-1048.
3. Baehr G, Klemperer P, Schrifrin A. A diffuse disease of the peripheral circulation usually associated with lupus erythematosus and endocarditis. *Trans Assoc Am Phys* 1935;50:139-155.
4. Hargraves MM, Richmond H, Morton R. Presentation of two bone marrow elements: The "tart cell" and the "LE" cell. *Proc Staff Meet Mayo Clin* 1948;23:25-28.
5. Ward MM, Pyun E, Studenski S. Long-term survival in systemic lupus erythematosus. Patient characteristics associated with poorer outcomes. *Arthritis Rheum* 1995;38:274-283.
6. Tan EM, Cohen AS, Fries JF, et al. The 1982 revised criteria for the classification of systematic lupus erythematosus (SLE). *Arthritis Rheum* 1982;25:1271-1277.
7. Liang MH, Partridge AJ, Daltroy LH, et al. Strategies for reducing morbidity and mortality in blacks with systemic lupus erythematosus. *Arthritis Rheum* 1991;34(9):1187-1196.
8. Agnello V. Association of systemic lupus erythematosus and systemic lupus erythematosus-like syndromes with hereditary and acquired complement deficient states. *Arthritis Rheum* 1978;21:S146.
9. Strasser A, Harris AW, Cory S. bci-2 transgene inhibits T cell death and perturbs thymic self-censorship. *Cell* 1991;67:889-899.
10. Boumpas DR, Fessler BJ, Austin HA, et al. Systemic lupus erythematosus: Emerging concepts. Part 2: Dermatologic and joint disease, the antiphospholipid antibody syndrome, pregnancy and hormonal therapy, morbidity and mortality, and pathogenesis. *Ann Intern Med* 1995;123:42-53.
11. Cheng J, Zhou T, Liu C, et al. Protection from *Fas*-mediated apoptosis by a soluble form of the *Fas* molecule. *Science*

1994;263(5154):1759-1762.

12. Tan EM. Antinuclear antibodies: Diagnostic markers for autoimmune diseases and probes for cell biology. *Adv Immunol* 1989;44:93-151.
13. Laman SD, Provost TT. Cutaneous manifestations of lupus erythematosus. *Rheum Dis Clin North Am* 1994;20(1):195-212.
14. Sontheimer RD, Gilliam JN. Systemic lupus erythematosus and the skin. In: Lahita RG, ed. *Systemic Lupus Erythematosus.* 2nd Edition. New York: Churchill Livingstone; 1992:657-681.
15. David-Bajar KM, Bennion SD, DeSpain JD, et al. Clinical, histologic, and immunofluorescent distinctions between subacute cutaneous lupus erythematosus and discoid lupus erythematosus. *J Invest Dermatol* 1992;99:251-257.
16. Pistiner M, Wallace DJ, Nessim S, et al. Lupus erythematosus in the 1980s: A survey of 570 patients. *Semin Arthritis Rheum* 1991;21:55-64.
17. Cronin ME. Musculoskeletal manifestations of systemic lupus erythematosus. *Rheum Dis Clin North Am* 1988;14:99-116.
18. Panush RS, Edwards NL, Logley S, et al. "Rhupus" syndrome. *Arch Intern Med* 1988;148:1633-1636.
19. Golbus J, McCune WJ. Lupus nephritis. Classification, prognosis, immunopathogenesis, and treatment. *Rheum Dis Clin North Am* 1994;20:213-242.
20. Gladman DD, Urowitz MB, Cole E, et al. Kidney biopsy in SLE. I. A clinical-morphologic evaluation. *Quart J Med* 1989;73:1125-1153.
21. Hahn BH, Tsao BP. Antibodies to DNA. In: Wallace DJ, Hahn BH, eds. *Dubois' Lupus Erythematosus.* 4th Ed. Philadelphia: Lea & Febiger; 1993:195-201.
22. Foster MH, Cizman B, Madaio MP. Nephritogenic autoantibodies in systemic lupus erythematosus: Immunochemical properties, mechanisms of immune deposition, and genetic origins. *Lab Invest* 1993;69:494-507.
23. Schneebaum AB, Singleton JD, West SG, et al. Association of psychiatric manifestations with antibodies to ribosomal P proteins in systemic lupus erythematosus. *Am J Med* 1991; 90:54-62.
24. Tzioufas AG, Kokori SI, Petrovas CI, et al. Autoantibodies to human recombinant erythropoietin in patients with systemic lupus erythematosus: Correlation with anemia. *Arthritis Rheum* 1997;40:2212-2216.
25. Alarcon-Segovia D, Deleze M, Oria CV, et al. Antiphospholipid antibodies and the antiphospholipid syndrome in systemic lupus erythematosus. A prospective analysis of 500 consecutive patients. *Medicine* 1989;68:353-365.
26. Reveille JD, Bartolucci A, Alarcon GS. Prognosis in systemic lupus erythematosus: Negative impact of increasing age at onset, black race, and thrombocytopenia, as well as causes of death. *Arthritis Rheum* 1990;33:37-48.
27. Laurence J, Wong JE, Nachman R. The cellular hematology of systemic lupus erythematosus. In: Lahita RG, ed. *Systemic Lupus Erythematosus.* New York: Churchill Livingstone; 1992:871-906.
28. Petri M, Perez-Gutthan S, Spence D, et al. Risk factors for coronary artery disease in patients with systemic lupus erythematosus. *Am J Med* 1992;93:513.
29. Schwab EP, Schumacher Jr HR, Freundlich B, et al. Pulmonary alveolar hemorrhage in systemic lupus erythematosus. *Semin Arthritis Rheum* 1993;23:8-15.
30. Gladman DD, Urowitz MB. Clinical and laboratory features. In: Klippel JH, Weyand CM. Wortmann RL, eds. *Primer on Rheumatic Diseases.* 11th Ed. Atlanta: Arthritis Foundation; 1997:251-257.
31. Lee LA. Neonatal lupus erythematosus. *J Invest Dermatol* 1993;100:95-135.
32. Asherson RA, Cervera R. Antiphospholipid syndrome. In: Kelley WN, Harris ED, Ruddy S, et al, eds. *Textbook of Rheumatology.* Philadelphia: W.B. Saunders; 1997:1057-1064.
33. Petri M. Systemic Lupus Erythematosus. In: Weisman MM, Weinblatt ME, eds. *Treatment of the Rheumatic Diseases.* Philadelphia: W.B. Saunders; 1995:93-108.
34. Hess EV, Mongey AB. Drug-related lupus. *Bull Rheum Dis* 1991;40:1-8.
35. Ginzler EM, Diamond HS, Weiner M, et al. A multi-center study of outcome in systemic lupus erythematosus. *Arthritis Rheum* 1982;25:601-611.
36. Dinant HJ, Decker JL, Klippel JH, et al. Alternative modes of cyclophosphamide and azathioprine therapy in lupus nephritis. *Ann Intern Med* 1982;96(6 Pt 1):728-736.
37. Ginzler EM. Renal diseases in SLE. In: Weisman MM, Weinblatt ME., eds. *Treatment of the Rheumatic Diseases.* Philadelphia: W.B. Saunders; 1995:109-127.
38. Jones JV, Robinson MF, Parciany RK, et al. Therapeutic plasmapheresis in systemic lupus erythematosus: Effect on immune complexes and antibodies to DNA. *Arthritis Rheum* 1981;24:1113.
39. Lin C-Y, Hsu H-C, Cliang H. Improvement of histological and immunological change in steroid and immunosuppressive drug-resistant lupus nephritis by high-dose intravenous gamma globulin. *Nephron* 1989;53:303.
40. Favre H, Miescher PA, Huang YP, et al. Cyclosporin in the treatment of lupus nephritis. *Am J Nephrol* 1989;9 (Suppl 1): 57-60.
41. Stone JH, Millward CL, Olson JL, et al. Frequency of recurred lupus nephritis among ninety-seven renal transplant patients during the cyclosporine era. *Arthritis Rheum* 1998;41:678-686.
42. Goss JA, Cole BR, Jendrisak MD, et al. Renal transplantation for SLE and recurrent lupus nephritis. *Transplantation* 1991;52:805.
43. Bluestein, HG. The neuropsychiatric manifestations of SLE. In: Weisman MM, Weinblatt ME, eds. *Treatment of the Rheumatic Diseases.* Philadelphia: W.B. Saunders; 1995:128-136.
44. Futrell N, Millikan C. Frequency, etiology, and prevention of stroke in patients with systemic lupus erythematosus. *Stroke* 1989;20:583.
45. Khamashta MA, Ruiz-Irastorza G, Hughes GRV. Systemic lupus erythematosus flares during pregnancy. *Rheum Dis Clin North Am* 1997;23:15-30.
46. Asherson RA, Cervera R. The antiphospholipid syndrome: A syndrome in evolution. *Ann Rheum Dis* 1992;51:147-150.
47. Cowchock FS, Reece EA, Balaban D, et al. Repeated fetal losses associated with antiphospholipid antibodies: A collaborative randomized trial comparing prednisone with low-dose heparin treatment. *Am J Obstet Gynecol* 1992;166:1318-1323.
48. Many A, Pauzner R, Carp H, et al. Treatment of patients with antiphospholipid antibodies during pregnancy. *Am J Reprod*

Immunol 1992;28:216-218.

49. van Vollenhoven RF, Engleman EG, McGuire JL. Dehydroepiandrosterone in systemic lupus erythematosus. Results of a double-blind, placebo-controlled, randomized clinical trial. *Arthritis Rheum* 1995;38:1826-1831.
50. Reveille JS, Bartolucci A, Alarcon GS. Prognosis in systemic lupus erythematosus: Negative impact of increasing age at onset, black race, and thrombocytopenia, as well as causes of death. *Arthritis Rheum* 1990;33:37.

Upper Extremity Fractures and Dislocations

William J. Brady, MD
Gregory G. Degnan, MD
Leslie P. Buchanon, RN, MSN, ENP
Susan Schwartz, RN, MSN, ENP
Abhinav Chhabra, MD

The majority of orthopedic injuries encountered by the emergency physician are diagnosed promptly and treated appropriately. In these cases, the mechanism of injury is well delineated, the symptoms are strongly suggestive of a specific diagnosis, the physical examination pinpoints the nature of the injury, and routine radiographic studies identify the expected lesion. However, there is a spectrum of orthopedic injuries—including subtle fractures and difficult-to-identify dislocations—that present a formidable diagnostic challenge for the emergency physician.

These orthopedic "pitfalls" frequently involve such areas as the wrist, shoulder, and hand, anatomic regions where trauma can produce a diverse, unusual, and sometimes unexpected range of clinically signficant dislocations and fractures that are extremely difficult to pinpoint during the initial emergency department (ED) encounter. Unfortunately, delays in diagnosis can lead to non-union of fractures, neurovascular compromise, functional impairment, chronic deformity, and the need for surgical correction of unnecessary complications.

Despite the assessment and treatment challenges presented by these entities—among them, posterior and inferior glenohumera dislocations, fracture/dislocations of the wrist bones, and carpo-metacarpal dislocations—there are step-by-step strategies for minimizing misdiagnosis, reducing medico-legal risks, and optimizing clinical results. Almost without exception, this requires a thorough understanding of the clinical anatomy, maintaining a high index of suspicion for specific fractures and/or dislocations based on mechanism of injury, knowing how to interpret the physical examination, and customizing radiographic studies (including number and angles of different views) to increase the sensitivity of this diagnostic tool.

In this chapter, the author elucidates diagnostic and treatment pitfalls for orthopedic injuries involving the upper extremity.

Shoulder Injuries

Posterior Glenohumeral Dislocation. As a rule, acute shoulder dislocations are correctly diagnosed and appropriately managed in the ED. The majority of these shoulder dislocations, however, are anterior.[1] Acute traumatic posterior dislocation is rare and, despite its infrequent occurrence, it is the most commonly missed joint dislocation in the body. In fact, more than 50% of posterior dislocations are incorrectly diagnosed and/or poorly managed at the time of the initial encounter, and even emergency physicians may find this orthopedic condition problematic.[1,2] Reflecting the widespread problem of initial mismanagement of posterior glenohumeral dislocation, the orthopedic literature is replete with discussions outlining the treatment of chronic, unreduced posterior shoulder dislocations. From a clinical perspective, the diagnosis is often missed because the examining physician does not have a sufficiently high index of suspicion to seek out the classic physical findings. However, even if the

Figure 1

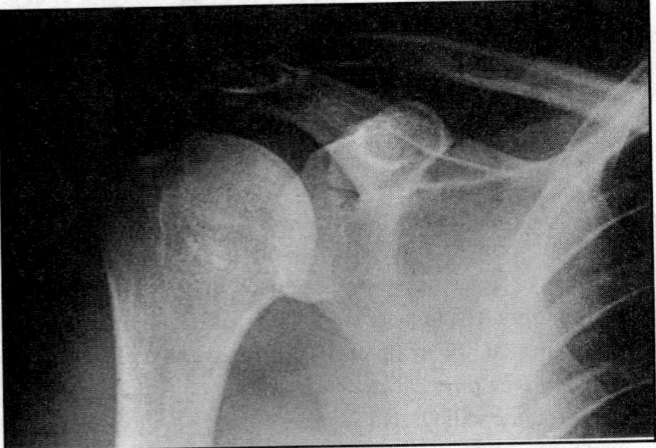

Normal AP view of the glenohumeral joint. Note the overlap shadow of the humeral head superimposed on the glenoid rim—this overlap is lost in the posterior shoulder dislocation.

Figure 2

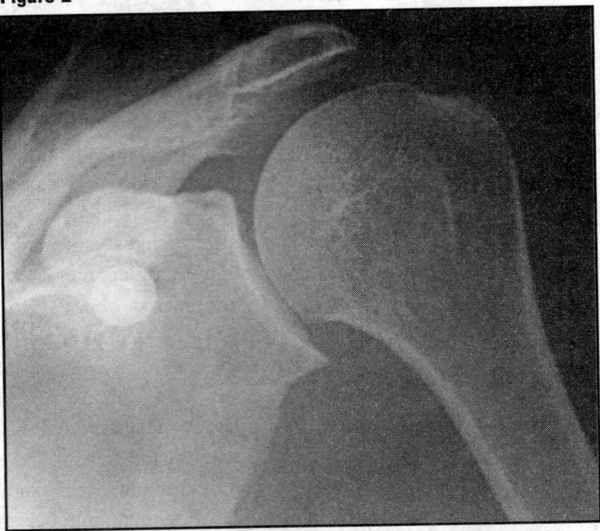

Posterior shoulder dislocation. AP radiograph of a posterior shoulder dislocation. This film could easily be interpreted as normal if some form of lateral radiograph is not obtained. On the routine AP view, there is usually an overlap shadow created by the head of the humerus superimposed on the glenoid fossa. The shadow is a smooth bordered ellipse. In posterior dislocations, the articular surface of the humeral head is posterior to the glenoid and the elliptical overlap shadow is distorted. Also note that the glenoid appears partially vacant—the so called "rim sign." Finally, note the hollowed out appearance of the humeral head.

clinician does not initially consider the problem and misses the diagnosis on physical examination, appropriate radiographs will clearly delineate the problem. Put simply, these injuries should be suspected in all patients who present with shoulder injuries and in all individuals who have suffered a seizure or electrical shock.[3]

History. When obtaining the history in a patient with shoulder trauma, it is important to obtain specific information about the mechanism of injury and the position of the arm at the time of injury. In this regard, posterior glenohumeral dislocations generally occur when the arm is forward flexed and slightly internally rotated. The dislocation can occur when an axial load is applied in this position. Hitting a heavy punching bag or striking the dashboard with the arm extended to the front are examples of mechanisms of injury consistent with this type of dislocation. As a rule, posterior dislocations frequently are the result of indirect forces producing a combination of internal rotation, adduction, and flexion. This injury can be encountered in the patient with seizures, alcohol withdrawal, or electrical shock. In these patients, the diagnosis should be immediately considered and actively ruled out, even if shoulder pain is not part of the presenting complaint.

Examination. There is a constellation of classic physical findings associated with posterior dislocation that may be found on shoulder examination. Generally, the patient will complain of severe pain; as a rule, these injuries tend to be more painful than anterior dislocations. The patient usually will be sitting with the arm held tightly across the front of the trunk. The arm is fixed in a position of adduction and internal rotation; external rotation, whether active or passive, is blocked and abduction is severely limited. The posterior aspect of the shoulder is rounded and more pronounced than the normal shoulder. In contrast, the anterior aspect of the shoulder is flattened, and the coracoid process is prominent if compared to the uninjured side. These contour changes in the shoulder can best be viewed with the patient sitting on a low stool as the examiner stands behind him or her and the gown is draped beneath the patient's shoulders in the axillae. This permits simultaneous visualization of the front and back of the shoulders (bilaterally) for comparison. A more subtle finding, which is always present, is lack of wrist supination on the affected side when the arms are forward flexed.

Radiographs. Appropriate radiographs should be obtained in order to confirm the diagnosis and to identify associated fractures; nevertheless, the initial diagnosis should be made primarily based on findings generated from physical examination of the patient. A routine anteroposterior (AP) shoulder film usually is sufficient to detect a variety of anterior dislocations. Unfortunately, this radiograph is rarely sufficient to diagnose posterior glenohumeral dislocation. It should be stressed that this type of dislocation may look deceptively normal on the AP radiograph because a "routine" AP film of the shoulder does not afford a true AP view of the glenohumeral joint. *(Please see Figures 1 [normal] and 2 [dislocation] at left.)* A routine AP view of the shoulder is taken anteroposteriorly to the plane of the chest. The scapula lies on the posterolateral chest wall at an angle of 45° from the frontal plane; the glenoid, therefore, anteriorly faces 45°. As a result, the routine AP radiograph projects a significant overlap shadow of the humeral head superimposed on about three-fourths of the glenoid. This orientation of the glenohumeral joint to the plane of the AP radiograph prevents visualization of the normal joint space; as a result, loss of this joint space, which is not visualized on the standard AP view of the shoulder, is lost in a posterior dislocation, which presents a significant radiographic pitfall.

Another radiographic problem in the evaluation of posterior shoulder dislocation is associated with the lack of perpendicular views. It is essential that injured portions of the skeleton be imaged with two views oriented perpendicular to one another. The "standard" trauma shoulder series in many institutions includes AP views in internal and external rotation. Such an approach merely provides two oblique views of the same projection rather than views aligned at 90°; the oblique orientation is not sufficient for diagnosing posterior shoulder dislocations. Either an axillary lateral or scapular lateral view is required for adequate evaluation of the shoulder. The scapular lateral is slightly more difficult to interpret for those not familiar with this projection and, therefore, the axillary lateral is preferred by most physicians.

The point should be made that no AP film made in the plane of the chest is diagnostic of posterior dislocation—these films may only be suggestive of the diagnosis. However, there are specific radiographic signs seen on the routine AP view that point toward this injury.

Absence of the normal elliptical shadow. On the routine AP view, there is usually an overlap shadow created by the head of the humerus superimposed on the glenoid fossa. The shadow is a smooth bordered ellipse. In posterior dislocation, the articular surface of the humeral head is posterior to the glenoid and the elliptical overlap shadow is distorted. *(Please see Figure 2.)*

Vacant glenoid sign. In the normal shoulder, the humeral head occupies the majority of the glenoid cavity. In posterior dislocations, the head rests behind the glenoid; as a result, the glenoid fossa appears to be partially vacant. This finding has also been referred to as the positive rim sign. If the space between the anterior rim and the humeral head is greater than 6 mm, a posterior dislocation is likely. *(Please see Figure 2.)*

The "trough line." A "trough line" is noted on the AP radiograph; this is the result of an impaction fracture of the humeral head caused by the posterior rim of the glenoid. It is analogous to the Hill-Sachs impaction fracture seen in anterior dislocations. Radiographically, two parallel lines of cortical bone are visible on the medial cortex of the humeral head. One line represents the medial cortex of the humeral head while the other represents the margin of an impaction fracture. *(Please see Figure 3.)*

"Hollowed out" or "cystic" humeral head. In posterior dislocation, the arm is locked in internal rotation. The x-ray beam, therefore, passes through both the greater and lesser tuberosities, creating the image of a hollow or cystic humeral head.[1,2,4] *(Please see Figure 4.)*

The scapular lateral radiograph is, perhaps, the most clinically useful and patient-friendly shoulder film necessary for diagnosis of posterior dislocation; however, it is used infrequently. *(Please see Figure 5.)* This film can be taken with the patient standing, sitting, or supine, without moving the arm away from the side. It is virtually diagnostic of posterior dislocation. The technique for shooting this film is relatively easy. The arm is left undisturbed in the position of comfort for the patient. The anterolateral portion of the injured shoulder is placed against the cassette. The x-ray beam passes tangentially across the posterolateral chest parallel to and down from the spine of the scapula onto the cassette. The resulting image represents a true lateral of the scapula and, therefore, of the glenohumeral joint. In order to properly interpret the view, one must understand the three-dimensional anatomy of the scapula. In the lateral view, the scapula projects as the letter "Y." The vertical stem of the "Y" is the body of the scapula, and the upper fork is formed by the juncture of the coracoid and the acromion processes. The glenoid is located at the junction of the stem and the apex of the fork, which is visible as a dense circle of bone. In the normal shoulder, the humeral head should be centered on the point of intersection of the stem and branches of the upper fork.

Figure 3

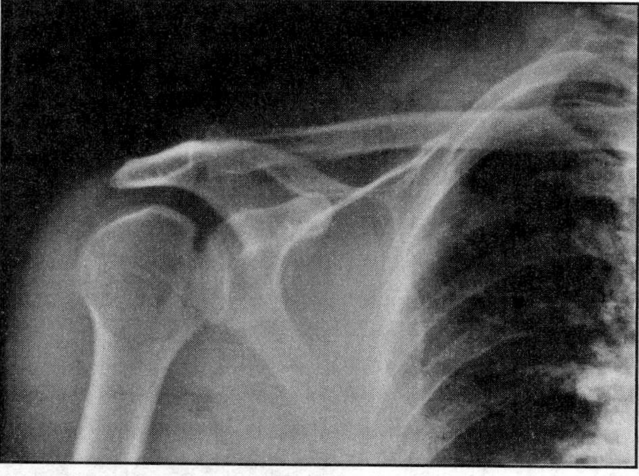

Posterior shoulder dislocation with double cortical line or trough line. A trough line is noted on the AP radiograph, the result of the impaction fracture of the humeral head caused by the posterior rim of the glenoid; it is analogous to the Hill-Sachs impaction fracture seen in anterior dislocations. Radiographically, two parallel lines of cortical bone are visible on the medial cortex of the humeral head. One line represents the medial cortex of the humeral head, while the other represents the margin of an impaction fracture.

Figure 4

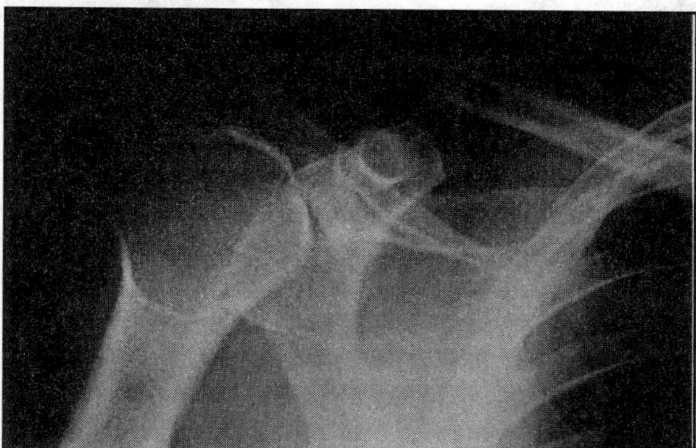

Posterior shoulder dislocation with hollow or cystic humeral head. In posterior dislocation, the arm is locked in internal rotation. The x-ray beam, therefore, passes through both the greater and lesser tuberosities, creating the image of a hollow or cystic humeral head. Also note the increased overlap of the humeral head on the glenoid.

this painful position. There are two commonly used and relatively painless variations of the classic axillary radiograph that also provide an adequate lateral view. A camera axillary lateral view can be obtained without abducting the injured shoulder. In this view, the humerus is forward flexed 20-30°, the cassette is placed superior to the shoulder, and the x-ray tube is inferior to the elbow. The Velpeau axillary lateral projection is another view that does not require abduction of the painful shoulder.[2] In this view, the patient is placed in a Velpeau dressing and asked to lean backward 30° over the cassette on the table. The tube is then positioned above the shoulder and the beam is directed vertically down onto the cassette. This view is

Figure 5

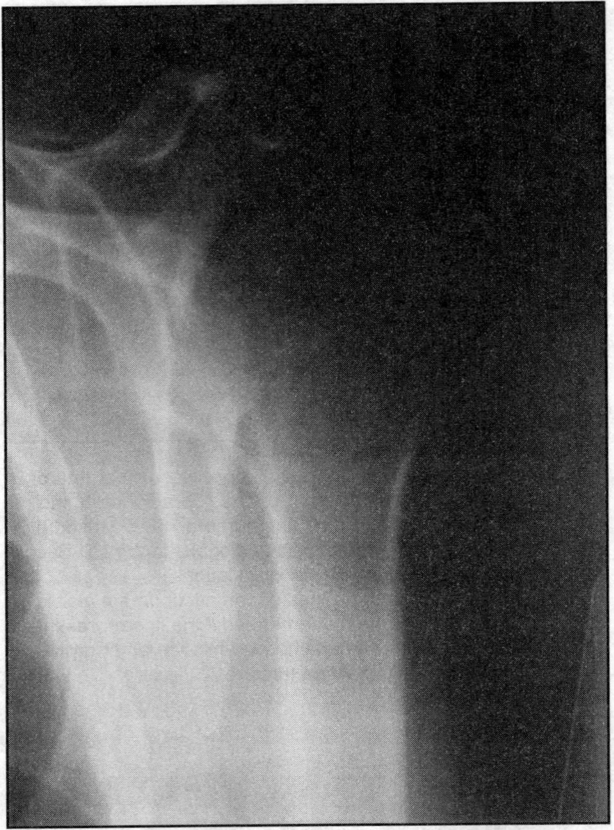

Posterior shoulder dislocation. Scapular lateral radiograph of a posterior dislocation. The glenoid is clearly visible at the junction of the stem and apex of the upper fork of the "Y." The humeral head is clearly not centered in the glenoid.

Figure 6

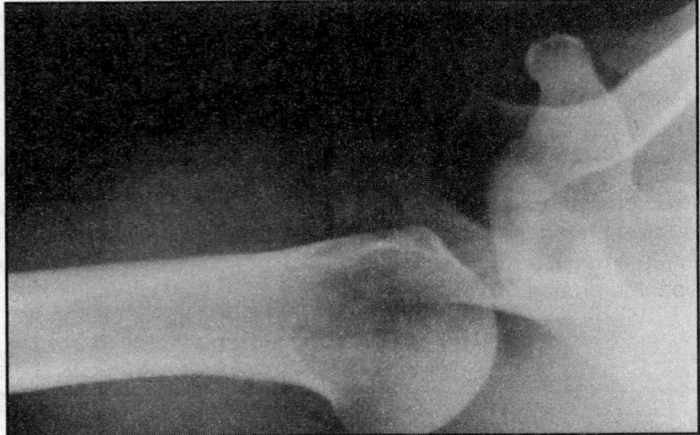

Posterior shoulder dislocation. Axillary lateral view of a posterior dislocation. The humeral head is clearly posterior to the glenoid.

The axillary lateral radiograph is the most commonly ordered lateral view and is also the easiest to interpret. *(Please see Figure 6.)* Unfortunately, as it is classically described, it requires the patient to lie supine and his or her arm to be abducted 70-90° with the cassette above the shoulder and the tube positioned near the hip. Radiology technicians are understandably reluctant to position the patient in particularly helpful following reduction when the patient is in a shoulder immobilizer.

Management. Patients with acute traumatic posterior dislocations are generally in more severe pain than those with anterior dislocations. The use of intravenous sedation and muscle relaxants, while almost always successful in the reduction of anterior dislocations, may be insufficient for posterior dislocations. Not infrequently, these patients require general anesthesia. However, reduction in the ED should be attempted under sedation, with muscle relaxation prior to subjecting the patient to general anesthesia. The patient should be placed supine, and traction should be applied to the adducted arm in the line of deformity. While applying traction, the humeral head should be gently lifted back into the glenoid fossa. The arm should not be forced into external rotation. If the head is locked on the glenoid rim, forced rotation may fracture the head or shaft of the humerus. If the pre-reduction radiographs reveal the head to be locked on the glenoid rim, distal traction should be combined with lateral traction on the upper arm. This combined traction approach can be accomplished by an assistant using a folded towel to apply the lateral contribution.

The type of post-reduction immobilization depends on the stability of the shoulder after reduction. If the shoulder is stable, a sling and swathe or standard immobilizer are adequate. If, however, the shoulder tends to sublux in the sling and swathe, a shoulder spica cast will need to be applied, with the shoulder positioned in external rotation. When available, orthopedic consultation should be obtained in the ED; if it is not available and reduction is correctly performed, prompt outpatient orthopedic follow-up is necessary. Fractures of the glenoid rim, humeral head, tuberosities, and upper humeral shaft are commonly associated with the posterior shoulder dislocation. The incidence of coexistent fractures is approximately 50%.[5] These fractures contribute to the frequency of misdiagnosis as they lead the physician to believe that he or she has identified a source of the pain and motion loss. Posterior dislocation should be considered in all proximal humerus or glenoid fractures; a lateral film must be obtained. Neurologic injuries are far more common with anterior dislocation but still must be ruled out with posterior dislocation. These injuries generally spontaneously recover. Vascular injuries are also rare in glenohumeral dislocations, but must be considered. This is particularly true in the elderly patient who has atherosclerotic vascular disease with loss of vessel elasticity. Oftentimes, the only physical finding in these cases is asymmetry of pulses compared with the normal side.

Inferior (Luxatio Erecta) Glenohumeral Dislocation

Inferior shoulder dislocation, also known as luxatio erecta, is a rare form of shoulder dislocation. The incidence of luxatio erecta is reported to be 0.5% of all shoulder dislocations. Luxatio erecta can occur in any age group. The injury is most often unilateral; simultaneous bilateral luxatio erecta has been reported.

Luxatio erecta presents in a unique and unusual fashion. The initial impression may suggest hysteria. Careful attention must be directed toward making the distinction between anterior and inferior shoulder dislocations. A recent report describing luxatio erecta suggests it is initially misdiagnosed as an anterior dislocation.[6] In this case, standard approaches to reduction of anterior dislocation were unsuccessful. Only after orthopedic referral and complete radiographic evaluation was the correct diagnosis made. Multiple attempts at reduction carry the risks of iatrogenic injury. Consequently, the suspicion of luxatio erecta must be present when examining all shoulder dislocations.

The mechanism of injury involves hyperabduction of the arm at the shoulder with extension at the elbow. The forearm is pronated. Direct or violent force is applied to the shoulder from a superior direction, causing inferior movement of the humeral head relative to the glenoid fossa. The inferior portion of the glenohumeral capsule is then disrupted, and inferior glenohumeral dislocation occurs. Alternatively, leverage of the humeral head across the acromion by a hyperabduction force also can result in inferior dislocation of the humeral head.

Clinical Presentation. The presentation of inferior dislocation of the shoulder is unique. The patient usually presents in distress with the involved arm hyperabducted at the shoulder and flexed at the elbow. The forearm frequently rests behind the head. An anxious patient presenting with either one or both arms raised above the head can suggest hysteria. Patient or physician attempts at adduction are extremely painful. The glenoid fossa is empty and the humeral head is palpitated in the axilla adjacent to the lateral chest wall. Skin creases are noted on the superior aspect of the shoulder, indicating the acute angle formed by the acromion and humerus. Neurovascular compromise may be found. Radiographic examination of the shoulder in cases of suspected luxatio erecta includes the following views: AP views in both internal and external rotation and lateral views including the "Y" or axillary approaches. The AP view often will demonstrate an inferior displacement of the humeral head relative to the glenoid; furthermore, the arm is hyerabducted at the shoulder. *(Please see Figure 7A.)* The lateral views, in particular the axillary view, closely defines the relationship of the humeral head and glenoid fossa and are of significant use in difficult cases.

Treatment in the ED most frequently involves closed reduction with adequate muscle relaxation and anesthesia. *(Please see Figure 7B.)* In-line traction should be applied to the fully abducted arm while firm, cephalad pressure is maintained on the humeral head. Counter-traction is used with a rolled bed sheet placed superior to the shoulder.[7] When the humeral head is reduced into the glenoid fossa, the arm is adducted toward the body and the forearm is supinate. Post reduction, the shoulder is immobilized in the typical fashion (either a sling and swathe or shoulder immobilization), and outpatient orthopedic referral should be arranged.

Associated injuries are common and include: disruptions of various shoulder muscles (supraspinatus, infraspinatus, subscapularis, and pectoralis major); fractures of the clavicle, coracoid, acromion, inferior glenoid, and greater tuberosity of the humerus; and neurovascular compromise involving the brachial plexus and the axillary artery. Concomitant fracture or rotator cuff injury is reported in 80% of cases. Additionally, 60% of these patients manifest neurologic injury on presentation, most commonly to the axillary nerve. The neurologic deficits usually resolve in rapid fashion. A small percentage of cases are complicated by vascular injury. Fracture of the greater tuberosity of the humerus reportedly spares injury to the rotator cuff. The prognosis for normal shoulder function in complicated cases is usually favorable. Recurrent inferior dislocation of the shoulder is very unusual. Violent injuries have resulted in open fractures complicating the inferior dislocation.

Figure 7A

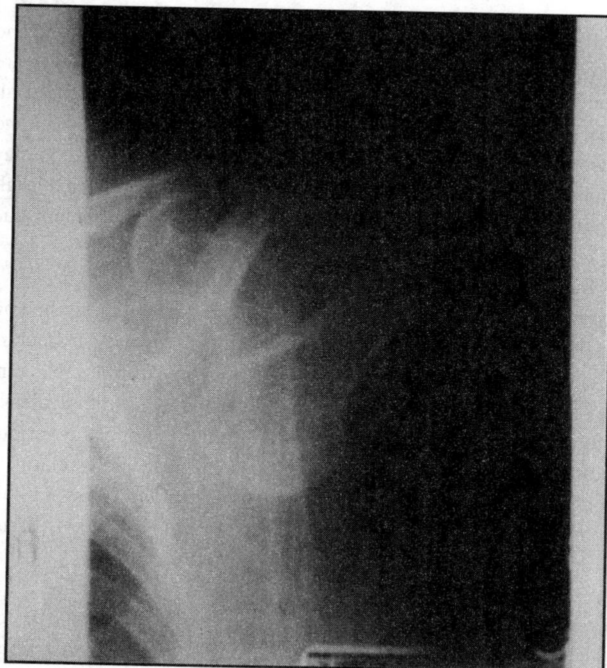

Inferior shoulder dislocation. Left shoulder radiograph demonstrating inferior dislocation of the humeral head. Note the inferior position of the humeral head relative to the glenoid. The arm is hyperabducted at the shoulder.

Figure 7B

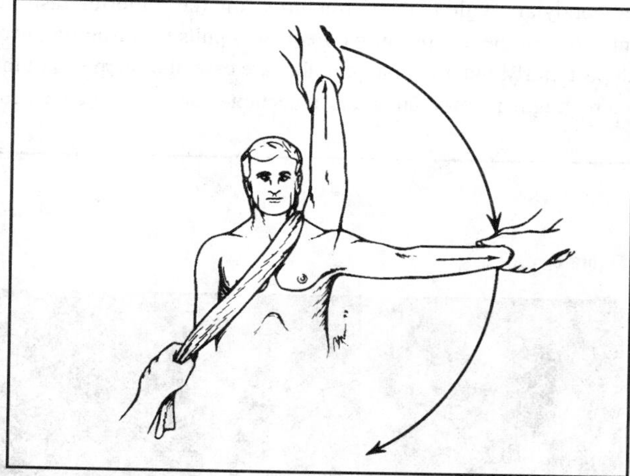

Reduction technique in the patient with inferior glenohumoral dislocation. The patient is placed in the supine position and given intravenous sedation, analgesia, and muscle relaxation. In-line traction is applied to the fully abducted arm while firm cephalad pressure is maintained on the humeral head. Counter-traction is used with a rolled bed sheet placed superior to the shoulder. When the humeral head is reduced into the glenoid fossa, the arm is adducted toward the body and the forearm supinated.
Reproduced with permission from Brady WJ, Knuth CJ, Pirrallo RG. Bilateral inferior glenohumeral dislocation: Luxatio Erecta, an unusual presentation of a rare disorder. *J Emerg Med* 1995;13:37-42.

Elbow Fractures

Injuries involving the elbow usually are correctly diagnosed and appropriately managed in the ED. Two specific injuries, however, are frequently missed: the pediatric supracondylar fracture and the adult radial head fracture. Both injuries present with significant pain and nonspecific soft-tissue swelling and tenderness. The radiograph may be unrevealing, since, in children, the elbow is a difficult area to evaluate roentgenographically with the multiple ossification centers, and the adult elbow often "hides" fracture.

Supracondylar Fracture. The supracondylar fracture is a bony injury of the distal humerus that is found proximal to the epicondyles. The vast majority of patients with supracondylar fracture are children, with a mean age of 7 years; this type of fracture is rare after the patient reaches 15 years of age. This pediatric prevalence results from a mismatch in structural strength among the various elbow tissues. The ligamentous and capsular tissues are relatively stronger than the bony structures. Consequently, stress in this region is more likely to produce bony injury rather than soft-tissue disruption; the converse is true with the adult, in that a similar injury mechanism results in posterior elbow dislocation. Supracondylar fractures are described as either flexion or extension type; flexion fractures account for a small percentage of supracondylar injuries, while extension-mediated lesions occur in more than 95% of cases.

As a rule, extension supracondylar fractures result from a fall on the outstretched arm with the elbow fully extended or hyperextended. The force of impact is usually directed in forward fashion, producing a torque force at the elbow. The distal humerus in the supracondylar region then fractures in the anterior aspect. Contraction of the triceps muscle frequently pulls the distal fragment both posteriorly and proximally. In the rare case, the sharp end of the fracture fragment may enter the antecubital area, producing neurovascular injury to the brachial artery and median nerve; most often, soft-tissue protects the neurovascular structures from laceration.

Clinical Presentation. Examination will reveal a child in significant distress, holding the arm extended at the elbow in the usual "S"-shaped position. Soft-tissue swelling and tenderness are found about the elbow, and limited range of motion is noted on examination. With complete fractures, the olecranon, which is attached to the fracture fragment, is palpable. Incomplete fractures produce less obvious deformity; soft-tissue swelling and nonspecific tenderness may be the only findings. The neurovascular status must be evaluated.

Radiographically, complete injuries are obvious on the film. On the lateral view, the fractured fragment is displaced proximally and posteriorly; the AP film may reveal medial or lateral displacement of the fragment. Since these fractures predominantly occur in children with elastic bony structures, incomplete injuries are common and represent a diagnostic challenge. In fact, approximately one-quarter of supracondylar fractures are of the greenstick variety—disruption occurs along the anterior aspect of the humerus while the posterior portion remains intact. The lateral view may demonstrate only abnormal fat pads while the AP film may be negative, particularly if the fracture line is transversely oriented. Fractures may be divided as follows: Type I, minimal to no displacement; Type II, incomplete injury with minimal to moderate displacement and/or intact posterior cortex; and Type III, complete displacement of fragment with posterior cortical disruption. In most instances, the fracture is apparent on the film; certain patients, however, will have occult bony injury. Two radiographic markers are useful in this setting—the anterior humeral line *(please see Figures 8 and 9)* and the fat pad signs. *(Please see Figure 10.)* The anterior humeral line is helpful in evaluating possible supracondylar fracture in the pediatric patient. A line is drawn along the anterior aspect of the distal humerus extending through the elbow. In the normal state, the line will bisect the middle of the capitellum. *(Please see Figure 8.)* In the child with a supracondylar

Figure 8

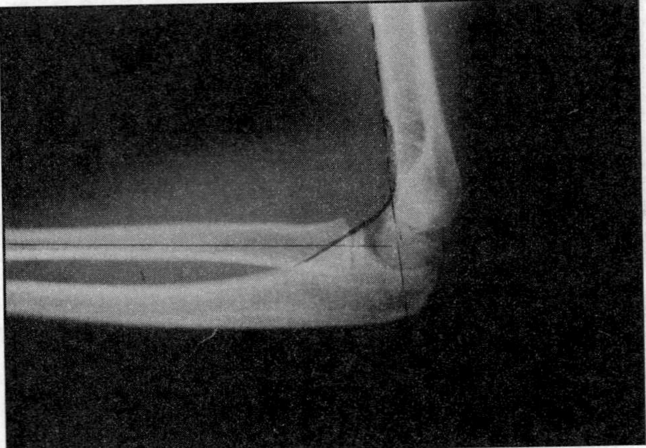

The anterior humeral line. The anterior humeral line is useful in evaluating possible supracondylar fracture in the pediatric patient. A line is drawn along the anterior aspect of the distal humerus extending through the elbow. In the normal state, the line will bisect the middle third of the capitellum.

Figure 9

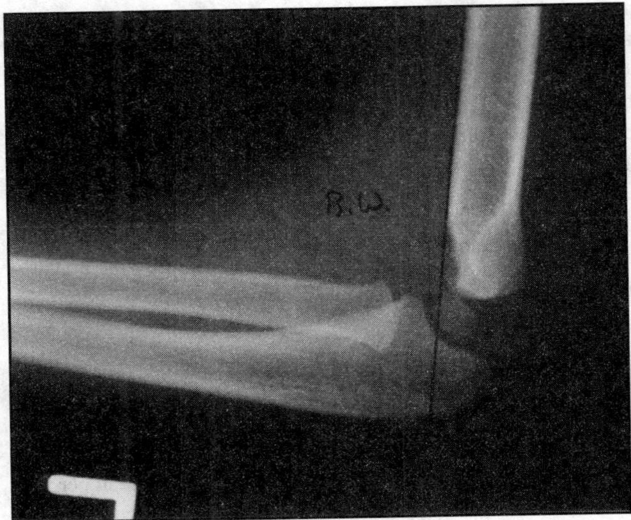

The child with supracondylar fracture. In the child with supracondylar fracture, this line will either strike the anterior third of the capitellum or miss it entirely—anterior to the capitellum.

fracture, this line will either strike the anterior third of the capitellum or miss it entirely, appearing anterior to the capitellum. *(Please see Figure 9.)*

The fat pad sign results from swelling adjacent to the distal humerus. In the uninjured elbow, fat located about the elbow joint found in bony recesses and is essentially radiographically hidden. The anterior fat pad is often present in the normal patient as a narrow strip of radiolucency along the distal humerus; the posterior fat pad is not seen in the uninjured patient. With fractures involving intra-articular structures about the elbow, hemorrhage and/or edema fluid will distend the joint capsule and displace the fat out of the bony concavities, producing the radiographically evident fat pad signs. The abnormal anterior fat pad is seen as a triangular structure resembling a sail boat spinnaker along the anterior aspect of the distal humerus. The appearance of a posterior fat pad of any morphology is considered abnormal. In the patient with traumatic elbow pain, an abnormal fat pad is associated with fracture in 90% of cases. The presence of a fat pad should prompt the emergency physician to strongly consider an occult fracture, especially an incomplete supracondylar fracture in a child or a radial head fracture in the adult.

Management. Treatment in the ED should be tailored according to radiographic injury type listed above. Type I fractures are mechanically stable; splinting may be used primarily for pain control and comfort. Type II injuries should be reduced, preferably by an orthopedist. After reduction, splinting or casting at 120° of flexion is recommended in most cases; the exception is the patient with significant soft-tissue swelling who is at risk for vascular compromise at the elbow. A rare patient with Type II injury may require surgical stabilization.

Type III fractures require ED reduction, once again, by an orthopedist. These fractures are associated with loss of arm length, various deformities, and neurovascular compromise. The emergency physician may attempt reduction if vascular compromise is encountered; otherwise, this maneuver should be performed by an orthopedic surgeon in the ED at the time of initial visit. Closed reduction can be accomplished after adequate conscious sedation (muscle relaxation/pain control) has been achieved. The physician applies traction at the wrist in line with the upper extremity, with the thumb in the "up" position. Any medial or lateral deformity is corrected. With restoration of the arm's length, the elbow is slowly and gently flexed to 100°. Any angulation is corrected at this stage. Supracondylar fractures with medial displacement are immobilized with the forearm pronated; laterally displaced fractures are immobilized with the arm supinate. Post-reduction radiographs should be obtained while a repeat neurovascular examination is performed. If this reduction attempt is unsuccessful, further attempts should not be made. Circulation may be restored with traction applied to the arm with the elbow extended while the orthopedist is en route to the ED. Admission to the hospital should be considered with a displaced supracondylar fracture since these patients are prone to vascular compromise. Inpatient disposition allows close observation of the perfusion status of the arm. In most cases of compromised perfusion, edema rather than arterial injury is the usual culprit force.

Radial Head Fracture

The radial head fracture usually results from a fall on the outstretched hand in an adult patient. The impact is transmitted axially

Figure 10

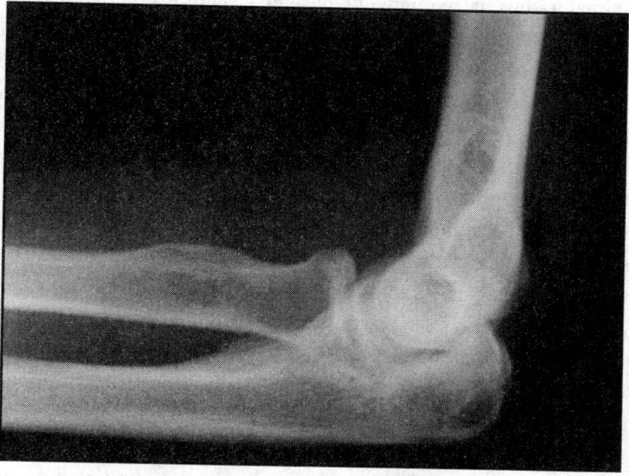

Fat pad signs. The anterior fat pad is often present in the normal patient as a narrow strip of radiolucency along the distal humerus; the posterior fat pad is not seen in the uninjured patient. With fracture about the elbow involving intra-articular structures, hemorrhage and/or edema fluid will distend the joint capsule and displace the fat out of the bony concavities, producing the radiographically evident fat pad signs. The abnormal anterior fat pad is seen here as a triangular structure resembling a sail boat spinnaker sail along the anterior aspect of the distal humerus. The appearance of a posterior fat pad of any morphology is considered abnormal. The presence of a fat pad should prompt the emergency physician to strongly consider an occult fracture—particularly the incomplete supracondylar fracture in a child or the adult radial head fracture (as seen in this example).

Figure 11

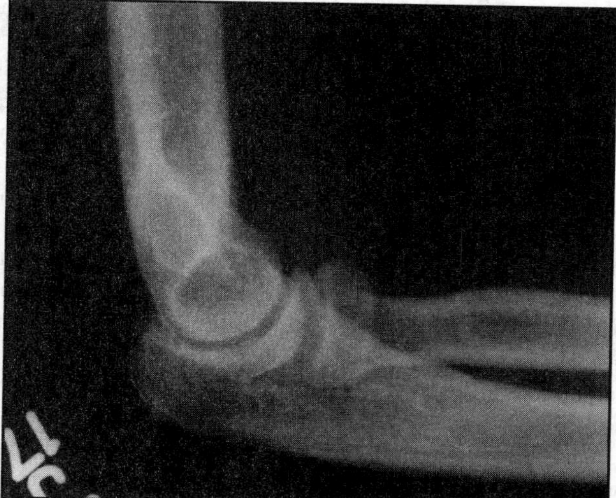

Radial head fracture. Undisplaced radial head fractures are difficult to detect radiographically. The normal cortex of the radial head is smooth with a continuous concave morphology. Any irregularity of the radial head, particularly in association with an abnormal fat pad, is a radial head fracture until proven otherwise. An abnormal anterior fat pad (triangular shape) is seen here as well.

through the radius, forcing the radial head against the capitellum; the proximal radius is a relatively weaker structure compared to the capitellum, resulting in a fracture. The examination is nonspecific, revealing tenderness and soft-tissue swelling at the elbow. The radiograph may demonstrate either an obvious fracture or only the presence of pathologic fat pads, which are strongly suggestive of an occult fracture. Undisplaced radial head fractures are difficult to detect radiographically. The normal cortex of the radial head is smooth with a continuous concave morphology. Consequently, any irregularity of the radial head, particularly in association with an abnormal fat pad, is a radial head fracture until proven otherwise. *(Please see Figure 11.)* As with the supracondylar fracture, the radial head fracture may be classified along the following lines: Type I, undisplaced; Type II, minimal displacement; Type III, comminuted fracture; and Type IV, any fracture with dislocation.

Type I injuries are symptomatically treated with sling support and early application of range-of-motion exercises (initiated on day two). Joint aspiration with infusion of an anesthetic agent may drastically reduce pain, although this maneuver has no effect on outcome. Most patients will return to preinjury functional status, although a minority of patients will experience long-term disability (pain and contracture). Type II injuries may be treated in similar fashion; such patients may require surgery with excision of the radial head if patients fail range-of-motion maneuvering. Type III injuries should receive a similar approach in the ED with early orthopedic follow-up for surgical removal of the radial head. Type IV fractures are managed with reduction of dislocation and early surgical excision of the radial head. Outcomes of patients with Types III and IV fractures are excellent.

Wrist Injuries

One of the most common but inaccurate diagnoses made in the injured extremity is wrist sprain. Although wrist sprains do occur, the diagnosis should only be considered *after* careful physical and radiographic examinations have ruled out fracture and dislocation in this anatomic region. In fact, the diagnosis of *wrist* sprain usually is one of *exclusion*. Accurate diagnosis of wrist injuries is dependent on a thorough knowledge of the topographical anatomy of the wrist and careful, systematic evaluation of the extremity and appropriate radiographs. Although the wrist fracture/dislocation is a rare entity among all cases of extremity trauma, several injuries deserve attention, including scaphoid fractures, scapholunate dissociations, distal radioulnar joint dislocations, hamate hook fractures, and triquetral avulsion fractures. These injuries are easily missed in the ED and have significant morbidity associated with delayed diagnosis.

Since demonstration of specific point tenderness within the carpus is the most important diagnostic test in assessing injuries to the wrist, it is critical that physicians be comfortable with the anatomy of this area. The wrist bones should be palpable in the normal uninjured wrist. Radially, the anatomic snuffbox is the area between the tendons of the first and third dorsal compartments on the radial side of the wrist. This area is best palpated by bringing the thumb into radial abduction (the hitchhiker's position), defining the hollow situated between the extensor pollicus longus, the abductor pollicus longus, and extensor pollicus brevis. The radial styloid is palpable at the base of the snuffbox, and the body of the scaphoid is palpable in the depths of this area. On the ulnar aspect of the wrist, the ulnar head and styloid are palpated. The position of these structures varies with pronation and supination of the forearm. In a neutral position, the ulnar styloid is prominent at the ulnar side of the wrist. The ulnar head is palpable dorsally in pronation and palmarly in supination.

On the palmar aspect, the distal wrist crease is the visible landmark that defines the underlying anatomy. Radially, at the intersection of the flexor carpi radialis tendon and the wrist crease, the scaphoid tuberosity is palpable as a bony prominence at the base of the thenar muscles. Ulnarly, the pisiform is palpable at the junction of the flexor carpi ulnaris and the wrist crease. Immediately distal and radial to the pisiform is the hook of the hamate. The area between the scaphoid tuberosity and the pisiform contains the contents of the carpal tunnel, the area where abnormal prominences will be palpable in perilunate dislocations. The area just proximal to the proximal wrist crease is where the ulnar head will be palpably prominent in a volar dislocation of the distal radioulnar joint.

On the dorsum of the wrist, Lister's tubercle is the most significant landmark. Just distal to this bony ridge is the scapholunate junction. Just distal to the ulnar head and radial to its styloid lies the lunotriquetral junction. These two areas are common sites of injury. Dorsally, abnormal bony prominences usually represent the dorsally displaced rim of the distal radius or the proximal row of carpal bones that are palpable because of the dorsal collapse of the fractured distal radius. The distal ulna will also seem prominent relative to a shortened distal radius. The metacarpal shafts are easily palpable on the dorsum of the hand, and, when followed proximally, they lead to the easily palpable prominences of the carpometacarpal joints, which are the most distal structures of the wrist.

Familiarity with this anatomy is critical since the best and most dependable sign of carpal injury is specific and well-localized point tenderness. Fractures of the scaphoid demonstrate point tenderness in the anatomic snuffbox and over the scaphoid tuberosity. Scapholunate and lunate injuries will be maximally tender just distal to Lister's tubercle on the dorsum of the wrist. Triquetral and lunotriquetral injuries will be tender over the dorsum of the appropriate bone one fingerbreadth distal to the ulnar head. The diagnosis of a hamate hook fracture is almost always made clinically by eliciting tenderness over the area just distal and radial to the pisiform.

Scaphoid Fracture. Of all wrist injuries, fracture of the scaphoid is the most commonly missed diagnosis. Fractures of the scaphoid account for 60-70% of all diagnosed carpal injuries. Radiographic findings are either subtle or absent, making the diagnosis difficult in the absence of a thorough clinical examination by an informed clinician who has a high index of suspicion. Accurate, early diagnosis is critical, as the morbidity associated with a missed or late diagnosis is significant.

The classic history for scaphoid fracture is a fall on the outstretched hand (FOOSH). The patient generally has immediate pain, but may have little or no swelling and is able to continue his or her activity. Not uncommonly, these injuries are associated with other injuries about the upper extremity; the wrist complaint may actually be a lower priority from the patient's perspective. Proper palpation during physical examination, however, will exacerbate pain, prompting the physician to obtain the proper films. The patient's degree of swelling, discomfort, and motion loss are variable. Palpation of the scaphoid body in the anatomic snuffbox is the most reliable diagnostic maneuver. Additionally, however, direct palpation of the scaphoid tuberosity palmarly should also elicit complaints of tenderness.

Radiography. Although the diagnosis of scaphoid fracture is suggested by the history and physical examination, in a majority of cases it is confirmed only by radiographic evaluation. It is critical to visualize the bone with two views oriented perpendicularly. On the AP view, it is best to align the longitudinal axis of the scaphoid parallel with the film; this alignment is best accomplished by positioning the wrist in ulnar deviation, placing the scaphoid in an extended position. Performing this view with the fist clenched will also provide an axial load and accentuate any scapholunate diastasis that may be present as part of a scapholunate dissociation. Even with appropriate films, these fractures can be subtle and difficult to see. A significant percentage of these fractures will not be acutely visible on any view. *(Please see Figures 12 and 13.)* In the acute management of these injuries, the films are actually more important for ruling out concomitant injuries than for accurately diagnosing the scaphoid fracture itself.

All suspected scaphoid fractures initially should be treated as though a fracture exists (i.e., splint and refer to an orthopedist for repeat evaluation). Since a number of these fractures are not radiographically detectable on initial presentation, any patient with an appropriate history and snuffbox or tuberosity tenderness should be treated with a thumb spica splint and evaluated by an orthopedist in 10-14 days for repeat studies. Strict adherence to this policy will ensure that any fracture with subtle or absent radiographic initial findings will still be appropriately treated without delay. An undiagnosed and improperly treated scaphoid fracture is complicated by chronic pain, reduced functional ability, and early arthritis due to the ischemic necrosis and malunion. *(Please see Figure 13.)*

Figure 12

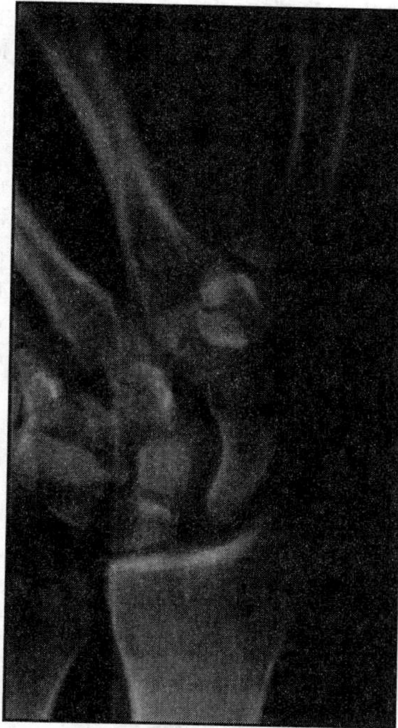

Occult scaphoid fracture. AP view of the wrist in ulnar deviation taken at the time of injury. Note that there is no fracture line visible. Despite a suggestive mechanism (FOOSH) coupled with anatomical snuffbox tenderness, the patient was not appropriately treated for a scaphoid injury (thumb spica splint and orthopedic follow-up). The undiagnosed, radiographically occult scaphoid fracture resulted in chronic pain and ultimate functional instability of the wrist due to nonunion, as noted in Figure 13.

Figure 13

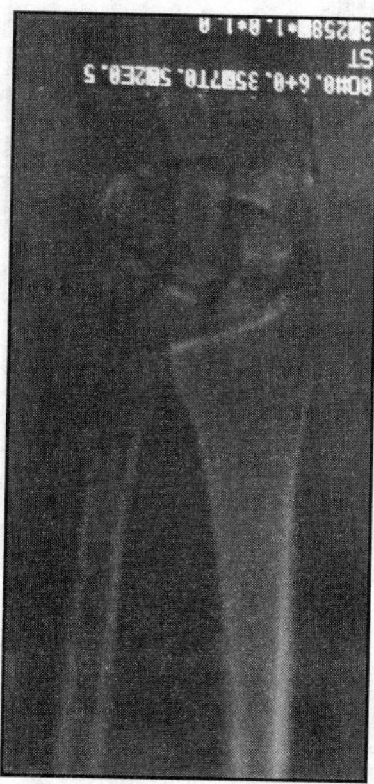

Initially occult scaphoid fracture with ultimate nonunion. Patient from Figure 12 presented several months later complaining that the "sprain" had never gotten better. Note the established nonunion.

Scapholunate Dissociation

Scapholunate dissociation is the most common form of carpal instability. Despite the literature supporting the importance of early diagnosis and treatment, this problem is rarely recognized on initial presentation. With the growing awareness of the problem of occult scaphoid fracture, scapholunate dissociation seems to have replaced this carpal fracture as the most commonly misdiagnosed cause of the wrist sprain diagnosis. If recognized initially and treated appropriately, this condition has a very good prognosis for recovery of both motion and function. If treatment is delayed, however, chronic disability is inevitable. These patients do not necessarily have tenderness in the anatomic snuffbox and their symptoms resolve rapidly; consequently, if the diagnosis is not made or suspected in the ED, the patient may never see an orthopedist until the condition becomes chronic and the outcome much less favorable.

These injuries occur with hyperextension and/or the FOOSH mechanism. Subjectively, the complaints of pain vary from minimal to excruciating. Patients will often complain of weakness and possibly a "click" or "clunk" with gripping activity. Additionally, the patient who presents to the ED with complaints of a growing dorsal wrist mass should be evaluated with radiographs as a dorsal ganglion can be associated with the chronic form of this condition. The most important aspect of the physical examination, as with all wrist injuries, is precise localization of the point of maximal tenderness. These patients will localize their tenderness to the scapholunate junction, which is palpable just distal to Lister's tubercle. They may or may not also have snuffbox or tuberosity tenderness. Wrist motion is variable and may be extremely limited or may be nearly normal; the degree of swelling is also very variable.

Radiographs. The radiographic findings in this condition are numerous and readily visible on three films. The supinate AP, clenched fist AP, and lateral views will demonstrate the following characteristic findings: 1.) widening of the scapholunate gap greater 3 mm, the Terry Thomas sign (an indicator of scapholunate dissociation that is best visualized on a is supinate AP or clenched fist AP view) *(Please see Figure 14.)*; 2.) foreshortened appearance of the scaphoid in palmar flexed position on the AP view; 3.) cortical ring sign seen in the AP view, representing a double density shadow produced by the axial projection of the abnormally oriented scaphoid upon itself; 4.) on the lateral view, the scaphoid lies more perpendicular to the axis of the radius rather than at its usual angle of 45-60°; 5.) trapezoidal lunate as seen on the AP view is produced by a trian-

Figure 14A

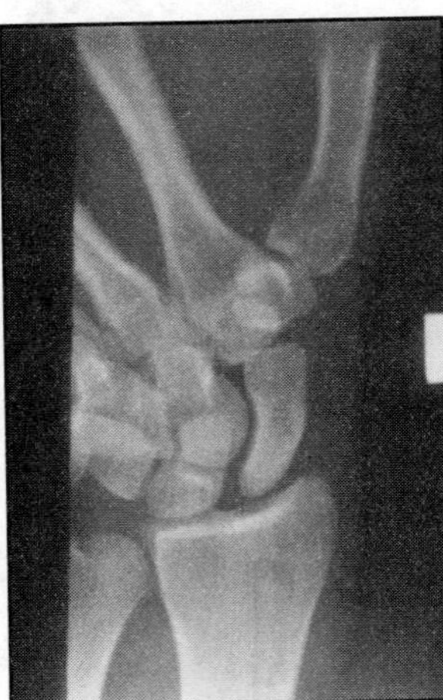

Scapholunate dissociation. Widening of the scapholunate gap to greater than 3 mm, the Terry Thomas sign, is an indicator of scapholunate dissociation, which is best visualized on a supinated AP or clenched fist AP view.

Figure 14B

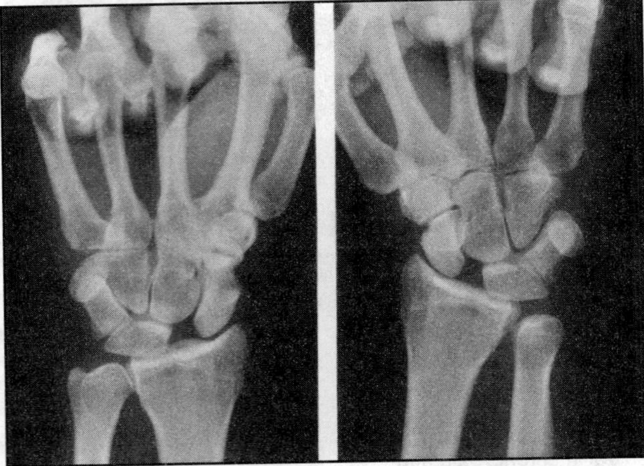

AP of the wrist demonstrates a scapholunate dissociation. Note the increased scapholunate gap, the flexed position of the scaphoid, the cortical ring sign, and the trapezoidal shape of the lunate.

Figure 14C

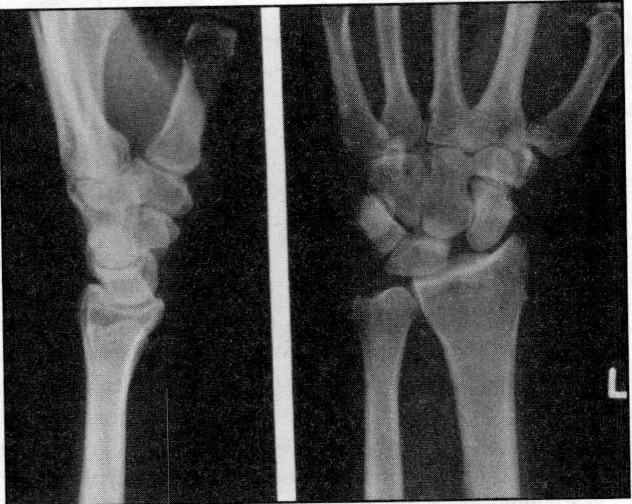

Lateral view of the wrist in scapholunate dissociation. Note the increased scapholunate angle and the extended position of the lunate relative to the radius and the capitate.

gular shape of the lunate as it overlaps the capitate, an indicator of the rotation of the lunate into an extended position; and 6.) Taleisnik's "V" sign is produced by palmar flexion of the scaphoid leading to a more acute angle between the distal radius and scaphoid forming a sharper "V" shaped pattern rather than the broad, c-shaped arc seen in the normal wrist.

Treatment for this disorder is relatively simple in the ED. A thumb spica splint is applied acutely and referral is made to an orthopedic or hand surgeon for operative repair. This referral is not emergent, although the patient should be seen within 10 days to facilitate early repair. The real key for ensuring appropriate treatment for this potentially disabling condition is to have a high index of suspicion and to make the diagnosis acutely so that early repair is possible.

Dislocations of the Distal Radioulnar Joint

Isolated dislocation of the distal radioulnar joint is uncommon; unfortunately, however, it may not be initially recognized in the ED. Delay in the treatment of this injury leads to significant disability, since treatment options for chronic distal radioulnar joint are limited and suboptimal. However, this injury is relatively easy to treat and carries a reasonable prognosis if recognized early.

Isolated subluxations or dislocations of this joint occur from falls, twisting injuries, or suddenly lifting heavy loads with the wrist outstretched. Although the ulna actually stays fixed in space, it is actually the radius and carpus that dislocate about the ulna; convention dictates that these injuries be classified according to the position of the ulna relative to the radius. Dorsal dislocations of the ulna occur with hyperpronation injuries, while palmar or volar dislocations occur with hypersupination injuries. Patients complain of a painful loss of rotation of the forearm. The clinical examination, therefore, is critical for diagnosing the condition. Dorsal dislocations present with an asymmetrically prominent distal ulna dorsally associated with a painful loss of supination. Palmar dislocation manifests with a wrist that is narrowed in its AP diameter and full on the palmar ulnar aspect; a corresponding dorsal sulcus (i.e., an empty space) where the ulnar head should be palpable. Pronation is painfully limited or impossible.

Radiographs. Subluxations and dislocations of the distal radioulnar joint can be difficult to detect radiographically. The signs are often subtle and only are apparent if there is a high index of suspicion. Inability of the technician to obtain what you believe to be adequate AP and lateral films should trigger suspicion of this injury. It is very difficult to obtain true laterals in this condition. Dorsal dislocations, in particular, are difficult to recognize. The appearance of the ulnar head dorsally above the radius can be misleading. When the head of the ulna appears dorsally, the clinician should evaluate the alignment of the triquetrum with the ulna on the lateral view; if the triquetrum is not aligned with the ulna, a dorsal dislocation is likely. Palmar dislocation is somewhat easier to recognize. On the AP view, the ulnar head lies partially superimposed on the radial metaphysis, the forearm is narrowed, the sigmoid notch is empty, and the ulnar styloid is often fractured near its base. *(Please see Figure 15.)* On the lateral view, the ulna is displaced beneath the radial metaphysis. *(Please see Figure 16.)*

Figure 15

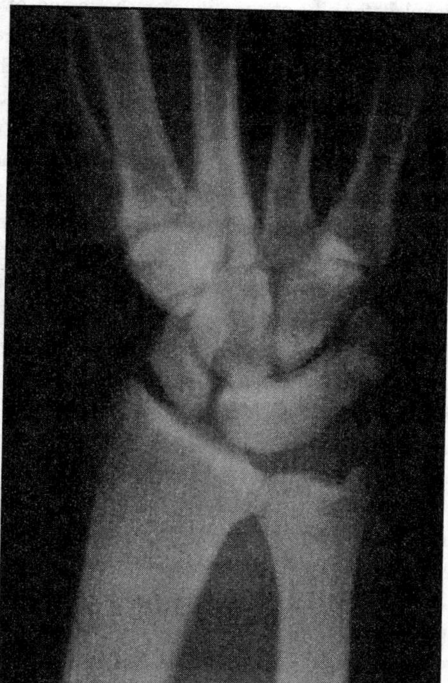

Distal radioulnar joint dislocation. AP view of the wrist in a volar DRUJ dislocation. Note the narrowed appearance of the wrist and the empty appearance of the sigmoid notch.

Figure 16

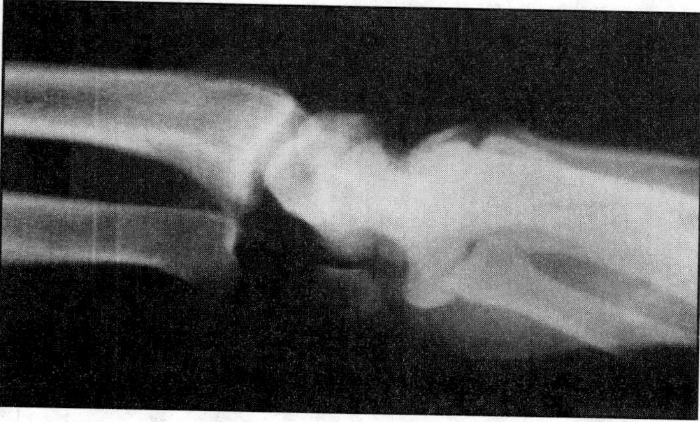

Distal radioulnar joint dislocation. Lateral of the wrist from Figure 15. Note that the ulna is clearly volar to the radius and is in line with the pisiform—an abnormal position for the ulna on the lateral wrist projection.

Management. Acute dorsal subluxation should be managed by reducing the ulnar head and immobilizing the forearm in full supination with a sugartong splint or volar and dorsal splints that cross the elbow. Palmar dislocation is often locked and usually cannot be reduced without regional anesthesia, although an attempt can be made using conscious sedation. Direct pressure on the ulnar head with counter-pressure over the distal radius may allow reduction. Hypersupination may be necessary to unlock the ulnar head. Once reduced, the forearm should be immobilized in pronation. The volar dislocation is generally stable after reduction. Prompt referral to an orthopedic or hand surgeon is indicated for definitive care.

Fractures of the Hook of the Hamate. Fractures of the hook of the hamate are uncommon injuries that are commonly missed. If detected early and immobilized, they have a reasonable chance of healing without sequelae. Usually, however, the diagnosis is delayed and these fractures progress to nonunion. Treatment for nonunion is surgical excision of the fragment. This fracture may occur from a fall on the dorsiflexed wrist with tension exerted through the transverse metacarpal ligament and the pisohamate ligament. More commonly, however, this fracture occurs when patients are involved in sports that require use of clubs, bats, or racquets; these objects fracture the hamate through direct forces applied to the hypothenar eminence. The history and mechanism provide clues that raise the index of suspicion for these fractures. Patients will complain of weak and painful grip and report discomfort with direct pressure over the hypothenar eminence.

These patients will generally have a full range of motion and minimal, if any, swelling. They will have a weak grip compared with the opposite side. The definitive physical finding is identifying the point of maximal tenderness to deep palpation. Usually, the point of maximal tenderness will be just distal, radial, and deep to the pisiform. When a hamate hook fracture is suspected, standard AP and lateral views should be obtained to rule out other injuries. These views, however, will not assist in the diagnosis of the hamate hook fracture. A carpal tunnel view is the best plain radiograph for identifying this injury. Even this view, however, may not demonstrate the fracture and, if clinical suspicion is high, a CT scan is the definitive study.

Treatment for this injury is a short arm cast for 4-6 weeks. In the ED, a short-armed volar splint, which leaves the metacarpal phalangeal joints free to flex, is appropriate. Referral to an orthopedist is indicated for definitive treatment.

Dislocations of the Carpometacarpal Joints. The carpometacarpal (CMC) joints of the hand, excluding the thumb, are extremely stable joints with relatively limited motion. They have significant bony and ligamentous supports that fix them in position. As a result, isolated dislocations are not common. Dislocations are usually associated with significant trauma and frequently are associated with fractures of the base of the metacarpal. Isolated dislocations do occur, however, and the fourth and fifth CMC joints are the most common sites, since they have the greatest degree of motion and related laxity. Numerous attempts in the laboratory have failed to produce a precise reproducible mechanism for isolated dislocations to these joints. Usually, however, they result from extreme violence, such as motor vehicle accidents or direct blows from heavy, falling objects. Alternatively, on occasion, they are associated with direct blows with a closed fist against an immovable object such as a brick

Figure 17

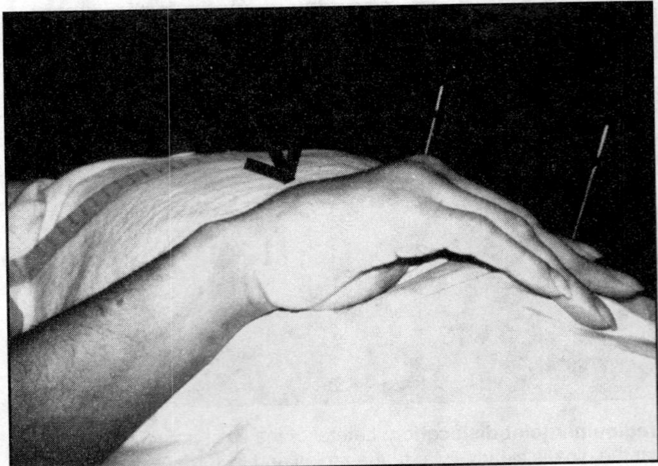

Carpometacarpal (CMC) dislocation. The gross deformity of the subluxed or dislocated joint is often obscured by the severe swelling present on the dorsum of the hand. An obvious step-off deformity may be observed and/or palpated at the level of the dislocation (i.e., note the proximal end of the metacarpal as it overrides the distal carpus).

Figure 18

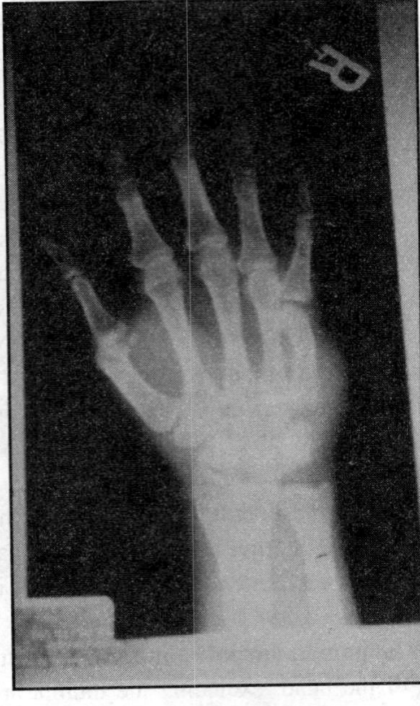

CMC dislocation. AP view of the hand from the patient seen in Figure 17 demonstrating CMC dislocation of the fifth metacarpal-carpal interface. The loss of the joint space is seen here.

wall. These dislocations are high-energy injuries and should alert the physician to search for other associated injuries to the hand and wrist. They are commonly associated with fractures of adjacent metacarpals.

The gross deformity of the subluxed or dislocated joint is often obscured by the severe swelling present on the dorsum of the hand. An obvious step-off deformity may be observed and/or palpated at the level of the dislocation (i.e., note the proximal end of the metacarpal as it overrides the distal carpus. *(Please see Figure 17.)* The points of maximum tenderness will be over the metacarpal bases and any areas of corresponding fractures. There may be rotational deformity of the digits or shortening of the metacarpal with attempted fisting. In all these injuries, a careful assessment should be made of the neurovascular status of the hand. In dislocations of the fifth CMC joint (the most common injury pattern), specific attention should be directed to the status of the deep branch of the ulnar nerve in that it lies immediately volar to the fifth CMC joint where it winds around the hook of the hamate. The median nerve may also be injured, particularly with dislocation patterns resulting from a direct blow to the hand. Vascular compromise, particularly in patients with injury to the third metacarpal, may involve the deep palmar arterial arch that lies directly beneath the third CMC joint. Integrity of the wrist extensor tendons must also be assessed in these dislocation injuries, since disruption of these structures may occur. Additionally, those patients who have suffered a direct blow are at risk for compartment syndrome in the hand.

Radiographs. The radiographic series for assessing these injuries should include an AP, lateral, and oblique view of the wrist. The AP view may reveal an overlap of the carpal bones over the proximal metacarpals. *(Please see Figure 18.)* The lateral radiograph often is diagnostic, demonstrating obvious dislocation of the CMC joint. *(Please see Figure 19.)* The oblique films should be taken with the hand pronated and is supinate, respectively, from the true lateral perspective. The critical factor for the physician reviewing the films is to recognize the potential for this injury any time there is a displaced fracture of a metacarpal. The metacarpals are tightly tethered together, and these injuries can be analogous to Galleazi and Monteggia fractures in the forearm. Any displaced metacarpal fracture should, therefore, elicit concern about injury to the adjacent CMC joints.

Acute treatment in the ED consists of ruling out compartment syndrome and attempting closed reduction. This can usually be accomplished with longitudinal traction, which is most easily accomplished by hanging the patient in finger traps with 5-10 lbs of weight suspended from the arm. The hand should then be splinted, with digital motion encouraged to prevent stiffness associated with swelling. The patient must be referred for definitive care, since these injuries often require percutaneous pinning or open reduction/internal fixation.

Closed Tendon Injuries of the Hand. In Rockwood and Green's textbook on fractures, it is stated that "... the initial evaluation and care of the injured hand are critical, for at that time the surgeon has his best opportunity to assess accurately the extent of damage and to restore the altered anatomy." They further state that "... many authors have observed that the fate of the hand largely depends on the judgment of the doctor who first sees the patient." The surgeon is rarely the one who first sees the patient, and the ultimate outcome in these injuries often depends on the appropriateness of the diagnosis and treatment provided in the ED.

Closed tendon injuries of the hand frequently are not treated with the same respect as other injuries. When there are no open wounds and no fractures present on x-ray, these injuries are often viewed as minor. In fact, these injuries can result in debilitating deformities if left untreated. As with many hand injuries, treatment is relatively simple and successful if instituted early. If the diagnosis is initially missed, however, the resultant deformities may require

Figure 19

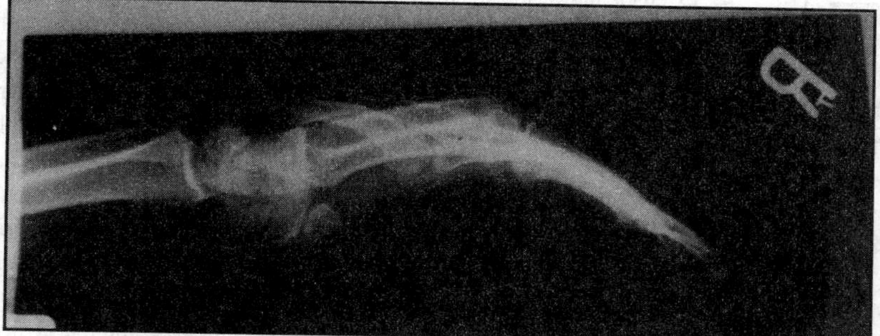

CMC dislocation. Lateral view of CMC dislocation from Figure 18 revealing obvious dorsal displacement of the proximal portion of the fifth metacarpal.

Figure 20

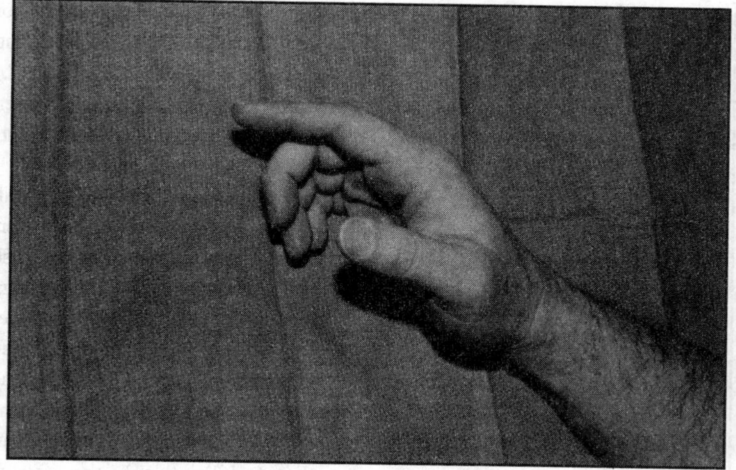

Flexor digitorum profundus rupture. On clinical examination, the patient will have inability to flex the distal IP joint actively when the proximal IP joint is blocked in extension; loss of the normal flexion cascade is seen with the involved digit remaining in either partial or complete extension in comparison to the other fully flexed digits.

Figure 21

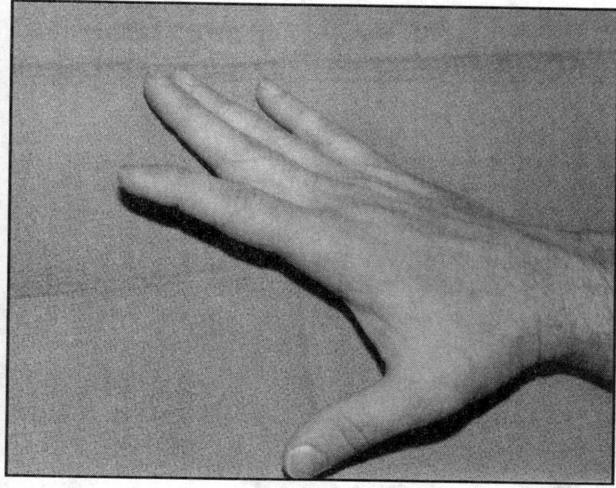

Mallet finger. Mallet finger is produced by a closed injury resulting in disruption of the distal extensor apparatus of the digit and manifested by a flexion deformity at the distal IP joint. Acutely, patients may have ecchymosis over the dorsum of the distal IP joint and always demonstrate an extensor lag at the distal IP joint.

surgical reconstruction or joint arthrodesis. These injuries occur at all three joints of the digits and on both the flexor and extensor aspects of the hand.

Flexor Digitorum Profundus Rupture. Injuries to the flexor digitorum profundus tendon of the digits are often called "rugger jersey" injuries, a relatively uncommon mishap that is often missed on initial evaluation. A high index of suspicion is necessary, for in most cases early surgical repair will provide a good result. Avulsion of the profundus tendon is caused by forceful hyperextension of the distal interphalangeal (IP) joint while the profundus tendon is maximally contracted. It is most commonly seen in athletic events when a player grabs at an opposing player's jersey. The ring finger is most commonly involved but all fingers are susceptible. The tendon may pull directly off the distal phalanx or it may avulse a bone fragment of variable size. Because the tissue is torn and not lacerated, the degree of soft tissue injury and hemorrhage is greater than that seen with a laceration in the same zone. As a result, the scarring within the sheath is often significant and the adjacent superficialis tendon may become secondarily involved. Additionally, the avulsed fragment may catch at the level of the superficialis chiasm and a flexion contracture may develop at the proximal IP joint. These injuries often go unnoticed or ignored by the patient and he or she may come to the ED late because of persistent pain and swelling of the proximal IP joint. Patients may also complain of the inability to make a complete fist.

Since the radiographs are often normal in this condition, the diagnosis must be made on physical examination. The deformity is a subtle one with only a slight loss of the normal flexion cascade of the fingers. On clinical examination, the patient will have inability to actively flex the distal IP joint when the proximal IP joint is blocked in extension *(please see Figure 20.)*; loss of the normal flexion cascade is seen with the involved digit remaining in either partial or complete extension in comparison to the other fully flexed digits. *(Please see Figure 20.)* A tender fullness at the proximal IP joint or proximal digital crease where the tendon has retracted is often demonstrated. AP and lateral views of the digit (not the hand) should

Figure 22

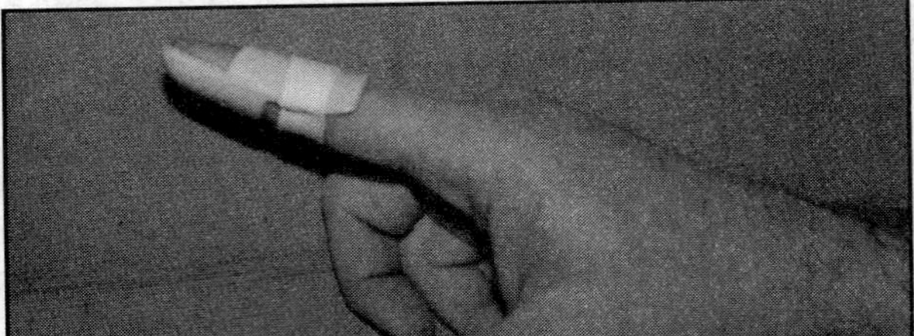

Mallet finger. Soft tissue mallet fingers should be immobilized in extension continuously for eight weeks.

Figure 23

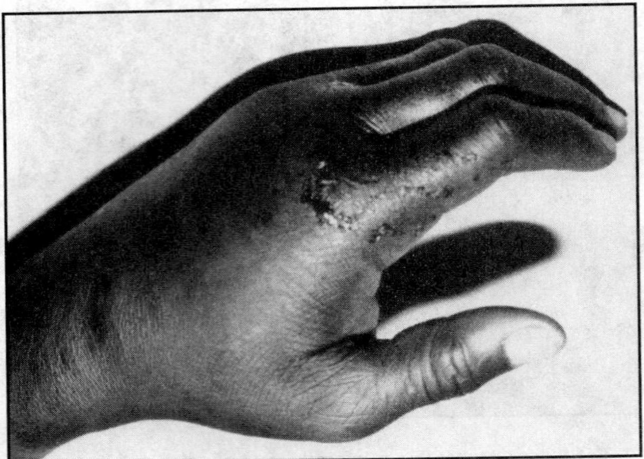

Closed fist injury with hand infection due to fight bite wound. Human saliva contains as many as 42 species of bacteria. Traumatic injury with joint space and/or deep space involvement will produce an infection that is aggressive and rapidly destructive. Improper initial care results in significant hand infection with deep space penetration and purulent tenosynovitis as seen here.

be obtained to evaluate the injury for bony involvement. Fracture may have an effect on both the timing and type of surgical repair. Most of these injuries, however, will have normal films.

Definitive treatment of these injuries must be individualized according to the needs and desires of the patient. From an ED standpoint, however, all of these patients should be considered surgical candidates. In order to ensure that repair is a viable option, all patients should be placed in a dorsal splint and referred to a surgeon within 7-10 days of injury. The position of splinting is at 30° of wrist flexion, 70° of metacarpalphalangeal joint flexion, and 30-45° of IP flexion.

Mallet Finger. Mallet finger is produced by a closed injury resulting in disruption of the distal extensor apparatus of the digit. A flexion deformity at the distal IP joint is noted. This injury generally results from a direct blow that forcibly flexes an extended finger. It can, however, occur with relatively minor trauma to the fingertip or even a direct blow to the dorsum of the finger. Additionally, the extensor lag at the distal IP joint may not appear for several days. This is rarely a painful condition, which is why patients frequently seek help late in the course. Patients will rarely complain of functional disability since there are relatively few activities that require full digital extension. This injury is one that patients commonly choose to ignore when faced with a prolonged treatment plan. What they fail to realize, however, is that, if left untreated, the chronic mallet finger may go on to develop a swan neck deformity of the digit. Unfortunately, many patients are also led to believe at their ED encounter that this is a simple problem to treat and that these injuries universally do well. Unfortunately, that is not the case and it is always best if the patient hears the correct information from the first physician whom they encounter.

Acutely, patients may have ecchymosis over the dorsum of the distal IP joint but there may be no tenderness, swelling, or discoloration. *(Please see Figure 21.)* All patients will exhibit an extensor lag at the distal IP joint, with the magnitude of the lag varying depending on the type and severity of injury. *(Please see Figure 21.)* Be aware that, on rare occasions, a locked trigger finger has been misdiagnosed as a mallet finger; mallet fingers are passively correctable to full extension, without catching or triggering.

Soft-tissue mallet fingers should be immobilized in extension full time for eight weeks. *(Please see Figure 22.)* The patient must understand that if he or she takes the finger out of immobilization to wash or air it out that he or she cannot let the distal IP joint fall into flexion. Each time the distal IP joint flexes, the treatment clock starts over again at time zero. Skin breakdown can be a significant problem, and patients should be instructed to remove the splint daily while holding the joint in extension, resting the joint on a flat surface to allow the skin to dry and reduce the chance of maceration. The vast majority of hand surgeons would recommend immobilizing only the affected joint. Routine referral to an orthopedist for definitive care is indicated.

Acute Rupture of the Central Slip (Extensor Mechanism). Injuries to the proximal IP joint are extremely common; associated proximal extensor apparatus disruption also is frequently noted. Dislocations of this joint occur frequently in athletes and are often reduced on the field by coaches, trainers, or the players themselves. This "field" correction prevents the treating physician from observing the position of the dislocation. The injured structures should be assessed by physical examination.[8] Failure to recognize a central slip rupture acutely can result in a boutonniere deformity. This is one of the most difficult, least gratifying hand deformities to treat. Early recognition and treatment in the ED is critical to prevent this late and problematic deformity.

Acute central slip ruptures occur by one of two mechanisms, the most common of which is forced flexion of the proximal IP joint that is held rigidly in extension. This mechanism is seen in basketball players and martial artists who use open hand-blocking techniques. Volar dislocations of the proximal IP joint are also a cause of central slip rupture; these are rare injuries that are accompanied by central slip disruption. An unreduced volar dislocation will present with the obvious deformity of the proximal IP joint. The middle phalanx will be palmar to the proximal phalanx. Some patients present with an acute boutonniere (button-hole) deformity with flexion of the proximal IP joint and hyperextension of the distal IP and metacarpophalangeal joints.[8] In these patients, the proximal IP joint can be passively brought to full extension, but active extension is not possible. The patient who presents, however, with a painful, swollen proximal IP joint *without* gross deformity is the one who requires careful examination. Once again, it is the area of maximum tenderness that will lead the physician to the proper diagnosis. The patient will usually have tenderness near one or both of the collateral ligaments and only mild to minimal tenderness over the volar plate. The area of maximum tenderness will be over the central slip on the dorsal aspect of the proximal IP joint. Generally, this area will also be ecchymotic. Acutely, the patient may or may not be able to fully extend the proximal IP joint. Do not be reassured by full, active extension, since this movement does not assure the integrity of the central slip. In the acute setting, the patient may be able to fully extend through the action of the lateral bands despite a complete rupture of the central slip.

Radiographs. AP and lateral radiographs of the digit should be obtained when this injury is suspected. In a volar dislocation, the base of the proximal phalanx is volar relative to the head of the middle phalanx. If the dislocation has been reduced, or if the rupture is isolated without dislocation, the radiographs will be normal.

Physical examination will help make the diagnosis of central slip injury but may not clarify whether the structure is partially or completely torn, since active extension may still be present. The prudent course, therefore, is to initially treat all central slip injuries as though they are complete ruptures. The proximal IP joint should be splinted in extension, leaving the distal proximal IP and metacarpophalangeal joints free to move. The patient should be instructed to aggressively move the distal IP joint so as not to develop an extension contracture. Referral should be made to an orthopedist or hand surgeon at 10-14 days to re-evaluate the degree of the injury. Definitive treatment will consist of 3-4 weeks of static extension splinting, followed by 2-3 weeks of dynamic extension splinting.

Traumatic Rupture of the Extensor Hood. Subluxation or dislocation of the extensor hood may occur at the metacarpophalangeal joint secondary to acute rupture of the extensor mechanism. This injury occurs following a forceful flexion or extension injury of the digit and is often called the "flea flicker" injury because it occurs when the finger is used to forcefully flick something away. The patient presents with a history of forced flexion or extension at the metacarpophalangeal joint with immediate pain and loss of extension. Patients will complain of a persistent loss of extension or of painful popping over the dorsum of the joint with attempts at motion. The middle finger is most commonly involved, followed by the index finger.

Examination reveals loss of active extension of the metacarpophalangeal joint. When the joint is passively brought into extension, the tendon can be seen to centrally relocate over the joint, and the patient will then be able to maintain extension actively. The tendon is usually subluxed ulnarly due to tearing of the sagittal fibers on the radial side. Passive range of motion at the joint should be normal, although the patient may report pain as the metacarpophalangeal joint is brought into extension with tendon relocation. AP, lateral, and oblique radiographs should be obtained.

These injuries are usually treated with acute surgical repair; however, some authors advocate nonoperative management with extension splinting. Splinting of the metacarpophalangeal joint in full extension is not recommended because of the potential for developing an extension contracture. In this case, the metacarpophalangeal joint should be passively brought into extension just until the tendon is seen to relocate. The joint should then be splinted in that position. The other MP joints should be left free, however, to ensure that no contractures develop in adjacent digits.

Ulnar Collateral Ligament Rupture. Rupture of the ulnar collateral ligament of the metacarpophalangeal joint of the thumb is a common athletic injury. Patients are often anxious to return to their normal activity level and will actively seek such reassurance. Therefore, it is critical that the clinician understand that *all* injuries to this ligament warrant referral to an orthopedic surgeon. Even incomplete lesions require casting or customized bracing due to the high potential for long-term morbidity.

A sudden valgus stress, usually associated with hyperextension, applied to the thumb results in partial or complete tearing of the ulnar collateral ligament that is frequently associated with injury to the volar plate. Ulnar collateral ligament injury often occurs with ski poles, resulting in the term "skier's thumb."[9] It is also very common among basketball players and in the "grappling" sports such as wrestling or the martial arts. Patients will often give the history that they saw the thumb "pointing away" from the hand and will note pain, swelling, and weakness of pinch/grip.

The thumb will be swollen, painful with motion, and may have a gross deviation radially. The point of maximal tenderness is elicited over the ulnar aspect of the metacarpophalangeal joint. Differentiating complete from incomplete ruptures requires stressing of the joint, but this should never be done prior to x-ray.[10] If the ligament has avulsed a piece of bone off the proximal phalanx, stress testing could displace the fragment. AP and lateral radiographs should be obtained. The AP is assessed for bony injury at the phalangeal or metacarpal attachment of the ligament. A displaced or rotated fragment off the phalanx is a definite indication for surgery. The lateral film is often overlooked or ignored. Any evidence on this film of volar subluxation of the phalanx is an indicator of significant ligamentous injury to the volar plate complex.

As previously emphasized, treatment of complete injuries is somewhat controversial. Even incomplete lesions, however, require casting or custom splinting for several weeks. All patients should be referred to an orthopedist for definitive care. Treatment in the ED should consist of the application of a thumb spica splint leaving the distal joint free to flex. This is crucial as the IP joint will start to scar early in the healing process unless it is free to move.

Closed Fist Injuries. Closed fist injuries result from striking another individual in the mouth region with the fist; such blunt impact on the aggressor's hand likely produces soft-tissue and bony injury to the hand. If the soft-tissue injury includes a break in the integrity of the skin on the dorsum of the hand, infection may complicate the original injury. As such, these injuries should be approached with great respect.

Although these injuries are common, they are frequently mismanaged. Mismanagement results from a number of factors. Patients who suffer these injuries are often intoxicated, making an adequate history and thorough examination difficult. They may also be reluctant to reveal the cause of injury and provide misleading histories. The physician must have a high index of suspicion in any injury where there are lacerations, abrasions, or bruising over the metacarpophalangeal joints. Closed fist injuries fall into two basic categories: 1.) those that involve the bony structures; and 2.) those with open wounds. Closed fist injuries with open wounds are among the most dangerous because they usually involve a human bite—the so-called fight-bite wound.

Metacarpal Head Fractures. These intra-articular fractures result from significant impact force on the fist.[11] These bony injuries more commonly occur in the index and long fingers; the fractures are usually comminuted. Fractures are frequently missed on the radiograph as the focus of attention is often on the metacarpal shaft. Additionally, they are difficult to see on the lateral view because of overlap of the metacarpal heads. Oblique radiographs are often very useful in identifying the fracture as well as the degree of comminution.

These are intra-articular fractures and can lead to early joint arthrosis if not properly diagnosed and managed. These injuries should be treated with a splint that immobilizes the metacarpophalangeal joint in 70-90° of flexion. Unquestionably, the most common and clinically significant error made in treating these fractures in the ED is poor positioning of the metacarpophalangeal joints in the splint. Meticulous attention to proper splinting is mandatory for the clinician in that improper splinting allows the ligaments to remain in a relaxed position; such lax ligaments may result in contractures at the MP joint and represent one of the most difficult problems faced by the hand surgeon.[12] Early referral to an orthopedist after splinting is appropriate.

Metacarpal Neck Fractures. Fractures of the metacarpal neck represent the most common associated fracture in the patient with a closed fist injury. Fracture of the fifth metacarpal neck, the "boxer's fracture," is the most frequently encountered "closed fist" bony injury. Fractures of the metacarpal neck are generally unstable because of volar comminution, more so for the radial metacarpals than the ulnar bones. The two radial metacarpals can tolerate almost no residual angulation without functional loss, while the ulnar two digits can tolerate some angulation without functional problem. These fractures can again be difficult to assess adequately on a lateral x-ray because of overlap; oblique views may be helpful. Associated CMC joint injury is common in patients with metacarpal neck fracture. Metacarpal neck fractures should be treated acutely in the same manner as the metacarpal head fractures. A splint with the metacarpophalangeal joints held in 70-90° of flexion should be applied and the patient referred for definitive orthopedic care.

Metacarpal Shaft Fracture. Metacarpal shaft fractures present more of a treatment challenge to the orthopedist than the neck fracture; yet, from the standpoint of the emergency physician, they can be treated in similar fashion. It should be noted, however, that associated carpometacarpal joint injuries are more common with these fractures and should be suspected and aggressively ruled out.

Metacarpal Base Fractures. Fractures of the base of the metacarpal are commonly missed. The overlap of the metacarpal bases on standard radiographic views can make it difficult to detect these injuries; oblique views will confirm the diagnosis if the AP films are equivocal.[13] Physical examination, however, with demonstration of the area of maximum tenderness should suggest to the physician the probability of the injury. Early diagnosis and referral for treatment will usually lead to a satisfactory result. These injuries should be treated with the standard metacarpal splint with the metacarpophalangeal joints flexed downward.

Fight-Bite Wounds Complicated by Infection. Human saliva contains as many as 42 species of bacteria with a microbe concentration of 1×10^8 organisms/mL.[14,15] Fist-to-mouth contact is perhaps the most common cause of human bite wounds. These fight-bite wounds have the highest incidence of complications of any closed fist injury and of any type of bite wound. These injuries usually occur over the dorsal aspect of the third, fourth, or fifth metacarpophalangeal joints, an area that is susceptible to deep infection because the thin skin overlying the joint provides little protection to the underlying ligaments, synovium, and cartilage.[16] Joint space infections resulting from a human bite wound are aggressive and rapidly destructive. They usually occur in young people, and the resulting destructive changes of the MP joint can be devastating as there is no good surgical option to reconstruct the MP joint of a young person. For these reasons, it is a commonly accepted axiom in the world of hand surgery that all open wounds over the metacarpophalangeal joints are considered to be probable fight bites; such an approach will ensure that all patients will receive appropriate therapy.

The wound must be thoroughly explored to rule-out joint capsule violation as well as a retained foreign body, such as a tooth fragment or piece of jewelry. The wound should be copiously irrigated. If the joint space was violated, this area should be thoroughly irrigated as well. After aggressive care has been completed, the wound should be left open (i.e., no primary closure should be attempted in that such an approach will increase the possibility of infection). Further, the patient should receive a parenteral, broad-spectrum antibiotic in the ED with continued outpatient oral antimicrobial agents. Early follow-up (at 24-48 hours) with a physician skilled in the management of such injuries is encouraged. If the patient appears noncompliant, consideration should be made for initial inpatient care. Early range of motion is initiated and the wound is allowed to heal secondarily or closed as a delayed primary closure. Improper initial care—frequently due to either the lack of physician knowledge of the potential infectious complications or patient claims stating the wound did not occur with fist-to-mouth contact—will result in significant hand infection with deep space penetration and purulent tenosynovitis. *(Please see Figure 23.)*

References

1. Paton DF. Posterior dislocation of the shoulder: A diagnostic pitfall for physicians. *Practitioner* 1979;223:111-112.
2. Bloom MH, Obata WG. Diagnosis of posterior dislocation of the shoulder with use of velpeau axillary and angle-up roentgenographic views. *J Bone Joint Surg* 1967;49A:943-949.
3. Ahlgren O, Lorentzon R, Larsson SE. Posterior dislocation of the shoulder associated with general seizures. *Acta Orthop Scand* 1981;52:694-695.
4. Cisterno SJ, Rogers LF, Stufflebaum BC, et al. The trough line: A radiographic sign of posterior shoulder dislocation. *Am J Roent* 1978;130:951-954.
5. Messner DG. Posterior dislocation of the shoulder: With or without associated fracture. *J Bone Joint Surg* 1966;48A:1220-1221.
6. Pirrallo RG, Bridges TP. Luxatio erecta: A missed diagnosis. *Am J Emerg Med* 1990;8:315-317.
7. Brady WJ, Knuth CJ, Pirrallo RG. Bilateral inferior glenohumeral dislocation: Luxatio erecta, an unusual presentation of a rare disorder. *J Emerg Med* 1995;13:37-42.
8. Carducci AT. Potential Boutonniere deformity: Its recognition and treatment. *Orthop Rev* 1981;10:121-123.
9. Morgan JV, Davis PH. Upper Extremity Injuries in Skiing.

Clin Sports Med 1982;1:295-308.

10. Frank WE, Dobyns J. Surgical pathology of collateral ligament injuries to the thumb. *Clin Orthrop* 1972;83:102-114.
11. McElfresh EC, Dobyns JH. Intra-articular metacarpal head fractures. *J Hand Surg* 1983;8:383-393.
12. Akeson WH, Amiel DI, Abel, MF, et al. Effects of immobilization on joints. *Clin Orthrop* 1987;219:28-37.
13. Kaye JJ, Lister GD. Another use for Brewerton view. *J Hand Surg* 1978;3:603-607.
14. Faciszewski T, Coleman DA. Human bite wounds. *Hand Clin* 1989;5:561-569.
15. Rayan GM, Flournoy DJ. Hand infections. *Contmep Orthop* 1990;20:41-54.
16. Mann RJ, Hoffeld TA, Farmer CB. Human bites of the hand: Twenty year's experience. *J Hand Surg* 1977;297:104-111.

Lower Extremity Fractures and Dislocations

William J. Brady, MD
Gregory G. Degnan, MD
Leslie P. Buchanon, RN, MSN, ENP
Susan Schwartz, RN, MSN, ENP
Abhinav Chhabra, MD

This chapter on difficult-to-diagnose and challenging orthopedic injuries focuses on lower extremity fractures, dislocations, and tendon disruptions, as well as pediatric injuries. The role of ancillary MRI and CT scanning techniques for evaluation of hip fractures and pediatric orthopedic trauma are outlined in detail.

Because orthopedic injuries involving the lower extremity—from talar and calcaneal fractures to tendon ruptures and occult epiphyseal disruptions in children—are associated with function-threatening complications, the approach to these anatomic regions must be systematic. When evaluating fractures of the lower foot, in particular, the emergency physician must maintain a high index of suspicion for associated tendon and soft-tissue injuries. Complicated fractures may be associated with compartment syndrome, a limb-compromising complication that requires prompt recognition and urgent management.

Because radiographic evaluation is key to optimal management, we have provided a supplement featuring x-rays that characterize difficult-to-identify fractures and suggest which views will enhance recognition of elusive injuries.

Occult Hip Fracture in the Elderly

Acute fractures of the proximal femur are among the most common orthopedic injuries encountered by the emergency physician. From an anatomical perspective, these fractures include bony injury to the following structures: femoral head, neck, or proximal shaft; intertrochanteric or subtrochanteric regions; and isolated less or greater trochanteric areas. In the elderly patient who has fallen, femoral neck, intertrochanteric and subtrochanteric fractures are the most common bony hip injuries seen; the common mechanistic denominator in these injuries is weakened bone, most often osteoporosis. The elderly patient who sustains a fall and presents to the ED with severe hip pain usually does not present a diagnostic dilemma. Typically, the physical examination will reveal significant tenderness in the hip region with marked discomfort associated with any degree of movement of the affected extremity. Attempts at ambulation are difficult, if not impossible; if ambulation is possible, the gait is usually antalgic. The hip radiographs in these patients invariably demonstrate the suspected fracture.

In certain situations, however, the radiograph does not demonstrate a fracture *(please see Figure 1)*; in these cases, the emergency physician is then left with an osteoporotic patient who has experienced trauma and is unable to ambulate. The majority of these patients have inconsequential soft tissue injuries; however, the minority of elderly patients with this presentation, in fact, will have a fracture of the proximal femur that is not visualized on the radiograph—the so-called occult hip fracture. When this fracture is not detected, occult fracture has an even higher rate of morbidity and mortality; in particular, the orthopedic outcome may be compromised as

Figure 1

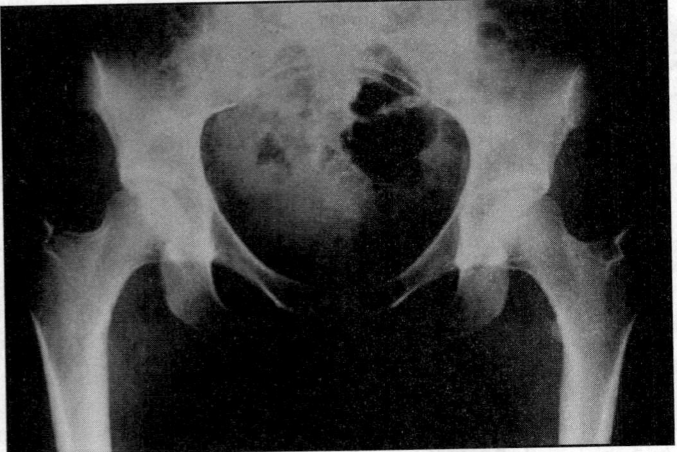

Figure 2

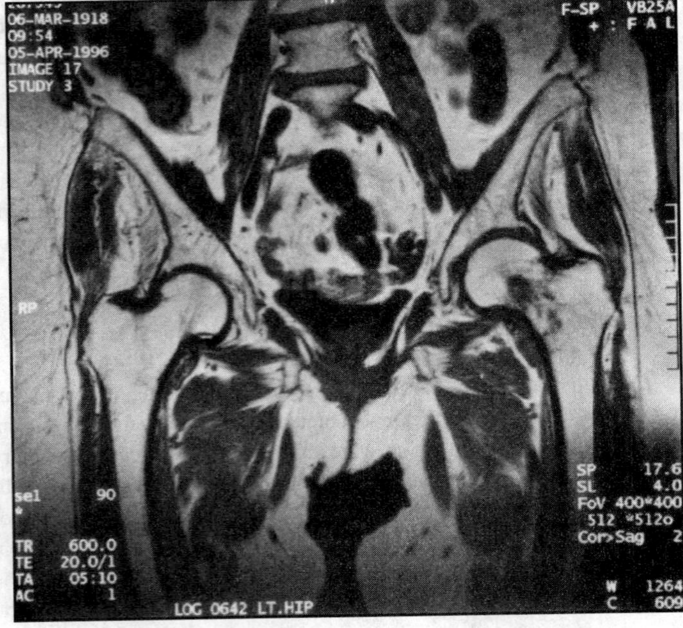

Occult Hip Fracture in the Elderly Noted by MRI. MRI of the patient in Figure 1 revealing the left femoral neck fracture; the MRI was performed on the initial ED presentation, allowing for timely diagnosis and appropriate therapy in this patient.

a result of avascular necrosis. Numerous strategies have been recommended for evaluating these patients, including bed rest with repeat plain-film radiography in 7-10 days, and, if required, computed tomographic scanning, bone scan, and/or magnetic resonance imaging (MRI). Perhaps, the most appropriate diagnostic approach involves early application of the MRI *(please see Figure 2)*.[1-3] This approach has been employed in many EDs with substantial success. A sound strategy includes use of MRI in the patient with a suggestive mechanism of injury and significant pain with hip movement and/or ambulation (i.e., a reasonably strong clinical impression of hip fracture coupled with a negative plain film). The time window during which the MRI will reliably demonstrate occult fracture is unknown, although many series suggest this injury may be identified as early as four hours after occurrence.[1-3]

Tibial Plateau Fractures

The medial and lateral tibial condyles form a plateau that transmits the weight of the body from the femoral condyles to the tibial shafts. Proximal tibial fractures include fractures above the tibial tuberosity. These fractures may be described as extra-articular, among them tibial spine, tubercle, and subcondylar fractures, or articular fractures, including the condylar injuries. Proximal tibial fractures may be divided into five categories on the basis of anatomy.

The normal forces that are applied to the tibial plateau include axial compression and rotation. Fractures occur when these forces exceed the strength of the bone. Automobile-pedestrian accidents in which the automobile bumper makes direct impact over the proximal tibia represent the most frequent mechanism of injury. A direct blow, such as a fall from a significant height, is responsible for approximately 20% of condylar fractures.[4] The remaining 30% of the fractures result from a combination of axial compression and rotational strain. Fractures of the lateral tibial plateau are the result of an abduction force on the leg. Medial plateau fractures usually result from an adduction force applied to the lower leg. If the knee is in extension at the time of injury, the fracture tends to be anterior. Conversely, if the knee is flexed at the time of impact, the fractures tend to involve the posterior condyle.

Clinical Presentation. The patient with tibial plateau fracture will present with a history consistent with the aforementioned mechanism of injury, and will complain of pain and swelling; the knee may be slightly flexed. On inspection, there may be an abrasion, laceration, or area of ecchymosis indicating the point of impact. Typically, an effusion and decreased active range of motion are present. A varus or valgus deformity indicates a depressed fracture. Tibial plateau fractures frequently are associated with soft-tissue injuries to the collateral and cruciate ligaments, menisci, and/or surrounding neurovascular structures. One study evaluated 30 tibial plateau fractures and found a 56% rate of associated soft-tissue injuries, including involvement of the medial collateral ligaments (20%), the menisci (20%), the anterior cruciate ligaments (10%), the lateral collateral ligaments (3%), and the peroneal nerve (3%).[4] The physical examination should include assessment of joint laxity. Distal neurovascular status should be assessed and documented.

Radiographs. Anteroposterior (AP), lateral, and oblique radiographic views of the knee usually are adequate for demonstrating a tibial plateau fracture. A specific film, the tibial plateau view, is helpful for assessing the degree of depression. Anatomically, the tibial plateau slopes from the anterior aspect superiorly to the posterior area inferiorly. Routine AP views may not detect this slope and, therefore, may not demonstrate some depression fractures. Plain film tomography, CT scanning, or MRI may be necessary to detect occult fractures or to assess the degree of depression of a fracture that is apparent on regular films. Multiple studies have compared MRI, CT, tomography, and plain-film radiography. One study found that MRI was more accurate than standard radiography in classification of the fracture, identification of occult fracture, and accurate measurement of the displacement and depression of fragments.[5] MRI also provides reliable identification of associated intra- and periarticular soft-tissue injuries pre-operatively.[5] Another trial investigated 30 patients with 31 tibial plateau fractures that were diagnosed with standard radiography, comparing tomography and MRI. MRI was found to be as effective as tomography in quantitating the amount of articular depression and was found to be more effective in determining the extent of comminution. Again, it was noted that MRI demonstrated associated ligamentous and meniscal injuries.[6]

Management. The therapeutic goal in managing tibial plateau fractures is precise reconstruction of the articular surfaces, stable fragment fixation allowing early motion, and repair of all concomitant lesions. The four most common treatment modalities include 1) compressive dressing; 2) closed reduction and casting; 3) skeletal traction; or 4) open reduction and internal fixation. Therapy depends upon on the type of fracture. A type I, nondisplaced fracture in an ambulatory patient with no associated ligamentous injuries may be managed with aspiration of the hemarthrosis, application of a compressive dressing, ice, and elevation for 48 hours. The patient will have to remain non-weight bearing until healing is complete. If after 48 hours x-rays remain unchanged, range of motion exercises and quadriceps exercises may be initiated. Casting is not recommended at the time of injury until 4-6 weeks because of the high incidence of knee stiffness. Early orthopedic consultation is advised.

Emergency management of Type II, local compression fractures depends upon the presence of associated ligamentous injuries, the location of the fracture, and the degree of depression. A depression of 8 mm or more requires operative intervention to elevate the fragment. Anterior or middle depression injuries are more ominous than posterior fractures. Conservative therapy of nondisplaced local compression fractures without ligamentous injuries includes aspiration of the hemarthrosis, compression dressing or posterior splint, and non-weight bearing for up to three weeks. Early orthopedic consultation is recommended.

Primary management of Type III, local compression, Type IV, total condylar depression, and Type VI, comminuted fractures includes ice, elevation, aspiration of hemarthrosis, and immobilization in posterior splint. The patient must remain non-weight bearing. Accurate radiographic assessment of the degree of displacement will determine therapy by the orthopedist. Type V split fractures will need immediate consultation, since open reduction with internal fixation is the recommended therapy.

Complications. Tibial plateau fractures are prone to the development of several serious complications. Because loss of full range of motion of the knee may follow prolonged immobilization, the importance of early non-weight bearing range of motion and quadriceps exercises cannot be overemphasized. Angular deformity of the knee may develop in the first several weeks, even with nondisplaced fractures. Early orthopedic referral and follow-up are essential. Persistent subluxation or instability may complicate these injuries if there is ligamentous damage. Post-operative infection is a risk to open reduction and internal fixation or hemarthrosis.

Degenerative arthritis is a potential, long-term complication of tibial plateau fractures. Secondary osteoarthritis after tibial plateau fracture is found in approximately one-half of patients 10 years after the initial injury.[7] Narrowing of the joint space was noted during the first seven years after injury, usually in the same compartment as the fracture. The incidence increases with age of the patient at the time of the injury. Removal of the meniscus resulted in secondary degeneration in 74% of the patients. When the meniscus was intact or repaired, the percentage of degenerative changes decreased to 37%.[7] Normal or slight valgus alignment of the tibial plateau with an intact meniscus protected best against degenerative disease. However, medial or lateral tilt of the plateau after removal of a meniscus was complicated by osteoarthritis in many cases. Associated ligamentous injuries and postoperative infection increased the incidence of secondary degeneration. Neurovascular complications usually are the result of compartment syndromes.[7,8] The complication of compartment syndrome after tibial plateau fracture is relatively rare because of the dissipation of tissue pressures into the knee joint compartments.

Knee Extensor Mechanism Disruptions

The extensor mechanism disruptions involving the knee include rupture of the quadriceps tendon, patellar fracture, patellar tendon rupture, and tendon avulsion at the tibial tubercle. The most commonly encountered disruption involves rupture of the patellar tendon. *(Please see Figure 3.)* Extensor mechanism disruption generally occurs as the result of the quadriceps muscle suddenly contracting forcefully against a slightly flexed knee; biomechanical study has shown that when the knee is slightly flexed, the forces across the patellar tendon are maximal. Direct trauma to either the patella or the proximal tibia may also result in extensor mechanism disruption, which usually involves a patellar fracture or avulsion of the patellar tendon. Misdiagnosis by the primary care provider has been reported to be as high as 38%.[9] Accurate early diagnosis is essential to ensure the best outcome, which requires early surgical repair and intensive physical therapy.

Quadriceps tendon rupture is more common in patients with systemic disease, such as chronic renal failure, gout, hyperparathyroidism, diabetes, and obesity; patients with degenerative arthritic changes in the knee also are susceptible. Patellar tendon injuries in this patient group are less common; in general, individuals with this injury tend to be younger and less likely to have degenerative disease or systemic illness. Bilateral patellar tendon rupture has been reported and is associated with systemic lupus erythematosus and rheumatoid arthritis. Extensor mechanism disruption has been reported as an unusual complication of Paget's disease; the patellar tendon usually is avulsed from the tibial tubercle in the region of pagetic bone.[9] In other cases, rupture of the tendon occurs through a pathologic area of the tendon; several studies have implicated steroid injections and microscopic damage to the tendon's vascular supply as a cause of failure.[9]

The clinical presentation of extensor mechanism disruption generally includes complaints of acute onset of knee pain accompanied by loss of function. The history includes either stumbling or jumping followed by sudden buckling of the knee and extreme pain. The patient usually gives a history characterized by forceful axial loading on a partially flexed knee; the inability to extend the knee results in loss of function. Furthermore, a careful medical history is essential to alert the examiner to associated systemic illnesses.

Physical examination may reveal a palpable defect in the quadriceps or patellar tendon; accordingly, the position of the patella should be assessed. Quadriceps tendon ruptures will present with inferior displacement of the patella (patella baja), proximal ecchymosis, and

Figure 3

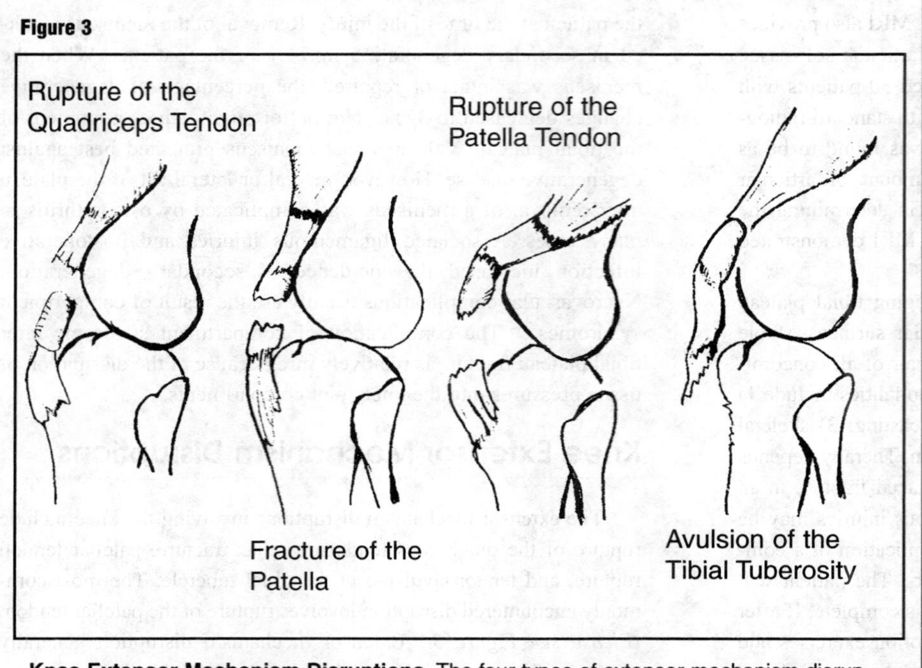

Knee Extensor Mechanism Disruptions. The four types of extensor mechanism disruption at the knee joint.

swelling. In contrast, proximal patellar displacement (patella alta), inferior pole tenderness, and swelling indicate patellar tendon rupture. Evaluation of range of motion will reveal markedly depressed active extension at the knee, inability to maintain passive extension against gravity, or complete loss of knee extension. Patients with partial ruptures may have active extension, but it will be markedly weakened. Hematoma or hemarthrosis may mask these clinical signs. In most cases, the diagnosis is made on the basis of the patient's inability to extend the knee in the setting of an appropriate mechanism of injury.

Radiographs. Radiographic findings in patients with quadriceps tendon rupture include inferior patellar displacement (patella baja), superior pole boney avulsion fragment, and degenerative spurring of the patella seen on the tangential view (tooth sign). Complete disruption of the patellar tendon is suggested by superior displacement of the patella *(please see Figure 4)* and inferior boney avulsion fragment. Comparison views may be necessary for diagnosing subtle patellar displacement. In cases involving bony injury, either a patellar fracture or an avulsed bone fragment will be seen on the radiograph. In many cases, the radiograph may be entirely normal; this finding should not dissuade the clinician from the diagnosis of patellar tendon rupture.

Additional radiographic imaging may be required, usually after referral to the orthopedic surgeon. The quadriceps and patellar tendons are easily visualized using MRI. Partial tears and tendinosis may be difficult to diagnose, but complete tears are easily visualized. Patellar fractures, bone bruises, and avulsion of the tibial tubercle are revealed as changes in marrow signal intensity. MRI is also extremely useful for identifying associated meniscal tears and chondromalacia patella. Ultrasound and CT have also been used to evaluate continuity of the extensor mechanism.

Accurate diagnosis of partial or complete patellar tendon ruptures, avulsion fractures of the patella or tibial tubercle, and complete quadriceps tendon tears is essential because optimal outcomes are obtained with early surgical repair. The primary treatment issues for the emergency physician include accurate diagnosis and timely orthopedic referral. Orthopedic consultation should be initiated at the time of injury or within 24 hours of presentation. Knee immobilization with crutch walking should be advised until orthopedic follow-up is accomplished. Definitive repair usually involves surgery. Delay in treating a quadriceps tendon tear for 4-6 weeks may result in the tendon being difficult to mobilize. Patients with patellar tendon ruptures that have gone undetected for more than two weeks may develop significant proximal retraction of the patella, with quadriceps contracture and adhesion. Most surgical repair techniques are followed by immobilization in a long leg cast in extension for 4-6 weeks, with partial weight bearing using crutches. Intensive physical therapy is prescribed, beginning with active flexion and passive extension exercises. Strengthening exercises are advanced as knee flexion returns. Patients can return to sporting activities in 4-6 months, when knee flexion is at least 120° and strength deficits are less than 10%.

Achilles Tendon Rupture

Emergency physicians are often the first to evaluate Achilles tendon injuries. The diagnosis of Achilles tendon rupture is missed in about 25% of cases.[10] An overlooked rupture can lead to discernible loss of long-term function. Achilles tendon is the most commonly ruptured tendon, accounting for 40% of all surgically repaired tendon ruptures.[10] A Scandinavian study of 111 closed Achilles tendon ruptures from 1979 through 1994 demonstrated a mean age of 40, and a division by sex of 85% men to 17% women. Seventy percent of the patients were recreational athletes, 18% competitive athletes, and 12% practiced no sport.[11]

Achilles tendon rupture occurs when stress is applied to a previously contracted muscle/tendon. A rapid push off with the knee extended or a sudden unexpected dorsiflexion have been suggested as mechanisms of injury. These injuries occur most frequently (81%) while playing sports, usually during an activity requiring sudden acceleration or jumping.[11] Rarely does the rupture occur from a direct blow to the tendon. Typically, the injury occurs to middle aged men who are weekend athletes. The tendon most often ruptures 2-6 cm proximal to the calcaneus, the area of the tendon with minimal blood supply.[12] Although patients may describe symptoms related to Achilles tendinitis prior to the injury, this prodromal complaint is generally not the case. Histologically, however, virtually all patients with acute Achilles tendon rupture have preexisting degenerative changes of their tendon; specifically, these include hypoxic, mucoid, lipomatous, and calcific changes.

The history of the injury frequently is pathognomonic. Typically, patients describe a sudden, audible bang or pop, with immediate burning or searing pain in the posterior ankle. Patients describe a sensation of having been shot or kicked in the heel and often turn around to search for an assailant. Most patients seek immediate medical care since they are unable to walk normally on the affected foot. The initial sharp pain is replaced by a dull ache and stiffness in the ankle. Physical examination of the ankle should include active range of motion, palpation of the length of the tendon from the gastrocnemius muscle to the calcaneus, and the Thompson's squeeze test. The range of motion may or may not reveal an inability to plantar flex the foot, as the posterior tibialis and intact toe flexors may compensate for the completely ruptured tendon. A palpable defect in the tendon and tenderness at the site of rupture are characteristic of a ruptured Achilles tendon. The most reliable sign of a completely ruptured tendon is a positive Thompson's squeeze test. *(Please see Figure 5.)* The patient is placed with the knees flexed to 90°—a squeeze of the calf muscles will produce passive plantar flexion of the foot in the unaffected tendon. A positive, or abnormal, Thompson's squeeze test is an absence of passive plantar flexion.

Most often, the diagnosis of a ruptured Achilles tendon usually is made based on the history and physical examination. Radiographic examination is a simple and relatively inexpensive adjunct to diagnosis when the physical examination is equivocal.[13] A lateral x-ray view will help identify Kager's Triangle. A normal Achilles tendon is demonstrated by a clearly perceptible Kager's triangle, with easily identified smooth edges. Patients suffering from ruptured Achilles tendons demonstrate a smaller, less transparent, fuzzy triangle.[12] The utility of MRI in the ED is very limited; however, it does provide a very clear picture of the Achilles tendon and may be employed in difficult cases either in the ED or in the orthopedic office at follow-up.

Management. In the acute setting, at time of initial presentation, two approaches for management of a ruptured Achilles tendon are described in the orthopedic literature.[14,15] Lea and Smith[14,15] have been advocates for non-operative management with a cast for eight weeks. The patient is initially placed in a posterior splint with the ankle placed in gravity equines (not forced equines). This conservative method of management, however, is complicated by a recurrent rupture in 10-35% of cases. The second option for initial management is surgical repair, using one of many techniques. Surgical repairs are complicated by a much lower re-rupture rate (i.e., less than 6%). Proponents of surgical repair argue that the decreased risk of re-rupture, coupled with a stronger tendon outweighs the risks associated with surgery. Nonetheless, for the emergency physician, either orthopedic consultation in the ED or very close orthopedic follow-up within several days of presentation is required in all suspected cases. Although the patient faces a prolonged convalescence regardless of therapy, the correct initial diagnosis and appropriate management by the emergency physician will have a major impact on the long-term recovery.

Posterior Malleolar (Ankle) Fracture

Isolated posterior malleolus fractures, although rare, have been reported as "frequently overlooked radiographically."[16] Fractures of the posterior malleolus, however, are most often seen in association with lateral and/or medial malleolar fractures of the ankle. Avulsion fractures of the posterior tibial tubercle are seen in association with

Figure 4

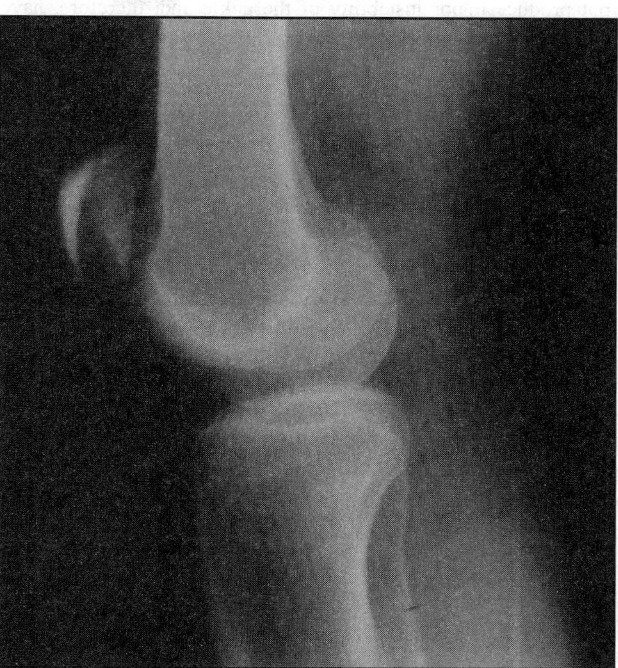

Knee Extensor Mechanism Disruptions (Patella Alta). Knee radiograph of a patient with patellar tendon disruption manifested by patella alta. The patella is high riding. Correct position of the patella may be judged by the following: The distance from the inferior pole of the patella to the proximal portion of the tibial tuberosity should equal the vertical length of the patella itself ± 20% of this distance.

Figure 5

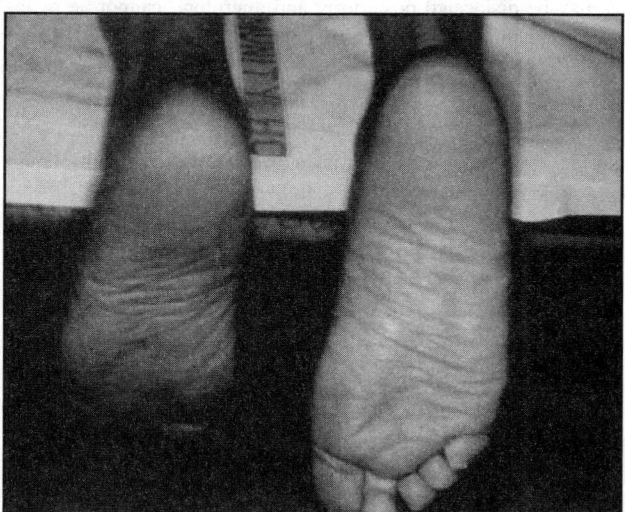

Achilles Tendon Rupture. The most reliable sign of a completely ruptured tendon is a positive Thompson's squeeze test. The patient is placed with the knees flexed to 90°—a squeeze of the calf muscles will produce passive plantar flexion of the foot in the unaffected tendon. A positive or abnormal Thompson's squeeze test is an absence of passive plantar flexion.

injuries of the posterior tibio-fibular ligament. Fractures of this kind do not produce major instability of the ankle and, therefore, have minimal clinical significance. Fractures of the posterior process of the tibia (posterior lip), however, represent significant injuries. These fractures, through the articular surface, frequently lead to subluxation of the talus. According to the Lauge-Hansen classification of ankle fractures, avulsions or ruptures of the posterior tibio-fibular ligament occur when an eversion force is applied to a supinated ankle. Posterior lip fractures of the tibia are most often seen when the eversion force is applied to a pronated ankle through axial force. These serious fractures, however, may be associated with any mechanism of injury producing a malleolar fracture. Other factors that predispose to a posterior lip fracture include obesity and osteoporosis.

Presentation. Patients with posterior malleolus fractures usually give a history describing a forced ankle twist. Isolated, posterior malleolus fractures most often present with swelling, tenderness, and ecchymosis around the Achilles tendon. Posterior malleolus fractures associated with medial and/or lateral malleolar fractures present with significant, generalized soft tissue swelling and pain and, in some cases, with talar dislocations. Initially, standard radiographs of the ankle including AP, lateral, and mortise views are required for accurate assessment. Often, posterior malleolar fractures are seen only as double densities that are superimposed on the tibial metaphysis; as a result, they may be missed. Patients who present with a high degree of suspicion should have a CT scan performed that can provide explicit imaging of the size, location, and displacement of fractures.

Avulsions of the posterior tibio-fibular ligament (which does not contribute to the stability of the ankle) do not require fixation. Initial management consists of an ankle immobilization device and other symptom-based therapy. Conversely, fractures of the posterior lip of the tibia frequently are associated with significant instability; the talus may be dislocated posteriorly and, therefore, cannot be maintained in reduction. Dorsiflexion of the foot aggravates the inclination to dislocate. Patients with posterior malleolus fractures should be placed in a Robert Jones dressing—dorsiflexion should be avoided—to reduce soft tissue swelling. If more than 25-30% of the joint surface is involved, most authors agree that the fragment should undergo open fixation in order to stabilize the ankle.[17]

Calcaneal and Talar Fractures

The talus and the calcaneus make up the hindfoot; a major structural determinant of normal gait. In combination, the tibiotalar (ankle joint) and talocalcaneal (subtalar joint) comprise a universal joint. The tibiotalar joint provides for flexion and extension, whereas the subtalar joint is responsible for up to 65° of inversion/eversion movements. This universal joint provides a "shock absorber" effect for the hindfoot during normal gait, as well as the ability to ambulate on uneven surfaces (i.e., the off-center heel strike). Loss of universal joint function will cause the talus to bind in the ankle mortise, increasing sheer stress and decreasing efficiency of gait. As a result, fractures of the hindfoot are common and are associated with significant morbidity if missed or treated inappropriately. Avascular necrosis of the talus or subtalar arthrosis are potentially devastating sequelae of these fractures, which can be prevented with early diagnosis and proper treatment. Unfortunately, assessment can be difficult, inasmuch as radiographs of this area can be difficult to interpret.

Stress Fractures. Stress fractures of the foot were once encountered almost exclusively in military recruits. However, recent interest in physical fitness and running has made this fracture much more common in the general population. Running and athletic activity are not the only risk factors for stress fracture. Any new mechanical stress applied to the foot can produce this injury. Stress fractures have even been reported in patients following bunionectomy. Accordingly, any patient with foot pain and a recent history of increased or altered activity should be considered a possible candidate for stress fracture.

Although the most common sites for stress fracture of the foot are the second metatarsal and the calcaneus, any bone can be involved. Interestingly, calcaneal stress fractures have been noted to be bilateral in approximately one-quarter of all cases.[18] Moreover, it is not uncommon to have multiple sites of stress fracture in the same foot. The typical underlying mechanism of injury is excessive, repetitive stress applied to a bone that does not have sufficient structural strength to withstand such stress. Under such circumstances, especially if the stress is applied long enough, the bone will fatigue and break. Bone resists fatigue fracture by remodeling—strength is enhanced by adding trabeculae along lines of stress. This process, however, is slow and requires up to two weeks to resorb the old trabeculae in vulnerable areas. As might be expected, if excessive stress is applied before the new trabeculae form, a fracture occurs. Since the calcaneus is primarily cancellous bone, the typical result is a compression fracture at the junction of the body and the tuberosity.

In the initial stages of this condition, the patient will develop mild to moderate pain accompanied by localized swelling. It is unusual for the physician to see the patient at this stage, since the individual usually will try to work through the pain. At this point, the physical findings are nonspecific. With careful examination, however, a discreet area of point tenderness can be localized. Plain x-ray will be normal at this stage. Bone scan, however, the diagnostic study of choice, will demonstrate increased uptake at the fracture site as early as two days after the onset of symptoms.[18] Treatment during the early stages consists of protecting the extremity from stress until the symptoms resolve, which usually requires about 1-3 weeks. Protection against future injury can be achieved by eliminating stressful activity, putting the patient on crutches, or application of a walking cast. Orthopedic or primary care follow-up is recommended. When symptoms resolve, the patient may be allowed to gradually return to his or her normal activities.

Patients who present more than two weeks after the onset of symptoms usually will have more definitive physical and radiographic findings. Swelling and tenderness are invariably present. Radiographs will usually show bone resorption, a transverse fracture line, or new periosteal bone formation. *(Please see Figure 6.)* ED treatment at this stage consists of rest to the foot to facilitate healing of the fracture, a posterior splint and crutch walking, and prompt orthopedic outpatient follow-up. Some authors advocate immobilization in a non-weight-bearing cast. Generally, however, immobilization in a weight-bearing cast is sufficient. Protection should continue until the fracture is non-tender, which usually requires about 4-6 weeks. The patient may then begin gradual, progressive return to normal activities.

Talar Neck Fractures. The talus is one of the most important bones in the foot because it both supports and distributes the body's weight. It permits motion between the tibia and the foot, and is the pivot point for tibiotalar and subtalar motion. The talus is the sec-

Figure 6

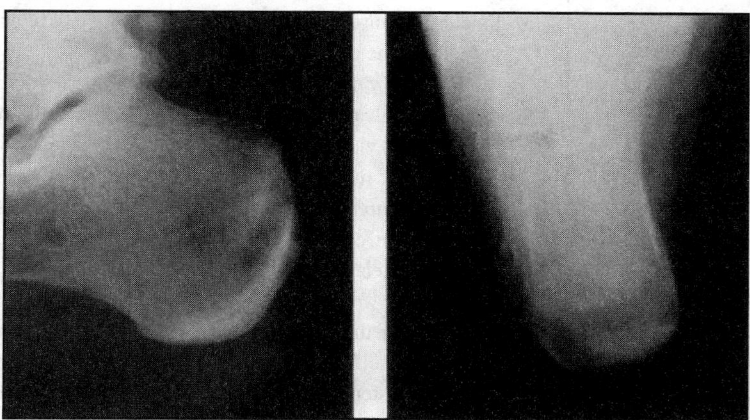

Calcaneal Stress Fracture. Stress fracture of the calcaneus. Note that the fracture line is perpendicular to the normal trabeculae and that it occurs at the junction of the body and the tuberosity. Also note the new bone formation.

Figure 7

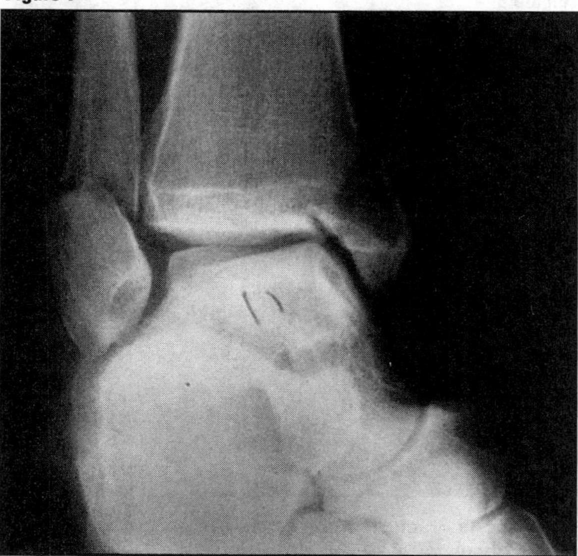

Talar Neck Fracture. Mortise view of the ankle demonstrates the talus fracture, an associated bimalleolar fracture (medial and lateral malleoli), and the alignment of the ankle joint.

ond most commonly fractured tarsal bone. These fractures are important because of the potential loss of function associated with talar injuries and because of poor blood supply to this bone. Three-fifths of the bone is covered with articular cartilage, and fractures through the neck have a high incidence of avascular necrosis. The most common mechanism of injury producing talar neck fracture is hyperdorsiflexion of the foot; rarely, however, a direct blow to the dorsum of the foot may produce a neck fracture. The typical sequence of injury usually occurs as follows: 1) with hyperdorsiflexion of the foot, the posterior capsular ligaments of the subtalar joint rupture; 2) the neck of the talus makes an impact against the anterior edge of the distal tibia; and 3) a fracture line develops at the neck of the talus.

The history usually involves one of a severe, high-energy injury in which the foot is driven into dorsiflexion, as might occur in a motor vehicle accident in which the foot is driven against the brake pedal or in a fall from a great height. The patient will complain of severe pain in the foot and ankle and, usually, will not be able to bear weight. They will note immediate and significant swelling. On examination, the foot and ankle will be grossly swollen, with loss of normal contours of the ankle and hindfoot. The foot and ankle should be assessed for open wounds; tented skin with ischemic appearance should be noted, and neurovascular integrity evaluated. The examining physician should identify associated injuries, which are common because of the high-energy mechanism; in fact, associated lower-extremity injuries have been reported in approximately two-thirds of talar neck fractures.[19] All structures should be palpated and assessed for tenderness or swelling. All suspected talus fractures should be evaluated with AP, lateral, and mortise views of the ankle, as well as AP and lateral films of the foot. The AP and mortise views of the ankle will demonstrate alignment of the talus in the mortise and will identify associated ankle fractures. The lateral x-ray of the ankle and foot is used to demonstrate a fracture line through the talar neck and to evaluate the alignment of the subtalar joint.

In the ED, the key to optimizing outcomes in these injuries is maintaining a high index of suspicion, which permits early recognition and treatment. Immediate orthopedic consultation usually is indicated since definitive treatment involves early, open reduction and internal fixation. When an orthopedist is not immediately available, an attempt at closed reduction should be made. Closed reduction is accomplished by manipulating the foot so that it is realigned with the body fragment. Sedation and/or ankle block should be administered as gentle traction is applied. While traction is initiated, the foot is plantar flexed to bring the head fragment in line with the body, and AP and lateral x-rays should be obtained. *(Please see Figure 7.)* If reduction is achieved the foot should be splinted, not acutely casted, in plantar flexion. Urgent consultation should be arranged.

Fractures of the Calcaneus. The calcaneus is the most commonly fractured tarsal bone. Intra-articular fractures account for 75% of calcaneus fractures. Almost always, this injury is the result of from a fall from a significant height. Typically, the patient lands on the heels, with the entire weight of the body absorbed by the calcaneus, a primarily cancellous bone lacking cortical strength. Consequently, the fall does not have to be from a great height. The severity of the injury depends more on the exact location of the point of impact than on the height of the fall. It is critical to appreciate that these injuries have a significant potential for producing soft tissue complications if not recognized and treated properly in the acute setting. In addition, the ED physician must be aware of the high incidence of associated spine injuries.

Clinical Presentation. The patient with a calcaneus fracture will present with heel pain and swelling. Unlike those with a talar neck fracture, these patients may be able to bear weight despite consider-

Figure 8

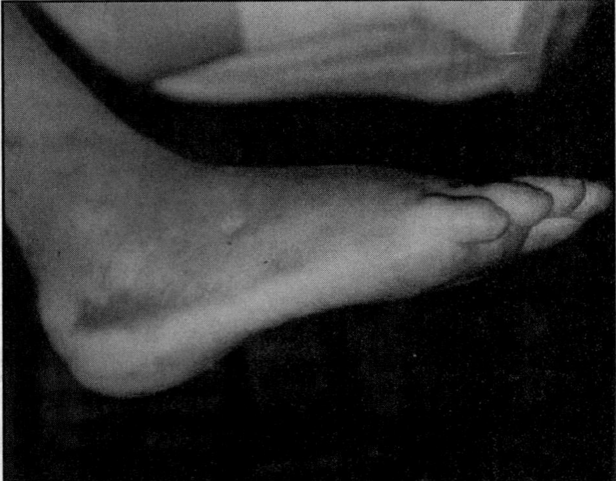

Calcaneus Fracture. Appearance of the foot in a patient with a calcaneus fracture. Note the ecchymosis, the loss of normal contour, and the shortened, widened hindfoot.

Figure 9

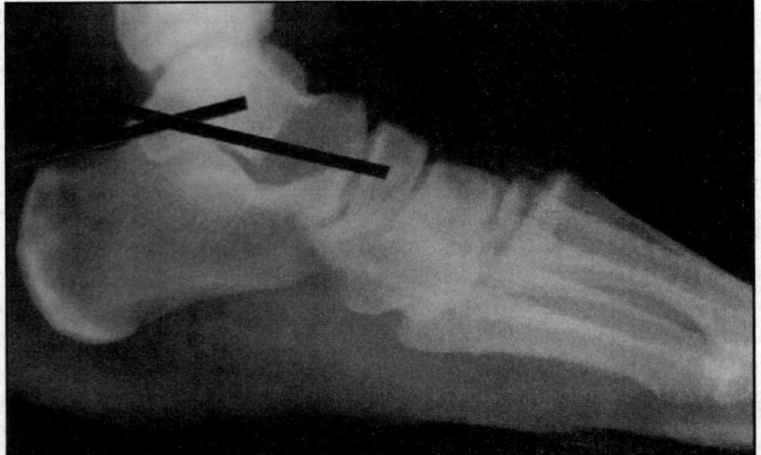

Bohler's angle. Bohler's angle, measured on this normal lateral view, is used in this instance to detect a radiographically occult calcaneal compression fracture. The angle itself is obtained by drawing two lines, one from the posterior tuberosity to the apex of the posterior facet and the other from the apex of the posterior facet to the apex of the anterior process. Bohler's angle may vary from 20° to 40°; a compression fracture is suggested with an angle less than 20°.

able pain. It should be stressed that this injury is associated with other lower extremity injuries in 70% of cases and spine fractures in 10%; moreover, these other injuries can be painful enough to overshadow the foot injury and the patient may not even complain of significant heel pain. Accordingly, all patients who sustain a fall from a height should have a comprehensive examination directed at the heel to the thoracic spine. Calcaneus fractures present with tenderness, swelling, and ecchymosis of tissues surrounding the calcaneus; ecchymosis extending onto the arch of the foot is felt to be pathognomonic of a calcaneus fracture. The normal contour of the heel is lost and the heel appears widened and shortened. *(Please see Figure 8.)* Open fractures are common and the skin should be carefully examined for small puncture wounds. Finally, fracture blisters can develop very quickly and may affect the course of treatment.

Radiography. The basic radiographic series for a suspected calcaneus fracture includes AP, lateral, and Harris axial views of the foot. The lateral view will demonstrate most intra-articular fractures. Bohlers' angle, measured on the lateral view, is used to assess the degree of compression of the calcaneus; it also is useful in detecting a radiographically occult calcaneal compression fracture, as well as in determining the congruity of the posterior facet of the subtalar joint. The angle itself is obtained by drawing two lines—one from the posterior tuberosity to the apex of the posterior facet, and the other from the apex of the posterior facet to the apex of the anterior process. *(Please see Figure 9.)* Bohlers' angle may vary from 20 to 40°; a compression fracture is suggested with an angle less than 20°. *(Please see Figure 10.)* If a fracture is identified, a lateral x-ray of the opposite foot is necessary in order to compare the angles. The axial view of the foot demonstrates the amount of widening of the heel and is critical for guiding definitive treatment. The AP of the foot will reveal extension of the fracture into the calcaneocuboid joint or associated subluxation of the talonavicular joint.

The acute ED treatment of these fractures requires careful management of the soft tissues. Soft-tissue swelling and fracture blisters frequently accompany this injury during the first hours after injury. Immediate application of a bulky, compressive dressing with a posterior splint, combined with elevation and ice application, can prevent fracture blisters and skin sloughing; surgical intervention may be required.

Lisfranc Fracture/Dislocation

The articulation between the tarsal and metatarsal bones in the foot is named after the French physician, Jacques Lisfranc, a field surgeon in Napoleon's army who first described amputations through this joint. Injuries to this anatomic region result from falls and motor vehicle or industrial accidents, and range from mild sprains to severe dislocations, as well as fracture/dislocations. Historically, Lisfranc injuries were thought to be rare, accounting for less than 1% of all orthopedic trauma; the overall incidence, however, is increasing and these fractures are more common than initially recognized.[20] The complex bony and ligamentous anatomy of this joint and the multiple patterns and mechanisms of injury make radiographic interpretation challenging and the diagnosis difficult. In fact, the diagnosis is missed on initial presentation to the emergency department in about 20% of cases.[20-23] Failure of diagnosis, misdiagnosis, or inappropriate treatment is associated with an increased risk for chronic disability.[20] As a result, emergency physicians should be familiar with the presentation of Lisfranc injuries, and recognize that early diagnosis and timely orthopedic referral are essential for optimal treatment and outcome.

Lisfranc injuries are caused by either direct or indirect trauma. Direct or crush injuries to the dorsum of the foot are rare and may be complicated by contamination, vascular compromise, or compartment syndrome.[20] Displacement of the metatarsal bases may occur in either the plantar or dorsal direction depending on the direction of force at the time of injury. Indirect forces are responsible for the largest group of injuries, which result from either a rotational force applied to the forefoot with a fixed hindfoot or axial loading on a plantar flexed, fixed foot. The longitudinal force results in metatarsal dislocation dorsally at the site of least resistance, while the rotational force causes dislocation medially or laterally. Inasmuch as significant energy is required to produce dislocation, these injuries frequently are associated with multiple fractures and significant soft-tissue injury.[24] Common causes of indirect trauma include falls from a height, motor vehicle or motorcycle accidents, equestrian accidents, and athletic injuries.

Lisfranc injuries range from mild, undetectable subluxations to obvious fracture/dislocations. The clinical presentations are as varied as the patterns of injury. Consequently, the emergency physician should always maintain a high index of suspicion when evaluating an injured foot. Patients with a significant tarsometatarsal injury, generally present with complaints of midfoot pain, swelling, and difficulty bearing weight. In mild injuries, patients may be able to bear weight acutely and may be surprisingly active despite the pain. Tenderness along the Lisfranc joint is common and passive pronation with abduction of the forefoot with the hindfoot held fixed elicits pain; this maneuver is specific for tarsometatarsal injuries.[24] The foot may appear normal or markedly deformed, depending on the severity of the injury. However, significant swelling of the foot may mask a deformity. If the mechanism of injury is severe or deformity is obvious, manipulation of the foot should be kept to a minimum to prevent further displacement.

A broadened foot, shortening in the anteroposterior plane, or a pathologic range of motion suggest severe fracture dislocation.[22] One study reported the potential for injury to the terminal branch of the dorsalis pedis artery as it passes to the plantar surface of the foot between the first and second metatarsal.[22] Vascular compromise at this level rarely results in ischemic necrosis of the foot, but severe fracture dislocations can damage vessels or cause vascular spasm at the level of the ankle (posterior tibial artery). Serial vascular exams are important if this injury is suspected. Tense swelling of the foot with diminished pulses suggests compartment syndrome; in these cases, immediate surgical intervention is necessary to save the extremity.[20,24] In a multiply injured, unconscious patient, the injury is easily missed because more life-threatening issues preclude full evaluation of the extremities. After the patient's condition has improved, stability of the tarsometatarsal joint should be evaluated.

Figure 10

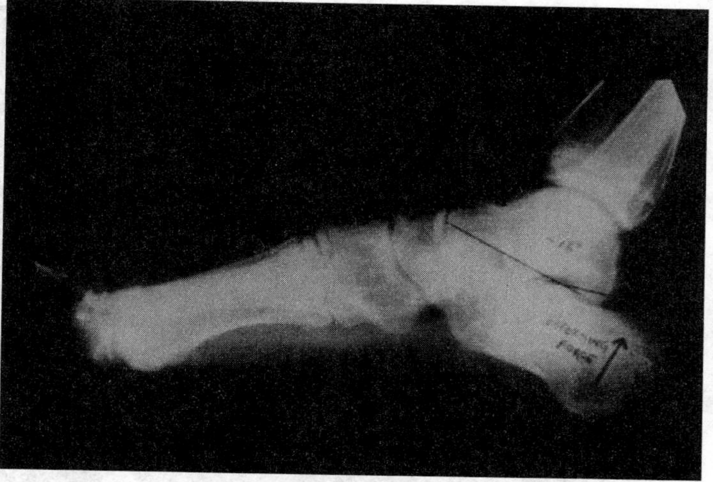

Calcaneus fracture with abnormal Bohler's angle. Lateral view of a calcaneus fracture. Note the loss of Bohler's angle—here, the angle is approximately 16°, confirming the clinical impression of calcaneal fracture in this patient who fell 16 feet, landing on his feet; he also a tibial plateau fracture and lumbar compression fracture.

Figure 11

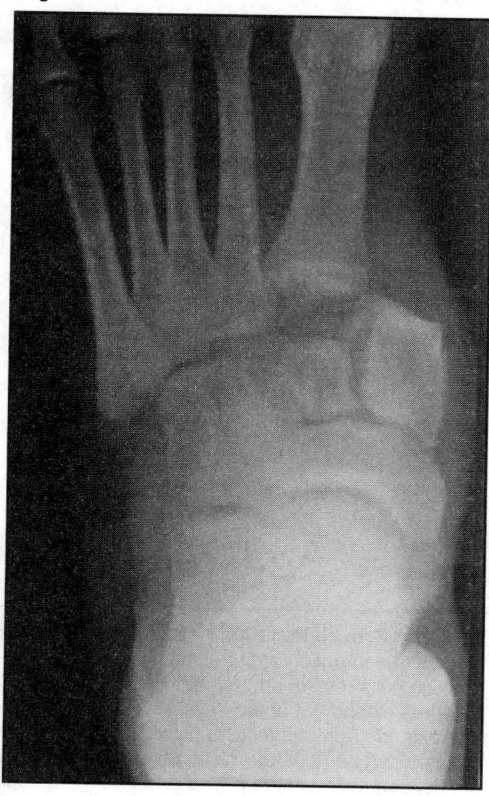

Lisfranc Fracture/Dislocation. AP view of a fracture/dislocation. Note the malalignment of the medial border of the second metatarsal and the medial aspect of the middle cuneiform.

Radiography. Proper radiographic evaluation of the foot is essential for the diagnosis of Lisfranc injuries. The tarsometatarsal trauma series should include accurate radiographs of three planes of the injured foot—anteroposterior, lateral, and oblique views. Comparison radiographs of the contralateral foot may be helpful in detecting subtle injuries. Major fracture/dislocations are easily recognized and are rarely missed. Sprain injuries without dislocation, however, are difficult to diagnose radiographically even though physical examination findings are highly suggestive of tarsometatarsal involvement. Roentgenograms of the tarsometatarsal joint can be difficult to interpret because of the overlapping bony articulations.

Figure 12

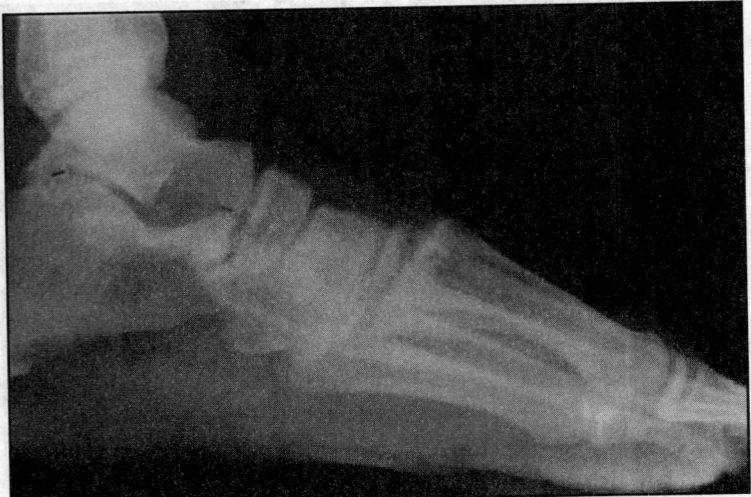

Lisfranc Fracture/Dislocation. Lateral view of the patient from Figure 11 demonstrating the dislocation at the level of the tarsal-metatarsal interface. Note the over-riding metatarsal bone with dorsal displacement relative to the remainder of the foot.

Figure 13

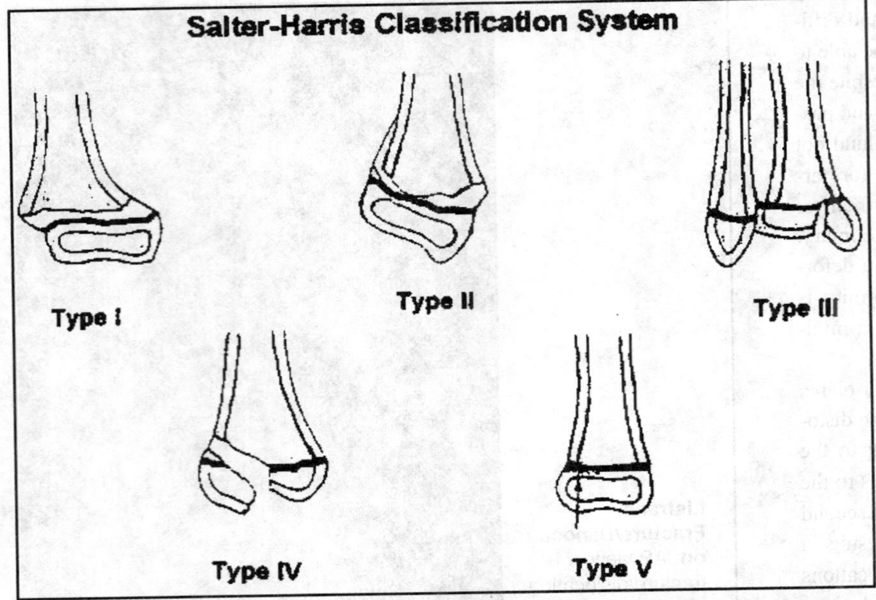

Pediatric Growth Plate Injuries According to the Salter-Harris Description. *Type I*: Complete separation of the epiphysis from the metaphysis without osseous fracture. The growing cells remain on the epiphysis. *Type II*: The most common growth plate injury, these fractures extend out of the physis through the metaphysis. *Type III*: This intra-articular fracture extends from the joint surface to the epiphyseal plate, then along the plate to the perimeter. *Type IV*: Intra-articular fractures extending from the joint surface through the epiphysis, across the entire physis and through a segment of the metaphysis. *Type V*: Type V injuries are crush injuries of the epiphysis.

Lisfranc injuries will not be missed if the clinician is familiar with the consistent anatomical relationships of the normal foot. The second metatarsal base should always be carefully evaluated for fracture, avulsions, and displacement. On AP and oblique radiographs, the medial border of the second metatarsal base and the middle cuneiform and the medial border of the fourth metatarsal base and cuboid should form a straight, unbroken line.[20] Any disruption of these lines or fracture fragments around the base of the second metatarsal or along the lateral border of the cuboid indicates significant tarsometatarsal injury. *(Please see Figure 11.)* Other normal findings include a straight line formed by the lateral border of the base of the third metatarsal and lateral border of the lateral cuneiform. On the lateral film, a metatarsal shaft should never be more dorsal than its respective tarsal bone.[21] *(Please see Figure 12.)* A fracture of the cuboid, cuneiforms, navicular, or metatarsal shafts is suggestive of disarticulation of the tarsometatarsal joint. In minor subluxation injuries, the key to diagnosis is the mortise configuration of the second metatarsal. Separation between the base of the first and second metatarsal or between the medial and middle cuneiforms is strongly suggestive of subluxation.[22,24] Widening can also occur between the second and third metatarsal or middle and lateral cuneiforms. A minor displacement of the three lateral metatarsal bones may be missed on AP and lateral films but should be obvious on 30° oblique views.[22]

Definitive treatment of these fractures involves surgical intervention. The ED physician should suspect the diagnosis, confirm the injury radiographically, and recognize that compartment syndrome may accompany this fracture. If orthopedic consultation is not immediately available, the emergency physician should attempt closed reduction by hanging the foot by the toes using finger traps. If reduced, a bulky compressive dressing should be applied with a posterior splint. These injuries warrant acute orthopedic evaluation.

Compartment Syndrome

Compartment syndrome is a serious life- and limb-threatening complication of extremity trauma. Fracture, crush injury, burn, and arterial injuries can result in increased tissue pressure within a closed compartmental space.[25] Compartment syndrome develops when there is increased pressure in a limited space, such as muscle compartments bound by dense fascial sheaths. Compartments in the arm and leg are most vulnerable to this syndrome. The upper arm contains anterior (the biceps-brachialis muscle and the radial, ulnar, and median nerves) and posterior (the triceps muscle) compartments. The forearm has a

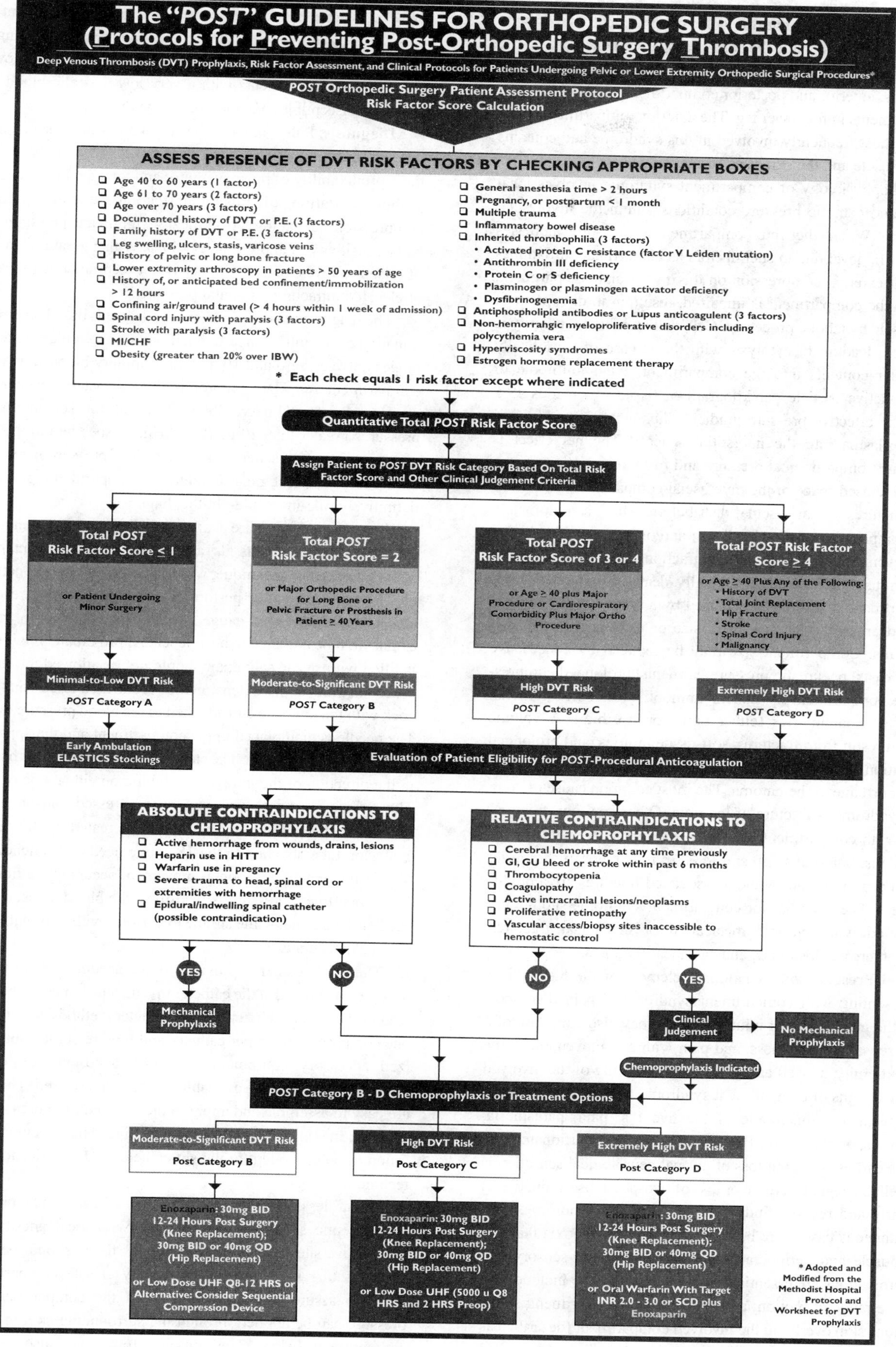

The "POST" GUIDELINES FOR ORTHOPEDIC SURGERY
(Protocols for Preventing Post-Orthopedic Surgery Thrombosis)
Deep Venous Thrombosis (DVT) Prophylaxis, Risk Factor Assessment, and Clinical Protocols for Patients Undergoing Pelvic or Lower Extremity Orthopedic Surgical Procedures*
POST Orthopedic Surgery Patient Assessment Protocol
Risk Factor Score Calculation
ASSESS PRESENCE OF DVT RISK FACTORS BY CHECKING APPROPRIATE BOXES
Age 40 to 60 years (1 factor)
Age 61 to 70 years (2 factors)
Age over 70 years (3 factors)
Documented history of DVT or P.E. (3 factors)
Family history of DVT or P.E. (3 factors)
Leg swelling, ulcers, stasis, varicose veins
History of pelvic or long bone fracture
Lower extremity arthroscopy in patients > 50 years of age
History of, or anticipated bed confinement/immobilization > 12 hours
Confining air/ground travel (> 4 hours within 1 week of admission)
Spinal cord injury with paralysis (3 factors)
Stroke with paralysis (3 factors)
MI/CHF
Obesity (greater than 20% over IBW)
General anesthesia time > 2 hours
Pregnancy, or postpartum < 1 month
Multiple trauma
Inflammatory bowel disease
Inherited thrombophilia (3 factors)
• Activated protein C resistance (factor V Leiden mutation)
• Antithrombin III deficiency
• Protein C or S deficiency
• Plasminogen or plasminogen activator deficiency
• Dysfibrinogenemia
Antiphospholipid antibodies or Lupus anticoagulent (3 factors)
Non-hemorrahgic myeloproliferative disorders including polycythemia vera
Hyperviscosity symdromes
Estrogen hormone replacement therapy
* Each check equals 1 risk factor except where indicated
Quantitative Total POST Risk Factor Score
Assign Patient to POST DVT Risk Category Based On Total Risk Factor Score and Other Clinical Judgement Criteria
Total POST Risk Factor Score ≤ 1
or Patient Undergoing Minor Surgery
Minimal-to-Low DVT Risk
POST Category A
Early Ambulation
ELASTICS Stockings
Total POST Risk Factor Score = 2
or Major Orthopedic Procedure for Long Bone or Pelvic Fracture or Prosthesis in Patient ≥ 40 Years
Moderate-to-Significant DVT Risk
POST Category B
Total POST Risk Factor Score of 3 or 4
or Age ≥ 40 plus Major Procedure or Cardiorespiratory Comorbidity Plus Major Ortho Procedure
High DVT Risk
POST Category C
Total POST Risk Factor Score ≥ 4
or Age ≥ 40 Plus Any of the Following:
• History of DVT
• Total Joint Replacement
• Hip Fracture
• Stroke
• Spinal Cord Injury
• Malignancy
Extremely High DVT Risk
POST Category D
Evaluation of Patient Eligibility for POST-Procedural Anticoagulation
ABSOLUTE CONTRAINDICATIONS TO CHEMOPROPHYLAXIS
Active hemorrhage from wounds, drains, lesions
Heparin use in HITT
Warfarin use in pregancy
Severe trauma to head, spinal cord or extremities with hemorrhage
Epidural/indwelling spinal catheter (possible contraindication)
RELATIVE CONTRAINDICATIONS TO CHEMOPROPHYLAXIS
Cerebral hemorrhage at any time previously
GI, GU bleed or stroke within past 6 months
Thrombocytopenia
Coagulopathy
Active intracranial lesions/neoplasms
Proliferative retinopathy
Vascular access/biopsy sites inaccessible to hemostatic control
YES
NO
NO
YES
Mechanical Prophylaxis
Clinical Judgement
No Mechanical Prophylaxis
Chemoprophylaxis Indicated
POST Category B - D Chemoprophylaxis or Treatment Options
Moderate-to-Significant DVT Risk
Post Category B
Enoxaparin: 30mg BID 12-24 Hours Post Surgery (Knee Replacement); 30mg BID or 40mg QD (Hip Replacement)
or Low Dose UHF Q8-12 HRS or Alternative: Consider Sequential Compression Device
High DVT Risk
Post Category C
Enoxaparin: 30mg BID 12-24 Hours Post Surgery (Knee Replacement); 30mg BID or 40mg QD (Hip Replacement)
or Low Dose UHF (5000 u Q8 HRS and 2 HRS Preop)
Extremely High DVT Risk
Post Category D
Enoxaparin: 30mg BID 12-24 Hours Post Surgery (Knee Replacement); 30mg BID or 40mg QD (Hip Replacement)
or Oral Warfarin With Target INR 2.0 - 3.0 or SCD plus Enoxaparin
*Adopted and Modified from the Methodist Hospital Protocol and Worksheet for DVT Prophylaxis

volar and dorsal compartment; the volar compartment contains the wrist and finger flexors, while the dorsal compartment holds the wrist and finger extensors. In the lower extremity, there are three gluteal compartments, anterior and posterior compartments in the thigh, and four compartments in the lower leg. The anterior compartment of the lower leg is most frequently involved in this syndrome and contains the tibialis muscle and the extensors of the toes.

The pathophysiology of compartment syndrome involves local hydrostatic and osmotic pressure conditions within the myofascial compartment. When the intracompartmental pressure increases above a specific level due to such factors as hemorrhage, inflammatory fluid, or external compression on the myofascial compartment, perfusion to the compartment is impaired, resulting in disruption of skeletal muscle metabolic processes. Cell wall membrane integrity is compromised, leading to cytolysis with the release of osmotically active cellular contents into the compartment. Each millimole of osmotically active particle per kilogram of tissue water adds 19.5 mmHg to the effective pressure gradient, thus attracting additional fluid from plasma into the interstitial space.[26] The net effect is increased intracompartmental pressure and further disruption of perfusion to the closed space of the myofascial compartment, as well as to distal structures of that vascular distribution, which can ultimately lead to a compromise of the circulation and/or nerve conduction as well as irreversible muscle injury, contractions, loss of limb, myoglobinuria, renal failure, and, occasionally, death.[27]

Compartment syndromes are caused by a number of conditions that either decrease the compartment size or increase the compartment contents. Compartment size may be reduced by constrictive dressing or casts, pneumatic pressure garments, prolonged compression of the compartment by patient immobility, closure of fascial defects, or thermal injuries (either burns or frostbite). A volume increase can result from fractures, soft-tissue injuries, and prolonged immobilization with limb compression, vessel lacerations, exertion, edema, hemorrhage, or hematoma. The most common cause of compartment syndrome is fracture of the tibia. Other common fractures associated with compartment syndrome are supracondylar fractures of the humerus, humoral shaft, and forearm fractures. Crush injuries to the hand or foot with or without associated fractures are a predisposing factor. The potential for compartment syndrome should also be considered with multiple metacarpal or metatarsal fractures, Lisfranc fractures/dislocations, and calcaneal fractures.

Clinical Presentation. A hallmark element of the history in a patient presenting with compartment syndrome is pain disproportionate to the mechanism of injury. Patients may also complain of a change in sensation, weakness, and pain with any movement of the involved extremity, as well as tightness and swelling of the involved area. Clinical signs of compartment syndrome can easily be remembered by using the mnemonic of the five P's: pain, paresthesia, paresis, pulses, and pressure. Pain, especially disproportionate pain, is often the earliest sign, but loss of normal neurological sensation is the most reliable sign. Decrease or loss of two-point discrimination is also an early and reliable finding of compartment syndrome. Skin and subcutaneous tissues are better able to survive hypoxia than are skeletal muscle and peripheral nerves. Careful serial sensory and motor examinations are essential. Clinical findings also include pain with passive range of motion; a palpable, tense compartment; shiny, erythematous skin overlying the involved compartment (described as a "woody" feeling); and excessive swelling. A thready or diminished pulse is not a very reliable early sign. Intra-compartmental tissue pressure is usually lower than arterial blood pressure, making peripheral pulses and capillary refill poor indicators of blood flow within the compartment. Patients with a very low diastolic blood pressure are more susceptible to compartment syndrome.

Diagnosis. Pulse oximetry has been advocated as a simple, noninvasive indicator of vascular compromise. One study investigated the reproducibility of pulse oximetry and the effect on arterial hemoglobin saturation of raising intracompartmental pressure by compression bandaging. At clinically significant pressures, the test had a sensitivity of approximately 40%. With a greater then 50% risk of false negatives, pulse oximetry is not recommended for detection of elevated intracompartmental pressure.[28]

The diagnosis of compartment syndrome is based on direct determination of the intracompartmental pressure. Normal tissue pressure ranges between zero and 10 mmHg. Capillary blood flow within the compartment may be compromised at pressures greater than 20 mmHg. Muscle and nerve fibers are at risk for ischemic necrosis at pressures greater than 30 to 40 mmHg. Tissues within the compartment may become ischemic and necrotic if pressure is not promptly reduced. The direct measurement of compartment pressures will definitively rule-in or rule-out the diagnosis.

Several techniques are available for intracompartmental pressure determination; each has its advantages and disadvantages. They include the needle technique, wick catheter, and the slit catheter. The needle technique can be performed with items that are readily available in the ED. An 18-gauge needle is attached to an intravenous extension tube and then to a stopcock. Approximately half the tubing is filled with sterile saline; air should not be allowed into the tubing. A second intravenous extension tube is attached to the four-way stopcock with the opposite end attached to the blood pressure manometer. The needle is then placed in the compartment and the apparatus kept at the level of the needle. The stopcock is then turned so that it is open in the direction of the intravenous tubing on either side of a syringe. The syringe filled with air is slowly compressed, causing air to move into both extension tubes. The meniscus created by the saline in the extension tube attached to the 18-gauge needle is watched carefully for any movement. As soon as movement occurs in the fluid column, the compartment pressure is read from the blood pressure manometer. This technique, while simple to perform with minimal equipment, may be inaccurate.

The wick catheter provides more accurate readings, but can become coagulated at the catheter tip and leave material behind in the wound. The wick catheter and slit catheter methods can only measure one compartment site per catheter and require cumbersome, specialized accessory equipment. Portable, hand-held tissue pressure monitoring systems are available and are widely used. These systems are easy to assemble and apply in the ED; multiple uses are possible per unit, making the system cost effective. Their accuracy has been found to be equivalent to the slit catheter and superior to the needle technique.

Regardless of the method used, the skin should be prepped with an antiseptic solution and infiltrated with local anesthesia at the prospective site. Only the subcutaneous tissue should be infiltrated. Intramuscular injection may artificially elevate compartment pressure. To assure that the needle is in the compartment, external pressure can be applied through the surrounding skin to the muscle compartment below. The muscle group may also be passively stretched to transiently increase compartment pressure. The site of pressure measurement is important. In a study of 25 patients with closed tibial fractures, failure to measure tissue pressure within a few centimeters of the zone of peak pressure can result in underestimation of the maximum compartment pressure. Measurements should be taken in both the anterior and deep posterior compartments at the level of the fracture as well as at locations proximal and distal to the zone of the fracture to determine the locations of highest tissue pressure in a lower extremity.

Treatment. The goal of treatment of compartment syndrome is to decrease tissue pressure, restore blood flow, and minimize tissue damage and related functional loss. External pressure from casts or dressings should be removed immediately. It has been shown that if a cast is bivalved, the compartment pressures may decrease as much as 55%, and if a cast is completely removed, the pressure may decrease as much as 85%. The affected limb should be elevated to the level of the heart to promote arterial blood flow and not decrease venous return. Elevation above the heart can result in decreased perfusion. Ice is contraindicated because it may compromise the microcirculation. Steroids and vasodilating agents have not been shown to be of benefit.

Acute compartment syndrome is a surgical emergency. Fasciotomy is definitive therapy and should be performed as soon as possible. Delays of more than 24 hours can have devastating consequences, including significant muscle mass damage resulting in myoglobinuria, renal failure, metabolic acidosis, hyperkalemia, and, ultimately, contracture formation or loss of the limb. Absolute indications for fasciotomy are: 1) clinical signs of acute compartment syndrome, 2) raised tissue pressure greater than 30 mmHg in a patient with the clinical picture of compartment syndrome, and 3) interrupted, arterial circulation to an extremity for greater than four hours.

Pediatric Fractures—Growth Plate Injuries

The epiphyseal plate (physis) is the growth cartilage of the long bones of children. It is most frequently injured after the age of 10. Physeal injuries have been reported to account for between 15% and 30% of all skeletal injuries in children.[29-31] One study suggested that 15% of these injuries result in physeal arrest.[32] Another study, however, demonstrated that proper therapy of these injuries reduced the incidence of physeal arrest to 1.4%.[30] The generation of the fracture line through the growth plate is used to categorize fractures using the Salter-Harris Classification System described in 1963.[32] *(Please see Figure 13.)*

- Type I. Complete separation of the epiphysis from the metaphysis without osseous fracture. The growing cells remain on the epiphysis.
- Type II. The most common growth plate injury; these fractures extend out of the physis through the metaphysis.
- Type III. This intra-articular fracture extends from the joint surface to the epiphyseal plate, then along the plate to the perimeter.
- Type IV. Intra-articular fractures extending from the joint surface through the epiphysis, across the entire physis and through a segment of the metaphysis.
- Type V. Type V injuries are crush injuries of the epiphysis.

AP and lateral radiographic views are required to diagnose growth plate injuries; comparison views of the contralateral bone may often assist in determining the difference between an irregular physis and a fracture. Complex fractures may require plain tomography or CT scan, especially those of the distal tibia or those Type III and IV fractures in which the degree of displacement may be the deciding factor for open reduction and fixation.

Type I fractures are most frequently encountered in infants and toddlers. The injury mechanism generally involves a shearing, torsion, or avulsion movement, which essentially produces a separation through the growth plate. Closed reduction of Type I fractures is relatively easy, if diagnosed early. The prognosis for ensuing growth is good unless there has been damage to the arterial supply of the epiphysis, which is seen with injuries involving displacement of the capital femoral epiphysis or the epiphysis of the head of the radius. Type II injuries occur most often in children older than 8 years of age and involve a fracture line that passes through the epiphyseal plate; the epiphysis is laterally displaced, tearing the periosteum on one side while leaving it intact on the side of the metaphyseal fracture. Type II fractures are easily reduced due to the intact periosteum on the fracture side. Because circulation to the epiphysis remains intact, the prognosis for growth is good. Displaced Type I or II fractures that require reduction are treated with complete limb splint for 6-8 weeks.

Type III fractures are uncommon, and occur at the upper or lower tibial physis. Intra-articular shearing forces cause the injury; the fracture line passes through the epiphysis. Accurate reduction of a Type III fracture is essential to restore the joint surface. Prognosis for growth is good provided that the blood supply to the fractured epiphysis remains intact. More than 2 mm of displacement suggests the need for surgery with open reduction. Type IV injuries are most commonly seen at the lower end of the humerus, with the fracture line passing through the metaphyseal and epiphyseal portions of the bone. Unless the fracture is non-displaced, open reduction is always necessary to restore the smooth joint surface. The physis must be perfectly aligned to prevent premature closure of the growth plate. Type V fractures are severe crush injuries through the epiphysis damaging a portion of the physis. These injuries are uncommon but can lead to severe growth reduction problems. Because of minimal displacement, this fracture is often difficult to detect radiographically. As the prognosis for continued bone growth is poor, localized physeal tenderness should increase suspicion for a Type V fracture. Maintaining non-weight-bearing for three weeks can reduce the risk of premature growth arrest.

References

1. Bogost GA, Lizerbram EK, Crues JV. MR imaging in evaluation of suspected hip fracture: Frequency of unsuspected bone and soft-tissue injury. *Radiol* 1995;197: 263-267.
2. Pandey R, McNally E, Ali A, et al. The role of MRI in the diagnosis of occult hip fractures. *Injury* 1998;29:61-63.
3. Mlinek EJ, Clark KC, Walker CW. Limited magnetic resonance imaging in the diagnosis of occult hip fracture. *Am J Emerg Med* 1998;16:390-392.
4. Bennett WF, Browner B. Tibial plateau fractures: A study of associated soft-tissue injuries. *J Orthop Trauma* 1994;8: 183-188.
5. Holt MD, William LA, Dent CM. MRI in the management of

tibial plateau fractures. *Injury* 1995;26:595-599.
6. Barrow BA, Fajman WA, Parker LM, et al. Tibial plateau fractures: Evaluation with MR imaging. *Radiographics* 1994;14:553-559.
7. Honkonen SE. Degenerative arthritis after tibial plateau fractures. *J Orthop Trauma* 1995;9:272-277.
8. Andrews JR, Tender JL, Godbout BP. Bicondylar tibial plateau fracture complicated by compartment syndrome. *Orthop Rev* 1992;219:317-319.
9. Lapinsky AS, Padgett DE, Hall FW. Disruptions of the extensor mechanism in Paget's disease. *Am J Orthop* 1995; 24:165-167.
10. Jozsa L, Kvist M, Balint BJ, et al. The role of recreational sport activity in Achilles tendon rupture. A clinical, pathoanatomical, and sociological study of 292 cases. *Am J Sports Med* 1989;17:338-343.
11. Leppilahti J, Puranen J, Orava S. Incidence of Achilles tendon rupture. *Acta Orthop Scand* 1996;67:277-279.
12. Kvist H, Kvist M. The operative treatment of chronic calcaneal paratendinitis. *J Bone Joint Surg* 1980;62B: 353-356.
13. Cetti R, Andersen I. Roentgenographic diagnoses of ruptured Achilles tendons. *Clin Orthop Related Research* 1993;286: 215-221.
14. Lea RB, Smith L. Rupture of the Achilles tendon nonsurgical treatment. *Clin Orthop* 1968;60:115-119.
15. Lea RB, Smith L. Non-surgical treatment of Achilles rupture. *J Bone Joint Surg* 1972;54A:1398-1404.
16. Freed H, Shields NM. Most frequently overlooked radiographically apparent fractures in a teaching hospital emergency department. *Ann Emerg Med* 1984;13:900-904.
17. Trafton PG, Bray TJ, Simpson LA. Fractures and soft-tissue injuries of the ankle. In: Browner B, Jupiter J, Levine A, et al (eds). *Skeletal Trauma,* vol 2. WB Saunders: Philadelphia; 1992.
18. Geslian GE, Thrall JH, Espinoza JL, et al. Early detection of stress fractures using 99mTC-poly-phosphate. *Radiol* 1976; 121:683-687.
19. Hawkins LG. Fractures of the neck of the talus. *J Bone Joint Surg* 1970;52A:991-1002.
20. Arntz CT, Hansen ST. Dislocations and fracture dislocations of the tarsometatarsal joints. *Orthop Clin North Am* 1987; 18:105-114.
21. Englenhoff G, Anglin D, Hutson HR. Lisfranc fracture dislocation: A frequently missed diagnosis in the emergency department. *Ann Emerg Med* 1995;26:229-233.
22. Goosens M, DeStoop N. Lisfranc's fracture dislocations: Etiology, radiology, result of treatment. *Clin Orthop* 1983;176:154-162.
23. Vuori JP, Aro HT. Lisfranc joint injuries: Trauma mechanisms and associated injuries. *J Trauma* 1993;35:40-45.
24. Myerson M. The diagnosis and treatment of injuries to the Lisfranc joint complex. *Orthop Clin North Am* 1989;20: 655-664.
25. Mabee JR. Compartment syndrome: A complication of acute extremity trauma. *J Emerg Med* 1994;12:651-656.
26. Linjen P, Hespel P, Eynde EV, et al. Biochemical variables in plasma and urine before and after prolonged physical exercise. *Enzyme* 1985;33:134-142.
27. Dalismer D. Case of delayed onset compartment syndrome. *Am J Emerg Med* 1994;12:176-177.
28. Mars M, Maseko S, Thompson S, et al. Can pulse oximetry detect raised intro compartmental pressure? *So Afr J Surg* 1994;32:48-50.
29. Mann DC, Rajmaira S. Distribution of physeal and nonphyseal fractures in 2650 long bone fractures in children aged 0-16 yrs. *J Pediatr Orthop* 1990;10:713-716.
30. Mizuta T, Benson W M, Foster BK, et al. Statistical analysis of the incidence of physeal injuries. *J Pediatr Orthop* 1987;7:518-523.
31. Ogden J A. Skeletal growth mechanism injury patterns. *J Pediatr Orthop* 1982;2:371-377.
32. Salter RB, Harris WR. Injuries involving the epiphyseal plate. *J Bone Joint Surg* 1963;45A:587-522.

Winter Sports-Related Injuries

Charles Stewart, MD, FACEP

Each winter, ice and snow provide abundant opportunities for recreation and enjoyment. Skiing, snowboarding, sledding, tobogganing, and skating are enjoyed by millions of adults and children. Unfortunately, these sports also have a legacy of producing serious injuries and, occasionally, even death.

Etiological and predisposing factors associated with winter sports-related injuries are well-documented. Skiers glide gracefully downhill on groomed slopes at speeds that can exceed 60 mph. Typically, these slopes are littered with other skiers, trees, rocks, moguls, and precipices. Advanced skiers revel in these hazards and go out of their way to find "maximum" vertical slopes to increase both the speed and the feeling of danger. Snowboarders revel in edged turns and jumps, whereas sledders and tobogganers seek maximum speed and jumping opportunities to add excitement to their runs.[1-4]

Each year, downhill skiers make about 50-60 million visits to their favorite slopes. For every 1000 visits, about three will result in an injury serious enough to require immediate medical care. Unfortunately, many of these individuals will seek definitive care after they have returned home, where practitioners may not be familiar with the spectrum or potential seriousness of injuries sustained during such activities. In addition, it is estimated that as many as 40% of alpine ski-related injuries, especially those of minor severity, are never reported to a physician.[1-3]

This review provides a practical and comprehensive review of both minor and serious injuries associated with such winter sports as alpine skiing, cross-country skiing, sledding, snow-boarding, and tobogganing. Emphasizing mechanism of injury, historical features of the accident, and physical evaluation, this article guides emergency physicians toward specific diagnoses and strategies for definitive management.

Downhill Ski Injuries: Demographics, Risk Factors, and Environmental Precipitants

Demographics. The recent deaths of Michael Kennedy and U.S. Rep. Sonny Bono from head trauma associated with skiing have focused attention on skiing injuries. Despite this adverse publicity, skiing remains safe when appropriate precautions are taken.

Not surprisingly, it is difficult to determine the "real" injury rate on recreational ski slopes. First, many accidents sustained by skiing enthusiasts are simply not reported; second, skiers may seek initial care somewhere else for minor, and sometimes even major, injuries. In some ski areas, when given a choice between an exorbitant medical bill and a bit of pain and suffering while the patient is evacuated by family and friends, many patients will prefer to be treated at facilities far from the slopes.

There are other confounding variables. For example, some injuries are not thought to be "that bad" until the following day, when the patient seeks medical care off the slope. In some cases, experi-

Table 1. Incidence of Selected Injuries Due to Downhill Skiing

INJURY	INCIDENCE
Sprains, strains	45.0%
Cold injury	20.0%
Lacerations, abrasions	11.5%
Fractures	9.5%
Contusions	5.0%
Dislocations	3.0%

Adapted from: Foster CR, Garrick JG, Steadman JR, et al. When skier turns tumbler. *Pat Care* 1987;21:24-44.

enced skiers may consider the injury to be part of the sport, while "softer" novices seek medical care for equivalent injuries. Consequently, injury figures provided by a ski patrol reflect only those patients who seek medical care from the patrol, rather than all who eventually require medical care.[2,3]

Injury Rates. Given the aforementioned limitations, it is estimated that males have an injury rate of about 4.9 injuries per 1000 days of skiing, whereas the rate for females is 7.9 injuries per 1000 days.[5] Juvenile skiers have at least three times the injury rate of adult skiers,[6] with at least one-third of all injuries occurring among skiers who are under the age of 16.[7] The highest rate of head and neck injuries is reported in the 11-13-year age group.[8]

Experience and athletic proficiency appear to be major factors in reducing the risk of injury associated with skiing. For example, entry-level skiers have 2-3 times the injury rate observed in more experienced skiers.[7] Not only is the inexperienced skier more likely to sustain injury, but he or she is more likely to cause injury to another skier.[9] When asked to identify the reason for their injuries, one-third of all skiers injured felt that they were going too fast for their expertise and/or the condition of the slopes.[9]

Snow Conditions. Environmental conditions play a major role in ski-related injuries. Skis are more likely to get entrapped in heavy, wet snow, in which twisting knee and ankle injuries are more likely to occur. In contrast, during icy conditions, upper-extremity injuries are more likely to occur because skis slide out from under the skier. In these accidents, the skier may fall on the face, shoulders, and upper body in the process of trying to break a fall. As might be expected, powder snow is associated with the lowest frequency of injuries. Groomed powder-covered slopes have a higher incidence of injuries than ungroomed slopes, but skilled skiers use ungroomed slopes more frequently than beginners.

Fatigue. Temporal considerations also play a role. For example, more injuries occur in afternoons—between 1 p.m. and 4 p.m.—when skiers are tired and hungry.[10] The last run of the day is typically the most dangerous and is the time when most accidents occur. Not only is the skier fatigued at this point, but there is sometimes a mad frenzy to get in "just one more run" before the slopes close for the day. From a prevention point of view, skiers should recognize their physical limits and not ski when exhausted. Many slopes now offer a service known as "downloading," in which a skier can take a chairlift down the slope instead of skiing if he or she feels tired.

Alcohol. Injuries are reported at a higher rate and tend to be more serious if alcohol consumption prevents the skier from being able to concentrate on the mechanics of skiing.[11,12] Alcohol promotes fluid losses by diuresis. Heat loss is accentuated by peripheral vasodilation caused by alcohol. These two effects of alcohol make skiers more prone to cold and dehydration.

Prevention: Protective Equipment and Safety

As might be expected, innovations in the design of skiing equipment have made a dramatic impact on ski-related trauma.

Boots. The contemporary ski boot consists of a high, hard-plastic outer shell coupled to a soft inner liner. The plastic outer shell is designed to transmit foot and leg forces to the ski in order to increase control over the ski. The liner is a thick sock-like bootie that surrounds the foot with a moldable form. The body heat molds the liner around the foot so that the bony parts of the foot are protected from the hard outer shell. Padding is provided for the anterior shin with a wide, thick foam tongue on the boot liner. Forces from the skis are transmitted through the boots and are applied at the mid-third of tibia.

Because the ankle and foot are reinforced, there are fewer ankle and foot injuries. Over the past 25 years, the incidence of tibial and fibular fractures has been reduced by 72% and 43%, respectively, because of improvements in boot design.[7] Low boots similar to old-style downhill boots are often used with cross-country skis, particularly in Telemark skiing. These boots allow the stresses of a fall to be absorbed by the relatively weak ligaments of the ankle and lower portion of the tibia and fibula. Ankle movement is freer and rotation abduction of the leg can occur about the ankle. This can result in both ankle injuries and mid-distal-third tibia fractures.

Bindings. Of all of the factors that determine whether the skier will still be skiing at the end of the day, the type and appropriate function of the bindings are most significant. Bindings have two competing functions. First, they must rigidly attach the skier's foot to the ski. Second, they must release this attachment under any stress that could injure the skier. Current dual-mode bindings release in two different directions: toe rotation and heel lift. This protects the skier from most rotation-based injuries. When combined with high-topped boots, the ankle is almost completely protected.

Unfortunately, the knee then becomes the main shock absorber in trauma to the lower extremity. The knee is quite vulnerable to this trauma for the following reasons:[13,14] Rotational forces that used to cause ankle injuries are transferred to the knee by the high boots as described above. Forces that are not protected by the dual-mode binding can cause injury to the knee. (Upward release at the toe would decrease some of these injuries.) Criteria for protection of the tibia from injury are based on cadaver studies on fractures of the tibial plateau. Unfortunately, this protection does not extend to the ligaments of the knee. Finally, the binding may fail to protect the patient in deep and wet snow conditions.

Probably the most significant failing of the bindings occurs before they are put on, when the skier adjusts the tightness. If the binding is too tight, then it will not release under forces that will

Figure 1. External Rotation in Downhill Skiing

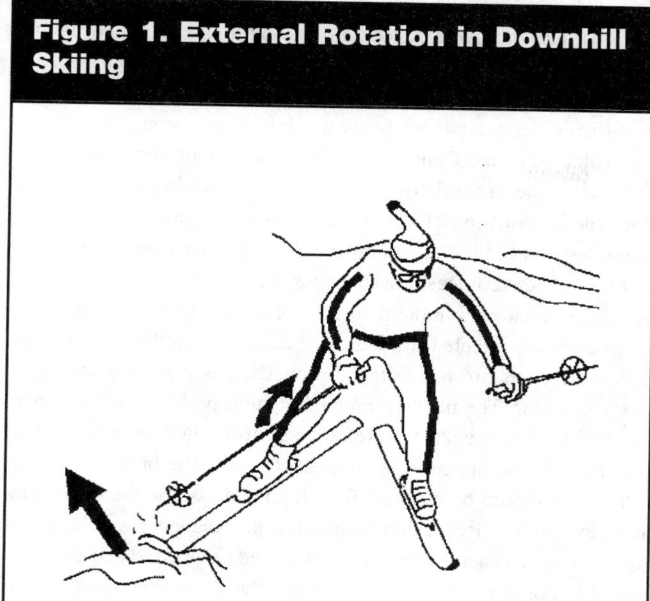

Figure 2. Forward Fall in Downhill Skiing

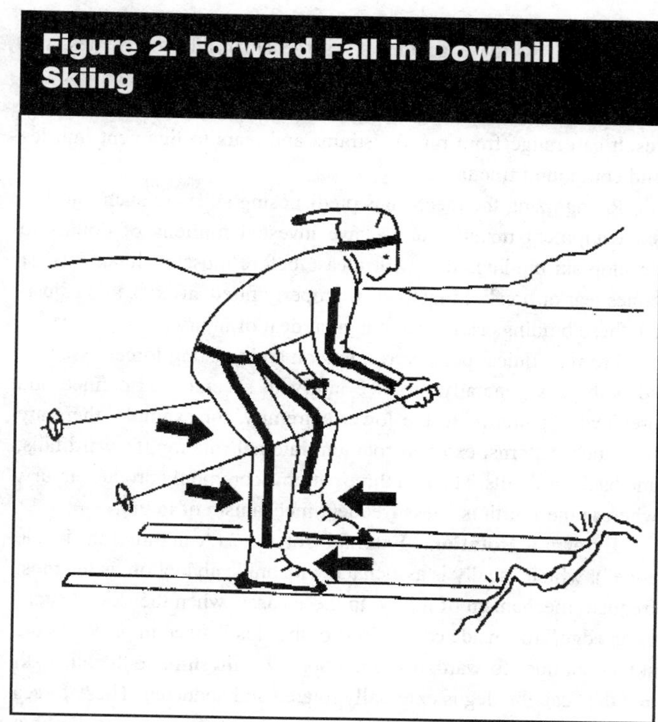

fracture or seriously damage the knee. Failure of the release mechanism accounts for 44% of downhill injuries and 70% of lower leg fractures and serious knee injuries.[15] This may be due to either improper maintenance or improper adjustment of the bindings.[7,16]

Mechanisms and Categories of Injury: General Principles

From a practical perspective, skiing accidents can be grouped into two main categories—falls and collisions. In addition, skiers may also develop so-called "overuse" injuries of unprepared muscles, ligaments, and joints. *(See Table 1.)*

Collisions. Collisions account for only 5% of all injuries sustained on the slopes but more than 67% of all admissions.[17] In particular, high-speed collisions with immovable objects such as trees, buildings, support towers, or even snow-grooming machines can cause massive blunt trauma and impalement injuries.[17] The typical fatal ski crash is exactly what happened to Kennedy and Bono; the skier slams into a tree and dies of head injury.[18,19] The nature of collision injuries is not predictable and varies widely depending on the part of the body involved and the speed. Impact at speeds as slow as 20 mph can be fatal. In 1995, there were 6500 known skiing head injuries in the United States, including 3315 concussions, and 451 ski concussions that required hospitalization. According to the National Safety Council, there were 36 skiing deaths in the 1996-1997 ski season. During 1996, there were 716 boating deaths and 800 bicyclist deaths. Major skiing injuries in children included injuries to the head in nearly 80% of cases.

There is little data on the effectiveness of ski helmets in prevention of ski deaths. A group of researchers in the Department of Industrial and Manufacturing Engineering at Rochester Institute of Technology estimated that helmets could prevent 60-80% of skiing head injuries. There are arguments against helmet use; The skier is overconfident because of the protection, the helmet obstructs visibility, and the helmet will lead to increased neck injury. The same arguments have been advanced in cycling and statistics show marked reduction in death and serious head injury when helmets are used by cyclists.

Overuse Injuries. Overuse syndromes are probably the most common type of injury sustained by skiers. These injuries are common and, because they are usually minor, are often ignored by both novice and experienced skiers. Since symptoms associated with overuse injuries usually do not declare themselves until the following day, estimates on their incidence are inaccurate. The most common overuse injuries are characterized by muscle discomfort and pain in the quadriceps femoris, the gastromelus, and the paravertebral muscles of the back. Aggressive use of ski poles may also lead to triceps tendinitis. Treatment of overuse injuries includes reduction in intensity of activity, strengthening exercises, nonsteroidal anti-inflammatory drugs (NSAIDs), and application of ice. Although frequency, duration, and intensity of exercise should be reduced, complete cessation of activity usually is not necessary.

Falls and Lower-Extremity Injuries. More than 87% of all reported ski injuries are caused by a fall.[20] Fortunately for emergency care providers, injury patterns resulting from ski-related falls are predictable, well-studied, and permit a systematic approach to patient evaluation and management. The most common injuries, in order of occurrence, are: thumb injuries, knee injuries, lacerations of the face and head, leg contusions, shoulder injuries, ankle sprains, tibia fractures, knee contusions, and dislocations of the shoulder.

As many sports medicine experts have noted, strapping a ski onto the foot produces an increased lever arm and, in turn, "enhances" the chances of an injury with any given fall. If the tip of the ski becomes fixed in deep snow or is lodged against a tree, the resultant forces can be enormous and cause massive musculoskeletal damage. In these accidents, as the skier falls or rotates, the increased lever arm of the ski-foot-leg combination will exceed the tensile strength of the human musculoskeletal system. The clinical result can range from muscle strains and tears to ligament injuries and compound fractures.

Recognizing the mechanics predisposing skiers to such injuries, ski equipment manufacturers have invested millions of dollars to develop ski bindings that will release before muscles, ligaments, or bones tear or break. In fact, when properly fitted, affixed, and adjusted, these bindings can prevent a great deal of injury.

From a clinical perspective, torsion and twisting forces associated with falls generally produce injury in several well-defined and predictable patterns. In the lower extremity, for example, there are four such patterns: external rotation, internal rotation, forward falls, and backward falls. The first three patterns commonly produce injury, whereas the fourth is a less frequent mechanism of injury.

External Rotation. External rotation ("catching an inside edge"), which usually is associated with ankle abduction, is the most frequent mechanism of injury. In these cases, when the skier "catches an edge," the inside edge of one of the skis is fixed in place. As the skier continues forward, his or her body weight shifts to the other ski and the "caught" leg is externally rotated and abducted. These forces may fracture the lateral malleolus, cause spiral fractures of the tibia and fibula, or produce ankle sprains and knee sprains. *(See Figure 1.)*

Internal Rotation. Internal rotation ("catching an outside edge") injuries occur in exactly the opposite manner from that described for external rotation injuries. The skier, who is usually a novice, will catch the outside edge of the ski during a turn or when the skis cross. The internal rotation forces that result can produce an ankle sprain of the anterior talofibular ligament, a medial malleolus fracture, or a tibial fracture.

Forward Fall. Forward falls most often occur when the skier digs a tip of the ski into the snow and continues in forward motion as the ski stops. The lower leg angulates over the boot top as the skier's forward momentum is terminated abruptly by the ski, which remains wedged in the snow. If the binding fails to "give," the musculoskeletal system will be disrupted and produce one of three injuries: boot-top fractures, Achilles tendon ruptures, or dislocation of the peroneal tendon. If the skier extends the arms to protect the face, upper-extremity injuries also may occur. *(See Figure 2.)*

Specific Injuries of the Leg, Foot, and Ankle

Midfoot Sprains. Midfoot sprains occur when the skier digs a ski tip into the snow. The resulting hyperflexion of the foot can cause pain over the dorsum of the foot as well as swelling and tenderness. Midfoot sprains are more common with poor-fitting boots and when skiers have loosened their boot buckles.

Pressure Injuries. Pressure injuries to the foot occur when the skier is wearing boots that are either too small or buckled too tightly. Even with integral padding, the pressure of tight-fitting boots may decrease distal circulation and exacerbate cold-mediated injuries. Because anesthesia of the area may accompany this type of injury, the skier may not notice the problem until the boots are removed and the pressure is relieved. Subungual hematomas (skier's toes) and injuries to the bony prominences are common signs of direct pressure trauma. In extreme cases, anesthesia may persist due to pressure-mediated peroneal nerve palsy.

Rest, elevation, and cessation of skiing until healing occurs are appropriate therapeutic maneuvers. Unfortunately, convincing a skier who has booked a "once-in-a-lifetime" vacation to avoid skiing may be difficult. Recovery is relatively quick in most cases.

Ankle Sprains. Contrary to what many clinicians think, ankle sprains have become relatively uncommon injuries in downhill skiing since the introduction of high-padded boots. Overall, they now represent less than 1% of all ski injuries.[1-3] However, when older boots and less-effective release mechanisms were in common use, ankle injuries accounted for more than 25% of all ski-related injuries.[3,4]

Prevention-oriented measures should be emphasized to the patient. If boots are not fastened properly, ankle sprains are more likely to occur. The most common fastening problem occurs when the skier unfastens buckles to relieve a tight-fitting boot or ankle discomfort. To minimize the likelihood of injury, the buckle over the ankle joint should be fastened first. It should also be the tightest in order to keep the heel seated during downhill maneuvers.[21] All other buckles can be fastened to comfort. It should be stressed that even the best ski boot available does not protect the ankle completely from severe rotational forces. Fortunately, however, dual-mode bindings release easily with rotational stress and protect the ankle from these potentially destructive forces.

Most ankle sprains associated with properly adjusted boots occur when the skier catches the inside edge of the ski and both abducts and externally rotates the ankle. Anatomically, the talus is forced against the lateral malleolus and stretches the anterior talofibular ligament. If the ligament is disrupted, an unstable ankle injury may result. Treatment depends on the severity of the sprain. Grade I sprains are treated with rest, ice to the area, compression dressings, and elevation (RICE). Weight-bearing may be resumed when pain is no longer present.

Grade II and III sprains may show evidence of instability. If the patient complains of pain without weight-bearing and has severe swelling, suspect a grade II sprain. A grade III sprain represents complete ligamentous disruption, which requires fixation with plaster and, in some cases, may even necessitate surgical repair. Patients with either grade II or grade III sprains are treated with ankle immobilization and should be referred to an orthopedic surgeon for further treatment.

Lateral Malleolus Fracture. In the setting of ski-related trauma, the lateral malleolus fracture is often produced by a forward fall, particularly if the fall is combined with external rotation. The most serious injuries occur when the skier catches a ski tip and falls forward and rotates the ankle during forward movement. Most of these orthopedic injuries are isolated lateral malleolar fractures, although medial malleolus and comminuted fractures may also be seen. Not uncommonly, tibiofibular ligament sprains are be associated with the injury, and, occasionally, the neck of the talus may be fractured rather than the medial malleolus. Since these fractures are easy to miss, a high index of suspicion is required for their detection.

On physical examination, lateral malleolar fractures present with the usual swelling, pain, and tenderness on palpation of the fracture site. Ecchymosis may or may not be present. Deformity should suggest a displaced and unstable fracture. Fractures of the neck of the talus are characterized by tenderness on both sides of the ankle, in a location anterior to the medial and lateral malleolus.

Diagnosis of a fracture of the ankle is best made with appropriate radiographs. If a fracture of the neck of the talus is suspected, ask

Table 2. Classification of Skier's Thumb

INJURY CLASSIFICATION	FINDINGS	TREATMENT
Grade 1	Pain without instability of UCL on stress testing	Symptomatic treatment, protect the thumb from re-injury
Grade 2	Instability on stress testing with a firm endpoint Undisplaced or chip fracture	Cast for 2-4 weeks and follow-up with orthopedic surgeon
Grade 3	Instability on stress testing with a firm endpoint Displaced fracture fragments	Immediate referral to orthopedic surgeon

Adapted from: Rettig AC, Wright HH. Skier's thumb. *Phys Sports Med* 1989;17:65-75; Rettig AC, Wright HH. Skier's thumb. *Phys Sports Med* 1989;17:65-75.

for a tangential view of the neck of the talus. This view is taken with the foot placed flat on the film. Treatment requires appropriate immobilization in a splint, ice, elevation of the extremity, and orthopedic referral.

Achilles Tendon Rupture. This injury occurs when the skier runs into a mogul or other object and the skis stop while the skier continues in forward motion. This produces a forward fall, which is accompanied by marked dorsiflexion of the ankle. The patient may note a tearing or popping sound as the tendon rips. Males older than 35 are at high risk for this injury.

Following the accident, the patient may be able to walk, have little or no pain, and be able to plantar flex the foot despite a tear of the Achilles tendon. On physical examination, however, the patient will have tenderness and swelling along the tendon sheath, with a palpable defect present about 2-3 cm proximal to the calcaneus. In some cases, the patient will have a obvious foot drop and will be unable to plantar flex the foot. Thompson's test of the calf, which may demonstrate disruption of the Achilles tendon, is performed on a sitting patient with legs in a dangling position. When the middle third of the calf is squeezed, the foot should plantar flex. If there is no plantar flexion, suspect an Achilles tendon tear.

If an Achilles tendon tear is strongly suspected, the patient should be immobilized in a long leg splint and referred to an orthopedic surgeon. Partial tears can be treated with immobilization alone but still require evaluation by an orthopedic surgeon.

Peroneal Tendon Rupture. Although dislocation of the peroneal tendon is considered a rare injury in a typical orthopedic practice, it is considered one of the more common ski-related ankle injuries.[22] Moreover, peroneal tendon rupture or dislocation is also one of the most under-reported and over-looked skiing injuries.[23] Dislocation can occur when the skier forcefully edges the downhill ski during a turn. At this point, because the peroneal tendon is supporting the full weight of the ski and foot, the peritoneal retinaculum is subject to tears.[22] If the tendon sheath alone is torn, the tendon may dislocate anteriorly.[24]

About 1% of all reported skiing injuries involve the peroneal tendon.[22] This injury also can occur when the skier hits a mogul or some other object and continues in forward motion while the skis stop. If the skier falls forward with the foot in dorsiflexion and external rotation, the peroneal retinaculum or the peroneal tendon may be torn. Typically, the patient will describe the fall, followed by pain, swelling, ecchymosis, and tenderness that occur posterior to the lateral malleolus.

On physical examination, the physician should palpate for tenderness on the lateral and posterior aspect of the malleolus. If the peroneal tendon subluxes during dorsiflexion and external rotation, the diagnosis is confirmed. Radiographs may demonstrate little more than a small avulsion fracture of the posterior lateral malleolus, right at the attachment of the peroneal retinaculum (a fracture fragment may be demonstrated on an overrotated lateral view of the ankle).[25] When detected, this subtle fracture is highly suggestive of a torn peroneal ten-don or sheath.

These patients require surgical repair of the tendon and/or tendon sheath. In the emergency setting, the patient requires immobilization, ankle elevation, and referral to an orthopedic surgeon.

Tibia Fractures. Fractures of the tibia are common and dramatic reminders of the magnitude—and potential destructiveness—of forces that act on the falling skier. If a prominent rotatory component is present, a spiral fracture of the tibia and fibula may result. However, when the primary force is a bending motion at the top of the boot, a boot-top fracture should be suspected. If some combination of both forces is present, elements of both injuries may be found. These fractures are usually easy to diagnose with AP and lateral x-rays of the lower leg.[7]

The incidence of these fractures has remained constant or slightly increased in frequency.[26] Spiral fractures have decreased markedly since the 1960s. Since torque at the toe will release current dual-mode bindings, these are precisely the fractures that modern bindings are designed to prevent.

Children who fall and develop shin pain should be assumed to have a tibial or fibular fracture.[27] In childhood, ligaments and muscles are strong and do not easily give. Special attention should be paid to the joints and epiphysis in children. Fractures at this age are more common than sprains. Isolated tibial fractures are more common in children than adults. If the child has tenderness near the joint, look for an epiphyseal fracture.

Standard care for fractures includes immobilization and referral to an orthopedic surgeon. Appropriate elevation and pain medication are essential. Open fractures should be cultured and the patient should be started on IV antibiotics.

Table 3. Incidence of Shoulder Injuries in Downhill Skiing

INJURY	INCIDENCE
Anterior dislocation	52%
External rotation and abduction from the ski pole	60%
Direct fall on the shoulder	40%
Rotator cuff tear	20%
Direct impact (AC separation)	18%
Fractures	4%

Adapted from: Weaver JK. Skiing-related injuries to the shoulder. *Clin Orthop Rel Res* 1987;216;24-29.

Fibula Fractures. Most fibular fractures are found in association with fractures of the tibia. If an isolated fibular fracture is confirmed, the emergency physician should assume there is an associated severe ankle injury until proven otherwise. If a spiral fracture is found, a major ankle injury is extremely common. A backward or lateral fall may cause a boot-top fracture of the fibula alone, but this is unusual. Radiographs of the lower leg will usually confirm presence of the injury. Boot-top fractures of the fibula are often subtle, hair-line fractures; therefore, detection of these injuries may require a magnifying glass.[28]

Treatment requires immobilization of the ankle and lower leg. If an isolated boot-top fracture is confirmed, a compression dressing, ice, NSAIDs, elevation, and limitation of weight-bearing are adequate therapy. Weight bearing can be resumed when the patient is pain-free.

Knee Injuries

About 20% of all downhill ski injuries involve the knee.[29] Although overall injury rates have been reduced, knee injuries have increased in the last 20 years.[28] Fortunately for skiers, 90% of these knee injuries are minor.[29] Most are ligament sprains, but bony fragments may be torn free. Skiers may also sustain lacerations, contusions, or patellar injuries if the knee strikes other objects or the ground. Dislocations of the knee are rare.

Medial Collateral Ligament Sprains. Catching the inside edge of the ski will rotate the ski and attached foot externally, a motion that will stress the medial collateral ligament of the knee on the same side. This is a common injury in skiers and—with or without rupture of other ligaments—may account for as many as 60% of all ski-related knee injuries and 83% of all knee ligament injuries.[30] If the external rotation and lateral forces are pronounced, then the anterior cruciate ligament also may be involved. Both medial and lateral collateral ligament strains may demonstrate tenderness around the involved ligament. It should be emphasized that if the ligament is completely torn, laxity of the knee with medial (varus) and lateral (valgus) knee stress will be noted on exam. Evaluation is enhanced if the knee is examined both in full extension with 20-30 of flexion.

The acute injury should be treated with immobilization, ice, and decreased weight-bearing. Referral to an orthopedic surgeon for management of rehabilitation is appropriate. Lateral collateral ligament sprains are far less common, probably because it is more difficult for skiers to catch an outside edge at high speed. Consequently, this injury accounts for about 4% of all knee sprains.[28,30]

Anterior Cruciate Injuries. During early surveys of skiing injuries, only 7% of knee sprains involved the anterior cruciate ligament (ACL).[29] However, as a result of improved bindings and boots designed to protect the tibia, ACL injuries have rapidly increased in incidence and now account for more than 33% of all skiing injuries.[7] In fact, the ACL is now the most frequently injured part of the lower extremity.

As might be expected, this injury is produced when the skier hyperextends the knee and stresses the ACL. Typically, this mechanism of injury is encountered in the following ski-related movements: 1) When the skier catches the inside edge of the ski with the tip pointed outward and continues traveling forward.[13,14] This rotates the skier's knee internally and places valgus (lateral) stress on the knee. In this case, the medial collateral ligament and the medial meniscus may also be involved. 2) When the skier sits down to stop or regain control of forward motion. This is a common technique used by less-experienced skiers. In this case, a single ski may slide forward and the other knee flexes. The boot top forces the tibia forward, and the ACL is torn by anterior "drawer" loading. 3) When the skier lands on the tails of the skis from a jump or fall and one of the skis shoots forward. This is analogous to the novice's stopping technique and also forces the tibia forward and stretches the ACL. Finally, "isolated" ACL injuries may also occur with these mechanisms, which tend to occur when the skier is wearing high and stiff boots.

It should be stressed the ACL tear may be a very subtle injury; consequently, the emergency physician must carefully consider an ACL whenever the patient presents with knee pain after skiing. The skier will often describe both feeling and hearing a "pop" in the knee during the injury. Immediately following the accident, a joint effusion is often found on physical examination and, if aspirated, it will usually be bloody. In fact, the presence of a rapidly evolving effusion after a fall while skiing is associated with a 75% or greater chance of an ACL sprain.[31,32] An anterior "drawer" sign also may be positive. This test is performed on a supine patient. The hip is bent at a 45° angle and the knee is bent to 90°. The foot should be immobilized by sitting on it. The calf is pulled forward while the examiner palpates the anterior knee. Anterior motion of the tibia is found with an ACL injury.

There is substantial controversy regarding treatment of ACL injuries. Generally, ACL injuries are most often treated with surgical repair and may involve a protracted recovery period. Rarely, ACL injuries result in permanent disability of the skier. Emergency treatment of the injury is immobilization, ice, and relief of pain, followed by prompt orthopedic referral.

Posterior Cruciate Injuries. Only 1% of knee sprains are posterior cruciate ligament injuries.[33] These injuries most frequently occur when the skier hits a fixed object with knee flexed.

Meniscus Injuries. About 7% of knee injuries involve the meniscus.[33] Patients with these injuries often present with complaints of intermittent locking or giving way of the joint. Pain, clicks, and effusions are also associated with these injuries. Meniscal tears may occur without any other significant knee injury. These isolated meniscal tears may occur when an aggressive skier lands during mogul skiing or jumping over small hills. In many cases, the skier doesn't even fall. Orthopedic consultation and arthroscopy will improve diagnostic accuracy.

Patellar Injuries. Lateral dislocations of the patella occur when the skier catches the inside edge of the ski and externally rotates the leg. Contraction of the quadriceps muscle forces the patella laterally and out of the femoral groove. Diagnosis and treatment of this injury are straightforward. The patella may be relocated with medial pressure and passive extension of the knee. Immobilizing the knee in a cylindrical plaster cast for four weeks has been advocated. In most cases, a knee immobilizer is sufficient.

As with dislocation of the patella, treatment of patellar fracture requires routine immobilization of the knee. The clinician should exclude complete disruption of the patellar ligament by having the patient lift the straightened leg off of the bed. Inability to perform this motion usually means that the patient will require urgent surgical repair.

Ski-Related Injuries of the Upper Extremity

Equipment improvements have made the sport far safer for the ankle and lower leg. Unfortunately, the upper extremity and hand have not had the same protection.

Skier's Thumb. The term "skier's thumb" has been used since 1981 to denote a tear of the ulnar collateral ligament of the metacarpophalangeal joint of the thumb.[34] Prior to 1981, this injury was often called a gamekeeper's thumb, which was a chronic laxity rather than an acute injury.[35] In any event, a tear of the ulnar collateral ligament of the metacarpophalangeal joint of the thumb may be the most common injury sustained in skiing, with a reported incidence of up to 9% of all skiing injuries.[35,36] On indoor (dry) training slopes, as many as 70% of all injuries sustained are to the hand and thumb.[37]

Various mechanisms of injury have been proposed to explain ulnar collateral ligament injuries in skiers.[38] In general, however, it is agreed that these injuries occur when the skier sustains forced abduction of the thumb, which, in the context of skiing, is most likely to occur when the skier attempts to break a fall with an outstretched hand while the hand is still inter-locked with the ski pole and strap. Alternatively, this injury may also occur when the skier strikes the ground or has the thumb entangled in the strap,[39] in which case the pole, ground, or strap will push the thumb backward and outward. In the process, the ligament will be stretched, torn, or avulsed from the base of the first phalanx.

When the thumb is examined, the clinician will note tenderness over the ulnar collateral ligament. If the ligament has been displaced, there may be a bulge over the site of the ulnar collateral ligament. The physician should be gentle when examining sprains of the ulnar collateral ligament since the ligament may be further displaced by a vigorous examination and, in rare cases, may subject the patient to surgery. Prudent care dictates that an x-ray of the thumb be obtained in all thumb sprains, even if they appear minor. A fracture may be associated with the sprain in up to 30% of cases.[40] Surgery is required if the fracture is significantly displaced or if it involves a significant portion of the articular surface.

A significant complication results when the ulnar collateral ligament is completely torn and displaced. In some cases, the torn end may be displaced outside of the adductor aponeurosis. When the thumb heals in this position, the patient develops a pinch grip instability. This complication is called a Stener's lesion and must be surgically reduced.[41] Unfortunately, there is no generally accepted nonsurgical method that will distinguish an undisplaced, torn ulnar collateral ligament from one that has significant displacement.[42]

Table 4. Ten Tips for Safe Skiing and Snowboarding

Get into shape early
Have your equipment checked by a qualified technician before you go skiing.
Take ski lessons
Wear sunblock and either glasses or goggles
Dress in layers
Don't drink when skiing
Warm up before you start
Don't exceed your capabilities
Don't ski the hardest runs first
Don't take the last run.
Consider a helmet

Probably the best diagnostic technique is stress examination of the ligament. The normal amount of lateral motion of the metacarpophalangeal joint ranges from 0-30 in extension. With the joint in full flexion, there is an average of about 1 of radial deviation.[42] It is important to examine the uninvolved thumb and note whether the skier has had an injury to the uninvolved thumb. To test the integrity of the ulnar collateral ligament, first stabilize the metacarpal with the thumb and index finger. Then apply radial stress to the distal phalanx. This should be checked with the thumb both flexed and fully extended. When the thumb is fully flexed, the ulnar collateral ligament is assessed. When the thumb is fully extended, the accessory collateral ligament and the volar plate are tested. The injury may be graded from 1-3. *(See Table 2.)*

If the patient wishes to continue skiing with a grade 1 injury, a thumb spica splint should be molded to fit around the ski pole to prevent any further damage. The patient may remove the splint daily and use ice and range-of-motion exercises. An unstable injury should not be treated in this manner. If the patient has significant pain or swelling, then more conservative therapy is indicated.

A thumb spica cast is used for patients with either an incomplete tear or an avulsion fracture. After adequate immobilization in a thumb spica splint, these patients should be referred to an orthopedic surgeon familiar with this injury. A delay of more than three weeks before surgery increases the risk of diminished thumb function.[5] Treatment of a serious (grade 2 or 3) injury is either surgical repair or immobilization in a thumb spica cast. Surgical repair is usually reserved for those with displaced fractures and completely torn ligaments (grade 3). These patients should be referred on an immediate basis to an orthopedic surgeon for further management.

Shoulder Injuries. The most common type of shoulder injury sustained in downhill skiing is the anterior dislocation (52%), followed by rotator cuff tears (20%).[43] Acromioclavicular separations account for an additional 18% of shoulder injuries.[43] *(See Table 3.)* Two different mechanisms of injury account for these dislocations. Most (60%) have the arm externally rotated and forcibly abducted; the ski pole is implicated in 50% of these hyperabduction shoulder injuries.[3,4] About 40% of patients fall directly onto the shoulder and sustain a dislocation from this mechanism.[43] Ten percent of shoulder dislocations have a minimally displaced fracture of the greater tuberosity.[4,5] Dislocations are best managed with immediate reduction. The patient should be carefully examined for associated fractures and upper extremity neurological problems.

Rotator Cuff Tears. Rotator cuff tears occur when the skier falls on his or her side with the arm in abduction to ward off the impact from a fall. Since partial rotator cuff tears are not always easy to diagnose, these injuries are probably under-reported. However, they are more likely to occur in older patients (40 years or older) and in patients who have had a previous shoulder injury. The most important physical finding elicited in a rotator cuff tear is the inability to actively abduct the arm.

Acromioclavicular (AC) Separation. Patients who sustain an AC separation universally describe a fall directly on the point of the shoulder. Physical findings and treatment of AC separations are unchanged from any other mechanism that produces these injuries. Fractures of the area around the shoulders are relatively rare. The most common ski fracture of the shoulder is a fracture of the greater tuberosity, usually minimally displaced. This may occur when the patient falls on the elbow and the force is directly transmitted to the shoulder. Fractures of the clavicle may occur from direct trauma to the area.

Clavicle Fractures. Clavicle fractures result from direct trauma to the clavicle or from falls on the outstretched arm. If the skier falls with the ski pole held diagonally across the body, then the pole may produce impact against the clavicle and fracture it. Neither the diagnosis nor the treatment differ from usual management of clavicle fractures associated with other causes.

Snowboarding Injuries

Snowboards are large, flat boards that resemble oversized skateboards. They vary from about 140-190 cm and are about 30-40 cm wide. The skier is firmly fixed to the board in non-releasable boots and bindings. The front foot is set at 45° to the board, and the rear foot is positioned perpendicular to the board. Snowboard riding techniques are similar to those of surfing and skateboarding. The rider's weight is mostly over the front foot and turns are made by shifting weight and swinging the back end of the board around and then setting the edges.

Most snowboarders are well-conditioned males with an average age of about 21 years.[44] Nearly 50% of injuries will occur in beginners, as opposed to only 18% of skiers.

Injuries occur at a similar rate to skiing with 3 to 4 injuries per 1000 exposure days. Aerial maneuvers are associated with increased risk of injury to the head, spine, face, and abdomen. As in alpine skiing, collisions are associated with increased severity of injury. The rate of fractures is markedly higher in snowboarders with 38% of injuries in snowboarders and 15% in skiers. The most common mechanism of injury is direct impact of the rider against the slope. Typically, the full impact of the fall is absorbed by the upper extremities, a mechanism that can produce damage to the shoulder, elbow, wrist, or hand. Over 40% of injuries are found in the upper extremities.

If the lower extremity is injured, the front leg is involved in about 75% of cases.[44] Because both feet are fixed to the same board, far fewer torsion injuries to knee and ankle are found. Snowboarders are also less likely to sustain lacerations, boot-top contusions, and thumb injuries. Ulnar collateral ligament injuries also are far less frequent. Unfortunately, they are more likely to have buttock contusions, spinal injuries, and distal radius fractures than downhill skiers.[45]

The most common non-impact injuries to snowboarders are caused by hyperdorsiflexion of the ankle as the rider falls forward.[45] This can cause Achilles tendon and gastrocnemius injuries. The rider is also more likely to sustain hyperplantarflexion foot and inversion and eversion ankle injuries, since these individuals are falling with a soft boot that is rigidly fixed to the board. Hard-shelled boots or inserts as well as ankle supports help to prevent these injuries. Unfortunately, these new boots also are often affixed to the snowboard with rigid metal non-release bindings. The lower extremity injuries associated with these boards and bindings are quite similar to those found in the older style non-release ski bindings.

Cross-Country Skiing Injuries

In general, cross-country (Nordic) skiing can be performed wherever there is snow. Downhill skiing, on the other hand, requires a lift up the slope before skiing down it. This lift requirement limits the areas servicing alpine skiers to those around resorts. In contrast, the cross-country skier can travel to quite isolated areas. For this reason, there are significant differences in both skiing styles and equipment favored by these two types of skiers.

In spite of the growing interest in Nordic skiing, there is much less documentation in the literature about the injuries that can be sustained by the cross-country skier. There are several reasons for this paucity of literature. It is suspected that cross-country skiers are injured less frequently than their alpine counterparts, and that these injuries are often less severe. Unfortunately, if under-reporting is a problem when the alpine skier is injured at the resort, it is far worse for injuries resulting from cross-country skiing.

Cross-country skiers are often superior athletes. Nordic skiing is "real work." Caloric expenditures for cross-country skiers range from 0.098 Kcal/min/kg for leisurely skiing on level ground to 0.274 Kcal/min/kg for maximal uphill skiing on hard snow.[46] This corresponds to an energy expenditure of 446 to 1244 Kcal/hour for the standard 70 kg body weight.[47] Athletes at this level of experience and conditioning often will take care of their minor injuries with self-care. These well-conditioned athletes will often not be involved in the same kind of accidents that afflict less-conditioned novices.

Risk Factors. In the few reports that are available, it appears that cross-country skiers are injured at one-tenth the rate seen in downhill skiers.[48] Generally speaking, more gentle slopes are used by Nordic skiers than are used by alpine skiers. Nevertheless, injuries from Nordic skiing are becoming more severe than in the past, in large part because of the popularity of faster, more rigid skis and heel fixation devices that give more edge control.[48] In many respects, the modern Nordic skier has merely replicated injury patterns observed in alpine skiing prior to the extensive development of safer equipment. Heel fixation devices, lower boots, and more rigid skis used in Nordic skiing are similar to those used by downhill skiers 20-30 years ago, but permit faster speeds than these skiers were able to achieve.

Not surprisingly, 88% of all acute injuries to cross-country skiers occur on downhill terrain.[49,50] Telemark skiing, a down-hill variant of cross-country skiing, brings the skier full circle to downhill skiing with older-style bindings and lower boots. Knee injuries sustained by telemark skiers are less severe than those found in alpine skiers, with less duration of disability and lower surgical rates. Cold injuries comprise about 20% of reported injuries,[51] an incidence much higher than found in alpine skiers, probably due to the remote terrain sought by cross-country skiers. The most common fatalities associated with cross-country skiing are from avalanche and hypothermia.[52] To all of these troubles must be added the problem of evacuation. Since many cross-country skiers seek remote areas for their avocation, this is often a major problem. These skiers, unlike those found in alpine resorts, do not have the services of a paid or highly trained volunteer ski patrol for evacuation and care.

Overuse Injuries. Since cross-country skiing is "real work," most cross-country skiing injuries are due to overuse.[51]

Diagonal Stride Overuse Injuries. With the classic stride (also called the diagonal stride), the most common overuse syndromes are shin splints, Achilles tendinitis, and low back pain.[7] Since this is the most common stride used by recreational skiers, these injuries are most often encountered in the less-conditioned skier.

Skating Overuse Injuries. A "freestyle" or skating stride is often used by racing skiers. Freestyle skiers or those using a skating technique will have more trouble with the adductors and internal rotators of the hip.[53,54] The anterior and medial compartment muscles of the lower leg will also be stressed.[55] Longer ski poles put additional stress on the wrist and carpal tunnel, increasing the incidence of extensor tendinitis and carpal tunnel syndrome.

Skier's Toe. Increased stress to the flexor hallucis longus muscle during the pushoff part of the skating technique (dorsi-flexion of foot) can cause a stress injury. This injury of the flex-or hallucis longus muscle is termed "skier's toe." Most of these injuries are neither reported nor come to formal medical attention, and treatment is simple: Reduce the stress by decreasing the intensity or duration of the exercise; apply ice to the area for 10-20 minutes after the exercise. Stretching and strengthening exercises are often helpful. NSAIDs will both reduce the inflammation and relieve the pain in acute injuries.

Lower-Extremity Injuries. The knee is the joint injured in about 31% of cross-country ski injuries.[49] Since the ankle remains free, the number of ACL injuries is lower, but the medial collateral ligament is injured more frequently.[56] Heel fixation with cross-country bindings increases the number of twisting, lower extremity injuries. With these devices, sprains of the ankle are common. Fortunately, cross-country skiing is not associated with the high incidence of ankle fractures described with older skiing equipment. This may change as Telemark skiing gains popularity.

Upper-Extremity Injuries. Upper extremity injuries associated with cross-country skiing can be divided into overuse injuries and injuries due to falls.

Upper-Extremity Overuse Injuries. As noted earlier, cross-country skiers have an increased incidence of both extensor tendinitis of the wrist and carpal tunnel syndrome. This is thought to be due to the high position of the wrists when using properly adjusted Nordic ski poles. Ulnar collateral ligament sprains of the thumb occur in the same manner as described for alpine skiers and are the single most common hand injury.[56]

Falls. The most common shoulder injury encountered in cross-country skiing accidents is anterior shoulder dislocation. Shoulder dislocations are usually caused by catching the arm or pole in underbrush as the skier passes by. The arm is then forced into abduction and external rotation with resultant dislocation.

Treatment of this injury in the field is a dilemma. Most providers are simply not adequately trained in how to reduce a dislocated shoulder. On the other hand, the injured skier, especially in the remote wilderness, is a distinct liability. Probably, a single attempt at shoulder reduction in the field by an appropriately trained provider is reasonable. If this is not successful, repeated attempts without x-ray are unlikely to be beneficial. The patient should be transported to a medical facility. Acromioclavicular separations are usually caused by direct trauma and are the second major shoulder injury found in the Nordic skier.[56]

Ski Jumping

Although ski jumping is quite spectacular and gives the appearance of being very dangerous, it has a surprisingly low injury rate.[57] Injury rates for non-World Cup competitions and World Cup competitions were 4.3 and 1.2 injuries per 1000 skier days, respectively.[57] Ski jumpers tend to be young, aggressively trained athletes in outstanding physical condition. The sport is rigidly controlled, and those who have not been properly trained essentially are not allowed on the jump. These well-supervised conditions result in exceptionally low injury rates. Moreover, the jump is controlled so that the skier lands on the steep downhill portion of the hill. As long as the jumper lands in this part of the hill, the kinetic energy can be dissipated by sliding. On the other hand, if the fall is very long or very short, the jumper can be badly injured by a failed jump.

Ten percent of ski-jump injuries involve visceral organ damage due to the impact.[57] The most common injuries are contusions, abrasions, and dislocations, primarily of the shoulder. Fractures account for about 15% of the total injuries, most of which involve the upper extremity injuries.[57]

Sledding

Generally considered to be a benign winter sport,[58] downhill sledding is a common recreational activity for children and adults. Sledders may use commercial sleds, toboggans, or saucers, and makeshift cardboard boxes or inner tubes can be recruited. Injury statistics suggest that younger people are at higher risk for injury.[59] Since this is a traditional children's sport, younger children are often supervised by only slightly older children. Poor judgment is commonly implicated in cited injuries. Children will often choose a "quiet" street on a hill for their course with potentially disastrous results if a vehicle is on the street at the wrong time.[60]

Sledding and tobogganing require relatively little snow. A sunny day followed by a cold night may produce a fast course on icy slopes with hard ground. During icy conditions, the rider may have high-velocity impacts with hidden obstacles such as rocks, stumps, and moguls.

The most common injuries are lacerations, followed by contusions and strains. The standard sled can be steered when ridden in the prone position. This is the most common position of riding. The rider can also sit upright and control steering with the feet. When the rider is prone, head and facial injuries are more common.[61]

Serious injuries occur in as many as 21% of sledding injuries.[62] Abdominal injuries result from bumps or after impact with the ground. When the rider sits erect, the spine is more susceptible to hyperflexion injuries.

Toboggan injuries usually produce injury to the lower extremities. Toboggans and inner tubes are ridden in the seated position, with riders often leaning forward with their back arched. It is thought that this position enhances the likelihood and severity of a spinal injury. Even more life-threatening injuries have been reported in tubing than in tobogganing.[59,63] It is possible that these devices can be made somewhat safer for our children. Steerable devices, such as sleds and toboggans, are safer than nonsteerable devices, such as saucers, tubes, or cardboard boxes. Finally, a bicycle helmet may provide impact protection while riding a sled in the prone position.

Summary

Winter sports are associated with a distinct spectrum of orthopedic injuries. Diagnosis of these injuries is facilitated by recognizing specific mechanisms of injury and performing appropriate radiographic studies. In general, treatment is similar to that required for fractures, strains, and ligamentous tears seen in non-skiing injuries. Finally, prevention of these injuries is possible if newly developed equipment is used appropriately.

References

1. Clifford PS. Scientific basis of competitive cross-country skiing. *Med Sci Sports Exerc* 1992;24:1007-1009.
2. Requa RK, Toney JM, Garrick JG. Parameters of injury reported in skiing. *Med Sci Sports Exerc* 1977;9:185.
3. Eckert WR. Diagnosis and initial management of common alpine ski injuries. *Emerg Med Rep* 1987;8:9-16.
4. Johnson RJ, Ettlinger CF, Campbell RJ, et al. Trends in skiing in-juries: Analysis of a six-year study. *Am J Sports Med* 1980;8:106-113.
5. Clancy WG, McConkey JP. Nordic and alpine skiing. In: Schneider RC, eds. *Sports Injuries: Mechanisms, Prevention, and Treatment.* Baltimore: Williams & Wilkins, 1985;247-249.
6. Kristiansen TK, Johnson RJ. Fractures in the skiing athlete. *Clin Sports Med* 1990;9:215-224.
7. Johnson RJ. Skiing and snowboarding injuries: When schuss-ing is a pain. *Postgrad Med* 1990;88:36-51.
8. Myles ST, Mohdadi NGH, Schnittker J. Injuries to the nervous system and spine in downhill skiing. *Can J Surg* 1992;35:643-648.
9. Bouter LM, Knipschild PG, Volovics A. Personal and environmental factors in relation to injury risk in downhill skiing. *Int J Sports Med* 1989:10:298-301.
10. Blankenstein A, Salai M, Israeli A, et al. Ski injuries in 1976-1982: Ybrig region, Switzerland. *Int J Sports Med* 1985;6:298-300.
11. Baranas C, Miller CH, Sperner G, et al. The effects of alcohol and benzodiazepines on the severity of ski accidents. *Acta Psych Scand* 1992;86:296-300.
12. Rogers CC. Some skiers get lifts from drinks. *Phys Sports Med* 1985;13:27.
13. McConkey JP. Anterior cruciate ligament rupture in skiing: A new mechanism of injury. *Am J Sports Med* 1986;14:160-164.
14. Fritschy D. An unusual injury in top skiers. *Am J Sports Med* 1989;17:282-286.
15. Ekeland A, Holtmoen A, Lystad H. Lower extremity equipment-related injuries in alpine recreational skiers. *Am J Sports Med* 1993;21:201-205.
16. Bouter LM, Knipschild PG, Volovics A. Binding function in relation to injury risk in downhill skiing. *Am J Sports Med* 1989;17:226-233.
17. Pliskin M, D'Angelo M. Atypical downhill skiing injuries. *J Trauma* 1988;29:520-522.
18. Morrow PL, McQuillen EN, Eaton LA, et al. Downhill ski fatalities: The Vermont experience. *J Trauma* 1988;28:95-100.
19. Tough SC, Butt JC. A review of fatal injuries associated with downhill skiing. *Am J Forensic Med Pathol* 1993;14:12-16.
20. Johnson RJ, Pope MH, Ettlinger C. Ski injuries and equipment function. *J Sports Med* 1974;2:229.
21. Santoro JP, Kirby KA. Boot fitting problems in the skier. *J Am Pod Med Assoc* 1986;76:572-576.
22. Oden RR. Tendon injuries about the ankle resulting from skiing. *Clin Orthop Rel Res* 1987;216:63-69.
23. Leach RE, Lower G. Ankle injuries in skiing. *Clin Orthop* 1985;198:127.
24. Eckert WR, Davis EA. Acute rupture of the peroneal retinaculum. *J Bone Joint Surg* 1976;58:670.
25. Trevino SG, Alveraz R. The spectrum of lower leg injuries in skiing. *Clin Sports Med* 1982;1:263.
26. Freeman JR, Weaver JK, Oden RR, et al. Changing patterns in tibial fractures resulting from skiing. *Clin Orthop Rel Res* 1987;216:19-23.
27. Ungerholm S, Gierup J, Lindsjo U, et al. Skiing injuries in children: Lower leg fractures. *Int J Sports Med* 1985;6:292-297.
28. Garrick JG. Symposium on ankle and foot problems in the athlete: Epidemiologic perspective. *Clin Sports Med* 1982;1:13.
29. Taunton JE, McKenzie DC, Clement DB. The role of biomechanics in the epidemiology of injuries. *Sports Med* 1988;6:107120.
30. Howe J, Johnson RJ. Knee injuries in skiing. *Orthop Clin North Am* 1985;16:303.
31. McConkey JP. The toll on skiers' knees. *Emerg Med* 1986;(Dec 15):25-44.
32. Perko MMJ, Cross MJ, Ruske D, et al. Anterior cruciate ligament injuries: Clues for diagnosis. *Med J Aust* 1992;157:467-470.
33. Howe J, Johnson RJ. Knee injuries in skiing. *Orthop Clin North Am.* 1985;16:303.
34. Gerber CL, Sena E, Matter P. Skier's thumb. *Am J Sports Med* 1981;9:171-177.
35. Newland CC. Gamekeeper's thumb. *Orthop Clin North Am* 1992;23:41-48.
36. Fairclough JA, Mintowt-Czyz WJ. Skier's thumb—a method of prevention. *Injury* 1986;17:203-204.
37. Smith E, Rowles J. An increasing seasonal sports injury. *Practitioner* 1988;232:1385-1386.
38. Miller RJ. Dislocations and fracture dislocations of the metacarpophalangeal joint of the thumb. *Hand Clin* 1988;4:45-65.

39. Primiano GA. Skier's thumb injuries associated with flared ski pole handles. *Am J Sports Med* 1985;13:425-427.
40. Ferlic D. Skier's thumb. *Prim Care Bull* 1992;7:36-39.
41. Stener B. Displacement of the ruptured ulnar collateral ligament of the metacarpophalangeal joint of the thumb. A clinical and anatomical study. *J Bone Joint Surg* 1962;44B:869-879.
42. Wadsworth LT. How to manage skier's thumb. *Phys Sports Med* 1992;20:69-78.
43. Weaver JK. Skiing-related injuries to the shoulder. *Clin Orthop Rel Res* 1987;216;24-29.
44. Pino EC, Colville MR. Snowboard injuries. *Am J Sports Med* 1989;17:778-781.
45. Abu-Laban RB. Snowboarding injuries: An analysis and comparison with alpine skiing injuries. *Can Med Assoc* J 1991;145:1097-1103.
46. McArdle WD, Katch FI, Katch VL. Exercise Physiology: Energy, Nutrition, and Human Performance. 2nd ed. Philadelphia: Lea & Febirger; 1986:126-127, 648.
47. Goss FL, Robertson RJ, Spina RJ, et al. Aerobic metabolic requirements of simulated cross-country skiing. Ergonomics 1989;32:1573-1579.
48. Street G. Technological advances in cross-country ski equipment. *Med Sci Sports Exerc* 1992;24:1048-1054.
49. Boyle JJ, Johnson RJ, Pope MH. Cross-country injuries: A prospective study. *Iowa Orthop* J 1981;1:41.
50. Scott D. Ski injuries. *Minnesota Med* 1978;129. Letter.
51. Renstrom P, Johnson RJ. Cross-country skiing injuries and biomechanics. *Sports Med* 1989;8:346-70.
52. Tough SC, Butt JC. A review of 19 fatal injuries associated with back country skiing. *Am J Forens Med* Pathol 1993;14:17-21.
53. Johnson RJ, Incavo SJ. Cross-country injuries. In: Casey MJ, eds.*Winter Sports Medicine.* Philadelphia: FA Davis; 1990;302-307.
54. Dorsen PJ. Overuse injuries from Nordic ski skating. *Phys Sports Med* 1986;14:34.
55. Lawson SK, Reid DC, Wiley JP. Anterior compartment pressure in cross-country skiers: A comparison of classic and skating skis. *Am J Sports Med* 1992;20:750-753.
56. Renstrom P, Johnson RJ. Cross-country ski injuries and biomechanics. *Sports Med* 1989;8:346-370.
57. Wright JR, Hixson EG, Rand JJ. Injury patterns in Nordic ski jumpers. *Am J Sports Med* 1986;14:393-397.
58. Fiennes A, Melcher G, Ruedi TP. Winter sports injuries in a snowless year: Skiing, ice skating, and tobogganing. *BMJ* 1990;300:659-661.
59. Reid DC, Saboe L. Spine fractures in winter sports. *Sports Med* 1989;7:393-399.
60. Shugerman RP, Rivara FP, Wolf ME, et al. Risk factors for childhood sledding injuries: A case-control study. *Ped Emerg Care* 1992;8:283-286.
61. Landsman IS, Knapp JF, Medina F, et al. Injuries associated with downhill sledding. *Ped Emerg Care* 1987;3:277-280.
62. Dershewitz R, Gallagher SS, Donahoe P. Sledding-related injuries in children. *Am J Dis Child* 1990;144:1071-1073. Letter.
63. Lehman LB. Neurologic injuries from winter sporting accidents. *Postgrad Med* 1986;80:88-98.

Knee Injuries

Charles Stewart, MD, FACEP

The knee is one of the most frequently injured joints in the body and can have a bewildering array of injuries.[1] Since it is a weight-bearing joint, it is constantly subjected to substantial force. Unfortunately, the knee is found at the end of two relatively long lever arms, so a modest amount of force beyond "design limits" can cause a major disruption of the joint. Falls, automobile accidents, and virtually any sports activity can result in an acute knee injury. Despite the frequency of injuries and the resultant wide experience with their management, consensus standards for the treatment of many acute knee injuries do not exist. In addition, the initial bedside diagnosis of intra-articular ligamentous and cartilaginous injuries is imprecise. As such, the expeditious diagnosis and referral of patients with traumatic hemarthrosis and/or suspected ligamentous injury is most likely to yield optimal results.[2] The emergency physician is in an ideal position to facilitate early diagnosis and surgical repair when appropriate.

This review of acute knee trauma will focus on anatomic essentials and examination and imaging techniques. Special attention will be given to ligamentous, meniscus, and fracture/dislocation injuries.

Anatomy

The knee is a hinge joint with a range of motion from about 0° in full extension to about 130° of flexion. There is some rotational flexibility in the knee joint, but this varies from patient to patient. There are three bones, four ligaments, and two cartilages included in the knee. These are augmented by the extensor and flexor mechanisms. The bony knee is formed by the articulation of the distal femur, the proximal tibia, and the posterior aspect of the patella. Although the proximal fibula is an attachment for ligaments that support the joint, it is not part of the knee joint articulation. *(Please see Figure 1.)*

There is no inherent stability to the knee joint. All stability is provided by the ligamentous structures that surround the knee. Anterior and posterior stability is provided by the two cruciate ligaments, with the posterior cruciate providing most of this stability. The medial and lateral collateral ligaments stabilize the knee in side-to-side motion. Finally, the meniscal cartilages provide some stability, but they mostly act as shock absorbers for the knee.

The extensor mechanism of the knee is the quadriceps femoris muscles, the quadriceps tendon, the patella, the patellar tendon, and the insertion of the patellar tendon into the tibial tubercle. Four muscle groups comprise the quadraceps femoris: the superficial rectus femoris, the vastus medialis, vastus lateralis, and the deeper vastus intermedius muscles. Fibers of the rectus femoris invest the patella and contribute to the patellar tendon. The patellar tendon inserts into the anterior lip of the tibia and the tibial tubercle.

Table 1. Minimum Essentials to Document in All Knee Injuries

- Neuromuscular evaluation
- Documentation sufficient to exclude dislocations and fractures
- Results of valgus and varus stress test examination in 20° flexion.
- Lachman's test
- Extensor mechanism function

Clinical Presentation

The approach to an acute knee injury depends, in part, on when the patient presents to the ED. In most cases, there is little problem with the history. The patient comes to the department with a history of force applied to the leg or knee directly. This may be caused by a sporting accident, an automobile accident, or a fall. Certain mechanisms provide clues to diagnosis: "catching a tip" while skiing leads to anterior cruciate ligament (ACL) tear; a side tackle in football leads to a medial collateral tear; a head-on motor vehicle accident (MVA) may produce rupture of the posterior cruciate.

Many of the injuries that occur to the knee involve more than one ligament. It is essential to appreciate this fact before attempting to diagnose the condition.

If the emergency physician is careful in obtaining a mechanism of injury and appropriate history, then the diagnosis may be obvious prior to examination of the knee. Acute swelling may mean bleeding from a fracture or torn ligament. Immediate loss of extension may indicate a cartilaginous tear, a loose foreign body, or rupture of the extensor mechanism (quadriceps or patellar tendon). Contact injuries may involve a valgus load that will first tear the medial collateral ligament (MCL), then the posterior medial capsule of the knee and, finally, the ACL. This is known as O'Donaghues' triad.[3] A force that produced hyperextension will first disrupt the ACL, then the posterior cruciate ligament.

The examiner should be wary of hip problems (such as slipped capital femoral epiphysis) that present with knee pain, especially in children. A complete examination should include palpation of the hip and complete range of motion of the hip. Pain with flexion, internal rotation, or external rotation should suggest a possible hip fracture, Legg-Perthe's disease, avascular necrosis, or arthritis of the hip. If there is any question of referred pain or concomitant hip injury, then radiographs of the hip should also be obtained.

Examination of the Knee

Most acute knee injuries can be completely evaluated with an adequate history that includes mechanism of injury and careful examination of the knee. The emergency physician must master the physical examination of the acutely injured knee. *(Please see Table 1.)*

When examining the patient's knee, the patient should be supine, since this relaxes the muscles of the leg.[4] Sitting up will contract the quadriceps. Hanging the leg off of the side of the bed will obscure many findings but does allow for visualization of active flexion beyond 90°. Examination of the patient in a wheelchair is completely inadequate.

Inspection of the knee joint may reveal ecchymosis about specific structures. Areas of ecchymosis should be examined closely to check the underlying structures. The most common areas are the tibial tubercle, the MCL, the patella, the iliotibial band, and the postero-lateral aspect of the knee. Inspection may reveal lacerations that can potentially invade the knee joint, as well as evidence of swelling or patellar dislocation.

Palpation. Palpation is one of the most important sections of the physical examination of the knee. It is wise to start away from the area of injury and work toward the injury. This will allow the examiner to establish a rapport before starting the painful part of the examination. If a fracture is strongly suspected, the emergency physician should defer stressing the knee until after radiographs are taken. If a significant fracture is present, stressing the knee to determine ligamentous laxity is unnecessary and potentially harmful.

Palpate the course of the collateral ligaments and the posterior corners of the joint capsule. Tenderness along the course of the collateral ligament should point the examiner toward an injury of that ligament, while tenderness in the joint line may mean a meniscal tear. Patellar tendinitis and chondromalacia patella may be associated with tenderness at the inferior portion of the patella. Palpate the epiphyseal plates in children and adolescents so that a nondisplaced epiphyseal injury is not missed.

An acute hemarthrosis may be found on examination of the knee. This finding usually indicates serious injury to one or more structures of the knee. The most common injury is to the ACL (about 70% of cases). Peripheral meniscal tears make up another 10% of cases. Patellar subluxation is seen in about 10-15% of cases, and osteochondral fracture fragments occur about 5% of the time.[5] Meniscal and cruciate ligament tears may co-exist in as many as 60% of the cases.[5] Osteochondral fractures are the predominant injury associated with ACL tears in children.

Extensor Mechanism. Determine whether the patient can raise the leg straight against gravity. If the patient cannot do this, then look for a fracture of the patella or rupture of the quadriceps tendon. Quadriceps rupture occurs when there is a sudden stop during active extension, as in stumbling forward. Patellar tendon ruptures and fractures of the tibial tubercle should also be considered.

McMurray Test. A positive McMurray test is indicative of a cartilaginous tear. It is performed by hyperflexing the knee, internally rotating it, and extending the knee while palpating the knee joint. The knee is then hyperflexed and externally rotated. If the examiner feels a crunch, grind, or pop in the joint line, the test is positive.

Drawer Test. The drawer test determines the integrity of the ACL. Have the patient lie supine on the examination table and flex the knee to 90° with the foot planted flat on the table. Stabilize the foot with your body. Wrap your hands around the knee with the fingers in the areas of insertion of the medial and lateral hamstrings and the thumbs on the joint line. Put the thumbs in the joint line to feel a step-off. Draw the tibia toward you. If it slides under the femur toward you, the ACL may be torn. A little anterior draw is normal if present on both sides. The anterior drawer test is unreliable in the acutely injured knee because of pain and swelling.

It the test is positive, repeat with the leg in internal and external rotation. External rotation will tighten the postero-medial portion of

Figure 1. Ligaments of the Knee Joint

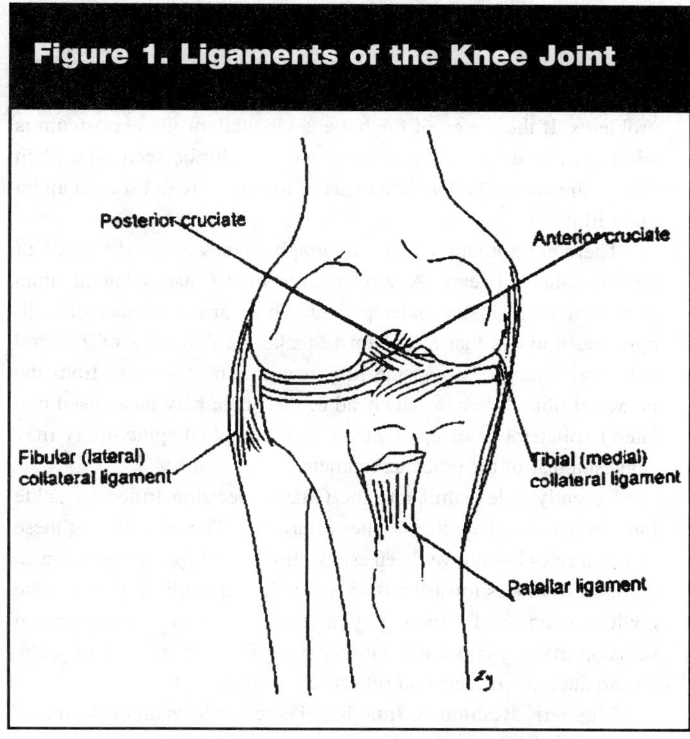

Figure 2. Lachman's Test

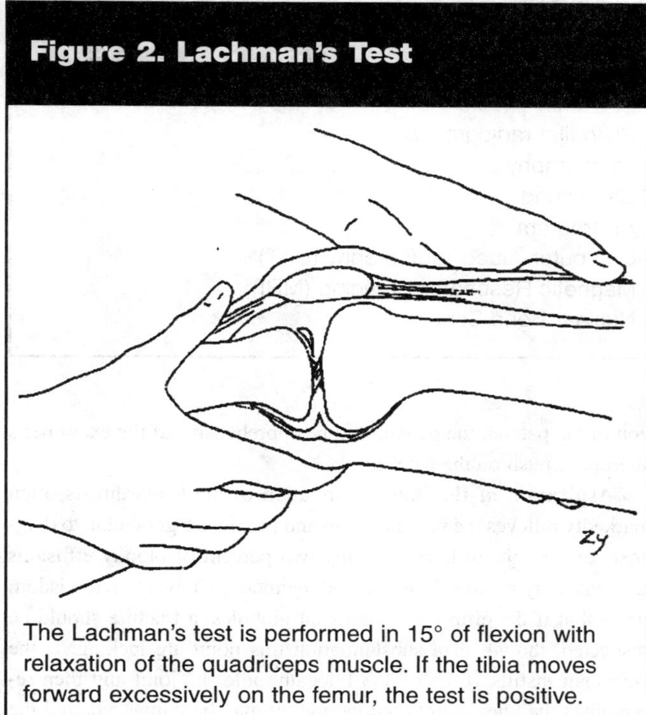

The Lachman's test is performed in 15° of flexion with relaxation of the quadriceps muscle. If the tibia moves forward excessively on the femur, the test is positive.

the joint capsule, so there should be reduction of the motion, even when the anterior cruciate is torn. When there is no reduction of the motion, suspect that both the anterior cruciate and the posterior medial potion of the joint capsule were damaged. Internal rotation demonstrates tears of the postero-lateral joint capsule.

The posterior cruciate (posterior-drawer test) is tested by pushing on the tibia rather than pulling. If it moves posteriorly, then the posterior cruciate may be damaged. Isolated tears of the posterior cruciate ligament are not common. Normal knees have no posterior excursion.

Lachman's Test. The Lachman's test is more sensitive than the anterior drawer test for acute rupture of the ACL. *(Please see Figure 2.)* The knee is placed in full extension while the distal femur is elevated, thereby permitting the knee to flex. Next, the proximal tibia is pulled anteriorly in an attempt to displace the tibia on the femur. If the tibia moves forward excessively on the femur, the test is positive. The result that should be noted on the chart is the maximum displacement of the knee at the joint line. This should be compared to the opposite side. A difference of more than 2.5 mm from side to side is diagnostic of a tear of the ACL in most cases.[6] A partial tear may allow an elastic rebound to the pull rather than a full, firm stop. The Lachman's test is much more sensitive for an anterior cruciate tear than the standard drawer test. The Lachman's test can also be done for a posterior cruciate injury by pushing rather than pulling.

Pivot-shift Test. The pivot-shift test reproduces the instability experienced by the patient. The knee is examined in full extension, the tibia is internally rotated, with one hand grasping the foot and the other hand applying lateral (valgus) stress at the knee joint. The knee is then flexed to about 20-30°. The examiner will feel a jerk at the anterolateral corner of the proximal tibia. The Lachman's test is probably a better test for ACL insufficiency than the pivot-shift test.

Like the Lachman's and the anterior drawer tests, the posterior cruciate ligament can be tested by reversing the directions above. The examiner supports the limb with a hand under the heel, the knee in full extension, and then applies a mild valgus stress with the other hand on the patient's lateral calf and flexes the knee. If the test is positive, the tibia will externally rotate and the lateral tibial plateau will subluxate. When the knee is extended, the tibia will reduce. Unlike the Lachman's and anterior drawer tests, the reverse pivot-shift test is probably the best test for a posterior cruciate ligament injury.

Collateral Ligaments. To test the medial aspect of the knee for stability, push medially against the knee and laterally against the knee to open the knee joint on the medial side. Palpate the medial joint line for gaps. If there is a gap, then the medial collateral ligament is torn. These gaps may be either palpable or visible. When the stress is released, the examiner may feel a "clunk" as the tibia and femur close.

Palpate the medial surface of the medial femoral condyle for tenderness. This is the area where the MCL is most often torn.

Since the MCL is more crucial to stability than the lateral collateral ligament, a complete tear may cause joint instability. Most collateral ligament tears are medial.

To test the lateral aspect of the knee for stability, push laterally against the knee and medially against the knee to open the knee joint on the lateral side. Palpate the lateral joint line for gaps. These gaps may be either palpable or visible. When the stress is released, the examiner may feel a "clunk" as the tibia and femur close. Both lateral and medial stability should be tested with the leg in full extension and in 20° flexion. The extended-knee exam tests the posterior capsule. By flexing the knee, the posterior capsule becomes lax, and the collateral ligaments are tested in isolation.

Patellar Apprehension Test. To perform the patellar apprehension test, the examiner will attempt to laterally displace the patella in extension, at full hyperextension, and at 30° of flexion. This test is sensitive but not always specific. If there has been a recent disloca-

Table 2. Diagnostic Imaging Techniques for Knee Injuries

Plain film radiographs
Tomography
Ultrasound
Arthrogram
Computer-Aided Tomography (CAT)
Magnetic Resonance Imaging (MRI)
Nuclear Bone Scan

tion of the patella, the patient will be apprehensive of the examiner's attempt to push on the patella.

Aspiration of the Knee. Aspiration of the hemarthrosis often markedly relieves the patient's pain and provides a good clue to diagnosis of the injured knee. Seventy-two percent of bloody effusions are caused by a tear of the cruciate ligament.[7] Conventional wisdom states that if the effusion contains fat globules, a fracture should be suspected, though data substantiating this point are lacking. If the physician instills 10 cc of 1% lidocaine into the joint and then reexamines the knee, additional pathology may be unmasked, and the patient will be far more comfortable. A combination of marcaine and morphine in the joint gives up to 48 hours of pain relief. A Lachman's or pivot-shift test may be possible to perform after the patient's knee has been aspirated and the hemarthrosis drained.

The technique is simple and rapid. Although the effusion may reaccumulate, it can be slowed by ice, elevation, and a compression dressing of the knee. The emergency physician should not hesitate to perform this diagnostic and therapeutic technique.

Imaging Knee Injuries

When the patient presents with a possible knee injury, the evaluating physician can choose from conventional radiography, imaging with tomography, skeletal scintigraphy, arthrograms, arthroscopy, computed tomography, and magnetic resonance imaging (MRI). The costs, capabilities, and limitations of these techniques must be appreciated by the diagnostician. Each of these techniques gives additional information at an incremental cost to the patient. The emergency physician should realize that only rarely will his or her emergency therapy be changed by one of these advanced techniques. *(Please see Table 2.)*

Plain Film Radiographs. The standard knee series varies from institution to institution. The ideal approach involves establishing a presumptive diagnosis after a careful examination before ordering radiographs. A standing anteroposterior (AP) view of the injured knee, or a regular AP if the patient cannot stand, is standard. Lateral, oblique, and notch views may also be obtained. The cross-table lateral view may reveal a blood/fat level in the joint which is pathognomonic of a fracture. The oblique view may demonstrate a fracture or loose foreign body in the joint. The notch view will allow evaluation of an osteochondral fracture. The sunrise view demonstrates the patella. If a plateau fracture is suspected despite normal films, consider a plateau view of the knee.

The plain films can show intra-articular effusions, fractures, tendinous calcifications, and most foreign bodies. They are not particularly helpful in diagnosis of soft-tissue and many cartilaginous and osseous abnormalities. In part, abnormalities of movement are often rotatory, and the conventional films will not demonstrate these problems. If the cortex of the bone is violated, or the periosteum is stimulated or displaced, the injury will usually be seen on a plain film of the knee. The five ligaments of the knee are not seen at all on plain films.

There are not significant radiographic clues to the diagnosis of medial collateral tears. A valgus force may cause a lateral tibial plateau fracture in the older patient. There are a number of radiographic findings that may help to make the diagnosis of a lateral collateral injury. The capsule may tear a bony fragment from the proximal tibia. Likewise, the head of the fibula may be avulsed in a lateral collateral or biceps femoris injury. A tibial spine injury may suggest a tear of the cruciate ligament.

Recently, rules similar to the Ottawa Decision Rules for ankle injuries have been applied to knee injuries.[8-11] The reliability of these decision rules has not yet been established in multiple settings. Given the current moves toward cost-containment in medical care and the obvious overuse of radiography, a reliable tool to support clinical decision making is needed. Further work is necessary before widespread adoption of decision rules is appropriate.

Magnetic Resonance Imaging. There has been an explosion of interest in MRI since 1985. The major reason for the rapid acceptance of MRI in the diagnosis of acute and chronic knee injuries is that it provides additional clinical information that is not easily obtained by any other imaging technique, including arthrograms and arthroscopy.[12] This should be considered an advanced imaging technique. Only rarely should the emergency physician even consider employing MRI in the emergency management of the acute knee injury.

In many centers, MRI has completely replaced arthrograms for the investigation of the internal disorders of the knee, since MRI has superior tissue-contrast resolution and is totally noninvasive.[13] There is no need for intra-articular contrast injection and no use of ionizing radiation. MRI is not limited to the surface of the joint or only to the surfaces that can be exposed by arthroscopy. Using MRI, the physician can evaluate more structures than just the bones, cruciate ligaments, and the surfaces of the menisci. The MRI can show both internal and external meniscal abnormalities. Osteochondral injuries, such as osteochondritis dissicans or traumatic osteochondral fracture, can be easily seen on MRI. MRI can also show acute or chronic damage to the articular cartilages of the tibia, femur, and patella. Tears of the anterior cruciate that are difficult to diagnose in the presence of a significant joint effusion are easy to find on MRI. These cruciate ligament tears are diagnosed on physical examination about 85% of the time but are seen 95% of the time on MRI. Rupture of the extensor tendon mechanism at either the patellar tendon or the quadriceps femoris is most easily diagnosed by MRI.[14]

The major disadvantage of MRI is its high cost. Since the MRI is both new and fairly expensive, cost-benefit ratios in the evaluation of acute knee injuries have not yet been determined. A more detailed knowledge of the anatomy and pathology is required as more anatomic areas are now visible and more diseases able to be diagnosed in the knee.

Arthroscopy of the Knee. The knee is the largest joint in the body and, as such, is the most amenable to both visualization and operative repair of lesions. Initially, diagnostic arthroscopy allows assessment of meniscal and cruciate ligament injuries. Arthroscopy of the knee is usually accomplished through an anterolateral port, and evaluation of the inferior surface of the posterior part of the medial meniscus is quite difficult.[15] Other areas that are difficult to see with an arthroscope include the peripheral attachments of the meniscus on both sides and the posterior section of the lateral meniscus. Evaluation may include performance of a drawer test during the arthrogram.

The arthroscope can be used not only to diagnose knee injuries but, in skilled hands, repair them. The resulting morbidity of the athlete is markedly reduced, with far shortened times in both hospital and recuperation. Meniscal repair through the arthroscope allows the patient to return to full activity sooner and, possibly, with a decreased likelihood of complications than with open surgery.[16] Needless to say, arthroscopy is not an emergency medicine procedure.

Ultrasound. Ultrasound scanning can display lesions in ligaments with considerable accuracy. It is more accurate than CT scanning but somewhat less accurate than MRI.[17] With the availability of relatively inexpensive and more accurate MRI, ultrasound examination of the knee has been largely supplanted.

Ligamentous Injuries

Anterior Cruciate Ligament Sprain. *Incidence.* The ACL is the most commonly injured major ligament of the knee, with these injuries occurring predominantly during non-contact sports. It also has the potential for causing the greatest disability. Early diagnosis decreases further injury and shortens the time until resumption of normal activity.

Anatomy and Function. The ACL attaches to the posterior aspect of the lateral femoral condyle and to a fossa just anterior and lateral to the anterior tibial spine. The tibial attachment is broad and extends into the lateral meniscus. The femoral attachment is a semicircle, with the anterior border straight and the posterior border convex. There are two major bundles within the ligament—the anteromedial and the posterolateral. The anteromedial bundle tightens during flexion, and the posterolateral bundle tightens during extension. This means that the ligament is under tension, and hence, at risk during all motions of the knee.

The vascular supply is almost exclusively from the synovial covering. There is little blood supply from the bony attachments. The nerve supply is mechanoreceptors with only scant pain fibers.[7] Since there are few pain fibers, ACL tears may not hurt much.

The ACL has five major functions: controling and resisting internal rotation of the femur and the tibia, resisting displacement of the tibia anteriorly on the femur, preventing hyperextension of the knee, acting as fine-tuning for the locking mechanisms of the knee, and restraining against valgus and varus strain in flexion of the knee. Of these functions, perhaps the prime role is to prevent internal rotation of the flexed knee on the femur.

History. The ACL is the most frequently injured ligament in the knee.[18] No single common mechanism causes rupture of the ACL, although a twisting motion of the knee is a common one. *(Please see Table 3.)* Basketball, football, soccer, and, to a lesser extent, rugby are common sports in which this injury occurs. Failure of ski binding to release may be associated with an anterior cruciate tear. The patient may note a "pop" or tear at the time of the injury.[19]

The patient may describe hyperextension of the knee by falling while playing basketball or missing a dismount in gymnastics. Basketball, football, soccer, and rugby players may attempt to stop suddenly in order to change directions. This appears to produce a quadriceps contraction that displaces the tibia anteriorly. Skiers may injure the ACL when they catch the outside edge of a downhill ski and both extend and internally rotate the tibia on the femur.

The patient will usually complain of posterolateral knee pain, immediate swelling of the knee, and varying degrees of knee instability. The patient may be unable to continue to play or walk but may also have sufficient stability of the knee to walk off of the field. A tense, bloody knee effusion is common, but if there is sufficient disruption of the joint capsule, the blood may extravasate into the surrounding tissues. Early application of ice may delay the hemarthrosis. Intense pain may develop within hours as the swelling from hemarthrosis ensues.

Examination of the acutely swollen knee is usually difficult and often unrewarding. A positive anterior drawer or Lachman's test is strongly suggestive. The anterior drawer test is often normal in acute injuries because the meniscus may block the forward motion of the tibia, or the hamstring spasm may prevent forward motion in the patient with a tense effusion of the knee.

Classic symptoms and signs of complete ACL tear are: the knee gave way, buckled, or "popped," there is a question of the patient being able to continue activity, or there is acute hemarthrosis within the first few hours.

Unfortunately, some athletes will have a tear of the ACL and not only have minimal symptoms but may return to the game rapidly.[7] In these patients, diagnosis may be difficult. Some patients will develop a secondary degenerative arthritis of the knee, while others will show little joint deterioration. Since the presentation of the ACL injury is so variable and the long-term prognosis is equally difficult to predict, the results of surgical procedures and nonoperative treatment alike are open to question.[20]

X-Rays. The astute physician should carefully examine the knee series. The standard radiographs are often normal or may simply demonstrate an intra-articular effusion. A small avulsion fracture of the lateral tibial condyle just below the joint line is a sign of an ACL tear. This is often called the "lateral capsular sign."[21]

MRI may be required for an accurate diagnosis. With the advent of noninvasive MRI studies, arthroscopy is now employed less often. MRI may show concomitant subchondral bone lesions (fractures or bruises) with ACL injuries.[22]

Treatment. Treatment of the isolated ACL injury is both individualized and controversial.[17,23] There is no convincing study demonstrating that immediate surgery is essential to long-term usefulness and decreased morbidity. Both conservative non-operative approaches and operative approaches are currently recommended by significant numbers of physicians who claim advantages for their therapy.

Consider the acuteness of injury, age, instability, degree, type of injury to the ACL, ability to rehabilitate, and, most importantly, the desired level of future activity in recommending one or the other therapy. Early surgical intervention is favored in athletes who desire to return to sports that place high functional demands on the knee.[24] The patient who has a positive pivot-shift examination is likely to develop functional instability and require surgical repair.[3]

If the patient has a tense, painful hemarthrosis, it may be aspirated and the patient placed in a knee immobilizer or other splinting device. Aspiration of the hemarthrosis will provide both a significant clue to the diagnosis and substantial pain relief for the patient. This should be followed by ice to the area, adequate pain management, and expeditious orthopedic referral.

Complications. Complications of ACL injuries include knee dislocation and functional loss that produces abnormal knee motions and major degenerative changes.

Posterior Cruciate Ligament Sprain. *Mechanisms of Injury.* The posterior cruciate ligament is rarely injured alone. Sports-related trauma and motor vehicle accidents (MVAs) are the most common causes of injury to the posterior cruciate ligament, but these injuries are often associated with simultaneous injuries to other ligaments in the knee. Isolated injuries to the posterior cruciate can occur with a fall on a flexed knee or a dashboard injury to the flexed knee.[25] *(Please see Table 3.)* Hyperextension of the knee tears the posterior cruciate ligament only after the ACL has been destroyed. The resultant dislocation of the knee may be reduced by the time that the patient presents to the ED. A severe varus or valgus bending movement of the knee will injure the posterior cruciate ligament together with the anterior cruciate and or the collateral ligaments. A "clipping" injury can disrupt the posterior-lateral structures, including the posterior-cruciate ligament.

Table 3. Mechanisms of Injury and the Possible Joint Structures Involved

MECHANISM	STRUCTURES
Varus or valgus contact	Collateral ligaments Epiphyseal fracture Patellar dislocation
Varus or valgus contact with rotation	Collateral and cruciate ligaments Collateral ligaments and patellar dislocation Meniscus tear
Blow to patellofemoral joint with fall on flexed knee	Patellar articular injury or fracture
Blow to tibial tubercle with fall on flexed knee	Posterior cruciate ligament
Anterior blow to tibia with hyperextension	Anterior cruciate ligament
Noncontact hyperextension	Anterior cruciate ligament
Deceleration	Anterior cruciate ligament
Deceleration with tibial medial rotation, or femoral lateral rotation on fixed tibia	Anterior cruciate ligament
Turn with tibia rotated in opposite direction	Patellar dislocation
Rotation with varus or valgus loading	Meniscus injury
Compressive rotation without contact	Meniscus injury Osteochondral fracture

Magee DJ. *Orthopedic Physical Assessment.* Philadelphia: W.B. Saunders; 1987.

Symptoms and Signs. Abrasions, lacerations, or ecchymosis about the tibial tubercle should invoke suspicion of a posterior cruciate injury. The patient may walk with a slightly flexed knee to avoid a terminal extension of the knee. A thorough neurovascular examination and consideration of the possibility of an acute popliteal artery injury are essential if this injury is found, since the patient may have had a dislocation of the knee that has been reduced in the field.

The most accurate assessment of the posterior cruciate ligament is either the posterior drawer test in 90° of flexion or the reverse pivot-shift test. The posterior drawer test is performed exactly like the anterior drawer test except that the tibia is pushed posteriorly instead of pulling on it. Some authors also feel that the test should be performed at 45° to increase the sensitivity of the examination.[26]

Insall and Hood described the posterior sag sign associated with posterior cruciate ligament injuries. If the patient is supine and the knee is flexed 90°, the tibia will sag into posterior subluxation if the patient has a complete tear of the posterior cruciate ligament.[27]

The diagnosis can be confirmed by MRI. This test is essentially 100% specific and sensitive in the diagnosis of an acute posterior cruciate ligament injury.[22] There may be some chronic injuries of the posterior cruciate ligament that are not noted on MRI.

Treatment. Treatment of the isolated tear of the posterior cruciate ligament is under debate. Since the posterior-cruciate ligament is often not damaged alone, orthopedic literature has focused on these combined injuries. Some authors feel that patients with slight-to-moderate posterior instability are often able to compensate adequately with good quadriceps function.[26] Others feel that there is substantial long-term disability associated with isolated injuries of the posterior cruciate ligament; and these orthopedic surgeons are re-thinking the non-operative treatment currently rendered.[25]

If the patient has a posterior cruciate ligament injury combined with other ligament injuries, then the patient should be suspected of having a dislocation of the knee that has been reduced in the field. This patient should be treated as if he or she has had a dislocation, and the neurovascular status should be carefully evaluated by frequent examinations or arteriogram.[28]

Collateral Ligament Tears. *Incidence.* Collateral ligament strains and sprains are common. The vast majority of collateral ligament injuries result from sports. Although contact sports such as soccer and football are most often implicated, skiing is an important cause of knee injuries.[29] In a study of 160 knee injuries in athletes,

12% were collateral ligament tears, and all but one occurred on the medial side.[30]

Mechanisms of Injury. The patient with a collateral ligament injury usually has trauma to the contralateral side of the knee or has had excessive forces applied to the knee in a valgus or varus direction. *(Please see Table 3.)* The skier may have the ski rotate without a binding release or with the boot catching in the snow after the binding releases. Combined injuries of the ACL and the MCL are common.

Symptoms and Signs. The patient may report a tearing sensation and immediate pain at the time of the injury. The amount of swelling and ecchymosis depends on the severity of the injury. If the capsular portion of the medial collateral ligament is torn, or if the patient has a concomitant cruciate injury, then a hemarthrosis may be found. Complete capsular disruption may allow blood to extravasate into the tissues.

The patient is usually tender about the distal femur at the femoral condyle and extending to the joint line because the injury most often involves the proximal portion of the MCL. If the patient is tender about the medial side of the patella, then look for a tear of the medial retinaculum.

Since lateral collateral ligament injuries are uncommon, they may be missed. When there is lateral collateral tenderness, swelling, or ecchymosis, the examiner must carefully elicit the mechanism of injury in order to ensure that the lateral collateral ligament is not involved. MCL injuries cause joint instability more frequently than do lateral collateral ligament injuries. The wider, lateral collateral ligament is most often partially torn; hence, no instability is found.

Treatment. The treatment for a grade I or grade II collateral sprain is ice to the area, compression, elevation, and rest. *(Please see Table 4.)* A non-steroidal anti-inflammatory medication may both relieve pain and decrease swelling. A knee brace for 4-6 weeks will decrease the chance of a re-injury.

Treatment of a grade III injury is somewhat controversial. Most orthopedic surgeons favor nonoperative therapy and short-term immobilization. The knee should be adequately braced during the rehabilitation. Prospective studies show no benefit from surgical management, but some orthopedic surgeons still feel that a surgical repair is indicated in these cases.[31,32]

Meniscus Injuries

The menisci are semilunar fibrous cartilages in the capsule of the knee joint. In cross-section, the meniscus is triangular in shape, with the apex of the triangle directed central and the base of the triangle at the joint margin. They act as shock absorbers, provide lubrication, and more evenly distribute weight to the femoral condyles and the tibial plateau. They also act as spacers to increase the stability of the knee. The medial meniscus is attached to the capsular portion of the MCL. If the MCL is damaged, then the medial meniscus may also be disrupted. The attachments of the lateral meniscus have the popliteal tendon passing through them posteriorly and laterally. Like the lateral collateral tendon, the lateral meniscus is less frequently damaged than the medial meniscus.

The peripheral portion of the meniscus is vascular, while the central portion of the meniscus is relatively avascular. Both menisci receive their entire blood supply from their peripheral attachments, so a torn meniscus may become avascular and degenerate rapidly. The medial avascular portion of the meniscus does not heal well, even if repaired.

Table 4. Classification of Ligament Sprains

STRETCH—GRADE I
A first-degree sprain is really a microscopic tear and can be treated with rest, ice, and protection with crutches and/or a splint.
PARTIAL TEAR—GRADE II
A second-degree sprain should be immobilized to prevent the ligament from tearing completely.
COMPLETE TEAR—GRADE III
Third-degree sprains may require surgery. Therapy is somewhat controversial.

The majority of patients with a meniscus tear are in their 20s.[33] Because the meniscus has such important functions in load bearing and stability of the knee, a loss of this structure in the young athlete is associated with significant degenerative changes. When the meniscus is removed or becomes avascular and degenerates, the mechanics of the knee will change.[34] The articular surface contact forces rise 2-3 times, and substantial degenerative changes in the contact surfaces of the joint result.

The two meniscal cartilages are easily injured, often with seemingly trivial trauma.[35] The menisci can be injured as a result of twisting, hyperflexion of the knee, and rotatory instability of the knee. Patients may note that they planted the foot and twisted the knee or fell on the hyperflexed knee. This combination is often found in the martial arts.

There is no generally accepted classification of meniscal tears. They can be classified by shape, position in relation to the anterior or posterior "horn" of the meniscus, and by whether or not they have been displaced from the normal position. They can also be graded by whether or not they occur due to trauma, degeneration, or are in association with ligamentous knee instability. The most common types of meniscal tear are the "bucket handle" tear and a flap tear, where one end of the "bucket" handle has been torn free. These are both vertical lesions that occur following injuries, and are often displaced. Medial tears are more common than lateral tears. Medial bucket-handle tears may be associated with a chronic ACL tear.

When they are torn, meniscal injuries frequently present with a clear effusion and delayed swelling. The patient often notes swelling the day after the injury. If the meniscus is torn in the vascular peripheral third of the meniscus, the effusion may be both bloody and immediate. However, the acuity of the hemarthrosis is of limited help in differentiating meniscal from ligamentous injuries. Occasionally, the patient may complain that the knee "locks." Later in the course, the patient may note pain during activity (turning and pivoting) and morning stiffness.

The examiner may note tenderness in the medial or lateral joint line. This may be the most predictive clinical finding of meniscal injury.[36] If the tear is posterior, then hyperflexion of the knee will increase the pain. Likewise, hyperextension of the knee will be painful if the tear is anterior. A spongy block to full knee extension may be noted when the patient has a displaced bucket-handle tear that is in the intercondylar notch. A chronic injury may be accompanied by visible quadriceps atrophy or may be documented by measuring thigh circumference about one hand-breath above the patella in both thighs.

Definitive diagnosis of a meniscal tear may be made with arthroscopy or MRI. Arthroscopy has the advantage of simultaneous repair if indicated, while MRI is completely non-invasive.

Meniscus tears may be managed nonoperatively, by meniscectomy (both open and by arthroscopy), and by repair of the meniscus by various means.[37] In general, the smaller tears, or those that are only partial thickness, may best be managed by leaving them alone. Meniscectomy, by either arthroscopy or open surgery, still causes significant long-term disability in many cases, beginning after only a few years.[38,39] Disability is markedly reduced if the repair is done within two months of the injury.[33]

Fractures

Distal Femur Fractures. Fractures of the distal femur are usually caused by axial loading combined with varus or valgus stress and rotation. They may be classified as supracondylar, intercondylar, or condylar fractures.

Supracondylar fractures are often transverse or slightly oblique, with varying degrees of displacement and/or comminution of the fracture fragments. Like all fractures, they may be open or closed. If there is a posterior component, the popliteal artery may be involved. If there is sufficient force, then the patient may have also sustained damage to the four major ligaments at the same time. Some supracondylar fractures can extend into the knee to form an intercondylar fracture.

Condylar fractures result from varus or valgus force. These fractures are more difficult to detect on routine radiographs. MRI or CT scan may demonstrate the fracture site. In children and adolescents, the attachment of the adductor muscle group may be avulsed, leaving a cortical irregularity.

Proximal Tibia Fractures. *Mechanism.* Mechanisms that can cause a tibial plateau fracture include axial loading (fall from a height), varus or valgus forces, and/or rotation. Sports that can cause these injuries include football, soccer, rugby, hang gliding, gymnastics, and sport parachuting. Common features of these fractures include a very stable fracture and intact ligaments of the knee.

Violent, twisting movements or abduction-adduction injuries can cause fractures of the tibial spine or the intercondylar eminence. These injuries are often combined with significant soft-tissue and ligamentous lesions and may be classified as a "fracture dislocation" of the knee. Needless to say, these injuries may also cause simultaneous arterial or nerve damage.

Signs and Symptoms. Signs and symptoms include tenderness and swelling over the fracture site, instability of the knee with stress testing, and the inability to bear weight.

Diagnosis. Intra-articular fractures of the proximal tibial plateau may be quite subtle. In addition to the conventional radiographic series of the knee, computerized tomography may be required for diagnosis. The films should be carefully examined for disruption of the articular surface, effusions, and avulsion fractures at the sites of ligamentous attachments in the femoral condyles, fibular head, and intercondylar eminence. Tibial plateau fractures should be suspected in the presence of localized bony tenderness, effusion, and pain with axial loading.

Treatment. Conservative treatment with long-leg splinting is appropriate unless the fracture is depressed or displaced by more than a centimeter. These fractures may require operative reduction with internal fixation (ORIF) if the fragments are widely separated or depressed. If there is a depressed fragment in an area of weight bearing, then operative intervention may be indicated.

Deep vein thrombosis is a common complication in tibial plateau fractures.[40] Doppler studies are indicated in these patients at the slightest suspicion of DVT.

Complex trauma involving the proximal tibia may also cause compartment syndrome. If there is any suspicion that the patient has a compartment syndrome, then compartmental pressures should be measured promptly.

Fibular Fractures. The fibula is rarely fractured in isolation. These injuries may result from direct trauma to the head or neck of the fibula (bumper injuries), varus forces that avulse a fragment of the proximal pole or styloid process of the fibula, valgus forces that also produce lateral tibial plateau fractures or medial collateral ligament injuries, or twisting injuries at the ankle with pronation and external rotation. Detection of a fracture of the fibula should prompt evaluation of the ankle or a simultaneous ligamentous injury.

The fibular fracture may be accompanied by rupture of the lateral capsule and ligamentous structures and stretching of the peroneal nerve. Other complications of the proximal fibular fracture include arterial injury to the nearby anterior tibial artery or contusion of the biceps tendon.

Fractured Patella. *Mechanism.* Fractures of the patella are caused by either direct trauma or indirect forces caused by forcible quadriceps tendon contraction. Direct trauma is the most common mechanism of injury. Unilateral injuries are very common, but some bilateral fractures occur. There is a 2:1 predominance in males over all age groups. About 50-80% of patellar fractures are transverse.[41] Longitudinal (25%) or stellate fractures (20-35%) usually result from direct trauma, such as "dashboard knee."[42] Patellar fractures caused by quadriceps traction may break the bone into equal-sized components or avulse either pole of the patella. Fractures of the inferior portion of the patella are more common.

The most important clinical feature is whether the patient can actively raise the leg off the bed in full extension. Any injury causing complete disruption of the extensor mechanism, including fracture of the pelvis and the surrounding retinaculum, will prevent this motion.

Severely comminuted fractures may require surgical removal of the patella, as degenerative arthritis is found in 39% of the cases.[43] Fractures that are so disrupted that the leg cannot be raised require surgical repair of the patella for functioning of the quadriceps tendon.

Signs and Symptoms. The examiner may find tenderness and swelling over the patella or an inability to extend the knee. If the extensor mechanism is disrupted, the patient may be able to stand but not walk with a normal gait. Walking may be accomplished by leaning forward over the injured leg and allowing gravity to drop the leg. A palpable defect or a bloody joint effusion may also be noted.

X-Ray. Most patellar fractures are readily apparent in normal overhead radiographs. Be sure to get the sunrise (axial/skyline) view to ensure an adequate view of the patella if standard views are non-diagnostic in the setting of strong clinical suspicion.

Treatment. If the fragments are displaced more than 4 mm, or if the patient is unable to raise the extended leg off of the bed, then operative intervention is needed. If there is no displacement, then a long-leg cylinder cast or knee immobilizer is appropriate. Unless there is a complication requiring immediate intervention, orthopedic referral can be in the office over the next few days.

Dislocation of the Knee

Traumatic dislocation of the knee (referring to the tibia and femur) is rare.[44] It requires violent trauma to dislocate the knee, and even large teaching institutions see only a few of the these serious injuries in a year. If it is not properly and promptly managed, significant long-term disability or loss of the limb can result.[45]

Complete dislocation of the knee is caused by direct or indirect violence. Dislocations may be classified as anterior, posterior, lateral, medial, or rotatory. The type of dislocation will depend on the direction and location of the forces applied. Since a severe force is required to dislocate the knee, most are caused by automobile accidents, car vs. pedestrian accidents, motorcycle injuries, and contact sports.[46] Motor vehicle accidents are the most common cause, with athletic injuries being a distant second.

Hyperextension of the Knee. Anterior knee dislocations are produced by hyperextension. As the knee is hyperextended, the posterior capsule ruptures at about 30°. The anterior and posterior cruciate ligaments follow shortly thereafter.[47] When the posterior cruciate ligament ruptures, the tibia rides forward on the femur, producing the anterior dislocation. As the hyperextension continues, the popliteal artery is stretched, and then ruptured, at about 50°. These figures were measured in cadavers, but less hyperextension was thought to be needed for the same injury in living subjects.[48]

Medial, Lateral, and Posterior Dislocations. Medial, lateral, and posterior dislocations are much more difficult to produce experimentally. The experimental procedures used to produce them cause tibial plateau and supercondylar fractures more frequently than they dislocate the knee.[46] This is the same pattern found in clinical practice. These dislocations are usually caused by extreme direct violence applied to the lower end of the femur with a fixed tibia, or the upper end of the tibia when the femur has been fixed in place. Medial dislocation tears the cruciate and lateral ligaments. Lateral dislocation tears the medial and cruciate ligaments. Posterior dislocation is caused by a direct force to the proximal anterior tibia.[49]

Rotary dislocations are caused by a rotation of the foot about the knee. The most common rotatory dislocation is the posterolateral dislocation. Surgical reduction may be required if closed reduction fails.

Signs and Symptoms. Unfortunately, evaluation of the traumatic dislocation may not reveal any deformity.[46] Frequently, either spontaneous reduction or reduction at the scene by trainers or EMS providers occurs. If severe ligamentous injury is found in the knee and there is a compatible mechanism recounted by patient or spectators, then a reduced dislocation should be suspected. A knee with a torn ACL, posterior cruciate ligament, and a collateral ligament tear on one side should be considered a dislocation that has been reduced.[50] Dislocations of the knee that cannot be easily reduced in the ED are quite rare indeed.[51]

A detailed assessment of the lower extremity and knee, including evaluation for signs of compartment syndrome, is vitally important. Particular attention should be directed to the distal pulses, the sensation of the great toe and first web space, the ability to move the toes, and examination of the knee. Swelling, coolness, lack of distal pulses, distal skin coolness, or decreased sensation should prompt rapid evaluation of the patient's arterial supply to the lower leg.

Since it is difficult to differentiate between neural and vascular injury in the lower extremity, evaluation of the blood supply with an angiogram is almost always needed. If the patient develops a gradual loss of sensation over the digits, then critical ischemia may be present. An obvious temperature difference between the two feet should strongly suggest an arterial occlusion. If the pulses are absent, then immediate evaluation and treatment is imperative.

Complications. *Open Dislocations.* Dislocations also may be open or closed. A less favorable prognosis is found in open dislocations, but this may be because there is extensive soft-tissue damage and associated injuries in many of these cases.

Popliteal Artery Injury. The blood supply to the foot and leg is very dependent on the popliteal artery, and very little collateral circulation exists. Damage to the popliteal artery is the single most devastating complication of traumatic dislocation of the knee. It occurs in about 40% of all knee dislocations.[52] Collateral circulation around the knee is clearly inadequate to supply the foot and lower distal leg, and the extremity will be ischemic if the popliteal artery is damaged. If it is not treated promptly and adequately, then the patient will require amputation of the lower extremity more than 90% of the time.[52]

An arteriogram should be obtained if there is even the remotest suspicion of vascular injury or if there is any neurologic injury. This procedure cannot wait, since the blood vessel must be repaired within 6-8 hours to maintain viability of the extremity. A good rule of thumb is that the patient needs an arteriogram if three out of four ligaments are torn.

Peroneal and Tibial Nerve Injury. Fortunately, nerve injuries associated with dislocation of the knee are less frequent than vascular injuries. The tibial and common peroneal nerves are less prone to injury because they are not as firmly attached to the structures in the back of the knee. When injury occurs, there is often extensive longitudinal damage from the traction on the nerves. Peroneal nerve injury has a poor prognosis. There appears to be no help from any operative procedure. If the patient has signs of peroneal nerve injury, an arteriogram is needed to discover any concomitant or causative vascular injury.

Treatment. The dislocated knee must be reduced promptly. If there is any vascular compromise, immediate reduction prior to radiographs is indicated. The knee is reduced by longitudinal traction, while simultaneously lifting the femur into place. Avoid pressure in the popliteal fossa during reduction. Have an assistant provide counter-traction by holding onto the shoulders or hips. Simple traction and counter-traction will usually suffice for reduction and provide significant pain relief. Supplemental intravenous pain medication is generally needed, however. Following reduction, a posterior leg splint should be placed at 15° flexion to avoid stretching the popliteal artery. An arteriogram to evaluate the popliteal artery should then be obtained. Surgery will be needed if there is an open fracture, if the dislocation cannot be reduced, or if there is evidence of popliteal artery injury.

Dislocated Patella

Mechanism. Dislocation of the patella is quite common. Lateral dislocation is most common and may be caused by flexion, external rotation, and simultaneous contraction of the quadriceps tendon. Quadriceps contraction pulls the patella lateral during push off or step. Direct trauma may also cause a dislocation. Dislocations are unlikely if the patient has normal patello-femoral anatomy.

Signs and Symptoms. Clinically, the patient will have an obvious lateral deformity and swelling. If spontaneous reduction occurs, tenderness on medial patellar and lateral femoral-line palpation can be noted.

If recurrent dislocation is suspected, check the "apprehension" test. Ask the patient to lie supine on the examination table with legs flat and the quadriceps relaxed. Press against the medial border of the patella. The patient will start to show apprehension and distress. In addition, the underside of the patella may be tender.

Complications. Osteochondral fracture with intra-articular fragments may be present and cause degenerative arthritis. This is more common when the patella is dislocated by direct trauma. Since 28-50% of patients with patellar dislocation have an associated fracture, radiographs of the patella are needed even when the dislocation has been reduced.[53,54]

The patient may develop a hemarthrosis following dislocation of the patella. Aspiration of the joint may be needed if reduction is obstructed by the hemarthrosis.

Recurrent dislocation is a significant problem. The younger the patient is at the time of the initial injury, the more likely a recurrent dislocation becomes.[54] Recurrence of dislocation may be lessened by strengthening of the vastus medialis, oblique, and gluteus muscles.

Treatment. Treatment includes immediate reduction of the patella by simply extending the knee and moving the patella medially. The patient will be more comfortable if a hemarthrosis is aspirated when present. The patient may be treated with either a cylinder cast or a knee immobilizer with follow up in the consultant's office. Recurrent dislocations or fractures that are associated with dislocations may require an operation.

Miscellaneous Injuries

Quadriceps and Patellar Tendon Rupture. Rupture of the quadriceps tendon is relatively uncommon.[55] Like the disruption of the patella associated with a patellar fracture, the patient is unable to maintain the knee in full extension against gravity. The patient will be unable to climb stairs or to walk up an incline. A palpable soft-tissue defect may be found above the patella proximal to the superior pole of the patella. A complete rupture is usually found, but partial ruptures may also be found.

Quadriceps tendon rupture can present in a deceptively mild fashion. About half of patients are initially misdiagnosed. The patient may have little swelling and pain and is simply unable to raise the leg against gravity. If the patient is not asked to perform a straight-leg raise or to walk, the patient's problem may be missed. If the patient is treated with a knee immobilizer, then he or she is able to walk because the immobilizer takes the place of the torn quadriceps tendon.[56]

Radiographs may occasionally show an avulsion chip fracture, but are most often normal. Quadriceps rupture may be noted on ultrasound or MRI, but neither is usually ordered from the ED.

Treatment of rupture of the quadriceps tendon is usually early surgical repair. Following repair of the tear, the patient is treated with cast immobilization. Most patients regain full function of the knee. If the treatment is delayed, then the quadriceps tendon will retract and atrophy, making successful reapproximation of the ends more difficult.[57]

Rupture of the patellar tendon is less common than either fracture of the patella or rupture of the quadriceps tendon. It is more often seen in basketball and volleyball players, who have repetitive violent contraction of the quadriceps muscles.[58] An abnormally high position of the patella may be helpful in diagnosis. A knee radiograph may show an avulsion of the tibial tubercle and displacement of the patella superiorly.

Summary

The emergency physician is often the initial health care provider evaluating patients with acute knee injuries. Using basic examination techniques and selected imaging studies, identification of specific diagnoses may be possible. Many serious injuries may not be able to be diagnosed acutely; however, careful evaluation will generate appropriate suspicion and should result in early orthopedic referral such that optimal long-term management and surgical repair, as indicated, result.

References

1. Dehaven K, Litner DM. Athletic injuries: Comparison by age, sport, and gender. *Am J Sports Med* 1986;14:218-224.
2. Tubbs N. Injured ligaments of the knee. *Injury* 1990;21: 291-293.
3. Gersoff WK, Clancy WG Jr. Diagnosis of acute and chronic anterior cruciate ligament tears. *Clin Sports Med* 1988;7: 727-738.
4. Lombardo JA. The athlete's knee: An orderly examination. *Emerg Med* 1984;16:34.
5. Baker CL. Acute hemarthrosis of the knee. *J Med Assoc Georgia* 1992;81:301-305.
6. Daniel DM, Malcom LL, Losse G, et al. Instrumented measurement of anterior laxity of the knee. *J Bone Joint Surg* 1985;67A:720-726.
7. King JB, Aitken M. Treatment of the torn anterior cruciate ligament. *Sports Med* 1988;5:203-208.
8. Stiell IG, et al. Derivation of a decision rule for the use of radiography in acute knee injuries. *Ann Emerg Med* 1995;26: 405-413.
9. Weber JE, et al. Clinical decision rules discriminate between fractures and non-fractures in acute isolated knee trauma. *Ann Emerg Med* 1995;26:429-433.
10. Bauer SJ, Hollander Je, Fuchs SH, et al. A clinical decision rule in the evaluation of acute knee injuries. *J Emerg Med* 1995;13:611-615.
11. Stiell IC, Greenberg GH, Wells GA, et al. Prospective validation of a decision rule for the use of radiography in acute knee injuries. *JAMA* 1996;275:611-615.
12. Herzog RJ. Imaging of the knee. *Orthop Rev* 1992:21: 421-424.
13. Mink JH, Deutsch AL. Magnetic resonance imaging of the

knee. *Clin Orthop and Rel Res* 1989;244:29-47.
14. Yu JS, Petersilge C, Sartoris D, et al. MR imaging of the injuries of the extensor mechanism of the knee. *Radiographics* 1994;14:541-551.
15. Ekstrom JE. Arthrography: Where does it fit in? *Clin Sports Med* 1990;9:561-566.
16. Sonnaben DH, Collican MRJ. Recent advances in arthroscopy. *Aust Fam Pract* 1993;21:421-424.
17. King JB. Focal points in orthopaedics. *Br Med Bull* 1992;48:651-667.
18. Swenson TM, Hamer CD. Knee ligament and meiscal injuries. *Orthop Clin North Am* 1995;26:529-546.
19. Perko MMJ, Cross MJ, Ruske D, et al. Anterior cruciate ligament injuries: Clues for diagnosis. *Med J Aust* 1992;157:467-470.
20. Daniel DM, Fithian DC. Indications for ACL surgery. *Arthroscopy* 1994;10:434-441.
21. Woods GW, Stanley RF, Tullos HS. Lateral capsular sign: X-ray clue to a significant knee instability. *Am J Sports Med* 1979;7:29-33.
22. Fowler PJ. Bone injuries associated with anterior cruciate ligament disruption. *Arthroscopy* 1994;10:453-460.
23. Noyes FR, McGinnis GH. Controversy about treatment of the knee with anterior cruciate laxity. *Clin Orthop* 1985;198: 61-76.
24. Gooch JI, Geiringer SR, Akau CK. Sports medicine. 3: Lower extremity injuries. *Arch Phys Med Rehabil* 1993;74: S438-S442.
25. Covey DC, Sapega AA. Current concepts review: Injuries of the posterior cruciate ligament. *J Bone Joint Surg* 1993;75A: 1376-1384.
26. Whipple TL, Ellis FD. Posterior cruciate ligament injuries. *Clin Sports Med* 1991;1:515-527.
27. Insall JN, Hood RW. Bone-block transfer of the medial head of the gastrocnemius for posterior cruciate insufficiency. *J Bone Joint Surg* 1982;64A:691-699.
28. Bratt HD, Newman AP. Complete dislocation of the knee without disruption of both cruciate ligaments. *J Trauma* 1993;34:383-389.
29. Steadman JR, Sterett WI. The surgical treatment of knee injuries in skiers. *Med Sci Sports Exerc* 1995;27:328-333.
30. Jensen JE, Conn RR, Hazelrigg G, et al. Systematic evaluation of acute knee injuries. *Clin Sports Med* 1985;4: 295-312.
31. Indelicato PA. Non-operative management of complete tears of the medial collateral ligament of the knee. *J Bone Joint Surg Am* 1983;65:323-329.
32. Smith BW, Green GA. Acute knee injuries part II. Diagnosis and management. *Am Fam Phys* 1995;51:799-806.
33. Henning CE. Current status of meniscus salvage. *Clin Sports Med* 1990;9:567-576.
34. Renstrom P, Johnson RJ. Anatomy and biomechanics of the menisci. *Clin Sports Med* 1990;9:523-538.
35. Hardin GT, Farr J, Bach BR. Meniscal tears: Diagnosis, evaluation, and treatment. *Orthopedic Rev* 1992;21: 1311-1317.
36. Hede A. Treatment of meniscal lesions in the knee. *Dan Med Bull* 1993;40:317-331.
37. Muckle DS. Meniscal repair in athletes. *Sports Med* 1988;5: 1-5.
38. Henning CE. Semilunar cartilage of the knee: Function and pathology. *Exer Sport Sci Rev* 1988;16:205-213.
39. DeHaven KE, Sebastianelli WJ. Open meniscus repair: Indications, technique, and results. *Clin Sports Med* 1990;9: 577-586.
40. Tscherne H, Lobenhoffer P. Tibial plateau fractures: Management and expected results. *Clin Orthop Rel Res* 1993;292:87-100.
41. Calkins C, Sartoris DJ. Imaging acute knee injuries. *Phys in Sports Med* 1992;20:91-99.
42. Duncan GF, Meals R. One hundred years of automobile induced orthopedic injuries. *Orthopedics* 1995;18:167-170.
43. Crenshaw AH, Wilson FD. The surgical treatment of fractures of the patella. *South Med J* 1954:47:716.
44. Hoover NW. Injuries of the popliteal artery associated with fractures and dislocations. *Surg Clin North Am* 1961;41: 1099-1112.
45. Kremchek TE, Welling, RE, Kremchek EJ. Traumatic dislocation of the knee. *Orthop Rev* 1989;18:1051-1057.
46. Roman PD, Hopson CN, Zenni EJ. Traumatic dislocation of the knee: A report of 30 cases and literature review. *Orthop Rev* 1987;16:917-924.
47. Girgis M. The cruciate ligaments of the knee joint. *Clin Orthop* 1975;106:216-231.
48. Kennedy J. Complete dislocation of the knee joint. *J Bone Joint Surg* 1963;45A:889-904.
49. Taylor AR, Arden GP, Rainey HA. Traumatic dislocation of the knee: A report of 43 cases with special reference to conservative treatment. *J Bone Joint Surg* 1972;54B:96-102.
50. Merrill KD. Knee dislocations with vascular injuries. *Orthop Clin North Am* 1994;25:707-173.
51. Nystrom M, Samimi S, HaEri GB. Two cases of irreducible knee dislocation occurring simultaneously in two patients and a review of the literature. *Clin Orthop Rel Res* 1992;277: 197-200.
52. Green A. Vascular injuries associated with dislocation of the knee. *J Bone Joint Surg* 1977;59A:236-239.
53. Garrick JG. Knee problems in adolescents. *Pediatr Rev* 1983;4:235-243.
54. Cash JD, Hugston JC. Treatment of acute patellar dislocation. *Am J Sports Med* 1988;16:244-249.
55. Ramsey RH, Muller GE. Quadriceps tendon rupture: A diagnostic trap. *Clin Orthop Rel Res* 1970;70:161.
56. Roberts J. Quadriceps tendon rupture. *Emerg Med News* 1993;July:14-16.
57. Siwek CW, Rao JP. Ruptures of the extensor mechanism of the knee joint. *Am J Bone Joint Surg* 1981;63:932-937.
58. Nance EP, Kaye JJ. Injuries of the quadriceps mechanism. *Radiology* 1982;142:301-307.

The Injured Ankle

Earl J. Reisdorff, MD, F ACEP
Kathleen M. Cowling

Cost-effective and therapeutically targeted management of ankle injuries has become one of the most interesting challenges in the day-to-day practice of emergency medicine. While many ankle injuries are benign in appearance and resolve without sequelae, emergency physicians are faced with the difficult task of identifying more subtle but serious injuries that have the potential of producing long-term complications that range from joint pain to gait dysfunction.

There is no dearth of pathology. The fact is, ankle injuries are among the most common injuries seen in the emergency department (ED), accounting for 3-12% of all ED visits.[1-3] In fact, ankle sprains are the most frequently incurred sports-related orthopedic injury, especially in competitive athletics.[4,5] From a radiographic perspective, ankle radiographs may account for 10% of all x-rays taken through the ED.[6] Given the significant costs associated with evaluation of what are sometimes only minor injuries, indications for cost-effective radiographic evaluation of ankle injuries have recently been defined.[2] Despite the potential usefulness of these clinical guidelines, application of such highly sensitive criteria to emergency medicine practice in the United States has been limited.

Although ankle injuries may appear to be minor at first glance, up to 44% of patients may have persistent symptoms one year after the injury.[7] Given the potential morbidity associated with ankle strains, dislocations, and fractures, emergency physicians must be skilled at recognizing severe injuries and initiating appropriate therapies that will accelerate recovery and limit chronic joint dysfunction.

This chapter presents an organized approach for physical examination of the acutely injured ankle, defines clinical indications for radiographic study, and outlines acute treatment modalities that facilitate pain relief and rehabilitation of the involved extremity.

Anatomic Consideration and Mechanism of Injury

The ankle is a modified hinge joint formed by three bones-the tibia and fibula superiorly and the talus inferiorly. *(Please see Figure 1.)* The tibia forms the joint plafond (French for "ceiling") and the medial malleolus. The fibula forms the lateral malleolus. The posterior lip of the distal tibia is sometimes referred to as the posterior malleolus. The tibia and fibula are held in relationship to one another by the anterior tibiofibular ligament, the posterior tibiofibular ligament, and the interosseous membrane, which forms a fibrous joint between the distal tibia and fibula called the syndesmosis.

The most proximal tarsal bone, the talus, superiorly, assumes a rounded trapezoid shape called the dome or trochlea. The articulation of the talar dome and the tibia is called the tibiotalar joint, creating a structure that resembles a mortise-tenon joint, much like that used by carpenters. *(Please see Figure 2.)* As a consequence, the element of

Figure 1. The Bones That Form the Ankle

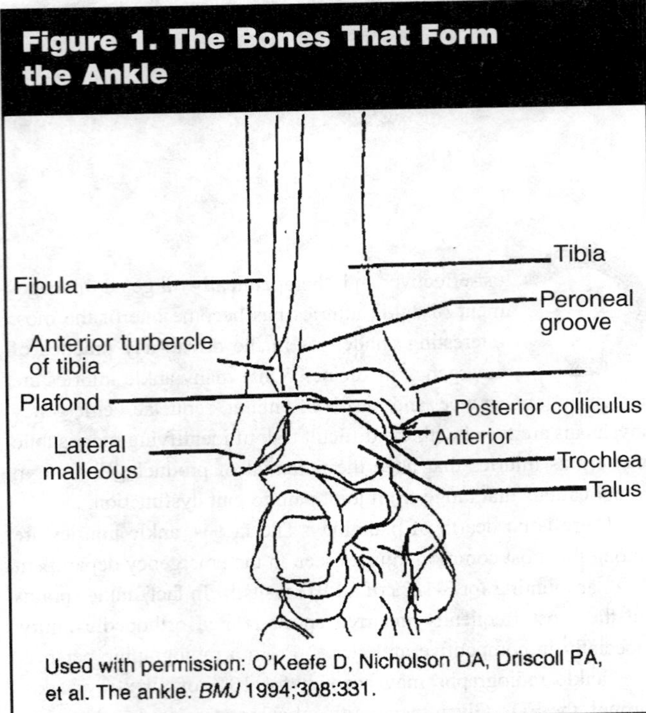

Used with permission: O'Keefe D, Nicholson DA, Driscoll PA, et al. The ankle. *BMJ* 1994;308:331.

Figure 2. The Mortise-Tenon Joint

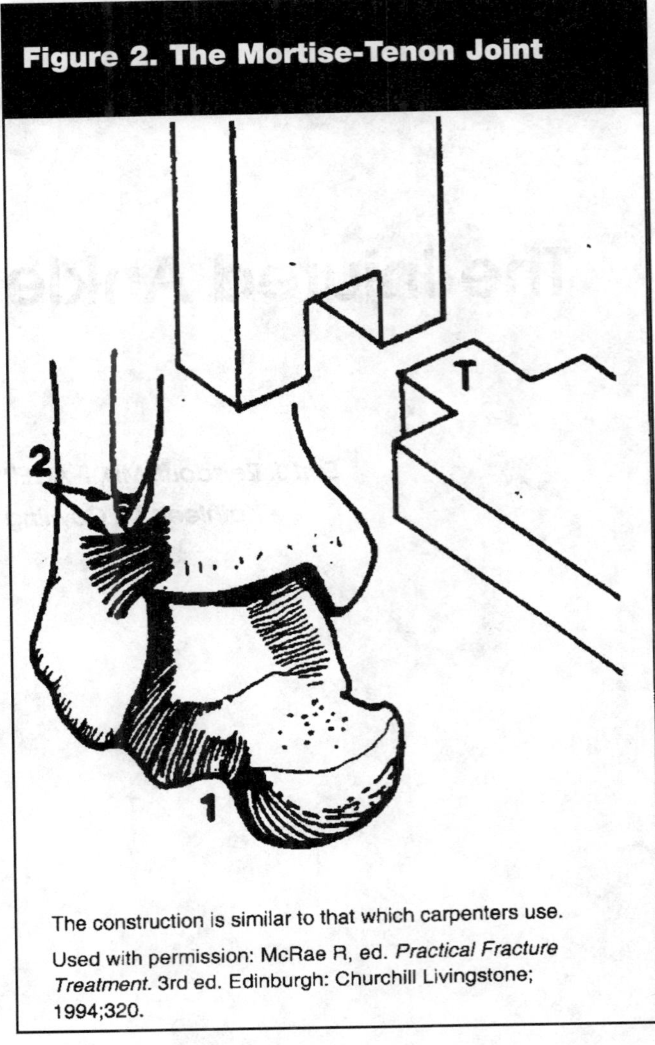

The construction is similar to that which carpenters use.

Used with permission: McRae R, ed. *Practical Fracture Treatment*. 3rd ed. Edinburgh: Churchill Livingstone; 1994;320.

the joint that accepts the talar dome is called the mortise, an orientation that permits dorsiflexion (upward) and plantar flexion (downward). Because the trapezoid shape of the talar dome is wider anteriorly, in dorsiflexion the talus wedges between the malleoli more tightly and the attached ligaments become taut. Correspondingly, plantar flexion is a more unstable position, relying on the ligaments to a greater measure for stability. Most other motions of the ankle, primarily inversion (rotating inward) and eversion (rotation outward), occur at the subtalar joint.

Anatomic positions of ankle bones are maintained by major ligament groups including the collateral ligaments, which attach at the lateral and medial malleoli and lock the talus into the mortise. *(See Figure 3.)* On the other hand, the lateral collateral grouping is composed of three ligaments-the anterior talofibular (ATFL), the posterior talofibular, and the calcaneofibular ligaments (CFL). The ATFL, which is the primary stabilizing ligament of the lateral group, originates at the anterior tip of the lateral malleolus, runs in line with the foot, and attaches to the neck of the talus. The medial collateral group of ligaments is collectively called the deltoid ligament, which is extremely strong and less prone to injury. In general, stability of the ankle is lost when two separate anatomic sections are disrupted.

Neuromotor function of the ankle is supplied by the anterior, medial, and posterior crural (leg) compartments. Anterior crural muscles, which are innervated by the deep peroneal nerve (L4-S1), are primarily involved in inversion and dorsiflexion. The posterior crural muscles are involved in plantar flexion and foot inversion, and are innervated by the tibial nerve (L4-S3). Innervated by the superficial peroneal nerve (L5-S2), the lateral crural muscles affect plantar flexion and foot eversion.

Determining the mechanism of injury is critical for diagnosis of ankle injuries. Generally speaking, the magnitude and the direction of the forces will determine the most likely injury pattern. For example, low-velocity injuries (e.g., low-impact sports) usually result in injuries involving only the nonbony elements, whereas a high-velocity impact tends to cause fractures. It should be stressed that the ankle sustains the greatest loading force per surface area of any joint,[8] and during normal ambulatory function, the forces applied to the ankle joint approach five times body weight. Consequently, even with moderate activities (e.g., landing jump on one foot while inverting the ankle), abnormally high forces are applied, predisposing to significant tissue destruction.

Clinical Evaluation

A detailed history of the trauma is essential, since ankle injuries generally follow patterns determined by the mechanism of injury. A reasonable historical profile would include; 1) date and time of the traumatic episode; 2) any previous trauma to the ankle; 3) relevant medical conditions (e.g., osteoarthritis. osteopenia); and 4) any treatment that has already been initiated. Moreover, the emergency physician should determine the onset of symptoms (e.g., pain, swelling, weakness, stiffness), sensations suggesting ankle instability, sounds ("snap" or "pop") heard during the traumatic event, and the patient's ability to continue ambulating or playing following the event. Specifically, whether the patient was unable to bear weight within one hour of injury should be ascertained. Factors that increase

The Ottowa Ankle Rules: A Consultant's Perspective

Abstract & Commentary
By David J. Karras, MD

Editor's note: Ankle injuries are a common presenting complaint in the emergency department, yet radiographs frequently fail to reveal a significant fracture. In addition, about $500 million is spent annually in North America to evaluate blunt ankle trauma. The Ottawa ankle rules can be a cost- and time-saving asset to emergency physicians. David J. Karras, MD, Assistant Professor of Medicine at Temple University School of Medicine and Director of Emergency Medicine Research at Temple University Hospital in Philadelphia, offers additional insight into these clinical practice guidelines.

The onslaught of clinical practice guidelines has struck terror into the hearts of many emergency physicians who view them as unwieldy bureaucratic intrusions. A recent study by Stiell and colleagues focuses on one guideline that is practical and sensitive as well as cost- and time-saving: the Ottawa ankle rules.

Ankle injuries are a common presenting complaint in the ED, yet less than 15% of radiographs actually reveal a significant fracture. In 1992, Stiell and associates (Stiell IG, et al. *Ann Emerg Med* 1992;21:384-390) published a clinical decision rule designed to markedly reduce the number of unnecessary ankle and foot radiographs, but the rule had not been validated—until now. The resulting guideline, known as the "Ottawa ankle rules," has since been further refined and states that radiographs of the ankle are necessary only if there is pain in the malleolar region and there is either tenderness in the distal 6 cm of the posterolateral medial or lateral malleolus or inability to bear weight both immediately after the injury and in the ED. Radiographs of the foot are necessary only if there is pain in the midfoot and there is either tenderness, or inability to bear weight.

Table. The Ottawa Ankle Rules

An ankle radiographic series is only required if there is any malleolar pain and any of the following findings:

- bone tenderness at the posterior edge or tip of the lateral malleolus (distal 6 cm) **or**
- bone tenderness at the posterior edge or tip of the medial malleolus (distal 6 cm) **or**
- instability to bear weight both immediately and in the emergency department.

Adapted with permission: StiellIG, et al. *JAMA* 1993;269: 1127-1132.

The current findings are derived from a prospective, non-randomized, controlled study designed to validate the Ottawa ankle rules' ability to predict the need for radiography in evaluating acute blunt ankle injuries. The study was performed at a university hospital, and, using a community hospital as a control, assessed the effect on clinical practice before and after dissemination of the ankle rules. A total of 2342 adult patients (mean age, 36; range, 18-92 years) were evaluated. Using the rules in the ED, 100% of clinically significant fractures were detected, the number of radiographs per patient was reduced by 24%, and the number of patients who received no radiographs at all rose from 4% to 24%.

Physicians felt very comfortable using the rules and ordered radiographs "unnecessarily" in only 4% of cases (all were negative). Compared to nonfracture patients at the control hospital who underwent radiographs, the patients not undergoing radiographs did not differ in tenus of satisfaction with their medical care or in number under-going follow-up radiographs, but medical costs were reduced by 36% and waiting time was reduced by 69%.

Use of the Ottawa ankle rules minimizes the use of radi-ographs, lowers costs, and reduces waiting time for patients without missing significant fractures. (Stiell IG, et al. Implementation of the Ottawa ankle rules. *JAMA* 1994;271:827-832.)

COMMENT BY DAVID J. KARRAS, MD

This study bears out earlier findings that the prediction rule is 100% sensitive in detecting clinically significant ankle fractures (defined as having bony fragments > 3 mm in breadth). It is important to note that patients younger than 18 years were not studied, and no attempt should be made to generalize the findings to the pediatric population. Interestingly, the original prediction rule used age greater than 55 years as an indication for obtaining radiographs; this criterion has been dropped without any loss of sensitivity.

The perceived risk of malpractice liability is frequently cited as a major factor in physicians' overordering of radiographs for ankle injuries, even when clinical judg-ment tells the practitioner that the risk of fracture is van-ishingly small. Decision rules such as these can be used by emergency physicians to support clinical decisio making and to justify, whether to the patient or to them-selves, a decision not to obtain radiographs when not warranted by physical examination. This study went the extra step by anticipating the objection that patients would be dissatisfied if no radiographs were obtained. When given a careful explanation by the physician of the rationale for not obtaining radiographs, it was found that patient dissatisfaction was actually extremely low.

the risk or incidence of ankle injury include age (< 18 or > 65 years), male sex, and warmer months, which are associated with increased intensity of recreational activity. Though age extremes have an increased risk of fracture, the greatest number of ankle injuries occurs in people 21-30 years of age.[6]

Physical examination, which must be thorough and conducted in an organized fashion, is useful for assessing ligament disruption, joint instability, neurovascular compromise, and the extent of soft-tissue injury. First, the physician should visually compare the injured side to the uninjured side, inspecting for ecchymosis, swelling, deformity,

Figure 3. The Ligaments of the Ankle

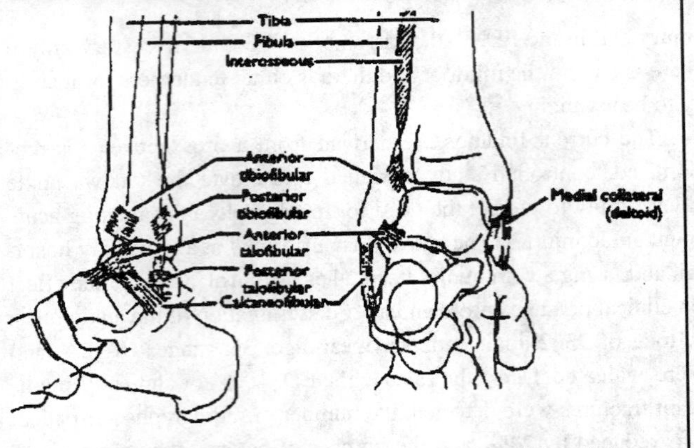

Used with permission: O'Keefe D, Nicholson DA, Driscoll PA, et al. The ankle. *BMJ* 1994;308:333.

and interruptions in the integrity of the skin. Swelling alone is an unreliable indicator of injury severity.[3] Nonetheless, a fracture is almost always associated with soft-tissue swelling.[2] A marked deformity may indicate an ankle dislocation, which may require immediate reduction, especially if there is skin blanching or neurovascular compromise. Circulation should be assessed by inspecting for capillary refill and intensity of distal pulses of the posterior tibial and the dorsalis pedis arteries.

Range of motion is best determined by evaluating the uninjured side first. Often, range of motion is limited due to pain and edema. Nonetheless, one should attempt to estimate the amount of dorsi-flexion and plantar flexion of the injured ankle. Generally speaking, the range of motion of the ankle is 13-16° dorsiflexion and 31-44° plantar flexion.[9] The neutral (anatomic) position of the ankle is 90° as defined by the foot in relation to the long axis of the tibia.

Palpation should begin at a site away from that presumed to be tender. Some examiners first test remote areas (the proximal tibiofibular joint, the calf, and the foot) to detect atypical or associated injuries. Palpation of the foot (especially the fifth metatarsal, the calcaneus, and midfoot) may also assist in determining which radiographic studies should be performed. Evaluating remote areas is especially critical because they are not visualized by the routine ankle radiograph series. Gradually, the examiner should approach the areas presumed to be most tender, carefully palpating both malleoli (especially the distal 6 cm) at the tips as well as the posterior edges. The proximal fibula should always be evaluated for possible fracture; in children, the physes (growth plates) are palpated to determine the likelihood of fracture.

Because of limitations (patient anxiety, extreme pain) in performing a thorough examination in the moderately to severely injured patient, ligamentous instability may go undetected in the ED. Although some experts suggest injecting the injured area with a local anesthetic in order to facilitate examination of stressed ligaments,[10,11] this method is rarely practiced in the ED. Stress testing the ligaments in a painful ankle is probably unnecessary in the ED if the patient will be re-examined in 3-5 days. In addition, the reliability of ED ankle stress testing is questionable, since examiner techniques vary widely. Nevertheless, ligamentous instability must be assessed at follow-up

Figure 4. The Anterior Drawer Test

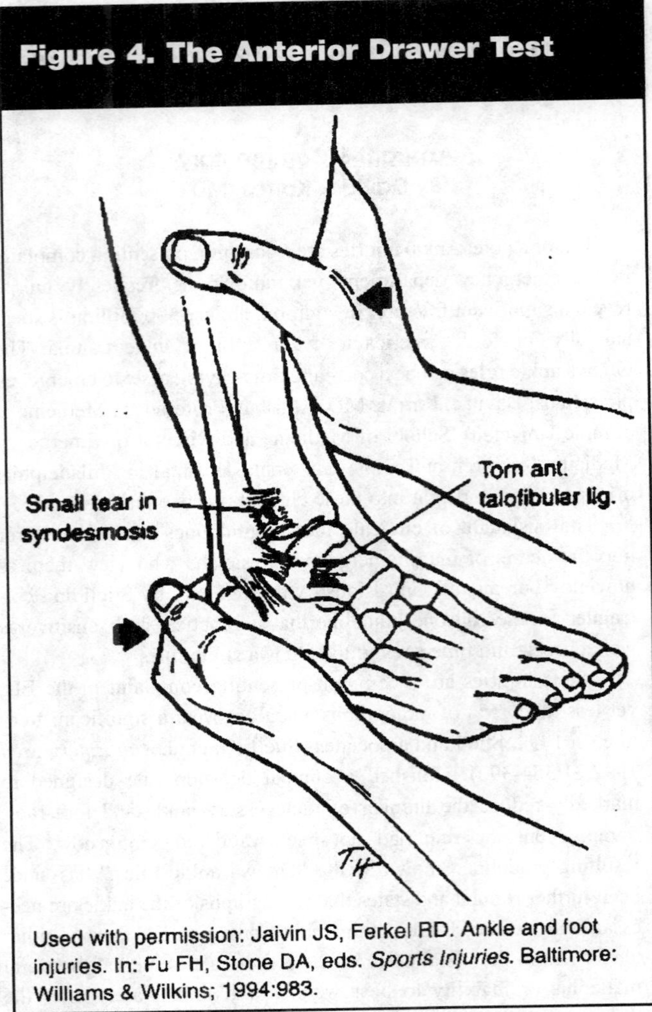

Used with permission: Jaivin JS, Ferkel RD. Ankle and foot injuries. In: Fu FH, Stone DA, eds. *Sports Injuries*. Baltimore: Williams & Wilkins; 1994:983.

so that appropriate definitive orthopedic care can be initiated.

Specific Testing Maneuvers. The anterior drawer test (sagittal stress test) is most useful for assessing the ATFL. *(Please see Figure 4.)* The maneuver is performed while holding the heel steady, with the foot partially plantar flexed (0-10°). One attempts to shift the distal tibia posteriorly while pulling the foot anteriorly. Clinically, scoring ligamentous instability is subjective and usually is characterized as mild, moderate, or marked.

The talar tilt test (inversion stress test) evaluates integrity of the lateral collateral ligaments, especially the CFL. The test is performed with the ankle in neutral (anatomic) position. The heel and the distal tibia are held stationary while the foot is inverted. *(Please see Figure 5.)* When the CFL is disrupted, the talar dome (trochlea) will separate from the tibial plafond. The examination results are usually described as a mild, moderate, or marked talar tilt angle. Ligamentous laxity with eversion suggests a deltoid ligament disruption.

The squeeze test is a somewhat subjective maneuver to determine whether the syndesmosis (the fibrous joint formed by the distal fibula, tibial, and surrounding ligaments) has been injured. The test is Performed by grabbing the calf and compressing the distal tibia and fibula together. The test is "positive" if the maneuver causes pain at the distal interosseous membrane. The ankle examination is concluded by testing weight-bearing. To "bear weight, " the patient must take at least two unassisted steps with each foot.

Radiographic Evaluation

The Ottawa Ankle Rules. Routine radiographic evaluation of all blunt ankle trauma has long been regarded as the "standard of care" by many clinicians. Of radiographs taken to evaluate blunt ankle trauma, 85% show no fracture.[12-14] In addition, it is estimated that $500 million is spent on ankle radiographs in North America each year.[15] These factors have led to the development of guidelines, frequently referred to as the Ottawa ankle rules, which were generated by a group of Canadian physicians for ordering ankle and foot radiographs. *(Please see Table.)*

When appropriately applied, these rules led to a 28% reduction in ordering ankle radiographs at the participating institution.[15] Patients who underwent radiographic study spent 116 minutes in the ED at a cost of $173 compared to 80 minutes at a cost of $62 for those who did not receive an x-ray study. Application of the Ottawa ankle rules yielded a sensitivity of 100% for clinically significant fracture. Small avulsion fractures that do not change initial ED management were considered clinically insignificant.[42] Because the criteria have been designed to have a high sensitivity, the specificity is poor-about 40%. Even using the Ottawa ankle rules, 77% of studies showed no fracture. Radiographs should also be considered, despite the Ottawa guidelines, in the patient who has altered sensorium, diminished peripheral limb sensation, or multiple painful and distracting injuries.

Patients excluded from the application of the Ottawa ankle rules included individuals younger than 18 years old, pregnant patients, those with isolated skin injuries, patients with injuries that occurred 10 days prior to evaluation, and those returning for recheck visits. When the Ottawa ankle rules were applied in a small physician study in the United States, the sensitivity was also 100%.[16]

Despite the usefulness and general acceptance of the Ottawa guidelines, it should be stressed that one trial failed to validate the Canadian findings.[17] A multicenter trial in New Zealand found a sensitivity of 93%, a specificity of 11%, and a positive predictive value of 22%. Of 75 fractures, five would have been missed by strict application of the Ottawa ankle rules, yielding a false-negative rate of 14%. One of the fractures was defined as "an unstable fracture of the distal fibula." The clinical significance of the other missed injuries was not characterized.

Radiographic Modalities

The ankle should be radiographically evaluated using at least the lateral and the anteroposterior (AP) views, which are capable of detecting virtually all fractures.[2] Nevertheless. some fractures are more easily visualized using an oblique or mortise view. In fact, most radiographic series in the United States include three views—the AP, the lateral, and the mortise view. The mortise view is taken with the leg rotated inwardly at 15-20° and provides the best view of the mortise. Sometimes, an oblique view is taken with the leg held in 45° of inward rotation. The use of three projections (AP, lateral, and mortise) allows for examination of both malleoli, the talar dome, the tibial plafond, and the anatomic spacing of the joint and bony relationships to assess for diastasis.

The articular space seen on an oblique view should be uniform in width. Widening beyond 4 mm between the medial malleolus and the medial aspect of the talus indicates diastasis and most likely rupture of the deltoid ligament. Other views should be considered when clinically indicated. For example, a mechanism of injury and tenderness consistent with a Maisonneuve fracture (see below) warrants an AP and lateral view of the entire leg to check for a proximal fibula fracture. Tenderness in the foot requires standard radiographic views of the foot for evaluation. The Ottawa group has developed similar clinical decision rules for radiographic evaluation of minor foot injuries.[14-16]

Figure 5. The Talar Tilt Test

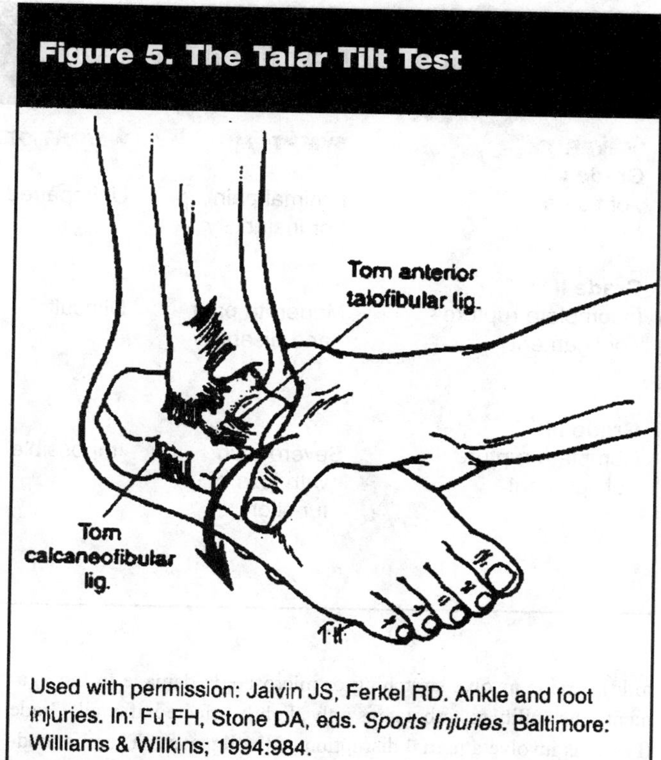

Used with permission: Jaivin JS, Ferkel RD. Ankle and foot injuries. In: Fu FH, Stone DA, eds. *Sports Injuries.* Baltimore: Williams & Wilkins; 1994:984.

Stress radiographs of the ankle are usually unnecessary in the ED, although these views assist the orthopedist in accurately quantifying the degree of ligamentous laxity. In general, clinical estimates of tibiotalar mobility exaggerate the actual amount as determined by radiograph.[9] Essentially, all manual stress tests performed to assess the ankle can be recorded radiographically. Since anterior subluxation is more common than talar tilt, a lateral radiograph should be performed to evaluate all unstable ankles.[18] Using radiographic evaluation, an anterior drawer test demonstrating 6 mm slippage is abnormal, as is a change of 6° in the angle during the talar tilt test.[19] One author has reported that 10° on talar tilt suggests a tear of the ATFL, whereas greater than 20° suggests that the CFL is also ruptured.[20]

Other diagnostic techniques for imaging the ankle include CT, MRI, arthrography, and bone scan, all of which are most appropriately ordered in consultation with an orthopedic specialist. CT and MRI are most helpful in defining intra-articular pathology, pediatric epiphyseal injuries, and soft-tissue pathology.

Sprains

Of all ankle injuries, 85% are sprains.[5] Classification of sprains is typically defined in three grades (or "degrees") and is based on the amount of ligamentous damage. *(Please see Table 1.)* Grade I (or

Table 1. Ankle Sprain Grading System

SEVERITY	SYMPTOMS	WEIGHT-BEARING	SIGNS	STRESS RADIOGRAPHS
Grade I of fibers	Minimal pain or instability	Unimpaired	Slight edema Anterior drawer and talar tilt test negative	Normal
Grade II Incomplete rupture of ligament	Moderate pain and disability	Difficult	Moderate edema and ecchymosis Anterior drawer and talar tilt test positive	Anterior drawer 4-14 cm Talar tilt > 5-10 degrees
Grade III Complete rupture of ligament	Severe pain with loss of function	Impossible	Severe edema and ecchymosis Anterior drawer and talar tilt test positive Possible avulsion fracture	Anterior drawer > 15 mm Talar tilt > 20 degrees

mild) sprains involve stretching or microscopic damage to the ligament. The ability to ambulate is only slightly affected, if at all. Grade II sprains involve a partial disruption of the ligament. There is moderate loss of function with an increased difficulty in the ability to walk. The localized edema that occurs can be pronounced. With a Grade III sprain, there is complete disruption of the ligament. There is usually hemorrhage into the surrounding soft tissues, resulting in a dramatic local or generalized swelling. This is accompanied by marked joint instability, pain, and the inability to walk. As previously mentioned, clinical and radiographic evaluation of joint stability is usually not performed on the acutely injured ankle.

Although ligamentous tears cannot be visualized directly on radiographic examination, the absence of a fracture, the position of the bony elements, and the pattern of soft-tissue swelling can indirectly suggest ligamentous disruption. Of all ankle sprains, 85% involve the lateral ligaments[21] with the ATFL being the most commonly injured ligament[22] The ATFL is particularly vulnerable to injury because its course changes during motion. At rest, the ATFL runs parallel to the foot; during plantar flexion, it runs parallel to the leg.[23] In addition, the ATFL has less elasticity, also making it more injury-prone.[19]

With ATFL rupture, the midpart of the ligament is completely disrupted. Usually, when the ligament is completely torn (ruptured), the joint capsule will also be interrupted. If the ankle is injured while in a neutral position, the CFL is more vulnerable to injury. If the ankle is dorsiflexed during the injury, the syndesmosis is more easily injured. In 20% of sprains, both the ATFL and the CFL are involved.[22]

Although the lateral ligaments are injured far more frequently than the medial ligaments, isolated medial ligament injuries can occur. Medial ligament injuries usually result from an eversion stress. Because the deltoid ligament is so strong, it is rarely injured in isolation but rather in association with a lateral malleolus fracture.[22] In this case, the ligament may rupture or be avulsed away from its attachment to the medial malleolus or talus. When a deltoid sprain is suspected, one must exclude an associated fracture (often of the proximal fibula) or concomitant syndesmosis rupture.

Syndesmosis sprains (interosseous membrane injuries) typically result from axial loading, in which the talar dome is forced upward, separating the tibia from the fibula. This action splits the tibia and fibula apart, tearing the interosseous membrane. Significant injuries to the syndesmosis are rarely isolated. More often, they are associated with a fracture of the lateral, medial, or posterior malleolus. In addition to the aforementioned squeeze test, the integrity of the syndesmosis can also be assessed by the Cotton test, which evaluates mediolateral movement of the talus within the ankle mortise. For the Cotton test, the distal leg is held with the ankle in a neutral position, while the foot is rotated from a medial to lateral position. During this maneuver, the examiner also feels for crepitus and instability .Any additional movement greater than 3 mm suggests a diastasis.[24]

Physicians sometimes fail to appreciate the chronic disability that can result from an ankle sprain. In particular, degenerative arthritis is common sequelae of chronic lateral ankle ligament instability,[25] with almost one-half of patients complaining of pain one year after ankle injury.[7]

Dislocations

Ankle dislocation results from complete disruption of articular elements in the ankle. When dislocated, the joint can no longer move in an anatomically normal fashion. Abnormal shifting of the talus in relation to the tibia that is incomplete is called a subluxation. An isolated ankle dislocation without associated fracture is quite rare. However, when ankle dislocation without fracture does occur, the overlying skin is usually tom or lacerated; the dislocation is open.[26] Joint stability after reduction and rehabilitation is surprisingly good, even though most patients will require surgical repair of the lateral ligaments. Due to the structure of the mortise and the strength of the surrounding ligaments, most dislocations will result in an associated fracture.

Posterior dislocation of the talus is the most frequent type of ankle dislocation and usually results from forced plantar flexion with inversion. This action distracts the joint anterolaterally, resulting in rupture of the lateral ligaments. Treatment may require rapid reduction if the anterior lip of the tibia is causing skin blanching. This finding indicates an ischemic area of skin and imminent skin perforation from pressure necrosis, which has the potential of converting this injury to an open fracture-dislocation. There can also be injury to the neurovascular structures and extensor tendons, especially if the injury is open. Non-posterior dislocations of the ankle are rare.

Fractures

Ankle fractures are usually defined as single malleolar, bimalleolar, or trimalleolar. A useful method for characterizing ankle fractures, the Lauge-Hansen system, divides the injury pat-tern into five major categories based on mechanism of injury.[27] There are 15 basic types of injury patterns grouped into these five main categories. The Lauge-Hansen system defines injury mechanism by two-word phrases. The first word refers to the position of the foot prior to the application of force, and the second word characterizes the direction of the talus within the mortise causing the fracture (e.g., supination-external rotation).

A more commonly used classification method is the Danis-Weber system, which focuses on the distal fibula to define the injury.[28] For example, a Type A fracture involves the fibula below the level of the tibiotalar joint, whereas Type B fractures occur at the level of the tibiotalar joint and involve partial rupture of the tibiofibular syndesmosis. A Type C fracture occurs above the level of the tibiotalar joint and disrupts the ligamentous connections between the tibia and the fibula up to the level of the fracture. Type A fractures tend to be stable; Type C fractures are unstable.

Isolated fibular fractures are the most common type of fracture and, without displacement, usually requires 4-6 weeks to heal.[6] Lateral malleolus fractures that occur above the level of the mortise are more unstable, more likely to be displaced, and should be referred to an orthopedist. Small lateral malleolus avulsion fractures occurring below the level of the talar dome are less likely to displace and, in some cases, can be treated with an orthopedic device called an orthosis (e.g., DonJoy Walker). Most displaced bimalleolar and trimalleolar fractures require open reduction to ensure an optimal functional result. Bimalleolar and trimalleolar injuries often involve concurrent injury to the syndesmosis.

Tibial plafond fractures are usually the result of high-energy injuries and involve intra-articular sites. With plafond fractures, the ankle is quite unstable and the resultant diastasis at the medial joint space usually requires operative repair. There is a high incidence of post-traumatic arthritis.

Proximal fibular fractures can occur from either dorsiflexion or eversion, which can occur when a jumping athlete lands on another player's foot. These fractures are frequently combined with a rupture of the anterior tibiofibular ligament and disruption of the interosseous ligament. When a fracture occurs 7-10 cm above the ankle, it is called a Dupuytren's fracture. In contrast, a Maisonneuve fracture is found proximally at the fibular neck. Some Maisonneuve fractures are associated with a medial malleolus fracture or a Grade III sprain to the deltoid ligament. Because of the proximity of the peroneal nerve to the fractured fibular neck, direct operative repair is generally avoided.[29] However, a syndesmotic screw is frequently placed.

Because the talus has a tenuous, "retrograde" blood supply, similar to that of the wrist's navicular (scaphoid) bone, fractures of this bone can lead to chronic disability. Consequently, when the distal or midportion of the talus is fractured, the dome is subject to osteonecrosis. Some small talar dome fractures can result in osteochondritis. The separate-appearing fragment "floating" in the joint is sometimes called a "joint mouse." Occasionally, the osteochondral fragment requires arthroscopic surgical removal.

Overlooked Injuries

Several disabling injuries pose diagnostic challenges for the physician evaluating patients with ankle problems. These subtle, often unrecognized injuries include: 1) fractures of the os trigonum; 2) Achilles tendon injuries; 3) dislocating peroneal tendons; 4) fractures of the fifth metatarsal; 5) transchondral talar-dome fractures; and 6) ankle diastasis.

The os trigonum is an accessory bone (sesamoid) located posterior to the posterior tubercle of the talus. It is present in 5-14% of the population and is frequently unilateral.[30] This accessory bone may be fused to the talus, calcaneus, or both. Patients with a fracture of the os trigonum often give a history of having sustained an ankle sprain weeks to months earlier, at which time radiographs were interpreted as normal. They give a history of persistent posterior and posterolateral ankle pain, swelling, and giving way of the ankle. Paulos and colleagues noted that the physical examination of these patients was consistently diagnostic.[31] All had a 25° decrease in plantar flexion of the ankle and pain to palpation posterior to the tibia but anterior to the Achilles tendon. The pain was enhanced by forced plantar flexion of the ankle or resisted plantar flexion of the great toe.

Physicians miss injuries to the Achilles tendon in 25% of cases, most often due to preservation of foot plantar flexion by the posterior tibial, peroneal, and toe flexor muscles? Patients will often describe the sensation of being kicked or "shot" in the back of the ankle with an immediately ensuing intense pain. Physicians should look for a palpable gap in the tendon and a positive Thompson test, since these are readily apparent in patients with complete rupture. With the patient in a prone position, instruct the patient to flex his knee. When the calf muscles are squeezed against the tibia and fibula, mechanical contraction of the gastrocnemius and soleus muscles occurs. If the Achilles tendon is ruptured, then contraction of the calf muscles will not plantar flex the foot. Incomplete ruptures may present greater diagnostic difficulties. In patients with these injuries, posteriorly located pain, swelling, and ecchymosis may be the only clue.

Like Achilles tendon injuries, damage to the peroneal tendons is easy to overlook. Unfortunately, this can result in tendon instability and chronic subluxation or actual dislocation of the tendons. This injury involves the peroneal tendons where they pass behind and beneath the lateral malleolus. With sudden, forceful dorsiflexion and eversion of the ankle and the simultaneous, forceful contraction of the peroneal muscles, the peroneal retinaculum is torn and the tendons dislocate anteriorly to a position where they overlie the lateral malleolus.[33] Patients with this type of injury usually present with Posterolateral or retromalleolar swelling, ecchymosis, and tenderness. This is in contrast with most lateral ligament injuries in which these signs occur anterior or inferior to the lateral malleolus. In addition, plantar flexion, eversion, and dorsiflexion against resistance increase the patient's pain in this area and may reproduce the injury in those patients in whom dislocation with spontaneous relocation occurs. Therapy for peroneal tendon subluxation or dislocation is controversial. Casting appears to work best in patients who are not

Figure 6. The Salter-Harris Classiffication of Growth-Plate Fractures

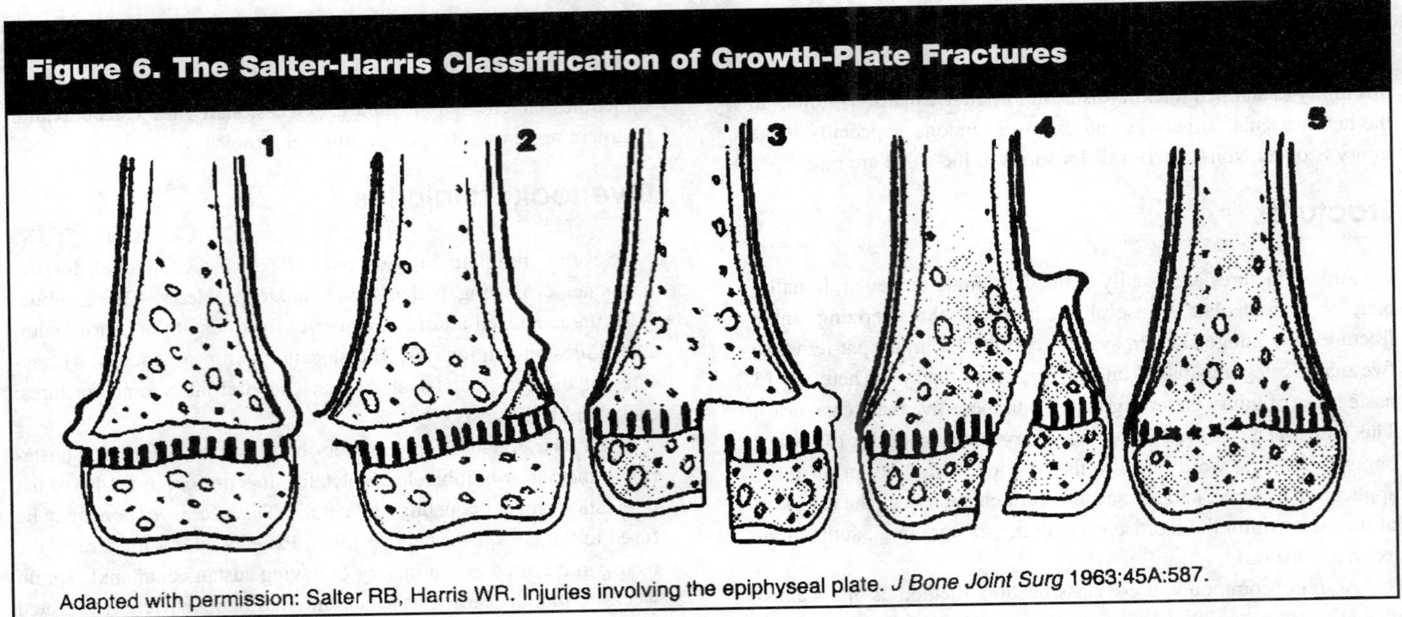

Adapted with permission: Salter RB, Harris WR. Injuries involving the epiphyseal plate. *J Bone Joint Surg* 1963;45A:587.

seriously injured in athletics. But in very athletic patients and those who have associated avulsion fractures, operative repair prevents ankle instability, recurrent dislocation, and chronic pain.[34]

A vulsion of the fifth metatarsal by the peroneus brevis tendon is an injury caused by virtually the same mechanism that causes ankle injuries. In the process of ankle inversion, the tendon, which loops under the lateral malleolus, is stretched and avulses its osseous attachment. These avulsion injuries are typically manifested by discrete tenderness over the fifth metatarsal head in association with local swelling. Often incorrectly called a Jones' fracture, tuberosity fractures heal with minimal, if any, treatment.

Transchondral talar-dome fractures occur with inversion and eversion injuries of the ankle but frequently are not diagnosed when the injury occurs because the radiographs do not show the fracture. The injury causes a compression fracture of the articular surface of the talus and secondary changes in the subchondral bone that may not be radiographically evident for many weeks. Although the acute pain and generalized swelling associated with the injury resolve in 2-3 weeks, the patient experiences persistent stiffness. intermittent joint pain, instability, or catching or locking of the ankle. If the patient returns for evaluation six weeks or more after the initial injury, x-rays may reveal a fracture of the talar dome.[33]

Finally, diastasis of the ankle at the distal tibiofibular joint can occur without fracture.[35] This may result from complete or partial disruption of the ligament complex that forms the tibiofibular syndesmosis. Usually, the interosseous ligament is injured, often in combination with either the ATFL, deltoid ligament, or both.

In an injury at the tibiofibular syndesmosis, an oblique x-ray is most informative; look for widening of the syndesmosis beyond the normal 1-2 mm.

The Child's Ankle

Ankle fractures in children most often involve the physis (growth plate), which can produce a growth plate injury and chronic deformity. Fractures involving the physis are classified using the Salter-Harris system. *(Please see Figure 6.)* Most fractures of the distal fibula are simple Salter-Harris I fractures, whereas most fractures of the distal tibia involving the physis are usually Salter-Harris types II, III, and IV.

Since the ligaments of the ankle are quite strong. the growth plate is the Structure most likely to be disrupted in children younger than 10 years of age. Therefore, a simple Salter-Harris I fracture of the distal fibula is more likely to occur in the child than is disruption of the ATFL. The growth plates of the distal tibia and fibula account for 15-25% of all physeal injuries in the child, second only to distal radius physis injuries.[36]

The distal tibial growth plate fuses first on the medial side, then fuses progressively more laterally. Eversion and lateral rotation can lead to a Salter-Harris type III injury of the lateral tibial epiphysis. This is often called the Tillaux fracture. *(Please see Figure 7.)* Fractures of the lateral plafond (epiphysis) of the tibia can be difficult to see radiographically due to the overlap of the fibula and from an incomplete radiographic study. For these reasons, this fracture is often missed in the ED. A Tillaux fracture usually requires surgery for anatomic reduction.

The triplane fracture is an unusual fracture of the distal tibia occurring prior to the closure of the physis. It is named "triplane" because the fracture lines traverse three discrete planes—coronal, transverse, and sagittal. *(Please see Figure 8.)* The triplane fracture accounts for 5-10% of pediatric intra-articular fractures.[37] The complex patterns of triplane fractures result because the growth plate fuses in a mediolateral direction, leaving the lateral aspect of the tibia vulnerable to injury, especially during adolescence. Evaluation of the triplane fracture requires an oblique radiograph to avoid mistaking it by the overlapping shadow of the fibular. Frequently, CT scan is required to define the fracture lines. Closed reduction is initially attempted and often leads to a good result if anatomic reduction can be obtained and maintained.

Treatment Considerations

The RICE regimen (rest, ice, compression, and elevation) is always indicated with acute ankle trauma. Elevation enhances the

Figure 7. The Tillaux Fracture

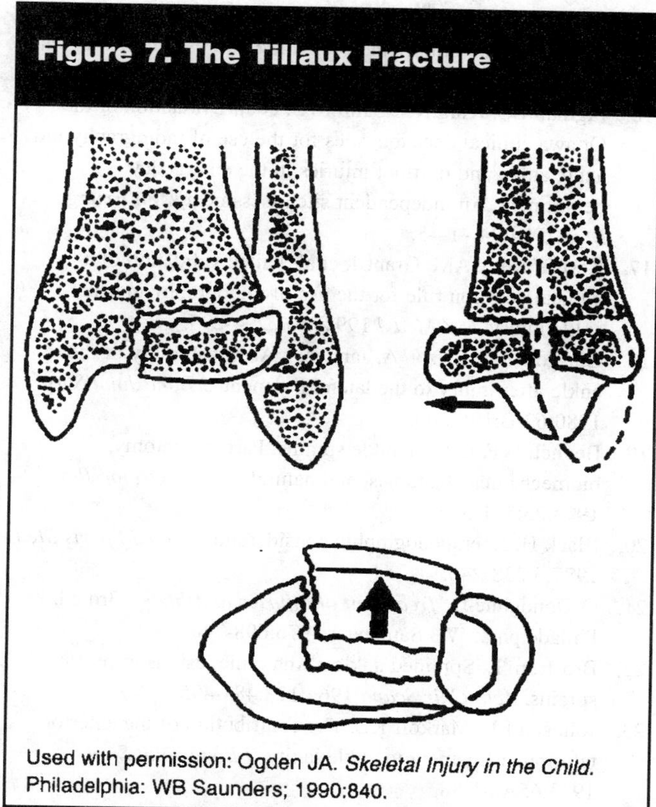

Used with permission: Ogden JA. *Skeletal Injury in the Child.* Philadelphia: WB Saunders; 1990:840.

Figure 8. The Triplane Fracture

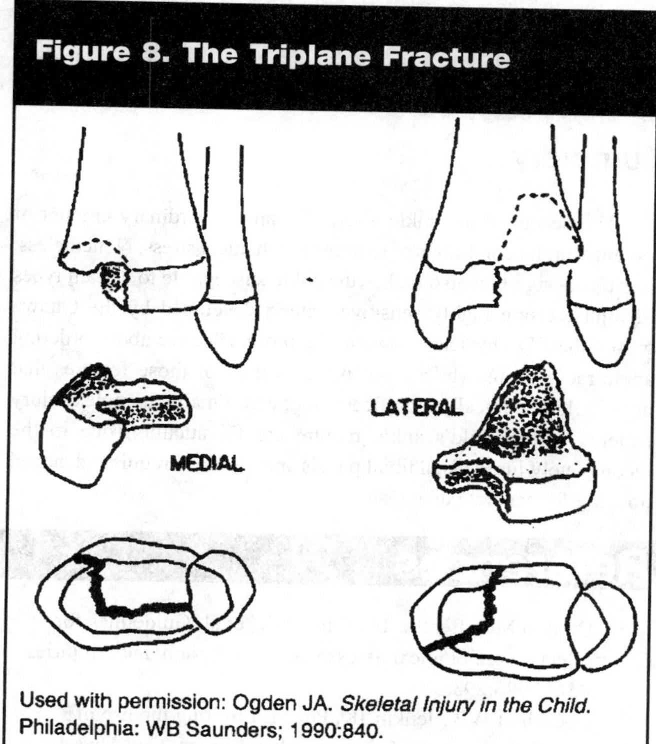

Used with permission: Ogden JA. *Skeletal Injury in the Child.* Philadelphia: WB Saunders; 1990:840.

venous return to reduce swelling. Cryotherapy is recommended for up to 20 minutes three times daily followed by compressive dressings. Although cold therapy causes initial vasoconstriction, discontinuation of cold therapy causes vasodilation and leakage of capillaries due to cold-induced vascular damage. It is for this reason that compression and elevation are advised after cold therapy—to minimize cold-induced reflex swelling.[38,39] Beyond these measures, the specific treatment depends on the injury. Some form of immobilization is typically used; for severe injuries, surgery may be indicated.

Grade I and II ligamentous injuries initially require non-weight-bearing, with a gradual progression of increased weight-bearing over a two- to four-day period. Functional support such as a gel splint, air splint, or a Swedo boot limits eversion-inversion and provides early mobilization. For rehabilitation, some clinicians recommend early active and gentle passive range of motion in plantar flexion and dorsiflexion; eversion and inversion should be avoided.

For more severe injuries, immobilization with a plaster posterior ankle splint or a Sugar-tong splint, which limits all motion and weight-bearing, and orthopedic evaluation may be necessary.

Most fractures require cylindrical casting. However, there is a growing tendency to avoid casting and to use less restrictive orthotic devices that provide protective support and allow early mobility and enhanced rehabilitation. A nondisplaced malleolus fracture usually requires a short leg cast with the ankle in a neutral position, whereas a nondisplaced bimalleolar fracture is often treated with a long leg cast with the knee in 30° flexion. As a rule, casting should be performed within two days of the injury or as soon as reduction of tissue swelling permits cast placement to occur with minimal discomfort to the patient and with minimal risk for skin compression injuries. A displaced bimalleolar fracture or a displaced medial malleolus fracture should be splinted. Urgent surgery is usually required for open reduction and fixation of displaced fractures, and immediate orthopedic consultation is usually advisable. A fracture-dislocation should be emergently reduced, especially if there is any sign of tissue ischemia or neurovascular compromise. Once reduced, the ankle is splinted and the patient frequently undergoes surgery. To reduce an ankle dislocation, one maneuvers the foot and ankle in a way that reverses the forces applied during the injury, while applying longitudinal traction. This will result in adequate reduction, decreasing the risk of skin ischemia and restoring the neurovascular integrity.

Most minor injuries do not require orthopedic referral. However, injuries that are complex, fractures that have a significant morbidity, injuries with delayed recovery, presentations with diagnostic uncertainty , and patients in whom the risk of disability must be minimized (e.g., competitive athletes) should be considered for prompt orthopedic referral. For minor injuries, patients should be encouraged to return to the ED or visit an orthopedist should pain persist beyond 3-5 days. Patients should also be encouraged to obtain a final x-ray report by the radiologist within 2-3 days of their ED visit.

Drug therapy is usually confined to acetaminophen or nonsteroidal anti-inflammatory drugs (NSAIDs). NSAIDs provide good analgesia, but their role in attenuating the acute inflammatory response remains uncertain. Acetaminophen with codeine or other codeine congeners can be used should greater analgesia be required.

If there is an open fracture and a high risk of infection, immediate administration of antibiotics should be considered. In all cases, a sterile dressing using sterile saline or an iodine solution should be applied to the disrupted skin site, which should be manipulated as little as possible.[29] A reasonable initial antibiotic regimen in the ED for adults is cefazolin (1-2 g IV). Additional antibiotic coverage for gram-negative and anaerobic organisms may be necessary depending on the environmental exposure and potential contaminants. All open ankle fractures require immediate orthopedic consultation.

Summary

The design of the ankle allows for an extraordinary amount of mobility under conditions of extreme mechanical stress. Nonetheless, it is this design that also makes the ankle susceptible to certain types of injury. Using highly sensitive criteria developed by the Ottawa group, the ED physician now can be more selective about ordering ankle radiographs while being more assured of those features that help exclude clinically significant fractures. Finally, complex injury patterns in the child's ankle require careful attention due to the incompletely fused distal tibial physis and also may require advanced imaging for accurate diagnosis.

References

1. Dunlop MG, Beattie TF, White GK, et al. Guidelines for selective radiological assessment of inversion ankle injuries. *BMJ* 1986;293:603.
2. Cockshott WP , Jenkin JK, Pui M. Limiting the use of routine radiography for acute ankle injuries. *Can Med Assoc J* 1983;15:129-131.
3. Sujitkumar ,. Hadfield JM, Yates DW. Sprain or fracture? An analysis of 2000 ankle injuries. *Arch Emerg Med* 1986;3: 101-106.
4. Garrick JG, Requa RK. The epidemiology of foot and ankle injuries in sports. *Clin Sports Med* 1988;7:29-36.
5. Garrick JG. The frequency of injury, mechanism of injury, and epidemiolo logy of ankle sprain. *Am J Sports Med* 1977; 5:241-242.
6. Vargish T, Clarke WR, Young RA, et al. The ankle injury-indications for the selective use of x-rays. *Injury* 1983;14: 507-512.
7. Dettori JR, Basmania CJ. Early ankle mobilization, Part II: A one-year follow-up of acute, lateral ankle sprains (a randomized clinical trial). *Mil Med* 1994;159:20-24.
8. Sartoris DJ. Diagnosis of ankle injuries: The essentials. *J Foot Ankle Surg* 1994;33:101-107.
9. Backer M, Kofoed H. Passive ankle mobility. Clinical measurement compared with radiography. *J Bone Joint Surg* 1989;71:696-698.
10. Staples OS. Result study of ruptures of lateral ligaments of the ankle. *Clin Orthop* 1972;85:50-58.
11. Mack RP. Ankle injuries in athletics. *Clin Sports Med* 1982; 1:71-84.
12. Brand DA, Frazier WH, Kohlhepp WC, et al. A protocol for selecting patients with injured extremities who need x-rays. *N Engl J Med* 1982;306:333-339.
13. Dunlop MG, Beattie TF, White GK, et al. Guidelines for the selective radiological assessment of inversion ankle injuries. *BMJ* 1986;293:603-605.
14. Stiell IG, McDowell I, Naif RC, et al. Use of radiography in acute ankle injuries; physician's attitudes and practice. *Can Med Assoc J* 1992;147:1671-1678.
15. Stiell IG. McKnight RD, Greenberg GH, et al. Decision rules for use of radiography in acute ankle injures: Refinement and prospective validation. *JAMA* 1993;269:1127-1132.
16. Pigman EC, Klug RK, Sanford S, et al. Evaluation of the Ottawa clinical decision rules for the use of radiography in acute ankle and midfoot injuries in the emergency department: An independent site assessment. *Ann Emerg Med* 1994;24:41-45.
17. Kerf L, Kelly AM, Grant J, et al. Failed validation of a clinical decision rule for the use of radiography in acute ankle injury. *N Z Med J* 1994; 107:294-295.
18. Glasgow M, Jackson A, Jamieson AM. Instability of the ankle after injury to the lateral ligament. *J Bone Joint Surg* 1980;62-B:196-200.
19. Bennett WF. Lateral ankle sprains. Part I: Anatomy, biomechanics, diagnosis, and natural history. *Orthop Rev* 1994;23:381-387.
20. Black H. Roentgenographic considerations. *Am J Sports Med* 1977;5:238-240.
21. O'Donoghue D. *Treatment of Injuries to Athletes.* 3rd ed. Philadelphia: WB Saunders; 1976:698-746.
22. Brostrom L. Sprained ankles: Anatomic lesions in recent sprains. *Acta Chir Scand* 1964;128:483-495.
23. Johnson EE, Markolf KL. The contribution of the anterior talofibular ligament to ankle laxity. *J Bone Joint Surg* 1983;65A:81-88.
24. Renstrom PAFH, Kannus P. lnjuries of the foot and ankle. ln: DeLee JC, Drez D Jr., eds. *Orthopaedic Sports Medicine. Principles and Practice.* Vo1 2. Philadelphia: WB Saunders: 1994: 1731.
25. Harrington KD. Degenerative arthritis of the ankle secondary to long-standing lateral ligament instability *J Bone Joint Surg* 1979;61A:354-361.
26. Moehring HD. Tan RT, Marder RA. et al. Ankle dislocation. *J Orthop Trauma* 1994;8:167-172.
27. Lauge-Hansen N. Fractures of the ankle. II Combined experimental-surgical and experimental-roentgenologic investigation. *Arch Surg* 1950;60:957.
28. Weber BG. *Die Verletzungen des Oberen Sprunggeleukes* Bern; Hans Huber: 1966.
29. Chandler RW. Management of complex ankle fractures in athletes. *Clin Sports Med* 1988;7:127-141.
30. Davis AW, Alexander IJ. Problematic fractures and dislocations in the foot and ankle of athletes. *Clin Sports Med* 1990;9: 163-181.
31. Paulos LE, Johnson CL, Noyes FR. Posterior compartment fractures of the ankle. *Am J Sports Med* 1983;11:439-443.
32. Abraham E. Neglected rupture of the peroneal tendons and recurrent ankle sprains. *J Bone Joint Surg* 1979;6IA: 1247-1251.
33. Keene IS, Lange RH. Diagnostic dilemmas in foot and ankle injuries. *JAMA* 1986;256:247-251.
34. McLennan JG. Treatment of acute and chronic luxations of the peroneal tendons. *Am J Sports Med* 1980;8:432-436.
35. Edwards GS Jr., DeLee JC. Ankle diastasis without fracture. *Foot Ankle* 1984;4:305-312.
36. Sloan EP, Rittenbeny TJ. Ankle and foot injuries. In: Reisdorff EJ, Roberts MR, Wiegenstein JG, eds. *Pediatric*

Emergency Medicine. Philadelphia: WE Saunders; 1993:978.

37. Whipple TL, Martin DR, McIntyre LF, et al. Anhroscopic treatment of triplane fractures of the ankle. *J Arthroscopic Rel Surg* 1993;9:456-463.
38. Hocun lE, Jaffe R, Rylander CR. Cryotherapy in ankle sprains. *Am J Sports Med* 1982;10:316-319.
39. Fany PJ, Prentice NG, Hunter AC, et al. Ice treatment of injured ligaments: An experimental model. *N Z Med J* 1980; 91:12-17.

The Limping Child

Kelley A. Hails, MD
Earl J. Reisdorff, MD, FACEP

The child who limps, refuses to walk, or complains of limb pain presents a diagnostic challenge. Very young children may not be able to communicate their problem. Children who can talk often cannot localize the exact site of pain, and referred pain is common. Although the differential diagnosis is diverse, certain causes of limping must be excluded during the initial emergency department evaluation.

The following chapter provides a systematic approach to the child who presents with limping. The review begins by discussing the mechanics of normal and abnormal gait patterns. Next, the authors present an approach to the clinical evaluation of the child with limb pain, with emphasis on the history and physical examination along with guidelines for the use of simple diagnostic aids in the emergency department (ED). Specific age-related conditions that cause limping in children are discussed, and the emergency evaluation and treatment of each is reviewed.

Developmental Milestones and Abnormal Gait Patterns

Walking is a complex skill requiring integrity of the lumbar spine, pelvis, and the entire lower extremity, as well as balance, coordination, and strength. Children typically "cruise" or walk holding onto objects at 10 months of age and walk independently by 12 to 18 months of age. A mature walking pattern evolves by age 3 years.[2]

Although achieving these developmental milestones of gait varies somewhat among children, sudden deterioration in walking abilities may indicate neuromuscular disease or a central nervous system (CNS) disorder.

Any alteration of a normal gait pattern is a limp. Gait may be affected by numerous conditions, including limb pain, bone or joint trauma, infection, inflammation, congenital deformity, and neoplasm. *(Please see Table 1.)*

A limp may take one of several forms. An antalgic limp, caused by pain, is characterized by shortened weight-bearing time on the painful limb. A stiff-legged gait is used to reduce motion in a painful knee. A child may walk on the heel if the ball of the foot has a puncture wound.

A child with vertebral osteomyelitis or disc space infection (discitis) walks slowly to avoid jarring the spine. A side-lurching or Trendelenburg limp may be caused by congenital dislocation of the hip (CDH), Legg-Calvé-Perthes disease (LCP), or a slipped capital femoral epiphysis (SCFE). Muscular dystrophy results in hip girdle weakness and a lordotic gait.

Clinical Evaluation

Physicians must develop a systematic approach to the evaluation of the limping child. In most cases, the diagnosis can be established

Table 1. Differential Diagnosis of Limb Pain in Children

Organic Conditions

Traumatic
- Stress fracture
- Myohematoma
- Myositis ossificans

Orthopedic
- Chondromalacia patellae
- Osteochondritis dissecans
- Osgood-Schlatter disease
- Slipped captial femoral epiphysis
- Legg-Calve-Perthes disease
- Hypermobility syndromes

Collagen-Vascular
- Juvenile rheumatoid arthritis
- Systemic lupus erythematosus
- Dermatomyositis
- Mixed connective tissues disease
- Henoch-Schonlein purpura
- Familial Mediterranean fever
- Palindromic rheymatism
- Rheymatic fever
- Inflammatory bowel disease

Infectious
- Bacterial
  - Osteomyelitis
  - Discitis
- Septic
  - Septic arthritis
- Pyogenic
- Pyogenic myositis
- Viral
  - "Toxic" synovitis
  - "Transient" synovitis
  - Rubella vaccination
  - Viral myositis

Endocrine
- Hypercortisolism
- Hyperparathryoidism
- Hypothyroidism
- Osteoporosis
- Myopathies

Neoplastic
- Leukemia
- Lymphoma
- Neuroblastoma
- Histiocytosis X
- Bony tumors
  - Osteogenic sarcoma
  - Ewing's sarcoma
  - Chrondrosarcoma
- Soft tissue tumors
  - Rhabdomyosarcoma
  - Fibrosarcoma
  - Synovial cell sarcoma

Hematologic
- Sick cell anemia
- Hemophilia

Nutritional
- Scurvy (vitamin C)
- Rickets (vitamin D)
- Hypervitaminosis A
- Hypercholesterolemia

Miscellaneous
- Storage diseases
  - Mucopolysaccharidoses
  - Mucolipidoses
- Recurrent arthralgias/myalgias associated with strep and other infections

Syndromes of Unknown Origin
- Fibromyalgia
- Growing pains

Psychosomatic
- Hysteria/conversion reactions
- Reflex neurovascular dystrophy
- School phobia

Used with permission. Bowyer SL, Hollister JR. Limb pain in childhood. *Pediatr Clin North Am* 1984;31:1054.

by a careful, complete history; a detailed physical examination; and proper use of selected laboratory and radiographic studies.

History. In the initial evaluation of the limping child, the physician should determine when and how the limp started, the progression of the symptoms, and whether the limp is painful. Pain tends to be severe with fractures, dislocations, septic arthritis, acute rheumatic fever, and osteomyelitis. Conversely, patients with juvenile rheumatoid arthritis (JRA), LCP, SCFE, Osgood-Schlatter disease, and transient synovitis may have minimal to moderate pain. Pain that is worse in the morning suggests JRA, whereas pain that worsens throughout the day is consistent with muscle fatigue. Stress fractures also may cause painful limping that worsens with activity.

Clinicians must ascertain whether extremity pain is originating from the painful site or is referred from another site. For example, children with hip pathology commonly have pain referred to the knee and may present with a chief complaint of knee discomfort. Likewise, pain secondary to pelvic osteomyelitis, lumbar discitis, and spinal cord lesions also may be referred to the lower extremity.

Constitutional symptoms may provide additional clues to the underlying process. Fever and chills frequently suggest joint infection or osteomyelitis.[3] A low-grade fever may occur with more indolent infections. Malaise, weight loss, and mild fever may accompany rheumatoid disease or occult malignancies.

Physical Examination. After performing a general examination, the physician should evaluate the child's gait with the patient wearing little clothing. First, examine the child's stance and note the presence of pelvic tilting or scoliosis and any compensatory postures, such as knee flexion. Observe the child walking, running, and squatting while barefoot, and ask the parent to indicate what concerns them about the child's gait. Children age 3 years or older should be able to stand on one leg; older children should be able to perform heel and toe walking.

Carefully inspect the extremities for erythema, rashes, ecchymosis, puncture wounds, and deformities. Palpate all bones and joints for warmth, effusion, masses, irregular contour, and tenderness. Evaluate passive and active range of motion of the feet, ankles, knees, hips, and back, noting any limitation or pain. Assess strength in all muscle groups and measure the circumference of each thigh (two inches above the patella) and each calf (at the fullest point) to determine unilateral muscle atrophy.

Carefully evaluate neurologic function in both extremities, noting any weakness, sensory deficits, or reflex abnormalities. Finally, assess circulation, checking peripheral pulses, temperature, color, and capillary refill.

Radiologic Studies. The need for radiographic evaluation is determined by the physical examination. Areas of suspected pathology should be evaluated by radiographic views from perpendicular planes. Comparison views of the uninvolved side occasionally are necessary. For small children in whom a specific site cannot be localized, screening views of both lower extremities should be obtained, including the pelvis and both complete lower extremities on a single film. These views are taken in the anteroposterior and frog-leg position with the patient supine. For older children with suspected SCFE, anteroposterior and frog-leg lateral views of the hips and pelvis are required.

Persistent knee pain is evaluated radiographically by anteroposterior, lateral, and notch views of the knees and anteroposterior and lateral views of the hips. Follow-up radiographic studies may be necessary because nondisplaced and stress fractures may become apparent when periosteal reactions occur after two weeks.

Bone scans are helpful in detecting stress fractures, osteomyelitis, and metastatic or infiltrative bone disease even when initial radiographs are interpreted as normal. Other imaging studies

Table 2. Synovial Fluid Analysis in Children

	Normal	Traumatic (Hemorrhagic) Arthritis	Acute Rheumatic Fever	Juvenile Rheumatoid Arthritis	Septic Arthritis
Appearance	Clear, yellow to colorless	Bloody, xanthochromic, or straw-colored	Cloudy yellow	Cloudy yellow	Cloudy yellow to purulent
Mucin clot	Good	Variable	Variable	Fair to poor	Poor
WBC*	< 200	< 5,000	5,000 to 50,000	5,000 to 80,000	50,000 to 200,000
PMNs**	< 25%	<25%	50%	50% to 75%	75% to 100%
Comments	No fibrin clot	High number of RBCs	Large fibrin clot	Large fibrin clot	Bacterial culture positive

*White blood cell counts can vary greatly
**Polymorphonucleocytes can vary somewhat
RBCs = red blood cells

Used with permission: Reisdorff W, Roberts MR, Wiegenstein JG. *Pediatric Emergency Medicine*. Philadelphia; WB Saunders; 1992:997.

such as computed tomography, magnetic resonance imaging, myelography, and arthrography may be diagnostic and usually are ordered in consultation with the orthopedic specialist.

Laboratory Evaluation. A complete blood count (CBC) and erythrocyte sedimentation rate (ESR) should be obtained on any limping child in whom an obvious cause has not been identified. An elevated serum white blood cell (WBC) count usually indicates an infection or inflammatory process. Nevertheless, in newborns with joint and bone infections, the WBC count may be normal.

An elevated ESR suggests septic arthritis, osteomyelitis, rheumatoid arthritis, collagen vascular disease, or an occult malignancy. The ESR is normal in trauma, LCP, SCFE, and osteochondritis dissecans.

Blood cultures should be obtained when infection is considered. Additional studies such as rheumatoid factor, antinuclear antibodies, serum immunoglobulins, and creative phosphokinase may be indicated if symptoms have persisted for longer than two weeks and the diagnosis is uncertain.

If septic arthritis is suspected, arthrocentesis is essential. *(Please see Table 2.)* Arthrocentesis of the knee or ankle is relatively easy to perform. Arthrocentesis of an infected hip is more difficult and should be performed by the orthopedic consultant.

Joint fluid should be cultured, Gram-stained, and analyzed for appearance, crystals, cell count, protein level, and glucose level.

Urgent and Age-Specific Conditions

Certain disease processes must be excluded during the initial evaluation of the limping child. Fractures, child abuse-related injuries, septic arthritis, osteomyelitis, congenital dislocation of the hip, SCFE, and neoplasm (e.g., osteosarcoma, leukemia, spinal cord tumor) require urgent orthopedic consultation. Other conditions that alter gait and require immediate recognition and therapy include paraspinal abscess, Guillain-Barre syndrome, tick paralysis, CNS infection, and appendicitis.[5]

Particular conditions tend to be more prominent at different ages. From birth until age 2 years, septic arthritis, osteomyelitis, and congenital dislocation of the hip are the most serious conditions. From age 2 to 10 years, osteomyelitis and septic arthritis still are common, but LCP, toxic synovitis of the hip, and juvenile rheumatoid arthritis also occur. In children age 10 to 18 years, fractures are more common along with toxic synovitis, SCFE, and tumors.

Trauma

Given the active nature of children, injuries are a common cause of limping. Children younger than age 5 years are susceptible to the toddler's fracture, a non-displaced oblique fracture of the distal tibial shaft. Tibial-fibular fractures cause 10% of all limping in this age group. Child abuse should be considered in any child with a femur or tibia fracture, when the history is inconsistent with the injury, or when there are injuries in various stages of healing. Young children also may limp due to pain from puncture wounds, splinters or foreign bodies, insect bites, or any irritation of the feet such as from poorly fitting shoes.

Older children and adolescents are susceptible to sports-related injuries, including contusions, sprains, fractures, and overuse injuries. Even though non-displaced epiphyseal plate fractures may not be apparent on radiographs, epiphyseal plate injury should be suspected if there is local trauma and tenderness circumferentially around the physis. Stress fractures most commonly involve the fibula and tibia, but also may occur in the metatarsals, femur, and pelvis.

Table 3. Septic Arthritis: Etiologic Approach to Therapy

Age Group	Common Pathogens	Uncommon Pathogens	Rare Pathogens	Parenteral Antibiotic Considerations
Neonate to 6 weeks	*S. aureus* Group B streptococci	*Enteric bacilli* *Candida* *N. gonorrhoeae*	*H. influenzae*	Nafcillin or oxacillin + aminoglycoside Ceftriaxone Cefotaxime Cefuroxime
6 weeks to 3 years	*S. aureus* *H. influenzae* Group B streptococci Group A streptococci	Gram-negative bacilli		Cefuroxime Ceftriaxone Cefotaxime
> 3 years	*S. aureus* Hemolytic streptococci	Gram-negative bacilli *N. gonorrhoeae*	*S. pneumoniae* *H. influenzae*	Nafcillin Oxacillin Cefazolin

Used with permission: Tachdjian MO. *Pediatric Orthopedics.* 2nd ed. Philadelphia: WB Saunders; 1990:1417.

Septic Arthritis

More than 90% of cases of septic arthritis affect the joints of the lower extremity, with the knee most commonly involved.[8,9] The most common pathogens include *Staphylococcus aureus, Streptococcus pneumoniae, Hemophilus influenzae* (in children younger than 2 years), *Neisseria gonorrhoeae* (especially in adolescents), and *Salmonella* (especially in sickle cell disease). *(Please see Table 3.)*

H. influenzae type b is a leading cause of septic arthritis in infants and children 1 month to 3 years old, yet is rare in children older than 6 years.[10,11] *H. influenzae* arthritis is associated with extra-articular infection, including otitis media (35%), meningitis (30%), osteomyelitis (26%), and overlying cellulitis (22%).[12]

S. pneumoniae infections are more common in children younger than 2 years of age. Group A streptococcus and *S. aureus* infections predominate in children older than 2 years. In children older than 3 years, joint infections usually are caused by the same organisms as those found in adults: *S. aureus* (33%), hemolytic streptococci (18%), *N. gonorrhoeae* (7%), and "unknown" (34%).[13]

Acute joint infection causes synovial edema and increased synovial fluid production. After a few days, pus accumulates and causes destructive changes in the joint space. Fibrin adhesions form within the joint space, producing loculations of pus and limitation of joint motion.

Most children with septic arthritis have fever, joint pain, joint swelling, and limitation of motion. The fever may be as high as 40.0 to 40.5°C (104° to 105°F), although some children are afebrile. The infected joint often will be partially flexed to minimize discomfort. The hip may be in 30" to 60" of flexion and 15" abduction as well as external rotation. In fact, early on, the only physical finding of septic arthritis of the hip may be slight limitation of internal rotation with the hip in flexion. At times, the hip joint capsule may be so distended that the femoral head is pushed laterally and may even dislocate.[14]

In the neonate, the clinical manifestations of septic joint may be vague. The peripheral white blood cell count and differential may be normal. However, the hip joint usually is tender, a finding that may be noticed first during diaper changes.

Radiographic findings in patients with septic hip include increased joint opacity due to increased synovial fluid, distortion of periarticular fat and muscle shadows, and lateral displacement of the femoral head. The white blood cell count and ESR are elevated in the majority of cases. Blood cultures should be obtained if joint infection is suspected.

Any joint suspected of being infected should be aspirated. The gross appearance of the joint fluid is an unreliable indicator of infection. Turbid fluid may be seen in inflammatory arthritis; clear-appearing fluid may have a high bacteria count. It can be difficult to distinguish an infectious process from a noninfectious, inflammatory process by the synovial fluid cell count alone.

The diagnosis of septic arthritis is confirmed by the recovery of organisms from the joint fluid. Joint cultures are positive in 80% of patients, although antibiotic use may decrease the yield to 38%.[15] The Gram stain suggests a causative organism in one-third of cases. Latex agglutination techniques can rapidly detect antigens for *H. influenzae, N. meningitides, S. pneumoniae,* and Group B streptococcus.[16]

The management of suppurative joint infections includes surgical drainage of the purulent material from the joint as well as antibiotic therapy. Antibiotic therapy is determined, in part, by the age of the patient and the likely causative organism. *(Please see Tables 3 and 4.)*

Juvenile Rheumatoid Arthritis

Juvenile rheumatoid arthritis is the most common chronic pediatric rheumatologic disease. JRA is a chronic nonsuppurative synovitis that occurs in children younger than 16 years of age. The arthritis is frequently symmetric and predominantly affects larger joints (knees, wrists, and ankles). By definition, JRA persists longer than six weeks.

There are three JRA subgroups: pauciarticular, polyarticular, and systemic. Pauciarticular JRA, the most common type, involves four or fewer joints. It begins in a single joint, usually the knee, elbow, or ankle. These children may develop ankylosing spondylitis, Reiter's syndrome, or inflammatory bowel disease.

Polyarticular JRA affects five or more joints, occurs primarily in females, and affects large and small joints. Rheumatoid factor-positive patients may have long-term morbidity due to joint destruction, primarily in the hips.

Systemic JRA is the least common type, occurs in 20% of patients, and is associated with a fever and rash. The fever approaches 39.4°C (103°F), is intermittent, and may be accompanied by shaking chills. The rash is a coalescent, pale, erythematous macular eruption that occurs primarily in a central distribution but may include the palms and soles. Pleuritis, pericarditis, and hepatosplenomegaly occur frequently. Joint inflammation may progress to joint destruction and long-term disability in 25% of patients.

JRA is associated with elevated serologic acute phase reactants such as ESR and C-reactive protein. Synovial fluid contains 5,000 to 80,000 WBCs/mm3, predominantly polymorphoneucleocytes without bacteria. Early radiographs show soft tissue swelling, but later in the disease, joint destruction may be seen. Antinuclear antibody and rheumatoid factor testing assists in defining the type of JRA and prognosis.

Treatment attempts to control extra-articular manifestations and maintain joint function. Drug therapy begins with nonsteroidal anti-inflammatory drugs (NSAIDs). Aspirin is the drug of choice in doses sufficient to maintain therapeutic serum levels of 20 to 30 mg-percent. Corticosteroids are indicated for severe systemic JRA unresponsive to aspirin, decompensated pericarditis, myocarditis, and iridocyclitis unresponsive to other ophthalmologic drugs. Intra-articular steroid injections are not indicated in the ED.

Table 4. Intravenous Antibiotic Doses for Bone and Joint Infections in Infants Beyond the Newborn Period*

	Dose (mg/kg/day)	Maximum (gm/day)	Dosing Interval
Ampicillin	150-200	6-12	q 6
Nafcillin	150-200	4-12	q 6
Oxacillin	150	4-12	q 6
Gentamicin	6.0-7.5	**	q 8
Ceftriaxone	50-75	4	q 12-24
Cefuroxime	75-150	4*6	q 8
Cefotaxime	100-150	8-10	q 8
Cefazolin	75-100	4-6	q 8
Vancomycin	40	2-4	q 6
Clindamycin	25-30	1.2-2.7	q 8

*Orthopedic or infectious disease specialist should be consulted for antibiotic dosing

**No maximum dose given; serum levels should be monitored

Used with permission: Reisdorff EJ, Roberts MR, Wiegenstein JG. *Pediatric Emergency Medicine*. Philadelphia: WB Saunders; 1992:1003.

Osteomyelitis

Osteomyelitis is a pyogenic infection of bone caused by hematogenous spread, direct extension from an adjacent infection (e.g., septic arthritis), or by inoculation from a puncture wound or open fracture. Osteomyelitis most commonly occurs in the metaphysic of the distal femur and proximal tibia. The infected bone becomes inflamed and may form an abscess. Elevation of the periosteum denudes cortical bone of its blood supply causing bony destruction.

Osteomyelitis most commonly is caused by *S. aureus*, although *S. pneumoniae*, *Salmonella*, and other pyogenic organisms may be involved. Puncture wounds of the foot are susceptible to *Pseudomonas aeruginosa* osteomyelitis. Sickle cell patients are at increased risk for *Salmonella* osteomyelitis,[19,20] which frequently involves multiple sites and creates punched out, destructive lesions of the metaphysic and diaphysis. *H. influenzae* osteomyelitis may occur in infants and children, but is uncommon. Children with *H. influenzae* osteomyelitis have fevers, and most demonstrate localized swelling and concomitant joint infection.[21]

The vast majority of patients with osteomyelitis will have a single bone infected. Pain may be severe, constant, and aggravated by motion. High fever, chills, and vomiting may occur in older infants and young children. Localized swelling and warmth may be discernible, but extreme erythema is unlikely until late in the infection. The adjacent joint may be held in partial flexion due to protective muscle spasm.

In early osteomyelitis, radiographic changes are limited to subtle soft tissue changes.[22] After 10 to 14 days, purulent exudate in the medullary cavity creates a hazy appearance of the metaphysic. Irregular areas then appear, as trabecular necrosis and absorption occurs. Finally, subperiosteal new bone formation occurs as infection spreads through the cortex. Dense areas with a sharp outline represent sequestered dead bone. A bone scan usually will diagnose osteomyelitis in the first 24 to 48 hours. Laboratory testing may show peripheral leukocytosis and an elevated ESR. A bacterial diagnosis can be established by aspiration of the affected bone.[23,24]

Treatment of osteomyelitis includes parenteral bactericidal antibiotics. *(Please see Table 5.)* In neonates, Group B beta hemolytic streptococcus infection is common has an indolent course, and has a predilection for involving the proximal humerus. Gram-negative enteric bacilli also cause osteomyelitis in this age group. Children 2 months to 3 years of age most commonly develop osteomyelitis caused by *Staphylococcus*, although *Streptococcus* and *H. influenzae* also can cause infection in this age group. In children older than 3 years of age, *S. aureus* and *Streptococcus* are the most common causes of osteomyelitis. Older children or adolescents using intravenous drugs may develop osteomyelitis due to *Pseudomonas* or *Serralia marcescens.*

Congenital Dislocation of the Hip

The diagnosis of congenital dislocation of the hip should be made as early as possible. Most affected infants are firstborns and the left hip is involved more commonly than the right. Dislocation is detected by the Ortolani test, which is performed with the infant relaxed and supine.

Table 5. Etiologic Approach to Therapy for Osteomyelitis

Age Group	Common Pathogens	Uncommon Pathogens	Rare Pathogens	Parenteral Antibiotic Considerations
Neonate to 6 weeks	*S. aureus* Group B streptococci Enteric baccili	*H. influenzae*	*Candida*	Nafcillin or oxacillin + aminoglycoside Ceftriaxone Cefuroxime Cefotaxime
6 weeks to 3 years	*S. aureus* Streptococci	*H. influenzae* *Pseudomonas* species	*Candida* *M. tuberculosis*	Ceftriaxone Cefuroxime Cefotaxime Nafcillin + ampicillin
> 3 years	*S. aureus* Streptococci	*Pseudomonas* species	*M. tuberculosis* *Candida*	Nafcillin Oxacillin Cefazolin Clindamycin Vancomycin

Used with permission: Tachdjian MO. *Pediatric Orthopedics*. 2nd ed. Philadelphia: WB Saunders; 1990:1417.

Examine each hip separately. The examiner stabilizes the pelvis with one hand and positions the long finger of the other hand on the posterior hip over the greater trochanter. Place the thumb anteriorly over the lesser trochanter. With the knee and hip flexed 90°, gently abduct the thigh while lifting the femoral head anteriorly. A palpable "clunk" is felt with reduction of the dislocated hip into the acetabulum. *(Please see Figure 1.)*

The Barlow test detects a subluxable or dislocatable hip. With the infant in the same position, gently abduct the thigh and apply pressure with the thumb. The head of the femur will be felt to move partially or completely out of the acetabulum when CDH exists.

The ambulatory child with CDH has a short leg gait with an abductor lurch. If both hips are dislocated, the perineal space is widened and the child will have a waddling, lordotic gait.

Any patient with suspected CDH should be referred to an orthopedic specialist. The use of double or triple diapers to reduce a subluxing femoral head is insufficient.[26]

Legg-Calvé-Perthes Disease

Legg-Calvé-Perthes disease is idiopathic avascular necrosis of the femoral head complicated by a subchondral stress fracture. It primarily occurs in males 4 to 9 years of age. Limping is the predominant symptom. Pain is minimal to absent, may be referred to the thigh or knee, and is worsened by activity. The child will appear nontoxic with an antalgic limp, internal rotation of the hip, and limited hip abduction.

Laboratory tests are nondiagnostic, although radiographic findings are suggestive of the diagnosis. In the initial phase, avascularity creates a smaller, more radiodense, ossific nucleus of the femoral head on radiograph. There is widening of the medial joint space. Epiphyseal stress fracture creates a subchondral radiolucent zone (crescent sign). In the second phase, the fragmentation phase, epiphysis fragments, creating areas of radiodensity and radiolucency. In the reparative or reossification phase, bone density returns to normal but the proximal femur has an abnormal shape. The final, healed phase is seen after the repair process is complete. A bone scan is useful in the early diagnosis of LCP disease. When LCP disease is suspected, immediate orthopedic referral is necessary.

Slipped Capital Femoral Epiphysis

Any adolescent who limps should be evaluated for slipped capital femoral epiphysis. SCFE occurs when the capital femoral epiphysis is displaced posteriorly and inferiorly relative to the femoral neck. The femoral head remains in its normal position relative to the acetabulum. Obese males are at the highest risk for SCFE.[27]

Symptoms include dull, aching pain in the thigh, hip, groin, or knee that is worsened by activity. The patient limps with an antalgic, Trendelenburg gait. The hip may be tender anteriorly, and classically, externally rotates with flexion. Flexion, internal rotation, and abduction may be limited.

Anteroposterior and lateral radiographs of the hip should be obtained. In the anteroposterior view, a line drawn along the superior border of the femoral neck should transect the epiphysis by at least 20%.

If the diagnosis of SCFE is missed, further weight bearing may convert a mild slip to a severe slip and increase the risk of avascular necrosis. Treatment includes immediate hospitalization for bed rest, traction, and surgical fixation of the femoral head onto the neck. The unaffected side also may need to be surgically fixed, because it is prone to slip as well.

Transient Synovitis

Transient or "toxic" synovitis is a common hip disorder occurring in children 18 months to 12 years of age. The cause is unknown,

Figure 1. Examination for Congential Dislocation of the Hip

Examination technique for the Barlow test to screen for congenital dislocation of the hip.

Used with permission: Burnside JW. *Physical Diagnosis: An Introduction to Clinical Medicine.* 16th ed. Baltimore: Williams and Wilkins; 1981: 246.

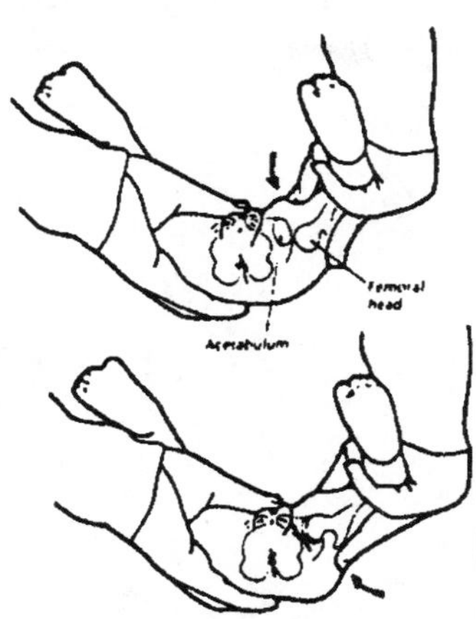

but patients frequently have a history of preceding upper respiratory infection," a recent streptococcal infection, or recent mild trauma. Symptoms (mainly pain) are usually less than two weeks in duration and may involve the hip, thigh, or knee. Pain is variable, ranging from mild discomfort to an inability to bear weight. Temperature may be normal or slightly elevated. Transient synovitis is a diagnosis of exclusion. The WBC count and ESR are normal or slightly elevated. A WBC count of greater than 15,000/mm^3 is unusual. Radiographs are normal or may show a hip joint effusion. Ultrasound of the hip will detect hip joint effusion in up to 95% of cases with synovitis.[29] Treatment is directed toward symptomatic relief (usually with NSAIDs), and surveillance for early LCP disease.

Osgood-Schlatter Disease

Adolescents of both sexes are affected by Osgood-Schlatter disease, osteochondrosis of the anterior tibial tubercle. The disorder is thought to occur from overuse of the quadriceps muscle, resulting in injury to the tibial tuberosity epiphysis. It may occur bilaterally. Patients complain of pain over the tibial tuberosity, which worsens with leg extension against resistance.

The diagnosis is determined by the clinical examination. There is tenderness over the tibial tuberosity which may be enlarged. Radiographs may be normal or may show tuberosity fragmentation or a normal variant. Radiographs are necessary to exclude tumors or stress fractures. Therapy is aimed at the avoidance of pain by restricting activity for about six weeks. Immobilization is unnecessary. Once the apophysis becomes fused, the condition resolves.

Neoplasms and Hematologic Conditions

Children with neoplasms may limp due to local pain from tumors, from the nonspecific pain of leukemia, or from a gradual deterioration of gait because of a CNS tumor. Leukemic bone infiltrates may produce radiographic changes such as osteolytic lesions or periosteal elevation in 40% to 75% of patients. Bone tumors are generally uncommon in children, with osteosarcoma being the most common type.[31]

Osteosarcoma usually affects the distal femur or proximal tibia in adolescents. The most common symptom is knee pain, which is worse at night and unrelated to activity.

Osteosarcoma may be associated with an elevated serum alkaline phosphatase. Radiographs should be taken of all the bones and joints of the affected extremity. A bone tumor destroying or replacing bone creates a radiolucent defect. Occasionally, the tumor may produce an organized, radiodense ossification or a disorganized radiodense calcification pattern.

Some hematologic disorders also may cause limb pain or a limp. Lower extremity hemarthrosis in hemophilia may cause a limp. Patients with sickle cell disease have vaso-occlusive episodes which may cause severe limb or joint pain. Infarction of the humerus, tibia, and femur creates limb pain.[32] Repetitive vaso-occlusive episodes may result in bony sclerosis, periosteal reaction, and infarction.

Ensuring An Organized Approach to Diagnosis

For most conditions that cause a child to limp, a delay in diagnosis does not endanger the child. However, fractures, child-abuse related injuries, septic arthritis, osteomyelitis, CDH, neoplasm, and slipped capital femoral epiphysis require emergent treatment. The emergency physician must exclude these conditions at the time of initial presentation of the limping child, and usually can identify these disorders by a thorough history and physical examination, appropriate radiographs, and when needed, a CBC and ESR.

References

1. Chung SMK. Identifying the cause of acute limp in childhood. *Clin Pediatr* 1974;13:769-772.
2. Sutherland DH, Olshen R, Cooper L, Woo SL. The development of mature gait. *J Bone Joint Surg* 1980;62: 336-353.
3. McCarthy PL, Wasserman D, Spiesel SZ, et al. Evaluation of arthritis and arthralgia in the pediatric patient. *Clin Pediatr* 1980;19:183-190.
4. Money BF, Bianco AJ, Rhodes KH. Septic arthritis in children. *Orthop Clin North Am* 1975;6:923-934.
5. Singer JI. The cause of gait disturbance in 425 pediatric patients. *Pediatr Emerg Care* 1985;1:1-10.
6. Dunbar JS, Owen HF, Nogrady MB, et al. Obscure tibial fracture of infants—The toddler's fracture. *J Can Assoc* Radiol 1964;15:136-144.
7. Roberts MR, Reisdorff EF. Limping arthritis and orthopedic infections. In: Reisdorff EJ, Roberts MR, Wiegenstein JG, eds. *Pediatric Emergency Medicine*. Philadelphia: WB Saunders; 1992:991-1005.
8. Nade S. Choice of antibiotics in management of acute osteomyelitis and acute septic arthritis in children. *Arch Dis Child* 1977;52:679-682.
9. Wiley JJ, Fraser GA. Septic arthritis in childhood. *Can J Surg* 1979;22:326-330.

10. Nelson JD. The bacterial etiology and antibiotic management of septic arthritis in infants and children. *Pediatrics* 1972;50: 437-440.
11. Welkon CJ, Long SS, Fisher MC, et al. Pyogenic arthritis in infants and children: A review of 95 cases. *Pediatr Infect Dis* 1986;5:669-676.
12. Rotbart HA, Glode MP. Haemophilus influenzae type b septic arthritis in children: Report of 22 cases. *Pediatrics* 1985;75:254-259.
13. Tachdjian MO. *Pediatric Orthopedics*. 2nd ed. Philadelphia: WB Saunders; 1990:14 16.
14. Chung SMK, Pollis RE. Diagnostic pitfalls in septic arthritis of the hip in infants and children. *Clin Pediatr* 1975;14: 758-767.
!5. DeLuca PA, Gutman LT, Ruderman RJ. Counterimmuno-electrophoresis of synovial fluid in the diagnosis of septic arthritis. *J Pediatr Orthop* 1985;5:167-170.
16. Speiser JC, Moore TL, Osborn TG, et al. Changing trends in pediatric septic arthritis. *Semin Arthritis Rheum* 1985;15: 132-138.
17. Mosca VS, Sherry DD. Juvenile rheumatoid arthritis and the seronegative spondylo arthropathies. In: Morrisy RT, ed. *Lovell and Winter's Pediatric Orthopaedics*. 3rd ed. Philadelphia: JB Lippincott; 1990:297-324.
18. Miller EH, Semian DW. Gram-negative osteomyelitis following puncture wounds of the foot. *J Bone Joint Surg* 1975;57:535-537.
19. Barrett-Connor E. Bacterial infection in sickle cell anemia. Medicine (Baltimore) 1971;50:97-112.
20. Ortiz-Neu C, Marr JS, Cherubin CE, et al. Bone infections due to Salmonella. *J Infect Dis* 1978; 138:820-828.
21. Lebel MH, Nelson JD. Haemophilus influenzae type b osteomyelitis in infants and children. *Pediatr Infect Dis* 1988;7:250-254.
22. Bonakdar-Pour A, Gaines VD. The radiology of osteomyelitis. *Orthop Clin North Am* 1983;14:21-37.
23. Dich VQ, Nelson JD, Haltalin KC. Osteomyelitis in infants and children. *Am J Dis Child* 1975;129:1273-1278.
24. Winters JL, Cahen 1. Acute hematogenous osteomyelitis. *J Bone Joint Surg* 1960;42:691.
25. Edwards MS, Baker CJ, Wagner ML, et al. An etiologic shift in infantile osteomyelitis: The emergence of the group B streptococcus. *J Pediatr* 1978;93:578583.
28. Chung SMK. Diseases of the developing hip joint. *Pediatr Clin North Am* 1986;33:1457-1473.
27. Bowyer SL, Hollister JR. Limb pain in childhood. *Pediatr Clin North Am* 1984;31:1053-1081.
28. Illingworth CM. 128 limping children with no fracture, sprain, or obvious cause. *Clin Pediatr* 1978;17: 139-142.
29. Marchal GJ, Van Holsbeeck MT, Raes M, et al. Transient synovitis of the hip in children: Role of US radiology 1987; 162:825828.
30. Brower AC. The osteochondroses. *Orthop Clin North Am* 1983;14:99-117.
31. Conrad EU. Pitfalls in diagnosis: Pediatric musculoskeletal tumors. *Pediatr Ann* 1989;18:45-52.
32. Keeley K, Buchanan GR. Acute infarction of long bones in children with sickle cell anemia. *J Pediatr* 1982;101:170-175.

Wrist Injuries

Barbara J. Dwyer, RN, MA

Although wrist trauma is a common complaint, specific lesions often go undiagnosed in the emergency setting. In fact, the wrist's complex anatomy and physiology make it one of the three most common sites at which physicians overlook fracture-dislocations.[1,2]

It is relatively easy to underestimate the seriousness of injuries in patients who have sustained wrist trauma. Common diagnostic pitfalls typically include missed injuries to the carpal bones, which are often difficult to see on routine films and may not be visible for a week or two. Discharging these patients with a diagnosis of sprained wrist without adequate immobilization and follow-up risks serious long-term complications.

Although open reduction and exploration of complicated wrist injuries fall within the purview of orthopedic and hand specialists, emergency physicians can do much to minimize disability by making early, accurate diagnoses; initiating proper treatment; and obtaining specialist referral when appropriate.

After providing a review of the normally functioning wrist, this chapter reviews common mechanisms of injury. It discusses evaluation of the acutely injured wrist, including specific aspects of the history and physical examination, as well as radiographic findings. The author then discusses the emergency management of commonly encountered traumatic wrist lesions, including distal radius and ulnar fractures, carpal bone injuries, penetrating trauma, and sprains.

The Normal Wrist: Anatomic and Functional Considerations

The numerous activities for which the hands are used make the surrounding joints vulnerable to trauma.[4] When a wrist exceeds the normal limits of flexion, extension, or direct force, fracture, dislocation, or ligament rupture can occur, depending on the amount of trauma sustained.

Wrist Anatomy and Normal Movement. The wrist (radiocarpal joint and midcarpal joint) consists of the distal end of the radius and the articular disc, the distal surface of which articulates with the convex, proximal surfaces of the scaphoid, lunate, and triquetrum carpal bones.[5] The palmar surface of the triquetrum and the neck of the capitate contain two arcades of fibers that join the pisotriquetral areas. The scaphoid, the trapezium, the trapezoid, and the carpometacarpal joints also are linked by strong ligaments.[4] The proximal carpal row includes the lunate and the triquetrum, and the distal carpal row consists of the trapezoid, hamate, and capitate. *(Please see Figures 1A and 1B.)*[1,5] The two carpal rows are joined by the scaphoid, which not only provides support for the metacarpal of the thumb, but also, by virtue of its position, is susceptible to numerous injuries.[4]

The distal ulna has several functions, including: 1) it suspends the ligaments that stabilize the wrist's ulnar border; 2) it: contains

Figure 1A. Vertical Section Through the Articulations at the Wrist

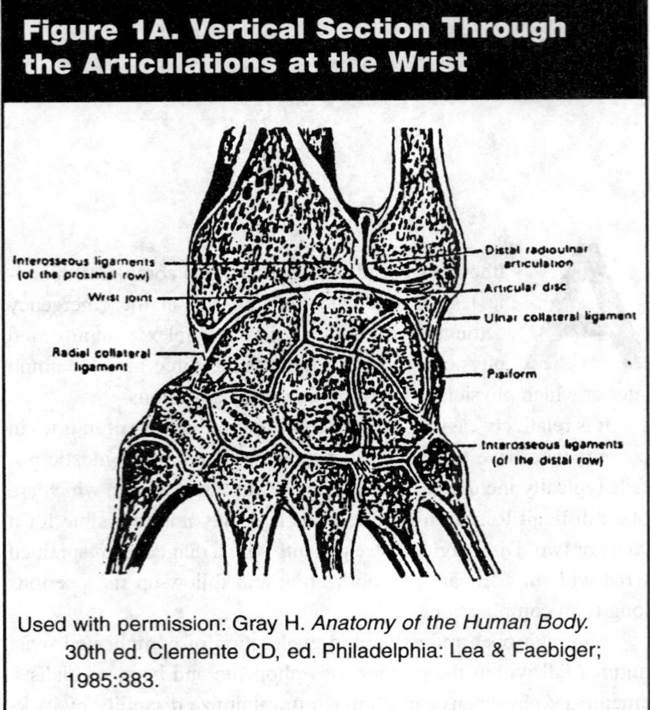

Used with permission: Gray H. *Anatomy of the Human Body.* 30th ed. Clemente CD, ed. Philadelphia: Lea & Faebiger; 1985:383.

Figure 1B. Ligaments of the Left Wrist and Metacarpals (Palmar Aspect)

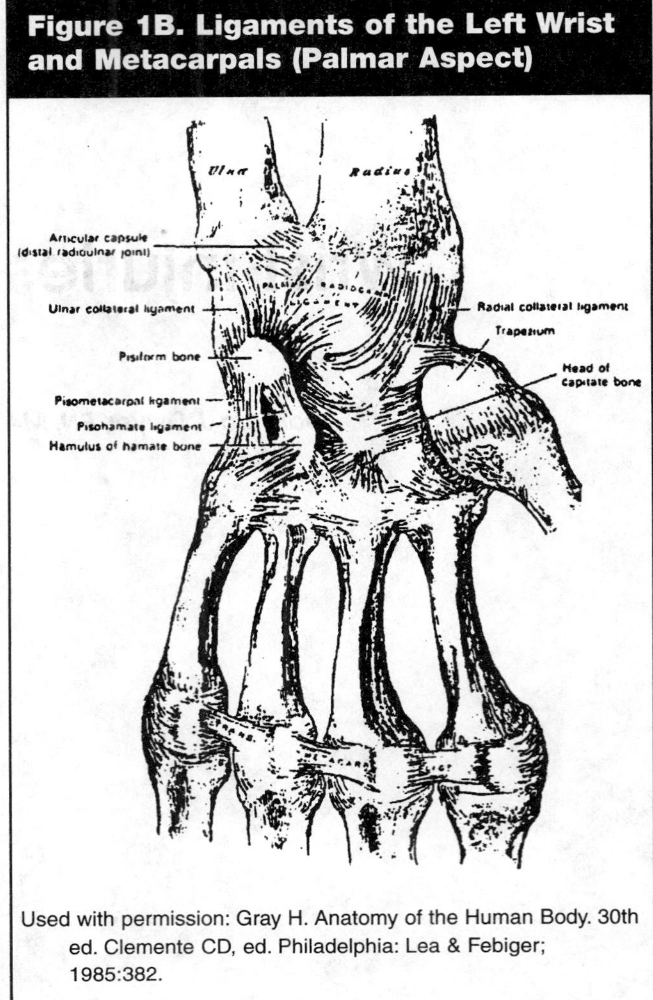

Used with permission: Gray H. Anatomy of the Human Body. 30th ed. Clemente CD, ed. Philadelphia: Lea & Febiger; 1985:382.

the load-bearing triangular fibrocartilage complex on its distal midportion; and 3) it articulates with the radius and facilitates forearm rotation at its proximal portion.[6]

Wrist movements depend on radiocarpal and intercarpal joint integrity. The radiocarpal joint contributes to the hand's mobility by allowing flexion, extension, adduction, and abduction to occur.[7,8] The volar ligaments form a double arcade structure that arches from the distal radius and ulna to the proximal carpal rows and then back again into the ulnar compartment: This structure allows for a wide range of motion in two planes while restricting abnormal motion.[4]

Neurovascular Function. The radial, ulnar, and median nerves supply the wrist and are injured more frequently by carpal dislocation or fracture than with fractures of the radius or ulna. The ulnar nerve, which runs deep to the flexor carpi ulnaris tendon through Guyon's canal, provides motor innervation to 15 of the 20 intrinsic hand muscles, and generally is responsible for fine manipulation. The ulnar nerve supplies sensation to the little finger and the ulnar half of the ring finger,[4] with the purest sensory area over the volar surface of the tip of the little finger. *(Please see Figure 2.)*

The median nerve runs between the flexor carpi radialis and palmaris longus tendons through the carpal tunnel. The media nerve innervates five intrinsic hand muscles, including the two radial lumbricals, the abductor pollicis brevis, the opponens pollicis, and the superficial head of the short thumb flexor. The median nerve permits thumb opposition and pronation. The median nerve provides sensory innervation to the radial half of the palm and the palmar surfaces of the thumb, index finger, middle finger, and radial aspect of the ring finger. Median nerve innervation is purest over the volar tip of the index finger. Because of its location, the median nerve is susceptible to injury by lacerations and penetrating trauma involving the volar surface of the wrist.

The radial nerve supplies motor function to the extrinsic wrist and finger extensors and provides sensation to the dorsal hand over the three and one-half radial digits. The dorsal surface of the web space between the thumb and index finger is supplied almost exclusively by the radial nerve.

Circulation is supplied by the radial and ulnar arteries and the anterior and posterior interosseous arteries. Distally, these arteries join to form the carpal arch, which supplies the scaphoid and lunate bones from their distal ends. By virtue of this unique vascular anatomy, injury to these carpal bones is associated with the danger of avascular necrosis.

An Overview of Common Wrist Injuries

Most wrist injuries result from stress (such as a fall) on an outstretched hand. Failures of bone, ligament, or both account for the most common injuries, including Colles' fractures, scaphoid fractures, and fracture-dislocations of the lunate. Palmar-flexion stress also causes volarly displaced and angulated fractures of the distal radius (Smith fracture) and carpal bone dislocations.

Although no age or socioeconomic group is exempt from sports- or work-related wrist trauma, certain occupations and activities make some individuals more susceptible than others. Children, because of their natural exuberance and fearlessness, commonly fracture their wrists. Athletes may sustain any type of wrist injury,

Figure 2. Sensory Distribution of the Wrist and Hand

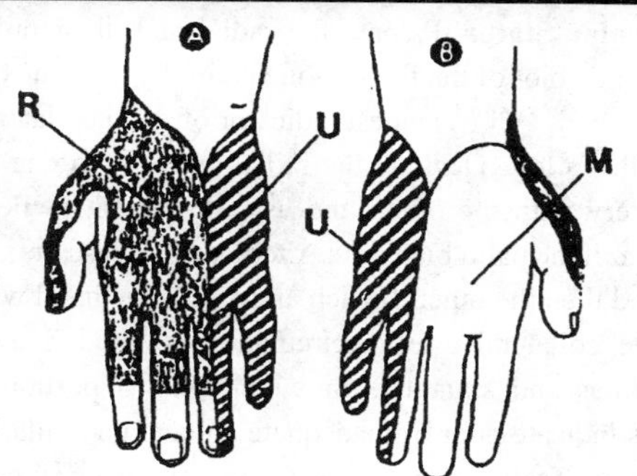

Dorsal (A) and palmar (B) sensation of hand. R = radial nerve; U = ulnar nerve; M = median nerve.

Taken from: Mercier LR. The forearm, wrist and hand. In: Practical Orthopedics, 3rd ed. St. Louis: CV Mosby; 1991:100.

and frequently continue to play despite significant wrist trauma.[9-11] Wrestlers, skiers, and basketball players often fall on their outstretched hand, whereas football players and martial arts enthusiasts commonly sustain injury by striking an opponent with the palm of the dorsiflexed hand.[12]

Open and penetrating wrist injuries commonly occur during accidents, wrist-slashing suicide attempts, and in patients who accidentally or purposefully put their hands through plate glass. Overuse injuries, such as tendinitis and nerve entrapment syndromes, typically develop in people who perform repetitive movements, such as office workers who use computers[10,12] or gymnasts.[13]

Some special considerations apply in children with acute wrist injuries. Children's bones are soft and porous, but their ligaments are stronger than the metaphysic and growth plates to which they are attached. Joint injuries account for 15% of all childhood trauma and usually result in a fracture or separation of the growth plate, rather than a sprain.[14,15] Separations of the distal radial epiphysis occur most often in children between ages 10 and 16 years old, whereas transverse fractures of the distal radius and ulna are more common in children between 4 and 10 years of age.

Clinical Evaluation

The goals of the ED evaluation of the injured wrist are to diagnose fractures and ligamentous injury, detect subtle injuries, identify neurovascular compromise, and prevent long-term disability. Some bony injuries are not immediately apparent on clinical examination or radiography and require careful, timely follow-up for reassessment.

History. Sprains, fractures, and fracture dislocations all produce complaints of pain and tenderness. During evaluation, physicians should ascertain the mechanism of trauma, because it often provides valuable clues to which anatomical structures are injured. *(Please see Table 1.)* For wrist injuries resulting from falls, important questions to ask include:

- Was the wrist flexed or extended?
- Was the arm supinated or pronated?
- Did the point of contact involve the radial or ulnar side of the wrist?
- What was the patient's activity at the time of injury?

Falling on an extended wrist should raise suspicion of a distal radius fracture, scaphoid fracture, or, on occasion, a transscaphoid perilunate dislocation. Falling onto a flexed wrist increases the risk of rupture of the dorsal radiocarpal ligaments, especially if the wrist was pronated at the time of impact. Patients who fail onto their fingers or distal palms are at risk for scaphoid fracture, whereas those who catch themselves with the heel of the hand are susceptible to either a fracture of the distal radius or carpal dislocation near the Innate.

The mechanism of injury with penetrating trauma is also important. Patients who lacerate their hands by placing them through plate glass windows often sustain volar and dorsal trauma from shattered glass. Self-inflicted razor or knife slashes often are attempted with the wrist in hyperextension, and therefore may cause partial or complete arterial lacerations. Associated nerve and tendon injuries are common, with the palmaris longus tendon frequently involved.

Physical examination should be performed with the injured arm entirely exposed. Remove all rings and bracelets before edema compromises circulatory status. Comparison with the uninjured extremity establishes a baseline status of the skin, bony prominences, and neurovascular structures.[16] Also, examine the patient's ipsilateral elbow joint, proximal radius, and entire forearm.

Inspection. Begin the examination away from the point of maximum pain and evaluate the wrist in a systematic manner. Inspect both the dorsal and volar surfaces of the extremity for deformity, lacerations, hematoma, edema, and abnormal posture.

Palpation produces tenderness in most patients with wrist injuries, but localizing the site of maximum pain often points to a specific lesion. First, identify the dorsal pole of the lunate (a key topographic point). As the patient palmar flexes the wrist, the examiner should palpate the point of rounded prominence of the dorsum of the carpus using the volar pad of the thumb or index finger to apply pressure to the area being assessed.

To evaluate the palmar aspect of the wrist, apply pressure over the radial styloid and carpal bones. Tenderness with direct pressure over the radial styloid may signify a distal radius fracture, whereas tenderness elicited with firm pressure applied at the hypothenar eminence suggests fracture of the hook of the hamate. (In some cases, the patient may feel pain dorsally.)[1,17] Look for a fracture of the triquetrum or pisiform if palpation produces tenderness over the prominence of the pisiform.

Evaluate the dorsal wrist by attempting to elicit tenderness over the radial styloid (which suggests contusion or fracture). Then, palpate the anatomical "snuffbox," located just beyond the radial styloid, between the tendons of the extensors pollicis brevis and pollicis longus. The snuffbox contains the scaphoid, the radial artery, the scapho-trapezial joint, and the radial collateral ligament. Local tenderness in this area should raise suspicion of a scaphoid fracture. Tenderness accompanied by a sensation of "clicking" or "giving" on firm palpation suggests scapho-lunate ligamentous injury. The trapezium, which is just distal to the snuffbox, is located by passive flexion of the thumb and may be tender in patients with radial collateral ligament injury or, rarely, trapezium fracture.

Table 1. Wrist Injuries: Cost Considerations and Legal Concerns

- Be judicious when ordering non-standard radiographic views. These are cost-effective only when posterior-anterior, lateral, and oblique views reveal no abnormality.
- Always obtain x-rays of a suspected wrist fracture-dislocation before attempting reduction. Also, obtain postreduction films (including comparison veiws if necessary) to rule out injury secondary to reduction.
- Document neurovascular status of the hand and upper extremity in all patients with wrist trauma before and after therapeutic manipulation.
- Avoid circumferential casts in the immediate post-injury phase due to the likelihood of edema development and circulatory constriction.
- Provide follow-up care within 24 hours in all patients to ascertain that there is no neurovascular compromise.
- If patients complain of severe pain beneath a casted or splinted site, the splint must be removed completely. Adequate capillary refill in the nail beds is *not* a reliable sign of adequate circulation.
- Children with wrist fractures, especially those involving the epiphyses, may have complications of bone foreshortening because of growth arrest. Inform the parents of this possibility, and document this information.

Ligament Assessment. Ligament trauma is caused by forced palmar flexion injuries and may occur with or without associated fractures of the carpometacarpal joints. During examination, support the metacarpals and apply direct pressure to the bases of the metacarpals. The Linschied test helps identify the presence of joint instability due to ligamentous injury. Support the metacarpals over their shafts and press distally over the metacarpal heads in the palmar and dorsal direction. Localized pain to the carpometacarpal joint constitutes a positive test.[18]

Suspect distal dorsal radio-lunar disruption in patients with discrepancies of volar or dorsal motion and a click when pressure is applied just distal to the ulnar styloid during radial deviation of the wrist. This maneuver pushes the triquetrum into the sulcus, and will help reveal ligamentous disruption.

Motor Function. If possible, compare flexion and extension as follows: To judge the range of wrist extension, have the patient place the palms and fingers of the hands together in the vertical plane and lift the elbows as far as possible while keeping the heels of the hands together.[8] It is easy to compare the angle between the hand and forearm on either side.

To evaluate the range of wrist flexion, ask the patient to reverse the maneuver by placing the backs of the hands together with the fingers directed vertically downward, while lowering the elbows as far as possible.[8] Compare the angle between the hand and the forearm on both sides.

To determine the range of motion of the distal radio-ulnar joint, have patients flex their elbows at a right angle in order to eliminate rotation at the shoulder.

Vascular Status. Palpate the radial and ulnar pulses, note the warmth and color of the fingers, and carefully evaluate capillary refill at the nail beds.[8,16,19] The best indicator of good collateral circulation is the Allen's test. Occlude the radial artery with one hand and the ulnar artery with the other, and ask the patient to flex the fingers rapidly until the palm blanches. Alternately release pressure from one artery and then the other. If each artery fills the hand within five seconds, the collateral arterial circulation is good. However, slower filling times and situations in which only a portion of the hand responds indicate poor or inadequate collateral circulation.

Sensory Testing. Careful evaluation of sensory function is essential in all patients with wrist injuries. Sensation should be checked over the volar, dorsal, radial, and ulnar aspects of all digits, as well as over the entire palm and dorsum of the hand. Sensation in the isolated areas supplied by the radial, median, and ulnar nerves also should be assessed.

Light touch and pinprick testing may reveal most sensory deficits, although two-point discrimination is helpful to reveal subtle sensory abnormalities. Sensory deficits may result from direct injury to nerves supplying the hand, or may be secondary to compressive effects or vascular compromise. In addition to an intact afferent pathway, normal sensation in the digits requires adequate circulation to conduct impulses, and interruption of the blood supply quickly results in sensory loss.

Serial Evaluation. Following wrist injuries, check regularly for adequate neurovascular status and document the findings carefully. Only about 3% of patients with Colles' fractures develop median nerve compression. However, patients may develop post-traumatic ischemia from radial or ulnar arterial laceration or compression due to hematoma or edema formation. Rapid wrist swelling or pulsatile hemorrhage suggests arterial injury, particularly in patients who have penetrating wrist injuries or fractures with displaced bony fragments. Diminished arterial pulses or sensory loss requires immediate intervention by a specialist.

Radiographs Pivotal for Diagnosis

Radiographic evaluation of the injured wrist consists of three standard views, in addition to special projections as clinical findings dictate. All patients require: 1) posteroanterior (PA) view in neutral forearm rotation, 2) a lateral view in neutral rotation, and 3) oblique views with 45° each of partial supination and pronation from the position of the PA radiograph.[8,12,19-24]

For patients with suspected carpal fractures, obtain a scaphoid view, which is performed by ulnar deviation of the wrist to elongate the scaphoid, or by angling the radiographic tube < 5° cranially to visualize the long axis of the scaphoid bone. Comparison views of the uninjured wrist usually are unnecessary, but may be helpful if the diagnosis is in doubt.

Stress radiographs are superior to plain views to detect subtle fracture dislocations of the carpal bones.[12,21,35] PA and lateral views with the arm in neutral rotation, supplemented by fist clenching, radial and ulnar deviation, and flexion and extension, reproduce the positions that facilitate normal gliding of the carpal bones over one another. Therefore, fractures, joint widening, scapholunate dissocia-

Figure 3. Fractures of Distal Forearm Bones

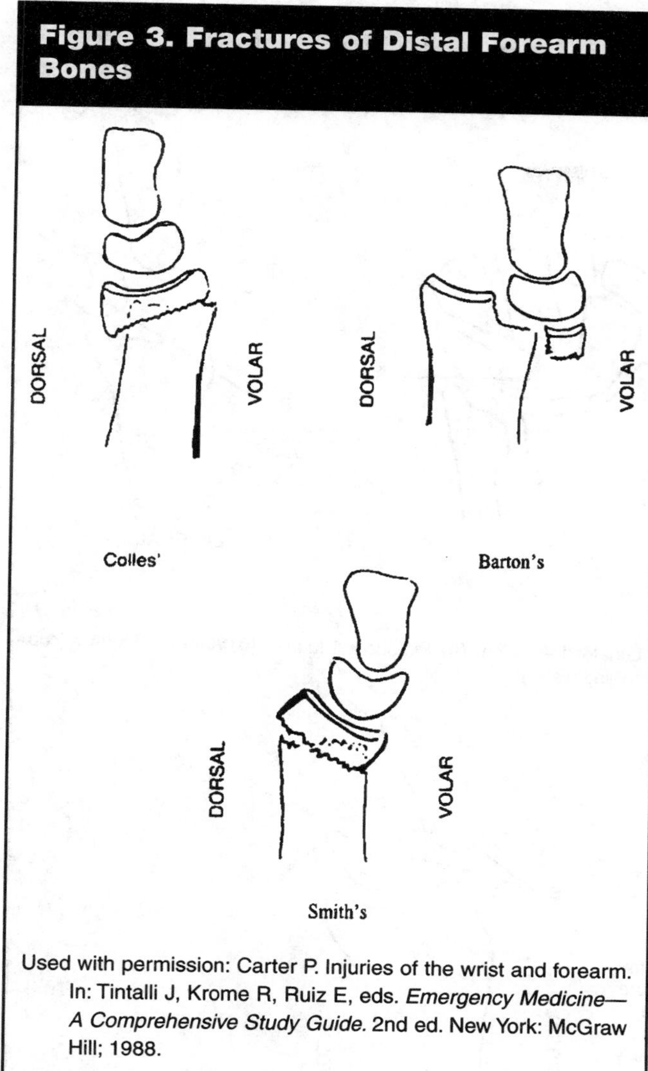

Used with permission: Carter P. Injuries of the wrist and forearm. In: Tintalli J, Krome R, Ruiz E, eds. *Emergency Medicine—A Comprehensive Study Guide.* 2nd ed. New York: McGraw Hill; 1988.

Figure 4. Reduction of Colles' Fracture

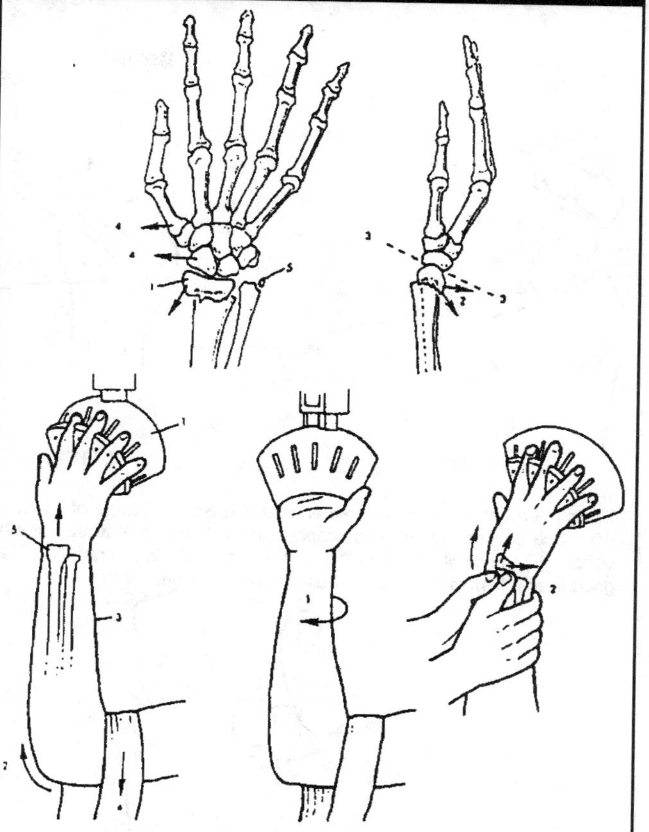

Used with permission: Orban DJ. Forearm and wrist. In: Rosen P, Baker FJ, Barkin RM, et al, eds. Emergency Medicine: Concepts and Clinical Practice. 2nd ed. St. Louis: CV Mosby; 1988:767.

tion, and the relationship of the carpal bones to one another will be detected more easily.

Other radiographic imaging studies, such as bone scans, computed tomography, and magnetic resonance imaging, generally are not helpful for the ED diagnosis of acute wrist injury.[19,21,26,27] However, these diagnostic adjuncts may be necessary on occasion, particularly in the evaluation of chronic wrist pain or significant wrist pain and disability with normal plain films, but generally are arranged in consultation with the orthopedic surgeon.

Distal Radius Fractures

Common fractures of the distal radial metaphysic include Colles' and Smith's fractures, epiphyseal separation (in children), and the intra-articular Barton's fracture. Accurate and early diagnosis helps to prevent development of serious sequelae such as malunion or osteonecrosis, with their problems of chronic pain and disability.[31] Uncomplicated lesions usually can be treated safely in the emergency setting, but comminuted or intra-articular fractures and those occurring in children require specialty consultation.

Colles' fracture is one of the most commonly encountered wrist injuries in the emergency setting. A history of a fall on an outstretched hand with resultant pain, edema, limited range of motion, and the characteristic "dinner fork" deformity of the wrist suggests the diagnosis.[4,7]

On PA films, look for a transverse or comminuted distal radius fracture with extension of the fracture lines into the radial joint.[32] Proximal displacement of the distal radial fragment with deviation of the carpus and hand toward the radius may be evident. The ulnar styloid is fractured through the base in approximately 60% of patients.[33] The lateral view also may reveal dorsal and proximal displacement of the distal radial fragment, as well as dorsal inclination of the articular surface of the radial fragment (normally a palmar inclination of 15°). In all cases, concomitant carpal and elbow fractures should be ruled out.[4] *(Please see Figure 3.)*

Most closed reductions of mild to moderately displaced Colles' fracture can be done in the ED. For minimally displaced fractures, splinting may suffice. Before attempting reduction, inject the hematoma over the fracture site with approximately 5 ml of lidocaine, and apply finger traps to achieve distraction.

After suspending approximately 10 pounds of countertraction from the elbow, apply thumb pressure dorsally to the distal fragment and exert counterforce on the palmar aspect of the distal fragment.[4]

Figure 5. Lunate and Perilunate Dislocations

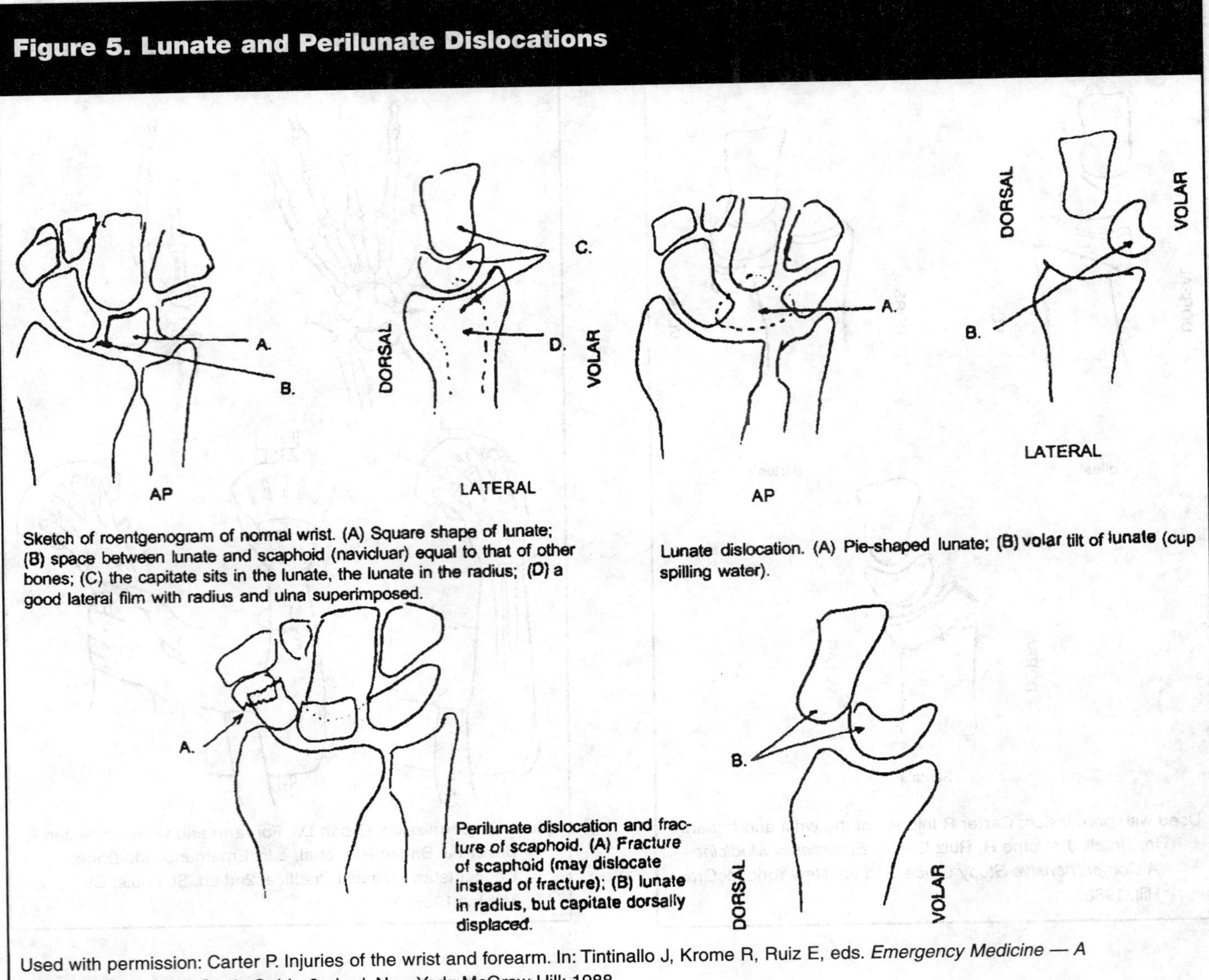

Sketch of roentgenogram of normal wrist. (A) Square shape of lunate; (B) space between lunate and scaphoid (navicluar) equal to that of other bones; (C) the capitate sits in the lunate, the lunate in the radius; (D) a good lateral film with radius and ulna superimposed.

Lunate dislocation. (A) Pie-shaped lunate; (B) volar tilt of lunate (cup spilling water).

Perilunate dislocation and fracture of scaphoid. (A) Fracture of scaphoid (may dislocate instead of fracture); (B) lunate in radius, but capitate dorsally displaced.

Used with permission: Carter P. Injuries of the wrist and forearm. In: Tintinallo J, Krome R, Ruiz E, eds. *Emergency Medicine — A Comprehensive Study Guide.* 2nd ed. New York: McGraw Hill; 1988.

This action reduces the distal fragment volarly and pronates it onto the proximal fragment. *(Please see Figure 4.)*

Splint the arm in 20° of flexion using a sugar-tong splint molded dorsally and volarly over the hand and forearm around the flexed elbow. Complications include: 1) injury to the median nerve, which requires orthopedic intervention, and 2) edema and vascular compromise, which contraindicate the use of a cylindrical cast. Following acceptable reduction, Colles' fractures are inherently unstable and susceptible to malalignment secondary to tearing of the interosseous ligaments. Patients should therefore be followed by an orthopedist until healing has occurred. Likewise, if the reduction is unsatisfactory or fails to hold with splinting, orthopedic consultation is required.

Epiphyseal Fracture-separation. Children and adolescents who fall on an outstretched hand frequently sustain distal radial epiphyseal separation, which is the pediatric equivalent of the Colles' fracture. Diagnosis may be difficult if the injury is nondisplaced. However, clinicians should bear in mind that wrist sprains are uncommon in children because the epiphyseal plate is weaker than are the surrounding ligaments, and therefore should maintain a high suspicion for this injury.

Tenderness over the epiphysis strongly suggests a fracture. Separation usually occurs on the metaphyseal side of the epiphyseal plate with concomitant displacement of the triangular portion of the metaphysis.[1] Radiographically, the PA view may show only mild radial or ulnar epiphyseal displacement, and the shadow of the dorsal metaphyseal fragment may be eclipsed by neighboring bone. A lateral view should clearly reveal the displaced ossification center and dorsal metaphyseal fragment in most cases.

Because of the potential for growth deformities, refer all children with epiphyseal fracture-dislocations to an orthopedist. Fragmentation of the radial epiphysis may result in premature physeal closure with subsequent shortening and deformity of the radius. It is essential to explain the possibility of complications to the parents and to document such explanation in the chart. Urgent referral is mandatory if angulation or displacement exceeds 25°. For patients with stable fractures, apply a short-arm splint, with the forearm supinated and the wrist in slight extension, and arrange for orthopedic follow-up within one to two days.

Smith's Fracture. Smith's fracture (sometimes referred to as a "reverse Colles" fracture) is a metaphyseal fracture with volar displacement of the distal radius, and radial shortening.[3,30] Compared with Colles' fracture, Smith's is about one-tenth as common in emergency practice.[4,7] *(Please see Figure 5.)*

Suspect this lesion in patients who 1) have fallen on the supinated forearm with the hand extended; 2) present with wrist pain and swelling after punching someone; or 3) receive a direct blow to the dorsum of the wrist with the hand flexed and forearm prorated.[1,34] Motorcycle accident victims whose wrists are hyperextended before being thrown over the handlebars are susceptible, particularly if they receive a direct blow to the dorsum of the hand.

Radiographic findings relate to the direction of the fracture line and concomitant articular involvement.[32] Type 1 lesions are transverse fractures, whereas type 2 fractures are oblique. Type 3 Smith's fractures are characterized by an oblique fracture line with articular displacement. On the PA view, look for volar and proximal displacement with the fracture line running transversely or obliquely through the metaphyseal bone about 1 cm to 2 cm proximal to the articular surface. The lateral film may show volar displacement of the distal fragment. Characteristically, the fracture extends over the entire metaphysic with volar displacement and volar angulation of the radial articular surface of the distal fragment.

For types 1 and 2 Smith's fractures, reduce in a fashion similar to Colles', using different forces and methods of immobilization (type 3 requires open reduction and internal fixation). Apply longitudinal distraction while manipulating the distal fragment dorsally against counterpressure on the proximal dorsal forearm. An assistant should steady the arm with the forearm in 90° of supination while holding the patient's hand and placing the wrist in 25° of dorsiflexion and maximum ulnar deviation.

Following reduction, immobilize the arm in a molded sugar-tong splint, with ulnar pressure applied to the hand and dorsal forces to the distal fragment against a counterforce of the middle forearm. Patients with satisfactory reductions may be discharged with appropriate analgesics and arrangements for timely orthopedic follow-up. All patients should be reevaluated within five days to determine whether reduction is still acceptable.

Barton's Fracture. Essentially the reverse of the intra-articular Smith's fracture, Barton's fracture involves an oblique fracture-dislocation through the articular portion of the distal radius. Most commonly, the volar rim of the radius fractures, resulting in an unstable lesion. Patients who fracture the dorsal rim have a wedge-shaped articular fragment separated from the dorsal surface of the radius. For both volar and dorsal rim fractures, lateral radiographs show radiocarpal subluxation or dislocation. The distal radius typically is obscured by the proximal row of carpal bones on the PA view.

Because Barton's fractures involve the intra-articular surface, accurate reduction is essential. Immobilize the extremity in a long-arm bivalved splint, and consult an orthopedist. Open reduction is often necessary.

Carpal Fractures and Dislocations

There are many types of fractures and dislocations of the carpal bones. The physical examination and radiographs—particularly stress views[12,21,22,25]—establish the diagnosis. Because the articulations of the carpal bones are complex and subtle, comparison views may be helpful to identify specific lesions.

Nondisplaced Carpal Bone Fractures. Treatment for nondisplaced carpal fractures is similar to nondisplaced distal radius fractures and is achieved by immobilization, whereas open fractures are a surgical emergency. The high likelihood of complications and disability requires that all patients be seen by a hand specialist or orthopedist. If consultation is not immediately available, immobilize the hand in a bivalved, long-arm splint, provide adequate analgesia, and arrange for early referral.

Scaphoid (navicular) fractures are the most common type of carpal bone injuries and among the easiest to miss.[1,7,16,35-37] Any "wrist sprain" that is severe enough to require radiographic evaluation of the scaphoid should be treated initially as a scaphoid fracture and then re-evaluated at two weeks, even if initial radiographs are negative. This is because: 1) vascular supply is through the bone's distal portion, and missed diagnosis of a midscaphoid fracture can result in avascular necrosis of the proximal fragment; 2) non-union is frequent following scaphoid fracture; and 3) 17% of scaphoid fractures are associated with other fractures of the carpus and forearm.[7,35]

Patients usually relate a history of a fall on the outstretched palm. Impact on the fingers or distal palm suggests a scaphoid fracture, whereas landing on the heel of the hand is more likely to result in a fracture of the distal radius.[4] The only symptom of a scaphoid fracture may be pain and swelling over the snuffbox area, which increase with use of the wrist.

With nondisplaced fragments, wrist radiographs may be negative for up to several weeks after injury until decalcification around the fracture line occurs. Scaphoid fractures that are visible on PA views are frequently transverse or minimally oblique to the long axis of the bone, and the fragments usually are undisplaced. The more proximal the fracture line (if present), the higher the risk of avascular necrosis in the proximal fragment. A vertical fracture suggests delayed healing. Oblique projections are best for detecting fractures of the waist, whereas oblique and lateral films may reveal fractures of the tuberosity. A positive scaphoid "stripe" sign is characteristic of, but not diagnostic for, scaphoid fracture. Estimate the fracture's stability by looking for displacement or shortening of any of the fragments and angulation or shortening of the bone.

Treatment of scaphoid fracture is by casting, initially with a bivalved splint that incorporates the thumb. If the diagnosis is suspected, even if the radiographs do not repeal a fracture, splint the hand and forearm. Advise the patient to follow up with an orthopedist in seven to 10 days, at which time a thumb-spica cast may be sufficient. Orthopedic follow-up is prudent in all cases.

Lunate and perilunate dislocations are uncommon injuries, but commonly missed on initial evaluation.[16] Patients who fall on the heel of the hand are particularly susceptible to these injuries.

Common presentations include acute wrist deformity and limitation of motion. On examination, patients complain of pain when the examiner applies volar pressure proximal to the dorsal pole of the Innate. Wrist flexion is markedly reduced and the patient may report numbness in the median nerve distribution.

The diagnosis of lunate and perilunate dislocations rests on careful interpretation of wrist radiographs, with particular attention to the relationship among the radius, lunate, and capitate as depicted on the true lateral wrist radiograph. Normally, the PA view reveals a square-shaped lunate, with the spacing between the lunate and scaphoid equal to that of the other carpal bones. On the lateral radiograph, the proximal aspect of the "moon-shaped" lunate articulates with the curved portion of the distal radius. Likewise, the dorsal aspect of the lunate articulates with the proximal portion of the capitate. *(Please see Figure 5.)*

With lunate dislocation, the lunate appears triangular shaped on the PA film, whereas on the lateral view the lunate no longer articulates with the capitate, but is tilted volarly. With perilunate dislocation, the radius and lunate maintain their normal relationship, but the capitate and the remainder of the proximal carpal bones have dislocated dorsally around the lunate. Perilunate dislocation may occur with or without an associated scaphoid fracture.

Patients with lunate or perilunate dislocations require orthopedic consultation and frequently must undergo open reduction. Because of the force required to produce these injuries, associated skin and neurovascular trauma is common.[16]

Penetrating Wrist Trauma

Whether emergency physicians attempt repair of penetrating wrist injuries depends on their levels of experience and comfort and the nature of the injury. All open fractures or penetrating wounds with vascular compromise or neurologic deficits constitute an orthopedic emergency and require orthopedic or hand surgery consultation.

All wrist wounds require careful and complete exploration, thorough cleansing, and copious irrigation. For uncomplicated skin lacerations, primary closure by the emergency physician is appropriate. For penetrating injuries involving underlying structures, hand surgery or orthopedic consultation is indicated, along with parenteral administration of broad-spectrum antibiotics (such as a cephalosporin with anti-staphylococcal coverage) and tetanus immunization according to the patient's needs. *(Please see Table 2.)*

There are few instances in which arterial bleeding cannot be controlled with direct pressure. If the radial artery is transected, bleeding is relatively easy to control. In contrast, hemorrhage can be difficult to arrest with a partial arterial wound. In all cases, application of direct pressure should be the initial attempt to arrest bleeding, possibly augmented with brief use of a blood pressure cuff placed on the upper arm and inflated, if necessary. Physicians never should attempt to clamp the artery blindly, because significant injury to nerves and tendons may result.

Any injury that requires open repair or exploration should be cleansed and splinted and referred immediately to a hand surgeon. With the possible exception of palmaris longus repairs (when both ends are visible), tendon, nerve, and vascular repairs fall within the specialist's purview.

Acute Wrist Sprains

Patients who present with swollen, painful wrist joints and limitation of motion following a history of trauma require careful evaluation for the presence of bony injury. Negative radiographic findings do not necessarily rule out a fracture or clinically significant ligamentous injury. Patients who have maximal tenderness and swelling in the anatomic snuffbox (especially when compared with the opposite wrist) are at high risk for a nondisplaced navicular fracture. In all cases, physicians should not diagnose "wrist sprain" without carefully ruling out the possibility of a scaphoid fracture or ligamentous injury.

The majority of "wrist sprains" involving the radial aspect of the carpus should be treated as navicular fractures until proved otherwise by radiographic and physical examination two weeks after the injury.[16,29] After ruling out neurovascular compromise, apply a short-arm thumb-spica splint and arrange for early orthopedic follow-up.[7-30] Other injuries to consider in patients with apparent wrist sprain include nondisplaced epiphyseal fractures of the distal radius in children; fracture of the hook of the hamate after a direct blow to the palm; and avulsion fracture of the triquetrum.[7]

Table 2. Pharmacologic Considerations for Wrist Injuries

Local anesthesia: Inject 1 to 3 ml of 1% xylocaine into the fracture hematoma (aspirating dark bood ensures that the needle is placed correctly).

Pain relief: Adequate pain relief assumes high priority. In the ED, IV or IM narcotics frequently are necessary; clinicians also may administer an anxiolytic such as IV diazepam. For outpatient use, oral analgesics (NSAIDS or oral narcotics as dictated by level of pain and edema). Avoid aspirin-containing compounds to avoid increasing the size of fracture hematomas.

Tetanus booster: Provide as indicated for patients with open fractures, puncture wounds, or lacerations.

Antibiotics: Are essential for patients with open wrist fractures or "dirty" penetrating injuries. Broad-spectrum antibiotics such as IV cephalosporins are the agents of choice.

Neuropathy and Tendinitis

Carpal Tunnel Syndrome. This common condition results from compression of the median nerve between the transverse carpal ligament and the flexor tendons with their enlarged synovium.[7] *(Please see Figure 6.)* Carpal tunnel syndrome develops most commonly in patients who perform repetitive movements, although the disorder also has been associated with hypothyroidism, rheumatoid and gouty arthritis, and, occasionally, pregnancy.

The onset of pain is usually spontaneous, increases at night, is located in the median nerve distribution, and may be accompanied by paresthesias in the thumb, index, and long fingers. Suggestive findings include Tinel's sign, which consists of reproduction of pain and tingling with percussion over the median nerve, and Phalen's test, which involves reproduction of symptoms following one minute of wrist flexion against resistance.[1,7] Plain radiographs are nonspecific, but usually are obtained to rule out bony abnormality. In some cases, high-resolution ultrasonography may be diagnostic.[26]

Treatment consists of eliminating the cause of compression. Temporarily splinting the wrist and prescribing anti-inflammatory medications help to reduce discomfort. Pregnant patients usually

Figure 6. Carpal Tunnel Syndrome

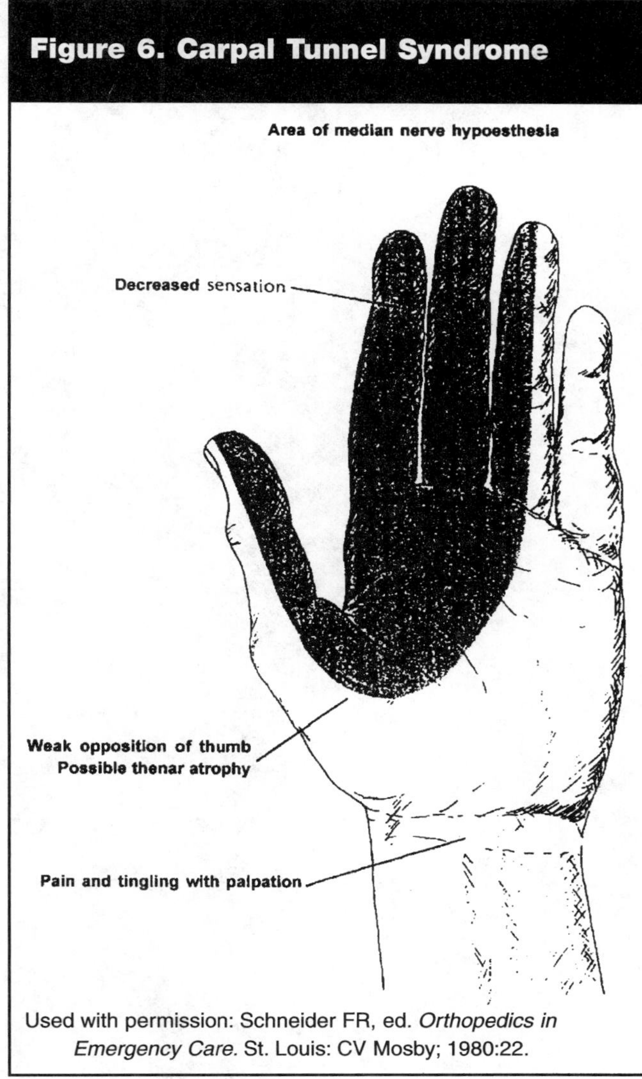

Used with permission: Schneider FR, ed. *Orthopedics in Emergency Care.* St. Louis: CV Mosby; 1980:22.

experience resolution of symptoms with delivery, although some authors suggest diuretics for symptomatic relief. Local injection of steroids or xylocaine can cause extreme pain and further damage the nerve, and arc not recommended. If conservative measures fail and the diagnosis is confirmed, surgical carpal tunnel release may be required.

Ulnar Tunnel Syndrome. This syndrome is much less common than median nerve compression and is caused by ulnar nerve compression by soft-tissue tumors, ganglia, or ulnar artery thrombosis. Signs and symptoms are similar to those of carpal tunnel syndrome but manifest in the ulnar nerve distribution. Treatment is the same as for carpal tunnel syndrome, and surgical release is frequently necessary.

de Quervain's Tenosynovitis. This disorder affects the first extensor compartment involving the abductor pollicis longus and extensor pollicis brevis tendons at the level of the radial styloid.[28] Patients complain of pain in the radial aspect of the wrist, which is aggravated by ulnar deviation of the hand with the thumb flexed (such as turning a doorknob). On physical exam, tenderness is localized to the involved tendons, and examiners occasionally can palpate a thickening or nodule in the sheath.[30] The Finklestein maneuver (passively placing the thumb in the palm, covering it with the fingers, and performing passive ulnar deviation of the wrist) increases pain in the affected area.

Initial management of tenosynovitis includes immobilization with a thumb silica splint and prescribing oral nonsteroidal anti-inflammatory agents. Steroid injections into the tendon sheath may provide symptomatic relief, but increases the risk of tendon rupture. In some cases of de Quervain's tenosynovitis, surgical intervention may be necessary.

References

1. Bukata WR, Orban D, Newmeyer WL, Karkal S. Reducing pain and disability from common wrist injuries. *Emerg Med Reports* 1986;7:138.
2. Freed HA, Shields NN. Most frequently overlooked radiographically apparent fractures in a teaching hospital emergency department. *Ann Emerg Med* 1984;29:153.
3. Cooper MA. Upper-extremity injuries: Shoulder, arm, and wrist. In: Chipman C, ed. *Emergency Department Orthopedics.* Rockville, Aspen 1982:13-25.
4. Orban DJ. Forearm and wrist. In: Rosen P, Baker FJ, Barkin RM, et al., eds. *Emergency Medicine: Concepts and Clinical Practice.* 2nd ed. St. Louis: CV Mosby; 1988:761-773.
5. Gray H. *Anatomy of the Human Body.* 30th ed. Clemente CD, ed. Philadelphia: Lea & Febiger; 1985:382-383.
6. Braun RM. The distal joint of the radius and ulna. Diagnostic studies and treatment rationale. *Clin Orthop* 1992;275:74.
7. Mercier LR. The forearm, wrist, and hand. in: *Practical Orthopedics.* 3rd ed. St. Louis: CV Mosby; 1991:99-134.
8. Adams JC. The forearm, wrist and hand, in: *Outline of Orthopaedics.* 9th ed. London: Churchill Livingstone; 1981:267-300.
9. Culver JE. Sports-related fractures of the hand and wrist. *Clin Sports Med* 1990;9:85.
10. Klefhaber TR, Stern PJ. Upper extremity tendinitis and overuse syndromes in the athlete. *Clin Sports Med* 1992; 11:39.
11. Rettig AC. Closed tendon injuries of the hand and wrist in the athlete. *Clin Sports Med* 1992;11:77.
12. Garrick J. Emergencies in sports. In: Schwartz GR, Safar P, Stone JH, et al, eds. P*rinciples and Practices of Emergency Medicine.* 2nd ed. Philadelphia: WB Saunders; 1986;11446.
13. Weiker GG. Hand and wrist problems in the athlete. *Clin Sports Med* 1992;11:189
14. Ogden JA. The uniqueness of growing bones. In Rockwood CA, Wilkens KE, King RE, eds. *Fractures in Children.* Philadelphia: JB Lippincott; 1984:5.
15. Kennington RT, Dwyer BJ, Phillips WA. Avoiding misdiagnosis with pediatric arm injuries. *Emerg Med Reports* 1990;11:189.
16. Simmons DP, MacAusland WR. Trauma to the extremities and soft tissues. In: Schwartz GR, Safar P, Stone JH, et al., eds. *Principles and Practices of Emergency Medicine.* 2nd ed. Philadelphia: WB Saunders; 1986:14121417.
17. Gittlen WB. Hamulus fracture. *Ann Emerg Med* 1984;13:122.
18. Beckenbaugh RB. Accurate evaluation and management of the painful wrist following injury. An approach to carpal

instability. *Orthop Clin North Am* 1984;15:289.

19. Pin PG, Young VL, Gilula, Weeks PM. Wrist pain: A systematic approach to diagnosis. *Plast Reconstr Surg* 1990; 83:42.
20. Sternbach GL, Doris PE, Rosen P. In: *Diagnostic Radiology in Emergency Medicine*. St. Louis: CV Mosby; 1992:11.
21. Levinson EM. Imaging of the wrist. *Radial Clin North Am* 1990;28:905.
22. Schernberg F. Roentgenographic examination of the wrist: A systematic study of the normal, lax, and injured wrist. Part 1: The standard and positional views. *J Hand Surg* 1990; 15B:210.
23. Larsen CF. Mathiesen FK, Lindequist A. Measurements of carpal bone angles on normal wrist radiographs. *J Hand Surg* 1991;16:888.
24. Fitzrandolph RL. Radiographic and orthopedic evaluation of wrist trauma. *Curr Probl Diag Radiol* 1991;20:1.
25. Schernberg F. Roentgenographic examination of the wrist: A systematic study of the normal, lax, and injured wrist. Part 2. Stress views. *J Hand Surg* 1990;158:220.
26. Buchberger W, Schon G, Strasser K, Jungwirth W. High-resolution ultrasonography of the carpal tunnel. *Ultrasound Med* 1991;10531.
27. Gundry CR, Schils JP, Resnick D, Sartoris DJ. Arthrography of the post-traumatic knee, shoulder, and wrist. *Radial Clin North Am* 1989;27:957.
28. Kursunoglu-Brahme S, Grundry CR, Resnick D. Advanced imaging of the wrist. *Radial Clin North Am* 1990;28:307.
29. Moonev JF III, Seigel DB, Kaman LA. Ligamenlous injuries of the wrist in-athletes. *Clip Sports Med* 1992;11:129.
30. Schneider FR, ad. *Orthopedics in Emergency Care.* St. Louis: CV Mosby; 1980;2023:85-101.
31. Barnaby W. Fractures and dislocations of the wrist. *Emerg Med Clin North Am* 1992;10:133.
32. Rogers LF. *Radiology of Skeletal Trauma*. Vol 1. New York: Churchill Livingstone; 1982.
33. Hamlin C. Diagnosis of wrist injuries. *Emerg Med Clin North Am* 1985;3:311.
34. Simon RR, Koenigsknecht SJ. *Orthopedics in Emergency Medicine: The Extremities.* New York: Appleton Century-Crofts; 1982.
35. Milford L. The hand: Fractures and dislocations. In: Crenshaw AH, ed. *Campbells Operative Orthopaedics*. 7th ed. Vol 1. St. Louis: CV Mosby; 1987.
36. Mittal RL, Dargan SL. Occult scaphoid fracture: A diagnostic enigma. *J Orthopedic Trauma* 1989;3:306.
37. Jones WA. Beware the sprained wrist. The incidence and diagnosis of scapholunate instability. *J Bone Joint Surg* 1988; 70:293.

Adult and Pediatric Hip Injuries

Charles Stewart, MD, FACEP

Although hip fractures are considered to be a meat-and-potatoes problem that is usually approached in a cookbook fashion, clinical experience has taught us that managing patients with hip injuries is much more treacherous than it may seem. Despite the pitfalls of diagnosing and triaging patients with hip problems, the approach to patients with possible hip fractures in the emergency setting is often cavalier. This can lead to sketchy evaluations, failure to detect associated injuries, and incomplete radiographic studies. From an emergency perspective, individuals suspected of having a hip fracture require prompt and comprehensive evaluation. Special attention should be paid to uncovering risk factors that maybe have contributed to the injury. In particular, the possibility of blood loss, cardiovascular instability, and central nervous system (CNS) compromise must always be considered during the initial evaluation. An electrocardiogram (ECG), complete blood count (CBC), electrolytes, and IV access should be obtained upon arrival, and measures to relieve pain and stabilize volume loss secondary to hemorrhage should be implemented early in the clinical course.

Injuries to the hip and pelvis are common and constitute a major financial and health care burden in the United States. Two hundred fifty thousand hip fractures occur annually, resulting in health care expenditures in excess of $1.25 billion, and there has been a marked increase in the incidence of hip fractures over the last 25 years.[2] Between 1965 and 1995, the number of hip fractures will quadruple. And with the general population aging, the incidence of these fractures may double again within the next 50 years.[3] In some regions of the world, as many as half of all women will suffer a fracture and [4] about one in six will suffer a hip fracture.[4] In addition, hip fractures significantly tax the limited physical reserves of elderly patients and can lead to prolonged and costly rehabilitation programs.[5] Moreover, when fractures do occur in this patient subgroup, they are associated with a mortality rate ranging from 13-30% within the first year of injury.[6,7]

Because many patients with hip injuries are elderly, a meticulous search should be made for life-threatening, underlying disorders known to increase the risk of falling, such as cardiac arrhythmias, gastrointestinal tract hemorrhage, infection, metabolic disorders, and acute cerebrovascular events.[8] And while the diagnosis of most hip injuries can readily be made with standard radiography, femoral neck and subcapital hip fractures can present with very subtle or, sometimes, undetectable radiographic abnormalities.

The purpose of this chapter is to provide a comprehensive review of the pearls and pitfalls associated with the evaluation and management of hip injuries. Classification of hip fractures, assessment of precipitating causes, and strategies for improving outcomes with radiographic studies will be emphasized.

Table 1. Frequent Causes of Hip Fractures in the Elderly

Osteoporosis	**Osteomalacia**
Estrogen/testosterone deficiency	Vitamin D deficiency
Calcium deficiency	
	Drug-Induced Side Effects and Hypotension
Syncope	Tricyclic antidepressants
Postural hypotension	Long-acting benzodiazepines
Arrhythmias	Antipsychotics
Hypoglycemia	Scopolamine-containing antidiarrheal agents
Polypharmacy	
Heart disease	Anti- Parkinsonian drugs
Drop attacks	Antihypertensive agents
Gastrointestinal tract hemorrhage	
	Increased Risk of Falls
	Decreased muscle strength
Cardiac Arrhythmias	Gait abnormalities
Bradyarrhythmias	Obesity
Sick sinus syndrome	Lower-extremity weakness
Supraventricular tachyarrhythmias	Malnutrition
	Cognitive impairment
Syncope associated with aortic stenosis	Reduced soft tissue padding
	Podiatric deformities
Environmental Hazards	**Mechanics of Fall and Landing**
Ice and snow	
Throw rugs	Slowed reaction time
Poor quality shoes	Decreased muscle strength
Phone cords	Alterations of balance
Lack of supervision	Female pelvic and femur shape

Hip Fracture: Clinical Presentation

Fractures of the hip occur by one of three mechanisms: l) osteoporosis; 2) high-impact trauma; and 3) intrinsic defects in the bone.

In the elderly, significant reductions in bone density associated with osteoporosis permit fractures to occur from minor trauma, such as low-impact falls. With increasing age, sedentary lifestyle habits, and metabolic bone disease, there is a progressive loss of trabecular bone from the proximal femur, which increases the risk of hip fracture.[9,10] The risk of these fractures increases with age, with a peak incidence observed in the 70- to-80-year-old age group.[11] Occasionally, an osteoporotic proximal femur fracture can occur with no identifiable trauma.[12] Because the incidence of osteoporosis is greater in women, they are five times more likely than men to sustain hip fractures. Other predisposing factors to fractures in the elderly include lean body habitus, low calcium intake, smoking, alcohol ingestion, inactivity, and medication reactions.[13,14] *(Please see Table 1.)*

Hip fractures in younger patients tend to be associated with high-energy trauma such as motor vehicle accidents. Comminution, soft-tissue damage, open wounds, and multiple associated injuries are frequently associated with these fractures, which are most likely to occur in young male adults. Because of the high-energy forces required to produce hip disruption in young patients, femoral neck fractures in these individuals may be associated with ipsilateral shaft fractures of the femur.[15]

The third precipitant of hip fractures is metastatic disease to bone, which occurs most commonly in the proximal femur and head and is associated with breast, lung, colon, and prostate carcinomas. Pathologic fractures require accurate assessment and orthopedic intervention, as well as therapeutic—or palliative—management of the underlying neoplastic process.

Prognosis following a fracture of the hip is determined by the age and overall condition of the patient, the stability of the fracture, and the degree of osteoporosis of the proximal femur.[16,17]

Physical Examination

Pain is the most common chief complaint in elderly patients who have sustained a fracture of the hip. Initial assessment may reveal that the affected extremity is slightly flexed, shortened, and in some external rotation. Gross bony abnormalities are uncommon. The level and position of the greater trochanters should be palpated and the femoral pulses noted. Passive range of motion of the hip should be attempted unless a fracture or dislocation is obvious. The physician should inspect for contusions and document range of motion. Although rarely used, auscultatory percussion is, nevertheless, a sensitive test for detecting fractures of the femur and pubic ramus.[18]

Physical examination of younger patients with hip fractures produced by high-energy trauma should proceed along guidelines mandated for victims of major trauma. Long-bone fractures are common[19] in this group of patients, and associated injuries to the head, abdomen, and chest frequently require priority.

Radiographic Examination

The most helpful radiologic view for the emergency practitioner in examining for hip fracture is a straight anterior-posterior (AP) view of the pelvic area that includes both femoral necks and trochanters, and a lateral view of the affected hip. There are several strategies that enhance the physician s interpretation of this radiograph and that will help detect occult fractures. First, the clinician should be aware that the neck of the femur forms an inferior angle of approximately 135° with the shaft of the femur and that the neck of the femur of the affected side should be compared with the non-affected side. These angles should be very nearly equal if the patient has not been rotated during the radiologic exam. Second, the physician should follow Shenton's line, which, in a straight AP view, consists of the smooth line formed by the inferior border of neck of the femur and which is almost continuous and unbroken with that line formed by the superior margin of the obturator foramen. Third, the physician should attempt to identify faint shadows around the neck of the femur superiorly and inferiorly formed by the iliopsoas muscles bilaterally. These shadows will appear distended or bulging if a patient has suffered a fracture that has caused bleeding into the capsule surrounding the neck of the femur. Fourth, and perhaps most important, close examination must be made of the cortex of the femoral both superiorly and inferiorly and along both trochanters. If this cortical line appears to be broken or not contiguous in any portion, additional views must be obtained. Finally, the relative absence of trabecular patterns through the femoral neck should be noted.

Classification of Hip Fractures

Fractures of the hip are usually classified according to the following anatomic locations: 1) subcapital; 2) femoral neck; 3) intertrochanteric; 4) subtrochanteric. Within each anatomic category, numerous classification systems have been proposed to identify fracture stability and healing rates. For example, because bony fragments associated with intertrochanteric fractures have an adequate blood supply, these fractures will often unite without complications after simple reduction and fixation. On the other hand, because fractures of the femoral neck are infra-articular and have a poor blood supply to a thin periosteum, these fractures are troubled with high rates of avascular necrosis and late degenerative changes. Subtrochanteric fractures are associated with high mechanical stresses, which are likely to produce complications.

Femoral Head Fractures

Although femoral head fractures are uncommon, when they do occur, they are most often associated with hip dislocation in the setting of high-energy trauma.[20,21] In addition, if a patient presents with a traumatic dislocation of the hip, the examiner should be aware that an associated fracture of the head of the femur may be present. If the hip dislocates anteriorly, the superior portion of the femoral head can be sheared off. When a posterior dislocation occurs, the inferior portion of the femoral head may be damaged, and, in most cases, disrupted fragments can be seen on standard AP and lateral radiographs.

Because of the mechanism of injury associated with femoral head fractures, the physician should search for other orthopedic injuries associated with high-energy trauma. In particular, special care should be taken to exclude fractures of the pelvis, ipsilateral femur, and knee. Management of femoral head fractures associated with dislocation is controversial, probably because of the small number of cases and the high morbidity associated with this injury. However, generally speaking, if fragments are noted, preparations should be made for operative reduction.[21] On the other hand, if the patient is elderly, the orthopedist may initially elect a closed reduction, which can then be followed by arthroplasty in the event of an unsatisfactory result.

Femoral Neck (Subcapital) Fractures

The most common type of hip fracture, femoral neck fractures are most likely to occur in elderly females. An estimated 200,000 cases of femoral neck fractures occur in the United States each year.[22] In the elderly, these fractures are associated with osteoporosis or osteomalacia.[9]

Typically, the patient will give a history of tripping over an object, slipping on a slick surface, or being knocked down. In many cases, it is uncertain whether the patient had a fall that caused the fracture or whether a spontaneous fracture caused the fall. If abduction forces are more prominent, then the fracture line is more horizontal across the neck of the femur. Conversely, if the forces of adduction are more prominent, the fracture line is oriented more vertically through the neck of the femur. A fall that has a lateral component may cause impaction of the femoral head on the neck of the femur. In the young, subcapital fractures are most often associated with high-kinetic-energy injuries. In these patients, there is often marked soft-tissue injury and comminution of the bony fragments.

Signs and Symptoms. Clinical signs of a femoral neck fracture may range from localized hip pain to dramatic shortening and external rotation. When a femoral neck fracture is incomplete, impacted, or nondisplaced, symptoms may be minor, with the patient complaining of little more than groin discomfort, pain on pressure over the greater trochanter, or pain on light heel punch (anvil test). In general, if the fracture is impacted, it is more stable and the patient may even be able to ambulate. In fact, the only indication of injury may be a bruise over the greater trochanter.[23] On the other hand, if the fracture is not impacted, crepitus may be palpated when the hip is moved. These unstable fractures will generally demonstrate more shortening and rotation on physical examination.

Radiography. Interpretation of femoral neck radiographs may be difficult. Normally, subtle osteophytic lipping can be seen at the femoral head and neck junction; this finding is sometimes difficult to differentiate from a nondisplaced fracture. However, on close inspection, some disruption of the trabecular latticework is usually apparent, a finding that can be accentuated by obtaining views of the hip with slight external or internal rotation. For the most part, although displaced fractures are readily visible on standard AP and lateral films of the hip, impacted fractures may be quite subtle and visible only on tomography or with special views. A subtle displacement of the normal angle of the femoral neck may be the only clue to hip fracture. Indeed, if the fracture is not displaced on x-ray, a bone scan may be necessary to identify a fracture. If a fracture is strongly suspected, but there is no radiographic evidence on plain films, tomograms may be helpful. Magnetic resonance imaging (MRI) will verify the diagnosis. If the MRI is negative, the likelihood of bone injury is virtually excluded.[24]

Treatment. The treatment of choice is operative reduction and internal fixation. In general, the more proximal the fracture (i.e., the closer it is to the head of the femur), the greater the incidence of complications, with nonunion occurring in up to 22% of all femoral neck fractures.[25] Subcapital fractures of the femoral neck are at risk for vascular disruption. Accordingly, osteonecrosis is also common, with an incidence that ranges from 440%.[25]

Trochanteric and Intertrochanteric Fractures

Signs and Symptoms. Less common in elderly patients, trochanteric fractures are most often found in young adults. Not surprisingly, the mechanism of injury is almost always direct trauma. In general, greater trochanteric fractures present with tenderness and pain that are exacerbated by active abduction of the thigh. On the other hand, lesser trochanteric fractures are usually the result of an avulsion injury and typically present with tenderness and pain that is increased with flexion and rotation of the hip. Treatment of trochanteric fractures is usually conservative, and only rarely will surgery be needed.

Table 2. Complications of Hip Fracture

Venous thrombosis
Nonunion
Inadequate fixation
Avascular necrosis of femoral head
Pressure sores
Arthritis
Debilitation

Intertrochanteric fractures are the second most common type of hip injury. As a rule, these are extracapsular fractures with cancellous bone and a good blood supply.[26] Most intertrochanteric fractures involve higher injury energy than fractures through the surgical neck of the femur. Clinical signs of intertrochanteric fractures may range from minimal pain to marked shortening and external rotation. Swelling is frequently extensive and may be associated with hematoma formation caused by bleeding and muscle injury. A rotational deformity is more likely than with femoral neck fractures.

Almost all intertrochanteric fractures are unstable, which explains why patients usually are unable to walk or stand after the injury.[27] AP and lateral radiographs of the hip will readily provide the diagnosis in most cases. Factors that make an intertrochanteric fracture unstable include comminution of the fragments between the greater trochanter and the proximal femur, steep vertical fracture lines, or subtrochanteric extension of the fracture.[28-30]

The mortality rate after an intertrochanteric fracture is more than twice that reported for fractures of the femoral neck. There are several reasons for this adverse prognosis: Patients with intertrochanteric fractures are slightly older, blood loss is slightly greater, more severe trauma is required to produce this kind of fracture, and patients require a longer operative procedure.[5,31]

Management. Most intertrochanteric fractures are treated with urgent operative reduction and external fixation. Both mortality and morbidity increase after delays of more than 48 hours.[32] Occasionally, patients who are extremely poor operative candidates will be managed conservatively. Although this fracture may respond to nonoperative management, long periods of immobility are required, and consequently, the risk of complications is increased.

Subtrochanteric Fractures

The subtrochanteric area extends from the lesser trochanter to about 5 cm distal to the hip. Fractures that involve the area just distal to the hip are called subtrochanteric fractures. Because of the high mechanical stress in this region, subtrochanteric fractures are associated with high rates of nonunion as well as metal fatigue failure of implants. Moreover, these fractures often have a rotational component or a spiral configuration.

Mechanism of Injury. Like the other orthopedic injuries to the hip, subtrochanteric fractures are classified according to mechanism of injury, anatomy, number of comminuted fragments, and stability.[33] Of all of the classifications, mechanism of injury is most useful to emergency practice and includes the following categories: 1) low-energy fall in patients with osteoporosis; 2) linear fractures through bony defects; and 3) high-speed trauma.

In the elderly with osteoporosis, subtrochanteric fractures are often due to a low-energy fall. Frequently spiral fractures with little comminution, subtrochanteric fractures occur much more often in men than in women, in large part because the male femoral neck is stronger in construction.[34] A second mechanism involves a linear fracture through a bony defect such as a metastatic lesion. Therapy of this condition depends as much on the underlying process as on fracture anatomy. The third mechanism of producing fractures of this type is high-speed trauma, such as a motor vehicle accident, pedestrian accident with a motor vehicle, or a fall from a high place. These fractures are frequently comminuted, they may have extensive soft-tissue damage, and they may be associated with head, thoracic, or abdominal trauma.

Management. Treatment is almost always operative reduction and internal fixation. If the bone is so fragmented that reduction is impossible, then skeletal traction may be used. Generally, about three months of traction will be required before limited weight-bearing can be tolerated.

Osteonecrosis of the head of the femur, which is characterized by mottling of normal bone density, is a common sequela of hip trauma. This complication, which occurs in about 85% of displaced fractures and 15-25% of nondisplaced fractures involving the femoral neck,[35-37] can follow intracapsular fracture of the neck of the femur, dislocation of the hip, and compression fracture of the head of the femur. Bone death results when vessels entering the periosteum are crushed or sheared, a disruption that will deprive the head of the femur of its blood supply within eight hours of the injury. *(Please see Table 2.)*

Hip Dislocation: Posterior Hip Dislocation

Mechanism of Injury. Of all hip dislocations, about 80-90% are posterior in location, the majority of which result from motor vehicle accidents. When the hip is flexed about 90° and slightly adducted, it is at greatest risk from a force along the longitudinal axis. In unrestrained patients, the impact of the knee on the dashboard pushes the femoral head posteriorly through the capsule.

Clinical Findings. A posteriorly dislocated hip produces classical signs and symptoms. The thigh is partially flexed, adducted, shortened, and internally rotated. The joint space is widened and an acetabular fracture may be present. The femoral head is posterior to the acetabulum and locked in place. This is best seen in the true lateral view of the hip. An oblique view may also show the dislocation. Computerized tomography can provide better evaluation of the acetabulum and the femoral head. The clinician should look for evidence of acetabular or femoral fractures as well as knee injury, since as many as 50% of patients with posterior dislocation of the hip will have an associated fracture.

Sciatic nerve injury complicates 10-15% of posterior dislocations. The physician should search for decreased muscle function below the knee, impairment of knee flexion, and decreased sensation on the posterolateral leg and sole of the foot. Up to 50% of patients with a posterior hip dislocation will develop post-traumatic arthritis. It should be emphasized that sciatic nerve involvement represents a true orthopedic emergency.

Management. Treatment consists of prompt closed reduction, which will require excellent analgesia and muscle relaxation. The hip can frequently be reduced with manual traction in the ED but can require operative anesthesia. When departmental reduction is attempted, the emergency physician should stand astride the involved hip, which should be flexed 90° and positioned in about 15° of adduction. The pelvis should be stabilized by another person as traction is applied along the axis of the femur. The hip should be gently rotated through internal and external rotation. With these small rotational movements and traction, the hip can usually be reduced. If the hip cannot be reduced with IV sedation, then general anesthesia is needed. No sudden movements or excessive force should be applied since it is possible to break the head of the femur.

Complications. Avascular necrosis is not uncommon with posterior dislocation of the hip. Since the incidence of avascular necrosis increases markedly after about eight hours, the dislocated hip should be reduced as soon as possible.[38] Consequently, orthopedic follow-up after reduction of the hip is essential. X-rays of the hip should be obtained every three months for the first year and every six months for two more years to identify avascular necrosis, which may be delayed in presentation.

Anterior Dislocation

Mechanism of Injury. Responsible for 10-25% of all hip dislocations, anterior dislocation requires the hip to be slightly flexed as it withstands extreme abduction (hyperextension) forces that produce extreme, unopposed external rotation. These forces and anatomic configurations permit the femoral head to be pushed out through a tear in the anterior capsule superiorly through the iliofemoral ligament. The most common causes of this injury include auto accidents, falls, a blow to the back while squatting, and running with sudden turning.

Physical Examination. Patients usually present with an adducted hip that is externally rotated and slightly flexed. The patient almost always cannot actively flex the hip, and the femoral head is palpable in the area of the anterosuperior iliac spine or just deep to the femoral artery. AP and cross-table lateral views of the hip should show the displacement of the head of the femur from the acetabulum up into the pubic or supraspinous region. The femur is externally rotated.

Management. Reduction of this dislocation is accomplished by further extension of the hip, followed by a push-down motion on the displaced femoral head in order to return it through the capsular tear. The extension motion will release the tight posterior capsule. Diminishing femoral or distal pulses (or progressive swelling of the leg) indicates an emergent need for reduction of the hip. If the femoral nerve is involved, there is decreased strength in the quadriceps, decreased deep-tendon reflex, and decreased sensation on the anteromedial thigh.

Obturator (Central) Dislocations

Caused by hyperabduction of the hip in neutral position, obturator dislocations are uncommon. In this injury, the greater trochanter is pushed against the pelvis, thus serving as a fulcrum against which to lever the femoral head out of the acetabulum. This forces the head of the femur inferiorly into the obturator foramen. AP radiographs show the femoral head in the obturator foramen. Lateral views confirm that the femoral head is neither anterior nor posterior to the obturator foramen. Hip abduction may be quite pronounced. Because the hip is dislocated into the obturator foramen, blood vessels are not disrupted, and avascular necrosis is an uncommon complication.

Table 3. Complications of Hip Dislocations

Early Complications:

Posterior dislocations — Sciatic nerve injury (10% of patients)

Anterior dislocation — Femoral artery, vein, and nerve injury

Late Complications:

All dislocations — Osteoarthritis

Posterior dislocations — Avascular necrosis of the femoral head (15-30% of patients)

Anterior dislocations — Femoral artery/vein thrombosis, pulmonary embolism, avascular necrosis of the femoral head

Prosthesis Dislocation and Fracture

Dislocation of a prosthetic hip occurs in about 10% of patients with hip replacements.[39] Increased range of motion, loss of the abductor mechanism, shortening of the limb, and malorientation of the prosthesis components are all important causes of this type of dislocation.[40] As the number of patients who have had replacement of all or part of the hip joint increases, the chances of fracture of and around the hip prosthesis also increases.[41]

Although prosthesis dislocation is not common, it does occur and can be difficult to detect unless careful comparison is made with older films. A prosthesis that is cemented into place may also have the cement fragment or loosen.[41]

Chronic Dislocation

Chronic hip dislocations are infrequently missed. But when they are, it is usually in patients who are unconscious, in those with multiple injuries, and in patients who have another injury to the opposite hip. Dislocations may also be masked by a concomitant fracture of the femoral shaft. If a chronic dislocation has been present for less than three months, then closed reduction with skeletal traction may be successful. Traction may be needed for up to one week before the reduction is attempted; rarely is this performed as an emergency procedure. There is a high incidence of avascular necrosis in this injury. If closed reduction is not successful, if there is a fracture of the acetabulum or the femoral head, or if the dislocation has been present for longer than three months, open reduction with primary total hip replacement may be required. *(Please see Table 3.)*

Pediatric Hip Injuries

Hip fractures are uncommon in children, accounting for only 1 % or fewer of all fractures in this age group.[42] However, when they do

The "*POST*" GUIDELINES FOR ORTHOPEDIC SURGERY
(Protocols for Preventing Post-Orthopedic Surgery Thrombosis)

Deep Venous Thrombosis (DVT) Prophylaxis, Risk Factor Assessment, and Clinical Protocols for Patients Undergoing Pelvic or Lower Extremity Orthopedic Surgical Procedures*

POST Orthopedic Surgery Patient Assessment Protocol
Risk Factor Score Calculation

ASSESS PRESENCE OF DVT RISK FACTORS BY CHECKING APPROPRIATE BOXES

- ❑ Age 40 to 60 years (1 factor)
- ❑ Age 61 to 70 years (2 factors)
- ❑ Age over 70 years (3 factors)
- ❑ Documented history of DVT or P.E. (3 factors)
- ❑ Family history of DVT or P.E. (3 factors)
- ❑ Leg swelling, ulcers, stasis, varicose veins
- ❑ History of pelvic or long bone fracture
- ❑ Lower extremity arthroscopy in patients > 50 years of age
- ❑ History of, or anticipated bed confinement/immobilization > 12 hours
- ❑ Confining air/ground travel (> 4 hours within 1 week of admission)
- ❑ Spinal cord injury with paralysis (3 factors)
- ❑ Stroke with paralysis (3 factors)
- ❑ MI/CHF
- ❑ Obesity (greater than 20% over IBW)
- ❑ General anesthesia time > 2 hours
- ❑ Pregnancy, or postpartum < 1 month
- ❑ Multiple trauma
- ❑ Inflammatory bowel disease
- ❑ Inherited thrombophilia (3 factors)
  - Activated protein C resistance (factor V Leiden mutation)
  - Antithrombin III deficiency
  - Protein C or S deficiency
  - Plasminogen or plasminogen activator deficiency
  - Dysfibrinogenemia
- ❑ Antiphospholipid antibodies or Lupus anticoagulent (3 factors)
- ❑ Non-hemorrahgic myeloproliferative disorders including polycythemia vera
- ❑ Hyperviscosity symdromes
- ❑ Estrogen hormone replacement therapy

* Each check equals 1 risk factor except where indicated

Quantitative Total *POST* Risk Factor Score

Assign Patient to *POST* DVT Risk Category Based On Total Risk Factor Score and Other Clinical Judgement Criteria

Total *POST* Risk Factor Score ≤ 1
or Patient Undergoing Minor Surgery
→ Minimal-to-Low DVT Risk — *POST* Category A
→ Early Ambulation ELASTICS Stockings

Total *POST* Risk Factor Score = 2
or Major Orthopedic Procedure for Long Bone or Pelvic Fracture or Prosthesis in Patient ≥ 40 Years
→ Moderate-to-Significant DVT Risk — *POST* Category B

Total *POST* Risk Factor Score of 3 or 4
or Age ≥ 40 plus Major Procedure or Cardiorespiratory Comorbidity Plus Major Ortho Procedure
→ High DVT Risk — *POST* Category C

Total *POST* Risk Factor Score ≥ 4
or Age ≥ 40 Plus Any of the Following:
- History of DVT
- Total Joint Replacement
- Hip Fracture
- Stroke
- Spinal Cord Injury
- Malignancy

→ Extremely High DVT Risk — *POST* Category D

Evaluation of Patient Eligibility for *POST*-Procedural Anticoagulation

ABSOLUTE CONTRAINDICATIONS TO CHEMOPROPHYLAXIS

- ❑ Active hemorrhage from wounds, drains, lesions
- ❑ Heparin use in HITT
- ❑ Warfarin use in pregancy
- ❑ Severe trauma to head, spinal cord or extremities with hemorrhage
- ❑ Epidural/indwelling spinal catheter (possible contraindication)

YES → Mechanical Prophylaxis
NO → *POST* Category B - D Chemoprophylaxis or Treatment Options

RELATIVE CONTRAINDICATIONS TO CHEMOPROPHYLAXIS

- ❑ Cerebral hemorrhage at any time previously
- ❑ GI, GU bleed or stroke within past 6 months
- ❑ Thrombocytopenia
- ❑ Coagulopathy
- ❑ Active intracranial lesions/neoplasms
- ❑ Proliferative retinopathy
- ❑ Vascular access/biopsy sites inaccessible to hemostatic control

NO → *POST* Category B - D Chemoprophylaxis or Treatment Options
YES → Clinical Judgement → No Mechanical Prophylaxis / Chemoprophylaxis Indicated → *POST* Category B - D Chemoprophylaxis or Treatment Options

POST Category B - D Chemoprophylaxis or Treatment Options

Moderate-to-Significant DVT Risk — Post Category B
Enoxaparin: 30mg BID 12-24 Hours Post Surgery (Knee Replacement); 30mg BID or 40mg QD (Hip Replacement)
or Low Dose UHF Q8-12 HRS or Alternative: Consider Sequential Compression Device

High DVT Risk — Post Category C
Enoxaparin: 30mg BID 12-24 Hours Post Surgery (Knee Replacement); 30mg BID or 40mg QD (Hip Replacement)
or Low Dose UHF (5000 u Q8 HRS and 2 HRS Preop)

Extremely High DVT Risk — Post Category D
Enoxaparin: 30mg BID 12-24 Hours Post Surgery (Knee Replacement); 30mg BID or 40mg QD (Hip Replacement)
or Oral Warfarin With Target INR 2.0 - 3.0 or SCD plus Enoxaparin

* Adopted and Modified from the Methodist Hospital Protocol and Worksheet for DVT Prophylaxis

occur, hip fractures are more devastating in pediatric patients than in adults, because the growth plate can be disrupted and because blood vessels in the rapidly growing femoral head are more easily compromised. In addition, the periosteal tube in a child is much stronger than that of an adult, so about 50% of these fractures are nondisplaced. Appropriate radiographs for detecting hip pathology in children include a standing AP and supine frog lateral view of both hips.

According to the most commonly used classification of hip fractures in children,[43] four categories of injury are identified: l) type I, a separation of the epiphysis with or without dislocation of the femoral head; 2) type II, fractures across the neck of the femur (transcervical); 3) type DI, cervicotrochanteric fractures; and 4) type IV, intertrochanteric fractures.

Management of hip injuries in children is different than in elderly adults. There is no prosthesis that can accommodate the growing child. Fortunately, children can tolerate immobility better than adults. Consequently, traction, immobilization with casting, and bed rest are viable means of therapy.

Complications

The most common complication of hip fractures in children is avascular necrosis. As in adult fractures, displacement of the fragments is a key factor producing disruption of the blood supply to the head of the femur. In younger children, avascular necrosis is not always treated with surgery, since a prosthesis is not often available. Premature closure of the epiphysis can occur. It is usually not significant since the capital epiphysis contributes only about 15% of the femur s length. Nonunion of fragments occurs less frequently in children than in adults.

Osteochondrosis of the Femoral Head (Legg-Calve-Perthes Disease). This disease of children is characterized by ischemic necrosis of the femoral head. It is more common in males than in females and has a peak incidence in 6-to-7-year-old age group. Frequently associated with steroid therapy, this condition can also be seen with blood dyscrasias, juvenile rheumatoid arthritis, and diabetes.[44] The patient is afebrile, and the white blood cell count and sedimentation rate are normal. Typically, the patient presents with hip pain, spasm of the muscles, a limp, and limitation of both internal rotation and abduction. X-rays show flattening of the femoral head, necrosis of the ossification center, and widening of the neck of the femur. On the frog lateral view, a crescent sign may be visible as a thin area of lucency just below the subchondral bone in the anterolateral portion of the head. Later findings may include fibrosis and slow ossification of the fibrous tissue.

Traumatic Epiphyseal Slip (Type I Fractures). Separation or slippage of the femoral epiphysis is almost always due to an acute injury. Most often, it follows an upward blow transmitted through the shaft of the femur. Pain may be localized to the hip, but, not uncommonly, it is referred to the knee or groin. The leg may be shortened, externally rotated, and abducted. Pain is noted with movement, and, almost without exception, internal rotation and abduction are limited. A slipped capital femoral epiphysis is most often encountered in preadolescent or adolescent boys who present with knee pain and have normal knee x-rays. It also can occur during reduction of a hip dislocation in a child with an open epiphysis, which is a true orthopedic emergency that demands early care and open reduction of the fragments.[42] Avascular necrosis occurs in 80-100% of cases, and the family should be counseled on the probable need for further reconstructive procedures.[45]

Fractures of the Neck of the Femur (Type II). Transcervical fractures are the most common type of hip fracture in children.[42] Most of these fractures are displaced and the amount of displacement appears to correlate with the rate of avascular necrosis. Early evacuation of the perifracture hematoma may decrease the incidence of avascular necrosis.[46] Internal fixation is recommended for all type II fractures because of the high incidence of fracture instability.

Stress fractures of the neck of the femur occur in children. These may be divided into displaced transverse fractures and compression fractures. Compression fractures are treated with a decrease of weight-bearing and limitation of activity. Displaced fractures are treated with surgical fixation.

Cervicotrochanteric Fractures (Type III). Cervicotrochanteric fractures in children are similar to those that occur at the base of the neck of the femur in adults. The incidence[42] of avascular necrosis is somewhat higher in children. The fracture may usually be treated with a spica cast if it is nondisplaced. Displaced fractures often require open reduction and internal fixation.

Intertrochanteric Fractures (Type IV). Intertrochanteric fractures in children are usually not complex. Because young children heal rapidly, skeletal traction is viable for treatment of this disease. Internal fixation is not usually needed. In older children, open reduction and internal fixation may be used. Isolated fractures of the greater or lesser trochanter are not common and rarely require surgery.

Summary

The clinical spectrum of hip injuries in adults and children is extensive, diverse, and diagnostically challenging. Elderly patients with hip fracture, almost without exception, are unable to walk. Occasionally, however, these patients may have little or no pain. Most patients with isolated hip fractures have stable vital signs and are not clinically in shock. However, if there is any doubt about hemodynamic status, an IV line should be established early. The general approach to hip fracture in adults includes a comprehensive assessment, and if the emergency physician is confident there are no other serious associated injuries, the patient should be made as comfortable as possible before proceeding further. Meperidine (Demerol) in combination with an anti-emetic is usually sufficient to control muscle spasm and pain.

If the patient remains stable, he or she may go to the radiology department for appropriate x-rays, which include an AP and lateral view of the hip that includes the femoral neck and both trochanters. A routine chest x-ray is also advisable in the event that admission is likely. It should be stressed that occult fractures are possible and that, even in the absence of hard radiographic abnormalities, a nonambulatory patient should almost always be hospitalized for a short observation period and further diagnostic testing, including MRI scanning and orthopedic consultation.

References

1. Hay EK. That old hip: The osteoporosis process. *Nurs Clin North Am* 1991;26:43-51.

2. Pierron RL, Perry HM III, Grossberg G, et al. The aging hip. *J Am Geriatr Soc* 1990;38:1339-1352.
3. LaCroix AZ. Thiazide diuretic agents and prevention of hip fractures. *Compr Ther* 1991;17:30-39.
4. Cummings SR, Black DM, Rubin SM. *Arch Int Med* 1989;149:2445.
5. Lindberg EL Macias D, Gipe BT. Clinically occult presentation of comminuted intertrochanteric hip fractures. *Ann Emerg Med* 1992;21:15111514.
6. Scott JC. Osteoporosis and hip fractures. *Rheum Dis Clin* North Am 1990;16:717-740.
7. Cooper C. Bone mass, muscle function and fracture of the proximal femur. *Br J Hosp Med* 1989;42:277-280.
8. Finsen V. Improvements in general health among the elderly: A factor in the rising incidence of hip fractures. *J Epidem Comm Health* 1988;42:200203.
9. Cummings SR. Prevention of osteoporotic fractures: What we need to know. *Baillieres Clin Obstet Gynaecol* 1991; 5:935-942.
10. Russell TA. Fractures of hip and pelvis. In: Crenshaw AIL ed. Campbell's Operative Orthopedics 8th ed. St. Louis: Mosby; 1992:895-987.
11. Barter HRK. Osteoporosis: The challenge of protection. *Geriatrics* 1985;40:19.
12. Hofeldt F. Proximal femoral fractures. *Clin Orthop* 1987; 218:12-18.
13. Risk factors in postmenopausal osteoporosis. *Lancet* 1985; June15:1370-1372. Editorial.
14. Jackson TK, Which IH. Understanding osteoporosis. *Postgrad Med* 1984;75:118.
15. Protzman RR, Burkhalter WE. Femoral-neck fractures in young adults. *J Bone Joint Surg* (Am) 1976;58:689-695.
16. Law MR, Wald NJ, Meade TW. Strategies for prevention of osteoporosis and hip fracture. *BMJ* 1991;303:453-460.
17. Sorock GS. Falls among the elderly: Epidemiology and prevention. *Am J Prev Med* 1988;4:282-288.
18. Berger EY. More on diagnosing fractures of the hip or pelvis. *N Engl J Med* 1982;308:971-973.
19. Kyle RF. Techniques of fixation for femoral neck fractures in young adults. *Techniques Orthop* 1986;1:33-38.
20. Pipkin G. Treatment of Grade VI fracture dislocation of the hip. *J Bone Joint Surg* 1957;39A:1027.
21. Lang-Stevenson A, Getty CJM. The Pipkin fracture-dislocation of the hip. *Injury* 1987;18:264-269.
22. Hofmann A, Wyatt R. Missed subcapital fractures. *Ann Emerg Med* 1984;13:951-955.
23. Hoffman A, Wyatt R. Missed subcapital fractures. *Ann Emerg Med* 1984;13:951-955.
24. Hiehle JF, Kneeland JB, Dalinka MK. Magnetic resonance imaging of the hip with emphasis on avascular necrosis. *Rheum Dis Clin North Am* 1991;17:669-693.
25. Fielding JE, Wilson, SA, Ratzan S. A continuing end result of displaced intracapsular fractures of the neck of the femur treated with the Pugh nail. *J Bone Joint Surg* [Am] 1974;56: 1464-1472.
26. Evans EM. The treatment of trochanteric fractures of the femur. *J Bone Joint Surg* 1951:33B:192-204.
27. Zuckerman JD, Schon, LC. Hip fractures. In: Zuckerman JD, ed. *Comprehensive Care of Orthopedic Injuries in the Elderly.* Baltimore: Urban & Schwarzenberg; 1990:23-111.
28. Kyle RF, Gustilo RB, Premer RF. Analysis of six hundred twenty-two intertrochanteric hip fractures. *J Bone Joint Surg* 1979;61A:216-221.
29. Harrington KD, Johnston JO. The management of comminuted unstable intertrochanteric fractures. *J Bone Joint Surg* 1973;57A:1367-1376.
30. Caudle RJ, Hopson CN, Clarke RP. Unstable intertrochanteric fractures of the hip. *Orthopaedic Rev* 1987; 16:538-549.
31. Russell TA. Fractures of the hip and pelvis. In: Crenshaw AH, ed. *Campbell's Operative Orthopedics*. St. Louis: Mosby; 1992:896.
32. DeLee JC. Fractures and dislocations of the hip. In: Rockwood CA, Green DP, eds. *Fractures*. Philadelphia: JB Lippincott Co; 1984:1211-1356.
33. Trafton PG. Subtrochanteric-intertrochanteric femoral fractures. *Orthop Clin North Am* 1987;18:59-71.
34. Kumar VN, Redford JB. Rehabilitation of hip fractures in the elderly. *Am Fam Physician* 1984;29:173-180.
35. Sevitt S. Avascular necrosis and revascularization of the femoral head after intracapsular fracture. *J Bone Joint Surg* 1964;46B:270.
36. Sevin S, Thompson RG. The distribution and anastomosis of arteries supplying the head and neck of the femur. *J Bone Joint Surg* 1965;47B:560.
37. Meyers MH. Osteonecrosis of the femoral head. Pathogenesis and longterm results of treatment. *Clin Orthop Rel Research* 1988;231:51-61.
38. Pietrafesa CA, Hoffman JR. Traumatic dislocation of the hip. *JAMA* 1983;249:3342-3346.
39. Gregory RJH, Gibson MJ, Moran CG. Dislocation after primary arthroplasty for subcapital fracture of the hip. *J Bone Joint Surg* 1991;73B:11-12.
40. Fraser GA, Wroblewski BM. Revision of the Charnley low-friction arthroplasty for recurrent or irreducible dislocation. *J Bone Joint Surg* [Br] 1981;63B:552-555.
41. Serocki JH, Chandler RW, Dorr LD. Treatment of fractures about hip prostheses with compression plating. *J Arthroplasty* 1992;7:129-135.
42. Canale ST. Fractures of the hip in children and adolescents. *Orthop Clin North Am* 1990;21:341-352.
43. Colona PC. Fracture of the neck of the femur in children. *Am J Surg* 1993;6:793.
44. DeLuca SA, Rhea IT. Legg-Calvé-Perthes disease. *Am Fam Physician* 1983;28:147-148.
45. Walls JP. Hip fracture-dislocation with transepiphyseal separation: Case report and literature review. *Clin Orthop* 1992;284:170-175.
46. Boitzy A. Fractures of the proximal femur. In: Weber BG, Brunner CH, Freuler F, eds. *Treatment of Fractures in Children and Adolescents.* Berlin: Springer-Verlag; 1980.

Inflammatory Disorders of the Shoulder

Charles Stewart, MD, FACEP

Common in both younger and older adults, shoulder injuries are among the most painful and often encountered of all orthopedic problems presenting to the emergency department (ED). Although diagnosis is frequently straightforward, radiographic evaluation often requires complementary techniques or views, and alleviation of pain is a clinical priority. Associated complications must be suspected, neurovascular status must be documented, and diagnostic assessment may require more than one radiographic modality.

Perhaps the most challenging part of managing patients with acute shoulder pain is differentiating among many diagnostic possibilities that run the gamut from bursitis and supraspinatus tendinitis to rotator cuff tears and anterior shoulder dislocations. Although each entity is associated with physical findings that can help suggest a specific anatomic defect, definitive evaluation is complicated by the fact that the shoulder girdle is a complex structure that may require magnetic resonance imaging (MRI) scanning or arthroscopy to delineate clinical abnormalities.

This review outlines strategies for shoulder evaluation that will improve diagnostic yields. It also presents a step-by-step approach to specific diagnostic and management techniques that can be performed by the emergency physician in the acute ambulatory environment.

Clinical Anatomy

Clinical evaluation of shoulder injuries is enhanced by a thorough understanding of the relationship between primary and supporting anatomic structures. *(Please see Figure 1.)* The shoulder is an extremely complex joint that comprises the clavicle, humerus, and scapula. Mobility depends on the glenohumeral, scapulothoracic, sternoclavicular, and acromioclavicular (AC) joints. Both the AC and the sternoclavicular joints have internal intraarticular menisci. The scapula forms the posterior and medial portion of the shoulder joint—the "saucer" in which the cup of the humerus sits. The glenoid fossa is a shallow cavity deepened by the fibrous glenoid lip that forms the capsule of the glenohumeral joint and extends from the glenoid lip and attaches to the anatomic neck of the proximal humerus.

A dense musculotendinous structure, the rotator cuff helps to keep the cup in the saucer, whereas the coracoacromial arch prevents upward displacement of the humerus. Formed by the subscapularis, supraspinatus, infraspinatus, and the teres minor muscles, the rotator stabilizes the glenohumeral joint. From a functional perspective, the rotator cuff moves the shoulder downward and inward, whereas the trapezius and the serratus anterior rotate the scapula. The shoulder's nerve supply is provided by the axillary and suprascapular nerves of the fifth cervical root (C5). As a result, pain from any shoulder structure may be perceived as lateral arm or shoulder pain.

Figure 1. Bones and Joints of the Shoulder Girdle

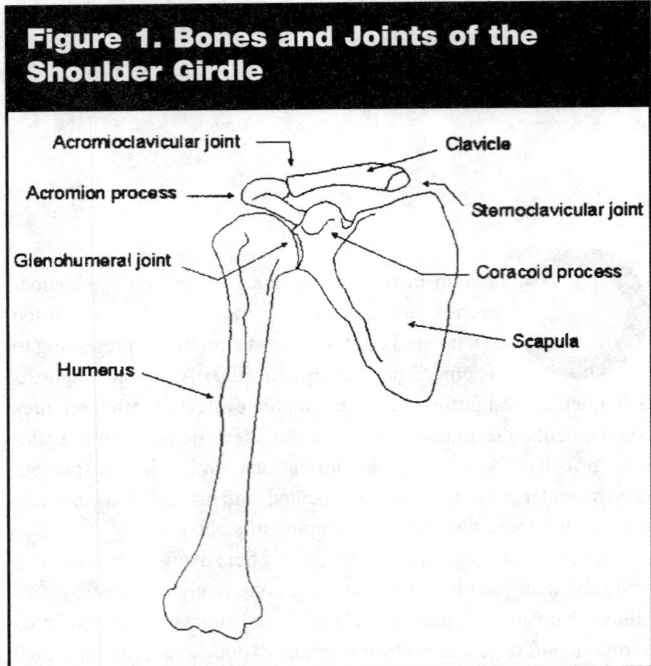

Table 1. Shoulder Motions

TYPE OF MOVEMENT	MANEUVER
Abduction	Laterally raise the arms above the head
Abduction	Laterally lower the arms
Flexion	Raise hands forward above the head
External Rotation	Place hand behind head
Internal Rotation	Place hand behind back as high as possible ("parade rest" position)

Evaluation of the Injured Shoulder

History. Differential diagnosis of shoulder pathology is facilitated by acquisition of a thorough, detailed history and proper interpretation of clinical clues, mechanism of injury, and presenting symptoms. For example, acute onset of generalized shoulder pain should suggest either rupture of the supraspinatus muscle or separation of the AC joint. Rotator cuff lesions are frequently characterized by pain that occurs only during a specific portion of the range of motion examination. In contrast, arthritis or inflammation of the joint capsule will produce pain during all phases of shoulder movement. Pain that accompanies an overhead motion may signal an impingement syndrome, whereas a snap or catch associated with ball throwing may indicate a rotator cuff tear or damage to the biceps tendon.

Tendinitis of the infraspinatus muscle frequently produces posterior shoulder pain, whereas patients with biceps tendinitis tend to localize pain anteriorly at the biceps groove. Discomfort over lateral shoulder structures, sometimes accompanied by radiation, are suggestive of glenohumeral arthritis, supraspinatus tendinitis, or subacromial bursitis. A constant, unremitting pain should arouse suspicion of a malignancy. Finally, it should be stressed that abdominal pathology can produce referred pain that radiates to the shoulder.

Physical Examination. *(Please see Table 1.)* The emergency physician frequently can make the correct diagnosis with careful inspection of the shoulder joint. For example, the high wing of a complete AC separation and the squared-off, boxed-shaped shoulder associated with anterior shoulder dislocations are well-described findings. The position of the arm, shoulder asymmetry, muscle wasting, and obvious deformities should be noted in the record. Moreover, both active and passive range of motion exercises should be attempted, but only as tolerated by the patient. In this regard, passive range of motion is often more painful in patients with acute injuries, arthritis, and bursitis, whereas active range of motion is more painful in patients with tendinitis. It is frequently more informative to have the patient execute a set of movements with both arms simultaneously in order to note differences in arc, pattern, and range of motion between the injured and normal shoulder.

Because patients with shoulder injuries are frequently in severe pain, a systematic range of motion exam should be performed expeditiously. First, ask the patient to reach straight forward, with arms in a horizontal position relative to the ground. This is followed by having the patient reach overhead and then back past the ears as far as possible. Next, instruct the patient to put a hand on the small of the back, and then the head, as high as he or she can reach. Permit the patient to drop his or her arms to a resting position at his or her side and then have the patient hold his or her elbows against the body as he or she rotates outward with both hands. The physician should abduct the arms to 90°, after which the patient should attempt to perform the same maneuver. If the patient cannot bring the arm away from his or her side or if abduction is limited to no more 20-30°, a rotator cuff tear should be suspected.

Resistance testing requires slightly more time. Instruct the patient to hold both arms at 90° abduction (i.e., straight out at the sides with hands in a neutral position and palms downward). Push down on the elbow and ask the patient resist this maneuver. A rotator cuff tear is associated with significant weakness of the involved arm. Axillary nerve damage will produce deltoid paresis and decreased strength in the involved arm. With the arms still in the abducted position, rotate the palm against resistance. Internal and external rotation weakness may indicate damage to the external rotator cuff or internal rotator tendons.

Finally, the patient should be evaluated using pain-provoking maneuvers. *(Please see Table 2.)* One of the most useful involves extending the elbow as the arm is brought back in an arc of extension behind the trunk. Called the Speed test, this maneuver stretches the biceps tendon and pulls it into the biceps groove. Patient with biceps tendinitis will report significant pain induction with this provocative test.

Radiography. Precise interpretation of plain radiographs is pivotal to optimizing management of shoulder injuries. Without exception, comprehensive evaluation of the glenohumeral joint requires at least two views of the shoulder girdle, including an anteroposterior (AP) film, and one additional view at either 90° or some other angle relative to the AP projection. It should be stressed that the AP view does not provide all the information required to interpret shoulder trauma; therefore, reliance on a single radiographic view is not recommended.

The complementary view may include a transthoracic lateral or an axillary projection. The transthoracic x-ray is especially useful in suspected dislocations, whereas the axillary view is tailored not only for evaluation of shoulder dislocations, but for detection of subtle, scapular fractures and coracoid abnormalities. The scapula-Y view provides a 60° anterior oblique view of the shoulder in the upright position, which is useful not only for confirmation of dislocation, but for subluxation of the humerus and scapular fractures. In the case of dislocation, the scapula-Y view will demonstrate inferior displacement of the humeral head and subluxation of the humerus in the absence of posterior or anterior displacement.

Other views include the "West Point" axillary, Stryker notch, and Neer views. The Stryker view is particularly helpful for demonstrating a Hill-Sachs humeral head defect, which is seen in dislocations and recurrent subluxations. The Neer view is simply an AP with about 15-25° of cephalad angulation and is useful for evaluation of the acromion process.1

Many radiologists also include AP views with internal and external rotation. Although soft tissue (muscolotendinous) injuries are not well visualized on plain film radiographs, both computerized tomography (CT) and MRI may be used to delineate these injuries. MRI can demonstrate the rotator cuff and the supraspinatus muscle, with some studies suggesting that MRI may be more accurate in these conditions than simple arthrograms.[1] CT scanning may be combined with an arthrogram to demonstrate abnormalities of the rotator cuff.

Soft-Tissue Injuries

Tendinitis. Although tendinitis may involve any of the structures that stabilize, traverse, or insert into the shoulder, the two most frequent sites of occurrence include the supraspinatus and biceps tendons.[2] In fact, supraspinatus tendinitis may be the most common cause of acute shoulder pain in patients presenting to the ED.[2,3] The distal part of the tendon is particularly susceptible to inflammation, degeneration, and calcification, especially in middle-age and older individuals. Recurrent stress of the tendon increases the likelihood of injury, and the condition may be either chronic or acute.

Rotator cuff tendinitis characteristically produces pain in the back of the arm and at the insertion of the deltoid muscle. Physical findings include pain that is elicited during active abduction and that is most intense from 70-120° of abduction.[3] The pain usually decreases with motion beyond this range, and the patient may be tender in the area around the supraspinatus muscle, beneath the acromion laterally and anteriorly.

Biceps tendinitis is associated with pain that radiates down the anterior arm, increases with abduction, and is most severe when the arm is laterally rotated and abducted. The examiner may provoke discomfort by flexing the biceps against resistance. Moreover, during elevation of the biceps, the tendon may slip out of the biceps groove. Because the long head of the biceps tendon is continuous with the capsule, symptoms of biceps tendinitis may mimic those of rotator cuff injury.

Initial Management. Initial treatment of tendinitis involving shoulder structures consists of rest, a short (2-3 days) period of shoulder immobilization, ice for the first 12-24 hours, and non-steroidal anti-inflammatory drugs (NSAIDs). After pain relief has been achieved, the patient should be instructed in range-of-motion exercises with the arm hanging in a dependent position (i.e., pendulum exercises). In addition, the patient should be introduced to the idea of "active rest"—cessation of motions that cause pain, but continuation of exercises and activities that do not produce extreme discomfort. Gradual return to full activity should be started only after the patient is entirely free of pain.

Table 2. Pain-Provoking Maneuvers

BICEPS TENDINITIS

Flex elbow to 90° and palpate biceps groove
Pain with resistance of supination (Yergason's sign)[3]
Extending the elbow and bringing the arm back behind the trunk (external rotation) will cause pain (Speed test)

SUPRASPINATUS TENDINITIS

Palpate tendon during resisted abduction
External rotation of the arm is limited by pain

IMPINGEMENT

Bring the arm up into maximum flexion (start of an overhead tennis serve)

INFRASPINATUS TENDINITIS

Flex the elbow to 90° and bring the arm to 90° of abduction, then palpate the posterior aspect of the greater tuberosity

SUBSCAPULARIS TENDINITIS

Flex the elbow 90° and have the patient attempt medial rotation against resistance. Then palpate medial to the lesser tuberosity.

Subacromial Impingement Syndrome. Motions that push the humerus against the acromion produce a mechanical impingement syndrome, which is characterized by pain in the anterior shoulder that is exacerbated by overhead shoulder movements such as those required for swimming, tennis, and baseball. Manual laborers who work overhead, including electricians, sheet rockers, and painters, also are at risk for developing this injury,[4] which may lead to inflammation of the supraspinatus ligament.

This condition has been classified into three stages: Stage 1, which consists of edema and hemorrhage in the subacromial space; Stage 2, characterized by thickening and fibrosis of the subacromial bursa; and Stage 3, characterized by a full-thickness tear of the rotator cuff.[5]

In the early stages, the patient will report a dull, aching pain after exercise. There is often point tenderness over the anterior of the acromion and greater tuberosity. If the patient reaches for the sky and brings the hands forward, the pain will be intensified. Later in the course of this injury, the patient may note a "catch" as the arm is elevated or lowered from an abducted position.

NSAID therapy should be initiated, ice should be applied to the area, the shoulder should be immobilized, and the patient should be instructed to avoid maneuvers that reproduce the pain.

Figure 2. Anterior Muscles of the Rotator Cuff

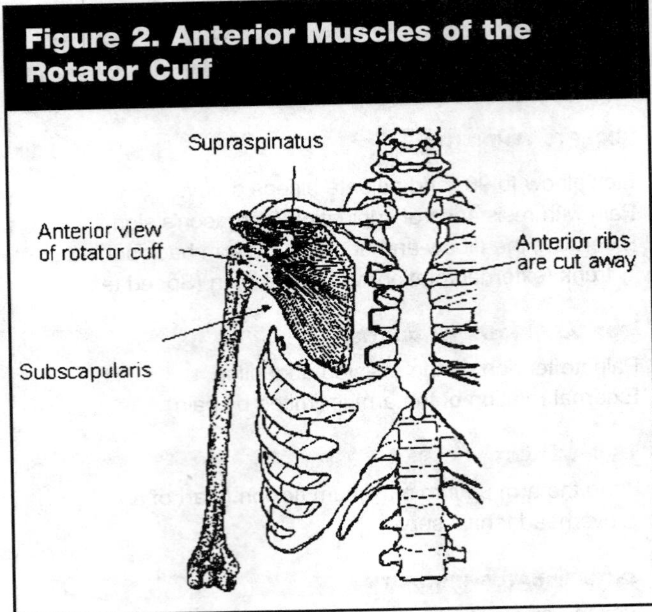

Figure 3. Posterior Muscles of the Rotator Cuff

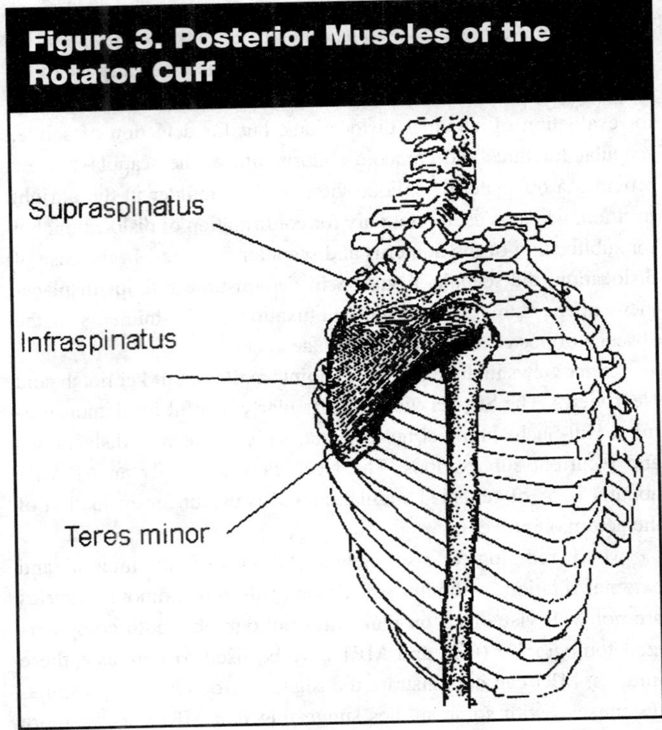

Physical therapy and follow-up with an orthopedic surgeon are recommended.

Rotator Cuff Tears. *(Please see Figure 2 and Figure 3.)* Rotator cuff tears, which most often involve the supraspinatus tendon, may be seen with or without trauma. Although trauma is usually implicated in younger patients, in older patients, the incidence of rotator cuff injuries without trauma increases dramatically. Because of the morbidity associated with this condition, recognition of a complete rupture of the supraspinatus tendon is essential.

Clinical Findings. Although pain in the the deltoid muscle is often the first indication of a rotator cuff tear, this symptom is rarely diagnostic.[6] However, if the patient experiences pain on abduction of the shoulder, then a rotator cuff tear should be suspected. With partial tears of the rotator cuff, the patient may still be able to abduct the arm, but only with significant pain. With a complete tear of the rotator cuff, the patient cannot abduct or externally rotate the arm. Complete tears of the remaining rotator cuff tendons may not cause shoulder instability,[7] but if the patient attempts to abduct the arm, the deltoid muscle will elevate the humerus under the overhanging acromion.

The patient may be able to abduct the shoulder by rotation of the scapula. Because the supraspinatus muscle initiates abduction, pain occurs when abduction is initiated. A characteristic position is assumed with the neck angled toward the injured shoulder, which may be hunched up in order to produce the requested abduction. The shoulder will usually hurt at this point, and to compensate, the patient may try to whip the arm above this point and let the more powerful deltoid muscle stabilize the abduction. If the patient has had a chronic injury, this maneuver may be so slick that the patient appears to have almost normal function.

In the case of a partial tear of the rotator cuff, the patient may complain of the arm "catching" at a certain angle of abduction. The arm can be elevated beyond this point with some pain as this critical point is reached. However, once beyond the "catch," the arm can be elevated normally. As the arm is lowered, there may be a similar "catch" on the way down. This phenomenon is thought to be caused by a nodule of collagen fibers—which is caught between the acromion and the greater tubercle during active abduction—positioned along the supraspinatus tendon at the site of the partial tear.[6]

Imaging. Imaging of rotator cuff tendons is accomplished with shoulder arthrograms, ultrasound, CT, and MRI. The gold standard for diagnosis of a complete rotator cuff tear is arthroscopy.[8] MRI is considered an excellent tool for detection of rotator cuff tears.[9]

Initial Management. Early repair of tendon tears increases the chances of complete recovery. Consequently, if the patient is suspected of having an acute rotator cuff tear, immobilization, ice, analgesia, and prompt referral to an orthopedic surgeon are essential. If the patient has a chronic cuff tear, then a sling or shoulder immobilizer, NSAIDs, and referral to an orthopedic surgeon are appropriate.

Subacromial Bursitis. The supraspinatus tendon passes along the subacromial bursa. Consequently, subacromial bursitis is often secondary to tendinitis of the rotator cuff or biceps. If the supraspinatus tendon becomes inflamed, the adjacent bursa is frequently involved. As inflammation increases, the bursa may even rupture. And if the inflammatory process becomes chronic, calcium deposition may produce a chronic bursitis and adhesive capsulitis.

Unfortunately, it is almost impossible to clinically distinguish acute subacromial bursitis from supraspinatus tendinitis. Radiographs taken later in the patient's course may show calcification of the bursa in the region of the greater tuberosity. Most patients will respond to ice, brief immobilization of the shoulder, and NSAIDs. Injection of cortisone and lidocaine mixture into the subacromial bursa will decrease the pain considerably. In general, no more than two cortisone injections should be administered in order to avoid damage to the rotator cuff.[9] The shoulder should not be immobilized for longer than a few days, because this will increase the chances of an adhesive capsulitis. The patient should be referred to an orthopedic surgeon for further follow-up.

Shoulder (Glenohumeral) Dislocations

A shoulder dislocation is defined as complete separation of the humeral head from the glenoid fossa. The humeral head can be dislocated inferiorly, anteriorly, or posteriorly. Because the acromion prevents upward movement of the humerus, it is not possible to have a superior dislocation of the shoulder.

Anterior Dislocation. The most common dislocation in the body,[10,11] anterior dislocation of the shoulder is most often caused by external forces pushing the arm into abduction, extension, and external rotation. The head of the humerus may be displaced into the subglenoid, subcoracoid, or subclavicular regions. Following anterior shoulder dislocation, the humeral head is always pulled to the medial portion of the shoulder by the muscles of the rotator cuff. *(See Figure 4.)* As a result, the patient's shoulder will be squared off and the head of the humerus can be palpated anteriorly. Since these forces also stretch the muscles of the rotator cuff, associated tears are common.

In addition, anterior dislocation of the shoulder can compromise the axillary nerve. When this occurs, physical examination will demonstrate weakness in the deltoid muscle and poor strength in shoulder abduction. A sensory deficit may be detected in the upper lateral arm and shoulder. Because of the intense pain associated with shoulder dislocation, these findings are often missed. Return of axillary nerve function is likely if there is prompt reduction.

Radiographs. Anterior dislocation is best visualized on the AP view. If there is any question as to whether the dislocation is anterior or posterior, the axillary or Y-scapular views will provide resolution. About 5-15% of anterior dislocations will have an associated greater tuberosity fracture.[12] Post-reduction x-rays may show a Hill-Sachs compression fracture of the posterior and lateral surface of the humeral head,[13] which results when the soft humeral head impinges on the glenoid rim during either reduction or dislocation. This associated injury is found in about 35-40% of cases.[14] Anterior glenoid fractures may occur by the same mechanism.

Initial Management. Because shoulder dislocation is extremely painful, appropriate analgesia, ice, and immobilization of the injured shoulder should be instituted expeditiously. Following successful reduction (see below), the shoulder should be immobilized for a minimum of three weeks with either a sling and swath or a commercial shoulder immobilizer. The patient should be referred to an orthopedic surgeon for follow-up within 2-3 days. Judicious use of postreduction NSAIDs, ice to the area, and elevation will decrease swelling and subsequent pain.

Reduction Methods. Because no single shoulder reduction technique is infallible, the emergency physician should be proficient in several methods. *(Please see Table 3.)* Only 5-10% of anterior shoulder dislocations cannot be reduced in the ED.[15] Three basic methods, including traction, leverage, manipulation of the scapula—as well as methods that combine all three strategies—are recommended and will achieve a 70-90% success rate for a first reduction attempt.[15]

Although some operators feel that a shoulder may be reduced "painlessly," all of the techniques described below will be facilitated by use of appropriate analgesia (meperidine), antiemetics, and muscle relaxation agents (benzodiazepines).

Figure 4. Anterior Shoulder Dislocations

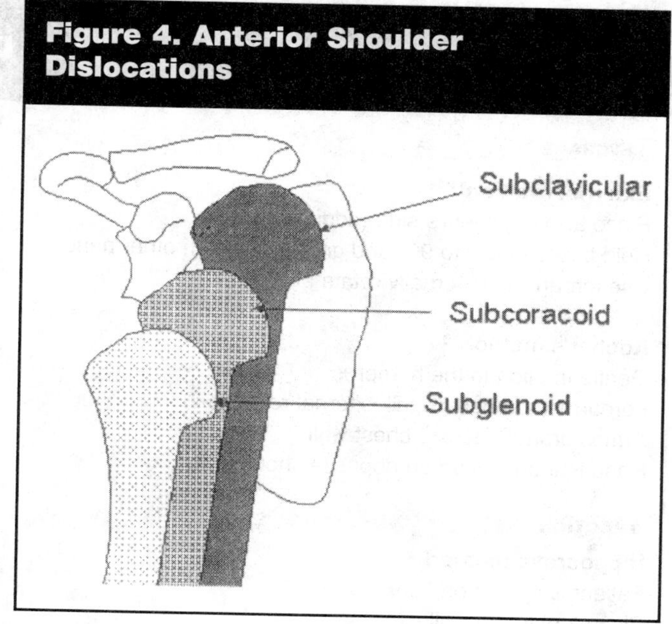

Traction. Traction methods require stretching the muscles that hold the humeral head in the dislocated position. As these muscles are stretched, the humeral head moves to the edge of the glenoid fossa and then springs back into a normal position. In the abduction or Hippocratic maneuver, the physician's foot is placed into the axilla and then pulls along the axis of the arm and leans backward. The foot acts as a lever to push the humeral head laterally, while the physician pulls the head toward the patient's foot along the surface of the glenoid. Although frequently successful, this method can cause brachial plexus palsy or damage to the brachial vessels.

In the traction-countertraction technique, a sheet is placed around the torso and an assistant provides countertraction in the direction of the opposite shoulder. The examiner bends the patient's elbow 90° to provide a traction point. A second sheet around the examiner's waist and the patient's arm will allow substantial force to be developed by simply leaning back. With a gradual increase in traction and gentle external rotation of the arm, the head of the humerus will "pop" back into place. In difficult reductions, the assistant may push upward (anteriorly) on the underside of the humeral head.

In the Stimson method, which is advocated for the frail or obese individual, the patient is placed prone on a cot. The affected arm is allowed to hang over the edge of the cot. A heavy weight (10-pound sandbag or bucket of water) is placed and taped into the hand. This gradually lengthens and relaxes the contracted muscles and, eventually, the shoulder reduces spontaneously. It should be stressed that substantial patience is needed, since this method may require 15-20 minutes or longer in muscular individuals. The most common problem associated with the Stimson method is that the cot is not high enough for the weights to clear the floor. Stimson's method is ideal for the very apprehensive patient as it is simple, atraumatic, and does not require unfamiliar maneuvers.[15]

The Milch/Cooper method is arguably the least painful method for reducing an anterior shoulder dislocation.[15] The physician places a hand on the shoulder with the thumb against the dislocated humeral head. The patient's arm is gently abducted to the overhead position, and the head of the humerus is supported so that it cannot move

Table 3. Reduction Methods for Shoulder Dislocations

LEVERAGE

External rotation[11,16]
Place arm at patient's side (adduction).
Hold flexed elbow to 90° and grasp wrist with other hand
Use forearm to externally rotate arm

Kocher's method[10]
Gentle traction to the humerus
Forearm is brought to full external rotation
Arm is brought across chest wall
Hand is then placed on opposite shoulder

TRACTION

Hippocratic method
Patient is supine on floor
Place foot in the axilla
Lift arm and pull by leaning back

Traction-countertraction
Patient is supine on bed
Place sheet around torso
Assistant pulls on sheet toward point of opposite shoulder
Elbow flexed 90°

Traction and external rotation of arm
Stimson (hanging weight)[39]
Patient is prone on cot
Arm is hanging over the cot (forward flexion)
10-pound sandbag is attached to the hand
Apply patiently to the patient (15-20 minutes)

Eskimo method (hanging patient)[40]
Patient lies on unaffected side on the floor
Physician (and assistant) lift patient upward by arm

Milch/Cooper method[41]
Patient is supine
Hold the head of the humerus in place with a thumb
Abduct the arm to the overhead position
As the arm is abducted, it is externally rotated
Apply traction along the axis of the humerus
Push the head of the humerus over the glenoid rim with the thumb

SCAPULAR MANIPULATION[42]
Patient is prone on table with arm hanging over side
5-10 pounds of weight are placed on arm for about five minutes
Superior border of scapula is stabilized
Inferior tip of scapula is rotated medially

downward. As it is abducted, the arm is gently externally rotated. When the arm is overhead, the physician pushes the head of the humerus over the glenoid rim and into the fossa. Often, analgesia is not required, and there are few failures.

Leverage Methods. This technique is based on various maneuvers that can leverage the head of the humerus back into the glenoid fossa. In the Kocher method, gentle traction is applied to the head of the humerus in a supine patient. The forearm is externally rotated to about 60°. While the forearm is held in external rotation, the entire arm is brought across the chest. Unfortunately, this method has been associated with fractures of the humerus and damage to surrounding soft tissue.[10]

This approach is not appropriate in an elderly patient due to the high stress placed on the humeral neck. Moreover, it is much more difficult to employ in obese and heavy patients. A less traumatic variant of the leverage technique involves externally rotating the arm, abducting it to the patient's side, and then applying traction to the humerus.[11] Far fewer complications are noted with this method than with the Kocher method.[16,17]

Scapular Manipulation. At first, scapular manipulation appears to be a variant of the Stimson maneuver. But unlike the Stimson maneuver, the primary focus is not to move the head of the humerus, but to manipulate the glenoid back into the usual position.[18] The patient is placed in a prone position with the arm hanging off of the table. A weight of 5-10 pounds is placed in the hand. After 5-10 minutes of hanging, the physician pushes the tip of the scapula medially and stabilizes the superior and medial surface of the scapula.[19] The scapula is rotated around the superior portion. It is thought that traction on the externally rotated humerus elevates the humeral head from the glenoid fossa. The scapula is then manipulated back into an anatomic position and the humeral head is carried into reduction. In many patients, this technique may be performed without anesthesia or sedation.[20] As a rule, it is gentle and has few complications.

Complications. The most common complication of anterior dislocation is tear of the glenoid labrum.[14] Recent studies show that there may be a significant relationship between this lesion and recurrent dislocation of the shoulder in younger patients.[21,22] Unfortunately, there is little in the literature on the diagnosis and treatment of this lesion.

Shoulder dislocations complicated by fractures of the humeral head—including fractures of the surgical neck as well as those of the tuberosities—are the most difficult to reduce. Fracture dislocations are rare in children.[23] When fractures and dislocations coexist, urgent orthopedic referral is mandatory.

Nerve Injury. Injuries to the brachial plexus and peripheral nerves can occur with a shoulder dislocation. Elderly patients and those with obvious hematomas have a higher incidence of nerve palsy.[24] Axillary nerve palsy is the most frequent nerve injury and can produce hypoesthesia or sensory loss over the deltoid area. The most commonly involved peripheral nerve, musculocutaneous nerve injury causes sensory loss over the radial aspect of the forearm. The prognosis for recovery of function is usually good if only one nerve is involved, but is less favorable if the brachial plexus or multiple peripheral nerves are involved.

Vascular Injuries. Arterial damage may include intimal damage, thrombosis, avulsion of a branch of the axillary artery, or rupture of the main trunk of the axillary artery. The subscapular or circumflex arteries are the most commonly avulsed branches of the axillary artery.

Recurrent Dislocation. Recurrent shoulder dislocation is a frequent long-term complication of patients who are younger than 20 years, in whom there is an 80-90% dislocation recurrence rate.[25] An associated avulsion fracture of the tuberosity decreases the likelihood of a recurrence. If the patient's shoulder is not appropriately immobilized after the injury, the rate of recurrent dislocation increases at all ages. A Hill-Sachs compression fracture of the posterior humeral head or a fracture of the glenoid rim is associated with a higher rate of recurrent dislocations.[22]

Posterior Dislocation. Forceful adduction and internal rotation of the shoulder may occur following direct trauma or a seizure. The humeral head is trapped and caught on the posterior rim of the glenoid fossa at the concave portion of the humeral head. This concavity is medial to the lesser tuberosity. The patient presents with the arm locked in internal rotation and adduction and, therefore, can neither abduct nor externally rotate the shoulder. The coracoid process is prominent and the head of the humerus can be palpated posteriorly under the acromion.

Radiography. The principal diagnostic pitfall is excessive dependence on the AP film of the shoulder, because the humeral head can be obscured by the overlying scapula on this view. The single best view to demonstrate a posterior dislocation is probably the scapula-Y view of the shoulder, in which the anterior glenoid fossa can be visualized at the center of the Y-shaped scapula. The head of the humerus will overlap the posterior rim and and will be inferior to the acromion.

Initial Management. In most cases of posterior dislocation, immediate orthopedic consultation is appropriate. It is probably best to reduce posterior dislocations under general anesthesia rather than conscious sedation. Posterior dislocations are quite painful and require greater muscle relaxation for reduction.

Inferior Dislocation (Luxatio Erecta). Inferior dislocation of the glenohumeral joint is rare. The mechanism is usually hyperabduction and extension of the arm with the arm pronated. This type of shoulder dislocation differs from anterior and posterior dislocations in that the superior aspect of the head of the humerus is directed inferiorly. The glenohumeral capsule is often ruptured and a "buttonhole" effect occurs where the humeral head is driven through the capsule inferiorly.

The classic finding is an abducted arm with the elbow flexed and the hand above the head. A depression or crease on top of the shoulder demonstrates the acute angle of the humerus with the acromion. The head of the humerus can often be palpated on the chest wall, and the patient often has a radial nerve palsy with decreased sensation in the distribution of the axillary nerve. Most inferior glenohumeral dislocations are associated with rotator cuff tears. In addition, the greater tuberosity, acromion, and the inferior glenoid fossa may be fractured with the force of the inferior dislocation.[26]

Initial Management. Closed reduction may be attempted with traction-countertraction if there is no fracture. This should be followed by shoulder immobilization and a surgical consult. The patient may require surgical repair of the rotator cuff following reduction. If a buttonhole effect occurs, closed reduction will be unsuccessful and operative reduction is needed.[26]

Shoulder Fractures

Clavicular Fractures. Clavicle fractures account for about 40% of all shoulder injuries and about 5% of all fractures.[27,28] The mechanism of injury may include a fall onto the shoulder with a forward roll. Sudden force on the medial end of the clavicle can also dislocate the clavicle at the sternum.[29] Generally speaking, the patient will complain of pain in the region of the fracture; swelling and tenderness are usually found at the fracture site. Swelling, tenderness, and crepitus are found in the region of the fracture. The patient often will carry the shoulder slumped downward and forward and support the elbow with the opposite hand. However, precise localization may be difficult, especially in children.

Fractures of the proximal third of the clavicle are the least common and account for about 6% of all clavicular fractures,[28] most of which are due to blunt trauma. Fortunately, complications of clavicle fractures are rare. However, if the fracture is displaced posteriorly, it can endanger structures of the superior mediastinum. Middle third fractures are most common, accounting for about 75-80% of clavicular fractures.[27,28] Fracture fragments may be widely displaced due to the weight of the arm and the pull of the muscles on the clavicle. Since the neurovascular bundle is located beneath the bone, there is a potential for associated neurovascular complications. Lateral third fractures account for only 10-15% of clavicle fractures but are associated with the highest risk of complications.[27,28]

Shoulder pain, stiffness, nonunion of fragments, and osteoarthritis of the AC joint have been reported following a fracture of the distal third of the clavicle.[27,28] Intra-articular fractures of the clavicle are associated with osteoarthritis of the AC joint and are frequently missed on initial radiographs. Fractures with displacement of the distal fragment and disruption of the coraco-clavicular ligaments are associated with frequent nonunion of fracture fragments. This may be due to the increased forces on the fragments at this site. Undisplaced lateral clavicle fractures tend to have fewer complications.

Initial Management. To some degree, initial management of clavicular injuries will depend on the location of the fracture site. Without exception, however, the fracture should be immobilized and supported. Appropriate pain management, ice to the area, and gentle evaluation of the fracture are required. Although vascular complications are rare, every patient deserves evaluation of the neurovascular status of the hand. Comminuted, widely displaced fractures should be referred emergently to an orthopedic surgeon for possible open reduction. A fracture associated with pneumothorax, vessel damage, or nerve palsy requires immediate consultation.

Stable distal clavicle fractures can be treated with a sling; range-of-motion exercises can be started as soon as the patient is able. Fractures that are distal to the coracoclavicular ligament may also need operative reduction, particularly if the fragments are displaced. These unstable fractures of the distal clavicle should be referred to an orthopedic surgeon for further care. For fractures involving the middle third of the clavicle, immobilization is best accomplished with a padded cloth figure-of-eight bandage. The figure-of-eight bandage wraps over the anterior shoulder and goes under the axilla posteriorly. These devices attempt to draw the shoulders up and back to bring the distal fragment to the proximal fragments. Although they support the fracture sufficiently to prevent subsequent pain and to maintain an acceptable position, they do not reduce the fracture.

Humeral Fractures. Proximal fractures of the humerus can cause bone necrosis, osteoarthritis, and chronic shoulder pain. Fractures of the proximal humerus are more common in older adults. Since the major blood supply of the proximal humerus is fed through both tuberosities, a fracture must involve both tuberosities in order to cause an avascular head.

Fractures with minimal displacement usually have a good outcome and are stable. If the tuberosities are displaced from the humeral head, then there is a substantial chance of subsequent osteonecrosis. Fracture dislocations are associated with substantial trauma and have a higher incidence of neurovascular complications.

Clinical Findings. In most cases, the patient will present with shoulder pain and significant tenderness in the shoulder and upper arm. The patient will not move the shoulder and will resist any attempt at either active or passive motion. Patients who present soon after the fracture may have little or no swelling, although there may be contusions or abrasions noted on the upper arm or shoulder. Delayed presentations may be accompanied by a substantial hematoma or ecchymosis.

Initial Management. Acute management of these fractures should be directed toward immobilization and pain control. A sling and swath or commercial shoulder immobilizer are usually adequate. In addition, the shoulder should be carefully evaluated for a concomitant dislocation and neurovascular damage. Epiphyseal fractures in children and widely displaced fragments at any age should mandate an orthopedic consult. The presence of a concomitant dislocation or involvement of both tuberosities also calls for an orthopedic consultation.

Scapular Fractures. Fractures of the scapula are uncommon, probably because the scapula is strong, not easily disrupted, and not subject to bending during falls. When these fractures do occur, it is because a significant amount of force has been directly applied to the area. This makes the scapular fracture notable for the following associated injuries: pulmonary contusion, rib fractures, clavicular fractures, or brachial plexus injuries.[30] Injury to the brachial plexus is extremely rare following blunt trauma unless the patient has a scapular fracture. In general, a major scapular fracture will be visible on any AP view of the chest. The AP film may not be sufficient for small isolated fractures of the body of the scapula or glenoid fossa, however. If a major fracture of the scapula is present, then a diligent search for associated severe injuries is indicated.

Miscellaneous Shoulder Injuries

Subluxation of the Shoulder. A shoulder subluxation is defined as increased excursion of the humerus around the glenoid fossa. This may occur after a dislocation or as a primary disease process. The shoulder may be displaced when the inferior capsule or the lip of the glenoid is stretched or torn. In contrast, superior subluxation may occur when a sudden weight is placed on an arm that is extended upward (e.g., someone who is falling tries to stop the fall by grabbing at a ledge or branch with one hand). The body weight forces the shoulder upward and tears the insertion of the rotator cuff from the greater tuberosity. Inferior subluxation occurs when the muscles of the rotator cuff are torn or atrophy after a prolonged immobilization. A serious rotator cuff tear is can be associated with inferior subluxation.

Clinical Findings. A patient with a subluxation will often complain of a sensation of the shoulder slipping in and out of joint. He or she may feel or hear cracking or popping sounds in the joint. In other cases, the patient may experience a sudden, sharp pain and note that the limb feels weak or "goes dead." This is particularly common after excessive throwing or serving in tennis or racquetball. In addition, the patient may complain of loss of control of the arm or dropping of objects. In anterior subluxation, the patient will report loss of external rotation with the arm at the side or when raised 90°. The patient may be tender in the posterior humeral head, especially when the arm is adducted across the chest. The patient may also guard when asked to abduct and externally rotate the arm. In a posterior subluxation, the patient is unable to internally rotate the arm when it is at 90°. A backward push, elevation of the arm forward to 90°, or internal rotation may cause the patient to guard.

Acromioclavicular Separations and Dislocations. Acromioclavicular injuries, which are commonly encountered in the ED, often result from a fall directly on the shoulder or a fall on an outstretched hand. This injury is frequently found in skiers and football, rugby, or soccer players. The patient often presents to the ED with the injured arm cradled in the opposite hand.

Acromioclavicular separation is divided into several grades.[31] A grade I sprain is a minor tear of the AC ligaments without any damage to the coracoclavicular (CC) ligaments. A grade II injury is a rupture of the AC ligament with stretching of the CC ligaments. A grade III injury indicates a complete tear of both the AC and CC ligaments. Grade IV injuries, with posterior clavicular displacement, and grade V injuries, with marked superior clavicular displacement, have been described but are rare.[32]

Clinical Findings. The most consistent physical finding in an AC separation is pain in the AC joint. Pain is increased with most manipulations of the clavicle. Patients will limit range of motion with both active and passive range of motion. A prominent bulge is often present where the distal clavicle rides above the acromion in a grade III AC separation. Temporary reduction of the bulge may or may not be possible, depending on the degree of soft-tissue swelling between the acromion and the distal clavicle. In some grade II separations there is a slight bulge, but grade I separations have no bulge.

It is important to compare the injured side with the opposite side because the normal clavicle may be prominent. It is also important to note whether the patient has had a prior AC separation or injury, because a distal clavicular prominence may represent old injury. The most confusion results when the patient has an old AC separation on the opposite side and a new lesion on the acutely injured side.

Radiographs. Although many experts recommend both plain films of the shoulder and stress radiographs (weighted shoulder films), this is controversial. A consistent x-ray finding in grade III AC separations is visible widening of the AC joint on normal views of the shoulder. The extra weighted films of the shoulder are designed to "unmask" otherwise unapparent grade III AC strains. Stress views have a low diagnostic yield, and it is uncertain how frequently these extra films are needed.[32] They do cause extra radiation exposure and expense to the patient, so they should be ordered judiciously. The single most important complication associated with this injury is a displaced fracture of the coracoid process of the scapula.

Initial Management. More than 50 different bandaging techniques and 30 different surgical procedures have been recommended for this injury in the literature.[33] More recent studies suggest that a nonoperative approach is preferable for most patients.[33-36] Immediate treatment of an AC separation includes a shoulder immobilizer, ice to the area, appropriate pain relief, and referral to an orthopedic surgeon. If the patient has a grade II or III injury, then the referral should be more urgent.

Sternoclavicular Dislocations and Strains. Although the sternoclavicular joint is not part of the shoulder, it is essential to mobility of the shoulder joints. Dislocation of the sternoclavicular joint is relatively rare but is easy to diagnose once suspected.[37] Because posterior dislocations may precipitate a pneumothorax or injury to the superior mediastinal contents, prompt diagnosis is essential.

Clinical Findings. When a patient who has injured the shoulder guards the upper arm and also tilts the head toward the injured side, trauma to the medial clavicle should be suspected. The patient may complain of pain and point tenderness about the medial end of the clavicle. Inspection of the chest may demonstrate an elevation or depression of the skin over the injured joint, ecchymosis near the medial third of the clavicle, or swelling of the medial portion of the clavicle.

Anterior dislocations are far more frequent than posterior dislocations.[38] Because the injury may be difficult to identify on standard chest x-rays or clavicle series, a CT scan may be needed to identify this dislocation.

Initial Management. Sternoclavicular joint strains should be treated with a shoulder immobilizer, ice, NSAIDs, and non-urgent referral to an orthopedic surgeon. Closed reduction of a dislocation of the sternoclavicular joint can be performed by placing a sandbag in the middle of the back between the scapulae and extending the arm with lateral traction. The medial end of the clavicle is then reduced with direct pressure or traction as appropriate. If this maneuver is not successful, operative reduction is required. A delay in attempting closed reduction will mean a higher failure rate.

Summary

Acute evaluation of the injured or painful shoulder requires a careful, detailed physical examination. Pain management is an important clinical priority, and orthopedic referral is necessary in the majority of patients. Diagnostic errors can be avoided by a directed radiographic examination that includes appropriate views, comparison studies, and provocative maneuvers, when necessary. Finally, experience with shoulder reduction techniques is mandatory for the management of shoulder dislocations, the majority of which can be reduced in the emergency setting.

References

1. Pope TL, Chen MYM. Imaging the acutely painful shoulder. *Emerg Med* 1992;Sept 15:122.
2. Riley GP, Harral RL, Constant CR, et al. Glycosaminoglycans of human rotator cuff tendons: Changes with age and in chronic rotator cuff tendinitis. *Ann Rheum Dis* 1994;53: 367-376.
3. Bonafede RP, Bennett RM. Shoulder pain: Guidelines to diagnosis and management. *Postgrad Med* 1987;82:185.
4. Hunting KL, Welch LS, Cuccherini BA, et al. Musculoskeletal symptoms among electricians. *Am J Indust Med* 1994;25:149.
5. Neer CS. Anterior acromioplasty for the chronic impingement syndrome of the shoulder. *J Bone Joint Surg* (Am) 1972;54:41.
6. Bigiliani LU, Kimmel, J, McCann PD, et al. Repair of rotator cuff tears in tennis players. *Am J Sports Med* 1992; 20:112.
7. Gerber C, Krushell RJ. Isolated rupture of the tendon of the subscapularis muscle. *J Bone Joint Surg (Br)* 1991;73B:389.
8. Neer CS. *Shoulder Reconstruction*. Philadelphia: WB Saunders; 1990.
9. McCann PD, Bigliani LU. Shoulder pain in tennis players. *Sports Med* 1994;17:53.
10. Nash J. The status of Kocher's method of reducing recent anterior dislocation of the shoulder. *J Bone Joint Surg* 1934; 16A:535.
11. Leidelmeyer R. Reduced! A shoulder, subtly and painlessly. *Emerg Med* 1977;9:233.
12. DePalma AF, Flannery GF. Acute anterior dislocation of the shoulder. *Am J Sports Med* 1973;1:6-15.
13. Harvey RA, Trabulsy ME, Roe L. Are postreduction anteroposterior and scapular Y views useful in anterior shoulder dislocations? *Am J Emerg Med* 1992;10:149.
14. Baker CL, Uribe JW, Whitman C. Arthroscopic evaluation of acute initial anterior shoulder dislocations. *Am J Sports Med* 1990;18:25.
15. Riebel GD, McCabe JB. Anterior shoulder dislocation: A review of reduction techniques. *J Emerg Med* 1991;9:180.
16. Mirick MJ, Clinton JE, Ruiz E. External rotation method of shoulder dislocation reduction. *JACEP* 1979;8:528.
17. Danzl DF. Closed reduction of anterior subcoracoid shoulder dislocation, evaluation of an external rotation method. *Orthoped Rev* 1986;15:75-79.
18. Kothari RU, Dronen SC. Prospective evaluation of the scapular manipulation technique in reducing anterior shoulder dislocations. *Ann Emerg Med* 1992;21:1349.
19. Kothari RU, Dronen SC. Prospective evaluation of the scapular manipulation technique in reducing anterior shoulder dislocations. *Ann Emerg Med* 1992;21:1349-1352.
20. McNamara RM. Reduction of anterior shoulder dislocations by scapular manipulation. *Ann Emerg Med* 1993;22:1140.
21. Altchek DW, Warren RF, Wickiewicz TL, et al. Arthroscopic labral debridement: A three year follow-up study. *Am J Sports Med* 1992;20:702.
22. Vermeiren J, Handelberg F, Casteleyn PP, et al. The rate of recurrence of traumatic anterior dislocation of the shoulder. *Int Orthoped* 1993;17:337-341.
23. Obremsky W, Routt MLC. Fracture-dislocation of the shoulder in a child: Case report. *J Trauma* 1994;36:137.
24. DeLaat EA, Visser CP, Coene LN, et al. Nerve lesions in primary shoulder dislocations and humeral neck fractures. *J Bone Joint Surg* (Br) 1994;76B:381-383.
25. McLaughlin HC, Cavallaro WN. Primary anterior dislocation of the shoulder. *Am J Surg* 1950;80:615.
26. Saxena K, Stavas J. Inferior glenohumeral dislocation. *Ann*

Emerg Med 1983;12:718.

27. Moore TO. Internal pin fixation for fracture of the clavicle. *Am Surg* 1951;17:580.
28. Rowe CR. An atlas of anatomy and treatment of midclavicular fractures. *Clin Orthop* 1968;58:29.
29. Selesnick FH, Jablon M, Frank C, et al. Retrosternal dislocation of the clavicle. Report of four cases.*J Bone Joint Surg* 1984;66-A:287.
30. Thomson DA, Flynn TC, Miller PW, et al. *J Trauma* 1985;25:974.
31. Allman F. Fractures and ligamentous injuries of the clavicle and its articulation. *J Bone Joint Surg* 1967;49A:774.
32. Bossart PJ, Joyce SM, Manaster BJ, et al. Lack of efficacy of "weighted" radiographs in diagnosing acute acromioclavicular separation. *Ann Emerg Med* 1988;17:20.
33. Larsen E, Bjerg-Nielsen A, Christensen P. Conservative or surgical treatment of acromioclavicular dislocation. *J Bone Joint Surg* 1986;68A:552.
34. Post M. Current concepts in the diagnosis and management of acromioclavicular dislocations. *Clin Orthop* 1985;200: 234.
35. Darrow JC Jr, Smith JA, Lockwood RC, et al. A new conservative method for treatment of type III acromioclavicular separation. *Orthop Clin North Am* 1980; 11:727.
36. Tibone J, Sellers R, Tonino P. Strength testing after third-degree acromioclavicular dislocations. *Am J Sports Med* 1992;20:328.
37. Wickiewicz TL. Acromioclavicular and sternoclavicular joint injuries. *Clin Sports Med* 1983;2:429.
38. Szalay EA, Rockwood CA. Injuries of the shoulder and arm. *Emerg Med Clin North Am* 1984;2:279.
39. Stimson LA. An easy method of reducing dislocations of the shoulder and hip. *Med Rec* 1900;57:356.
40. Poulson SR. Reduction of acute shoulder dislocation using the Eskimo technique: A study of 23 consecutive cases. *J Trauma* 1988;28:1382.
41. Milch H. Treatment of dislocation of the shoulder. *Surgery* 1938;3:732.
42. Anderson D, Zvirbulis R, Ciullo J. Scapular manipulation for reduction of anterior shoulder dislocations. *Clin Orthop* 1982;164:181-183.

Hand Injuries

Charles Stewart, MD, FACEP

More than 30% of industrial accidents and approximately three-fourths of industrial injuries that cause partial disability involve the hand or hands.[1] Each year, more than 16 million people in the United States seek emergency care for hand injuries, including amputations, fractures, infections, and ligamentous lacerations.

Successful evaluation and treatment of these injuries requires both knowledge of the relevant clinical anatomy of the hand and an understanding of the mechanism of injuries, complications, presentations, and disabilities the injuries produce. From an outcomes perspective, it should be stressed that the hand can only be fully functional if both sensation and appropriate motion are preserved.

With these considerations in clear focus, the purpose of this chapter is to review common injuries and infections of the hand. The goal is to provide a systematic, step-by-step approach that will guide the emergency physician through assessment and early therapy of the hand injury.

Evaluation of the Injured Hand

When it comes to hand injuries, appearances are often deceiving. Consequently, a comprehensive history of the injury and the patient's general condition are essential. Ensure that the ABCs of good emergency medical care are attended to, and do not be distracted from more serious injuries by a bleeding or deformed hand.

Two tasks should be given priority consideration. First, remove any rings, watches, or other jewelry with a ring cutter if necessary. This is important, because if the finger swells, the unstretchable metal ring will compromise circulation. Some patients may refuse to allow removal of a ring because of financial or sentimental value. If a patient persists in their refusal to have rings removed, you must warn them about the danger of vascular compromise and then have them sign an "against medical advice" form that documents this warning.

The second immediate task is to remove all clothing up to and including the chest. Some well-meaning bystander may have applied a tourniquet or the patient may have a more proximal injury. In extreme cases, the patient may have a chest injury. If the patient has been in a motor vehicle accident or industrial accident, be certain that no other injury exists or is masked by the pain of the hand injury.

History of the Injury. The patient's age, occupation, and dominant hand should be recorded. The ED physician needs to document whether the injury occurred in a clean or dirty environment. The circumstances in which the injury occurred also need to be recorded. Particular attention should be paid to injuries sustained in a fight; injuries involving crushing forces; injuries involving high-pressure air, paint, grease, or water hoses; burns caused by chemicals, steam, or electricity; and ring or jewelry injuries.[2]

The following points should be documented:

- Exactly what happened;
- Any prior injury or illness to the involved arm or hand;
- Dominant hand;
- Occupation and important avocations;
- Current medications and allergies (include any previously prescribed or "loaner" antibiotics);
- Tetanus prophylaxis status;
- Concurrent medical illnesses (risk factors that may compromise healing);
- Last meal and drink (if patient is to go to surgery).

Anytime the patient hears a snap or pop during the injury, the examiner should consider the injury to be serious. Certain activities or sports should increase the suspicion of specific injuries. Football, baseball, volleyball, and basketball can have direct impact of the ball on a finger with resultant proximal interpharangeal (PIP) fractures or dislocations. Skiers and, to a lesser degree, baseball players may have thumb collateral ligament ruptures.

Initial Examination of the Hand Injury. The hand consists of five fingers (four fingers and the thumb), 14 finger joints, three major nerves, intrinsic and extrinsic muscles, and multiple intercarpal wrist joints among the ten carpal bones and the two bones of the forearm. Tissues specifically adapted for the function of the hand cover the hand. On the dorsum of the hand, the skin is thin and mobile. This skin stretches to completely cover without tension when the fist is clenched. The thin skin of the dorsum of the hand may be easily damaged in shearing type injuries. The palmar skin is adherent to the supportive fascia, and the fascia is adherent to the underlying skeleton. Even the fingerprint serves to increase friction and hence a more secure grasp of an object.

Frequently, injured hands are soiled and need to be cleaned before an adequate examination can be performed. Unfortunately, cleansing appropriately may require anesthesia. The safest approach is to check sensation before any anesthesia is used—even topical. If at all possible, get the patient comfortable in the supine position before starting the examination. Ensure that all jewelry is removed and that the patient's clothing is removed at least to the shoulder. Place the patient's hand on a firm support.

Start the examination by comparing the two hands for symmetry. Comparison with the uninjured extremity may show swelling from an infection, abnormal positioning from tendon or bone injury, color changes, or even lack of sweating. Note the presence of cyanosis, pallor, edema, erythema, ecchymosis, or blistering.

The location of the injury should be described as being on the radial or ulnar side and on the volar or dorsal (flexor or extensor) surface. Remember that the palmar aponeurosis and lymphatic drainage from palmar surface to the dorsum will cause infection or other palmar processes to be visible in the dorsum of the hand. If the patient has swelling of the dorsum of the hand, but is otherwise normal, turn the hand over. Often, a palmar puncture wound or other lesion will be found.

If the patient has an infected wound in the flexor tendon sheath of the digit, the palm of the hand may be quite tender. The flexor tendon sheath may conduct infection from these wounds directly into the palm of the hand. With fresh tendon injuries, blood in the flexor tendon sheath may cause pain on palpation of the sheath.

Vascular Status. The history of the injury may be helpful in suggesting the presence of vascular injuries. For example, a deep penetrating injury with subsequent pulsatile bleeding suggests arterial injury. This may be the only indicator of arterial injury, particularly in young, healthy patients. It should be noted that bleeding may stop rapidly in these patients due to spontaneous arterial retraction and constriction.

Check the skin color and then check for capillary refill. Repeat the test on an uninjured digit for comparison. The best place to test may be near the nail ridge. The pulp may be callous, or you may not be able to see refill in the pulp in patients with dark skin. Radial and ulnar pulses are often helpful if they are present and the patient has good color and capillary fill. If the radial and ulnar pulses are present and the patient has any signs of vascular trauma, use a Doppler probe. Doppler probes measure flow, while pulses indicate a pressure wave. The distinction is immaterial unless a flap or clot prevents flow but allows the pulse pressure wave to be transmitted. Digital pulses may not be palpable, but they may be auscultated with a Doppler probe.

The Allen test confirms that the patient has both ulnar and radial circulation and that there is collateral circulation between the two vessels through the palmar arch. Have the patient forcefully open and close the fist 10-20 times. The examiner should then compress the radial and ulnar arteries simultaneously as the patient opens the hand. When the ulnar artery is released, the patient's skin pallor should rapidly resolve. The process should also be reversed to ensure that the radial artery can perfuse the entire hand.

If the patient is bleeding, first try elevating the arm and applying a sterile wet-compression dressing. If bleeding continues despite elevation, a blood pressure cuff can be inflated to about 100 mmHg above the patient's systolic blood pressure. Never leave this cuff on for more than 30 minutes.

Since the nerves follow vessels, never ligate a hand vessel without directly visualizing the bleeding vessel and all surrounding structures. This will require better exposure, lighting, and instruments than are available in most EDs. Never blindly clamp a bleeding vessel. This invites trauma to nerve, tendon, or even associated vessels.

Neurologic Evaluation. Accurate diagnosis of a nerve injury in the hand requires knowledge of the distribution of the major nerves and a disciplined thought process. Be sure to examine the patient's sensation prior to instilling anesthesia. Lacerated nerves are common, particularly when the patient sustains a laceration over the known position of a mixed or sensory nerve.

The hand is supplied by three major nerves: the median, ulnar, and radial nerve. *(Please see Figure 1 and Figure 2.)* The ulnar and median nerve enter the hand on the palmar side. The radial nerve crosses the radial styloid from the volar to the dorsal surface at the wrist. These nerves control the wrist, fingers, and thumb's motion and sensation. *(Please see Figure 1.)* Loss of a major nerve at any level can compromise function of the hand.

Clinical tests for sensation and motor function should always be done to test integrity of the nerve. Although the patient's cooperation is helpful, most of these tests can be done without complete cooperation. Sensation should be assessed without disturbing the injured hand whenever possible. Digital nerve transection may result in a painful neuroma as well as insensitivity of the finger distal to the nerve injury. Using appropriate microsurgical techniques may minimize these complications, so referral for digital nerve injuries is mandatory.

Nerve repair need not be done emergently but can be delayed for a more complete evaluation within the first week following the injury. If a surgeon is available to repair the nerve within a day or so, then

Figure 1. Innervation of Dorsal Surface of Hand

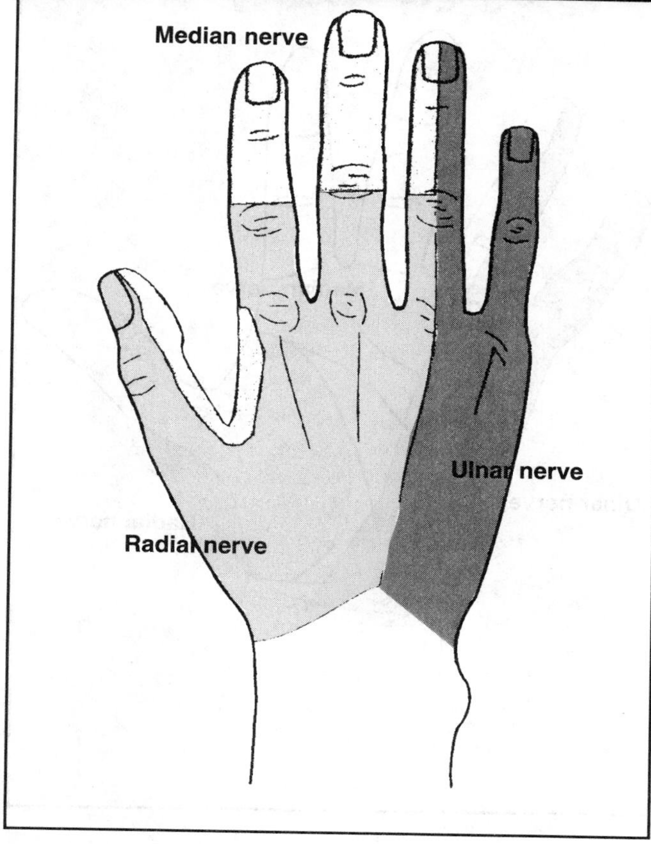

the wound can be cleaned and dressed without suturing or with loose suturing of the wound. A splint should be applied and the patient sent promptly to the surgeon for repair.

Sensory Examination. A major clue to loss of sensation in the hand that does not require the patient's cooperation is loss of sweating. The skin supplied by an injured nerve dries rapidly. Another test for the uncooperative patient may be O'Riain's wrinkle test. The hand can be immersed in hot water for about 10 minutes. The skin will not wrinkle if the nerve supplying it was severed.

If the patient can cooperate, two-point discrimination is quick and reliable. This test can be rapidly and inexpensively performed with a bent paper clip. Normally, patients should be able to discriminate two points at somewhat less than 5 mm. Ensure that the two points are oriented in line with the digital nerve, rather than transversely across two nerves' distribution. Pinprick (sharp/dull) testing may be misleading and may make other parts of the exam unreliable in children.

Three key locations will allow rapid sensory testing of the major nerves.

- The ulnar nerve supplies the fifth finger.
- The median nerve supplies the web space between the thumb and first finger.
- The radial nerve supplies the dorsal surface of the proximal first and second fingers.

Motor Examination. A simple screening test of motor function can be performed by having the patient bring the tips of the thumb and all fingers in a circle around the examiner's pen. Then ask the patient to spread the fingers widely. Finally, ask the patient to spread the thumb away from the palm. It's not possible to do all of these maneuvers unless the ulnar, radial, and median nerve are all intact. If the patient can't do these, you must look for the specific deficit.

Table 1. Tests of Muscle Innervation in the Hand

Look for the demon RUM to be opposed by the WCTU.

Nerve	Opposing Feature
Radial	Wrist extenders
Ulnar	Claw hand
Median	Thumb-up maneuvers

Simple and quick tests can be performed that correspond to the major patterns of muscle innervation. A mnemonic can be used to remember this simple battery of tests. "Look for the demon RUM to be opposed by the WCTU." RUM stands for the Radial, Ulnar, and Median nerves that are respectively opposed by Wrist extenders, Claw hand, and Thumb Up maneuvers.

The radial nerve innervates the extrinsic wrist and fingers in extension, the ulnar deficit will cause a claw hand formation, and the median nerve is needed for the thumb up maneuver. Having the patient cock the wrist back (dorsiflexion) against resistance and then completely extend all fingers can check the radial nerve. *(Please see Table 1.)* If the patient can't extend at all, then look for nerve damage. If the patient can move it, but does so weakly, then painful range of motion may be at fault rather than nerve injury.

A wrist drop should clue the examiner that there may be a problem with the radial nerve. The radial nerve is close to the brachioradialis and the flexor carpi radialis tendons in the proximal wrist. If these tendons are damaged, look for injury to the radial nerve. If the little and ring fingers claw, look for damage to the ulnar here.

The ulnar nerve innervates all the intrinsic muscles of the ring and little fingers. *(Please see Figure 2.)* If the index and middle fingers claw, both the ulnar and median nerve must be damaged, since some intrinsic muscles are innervated by each.

Another important test of ulnar nerve function is to ask the patient to form an "O" with thumb and index finger. If the circle is askew (caved in), look for ulnar nerve damage with loss of thumb adductor function. This is called "Froment's sign."

Check for contraction of the second dorsal interosseous muscle as a further test of the integrity of the ulnar nerve. Ask the patient to abduct the extended index finger against resistance and palpate the webspace of the radial side of the second (index finger) metacarpal. Since the ulnar nerve is just deep to the flexor carpi ulnaris, suspect an ulnar nerve injury if the tendon is damaged. Having the patient bring the thumb out of the palm (toward the ceiling when the dorsal surface of the hand is flat on the exam table), while you palpate the thenar eminence and check function of the median nerve.

If the patient can't point the thumb up, then the intrinsic opponens and abductor function is lost. *(Please see Table 1.)* Remember that the median nerve supplies half a LOAF—half of the Lumbricals (the index and middle fingers) the Opponens, Abductors, and superficial half of the Flexor muscles of the thumb. It also supplies the flexor side of the forearm, so if the median nerve is damaged anywhere above the wrist, the patient will not be able to pronate the palm down. The median nerve is superficial right around the carpal tunnel. Lacerations about this area may point to damage to the median nerve.

Repair of a lacerated nerve demands an operating room, an experienced hand surgeon, good microinstruments, and an operating microscope. These techniques are beyond the scope of most emergency physicians and should usually be referred. Never "tag" nerve ends; if the surgeon needs a "tag" to find the nerve, find another surgeon.

A laceration of a mixed motor and sensory nerve such as the ulnar or median nerve should be repaired as a primary procedure if at all possible. Isolated lacerations of sensory nerves such as a digit may often be best repaired three or four days later. In some cases, sensation will return if the nerve is bruised (neuropraxia), and, in others, a better exam with a less painful hand will be more accurate.

Range of Motion. Recognition of tendon injuries requires a systematic examination of the flexion and extension of each finger at each joint. Although some tendon injuries can be seen in the depths of the wound, the most reliable way to detect injuries is functional testing of the hand. It is sometimes helpful to demonstrate the various normal motions and then have the patient mimic them. This is particularly helpful in examination of children.

Patients who are unable to flex one finger together with the others will often be found to have a tendon injury. Weak movement of the joint may mean that the tendon injury is incomplete. (It also may mean that the patient has too many other injuries and is simply moving the finger inadequately. This is a difficult judgment call.) Remember that some uninjured parts of the hand may not move normally if there is an injury close by. Some injured structures may be moved by uninjured parts of the hand. Occasionally, the fifth digit may be extended by the extensor communis, despite a fifth digit extensor tendon laceration.

Rarely, a partially lacerated tendon will rupture during or after the examination and leave a complete tendon laceration. This can be appropriately repaired. Pain along the course of a tendon during motion is a nonspecific indication of injury. Because the vessels and nerves are so close to the flexor tendons, any injury that clearly involves one of these is likely to involve the others. Before any direct examination of the wound, ensure that both sensation and vascular status are recorded.

Flexion. There are two flexor tendons to each digit and one to the thumb. The deep digital flexor tendon inserts on the distal phalanx and flexes all joints during motion. It is the most important of the flexors and is tested by strong flexion of the distal joint. The profundus tendon produces all of the flexor strength at the distal interphalangeal (DIP) joint and more than half of the strength at the PIP joint. To test the deep digital flexor tendon, restrain the PIP joint and have the patient attempt to flex the DIP joint.

The superficial digital flexor tendon attaches to the middle phalanx. The tendons are formed in the forearm, pass through the carpal tunnel at the wrist superficial to the profundus tendons, and through the digital fibroosseous sheaths to a broad insertion on the middle phalanx.[3]

Movement of this tendon causes flexion of the proximal interphalangeal joint. Isolated injuries of this tendon are uncommon. To test this, hold three fingers and have the patient attempt to flex the fourth at the PIP joint. Test each finger in this way. Often the fifth digit superficial tendon may not be independent, small, or even absent. About 15% of people cannot actively flex the PIP of the fifth digit without flexing the adjacent ring finger PIP simultaneously.[4]

Figure 2. Innervation of Palmar Surface of Hand

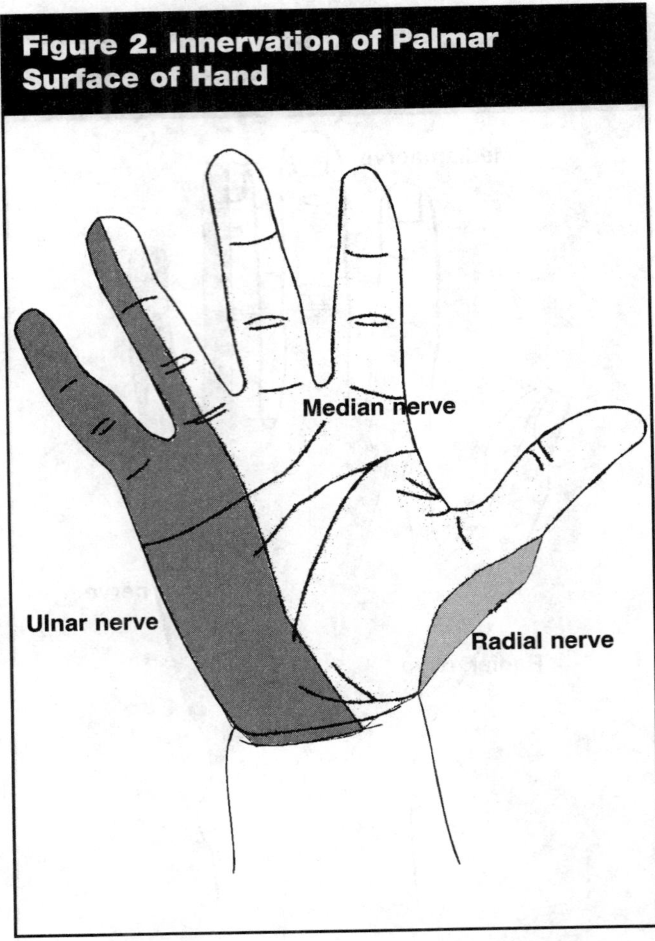

If there is a laceration of the flexor tendon sheath, then it should be assumed that the patient has a laceration (partial or complete) of the flexor tendon until proven otherwise. The wound should be carefully examined, including examination with the hand flexed as it was during the injury. If the digit was flexed at the time of the injury, then skin, tendon, and sheath will all be lacerated at different levels when the digit is extended.

Extension. Have the patient place the hand palm-down on a table and extend the fingers off the table one at a time. If you suspect an extensor tendon laceration but can't see one in the wound, try putting the hand in the position it was in when the injury occurred. This often shows an extensor tendon injury. Moving the appropriate finger also increases the chances of seeing a tendon injury in the wound.

Repair of Tendon Injuries. The extensor tendons are superficial and not constrained by a tight tendon sheath. This means that they can be relatively easily located and repaired, unlike flexor tendons. If the emergency physician has experience, training, appropriate tools, lighting, and exposure, and has a patient with a clean wound, then repair in the ED is possible. If all of these are not available, then the patient should be referred to a hand surgeon for repair in an operating room.

Flexor tendon injuries are not suitable for emergency repair. Although these injuries have been divided into several zones to identify complications associated with repair, classification of the injury does not change the appropriate emergency management of the patient.[5] These injuries should be referred to a qualified hand or orthopedic surgeon for repair. This may be done within a few days if the wound is carefully cleansed and the skin is loosely closed over the injury.

Splint the hand and carefully counsel the patient that the skin repair does not repair the underlying tendon injury.

Cleansing the Injured Hand. Do not use scrubs and cleanser solutions such as iodine and hexachlorphene directly on a wound. These substances may delay healing by shortening the life span and decreasing the migration ability of the polymorphoneucleocyte. These solutions may be used to disinfect the surrounding epidermis.

Large volumes of water delivered at high pressure are the best way to remove debris in the wound. There are many opinions about the best way to irrigate a wound, but almost all of these methods are controversial. There are multiple commercial aids to help with this irrigation, but all add expense to the procedure. About the only non-controversial method of irrigation is to use an 18g or 19g needle and a 30cc syringe full of saline with rapid firm pressure.

Imaging Hand Injuries

Plain Film Radiographs. In all but the most minor lacerations or contusions of the hand, a standard series of radiographs should be obtained. These radiographs help to identify joint injury, fractures, or dislocations. They also help to locate retained foreign bodies. A laceration from glass or other foreign body such as porcelain should almost always have a radiograph of the hand to insure that no foreign body remains. X-rays should be obtained for all gunshot wounds.

Three views of the hand should always be obtained. These include a posteroanterior (PA), a true lateral, and an oblique presentation. Oblique views are essential to identify the metacarpal heads. The Brewerton view can demonstrate small fractures of the head of the second through the fifth metacarpals.[6]

If a phalanx is injured, then the beam should be centered on the phalanx and a PA of the entire hand and a true lateral and oblique projection of the injured digit. Eccentric soft-tissue swelling noted on one side of an interphalangeal joint is suggestive of a collateral ligament injury to that joint.

Small avulsion fractures may be noted with a mallet finger, avulsion of the profundus tendon from the insertion, or avulsion of the palmar plate of the phalanx. Scaphoid views show the entire length of the scaphoid bone. The fingers are flexed into a fist and the thumb is held straight. Both the wrist and the fist lie flat on the film. This dorsiflexes the long axis of the scaphoid into a plane that is parallel to the film. A second view is added with ulnar deviation of the wrist.[7] Some acute fractures, particularly scaphoid fractures, are difficult to visualize. Osteolysis causes the fracture line to be more radiolucent some 7-10 days after the fracture.

It is often appropriate to splint patients based on the history and physical examination, even if the radiographs appear normal. A key to the identification of dislocations of the carpal bones is the position of the lunate in the lateral projection. The capitate rests in the concavity of the lunate, which in turn rests in the distal concavity of the radius. In a dorsal perilunate dislocation, the capitate is dorsally displaced out of its normal position in the lunate. In the palmar dislocation of the lunate, the capitate remains in line with the radius, but the lunate bone is displaced towards the palmar surface.

Other occult fractures and some dislocations may be heralded by loss of fat pads, soft tissue swelling, or changes in the angulation of the carpal bones. A gap greater than 2 mm between the scaphoid and the lunate is diagnostic of scapholunate dislocation.[8]

Special Studies. If initial films of hand injuries do not visualize an opaque foreign body, consider a xeroradiogram of the hand. These are better for wood and plastic foreign bodies than plain film radiograms. In patients with persistent pain from an injury to the hand, computed tomography (CT), scintigraphy, or MRI may be used to identify an occult fracture.[9] In occult fractures of the radius, scaphoid bone, or the hook of the hamate bone, MRI may allow early evaluation of avascular necrosis.[10]

MRI may also be used to evaluate the soft tissue injury of distal avulsion fractures in patients with suspected trigger finger injuries or gamekeeper's thumb. Both MRI and CT can be used for identification of foreign bodies in the hand. An emergency physician would rarely order these studies.

Specific Hand Injuries

Amputations. Amputations represent about 5% of upper extremity injuries and involve about 150,000 people in the United States each year.[11] Reimplantation of amputated digits has become commonplace. Survival and function depend on many factors including the type of injury, ischemia of the injured part (particularly if warm), and the patient's general condition and prior medical illnesses. Most surgeons would recommend reimplantation of a thumb, the index finger proximal to the PIP joint, multiple digits, and single amputated digits in children.[12]

Generally, sharp injuries do much better than crush or avulsion injuries.[13] Hemophilia and sickle cell disease are strong relative contraindications. Remember that replantation of an amputation means that there is a prolonged healing time of many months.

Amputated or devascularized digits should be cooled as quickly as possible. Proper cooling of the amputated digit or extremity markedly extends the time that the amputated part can survive before revascularization. The amputated part should be placed in saline soaked gauze and put in a sealed container such as a baggie, on ice. The parts should not be immersed in nonphysiologic solutions and should never be frozen.

The injured extremity should be dressed, splinted, and elevated without an attempt to clean the injury. (Cleansing can be done at the time of the repair.)

Survival rates of amputated parts may approach 90% in some centers, but survival of the digit does not necessarily mean that full function has been restored. To avoid unrealistic expectations on the part of patient and family alike, ensure that all understand that the decision to replant a digit or hand will be made by the surgeon at the referral center after a thorough examination.

Ring avulsion injuries may run the spectrum from a minor skin injury to complete avulsion of the digit with flexor tendon from the forearm.[14] Simple avulsions with small amounts of skin may be safely repaired. If the skin is denuded from the finger, there may be a great desire to simply roll the skin envelope back onto the digit and suture it into place. This, unfortunately, may not restore sensation or blood flow to the skin. A hand surgeon should see these complex injuries.

Crush Injuries. A crush injury to the hand is one of the most unpredictable and potentially devastating injuries. Because of the unique functions of the hand and the lack of protective muscle mass, the hand is particularly vulnerable to crush injuries. These injuries may involve multiple tissues and may have both normal and irreversibly damaged tissues side by side. Open wounds, massive levels of contamination, and thermal injuries often complicate these injuries.[15,16]

Ischemia may result from damage to local microcirculation from the crush, from damage to major blood vessels, or a combination of these. Severely mangled hands may require amputation or revascularization.[17]

Closed Injuries. Closed or "roller" or "wringer" injuries of the hand and forearm are often much more serious than initially suspected. When the patient's hand is caught between two compressing rollers, hemorrhage deep within the muscle and fascial planes may be found. If the patient has pain on passive extension of the digits, then deep hemorrhage may be causing compression in the muscle compartments. In this case, decompression by a hand surgeon is indicated.

Forearm muscle compartment pressure may be monitored with Wick catheters. If immediate decompression is not needed, then the patient should be admitted to the hospital for hourly neurovascular monitoring for 24 hours. A bulky dressing with the elbow flexed, the wrist slightly extended, and the MP joints slightly flexed (anatomic position) should be applied. The arm should be elevated and ice applied.

Dislocations. Fingers can dislocate in a variety of directions. Dislocations, fractures, and ligament disruptions may present with identical deformities. Ensure that the patient has "only" a dislocation and not a fracture or fracture dislocation with a radiograph prior to any reduction maneuver.

Many patients will report that they have "jammed" their finger. This inaccurate terminology may be adequate for the coach, but not for the emergency physician.

Be certain that an adequate history of the injury is obtained. A finger that is forced upward may cause a volar plate rupture or dorsal dislocation. A finger that has been compressed is more likely to have a fracture or mallet finger. A joint that is pushed sideways should prompt the emergency physician to think of a collateral ligament injury.

Dorsal dislocation of the PIP joint produces a characteristically excessive prominence of the middle phalanx. This causes a distal rupture of the volar plate. It is often termed a simple dislocation since non-operative management is almost uniformly successful.

Reduction may be done with direct traction to the digit, followed by mild hyperextension. The physician may add direct pressure over the base of the middle phalanx as traction is applied. It may be remarkably easier and much less painful for the patient to use a digital block prior to the reduction maneuver. Ensure that the finger is well-aligned after the reduction.

The reduction is stable if the patient does not displace with usual range of motion or gentle lateral stressing. The joint should be splinted for three weeks with a foamed aluminum dorsal splint. After three weeks, unrestricted motion should be encouraged.

In some patients, rupture of the volar plate does not result in dislocation. The usual deformity is absent and only a small avulsion fracture is found at the base of the middle phalanx. These patients require splinting and referral to a hand surgeon. If there is a large fragment, then the patient may need operative reduction and stabilization of the fragments.

Anterior dislocation of the PIP joint is more easily overlooked on physical examination. The classic deformity of the dislocation is missing and the patient may be holding the finger in flexion. This should be suspected if the patient has a tender joint on palpation and is unable to extend the finger. In these patients, the extensor mechanism is often damaged and operative repair is often needed. These injuries should be splinted and the patient referred to a hand surgeon. If the injury is misdiagnosed because no radiograph was obtained, the patient may develop the boutonniere deformity.

Dislocation of the metacarpal joint may result in a proximal rupture of the volar plate and dorsal displacement of the proximal phalanx. In some patients, the volar plate becomes trapped in the joint space and simple reduction is not possible. Reduction of the simple metacarpal joint dislocation requires flexion of the wrist to relax the flexor tendons. Steady pressure is applied on the dorsal surface of the proximal phalanx. The phalanx is lifted up and over the metacarpal head into the reduced position. Excessive traction may cause the volar plate to enter the joint space and convert a simple dislocation into one that requires operative reduction.[18]

Fractures of the Hand

Phalangeal fractures are among the most common of hand fractures. The majority of these are stable injuries that can be adequately treated by simply buddy-taping them to the adjacent finger. Simple splinting with foam and aluminum splints for 14-21 days is another option.

Distal Phalanx. The most common distal phalanx fracture is the comminuted tuft fracture. Usually, angulation and distraction of the fragments is minimal because the phalanx is splinted dorsally by the nail matrix and volarly by the fibrous septa of the pulp. These fractures may be treated by splinting the finger. A foam and aluminum splint that extends from dorsal to volar surface up and over the distal tuft will provide more protection for the patient's distal fingertip than a dorsal or volar splint alone. Splint from the proximal phalanx to proximal phalanx and instruct the patient to keep the splint in place for 14-21 days.

Subungual hematomas may produce significant throbbing pain from the pressure on the nail bed. Small subungual hematomas may be relieved by simple decompression of the hematoma.[19] If the subungual hematoma is more than about 25%, then elevation of the nail and inspection of the underlying nail bed is more appropriate therapy. If there is a transverse fracture with displacement of the fragments, then a nail bed injury is common. Nail bed lacerations should be repaired by elevation of the nail and repair of the nail bed.

Volar and Dorsal Fracture Dislocations. Volar and dorsal fracture dislocations occur when the distal interphalangeal joint is not only fractured but also dislocated. In volar fracture dislocations, the distal phalanx is subluxed volarly and the dorsal fragment is displaced by the tension of the extensor tendon. In dorsal fracture dislocations, the distal phalanx is subluxed dorsally and the deep flexor tendon displaces the volar fragment. These injuries will often require open reduction and internal fixation of the fracture fragments.

Dorsal articular fractures in adults can cause a "mallet finger" deformity or "drop finger" as described above. There is considerable controversy about the best method of treatment for these injuries and options range from surgical exploration and fixation of the fragments to splinting alone. Certainly, the emergency physician's best course of action is to splint the injury and allow the hand surgeon to weather the controversy.

Proximal Phalangeal Fractures. These fractures may be treacherous and require open fixation and immobilization. Often the oblique x-ray does not show the true nature of the fracture, and a true lateral radiograph is needed to show the anterior angulation of the fracture. If this angulation is present, then the function of the tendon will be significantly impaired. Unstable fractures are usually rotated, spiral, or comminuted fractures.

Metacarpal Fractures. Metacarpal neck fractures are very common, particularly neck fractures of the fourth and fifth metacarpal (Boxer's fracture). They are usually the result of crush or direct impact injuries.

Most of these metacarpal neck fractures can be treated with closed reduction and casting. If there are several large fragments, open reduction and internal fixation are often recommended.[20] Assess for rotational deformity by having the patient slowly make a fist with the palm facing upward.

With a rotational injury, the nails will no longer be in line and the finger may be obviously rotated. If there is any significant rotational deformity, this must be corrected. The fourth and fifth metacarpals may have up to 30° of rotation before reduction is necessary, but little rotational deformity is tolerated for the second or third metacarpal. Reduction of the fracture is generally beyond the training of most emergency physicians, and referral to an orthopedic or hand surgeon is appropriate.

For fractures of the fourth and fifth metacarpals, an ulnar gutter splint with the joints in about 60° of flexion is appropriate. Fractures of the second and third metacarpals can be treated with a radial gutter splint. For these splints, a hole must be made in the splint for the thumb.

Metacarpal shaft fractures can be transverse, oblique, or comminuted. Transverse fractures are usually due to a direct blow to the hand, while oblique fractures are the result of rotational forces to the hand. Transverse fractures may have unacceptable angulation, while rotational deformity may complicate oblique fractures. Either may be unacceptable and require reduction and fixation. This is best done by an orthopedic or hand surgeon.

Comminuted fractures of the metacarpal shaft are often associated with significant soft-tissue injury to the hand. These lesions should be treated by a hand or orthopedic surgeon and may require substantial surgical repair of the other lesions.

Metacarpal base fractures are usually the result of compression in line with the bone or from a direct blow. They may involve the joint, may be rotated, and may be stable or unstable. If the fracture is stable and does not have joint involvement, splinting followed by routine orthopedic referral is appropriate.

Unstable fractures of the metacarpal usually involve the fifth metacarpal with its unopposed pull by the extensor carpi ulnaris. These will often require surgical reduction.

Displaced fractures of the metacarpal base or shaft are also unstable. Intra-articular fractures should be referred to an experienced orthopedic surgeon for management. Fractures of the thumb metacarpal are most common at the base of the thumb. The two most common intra-articular fractures of the thumb are Bennett's fracture and Rolando's fracture of the thumb.[21,22] Bennett's fracture is a fracture dislocation that characteristically has an intra-articular fracture through the base of the metacarpal bone with an ulnar fragment that is pulled medially and ulnarward.

The rest of the bone is dislocated dorsally and radially by the pull of the abductor pollicis longus muscle and the adductor pollicis muscle. These fractures often require closed reduction and percutaneous pinning or open reduction and internal fixation.

Occasionally, the force that would cause a Bennett's fracture will produce a dislocation by rupturing the anterior oblique ligament that bridges the metacarpal base and the trapezium. The treatment is immobilization, but the injury may still cause an unstable joint and traumatic arthritis.

Rolando's fracture is similar to a Bennett's fracture but there is a comminuted Y or T fracture pattern. These complicated fractures deserve the prompt attention of a hand surgeon to maximize function of the thumb.

Infections and Simple Lacerations of the Hand

The hand has a unique anatomic arrangement that makes it possible for infections to extend throughout the various planes of the hand without resistance. Infections that start in the fingers may proceed through the flexor tendon sheath and enter the mid-palmar space. Pressure in the mid-palmar space extends rapidly into the thenar space. The resulting infection may be devastating for the entire hand and may occur despite massive treatment with antibiotics. These patients will require incision and drainage in the operating room.

The four cardinal signs of a flexor tenosynovitis are tenderness over the flexor tendon, swelling of the finger, pain on passive extension, and a flexed posture of the digit. The tendons have scanty blood supply and blood flow is easily interrupted by relatively little edema. An infection within the tendon sheath decreases this blood supply, and often destroys the underlying tendon. Peritendonous scarring may result in subsequent loss of function of the hand. These patients require prompt drainage in the operating room and should be admitted with appropriate intravenous antibiotic therapy.

In about half of the patients, there is communication between the ulnar and the radial bursae. This may cause a horseshoe shaped abscess in the palm. An additional concern is the "collar button" abscess. A palmar infection may extend through the intermetacarpal spaces to the dorsum of the hand. These abscesses may "point" both dorsal and volar.

Most hand infections require intravenous antibiotics and surgical drainage of the infection. This is not the usual province of the emergency physician, and these patients should have a hand or orthopedic surgical consult. Three specific types of hand infections may be treated by the emergency physician: the paronychia, the herpetic whitlow, and the felon.

Paronychia. An infection around the margin of the nail bed is a paronychia. The portal of entry is often between the nail and the soft tissue of the nail gutter. The collection of pus may extend under the nail and damage the nail bed. If treated early, a simple incision with a pointed blade along the nail fold will allow this infection to drain adequately. If there is pus under the nail, then the proximal end of the nail must be elevated and incised to expose the entire area of infection. The wound is left open, and antibiotics are only rarely needed for successful treatment of this infection. Warm soaks may be helpful. The most common organisms are *Staphylococcus aureus* and *Streptococcus* species.

Felon. A felon is a subcutaneous infection of the pulp space of the fingertip. This anterior closed space often can become infected after a puncture wound. The resulting infection is extremely uncomfortable. The swelling that ensues can compromise perfusion predisposing the patient to necrosis of the pulp, infection of the bone, and a chronic infection. A felon must be drained by a longitudinal incision along the lateral nail margin and extending along the tip of the finger just below the distal nail margin.

This will allow drainage of all of the septal spaces in the anterior closed space and adequate decompression of the wound. A "fishmouth" incision is not necessary for complete healing of this lesion. The most common organism is *Staphylococcus aureus*, and appropriate antibiotics are indicated.

Herpetic Whitlow. Herpetic whitlow is a viral infection of the fingertip. The lesions will be cutaneous bullae. The most common organism is *Herpes* species, but multiple digital involvement may also be seen with *Coxsackie* virus. The patient may be treated with antiherpetic agents such as Zovirax. A dry dressing should be used. These lesions may occasionally be misdiagnosed as a felon.

Lacerations; and Fingertip, Nail Bed, and Ligamentous Injuries

Lacerations. Simple, tidy, superficial hand lacerations can be readily closed.[23] The wound must be cleansed as earlier described, cleared of dirty tissue, and closed. Even if the laceration is 6-10 hours old, infection is unlikely. Contaminated wounds are a different matter, of course. If the wound cannot be debrided to the appearance of an elective surgical wound, then it should be left open, packed with fine mesh gauze, and closed in 3-5 days. (This is known as delayed primary closure or DPC.) If there is any doubt about the cleanliness of a wound, then DPC is safest.

Fingertip Injuries. Distal fingertip amputations can be treated openly without grafting and preserve the maximum amount of length. Healing by secondary intention can be accomplished without infection, with good return of normal sensation, and with preservation of joint mobility.[24] The healing tissue will pull normal tissue from the pulp to the very tip of the finger. This means that the pulp is free of scar tissue and is markedly less tender. The tip may have an adherent tender scar, but the pulp with grip and sensation is not tender.[25]

Fingertip Amputation. One of the most common problems in any ED is the amputated fingertip. The major object of our treatment must be the early rehabilitation of the hand with a painless and durable skin cover. There are a multitude of techniques that may involve complicated and novel skin flaps that have been developed for these injuries.

Nail-bed Injuries. The fingernail is a vital component of the hand, protecting and supporting the fingertip. It acts as a firm base so that our fingertips have enhanced sensation. Appropriate initial treatment of nail bed injuries will decrease deformity, discomfort, and help the nail heal. Nail-bed injuries can include lacerations, crush injuries to the nail, and avulsions of the nail. An avulsion may be incomplete with nail remaining attached to the underlying nail bed or complete separation of nail from nail bed. If the nail remains intact, it can obscure the extent of the underlying damage. Likewise, an extensive subungual hematoma can obscure deeper damage to the nail bed. In these cases, removal of the nail and repair of the nail bed is appropriate.[26]

The radiograph may show a transverse fracture of the distal phalangeal tuft or an epiphyseal growth plate separation injury. This should be considered as an open fracture and the patient's wound should be irrigated and thoroughly debrided then fracture fragments reduced as appropriate. Suspect a nail bed laceration if the fragments are separated.

If the fracture fragments are unstable, then they need to be fixed in place with a fine Kirschner wire. This is best left to an orthopedic or hand surgeon unless the emergency physician has the training, time, and tools available to repair the injury appropriately.

The nail bed should be carefully inspected and any fragments restored to position. The nail bed margins need to be accurately approximated with 6-0 or 7-0 absorbable sutures. Lacerations of the fold and the fingertip pulp should be approximated and repaired.

If available, the nail is cleansed, trimmed, and replaced within the nail fold as both an organic splint and dressing. If the nail is not available or too damaged, then non-adherent dressing should be used. Without support of the palmar pulp tissue, about 25% of patients will have a tendency for the nail to grow over the end of the finger (a hooked nail). Routine nail grooming should provide relief for this injury.

Ligamentous Injuries: Collateral Ligament Injuries (Gamekeeper's Thumb). Stability of the metacarpophalangeal joint of the thumb is maintained by an arrangement of capsular, ligamentous, and musculotendinous supporting structures. Mediolateral stability is principally provided by the strong collateral ligaments, which start at the metacarpal condyles and pass obliquely toward the palm and attach on the volar third of the proximal phalanx and volar plate. Ulnar collateral ligament injuries of the thumb are particularly common among skiers and ball players. They occur more frequently than radial collateral injuries. Injuries are often termed "gamekeeper's thumb."

This term is derived from anecdotal reports of British gamekeepers breaking small animal's necks by using the thumb as a wedge.[27] The mechanism of injury is forced radial deviation-abduction often combined with hyperextension of the metacarpophalangeal joint. This can cause a complete or partial rupture of the ligament. This injury may be accompanied by an avulsion fracture at the site of the insertion of the collateral ligament at the volar base of the proximal phalanx. In most cases, however, the injury is purely ligamentous and the radiographs are normal.

Joint effusion and tenderness over the collateral ligaments are nonspecific indicators of collateral ligament tear. If the patient's joint opens with stress testing, there is no question of the collateral ligament injury, but pain and muscle spasm may limit passive abduction of the thumb and give a false-negative result. Examination under anesthesia may reveal an injury when pain and muscle spasm intervenes, but this is usually left to the orthopedic or hand surgery consultant.[28,29]

Emergency therapy is a thumb Spica splint and referral to a hand or orthopedic surgeon for definitive care. The final treatment depends on whether the ligament tear is partial or complete. Partial tears respond well to immobilization for 3-6 weeks in a thumb Spica cast. Surgery is often recommended for complete tears. Associated fractures are also indications for repair if they involve 25% or more of the articular surface or if an avulsion fracture is displaced more than 5 mm.

Sprained Finger. Sprained finger is a diagnosis often made. Unfortunately, it should be reserved for patients who have had a thorough physical and radiographic evaluation of their injury. Several injuries that require more definitive treatment masquerade as a sprain.

Mallet Finger. Disruption of the terminal extensor tendon mechanism can occur when a baseball or other object strikes the end of the finger. Three types of "mallet or baseball finger" can occur: disruption of the extensor tendon, avulsion fracture at the base of the distal phalanx (clinically this injury is indistinguishable from a laceration of the extensor tendon.), and a volar fracture subluxation of the distal joint. All three will have the classic drooping finger deformity. The difference can only be seen on x-ray.

Treatment ranges from simple splinting of the joint in extension for extensor tendon disruptions to open reduction and internal fixation of the bony fragments.

Boutonniere Finger. A sharp force against the tip of the partially extended finger will result in hyperflexion of the middle joint and may rupture the insertion of the central slip of the extensor tendon into the base of middle phalanx. The middle joint becomes "buttonholed" between the two lateral extensor tendons. On examination, the emergency physician should look for point tenderness about the base of the middle phalanx and for diminished extensor tendon strength with increased pain when the middle joint is extended against resistance.

These lesions are often missed and a diagnosis of sprained finger is made. On resuming active motion, the patient notes difficulty flexing the distal joint.

Treatment is splinting the joint in complete extension for four weeks. Surgical consultation for continued care is appropriate. Flexor digitorum profundus avulsion. The patient may also avulse the insertion of the flexor digitorum profundus tendon by forced extension of the finger when the flexor profundus is contracting. This happens when the finger is caught in a loop or pocket. The patient is simply unable to flex the tip of the finger. X-ray findings are usually normal, although a small avulsion fracture may be noted.

Treatment of this injury is surgical. A removable wire may be inserted to refix the tendon in place.

Collateral Ligament Injuries. Collateral ligament injuries of the fingers are less common than of the thumb as described above. In most cases, these can be splinted to an adjacent digit. If there is obvious deformity or instability, then operative repair and referral to a hand surgeon is indicated.

Miscellaneous Injuries

Foreign Bodies. When evaluating a puncture wound or laceration of the hand, the emergency physician must consider the possible presence of a residual foreign body in the tissues. The physician often misses initial diagnosis of the foreign body.[30] The best defense for missing a foreign body is to document an adequate history, adequately explore the wound, and obtain a radiograph of the hand. In general, foreign bodies of the hand require removal. The major question is when to remove them. Circumstances under which foreign bodies should be removed within the first 96 hours include:

- foreign bodies in the finger;
- history or evidence of significant contamination (wounds with heavy contamination and a residual foreign body need acute surgical debridement);
- foreign bodies that are within a bone or adjacent to a fracture and may contribute to an osteomyolitis;
- anticipation of progressive injury to adjacent vessel, nerve, or tendon (sharp-edged foreign bodies next to these structures may need removal acutely);
- intra-articular foreign bodies need acute surgical debridement of the foreign body;
- patients with known allergies to the foreign body;
- the presence of infection that requires immediate intervention.

Considerations for timing of the removal include the location of the foreign body, the material of the foreign body, the existence or anticipation of infection, the functional or anticipated impairment, and the general condition of the patient. Unfortunately, removal of foreign bodies in the hand can be time-consuming and even dangerous when attempted without adequate anesthesia, hemostasis, exposure, and lighting.

It is equally unfortunate that unplanned delayed removal of a foreign body may be associated with more legal complications than medical. Ensure that a radiograph is obtained whenever there is a suspicion of a retained foreign body. Metallic foreign bodies are generally non-reactive and easily visualized on radiographs. Glass fragments are notoriously difficult to see in tissues but are quite easy to see on a radiograph.

Small fragments of these two materials may usually be removed on a delayed basis without significant complication. Wooden splinters are often parallel with the skin surface and can be either deep or parallel to the skin surface. In many cases, the splinter can be palpated. Unfortunately, the patient or well meaning friend may grasp the splinter with pliers or even forceps and attempt to remove it. This will often leave behind fragments of wood or thorn deep within the tissues.

The appropriate treatment is to open the entire tract and remove the foreign body with direct visualization. In general, wooden foreign bodies should be removed as soon as practical. Subungual splinters are a special case. These are often quite painful and may be wood, metal, or even plastic. Often the patient is seen after several home attempts to remove the splinter have occurred. These attempts may either leave fragments of the splinter behind, or may push fragments deeper under the nail. At this point, it is often easier on the emergency physician and the patient alike to instill a digital block, sharply incise a window of nail plate above the splinter and remove the splinter with direct visualization.

Puncture Wounds. The surface wound may be misleading when dealing with puncture wounds. Simple puncture wounds may be cleaned both before and after the removal of the penetrating object. Wounds produced by staples, nails, and needles may penetrate bone or introduce gross contamination into the hand. Tetanus immunization is particularly important in these wounds.

If the penetrating body punctures bone, carries in a plug of skin or a contaminating foreign body, then formal exploration is also required. These wounds must be opened, irrigated, debrided if necessary, and allowed to heal by secondary intention. If the flexor tendon sheath is penetrated, then surgical consultation is indicated and the patient should be referred.

Fight Bites. Human bites (fight bites) are among the most dangerous contaminated wounds that an emergency physician treats. They require thorough surgical debridement and excision to prevent any deep infection. Fight bites must be treated with antibiotics because they have an infection rate as great as 50%.[31] *Staphylococcal* species, *Streptococcus species,* and *Eichenella corrodens* are the most common isolates.[32] *Eichenella corrodens* will cause rapidly spreading cellulitis with profound tendon damage if present. Treatment is a first generation penicillin or amoxicillin/clavulanate or cephalosporin. Antistaphylococcal penicillins will not adequately cover this organism.

High-Pressure Injection Injuries. Grease gun, paint sprayers, or compressed air devices may produce serious penetrating injuries that require wide debridement.[33] High-pressure injection devices may generate pressures that range from 1500 to 7000 psi and deposit substantial quantities of material into tendon and synovial sheaths.[34] The most common site of injection is the index finger followed by the palm and long finger.[35] The patient may develop intense throbbing and pain shortly after the injury.

Chemical properties of the substance injected may contribute to the severity of the injury. Paint and paint solvents appear to be the most irritating to tissue. Swelling due to injury, substance induced irritation, and material deposited within the sheath may rapidly compromise circulation to the digits.

The classic treatment of these injection injuries is early extensive surgical debridement and decompression of the wound. Prophylactic broad-spectrum antibiotics are often used in these patients, but there is no controlled data about their efficacy and cultures are frequently negative.[36] Corticosteroids have been used, but again there is no controlled data about efficacy or complications.

Summary

Hand injuries result from many different traumatic events, including crush injuries, amputations, fractures, and dislocations. Much of the treatment of hand injuries falls within the province of the emergency physician. Initial assessment and stabilization can change the course and decrease morbidity in a patient with a significant hand injury.

A thorough examination should always be both performed and documented. The emergency physician should closely inspect the hand and then perform a thorough sensation, ligament, and motion examination of the injured hand. Remember that examination for tendon injuries can be misleading due to partial tendon injuries. Copiously irrigate all open wounds and explore them for tendon, tendon sheath involvement, and foreign bodies.

Administer appropriate antibiotics for bites, contaminated wounds, and wounds that involve open fractures, amputations, and tendon injuries. Admit those patients with a tendon or joint infection and those with palmar infections. Seek hand surgery consultation when the patient has an amputation, a deep space infection, flexor tendon lacerations, or an unstable or angulated fracture.

References

1. Markovick VJ, Pons PT, Wolfe RE. *Emergency Medicine Secrets* Philadelphia: Hanley and Belfus, Inc; 1993.
2. Gillespie CA, Rodeheaver GT, Smith S, et al. Airless paint gun injuries: Definition and management. *Am J Surg* 1974; 128:383-391.
3. Rooks MD. Rock climbing injuries. *Sports Med* 1997;23: 261-270.
4. Rooks MD. Rock climbing injuries. *Sports Med* 1997;23: 261-270. OP CIT.
5. Herndon JH. Tendon injuries—flexor surface. *Emerg Med Clin North Am* 1985;3:341-349.
6. Brewerton DA. A tangential radiographic projection for demonstrating involvement of metacarpal heads in rheumatoid arthritis. *Br J Radiol* 1967;40:233-235.
7. Stecher WR. Roentgenography of the carpal navicular bone. *Am J Roentgenol* 1937;37:704-705.
8. Frankel VH. The "Terry Thomas" sign. *Clin Orthop* 1977; 129:321-322.
9. Eustace S, Denison W. Pictoral review: Magnetic resonance imaging of acute orthopedic trauma to the upper extremity. *Clinical Rad* 1997;52:338-344.
10. Horton MG, Timins ME. MR imaging of injuries to the small joints. *Imaging Orth Trauma* 1997;35:671-700.
11. Cunningham BL, Shons AR. Upper extremity replantation surgery. *Minn Med* 1982;65:463-466.
12. Moore JR, Weiland AJ. Current concepts of digit replantation. *Am Fam Phys* 1981;24:121-125.
13. Stevanovic MV, Vucetic C, Bumbasirevic M, et al. Avulsion injuries of the thumb. *Plast Reconstr Surg* 1991;87: 1099-1104.
14. Burkhalter WE. Ring avulsion injuries, care of amputated parts, replants, and revascularization. *Emerg Med Clin North Am* 1985;3365-3371.
15. Buchler U, Hastings H II. *Combined Injuries in Operative Hand Surgery* New York: Churchill Livinston; 1993.
16. Muir L, Foucher G, Marin-Braun F. Ax injuries of the hand. *J Trauma* 1997;42:928-932.
17. Bomar KS, Calandruccio JH. Crush injuries to the hand and forearm. *Orthop Nurs* 1996;15:56-65.
18. Melone CP. Joint injuries of the fingers and thumb. *Emerg Clin North Am* 1985;3:319-331.
19. Zook EG. Injuries of the fingernail. In: Green DP, ed. *Operative Hand Surgery*. New York: Churchill-Livingston; 1982:902.
20. Coleman DA. Metacarpal and phalangeal fractures. *Top Emerg Med* 1988;10:39-64.
21. Bennett EH. Fractures of the metacarpal bones. *Dublin J Med Sc* 1882;73:72-75.
22. Rolando S. Fracture de la base du premier metacarpien, et principalement sur une variete non encore decrite. *PressMed* 1910;33:303.
23. Altman RS, Harris GD, Knuth CJ. Initial management of hand injuries in the emergency patient. *Am J Emerg Med* 1987;5:400-404.
24. Lamon RP, Cicero JJ, Frascone RJ, et al. Open treatment

offingertip amputations. *Ann Emerg Med* 1983;12:358-360.
25. Burkhalter WE. Fingertip injuries. *Emerg Clin N Am* 1985;3:245-253.
26. Zook EG, Guy RG, Russell RC. A study of nail bed injuries: Causes, treatment, and prognosis. *J Hand Surg* 1984;9:247.
27. Hankin FM, Wylie RJ. Gamekeeper's thumb. *Am Fam Phys* 1988;38:127-130.
28. Louis DS, Huebner JJ Jr, Hankin FM. Rupture and displacement of the ulnar collateral ligament of the metacarpophalangeal joint of the thumb. Preoperative diagnosis. *J Bone Joint Surg* 1986;68:1320-1326.
29. Bowers WH, Hurst LC. Gamekeeper's thumb. Evaluation by arthrography and stress roentgenography. *J Bone Joint Surg* 1977;59:519-524.
30. Smoot EC, Robson MC. Acute management of foreign body injuries of the hand. *Ann Emerg Med* 1983;12: 434-437.
31. Galloway RE. Mammalian bites. *J Emerg Med* 1988;6: 325-331.
32. Stewart CE. Mammalian bites. In: Stewart CE. *Environmental Emergencies.* Williams and Wilkins; Baltimore; 1990
33. Parks BJ, Horner RL, Trimble C. Emergency treatment of high pressure injection injuries of the hand. *JACEP* 1975;4:216-217.
34. Lewis RC. High compression injection injuries to the hand. *Emerg Med Clin North Am* 1985;3:373-381.
35. Kaufman HD. The clinicopathological correlation of high pressure injection injuries. *Br J Surg* 1968;55:214-218.
36. Curca PA, Chisholm CD. High-pressure water injection injury to the hand. *Am J Emerg Med* 1989;7:165-167.

COX-2 Specific Inhibitors

Keith K. Colburn, MD
Raymond Flores, MD
John Rambharose, MD

Despite their well-documented renal and gastrointestinal side effects, nonsteroidal anti-inflammatory drugs (NSAIDs) are among the most widely prescribed medications in clinical practice. Gastrointestinal (GI) toxicities represent some of the most serious side effects of this drug class, and common complications include gastric mucosal ulceration, hemorrhage, or perforation. The analgesic and anti-inflammatory mechanism of action of NSAIDs has been attributed to their capacity for inhibiting the enzyme cyclooxygenase (COX). Recently, two isoforms of cyclooxygenase have been identified. COX-1 is believed to have a gastroprotective effect, while COX-2 specific inhibition is responsible for the production of proinflammatory mediators.

Pharmacological differences among NSAIDs are playing an increasingly important role in drug selection, and clinicians must be aware of the potential advantages and disadvantages of drugs that belong to this large and potentially problematic therapeutic class. For example, generally speaking, older NSAIDs such as ibuprofen and ketoprofen are relatively more potent inhibitors of COX-1 than COX-2, whereas newer NSAIDs, such as nabumatone and etodolac, have more balanced inhibition. A new and recently approved class of selective COX-2 inhibitors—represented by celecoxib (Celebrex®) and rofecoxib (Vioxx®)—offer new opportunities for high-benefit/low-risk therapy in appropriately selected and risk-stratified patients previously requiring conventional NSAID therapy.

It is estimated that NSAIDs currently are taken by approximately 17 million Americans every day.[1] Overall, NSAIDs account for about 4.5% of all prescriptions written in the United States and approximately 22-31% of prescriptions written in the outpatient and/or emergency department.[2] Worldwide, it has been estimated that 100 million prescriptions are written annually, accounting for more than $2 billion in sales, excluding over-the-counter (OTC) purchases.[3] These usage patterns reflect a large segment of the population suffering from such conditions as osteoarthritis (OA) and rheumatoid arthritis (RA), in whom NSAIDs represent initial therapy for control of inflammation and relief of pain and stiffness.

Not surprisingly, more than 50% of NSAID prescriptions are written for individuals older than 60 years of age for the management of OA.[2,4] However, in the acute, outpatient, and emergency practice environments, NSAIDs have become a bulwark of defense against pain syndromes linked to non-rheumatic conditions, among them migraine headache, muscle tension, ureteral and biliary colic, dysmenorrhea, and trauma.

As a therapeutic class, NSAIDs exhibit analgesic, anti-inflammatory, antipyretic, and platelet inhibitory properties.[1] Generally speaking, analgesic effects are obtained at lower doses than those required for anti-inflammatory activity. Although there is some controversy surrounding the issues of relative effectiveness, most experts agree—and clinical experience supports the observation—that when prescribed at equipotent doses, NSAIDs are purported to show similar clinical efficacy. Clinical responses, however, may vary among individuals.[5]

Table 1. Risk Factors for NSAID-Induced Ulcers

DEFINITE

- Age older than 65
- Previous ulcer or GI bleeding
- Concomitant corticosteroid therapy
- High-dose or multiple NSAID therapy
- Duration of therapy

POSSIBLE

- Smoking
- Alcohol
- *Helicobacter pylori*
- Comorbid conditions

Unfortunately, complications associated with NSAID use in the United States result in approximately 100,000 hospitalizations a year at a cost of $4 billion; moreover, it is estimated that NSAIDs are directly linked to about 10,000-20,000 deaths each year.[6] Among the elderly alone, an estimated 41,000 hospitalizations and 3300 deaths annually are thought to be secondary to NSAID therapy.[7] Studies comparing diclofenac, naproxen, and acetaminophen showed that NSAID use in the elderly increased GI complications three- to five-fold as compared with non-NSAID use.[8-13] As the geriatric population has grown, the incidence of OA has increased. As might be expected, elderly patients with OA and RA have been identified as being at high risk for NSAID toxicity. As a result, the search has been ongoing for NSAIDs that specifically target molecules that generate pain and inflammation, but without compromising the cytoprotective effects of prostaglandins. (Please see Table 1.) NSAID toxicity is greater during the first month of therapy and is potentiated by higher doses.[15,16]

Given the frequency with which NSAIDs are used in acute outpatient and emergency practice, a thorough understanding of the benefit-to-risk ratio associated with specific agents is essential for outcome-effective, toxicity-minimizing therapy. Moreover, recent guidelines from the American College of Rheumatology mandate GI protection in patients with OA of the knee and hip who are at increased risk for adverse GI events, i.e. gastrointestinal erosions, ulcerations, and associated hemorrhagic complications.[17] These include individuals 65 years of age or older, those with comorbid conditions, chronic oral corticosteroid use, previous history of gastric or duodenal ulceration or UGI bleeding, and anticoagulant use. Because these guidelines are becoming the standard of care, primary care physicians must be aware of therapeutic options, among them, COX-2 specific inhibitors, that reduce the risk of GI complications in the aforementioned high-risk subgroups.[17-19]

With these issues in clear focus, the purpose of this detailed review is to outline the current status of NSAIDs (i.e., clinical options, risks, pearls, pitfalls, and solutions) in emergency and acute outpatient practice. To this end, the authors discuss the pharmacological properties of NSAIDs, their potential side effects and drug interactions, as well as their risks and benefits in specific clinical settings and for well-established indications. Because the NSAID landscape is undergoing a rapid shift toward COX-2 specific inhibiting agents, "traditional" NSAIDs are compared with currently available COX-2 specific inhibitors with respect to efficacy, mechanism of action, and relative toxicities.

Table 2. History

- Ancient Egyptians, Greeks, and Romans used salicylate extracts derived from myrtle leaves, poplar tree juices, and willow leaves as analgesics and antipyretics.
- Medicinal herb gardens in the Middle Ages and Renaissance featured salicylate containing wintergreen and meadowsweet plants.
- 1763: The Rev. Edward Stone reported on use of willow bark powder as an antipyretic.
- 1853: Charles Frederic Von Gerhardt synthesized acetylsalicyclic acid.
- 1860: Felix Hoffman, using a modified Von Gerhardt method, synthesized acetylsalicyclic acid.
- 1949: Phenylbutazone introduced.
- 1963: Indomethacin introduced.
- 1971: Vane and Piper demonstrated NSAIDs inhibit prostaglandin production.
- 1974: Ibuprofen introduced.
- 1976: Miyamoto et al purified the COX enzyme.
- 1982: Piroxicam introduced.
- 1989: Simmons et al identified the COX-2 enzyme.
- 1999: Celecoxib introduced.
- 1999: Rofecoxib introduced.

Therapeutic History of NSAIDs: An Overview

Dating as far back as ancient Greece and Egypt, salicylic acid and salicylates extracted from myrtle leaves and willow bark were used as therapeutic agents to treat fever, pain, and swelling. In 1860, salicylic acid was chemically synthesized in Germany, where it was used as an external antiseptic and antipyretic, and as a treatment for "rheumatism." In 1899, Felix Hoffman, a chemist who worked for Bayer, synthesized acetyl salicylic acid, or aspirin (a palatable form of salicylic acid), which was introduced for public consumption by its research director, Herman Dresser.[20]

Other early, anti-rheumatism drugs included antipyrene, phenacetin, phenyl-butazone (introduced in 1949), and indomethacin (introduced in 1967). Because these drugs had similar therapeutic

Table 3. Comparison of COX-1 and COX-2

	COX-1	COX-2
Tissue Localization	Most tissues except RBCs	CNS, kidney, and areas of inflammation
Gene	Chromosome 9	Chromosome 1
Stimuli	Basal expression under physiologic conditions—may have increased expression in response to some hormones or growth factor	Basal expression in kidney and brain-mitogens, growth factors, proinflammatory cytokines, and tissue injury
Function	Prostaglandin production, renal blood flow, platelet aggregation, gastric cytoprotection, vascular tone, and-fetal development	Ovulation, parturition, renal development, salt and blood pressure regulation, response to tissue injury, colon cancer pathogenesis, and defense against GI pathogens
Inhibitors	Aspirin, NSAIDs	Glucocorticoids, aspirin, NSAIDs
Homology	60% sequence homology for both enzymes	

effects, they were grouped under the "aspirin-like" drug category. And because these medications were clearly distinct from glucocorticoids, they were categorized as nonsteroidal anti-inflammatory drugs or NSAIDs. In 1971, it was demonstrated that inhibition of prostaglandin synthesis is the primary mechanism of action for NSAIDs.[21] Cyclooxygenase was synthesized in 1976, identifying the key pathway in prostanoid synthesis inhibited by NSAIDs.[22] In 1989, a second enzyme with COX activity was identified, and the two isoforms were designated as "COX-1" and "COX-2."[23] *(Please see Table 2.)*

NSAIDs: Mechanism of Action

First and foremost, NSAIDs are COX inhibitors. Accordingly, the majority of NSAID-related side effects, in large part, can be attributed to inhibition of prostaglandin production.[24,25] The actions, properties, and tissue characteristics of two forms of cyclooxygenase, COX-1 and COX-2, are described in *Table 3*. The COX-1 isoform is located in all tissues, except red blood cells, and is constitutively expressed in the stomach, kidneys, platelets, and endothelial cells under normal physiologic conditions. In contrast, COX-2 production is induced by proinflammatory substances *(see Table 4)*, such as lipopolysaccharides, tumor necrosis factor alpha (TNF-a), interleukin-1 (IL-1), platelet-derived growth factor (PDGF), and other growth factors.[24,26,27]

In addition, COX-2 production is decreased by glucocorticoids, interleukin-4 (IL-4), and interleukin-13 (IL-13).[24] COX-2, which is constitutively expressed in the brain and kidney, is found in significant quantities in other tissues only in areas undergoing active inflammation, and is undetectable under basal conditions in other tissues.[26-29] Both COX isoforms share a 60% amino acid sequence homology and differ in their tertiary structures. For example, unlike the COX-1 enzyme, COX-2 has valine at position 523 instead of isoleucine. This substitution allows COX-2 inhibitors access to the secondary internal side pocket of the molecule that is obstructed by isoleucine in the COX-1 isoform.[24,29-32]

Tissue Activity. Clinical effects produced by COX-1 and COX-2 differ because each has a distinctive pattern of expression. In this regard, COX-1 is a "constitutive" enzyme, which means that it is always present, it is found in most tissues, and it is involved in physiologic, homeostatic functions (i.e., maintaining the integrity of gastric and duodenal lining, as well as playing an integral, vasoactive role in the renal and vascular systems). COX-1 activation leads to the production of prostacyclin, which is cytoprotective when released by the gastric mucosa. Hence, the inhibition of COX-1 can lead to GI ulcerations and erosions.

Moreover, the COX-1 enzyme does not appear to be involved in the mediation of the inflammatory response and associated pain. Studies using a rat air pouch model of lipopolysaccharide-induced inflammation revealed that the COX-1 specific inhibitor investigational drug, SC-560, did not significantly inhibit the production of prostaglandin E2 (PGE 2) in the air pouch, while COX-1 derived PGE 2 production in the gastric mucosa was significantly diminished.[33] This study also demonstrated that SC-560 had no significant effect on pain or edema in a carrageenan-inflamed rat foot pad model, while celecoxib, a COX-2 specific inhibitor, significantly reduced both pain response and paw edema, indicating that COX-2 was the primary enzyme mediating inflammation.[33] When human synovial tissue from patients with RA, ankylosing spondylitis, and psoriatic arthritis was compared with patients with OA, there was increased expression of COX-2 enzyme but not COX-1, providing additional confirmation of the importance of this enzyme in inflammatory diseases.[34]

Anti-Inflammatory Effects. The COX-2 isoform is an "inducible" enzyme, meaning that it is normally not detected unless stimulated or, if it is expressed, it is found in low levels. One study demonstrated up-regulation of COX-2 mRNA and increased

PGE 2 production using mycobacterial adjuvant-induced arthritis and inflamed rat foot pad models.[35] Conversely, there was no increase in COX-1 mRNA. Like COX-2 mRNA, the mRNAs of the proinflammatory cytokines, IL-6 and TNF-a, also were elevated in the affected paws. In this experimental model, treatment with either celecoxib or indomethacin resulted in reversal of paw edema and a reduction of PGE 2 levels to the baseline. The expression of paw COX-2 mRNA was decreased in animals treated with celecoxib. The inhibition of COX-2 activity was associated with a decline in PGE 2 levels along with a decrease in paw and serum IL-6, suggesting that COX-2 derived prostaglandins provide a partial stimulus for the local and systemic production of proinflammatory cytokines.[35] *(Please see Table 4.)*

Table 4. Cytokines that Interact with COX-2

CYTOKINES	SOURCE	ACTION OF CYTOKINES
IL-1	Macrophages, monocytes	T- and B-cell activation increases body temperature, bone resorption, neutrophil mobilization, and early inflammatory response
IL-4	T-cells and mast cells	B-cell activation IgE isotype switching
IL-6	T-cell, macrophages	Early inflammatory response T- and B-cell growth factor Pyrogen
IL-13	T-cells	B-cell growth and differentiation

In human synovium, the generation of COX-2 occurs at inflammatory sites in the presence of macrophages and endothelial cells up-regulated by cytokines and in the presence of bacterial products such as lipopolysaccharide. COX-2 is found in the synovial membrane of patients with RA; however, in healthy patients as well as those individuals with OA, COX-2 is found at low levels or is not detectable.[36] Accordingly, an NSAID selective for selective COX-2 inhibition has the potential of being an "ideal" anti-inflammatory drug, since it spares COX-1 activity, and therefore, has the potential to minimize or prevent GI , and possibly renal, toxicity.

NSAIDs and COX Selectivity

Different NSAIDs vary in their relative COX-1 and COX-2 specific selectivity, a pharmacological property that has important clinical implications. The capacity of any NSAID to inhibit prostanoid production by these enzymes is expressed as the inhibitory concentration of 50% of an enzyme (IC50). The ratio of the IC50 of COX-2 to COX-1 defines COX-2 selectivity. Therefore, the smaller the ratio, the more COX-2 selective the drug.[37] For example, a ratio of less than 1 would signify greater COX-2 inhibition than a ratio greater than 1, while an IC50 of 1 reflects equal selectivity.

Interestingly, the IC50 results depend on the assay that is being used. Salicylates do not significantly inhibit either COX isoform in pure cell free recombinant enzyme systems, but they demonstrate significant inhibition of both enzymes in a cell membrane system.[34.38] Most NSAIDs inhibit the COX-1 isoform and exhibit a variable ability to inhibit the COX-2 enzyme.[34,37] NSAIDs such as etodolac (Lodine®) and nambumetone (Relafen®) demonstrate some COX-2 specificity at lower doses and are more COX-1 selective at higher anti-inflammatory doses. As a result, these NSAIDs have been referred to as COX-2 "preferential."

Drugs that demonstrate consistent COX-2 specific inhibition throughout their dose ranges are called COX-2 "selective."[25,29] *Table 6* ranks NSAIDs at usual therapeutic doses from the least to the most COX-2 selectivity; this ranking reflects NSAIDs that were available prior to the introduction of the COX-2 specific inhibitors.[39] From a clinical perspective, it should be noted that NSAIDs introduced prior to celecoxib are capable of GI mucosal prostaglandin depletion at recommended therapeutic doses. In contrast, early studies showed no prostaglandin inhibition with NS-398, an experimental COX-2 specific inhibitor, and nonacetylated salicylic acid.[39]

In order to completely inhibit COX-2 without affecting the COX-1, an NSAID should be about 100 times more potent against COX-2 than COX-1 and it should have an IC50 COX-2/IC50 COX-1 ratio of 0.01 or lower. Celecoxib and rofecoxib far exceed this standard for a selective COX-2 inhibitor.

Specifically, celecoxib demonstrates a 375-fold selectivity for COX-2, while rofecoxib has approximately an 800-fold selectivity for COX-2 in human enzyme systems.[27,40] The clinical significance of the differences in COX-2 selectivity between these drugs has not been determined. Celecoxib was introduced into the market in February 1999. Rofecoxib was released in June 1999. A recent review comparing celecoxib, meloxicam, and nabumetone in dogs demonstrated GI and renal injury in all the subjects given nabumetone, in some given meloxicam, and in none of the subject in the celecoxib group.[41]

Celecoxib

Celecoxib is indicated for the relief of the signs and symptoms of OA and RA in adults. Specifically, for the relief of the signs and symptoms of osteoarthritis, the recommended dose is 200 mg daily administered as a single dose or as 100 mg twice daily. For the relief of the signs and symptoms of rheumatoid arthritis, the recommended dose is 100-200 mg twice daily. Celecoxib is priced similar to other branded NSAIDs.

Borderline elevation of one or more liver tests may occur in up to 15% of patients. Significant elevation (> 3 times the upper limits of normal) has been reported in only 1% of patients in clinical trials. Celecoxib is contraindicated in patients with a known allergy to aspirin or to other NSAIDs. Because celecoxib is a 4 benzenesulfonomide, it is also contraindicated in patients with documented sulfonamide allergy.[42]

This COX-2 specific inhibitor is rapidly absorbed, reaching a maximum serum concentration in three hours with a half-life of 11 hours. The drug is metabolized in the liver by the cytochrome P450 enzyme, CYP2C9, and excreted in feces and urine. Celecoxib also inhibits CYP2D6 in vitro.[42] Therefore, there is a potential for an in vivo drug interaction.[44] Higher than recommended doses of celecoxib (600 mg bid for 7 days) have no effect on platelet aggregation and bleeding time. A single dose of 800 mg of celecoxib did not inhibit platelet COX-1 dependent aggregation. Celecoxib does not appear to affect the anticoagulant effect of warfarin, although caution should be exercised if coadministration is considered.

The GI safety of celecoxib has been evaluated in several excellent studies.[17-19,43-45] In comparative trials between celecoxib and ibuprofen or naproxen, celecoxib was associated with a statistically significant lower incidence of endoscopic ulcers evaluated at 12 weeks. The incidences were 9.9%-17.6% with naproxen (500 mg bid) and 9.6% for ibuprofen (800 mg tid), compared to 1.5-4% and 1.5-5.9% for celecoxib at 100 mg bid and 200 mg bid, respectively. Moreover, among 5285 patients studied who received celecoxib over a 1-6 month period, only two patients (0.04%) experienced significant upper GI bleeding, at 14 and 22 days after initiation of therapy. The discontinuation rate for celecoxib (7.1%) was similar to that for placebo (6.1%). [14B]

In initial studies evaluating tolerability of celecoxib, it was found that the occurrence rate of dyspepsia and abdominal pain with celecoxib was lower than that of naproxen, ibuprofen, and diclofenac but slightly higher than placebo. The occurrence rates were 8.8% for dyspepsia and 4.1% for abdominal pain compared to 6.2%/2.8%, 12.2%/7.7%, 10.9%/9%, and 12.8%/9% for placebo, naproxen, ibuprofen, and diclofenac, respectively. Dyspepsia and abdominal pain were the most common side effects of celecoxib which led to discontinuation in clinical trials.[44]

A more recent study was designed to determine the upper gastrointestinal tolerability of celecoxib as compared to naproxen and placebo in patients with OA and RA.[46] The symptom-based GI endpoints evaluated included severe abdominal pain, dyspepsia, and nausea. The investigators of this study concluded that OA and RA patients treated with celecoxib were significantly less likely to report common upper GI symptoms than were OA and RA patients treated with the traditional NSAID naproxen. In addition, the cumulative incidence of common upper GI symptoms experienced by celecoxib users did not differ significantly from that of patients receiving placebo. Finally, this clinical trial did not find a dose-response relationship between celecoxib and common upper GI symptoms.[46]

Until recent studies, the correlation between endoscopic findings or symptoms and serious GI side effects and prediction of clinically significant GI complications had not been precisely established. However, with publication of the CLASS study, this relationship has been clarified. Endoscopically observed ulcers may not be reliable predictors of severe GI events. Endoscopic ulcers tend to be smaller, superficial, and predominately gastric, while serious events tend to be both gastric and duodenal.[44] However, available endoscopic data showing reduction in ulcers as well as reduction in dyspepsia and abdominal pain are sufficiently compelling to recommend COX-2 specific inhibitors such as celecoxib as initial therapy for pain management in patients with OA.

Newer studies (CLASS, VIGOR) have been even more encouraging and explicit in evaluating the relationship between COX-2 specific inhibitors and upper GI complications. Primary care practitioners now appear to have a new, safer treatment paradigm for this patient population.[19] From a risk management and therapeutic upgrade perspective, celecoxib was associated with a statistically significant reduction in ulcer complications and symptomatic ulcers. For all patients, the annualized incidence rates of upper GI ulcer complications alone and combined with symptomatic ulcers for celecoxib vs NSAIDs were 0.76% vs 1.45% (P=.09) and 2.08% vs 3.54% (P=.02), respectively. Accordingly, the relative reduction in the celecoxib treatment arm as compared to the conventional NSAID group, for the combined UGI complication/symptomatic ulcer endpoints was 60%. For patients not taking aspirin, the annualized incidence rate of upper GI ulcer complications alone and combined with symptomatic ulcers for celecoxib vs NSAIDs were 0.44% vs 1.27% (P = 0.04) and 1.40% vs 2.91% (P = 0.02), reflecting a 64.2% relative reduction in upper GI complications alone among non-aspirin celecoxib users vs non-aspirin users of conventional NSAIDs.[19]

For patients taking aspirin, the annualized incidence rates of upper GI ulcer complications alone and combined with symptomatic ulcers for celecoxib vs NSAIDs were 2.01% vs 2.12% (P = 0.92) and 4.70% vs 6.00% (P = 0.49). Of special clinical significance is the fact that fewer celecoxib-treated patients than NSAID-treated patients experienced chronic GI blood loss, GI intolerance, hepatotoxicity, or renal toxicity. Moreover, no difference was noted in the incidence of cardiovascular events between celecoxib and NSAIDs, irrespective of aspirin use. Put simply, the clinical superiority and safety benefits of celecoxib over two commonly prescribed traditional NSAIDs—as measured by improved GI outcome, toleration, and safety endpoints—has been firmly established by the landmark CLASS trial and other recent investigations.[17-19,45,46]

Rofecoxib

Rofecoxib inhibits COX-2 without evidence of COX-1 inhibition, even at oral doses of up to 1000 mg.[17] This COX-2 inhibitor is approved for treatment of OA pain in adults and conditions such as pain from postoperative dental and orthopedic surgical procedures and primary dysmenorrhea. Rofecoxib does not have approval for RA treatment.[48] Oral doses of rofecoxib 12.5-50 mg daily have been found to be as effective for the treatment of OA as diclofenac (Voltaren) 50 mg po three times a day.[49]

Rofecoxib is contraindicated in patients who exhibit an allergic reaction to aspirin and NSAIDs. The drug is metabolized by reduction with cytosolic enzymes. CP450 plays a minor role in the metabolism of rofecoxib. A general enzyme inducer, rifampin, has been reported to produce a 50% decrease in the plasma concentration of rofecoxib. Rofecoxib has no effect on platelet function. Dosages up to 375 mg given daily for up to 12 days did not affect bleeding time relative to placebo.[48-50]

Adverse effects experienced by patients on rofecoxib include diarrhea, headache, insomnia, and edema.[50]

This COX-2 specific inhibitor is available as 12.5 mg or 25 mg tablets and as an oral suspension containing 12.5 mg or 25 mg per 5 mL. The recommended initial dose for osteoarthritis is 12.5 mg once daily. Some patients may achieve added benefit at a dose of 25 mg once daily, which is considered the maximum dose for this indication. It may be taken without regard to meals.

Rofecoxib, 25 mg or 50 mg daily, has been reported to produce a lower percentage of endoscopic gastroduodenal ulcers than ibuprofen 2400 mg daily. The difference was statistically significant at 12- and 24-week assessments. Rofecoxib also appears to be well tolerated in terms of GI adverse events. In a clinical trial, the percent of patients experiencing diarrhea was 6.8% vs. 6.5% for placebo, 3.5% vs. 2.7% for dyspepsia, 3.8% vs. 2.8% for epigastric discomfort, and 4.2% vs. 3.6% for heartburn. In the VIGOR trial, with respect to clinical UGI endpoints, rofecoxib significantly decreased annualized risk of clinically important GI events by 54-62% ($P < 0.001$ for clinical UGI events as compared to naproxen 500 mg po bid [$P = 0.005$ for complicated GI events, and $P < 0.001$ for any GI bleeding]). Prior clinical UGI events, steroid use, and lack of prior NSAID use were significant risk factors for development of clinical UGI events. From a GI safety perspective, the VIGOR trial, as CLASS did for celecoxib, confirms the potential GI safety advantages of rofecoxib as compared to NSAIDs.

Rofecoxib is approved for OA but not for RA. The renal effects of rofecoxib are similar to those of other NSAIDs. The use of rofecoxib for the relief of pain at the 50 mg dose is not recommended beyond five days, because prolonged administration of this agent at the 50 mg dose has been shown to be associated with an increased incidence of peripheral edema and hypertension. Specifically, when the 50 mg dose has been used in OA trials for extended periods of time, the rate of hypertension increased from 3.5% to 8.2%, and the peripheral edema rate increased from 3.7% to 6.3%. Coadministration of rofecoxib and warfarin has resulted in an increase of 8-11% in INR. Therefore, monitoring of INR is recommended with coadministration.

In OA, rofecoxib (12.5-25 mg) has been reported to be similar in effectiveness as ibuprofen 800 mg tid over six weeks or diclofenac 50 mg tid over six months. Study patients included patients with OA of the hip or knee. Ninety percent had an increase in pain following withdrawal of NSAIDs and 10% had moderate symptoms while taking acetaminophen. Rofecoxib, ibuprofen, and diclofenac all showed about a 50% reduction in the WOMAC (Western Ontario and McMaster Universities OA index) visual analog scale walking on a flat surface. This is a composite of pain, stiffness, and functional measures in OA. Like celecoxib, rofecoxib (25 mg-50 mg) has been associated with fewer endoscopic ulcers than ibuprofen 2400 mg daily (4.1-8.8% vs 27.7-29.2%). This compares favorably to placebo (5.1-9.9%).[44,48-50] Rofecoxib (12.5-25 mg daily) is priced competitively with celecoxib when used for OA.

Efficacy and Safety of COX-2 Specific Inhibitors

In the United States, two COX-2 selective agents, celecoxib (Celebrex®) and rofecoxib (Vioxx®), have received FDA approval. The potential for this new class of NSAIDs to affect prescribing of anti-inflammatory drugs by primary care physicians should not be minimized. Early studies comparing side effects safety of the COX-2 specific inhibitors with other NSAIDs are impressive, especially in the GI system.

In this regard, the safety and efficacy of celecoxib in RA was reported in both phase II and phase III clinical trials. In a four-week phase II trial, 330 RA patients received celecoxib at doses of 40 mg bid, 200 mg bid, 400 mg bid, or a placebo. At the end of the trial, 18% of the patients had withdrawn from the placebo group due to lack of efficacy compared with 17% for the 40 mg group, 4% from the 200 mg group, and 6% from the 400 mg group. A statistically significant difference ($P < 0.005$) was seen in the higher-dose celecoxib groups at weeks 1, 2, and 4 when compared with placebo.[40]

In a 12-week, double-blind, placebo-controlled trial, 1149 subjects with active RA received celecoxib at doses of 100 mg, 200 mg, or 400 mg bid, or naproxen 500 mg bid, or placebo.[43] Celecoxib at 200 mg bid and 400 mg bid was as effective as the naproxen 500 mg bid. All were statistically better than placebo ($P < 0.05$) in demonstrating improvement of the ACR 20 responder.[43] *(Please see Table 7.)*

Celecoxib demonstrated safety and efficacy in a two-week placebo-controlled study of 293 subjects with OA.[40] Patients were randomized to receive celecoxib in doses of 40 mg, 100 mg, 200 mg bid, or placebo. Withdrawals due to lack of efficacy were greater in the placebo group (14%) vs. subjects in the 100 mg group (1%) and the 200 mg group (4%).[40] Except for the group on 40 mg celecoxib bid, the patient assessment of pain using a visual analog scale (VAS) was statistically significant ($P < 0.048$) at both weeks 1 and 2 for the treatment groups compared to placebo.[40]

No effect on collagen-induced platelet aggregation was seen in a study of six healthy male subjects receiving celecoxib 400 mg bid. Results of pre- and post-treatment collagen-induced platelet aggregation were not statistically significant. This same group subsequently received a single dose of 650 mg aspirin. The post-dose values were significantly different from predose values ($P = 0.031$).[85] In another study, bleeding time was affected slightly by celecoxib 600 mg qd when compared to naproxen 500 mg bid after 10 days. The mean increase in bleeding time for naproxen was 244.7 seconds vs. 60.5 seconds for celecoxib.

Hypertensive Effects

A six-week, multi-center, double-blind parallel study of approximately 800 hypertensive patients with OA—all of whom were being treated with antihypertensive medication(s) and were > 65 years of age—was designed to compare the incidence of clinically significant cardiorenal events associated with celecoxib (200 mg po qd) with that of rofecoxib (25 mg po qd). Half of the study's patients were between the ages of 65 and 74, and the other half were ≥ 74 years of age. Clinical assessments were conducted at baseline and then at weeks one, two, and six to determine key measures of cardiorenal safety such as edema and systolic blood pressure.

The results of the this study show hypertensive patients with OA who were taking rofecoxib experienced significantly more increases in edema and systolic hypertension than those taking celecoxib. Specifically, those OA patients taking the usually prescribed OA dose (25 mg po qd) of rofecoxib experienced a two-fold increase in clinically significant edema compared to the celecoxib-treated group ($p < 0.05$). Of special clinical importance was the finding

Table 5. Adverse Effects of NSAID Therapy

GI	Gastroduodenal ulcers, strictures, esophagitis, gastritis, colitis, small and large bowel erosions
Renal	Acute and/or chronic renal failure, fluid and electrolyte imbalances, hyperkalemia, hematuria, nephrotic syndrome with interstitial nephritis, papillary necrosis
Cardiovascular	Exacerbation of hypertension, exacerbation of congestive heart failure, arrhythmia
Hepatic	Elevated transaminases, choleostasis, hepatic failure (rare)
CNS	Headache, tinnitus, vertigo, tremor, depression, somnalence, altered mental status, aseptic meningitis
Hematologic	Thrombocytopenia, hemolytic anemia, agranulocytosis, leukopenia, eosinophilia, aplastic anemia
Pulmonary	Exacerbation of asthma, cough, respiratory depression, laryngeal and pharyngeal edema
Dermatologic	Skin rash, photosensitivity, Stevens Johnson syndrome, pemphigoid reaction, erythema multiform, urticaria, angioedema
Bone/Cartilage	Joint erosions, decreased repair of cartilage damage

that within two weeks of the start of the study, significantly more rofecoxib patients had clinically important increases in systolic blood pressure (≥ 20 mmHg) vs. those on celecoxib. Investigators also reported that by the six-week endpoint, almost 60% more patients on rofecoxib than on celecoxib experienced systolic blood pressure elevations of 20 mmHg or more, a measure of clinically significant hypertension. The statistical difference between celecoxib and rofecoxib was observed as early as week two of the study and confirmed again at the six-week endpoint. Systolic hypertension has been shown to be an important risk factor for MI and stroke. Therefore, the reported increases in systolic BP have the potential for adversely affecting a patient's cardiovascular risk profile, and should be considered when selecting these agents.

Toxicity of Traditional NSAIDs vs. COX-2 Specific Inhibitors: Incentives for Risk Management Upgrades

The therapeutic shift—or risk management upgrade—from traditional NSAIDs to selective COX-2 inhibitors is justified by the relative benefit-to-risk advantage that appears to be associated with the newly introduced agents. Currently, NSAIDs play an important role in the management of various types of arthritis and are often the primary treatment used for patients with OA. These drugs are used for a variety of inflammatory arthritides, supplementing disease-modifying antirheumatic drugs (DMARDs) to reduce pain and inflammation. Unlike DMARDs, however, NSAIDs do not slow the progression of the disease process. Their primary benefits frequently are related to pain relief but, on the downside, NSAIDs also may be responsible for significant, and even fatal, side effects.[51] *(See Table 5.)*

Adverse Gastrointestinal Effects. GI side effects associated with NSAID therapy are common. Approximately 30-60% of NSAID users experience some abdominal discomfort, or dyspepsia.[52,53] These symptoms do not necessarily correlate with endoscopic findings. Approximately 40% of persons with erosive gastritis are asymptomatic, while almost 50% of patients with dyspepsia have no evidence of mucosal damage on endoscopy.[48]

Endoscopic studies of arthritic patients receiving chronic NSAID therapy revealed that 50-75% of subjects have gastroduodenal lesions ranging from small subepithelial hemorrhages and mucosal erosions to ulcers.[52] The majority of these lesions are of little clinical significance.[53,54] Studies showed the prevalence of peptic ulcers in patients on chronic NSAIDs to be about 25%.[55] Gastric ulcers were seen in 15% of patients, while duodenal ulcers were present in 10%.[53]

Strategies used to avoid GI mucosal injury from NSAIDs included the use of enteric-coated NSAIDs, rectal suppositories, injectable NSAIDs, and the use of pro-drugs such as sulindac. Unfortunately, GI mucosal damage and ulcers still occurred with all of these formulations.[52,56,57]

Another commonly used strategy is to recommend ingestion of NSAIDs with food. A study of healthy volunteers failed to support the outcome-effectiveness of this approach.[58] In one study, the participants, who took ranitidine and aspirin with meals, had significantly more gastric erosions than those who ingested these medications two hours before meals.[58] Misoprostol, a synthetic PGE1 analog with antisecretory and cytoprotective effects, was shown to prevent both gastric and duodenal ulcers in chronic NSAID users.[59] One trial found that misoprostol 200 mg qid decreased upper GI tract NSAID complications such as perforated ulcers, obstruction, and bleeding ulcers by 40%; however, 42% of study patients had to withdraw because of side effects from misoprostol including diarrhea and abdominal discomfort.[60]

The ability of the proton pump inhibitor, omeprazole, to decrease the incidence of gastroduodenal ulcers in NSAID users was demonstrated in four recent large, randomized, controlled trials.[61-64] Omeprazole 20 mg/d was superior to ranitidine 150 mg bid in the treatment and prevention of gastroduodenal ulcers.[61] At the end of the eight-week healing phase in this six-month trial, 80% of patients in the omeprazole group had been successfully treated compared to 63% of patients in the ranitidine group.

Upon completion of the trial, 72% of subjects taking omeprazole remained in remission vs. 59% of those given ranitidine.[61] Another study showed that omeprazole 20 mg daily exhibits greater efficacy in gastroduodenal ulcer prevention than placebo or misoprostol 200 mg bid.[62] Healing rates at eight weeks were 87% for gastric ulcers and 93% for duodenal ulcers in the omeprazole group, while healing rates for the misoprostol subjects were approximately 73% for gastric ulcers and almost 77% for duodenal ulcers. Sixty-one percent of patients remained in remission in the omeprazole group vs. 48% receiving misoprostol and 27% on placebo.[62]

Lower GI complications, while not as common as those seen in the upper GI tract, are potentially serious. NSAID use can be associated with colonic ulceration, perforation, inflammation, strictures, and diarrhea.[56] Patients with quiescent inflammatory bowel disease could suffer an exacerbation of their disease by taking NSAIDs.[65]

Recent reports suggest that NSAIDs suppress the development of colon polyps.[66,67] COX-2 specific inhibitors may be helpful only in preventing tumors that have increased expression of COX-2 enzymes. Two separate reports found that the expression of COX-2 increases during the formation of colorectal adenomas and adenocarcinomas.[68,69] A recent, large population-based study reported that chronic NSAID use reduced the risk of colon cancer by approximately one-half. Celecoxib has been approved for prevention of polyps in individuals with familial polyposis of the colon. Most non-aspirin NSAIDs have demonstrated the ability to prevent colon cancer.[70] COX-2 generation was mapped to chromosome No. 1 at one of the loci associated with colon cancer.[68] COX-2 is present in pancreatic islet cells under both basal and cytokine stimulated conditions.[71,72] The effects of the new COX-2 selective drugs on the GI system will be addressed under the heading, "Safety and Efficacy of COX-2 Inhibitors."

Renal Effects. As previously discussed, the COX-2 enzyme is constitutively expressed in endothelial and smooth muscle cells of the renal vasculature and in the podocytes of the glomerulus. COX-1 is present in the podocytes of the fetal kidney but absent in adult glomeruli.[73] Prostacyclin and PGE2 maintain renal blood flow in states of effective volume depletion such as congestive heart failure (CHF), liver cirrhosis, and true volume depletion seen with chronic diuretic therapy.[74] Prostacyclin and PGE2 preserve renal blood flow by antagonizing the vasoconstrictive effects of angiotensin II and norepinephrine.

Because of these properties, NSAID use maybe associated with peripheral edema, hyperkalemia, acute renal failure in patients with hypovolemia, altered intrarenal plasma flow, nephrotic syndrome with interstitial nephritis, and papillary necrosis.[75] Apart from peripheral edema, there are no studies implicating COX-2 specific inhibitors with the aforementioned adverse renal complications from NSAID use. Animal models demonstrated that high doses of celecoxib do not impair renal prostaglandin synthesis.[76] Future studies will clarify the potential renal-sparing effects of COX-2 specific inhibitors.

For now, short-term studies of patients with RA and OA taking celecoxib have reported no renal dysfunction. In this regard, small randomized, single-blinded crossover investigations[77] have been reported suggesting that both therapeutic (200 mg po bid) and supra-therapeutic (400 mg po bid) doses of celecoxib, as compared to naproxen (500 mg po bid), are not associated with detrimental changes in GFR in healthy elderly subjects. This suggests that celecoxib may afford benefits in elderly patients susceptible to acute, NSAID-mediated changes in renal hemodynamic function.[77]

Table 6. COX-1/COX-2 Ratios for a Variety of NSAIDs

RANK	DRUG	RATIO*
1	Flubiprofen	10.17
2	Ketoprofen	8.16
3	Fenoprofen	5.14
4	Aspirin	3.12
5	Oxaprofin	2.52
6	Tolmetin	2.09
7	Indomethacin	1.78
8	Ibuprofen	1.69
9	Naproxen	0.88
10	Piroxicam	0.79
11	Ketorolac	0.68
12	6-MNA	0.64
13	Nabumetone	0.62
14	Sulindac	0.61
15	Bismuth (subsalicylate)	0.50
16	Salsalate	0.29†
17	Acetaminophen	0.25
18	Salicylic acid	0.13†
19	Etodolac	0.12
20	Mefenamic acid	0.08
21	Diclofenac	0.05
22	NS-398	0.042
23	Nimesulide	0.017
24	Dexamethasone	0.002
25	Valeryl salicylate	0.001

* Ratios more than 1 indicate drug is more COX-1 selective; ratios less than 1 indicate drug is more COX-2 selective.

† Since actual IC_{50} for COX-1 in blood was more than 100 μM, a value of 100 μM was used in calculation of ratio; therefore, these ratios represent a maximum possible ratio of IC_{50} COX-2/ IC_{50} COX-1 in blood.

Studies have suggested that peripheral edema was minimally higher in the celecoxib group of patients than in the placebo group, implying a role for COX-2 in maintaining fluid and electrolyte balance.[28,78] Interstitial nephritis caused by NSAIDs was extremely rare and, most likely, idiosyncratic in nature.[79,80] Mice deficient in COX-2 enzymes developed kidney abnormalities including inflammation, fibrosis, and papillary mineralization.[81]

Hepatic Effects. Liver injury from NSAIDs ranges from asymptomatic transaminase elevation to clinical hepatitis.[82] Fatal liver damage may rarely occur. Liver function tests are advised at the beginning of treatment and three months later, since side effects fre-

Table 7. ACR-20 Responder Index

PATIENT MUST SHOW A 20% IMPROVEMENT IN:
- Number of tender/painful joints
- Number of swollen joints

AND IN THREE OR MORE OF THE FOLLOWING:
- Physician's global assessment of arthritic condition
- Patient's global assessment of arthritic condition
- Visual analog scale
- Health assessment questionnaire of patient activities of daily living
- C-reactive protein

quently appear during the initial three months of therapy.[82] NSAIDs should be discontinued when alanine transferase (ALT) and asparate transferase (AST) are elevated 2-3 times normal levels. A recent review identified the three NSAIDs most commonly associated with hepatic toxicity as sulindac, diclofenac, and aspirin.[83]

Differences in the IC50 of these NSAIDs do not appear to directly correlate with increased risk of liver injury.[40] According to one group of investigators, the risk of liver toxicity ascribed to certain NSAIDs may be biased because estimates are based on spontaneous reports from physicians or patients.[41]

Hematologic Effects. Adverse hematologic side effects from NSAIDs are rare. Agranulocytosis and aplastic anemia are the most serious.[41] Phenylbutazone (not available in the United States) and indomethacin are the NSAIDs most commonly associated with agranulocytosis. The potential for hematologic side effects with COX-2 inhibiting drugs is not yet clear.

Coagulation Effects. There are several mechanisms by which NSAIDs increase the risk and severity of bleeding, especially in a patient already taking warfarin. A direct hypoprothrombinemic effect occurs by depressing the vitamin K-dependent synthesis of clotting factors VII, IX, and X. Second, NSAIDs displace warfarin from plasma albumin, which is a transient effect, since there is an increase in the clearance of unbound warfarin until the previous concentration is again reached.[41]

Because platelets contain COX-1 but not COX-2, non-COX-2 selective NSAIDs demonstrate antiplatelet effects by inhibiting COX-1. COX-2 selective agents do not interfere with platelet activity.[41,84] Celecoxib administered at doses of 600 mg bid does not interfere with serum thromboxane, bleeding time, or platelet aggregation as is seen with naproxen.[85] Moreover, celecoxib, when combined with 2-5 mg per day of warfarin, does not prolong the prothrombin time.[86] A role for celecoxib as prophylaxis for myocardial infarction and stroke is not likely, due to its lack of antiplatelet activity.

Cartilage Effects. Prostaglandins are well-documented modulators of articular cartilage metabolism and bone resorption.[87] According to some reports, NSAIDs can exacerbate cartilage erosion, produce bony destruction of the femoral head in OA patients, and accelerate the progression of joint damage.[88-90] COX-2 was recently shown to play a part in the bone loss induced by interleukin-1. *(Please see Table 7.)* Interleukin-1 functions to stimulate osteoclast formation.[91] However, an increase in COX-2 production in cartilage explants suggests it may have a role in cartilage repair.[92]

Pulmonary Effects. A four- to 14-fold increase in COX-2 levels in asthmatic subjects has been reported, suggesting a possible COX-2 role in the pathogenesis of asthma.[93] As might be expected, COX-2 blockade may be therapeutic in asthma, whereas older NSAIDs can cause bronchoconstriction and edema, especially in aspirin-sensitive patients. The authors, however, are not aware of studies evaluating COX-2 inhibitors for asthma treatment.

Central Nervous System Effects. NSAIDs can cause headaches, confusion, and dizziness, and aggravate psychiatric illness, epilepsy, and parkinsonism. Ingestion of indomethacin is associated with the highest incidence of NSAID-associated CNS symptoms. There are anecdotal reports of aseptic meningitis in SLE patients using ibuprofen.[94]

The presence of the COX-2 protein in neuronal and glial cells following ischemic injury has been reported, suggesting a possible pathologic role for COX-2.[94] Epidemiologic studies suggest that COX-2 inhibition delays the development of Alzheimer's disease, possibly by blocking neuro-inflammation; however, the precise mechanism is not known.[74,95] COX-2 is reported to be the predominant isoform in the neocortex and hippocampus areas of the brain, the same areas affected by Alzheimer's disease.[96] No consistent association is found between COX-2 expression and neurologic abnormalities.

Reproductive Tract Effects. The COX-2 enzyme is apparently induced in ovulation. Mice deficient in COX-2 are noted to be infertile.[97] COX-2 expression is prominent in the human amnion at term by 100-fold compared with earlier in gestation, suggesting a possible role for COX-2 inhibiting preterm labor.[41] COX-2 specific inhibitors are contraindicated at or near term. Recent data showed that the fetus produces PGF2a-inducing luteolysis, leading to uterine contractions. This process reduces maternal progesterone levels and induction of oxytocin receptors in the myometrium, leading to parturition.[98] COX-2 also influences fertilization and implantation. This enzyme is required for normal oocyte development and probably for generation of the enzymes necessary to rupture the follicle.[99] Following fertilization, COX-1 prepares the wall for interaction with the embryo, while COX-2 and prostaglandin receptors mediate implantation.[100-102]

Cardiovascular Effects. Cardiovascular side effects of NSAIDs occur more frequently than previously recognized. NSAIDs have increased the blood pressure of subjects in several trials. By inhibiting prostaglandin synthesis, NSAIDs interfere with systemic and renal vasodilation, glomerulo-filtration, tubular secretion of fluids and electrolytes, adrenergic neurotransmission, and the renin-angiotensin-aldosterone system, leading to hypertension.[103]

A recent meta-analysis of 50 studies reported that NSAIDs increased the mean blood pressure by approximately 5 mmHg.[104] Investigators also found that hypertensive patients taking blood pressure-lowering drugs were more severely affected by NSAID use than normotensive volunteers given antihypertensives. The hypertensive effect of NSAIDs appears to be most pronounced in patients taking angiotensin-converting enzyme inhibitors, diuretics, and beta-blockers.[105] However, the anti-hypertensive effect of calcium channel blockers does not appear to be affected by NSAIDs.[105]

The American College of Rheumatology (ACR) recommends that for patients taking NSAIDs, a baseline CBC, creatinine, AST, and ALT should be done and repeated yearly.[106] It is also advisable to check a patient's blood pressure within a few weeks of initiating NSAID therapy and 2-3 times a year, as indicated, thereafter.[105] Other cardiovascular effects of NSAIDs include exacerbation of CHF and isolated peripheral edema.[105] NSAIDs are beneficial in relieving the pain of post-pericardectomy syndrome and pericarditis.[105] The extent to which COX-2 selective drugs affect the cardiovascular system requires further study.

Summary

The decision to use NSAIDs for treatment of inflammatory arthritides and pain-producing conditions must weigh the potential clinical benefits of COX-2 specific inhibitors such as celecoxib against the potential short- and long-term adverse effects and/or discomfort that may be associated with "traditional" COX-1 inhibitors. Until the recent introduction of selective COX-2 inhibitors such as celecoxib, the risks of using traditional NSAIDs such as ibuprofen, naproxen, and ketoprofen frequently outweighed the possible benefits, especially in high-risk populations (i.e., the elderly; individuals with CHF and/or hypertension; patients with renal disease; patients on warfarin; and most importantly, patients at risk for gastric or duodenal ulceration).

The introduction of COX-2 specific inhibitors has dramatically changed the therapeutic landscape for anti-inflammatory treatment in the emergency department and acute care clinic. The mandate to use COX-2 specific inhibitors is now established, especially for the aforementioned high-risk subgroups, in whom the benefits of pain relief and inflammation management can now potentially be accomplished with a significant reduction in gastrointestinal complications, at least based on initial endoscopic surveillance studies and associated comparative data suggesting a 40- to 100-fold reduction in significant GI tract hemorrhage in patients taking selective COX-2 inhibitors.

Although both COX-2 specific inhibitors appear to be associated with a high benefit-to-risk ratio, celecoxib appears to have features and flexibility that make it especially useful in the elderly patients with co-morbid conditions, especially in individuals with known risk factors for or with active heart disease. It has dual indications for both OA and RA, it can be administered safely in combination with aspirin or warfarin, and toleration is excellent. However, it should be stressed that caution is advised for patients who are taking NSAIDs or COX-2 specific inhibitors in combination with warfarin, and that patients should be carefully monitored. In addition, a recent study suggests that celecoxib is not associated with an increased risk of thromboembolic events.[19]

Based on evidence-based trial data evaluating adverse GI, cardiovascular, and renal endpoints, expert consensus opinion, medico-legal considerations, and available post-marketing experience, the "risk management" upgrade from NSAIDs to COX-2 specific inhibitors such as celecoxib makes excellent clinical sense. A "First, do no harm" medication that has a high-benefit and low-risk ratio should be considered a milestone in modern medicine. We've come a long way from aspirin.

References

1. Pollison R, ed. *Rheumatology MKSAP*. 2nd ed. Philadelphia, PA: American College of Physicians; 1997:74.
2. Elashoff JD, Grossman MI. Trends in hospital admission and death rates for peptic ulcer in the United States from 1970 to 1978. *Gastroenterology* 1980;78:280-285.
3. Winzeler S, Rosenstein B. Non-steroidal antiinflammatory drugs—A review. *AAOHN J* 1998;46:253-259.
4. Hawker G. Prescribing nonsteroidal anti-inflammatory drugs—What,s new? Editorial. *J Rheumatol* 1997;24:243-244.
5. Simon LS, Strand V. Clinical response to non-steroidal anti-inflammatory drugs. *Arthritis Rheum* 1997;40:1940-1943.
6. Scheiman JM. Gastrointestinal effects of NSAIDs therapeutic implications of COX-2 selective agents. *Postgrad Med Special Rep* 1998;17-22.
7. Ray WA, et al. Adverse drug reactions and the elderly. *Health Aff* (Millwood) 1990;9:114-122.
8. Dieppe P, et al. A two year placebo-controlled trial of non-steroidal anti-inflammatory therapy in osteoarthritis of the knee joint. *Br J Rheumatol* 1993;32:595-600.
9. Williams HJ, et al. Comparison of naproxen and acetaminophen in a two year study of treatment of osteoarthritis of the knee. *Arthritis Rheum* 1993;36:1196-1206.
10. March LM, et al. N-of-1 trials comparing a non-steroidal anti-inflammatory drug with paracetamol in osteoarthritis. *BMJ* 1994; 309:1041-1046.
11. Henry D, et al. Variability in risk of gastrointestinal complications with individual non-steroidal anti-inflammatory drugs: Results of a collaborative meta-analysis. *BMJ* 1996;312:1563-1566.
12. Gabriel SE, et al. Risk for serious gastrointestinal complications related to use of nonsteroidal anti-inflammatory drugs: A meta-analysis. *Ann Intern Med* 1991;115:787-796.
13. Bollini P, et al. The impact of research quality and study design on epidemiologic estimates of the effect of nonsteroidal anti-inflammatory drugs on upper gastrointestinal tract disease. *Arch Intern Med* 1992;152:1289-1295.
14. Health Management Bulletin. *Clinical Issues in Drug Management*. American Medical Association. July 1997;1-8.
15. Bolten WW. Scientific rationale for specific inhibition of COX 2. *J Rheumatol* 1998;51(Suppl):2-7.
16. Garcia Rodriguez LA, Jick H. Risk of upper gastrointestinal bleeding and perforation associated with individual non-steroidal anti-inflammatory drugs [published erratum appears in Lancet 1994;343:1048]. *Lancet* 1994;343:769-772.
17. American College of Rheumatology Subcomittee on Osteoarthritis Guidelines; Recommendations for the Medical Management of Osteoarthritis of the Knee and Hip. Arthritis and Rheumatism, 2000, Vol 43, No 9; 1905-1915.
18. Goldstein, J.L. Silverstein, FE et al, Reduced Risk of Upper Gastrointestinal Ulcer Complication With Celecoxib, A Novel COX-2 Inhibitot. *Am J Gastroenterol* 2000;95:1681-1690.
19. Silverstein FE, Faich G, et al. The CLASS Study. (Celebrex Long-term Arthritis Safety Study), *JAMA* 2000;284;10.
20. Vane JR, Botting RM. Mechanism of action of nonsteroidal anti-inflammatory drugs. *Am J Med* 1998;104(3A):2S-8S.
21. Vane JR. Inhibition of prostaglandin synthesis as a mechanism of

action for aspirin-like drugs. *Nature* 1971;231:232-235.

22. Miyamoto T, et al. Purification of prostaglandin endoperoxide synthetase from bovine vesicular gland microsomes. *J Biol Chem* 1976;251:2629-2636.
23. Simmons DL, et al. Identification of a phorbol ester-repressible v-src.-inducible gene. *Proc Natl Acad Sci USA* 1989;86: 1178-1182.
24. Vane J. Differential inhibition of cyclooxygenase isoforms: An explanation of the action of NSAIDs. *J Clin Rheumatol* 1998; 4(5)(Suppl):S3-S10.
25. Simon LS, Smith TJ. NSAID mechanisms of action, efficacy, and relative safety. Postgrad Med Special Rep 1998;12-16.
26. Silas S, Clegg DO. Selective COX-2 inhibition. *Bull Rheum Dis* 1999;40:1-4.
27. Crofford LJ. COX-1 and COX-2 tissue expression: Implications and predictions. *J Rheumatol* 1997;24(Suppl 49):15-19.
28. Furst DE. Perspectives on the cyclooxygenase-2/cyclooxygenase-1 hypothesis. *J Rheumatol* 1998;4(5)(Suppl):40-48.
29. Dewitt DL, et al. PGH synthease isoenzyme selectivity: The potential for safer nonsteroidal antiinflammatory drugs. *Am J Med* 1993;96(Suppl 2A):40-44.
30. Kurumbail RG, et al. Structural basis for selective inhibition of cyclooxygenase-2 by anti-inflammatory agents. *Nature* 1996; 384:644-648.
31. Luong C, et al. Flexibility of NSAID binding site in the structure of human cyclooxygenase-2. *Nat Struct Biol* 1996;3:927-933.
32. Gierse JK, et al. A single amino acid difference between cycloxygenase-1 (COX-1) and -2 (COX-2) reverses the selectivity of COX-2 specific inhibitors. *J Biol Chem* 1996;271: 15810-15814.
33. Smith CJ, et al. Pharmacological analysis of cyclooxygenase-1 in inflammation. *Proc Natl Acad Sci USA* 1998;95: 13313-13318.
34. Siegle I, et al. Expression of cyclooxygenase 1 and cyclooxygenase 2 in human synovial tissue. *Arthritis Rheum* 1998; 41:122-129.
35. Anderson GD, et al. Selective inhibition of cyclooxygenase (COX)-2 reverses inflammation and expression of COX-2 and interleukin-6 in rat adjuvant arthritis. *J Clin Invest* 1996; 97:2672-2679.
36. Crofford LJ, et al. Cyclooxygenase-1 and -2 expression in rheumatoid synovial tissues. Effect of interleukin 1b, phorbol esters, and corticosteroids. *J Clin Invest* 1994;93:1095-1101.
37. Hawkey CJ. COX-2 inhibitors. *Lancet* 1999;353:307-314.
38. Mitchell JA, et al. Selectivity of nonsteroidal antiinflammatory drugs as inhibitors of constitutive and inducible cyclooxygenase. *Proc Natl Acad Sci USA* 1994;90:11693-11697.
39. Cryer B, Feldman M. Cycloxygenase-1 and cycloxygenase 2 selectivity of widely used nonsteroidal anti-inflammatory drugs. *Am J Med* 1998;104:413-421.
40. Simon LS, et al. Preliminary study of the safety and efficacy of SC-58635, a novel cyclooxygenase 2 inhibitor. *Arthritis Rheum* 1998;41:1591-1602.
41. Furst DE, Hilson JL. What is the role of selective COX-2 inhibitors in the spectrum of NSAID therapy? *Rheum Grand Rounds* 1998;1:1-12.
42. Abramowicz M, ed. Celecoxib for arthritis. *Med Lett Drugs Ther* 1999;41(Issue 1045):11.
43. Geis GS, et al. Safety and efficacy of celecoxib, a specific COX-2 inhibitor in patients with rheumatoid arthritis. *Arthritis Rheum* 1998;41(Suppl 9):s364 [Abstract 1990].
44. Celebrex. Package insert. Searle Pharmaceuticals. 2000
45. The CLASS Study, Presented at EULAR. June 22nd Nice, France.
46. Benson, WG, Zhao, SZ, Burke, T, et al. Upper Gastrointestinal Tolerability of Celecoxbib, a COX-2 Specific Inhibitor, Compared to Naproxen and Placebo. *J Rheumatol* 2000;27: 1876-1883.
47. Ehrich EW, et al. Characterization of rofecoxib as a cyclooxygenase-2 isoform inhibitor and demonstration of analgesia in the dental pain model. *Clin Pharmacol Ther* 1999;65:336-347.
48. Clinical data overview of Vioxx (Rofecoxib) presented by Merck to FDA. FDA-gov.org (Vioxx, 1999, April 24).
49. Cannon G, et al. MK-0966, a specific COX-2 inhibitor, has clinical efficacy comparable to diclofenac in the treatment of knee and hip osteoarthritis (OA) in a 26-week, controlled clinical trial. *Arthritis Rheum* 1998;41(Suppl 9):983 [abstract].
50. Rofecoxib drug evaluation monograph. Available at https://www.micromedex.com/de/rofec.htm. Accessed Feb. 4, 1999.
51. Brooks P. Use and benefits of nonsteroidal anti-inflammatory drugs. *Am J Med* 1998;104(3A):9S-13S.
52. Lichtenstein DR, Syngal S, Wofe MM. Nonsteroidal antiinflammatory drugs and the gastrointestinal tract. *Arthritis Rheum* 1995;38:5-18.
53. McCarthy D. Nonsteroidal anti-inflammatory drug-related gastrointestinal toxicity: Definitions and epidemiology. *Am J Med* 1998;105(5A):3S-9S.
54. Sheiman JS. Pathogenesis of gastroduodenal injury due to nonsteroidal antiinflammatory drugs: implications for prevention and therapy. *Semin Arthritis Rheum* 1992;21:201-210.
55. Morham SG, et al. Prostaglandin synthase 2 gene disruption causes severe renal pathology in the mouse. *Cell* 1995;83: 473-482.
56. Cryer B, Kimmey MB. Gastrointestinal side effects of nonsteroidal anti-inflammatory drugs. *Am J Med* 1998;105(1B): 20S-30S.
57. Rothstein R. Safety profiles of leading non-steroidal anti-inflammatory drugs. *Am J Med* 1998;105(5A):39S-43S.
58. Cole AT, et al. Ranitidine, aspirin, food and the stomach. *BMJ* 1992;304:544-545.
59. Silverstein FE, et al. Misoprostol reduces serious gastrointestinal complications in patients with rheumatoid arthritis receiving nonsteroidal anti-inflammatory drugs. A randomized, double-blind, placebo-controlled trial. *Ann Intern Med* 1995;123: 241-249.
60. Baskin JB, et al. Misoprostol dosage in the prevention of nonsteroidal anti-inflammatory drug-induced gastric and duodenal ulcers: A comparison of three regimens. *Ann Intern Med* 1995; 123:344-350.
61. Yeomans ND, et al. A comparison of omeprazole with ranitidine for ulcers associated with nonsteroidal antiinflammatory drugs. *N Engl J Med* 1998;338:719-726.
62. Hawkey CJ, et al. Omeprazole compared with misoprostol for

ulcers associated with nonsteroidal antiinflammatory drugs. *N Engl J Med* 1998;338:727-734.

63. Ekstrom P, et al. Prevention of peptic ulcer and dyspeptic symptoms with omeprazole in patients receiving continuous non-steroidal anti-inflammatory drug therapy—a Nordic multicentre study. *Scand J Gastroenterol* 1996;31:753-758.
64. Cullen D, et al. Primary gastroduodenal prophylaxis with omeprazole for non-steroidal anti-inflammatory drug users. *Aliment Pharmacol Ther* 1998;12:135-140.
65. Kaufmann HJ, Taubin HL. NSAID activate quiescent inflammatory bowel disease. *Ann Intern Med* 1987;107:513-516.
66. Zakim SK. Inhibition of cyclooxygenase: A novel approach to cancer prevention. *Proc Soc Exp Biol Med* 1997;216:201-210.
67. Smalley WE, DuBois RN. Colorectal cancer and nonsteroidal anti-inflammatory drugs. *Adv Pharmacol* 1997;39:1-20.
68. Eberhardt CE, et al. Up regulation of cyclooxygenase 2 gene expression in human colorectal adenomas and adenocarcinomas. *Gastroenterology* 1994;107:1183-1188.
69. Kargman SL, et al. Expression of prostaglandin G/H synthase-1 and -2 protein in human colorectal cancer. *Cancer Res* 1991; 55:2556-2559.
70. Smalley W, et al. Use of nonsteroidal anti-inflammatory drugs and incidence of colorectal cancer. *Arch Intern Med* 1999; 159:161-166.
71. Sorli CH, et al. Basal expression of cylooxygenase-2 and nuclear factor-interleukin 6 are dominant and coordinately regulated by interleukin 1 in the pancreatic islet. *Proc Natl Acad Sci USA* 1998;95:1788-1793.
72. Kwon G, et al. Evidence for involvement of the proteasome complex (26S) and NFkappaB in IL-1beta-induced nitric oxide and prostaglandin production by rat islets and RINm5F cells. *Diabetes* 1998;47:583-591.
73. Komhoff M, et al. Localization of cyclooxygenase-1 and -2 in adult and fetal human kidney: Implication for renal function. *Am J Physiol* 1997;272(4 Pt 2):F460-468.
74. Davies NM, Wallace JL. Selective inhibitors of cyclooxygenase-2. Potential in elderly patients. *Drugs Aging* 1996;9:406-417.
75. Whelton A. Nephrotoxicity of non-steroidal anti-inflammatory drugs: Physiologic foundations and clinical implications. *Am J Med* 1999;106(5B):13S-24S.
76. Reitz DB, et al. Selective cyclooxygenase inhibitors: Novel 1,2 diarylcyclopentenes are potent orally active COX-2 inhibitors. *J Med Chem* 1994;37:3878-3881.
77. Whelton A, Schulman G, et al; Effects of Celecoxib and Naproxen on Renal Function in The Elderly. *Arch Intern Med* 2000;160:1465.
78. Hubbard RC, et al. Pilot efficacy of SC-58638. A COX-2 selective inhibitor in rheumatoid arthritis. Abstract. *Arthritis Rheum* 1997;40:s125.
79. Lipsky PE, Isakson PC. Outcome of specific COX-2 inhibition in rheumatoid arthritis. *J Rheum* 1997;24:9-14.
80. Lane NE. Pain management in osteoarthritis: The role of COX-2 inhibitors. *J Rheumatol* 1997;24:20-24.
81. Morham SG, et al. Characterization of prostaglandin H synthase 2 deficient mice and implications for mechanisms of NSAID action. *Adv Ex Med Biol* 1997;407:131-138.
82. Winzeler S. Non-steroidal antiinflammatory drugs. A review. *AAOHN J* 1998;46:253-259.
83. Bjorkman D. Nonsteroidal anti-inflammatory drug-associated toxicity of the liver, lower gastrointestinal tract, and esophagus. *Am J Med* 1998;105(5A):17S-21S.
84. Vane J. Towards a better aspirin. *Nature* 1994;367: 215-216.
85. Mengiei-Gaw L, et al. A study of platelet effects of SC-58635. A novel COX-2 selective inhibitor. [Abstract]. *Arthritis Rheum* 1997;40:s374.
86. Karim A, et al. Celecoxib, a specific COX-2 inhibitor, lacks significant drug-drug interactions with methotrexate or warfarin. *Arthritis Rheum* 1998;41(9 Suppl):S-315 [abstract].
87. Milner JC. Osteoarthritis of the hip and indomethacin (abstract). *J Bone Joint Surg Am* 1971;54B:752.
88. Ronningen H, Langeland N. Indomethacin treatment in osteoarthritis of the hip joint. *Acta Orthop Scand* 1979;50: 169-174.
89. Brooks PM, et al. NSAID and osteoarthritis: Help or hindrance? *J Rheumatol* 1982;9:3-4.
90. Dingle JT. The interactions of cytokines, NSAIDs and prostaglandins in cartilage destruction and repair. *Adv Prostaglandin Thromboxane Leukot Res* 1990;21:955-965.
91. Sato T, et al. Involvement of cyclooxygenase-2 in bone loss induced by interleukin-1. *Adv Prostaglandin Thromboxane Leukot Res* 1995;23:445-447.
92. Amin AR, et al. Superinduction of cyclooxygenase-2 activity in human osteoarthritis-affected cartilage. *J Clin Invest* 1997; 99:1231-1237.
93. Sousa AR, et al. Enhanced expression of cyclooxygenase isoenzyme 2 (COX-2) in asthmatic airways and its cellular distribution in aspirin-sensitive astham. *Thorax* 1997;52: 940-945.
94. Sairanen T, et al. *Cyclooxygenase-2* is induced globally in infarcted human brain. Ann Neurol 1998;43:738-747.
95. Stewart WF, et al. Risk of Alzheimer,s disease and duration of NSAID use. *Neurology* 1997;48-626-632.
96. Lukiw WJ, Bazan NG. Cyclooxygenase 2 RNA message abundance, stability, and hypervariability in sporadic Alzheimer neocortex. *J Neurosci Res* 1997;50:937-945.
97. Lim H, Paria BC, Das SK, et al. Multiple female reproductive failures in cyclooxygenase 2-deficient mice. Cell 1997;91: 197-208.
98. Lipsky PE. Specific COX-2 inhibitors in arthritis, oncology, and beyond: Where is the science headed? *J Rheumatol* 1999; 26(Suppl 56):25-30.
99. Tsafriri A. Ovulation as a tissue remodelling process. Proteolysis and cumulus expansion. *Adv Exp Med Biol* 1995; 377:121-140.
100. Chakraborty I, et al. Developmental expression of the cyclo-oxygenase-1 and cyclo-oxygenase-2 genes in the peri-implantation mouse uterus and their differential regulation by the blastocyst and ovarian steroids. *J Mol Endocrinol* 1996;16:107-122.
101. Yang ZM, et al. Potential sites of prostaglandin actions in the periimplantation mouse uterus: Differential expression and regulation of prostaglandin receptor genes. *Biol Reprod* 1997; 56:368-379.
102. Lim H, Dey SK. Prostaglandin E-2 receptor subtype EP2 gene expression in the mouse uterus coincides with differentiation of the luminal epithelium for implantation. *Endocrinology* 1997;

138:4599-4606.

103. Houston MC. Nonsteroidal anti-inflammatory drugs and antihypertensives. [Review]. Am J Med 1991;90(5A):42S-47S.
104. Johnson AG, Nguyen TV, Day RO. Do nonsteroidal anti-inflammatory drugs affect blood pressure? *Ann Intern Med* 1994; 121:289-300.
105. Yost JH, Morgan GJ. Cardiovascular effects of NSAIDs. *J Musculoskel Med* 1994;11:22-34.
106. American College of Rheumatology Ad Hoc Committee on Clinical Guidelines. Guidelines for monitoring drug therapy in rheumatoid arthritis. *Arthritis Rheum* 1996;39:723-731.

Acute Back Pain: Part I

Jonathan A. Edlow, MD
Gideon Bosker, MD, FACEP

Back pain is one of the most common symptoms that brings patients to the emergency department (ED). Assessment of these patients is complicated by the fact that human beings have a propensity to suffer from mechanical low back pain. Most likely, this is an intrinsic "side effect" of our evolution into bipeds, yet this evolutionary effect can be difficult to distinguish from life-threatening causes of this symptom complex. While the elderly patient with back pain and osteophytes may have an acute exacerbation of osteoarthritis, the same patient also must have more serious conditions, such as aortic aneurysm and spinal malignancy, considered in the differential diagnosis. And while the young athlete with pain caused by back trauma may have a musculoskeletal contusion, the possibility of epidural hematoma must be considered when focal neurologic deficits suggest this diagnosis.

From a clinico-economic perspective, between 70% and 90% of all individuals experience back pain at some point in their lives,[1,2] extracting an enormous productivity toll, as well as annual medical costs estimated to be $24 billion.[1,2] If lost work, disability, and other indirect costs are factored into the equation, the total annual dollar cost of back pain-related illness has been estimated at between $50 and $100 billion.[2,3] Each year, 2% of all Americans receive some form of compensation for back problems and 14% miss at least one day of work because of back pain.[2]

As with most symptoms that emergency physicians must evaluate, there are many potential causes of acute back pain. A small but significant minority of this vast group of patients will be afflicted with serious life- or limb-threatening conditions. Because of the potential adverse sequelae of these potentially treatable diseases, they can be classified as "cannot miss diagnoses." For example, in the primary care setting, about 0.7% of patients who present with back pain have a spinal malignancy and about 0.01% have spinal infections, including such conditions as epidural abscess or vertebral osteomyelitis.[1]

Unfortunately, disease-specific incidence figures for the spectrum of patients presenting to an ED with back pain are not currently available, but it is likely that a higher percentage of individuals with serious conditions present to the ED than they do in a primary care practice. Nevertheless, the ratio of the percentage of patients with serious disease vs. those suffering from common mechanical or simple low back pain is low, a fact that makes diagnosis potentially problematic and challenging.

As is the case in other conditions, in which the objective is to identify serious conditions that underlie common symptomatology, the emergency physician's goal is to correctly diagnose the small group of patients with potentially life-compromising disease while simultaneously minimizing expensive diagnostic testing. Although there is no uniformity of opinion regarding critical pathways for back pain evaluation in the ED, one excellent and authoritative source of information for physicians evaluating patients with back pain is to consult Guidelines #14, produced by the Agency for Health Care Policy and Research (AHCPR); these protocols can be accessed and downloaded via the Internet (http://text.nlm.nih.gov). At this Web site, physicians can navigate through a 133-page document, with an extensive bibliography, that painstakingly details the most significant body of the research prior to 1994, when the Guidelines document was published.[4]

With these issues and challenges in mind, the purpose of this review is to present a practical approach to evaluating nontraumatic, acute back pain in patients presenting to the ED. One of the principal goals of this comprehensive monograph is to discuss strategies that help the clinician distinguish common, mechanical back pain from serious, "cannot miss" diagnoses requiring prompt, aggressive management. In addition, new treatment strategies will be highlighted, among them, the use of cyclooxygenase-2 (COX-2) inhibitors for osteoarthritis-induced back pain.

The Diagnostic Imperative

The diagnostic approach to patients with back pain must be systematic, focused, and targeted. Above all, the clinician must pursue a fail-safe diagnostic algorithm that, even in the absence of yielding an organ-specific diagnosis, will help distinguish patients who are likely to harbor a serious life- or limb-threatening entity from those whose back pain has been precipitated by more benign pathology.

As with patients who have an acute surgical abdomen or ventricular fibrillation, it is sometimes more important initially to determine the correct course of action in terms of procedural or pharmaco-therapeutic intervention, or more aggressive diagnostic evaluation, than establishing an organ- or disease-specific diagnosis. This is certainly true for patients with back pain. In fact, one landmark publication has systematized the approach to back pain evaluation by suggesting that clinicians determine answers to the following three questions in all patients who present with back pain:

1. Is there likely to be a serious systemic disease causing the pain?
2. Does the patient have a neurologic disease requiring neurosurgical evaluation?
3. Is there psychological stress that might be exacerbating the patient's condition?

Although in some ways simplistic, the wisdom of this approach is also evident. If the physician can answer all three questions with some degree of accuracy, the next steps, from a diagnostic and interventional perspective, are clear. For example, if there is objective neurological compromise, the patient needs a neuro-imaging study and a neurosurgical consultation, regardless of whether the ultimate pathology is a central disk herniation or a spinal metastasis. On the other hand, if the patient is known to have systemic manifestations of osteoarthritis, the gradual onset of back pain, in the absence of neurologic findings and in the presence of confirmatory radiologic studies, is strongly suggestive of osteoarthritis as a likely etiology.

It should be stressed that despite extensive trials and a vast body of literature, there still is no consensus of opinion on how patients with acute back pain should be evaluated and risk-stratified in the acute care setting. Moreover, there are no prospective clinical instruments or decision support tools confirming the outcome-effectiveness of one approach vs. another. For example, another strategy for separating patients with serious back-related conditions from those with benign precipitants is recommended by the AHCPR Guidelines #14 document, which suggests that the clinician's goal should be to classify the patient's back pain into one of the three following categories:

1. Those patients with serious spinal conditions (referred to in this review as "cannot miss diagnoses").
2. Those patients with sciatica, suggesting nerve root compression.
3. Those patients with nonspecific symptoms who fit into neither of the above categories.

Naturally, implicit in any set of goals, especially in this era of increased managed care, is cost-effectiveness. A corollary to this is that frequently no diagnostic studies are required in the emergency setting. In addition, it is more outcome-effective to manage the vast majority of patients who do not have one of the "cannot miss" diagnoses in a manner that returns them to their baseline activities as rapidly as possible. Finally, it is important for the physician to understand that patient satisfaction in the setting of back pain is not related to what specific tests are performed but rather to the patient-physician interaction as a whole. Providing a likely diagnosis, a discussion of maneuvers that will restore functional status, a brief explanation of the prognostic implications of the underlying condition, and a plan directed at pain management are critical components of this interaction.

Anatomic and Physiological Considerations

Optimal and rational care of patients presenting with back pain requires a fundamental, clinically relevant knowledge base as it pertains to spinal and neuroanatomy. A complete review is not possible within the scope of this monograph. However, an essential primer of relevant clinical anatomy is essential for diagnostic purposes and will be presented.

A protective bony column surrounds the canal in which the spinal cord and nerve roots are enclosed. Anteriorly, the vertebral bodies provide protection, whereas laterally, the pedicles and transverse processes serve this function; on the posterior aspect, the laminae and spinous processes protect neural tissue. Between the vertebral bodies are positioned the intervertebral disks, which are formed by an outer anulus fibrosis and an inner gelatinous nucleus pulposis. This combination of rigid bone and the softer disks facilitates weight bearing as well as shock absorption, flexibility, and protection of vital neural structures. The spinal cord itself ends at the L1-L2 interspace, below which lie the lower roots that form the cauda equina.

Intervertebral disks are a common site for back pain-related pathology. For example, the pressure within the disks increases with cough, straining, bending, and sitting. At about 30 years of age, these disks often begin to degenerate,[2] most often posterolaterally, in the area where the nerve roots exit the spinal column via the intervertebral foramina. Over time, even the nucleus pulposis begins to fibrose, which is why it is less likely to herniate in older patients.

The epidural space lies between the vertebral periosteum and the dura that envelops the cord and cauda equina and then extends into the intervertebral foramina along with the exiting spinal nerves.

The space contains fat, connective tissue, and an extensive venous plexus. In general, it requires about a 50% reduction in the anterior-posterior diameter of the spinal canal to produce neurological symptoms.[5] There is more space in the spinal canal located in the lumbar segment as compared to the thoracic area.

Differential Diagnosis. From an anatomic perspective, there are two major strategies for working through the extensive differential diagnosis of back pain. In this regard, back pain can result from pathological processes involving all contiguous anatomic areas, as well as systemic disease. Accordingly, the clinician can group the diagnostic possibilities according to contiguous structures and "regional" anatomic sites that might involve the spine, canal, and soft tissues. These can be grouped according to abdominal, pulmonary, retroperitoneal, spinal, and systemic causes. *(Please see Table 1.)*

Another approach is to break down the differential diagnosis of back pain according to underlying causes. For example, is the pain neurologic in etiology, vascular, visceral, or due to musculoskeletal causes? As with any problem, developing the habit of thinking through this list in all patients will help avoid missing serious disease. Consistency is more important than the specific method chosen.

Table 1. Causes of Low Back Pain by Region

SPINAL CAUSES
- Central disk herniation
- Tumor
- Infection—vertebral osteomyelitis, epidural abscess, brucellosis, tuberculosis
- Epidural hematoma
- Transverse myelitis
- Ankylosing spondylitis
- Spinal stenosis

ABDOMINAL CAUSES
- Biliary disease—cholecystitis, pancreatitis
- GI—posterior penetrating ulcer, esophageal disease
- GYN disease—ovarian torsion, mass, abscess

RETROPERITONEAL CAUSES
- Vascular—AAA, dissection, RPH
- Renal—stone, tumor, abscess, obstruction
- Pancreatic—abscess, pancreatitis, mass

PULMONARY CAUSES
- Any process inflaming the posterior parietal pleura—tumor, infarction, infection, pleurisy

SYSTEMIC CAUSES
- Endocarditis and bacteremia
- Transfusion reactions

Clinical Approach to the Patient with Back Pain

History. Given the diagnostic objectives to identify potential serious causes of back pain that require urgent neuroradiological evaluation and possibly, procedural intervention, it is imperative that the physician extract as much information as possible from the history and physical examination. In combination, they can provide essential clues that frequently suggest the correct diagnosis, even prior to radiological imaging. Moreover, epidemiological context is also important. For example, sudden onset of acute back pain in an older patient is more likely due to a serious cause than pain in a younger patient.

A history of cancer suggests the possibility of metastatic disease to the spine, which is common in prostate cancer, lung cancer, and breast malignancy. A dissecting aortic aneurysm is more common in elderly patients with hypertension. A history of a known aortic aneurysm may signify aneurysmal expansion or impending rupture. A history of peptic ulcer disease may suggest a posteriorly penetrating ulcer. Other medical conditions, such as diabetes, intravenous drug use, or infection with the human immunodeficiency virus (HIV) should cause the physician to search compulsively for a serious cause, including epidural infection. Systemic anticoagulation may predispose to epidural hemorrhage, whereas recent back surgery should raise the suspicion of infection or expanding mass.

The history in patients with back pain should include the onset of pain, its duration, character, and factors that either exacerbate or ameliorate the pain. The presence or absence of trauma is especially important. A history of fever or chills may be a clue to an infection such as epidural abscess. Likewise, recent urinary tract, soft tissue, or bacteremic infection or recent spinal anesthesia may predispose to abscess. Back pain that is worse at night or with rest also is an ominous sign, since it indicates ongoing inflammation in the absence of mechanical stress.

Radiation of pain can sometimes pinpoint the anatomic origin of back-related symptoms. Pain that affects the abdomen suggests an intra-abdominal source or a lesion in the thoracic spine affecting a nerve root. Pain radiating in a unilateral distribution into the buttock or leg below the knee in a radicular pattern suggests irritation of the sciatic nerve known as sciatica.[2] Bilateral sciatica, on the other hand, frequently indicates more serious, extensive disease involving the nerve roots.

Duration of symptoms is another important feature that can help exclude a more benign diagnosis. For example, the natural history of mechanical low back pain and sciatica tends to be characterized by spontaneous improvement over a period of weeks. Accordingly, pain that persists beyond this time frame or worsens over time is frequently not related to a musculoskeletal process. Co-existing symptoms such as fever, chills, weight loss, and anorexia also connote a more serious etiology for back pain. Finally, a careful history that elicits dysfunction of either the urinary or rectal sphincters points strongly to a neurological etiology.

The social history also can be important. An older person who lives alone should be questioned about frequent falls or recent use of a walking aid. Any discharge plan must be consistent with the patient's home situation.

Physical Examination. The physical examination is extremely important in evaluating patients with back pain. In this regard, a careful and meticulous neurological examination of the lower extremities is essential. The back should be inspected for ecchymosis and deformity. Muscle spasm, as well as midline and paravertebral tenderness, should be elicited, although the interobserver reliability is fair to poor for these tests in published studies.[6]

The physician should also test for range of motion (ROM). In one study, the straight leg raise test (SLR) was used to identify lesions that stretched the sciatic nerve. With the patient lying supine, the examiner passively flexes the hip, with the knee straight, to see if radicular symptoms can be reproduced. The nerve is not stretched until the hip has been flexed about 30 degrees; therefore, pain occurring prior to this arc of movement suggests a psychological component or that the patient is actively using the iliopsoas muscles. The clinician should record the angle at which pain begins. If the examiner lowers the leg a few degrees from where the pain was elicited, the pain should disappear. Passive dorsiflexion of the foot at that lower angle should then elicit the pain again. Crossed SLR (performing the test on the opposite side of the patient's symptoms) provides increased specificity for a sciatic nerve lesion, but at the cost of sensitivity.

As far as the neurological examination of the lower extremities, the clinician should first determine if the motor, sensory, and reflex examinations are normal. If they are not normal, the emergency physician should try to localize the lesion. Is it in the spinal cord, the cauda equina, the nerve plexus, or the nerve root? It should be stressed that an acceptable examination requires 1) that the patient be properly exposed, including the feet and toes, and 2) that no lower extremity neurological/physical examination is complete without removal of shoes and socks.

About 95-98% of all lumbar disk herniations involve the L5 and S1 roots, whereas the majority of other herniations affect the L3 and L4 roots (the femoral nerve).[1,7] The motor and sensory functions and reflexes supplied by these roots can be rapidly tested in cooperative patients. A matrix can be used to facilitate anatomic localization. An L5 lesion will produce the motor, sensory, and reflex impairments or manifestations as follows: impaired extension of the great toe, decreased sensation of the first dorsal web space, and no reflex changes. An S1 lesion will be characterized by weakened plantar flexion of the foot, decreased sensation in the lateral aspect of the fifth toe, and decreased or absent ankle jerk. An L3-L4 lesion is manifested by decreased strength of knee extension, decreased sensation of the medial knee, and a compromised knee reflex.

Although usually useful and essential, a rectal examination need not be performed in every patient with back pain. However, it should be performed in four subgroups of patients with back pain: 1) those with extreme pain; 2) those whose history suggests sphincter abnormalities; 3) those with any abnormality found by neurological examination; and 4) those at risk for serious, "cannot-miss" diagnoses. Urinary retention is encountered in 90% of cases and diminished anal sphincter tone is seen in about 70% of cases of cauda equina syndrome.[1] Finally, assessing the ability of the patient with back pain to ambulate is essential. Rapid deterioration in ambulation without an identifiable cause is an indication for urgent imaging. It also should be emphasized that a normal neurological examination does not exclude serious illnesses such as abscess or tumor, since these processes usually cause back pain prior to production of neurological deficits.

Laboratory and Radiographic Studies

Once the history and physical examination are complete, the physician must decide whether or not to order laboratory or imaging studies. Clearly, the presence of neurological abnormalities, the presence of back pain in a patient with known malignant disease, HIV infection or other immunocompromise, or back pain in an elderly patient with progressive systemic symptoms will mandate radiographic evaluation and selected laboratory tests.

For the most part, laboratory testing plays a small role in the evaluation of patients with back pain. If historical or physical examination points to the urinary tract as a source of the patient's back pain, a urinalysis may be revealing. The complete blood count may not be helpful unless the patient has multiple myeloma or evidence of chronic anemia associated with a systemic disease. Even in patients with epidural abscess, in one study 68% (27 of 40) had an elevated white blood cell count.[8]

The only blood test that may play a role in selected cases is the erythrocyte sedimentation rate (ESR). In an analysis of patients older than 50 years of age seen in the practice of one orthopedic surgeon, the ESR was elevated in all (12 of 12) of patients with metastatic disease and most (3 of 4) patients with primary spinal tumors.[9] Based on these findings, this author recommended an ESR, as well as serum calcium and alkaline phosphatase levels, and found that one of the three tests was positive in all patients with back pain from cancer.[9] In a much larger study of nearly 2000 patients presenting to an outpatient clinic with back pain, an elevated ESR was also useful.[10] The likelihood ratios for patients with back pain having cancer were 2.4 (for ESR > 20 mm/h), 19.2 (for ESR > 50), and 55.5 (for ESR > 100). The presence of anemia in that study (normal hematocrit > 40 for men; > 38 for women) also was somewhat predictive, with a cancer likelihood ratio of 4 in those with anemia; however, the specificity was extremely low.[10]

Despite evidence suggesting the possible predictive value of the ESR and other ancillary tests, laboratory testing is not recommended on a routine basis for all patients with back pain. However, the data are strongly suggestive that the ESR may be useful in specific patients (especially the elderly) who are at risk for tumor, infection, or ankylosing spondylitis.

Imaging. The decision to image patients with nontraumatic back pain is affected by a number of considerations, including historical and physical findings, the patient's age, the presence of systemic disease, and the likelihood that a "cannot miss" diagnosis is the most likely explanation for the patient's back pain. A wide variety of tests are available, among them plain films, radionuclide scans, computerized tomographic (CT) scans, magnetic resonance (MR) scans, and conventional myelography.

Each imaging modality has its unique advantages and disadvantages. And even though obtaining routine plain films of the spine is a common practice, this approach to patient assessment on a routine basis is difficult to justify.[11] Nevertheless, this practice continues for two reasons: 1) as a result of patient pressure "to know what the problem is"; and 2) physician discomfort with "not knowing what the problem is." Unfortunately, the information pro-

Table 2. Risk Stratification for Imaging in Patients with Low Back Pain

HISTORY

1. Duration > 4 weeks
2. Failure of conservative therapy or increasing symptoms during conservative therapy
3. Bilateral radicular symptoms
4. Focal lower extremity weakness (recent use of walking aid, frequent falls)
5. History of malignancy (or suspicion of recent nonintentional weight loss)
6. HIV infection with CD4 counts of < 200
7. Urinary urgency or loss of sphincter control
8. Fever (without alternative source), recent infections
9. Claudication—neurogenic or vascular
10. Drug history
    - Immunosuppressive drugs or chronic steroids
    - IVDA
    - Anticoagulation with INR > 3.0
11. Recent back surgery or spinal anesthesia *and* on anticoagulants

PHYSICAL EXAMINATION

1. Fever (without alternative source)
2. Abdominal mass or tenderness
3. Abnormal neurological findings
    - Cord lesion
    - Cauda equina lesion
    - Nerve plexus lesion
    - Nerve root (radicular) lesion

vided by many of these studies usually does not provide the answers that either party is seeking.

Regarding patient satisfaction, one study evaluated 1555 patients with back pain treated by several groups of health providers, including family physicians, internists, chiropractors, and orthopedic surgeons.[12] The investigators found that satisfaction was not specifically correlated with radiological tests that were performed. Rather, there were three determinants of patient satisfaction: 1) the patient's perception of having had a complete history; 2) the patient's perception of having had a thorough physical examination; and 3) the patient's feeling that the physician provided a clear explanation of the problem.

The physician side of this equation also has been studied. Regarding plain films, clinic-pathologic correlation can be difficult. For example, there are numerous radiologic findings that may be present on x-ray, but are not directly responsible for causing the patient's pain. Such findings include degenerative changes, spondylolysis and spondylolisthesis, Schmorl's nodes, transitional vertebrae, and others.[13] In addition, plain films may fail to reveal such serious problems as tumor, infection, or central disk herniation, even though they may be present and responsible for the clinical presentation. In this regard, approximately 30-50% of a vertebral body must be destroyed before one can detect abnormalities on a plain film.[3,14] Therefore, the plain films can be normal early in the course of destructive lesions. In many other cases, plain radiographs are neither sensitive nor specific.

Bone scans are sensitive for patients with cancer (except for multiple myeloma) but they are very non-specific.[15] Degenerative changes give a similar appearance to metastatic lesions and are common in the age-group that is often being tested for cancer.[15] CT scans show greater detail of the disks and soft tissues surrounding the spine. However, without the administration of intrathecal contrast, the subarachnoid space is poorly visualized and intradural lesions may be missed.[7] In general, these two tests have been supplanted by MR imaging.

However, even MR imaging is not perfect. Multiple studies evaluating MR imaging of the lumbar spine have shown that this technique has the potential for providing misleading information, especially in patients with minimal symptoms.[16,17] In MR scans of 98 asymptomatic people with no history of back pain, only 36% had normal disks at all levels. Fifty-two percent had at least one bulging disk, 27% had disk protrusions, and 1% had frankly herniated disks.[17] In this same study, 19% of patients had Schmorl's nodes, 14% had annular defects in the disk, and 8% had facet joint arthropathy. As with any radiological study, inter-observer reliability is an important issue.[18]

Since the overwhelming majority of patients with low back pain improve with conservative therapy, routine MR scans—with their propensity for demonstrating abnormalities even in asymptomatic patients—may direct physicians toward unneccesarily aggressive treatment plans. This may adversely affect the patient and lead to unnecessary cost of care. Clearly, a risk stratification strategy based on history and physical examination that identifies which patients with back pain should be imaged with MR scanning is essential for optimizing outcomes. *(Please see Table 2.)* This issue is discussed in more detail in subsequent sections.

Simple and Mechanical Causes of Back Pain

By far, the most common causes of nontraumatic low back pain are musculoskeletal in origin, only a few percent of which are sciatica.[1] In the majority of cases with musculoskeletal etiologies, the physician will not be able to make a specific anatomic diagnosis (e.g., muscle strain vs ligamentous injury vs facet joint inflammation). The typically benign natural history of patients with low back pain allows such imprecision without producing poor outcomes. The vast majority of these patients, even those with herniated disks, will improve spontaneously or with conservative interventions such as nonsteroidal anti-inflammatory drugs (NSAIDs) and a few days of rest. The favorable natural history of musculoskeletal back pain emphasizes the importance of taking a careful history and performing a comprehensive physical examination that will distinguish those patients who need further evaluation from those who do not.

Because imaging studies may provide misleading information, and given the benign natural history of mechanical back pain in most patients, a strategy of highly selective imaging in patients with back pain is desirable. When imaging is not indicated, the clinician may find it advantageous to have a brief but focused discussion with the patient in order to explain and provide reassurance about three important features of their assessment: 1) the clinician should explain that based on a careful history and physical examination (this assumes a careful history and physical examination were performed), there is nothing to suggest a serious cause of the back pain; 2) the physician should explain that plain x-rays frequently do not show the relevant structures that may be causing back pain; and 3) that MR scanning, while it will show those details, is so sensitive that it often shows potentially misleading abnormalities even in asymptomatic individuals. This discussion can help produce patient satisfaction and reduce unnecessary expenditures.

Management. For management, there is a growing body of literature that provides guidance for the individual physician in developing a treatment plan for these patients. Traditionally, bed rest has been the cornerstone of therapy for simple, mechanical low back pain or a herniated disk without neuromotor signs. However, in one landmark study that compared two days vs. seven days of prescribed "bed rest," there were no differences in the functional, physiologic, or perceived outcomes between the groups.[19] Another group of investigators compared three treatment regimens for simple, mechanical back pain: 1) bed rest for two days; 2) back-mobilizing extension exercises; and 3) continuation of normal activities as tolerated.[20] The latter group (i.e., those who continued normal activities) had a more rapid recovery than the treatment groups. Another study comparing physical therapy, chiropractic therapy, and a simple patient instruction booklet found only minimal differences between the two active therapies and the instruction booklet.[21] The costs for the booklet were much less than for the physical therapy or chiropractic care.

From a clinical, outcome-sensitive perspective, the preponderance of the evidence suggests that most patients can be effectively treated with early resumption of normal activities. Common sense would dictate that strenuous activities or heavy lifting, even if "normal" for an individual patient, should be limited until recovery is well under way. Moreover, prolonged sitting may cause increased discomfort. If bed rest is prescribed, it should be only for a short period. While patients may benefit from physical therapy and chiropractic treatments, there is no convincing evidence that these are superior to simple time, reasonable resumption of activity, and "Mother Nature."

With respect to pain management with medications, the AHCPR Guidelines, which examined a large body of medical literature, generated several conclusions.[4] It should be noted that many of the studies upon which this council based its opinions were judged to be methodologically weak. First, acetaminophen, aspirin, and other NSAIDs are acceptable therapy. The Guidelines further recognized the potential adverse side effects of the NSAIDs and specifically cautioned against phenylbutazone, which has serious bone marrow toxicity. The introduction of the cyclooxygenase-2 (COX-2) inhibitor class of NSAIDs offers evidence-based advantages in managing osteoarthritic back pain, especially in the elderly.

Second, they concluded that muscle relaxants, while probably more effective than placebo, are no better than NSAIDs and that there is no benefit from combining muscle relaxants with NSAIDs. The potential drowsiness associated with muscle relaxants was highlighted. Third, the group recognized that, while narcotics were an option in the short term, the physician needed to be aware of side effects and issues of dependency. The evidence did not favor use of steroids, colchicine, or antidepressants.

The Guidelines also recommended against injections of facet joints and trigger points. Physical manipulation (chiropractic therapy) was deemed to be helpful in patients without radiculopathy during the first month of symptoms. Epidural injections were only recommended for patients with radiculopathy and then, only after a failure of conservative management and when there was an attempt to prevent surgery. Subsequent to publication of the AHCPR Guidelines, a randomized, double-blinded trial of epidural steroid injections for sciatica from herniated disk showed neither functional benefit at three months nor reduction in need for surgery.[22]

Despite documented success with conservative therapy, the occasional patient with a herniated disk will require surgery, the referral for which generally falls under the purview of the primary care physician. The AHCPR Guidelines recommend such referral if all three of the following conditions are met: 1) sciatica is both severe and disabling; 2) symptoms of sciatica persist without improvement or show progression; and 3) there is clinical evidence of nerve root compromise.[4]

References

1. Deyo RA, Rainville J, Kent DL. What can the history and physical examination tell us about low back pain? *JAMA* 1992;268:760-765.
2. Wipf J, Deyo R. Low back pain. *Med Clin North Am* 1995; 9:231-246.
3. Borenstein D. A clinician's approach to acute low back pain. *Am J Med* 1997;102(suppl 1A):16S-22S.
4. AHCPR. Acute Low Back Pain in Adults: Clinical Practice Guideline #14, AHCPR Publication #95-0642, Rockville, MD, 1994. Agency for Health Care Policy and Research.
5. Boogerd W, Van der Sande J. Diagnosis and treatment of spinal cord compression in malignant disease. *Cancer Treat Rev* 1993;19:129-150.
6. McComb P, Fairbank J, Cockersole B, et al. Reproducibility of physical signs in low-back pain. *Spine* 1989;14:908-918.
7. Deen H. Concise review for primary care physicians—Diagnosis and management of lumbar disk disease. *Mayo Clin Proc* 1996;71:283-287.
8. Darouiche R, Hamill R, Greenberg S, et al. Bacterial spinal epidural abscess—Review of 43 cases and literature survey. *Medicine* 1992;71:369-385.
9. Fernbach J, Langer F, Gross A. The significance of low back pain in older adults. *CMA Journal* 1976;115:898-900.
10. Deyo R, Diehl A. Cancer as a cause of back pain: Frequency, clinical presentation, and diagnostic strategies. *J Gen Intern Med* 1988;3:230-238.
11. Carey TS, Garrett J. Patterns of ordering diagnostic tests for patients with acute low back pain. The North Carolina Back Pain Project. *Ann Intern Med* 1996;125:807-814.
12. Carey T, Garrett J, Jackman A, et al. The outcomes and costs of care for acute low back pain among patients seen by primary care practitioners, chiropractors, and orthopedic surgeons. *N Engl J Med* 1995;333:913-917.
13. Deyo RA, Bigos SJ, Maravilla KR. Diagnostic imaging

procedures for the lumbar spine. *Ann Intern Med* 1989;111: 865-867.

14. Dixon A. Imaging the bad back: Increasing reliance on MRI. *Hosp Med* 1998;49:496-498.
15. Byrne T. Spinal cord compression from epidural metastases. *N Engl J Med* 1992;327:614-619.
16. Boden SD, Davis DO, Dina TS, et al. Abnormal magnetic-resonance scans of the lumbar spine in asymptomatic subjects. A prospective investigation. *J Bone Joint Surg* [Am] 1990;72:403-408.
17. Jensen MC, Brant-Zawadzki MN, Obuchowski N, et al. Magnetic resonance imaging of the lumbar spine in people without back pain. *N Engl J Med* 1994;331:69-73.
18. Smith B, Hurwitz E, Solsberg D, et al. Interobserver reliability of detecting lumbar intervertebral disc and high-intensity zone on magnetic resonance imaging and association of high intensity zone with pain and anular disruption. *Spine* 1998;23:2074-2080.
19. Deyo R, Diehl A, Rosenthal M. How many days of bed rest for acute low back pain? A randomized clinical trial. *N Engl J Med* 1986;315:1064-1070.
20. Malmivaara A, Hakkinen U, Aro T, et al. The treatment of acute low back pain—Bed rest, exercises, or ordinary activity? *N Engl J Med* 1995;332:351-355.
21. Cherkin D, Deyo R, Battie M, et al. A comparison of physical therapy, chiropractic manipulation, and provision of an educational booklet for the treatment of patients with low back pain. *N Engl J Med* 1998;339:1021-1029.
22. Carette S, Leclaire R, Marcoux S, et al. Epidural corticosteroid injections for sciatica due to herniated nucleus pulposus. *N Engl J Med* 1997;336:1634-1640.

Acute Back Pain: Part II

Jonathan A. Edlow, MD
Gideon Bosker, MD, FACEP

Accurate assessment of acute back pain is essential for preventing negative patient outcomes. Although back pain is frequently the result of simple, mechanical factors producing musculoskeletal strain (or, in the elderly, a consequence of osteoarthritis and osteophyte formation), there are a number of serious, life-threatening conditions that require prompt diagnosis and immediate intervention. These so-called "cannot miss" diagnoses include abdominal aortic aneurysm (AAA), vertebral osteomyelitis, epidural abscess, spinal malignancy, and epidural hematoma.

These problems are common, especially in elderly patients, but this subgroup may suffer from spinal stenosis, and back pain also may be a manifestation of osteoarthritis. Historical features and radiographic examination will help identify patients who can be treated with pain management alone, including traditional NSAIDs or cyclooxygenase-2 (COX-2) inhibitors, when the etiology is osteoarthritis.

With these issues in mind, this review of acute back pain discusses high-risk conditions, with a special emphasis on diagnostic procedures and clinical findings that will direct the clinician toward life- and/or limb-threatening conditions. A detailed section on back pain in the elderly outlines a clinically useful pathway for differential diagnosis and analyzes pharmacotherapeutic strategies directed at pain management.

'Cannot Miss' Conditions

Nonspinal Causes. A comprehensive discussion of the many nonspinal causes of low back pain is beyond the scope of this article. Nevertheless, it is mandatory that the primary care physician consider these conditions as part of the differential diagnosis, since they will be encountered in primary care. Perhaps the most most important condition, from a morbidity and mortality standpoint, that must be considered in patients with back pain is aortic dissection and expansion or rupture of an abdominal aortic aneurysm (AAA). These vascular causes of back pain occasionally can present in a less-than-dramatic manner, and their subtle findings frequently are inappropriately ascribed to musculoskeletal or benign causes of back pain. Moreover, pain referred to the back can be precipitated by abdominal disease, including that localized to the biliary tract, pancreas, gastrointestinal tract, and gynecological structures.

While all the aforementioned entities are considered "cannot miss" diagnoses, the remainder of this review will focus on those conditions that can lead to permanent neurologic disability if not promptly diagnosed and treated. Most of these conditions are relatively uncommon disorders; therefore, each is considered separately. Musculoskeletal causes, including central herniated disk and ankylosing spondylitis, are addressed first. Spinal stenosis will be discussed separately in the section on back pain in the elderly, although it is worth noting that in one study of 145 patients, one-third of individuals with spinal stenosis presented before age 50.[1]

Disk Herniation. The vast majority of herniated disks rupture posterolaterally and impinge on the spinal nerve as it exits the foramen. Fewer than 1% of patients with herniated disks that require surgery will displace directly posteriorly (or centrally).[2] In this scenario, disk fragments impinge on the cauda equina, causing dysfunction to the spinal nerves not as they exit, but as they traverse the spinal canal. Back and bilateral leg pain, as well as numbness and sphincter dysfunction, mark the cauda equina syndrome. Urinary retention and anal sphincter dysfunction occur in 90% and about 70% of patients, respectively.[2] Anesthesia of the perineum (saddle anesthesia) and of the posteromedial thigh (innervated by S-3 and 4) is found in 75% of patients.[3]

The clinical findings do not pinpoint the etiology, which can be metastatic disease, idiopathic, or infectious. Patients who rapidly develop neurologic dysfunction must be decompressed surgically if permanent dysfunction is to be prevented. Thus, prompt recognition and treatment are essential.

Ankylosing spondylitis is another important, though uncommon disease that presents with back pain. This inflammatory process usually affects young males and presents with slowly progressive back ache and stiffness that is worse in the morning and improves over the course of the day. Gradually, these patients develop diminished range of motion of the back. This is one of the HLA-B27-related inflammatory arthropathies that include psoriatic, Reiter's, and inflammatory bowel disease-related syndromes. Physical examination reveals diminished excursion of the lumbar spine and chest. This is one situation in which plain films and the erythrocyte sedimentation rate (ESR) are helpful.

Abdominal Aortic Aneurysm

Overview. Abdominal aortic aneurysm (AAA) must always be considered in older, hypertensive patients who present to the primary care physician (PCP) with back pain, high blood pressure, and a pulsatile abdominal mass. It is clear that clinical strategies for improving the often dismal outcome of these patients should be explored in earnest. Complicating the diagnosis of patients with this disorder is the fact that clinical features in patients with ruptured or expanding aneurysms can be extremely subtle. For example, most patients with a ruptured AAA have no prior manifestations, and a significant percentage of these patients are unaware that they are harboring an aneurysm.[4,5] On the other hand, when abdominal or flank pain, shock, and a pulsatile abdominal mass are present, the diagnosis of ruptured AAA is relatively straightforward.

Unfortunately, this triad of features is present only in 24-42% of all patients with this condition.[6] Because these "textbook" features are frequently absent, misdiagnosis is a common problem, occurring in nearly one-third of cases.[6-8] Accordingly, PCPs should be aware that ruptured AAA may present with atypical signs and symptoms, many of which will mimic other disorders such as osteoarthritic back pain, renal colic (acute flank pain with hematuria), acute diverticulitis (left lower quadrant pain), and GI bleeding.[9]

Physical Examination. The abdominal examination is highly unreliable for diagnosing an AAA. Nevertheless, several clues on physical examination should heighten the clinical suspicion for AAA in patients who present to the PCP with back pain. First, the presence of an abdominal bruit is an important finding. An AAA generally can be palpated above the umbilicus and to the right of the midline. If it does not cross the midline, it may be a tortuous aorta.[10] Although there is a widely held premise that repetitive palpation of the abdominal aorta may result in rupture of an AAA, there are no studies confirming this fear. When palpating the aorta, the physician should note the position of the pulse wave, which, in the normal aorta, will expand in an anterior direction. When palpation of the aorta reveals lateral displacement of the pulse wave, AAA should be suspected.[10] Other clues include diminished lower extremity pulses and evidence of peripheral emboli or arterial occlusive disease (e.g., cool skin, poor hair growth, poor capillary refill).[5]

Misdiagnosis of AAA. Unfortunately, the vast majority (> 80%) of patients who present with ruptured aneurysms have never been diagnosed as having an AAA.[4,5] Abdominal, flank, or back pain are the most common symptoms in patients with a rapidly expanding or ruptured AAA.[4,5] In addition, some patients may become syncopal due to sudden hemorrhage. Complicating the diagnosis of AAA is the fact that physical findings in patients with AAA can be subtle. Consequently, physicians may attribute such symptoms as back pain, abdominal pain, flank pain, lower extremity ischemic symptoms, or hypotension to other, more common disorders seen in the elderly.

In fact, 24-42% of patients with ruptured AAAs are misdiagnosed when they first seek medical care.[6-8,11] These patients have almost double the mortality rate of those who are diagnosed correctly at the time of their initial complaints.[12] Common misdiagnoses include renal colic, diverticulitis, GI bleeding, myocardial infarction, and musculoskeletal or osteoarthritic back pain.

The misdiagnosis rate is not surprising, considering that each of these disorders occurs more frequently than AAA in the elderly population and features of each overlap with signs and symptoms (i.e., abdominal, back, and flank pain, as well as hypotension) seen in AAA.[13,14] Nevertheless, clinical features in misdiagnosed patients differ in several important ways from those who are correctly diagnosed at the time of initial presentation. For example, only 9% of patients in one series of misdiagnosed patients presented with the triad of abdominal or back pain, shock, and a pulsatile mass.[6] A pulsatile abdominal mass was present in only 26% of misdiagnosed patients compared to greater than 70% who were correctly diagnosed, while back pain was present in only 12% of misdiagnosed patients.[6,11]

Musculoskeletal complaints also can be seen in patients with ruptured AAAs. In particular, back and leg pain from an AAA may be due to sudden expansion, intrinsic vessel wall pathology, pressure on adjacent neurosensory structures, or vertebral body erosion.[15] Because the diagnosis of AAA can be elusive, mimicking many common diseases seen in the elderly, physicians should consider this disorder in every elderly patient with hemodynamic instability or abdominal, back, GI, or lower extremity musculoskeletal symptoms.

Diagnostic Modalities. Ultrasonography (US) is essentially 100% sensitive in detecting an AAA.[16] In addition, it has the advantage of being a noninvasive, relatively inexpensive, and accurate test within 3-4 mm with respect to assessing the diameter of the aorta.[10] Moreover, in the unstable patient ultrasonography can distinguish free intraperitoneal blood as well as the presence of an AAA—findings that confirm that diagnosis.

Unfortunately, US is not particularly helpful for assessment of aneurysmal rupture, nor is it ideal for evaluating complications such as visceral or renal artery involvement.[16] Furthermore, US is not useful for imaging the thoracic or suprarenal aorta because of interference from overlying lung.[17] It should be stressed that aneurysmal involvement of these aortic segments can also present with back pain and should be considered in the differential diagnosis. Obesity, intestinal gas, adjacent lymph nodes, and barium within the bowel also interfere with US imaging.[17] Because of these limitations, US is primarily used to screen patients at risk for AAA and to follow AAA growth over time. If patients are unstable and cannot be safely moved, portable bedside US may provide an immediate answer to the question of whether an aneurysm is present.[17,18]

Computerized tomography (CT) has the advantage of being able to measure the size, as well as the full anatomic involvement of an abdominal or thoracic aneurysm. Because CT can generate two-dimensional, cross-sectional images of the aorta and other intra-abdominal structures, it is more accurate than US at detecting rupture and visceral involvement. Modern CT scanners are able to identify the entire aorta, including the suprarenal and thoracic aorta, in addition to the celiac, superior mesenteric, renal, and iliac arteries and adjacent organs.[19,20] Intravenous contrast enhancement allows for evaluation of the aortic lumen size, the presence of mural thrombus, hematoma (from rupture), dissection, and retroperitoneal structures.[19]

Spiral CT provides a rapid, three-dimensional reconstruction of intra-abdominal organs, a feature that further increases the ability of CT to identify complications of aortic aneurysms, including adjacent organ and branch vessel involvement.[20] The major drawbacks of CT include expense, time requirements, and the need for patient stability.[19,20] However, the high resolution of CT makes it superior to US in the assessment of stable patients with aneurysmal disease.

Management. Patients in whom AAA is strongly suspected must be managed in a rapid, directed manner. Measures to stabilize and monitor the patient's hemodynamic status, as surgical and radiologic consultants are being mobilized, must be instituted promptly. It should be stressed that for patients who are clinically unstable and who present with features highly suspicious for a ruptured abdominal aneurysm, radiological evaluation can waste valuable time, as the patient undergoes clinical deterioration. Consequently, unstable patients should be taken directly to the operating room. On the other hand, those patients who have less urgent symptoms are appropriate candidates for expedient diagnostic evaluation.

Infections of the Spine and Spinal Canal

The two most important spinal infections that must be considered in patients with back pain are vertebral osteomyelitis and epidural abscess. Another rare infection is intramedullary abscess.[21] In all of these conditions, the cord, cauda equina, and nerve roots are at risk, and once the diagnosis is made or strongly suspected, immediate consultation with a neurologist or neurosurgeon should be initiated. All of these patients will be hospitalized, some may require biopsy to obtain the causative organism, and surgical treatment is the rule rather than the exception. Early diagnosis and definitive therapy lead to improved outcomes.

Vertebral Osteomyelitis. Various types of infections can invade the spinal column and canal. The pathophysiology of vertebral osteomyelitis has special clinical importance. The vertebral bodies have a rich, but sluggish blood supply. In the embryo, one artery supplies two vertebrae (the lower portion of the superior body and the upper part of the inferior vertebral body) along with the intervening disk.[22] Therefore, vertebral osteomyelitis of the spine typically involves two adjacent vertebral bodies, whereas tumor infiltration may involve only a single vertebral body; this may be an important differential point. Vertebral osteomyelitis can develop from hematogenous or contiguous spread of infection. In some cases, no obvious source is identified.

Back pain is the symptomatic hallmark of patients with vertebral osteomyelitis. Other symptoms include fever and radicular pain, including hip pain.[22] The pain often had been present for weeks to months. Depending on the location, other symptoms referable to the GI tract (dysphagia) or pleural spaces (effusions) may develop. Fever is only present in about one-half of cases.[22,23]

The physical exam may demonstrate spinal tenderness, diminished ROM, and positive straight leg raising (SLR) test. Neurologic deficits related to the cord, cauda equina, or individual nerve roots may also be found. Because this process usually involves the anterior vertebral body, the back pain can precede onset of neurologic findings by some time. The progression from back pain to root, cord, or cauda equina compression can be gradual or abrupt. Pyogenic vertebral osteomyelitis of the posterior elements has been reported but is far less common.[24]

Staphylococcus aureus is the most common offending organism, followed by gram-negative enteric species. Salmonella has classically been associated with sickle cell disease or infected vascular tissue but is otherwise uncommon. In some areas of the world, tuberculosis and brucellosis must be considered.[22] The lumbar, thoracic, and cervical spine are involved in 50%, 35%, and 15% of cases, respectively, for bacterial cases, while the thoracic spine is much more common in tuberculous cases.[22]

An elevated white blood cell count is found in less than one-half of cases and the ESR, while usually elevated, lacks specificity.[22] Plain films are abnormal in as many as 95% of cases of vertebral osteomyelitis although in intravenous drug abusers (IVDA), this figure drops to 80%. Magnetic resonance scanning, while more expensive than plain films, is nevertheless very sensitive and adds more information about the state of the cord and nerve roots as well as other diagnostic information.

Epidural Abscess. Epidural abscess is another rare, but important, infection that can create serious morbidity and mortality. Epidural abscess can result from vertebral osteomyelitis and genitourinary and soft-tissue infections, or it can follow epidural anesthesia, back surgery, and trauma.[22,25-27] Diabetes, IVDA, and alcoholism are frequent comorbid conditions that accompany epidural abscess.[25-26,28] However, about 20% of patients have no predisposing factors identified.[25,28] Back pain is the presenting symptom in the majority of cases,[25,28-29] while no other symptoms were present in more than 50% of cases in the largest recent series.[25] Other symptoms include radicular pain; motor, sensory, or sphincter symptoms; and back (or neck) stiffness. Fever is present in about 75% of cases.[25,29] Spinal tenderness is often present, but the neurological examination is normal in approximately one-half of patients on the day of presentation.[28] When abnormal, the exam may show root, cord, or cauda equina signs.

In one large series, the white blood cell count was greater than 11,000 in less than 70% of cases; neither fever nor leukocytosis was present in 7%.[25] The ESR is usually elevated but depends upon the cut-off level used. *Staphylococcus aureus* is by far the most common organism implicated, followed by various streptococcal and gram-negative enteric organisms. Blood cultures were positive in as many as 95% of cases in one series[25] but in only about 60% in most other series.[26,28]

The location of epidural abscess in the spine has been divided equally between posterior and anterior in most series,[8,44] although one study found a preponderance of abscesses posteriorly.[29] Cervical location is not uncommon.[25,26] The abscess usually extends over multiple vertebral segments (over four segments, on average).[25] Plain x-rays are positive in 44-65% of cases[25,28] and do not predict CT or magnetic resonance (MR) findings.[25] MR imaging (MRI) has emerged as the diagnostic modality of choice[29] and has largely replaced bone scanning, CT, and conventional myelography. In cases where MR is not available, the latter two methods are still useful.

The mainstay of treatment is intravenous antibiotics and surgical decompression. Early neurosurgical consultation is important, as neurologically intact patients can deteriorate abruptly, usually as a result of vascular factors rather than mechanical cord compression.[25,28] Deterioration on intravenous antibiotics while awaiting surgery can occur,[28] although some patients have done well when treated with antibiotics alone.[25] Appropriate antibiotics would cover *S. aureus* and gram-negative enteric organisms. The choice of which antibiotics to use depends on hospital and regional resistance patterns.

Patient outcomes are largely a function of the neurologic condition at time of presentation and the duration of neurological deficits prior to examination. Patients who are diagnosed while still ambulatory generally remain so; the mortality rate ranges from 5% to 23%.[25,28-29]

Spinal Cancer

The incidence of spinal malignancy is low in unselected populations of outpatients with back pain; however, metastatic disease in the spine is a common diagnosis in patients with known cancer. In one series of 851 cancer patients seen for neurological symptoms, 18.2% had back pain.[30] Of the 133 patients in this series with back pain, 30% of the cases were due to bony metastases, 33% were due to epidural metastases, and in 20% other metastases (meninges, paravertebral soft tissues, and to the nerve plexuses) were found.

Lung, breast, and prostate were the most common primary sites of cancers associated with back pain. Other frequent primary malignancies included lymphoma, renal cell carcinoma, melanoma, sarcoma, and multiple myeloma.[31] Thyroid cancer frequently spreads to bone; it may be the cause of epidural metastasis.[32] Epidural tumor is the first manifestation of cancer in about 10% of patients with spinal metastases; accordingly, all patients with spinal metastases will not have a history of cancer.[33]

Spread of cancer to bone is second only to lung cancer in frequency. Among cases of metastatic bone involvement, the spine is the most commonly involved site.[33] The vertebral body is usually involved first; therefore, spinal metastatic disease is most commonly found anteriorly.[31,33] Experimentally, cancer cells invade the spinal canal via the foramina of vertebral veins rather than by bony destruction; therefore, radiographic evidence of vertebral metastatic disease can be a late event.[34]

The pathogenesis of metastatic spine disease in humans results from direct epidural extension from a vertebral lesion in 85% of cases. Other possibilities include extradural extension from paravertebral tumor (especially common in lymphoma), or impingement of bony fragments, or angulation of the cord from pathologic vertebral fracture.[31,33] The degree to which vascular factors play a role is incompletely understood.

Location. A thoracic location is most common (about 60-70% of all cases), followed by lumbar involvement.[2,33] Prostate and colon cancer tend to spread to the lumbar area, whereas lung cancer preferentially affects the thoracic spine. Breast and prostate cancer tend to spread to multiple (although they are not always symptomatic) areas, while lung cancer often produces a single lesion.[33] As with most causes of spinal cord compression, the rate of development of compression is an important factor in the prognosis; the more rapid the development, the worse the outcome.

Diagnosis. Pain is the most common symptom of spinal cancer.[31,33] There is often a progression of symptoms from back pain (vertebral metastases) to radicular pain (caused by nerve root compression) to neurological signs resulting from cord or cauda equina compression.[33] The pain produced by spinal metastatic disease is similar to that described in patients with a herniated disk: both increase with activities that produce a Valsalva maneuver (coughing, sneezing, etc.).[31,33] The SLR test will be positive in both herniated disk and cord compression.[2,33]

Other symptoms help distinguish the two processes. Pain from cancer tends to be unaffected or worse with rest or at night, whereas pain from sciatica or degenerative disease behaves in the opposite manner. Cancer pain can occur at any area in the spine, whereas benign disease tends to cluster in the lower neck and lower back. Weakness, sensory, and sphincter symptoms tend to follow isolated pain.[31] The high frequency in which neurological symptoms are found at presentation in many series may be a reflection of delayed diagnosis.[33]

As previously outlined, there is evidence to suggest that ordering an ESR in this setting can be helpful.[35] The important question is, if the ESR is not elevated, should one proceed further? In one study, the combination of plain films and ESR along with careful history identified all patients with cancer.[35] There were some patients in that study who were proven to have cancer but who did not have either or both studies done. Therefore, the question is who should be imaged, when, and with what study?

One investigation divided cancer patients with back pain into three groups. It is important to note that this study was published in 1987, prior to widespread use of MR and prior to the current economic conditions.[36] In Group 1 (patients with new signs of symptoms of cord or cauda equina disease), plain films were recommended while waiting for myelography. For Group 2 (patients with evidence of "stable or mild" spinal cord compression or those with radiculopathy or plexopathy), they recommended CT scan followed by plain films and myelography for patients with suspected coexistent radiculopathy. For those without suspected radiculopathy, the algorithm called for CT along with plain films or radionuclide scan and myelography for any positive finding. In Group 3 patients (those with back pain alone), the algorithm calls for sequential plain films, followed by radionuclide scanning, and then a CT scan. A positive on any test would lead to myelography.

MRI Scanning. Since 1987, the MRI scan has become the imaging method of choice in hospitals where it is available.[31,33] For patients with neurological findings, MR scanning is clearly indicated, the only issue being how urgently. For patients with no neurological signs or symptoms, should one directly proceed to MRI scan or should plain films be obtained as an initial screen? If plain films are positive, MRI scan is still indicated, in part, to plan for radiotherapy fields. The question becomes, in cancer patients with back pain and normal plain films, how likely is there to be a spinal metastasis?

In one autopsy study of 832 consecutive patients with a "terminal" diagnosis of cancer, the spines were examined grossly, radiographically, and histologically.[32] The investigators found that 26% of metastatic deposits were not seen on plain films and conversely, 22% of cases of vertebral collapse were not due to the malignancy. In the former group, it is not known if the occult metastatic lesions were clinically relevant.

Knowledge of the primary tumor may assist in decision-making; 94% of patients with breast cancer have abnormal plain films, as do 74% of those with lung cancer. In patients with lymphoma and pediatric neoplasms, on the other hand, only one-third demonstrated abnormal plain films.[31] Two authorities conclude that while the risk of metastases may be low, in cancer patients with back pain, even those with no neurological signs or symptoms and normal plain films, MRI scanning may be useful.[31,33] The issue and approaches to the work-up of cancer patients with back pain are still a matter of debate and must be considered controversial.

The authors' opinion, based on the existing evidence, is that the rapid advances in technology and the decrease in real costs justify proceeding to MRI scanning directly as the best policy. If such patients are not imaged with MRI, they must be followed extremely closely. Remember that this controversy applies only to patients with no signs or symptoms of neurological disease. Cancer patients with neurological signs or symptoms clearly should have an MRI scan immediately. Twenty-five percent of cancer patients whose symptoms or signs suggest radiculopathy, and who have normal plain films, have metastatic epidural cord compression.[31]

In cases where MRI scanning is unavailable or if it is contraindicated (claustrophobia or metallic clips or pacemakers), conventional CT scan or myelography should be performed. Rarely, in a patient with a high suspicion for a lesion and a nondiagnostic MRI scan, conventional myelography may show the lesion.[31,33] Needle biopsy may also be indicated in patients whose primary tumor is unknown.

Regarding timing of the study, patients with signs of cord or cauda equina lesions should be imaged within hours; those with root or plexus lesions and with isolated back pain can be imaged urgently, preferably within 24 hours.

Consultation with the patient's oncologist, as well as with a radiation oncologist and neurosurgeon, should be initiated early. Steroids and radiation therapy are the mainstays of therapy, although decompressive surgery is undertaken in selected patients.[33] For patients with severe compression or rapid progression, 100 mg of intravenous dexamethasone is recommended; pain relief often occurs over hours. Lower doses may be just as effective and are used for patients with less dramatic presentations.[31,33]

Spinal Hematomas

Spontaneous spinal epidural hematoma is another rare but serious disease that can lead to poor outcomes if not promptly diagnosed and treated. While there is a peak incidence of this entity between 50 and 80 years of age, cases were found in all age groups at a frequency not much lower than the peak.[37] Almost all are posterolateral in location and are thought to be due to rupture of veins in the spinal epidural plexus.[37] Anticoagulation of any type, recent spinal surgery, or spinal anesthesia are important risk factors, especially in combination. Moreover, spontaneous spinal epidural hematoma is a rare complication of lumbar puncture.[38]

Magnetic resonance scanning permits prompt diagnosis.[39,40] Surgical therapy is indicated in most cases, although conservative therapy has worked in selected cases.[40,41]

Back Pain in the Elderly

Patients older than the age of 50 years have a higher incidence of "cannot miss" diagnoses. This is in part because many of these conditions are more common in older patients and because herniated disk is less common, owing to age-related fibrosis of the nucleus pulposis. The Agency for Health Care Policy and Research (AHCPR) Guidelines does list age older than 70 as a risk factor for spinal fracture.[42] Patients older than the age of 50 with new or different back pain must be approached with a high degree of suspicion for serious disease.

Other than the "cannot miss" diagnoses, another important condition causing back pain in the elderly is spinal stenosis, a narrowing of the spinal canal or exit foramina of the spinal nerves. The stenosis can be of the central canal (diameter of less than 11 mm) or the lateral recesses (depth less than 3 mm).[1] While this stenosis can be congenital, it is the acquired type that results from hypertrophic soft tissue and bony degenerative changes that is most commonly seen.

The classic symptom suggesting spinal stenosis is neurogenic claudication. This typically consists of pain in the legs, with or without other neurologic symptoms (especially paresthesias), that occurs with walking, exercise in the erect posture, and even standing.[1,2] The pain can be sharp, aching, or cramping. Extension of the back increases the pain and impotence and cauda equina symptoms can be seen as sequelae.[1] The sensitivity of neurogenic claudication as an indicator of spinal stenosis has ranged from 60% to 100%.[1,2]

As compared to vascular claudication, the neurogenic variety is more commonly seen with standing alone, it may be increased by Valsalva (cough and sneeze), and it is associated with normal arterial pulses.[2] The increase in pain with extension also distinguishes the pain from herniated disk, which usually is exacerbated by flexion.[2]

Precise diagnostic criteria and therapeutic options are not clear at the present time. Measurements of the size of the spinal canal by CT scan were used in one study, which also concluded that conservative treatment with physical modalities and salmon calcitonin led to improvement in many patients.[1] Indications for surgery are unclear, but patients who have increasing symptoms or incapacitation should be referred for consultation with a skilled spine surgeon.

Osteoarthritis

Although many of the aforementioned conditions (from spinal abscess to epidural malignancy) can cause back pain in the geriatric patient, the clinician must always consider osteoarthritis in the differential diagnosis of elderly patients presenting to the primary care setting. Overall, osteoarthritis is the most commonly diagnosed joint disorder in the elderly population. If radiographic criteria are used exclusively (including joint space narrowing, bony sclerosis, cyst formation, and osteophyte formation), the prevalence of osteoarthritis by age 70 approaches almost 100%.[43] However, the number of people in this age group with functional loss or symptomatic osteoarthritis at any given time is less than 50%.[43,44]

Disease Categorization. Osteoarthritis can be divided into a) primary osteoarthritis, in which a precipitating cause of the arthritis is unknown; and b) secondary osteoarthritis, in which an initiating set of factors can be discerned. In general, osteoarthritis can be thought of as a "final common pathway" rather than as a discrete clinical entity with a consistent set of clinicopathologic correlations. Most patients, it should be stressed, have primary osteoarthritis, which is a disease of aging and is more prevalent symptomatically in females than males. Moreover, it is a disease of all races, and while various risk factors, such as obesity, have been proposed, none is conclusively established as a cause of this condition.

Secondary osteoarthritis can be precipitated by numerous underlying etiologies, most of which can be identified from a detailed history. Causes of secondary osteoarthritis can be broken down into three major categories: mechanical, congenital or developmental disorders, and systemic diseases. Trauma, including vertebral fractures, is one of the leading mechanical factors for the development of secondary osteoarthritis. This mechanical factor includes fractures that enter the joint space with disruption of the joint surface, post-operative degeneration, and major injury to the supportive structures of a joint.

Figure. Neuro-imaging of Back Pain Patients

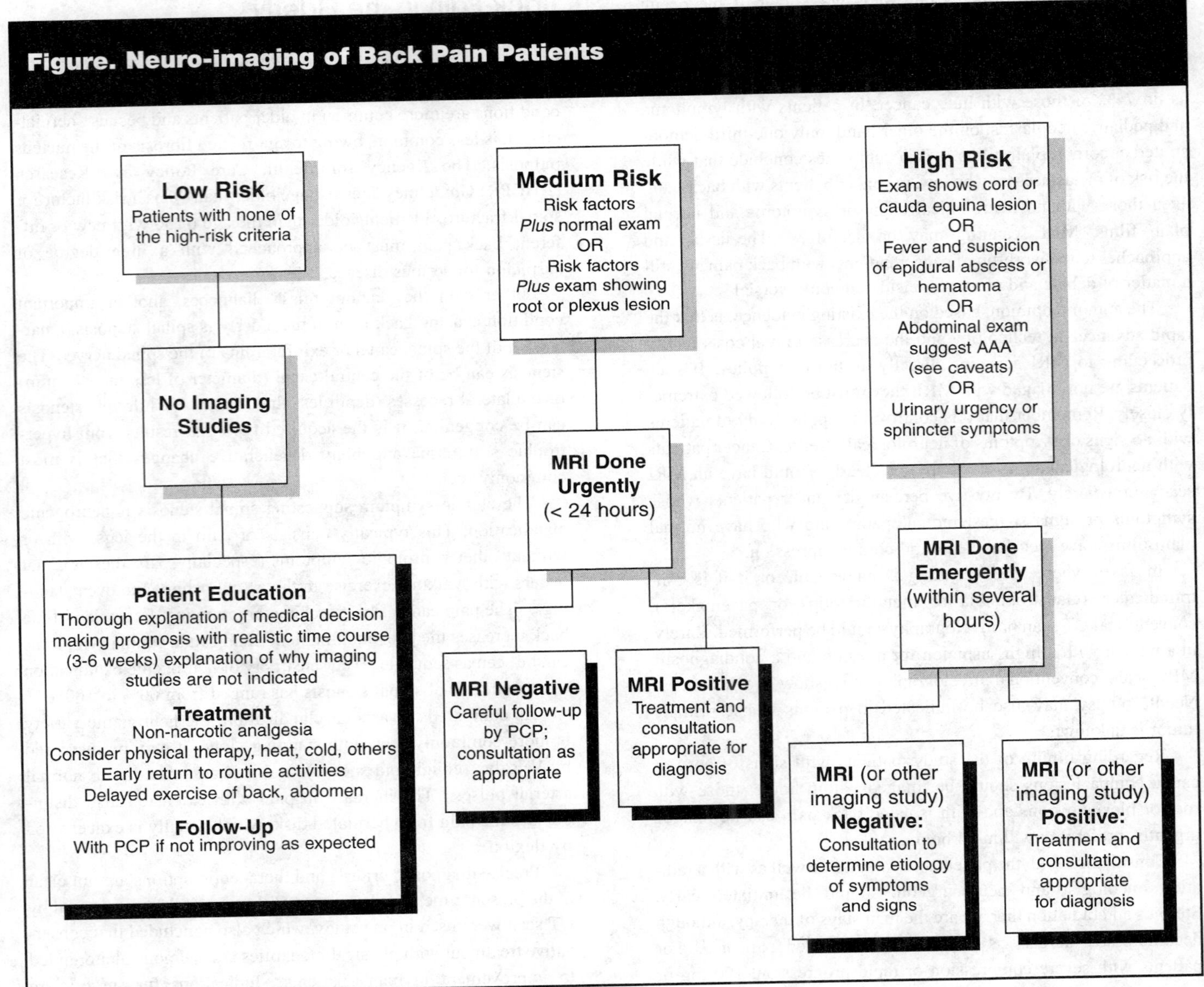

Diagnosis. Ascribing acute or chronic low back pain to osteoarthritis requires historical support and radiographic confirmation of osteophytes as well as other changes and symptoms consistent with established osteoarthritis. The usual presenting complaint of osteoarthritis is joint pain, which is often characterized by pain with use and relief with rest. The pain is usually aching, and will progress to chronic pain, including nocturnal joint pain, with exacerbation from activity. The etiology of recurrent, chronic, and/or intermittent back pain is thought to be a combination of periosteal elevation and damage by osteophyte formation, and possibly even microfractures in areas of weakened cystic bone. Morning joint stiffness that is relieved rapidly with use is the cardinal symptom of osteoarthritis.

The disease is insidious and usually takes months to years to develop. There are no systemic symptoms associated with osteoarthritis unless the condition has been caused by an underlying secondary disorder. In its early presentation, osteoarthritis is usually monoarticular, but with advancing disease the cervical and lumbar spine, hips, knees, and the interphalangeal joints of the hand become involved. Involvement of the wrist, shoulder, or elbow is uncommon in osteoarthritis.

Osteoarthritic involvement of the spine, at least by radiographic criteria, is present in almost 100% of adults 70 years of age or older. This should be contrasted with rheumatoid arthritis, which usually has a more rapid polyarticular onset, and in which lumbar pain is much less common. The presenting symptoms of vertebral involvement include the insidious onset of pain, usually most prominent in the morning and with development of stiffness.

Treatment. Once the clinician has determined that the cause of back pain is osteoarthritis, pain management and functional improvement are principal goals of therapy. Acetaminophen has been used in mild cases, but the mainstay of therapy has been nonsteroidal anti-inflammatory drugs (NSAIDs), among them ibuprofen, naproxen, and a number of other agents, including once-daily preparations.

Unfortunately, NSAIDs, especially the cyclooxygenase-1 (COX-1) isoenzyme inhibitors, have been an important cause of drug-related morbidity and mortality in the elderly population. This is because, until recently, the available NSAIDs generally inhibited both COX-1 and cyclooxygenase-2 (COX-2) pathways. Inhibition of COX-2 is believed to provide the therapeutic anti-inflammatory and analgesic benefit of traditional NSAIDs, while inhibition of COX-1 may contribute to upper gastrointestinal adverse effects, such as ulcers, and also mediates the antiplatelet aggregation effects of NSAIDs.

NSAIDs are among the most commonly prescribed drugs and many are also available over the counter (OTC). Gastrointestinal toxicities are among the most serious side effects of the drugs, including ulceration, hemorrhage, or perforation. The mechanism of action of NSAIDs has been explained largely on their ability to inhibit the enzyme cyclooxygenase (COX). COX-1 is believed to have a gastroprotective effect, while COX-2 is responsible for the production of proinflammatory mediators.[45,46] Older NSAIDs are generally better inhibitors of COX-1 than COX-2, whereas newer NSAIDs, such as nabumetone and etodolac, have more balanced inhibition.[45]

The treatment landscape for pain associated with osteoarthritis is now changing. When managing back pain that is clinically linked to osteoarthritis, practitioners have the option of using COX-2 inhibitors, which, on the basis of comparative endoscopic data evaluating gastric erosion and ulcer formation, appear to reduce the possible risk of gastrointestinal hemorrhage. The two COX-2 agents currently available for osteoarthritis include celecoxib (Celebrex) and rofecoxib (Vioxx).

Celecoxib. Celecoxib is a NSAID but, unlike most other NSAIDs previously used to manage osteoarthritis, it is a selective inhibitor of COX-2. At therapeutic concentrations, celecoxib does not inhibit COX-1. Celecoxib is indicated for the relief of the signs and symptoms of osteoarthritis and rheumatoid arthritis in adults. For the relief of the signs and symptoms of osteoarthritis, the recommended dose is 200 mg daily administered as a single dose or as 100 mg twice daily.[47] For the relief of the signs and symptoms of rheumatoid arthritis, the recommended dose is 100-200 mg twice daily.

In elderly patients (> 65 years of age), consideration should be given to starting celecoxib at a lower dose.[47] Celecoxib can be taken without regard to meals. However, a high-fat meal delays the absorption by about 1-2 hours, with an increase in total absorption of 10-20%. Coadministration with an aluminum- and magnesium-containing antacid reduces the peak plasma level by 37% and total absorption by 10%. Celecoxib is supplied as 100-mg and 200-mg capsules. Celecoxib should not be taken by patients who have demonstrated allergic-type reactions to sulfonamides.

In comparative trials between celecoxib and ibuprofen or naproxen, celecoxib was associated with a statistically significantly lower incidence of endoscopic ulcers evaluated at 12 weeks.[47] The incidences were 9.9-17.6% with naproxen (500 mg bid) and 9.6% for ibuprofen (800 mg tid), compared to 1.5-4% and 1.5-5.9% for celecoxib at 100 mg bid and 200 mg bid, respectively.[47] Moreover, among 5285 patients studied who received celecoxib over a 1-6 month period, only two patients (0.04%) experienced significant upper GI bleeding, one at 14 and another at 22 days after initiation of therapy. The discontinuation rate for celecoxib (7.1%) was similar to that for placebo (6.1%). Higher than recommended doses of celecoxib (600 mg bid for 7 days) had no effect on platelet aggregation and bleeding time. A single dose of 800 mg of celecoxib did not inhibit platelet COX-1 dependent aggregation.[48] Celecoxib does not appear to affect the anticoagulant effect of warfarin, although caution should be exercised if coadministration is considered.

It should be noted that the effect of celecoxib on the anticoagulant effect of warfarin was studied in a group of healthy subjects. In these subjects, celecoxib did not alter the anticoagulant effect of warfarin as determined by prothrombin time. However, there have been infrequent reports of increases in prothrombin time, sometimes associated with bleeding events, predominantly in the elderly. Therefore, anticoagulant activity should be monitored when therapy with celecoxib is initiated or changed in patients taking warfarin, particularly in the first few days. Celecoxib, by itself, has no effect on platelet aggregation or bleeding time at therapeutic doses and may be an appropriate treatment option in patients taking warfarin, when anti-inflammatory therapy is indicated.

The occurrence rate of dyspepsia and abdominal pain with celecoxib appears to be numerically lower than that of naproxen, ibuprofen, and diclofenac but slightly higher than placebo. The occurrence rates were 8.8% for dyspepsia and 4.1% for abdominal pain compared to 6.2% and 2.8%, 12.2% and 7.7%, 10.9% and 9%, 12.8% and 9% for placebo, naproxen, ibuprofen, and diclofenac, respectively.[47] Dyspepsia and abdominal pain were the most common side effects of celecoxib that led to discontinuation in clinical trials (0.8% and 0.7% for celecoxib compared to placebo, 0.6% and 0.6% for each symptom, respectively). Borderline elevation of one or more liver tests may occur in up to 15% of patients. Significant elevation (> 3 times the upper limits of normal) has been reported in only 1% of patients in clinical trials.[47]

Celecoxib is metabolized by cytochrome P450 2C9, and fluconazole, an inhibitor of this isoenzyme, causes a two-fold increase in plasma level. In vitro studies suggest that celecoxib is an inhibitor of P450 2D6 and there are potential interactions with substrates of this isoenzyme. Celecoxib increases the plasma level of lithium, and monitoring is recommended with coadministration.[47] Celecoxib does not appear to be renal sparing, as the renal effects are similar to other NSAIDs.

The potential superiority of celecoxib over other NSAIDs in terms of serious upper GI side effects has not been clearly established. In the celecoxib trials, endoscopic ulcers were used as surrogate markers. The correlation between endoscopic findings or symptoms and serious GI side effects has not been established. Although this method has been widely used in clinical studies, endoscopically observed ulcers may not be reliable predictors of severe GI events.[49-51] Endoscopic ulcers tend to be smaller, superficial, and predominantly gastric while serious events tend to be both gastric and duodenal.[49,50]

Despite the present lack of conclusive, prospective post-marketing studies confirming the gastrointestinal-sparing effects and safety advantages of COX-2 inhibitors such as celecoxib over other NSAIDs, the available endoscopic data showing reduction in ulcers, as well as the reduction in dyspepsia and abdominal pain, are sufficiently compelling to recommend COX-2 inhibitors such as celecoxib as initial therapy for pain management in patients with osteoarthritis. Celecoxib is priced similar to branded NSAIDs. The average wholesale price is $2.42 for the 200-mg capsules and $1.43 for the 100-mg capsules. These are similar to nabumetone (1000 mg/d) and oxaprozin (1200 mg/d).

Rofecoxib. Another COX-2 inhibitor, rofecoxib is approved for the relief of the signs and symptoms of osteoarthritis, for the management of acute pain in adults, and for the treatment of dysmenorrhea. Rofecoxib is available as 12.5-mg or 25-mg tablets and as an oral suspension containing 12.5 mg or 25 mg per 5 mL. The recommended initial dose for osteoarthritis is 12.5 mg once daily. Some patients may achieve added benefit at a dose of 25 mg once daily, which is considered the maximal dose for this indication. It may be taken without regard to meals. Rofecoxib should not be taken by patients who have experienced allergic-type reactions to aspirin or other NSAIDs.

Rofecoxib, 25 mg or 50 mg daily, has been reported to produce a lower percentage of endoscopic gastroduodenal ulcers than ibuprofen 2400 mg daily. The difference was statistically significant at 12- and 24-week assessments.[52] Rofecoxib also appears to be well tolerated in terms of GI adverse events. In a clinical trial, the percent of patients experiencing diarrhea was 6.8% vs. 6.5% for placebo, 3.5% vs. 2.7% for dyspepsia, 3.8% vs. 2.8% for epigastric discomfort, and 4.2% vs. 3.6% for heartburn.[52] The metabolism of rofecoxib does not involve the cytochrome P450 enzymes, thus minimizing potential drug interactions. A general enzyme inducer, rifampin, has been reported to produce a 50% decrease in the plasma concentration of rofecoxib.[52] Rofecoxib has no effect on platelet function. Dosages of up to 375 mg given daily for up to 12 days did not affect bleeding time relative to placebo.[52]

Rofecoxib is approved for osteoarthritis but not for rheumatoid arthritis. The renal effects of rofecoxib are similar to those of other NSAIDs. The use of rofecoxib for the relief of pain at the 50-mg dose is not recommended beyond five days.[52] Coadministration of rofecoxib and warfarin have resulted in an increase of 8-11% in INR. Therefore, monitoring of INR is recommended with coadministration.[52]

In osteoarthritis, rofecoxib (12.5-25 mg) has been reported to be similar in effectiveness to ibuprofen 800 mg tid over six weeks or diclofenac 50 mg tid over six months.[52-54]

Although rofecoxib does carry an indication for management of acute pain, practitioners should note the following possible parameters, findings, and/or limitations regarding its use for this population. The recommended initial dose for acute pain is 50 mg once daily, and subsequent doses should also be 50 mg once daily as needed. Moreover, use of refecoxib for more than five days for management of pain has not been studied. Finally, in clinical osteoarthritis trials of up to six months, the general safety profile of the rofecoxib 50 mg qd dose was similar to the recommended 12.5 and 25 mg qd dose, although there was a higher incidence of dose-related gastrointestinal symptoms (abdominal pain, epigastric pain, heartburn, nausea, and vomiting), lower extremity edema (6.3%), and hypertension (8.2%). The additional cost of the 50-mg dose for acute pain is also a deterrent to routine use.

Summary and Diagnostic Algorithm

The algorithm proposed in the Figure is based on the authors' interpretation of evidence-based literature. It would be expected to identify the vast majority of back pain patients with serious disease, while simultaneously avoiding unnecessary imaging studies in patients whose clinical management plan would be unchanged. However, this algorithm has not been prospectively validated, and therefore its accuracy remains conjectural.

Whatever algorithm is chosen, the PCP must remain alert for patients whose back pain falls into the "cannot miss" group. Since back pain is such a common symptom, the history and physical examination, coupled with a detailed knowledge of the differential diagnosis and risk factors for serious causes will assist the PCP in arriving at the correct diagnosis.

References

1. Onel D, Sari H, Donmez C. Lumbar spinal stenosis: Clinical/radiologic therapeutic evaluation in 145 patients. Conservative treatment or surgical intervention? *Spine* 1993;18:291-298.
2. Deyo RA, Rainville J, Kent DL. What can the history and physical examination tell us about low back pain? *JAMA* 1992;268:760-765.
3. Wipf J, Deyo R. Low back pain. *Med Clin North Am* 1995;9:231-246.

4. Darke SG, Eadie DDG. Abdominal aortic aneurysmectomy: A review of 60 consecutive cases contrasting elective and emergency surgery. *J Cardiovasc Surg* 1973;14:484-491.
5. Vohra R, Reid D, Groome J, et al. Long-term survival in patients undergoing resection of abdominal aortic aneurysm. *Ann Vasc Surg* 1990;4:460-465.
6. Marston WA, Ahlquist R, Johnson G, et al. Misdiagnosis of rup-tured abdominal aneurysms. *J Vasc Surg* 1992;16:17-22.
7. Banerjee A. Atypical manifestations of ruptured abdominal aortic aneurysms. *Postgrad Med J* 1993;69:6-11.
8. Bengtsson H, Bergqvist D. Ruptured abdominal aortic aneurysm: A population-based study. *J Vasc Surg* 1993; 18:74-80.
9. Dixon A. Imaging the bad back: Increasing reliance on MRI. *Hosp Med* 1998;49:496-498.
10. Kiell CS, Ernst CB. Advances in management of abdominal aortic aneurysm. *Adv Surg* 1993;26:73-98.
11. Zimmer T. Absence of back pain and tachycardia in the emer-gency presentation of abdominal aortic aneurysm. *Am J Emerg Med* 1988;6:316-321.
12. Hoffman M, Avellone JC, Plecha FR, et al. Operations for rup-tured abdominal aortic aneurysms: A community-wide experience. *Surgery* 1982;91:597-602.
13. Rothrock SG, Greenfield RH, Falk JL. Acute abdominal emergen-cies in the elderly: Clues to identifying serious illness. Part I-Clinical assessment and diagnostic studies. *Emerg Med Reports* 1992;13:177-184.
14. Rothrock SG, Greenfield R, Falk JL. Acute abdominal emergencies in the elderly: Clinical evaluation and management. Part II-Diagnosis and management of common conditions. *Emerg Med Reports* 1992;13:185-192.
15. Tsolakis I, Korovessis P, Spastris P, et al. Acute rupture of an aortic aneurysm mimicking the discus hernia syndrome. A case report. *Internat Angiol* 1992;11:142-144.
16. Earnst CB. Abdominal aortic aneurysms. *N Engl J Med* 1993;328:1167-1172.
17. LaRoy LL, Cormier RJ, Matalon TA, et al. Imaging of abdominal aortic aneurysms. *Am J Roentgenol* 1989;152: 785-792.
18. Swedenborg J. Optimal method for imaging of abdominal aortic aneurysms. *Ann Chir Gynaecol* 1992;81:158-160.
19. Bower TC, Cherry KJ, Pairolero PC. Unusual manifestations of abdominal aortic aneurysms. *Surg Clin North Am* 1989; 69:745-754.
20. Stanford W, Rooholamini SA, Galvin JR. Ultrafast computed 4237 screened patients: Prevalence, development and management over 6 years. *Br J Surg* 1991;78: 1122-1125.
21. Chan C, Gold W. Intramedullary abscess of the spinal cord in the antibiotic era: Clinical features, microbial etiologies, trends in pathogenesis and outcomes. *Clin Infect Dis* 1998; 27:619-626.
22. Sapico F, Montgomerie J. Vertebral osteomyelitis. *Infect Dis Clin North Am* 1990;4:539-550.
23. Bass S, Ailani R, Shekar R, Gerblich A. Pyogenic vertebral osteomyelitis presenting as exudative pleural effusion: A series of five cases. *Chest* 1998;114:642-647.
24. Babinchak T, Riley D, Rotheram Jr. E. Pyogenic vertebral osteomyelitis of the posterior elements. *Clin Infect Dis* 1997;25:221-224.
25. Darouiche R, Hamill R, Greenberg S, et al. Bacterial spinal epidural abscess—Review of 43 cases and literature survey. *Medicine* 1992;71:369-385.
26. Danner R, Hartman B. Update of spinal epidural abscess: 35 cases and review of the literature. *Rev Infect Dis* 1987;9: 265-274.
27. Kindler C, Seeberger. M, Staender S. Epidural abscess complicating epidural anesthesia and analgesia. An analysis of the literature. *Acta Anaesthesiol Scandinavia* 1998;42: 614-620.
28. Hlavin M, Kaminski H, Ross J, Ganz E. Spinal epidural abscess: A ten-year perspective. *Neurosurgery* 1990;27: 177-184.
29. Mackenzie A, Laing R, Kaar G, et al. Spinal epidural abscess: The importance of diagnosis and treatment. *J Neurol Neurosurg Psychi* 1998;65:209-212.
30. Clouston P, DeAngelis L, Posner J. The spectrum of neurological disease in patients with systemic cancer. *Ann Neurol* 1992;31:268-273.
31. Byrne T. Spinal cord compression from epidural metastases. *N Engl J Med* 1992;327:614-619.
32. Wong D, Fornasier V, MacNab I. Spinal metastases: The obvious, the occult and the impostors. *Spine* 1990;15:1-4.
33. Boogerd W, Van der Sande J. Diagnosis and treatment of spinal cord compression in malignant disease. *Cancer Treat Rev* 1993;19:129-150.
34. Arguello F, Baggs R, Duerst R, et al. Pathogenesis of vertebral metastasis and epidural spinal cord compression. *Cancer* 1990;65:98-106.
35. Deyo R, Diehl A. Cancer as a cause of back pain: Frequency, clinical presentation, and diagnostic strategies. *J Gen Intern Med* 1988;3:230-238.
36. Portenoy R, Lipton R, Foley K. Back pain in the cancer patient: An algorithm for evaluation and management. *Neurology* 1987;37:134-138.
37. Groen R, Ponssen H. The spontaneous spinal epidural hematoma—A study of the etiology. *J Neurological Sci* 1990;98:128-138.
38. Egede L, Moses H, Wang H. Spinal subdural hematoma: A rare complication of lumbar puncture. Case report and review of the literature. *Maryland Med J* 1999;48:15-17.
39. Sklar E, Post J, Falcone S. MRI of acute spinal epidural hematomas. *J Computer Ass Tomograph* 1999;23:38-43.
40. Alexiadou-Rudolf C, Ernestus R, Nanassis K, et al. Acute nontraumatic spinal epidural hematomas: An important differential diagnosis in spinal emergencies. *Spine* 1998;32:1810-1813.
41. Pahapill P, Lownie S. Conservative treatment of acute spontaneous spinal epidural hematoma. *Canadian J Neurol Sci* 1998;25:159-163.
42. AHCPR. Acute low back pain in adults: Clinical Practice Guideline #14, AHCPR Publication #95-0642, Rockville, MD, 1994. Agency for Health Care Policy and Research.
43. Bergstrom G, et al. Joint disorders at ages 70, 75, and 79 years: A cross sectional comparison. *Br J Rheumatol* 1986;25:333-341.

44. Spiera, H. Osteoarthritis as a misdiagnosis in the elderly. *Geriatrics* 1987;42:37-42.
45. Jouzeau JY, et al. Cyclo-oxygenase isoenzymes. How recent findings affect thinking about nonsteroidal anti-inflammatory drugs. *Drugs* 1997;53:563-584.
46. Lipsky PE, Isakson PC. Outcome of specific COX-2 inhibition in rheumatoid arthritis. *J Rheumatol* 1997; 24(suppl 49):9-14.
47. Celebrex Product Information. G.D. Searle & Co. December 1998.
48. McAdam BF, et al. Systemic biosynthesis of prostacyclin by cyclooxygenase (COX)-2: The human pharmacology of a selective inhibitor of COX-2. *Proc Natl Acad Sci* 1999;96: 272-277.
49. Walt RP. Misoprostol for the treatment of peptic ulcer and anti-inflammatory-drug-induced gastroduodenal ulceration. *N Engl J Med* 1992;327:1575-1580.
50. McCarthy D. Nonsteroidal anti-inflammatory drug-related gastrointestinal toxicity: Definitions and epidemiology. *Am J Med* 1998;105(5A):3S-9S.
51. Kimmey MB. Role of endoscopy in nonsteroidal anti-inflammatory drug clinical trials. *Am J Med* 1998;105(5A): 28S-31S.
52. Vioxx Product Information. Merck & Co. May 1999.
53. Saag K, et al. *Arthritis Rheum* 1998;41(suppl 9):984.
54. Cannon G, et al. *Arthritis Rheum* 1998;41(suppl 9):985.

Part XII

Toxicologic Emergencies

Over-the-Counter Medications: Toxic Effects and Adverse Reactions: Part I

Richard Y. Wang, DO, FACEP, FACMT
Daren D. Girard, MD

Recent advances in consumer marketing have fueled the creation of a proliferation of self-treatment products. These products, known as "over-the-counter" or OTC agents, include traditional remedies, new formulations, and combinations, as well as reduced-strength versions of prescription medications. Examples of OTC formulations of prescription drugs include cimetidine, nonsteroidal anti-inflammatory drugs (NSAIDs), and antihistamines.

In 1998, the American Association of Poison Control Centers Toxic Exposure Surveillance System (AAPCC TESS) registered more than 500,000 exposures to OTC formulations.[1] *(Please see Table 1.)* While the majority of these produced no serious harm, some OTC exposures resulted in significant morbidity and mortality. *(Please see Table 2.)* The recent withdrawal of phenylpropanolamine-containing flu remedies suggests increasing vigilance in review of OTC products to prevent toxicity. As a result, it is important that emergency health care providers be familiar with these agents so they can optimize care for their patients. With these issues in focus, this detailed chapter outlines the clinical manifestations and management of important OTC exposures caused by various routes of administration. Part I of this two-part series will review topical preparations.

Dermatologic Preparations: Topical Products

Dermatologic preparations include formulations of creams, ointments, gels, liquids, and aerosols; the principal difference among these products is the base or vehicle. Vehicles determine the rate of absorption at the site of action. Creams are water-in-oil emulsions and permit absorption into the subdermal and subcutaneous layers. Ointments are hydrophobic mixtures, usually hydrocarbon based (e.g., petrolatums), and are intended to remain at the site of application, with minimal absorption. Gels are water-based vehicles, allowing rapid dissolution and absorption.

Inadvertent ingestion of any of the vehicles may produce toxic effects similar to mild anionic and nonionic surfactants (e.g., soaps), which produce both emetic and laxative effects. Although toxicity is unusual during therapeutic use, applying these agents to large areas of abraded or denuded skin increases the amount of vehicle absorbed, as well as the potential for symptoms.[2] Increasing absorption with occlusive dressings, repeat application, or application to a large percentage of body surface area also may lead to toxicity.

Rubefacients. Rubefacient preparations are intended to produce mild local irritation, creating an increase in blood flow, and subsequently, erythema. The result of this process is the sensation of warmth. Camphor and menthol combinations are traditional formulations that have been around for decades. *(Please see Table 3.)* A druggist's handbook, circa 1877, identifies 10 different formulas

Table 1. Incidence of OTC Exposures in 1998[1]

OVER THE COUNTER PREPARATION	NUMBER OF EXPOSURES	NUMBER OF MORBIDITIES	NUMBER OF MORTALITIES
Analgesics (acetaminophen, NSAIDs, salycilates)	133,899	5,383	107
Cosmetics and personal care products	210,224	33,769	3
Cough and cold formulations (antihistamines, decongestants)	118,280	23,050	16
Topicals (dermal, nasal, ocular, oral, rectal, vaginal)	83,455	9,702	1
Vitamins and iron supplements	53,657	4,237	1
Gastrointestinal formulations (antacids, antidiarrheals, laxatives)	45,696	4,355	6

using various combinations.[3] Typically, camphor and menthol are mixed together to form an eutectic mixture that is then incorporated into a vehicle, commonly petrolatum. The concentrations of camphor and menthol range from 2% to 5% and 1% to 16%, respectively.[4] Camphor is still available, however, in a solid, block form, usually in a 1-ounce size.[4]

Toxicity is characterized initially by gastrointestinal (GI) symptoms, including: nausea, vomiting, and abdominal distress. More significant exposures may demonstrate such central nervous system (CNS) effects as delirium, excitement, and seizures. Onset of symptoms usually occurs within 5-20 minutes and peaks within 90 minutes. Camphor is readily absorbed, and death has occurred from ingestion of as little as 1 gram.[5]

Menthol is the major constituent of peppermint oil. It also causes such gastrointestinal symptoms as nausea, vomiting, and abdominal pain. After a significant exposure (i.e., pure peppermint oil or a large ingestion of high concentration product), CNS effects, including ataxia, drowsiness, or coma, may be seen.[6] Acute toxic effects from ingestion of small amounts are unlikely given the available formulations, but significant toxicity may occur with ingestion of even a small amount of either agent in its pure form. Trivial (a mouthful or less) ingestions of the combination forms are treated by dilution, in conjunction with observation for local oral and GI irritant effects.

Capsaicin. Another counter irritant ingredient approved for OTC use is capsaicin. Previously available in prescription strengths of 0.025% and 0.075%, it was converted to OTC status in 1990.[7] Used in combination with camphor and menthol in 0.025% concentrations, capsaicin is derived from capsicum oleoresin, the irritant oil from the pepper plants of the *Solanacae* family. The clinical effects range from a feeling of warmth to burning, depending on the concentration applied.[8] Ingestion of the agent causes nausea and vomiting secondary to gastric irritation. Treatment consists of dilution or irrigation; symptoms abate after 30-60 minutes.

Ingredients in various rubefacient products include eucalyptol, thymol, cajput oil, and turpentine. They are present in very low concentrations and their toxicity is limited to minor irritation in the amounts available.

Topical Analgesics. Topical analgesics are used for muscle or joint pain. Like rubefacients, these agents are counter irritants, stimulating circulation and a feeling of warmth. Topical analgesics usually contain methyl salicylate (e.g., oil of wintergreen), or other salt forms of salicylate (e.g., trolamine salicylate). Commonly used in combination with other ingredients, especially camphor and menthol, the concentration of methyl salicylate may be as high as 35%.[9] Oil of wintergreen contains approximately 98 gm/100 mL of methyl salicylate, and the purified oil can be highly toxic; in fact, an ingestion of as little as 7 gm (7.5 mL) has produced significant morbidity in a 2-year-old child.[10] Since methyl salicylate is the methyl ester form of salicylate, symptoms of salicylate intoxication can be seen with ingestion or chronic application of more concentrated products.

Keratolytics. Other formulations that use concentrated salicylates include the keratolytics. These agents produce desquamation of the skin and are used as wart and corn removers. These products contain salicylic acid in concentrations ranging from 17% to 40% in liquid, solution, gel, patch, plaster, and cream form. The creams utilize the higher concentrations, with the liquid, gel, and solution products limited to less than 30%.[11] The liquid formulations commonly use flexible collodion (e.g., nitrocellulose) as a vehicle. These products can produce oral irritation, or potentially a burn if they have prolonged contact with skin. Nitrocellulose is water resistant and may cause adherence to mucus membranes. Due to the high concentrations of salicylate available in these OTC formulations, significant or chronic misuse can result in intoxication. Patient management includes monitoring serum salicylate levels, initiating urinary alkalinization, and hemodialysis, as would be indicated in salicylate poisoning.

Local Anesthetics. Topical anesthetics are used for local analgesia on intact dermis and to treat pruritic conditions such as insect bites, plant poisonings, eczema, and minor burns. These agents interrupt nerve impulse conduction by altering cell membrane ion flux, and as a result, produce an anesthetic effect. Most local anesthetic agents are poorly absorbed through intact dermis, but readily absorbed through the mucous membranes. Abraded skin augments the effectiveness of local anesthetics by increasing absorption. Anesthetic agents are classified according to their structure. Most agents belong to one of two classes: 1) benzoate esters; or 2) amides. Benzoate esters include benzocaine, tetracaine, and butamben picrate. The amides are dibucaine and lidocaine. Another topical anesthetic agent, pramoxine, is structurally unique.

Adverse effects of local anesthetics during therapeutic use include local irritation, burning, sloughing, interaction between other drugs, and hypersensitivity reactions.[12,13] The toxicity of these agents affects the cardiovascular, neurologic, and hematologic systems. Cardiac dysrhythmias, seizures, and coma can be seen with severe toxicity. Additionally, benzocaine and lidocaine can produce methemoglobinemia.[14]

Table 2. OTC Agents with Reported Clinical Toxicity

AGENT	OTC APPLICATION	CLINICAL MANIFESTATION
Acetaminophen	Analgesic, Antipyretic	Hepatic failure
Antihistamine (H1 receptor) (diphenhydramine, chlorpheniramine, brompheniramine, doxylamine)	Decongestant, Antipruritic, Sleep aid	Anticholinergic syndrome
Caffeine	Stimulant	Agitation, seizure, nausea, vomiting, tachydysrhythmia, hypotension, hypertension
Camphor	Rubefacient	Seizures
Dextromethrophan	Antitussive	Altered mental status, hypoventilation
Ethanol	Mouthwash/ Germicide	Depressed mental status, hypoventilation, hypoglycemia
Imidazoline (tetrahydrolozine, naphazoline, oxymetazoline, xylometazoline)	Topical decongestant	Depressed mental status, miosis, hypoventilation, bradycardia, alteration of blood pressure
Inorganic salts (magnesium, calcium, aluminum, sodium bicarbonate)	Antacid Laxative	Dehydration, electrolyte abnormalities
Iodine (povidone-iodine)	Antiseptic/Germicide Vaginal douche	Nausea, vomiting, abdominal pain, gastrointestinal tract burns
Iron salts (e.g., ferrous sulfate, ferrous gluconate, etc.)	Mineral supplement	Nausea, vomiting, abdominal pain, gastrointestinal bleeding, metabolic acidosis, hypotension, decreased mental status
Local anesthetics (benzocaine, dibucaine, dyclonine, lidocaine)	Topical analgesic	Depressed mental status, seizure, bradycardia, methemoglobinemia
Loperamide	Antidiarrheal	Depressed mental status, hypoventilation
Nonsteroidal anti-inflammatory agents (ibuprofen, ketoprofen, naproxen)	Analgesic, anti-inflammatory, antipyretic	Gastrointestinal distress, CNS depression
Permethrin	Pediculocide	Hypersensitivity
Pyrethrin	Scabicide	Keratitis
Quartenary ammonium compounds (alkyldimehtylbenzylammonium chlorides)	Antiseptic/Germicide	Nausea, vomiting, abdominal pain, gastrointestinal tract burns
Salicylate	Analgesic, antipyretic rubefacient, keratolytic	Nausea, vomiting, tinnitus, altered mental status, mixed acid/base disorder, pulmonary edema
Sympathomimetics (ephedrine, psuedoephedrine, phenylephrine, phenylpropanolamine)	Decongestant Appetite suppressant	Sympathomimetic syndrome

Lidocaine is available in gel, cream, ointment, liquid, and spray formulations. OTC preparations are limited to concentrations of 2.5% or less. Oral ingestions of 5-30 mL of a 2-4% viscous lidocaine solution have resulted in seizures in children.[15-17] Lidocaine has the potential to produce systemic effects, and repeated applications can lead to accumulation of the drug and its metabolites. It should be used with caution in patients who are taking Class I antiarrhythmic agents (e.g., tocainanide, mexilitene), due to a potential for synergism.

Lidocaine is readily absorbed if ingested, and it may accumulate in patients with hepatic impairment. Systemic effects, which can be seen with toxic plasma levels, include seizures, metabolic acidosis, heart block, bradycardia, hypotension, and methemoglobinemia. Very young patients, as well as patients with G6PD-deficiency, are more susceptible to methemoglobinemia.[18] General treatment is supportive; methylene blue is used to treat methemoglobinemia.

Benzocaine is available in creams, ointments, lotions, sprays, and liquids in concentrations ranging from 0.5% to 20%. It also is available in several combination products with menthol, phenol, camphor, alcohol, and antiseptic agents. Benzocaine's principal toxic effect is methemoglobinemia. It does not produce the CNS or cardiovascular effects observed with lidocaine.[19] Methemoglobinemia may be dose-related or idiosyncratic. Onset is usually within 20-60 minutes of application. Clinical symptoms of methemoglobinemia are related to the percentage of hemoglobin involved; dyspnea and tachycardia are

Table 3. Topical OTC Preparations and Their Ingredients

OTC PREPARATION	ACTIVE AGENTS
DERMAL (GELS)	
Acne	Benzoyl peroxide, sulfur, salicylic acid
Analgesics	Salicylates
Anti-infectives	Bacitracin, polymyxin B, neomycin, clotrimazole, miconazole
Cleansers	Benzalkonium choride, benzoyl peroxide, chlorhexidine, ethanol, povidine iodine, salicylic acid, sulfur
Corticosteroids	Hydrocortisone
Keratolytics	Salicylate
Local anesthetics	Benzocaine, tetracaine, dibucaine, lidocaine, pramoxine
Lotions (e.g., sunscreens, skinsofteners, scalp care)	PABA, kaolin, lanolin, mineral oil
Rubefacients	Essential and volatile oils (e.g., camphor, capsaicin, chamomile, eucalyptus, menthol, wormwood)
Miscellaneous (diaper rash, poison ivy)	Zinc oxide, calamine, local anesthetics, essential oils, diphenhydramine
DERMAL (LIQUIDS, POWDERS)	
Antiperspirant	Aluminum chloride, talc
Antiseptics, germicides	Iodide, inorganic mercury, quarternary ammonium chloride, chlorhexidine gluconate
Astringents	Calamine
Pediculocide, scabicide	Pyrethrin, piperonyl butoxide
ORAL	
Anesthetics (teething, dental pain)	Benzocaine, lidocaine
Mouthwashes	Ethanol
Toothpaste	Fluoride
OCULAR	
Vasoconstrictors	Imidazolines, phenylephrine
NASAL	
Decongestants	Imidazolines, propylhexedrine
VAGINAL AND RECTAL	
Analgesics	Acetaminophen, local anesthetics, salicylate
Antifungal	Clotriamazole, miconazole, butoconazole
Douches	Iodine (povidone-iodine)

present at high methemoglobin levels.[20] Methemoglobinemia is treated with methylene blue.

Dibucaine is available in cream or ointment forms in 0.5% or 1% concentrations. It is a potent amide-type anesthetic and can cause seizures and dysrhythmias in children, leading to fatality.[21] Photosensitivity and allergic dermatitis also have occurred with therapeutic use.[22,23] Pramoxine is available in creams, lotions, gels, and a spray, all of which are available in a 1% concentration. Its reported systemic toxicity is low, and the incidence of hypersensitivity reactions to pramoxine is less than that of other local anesthetics.[13]

Topical Anti-Infectives. Topical anti-infective agents include antibiotics such as neomycin, polymixin B, and bacitracin zinc; and antifungal agents such as clotrimazole, miconazole, undecyclenic acid derivatives, tolnaftate, and gentian violet. Anti-infective agents are available in formulations that include creams, ointments, gels, lotions, and powders. They are used to treat various minor infections. The relative toxicity of any of these agents is low; toxic effects from ingestion are limited to the GI tract, principally diarrhea, especially with the non-absorbable antibiotics. Hypersensitivity reactions are always possible, although the incidence of systemic reactions from ingestion is very low.

Corticosteroid. Topical corticosteroids are used for treatment of inflammatory and pruritic conditions. They are used alone or in combination with an antibiotic or antifungal agent. The only available OTC topical corticosteroid is hydrocortisone. It is available in creams, ointments, and lotions in 0.5% and 1% concentrations. The relative toxicity of hydrocortisone, even when large amounts (a mouthful) are ingested, is minimal. Dermal absorption occurs with topical application and hypothalamic-pituitary-adrenal axis suppression is possible, especially if an occlusive dressing is applied over a large surface area, or with chronic application over large areas of abraded skin.[24]

Soaps. Soaps for personal use are comprised almost entirely of anionic and nonionic surfactants. The balance of ingredients depends upon the particular form (liquid, bar, shampoo, etc.), and may include such additives as perfumes, stabilizers, and antibacterial agents. Used for personal cleaning and disinfecting, the number and variety of products available are staggering. Fortunately, the toxicity of soaps, whether liquid or solid, is very low. However, they are irritating to all mucus membranes—nasal, ocular, oral, rectal, and vaginal. Ingestion of even small amounts usually produces immediate emesis.[25] Treatment is symptomatic, with irrigation of exposed, irritated areas. Dilution is recommended with ingestion, and resolution of symptoms occur within minutes.

Lotions. Hand and body lotions are comprised of emulsions of oil in water or water in oil. As such, their toxic potential is low. High viscosity, a desirable property in a lotion, minimizes the aspiration potential on ingestion. Ingestion of significant amounts can cause emesis and also can have a laxative effect similar to that of other emollient laxatives (e.g., mineral oil or glycerine). Additives, such as perfumes, preservatives, stabilizers, emulsifiers, and thickeners, are present in negligible amounts. Ocular exposures cause irritation and conjunctival inflammation, and treatment should include dilution and irrigation, with ophthalmologic referral if prolonged or significant irritation occurs.

Acne Preparations. Acne preparations use benzoyl peroxide or sulfur as antibacterial agents. Benzoyl peroxide also has keratolytic and irritant effects and is available in creams, gels, or lotions in concentrations ranging from 2.5% to 20%. Likewise, sulfur has a keratolytic effect and is commonly available as either precipitated sulfur or colloidal sulfur in concentrations of 0.5-10%. Patient tolerance may limit the concentration of product applied.

The relative toxicity of acne preparations is low. Ocular and GI irritation can occur with significant exposures to either benzoyl peroxide or sulfur compounds.[26] Superficial corneal opacification may occur with benzoyl peroxide in concentrations greater than 5%.[27] Irrigation and dilution are recommended for these exposures, with ophthalmologic referral for persistent eye irritation. Make up or cosmetic products include mascaras, lipsticks, facial cremes, blushes, eye shadows, etc. Although multiple ingredients are involved, they are considered non-toxic.

Zinc Oxide. Zinc oxide is used for the treatment of diaper rash, abrasions, burns, and minor skin irritations. When used for the treatment of diaper rash, it forms a protective barrier against further irritation. It is available as an ointment in concentrations of 20% and is very often combined with other ingredients (e.g., zinc oxide and calamine for the treatment of poison ivy). Its systemic toxicity is low and needs no GI decontamination other than dilution.[28]

Poison Ivy Products. There are numerous products available for the symptomatic treatment of poison ivy exposure. These are all combination products, with the relative toxicity of each determined by its specific ingredients. They employ astringent agents such as calamine and zinc oxide, local anesthetic agents (e.g., benzocaine, pramoxine), antipruritic agents (e.g., diphenhydramine), and counterirritants (e.g., menthol, phenol, and camphor). They come in creams, ointments, and lotions. Their relative toxicity is low. Diphenhydramine in combination with calamine has caused severe anticholinergic toxicity in children and is no longer available OTC.[29,30]

Pediculocides/Scabicides. These products are used for the treatment of *Sarcoptes scabiei* (scabies) and *Pediculus capitus, pubis,* and *humanus* (head, pubic, or body lice, respectively), and their nits or eggs. The OTC products available for these conditions contain pyrethrins or permethrin, a synthetic pyrethroid, and piperonyl butoxide. Pyrethrins are obtained from the chrysanthemum plant, and are extremely effective against many insects. Hypersensitivity to the chrysanthemum plant, or any member of the *Asteracaea* (daisy) family, is a contraindication to the use of pyrethrin/pyrethroid-containing products. Permethrin is available as a 5% prescription cream for the treatment of scabies or a 1% cream rinse for the treatment of lice. Combination products containing pyrethrins and piperonyl butoxide are available OTC in concentrations ranging from 0.1% to 0.3%, and 2% to 4%, respectively. These are formulated into liquids, gels, and shampoos.

The relative toxicity of pyrethrins and pyrethroids is low; hypersensitivity is the primary concern.[31] Serious systemic hypersensitivity reactions are rare.[32] A fatality attributed to an asthma attack that was precipitated by the use of a pyrethrin-based dog shampoo has been reported.[32] CNS symptoms have occurred, especially in children exposed to the more potent pyrethroids.[33] It has been suggested that children are less able to metabolize pyrethrins efficiently, making them more susceptible to symptoms of toxicity, especially with application to large areas of skin. CNS depression and stimulation and dizziness, as well as periorbital paresthesias and dysesthesias have been reported.[33,34] Seizures have occurred with accidental and intentional exposure to products containing higher concentrations of pyrethrins/pyrethroids. No case reports could be found in the primary literature documenting these CNS effects after exposure to the OTC-strength topical products.[35]

Ocular exposure with subsequent corneal damage can result from the use of shampoo containing pyrethrin.[36] Irritation and contact dermatitis can be seen, especially with chronic, prolonged exposure; severe allergic reactions have been reported.[37] Treatment is primarily symptomatic and supportive. Thorough irrigation is indicated for dermal and ocular exposures. Fluorescein staining to assess corneal patency is indicated if there is continued eye pain after adequate irrigation.

Antiseptics and Germicidals. Antiseptics and germicidals are used to clean and disinfect cuts and abrasions and to cleanse an area prior to a medical procedure, such as intravenous catheter insertion or phlebotomy. OTC products available for this use are identical to those used in the hospital setting, with the exception of hexachlorophene. The use of this agent has declined with the discovery of its neurotoxic potential. Products available OTC for antisepsis and disinfection comprise agents containing mercury and iodine compounds, quaternary ammonium compounds, and chlorhexidine gluconate.

When mercury is used, it is in the organic form of merbromin or thiomerosal. Mercurochrome contains 2% merbromin, which is 24-27% mercury and 18-22% bromine. It is available as an aqueous solution and has very limited bacteriostatic activity. Thiomerosal (merthiolate) is comprised of 49% organically bound mercury. Although more effective than merbromin, thimerosal shares the disadvantage of poor tissue penetration and tissue fixation and therefore has limited bacteriostatic activity.[38] Thiomersal is available in solutions, tinctures (with a vehicle containing as much as 50% alcohol), and sprays.

The toxicity of mercury compounds is low with normal or recommended use. Ingestion of merbromin (mercurochrome) or thimerosal (merthiolate) causes nausea and vomiting. Serious poisoning is unlikely, due to the small volumes available in OTC formulations and the relatively low mercury content. Applications to large areas of abraded skin or frequent or prolonged use could potentially lead to absorption and mercury poisoning (mercurialism). This syndrome is characterized by acrodynia (pain and erythema of the palms and soles), polyneuritis, irritability, diaphoresis, and GI symptoms, especially anorexia.[39] The most common toxicity from application of these OTC preparations is sensitization, either from the mercury or thio radical (in merthiolate). This is evidenced by erythematous, papular, and vesicular lesions where applied.

Treatment depends on the extent of poisoning. Dermal reactions are managed supportively and resolve after discontinuation of use. More serious systemic poisonings may require chelation with British

Anti-Lewisite (BAL, dimercaprol), dimercaptosuccinic acid (DMSA), or D-penicillamine after initial stabilization.[40] This degree of poisoning is not expected with common misuse of OTC mercurials and requires consultation with a regional poison control center or medical toxicologist.

Iodine. Iodine is an effective and inexpensive germicidal, with low tissue toxicity. Iodine compounds include solutions, tinctures, and povidone-iodine, a water soluble complex. The solutions of iodine contain free-iodine and potassium iodide for increased solubility. The tinctures are composed of free-iodine, potassium iodide, sodium iodide for increased miscibility, and alcohol. Tinctures come in strengths of 2% and 7% iodine. Povidone-iodine complexes contain 9-12% iodine and are available as 5% creams; 10% gels; 4-10% ointment; 10% solutions in aerosols, perineal washes, saturated gauze pads, and swabs; and a 0.5% mouthwash.

Iodine's toxicity is related to its corrosive nature. Local inflammatory reactions can occur secondary to the application of strong tincture to wounds. Upon ingestion, symptoms of vomiting, hypotension, and circulatory collapse can occur, though death is rare following acute exposure.[41] Iodine is rapidly inactivated by the presence of food in the stomach, particularly starches. In the vomiting patient, iodine ingestion is suggested by a blue colored emesis (due to the conversion of iodine to iodide). Serious systemic symptoms have occurred after irrigation of wounds with iodine compounds.[42] These include hypothyroidism, renal failure, metabolic acidosis, leukopenia, and hemolysis.[43] Estimates of the mean lethal dose range from 2 to 4 grams of free iodine.[44]

Treatment is primarily symptomatic and supportive. Induction of emesis is, and lavage may be, contraindicated with ingestion of concentrated solutions, due to iodine's corrosive nature. Although iodine is adsorbed by activated charcoal, the presence of charcoal in the gut limits the endoscopist's ability to assess the extent of caustic injury.[45] Cornstarch (15 gm/ 500 mL water) is a better alternative for limiting gut iodine absorption. Starch converts iodine to iodide and then binds to the iodide salt. Further evaluation of the corrosive injury must be performed, including timely esophagoscopy.

Quaternary ammonium compounds are cationic surfactants comprised of mixtures of alkyldimethylbenzylammonium chlorides with alkyl chains varying in length from C_8H_{17} to $C_{18}H_{37}$. The aqueous solutions are used for cleansing of skin, mucous membranes, and wounds; irrigation of bladder, urethra, body cavity; and vaginal douching. Quaternary ammonium compounds are effective against bacteria, some viruses, protozoa, and fungi and have a sustained duration of action.[46] Composition of product is usually expressed in percentages of alkyl chain length, but this is less important than the concentration of the mixture. Concentrations of greater than 7% are potentially corrosive.

At lower concentrations, local irritation is the only adverse effect.[47] Dilute solutions used for irrigation and antisepsis can be more irritating to inflamed or abraded skin and sensitization has occurred.[48] Nausea, vomiting, and diarrhea are expected after trivial ingestions of even dilute solutions. Gastrointestinal tract burns have been reported with small volume ingestions of concentrated solutions.[49] CNS depression progressing to coma, seizures, and shock also have been reported after ingestion of concentrated solutions.[50] Serious corneal injury may occur with ocular exposure to concentrated solutions.[51]

Treatment depends on the concentration and circumstances of the exposure. Ingestion of small amounts of dilute solutions is managed with dilution and observation alone; more concentrated solutions are diluted and evaluated in a health care facility for potential GI tract burns. Emesis is contraindicated, as is gastric lavage, due to the caustic nature of this agent and the potential for pulmonary aspiration from rapid CNS deterioration and loss of protective airway reflexes. Treatment consists of dilution, supportive care, and hospital admission as needed for esophagoscopy.

References

1. Litovitz TL, Klein-Schwartz W, Caravati EM, et al. 1998 Annual report of the American Association of Poison Control Centers Toxic Exposure Surveillance System. *Am J Emerg Med* 1999;17: 435-487.
2. Lie RL, Vermeer BJ, Edelbroek PM. Severe lidocaine intoxication by cutaneous absorption. *J Am Acad Dermatol* 1990;23: 1026-1028.
3. Nelson JH. *A Druggists Handbook of Private Formulas,* 5th ed. Cleveland, OH; 1880:102-127.
4. *Drug Facts and Comparisons,* 54th ed. St. Louis, MO: Facts and Comparisons; 2000:1718.
5. Smith AG, Margolis G. Camphor poisoning. *Am J Pathol* 1954; 30:857.
6. Eickholt TH, Box RH. Toxicities of peppermint and pycnanthemum albescens oil, fam. *Labiateae*. *J Pharm Sci* 1965;54: 1071-1072.
7. Product Infomation: Zostrix, capsaicin. GenDerm Corporation, Lincolnshire, IL, 1997.
8. Tominack RL, Spycker DA. Capsicum and capsaicin—A review: Case report to the use of hot peppers in child abuse. *J Toxicol Clin Toxicol* 1987;25:591-601.
9. Chan TYK. Medicated oils and severe salicylate poisoning: Quantifying the risk based on methyl salicylate content and bottle size. *Vet Hum Tox* 1996;38:133-134.
10. MacCready RA. Methyl salicylate poisoning: A report of five cases. *N Engl J Med* 1943;228:155-156.
11. *Drug Facts and Comparisons,* 54th ed. St. Louis, MO: Facts and Comparisons; 2000:1663-1664.
12. Altman RS, Smith-Coggins R, Ampel LL. Local Anesthetics. *Ann Emerg Med* 1985;14:1209-1217.
13. Fisher AA. Allergic reactions to topical (surface) anesthetics with reference to the safety of tronothane (pramoxine hydrochloride). *Cutis* 1980;25:584-591.
14. Bun D, Doughty A. Methaemoglobinemia follows lignocaine. *Lancet* 1974;2:971.
15. Bowman S, Francillo R, Gibbons W. Correspondence: CNS toxicity after ingestion of topical lidocaine. *N Engl J Med* 1982; 306:426-427.
16. Rothstein P, Dornbusch J, Shaywitz BA. Prolonged seizures associated with the use of viscous lidocaine. *J Pediatr* 1982;101:461-463.
17. Sakai R, Lattin J. Lidocaine ingestion. *Am J Dis Child* 1980; 134:323.
18. Olson ML, McEvoy GK. Methemoglobinemia induced by local anesthetics. *Am J Hosp Pharm* 1981;38:89-93.
19. Rodriguez LF, Smolik LM, Zbehlik AJ. Benzocaine-induced methemoglobinemia: Report of a severe reaction and review of the literature. *Ann Pharmacother* 1994;28:643-649.
20. Eldadah M, Fitzgerald M. Methemoglobinemia due to skin application of benzocaine. *Clin Pediatr* 1993;32:687-688.
21. Dayan P, Litovitz TL, Crouch BI, et al. Fatal accidental dibucaine poisoning in children. *Ann Emerg Med* 1996;28:442-445.

22. Horio T. Photosensitivity reaction to dibucaine: Case report and experimental induction. *Arch Dermatol* 1979;115:986-987.
23. Lee AY. Allergic contact dermatitis from dibucaine in Proctosedyl ointment with cross-sensitivity. *Contact Dermatitis* 1998;39:261.
24. Cornell RC, Stoughton RB. The use of topical steroids in psoriasis. *Dermatol Clin* 1984;2:397-409.
25. Coppack RW, Mostrom MS, Lillie LE. The toxicology of detergents, bleaches, antiseptics, and disinfectants in small animals. *Vet Hum Tox* 1988;30:463-473.
26. Lin AN, Reimer RJ, Carter DM. Sulfur revisited. *J Am Acad Dermatol* 1988;18:553-558.
27. Jackson EM. Editorial: Benzoyl peroxide: An old dog with new problems. *J Toxicol Cutan Ocul Toxicol* 1986;5:161-163.
28. Anonymous. Position statement: Gastric lavage (cathartics, ipecec syrup, single-dose activated charcoal). American Academy of Clinical Toxicology/European Association of Poison Centres and Clinical Toxicologists. *Clin Toxicol* 1997; 35:711-719.
29. Tomlinson G, Helfael M, Wiedermann BL, et al. Diphenhydramine toxicity mimicking Varicella encephalitis. *Ped Infect Dis J* 1987; 6:220-221.
30. Goetz CM, Lopez G, Dean BS, et al. Accidental childhood death from diphenhydramine overdosage. *Am J Emerg Med* 1990;8: 321-322.
31. Culver CA, Malina JJ, Talbert RL. Probable anaphylactoid reaction to a pyrethrin pediculocide shampoo. *Clin Pharm* 1988;7: 846-849.
32. Wax PM, Hoffman RS. Fatality associated with inhalation of a pyrethrin shampoo. *Clin Toxicol* 1994;32:457-460.
33. He F, Wang S, Liu L, et al. Clinical manifestations and diagnosis of acute pyrethroid poisoning. *Arch Toxicol* 1989;63:54-58.
34. Le Quesne PM, Maxwell UC, Butterworth ST. Transient facial sensory symptoms following exposure to synthetic pyrethroids: A clinical and electrophysiological assessment. *Neurotoxicol* 1980;2:1-11.
35. He F. Synthetic pyrethroids. *Toxicol* 1994;91:43-49.
36. Grant WM, ed. *Toxicology of the Eye*, 4th ed. Springfield, IL; Thomas: 1993:39.
37. Lisi P. Sensitization risk of pyrethroid insecticides. *Contact Dermatitis* 1992;26:349-350.
38. Harvey SC. Antiseptics and disinfectants; fungicides and ectoparasiticides. In: Gilman AG, Goodman L, Gilman A, eds. *The Pharmacological Basis of Therapeutics*. 6th ed. New York: Macmillan; 1980:976.
39. Warkany J, Husband DM. Acrodynia and mercury. *J Pediatr* 1953; 42:365.
40. Fournier L, Thomas G, Garnier R, et al. 2,3-dimercaptosuccunic acid acid treatment of heavy metal poisoning in humans. *Med Toxicol* 1988;3:499-504.
41. Kurt TL, Morgan ML, Hnilica V, et al. Fatal iatrogenic iodine toxicity in a nine-week-old infant. *Clin Toxicol* 1996;34:231-234.
42. Campistol JM, Abad C, Nogue C, et al. Acute renal failure in a patient treated by continuous povidone-iodine mediastinal irrigation. *J Cardiovasc Surg* 1988;29:410-412.
43. Lavelle KJ, Doedens DJ, Kleit SA, et al. Iodine absorbtion in burn patients treated topically with povidone-iodine. *Clin Pharmacol Ther* 1975;17:355-372.
44. Therapeutics Index. In: Gosselin RE, Smith RP, Hodge HC, eds. *Clinical Toxicology of Commercial Products*. 5th ed. Baltimore: Williams and Wilkins; 1984:213-214.
45. Anonymous. Position statement: Single dose activated charcoal. American Academy of Clinical Toxicology; European Association of Poison Centres and Clinical Toxicologists. *Clin Toxicol* 1997;35:721-736.
46. Harvey SC. Antiseptics and disinfectants; fungicides and ectoparasiticides. In: Gilman AG, Goodman L, Gilman A, eds. *The Pharmacological Basis of Therapeutics*. 6th ed. New York: Macmillan; 1980:978-979.
47. Coulston F, Drobeck HF, Mielens ZE, et al. Toxicology of benzalkalonium chloride given orally in milk or water to rats and dogs. *Toxicol Appl Pharmacol* 1961;3:584-594.
48. Bernstein JA, Stauder T, Bernstein DI, et al. A combined respiratory and cutaneous hypersensitivity syndrome induced by work exposure to quaternary amines. *J Allergy Clin Immunol* 1994; 94:257-259.
49. Wilson JT, Burr IA. Benzalkalonium chloride poisoning in infant twins. *Am J Dis Child* 1975;129:1209-1209.
50. Van Berkel M, De Wolff FA. Survival after acute benzalkalonium chloride poisoning. *Human Toxicol* 1988;7:191-193.
51. Grant WM, ed. *Toxicology of the Eye*, 4th ed. Springfield, IL; Thomas: 1993:774.

Over-the-Counter Medications: Toxic Effects and Adverse Reactions: Part II

Richard Y. Wang, DO, FACEP, FACMT
Daren D. Girard, MD

Medications available from over-the-counter (OTC) sources have the capacity to produce adverse reactions, serious side effects, and problematic drug-drug and drug-disease interactions. Examples of OTC formulations of prescription drugs that have the potential to cause such complications include cimetidine, non-steroidal anti-inflammatory drugs (NSAIDs), and antihistamines.

The first part of this two-part series focused on formulations delivered topically and by mucosal routes of administration. This, the second and final part of the series, focuses on agents that are consumed orally and have the potential to cause serious toxicity, especially if taken inappropriately by the patient.

Oral Topical Products

Toothpastes. Toothpastes and gels contain fluoride, which is added for dental caries protection. Studies conducted in the 1950s showed that fluoride was beneficial to dental health and the variable availability of fluoridated water prompted its addition to dentifrices.

Fluoride usually is present in dentifrices as a salt, including sodium fluoride, stannous fluoride, and sodium monofluorophosphate. The maximum amount of fluoride allowed in a tube of toothpaste is 260 mg.[1] Generally, estimates of elemental fluoride concentration in toothpastes and gels is a maximum of 1 mg/g.[2] The dose is calculated based on the amount of elemental fluoride present, regardless of the salt form. Symptoms have occurred with ingestion of 3-5 mg/kg. An acute toxic exposure is estimated to be between 5 mg and 10 mg of elemental fluoride/kg—a dose that is certainly possible in the case of toothpaste ingestion by a small child.[3]

Trivial ingestions of mouthful amounts are unlikely to cause symptoms, but calculations of potential fluoride dose should be done for ingestions of larger amounts. If the specific fluoride salt concentration is unknown, then the elemental fluoride concentration (1 mg/g) may be used to determine exposure risks. Acute ingestion commonly causes gastrointestinal (GI) upset, with nausea and vomiting; the response is thought to be caused by the conversion of fluoride to hydrofluoric acid in the acidic environment of the stomach.[4] Diarrhea also is a possible reaction, due to both the fluoride content and the vehicle (which commonly uses sorbitol as a sweetener to improve palatability). The more serious symptoms seen with significant fluoride ingestion are hypocalcemia and hyperkalemia, with resultant tetanic spasms and dysrhythmias.[5,6] In severe poisoning, dysrhythmias and hypotension can develop, progressing to cardiac or respiratory failure.[2] This is unlikely with over-the-counter (OTC) dentifrices.

Management of ingestion of fluoride-containing toothcare products depends on the estimated dose ingested. Asymptomatic patients who have ingested fewer than 8 mg/kg are managed with dilution, preferably with milk (calcium binds the fluoride ion).[7] Observation for development of GI symptoms and disposition after

Table 1. Incidence of OTC Exposures in 1998[24]

OVER-THE-COUNTER (OTC) PREPARATION	NUMBER OF EXPOSURES	NUMBER OF MORBIDITIES	NUMBER OF MORTALITIES
Analgesics (acetaminophen, NSAIDs, salycilates)	133,899	5,383	107
Cosmetics and personal care products	210,224	33,769	3
Cough and cold formulations (antihistamines, decongestants)	118,280	23,050	16
Topicals (dermal, nasal, ocular, oral, rectal, vaginal)	83,455	9,702	1
Vitamins and iron supplements	53,657	4,237	1
Gastrointestinal formulations (antacids, antidiarrheals, laxatives)	45,696	4,355	6

4-6 hours are usually sufficient for patient treatment.[8] Development of GI symptoms or the potential ingestion of greater than 8 mg/kg requires determination of baseline serum electrolyte and calcium levels and the administration of calcium- and magnesium-containing antacids after initial dilution.

Mouthwashes and Gargles. Mouthwashes and gargles are a routine part of oral hygiene. These formulations are generally composed of water, ethanol, and flavoring agents, which may include sorbitol, saccharin, and essential oils. The germicidal activity of these products is primarily due to the ethanol content, which may be as high as 30%, although other agents with mild antibacterial activity may be present in low concentrations (e.g., cetylpyridinium).

Mouthwashes are made to have an agreeable taste; therefore, ingestion by unassuming children is a special concern because ethanol is particularly toxic in this age group.[9] Acute ingestion can produce coma, respiratory and cardiac depression, hypothermia, hypotension, and hypoglycemia. Mouthful or greater ingestions of the products containing higher concentrations of ethanol have the potential to produce clinically significant serum ethanol levels.[10] Due to rapid absorption, peak levels are reached between 20 minutes and 60 minutes after ingestion; the presence of food delays absorption.[11] Children presenting to the emergency department (ED) may be hypoglycemic, even with serum ethanol levels as low as 20-30 mg/dL; fatal complications have been seen with concentrations as low as 50 mg/dL.[10] Often, the initial clinical presentation is marked sleepiness with ataxia. This can progress to coma, respiratory depression, and seizures. Blood glucose should be determined immediately, with administration of an intravenous dextrose bolus in symptomatic patients. Supportive care is essential.

Antiseptics. The mild antiseptics employed in OTC lozenges, sprays, and gargles are cetylpyridinium, hexylresorcinol, thymol, and eucalyptol. Cetylpyridinium is a cationic detergent/surfactant (one of the quaternary ammonium compounds discussed previously in Part I). Used in low concentrations of 0.05-0.45%, ingestion of even large amounts would be expected to cause only nausea and vomiting. Phenol and the phenolic derivative hexylresorcinol are found in sprays and lozenges. Applied topically, they have local anesthetic effects—hence their use in oral sprays and lozenges. The concentrations in sprays range from 0.3% to 1.4%, levels that are too low to have a caustic effect on tissues. Hypersensitivity is the only toxicity of the phenols and their derivatives at these concentrations.[12] Thymol is another phenolic compound often used in lozenges and mouthwashes. It is used in such low concentrations (usually unspecified), that it is ineffective as a therapeutic agent and is non-toxic. Eucalyptol is derived from oil of eucalyptus, and also is used in very low, non-toxic concentrations.

Anesthetic Agents. Oral anesthetic agents are used for their analgesic and mild antiseptic properties. They are available in gels and liquids and are used for teething, denture/dental pain, and minor ulcers and irritations of the buccal mucosa. Lozenges and troches are used for mild cases of pharyngitis, as are sprays and gargles.

OTC anesthetics include benzocaine (see section on local anesthetics in Part I of this two-part series) and dyclonine. The counterirritants, menthol, camphor, and phenol, also may be found in low concentrations in OTC anesthetics. These agents are commonly used in a population of teething-age children, and misuse or accidental poisoning is a possibility. Dyclonine is a synthetic anesthetic, with an onset and a duration of action similar to that of procaine.[12] It is readily absorbed into mucus membranes, and has a low order of toxicity. Dyclonine is available OTC in lozenge form, with a maximum adult dose of 3 mg/lozenge, and as a 0.1% spray.[13] Higher concentration sprays (0.5% and 1%) are used to provide relief from mouth ulcers secondary to chemotherapy.[14] These higher concentration products are not available OTC.

The primary toxicity of OTC dyclonine is hypersensitivity, with isolated case reports of contact dermatitis.[15] The more concentrated prescription products have produced adverse effects in the cardiovascular and central nervous systems. These include hypotension, hypertension, bradycardia, and cardiac arrest, as well as variable central nervous system (CNS) effects.[14] This degree of toxicity is unlikely given the concentrations found in these OTC products, but is a possibility that clinicians should anticipate in cases of excessive use.

Vaginal and Rectal Preparations

Vaginal products are available OTC to treat vaginal candidiasis (moniliasis). These are limited to the imidazole antifungals: clotrimazole, miconazole, and butoconazole. The antifungals terconazole, tioconazole nitrate, and nystatin (a polyene antibiotic) are still available by prescription only. These products are formulated as creams, suppositories, and vaginal tablets. The tablets use lactose as an excipient and the suppositories use hydrogenated vegetable oil. All have a very low order of toxicity. The only adverse effect that has been reported is hypersensitivity.[16] There have been no reports of oral toxicity.

Other OTC vaginal products include douches, spermicides, vaginal lubricants, and miscellaneous items. Vaginal douches are used for general cleaning and removal of secretions, deodorizing, and relief of pruritis. They reflect a combination of ingredients, including phenol, methyl salicylate, menthol, eucalyptol, thymol, cetylpyridinium, surfactants, and pH-altering agents. All of these components are present in essentially non-toxic concentrations. The only potentially toxic products are concentrated povidone-iodine douches. These come in concentrations as high as 12% and are designed to be diluted prior to use to a final concentration of 0.3%. Povidone-iodine is absorbed from the vaginal tissue and, therefore, may affect thyroid function with continued or prolonged use.[17] The toxicity of povidone-iodine was discussed in Part I.

Topical spermicides are used to prevent conception. Nonoxynol-9 is the only approved spermicide. It is available in foams, suppositories, gels, jellies, and a vaginal film. Concentrations used are: 8-12% in the foams, 3-5% in the gels and jellies, a 28% concentration in the film , and 100-150 mg strengths in suppositories. The only potential toxicity of nonoxynol-9 is hypersensitivity.

Miscellaneous vaginal products are used as moisturizers, lubricants, and antipruritics. Some products contain benzocaine or counterirritants, such as resorcinol. They are available in creams, gels, and suppositories. The products containing benzocaine (some in concentrations as high as 20%) have some potential for toxicity. All of the moisturizers and lubricants are non-toxic, with essentially water soluble or water-miscible ingredients such as glycerine, hydroxyethylcellulose, or propylene glycol.

Anorectal combination products are used primarily for relief of pruritis and irritation secondary to hemorrhoids. They contain topical anesthetics such as benzocaine and pramoxine, counterirritants such as camphor, or astringents such as zinc oxide and witch hazel. None of these OTC products contain steroids. Other ingredients in these preparations are emollients, mild antiseptics (e.g., benzalkalonium chloride, phenylmercuric nitrate), local vasoconstrictors (e.g., ephedrine, phenylephrine), or wound healing agents (e.g., peru balsam, yeast-cell extract).[18] The local anesthetic products are available in the forms of creams, foams, and ointments. The benzocaine and pramoxine concentrations may be as high as 20% and 1%, respectively. Although toxicity has not been described, the potential exists if the products containing local anesthetics are misused or ingested, since these products are highly concentrated.[18] All other products are more likely to produce symptoms relative to the vehicle rather than the active ingredients.

Oral and Over-the-Counter Preparations

Analgesic Preparations. Analgesic preparations available for self-treatment include acetaminophen, aspirin, and nonsteroidal anti-inflammatory drugs (NSAIDs). Because of their routine use for fever and pain control, these agents are readily accessible to many patients. Wide availability has created a high rate of toxic exposure to these drugs. *(Please see Table 1.)* This discussion will focus on the NSAIDs.[19,20]

The number of NSAIDs available as OTC formulations has increased over recent years and includes: ibuprofen in 100 mg and 200 mg tablets, and 100 mg/5 mL suspension; naproxen in 200 mg tablets; and ketoprofen in 12.5 mg tablets. Among these agents, exposure to ibuprofen has been the most extensively studied. Ibuprofen ingestions of fewer than 100 mg/kg are unlikely to result in clinical symptoms.[21] However, the onset of symptoms in patients with significant ibuprofen exposures occurs within four hours of ingestion. In the majority of these patients, toxicity is mild and consists of GI distress and CNS depression. Significant toxicity is uncommon and is manifested by seizures, metabolic acidemia, and renal insufficiency.[22] Patients with manifestations of mild toxicity can be managed in the ED with intravenous fluid hydration, antiemetics, and repeat serum electrolytes after four hours. Standard supportive treatment is required for more serious symptoms. Serum ibuprofen concentrations lack clinical correlation and are not necessary to determine toxicity.[23]

Despite their well-documented renal and GI side effects, NSAIDs are among the most widely prescribed medications and OTC agents used for pain relief. GI toxicities represent some of the most serious side effects of this drug class, and common complications include gastric mucosal ulceration, hemorrhage, or perforation. The analgesic and anti-inflammatory mechanism of action of NSAIDs has been attributed to their capacity for inhibiting the enzyme cyclooxygenase (COX). Recently, two isoforms of cyclooxygenase have been identified. COX-1 is believed to have a gastroprotective effect, while COX-2 specific inhibition is responsible for the production of pro-inflammatory mediators.

Pharmacological differences among NSAIDs are playing an increasingly important role in drug selection, and clinicians must be aware of the possible advantages and disadvantages of drugs that belong to this large and potentially problematic therapeutic class. For example, generally speaking, older NSAIDs, such as ibuprofen and ketoprofen, are relatively more potent inhibitors of COX-1 than COX-2, whereas newer NSAIDs, such as nabumatone and etodolac, have more balanced inhibition. A new and recently approved class of selective COX-2 inhibitors (represented by celecoxib [Celebrex] and rofecoxib [Vioxx]) offer new opportunities for high-benefit/low-risk therapy in appropriately selected and risk-stratified patients who would have previously required conventional NSAID therapy.

It is estimated that NSAIDs are taken by approximately 17 million Americans every day.[24] Overall, NSAIDs account for about 4.5% of all prescriptions written in the United States and approximately 22-31% of prescriptions written in the outpatient setting and/or ED.[25] Worldwide, it has been estimated that 100 million prescriptions are written annually, accounting for more than $2 billion in sales (excluding OTC purchases). These usage patterns reflect a large segment of the population suffering from such conditions as osteoarthritis (OA) and rheumatoid arthritis (RA), for whom NSAIDs represent initial therapy for control of inflammation and relief of pain and stiffness. Not surprisingly, more than 50% of NSAID prescriptions are written for individuals older than 60 years of age for the management of OA.

As a therapeutic class, NSAIDs exhibit analgesic, anti-inflammatory, antipyretic, and platelet inhibitory properties.[24] Generally speaking, analgesic effects are obtained at lower doses than those required for anti-inflammatory activity. Although there is some controversy surrounding the issues of relative effectiveness, most experts agree—and clinical experience supports the observation—that when prescribed at equipotent doses, NSAIDs are purported to show similar clinical efficacy. Clinical responses, however, may vary among individuals.

Unfortunately, complications associated with NSAID use in the United States result in approximately 100,000 hospitalizations a year at a cost of $4 billion; moreover, it is estimated that NSAIDs are directly linked to about 10,000-20,000 deaths each year. Among the elderly alone, an estimated 41,000 hospitalizations and 3300 deaths

Table 2. Oral OTC Preparations and Their Ingredients

OTC PREPARATION	ACTIVE AGENTS
Antacids	Aluminum salts, calcium carbonate, magnesium hydroxide, sodium bicarbonate
Antidiarrheals	Bismuth subsalicylate, loperamide
Antihistamines	
Histamine (H1) receptor	Brompheniramine, chlorpheniramine, cyproheptidine, diphenhydramine, doxylamine, phenindamine, pheniramine
Histamine (H2) receptor	Cimetidine, famotidine, ranitidine
Antispamodics	Attapulgite (e.g., Donnagel), Kaolin/pectin
Decongestants	Ephedrine, phenylephrine, phenylpropanolamine, pseudoephedrine
Iron salts	Elemental iron
Laxatives (e.g., saline, bulk, stool softener, stimulants)	Lactulose, phenophtalein, magnesium salts, mineral oil
Nonsteroidal anti-inflammatory agents	Ibuprofen, ketoprofen, naproxen
Vitamins	A, B complex, C, D, E, K

annually are thought to be secondary to NSAID therapy.[26] Studies comparing diclofenac, naproxen, and acetaminophen showed that NSAID use in the elderly increased GI complications three- to five-fold as compared with non-NSAID use.

As the geriatric population has grown, the incidence of OA has increased. As might be expected, elderly patients with OA and RA have been identified as being at high risk for NSAID toxicity. GI intolerance has been reported in up to 50% of patients on long-term NSAIDs. Among long-term users of NSAIDs, endoscopic ulcers have a reported incidence of 15-25% per year, with an estimated complication rate of 1-2%. Overall, the incidence rate of symptomatic ulcers and/or ulcer complications has been reported to be in the range of 2% to 4%, with similar rates observed in patients with RA and OA.

Although GI side effects and complications occur with the greatest frequency, adverse renal and/or cardiovascular effects of NSAIDs and COX-2 inhibitors also have been well-recognized and play an equally important role in drug selection and identifying risk management upgrades for specific patient subgroups. A prudent and rational selection process among NSAIDs and COX-2 specific inhibitors requires a comparative, evidence-based evaluation of drug efficacy as well as a comparative analysis of the full range of safety end points, including GI, cardiovascular, and renal organ systems.

Cough and Cold Preparations

Antihistamines. Antihistamines block one of the two major histamine receptor types (H1 or H2), which in turn determines their clinical use. H1-receptor antagonists are used alone or in combination with other agents for the suppression of motion sickness and vertigo, sedation, and the treatment of hypersensitivity reactions and cold symptoms.[27] In 1998, nearly 90% of exposures to antihistamines were to H1-receptor antagonists.[24] Diphenhydramine (DPH) was involved in 25,000 exposures and 16 deaths. Some of the other H1-receptor antagonists available OTC include brompheniramine, chlorpheniramine, cyproheptadine, doxylamine. *(Please see Table 2.)*

In addition to relief of allergic symptoms, antihistamines have other important pharmacologic properties that are variably manifested at therapeutic and toxic concentrations. Central H1-receptor antagonism causes both CNS stimulation and depression. Decreased alertness and sedation are common, but restlessness, agitation, insomnia, and seizures occur in some. These excitatory effects are more likely to occur in children and in patients with large exposures.[27] Many H1-receptor antagonists have anticholinergic effects and cardiac membrane stabilizing activity, both of which bear toxicity in overdose. Second-generation, or non-sedating, H1-receptor blockers have less CNS activity, but have been associated with serious cardiac dysrrhythmias, including torsades des pointes.[28] These preparations are available only by prescription.

Acute overdose of DPH is most commonly associated with some degree of impaired consciousness, including coma.[29] Psychomotor agitation, hallucinations, and seizures also can occur.[30] Anticholinergic signs can be prominent and include: impaired vision, dry mouth, tachycardia, hypertension, decreased GI motility, and urinary retention. Increased heart rate, significant QTc prolongation, and wide-complex tachycardia are documented cardiac complications of DPH overdose.[27,31,32] Death has been the result of cardiovascular collapse and respiratory failure.[31,33] In the pregnant patient, DPH poisoning may produce uterine contractions by an oxytocin-like effect.[34]

Laboratory evaluation of antihistamine overdose includes a 12-lead ECG with continuous monitoring as needed. Because aspirin, acetaminophen, and ethanol are frequently combined with antihistamines in OTC preparations, co-ingestions of these compounds should be assessed. Treatment is generally supportive, with initial efforts focused on stabilization of vital signs. Gastric lavage is recommended for the patient presenting within an hour of the ingestion or with significant clinical toxicity and an unknown time of ingestion. Activated charcoal may be useful. Attempts to control seizures begin with benzodiazepines. Wide complex tachycardia is treated with serum alkalinization by intravenous sodium bicarbonate.[32] Physostigmine, an anticholinesterase inhibitor, is considered only in cases of significant central anticholinergic symptoms (e.g., psychomotor agitation and seizures refractory to standard therapies). This treatment should be avoided if co-ingestion of tricyclic antidepressants is suspected or if cardiac conduction abnormalities are observed.

Antitussives. The antitussive dextromethorphan is found in a number of cough and cold preparations, cough drops, and throat lozenges. Dextromethorphan is the opposite stereoisomer of codeine. Unlike codeine, it is an effective cough suppressant and has few analgesic or addictive properties.[35] The dextromethorphan concentrations in OTC products vary, with the usual adult dose being 10-30 mg every 4-6 hours. This agent is generally safe, but children taking large doses may experience toxicity. The most common toxic effect is CNS depression, manifesting as drowsiness, stupor, and coma.[36] Respiratory depression, which can be fatal, also is seen in overdose.[36-38] These symptoms are reversed by the administration of naloxone.[36]

If dextromethorphan is co-administered with monoamine oxidase inhibitors or serotonin-reuptake inhibitors, such as fluoxetine and paroxetine, a serious interaction, known as the serotonin syndrome, can occur. This syndrome is characterized by hypertension, hyperthermia, muscular rigidity, and mental status changes.[39-41] Symptoms can rapidly progress to include seizures, cardiovascular collapse, and death. Treatment is generally supportive and includes controlling hypertension with intravenous nitroprusside or nitroglycerin, intravenous fluids and vasopressors for hypotension, benzodiazepines for myoclonous and seizures, and aggressive cooling to enhance evaporative heat loss.

Decongestants. Decongestants are widely available in nonprescription cough and cold preparations. Their decongestant effect is secondary to sympathomimetic agents that are supplied as either oral or topical (ocular, nasal) formulations. Common oral agents are ephedrine, psuedoephedrine, phenylephrine, and phenylpropanolamine (PPA), which recently was removed from the market. These agents produce arteriolar vasoconstriction by stimulation of the alpha-adrenergic system. Vasoconstriction of engorged nasal mucosa leads to relief of congestion. Combined with antihistamines, analagesics, and antitussives, these drugs help to alleviate the symptoms of the common cold. Topical decongestants in the form of ophthalmic and nasal solutions are used for the treatment of sinusitis, hayfever, colds, and ocular irritations.[42] The imidazoline compounds found in these topical preparations cause local vasoconstriction by their action on alpha-adrenergic receptors. These compounds, which are structurally related to clonidine, include tetrahydrozoline, naphazoline, oxymetazoline, and xylometazoline.

The toxic effects of this group are related to excessive adrenergic stimulation, with hypertension being the most serious result. Co-ingested antihistamines can potentiate hypertension by preventing reflex reduction of heart rate.[43] Three times the single therapeutic dose of PPA (85 mg in an adult) can increase the diastolic blood pressure to greater than 100 mmHg.[44] With larger exposures (e.g., overdose) hypertensive emergencies can ensue.[43] Severe headache, mental status changes, seizures, intracranial hemorrhage, myocardial infarction, and death are all possible complications.[45-47] Evaluation of the hypertensive patient includes measurement of cardiac isoenzymes and an ECG. A computer tomography scan of the brain may be required to evaluate for intracranial hemorrhage. GI decontamination is accomplished with oral activated charcoal. Treatment is directed at controlling elevated blood pressure. Intravenous nitroprusside, phentolamine, or labetalol may be used for this purpose.[46]

Table 3. Serum Magnesium Levels and Clinical Manifestations of Toxicity

SERUM MAGNESIUM LEVEL (mEq/L)	CLINICAL MANIFESTATIONS
4	Depression of deep tendon reflexes
4-7	CNS depression, bradycardia, hypotension, nausea, vomiting, diarrhea, skin flushing
8-10	Paralysis, respiratory depression
15	Asystole

The pediatric population is at greatest risk for imidazole decongestant toxicity. A retrospective review of tetrahydrozoline exposures showed that 89% involved children younger than 2 years of age.[48] Most of these cases resulted from unintentional oral ingestions of either ophthalmic or nasal solutions. The ingestion of 2.5 mL of 0.05% tetrahydrozoline eyedrops can produce serious toxicity in toddlers, including miosis, bradycardia, hypotension or hypertension, agitation, and coma. An adult who ingested 30 mL of 0.05% tetrahydrozoline developed chest pain, bradycardia, and mental status changes.[49]

The systemic toxicity of imidazole decongestants appears to be related to stimulation of central alpha2 adrenergic-receptors. Stimulation of these receptors results in a decreased output from central vasomotor centers and a reduction in heart rate and blood pressure.[42,49-51] CNS depression is manifested by lethargy and obtundation, but fluctuations of consciousness, such as stupor alternating with psychomotor agitation, have been observed.[50] Respiratory depression also is a common finding. Due to the rapid gut absorption of these liquid preparations upon ingestion, GI decontamination is not recommended. Treatment is otherwise supportive.

Gastrointestinal Agents

Antacids. Antacids are salts (e.g., magnesium hydroxide, aluminum hydroxide, aluminum phosphate, calcium carbonate, and sodium bicarbonate) that react with gastric acid to increase the pH in the stomach and the duodenal bulb. Current uses include the treatment of gastritis, gastroesophageal reflux, peptic ulcer disease, hyperphosphatemia, calcium deficiency states, and hypomagnesemia. Oral doses are 15-30 mL four times a day in adults, and 0.5-5 mL four times a day in children.

Acute ingestion of antacids rarely contributes to toxicity because of their limited gut absorption, although calcium carbonate and sodium bicarbonate require some monitoring.[52] The long-term administration of these agents or excessively large exposures can result in GI disorders and electrolyte abnormalities, which commonly manifest as cardiovascular and CNS disturbances. GI decontamination is not necessary unless co-ingestants are involved. Serum electrolytes, blood pH, serum aluminum, calcium, and magnesium should be monitored in patients with renal insufficiency.

Most reported cases of hypermagnesemia occur in patients with renal insufficiency who use magnesium-containing antacids. Toxicity can occur within one week of standard use, especially in patients with a creatinine clearance of less than 10-30 mL/min.[53] Aside from patients with renal insufficiency, elderly patients also are at risk for increased serum magnesium toxicity. Increased serum magnesium

Table 4. Potentiated Drug Effects When Used with Cimetidine[28]

DRUG	CLINICAL MANIFESTATIONS
Benzodiazepine (alprazolam, chlordiazepoxide, clonazepam, clorazepate, diazepam, flurazepam)	Sedation, impaired psychomotor function and cognition
Beta adrenergic antagonists (labetolol, metoprolol, propanolol)	Hypotension, bradycardia (possible)
Calcium channel blockers (diltiazem, nifedipine)	Hypotension, tachycardia, bradycardia
Carbamazepine	Ataxia, nystagmus, diplopia, headache, vomiting, seizures, coma
Phenytoin	Ataxia, nystagmus, tremor
Theophylline	Tachycardia, nausea, vomiting
Tricyclic antidepressants	Anticholinergic syndrome
Warfarin	Hypoprothrombinemia

impairs nerve conduction and depresses peripheral neuromuscular function to cause muscle weakness and paralysis.[54] The manifestations of hypermagnesemia correlate with serum concentrations and include neuromuscular paralysis, respiratory failure, bradycardia, and hypotension. *(Please see Table 3.)* The initial clinical finding in hypermagnesemia is diminished deep tendon reflexes, which occurs at a serum magnesium level of 4 mEq/L.[55] Respiratory depression can be seen at 10 mEq/L in adults and at lower concentrations in infants.[56] Laboratory findings associated with hypermagnesemia include decreased anion gap, hypocalcemia, and prolonged QT interval.[57]

Treatment of hypermagnesemia begins with stabilization of the airway and mechanical ventilation as needed. Cardiac monitoring is needed when the serum magnesium concentration is greater than 5 mEq/L. Patients without life-threatening symptoms and normal renal function can be managed with saline loading and furosemide-induced diuresis to promote renal clearance of magnesium. Calcium infusion (0.2-0.5 mL/kg of 10% calcium gluconate up to 10 mL over 10 minutes) displaces magnesium from cell membranes and antagonizes respiratory depression. Hemodialysis is indicated for symptomatic hypermagnesemia with either diminished renal clearance, pulmonary edema, failure of forced diuresis, or resistant cardiotoxicity.

Aluminum toxicity is observed in patients with decreased renal clearance and chronic use of aluminum salt antacids.[58,59] The manifestations are neurologic and include myoclonus, encephalopathy, and seizures.[60] Additionally, constipation, bowel obstruction, bezoar formation, and electrolyte abnormalities, such as hypocalcemia and hypophosphatemia, can occur with the chronic use of aluminum salts.[61-64] Along with phosphate loss, there is the potential for development of osteomalacia and osteoporosis. This occurs because aluminum binds to phosphate in the gut, which in turn prevents phosphate absorption.[65] Phosphate depletion leads to bone demineralization. Patients who use aluminum hydroxide on a regular basis and complain of weakness or bone pain should be evaluated for calcium and phosphate depletion. In addition, these patients should have directed skeletal radiographs to look for osteomalacia and pathologic fractures.[66] Aluminum toxicity is treated with chelation therapy and hemodialysis.[67]

Metabolic alkalosis can result from the long-term use of antacids containing sodium bicarbonate or calcium carbonate.[68] This state is secondary to nephrocalcinosis, which causes renal insufficiency and diminished bicarbonate ion excretion.[69] Patients may present with hypotension due to dehydration from GI fluid losses, a compensatory hypoventilatory response to the alkalemia, and myalgia and muscle spasms from hypokalemia and hypocalcemia. Neurologic manifestations include seizures, increased deep tendon reflexes, and mental status changes. Severe alkalemia (i.e., pH > 7.60) can cause serious cardiac dysrhythmias.[69] Electrolyte disorders associated with metabolic alkalosis include hypochloremia, hypocalcemia, and hypokalemia. Increased sodium load from sodium bicarbonate can exacerbate congestive heart failure.[70] In addition, hypercalcemia can be seen with calcium carbonate use and initially is treated with saline diuresis.[71]

When the blood pH is greater than 7.50, treatment is advised. Hypovolemic patients should be rehydrated with intravenous normal saline containing potassium chloride. This promotes renal excretion of bicarbonate and the retention of chloride. When the patient is euvolemic, intravenous fluid therapy is reduced and hypokalemia is corrected. Severe alkalemia (i.e., > 7.60) can be corrected by endotracheal intubation with careful hypoventilation, provided that adequate oxygenation is maintained. Ammonium chloride may be administered intravenously as an acidifying agent (100-200 mEq of ammonium chloride may be administered in 500-1000 mL normal saline (NS) and infused at a rate below 5 mL/min). In renal failure patients, hemodialysis may be needed to remove bicarbonate ions.

The "milk alkali" syndrome is associated with the chronic use of antacids (e.g., sodium bicarbonate or calcium carbonate) and milk.[72] The manifestations include hypercalcemia, nausea, vomiting, anorexia, reduced parathyroid hormone secretion, precipitation of calcium in the kidneys leading to renal insufficiency, and metabolic alkalosis. Treatment is primarily supportive. Further antacid and calcium use must be discontinued and other causes of hypercalcemia evaluated.

H2-receptor antagonists also are used in the treatment of peptic ulcer disease and gastroesophageal reflux disease. These agents decrease the production of gastric acid by their antagonism of H2-receptors. OTC formulations include cimetidine, famotidine, and ranitidine. H2-receptor antagonists, particularly cimetidine, cause adverse effects by interfering with the metabolism of other potentially dangerous drugs. Cimetidine inhibits hepatic metabolism by its interaction with cytochrome P-450 and may thereby increase certain drug concentrations.[73] *(Please see Table 4.)* In addition, H2-receptor antagonists have been implicated in producing acute confusional states, especially in the elderly.[74]

Antidiarrheals. Loperamide is a meperidine analogue, and it is available OTC as Imodium. Opioid toxicity is a concern in large exposures and can be observed at a dose of 0.1-0.2 mg/kg. Other

manifestations include bradycardia, nausea, and vomiting. Children are more susceptible to the drug's effects, and deaths have been reported.[75] Ingestions of up to 0.4 mg/kg in children older than 6 months of age can be safely monitored at home.[76] Peak serum levels occur within four hours of ingestion, and the administration of activated charcoal can limit GI drug absorption. Naloxone is effective in reversing the manifestations of opioid toxicity from loperamide.[77,78]

Bismuth salts are used medicinally for GI disorders (diarrhea, dyspepsia, ulcerogenic therapy) and as a skin protectant. They work as antidiarrheal agents due to their antimicrobial and anitsecretory properties.[79] They are clinically differentiated by their solubility.[80] The inorganic salts and subsalt forms (e.g., bismuth subsalicylate) are water insoluble and have minor gut absorption.[81] The dermal preparations are generally non-soluble (e.g., bismuth subgallate) and are less concerning from a toxicological point of view.

The salicylate component of bismuth subsalicylate is extensively absorbed; however, systemic salicylate toxicity is not a concern during recommended use of this product since peak plasma levels are below the toxic range even after maximum daily dosing.[82] In contrast, little bismuth is absorbed from intact gut epithelium. Thus, patients at risk for salicylate or bismuth toxicity from bismuth subsalicylate are those who exceed the recommended daily dose or those with enteropathies (e.g., inflammatory bowel disease, HIV enteropathy).[83]

The primary manifestation of bismuth toxicity is neurologic toxicity. Central neurologic findings include cognitive and affective disorders and can progress to clonic jerks, dysarthria, and ataxia.[84,85] The onset of symptoms varies from weeks to years.[84,85] Treatment for bismuth toxicity includes chelation and hemodialysis for patients in renal failure. Consultation with a regional poison center or medical toxicologist is recommended for the management of these patients.

Laxatives. Clinical toxicity from acute exposure to laxatives is uncommon because of their limited gut absorption. However, when ingested in large amounts, fluid and electrolyte disorders can occur. There are several preparations, including irritants, bulk formers, osmotic agents, stimulants (e.g., castor oil, phenolphthalein, bisacodyl, phenisatin, cascara sagrada, and senna), and emollients. Mineral oil, an example of the latter category, has the potential to cause aspiration pneumonitis upon ingestion.[86] Patients at risk for chronic misuse of these agents are those with eating disorders (e.g., anorexia, bulimia) and factitious disorders (e.g., Munchausen's). Nausea, vomiting, abdominal pain, and diarrhea are frequent findings in laxative abuse.

The clinically important agents in this category are those containing lactulose (e.g., Cephulac, Chronulac), magnesium salts (magnesium citrate, magnesium sulfate), and phenophthalein (Ex-Lax). Lactulose causes an osmotic load in the gut that draws water into the intestinal tract. In excessive amounts, lactulose can cause hypovolemia, hypokalemia, and hypernatremia. Lactic acid is a byproduct of gut bacterial metabolism of lactulose and can be absorbed systemically in the presence of bowel ileus.[87] Magnesium causes increased gut motility by inducing the secretion of cholecystokinin. Significant hypermagnesemia can occur from increased use of magnesium salts, or use of these agents by patients with either renal insufficiency or bowel motility disorders. Phenolphthalein directly stimulates the gut to increase motility. Toxicity from this agent is uncommon, but appears to include GI bleeding, pancreatitis, liver failure, and hypotension.[88-90]

Table 5. Elemental Iron Equivalents for Iron Salts⁺

COMPOUND	PERCENTAGE OF ELEMENTAL IRON
Ferrous carbonate	48
Ferrous cholinate	12
Ferrous fumarate	33
Ferrous gluconate	12
Ferric phosphate	37
Ferric sulfate (hydrate)	20

⁺ To determine risk of toxicity, calculate dose of elemental iron ingested.

Total dose of elemental iron ingested (mg/kg) = [Number of tablets x Amount of iron compound (mg) in one tablet*] x Percentage of elemental iron in compound/Patient weight (kg)

* See product labeling.

Phenolphthalein can cause red colored stools, which are not secondary to bleeding. Children ingesting more than 1 gram of phenolphthalein should be evaluated at a health care facility and receive activated charcoal for GI decontamination. Symptomatic patients require monitoring of serum electrolytes and are managed supportively.

Miscellaneous Oral Agents

Caffeine. Caffeine is a socially accepted stimulant that is available in numerous beverages and foodstuffs (e.g., soda, coffee, tea, cocoa, chocolate), and as an OTC formulation. Caffeine is a methylxanthine compound, similar to theophylline and theobromine. These agents stimulate the cardiovascular, GI, and central nervous systems by increasing cyclic adenosine monophosphate (cAMP) activity and increasing intracellular calcium concentration. The amount of caffeine varies in different products. The maximum allowable caffeine concentration is 72 mg in a 12-ounce can of soda. Coffees and teas contain between 50 mg and 200 mg of caffeine in 5 ounces. Various OTC preparations contain between 32 mg and 200 mg of caffeine in a single tablet.

Caffeine is generally considered safe. However, serious toxicity, including death, can occur in overdose. Caffeine toxicity is primarily due to sympathomimetic effects, but clinical manifestations can be variable and include nausea, vomiting, psychomotor agitation, seizures, and tachydysrhythmias. Leukocytosis, hypokalemia, hyperglycemia, lactic acidosis, and metabolic acidemia can be found as well. CNS hyperactivity, tachycardia, and tachypnea were reported after ingestion of approximately 3 grams of caffeine by an infant.[91] A fatality in an adult occurred after ingestion of only 6.5 grams,[92] while others have survived much larger ingestions.[93]

Treatment of caffeine toxicity is similar to theophylline exposure and includes GI decontamination with repeat doses of oral activated charcoal, stabilization of the vital signs, and enhanced elimination with hemoperfusion. Adenosine is not effective in treating supraven-

Table 6. Clinical Manifestations of Hypervitaminosis[114]

VITAMIN	RDA⁺	TOXIC DOSE	CLINICAL MANIFESTATIONS
A			
	1000 IU/ day	*Acute:* 150,000 IU to 1.5 million IU *Chronic:* 10 times the RDA for a period of weeks	Altered mental status, dermatitis, hepatitis, cerebral edema, hypercalcemia
B_1 (THIAMINE)			
	1.5 mg/day	Undefined	
B_2 (RIBOFLAVIN)			
	1.7 mg/day	Undefined	
B_3 (NIACIN)			
	19 mg/day	*Acute:* 2 gm/kg	Skin flushing, hepatitis
B_6 (PYRIDOXINE)			
	2 mg/day	*Acute:* 2 gm/kg	Peripheral neuropathy
B_{12} (COBALAMIN)			
	2 mcg/day	Undefined	
C (ASCORBATE)			
	60 mg/day	*Acute:* > 4 g	Diarrhea, hemolysis
D			
	200 IU/ day	*Acute:* > 1000 IU/kg	Altered mental status, anorexia, nausea, vomiting, hypercalcemia
E			
	10 mg/day	*Acute:* > 200 mg/kg	Increased bleeding tendency
K			
	80 mcg/day	Undefined	Reversal of therapeutic anticoagulation (PT) therapy

⁺ Recommended daily allowance for 25- to 50-year-old male

tricular tachycardia because the methylxanthines are adenosine receptor antagonists.[94] Supraventriclur tachydysrhythmias can be rate controlled with either calcium channel blocking or beta adrenergic receptor-blocking agents.[95] Patients with hypotension should be administered an intravenous fluid challenge before receiving these agents. Seizures can be refractory to standard supportive care and may require consultation with either a regional poison center or a medical toxicologist to arrange for hemoperfusion.

Iron. Iron is a popular dietary supplement that is available as individual iron salts and in combination with multivitamins. There are nearly 100 iron-containing preparations, and more than 20 of these are available for purchase without a prescription.[96] Due to the high prevalence of these supplements, iron poisoning is common, particularly in the pediatric population. The annual incidence of iron poisoning in children is estimated to be about 22,000 and usually represents about 80% of all iron exposures. Each year, iron accounts for approximately 2% of all toxic exposures in children younger than 6 years of age.[97]

The dose of ingested elemental iron determines toxicity. *(Please see Table 5.)* Elemental iron ingestions of less than 20 mg/kg are considered non-toxic, and ingestions of greater than 60 mg/kg are associated with significant systemic toxicity. The toxic effects of iron burden the GI, cardiovascular, and central nervous systems. Excess iron in the GI tract exerts a local corrosive effect on the mucosa that can cause hemorrhage, necrosis, and perforation. The clinical manifestations of this local GI irritation include abdominal pain, nausea, vomiting, hematemesis, bloody diarrhea, and even hypovolemic shock.[96,97] The development of hypotension is multifactorial, including hypovolemia from GI losses, iron-mediated vasodilation, and myocardial depression.[98,99] The CNS effects of iron poisoning are variable and range from minor alterations of consciousness to coma.

Laboratory assessment in toxic patients includes CBC, serum electrolytes, blood urea nitrogen (BUN), creatinine, glucose, liver function tests, coagulation studies, and a serum iron level. An abdominal radiograph can assist in identifying iron pills.

Treatment begins with support of vital functions. Cardiovascular status should be optimized with intravenous fluids, blood and blood products, and vasopressors. Activated charcoal does not absorb iron and is not recommended. GI decontamination with gastric lavage and whole bowel irrigation is indicated in symptomatic patients with large gut iron load.[96,100] Patients with systemic toxicity require deferoxamine, an iron chelator, to remove excess free iron from the body. Indications for its use include significant GI symptoms, altered mental status, metabolic acidosis, and hypotension.[96,97] Also, the finding of an elevated serum iron level (> 500 (g/dL) is an indication for deferoxamine treatment.[97]

Vitamins. An estimated 40% of the U.S. population take vitamins on a regular basis.[101] This practice is generally safe, but vitamin intoxication does occur. Vitamins are available in a wide range of oral formulations designed for dietary supplementation. The fat-soluble vitamins A, D, E, and K have a greater potential for toxicity than the water-soluble vitamins B and C, which are readily eliminated by the kidneys and, therefore, rarely accumulate to dangerous levels. *(Please see Table 6.)*

Vitamin A is required for normal development of epithelial cells and for maintenance of night vision.[102] Toxicity occurs in the setting of both acute and chronic over exposure. Acute overdose was documented in individuals who had consumed polar bear, seal, dog, and halibut livers. Additionally, doses of 500,000 IU to 4 million IU of vitamin A have resulted in acute toxic symptoms, including: nausea, vomiting, fatigue, lethargy, headache, increased intracranial pressure, and papilledema.[103] Chronic intoxication is more common and generally requires the intake of more than 100,000 IU/day over a period of weeks to months.[103]

Toxicity involves multiple organ systems: skin changes include dryness, desquamation, and pruritis; musculoskeletal irregularities resemble the clinical spectrum of the seronegative spondylarthropathies; liver involvement is evidenced by elevated transaminase levels, ascites, and jaundice; CNS abnormalities manifest as benign intracranial hypertension, diplopia, and psychosis; and metabolic alterations are observed, especially hypercalcemia.[103-107] Laboratory assessment includes measurement of serum calcium and liver function studies. Therapy generally is supportive and begins with discontinuation of the vitamin supplement. Hypercalcemia may require specific treatment with forced saline diuresis, intravenous furosemide, and corticosteroids as necessary. Increased intracranial pressure may require aggressive management.

Vitamin D is an important regulator of calcium and phosphorous homeostasis. Over-supplementation causes hypercalcemia. Hypercalcemia was observed in 21 patients who had been taking milligram doses (range equivalent to 25,000 IU and 400,000 IU) of vitamin D/day.[108] Prolonged daily intake of 75,000 IU (almost 200 times the RDA) significantly increases serum calcium in most patients. The pathophysiologic mechanisms for this process include increased resorption of calcium from bone, increased gut absorption of dietary calcium, and increased renal calcium reclamation.[109]

The symptoms of hypercalcemia are non-specific: anorexia, nausea, vomiting, generalized weakness, mental status changes, polydipsia, and polyuria. Metastatic calcifications and cardiac dysrythmias also can occur.[108,110] Laboratory evaluation reveals elevated serum calcium and phosphorus. Hypercalciuria can be seen on urine analysis. Activated charcoal is recommended for acute ingestions that are 100 times greater than the RDA. Otherwise, treatment is largely directed at correcting hypercalcemia. Bisphosphonates and calcitonin may be necessary to inhibit bone resorption.

Daily vitamin E ingestions as high as 3200 mg (nearly 10 times the RDA) have produced few adverse effects.[111] In the 1980s, hepatotoxicity, necrotizing enterocolitis, and sepsis were observed in premature neonates given high-dose vitamin E to prevent retinopathy of prematurity.[103] Excess vitamin E can augment anticoagulation in patients who also are taking warfarin. This effect is due to vitamin E-mediated inhibition of vitamin K-dependent carboxylases. Significant coagulopathy is not observed in normal adults who take high doses of vitamin E and probably is not important in warfarin-treated patients if daily intake is less than 100 mg.[103,111] Nevertheless, laboratory evaluation of significant overdose should include coagulation studies. Treatment is supportive and includes vitamin E withdrawl and cessation. Intramuscular vitamin K reverses coagulopathy.[103]

Vitamin K is necessary for the synthesis of clotting factors 2, 7, 9, and 10. These same factors are inhibited by anticoagulation therapy with warfarin. Vitamin K is available in some multivitamins and as single oral supplements. Additionally, a significant amount of vitamin K is found in several foods, such as green tea, turnip, broccoli, spinach, cabbage, asparagus, and lettuce. Excess vitamin K from these sources can inhibit or reverse the therapeutic effects of warfarin. This supplement has not been shown to have other major toxicities.

The vitamin B complex is made up of the following compounds: thiamine (B_1), riboflavin (B_2), niacin (B_3), pyridoxine (B_6), and cobalamin (B_{12}). These supplements are essential for a range of vital processes, from DNA and amino acid synthesis to important redox reactions that power cellular metabolism. Deficiencies of these vitamins have been characterized in well-known clinical syndromes. Toxicity is extremely rare. Niacin routinely causes skin flushing and pruritus at therapeutic doses. Daily doses of time-release preparations of niacinamide greater than 1 g have resulted in lactic acidosis, myopathy, and extensive liver damage.[112] Excess of pyridoxine has been associated with sensory neuropathy.[113] Treatment for these conditions is supportive and toxic effects generally improve after removal of the vitamin supplement.

Vitamin C is involved in the production of collagen and also has antioxidant properties. Vitamin C is considered safe at doses up to 2 grams/day.[103] Greater daily intake most commonly results in an osmotic diarrhea. Additional adverse effects of high-dose vitamin C are renal calculi and decreased prothrombin time in patients who also are taking warfarin.[103] Treatment is supportive.

Summary

A wide range of products are available for OTC use. These products are designed for administration by a variety of routes. Exposures to OTC agents can produce a significant and wide range of toxicities that must be recognized and managed by emergency health care providers. Although fatalities are rare, more than 500,000 OTC exposures were reported to the American Association of the Poison Control Centers Toxic Exposure Surveillance System (AAPCC TESS) in 1998, a number that certainly underestimates the actual incidence. The pediatric patient, the elderly, and those with co-morbid conditions are at greater risk for serious toxicity from these products. The ED history should include detailed questions regarding OTC products, which should be considered in all cases of intentional overdose. Per protocol, treatment begins with advanced life support of the unstable patient. Consultation with a regional poison control center is necessary to determine the proper method of decontamination and the need for specific therapies, including potential antidotes.

References

1. American Conference of Governmental Industrial Hygienists. 1998 Threshold Limit Values (TLV's) for Chemical Substances and Physical Agents and Biological Exposure Indices (BEIs). Cincinnati, OH: 1998.
2. Heifetz SB, Horowitz HS. Amounts of fluoride in self-administered dental products: Safety considerations for children. *Pediatrics* 1986;77:876-882.
3. Eichler HG, Lenz K, Fuhrmann M, et al. Accidental ingestion of NaF tablets by children: Report of a poison control center and one case. *Int J Clin Pharmacol Ther Toxicol* 1982;20:334-338.
4. Spak CJ, Sjöstedt S, Eleborg L, et al. Tissue response of gastric mucosa after ingestion of fluoride. *BMJ* 1989;298:1686-1687.
5. Baltazar RF, Mower MM, Reider R, et al. Acute fluoride poisoning leading to fatal hyperkalemia. *Chest* 1980;78:660-663.
6. Swanson L, Filandrinos DT, Shevlin JM, et al. Death from accidental ingestion of an ammonium and sodium bifluoride glass etching glass etching compound (abstract). *Vet Human Toxicol* 1993;35:351.
7. Larsen MJ, Jensen SJ. Inactivation of hydrofluoric acid by solutions intended for gastric lavage. *Pharmacol Toxicol* 1990;67:447-448.
8. Augenstein WL, Spoerke DG, Kulig KW, et al. Fluoride ingestion in children: A review of 87 cases. *Pediatrics* 1991;88:907-912.
9. Hornfelt CS. A report of acute ethanol poisoning in a child: Mouthwash versus cologne, perfume and aftershave. *Clin Toxicol* 1992;30:115-121.
10. Vogel C, Caraccio T, Mofensen H, et al. Alcohol intoxication in young children. *J Toxicol Clin Toxicol* 1995;33:25-33.
11. Holt S, Stewart MJ, Adam RJ, et al. Alcohol absorbtion, gastric emptying, and a breathalyser. *Br J Clin Pharmacol* 1980;9: 205-208.
12. Ritchie JM, Greene NM. Local anesthetics. In: Gilman AG, Goodman L, Gilman A, eds. *The Pharmacological Basis of Therapeutics*. 6th ed. New York: Macmillan; 1980:310.
13. Product Information: Sucrets Children's Lozenges. Beecham Products, USA, Pittsburgh, PA: 1991.
14. Product Information: Dyclone, dyclonine topical tolpical solutions 0.5% and 1%. Westboro, MA: Astra Pharmaceuticals;1997.
15. Purcell SM, Dixon SL. Allergic contact dermatitis to dyclonine hydrochloride simulating extensive herpes simplex labialis. *J Am Acad Dermatol* 1985;12:231-234.
16. Jelen G, Tennestedt D. Contact dermatitis from topical imidazole antifungals: 15 new cases. *Contact Dermatitis* 1989;21:6-11.
17. Danziger Y, Pertzelan A, Mimouni M. Transient congenital hypothyroidism after topical iodine in pregnancy and lactation. *Arch Dis Child* 1987;62:295-296.
18. *Drug Facts and Comparisons.* 54th ed. St. Louis: Facts and Comparisons; 2000:1669-1673.
19. Chiang WK, Wang RY. Evaluation and management of acetaminophen toxicity. *Emerg Med Reports* 1993;14:83-90.
20. Spitalnic S, Wang RY. Update: Salicylate toxicity. *Emerg Med Reports* 1993;14:174-180.
21. Smolinske SC, Hall AH, Vandenber SA, et al. Toxic effects of nonsteroidal anti-inflammatory drugs in overdose: An overview of recent evidence on clinical effects and dose-response relationships. *Drug Saf* 1990;5:252-274.
22. Hall AH, Smolinske SC, Conrad FL, et al. Ibuprofen overdose: 126 cases. *Ann Emerg Med* 1986;15:1308-1313.
23. McElwee NE, Veltri JC, Bradford DC, et al. A prospective, population-based study of acute ibuprofen overdose: Complications are rare and routine serum levels not warranted. *Ann Emerg Med* 1990;19:657-662.
24. Litovitz TL, Klein-Schwartz W, Caravati EM, et al. 1998 Annual report of the American Association of Poison Control Centers Toxic Exposure Surveillance System. *Am J Emerg Med* 1999;17:435-487.
25. Lie RL, Vermeer BJ, Edelbroek PM. Severe lidocaine intoxication by cutaneous absorption. *J Am Acad Dermatol* 1990;23: 1026-1028.
26. Product Infomation: Zostrix, capsaicin. Lincolnshire, IL: GenDerm Corporation; 1997.
27. Garrison JC. Histamin, Bradykinin, 5-Hydroxytryptamine, and Antagonists. In: Gilman AG, Goodman L, Gilman A, eds. *The Pharmacological Basis of Therapeutics.* 8th ed. New York: Pergamon Press; 1990:582-588.
28. Zareba W, Moss AJ, Rosero SZ, et al. Electrocardiographic findings in patients with diphenhydramine overdose. *Am J Cardiol* 1997;80:1168-1173.
29. Koppel C, Ibe K, Tenczer J. Clinical symptomatology of diphenhydramine overdose: An evaluation of 136 cases in 1982 to 1985. *J Toxicol Clin Toxicol* 1987;25:53-70.
30. Lavenstein BL, Cantor FK. Acute dystonia: An unusual reaction to diphenhydramine. *JAMA* 1976;236:291.
31. Mullins ME, Pinnick RV, Terhes JM. Life-threatening diphenhydramine overdose treated with charcoal hemoperfusion and hemodialysis. *Ann Emerg Med* 1999;33:104-107.
32. Clark RF, Vance MV. Massive diphenhydramine poisoning resulting in a wide-complex tachycardia: Successful treatment with sodium bicarbonate. *Ann Emerg Med* 1992;21:318-321.
33. Freedberg RS, Friedman GR, Palu RN, et al. Cardiogenic shock due to antihistamine overdose. *JAMA* 1987;257:660-661.
34. Brost BC, Scardo JA, Newman RB. Diphenhydramine overdose during pregnancy: Lessons from the past. *Am J Obstetr Gynecol* 1996;175:1376-1377.
35. American Academy of Pediatrics. Committee on Drugs. Use of codeine and dextromethorphan containing cough syrups in pediatrics. *Pediatrics* 1978;62:118-122.
36. Schneider SM, Michelson EA, Boucek CD, et al. Dextromethorphan poisoning reversed by naloxone. *Am J Emerg Med* 1991;9:237-238.
37. Shaul WL, Wandell M, Robertson WO. Dextromethorphan toxicity: Reversal by naloxone. *Pediatrics* 1977;59:117-119.
38. Rammer L, Holmgren P, Sandler H. Fatal intoxication by dextromethorphan: A report on two cases. *Forensic Sci Int* 1988;37:233-236.
39. Rivers N, Horner B. Possible lethal reaction between nardil and dextromethorphan (letter). *Can Med Assoc J* 1970;103:85.
40. Sovner R, Wolfe J. Interaction between dextromethorphan and monoamine oxidase inhibitor therapy with isocarboxazid (letter). *N Engl J Med* 1988;319:1671.
41. Skop BP, Brown TM, Mareth TR. The serotonin syndrome associated with paroxetine. *Am J Emerg Med* 1995;13:606-607.
42. Liebelt EL, Shannon MW. Small doses, big problems: A selected review of highly toxic common medications. *Pediatr Emerg Care* 1993;9:292-297.
43. Pentel P. Toxicity of over-the-counter stimulants. *JAMA* 1984;252:1898-1903.
44. Horowitz JD, Lang WJ, Howes LG, et al. Hypertensive responses induced by phenylpropanolamine in anorectic and decongestant preparations. *Lancet* 1980;1:60-61.
45. Glick R, Hoying J, Cerullo L, et al. Phenylpropanolamine: An over-the-counter drug causing entral nervous system vasculitis and intracerebral hemorrhage. *Neurosurgery* 1987;20:969-974.

46. Mariani PJ. Pseudoephedrine-induced hypertensive emergency: Treatment with labetalol. *Am J Emerg Med* 1986;4:141-142.
47. Centers for Disease Control and Prevention. Adverse events associated with ephedrine-containing products. *MMWR Morb Mortal Wkly Rep* 1996;45:689-693.
48. Klein-Schwartz W, Gorman R, Oderda GM, et al. Central nervous system depression from ingestion of nonprescription eyedrops. *Am J Emerg Med* 1984;2:217-218.
49. Lev R, Clark RF. Visine overdose: Case report of an adult with hemodynamic compromise. *J Emerg Med* 1995;13:649-652.
50. Higgins GL, Campbell B, Wallace K, et al. Pediatric poisoning from over-the-counter imidazoline-containing products. *Ann Emerg Med* 1991;20:655-658.
51. Tobias JD. Central nervous system depression following accidental ingestion of visine eye drops. *Clin Pediatr* 1996;35:539-540.
52. Fleming LW, Prescott A, Stewat WK, et al. Bioavailability of aluminum. *Lancet* 1989;1:433.
53. Jameson S. Magnesium-containing antacids to patients with uremia–An intoxication risk. *Scand J Urol Nephrol* 1972;6:260-264.
54. Layzer RB. Neuromuscular manifestations of systemic disease. Philadelphia, PA: FA Daves Co; 1985:62-63.
55. Woodard JA, Shannon M, Lacouture PG, et al. Serum magnesium concentrations after repetitive magnesium cathartic administration. *Am J Emerg Med* 1990;8:297-300.
56. Fessler HE, Brower RG, Permutt S. CPAP reduces inspiratory work more than dyspnea during hyperinflation with intrinsic PEEP. *Chest* 1995;108:432-440.
57. Clark BA, Brown RS. Unsuspected morbid hypermagnesemia in elderly patients. *Am J Nephrol* 1992;12:336-343.
58. Puntis JWL, Ballantine NE, Durbin GM. Raised plasma aluminum in an infant on antacid. *Lancet* 1989;2:923.
59. Kaehny WD, Hegg AP, Alfrey AC. Gastrointestinal absorption of aluminum from aluminum-containing antacids. *N Engl J Med* 1977;296:1389-1390.
60. Nathan E, Pedersen SE. Dialysis encephalopathy in a non-dialysed uraemic boy treated with aluminum hydroxide orally. *Acta Paediatr Scand* 1980;69:793-796.
61. Brettschneider L, Monafo W, Osborne DP. Intestinal obstruction due to antacid gels: Complication of medical therapy for gastrointestinal bleeding. *Gastroenterology* 1965;49:291.
62. Adams PL, Rutsky EA, Rostand SG, et al. Lower gastrointestinal tract dysfunction in patients receiving long-term hemodialysis. *Arch Intern Med* 1982;142:303-306.
63. Sinaasappel M, Ouden WJ, Luyednijk I, et al. Increased vomiting induced by an antiemetic drug. *Arch Dis Child* 1984;59:272-274.
64. Spencer H, Kramer L, Norris C, et al. Effect of small doses of aluminum-containing antacids on calcium and phosphorous metabolism. *Am J Clin Nutr* 1982;36:32-40.
65. Neumann L, Jensen BG. Osteomalacia from Al and Mg antacids: Report of a case of bilateral hip fracture. *Acta Orthop Scand* 1989;60:361-362.
66. Monteagudo FSE, Cassidy MJD, Folb PI. Recent developments in aluminum toxicology. *Med Toxicol* 1989;4:1-16.
67. Wills MR, Savory J. Aluminum poisoning: Dialysis encephalopathy, osteomalacia, and anemia. *Lancet* 1983;2:29-34.
68. Korenmen MD, Stubbs MB, Fish JC. Intestinal obstruction from medication bezoars. *JAMA* 1978;240:54-55.
69. Shapiro JI, Kaehny WD. Pathogenesis and management of metabolic acidosis and alkalosis. In: Schrier RW, ed. *Renal and Electrolyte Disorders*. 4th ed. Boston, MA: Little Brown; 1992:161-210.
70. Rimer DG, Franklin M. Sodium content of antacids. *JAMA* 1960;173:995
71. Stiel J, Mitchell CA, Radcliff FJ, et al. Hypercalcemia in patients with peptic ulceration receiving large doses of calcium carbonate. *Gastroenterol* 1967;53:900.
72. Kapsner P, Langsdorf L, Marcus R, et al. Milk-alkali syndrome in patients treated with calcium carbonate after cardiac transplantation. *Arch Intern Med* 1986;146:1965-1968.
73. Sedman AJ. Cimetidine-drug interactions. *Am J Med* 1984;76: 109-113.
74. McMillen MA, Ambis D, Siegel JH. Cimetidine and mental confusion (letter). *N Engl J Med* 1978;298:284-285.
75. Bhutta TI , Tahir KI. Loperamide poisoning in children (letter). *Lancet* 1990;335:363.
76. Litovitz TL, Clancy C, Korberly BH, et al. Surveillance of loperamide ingestions: Analysis of 216 poison center reports (abstract). *Vet Hum Toxicol* 1993;35:369.
77. Minton NA, Smith PGD. Loperamide toxicity in a child after a single dose. *BMJ* 1987;294:1303.
78. Friedli G, Haenggeli CA. Loperamide overdose managed by naloxone (letter). *Lancet* 1980;1:1413.
79. Lambert JR. Pharmacology of bismuth-containing compounds. *Rev Infect Dis* 1991;13(S8):691-695.
80. Serfontein WJ, Mekel R. Bismuth toxicity in man II. Review of bismuth blood and urine levels in patients after administration of therapeutic bismuth formulations in relation to problems of bismuth toxicity in man. *Res Commun Chem Path Pharmacol* 1979;26: 391-411.
81. Ericsson CD, DuPont HL, Pickering LK. Bismuth preparations for diarrhea. *JAMA* 1980;244:1435-1436.
82. Bierer DW. Bismuth subsalicylate: History, chemistry, and safety. *Rev Infect Dis* 1990;12:S3-S8.
83. Mendelowitz PC, Hoffman RS, Weber S. Bismuth absorption and myoclonic encephalopathy during bismuth subsalicylate therapy. *Ann Intern Med* 1990;112:140-141.
84. Winship KA. Toxicity of bismuth salts. *Adv Drug React Ac Pois Rev* 1983;2:103-121.
85. Jones JA. Bipp: A case of toxicity? *Oral Surg Oral Med Oral Pathol* 1990;69:668-671.
86. Ferguson GT, Miller YE.: Occult mineral oil pneumonitis in anorexia nervosa. *West J Med* 1988;148:211-213.
87. Mann NS, Russman HB, Mann SK, et al. Lactulose and severe lactic acidosis. *Ann Intern Med* 1985;15:177-181.
88. Lambrianides AL, Rosin RD. Acute pancreatitis complicating excessive intake of phenolphthalein. *Postgrad Med J* 1984;60: 491-492.
89. Weiss BD, Wood GA. Laxative abuse causing gastrointestinal bleeding. *J Fam Pract* 1982;15:177-181.
90. Sidhu PS, Wilkinson ML, Sladen GE, et al. Fatal phenolphthalein poisoning with fulminant hepatic failure and disseminated intravascular coagulation. *Human Toxicol* 1989;8:381-384.
91. Fligner CL, Opheim KE. Caffeine and its dimethylxantine metabolites in two cases of caffeine overdose: A cause of falsely elevated theophylline concentrations in serum. *J Anal Toxicol* 1988;12: 339-343.
92. Alstott RL, Miller AJ, Forney RB. Report of a human fatality due to caffeine. *J Forensic Sci* 1973;18:135-137.
93. Lesson CL, McGuigan MA, Bryson SM. Caffeine overdose in an adolescent male. *Clin Toxicol* 1988;26:407-415.
94. Fredholm BB, Abbrocchio MP, Burnstock G, et al. Nomenclature and classification of purinoceptors. *Pharmacol Rev* 1994;46: 143-156.
95. Nagesh RV, Murphy KA. Caffeine poisoning treated by hemoperfusion. *Am J Kidney Dis* 1988;4:316-318.
96. Morse SB, Hardwick WE, King WD. Fatal iron intoxication in an

infant. *South Med J* 1997;90:1043-1047.
97. McGuigan MA. Acute iron poisoning. *Ped Ann* 1996;25:33-38.
98. Tenenbein M, Kopelow ML, deSa DJ. Myocardial failure and shock in iron poisoning. *Human Toxicol* 1988;7:281-284.
99. Vernon DD, Banner W, Dean JM. Hemodynamic effects of experimental iron poisoning. *Ann Emerg Med* 1989;18:863-866.
100. Tenenbein M. Whole bowel irriation in iron poisoning. *J Pediatr* 1987;111:142-145.
101. Stewart ML, McDonald JT, Levy AS, et al. Vitamin/mineral supplement use: A telephone survey of adults in the United States. *J Am Diet Assoc* 1989;89:383-386.
102. Wilson JD. Vitamin deficiency and excess. In: Isselbacher KJ, Braunwald E, Wilson JD, et al, eds. *Harrison's Principles of Internal Medicine*. 13th ed. New York: McGraw-Hill; 1994: 4732-4739.
103. Meyers DG, Maloley PA, Weeks D. Safety of antioxidant vitamins. *Arch Intern Med* 1996;156:925-935.
104. Katz CM, Tzagournis M. Chronic adult hypervitaminosis A with hypercalcemia. *Metabolism* 1972;21:1171-1176.
105. Lombaert A, Carton H. Benign intracranial hypertension due to A-hypervitaminosis in adults and adolescents. *Eur Neurology* 1976;14:340-350.
106. Nesher G, Zuckner J. Rheumatologic complications of vitamin A and retinoids. *Semin Arthritis Rheum* 1995;24:291-296.
107. Inkeles SB, Connor WE, Illingworth DR. Hepatic and dermatologic manifestations of chronic hypervitaminosis A in adults. *Am J Med* 1986;80:491-496.
108. Paterson CR. Vitamin-D poisoning: Survey of causes in 21 patients with hypercalcemia. *Lancet* 1980;1:164-165.
109. Holick MF, Stephen KM, Potts JT. Calcium, phosphorous, and bone metabolism: Calcium-regulating hormones. In: Isselbacher KJ, Braunwald E, Wilson JD, et al, eds. *Harrison's Principles of Internal Medicine*. 13th ed. New York: McGraw-Hill; 1994: 2137-2151.
110. Deftos JL. Hypercalcemia: Mechanisms, differential diagnosis, and remedies. *Postgrad Med* 1996;100:119-126.
111. Bendich A, Machlin J. Safety of oral intake of vitamin E. *Am J Clin Nutr* 1988;48:612-619.
112. Rader JI, Calvert RJ, Hathcock JN. Hepatic toxicity of unmodified and time-release preparations of niacin. *Am J Med* 1992;92:77-81.
113. Schaumburg H, Kaplan J, Windebank A, et al. Sensory neuropathy from pyridoxine abuse. *N Engl J Med* 1983;309:445-448.
114. Marcus R, Coulston AM. The vitamins. In: Gilman AG, Goodman L, Gilman A, eds. *The Pharmacological Basis of Therapeutics*. 8th ed. New York: Pergamon Press; 1990:1525.

Bioterrorism

W. Paul McKinney, MD
Frank J. Bia, MD, MPH
Chuck Stewart, MD
Gideon Bosker, MD, FACEP

Recent reports of anthrax exposure and disease have prompted a serious assessment of clinical strategies related to bioterrorism. Few natural or intentional threats generate more concern of among emergency management planners, physicians, and toxicologists in this country than the use of biological agents as an act of war or terrorism against citizens of the United States. Although a vast array of first responders, including elements of the military, police, fire departments, emergency medicine services, and hazardous materials units have been preparing to respond to such emergencies, relatively few physicians or pharmacists have been involved in comprehensive efforts to defend against possible acts of bioterrorism.

Especially in a covert attack, however, primary care physicians, emergency medicine specialists, and departments of pharmacy—which would be responsible for maintaining adequate inventories of antidotes, vaccines, and antimicrobials required for such a contingency—would play a front-line role in the detection, evaluation, and response to this threat. Formal educational curricula informing clinicians and pharmacist about the likely agents of bioterrorism (BT) are essential to ensure that cases are identified, reported, treated, and monitored as rapidly and efficiently as possible.

As physicians and pharmacists are well aware, the current bioterrorist threat remains a fluid, uncertain situation. In light of rapid changes in both our understanding and approach to bioterrorist activities, and, as new patterns of infection are recognized, the treatment options, epidemiology, and approaches to management and prophylaxis of these conditions are being closely monitored by medical, military, and governmental agencies.

This has important implications for clinical practice. Because diagnostic and management strategies are under constant review and evaluation, clinicians are advised to consult and monitor the most recent recommendations, reports, and advisories issued by such expert bodies as the Centers for Disease Control and the Food and Drug Administration, as well as such publications as the *Morbidity and Mortality Weekly Report* (MMWR) and *Biological Warfare Defense General Information Sheet.* Regional Poison Control Centers are also excellent sources of current information regarding bioterrorist threats, and may also be accessed for up-to-date information.

With these concerns in mind, this chapter will review recent clinical and pharmacological developments in the field of bioterrorism. Special emphasis is devoted to antimicrobial preparedness, recent developments concerning anthrax management, and current programs under development for responding to bioterrorist activities.

Table 1. Clinical Syndromes Suggestive of Bioterrorism-Associated Illness

AGENT	CLINICAL PRESENTATION
Anthrax	Widened mediastinum, not associated with chest trauma
Smallpox	Characteristic vesiculopustular rash, with eruption of palms and soles, involving face sore than chest, and all lesions in same phase of development
Botulism	Prominent neurologic symptoms: descending paralysis beginning with cranial nerve palsies
Plague, Tularemia	Increased incidence of atypical pneumonia in population

Introduction

Background. Evidence of attempts to induce fatal infectious illnesses among enemy combatants is hardly a recent concept and actually dates back in time to an era long before the acceptance of the germ theory of disease. The intentional use of biological agents as a weapon of warfare first occurred no later than the Middle Ages, when attacking 14th-century Tatar forces in what is now Ukraine catapulted the corpses of their troops who had died from plague into a besieged stronghold in an attempt to induce an outbreak of plague among their enemy.[1] Other evidence of such intentional use of biological agents as a weapon can be found in North America during the mid-18th century, when British commander Sir Jeffrey Amherst ordered the transfer of blankets used by British smallpox victims to Native American tribal members, ostensibly as a gesture of goodwill, with the intention of inducing illness.[1]

Indeed, the United States had a program of developing biological agents for use in warfare well into the Vietnam War era until that strategy was abandoned and the offensive use of such weapons was forbidden by U.S. policy under executive orders of President Richard Nixon in 1969-1970.[1]

International Threats. Since the Persian Gulf conflict of the early 1990s, attention has focused on the arsenals of biological warfare agents amassed by Iraq and by the nations comprising the former Soviet Union. During the Cold War era, Soviet military experts oversaw the weaponization of a variety of bacteria and viruses; unfortunately, the whereabouts of much of this material is currently unknown.[2] Moreover, in the 1990s, Japan's quasi-religious Aum Shinrykyo cult planned attacks using biological agents, specifically, anthrax and botulinum toxin.[3] While these biological attacks were not successful, cult members later implemented the release of sarin nerve gas in the Tokyo subway system, killing 12 persons, producing illness in almost 1000 persons, and inducing panic in the population.[4]

Incidents and Hoaxes in the United States. The United States has not escaped such assaults, as biological agent attacks against American citizens have already occurred, and plans for others were discovered before their successful implementation. In 1984, members of the Rajneesh cult contaminated salad bars in Oregon with salmonella, resulting in the infection of 751 persons.[5] Moreover, a variety of feigned exposures to anthrax spores occurred in several U.S. cities in 1998, including Cincinnati, Louisville, and Indianapolis.[6] In Indianapolis, a full-scale response by emergency services and public health personnel occurred before the episode was proven to be a hoax.

These exposures point out the need for a high level of preparedness in this country against bioterrorist activities. Currently, the network of local and state health departments, with support of the Centers for Disease Control and Prevention (CDC), forms the backbone of the surveillance and response system for such events. A variety of other federal entities, including the Department of Defense, the Office of Emergency Preparedness, the Federal Emergency Management Agency (FEMA), the Department of Veterans Affairs, the Central Intelligence Agency (CIA), and the Federal Bureau of Investigation (FBI), are also actively nvolved in integrated planning efforts on the national level. In addition, the national surveillance arm is supplemented by arrangements with three elements of the medical care delivery system: emergency department physicians from hospitals serving selected large metropolitan areas, a network of infectious disease physicians, and selected international travel clinics.

Antimicrobial Preparedness for Anthrax-Mediated Bioterrorist Threats: Rationale, Indications, and Guidelines for Ciprofloxacin Therapy and Inventory Strategies

Although this review will examine many aspects of responding to and managing a variety of potential bioterrorist threats, recent approval of one antimicrobial for post-exposure treatment of patients exposed to anthrax is a most recent development, and therefore, deserves discussion.

Fear of Bioterrorist Threats and Studies Leads To New Indication For Ciprofloxacin. Preparation for defense against infection-based biological weapons requires maintenance of adequate inventories of antibiotics that can be used to either prevent infection after exposure (post-exposure treatment) or treat the acute disease after manifestation of symptoms. Gaining FDA approval for such indications has been hampered by the inability to perform studies in human populations. Consequently, although such conditions as anthrax may be life-threatening, the incentives and rationale for stockpiling effective antimicrobials that can play an integral role in public health preparedness have been slow in coming.

The landscape for antibiotic-mediated post-exposure treatment is quickly changing. In one of the first antimicrobial drug applications submitted to the Food and Drug Administration to

Table 2. Agents With Risk for Secondary Transmission of Illness

AGENT	SECONDARY TRANSMISSION RISK
Smallpox	Yes
Anthrax	No
Botulism	No
Tularemia	No
Plague	Yes
Brucellosis	No

respond to and manage the intentional use of a biological agent, the federal government has approved the antibiotic, ciprofloxacin (Cipro®), to use in people exposed to inhaled anthrax. Ciprofloxacin is indicated for reducing the incidence or progression of inhalational anthrax following exposure to aerosolized *Bacillus anthracis*, the bacterium that causes anthrax.

Inhalational anthrax is an extremely rare disease that results from exposure to contaminated animal hides and hairs, with most transmissions usually occurring in an industrial setting. However, the causative organism, *Bacillus anthracis*, is a spore-forming, gram-positive rod that can also be used as a biological weapon. According to military and infectious disease experts, inhalational anthrax is considered the most likely form of infection from intentional use of an aerosolized preparation of spores of *Bacillus anthracis*.

Anthrax and Animal Testing: Ciprofloxacin Efficacy Established. On July 28, 2000, the FDA approved ciprofloxacin under accelerated approval regulations, based on the use of a surrogate endpoint and ciprofloxacin serum concentrations in humans. Because high mortality rates in anthrax precludes performing studies in humans, the use of a surrogate endpoint was supported by ciprofloxacin serum concentrations in the rhesus monkey model of post-exposure inhalational anthrax.

Investigational studies employing this model demonstrated a significantly improved survival rate for animals receiving ciprofloxacin as compared to animals that did not receive this antimicrobial after exposure to aerosolized Bacillus anthracis. Moreover, the serum levels measured in monkeys that survived exposure to anthrax bacteria can be achieved or exceeded in humans receiving the recommended doses of ciprofloxacin.

Support for ciprofloxacin-based post-exposure prophylaxis in this model is based on the similarities between experimental animals and humans regarding the pathogenesis, clinical course, and tissue pathology of inhalational anthrax. Although ciprofloxacin is currently not approved for children (for non-anthrax related disorders) due to its potential adverse effects on cartilage, this effect has never been conclusively proven in humans. In addition, recent safety data in the elderly have shown ciprofloxacin to be as safe and efficiacious in the elderly as it is in younger adults for management of urinary tract infection.

Clearly, the risk-benefit equation for ciprofloxacin therapy in the case of anthrax post-exposure prophylaxis justifies use of this antimicrobial for the pediatric population. The recommended adult dose of ciprofloxacin for post-exposure prophylaxis of inhalational anthrax is 500 mg given orally twice daily. The recommended pediatric dose of ciprofloxacin for post-exposure inhalational anthrax is 15 mg/kg given orally twice daily. The adult intravenous dose is 400 mg BID; the pediatric intravenous dose is 10 mg/kg BID.

Prophylaxis with ciprofloxacin should begin as soon as possible after suspected exposure and the drug should be administered for 60 days. The most common adverse drug reactions from ciprofloxacin include nausea, vomiting, diarrhea, abdominal pain, rash, headache, and restlessness. It should be emphasized that in patients who have received ciprofloxacin for 60 days or longer, no new or unexpected adverse reactions were identified, as compared with patients receiving shorter courses of approved regimens.

Medical, Antimicrobial, and Organizational Preparedness for Bioterrorism (BT): Educational Deficiencies and POLICY Objectives

The use of biological agents as part of a terrorist threat or as an unsanctioned modality for warfare has gained increasing attention in recent months. If, some day, infectious or biological weapons are ever employed against civilian or military populations, primary care clinicians, emergency department physicians, and nurses on the front lines will face the challenge of responding to such hostile acts. As a proactive measure, pharmacists may be required to stockpile agents that are effective in treating or preventing the adverse consequences of toxic biological agents. Consequently, health care providers must be educated about methods of detection, prevention, preparedness, and, in general, strategies for responding to a bioterrorism (BT) attack.

BT is defined by the Atlanta-based Centers for Disease Control and Prevention (CDC) as "The intentional or threatened use of viruses, bacteria, fungi, toxins from living organisms, or other chemicals, to produce death or disease in humans, animals, or plants." BT agents can be "deliberately released into the population, the food supply, or into the air, or they may be disseminated through infected persons," explains Scott Lillibridge, MD, director of the CDC's Bioterrorism Preparedness and Response Program. "And the first responders will be health care providers." The CDC director offered this analysis during the International Conference on Emerging Infectious Diseases 2000, held in Atlanta July 16-19. The conference was organized by the CDC, the Council of State and Territorial Epidemiologists, the American Society for Microbiology, the Association of Public Health Laboratories, and the National Foundation for CDC.

"Initial detection and initial response will be local," added Ali S. Kahn, MD, MPH, who is also affiliated with the Bioterrorism Preparedness and Response Program. "Clinical diagnostics at the point of care will be critical; astute clinicians will be invaluable. We need physician education." Emergency department

Table 3. Availability of Licensed, Pre-exposure Vaccines for Prevention of Bioterrorism-Associated Disease

AGENT	VACCINE
Smallpox	**Yes** Currently approved on as-needed basis for lab workers
Anthrax	**Yes** Vaccine for civilian use must be approved by Dept. of Defense
Botulism	**No**
Tularemia	**No**
Plague	**Yes** But not proven effective against pneumonic plague
Brucellosis	**No**

Table 4. Prophylaxis and/or Treatment Regimens for Agents of Bioterrorism[9]

AGENT	VACCINE
Variola	Treatment of active smallpox can be attempted with cidofovir, an agent with activity against many pox viruses; three other agents—adefovir dipivoxide, cyclic cidofovir, and ribavirin—may also be candidates for use in this setting.
Anthrax	IV administration of ciprofloxacin 400 mg every 8-12 hrs (post-exposure prophylaxis)
Botulism	Trivalent equine antitoxin if the disease is in a phase of progression. Contact the CDC for release of antitoxin. Skin testing should be done first to avoid the occurrence of anaphylaxis or serum sickness.
Tularemia	Streptomycin given 30 mg/kg/day IM in two divided doses for 10-14 days.
Plague	Streptomycin 30 mg/kg IM per day in two divided doses. (Gentamicin is considered a substitute agent.) IV chloramphenicol may be given for plague meningitis or in sepsis syndrome. IV doxycycline (100 mg every 12 hours for 10-14 days, after an initial loading dose of 200 mg) is also effective.
Brucellosis	Preferred for severe brucellosis (bone, joint, heart, CNS infection) is a combination of doxycycline (100 mg BID) plus rifampin 600-900 mg/day orally for six weeks.

visits will be a critical point of identification, Kahn noted, adding: "We will be very dependent on calls from individuals such as infection control nurses."

Other experts at the conference concurred that the initial victims will be managed in traditional clinical environments. "The first place BT victims will be treated will be in emergency departments and clinics," said Stephen S. Morse, PhD, a program manager in the Defense Sciences Offices of DARPA, the Defense Advanced Research Project Agency of the Defense Department, based in Arlington, Virginia.

Management of BT victims is especially difficult because BT presents the prospect of a disaster with which most emergency responders and pharmacists are not familiar. CDC expert Lillibridge noted that, "Whole cities and regions could be in peril," and underscored that this type of major medical emergency may be much different from those that FEMA [Federal Emergency Management Agency], for example, has been dealing with, and with which we are more familiar."

The most likely biological agents that would be used in an attack include anthrax, smallpox, plague, botulism, tularemia, or VHF. These agents have been identified by the CDC as "Critical Biologic Agents," said Kahn. This is not necessarily because a terrorist would more likely choose these over other agents, but because "if released, we would have a major public health issue." The treatment and outcomes, noted Lillibridge, may not be that different from what would be seen with an emerging infectious disease. "But it's been a long time since we've had to respond to a situation like this; we've had little experience here with epidemics involving a large population and that would constitute a major federal outbreak."

Yet Lillibridge is convinced the threat is very real. He noted the accessibility of biotechnology information to terrorist groups such as Aum Shinrykyo, "which, in addition to releasing nerve gas in Tokyo's subway, experimented with botulism and anthrax," he said in a September 22, 1999, statement before the Subcommittee on National Security, Veterans Affairs and International Relations Committee on Government Reform, U.S. House of Representatives. "An attack with an agent such as smallpox could pose threats to large populations because of the potential for person-to-person transmission, enabling spread to other cities and states. This would quickly culminate in a nationwide emergency. International involvement would be sure to follow," he said in his statement.

He went on to note that vaccine and quarantine have worked well in combination against smallpox, since history shows an average of 1.48 people infected by each initially infected person. Nevertheless, he added, rapid response is essential. "The difference between 25 days and 45 days is unbelievable," he said. "We have to be prepared." The subsequent "Q&A" session demonstrated that even the experts are not clear on what it would take to win such a war. Meltzer suggested that 40 million doses of vaccine should be stockpiled to be adequately prepared for a BT attack using smallpox. But he also suggested that individuals vaccinated more than 30 years ago still have sufficient immunity so that the virus would not kill them. "I believe 80% of the individuals are susceptible in this population," argued a questioner. "And

Table 5. Post-exposure Prophylaxis Against Agents of Bioterrorism[9]

Agent	Prophylaxis
Variola virus	Smallpox vaccine is effective in preventing death if given up to five days after exposure and in preventing illness if given within 72 hours.
Anthrax	Ciprofloxacin 500 mg orally bid. Also initiate anthrax immunization, if available. Antibiotic prophylaxis should continue for at least four weeks and until three doses of vaccine have been given.
Botulism	Trivalent equine antitoxin, available from CDC
Tularemia	Doxycycline 100 mg orally bid for 14 days
Plague	Doxycycline 100 mg orally bid for seven days
Brucellosis	Doxycycline 100 mg bid plus rifampin 600-900 mg/d for three weeks

Postexposure Prophylaxis: Prophylaxis immediately after recognized exposure may be given with doxycycline 100 mg b.i.d. for 14 days.[9] For long-term advanced prophylaxis, a live attenuated vaccine is available in the United States under an investigational new drug protocol.[29]

40 million doses is not enough." In either case, with the virus "eradicated" years ago, the current stockpile is negligible.

Complicating the issue is that in the early stages of infection, BT agents are difficult to identify. "Many of the early symptoms are flu-like," said Morse, noting that they can include headache, muscle aches, chills, and loss of appetite. "Biological warfare agents are often indistinguishable from the flu and from each other." Morse then added this chilling admission: "By the time the symptoms appear, it may be too late to save the patient; we need to determine who was exposed before the symptoms appear." All of this makes the case for better education in the area of BT a national priority.

A Nationwide Effort. With the CDC at the helm, a growing group of federal public health and military agencies is working together to better identify and respond to possible BT outbreaks. For example, the National Notifiable Disease Surveillance System (NNDSS) reports weekly to the CDC.

Armed with data on previous outbreaks of infectious diseases, they are alerted by infections that occur "outside normal areas, or with unusual or unexplained [population] distribution," explained the CDC's Man-huei Chang, MPH. Chang reported, however, that there is no single U.S. system for baseline data that are needed, underscoring the fact that national preparedness efforts are also in a race against time.

Since 1973, at least 30 new viral agents have been identified, and there are new threats being introduced all the time," noted Lillibridge, who cited HIV, resistant TB, and West Nile virus as some of the more recent threats. "The tools of bioscience are increasingly available for altering existing pathogens or creating new ones, and we are not prepared." Kahn noted that several medical groups, including the American Medical Association and the American College of Emergency Physicians, are taking the lead in working with the CDC to educate their members and to help prepare for an event that may be more likely than many would like to admit. A high state of preparedness could help ensure the public safety on more than one level, he said. Lillibridge. "After all," he noted, "in a BT attack, the health care provider population could be decimated as well."

Recent Programs and Strategies Established Against Bioterrorist Threats

Recent media coverage and anthrax exposures have revealed grave concerns about potential bioterrorism against the United States and national vulnerability. In this regard, announcements of new funding for efforts to bolster national defenses continue to be issued by private companies, academic institutions and government agencies. These are likely to continue, as fears of bioterrorism have little reason to abate.

Carnegie Mellon University and the University of Pittsburgh announced the creation of the Biomedical Security Institute (BMSI), a partnership between the two universities, and of two awards to BMSI—one from the Agency for Healthcare Research and Quality (AGRQ) and one from the Centers for Disease Control (CDC). The BMSI was established to advance capabilities to detect, analyze, prevent and respond to acts of terrorism and natural events involving biological agents.

One major concern is the use of smallpox for bioterrorist activities. The United States is extremely susceptible to smallpox, as it was eradicated in this country in the 1960s and no immunizations have been given in 40 years. SIGA Technologies, Inc. announced its receipt of a $600,000 research grant from the Department of Health and Human Services (DHHS), which it will share with Oregon State University, to develop a drug for treating or preventing disease caused by poxviruses, should they be used during biological warfare or emerge in nature. Over a three-year period, SIGA and Oregon State University will work together to identify the viral gene product responsible for catalyzing core protein maturation and use genetic approaches to validate it as an antiviral target. Lead compounds identified by the research will be tested for the ability to inhibit the replication of various orthopoxviruses in tissue culture cells.

The Senate Health, Education, Labor and Pension Committee reported out S. 2731, the "Public Health Threats and Emergencies Act" which had been introduced by Senators Frist (R-TN) and Kennedy (D-MA) on June 14, 2000. The bill is designed to increase the ability of the federal, state, and local governments to respond to public health threats, including significant outbreaks of infectious diseases, bioterrorist attacks, or antimicrobial resistance problems.

The Clinician's and Pharmacist's Role in Bioterrorism

The threat of bioterrorist actions has generated extensive plans for detection and response involving several elements of our health care system. The rationale for such planning is straightforward: failure to make the diagnosis as early as possible during the first wave of illness following covert exposure risks substantially loss of human life.

In an era characterized by increased penetration of managed care and emphasis on the provision of care in rural areas, persons with acute infectious diseases are less likely to have direct access to infectious disease specialists. As a result, many patients exposed to a bioterrorist-associated infection are more likely to be seen first by primary care physicians or emergency medicine specialists. The fact, is, referring such exposed individuals to infectious disease specialists would consume additional time, and potentially, could result in many more infected cases or deaths before the source could be identified and contained. Moreover, in the event of a large-scale exposure, these clinicians would necessarily be called upon to support the civilian health sector response. The CDC has issued interim recommendations for postexposure prophylaxis for prevention of inhalation anthrax after intentional exposure to *Bacillus anthracis*. (*Please see Table 6*.) Finally, the optimal response to such exposures requires maintenance of adequate stockpiles of antidotes, antimicrobials, and vaccines.

Detection and Management of Bioterrorism-Associated Illness

Clearly, it is necessary to involve the full spectrum of primary care clinicians and pharmacists in preparing for the possibility of bioterrorist events. A systematic approach to this problem would involve the following strategies: (1) integrating physicians into an established national surveillance network to enhance the capacity for early detection and large-scale response; (2) educating clincians them through enhanced curricula during medical school and residency training regarding syndromes or disease patterns that are suspicious for biological warfare agent exposures; and (3) educating clinicians about preferred immunobiologic and pharmaceutical management strategies.

Given these objectives and concerns, this review article will discuss diagnostic approaches and management strategies for the six agents most likely be involved in a bioterrorist event: anthrax, smallpox, botulism, tularemia, plague, and brucellosis.

Anthrax

One of the great infectious diseases of antiquity, anthrax is caused by Bacillus anthracis. Anthrax is also known as woolsorters' disease or the black bane. The anthrax bacillus was the first organism shown to be the cause of a disease in 1877, and five years later, the first bacterial disease for which an immunization was available.

Anthrax produces three proteins that enhance the lethality of this organism. These proteins are known as edema factor (EF), lethal factor (LF), and protective antigen (PA). Edema toxin results from the combination of EF + PA, and lethal toxin results from combining LF + PA. These toxins result in necrosis of lymphatic tissue and release of large numbers of bacteria from the tissue. The organisms gain access to the circulation and produce overwhelming fatal septicemia. Death is often sudden and unexpected. A cell-free plasma of animals dying of anthrax injected into healthy animals will cause symptoms of anthrax in the healthy animals.

Under normal (non-wartime) conditions, humans become infected by contact with an infected animal or contaminated animal byproducts. Certain environmental conditions appear to produce anthrax zones where the soil is heavily contaminated with spores. Anthrax zones in the United States closely parallel the cattle drive trails of the 1800s. Domestic herbivores can acquire the disease while grazing in areas of high soil contamination.

There are three forms of anthrax: cutaneous, inhalation, and gastrointestinal. Almost all naturally occurring cases of anthrax are cutaneous or gastrointestinal. Cutaneous anthrax is readily recognizable, easily diagnosed, and is amenable to therapy with many antibiotics. Gastrointestinal anthrax is quite rare. Inhalation anthrax is likewise quite rare, but may be found in those who handle wool (hence, the name wool sorters' disease). Although anthrax is rare in the United States, large anthrax outbreaks have occurred in other countries during the modern era. More than 6000 cases occurred between October 1979 and March 1980 in Zimbabwe.[35B] In 1987, 25 cases in Paraguay were traced to meat from a single cow.[42]

In the minds of most military and counterterrorism planners, Anthrax is thought to represent the single greatest biowarfare threat.[37B] Anthrax spores easily can be made into an aerosol, resist environmental degradation, and are the ideal size (2-6 microns) for lodging in the lower respiratory mucosa. Anthrax has a fairly high dose of 8,000-10,000 spores required to produce death.

Anthrax has been proposed and investigated as a bioweapon by both allies in WWII, and by the communists in the former USSR. An epidemic that caused 96 cases of human anthrax in the city of Ekaterinburg (formerly Sverdlovsk) in 1979 was traced to a Russian bioweapon strain of anthrax. In these patients, the pathogen was airborne. The epidemiology of this release was unusual. None of the victims were children. Whether this is due to a difference in susceptibility between children and adults or the possibility that children weren't outdoors during the release is not known.

Because it has been thought by both civilian and military authorities to present a significant threat, anthrax is also a bioterrorist hoax of choice. There have been multiple threats of bioterrorism involving anthrax.[43,44] As a result, it is increasingly likely that emergency physicians will be confronted with patients who have been theoretically exposed to anthrax spores.

Presentation. Anthrax is most likely to be disseminated as an aerosol of the very persistent spores. The inhalational form of anthrax is uncommon but it is particularly lethal. Inhalation anthrax has an incubation time from 1 to 6 days. Anthrax may have a prolonged incubation period of up to two months. The longer incubation periods are seen most frequently when partial

Table 6. Interim Recommendations for Postexposure Prophylaxis for Prevention of Inhalation Anthrax After Intentional Exposure to *Bacillus anthracis*

CATEGORY	INITIAL THERAPY	DURATION
Adults (including pregnant women and immunocompromised persons)	Ciprofloxacin 500 mg po BID or Doxycycline 100 mg po BID	60 days
Children	Ciprofloxacin 10-15 mg/kg po Q12 hrs* or Doxycycline: > 8 yrs and > 45 kg: 100 mg po BID > 8 yrs and ≤ 45 kg: 2.2 mg/kg po BID ≤ 8 yrs: 2.2 mg/kg po BID	60 days

* Ciprofloxacin dose should not exceeed 1 gram per day in children

treatment has been given. The spores can be quite stable, even in the alveolus.

After the incubation period, a nonspecific flu-like illness develops with fever, myalgias, cough, headache, and mild chest discomfort. In its early presentation, inhalation anthrax may be confused with a plethora of viral or bacterial respiratory illnesses. The patient may have a brief period of improvement, but rapid deterioration follows.

The second phase is marked by high fever, dyspnea, stridor, cyanosis, and shock. Widening of the mediastinum on chest radiograph is common. Evidence of infiltrates on the chest x-ray are uncommon. Other suggestive findings include chest wall edema, hemorrhagic pleural effusions, and hemorrhagic meningitis. Death is universal in untreated cases and may occur in 80% of treated cases if the therapy is started more than 48 hours after the onset of symptoms.

Diagnosis. Pulmonary anthrax is a rare form of anthrax. The disease is difficult to diagnose within the treatable stage. Diagnosis can be made by culture of blood, pleural fluid, or cerebrospinal fluid. The blood culture is most often positive and the bacillus can be seen in blood smears. In fatal cases, impressions of mediastinal lymph nodes or spleen will be positive. A preponderance of gram-positive bacilli in swabs of the nose or from environmental samples would support a diagnosis of inhalational anthrax.

Anthrax toxin may be detected in blood by immunoassay. Diagnosis also can be made by direct fluorescent antibody testing by the United States Army Medical Research Institute for Infectious Diseases (USAMRIID) at Fort Detrick in Maryland.

The cases in Ekaterinburg were diagnosed on autopsy by a pathologist who noted a peculiar "cardinal's cap" meningeal inflammation, which is typical in anthrax.[45] All victims had hemorrhagic mediastinitis. The presentation of multiple patients with chest x-rays showing mediastinal widening in the absence of other obvious explanations should clue the physician to the diagnosis. Unfortunately, this is a late finding in the course of the disease. Multiple cases seen in one city are prima facie evidence that biological warfare is being waged.

Antimicrobial Management. Penicillin is considered the drug of choice for treatment of naturally occurring anthrax. However, penicillin-resistant strains do exist, and one would expect that anthrax developed as a biologic weapon would be penicillin resistant. Therefore, prophylaxis of anthrax with a non-penicillin antimicrobial (ciprofloxacin—see below) is recommended in the setting of biological threats.

As mentioned earlier, the Food and Drug Administration has approved ciprofloxacin (Cipro®) as the antimicrobial agent of choice to respond to and manage the intentional use of anthrax as a biological agent for post-exposure prophylaxis in people exposed to inhaled anthrax. Ciprofloxacin is indicated for reducing the incidence or progression of inhalational anthrax following exposure to aerosolized Bacillus anthracis, the bacterium that causes anthrax.

The recommended adult dose of ciprofloxacin for post-exposure inhalational anthrax is 500 mg given orally twice daily. The recommended pediatric dose of ciprofloxacin for post-exposure inhalational anthrax is 15 mg/kg given orally twice daily. The adult intravenous dose is 400 mg BID; the pediatric intravenous dose is 10 mg/kg BID.

It is imperative that prophylaxis with ciprofloxacin should begin as soon as possible after suspected exposure and the drug should be administered for 60 days. The most common adverse drug reactions from ciprofloxacin include nausea, vomiting, diarrhea, abdominal pain, rash, headache, and restlessness. It should be emphasized that in patients who have received ciprofloxacin for 60 days or longer, no new or unexpected adverse reactions were identified, as compared with patients receiving shorter courses of approved regimens.

Tetracycline and erythromycin have been used for patients who are allergic to penicillin. Induction of resistance to these antibiotics is an easy exercise in genetic manipulation and warfare strains should be presumed to be resistant to these antibiotics until proven otherwise. The logistics of trying to provide antibiotics to tens or thousands or even hundreds of thousands of people who might have been exposed to anthrax would be a formidable challenge. As a result, military clinics, disaster response centers, major medical centers, and pharmacy warehouses should maintain adequate inventories of approved antimicrobials such as ciprofloxacin as part of a preparedness strategy.

Prophylaxis. Anthrax has little potential for person-to-person spread. Standard infection precautions are all that is required for safe treatment of these patients. Anthrax has an incubation period of more than 24 hours and requires a rather large exposure to produce infection. This means that decontamination is not necessary in most patients. If there is a known exposure to dust or powder that contains anthrax spores, then decontamination may be appropriate.

Two types of anthrax vaccine for human use are available in the United States and United Kingdom, albeit in totally insufficient quantities for a civilian BW challenge. Both are based on the partially purified protective antigen of B. anthracis absorbed to an aluminum adjuvant. The usual immunization series is six 0.5 mL doses over a span of 18 months. The military feels that a primary series of three 0.5 mL doses (0, 2, and 4 weeks) will be protective against both cutaneous and inhalation anthrax for about six months after the primary series.[46] These immunizations were given to many coalition troops during the Gulf War in anticipation of Saddam Hussein's employment of this agent. Large quantities of antigen are presumed to be stockpiled for military use since this agent has been a recurring threat.

Unless civilian immunizations start about one month prior to a terrorist attack, EMS and medical providers will be essentially unprotected. Post exposure chemoprophylaxis to all exposed persons is appropriate when anthrax exposure is confirmed. If appropriate antibiotics are available, these antibiotics should be given for four weeks or until protection is achieved with three doses of the vaccine.[43]

Although minor reactions to the vaccine are common (6% of immunized population), major reactions are uncommon. Obviously, the vaccine is contraindicated for those who are known to be sensitive to it and those who have already had clinical anthrax. The choice between immunization and some allergic reaction and no immunization in the face of a serious biowarfare threat will present a difficult clinical dilemma. The vaccine has not been evaluated for safety and efficacy in children younger than 18 years or adults older than 60 years.[46] If there is true exposure to anthrax, the risk of anthrax may well be much more compelling than the risks posed by vaccination in these age groups.

A live anthrax vaccine is used in Russia to immunize both livestock and human beings. It is a spore vaccine with both STI-1 and strain 3 mixtures. The Russians feel that this vaccine is superior at stimulating cell-mediated immunity[47] There would be considerable resistance to use of the Russian vaccine in Western countries because of concerns about purity and residual virulence of a live vaccine.

There is no available evidence that these vaccines will adequately protect against an aerosol challenge. New vaccines with a highly purified protective antigen or designer attenuated strains have both been used in laboratories but are not commercially available.[48,49]

Antibiotic prophylaxis with ciprofloxacin (500 mg PO bid), or doxycycline (100 mg PO bid) is also recommended by the U.S. military for imminent attack by a biological weapon. Should the attack be confirmed as anthrax, then antibiotics should be continued for at least 60 days for all who are exposed. Those exposed should also be started on anti-anthrax vaccine with the standard schedule (if it is available), if they have not been previously immunized. Those who have received fewer than three doses of vaccine prior to exposure should receive a single booster injection. If vaccine is not available, then antibiotics should be continued until the patient can be safely and closely observed after the antibiotics are discontinued. (Inhaled spores are not destroyed by antibiotics and may persist beyond the course of antibiotics recommended.) Animal carcasses should be burned, not buried, to prevent long-term environmental contamination. Human remains should be cremated.

Smallpox

Perhaps the worst-case scenario in bioterrorism in terms of both immediate consequences and the potential for secondary and further generations of infection is exposure to smallpox. Most physicians in practice have received lectures about the disease and many will remember being immunized; however, few have hadSignificant experience in diagnosis, and even fewer have seen even one case of illness in the past 40 years. Therefore, the potential for the failure of physicians to recognize this disease in its first wave is great, allowing the propagation of further waves of infection.

Epidemiology and Clinical Features of Smallpox. Transmission of smallpox to humans may occur via fomites, but the risk of infection is greatest when aerosolized particles enter the respiratory tract. Following an incubation period of 12-14 days, symptoms begin with the abrupt onset of chills, fever, malaise, vomiting, headache, backache, and occasionally mental status changes or an erythematous macular rash. After 2-3 more days, an enanthem and discrete papular rash of the face, hands, and arms begin, later spreading to the legs and finally the trunk.[7] The papules evolve into vesicles and finally pustules as fever and pain persist. Most lesions develop on the face and extremities and all are synchronous, that is, in the same phase of development at a given time. The pustules form scabs that are infectious until separation, and form deep, depigmented scars.[7]

Mortality from smallpox is 3% among vaccinated persons and 30% overall among those unvaccinated.[8] Among those with a secondary bacterial pneumonia, mortality rises to 50%.[9] Death usually occurs in the second week of illness, although 5-10% of cases with a more fulminant course progress to death within seven days. It is absolutely critical to distinguish smallpox from primary varicella, or chickenpox. As opposed to smallpox, the lesions of chickenpox are more superficial and appear in crops or waves and thus are asynchronous in development, with groups of vesicles, pustules, and scabs appearing adjacent to one another. The lesions of chickenpox are clustered much more densely over the trunk and do not appear on palms or soles.[7] Also to be distinguished are monkeypox, which typically causes cervical and inguinal adenopathy, and skin eruptions from exposures to certain drugs or skin contact agents, such as erythema multiforme and allergic dermatitis.[9]

Postexposure Management. Any person exposed to smallpox should be immunized immediately with either the calf-lymph-derived or cell culture vaccine developed by the Department of Defense.[9] Vaccination against smallpox is effective in preventing death if given up to five days after exposure and in preventing illness if given within 72 hours. Quarantine of those exposed should continue for 17 days, as they may transmit infection asymptomatically through oral and pharyngeal secretions.[9]

Treatment. There are currently no agents with proven efficacy against active smallpox infection in humans. Treatment of active smallpox might be attempted with cidofovir, an agent with activity against many pox viruses; three other agents, adefovir dipivoxide, cyclic cidofovir, and ribavirin, may also be candidates for use in this setting.[9]

Botulism

On a per gram basis, botulinum toxin is one of the most toxic substances known. Practitioners are perhaps most familiar with botulism as a food-borne illness from instruction in microbiology and the immediate attention the illness receives following consumption of prepared food or restaurant exposure. However, natural clinical illness may also follow exposure from wounds or ingestion of certain uncooked food products by infants.

Epidemiology and Clinical Features of Infection. Botulinum toxin causes illness in humans by binding to presynaptic nerve endings and blocking acetylcholine release, thus interrupting neurotransmission and causing weakness of muscles supplied by the affected nerves.[18] While natural intoxication most often follows ingestion, the inhalation route is expected to be the target of bioterrorists.[9] Symptoms will begin within 24-36 hours to several days of respiratory exposure, depending on the magnitude of the dose,[19,20] starting with abnormalities of cranial nerve function. These manifest by ocular symptoms, with blurred and double vision as well as light-induced pain; disordered speech, as evidenced by articulation problems, hoarseness, and trouble swallowing; and a descending, symmetrical,skeletal muscle paralysis.[9]

The clinical examination of persons with botulism reveals them to be alert, awake, and oriented, with no fever or sensory findings. Involvement of the autonomic nervous system may be evidenced by orthostatic hypotension. Eyes may show disconjugate gaze, pupillary dilatation, and eyelid drooping. The gag reflex is absent. Constipation and urinary retention are common.[21] Cyanosis with advancing respiratory compromise signals severe impairment of phrenic nerve function and the need for immediate ventilatory support. Fortunately, less than 5% of cases are fatal if adequate treatment of respiratory failure is instituted promptly.[9]

A variety of clinical conditions may be confused with botulism. Guillain-Barre syndrome typically causes an ascending paralysis with notable sensory findings and elevated protein in the cerebrospinal fluid. Myasthenia gravis is usually, but not always, distinguished by a positive edrophonium (Tensilon) test, has a typical electromyographic profile, and induces antibodies to acetylcholine receptors. Additionally, the Eaton-Lambert syndrome, acute poliomyelitis, tick paralysis, diphtheria, hypermagnesemia, and mushroom or chemical intoxications all may induce similar neurologic manifestations and may be confused with botulism.[21]

Prophylactic Management. The horse-serum-derived antitoxin against botulism is most effective if given immediately postexposure, before the appearance of clinical symptoms,[19] though in clinical practice such opportunities rarely arise. A trivalent antitoxin is available from the CDC and a heptavalent product developed by the U.S. Army of as-yet-undetermined efficacy in humans[19] is available as an investigational new drug.

Treatment of Cases. Treatment of active botulism involves the use of the equine antitoxin if the disease is in a phase of progression. For treatment of one or a small number of cases, direct contact of the CDC for release of antitoxin is most efficient. If large quantities are required, local, regional, or national stockpiles will need to be tapped. All antitoxin products are of equine origin, so skin testing should be done first to avoid the occurrence of anaphylaxis or serum sickness.

Tularemia

Named for the first recognition of clinical cases from Tulare County, California, tularemia is an organism understandably feared by microbiologists for its potential to cause infection of laboratory workers via aerosolization. An endemic infectious disease primarily of the western United States, tularemia is a well-known risk for hunters and persons venturing into wilderness areas. Its ability to cause severe disease following respiratory exposure has made it a target for biological weapons developers.

Epidemiology and Clinical Features of Infection. The forms of Francisella tularensis infection recognized in humans include glandular/ulceroglandular/oculoglandular, pulmonary, gastrointestinal, and typhoidal. These result from direct penetration of the skin or exposure of mucous membranes with blood or tissue of infected animals or indirectly from bites of deerflies, ticks, or mosquitoes; inhalation; or ingestion of contaminated food or water.

The typhoidal and pulmonary forms result primarily from aerosol exposures.[22] After an incubation period of 2-10 days, patients present with fever, headache, myalgias, weight loss, fatigue, but no lymphadenopathy.[23-25] Chest pain, nonproductive cough, and Pneumonia with pleural effusions may occur. Radiographically, such infection may result in patchy, lobar, or cavitary infiltrates; mortality in such cases that go untreated is about 35%.[23,26] Despite evident pulmonary involvement, secondary human-human transmission is unusual. High fever, meningitis, hepatitis, endocarditis, osteomyelitis, and septic shock may occur in the final stages of typhoidal tularemia.

The differential diagnosis of pulmonary tularemia should include all the atypical pneumonias, including psittacosis, Legionellosis, Q fever, mycoplasma, and C. pneumoniae infections.[22]

Treatment of Clinical Cases. Beta lactam antibiotics are not ineffective in tularemia. The drug of choice for severe infections is streptomycin given 30 mg/kg/d IM in two divided doses for 10-14 days.[27] Gentamicin may also be used.[25,28]

Plague

A well-recognized risk for residents of the four corners region of the Southwest and contiguous areas, Yersinia pestis is thought of in this country primarily as a flea-borne illness and is perhaps easiest to recognize in its bubonic form. Sometimes a complication of other routes of exposure, the pneumonic form is transmissible from person to person and could result in secondary infection following a bioterrorist event.

Epidemiology and Clinical Features of Infection. Three forms of plague infection are recognized in the human host: 1) Bubonic, transmitted by the bite of infected fleas, leading to regional lymph node infection with pain, tenderness, swelling, and, rarely, to meningitis; 2) Septicemia, beginning commonly with gastrointestinal symptoms, then proceeding to systemic symptoms with disseminated intravascular coagulation (DIC), adult respiratory distress syndrome (ARDS), and circulatory collapse; and 3) Pneumonic, the form following respiratory exposure and that most likely to be targeted by a bioterrorist attack.[30,31]

Following an incubation period of 2-3 days, primary respiratory infection with plague bacilli causes the rapid onset of fever, chills, malaise, myalgia, and headache and an acute pneumonia syndrome, accompanied by chest pain, dyspnea, and cough.9 Sputum production is usually watery and blood-tinged, but may be frankly bloody.[32] Therefollows a rapid progression to respiratory failure and shock. The chest x-ray of pneumonic plague victims shows patchy or consolidated airspace disease with involvement of a single lobe or multiple lobes on both sides of the chest; cavitation of the pneumonia may be evident early on in the course of disease.[32]

Treatment of Clinical Cases. Pneumonic plague is fatal if not treated in the first 24 hours. Appropriate antibiotic therapy includes streptomycin 30 mg/kg IM per day in two divided doses or gentamicin IV for 10 days. IV chloramphenicol may be given for plague meningitis or in sepsis syndrome. IV doxycycline (100 mg every 12 hours for 10-14 days, after an initial oading dose of 200 mg) is also effective.[9]

Postexposure Prophylaxis. Unfortunately, there is no proven benefit of the plague vaccine against pneumonic infection.[33] Exposed individuals should be treated prophylactically with 100 mg of doxycyline orally every 12 hours for seven days.[9]

Brucellosis

Epidemiology and Clinical Presentation of Illness. Human brucellosis may occur following enteric, percutaneous, or respiratory exposure, and subsequent patterns of illness are similar in all forms of infection. This fact reflects the distribution of these intracellular organisms to macrophages in bone, joints, brain, liver, spleen, and lung, and accounts for the wide range of involved systems and the protean manifestations of illness. After an incubation period ranging from 5-60 days, fever, chills, diaphoresis, headache, myalgia, fatigue, anorexia, joint and low back pain, weight loss, constipation, sore throat, or dry cough are common.[34]

Although respiratory symptoms of cough and pleuritic chest pain occur in 20% of patients, overt pneumonia is uncommon.9 Skeletal involvement is evidenced by osteomyelitis of the vertebrae as well as by major joint infections including the knees, hips, shoulders, and sacroiliac joints.[35-37] While bone marrow involvement with declines in all hematopoietic cell lines, hepatitis, and genitourinary tract infections may also occur, most fatalities result from CNS infection and endocarditis, which occur in only 5% of untreated patients.[38] Symptoms may persist for weeks to months, but most patients will eventually recover within a year, regardless of treatment[39]; however, subsequent relapses are frequent.

Treatment of Clinical Cases. The treatment of choice for severe brucellosis (bone, joint, heart, CNS infection) is a combination of doxycycline (100 mg b.i.d.) plus an aminoglycoside for four weeks, followed by the same dose of doxycycline plus rifampin 600-900 mg/d for six weeks.[40,41]

Postexposure Prophylaxis. The latter regimen may be used as prophylaxis for three weeks following recognized exposure. At present, no vaccine is licensed in the United States for prevention of brucellosis among high-risk individuals.[9]

Off-Label Use of Therapeutic Agents—A Cautionary Note. It should be stressed that many bioterrorist-mediated infections are rare and fatal. Therefore, it is virtually impossible to conduct rigorous, controlled studies in humans evaluating the safety and efficacy of antimicrobial agents. As a result, some agents (i.e., spectinomycin) may not carry formal FDA indications for bioterrorist-mediated infections (i.e., tularemia), although they are still considered by military and infectious disease experts—and according to accepted general medical practice standards—as the agents of choice for managing specific infections. However, to ensure that the highest clinical standards are being met, clinicians and pharmacists are strongly advised to review formal indications for specific agents cited in this review. When antimicrobials are recommended for treatment, clinicians should review their specific indications. When agents do not have formal FDA approval, it is advised that infectious disease experts—as well as such bodies as the Centers for Disease Control and the Food and Drug Administration—be consulted for clarification and/or current strategies for optimal therapy.

Summary

A bioterrorist attack against Americans could result in morbidity and mortality on a scale unknown to this nation since the influenza pandemic of 1918-1919. The inclusion of emergency medicine specialists, pharmacists, military personnel, CDC epidemilogists and planners, and primary care clinicians as first responders in strategic planning for the defense against bioterrorism is essential.

It is imperative that the nation's professional organizations, academic health centers, and governmental agencies work together to ensure the appropriate education of clinicians at all levels of training to reduce the likelihood of catastrophic consequences of such an event. Stockpiling of appropriate antimicrobials and vaccines represents prudent response to such a threat.

(Editor's Note: For more information about the CDC's Bioterrorism Preparedness and Response Program, visit their Web site at: http://www.bt.cdc.gov/index.asp. Or, contact: Centers for Disease Control and Prevention, 1600 Clifton Road, Atlanta, GA 30333. Telephone: (404) 639-3311.)

References

1. Christopher GW, et al. Biological warfare: A historical perspective. *JAMA* 1997;278:412-417.
2. Alibek K. Biohazard. New York, NY: Random House; 1999:107-122.
3. Henderson DA. Bioterrorism as a public health threat. *Emerg Infect Dis* 1998;4:488-492. www.cdc.gov/ncidod/eid/vol4no3/hendersn.htm.
4. Centers for Disease Control. Statement of Richard Jackson, MD, MPH, Director, National Center for Environmental Health, CDC, DHHS, before the Subcommittee on Labor, HHS, and Education Committee on Appropriations, US Senate, June 2, 1998. URL:www.cdc.gov/ncidod/diseases/jackson.htm.
5. Torok TJ, et al. A large community outbreak of salmonellosis caused by intentional contamination of restaurant salad bars. *JAMA* 1997;278:389-395.
6. Centers for Disease Control and Prevention. Bioterrorism alleging use of anthrax and interim guidelines for management'United States, 1998. *MMWR Morb Mortal Wkly Rep* 1999;48:69-74.
7. Henderson DA. Smallpox: Clinical and epidemiologic features. *Emerg Infect Dis* 1999; 5:537-539.
8. Fenner F, et al. Smallpox and its Eradication. Geneva: World Health Organization 1988:1341.
9. Franz DR, et al. Clinical recognition and management of patients exposed to biological warfare agents. *JAMA* 1997; 278:399-411.
10. Centers for Disease Control and Prevention. Summary of notifiable diseases, US, 1997. *MMWR Morb Mortal Wkly Rep* 1998;46:3-87.
11. Brachman PS, Friedlander AM. Anthrax. In: Plotkin SA, Mortimer EA Jr., eds. Vaccines. Philadelphia, PA: WB Saunders 1994:729-739.
12. Friedlander AM. Anthrax. In: Zajtchuk R, ed. Textbook of Military Medicine: Medical Aspects of Chemical and Biological Warfare. Washington, DC: U.S. Department of the Army, Surgeon General, and the Borden Institute 1997:467-478.
13. Brachman PS. Inhalation anthrax. *Ann NY Acad Sci* 1980; 353:83-93.
14. Abramova FA, et al. Pathology of inhalational anthrax in 42 cases from the Sverdlovsk outbreak of 1979. *Proc Natl Acad Sci USA* 1993;90:2291-2294.
15. Dutz W, Kohout E. Anthrax. *Pathol Annu* 1971;6:209-248.
16. Cieslak TJ, Eitzen EM Jr. Clinical and epidemiologic principles of anthrax. *Emerg Infect Dis* 1999;5:552-555.
17. Friedlander AM, et al. Postexposure prophylaxis against experimental inhalation anthrax. *J Infect Dis* 1993;167:1239-1243.
18. Simpson LL. Peripheral actions of the botulinum toxins. In: Simpson LL, ed. Botulinum Neurotoxin and Tetanus Toxin. New York, NY: Academic Press, Inc. 1989:153-178.
19. Franz DR, et al. Efficacy of prophylactic and therapeutic administration of antitoxin for inhalation botulism. In: Das Gupta B, ed. *Botulinum and Tetanus Neurotoxin and Biomedical Aspects.* New York, NY: Plenum Press 1993:473-476.
20. Middlebrook JL. Contributions of the U.S. Army to botulinum toxin research. In: Das Gupta B, ed. *Botulinum and Tetanus Neurotoxin and Biomedical Aspects.* New York, NY: Plenum Press 1993:515-519.
21. Abrutyn E. Botulism. In: Fauci AS, et al, eds. *Harrison's Principles of Internal Medicine.* 14th ed. New York, NY: McGraw Hill 1998: 904-906.
22. Jacobs RF. Tularemia. In: Fauci AS, et al, eds. *Harrison's Principles of Internal Medicine.* 14th ed. New York, NY: McGraw Hill 1998: 971-975.
23. Evans ME, et al. Tularemia: A 30-year experience with 88 cases. *Medicine* 1985;64:251-269.
24. McCrumb FR, Jr. Aerosol infection of man with Pasteurella tularensis. *Bacteriol Rev* 1961;25:262-267.
25. Miller RP, Bates JH. Pleuropulmonary tularemia. A review of 29 patients. *Am Rev Respir Dis* 1969;99:31-41.
26. Evans ME, Friedlander AM. Tularemia. In: Zajtchuk R, ed. Textbook of Military Medicine: Medical Aspects of Chemical and Biological Warfare. Washington, DC: U.S. Dept. of the Army, The Surgeon General, and the Borden Institute 1997:503-512.
27. Penn RZL. Francisella tularensis (tularemia). In: Mandell GA, et al, eds. *Principles and Practices of Infectious Diseases.* New York, NY: Churchill Livingstone, Inc 1995:2060-2078.
28. Sawyer WD, et al. Antibiotic prophylaxis and therapy of airborne tularemia. *Bacterial Rev* 1966;80:542-548.
29. Burke DS. Immun. against tularemia. *J Infect Dis* 1997; 135:55-60.
30. Butler T. *Plague and Other Yersinia Infections.* New York, NY: Plenum Press, 1983.
31. McGovern TW, Friedlander AM. Plague. In: Zajtchuk R, ed. *Textbook of Military Medicine Medical Aspects of Chemical and Biological Warfare.* Washington, DC: U.S. Dept. of the Army, Surgeon General, and the Borden Institute 1997:479-508.
32. Campbell GL. Plague. In: Fauci AS, et al, eds. *Harrison's Principles of Internal Medicine.* 14th ed. New York: McGraw Hill 1998:975-980.
33. Cavanaugh DC, et al. Plague immunization. *J Infect Dis* 1974; 129:S37-S40.
34. Madkour M. Brucellosis. In: Fauci AS, et al, eds. *Harrison's Principles of Internal Medicine.* 14th ed. New York, NY: McGraw Hill 1998:969-971.
35. Gotuzzo E, et al. Articular involvement in human brucellosis: Retrospective analysis of 304 cases. *Semin Arthritis Rheum* 1982;12:245-255.
36. Mousa AR, et al. Osteoarticular complications of brucellosis: A study of 169 cases. *Rev Infect Dis* 1987;9:531-543.
37. Ariza J, et al. Brucellar spondylitis: A detailed analysis based on current findings. *Rev Infect Dis* 1985;7:656-664.
38. Peery TM, Belter LF. Brucellosis and heart disease. *Am J Pathol* 1960;36:673-697.
39. Evans AC. Comments on the early history of human brucellosis. In: Larson CH, Soule MH, eds. Brucellosis. Baltimore, MD: Waverly Press 1950:1-8.
40. Luzzi GA, et al. Brucellosis. *Trans R Soc Trop Med Hyg* 1993; 87:138-141.
41. Joint FAO/WHO expert committee on brucellosis. *World Health Organ Tech Rep Ser* 1986;740:1-132.
42. Harrison LH, Ezzell JW, Abshire TG, et al. Evaluation of serologic tests for diagnosis of anthrax after an outbreak of cutaneous anthrax in Paraguay. *J Infect Dis* 1989;160:
43. Centers for Disease Control and Prevention: Bioterrorism alleging use of anthrax and interim guidelines for management - United States 1998. *MMWR Morb Mortal Wkly Rep* 1999;48:69-74.
44. Swanson ER, Fosnocht DE. Anthrax threats: A report of two inci-

dents from Salt Lake City. *J Emerg Med* 2000;18:229-232.

45. Personal interviews during visit to University of Urals, Ekatrinburg, 1996.
46. Friedlander AM, Pittman PR, Parker GW. Anthrax vaccine: Evidence for safety and efficacy against inhalational anthrax. *JAMA* 1999;282:2104-2106.
47. Shlyakhov EN, Rubinstein E. Human live anthrax vaccine in the former USSR. *Vaccine* 1994;12:727-730.

Volatile Substance Abuse

Earl J. Reisdorff, MD, FACEP
Mary Beth Miller, DO

Although volatile substance abuse (VSA) with toluene, aromatic hydrocarbons, or butane does not make the same splashy headlines as the recreational abuse of cocaine, marijuana, or heroin, the problems associated with solvent inhalation are potentially destructive and must be recognized by the emergency practitioner. *(Please see Table 1.)*

Although most abusers of solvent substances never access the emergency department (ED) for medical attention, severe cases of volatile substance abuse can produce ventricular fibrillation, asphyxiation, noncardiogenic pulmonary edema, and various neuropsychiatric syndromes. Considering that volatile substances capable of producing euphoria and intoxication are so ubiquitous that they can be found in such common household products as glue, typewriter correction fluid, and cigarette lighters, it is not surprising that up to 20% of American high school students have reported experimentation with these types of "recreational" substances.[1]

This chapter presents a clinically useful outline of the demographic patterns associated with VSA as well as a substance-by-substance discussion of the clinical manifestations and toxicological consequences of acute and chronic abuse. A detailed discussion of the presenting signs and symptoms as well as the potential life-threatening cardiac complications associated with solvent inhalation will prepare the ED physician to treat patients who present with volatile substance abuse syndromes.

Background

Solvents are volatile hydrocarbons that evaporate rapidly at room temperature. These chemicals are absorbed into the blood through the lungs. Because solvents are extremely lipid soluble, they rapidly enter organs with a high fat content, including the brain. Metabolism and excretion are determined by the type of agent inhaled. Most agents are excreted directly through the lungs, although isolated substances are excreted in the urine after hepatic metabolism. For example, methylene chloride is metabolized in the liver, producing carbon monoxide. Carbon monoxide binds avidly to hemoglobin and is slowly excreted during respiration. Some inhalants, such as freons, leave the body through respiration essentially unchanged.

The abuse of inhaled solvents is most appropriately called volatile substance abuse (VSA). It should be stressed that many other drugs of abuse, including marijuana, cocaine, and methamphetamine, are also inhaled for their stimulatory effects. Even fentanyl patches have been heated and the vapors inhaled for illicit purposes. These drugs, however, are not solvents, and therefore do not share the same chemical and physical properties of commonly abused inhalant agents.

From a clinical perspective, VSA involves solvents that readily vaporize at room temperature. Because inhalants are inexpensive, readily found in the home, and can be legally purchased by people of all ages in some states, the potential for VSA is significant. With the

Table 1. Warning Signs of Substance Abuse

- sudden increase or decrease in appetite
- weight loss or gain
- anorexia
- increased pulse rate, blood pressure, diaphoresis, fever
- flushed face
- nystagmus
- abdominal pain/muscular ache
- rhinitis/rhinorrhea
- photophobia
- dilated or constricted pupils
- ataxia
- odor of alcohol
- fatigue
- recurrent trauma
- poor hygiene/grooming
- depression/isolation
- mood swings
- tearfulness
- irritability
- anxiety
- agitation
- talkativeness/rapid speech
- sleep problems
- daytime drowsiness
- resisting medication
- demanding medication
- cheeking medication (Certain patients may tend to hide pills in their buccal mucosa crevices rather than swallow them, then retrieve them and accumulate them for a later "high.")
- frequent visits to doctor to obtain medications for insomnia, anxiety, tension, vague pain
- persistent pain after tissue repair
- trouble concentrating
- impaired learning skills
- distraction
- confusion
- suicidal ideation
- verbal or physical threats
- desire to hurt others or self
- angry outbursts
- destruction of property
- legal problems

exception of the nitrite group (e.g., amyl nitrite), abused inhalants have potent psychoactive properties.

Commonly abused agents include typewriter correction fluid (trichloroethane), gasoline, toluene, nitrites, and acetone (nail polish remover). In addition, such ordinary household products as all-purpose cleaning fluids, acrylic spray paints, paint thinners, model glue, and aerosol propellants (e.g., hair spray, room deodorizers, insecticides, and deodorants) also have abuse potential. Other agents that are frequently used for inducing psychoactive effects include "magic" marker and highlighter pens, lighter fluid, and antifreeze. Among Native American youths, gasoline is a commonly inhaled abuse agent.[2]

Epidemiology

Demographic Patterns. From a recreational perspective, solvents are inhaled for their inebriating effects, which range from lightheadedness and euphoria to disorientation and frank intoxication. The use of solvents as euphoria-inducing agents became widespread in the 1960s. In this regard, VSA became entrenched as a recreational pursuit in California with the advent of gasoline sniffing.[2] Soon thereafter, glue sniffing emerged as a common practice among adolescents, a practice that became widely reported in the United States and Great Britain.[3,4]

Although VSA extends into all demographic groups, it is most prevalent among urban adolescents of lower socioeconomic levels, especially among those individuals who have poor school performance.[3,4] Among adolescents in Mexico, there is a specific association between inhalant abuse and juvenile delinquency, with some studies reporting that 23% of Mexican juvenile offenders have used inhalants.[5] In fact, among eighth graders in certain geographic areas, VSA is more common than smoking marijuana. Not surprisingly, patterns of abuse are characterized by specific features. For example, VSA is frequently carried out in groups, primarily among adolescent boys.[6] In this setting, abuse of multiple agents is a common practice. A number of volatile substances may be passed around, or an inhalant may be used in combination with other drugs such as marijuana or alcohol.

Generally, VSA tends to be limited to brief periods of experimentation. However, some abusers continue this destructive practice well into adulthood, sometimes abusing a series of different drugs. There is a tendency for users to migrate from abuse of solvents to chronic ethanol abuse.[7] In fact, some studies suggest that inhalant abuse may be an independent risk factor for intravenous (IV) drug use. Even when adjusting for sex, age, race, socioeconomic status, and marijuana use, inhalant users were still 5.3 times more likely than nonusers to have injected drugs.[8]

Unfortunately, the prevalence of VSA is very difficult to quantitate, as are the actual number of deaths from the intentional inhalation of solvents. In England, however, the mortality rate from VSA appears to be increasing.[9] Between 1970 and 1991, 91 deaths were reported in Great Britain. During the period 1991 to 1993, 185 deaths were reported. Among these fatalities, 51% were caused by direct toxic effects from the inhalant. In addition, 21% of deaths were associated with asphyxia, 18% with aspiration, and 11% were caused by trauma-related circumstances (e.g., drowning, autoerotic strangulation).

Morbidity and Mortality Features. In the United States, the majority of deaths linked to VSA have been reported in males 15-19 years old.[10] Fuel gases (butane, propane, gasoline), trichloroethane (typewriter correction fluid, dry cleaning fluids), and freons (especially bromochromodifluoromethane found in yellow fire extinguishers) are responsible for 60% of these deaths.[10] Deaths can also occur from the unintentional inhalation of these agents, such as when a fire extinguisher is discharged inside of a battle tank.[11] Habitual abusers generally prefer toluene-based solvents for the high degree of euphoria that they allegedly produce. Another agent commonly found among abusers is gold acrylic spray paint. Gold acrylic spray paint is alleged to produce unique psychoactive effects not found in other colors of paint. Typewriter correction fluid (trichloroethane) is a popular substance of abuse among adolescents.

The National Institute of Drug Abuse's annual survey of high school graduates suggests a lifetime incidence of about 15-20%.[1] Although one British report suggests that as many as 13% of adolescents routinely abuse inhalants, a more recent study from England suggests that 3.5-10% of current adolescents have at least experimented with solvents.[12,13] One U.S. survey of 10,198 middle school and high school students showed a lifetime volatile substance usage rate of 12.8%, with 4.8% of students reporting they had used inhalants for a euphoric effect in the previous month. Interestingly, inhalant use increases during grades 6-8 and begins to decline in grades 10-12.[14] Since 1988, inhalant use has become more common than marijuana use among eighth graders.[15] Of all calls made to a regional poison center that originate in schools, 7% involve inhalant-related questions or problems.[16]

Attempts to curb VSA have met with variable success. Warning labels that indicate what materials are inhalants may actually serve to draw the abuser's attention to the product.[17] Some manufacturers have added mucosal irritants such as oil of mustard to deter abuse.

Methods of Abuse

Abuse of solvents occurs through three primary activities: sniffing, bagging, and huffing. *Sniffing* is the act of inhaling the solvent directly from an open container such as a can or jar. Gasoline is commonly abused in this manner. The *bagging* technique requires the solvent to be poured or sprayed into a bag (e.g., a potato chip bag). The bag is then placed over the mouth and nose and the person breathes deeply. Solvent vaporization is enhanced by shaking the plastic bag. As might be expected, bagging is the most dangerous method of inhalation, because increased solvent levels are achieved and hypoxia is more likely. Complications include suffocation, which can occur if the bag adheres to the face of a lethargic patient. Another danger is aspiration, which results if the person vomits into the bag. Despite these hazards, bagging is the preferred method of abuse since the highest amount of solvent vaporization is achieved. *Huffing* is the practice of inhaling vapors by placing a solvent-soaked cloth (e.g., a rag or sock) over the mouth and nose. One variant of huffing involves breathing fumes from solvent-soaked cotton balls that are placed in the reservoir of a dust protection mask or gas mask. This is particularly dangerous because of the high risk of hypoxia as well as vomiting and aspiration.

Toxicology and Clinical Effects

Overview. The toxicological and clinical effects of volatile substances are variable. The majority of inhalants can produce neurologic dysfunction, asphyxia, and cardiovascular abnormalities that range from rhythm disturbances to myocardial suppression. Typically, abusers can be expected to develop some degree of inebriation, ranging from mild euphoria to frank psychosis. Other clinical signs and symptoms include blurred vision, photophobia, tinnitus, slurred speech, headache, conjunctival injection, and abdominal pain. Transient hypertension, salivation, persistent sneezing and coughing, chest pain, and bronchospasm have also been described.

Cardiac arrhythmia is the primary cause of death from VSA. Other contributing mechanisms include myocardial sensitization to catecholamines, hypoxemia, respiratory depression, vagal stimulation, aspiration, laryngospasm (especially with butane inhalation), and associated trauma (e.g., drowning).[10]

Neurologic Manifestations. The primary effect of abused inhalants is central nervous system (CNS) depression. Predictably, an inebriated or intoxicated state is produced that is similar to that seen with ethanol or marijuana use. Initially, there is a state of euphoria that is quickly followed by progressive CNS depression. Other reported effects include excitement, tinnitus, slurred speech, bizarre behavior, syncope, and seizures. Visual and auditory hallucinations have been reported with gasoline, lighter fluid, and toluene use.

It is postulated that the euphoria accompanying VSA provides the psychological reinforcement that leads to long-term abuse. Whether or not VSA leads to physical addiction is unclear. Generally speaking, however, physical dependence characterized by a physical withdrawal syndrome has not been described for most volatile substances. One exception is toluene habituation, a syndrome in which sudden cessation of the solvent can produce a syndrome similar to that encountered with alcohol withdrawal. A similar withdrawal syndrome has been suggested for butane abuse.[18]

Patients suffering the acute effects of volatile substances usually appear drunk; consciousness is almost always clouded in moderate to severe inhalations. Typically, a state of inebriation occurs within a few seconds of inhalation. Hypoxia and hypercapnia, which result from bagging, accentuate the CNS depressive effects. Intoxication lasts from 10 minutes to three hours depending on the type of agent, the exposure concentration, the duration of exposure, and the rate of detoxification (metabolism) by the patient. It is possible to induce general anesthesia in humans with toluene after one minute of steady inhalation with high concentrations attained while bagging.

Long-term CNS effects related to solvent abuse—particularly in individuals with chronic toluene inhalation—include encephalopathy, cerebellar degeneration, and disorders of equilibrium.[19,20] Irreversible structural changes may also occur. For example, the neuropathologic effect in people who chronically sniff paint, so-called "spray heads," is neuronal demyelination. Because of their chemical properties, many solvents also have the capacity for "liquefying" fat. Because the brain is a lipid-rich organ, chronic solvent abuse essentially "dissolves" brain cells. This appears as brain atrophy and discoloration of cerebral and cerebellar white matter. Microscopic analysis reveals unique oval membrane-bound cytoplasmic bodies filled with inclusions.[21]

On neuroimaging studies, the manifestations of chronic paint sniffing appear as a loss of cerebral and cerebellar gray-white matter discrimination, scattered multifocal deep white-matter lesions, and gross generalized atrophy of the cerebrum, cerebellum, and the corpus callosum.[22] Specifically, MRI findings in chronic toluene abusers include abnormalities in the middle cerebellar peduncle and the cerebellar white matter. Lesions also are observed in the deep cerebral white matter, the posterior limb of the internal capsule, thalamus, and basal ganglia.[23]

In addition, VSA can produce a syndrome similar to Parkinson's disease. This complication occurs most often with lacquer thinner.[24] The symptoms can be indistinguishable for idiopathic parkinsonism (Parkinson's disease). Clinical findings may persist for months and, in some cases, respond to levodopa therapy.[24] Cerebral infarction and hemiplegia also have occurred as a result of vasospasm associated with VSA.[25] Peripheral neuropathies, such as those seen with hexane, can also occur.[26]

Other findings encountered in chronic inhalant abusers (particularly those who abuse toluene) include persistent paranoid psychosis and, perhaps, an increased risk of temporal lobe epilepsy.[27] In particular, ototoxicity has been associated with toluene.[28] Finally, poor school performance and behavioral disorders are associated with VSA. However, it is argued that many of the neuropsychiatric disturbances associated with VSA result from social disadvantages and a history of delinquency. When controlled for these variables, neuropsychiatric sequelae may not be a direct result of substance abuse.[29]

Pulmonary Complications. All solvents are simple asphyxiants. The vapor displaces oxygen from the alveoli and, in the process, decreases the amount of oxygen that is available to pass across the alveolar membrane and into the blood. In addition, the various practices by which solvents are inhaled (especially bagging) can exacerbate hypoxia. The hypoxic effect, by itself, is sufficient to cause death.[30]

Other pulmonary effects result primarily from direct alveolar damage. In this regard, inhalation of high concentrations of hydrocarbon vapors—especially toxic hydrocarbons—can produce severe chemical pneumonitis. Alveolar membrane damage can cause cardiogenic pulmonary edema, further exacerbating hypoxemia. In some cases, VSA can cause acute eosinophilic pneumonia. The clinical presentation is identical to idiopathic acute eosinophilic pneumonia and may require mechanical ventilation.[31]

Cardiovascular Effects. Cardiac arrhythmia is the most common cause of sudden, VSA-related mortality. Although the exact mechanism by which volatile abused substances produce arrhythmias is unclear, sensitization of the myocardium to endogenous catecholamines is a likely cause. Other factors that may have a role in the genesis of cardiac arrhythmias include electrolyte imbalances, hypoxia, acidosis, coronary artery spasm, and myocardial infarction.

A bizarre and, unfortunately, fatal phenomenon associated with VSA is called *sudden sniffing death*. In these cases, the affected individual typically acts startled, jumps up, runs about, and then collapses in ventricular fibrillation. This syndrome occurs without a subjective prodrome, giving the abuser no warning that death may occur. As a result, the substance abuser is unable to detect warning signs that might caution him or her to stop before the fatal event ensues. In Great Britain, sudden sniffing death syndrome is responsible for 55% of the deaths associated with VSA.[32] As an explanation for sudden sniffing death, it is theorized that the inhalants sensitize the myocardium to endogenous epinephrine. When the level of circulating epinephrine suddenly increases, such as when one is startled, the irritable myocardium fibrillates. The exact mechanism by which this occurs remains unknown.

Among commonly abused volatile substances, fluorinated hydrocarbons (freons) are commonly implicated as a cause of arrhythmias associated with VSA. Bretylium may have a theoretical advantage over other antiarrhythmics for treating ventricular fibrillation. Of the halogenated hydrocarbons, trichloroethane (typewriter correction fluid) is also known to precipitate fatal cardiac dysrhythmias. Acute myocardial infarction has occurred from coronary vasospasm caused by toluene sniffing. Finally, *glue sniffer's heart*, a dilated cardiomyopathy, can result from chronic VSA.

Miscellaneous Effects. Long-term toxic sequelae caused by VSA involve almost every organ system. Primary sites of injury include the liver, kidneys, central and peripheral nervous systems, and bone marrow. *(Please see Table 2.)* With respect to neuropsychiatric symptoms, chronic inhalant abuse can cause anorexia, listlessness, and extreme moodiness. Although somewhat rare, acute tubular necrosis, renal failure, glomerulonephritis, and nephrotic syndrome can also occur. The renal insult may result in permanent renal dysfunction.

Hepatic damage also occurs, especially in the setting of toluene, trichloroethylene, chloroform, and carbon tetrachloride abuse. Bone marrow depression, aplastic anemia, and leukemia are associated with sniffing certain glues,[33] whereas lead poisoning can develop from inhaling leaded gasoline. This is more common on Native American reservations where leaded gasoline is still widely available. Patients abusing acetone can present in a fashion similar to diabetic ketoacidosis; in these patients, however, the ketonemia is more pronounced than the acidosis.

Table 2. Long-Term Effects of Solvent Inhalation Abuse

CARDIOVASCULAR/HEMATOLOGIC
Aplastic anemia
Leukemia
Dilated cardiomyopathy ("glue sniffer's heart")
Dysrhythmia
RENAL
Glomerulonephritis
Goodpasture's syndrome
Renal tubular acidosis
Tubulointerstitial nephritis
Nephrotic syndrome
HEPATIC
Hepatic necrosis
Hepatic carcinomas
CENTRAL NERVOUS SYSTEM
Peripheral neuropathies
Dementia (organic brain syndrome)
Cerebellar degeneration, ataxia
Cranial nerve damage (oculomotor palsies, optic atrophy, deafness)
Parkinson-like syndrome, tremors, choreiform movements
Diffuse motor weakness, flaccid paralysis
Vestibular dysfunction, dizziness
Lead encephalopathy

Adapted from: Prendergast MC. Hydrocarbons and inhalants. In: Reisdorff EJ, Roberts MR, Wiegenstein JG. *Pediatric Emergency Medicine*. Philadelphia: W.B. Saunders Co; 1993:713.

Common Inhalants and Management Issues

Glue-Sniffing (Toluene). Generally speaking, only glues containing aromatic hydrocarbons (e.g., toluene) have the potential for abuse. As far as availability, toluene is found in household plastics, model cement, and lacquer thinner. It is an extremely potent neurotoxin and can produce a peripheral, sensorimotor neuropathy with a stocking-glove distribution. This is especially likely to occur when N-hexane is combined with toluene. Muscle weakness of the lower extremities has also occurred after sniffing pure toluene.[34] The dramatic clinical presentation of motor weakness associated with VSA can be confused with Guillain-Barré syndrome.[35]

Chronic toluene abuse can lead to permanent cerebellar ataxia, chronic encephalopathy, headaches, and personality changes. Toluene abuse during pregnancy has been implicated in intrauterine growth retardation, premature delivery, and congenital malformations (renal and skeletal).[36] Renal abnormalities linked to glue sniffing include nephrotic syndrome, nephritis, and renal tubular acidosis. Adult glue sniffers commonly present with neuropsychiatric disorders, gastrointestinal disorders, or muscle weakness. Toluene can also cause a hyperchloremia and acidosis accompanied by impaired urinary acidification.[34] The anion gap may be normal or elevated. Hypokalemia can be severe and contribute to both weakness and arrhythmias. Though some effects may be transitory, proximal and distal tubular dysfunction may persist.[34]

Gasoline. Gasoline abuse is frequently seen among the displaced native peoples in the United States, Canada, Mexico, South Africa, and Australia.[37] Gasoline is a complex mixture of hydrocarbons, some of which have powerful narcotic-like properties. Other unsaturated hydrocarbons contained in gasoline have anesthetic properties and can cause nausea, ataxia, and coma. While inhaling gasoline, the abuser may experience intense excitement followed by coma. Profound intoxication can cause marked respiratory depression and cardiac irritability that can be fatal.[38]

Abuse of gasoline usually involves inhalation directly from a can or glass jar. Intoxication occurs after 10-20 breaths and lasts for 3-5 hours. Intoxication is frequently accompanied by nausea and vomiting, which increases the risk of aspiration during the inebriated state. Where "leaded" gas is still available, lead toxicity can occur. The primary additive is tetraethyl lead. Tetraethyl lead and its metabolites are extremely neurotoxic and can produce a syndrome of ataxia, tremor, and encephalopathy in chronic users.[39,40]

Butane. Butane is the major flammable ingredient of cigarette lighter refills, camping stoves, and small blowtorches. It is commonly mixed with propane and can cause toxicity as a result of simple asphyxiation. The gas from cigarette lighter refills is released by using the teeth to press the nozzle. This practice can easily cause a fire, resulting in orofacial burns and laryngoedema.

Halogenated Hydrocarbons. Halogenated hydrocarbons include chlorinated as well as fluorinated hydrocarbons (freons). Chlorinated hydrocarbons include carbon tetrachloride, trichloroethane , and trichloroethylene. These agents initially cause euphoria and a sense of excitement that is promptly followed by headache, dizziness, nausea, and vomiting. Intoxication can eventually lead to stupor, coma, and seizures. Typewriter correction fluid, which contains 52% trichloroethane, is one of the most commonly abused substances among teenagers. Of special concern is the fact that chlorinated hydrocarbons cause acute renal failure and hepatic necrosis. Since the hepatic damage is centrilobular, N-acetylcysteine (Mucomyst) has been suggested as a possible treatment modality. Its effectiveness in this setting, however, is unproven. Trichloroethylene causes optic nerve atrophy and cranial nerve damage.

Freons, which are responsible for an alarming number of VSA-related deaths, can produce ventricular dysrhythmias including ventricular fibrillation. Freons have been used extensively as propellants and in cooling systems such as refrigerators and air-conditioning units. They are also used in yellow fire extinguishers and in some upholstery protection agents. In one reported case, a 15-year-old boy developed ventricular fibrillation after intentionally inhaling freon from an automobile air conditioner recharge unit. Cardiopulmonary resuscitation was started, and, after administering bretylium, a sinus tachycardia resulted; neurologic recovery was complete.[41]

Methylene Chloride. Methylene chloride, which has been associated with a unique constellation of problems, is commonly found in paint thinners and is metabolized by the liver to carbon monoxide. Although the primary toxic effects result directly from the agent, the amount of carbon monoxide produced is significant and can adversely affect an already compromised patient.[42] As opposed to exposure by direct inhalation, carbon monoxide is produced even after removal from the source of exposure and has a half-life 2.5 times that of inhaled carbon monoxide at room air.[43] The toxic effects of carbon monoxide, such as hemoglobin binding, myoglobin binding (including cardiac myoglobin), and suppression of mitochondrial respiration, can further exacerbate the effect of the parent compound.

Nitrous Oxide. Nitrous oxide was first used as an inhalational anesthetic and is still used as an anesthetic-analgesic. It is used commercially in the cartridges for whipped cream dispensers. Referred to as *whippets* among the drug culture, these can be obtained legally. Whippets are used for their mild intoxicating effects. The primary clinical concern associated with nitrous oxide is its propensity for causing fatal hypoxia. Chronic abuse may cause demyelination and neuropathy.

Nitrites. Although nitrites are commonly abused inhalants, they are neither solvents nor are they psychoactive agents. Their primary effects are cardiovascular (vasodilation). In fact, since 1867, amyl nitrite had been used medicinally to relieve angina pectoris. Slang terms for nitrites are *bullet*, *hardware*, *lightning bolt*, *locker room*, *rush*, *sweat*, and *thrust*. Amyl nitrite pearls are found in cyanide treatment kits and are called *poppers* or *snappers*. Amyl nitrite is available in cotton-wrapped ampules designed to be crushed, and then inhaled. Patients describe feeling light-headed and having a throbbing, vascular, migraine-like headache.

Nitrites can cause methemoglobinemia, cyanosis, and hypotension. Though the methemoglobinemia usually results from *ingestion* of amyl, butyl, or isobutyl nitrites, inhalation of amyl nitrite can cause symptomatic methemoglobin levels.[44] Fatal methemoglobinemia from inhalation of isobutyl nitrite has also been reported.[45] Methemoglobinemia is managed by administering methylene blue in an initial dose of 2 mg/kg IV push over 3-5 minutes. Inhaling volatile nitrites has also caused hemolytic anemia.[46]

Nitrites are frequently abused by homosexual men, who use the drug for its alleged aphrodisiac effects. The drug reportedly causes relaxation in the anal sphincter. Amyl nitrite does cause some smooth muscle relaxation. Some studies suggest a tenuous association between the HIV virus and nitrite abuse in the clinical expression of AIDS. Clearly, however, abuse of nitrite inhalants has been epidemiologically associated with Kaposi's sarcoma.[47] Transient, reversible hematologic and immune suppression are seen with inhalational exposure to isobutyl nitrite.[48,49]

Clinical Assessment and Differential Diagnoses

There are no clear identifying features of VSA, nor does the clinical presentation follow any distinct toxidrome pattern. In the ED, the patient appears inebriated. The odor of gasoline or solvents on the

Table 3. Selected Inhalants and Solvents

SOLVENT	SOURCE	SPECIAL FEATURES	TREATMENT CONSIDERATIONS
Butane	Cigarette lighter refills	burns, laryngeal edema laryngospasm	airway protection burn care
Gasoline (leaded)	—	contains tetraethyl-lead	consider use of Dimercaprol (BAL)
Methylene chloride	paint stripper	metabolized to carbon monoxide	100% oxygen, prolonged observation
Nitrites	ampules	may cause methemoglobinemia	Methylene blue 2 mg/kg IV
Trichloroethane	typewriter correction fluid	centrilobular liver necrosis	consider use of N-acetylcysteine (Mucomyst)

hair, breath, or clothing may suggest the diagnosis. Because many solvents are excreted through the lungs, the odor of solvents is strongest on the breath, where it may be detected for hours.[50]

On physical examination, the midface may be marked with an acrylic paint, typewriter correction fluid, or glue. An erythematous rash may be present around the mouth as a result of repetitive inhalation. This is commonly referred to as *glue sniffer's rash*. EMS personnel, family, or friends may report empty adhesive tubes, aerosol spray cans, cigarette lighter refills, or potato chip bags at the scene.[51] Patients may present with thermal burns, denying that an errant episode of solvent abuse led to the injury.

If the aforementioned clinical clues are lacking, a thorough, systematic search to uncover the etiology of the patient's altered mental status must be initiated. Metabolic, infectious, traumatic, or drug-induced causes should be excluded.

Emergency Management

The primary treatment for inhaled solvents focuses on eliminating the offending toxin and treating the acute symptoms. *(Please see Table 3.)* The airway, breathing, and circulation must be evaluated and stabilized as necessary. The majority of people recover rapidly from VSA intoxication and, therefore, never seek medical consultation. Most cases are adequately treated by simply removing the inhalant and providing oxygen. However, endotracheal intubation and mechanical ventilation may be required in the comatose patient.

Because myocardial irritability can be a problem, great caution should be used when considering the use of epinephrine and other catecholamines. If the patient already presents in ventricular fibrillation, standard ACLS protocols should be initiated. Successful suppression of ventricular dysrhythmia—albeit anecdotal—has been reported using phenytoin as an antiarrhythmic.[52] Brady proposes a theoretical advantage to bretylium as an agent to treat freon-induced ventricular fibrillation.[41] The adrenergic (ganglionic) blocking effect as well as the antiarrhythmic effect of bretylium may present an advantage over Class 1 antiarrhythmics.

Burns have been reported more frequently with butane cigarette lighter fluid abuse. They tend to be fairly minor, with an average hospital stay of two days, but may be particularly severe if the patient is stuporous at the time the fire begins.[53,54] Any thermal burns should be treated in the standard manner.

If the patient has had extended loss of consciousness and has been lying on the floor, rhabdomyolysis may be present.[41] The diagnosis is made by obtaining a serum myoglobin level and urinalysis for myoglobinuria. Tea-colored urine or a urinalysis with chemical markers suggesting a large amount of blood yet few red blood cells on microscopic examination suggests rhabdomyolysis.

Profound metabolic acidosis and severe electrolyte disturbances may be life-threatening. An arterial blood gas should be performed to determine the degree of hypoxia; a carboxyhemoglobin level should be obtained, and the presence of methemoglobin should be evaluated. In the hypoxic patient, or in the patient with abnormal auscultatory findings, a chest radiograph should be performed to exclude noncardiogenic pulmonary edema.

Carboxyhemoglobin is treated with oxygen and methemoglobin with methylene blue. The emergency physician may consider a more comprehensive evaluation of the patient to detect long-term pathophysiologic effects by assessing a complete blood count, urinalysis, electrolytes, blood urea nitrogen (BUN), creatinine, and liver function studies. The blood count helps determine hematologic toxicity; the urinalysis, BUN, and creatinine assess renal impairment; electrolytes are essential for measuring an anion gap acidosis; and the liver studies define any hepatotoxicity. Routine urine and serum drug screens do not detect these substances of abuse. Levels of salicylate and toxic alcohols should be considered if the diagnosis is unclear.

Summary

Volatile substance abuse has become a serious health concern, especially among young adolescents. Inhalants are easily obtained. Both immediate and long-term effects are associated with considerable morbidity and, in some cases, can cause death. Emergency physicians should consider VSA and its complications in patients who present to the ED in an inebriated state.

References

1. Johnston LD, O'Malley PM, Bachman JG. Prevalence of drug user among 8th, 10th, and 12th grade students. In: *National Survey Results on Drug Use from Monitoring the Future Study, 1975-1992*. Rockville, MD: National Institute

on Drug Abuse-U.S. Dept of Health and Human Services; 1993.

2. Bass M. Sudden sniffing death. *JAMA* 1970;212:2075-2079.
3. Glaser HH, Massengale ON. Glue sniffing in children: Deliberate inhalation of vaporized plastic cements. *JAMA* 1962;181:300-303.
4. Merry J, Zachariadis N. Addiction to glue sniffing. *BMJ* 1962;2:1448.
5. Tapia-Conyer R, Cravioto P, De La Rosa B, et al. Risk factors for inhalant abuse in juvenile offenders: The case of Mexico. *Addiction* 1995;90:43-49.
6. Masterton G, Sclare AB. Solvent abuse. *Health Bull (Edinb)* 1978;36:305-309.
7. Cohen S. Glue sniffing. *JAMA* 1975;231:653-654.
8. Schutz CG, Chilcoat HD, Anthony JC. The association between sniffing inhalants and injecting drugs. *Compr Psychiatry* 1994;35:99-105.
9. Anderson HR, Macnair RS, Ramsey JD. Deaths from abuse of volatile substances: A national epidemiologic study. *BMJ* 1985;290:304-307.
10. Adgey AA, Johnston PW, McMechan S. Sudden cardiac death and substance abuse. *Resuscitation* 1995;29:219-221.
11. Lerman Y, Winkler E, Tirosh MS, et al. Fatal accidental inhalation of bromochlorodifluoromethane (Halon 1211). *Hum Exp Toxicol* 1991;10:125-128.
12. Gay M, Meller R, Stanley S. Drug abuse monitoring: a survey of solvent abuse in the county of Avon. *Hum Toxicol* 1982; 1:257-263.
13. Langa A. Volatile substance abuse: A brief report. *Br J Clin Pract* 1993;47:94-96.
14. Hansen WB, Rose LA. Recreational use of inhalant drugs by adolescents: A challenge for family physicians. *Fam Med* 1995;27:383-387.
15. Edwards RW. Drug use among 8th grade students is increasing. *Int J Addict* 1993;28:1613-1620.
16. Perry PA, Dean BS, Krenzelok EP. A regional poison center's experience with poisoning exposures occurring in schools. *Vet Hum Toxicol* 1992;34:148-151.
17. Liss BI. Government, trade, and industry and other preventative responses to volatile substance abuse. *Hum Toxicol* 1989; 8:327-330.
18. Evans AC, Raistrick D. Phenomenology of intoxication with toluene-based adhesives and butane gas. *Br J Psychiatry* 1987;150:769-773.
19. Knox JW, Nelson JR. Permanent encephalopathy from toluene inhalation. *N Engl J Med* 1966;275:1494-1496.
20. Sera M, Igarashi S, Miyazaki T, et al. Equilibrium disorders with diffuse brain atrophy in long-term toluene sniffing. *Arch Otorhinolaryngol* 1978;221:163-169.
21. Kornfeld M, Moser AB, Moser HW, et al. Solvent vapor abuse leukoencephalopathy: Comparison to adrenoleukodystrophy. *J Neuropathol Exp Neurol* 1994;53:389-398.
22. Xiong L, Matthes JD, Li J, et al. MR imaging of "spray heads": Toluene abuse via aerosol paint inhalation. *AJNR Am J Neuroradiol* 1993;14:1195-1199.
23. Kojima S, Hirayama K, Furumoto H, et al. Magnetic resonance imaging in chronic toluene abuse and volitional hyperkinesia. *Rinsho Shinkeigaku* 1993;33:477-482.
24. Uitti RJ, Snow BJ, Shinotoh H, et al. Parkinsonism induced by solvent abuse. *Ann Neurol* 1994;35:616-619.
25. Prendergrast MC. Hydrocarbons and inhalants. In: Reisdorff EJ, Roberts MR, Wiegenstein JG, eds. *Pediatric Emergency Medicine* Philadelphia: WB Saunders; 1993:712.
26. Byrne A, Kirby B, Zibin T, et al. Psychiatric and neurological effects of chronic solvent abuse. *Can J Psychiatry* 1991;36: 735-738.
27. Tenenbein M, DeGroot W, Rajani KR. Peripheral neuropathy following intentional inhalation of naphtha fumes. *Can Med Assoc J* 1984;131:1077-1079.
28. Pryor GT, Rebert CS, Dickinson J, et al. Factors affecting toluene-induced ototoxicity in rats. *Neurobehav Toxicol Teratol* 1984;6:223-238.
29. Chadwick OF, Anderson HR. Neuropsychological consequences of volatile substance abuse: A review. *Hum Toxicol* 1989;8:307-312.
30. Winek CL, Wahba WW, Rozin L. Accidental death by nitrous oxide inhalation. *Forensic Sci Int* 1995;73:139-141.
31. Kelly KJ, Ruffing R. Acute eosinophilic pneumonia following intentional inhalation of Scotchguard. *Ann Allergy* 1993;71: 358-361.
32. Ramsey J, Anderson HR, Bloor K, et al. An introduction to the practice, prevalence and chemical toxicology of volatile substance abuse. *Hum Toxicol* 1989;8:261-269.
33. Powars D. Aplastic anemia secondary to glue sniffing. *N Engl J Med* 1965;273:700-702.
34. Kamijima M, Nakazawa Y, Yamakawa M, et al. Metabolic acidosis and renal tubular injury due to pure toluene inhalation. *Arch Environ Health* 1994;49:410-413.
35. Streicher HZ, Gabow PA, Moss AH. Syndromes of toluene sniffing in adults. *Ann Intern Med* 1981;94:758-762.
36. Donald JM, Hooper K, Hopenhayn-Rich C. Reproductive and developmental toxicity of toluene: A review. *Environ Health Perspect* 1991;94:237-244.
37. Chalmers EM. Volatile substance abuse. *Med J Aust* 1991; 154:269-274.
38. Poklis A, Burkett CD. Gasoline sniffing: A review. *Clin Toxicol* 1977;11:35-41.
39. Valpey R, Sumi SM, Copass MK, et al. Acute and chronic progressive encephalopathy due to gasoline sniffing. *Neurology* 1978; 28:507-510.
40. Ross CA. Gasoline sniffing and lead encephalopathy. *Can Med Assoc J* 1982;127:1195-1197.
41. Brady WJ, Stremski E, Eljaiek M, et al. Freon inhalation abuse presenting with ventricular fibrillation. *Am J Emerg Med* 1994;12:533-536.
42. Horowitz BZ. Carboxyhemoglobinemia caused by inhalation of methylene chloride. *Am J Emerg Med* 1986;4:48-51.
43. Stewart RD, Hake CL. Paint-remover hazard. *JAMA* 1976;235:398-401.
44. Machabert R, Testud F, Descotes J. Methaemoglobinaemia due to amyl nitrite inhalation: A case report. *Hum Exp Toxicol* 1994;13:313-314.
45. Bradberry SM, Whittington RM, Parry DA, et al. Fatal methemoglobinemia due to inhalation of isobutyl nitrite. *J Toxicol Clin Toxicol* 1994;32:179-184.
46. Bogart L, Bonsignore J, Carvalho A. Massive hemolysis fol-

lowing inhalation of volatile nitrites. *Am J Hematol* 1986;22:327-329.

47. Newell GR, Mansell PW, Spitz MR, et al. Volatile nitrites: Use and adverse effects related to the current epidemic of the acquired immune deficiency syndrome. *Am J Med* 1985;78: 811-816.
48. Soderburg LS, Flick JT, Barnett JB. Acute inhalation exposure to isobutyl nitrite causes nonspecific blood cell destruction. *Exp Hematol* 1996;24:592-596.
49. Dax EM, Adler WH, Nagel JE et al. Amyl nitrite alters human in vitro immune function. *Immunopharmacol Immunotoxicol* 1991;13:577-587.
50. Meredith TJ, Ruprah M, Liddle A, et al. Diagnosis and treatment of acute poisoning with volatile substances. *Hum Toxicol* 1989;8:277-286.
51. Flanagan RJ, Ives RJ. Volatile substance abuse. *Bull Narc* 1994;46:49-78.
52. Katz RL, Bigger JT. Cardiac arrhythmias during anesthesia and operation. *Anesthesiology* 1970;33:193-213.
53. Scerri GV, Regan PJ, Ratcliffe RJ, et al. Burns following cigarette lighter fluid abuse. *Burns* 1992;18:329-331.
54. McGill-Rizer B. The 38-cent high. *J Michigan Pharmacist* 1994;32:138.

Office Diagnosis of Alcoholism

Mark A. Hurst, MD

Alcoholism is one of the most common medical illnesses found in U.S. society. Each year, millions of individuals with alcoholism are seen in primary care settings for a variety of complaints, some of which are related to the effects of alcohol and some of which are not. These "routine" visits provide the primary care physician (PCP) a unique opportunity to identify the patients with alcoholism and assist them in obtaining treatment. Such intervention can be effective and diminish the needless morbidity and mortality caused by this devastating disorder.

This chapter provides an overview of alcoholism and gives pragmatic information to help us assist our patients in recovering from this treatable illness.

Introduction

Alcoholism and other substance-use disorders have been recognized as major societal problems for millennia. There are numerous references to drunkenness and the untoward effects of alcohol in ancient writings, and historically, individuals with alcoholism were considered to be weak-willed, immoral, insane, or some combination thereof. These individuals were felt to be beyond help and often were rebuked by society.[1]

In 1956, the American Medical Association (AMA) officially recognized alcoholism as a disease.[2] Since then, evidence that alcoholism is a true biomedical illness has accumulated, and many individuals with alcoholism have been successfully treated using Alcoholics Anonymous (AA) and other treatment modalities.[3]

Alcohol is one of the most available substances of abuse in our society, the most commonly used substance, and the most frequent substance of dependence. More than two-thirds of men and approximately half of all women drink on a regular basis, with peak ages of alcohol consumption from the late teens to mid-twenties. The highest rates of *alcohol consumption* (*not* alcoholism) are among those with higher education and higher socioeconomic status. Up to one-third of all young men may have some temporary life problems related to the use of alcohol, but only a subset of these individuals will go on to develop alcoholism.[4,5]

Alcohol is also a major problem in teenagers. Alcohol is the most readily available substance to adolescents and is also the most commonly used and abused substance in this age group. Studies indicate that as many as 90% of all high school seniors have tried alcohol, 50% drink at least twice weekly, and 10% are daily drinkers. This clearly has implications for not only clinical practice, but also for public health intervention and prevention.[6]

Table 1. Recommendations for Low-Risk Drinking[15]

Men:	4 or fewer drinks per week Never more than 4 drinks per occasion
Women:	7 or fewer drinks per week Never more than 3 drinks per occasion
For individuals older than age 65, the above quantities should be halved.	
Pregnant Women:	NO ALCOHOL
Alcoholics:	NO ALCOHOL

Table 2. The CAGE Questions[18]

- Have you ever felt that you should **cut down** on your drinking?
- Have people **annoyed** you by criticizing your drinking?
- Have you ever felt bad or **guilty** about your drinking?
- Have you ever had a drink first thing in the morning to steady your nerves or get rid of a hangover (**eye opener**)?

Two or more positive responses are considered a positive screen.

Even one positive response warrants further evaluation.

With regard to *alcohol dependence* (the terms "alcoholism" and "alcohol dependence" will be used interchangeably in this article), most studies find that between 12% and 16% of the male population and 2-5% of the female population will have lifetime histories of alcoholism. Alcoholism is more common among those with lower education and lower socioeconomic status. It should be kept in mind, however, that alcoholism is truly a disease that affects individuals of all socioeconomic, educational, ethnic, and age groups. Unfortunately, less than one-third of those affected will seek help during their lives. Additionally, alcoholism is even more common among individuals with medical illness or psychiatric problems.[7]

The consequences of alcoholism are great. Hundreds of thousands of people die in this country as a consequence of alcohol, nicotine, and other drug dependence and it is estimated that the annual cost of substance abuse in the United States exceeds $250 billion. These costs are not only due to the associated costs of health care, but also law enforcement and lost work productivity.[8,9] Given these factors, it is obvious that all physicians should have knowledge in the identification and treatment of alcoholism and other substance-related disorders.

At-Risk Populations

One of the first challenges that a PCP faces in dealing with alcohol-related issues is determining which specific patients are at risk, and then assisting them in changing their drinking habits. Some individuals may clearly be alcohol dependent. Others may be engaging in "high-risk" drinking behavior, yet not be able to be diagnosed as alcohol dependent, and others may be at high risk for developing alcoholism by virtue of their family history or responses to alcohol. It is important to determine whether a patient falls in one of these groups to appropriately intervene and minimize the risk of alcohol-related difficulties.

Ideally, it would be possible to identify individuals at high risk for alcoholism before they begin drinking and suffer the devastating effects of this illness. Although this cannot currently be done with a high degree of diagnostic certainty, alcoholism is much more common in individuals with certain characteristics. These characteristics include a positive family history (children of alcoholics are 3-4 times more likely to develop alcoholism),[10] "innate tolerance" (having a less than expected behavioral response to alcohol when first exposed to alcohol, e.g., more than 3-4 drinks),[11] and beginning to drink alcohol at an earlier age (i.e., age 10-12).[12] If such factors are known, the patient should be counseled about this and be informed that alcohol use may carry a higher risk in them than in other individuals.

It has also been discovered that individuals at high risk for alcoholism have an enhanced response to pituitary β-endorphin when exposed to alcohol compared to low-risk individuals.[13] Although this currently is not of clinical relevance for diagnostic or predictive purposes, it has reinforced the biological nature of alcoholism and has been of great importance in the development of effective pharmacological treatments.

Screening for Alcoholism

When assessing a person's current drinking behavior, the PCP should first ascertain if the patient consumes any alcohol at all. If the patient is, and always has been a total abstainer ("teetotaler"), then a need for a family history of alcoholism is needed. If the patient does drink, then the physician should try to determine the frequency of drinking ("How many days in a week do you drink?"), the quantity ("How many drinks on those days?"), and the presence or absence of binge drinking ("What is the most you've drunk on any day over the past month?").[14] Patients who exceed "low-risk drinking" guidelines may be at risk for developing alcohol-related problems (*please see Table 1*). Such patients should be more thoroughly assessed for possible presence of alcoholism. If they do not meet criteria for alcoholism, they should be advised to adhere to the recommendations for "low-risk drinking."[15,16] The physician should be certain to follow-up on this at subsequent appointments, giving positive feedback for successful reduction in alcohol use, and being attentive to the possibility that some of these individuals may develop alcoholism and/or revert to "high-risk" drinking.

When evaluating a patient's alcohol use, quantities consumed should be standardized. A "standard drink" contains 12 g of absolute alcohol. This is equivalent to the amount found in a 12 oz beer, a 5 oz glass of wine, or 1.5 oz (a "shot") of 80-proof liquor. If a patient drinks "tall boy" beers or "double" mixed drinks, this should be adjusted accordingly.

Screening Instruments

After evaluating a person's current use of alcohol, it is then appropriate to proceed with a screening tool.

It would be cumbersome for a PCP to do an intensive diagnostic interview for alcoholism on all patients seen, but given the high prevalence of alcoholism, it is critical that all patients be screened. There are a number of screening tools that can be used, such as the "CAGE" questionnaire, the Michigan Alcohol Screening Test (MAST), and the Alcohol Use Disorders Identification Test (AUDIT). All have been validated in primary care settings, are quick and easy to administer, and have reasonably high sensitivity and specificity.[17] It is generally advisable to complete an alcohol screening as part of routine health assessments, when prescribing medication that could interact with alcohol (i.e., opiates, benzodiazepines, barbiturates, antidepressants), or when dealing with problems that could be caused or exacerbated by alcohol[15] (such as gout, peptic ulcer disease, depression, hypertension or insomnia).

Many clinicians favor the use of the CAGE questionnaire as a screening tool (*please see Table 2*).[18] It is widely used in clinical practice, takes less than a minute to administer, and can be used unobtrusively during routine history taking. An affirmative response to two or more questions is highly suggestive of an alcohol problem, and even one positive response should alert the physician to potential problem drinking and need for further assessment and continued follow-up. It should be noted that neither the CAGE nor any other screening test diagnoses alcoholism. This can only be done with a complete diagnostic assessment using standard diagnostic criteria.

The Michigan Alcohol Screening Test (MAST) is also widely used and provides reliable results.[19] This is generally administered as a paper-and-pencil test and consists of 25 yes-or-no questions, which examine the patient's pattern of alcohol use and any associated life problems. The questions are given weighted scores based upon their importance. A score of 4 or less is not associated with problem drinking. Scores of 7 or more indicate a high likelihood of alcoholism, and scores of 5 or 6 are "borderline" and indicate a need for further assessment.

In recent years, the Alcohol Use Disorders Identification Test (AUDIT) has gained increasing favor as a screening tool for alcoholism.[20] It was developed by the World Health Organization specifically for use in primary care and has a high sensitivity and specificity. It may be superior to the CAGE and MAST in identifying alcohol problems in the early stages. If the physician prefers a "paper-and-pencil" screen, the AUDIT is probably superior to the MAST.

Diagnosing Alcoholism

Alcoholism has been defined in many ways. The terms "alcoholism," "alcohol dependence," and "alcohol abuse" are all used when describing alcohol-related problems. In 1990, the American Society of Addiction Medicine and the National Council on Alcoholism and Drug Dependence defined alcoholism as follows:

"Alcoholism is a primary chronic incurable disease with genetic, psychological, and social factors influencing its development and manifestations. It is often progressive and fatal. It is characterized by periodic or continuous:

- impaired control over drinking;
- preoccupation with alcohol;
- use of alcohol despite adverse consequences;
- distortions in thinking, most notably denial."[21]

Although this is a very accurate and comprehensive definition of alcoholism, it is difficult to apply this to individual patients. Currently, the most commonly used diagnostic criteria are those found in the *Diagnostic and Statistical Manual of Mental Disorders, Fourth Edition* (DSM-IV).[22] They can be applied objectively to a variety of individuals in different settings, enhancing diagnostic reliability. In order to be considered *alcohol dependent* by DSM-IV, an individual must have a maladaptive pattern of alcohol use characterized by three of the following occurring at any time in the same 12 consecutive month period:

- **Tolerance.** Either needing increased amounts of alcohol to attain the desired effect *or* having a significantly decreased effect when using the same amount.
- **Withdrawal.** Developing alcohol withdrawal symptoms (*please see Table 3*) after stopping or reducing alcohol consumption *or* taking alcohol or another sedative with cross-tolerance to alcohol (e.g., benzodiazepines) to treat or avoid withdrawal symptoms. An example of this would be someone who always drinks (or takes 5 mg of diazepam) at lunch to relieve a withdrawal tremor.
- **An Inability to Control the Use of Alcohol.** Social drinkers can stop using at anytime of their choosing. Individuals with alcoholism often have times when they attempt to control the amount of alcohol they consume but are unsuccessful in doing so (consistently or predictably).
- **Unsuccessful Attempts to Cut Down or Stop the Use of Alcohol.** Alcoholics will often have periods of self-imposed abstinence, only to return to alcohol use again.
- **Spending Long Periods of Time Procuring, Taking, or Recovering from the Effects of the Substance.** The alcoholic may become preoccupied with alcohol, always be sure he or she has a supply available, and spend large amounts of time in alcohol-related activities.
- **Reducing Important Activities Due to Alcohol Use.** The alcoholic begins to give up time with family, hobbies, and vocational activities in favor of alcohol use.
- **Continuing the Use of Alcohol Despite Adverse Consequences Relating to Its Use.** A person with alcoholism may be arrested for drunken driving, yet continue to drink and drive, or may be advised to quit drinking by his physician due to elevated liver enzymes, yet continue to do so.

Table 3. Common Symptoms of Alcohol Withdrawal*[22]

- Tachycardia
- Hypertension
- Diaphoresis
- Tremor
- Insomnia
- Nausea or vomiting
- Anxiety/agitation
- Transient hallucinations (usually visual)
- Withdrawal seizures

* *Developing within 24 hours of stopping or reducing use*

Alcohol dependence is a heterogeneous disorder, and not all of these criteria will apply to all individuals with alcoholism. Additionally, tolerance and withdrawal are *not required* for someone to be considered alcohol dependent. Individuals with no tolerance or withdrawal, but other symptoms such as an inability to control use of alcohol, unsuccessful attempts at abstinence, and multiple psychosocial consequences *would* be considered alcoholic as much as the individual who consumes prodigious amounts of alcohol and can attain high blood alcohol levels without evidence of intoxication. In fact, tolerance *alone* is inadequate to diagnose alcohol dependence—other diagnostic criteria must also be met.

Individuals who exhibit a pattern of pathological alcohol use but have never met diagnostic criteria for alcohol dependence are considered to have *alcohol abuse*. An individual with alcohol abuse must have *one* of the following within any 12-month period:

- repeated inability to fulfill major role obligations due to alcohol use (such as missing work due to substance use)
- repeated substance use in situations where it is physically hazardous (such as drinking and driving, or drinking and rock climbing)
- recurrent legal problems relating to substance use (such as multiple drunk driving charges)
- continued substance use despite interpersonal problems or social problems related to use (marital problems secondary to substance use for example).

Many individuals who are diagnosed with alcohol abuse will subsequently develop alcohol dependence, though a subset will continue to abuse without becoming dependent and others will spontaneously revert to "low-risk" drinking.

Assessment

All individuals with positive screens and those individuals who exceed "low-risk drinking" limits should be thoroughly assessed for the presence of an alcohol use disorder. Although some physicians prefer to obtain "expert" consultation from an alcohol counselor or mental health professional, physicians are uniquely qualified to diagnose alcoholism due to the nature of their relationship with patients and ability to obtain and interpret information that is not available to nonmedical professionals, such as physical and laboratory information. Additionally, patients usually feel more comfortable interacting with their PCP, which may permit them to be more forthcoming with information about alcohol use and its consequences. Finally, there is less stigma associated with a primary care visit than a trip to an alcohol treatment or mental health facility. Accordingly, involvement of the PCP is important for accurate diagnosis and successful outcome.

History

Gathering historical information and clinical interviews are the most important procedures in assessing for alcoholism.[14] The physician should approach the patient in a caring and professional manner, taking care not to raise the defensiveness of the patient.[23] Although information is being obtained for assessment purposes, this is also an important therapeutic contact. Every attempt should be made for this to be a positive experience for the patient in order for him to develop trust and have a willingness to accept the physician's conclusions and recommendations. A highly confrontational approach will almost always compromise the interview and the therapeutic relationship, serving the patient poorly. If we genuinely believe that alcoholism is a potentially fatal, but treatable, illness, we should approach individuals afflicted with it with the same dignity and respect with which we approach all other patients.

For the PCP, assessment for alcoholism is rarely a single event. Alcoholism is a chronic illness, and as a result, a patient may present with different symptoms and signs of alcoholism at different times during the treatment relationship. A single appointment often provides incomplete cross-sectional information and could lead to erroneous conclusions. Conversely, a longitudinal perspective gives more complete information. If a physician has a high index of suspicion and reflects on previous treatment contacts, the diagnostic picture may become clearer, especially when both medical and non-medical information is considered and correlated.

All aspects of the history are important, including chief complaint, present illness, medical history, psychiatric history, medications, allergies, family history, social history, and systems review. Patients with alcoholism rarely complain of problems with alcohol use, but more commonly present with problems such as abdominal pain, gout, or as victims of trauma. It is only after pursuing an alcohol history that the physician becomes aware that the presenting complaint is a consequence of alcohol use. This includes not only medical problems, but also psychiatric problems such as depression, insomnia, or anxiety, as well as social problems such as marital discord, legal problems, or employment concerns.[24]

Medication history and allergies are often overlooked as potential sources of diagnostic information. If an individual has a history of extensive exposure to controlled drugs, the physician should ascertain the reason for this and attempt to determine their pattern of use. Specific concerns should be raised if the person has taken controlled drugs in high doses and/or for long periods for relatively minor complaints, if they run out of medication prematurely, or if they drink when taking drugs, which may adversely interact with alcohol. A complaint of "allergies" to multiple controlled drugs should raise similar suspicions. Although certainly there are individuals who are particularly sensitive to a particular class of controlled drugs, one should also consider the possibility that such an individual is seeking a "drug of choice" in that particular class.

Physical and Laboratory Findings

Physical examination, laboratory testing, and mental status assessment are also helpful in detecting possible complications of alcohol use.[24] A brief summary of some common physical and laboratory findings associated with alcoholism may be found in Table 4.

A number of physical illnesses are highly correlated with alcoholism, and alcohol affects virtually every organ system in the human body.[25] Individuals with medical problems that may be alcohol induced should be closely questioned about their use. Early intervention on drinking habits in affected individuals can frequently stop the progression of almost all alcohol-related medical illnesses and often reverse it, further emphasizing the importance of effective alcohol screening and early diagnosis.

Physical Complications of Alcoholism

Alcohol dependence is associated with a significantly reduced life expectancy, with the average age of death of alcoholics being between ages 55 and 60 (20 years younger than the general population). The leading causes of death among alcoholics are cardiovascular and neoplastic diseases with certain cancers (head and neck, esophageal, and gastric) being over-represented. Accidental deaths and suicide are also greatly increased in alcoholics, with the rate of suicide being as high in alcoholics as it is in individuals suffering from major depression.[26]

Gastrointestinal System. Alcohol also may cause esophagitis, gastritis, duodenitis, and gastric and duodenal ulcers. Additionally, one-half of all cases of pancreatitis are related to alcohol use. Alcohol also has a significant effect on the liver including fatty liver, alcoholic hepatitis, and cirrhosis. Patients with hepatitis C should not use alcohol. Women are significantly more sensitive to the hepatic effects of alcohol than are men, with decreased quantities and lower durations of consumption leading to development of cirrhosis of the liver.[25]

Cardiovascular System. Alcohol is also one of the leading causes of cardiomyopathy.[25] In the past, alcoholics were not considered to be candidates for cardiac or hepatic transplantation; however, with further recognition of the disease nature of alcohol dependence, individuals who are in remission from alcohol dependence and meet certain criteria may be appropriate transplant candidates.

Recent research has indicated that moderate alcohol consumption decreases the risk of cardiovascular disease,[27] and some patients will use this as a rationale to continue drinking. While it is true that *moderate* use *decreases* cardiovascular risk, *excessive* use *increases* risk, with higher rates of cardiac arrythmias, hypertension, and stroke.[25] There are many other things that patients can do to decrease the risk of cardiovascular disease, such as following a prudent diet, stopping smoking, and exercising. No one needs to drink solely for its cardioprotective effect.

Reproductive System. Alcohol also has a significant effect on the reproductive system. Impotence is common among male alcoholics, as is infertility in both male and female alcoholics. Spontaneous abortions are increased among women who are actively drinking. Low birthweight offspring are seen in pregnant women who are actively drinking, as well as in abstinent nonalcoholic women who are married to alcoholic husbands. This may be due to both the stress of living with an actively drinking alcoholic, as well as possible effects on sperm motility and sperm morphology.[25,28]

Fetal alcohol syndrome is a common birth defect, which is due to the effect of alcohol on the developing fetus. Other factors may also be involved such as nutritional deficits, lack of prenatal care and vitamin deficiencies, but it is clear that alcohol is a major teratogen. There is a dose-response relationship, with higher amounts of alcohol being associated with more severe pathology in the affected children. Typical features include growth retardation, microcephaly, microphthalmia, absent philtrum, a broad bridge to the nose, and learning disabilities. *No amount of alcohol is proven safe in pregnancy* and pregnant women should consume no alcohol at all. Additionally, women who are breastfeeding should also avoid the consumption of alcohol to avoid potential effects in the newborn.[28,29]

Central Nervous System. Neurological sequelae of alcoholism are not uncommon, including alcoholic cerebellar degeneration and the Wernicke-Korsakoff syndrome. Individuals affected by Wernicke's syndrome have a broad-based gait, ataxia, abnormalities of eye movements (particularly of the sixth cranial nerve), and some memory deficits caused by thiamine deficiency. All alcoholics should be given oral thiamine as part of their treatment regimen, and those individuals experiencing symptoms of Wernicke's syndrome should be given intravenous thiamine.

Following Wernicke's syndrome, a Korsakoff's syndrome may develop. This is associated with all of the signs of Wernicke's syndrome and marked memory impairment, most notably in recent memory (although memory is globally affected). Patients often will confabulate to fill in memory gaps. This disorder may also be treated with intravenous thiamine, although less successfully than Wernicke's syndrome. Alcoholic cerebellar degeneration causes a broad-based gait, nystagmus, and intention tremor. This condition is irreversible and its neuropathology differs from Wernicke-Korsakoff syndrome.[5]

There are a variety of psychiatric complications of alcohol dependence as well. Individuals who are alcohol dependent

Table 4. Common Physical and Laboratory Findings in Alcoholism

Physical Findings
- Unexplained bruises and abrasions
- Frequent trauma
- Acne rosacea
- Hepatomegaly
- Tremor
- Alcohol on breath
- Cigarette burns on chest or between fingers
- Peripheral neuropathy
- Memory deficits

Laboratory Findings
- Increased mean corpuscular volume (MCV)
- Increased hepatic enzymes (GGT, SGOT, SGPT)
- Elevated triglycerides, high-density lipoprotein (HDL)-cholesterol
- Elevated uric acid
- Incidental rib fracture on chest x-ray

may suffer from anxiety, hallucinosis, comorbid drug addiction, comorbid personality disorders (with a clear over-representation of antisocial personality disorder), and depression. These symptoms may occur in the course of the alcohol dependence and be clearly secondary to it, or may be true comorbid psychiatric conditions that are in need of separate treatment. Substance-dependent individuals who are suffering from significant psychiatric symptomatology should have a thorough assessment for associated psychiatric illness and receive appropriate treatment when indicated. Individuals with alcoholism and associated psychiatric illness have a significantly higher relapse rate and should have this addressed in the course of their treatment.[30]

For a further review of the physical and laboratory findings in individuals with alcohol dependence, the reader is referred to comprehensive textbooks of internal medicine such as *Harrison's Textbook of Internal Medicine*.

Initiating Treatment

After all historical and physical information is obtained, it should be summarized in a cohesive manner and presented to the patient in a kind and empathetic manner. It often is helpful to use the patient's chief complaint and any physical data to impress upon them the seriousness of the problem. Options for treatment can then be outlined.

It would be ideal if the patient then accepted the diagnosis, entered treatment, and had life-long sobriety. Unfortunately, this rarely occurs. Individuals often have significant denial and initially may have little insight or motivation to pursue treatment. Although this is frustrating to the physician, it should be seen as another facet of the illness to be dealt with, not as a character flaw of the patient or a personal affront to the treatment provider.

If the patient is not receptive to the diagnosis or treatment recommendations, the physician might consider either a second opinion with another physician with expertise in substance dependence or suggest an "abstinence contract." With an abstinence contract, the treatment provider would ask the patient to be abstinent from alcohol and all drugs of abuse for a fixed period of time (60 or 90 days). The patient has regular appointments with the physician during this period and the course of his or her recovery is followed. Should the patient use alcohol or other drugs during this period, this gives further diagnostic information. Should the patient be successful in abstaining from alcohol and other drugs, often he or she will note positive changes and be willing to continue to abstain.

If the patient continues to drink, regular follow-up appointments should still be made, as would be done with any chronic and progressive disease. At these appointments, the physician should continue to address the alcohol issue, focusing on the development of insight and motivation to change behavior. Eliciting the *patient's* reasons for changing their drinking behavior is often helpful in this respect.

Active Alcohol Treatment

There are a variety of intensities of treatment varying from medically monitored inpatient treatment in a general medical hospital, to outpatient treatment with little counseling and an agreement to abstain totally from all substances of abuse (*please see Table 5*). The preferred level of care is the least restrictive setting in which the patient can successfully maintain abstinence and maintain medical stability. There is some evidence that many people with alcohol problems can stop alcohol use on their own,[31] although many others will require a formal rehabilitation program.

Most alcoholism treatment providers in the United States use the same basic principles. These include a disease model of addiction (treating a true biomedical illness), absolute abstinence from all drugs of abuse (unless absolutely medically necessary), education, and 12-step programs such as AA. The patient may be involved with a variety of other therapeutic modalities depending upon his or her individual needs including individual counseling, group counseling, family and marital counseling, medical management, and psychiatric treatment. The focus of this phase of treatment is to help individuals achieve substance-free lives and to rebuild those areas that have been adversely affected by their illness. Virtually all life areas are affected by alcoholism and each of these areas should be addressed in each patient.[32,33]

One of the most important interventions that a physician can make in this stage of treatment is to stress the importance of absolute abstinence. Outcome research is very clear. In a 50-year prospective study of individuals with alcoholism, Dr. George Vaillant found that only 11% were successful in return-

Table 5. Levels of Treatment Intensity for Alcoholism

- Medically-monitored inpatient (most intensive)
- Medically-supervised inpatient
- Residential treatment
- Partial hospital treatment
- Intensive outpatient (3 h, 3 times weekly)
- Counseling (group, family, individual)
- Support groups alone (least intensive)

ing to sustained "controlled drinking." The remainder were either still abusing, fully abstinent, or dead. In short, it is exceedingly unlikely that an alcoholic will be successful in attempting to return to "controlled" (or social) drinking.[34]

Physicians should also avoid prescribing benzodiazepines, opioids, or other controlled drugs to known alcoholics or addicts, unless absolutely necessary (such as when using benzodiazepines for treatment of alcohol withdrawal).

Relapse Prevention

Most research finds that between 40% and 50% of substance-dependent individuals will have a relapse within the first three months of leaving active treatment. Therefore, it becomes important to assist individuals in minimizing both the likelihood of relapse and the duration of relapse should it occur. Preventing relapse on substances should begin with the initiation of treatment. The individual should be assisted in identifying situations and stressors that may lead to relapse and developing coping strategies to help deal with these situations. A variety of modalities may be used including counseling, self-help groups, written homework assignments, behavioral and cognitive therapies, and pharmacotherapy.[35]

Pharmacological treatments to reduce the likelihood of alcohol relapse may be helpful but are only a small part of a recovery program. Disulfiram (Antabuse) previously was one of the few available options. It is an irreversible inhibitor of aldehyde dehydrogenase and when individuals consume alcohol when taking this medication, they experience an unpleasant reaction due to acetaldehyde accumulation. A large multicenter Veterans Administration study, which was done in the 1980s, revealed little difference in treatment outcome between individuals taking Antabuse and control groups. Nonetheless, certain individuals may respond well to disulfiram and it may be a valuable tool in this treatment process.[36]

An important advance in treatment of alcohol dependence has been the development of naltrexone for use in alcohol dependence. Naltrexone is an opioid antagonist and has been used due to observable differences in endogenous opioid activity in individuals at high risk and low risk for alcohol dependence. In replicated studies, alcohol-dependent individuals taking naltrexone at a dose of 50 mg per day had a 50% lower relapse rate than individuals taking placebo and receiving the same psychosocial treatments. Furthermore, the group treated with naltrexone had decreased craving for alcohol and if they did consume alcohol, were less likely to proceed to a major relapse of uncontrolled drinking than those taking the placebo.[37,38] Although no pharmacological "magic bullet" exists for the treatment of alcohol dependence (or any other substance-dependence disorder) at this point, naltrexone is an important addition to the therapeutic armamentarium. All pharmacological treatments should be combined with a comprehensive biopsychosocial treatment process to fully address the needs of the individual with alcohol dependence. Even more importantly than medication, encouragement from the physician to attend AA, contact with an AA sponsor, and maintain a commitment to sobriety can be of great value.

Summary

Substance-related disorders are extremely common in our society. All physicians will come in contact with individuals who are suffering from alcoholism and should have some knowledge of its identification and treatment. In the future, there will be better methods of prevention, intervention, and treatment in order to decrease the associated morbidity and mortality in our society. Individuals who suffer from these disorders are certainly not "hopeless" and many individuals do lead happy and productive lives after receiving appropriate intervention and treatment.

References

1. Musto DF. Historical Perspectives. In: Lowinson JE, et al, eds. *Substance Abuse—A Comprehensive Textbook*. 3rd ed. Baltimore, Md: Williams & Wilkins; 1997:1-10.
2. Report of Officers. Hospitalization of patients with alcoholism. *JAMA* 1956;162:750.
3. U.S. Department of Health and Human Services. Treatment of alcoholism and related problems. In: *Ninth Special Report to Congress on Alcohol and Health*. Rockville, Md: National Institutes of Health; 1997:337-371.
4. Winick C. Epidemiology. In: Lowinson JE, et al, eds. *Substance Abuse—A Comprehensive Textbook*. 3rd ed. Baltimore, Md: Williams & Wilkins; 1997:10-16.
5. Schuckit MA. Alcohol and Alcoholism. In: Isselbachecks, et al, eds. *Harrison's Principles of Internal Medicine*. 13th ed. New York, NY: McGraw-Hill; 1994:2420-2425.
6. Adger H, Werner MJ. The pediatrician. *Am J Addict* 1996;5: 520-529.
7. U.S. Department of Health and Human Services. Epidemiology of Alcohol use and alcohol-related consequences. In: *Ninth Special Report to Congress on Alcohol and Health*. Rockville, Md: National Institutes of Health; 1997:1-31.
8. Goodwin DW, Gabrielli WF. Alcohol: Clinical aspects. *JAMA* 1956;162:142-148.
9. U.S. Department of Health and Human Services. Economic aspects of alcohol use and alcohol-related problems. In: *Ninth Special Report to Congress on Alcohol and Health*. Rockville,

Md: National Institutes of Health; 1997:275-299.
10. Dawson DA, et al. Family history as a predictor of alcohol dependence. *Alcohol Clin Exp Res* 1992;16:572-575.
11. Schuckit MA. Low level of response to alcohol as a predictor of future alcoholism. *Am J Psychiatry* 1994;151:184-189.
12. DeWit DJ, et al. Age at first alcohol use: A risk factor for the development of alcohol disorders. *Am J Psychiatry* 2000;157: 745-750.
13. Gianoukalis C, et al. Enhanced sensitivity of pituitary β-endorphin to ethanol in subjects at high risk of alcoholism. *Arch Gen Psychiatry* 1996;53:250-257.
14. O'Connor PG. The general internist. *Am J Addict* 1996;5:59.
15. National Institute on Alcohol Abuse and Alcoholism. *The Physician's Guide to Helping Patients with Alcohol Problems*. Rockville, Md: National Institutes of Health; 1998:11.
16. Sanchez-Craig M, et al. Empirically based guidelines for moderate drinking: 1-year results from three studies with problem drinkers. *Am J Public Health* 1995;85:823-828.
17. Nilssen O, Cone H. Screening pateints for alcohol problems in primary health care settings. *Am J Addict* 1996;5:53-56.
18. Ewing JA. Detecting alcoholism: The CAGE questionnaire. *JAMA* 1984;252:1905-1907.
19. Selzer ML. The Michigan Alcohol Screening Test: The quest for a new diagnostic instrument. *Am J Psychiatry* 1971;127: 1653-1698.
20. Babor TF, Grant M. From clinical research to secondary prevention: international collaboration in the development of The Alcohol Use Disorders Identification Test (AUDIT). *Alcohol Health Res World* 1989;13:371-374.
21. Morse RM, Flavin DK. The definition of alcoholism. *JAMA* 1992;268:1012-1014.
22. *Diagnostic and Statistical Manual of Mental Disorders*. 4th ed. Washington, DC: American Psychiatric Association; 1994.
23. Schottenfeld RS. Assessment of the patient. In: Galanter M, Kleber HD, eds. *American Psychiatric Press Textbook of Substance Abuse Treatment*. Washington, DC: 1994:25-34.
24. Senay EL. Diagnostic interview and mental status examination. In: Lowinson JE, et al, eds. *Substance Abuse—A Comprehensive Textbook*. 3rd ed. Baltimore, Md: Williams & Wilkins; 1997: 364-369.
25. U.S. Department of Health and Human Services. Effects of alcohol on health and body systems. In: *Ninth Special Report to Congress on Alcohol and Health*. Rockville, Md: National Institutes of Health; 1997:131-191.
26. Schuckit MA. Drug and Alcohol Abuse. *A Clinical Guide to Diagnosis and Treatment*. 4th ed. New York, NY: Plenum Medical Book Company; 1995.
27. Klatsy AL. Epidemiology of coronary heart disease—Influence of alcohol. *Alcohol Clin Exp Res* 1994;18:88-96.
28. U.S. Department of Health and Human Services. Effects of alcohol on fetal and postnatal development. In: *Ninth Special Report to Congress on Alcohol and Health*. Rockville, Md: National Institutes of Health; 1997:193-246.
29. Streissguth AP, et al. Fetal alcohol syndrome in adolescents and adults. *JAMA* 1991;265:1961-1965.
30. Beeder AB, Millman RB. Patients with psychopathology. In: Lowinson JE, et al, eds. *Substance Abuse—A Comprehensive Textbook*. 3rd ed. Baltimore, Md: Williams & Wilkins; 1997: 551-563.
31. Tucker JA, Gladsojo JA. Help-seeking and recovery by problem-drinkers: Characteristics of drinkers who attended Alcoholics Anonymous or formal treatment or who recovered without assistance. *Addict Behav* 1993;18:529-542.
32. Geller A. Comprehensive treatment programs. In: Lowsin JE, et al, eds. *Substance Abuse—A Comprehensive Textbook*. 3rd ed. Baltimore, Md: Williams & Wilkins; 1997:425-429.
33. Schuckit MA. Goals of treatment. In: Galanter M, Kleber HD, eds. *American Psychiatric Press Textbook of Substance Abuse Treatment*. Washington, DC: 1994:3-10.
34. Vaillant G. A long-term follow-up of male alcohol abuse. *Arch Gen Psychiatry* 1996;53:243-249.
35. Marlatt GA, Barrett K. Relapse prevention. In: Galanter M, Kleber HD, eds. *American Psychiatric Press Textbook Of Substance Abuse Treatment*. Washington, DC: American Psychiatric Press; 1994:25-34.
36. Fuller RK, et al. Disulfiram treatment of alcoholism: A Veteran's Administration cooperative study. *JAMA* 1986;256:1449-1455.
37. Volpicelli JR, et al. Naltrexone in the treatment of alcohol dependence. *Arch Gen Psychiatry* 1992;49:876-880.
38. O'Malley SS, et al. Naltrexone and coping skills therapy for alcohol dependence. *Arch Gen Psychiatry* 1992;49:881-887.

Alcohol Withdrawal Syndromes

Phillip A. Brewer, MD
Gail D'Onofrio, MD, FACEP

Perhaps more than any other specialist, the practicing emergency physician (EP) encounters the entire gamut of alcohol-related problems on a regular basis and should be well-versed in their recognition and management.

The problems of recognition, prevention, treatment, and appropriate disposition, can be all the more challenging because of the patients' background of substance abuse and the need to differentiate between overlapping causes of mental status changes. Probably the two most important tasks in caring for this population are recognition of the need for immediate evaluation to rule out traumatic or infectious CNS condition, and deciding whether to admit to a hospital, refer to an in-patient substance-abuse treatment unit, or refer for out-patient management that includes alcohol counseling.

Alcohol abuse and the risk of alcohol withdrawal syndrome are under-recognized by physicians. This is illustrated in a study of 100 acute orthopedic admissions that found that only 37% of patients had an adequate drinking record correctly identifying alcohol problems.[1] In the population that was identified as problem drinkers, action was taken in only 36% of cases, usually after withdrawal symptoms appeared. Otherwise, no action was taken, even when it was recognized that the admission was the direct consequence of drinking.

This chapter deals with a spectrum of alcohol-related complications that are grouped under the term alcohol withdrawal syndromes (AWS). These complications range in severity from hangover and insomnia, tremor and tachycardia, to life-threatening delirium tremens. Their common mechanism is rebound of the altered metabolic and neurohormonal physiology of ethanol exposure when ethanol is abruptly withdrawn or reduced. Chronic effects of ethanol, such as congestive cardiomyopathy and alcoholic neuropathy, lie outside the scope of this article and will not be discussed unless they have a direct bearing on AWS.

Epidemiology

Approximately 111 million Americans age 12 and over are current alcohol users.[2] There are an estimated 22 million alcoholics in the United States and more than 107,000 alcohol-related deaths per year.[2,3] Up to one-third of adult inpatients have problems related to alcohol, and 20% of the total national expenditure for hospital care is related to alcohol abuse.[4,5] Alcoholism is the leading cause of morbidity and mortality in the United States. One study determined that 40% of all patients presenting to the ED in the evening had been drinking and had blood alcohol concentrations (BAC) greater than 80 mg/dL.[6] The economic impact of alcohol abuse and alcoholism is monumental. It is estimated that the cost to the nation is anywhere from $130 billion to $200 billion per year.[5]

Table 1. The CAGE Questionnaire

1. Have you ever felt you should **C**ut down on your drinking?
2. Have people ever **A**nnoyed you by criticizing your drinking?
3. Have you ever felt bad or **G**uilty about your drinking?
4. Have you ever had a drink first thing in the morning to steady your nerves or to get rid of a hangover (**E**ye-opener?)

Two positive answers indicate a high likelihood of alcohol dependency.

Definitions

Alcohol abuse refers to patterns of problem drinking that result in health consequences, social problems, or both.[3] *Alcohol dependence*, often called alcoholism, refers to a disease that is characterized by abnormal alcohol-seeking behavior that leads to impaired control over drinking.[3]

Alcohol dependence by *DSM-IV*[7] criteria is characterized by development of three or more of the following symptoms over a 12-month period: loss of control over use, development of tolerance or withdrawal symptoms, inability to fulfill roles, neglect of activities, and continued use despite problems.

The National Institute on Alcohol Abuse and Alcoholism (NIAAA) defines a patient at risk for alcohol-related problems as: a man who consumes more than 14 drinks per week or four drinks per occasion, a woman who consumes more than seven drinks per week or more than three drinks per occasion; or anyone who gives one or more positive answers to the CAGE that have occurred in the past year.[8] *(Please see Table 1.)*

Assessment of Alcohol Use and Abuse

Assessment of individuals presenting to the ED should include questions regarding alcohol use. The physician is then able to recognize not only the patient who is presenting in a withdrawal state but also those who are at risk. Relying on breath alcohol and self-report alone have been shown to be inadequate screening tests for alcohol abuse, with sensitivities as low as 20% to 29%, respectively.[9]

Screening and assessment tools, such as the CAGE and the brief MAST surveys, are helpful in establishing patterns of alcohol use and the presence of physiological dependency.[10,11] *(Please see Tables 1 and 2.)* CAGE is a short, four-item survey that assesses lifetime consumption of alcohol and is easy to remember and administer. One or more positive answers requires further assessment. The brief MAST (Michigan Alcoholism Screening Test) survey is a 10-item subset of the original 25-item MAST, with weighted responses. Cherpitel found that when used to identify alcohol dependence in patients in an ED setting, a cutoff of two or more positive answers on the CAGE had an accuracy of 84%, with a sensitivity of 76% and a specificity of 90%. When using a cutoff score of 4 with the brief MAST, she reported an accuracy of 67%, with a sensitivity of 48% and a specificity of 89%.[12]

Cyr and Wartman reported a 91.5% sensitivity in identifying alcohol dependency when the two following questions from the MAST survey were used: "Have you ever had a drinking problem?", and "Have you had a drink within the last 24 hours?"[13]

After screening for alcohol abuse and dependency, the EP should make an assessment of the risk of progression to AWS. It is preferable to predict and prevent AWS rather than wait for the onset of symptoms.

Pathophysiology of Ethanol Exposure

Ethanol produces long-term metabolic and histologic changes in a variety of organ systems. These changes account for most of the effects of withdrawal from chronic ethanol exposure, and many have direct implications for prevention and treatment of withdrawal syndromes.

Metabolism of Ethanol. Ethanol (ETOH) is rapidly absorbed by the gastric and intestinal mucosa and enters the bloodstream. It is eliminated in small quantities by the lungs and kidneys but is primarily metabolized by the liver. With repeated exposure, alcohol dehydrogenase is induced, and, at higher concentrations, the microsomal P_{450} enzyme system is also engaged in ETOH metabolism. The quantity of alcohol present in one shot of spirits, one 4 oz. glass of wine, or one 12 oz. beer will raise the blood alcohol level by approximately 25 mg/dL in the average adult, who will metabolize ETOH at the rate of about 15-25 mg/dL/h, assuming normal liver function. The time at which the BAC begins to fall depends on the quantity of ethanol present in the gut and the point at which there is no further absorption. Repeat breath analysis of ETOH concentration may actually show a rise during the first hour or two after presentation.

Chronic CNS Effects. Long-term exposure to ethanol modifies certain neurotransmission sites in the CNS. Withdrawal from alcohol results in rebound hyperstimulation and some degree of neuronal death.[14]

The N-methyl-D-aspartate (NMDA) type of glutamate receptor, which is specifically inhibited by ethanol, plays a role in neuronal development. Its inhibition is thought to be the mechanism underlying fetal alcohol syndrome as well as neuronal demise by up-regulation of chronically ethanol-inhibited hippocampal cells.[15] Compensatory glutamate-mediated hyperstimulation of the NMDA receptor during withdrawal produces excitotoxic cell death and may cause epileptiform seizure activity. This is particularly true following drinking binges, and administration of antagonists of NMDA may be protective. Withdrawal-induced synaptic excitation mediated by the NMDA receptor is accompanied by increased calcium spikes. Some calcium-channel antagonists are effective in preventing withdrawal seizures.[16,17]

Alcohol also potentiates the inhibitory neurotransmitter gamma-aminobutyric acid (GABA). The activity of the neuronal chloride ion channel linked to the A-type GABA receptor is increased during acute exposure to high alcohol levels.[18] This receptor is the site of action of benzodiazepines and may partly explain their benefit in alcohol withdrawal. Alcohol's affect on $GABA_A$ may contribute to alcohol's anxiolytic, sedative, and motor impairment actions.[3] Hyperexcitability and seizures may develop in alcohol withdrawal from a compensatory change in the number or function of $GABA_A$ receptors following chronic alcohol exposure.[3] Growth hormone and

Table 2. The Brief Michigan Alcoholism Screening Test (MAST)

QUESTIONS	ANSWERS (Y/N)	POINTS
1. Do you feel you are a normal drinker?	Yes/No	N2
2. Do friends or relatives think you are a normal drinker?	Yes/No	N2
3. Have you ever attended a meeting of Alcoholics Anonymous?	Yes/No	Y5
4. Have you ever lost friend/boyfriend/girlfriend because of drinking?	Yes/No	Y2
5. Have you ever gotten into trouble at work because of drinking?	Yes/No	Y2
6. Have you ever neglected your obligations, your family, your work for two or more days in a row because of drinking?	Yes/No	Y2
7. Have you ever had delirium tremens or severe shaking, or heard voices or seen things that weren't there after heavy drinking?	Yes/No	Y2
8. Have you ever gone to anyone for help about your drinking?	Yes/No	Y5
9. Have you ever been in a hospital because of drinking?	Yes/No	Y5
10. Have you ever been arrested for drunk driving or driving after drinking?	Yes/No	Y2

corticosterone are also implicated in the mediation of withdrawal syndromes.[19,20]

Effects on the Liver. Eventually, the toxic effects of ethanol metabolism produce hepatic steatosis and hepatocellular degeneration, which leads to cirrhosis and hepatic insufficiency in some cases.

Effects on the Heart and Cardiovascular System. Alcoholism is often associated with the abuse of tobacco as well as cocaine, which cause coronary artery disease and hypertension. Both adrenaline and noradrenaline secretion are increased during withdrawal from alcohol in dependent subjects, resulting in the tachycardia and hypertension seen in withdrawal states. Acute myocardial ischemia may ensue.[21]

Alcoholic Ketoacidosis. Alcoholic ketoacidosis (AKA) is defined as a wide anion gap metabolic acidosis, with ketonemia occurring in the dehydrated, fasting, chronic alcoholic who is undergoing withdrawal from ethanol and in whom other causes of metabolic acidosis have been ruled out.[22] *(Please see Table 3.)* It is rapidly reversible and has a low mortality when recognized.

When glucose and glycogen are depleted, free fatty acids are mobilized as a secondary source of energy. The Krebs cycle is inhibited by a high NADH/NAD ratio. This further increases fatty acid production, most of which is converted from acetoacetate to beta-hydroxybutyrate. The former, but not the latter, is detected by urine ketone reagent strips, Acetest tablets, or the nitroprusside test. Combined with preexisting dehydration, an anion gap acidosis ensues.

Description of Alcohol Withdrawal Syndromes

The hallmarks of AWS constitute a continuum of signs and symptoms, ranging from tremulousness to delirium tremens. At one time, alcohol withdrawal was divided into stages.[23] However, since the full spectrum of symptoms varies greatly and overlaps in duration and temporal sequence, it is more clinically helpful to define a constellation of signs and symptoms ranging from mild/minor phenomena to severe/major phenomena.[76]

Mild Alcohol Withdrawal. Mild withdrawal usually occurs less than 24 hours after cessation of or decrease in alcohol intake. It may include tremulousness, anxiety, nausea, vomiting, diaphoresis, hyperreflexia, and minor autonomic hyperactivity.

Severe Alcohol Withdrawal. Severe withdrawal occurs more than 24 hours and up to five days after cessation of or decrease in alcohol intake. It is characterized by disorientation, agitation, hallucinations, and severe autonomic derangement.

Moderate Alcohol Withdrawal. Moderate withdrawal is an intermediate position along the continuum with the hallmark of hallucinosis but an otherwise clear sensorium.

Seizures, hallucinations, and DTs are considered major phenomena. Seizures can occur with any severity level of withdrawal.

Table 4 summarizes the characteristics of mild, moderate, and severe withdrawal that are useful for ED diagnosis and assessment. The Clinical Institute Withdrawal Assessment for Alcohol (CIWA-Ar) scale is a well-validated instrument for the assessment of severity of alcohol withdrawal for use in inpatient settings. Points are assigned for categories of symptoms and signs including: nausea and vomiting, tremor, sweats, anxiety, agitation, tactile and visual disturbances, headache, and an abnormal orientation and sensorium.[24] Higher scores reflect more serious withdrawal states. A quantitative score also allows for objective monitoring and evaluation of interventions.

A variety of circumstances may lead to cessation of drinking, including incarceration, acute illness or injury, depletion of funds, retail closings on Sundays, nausea and vomiting, and, finally, a decision to quit drinking. Whatever the circumstance, the progression to AWS is frequently predictable, and the EP must recognize the symptoms of withdrawal as well as the situations in which the patient is at risk for developing AWS.

A description of the various alcohol withdrawal syndromes follows.

Hangover. Hangover is often overlooked in classifications of alcohol withdrawal, perhaps because it occurs after acute as well as chronic alcohol exposure. It is the mildest form of withdrawal, occurring within several hours of cessation. It consists of a period of

Table 3. Causes of Metabolic Acidosis in the Alcoholic Patient

HIGH ANION GAP ACIDOSIS
Alcoholic ketoacidosis
Diabetic ketoacidosis
Lactic acidosis
Sepsis
Seizure/agitation
Prolonged hypotension
Hypothermia
Ingestions
Biguanides*
Isoniazid*
Salicylates*
Ethylene glycol
Methanol
Solvents (Tolulene)
Starvation ketoacidosis
NORMAL ANION GAP ACIDOSIS
Cirrhosis-related renal tubular acidosis
Diarrhea

* Cause lactic acidosis

psychomotor impairment that follows an acute exposure to inebriating quantities of alcohol. Severity of hangover symptoms is a risk factor for subsequent alcohol dependency, perhaps because individuals prone to severe hangover develop a pattern of relieving symptoms by further drinking, known as an "eye-opener."[25]

Even in the naive drinker, such exposure may result in neurochemical changes that persist for up to 48 hours. Performance on discrimination tasks was tested in rats and found to be impaired 18 hours after a single exposure to 4 g/kg of ETOH.[26] Three rebound hypotheses were proposed: an opponent-process physiological rebound from intoxication; a toxic reaction to ethanol or its metabolites; and, circadian dysrhythmia induced by acute ethanol intoxication.[27] In addition to these hypotheses, dehydration secondary to the diuretic effect of ethanol is also a likely factor.

Alcohol Withdrawal Tremor. Barring additional alcohol intake, the chronic drinker develops increasing tremors and craving for alcohol during the first 8-12 hours of observation, which peaks at 24-48 hours. The patient may also experience insomnia, tachycardia, anxiety, and nausea at this stage. The drinker may calm "the shakes" at this point by consuming additional alcohol.

Alcohol Withdrawal Hallucinations. Alcohol withdrawal hallucinations are noted as early as 24 hours after the last drink and last approximately as long. They occur in about a quarter of cases and are usually visual but less frequently will be auditory or combined auditory and visual.[28] Binding of mediator analogs by dopaminergic receptors in the visual cortex in rats is altered during withdrawal from alcohol, and this may account for the visual disturbances that accompany AWS.[29] They are not necessarily linked to other aspects of the syndrome, such as adrenergic hyperstimulation, and may occur as an isolated phenomenon. In early-stage AWS, they are recognized by the patient as hallucinations. In late-stage AWS, they are perceived as real and may provoke extreme fear and anxiety.

Delirium Tremens. Delirium tremens (DT) is a severe, life-threatening complication of alcohol withdrawal. It is characterized by increasingly pronounced disorientation, agitation, and autonomic stimulation, with hypertension, tachycardia, hyperthermia, and profound diaphoresis. Mortality rates of up to 20% have been noted in the past but have improved gradually with the development of intensive care units, more aggressive investigation of traumatic and infectious complications, better fluid replacement, rapid cooling of critical hyperthermia, and the advent of benzodiazepines.[23, 30-32]

Onset typically occurs approximately 48 hours after cessation of drinking. The mild tremor and lucid hallucinations of early withdrawal give way to delirium and agitation. The patient begins to pull at imaginary objects or at his or her clothing and sheets. Life-threatening hyperthermia, which results from increased motor activity and is exacerbated by volume depletion may develop, with temperatures reaching 104°F or greater.

Dehydration is a critical factor in the appearance of DT and may be severe. Of the 39 fatalities described by Tavel et al, dehydration was a factor in all cases in which volume status was noted.[31] Mechanisms of fluid depletion include profuse diaphoresis, increased pulmonary losses related to fever and tachypnea, nausea, vomiting, diarrhea, and decreased oral intake secondary to increasing confusion. A recent study found elevated alpha-atrial natriuretic peptide in every patient who went on to develop DT.[33] This suggests an even greater need for aggressive fluid and electrolyte replacement in DT.

The emergency physician cannot assume that alcohol withdrawal accounts for the entire clinical picture of a patient who presents with these symptoms. The following illnesses must be considered, particularly those which can also produce any or all of the symptoms of DT: alcohol intoxication, other toxins, hypoglycemia, sepsis, severe dehydration, CNS infection, hepatic insufficiency, cerebral injury and/or hemorrhage, and seizure (post-ictal).

Alcohol-Related Seizure. Seizures related to alcohol are a common cause of adult convulsions presenting to the ED. The term "alcohol withdrawal seizures" was originally described by Victor and Brausch in adult patients who were confirmed alcoholics of many years' duration.[28] They reported these seizures as occurring in approximately 10% of people withdrawing from alcohol. They found them to be generalized tonic-clonic (95%), often multiple (60%), and usually occurring 7-48 hours after cessation of drinking (90%). Most were noted to have normal EEGs (90%). They reported the time interval from first to last seizure was less than six hours in 85% of patients. Other studies substantiate the withdrawal component of seizures in the alcohol-dependent patient. Hillbom and Hjelm-Jager and Rathlev et al reported increased seizure frequency with decreased access to alcohol.[34,35] Rathlev et al found that 66% of patients seized during the time when alcohol was not available due to state laws, suggesting decreasing alcohol intake may be a precipitating factor, and that patients who seize with elevated alcohol levels may, in fact, be at lower levels than they are accustomed to.

In addition, other factors independent of abstinence may predispose the alcohol-dependent patient to seize. Recently, Ng et al reported that alcohol itself may induce seizures.[36] The fact that patients seize who have high blood alcohol levels, and that many patients with seizures related to alcohol do not exhibit other signs or symptoms of withdrawal, support this possibility.

Alcohol itself may also exacerbate other existing conditions, such as epilepsy.[37-39] To add to the complexity, chronic alcohol abusers have an increased frequency of structural alterations, including brain infarction, hemorrhagic stroke, and subarachnoid hemorrhage, that may contribute to seizures.[40-43] Because of the multifactorial origin of seizures in the setting of acute and chronic alcoholism, the term alcohol-related seizure (ARS) is frequently used instead of alcohol withdrawal seizure.[44]

Repeated episodes of alcohol withdrawal may lead to an increase in the severity of subsequent episodes and a lower seizure threshold through a process known as kindling.[45-47] Individuals who have had five or more alcohol detoxifications have a greater risk of withdrawal seizures.[48]

Management of Alcohol Withdrawal Syndrome

The goals of ED management of AWS include prevention, recognition of risk factors, control of symptoms of withdrawal states, and recognition of associated conditions.

Assessment and management are often made difficult by acute intoxication or the altered mentation associated with chronic alcoholism and withdrawal states. This is never an excuse for substandard care, and timely use of sedating drugs may facilitate delivery of care. In the patient who appears to be inebriated, alcohol intoxication must be confirmed by measuring breath or blood alcohol levels.

Evaluation of the Patient with Symptoms of Alcohol Withdrawal Syndrome. *Initial Assessment.* As with all patients presenting acutely to the ED, a quick assessment of airway, breathing, and circulatory status must begin the evaluation. Tachycardia, fever, and hypertension or hypotension may be found. In the patient with moderate to severe signs of withdrawal, a secure IV should be placed. In case of frank mental status changes with CNS depression, administer naloxone 2 mg IV. A rapid blood glucose determination should be made; and if necessary 25 mL of D_{50} may be given IV, preceded by thiamine 100 mg IV to prevent precipitating acute Wernicke's encephalopathy.

The AWS may be confused with a variety of illnesses, including hypoglycemia, acute schizophrenia, head trauma, infection, thryotoxicosis, anticholinergic poisoning, withdrawal from other sedative-hypnotic type drugs, and drug-induced psychosis. The EP should keep this differential diagnosis in mind when eliciting the history, performing the physical exam, and ordering lab tests.

History. Obtain as thorough a history as possible. In the uncooperative, confused, or comatose patient, interview secondary sources (i.e., family, friends, police, or EMS personnel) and search medical records. In particular, look for prior episodes of AWS. Pay particular attention to a history of recent trauma, known seizure disorder unrelated to alcohol use, use of prescription or street drugs (such as anticholinergic agents including neuroleptics and decongestants/OTC sedatives, cocaine, and stimulants), and psychiatric illness.

Table 4. Alcohol Withdrawal Severity Assessment

SYMPTOM	WITHDRAWAL CATEGORIES		
	Mild	**Moderate**	**Severe**
Delirium Disorientation Abnormal sensorium Agitation	None	None	Present
and			
Hallucinosis Auditory Visual Tactile	None	Present	Present
and (2 of 3)			
Temperature	<100°F po	100-101°F po	>101°F po
Pulse	<100 bpm	100-120 bpm	>120 bpm
Diastolic Blood Pressure	100 mmHg	100-110 mmHg	>110 mmHg
and any of:			
Tremulousness Anxiety Hyperreflexia Nausea/vomiting Diaphoresis	Present	Present	Present

Alcohol Withdrawal Severity Assessment (AWSA)*

MILD—No delirium, no hallucinosis; at least two of three vital signs as noted; any combination of minor withdrawal symptoms

MODERATE—No delirium but hallucinosis present; or at least two of three vital signs as noted and any combination of minor withdrawal symptoms.

SEVERE—Delirium present; or hallucinosis present and at least two of three vital signs as noted and any combination of minor withdrawal symptoms.

Recommended disposition—Intensive care evaluation for any patient with: 1) SEVERE withdrawal; or 2) MODERATE withdrawal with any of the following symptoms: head or other major trauma, pneumonia, asthma exacerbation, moderate/severe COPD, ischemic heart disease, CHF, age > 50, significant GI hemorrhage, significant pericarditis, drug/med intoxication, major metabolic derangement, recurrent seizures, hepatic or renal failure, significant volume depletion.

Medical floor for uncomplicated MODERATE withdrawal and potentially for the first episode of MILD withdrawal. **Community detox bed** for MILD withdrawal or isolated seizure after six hours of observation.

*Seizures may occur at any severity level

Adapted from a protocol developed by the Boston City Hospital Departments of Emergency Medicine and Medicine, 1991.

Physical Examination. The examination of the alcoholic patient can be a taxing exercise, particularly if the patient is abusive, violent, or unkempt. However, it must be done rigorously in order to reveal

Table 5. Differential Diagnosis of Seizures in the Alcohol-Dependent Patient

Withdrawal of ethanol or other sedative hypnotics
Exacerbation of idiopathic or post-traumatic epilepsy
Acute overdose (amphetamines, anticholinergics, cocaine, isoniazid, phenothiazines, tricyclics)
Metabolic disorders (hypoglycemia, hyponatremia, hypomagnesemia, hypocalcemia)
CNS:
- Infections (meningitis, encephalitis, brain abscess)
- Head trauma
- Stroke
- Noncompliance with anticonvulsant medications

occult, potentially life-threatening injuries or illness. A systematic evaluation of fluid status, degree of withdrawal, and search for signs consistent with precipitating or concomitant illness must be performed. Early sedation may be necessary in order to perform the exam and proceed with further care.

The neurological exam should look for dilated pupils consistent with catecholamine surge, focality of seizures indicative of intracerebral lesions, degree of tremor, and orientation. Examine the head, neck, and musculoskeletal system for signs of trauma. Any sign of hepatic insufficiency, including bleeding or bruising, roving eye movements, jaundice, and hepatomegaly or ascites, must be noted. Tongue injury and soiled clothes may signal the post-ictal state.

Laboratory Tests. Specific tests should depend upon the presentation of the patient and potential for co-existing medical illnesses. All patients need rapid blood glucose determinations. Depending on the clinical situation, electrolytes determinations, including phosphorus, magnesium, and calcium, renal and liver function tests, amylase, coagulation studies, specific toxicologic screens, and urine analysis may be necessary. Lumbar punctures may be necessary to rule out infection and encephalitis. Chest x-rays and head CTs may be of value in diagnosing infection or trauma in selected patients.

Assessment of Alcohol-Related Seizures. As with other conditions, a complete history must be obtained for all patients presenting with a seizure. The patient, family, bystanders, and/or paramedics should be interviewed. Identification and treatment of life-threatening causes of seizures is a priority. *(Please see Table 5.)* The physical exam includes obtaining vital signs, including core temperature, inspection for signs of trauma, and a careful neurological examination to detect focal deficits. The importance of serial neurological examinations cannot be overemphasized.

Emergent head CT scans should be performed on those patients who present with new-onset seizures, a change in pattern from previous seizures, and a focal or deteriorating neurological exam. In a study that followed CT scans in 259 patients with new-onset AWS, 10 (3.9%) had unsuspected intracranial lesions leading to altered clinical management.[49]

Laboratory tests should include a fingerstick for glucose determination and a rapid alcohol breath analysis as part of the initial screening. A complete electrolyte panel, including magnesium, calcium, creatinine, and blood urea nitrogen, should be obtained in new-onset seizures. Cocaine use is associated with seizures, and a urine assay for cocaine metabolites should also be considered. In recurrent ARS, laboratory studies may be limited to glucose, alcohol, and, if appropriate, anticonvulsant levels.

Treatment Regimens. Benzodiazepines are the mainstay of therapy due to their rapid absorption and cross-tolerance with alcohol. They have been shown in randomized trials to treat the symptoms of withdrawal and reduce the frequency of seizures and delirium tremens.[50-57] The benzodiazepines have anticonvulsant activity, minimal respiratory and cardiac depression, and can be administered parenterally. Long-acting benzodiazepines, such as diazepam and chlordiazepoxide, have active metabolites that offer a tapering effect and often preclude additional dosing. For patients unable to take oral medications, the elderly, or those with a prolonged prothrombin time secondary to hepatic dysfunction, lorazepam may be an alternative. Multiple dosing schedules have been used, ranging from front-loading with large amounts of drug, to fixed-schedule dosing, to only symptom-triggered therapy.[55,56,58,59] Other drug therapies, such as beta-blockers and clonidine, have been used for the treatment of AWS but have not been shown to be as effective as monotherapy in moderate/severe withdrawal, nor in patients with significant underlying medical problems. *Table 6* refers to treatment strategies for ED patients with mild to moderate withdrawal, with and without intact oral intake, and severe withdrawal. Specific problems to correct are addressed: adrenergic hyperactivity, dehydration, nutritional deficiency, hypoglycemia, and hyperthermia.

In mild AWS with intact oral intake, control of symptoms is readily obtained. Once concurrent medical problems have been addressed, an appropriate disposition may be determined.

Severe AWS is a true medical emergency requiring rapid intervention. All aspects of treatment listed in Table 6 must be addressed. Physical restraints must be applied to prevent injury pending adequate sedation, which must be accomplished quickly in order to allow an adequate assessment of underlying conditions. In addition to sedation, rehydration is extremely important because dehydration is a significant contributing factor to mortality in AWS. Proper fluid management also protects the restrained, hyperthermic, agitated patient from possible acute tubular necrosis (ATN) due to rhabdomyolysis. Light and noise exacerbate the agitation and delirium of AWS, and the patient should be placed in a quiet room with subdued lighting under constant, direct observation. Significant control of symptoms should be obtained in the ED, and aggressive therapy must continue during and after the transition to an inpatient unit.

Seizures in the Alcohol-Dependent Patient. Currently, there is no uniform standard of care for the patient who presents to the ED with an alcohol-related seizure (ARS). There is great variation in practice patterns, ranging from early discharge at resolution of the post-ictal state, to admission either to six-hour observation units based on Victor and Brausch's data on inpatient beds.[28]

The ideal drug for the prevention and treatment of ARS would exhibit a rapid onset of action, cross-tolerance with ethanol, metabolism independent of liver function, and yet still be safe with little or no abuse potential. Benzodiazepines possess many of these qualities, and, with short-acting agents such as lorazepam now available, their administration accompanied by proper oxygen and cardiac monitoring has been proven to be safe and effective with few adverse reactions.[60,61] Several studies have suggested that benzodiazepines

Table 6. Treatment of Alcohol Withdrawal

PROBLEM TO CORRECT	MILD/MODERATE AWS PO INTACT	MILD/MODERATE AWS INADEQUATE PO INTAKE	SEVERE AWS†
Adrenergic Hyperactivity	Diazepam* 20 mg po q1-2h until symptoms resolve (total dose of 60 mg)	Diazepam 5-10 mg IV Lorazepam 1-2 mg IM/IV q1-2h as needed	Diazepam 5-10 mg IV q 5-10 min; lorazepam 1-2 mg IV q 5-10 min✧
Dehydration	Water, juice po	D_5NS 200-1000 mL/h as indicated	Aggressive hydration with D_5NS/NS
Nutritional Deficiency	• Thiamine 100 mg po • multivitamins • milk of magnesium 30 mL po • folate 1 mg po	• Thiamine 100 mg IV • multivitamins 1 amp in first liter of IV fluids • folate 1 mg IV in first liter of IV fluids • Magnesium sulfate 2 g/L of IV fluid × 2-3 doses over 3-4 hours	• Thiamine 100 mg IV • multivitamins 1 amp in first liter of IV fluids • folate 1 mg IV in first liter of IV fluids • Magnesium sulfate 2 g/L of IV fluid × 2-3 doses over 3-4 hours
Hypoglycemia	High fructose solution po	25 mL D_{50} IV (repeat as necessary)	25 mL D_{50} IV (repeat as necessary)
Hyperthermia			Cooling blankets
Seizures (can occur at any level of severity)	Lorazepam 2 mg IV	Lorazepam 2 mg IV	Lorazepam 2 mg IV

*Lorazepam 2 mg po q2h or chlordiazepoxide 25-100 mg po q6h are alternatives. However, without severe hepatic/renal dysfunction, diazepam is a better choice. Its rapid onset and longer half-life due to active metabolites often precludes further dosing. Avoiding chlordiazepoxide prevents polydrug use if parenteral dosing becomes necessary.

† Requires continuous cardiac and oxygen saturation monitoring in the ED. Admission to intensive care unit is required.

✧ Total dosing of IV diazepam should not routinely exceed 100 mg/h or 250 mg in eight hours. Total dosing of IV lorazepam should not routinely exceed 20 mg/h or 50 mg in eight hours.

alone are sufficient to prevent ARS.[50-52] Lorazepam is well-suited to the treatment of ARS because of its unique pharmacological and pharmacokinetic properties. It has been shown to be a potent anticonvulsant with minimal depressant effects on respiration and circulation.[53,62,63] Lorazepam's duration of seizure control is longer than diazepam. The elimination half-life is approximately 13 hours, without active metabolites. Lorazepam is conjugated to form an inactive glucuronide that is excreted in the urine. Therefore, its elimination half-life is not substantially prolonged in patients with liver dysfunction such as cirrhosis.[64,39] The combination of minimal accumulation in the plasma after multidose therapy, metabolism that is unaffected by concurrent drug therapy (i.e., cimetidine, disulfiram, ethanol), disease states such as cirrhosis, its lower abuse potential compared to other benzodiazepines, and the fact that its metabolism is not altered in the elderly, make it an ideal drug for the population of patients with ARS.[53,65-68]

D'Onofrio et al recently demonstrated the superiority of IV lorazepam over placebo in the ED treatment of recurrent ARS.[69]

In light of the above, patients presenting with an ARS should receive an IV dose of 2 mg of lorazepam as soon as possible. The heart rate, blood pressure, and oxygen saturation for the initial one hour after drug administration should be monitored. Additional doses of lorazepam may be administered for recurrent seizures. Treat other conditions such as hypoglycemia as they are identified. Observe the patient for six hours after the first seizure. Those patients with recurrent seizures after treatment with lorazepam or who appear to develop other symptoms of AWS should be considered as for hospital admission.

Several studies have shown phenytoin to be ineffective in the treatment of recurrent ARS.[70-72] However, patients with known CNS structural defects or positive EEGs indicating an epileptogenic focus should be placed on long-term anticonvulsant therapy and encouraged to be compliant with their medication.[73] Patients who are noncompliant with their anticonvulsants and take them erratically may be at increased risk for seizures.[74] Repeated ED visits by alcohol-dependent patients with documentation indicating poor compliance with long-term anticonvulsant therapy should prompt consultation with the primary care provider and neurologist regarding discontinuation of the therapy.

Alcoholic Ketoacidosis. Fluid and glucose deficiencies are involved, and therapy is aimed at their replacement.[23] IV hydration with 5% dextrose in normal saline, or in 0.5N saline, will both replenish fluid losses and provide necessary glucose; along with nutritional meals, this will eliminate further production of fatty acids and allow for reconstitution of normal NADH/NAD ratios.

Disposition

Hospitalization. The two indications for hospital admission of the patient in or at risk for AWS are the presence of any condition requiring inpatient management, and any condition that, if not properly treated as an outpatient, is likely to worsen and require subsequent admission at a higher level of care. In severe AWS, admission to an intensive care unit is obligatory.

In the presence of alcohol dependency and an illness interfering with the patient's mobility or ability to maintain oral intake of food and fluids, hospitalization is indicated unless it can be clearly demonstrated that the patient has an adequate support system ensuring his or her ability to return for admission should outpatient therapy fail.

If admission is indicated for reasons other than alcohol use, every effort should be made to screen the patient for dependency, and this information must be transmitted to the admitting physician. Adequate surveillance for and prevention of AWS may then be instituted.

The following conditions require hospitalization:[73]

1. Any medical or surgical condition requiring inpatient treatment;
2. Medical condition requiring treatment combined with any mental status changes or when it is unlikely for financial or social reasons that the patient will follow through;
3. Intractable nausea and vomiting or evidence of dehydration;
4. Severe withdrawal including delirium tremens;
5. Fever.

Referral to Inpatient or Outpatient Detoxification. Patients with a diagnosis of alcohol dependency and no life-threatening signs of withdrawal requiring hospitalization should be considered for admission to an outpatient or inpatient detoxification unit. Availability of such treatment, particularly for the uninsured patient, is variable depending on the locale. In some areas, there are state-operated or state-financed facilities which offer both voluntary and involuntary treatment for alcohol detoxification. In addition, there are many privately run detoxification facilities, but most do not accept patients without insurance. The severely dependent alcoholic, who is often described as the "frequent flyer," is capable of recovery given the right circumstances— if left in the cycle of recurrent binges, has a high five-year mortality rate.[75]

Programs for outpatient detoxification from alcohol do exist but require a structured environment and a motivated, oriented patient. Close monitoring is required in order to transfer to inpatient care if needed. Unless admission to such a program can be arranged and all of the above are criteria met, discharge of the emergency patient who is withdrawing or at risk for withdrawal is not advisable. It will invariably result in a continuation of drinking, complicated withdrawal, or a return to the ED in a more advanced withdrawal state.

Programmatic Approach to AWS

The "upstream" approach to emergency medicine states that rather than standing by the river bank and attempting to save drowning people, one can go upstream and attack the problem at its origin. Repeated short-term, ED-based management of alcoholics without proper referral to treatment programs is the "downstream" approach and is destined to perpetuate the problem of recurrent presentation of alcoholic patients to the ED with increasingly life-threatening symptoms. A major impediment to referral is the scarcity of resources. As the frontline physicians in the management of patients with alcohol-related problems, EPs must work collectively and individually to improve the availability of substance abuse treatment services, including creating and operating short-term detoxification facilities.

Summary

AWS is a spectrum of minor to life-threatening complications of cessation of alcohol intake after heavy, usually chronic, exposure to ethanol. Because many ED patients either have active or impending AWS, it is incumbent upon the emergency physician to screen for patients who are at risk for AWS, to recognize ongoing symptoms of AWS, and to treat accordingly.

With proper treatment, mortality and morbidity from AWS can be reduced to a minimum, provided AWS is anticipated or recognized and managed appropriately. ED administrators can reduce hospital admissions and ED length of stay by actively promoting the creation and ongoing support of detoxification beds.

References

1. Hamilton MR, Menkes DB. How alert are hospital doctors to alcohol misuse among acute orthopedic patients? *N Z Med J* 1992;105:167-169.
2. NCADI. *1995 National Household Survey of Alcohol and Drug Abuse.* Advanced Data: 1996;275:1-15.
3. U.S. Secretary of Health and Human Services. Eighth Special Report to the U.S. Congress on Alcohol and Health. 1993.
4. Rice DP, Kellman S, Miller LS, et al. Estimates of economic costs of alcohol and drug abuse and mental illness, 1985 and 1988. *Pub Health Rep* 1991;106:280-292.
5. Burke TR. The economic impact of alcohol abuse and alcoholism. *Pub Health Rep* 1988;103:564-568.
6. Holt S, Stewart IC, Dixon JMJ, et al. Alcohol and the emergency services patient. *BMJ* 1980;281:638-640.
7. American Psychiatric Association. *Diagnostic and Statistical Manual of Mental Disorder.* 4th ed. Washington, DC:1994.
8. U.S. Department of Health and Human Services, National Institutes of Health, National Institutes of Alcohol Abuse and Alcoholism. *The Physician's Guide to Helping Patients with Alcohol Problems.* NIH Publication N. 95-3769; 1995.
9. Cherpitel CJ. Screening for alcohol problems in the emergency department. *Ann Emerg Med* 1995;26:158-166.
10. Mayfield DG, McLeod G, Hall P. The CAGE questionnaire: Validation of a new instrument. *Am J Psychiatr* 1974;131: 1121-1123.
11. Pokorny AO, Miller BA, Kaplan HB. The brief MAST: A shortened version of the Michigan Alcoholism Screening Test. *Am J Psychiatry* 1972;129:342-345.
12. Cherpitel CJ. Screening instruments for alcohol problems in the emergency room. *J Stud Alcohol* 1995;56:695-700.
13. Cyr MG, Wartman SA. The effectiveness of routine screening questions in the detection of alcoholism. *JAMA* 1988;259: 51-54.
14. Hunt WA. Are binge drinkers more at risk of developing brain damage? *Alcohol* 1993;10:559-561.
15. Hoffman PL, Tabakoff B. The role of the NMDA receptor in

ethanol withdrawal. *EXS* 1994;71: 61-70.

16. Whittington MA, Lambert JD, Little HJ. Increased NMDA receptor and calcium channel activity underlying ethanol withdrawal hyperexcitability. *Alcohol Alcohol* 1995;30: 105-114.
17. Watson WP, Little HJ. Interactions between diltiazem and ethanol: Differences from those seen with dihydropyridine calcium channel antagonists. *Psychopharmacology.* 1994; 114:329-336.
18. Aguayo LG. Ethanol potentiates the $GABA_A$ activates Cl^- currents in mouse hippocampal and cortical neurons. *Eur J Pharmacol* 1990;187:127-130.
19. Dettling M, Heinz A, Dufeu P, et al. Dopaminergic responsivity in alcoholism: Trait, state, or residual marker? *Am Rev Psych* 1995;152:1317-1321.
20. Roberts AJ, Crabbe JC, Keith LD. Corticosterone increases severity of acute withdrawal from ethanol, pentobarbital, and diazepam in mice. *Psychopharmacol* 1994;115:278-284.
21. Dennison H, Jern S, Jagenburg R, et al. Influence of increased adrenergic activity and magnesium depletion on cardiac rhythm in alcohol withdrawal. *Br Heart J* 1994;72:554-560.
22. Wrenn KD, Slovis CM, Minion GE, et al. The syndrome of alcoholic ketoacidosis. *Am J Med* 1991;91:119-28.
23. Victor M, Adams RD. The effect of alcohol on the nervous system. *Res Publ Assoc Nerv Ment Dis* 1953;32:526.
24. Sullivan JT, Sykora K, Shneiderman, et al. Assessment of alcohol withdrawal: The revised Clinical Institute Withdrawal Assessment for Alcohol scale (CIWA-Ar). *Br J Addict* 1989; 84:1353-57.
25. Earlywine M. Personality risk for alcoholism covaries with hangover symptoms. *Addict Behav* 1993;18:415-420.
26. Gauvin DV, Goulden KL, Holloway FA. State-dependent stimulus control: Cueing attributes of ethanol hangover in rats. *Alcohol Clin Exp Res* 1993;17:1210-1214.
27. Gauvin DV, Change EY, Holloway FA. Recent developments in alcoholism: Biobehavioral correlates. *Recent Dev Alcohol* 1993;11:281-11304.
28. Victor M, Brausch C. The role of abstinence in the genesis of alcoholic epilepsy. *Epilepsy* 1967;8:1-20.
29. Gil-Martin E, Fernandez-Briera A, Fernandez-Lopez A, et al. Effect of chronic treatment with ethanol and withdrawal of ethanol on binding of [3H]SCH23390 to D1 dopamine receptors in rat visual cortex and hippocampus. *Neuropharmacol* 1994;33:1203-1209.
30. Isbell H, Fraser HF, Wikler A, et al. An experimental study of "rum fits" and delirium tremens. *Q J Stud Alcohol* 1955;16: 1-33.
31. Tavel ME, Davidson W, Batterton TD. A critical analysis of mortality associated with delerium tremens: review of 39 fatalities in a nine-year period. *Am J Med Sci* 1961;242: 18-29.
32. Victor M, Adas RD. The effect of alcohol on the nervous system. *Res Publ Assoc Nerv Ment Dis* 1953;32:526.
33. Bezzegh A, Nyuli L, Kovacs GL. Alpha-atrial natriuretic peptide, aldosterone secretion and plasma renin activity during ethanol withdrawal: A correlation with the onset of delerium tremens. *Alcohol* 1991;8:333-336.
34. Hillbom M, Hjelm-Jager M. Should alcohol withdrawal seizures be treated with anti-epileptic drugs? *Acta Neurol Scand* 1984;69:39-42.
35. Rathlev N, Shieh T, Callum M. Etiology of alcohol withdrawal seizures and their occurrence in relation to the decreased availability of alcohol. *Ann Emerg Med* 1992;21:663. Abstract.
36. Ng SKC, Hauser WA, Brust JCM, et al. Alcohol consumption and withdrawal in new-onset seizures. *N Eng J Med* 1988; 319:666-673.
37. Chan A. Alcoholism and epilepsy. *Epilepsia.* 1985;25:323. Abstract.
38. Devetag F, Mandich G, Zaiotti G, et al. Alcoholic epilepsy: Review of a series and proposed classification and etiopathogenesis. *Ital J Neurol Sci* 1983;3:275.
39. Lennox WG. Alcohol and epilepsy. *Q J Stud Alcohol* 1941; 2:1.
40. Gill JS, Shipley MJ, Tsementzis SA, et al. Alcohol consumption—a risk factor for hemorrhagic and non-hemorrhagic stroke. *Am J Med* 1991;90:489-497.
41. Hillbom M, Kaste M. Alcohol intoxication: A risk factor for primary subarachnoid hemorrhage. *Neurology* 1982;32:706.
42. Hillbom M, Kaste M. Does ethanol intoxication promote brain infarction in young adults? *Lancet* 1978;2:1181-1183.
43. Weisberg L. Alcoholic intracerebral hemorrhage. *Stroke* 1988; 19:1565-1569.
44. McMicken, D, Freedland E. Alcohol-related seizures: Pathophysiology, differential diagnosis, evaluation, and treatment. *Emerg Clin North Am* 1994;12:1057-1079.
45. Browne M, Anton R, Malcolm R, et al. Alcohol detoxification and withdrawal seizures: Clinical support for a kindling hypotheses. *Biol Psychiatry* 1988;23:507-514.
46. Pinel J. Alcohol withdrawal seizures: Implications of kindling. *Pharmac Biochem Behav* 1980;13:225-231.
47. Lechtenberg R, Worner T. Seizure risk with recurrent alcohol detoxification. *Arch Neurol* 1990;47:535-538.
48. Lechtenberg R, Worner TM. Relative kindling effect of detoxification and non-detoxification admissions in alcoholics. *Alcohol Alcohol* 1991;26:221-225.
49. Earnest M, Felman H, Marx J, et al. Intracranial lesions shown by CT in 259 cases of first alcohol-related seizures. *Neurol* 1988;38:1 561-1562.
50. Devenyi P, Harrison M. Prevention of alcohol withdrawal seizures with oral diazepam loading. *Can Med Assoc J* 1985; 132:798-800.
51. Haddox VO, Bidder TG, Waldron LE, et al. Clorazepate use may prevent alcohol withdrawal convulsions. *West J Med* 1987;146:695-696.
52. Marx JA, Berner J, Bar-Or D, et al. Prophylaxis of alcohol withdrawal seizures: A prospective study. *Ann Emerg Med* 1986;15:637. Abstract.
53. Greenblatt D, Shader R. *Benzodiazepines in Clinical Practice.* New York: Raven; 1974.
54. Turner RC, Lichstein PR, Peden JG, et al. Alcohol withdrawal syndromes: A review of pathophysiology, clinical presentation, and treatment. *J Gen Intern Med* 1989;4: 432-444.
55. Greenblatt DJ, Shader RI, Abernethy DR. Current status of benzodiazepines. *N Engl J Med* 1983;309:410-416.

56. Kaim SC, Klett CJ, Rothfeld B. Treatment of acute alcohol withdrawal state: A comparison of four drugs. 1969;125:1640-1646.
57. Institute of Medicine. *Prevention and Treatment of Alcohol Problems.* Washington, DC: National Academy Press; 1990:268-269.
58. Saitz R, et al. Individualized treatment for alcohol withdrawal: A randomized, double-blind controlled trial. *JAMA* 1994;272:519.
59. Saitz R. Alcohol withdrawal: A nationwide survey of inpatient treatment practices. *J Gen Intern Med* 1995;10: 479-487.
60. Comer WH, Elliott HW, Nomof N. Pharmacology of parenterally administered lorazepam in man. *J lnt Med Res* 1973;1:216.
61. Elliott HW, Nomof N, Navarro G, et al. Comer WH. Central nervous system and cardiovascular effects of lorazepam. *Clin Pharmacol Ther* 1971;12:468-481.
62. Walker JE, Homan RW, Vasko MR, et al. Lorazepam in status epilepticus. *Ann Neurol* 1979;6:207-213.
63. Leppik IE, Derivan AT, Homan RW, et al. Double-blind study of lorazepam and diazepam in status epilepticus. *JAMA* 1983; 249:1452-1454.
64. Miller WC, McCurdy L. A double-blind comparison of the efficacy and safety of lorazepam and diazepam in the treatment of the acute alcohol withdrawal syndrome. *Clin Ther* 1984;6:364-370.
65. Sellers R et al. Diazepam loading: Simplified treatment of alcohol withdrawal. *Clin Pharmacol Ther* 1983; 34:822.
66. Hoyumpa AM. Disposition and elimination of minor tranquilizers in the aged and in patients with liver disease. *South Med J* 1978;71:23-28.
67. Kraus JW, Desmond PV, Marshall JP, et al. Effects of aging and liver disease on disposition of lorazepam. *Clin Pharmacol Ther* 1978;24:411.
68. Kraus JW, Marshall JP, Johnson R, et al. Lorazepam elimination in liver disease. *Gastroenterol* 1977;73:1228.
69. D'Onofrio G, Rathlev NK, Ulrich AS, et al. Lorazepam prevents recurrent alcohol related seizures. *Acad Emerg Med* 1995;2:366.
70. Alldredge B, Lowenstein D, Simon R. Placebo-controlled trial of intravenous diphenylhydantoin for short-term treatment of alcohol withdrawal seizures. *Am J Med* 1989;87: 645-648.
71. Chance J. Emergency department treatment of alcohol withdrawal seizures with phenytoin. *Ann Emerg Med* 1991; 20:520-522.
72. Rathlev NK, D'Onofrio G, Fish SS, et al. The efficacy of phenytoin in the prevention of recurrent alcohol withdrawal seizures. *Ann Emerg Med* 1992;21:661-662. Abstract.
73. Sellers E. Alcohol, barbiturate and benzodiazepine withdrawal syndromes: Clinical management. *Can Med Assoc J* 1988;39:11311-11318.
74. Sellers EM, Giles HG, Greenblatt DJ, et al. Differential effects on benzodiazepine disposition by disulfiram and ethanol. *Arzneimittelforsch* 1980;30:882-886.
75. Saadi H. *Presentation Pattern of Recurrent Alcoholic Patients in the Emergency Department.* New Haven: Yale University School of Public Health; 1995.
76. McMicken DB. Alcohol withdrawal syndromes. *Emerg Med Clin North Am* 1990;8:805-816.
77. Saitz R. Recognition and management of occult alcohol withdrawal. *Hosp Pract* 1995;30.

Poison Antidotes

Robert O. Wright, MD
Richard Y. Wang, DO, FACEP

As recently as 25 years ago, the universal recipe for poison management could be summarized as follows: "One part activated charcoal, one part magnesium oxide, and one part tannic acid." Fortunately, more effective and potentially less toxic therapies have been developed.[1] More specific and targeted, current antidotes employ a variety of biochemical strategies, such as preventing production of toxic metabolites, exerting direct antagonistic effects against the poison, or binding to the poison to make it ineffective or enhance its elimination. In addition, antibody therapy is currently available to manage toxicity caused by certain venoms, cardiac glycosides, clostridial toxin, and colchicine.[2]

Unfortunately, the number of antidotes that are specific for certain drugs or poisons is limited. Nevertheless, when used in the correct setting, they can be life-saving. Despite their efficacy, the initial approach to the patient must always include assessment and stabilization of the airway, breathing, and circulation. Antidotal therapy is secondary. Moreover, because of the potential for adverse reactions, these agents should not be used indiscriminately. Patients must be evaluated clinically with appropriate laboratory tests (if available), and the expected action/outcome of the toxin should be considered carefully.

Generally speaking, consultation with a regional poison center is recommended in almost all clinical encounters requiring antidote administration, especially if the diagnosis is in doubt or if the practitioners lack clinical experience with the antidote. Decontamination procedures, though not toxin-specific, also may be useful. Gastric lavage, activated charcoal, and whole bowel irrigation may decrease the toxic burden and reduce the amount of antidote needed and the duration of therapy required for definitive management.

With these issues in mind, this chapter reviews commonly used antidotes for specific poisons. *(Please see Table 1 and Table 2.)*

Acetaminophen

When ingested in toxic quantities, acetaminophen causes centrilobular hepatic necrosis. Cellular damage occurs when free radicals accumulate because of a depletion of the reducing substance, glutathione. In the acute setting, a toxic ingestion is 140 mg/kg. In multiple-dose ingestions or in sustained-release form, toxic amounts are not well-defined and depend on host factors and other considerations.

N-acetylcysteine. N-acetylcysteine (NAC) is the antidote for acetaminophen toxicity. Four mechanisms have been postulated to explain the efficacy of NAC.[3] These include: 1) enhancing the synthesis of glutathione; 2) acting intracellularly as a glutathione substitute; 3) providing substrate to enhance nontoxic sulfation metabolism; and 4) acting as an antioxidant.

The Rumack-Matthew nomogram determines NAC therapy in acetaminophen overdoses associated with single-dose ingestions of

Table 1. Poisons and Their Antidotes

POISON	ANTIDOTE
Acetaminophen	N-acetylcysteine
Anticholinergics (e.g., diphenhydramine, benzotropine)	Physostigmine
Anticoagulants	
Coumarin derivatives	Vitamin K_1
Heparin	Protamine
Benzodiazepines	Flumazenil
Botulism	Botulinim antitoxin
Carbon monoxide	Oxygen
Cardiac medications	
Beta-adrenergic blockers	Glucagon
Calcium-channel blockers	Calcium
Digoxin	Digoxin Fab antibodies
Cholinergics	
Organophosphates, carbamates	Atropine, pralidoxime
Cyanide	Amyl nitrite, sodium nitrite, sodium thiosulfate, hydroxocobalmin
Hypoglycemia	Glucose, hydrocortisone, diazoxide
Iron	Deferoxamine
Isoniazid	Pyridoxine
Lead	BAL (British anti-Lewisite), $CaNa_2EDTA$, DMSA (dimercapto succinic acid)
Methemoglobinemia	Methylene blue
Opioids	Naloxone
Toxic alcohols	
Ethylene glycol	Ethanol, pyridoxine, thiamine
Methanol	Ethanol, folinic acid
Tricyclic antidepressants (TCAs)	Sodium bicarbonate
Venoms	
North American rattlesnakes	Crotalidae antivenin
Eastern, Texas coral snake	Elapidae antivenin
Black widow spider	Lactrodectus antivenin

immediate-release formulations.[4] *(Please see Figure 1.)* Serum acetaminophen levels between four and 24 hours post-ingestion are plotted on the nomogram, and those that fall below the lower line require no treatment. In contrast, levels at or above the lower line require NAC therapy. For extended-release formulations of acetaminophen, the manufacturer's recommendation is to obtain a four- and eight-hour post-ingestion acetaminophen level.[5] If either level falls on or above the lower nomogram line, the patient should be treated with NAC. Consultation with the regional poison center is recommended for unusual exposures that fall outside of these well-defined parameters.

It should be stressed that therapy must be started as soon as possible and is most efficacious if initiated within eight hours of ingestion.[6] The standard NAC dosing regimen for patients meeting nomogram criteria is as follows: loading dose, 140 mg/kg po; maintenance dose, 70 mg/kg po q4h for a total of 17 doses. The NAC can be chilled and diluted to a 5% concentration with a beverage to ensure compliance. All patients are treated for the full course, regardless of declining acetaminophen levels. Patients with fulminant liver failure may benefit from late and continual NAC therapy.[7]

Activated charcoal can be used with NAC when coingestants are present. For routine acetaminophen overdoses, the amount of NAC that is bound by charcoal is not of clinical significance and the standard NAC dosing is adequate.[6] Otherwise, the NAC dose may be either increased by 40% when used in conjunction with activated charcoal or staggered by two hours with the charcoal dose.[8]

Although there is still a debate about oral vs. IV use of NAC, IV NAC has been used successfully in Great Britain and Canada, and this route is still being evaluated in the United States.[9,10] Anaphylactoid reactions have been reported with IV administration.[11]

Amanita phalloides

The *A. phalloides* mushroom contains a number of hepatotoxic cyclopeptides. Onset of symptoms typically occurs more than six hours after ingestion and consists of vomiting, diarrhea, and abdominal pain. Fulminant hepatic failure may ensue. Less than 0.1 mg/kg of amatoxin is considered lethal.[12]

Penicillin. A variety of antidotes have been used for *A. phalloides* poisoning, including penicillin, thicotic acid, and silibinin. However, none of them has been shown to be more effective than good supportive care. Thicotic acid, which was thought to work as a free radical scavenger, has not been shown to be effective in experimental trials.[13] High-dose penicillin and silibinin may inhibit hepatocyte uptake of the cyclopeptides.[14] Despite its questionable efficacy, penicillin therapy is safe and can be started at 300,000 to 1,000,000 U/kg/d. Thicotic acid and silibinin are not available in the United States.

Anticholinergic Toxicity

Anticholinergic effects can be produced by a number of pharmacologic agents, including antihistamines, antiparkinsonian medications, antipsychotics, belladonna alkaloids, antispasmodics, cyclic antidepressants, and certain plants and mushrooms. Clinical toxicity is characterized by confusion, agitation, fever, mydriasis, diminished bowel activity, urinary retention, and

Table 2. Antidotes: Dosages and Routes of Administration

ANTIDOTE	DOSAGE
Atropine	Initial: 0.5-2.0 mg IV
Amyl nitrite	Inhale pearls for 30 sec/min
BAL	Initial: 3-5 mg/kg IM
$CaNa_2EDTA$	50-75 mg/kg/d IV
Calcium salts	
10% calcium chloride	Adults: 1-2 g IV Pediatric: 0.2-0.25 mL/kg IV
10% calcium gluconate	Adults: 3 g IV
Deferoxamine	90 mg/kg IM (maximum: children, 1 g; adults, 2 g) 15 mg/kg/h IV
Dextrose	
50% solution	Adult: 50-100 mL IV
25% solution	Children: 2-4 mL/kg IV
Digoxin Fab antibodies	Empirical therapy
Acute toxicity	5-10 vials
Chronic toxicity	2-5 vials
Dimercaptosuccinic Acid (DMSA)	10 mg/kg po tid for 5 days, then 10 mg/kg po bid for 14 days
Ethanol	Load: 1g/kg Maintenance: 0.1g/kg/h
Folinic acid	Adult: 50 mg IM/IV
Flumazenil	Adults: 0.2 mg IV over 15 seconds. May be repeated every 60 sec. up to a total dose of 1 mg
Glucagon	Load: 2-10 mg IV in adults Start 50 mcg/kg IV in children Maintenance: 2-5mg/h IV
Methylene blue	Initial: 1-2 mg/kg IV

ANTIDOTE	DOSAGE
N-acetylcysteine	Load: 140 mg/kg po Maintenance: 70 mg/kg po for 17 doses
Naloxone	2-10 mg IV/IM/endotracheal
Oxygen	100% through a tight-fitting non-rebreather mask
Physostigmine	Adult: 1-2 mg IV Children: 0.2-0.6 mg IV
Pralidoxime	Adult: 1-2 g IV Children: 25-50 mg/kg IV
Protamine	1 mg IV for every 100 units of heparin
Pyridoxine	
Isoniazid	Empirical therapy Adult: 5 g IV Children: 70 mg/kg IV
Ethylene glycol	Adult: 50 mg IM/IV
Sodium bicarbonate	Load: 1-2 mEq/kg IV Maintenance: 0.2-0.4 mEq/kg/h IV
Sodium nitrite	
3% solution	Adult: 10 mL IV Children: 0.15-0.33 mL/kg IV for a hemoglobin of 12 g/dL
Sodium thiosulfate	
25% solution	Adult: 50 mL IV Children: 1.10-1.95 mL/kg IV for a hemoglobin of 12 g/dL
Thiamine	Adult: 100 mg IM/IV
Vitamin K_1	Initial: Adult: 10 mg SQ

dry mucocutaneous membranes. Dysrrhythmias, coma, and seizures may also occur in severe cases.

Physostigmine. Antidotal therapy with physostigmine can achieve remarkable results and facilitates the medical management of patients with anticholinergic poisoning. Physostigmine is a reversible cholinesterase inhibitor that prolongs the action of acetylcholine at cholinergic receptors, an action that permits it to protect against anticholinergic effects. Moreover, this agent crosses the blood-brain barrier, a property that makes it useful for reversing coma, treating agitated delirium, and reducing seizure activity. However, despite the availability and effectiveness of this antidote, most patients with anticholinergic poisoning can be adequately treated with supportive measures alone.

Moreover, potentially serious complications can result from the incorrect use of physostigmine. In some case series, as many as 12% of patients receiving physostigmine developed seizures, cholinergic crisis, bradycardia, or even asystole.[15] The majority of patients with complications had overdosed on medications with the potential for seizures and dysrhythmias (e.g., tricyclic antidepressants). Consequently, physostigmine should only be given in the face of significant neurologic toxicity caused by drugs with known anticholinergic properties (e.g., diphenhydramine, benzotropine).

Indications for its use include intractable seizures and pronounced agitation during which the patient may be dangerous to himself or to others. Relative contraindications to use are active asthma, gangrene, cardiovascular disease, and gastrointestinal or urinary obstruction. An ECG showing conduction abnormalities precludes the use of this antidote. Patients should be on a cardiac monitor, and atropine must be available at the bedside in the event that cholinergic crisis ensues. Initial doses of physostigmine are 0.2-0.6 mg/kg IV for children and 1-2 mg IV for adults. The dose should be given slowly over five minutes and may be repeated every 10 minutes until the desired effects are achieved. The maximum total dose should not exceed 4 mg. Patients may require repeat treatment when the physostigmine wears off (usually in about 45 minutes).

Anticoagulants

The oral anticoagulants include warfarin, acenocoumarin, phenprocoumon, biscoumacetate, and bishydroxycoumarin. Because these compounds are similar in structure to vitamin K, they competitively inhibit the enzymatic activation of vitamin K-dependent clotting factors (II, VII, IX, and X). Heparin catalyzes the binding of antithrombin III to thrombin and other proteases in order to inhibit clot formation.

Vitamin K_1. Patients with life-threatening hemorrhage require factor replacement with fresh frozen plasma (4-6 units in adults, 20 mL/kg in children). This approach is preferred initially because it is the most rapid method of reversing anticoagulation. Vitamin K_1 is indicated when there is evidence of hypoprothrombinemia associated with oral anticoagulant toxicity; this antidote requires 6-12 hours to produce reversal of anticoagulation. Because of its delay in onset of action, it is not the mainstay of therapy in actively bleeding patients.

Vitamin K_1 may be administered orally, intramuscularly, subcutaneously, or intravenously. Although the IV route works most rapidly, it has been associated with life-threatening anaphylactoid reactions.[16] In situations requiring IV therapy, vitamin K_1 should be administered no faster than 1 mg/min. In general, the subcutaneous or oral route is preferred. The dose of vitamin K_1 in the adult is initially 10 mg SQ, with subsequent dosages requiring adjustment according to the prothrombin time. Because of the antidote's short half-life, the dose may have to be repeated every 6-8 hours. In this regard, it should be emphasized that overdoses with the superwarfarins (e.g., brodifacoum) require high doses of vitamin K_1 for a prolonged duration.[17]

Protamine. The protamines, proteins derived from fish sperm, bind to heparin and, in the process, inactivate it. The dose of protamine depends on the dose of heparin requiring inactivation. In general, approximately 1 mg of protamine will neutralize 100 units of heparin. The maximum dose of protamine is 50 mg and the antidote should be infused intravenously at a 10 mg/mL concentration over 10 minutes. Since anaphylactic/anaphylactoid reactions are associated with the use of this antidote,[18] and the half-life of heparin is short (1-3 hours), protamine is not indicated if bleeding is minor, and the site can be compressed in order to achieve hemostasis.

Benzodiazepines

Benzodiazepine overdose may cause sedation, amnesia, or lethargy. When taken alone, mortality from this drug class is extremely low. However, when taken in combination with other sedative-hypnotic agents, coma and respiratory failure can occur. All patients managed with timely respiratory support can be expected to do well.

Flumazenil. Flumazenil will reverse the sedative, ataxic, muscle relaxant, anxiolytic, and anticonvulsant effects of benzodiazepines.[19] The reversal of anticonvulsant effects can be problematic in co-ingestions involving tricyclic antidepressants. This agent competitively binds to CNS benzodiazepine receptors. In addition to intentional ingestions, flumazenil also can be used to treat patients who have inadvertently overdosed with benzodiazepines after conscious sedation. Patients respond with dramatic improvement in state of consciousness and respiratory status within 1-5 minutes after administration. The initial dose is 0.2 mg IV and may be titrated as 0.2-0.5 mg/min to effect. No more than 3 mg should be given over an hour, and if no results are observed after 5 mg, then the diagnosis of benzodiazepine toxicity should be questioned.

Generally speaking, flumazenil has been used in the ED to successfully treat and diagnose benzodiazepine ingestions, with few reported complications.[20] There have been, however, case reports of death from seizures when flumazenil was administered to patients with combined tricyclic antidepressant/benzodiazepine ingestions.[20,21] Presumably, in these cases the benzodiazepine provides a protective effect against the CNS toxicity (i.e., epileptogenic properties) of the antidepressant. Flumazenil is not recommended for reverse respiratory compromise due to benzodiazepines because of the short duration of action of the antidote. In these cases, interventional approaches directed toward stabilization of the airway are preferred.

Because of the questionable histories obtained from comatose overdose patients, and the chance of precipitating sedative-hypnotic withdrawal and seizures, flumazenil should not be used *routinely* in comatose patients and should be used with extreme caution in patients with presumed benzodiazepine overdose. Clinical judgment must dictate the suitability of this antidote on a patient-by-patient basis.

Botulism

Botulism is characterized by cranial nerve palsies and gastrointestinal symptoms. In severe cases, progressive muscle paralysis leads to respiratory failure and death. The toxin—of which there are eight varieties (A-G)—is produced by *Clostridium botulinum.* Toxicity results either from ingestion of preformed toxin or from wound bacterial contamination. The toxin causes paralysis by blocking the release of acetylcholine at neuromuscular receptors. As little as 0.5 mcg of the toxin can be lethal.

Botulinum Antitoxin. Airway assessment and management with intubation and mechanical ventilation, if necessary, are the initial approaches to the treatment of botulism. The antitoxin binds only to circulating toxin and has no effects on toxin already bound to neuromuscular receptors. Consequently, the antitoxin can *prevent* and *limit* paralysis, but cannot *reverse* it.[22] Infant botulism does not require antitoxin therapy because the amount of circulating toxin is very low.

Once the disease process is recognized, antitoxin should be administered. If the variety of toxin is not known, the trivalent type (A, B, E) is used. A single vial contains 10 mL of antitoxin, which is given as a 1:10 dilution in 0.9% normal saline IV over 30 minutes. This dose may be supplemented with an IM dose, and subsequent IV doses given every 2-4 hours may follow. The antitoxin is derived from horse serum, and complications include anaphylaxis and serum sickness. Serum sickness is more commonly seen with higher doses, (i.e., those in the 40 mL range).

Figure 1. Nomogram: Plasma or Serum Acetaminophen Level vs. Time Post-Acetaminophen Ingestion

Estimating potential for hepatotoxicity: The following nomogram has been developed to estimate the probability that plasma levels in relation to intervals post ingestion will result in hepatotoxicity.

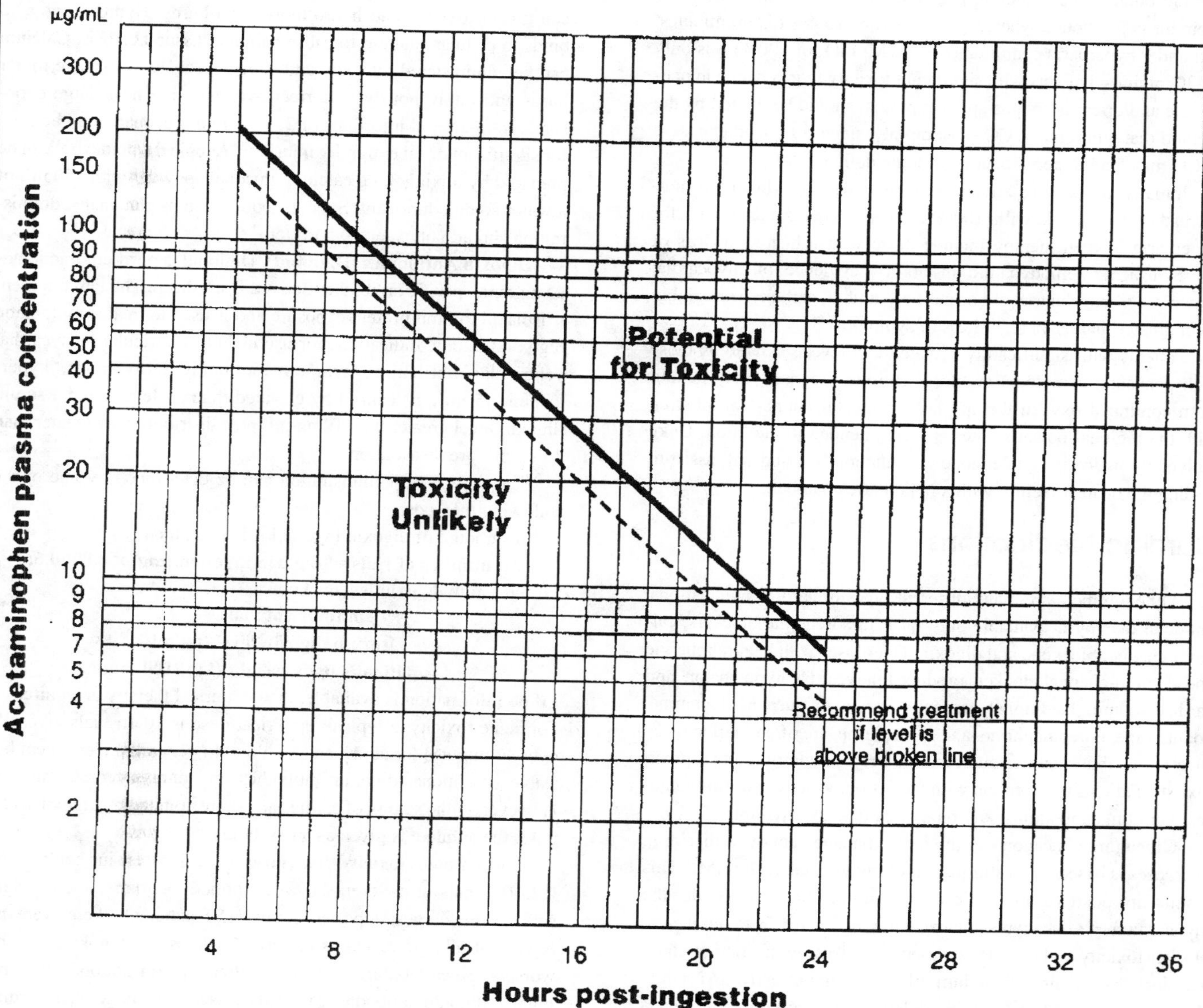

Cautions for use of this chart:

1. The time coordinates refer to time post ingestion.
2. The graph relates only to plasma levels following a single acute overdose ingestion.
3. The broken line, which represents a 25% allowance below the solid line, is included to allow for possible errors in acetaminophen plasma assays and estimated time from ingestion of an overdose.

Adapted from: Rumack BH, Matthew H. Acetaminophen poisoning and toxicity. *Pediatrics* 1975;55:871-876.

A human-derived botulism immune globulin is presently being studied. This immune globulin is pentavalent (A, B, C, D, E) and is harvested by plasmapheresis from human donors vaccinated with botulinum toxoid.[23] For assistance with antitoxin availability and dosage, contact the local department of health or the Centers for Disease Control and Prevention.

Carbon Monoxide

Carbon monoxide (CO) is the product of incomplete combustion of fuel-powered engines. It binds to hemoglobin with an affinity 200-250 times greater than oxygen and inhibits oxygen transport. At the cellular level, CO may bind to mitochondrial enzymes and cause cellular hypoxia. Early symptoms are often "flu-like" (headache, malaise, weakness, etc.); consequently, the toxic syndrome is often not recognized. Prolonged exposure can result in coma, seizures, residual neurologic deficits, and death.

Oxygen. Administration of pure oxygen shortens the time CO remains bound to hemoglobin. The half-life of carboxyhemoglobin at room air is 5-6 hours, whereas at an FiO_2 of 100% it is 90 minutes, and under hyberbaric conditions (2.8 ATM, FiO_2 of 100%) it is only 20-30 minutes. Patients with significant toxicity (e.g., change in neurologic and/or cardiac signs and symptoms) should be treated by the method that will remove CO most rapidly, since continued exposure to CO may lead to permanent neurologic deficits.[24]

Initially, all patients should be treated with a tight-fitting non-rebreather face mask with 100% oxygen. Patients considered for hyperbaric oxygen therapy include those with a history of loss of consciousness, hemodynamic instability, evidence of myocardial injury, neuropsychiatric abnormalities, and a carboxyhemoglobin level greater than 25% regardless of symptoms.[25]

Patients with significantly elevated CO levels, as well as those with persistent symptoms or those who are pregnant, may benefit from continued oxygen therapy lasting several hours. Consultation with the regional poison center is recommended. In addition, Duke University maintains a telephone consultation line and will assist in finding the nearest facility with a hyperbaric chamber..

Cardiac Medications

Although there are many different types of cardiac medications, antidotal therapy is available only for beta-adrenergic blockers, calcium-channel blockers, and digoxin. Overdoses with beta-adrenergic and calcium-channel blockers produce bradycardia, hypotension, and cardiac failure. Traditional vasoactive pressors, such as dopamine, dobutamine, norepinephrine, and epinephrine, are often ineffective.[26] Electrolyte abnormalities and renal failure can contribute to digoxin toxicity. Patients may present with confusion, visual aberrations, nausea, vomiting, and almost any type of cardiac dysrhythmia.

Glucagon. Glucagon's utility in the management of cardiac drug overdoses is based on its stimulation of myocardial cyclic AMP. This results in positive inotropic and chronotropic effects on the myocardium.[27] Glucagon is indicated in *symptomatic* beta-adrenergic blocker toxicity and can also be used in patients with calcium-channel blocker poisoning if calcium infusion is not effective. An initial IV dose of glucagon of 2 mg for adults and 50 mcg/kg for children is recommended. Therapy is quickly titrated to a total loading dose of 10 mg before glucagon is considered ineffective. A beneficial response is followed by a continuous drip at 2-5 mg/h in D_5W. Nausea, vomiting, and hyperglycemia may be seen with glucagon therapy. When more than 2 mg of glucagon is used, the phenol diluent supplied by the manufacturer should be replaced with sterile water.[28]

Calcium. Calcium-channel blockers selectively block voltage-dependent L channels in cardiac and smooth muscles. The inhibition of these channels can be overcome with administration of IV calcium. The initial dose in an adult is 1 g of calcium chloride or 3 g of calcium gluconate, both of which are given as a 10% solution. This dose may be repeated every 10 minutes up to a total of four doses. In children, the dose of calcium chloride is 0.2-0.25 mL/kg given as a 10% solution, and may be repeated once in 10 minutes. If multiple doses are given, serum calcium should be monitored in order to avoid hypercalcemia. Calcium should not be given to patients with digoxin toxicity because of concern for raising myocardial calcium levels and, therefore, potentiating digoxin-mediated cardiac toxicity.

Calcium therapy may also be of benefit in the management of hypermagnesemia, hyperkalemia, black widow envenomation, ethylene glycol toxicity, and hydrofluoric acid burns. Hydrofluoric acid binds to cellular calcium to cause pain and tissue necrosis. Calcium can be administered topically and subcutaneously to manage minor burns and intravenously to correct hypocalcemia from large exposures. Intra-arterial injections of 2% calcium gluconate may be used for significant distal extremity injuries.[29] A topical calcium gel can be prepared by mixing 3.5 g calcium gluconate powder with 150 mL of a water-soluble lubricant. Subcutaneous calcium gluconate administration should not exceed 0.5 mL/cm².

Digoxin Antibodies (Digibind). Digibind is purified, fractionated digoxin-specific antibodies derived from sheep. The Fab fragment is isolated to limit protein exposure and is used to treat symptomatic digoxin toxicity. Indications for use include ventricular tachycardia, ventricular fibrillation, symptomatic bradydysrhythmias, hyperkalemia (5 mEq/L) caused by elevated digoxin levels, and a serum digoxin level greater than 10 ng/mL post distribution or greater than 15 ng/mL pre distribution.[30]

The dosage of administration can be determined by one of the following methods:

1) if the amount of digoxin ingested is known, then

number of vials = [digoxin ingested (mg) × 0.80]/0.6;

2) if the serum digoxin level is known, then

number of vials =
[serum digoxin level (ng/mL)
× patient's body weight (kg)]/100; and

3) if no information is available, then empirical therapy is required. For acute toxicity, a typical, empirical dose is 10-15 vials given IV over 30 minutes for adults and children. In general, under urgent but stable conditions, digoxin antibodies are given over 30 minutes. However, in the setting of cardiac arrest precipitated by digoxin overdose, the antidote is given as an IV bolus.

For chronic toxicity, the dose is 2-5 vials in adults, and 0.25-0.5 vials in children. Digoxin antibody administration is very safe. In the largest reported series (150 patients), there were no reports of allergic reactions or serum sickness.[31] Hypokalemia and worsening heart failure may occur after digoxin antibody therapy. Finally, digoxin antibodies can also be used to manage plant cardiac glycoside (e.g., *Nerium oleander)*-induced dysrhythmias.[32]

Cholinergics

Organophosphate and carbamate pesticides inhibit acetylcholinesterase, an enzyme that breaks down acetylcholine in synaptic junctions. Acetylcholine accumulates and excessively stimulates cholinergic nervous transmission. Physiologic manifestations of muscarinic stimulation are salivation, lacrimation, urination, diaphoresis, emesis, miosis, bradycardia, and bronchorrhea. Nicotinic effects are fasciculations, weakness, and paralysis. The most common presenting symptoms are "flu-like"; therefore, this form of toxicity may be misdiagnosed as gastroenteritis.

Atropine. Atropine blocks acetylcholine at the post-synaptic receptors and serves as a physiologic antidote for organophosphate and carbamate poisonings. It is only effective in treating the *muscarinic* manifestations of cholinergic toxicity. An initial, empirical adult dose is 2 mg IV and should be repeated if there is no effect. The dose may be increased to 5 mg every 15 minutes in the critically ill adult patient. The initial pediatric dose is 0.02 mg/kg (minimum dose, 0.1 mg). Atropine therapy is titrated to the drying of bronchial secretions.

Atropine is also effective in the treatment of other cholinergic poisonings, such as the clitocybe or inocybe mushroom, synthetic cholinergic agonists (bethanecol), and physostigmine.

Pralidoxime. Pralidoxime (2-PAM) is a specific antidote for organophosphate poisoning. It improves muscarinic and nicotinic symptoms by removing the organophosphate moeity from the acetylcholinesterase enzyme. Pralidoxime's other beneficial effects include its direct detoxification of the organophosphate molecule and its synergistic activity with atropine.[33] Pralidoxime is indicated whenever atropine is used in these poisonings. Patients with delayed and prolonged nicotinic manifestations of toxicity may benefit from continued pralidoxime therapy.[34,35] The initial adult dose of pralidoxime is 1-2 g IV given over 15-30 minutes. The pediatric dose is 25-50 mg/kg IV. The dose is repeated every 6-12 hours for 24-48 hours. Pralidoxime generally has minimal toxic side effects.

Cyanide

Cyanide causes cellular hypoxia by binding to iron (Fe^{+3}) at the mitochondrial cytochrome oxidase and inhibiting aerobic metabolism. The heart and brain are most sensitive to the lack of oxygen and are the first to show manifestations of toxicity. Symptoms begin as headache and dyspnea and can progress rapidly to coma, convulsions, shock, respiratory failure, and death.

Cyanide Antidote Kit. Patients manifesting cyanide toxicity with persistent metabolic acidosis warrant emergency treatment with the Eli Lilly antidote kit. The kit contains amyl nitrite pearls, sodium nitrite, and sodium thiosulfate. Nitrites will induce a methemoglobinemia, which attracts cyanide away from the mitochondria, so that aerobic metabolism can resume. Thiosulfate combines with cyanide to form the nontoxic thiocyanate, which is eliminated renally.

Although the nitrites and thiosulfate can be effective when given alone, they should be administered together if possible. The amyl nitrite pearls are intended for use by first responders and when IV access is not available. The small ampules (pearls) are broken into a gauze and held close to the nose of breathing patients to induce a methemoglobinemia. Alternatively, the pearls may be placed in the lip of the face mask or within the resuscitation bag of patients with respiratory compromise. Patients should inhale the pearls for 30 seconds of each minute until IV access is obtained. Once IV access is obtained, 10 mL of sodium nitrite as a 3% solution is given over 2-4 minutes in adults. The goal of nitrite therapy is to achieve a methemoglobin level of approximately 30%. In children, there is potential for causing methemoglobin toxicity, and the sodium nitrite dose is adjusted according to the patient's hemoglobin level, if available.

The average child should receive 0.15-0.33 mL/kg (max, 10 mL) of sodium nitrite. The nitrite infusion can cause rate-dependent hypotension and is administered over a period of at least five minutes. The IV dose of the sodium thiosulfate is also adjusted in children, and the range is 1.10-1.95 mL/kg of a 25% solution. In adults, 50 mL of the thiosulfate is administered over 10-15 minutes. One kit can treat two adult patients, or one ill patient twice. Repeat nitrite and thiosulfate therapy will be dependent on clinical response. Patients with suspected cyanide and CO poisoning from smoke inhalation should be initially treated with thiosulfate alone until the carboxyhemoglobin level is known.

Hydroxocobalamin. This antidote is used in Europe for treatment of cyanide toxicity. The advantage of this antidote is that it does not induce a methemoglobinemia. Hydroxocobalamin (B_{12a}) binds to cyanide and forms the nontoxic cyanocobalamin (B_{12}), which is excreted renally. However, the limitation of this therapy is the large quantity of antidote necessary to treat poisoned patients. Fifty grams of hydroxocobalamin are needed to bind one gram of cyanide. A "new" cyanide antidote kit containing hydroxocobalamin and thiosulfate is being evaluated in Europe.[36] Thiosulfate should reduce the amount of hydroxocobalamin required.

Hypoglycemia

Hypoglycemia may be induced by a number of drugs, most commonly oral hypoglycemic agents and insulin. Ketotic hypoglycemia can be caused by agents that disrupt oxidative phosphorylation, such as aspirin, or by agents that interfere with glucose metabolism, such as ethanol. Any patient with symptomatic hypoglycemia requires glucose administration.

Dextrose. To treat hypoglycemia, the adult IV dose is 50-100 mL of $D_{50}W$. In children, the dose is 2-4 mL/kg IV of $D_{25}W$. A maintenance drip of $D_{10}W$ can be titrated according to clinical symptoms and serum glucose levels for longer-acting hypoglycemic agents. When hypoglycemia is refractory to glucose therapy, hydrocortisone and diazoxide are indicated to increase serum glucose levels.[37] Dextrose, in conjunction with insulin, is also used to treat hyperkalemia.

Iron Toxicity

Iron toxicity can present with nausea, vomiting, abdominal pain, gastrointestinal bleeding, and hypovolemic shock. Metabolic acidosis and cardiac, renal, and hepatic failure may also be seen. Serum total iron binding capacity (TIBC) can help in the assessment of free iron toxicity. However, artifactual TIBC elevations may occur and yield a false sense of security.[38] Symptomatology should be the major consideration in the initiation of chelation therapy.

Deferoxamine. The mainstay of treatment is deferoxamine, a chelating agent that binds free iron to form ferrioxamine. Ferrioxamine is nontoxic and is excreted in the urine, where its presence is noted by a "vin rose" color. In potentially toxic ingestions, an initial deferoxamine dose of 90 mg/kg IM (maximum, 1 g in children, 2 g in adults) may be given and the urine examined for vin rose coloration. Upon confirmation of toxicity, deferoxamine is continued at the same dose IM every eight hours until the resolution of clinical toxicity, fall of serum iron to less than 150 mcg/dL, and return of urine color to normal. Patients with shock require IV deferoxamine therapy.

The starting dose is 5 mg/kg/h and subsequent administration is quickly titrated over several minutes to 15 mg/kg/h. Initiation of IV therapy at the higher rate or a too-rapid rate of infusion may cause hypotension or an anaphylactoid reaction. If these adverse events occur, therapy should be suspended temporarily and the infusion restarted when the patient is stable. Slowing the rate of infusion and adequate hydration may prevent hypotension. Antihistamines, epinephrine, and steroids can be used treat anaphylactoid reactions.

Isoniazid

Isoniazid (INH) is a hydrazine antibiotic used for the treatment of tuberculosis. Acute ingestions of 35-40 mg/kg can produce seizures. INH inhibits pyridoxine-dependent enzymes that are involved in the production of the central inhibitory neurotransmitter, gamma-amino-butyric acid (GABA). Toxic INH ingestions decrease the levels of GABA and induce seizures that can be difficult to manage with standard anticonvulsant therapy.

Pyridoxine. Pyridoxine (B_6) is the antidote of choice for INH-induced seizures. The dose is mg to mg equivalent to the dose of INH ingested. If the amount ingested is unknown, an empirical dose of 5 g IV is given to adults, and 70 mg/kg to children. Repeat doses may be necessary if seizures recur. Patients treated with pyridoxine for INH toxicity are admitted for a 24-hour period of observation. Hospitals should have contingency plans for obtaining more pyridoxine because one significant INH ingestion may deplete the pharmacy's supply.[39] Benzodiazepines are GABA agonists and act synergistically with pyridoxine to stop INH-induced seizures.

Hydrazines in the false morel *(Gyromitra esculenta)* mushroom can also cause toxic seizures. These can be treated with pyridoxine at 25 mg/kg IV.

Lead Toxicity

Lead is the most common form of heavy metal poisoning encountered in clinical practice. Contamination results mainly from the ingestion of lead-based paint. Soil, water, and household dust represent other sources of exposure. The principal areas of the body affected are the bone marrow and the nervous system. Symptoms of lead poisoning are diverse and include lethargy, irritability, abdominal pain, constipation, and anorexia. Anemia is a common finding in chronic poisoning.

Chelation. The most important component of treatment of lead poisoning is to identify and remove the source. Chelating agents used for lead toxicity are calcium disodium EDTA ($CaNa_2EDTA$), BAL (British anti-Lewisite), and dimercaptosuccinic acid (DMSA). Indications for chelation therapy include either a venous blood lead level greater than 45 mcg/dL, a venous blood lead level of 25-44 mcg/dL with an erythrocyte protoporphyrin greater than 125 mcg/dL, or a venous blood lead level of 25-44 mcg/dL in a symptomatic patient.[40] The treatment for certain cases may vary and the regional poison center should be consulted.

Initial inpatient chelation consists of BAL and $CaNa_2EDTA$ therapy. BAL is suspended in peanut oil and administered at 3-5 mg/kg IM every 4-8 hours. This agent should not be given to patients with either peanut sensitivity, hepatic insufficiency, or glucose 6 phosphate dehydrogenase (G6PD) deficiency.[41] In general, it is preferable to administer $CaNa_2EDTA$ as a continuous IV infusion at 50-75 mg/kg/d. Asymptomatic patients with lead levels of 45-70 mcg/dL may be treated with $CaNa_2EDTA$ alone.

For patients with symptoms or levels greater than 70 mcg/dL, $CaNa_2EDTA$ is given in combination with BAL. The first dose of BAL is given about four hours prior to the start of $CaNa_2EDTA$. Most patients should be started on DMSA as inpatients and continued on DMSA after discharge. The starting dose for DMSA is 10 mg/kg po tid for five days, and therapy is continued at the same dose bid for 14 days. DMSA is approved for use only in children with lead toxicity and may be used in G6PD-deficient patients. Lead encephalopathic patients are not to be treated with DMSA. Currently, DMSA is being used in the outpatient management of patients with mild lead toxicity.

BAL can also be used as chelation therapy for inorganic mercury, arsenic, gold, and copper toxicity. Similarly, $CaNa_2EDTA$ may be used in the treatment of chromium, cobalt, manganese, and zinc toxicity.

Methemoglobinemia

Methemoglobin is an abnormal hemoglobin in which iron is oxidized from the Fe^{+2} to the Fe^{+3} state. In poisoned patients, oxygen transport is impaired because methemoglobin is incapable of binding oxygen. Acquired methemoglobin may be induced by a number of oxidizing agents, such as nitrites, nitrates, aniline dyes, lidocaine, pyridium, and dapsone. Methemoglobin levels of 15% are associated with visible cyanosis and few, if any, symptoms. Levels between 30% and 55% are associated with headache, fatigue, weakness, and dizziness. Levels above 55% may cause profound acidosis, dyspnea, bradycardia, and coma. Symptoms may be seen at lower levels in patients with anemia, heart disease, or lung disease.

Methylene Blue. This antidote is indicated for the treatment of patients with symptomatic methemoglobinemia or with levels greater than 20%. Methylene blue serves as a cofactor in the NADPH-methemoglobin reductase pathway to enhance the conversion of hemoglobin back to the Fe^{+2} state. Patients with G6PD deficiency may not respond to methylene blue therapy because they cannot produce enough NADPH to support the reductase pathway. The dose of methylene blue is 1-2 mg/kg IV given as a 1% solution over five minutes. A significant drop in methemoglobin levels should be seen in approximately one hour. Repeat doses may be given up to a maximum total dose of 7 mg/kg. When excess methylene blue is administered, the reverse reaction is favored and methemoglobin production can increase.[42] The following should be considered if the patient does not respond to therapy: ongoing absorption of toxin, inadequate dosing of antidote, G6PD deficiency, hemoglobin M disorder, and sulfhemoglobinemia toxicity. This antidote will cause a bluish discoloration of bodily fluids, and, in some cases, hemolytic anemia is produced in patients with G6PD deficiency.

Opioids

Classic opioid toxicity, such as that seen with heroin, produces the clinical triad of miosis, respiratory depression, and CNS depression. The routes of exposure are varied and include oral, intravenous, insufflation, and transdermal. Patients with clonidine toxicity can present in a similar fashion, and the syndrome may be accompanied by bradycardia, hypotension, and periodic respiratory apnea.

Naloxone. Naloxone was the first pure opiate antagonist developed. It can be given intravenously, intramuscularly, sublingually, or via an endotracheal tube.

Administration will reverse almost all effects of the opioid, including respiratory and CNS depression, analgesia, miosis, and decreased peristalsis.[43] The duration of action of naloxone is short (i.e., only 30-60 minutes). Since most opioid agents last longer than 30 minutes, a continuous infusion of naloxone is usually necessary. The initial dose of naloxone is 2-10 mg, regardless of age. Synthetic opiates will require more antidote. If a positive response is noted, a naloxone maintenance infusion of two-thirds the initial dose per hour should be started and titrated to effect.[44] Patients should be monitored for at least 90 minutes prior to discharge from the ED. Longer-acting opioid antagonists are now available (e.g., nalmefene, naltrexone), but their role in the acute care setting needs to be defined. Naloxone can sometimes be effective in reversing clonidine toxicity.

Toxic Alcohols

Methanol and ethylene glycol are metabolized by alcohol dehydrogenase to their respective toxic metabolites, formic acid and oxalic acid. Patients with toxicity usually present with confusion, coma, ataxia, nausea, vomiting, and abdominal pain. High anion gap metabolic acidosis and increased serum osmols may also be seen. Antidotes include ethanol, folinic acid, thiamine, pyridoxine, and 4-methyl pyrazole. Dialysis may be required.

Ethanol. Ethanol acts as a competitive substrate with methanol and ethylene glycol for alcohol dehydrogenase. Because ethanol has a higher affinity for the enzyme, it is able to inhibit the production of the toxic metabolites.[45] Patients with either clinical evidence of toxicity or a methanol/ethylene glycol level greater than 20 mg/dL should be started on ethanol therapy. The therapeutic serum ethanol level is 100 mg/dL, or a ratio of at least 1:4 of ethanol to methanol or ethyleneglycol, whichever is greater. Ethanol can be given either orally or intravenously. Intravenous administration is preferred as it avoids gastritis and can be given to the unconscious or uncooperative patient.

The loading dose of ethanol is 1 g/kg. It is given intravenously as a 10% solution in D_5W over a period of 30 minutes. An ethanol maintenance drip is then started at a rate of 0.1 g/kg/h as a 10% solution and titrated to the desired serum ethanol level. Complications of ethanol treatment are hypoglycemia, CNS depression, hypotension, and electrolyte abnormalities.

Cofactors. Thiamine (B_1), pyridoxine (B_6), and folinic acid are also used in the management of methanol and ethylene glycol toxicity. Thiamine and pyridoxine are used for ethylene glycol toxicity, and their initial doses are 100 mg and 50 mg, respectively. Folinic acid assists methanol metabolism and is administered as an initial dose of 50 mg. These cofactors may be given IV or IM.

Folinic acid is also used as rescue therapy to limit methotrexate-induced bone marrow, gastrointestinal, and renal toxicity.

4-Methylpyrazole. This compound is a potent inhibitor of alcohol dehydrogenase and prevents the metabolism of methanol and ethylene glycol. Several case reports have documented successful treatment of ethylene glycol intoxication.[46,47] This compound has the advantage of not producing CNS depression and has not been associated with significant toxicity. It is at present investigational, and clinical trials in the treatment of methanol and ethylene glycol toxicity are currently in progress.

Tricyclic Antidepressants

Tricyclic antidepressants (TCAs) produce myriad pharmacologic effects, the most worrisome of which is their ability to cause myocardial membrane stabilization. In essence, these agents behave as Type IA antidysrhythmics; they inhibit sodium transmission in phase 0 of ventricular depolarization, which is manifested by prolongation of the QRS complex on the ECG.

Sodium Bicarbonate. The mainstay of treatment for cardiac dysrrhythmias with QRS prolongation and seizures is sodium bicarbonate. The sodium serves to overcome the inhibitory effects of the TCAs on the sodium channels and, by raising the serum pH, bicarbonate promotes the *unbinding* of the TCAs from the myocardium.[48] Patients with a QRS greater than 0.1 seconds should be considered strong candidates for bicarbonate therapy. Sodium bicarbonate is administered intravenously as a loading dose (1-2 mEq/kg) and then as a continuous drip (0.2-0.4 mEq/kg/h). The goal is to maintain a serum pH between 7.45 and 7.55. Excessive serum alkalinization, fluid overload, and hypokalemia should be monitored and avoided.

Venoms

Venoms consist primarily of proteins, such as proteinase, phospholipases, cholinesterases, and hyaluronidases. Snake envenomations are the most notable, and there are two major varieties in the United States. Pit viper (e.g., rattlesnake) venom causes tissue necrosis and coagulopathy. The venom of elapidaes (e.g., coral snakes) causes neuromuscular paralysis, which can present in a delayed fashion.

Antivenin. Antivenins bind to components of the venoms and inhibit their toxic activity. They are commercially prepared from animals inoculated with the venoms. Snake antivenins are currently prepared from horses and have the potential of causing anaphylaxis. An intradermal test kit is provided with the antivenin to evaluate the sensitivity of the patient prior to therapy. This kit should only be used after it has been determined that antivenin therapy will be given. False-negative results have been reported from this test, and the emergency physician should be prepared with epinephrine, antihistamine, and steroid therapy.[49] If an allergic reaction is likely, the patient should be pretreated with antihistamines and a steroid, and the antivenin should be given slowly.

There are three FDA-approved, commercially available antivenins in the United States: Crotalidae polyvalent (rattlesnake), coral snake, and *Lactrodectus mactans* (black widow spider). The Crotalidae antivenin is active against the water moccasin, copperhead, North American rattlesnakes, some Asian snakes, and Central and South American pit vipers. The indications for its use is dependent on the patient's clinical manifestations and progression.[50]

Mild envenomations with minor localized swelling and no systemic or laboratory findings are supportively managed. Moderate envenomations with advancing edema, bleeding and ecchymosis at the site, and mild systemic and laboratory findings are treated with 4-10 vials. Severe envenomations, with either rapidly advancing edema along the extremity, significant systemic toxicity (i.e., hypotension), or laboratory findings of coagulopathy, will require 10-40 vials.

The coral snake antivenin is effective for the Eastern and Texas coral snakes but not for the Western (Sonoran) coral snake. Antivenin therapy is initiated early, with 3-5 vials, as respiratory failure can occur suddenly or in a delayed fashion.[51] The black widow antivenin is reserved for infants, the elderly, pregnant women, and those with significant underlying cardiopulmonary disease.

Summary

Management of life-threatening overdoses requires prompt recognition and meticulous attention to the ABCs. Unfortunately, histories associated with toxic ingestions are often less than reliable, which may require the practitioner to administer antidotes based on the clinical presentation alone. Adherence to established guidelines and recognition of possible adverse reactions will reduce toxicity associated with therapy and improve patient outcomes.

References

1. Dean BL, Peterson RC, Garrettson LK, et al. American Association of Poison Control Centers and American Academy of Clinical Toxicology policy statement: Universal antidote. *J Toxicol Clin Toxicol* 1982;19:527-529.
2. Baud FJ, Sabouraud A, Vicaut E, et al. Brief report: Treatment of severe colchicine overdose with colchicine-specific Fab fragments. *N Engl J Med* 1995;332:642-645.
3. Linden CH, Rumack BH. Acetaminophen overdose. *Emerg Med Clin North Am* 1984;2:103-119.
4. Rumack BH, Matthew H. Acetaminophen poisoning and toxicity. *Pediatrics* 1975;55:871-876.
5. McNeil Consumer Products Company. Letter to physicians: Tylenol Extended-Relief product information. January 3, 1995.
6. Smilkstein MJ, Knapp GL, Kulig KW, et al. Efficacy of oral N-acetylcysteine in the treatment of acetaminophen overdose. *N Engl J Med* 1988;319:1557-1562.
7. Keays R, Harrison PM, Wendon JA, et. al. Intravenous acetylcysteine in paracetamol-induced fulminant hepatic failure: A prospective controlled trial. *BMJ* 1991;103:1027-1029.
8. Ekins BR, Ford DC, Thompson MB, et al. The effects of activated charcoal on N-acetylcysteine absorption in normal subjects. *Am J Emerg Med* 1987;15:483-487.
9. Prescott KF, Illingworth RN, Crithcley JA, et al. Intravenous N-acetylcysteine: The treatment of choice for paracetamol poisoning. *BMJ* 1979;2:1097-1100.
10. Smilkstein MJ, Bronstein AC, Linden C, et al. Acetaminophen overdose. A 48-hours intravenous N-acetylcysteine treatment protocol. *Ann Emerg Med* 1991;20:1058-1063.
11. Mant TG, Tempowsi JH, Volans GN, et al. Adverse reactions to acetylcysteine and effects of overdose. *BMJ* 1984;289: 217-219.
12. Lampe KF, McCann MA. Differential diagnosis of poisoning by North American mushrooms with particular emphasis on *Amanita phalloides*-like intoxication. *Ann Emerg Med* 1987; 16:956-962.
13. Alleva FR, Balazs T, Sager AO, et al. Failure of thicotic acid to cure mushroom-poisoned mice and dogs. Presented at 14th Annual meeting of the Society of Toxicology, Williamsburg, Virginia, 1975. Abstract 155.
14. Goldfrank LR. Mushrooms: Toxic and hallucigenic. In: Goldfrank LR, et al, eds. *Goldfrank's Toxicologic Emergencies.* East Norwalk, CT: Appleton & Lange; 1994:955.
15. Walker WE, Levy RC, Henenson IB. Physostigmine—its use and abuse. *J Am Coll Emerg Phys* 1976;5:335.
16. Barash P, Kitahata LM, Mandel S. Acute cardiovascular collapse after intravenous phytonadione. *Anesth Analg* 1976; 55:304.
17. Hoffman, RS, Smilkstein MJ, Goldfrank LR, et al. Evaluation of coagulation factor abnormalities in long-acting anticoagulant overdose. *Clin Toxicol* 1988;26:233-248.
18. Weiss, ME, Nyhan D, Zihuky P. Association of protamine IgG and IgE antibodies with life-threatening reactions to intravenous protamine. *N Engl J Med* 1989;320:886-892.
19. Sugarman J, Paul R. Flumazenil: A review. *Pediatr Emerg Care* 1994;10:37-43.
20. Spivey WH, Roberts JR, Derlet RW. A clinical trial of escalating doses of flumazenil for reversal of suspected benzodiazepine overdose in the emergency department. *Ann Emerg. Med* 1993; 22:1813-1821.
21. McDuffee AT, Tobias JD. Seizure after flumazenil administration in a pediatric patient. *Pediatr Emerg Care* 1995;11:186-187.
22. Grabenstein JD. Immunoantidotes: II. One hundred years of antitoxins. *Hosp Pharmacol* 1992;27:637-646.
23. Frankovitch TL, Arnon SS. Clinical trial of botulism immune globulin for infant botulism. *West J Med* 1991;154:103.
24. Thom SR, Taber RL, Mendiguren II, et al. Delayed neuropsychologic sequelae after carbon monoxide poisoning: Prevention by treatment with hyperbaric oxygen. *Ann Emerg Med* 1995; 25:474-480.
25. Tomaszewski C. Carbon monoxide. In: Goldfrank LR, et al, eds. *Goldfrank's Toxicologic Emergencies.* East Norwalk: Appleton & Lange; 1994:1200.
26. Critchley J, Ungar A. The management of poisoning due to beta-adrenoreceptor antagonists. *Med Toxicol* 1989;4:32-45.
27. Braunwald E, Sonnenblick EH, Ross J. Mechanisms of cardiac contraction and relaxation. In: Braunwald E, ed. *Cardiovascular Medicine.* Philadelphia: W.B. Saunders Co; 1992:351-392.
28. Brancat DJ. Recognizing potential toxicity of phenol. *Vet Hum Toxicol* 1982;24:29-30.
29. Vance MV, Curry SC, Kunkel DB, et al. Digital hydrofluoric acid burns: Treatment with intra-arterial calcium infusion. *Ann Emerg Med* 1986;15:890-896.
30. Howland MA. Digoxin-specific antibody fragments. In: Goldfrank LR, et al, eds. *Goldfrank's Toxicologic Emergencies.* East Norwalk: Appleton & Lange; 1994:695.
31. Antman EM, Wenger TL, Butler VP, et.al. Treatment of 150 cases of life-threatening digitalis intoxication with digoxin-specific Fab antibody fragments. *Circulation* 1990;81:1746-1750.
32. Shumaik GM, Wu AU, Ping AC. Oleander poisoning: Treatment with digoxin-specific Fab antibody fragments. *Ann Emerg Med* 1988;17:732-735.
33. Natoff IL, Reif B. Effect of oximes on the acute toxicology of acetylcholinesterase carbamates. *Toxicol Appl Pharmacol* 1973;25:569-575.
34. Borowitz SM. Prolonged organophosphate toxicity in a twenty-six-month-old child. *J Pediatr* 1988;112:303-304.
35. Merrill D, Mihn F. Prolonged toxicity of organophosphate poi-

soning. *Crit Care Med* 1982;10:550-551.

36. Hall AH, Rumack BH. Hydroxocobalamin/sodium thiosulfate as a cyanide antidotes. *J Emerg Med* 1987;5:115-121.
37. Palatnick W, Meatherall RC, Tenenbein M. Clinical spectrum of sulfonylurea overdose and experience with diazoxide therapy. *Arch Intern Med* 1991;151:1859-1862.
38. Tennenbein M, Yatscoff RW. The total iron binding capacity in iron poisoning. *Am J Dis Child* 1991;145:437-439.
39. Scharman EJ, Rosencrance JG. Isoniazid toxicity: A survey of pyridoxine availability. *Am J Emerg Med* 1994;12:386-387.
40. Preventing Lead Poisoning in Young Children. U.S. Department of Health and Human Services; Centers for Disease Control and Prevention. 1991:51-64.
41. Janakirane, N, Seeler, RA, Royal JE. Hemolysis during BAL chelation therapy for high blood lead levels in glucose G-6-PD deficient children. *Clin Pediatr* 1978;17:485-487.
42. Harvey JW, Keitt AS. Studies of the efficacy and potential hazards of methylene blue therapy in aniline-induced methaemoglobinemia. *Br J Haematol* 1983;54:29-41.
43. Moore RA, Rumack BH, Conner CS, et. al. Naloxone: Underdosing after narcotic poisoning. *Am J Dis Child* 1980; 134:156-158.
44. Goldfrank LR, Weisman RS, Errick JK, et al. A dosing nomogram for continuous infusion naloxone. *Ann Emerg Med* 1986;15:566-570.
45. Jacobsen D, McMartin KE. Methanol and ethylene glycol poisonings: Mechanism of toxicity, clinical course, diagnosis, and treatment. *Med Toxicol* 1986;1:309-334.
46. Blomstrand R, Theorall H. Inhibitory effect on methanol metabolism in man after administration of 4-methylpyrazole. *Life Sci* 1970;9:631-640.
47. Baud F, Bismuth C, Garnier R, et al. 4-methylpyrazole may be an alternative therapy for ethylene glycol intoxication in man. *J Toxicol Clin Toxicol* 1986;24:463-483.
48. Sasyniuk BI, Jhamandas Y. Mechanism of reversal of toxic effects of amitriptylene on cardiac purkinje fibers by sodium bicarbonate. *J Pharmacol Exp Ther* 1984;231:387-394.
49. Jurkovich GJ, Luterman A, McCullar K, et al. Complications of Crotalidae antivenin therapy. *J Traum* 1988;28:1032-1037.
50. Roberts J, Otten EJ. Snakes and other reptiles. In: Goldfrank LR, et al, eds. *Goldfrank's Toxicologic Emergencies.* East Norwalk: Appleton & Lange; 1994:1306.
51. Kitchen CS, Microp LHS. Envenomation by the Eastern coral snake. *JAMA* 1987;258:1615-1618.

Digitalis Intoxication

Shivanand S. Karkal, MB, HS, MD

More than 200 years after William Withering's succinct description of digitalis toxicity, the glycoside continues to be the source of the most prevalent iatrogenic intoxication.[1,2] Although the true incidence is currently unknown, studies in the 1960s and 1970s indicated that about 20% of hospitalized patients suffered definite digitalis toxicity, of which as many as 41% died.[3-5] Authorities have criticized these older studies and point out that factors such as better understanding of digitalis pharmacokinetics and drug interactions, smaller maintenance doses, and better utilization of serum levels have since reduced the prevalence of toxicity.[2,6-9]

A major reason for the continuing morbidity and mortality from digitalis intoxication, especially that of the more common chronic form of the syndrome, is the difficulty of rapid diagnosis. Early manifestations are subtle and non-specific and may simulate exacerbation of underlying congestive heart failure or a variety of other illnesses. In fact, 28% of patients have extracardiac symptoms for more than three weeks before the correct diagnosis is suspected; conversely, in 50% of patients, no extracardiac symptoms precede cardiac dysrhythmias.[10,11]

Moreover, there are no protean rules to the ECG manifestations of digitalis intoxication. Some patients develop ventricular ectopy and tachycardia, whereas others present with varying degrees of blocks and progress to asystole without ever having a tachydysrhythmia.[12] No cardiac dysrhythmia is unique to digitalis poisoning, and the same dysrhythmia may arise from preexisting cardiac disease, other concomitantly administered drugs, or even non-cardiac processes.[13,14]

These clinical uncertainties are compounded by the difficulty in interpreting serum digitalis levels.[15-17] Even if correctly drawn and accurately reported, no specific level reliably separates the patient with and without digitalis toxicity. A significant overlap between toxic and therapeutic levels, as well as numerous extracardiac factors predispose individual patients to toxicity even though their serum levels are well below 2 ng/mL, long believed to be the upper limit of normal.[17]

Management of digitalis-toxic dysrhythmias poses other unique problems. Pharmacological therapy and electrical measures may prove either ineffective or, more alarmingly, can precipitate refractory tachydysrhythmias or even asystole.[16]

Until recently, clinicians also lacked a simple means of promptly reversing cardiac toxicity by enhancing digitalis excretion and metabolism. The extensive tissue distribution of digitalis limits the use of such measures as forced diuresis, hemodialysis, hemoperfusion, and exchange transfer.[17,18] The recent introduction of digoxin-specific antibody fragments (Fab) provides a safe and effective means of overcoming this hurdle, but its cost—$175 to $7,000 per patient—mandates judicious and selective use.[19-24]

To facilitate keener appreciation of the syndrome's clinical vagaries, the following article first provides a short account of how

Table 1. Signs and Symptoms of Digitalis Toxicity

MANIFESTATION	PREVALENCE (%)
Fatigue	95
Visual symptoms	95
Weakness	82
Nausea	81
Anorexia	80
Psychic complaints	65
Abdominal pain	65
Dizziness	59
Abnormal dreams	54
Headache	45
Diarrhea	41
Vomiting	40

Used with permission: Smith TW, Antman EM, Friedman PL. Digitalis glycoddes: Mechanisms and manifestations of toxicity. *Prog Cardiovusc Dis* 1984;26:413.

the digitalis toxidrome evolves. Next, the authors review the utility and limitations of specific laboratory tests in suspected digitalis intoxication. Finally, the review discusses the therapeutic modalities available to counter the various cardiac manifestations of digitalis toxicity. Analysis and synthesis of this information will enable clinicians to secure a better outcome for individual patients with this potentially lethal toxidrome.

Evolution of the Digitalis Toxidrome

No two patients with digitalis intoxication present identically. Nevertheless, a clear understanding of the pharmacology and electrophysiology of digitalis toxicity will help clinicians anticipate this common syndrome.

Digitalis and the Normal Heart.[25-27] Although digitalis glycosides have numerous and complex cardiovascular effects, a key electrophysiological property is inhibition of the myocardial sodium-potassium-adenosine triphosphatase (Na-K-ATPase) "pump." Inhibition of this pump leads to intracellular gain of sodium and calcium and loss of potassium. Increased intracellular calcium promotes increased myofibrillar interaction, producing a positive inotropic action. A second basic property shared by cardiac glycosides is their ability to increase vagal tone and depress conduction through the AV node, which results in a negative chronotropic effect.

Pathophysiology. Researchers have only recently elucidated the complex electrophysiology of digitalis cardiotoxicity.[13,28] Essentially, high levels of digitalis poison the myocardial Na-K-ATPase pump and cause abnormally enhanced intracellular entry of sodium and calcium, along with egress of potassium. The excessive entry of intracellular potassium increases myocardial automaticity, enhances excitability, and may lead to the formation of delayed after depolarizations (DADs)—oscillations in transmembrane potentials following full repolarization. Digitalis-induced enhanced automaticity, excitability, and DADs contribute to the development of ectopy and tachydysrhythmias. On the other hand, the vagal effect and AV node depression produced by the glycosides result in bradydysrhythmias and AV blocks.

Both hypo- and hyperkalemia can exacerbate digitalis cardiotoxicity.[10,29] Hypokalemia—especially at serum levels less than 2.5 mEq/L—inhibits Na-K-ATPase activity and adds to the pump inhibition induced by toxic levels of digitalis. In addition, hypokalemia enhances myocardial automaticity and is potentially arrhythmogenic. The net effect of hypokalemia is intensification of digitalis-related tachydysrhythmias. In contrast, hyperkalemia—especially at serum levels exceeding 5.4 mEq/L,—leads to hyper-polarization of myocardial cells, especially in conductive tissue such as the AV node, aggravating digitalis-induced bradydysrhythmias and conduction delays.

Focused Clinical Evaluation

Timely diagnosis and management of digitalis toxicity demands a high degree of suspicion. In addition to the specific clinical setting, knowledge of certain epidemiological features and drug interactions will help clinicians identify this potentially fatal cardiotoxic syndrome.

Incompletely Understood Epidemiology. The most common source of digitalis toxicity is iatrogenic administration, which stems from chronic treatment with digoxin, (Digitoxin, the other major preparation, is rarely used in the United States, unlike in Europe.) Although uncommon, digitalis toxicity also can arise from accidental ingestion of cardiac glycoside-containing plants such as oleanders, foxglove, lily of the valley, and redskill.[30] The yew plant also contains an arrhythmogenic alkaloid that although chemically unrelated, has actions similar todigitalis [31,32]

The precise incidence and mortality of digitalis intoxication remain unknown. However, authorities believe the current incidence and mortality of digitalis intoxication in hospitalized patients are much lower than previously reported.[9] In one recent survey, researchers attempted to more clearly delineate these statistics.[2] Of hospitalized patients diagnosed with digitalis toxicity, only 20% were definitely digitalis toxic; 60% were re-classified as possibly digitalis toxic; and 20% had no clinical evidence to support this diagnosis. Moreover, the mortality rate in the definite toxicity subgroup was 4.6% (compared to 41% in 1971)[3]

Symptoms of digitalis intoxication are non-specific and primarily involve the gastrointestinal and central nervous systems. *(Please see Table l.)* Patients with either acute or chronic intoxication commonly report anorexia, nausea, and vomiting.[33] In contrast, clinicians will likely encounter neuropsychiatric manifestations more frequently in chronic digitalis intoxication. Neurologic features range from headache, malaise, drowsiness, and muscle weakness to vertigo, syncope, lethargy, and even seizures.[34] Impaired memory, confusion, disorientation, delusions, depression, and delirium also can occur.[35]

Visual hallucinations, which are less common and more characteristic of chronic digitalis poisoning, result from retinal dysfunction that chiefly involves the cones rather than the rods.[36,37] Affected individuals may report a variety of visual disturbances, including yellow or green vision, halos or borders around objects, as well as blurred vision, photophobia, and transient amblyopia.

Key clinical parameters that help guide management and estimate the prognosis in individual cases include the patient's age; the presence of underlying cardiac and other systemic diseases; and in

Table 2. Predisposing Factors to Digitalis Intoxication

PATIENT ABNORMALITIES
Old age
Severe heart disease
Myocardial infarction
Myocarditis
Recent cardiac surgery
Cor pulmonale
Renal failure
Hemodialysis
Hypothyroidism
Hypoxemia
ELECTROLYTE ABNORMALITIES
Hypokalemia
Hypernatremia
Hypercalcemia
Hypomagnesemia
Alkalosis
DRUGS
Diuretics
Steroids
Reserpine
Catecholamines
Quinidine
Verapamil

Used with permission: Goodman LS. Digitalis. In: Haddad LM, Winchester JF, eds. *Clinical Management of Poisoning and Drug Overdose.* Philadelphia: WB Saunders; 1990.

Table 3. Electrolyte Abnormalities and Cardiac Glycoside Toxicity

INCREASED SENSITIVITY	DECREASED SENSITIVITY
Hypokalemia	Hyperkalemia
Hypercalcemia	Hypocalcemia
Hypomagnesemia	Hyponatremia
Alkalosis	Acidosis

ACUTE POTASSIUM ADMINISTRATION IN SUSPECTED DIGITALIS TOXICITY

Indications

- Serum potassium x 4.0 mEq/L and
  - VPCs and ventricular tachycardia
  - SVT with AV block
- Serum potassium ~3.0 mEq/L and
  - Type I or Type II AV block

Contraindications

- Serum potassium z-4.5 mEq/L
- Serum potassium > 3.5 mEq/L and AV block

AV = atrioventricular; SVT = supraventricular tachycardia; VPC = ventricular premature complexes

Adapted with permission: Kelley RA. Cardiac glycosides and congestive heart failure. *Am J Cardiol* 1990;65:10E.

acute overdoses, the amount of drug and time since exposure.[38] *(Please see Table 2.)*

In general, expect to encounter digitalis toxicity most often in elderly patients. Age-related factors contributing to digoxin accumulation include the following: 1) decreased muscle mass to bind digitalis, 2) decreases in renal excretion of digoxin, and 3) alterations in the sodium pump and its binding capacity for digoxin. Conversely, children and infants tolerate higher serum levels of digoxin.[10] Indeed, children may only be mildly symptomatic at levels that would otherwise produce serious cardiac sequelae in elderly patients.

Pre-existing cardiac disease also must be borne in mind while evaluating a patient for possible digitalis toxicity. Patients with acute myocardial ischemia or infarction are more likely to suffer digitalis toxicity. Less common predisposing cardiac factors include myocarditis, cardiomyopathy, amyloidosis, and recent cardiac surgery.[38]

Systemic diseases also predispose older individuals to digitalis toxicity. Patients with chronic obstructive lung disease are at increased risk for ventricular dysrhythmias because of a complex interplay of hypoxemia, beta-adrenergic agents, and methylxanthines.[30] Patients with renal dysfunction are at greater risk because of reduced excretion and increased volume of distribution of digoxin. Hypothyroid patients are more likely to develop increased serum digoxin levels because of reduced glomerular filtration rate and enhanced myocardial sensitivity to digitalis.[39] Individuals with a recent cerebrovascular accident are more likely to develop digoxin toxicity because of the superimposed arrhythmogenic potential of the accompanying hyperadrenergic state.[38]

In acute digitalis overdose, attempt to estimate the amount ingested and the time since exposure. Although the lethal dose varies with age and underlying cardiac status, in a general, an acute ingestion of more than 10 to 20 mg in a previously healthy adult can prove fatal.[40] In older patients with underlying heart disease or hypokalemia, smaller doses can be lifethreatening: Several deaths have occurred in patients on chronic digitalis treatment who acutely ingested 6 mg of digoxin.[40]

Drug interactions facilitate digoxin toxicity through various mechanisms and are especially relevant in chronic digitalis intoxication. For example, antacids, cholestyramine, colestipol, and sulfasalazine decrease digoxin absorption. Patients receiving digoxin and one or more of these agents may develop acute digitalis toxicity if they abruptly stop taking the other agent and do not have their maintenance digoxin dose reduced.[8]

Clinicians must be especially alert to the possibility of iatrogenic digoxin toxicity in patients taking the glycoside and another cardiac medication. Antiadrenergic agents such as clonidine, methyldopa, and beta blockers can predispose to bradydysrhythmias when used concomitantly with digoxin, especially in individuals with underlying sinus node disease.[8]

Concomitant use of numerous antiarrhythmic agents can elevate digoxin levels and precipitate toxicity. Quinidine, for example, produces a variable increase in serum digoxin level in over 90% of patients.[41] Quinidine reduces digoxin's volume of distribution by displacing the glycoside from muscle-binding sites and reducing its non-renal clearance." Serum digoxin levels may reach six times baseline values, although clinicians should anticipate an average of a twofold elevation.[10]

Concurrent use of calcium channel blockers also carries the potential for precipitating digoxin toxicity. Verapamil can raise serum digoxin levels by up to 70% via changes in renal and extrarenal clearance.[8] Moreover, verapamil also reduces AV nodal conduction. These combined effects can lead to dramatically elevated digoxin levels, with resulting brady-systolic manifestations of cardiac toxicity. Investigators have not commonly reported major clinical interactions with other calcium channel blockers, such as diltiazem and nifedipine, and digoxin.[10]

Amiodarone exhibits a dose-related property of elevating serum digoxin levels via inhibition of renal tubular secretion of the glycoside. Patients taking both amiodarone and digoxin may demonstrate a 25% to 70% increase in digoxin levels.[8] As in those with the verapamil-digoxin interaction, patients with amiodarone-related digoxin cardiotoxicity are more likely to experience bradydysrhythmias and varying degrees of AV block.

In contrast to the above antiarrhythmics, patients taking digoxin with procainamide, disopyramide, mexiletine, tocainide, flecainide, or encainide do not appear to be at increased risk of elevated digoxin levels due to drug interaction. However, because class I agents (procainaminde and disopyramide) depress AV conduction, they may contribute to digoxin cardiotoxicity.[10,15]

Optimizing Laboratory Utility in Suspected Digoxin Toxicity

Successful management of digitalis toxicity mandates that clinicians provide themselves with certain baseline biochemical parameters, in addition to serum digoxin levels, and a 12-lead ECG.

Laboratory studies. A variety of electrolyte abnormalities may occur in digitalis poisoning. *(Please see Table 3.) Hyperkalemia* usually signals acute digitalis toxicity. Digitalis-induced inhibition of the Na-K-ATPase pump produces egress of large amounts of potassium from intracellular to extracellular sites.[42] Initial *hyperkalemia* may have prognostic significance in acute digitalis overdose. In some series, serum potassium levels are a better index of subsequent mortality than either initial ECG changes or serum digitalis concentrations.[43]

In contrast, clinicians will usually encounter hypokalemia in the setting of chronic digitalis intoxication. In these patients, hypokalemia, which stems from concomitant diuretic usage, enhances the arrhythmogenic potential of digitalis and predisposes to ventricular ectopy and tachydysrhythmias.[36]

Hypomagnesemia has a similar potential for exacerbating digitalis cardiotoxicity. Hypomagnesemia increases myocardial digoxin uptake, decreases cellular Na-K-ATPase activity, increases the amplitudes of digitalis-induced DADs,[44] and can cause intracellular hypokalemia refractory to potassium replacement. Moreover, some patients may have depletion of total body magnesium but have apparently normal serum magnesium levels. Patients with hypomagnesemia, hypokalemia, or both may become cardiotoxic even with "therapeutic" digitalis levels.

Several other *metabolic abnormalities* that may be associated with or exacerbate digitalis cardiotoxicity include hypoxia, hypercalcemia, and metabolic alkalosis.[45] Finally, given the predominant renal role in digitalis clearances 60% to 80% of digoxin is excreted unchanged by the kidneys- baseline serum BUN and creatine values are helpful to gauge possible toxicity in individuals with "therapeutic".

Serum *digoxin* levels are often not easily interpretable in the emergent situation because of a number of factors. For example:

1) Significant overlap exists among assays of different digitalis formulations."[36]

2) Levels should be drawn at least four hours after an IV dose or six hours following an oral dose. If drawn earlier before steady levels are reached—values may be misleadingly high.

3) Patients may have a false-positive assay from such disparate factors as concomitant spironolactone therapy, hyperbirubinemia, chronic renal failure (60% of such patients possess an endogenous circulating digitalis-like substance), and circulating gamma-emitting radioactive substances.[10,46,47]

4) Although the therapeutic range has long been regarded as 0.5 to 2 ng/ml for digoxin, significant overlap exists between levels in toxic and non-toxic patients: About 10% of patients who have apparently normal serum digoxin levels demonstrate cardiac toxicity; conversely, about 10% of those without toxicity have serum levels between 2 and 4 ng/ml.[10]

Even so, a review of 43 reports on digitalis toxicity revealed that patients with intoxication had a mean serum level of 3.3 ng/ml.[48] Indeed, the higher the serum levels, the greater the likelihood of toxicity. Patients with levels exceeding 3 ng/ml are twelvefold more likely to be digitalis-toxic than those with levels less than 0.99 ng/ml.[49] Conversely, patients with serum levels less than 1.5 ng/ml in the absence of hypokalemia are unlikely to have digitalis toxicity, and serum levels less than 1 ng/ml in the absence of hypokalemia essentially rule out digitalis toxicity.[12]

ECG manifestations. Although virtually any rhythm disturbance can occur secondary to digitalis cardiotoxicity, clinicians will, in general, encounter different types dysrhythmias in chronic, compared with acute toxicity. *(Please see Tables 4 and 5.)*

In *older individuals with chronic digitalis intoxication*, characteristic dysrhythmias result from both enhanced myocardial automaticity and impaired conduction.[29] Classically, this electrophysiologic combination manifests as non-paroxysmal junctional tachycardia with AV block, which many authorities believe is virtually diagnostic of digitalis toxicity. AV dissociation with accelerated junctional rhythm and non-paroxysmal atrial tachycardia with AV block (often mislabeled as paroxysmal atrial tachycardia with block) are less common but are likewise highly suggestive of digitalis toxicity.[50] Premature ventricular contractions, often multifocal, are the most frequent isolated rhythm disturbance, although premature atrial contraction and premature junctional contractions are also common. Ventricular bigeminy or bidirectional ventricular tachycardia (VT) are highly indicative of chronic digitalis toxicity.[13]

In contrast, *in the younger patient with a normal heart and acute digitalis overdose*, the vagal and AV nodal depressive effects of the glycoside tend to predominate.[13,33] As a result, acute digitalis cardiotoxicity manifests with various forms of bradydysrhythmias, AV blocks, or both, with ventricular ectopy and tachydysrhythmias ocurring less frequently.

Table 4. Differences in Acute and Chronic Digoxin Poisoning

	Acute Intoxication	Chronic Toxicity
Types of patients most commonly involved	In many cases, the patients are normal with no history of cardiac disease.	Patients are ill with cardiac abnormalities underlying the toxic state. The symptoms may mimic the condition for which the drug is being used.
Symptoms on admission	Nausea and vomiting are the most consistent findings. Diarrhea is occasionally observed.	Anorexia, nausea, vomiting, headache, malaise, fatigue, weakness, and drowsiness are common. Diarrhea is less commonly seen. Paresthesias and neuritic pain along with confusion, disorientation, aphasia, delirium, hallucinations, and rarely convulsions are all reported. Visual changes and skin rashes also are noted.
Findings on admission	ECG findings indicate supraventricular arrhythmias, in general, with heart block and bradycardia most commonly noted. There is a general lack of ventricular arrhythmias.	All types of arrhythmias have been attributed to digitalis glycosides. The most common arrhythmias are non-paroxysmal nodal tachycardia, atrial tachycardia with AV dissociation, and bidirectional ventricular tachycardia.
Serum potassium	Normal or increased depending on the magnitude of the overdose and the relative time course.	Normal to decreased depending on the use of potent loop diuretics, nutrition status of the patient, and the presence of other factors known to affect the potassium level.
Serum digoxin determinations	High levels are always expected and seem to roughly correlate with the magnitude of the rise in serum potassium and presence of serum cardiac arrhythmias.	The levels may not clearly identify therapeutic ranges but are generally elevated in any prominent toxic state. Borderline normal values may represent toxicity.

Used with permission: Elkins BR. Management of acute digoxin overdosage. *Clin Tox Consult* 1979;4:96.

Finally, clinicians will rarely encounter certain dysrhythmias in patients with either acute or chronic digitalis toxicity.[51] These include Mobitz 11 AV block, parasystole, multifocal atrial tachycardia, and atrial flutter or fibrillation with a rapid ventricular response.

Management of a Complex Cardiotoxic Syndrome

A variety of pharmacological and electrical measures is readily available to the clinician managing a patient with digitalis toxicity. *(Please see Table 6.)* In order to optimize outcome in individuals cases physicians should be able to weigh the pros and cons of gastrointestinal decontamination; pharmacological agents such as atropine, phenytoin, lidocaine, potassium, and magnesium; electrical measures such as transvenous pacing and cardioversion; and last but not least, digoxin-specific antibodies (Fab).

Gut decontamination, as in most other poisonings, is more relevant to patients with acute digitalis intoxication who present to the emergency department within the first few hours of ingestion. In these cases and in the absence of such contraindications as impaired consciousness, clinicians should attempt *gastric evacuation* using ipecac-induced emesis, followed by lavage. Keep in mind, though, that in digitalisintoxicated patients with AV blocks or bradydysrhythmias, measures aimed at gastric evacuation can potentially increase vagal tone and exacerbate the problem. (In one case study, gastric lavage in a patient with digoxin overdose and a functional rhythm precipitated asystole.)[52] In such cases, clinicians should consider pretreatment with atropine before attempting gastric evacuation.

Activated charcoal does not have a clear-cut use in digitalis

Table 5. Cardiac Manifestations of Digitalis Intoxication

ACUTE INTOXICATION
Atrioventricular conduction disturbances
First-degree block
Sinus impulse formation disturbances
Sinus bradycardia
Sinus arrest
Sinoatrial block
Second-degree atrioventricular block
Third-degree atrioventricular block
CHRONIC INTOXICATION
Non-paroxysmal atrial tachycardia with block
Non-paroxysmal junctional tachycardia
Atrioventricular dissociation
Second-degree atrioventricular block (Type I)
Premature ventricular contractions
Ventricular bigeminy
Ventricular tachycardia
Bidirectional ventricular tachycardia
Ventricular fibrillation

Adapted with permission: Bryson PD, ed. Cardiac Glycosides. In: *Comprehensive Review in Toxicology*. Rockvilie: Aspen; 1989.

Table 6. Management of Digitalis Toxicity

GENERAL THERAPY
Discontinue digitalis
Monitor cardiac rhythm
Determine electrolytes and serum digoxin concentration
Observe for hemodynamic compromise
In massive digitalis overdose, activated charcoal or cholestyramine orally
MANAGEMENT OF DYSRHYTHMIAS
Potassium and magnesium replacement, indicated in the presence of hypokalemia and contraindicated in the presence of pre-existing hyperkalemia, bradycardia, and atrioventricular block
Phenytoin or lidocaine for ventricular arrhythmias in the presence of atrioventricular block
Atropine for sinoatrial and atrioventricular conduction anomalies
Pacemaker therapy for persistent bradycardia and atrioventricular block
Cardioversion with lowest effective energy for immediate therapy of ventricular tachycardia or fibrillation
Drugs to be avoided: procainamide, quinidine, disopyramide, beta-blocking agents, isoproterenol, bretylium, and verapamil
FAB-digoxin therapy
Life-threatening arrhythmias (ventricular tachycardia)
Hyperkalemia (serum potassium > 5.5 mEq/L)
MANAGEMENT OF HYPOTENSION AND LOW-OUTPUT STATE
Vasopressor to maintain arterial pressure
FAB-digoxin therapy
Control-associated dysrhythmias

Used with permission: Chatterjee K. Digitalis, catecholamines, and other positive inotropic agents. In: Parmlesy WW, Chaterjee K, eds. *Cardiology.* Baltimore: JB Lippincott; 1989.

poisoning, especially in chronically intoxicated individuals. Its advocates claim that repeated doses of charcoal—50 to 100 g initially, followed by 50 g every six hours—may reduce the half-life of digitalis, especially in those with massive overdose, by reducing its absorption from the GI tract.[53] Activated charcoal not only binds digitalis directly and prevents its primary absorption, but also accentuates the transluminal digitalis concentration gradient and promotes more rapid diffusion of digitalis into the GI tract. Prevention of this delayed absorption may be beneficial even in patients administered activated charcoal one to four hours post-ingestion.[54] (Given the significant enterohepatic circulation of digitoxin compared with digoxin, this secondary prevention may be more relevant to those poisoned with digitoxin.)

Resins such as cholestyramine have variable benefits in digitalis poisoning. As with activated charcoal, the proposed rationale for their use is that they may decrease the serum halflife of digitalis by binding and excretion via the gut—an effect that, again, may be more effective in those poisoned with digitoxin, which undergoes enterohepatic recirculation. Choiestyramine—4 to 8 g every six hours—has no advantage over activated charcoal except that it is more palatable and is used currently only as an adjunct in non-lifethreatening digitalis intoxication's.[55]

Atropine—0.5 mg IV repeated at five-minute intervals if effective—is the initial treatment of choice in digitalispoisoned patients who are hemodynamically compromised by sinus bradycardia, high-degree AV block, and sinus exit block.[10,54] The effectiveness of atropine stems from its ability to reverse digitalisinduced vagal effects on the sinoatrial and atrioventricular nodcs. Howcvcr, bccause these effects are only partially vagally mediated, atropine does not consistently abolish AV blocks and bradydysrhythmias in digitalis toxicity.[57] In general, atropine is more likely to be effective in acute poisoning than in chronic intoxication." In patients with nonresponsive bradydysrhythmias, other cardiac stimulants, including beta agonists (i.e., isoproterenol), are contraindicated because they may prove more arrhythmogenic.

Temporary transvenous pacing is the next step in digitalisinduced bradydysrhythmias or AV block unresponsive to atropine. Bear in mind, however, that the digitalis-toxic myocardium may not respond normally to electrical pacing: These patients have a lowered threshold for pacemaker-induced extrasystole, and the procedure may precipitate more serious tachydysrhythmias.[33]

Anti-arrhythmic agents most likely to be effective in digitialis intoxication are phenytoin and lidocaine. Of these, phenytoin has long been the agent of choice to suppresss digitalis-related enhanced automaticity as well as AV nodal and sinoatrial conduction depres-

Table 7. Calculation of Fab Dose Requirements

I. Calculation of Body Load:

A. Amount ingested (me) x F

B. Serum glycoside conceitrration (ng/mL)[b] x Vd[c] x weight (kg) / 1,000

II. Calculation of Equimolar Dose of Fab Determined from Glycoside Body Load:

A. Body load of glycoside (mg) / 0.6 mg/vial = Fab dose (# of vials)

Or

B. If amount ingested is unknown, administer 800 mg (20 vials)

[a] F (bioavailability factor) = 0.8 for digoxin tablets; 1.0 for digoxin elixir, capsules, or digitoxin

[b] q/mL = pg/L

[c] Vd = 5.6L /kg for digoxin and 0.56 L/kg for digitoxin

Used with permission: Martiny SS, Phelps SJ, Massey KL. Treatment of severe digitalis intoxication with digoxin-specific antibody fragments: A clinical review. *Crit Care Med* 1988;16:6.

sion. Phenytoin can counter ventricular tachydysrhythmias, atrial tachycardia with block, and non-paroxysmal junctional tachycardia.[10] The initial IV loading dose is 5 mg/kg administered at 50 mg/min, followed by 100 mg orally every four to six hours if a beneficial effect occurs.

Lidocaine is chiefly used to treat digitalis-related ectopic rhythms. In general, this agent is effective for ventricular tachycardia and atria] tachycardia with block, but not for functional tachycardia with block.[59] Clinicians most commonly use an initial bolus dose of 1.0 to 1.5 mg/kg IV, with subsequent maintenance administration of 2 to 4 mg/min IV infusion. Unlike phenytoin, lidocaine's brief duration of action (15 to 20 minutes) is a major advantage should there be deterioration of the baseline cardiac rhythm."

Amiodarone (300 mg IV) has been used successfully in a refractory digitalis-toxic tachydysrhythmia.[60] However, limited experience with this agent precludes its routine use in digitalis intoxication.[40]

Magnesium. Although precisely how intravenous magnesium is effective in digitalis poisoning remains unknown, authorities have proposed numerous mechanisms to explain its effectiveness in such patients. These hypotheses range from blockade of the transient inward calcium current, antagonism of calcium at intracellular binding sites, amelioration of digitalis-related ventricular irritability, and counteracting hyperkalemia via blockade of potassium egress from digitalispoisoned cells.[61-64]

For adults with digitalis toxicity, administer 2 g magnesium sulfate (10%) IV over 20 minutes.[65] (No standard recommendations currently exist for pediatric patients, although some authorities suggest 20 mg/kg IM or IV over 20 minutes.) Because the effect of the magnesium bolus injection may be transient secondary to rapid renal clearance in those with normal kidneys, follow the initial dose with an infusion of 1 to 2 g/hr. Carefully monitor the patient for clinical and laboratory evidence of hypermagnesemia. Obtain a pre-treatment magnesium level in patients with renal dysfunction and those who may have pre-existing hypermagnesemia.[66] In all cases, check a serum magnesium level every two hours, and titrate the infusion to maintain a level of 4 to 5 mEq/L.

In addition, clinicians should closely monitor patients for neuromuscular dysfunction or respiratory compromise or both during IV magnesium administration. Depression of deep tendon reflexes or respiration mandates prompt cessation of the infusion and a repeat serum magnesium level.[65] Other potential problems with IV magnesium in digitalis-toxic patients include precipitation of hypotension and advanced AV block.[10]

Hyperkalemia associated with digitalis toxicity may be refractory to traditional measures such as resins, IV calcium, or dextrose-insulin or HCO, infusions. In fact, calcium administration for hyperkalemia secondary to digitalis toxicity can potentiate underlying cardiotoxicity and is contraindicated.[43] In hemodynamically stable patients with hyperkalemia, sodium polysterone sulfonate—1 g/mEq of excess serum potassium—with 70% sorbitol orally or as a retention enema may provide a gradual correction of serum potassium levels.

Until recently, hemodialysis was the treatment of choice for refractory hyperkalemia in digitalis intoxication. Even this modality, however, may only transiently reduce serum potassium without diminishing endogenous digitalis levels. The NaK-ATPase pump remains "poisoned," and cardiac membrane potentials are essentially unchanged.[67]

Hypokalemia. IV potassium chloride has long been the agent of choice for rapid correction of ventricular and supraventricular tachydysrhythmias due to chronic digitalis intoxication in hypokalemic patients.[10] Replenishing potassium in such patients helps counter ventricular tachycardia, paroxysmal atrial tachycardia with block, and non-paroxysmal functional tachycardia, although digitalis-related ventricular tachydysrhythmias are more responsive to intravenous potassium.[51] Potassium may also be useful in chronic digitalis-toxic rhythms inpatients with normal serum potassium levels.[21]

Given the potential for exacerbating certain digitalis-toxic dysrhythmias, administer IV potassium under close clinical and ECG monitoring. Also be aware of several specific cautions: First, potassium has a bimodal effect on AV conduction hypokalemia exacerbates digitalis-related AV block, whereas hyperkalemia reduces AV conduction,[29] and hyperkalemia also can exacerbate sinoatrial conduction delays. Hence, potassium administration in those with first- or second-degree AV blocks may prove hazardous.

Second, co-administration of glucose drives potassium ions intracellularly and may decrease extracellular potassium levels, enhance digitalis sensitivity, and exacerbate dysrhythmias.[51] Therefore, administer potassium in normal or half-normal saline, but avoid large amounts of saline, which can be detrimental in patients with congestive heart failure.

Third, be certain that IV potassium solutions do not exceed 120 to 160 mEq/L because higher concentrations produce severe pain at the injection site.[15]

Fourth, do not exceed infusion rates of more than 0.5 to 1.0 mEq/min. Ventricular tachydysrhythmias likely to be countered by IV potassium usually subside following administration of 40 mEq.[15,51] Finally, some authorities recommend that clinicians avoid infusing potassium via central venous lines because of a possibly heightened risk of cardiac arrest.

Electrical Cardioversion. Clinicians traditionally believed that digitalis substantially reduced the threshold for cardioversion-

Table 8. Fab Antibody Dosage Calculation Chart

Approximate Digibind dose for reversal of single-ingestion digoxin overdose

Number of Tablets or Capsules of Digosin ingested			*Digibind Dose*
0.05 mg capsules	0.125 mg tablets or 0.1 mg capsules	0.25 mg tablets or 0.2 mg capsules	0.5 mg tablets
25	12-13	6	3
50	25	12-13	6
100	50	25	12-13
200	100	50	25
300	150	75	37-38
400	200	6	50
		100	

Estimated adult doses in vials (v) from serum digoxin concentration (ng/mL)

	Serum Digoxin Concentration (ng/mL)						
Patient weight (kg)	1	2	4	8	12	16	20
40	0.5v	1v	2v	3v	5v	6v	8v
60	0.5v	1v	2v	5v	7v	9v	11v
70	1.0v	2v	3v	5v	8v	11v	13v
80	1.0v	2v	3v	6v	9v	12v	15v
100	1.0v	2v	4v	8v	11v	15v	19v

Estimated pediatric doses in vials (v) from serum digoxin concentration (ng/mL)

	Serum Digoxin Concentration (ng/mL)							
Patient weight (kg)	1	2	4	8	8	12	16	20
1	0.5 mg	1.0 mg	1.5 mg	2.9 mg	3.0 mg	5 mg	6 mg	8 mg
3	1.0 mg	2.0 mg	5.0 mg	9.0 mg	9.0 mg	13 mg	18 mg	22 mg
5	2.0 mg	4.0 mg	8.0 mg	15.0 mg	15.0 mg	22 mg	30 mg	40 mg
10	4.0 mg	8.0 mg	15.0 mg	30.0 mg	30.0 mg	50 mg	50 mg	80 mg
20	8.0 mg	15.0 mg	30.0 mg	50.0 mg	60.0 mg	120 mg	120 mg	160 mg

Adapted from Digibind, Product Information, Burroughs Wellcome, Research Triangle Park, NC, 1986.

induced dysrhythmias and synchronized cardioversion often produced refractory supraventricular and ventricular ectopic rhythms in digitalized patients.[16] Recent studies, however, have disproved these beliefs in individuals with therapeutic digitalis levels.[56,58]

In contrast, patients with overt digitalis toxicity are more likely to suffer refractory ventricular tachydysrhythmias after receiving electrical therapy at any energy levels. Hence, although cardioversion appears safe in therapeutically digitalized patients, most authorities advise extreme caution in patients with digitalis toxicity. Nonetheless, clinicians may have to use electrical cardioversion in hemodynamically unstable patients with digitalis-related tachydysrhythmas when therapeutic measures discussed previously fail to restore normal sinus rhythm. To minimize the risk of precipitating refractory dysrhythmias, initiate cardioversion at the lowest possible energy level.[43]

Antidotal therapy with digoxin-specific antibody fragments (Fab) is the single most signficant recent development in the management of this toxidrome. So far, authorities have successfully used Fab therapy in more than 1,000 patients.[2,20-24]

Essentially, Fab treatment is based on a simple mechanism of action. Following IV infusion, Fab binds free digoxin intravascularly, forming a pharmacologically inert compound that is rapidly eliminated via the kidneys.[69] Subsequently, Fab antibodies diffuse out of the intravascular space to bind free digoxin in the extracellular space. These events produce a concentration gradient that facilitates egress of digoxin from intracellular (and more specifically, intramyocardial) sites into the extracellular and intravascular spaces, where it is promptly complexed by Fab. Fab also possess a much closer affinity for digoxin than the glycoside's affinity for the myocardial Na-KATPase receptor. Together, all these factors relieve the "poisoning" of the myocardial Na-K-ATPase pump, and the subsequent return of pump function ameliorates cardiotoxicity.[36]

Indications for Fab therapy primarily include potentially or immediately life-threatening dysrhythmias induced by digitalis intoxication.[15,23] In chronic intoxication, this includes ventricular fibrillation or tachycardia, bradydysrhythmias, or AV block with hemodynamic compromise or unresponsiveness to standard measures discussed before.

In acute digitalis overdose, authorities recommend a more liberal use of Fab. Specific indications include the following:

- elderly patients with underlying cardiac and systemic diseases who have ingested large amounts of digitalis;
- ingestion of more than 10 mg digitalis in previously healthy adults or 4 mg in children;[15]
- a six- to eight-hour post-ingestion serum digitalis concentration greater than 10 to 15ng/ml of digoxin or 150 ng/ml of digitoxin;"
- initial serum potassium greater than 5 mEq/L (some studies have reported a mortality of up to 50% in initially hyperkalemic patients not administered Fab).[15,40]

In the above groups of patients, current recommendations are to use Fab therapy even if apparently benign dysrhythmias are present on initial presentation. Rather than awaiting more dangerous dysrhythmias, early use of Fab decreases morbidity and mortality and provides cost-effective treatment in such cases.

Finally, in assessing the need and dosage of Fab in individual cases, consider the various conceptual limitations of the "minimal lethal dose" in digitalis poisoning. Authorities have recorded survival in acute overdoses of 20 mg, even though 15 mg is traditionally regarded as the minimal adult lethal dose.[52,70]

Administration of Fab is guided by certain principles. Each vial contains 40 mg of Fab; each 40 mg binds 0.6 mg of digoxin or digitoxin.[71] Hence, in a given patient with digitalis intoxication, number of vials = digitalis body load (DBL) (mg)/ 0.6 (mg/vial). *(Please see Tables 7 and 8.)*

To estimate the DBL, use either the estimated amount ingested (in acute overdoses) or the serum digitalis concentration (in chronic intoxication). In acute overdoses, the DBL approximates the dose ingested multiplied by a bioavailability factor of 0.8 for digoxin tablets. For those exposed acutely to digoxin elixir or capsules, or digitoxin, use a bioavailability factor of 1.

In chronic intoxication, clinicians may use the serum digitalis concentration to estimate the Fab dose.[19] However, obtain the serum concentration at least eight hours after the last dose, multiply the serum concentration by the volume of distribution (Vd) and divide by 1,000 to convert (mu)g to mg. (Currently recommended mean Vd for digoxin is 5.6L/kg and for digitoxin, 0.56 L/kg.) No standard recommendations for altered dosing in pediatric patients and in patients with renal failure currently exist.[21]

If neither the amount acutely ingested nor a serum digitalis level is available, authorities recommend administering an initial dose of 800 mg of Fab (20 vials) in both children and adults?*

After calculating the estimated dose, reconstitue the Fab vials with sterile water or sterile isotonic saline to a 10 mg/ml concentration. Next, infuse the dose IV over 30 minutes through a 0.22-micron filter. Alternatively, in an emergent situation, administer the dose as an IV bolus. Concentrations exceeding 10 mg/ml may be necessary in certain individuals to prevent exacerbation of congestive failure. In infants and young children, dilute to a concentration of 1 mg/mL.

Fab successfully counters digitalis-related cardiotoxic rhythms in more than 70% of individuals, often in a dramatic fashion within 30 to 60 minutes of initial administration.[24] In fact, within one minute of IV administration in most patients, free digoxin levels become unmeasurable. This produces a potential problem with subsequent monitoring and follow-up because conventional immunoassays for digoxin (which measure both the bound and unbound agent) are unreliable for at least the next seven days and may reveal values of 10 to 20 times baseline concentrations. Researchers have used equilibrium dialysis to estimate free serum digoxin concentrations after Fab therapy. However, because this cannot be routinely performed, physicians must rely on clinical grounds rather than serum digitalis levels to determine not only the need for more Fab doses in the acute setting, but also the appropriate maintenance dose of digoxin on discharge.

Side effects of Fab therapy are, in general, minor. About 10% or less of patients may suffer exacerbation of pre-existing congestive failure, increased ventricular response in atrial fibrillation, or hypokalemia.[24] About 1% of recipients may develop minor idiosyncratic allergic reactions. Researchers have not reported major allergic reactions such as anaphylaxis, and routine pre-administration skin testing is'not currently recommended.

Laboratory and ECG Data Are Key to Early Diagnosis

Digitalis toxicity, especially its chronic form, is a largely iatrogenic toxidrome that continues to occur commonly. Although authorities have recently unraveled its complex cardiac electrophysiology, prompt recognition of digitalis toxicity is hampered by its frequently variable and non-specific signs and symptoms. A high index of suspicion, however, as well as judicious utilization of key laboratory and ECG data will help clinicians achieve early diagnosis in individual cases. Subsequently, selective utilization of both nonspecific measures, such as electrolyte replenishment, as well as specific modalities, such as Fab antidotal therapy, will help reduce the morbidity and mortality from this potentially lethal syndrome.

References

1. Smith TW, Amman EM, Friedman PL. Digitalis glycosides: Mechanisms and manifestations of toxicity. *Prog Cardiovasc Dis* 1984;26:413.
2. Mahdyoon H, Battilana G, Goldstein S. The evolving pattern of digoxin intoxication: observations at a large urban hospital from 1980 to 1988. *Am Heart J* 1990;20:5.
3. Beller GA, Smith TW, Abelman WH. Digitalis intoxication: A prospective clinical study with serum level correlations. *N Engl J Med* 1971;284:1989.
4. Hurwitz N, Wade OL: Intensive hospital monitoring of adverse reactions to drugs. *Br Med J* 1969;1:531.
5. Storstein 0, Hansteen V, Hatle L. Studies on digitalis. XIII. A prospective study of 649 patients on maintenance treatment with digitoxin. *Am Heart J* 1977;93:434.
6. Vitti TG, Banes D, Byers TE. Bioavailability of digoxin. *N Engl J Med* 1971;285:1433.

7. Duhme DW, Greenblatt DJ, Koch-Weser J. Reduction of toxicity associated with measurement of serum levels. *Ann Intern* 1974;516. .
8. Marcus FI. Pharmacokinetic interactions between digoxin and other drugs. *J Am Coll Cardiol* 1985;5:82A.
9. Smith TW. Should digoxin be the drug of first choice after diuretics in chronic congestive heart failure? Protagonist's viewpoint. *J Am Coll Cardiol* 1988;12:267.
10. Chatterjee K. Digitalis, catecholamines, and other positive inotropic agents. In: Parmlesy WW, Chatterjee K, eds. *Cardiology*. Baltimore: JB Lippincott; 1989.
11. Lely AH, VanEnter CHJ. Noncardiac symptoms of digitalis intoxication. *Am Heart J* 1972;83:149.
12. Marcus Fl, Huang SK. Digitalis. In: Hurst JW, Schlant RC, Rackley CE, et al, eds. *The Heart Arteries and Veins*. New York: McGraw-Hill; 1990.
13. Bigger J. Digitalis toxicity. *J Clin Pharmacol* 1985;25:514.
14. Fisch C. Digitalis intoxication. *JAMA* 1971;1:216.
15. Goedman LS. Digitalis. In: Haddad I M, Winchester JF, eds. *Clinical Management of Poisoning and Drug Overdose*. Philadelphia: WB Saunders; 1990.
16. Lown B, Kleiger R, Williams J. Cardioversion and digitalis drugs: Changes in threshold to electric shock in digitalized animals. *Circ Res* 1965;57:519.
17. Ellenhom MJ, Barceloux DG, eds. Digitalis. In: *Medical Toxicology Diagnosis and Treatment of Human Poisoning*. New York: Elsevier; 1988.
18. Bismuth C, Wattel F, Gosselin B, et al. L'Hemoperfusion sur charbon active enrobe experience des centres antipoisons francais: 60 intoxications. *Nouv Presse Med* 1979;8:1235.
19. Mattiny SS, Phelps SJ, Massey KL. Treatment of severe digitalis intoxication with digoxin-specific antibody fragments: A clinical review. *Crit Care Med* 1988;16:6.
20. Smith TW, Haber E, Yeatman L. Reversal of advanced digoxin intoxication with Fab fragments of digoxin-specific antibodies. *N Engl J Med* 1976;294797.
21. Wenger T, Butler VP, Haber E. Digoxin-specific antibody treatment of digitalis toxicity: Update. In: Erdmann E, Greef K, Skou JC, eds. Darmstadt: *Cardiac Glycosides* 1785-1985. New York: Springer; 1986.
22. Friedman PL. Foxglove and Fab: Immunological approaches to digitalis intoxication. *Int J Cardiol* 1983;3:237.
23. Wenger TL, Butler VP, Haber E. Treatment of 63 severely digitalis toxic patients with digoxin-specific antibody fragments. *J Am Coll Cardiol* 1985;5:118A.
24. Antman EM, Wenger TL, Butler VP. Treatment of 150 cases of life-threatening digitalis intoxication with digoxin-specific Fab antibody fragments. *Circulation* 1990;81:1744.
25. Fozzard HA, Sheets ME. Cellular mechanisms of action of cardiac glycosides. *J Am Coll Cardiol* 1985;5:10A.
26. Katz AM. Effects of digitalis on cellular biochemistry: Sodium pump inhibition. *J Am Coll Cardiol* 1985;5:16A.
27. Smith TW. Digitalis: Mechanisms of action and clinical use. *N Engl J Med* 1988;318:358.
28. Rosen MR. Cellular electrophysiology of digitalis toxicity. *J Am Coll Cardiol* 1985;5:22A.
29. Kelley RA. Cardiac glycosides and congestive heart failure. *Am J Cardiol* 1990;65:10E.
30. Haynes BE, Bessen HA, Wightman WD. Oleander tea: Herbal draught of death. *Ann Emerg Med* 1985;14:350.
31. Cummins RO, Haulman J, Quan L, et al. Near fatal cardiac arrhythmias and shock following yew leaves ingestion. *Ann Emerg Med* 1990;19:1.
32. Yersin B, Frey J-G, Schaller M-D, et al. Fatal cardiac arrhythmias and shock following yew leaves ingestion. *Ann Emerg Med* 1987;16:1396.
33. Sharff J, Bayer M. Acute and chronic digitalis toxicity: Presentation and treatment. *Ann Emerg Med* 1982;11:327.
34. Jefferson JW, Marshall JR. Digitalis neurotoxicity. *Medical Grand Rounds* 1982;1:360.
35. Wamboldt FS, Jefferson JW, Wamboldt MZ. Digitalis intoxication misdiagnosed as depression by primary care physicians. *Am J Psychiatry* 1986;143:2.
36. Bryson PD, ed. Cardiac Glycosides. In: *Comprehensive review in Toxicology.* Rockville: Aspen; 1989.
37. Chuman M, LeSage J. Color vision deficiencies in two cases of digoxin toxicity. *Am J Oplithalmol* 1985;100:682.
38. Surawicz B. Factors affecting tolerance to digitalis. *J Am Coll Cardiol* 1985;5:69A.
39. Doherty JE, Perkins WH. Digoxin metabolism in hypoand hyperthyroidism. Studies with titrated digoxin in thyroid disease. *Ann Intern Med* 1966;64:489.
40. Manolio TA. Digitalis. In: Nioji EK, Kelen GD, Goessel TK, eds. *Manual of Toxicologic Emergencies.* Chicago: Year Book; 1989.
41. Leahy EG. Digoxin-quinidine interactions: Current status. *Ann Intern Med* 1980;93:775.
42. Doherty J. Digitalis glycosides. *Ann Intern Med* 1973; 19:229.
43. Goldfrank LR, Lewin NA, Howland MA, et al. Digitalis, beta blockers, calcium channel blockers, and clonidine. In: Goldfrank LR, Flomenbaum NE, Lewin NA, et al, eds. *Goldfranks' Toxicologic Emergencies*. Norwalk: Appleton Century-Crofts; 1990.
44. Goldman RH, Kleiger RE, Schweizer E. The effect on myocardial 3-H digoxin of magnesium deficiency. *Proc Exp Biol Med* 1971;136:747.
45. Brater DC, Morelli HF. Systemic alkalosis and digitalis related arrhythmias. *Acta Med Scand* 1981;647:79.
46. Craver JL, Valdes R: Anomalous serum digoxin concentration in uremia. *Ann Intern Med* 1983;98:483.
47. Graves SW, Brown B, Valdes R. An endogenous digoxin like substance in patients with renal impairment. *Ann Intern Med* 1983;99:604.
48. Lee TH, Smith TW. Serum digoxin concentration and diagnosis of digitalis toxicity: Current concepts. *Clin Pharmacokinet* 1983;8:279.
49. Eraker SA, Sasse L. The serum digoxin test and digoxin toxicity: A bayesian approach to decision making. *Circulation* 1981;2:604.
50. Moorman JR, Pritechett ELC: The arrhythmias of digitalis intoxication. *Arch Intern Med* 1985;145:1289.
51. Doherty JE: Principles and practice of digitization. In: Messerli FH, ed. *Cardiovascular Drug Therapy*. Philadelphia: WB Saunders; 1990.
52. Hobson JD, Zettner A. Digoxin serum half life following

suicidal digoxin poisoning. *JAMA* 1973;223:147.

53. Lalonde RL, Deshpande R, Hamilton PP, et al. Acceleration of digoxin clearance by activated charcoal. *Clin Pharmacol Ther* 1985;37:367.
54. Reissel P, Manninen V. Effect of administration of activated charcoal and fibre on absorption, excretion and steady state blood levels of digoxin and digitoxin. Evidence for intestinal secretion of the glycosides. *Acta Med Scand* 1982; 668(Suppl):88.
55. Henderson RP, Solomon CP. Letter. *Arch Intern Med* 1989; 149:2603.
56. Doherty JE: Conventional drug therapy in the management of heart failure. In: Chon JN, ed. *Drug Treatment of Heart Failure.* New York: York Medical; 1983.
57. Hansteen V, Jacobsen D, Knudsen K, et al. Acute, massive poisoning with digitoxin. Report of seven cases and discussion of treatment. *Clin Toxicol* 1981;18:679.
58. Bigger JT, Strauss WC. Digitalis toxicity—drug interactions promoting toxicity and the management of toxicity. *Sem Drug Treatment* 1972;2:147.
59. Castellenos A, Ferreiro J, Pefkaros K, et al. Effects of lidocaine on bidirectional tachycardia and on digitalis induced atria] tachycardia with block. *Br Heart J* 1982; 48:27.
60. Maheshwaran R, Bramble MA, Hordisty CA. Massive digoxin overdose. Successful treatment with intravenous amiodarone. *Br Med J* 1983;287:392-393.
61. French JH, Thomas RG, Siskind AP, et al. Magnesium therapy in massive digoxin intoxication. *Ann Emerg Med* 1984;13:562.
62. Seller RH. The role of magnesium in digitalis toxicity. *Am Heart J* 1971;82:551.
63. Spechter MJ, Schweizer E, Goldman RH. Studies on magnesium's mechanism of action in digitalis induced arrhythmias. *Circulation* 1975;52:1001.
64. Wang R, Aikawa J. Magnesium deficiency and refractoriness to potassium repletion. *J Chron Dis* 30:65, 1977.
65. Reisdorff El, Clark MR, Walters BL: Acute digitalis poisoning: The role of intravenous magnesium sulfate. *Ann Emerg.Med* 1986;4:463.
66. Beller GA, Hood WB, Smith TW, et al. Correlation of serum magnesium level and cardiac digitalis intoxication. *Am J Cardiol* 1974;33:225.
67. Murphy D, Bremmer F, Haber E, et al. Massive digoxin poisoning treated with Fab fragments of digoxin-specific antibodies. *Pediatrics* 1982;70:472.
68. Ditchey RV, Curtis GP. Effects of apparently nontoxic doses of digoxin on ventricular ectopy after direct current electrical shocks in dogs. *J Pharmacol Exp Ther* 2 1981;18:212.
69. Rollins D, Brizgys M. Immunological approach to poisoning. *Ann Emerg Med* 1986;15:1046.
70. Wharton CFP. Attempted suicide by digoxin self administration and its management. *Guys Hosp Rep* 1970; 119:243.
71. Schmidt DH, Butler VP. Immunologic protection against digoxin toxicity. *J Clin Invest* 1971;50:866.
72. Digibind, Product Information, Burroughs Wellcome, Research Triangle Park, NC, 1986.

Mushroom Toxicity

Ginger W. Wilhelm, MD, FACEP

Proper medical care of a patient who has ingested a wild mushroom that may be toxic can seem like a daunting task for the emergency physician. Many issues must be considered depending upon the patient's age, site of contamination, and presenting symptoms. For example, is gastric decontamination warranted for the toddler who took a bite of the little brown mushroom ("LBM") found on the lawn? What is a logical approach to the teenager who thought he ingested a hallucinogenic psilocybe mushroom, but who is instead stricken with profuse vomiting and diarrhea two hours later? What type of treatment and referral is warranted for the mushroom forager who presents with delayed hepatotoxicity following ingestion of freshly picked field mushrooms?

In this chapter reviewing of mushroom toxicity and poisoning, the authors provide a logical framework for approaching the patient with possible toxic mushroom ingestion. At the outset it should be stressed that in any given mushroom ingestion, the odds are in favor of a benign outcome unless the patient was intent upon suicide. Of the 5,000-10,000 species of mushrooms in North America, only about 100 are toxic, and only about 10 species are considered deadly.[1,2] However, even the most feared of all, *Amanita phalloides* (the "death cap"), has been found growing in urban yards. As a result, in each case, an attempt should be made to identify the mushroom. Sources for identification will be presented in this review.

Prediction of patient outcome also can be based upon a symptoms approach. A symptom complex that is predictably associated with a toxin or group of toxins is known as a toxidrome. A good example of a toxidrome is the symptom complex associated with an organophosphate poisoning. Those symptoms of cholinergic nervous system excess, often given the acronym "SLUDGE," consist of salivation, lacrimation, urination, diarrhea, gastrointestinal distress, and emesis. One of the mushroom toxin groups that contains muscarine causes a very similar symptom complex.

The currently known mushroom toxins can be categorized into eight groups, each with a characteristic symptom complex. The most deadly *Amanita* species, with their potential for delayed hepatic failure, fall into the first group. The hallucinogenic psilocybe is an example of another. The last group contains the miscellaneous gastrointestinal irritants, which cause unpleasant symptoms, but usually have benign outcomes, particularly with appropriate fluid resuscitation. This review outlines the epidemiology of mushroom poisoning and highlights the "at risk" populations. Each toxin group is discussed with respect to pathophysiology and specific treatments.

Finally, a general approach to mushroom ingestions is provided, including questions that should be asked about each ingestion.

Epidemiology and Mushroom Identification

The American Association of Poison Control Centers (AAPCC) maintains a database of toxic exposures known as the Toxic Exposure Surveillance System (TESS). In 1998, of the 2.2 million reported human exposures to toxins, approximately 10,000 were mushroom exposures (0.5% of total exposures).[3] This percentage has remained constant for several years.[4] It is of interest to note that the number of ingestions of hallucinogenic mushrooms doubled between 1989 and 1998.[4,5]

Identification. Fortunately, the majority of mushroom exposures will have a benign outcome. However, many cases go unreported, so that the actual number of cases with a benign outcome may be considerably higher. Although a positive identification of the involved mushrooms is not made in the majority of cases, this should not deter the clinician from trying to make an identification in each case. Most exposures occur in children younger than 6 years, and they occur as a result of "backyard grazing" of LBM's. However, deadly species of *Amanita* have been found in backyards, so any given ingestion should be considered potentially toxic, and an attempt should be made at definitive identification.

A mycologist can prove invaluable for identification of mushrooms. Accordingly, the emergency physician should know how to contact a mycologist in his or her area. These individuals usually are listed with the local Poison Control Center, or they may be contacted through the Rocky Mountain Poison Control and Drug Center (303-739-1123). Other sources include local universities, botanical organizations, museums, mycological societies, commercial growers, or the U.S. Department of Agriculture.[5] If a mycologist is not available, field guidebooks, Certified Poison Centers, and the Poisondex database may be helpful for mushroom identification.[6] A useful Internet site for contacting mycological societies in the United States and Canada is http://namyco.org (North American Mycological Association). A guide to mushroom databases also can be found at http://molbiol.soton.ac.uk/msdn/web.html.

Because mushroom identification can be complex, it is preferable to consult with experts. Mushroom identification keys can be helpful, but can be difficult to interpret.[7] To use a key requires familiarity with mushrooms and their anatomy. Identification of a mushroom can be foiled if a component of the fungus, such as the annulus or volva (please see Figure 1) has been removed from an *Amanita* specimen. Moreover, individual specimens in the same species may vary considerably in color, shape, and odor.

A sample mushroom of the type ingested should be retrieved if possible; even uneaten portions of a meal may prove helpful. Emesis and stool can also be saved for potential spore and chemical analysis. Uneaten mushroom specimens are best transported by courier to the mycologist in a dry paper bag, as transportation in plastic will hasten decomposition.[8] There can be other pitfalls to correct mushroom identification. More than one type of mushroom may have been ingested, compromising the reliability of diagnosis according to symptom complex and onset of symptoms. Furthermore, bacterial contamination may be the cause of gastrointestinal symptoms. A few individuals may experience idiosyncratic or allergic symptoms instead of true toxin ingestion.

Epidemiology and Ingestion Patterns. A mushroom is actually the fruiting body of a much larger organism, the mycelium, which is underground. The mushroom fruiting bodies often emerge from the mycelium, yielding the "fairy rings" of legend and folklore. Because fungi have no chlorophyll, they must extract nutrients from other sources; as a result, they live in symbiosis with trees or are found on cow dung. Mushrooms change shape as they emerge from the ground, starting as egg shaped inside a veil, and then maturing with fully extended umbrella-like cap with the spores underneath. Some species have remnants of the veil remaining as "warts" on top.[9] *(Please see Figure 1.)*

Both recreational and commercial mushroom hunting have increased in the last few years.[10] In the Pacific Northwest, mushroom hunting has been nicknamed "a new gold rush," and exportation of mushrooms such as the matsutake or "pine mushroom" to Japan (where supplies have diminished) has become a multimillion-dollar industry. *Amanita smithiana*, which has been associated with renal failure, has been mistaken for the matsutake by amateurs.[12,13] The highly prized chanterelle can be confused with the American Jack O' Lantern, which is toxic. Because mushrooming is more common in Europe, several hundred deaths are reported annually from this part of the world.[10] Immigrants from Asia and Europe are considered potential "at risk" populations for making errors with mushroom identification. However, no ethnic group should be excluded as "at risk" because mushrooms have always been a food source, especially during times of war and in periods of deprivation.[14]

In a case report from 1989, a group of four illegal aliens who had been without food for several days were fatally poisoned after consuming *Amanita phalloides* picked in a field in southern California. It is notable that they did not seek medical care until about three days after the ingestion.[15] A 1996 study of patients with serious mushroom poisonings who were hospitalized in California showed that poisoning rates between ethnic groups did not vary significantly. This report also mentioned another death, in a migrant farm worker, which also appeared to be linked to *Amanita* ingestion. The authors noted that their study might have been limited by the fact that not all groups presented themselves for medical care. They also concluded that children younger than age 5 had a higher rate of hospitalization than other age groups.[10]

Mushroom Toxin Classification System

Mushroom toxins have been classified into several groups. Unfortunately, different authorities use slightly different classification systems. This review uses the classification system outlined by the Poisondex database by Micromedex and the Handbook of Mushroom Poisoning, edited by Spoerke and Rumack.[6,7] Mushroom toxins generally fall into one of eight groups, as listed below:

I. Cyclopeptide-containing group (e.g., *Amanita phalloides*)
IA. Cyclopeptides/Orellanine (Cortinarius mushrooms)
II. Muscimol/Ibotenic Acid-containing group
III. Gyromitrin-containing group (monomethyl-hydrazine)
IV. Muscarine-containing group
V. Coprine-containing group
VI. Psilocybin-containing group
VII. Miscellaneous/gastrointestinal irritants

A few exceptions to the aforementioned classification systems do occur, and it is likely that more will be discovered as knowledge of the chemistry of mushroom toxins expands. For example, in the Pacific Northwest there have been recent case reports of acute renal failure associated with ingestion of *Amanita smithiana* as mentioned above. However, the toxidrome of renal failure is more typically associated with *Cortinarius* mushrooms, rather than with members of the *Amanita* genus. The implicated toxins, pentynoic acid and allenic norleucine, are distinct from both groups I and IA.[13] Please refer to Table 1, which provides an overview of mushroom toxins, their associated symptoms, and treatment strategies.

Figure 1. Structural Characteristics of a Mushroom

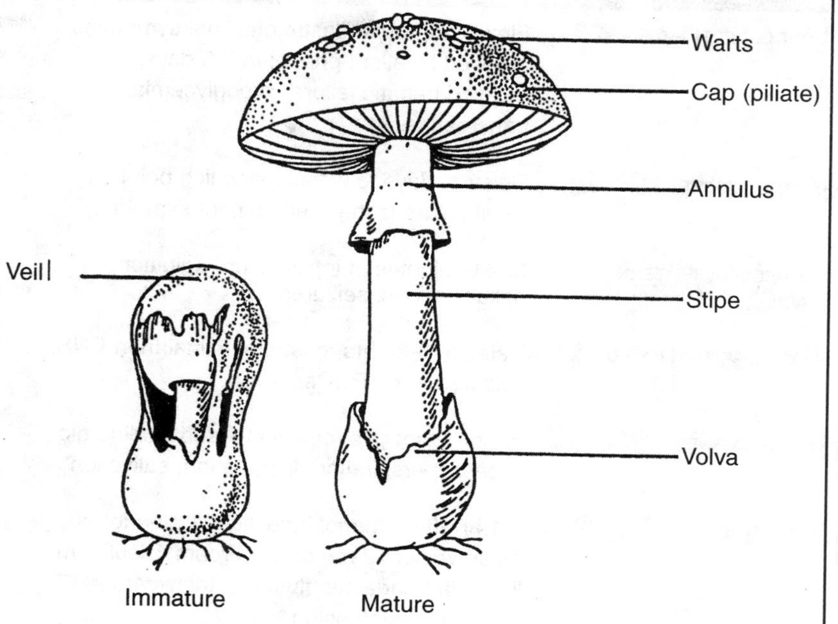

Reproduced with permission from: Schneider S. Mushroom Toxicity. In: Wilderness Medicine, 3rd. ed. Auerbach P, ed. St. Louis, MO; Mosby-Yearbook; 1995:892.

Cyclopeptide-Containing Mushrooms

Although exposures to cyclopeptide-containing mushrooms are uncommon, they account for 95% of all mushroom fatalities in North America and a significant percentage of mushroom-related deaths in Europe.[8,16,17] In this regard, the *Amanita* genus is associated with the greatest number of fatalities, and three of the most common species are *A. phalloides* (the "death cap"), *A. verna*, and *A. virosa* (the "destroying angel"). However, not all members of the genus *Amanita* contain the highly toxic cyclopeptide toxins; some are associated with other toxidromes (see group II below) and others are listed in some field guides as edible.[18]

Moreover, the toxic cyclopeptides have been reported in other genera, including selected species of *Galerina* and *Lepiota* genera. Interestingly, cyclopeptide-containing mushrooms exist on all continents except Antarctica. *Amanita phalloides* is known to be indigenous to the gulf coastal regions of the United States, and *Amanita* species have been found throughout the United States including urban yards, although they are more commonly found in temperate forests, especially in symbiosis with oak trees.[19]

In addition to the cap and stem, members of the *Amanita* group usually have both an annulus (ring) around the stem and a cup (volva) at the base.[19,20] *(Please see Figure 1.)* It is important to remember that these distinguishing features for identifying an *Amanita* mushroom might be separated from an individual specimen. A typical *A. phalloides* has no warts on the cap, is light to olive green or brown, but also can be off-white. It has white gills on the undersurface on the cap and white spores (spore color must be determined by spore print).[18,20] A single death cap contains enough toxins to be fatal to an adult.[18,19]

Clinical Syndrome. The offending toxins are small cyclopeptides, among them amatoxins, phallotoxins, and virotoxins.[8] Phalloidins or phallotoxins impair cell membrane function, but have limited gastrointestinal (GI) absorption, so it is postulated that the phalloidin's toxicity is primarily gastrointestinal in nature.[16,21,22] The amatoxins are heat stable, and therefore, cooking does not diminish toxicity. Amatoxins are absorbed systemically and cause severe hepatic, renal, and central nervous system (CNS) damage.[23] The cyclic structure of amatoxin resists digestive peptidases.[24] Alpha-amanitin is cytotoxic because it interferes with RNA polymerase II, an enzyme required for protein synthesis.[25] The liver and kidneys are primary target organs because of their high rate of protein synthesis.[21] Toxins are eliminated in the urine and feces for several days following ingestion; they can be detected by various chemical analyses of serum, urine, gastrointestinal fluid, and liver and by kidney biopsy.[8,19] Serum amatoxin levels do not correlate well with the severity of illness.[19,21,26,27]

The initial phase of a cyclopeptide poisoning is similar to several other mushroom toxicities and may be indistinguishable from gastroenteritis. Typically, there is a delay of 6-10 hours after ingestion before the onset of severe abdominal pain, vomiting, and cholera-like diarrhea.[5,8,27] The stools may progress to contain blood and mucus. This phase usually lasts several hours, and if the patient is not identified as a potential amatoxin victim, he or she may be inadvertently discharged without adequate follow-up. The stages of toxicity that follow, which are somewhat analogous to acetaminophen toxicity, include a second quiescent phase in which the patient feels well but the liver enzymes begin to rise.

The second phase is followed by a third phase at 3-5 days post ingestion and is characterized by potentially severe hepatic, renal, and occasionally, pancreatic involvement.[8,19] The patient may manifest fever, fatigue, malaise, loss of appetite, nausea, abdominal pain, dark urine, and jaundice.[26] Lab abnormalities include elevated liver function tests, hyperbilirubinemia, abnormal clotting studies, hypoglycemia, hypocalcemia, and elevated creatinine, and blood urea nitrogen.[5,8,16] Hepatic necrosis, which is primarily centrilobular, may rapidly progress to clinical hepatic failure and encephalopathy. Renal

Table 1. Mushroom Toxins, Symptoms, and Treatment Strategies

TOXIN	ONSET & SYMPTOMS	TREATMENT	PROGNOSIS
I. CYCLOPEPTIDES	First 6-10 hours: gastrointestinal symptoms, followed by silent phase; In 2-3 days, delayed hepatic failure, hypoglycemia, pancreatitis	Admission to the ICU, fluids, activated charcoal, high-dose penicillin-G, silibinin, cimetidine, liver transplant	20-30% mortality
IA. ORELLANINE	Delay of days to weeks, at which point renal failure is the predominant symptom	Hemodialysis, renal transplant	Mortality rare with dialysis
II. MUSCIMOL/IBOTENIC ACID	30-90 minutes of intoxication, agitation, hallucinations, seizures	Supportive treatment, benzodiazepines	Full recovery
III. MONOMETHYLHYDRAZINE	Delay of 6-24 hrs, gastrointestinal then CNS, seizures, liver, RBCs.	Supportive, benzodiazepines, pyridoxine 25 mg/kg	Mortality 15-35%
IV. MUSCARINE	< 2 hr onset gastrointestinal and cholinergic excess: perspiration, lacrimation, salivation	Atropine and fluids	Full recovery
V. COPRINE	< 1 hr after ethanol ingestion, if ethanol taken within 72 hrs of mushroom. Disulfiram-like with headache, flushing, tachycardia, vomiting, hypotension	Fluids, vasopressors	Full recovery
VI. PSILOCYBIN	< 1 hr of euphoria, hallucinations	Reassurance, calm environment, benzodiazepines	Full recovery
VII. MISCELLANEOUS GASTROINTESTINAL IRRITANTS	< 2 hr onset of gastrointestinal symptoms	Charcoal, fluids	Full recovery

Adapted from: Goldfrank LR, Flomenbaum NE, Lewis NA, eds. *Goldfrank's Toxicologic Emergencies.* 6th ed. Stamford, Conn: Appleton & Lange; 1998:1209; and Schneider SM, Cochran KW, Krenzlok EP. Mushroom poisoning: Recognition and management. *Emerg Med Reports* 1991;12:83.

failure also may ensue by direct toxic effect or by the hepatorenal syndrome.[25] Bone marrow suppression also has been noted.[22] Death from fulminant hepatic failure typically occurs at an average of eight days post ingestion.[19,22]

Treatment. Current therapy has reduced mortality associated with *A. phalloides* ingestion from the 50-60% rate of previous years to 20-30%.[8,19,22,25] Children, it should be noted, have a predictably higher mortality rate.[8,22] Any patient in whom cyclopeptide ingestion is suspected should be admitted to the hospital. Initial management should include vigorous monitoring and replacement of expected fluid and electrolyte losses, which may be several liters per day.[22] Emesis and lavage are usually not indicated because of the emesis induced by the toxin itself.[8] Because amatoxin undergoes enterohepatic circulation, oral multidose activated charcoal is indicated.[8,19] The initial dose is 30-100 grams of charcoal in 240 mL diluent orally, with repeat doses of 20-50 grams every 2-6 hours. For children, a dose of 1-2 gm/kg in 4 mL/kg diluent is recommended.[19] A cathartic is ill-advised if the patient has diarrhea. The patient should be hemodynamically monitored and lab parameters also followed closely.

Other therapeutic approaches also are used. High-dose penicillin G in doses of 300,000 to 1,000,000 U/kg per day by intravenous infusion has been shown in experimental studies to inhibit liver uptake of amatoxin and is used in several centers.[8,19,21,22,26] Another drug, Silibinin, available in Europe for parenteral use, is derived from the milk thistle plant and has fewer side effects than penicillin.[27] The oral form, silymarin, is more available in the United States. Silibinin and silymarin are thought to work by a mechanism similar to that of high-dose penicillin.

High-dose cimetidine, a cytochrome P-450 inhibitor, is often used for its theoretical role in preventing toxic metabolites.[5,19,28,29] Thioctic (alpha-lipoic) acid is another experimental therapy. It is an antioxidant that may be of benefit in some case series but is unproven.[8,19] Some of the therapies listed above have become part of many centers' standard treatment regimens, even though they have not been subjected to well controlled studies; consequently, their precise benefit may be difficult to determine.

If a patient begins to manifest significant hepatotoxicty, he or she should be transferred to a liver transplantation center. Indications for liver transplantation include markedly prolonged prothrombin time and other clotting abnormalities, hypoglycemia, acidosis, and hyperbilirubinemia.[16,22,29] Generally, liver transplantation is advised before the onset of advancing hepatic encephalopathy because of the associated poorer prognosis once hepatic encephalopathy has been established.[16,26] Recent case series report good results when liver transplantation is performed according to the aforementioned criteria.[16,22,30]

Orellanine- and Cortinarin-Containing Mushrooms

Orellanine and related compounds are found in some of the *Cortinarius* species of mushrooms. Cortinarius mushrooms are widespread in Europe and have been reported in North America, but ingestions of this genus are much more rare in the United States.[3,29,31,32] *Cortinarius orellanus* is a large handsome mushroom with a vivid orange and brown cap that flourishes in late summer through fall.

The world literature's first large case series was reported in the 1950s from Poland (where "mushrooming" is very common) by Gryzmala, who also did work to isolate the toxins.[32] Orellanine has a bipyridyl structure similar to the deadly herbicide paraquat but has a different mode of action and exerts it principal effects on the kidneys.[8,21,31,33] Poisonous *Cortinarius* species also have been reported to contain cyclopeptides that are closely related to the amatoxins. These are called cortinarins A, B, and C. Cortinarins A and B have been shown to be nephrotoxic in laboratory animals.[24]

Clinical Syndrome. The target organ of *Cortinarius* toxicity is the kidney. The delay of symptoms is one of the longest of all mushroom poisonings: from 3 to 20 days, with the more severe cases presenting closer to three days.[34] Because of this delay in the onset of symptoms, the patient may not make the association between symptoms and the mushroom ingestion. In some cases, the diagnosis is often not made until renal failure has already started.[33]

The typical symptoms of *Cortinarius* or orellanine poisoning consist of severe thirst, headache, chills, polyuria or oliguria, and back pain.[21,32,33] On laboratory examination, signs of renal failure are evident, including elevation of blood urea nitrogen and creatinine; the urinalysis may show hematuria, red cell casts, and proteinuria. Other lab parameters usually are normal, including liver enzymes.[32]

Treatment. Treatment of orellanine poisoning is supportive, with hemodialysis being indicated for cases with severe renal impairment. Approximately 50% of patients requiring hemodialysis will eventually recover renal function and will not require permanent dialysis or renal transplant.[33] Extracorporeal hemoperfusion in combination with hemodialysis also has been suggested by some authors.[21,32]

Muscimol/Botenic Acid-Containing Mushrooms

Muscimol, and its derivative, ibotenic acid, are stereochemically related to gammaminobutyric acid (GABA) and glutamic acid, respectively. As a result, muscimol is a strong GABA agonist and has sedative properties; ibotenic acid is a CNS stimulant.[8,21]

These compounds are found in a few species of *Amanita*, but not in *Amanita phalloides* as they are group I toxins. Examples of muscimol/ibotenic acid-containing mushrooms include *Amanita muscaria* and *A. Pantherina* (the "panther" because it is brown with white spots).[18] The toxidrome is sometimes known as the "pantherina syndrome." *Amanita muscaria* is a large, bright orange mushroom with white spots on the cap. Both types of mushrooms are distributed worldwide, and *A. muscaria* has the nickname "fly agaric" for its ability to attract and kill flies (agaric means mushroom).[35] These mushrooms contain other chemicals in smaller amounts such as muscarine, which was isolated first from *A. muscaria* in 1869 and used in the elucidation of cholinergic receptors.

Clinical Syndrome. The CNS effects of the muscaria mushroom have been known for centuries. In the 16th century, Siberians would drink the urine of other people who had become intoxicated from eating the mushroom, with similar intoxicating effects; suggesting that the toxins are excreted at least partially unchanged in the urine.[35]

After ingestion of the mushroom, symptoms begin rapidly, usually within 30-90 minutes, and they are similar to ethanol intoxication.[2,21,36] There is often a mixture of CNS depression and stimulation, causing drowsiness alternating with agitation, ataxia, and mild hallucinations. Occasionally, patients may become comatose or have seizures. Gastrointestinal symptoms usually are mild.

Treatment of the muscimol/ibotenic acid group is supportive, and symptoms usually resolve within a few hours. Gastrointestinal decontamination with oral activated charcoal is reasonable if the patient is seen early after the ingestion. Severe cases may warrant airway control or anti-seizure therapy with benzodiazepines.

Monomethylhydrazine-Containing Mushrooms

The mushroom genus *Gyromitra* is found during the spring months in North America and Europe. These unusual-appearing mushrooms with irregularly convoluted caps are known as false morels and are occasionally mistaken for true morels, which are considered a delicacy. Despite a potential for significant toxicity, *Gyromitra* have been canned and sold in eastern Europe, but are banned now in some countries.[24]

Gyromitras contain precursors to a toxin known as gyromitrin. Gyromitrin is N-methyl-N-formyl hydrazine, which is unstable, and upon hydrolysis in the body yields monomethylhydrazine (MMH). MMH is a highly reactive compound used in industry as a solvent and rocket fuel![37] These chemicals are highly volatile and, as a result, boiling will eliminate a significant percentage, but not all, of the toxins. Vapors definitely pose a hazard to the cook and, until recently, have been a hazard in the canning industry.[24,38]

Similar to the clinical effects of isoniazid, which is chemically related to MMH and is a hydrazine derivative, the hydrazine toxins of *Gyromitra* interfere with pyridoxine dependent enzymes used for the production of acid GABA in the brain. This leads to lack of GABA, which can result in seizures.[8,38-40]

Clinical Syndrome. Like the mushroom toxins in group I and IA, *Gyromitra* ingestions often have a delay prior to onset of toxic symptoms for 6-24 hours or longer.[39] Initial symptoms are gastrointestinal, with abdominal pain, bloating, vomiting, and diarrhea lasting a few days.[39,40] Other target involved include the liver, red blood cells, and the CNS. Late findings may include jaundice and elevation of liver enzymes. Because of its reactivity, MMH can cause oxidation of hemoglobin to methemoglobin and cause hemolysis. The CNS effects include headache, ataxia, depressed sensorium, and seizures.[40]

Treatment. General decontamination methods will be addressed in the final section. Seizures initially should be treated with benzodiazepines. Like isoniazid toxicity, the seizures induced by monomethylydrazine also can be treated with pyridoxine in doses of 25 mg/kg intravenously to restore GABA production in the CNS.[8] Very large doses of pyridoxine can result in delayed peripheral neuropathies. Intravenous methylene blue can be used in cases with severe methemoglobinemia. Patients should be followed closely for evidence of hypoglycemia and delayed hepatotoxicity. Mortality rates have been reported to be in the range of 15% to 35%.[29,39]

Muscarine-Containing Mushrooms

Although muscarine was initially discovered in *Amanita muscaria*, much greater quantities of this toxin are present in many species of *Inocybe* mushrooms, and some species of *Clitocybe*, which are distributed worldwide. The orange luminous Jack-O-Lantern mushroom (*Omphalotus illudens* and *O. oleareus*), which is often mistaken for the yellow edible chanterelle, has previously been classified in the genus *Clitocybe*. The Jack-O-Lantern has not been definitely shown to contain muscarine, but is associated with a very similar symptom complex of acute gastrointestinal irritation, and therefore, it is mentioned in this discussion.[41,42]

Stimulating these receptors causes perspiration, salivation, and lacrimation (PSL syndrome) along with vomiting, diarrhea, urination, bronchorrhea, bradycardia, and pupillary constriction.[41] This complex is similar to that encountered in organophosphate poisoning, but without the nicotinic effects on striated muscles. Although the GI symptoms are common to most mushroom intoxication syndromes, the PSL syndrome is unique to this group of mushrooms; fortunately, it is self-limited to less than a day.[43] If a patient clearly has symptoms of cholinergic excess, the specific antidote atropine may be titrated to block the symptoms. The dose of atropine for an adult is 1-2 mg given IV slowly. For children the dosage is 0.05 mg/kg.[6,41]

Coprine-Containing Mushrooms

Various members of the widely disseminated genus *Coprinus*—in particular *C. atramentarius*—have the peculiar feature of only causing toxicity if consumed with alcohol. The resultant toxic symptom complex is similar to a disulfiram reaction, causing several hours of extreme unpleasantness for the victim, but is seldom life threatening. The light-colored *Coprinus atramentarius* is known as the "inky cap," and gets its name from its association with dung ("Coprinus") and the phenomenon of autodigestion of the gills into an inky black residue ("atramentarius") when the specimen begins to age.

The offending protoxin is coprine, an atypical amino acid. Coprine is metabolized in the body to 1-aminocyclopropanol, which is further metabolized to an intermediate that blocks the function of the enzyme aldehyde dehydrogenase.[44] If ethanol is consumed, the acetaldehyde that is a normal intermediate in ethanol's metabolism will accumulate, leading to the toxic symptoms. Coprine is not inactivated by cooking.[45,46]

The patient is vulnerable to the effects of coprine if alcohol is consumed shortly before and up to 72 hours after the mushroom is ingested.[45] Symptoms include throbbing headache and upper body flushing from the vasodilatory effects, as well as nausea and vomiting, a metallic taste in the mouth, tachycardia, and hypotension.[44] Occasional cases of atrial fibrillation are reported.[46] The symptoms are self-limited, but the patient should be warned not to ingest any more alcohol for a few days.

Gastrointestinal decontamination is not necessary and syrup of ipecac, because it may contain ethanol, should be avoided. Isotonic fluid resuscitation is indicated and diphenhydramine may help the flushing. Vasopressors may occasionally be indicated. An antidote, which sould theoretically work, but has not been FDA approved is 4-methylpyrazole (4-MP).[46] 4-MP, which is approved for toxic alcohol ingestion (e.g., methanol), works by blocking the metabolic step before aldehyde dehydrogenase. That step is alcohol dehydrogenase; as a result, acetaldehyde is not produced after alcohol consumption.[47]

It should be noted there are several other drugs and chemicals that have a disulfiram-like reaction when taken with ethanol. One of the most familiar is metronidazole. Workers in the rubber industry who are exposed to tetramethylthiuram disulfide can have the same reaction if they ingest a beer after work.[47] Coprine was investigated as a potential therapeutic agent for alcoholism, but was found to be carcinogenic when used long term.[44]

Psilocybin-Containing Mushrooms

Psilocybin-containing, or hallucinogenic, "magic" mushrooms have been popular in the drug culture for the past last 30 years. Their popularity was a consequence of the rediscovery during the 1950s of "teonanacatl" ("flesh of the gods"), which was the psilocybe mushroom used in Mexican Aztec religious rituals as long as 2000 years ago. The discoverer of lysergic acid diethylamide (LSD), the organic chemist Dr. Albert Hofman, also isolated psilocybin and psilocin, the active hallucinogens in some *Psilocybe, Panaeolus*, and *Gymnopilus* species of mushrooms. These mushrooms are distributed worldwide, and *Gymnopilus spectabilis* is known as the "big laughing mushroom" in Japan.[48] Hallucinogens were briefly used in legitimate psychiatric research in the 1950s and 60s but became rapidly adapted as pleasure drugs in the hippie movement of the 1960s.[49]

Magic mushroom growing spore kits have been available through mail order in drug-oriented periodicals for many years, and they are now available for credit card purchase at various Web sites on the Internet. Possession of psilocybin mushrooms is illegal but possession or shipment of spores may not be.[50] Various surveys of college students indicate 10-15% of them have tried "shrooms" at least once.[50,51]

Several species of psilocybe mushrooms are indigenous to the United States, particularly in moist fertile areas of the Northwest and Southeast. "Magic" mushrooms sold on the street often contain no psilocybin, but instead may represent commercial mushrooms laced with LSD or phencyclidine.[48] The largest percentage of mushroom exposures reported to poison control centers, other than unknowns, are hallucinogenic.[3,52] There are a few hundred reports of hallucinogenic mushrooms ingestions to poison centers yearly, but this represents only a tiny fraction of the actual ingestions.

Hallucinogenic mushrooms vary widely in their psilocybin content, some requiring ingestion of only a few specimens; and some, like *Psilocybe semilanceata* (Liberty caps), 20-40 fresh specimens must be ingested for an adequate dose.[48] This explains the frequent gastrointestinal symptoms associated with these ingestions, inasmuch as large quantities of mushrooms may be difficult to digest or may contain other toxins. Several species of hallucinogenic mushrooms have the characteristic of turning blue when bruised, but this neither necessarily indicates hallucinogen content nor confirms lack of other toxicity.[48,50,53]

Clinical Syndrome. Psilocybin and psilocin are indole derivatives, and therefore, are closely related to serotonin, LSD, and tryptophan. Symptoms begin shortly after ingestion, usually within one hour, and typically last 2-4 hours.[48] Gastrointestinal side effects are common. Sympathomimetic effects also accompany the perceptual changes, and include tachycardia, mydriasis, and occasional hypertension.[48,54] The hallucinations produced by psilocybin and other psychedelic "mind-expanding" drugs are distinct from those produced by toxic amounts of other drugs such as anticholinergics and cocaine and withdrawal states. The hallucinations consist of altered or heightened sensory perceptions ("hearing colors" or "seeing music"), altered time, or visual distortions. The individual may experience these perceptions with a sense of religious exhalation or may become very frightened.

Commonly cited is the feeling of being outside one's self, observing; also commonly reported is the sensation or feeling of a union with mankind or the cosmos.[55]

The effects last a few hours. Occasional overdoses may result in a more prolonged toxic psychosis. Seizures and hyperthermia have been occasionally reported in children.[48] Accidental trauma such as jumping off a roof while thinking one can fly is another consequence. Treatment of the ingestion usually is not necessary. Assurance and a calm environment often suffice. Benzodiazepines are the drugs of choice for agitation.[54]

Gastrointestinal Irritants

This final and largest category also qualifies as a "miscellaneous" since many varieties of mushrooms that have not been mentioned in previous categories may lead to GI upset. The most commonly ingested mushroom from this group is *Chlorophyllum molybdites* (also known as *Lepiota morgani* or the green parasol mushroom), which grows throughout the United States and much of the southern hemisphere. This is a large, light-colored mushroom with grayish green gills and is often mistaken as edible or is eaten by young children. This mushroom produces symptoms that begin quickly (within 30 minutes to two hours after ingestion), and are characterized by intense nausea, vomiting, and diarrhea. Clinical shock from severe dehydration is possible.[56,57]

Chlorophyllum can occasionally cause disseminated intravascular coagulation and obtundation but these are rare.[56,58] The toxins involved have not been elucidated. Most cases are self-limited and require only fluid resuscitation, electrolyte monitoring, and symptomatic treatment. There is variable susceptibility among individuals, so some may become ill when others do not.[5]

Approach to Mushroom Ingestion

There are several questions that should be asked in cases of suspected mushroom poisoning:[1,2,6]

1. How long after mushroom consumption did symptoms begin? *(A latency period of six hours or greater suggests exposure to the more poisonous groups: I, IA, or III.)*
2. Was more than one type of mushroom consumed? *(The prolonged latency period of a more toxic mushroom could be masked, leading to a false sense of security.)*
3. What were the initial symptoms? *(Autonomic symptoms, inebriation, or hallucinations suggests groups: II, IV, V, or VI.)*
4. Was alcohol consumed within 72 hours after mushroom ingestion? *(Autonomic symptoms and GI upset suggest group V.)*
5. Did everyone who ate the mushrooms become ill? *(If only one person became ill, this might represent food sensitivity or an unrelated illness.)*
6. Did anyone who did not eat the mushrooms become ill? *(This suggests food poisoning or infectious gastroenteritis.)*
7. How were the mushrooms collected, prepared, and stored? *(Again, consider the possibility of bacterial contamination.)*
8. Were the mushrooms collected on a golf course, public park, or transportation right-of-way? *(Mushrooms can cause illness if contaminated by fertilizers, insecticides, or herbicides.)*

Symptomatic patients should be admitted for observation until symptoms resolve. Patients with delayed symptoms should be admitted to the hospital for monitoring and treatment while an attempt is made to identify the mushroom, to exclude cyclopeptide, orellanine, or gyromitrin poisoning. If follow-up of a patient cannot be assured, admission for 3-5 days also should be considered.[6,8]

Gastrointestinal decontamination methods should be individualized to each patient's circumstance. Only very recent ingestions (1-2 hours) would have any benefit from ipecac or gastric lavage. Administration of ipecac will confuse the clinical picture by causing vomiting, yet it maybe more efficacious than lavage at retrieving larger undigested pieces of mushroom. Administration of activated charcoal is a very reasonable, and perhaps preferable, alternative.[1,5,59]

Close attention should be paid to the patient's vital signs, glucose, and fluid and electrolyte status. Fluid resuscitation and symptomatic treatment will be adequate in the majority of cases. Thorough discharge instructions alerting the patient to delayed symptoms and follow-up arrangements should be provided.[8]

As mushroom hunting for food and thrill seeking is rising, emergency physicians will continue to be called upon to treat these patients. Knowledge of the types of toxins and their clinical features, along with a plan for mushroom identification and appropriate treatment will contribute to a successful outcome.

References

1. McPartland JM, Vilgalys RJ, Cubeta MA. Mushroom poisoning. *Am Fam Physician* 1997;55:1797-1800, 1805-1809, 1811-1812.
2. Blackman JR. Clinical approach to toxic mushroom ingestion. *J Am Board Fam Pract* 1994;7:31-37.
3. Livovitz TL, Klein-Schwartz W, Caravati EM, et al. 1998 Annual Report of the American Association of Poison Control Centers Toxic Exposure Surveillance System. *Am J Emerg Med* 1999;17:435-487.
4. Trestrail JH. Mushroom poisoning in the United States—An analysis of 1989 United States Poison Control Center data. *J Toxicol Clin Tox* 1991;29:459-465.
5. Schneider SM, Cochran KW, Krenzlok EP. Mushroom poisoning: Recognition and emergency management. *Emerg Med Rep* 1991;12:81-88.
6. Poisondex System: Toxicologic Management. Mushrooms. In: Rumack BH, Sayre NK, Gelman CR, eds. Poisondex System. Englewood, Colorado: Micromedex; Ed expires 6-30-99.

7. Spoerke DG. Introduction to Identification and Toxicology. In: Spoerke DG, Rumack BH, eds. *Handbook of Mushroom Poisoning, Diagnosis and Treatment.* Boca Raton, FL: CRC Press; 1994:1-8.
8. Goldfrank LR. Mushrooms: Toxic and Hallucinogenic. In: Goldfrank LR, Flomenbaum NE, Lewis NA, eds. *Goldfrank's Toxicological Emergencies.* 6th ed. Stamford Conn: Appleton and Lange; 1998:1207-1220.
9. Grimes GL. Principles of Mushroom Identification. In: Spoerke DG, Rumack BH, eds. *Handbook of Mushroom Poisoning, Diagnosis and Treatment.* Boca Raton, FL: CRC Press; 1994: 65-96.
10. Jacobs J, VonBehren J, Kreutzer R. Serious mushroom poisoning in California requiring hospital admission, 1990 through 1994. *West J Med* 1996;165:318-319.
11. Lipske M. A new gold rush packs the woods in Central Oregon. *Smithsonian* 1994;24:35-45.
12. Warden CR, Benjamin DR. Acute renal failure associated with suspected *Amanita smithsonia*. Mushroom Ingestions: A case series. *Acad Emerg Med* 1998;5:808-812.
13. Leathem AM, Purssell RA, Chan VR et al. Renal failure caused by mushroom poisoning. *Toxicol Clin Tox* 1997;35:67-75.
14. Shaw M. Amateur Opportunity. In: Spoerke DG, Rumack BH, eds. *Handbook of Mushroom Poisoning, Diagnosis and Treatment.* Boca Raton, FL: CRC Press; 1994:9-38.
15. McClain JL, Hause DW, Clark MA. *Amanita phalloides* mushroom poisoning: A cluster of four fatalities. *J Forensic Sci* 1989;34:83-87.
16. Klein AS, Hart J, Brems JJ, et al. *Amanita* poisoning: Treatment and the role of liver transplantation. *Am J Med* 1989;86:187-193.
17. Larrey D, Pageaux GP. Hepatotoxicity of herbal remedies and mushrooms. *Semin Liver Dis* 1995;15:183-188.
18. Pacioni G, Lincott G. *Simon & Schuster's Guide to Mushrooms.* New York: Simon & Schuster; 1981.
19. Poisondex System: Toxicologic Management. Mushrooms-Cyclopeptides. In: Rumack BH, Sayre NK, Gelman CR, eds. Poisondex System. Englewood, CO., Micromedex, Ed expires 6-30-99.
20. Gillman L. Identification of Common Poisonous Mushrooms. In: Spoerke DG, Rumack BH, eds. *Handbook of Mushroom Poisoning, Diagnosis and Treatment.* Boca Raton, Fla: CRC Press; 1994: 97-130.
21. Köppel C. Clinical symptomatology and management of mushroom poisoning. *Toxicon* 1993;31:1513-1540.
22. Pinson CW, Daya MR, Benner KH, et al. Liver transplantation for severe *Amanita phalloides* mushroom poisoning. *Am J Surg* 1990;159:493-499.
23. Vetter J. Toxins of Amanita phalloides. *Toxicon* 1998;36:13-24.
24. Chilton WS. The Chemistry and Mode of Action of Mushroom Toxins. In: Spoerke DG, Rumack BH, eds. *Handbook of Mushroom Poisoning, Diagnosis and Treatment.* Boca Raton, FL: CRC Press; 1994:165-233.
25. Cappell MS, Hassan T. Gastrointestinal and hepatic effects of *Amanita phalloides* ingestion. *J Clin Gastroenterol* 1992;15: 225-228.
26. Shakil AO, Mazariegos GV, Kramer DJ. Fulminant hepatic failure. *Surg Clin North Am* 1999;79:77-108.
27. Faulstich H, Zilker TR. Amatoxins. In: Spoerke DG, Rumack BH, eds. *Handbook of Mushroom Poisoning, Diagnosis and Treatment.* Boca Raton, FL: CRC Press; 1994:233-249.
28. Schneider SM, Borochovitz D, Krenzlok EP. Cimetidine protection against alpha-Amanitin hepatotoxicity in mice: A potential model for the treatment of *Amanita phalloides* poisoning. *Am Emerg Med* 1987;16:1136-1140.
29. Schneider SM. Mushroom Toxicity. In: Auerbach PS. *Wilderness medicine, Management of Wilderness and Environmental Emergencies.* 3rd ed. St. Louis: Mosby; 1995:891-907.
30. Meunier B, Camus CM, Houssin DP, et al. Liver transplantation after severe poisoning due to Amatoxin-containing Lepiota—Report of three cases. *J Toxicol Clin Txi* 1995;33:165-171.
31. Horn S, Horina JH, Krejs GJ, et al. End-stage renal failure from mushroom poisoning with *Cortinarius orellanus*: Report of four cases and review of the literature. *Am J Kidney Dis* 1997;30: 282-286.
32. Poisondex System: Toxicologic Management. Mushrooms-Cyclopeptides. In: Rumack BH, Sayre NK, Gelman CR, eds. Poisondex System. Englewood, CO: Micromedex; Ed expires 6-30-99.
33. Jaeger A. Orellanine Mushrooms. In: Spoerke DG, Rumack BH, eds. *Handbook of Mushroom Poisoning, Diagnosis and Treatment.* Boca Raton, FL: CRC Press; 1994:249-264.
34. Bouget J, Bousser J, Pats B. Acute Renal Failure following collective intoxication by *Cortinarius orellanus. Intens Care Med* 1990;16:506-510.
35. Hall AH, Hall K. Ibotenic Acid/Muscimol Containing Mushrooms. In: Spoerke DG, Rumack BH. eds. *Handbook of Mushroom Poisoning, Diagnosis and Treatment.* Boca Raton, FL: CRC Press; 1994:265-278.
36. Poisondex System: Toxicologic Management. Mushrooms-Muscimol/Ibotenic Acid. In: Rumack BH, Sayre NK, Gelman CR, eds. Poisondex System. Englewood, CO: Micromedex; Ed expires 6-30-99.
37. Sullivan JB. Cryogenics, Oxidizers, Reducing Agents and Explosives. In: Sullivan JB, Krieger GR, eds. *Hazardous Materials Toxicology, Clinical Principles of Environmental Health.* Baltimore, MD: Williams & Wilkins; 1992:1192-1201.
38. Michelot D, Toth B. Poisoning by Gyromita esculenta—A Review. *J Appl Toxicol* 1991;11:235-243.
39. Poisondex System: Toxicologic Management. Mushrooms-Monomethylhydrazine. In: Rumack BH, Sayre NK, Gelman CR, eds. Poisondex System. Englewood, CO: Micromedex; Ed expires 6-30-99.
40. Trestrail JH. Monomethylhydrazine-Containing Mushrooms. In: Spoerke DG, Rumack BH, eds. *Handbook of Mushroom Poisoning, Diagnosis and Treatment.* Boca Raton, FL: CRC Press; 1994: 279-288.
41. Young A. Muscarine-Containing Mushrooms. In: Spoerke DG, Rumack BH, eds. *Handbook of Mushroom Poisoning, Diagnosis and Treatment.* Boca Raton, FL: CRC Press; 1994:289-302.
42. French AL, Garrettson LK. Poisoning with the North American Jack O'Lantern Mushroom, *Omphalotus illudens. J Toxicol Clin Tox* 1988:26:81-88.
43. Mitchell DH, Rumack BH. Symptomatic Diagnosis and Treatment of Mushroom Poisoning. In: Rumack BH, Salzman E, eds. *Mushroom Poisoning: Diagnosis and Treatment.* West Palm Beach, FL: CRC press; 1978:171-180.

44. Michelot D. Poisoning by *Coprinus atramentarius*. Natural Toxins 1992;1:73-80.
45. Kunkel DB, Connor DA. Coprine-Containing Mushrooms. In: Spoerke DG, Rumack BH. eds. *Handbook of Mushroom Poisoning, Diagnosis and Treatment.* Boca Raton, FL: CRC Press; 1994:303-308.
46. Poisondex System: Toxicologic Management. Mushrooms-Coprine. In: Rumack BH, Sayre NK, Gelman CR, eds. Poisondex System. Englewood, CO: Micromedex, Ed expires 6-30-99.
47. Goldfrank LR. Disulfiram and Disulfiram-like Reactions. In: Goldfrank LR, Flomenbaum NE, Lewin NA, et al. *Goldfrank's Toxicologic Emergencies.* 6th ed., Stamford, Connecticut: Appleton and Lange; 1998:1043-1048.
48. Smolinske SC. Psilocybin-Containing Mushrooms. In: Spoerke DG, Rumack BH, eds. *Handbook of Mushroom Poisoning, Diagnosis and Treatment.* Boca Raton, FL: CRC Press; 1994: 309-324.
49. Hofmann A. LSD, My Problem Child. New York, NY: JP Tarcher/Perigree Books; 1983.
50. Schwartz RH, Smith DE. Hallucinogenic mushrooms. *Clin Peds* 1988;27:70-73.
51. Webb E, Ashton CH, Kelly P. Alcohol and drug use in UK University Students. *Lancet* 1996;348:922-925.
52. Litovitz TL, Klein-Schwartz W, Dyer KS, et al. 1997 Annual Report of the American Association of Poison Control Centers Toxic Exposure Surveillance System. *Am J Emerg Med* 1998; 16:443-490.
53. Lincoff G, Mitchel DH. *Toxic and Hallucinogenic Mushroom Poisoning, A Handbook for Physicians and Mushroom Hunters.* New York: Van Nostrand Reinhold Co.; 1977:100-136.
54. Poisondex System: Toxicologic Management. Mushrooms-Hallucinogenic. In: Rumack BH, Sayre NK, Gelman CR. eds: Poisondex System. Englewood, CO: Micromedex; Ed expires 6-30-99.
55. Jaffe JH. Drug Addiction and Drug Abuse. In: Goodman Gilman A, Rall TW, Nies AS, et al, eds. *Goodman and Gilman's The Pharmacologic Basis of Therapeutics,* 8th ed. New York: Pergamon Press; 1990:522-573.
56. Poisondex System: Toxicologic Management. Mushrooms-Chlorophyllum. In: Rumack BH, Sayre NK, Gelman CR, eds. Poisondex System. Englewood, CO: Micromedex; Ed. expires 6-30-99.
57. Stenklyft PH, Augenstein WL. *Chlorophyllym molybdites*—Severe mushroom poisoning in a child. *J Toxicol Clin Tox* 1990;28:159-168.
58. Augenstein WL. Chlorophyllum molybdites. In: Spoerke DG, Rumack BH, eds. *Handbook of Mushroom Poisoning, Diagnosis and Treatment.* Boca Raton, FL: CRC Press; 1994:325-338.
59. Rumack BH. Symptomatic Diagnosis and Treatment of Mushroom Poisoning. In: Spoerke DG, Rumack BH. eds. *Handbook of Mushroom Poisoning, Diagnosis and Treatment.* Boca Raton, FL: CRC Press; 1994:149-164.

Acetaminophen Toxicity

William K. Chiang, MD
Richard Y. Wang, DO

Acetaminophen is one of the most widely used analgesics and antipyretics in the United States. It is available without prescription, and is marketed under at least 50 brand names and contained in more than 200 proprietary drug combinations.[1-2] Perhaps not surprisingly, by virtue of its wide spread popularity and availability, ingestion of acetaminophen, either alone or in combination with other agents, has become a common toxicological problem, accounting for more than 80,000 drug exposures and approximately 60 deaths annually.[3] With prompt treatment, emergency physicians can help to limit hepatotoxicity and prevent mortality associated with this frequent toxicological emergency.[4-6]

The following chapter provides emergency medicine clinicians with an effective strategy for accurate evaluation and effective management of patients with acute acetaminophen ingestion. After briefly reviewing the pharmacokinetics, pathophysiology, and stages of acetaminophen poisoning, the authors describe key clinical features necessary to determine the severity of acetaminophen ingestion, emphasizing the optimal time to obtain acetaminophen levels and proper interpretation of the acetaminophen nomogram. The article also presents specific recommendations for appropriate therapeutic intervention, including guidelines for preventing further drug absorption, detailed indications and dosages for administration of antidote therapy, and special considerations regarding acetaminophen toxicity in certain high-risk groups.

Pharmacokinetics and Pathophysiology

Acetaminophen is a weak acid (pKa of 9.5) and is rapidly absorbed in the small intestine. After a therapeutic dose, peak levels are reached within 30-120 minutes and the half-life is approximately two hours.

Upon absorption, 90% of acetaminophen is conjugated via glucuronidation (60%) and sulfation (30%) by the liver. Another 4% is metabolized by the cytochrome P450 enzymes into a toxic intermediate, N-acetyl-p-benzoquinoneimine (NAPQI), which then normally is detoxified by glutathione into mercapturic acid and cysteine conjugates.[9-11]

After an overdose, both the glucuronidation and the sulfation processes become saturated, shunting more acetaminophen toward the P450 enzyme system and increasing NAPQI formation. Once glutathione is depleted to less than) 30% of normal, NAPQI accumulates.[8,12] *(Please see Figure 1.)*

NAPQI is an extremely electrophilic molecule that reacts with sulfhydryl groups in cellular proteins to produce liver toxicity.[10,13] The typical histologic finding of liver toxicity is centrilobular necrosis with minimal inflammation, which reflects the corresponding increased activity of the hepatic p450 enzyme system.[13,15]

Similar metabolic mechanisms also are responsible for the occasional renal toxicity associated with acetaminophen overdose.[11]

Figure 1. Acetaminophen Metabolism

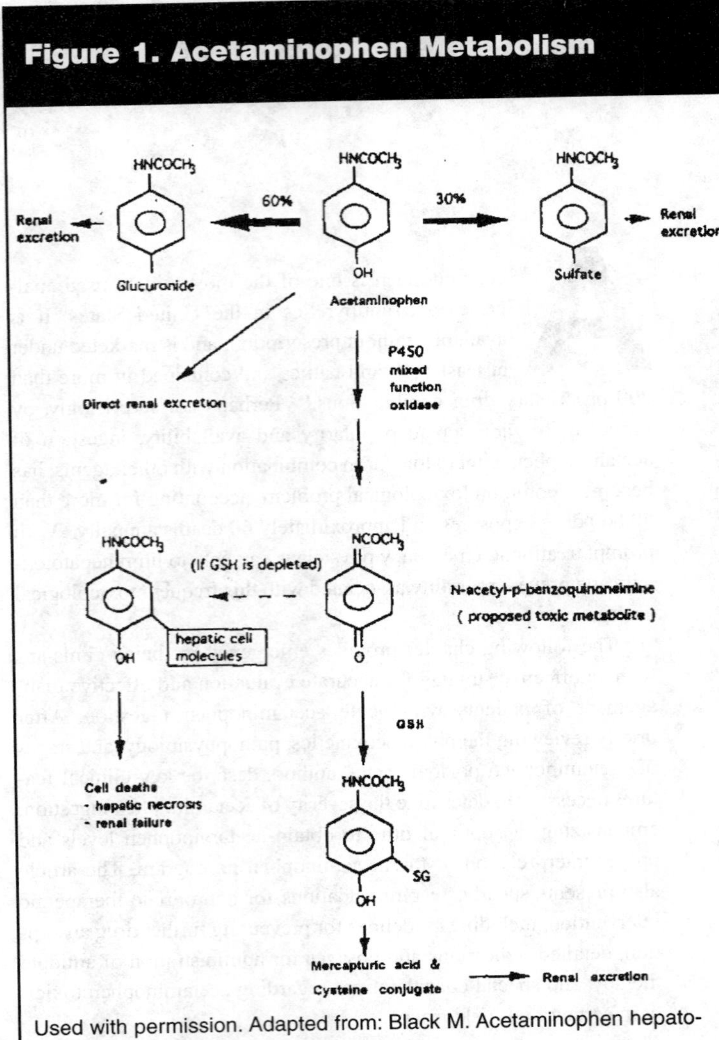

Used with permission. Adapted from: Black M. Acetaminophen hepatotoxicity. *Gastroenterology* 1980; 78:385.

Phases of Acetaminophen Toxicity

The best way to summarize the signs and symptoms of acetaminophen toxicity are to describe those of delayed hepatotoxicity. Unfortunately, by the time significant hepatotoxicity can be recognized easily, the usefulness of any antidote is limited. The characteristic features of untreated acetaminophen toxicity can be classified into four phases.[16,17] *(Please see Table 1.)*

Phase 1 of acute acetaminophen toxicity begins within 30 minutes of ingestion and may last for 12-24 hours. Anorexia, nausea, and vomiting are the most common symptoms and are due to local effects of acetaminophen on the gastrointestinal tract. Diaphoresis also may be noted and is attributable to the effects of acetaminophen on hypothalamic temperaturere-gulating centers. Clinicians should be aware that many patients can be completely asymptomatic during the first phase of acetaminophen toxicity, even following ingestion of significant amounts of the drug.

On occasion, lethargy, coma, and significant metabolic acidosis may occur with massive acetaminophen ingestions.[3,11] However, these symptoms are so uncommon during Phase I, that they can be attributed to acetaminophen only when co-ingestion of depressant-type drugs and other etiologies for central nervous system (CNS) depression have been excluded.

Phase 2 of acute acetaminophen toxicity occurs 24-72 hours following ingestion and is a relatively asymptomatic period. Most of the gastrointestinal symptoms observed during Phase 1 will have subsided, but the patient may complain of right upper quadrant abdominal pain as a result of early hepatic necrosis. Laboratory evidence of abnormal hepatic function may appear, including increased levels of liver enzymes and bilirubin and prolonged prothrombin time.[16]

The kidneys are the second most common major organ involved in acute acetaminophen toxicity. Renal involvement is almost always associated with liver toxicity and is evidenced by creatinine elevation. The BUN may remain low as a result of decreased formation of hepatic urea. Other Phase 2 complications, such as pancreatitis and myocardial necrosis are uncommon in acetaminophen toxicity but have been described occasionally.[13,18]

Phase 3 of acute acetaminophen toxicity occurs at 72-96 hours after ingestion and represents the manifestation of hepatic necrosis. Patients with extensive hepatic necrosis develop nausea, vomiting, jaundice, and hepatomegaly, and hepatic encephalopathy and coagulopathy may ensue. Laboratory findings include marked elevations of liver enzymes and bilirubin, and prolonged prothrombin time.[16]

Patients with irreversible liver damage secondary to acetaminophen toxicity may develop progressive clinical deterioration and a variety of severe complications, including hypotension, renal failure, lactic acidosis, hemorrhage, hypoglycemia, and markedly prolonged prothrombin time. Mortality usually is related to fulminant hepatic failure and increased intracranial pressure.[19]

Phase 4. Patients surviving Phase 3 of acute acetaminophen toxicity enter Phase 4 (the recovery phase) which occurs from day four to two weeks following acute ingestion. For patients with reversible hepatic necrosis, complete resolution of liver damage and hepatic dysfunction occurs during this time frame.

Clinical Assessment

Amount of Ingestion. Historical information regarding the amount of drug ingestion is frequently inaccurate. However, many authorities suggest that a conservative estimate of the toxic dose for an acute acetaminophen ingestion is 7.5 gm for adults and 150 mg/kg for children.[16-20] Since the widespread availability of rapid serum acetaminophen analysis, the history of the amount ingested is less important in predicting toxicity. In addition, as with any overdose, clinicians should also consider the possibility of co-ingestion of other agents.

Time of Ingestion. The single most important question in the assessment of acetaminophen ingestion is the accuracy of the time of the ingestion. Furthermore, the time of ingestion is essential for decision-making concerning initial patient management, particularly with regard to selecting the most appropriate decontamination procedure and determining whether antidotal therapy is required immediately.[21]

Laboratory Analysis. Acetaminophen is one of the few drugs for which the serrum concentration is the major determinant of acute toxicity. The acetaminophen nomogram was developed in 1975 and has remained the well-tested standard for the determination of acute acetaminophen toxicity.[21,22] *(Please see Figure 2.)* A single acetaminophen level obtained at least four hours postingestion is sufficient to determine toxicity.

Acetaminophen levels greater than 150 μg/ml at four hours postingestion or levels above the nomogram line should be considered toxic. Repeat acetaminophen levels are not helpful and are unnecessary. Additional diagnostic studies, such as serum electrolytes and an electrocardiogram should not be affected by acetaminophen, but should be obtained for all overdoses to help exclude significant co-ingestions not reported by the patient.

There are two potential errors that should be noted in determining acute acetaminophen toxicity. First, the units in which the acetaminophen level is reported should be confirmed. Some laboratories may report the result in μg/dl instead of μg/ml, which may lead to a ten-fold underestimation error. The second source of error involves is the method of the acetaminophen assay. The most reliable methods for determining acetaminophen levels are radioimmunoassays, high pressure liquid chromatography, and gas chromatography, Assays using rapid colorimetric techniques may be unreliable in the presence of hyperbilirubinemia, salicylates, methyldopa, and renal failure.[23,24]

Table 1. Phases of Acute Acetaminophen Toxicity

Phase 1
(30 minutes to 24 hours)
- Anorexia
- Nausea
- Vomiting
- Pallor
- Diaphoresis
- Patient also may be symptomatic

Phase 2
(24-72 hours)
- Symptomatology from Phase 1 becomes less pronounced
- Right upper quadrant pain from liver damage
- Liver enzyme abnormalities
- PT and creatinine abnormalities

Phase 3
(72-96 hours)
- Sequelae of hepatic damage
- Jaundice
- Coagulopathy
- Encephalopathy
- Renal failure
- Cardiomyopathy
- Death

Phase 4
(4 days to 2 weeks)
- Resolution of symptoms and lab abnormalities, with complete resolution of liver damage

or

- Continued worsening of liver function and death

Used with permission. Adapted from: Linden C, Rumack BH. Acetdminophen overdose. WB Saunders Co. *Emerg Med Clin North Am* 1983;2:110.

Initial Treatment of Acute Acetaminophen Ingestion

Gastrointestinal Decontamination. The method of gastrointestinal decontamination is largely determined by the approximate timing and estimated amount of acetaminophen ingested, any suspected co-ingestions, and the patient's mental status. When acetaminophen is the only substance ingested, gastric lavage or ipecac administration may be beneficial for large ingestions in patients who present within two hours of ingestion. Gastric emptying procedures are less effective if more than two hours have elapsed because absorption is nearly complete by this time. Ipecac is contraindicated in the setting of altered mental status, or a co-ingestion that potentially can cause seizures or rapid deterioration of mental status. Protracted vomiting induced by ipecac also may cause difficulty with the subsequent administration of activated charcoal or acetaminophen antidote.

Activated Charcoal. Acetaminophen is adsorbed well by activated charcoal. Therefore, to bind any residual acetaminophen in the gastrointestinal tract, activated charcoal (1 gm/kg) should be administered. Repeat doses of activated charcoal have no significant effect on acetaminophen ingestion because of its rapid absorption and limited enterohepatic excretion. Similarly, concomitant use of cathartic agents (such as sorbitol, magnesium citrate, or magnesium sulfate) is common but probably does not affect acetaminophen absorption. Proper gastrointestinal decontamination may decrease the severity of the effects of the ingestion and potentially make an otherwise toxic acetaminophen ingestion nontoxic.

Antidote Therapy for Acetaminophen Toxicity

Once scientists determined that glutathione depletion and binding of toxic metabolites to sulfhydryl groups were important processes for acetaminophen toxicity, different amino acids containing sulfhydryl groups were tested as potential antidotes.[11,25] Glutathione was an immediate choice but was expensive and had poor penetration into cells. Although cysteamine and methionine were found to be effective antidotes, Nacetylcysteine (NAC) was more effective and had fewer adverse effects.[13,25,28]

Mechanism of Action. N-acetylcysteine is the antidote of choice for acetaminophen toxicity. Several different mechanisms of action have been postulated for the antidotal effect of NAC, including: 1) NAC is a glutathione precursor that repletes glutathione storage; 2) NAC reacts directly with NAPQI and prevents cellular damage; 3) NAC acts as a sulfur donor to enhance the non-toxic sulfation elimination of acetaminophen;[29] and 4) NAC has some non-specific cellular protective effects, which may be related to anti-oxidizing effects in the microcirculatory system.[23,26,30]

Administration. In the United States, only the oral form of NAC (MucomystR) is approved by the FDA. Oral NAC is slightly different from the intravenous form used in Canada and Great Britain in that it is sterile but not pyrogen-free. The loading dose of NAC is 140 mg/kg; the maintenance dose is 70 mg/kg every four hours for an additional 17 doses (72 hours total).[22] *(Please see Table 2.)*

The primary side effects of oral NAC are nausea and vomiting, which are due to the hyperosmolarity and disagreeable "rotten egg" odor of NAC. To minimize these gastrointestinal symptoms, NAC should be diluted to a 5% solution with a sweet beverage to make it more palatable. Alternatively, NAC may be administered through a nasogastric tube.[23] Occasionally, an antiemetic agent such as metoclopromide (0.1-1.0 mg/kg intravenously) may help to relieve GI side

Figure 2. Plasma or Serum Acetaminophen Concentration Vs. Time Postingestion

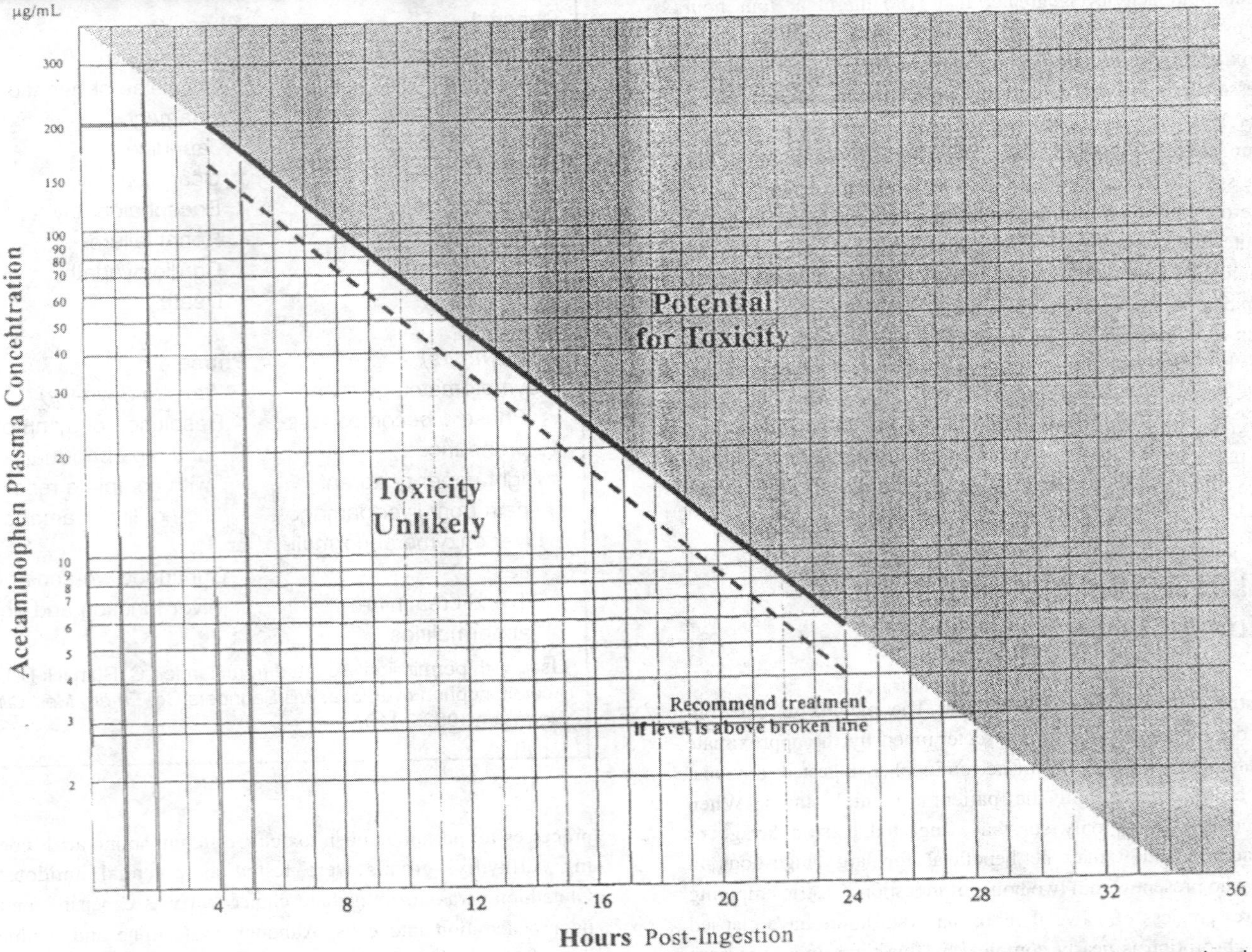

Cautions for use with this chart:

1. The time coordinates refer to time postingestion.
2. The graph relates only to plasma levels following a single acute overdose ingestion.
3. The broken line, which represents a 25% allowance below the solid line, is included to allow for possible errors in acetaminophen plasma assays and estimated time from ingestion of an overdose.

Used with permission: McNeil Consumer Products Co. Adapted from: Rumack BH, Matthews H. Acetaminophen poisoning. *Pediatrics* 1975;55:871-876.

effects. Anaphylactoid reactions are rare with oral NAC, although rash, angioedema, and bronchospasm have been reported with intravenous NAC.[26,31]

In special circumstances when NAC is indicated and oral administration is not possible (such as with corrosive ingestion; upper gastrointestinal bleeding, or severe, uncontrollable vomiting), NAC may be given intravenously using the same dosing regimen. The NAC preparation should be infused over 60 minutes using a micropore filter attachment to the intravenous tubing. It is advisable to obtain patient consent and to consult with the local poison control center. Oral NAC should be re-instituted as soon as possible.

Timing of NAC Administration. The optimal time for NAC administration is within the first eight hours following acetaminophen ingestion. During this period and regardless of the amount ingested and the acetaminophen level, NAC is uniformly effective. After the eight-hour postingestion period, the efficacy of NAC decreases progressively.[22] If a patient with acetaminophen overdose presents more than eight hours after ingestion, an acetaminophen level should be sent to the lab, and NAC should be started immediately for those with suspected significant ingestions while awaiting the result. Decisions regarding whether NAC therapy should be continued or discontinued depend on the result of the acetaminophen level. *(Please see Figure 3.)*

Efficacy of NAC. Results of the Multi-center Oral N-Acetylcysteine Trial suggest that NAC is beneficial up to 24 hours after ingestion. Other studies comparing a 48-hour oral protocol in the United States vs. a 20-hour intravenous NAC protocol in Britain found that both modalities were effective if started within 8-10 hours of ingestion.[22,32,33] However, a 72-hour oral NAC protocol appeared to be more effective for high-risk patients presenting late (i.e., 16-24 hours following ingestion).[22,32,33]

Table 2. Guidelines for N-Acetylcysteine Administration

1. Preparation
   a. N-acetylcysteine 20% solution. Sterile vials of 4 ml, 10 ml, and 30 mL
   b. N-acetylcysteine 10% solution. Sterile vials of 4 ml, 10 ml, and 30 mL
2. Dosage Schedule for NAC as an Antidote for Acetaminophen Overdose
   a. Loading dose: 140 mg/kg.
   b. Maintenance dose: 70 mg/kg administered four hours after the loading dose and every four hours thereafter over a period of 68 hours (i.e., 17 maintenance doses), If the patient vomits a loading or maintenance does within one hour of dosing, repeat the dose. Once toxic levels are confirmed, the whole 17-dose course must be administered.
3. Preparation of Antidote Solution
   The 20% solution of NAC is recommended for preparing the antidote for administration to the patient. NAC should be diluted with cola, orange juice, or water to achieve a 5% solution, which is approximately isotonic. The mixture should be consumed within one hour of preparation.

BODYWEIGHT (kg)	20% NAC (mL)	DILUENT (mL)	5%SOLUTION (total mL)
Loading dose			
100-110	75	225	300
90-99	70	210	280
80-89	65	195	260
70-79	55	165	220
60-69	50	150	200
50-59	45	120	160
40-49	35	105	140
30-39	30	90	120
Maintenance dose			
100-110	38	113	150
90-99	35	105	140
80-89	33	98	130
70-79	28	83	110
60-69	25	75	100
50-59	20	60	80
40-49	18	53	70
30-39	15	45	60

Used with permission. Adapted from: Ellenhorn MJ, Barceloux DG. *Acetaminophen (Paracetamol).* Medical Toxicology. P. 163 Elsevier Science Publishing.

Prior to the advent of an antidote, the mortality rate of patients at probable risk of hepatotoxicity (> 200 μg/ml at four hours) was reported between 5.3% and 24%.[5] The overall mortality rates reported with the 20-hour intravenous NAC protocol and the 72-hour oral protocol were 2% and 0.68%, respectively.[22,32] However, no fatalities were reported in any protocol in which NAC therapy was instituted within 10 hours of ingestion.

Delayed NAC Therapy. Recently, a randomized blinded trial from Britain evaluated the efficacy of late NAC therapy in patients with fulminant liver failure and Grade III or IV hepatic encephalopathy. The investigators demonstrated significant improvement in survival rate (48% vs 20%) with NAC therapy and decreased incidence of elevated intracranial pressure and systemic hypotension.[34]

In another study examining effects of NAC on the microcirculation of different organs in patients with either Grade III or IV hepatic coma and fulminant liver failure from different etiologies, the authors discovered that NAC increased cardiac index, decreased vascular resistance, and improved oxygen delivery and extraction.[30] Although this evidence appears to support NAG therapy for acetaminophen-toxic patients regardless of the time of ingestion, the optimal dose and duration of late NAC therapy remains undefined.

NAC and Activated Charcoal. Binding of NAG to activated charcoal has been demonstrated in both in-vitro and in-vivo studies.[35,36] Administration of 60 gm of activated charcoal with NAC decreases the bioavailability of NAC by approximately 20%.[36] However, the current evidence suggests that a small decrease in NAC does not alter its efficacy.[22,23] If multiple doses of activated charcoal are required because of co-ingestions, it would be prudent to separate NAC and activated charcoal dosing by 1-2 hours.

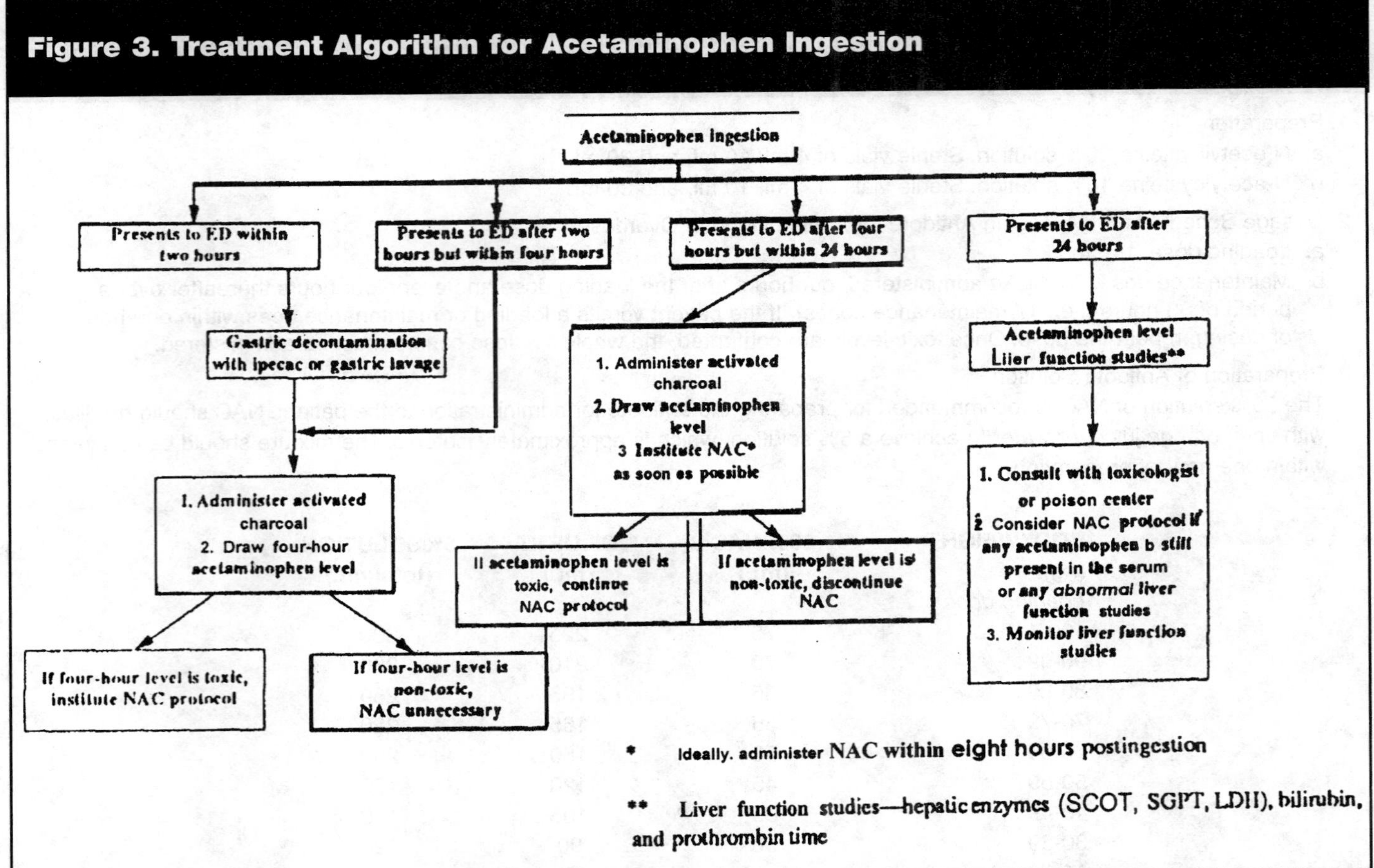

Figure 3. Treatment Algorithm for Acetaminophen Ingestion

Other Therapies for Acetaminophen Toxicity

Extracorporeal Removal. Hemodialysis removes only small amounts of acetaminophen. When charcoal hemoperfusion is used, acetaminophen clearance is better than hemodialysis although the amount of drug removal is quite variables.[23] However, charcoal hemoperfusion does not remove any toxic intermediates formed in the liver or the kidney and currently has no role in the management of acetaminophen toxicity.

Cimetidine. By virtue of its ability to inhibit cytochrome P450 enzymes, cimetidine was postulated to have a role in the treatment of acetaminophen toxicity. An initial animal study suggested a reduction of hepatotoxicity and mortality when cimetidine was combined with NAC therapy.[37] However, cimetidine has not been proved to affect the metabolism of acetaminophen in humans.[38] In one investigation the use of IV cimetidine as adjunctive therapy with NAC in patients presenting more than eight hours after acetaminophen ingestion did not affect the incidence of hepatotoxicity.[39] Currently, there is no established role for cimetidine in the treatment of acetaminophen toxicity.

Liver Transplant. Liver transplantation maybe the last viable option in patients with fulminant hepatic failure from acetaminophen. However, the shortcomings of this practice include deciding the optimal timing for referral and the relatively limited experience with liver transplantations for acetaminophen hepatic damage. In a study examining liver transplant for patients with fulminant hepatic failure, advanced hepatic coma, severe acidosis, markedly prolonged prothrombin time, and evidence of significant renal failure, four of six patients undergoing liver transplantation survived for one year, whereas only four of 23 patients with the same clinical indications but who did not receive liver transplantation survived for the same period of time.[40,41] In fact, the survival rate for patients with acetaminophen hepatic toxicity does not appear to be significantly different from the one-year survival rate observed in liver transplants for other causes.

Special Risk Groups in Acetaminophen Toxicity

Children. Compared with adults, children younger than 6 years of age have an increased sulfation capacity to metabolize acetaminophen and a higher turnover rate of glutathione. Consequently, it has been suggested that children may be less susceptible to acetaminophen toxicity, although current data exploring this concept are limited and inconclusive.[42-44] Another potential factor resulting in a relatively reduced degree of acetaminophen toxicity observed in children is that children are more likely to ingest a smaller toxic dosage compared with adults.

In contrast, several case reports have suggested that the therapeutic index of acetaminophen dosing in children may be small. In fact, simply doubling the therapeutic dose of acetaminophen for several days has resulted in cases of liver toxicity. Currently, children with suspected acetaminophen ingestion should not be treated differently than adults.

Alcoholism. Alcoholics may be at increased risk of acetaminophen toxicity due to increased P450-mixed function oxidase activity and decreased glutathione storage.[48,49] Theoretically, acute ethanol intake may have a protective role against acetaminophen toxicity by competing for P450 enzymes.[17] However, fulminant liver failure has been documented in alcoholic patients taking chronic therapeutic doses of acetaminophen.[49] In these cases, acetaminophen levels and liver biopsies were not performed, and consequently it is uncertain if these patients had progression of alcoholic liver disease or acetaminophen hepatotoxicity. Likewise, the oral NAC trial was unable to correlate the effects of alcohol with acetaminophen toxicity.[22]

Pregnancy. Acetaminophen can cross the placenta and cause fetal liver toxicity and fetal demise. In a study assessing acetaminophen toxicity and NAC therapy in 113 pregnant patients, there were no fetal malformations associated with either acetaminophen ingestion or NAC therapy. However, delay in NAC therapy was associated with fetal toxicity and spontaneous abortion. In a bovine placental model, NAC was shown to have minimal penetration into the fetal circulation, leading the authors to speculate that NAC is unlikely to be of significant benefit to the fetus once fetal toxicity has occurred. However, because NAC appears to be safe in pregnancy and because delaying therapy can lead to dire consequences, NAC should be started early in the pregnant patient with acetaminophen toxicity.

Multiple-Dose Ingestions. Currently, there are no standard guidelines for the evaluation and treatment of multiple dose acetaminophen ingestions occurring over a period of time. The acetaminophen nomogram is applicable for acute acetaminophen ingestion and may not be accurate for repeated or prolonged ingestions. However, because of the potentially beneficial action of NAC, therapy with this agent appears reasonable in this setting. NAC should be considered if the total dose of acetaminophen ingested over a 24-hour period exceeds 150 mg/kg, if the acetaminophen half-life is greater than four hours, or if liver enzymes are elevated. For these and other situations for which therapy is not well defined, physicians should contact toxicology experts or local or national poison control centers for assistance.

References

1. Acetaminophen. In: Bryson PD. *Comprehensive Review in Toxicology*, 2nd ed. Rockville, MD: Aspen Publishers; 1989:415426.
2. Acetaminophen (Paracetamo). In: *Ellenhorn MD, Barceloux DG. Medical Toxicology—Diagnosis and Treatment of Human Poisoning.* New York: Elsevier Science Publishers; 1991:156-164.
3. Litovitz TL, Holm KC, Bailey KM, et al. 1991 Annual report of the American Association of the Poison Control Centers national data collection system. *Am J Emerg Med* 1992;10: 452-489.
4. Henry J, Volans G. ABC of poisoning. Analgesics: II Paracetamol. *Br Med J* 1984;289:907.
5. Meredith TJ, Vale JA, Goulding R. The epidemiology of acute acetaminophen poisoning in England and Wales. *Arch Intern Med* 1981;141:397-400.
6. Janes J, Routledge PA. Recent developments in the management of paracetamol (acetaminophen) poisoning. *Drug Safety* 1992;7:170-177.
7. Prescott LF. Kinetics and metabolism of paracetamol and phenacetin. *Br J Clin Pharmacol* 1980;10:291S-298S.
8. Black M. Acetaminophen hepatotoxicity. *Gastroenterol* 1980;78:382-392.
9. Dahlin DC, Nelson SD. Synthesis, decomposition kinetics, and preliminary toxicological studies of pure N-acetyl-p-benzoquinoneimine, a proposed toxic metabolite of acetaminophen. *J Med Chem* 1992;25:885-886.
10. Corcoran GB, Mitchell JR, Vaishnav YN, et al. Evidence that acetaminophen and N-hydroxyacetaminophen form a common arylating intermediate, N-acetyl-p-benzoquinoneimine. *Mol Pharmacol* 1980;18:536-542.
11. Huggett A, Blair IA. The mechanism of Paracetamol-induced hepatotoxicity: Implication for therapy. *Human Toxicol* 983;2:399-405.
12. Mitchell JR, Jollow DJ, Potter WZ, et al: Acetaminophen-induced hepatic necrosis. Protective role of glutathione. *J Pharmacol Exp Ther* 1973;187:21 I-217.
13. Precott LF. Paracetamol overdose. Pharmacological considerations and clinical management. *Drugs* 1983;25: 290-314.
14. Mitchell JR, McMurtry RJ, Statham CN, et al. Molecilar basis for several drug-induced nephropathies. *Am J Med* 1977;62:518-526.
15. Clark R, Borirakehanyavat V. Davidson AR, a al. Hepatic damage and death from overdose of paracetamol. *Lancet* 1973;1:66-69.
16. Linden C, Rumack BH. Acetaminophen overdose. *Emerg Med Clin North Am* 1984;2:103-119.
17. Rumack BH, Koch G, Amara I. Acetaminophen overdose - 662 cases with evaluation of oral acetycysteine treatment. *Arch Intern Med* 1981;14 1:380-385.
18. Mann JM, Pierre-Louis M, Kragel PJ, et al. Cardiac consequences of massive acetaminophen overdose. *Am J Cardiol* 1989;63:1018-1021.
19. O'Grady JO, Williams R. Acute liver failure. *Bailliere's Clin Gastroenterol* 1989;3:75-89.
20. Prescott I.F,Roscoe R. Wright N. et al. Plasma-paracetamol half-life and hepatic necrosis in patients with paracetamol overdose. *Lancet* 1971;1:519-522.
21. Rumack BH, Matthew H. Acetaminophen poisoning and toxicity. *Pediatrics* 1975;55:871-876
22. Smilkstein M1, Knapp GL, Kulig KW. et al. Efficacy of oral Nacetylcysreine in the treatment of acetaminophen overdoses. Analysis of the national multicenter study (1976-1985). *N Engl J Med* 1988;319:15571562.
23. Goldfrank LR, Howland MA, Weisman KS, et al. Analgesics and over-the counter preparations. In: *Goldfrank's Toxicologic Emergencies.* 4th ed. Norwalk, Connecticut: Appleton S Lange; 1990:251-258.
24. Osterloh J. Limitation of acetaminophen assays. *J Toxicol Clin Toxicol* 1983;20:19.
25. Prescott LF. Newton RW, Swainson CP, et al. Successful

treatment of severe paracetamol overdose with cysteamine. *Lancet* 1974;1:588-592.

26. Flanagan RJ. The role of acetylcysteine in clinical toxicology. *Med Toxicol* 1987;2:93-104.
27. Vale JA. Meredith TJ, Goulding R. Treatment of acetaminophen poisoning, The use of oral methionine. *Arch Intern Med* 1981;14l:394-396.
28. Piperno E, Brrssenbruegge DA. Reversal of experimental paracetamol toxicosis with N-acetylcysteine. *Lancet* 1976; 2:738-739.
29. Lin JH, Levy G. Sulfate depletion after acetaminophen administration and replenishment by infusion of sodium sulfate or N-acetylcysteine in rats. *Biochem Pharmacol* 1981;19:2273-2725.
30. Harrison PM, Wendon JA, Gimson AES. Improvement of acetylcysteine of hemodynamics and oxygen transport in fulminant hepatic failure. *N Engl J Med* 1991;324: 1852-1957.
31. Mant TGK, Tempowski JH, Volans GN, et al. Adverse reactions to acetylcysteine and effects of overdose. *Br Med J* 1984;289:217-219.
32. Prescott LF, Illingworth RN, Critchley JAJH, et al. Intravenous NAcetylcysteine: The treatment of choice for paracetamol poisoning. *Br Med J* 1979;2:1097-1 100.
33. Smilkstein MJ, Bronstein AC, Linden C, et al. Acetaminophen overdose: A 48-hour intravenous N-acetylcysteine protocol. *Ann Emerg Med* 1991;20:1058-1063.
34. Keays R, Harrison PM, Wendon JA, et al. Intravenous acetylcysteine in paracetamol induced fulminant hepatic failure: a prospective controlled trial. *Br Med J* 1991;303: 1026-1029.
35. Ekins BR. Ford DC, Thompson MIB, et al. The effect of activated charcoal on Nacetylcysteine absorption in normal subject. *Am J Emerg Med* 1987;5:483-487.
36. Renzi RP, Donovan JW, Martin TG, et al. Concomitant use of activated charcoal and N-acetylcysteine. *Ann Emerg Med* 1985;14:568-572.
37. Speeg KV, Mitchell MC, Maldonado AL. Additive protection of cimetidine and Nacetylcysteine treatment against acetaminophen-induced hepatic necrosis in the rat. *J Pharmacol Exp Ther* 1985;234:550-554.
38. Slattery JT, McRorie TI, Reynolds R, et al. Lack of effect of cimetidine on acetaminophen disposition in humans. *Clin Pharmacol Ther* 1989;46:59 1-597.
39. Burkhart K, Janco N, Kulig K. et al. Cimetidine as adjunctive treatment for acetaminophen overdose (abstract). *Vet Hum Toxicol* 1989;31:337.
40. O'Grady JG, Alexander GJM, Hayllar KM, et al. Early indicators of prognosis in fulminant hepatic failure. *Gastroenterol* 1989;97:439-435.
41. O'Grady JIG, Wendon J, Potter D, et al. Liver transplantation after paracetamol overdose. *Br Med J* 1991;303:227-223.
42. Rumack BH. Acetaminophen overdose in young children: Treatment and effects of alcohol and other additional ingestant in 417 cases. *Am J Dis Child* 1984;138:428433.
43. Peterson RG, Rumack BH. Age as a variable in acetaminophen overdose. *Arch Intern Med* 1981;141: 390-393.
44. Penny A, Buchanan N. Paracetamol poisoning in children and hepatotoxicity. *Br J Clin Pharmacol* 1991;32:143-149.
45. Henretig F, Selbst SM. Forrest C, et al. Repeated acetaminophen overdosing. Causing hepatotoxicity in children. *Clin Ped* 1989;28:525-528.
46. Swetnam SM. Florman AL. Probable acetaminophen toxicity in an 18-month-old infant due to repeated overdosing. *Clin Ped* 1984;23:1114-1 OS.
47. Greene JW, Craft L, Ghishan F. Acetaminophen poisoning in infancy. *Am J Dis Child* 1983;13&:386-387.
48. Lauterburg BH, Velez ME. Glutathione deficiency in alcoholics: Risk factor for Paracetamol hepatotoxicity. *Gut* 1988;29:1153-1157.
49. Seeff LB, Cuccherini BA, Zimmerman HJ, et al. Acetaminophen hepatotoxicity in alcoholics: A therapeutic misadventure. *Ann Intern Med* 1986:104:399-404.
50. Riggs HS, Branstein AC, Kulig K, et al. Acute acetaminophen overdose during pregnancy. *Obstet Gynecol* 1989;74:247-253.
51. Seiden BS. Curry SC. Clark RF, et al. Transplacental transport of Nacetylcysteine in an ovine model. *Ann Emerg Med* 191;20:1069-1072.

Salicylate Toxicity

Stuart J. Spitalnic, MD
Richard Y. Wang, DO

Salicylate ingestion is one of the most common causes of drug exposure in the United States and is among the top 10 causes of fatal pediatric poisonings. In 1991, 23,000 cases were reported, the vast majority of which involved aspirin, either alone or as a combination preparation. Although these ingestions represent a large number of drug exposures, the true extent of salicylate ingestion is underestimated because many cases may be unrecognized or unreported. Clearly, the frequency with which patients with salicylate ingestion present to health care facilities requires that emergency physicians have a firm under standing of the significant toxicity of these agents.

Here, the authors review the pharmacology of salicylates and the clinical manifestations of salicylate toxicity, including the typical findings encountered in acute intentional overdoses as well as subtle, atypical manifestations that may occur in chronic salicylate exposures. Current management strategies are discussed so that physicians can institute immediate and appropriate therapy.

The Ubiquitous Nature of Salicylates

Salicylates are ubiquitous agents that can be found in hundreds of over-the-counter medications and in numerous prescription drugs. More than 10,000 tons of aspirin are consumed in the United States each year.[2] Salicylic acid and its derivatives are active ingredients in a wide variety of readily available topical preparations used for the treatment of pain, warts, and acne.[3] Pepto-Bismol, a commonly employed antidiarrheal agent, contains 131 mg of salicylate per tablespoon and is an easily overlooked source of systemically available salicylate.[4] Oil of wintergreen, which is used in home and industry as a candy flavoring and liniment, is a potent source of methyl salicylate. One teaspoon of the concentrated solution contains the equivalent of about 7 grams of aspirin or approximately 22 adult-strength aspirin tablets.[5]

The prevalence of aspirin-containing analgesic products in virtually every household makes these agents common sources of both accidental and suicidal ingestion. However, because many derivatives of salicylates besides aspirin are available, it may be helpful to express their potential for toxicity in more familiar terms. To assist with this determination, "aspirin conversion factors" or "aspirin equivalent doses" have been developed for a variety of preparations.[6] The usual adult dose of aspirin for fever control or analgesia is 325-650 mg orally every four hours; for children, the dose is 65 mg/kg/day in divided doses administered every 4-6 hours, to a maximum daily dose of 3.6 gm.[2] Toxicity is anticipated when the amount of aspirin ingested is greater than 150 mg/kg.[7] *(Please see Table 1.)*

Salicylate Pharmacokinetics

Absorption. Absorption characteristics of salicylates vary with the dose, formulation, and route of administration. The absorption of

Table 1. Assessment of the Severity of Salicylate Intoxication Based on Ingested Dose

Dose (mg/kg)	Estimated Severity
< 150	No toxic reaction expected
150-300	Mild-to-moderate toxic reaction
300-500	Serious toxic reaction
> 500	Potentially lethal

Adapted from: Temple AR. Acute and chronic effects of aspirin toxicity and their treatment. *Arch Intern Med* 1981;141:364-369.

topical salicylates is proportional to the body surface area involved, duration of exposure, concentration, and skin integrity. Acetylsalicylic acid (ASA) is hydrolyzed to salicylic acid in the stomach, is then quickly absorbed, and is responsible for the clinical effects of aspirin. Unlike liquid preparations, the time for complete absorption of pill forms can be delayed for many hours in acute overdoses, due to concretion formation or enteric coatings.[8,9] In addition, large doses of aspirin can induce pylorospasm that can further delay gastric emptying and prolong drug absorption.

Distribution. The distribution of salicylic acid in body tissues is based on pH-dependent passive transport and the degree of protein binding. Salicylic acid is considered to be highly protein-bound (80-90%). However, as serum salicylate levels increase, the fraction of drug bound to protein decreases.[10,11,12]

Therefore, at increased serum levels, a higher percentage of free (unbound) salicylic acid is available for distribution, a factor that can worsen systemic toxicity.[13] This effect may be particularly important in patients with hypoproteinemia, such as the elderly, those with liver or renal disease, or those suffering from inadequate nutrition. [14,15,16]

Salicylic acid is considered a weak acid and has a pKa of approximately 3.5. In acidemia, distribution is increased because the non-ionized fraction of drug increases and is readily permeable across cell membranes.[17] Conversely, alkalemia favors the ionized state and results in trapping the salicylate ion within body compartments. This principle forms the theoretical basis for both increased tissue toxicity at low pH and the use of urinary alkalization to enhance elimination.

The perinatal use of aspirin should be cautioned against because salicylic acid crosses the placenta and may affect fetal circulation through inhibition of prostaglandin synthesis.[18-19] Salicylic acid has been demonstrated to have a longer half-life in newborn infants than in their mothers, a fording that may be due to preferential shunting of blood away from the liver by the ductus venosus.[20]

Clearance. At therapeutic levels, the half-life of salicylic acid is 2-4 hours. As salicylate levels increase into the toxic range, the half-life can be greater than 18 hours.[21] Beginning at moderately toxic levels, the predominant metabolic pathways become saturated. As a result, in patients receiving chronic salicylate therapy, small dose increases may raise the serum level disproportionately into the toxic range.

Renal elimination of salicylic acid is the sum of the net effects of glomerular filtration, tubular secretion, and passive tubular resorption.[23] Salicylate clearance is strongly dependent on pH. For example, if urinary pH increases from 5 to 8, the amount of salicylate eliminated in the urine increases from 3% to more than 80%.[23,24]

Clinical Manifestations of Toxicity

Respiratory. Salicylates result in direct and indirect stimulation of respiration. Direct medullary stimulation results in a dose-dependent increase in both depth and rate of respiration that begins at a serum salicylate level of about 35 mg/dL.[25] High serum levels or prolonged exposure may result in central respiratory paralysis. The uncoupling of oxidative phosphorylation by salicylates causes an increased metabolism and production of CO_2 that may also increase respiratory drive [26]

A small percentage of patients with salicylate toxicity will develop noncardiogenic pulmonary edema. Although the precise mechanism is unclear, hypoxia or loss of cell membrane integrity from the inhibition of prostaglandin synthesis may play an important role. Risk factors for the development of pulmonary edema include metabolic acidosis, age greater than 30 years, history of smoking, chronic ingestion, neurologic symptoms, and high altitude exposures.[28]

Metabolic. Salicylic acid has several important metabolic effects that contribute to its toxicity. The net effects of salicylate as a metabolic poison are an increase in metabolic activity with the production of heat, generation of metabolic acidosis and ketoacidosis, and increased glucose utilization.

The uncoupling of oxidative phosphorylation results in impaired production of adenosine triphosphate and the liberation of heat. [26] This decreased efficiency of energy generation causes increased reliance on anaerobic metabolism for the maintenance of cellular activity. Additionally, salicylic acid interferes with several Kreb's Cycle enzymes.[29] These effects on cellular metabolism lead to the production of organic acids and metabolic acidosis.[30] Increased energy demand leads to the breakdown of fatty acids and the production of ketoses.[31]

A variety of glucose responses can occur with salicylate toxicity.[32] Hyperglycemia may result from salicylate-induced glucose-6-phosphatase activity and epinephrine release. Children and severely intoxicated adults are prone to hypoglycemia secondary to increased energy requirements, impaired gluconeogenesis, and depletion of glycogen stores. Increased cellular metabolic activity due to uncoupling of oxidative-phosphorylation may produce clinical hypoglycemia as intracellular glucose is depleted, even though serum levels may remain within normal limits.[33]

The combined influences of respiratory and metabolic abnormalities determine the acid-base status of the patient, which varies with the severity and duration of salicylate exposure. The initial increase in respiratory drive results in alkalemia. The pH may normalize as alkalosis from hyperventilation is countered by the developing metabolic acidosis. With severe toxicity, increased carbon dioxide production and retention can result from central nervous system (CNS) dysfunction and pulmonary damage. Increased carbon dioxide levels in conjunction with ongoing metabolic acidosis can lead to acidemia. When interpreting the pH on an arterial blood gas (ABG) analysis, clinicians must consider both the metabolic and respiratory contributions. For example, a normal pH in a hyperventilating patient should be considered a worrisome sign.

Fluid and Electrolytes. Patients with salicylate toxicity demonstrate varying degrees of dehydration secondary to increased gastrointestinal and insensible fluid losses.[35] Salicylate-toxic patients develop hyperpnea, hyperthermia, and vomiting. Dehydration decreases renal clearance of salicylate and organic acids and can prolong and worsen toxicity.

The primary respiratory alkalosis characteristic of early salicylate toxicity contributes to hypokalemia and hypocalcemia. The change in pH causes intracellular movement of potassium and calcium ions; the latter may manifest as tetany.[36] Renal compensation for alkalosis produces an increase in the excretion of bicarbonate with a concurrent loss of potassium.

Patients who either have chronic salicylate intoxication or those who are at the extremes of age are more likely to develop profound electrolyte derangements than are previously healthy adults with acute ingestions.[37,38]

Central Nervous System. Tinnitus is an early manifestation of neurotoxicity from increasing salicylate levels. Before the wide availability of salicylate levels, physicians used the presence of tinnitus to guide aspirin therapy of diseases such as rheumatic fever and gout.[39]

Some of the more significant signs and symptoms of CNS toxicity include nausea, vomiting, hyperpnea, and lethargy.[40] With increasing severity, these findings can progress to disorientation, seizures, cerebral edema, hyperthermia, coma, and death.

The CNS effects of salicylates are proportional to the amount of drug bound to the CNS tissue.[41] Acidemia worsens CNS toxicity due to increased distribution of the drug across the blood brain-barrier[13] Because tissue levels may be sustained within the CNS compartment after the start of alkalization therapy, a more aggressive therapeutic approach is warranted in the presence of neurologic symptoms.

Gastrointestinal (GI). Nausea and vomiting induced by salicylates occur from the combined effects of local GI tract irritation and central stimulation of the medullary chemoreceptor trigger zone.[42] Other GI effects induce gastritis, exacerbation of peptic ulcer disease, and gastric ulceration. Painless GI bleeding can occur with anti-inflammatory doses of salicylates. Adults using salicylates regularly will lose approximately 3-8 mL of blood per day into the GI tract (compared with normal GI loss of 0.6 mL/day).[43] When large doses of aspirin are ingested, pylorospasm and decreased GI motility also can occur.

Hepatic. Liver injury from acute salicylate toxicity is rare, however dose-dependent hepatitis may develop during salicylate therapy for connective tissue disorders.[44,45] Although hepatic dysfunction can occur at any salicylate level, the incidence increases when levels are greater than 25 mg/dL. The majority of patients with salicylate-induced hepatitis-will only have elevated aminotransferases. Some patients develop more prominent signs and symptoms of liver disease including hepatomegaly, hyperbilirubinemia, and prothrombin time prolongation. Salicylic acid also can promote bleeding by inhibiting either vitamin K-dependent enzymes or by the formation of thromboxane A_2.

Table 2. Clinical Manifestations of Salicylate Toxicity

Metabolic	**CNS**
Hyperthermia	Tinnitus
Hyperpnea	Decreased hearing
Anion gap elevation	Lethargy
Metabolic acidosis	Cerebral edema
Ketosis	Convulsions
Altered glucose metabolism	Coma
Dehydration	**Coagulation**
Respiratory	Factor inhibition
Hyperpnea	Platelet dysfunction
Tachypnea	**Gastrointestinal**
Noncardiogenic pulmonary edema	Nausea
Respiratory alkalosis	Vomiting
Hepatic	Gastritis
Elevated liver enzymes	GI bleeding
Hepatitis	Decreased GI motility
	Pylorospasm

Adapted from: Goldfrank LR, Bresnitz EA. Hartnett L. Salicylates. In: Goldfrank LR, ed. *Goldfrank's Toxicologic Emergencies*. East Norwalk, CT: Appleton & Lange;1990:261-270.

Clinical Assessment

Initial Evaluation. The purpose of the initial patient encounter is not only to decide if the patient is symptomatic from the acute ingestion but also to obtain information that may affect immediate and subsequent management. Key data to obtain include the type of salicylate involved, the amount ingested, the approximate time of ingestion, the chronicity of ingestion, potential co-ingestants, and the presence of any complicating medical conditions such as cardiac or renal disease. The presence of renal disease in the salicylate-intoxicated patient should prompt early consultation with the nephrologist because the capability for aggressive fluid management and urinary alkalization therapy are limited.

Unstable patients require immediate stabilization of airway, breathing, and circulatory status. Respiratory distress from non-cardiogenic pulmonary edema should be managed with early intubation, high-flow oxygen, and positive-end expiratory pressure (PEEP). Adequate ventilation must be ensured because increasing pCO_2 levels and resulting respiratory acidosis increase toxicity.

A fluid bolus with crystalloid should be administered to all patients with hypotension and tachycardia. Patients who are hypotensive and bradycardic should be evaluated for associated medical conditions (e.g., underlying cardiac disease) and other types of ingestions (e.g., beta-blocker ingestion) before attributing the clinical findings to salicylates alone.

Patients with altered mental status and suspected salicylate or other drug ingestion should receive intravenous dextrose, thiamine, and naloxone as indicated. Dextrose administration should be considered even for patients who are euglycemic because CSF glucose may be abnormally low.[33]

Clinical Evaluation. Patients symptomatic from a salicylate ingestion should not have therapy withheld because of pending serum levels. Salicylism is a diagnosis that can be made at the bedside with a few readily available laboratory studies. The patient should be questioned for the presence of tinnitus, hearing impair-

Table 3. Characteristics of Patients with Acute or Chronic Salicylism

	Acute	Chronic
Age	Young	Older
Etiology	Overdose (mixed) intentional	Iatrogenic (may have other medications)
Diagnosis	Usually obvious	Often unrecognized
Other disease states	None	Underlying disorder(s)
Suicidal	Yes	No
Clinical differences		Pulmonary edema CNS abnormalities
Serum concentrations	Significant elevation	Intermediate elevation
Mortality	Rare	25% rate

Modified from: Goldfrank LR, Bresnitz EA. Harmett L. Salicylates. In: Goldfrank LR, ed. *Goldfrank's Toxicologic Emergencies.* East Norwalk, CT: Appleton & Lange;1990:261-270.

ment, and gastrointestinal symptoms. The vital signs may reflect salicylate toxicity by the presence of tachypnea, tachycardia, or an elevated temperature. Tachypnea or hyperpnea also can result from central stimulation of the respiratory drive, or occasionally, from pulmonary edema. However, salicylate-induced hyperventilation may cause an increased tidal volume and a normal respiratory rate.[25] The presence of the above findings, along with a history of salicylate ingestion, allows the clinician to make a bedside diagnosis of toxicity. In order to complete the diagnosis, short of obtaining a salicylate level, a urine analysis and ABG analysis are required. *(Please see Figure 1.)*

Recognizing Chronic Toxicity. The diagnosis of chronic salicylate toxicity is often delayed by lack of clinical suspicion. Abnormalities consistent with salicylate toxicity, such as hearing loss, mental status changes, or metabolic derangements may be attributed to age or other disease processes and not to the drug itself. In a review of adults admitted with a delayed diagnosis of salicylate intoxication, 30% were chronically intoxicated.[38] The mortality rate and mean age for this group were significantly greater than for patients admitted with acute salicylate exposure.

The elderly are particularly at high risk for the development of chronic salicylate toxicity because of decreasing renal function and a tendency for dehydration from poor nutrition.

In addition, neurologic and pulmonary manifestations are more common in chronically intoxicated patients than in patients with acute salicylate overdose. *(See Table 3.)* In fact, therapy for chronic salicylate toxicity is based more on clinical signs and symptoms than on serum levels.

Use of the Laboratory

Bedside Testing. Qualitative determination for the presence of salicylates can be performed rapidly in the emergency department (ED) by combining 1.0 mL of the patient's urine with a few drops of 10% ferric chloride.[6] If salicylates arc present, the solution will turn a brown-purple color.

The ferric chloride test is useful when evaluating a patient with an unknown overdose and metabolic acidosis when the salicylate level is not readily available. A positive urine ferric chloride test necessitates obtaining a quantitative serum salicylate level because even the ingestion of one aspirin tablet can result in a positive test. The urine should also be evaluated for pH level and the presence of ketones. The pH level will guide alkalization therapy.

Arterial Blood Gases. ABG should be evaluated for the presence of a mixed acid-base disturbance.[38] Early in salicylic acid toxicity, a primary respiratory alkalosis is observed. As toxicity continues, concomitant primary metabolic acidosis develops due to tie production of lactic acid, metabolites, and other organic acids. In severe and late toxicity, primary metabolic and respiratory acidosis is observed. Depression of respiratory drive from either direct CNS toxicity or cerebral edema accounts for the respiratory acidosis. Children, who have limited respiratory reserves, tend to pass quickly through the hyperventilation phase and may present with an early metabolic acidosis. In mixed overdoses, the expected sequence of acid-base events may not be observed because CNS depressants (i.e., sedative-hypnotics, opioids) may blunt the respiratory response.[49] Based on the ABG findings, the urinalysis, history, and physical exam, therapy should be initiated without waiting for other laboratory studies.

Salicylate Levels. Initial and serial salicylate levels are important in the evaluation of the salicylate-intoxicated patient, although the absolute level should not detract from the importance of careful and repeated clinical evaluation. An abnormally high salicylate level or increasing serial levels should encourage aggressive treatment strategies, as should significant clinical manifestations in patients with moderate levels.[38] In general, salicylate levels less than 30 mg/dL are considered therapeutic, whereas those greater than 100mg/dL are considered markedly elevated.[50]

The Done nomogram was formulated in 1960 to assist clinicians in predicting the severity of salicylate intoxication based on a serum level and a known time of ingestion. However, there are several important limitations to its clinical applicability. First, the original nomogram was developed from pediatric patients with acute, non-mixed ingestion of plain aspirin. This means that the nomogram cannot be used with chronic intoxications and preparations that are either liquid or enteric-coated. Second, the pH of these patients was approximately 7.4. At a lower pH and with the same serum level, drug distribution is increased and clinical illness is more severe. This factor is not accounted for in the nomogram. Third, the categories of clinical illness that were established are not consistent with the current understanding of salicylate toxicity. Altered mental status, hyperthermia, and coagulopathy are considered as only mild to moderate manifestations of salicylate toxicity by the nomogram whereas,

Figure 1. Treatment Algorithm for Salicylate Ingestion

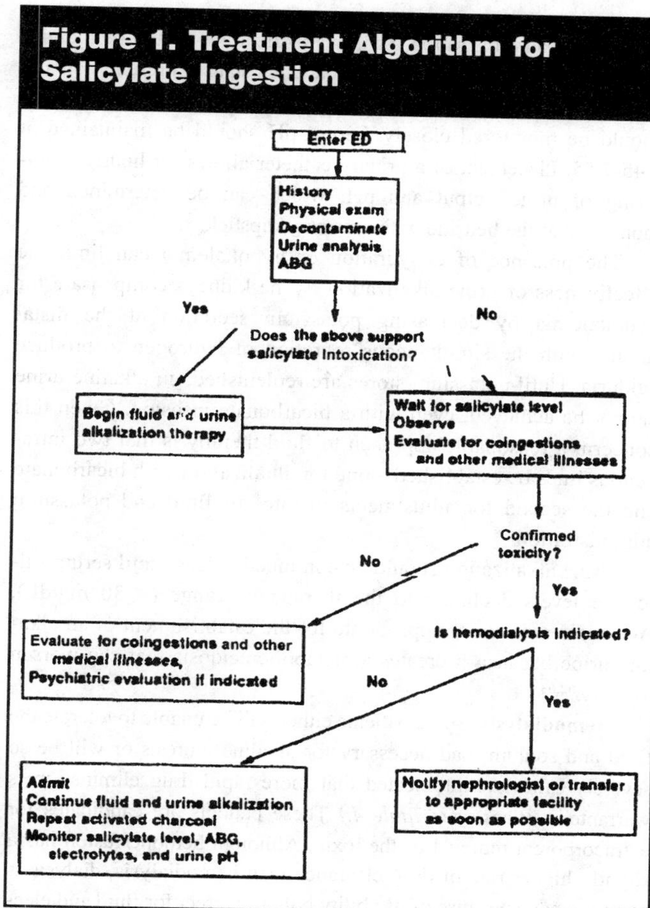

Figure 2. Protocol for Urine Alkalization

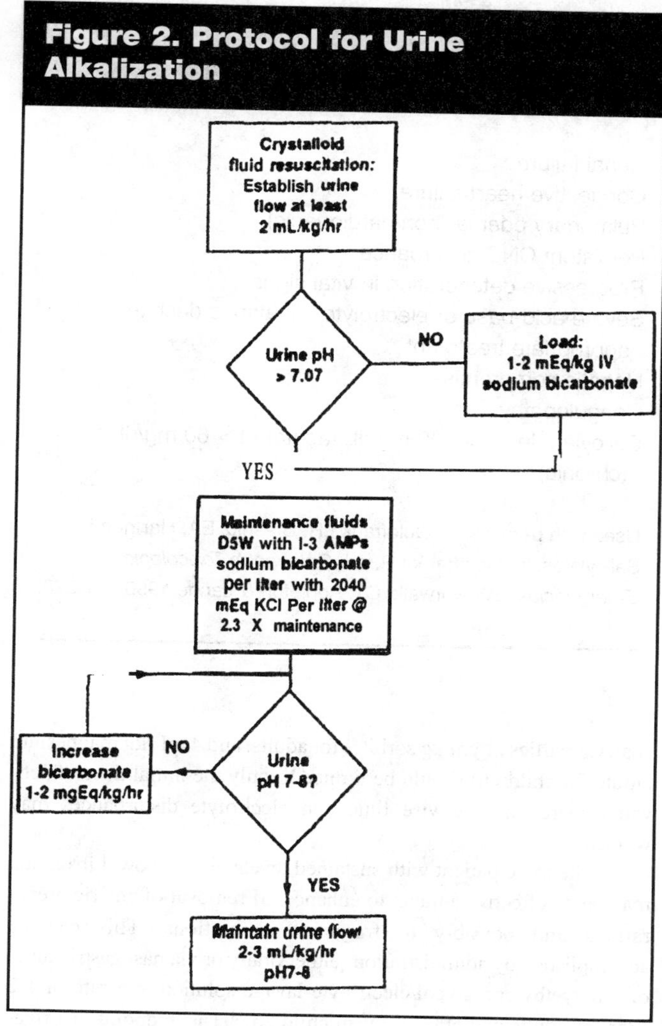

by current standards, these complications are considered to be severe.[52,53] Finally, inappropriate application of the nomogram can result in a misleading assessment of the severity of the poisoning. In fact, salicylate overdoses can be properly managed without ever referring to the nomogram.

Additional Studies. Other useful laboratory studies that should be obtained include electrolytes, renal function studies (blood urea nitrogen and creatinine), serum glucose level, as well as acetaminophen and other drug levels as indicated. Acetaminophen levels are particularly important because patients may use the word "aspirin" to refer to any number of over-the-counter analgesics, the true composition of which may be indeterminate from the history alone. Liver function studies and coagulation studies (e.g., prothrombin time and partial thromboplastin time) should be obtained in patients who are admitted or in whom hepatic involvement is considered. Patients with confirmed salicylate toxicity should have serum levels, ABG analysis, and electrolytes checked simultaneously every 2-4 hours (depending on the severity of the intoxication) in order to monitor the effectiveness of therapy and to detect on-going absorption.

Emergency Management of Salicylate Toxicity

Gastrointestinal Decontamination. The timing of GI decontamination in salicylate ingestion is important and should be performed in all overdose patients who present within one hour from the time of ingestion. Gastric emptying also may be beneficial for those presenting up to four hours after salicylate exposure. Some authorities recommend performing gastric emptying in all symptomatic patients regardless of their time of ingestion.

The use of syrup of ipecac is limited to alert children evaluated within 1-2 hours post-ingestion. This agent is contraindicated in patients with altered mental status and in those who may deteriorate within a short period of time. In most situations, lavage with a large-bore orogastric tube is the procedure of choice for gastric evacuation. This technique is more efficient than ipecac for achieving gastric emptying, and the delay in administering oral agents (i.e., charcoal, antidotes) due to persistent emesis from ipecac is avoided. The formulation of the salicylate also may determine the method of GI decontamination. Nasogastric tube lavage is appropriate for patients presenting early after ingestion of oil of wintergreen.

Activated charcoal can limit further gut absorption by binding to available salicylate.[55] Repeated doses of charcoal can enhance salicylate elimination and shorten the serum half-life.[56,57] An initial dose of activated charcoal (1 gm/kg) should be administered to all patients with possible salicylate overdoses. Repeat doses of 0.5 gm/kg should be given every 2-4 hours (depending on severity of toxicity) to those with confirmed toxicity. Metoclopramide (0.1 mg/kg IV every 30 minutes to a maximum of 1-2 mg/kg/day, titrated to effect) can be administered to control vomiting in patients unable to tolerate char-

Table 4. Indications for Hemodialysis

Renal failure
Congestive heart failure
Pulmonary edema (non-cardiogenic)
Persistent CNS disturbance
Progressive deterioration in vital signs
Severe acid-base or electrolyte imbalance despite appropriate treatment
Hepatic compromise
Coagulqpathy
Salicylate level: > 100 mg/dL (acute) or > 60 mg/dL (chronic)

Used with permission: Goldfrank LR, Bresnitz EA, Hartnett L. Salicylates. In: Goldfrank LR, ed. *Goldfrank's Toxicologic Emergencies.* EW Norwalk, CT: Appleton & Lange;1990:261-270.

coal. Cathartics (1 gm/kg sorbitol for adults, and 4 mL/kg magnesium citrate for children) should be limited to only the initial dose of activated charcoal; otherwise fluid and electrolyte disturbances may worsen.

In the toxic patient with sustained levels, whole bowel irrigation may be an effective adjunct to enhance GI removal of enteric preparations and possibly to fragment concretions. This can be accomplished by administration (either orally or via nasogastric tube) of a polyethylene glycol/electrolyte lavage solution at a rate of 1-2 L/hr for adults and 500 mL/hr in children.[58] The endpoint of irrigation is when the rectal effluent is clear and salicylate levels arc declining. Because the bowel irrigation preparation is isotonic and isoosmotic, its use is not associated with any fluid or electrolyte shifts.[59,60] Although bicarbonate lavage has been suggested to solubilize salicylate concretions, this solution can enhance absorption and therefore is not recommended. If persistently high levels remain in the setting of significant clinical toxicity, upper GI endoscopy is warranted to identify and break up salicylate concretions and affect their removal.

The presence of either salicylate concretions or ingestion of enteric-coated preparations poses a significant problem to clinicians because of the prolonged time of absorption and duration of toxicity. Consider the possibility of one of these situations when salicylate levels arc not declining despite adequate standard treatment.

Urinary Alkalization. Patients who arc symptomatic from salicylate toxicity should be managed with urine alkalization. *(Please see Figure 2.)* Alkaline diuresis is highly effective in increasing the clearance of salicylic acid and is the mainstay of therapy. By increasing urinary pH to 7.5 with intravenous bicarbonate, urine reabsorption of salicylic acid is prevented. Bicarbonate therapy is also beneficial in correcting acidosis, thereby limiting CNS distribution of the drug. Patients should be fluid-resuscitated to maintain adequate urine output (at least 2 mL/kg/hr) in order to ensure adequate drug delivery to the kidneys and to reduce urine concentration of salicylate and limit passive reabsorption. Fluid management and bicarbonate administration for urine alkalization should be individualized and adjusted based on the patient's state at presentation and response to therapy. Serum electrolytes, ABG analysis, and urine pH should be monitored closely. Serum pH should be maintained at 7.45-7.55. Placement of a urinary catheter allows for hourly monitoring of urine output and pH, which can be determined and monitored at the bedside with a urinary dipstick.

The presence of dehydration or hypokalemia can limit the effectiveness of urine alkalization.[61] The kidneys compensate for hypokalemia by decreasing potassium secretion at the distal tubule, with the simultaneous secretion of hydrogen to produce aciduria. Until potassium stores are replenished, an alkaline urine cannot be achieved, even with a bicarbonate infusion. Given this concern, a reasonable approach to fluid therapy is that two intravenous lines be established—one for alkalization with bicarbonate and the second for adjustments in rates of fluid and potassium administration.

Urine alkalization should be continued at least until serum salicylate levels decline into the therapeutic range (< 30 mg/dL). Acetazolamide is not appropriate for the establishment of an alkaline urine because it creates a metabolic acidosis that can worsen toxicity.[62,63]

Hemodialysis. Some patients either will be unable to tolerate the fluid and sodium load necessary for alkaline diuresis or will be so severely salicylate-intoxicated that more rapid drug elimination is warranted. *(Please see Table 4.)* These patients are candidates for extracorporeal removal of the toxin. Although hemoperfusion has a slightly higher rate of drug clearance than hemodialysis, dialysis is recommended because of its ability both to correct for fluid and electrolyte disorders and to remove salicylates.[64] Peritoneal dialysis is only 10-25% as effective as hemoperfusion or hemodialysis and is not recommended.

The institution of hemodialysis in the chronically intoxicated patient is dependent more upon the clinical manifestations than on the salicylate level. Generally, a patient with a chronic salicylate level of 60 mg/dL should be considered for hemodialysis.

When unsure of the need for hemodialysis, consultation with the regional poison center may be helpful. Physicians responsible for hemodialysis should be notified as soon as possible because there may be a delay of several hours before dialysis actually can be started.

Patient Disposition

Medical clearance from the ED for an acute salicylate overdose can be accomplished by demonstrating a decreasing salicylate level in the therapeutic range in a mildly symptomatic patient. If the ingestion was a suicide attempt, ensure adequate psychiatric evaluation before discharge.

Patients who have an altered level of consciousness, pulmonary edema, or other significant medical disorders as well as those who require hemodialysis should be admitted to an intensive care unit. Patients without these complicating factors can be managed on a medical floor with close attention to the salicylate levels and the patient's clinical and metabolic status. If the patient may require hemodialysis at a later time and the institution cannot provide for the procedure, early transfer to an appropriate facility is recommended.

References

1. Litovitz TL, Holm KC, Bailey KM, et al. 1991 annual report of the American Association of Poison Control Centers National Data Collection System. *Am J Emerg Med* 1992;10: 452-505.
2. Insel PA. Analgesic-antipyretics and anti-inflammatory agents; drugs employed in the treatment of rheumatoid arthritis and gout. In: Goodman LS, Gilman A, eds. *The Pharmacological Basis of Therapeutics*. 8th ed. Elmsford: Pergamon Press. Inc.; 1990:638-681.
3. Leist ER, Banwell JC. Products containing aspirin. *N Engl J Med* 1974;291:710-712.
4. Sainsbury SJ. Fatal salicylate toxicity from bismuth subsalicylate. *West J Med* 1991;155:637-639.
5. Cauthen WL, Hester WH. Accidental ingestion of oil of winter green. *J Fam Pract* 1989;29:680-681.
6. Vandenberg SA, Rumack BH. Non-aspirin salicylates: conversion factors for estimating aspirin equivalency. *Vet Hum Toxicol* 1989;31:49-50.
7. Krause DS, Wolf BA, Shaw LM. Acute aspirin overdose: Mechanisms of toxicity. *Ther Drug Monit* 1992;14:441-445.
8. Bogacz K, Caldron P. Enteric-coated aspirin bezoar: Elevation of serum salicylate level by barium study. *Am] Med* 1987;83:783-786.
9. Wortzman DJ. Delayed absorption following enteric-coated aspirin overdose. *Am Emerg Med* 1987;16:434-436.
10. Wosilait WD. Theoretical analysis of the binding of salicylate by human serum albumin. *Euro J Clin Pharmacol* 1976;9:285-290.
11. Ekstrand R, et al. Concentration dependent plasma protein binding of salicylate in rheumatoid patients. *Clin Pharmacokinetics* 1979;4:137-143.
12. Alvan G, et al. High unbound fraction of salicylate in plasma during intoxication. *Br J Clin Pharmacol* 1981;11:625-626.
13. Posner JB, Plum F. Spinal fluid pH and neurologic symptoms in systemic acidosis. *N Engl J Med* 1967;227: 605-613.
14. Windorfer A. The influence of age on the activity of acetylsalicylic acid esterase and protein salicylate binding. *Eur J Clin Pharmacol* 1974;7:227231.
15. Wallace S, Brodie MJ. Decreased drug binding in serum from patients with chronic hepatic disease. *Eur J Clin Pharmacol* 1976;9:429-432.
16. Borga O. Protein binding of salicylates in uremic and normal plasma. *Clin Pharmacol Ther* 1976;20:464-475.
17. Hill JB. Experimental salicylate poisoning: observation of the effects of altering blood pH on tissue and plasma salicylate concentrations. *Pediatrics* 1971;47:658-665.
18. Berman W. Pharmacokinetics of inhibition of prostaglandin syn thesis in the perinatal period. *Semin Perinatol* 1980;4: 67-72.
19. Garrettson LK, Procknal JA, Levy G. Fetal acquisition and neonatal elimination of a large amount of salicylate. Study of a neonate whose mother regularly took therapeutic doses of aspirin during pregnancy. *Clin Pharmacol Ther* 1975;17: 98-103.
20. Green TP. Determination of drug disposition and effect in the fetus. *Ann Rev Pharmacol Tax* 1979;19:285-322.
21- Levy G. Pharmacokinetics of salicylate elimination in man. *J Pharm Sci* 1965;54:959-967.
22. Levy G, Tsuchiya T. Salicylate accumulation kinetics in man. *N Engl J Med* 1972;287:430-432.
23 MacPherson CR, et al. The excretion of salicylate. *Br J Pharmacol* 1955;10:484-489.
24. Smith PK. Studies on the pharmacology of salicylate. *J Pharmacol Exp Ther* 1946;87:237-255.
25. Temple AR. Acute and chronic effects of aspirin toxicity and their treatment. *Arch Intern Med* 1981;141:36.1-369.
26. Miyahara JT, Karlen R. Effect of salicylate on oxidative phosphorylation and respiration of mitochondrial fragments. *Biochem J* 1965;97:194-198.
27. Hmicek G, Skelton J, Miller W. Pulmonary edema and salicylate intoxication. *JAMA* 1974;230:866-867.
28. Walters JS, Woodying JH, Stelling CR. et al. Salicylate-induced pulmonary edema. *Radiology* 1983;146:289-293.
29. Kaplan EH, Kennedy J, Davis J. Effects of salicylate and other benzoates on oxidative enzymes of the tricarboxylic acid cycle in rat tissue homogenates. *Arch Biochem Biophys* 1954;51:47-6 1.
30. Schwartz R, Landry G. Organic acid excretion in oxidative intoxication. *J Pediatr* 1965;66:658-666.
31. Bartels PD. Lund-Jacobsen H. Blood lactate and ketone body concentration in salicylate intoxication. *Hum Toxicol* 1986; 5:363-366.
32. Done AK, Temple AR. Treatment of salicylate poisoning. *Modern Treat* 1971;8:528-551.
33. Thurston JH, Pollock PG. Warren SK, et al. Reduced brain glucose With normal plasma glucose in salicylate poisoning. *Clin Invest* 1970;49:2139-2145.
34. Hall AH, Rumack BH. Diagnosis and treatment of poisoning. In: Shoemaker WC, Aynes S. Grenvik A, et al, eds. *Textbook of Critical Care*. 2nd ed. Philadelphia: WB Saunders Co.; 1989:1170-1181.
35. Temple AR, George DJ, Dow AK, et al. Salicylate poisoning complicated by fluid retention. *Clin Toxicol* 1976;9:6 t-68.
36. Fox GN. Hypocalcemia complicating bicarbonate therapy for salicylate poisoning. *West J Med* 1984;141:108-109.
37. Bailey RB, Jones SJ. Chronic Salicylate Intoxication. *JAGS* 1989;37:556-561.
38. Anderson RJ, Potts DE, Gabow PA, et al. Unrecognized adult salicylate intoxication. *Ann lntern Med* 1976;85: 745-748.
39. Halla JT. Atchison SL, Hardin JG. Symptomatic salicylate ototoxicity: a useful indicator of serum salicylate concentration? *Ann Rhea Dis* 1991;50:682-684.
40. Done AK. Aspirin overdosage: Incidence, diagnosis and man agement. *Pediatrics* 1978;62(Supplement):890-897.
41. Reed JR, Palmisano PA. Central nervous system salicylate. *Clin Toxicol* 1975;8:623-631.
42. Smith PK. The pharmacology of salicylates and related com pounds. *Am NY Acad Sci* 1960;86:36-63.
43. Leonards JR, Levy G. Gastrointestinal blood loss during prolonged aspirin administration. *N Engl] Med* 1973;289: 1020-1022.

44. Hamdan JA, Manasra K, Ahmed M. Salicylate-induced hepatitis in rheumatic fever. *Am J Dis Child* 1985; 139: 453-455.
45. Schaller JG. Chronic salicylate administration in juvenile rheumatoid arthritis: aspirin "hepatitis" and its clinical significance. *Pediatrics* 1978;62:916-925.
46. Broder JN. The ferric chloride screening test. *Ann Emerg Med* 1987;16:1188. Letter.
47. Gandreault P, Temple AR, Lovejoy FH. The relative severity of acute vs. chronic salicylate poisoning in children: A clinical comparison. *Pediatrics* 1982;70:566-569.
48. Winters RW, White JS, Hughes MC, et al. Disturbances of acid-base equilibrium in salicylate intoxication. *Pediatrics* 1959;23:260-285.
49. Gabow PA, Anderson RJ, et al. Acid base disturbance in the salicylate intoxicated adult. *Arch Intern Med* 1978;138:1481-1484.
50. Koch-Weser J. Serum drug concentrations as therapeutic guides. *N Engl J Med* 1972;287-231.
51. Done AK. Salicylate intoxication: significance of measurements of salicylate in blood in case of acute ingestion. *Pediatrics* 1960;26:800-807.
52. Goldfrank LR, Bresnitz EA. Hartnett L. Salicylates. In: Goldfrank LR, ed. *Goldfrank's Toxicologic Emergencies.* East Norwalk, CT: Appleton & Lange;1990:261-270
53. Proudfoot AT. Salicylates and salicylamide. In: Haddad LM, ed. *Clinical Management of Poisoning and Drug Overdose.* 2nd edition. Philadelphia: W.B. Saunders; 1990:909-920.
54. Matthew H. Gastric aspiration and lavage in acute poisoning. *Br Med J* 1966;1:1333-1337.
55. Levy G, Tsuchiya T. Effect of activated charcoal on aspirin absorption in man. *Clin Pharmacol Ther* 1972;13:317-322.
56. Kirshenbaum LA, Mathews SC, Sitar DS, et al. Does multipledose charcoal therapy enhance salicylate excretion? *Arch Intern Med* 1990;150:1281-1283.
57. Fillippone GA, Fish SS, Lacouture PG. et al. Reversible adsorption (desorption) of aspirin from activated charcoal. *Arch Intern Med* 1987;147:1390-1392.
58. Tenebein M. Whole bowel irrigation as a gastrointestinal decontamination procedure after acute poisoning. *Med Toxicol* 1988;3:7784
59. Brady CE, Dipalma JA, Morawaski SG, et al. Urinary excretion of polyethylene glycol 3350 and sulfate after gut lavage with a polyethylene glycol electrolyte lavage solution. *Gastroenterol* 1986;90:1914-1918.
60. DiPiro JT, Michael KA, Clark BA, et al. Absorption of polyethylene glycol after administration of a PEG electrolyte lavage solution. *Clin Pharm* 1986;5:153-155.
61. Tannen RL. Effect of potassium on renal acidification and acid base homeostasis. *Semin Nephrol* 1987;7:263-273.
62. Feuerstein RC, Finberg L, Fleishman BS. The use of acetazolamide in the therapy of salicylate poisoning. *Pediatrics* 1960;25:215-227
63. Heller I, Hal J, Cohen S, et al. Significant metabolic acidosis induced by acetazolamide: not a rare complication. *Arch Intern Med* 1985;145:1815-1817.
64. Jacobsen D, Wiik-Larsen E, Bredesen JE. Haemodialysis or haemoperfusion in severe salicylate poisoning? *Hum Toxicol* 1988;7:161-163.

Chemical Injuries to the Skin

Charles Stewart, MD, FACEP

Few dermatological emergencies are as unpredictable and destructive as chemical injuries to the .skin. There are more than 25,000 chemicals that can burn the skin or mucous membranes.[1,2] Most of these substances are acids and alkalies used as row materials and as cleaning, curing, extracting, and preserving agents for manufactured products.[3] Not surprisingly, the majority of chemical skin burns seen in the emergency department (ED) occur in the workplace, and in most cases, the agent producing the burn can be identified. In the domestic environment, skin burns associated with household chemicals are most commonly caused by contact with phenols (deodorants, sanitizers, disinfectants), sulfuric acid (toilet bowl cleaners), sodium hypochlorite (bleaches), and lye (drain cleaners and paint removers).

Fortunately, most chemical burns are minor and involve less than 15% of the body surface area.[4] Generally speaking, the amount of tissue destruction is determined by the size and anatomical location of the affected surface, the concentration of the agent, the duration of exposure, and the specific characteristics of the chemical. With some chemicals, the injury may appear to be deceptively mild on first appraisal. Over the ensuing 2436 hours, however, the damage may progress to produce extensive necrosis of the skin and underlying structures and, in some cases, can cause life-threatening systemic effects.

This chapter reviews the most common causes of chemical burns of the skin and outlines specific therapeutic strategies.

Etiology and Natural History of Chemical Burns

Unlike thermal burns, chemical injuries are often insidious, in large part because the burning process will continue until the substance is inactivated, removed from the area, or exhausts its capacity to cause tissue destruction. Consequently, if removal of the toxic substance is delayed, the severity of the burn may be markedly increased. Moreover, chemical burns are known for their slow course of healing.

Alkali agents commonly associated with chemical burns include sodium, ammonium, lithium, potassium, barium, and calcium hydroxides used in industrial processes. In contrast, the most commonly used industrial acids include sulfuric, nitric, acetic, hydrochloric, hydrofluoric, formic, picric, tungstic, tannic, sulfosalicylic, trichloroacetic, and cresylic. Chromic and hydrofluoric acids are widely used in the microinstrument and microelectronics industries, whereas sulfuric and nitric acid are used in the steel industry for casting iron and steel and removing slag wastes.[1-4]

Although any of these caustic agents can cause a skin burn, lye and sulfuric acid account for the majority of chemical injuries.[2,3,5-8] In certain high-tech industries, hydrofluoric acid (HF) is the most common causative agent. in military training areas, the most common agent encountered is white phosphorus, which is rarely seen in civilian life.[2,8]

There also are some unusual causes of chemical burns, including self-inflating automotive airbags, which contain sodium azide. When ignited, this chemical breaks down to sodium hydroxide, which can cause facial and hand burns if the airbag breaks. Patients should also be evaluated for the presence of corneal abrasions.[9-11] Rescuers can also sustain burns from released chemicals.

Alkali Burns. Alkali burns are usually caused by sodium or potassium hydroxide, i.e., the "lyes." These burns damage tissue by increasing the number of hydroxyl ions beyond the limits of protein stability. This is rapidly followed by dissolution of protein and collagen and results in the formation of gel-like alkaline proteinates.[1-3] Although strong alkaline corrosives are most often found in drain cleaners and paint removers, alkali burns can also result from calcium oxide contained in lime or cement.

Alkali burns of the eye merit special consideration, because they produce some of the most severe chemically mediated eye injuries encountered in emergency practice. When a strong alkali is instilled or spilled into the eye, the epithelium is destroyed and allows the alkali access to the corneal stroma. This produces immediate opacification of the cornea and coagulation of scleral and corneal proteins. The pH of the anterior chamber rises within 2-3 minutes, causing damage to the iris, lens, and ciliary body. This can lead to an irreversible loss of vision within three minutes of exposure.[1,7]

Among the common alkalies, ammonium hydroxide has the fastest rate of skin penetration, followed by sodium hydroxide, potassium hydroxide, lithium hydroxide, strontium hydroxide, barium hydroxide, tetraethylammonium hydroxide, calcium hydroxide, and magnesium hydroxide.[9] Oven cleaners often have very high concentrations of sodium hydroxide.

Acid Burns. In general, acid burns are not as serious as alkali burns, but they are more fulminant and produce more immediate destruction. Acids are water-soluble and easily penetrate into the subcutaneous tissues. Tissues coagulate soon after contact, and a tough, leathery eschar forms, limiting further spread of the agents. Some acids, such as fuming nitric or sulfuric, act as desiccants and create an even more impenetrable eschar.[4,12] Burns caused by different acids can produce different skin colors.

General Principles of Chemical Burn Management

Assessment of potential toxicity associated with chemical exposure requires a detailed history. Whenever possible, the physician should attempt to identify all toxic ingredients that may be involved in the burn, as well as concentrations. The time elapsed since the exposure should be documented. Although irrigation will be the mainstay of therapy for most chemical burns, specific antidotes are available for some chemical agents. *(Please see Table 1)*

In some chemical burns, systemic involvement can be severe and require attention to the ABCs. In particular, resuscitation may be needed in patients who experience exacerbations in their reactive airway disease due to associated inhalation of toxic substances as well as in those patients who experience anaphylactic reactions to the substance. In these individuals, a treatment regimen consisting of epinephrine, diphenhydramine, and corticosteroids may be used.

Table 1. Summary of Treatment Measures for Specific Chemical Burns

IRRIGATION WITH WATER	
Chromic acid	Cantharides
Lye and alkalies	Potassium hydroxide
Sodium hydroxide	Ammonium hydroxide
Barium hydroxide	Calcium hydroxide
Sulfosalicylic acid	Acetic acid
Cresylic acid	Potassium permanganate
Dimethyl sulfoxide (DMSO)	Sodium hypochlorites
Phenol	Hydrofluoric acid
Dichromate salts	Tungstic acid
Picric acid	Trichloroacetic acid
Formic acid	Gasoline
CALCIUM SALTS IRRIGATION OR INJECTION	
Hydrofluoric acid	
COVER BURN WITH OIL	
Sodium metal	Lithium metal
Potassium metal	
COVER BURN WITH WATER	
Phosphorus metal	
SPECIAL MEASURES FOR CERTAIN CHEMICALS	
Sodium, potassium, and lithium metals: pieces must be excised	
Phenol: polyethylene glycol wipes	
White phosphorus: copper sulfate irrigation	
Alkyl mercury agents: debride and remove vesicle fluid	
Mustard agents: detoxify with bleach	

The need for pain control cannot be overemphasized. Many chemical burns are extremely painful, especially alkali burns to the eye, and individuals who sustain such injuries require aggressive measures for analgesia, including morphine and meperidine therapy. Finally, the patient with chemical burns also should be carefully monitored in order to detect signs of respiratory distress, renal failure (dichromate), hepatic necrosis (chromic, formic, picric, and phosphorus exposure), as well as systemic metabolic complications, including hypocalcemia with oxacolic and hydrofluoric acid burns and methemoglobinia associated with sodium and potassium nitrate.

In most cases, however, the cornerstone of chemical burn management is removal of the noxious substance. This is initiated by removal of garments soaked with the chemical, followed by irrigation of the area with copious amounts of water. The patient's clothing and protective garments must be removed to prevent both further injury to the patient as well as possible injury to the medical team. *(Please see Table 2.)*

Irrigation of the burn with large volumes of water under low pressure dilutes the toxic agent and washes it from the tissues, i.e., "The solution to chemical pollution is dilution." Irrigation should be performed with low pressure and high volumes in order to prevent additional contamination of other body surfaces. In order to further limit tissue damage and reduce penetration of the offending agent, all particulate matter should be debrided from the wound before or during the irrigation process.

In chemical injuries to the cornea, irrigation with normal saline is the treatment of choice. irrigation should continue, and pH paper should be employed to ensure attainment of physiological pH. Topical alcaine or tetracaine is mandatory for initial pain control, and many patients will require systemic analgesics. Cycloplegics, mydriatics, or antibiotics should be considered in consultation with an ophthalmologist.

Severity of chemical injuries is directly proportional to the length of time that the substance remains on the skin. If removal of the substance is delayed, tissue damage is greater. Studies of acid and alkali burns confirm the importance of early irrigation.[13] When irrigation is initiated within one minute after contact, the burn is substantially less severe as compared to irrigation that is delayed for three minutes.[14] When irrigation is delayed for 15 minutes in acid burns, tissue pH is not altered by lavage. Likewise, when irrigation is delayed for one hour in alkali burns, the tissue pH remains in the alkaline range for several hours.[13,15]

Clinically relevant experimental studies show that irrigation of tissues for at least one hour is needed to reverse tissue pH changes due to alkali chemical injuries? Some studies have even suggested that severe alkali burns should be irrigated for 8-24 hours. A rational regimen using extended hydrotherapy includes two hours of shower alternated with two hours of rest? If an alkali burn has a soapy feeling or if the tissue pH has not returned to normal, irrigation must be continued. Burns of the eye may be treated with continuous irrigation through a Morgan irrigating contact lens. An alternative is a small-bore soft catheter fixed in the palpebral sulcus or the IV tubing held by an attendant.

Finally, neutralization of the chemical with a weak acid or base opposite is not recommended for at least two reasons: 1) Irrigation should not be delayed while waiting for a specific antidote, i.e., immediate irrigation provides the best removal of the agent; and 2) neutralization may produce an exothermic reaction, which can produce further tissue damage.[17]

Lime and Cement Burns

In the presence of water, lime (calcium oxide) is converted to calcium hydroxide, a strong alkali with a pH as high as 12.[2,18] Interestingly, perspiration and skin moisture are sufficient to initiate this reaction. Portland cement, for example, consists of lime, magnesium, metal oxides, and sand. Consequently, Portland cement has the potential to produce as much tissue damage as lime. In premixed cement, the reaction with water is already in progress, which explains why wet cement can produce third degree alkali burns after as little as two hours of contact time. This burn was first described in a patient who developed burns after kneeling in premixed cement.[19]

Professional cement workers are well aware of this potential for skin burns, but most non-professionals are not. As a result, most injuries occur in the setting of "do-it-yourself" home projects. In many cases, the patient will sustain either ankle (boot-cuff) injuries caused by wet cement collecting inside the shoes or knee injuries that result from kneeling in wet cement without protection.[20] The resulting burn is often serious-first, because it usually is not appreciated early in the clinical course, and second, because the material is allowed to remain in contact with the skin for prolonged periods.

Table 2. Management Guidelines for Chemical Burns

I. Ensure that you are adequately protected. *This must take precedence over all patient care.*
II. Evaluate ABCs.
III. Start decontamination.
   A. Remove all clothing (undress to access and assess).
   B. Wipe away or debride all solid chemical particles.
   C. Inspect hair, nails, and web spaces for collections of the chemical.
   D. Remove caked compounds with green soap solution (liquid soap and 10% isopropyl alcohol).
IV. Obtain history.
   A. Type and concentration of chemical.
   B. Nature and duration of exposure.
   C. Concomitant traumatic injuries.
   D. Pre-existing medical illnesses.
   E. Tetanus immunization and allergies.
V. Start treatment with specific antidotes if applicable.
VI. Identify hospitalization criteria.
VII. Check effectiveness of irrigation. Use pH paper; if the pH is not neutral, continue irrigating for an additional hour.
VIII. Arrange follow-up and consultation. Follow-up checks at 24 hours, 72 hours, and 7 days. Do not use a closed dressing on a chemical burn!

Because lime is often used for marking football and other sporting fields, players may be exposed to lime powder.[21] These patients can present with burns in skin folds where lime has been trapped after a tackle. Initial treatment of lime or cement spilled on the skin consists of brushing away the particulate matter and then irrigating with copious amounts of water. Wet cement burns should be flushed with copious amounts of water and lesions should be treated as alkali burns.[16]

Hydrofluoric Acid Burns

HF is used in the glass and semiconductor industries as an etching agent, in the plastic industries for production of various plastic materials, and as a solvent for uranium. Many household aluminum brighteners or rust removal agents also contain HF.[22,23]

General Principles. From a clinical toxicology perspective, HF is important because it can produce extensive tissue damage, even at low concentrations. Moreover, it can result in potentially lethal systemic manifestations. Although HF causes caustic injury to the skin, it is less caustic than hydrochloric or sulfuric acids. Solutions containing HF in a concentration greater than 50% will produce immediate pain and apparent tissue destruction. HF solutions with a concentration in the range of 20-50% will produce clinical signs of injury within hours of exposure. On the other hand, injuries will not be apparent for up to 24 hours with solutions of less than 20%.[23-29] Finally, fluoride ions may enter the body through the skin or any mucous membrane, including the respiratory and gastrointestinal system. Damage is not due to the hydrogen ion but results from release of toxic fluoride ions.

From a pathophysiological point of view, fluoride ions cause a breakdown in all calcium-dependent reactions in the cell membrane,[30] a process that results in liquefaction necrosis of the skin and subcutaneous tissues. Without specific treatment, damage will progress over many hours, because the fluoride ions are not neutralized by the normal body defenses against acids or bases. Because the salts continue to be bioactive, the fluoride ions must be inactivated by combining them with other cations, including calcium and magnesium, which will form insoluble and nontoxic salts with fluoride anions.[31] All other salts are soluble and dissociate completely, thereby permitting continued diffusion of ions into the tissues. In addition, it should be stressed that if calcium is not available from an exogenous source, it will be leached from the patient's bony calcium deposits, a process that can produce life-threatening hypocalcemia.

Presentation. Topical exposure to HF is associated with extensive skin damage, including deep tissue destruction. Most exposures involve the skin, eyes, respiratory tract, or oral mucosa; even rectal exposure has been documented.[32] The initial presentation usually consists of pain at the site of the exposure, which is uniformly described as excruciating, particularly after exposure to solutions with greater than 20% concentration. Regional nerve blocks may be required for relief. Local erythema and edema also may be present.

As the injury progresses, erythema and edema progress to blanching. Bullae denote a more severe burn that requires aggressive treatment. A grossly necrotic area may develop with subsequent tissue sloughing and a very slowly healing lesion. In severe cases, bone injury may be present and severe decalcification may be noted. HF burns have caused systemic hydrofluorosis with subsequent death.[33-35]

Initial Treatment. Immediately after exposure, the affected area should be flooded with copious amounts of water at low pressures. All clothing and shoes can be removed in the shower to decrease the possibility of further contamination to both patient and staff. If there is evidence of skin damage, including erythema, the assumption can be made that the skin has been penetrated by fluoride ions, which will require inactivation. It is equally appropriate to assume that all skin spills are still contaminated and that the patient will develop additional injury if these areas are not treated.

Before proceeding with decontamination, the physician must ensure that he or she is adequately protected against HF exposure. Either butyl rubber or nitrile gloves and apron are recommended and should be worn. Shoe covers will decrease both "tracking" and contamination. All contaminated clothing and bedding should be placed in heavy plastic garbage bags and labeled.

The involved skin should be copiously flushed with running water while further preparations are in progress. In particular, nail beds and skin folds must be scrupulously cleansed. All bullae and vesicles should be aspirated to remove fluoride-containing fluids. Care must be taken not to spill the aspirate on any other part of the skin. Finally, the lesions should be debrided.

Topical Agents. After the area has been flooded with water for at least 30 minutes, any remaining fluoride ions can be "fixed" with the application of magnesium oxide, calcium chloride, or calcium gluconate solutions or topical ointments. Unfortunately, there is no convincing evidence that any of the these compounds produce significant tissue penetration. Despite all of the manufacturers' claims, the inactivated complex with fluoride in deep tissues simply will not be formed if the solution or ointment doesn't penetrate deeply enough to bind with free fluoride ions.[36] Consequently, once the fluoride has penetrated the skin, topical agents generally will no longer be effective.

If calcium chloride or gluconate gel is used, however, the residual fluoride will combine with the calcium and probably will neutralize any residual fluoride still on the skin.[37] This reaction will produce insoluble calcium fluoride which precipitates and clouds the clear gel. These cloudy areas mark neutralization of fluoride deposits,[30] which prevent further damage, making topical therapy worthwhile even if deep penetration into tissue fails to occur.

Local Infiltration. After debridement of lesions, 10% calcium gluconate can be injected into the burn to further bind the fluoride ions. This slow and painful process deposits calcium directly into the tissues and eventually provides pain relief.

About 0.5 mL of solution should be injected intradermally for every square centimeter of tissue damage. The injection is extended about 0.5 cm into the margins of the burn to bind ions that may have already migrated to this distal location.[22,23,25,26] To ease the pain of injection, a 27- or 30-gauge needle should be used and the area should be infiltrated slowly. Unfortunately, the volume of calcium gluconate that can be administered is limited to only 0.5 cc per injection. This severely restricts the amount of calcium that can be injected therapeutically at one sitting. Recurrence of the pain is an indication of further fluoride ion migration and necessitates an additional injection. Caution is advised, however, because multiple injections may contribute to local tissue ischemia. Calcium chloride is corrosive and should not be used for local infiltration.[38]

Intra-arterial Infusion. Intra-arterial calcium may provide better distribution and less tissue distention than injections into the burn. The arterial catheter should be placed in the distribution system. Arterial infusion of calcium may provide relief from burns to the fingertips without loss of either nail or distal finger.[39,40] Calcium may be infused as either the gluconate or chloride over four hours.[41] If the patient complains of continued pain, additional calcium may be infused.

Dressings and Topical Agents. After the injection of calcium, the area may be covered with a topical agent. Topical agents that have been used include calcium gluconate or chloride gels and soaks, magnesium oxide gel, paste, or soaks, and benzethonium and benzalkonium chloride soaks. Magnesium oxide dressings are less expensive and easier to obtain but are not as effective as calcium-based dressings.[26,27] Calcium chloride soaks may also be used. Some authors recommend 2.5% calcium gluconate in a gel vehicle, but further clinical trials are indicated before advocating this more costly therapy.[28] A mixture of 2.5-5.0% calcium gluconate in KY jelly may be used as an inexpensive alternative.[29]

Some authorities also recommend the use of quaternary ammonia compounds such as Hibiclens or Zephiran. These ammonia compounds have a dubious effect upon fluoride skin poisoning.[23,42] They may also tend to irritate sensitive skin tissues like the face or eye.

HF can rapidly penetrate the nail bed and destroy the underlying nail bed and matrix. Infiltration of calcium ions into the subungual spaces is extremely painful and may cause vascular compromise in the restrictive space between nail and nail bed. When ungual areas are involved in a HF burn, the affected nail must usually be excised under regional anesthesia. Removal of the nail will allow regeneration after the injury.

The wound must be inspected frequently to determine whether there is any further damage. Recurrence of pain is an indication for reinspection and reinjection. A fluoride burn should always be reinspected at 24-hour intervals, no matter how small or innocuous it seems. Surgical debridement may be necessary to prevent continued necrosis or if the exposure is in an inaccessible area.[32]

Systemic Complications. *(Please see Table 3.)* Skin burns with HF may be associated with significant systemic absorption of fluoride ions. Systemic toxicity can also occur with ingestion of sodium fluoride and inhalation of HF vapors.[43] As earlier noted, the fluoride leaches calcium from all available tissues, a process that can cause decalcification of bone and systemic hypocalcemia.

The precipitous drop in serum calcium has been implicated in fluoride-induced sudden death and may be more life-threatening than the burn damage.[34,44] The first sign of hypocalcemia is a profound bradycardia with a prolonged QT interval, which usually occurs within 30-45 minutes after exposure.

Accordingly, patients who are suspected of having this complication should be admitted to a telemetry unit to monitor for QT prolongation and possible dysrhythmias, as ventricular fibrillation may soon follow. This dysrhythmia may respond to high doses of intravenous calcium and surgical excision of the burn wound.[45] Death may also be caused by respiratory distress due to airway edema.[46] Several authors have reported use of massive doses of calcium salts for relief of hypocalcemia.[47] If there is evidence of systemic fluorosis or the possibility of inhalation injury, the patient should be admitted to the hospital and observed for at least 24 hours. Monitoring of liver function studies, renal function studies, electrolytes, and serial serum calcium levels is indicated .[23]

Ocular Injuries. HIT solution or vapor in or around the eye causes more extensive damage than other acids in similar concentrations. Deep penetration and liquefaction necrosis make HF especially destructive to the eye. Eye burns should be treated with immediate and copious irrigation immediately after exposure. A Morgan contact irrigating lens is well suited for this procedure. Eyelid spasm may be decreased by use of tetracaine or other ophthalmologic anesthetic solutions.[22] Following this irrigation, a 1% calcium gluconate solution in isotonic sodium chloride can be used as drops and instilled every 2-3 hours.[23] Other authors feel that only irrigation with water, isotonic saline solution, or magnesium chloride solutions offered therapeutic benefit.[24,48] Prompt ophthalmologic consultation is essential.

Elemental Sodium, Potassium, and Lithium Burns

Sodium, potassium, and, to a lesser extent, lithium will spontaneously ignite when in contact with water, including water vapor in the air or on the skin. Using water to irrigate these burns will only intensify the combustion effects. When these metals combine with water, sodium, potassium, and lithium hydroxides are formed, which are among the strongest alkalies and are capable of causing severe caustic burns.[49]

To extinguish these burning metals, oxygen and water must be removed from the area. A class D fire extinguisher or sand may be used to smother the fire. After the fire is extinguished, the area should be covered with oil, such as mineral or cooking oil, in order to isolate the metal from water. Small metal pieces should be removed by debridement to fresh tissue. Particles can be disposed of by placing them in alcohol; embedded pieces must be removed surgically. Following debridement and confirmation that all pieces have been removed, the area must be irrigated with water, using the same techniques described as for an alkali burn.[49]

Table 3. Signs of Acute Systemic Fluoride Toxicity

Hypotension
Bradycardia, followed by tachycardia
Prolongation of the QT interval
Ventricular fibrillation (often intractable)
Respiratory depression
Pulmonary edema
Seizures
CNS depression
Carpopedal spasm or tetany (often not found)
Hypocalcemia, hypomagnesemia
Coagulation disorders (rare)

Phosphorus Burns

A waxy, translucent substance that ignites spontaneously on contact with air, white phosphorus is the most common form of phosphorus found in chemical burns.[50,51] It is usually preserved underwater and becomes a liquid at 44°C. White phosphorus is used in the construction of military weapons and fireworks and is a component in insecticides and rodent poisons.

Phosphorous pentachloride is a yellow-white fuming crystalline mass with a pungent odor. It is widely used as a catalyst and as a chlorinating and a dehydrating agent. Because there is only one report of phosphorus pentachloride chemical burn in the literature, this agent will not be discussed in detail.[52]

Following an explosion of white phosphorus munitions, flaming droplets of white phosphorus are disseminated, producing dense clouds of white smoke with a typical "garlic-like" smell. Flaming pieces of white phosphorus may also cause high-speed projectile injuries.[50] Smoke results from the oxidation of phosphorus to phosphoric acid, which can damage pulmonary structures as well as the skin. This chemical reaction in combination with thermal activity produces extremely painful second-degree burns.

Flaming white phosphorus is extinguished by immersing the pieces in water. Surface particles and particles embedded in clothing should be promptly removed. During transport, prehospital personnel should cover burned areas with moistened cloths to prevent further conflagration. Irrigation may help to remove surface particles but will not be effective against those particles driven deep into tissue by blast effects.

The wound may then be washed with a 1% copper sulfate solution, which should be applied for only a few minutes in order to avoid systemic toxicity since copper sulfate can produce significant morbidity. Copper sulfate solution combines with the phosphorus to form copper phosphate, the black particles of which permit rapid identification and debridement.[2] If the particles are not debrided, they will be absorbed, producing systemic effects.[53]

To further minimize copper absorption, the wound may be irrigated with a solution of 5% sodium bicarbonate and 3% copper sulfate suspended in 1% hydroxyethyl cellulose.[51] Wet dressings of copper sulfate in any form should never be applied to the wound. Following debridement, which must be performed expeditiously, the wound should be irrigated with copious amounts of water to remove the copper salts.

From the perspective of systemic toxicity, metabolic derangements have been noted with white phosphorus injuries, including hypocalcemia, hyperphosphatemia, and ECG abnormalities.[54] Electrocardiographic abnormalities include prolongation of the QT interval, bradycardia, and nonspecific ST-T-wave changes. Moreover, depletion of clotting factors may contribute to hemorrhage. Vitamin K therapy may improve the clotting disorders that result from exposure to phosphorus.

Phenol Burns

Phenol is an aromatic acid alcohol that is a highly reactive and corrosive contact poison.[55-57] Phenols denature and precipitate cellular proteins and have been used not only as bactericidal agents but as chemical bases for plastics and organic polymers. In the form of creosote, it is also used as a wood preservative.

Phenol is rapidly absorbed through skin surfaces, while phenol vapors are easily absorbed by the lungs in either liquid or vapor form. If skin absorption is significant, exposure may result in toxic effects, which may include central nervous system depression, hypotension, intravascular hemolysis, pulmonary edema, shock, and death.[56,57]

The most common manifestation of systemic phenol poisoning is profound, fulminant central nervous system depression accompanied by coma, hypothermia, loss of vasomotor tone, and respiratory arrest. In many cases, loss of consciousness may be noted within 30 minutes of skin contact. Cardiopulmonary collapse frequently accompanies this CNS presentation and is due to the cardiac depressant effects of phenol. In animal studies, as little as 0.625 mg/kg of phenol has caused death.[56,57]

Phenol skin burns are characterized by initial pain followed by numbness as the nerve endings are anesthetized.[58] Phenol penetration of the skin causes coagulation necrosis of the papillary dermis. The skin blanches and an eschar forms over the burned area during a period of hours. Phenols in strong concentrations rapidly produce a whitish slough, which turns to a greenish-black or copper-colored eschar. Although coagulation necrosis of the dermis will delay absorption, this delay is only temporary.

Treatment must be initiated immediately. Before washing the contaminated area, remove any liquid on the skin. Swabs, gauze pads, and clothing are acceptable for this maneuver. If the solute polyethylene glycol is not available, glycerol, isopropyl alcohol, or vegetable oils may aid in the removal. Removal of the liquid should not wait until these materials are available.

There is some concern about using water for initial irrigation of phenol burns. In severe phenol burns, the necrotic tissues may act as a temporary barrier that does not allow penetration of the water into the deeper layers of the injury. The water may also dilute the phenol and allow more rapid penetration into the skin. Nevertheless, if access to specific solutes of phenol is not available immediately, irrigation with water in large-volume lavage is advocated, because this is preferable to allowing toxic phenol substances to remain in contact with skin surfaces.[56,57]

Although water irrigation may be somewhat effective for phenol burn, wiping the skin with undiluted polyethylene glycol (PEG 300 or PEG 400) will dissolve and remove the phenols more quickly than water alone. Isopropyl alcohol and glycerol are also effective in removing phenols. Finally, olyethylene glycol solutions are not irritating to the tissues and may safely be used to irrigate facial burns and eye injuries.

Bleaches

Bleaches include a wide range of compounds, among them, calcium or sodium hypochlorite, sodium perborate, or sodium peroxide mixtures. These may range in danger from the relatively innocuous household sodium hypochlorite bleach to quite corrosive solutions. Granular bleaches are more concentrated. Sodium hypochlorite solutions are manufactured by adding chlorine gas to a 12-15% sodium hydroxide solution until the solution is neutral. If even a little excess chlorine is added to the mixture, it will be an unstable acidic hypochlorite solution. A typical household bleach is about 4-6% hypochlorite, while pool sanitizers are about 70% hypochlorite, which explains why pool sanitizer mixtures can be extremely corrosive. When heated, hypochlorite powder decomposes to free chlorine gas and oxygen.

External contact should be treated with copious water irrigation. Ingestion should be treated first with milk or water followed by transport to the ED as soon as possible. If the patient tries to mix hypochlorites with other chemicals, dangerous fumes may be produced. For example, hypochlorite mixed with a strong acid will produce chlorine gas, whereas if hypochlorite is mixed with ammonia, a chloramine gas will be formed. These gases may be very irritating to the lungs, producing pulmonary edema in patients with significant exposure.

Anhydrous Ammonia Injuries

Anhydrous ammonia is one of the most common chemicals implicated in serious burn injuries.[59] Used extensively as an agricultural fertilizer, anhydrous ammonia is also used in the manufacturing process for nylon, rayon, and explosives. Anhydrous ammonia is stored at about -28°F, so exposure to this substance may cause both frostbite and a chemical injury. The substance produces liquefaction necrosis characteristic of severe alkaline injuries. Skin injuries may range from superficial to deep and are sometimes accompanied by full-thickness tissue loss. Ocular and respiratory injuries often accompany the skin lesion and may be severe.

Treatment consists of decontamination with copious amounts of water after removal of all clothing. Ocular injuries must be flushed immediately to ensure optimal outcomes. For both skin and eye exposure, irrigation should be continued for an extended period of time during the first 24 hours.[60] Partial-thickness skin injuries may be treated with silver sulfadiazine, but other ointments and salves should be avoided. Small, full-thickness injuries may be excised and closed primarily.

Table 4. Indications for Hospitalization of Patients With Chemical Burns

High-risk patients (concurrent illnesses)
Burns of hand, foot, face, eye, or perineum
Burns of greater than 15% of total body surface
Deep burns (deep second- or third-degree burns)
Burns with substances that have systemic toxicity

Alcohol Burns

Commonly used as a disinfectant in hospital settings as well as for cleaning in home and industry, isopropyl alcohol can produce skin burns in adults as well as infants and small children .The mechanism of action is thought to be de-esterification of the skin.[61] The degree of burn is related to the concentration of the alcohol, the duration of the exposure, and the condition of the skin to which the alcohol has been applied. Premature infants are at greatest risk. Burns occur most often in areas of pressure and at sites (e.g., diapers) that permit alcohol to pool.[62] The systemic effects of isopropyl alcohol, which can include multiorgan failure and metabolic derangements, can be significant not only after ingestion but also as a result of transcutaneous exposure and absorption. Isopronalol causes an elevated osmolal gap, with predominantly CNS depression and (rarely) cardiovascular compromise. The anion gap typically remains normal unless a secondary process (hypotension, hypoventilatory hypoxia) intervenes, causing lactic acidosis.

Summary

Fortunately, chemical burns usually involve only a small part of the patient's body surface area. In most cases, these burns can be managed on an outpatient basis. Patients who require hospitalization include those with burns from chemicals that have long-term or distant effects, such as gasoline, phenol, or hydrofluoric acid. Admission is also required when the burn involves a critical area or a large surface, and, of course, when the patient has a concurrent severe illness. *(Please see Table 4.)* As a rule, most chemical injuries can be managed by irrigation with large quantities of water. This measure serves to both dilute and remove the agent. For elemental lithium, sodium, and potassium metals, the particles must be removed before irrigation. Special antidotes should be used, if available, in appropriate cases.

References

1. Rodheaver GT, Herbert JM, Edlich RE. Initial treatment of chemical, skin, and eye burns. *Compr Ther* 1982;8:37-43.
2. Curreri PW, Asch MJ, Pruitt BA. The treatment of chemical burns: Specialized diagnostic therapeutic and prognostic considerations. *J Trauma* 1970; 10:634-642.
3. Winemaker M, Douglas L, Peters W. Combination alkali/thermal burns caused by "black liquor" in the pulp and paper industry. *Burns* 1992;18:68-70.
4. Sawhney CP, Kaushish R. Acid and alkali burns: Considerations in management. *Burns* 1989; 15:132- 134.
5. Wolfort FG, DeMeester T, Knorr N, et al. Surgical management of cutaneous lye burns. *Surg Gynecol Obstet* 1970:873-876.
6. Jelenko C III. Chemicals that "burn." *J Trauma* 1974;14:65-72.
7. Beare JDL. Eye injuries from assault with chemicals. *Br J Ophthalmol* 1990;74:514-518.
8. Leonard LG, Scheulen JJ, Munster AM. Chemical burns: Effect of prompt first aid. *Trauma* 1982;22:420-423.
9. Swanson-Biearman B, Mvros R, et al. Airbags: Lifesaving with toxic potential? *Am J Emerg Med* 1993;11:38-39.
10. Ingraham H, Perry H, Donefeld ED. Airbag keratitis. *N Engl J Med* 1991;324:1599-1600.
11. Larkin L. Air-bag-mediated cornea 1 injury. *Am J Emerg Med* 1991;9:444-446.
12. Kunkel DB. Burning issues: Acids and alkalies. II. Skin and eye exposures. *Emerg Med* 1984:165-172.
13. Yano K, Hata Y, Matsuka O, et al. Experimental study on alkaline skin injuries-periodic changes in subcutaneous tissue pH and the effects exerted by washing. *Burns* 1993;4:320-323.
14. Gruber RP, Laub DR, Vistnes LM. The effect of hydrotherapy on the clinical course and pH of experimental cutaneous chemical burns. *Plast Reconstr Surg* 1975;55:200.
15. Bromberg BE, Sang IC, Walden RH. Hydrotherapy of chemical burns. *Plast Reconstr Surg* 1965;35:85.
16. Stewart CE. Chemical skin burns. *Am Fam Physician* 1985;31:151-157.
17. Davidson EC. The treatment of alkali and acid burns. *Ann Surg* 1927;85:481.
18. Peters WJ. Alkali burns from wet cement. *Can Med Assoc J* 1984;130:902-903.
19. Rowe W, Williams CH. Severe reaction to cement. *Arch Environ Health* 1963;7:709-711.
20. Fisher AA. Cement burns resulting in necrotic ulcers due to kneeling on wet cement. *Cutis* 1979;23:272-274.
21. Benmeir P, Lusthaus S, Weinberg A, et al. Chemical burn due to contact with soda lime on the playground: A potential hazard, for football players. *Burns* 1993;19:358-359.
22. Flood S. Hydrofluoric acid burns. *Am Fam Physician* 1988;37:175-182.
23. Trevino MA, Herrmann GH, Sprout WL. Treatment of severe hydrofluoric acid exposures. *J Occup Med* 1983;25:861-863.
24. McCulley JP. Ocular hydrofluoric acid burns: Animal model, mechanism of injury, and therapy. *Trans Am Ophthahmol* Soc 1990;88:649-684.
25. Caravati EM. Acute hydrofluoric acid exposure. *Am J Emerg Med* 1988;6: 143-150.
26. Iverson RE, Laub DR. Hydrofluoric acid burn. *Surg Forum* 1970;21:517-519.
27. Chick LR, Borah G. Calcium carbonate gel therapy for hydrofluoric acid burns of the hand. *Plast Reconstr Surg* 1990;86:935-940.
28. Milner JE. The office treatment of minor chemical skin burns. *Cubs* 1982;29:285-288.
29. Mistry DG, Wainright DJ. Hydrofluoric acid burns. *Am Fam*

Physician 1992;45: 1748-1754.

30. Hirsch RL, Dunjey SI. A hand burn from unmarked hydrofluoric acid. *Med J Aust* 1993;158:136-137. Letter.
31. Carney SA, Hall M, Lawrence JC, et al. Rationale of the treatment of hydrofluoric acid burns. *Br J Intern Med* 1974;31:317-321.
32. Foster DE, Barone JA. Rectal hydrofluoric acid exposure. *Clin Pharmacol* 1989;8:516-518.
33. Mayer TG, Gross PL. Fatal systemic fluorosis due to hydrofluoric acid burns. *Ann Emerg Med* 1985;14:149-153.
34. Tepperman PB. Fatality due to acute systemic fluoride poisoning following a hydrofluoric acid skin burn. *J Occup Med* 1980;22:691-692.
35. Burke WJ, Hoegg UR, Phillips RE. Systemic fluoride poisoning resulting from a fluoride skin burn. *J Occup Med* 1973;15:39-41.
36. Dibbel DG, Iverson RE, Jones W, et al. Hydrofluoric acid burns of the hand. *J Bone Joint Surg Am* 1970;52:93 1-936.
37. Bracken WM, Cuppage F, McLaury RL, et al. Comparative effectiveness of topical treatment for hydrofluoric acid burns. *J Occup Med* 1985;27:733-739.
38. Upfal M, Doyle C. Medical management of hydrofluoric acid exposure. *J Occup Med* 1990;32:726-731.
39. Edinburg M, Swift R. Hydrofluoric acid burns of the hands: A case report and suggested management. *Aust NZ J* Surg 1989;59:88-91.
40. Siegel DC, Heard JM. Jntra-arterial calcium infusion for hydrofluoric acid burns. *Aviat Space Environ Med* 1992;63:206-211.
41. Vance MV, Curry SC, Kunkel DB, et al. Digital hydrofluoric acid burns: Treatment with intra-arterial calcium infusion. *Ann Emerg Med* 1986;15:890-896.
42. Bracken WM, Cuppage F, McLaury PR, et al. Comparative effectiveness of topical treatments for hydrofluoric acid burns. *J Occup Med* 1985;27:733-739.
43. Manoguerra AS, Neuman TS. Fatal poisoning from acute hydrofluoric acid ingestion. *Am J Emerg Med* 1986;4:362-363.
44. Mayer TG, Gross PL. Fatal systemic fluorosis due to hydrofluoric acid burns. *Ann Emerg Med* 1985;14:149-153.
45. Buckingham FM. Surgery: A radical approach to severe hydrofluoric acid burns. *J Occup Med* 1988;30:873-875.
46. Chela A, Reig R, Sanz P, et al. Death due to hydrofluoric acid. *Am J Forensic Med Pathol* 1989; 10:47-48.
47. Bertolini JC. Hydrofluoric acid: A review of toxicity. *J Emerg Med* 1992;10:163-168.
48. McCulley JP, Whiting DW, Pettitt MG, et al. Hydrofluoric acid burns of the eye. *J Occup Med* 1983;25:447-450.
49. Clare RA, Krenzelok EP. Chemical burns secondary to elemental metal exposure: Two case reports. *Am J Emerg Med* 1988;6:355-357.
50. Konjoyan TR. White phosphorus burns: Case report and literature review. *Mil Med* 1983;148:881-884.
51. Ben-Hur N, Appelbaum J. Biochemistry, histopathology and treatment of phosphorus burns. *Isr J Med Sci* 1973;9:40-48.
52. Eldad A, Chaouat M, Weinberg A, et al. Phosphorus pentachloride chemical burn-a slowly healing injury. *Burns* 1992; 18:340-341.
53. Dempsy WS. Combat injuries of the lower extremities. *Clin Plast Surg* 1975;2:585-614.
54. Bowen TE, Whelen TJ Jr, Nelson TG. Sudden death after phosphorus burns: Experimental observations of hypocalcemia, hyperphosphatemia and electrocardiographic abnormalities following production of a standard white phosphorus burn. *Ann Surg* 1971;174;779-784.
55. Roberts HL. Chloracetic acids: A biochemical study. *Ann Surg* 1926;49:245-247.
56. Conning DM, Haynes MJ. The dermal toxicity of phenol: An investigation of the most effective first-aid measures. *Br J Ind Med* 1970;27:155.
57. Brown VKH, Box VL, Simpson BJ. Decontamination procedures for skin exposed to phenolic substances. *Arch Environ Health* 1975;20: 1.
58. Abraham AJ. A case of carbolic acid gangrene of the thumb. *Br J Plast Surg* 1972;25:282-284.
59. Millea TP, Koran J0, Smoot EC 111. Anhydrous ammonia injuries. *J Burn Care Rehabil* 1989;10:448-453.
60. Slot GMJ. Ammonia gas burns: An account of six cases. *Lancet* 1938;2: 1356-1357.
61. Hodgkinson DJ, Irons GB, Williams TJ. Chemical burns and skin preparation solutions. *Surg Gynecol Obstet* 1978; 147:534-536.
62. Schick JB, Milstein JM. Burn hazard of isopropyl alcohol in the neonate. *Pediatrics* 198 1;68(4):587-588.

Snake Venom Poisoning

Robert L. Norris, MD, FACEP

Fortunately, snake venom poisoning is a relatively uncommon toxicologic emergency in the United States. Consequently, few physicians receive extensive training or have the opportunity to gain experience managing this life-threatening problem. To complicate matters, the literature on this topic is replete with controversies stemming from the complicated nature of snake venom poisoning and its management. For example, research data from animal studies must be extrapolated cautiously to humans due to great interspecific differences in response to snake venoms. Furthermore, each venom is different, reflecting not only interspecies differences, but variability in venom characteristics between snakes of the same species. Finally, every individual's response is different and depends on such factors as age, body size, allergy states, and health.

The estimated mortality rate for pit viper envenomation in the United States is 0.28% when treated with antivenin and 2.61% when antivenin is not administered.[1] These outcomes represent a significant improvement over the 5-25% mortality rates observed during the pre-antivenin era. Morbidity due to viperid bites is more difficult to assess but it is certainly significant, especially following rattlesnake bites to the hand.[2]

This chapter reviews our current understanding of snake venom poisoning in Ihe United States and presents a logical approach for evaluation and management of these victims. While there are many pitfalls associated with snakebite management, the emergency physician who exercises sound clinical judgment and understands the potential for multisystem organ failure will be best prepared for achieving an optimal outcome.

Introduction

The most complete analysis of the incidence of venomous snakebite injuries in the United States was performed in the early 1960s by Dr. Henry Parrish.[3] Demographics and patterns of outdoor activity have changed over the last 30 years, factors that have probably affected the in.cidence of snake venom poisoning. However, lacking more current figures, it is estimated from Parrish's data that there are approximately 8000 cases of venomous snakebites in the United States each year, 10-20 of which are fatal.[3,4]

Venomous snakes indigenous to the United States are divided into two major groups: the pit vipers (family *Viperidae*; sub-family *Crotalinae*) and the coral snakes (family *Elapidae*). More than 98% of bites in this country are inflicted by pit vipers (rattlesnakes, copperheads, and cottonmouth water moccasins. Less than 1% of bites are caused by coral snakes and other exotic snakes that have been imported tor zoos, scientific institutions, or private hobbyists.

There is at least one species of venomous snake indigenous to each state of the United States, with the exception of Maine, Alaska, and Hawaii.[1] Because snakes are poikilothermic ("cold-blooded"), the number of species as well as the total number of snakes is greater

Table 1. Characteristics Used in Identifying Venomous Snakes Native to the United States

	NONVENOMOUS	PIT VIPERS	CORAL SNAKES
Head shape	Round or triangular	Triangular	Round
Pupils	Round	Elliptical	Round
Facial pits	Absent	Present	Absent
Fangs	None (regular teeth)	Anterior, elongated, retractable	Anterior, short, fixed position
Subcaudal scales*	Double row	Single row	Double row
Rattles	Absent	Usually present in rattlesnakes	Absent
Color	Variable	Variable	Red/yellow/black (red and yellow contiguous)

* Subcaudal scales: The row of scales on the ventral aspect of the tail just distal to the large anal plate scale

in southern climates. Not surprisingly, the incidence of reported snakebites also is greater as one moves in a southward direction in North America.[1] There are a number of characteristics that are helpful in identifying and distinguishing pit vipers (viperids) and coral snakes indigenous to this country. *(Please see Table 1.)*

Venom Apparatus and Venoms

Pit vipers possess a venom apparatus that is among the most sophisticated encountered in all snake species. Venom is produced and stored in large, bilateral primary venom glands located just below and behind the eyes, near the angles of the mandible. The venom is activated by an accessory gland before it is carried by a duct to the base of the needle-like fang on the anterior aspect of the mandible. This fang is long (up to 20 mm in North American pit vipers[5]) and mobile. When not in use, it is stored in a folded position against the roof of the mouth. When a pit viper strikes, it brings its fangs into an upright position and thrusts them into its prey at speeds of up to eight feet per second.[6]

Although not a part of the venom apparatus per se, the heat-sensing pits for which these snakes are named contain infrared receptors. They are part of an integral, finely calibrated feedback mechanism that is linked to the venom apparatus and that is designed to both aim the strike and determine the quantity of venom required to incapacitate the prey.[5] It is interesting to note that approximately 25% of bites by pit vipers in the United States result in no venom injection ("dry bites")[1], a phenomenon that is not entirely understood.

One of the most complex naturally occurring toxins,[5] pit viper venoms are a mixture of tissue-reactive enzymes, low molecular weight polypeptides, and myriad other macromolecules whose precise role has not been fully elucidated. Although an in-depth discussion of these components is beyond the scope of this review, information is available in many excellent sources.[5,7-9] From a clinical perspective, however, it should be stressed that venoms are extremely variable in their activity, and that to ascribe a single toxicological manifestation (i.e., hemo-toxicity or neurotoxicity) to any whole snake venom is to over-simplify the situation. Accordingly, the clinician must be prepared to recognize and manage a wide range of potential adverse effects in all cases of snake venom poisoning.

Toxic Effects of Viperid Poisoning

With the vast majority of pit vipers indigenous to the United States, a successful envenomation will result in rapid onset of burning or searing pain at the bite site. Within minutes, there will be local swelling and edema, which may progress along the involved extremity over the next several hours to days. Because most venoms possess anticoagulant properties, there may be persistent, bloody oozing from the puncture wounds. In addition, over the next several hours, subcutaneous ecchymoses may appear and spread along the extremity. Since a significant amount of venom distributes via the lymphatic system,[4] the individual who is bitten by a snake may rapidly develop lymphangitis with regional lymphadenopathy. Over the first several hours to days, hemorrhagic blebs and serum-filled vesicles frequently will appear on the extremity, especially if treatment is delayed.

Systemic manifestations of pit viper poisoning are diverse; therefore, optimal management requires anticipation of serious complications associated with snake envenomation. For example, with some venoms, the patient may note an odd taste in the mouth and tingling in the face, scalp, or extremities. Fine muscle fasciculations suggest a potentially severe envenomation. Muscle weakness or actual paralysis, although not common, may occur following bites by some North American viperids (e.g., Mojave rattlesnake [*Crotalus scutulatus*]).[5,10]

Abnormal vital signs, which are commonly encountered in serious cases, include an increase in respiratory rate and pulse. In addition, the blood pressure may be elevated initially, but in severe cases complicated by anaphylaxis or intravascular volume depletion, hypotension is common. The causes for poor tissue perfusion are diverse. Early hypotension may be due to direct intravascular envenomation or an anaphylactic reaction.[6] However, in most cases, it is due to pooling of blood volume in the pulmonary and splanchnic vasculature. With time, third spacing of fluid as edema in the bitten extremity or intravascular hemolysis also can play a contributory role in the production of hypotension,[5,6] as can the direct myocardial depressant associated with some venoms? Finally, pulmonary edema may follow severe poisoning.[7]

Consumptive coagulopathies are common and bleeding may be observed in almost any anatomic site. Moreover, even in the absence of clinically significant hemorrhage, it is not unusual for patients to

Table 2. Severity Grading Scale for Pit Viper Bites*

	NONENVENOMATION	MILD	MODERATE	SEVERE
Fang marks	±	+	+	+
Pain	None	Moderate	Severe	Severe
Edema	None	Minimal	Moderate	Severe**
Ecchymosis	None	±	+	+
Systemic findings	None	None	Mild	Early, severe
Laboratory findings	Normal	Normal	Mildly abnormal	Very abnormal
Approximate percentage of total bites	27%	37%	22%	14%

* This scale was designes for use in cases of bites by indigenous North American pit vipers only. Strict reliance on this scale should not replace sound clinical judgment.

** There may be minimal swelling if intramuscular or intravascular venom injection occurs.

have abnormal coagulation parameters.[12,13] *(Please see Table 2.)* Renal failure can occur in severe cases, sometimes as a sequela of prolonged hypotension, hemoglobin or myoglobin deposition in renal tubules, and/or direct venom-mediated nephrotoxicity.[14]

Prehospital Management

Aggressive, early, and precise management is required to achieve optimal clinical outcomes. Perhaps the most important variable determining outcomes in snake venom poisoning is the promptness with which victims receive definitive care. A quick attempt to get a look at the snake may be worthwhile, but only if there is minimal risk of incurring a second bite or producing a second victim. Attempting to kill the snake is not recommended because this is hazardous and may waste precious time. Furthermore, since there is currently only one approved antivenin for use in all native viperid envenomations in the United States, precise identification is unnecessary.

The victim should be taken by the most expeditious route possible to an emergency care center. When bites are sustained in a wilderness setting, there is no precise formula as to whether a victim should attempt to hike out to medical care or wait while someone summons a source of transportation (e.g., helicopter). Variables such as apparent severity of the bite, health of the victim, terrain, and weather must be considered.

Some experts contend that a constriction band applied within a few minutes several centimeters proximal to the bite site may decrease systemic spread of venom.[15] If employed, this band should inhibit only lymphatic and, perhaps, superficial venous flow; distal arterial flow must remain intact to permit adequate tissue perfusion. A wide band (such as a handkerchief) or ace wrap is applied about as tightly as required to perform a phlebotomy. If swelling subsequently compromises arterial flow, a second band is applied in a more proximal position relative to the bite and the initial band is then removed. The involved extremity is splinted to limit muscular movement with resulting central dispersio nof venom and should be kept at approximately heart level when feasible, although this may be difficult for logistic reasons. With serious bites, constriction bands placed in the field should remain in place until after antivenin infusion has been started (see below). Otherwise, the patient may go into shock from a bolus effect of venom entering the systemic circulation.

It is now generally accepted that the combination of incision and suction of the bite wound is not advisable. First, cutting open fang puncture wounds in an unsterile setting probably does little to augment extraction of venom from any tissue depot. It does, however, increase the risk of wound infection and tissue necrosis.[16] Moreover, in inexperienced and nervous hands this approach may risk violation of underlying vital structures (nerves, vessels, etc.). Nevertheless, applying suction without cutting probably does no harm, and preliminary evidence suggests it may be possible to recover some of the venom using a strong suction device such as the "Extractor" (Sawyer Products, Safety Harbor, FL).[17] For a device of this kind to be effective, it must be applied within minutes of the bite.

Finally, a number of first-aid measures that were once recommended have been shown to be ineffective. These approaches include application of heat, ice therapy, electric shock treatments, and a wide array of poultices and topical agents.[5,18-20]

Management in the Hospital Setting

Assessing the apparent severity of an acute envenomation is a prerequisite for targeted therapeutic intervention. A severity grading scale for viperid bites used in the United States is summarized in *Table 2.*[6] No grading scale, however, is a substitute for careful evaluation of the patient. In addition, it should be stressed that snake venom poisoning is a dynamic process and that what appears initially to be a mild case can rapidly evolve into a severe, life-threatening emergency.

Principles of Initial Management. As the emergency physician elicits a history and performs the physical examination, two large-bore IV lines with crystalloid (normal saline or Ringer's lactate) should be established; blood studies should be drawn at this time. Cardiac and pulse oximetry monitoring are established, and if there is evidence of hypoxia, oxygen is administered. Initially, hypotension is treated with IV crystalloid resuscitation, although if vital signs fail to normalize quickly, albumin may be beneficial.[21] Vasopressors should be reserved for hypotension that is unresponsive to fluid resuscitation.

Table 3. Management of Adverse Reactions to Antivenin

- Stop antivenin infusion
- Administer epinephrine, antihistamines, steroids, IV fluids and pressors (e.g., dopamine) as needed (standard doses)
- Reconsider the need for antivenin
- If poisoning is severe, may be able to restart antivenin in a more dilute fashion at a slower rate (preferably in a critical care setting—see below)
- Steroids (e.g., prednisone 40-100 mg/day) until symptoms resolve, then taper over 7-10 days (admission for IV steroids is occasionally necessary)
- Antihistamines for symptomatic relief

Table 4. Antivenin Administration Technique

- Obtain informed consent if possible
- Begin reconstitution as soon as possible with warm diluent
- Have epinephrine at the bedside
- If the decision is made to skin test (see text):
  —follow the instructions in the package insert
  —substitute reconstituted antivenin, further diluted 1:1, in place of the "normal horse serum" supplied with the product
- Expand intravascular volume with crystalloid (if no contraindication)
- Premeditate with IV antihistamines (both H,- and Hz-blockers)
  —e.g., diphenhydramine (1 mg/kg up to 50 mg) and cimetidine (5 mg/kg up to 300 mg)
- Dilute the antivenin in normal saline or Ringer's lactate (50-100 mL for each vial)
- Begin infusion slowly (the treating physician should be in immediate attendance) for the first several minutes
- If no reaction, increase the rate to complete infusion in 1-4 hours
- Reassess clinical response after the initial dose
  —If swelling or systemic abnormalities progress or recur, give l-5 more vials every 30 minutes to two hours as needed

Rapid, systematic laboratory evaluation of a victim with a presumed pit viper bite is important because, not infrequently, the earliest evidence of systemic involvement is suggested by abnormal laboratory findings. A complete blood count (CBC), coagulation studies (prothrombin time, partial thromboplastin time, fibrinogen and d-dimer levels), muscle enzyme assays, and renal function studies are obtained as part of the initial database. A specimen for blood typing and crossing is collected as soon as possible, because once hemolysis has occurred, these studies may be difficult to perform. Urine specimens are assessed for evidence of gross or microscopic blood, protein, or glucose, and stool samples are checked for blood. Arterial blood gases, an electrocardiogram, and chest radiograph are recommended in the elderly, in those with a history of significant underlying diseases, and patients who appear to be suffering from severe, systemic envenomation.

It is helpful to mark two or more locations proximal to the wound on the extremity and to measure the circumferences at these sites every 15 minutes during the early stages. If the circumferences are increasing rapidly, the envenomation is likely to be serious. Blood products (packed red blood cells, platelets, fresh frozen plasma, etc.) may be required to treat clinically significant bleeding in the face of decreased coagulation factors. Ongoing consumption coagulopathy needs to be treated with antivenin (see below) prior to transfusion.[22] Finally, patients with previous exposure to snake venoms via bites or other routes are also at significant risk for venom-induced allergic reactions.

Antivenin Administration. In addition to supportive care, antivenin administration is the only treatment proven efficacious in the management of serious cases of snake venom poisoning. There is currently one product (Antivenin [Crotalidae] Polyvalent-Wyeth-Ayerst) available in the United States for any significant, indigenous pit viper envenomation. This is an equine-derived antiserum that carries risks of serious adverse reactions and, therefore, must be used judiciously. *(Please see Table 3.)* Although effective for managing systemic effects produced by envenomation, the ability of antivenin to decrease local tissue damage is limited unless administered within two hours of the bite.[5,23-26]

Although use of antivenin in mild envenomations (i.e., those characterized by local findings only) is controversial, its utility for managing moderate-to-severe envenomations is more generally accepted. From a practical perspective, when indicated, antidote should be administered as soon as possible after envenomation, although it still may be of some benefit for ameliorating systemic complications when given at any point during the first 24 hours following the bite.[27] A technique for administration is outlined in Table 4, and appropriate starting doses are summarized in *Table 5.*[28] Envenomations by copperheads usually do not require antivenin therapy since most bites produce only minor pain and edema.

Adverse Reactions. Acute anaphylaxis is the most worrisome adverse reaction to antivenin administration. It is characterized by an immediate, IgE-mediated response to equine proteins; manifestations include hives, respiratory distress, bronchospasm, laryngospasm, hypotension, dysrhythmias, and, on rare occasions, death. A non-allergenic, anaphylactoid reaction caused by direct, antivenin-mediated activation of the complement system has also been reported.[28,30]

The most common adverse reaction to antivenin, however, is a delayed serum sickness reaction, which is characterized by myalgias, arthralgias, arthritis, fever, uticaria, and malaise, which can be seen l-2 weeks after treatment.[6,31] This reaction is observed in nearly 75% of patients who receive antivenin and in almost 100% of patients who receive more than seven vials! Management of these adverse reactions is summarized in *Table 3.*

Skin Testing. Many experts, as well as the antivenin product manufacturer, recommend performing a skin test in an attempt to

Table 5. Recommended Starting Doses for North American Antivenins*

Severity	Number of vials
ANTIVENIN [CROTALIDAE] POLYVALENT	
Nonenvenomation	0
Mild	0 *or* 5 (50 mL)
Moderate	10 (100 mL)
Severe	15 (150 mL)
NORTH AMERICAN CORAL SNAKE ANTIVENIN	
Begin with 3-6 vials	
Give 3-5 more vials if new findings appear or worsen (> 10 vials are rarely required)	

* Antivenins should only be administered intravenously. Children require the same doses of antivenin as adults and occasionally even larger doses (may need to reduce the volume of dilutent in small children)

identify those patients who are likely to suffer an acute allergic reaction to antivenin.[5,6,24] The skin-testing technique is outlined in the package insert. From a practical perspective, however, the skin test requires at least 20 minutes to apply and read; moreover, the test is compromised by a significant number of false-positive and false-negative reactions. False-positive readings (i.e., patients with a positive skin test who can receive antivenin without an acute reaction) are well-documented.[31-33] Conversely, as many as 10% of patients with a negative skin test will demonstrate an acute (and sometimes severe) reaction upon IV infusion.[31]

These inconsistencies may be explained by the fact that the protein content of antivenin is different from that of the "normal horse serum" included in the package for use as the skin test agent.[34] Another explanation for falsenegative skin tests is that a certain percentage of these acute reactions are actually anaphylactoid in nature.[30] In any event, even in the presence of a negative skin test, patients should be observed closely for early adverse reactions during the antivenin infusion. Finally, the skin test should be performed only after it has been determined, on clinical grounds, that antivenin therapy is indicated.

If the victim is suffering from a severe envenomation, it is reasonable (although controversial) to omit skin testing altogether so that antivenin therapy can be initiated at least 20 minutes earlier than would be possible if the skin testing procedure were employed. The physician should be in attendance at the patient's bedside in order to intervene at the first sign of any adverse reaction.

Management of a patient who is found to be allergic to antivenin and also is suffering from a life-threatening envenomation requires skill and judgment. One approach to this difficult situation is outlined in *Table 6*.[6,31,35]

Wound Care and Management. Management of the involved extremity requires updating the victim's tetanus status, applying a dry, sterile dressing over the wound, and elevating the immobilized limb above heart level. These interventions are performed after antivenin, if indicated, has been administered. Prophylactic antibiotics are controversial, but are used by many physicians in all but the most minor bites.[6,8,36,37] Treatment with any broad-spectrum agent that covers gram-negative bacteria (the most abundant organisms in the oral cavities of snakes) is acceptable.[38]

Surgical Intervention. Controversy regarding medical vs. surgical approaches to snakebite management, to a large degree, has been resolved. In this regard, it is clear that snake venom poisoning is primarily a medical emergency, and that routine, early wound exploration, debridement, or fasciotomy is of no benefit.[5,12]

Despite this consensus, there are definite, albeit limited, indications for surgical intervention following viperid envenomation. While most pit viper bites result in venom deposition into subcutaneous tissues,[5] the fangs of larger snakes (especially rattlesnakes) are long enough to penetrate muscle compartments of the extremities. If significant amounts of venom are deposited in the deep tissues, intracompartmental swelling may result in a compartment syndrome. As expected, differentiating between intracompartmental and subcutaneous swelling may be difficult by exam alone. If there is suspicion of a developing compartment syndrome, pressures should be checked, and if found to be significantly elevated, surgical fasciotomy is indicated (along with antivenin administration). Fortunately, this procedure is required only in rare circumstances.[2,13,39]

Other surgical interventions that are of benefit in selected cases include debridement of necrotic tissue and blebs or vesicles 3-5 days post-envenomation[5] and delayed tissue grafting, when required.

Monitoring and Disposition

Victims of snake envenomation should be admitted to the hospital and observed in a closely monitored setting for at least 24 hours. Vital signs, urine output (including serial checks for hematuria), and extremity circumferences must be monitored carefully. Laboratory studies, including clotting times, CBC, and muscle enzyme assays, should be rechecked at least every six hours until vital signs suggest that the patient is stable.

The patient with an apparent dry bite should be observed for 6-8 hours.[40] After that time, if the victim is still asymptomatic and all laboratory studies and vital signs are normal, discharge to a reliable home environment is reasonable.

Coral Snake Bites

Domestic coral snakes are relatively shy creatures responsible for only about 20 reported bites each year.[41] Two subspecies (the eastern and Texas coral snakes; *Micrurus fulvius fulvius* and *M.f. tenere*, respectively) are found in the southeastern United States from North Carolina to Texas. A third species, the Arizona coral snake (*Micruroides euryxanthus*), is found in Arizona and New Mexico.[5]

These snakes possess a much less sophisticated venom apparatus than the viperids. With their small, anterior fangs, these snakes must hang onto their prey's tissue and chew for a brief period of time in order to inject significant quantities of their highly toxic venoms.[41] Coral snake venoms have little effect on local tissues, so signs at the bite site are minimal. Major clinical findings are systemic in nature and reflect the venom's curare-like effect on neuromuscular transmission.[42-44] The earliest findings can be delayed for many hours and consist of alteration in mental status and signs of cranial nerve dysfunction (e.g., diplopia).[45] Ultimately, peripheral muscle weakness, paralysis, and respiratory failure may ensue.[41]

Table 6. A Management Option for a Victim of Severe Snake Venom Poisoning Who Has a Serious Allergy to Equine Antivenin

- Establish invasive monitoring (arterial line and pulmonary arterial catheter)
- Expand intravascular volume with crystalloid or albumin if safe to do so
- Maximally premeditate with 1V antihistamines (H,- and HZ-blockers) and steroids (e.g., methylprednisolone 2 mg/kg up to 125 mg)
- Hang an epinephrine drip in a line separate from the antivenin (e.g., 1 mL of 1:l000 epinephrine in 500 mL diluent)
- Maximally dilute the antivenin (total volume dependent on the patient's ability to handle an intravascular volume load)
- Begin the antivenin very slowly
- If a systemic reaction occurs, stop infusion and begin the epinephrine drip (e.g., start at 0.25 mL/min and titrate for effect)
- Once a sympathetic response is evident and the allergic reaction is halted, restart the antivenin very slowly
- Titrate the antivenin drip against the epinephrine drip until the total dose of antivenin is given or the patient is stabilized

Management. First-aid measures should concentrate on getting the victim to medical care as soon as possible and supporting ventilation, as may be required. Initial hospital evaluation is sirnilar to that for victims of pit viper bites. A rapid history and physical examination must be performed while at least one IV line is established; cardiac and pulse oximetry monitoring are recommended. The paucity of local changes obviates the need for limb circumference measurements. Special attention must be paid to the victim's airway and respiration, inasmuch as respiratory paralysis represents the major threat to life.[46]

Routine laboratory tests are unlikely to be abnormal in otherwise healthy-appearing patients. Coagulopathy is not an expected finding? Arterial blood gas testing should be performed if there is any question of impending respiratory failure. It is vital to secure a definitive airway before a victim suffers a respiratory arrest.[46]

Definitive management relies on the use of the only other snake antivenin commercially available in the United States (Wyeth-Ayerst's North American Coral Snake Antivenin). It is recommended that antivenin be administered early in all victims of documented eastern or Texas coral snake bite, even in the absence of systemic signs or symptoms.[46,47] *(Please see Table 5.)* Once systemic abnormalities appear, they may progress rapidly and be difficult to treat, even with antivenin. This product is of no benefit for bites caused by the much less dangerous Arizona coral snake.[23]

The same precautions and adverse reactions associated with pit viper antivenin administration apply to coral snake antivenin. Victims who are likely to be allergic to this equine product (those who have a positive skin test) can probably be managed successfully with aggressive supportive care alone, including prolonged intubation and ventilator-y assistance if necessary.

Fortunately, there have been no deaths reported in the United States due to coral snake bites since the Wyeth-Ayerst antivenin became available,[5] although the mortality rate in untreated bites has been estimated at 10%.[41] There has never been a recorded death due to the Arizona coral snake.[48]

Exotic Venomous Snakebite

Due largely to their uniqueness and beauty, hobbyists have started to include exotic venomous species in their collections. Consequently, it is conceivable that emergency physicians may encounter a victim bitten by a cobra, mamba, or death adder, for example. Basic management principles are similar in these cases to those used in managing bites by indigenous U.S. snakes. The major difference is that an appropriate antivenin must be identified, located, and obtained. A regional poison control center or local zoo can be helpful in this regard.

Future Advances

Currently, there is significant ongoing research around the world in an effort to produce safer, more effective antivenins. In the United States, researchers have begun clinical trials using a sheep-derived antivenin that has been modified using F(ab) fragment technology. This product may prove much less allergenic and more effective than currently available commercial antivenins.[49]

Summary

While snakebite emergencies are relatively uncommon in this country, emergency physicians must be prepared to implement a systematic approach for managing these cases. If sound clinical judgment is used, appropriate supportive measures are aggressively instituted, and consultation with a snakebite expert is obtained in difficult cases, the chances for an excellent outcome for envenomation victims will be maximized.

References

1. Parrish HM. *Poisonous Snakebites in the United States*. 1st ed. New York: Vantage Press; 1980:l-469.
2. Grace TG, Omer GE. The management of upper extremity pit viper wounds. *J Hand Surg* 1980;5:168-177.
3. Parrish HM. Incidence of treated snakebites in the United States. *Pub Health Rep* 1966;81:269-276.
4. Parrish HM. Analysis of 460 fatalities from venomous animals in the United States. *Am J Med Sci* 1963;245:129-141.
5. Russell FE. *Snake Venom Poisoning*. 2nd ed. New York: Scholium International; 1983:l-562.
6. Wingert WA, Wainschel J. Diagnosis and management of envenomation by poisonous snakes. *South Med J* 1975;68: 1015-1026.
7. Russell FE, Puffer HW. Pharmacology of snake venoms. In: Minton SA ed. *Snake Venoms and Envenomation*. New York:

Marcel Dekker; 1971:87-98.

8. Van Mierop LHS. Poisonous snakebite: A review 1. Snakes and their venom. *J Fla Med Assoc* 1976;63:19 l-200.
9. Minton SA, Minton MR. Venomous Reptiles. New York: Charles Scribners Sons; 1969:1-274.
10. Russell FE, Carlson RW, Wainschel J, et al. Snake venom poisoning in the United States: Experiences with 550 cases. *JAMA* 1975;233:341-344.
11. Wingert WA. Poisoning by animal venoms. *Top Emerg Med* 1980;2:89-118.
12. Arnold RE. Controversies and hazards in the treatment of pit viper bites. *South Med J* 1979;72:902-910.
13. Nelson B K. Snake envenomation: Incidence, clinical presentation and management. *Med Toxicol* 1989;4:17-3 1.
14. Chugh KS, Pal Y, Chakravarty RN, et al. Acute renal failure following poisonous snakebite. *Am J Kidney Diseases* 1984;4:30-38.
15. Burgess JL, Dart RC, Egen NB, et al. Effects of constriction bands on rattlesnake venom absorption: A pharmacokinetic study. *Ann Emerg Med* 1992;21:1086-1093.
16. Stewart ME, Greenland S, Hoffman JR. First-aid treatment of poisonous snakebite: Are currently recommended procedures justified? *Ann Emerg Med* 1981;10:331-335.
17. Bronstein AC, Russell FE, Sullivan JB. Negative pressure suction in the field treatment of rattlesnake bite victims. *Vet Hum Toxicol* 1986;28:485.
18. Watt CH. Poisonous snakebite treatment in the United States. *JAMA* 1978;240:654-656.
19. Watt CH. Treatment of poisonous snakebite with emphasis on digit dermotomy. *South Med J* 1985;78:694-699.
20. Bucknall NC. Electrical treatment of venomous bites and stings. *Toxicon* 1991;29(4&5):397-400.
21. Schaeffer RC, Carlson RW, Puri VK, et al. The effects of colloidal and crystalloidal fluids on rattlesnake venom shock in the rat. *J Pharmacol Experi Therap* 1978;206:687-695.
22. Burgess JL, Dart RC. Snake venom coagulopathy: Use and abuse of blood products in the treatment of pit viper envenomation. *Ann Emerg Med* 1991;20:795-801.
23. Otten EJ. Antivenin therapy in the emergency department. *Am J Emerg Med* 1983;1:83-93.
24. *Physicians' Desk Reference*. 48th ed. Oradell, NJ: Medical Economics; 1995.
25. Russell FE, Lauritzen L. Antivenins. *Trans Royal Sot Trop Med Hyg* 1966;60:797-810.
26. McCollough NC, Gennaro JF. Evaluation of venomous snakebite in the southern United States from parallel clinical and laboratory investigations: Development of treatment. *J Fla Med Assoc* 1963;49:959-967.
27. Komalik F, Taborska E. Cross reactivity of mono- and polyvalent antivenoms with Viperidae and Crotalidae snake venoms. *Toxicon* 1989;27:1135-1142.
28. Wingert WA, Chan L. Rattlesnake bites in southern California and rationale for recommended treatment. *West J Med* 1988;148:37-44.
29. Sutherland SK. Serum reactions: An analysis of commercial antivenoms and the possible role of anticomplementary activity in de novo reactions to antivenoms and antitoxins. *Med J Aust* 1977;1:613-615.
30. Heilpem KL. The treacherous clinical spectrum of allergic emergencies: Diagnosis, treatment, and prevention. *Emerg Med Reports* 1994;15:211-222.
31. Jurkovich GJ, Luterman A, McCullar K, et al. Complications of Crotalidae antivenin therapy. *J Trauma* 1988;28: 1032-1037.
32. Stueven H, Aprahamian C, Thompson B, et al. Cobra envenomation: An uncommon emergency. *Ann Emerg Med* 1983; 12:636-638.
33. Griffen D, Donovan JW. Significant envenomation from a preserved rattlesnake head (in a patient with a history of immediate hypersensitivity to antivenin). *Ann Emerg Med* 1986;15:955-958.
34. Sullivan JB, Kulig K, Rumack BH, et al. Quantitative comparison of horse serum skin test, Wyeth Crotalidae Polyvalent Antivenin and a purified affinity gel column antivenin. *Vet Hum Toxicol* 1982;24(suppl):192.
35. Riffler E, Curry SC, Gerkin R. Successful treatment with antivenin of marked thrombocytopenia without significant coagulopathy following rattlesnake bite. *Ann Emerg Med* 1987; 16:1297-1299.
36. Russell FE. Prevention and treatment of venomous animal injuries. *Experientia* 1974;30:8-12.
37. Rush BM, McDonald JC, Liles DN. Snake bites in north Louisiana. *J La State Med Soc* 1987;139:37-40.
38. Goldstein EJC, Citron DM, Gonzalez H, et al. Bacteriology of rattlesnake venom and implications for therapy. *J Infect Dis* 1979;140:818-821.
39. Garfin SR. Rattlesnake bites: Current hospital therapy. *West J Med* 1982;137:411-412.
40. Hurlbut KM, Dart RC, Spaite D, et al. Reliability of clinical presentation for predicting significant pit viper envenomation. *Ann Emerg Med* 1988;17:438.
41. Parrish HM, Khan MS. Bites by coral snakes: Report of 11 representative cases. *Am J Med Sci* 1967;253:561-568.
42. Lee CY. Elapid neurotoxins and their mode of action. *Clin Toxicol* 1970;3:457-472.
43. Lee CY. Chemistry and pharmacology of polypeptide toxins in snake venoms. *Ann Rev Pharmacol* l972;12:265-286.
44. Chang CC. The action of snake venoms on nerve and muscle. In: Lee CY ed. *Snake Venoms.* New York: Springer-Verlag; 1979:309-376.
45. McCollough NC, Gennaro JF. Treatment of venomous snakebite in the United States. *Clin Toxicol* 1970;3:483-500.
46. Kitchens CS, Van Mierop LHS. Envenomation by the eastern coral snake (*Micrurus fulvius fulvius*): A study of 39 victims. *JAMA* 1987;258:1615-1618.
47. Russell FE, Banner W. Snake venom poisoning. In: Rake1 RE ed. *Conn's Current Therapy*. Philadelphia: WB Saunders; 1988:1002-1005.
48. Boyden TW. Snake venom poisoning: Diagnosis and treatment. *Aria Med* 1980;37:639-641.
49. Sullivan JB, Wingert WA, Norris RL. North American venomous reptile bites. In: Auerbach PS, ed. *Management of Wilderness and Environmental Emergencies*. 3rd ed. St. Louis: C.V. Mosby Co; 1995:680-709.

Marcel Dekker, 1979:79–98.
8. van Mierop LHS. Poisonous snakebite: A review. 1. Snakes and their venom. J Fla Med Assoc 1976;63:191–200.
9. Minton SA, Minton MR. Venomous Reptiles. New York: Charles Scribner's Sons, 1969:1–34.
10. Russell FE, Carlson RW, Wainschel J, et al. Snake venom poisoning in the United States: Experiences with 550 cases. JAMA 1975;233:341–344.
11. Wingert WA. Poisoning by animal venoms. Top Emerg Med 1980;2:89–118.
12. Arnold RE. Controversies and hazards in the treatment of pit viper bites. South Med J 1979;72:902–910.
13. Nelson BK. Snake envenomation: Incidence, clinical presentation and management. Med Toxicol 1989;4:17–31.
14. Chugh KS, Pal Y, Chakravarty RN, et al. Acute renal failure following poisonous snakebite. Am J Kidney Dis 1984;4:30–38.
15. Burgess JL, Dart RC, Egen NB, et al. Effects of constriction bands on rattlesnake venom absorption: A pharmacokinetic study. Ann Emerg Med 1992;21:1086–1093.
16. Stewart ME, Greenland S, Hoffman JR. First-aid treatment of poisonous snakebite: Are currently recommended procedures justified? Ann Emerg Med 1981;10:331–335.
17. Bronstein AC, Russell FE, Sullivan JB. Negative pressure suction in the field treatment of rattlesnake bite victims. Vet Hum Toxicol 1986;28:485.
18. Wood CR. Poisonous snakebite treatment in the United States. JAMA 1978;240:654–656.
19. Watt CH. Treatment of poisonous snakebite with emphasis on digit dermotomy. South Med J 1985;78:694–699.
20. [illegible] NC. Electrical [illegible] of venomous bites and stings. Toxicon 1991;29(2):[illegible].
21. Schaeffer RC, Carlson RW, Puri VK, et al. The effects of colloidal and crystalloidal fluids on rattlesnake venom shock in the rat. J Pharmacol Exp Ther 1978;206:687–695.
22. Burgess JL, Dart RC. Snake venom coagulopathy: Use and abuse of blood products in the treatment of pit viper envenomation. Ann Emerg Med 1991;20:795–801.
23. Otten EJ. Antivenin therapy in the emergency department. Am J Emerg Med 1983;1:83–93.
24. Physicians' Desk Reference. 48th ed. Oradell, NJ: Medical Economics, 1994.
25. Russell FE, Lauritzen L. Antivenins. Trans R Soc Trop Med Hyg 1966;60:797–810.
26. McCollough NC, Gennaro JF. Evaluation of venomous snakebite in the southern United States from parallel clinical and laboratory investigations: Development of treatment. J Fla Med Assoc 1963;49:959–967.
27. Kornalik F, Taborska E. Cross-reactivity of mono- and polyvalent antivenoms with Viperidae and Crotalidae snake venoms. Toxicon 1989;27(11):1135–1142.
28. Wingert WA, Chan L. Rattlesnake bites in southern California and rationale for recommended treatment. West J Med 1988;148:37–44.
29. Sutherland SK. Serum reactions: An analysis of commercial antivenoms and the possible role of anticomplementary activity in de-novo reactions to antivenoms and antitoxins. Med J Aust 1977;1:613–615.
30. Heikkinen EL. The treacherous clinical spectrum of allergic emergencies: Diagnosis, treatment, and prevention. Crit Care Nurs Clin North Am 1995;7(2):281–292.
31. Jurkovich GJ, Luterman A, McCullar K, et al. Complications of Crotalidae antivenin therapy. J Trauma 1988;28:1032–1037.
32. Stueven H, Aprahamian C, Thompson B, et al. Cobra envenomation: An uncommon emergency. Ann Emerg Med 1983;12:636–638.
33. Griffen D, Donovan JW. Significant envenomation from a preserved rattlesnake head (in a patient with a history of immediate hypersensitivity to antivenin). Ann Emerg Med 1986;15:955–958.
34. Sullivan JB, [illegible] et al. [illegible] Crotalidae Polyvalent Antivenom and [illegible] antibody. Vet Hum Toxicol [illegible].
35. Kitchens CS, [illegible]. Successful treatment with antivenin of [illegible] thrombocytopenia without significant coagulopathy following rattlesnake bite. Ann Emerg Med 1987;16:1297–1299.
36. Russell FE. Prevention and treatment of venomous animal injuries. Experientia 1974;30:8–12.
37. [illegible]
38. Goldstein EJC, Citron DM, Gonzalez H, et al. Bacteriology of rattlesnake venom and implications for therapy. J Infect Dis 1979;140:818–821.
39. [illegible]. Rattlesnake bites: Current hospital therapy. West J Med 1982;137:1–7.
40. Hurlbut KM, Dart RC, Spaite D, et al. Reliability of clinical presentation for predicting significant pit viper envenomation. Ann Emerg Med 1988;17:438.
41. Burgess JL, [illegible]. Rattlesnakes: Report of [illegible]. West J Med [illegible].
42. Lee CY. Elapid neurotoxins and their mode of action. Clin Toxicol 1970;3:457–472.
43. Lee CY. Chemistry and pharmacology of polypeptide toxins in snake venoms. Annu Rev Pharmacol 1972;12:265–286.
44. Chang CC. The action of snake venoms on nerve and muscle. In: Lee CY, ed. Snake Venoms. New York: Springer-Verlag, 1979:309–376.
45. McCollough NC, Gennaro JF. Treatment of venomous snakebite in the United States. Clin Toxicol 1970;3:483–500.
46. Kitchens CS, Van Mierop LHS. Envenomation by the Eastern coral snake (Micrurus fulvius fulvius): A study of 39 victims. JAMA 1987;258:1615–1618.
47. Russell FE, Dart RC. Snake venom poisoning. In: Haddad LM, Winchester JF, eds. Clinical Management of Poisoning and Drug Overdose. Philadelphia: WB Saunders, [illegible].
48. Gold BS, Wingert WA. Snake venom poisoning in the United States: A review of therapeutic practice. South Med J 1994;87:579–589.
49. Sullivan JB, Wingert WA, Norris RL. North American venomous reptile bites. In: Auerbach PS, ed. Wilderness Medicine: Management of Wilderness and Environmental Emergencies. 3rd ed. St. Louis: CV Mosby, 1995:680–709.

Part XIII

Trauma

Foreign Body Removal

Charles Stewart, MD, FACEP

Foreign body removal can be one of the most satisfying procedures performed by emergency physicians. The patient and the physician may both leave the emergency department (ED) with a feeling of accomplishment and satisfaction. Unfortunately, removal of a foreign body also can be a terrifying ordeal for the patient and frustrating for the physician. Unskilled attempts at removal, numerous repetitions of painful techniques, extended searches, improper instrumentation, and inadequate lighting all contribute to both patient and physician dissatisfaction.

Once a foreign body is identified in a wound, most patients will understand when told that elective removal outside of the ED setting may be the optimal course of treatment. What most patients will not understand, however, is being told that a foreign body is not present in a wound, only to find one later at the site of a wound infection. Failure to diagnose a foreign body in a wound has emerged near the top of successful malpractice actions against emergency physicians.[1]

How can we avoid this frustration for both patient and physician? As with most things in medicine, the answer often can be found when performing a careful history. Pertinent questions include: How did this happen? What was inserted? Where and when did it happen? With the answers to these questions, a guided and careful physical examination will result in the best plan for foreign body removal. This chapter covers many common foreign body scenarios.

Locating Foreign Bodies

Diagnosing a soft-tissue foreign body can be quite simple, or it can be exceptionally difficult. The mechanism of injury provides the first clue that a foreign body is present in the wound. If a history of injury is not present, the diagnosis will be delayed. Even small, seemingly superficial wounds should be investigated for foreign bodies. As one author notes: "No wound is too small to harbor a foreign body."[2]

A careful visual inspection of all puncture wounds is appropriate. This should be done under good lighting with careful exposure of the wound. Local anesthesia and an ischemic tourniquet may be appropriate in some situations. The physician may palpate a superficial foreign body in the wound with a surgical instrument. Useful signs that a foreign body is in the wound include sharp pain with palpation over the wound, pain on movement, or a mass in the wound.

It is important to remember that if a wound heals poorly or is particularly painful, it should also be investigated for a foreign body.[2] Antibiotics may temporarily improve an infection, but it will recur if the foreign body remains. Any wound infection that gets better with antibiotics only to return when the antibiotics are stopped should be considered to have a foreign body until proven otherwise.

Complications of a retained foreign body include pain, infection, peripheral nerve damage, vascular damage, and synovitis.[3-7] Of these, pain and infection are the most common complications.

Table 1. Equipment Necessary for Fishhook Removal

Gloves
Hemostat
Wire cutters
Scalpel with #11 blade
18-gauge needle
Skin prep materials
Dressing materials
Anesthesia equipment:
25-gauge needle
5 cc syringe
Local anesthetic of choice

Foreign body reactions are quite common and are most frequently caused by wooden splinters, nylon fibers, cactus bristles, plastics, or other materials.

All methods for detecting a superficial foreign body have limitations. Radiopaque objects can be discovered easily, localized, and removed with the aid of radiographs. A needle or paper clip can be used to localize the wound entrance prior to getting the radiograph.[8] Needles at right angles can create a reference plane to localize the foreign body.

One common misconception is that glass must contain lead in order to be visible on an x-ray. Glass was first shown to be visible on x-ray in 1932 by Lewis.[9] Numerous subsequent studies have completely confirmed this for all types of glass in pieces as small as 0.5 mm.[10-12] Glass is visible regardless of pigment content or source. Because almost all fragments of glass are visible on x-ray, an x-ray should be obtained whenever there is any suspicion of imbedded glass fragments.

Standard x-rays, computerized tomography, and xeroradiography are not particularly useful if the foreign body is not radiopaque. If the foreign body was recently introduced, then there may be some gas introduced within the wound. This may suggest a foreign body but cannot conclusively identify one. Thin sections with multiplane reformatting may enhance wood visibility on CT scan.[13]

Wood, in particular, is not easy to see on standard radiographs. Painted wood may occasionally be identified by the pigments in the paint. Cloth, plastic, foam from tennis shoes, spines, and cactus bristles are also difficult to see on an x-ray. These radiolucent foreign bodies may be suspected by deep soft-tissue thickening, swelling, or bony changes seen on the radiograph. Soft tissue gas that accompanies the foreign body may outline wood fragments, thorns, and spines.

The identification of these materials may be enhanced by use of techniques such as ultrasonography, xeroradiographs, and magnetic resonance imaging.[14,15] Of these, ultrasound may combine both reliability and lower cost. If a superficial foreign body is suspected but not detected on conventional radiographs, ultrasonography should be considered.

Xeroradiographs may be used to search for foreign bodies because the Xerox process will enhance the contrast between the foreign body and the surrounding tissue (edge enhancement). Wood, plastic, rubber, and graphite are more easily seen with the xeroradiogram than by plain films.[16-18]

CT scan is quite useful for locating objects and approximating size. A three-dimensional picture that shows the location may be generated and used to accurately locate the foreign body. Unfortunately, CT scanning is costly and delivers a high radiation dose.

Cutaneous Foreign Bodies

There are several basic requirements for successful removal of a soft-tissue foreign body. Lighting, adequate instruments, and appropriate anesthesia will aid in visualization. Appropriate hemostasis either by tourniquet or local vasoconstrictor will help greatly in the search. Before the wound is anesthetized or opened, the neurovascular status of the patient should be noted and documented.

The physician should set a time limit on searches so that both the patient and the physician will not degrade over time. About 20-30 minutes is appropriate and should suffice for an adequate exploration. After that time, further searching is not likely to be successful and often increases the likelihood of damage.

A standard suture kit with a scalpel is normally enough equipment to remove most foreign bodies in most locations. Tissue retractors and Metzenbaum scissors may be useful additions.

In general, the foreign body should be removed under direct visualization. Never blindly grab something in a wound with a hemostat. Vital structures may be damaged by this technique.

The wound should be explored with Metzenbaum scissors or a hemostat using a spreading technique. The scissors or hemostat is introduced into the incision, spread to open the tissues, and used to locate the foreign body. Scissors may be used to widen the incision to better see and remove the object. Incisions should usually be made transverse to the suspected foreign body rather than linearly.

If a foreign body is difficult to see or grasp or if the material stains the surrounding tissue, then a block dissection may be appropriate. In some cases, a deep elliptical incision around the wound entrance can remove both foreign body and contaminated tissue. This technique must avoid vital structures. It is quite suitable for highly contaminated and vegetable foreign bodies.

Following removal of the foreign body, the area should be thoroughly cleansed. High-volume and low-pressure irrigation are best to clean these wounds. Significantly contaminated wounds may be managed with delayed primary closure.

Fishhooks. Fishhook injuries are commonplace in both sport and commercial fishing. Fishhooks come in many different sizes and are either barbed along the shaft or free of barbs.[19] Treble hooks have three sets of barbs and hooks on the same shank, while double hooks have two. Many lures have one or two treble hooks attached.

There are many methods for removing fishhooks, which means that there is no single perfect method. The following methods have been tried with varying degrees of success. If the hook is in or near the eye, then an ophthalmology consult should be obtained. Make sure all necessary equipment for foreign body removal is available. *(Please see Table 1.)* Ensure that the other barbs in multiple-barbed lures are either protected with tape or removed before starting any of these techniques. It is inelegant to remove a fishhook only to have another hook on the lure imbedded in another part of the patient, a parent, or the physician. If the fisherman is worried about an expensive lure, remind him that the lure can be repaired at a good sporting goods store.

Clean the area surrounding the puncture wound with Betadine. Do not soak the area.

Local anesthesia is generally needed to aid the removal of a fishhook. The site of entry should be anesthetized with a small wheal of local anesthetic. For fingers, a digital block may be more appropriate.

Once the hook has been removed, the area should be re-cleaned and a topical antibiotic applied. Systemic antibiotics are not usually needed unless the hook has impaled tendon or cartilage or the wound is particularly large. Tetanus status should be evaluated and a booster given if appropriate. Advise the patient about the risk of infection and give appropriate instructions about wound care and to return if signs of infection develop.

String-Pull Technique. The string pull technique has been well-described in the literature.[20,23] It is fast, relatively painless, and carries a high rate of success.[24,25] Theoretically, no anesthesia is needed.

First, tie a string about two feet long to the hook at the curve of the hook. Push the hook shank down (towards the barb) parallel to the skin. This should disengage the barb from the tissue. Hold the other end of the string and pull the string away with a 30° angle to the skin. If the wrist is snapped away from the embedded site, the hook will also be snapped out.

The major disadvantage of this technique is the potential for a flying foreign body that can be impaled in the examiner, witnesses, or the patient. If the examiner hesitates during the removal process, then this technique can inflict considerable pain.

Advance-and-Cut Technique. The oldest technique in the literature is to advance the barb through the skin and then cut the barb off. It is probably best reserved for cases in which the barb is already visible through the skin or when another technique has failed.[20] If the patient has an imbedded barbed shank fishhook, this technique may also be the most appropriate.

Grasp the fishhook with a needle holder or pliers and push it through the skin. Cut the fishhook behind the barb and remove the rest of the hook back out the entrance wound in a retrograde fashion. Needless to say, for this technique, local anesthesia is recommended.

Needle-Cover Technique. In the needle-cover technique, the practitioner should insert about an 18-gauge needle along the tract of the entry wound. The needle should be placed to sheathe the barb of the hook so that it doesn't catch on tissue. Small strands of tissue may be incised with the sharp edge of the needle. With the barb covered by the needle, back the needle and hook out as one unit.

This method is relatively painless even without anesthesia and has a high rate of success. Advantages of this technique are that there is no potential for flying objects and little secondary damage results. It does require a bit more coordination than the other techniques.

Simple Retrograde Technique. Some authors describe the string technique without the string, calling it the streamside technique or simple retrograde technique.[28] Use the index finger to depress the tip of the hook and disengage the barb. The fishhook is removed by using gentle pressure on the shank of the fishhook while backing out the hook. This technique is only useful if the fishhook is superficial and the barb is not caught on fibers in the skin.

Cut It Out. If all of the other techniques fail or are inappropriate because they may endanger vital structures, the hook may be surgically removed with direct visualization of the wound. Direct exposure does allow for a complete irrigation of the wound tract. This may be important for some patients to lessen the possibility of infection.

Use a scalpel to extend a small incision from the entrance wound to the barb. Use scissors to bluntly spread and dissect tissue until the barb is directly visible. Grasp the tip of the hook with a hemostat and lift it out. Thoroughly irrigate the wound after removal of the object.

Table 2. Necessary Equipment for Ring Removal

WRAPPING TECHNIQUE
String, umbilical tape, or stout silk suture
KY jelly
Digital block equipment
RING-CUTTER TECHNIQUE
Ring cutter
Needle-nose pliers or needle holders (2)
GLASS RINGS
Diamond glass scoring tool for glass objects

Splinters. Simply pulling the end of a superficial protruding splinter may leave small shreds of wood. This technique is often tried prior to arrival in the ED. Wood is very reactive and will cause inflammation if left in place, so even small pieces of wood must be completely removed from soft tissue. Some woods, such as redwood and cedar, fragment quite easily. Wood that fragments will require extra effort to ensure that no small pieces are left behind.

If the wood is palpable beneath the skin, it may be more appropriate to make an incision along the axis of the splinter rather than to try to drag the splinter out through the entrance wound. After removal of the splinter, the tract can be thoroughly cleaned and any small remaining pieces extracted.

Splinters that are beneath a nail pose additional problems. If they are not completely removed, then an infection is quite likely. In some cases, this may mean that a small wedge-shaped segment is removed from the nail and the underlying splinter curetted out. This small segment may be removed by shaving the nail with a scalpel blade until the splinter is found. Alternatively, sharp scissors may be used to excise the portion of nail. When these procedures are used, a digital block of the finger may be quite helpful.

Sea Urchin Spines. Sea urchins are elongated or globular echinoderms that have a thin calcified shell and long spines. The spines are brittle and may impale the unwary diver or swimmer, breaking off during the process. The most common injury is a puncture wound from the spines, when the victim steps on, handles, or brushes against the sea urchin.

Some species of sea urchins have venom sacs on the tips of the spines. Sea urchin venom includes cholinergic substances, serotonin, proteases, and hemolysins. Symptoms of the envenomation include severe burning pain and discoloration. In those species with venom, systemic symptoms may include malaise, weakness, paresthesias, hypoesthesias, paralysis, arthralgias, aphonia, and, rarely, respiratory distress, hypotension, or death.[27] In most cases, the pain will subside somewhat in 1-2 hours; localized muscle weakness, if present, may persist for 4-6 hours.

Delayed secondary infections and indolent ulcerations are common following punctures. Secondary granuloma formation may occur two or more months after the original injury. A more diffuse

Figure 1. Wrapping Technique for Ring Removal

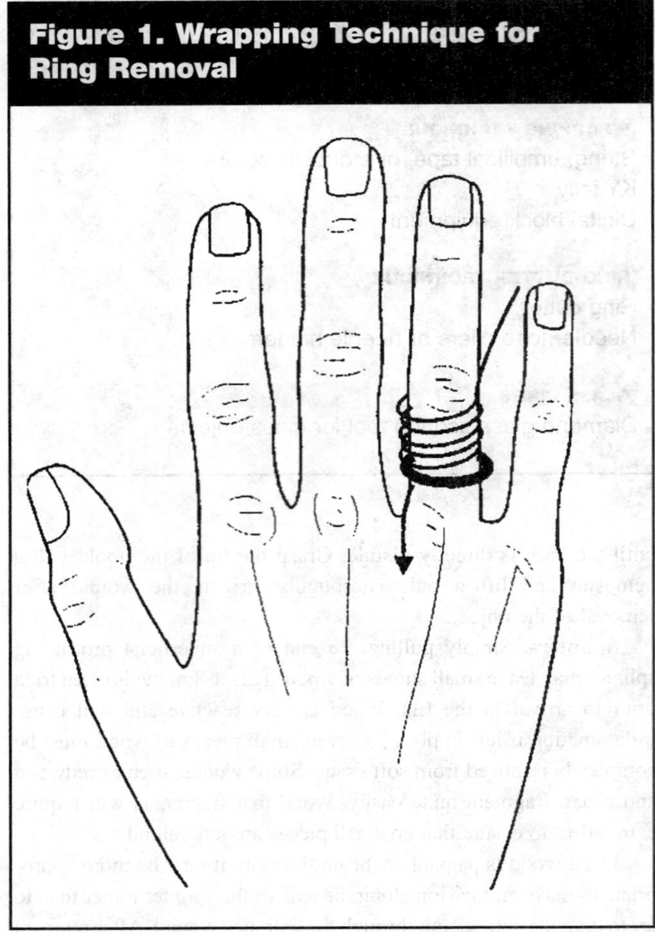

inflammatory process is often found in finger or toe lesions. Actual fusiform swelling and discoloration of the affected digit are noted.

Embedded spines should be removed if at all accessible. Radiographic localization of the spines should be accomplished before removal if possible. The spines are almost colorless and quite brittle. Use of operating microscopes and bloodless fields will greatly aid the removal process, particularly if the spine has entered a joint cavity or is in close proximity to neurovascular structures.

Some local "authorities" may recommend pounding the affected areas to break up the unremoved spines. This should be condemned as it increases the chances for foreign body reaction and infections. Subsequent removal of the spine fragments is far more difficult. A chronic inflammatory process resulting from the spine fragments in either hand or foot is disastrous.

Secondary granuloma formations should generally be excised, since there are few that heal spontaneously. Steroids injected into the granuloma are often recommended, but evidence is entirely anecdotal.

Hot water (110-115°F [43-46°C]) for 30-90 minutes will relieve the pain of the toxin. This therapy will inactivate heat-labile components of the venom and may reverse vasospasm from the toxin. Thorough cleansing of the wound is likewise beneficial in all cases.

Catfish Spines. Fish stings in fresh water are most often caused by catfish. The incidence is unknown, and most stings are probably not reported. Because catfish stings occur when the fish is handled or excited, they often involve the hands and arms.[28]

The venom apparatus is located in the anterior portion of the dorsal fin and the two pectoral fins, on a single spine in each location.[29] These spines are sharp, may have retroserrated teeth, and are fixed in the extended position when the fins are erected. Like the stingray's sting, these spines are enveloped in a sheath that encloses glandular toxin-producing tissues.

As the spine enters the skin, the enveloping sheath is ruptured. The venom-producing tissue is exposed and releases venom into the wound. The marine catfish is thought to have a more serious sting than the freshwater catfish, but this may be merely a factor of size.

The effects of catfish stings are comparable to a mild stingray envenomation. Variously described as stinging, burning, or throbbing, the pain is out of proportion to the small puncture wound usually found. The pain peaks in about 30 minutes, and small species may cause effects lasting only 2-3 hours. The wound generally has an ischemic, dusky margin that gradually resolves and progresses to a hyperemic reactive area about the site of the sting. Those species with recurved teeth may inflict significant lacerations.

Systemic effects include nausea, muscle spasm, sweating, and muscle fasciculations. Radicular pain in the affected limb is common. Rarely, and generally only with saltwater catfish stings, syncope, hypotension, respiratory distress, and death have been noted.[29,30]

Secondary infections are common, and lymphedema, lymphadenopathy, and lymphangitis may all be found. Localized necrosis due to infection may be seen in inadequately treated stings.

Hot water will inactivate the heat-labile toxin and will afford significant pain relief. Local infiltration of Lidocaine without epinephrine may also provide pain relief.

Radiographic identification and surgical exploration may be needed for removal of spine and investing sheath fragments. Primary closure of the wound is not recommended. Delayed primary closure may also afford the best cosmetic and surgical results.

Cactus Spines. The myriad visits for abrasions, scratches, and puncture wounds caused by plants are poorly documented. However, the perils of roses, brambles, briars, and cacti are well-known and documented in abundant folk literature. These thorns and spines may vary considerably in size, and the difficulty in removal is probably inversely proportional to the size of the object.

Best recorded in the literature is the trauma resulting from the spines of cacti.[27] These plants are ubiquitous in the Southwest. Cacti are also found as ornamental plants throughout cities, gardens, and homes. The typical patient will give a history of a fall from a ledge, horse, cross-country motorcycle, or all-terrain vehicle. Many patients will show up shortly after the fall, literally bristling with spines. Others will delay 7-10 days and present with multiple grouped pustular lesions, typically on the buttocks or lower extremities. Penetrations of thorns, spines, and cacti can lead later to an imbedded foreign body with subsequent foreign body granuloma.[31] These plant-induced granulomas must be differentiated from other causes of granulomatous disease by biopsy.

Usually, spines can be easily, but tediously, removed with forceps. Some physicians feel that these spines will be easier to remove a few days after the initial trauma, when a local reaction is present and the spines are more readily identified. For spines that are too fine to remove with forceps or splinter tweezers, apply rubber cement to the area.[27] Then immediately apply paper to the rubber cement. When the cement has hardened, the paper can be peeled off together with the spines. Alternatives that have been used include depilatory wax, commercial facial gels, and household glue.[32-35] Facial gels may require multiple applications in order to remove the spines.

Steroids will provide little relief for the foreign body reaction as long as the foreign body remains imbedded. Antibiotics should be reserved for areas of obvious infection.[36]

Rings

Injuries to the arm, hand, or the finger may cause swelling of fingers with rings on them. These injuries can include burns, lacerations, crush injuries, fractures, and bites. If the patient has an injury to the hand or arm, swelling of the finger should be anticipated and rings removed early in the patient's course. Rings that are somewhat tight may occlude venous flow and cause swelling, making ring removal quite difficult.

Remember that "rings" are not always jewelry and jewelry is not always gold, silver, or platinum. Children may try on pretty objects that look like rings, only to have difficulty removing them. "Pop-tops," in particular, have been used by children as jewelry. Some patients may use stainless steel for decoration, including rings. Ceramic-backed rings may be quite challenging to remove.

First lubricate the area with KY jelly and then try to remove the ring with a circular motion and traction on the ring. Elevation and cooling the involved digit for 10-15 minutes with either ice or very cold water may be of some help. If these simple techniques do not work, then it is time to try the string-wrap method or cut the ring off.

Wrapping Technique. About 15-20 inches of stout string, thin umbilical tape, or a thick silk suture must be passed under the ring.[37] *(Please see Table 2.)* A hemostat may be passed under the ring from the proximal side to grasp the wrapping.

The finger is then wrapped in spiral fashion from just proximal to the ring all the way past the distal interphalangeal joint. The wrap must be closely approximated so that no tissue bulges and the tissue is completely compressed beneath the wrap. The string is unwrapped by pulling on the proximal end and forcing the ring towards the end of the finger. *(Please see Figure 1.)*

This procedure may be painful and require a digital block. If there are injuries distal to the ring, the string technique is not appropriate. This technique results in varying degrees of success. It appears to work best on younger patients, when the size of the joint is close to the size of the digit. Severe arthritis may make the technique impossible. If the wrapping technique fails, do not continue to fruitlessly wrap and rewrap the finger.

Do not try to save a ring only to lose the digit. If the digit is ischemic, simply cut the ring off.

Ring-Cutter Technique. The quickest method of ring removal is to "simply" cut it off. *(Please see Table 2.)* For aluminum, pewter, and precious metal rings, this is quite simple. It becomes more difficult with copper, brass, or soft steel rings and may be very difficult with hardened steel washers used as rings. A standard ring cutter has a small hook that fits under the ring. This hook serves as a guide and tissue protector for a manual-powered saw wheel that cuts the metal. Select the thinnest site on the ring to cut (usually opposite stones or settings). Rotate this side away from any injury, if possible, or on the palmar surface of the ring. Spread the ring only enough to remove it without further trauma to the finger. A precious metal ring can be repaired if it is cut and removed in this manner.

Table 3. Equipment Necessary for Removal of Nasal Foreign Bodies

Topical anesthetic and decongestant
Light source
Suction tip
Right-angle hook
Curved forceps
Bayonet forceps
Nasal speculum
Alligator forceps
Nasopharyngeal mirror

Standard ring-cutter saws are designed for use on precious metals and simply do not cut hard metals well. Indeed, for some high-tensile-strength steel washers, only a diamond-backed hacksaw blade or a power tool will suffice (e.g., a Dremel Moto-tool operated at low speeds with a diamond-backed dental cutting tool). If the metal requires a hacksaw blade or power tool, be certain that the digit is padded and protected from slippage and from heat generated by friction. Allow plenty of time for cooling the object between cutting passes. Water cooling may be required in some cases to prevent burns. Although most textbooks will describe making only one cut, if a ring or washer of these harder metals is encountered, two cuts 180° apart are much more appropriate. Attempting to bend a high-tensile-strength washer or ring with a hemostat is a certain way to damage the hemostat and possibly both patient and physician as well.

Glass Rings. Ring cutters are also not effective for glass objects. *(Please see Table 2.)* Glass rings (and soda bottles) can be scored with a diamond cutter on two sides. A sharp rap with a small hammer will fracture the ring at the site of the score marks. Since the force vectors of this maneuver are away from the finger, no damage should result to the finger.

Zippers

The thin foreskin, abdominal skin, or vulva (rarely) may occasionally be caught in the mechanism of a zipper. This is exquisitely painful. If the zipper is unzipped, more tissue may be caught in the mechanism and the skin may be lacerated.

Using a bone cutter or pair of wire clippers, zippers are most easily removed by cutting the zipper "diamond" or median bar that holds the slider together. When this is done, the zipper will fall apart.

Ticks

A variety of plans, substances, and tools have been devised to aid in removing a tick, but with millions of years of evolution perfecting staying attached to moving animals, it is not surprising that the tick frequently remains attached despite our efforts.

The tick's mouth parts consist of two retractile jaws, a pair of short appendages (palps), and a central probe with recurved teeth (the hypostome). These structures are attached to a plate called the capitulum.[27] The tick attaches to the host with its mouth parts, which not only are imbedded in the skin but are also glued into place with a cement-like secretion. The tick can voluntarily detach from its host,

Table 4. Removal of Ear Foreign Bodies

NECESSARY EQUIPMENT
Light source (at a minimum an operating head otoscope)
Operating microscope if possible
Suction tips of various sizes (one with soft flexible funnel tip if possible)
Right-angle hook
Wire loop ear curette
Curved forceps
Alligator forceps (alternative Bayonet forceps)
Super glue
Microscope oil
COMPLICATIONS
Perforation of the tympanic membrane
Auditory canal lacerations
Ossicular bone damage

but when forced off, it may leave the capitulum and attached mouth parts imbedded in the skin. As long as the mouth parts are attached to the patient, the patient remains at risk for tick-borne illnesses.

There is no completely effective method for removal of ticks. One author evaluated five popular methods of removing ticks and concluded that the tick would best be removed by grasping the tick close to the skin and exerting a steady, even pressure.[38] However, grasping the body of the tick with fingers, forceps, or tongs and then pulling it off may leave the mouth parts behind. Likewise, twisting or jerking the tick may cause the mouth parts to break off. When the tick is grasped, the squeeze may inject additional saliva and more microorganisms through the mouth parts. Crushing or puncturing the body of the tick may release additional infective agents with the tick's body fluids. One author freezes the tick with ethyl chloride and then removes it with forceps to decrease the risk of injection.[39]

Common folk remedies include application of heat or organic solvents to the tick's body. Application of a lit match, cigarette, or cautery to the tick body will occasionally cause the tick to back out of the skin, but it is more likely to cause burns to the victim. Application of an organic solvent, such as chloroform, ether, gasoline, or fingernail polish, may also cause the tick to disengage itself, but it is more likely to result in the death of the tick. Needless to say, do not use a cautery or flame after application of such substances.

Finally, dead ticks (most often seen after one of the above methods has been tried and failed) should be removed by surgical excision of a small portion of the skin in order not to leave any mouth parts remaining. This can be done with an 18-gauge needle used as a scalpel.

Fingers should not be used to handle the tick or squeeze the tick, since tick feces and body fluids can also be contaminated. Gloves should always be worn.

Nasal Foreign Bodies

A multitude of various objects have been found in the nose. Common objects inserted in the nose include beans, corn, beads, buttons, paper wads, marbles, crayons, peas, sponges, and small toys. Almost all nasal foreign bodies are smooth, since rough, irregular, sharp objects are painful to insert. Objects such as beans, corn, peas, and paper swell when wetted by nasal secretions, which may make removal more difficult. Button batteries may cause caustic local tissue damage.[40,41] In warmer climates, many insects and larvae will attempt to set up residence in the patient's nose. Some of these animals can cause extensive tissue destruction.

Children with nasal foreign bodies frequently present with unilateral rhinorrhea. Initially, the discharge may be thin, serous, and without smell. It progresses to a foul-smelling mucopurulent discharge. Secondary infection may produce halitosis. Nasal foreign bodies are generally painless, so parents may detect no other signs or symptoms. If the history from the parents or child does not suggest the cause, looking in the nose often answers the question. Swelling and edema of the nose may be found. The swelling of the surrounding tissues may obstruct the nose or lead to sinusitis. If an insect is the foreign body, pain is more marked.

It is uncommon to see a child less than 18 months with a foreign body inserted into the nose due to lack of sufficient dexterity to insert the object. Older children (up to 5 or 6) often don't divulge the presence of these objects immediately because they fear parental retribution. Multiple foreign bodies are quite common.

Adult patients with nasal foreign bodies are much less common. Patients with a mental disorder may revert to this childhood behavior. Patients who are sniffing may get more than they bargain for in the process. Some patients who inhale sharply while snorting cocaine may get the coke spoon in the nose.

The single biggest clue to diagnosis of a nasal foreign body is a unilateral nasal discharge or obstruction. Indeed, if this is found, the patient should be considered to have a nasal foreign body until proven otherwise. The diagnosis is usually made by inspection of the nares. The most common location of the foreign body is adjacent to the inferior turbinate and below the middle turbinate. Examination of the posterior nasopharynx with a mirror may be appropriate but is difficult in children. Radiographs of the nose are often recommended but are more helpful in checking for surrounding sinusitis. X-rays are of little value when radiolucent foreign bodies (i.e., crayons, paper, food items) are noted, and these are the most common items found.

A patient with a foreign body in the nose is at risk for aspiration of that foreign body, so the problem must not be approached as casually as for a foreign body in the ear. The object must be removed. *(Please see Table 3.)* In truly uncooperative patients, endotracheal intubation and general anesthesia will ensure that aspiration does not occur.

Prior to removal of the foreign body, apply a decongestant such as topical phenylephrine and tetracaine, or Afrin nasal spray. This decreases the chances of blood obscuring the field and makes the removal much easier. Often the foreign body can be quite easily visualized after decongestant use.

The key to successful removal on the first pass is reassurance and adequate immobilization of the patient, good lighting, and use of appropriate instruments. A good headlamp is essential and an operating microscope with integral illumination is ideal. A variety of sizes of nasal speculums should be readily available.

A small nasal speculum should be used to spread the nares in order to see the object. Slow and gentle motions, together with abundant "verbal" anesthesia, are needed for the 18-month- to 5-year-old patient. If the foreign body is small, then a small alligator forceps can remove it easily. A hemostat may be useful to remove hard, rounded objects. A soft-tipped suction catheter can also be used for soft, rounded foreign bodies. Suction may be needed to remove excessive mucous or pus and may easily remove food items.

Other techniques that have been successfully employed include passing a Fogarty catheter above the foreign body, inflating the balloon, and tugging the foreign body out of the nose.[42,43] A small Foley catheter can also be used for the same technique. It is very important to ensure that the catheter neither wedges the foreign body further into the nose nor pushes it into the nasopharynx. A small right-angle blunt hook or a loop ear curette may be passed beyond the object and then turned to engage the object.[44] A calcium alginate swab (Calgiswab) bent to a 90° angle near the tip can be used as a field expedient for a right-angle blunt hook.[44]

For smaller children, parental positive pressure has been used quite successfully.[45,46] Have the parent push gently on the opposite side of the nose to occlude the nares, and place a gauze loosely over the unoccluded area. Have the parent puff gently into the patient's mouth. The positive pressure will make the foreign body pop out and the gauze will prevent the foreign body from hitting the parents face.

Ensure (and do not be terribly surprised) that multiple foreign bodies are not present. After the removal, bleeding may occur. This can be treated in the usual fashion for epistaxis. Residual inflammation of the nasal membranes will clear spontaneously over a few days. A follow-up visit in 2-3 days may be appropriate.

A significant potential complication is dislodging the object into the posterior pharynx resulting in subsequent aspiration. Bronchoscopy will be required in these cases to remove the object. Swallowing the object is usually harmless (button batteries are an exception). Mucosal lacerations can occur when attempting removal in an uncooperative child. Foreign bodies that are present for an extended time can erode into contiguous soft tissues, cause infections including sinusitis and otitis media, and serve as a nidus for formation of rhinoliths (nasal stones).[47]

If the foreign body cannot be removed easily, then an otolaryngologist should be consulted. Multiple attempts to remove a foreign body may result in both a difficult patient and an exasperated parent. Beans, corn, and other vegetable matter may swell with the nasal fluids and become very difficult to remove, even with anesthesia and an operating microscope. Animate foreign bodies may require curettage under anesthesia.

Ear Foreign Bodies

Foreign bodies in the external auditory canal are also quite common, but auricular foreign bodies are an entirely different matter than intranasal objects. The exact incidence of auricular canal foreign bodies is not known. Adult patients will usually be able to identify the foreign body and tell the examiner exactly when it was introduced. Children are often unable or unwilling to give any history at all. The event may be unnoticed, and the presentation may be a purulent discharge from the affected ear. If the patient has a perforated tympanic membrane, then bleeding, hearing loss, vertigo, or discharge from the ear may be noted.[48] The most common objects inserted in ears by children have been pebbles, beans, beads, corn, small toys, and folded pieces of paper.[49] Button batteries are the right size for insertion and may cause caustic damage to the canal and tympanic membrane.[50]

Foreign bodies in the ear can be extremely challenging to the emergency physician. Over 80% of foreign bodies can probably be removed by the emergency physician with readily available techniques.[51] Methods and equipment that have been used successfully include forceps removal, irrigation, suction, ear curettes, right-angle hooks, Fogarty catheters, magnets, and super glue. The least aggressive and invasive method should be attempted first. *(Please see Table 4.)*

The emergency physician should avoid aggressive or hurried attempts to remove foreign bodies. Particularly with children, a methodical, unhurried, and planned approach is essential to retain the child's cooperation. Emergency removal of foreign bodies in uncooperative children is necessary only if there are signs of obvious infection, disc batteries, and insects. An operating microscope and optimal sedation may be needed for some foreign bodies. Permanent damage to the ossicles or tympanic membrane can result from pushing the object further into the canal. Multiple attempts at removal are inappropriate. If the foreign body cannot be removed easily, then an otolaryngologist should be consulted.

The size, shape, and material of the foreign body have a large influence in the method of removal of the foreign body. Most foreign bodies will be located at the juncture of the bony and cartilaginous auricular canal. This means that the object will be in the outer two-thirds of the canal and away from the tympanic membrane. Smaller objects and insects may be directly against the sensitive tympanic membrane.

Attempt removal only under good lighting with direct visualization of the object. An operating microscope is ideal, and an operating head on an otoscope is minimal. Operating auricular speculums in various sizes and a head lamp are an appropriate compromise between cost and effectiveness.

Grossly assess the hearing both before and after removal of the object if at all possible. Ensure that there is only one foreign body.

Warn the patient or parents to avoid water both before and after removal of the foreign body. This is particularly important with vegetable materials such as beans, peas, and corn. Wetting these can cause them to swell or sprout and markedly increase the potential damage.

The patient's head should be stabilized during the procedure to prevent inadvertent movement while the examiner has an instrument near the tympanic membrane. An assistant or nurse should stabilize the patient's head. Hold the instruments loosely between thumb and forefinger while the tools are within the ear canal. If the patient does move, the loose grip will allow the instrument to move with the motion of the patient. Rigid instruments should be used with great caution in uncooperative patients. If the patient moves suddenly, the instrument can damage the middle ear structures.[52]

The cutaneous lining of the ear canal is quite sensitive rendering topical anesthetics of little use. Although many texts describe anesthesia techniques to remove foreign bodies in the ear, these techniques can be quite painful. There is little to be gained from this anesthesia over standard methods of conscious sedation, if such is required.

Insects. Insects are an interesting challenge. The movement, buzzing of the wings, and occasionally stinging or biting make these foreign bodies exceptionally irritating. Patients will often arrive panic-stricken to the ED. Commonly, immobilization of the insect is advocated to decrease these motions and to facilitate removal of the insect. Insects may be effectively immobilized with mineral oil, acetone, alcohol, or xylocaine.[53,54] Highly refined mineral oil is readily available in most hospitals as microscope immersion oil. Insects may fragment during removal, and irrigation may be the quickest way to get them out.

For patients who call and ask advice about this problem, baby oil and vegetable oil are readily available in many households. These are functionally equivalent to mineral oil and kill the insect en route to the ED. This markedly decreases the patient's suffering and expedites removal in the ED.

Removal. Small objects may be easily removed with forceps. Large objects should not be removed with forceps. As the forceps are advanced, the conical bony ear canal will cause them to close. Unless there is a protrusion on the object, this closure will likely push the object further into the bony canal. Beads with a hole may be grasped by putting an alligator forceps into the hole of the bead and spreading the end. Irrigation may be suitable for multiple small bodies, but the examiner must be certain that there is no perforation of the tympanic membrane.

Smooth, rounded objects can sometimes be removed using a small plastic suction catheter with a soft funnel-shaped tip. This greatly aids removal of the object. Small children may balk at the loud noise that this device makes, but it is easy to demonstrate that no harm will ensue. A similar device can be made by inserting a tympanostomy tube in the tip of a number 7 Frazier suction tube.[55]

A thin right-angle hook may be introduced gently and slowly around the object. The hook may be rotated behind the foreign body and traction applied. In a similar technique, a Fogarty catheter may be slid behind the object, the balloon inflated, and the catheter used for traction on the object. With the very small space within the ear canal, this may be dangerous to the tympanic membrane and quite painful if the balloon is overinflated.

Another technique that has not been extensively studied but shows promise is to affix the object with super glue.[56] A small drop of cyanoacrylate cement (super glue) is placed on the blunt end of a cotton swab. The stick is carefully introduced into the ear canal. No contact with the ear canal should be made. The stick is touched to the object and held in place for a minute. When the stick is removed, the object should be attached.

Do not attempt removal of an impacted smooth foreign body in an uncooperative child. Foreign bodies that are round and fit snugly into the canal can be quite difficult to remove under the best of circumstances with the best tools in a completely cooperative patient. The emergency physician will not help a fighting 2-year-old child by attempting to dig out a bead with inadequate tools under suboptimal lighting. Simply inform the parents that this object will best be removed under anesthesia by an otolaryngologist.

Summary

Using careful techniques, most foreign bodies can be removed successfully in the ED setting. Proper equipment and ancillary support are critical to the success of such endeavors. Some foreign bodies, however, cannot and should not be removed by the emergency physician without the support of professional colleagues. Maintaining the best interests of the patient in mind, the above guidelines can optimize not only patient satisfaction but also patient care.

References

1. Anonymous. Clinically and clinicolegally relevant: The problem of the glass foreign body. *Emerg Med Notes* 1991;4:1.
2. Anderson MA, Newymeyer WL, Kilgore ES. Diagnosis and treatment of retained foreign bodies in the hand. *Am J Surg* 1982;144:63.
3. Cutler CW. Injuries of the hand by puncture wounds and foreign bodies. *Surg Clin North Am* 1941;4:485-493.
4. Barnett JP, Fiddian NJ. Delayed median nerve injury due to retained glass fragments. *J Bone Joint Surg* 1985;67:382-384.
5. Cohen MA. False (traumatic) aneurysm of the facial artery caused by a foreign body. In: *J Oral Maxillofac Surg* 1986; 15:336-338.
6. Klein B, McGahan JP. Thorn synovitis. CT diagnosis. *J Comput Assist Tomogr* 1985;9:1135-1136.
7. Shah AS, Coldiron BM. Foreign-body granuloma due to an unsuspected wooden thorn. *Am Fam Physician* 1992;45: 673-674.
8. Anonymous. Embedded objects in perspective. *Emerg Med Clin North Am* 1985;3:104-105.
9. Lewis RW. A roentgenographic study of glass and its visibility as a foreign body. *Am J Roentgenol* 1932;27:853.
10. Couter BJ. Radiographic screening for glass foreign bodies—What does a "negative" foreign body series really mean. *Ann Emerg Med* 1990;19:997.
11. Pond GD, Lindsey D. Localization of cactus, glass, and other foreign bodies in soft tissues. *Ariz Med* 1977;34:700.
12. Tandberg D. Glass in the hand and foot: Will an x-ray film show it? *JAMA* 1982;248:1872.
13. Pyhtinen J, Ilkko E, Lahde S. Wooden foreign bodies in CT: Case reports and experimental studies. *Acta Radiol* 1995;36: 148-151.
14. Ginsberg MJ, Ellis GL, Flom L. Detection of soft-tissue foreign bodies by plain radiography, xeroradiography, computed tomography, and ultrasonography. *Ann Emerg Med* 1990;19:710-703.
15. Mizel MS, Steinmetz ND, Trepman L. Detection of wooden foreign bodies in muscle tissue: Experimental comparison of computed tomography, magnetic resonance imaging, and ultrasonography. *Foot Ankle Int* 1994;15:437-442.
16. Woesner ME, Sanders I. Xeroradiography. A significant modality in the detection of non-metallic foreign bodies in soft tissues. *Am J Roentgenol* 1972;115:636-640.
17. Bowers DG, Lynch JB. Xeroradiography for non-metalling foreign bodies. *Plast Reconstr Surg* 1977;60:470-471.
18. De Flaviis L, Scaglione P, Del Bo P, et al. Detection of foreign bodies in soft tissues: Experimental comparison of ultrasonography and xeroradiography. *J Trauma* 1988;28: 400-404.
19. Lantsberg L, Blintsovsky E, Hoda J. How to extract an indwelling fishhook. *Am Fam Physician* 1992;45:2589-2590.
20. Jastremski MS. Fishhook removal. In: Jastremski Ms, Dumas M, Penalver L, eds. *Emergency Procedures.* Philadelphia: WB Saunders; 1992:127.
21. Graham P. Removal of embedded fishhook. *Aust Fam*

Physician 1995;24:691.

22. Friedenberg S. How to remove an imbedded fishhook in 5 seconds without really trying. *N Engl J Med* 1971;284:733.
23. Barnett RC. Removal of fishhooks. *J Hosp Med* July 1980.
24. Doser C. Cooper WL, Ediger WM. Fishhook injures: A prospective evaluation. *Am J Emerg Med* 1991;9:413-415.
25. Anonymous. A few ways to unsnag a fishhook. *Emerg Med* 1981;13:22. Editorial.
26. Anonymous. To get a fisherman off the hook. *Emerg Med* 1992;24:179.
27. Stewart CE. Marine bites and stings. In: *Environmental Emergencies.* Baltimore: Williams & Wilkins; 1990.
28. Scoggin CH. Catfish stings. *JAMA* 1975;231:176-177.
29. Halstead BW, Vinci JM. Venomous fish stings (Ichthyoacanthotoxicoses). *Clin Dermatol* 1987;5:29-35.
30. Ratzan RM, Correia CJ, Cardoni AA. Poisoning by marine life: Recognizing and treating water-related stings and bites. *Consultant* 1983;23:29-41.
31. Epstein WL. Plant-induced dermatitis. *Ann Emerg Med* 1987;16:950-955.
32. Putnam MH. Simple cactus spine removal. *J Pediatr* 1981;98: 333.
33. Martinez TT, Jerome M, Barry RC, et al. Removal of cactus spines from the skin: A comparative evaluation of several methods. *Am J Dis Child* 1987;141:1291.
34. Schunk JE, Corneli HM. Cactus spine removal. *J Pediatr* 1987;110:667.
35. Lindsey D, Lindsey WE. Cactus spine injuries. *Am J Emerg Med* 1988;6:362.
36. Karpman RR, Sparks RP, Fried M. Cactus thorn injuries to the extremities: Their managment and etiology. *Ariz Med* 1980;37:849.
37. Smith R. Emergency ring removal. In: Jastremski M, Cantor R, Olson C, et al, eds. *The Whole Emergency Medicine Catalog.* Philadelphia: WB Saunders; 1985:365.
38. Needham GR. Evaluation of five popular methods for tick removal. *Pediatrics* 1985;75:997-1002.
39. Kumar RP. Tick trick. *Consultant* 1987;27:80. Letter.
40. Palmer O, Natarajan B, Johnstone A, et al. Button battery in the nose—An unusual foreign body. *J Laryngol Otol* 1994; 108:871-872.
41. Brown CRS. Intranasal button battery causing septal perforation: A case report. *J Laryngol Otol* 1994;108: 589-590.
42. Fox JR. Fogerty catheter removal of nasal foreign bodies. *Ann Emerg Med* 1980;9:37-38.
43. Nandapalan V, McIlwain JC. Removal of nasal foreign bodies with a Fogarty biliary balloon catheter. *J Laryngol and Otol* 1994;108:758-760.
44. Rudjinski M. A few brief tips: Nasal foreign bodies. *J Am Acad Phys Assist* 1990;3:156-157.
45. Stool SE, McConnel CS. Foreign bodies in pediatric otolaryngology: Some diagnostic and therapeutic pointers. *Clin Pediatr* 1973;12:113-116.
46. Backlin SA. Positive-pressure technique for nasal foreign body removal in children. *Ann Emerg Med* 1995;25:554-555.
47. Werman HA. Removal of foreign bodies of the nose. *Emerg Clin North Am* 1987;5:253-263.
48. Fritz S, Kelen GD, Sivertson KT. Foreign bodies of the external auditory canal. *Emerg Med Clin North Am* 1987;5: 183-192.
49. Virnig R. Nontraumatic removal of foreign bodies from the nose and ears of infants and children. *Minn Med* 1972;55: 1123.
50. Rachlin S. Assault with battery. *N Engl J Med* 1984;311: 921-922.
51. Baker MD. Foreign bodies of the ears and nose in childhood. *Pediatr Emerg Care* 1987;3:67-70.
52. Davidson BJ. Morris MS. The perforated tympanic membrane. *Am Fam Physician* 1992;45:1777-1782.
53. Leffler S, Cheney P, Tandberg D. Chemical immobilization and killing of intra-aural roaches: An in vitro comparative study. *Ann Emerg Med* 1993;22:1795-1798.
54. O'Toole K, Paris PM, Stewart RD, et al. Removing cockroaches from the auritory canal: Controlled trial. *N Engl J Med* 1985;312:1197. Letter.
55. Morris M, New device for foreign body removal. *Laryngoscope* 1984;94:980.
56. Pride H, Schwab R. A new technique for removing foreign bodies of the external auditory canal. *Pediatr Emerg Care* 1989;5:135-136.

Part XIV

Legal, Social, and Ethical Issues

Primary Care Medicine Medical/Ethical Issues

Brian P. Schwartz, MD
James J. Londis

Along with the explosion in medical science has come a similar explosion in ethical issues. The advances in medical science have engendered a corresponding increase in the ethical dilemmas facing physicians today. Additionally, the general public and special interest groups have become much more involved in these issues as medicine becomes less paternalistic and patients demand more autonomy and input into decision-making. This chapter, co-authored by an ethicist and a physician, examines the principles underlying ethical decision-making by practitioners and offers a practical guideline in dealing with ethical issues that face the clinician.

Introduction

The public holds physicians to a moral standard for their work that often exceeds legal requirements. As anyone knows from Ethics 101, the moral and the legal are different. Slavery, for example, was once legal in the United States even though it was immoral. Women were legally kept from voting for centuries, even though we would now acknowledge the evil of that prohibition. Physicians—whose life-and-death decision-making profession exposes them to enormous risks—must also distinguish between the legal and the ethical in their practice. As we have seen in recent years, some physicians are willing to challenge the law on certain issues because they believe the law is immoral. This article should help clinicians be more ethically aware in their treatment of their patients.

Case #1: A 34-year-old female has been under your care for the last 10 years. For the last three years, she has been fighting metastatic breast cancer. Despite her being on chemotherapy and hormonal therapy, recent scans indicate that the cancer has spread to her liver. She now asks you whether anything else can be done. You think about the possibility of further therapy with a bone morrow transplant but quickly realize that her HMO will not cover experimental therapies. Furthermore, you know that the chances of success with that therapy are marginal. Do you tell her about this option? Or, do you simply reassure her that every reasonable option has been tried?

Case #2: A 42-year-old male comes into your office complaining of no urine output for the last 24 hours. Three days ago, he was in your office with a muscle strain in his shoulder. At that time, you gave him an injectible non-steroidal medication. The blood work that you obtained in the office reveals creatinine levels of 3.4, and you suspect interstitial nephritis caused by the non-steroidal medication. Do you now tell him that the deterioration in his kidney function might be due to the medication that you prescribed several days before? Or, realizing that this may be self-limited, do you simply advise him to

Table 1. Glossery of Terms

- **Advance Directives**—Directions from a patient or surrogate to health care workers. They include living wills, durable powers of attorney for health care, and medical directives.
- **Bioethics**—The application of moral principles, rules, and reflection to medical care and research.
- **Descriptive Ethics**—The attempt to simply describe how individuals and groups make ethical and moral decisions and what behaviors they believe are consistent with their moral and ethical norms.
- **Do Not Resuscitate (DNR)**—More properly termed DNAR (do not *attempt* resuscitation) in the hospital chart which instructs medical personnel that if the patient's heart stops or if he stops breathing, no cardiopulmonary resuscitation should be performed. This order should only be put in charts after consultation with the patient or his surrogate.
- **Durable Power of Attorney for Health Care (DPAH)**—An advance directive that names a specific surrogate to make health care decisions for a patient if he is unable to do so.
- **Ethics Committee**—A representative and varied committee in any health care institution whose charter includes the development and review of ethically significant policies, the education of hospital staff on ethical matters, and the provision of services to resolve ethical disputes involving caregivers and their families. Such services may come in the form of a trained ethics consultant, a small subcommittee of the ethics committee, or the committee as a whole. Such committees are almost always advisory only.
- **Futility**—A patient so ill that, in the opinion of the attending physician, further medical treatment will almost certainly not improve the patient's situation and may cause needless discomfort or suffering. It is generally acknowledged that physicians have the right to refuse to continue treating a patient they believe cannot be helped any longer if their patient will be accepted by another physician.
- **Informed Consent**—The patient is provided all the relevant information regarding the risks and benefits of a particular procedure, gives evidence he understands them, and voluntarily agrees to undergo the procedure. Any physician who performs an invasive procedure in a nonemergency situation without the patient's (or appropriate surrogate's) consent commits legal "battery."
- **Living Will**—An advance directive instructing health care workers that in the event the patient cannot make decisions for himself, only certain actions may or may not be taken.
- **Normative Ethics**—Ethical reflection that deals with what we "ought" to do or not do in relation to our system of values. Unlike descriptive ethics, which merely describes, normative ethics "prescribes."
- **Surrogate**—Someone who makes decisions for another person. Such an individual is designated through a court, a statute, a common practice, or an advance directive.

come in for follow-up lab tests in hopes that this will resolve without causing further problems?

While the above cases are straightforward and unlikely to cause a major moral dilemma for most physicians, they do illustrate that physicians daily confront ethical issues. The principles that apply to straightforward cases will also help the physician address more complex ones.

A final case illustrates that an ethical dilemma may occur not with the physician but with the patient. For that reason, physicians also need to be adept at counseling and advising their patients who face their own ethical dilemmas.

Case #3: A 49-year-old Caucasian male presents to your office with penile discharge. A slide made of the discharge confirms that he has a chlamydia infection. You counsel him that he should inform his wife, as she may also need treatment. He confides in you that he has not had relations with his wife in several months but has been seeing a friend from work. He asks that you not tell his wife, who is also a patient in your practice and who is scheduled for an appointment in two weeks. What are your obligations to this man and his wife, both of whom are your patients? What counsel would you give to help him make the right decision in this dilemma?

As you read these cases typical of situations that confront the primary care physician, what mental steps did you take? What kind of reasoning did you employ to work through the issues? Did you start with the facts and details of the cases and then work toward a solution based on your general understanding of the moral atmosphere of our culture? Were you concerned more with the consequences than with the nature of the action itself? If so, you employed the kind of moral reasoning we call casuistry and may have employed a utilitarian method in your approach. Casuistry is an inductive approach that starts from the concrete facts of a case in the context of the moral rules people ordinarily use to make ethical decisions. It is not reasoning from general norms to particular cases. Using this approach, you would carefully weigh whether informing the female in case #1 about a bone marrow transplant would be appropriate given the facts of her case, her current feelings about her treatment, and the quality she wanted to have in the life remaining to her. There might be reason not to tell her about the bone marrow transplant option, although, even if it was hopelessly beyond her financial reach, we suspect that most physicians would mention it. Or, the physician might consider advocating on behalf of the patient with her insurance company, pressuring it to support this protocol.

Or, did you start with a theory of morality that would be applied to the facts? For example, if you assumed that every action is right or wrong in its own nature ("it is always wrong to lie, break a promise, steal, or commit a murder, regardless of the circumstances"), then you are probably a deductivist who thinks it relatively easy to determine right from wrong in a variety of situations, including those encountered in medicine. On this view, the physician would inform the patient in Case #1, regardless of the facts, on the basis that it is always a violation of patient autonomy to withhold important information as she tries to decide about her future.

Or, did you move between these two poles of moral decision-making in an effort to make them fit together and reinforce each other? Did you insist on having principles but not so inflexibly that they are imposed on the case without regard for its unique characteristics? Did you sense potential conflict between the principles and think about which of these principles would take precedence? If so, you are probably what is often referred to as a principlist.[1-3]

In more recent years, other ways of thinking about medical-ethical dilemmas have arisen, from a "care-based ethic"[4] to "feminist medical ethics."[5-7] Care-based theorists are working diligently on developing an ethic that arises out of the principle of "caring" rather than some of the more formal principles we will summarize momentarily. Feminist ethicists argue that the domination of medicine by males with their emphasis on competition, hierarchy, and abstract reasoning from formal principles cannot adequately resolve many of the moral dilemmas inherent in the care of patients. Further, they also insist that how one sees the patient and how one perceives the relationship between the physician and the care team, or the physician and the patient, is very different from the perspective of those historically at the "bottom" (females as nurses and physicians) in medicine than from those historically at the "top" (white male physicians). Feminists doing medical ethics want less hierarchy and more equality, a focus on the particularities of each case rather than on abstract principles, and each situation interpreted in terms of its effect on the relationships of the people involved.[8]

Because medicine often deals with people in extremis, or at least with people in pain and fearful about their health, every practicing primary care physician is familiar with the ethical challenges inherent in these cases. They are woven into the fabric of medicine so completely that it is difficult—if not impossible—to make any decisions or recommendations about patient care that do not have ethical implications. For that reason, it is helpful for physicians to familiarize themselves with how current medical-ethical thinking affects the challenges they face every day. While there are a number of principles that are important to medical ethics, most modern ethicists recognize that at least these four basic principles in medical-ethical reasoning form the basis for most of their work. They have been employed in one form or another since the time of the Greeks.

The Four Principles

1. Beneficence. Beneficence may be understood as that principle which impels the physician to "seek the patient's good," to put the patient's welfare above all that would compete with that welfare in the physician's eyes, most especially the physician's own good. Financial concerns, time constraints, managed care, government DRGs—nothing can trump the importance of the patient's welfare. In the fee-for-service system, one could afford to seek the patient's good without fear of being challenged, if "good" is taken to mean do everything possible for the patient. If a physician had the slightest doubt about a diagnosis, more tests could easily be ordered. No one would challenge a physician decision regarding diagnosis or treatment. Today, one must "do good" in a way that does not unduly waste resources. Now, clinical quality indicators and standards of care are invoked by medical institutions as well as HMOs to somewhat regulate the doctor's decisions about diagnosis and treatment. Recently, several celebrated cases in which HMOs refused to pay for either a lengthened hospital stay (obstetrics case) or for certain kinds of treatment modalities have been reviewed by the courts, thus reining in what some regard as excessive interference in medical treatment and patient care.

When a dispute is over what is in the patient's best interest, including how one achieves it, ethical issues naturally arise. In Case #3 concerning the man having an affair, the dilemma is particularly acute because one patient to whom the physician owes loyalty and confidentiality is asking the physician to protect him at the possible peril of another patient who also trusts him. Differences of opinion may exist on how best to address that dilemma. Or, physicians may feel that "doing good" requires a "compromise" when a patient is uncooperative with the care plan. When a patient suffers from dangerously high cholesterol, for example, the physician may feel compelled to prescribe a cholesterol-reducing drug that has unpleasant side effects because the patient will not change his lifestyle. In other words, there is no "list" of what is "best" for a patient that a physician can mindlessly apply to each condition or situation. Judgment, imagination, and sensitivity are also needed. In the dilemma of Case #3, the physician may feel either that the principle of beneficence is best upheld by assessing which course of action will most likely produce the best short- or long-term consequences for the female patient, or that one's obligation to the male patient requires that confidentiality be maintained.

2. Non-maleficence. Non-maleficence or "do no harm" is the second principle. This principle recognizes that when a patient places her very life in the physician's hands, she has the right to expect that the physician will not harm her, and that any risks associated with treatment will be reasonable ones in relationship to the desired outcome. This is also the principle used to support the view that under no circumstances may a physician assist a patient who wishes to die. Physicians may withhold or withdraw treatment; they may even prescribe pain-controlling drug therapies that can shorten life. Such practices fulfill the "do no harm" criterion.

3. Patient autonomy. Patient autonomy is the next principle. This means that we must give the competent patient or her designated surrogate final decision-making authority over what will or will not be done to and for her by the physician. That is, no one can ever be forced to accept treatment she does not want, even if it is in her best interest. In the history of medicine, the importance of this principle is a rather late arrival. For several centuries, a heavy-handed paternalism operated in medical culture. Patients could be treated against their will if the physician deemed it appropriate. Some will argue that our anti-paternalism is a uniquely American—or Western—principle given our highly individualistic democratic culture. Other parts of the world (Africa, for example) may not

Table 2. Suggested Reading

BOOKS

Beauchamp TL, Childress JF. *Principles of Biomedical Ethics,* 3rd ed. New York: Oxford University Press; 1989.

Holmes HB, Purdy LM (eds). *Feminist Perspectives in Medical Ethics.* Bloomington, IN: Indiana University Press; 1992 by Hypatia, Inc.

Iserson KV, Sanders AB, Mathieu D (eds). *Ethics in Emergency Medicine,* 2nd ed. Tucson, AZ: Galen Press, Ltd.; 1986.

Jonsen AR, Siegler M, Winslade W. *Clinical Ethics,* 4th ed. New York: McGraw-Hill; 1998.

Lo B. Resolving *Ethical Dilemmas: A Guide for Clinicians.* Baltimore, MD: Williams and Wilkins; 1995.

Monagle JF, Thomasma DC (eds) *Medical Ethics: A Guide for Health Professionals.* Rockville, MD: Aspen Publishers; 1988.

Pellegrino E, Thomasma D. *A Philosophical Basis of Medical Practice.* New York: Oxford University Press; 1981.

Reich WT, ed. *Encyclopedia of Bioethics.* Revised Edition. Vols. 1-5. New York: Simon & Schuster Macmillan; 1995.

Tong R. *Feminist Approaches to Bioethics.* Boulder, CO: Westview Press; 1997.

JOURNALS

Bioethics

Hastings Center Report

Journal of the American Medical Association

Journal of Clinical Ethics

New England Journal of Medicine

The Journal of Law, Medicine and Ethics

The Journal of Philosophy and Medicine

find this principle as compelling in their tribal or communal cultures. Because of our emphasis on autonomy, we have found it more difficult to deal with mentally ill people who refuse help and at the same time are not ill enough to be declared incompetent.

In 1840, John Stuart Mill argued against the absolute authority of a political sovereign and stated that he was sovereign over himself. This concept undergirds the contemporary bioethical principle of personal autonomy or self-determination, as well as much that is in American ethics and United States health care policy. This principle was applied in 1914 in the case of Mary E. Schloendorff v. The Society of New York Hospital which stated that ". . . every human being of adult years and sound mind has a right to determine what shall be done with his body; and a surgeon who performs an operation without his patient's consent commits an assault, for which he is liable in damages." The principle of autonomy suggests that physicians should see themselves engaged in a cooperative program with their patients which provides information to them about treatment possibilities and then helps patients achieve the care that best coincides with their values. It cannot be "the doctor knows best" without qualification. While the doctor may know best about specific treatment options, how those options fit into the person's life is best known by the patient. The ethical physician seeks to enhance a person's autonomy in all medically important decisions.

It must be emphasized that physicians and patients are not equal agents freely entering into a simple contract. Because vulnerable patients are in a "fiduciary" relationship with physicians who, because of their knowledge as professionals, must protect their patients, only physicians committed to their patients best interests can be truly ethical. For example, as patients struggle to make informed decisions in their own best interest, physicians must learn when and how to balance the importance of autonomy against their occasional need for protection and help. When physicians face a dilemma with respect to the competency of a patient, for example, they must know when to turn to another adult who might serve as the patient's decision-maker if the patient is unable to temporarily or permanently meet that goal.[9] The physician can certainly contribute to the decisions, and the surrogate does not need absolute control but can act as a third party who looks after the patient's interest.

A concept closely linked to patient autonomy is "competence." By definition, an autonomous or self-determining patient must be competent to understand his options and decide intelligently. To be competent, a patient must be able to understand the significance of the disease in question and its likely outcome. She must be able to process information about that disease and its treatment options. In order to be competent regarding a particular procedure or treatment plan, patients need only understand the implications for their particular treatment. They do not need to demonstrate competence in all aspects of their lives.

Many things can impair the patient's competence and, therefore, his autonomy. Examples include: drugs and alcohol, mental duress such as depression, a deficit in cognitive functioning such as dementia, and diseases that impair the ability to think and process information. On the other hand, certain diseases can mimic impairment, thus making it difficult to determine competence, such as expressive aphasia. In addition, a language barrier or different social norms can cause certain patients to feel unable to express themselves. A physician needs to sort through each of these possibilities and make sure that the patient is in fact able to process the information relevant to his care and make his own decisions. If he cannot, then competency must be in question. In those intractable cases that leave a physician in doubt, one must occasionally resort to the courts for final disposition. However, a court will typically appoint either a physician, psychologist, or social worker to assess the patient's ability to make decisions regarding her care. If it is felt that a mental illness is impairing a patient's ability to make a competent and informed decision, then it may be wise to have a psychiatric consult to identify the extent of the impairment. If a patient is found incompetent, then treatment may continue if he has given an advance directive such as a Living Will stating clearly how he would want to be treated in different situations. Or, one might instead look to a Durable Power of Attorney for Health Care (which is recognized in most states), in which a patient appoints another person to express his wishes regarding his care. It should be noted that the Durable Power of Attorney for Health Care does not confer unlimited decision-making power on the surrogate. The surrogate is expected to follow the directions either given by the patient at an earlier time or to judge what he would have wanted given the way he lived his life and the values he embraced.

Without that, input should be sought from the patient's next of kin, a practice typical in medicine and one supported by the courts. If there is a conflict about which person should exercise authority for the patient, one must resort to the court for appointment of guardianship. It is inappropriate for physicians to serve as surrogate decision makers because they are in a potential conflict-of-interest position. Like it or not, physicians have a vested interest and a natural bias in decisions that affect the life and well-being of their patients. We must also mention the importance of "listening" in the physician-patient encounter. Most of the time, patients reveal their values and wishes to their physicians in frequent and careful conversations.

Many primary care physicians will provide patient care in the "extended care" arena such as nursing homes. Patients in such settings are likely to feel an immediate loss of autonomy—all the more reason to help patients retain as much control over their own lives as is possible in a given situation. Naturally, end-of-life issues confront the physician in this setting most frequently. Sensitivity to the patient's and family's wishes will often prevent misunderstanding and frustration in the last years of the patient's life. For this population group it is especially important to have both a Living Will and a Durable Power of Attorney for Health Care. The Living Will does have limitations that may not address an individual patient's wishes or needs. It may clearly address these issues when a patient is in a terminal condition, but many patients can linger on for years supported by artificial nutrition or other interventions. For that reason, it is important to know something about the patient's values so that the following questions may be answered: What kind of life does this patient wish to live? If unable to reach those life goals, what type of interventions would he want? What type would he refuse?

Before we leave this subject, we should point out that there may be occasions when the patient's wishes cannot be respected with regard to treatment. For the physician to justify exercising some paternalism and coercion, one must be clear that the patientwhatever reason—is not competent to make such decisions.

While physicians may have a point of view and should feel free to express it, under no circumstances is it ethically appropriate for physicians to impose their personal values about medical treatment on their patients. Whatever is most appropriate will have to be consistent with the values of the patients themselves.

Ethical dilemmas may even arise over a critically ill patient's refusal of treatment when the physician knows that the patient can be helped. In such scenarios, as difficult as it may be, the physician's task is to give the best medical advice and then help the patient or surrogate integrate that advice with the patient's personal values. Thus, two patients with very similar problems may receive very different treatment based on their preferences.

It is therefore vital that primary care physicians spend some time reviewing with their patients how the patients' values might affect their decisions with respect to any life-threatening illness they might face.[10-11]

4. Justice. Justice is the fourth principle. It is concerned about the fair distribution of health care resources when it is impossible for everyone to have everything "possible." It is the principle that compels moral beings to be concerned about the tens of millions of Americans without health care coverage, with the fact that prenatal care among poor women is considerably below the national average, and with the fact that in some circumstances (e.g., a major earthquake or flood), resources may need to be "triaged" between those who need immediate care to survive, those who cannot survive, and those whose needs are real but not life-threatening. In other words, it is the principle that prevents us from neglecting the powerless and poor and from wasting resources.

Other Ethical Issues

Assisted Death. Human dignity and the principle of patient autonomy includes the right to refuse various interventions and to determine one's end-of-life needs.[12-13] Although not specifically legal in many states, the physician may be asked to assist the patient who wishes to end his life. A "not-so-secret" secret in medical circles is the phenomenon of patients asking physicians for help in bringing their suffering to an end not by withdrawing or withholding treatment (which are both legal) but by administering a drug in order to kill the patient. The use of potentially deadly levels of morphine to control suffering in end-stage cancer patients is common and considered both legal and ethical, since—as the "do no harm" principle illustrates—its intended purpose is to reduce suffering, not kill the patient. In the opinion of many legal and ethical scholars, when the intention is the death of the patient, a line has been crossed that should never be violated by a medical doctor. Those who do assist provide help through information or prescriptions but not by actively "doing" anything to the patient. While such behavior has been attacked both ethically and legally, no jury has convicted any physician of a crime. This suggests that large segments of the population perceive such "help" as meeting a genuine need in some terminally ill patients.

"Assisted Death" or what used to be called "Physician Assisted Suicide" (an inflammatory and prejudicial phrase in the opinion of many; hence, the change) will be with us for some time to come.[14-15] There are two primary reasons patients may ask for help in dying. The first is that in a very few instances, the physical pain cannot be relieved. In such a case, what is to be done? Some suggest that the patient "bear" the suffering bravely. Others believe that is cruel treatment. They assume that a "dignified" death is one made as tranquil as possible. A second, more widespread reason that people want help in dying is that they do not want to die a lingering death with the indignities associated with incontinence, memory loss, and dependence on family and health care workers. In their view, mercy and compassion require that we do all we can for people (or even animals) who are in suffering (physical, emotional, and spiritual) as they await their deaths.[16-18] The recent Supreme Court decision has made it clear that terminally ill patients do not have a "constitutional right" to assistance in suicide. On the other hand, the same decision also made it clear that it is not "unconstitutional" for states to have legislation permitting it. One may expect that this dilemma in bioethics and the law will undergo intense debate in the coming years.

Palliative Care. In recent years, the various medical associations have been promoting the benefits of palliative care. It is now widely accepted that physicians need to become both familiar and comfortable with relieving the suffering of patients in their last weeks or months of life. Well-administered comfort care is part of the art of healing to which physicians are committed. While it may not eliminate the perceived need of some patients for physician assisted death, aggressive palliative and supportive care would clearly diminish the number of requests for physician involvement with dying.[19-22]

Many of the issues discussed above are not a daily challenge for a typical primary care physician. Nevertheless, as we saw in the first three cases of this article, primary care physicians are confronted on a daily basis with ethically significant problems. They may be as simple as giving informed consent regarding the side effects of a particular medication; or notifying the Health Department and exposed adults about a sexually transmitted disease problem. Issues of domestic violence like child or spousal abuse impose obligations on the physician to report these activities. In doing a disability evaluation with patients who hope to benefit financially from having a particular disease, questions may arise. Patients with psychosomatic illnesses can make the physician wonder whether it would be appropriate to give a placebo as a treatment for the disease process. A typical procedure being questioned is a placebo intravenous saline solution that is administered to patients with pseudo seizures. The patient is told that this medication will in fact induce one of their seizures. If the patient then has one, this is thought to confirm the diagnosis of pseudo seizures induced by the patient himself. Since this "test" requires deceiving the patient, its ethics have recently come into question.

The Values and Obligations of Physicians

Physicians as Persons of "Virtue." A crucial point made repeatedly in contemporary ethics is that acting ethically requires not just reasoning from principles or being committed to caring in each case, but also that the physician be a person of "virtue," someone who has nurtured feelings and dispositions like compassion, prudence, self-sacrifice, and respect for the autonomy of patients. We need morally sensitized physicians.[14-15]

Bioethics asks of physicians at least three questions about virtue: How important are ethics and values in your personal life?; How central is ethics in your relationships with your patients?; and, how do your values define your relationship with the wider society?

Physicians as Protectors of Patients. Since, as we have seen, physicians' relationships with their patients almost always involve a power imbalance in which the patient is vulnerable, dependent, and often physically or emotionally "weak," the physician must be the kind of person who wields that power for the sake of the patient and not merely for his or her own benefit. It is for this reason that we say that in becoming a physician a person enters more than a career or means of employment. Rather, one adopts a vocation or "calling," which entails far more than the notion of a "contract." For many, the term "contract" sounds too impersonal and business-like. It fails to capture the almost "sacred" agreement made between the trained healer and the sick. For this reason, the agreement between the physician and the patient (and, by extension, the wider community) has even been characterized as a "covenant."[23]

One important way in which physicians and other healthcare providers protect their patients is by ensuring that their very personal medical information is kept as confidential as possible, something more and more difficult to do in the computer age. Patients can be harmed when their health problems are known by those who have no need nor right to know. Family integrity, job security, personal relationships, and self-esteem can suffer from a loss of confidentiality in the medical record. The need to maintain confidentiality is one of the strictest ethical and legal standards applied to healthcare institutions and the physicians who use them.

Physicians Have a Fiduciary Obligation. As professionals who possess knowledge and skills needed by the wider society, physicians offer their services in exchange for money. This places upon them a fiduciary responsibility that they cannot betray without betraying who and what they are as healers. That is one of the reasons why the sick must be treated regardless of their ability to pay. In recognition of this calling, physicians have traditionally taken an almost sacred oath that acknowledges the respect and trust vested in them by society.

One reason the physician has an almost "sacred" obligation to society is that no doctor gets his or her degree and license to practice without considerable sacrifice by a number of people. If one thinks of the mentors, professors, and teachers who sacrificed their time to instruct medical students, of an education heavily subsidized by public funds, and of the patients who allowed themselves to be "practiced on" for would-be physicians as they tried to understand the disease process and how to heal it, it seems clear that doctors owe a debt to society that only their best medical efforts can repay.

This trust from the public, which is so essential to the healer's art, is not impregnable, however. Only when physicians' lives and practices are governed by principles that will guide them through precarious situations can that trust remain strong. Because of the responsibility invested in physicians by the community, physicians must possess certain values and act on the basis of well-established principles.

The Physician's Obligations to Society

Traditionally, physicians were obligated almost exclusively to their patients. In more recent years, society has imposed its own obligations on physicians. In matters of health and public welfare, physicians now have many duties and obligations to either society at large, the local community, or third-party payers. Physicians may also incur obligations voluntarily, such as signing up with managed care organizations. Their obligations may be mandated by state and federal legislatures, such as conforming to what is considered reasonable standard of care for a local community. Physicians should be aware of these specific mandates for their particular states. Let us note a few that can create conflicts with the ethical principles discussed earlier.

Reporting. While it is expected that physicians will promote patient autonomy, dignity, and privacy, physicians may face patient illnesses with grave public health implications. In such cases, the principles of "do no harm" and "do good" would supersede the principle of patient autonomy and compel physicians to report their knowledge to the appropriate authorities. As already noted, respect for the patient's autonomy may be overridden when physicians can show that doing so either meets more important obligations to others or has far greater benefits for the larger society. Besides the issues surrounding sexually transmitted disease, suspected child abuse or neglect, patient threats against another person, or clearly impaired driving ability may also override the principle of patient autonomy. Further, some states require the notification of the Bureau of Motor Vehicles if a physician encounters an impaired patient. In all such instances, the physician's prima facie responsibility to the patient is superseded by his or her greater responsibility to others who are endangered and defenseless because of ignorance or immaturity. Another way to think through this issue is to point out that the burden imposed on the patient whose autonomy has been compromised is not as great as the burden placed on society if that autonomy is not set aside in these circumstances.

Signing Contracts. In this age of managed care, which has itself created numerous ethical dilemmas, physicians must be alert to the dangers that accompany the signing of managed care contracts which seek to control costs and care plans. Such contracts are filled with ethical issues.

It is incumbent upon physicians that they inform their patients of any and all limitations for treatment imposed on them by such contracts. This is becoming more acute in the managed care environment, which seeks to control costs by controlling treatment and care plans.

Use of Resources and Futile Care. Another socially significant ethical issue is this: When is it appropriate for physicians to refuse to give specific kinds of treatment which, medically, will "do no good" and waste valuable resources? This ethical challenge is not well understood because it is less frequently encountered by physicians than are end-of-life issues such as DNAR orders. It is often referred to as "futility" of care. When physicians believe that a treatment would be futile to administer at the same time the patient or the patient's surrogate insists that it be administered anyway, the physician is confronted with an ethical dilemma. If and when physicians invoke the argument from futility as a justification for not using a particular therapy, the notion of futility should be narrowly defined. If we remember that the physician's primary obligation is to the patient, then it may be difficult to justify withholding services out of a concern that resources not be wasted. While resource management is a legitimate concern that affects us all, it is a concern that must be addressed at the societal level through legislation. It is inappropriate for society to expect physicians by themselves to manage health care resources as they treat patients. This is not to deny that it may be justifiable for a physician to refuse to deliver a therapy or intervention. If, in the clinician's judgment, no benefit would accrue to the patient in relation to the patient's goals, this might justify refusal. The last point is crucial: What is the patient's goal? To get well? That may be impossible. To stay alive until his daughter arrives? That may be doable and, therefore, the treatment not futile. However, it is one's view of the sanctity of life that most affects his concept of what is "futile." Some believe that if the result of treatment will be life without self-awareness, it is futile. Others believe that life of any kind has quality, and it is therefore not futile. Clearly, this morally sensitive matter is reduced to a judgment call which can only be made by physicians in consultation with patients or their surrogates.

Besides the need to demonstrate that a planned therapy is of no benefit in treating a patient's disease process, we must also show that providing that therapy imposes a "burden" either on the patient, the family, the physician, society, or the institution involved. An example of a futile therapy may be the administration of an antibiotic for treating a viral upper respiratory infection. Let us suppose that the physician believes this therapy contains no benefit, but the patient wishes to proceed with it. The patient's desire alone may justify using it. But, since the therapy also exposes the patient to the risks associated with a medication's possible side effects and allergic reactions, and since the therapy may pose a public health risk by contributing to the adult antibiotic resistant bacteria, the physician may be justified in refusing to provide the antibiotic. Despite the demands of the patient, the arguments from futility and increased public risk might be sufficient. Alternatively, providing a ventilator therapy to a terminal patient may or may not be futile depending on the values of the patient. If the patient passionately values life, even diminished life, a few additional days on the ventilator may be justified regardless of the lack of any perceived benefit to the patient. Providing the ventilator imposes a burden on the caregivers and society at large, but whether removing that burden is of greater overall value than several days of additional (diminished) life for the patient is almost impossible to judge. This is all to say that at least in some instances physicians should not use the concept of futility to deny care to their patients.[25]

It is the conviction of some authors that the concept of "futility" is often misapplied.[26] Other ethicists believe that "futility" by itself is not a helpful concept. The physician must ask the patient and family: "What are your goals in treatment?" If the goal is lengthening of life to say goodbye to the family rather than "cure," a treatment might not be futile. If used at all, the concept should be used cautiously. However, there is no doubt that society must enter into serious discussion of how best to allocate our increasingly scarce resources. To do so will require a serious look at the issue of how we are to value one human life against another if we cannot save everyone. Is the dying elderly patient as or more important than the pregnant teenager who needs pre-natal care?

Resources for the Physician

Ethics Committees and Consultants. Because of the requirements of the Joint Commission on the Accreditation of Healthcare Organizations that some mechanism be established in hospitals and other healthcare institutions, many hospitals have established an ethics committee. Historically, such committees have provided policy development and oversight with respect to end-of-life decisions (e.g., DNR), ensured that adequate and continuing education on ethical issues takes place for the hospital staff and its physicians, and engaged in case review or case consultation to help mediate conflicts and resolve the ethical challenges facing families, patients, and their caregivers. Most of their time and effort is given to policy development and education, not consultations. These committees usually consist of physicians, nurses, chaplains, social workers, trustees, administrators, an "outside" impartial attorney, and community representatives.

The strength of the committees is their breadth of perspective as they wrestle with the issues and seek to educate themselves and then the rest of the institution. Physicians on the committee serve the role of educating the lay members about the clinical and ethical issues surrounding medicine and providing their unique insights and experience to the discussion. The weakness of the committees is that most cases for which a physician might seek counsel need prompt attention, something difficult to provide at the committee level. This has resulted in either a small subcommittee (available at a "moment's notice") responding to case inquiries or a consultant educated in medical ethics. Where there is a teaching hospital, very often a physician-ethicist or a philosopher-ethicist is available to help with the case, either informally or more formally by writing the consult in the medical chart. All physicians are exposed to the ethical dilemmas in medicine. Consultants are usually called for when disputes arise between the care team and the patient or family, or between care team members. They may mediate, arbitrate, educate or all three, depending on the situation. As primary care physicians, you are well advised to take advantage of whatever ethics resources exist in the institutions you serve. This will help you resolve delicate situations, stay within the law and the code of ethics, and give you the satisfaction of knowing you did all that was within your power to care for your patients in the most responsible and caring way.

Summary

The principles discussed above provide guidance to the practicing medical professional. They will help keep a physician from getting stuck in an ethical quagmire, with this caveat: Ethical principles are no substitute for the virtuous physician. Physicians may do the right thing for the wrong reason. When students begin their careers in medicine, we as a profession must model those virtues which are to govern the way a physician practices regardless of the restraints, legal system, or an ethics committee. If physicians foster a genuine respect for persons, especially the most disadvantaged members of society, if they manifest an interest in the patient as a person and not just as a diseased body, many modern healthcare dilemmas could be avoided. Further, because we live in a pluralistic society comprised of a bewildering plethora of cultures, religions, and value systems, the practice of quality medicine requires us to discuss seriously with our patients what their values and beliefs are. Even now, a program to teach spirituality and values in medical school is being funded by the Templeton Foundation. Because we can no longer treat every patient with a similar disease in the same way or assume we know what is best for each patient, it is imperative that physicians have a basic understanding of ethical principles and ethical reasoning and be able to articulate a justification for their actions in reference to a moral framework. The years of physicians "knowing what's best" are over. We can only claim to know what is "best" in treating disease, not what is best in treating the patient as a person. We can only know what is best in concert with our patients and their families and in cooperation with the society at large.

References

1. Beauchamp TL, Childress JF. Principles of Biomedical Ethics, 3rd ed. New York: Oxford University Press; 1989.
2. The Encyclopedia of Philosophy. USA: Macmillan; 1967;1:69-134.
3. Reich WT (ed). *Encyclopedia of Bioethics,* revised ed. Vol. 1-5. New York: Simon & Schuster Macmillan; 1995.
4. Fry ST, et al. Care-based reasoning, caring and the ethic of care: A need for clarity. *J Clin Ethics* 1996;7:41-47. See also *J Clin Ethics* 1992;3:8-20.
5. Tong R. Feminist Approaches to Bioethics. Boulder, CO: Westview Press; 1997.
6. Wolf SM (ed). *Feminism and Bioethics: Beyond Reproduction.* New York: Oxford University Press; 1996.
7. Holmes HB, Purdy LM (eds). *Feminist Perspectives in Medical Ethics.* Indianapolis, IN: Indiana University Press; 1992. See also *J Clin Ethics* 1996;7.
8. Gilligan C. *In a Different Voice: Psychological Theory and Women's Development.* Cambridge: Harvard University Press;

1982.

9. Parker LS, Buller TG. Case study: A hard policy to swallow. Hastings Center Report. 1994;July-August:23-24.
10. Zawacki BE. The "futility debate" and the management of Gordian Knots. *J Clin Ethics* 1996;6:112-127.
11. Callahan D. The Troubled Dream of Life. New York: Simon & Schuster; 1993.
12. Luce JM. Withholding and withdrawal of life support: Ethical, legal and clinical aspects. *New Horizons* 1997;5:30-37.
13. Medical Ethics Advisor. Nourishment or punishment: When should tube feeding stop? 1997;June.
14. Pelligrino ED, Thomasma DC. *The Christian Virtues in Medical Practice.* Washington, DC: Georgetown University Press; 1996.
15. Lown B. *The Lost Art of Healing.* Boston: Houghton Mifflin Co.; 1996.
16. Nelson HL. Death with Kantian dignity. *J Clin Ethics* 1996;7: 215-221.
17. Hendlin H, et al. Physician-assisted suicide and euthanasia in the Netherlands: Lessons from the Dutch. *JAMA* 1997;277:1720-1723.
18. Vorenberg J, Wanzer SH. Assisting suicide. *Harvard Magazine* 1997;March-April:30-ff.
19. The Journal of Law, Medicine & Ethics 1996;24:4.
20. Henry S. Should doctors help patients die? HIPPOCRATES 1997;August:26-28.
21. Weber DO. *Healthcare Forum Journal* 1995;March/April:14-25, 85.
22. Shapiro RS, Derse AR, Gottlieb M, Schiedermayer D, Olson M. Willingness to perform euthanasia: A survey of physician attitudes. *Arch Intern Med* 1994;March 14:575-584.
23. May WF. Testing the Medical Covenant. Grand Rapids, MI: William B. Eerdmans Co.; 1996.
24. The Protector. 1997;2nd Quarter:7.
25. Daniels N. Meeting the challenges of justice and rationing: Four unsolved problems. Hastings Center Report 1994;July-August:27-29.
26. Morreim EH. Profoundiy diminished life: The casualties of coercion. Hastings Center Report. 1994;January-February:33-42.

Preventive Ethics for the Managed Practice of Medicine

Laurence B. McCullough, PhD

American medicine has undergone a remarkable transformation in the past two decades, from a cottage-industry, fee-for-service practice in which physicians and institutions enjoyed considerable autonomy to a large-scale, institutionally based, mostly prepaid practice in which institutions now regulate the physician's clinical judgment, decision making, and behavior.[1] Medical ethics must respond to this change.[2,3]

Primary-care physicians can adopt one of two basic strategies in response to this change. First, primary care physicians can wait for the ethical conflicts inherent in the new practice of medicine to occur and then respond to them, just as they wait for acute and chronic diseases to occur in their patients and respond to them. Second, primary care physicians can anticipate the built-in potential for ethical conflict and adopt strategies designed to prevent those conflicts from occurring and managing them well when they sometimes do still occur. *(Please see Table 1.)* Primary care physicians, in short, can adopt the strategies of preventive ethics.[4] The reactive practice of ethics, like the reactive practice of medicine, takes a considerable toll on physicians, patients and their families, health care institutions, and society—far better for all involved that physicians adopt a proactive stance toward ethical issues in the new practice of medicine. The purpose of this paper is to identify preventive ethics strategies for the new, managed practice of medicine.[5] Preventive ethics has been proposed as a clinical tool in family medicine for the anticipation of conflicts about futile clinical management[6] and, in obstetrics and gynecology, for the anticipation of conflicts in the intrapartum period (e.g., cesarean delivery).[7]

The Emergence of Managed Practice

For centuries, physicians have practiced under what can usefully be called the cottage-industry model of medicine. (*Please see Table 2.*) In this way of practicing, physicians care for patients one at a time. The task of clinical judgment and practice is to identify each patient's problem and then to propose and implement clinical management of those problems. The physician turned his or her entire focus on the individual patient, did what was needed for that patient, and then moved on to the next patient to meet that patient's individual needs. Physicians made reference to populations of patients only insofar as doing so aided in diagnosis and treatment (e.g., awareness of viruses prevalent in one's community when the primary care physician worked a patient up for common upper respiratory problems during "cold season"). The community, however, is

Table 1. Preventive Ethics

- Identify built-in potential for ethical conflict in clinical practice and in institutional practice and policy.
- Identify strategies for preventing those conflicts from occurring.
- Manage well conflicts that do, nonetheless, occur.

not the physician's patient; this is the work of public health authorities. The physician-patient relationship formed the core of this enterprise, and the ethics of medicine responded to this relationship and the moral challenges that it posed to physicians (e.g., maintaining confidentiality, being honest with patients about the nature of their problems, and obtaining informed consent for the clinical management of those problems).

Physicians also practiced medicine on a fee-for-service basis. Conflicts of interest (i.e., conflicts between the physician's obligation to take appropriate care of patients and his or her self-interest) structured the physician-patient relationship.[8] With the rise of third-party, indemnity insurance after World War II and then Medicare in the 1960s, these conflicts of interest favored physicians' remuneration and job security. Especially in procedure-oriented specialties and sub-specialties, the more physicians did, the more they were paid. Primary-care physicians benefitted indirectly from this unusual economic phenomenon.

In the cottage industry model, by definition, physicians (especially primary care physicians) have little or no accountability to other physicians. The concept of accountability to non-physicians was essentially non-existent. Physicians enjoyed virtually unlimited autonomy in their clinical judgment, decision making, and behavior, especially in the out-patient settings of solo and small group primary care practice.

All of this occurred during more than two decades after World War II in the context of unparalleled economic abundance in the United States. We experienced levels of economic growth unlike those previously experienced in our national economy. Medicine and spending money on medicine became national priorities, and the nation expended enormous sums, with medical inflation regularly running at a multiplier of the consumer price index—sometimes at a multiplier of three.

In the mid-1970s, as global competition in heavy industry and then in consumer goods and services became a reality, our national economy returned to its historically normal growth rates. The ability to increase corporate profits by raising prices and by increasing market share became progressively more constrained. Cost-control became the only remaining business strategy to retain and grow profits. Therefore, private payers necessarily adopted the economically rational view that all costs of doing business, including employee benefits, had to be brought under control. The medical inflation of the 1970s and early 1980s had become unsustainable for private payers by the late 1980s.

In the public sector, the even more rapid increase in the costs of Medicare and Medicaid, as well as Veterans health affairs and military medicine, also became unsustainable, but for a different reason. The widespread resistance to increased taxation, which swept Ronald Reagan to the White House, finally made itself felt in Congress. Medicare was transformed from a fee-for-service, hospital-based, physician-controlled reimbursement system to a pre-paid, hospital-controlled system. (*See Table 2.*) Hospitals were put at risk, and those that were successful in changing the behavior of physicians and nurses did well—those that were not no longer exist.

The Medicare prospective payment system, based on diagnostic related groups, signaled a major change. Instead of conflicts of interest being built into the payment system and under the control of physicians, the federal government, in its role as a major payer, imposed conflicts of interest directly on institutions. The average length of stay for Medicare beneficiaries decreased by the end of the 1980s, and the rate of inflation in Medicare decreased as well. Prospective payment was given the credit and the effectiveness of a crucial management tool, imposing conflicts of interest that put incomes at risk, was taken to be demonstrated.

The private sector watched this change and adopted this management tool. Institutions, especially managed care organizations (MCOs), imposed economic conflicts of interest—withholding payments, discounted fee-for-service, and capitation—on physicians.[9,10] These institutions assumed that physicians, like hospitals, would change their behavior in the direction of less intensive use of resources when given the economic incentive (shared risk) for doing so.

Physicians have also been made more accountable for the quality and cost of patient care. As large-scale institutions have become responsible for patients, they directly employ or contract with physicians—introducing a level of accountability impossible when many physicians were self-employed. In addition, institutions now gather data on physician performance—in both the processes and outcomes of care—and they use these data to evaluate and manage physician performance (e.g., in profiling systems). Among those to whom physicians have now become accountable are both physician managers and non-physician managers. Both know a great deal more about aspects of a primary care physician's practice (e.g., cost and quality) than the physician does.

In making physicians accountable, institutions also began to regulate the clinical judgment, decision making, and behavior of physicians.[11] Both payer and provider institutions took note of the wide variation in the use of resources and that this variation does not result in improved outcomes.[12,13] Moreover, institutions took note of one of the important lessons of the Medicare prospective payment system: decreased use improved outcomes for many patients. Thus,

Table 2. Fee-for-Service, Cottage Industry Model vs. Prepaid, Large Institutional Model

Cottage Industry, Fee-for-Service	Prepaid, Large-Scale Institutional Model
Physician-patient relationship	Institution-population of patient's relationship
Built-in conflicts of interest that favor physicians	Conflicts of interest imposed that penalize and favor physicians
Little accountability to physician and lay managers	Increasing accountability to physician and lay managers
Economics of abundance	Economics of scarcity

the standard of care that prevailed in the fee-for-service, cottage-industry era of medicine lacks scientific justification to a considerable degree. That we can decrease use without necessarily harming patients became a management assumption and goal of institutional managers and private payers.

In summary, U.S. medicine has been transformed from an essentially unmanaged practice to the managed practice of medicine. Managed practice involves two elegant and powerful business tools:

Imposing conflicts of interest on physicians, putting income, job advancement, and job security at risk; and

Regulating the clinical judgment, decision making, and behavior of physicians.[14]

These two business tools aim for maximum economic efficiency. How they are used results in a heterogeneity of managed practice to which primary care physicians must respond.

At one end of the continuum, physicians confront institutions that aim only for cost control and cost reduction, with little attention to quality. These short-term market players intend to capture a sufficient market share to make themselves attractive take-over targets. They have no economic incentive to pursue quality, because their short-term time horizon means that they would not realize the economic returns of cost-benefit management.

At the other end of the continuum, physicians confront more responsible institutions with a long-term commitment to the market. They can realize the economic returns of cost-benefit management. Therefore, they pursue quality improvement as the means to gain cost-benefit advantages. They aim to increase quality and control costs.

At the present time, the private sector of managed practice has no public-policy mandate to maintain and even increase access. Such a mandate does exist in the public sector, especially for Medicaid and Veterans health affairs. The Veterans Administration (VA) now understands itself to be the nation's largest MCO operating out of federally funded medical centers. These MCOs aim to increase quality, control costs, and, therefore, maintain or even increase access. Current public policy (e.g., frequent open enrollment for Medicare MCOs makes a hash of this goal). A major public policy issue for the future will entail bringing enrollment practices, quality, and cost into more rational alignment.

Responding to the Business Tools of Managed Practice with Two Basic Ethical Concepts

The First Concept: The Physician and Institution as Moral Co-Fiduciaries of Populations of Patients. In the cottage-industry, fee-for-service model of medical practice, the physician could assert as a basic moral precept, "My patient comes first." This precept governed both out-patient and in-patient medical practice, at least in the private sector. It formed the core of the physician's moral fiduciary obligations to each patient. The physician as moral fiduciary: 1) makes the protection and promotion of each individual patient's health interests the physician's primary commitment; 2) blunts self-interest by this primary obligation, making self-interest a systematically secondary commitment; and 3) expects that income and prestige will follow from the first two commitments.[15] (*Please see Table 3.*)

In response to managed care, some have argued for the retention of the precept that "my patient comes first" and that physicians should resist population-based fiduciary obligations.[16-19] However, given the nature of the changes that have occurred, this line of reasoning will no longer do as the basis for the moral responsibilities of physicians because it will result in self-contradiction.

Institutions operate on fixed budgets, such that unnecessary expenditure for some patients may well mean that there will be insufficient resources available for other patients, who will then be harmed. No ethical theory supports the exercise of autonomy, including both the physician's and the patient's autonomy, in ways that put others at risk of serious harm without their consent. In an era of fixed institutional budgets, "My patient comes first" creates just such a risk and, therefore, jeopardizes the ability of each individual physician to put his or her patients first and the ability of an institution to meet its obligations to all of the patients in the population for which it is responsible. Making the protection and promotion of each individual patient's health related interests by some physicians means that other physicians in the institution will be denied the resources necessary to fulfill their moral obligation to their patients. Thus, moral fiduciary obligations come into conflict with each other. The solution to this problem is for physicians to adopt the concept appropriate to the new, large-scale institutional practice of medicine: physicians and

Table 3. The Physician as Moral Fiduciary of the Patient

- The physician's primary commitment is to protect and promote the interests of the patient.
- This commitment blunts the physician's own self-interests, making them a systematically secondary commitment.
- The physician should be confident that remuneration and prestige will follow from the first commitment and the self-regulation of self-interest.

Table 4. Physicians and Institutions as Moral Co-Fiduciaries of Populations of Patients

- Physicians and institutions cannot practice or allocate resources based on the old precept of cottage-industry medicine: "My patient comes first."
- Focusing on the interests of one patient at a time, in an era of fixed budgets, will result in some patients being harmed.
- Therefore, it will be impossible for physicians in an institutional setting to fulfill their moral fiduciary obligations to their patients, to protect and promote their health interests.
- Therefore, it will also be impossible for the institution to fulfill its moral fiduciary obligations to its population of patients, to protect and promote their health-related interests.
- Physicians and institutions share moral responsibility for protecting and promoting the health interests of populations of patients: they are moral co-fiduciaries of populations of patients.

institutions are moral co-fiduciaries of populations of patients. (*Please see Table 4.*)

Some institutions, especially MCOs, take the view that their decisions are simply business decisions. Thus, the decision to deny access to referral specialists or to parovide physicians with economic incentives to use such services sparingly are thought to be simply business decisions. This involves a serious conceptual mistake. Business decisions, like all decisions, have consequences. Institutions, like individuals, must be held responsible for the consequences of their decisions.

Moreover, the decisions of institutions, when they are based on the business tools of managed practice, are intended to have consequences in patient care. These institutions, therefore, bear moral responsibility for these consequences. Institutions must realize that they share responsibility for patient care for the population for which they are responsible: institutions and physicians are moral co-fiduciaries of populations of patients. (*Please see Table 4.*)

The Second Concept: Informed Consent as a Preventive Ethics Strategy. Informed consent has become a stable matter of medical ethics and law.[20] (*Please see Table 5.*) Informed consent obligates the physician to provide patients with information sufficient to make decisions based on awareness and understanding of their diagnosis, the medically reasonable alternatives for managing it, and the benefits and risks of each alternative. The goal of the consent process is for the patient to replicate for himself or herself the physician's clinical judgment and decision making and then decide whether to accept the clinical management that has been offered or recommended. Physicians, especially primary care physicians, should, in other words, make their clinical judgment and decision making "transparent" to the patient.[21] To do so, physicians should provide and explain information to the patient about the salient features of clinical judgment.[22]

The business tools of managed practice are designed and intended to be salient in the clinical judgment and decision making of physicians. Putting a physician's income at risk or requiring a physician to follow a practice guideline for the rapid discharge of a woman and her baby after an uncomplicated, singleton vaginal delivery, and the myriad other tactics of managed practice, surely become salient in the physician's clinical judgment and decision making. It follows logically, from the concept of transparency, that the existence, effects, benefits, and harms of the business tools of managed practice must be disclosed to patients. (*Please see Table 5.*)

There is also a shared fiduciary obligation of both institutions and patients. Disclosure and explanation of the business tools of managed practice should occur when patients first enroll ("upstream" consent) and when they later come under the care of the institution's physicians, especially its primary care physicians ("downstream consent").

Currently, it appears, few institutions provide sufficient information to patients about the existence and effects of the business tools of managed practice because of gag orders or an institutional culture that discourages disclosure.[23,24] As a consequence, physicians, especially primary care physicians, find themselves downstream from defective disclosure. They must not only explain the general nature of the business tools of managed practice but also their particular application to the patient's current condition and its clinical management. This approach will prevent the problem of patients first learning about both of these matters at the same time, compounding the risk of distrust within the physician-patient relationship.

This defective consent process appears to be having the following deleterious consequences. First, patients are angry and venting their anger at their physicians and nurses—the professionals who are the institution as far as the patient is concerned. Second, patients are beginning to withdraw trust from MCOs and physicians.[25-27] The fact that bills in Congress can be called the "Patients' Bill of Rights" further signals this withdrawal of trust. Third, physicians find themselves trapped downstream of defective disclosure by institutions. As a result, when physicians say nothing, they inadvertently further fuel distrust, and perhaps, even anger. Fourth, physicians and institutions exercise growing power over patients, especially in

Table 5. Informed Consent

- Physicians should make their clinical judgment and decision making transparent to patients, by disclosing and explaining salient features of clinical judgment and decision making.
- The business tools of managed practice are salient features of clinical judgment.
- Therefore, the existence and effects of the business tools of managed practice should be disclosed and explained to patients.
- Doing so gives moral authority to increasing the physician's and institution's power over patients.

MCOs and hospitals, without the moral authority that informed consent is intended to impart. Although large employers offer more options, many patients are employed by small businesses that offer limited or even no choice about which MCO will provide their health care. The more that patients' autonomy is constrained, the more morally important their autonomy becomes. When the exercise of autonomy through the consent process is absent, institutions and physicians wield absolute power. Lord Acton's famous dictum that power corrupts and absolute power corrupts absolutely applies to the current lack of informed consent from patients to be in managed practice settings.

This cycle must be broken, and primary care physicians should take the lead in doing so. A preventive ethics approach to informed consent can break this cycle by identifying the institution's and physician's "upstream" obligations and the physician's "downstream" obligations. (*Please see Table 6.*)

At enrollment, the institution, as the moral co-fiduciary of its population of patients, has an inescapable obligation to disclose and explain to patients the following information and to make a reasonable effort to determine that patients do indeed understand this information. First, patients should be told that their physicians, particularly their primary care physician who will control access to medical services, will have their incomes influenced by how many resources the physicians use (e.g., how often they make referrals, how often they prescribe expensive medications, and how often they hospitalize patients). Second, patients should be told that their physicians will not be free agents in how they think and act. Instead, the institution regulates or manages how its physicians think and act. Third, patients should be told that, to some extent, the changes in U.S. medicine constitute a social experiment and that institutions, while they intend to benefit patients, may inadvertently harm them. In addition, patients should be told that, as in any experiment, the law of unintended consequences applies—events may occur that no one could predict. Finally, patients should be provided with comparative information about available institutions, so that they can make an informed choice about enrollment or perhaps pressure their employers to offer them other choices.

Physicians have the important "upstream" obligation to see to it that the institution fulfills its moral fiduciary obligations in the consent process. (*Please see Table 6.*) Physicians should insist on adequate disclosure during enrollment and truth in advertising by the institution. Because primary care physicians bear most of the brunt of defective institutional disclosure, they should be especially vigorous in discharging these upstream obligations.

Once the patient comes into the primary care physician's office or examining room, that physician has "downstream" obligations. (*Please see Table 6.*) First, the primary care physician should remind the patient about the two key concepts that should have been disclosed "upstream:" that the physician's income is at risk and that the physician is not a free agent in the patient's care. Second, the particular applications of these concepts in the patient's current clinical circumstances should be explained. Thus, the obstetrician or family physician providing antenatal care to a pregnant woman with a singleton pregnancy that is expected to go to term and result in vaginal delivery should inform her that the timing of discharge from the hospital of her and her baby will be regulated by what is called a practice guideline. During the several antenatal visits, this guideline should be explained, including its scientific rationale and the experience of the MCO and hospital with it. The goal should be to provide the patient with sufficient information, so that the patient becomes willing to have intellectual trust in this regulation of her physician's clinical judgment, decision making, and behavior. If the institution uses financial incentives to encourage the primary care physician to follow such a guideline, then this should also be disclosed, so that the woman has enough information to decide whether to morally trust her primary care physician, as someone who is committed to her and the baby she intends to deliver, as their moral fiduciary, including the willingness to make economic sacrifice to see to that they receive appropriate care.

The same approach should be taken in other primary care settings. If the primary care physician considering referral to a specialist is paid, for example, on a withhold basis, this fact should be explained to the patient. The physician can point out that his or her compensation is influenced by the amount of referral services used, so that the patient can take this fact into account in the informed consent process for the management of the patient's problem. Such explanations should take little time, especially if they become commonplace.

A Preventive-Ethics Approach to Managing Conflicts of Interest

It is not enough to disclose and explain to patients the existence and effect of conflicts of interest. As a matter of integrity, physicians also have a moral fiduciary obligation to patients to manage conflicts of interest well, so that patients are not harmed by them.[28-33] Conflict of interest can now be more precisely defined: creating a conflict between the physician's moral fiduciary obligation to the patient to

Table 6. Informed Consent as a Preventive Ethics Strategy in Managed Practice

A. **The institution's "upstream" obligation to disclose adequate information about:**
- how its physicians are paid, including the concept of economic incentives to conserve expensive medical resources such as referral services and hospitalization;
- how the clinical judgment, decision making, and behavior of its physicians are regulated by the institution;
- the consequences of these two management tools, including the law of unintended consequences; and
- comparative results.

B. **The primary care physician's "upstream" obligations.**
- Insist on meeting the costs of informed consent as an essential business cost.
- Monitor consent process.
- Monitor marketing and advertising strategies, as well as tactics.

C. **The primary care physician's "downstream" obligations.**
- Remind patient that he or she is paid on an economic incentive to conserve expensive medical resources.
- Remind the patient that he or she is not a free agent in the use of such resources.
- Explain the particulars of how these two management tools apply in the patient's current clinical circumstances.

Table 7. Criteria for Moral Assessment of Conflicts of Interest

- Intensity
- Immediacy
- Individual vs. group
- Systematic in nature

provide care consistent with integrity on the one hand, and self-interest on the other hand. Integrity requires the physician to practice medicine according to intellectual and moral standards of excellence. These should not be equated with doing the most for patients; this standard, in fact, has often harmed patients (e.g., prolonging suffering and loss of quality of life in the intensive care unit for patients in the end-stages of chronic disease).

Conflicts of interest structure all current mechanisms for paying physicians in managed-practice settings. Therefore, as the first step of a preventive-ethics approach to managing conflicts of interest, primary care physicians should identify these conflicts of interest precisely: How and how much of a physician's compensation is put at risk? What is rewarded and why? Second, conflicts of interest should be assessed for their moral manageability according to the following criteria. *(Please see Table 7.)*[10,28]

1. How intense is the conflict of interest? *or* How much of the physician's total compensation is put at risk? The greater the intensity of a conflict of interest, given ordinary human weakness, the more likely it is to distort clinical judgment, decision making, and behavior in ways that could, in violation of moral fiduciary obligations to them, unnecessarily harm patients.
2. How immediate is the conflict of interest? *or* Is the conflict of interest the first thing that enters clinical judgment? To the extent that this is the case, clinical judgment does not start with the patient where it should for moral fiduciary physicians.
3. How systematic is the conflict of interest? *or* Is there no escape from its influence? The more aspects of clinical judgment, decision making, and behavior influencing the conflict of interest, the more systematic it is and the more likely it is to distort clinical judgment, decision making, and behavior in ways that could violate moral fiduciary obligations to patients.
4. Is the conflict of interest applied to physicians in isolation? It has been a staple of the world philosophical literature on the virtues that we do a better job of maintaining our integrity when we are accountable to others than we do when we are accountable only to ourselves.[14] The capacity for self-deception never should fail to surprise us. The best antidote to self-deception is the willingness to submit to fair-minded and rigorous moral peer review.

The higher any conflict of interest is on these four scales, the more primary care physicians should judge it to be morally unmanageable (i.e., likely to result in violation of moral fiduciary obligations to patients). Uncertainty about whether a conflict of interest is morally unmanageable should be resolved in the judgment that it will be morally unmanageable as a matter of prudence. In other words, imposing conflicts of interests on fiduciaries faces a burden of proof. Because they are inherently morally destabilizing for moral fiduciaries, conflicts of interest have to be shown by institutional managers to be morally acceptable. Institutional managers, physician and lay alike, should not assume that conflicts of interest have to be shown to be morally unacceptable.

If all conflicts of interest, after rigorous moral evaluation (a process in which primary care physicians must insist on playing a part—they should not work for institutions that disallow such a crucial role in preserving one's integrity), are reliably judged to be manageable, patients should be informed about them. Thus, in both the upstream and downstream informed consent process described, it should only be manageable conflicts of interest that are described and explained to patients. Unmanageable conflicts of interest are unethical. They should not be used by institutions, and primary care physicians should not sign contracts for employment or services that include them. Indeed, unethical conflicts of interest should be exposed by primary care physicians, even at the cost of considerable self-sacrifice.

Once a primary care physician has accepted employment or a contract for services that is reliably judged to include manageable conflicts of interest, that physician bears responsibility for protecting the patient from the consequences of that conflict of interest. When fiduciary obligations come into conflict with the physician's economic self-interest, integrity requires that the primary care physician accept that economic self-sacrifice. If doing so becomes unacceptable, the primary care physician should renegotiate these conflicts during the next contract period. This strategy involves some level of risk of deselection; however, this risk is unavoidable if integrity is to be maintained.

The preventive ethics of managing conflicts of interest also adds to the process of total quality management. Patterns of clinical management under all conflicts of interest must be monitored, both in their processes and their outcomes, for violations of integrity. This is a demanding scientific and moral standard and involves more than discomfort with change or a clinical impression that patients are being harmed. This clinical ethics judgment should, like all clinical judgment, be as evidence-based as possible. When such violations occur, they should be immediately corrected. Patients who have been adversely affected should be informed (even if this increases malpractice liability) and provided appropriate clinical management.

Preventive Ethics Approach to Rationing

It is not enough to inform patients about the regulation of clinical judgment, decision making, and behavior. This regulation, too, should be consistent with the integrity of the fiduciary practice of medicine by physicians and institutions.[34]

As noted, the wide and scientifically unexplainable variation in the use of medical resources, in which "geography is destiny," is not consistent with integrity. Many factors come together to explain this scientifically strange and unacceptable phenomenon. Fee-for-service payment of physicians surely had a distorting effect on how physicians have come to define the standards of care, just as the Scottish physician and philosopher, John Gregory (1724-1773), predicted that it would.[35-37] The economics of abundance after World War II and through the mid-1970s gave neither physicians, hospitals, nor private and public payers economic incentives to strive for greater scientific rigor and, therefore, economic efficiency in the use of medical resources. It is no surprise that "best" came to mean "doing everything possible" for patients. The language used by the scientific and medical communities, as well as patients, to win political and monetary support for medicine (e.g., "wars" and "cures") gave rise to scientifically unrealistic expectations for the capacity of medicine to manage our biology. This language is now being used to sell genetic treatment of disease in molecular medicine. Finally, the popular culture adopted and exaggerated these expectations—giving rise to the view that doing everything for patients was iatrogenically benign. However, experience teaches us that the intensity of utilization of medical resources can be lowered in many cases, without harming patients and often resulting in benefit for them, as we learned from Medicare's experiment with prospective payment.

Rationing of resources in medicine, therefore, almost always involves moving from a scientifically and morally unfounded "best = most" care to a scientifically and morally well founded concept of adequate medical care (i.e., clinical management that meets the medical needs of a population of patients adequately). Rationing below levels of adequacy makes little sense from an institutional point of view because it is economically irrational; inadequate care usually results in preventable worsening of the patient's condition and preventable, increased use of resources. Providing substandard care will, therefore, often be more expensive than providing adequate care. One exception might be Medicare MCOs from which early disenrollment is possible, which undermines this economic incentive to provide adequate care. Thus, even poorly managed MCOs have non-trivial economic incentives not to practice below acceptable standards of care. The malpractice law should be revised, as Texas has done, to provide statutory sanction for such irresponsible violation of fiduciary obligations—not only to patients, but to shareholders of for-profit MCOs.

A preventive ethics approach to rationing down to acceptable fiduciary standards of care for populations of patients involves the following. First, the outcomes expected to be achieved should be clearly identified and ethical justification for them should be given. If it is judged that it would be too expensive to try for marginal reduction in mortality or morbidity rates in a population of patients (e.g., by using a more expensive antibiotic), this economic judgment must be defensible. Second, the process of care in the rationing plan should be scientifically related to these outcomes (i.e., be reliably expected to produce them). Third, physicians must consent to practice under the rationing plan. After all, rationing alters clinical judgment and may increase the risk of harm to some patients. A rigorous consent process will allow physicians to test the rationing plan for its intellectual and moral integrity. Primary care physicians should insist on such a consent process and should carefully consider whether they should remain employed or contracted by institutions that refuse to adopt such a policy. Fourth, patients must be informed—especially of rationing of demand for services by primary care physicians, which is where the money is. Patients, especially those who have experienced only managed care (now millions of people) do not know when a level of intervention that might have occurred in the past is now being withheld by the primary care physician (e.g., referral to a specialist for the management of minor cardiac arrhythmia). Fifth, the institution should be prepared to resist gaming of rationing plans and should have clear policies that discourage, indeed prohibit, such gaming strategies (e.g., threatening to give one's primary care physician a bad quarterly "report card" if the primary care physician denies referral to a specialist, which the patient thinks is necessary).

This preventive ethics approach to rationing also adds to total quality management. Rationing plans should be intensely monitored for patterns of inadequate clinical management. These could easily occur, especially when rationing is coupled with imposition of conflicts of interest, without physicians noticing. When patterns of inadequate clinical management occur, they should be immediately corrected. Patients who have been adversely affected by such management should be informed and offered appropriate management for their problems.

The Role of Ethics Committees

A central theme of the preventive ethics approach to the managed practice of medicine described is the maintenance of integrity, both by physicians and by health care institutions, and, especially, MCOs, physician-hospital alliances, and institutions that will be invented in the coming years. Maintenance of integrity means that an institution creates a culture in which difficult and sometimes disturbing questions can routinely be asked about whether an institution and its physicians remain true to the intellectual and moral demands of being moral co-fiduciaries of patients. The institutional ethics committee can play a crucial role in creating such an institutional culture.[38-40]

Ethics committees have mainly been hospital-based and have mainly been concerned with clinical cases and policies. Lately, a trend of ethics committees has emerged, taking on development and evaluation of practices and policies that bear on the business tools of managed practice.[40] In addition, there appears to be a trend toward the creation of ethics committees within MCOs.

Primary care physicians should play an active role in encouraging the further development of these welcome trends. An active ethics committee that has familiarized itself with the topics discussed can help to develop and monitor practices and policies that implement a preventive ethics approach to the business tools of managed practice. Such committees could evaluate marketing and advertising strategies and materials for their conformance to the upstream obligations of institutions, such as MCOs in the informed consent. Ethics committees could review all contracts—both those written and those presented—for their conformance to preventive ethics criteria for morally manageable conflicts of interest. Practice guidelines, clinical pathways, appeals processes, and other utilization strategies could be evaluated for their conformance to preventive ethics standards of integrity. Physicians and others on such committees should be compensated to the extent that these tasks call for time-extensive time commitments. Maintaining integrity is an essential business cost of fiduciary institutions.

Tasking ethics committees with this important work also makes preventive ethics public within an institution and among its core values. It is difficult to maintain one's integrity in isolation and even more so in health care institutions without a public, core commitment to the integrity of physicians and institutions together acting as moral co-fiduciaries of populations of patients.

Summary

Primary care physicians have two alternatives for responding to the transformation of U.S. medicine from a fee-for-service cottage industry focused on one patient at a time to a pre-paid, large-scale institutional commitment to populations of patients. They can wait for ethical conflict built into the two business tools of managed practice to occur and respond in a reactive mode—until they are exhausted by the struggle to maintain their integrity as moral fiduciaries in isolation from like-minded physicians and without the support of a morally intact institutional culture. Or they adopt a proactive, preventive ethics approach that holds (I hope I have persuaded the reader) far greater prospect of maintaining integrity.

The stakes have become non-trivial. Under the influence of reforming, risk-taking physicians (such as John Gregory[35-37]), medicine began in the English-speaking world to become a profession in the late 18th century. It continued to become a profession, although the response of many physicians to the inherent conflicts of interest in the fee-for-service payment system impeded medicine's progress to fully becoming a moral fiduciary profession. The decisions that physicians make—especially primary care physicians who have the most contact with patients and increasing responsibility for their care—will decide whether medicine continues to become a profession or reverts to entrepreneurialism.[41] Self-sacrifice appears to be an unavoidable price that physicians will have to pay in order to maintain their integrity.[14] Gregory practiced medicine in such a world dominated by the self-interests of physicians and in which patients, therefore, could not and did not intellectually or morally trust their physicians. Gregory concluded that this self-interested medical practice constituted a moral disaster for patients and physicians alike. Patients now struggle to trust their physicians intellectually to know what they are doing or morally to be more concerned about their patients rather than their incomes. Adopting and institutionalizing a preventive ethics approach to the managed practice of medicine may help to prevent this moral disaster from occurring and keep medicine on the path of becoming a profession.

References

1. Starr P. *The Social Transformation of American Medicine*. New York: Basic Books; 1982.
2. Morreim EH. *Balancing Act: The New Medical Ethics of Medicine's New Economics*. Washington, DC: Georgetown University Press, 1995.
3. McCullough LB. Molecular medicine, managed care, and the moral responsibilities of patients and physicians. *J Med Philos* 1998;23:3-9.
4. McCullough LB. Preventive ethics, professional integrity, and boundary setting: the clinical management of moral uncertainty. *J Med Philos* 1995;20:1-11.

5. Chervenak FA, McCullough LB. The threat of the new managed practice of medicine to patient's autonomy. *J Clin Ethics* 1995;6:320-323.
6. Doukas JD, McCullough LB. A preventive ethics approach to counseling patients about clinical futility in the primary care setting. *Arch Fam Med* 1996;5:589-592.
7. Chervenak FA, McCullough LB. Clinical guides to preventing ethical conflicts between pregnant women and their physicians. *Am J Obstet Gynecol* 1990;162:303-307.
8. Morreim EH. *Conflicts of interest*. In: Reich WT (ed.) Encyclopedia of Bioethics. 2nd ed. New York: Macmillan, 1995:459-465.
9. Rodwin MA. *Medicine, Money, and Morals*. New York: Oxford University Press, 1993.
10. Khushf G. A radical rupture in the paradigm of modern medicine: conflicts of interest, fiduciary obligations, and the scientific ideal. *J Med Philos* 1998;23:98-122.
11 Lohr KN. Guidelines for clinical practice: What they are and why they count. *J Law Med Ethics* 1995;23:49-56.
12. Wennberg DE. Variation in the delivery of care: The stakes are high. *Ann Intern Med* 1998;128:866-868.
13. Wennberg J, Gittelsohn A. Small area variations in health care delivery. *Science* 1973;182:1102-1108.
14. Chervenak FA, et al. Responding to the ethical challenges posed by the business tools of managed care in the practice of obstetrics and gynecology. *Am J Obstet Gynecol* 1996;175: 523-527.
15. McCullough LB, Chervenak FA. *Ethics in Obstetrics and Gynecology*. New York: Oxford University Press, 1994.
16. Council on Ethics and Judicial Affairs AMA. Ethical issues in managed care. *JAMA* 1995;273:330-335.
17. Emanuel EJ, Dubler NN. Preserving the physician-patient relationship in the era of managed care. *JAMA* 1995;273:323-329.
18. Sorum PC. Ethical decision making in managed care. *Arch Intern Med* 1996;156:2041-2045.
19. Kassirer JP. Managing care—Should we adopt a new ethics? *N Engl J Med* 1998;339:397-398.
20. Faden RR, Beauchamp TL. *A History and Theory of Informed Consent*. New York: Oxford University Press, 1986.
21. Brody H. Transparency: Informed consent in primary care. *Hastings Cent Rep* 1989;19:5-9.
22. Wear S. *Informed Consent: Patient Autonomy and Physician Beneficence Within Clinical Medicine*, 2nd ed. Washington, DC: Georgetown University Press, 1999.
23. Woolhandler S, Himmelstein DU. Extreme risk: The new corporate proposition for physicians. *N Engl J Med* 1995;333: 1706-1708.
24. Brody H, Bonham VL Jr. Gag rules and trade secrets in managed care contracts: Ethical and legal concerns. *Arch Intern Med* 1997;157:2037-2043.
25. Mechanic D. The impact of managed care on patients' trust in medical care and their physicians. *JAMA* 1996;275:1693-1697.
26. Gray BH. Trust and trustworthy care in the managed care era. *Health Aff* 1997;16:34-39.
27. Blumenthal D. Effects of market reforms on doctors and their patients. *Health Aff* 1996;15:170-184.
28. Khushf G, Gifford R. Understanding, assessing, and managing conflicts of interest. In: McCullough LB, Jones JW, Brody BA (eds.): *Surgical Ethics*. New York: Oxford University Press, 1998: 342-366.
29. Wildes KW, Wallace RB. Relationships with payers and institutions that manage and deliver patient services. In: McCullough LB, Jones JW, Brody BA (eds.): *Surgical Ethics*. New York: Oxford University Press, 1998: 367-383.
30. Iserson KV, Jarrell BE. Financial relationships with patients. In: McCullough LB, Jones JW, Brody BA (eds.): *Surgical Ethics*. New York: Oxford University Press, 1998: 322-341.
31. Speece R, Shimm D, Buchanan A (eds.). *Conflicts of Interest in Clinical Practice and Research*. New York: Oxford University Press, 1996.
32. Emanuel EJ, Steiner D. Institutional conflict of interest. *N Engl J Med* 1988;319:262-267.
33. Latham SR. Regulation of managed care incentive payments to physicians. *Am J Law Med* 1996;22:399-432.
34. Capron AM. Practice guidelines: How good are medicine's new recipes? *J Law med Ethics* 1995;23:470-478.
35. Gregory J. Lectures on the Duties and Qualifications of a Physician. London: Strahan W and Cadell T (eds.): In: McCullough LB (ed.): *John Gregory's Writings on Medical Ethics and Philosophy of Medicine*. Dordrecht, The Netherlands and Boston: Kluwer Academic Publishers, 1998:161-245.
36. McCullough, LB. *John Gregory and the Invention of Professional Medical Ethics and the Profession of Medicine*. Dordrecht, The Netherlands and Boston: Kluwer Academic Publishers, 1998.
37. McCullough LB. John Gregory and the invention of professional relationships in medicine. *J Clin Ethics* 1997;8:11-21.
38. McCullough LB. Preventive ethics, managed practice, and the hospital ethics committee as a resource for physician executives. *HEC Forum* 1998;10:127-135.
39. Pentz RD. Expanding into organizational ethics: The experience of one clinical ethics committee. *HEC Forum* 1998;10:213-221.
40. Khushf G. The scope of organizational ethics. *HEC Forum* 1998;10:127-135.
41. McCullough LB, Chervenak FA. Ethical challenges in the managed practice of obstetrics and gynecology. *Obstet Gynecol* 1998; In press.

End of Life Challenges

Michael Sparacino, MD

Increasingly, we recognize death, dying, and end-of-life issues as important parts of our societal life cycle. As primary care physicians, we embrace these issues as profound, potentially beneficial areas of our patients' lives. We will be called upon to help guide our patients through these challenging life experiences. This chapter discusses end-of-life issues as they relate to primary care providers. It focuses on the concept of medical futility as it applies to the care of our dying patients. As with most issues dealing with medical ethics, there are very few unequivocal situations. Much more commonly, the question of whether medical care is futile arises in a scenario of extreme distress among family members, miscommunication, and subsequent conflict. Factors that may lead to futility situations are identified. Communication and negotiation skills directed at resolving conflict are discussed, as well as creating fair processes to resolve intractable conflict.

Introduction

Unfortunately, nearly every clinician will face the scenario where a dying patient's decision maker insists upon therapy that the physician thinks is futile. In fact, questions of medical futility constitute a significant number of ethics consults in hospitals.[1] Often these cases can be extremely frustrating and upsetting for the health care team as well as the patient's family. From the perspective of the health care team, the family can be seen as unrealistic, having the patient experience unnecessary pain and indignity before death. Professionals, feeling uncomfortable with conflict under such distressing circumstances, may feel the need to distance themselves from the patient and family, giving the impression that they are unconcerned. They may become accusatory toward family members and view family suggestions as unwanted encroachment on professional turf. Families, made especially sensitive during this life crisis, may perceive the health care team as uncaring. They may even accuse the team of being motivated by more malevolent considerations such as financial or racial aspects of the case. These circumstances make conflict nearly certain.

Like beauty, futility is in the eye of the beholder. Whether it is a physician who feels pressure to provide unjustified care or the family which is uncomfortable with continued aggressive care recommendations; no matter who is involved, the need to intervene, to do something, is intense. As physicians, we have been trained since medical school to intervene between a patient and his/her illness. Death is viewed as failure for physicians and an unacceptable outcome for our patients, no matter what the cause or illness.[2]

Illustrative Case

A 12-year-old male was struck by an automobile while riding his bicycle home from a Little League game. He has been your

Table 1. Examples of Medical Interventions That may be Considered Futile

- Life support in patients in a persistent vegetative state
- Resuscitation in patients with life-threatening illness
- Chemotherapy in patients with advanced refractory tumors
- Antibiotics and hydration for patients in the final stages of dying

patient since age four, when his family moved to town. He was stabilized in the emergency room and transferred to the intensive care unit, where he is being treated for a devastating brain injury. He has steadily deteriorated to the point to where, despite maximal therapy, he has developed multiple organ failure. He is currently receiving artificial ventilatory support and is on maximal pressor support. His parents are convinced he is aware of everything and expect him to wake up soon. They insist on continued aggressive treatment.

Defining Medical Futility

For the purpose of this chapter, the scenario assumed will be one in which the patient's family insists on care that the physician or other members of the health care team deems futile, as in the illustrated case. There have been a number of attempts to try and specifically define what exactly constitutes medical futility.[4] Which type of care being given must be answered. Of the several definitions put forth, some seem particularly appropriate for use by primary care providers. These include:

1. Medical care that does not meet the goals of the patient
2. Care that serves no legitimate goal of medical practice
3. Care that is ineffective more than 99% of the time
4. Care that does not conform to accepted community standards.[5]

Even with useful definitions to guide us, most medical futility cases are not straightforward and the potential for significant conflict between and among all participants in the discussion is common. In the case described above, the facts that the patient is so young patient and was injured so unexpectedly make it difficult for the health care team to withdraw therapy, even if clearly futile. Table 1 lists examples of medical interventions that may raise questions of futility.[5]

The issue of whether a specific medical intervention should be deemed futile is never clear cut. Some would argue that, in order to avoid conflict with a patient and his/her family, physicians ethically should not offer care that is unlikely to alter the course of the patient's illness. On the contrary, why should the physician's values override those of the patient and family, whose decisions and values may be religiously based? In response to this dilemma, and others like it, several groups have advocated to define medical futility on a case-by-case basis.[6]

Medical Futility as a Source of Conflict

Conflict is among the most common aspects of medical practice that physicians avoid. Unfortunately, conflict is common when dealing with cases of medical futility. When faced with conflict, one of the first things the physician must do is to try to resolve the conflict through negotiation with the patient and family. Successful negotiation can only come through a genuine understanding of the perceptions of the patient and family. The best way to deal with conflict initially is to find common ground that both parties can agree upon. In the case of medical futility, this is usually straightforward in that one of the herald obligations of the family physician is to support the patient and family as well as ease their suffering. Statements acknowledging commonalities such as "I think everybody wants what is best for your son" reinforce to the family that the physician is committed to doing what is best for the patient. It also allows an initial reference point in beginning negotiations on what types of therapy should or shouldn't be contemplated in dealing with the dying patient. In the illustrated case, building an alliance with the family to "do what is best" for the patient serves as a starting point. Through subsequent discussions and education, the specific definition of exactly what is best for the patient can be accomplished. Remember that during negotiation, the patient and family are partners, not opponents. It is absolutely imperative to understand why there is disagreement between the family and the primary care physician. When beginning the negotiating process with the patient and/or family, an important consideration is the degree of preparedness on the part of the primary care provider. Avoiding surprises during the negotiations is by far and away the best method of dealing with them. Table 2 lists some of the more important issues when negotiating with the patient and family.

Review the case, consider as many alternatives as possible, and think about the consequences of each prior to meeting with the patient and family. Try and have an understanding as to the particular needs of each of the family members. If possible, try and select a spokesperson for the family to maximize the quality of communication.[7]

Ideally, the patient should have had advanced care planning and would have his/her wishes clearly communicated to a trusted subordinate who would carry out those wishes without excessively emotional interplay.[8,9] Unfortunately, reality dictates that such communication can be lacking. In this case, determining why there is conflict can be addressed by asking a few questions. Table 3 lists appropriate questions to ask when conflict arises over medical futility.

If the patient lacks the capacity to make decisions for him/herself, the primary care provider must rely on another person to make decisions regarding medical care of the dying patient (i.e., the surrogate decision maker). In an ideal situation this person would be named by the patient in advanced directives and would have been educated by the patient as to what the patient would want to have happen in a variety of hypothetical situations. Several criteria exist for the ideal decision maker.[5] Table 4 lists these criteria.

It's always a good idea to be familiar with particular state statutes regarding the selection of surrogate decision makers.[8] In the rare instance when the primary care provider feels that the surrogate is not acting in the patient's best interests, he/she must go to court and have a court-appointed surrogate declared.[10]

Table 2. Important Negotiation Issues

- Be prepared
- Identify the central issue and break it into its simplest components
- Determine who should be involved
- Consider each party's real needs
- Develop and communicate your strategies

Table 3. Common Questions to Ask When Conflict Arises

- Is the surrogate decision maker the appropriate person?
- What are the specific misunderstandings?
- Are there personal factors involved?
- Is there a conflict in values?

A common theme that underlies conflict is miscommunication on one or more of several levels that result in misperception on the part of one of the parties. Several factors are involved in misperception and misunderstanding. Some of the more common ones are listed in Table 5.[8]

In order to best respond to misperceptions and subsequent conflict, the physician must first precisely understand what the patient and family are saying. One of the most widely quoted works in educating physicians on the communication of important information is Robert Buckman's *How to Break Bad News: A Guide for Health Care Professionals*. Using Buckman's six-step protocol is a good first step in maximizing the quality of communication.[11] Table 6 summarizes Buckman's six-step protocol.

Even before beginning a conversation with the patient and family an investment of a few moments to refamiliarize yourself with the major details of the case and confirm any controversial information is helpful. If rehearsal is needed, take the time to do it. It is also worthwhile to select an appropriate private, yet comfortable site to convey the information. While conversing with the patient and family, ensure to the best of your ability that interruptions are minimized (shut off beepers, hold calls, post the room as private, etc.).[12]

Despite the best preparation, misperceptions regarding futility of care are not uncommon. Table 7 lists some of the many things that can be done in response to misperceptions by patients and their families.[8]

In addition to the already contentious nature of medical futility disagreements, personal factors may also play important roles in aggravating disagreement.[13] As medicine has become increasingly exact in its scientific explanation of the nature of the diseases of humans, the physician's role as human companion has correspondingly become less important. Indeed, the proliferation of various "healers" mirrors society's need for interventions more dependent on human relationships rather than scientific explanation. Lack of effective human relationship in the practice of medicine leads to the possibility of mistrust among patients and their families. This mistrust stems from a lack of understanding of some of the more complex medical concepts present in the patient and the innate sense that practitioners who depend only on scientific explanation have more control of the situation. When information is presented by many providers in various formats, unintentional and inconsequential disparities may seem like unreliable (therefore untrustworthy) information from the family's perspective.[14] If the physician feels that mistrust is evident in the patient and/or family, active measures to restore trust must be carried out. Addressing the issue directly demonstrates concern to the patient and family. Listening and trying to understand patient and family issues is also important. Liberal use of second opinions by providers that the patient and family trust helps to alleviate mistrust.

Families of dying patients are actively grieving, whether or not they are in denial concerning the terminality of the patient. The use of a multidisciplinary team that includes clergy can help families manage the grieving process. Often, getting the family to realize what truly is in the best interest of the patient helps to minimize the chance that significant conflict will arise.[15]

The power of the family unit throughout the entire family life cycle is potent. This power can be used either productively or counterproductively by various family members, depending on the types of relationships that have developed between them over time.[16] Dysfunctional relationships between family members produce abnormal grief reactions and inappropriate guilt, which can lead to poor decision making. The stereotypic situation is the long-estranged relative who arrives late in the development of the crisis threatening legal action over any decision considering potentially futile therapy. Using Buckman's protocol could help focus on needs and fears of the family member in question, but typically communicating with such relatives requires skill and patience. Trying to successfully resolve longstanding intrafamily issues is probably overoptimistic, especially in time of crisis. Instead, try to recognize dysfunctional relationships in the context of the family and use this understanding to optimize communication. This could require input from the entire health care team, including nurses, social workers, and the clergy. Developing a family genogram may help to define relationships and provide context and insight into family dynamics.[17] This would also allow the physician to help more effectively in the decision making of a particular spokesperson who represents family views accurately and communicates well.

Particularly distasteful, and fortunately uncommon, is the scenario of a surrogate making decisions based on some selfish interest rather than the patient's good. This may stem from either the surrogate losing the financial support he/she had while the patient was alive or from the surrogate anticipating inheritance upon the patient's death.[18] Decision makers may also ask the physician to falsify insurance documents concerning the onset of illness or disability. This is particularly common in cases where the illness is sudden or unanticipated. Physicians should be sensitive to these problems and anticipate issues of secondary gain. When secondary

Table 4. Criteria for Surrogate Decision-Maker Selection

- Patient preference
- Legislated hierarchy for decision makers
- Likely to know what the patient would have wanted
- Able to reflect the patient's best interests
- Has the cognitive ability to make decisions

gain is suspected as a reason for decision making, asking for help from other disciplines such as social workers or, if the institution has one, an ethics committee. Ethics committees can be extremely useful to the clinician. They can add confidence to clinical decisions for dying patients as well as focus on other areas of care for the terminal patient. They may also help to avoid conflict between the health care team and the patient's family. Currently, the Joint Commission for Accreditation of Health Care Organizations (JCAHO) does not mandate the existence of ethics committees per se, though it does mandate many of an ethics committee's functions. Ethics committees are typically made up of physicians, nurses, social workers, community representatives, clergy, and legal experts. This breadth of expertise allows the committee to be sensitive to many social and cultural issues. It also allows a degree of empathy between the committee and the patient and family, helping to avoid conflict.[19]

Even with tools such as ethics committees, conflict still arises. Most legitimate conflict surrounds a disagreement over values between the physician and the dying patient's family. Specifically, parties usually disagree over either goals of therapy or benefit to the patient.[20] For example, the family's goal may simply be the preservation of life. Other considerations, such as the quality of life or the degree of pain and/or disability, are not a part of that goal. Health care workers may disagree with the notion that preservation of life as an end in itself is valid. In terms of differences over patient benefit, party positions may not be so clear. Probably the best example of this is the family's insistence that an experimental or miracle cure be continued despite the patient's lack of response to the protocol. Health care providers, realizing the lack of effect, may decide that palliative care would most benefit the patient, again setting the stage for conflict.

At the heart of many of the conflicts that arise over instances of medical futility is a difference in basic values of the patient, his/her family, and the health care provider/system. These value differences can be categorized broadly into three general areas—religious considerations, miracles, and value of life.[5]

Being sensitive to the patient's religious convictions can go a long way toward recognizing and avoiding conflict in cases of medical futility. Specifically addressing the patient's religious beliefs and the role they play in decision making can help the primary care physician more accurately assist the patient in making these decisions, including those concerning medical futility.[21] Often, a patient will respond to questions of further therapy with words to the effect, "It's God's will." Being specific about probable situations in which a decision had to be made by the health care staff can help provide insight into a patient's wishes. For example, saying, "If your heart should stop beating, would I be doing the right thing in doing CPR?" focuses on the specific issue at hand while at the same time lending insight into the patient's true wishes. If, after a careful assessment of the patient's wishes in the context of the patient's religious convictions, the physician feels his/her own religious beliefs are compromised, arrangements for transfer of care to another provider must be made as early in the situation as possible. It is sometimes difficult for physicians, or anybody else for that matter, to come to grips with personal religious beliefs as well as the realization of one's own morality. Thinking about and being comfortable with these issues will go a long way in helping the physician to address these same issues with his/her patients.

Sometimes the patient and/or family may advocate for medically futile care in hope of the occurrence of a miracle. By definition, miracles are rare, unpredictable, supernatural occurrences. Often, explaining to the patient that if a miracle were to happen, it would happen regardless of the types of medical decisions being made. Another approach would be to ask if the family was interfering with God's wish to "call the patient home" by continuing futile treatment. Again, these types of situations are perfect for formed ethics committees, which can help with communication and understanding. Having an ongoing relationship with local chaplaincy is essential in the care of the dying patient. Including the patient and/or family's personal religious consultant can increase the amount of trust between physician and patient.[22]

The foregoing discussion was meant to carefully consider the nature of situations that may lead to conflict over medical treatment between the physician and patient/family. Understanding the nature of the conflict often leads to obvious and acceptable solutions. But this is not always so. Table 8 summarizes a due process approach to conflicts that arise between the physician and patient.[23]

Many hospitals have policies related to the provision of futile care that use a step-by-step process of communication and problem solving to help resolve differences between the physician and the patient and/or family. This type of due process approach is strong-

Table 5. Common Factors Contributing to Misperceptions

- Decision maker is unaware of the diagnosis
- Language includes too much jargon
- Conflicting or rapidly changing information
- Unrealistic optimism by providers
- Stressful environment
- High emotional stress
- Unprepared psychologically
- Inadequate cognitive ability

Table 6. A Six-Step Protocol for Communicating Important Information

- Get started
- Find out what the patient/family knows
- Find out what the patient/family wants to know
- Share the information
- Respond to patient/family feelings
- Plan and follow-up

ly recommended by the AMA's Council on Ethical and Judicial Affairs, and should include the following steps.[5]

1. Attempt to negotiate an understanding between patient, surrogate, and physician about what constitutes futile care in advance of actual conflict. This step can preempt conflict.
2. To the maximum extent possible, joint decision-making should occur between the patient or surrogate and physician. Negotiate solutions to disagreements, if they arise, in order to reach a resolution satisfactory to all parties. Use the assistance of consultants as appropriate.
3. If disagreements persist, suggest the participation of other consultants, colleagues, and/or a group, such as an institutional ethics committee. These additional resources may provide a reasoned impartial assessment and evaluation of the conflict. The value of ethics committees has been well described in this article. The Joint Commission for Accreditation of Healthcare Institutions requires hospitals to have an ethics committee or a functional counterpart to aid its physicians, patients, and families to resolve difficult issues. The aim is to provide the maximum possible space for patient autonomy in the conduct of ethical medical practice.

Table 7. Responding to Misperceptions

- Choose a primary communicator
- Give information in manageable quantities
- Give information in different formats
- Use language that is understandable
- Frequently repeat information
- Do not hedge to soften the information
- Encourage written questions
- Provide support as needed
- Involve other professionals

Table 8. A Due Process Approach to Futility Situations

- Earnest attempts at negotiation in advance
- Joint decision making
- Negotiation of disagreements
- Involvement of an institutional ethics committee
- Transfer of care to another physician if necessary
- Transfer to another institution if necessary
- If unable to transfer, the intervention need not be offered

4. If the institutional review supports the patient's position and the physician remains unpersuaded, transfer of care to another physician within the institution may be arranged.
5. If the review supports the physician's position and the patient/surrogate remains unpersuaded, transfer to another institution can be carried out if both the transferring and receiving institutions agree. If transfer to another physician in another institution is not possible, the intervention need not be offered. However, there needs to be a diligent search for this option and legal input is suggested.
6. This process does not solve the problem when no receiving institution can be found. The issue of cost of medical care, both to patients and families as well as to the institution and the health care system, is implicit in many of these steps.

Summary

Situations involving true medical futility are uncommon. More often than not, the question of futility comes up when there is miscommunication and conflict. Sources of conflict may be identified as follows. The proxy may not be performing the role well. There may be misunderstandings over prognosis. There may be personal factors such as distrust or guilt. Or there may be differences in values. For intractable difficulties a fair process for conflict resolution is recommended. This process should include, if at all possible, prior discussion as to what constitutes futility, joint decision making with the patient/family and other parties, involvement of a consultant and/or ethics committee, and transfer of care to another physician or institution if necessary. Rarely, if no physician or institution can be found to provide the intervention, it may be necessary to withdraw or withhold what the patient and/or family has requested.

References

1. Halliday R. Medical futility and the social context. *J Med Ethics* 1997;23:148-153.
2. Harper W. The role of futility in improperly limiting the scope of clinical research. *J Med Ethics* 1998;24:308-313.

3. Spielman B. Bargaining about futility. *J Law Med Ethics* 1995;23:136-142.
4. Wiener RL, et al. A preliminary analysis of medical futility decision-making: Law and professional attitudes. *Behav Sci Law* 1998;16:497-508.
5. American Medical Association Institute for Ethics. Education for Physicians on End-of-Life Care (EPEC), Module 9, Medical Futility. Trainer's Guide. Chicago: American Medical Association; 1999. Supported by a grant from the Robert Wood Johnson Foundation.
6. Council on Ethical and Judicial Affairs. Medical Futility in End-of-Life Care. In: *Council on Ethical and Judicial Affairs Reports of End-of-Life Care*. Chicago, IL: American Medical Association; 1998:44-49.
7. Belzer EA. What the family physician needs to know about negotiation. *Fam Pract Man* 1995:66-75.
8. American Medical Association Institute for Ethics. *Education for Physicians on End-of-Life Care (EPEC), Module 1, Advance Care Planning.* Trainer's Guide. Chicago: American Medical Association; 1999. Supported by a grant from the Robert Wood Johnson Foundation.
9. American Medical Association Institute for Ethics. *Education for Physicians on End-of-Life Care (EPEC), Module 7, Goals of Care.* Trainer's Guide. Chicago: American Medical Association; 1999. Supported by a grant from the Robert Wood Johnson Foundation.
10. Olson E, et al. Treatment termination in long-term care: What about the physician? What about the family? *J Long Term Home Health Care* 1997;16:14-21.
11. Buckman R. *How to Break Bad News: A Guide for Health Care Professionals*. Baltimore, MD: The Johns Hopkins University Press; 1992:54-78.
12. Dunn PM, et al. Discussing futility with patients and families. *J Gen Intern Med* 1996;11:689-693.
13. Caplan AL. Odds and ends: Trust and the debate over medical futility. *Arch Intern Med* 1996;15:125:688-689.
14. Brett AS, et al. Beyond futility to an ethic of care. *Am J Med* 1995;99:443-444.
15. Jecker NS. Medical futility and care of dying patients. *West J Med* 1995;163:287-291.
16. Christie-Seely J. The family in family medicine. American Academy of Family Physicians, Home Study Self Assessment 1988;106:42-47.
17. Tong R. Toward a just, courageous, and honest resolution of the futility debate. *J Med Philos* 1995; 20:165-189.
18. Kopelman LM. Conceptual and moral disputes about futile and useful treatments. *J Med Philos* 1995;20:109-121.
19. Schwartz BP, et al. Primary care medicine and some medical/ethical issues. *Primary Care Reports* 1997;25: 231-239.
20. Rhodes R. Futility and the goals of medicine. *J Clin Ethics* 1998;9:194-205.
21. Hinds PS. Knowing when enough is enough. *J Pediatr Oncol Nurs* 1996;13:1.
22. Ebell MH. When everything is too much. *Arch Fam Med* 1995;4:352-356.
23. American Medical Association Institute for Ethics. *Education for Physicians on End-of-Life Care (EPEC), Module 9, Medical Futility,* pp. 15-16. Trainer's Guide. Chicago: American Medical Association; 1999. Supported by a grant from the Robert Wood Johnson Foundation.

Health Informatics

William F. Perry, MA, RN
Jane C. Buch, MLS

Health informatics is the practice of managing health care information with computers. Recording, storing, analyzing, and retrieving information to meet regulatory requirements, demonstrate quality improvement projects, and document complete patient care demands an ever increasing amount of physician time. This chapter will introduce the reader to computer-based practice management resources, the electronic medical record, e-mail, Internet resources, and security issues.

Computers are changing the face of primary care medicine. The electronic medical record can enhance a practice by improving legibility, improving documentation, and providing physicians with appropriate patient specific clinical reminders. Computers connected to the Internet offer the primary care practitioner an unprecedented opportunity for communication, collaboration, education, and research unhampered by the restrictions of time and distance.

Patients access many of the resources once primarily used by physicians. Health-related Internet sites appear and disappear rapidly. Consumers are inundated with ads urging them to visit drug-specific web sites and to ask their care providers if those drugs are appropriate for them. Patients are downloading information, e-mailing and chatting with others with similar symptoms, and bringing the results of their online investigations to their clinic appointments. If for no other reason, clinicians need to have an awareness of what is available to understand what their patients are reading.

Practice Management

Appointments, scheduling, and billing represent a major task for computers in the office setting. Patient demographics and insurance information are essential pieces of information to bill for services. Electronic certification of insurance participation is a timesaver for the clinician and patient. Computer resources can save practitioners and their office staff time while improving legibility, completeness, and maximizing reimbursement.

Clinically oriented systems can provide practitioners with documentation reminders to adequately justify appropriate diagnoses and interventions. By including the Health Care Financing Administration (HCFA) guidelines, billing and coding modules have reduced undercoding in some practices by 25-33%.[1] Plan-specific formularies may be available electronically. Prescriptions can be electronically written using an application such as eMD.com,[2] appointments made with consultants, and tests/procedures scheduled. These activities can result in efficiencies in patient care and time savings for all involved.

Business to business services give the primary care office the ability to order supplies and equipment electronically. This "just in time" approach saves money by minimizing the need to keep larger supplies on hand. Payment for goods is done through a secure system, and because of 24-hour availability, limitations imposed by time and geography decrease in significance.

Components of the Clinical Record

Searching for records, documenting care given, and providing copies of required documents takes time. An electronic medical record makes information available to whoever needs it, whenever they need it. In a multi-office practice, records do not have to be transported between offices, requests for information do not have to wait until the paper record is retrieved, forms do not have to be manually filed, and information duplication can be eliminated. Wireless technologies are being applied to the medical record with definite bottom line savings,[3] and patients are accepting computers in the exam room as a matter of routine. Physicians do not need to be tied to the office to complete or review records. Given the appropriate user identification and passwords, records can be viewed and worked on from any computer attached to the Internet, whether from home or a vacation hotel room.

In a summary of a 1998 *Lancet* panel, 12 advantages were noted to an electronic medical record:[4]

1. Simultaneous, remote access to patient data
2. Legibility of record
3. Safer data—protection from lost paper
4. Patient data confidentiality
5. Flexible data layout
6. Integration with other information resources
7. Incorporation of electronic data (electronic testing and recording equipment)
8. Continuous data processing (subject to user defined rules, interaction, and alerts criteria)
9. Assisted search
10. Greater range of data output modalities
11. Tailored paper output
12. Always up to date[5]

Approaches to an electronic medical record vary from complete systems for large, multisite and multiprovider practices to single physician offices. In the single provider office, systems can range from integrated clinical and administrative systems to a single-user clinical application. Some physicians have chosen to automate portions of their current practices for such tasks as creating forms for frequently used documents such as physicals and insurance forms. While not the computerized medical record per se, applications to process routine tasks such as form completion greatly enhance office productivity.[6]

Connected computers that share information form networks. Networks may consist of as few as two computers connected by a cable to millions of computers connected to the Internet. There are many small-office networking kits available that allow all the computers in an office or business to share information with each other. If an office is networked, data can be entered from any computer attached to the network whether in the physician's office or the exam room.

A relatively new approach to the electronic medical record involves an "application service provider" (ASP). Rather than purchasing the software, programs are leased and the vendor maintains the programs on their central computers. Information is entered into the systems using either a dedicated communications line or an Internet connection. With this method, savings are realized by outsourcing the technology component. The practice does not have to house the medical record software and the ASP takes care of hardware, security, and maintenance issues (such as backups), and patient copies of the medical record can be easily created. The patient medical record is password protected and can be viewed from any computer attached to the Internet. MedicaLogic offers a free trial of this approach.[7] As fast Internet connections using ISDN telephone lines, DSL connections, and cable modems become more readily available, the ASP model will be as efficient and responsive as an application housed within a local facility.

Patients are becoming more interested in having virtual copies of their health record. Services such as PersonalMD offer consumers the ability to create an online health record, which includes both text information and faxed documents such as EKGs, radiology, and lab reports.[8] The basic service is free to the consumer and any provider who has a need to see the recorded information; advertising and selling other value-added services supports the site. Access is via a secure Internet page and protected by a personal identification number (PIN). If a provider who does not have an Internet connection requires access to the information, a copy of the information can be automatically faxed to the requesting physician. If the patient's primary care physician assumes an active role in supplying information for this virtual patients' owned and oriented record, the benefits to the patient in an emergency situation could be life saving.

An evolving area in computerized health care information is where patients become participants in the documentation process by recording weights, medications taken, or transmitting information that originates from home monitoring devices. The health care provider reviews patient-transmitted information and appropriate interventions can be instituted early before they require vigorous intervention and hospitalization.

There are many vendors who supply the components to an electronic medical record. Prices and sophistication range considerably; the primary care practitioner who is contemplating an electronic approach can get an overview of various capabilities from such journals as *MD Computing*[9] or *Healthcare-Informatics*.[10] Single-user versions of a computerized record can be downloaded from such sites as PowerMed[11] or SOAPware.[12]

The electronic medical record is becoming an essential tool. Sooner or later it will touch your practice.

Security Issues and the Computerized Medical Record

The conveniences and efficiencies of computerized tools in health care are complicated by the threat of viruses and the need to protect patient information. Any computer system is vulnerable to unauthorized access and the most elaborate security system is only as effective as the least compliant user. The confidentiality of patients' electronic records is directly dependent on the security policies, procedures, and practices of the people using the system. Information becomes unprotected when passwords are shared, authorized users fail to log off a system when they are done using it, computers are left physically unprotected, or network safeguards such as firewalls are not implemented.

The Health Insurance Portability and Accountability Act of 1996 (HIPAA) proposes standardized approaches to the identification, transmission, storage, and security of electronic patient health care information. While still not finally released, any provider who stores patient information electronically will be affected. If a practitioner uses electronic mail to communicate with patients about health care issues, the e-mail files must also be protected. A list of suggested actions to prepare for implementation of these standards is on the American Academy of Family Practitioner's web site.[13] The proposed regulation and comments are posted on the Health and Human Services web site.[14]

Viruses are computer programs intentionally designed to cause damage to a computer or its resources. Viruses can be hidden in files downloaded from the Internet, from diskettes that have been used in an infected computer, or attached to e-mail messages. E-mail messages from unknown individuals, especially if they have attachments, should be deleted without opening them. Virus checking software should be installed on all computers. Trial software can be obtained safely from sources such as Symantec[15] or McAfee.[16] Comparisons between software packages can be made through web sites such as ZDNet[17] or Cnet.[18] The best way to protect a computer from viruses is to not allow anyone to run any software that is not a part of the office system.

In addition to good security practices, data must be backed up regularly to protect against electronic catastrophe. This is most often accomplished using tape backup systems or storing the files on CD-ROM. Internet-based storage is also becoming a popular way to store copies of electronic records away from the practice site. In the ASP model, the program vendor takes care of this function. In a locally housed system, it becomes a duty of the office staff. Even backups must be appropriately protected from unauthorized access.

Electronically Mediated Communication

In addition to the clinical record, the Internet-connected practice can expand communication with patients by allowing electronic mail requests for nonurgent clinical questions, appointments, and prescription refills. A practice web site can be a portal for these and other services such as patient education materials tailored to practitioner preferences. A 1999 Internet survey reported "the total number of health users"—those using the Internet for retrieval of health and medical information—as 24.8 million. Fifty percent of online users expressed interest in electronic communication with their physician or availability of information from their physician's web site.[19]

In 1998, The American Medical Informatics Association developed "Guidelines for the Clinical Use of Electronic Mail with Patients."[20] This document addressed concerns of clinicians regarding the medico-legal implications of such approaches and offers a set of protocols for the implementation of e-mail communication with patients. A successful approach to electronic communication begins with a documented agreement between the patient and their provider as to the services that may be requested, the types of problems that may be discussed, and the expected response time. In addition, it is critical there be the understanding that e-mail is a patient-provider interaction and is recorded in their medical record.

Electronic mail is not encrypted as a matter of routine and can be intercepted and read by anyone with the technical knowledge and equipment. In light of government regulations concerning the privacy of personal health care information, physicians must be very cautious when using unencrypted electronic mail. Encryption technologies exist, are available, and some are relatively inexpensive. A free, publicly available version of the encryption program Pretty Good Privacy (PGP) is available.[21] While relatively simple to use, they may prove difficult for patients who are using services such as America On Line to access the Internet. Secure e-mail services such as those provided by Salu.net[22] or Healinx[23] are user-friendly ways to provide security for physician-patient communications. A signed statement by the patient and provider waiving the requirement for secure electronic mail should be considered if a secure e-mail system is not available to both parties. Practical considerations and concerns regarding the use of e-mail and patients are outlined at the Informatics Review web site.[24]

Electronic mail from patients must be protected in the same manner as paper-based patient information. Administrative considerations include assigning the responsibility to triage e-mail, office protocols as to the review and filing of electronic communications, and assuring the confidentiality of electronic documents.

The Primary Care Practice Web Site

Given the number of health care consumers who use the Internet to search for health care information, a web site becomes a potential gateway for present and future patients to find, learn about, and interact with health care professionals. Internet web sites range from simple to complex and from free to tremendously expensive.

Information on a practice web site might include basic information about a practice such as physician names, office hours, location, telephone, and fax numbers. Internet-based maps such as MapBlast[25] or Expedia[26] can provide door to door directions for new or potential patients. Photographs of the staff and of the office building aid in personalizing the web site. Submitting the practice web site to various Internet search engines or linking with local hospital or city web sites becomes a marketing activity that expands practice exposure.

Expanded web site offerings could include e-mail links, patient education materials, survey forms, newsletters, or appointment request forms. Reminders or special announcements could be sent by electronic mail. Many types of patient-provider or patient-office staff interactions that currently occur via the telephone could potentially be replicated in a digital format, extending the potential number of clients.

Professional Collaboration

Collaboration, discussion, and other information exchange occurs constantly between health care professionals. Few, if any, practice in a state of professional isolation, but they may be limited in their opportunities for interaction with other physicians because of geographic location, practice responsibilities, or other time constraints. Internet-based discussion with professional peer groups can offer a means to a broader viewpoint on practice issues.

Professional organizations frequently have a web site that incorporates web-based discussion areas to facilitate professional communication and collaboration. One of the best resources to find peer discussion groups is located at the Medical Matrix web site.[27]

There are two kinds of computerized discussion areas: mailing lists, also frequently called listserves, and web-based discussion groups. Electronic communication can be synchronous, where both parties are connected to a site simultaneously such as a chat room, or asynchronous, where participants read the messages left by other group members at a time of their own choosing. The advantage of the listserv or web discussion group approach is the independence from time and place requirements. Professional communities exist for both forms of asynchronous group discussion and have been shown to be a viable method of professional communication and collaboration. E-mail or web-based discussions replicate informal conversations between practitioners centered on a common clinical topic or clinical specialty. Anyone is free to initiate a message thread, and the number of responses to the topic posted is limited only by the interest expressed by the readers. Posting, or sending an e-mail, is not a requirement to remain in the group. As in any conversational group, some prefer to listen while others do most of the talking.

In a mailing list, each member of the list receives copies of any message posted to the list membership. Messages a subscriber receives from a list membership can either be delivered singly or bundled together and delivered as a single message called a digest. Other commands can be sent to hold mail messages while the member is on vacation. Some e-mail lists generate a tremendous volume of e-mail messages. If ignored, they will continue to be delivered to the subscriber's electronic mailbox until the limit of the mailbox is reached and no other messages will be accepted.

In a discussion board, people wishing to read the posted messages go to the Internet site where the messages can be read as desired. No messages are delivered by electronic mail.

Continuing Medical Education

Continuing medical education opportunities abound on the Internet. Anytime, anywhere training is available to any practitioner with a computer and modem. Although electronically mediated CME lacks the personal interaction of a live professional meeting, the convenience of such approaches is drawing large numbers of practitioners. At some sites, interactivity may be encouraged making discussion boards available for participants.

Both fee based and free CME offerings are available. CMEweb.com offers more than 1100 hours in many areas of clinical interest, including internal medicine and primary care. Pharmaceutical manufacturers, hospitals, or medical schools and residency programs may sponsor free CME such as Helix.[28] Medscape offers a combination of free and fee based CME.[29]

Research

Even before the advent of a graphical interface (the World Wide Web), physicians with strong information technology backgrounds were using the Internet to gain access to research, especially that which was unpublished or not yet published. Often the search process involved hours of scrolling through menu screens without ever finding a primary source. Today the Internet offers a wide array of accessible resources for physicians. In fact, there are so many resources that physicians face a new problem: sifting through an overabundance of sites in an effort to distinguish trash from treasure.

PubMed

One of the undisputed treasures on the Internet is PubMed,[30] the National Library of Medicine's site for searching Medline and related databases. PubMed offers free access to anyone on the Internet. Technical support is available via e-mail or a toll-free number (800-338-7657).

Basic Search Techniques

Basic Searches are a good solution for searchers who are inexperienced, in a hurry, or who aren't getting any results with advanced search strategies.

Basic Search Steps.

1. At the PubMed home page, type your search terms in the query box at the top of the page. Use uppercase for Boolean connectors: AND, OR, NOT.
2. Press the Enter key or click the Go button.
3. After a few seconds, the results of your search will be displayed.

Displays.

1. The default for search results is a summary (citation) display of 20 items.
2. Click on the author's name to view the citation and abstract; use your browser's Back button to return to the list of citations.
3. To change the display on the results page, click on the drop down box next to the Display button and choose an alternate format, then click the Display button. The most commonly used formats are:
   - **Abstract:** includes citation and abstract

- **Citation:** includes citation, abstract, and medical subject headings
- **Link out:** includes an abbreviated citation and link to the journal web site when available

4. To change the number of items displayed on a single web page, click on the drop down box below the Display button, choose a different number, and click the Display button. It is sometimes easier to navigate with all the items displayed on one page rather than paging through the results.

Selecting Items, Using the Clipboard, and Printing.

1. There is a selection box to the left of each citation, no matter which display format you are using. When you click in this box to select the item, a check mark appears. To deselect the item, click in the box again and the check mark will disappear.
2. To save items to the clipboard, click on the Add to Clipboard button at any time in the selection process. Duplicate items are never added. If no selection boxes are marked, all of the items in the results (not just the items on the page) are added to the clipboard. Up to 500 items can be placed on the clipboard. They will remain there until they are deleted or until an hour has passed with no activity. This allows you to try as many search strategies as you like before printing.
3. To print selected items, click on the Clipboard link below the query box. On the clipboard page, choose the display format you want to print and click on your browser's Print button.
4. Before going onto a new search topic, it's a good idea to clear the clipboard by clicking on the Remove from Clipboard button. If no items are selected, all the items will be cleared.

Advanced Search Techniques.

Limits are a useful way to narrow the search when the retrieval is too large.

1. Click on the Limits link below the query box.
2. The limits page allows you to limit your search by:
   - common publication types;
   - language;
   - age groups;
   - human or animal studies;
   - gender;
   - publication date;
   - entrez date (the date the article was entered into the database); and
   - journal subsets such as Abridged Index Medicus, Nursing, Dental, PreMedline, and Publisher Supplied Citations.

Medical Subject Headings are Often the Starting Point for Experienced Searchers.

1. Click on Mesh Browser link on the blue bar on the left side of the home page.
2. Enter your first topic in the query box and Mesh Browser will try to identify a Medical Subject Heading related to it. For example, if you type "liver cancer," Mesh Browser will return the subject heading "liver neoplasms." If Browser can't map to an exact subject heading it will give you a list of headings from which to choose.
3. A definition of the term is usually displayed below the subject heading. Below that is an index section showing where the term fits into the subject heading scheme. At this point, you may click on a broader or narrower subject heading. Always remember to choose the narrowest or most specific subject heading appropriate to your topic when starting a search. For example, if you are more interested in liver cell adenoma than liver cancer in general, use that term rather than liver neoplasms.
4. Returning to the top of the screen, click on the Detailed Display link next to the subject heading. This will take you to the subheadings screen. Clicking on subheadings such as "diagnosis" or "drug therapy" will help you to further define your search. You may choose as many as you want; they will be OR'd together.
5. Detailed Display offers two further options:
   - Click in the box next to "Restrict Search to Major Topic headings only" when the subject heading you have chosen should be a major point of the article.
   - Click in the box next to "Do Not Explode this term" when you do not want narrower terms included in the search. For example, you want articles on liver cancer in general but not just on liver cell adenoma.
6. Click on the Add button to add your term to the search. A box will appear which contains your search strategy. At this point you may enter an intersecting term in the query box to add to the search strategy, or you may click on the PubMed Search button to complete the search.

Details.

The Details button appears on any page with search results, in the array at the top of the page. A link to Details also appears whenever a search strategy fails to produce any results. Click on it to see how PubMed has interpreted your search strategy and to edit your search strategy. If you have entered your search in plain text, this feature will show you whether PubMed has mapped it to a subject heading. If your search results are too broad, you can change your subject delimiter from "MeSH Terms" to "MAJR" for Major Topic headings. If your search results are too narrow, you can use the details dialog box to do the reverse. You can also add terms or delete them.

PreMedline and Publisher Supplied Records.

PreMedline records are citations that are so new they have not been completely processed. They usually don't include Medical Subject Headings. Publisher supplied records are citations that the National Library of Medicine includes only because the publisher supplies the information. These citations will never be assigned Medical Subject Headings. A search strategy that relies solely on Medical Subject Headings will exclude these citations, which often represent the newest information on a given topic. To make sure that PreMedline and Publisher Supplied records are included in your search, add terms with no qualifiers or with a [textword] qualifier to your strategy. For example: measles [MAJR] OR measles.

Other Features.

Clinical Queries uses built-in research filters to help you find clinically sound studies. The link to Clinical Queries is on the blue bar on the left side of the home page. On the Clinical Queries page, enter your search term(s) in the query box and click on one of these four categories: therapy, diagnosis, etiology, or prognosis. Then choose to emphasize either sensitivity or specificity and click on the Go button.

Citation Matcher aids you in completing partial citations. Click on the Single Citation Matcher link on the blue bar on the left side of the home page. Fill in as much of the citation as you know. You must use the full title of the journal unless you know the Medline abbreviation (which you can find using the Journal Browser link). PubMed will return any citations that match the information you input. You can use this feature to browse the contents of a journal issue by searching the journal title and volume/issue or date.

URL and Cubby are two separate functions, both of which allow you to save a search strategy. The URL function saves your search by bookmarking it. When you are satisfied that your strategy is producing the results you want, click on the details button and remove any publication date or entrez date references. Then click on the URL button below the dialog box. This will return you to the results page, but now the search strategy is embedded in the URL or web address. Use your browser's bookmark feature to bookmark the page. Every time you click on the bookmark, your search will be updated and run. With the new Cubby feature, you simply click on the Cubby link when your search is complete and name the search when prompted by PubMed. When you are ready to run the search again, go back to the Cubby link and click on the search name. The Cubby feature does require a brief, free registration and a log-in each time you use it.

Other Useful Sites

Clinical Trials. CenterWatch Clinical Trials is a division of the Medical Economics Company, publisher of *Physicians' Desk Reference*.[31] The site provides:

- a list of clinical trials arranged by disease category that gives brief information about the trials and a form to request further information;
- information on NIH studies;
- a clinical trial notification service; and
- information on newly approved drug therapies.

ClinicalTrials.gov, a new site sponsored by the NIH through the National Library of Medicine, allows users to search clinical trials using keywords or browse by disease/condition or sponsor.[32] The site provides information of the purpose of and eligibility for the studies, contact information, and a link to further information when it is available. There are also links to detailed information about participating in clinical trials.

Practice Guidelines. National Guideline Clearinghouse[33] is sponsored by the Agency for Healthcare Research and Quality (formerly the Agency for Health Care Policy and Research), the American Medical Association, and the American Association of Health Plans. The site expands on the AHCPR site for locating practice guidelines. In addition to keyword searches, the user may browse by disease/condition, treatment/intervention, or organization. Viewing formats include brief summary, full summary, and full text. A special feature of the Clearinghouse is the option to select guidelines and compare them in terms of adaptation, length, developer(s), funding source, committee, group composition, disease/condition, category, clinical specialty, intended users, objectives, target population, review methods, endorsers, outcomes considered, cost analysis, methods to collect evidence, methods to assess the quality and strength of the evidence, methods to analyze evidence, and availability of full text.

Instructions to Authors. Raymon H. Mulford Library of the Medical College Of Ohio hosts this page of links to more than 3000 journals in the health and life sciences that provide instructions to authors on the web.[34] Arrangement is alphabetical by journal title.

Drug Information. Gold Standard Multimedia's Clinical Pharmacology Online, previously a propriety product, is now available for free (registration is required).[35] This is the full product version and includes information on prescription, OTC, and investigational drugs; herbal products; drug photographs and product identification; drug interactions; and patient education.

The FDA Center for Drug Evaluation and Research's Drug Information page, updated daily, is a good resource for drug news, especially concerning recently approved drugs.[36] The link to New Drugs Approved for Cancer indications provides timely information on this rapidly changing topic.

Full Text Books. *The Merck Manual of Diagnosis and Therapy*[37] allows the user to do a keyword search or browse the table of contents of this core medical text.

Lexi-Comp's Diagnostic Procedures Handbook is part of the HealthGate site, one of the established medical malls on the Internet.[38] Entry is by keyword search or alphabetical index. This is a quick reference guide for diagnostic procedures that may include a section on what the procedure commonly includes, indications, contraindications, patient preparation, special instructions, equipment, technique, causes for rejection, turnaround time, normal findings, critical values, limitations, and references.

University of Iowa Family Practice Handbook is found on University of Iowa's Virtual Hospital site.[39] It is searchable by keyword or hyperlinked table of contents. The text is presented in outline form with hyperlinks to "see" references.

Virtual Hospital's Multimedia Textbooks offer electronic texts on a wide variety of topics.[40] As the name implies, these textbooks include graphics and sounds.

Full Text Journals. Brandon/Hill List of Journals is a National Library of Medicine site based on the "Brandon/Hill Selected List Of Books And Journals For The Small Medical Library."[41] A table lists all of the Brandon/Hill journals and indicates whether full text is available for each title and, if so, whether it is fee-based or free. Where full text is not an option, there is information on the availability of abstracts. Finally, the site provides start dates for online access.

MedWeb from Emory University lists more than 700 electronic medical journals.[42] There is no quick way to navigate through the alphabetic listing, but you can browse by subject or do a keyword search. The information offered about each journal is inconsistent; it may include a note on the publisher, a brief scope note, or full text options. Cost information is included for each title. Go to the Advanced Search and type "free" in the query box to get a list of titles that are offered gratis.

Patient Education. Clifford Stoll, noted computer security expert, wrote "Silicon Snake Oil" in 1996. Anyone who has spent any time searching the Internet for any type of information is confronted with an overwhelming number of choices in response to their queries. The dynamic nature of the Internet allows instantaneous publishing with a potential audience of millions. There is no censorship, quality assurance, or regulation of Internet resources.

The Miretek Organization, a nonprofit technology organization, is the home of The Health Information Technology Institute whose mission is "to ensure quality health care by conducting research in support of accessible, affordable, and appropriate health care in the public interest."[43] They have created an "Information Quality Tool," an online series of questions that helps users evaluate the content of a health care web site and returns a score based on the user's responses.

The federal government has a large number of web sites directed to health care consumer education. Professional organizations compile lists of peer-reviewed sites for both health care professionals as well as consumers. The Health on the Net Foundation is a voluntary group started in 1994 in Switzerland that encourages web site owners to post its logo if they agree to abide by their Code of Conduct.[44] The Code of Conduct is designed to make visitors to health care sites aware of that resource's approach to health care information. The areas addressed are authority, complimentarity, confidentiality, attribution, justifiability, transparency of authorship, transparency of sponsorship, and honesty in advertising and editorial policy.

Consumer discussion groups, both listserv and web bulletin boards, are common. The value of online support groups is well documented.

Patient Information Web Sites. MEDLINEplus, sponsored by the National Library of Medicine, is a good starting place for patient information.[45] It is not a primary source for disease/condition/procedure information, but it does provide links to excellent web resources. Users can do a keyword search or browse by topic. Pages are organized into two categories: government and other resources. Within those categories are such subgroupings as General/Overviews, Clinical Trials, Coping, Diagnosis/Symptoms, Pictures/Diagrams, Espanol/Spanish, Organizations, and Research. Nongovernment resources have been well-researched and evaluated. Other useful resources on MEDLINEplus include an illustrated medical encyclopedia, links to online medical dictionaries, and a guide to prescription and OTC drugs from the USP DI and Advice for the Patient.

The American Academy of Family Physicians' Health Information for Patients page offers 200 patient information handouts originally published in *American Family Physician*.[46] The AAFP Family Health & Medical Guide contains self-care flowcharts for common complaints.

Healthfinder contains an outstanding collection of consumer links that have been reviewed by federal librarians for accuracy and credibility.[47]

References

1. Kiel J. yourpractice.com: Making the leap to the Internet. 1999;16:27-29.
2. Douglas J. Online prescriptions from eMD.com. *MD Computing* 2000;17:11.
3. Holtzman S. Search for a workable EMR. *Physicians and Computers* 2000;17:14-17.
4. 1998 *Lancet* panel. http://www.informatics-review.com/thoughts/advantages.html.
5. Sittig D. Advantages of computer-based medical records. The Informatics Review. 1999. http://informatics-review.com/thoughts/advantages.html.
6. Levin M. (2000). How a salaried FP computerized his practice—on his own. *Family Practice Management* 1999. http://www.aafp.org/fpm/20000600/43howa.html.
7. MedicaLogic. http://www.medicalogic.com
8. PersonalMD. http://www.personalmd.com
9. MD Computing. http://www.mdcomputing.com
10. Healthcare-Informatics. http://www.healthcare-informatics.com
11. PowerMed. http://www.powermed.com
12. SOAPware. http://www.docs.com
13. American Academy of Family Practice. Chapter 1: Why do family physicians need computers?. http://www.aafp.org/fpnet/guide/ch01.html
14. Department of Health and Human Services Administrative Simplification. http://aspe.os.dhhs.gov/admnsimp/
15. Symantec. http://www.symantec.com
16. McAfee. http://www.mcafee.com
17. ZDNet. http://www.zdnet.com
18. Cnet. http://www.cnet.com
19. Reents S. Impacts of the Internet on the doctor patient relationship. *Cyber Dialogue*. http://www.cyberdialogue.com/pdfs/wp/wp-cch-1999-doctors.pdf
20. Kane B, Zands D. Guidelines for the clinical use of electronic mail with patients. *JAMA* 1998;5:104-111.
21. PGP Security. http://www.pgp.com
22. Salu.net (www.salu.net)
23. Healinx (www.healinx.com)
24. http://informatics-review.com/thoughts/pat-email.html
25. MapBlast. http://www.mapblast.com
26. Expedia. http://maps.expedia.com
27. The Medical Matrix. http://www.medmatrix.org
28. Helix. http://www.helix.com
29. MedScape. http://www.medscape.com
30. PubMed. http://www.ncbi.nlm.nih.gov/entrez
31. CenterWatch Clinical Trials. http://www.centerwatch.com
32. Clinical Trials.gov. http://clinicaltrials.gov
33. National Guideline Clearinghouse. http://www.guidelines.gov
34. Instructions to Authors in the Health Sciences. http://www.mco.edu/lib/instr/libinsta.html
35. Clinical Pharmacology Online. http://cp.gsm.com/
36. FDA Center for Drug Evaluation and Research. http://www.fda.gov/cder/drug/default.htm
37. *The Merck Manual of Diagnosis and Therapy*. 17th ed. http://www.merck.com/pubs/mmanual/
38. *Lexi-Comp Diagnostic Procedures Handbook*.

http://www.healthgate.com/dph/html/index.shtm
39. *University of Iowa Family Practice Handbook.* 3rd ed. http://www.vh.org/Providers/ClinRef/FPHandbook/FPContents.html
40. Virtual Hospital Multimedia Textbooks. http://www.vh.org/Providers/Textbooks/MultimediaTextbooks.html
41. Brandon/Hill List of Journals. http://www.nnlm.nlm.nih.gov/psr/outreach/branhill.html
42. MedWeb. http://www.medweb.emory.edu/Medweb/FMPro?-DB=Records.FP3&-Format=kw_records.htm&-error=search_kwerror.htm&-Max=25&-Op=cn&subject==*;Electronic_Publications:Journals*&-Token=Electronic_Publications:_Journals&-Sortfield=Lnk_txt&-Find)
43. The Health Information Technology Institute. http://hitiweb.mitretek.org
44. The Health on the Net Foundation. http://www.hon.ch
45. MEDLINEplus. http://www.nlm.nih.gov/medlineplus/
46. The American Academy of Family Physicians' Health Information for Patients page. http://www.aafp.org/family/patient.html
47. Healthfinder. www.healthfinder.gov

Other Suggested Resources

- Amatayakul M. Critical success factors. *Health Management Technology* 2000;21:14-16.
- Borowitz S, Wyatt J. The Origin, content, and workload of e-mail consultations. *JAMA* 1998;280:1321-1324.
- Danny's Clinical Use of Email (Electronic Patient Centered Communication) Page. http://clinical.caregroup.org/ePCC/
- Gruen J. The physician and the Internet—Observer or participant? *MD Computing* 1999;12:46-48.
- Jadad A, Gagliardi A. Rating health information on the Internet. *JAMA* 1998;279:611-614.
- Joch A. EMR the Web Way. E.MD Online. http://www.edot-md.com/s00/cover.htm
- Manteuffel T. Keeping e-mail secure for health care communication. *Internet Health Care Magazine* 2000;May/June:82-88.
- Noble S. PDAs and hand-helds: World without wires. *Health Management Technology* 2000;21:28-32.
- Spicer J. Practicing without paper. *Family Practice Management* 1999. http://www.aafp.org/fpm/990300fm/40.html
- Spielberg A. Oncall and online. *JAMA* 1998;280:1353-1359.
- Stevens L. Computer-based patient records. *Medicine on the Net* 1998;4(8):8-11.
- Tools for Your Visit to Your Doctor. http://www-med.stanford.edu/shs/smg/tools/index.html

Part XV

Diagnosis

Bedside Ultrasonography

Barbara J. Abrams, MD

Emergency physicians are charged with the mission to quickly recognize and treat a variety of acute clinical conditions. As medical technology has evolved, bedside evaluation with point-of-service testing has become increasingly important for the practicing emergency physician. Bedside ultrasound is a prime example of such a tool. As a diagnostic tool, the literature has affirmed bedside ultrasound's role as a portable, safe, noninvasive, rapid strategy in the evaluation of a select group of clinical conditions in the emergency department (ED) setting.

As more emergency physicians perform bedside ultrasound in the ED, it is imperative that the specific indications for, and limitations of, its use are understood. Ultrasound has six primary applications for use in the ED setting: acute gallbladder disease, obstructive uropathy, abdominal aortic aneurysm, traumatic hemoperitoneum, ectopic pregnancy, and pericardial tamponade.[4] Note that the latter four situations represent potentially life-threatening emergencies for which time is of the essence. In all applications, only highly focused, basic questions should be asked by the emergency physician performing bedside ultrasound:[4]

1. Is there evidence of cholecystitis?
2. Is there evidence of obstructive uropathy?
3. Is there an abdominal aortic aneurysm?
4. Is there blood in the abdomen?
5. Is there evidence of a living intrauterine pregnancy?
6. Is there a pericardial effusion?

Answers to these questions allow for specific clinical decisions to be made, but are not equivalent to a traditional ultrasound examination performed by a radiologist.

Viewed in this manner, bedside ultrasound in the ED can be a valuable clinical tool for emergency physicians, enhancing our ability to recognize and manage these conditions in a timely and effective manner. This chapter provides a basic understanding of the technology of ultrasound and discusses the potential uses of this technique in the setting of acute disease processes involving the gallbladder, aorta, intra-abdominal trauma, kidney, heart, and pelvic structures.

Physics and Image Production

The following introduction to the physics of sound and image production provides a basic understanding of the uses and limitations of ultrasound (US). With this information, it becomes clear why, for example, US works well for gallbladder imaging and why bowel gas can make imaging impossible.

Sound consists of compressions and decompressions of the material through which it travels. A hertz (Hz), or one cycle per second, consists of a single compression and decompression. Frequency describes the number of cycles over time. US represents those frequencies above human hearing or greater than 20,000 Hz.

Table 1. Frequencies Used for US Imaging

FREQUENCY	IMAGING USE
2.0-3.5 MHz	echocardiography
3-5 MHz	abdominal
5.0-7.5 MHz	TVS (transvaginal)
7.5-10.0 MHz	small parts

Table 2. Speed of Sound in Various Tissues

TISSUE	VELOCITY
air	331 m/sec
fat	1450 m/sec
soft tissue	1540 m/sec
muscle	1585 m/sec
bone	4080 m/sec

Typical frequencies used for diagnostic US are between 2-10 MHz (2 million-10 million cycles per second.)[1,2] *(Please see Table 1.)*

The distance traveled during one cycle is called the wavelength. Frequency and wavelength are inversely related; the higher the frequency, the shorter the wavelength. Although picture quality or resolution improves with higher frequencies, the imaging depth decreases.[1] Thus, the highest frequency transducer available that permits proper imaging in a particular patient is used. This explains why picture quality may be adversely affected when performing abdominal ultrasonography on an obese patient. The increased depth necessary for organ visualization often requires the use of a lower frequency probe with some loss of resolution.

The density and stiffness of materials either promotes or inhibits sound transmission.[1,3] Sound travels best in solids, and better in liquids, than in gaseous media. Thus, a filled bladder displaces gas-filled bowel loops and allows for good transmission of sound to view the deeper pelvic structures when performing transabdominal pelvic sonography. An empty bladder often does not allow proper, if any, visualization.

The probe or transducer converts electrical energy into mechanical energy and vice versa. This is done using one or more piezoelectric (or pressure electric) elements (PZ). The thickness and type of material of which the PZ is made determines the frequency of a transducer. These elements both transmit and receive sound. A single US probe may contain a single PZ, which can be observed as it oscillates in oil, or it may use hundreds of elements, which fire electronically and have no moving parts.

Alternating current applied to the PZ causes it to vibrate at its particular frequency. This emitted sound strikes an object or an organ and is "echoed" back to the transducer. Each returning echo is converted into electrical energy and displayed on the screen as a dot, the combination of which comprises an image. Echo strength is proportional to the brightness of the dot. Since the speed of sound varies in different materials, the time for sound transmission and echo return is calibrated for the sound speed in soft tissues (1540 m/sec) in most US machines. *Table 2* lists the speed of sound in various tissues.[1]

Terminology. An *acoustic window* is an organ or tissue that sound penetrates and allows for viewing of structures beyond it. For instance, the fluid-filled bladder serves as an acoustic window for deeper pelvic structures. *Echogenic* describes structures that cause echoes on the US monitor. Echoes are bright or white. A metallic foreign body would be described as echogenic. Relative differences in echogenicity are described as *hypoechoic* (darker than the structure to which it is being compared) or *hyperechoic* (causes more echoes to be returned than the area to which it is being compared). *Anechoic* describes structures that do not result in echo production and therefore appear black. The difference in acoustic densities between adjacent tissues provides for the variation of echogenicity, which forms the total image on the screen. The fluid-filled bladder is an example of an anechoic area.

There are different types or modes of US used for imaging. *A-Mode* is a graphic display of echo amplitude vs. depth. It is useful for determining whether a structure is cystic or solid. *B-Mode* displays an image where brightness is proportional to the echo strength. *M-Mode* displays B-mode dots over time and is typically used for echocardiographic studies.

Doppler measures change in frequency caused when sound returns to the probe after reflecting from a moving object. The change in frequency is proportional to the velocity of the object. *Real-time* describes cinematic movement of structures due to the number of images produced per second. *Duplex* describes simultaneous Doppler and real-time imaging. *Axial* and *lateral* resolution describe the ability of the transducer to distinguish between two closely spaced objects either along the axis of the beam or perpendicular to the beam, respectively.

Knobology. US machines, regardless of the type of equipment, have some standard features. These include the gain, time gain compensation (TGC), and the freeze frame controls. Gain is used to create an image from the artificial amplification of a returning signal that is relatively weak. The entire screen is affected equally, similar to the brightness control on a television set. Echogenicity is therefore affected. Excess gain results in artifactual echo creation. Thus, when assessing overall echogenicity, the gain must be adjusted appropriately.

The TGC acts like a graphic equalizer by allowing adjustments of gain settings for part of the overall image. The TGC is set so that a large organ without focal pathology appears homogeneous. The freeze frame creates a still image, which can typically be labeled while on the screen. A printed image is then made. Many US machines allow for the storage of a number of images that can be printed at a later time to allow for expedient scanning.

Probe Types. Transducers produce either a linear (square) or sector (pie-wedge-shaped) image. In addition, activation of the PZ can be done mechanically or electronically. Mechanical scanners are generally less expensive and PZ movement is both visible and palpable. Electronic scanners have no moving parts. Mechanical probes typically consist of 1-3 PZs within a fluid-filled scan head. The PZs either oscillate back and forth or spin on a wheel. Mechanical probes with multiple PZs may all be of the same frequency or of different frequencies.

Electronic scanning is accomplished with arrays, which are several PZs arranged in a line (linear array), either in a curved line (curvilinear array) or in concentric rings similar to a bull's eye (annular array). The PZs within the linear array probe fire in sequential groups, with each group operating like a separate transducer.[3] The image produced without moving the probe along the surface of the body is similar to that made by linear scanning with a manual probe with a single PZ. Unlike the mechanical scanners, focal length and beam direction can be altered. Overall, these probes tend to have long heads and require a large scanning surface.

Curvilinear arrays tend to be smaller and provide excellent images but are somewhat awkward to use while scanning over convex surfaces. Annular arrays focus electronically and optimize axial and lateral resolution over a larger area of interest.[1,3,4]

Organ Systems

The Gallbladder. The normal gallbladder is a pear-shaped, cystic structure measuring approximately 7-10 cm longitudinally and 2-3 cm in transverse section.[6] Ultrasonographically, any fluid-filled, anechoic structure (e.g., the filled bladder) is often described as cystic.[7] A large gallbladder may result from a prolonged fast or may represent gallbladder obstruction. It is best visualized after eight hours of fasting. Approximately 5-10% of the ED studies are unsuccessful secondary to postprandial contraction. Not all gallbladders are pear-shaped. About 15% of the normal population have irregular folds or bends in various parts of the gallbladder, called junctional folds and phyrigian caps.[4] When measuring the gallbladder, scan through the entire gallbladder in at least two planes and document the largest lumen obtained.

To image the gallbladder, a 3.5 or 5.0 MHz transducer is placed in the right subcostal area in the mid-clavicular line. Although patients are most often supine for the examination, the left lateral decubitus and upright positions can both detect pathology that might otherwise be missed (i.e., stones) and be used to demonstrate movement of stones or sludge. Sometimes intercostal imaging results in optimal imaging for a particular patient. Other techniques, such as having the patient hold a deep inspiration or push his or her abdomen outward, can also improve visualization.

Epigastric and right upper quadrant pain are common presenting complaints to the ED. The differential diagnosis includes gastritis, peptic ulcer disease, hepatitis, appendicitis, pneumonia, Fitz Hugh-Curtis syndrome, pancreatitis, and acute and chronic cholecystitis. Approximately 20 million Americans have cholelithiasis, with 1 million new cases each year, half of which are asymptomatic.[6] The incidence peaks during the fifth and sixth decades of life, with a female-male ratio of 3:1.[8]

Gallstones are associated with acute cholecystitis 90-95% of the time.[4,5] Sonographic criteria for acute cholecystitis include the presence of gallstones, sludge, wall thickening, pericholestatic fluid, gallbladder distention, abnormalities of the gallbladder wall, and a sonographic Murphy's sign (maximal tenderness and often inspiratory arrest with gentle probe pressure over the gallbladder).[9] Gallstones are the most common finding. Ultrasound can detect intraluminal stones as small as 1-2 mm. Sonography has an overall sensitivity for stones of 95%. [4,9]

Gallstones are typically echogenic with a well-delineated distal shadow. Intraluminal stones are usually dependent and will move with changes in patient position. Stones impacted in the common bile duct, cystic duct, and gallbladder neck are more difficult to image and do not move to dependent locations. Furthermore, some small stones may float and can be difficult to visualize.[8]

Acute cholecystitis is unlikely, however, if stones are present without any other findings. Stones in combination with wall thickening have a positive predictive value of 95.2% for acute cholecystitis.[8] The normal gallbladder wall measures less than 2 mm. Mean wall diameters for acute cholecystitis are 9 mm for acute cholecystitis and 5 mm for chronic cholecystitis. Wall thickness varies with probe placement and angulation. For greatest accuracy, the wall segment perpendicular to the ultrasound beam along the central, longest axis of the gallbladder is measured. Wall thickening is a nonspecific finding and can be seen with congestive heart failure, ascites, renal failure, multiple myeloma, hepatitis, hypoalbuminemia, cancer of the gallbladder, and, most commonly, with a partially contracted gallbladder.[8,10]

Bile stasis can result in the production of a viscous fluid, called sludge, that layers out with changes in position. It is an abnormal finding in ambulatory patients and is associated with acute cholecystitis in approximately 50% of cases.[4] An ultrasonic Murphy's sign is both sensitive and specific for acute cholecystitis. When it is present in combination with stones, it has a positive predictive value of 92.2% and a negative predictive value of 95% when neither stones nor a Murphy's sign is present.[8] Radionuclide studies are recommended when the ultrasound is equivocal for acute cholecystitis (i.e., wall thickening and stones present without a Murphy's sign or a positive Murphy's sign without other associated signs.)

Other abnormalities seen by ultrasound include: pericholecystic fluid, wall irregularities (i.e., intramural gas, pus, or hemorrhage), and a tense, dilated gallbladder.[8,10] Bile duct dilation greater than 7 mm (> 10 mm in patients with prior biliary surgery) can occur with duct obstruction.[4]

Acalculous cholecystitis occurs in 5-10% of the cases of acute cholecystitis and accounts for 47% of cases of postoperative cholecystitis.[8,9] Besides surgery, it is also associated with diabetes mellitus, bacterial and parasitic infections, burns, pancreatitis, and polyarteritis nodosa.[6] It is clinically indistinguishable from calculous cholecystitis. Without treatment, 52% of these cases can progress to gangrene and rupture.[8] Gallbladder enlargement, wall thickening, and a positive Murphy's sign can be appreciated; however, the sensitivity of ultrasound for the acalculous variety is 67-92%. Cryptosporidium and CMV are associated with a dilated, tender gallbladder with thickened walls in patients with AIDS.[8]

Gangrenous cholecystitis occurs in 2-38% of patients with acute cholecystitis, with perforation occurring in 10% of cases. There are no signs, symptoms, or laboratory values that differentiate this from uncomplicated cholecystitis.[8] Ultrasonographically, striations of the gallbladder wall that represent necrosis, hemorrhage, and microabscesses can be appreciated.[4,8] Although gangrenous cholecystitis only occurs in about 1% of patients with acute cholecystitis, it is associated with a significantly increased mortality rate. Diabetics are at risk for this as well as emphysematous cholecystitis. Emphysematous cholecystitis is acalculous 30% of the time.[8] Plain films may demonstrate air in the gallbladder or biliary tree.

Correct scanning techniques and gain settings help to prevent common errors such as missing a stone due to a fold or kink in the gallbladder and mistaking an intraluminal, echogenic density (e.g., polyp) for a stone. Knowing when the patient last ate, scanning through the entire gallbladder in longitudinal and transverse sections, and using the intercostal, upright, and lateral decubitus positions along with respiratory excursion can help prevent these pitfalls. Excessive gain can cause "pseudosludge," or artifactual echoes within the gallbladder that can be mistaken for sludge.

A stone-filled contracted gallbladder can be difficult to identify. It may appear as a dense, echogenic area with prominent posterior shadowing, similar to the gas-filled duodenum. This gas artifact can be mistaken for a gallstone. Another artifact created at the lateral edge of the gallbladder can also cause shadows when no stones are present. In addition, the valves of Heister in the gallbladder neck may shadow and therefore be confused with the presence of a stone.

To avoid these pitfalls, the stone should be visible in more than one plane and remain dependent despite patient positioning. Very small stones may not shadow and stones in the gallbladder neck must be looked for carefully since they can be difficult to visualize. A formal study should be ordered if the physician is unsure whether acute cholecystitis is present.

Overall, the use of bedside ultrasound can narrow the differential diagnosis in patients with upper abdominal pain, or confirm the diagnosis, allowing patient disposition in a more timely fashion. Furthermore, patient satisfaction is often improved when a definite etiology for the discomfort is determined.

The Aorta. The normal aortic diameter measures not more than 2.5 cm just below the diaphragm and gradually tapers to 1.5 cm at its bifurcation. The origins of the celiac axis and superior mesenteric artery can be seen arising from the aorta anteriorly when the US probe is placed in the epigastric area. Using a 3.5 MHz probe, the aorta should be imaged throughout its entire length in both the longitudinal and transverse planes. When measuring its diameter, the AP width in transverse section is the most accurate.

Bowel gas can interfere with imaging, but gentle probe pressure, visualization off the midline, and rescanning after a short time interval can help with this problem. The normal lumen is anechoic and its walls echogenic. If a thrombus is present, echoes may be present within the lumen depending on the age of the clot.

Dilations greater than 3 cm are abnormal and occur in about 2% of the population. Aneurysms are 5-10 times more common in males than females and typically occur after the fifth decade of life. Atherosclerosis is the most common etiology; however, other causes include syphilis, trauma, congenital abnormalities, and fungal infections. Ninety-seven percent are distal to the renal arteries. Since those involving the renal arteries have a more serious prognosis, documentation of an aneurysm's proximal and distal extent and relationship to major vessels is important. Operative candidates include those with aneurysms greater than 5-6 cm, since the rate of rupture increases with diameter.[6,11,12]

The extremes of presentation range from the incidental finding in an asymptomatic patient to hypotension and tachycardia in a patient with a pulsatile mass who complains of abdominal and/or back pain. In the latter type of patient, no confirmatory diagnostic studies are required. A more difficult problem is the apparently stable patient in whom suspicion for an abdominal aortic aneurysm (AAA) is not high. It is in this group that ultrasound can be most helpful for either confirming or ruling out the diagnosis, especially since the sensitivity of clinical detection for an AAA is low (14.7%).[13] The accuracy of US for AAA is 97%.[8]

Other advantages to US include its improved sensitivity over plain radiographs and the ability to perform the technique in the ED (vs CT scan and aortography), allowing optimal patient care should clinical deterioration occur.

Common pitfalls in aortic imaging include not using the aforementioned techniques for the displacement of bowel gas. Also, as with the gallbladder, the US beam must be perpendicular to the aorta to assure accuracy; hence, the aortic image should be in the center of the screen. The aorta should be scanned along its entire length in at least two planes and measurements taken from outer wall to outer wall while in transverse section. In addition, the aorta can be tortuous, and the probe must then move off the midline for adequate imaging.

Gain setting must be adjusted appropriately at the outset to avoid artifactual intraluminal echoes, which can be mistaken for thrombi. Finally, the inferior vena cava (IVC) can be confused with the aorta. Although it appears somewhat pulsatile, it has thinner walls than the aorta as well as being intrahepatic in location. Unlike the aorta, the IVC compresses with probe pressure. Scanning to the left and right in the sagittal plane will usually make identification of the aorta and IVC apparent.

Aortic dissection is 2-3 times more common than rupture of an AAA and has a 48-hour mortality rate of 50%.[14] Dissections are typically extensions of thoracic disease in patients with a history of hypertension. They are also seen in patients with coarctation, congenital abnormalities, Marfan's syndrome, and in pregnant women. Transesophageal echocardiography and aortography are superior studies to conventional US for this entity. Although a mobile, echogenic flap can sometimes be seen within the lumen, ultrasonography is not sensitive enough to rule out this diagnosis.

The advantages of US include its portability, safety, noninvasiveness, and its ability to reassess the patient at the bedside. US is accurate for detecting aneurysms; however, it is not sufficiently sensitive for detecting dissections. Aortic dilation prompts timely consultation with vascular surgeons, patient preparation for the operating room, arrangements for transfer; most importantly, patients are not discharged. Furthermore, referral for elective repair can be initiated for those patients in whom an aneurysm is discovered as an incidental finding, since the mortality with elective repair is preferable to that with emergent repair due to rupture (5% vs 70-100%, respectively.)[4,6]

Trauma. US has largely replaced diagnostic peritoneal lavage (DPL) for the evaluation of blunt abdominal trauma in Europe and Japan.[15-19] In the United States, however, DPL and CT are the primary diagnostic modalities used in patients who are neither emergent operative candidates nor patients who can be observed and re-examined. Although CT often delineates specific organ injury, it requires that the patient be transported outside the clinical setting of the ED. In addition, CT often requires expertise for interpretation and may necessitate patient sedation, which can interfere with subsequent neurologic and physical examinations.

Alternatively, DPL can be done rapidly on-site and has a low complication rate. Its disadvantages include its invasiveness, inability to assess the thorax and retroperitoneum, and oversensitivity for hemoperitoneum, particularly with concurrent pelvic fracture. In addition, it is relatively contraindicated in patients with prior laparotomies, pregnant women, and anticoagulated patients.

The ranges of sensitivity and specificity of US for free fluid are 82-98% and 88-100%, respectively.[15-24] Its advantages include those previously mentioned as well as its ability to assess the thorax, peri-

Table 3. Differential Diagnoses to be Considered in an Ultrasound Finding of Hydronephrosis

FALSE POSITIVES	FALSE NEGATIVES
Pregnancy	Staghorn calculi shadowing dilation
Acute and chronic pyelonephritis	Acute obstruction not yet dilated
Post-surgical dilation	Cysts with concurrent hydronephrosis
Tumors	Retroperitoneal fibrosis
Normal variants (e.g., congenital megacalyces)	Hydronephrosis presumed to be cysts or prominent pyramids
Overhydration	Dehydration with partial obstruction
Osmotic diuresis	Technical factors (e.g., obesity, gas)
Cysts or prominent pyramids confused with hydronephrosis	

cardial sac, peritoneal cavity, and retroperitoneum. Furthermore, US can assess the subcapsular and intraparenchymal areas of solid organs, unlike DPL. It can be performed in virtually any patient, including pregnant women and pediatric patients.

The multiple-view trauma examination typically uses a 3.5 MHz probe (or a 5.0 MHz probe in pediatric patients and very thin adults) and is generally completed in 4-5 minutes.[15,21-23,25]

The probe is initially placed over the epigastrum to assess overall cardiac contractility and to determine whether tamponade exists. The right upper quadrant, left upper quadrant, and pelvis are quickly scanned for any anechoic fluid collection that might be present. Free fluid in the thorax can be viewed when assessing the right and left upper quadrants. These four areas are rescanned to look for specific organ injury and again for evidence of hemoperitoneum. More recent studies assess a single view of Morison's pouch (the potential space between the liver and right kidney) with minimal degrees of Trendelenburg, since this examination can be done in a few seconds after minimal training and does not require Foley catheter placement.

Important questions to be answered concern the amount of fluid detectable with current technology, type of equipment used in the ED, and what amount of fluid should be considered significant. Approximately 250-300 cc of fluid appears to be readily detectable; however, some studies have concluded that this amount might be inconclusive and therefore comparable to an indeterminate DPL.[15,16]

The limitations of US include factors that can make imaging technically difficult, such as patient obesity, subcutaneous emphysema, areas with large, open wounds, poor equipment, and operator inexperience. US is not as sensitive as contrast CT for specific organ injury. In addition, due to adhesions from prior surgery and failure of clotted peritoneal blood to flow freely to dependent areas, free fluid may be present yet remain undetected. In addition, sonography cannot readily distinguish between different types of free fluid. Thus, differentiating between ascites and hemoperitoneum may not be possible.

Although US does not obviate the use of other modalities in equivocal cases, when the appropriate clinical picture and US identification of obvious free fluids exist, significant time is saved. Immediate feedback such as whether the blood is above or below the diaphragm or evidence of impending tamponade can provide the necessary information to formulate an appropriate treatment strategy for the patient.

The Kidney. The normal kidney is 9-12 cm long, 2.5-3.0 cm thick, and 4-5 cm wide. It appears football-shaped along its long axis and C-shaped in transverse section. Using a 3.5 or 5.0 MHz probe, the kidney can be viewed subcostally, intercostally, or in coronal section, with the patient in the supine, lateral decubitus, or prone positions. The liver and spleen are used as acoustic windows. The left kidney can be more difficult to image due to overlying ribs and lung and bowel gas.

The kidney is scanned for calculi, hydronephrosis, and perirenal fluid. Although patient preparation is not necessary, a small degree of hydronephrosis can be missed in a markedly dehydrated patient. Hydration also allows for examination of the ureterovesicular junction (UVJ) and the bladder for hydroureter and calculi.

The normal sonographic appearance of the kidney is so characteristic that it is recognized by the novice. A thin, echogenic capsule outlines its more hypoechoic cortex. The pyramids are anechoic and, if prominent, can be confused with both cysts and hydronephrosis. The pelvis and calyces form a central echogenic complex.

Renal colic is a common presentation to the ED. However, a number of serious entities can mimic colic (e.g., appendicitis, embolic disease, AAA, pelvic inflammatory disease, biliary colic, perforated peptic ulcer) and require different management.[4] Although intravenous pyelography (IVP) gives both functional information and can often identify the site of obstruction in the presence of renal colic, it is not suitable for patients with pregnancy, congestive heart failure, dehydration, diabetes mellitus, renal failure, renal insufficiency, or allergy to contrast material. Thus, in patients in whom the diagnosis of colic is in question, or where contrast dye might precipitate additional problems, US is a logical option that can be performed without delay at the bedside.[4]

The obstruction of urine outflow results in dilation of the renal pelvis and calyces. The normally echogenic central echo complex becomes anechoic. With time and higher degrees of hydronephrosis, renal atrophy and loss of the normal renal appearance occurs. The sensitivity of US in detecting obstructive uropathy ranges from 85-98%.[26-31] Pain with hydronephrosis has been shown to have a 100% sensitivity and a 95% specificity for obstructive uropathy. Only about 5% of patients with pain and no evidence of hydronephrosis will have obstructive uropathy, probably due to dehydration or a pre-existing renal disorder.[32]

Calcifications within the kidney, the bladder, or at the UVJ can be detected with US and appear similar to gallstones (in that they are highly reflective and may cause distal shadowing) but are much harder to visualize. Ureteral stones are generally small and obscured by bowel gas.

Several technical errors in scanning can result in erroneous conclusions. Patients are unlikely to have bilateral hydronephrosis in renal colic. Two possible explanations for this pseudohydronephrosis might include a full bladder and polycystic kidney disease. Thus, a complete examination includes scanning the bladder. If filled, rescan after having the patient void. Likewise, by scanning the opposite kidney and finding a similar appearance on the contralateral side, the diagnosis of colic is unlikely. Calculi can be missed if the bladder and UVJ are not scanned. Visualization of the renal artery can be confused with the ureter, which is not normally visible. *Table 3* contains a partial listing of conditions that might result in false-positive and false-negative examinations for hydronephrosis.[26,27]

Although US does not provide functional information about the kidney, it appears to be a good screening tool for obstructive uropathy. The appropriate clinical scenario and good scanning technique for intrarenal, bladder and UVJ calculi, unilateral hydronephrosis, and perirenal fluid (urinomas) provides indirect evidence that a patient has renal colic. Bedside US is preferred in those patients in whom IVP is not optimal, when IVP is not readily available, when the diagnosis is in question, in pregnancy, and in cases of contrast allergy.

The Heart. Cardiac imaging provides the emergency physician with a means for diagnosing a number of conditions for which no other practical means is readily available. Two distinct applications are differentiating between different causes of shock and assessment of pulseless electrical activity (PEA). Generally, a 3.5 MHz transducer is used with the patient in the supine or left lateral decubitus positions.

Four standard views are primarily used. With the subcostal view, the probe is placed in the subxiphoid region with the marker dot pointing toward the patient's right side. This view is useful in assessing both overall cardiac activity and the presence or absence of an effusion. It is a good all-purpose view for the ED since it can be used for patients who are noncompliant, on backboards, and it does not interfere with any concomitant interventions taking place in the thoracic area.

The left parasternal long and short axis views require a little more technical skill but are easily interpreted. With the probe in the 2nd-4th intercostal space (ICS) and the marker dot at the 4 o'clock position (beam plane is parallel to a line drawn from the right shoulder to the left hip), the ascending aorta, left atrium, and left ventricle can be visualized. With the probe in the same ICS, rotation of the marker dot to the 8 o'clock position permits imaging via the short axis view. This view is good for visualization of the mitral and aortic valves as well as overall global left ventricular function.[33,34]

The probe is placed over the maximal apical impulse to obtain the apical view. Patients often require left lateral decubitus positioning for this view. Often, multiple views must be attempted to find the view that meets the needs for that particular clinical scenario.

By assessing overall wall motion, chamber size, and pericardial fluid, one can distinguish between four causes of shock: cardiogenic, hypovolemic, tamponade, and right ventricular dysfunction (e.g., pulmonary embolus and right ventricular infarct). Not infrequently, patients arrive to the ED in shock with nonspecific cardiograms and inadequate histories. Cardiac imaging allows the emergency physician to tailor therapy toward a specific type of shock.

With cardiogenic shock, patients exhibit marked, diffuse wall motion abnormalities. Hypovolemic shock is characterized by a hyperdynamic heart with small, right-sided chambers. The echocardiographic hallmark of a massive right ventricular infarct or pulmonary embolism is a large, thin-walled hypokinetic right ventricle and a vigorously beating left ventricle.

Evaluation for pericardial tamponade remains one of the more important uses for echocardiography in the ED setting. The classic clinical findings (i.e., Beck's triad, electrical alternans, and pulsus paradoxus) are nonspecific and late findings. Pericardial fluid is anechoic, conforms to the heart, and is surrounded by the echogenic pericardial sac. Diastolic collapse of right-sided chambers can be seen. It is an invaluable tool for displaying pericardial fluid collections from traumatic etiologies (i.e., blunt and penetrating trauma) or secondary to pericarditis. Immediate determination of pericardial fluid allows for a formal study (if time permits), notification of surgical consultants, or an emergent pericardiocentesis, which can be performed with US guidance.

Echocardiography can reliably detect pericardial fluid. Limitations in this area include: patient cooperation, body habitus, type of equipment and operator experience. A large effusion can be detected by a novice, generally.

Another application is differentiating between cardiac and noncardiac causes of PEA. Often the subxiphoid view is sufficient for determining whether poor contractility and valve motion exist. With good cardiac activity, reversible etiologies can be sought. The distinctive appearances of hypovolemia, tamponade, and pulmonary embolus have been discussed in previous sections.

Some difficulties in cardiac scanning include patients who are noncompliant, have hyperinflated lungs secondary to COPD, or have difficulty changing position. Pericardial fat is hypoechoic and can be confused with an effusion. In the absence of diastolic collapse, a formal study might be appropriate. In addition, the effusion can be measured and the patient rescanned within a short time frame. When the study is suboptimal with one view, trying several other views and changing patient position, if possible, is helpful.

Cardiac imaging may require minimal expertise (e.g., identifying a large pericardial effusion) or may require additional technical skill (e.g., assessing wall motion abnormalities in patients with ischemic heart disease or for the presence of a thoracic dissection.) The topics mentioned here represent applications that can be of particular use for the emergency physician.

The Pelvis. Emergent pelvic sonography has long been accepted for the evaluation of pelvic pain and vaginal bleeding, both of which are frequent ED complaints. Both transabdominal sonography (TAS) and transvaginal sonography (TVS) provide an excellent means for the evaluation of the uterus and adnexa beyond the physical examination.

With TAS, a 3-5 MHz probe is placed above the pubic symphysis in the midline. The degree of bladder filling is critical since the bladder serves as the acoustic window to the pelvis. The bladder must extend above the fundus but not be overfilled or compression of the uterus and its contents results. Imaging is done in the longitudinal, transverse, and oblique planes. TAS can be difficult to perform in patients who are obese and have pelvic scarring.[35]

TVS avoids the difficulties of bladder filling, obesity, and scarring. Since the probe is closer to the imaged structures, higher resolution (up to 7.5 MHz) permits better detail. Studies comparing

TAS and TVS have found that TVS yields more information.[35,36] The transvaginal transducer is covered with a latex condom or examining glove into which US gel has been introduced. The TVS examination is performed after the pelvic examination has been completed. TVS should not be performed in the event of premature rupture of membranes. In this instance, translabial imaging is done. Orientation is initially more confusing than with TAS with images obtained in the sagittal, coronal, and oblique planes. TAS and TVS are complementary, with TAS providing a more global view of the pelvis and TVS able to focus in on areas of interest.

The uterus varies in size and shape depending on the patient's age and parity. Fallopian tubes are rarely seen with TAS unless they contain fluid; however, they are occasionally visualized with TVS at their junction with the cornua. Ovaries measure approximately 1 × 2 × 3 cm and are more difficult to image in the postmenopausal patient.[37]

Distinguishing between ectopic pregnancy and threatened abortion is a common and important theme for use in the ED. Formal, 24-hour, on-site sonography is not ubiquitously offered. Immediate bedside US often provides the basic information needed; either a definite intrauterine pregnancy (IUP) is present or it is not. Additional data such as fluid in the cul-de-sac, adnexal masses or extrauterine cardiac activity can also be obtained. Answering the question of whether a definite IUP exists can often permit immediate direction of patient management.

The earliest sonographic evidence of a normal pregnancy is an intrauterine round or oval gestational sac, a sonolucent structure surrounded by an echogenic ring. This can be identified transvaginally by about the fourth to fifth week from the last menstrual period. Although this sac is initially empty, soon afterwards the appearance of a yolk sac (5th week), cardiac activity (5th-6th week), and a fetal pole (6th week) appear.[38,39] In general, TVS permits visualization of structures one week earlier than TAS.

A "pseudosac" can occur with an ectopic pregnancy (about 10% of the time) and can be confused with a gestational sac. The appearance of a yolk sac, fetal pole, or cardiac activity effectively confirms that the intrauterine structure is truly a gestational sac. Intrauterine cardiac activity is considered the "gold standard" for a living IUP. The threshold for visualization of the gestational sac is reported to range from 600 to 1025 mIU/mL (IRP) HCG for TVS and 1800 mIU/IRP HCG for TAS. It is important to note that this threshold or discriminatory zone should be established for each institution since it varies with equipment and the examiner's skill. The frequency of a simultaneous IUP and extrauterine pregnancy is about 1 in 30,000 without the use of assisted reproductive technology. Thus, identification of an IUP effectively rules out an ectopic pregnancy.[4,38,40]

An ectopic pregnancy is confirmed when an extrauterine heart beat and an empty uterus are imaged. This occurs less than 25% of the time with TVS and 10% of the time with TAS.[4] More often, an empty uterus and an adnexal mass or fluid in the cul-de-sac is seen and considered highly likely for an ectopic pregnancy. An ectopic pregnancy is suspect when the quantitative HCG exceeds the institution's discriminatory threshold and no definite gestational sac is seen transvaginally. An empty uterus, a closed cervical os, and a quantitative HCG below the institution's discriminatory zone may signify an early IUP. In the appropriate clinical setting, the quantitative HCG is usually repeated in 48 hours since this level will double within 1.5-2.0 days in more than 85% of women.[40] With complete abortions, the uterus is either empty or contains both echogenic and sonolucent material, which, if measuring greater than 5 mm, makes the diagnosis of retained tissue likely.[4]

A few of the more important pitfalls have already been mentioned. Proper bladder filling is needed for TAS. Mistaking a pseudosac for a gestational sac can occur when the more developed embryologic structures are not imaged (e.g., yolk sac, fetal pole, etc.). Also, if the TVS study does not explain the patient's symptoms, TAS should be performed, and vice versa. A small amount of fluid in the cul-de-sac can appear large to the novice; however, TAS will often improve one's perspective. A quantitative HGC should be ordered to determine whether the threshold has been exceeded. If a definite gestational sac is identified, it must be within the uterus. Scanning in multiple planes will help determine this. Fluid in the rectum or within loops of bowel can be mistaken for either fluid in the cul-de sac or a cystic lesion. Uterine fibroids can obscure a gestational sac. Most importantly, if it has not been determined whether a definite IUP exists, a formal study is in order.[4,37]

There has been a marked increase in the number of ectopic pregnancies both in the United States and throughout the world. The inability to identify an ectopic pregnancy results in significant maternal morbidity and mortality. All women with positive pregnancy tests and pelvic pain and/or vaginal bleeding should be ruled out for ectopic pregnancy.[40,41] The use of US in the ED shortens time to diagnosis and permits more timely management of these patients.

Other Applications and Conclusion

The safety and recent improvements in technology make US a useful adjunct in the ED. The use of US to rule out deep venous thrombosis, a questionable case of appendicitis, or assess testicular pathology may become standard ED applications. The need for US-guided central venous access, foreign body identification and removal, paracentesis, and suprapubic aspiration represent other areas of interest.

The Society of Academic Emergency Medicine has published a curriculum for US training, and portable US is now a part of the core curriculum for residency training in emergency medicine.[42,43] The goal of this training is to guide the emergency physician through a limited, focused US examination that generally answers a yes/no question (e.g., yes/no AAA, yes/no IUP, etc.) An indeterminate study leaves the physician at the same point in the decision analysis that existed prior to the US examination. The decision can then be made to perform either additional diagnostic studies or a formal US.

The usefulness of US in confirming diagnoses such as cholecystitis, AAA, and pericardial effusion is well-established. Additional research is necessary to fully delineate the role of sonography as performed by properly trained emergency physicians. A safe, versatile bedside tool that would enable emergency physicians to provide more prompt, cost-effective care clearly has a role in the ED.

References

1. Pinkney N. *A Review of the Concepts of Ultrasound Physics and Instrumentation.* 4th ed. West Point: Sonicor, Inc.; 1990:1-34.
2. Thaler I, Bruck A. Transvaginal sonography and Doppler measurements—physical considerations. In: Timor-Tritsch IE,

Rottem S, eds. *Transvaginal Sonography.* 2nd ed. New York: Elsevier; 1991:1-27.
3. Kremkau FW. Ultrasound and transducers. In: Kremkau FW, *Diagnostic Ultrasound: Principles, Instruments and Exercises.* 3rd ed. Philadelphia: WB Saunders; 1989:9-104.
4. Heller M, Jehle D. *Ultrasound in Emergency Medicine.* Philadelphia: WB Saunders; 1995.
5. Grossman SJ, Joyce JM. Hepatobiliary imaging. *Radiol Clin North Am* 1991; 9:853-74.
6. Robbins SL, Cotran RS, Kumar V. *Pathologic Basis of Disease.* 3rd ed. Philadelphia: WB Saunders; 1984:529-535, 942-959.
7. Sanders RC. *Clinical Sonography: A Practical Guide.* Boston: Little, Brown and Co; 1984:27-34.
8. Mittelstaedt CA. Biliary system. In: Mittelstaedt CA, ed. *General Ultrasound.* New York: Churchill Livingstone; 1992:249-335.
9. Aufderheide TP, Brady WJ. Clolecystitis and biliary colic. In: Tintinalli JE, Ruiz E, Krome RL, eds. *Emergency Medicine: A Comprehensive Study Guide.* 4th ed. New York: McGraw-Hill, Inc; 1996:495-498.
10. Kane RA. The biliary system. In: Kurtz AB, Goldberg BB, eds. *Clinics in Diagnostic Ultrasound: Gastrointestinal Ultrasonography.* 1988; 23:75-137.
11. Glover JL. Thoracic and abdominal aneurysms. In: Tintinalli JE, Ruiz E, Krome RL, eds. *Emergency Medicine: A Comprehensive Study Guide.* 4th ed. New York: McGraw-Hill, Inc; 1996:382-386.
12. Vellman WP, Drake TR. Aortic aneurysms. In: Rosen P, Baker FJ, Barkin RM, et al, eds. *Emergency Medicine: Concepts and Clinical Practice.* 2nd ed. Washington DC: The C.V. Mosby Co; 1988:1197-1208.
13. Beede SD, Ballard DJ, James EM, et al. Positive predictive value of clinical suspicion of abdominal aortic aneurysm: Implications for efficient use of abdominal ultrasonography. *Arch Intern Med* 1990;150:549.
14. Feldman AJ. Thoracic and abdominal aortic aneurysms. In: Tintinalli JE, Ruiz E, Frome RL, eds. *Emergency Medicine: A Comprehensive Study Guide.* 2nd ed. New York: McGraw-Hill Book Co; 1988:240-242.
15. Goletti O, Ghiselli G, Lippolis PV, et al. The role of ultrasonography in blunt abdominal trauma: Results in 250 consecutive cases. *J Trauma* 1994;36:178-181.
16. Hoffman R, Nerlich M, Muggia-Sullam M, et al. Blunt abdominal trauma in cases of multiple trauma evaluated by ultrasonography: A prospective analysis of 291 patients. *J Trauma* 1992;32:452-458.
17. Tiling T, Bouillon B, Schmid A, et al. Ultrasound in blunt abdomino-thoracic trauma. In: Border JR, Allgoewer M, Hansen ST, et al, eds. *Blunt Multiple Trauma: Comprehensive Pathoshysiology and Care.* New York: Marcel-Dekker; 1990:415-433.
18. Tso P, Rodriguez A, Cooper C, et al. Sonography in blunt abdominal trauma: A preliminary progress report. *J Trauma* 1992;33:39-43.
19. Wening JV. Evaluation of ultrasound, lavage, and computed tomography in blunt abdominal trauma. *Surg Endosc* 1989;3:152-158.
20. Gruessner R, Mengtes B, Duber C, et al. Sonography versus peritoneal lavage in blunt abdominal trauma. *J Trauma* 1989;29:242-244.
21. Jehle D, Guarino J, Karamanoukian H. Emergency department ultrasound in the evaluation of blunt abdominal trauma. *Am J Emerg Med* 1993;11:342-346.
22. Kimura A, Otsuka T. Emergency center ultrasonography in the evaluation of hemoperitoneum: A prospective study. *J Trauma* 1991;31:20-23.
23. Ma OJ, Kefer MP, Mateer JR, et al. Single versus multiple views for rapid trauma ultrasound of the abdomen. *Ann Emerg Med* 1995;25:130.
24. Rozycki GS, Ochsner MG, Jaffin JH, et al. Prospective evaluation of surgeon's use of ultrasound in the evaluation of trauma patients. *J Trauma* 1993;34:516-522.
25. Sarkisian AE, Khondkarian RA, Amirbekian NM, et al. Sonographic screening of mass casualties for abdominal and renal injuries following the 1988 Armenian earthquake. *J Trauma* 1991;31:247-250.
26. Amis ES, Cronon JJ, Pfister RC, et al. Ultrasonic inaccuracies in diagnosing renal obstruction. *Urology* 1982;19:101-105.
27. Amis ES, Hartman DS. Renal ultrasonography 1984: A practical overview. *Radiol Clin North Am* 1984;22:315-332.
28. Ellenbogen PH, Scheible FW, Talner LB, et al. Sensitivity of gray scale ultrasound in detecting urinary tract obstruction. *Am J Roentgenol* 1978;130:731-736.
29. Erwin BC, Carroll BA, Sommer FG. Renal colic: The role of ultrasound in initial evaluation. *Radiology* 1984;152:147-150.
30. Malave SR, Neiman HL, Spies SM, et al. Diagnosis of hydronephrosis: Comparison of radionuclide scanning and sonography. *Am J Roentgenol* 1980;135:1179-1185.
31. Mittelstaedt CA. Kidney. In: Mittelstaedt CA, ed. *General Ultrasound.* New York: Churchill Livingstone; 1992:833-885.
32. Plummer D. Abdominal sonography. In: Tintinalli JE, Ruiz E, Krone RL, eds. *Emergency Medicine: A Comprehensive Study Guide.* 4th ed. New York: McGraw-Hill, Inc; 1996: 1390-1399.
33. Plummer D, Heller M. Cardiac applications. In: Heller M, Jehle D. *Ultrasound in Emergency Medicine.* Philadelphia: WB Saunders; 1995:126-134.
34. Plummer D. Other cardiac applications. In: Heller M, Jehle D. *Ultrasound in Emergency Medicine.* Philadelphia: WB Saunders; 1995:184-195.
35. Lavery MJ, Benson CB. Transvaginal versus transabdominal ultrasound. In: Timor-Tritsch IE, Rottem S, eds. *Transvaginal Sonography.* 2nd ed. New York: Elsevier; 1991:77-107.
36. Zimmer EZ, Timor-Tritsch, Rottem S. The technique of transvaginal sonography. In: Timor-Tritsch IE, Rottem S eds. *Transvaginal Sonography.* 2nd ed. New York: Elsevier; 1991:61-75.
37. Craig M. *Pocket Guide to Ultrasound Measurements.* New York: JB Lippincott Co; 1988:83-104.
38. Tessler FN, Perrella RR, Grant EG, et al. *Handbook of Endovaginal Sonography.* New York: Thieme Medical Publishers, Inc; 1992:38-90.
39. Timor-Tritsch IE, Blumenfeld Z, Rotten S. Sonoembryology. In: Timor-Tritsch IE, Rottem S, eds. *Transvaginal Sonography.* 2nd ed. New York: Elsevier; 1991:225-298.

40. Rottem S, Timor-Tritsch IE. Think ectopic. In: Timor-Tritsch IE, Rottem S, eds. *Transvaginal Sonography.* 2nd ed. New York: Elsevier; 1991:373-392.
41. Lee W, Comstock C. Pelvic ultrasonography. In: Tintinalli JE, Ruiz E, Krome RL, eds. *Emergency Medicine: A Comprehensive Study Guide.* 4th ed. New York: McGraw-Hill; 1996:1399-1410.
42. Mateer J, Plummer D, Heller M, et al. Model curriculum for physician training in emergency ultrasonography. *Ann Emerg Med* 1994;23:95-102.
43. Core content for emergency medicine. Developed by the American College of Emergency Physicians and the Society for Academic Emergency Medicine. *Ann Emerg Med* 1991;20:920-934.

Magnetic Resonance Imaging

Frank J. Edwards, MD, FACEP

In a 1977 issue of *Nature*, Waldo Hinshaw and colleagues published photographs of a wrist and hand that had been created by the induction of molecular resonance within a magnetic field. The images were astonishing in their clarity and heralded the arrival of a totally new diagnostic modality. Magnetic resonance imaging (MRI) began clinical use in 1981 and is arguably the most significant imaging advance since Roentgen's original work in the late 19th century.[1] The ability of MRI to create uncannily detailed soft-tissue images in multiple planes has revolutionized the evaluation of an ever-expanding list of diseases.

Many clinicians who desire an intellectual grasp of this technology find the physics and mathematics daunting and the terminology obscure. So do some radiologists, as one speaker at a radiology conference recently alluded to: "The only ones who really understand it," he stated, "are people who wear sandals and sleep until noon."

But, the practical uses for MRI continue to grow, and the emergency physician needs an understanding of how it works and when to consider using it instead of the CT scan. Despite superficial resemblances, the true natures of MRI and CT are as different as the moon and earth—an apt simile, for CT depends upon electrons to produce an image, and MRI the nucleus itself.[2]

This chapter discusses the physics and technology of MRI. Access to MRI technology is certain to become routine over the next decade. Those specific times when an emergency physician might now consider ordering an MRI study instead of a CT scan are highlighted. The use of both MRI and CT in head- and spine-injured patients is given special attention.

Background and Physics of MRI

Magnetic resonance imaging depends upon a phenomenon known as nuclear spin. In 1924, Wolfgang Pauli suggested that certain variations in atomic spectra could be explained with models in which nuclei were in rapid rotation. By the late 1940s, researchers studying the behavior of spinning nuclei in magnetic fields had opened up a novel way to investigate the universe—nuclear magnetic spectroscopy, a technique that led to Bloch and Purcell receiving the Nobel Prize in 1952.[2] In the late 1960s, Jasper Jackson first experimented with magnetic resonance in humans.

Creation of Images Through Nuclear Magnetic Resonance. MRI images depend upon the fact that the major isotope of hydrogen is abundantly found in all living tissues except bone, and that it possesses strong magnetic properties when spinning.[3,4] When tissue is exposed to a strong magnetic field, enough of the free and bound hydrogen atoms (protons) swing into alignment with the magnetic field to give the tissue a net magnetic vector.[3]

The protons (or any atom with a dipole), however, do not come into perfect alignment with the main magnetic axis of the external field but oscillate about it with a slight "wobble," known as precession. *(Please see Figure 1.)*

Figure 1. Precession

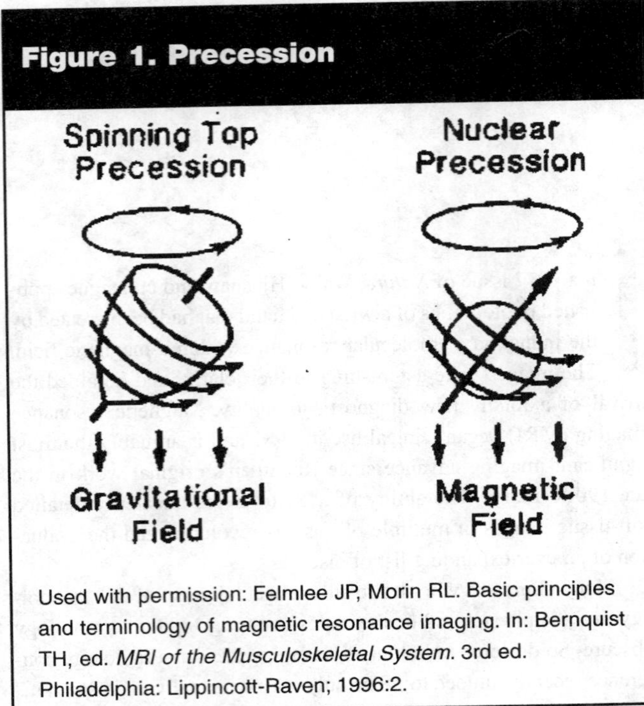

Used with permission: Felmlee JP, Morin RL. Basic principles and terminology of magnetic resonance imaging. In: Bernquist TH, ed. *MRI of the Musculoskeletal System*. 3rd ed. Philadelphia: Lippincott-Raven; 1996:2.

Figure 2. Generation of an MRI Echo by RF Excitation of Magnetized Tissue

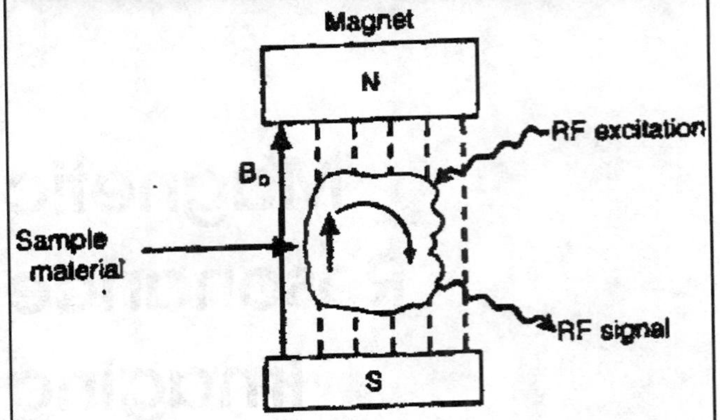

Used with permission: Felmlee JP, Morin RL. Basic principles and terminology of magnetic resonance imaging. In: Bernquist TH, ed. *MRI of the Musculoskeletal System*. 3rd ed. Philadelphia: Lippincott-Raven; 1996:3.

This precession generates an electromagnetic wave, the frequency of which is the Larmor frequency (L), per the equation below. The Larmor frequency for any given atom varies proportionately to the strength of the external magnetic field.

Larmor frequency (L) = (y/2p) ´ B

where y is the known gyromagnetic ratio for a given atom (a function of its charge balance and angular momentum), and B is the strength of the external magnetic field in Tesla units.

If a beam of radiofrequency (RF) energy is pulsed into the magnetized protons at the appropriate Larmor frequency, the energy states of atoms will rise and a spike of radio energy will echo from the tissue. *(Please see Figure 2.)*

Listening to Echoes. An early problem researchers faced was how to distinguish the RF echo from the RF excitation pulse itself, for both were at the same frequency and were almost simultaneous. It was discovered that if a second RF pulse were beamed into the tissue while the excited atoms were returning to baseline equilibrium , a distinct secondary echo would radiate from the tissue at a discrete time afterward. This scenario of initial pulse, second pulse, and echo return is called the "pulse-echo sequence."

The time it takes for atoms to relax back to baseline state has two components—T1 and T2, measured in milliseconds. T1, the spin-lattice relaxation time, measures intramolecular bonding. T2, the spin-spin relaxation time, is related to the magnetic pull of nearby precessing atoms. The important thing to remember is that each type of tissue has a very specific T1 and T2. *(Please see Table 1.)*

By varying the times between the pulses in the pulse-echo sequence, the operator can emphasize either the T1 or the T2 characteristics of a given tissue. The MRI operator can also manipulate the energy of pulses, the time of repetition (TR) between pulse-echo sequences, the magnetic gradient, and the echo time (TE). *(See Figure 3.)* The operator thus "weights" the image to take advantage of T1, T2, or hydrogen-atom density factors of the structure to be visualized.

Because, for example, cerebrospinal fluid (CSF) has a long T1, MRI device settings that maximize T1 and minimize T2 effects result in dark-appearing ventricles. Fat, on the other hand, with its short T1, appears as a bright area. Many newer MRI machines can reconstruct the image in any number of different planes.

Imaging in Head Injuries: MRI and CT

It is difficult to discuss the imaging of head-injured patients without discussing the use of computed tomography (CT). There are two issues of relevance to emergency physicians regarding the imaging of head injuries: 1) which ones require urgent imaging studies by CT; and 2) when might an MRI be the imaging method of choice? *(Please see Table 2.)*

With the exception of children under the age of 2 (where skull fracture complications such as leptomeningeal cysts and considerations of child abuse make assessment for simple fracture more important), plain skull x-rays are of little clinical value in most head-injury cases.[5,6] CT has become the method of choice for the evaluation of head-injured patients who may have lesions requiring neurosurgery.

There remains debate over where to set the threshold for performing CTs in patients with minor head injuries.[7-13] There is no doubt that a CT should be performed rapidly in patients displaying signs of significant neurologic impairment, such as unconsciousness or motor deficit, and in patients who have Glasgow Coma Scores (GCS) of 13 or less. As many as 40% of patients with GCSs of 13 in one series had CT abnormalities, 10% of which needed urgent neurosurgical intervention.[14] One recent prospective, multicenter study of head-injured patients found a greater prevalence of abnormal CTs in those younger than 2 or older than 60.[15] But for nonelderly adult patients with relatively minor injuries, the need for immediate imaging is less clear—and the issue more problematic in these times of shrinking budgets. A reasonable strategy, proposed by Stein and Ross

Table 1. Tissue Relaxation Constants (1.0 Tesla Magnet)

	BLOOD	FAT	BRAIN	MUSCLE	CSF
T1	900 ms	220 ms	860 ms	750 ms	3000 ms
T2	200 ms	60 ms	70 ms	55 ms	2000 ms

and endorsed by Jones in a recent review article, divides nonelderly adult patients with head injuries into minimal, mild, and potentially severe categories.[16,17] Patients with minimal injuries are those who do not lose consciousness, have no deficits, have a GCS of 15, and who are not taking anticoagulant drugs. These patients, all else being equal, can be discharged after a brief observation without imaging studies, as long as they are in the care of a responsible individual given standard head-injury precautions. Mildly injured patients are those with loss of consciousness (LOC) less than five minutes and a GCS of 14 or 15. These patients should receive a CT. If the CT is negative, they also can be discharged safely.

The evaluation of those with potentially severe injuries (i.e., patients with prolonged loss of consciousness, focal deficits, seizures, etc.) mandates not only immediate CT scanning but neurosurgical consultation as well.

Computed tomography offers many advantages over MRI in the head-injured patient. CT can be performed significantly faster, is less costly, and, compared to MRI, is generally much more available and less cumbersome to use with unstable patients. Metallic objects can become dangerous projectiles in the presence of an MRI's huge permanent magnet, which may also create serious problems with implanted ferrometallic devices such as aneurysm clips and pacemakers.

Both CT and MRI adequately detect the presence of hemorrhages significant enough to require surgery, but CT is more sensitive than MRI for the diagnosis of skull fractures and subarachnoid bleeding.[17-19] MRI, on the other hand, is significantly more sensitive in the detection of central nervous soft-tissue lesions, including diffuse axonal injury, shearing injury, contusions, brainstem injuries, sinus injuries, and small extra-axial blood collections.[18]

In 1991, Dozema and colleagues published a frequently quoted study that demonstrated MRI abnormalities in 10% of a sample of 58 patients discharged from the ED after suffering minor head injuries. Three patients had contusions, and three others had small subdural hematomas discovered by MRI. Two of the small subdural hematomas were not detected on the initial CT.[20] The clinical courses of these patients, however, were not altered by the MRI findings. This study and others have led to the suggestion that MRI may be an ideal way to evaluate head-injured patients with persistent symptoms and a negative CT.[21]

Imaging in Acute CVA

As evidence grows suggesting the possible value of thrombolytic agents in certain acute CVA patients, better ways of imaging the brain are needed to risk-stratify these patients, especially in terms of whether the stroke is ischemic or hemorrhagic. Two things are currently certain: 1) MRI has no significant advantage over CT in detecting hemorrhage; and 2) newer MRI strategies such as diffusion-weighted and perfusion imaging will provide heretofore unavailable information about the location and extent of ischemic strokes.[22,23] At this time, MRI has no significant advantage over CT in the detection of hemorrhagic stroke, and CT remains the study of choice to rule out hemorrhage in the patient with an acute CVA.

Figure 3. Basic MRI System

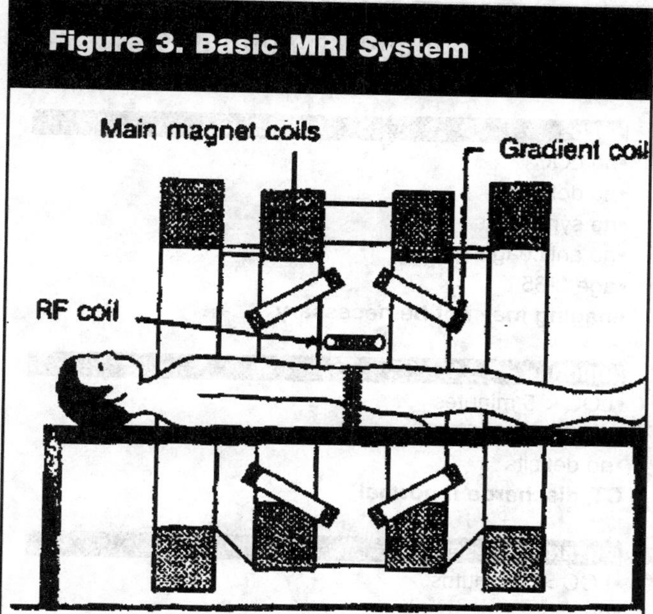

The "slice" of tissue visualized by MRI is created by an electromagnetic coil which imposes an adjustable gradient upon the field generated by the huge permanent magnet. Nuclear resonance will occur only where the magnetic gradient and the radiowave pulse frequency together satisfy the Larmor equation. The steeper the gradient, the thinner the slice. Move the gradient, so moves the slice. To obtain information about the echo returns from various depths within the slice, another magnetic gradient is intermittently pulsed briefly during the echo return phase of each spin-echo sequence. This slightly changes the oscillation frequency at each point along its gradient and "encodes" the echo from each level of the slice with a tiny but measurable shift in frequency.

Used with permission: Felmlee JP, Morin RL. Basic principles and terminology of magnetic resonance imaging. In: Bernquist TH, ed. *MRI of the Musculoskeletal System.* 3rd ed. Philadelphia: Lippincott-Raven; 1996:5.

Imaging of the Cervical Spine

Though MRI is far less sensitive than CT for the detection of bony spinal injuries (due to the paucity of hydrogen atoms in cortical bone), MRI is much better at detecting soft-tissue spinal injuries, including edema, transection, compression, hemorrhage, and disc herniation.[24] Therefore, MRI and CT are complementary in the evaluation of serious spinal injuries. CT delineates the bony

Table 2. Imaging in Head Injury

MILD
- no LOC
- no deficits
- no symptoms
- no anticoagulants
- age 2-65

Imaging may not be necessary

MINOR
- LOC < 5 minutes
- GCS 14 or 15
- no deficits

CT, discharge if normal

POTENTIALLY SEVERE
- LOC > 5 minutes
- deficits
- worsening in ED

Immediate CT and neurosurgical consult

PERSISTENT NEUROLOGIC SYMPTOMS POST HEAD INJURY

If CT is normal, do MRI

If CT was not done, consider CT first or go directly to MRI

injury; MRI displays extraordinary details and extent of soft-tissue damage.

Emergency evaluation of a potential cervical-spine injury obviously begins with the clinical evaluation. If a patient demonstrates any significant clinical risk factor for neck injury, plain radiography is undertaken.[25] If the plain radiographs suggest a fracture, or if clinical factors such as a neurologic deficit or unusual pain persist despite negative radiographs, CT is the next step.[26] If the CT is negative, but clinical suspicion of spinal pathology still remains, an MRI is justified.[27] In the case of known cervical spine injury, MRI will better display the extent of soft-tissue injury and may provide important prognostic and therapeutic information.

Back Pain

A significant percentage of patients with back pain who are treated in the ED require no imaging studies. Spinal radiographs have little value in the otherwise healthy adult who presents without neurologic deficit after an acute twisting or wrenching injury to the low back. Well-known risk factors for more serious problems include trauma and neurologic deficits, as well as symptoms that suggest malignancy or infection (e.g., age > 50, chronicity, lack of inciting event, and fever). In these patients, despite the lack of sensitivity, plain x-rays are an initial study of choice.

More sensitive diagnostic modalities include CT, myelography, and—more and more over the past decade—MRI. Both MRI and CT are equivalent in the detection of disc herniation, and both are better than myelography.[17] Though CT shows more bony detail than MRI, the MRI image can be reconstructed in a variety of planes, including the sagittal.

MRI is valuable in the diagnosis of infections of the spine, although it is not as sensitive as CT myelography at detecting epidural abscesses.[28] MRI is generally better at assessing spinal cord compression than plain CT, especially when the compression is secondary to a malignant process.[17] By calculating signal intensity ratios between diseased and normal structures, the MRI can differentiate between benign and malignant vertebral body compression fractures.

MRI can make the diagnosis of disc herniation as well as CT but it is more costly and less available. However, when the primary suspicion is that of a spinal infection or other soft-tissue abnormality, MRI should be considered after plain radiography.

Thoracic Aortic Dissection

A recent study in the *New England Journal of Medicine* compared noninvasive imaging methods for the evaluation of thoracic aortic dissection in 101 patients.[29] The sensitivities of MRI, transesophageal echosonography (TEE), and CT for the detection of this life-threatening condition were all high and relatively similar—98.3% for MRI, 97.7% for TEE, and 93.8% for CT. The authors of this study concluded that MRI should be the study of choice in hemodynamically stable patients. For unstable patients, TEE is the optimal method.

MRI has no clear role at this time in the evaluation of blunt trauma patients with possible thoracic aortic rupture. Aortic angiography remains the gold standard. This may change, however, as MRI devices become smaller and faster. A number of clinical studies have suggested that CT may be a useful and reasonably sensitive screening test prior to angiography in hemodynamically stable patients at risk for traumatic aortic tears.[30,31] For patients with signs of aortic injury on chest x-ray such as mediastinal widening and an apical cap, immediate angiography is indicated. If the chest x-ray is equivocal or suboptimal, or if the chest x-ray is normal but clinical suspicion is high for aortic injury, CT is indicated. If the CT is equivocal or positive for mediastinal hemorrhage, angiography is necessary.[32]

MRI Angiography

The attractiveness of MRI angiography lies in its potential to create vascular images without the radiation and invasiveness of angiography. It also demonstrates finer detail than echosonography. The primary mode of MRI angiography is called "time of flight" (TOF). Within a given slice of an MRI image, new volumes of blood (not exposed to the radiowave pulse) continually move into the slice. Ordinarily, the T1 of muscle and blood are very similar and have little MRI echo contrast. But the hydrogen atoms of the moving blood have not been "excited" by the radiowave pulse and, therefore, return little or no echo. Consequently, there is great contrast between the blood vessel and surrounding histologic environment, and images can be seen with TOF angiography that rival those of conventional angiography.[33,34]

In the assessment of carotid stenosis, MRI alone is not yet as accurate as conventional angiography. However, when carotid MRI angiography results are combined with sonography, the net information obtained is comparable to standard x-ray angiograms.[35]

To differentiate between venous and arterial flow, a technique in which blood upstream from the MRI slice is "presaturated" with radiowave frequency is used. When this "presaturated" blood enters the MRI slice, it too will resonate and display little contrast with the surrounding tissue. Blood coming from the opposite direction is "unsaturated" and will therefore appear in contrast to adjacent structures.[33]

MRI angiography is rapidly developing. As techniques improve and become more cost-effective, it is conceivable that one day an emergency physician might reach for this modality to evaluate carotid disease, abdominal aortic aneurysms, renal artery stenosis, portal vein disease, mesenteric ischemia, vena cava syndromes, and perhaps even the coronary arteries.[36] At present, however, its clinical utility for the evaluation of most ED patients seems limited.

Cardiac MRI

The recent medical literature contains a growing number of articles addressing the use of MRI in the evaluation of cardiac structure and function.[38-41] Clinically useful information regarding left and right ventricular ejection fractions, wall stress, wall mass, and valvular abnormalities can now be obtained by MRI.[37] Evaluation of the pulmonary vasculature is also now possible. This burst of progress is at least partly in response to the creation of ultrafast MRI devices that have reduced data acquisition times to the order of seconds.

Other cardiac study techniques involve the use of radio-tagged contrast materials.[42] Presently, the use of cardiac MRI studies in the ED is limited, but this is not likely to be the case in the future.

Miscellaneous MRI Applications

Multiple Sclerosis. MRI has become the single most important clinical tool in the evaluation of multiple sclerosis (MS). Its ability to show the plaques of MS within the central nervous system and to follow their changes over time has led to a greater understanding of the disease itself.[43] For ED patients suspected of having this condition, it may be reasonable to order an outpatient MRI examination after discussion with the primary care physician or neurologist.

Soft-Tissue Masses. Though MRI usually cannot determine the histologic features of a soft-tissue mass, it is frequently chosen by clinicians as the first test in the evaluation of such masses. Lipomas can be identified by MRI since their signal intensity (short T1) is identical to subcutaneous fat in all image weightings.[35]

Acute Joint and Musculoskeletal Problems. In recent years, MRI has become part of the diagnostic armamentarium for the evaluation of acute musculoskeletal injuries, including injuries of the knee, ankle, shoulder, elbow, major tendons, and muscles.[44-48] MRI can make anatomic diagnoses of such injuries with great accuracy and obviates the need for arthrography in many cases. For example, MRI of the wrist and hand can distinguish between navicular avascular necrosis, fractures, and tears of fibrocartilage, ligaments, and tendons. It can also aid in the diagnosis of carpal and tarsal tunnel syndromes.[35] In addition, MRI has great potential for the diagnosis of chronic musculoskeletal overuse syndromes, especially in athletes.

Table 3. MRI Safety Issues

- Ferromagnetic objects external to the body become projectiles.
- Ferromagnetic objects within the body (aneurysm clips, some prostheses including cochlear implants, certain types of heart valves, etc.) can torque and cause injury.
- Pacemaker dysfunction

MRI has become the test of choice over bone scintigraphy for the evaluation of osteomyelitis, since MRI can distinguish between soft-tissue and bone-marrow processes with greater sensitivity. In one study, MRI was 94% sensitive in making the diagnosis of osteomyelitis compared to 71% for scintigraphy.[35]

Peanut Foreign Bodies. A recent article from Japan described the successful use of MRI to localize peanut fragments aspirated by a child.[50] Peanuts are lucent on plain x-rays and are often ill-defined by CT images; but, with their high fat content (i.e., short T1), they give strong signals in T1-weighted MRI images. MRI should be considered among the options available to the emergency physician for the localization of select foreign bodies including peanut fragments.

MRI and the Hip. The superiority of MRI over bone scanning is also apparent in the evaluation of occult hip disorders. A recent British study evaluated the use of MRI in patients with hip injuries and negative plain x-rays. Although the number of patients in this study was too small to make statistically significant conclusions, MRI performed at least as well as bone scanning in the detection of occult femoral neck fractures. MRI was reported to have diagnosed two cases missed by scintigraphy.[51] MRI has become the premier diagnostic test for occult avascular necrosis of the hip.[35]

MRI and the Abdomen. MRI has an accuracy comparable to computed tomography for the detection of metastatic disease of the liver and may also be potentially better than CT at defining cavernous hemangiomas and distinguishing focal fatty infiltration from other conditions.[35] From a cost-effectiveness standpoint, however, a contrast-enhanced CT remains the test of choice for the assessment of liver metastases, provided the patient has no allergy to contrast material. Just as MRI angiography can demonstrate the fine detail of vasculature structure without the need for contrast injection, MRI can employ the same principle of flow-related resonance differences to the biliary tract.

The time may come when MRI "cholangiography" will be the initial study for patients with obstructive jaundice. It may become a supplement or a replacement for endoscopic retrograde cholangiopancreatography (ERCP).

Costs and Safety

Despite the extraordinary benefits of MRI, it has several obvious limitations. MRI is not universally available. The design of MRI devices makes the use of resuscitation equipment cumbersome or impossible in the MRI suite. In addition, MRI, by its very nature, will always raise major safety issues. *(Please see Table 3.)* Patients who possess ferromagnetic material within their bodies (e.g., pacemakers,

Table 4. Possible MRI Applications in the ED

- Evaluation of head injuries with normal CTs and persistent symptoms
- Disorders of the spine, including suspected spinal osteomyelitis or other infection, suspected malignancy, cord compression syndromes, or as an alternative to CT or myelography for evaluation of disc herniation
- In conjunction with CT for evaluation of cervical cord trauma
- Evaluation for multiple sclerosis
- To be considered an option in the evaluation of pediatric cases of peanut aspiration
- To be considered in the initial evaluation of suspected soft-tissue masses

clips, some prostheses, shrapnel, cochlear implants, etc.) are at risk of injury when exposed to the magnetic field. Individuals have been injured when metal objects were inadvertently brought close to the magnet. A screwdriver in the hand of a technician can become a high-energy projectile.

Finally, MRI is expensive. The cost of the magnet alone may exceed the price of an entire CT scanner. In 1990, the charges for MRI exams ranged from $540-$1308 (mean, $950), compared to charges for CT studies from $350-$600, and for ultrasound from $150-$300.[35]

MRI is reasonably sensitive at detecting anterior cruciate ligament tears, although a recent study argues that clinical examination is just as good or better, and the condition is treated conservatively anyway.[49] Increasingly, we must ask not only does a test or procedure work, but is it worth the expense?

Much of the cost, inconvenience, and potential danger of MRI devices are related to the size of the magnet. The tesla of the magnet of the average MRI device is 1000 times greater than the tesla of an ordinary household magnet. Smaller magnets would be cheaper, safer, and more convenient. However, image quality would be poorer, and the studies would take a longer time to perform. Technology is rapidly advancing toward the goal of smaller magnets, faster studies, and better images.

Conclusion

MRI is an imaging technique that capitalizes on the abundance of hydrogen atoms in living tissue and the natural propensity of these dipolar atoms to act like little magnets. When placed in a magnetic field and subjected to bursts of radiofrequency energy at an appropriate frequency, the hydrogen atoms briefly "resonate" and act like molecular radio transmitters. By varying the pulse sequences, differences between various types of soft tissue can be seen with far greater sensitivity than possible with x-ray beams.

Conventional radiography and CT scanning, however, remain the imaging methods of choice for bony injuries. However, just as CT and ultrasound have become part of the emergency physician's routine repertoire of diagnostic imaging options, the same will almost certainly hold true for MRI. *(Please see Table 4.)*

References

1. Wehrli FW. Principles of magnetic resonance. In: Stark DD, Bradley WG, eds. *Magnetic Resonance Imaging.* 2nd ed. St. Louis: Mosby; 1988:3-19.
2. Felmlee JP, Morin RL. Basic principles and terminology of magnetic resonance imaging. In: Berquist TH, ed. *MRI of the Musculoskeletal System.* 3rd ed. Philadelphia: Lippincott-Raven; 1996:1-35.
3. Balter S. An introduction to the physics of magnetic resonance imaging. *Radiographics* 1987;7:371-382.
4. Merritt CR. Magnetic resonance imaging—clinical perspective: Image quality, safety, and risk management. *Radiographics* 1987;7:1001-1016.
5. Yealy DM, Hogan DE. Imaging after head trauma: Who needs what? *Emerg Med Clin North Am* 1991;9:707-717.
6. Hackney DB. Skull radiography in the evaluation of acute head trauma: A survey of current practice. *Radiology* 1991; 181:711-714.
7. Duus BR, Lind B, Christensen H, et al. The role of neuroimaging in the initial management of patients with minor head injury. *Ann Emerg Med* 1994;23:1279-1283.
8. Reinus WR, Zwemer FL Jr. Clinical prediction of emergency cranial computed tomography results. *Ann Emerg Med* 1994; 23:1271-1278.
9. Sinclair DE, Kovacs G, Hillis M. Cranial CT scans—emergency department utilization. *J Emerg Med* 1993;11:643-646.
10. Reinus WR, Wippold FJII, Erickson KK. Practical selection criteria for noncontrast cranial computed tomography in patients with head trauma. *Ann Emerg Med* 1993;22: 1148-1155.
11. Reinus WR, Erickson KK, Wippold FJII. Unenhanced emergency cranial CT: Optimizing patient selection with univariate and multivariate analyses. *Radiology* 1993;186:763-768.
12. Mohanty SK, Thompson W, Rakower S. Are CT scans for head injury patients always necessary? *J Trauma* 1991;31: 801-805.
13. Pitts LH. The role of neuroimaging in minor head injury. *Ann Emerg Med* 1991;20:1387-1388. Editorial.
14. Stein SC, Ross SE. The value of computed tomographic scans in patients with low-risk head injuries. *Neurosurgery* 1990;26: 638-640.
15. Schynoll W, Overton D, Krome R, et al. A prospective study to identify high-yield criteria associated with acute intracranial computed tomography findings in head-injured patients. *Am J Emerg Med* 1993;11:321-326.
16. Stein SC, Ross SE. Minor head injury: A proposed strategy for emergency management. *Ann Emerg Med* 1993;22: 193-195.
17. Jones R. Advances in radiology in emergency medicine. *Top Emerg Med* 1994;16:34-44.
18. Orrison WW, Gentry LR, Stimac GK, et al. Blinded comparison of cranial CT and MR in closed head injury evaluation. *Am J Neuroradiol* 1994;15;351.

19. Skylar EM, Quencer RM, Bowen BC. Magnetic resonance applications in cerebral injury. *Radiol Clin North Am* 1992;30:350-366.
20. Doezema D, King J, Tandberg D, et al. Magnetic resonance imaging in minor head injury. *Ann Emerg Med* 1991;20: 1281-1285.
21. Olshaker JS, Whye DW. Head trauma. *Emerg Med Clin North Am* 1993;11:165-186.
22. Mohr JP, et al. Magnetic resonance vs. computed tomographic imaging in acute stroke. *Stroke* 1995;26:807.
23. Fisher M, Prichard JW, Warach S. New magnetic resonance techniques for acute ischemic stroke. *JAMA* 1995;274: 908-911.
24. Levitt MA, Flanders AE. Diagnostic capabilities of magnetic resonance imaging and computed tomography in acute cervical spinal column injury. *Am J Emerg Med* 1991;9:131.
25. Hoffman JR, Schriger DL, Mower W, et al. Low-risk criteria for cervical-spine radiography in blunt trauma: a prospective study. *Ann Emerg Med* 1992;21:1454-1460.
26. Murphey MD. Trauma oblique cervical spine radiographs. *Ann Emerg Med* 1993;22:728-730. Editorial.
27. Davis SJ, Khangure MS. A review of magnetic resonance imaging in spinal trauma. *Australas Radiol* 1994;38:241-253.
28. Post MJ. Spinal infections: Evaluation with magnetic resonance imaging and post-operative ultrasonography. *Radiology* 1988;169:765-771.
29. Nienaber CA, Kodolitsch Y, Nicolas V, et al. The diagnosis of thoracic aortic dissection by noninvasive imaging procedures. *N Engl J Med* 1993;328:1-9.
30. Raptopoulos V. Traumatic aortic tear: Screening with chest CT. *Radiology* 1992;182:667.
31. Hunink MG, Johanna JB. Triage of patients to angiography for detection of aortic rupture after blunt chest trauma: Cost-effectiveness analysis of using CT. *Am J Roentgenol* 1995;165:27-36.
32. Richardson P, Mirvis S, Scorpio R, et al. Value of CT in determining the need for angiography when findings of mediastinal hemorrhage on chest radiographs are equivocal. *Am J Roentgenol* 1991;156:273-279.
33. Sheppard S. Basic concepts in magnetic resonance angiography. *Radiol Clin North Am* 1995;33:91-112.
34. Atkinson D, Teresi L. Magnetic resonance angiography. *Magn Reson Q* 1994;10:149-172.
35. Edelman RR, Warach S. Magnetic resonance imaging (second of two parts). *N Engl J Med* 1993;328:785-790.
36. Muller MF, Edelman RR. Magnetic resonance angiography of the abdomen. *Gastroenterol Clin North Am* 1995;24:435-456.
37. Pattynama PM, DeRoos A, Van der Wall EE, et al. Evaluation of cardiac function with magnetic resonance imaging. *Am Heart J* 1994;128:595-607.
38. Wexler L, Higgins CB. The use of magnetic resonance imaging in adult congenital heart disease. *Am J Card Imag* 1995;9:15-28.
39. Vliegen HW, DeRoos A, Bruschke AV, et al. Magnetic resonance techniques for the assessment of myocardial viability: Clinical experience. *Am Heart J* 1995;129:809-818.
40. DeRoos A, Van der Wall EE. Evaluation of ischemic heart disease by magnetic resonance imaging and spectroscopy. *Radiol Clin North Am* 1994;32:581-592.
41. Wilke N, Jerosch-Herold M, Stillman AE, et al. Concepts of myocardial perfusion imaging in magnetic resonance imaging. *Magn Reson Q* 1994;10:249-86.
42. Henriksen O. MR spectroscopy in clinical research. *Acta Radiol* 1994;35:96-116.
43. Truyen L. Magnetic resonance imaging in multiple sclerosis: A review. *Acta Neuro Belg* 1994;94:98-102.
44. Haygood TM, Monu JU, Pope TL. Magnetic resonance imaging of the knee. *Orthopedics* 1994;17:1067-1072.
45. Beltran J. Magnetic resonance imaging of the ankle and foot. *Orthopedics* 1994;17:1075-1082.
46. Herzog RJ. Efficacy of magnetic resonance imaging of the elbow. *Med Sci Sports Exerc* 1994;26:1193-1202.
47. Brandser EA, El-Khoury GY, Saltzman CS. Tendon injuries: Application of magnetic resonance imaging. *Can Assoc Radiol J* 1995;46:9-18.
48. Steinbach LS, Fleckenstein JL, Mink JH. Magnetic resonance imaging of muscle injuries. *Orthopedics* 1994;17:991-999.
49. Liu SH, et al. The diagnosis of acute complete tears of the anterior cruciate ligament: Comparison of MRI, arthrometry and clinical examination. *J Bone Joint Surg Br* 1995;77B:586.
50. Imaizumi H, Kaneko M, Nara S, et al. Definitive diagnosis and location of peanuts in the airways using magnetic resonance imaging techniques. *Ann Emerg Med* 1994;23: 1379-1382.
51. Evans PD, et al. Comparison of MRI with bone scanning for suspected hip fracture in elderly patients. *J Bone Joint Surg Br* 1994;76B:158.

Cervical Spine Radiography

Raymond J. Roberge

Neurological sequel of cervical spine injury (CSI) may have a devastating impact upon a patient's future physical, social, emotional, and financial well-being. Consequently, physicians constantly must strive to improve diagnostic techniques when it comes to CSI. The past decade has witnessed a steady rise in the utilization of cervical spine radiography (CSR) to achieve such a goal.

Because blunt trauma is such a common entity, large numbers of trauma victims undergo CSR to rule out relatively infrequent CSIs. The decision to use CSR is influenced by many factors, such as triage protocols, patient expectations, uncertainty over the existence of asymptomatic[1] CSI, and fears of malpractice litigation.[2,3] However, recent concerns have surfaced over issues as diverse as health care cost containment, radiation exposure to patients and emergency department staff; patient flow patterns, and CSR interference with other necessary interventions,[3-5] forcing physicians to reconsider the role of CSR in blunt trauma.

Unfortunately, although the current guidelines for selective use of radiography in evaluating extremity[6] and pelvic trauma in alert patients possibly could be applied to CSR,[8] to do so remains too controversial. Current concepts regarding CSR utilization in blunt trauma have been based largely upon retrospective studies and anecdotal reports. The relatively recent appearance of prospective CSR studies has allowed a more in depth analysis of risk factors for CSI, and this, in turn, has led to the development of high-yield criteria for CSR in adult blunt trauma.

Many physicians are considerably (and understandably) anxious about radiographic selectivity for situations in which the failure to diagnose may result in potentially catastrophic consequences for both the patient and the practitioner. To alleviate some of the natural concerns over the selective utilization of CSR, this report focuses on the decision-making process for radiographic use in blunt trauma. The authors address the rationale for a selective approach to CSR in alert blunt trauma victims and outline potential medical and legal ramifications of employing such an approach. The result is a comprehensive guide to prudent CSR utilization in blunt trauma, which will serve the physician and patient equally well, while minimizing risk to both.

Gathering Essential Information

Ordering CSR on the basis of standing protocols results in many unnecessary radiographs and is discouraged.[1] For instance, the mere presence of a cervical immobilization device is not, of itself, a criterion for CSR. Physicians should determine the need for CSR in blunt trauma through historical and physical data gleaned from the initial survey of the trauma victim.[3]

For example, elicit from the patient details regarding the events that led to the injuries. If the patient is unable to provide this information, prehospital providers, police, family, or friends might be able

Figure 1. Posteior Cervical Spine Palpation

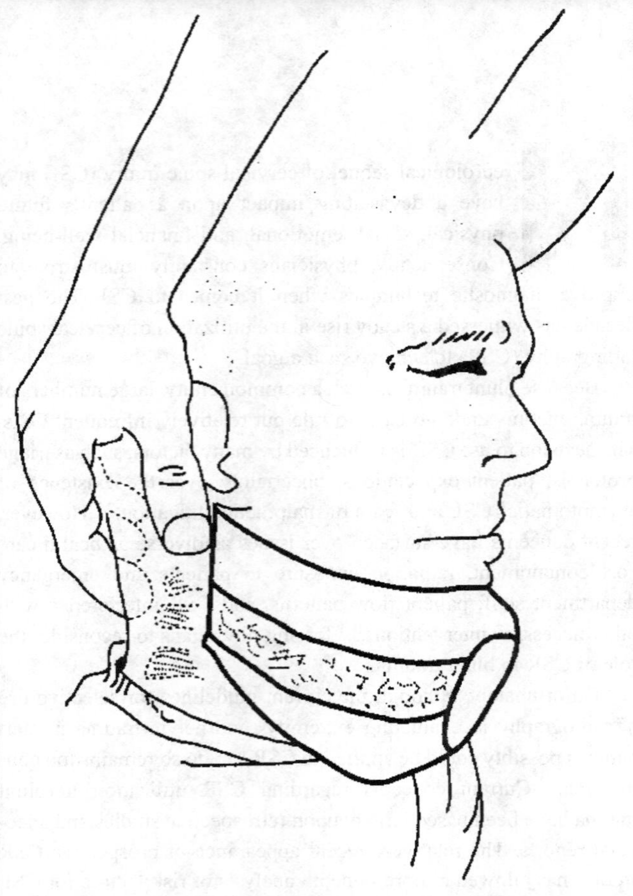

Posterior cervical spine palpation carried out while maintaining immobilization.

Figure 2. Ligamentous Cervical Spine Injury

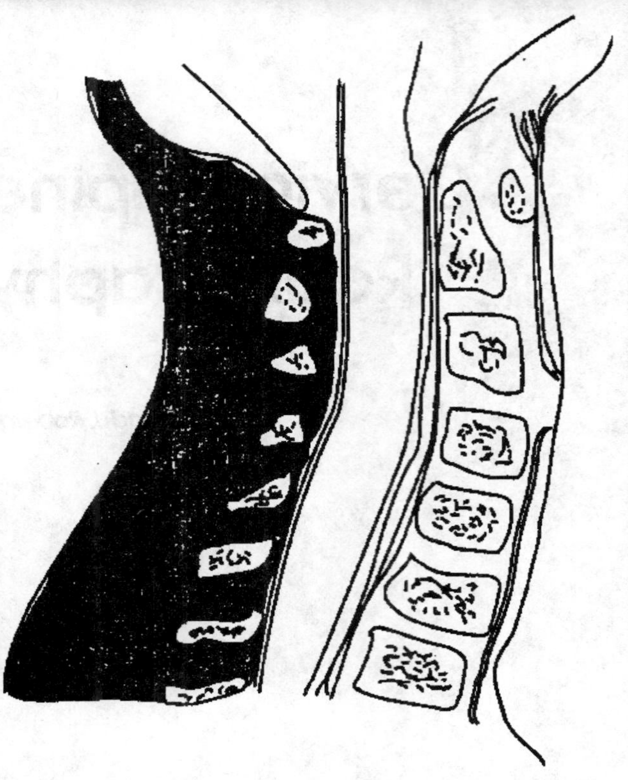

A cervical spine injury that may demonstrate normal radiography.

to do so. And during the physical survey, in addition to the usual mandatory assessment of the trauma victim's airway, breathing, and circulation, ascertain the victim's neurological status, including mental faculties and the possibility of drug involvement (e.g., breath odor, intravenous needle tracks, etc.).

There is little question that CSR is mandatory for any blunt trauma victim with neurological deficits or alteration of mental status for any reason (e.g., comatose state, hypoxia, intoxication).[4] The same holds true for patients who cannot reliably communicate (e.g., endotracheal incubation, mental retardation, psychiatric disorder, non-English speaking).[1,5]

Approach to the Alert Trauma Patient. In the alert trauma victim, specifically ask about any complaints (e.g., pain, aches, stiffness) referable to the cervical region.[10] This must include complaints in anterior, lateral, or posterior neck regions because some injuries (e.g., odontoid fractures) may not manifest classic posterior cervical region findings.[11] A positive response to questioning mandates CSR.

In the alert patient without cervical complaints, palpate the cervical spine with the posterior portion of the cervical immobilization device removed while the anterior portion continues to maintain the patient's neck in a neutral position. *(Please see Figure 1.)* Any positive cervical spine palpatory findings (e.g., tenderness, crepitus, spasm)[3,12] warrants replacing the cervical collar and obtaining CSR.

In the alert trauma victim without cervical signs or symptoms and a normal cervical spine palpatory examination, supervised painless unassisted range of cervical motion further supports exclusion of CSR.[13]

The patient with distracting injuries. CSR is required in alert blunt trauma victims without cervical signs and symptoms of neurologic deficits who have concomitant painful injuries. In these patients, the pain of concomitant injuries may distract the focus of attention away from the neck and mistakenly lull the clinician into assuming that no CSI exists.[5,11,14] This concept of "distracting" injuries, that is, competitive pain, is still poorly defined and has not received universal acceptance.[12]

Which concomitant injuries should be considered capable of diverting attention away from a CSI, and which are not? Unfortunately, studies focusing primarily on this topic do not exist" The majority of reported cases of "occult" CSI have been associated with major injuries in multiply-injured trauma victims. Injuries as diverse as bony fractures,[15] severe genital injuries,[5] multiple contusions and lacerations,[16] and severe internal injuries' have been labeled as "distracting"

The wide disparity in individual patient responses to painful stimuli make pain quantification extremely difficult. Certainly, major

Table 1. Objective Indications for Cervical Spine Radiography in Blunt Trauma

Alteration of mental status for any reason (e.g., hypoxia, comatose state, drugs, etc.)
Inability to communicate (e.g., comatose, intubated, non-English speaking, etc.)
Neurologic deficits
Concomitant, painful traumatic injuries
Pre-existent cervical disorders that impair spinal mobility (e.g., ankylosing spondylitis)
Complaints of neck discomfort
Positive palpatory findings (pain, spasm, crepitus)

concomitant injuries should prompt CSR. Apparently minor injuries that are disproportionally painful enough to alter the focus of attention away from the cervical spine also require CSR. Minor, minimally painful injuries in alert patients without cervical signs or symptoms do not require CSR.

Such injuries have been termed "occult" CSI because they may not be readily apparent on initial evaluation and therefore require a high index of suspicion.[1,11] In the often hectic environment of trauma evaluations, where multiple uncomfortable procedures may be ongoing (e.g., IV insertions, urinary catheter placement), it cannot be overemphasized that it is imperative for the clinician to receive the patient's undivided attention during questioning about cervical spine pain.

Underlying Cervical Spine Disease. Physicians also should be quite liberal in using CSR in patients with pre-existent cervical disorders that result in a rigid spine with impaired neck mobility (e.g., ankylosing spondylitis). These patients are at high risk for CSI from even minimal trauma.[1,14] Confounding the situation is that these patients may not report mild acute traumatic pain because they are accustomed to a daily existence of cervical discomfort.

Mechanism of Injury

Although the mechanism (e.g., hyperextension, hyperflexion, etc.) and mode (e.g., motor vehicle accident, fall, etc.) of injury frequently have been cited as indicators for CSR,[17,18] rarely have individual parameters been subjected to prospective analysis or statistical scrutiny.[11]

Correlating Mechanism of Trauma and CSI. Although it seems logical that patients involved in high-speed motor vehicle accidents are at increased risk for CSI, the asymptomatic, alert individual from such trauma has not been shown to be at a statistically higher risk for a cervical injury.[19]

Three prospective studies revealed no significant correlation between mechanisms of injury and CSI.[3,19,20] The only mode of injury to repeatedly demonstrate a statistically significant association with CSI in prospective studies is falls.[3,19,20] However, patients in these studies were not categorized according to mental status, neurologic involvement, or associated injuries.

The true value regarding the mechanism of injury may be in the evaluation of the alert, cervically symptomatic individual with subtle x-ray findings or normal CSR (e.g., hyperextension ligamentous injury).[18] *(Please see Figure 2.)* In these instances, knowledge of the forces involved will alert the physician to the possibility of a cervically inapparent serious CSI and prompt additional studies.

Delayed Presentation. A unique problem exists with regard to the ambulatory patient who presents in a delayed fashion with cervical complaints but no other associated injuries. Often, patients will report to the ED several hours or even days after the incident. Although cervical muscular and ligamentous strains commonly manifest in a delayed fashion following blunt trauma, rarely are these associated with CSI. Nonetheless, delayed presentations of CSI may occur in ambulatory patients because the injury was not diagnosed at the first ED presentation.[16] Also, if the patient was involved in a motor vehicle accident and was intoxicated at the time of injury, delayed presentation may occur either because symptoms were blunted by drugs or because the victim wished to avoid the legal ramifications of impaired driving. In general, evaluate delayed cervical complaints with exactly the same scrutiny as acute presentations.

"Asymptomatic" Cervical Spine Injuries

Indications for obtaining CSR in the majority of blunt trauma victims are based on objective, well-established criteria.[5,11,14,21] *(Please see Table 1.)* However, when physicians encounter alert, non-intoxicated, cooperative, blunt trauma victims with no cervical signs or symptoms and, at most, minor associated injuries, the question of whether to perform CSR becomes controversial.

"Asymptomatic" CSI. Intuitively, such patients are at low risk for CSI, and perhaps the major reason they are radiographed is that physicians fear missing what has been termed an "asymptomatic" CSI.[11] Early reports of symptomless or mildly symptomatic CSFI[10,22,25] encouraged liberal utilization of CSR in blunt trauma. This approach resulted in enhanced recognition of CSI that previously may have gone untreated. However, careful scrutiny reveals that some of these early articles were anecdotal[22,23] and others[10,24,25] reported patients who were, in fact, symptomatic at the time of pre-

Table 2. Symptomless Cervical Spine Injuries

Acute "occult" cervical spine injury
Associated with alterations of mental status, or painful concomitant injuries
Initially asumptomatic, but becomes symptomatic as the mental status clears or the pain of concomitant injuries lessens or abates
Rarely reported
Acute "asymptomatic" cervicalspine injury
The injury never is symptomatic
No such injury has yet been reported

Table 3. Injuries Reported as Distracting in Alert Trauma Victims[11]

Orthopedic injuries (fractures)
Severe internal injuries (e.g., fractured spleen, lacerated liver)
Genital injuries (i.e., severe scrotal lacerations)
Multiple contusions and abrasions

sentation. Nonetheless, the impact of these early reports persists and has perpetuated the concept of the asymptomatic CSI, a notion that is supported by some [9,22] and refuted by others.[26-28]

Asymptomatic CSI, by definition, implies a lesion that is never symptomatic.[11] No clear-cut cases of acute, asymptomatic CSI exist in the literature, leading some authorities to suggest that such an entity is no more than a myth.[1,26,27] Only one recent report even deserves consideration as an asymptomatic CST.[29] The case involved a patient with a pharyngeal infection in whom an asymptomatic odontoid fracture was discovered incidentally during radiography to evaluate a soft-tissue infectious process of the pharynx. However, the patient, an alcoholic, had no recollection of any recent trauma, so this injury may have represented a remote CSI that became asymptomatic with time.

Asymptomatic vs. Occult CSI. Confusion over the terms "occult" and "asymptomatic" CSI may be partially responsible for differences of opinion regarding symptomless CSI because these terms have incorrectly been used interchangeably. It is important for the clinician to understand the subtle, but important, differences in these two terms in order to more capably evaluate the literature of CSR and thus make a more informed decision with regard to employing CSR. *(Please see Table 2.)*

An occult CSI occurs in an alert patient in whom symptoms initially are masked by the pain of concomitant injuries.[26] Patients with occult CSI, whether stable or unstable, initially may not manifest cervical symptoms or signs, but subsequently become symptomatic as the pain of concomitant injuries lessens or abates. [9,11,21,30] Although occult CSIs are uncommon, several documented cases [9-11,21,30,31] of these injuries have been published in recent years. All cases have been associated with altered mental states, significant other injury, or both, which initially served to prompt CSR. *(Please see Table 3.)* In fact, two of these reports described patients who actually had cervical spine signs or symptoms at the time of presentation and thus did not warrant an occult designation.[10,31]

Selective Cervical Spine Radiography

Ideally, clinical decision making regarding CSR should be based upon sound scientific data that have been collected prospectively and are able to withstand statistical scrutiny. A number of prospective investigations evaluating the utilization of CSR in blunt trauma in several thousand patients have been published recently.[3,11,14,18,22,28,32] These studies have reported some remarkably similar findings namely, no CSI has been identified in any alert, acute blunt trauma patient without cervical signs and symptoms, neurological deficits, or the presence of distracting injuries.[11] Similar findings also have been reported for retrospective studies of CSR in several thousand blunt trauma victims.[4,5,8,12,33] Consequently, numerous authors suggest the elimination of CSR in this subgroup. [3,5,12,14,27,28,32,33] This low. risk subgroup probably encompasses no more than 10% to 15% of all blunt trauma victims.[3,11] Nonetheless, safely eliminating CSR in these patients may afford several theoretical benefits, but must be weighed against the possible disadvantages of employing a selective approach. *(Please see Table 4.)*

Unfortunately, diagnostic modalities with absolute sensitivity rarely exist in medicine, and CSR is no exception.[1] The physician, utilizing the current accepted standards of care, strives to offer the best possible care to the injured patient.

Table 4. Theoretical Advantages and Disadvantages of Selective Cervical Spine Radiography in Blunt Trauma

Advantages
Medical cost containment
Decreased radiation exposure to staff and patients
More effective utilization of staff
Enhanced patient flow in the emergency department
Diminished interference with other necessary, life-saving procedures
Disadvantages
Missed cervical spine injury with subsequent neurologic morbidity or mortality
Malpractice litigation
Disputes between specialists caring for trauma victimes (e.g., emergency physicians and trauma surgeons) regarding perceived standards of care
Paatient dissatisfaction with perceived lack of appropriate testing reflecting poorly on the physician or institution
Physician/institutional economic loss because perhaps as many as two-thirds of patients not initially radiographed will subsequently obtain cervical x-rays

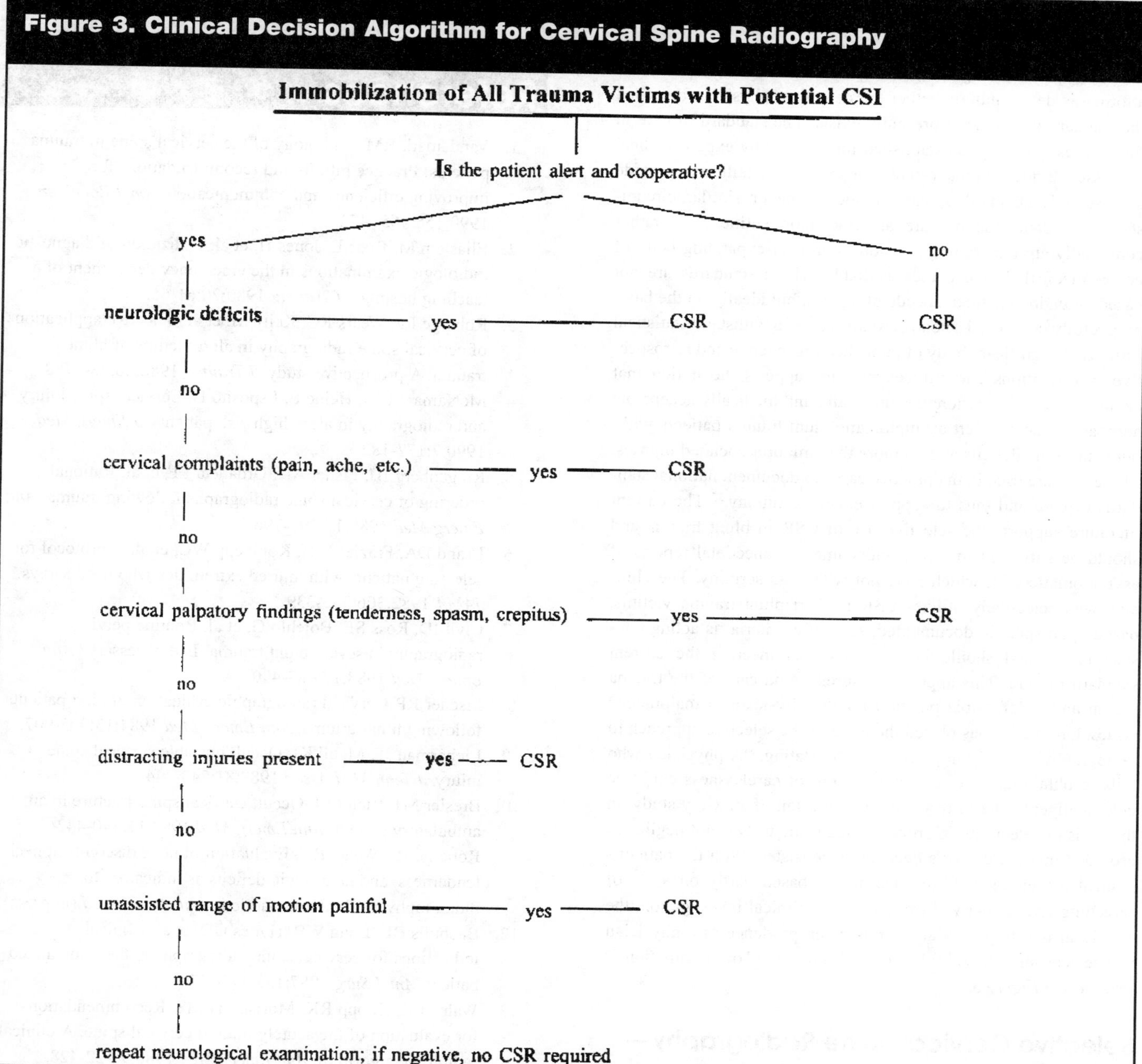

The majority of missed CSIs probably do not occur for lack of radiographs, but rather due to inadequate radiographs (e.g., failure to visualize the odontoid or the C_7T_1 interface[34]); faulty radiographic interpretation (clinician or radiologist);' careless histories and physical examinations; and the failure to consider the possibility of a CSI in the multiply-injured patient.[35] Radiographing every blunt trauma victim does not ensure the detection of every CSI because the sensitivity of CSR probably does not exceed 95%.[1] Some CSIs (e.g., hyperextension ligamentous injury, fractures of the anterior and posterior arches of C_1 linear vertical unilateral pillar fractures[36-38]) are not readily apparent on CSR. In such instances, information gleaned from the history and physical examination offers clues to radiographically inapparent injuries and should prompt further evaluation.[35] Thus, in the alert blunt trauma victim, selective use of CSR coupled with physical and historical data will ensure optimal diagnostic results.

Medical-Legal Concerns

Because of fears over malpractice, some clinicians may be wary of adopting a selective approach to CSR for fear that they may become the first to miss a truly asymptomatic CSI should such an injury subsequently be documented. It also might be argued that any cost containment brought about by selective CSR utilization would be more than offset by even one successful lawsuit. Clearly, CSI is a high-risk medical-legal area for emergency physicians. In fact, in a prospective follow-up study of post-traumatic neck pain, more than half of patients not receiving CSR at the initial evaluation went on to do so at a later date, and two-thirds of these individuals were involved in litigation.[36]

In malpractice litigation, an important issue for the plaintiff's attorney is determining whether the defendant physician breached the standard of care as it presently exists. The standard of care in these cases generally is established for the jury by expert medical witnesses. Evidence must establish a physician's failure to provide a reasonable standard of care in the "same or similar circumstances."[37] Standards of care are not static entities, but rather continually arc undergoing revision as an ever-expanding body of newer medical data becomes available. These standards are not based on undocumented, anecdotal reports, but ideally on the basis of carefully conducted scientific studies able to withstand statistical scrutiny. A significant body of published prospective and retrospective investigations currently exists and supports the notion that excluding CSR is a rational, sound, safe, and medically acceptable approach to acute, alert asymptomatic blunt trauma patients without neurologic deficits and no more than minor associated injuries. These data are used in malpractice cases to document national standards of care and thus to support expert testimony.[37] The current literature supports the selective use of CSR in blunt trauma and should be sufficient to refute undocumented anecdotal reports of asymptomatic CSI, which have not withstood scrutiny. The clinician who selectively utilizes CSR in alert blunt trauma victims, based upon specific documented, scientific criteria, is acting conscientiously and should be considered as meeting the current standard of care. This approach assures sound care of the trauma victim and a defensible position for the physician in malpractice issues. One expert has placed the issue of the selective approach to radiography squarely in perspective by stating, "A physician who fails to obtain an x-ray examination out of carelessness could be held negligent if harm resulted, but omission of an x-ray study on the basis of selectivity in ordering diagnostic tests is not negligent, provided that the doctor's decision is consistent with the patient's clinical presentation. If the decision is based partly on a set of screening criteria derived from a careful clinical investigation, the physician is acting with at least as much prudence as a physician whose decision is based solely on an 'impression' of the situation."[6] *(Please see Figure 3.)*

Selective Cervical Spine Radiography—Finding the Balance

Selective use of cervical spine radiography requires maintaining the proper balance among clinical findings, scientific data, and medical-legal considerations. Emergency physicians must individualize decision making regarding CSR for each patient, based primarily on a careful and complete clinical evaluation, but also taking into account mechanism of injury and patient expectations.

Among trauma victims, only those who are alert, non-intoxicated, and present acutely following blunt injury are candidates for selective use of CSR. An ever-increasing body of prospective, statistically scrutinized data indicates that in this subset of patients, those with no cervical spine symptoms or signs, no neurological deficits, and no "distracting" injuries represent a low-risk group for CSI and may forego CSR safely. Furthermore, because asymptomatic CSI has not been documented in patients presenting acutely after blunt trauma, CSR appears unwarranted in alert patients without cervical pain or tenderness and without concomitant injuries.

References

1. Vandemark RM. Radiology of the cervical spine in trauma patients: Practice pitfalls and recommendations for improving efficiency and communication. *Am J Roenigen* 1990;155:465- 472.
2. Eliastem M, Rose E, Jones H, et al. Utilization of diagnostic radiologic examinations in the emergency department of a teaching hospital. *J Trauma* 1980;20:61-66.
3. Roberge RJ, Wears RC, Kelly M, et al. Selective application of cervical spine radiography in alert victims of blunt trauma: A prospective study. *J Trauma* 1988;28:784-788.
4. McNamara RM, Heine E, Esposito B. Cervical spine injury and radiography in alert, high-risk patients. *J Emerg Med* 1990;7:177-182.
5. Ringenberg BJ, Fisher AK, Urdaneta LF, et al. Rational ordering of cervical spine radiographs following trauma. *Ann Emerg Med* 1988;17:792-796.
6. Brand DA, Frazier WH, Kohlhepp WC, et al. A protocol for selecting patients with injured extremities who need x-rays. *JAMA* 1982;306:333-339.
7. Civil ID, Ross SE, Botehlo G, et al. Routine pelvic radiography in severe blunt trauma: Is it necessary? *Ann Emerg Med* 1988;17:488-490.
8. Fischer RP. Cervical radiographic evaluation of alert patients following blunt trauma. *Ann Emerg Med* 1984;13:905-907.
9. Lieberman JF, Maull KI. Occult unstable cervical spine injury. *J Tenn Med Assoc* 1988;81:243-244.
10. Bresler MJ, Rich GH. Occult cervical spine fracture in an ambulatory patient. *Ann Emerg Med* 1982;11:440-442.
11. Roberge RJ, Wears RC. Evaluation of neck discomfort, neck tenderness, and neurologic deficits as indicators for radiography in blunt trauma victims. *J Emerg Med* (in press).
12. Bachulis BL, Long WB, Hynes GD, et al. Clinical indications for cervical spine radiographs in the traumatized patient. *Am J Surg* 1987;153:473-477.
13. Wales LR, Knopp RK, Morishima MS. Recommendations for evaluation of the acutely injured cervical spine: A clinical radiologic algorithm. *Ann Emerg Med* 1980;9:422-428.
14. Neifeld GL, Keene JG, Hevesy G, et al. Cervical injury in head trauma. *J Emerg Med* 1988;6:203-207.
15. Ogden W, Dunn JD. Cervical radiographic evaluation following blunt trauma. *Ann Emerg Med* 1986;15:604-605. Letter.
16. Walter J, Doris PE. Clinical presentation of patients with acute cervical spine injury. *Ann Emerg Med* 1984;13: 512-515.
17. Advanced Trauma Life Support Program for Physicians. Chicago: Committee on Trauma, American College of Surgeons; 1989: 163.
18. Cadoux CG, White JD. High-yield radiographic considerations for cervical spine injuries. *Ann Emerg Med* 1986;15:236-239.
19. Ross SE, O'Malley KF, DeLong WG, et al. Clinical

predictors of cervical spine injuries (CSI) in blunt high-energy transfer injuries (BHETI). *Ann Emerg Med* 1987;16:498-499. Abstract.

20. Jacobs LM, Schwartz R. Prospective analysis of acute cervical spine injury: A methodology to predict injury. *Ann Emerg Med* 1986;15:44-49.
21. McKee TR, Tinkoff G, Rhodes M. Asymptomatic occult cervical spine fracture: Case report and review of the literature. *J Trauma* 1990;30:623-626.
22. Maull KI, Sachatello CR. Avoiding a pitfall in resuscitation: The painless cervical fracture. *South Med J* 1977;70: 477-478.
23. Roberts JR. Trauma of the cervical spine. *Topics Emerg Med* 1979;1:63-77.
24. Thambyrajah K. Fractures of the cervical spine with minimal or no symptoms. *Med J Malaya* 1972;26:244-249.
25. Webb JK. McSweeney T, Park WM. Hidden flexion injury of the cervical spine. *J Bone Joint Surg* 1976;58B:322-327.
26. Gatrell CB. "Asymptomatic" cervical injuries: A myth? *Am J Emerg Med* 1985;3:263-264. Letter.
27. Mouw MW, Wolf CS, Zelenak RR, et al. A prospective study comparing cervical spine radiographic evaluations with clinical presentations. *Ann Emerg Med* 1988;17:879-880. Abstract.
28. Kreipke DL, Gillespie KR, McCarthy MC, et al. Reliability of indications for cervical spine films in trauma patients. *J Trauma* 1989;29a438-1439.
29. Mace SE. Unstable occult cervical-spine fracture. *Ann Emerg Med* 1991;20:1373-1375.
30. Maroon JC. "Burning hands" in football spinal cord injuries. *JAMA* 1977;238:2049-2051.
31. Haines JD. Occult cervical spine fractures: Illustrative cases and x-ray guidelines. *Postgrad Med* 1986;80:73-77.
32. Morse SD. Acute central cervical spinal cord syndromes. *Ann Emerg Med* 1982;11:436-439.
33. Bayless P, Ray VG. Incidence of cervical spine injuries in association with blunt head trauma. *Am J Emerg Med* 1989; 7:139-142.
34. Sumchai AP. Letter to the editor. *J Trauma* 1988;28:1686.
35. Rogers LF. Traumatic lesions of bones and joints. In: Juhl JH, Crummy AB (eds): *Paul and Juhl's Essentials of Radiologic Imaging*. 5th ed. Philadelphia: JB Lippincott; 1987:54.
36. McNamara RM, O'Brien MC, Davidheiser S. Posltraumatic neck pain: A prospective and follow-up study. *Ann Emerg Med* 1988;17:906-9 11.
37. Toth RS. Medical malpractice: Physician as defendant. In: *Legal Medicine: Legal Dynamics of Medical Encounters*. St. Louis: CV Mosby; 1988:488.
38. Vanden Hoek T, Propp D. Cervicothoracic junction injury. *Am J Emerg Med* 1990;8:30-33.

Sports Preparticipation Examinations

Steven Stahle, MD
Susan Stahle, MS, PNP

Sports participation is an exciting means of enhancing self esteem, increasing coordination, and boosting physical fitness. Athletics also can provide a positive experience in competition for young athletes. Amateur athletes in competition sports require a pre-participation physical exam (PPE). The screening exam performed today is much more sophisticated than the "general health" exam offered years ago. The family physicians who frequently work with young athletes should be knowledgeable about today's required elements in the preparticipation exam. This chapter specifically provides the goals and objectives of the PPE, routine testing in conjunction with the screening physical, and means of determining clearance in a private or station-based setting. This chapter does not include the special questioning or testing needed for athletes with disabilities. The ultimate determination in testing and clearance of the young athlete should be guided by each physician's clinical judgment.

Goals and Objectives

The overall goal of the PPE is to help maintain the health and safety of the athlete in training and competition.[1] It provides a practical means for the physician to educate the young athlete on a variety of health topics. Health education is an important aspect of the PPE with young athletes because this may be the only health maintenance exam they seek out all year. Athletes also may use this time to discuss overall health goals as they specifically relate to their own athletic performance. A strengthening or rehabilitation program may then be developed by coaches and trainers. The purpose of the PPE is not to disqualify athletes from competition, but to promote safety, identify ongoing injuries, and prevent future injuries. Only 0.3-1.3% of athletes are denied clearance during the PPE.[2]

The specific objectives of the PPE may vary slightly from physician to physician, but should always include: 1) detection of conditions that limit participation or may predispose to injury; 2) detection of conditions that may be life threatening or disabling; and 3) meeting legal requirements as set forth by the state or sponsoring school or club.[3] Other common objectives include determining the general health of the athlete, evaluating the athlete's fitness level, and optionally assessing the level of maturity.[4,5]

Timing and Setting

Healthcare professionals who wish to perform PPEs must be qualified based on specialty, training, and clinical expertise. Each state certifies healthcare practitioners qualified to perform PPEs at the secondary school level. College, professional, and

Table 1. Station Format and Personnel for Station-Based PPES

Station	Content / Personnel
Station 1	Review of Medical History Form
required	Physician or nurse
Station 2	BP, height, weight
required	Nurse, trainer
Station 3	Vision check
required	Nonspecialized personnel
Station 4	HEENT and skin
required	Physician or nurse
Station 5	Cardiovascular
required	Physician
Station 6	Abdomen, lymph, genitourinary
required	Physician
Station 7	Musculoskeletal and neurological
required	Physician
Station 8	Dental
optional	Dentist
Station 9	Nutrition
optional	Dietitian, nurse
Station 10	Flexibility
optional	Athletic trainer, physical therapist, exercise physiologist
Station 11	Body composition
optional	Athletic trainer, physical therapist, exercise physiologist
Station 12	Strength
optional	Athletic trainer, physical therapist, exercise physiologist
Station 13	Speed, agility, endurance
optional	Athletic trainer, coach, physical therapist, exercise physiologist
Station 14	Review of complete PPE for final determination
required	Physician

international competitors are governed by their own athletic boards as to specifically who may perform their PPE. The primary care physician is a well qualified candidate for performing the PPE due to his or her training in a broad range of problems. The primary care physician is also knowledgeable in consulting with specialty physicians when detected problems require further clinical expertise.

Timing. The PPE should be scheduled six weeks prior to the pre-season.[6] This allows adequate time for correction and rehabilitation of any problems detected. Timing for a collegiate athlete is often based on availability. Some athletes may return to school just days before pre-season begins. Physicians in this case may prefer to perform outgoing physicals at the end of the season with a follow-up review of the medical history just prior to the season. This would allow the physician to detect any conditions and the athlete to rehabilitate any injuries during his or her off season. Many schools will require one PPE for Fall/Winter sports and another for Spring/Summer sports. However, in general, an annual PPE is all that is required in high school athletes. Athletes who are minors are required to provide written permission from their legal guardian for the examination.

Settings. The two most common settings for performing PPEs are in a station-based environment or in the physician's office. Each setting has its own advantages and disadvantages in providing the best overall health screening to the athlete.

Station-Based Setting

Advantages. Station-based evaluations offer the athlete a group of clinical experts that can provide an extremely time-efficient and cost-effective examination Hundreds of PPEs can be performed in one day with a well-trained staff. Effective station-based setups will include the expertise of nurses, physical therapists, exercise physiologists, athletic trainers, and possibly dentists and nutritionists. Other assistants can be guided by physicians to efficiently administer sign in, vision checks, and weights and measurements. An athlete who receives care from a "team" setting may improve his communication with the medical personnel. Additionally, all members of the medical team and coaches will become more knowledgeable regarding each individual athlete.

Disadvantages. The disadvantages of a station-based format can be assessed simply by its requirements—precise training and coordination of staff members and a large physical space to set up the stations.[7] The setting itself can become confusing and noisy.

A lack of privacy may inhibit the athletes from discussing personal health matters. A feeling of being rushed may also decrease the health education and counseling offered by the physician. In addition, if a disqualifying condition is detected, an athlete and his or her parents may not fully understand the need for further evaluation or disqualification from play due to the lack of time and privacy.

Finally, the continuity of care may be compromised with a station-based evaluation.[8,9] Coordinating personnel and schedules can become difficult for the physician who is previously unknown to the athlete.

Station-Based Format

The station-based PPE can be divided into required and optional stations. Personnel best suited for each of the stations should be assigned by the physician. If more then one physician is present, the author suggests dividing the physical exam into two parts, medical and musculoskeletal. Female and male examining sites should be separated into two distinct areas. A suggested format of the stations is given in Table 1.

Office-Based Settings

Advantages. An office-based PPE performed by the athlete's own primary care physician offers the major advantage

Table 2. Components of Preparticipation Physicial Examination

Height

Weight

HEENT: Visual acuity, pupil size, visual correction

Cardiovascular: BP, pulses (radial & femoral), heart (rate, rhythm, murmurs)

Lungs: Breath sounds

Abdomen: Masses, tenderness, organomegaly

Genitourinary: Hernia, testicular mass, single or undescended testicles

Musculoskeletal: Contour, range of motion, stability, symmetry
- Neck
- Shoulder
- Elbow
- Wrist/hand
- Back: Flexion, extension, spondylolysis, spondylolisthesis
- Knee
- Ankle/foot
- Quadriceps/hamstrings

of familiarity. If the physician has treated the athlete throughout childhood, a complete medical history including previous physical examinations and medical records will provide a thorough review in comparison with the PPE screening evaluation form. The previously established working relationship may make it easier for the physician to educate and counsel the athlete on sensitive health issues such as drugs, alcohol, birth control, and sexually transmitted diseases. The continuity of care provided by the athlete's own physician can be crucial in detecting, evaluating, and treating any conditions discovered during the PPE.

Disadvantages. A physician's busy office schedule often only allows for a short general health screen. This is not an adequate amount of time to detect conditions that may predispose the athlete to injury or illness. Furthermore, many primary care physicians lack the interest or knowledge regarding sports-related medical problems. The physician may not be comfortable or qualified in determining clearance for an athlete.

We should not assume all athletes have an established primary care physician. In general, athletes represent a healthy population that may not seek medical attention unless required. Additionally, not all athletes can afford the cost of a private office-based PPE.

Office-Based Format

The office-based PPE follows the same examination procedure as any other primary care examination. The major difference between routine office-based examinations and the PPE is allowance of extra time for the PPE.

Routine Screening Testing

"Though issues surrounding routine laboratory screening tests are frequently discussed and often times controversial, the author societies concur that routine laboratory screening tests in asymptomatic athletes should not be required for the PPE."[10] Screening tests in the young athlete must be cost-effective. Studies thus far in evaluating the use of such tests as UA, CBC, Chemistry Profile, Lipid Profile Sickle Cell trait, and Ferritin Level in the PPE have not revealed any cost-effectiveness.[11-14] Extensive cardiopulmonary testing for routine screening in the PPE is also not recommended.[15-17] According to new AHA standards, a complete and careful personal and family history and physical examination designed to identify or raise the suspicion of cardiovascular lesions is the best available and most practical approach.[18] Symptomatic individuals and those athletes with significant familial medical history should be re-evaluated and scheduled for specific diagnostic tests. Individual symptoms and overall health should indicate to the physician whether or not clearance should be denied during the waiting period. In general, the athlete is allowed to continue participating.

Medical History

The most crucial portion of the PPE is the medical history. A complete history will identify approximately 75% problems affecting athletes.[19] It is important to remember that frequently a medical history completed by the athlete does not reveal the same results as one completed by the athlete's parent/guardian. Ideally, the athlete and parent will complete the form together prior to the exam. A sports screening evaluation form used by the U.S. Center for Sports Medicine for use with PPEs is shown in the supplement.

Questions in the medical history are arranged by their significance and emphasize the areas of greatest concern for sports participation. It is important to remember that these questions are screening questions and not all-inclusive.

Questions 1 and 2 are designed to signal the physician to the most common risks of sudden death (hypertrophic cardiomyopathy, anomylous vessels, arrhythmias, etc.) during exercise for young athletes.

Question 3 will assist the physician in assessing for exercise-induced bronchospasm (EIB), which will affect athletic performance.

Question 4 can also help screen for EIB due to an allergic link. The need for knowledge of specific allergies is obvious.

Question 5 identifies the need for possible neurologic evaluation along with recognizing significant risk for additional concussions.

Question 6 identifies the increased risk of heat injury.

Question 7 screens for previous sports-related injuries and significant joint trauma. This is important because prior injury that has not been rehabilitated is the most common reason athletes are not initially cleared for participation.[20]

Table 3. Medical Conditions and Sports Participation

Note: *This Table is designed to be understood by medical and nonmedical personnel. In the "explanation" section below, "needs evaluation" means that a physician with appropriate knowledge and experience should assess the safety of a given sport for an athlete with the listed medical condition. Unless otherwise noted, this is because of the variability of the severity of the disease or the risk of injury among the specific sports in Table 5.*

Condition	May Participate
Altantoaxial instability (instability of the joint between cervical vertebrae 1 and 2) *Explanation:* Athlete needs evaluation to assess risk of spinal cord injury during sports participation	Qualified Yes
Bleeding disorder *Explanation:* Athlete needs evaluation	Qualified Yes
Cardiovascular diseases	
Carditis (inflammation of the heart) *Explanation:* Carditis may result in sudden death with exertion	No
Hypertension (high blood pressure) *Explanation:* Those with significant essential (unexplained hypertension should avoid weight and power lifting, body building, and strenght training. Those with secondary hypertension (hypertension caused by a previously identified disease), or severe essential hypertension, need evaluation.	Qualified Yes
Congential heart disease (structural heart defects present at birth) *Explanation:* Those with mild forms may participate fully; those with moderate or severe forms, or who have undergone surgery, need evaluation.	Qualified Yes
Dysrhythmia (irregular heart rhythm) *Explanation:* Athlete needs evaluation because some types require therapy or make certain sports dangerous, or both.	Qaulified Yes
Mitral valve prolapse (abnormal heart valve) *Explanation:* Those with symptoms (chest pain, symptoms of possible dysrhythmia) or evidence of mitral regurgitation (leaking) on physical examination need evaluation. All others may participate fully.	Qualified Yes
Heart murmur *Explanation:* If the murmur is innocent (does not indicate heart disease), full participation is permitted. Otherwise the athlete needs evaluation (see congenital heart disease and mitral valve prolapse above).	Qualified Yes
Cerebral palsy *Explanation:* Athlete needs evaluation	Qualified Yes
Diabetes mellitus *Explanation:* All sports can be played with proper attention to diet, hydration, and insulin therapy. Particular attention is needed for activites that last 30 minutes or more	Yes
Diarrhea *Explanation:* Unless disease is mild, no participation is permitted, because diarrhea may increase the risk of dehydration and heat illness. See Fever.	Qualified No
Eating disorders **Anorexia nervosa** **Bulemia nervosa** *Explanation* These patients need both medical and psychiatric aassessment before participation.	Qualified Yes
Eyes **Functionally one-eyed athlete** **Detached retina** **Previous eye surgery or serious eye injury** *Explanation:* A functionally one-eyed athlete has a best corrected visual acuity of < 20/40 in the worst eye. These athletes would suffer significant disability if the better eye was seriously injured as would those with loss of an eye. Some athletes who have previously undergone eye surgery or had a seriuos eye injury may have an increased risk of injury because of weakened eye tissue. Availability of eye guards approved by the American Society for Testing Materials (ASTM) and other protective equipment may allow participation in most sports, but this must be judged on an individual basis.	Qualified Yes
Fever *Explanation:* Fever can increase cardiopulmonary effort, reduce maximum exercise capacity, make heat illness more likely, and increase orthostatic hypotension during exercise. Fever may rarely accompany myocarditis or other infections that may make exercise dangerous.	No
Heat illness, history of *Explanation:* Because of the increased likelihood of recurrence, the athlete needs individual assessment to determine the presence of predisposing conditions and to arrange a prevention strategy.	Qualified Yes
HIV infection *Explanation:* Because of the apparent minimal risk to others, all sports may be played that the state of health allows. In all athletes, skin lesions should be properly covered, and athletic personnel should use universal precautions when handling blood or body fluids with visible blood.	Yes

Table 3. Medical Conditions and Sports Participation *(continued)*

Condition	May Participate
Kidney, absence of one *Explanation:* Athlete needs individual assessment for contact/collision and limited contact sport.	Qualified Yes
Liver enlarged *Explanation:* If the liver is actually enlarged, participation should be avoided because of risk of rupture. If the liver is chronically enlarged, individual assessment is needed before collision/contact or limited contact sports are played	Qualified Yes
Malignancy *Explanation:* Athlete needs individual assessment.	Qualified Yes
Musculoskeletal disorders *Explanation:* Athlete needs individual assessment.	Qualifed Yes
Neurologic	
History of serious head or spin trauma, severe or repeated concussions, or craniotomy *Explanation:* Athlete needs individual assessment for collision/contact or limited contact sports, and also for noncontact sports if there are deficits in judgment or congnition. Recent research supports a conservative approach to management of concussion	Qualified Yes
Convulsive disorder, well controlled *Explanation:* Risk of convulsion during participation is minimal	Yes
Convulsive disorder, poorly controlled *Explanation:* Athlete needs individual assessment for collision/contact or limited contact sports. Avoid the following noncontract sports: archery, riflery, swimming, weight or power lifting, strength training, or sports involving heights. In these sports, occurence of a convulsion may be a risk to self or others.	Qualified Yes
Obesity *Explanation:* Because of the risk of heat illness, obese persons need careful acclimatization and hydration.	Qualified Yes
Organ transplant recipient *Explanation:* Athlete needs individual assessment.	Qualified Yes
Ovary, absence of one *Explanation:* Risk of severe injury to the remaining ovary is minimal.	Yes
Respiratory	
Pulmonary compromise including cystic fibrosis *Explanation:* Athlete needs individual assessment, but generally all sports may be played if oxygenation remains satisfactory during a graded exercise test. Patients with cystic fibrosis need accliminatization and good hydration to reduce the risk of heat illness.	Qualified Yes
Asthma *Explanation:* With proper medication and education, only athletes with the most severe asthma will have to modify their participation.	Yes
Aucte upper respiratory infection *Explanation:* Upper respiratory obstruction may affect pulmonary function. Athlete needs individual assessment for all but mild disease. See Fever.	Qualifed Yes
Sickle Cell Disease *Explanation:* Athlete needs individual assessment. In general, if status of the illness permits, all but high exertion, collision/contact sports may be played. Overheating, dehydration, and chilling must be avoided.	Qualified Yes
Sickle Cell Trait *Explanation:* It is unlikely that individuals with sickle cell trait (AS) have an increased risk of sudden death or other medical problems during athletic participation except under the most extreme conditions of heat, humidity, and possibly increased altitude. These individuals, like all athletes, should be carefully conditioned, acclimatized, and hydrated to reduce any possible risk.	Yes
Skin: boils, herpes simplex, impetigo, scabies, molluscum contagiosum *Explanation:* While the patient is contagious, participation in gymnastics with mats, martial arts, wrestling, or other collision/contact or limited contact sports is not allowed. Herpes simplex virus probably is not transmitted via mats.	Qualified Yes
Spleen, enlarged *Explanation:* Patients with acutely enlarged spleens should avoid all sports because of risk of rupture. Those with chronically enlarged spleens need individual assessment before playing collision/contact or limited contact sports.	Qualified Yes
Testicle, absent or undescended *Explanation:* Certain sports may require a protective cup.	Yes

Used with permission from: American Academy of Pediatrics. Medical Conditions and Sports. *Pediatrics* 1994;94:492-493.

Question 8 assesses for acute illness such as mononucleosis, hepatitis A, and febrile illnesses, which may temporarily restrict the athlete's ability to participate.

Question 9 and Question 10 are self-explanatory.

Question 11 reveals female maturation and identifies amenorrhea (which may be linked to stress fractures) and oligomenorrhea.

Question 12 is an effective screening question to help recognize eating disorders.

Question 13 is self-explanatory and is not necessarily a reason for disqualification.

Question 14 is an opportunity for education.

Question 15 is a variety of conditions that may or may not restrict an athlete's participation in play.

Item 16 provides an opportunity for the athlete to discuss sensitive issues with a qualified professional.

Physical Examination

The standard components of the preparticipation physical examination are shown in Table 2. This screening tool should be used to focus specifically on areas of concern in the particular athletic activity and areas identified as problems in the history. Males and females should be dressed in shorts, tank tops and athletic shoes.

Height and Weight. Height and weight should be recorded and reviewed yearly. Athletes who are extremely thin or obese should be questioned regarding sudden weight change, eating habits, and body image. Body composition determination is an optional station.

HEENT. Visual acuity should be 20/40 or better in each eye. Protective eyewear should be recommended for use with corrective eyewear, history of serious trauma, or absence of an eye. Protective eyewear should always be checked prior to play. Pupils should be checked for anisocoria. If found, this baseline information should be clearly recorded in the medical record and communicated to members of the athlete's medical team. This is a significant point of reference in assessing for head trauma. The general health of the remaining components of this exam should be assessed. Assessment of the ears should specifically check for scarring of the auditory canal, which may indicate the need for a hearing evaluation, and perforated tympanic membranes in athletes competing in water sports, which indicate the need for earplugs.[21] The oral cavity should be checked for ulcers and decreased enamel seen with bulimia; braces, which may indicate the need for a mouthguard; and a high-arched palate seen in those with Marfans.[22] Nasal polyps, deviated septum, and repeated trauma to the nose should be assessed for referral. Finally, any adenopathy should be assessed for infection or malignancy.

Cardiovascular. The American Heart Association (AHA) recently issued a new medical/scientific statement from the Sudden Death Committee and the Congenital Cardiac Defects Committee in which they believe that the standard preparticipation screening process for athletes appeared to be limited in their ability to identify cardiovascular lesions responsible for sudden death in young athletes.[23] As a consequence of this belief, the AHA statement recommends the development of a national standard for PPEs and strongly recommends that athletic screening be performed by health care workers who possess the requisite training, skill, and background to reliably obtain a detailed cardiovascular history, perform a related physical examination, and recognize heart disease.[24] The specific recommendation for a brachial artery blood pressure measurement was included in the statement. The new AHA statement should be reviewed for further recommendations by all sports medicine providers to insure their professional liability. Blood pressure that is initially high should be repeated a few minutes after the initial check. If the condition continues, the athlete should be questioned about stimulants such as caffeine, ephedrine, or nicotine.[25] A radial and femoral pulse should be palpated for rate and rhythm. Auscultation of the heart should be performed with the athlete in supine and standing positions.[26] A murmur of hypertrophic cardiomyopathy is best heard when the athlete is standing. Murmurs and the timing of murmurs should be assessed. Any detected murmur should be further clarified by instructing the athlete to perform deep

Table 4. Classification of Sports by Strenuousness

High-to-moderate dynamic and static demands	High-to-moderate dynamic and low static demands	High-to-moderate static and low dynamic demands
Boxing	Badminton	Archery
Crew/rowing	Baseball	Auto racing
Cross country skiing	Basketball	Diving
Cycling	Field hockey	Equestrian
Downhill skiing	Lacrosse	Field events (jumping)
Fencing	Orienteering	Field events (throwing)
Football	Ping-pong	Gymnastics
Ice hockey	Race walking	Karate or judo
Rugby	Racquetball	Motorcycling
Running (sprint)	Soccer	Rodeoing
Speed skating	Squash	Sailing
Water polo	Swimming	Ski jumping
Wrestling	Tennis	Water skiing
	Volleyball	Weight lifting
Low intensity (low dynamic and low static demands)		
	Bowling	
	Cricket	
	Curling	
	Golf	
	Riflery	

* Participation not recommended

Used with permission from: American Academy of Pediatrics. Medical Conditions and Sports. *Pediatrics* 1994;94:492-493.

Table 5. Classification of Sports by Contact

Contact/collision	Limited contact	Noncontact
Basketball	Baseball	Archery
Boxing*	Bicycle	Badminton
Diving	Cheerleading	Body building
Field hockey	Canoeing/kayaking (white water)	Bowling
Football (tackle, flag)	Fencing	Canoeing/kayaking (flat water)
Ice hockey	Field (high jump, pole vault)	Crew/rowing
Lacrosse	Floor hockey	Curling
Martial arts	Gymnastics	Dancing
Rodeo	Handball	Field (discus, javelin, shot put)
Rugby	Horseback riding	Golf
Ski jumping	Racquetball	Orienteering
Soccer	Skating (ice, inline, roller)	Power lifting
Team handball	Skiing (cross country, downhill, water)	Race walking
Water polo	Softball	Riflery
Wrestling	Squash	Rope jumping
	Ultimate frisbee	Sailing
	Volleyball	Scuba diving
	Windsurfing/surfing	Strength training
		Swimming
		Table tennis
		Tennis
		Track
		Weight lifting

* Participation not recommended

Used with permission from: American Academy of Pediatrics. Medical Conditions and Sports. *Pediatrics* 1994;94:492-493.

inspiration, squat-to-stand, and Valsalva's maneuver. In detecting aortic stenosis, the systolic murmur will decrease with Valsalva and increase with squatting. Conversely, with hypertrophic cardiomyopathy, squatting will decrease the intensity of the murmur, and Valsalva's will increase the intensity. Benign systolic murmurs are common in young athletes. Innocent murmurs will also increase with squatting and decrease with Valsalva but can be differentiated from aortic stenosis by volume, location, radiation, and duration.[27] Arrhythmias may require electrocardiographic evaluation. Any further cardiac evaluation should be referred to a cardiologist.

Lungs. Clear breath sounds should be revealed during the pulmonary exam.

Abdomen. The athlete should be supine during the assessment for masses, tenderness, and hepatosplenomegaly.

GU. The male should be assessed for singular or undescended testicles, testicular masses, and herniation. The female's GU exam should be deferred to a private primary care physician.

Musculoskeletal. The musculoskeletal system can be assessed by three different types of screening exams. The type and extent of musculoskeletal examination appropriate for the PPE is a widely debated topic. Asymptomatic athletes with no history of injury rarely reveal a musculoskeletal injury. In fact, history alone has been shown to be 92% sensitive in detection of significant musculoskeletal injuries.[28] This author supports the notion that a general screening examination is appropriate for asymptomatic athletes with no history of injury. If an athlete is currently symptomatic of an injury, or has a history of previous injury, weakness, or instability, the physician should perform a relevant joint-specific examination. If time is allowed, a joint-specific exam should be performed instead of a general screening; a sport-specific exam may be performed if time does not allow for a joint-specific exam.

General Screening Examination. A general screen will quickly assess range of motion, gross muscle strength, and muscle asymmetry along with identifying significant injuries.[29] The general screen will not allow for specific diagnosis or severity of injury.

Joint-Specific Testing. Joint-specific testing assesses individual joints by inspection, palpation, and maneuvers. It is much more thorough than the general screen but also significantly more time-consuming. A description of each joint-specific test is beyond the scope of this article but can be found in it's entirety in *Physical Examination of the Spine and Extremities*.[30]

Sports-Specific Testing. Sports-specific examinations include endurance, strength, and flexibility testing in addition to an orthopedic examination. The focus is indicated by the particular sport and the area of greatest stress. For instance, runners would be assessed for knee and ankle stability, strength, and flexibility by use of specific orthopedic maneuvers. The sports-specific exam is time-consuming and requires greater knowledge of particular sports than does the joint-specific testing. The author generally saves sports-specific examinations for highly competitive and professional athletes.

Neurologic. In general, a normal musculoskeletal examination denotes normal neurologic function. However, for athletes who have suffered severe or multiple concussions, an exam of cranial nerves along with cerebellar and cognitive function tests may be indicated. An athlete who has experienced recurrent nerve root or brachial plexus injuries ("stingers") should be assessed for deep tendon reflexes and upper extremity strength. Referral may be appropriate for any impairments noted.

Clearance

The culmination of the detailed medical history and lengthy physical examination in the PPE is the determination of clearance. Clearance can be divided into three categories: 1) unrestricted clearance for contact, limited contact, or noncontact play; 2) clearance upon further evaluation or rehabilitation; and 3) clearance deferred for a specific or all sports. If a condition is detected, the following questions should guide the physician to determining clearance for an athlete.[31]

1. Does the problem place the athlete at increased risk of injury?

2. Does the problem place any other participant at increased risk of injury?

3. Can the athlete safely participate with treatment?

4. Can limited participation be allowed while treatment is initiated?

5. If clearance is denied for specific sports, can other athletic activities be substituted?

Medical conditions affecting sports participation should be reviewed for clearance based on guidelines established by the 1994 American Academy of Pediatrics Committee on Sports Medicine and Fitness. *(Please see Table 3.)*[32] Cardiovascular abnormalities and congenital heart disease are thoroughly covered in the guidelines from the "26th Bethesda Conference: Recommendations for Determining Eligibility for Competition Athletes with Cardiovascular Abnormalities."[33] Furthermore, a review of the classification of sports by dynamic and static strenuousness should also assist in determining clearance for athletes with cardiovascular conditions. *(Please see Table 4.)* In consideration of potential for injury due to contact or collision, the physician should review the contact categories established by the AAP. *(Please see Table 5.)*[34] These published guidelines and recommendations in conjunction with the judgment of the physician provide an accurate means of determining clearance.

Medicolegal Considerations

Two very important medicolegal issues related to the PPE have been debated and should be reviewed. The primary legal issue is the athlete's right to participate. The right to make a final decision on whether to engage in athletics has been repeatedly recognized by the courts as resting with the athlete or with his or her parents.[35,36] A physician who is disqualifying an athlete from play should consult with expert physicians. Both the examining and the consulting physician should clearly review all reasons why the athlete should not participate with the athlete and his or her parents. Should the athlete choose to participate against medical advice, an exculpatory waiver stating the physician(s) has clearly informed the family of all risks accompanying the participation of play should be signed. An exculpatory waiver is a written form stating that the family recognizes and assumes the risk of injury and releases the physician(s) and the school from liability. The validity of these waivers is not nationally recognized, and legal counsel is recommended for the physician on an individual case basis.[37]

The other major legal issue is professional liability for physicians performing PPEs as volunteers. Until recently, Good Samaritan laws did not cover preparticipation evaluations even if performed without charge. Some states have now instituted protection for examiners for athletic programs under Good Samaritan statutes. The physician should become familiar with his or her own state's statutes. Physicians providing preparticipation evaluations should be familiar with standards set forth by significant medical committees such as those discussed throughout this article. After all, none of us can be protected from our own lack of knowledge.

Conclusion

The preparticipation physical examination can be successfully used to help our young athletes remain healthy and safe in sports. By encouraging young athletes to remain in athletics we may stimulate a personal commitment to physical fitness. Through continued contact with the athlete, we can also provide health education and physical care that may promote a healthy lifestyle for years to come

References

1. American Academy of Family Physicians (AAFP), American Academy of Pediatrics (AAP), American Medical Society for Sports Medicine (AMSSM), American Orthopaedic Medicine (AOASM). Preparticipation Physical Evaluation, 2nd ed. Minneapolis, MN: Phys Sportsmed; 1997:1-2.
2. Sallis R. The Preparticipation Examination. In: Sallis R, Massimino F. (eds): *ACSM's Essentials of Sports Medicine,* 1st ed. St. Louis: Mosby; 1997:151-160.
3. American Academy of Family Physicians (AAFP), American Academy of Pediatrics (AAP), American Medical Society for Sports Medicine (AMSSM), American Orthopaedic Society for Sports Medicine (AOSSM), and American Osteopathic Academy of Sports dicine (AOASM). Preparticipation Physical Evaluation, 2nd ed. Minneapolis, MN: Phys Sportsmed; 1997:1.
4. Snoddy RO. The Preparticipation Screening Examination. In: Baker CL (ed.): *The Hughston Clinic Sports Medicine Book,* 1st ed, Media: Williams & Wilkins; 1995:31-34.
5. ombardo J. Preparticipation Examination. In: Cantu R, Micheli L. (eds): *ACSM's Guidelines for the Team Physician,* 1st ed, Malvern, Lea & Febiger; 1991:71-94.
6. Ibid.
7. Snoddy RO. The Preparticipation Screening Examination. In: Baker CL. (ed): *The Hughston Clinic Sports Medicine Book,* 1st ed, Media: Williams & Wilkins; 1995:31-34.
8. American Academy of Family Physicians (AAFP), American Academy of Pediatrics (AAP), American Medical Society for Sports Medicine (AMSSM), American Orthopaedic Society for Sports Medicine (AOSSM), and American Osteopathic Academy of Sports Medicine (AOASM). Preparticipation Physical Evaluation, 2nd ed. Minneapolis: Physd Sportsmed; 1997:5.
9. Sallis R. The Preparticipation Examination. In: Sallis R, Massimino F. (eds): *ACSM's Essentials of Sports Medicine,* 1st ed. St. Louis: Mosby; 1997:151-160.
10. American Academy of Family Physicians (AAFP), American Academy of Pediatrics (AAP), American Medical Society for Sports Medicine (AMSSM), American Orthopaedic Society for Sports Medicine (AOSSM), and American Osteopathic Academy of Sports Medicine (AOASM). Preparticipation Physical Evaluation, 2nd ed. Minneapolis: Phys Sportsmed; 1997:7.
11. Lombardo JA, Robinson JB, Smith DM, et al: Preparticipation Physical Evaluation, ed.1. Kansas City, American Academy of Family Practice, American Academy of Pediatrics, American Medical Society for Sports Medicine, American Orthopaedic Association for Sports Medicine,and American Osteopathic Association for Sports Medicine; 1992.

12. Committee on Sports Medicine. Sports Medicine: Health Care for Young Athletes. Evanston, IL, American Academy of Pediatrics; 1983.
13. American Academy of Family Physicians (AAFP), American Academy of Pediatrics (AAP), American Medical Society for Sports Medicine (AMSSM), American Orthopaedic Society for Sports Medicine (AOSSM), and American Osteopathic Academy of Sports Medicine (AOASM). Preparticipation Physical Evaluation, 2nd ed. Minneapolis: Phys Sportsmed; 1997:7
14. Taylor WC III, Lombardo JA. Preparticipation screening of college athletes: Value of the complete blood cell count. *Phys Sportsmed* 1990;18:106-118.
15. Maron BJ, Isner JM, McKenna WJ: Task Force 3: Hypertrophic cardiomyopathy, myocarditis and other myopericardial diseases and mitral valve prolapse, in 26th Bethesda Conference: Recommendations for Determining Eligibility for Competition in Athletes with Cardiovascular Abnormalities. *Med Sci Sports Exerc* 1994;26 (10 suppl):S261-S267.
16. Ades PA. Preventing sudden death: Cardiovascular screening of young athletes. *Phys Sportsmed* 1992;20:75-89.
17. Feinstein RA, Colvin E, Oh MK. Echocardiographic screening as part of a preparticipation examination. *Clin J Sports Med* 1993;3: 149-152.
18. Herbert D. Pre-Participation screening: Competitive athletes and sudden death. *Sports Med Pri Care* 1996;2:90.
19. Johnson RJ. The sports qualifying screening evaluation.
20. Ibid.
21. American Academy of Family Physicians, American Academy of Pediatrics, American Medical Society for Sports Medicine, American Orthopaedic Society for Sports Medicine, and American Osteopathic Academy of Sports Medicine. Preparticipation Physical Evaluation, 2nd ed. Minneapolis: Phys Sportsmed; 1997:18.
22. Ibid.
23. Herbert D. Pre-participation screening: Competitive athletes and sudden death. *Sports Med in Pri Care* 1996;2:90.
24. Ibid
25. American Academy of Family Physicians, American Academy of Pediatrics, American Medical Society for Sports Medicine, American Orthopaedic Society for Sports Medicine, and American Osteopathic Academy of Sports Medicine. Preparticipation Physical Evaluation, 2nd ed. Minneapolis: Phys Sportsmed; 1997:18.
26. American Heart Association. Cardiovascular preparticipation screening of competititve athletes. Circulation 1996;94:850-856.
27. American Academy of Family Physicians, American Academy of Pediatrics, American Medical Society for Sports Medicine, American Orthopaedic Society for Sports Medicine, and American Osteopathic Academy of Sports Medicine. Preparticipation Physical Evaluation, 2nd ed. Minneapolis: Phys Sportsmed; 1997:19.
28. Gomez JE, Landry GL, Bernhardt DT. Critical evaluation of the 2-minute orthopedic screening examintion. *Am J Dis Child* 1993;147: 1109-1113.
29. Ibid
30. Hoppenfeld S. *Physical Examination of the Spine and Extremities.* Appleton-Centruty-Crofts; 1976.
31. American Academy of Family Physicians (AAFP), American Academy of Pediatrics (AAP), American Medical Society for Sports Medicine (AMSSM), American Orthopaedic Society for Sports Medicine (AOSSM), and American Osteopathic Academy of Sports Medicine (AOASM). Preparticipation Physical Evaluation, 2nd ed. Minneapolis: Phys Sportsmed; 1997;29.
32. Lombardo JE. Preparticipation Examination. In: Cantu R, Micheli L (eds). *ACSM's Guidelines for the Team Physician,* 1st ed. Malvern, Lea & Febiger; 1991:71-94.
33. 26th Bethesda Conference: Recommendations for determining eligibility for competition in athletes with cardiovascular abnormalitites. January 6-7, 1994. *Med Sci Sports Exerc* 1994;26 (10 Suppl):S223-S283 [published erratum appears in *Med Sci Sports Exerc* 1994;26(12): following table of contents]; also in *J Am Coll Cardiol* 1994;24:845-899.
34. American Academy of Family Physicians, American Academy of Pediatrics, American Medical Society for Sports Medicine, American Orthopaedic Society for Sports Medicine, and American Osteopathic Academy of Sports Medicine. Preparticipation Physical Evaluation, 2nd ed. Minneapolis: Phys Sportsmed; 1997:32-33.
35. Gallup EM. Law and the Team Physician. Champaign, IL: Human Kinetic Books; 1995:80-81.
36. Feinstein RA, Soileau EJ, Daniel WA, Jr. A national survey of preparticipation physical examination requirements. *Phys Sportsmed* 1988;16:51.
37. Gallup EM. Law and the Team Physician. Champaign, IL: Human Kinetic Books; 1995:76-77.

Anemia

David R. Little, MD, MS

Anemia is a clinical syndrome that presents many diagnostic and therapeutic challenges to the primary care physician. This chapter presents a series of algorithms that will enable the clinician to develop a focused approach to the diagnosis and avoid excessive laboratory testing.

Microcytic anemia commonly results from iron deficiency, chronic disease, lead toxicity, or disorders of hemoglobin synthesis. These conditions can usually be distinguished on the basis of serum iron, ferritin, and lead levels, along with an occasional hemoglobin electrophoresis.

The differential diagnosis for normocytic anemia includes acute blood loss, chronic disease, bone marrow failure, hypersplenism, and hemolytic anemia. The reticulocyte index provides key information about adequacy of bone marrow response to anemia, while the peripheral smear and the indirect Coombs' test are helpful in identifying hemolysis. Evidence of bone marrow failure will necessitate a marrow aspiration and biopsy.

Most cases of macrocytic anemia result from deficiency of vitamin B_{12}, folic acid, or both. Serum assays for these nutrients, along with the peripheral smear and the reticulocyte count, will clarify the diagnosis in most cases. The role of drugs and toxins in producing anemia is also essential to consider. Drugs may be responsible for a variety of types of anemia through various mechanisms, which are reviewed in this issue.

Once the precise etiologic diagnosis of anemia is confirmed, underlying causes must be determined. Anemia is often a sign of significant underlying illness. This chapter reviews the common causes of anemia, practical treatment approaches, and clinical implications associated with each condition.

Introduction

Anemia is a common clinical syndrome that primary care physicians are often called upon to diagnose and manage. The prevalence of anemia in the U.S. has been reported at 29-30 cases per 1000 in the female population across all age groups. In males, the prevalence is 6.0 cases per 1000 under age 45 and rises to a peak of 18.5 cases per 1000 men over age 75.[1] A targeted approach to the laboratory evaluation of the anemic patient will assist the clinician in achieving an efficient, cost-effective diagnosis. Accurate diagnosis for the underlying cause of anemia is critical, because it may be an indicator of significant underlying illness.

Anemia is defined as a reduction of the total red blood cell volume (hematocrit) or the concentration of blood hemoglobin.[2] The normal values for hematocrit and hemoglobin vary with age and gender. *(Please see Table 1.)* Results must also be interpreted in the context of coexisting medical

Table 1. Normal Hematologic Values

Age	Hemoglobin (g/dL)	Hematocrit (%)	MCV (fL)
1-3 days	14.5-22.5	45-67	95-121
6 months-2 years	10.5-13.5	33-39	70-86
12-18 years			
Male	13.0-16.0	37-49	78-98
Female	12.0-16.0	36-46	78-102
Adult			
Male	13.5-17.5	41-53	78-98
Female	12.0-16.0	36-46	78-98

Adapted from Reference 2.

conditions. For example, patients with severe pulmonary disease would be expected to have an elevated hematocrit. Normal values in this context may actually represent a reduction of the total RBC volume.

Clinical Features

The clinical presentation of anemia is widely variable. In some cases, it may present with non-specific signs and symptoms such as fatigue, shortness of breath, pallor, and tachycardia. The presence of conjunctival pallor was recently demonstrated to correlate well with severe anemia.[3] Many cases of anemia are discovered incidentally, or as a manifestation of another known disease process.

The medical history should focus on clues to the etiology of the anemia. Important questions include chronic blood loss from stool, urine, epistaxis, menstruation, or other foci. A history of exposure to drugs and toxins, including alcohol, is essential. A thorough family history will point to hereditary causes, and a complete review of systems may reveal other evidence of hepatic, renal, thyroid, or rheumatologic disease.

Physical examination should be directed toward clues to underlying illnesses. Specific evidence of rheumatologic disease, liver disease, endocrine disease, and malignancy should be sought. The presence of lymphadenopathy or splenomegaly is an important finding that may correlate with infection, leukemia, or lymphoma. Digital rectal exam is essential to detect mass lesions of the colon or prostate and to test for occult fecal blood loss. Suspected fecal blood loss may require multiple stool guaiac tests to detect.[4]

Laboratory Testing. The complete blood count (CBC) is the most commonly used laboratory test in evaluating anemia. The CBC will contain quantitative information about the contents of the blood (hemoglobin, hematocrit, and red blood cell count) and measures of the size and hemoglobin concentration of the red blood cells.[5] The measurements of red cell size and hemoglobin content are very useful in classifying cases of anemia and determining their potential causes. The white blood cell and platelet counts included in the CBC may also have implcations in the evaluation of certain causes of anemia.

The CBC will also contain the red cell distribution width (RDW), an index of the variability of red cell size. Larger values of the RDW indicate a more heterogenous red cell population. The RDW is an early indicator of some forms of anemia, particularly early iron deficiency.[6] In combination with the mean cell volume, the RDW can be used to classify causes of anemia.[7]

The peripheral blood smear may reveal characteristic abnormalities of RBC morphology that can be diagnostic of certain conditions, such as sickle cell disease, spherocytosis, and mechanical hemolytic anemias. Examples of other important diagnostic information available on the peripheral smear will be discussed throughout this chapter.

A wide variety of additional laboratory studies are available to assist the clinician in confirming the etiology of anemia. Selective use of these tests, as

Figure 1. Evaluation of Microcytic Anemia

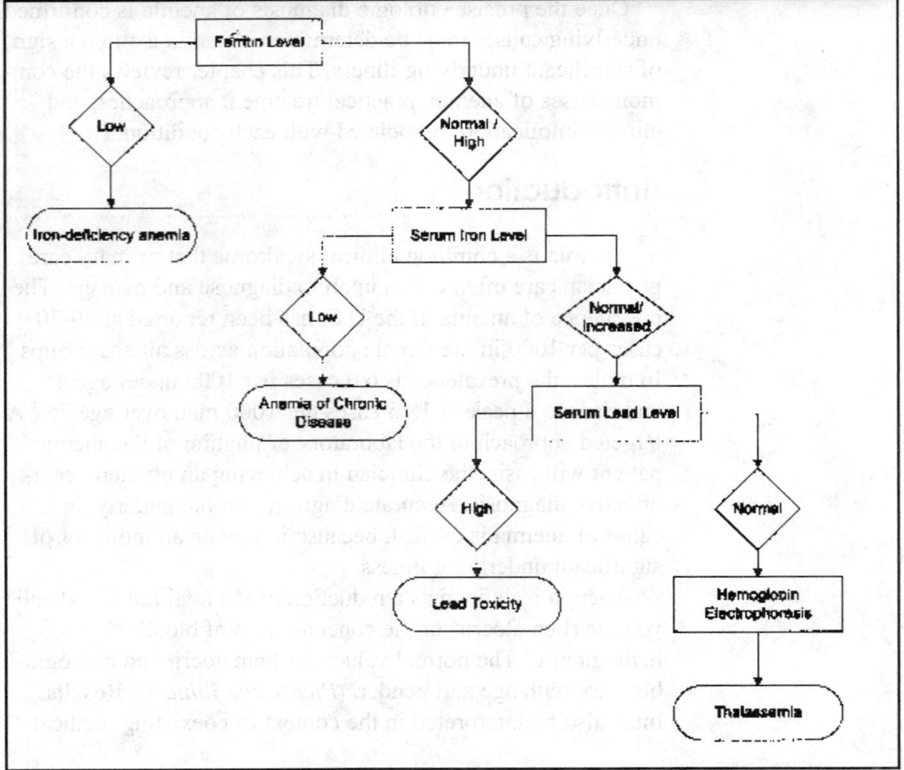

Ferritin Level
Low
Normal / High
Iron-deficiency anemia
Serum Iron Level
Low
Normal/ Increased
Anemia of Chronic Disease
Serum Lead Level
High
Normal
Lead Toxicity
Hemoglobin Electrophoresis
Thalassemia

described by the algorithms presented here, will aid in the diagnosis without resorting to a more costly, "shotgun" approach to laboratory testing.

Classification of Anemias. It is useful to classify anemias on the basis of the mean corpuscular volume (MCV). The normal range for MCV in adults is approximately 80-100 femtoliters (fL). Values of MCV within this range are termed normocytic. Values below 80 fL and above 100 fL are termed microcytic and macrocytic, respectively. RBCs are also classified according to hemoglobin content. Normochromic cells have a mean corpuscular hemoglobin concentration (MCHC) of 32-36 g/dL. Cells with an MCHC below 32 are termed hypochromic. Values above the normal range are seen only rarely, predominantly in spherocytic disorders.[2]

Microcytic Anemias

Iron-deficiency Anemia. A low ferritin level (< 30 ng/mL) confirms the diagnosis of iron deficiency.8 *(Please see Figure 1.)* Iron deficiency is the most common cause of anemia throughout the world.[2] When iron deficiency is discovered, the underlying cause must be sought. In children, this deficiency is typically dietary.[9] In adults, iron deficiency should be considered to represent chronic blood loss until proven otherwise. A list of potential causes of iron-deficiency anemia is presented in Table 2.

Table 2. Causes of Iron-Deficiency Anemia

Increased Requirements
Pregnancy
Growth spurts
Decreased Intake
Prematurity
Infancy
Early childhood
Decreased Absorption
Gastric surgery
Pernicious anemia with achlorhydria
Celiac or tropical sprue
Increased Blood Loss
NSAID therapy
Inflammatory bowel disease
Peptic ulcer disease
Gastroesophageal reflux disease
Intestinal parasites
Malignancy, especially gastrointestinal
Menstruation
Post-partum blood loss

Management. Once the underlying cause has been addressed, many cases of iron deficiency can be treated successfully with oral iron supplementation. A variety of oral iron preparations are available at relatively low cost. Sulfate, fumarate, and gluconate salts are most commonly used; none offers a distinct advantage in bioavailability.[10] Enteric-coated preparations are ineffective since the stomach is the optimum site of absorption. Optimum delivery of oral iron requires the capsule to dissolve rapidly in the stomach, so that the iron may be absorbed in the duodenum and upper jejunum. Enteric-coated tablets dissolve poorly and are ineffective for iron replacement.

Oral iron supplementation is best administered as a daily dose of ferrous sulfate, the least expensive preparation. A course of 150-200 mg elemental iron daily should be given for 4-6 months or until the target hemoglobin level has been achieved. Replacement therapy is usually continued for another 4-6 months or until the serum ferritin level reaches 50 ng/mL, reflecting adequate body iron stores.[11] Absorption of oral iron may be limited by antacids, H2 blockers, or proton pump inhibitors due to the reduced stomach acid content associated with these agents. Caffeine intake, particularly in the form of tea, also will reduce absorption.[10,12]

Failure of the patient to respond to oral iron supplementation may indicate an inability to absorb iron. This may be confirmed by measuring the serum iron level at two and four hours after an oral dose of 325 mg ferrous sulfate. Failure of the iron level to increase by 115 mcg/dL over pretreatment values indicates iron malabsorption.[10]

In the event of an inadequate response to oral iron supplementation, parenteral treatment with iron dextran should be considered. Specific indications for parenteral iron include: 1) inability to tolerate oral iron; 2) non-compliance with medication; 3) iron malabsorption after acid reduction surgery; or 4) continued blood loss.[13] Due to the unpredictable absorption and local complications of intramuscular administration, the intravenous route is preferred for parenteral iron treatment.

Parenteral iron dextran may be administered as a single dose. The total dose required to replenish body stores is based upon body weight and hemoglobin deficit. The dosage may be determined from standard nomograms accompanying the product.

The primary concern with intravenous iron dextran is the occurrence of adverse reactions. Immediate reactions may include headache; dyspnea; flushing; chest, abdominal, or back pain; nausea and vomiting; fever; hypotension; seizures; urticaria; and anaphylaxis. A small test dose should be given to observe the patient for an anaphylactic reaction.[14] If the test dose is tolerated, the full dose infusion may be given at a rate of 50 mg/min, up to a total daily dose of 100 mg.

Anemia of Chronic Disease. Anemia of chronic disease (ACD) is defined as "the anemia that accompanies chronic inflammatory, infectious, or neoplastic disorders."[15] Examples of conditions that may be associated with ACD are listed in Table 3. ACD is a common condition, second in incidence only to iron-deficiency anemia. It occurs as the result of decreased production of red cells in the context of an underlying illness. Although ACD is traditionally categorized as normochromic and normocytic, it can be microcytic in 30-50% of cases.

Some authors have subdivided ACD into separate categories according to differing pathophysiology. The anemia of chronic renal failure results from an absolute deficiency of erythropoi-

Table 3. Conditions Associated with Anemia of Chronic Disease

Malignancy
- Solid tumors
- Acute or chronic leukemia
- Hodgkin's or non-Hodgkin's lymphoma
- Multiple myeloma

Chronic Organ Failure
- Chronic renal failure
- Liver failure
- Hypothyroidism
- Hypoadrenalism
- Hypopituitarism
- Hypogonadism

Chronic Infections

Collagen Vascular Disease

etin. Anemias caused by endocrine dysfunction are often multifactorial, featuring a relative deficiency of erythropoietin. Anemia caused by malignancy, infections, and other inflammatory processes is the result of a "pseudo" iron deficiency. In these situations, iron is trapped within macrophages and becomes unavailable for erythropoiesis.

When ACD is microcytic, it is characterized by a relatively mild decrease in MCV, usually not less than 70 fL. This is accompanied by a normal or mildly elevated ferritin, low serum iron, low total iron-binding capacity, and low transferrin saturation. Differentiating ACD from iron-deficiency anemia may require additional testing. An elevated sedimentation rate is seen in ACD.[16] The serum transferrin receptor level is normal in ACD but markedly elevated in iron deficiency.[16,17] In some patients, iron-deficiency anemia may coexist with ACD. In this situation, a favorable response to iron supplementation will occur in the context of another chronic illness. Patients receiving dialysis may experience a microcytic anemia as the result of aluminum intoxication.

Management. The first objective in the management of ACD is to identify and treat the underlying cause. In many instances, no specific therapy will be necessary for the anemia. Transfusion therapy is the traditional standard for severe cases, but it is associated with significant costs and potential risks. A newer alternative to transfusion for patients with ACD is recombinant human erythropoietin (rhEPO).

Erythropoietin has been proven to be effective in correcting the anemia associated with many chronic conditions, including chronic renal failure,[18] rheumatoid arthritis,[19] cancer (with or without chemotherapy),[20] and AIDS.[21] The results of therapy include an improved hematocrit, less need for transfusions, and improvement in overall functional status.[15]

The preferred route of administration for rhEPO is subcutaneous. A dose of 25-250 U/kg is given three times weekly for 8-12 weeks. Treatment will result in an improvement of hemoglobin of 2 g/dL or more in greater than 50% of patients.[15]

Table 4. Variant Hemoglobin Forms

HEMOGLOBIN VARIANT	ASSOCIATED CONDITIONS
Hb S	Sickle cell disease or trait; sickle/thalassemia syndromes
Hb C	Forms of thalassemia
Hb F	Beta-thalassemia; Hereditary persistence of fetal hemoglobin; Sickly cell disease; Acquired disorders, including pernicious anemia, aplastic anemia, pregnancy, leukemia, chronic renal failure
Hb A_2	Beta-thalassemia, megaloblastic anemia
Hb H	Hb H disease (rare); alpha-thalassemia trait

Side effects are rare, but accelerated hypertension may occur in patients with renal failure. These individuals must be monitored closely during rhEPO therapy. There are no other contraindications to the use of rhEPO. The main factor limiting rhEPO treatment is cost. In our institution, the pharmacy cost for a single vial of rhEPO (10,000 Units, generally a single dose) is $193.

Lead Toxicity. Lead toxicity may present with a microcytic anemia. The characteristic feature of this anemia is the presence of basophilic stippling of RBCs on the peripheral blood smear. Blood lead testing will confirm the diagnosis. Generally, other symptoms of lead intoxication (neuro- and ototoxicity) will precede the appearance of the anemia.[22] Screening of other family members and a thorough investigation of the patient's environment should follow.

Hemoglobin Disorders. The presence of a microcytic anemia that is not attributable to iron deficiency, chronic disease, or lead toxicity suggests an underlying disorder of hemoglobin synthesis. These disorders may be categorized as hemoglobinopathies (production of abnormal hemoglobin) or thalassemia (underproduction of normal hemoglobin due to an absence or deficiency of normal variant chains).[23]

Most hemoglobin disorders present with a mild-to-moderate microcytic anemia with striking morphologic abnormalities. Electrophoresis will confirm the diagnosis, depending upon the precise hemoglobin variant discovered. *(Please see Table 4.)* These disorders may be difficult to distinguish from iron deficiency or may be exacerbated if iron deficiency is also present. Iron deficiency typically has an elevated RDW, while in hemoglobin disorders it remains normal. Other indices of RBC heterogeneity may also assist in the diagnosis.[24]

Severity of clinical illness is based upon the underlying genetic expression of the disorder. Homozygosity for hemoglobin disorders such as sickle cell disease and beta-thalassemia will result in severe illness. It is estimated that only 750-1000 patients with homozygous beta-thalassemia are present in North America, predominantly among

Figure 2. Evaluation of Normocytic Anemia

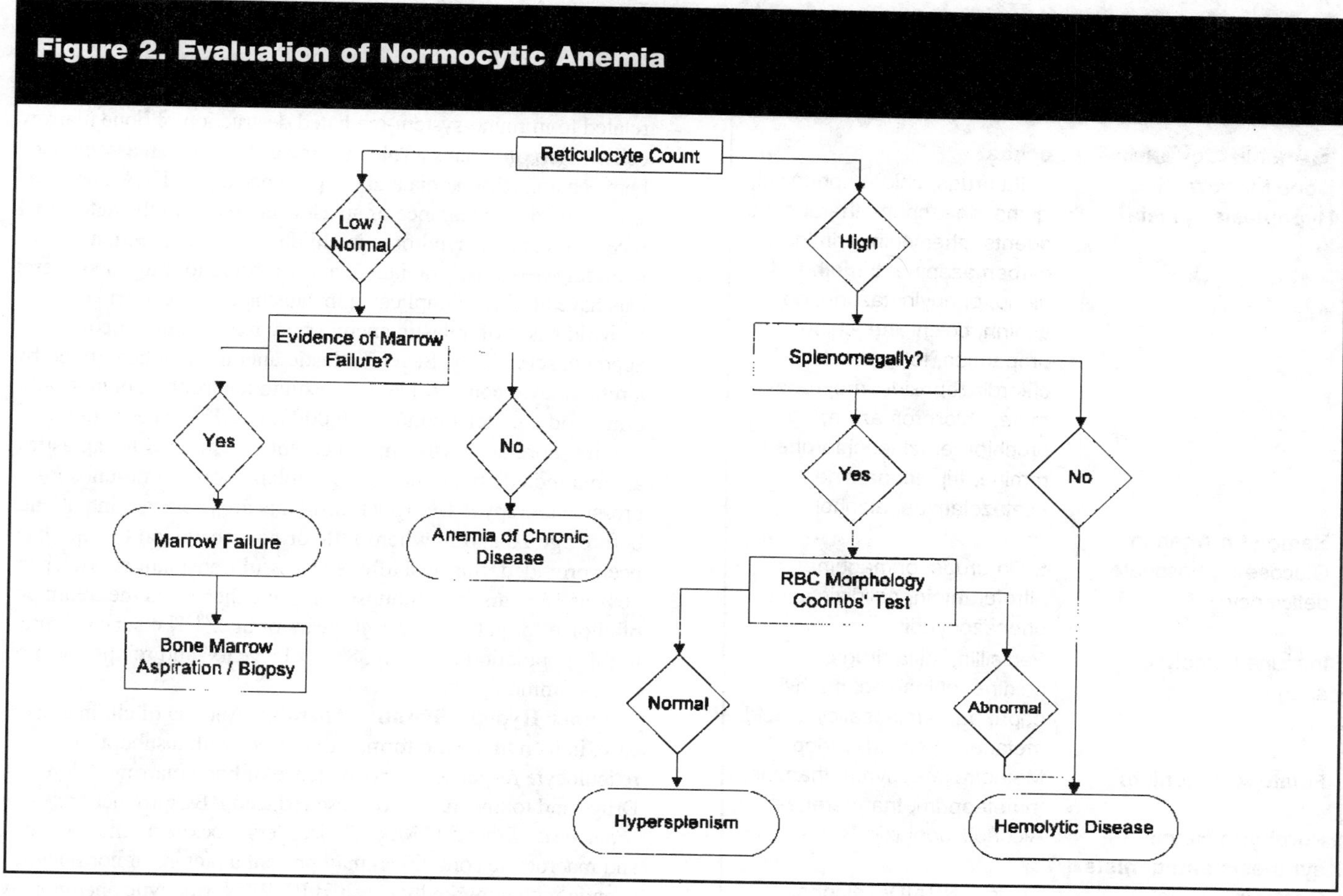

individuals of Mediterranean, Asian, or African descent.[25] Heterozygous expression of hemoglobin disorders (such as sickle cell trait and thalassemia trait) will present with a mild anemia which usually requires no further intervention. Alpha-thalassemia minor occurs primarily in Asian patients and may present periodically in areas with large Asian-American populations. Discovery of such a molecular defect should lead to screening of other family members and genetic counseling to explore the implications of potentially homozygous offspring.

Microcytic anemia also may be seen in some cases of RBC membrane defects such as hereditary spherocytosis (HS). HS may often be diagnosed directly from the peripheral smear.

Normocytic Anemia

The normocytic anemias may be divided into two broad etiologic categories: increased destruction (or loss) of red blood cells and decreased RBC production. The distinguishing feature between these categories is the reticulocyte count, which measures the compensatory response to the anemia. *(Please see Figure 2.)* Because the reticulocyte count is expressed as a percentage of total RBCs, it will increase in proportion to the severity of the anemia. For this reason, the count is usually corrected to a normal hematocrit of 45% using the following formula:[2]

Corrected Reticulocyte Count = Retic. Count ´ Hematocrit/45

Normocytic Anemias of Decreased RBC Production

Bone Marrow Failure. Bone marrow failure should be suspected in cases of normochromic, normocytic anemia accompanied by a markedly decreased reticulocyte count (< 0.5%), leukopenia and/or thrombocytopenia, or characteristic abnormalities of the peripheral blood smear including teardrop cells, nucleated RBCs, and immature granulocytes.[2] Involvement of multiple cell lines (red cells, white cells, and/or platelets), or the presence of abnormal cells point toward bone marrow failure. Precise pathologic diagnosis in these patients will require bone marrow aspiration and biopsy. Conditions that may cause bone marrow failure include aplastic anemia, myelodysplastic syndromes, and acute myelogenous leukemia,[5] metastatic disease of the bone marrow, myelofibrosis, pure red cell aplasia, and aplastic crises accompanying hemolytic anemias.

Aplastic Anemia. Aplastic anemia is the condition that most commonly causes bone marrow failure. It is defined as a failure of blood cell production resulting in pancytopenia with a markedly hypocellular bone marrow.[5] The documented incidence

Table 5. Drugs that Can Cause Anemia

MECHANISM OF ANEMIA	DRUGS
Bone Marrow Hypoplasia/aplasia	Sulfa drugs, chloramphenicol, quinacrine, chemotherapeutic agents, phenytoin, primidone, carbamazepine, trimethadione, phenylbutazone, gold, aspirin, colchicine, chlorpropamide, tolbutamide, chlordiazepoxide, meprobamate, chlorpromazine, prochlorperazine, chlorpheniramine, tripelennamine, acetazolamide, alcohol
Hemolytic Anemia	
Glucose-6-phosphate deficiency	Sulfa drugs, primaquine, nitrofurantoin, nalidixic acid, phenazopyridine
Immune hemolytic anemia	Penicillin, sulfa drugs, quinine, quinadine, methyldopa, paraaminosalicylic acid, mefanamic acid, levodopa
Folate Antagonists	Methotrexate, pyrimethamine, trimethoprim, triamterene
Porphyrin/Heme synthesis antagonists	Alcohol, isoniazid
Gastrointestinal blood loss	Aspirin, NSAIDs, alcohol

Adapted from reference 2.

of aplastic anemia in the United States and other developed countries is 5-10 cases per one million population per year. Most cases of aplastic anemia (65%) are idiopathic and appear to be related to immune-system-mediated destruction of bone marrow cells.[26] Heredity plays a role in some cases, with an association between aplastic anemia and the presence of the HLA-DR2 antigen,[27] and the appearance of aplastic anemia with the autosomal recessive Fanconi syndrome in childhood. Viral infections, including hepatitis,[28] radiation, and exposure to drugs and chemicals have also been implicated in causing aplastic anemia.

Mild cases of aplastic anemia may remit or may be managed conservatively. Severe aplastic anemia may be defined by a reticulocyte count < 1%, an absolute neutrophil count < 500 mm^3, and a platelet count < 20,000/mm^3. These cases may require more aggressive management. Treatments for aplastic anemia include bone marrow transplantation or immunosuppressive therapy.[29] Marrow transplants are preferred in patients before age 20 and in whom little or no transfusion therapy has been provided. Survival after successful transplant approaches 70% at 15 years.[30] Immunosuppressive therapy is the treatment of choice for patients over 40 years of age.[29] The survival rate in this population drops to 38% at 15 years, and relapse occurs more commonly.[30]

Other Hypoproliferative Anemias. Anemia of chronic disease, in its normocytic form, will present with a suboptimal reticulocyte response but no evidence of bone marrow failure. Drugs and toxins may also cause reduced RBC production. *(Please see Table 5.)* "Mixed" disorders (coexisting microcytic and macrocytic conditions) may present a picture of normocytic anemia with a markedly elevated RDW. Normocytic anemia may be idiopathic in 3-30% of cases, particularly in elderly patients.[31] This so-called "anemia of senescence" is a controversial entity.

Figure 3. Evaluation of Hemolytic Disease

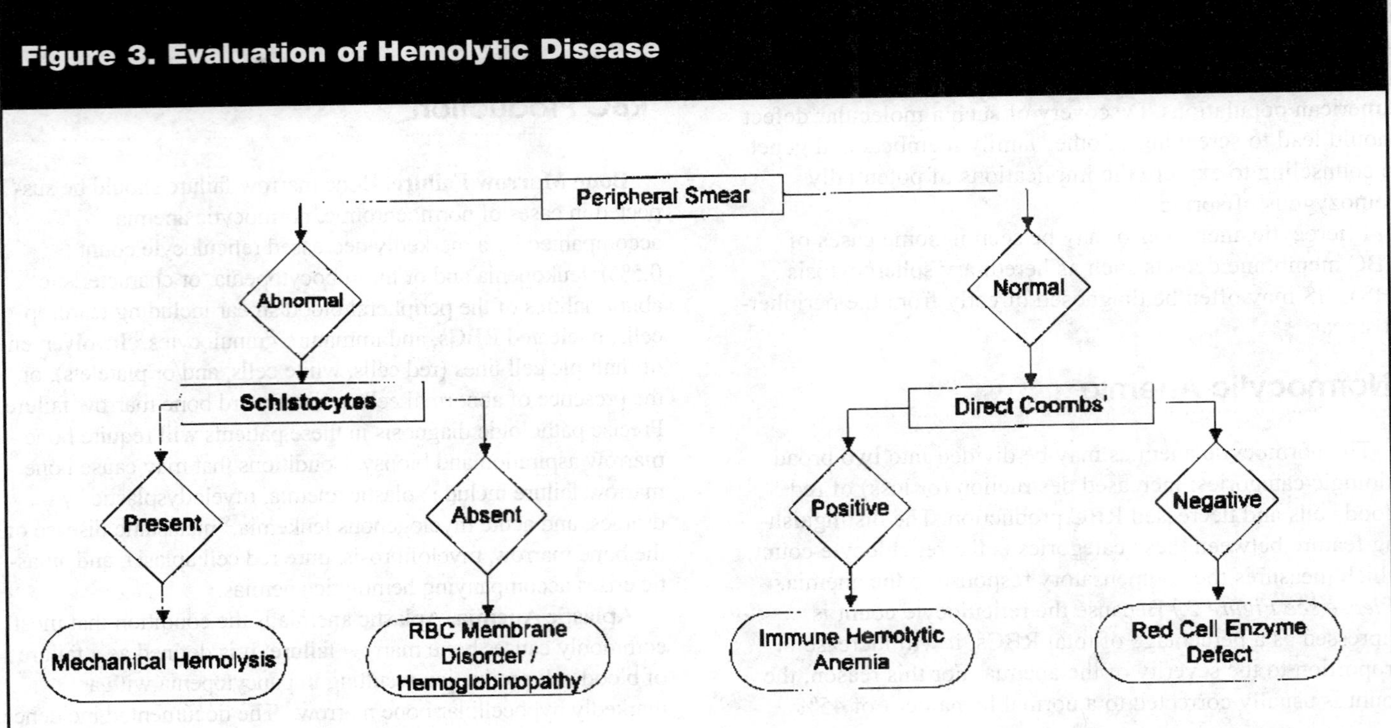

Table 6. Conditions Associated with Hemolytic Anemia

MECHANISM OF ANEMIA	ASSOCIATED CONDITIONS
Mechanical hemolysis	Valvular heart disease, coarctation of the aorta, aortic aneurysm, prosthetic valves, or vascular grafts
Intravascular hemolysis	Thrombotic thrombocytopenic purpura, hemolytic uremic syndrome, DIC, malignant hypertension, preeclampsia, eclampsia, drugs (Table 5), acute glomerulonephritis, polyarteritis nodosa, scleroderma, systemic lupus erythematosus, Wegener granulomatosis, march hemoglobinuria
Chemical agents	Arsenic, lead, copper, chlorates, formaldehyde, hyperbaric oxygen, insect venoms, heat
Infectious agents	Malaria, protozoan and parasitic infestations, *Clostridium welchii,* bacterial agents *(Haemophilus, Escherichia, Salmonella),* viral agents (Coxsackie, measles, cytomegallovirus, herpes viruses, HIV, varicella, influenza)
Warm-reacting autoantibiodies	Idiopathic (up to 60% of cases), chronic lymphocytic leukemia (CLL), lymphomas, systemic lupus erythematosus (often "mixed" warm- and cold-reacting antibiodies)
Cold-reacting antibiodies	Idiopathic, *Mycoplasma pneumoniae,* infectious mononucleosis
Alloimmune hemolytic disease of the newborn	Rh, ABO, or other red cell antigen incompatibility

These patients should be investigated for chronic blood loss and other underlying illnesses; however, bone marrow examinations in this situation have very low diagnostic yield.

Normocytic Anemia due to RBC Destruction/Loss

Acute Blood Loss. Normocytic anemia with increased RBC destruction may be due to acute blood loss. In most cases, the presentation will be fairly evident unless the source of blood loss is occult, such as a hip fracture or a retroperitoneal bleed. Reticulocyte counts require 3-5 days to mount a significant response to acute blood loss. It is useful diagnostically to observe the rate of fall of hemoglobin levels. A rapid drop is seen with acute blood loss, hemolysis, or hemodilution. Bone marrow failure, by contrast, will produce a much more gradual reduction.

Hypersplenism. Increased phagocytic activity within the spleen may lead to sequestration and destruction of red blood cells.[32] The result is the characteristic triad of anemia (and/or leukopenia), splenomegaly, and bone marrow hyperplasia. Hypersplenism may be the result of portal hypertension, myeloproliferative disorders, or chronic infections. Splenomegaly may also be present in hemolytic diseases and hemoglobinopathies as fragile RBCs are captured and destroyed. Splenectomy may be beneficial to correct anemia and reverse portal hypertension, but infectious and thrombotic complications may result.[5] Pneumococcal vaccine should be administered prior to splenectomy.

Hemolytic Anemia. Hemolytic anemia should be suspected in cases of normocytic anemia without acute bleeding, marrow insufficiency, or hypersplenism. *(Please see Figure 3.)* The presence of hemolysis will be further supported by increased indirect bilirubin and lactate dehydrogenase. Serum haptoglobin will be decreased in cases of intravascular hemolysis. There are many conditions that may cause hemolytic anemia, as listed in Table 6.

Hemolytic disease may be divided into two broad categories: 1) conditions caused by intrinsic red cell anomalies and 2) those resulting from extrinsic factors.

Intrinsic red cell anomalies include cell membrane defects (such as spherocytosis), red cell enzyme defects (such as G6PD and pyruvate kinase), and hemoglobinopathies. Many of these conditions may be identified by characteristic findings on the peripheral smear. A normal peripheral smear in the setting of a hemolytic anemia is most likely to be found in either an autoimmune hemolytic anemia or a red cell enzyme defect. Therefore, hemolysis in the presence of a normal peripheral smear and a negative Coombs test suggests an enzyme defect such as G6PD deficiency or pyruvate kinase deficiency.

Extrinsic conditions producing hemolytic anemia include mechanical factors, such as prosthetic heart valves, DIC, burns, neoplasms, or malignant hypertension.[2] The peripheral smear in these cases may reveal schistocytes (RBC fragments). Autoimmune antibodies are another extrinsic cause of hemolysis, as seen in transfusion reactions, Rh incompatibility, drug-induced hemolytic anemia, and warm or cold-reacting autoantibodies. Microangiopathic processes, infections, and chemical agents are other extrinsic factors that may be associated with hemolytic anemia. *(Please see Table 6.)*

Management. Management of hemolytic anemia should be directed at the underlying cause. Most patients with prosthetic heart valves will respond to administration of iron and folate supplementation. More severe cases may require replacement of the prosthesis. Recombinant erythropoietin has been successful in a few cases of mechanical hemolysis.[33] Offending drugs should be discontinued, and exposure to environmental agents strictly limited. Autoimmune hemolysis may respond to corticosteroids or other immunosuppressive agents.[5] Transfusion therapy and splenectomy may provide benefit in severe cases.

Macrocytic Anemia

Macrocytic anemia is defined by a mean corpuscular volume greater than 100 femtoliters. *(Please see Figure 4.)* The first issue to address in diagnosing macrocytic anemia is to determine whether it is megaloblastic or non-megaloblastic. The best way to make this distinction is to examine the peripheral smear. Macrocytic features that may be identified on the smear include hypersegmented neutrophils and oval macrocytes. Extremely high MCV values (> 120 fL) are usually associated with megaloblastic anemia.[34] An elevated LDH is suggestive of pernicious anemia as the result of hemolysis occurring within the bone marrow. On some occasions, megaloblasts may not appear in the peripheral smear. If the precise diagnosis of a macrocytic anemia cannot be achieved with B_{12} and folate assays, bone marrow examination may be necessary. The appearance of megaloblasts in the marrow may be so bizarre that the diagnosis may be mistaken for acute leukemia.

Megaloblastic Anemia. Megaloblastic anemia is most often the result of a deficiency of vitamin B_{12} and/or folic acid. These illnesses present a characteristic clinical picture which includes glossitis, gastrointestinal symptoms, and mild leukopenia and thrombocytopenia. The distinctive clinical feature of B_{12} deficiency is the presence of neurologic symptoms. Diagnosis of B_{12} or folate deficiency can be confirmed by the laboratory finding of decreased blood levels of these nutrients.

If a megaloblastic anemia does not appear to result from B_{12} or folate deficiency, it is important to take a careful history of medication use. Folate antagonists, antimetabolites, and other drugs may cause megaloblastic anemia. *(Please see Table 5.)* If nutrient deficiency cannot be confirmed and no drug use is apparent, referral to a hematologist is recommended for further evaluation.

Vitamin B_{12} Deficiency. Deficiency of vitamin B_{12} is generally the result of a prolonged failure of absorption, since body B_{12} stores are adequate for up to five years. Pernicious anemia, Crohn's disease, and drug therapy (please see Table 5) are the most frequent causes.[35] Post-surgical states, including post-total gastrectomy, surgical creation of a "blind loop," or ileal resection frequently result in an inability to absorb B_{12}. Strict vegetarianism may result in B_{12} deficiency, but, in general, nutritional intake is more than adequate to sustain bodily needs.

Figure 4. Evaluation of Macrolytic Anemia

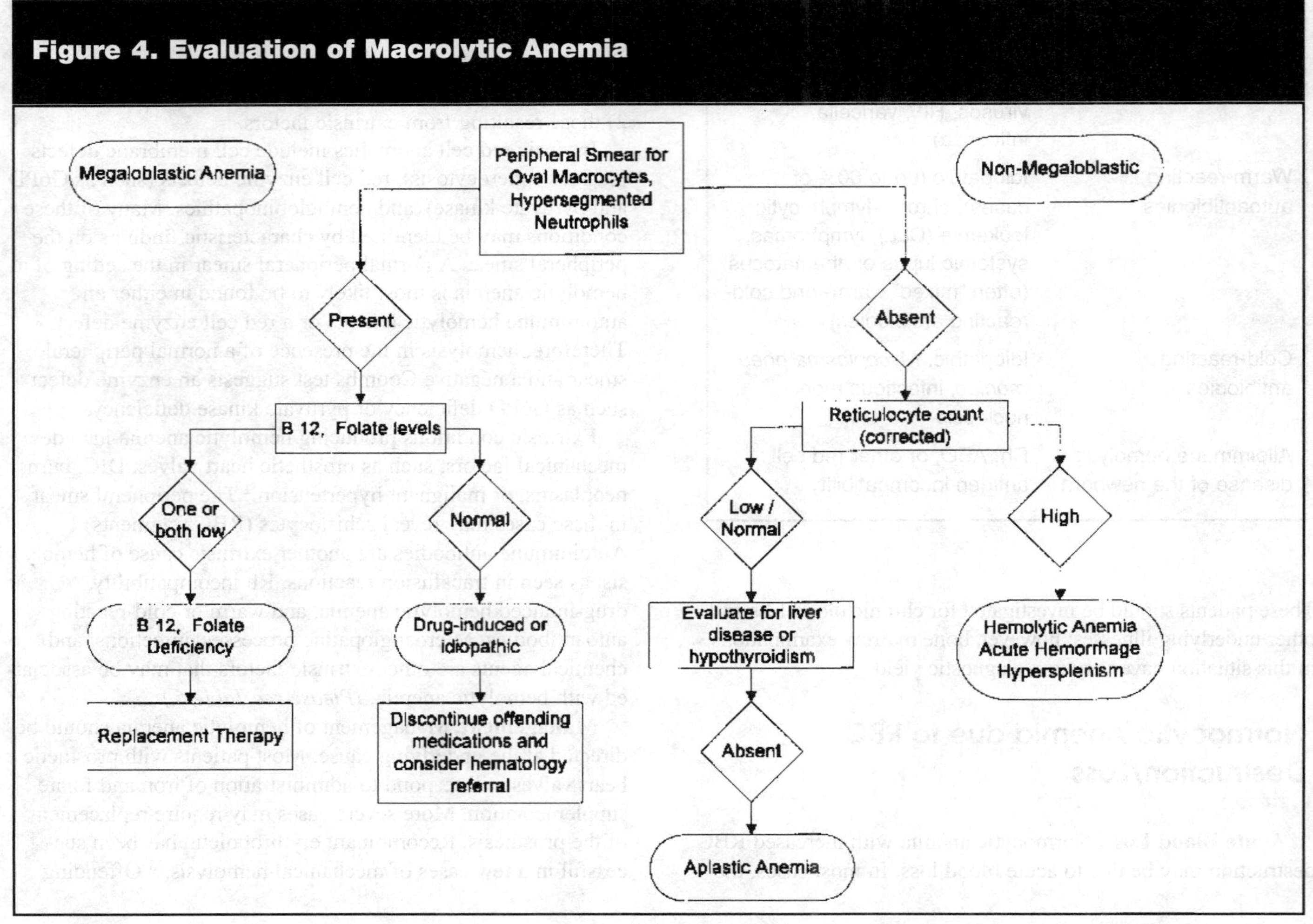

Laboratory diagnosis of B_{12} deficiency may be confirmed by the findings of increased urinary methylmalonic acid[36] and serum homocysteine.[37]

Pernicious Anemia. Pernicious anemia is by far the most common cause of B_{12} deficiency. This condition is especially common among the elderly, with an observed prevalence of up to 1.9%.[38] Pernicious anemia is caused by intestinal malabsorption due to atrophy of the gastric mucosa and decreased secretion of intrinsic factor. One recent hypothesis suggests an autoimmune mechanism, as illustrated by a case of spontaneous remission of pernicious anemia after corticosteroid therapy.[39] The question of a relationship between pernicious anemia and Helicobacter pylori has also been investigated, but evidence for this theory has not been conclusive.[40,41]

The diagnosis of pernicious anemia may be confirmed by the use of Schilling's test.[35] Failure to absorb radiolabelled B_{12} on the initial assay, followed by absorption when B_{12} is coadministered with intrinsic factor, establishes the diagnosis. Treatment of pernicious anemia consists of intramuscular injections of 1000 mcg of vitamin B_{12} at weekly intervals until B_{12} stores are replenished, followed by monthly injections for life.[42] Oral and intranasal preparations of B_{12} have been tried but without compelling success.[43]

Management of pernicious anemia should include surveillance for the development of gastric carcinoma. Preliminary reports suggest that routine endoscopic studies may be necessary for screening and early detection of this associated malignancy.[44,45]

Folate Deficiency. Folic acid deficiency is characterized by a megaloblastic anemia with a reduction in serum folate levels. Most cases of folate deficiency are a result of inadequate intake, increased folate requirements, or both.[35] Poor folate intake may occur with alcoholism, poverty, or advanced age. Body folate stores are marginally adequate, so reduced folate intake will result in a deficiency state in only 2-4 months. Increased folate demands are present during pregnancy and adolescence, especially during growth spurts. Drug therapy, including phenytoin, phenobarbital, sulfasalazine, and methotrexate, may also lead to folate deficiency.

Diagnosis of folate deficiency may require additional laboratory testing, due to the limitations of the serum folate assay.[46] Serum folate levels may transiently return to the normal range even after one folate-rich meal. Red blood cell folate levels are a more consistent measure of folate balance over a period of months. The homocysteine level will be increased, as in B_{12} deficiency; however, methylmalonic acid levels are normal in folate deficiency and elevated in B_{12} deficiency. The distinction between B_{12} and folate-deficient states is important, since B_{12} deficiency is associated with progressive neurologic deficits. Treating these patients with folic acid may produce transient hematologic improvements, masking the clinical symptoms of B_{12} deficiency while neurologic deterioration continues. This possibility has given rise to a debate over the value of food fortification with folic acid.[47]

Treatment of folate deficiency is straightforward. In the absence of a folate malabsorption state (such as tropical sprue), a daily dose of 1 mg folic acid given orally will replenish body stores in about three weeks.[35] Routine folic acid supplementation is recommended for women of child-bearing age to minimize the risk of fetal neural tube defects.

Non-megaloblastic Macrocytic Anemia. The most common cause of non-megaloblastic macrocytic anemia is alcoholism. The anemia may result from folate deficiency or from the direct toxic effects of alcohol upon the bone marrow. Macrocytosis may also appear as a result of reticulocytosis, since reticulocytes are larger than mature RBCs and their presence will cause a higher mean corpuscular volume. Hemolytic anemia, acute blood loss, or hypersplenism may cause this picture.

Non-megaloblastic macrocytic anemia with a low reticulocyte count may be seen with chronic diseases, most commonly liver disease and hypothyroidism. Aplastic anemia may also produce this picture, so bone marrow examination is advisable.

Myelodysplastic syndromes may produce an anemia characterized by the presence of macro-ovalocytes on the peripheral smear. Bone marrow examination will reveal dysplasia, sometimes with the presence of "megaloblastoid" cells.

Summary

Use of the algorithms presented here will assist the clinician in establishing the precise diagnosis for anemia in a cost-effective fashion, while avoiding the more expensive "shotgun" approach. Accurate diagnosis of anemia is essential, since it represents a clinical syndrome that is frequently associated with significant underlying illness.

References

1. Adams PF, Marano MA. Current estimates from the National Health Interview Survey, 1994. National Center for Health Statistics. *Vital Health Stat* 1995;10:83-84.
2. Brown RG. Anemia. In: Taylor RB (ed). *Family Medicine: Principles and Practice,* 4th ed. New York: Springer-Verlag; 1994:997-1005.
3. Sheth TN, et al. The relation of conjunctival pallor to the presence of anemia. *J Gen Int Med* 1997;12:102-106.
4. Mandel JS, et al. Reducing mortality from colorectal cancer by screening for fecal occult blood. *N Engl J Med* 1993;328: 1365-1371.
5. Beutler E, et al (eds). *Williams' Hematology,* 5th ed. New York: McGraw-Hill, Inc.; 1995. Chapters 1, 24, 59-67, 69.
6. McClure S, et al. Improved detection of early iron deficiency in nonanemic subjects. *JAMA* 1985;253:1021.
7. Bessman JD, et al. Improved classification of anemias by MCV and RDW. *Am J Clin Path* 1988;80:322-326.
8. Guyatt GH, et al. Laboratory diagnosis of iron-deficiency anemia: An overview. *J Gen Intern Med* 1992;7:145-153.
9. Centers for Disease Control and Prevention. Guidelines for school health programs to promote lifelong healthy eating. *MMWR Morb Mortal Wkly Rep* 1996;45:1-41.
10. Swain RA, et al. Iron deficiency anemia: When is parenteral therapy warranted? *Postgrad Med* 1996;100:181-193.
11. Cook JD. Iron deficiency anemia. In: Brain MC, Carbone P (eds). *Current Therapy in Hematology and Oncology,* 3rd ed. St. Louis:

Mosby-Year Book; 1987:9-11.

12. Gabrielli GB, De Sandre G. Excessive tea consumption can inhibit the efficacy of oral iron treatment in iron-deficiency anemia. *Haematologica* 1995;80:518-520.
13. Glass J. Iron deficiency anemia. In: Rakel RE (ed). *Conn's Current Therapy;* 1997:349-352.
14. Burns DL, et al. Parenteral iron dextran therapy: A review. *Nutrition* 1995;11:163-168.
15. Krantz SB. Pathogenesis and treatment of the anemia of chronic disease. *Am J Med Sci* 1994;307:353-359.
16. Ahluwalia N, et al. Iron deficiency and anemia of chronic disease in elderly women: A discriminant-analysis approach for differentiation. *Am J Clin Nutr* 1995;61:590-596.
17. Ferguson BJ, et al. Serum transferrin receptor distinguishes the anemia of chronic disease from iron deficiency anemia. *J Lab Clin Med* 1992;19:385-390.
18. Eschback JW, et al. Treatment of the anemia of progressive renal failure with recombinant human erythropoeitin. *N Engl J Med* 1989;321:158-163.
19. Peeters HR, et al. Effect of recombinant human erythropoeitin on anaemia and disease activity in patients with rheumatoid arthritis and anaemia of chronic disease: A randomised placebo controlled double blind 52 weeks clinical trial. *Ann Rheum Dis* 1996;55: 739-744.
20. Ludwig H, et al. Recombinant human erythropoeitin for the correction of cancer-associated anemia with and without concomitant cytotoxic chemotherapy. *Cancer* 1995;76:2319-2329.
21. Henry DA, et al. Recombinant human erythropoeitin in the treatment of anemia associated with human immunodeficiency virus (HIV) infection and zidovudine therapy: Overview of four clinical trials. *Ann Intern Med* 1992;117:739-748.
22. Chao J, Kikano GE. Lead poisoning in children. *Am Fam Phys* 1993;47:113-128.
23. Nguyen AN, et al. A rule-based expert system for laboratory diagnosis of hemoglobin disorders. *Arch Pathol Lab Med* 1996;120: 817-27.
24. Liu T, et al. The erythrocyte cell hemoglobin distribution width segregates thalassemia traits from other nonthalassemic conditions with microcytosis. *Am J Clin Path* 1997;107:601-607.
25. Pearson HA, et al. The changing profile of homozygous beta-thalassemia: Demography, ethnicity, and age distribution of current North American patients and changes in two decades. *Pediatrics* 1996;97:352-356.
26. Young NS, Barrett AJ. The treatment of severe acquired aplastic anemia. *Blood* 1995;85:3367-3377.
27. Nimer SD, et al. An increased HLA DR2 frequency is seen in aplastic anemia patients. *Blood* 1994;84:923-927.
28. Brown KE, et al. Hepatitis-associated aplastic anemia. *N Engl J Med* 1997;336:1059- 1064.
29. Fonseca R, Tefferi A. Practical aspects in the diagnosis and management of aplastic anemia. *Am J Med Sci* 1997;313:159-169.
30. Doney K, et al. Primary treatment of acquired aplastic anemia: Outcomes with bone marrow transplantation and immunosuppressive therapy. *Ann Intern Med* 1997;126:107-115.
31. Elis A, et al. A clinical approach to "idiopathic" normocytic-normochromic anemia. *J Am Geriatr Soc* 1996;44:832-834.
32. Shah SHA, et al. Measurement of spleen size and its relation to hypersplenism and portal hemodynamics in portal hypertension due to hepatic cirrhosis. *Am J Gastroenterol* 1996;91:2580-2583.
33. Kornowski R, et al. Erythropoeitin therapy obviates the need for recurrent transfusions in a patient with severe hemolysis due to prosthetic valves. *Chest* 1992;102:315.
34. Wallerstein RO, Jr. Laboratory evaluation of anemia. *West J Med* 1987;146:443-451.
35. Davenport J. Macrocytic anemia. *Am Fam Physician* 1996;53: 155-162.
36. Norman EJ, Morrison JA. Screening elderly populations for cobalamin (vitamin B_{12}) deficiency using the urinary methylmalonic acid assay by gas chromatography mass spectrometry. *Am J Med* 1993;589-594.
37. Stabler SP, et al. Clinical spectrum and diagnosis of cobalamin deficiency. *Blood* 1990;76:871-881.
38. Carmel R. Prevalence of undiagnosed pernicious anemia in the elderly. *Arch Intern Med* 1996;156:1097-1100.
39. Span J, et al. A reversible case of pernicious anemia. *Am J Gastroenterol* 1993;88:1277-1278.
40. Haruma K, et al. Pernicious anemia and Helicobacter pylori infection in Japan: Evaluation in a country with a high prevalrnce of infection. *Am J Gastroenterol* 1995;90:1107-1110.
41. Varis O, et al. Is Helicobacter pylori involved in the pathogenesis of the gastritis characteristic of pernicious anaemia? *Scand J Gastroenterol* 1993;28:705-708.
42. Swain R. An update of vitamin B12 metabolism and deficiency states. *J Fam Pract* 1995;41:595-600.
43. Pruthi RK, Tefferi A. Pernicious anemia revisited. *Mayo Clin Proc* 1994;69:144-150.
44. El-Newihi HM, et al. Gastric cancer and pernicíouc anemia appearing as pseudoachalasia. *Southern Med J* 1996;89:906-910.
45. Sjoblom SM, et al. Gastroscopic follow-up of pernicious anemia patients. *Gut* 1993;34:28-32.
46. Swain RA, St. Clair L. The role of folic acid in deficiency states and prevention of disease. *J Fam Pract* 1997;44:138-144.
47. Dickinson CJ. Does folic acid harm people with vitamin B_{12} deficiency? *Q J Med* 1995;88:357-364.

Part XVI

Renal Disease and Urological Conditions

Erectile Dysfunction

Gideon Bosker, MD

The clinical mandate to treat erectile dysfunction (ED) in primary care practice has never been more clearly or compellingly documented in the medical literature. Nor has the imperative to treat this condition ever been more pressing. Put simply, ED is an undertreated condition affecting about 30 million Americans, including up to 30% of men less than 50 years of age. Despite safe, cost-effective, and quality of life-improving therapy that is available with sildenafil (Viagra®), many primary care physicians nevertheless fail to pursue the diagnosis of ED, and to take full advantage of clinical support tools that are quick to administer, efficient, and can suggest effective treatment options.

Even in its mild form, both in the younger and older patient, ED is a bona fide medical condition that requires compassionate care, counseling, and full access to treatment options. And much like such common diseases as allergies, arthritis, and asthma, ED is a physically limiting and functionally compromising condition that prevents the individual patient from achieving maximum quality of life. Hence, treatment of ED should be viewed as an essential part of the primary care practitioner's role to heal, ameliorate pain (emotional or physical), and improve functional status.[1,2]

With increasing recognition of this clinical condition, the documented potential for patient satisfaction, and the proven efficacy and safety of sildenafil, the treatment imperative for ED now includes a younger population with milder forms of the disease. Of special importance is the recognition that even men between the ages of 25 and 50 years who report that they are sexually active require rapid and efficient evaluation for ED.

The mandate to treat this younger and active population, most of whom do not have co-morbid conditions that predispose to ED, is based on epidemiological studies and expert panel consensus reports. These studies confirm that a significant percentage of men who report they possess the capacity for and participate in sexual activity, upon further questioning, will nevertheless disclose objective evidence of ED requiring treatment. The qualitative symptoms suggesting ED may include, but are not limited to, the ability to achieve an erection, hardness of erection, ability to achieve an erection rapidly, maintaining an erection, maintaining an erection for sufficiently long periods to complete intercourse, and general level of satisfaction with sexual activity.

In this regard, it is estimated that even among such younger, sexually active individuals, the percentage of men with pharmacologically treatable ED meeting strict diagnostic criteria is about 32%.[3-7] A simple and quick-to-implement Sexual Health Inventory for Men (SHIM) will identify this receptive group within the framework of a simple, time-efficient outpatient evaluation. The screening test is easy to

Table 1. Risk Factors in Erectile Dysfunction
Diabetes
Obesity
Hypertension
Hyperlipidemia
Hypogonadism
Renal disease
Smoking
Alcohol or drug abuse
Trauma or surgery to the pelvis or spine
Coronary artery or peripheral vascular disease
Peyronie's disease
Depression or stress

administer and should be made available to all appropriate patients. It should be stressed that this subgroup which, because it is already sexually active—and therefore, meets the physiological, safety, and exercise stress criteria required for drug-based therapy—represents a unique opportunity for physicians to initiate a safe and outcome-effective sildenafil treatment program. Put another way, the sexually active individual, for all practical clinical purposes, has "cleared" himself as a physiologically safe—and therefore, very appropriate—candidate for drug therapy.

In addition, because younger men tend to be more sexually active, those with documented ED, even in its milder forms, are likely to derive greater benefits—from global patient satisfaction to improved mood and erectile function—over the long term than a cohort of elderly men with multiple comorbid conditions and in whom sexual activity may play a less important role in day-to-day life. Thus, the clinical importance of aggressive treatment of both younger and older individuals cannot be overemphasized.

From a mandate-to-treat perspective, new safety data demonstrating that there is no increased risk of cardiovascular adverse events, MI, stroke, or deaths in patients treated with sildenafil compared to placebo suggests that primary care physicians should incorporate ED screening techniques as part of the routine evaluation of all adult men who are sexually active, or who are prevented from sexual activity because of symptoms associated with ED.

With recent studies demonstrating efficacious and safe treatment with sildenafil (Viagra®), the mandate to manage this widespread condition in the primary care setting is now firmly established. Using a systematic and streamlined approach for the diagnosis and treatment of ED, primary care physicians can anticipate that the overall benefit-to-risk ratio for sildenafil-based treatment of ED will be more favorable than it is for the majority of common outpatient conditions they currently manage. For example, in a recent, independent study conducted by investigators at the University of Pittsburgh, it was reported that the cost of sildenafil fell well within the health insurance industry's cost guidelines when compared with its impact on quality of life for sufferers of ED. In particular, they found that sildenafil had a cost-effectiveness ratio of $11,290 per quality-adjusted life-year, compared favorably with such therapies as cholesterol-lowering medications, anti-hypertensive agents, antidepressants, kidney dialysis, and coronary artery bypass.

A number of other advantages may accrue to the practitioner from routine screening for and treatment of ED, including improvements in patient satisfaction, patient loyalty, patient retention, and an increased patient willingness to comply with other screening activities. Treatable, comorbid conditions such as heart disease, diabetes, prostate disease, depression, and neurovascular conditions may also surface as a result of routine, systematic approaches to ED detection. In conclusion, the necessity and relevance of treating ED is now no longer optional, but should be considered standard operating procedure in the setting of primary care. Because sildenafil is currently the only approved oral, medical therapy for ED, and because it is the most commonly used therapeutic option employed by primary care physicians, a comprehensive review of its clinical safety, relevance, and efficacy will help optimize treatment decisions and patient outcomes in primary care practice.

Introduction: Clinical Relevance of Treating ED in the Primary Care Setting

Erectile dysfunction is a potentially devastating ailment that affects not only men, but also their sexual partners. The Massachusetts Male Aging Study revealed that age is the single most important variable associated with erectile difficulty.[3] Currently, more than 30 million American men suffer some degree of erectile dysfunction (ED), with projections that up to 47 million individuals will have treatable erectile dysfunction by the year 2020.[4]

From a patient management perspective, there are a number of modalities for the treatment of erectile dysfunction. (*Please see Figure 1*). To maximize outcomes and account for patient flexibility, one group has introduced the concept of goal-directed therapy, in which the patient and his sexual partner have an active role in the decision-making process with respect to treatment.[8] A recent report revealed that most patients prefer the least invasive therapy even when the more invasive options are more effective.[9] With regard to these issues, there are essentially seven choices for impotence treatment: 1) accepting the loss of vaginal penetration with a rigid penis and using alternative sexual gratification methods; 2) medical therapy; 3) psychological sex therapy counseling; 4) vacuum/constriction devices; 5) home pharmacological penile injection therapy or urethral suppositories; 6) penile prosthesis; and 7) vascular surgery.[10] Consideration of advanced surgical techniques is beyond the scope of this review, which will focus on sildenafil, which rep-

Figure 1. Treatment Options for Erectile Dysfunction

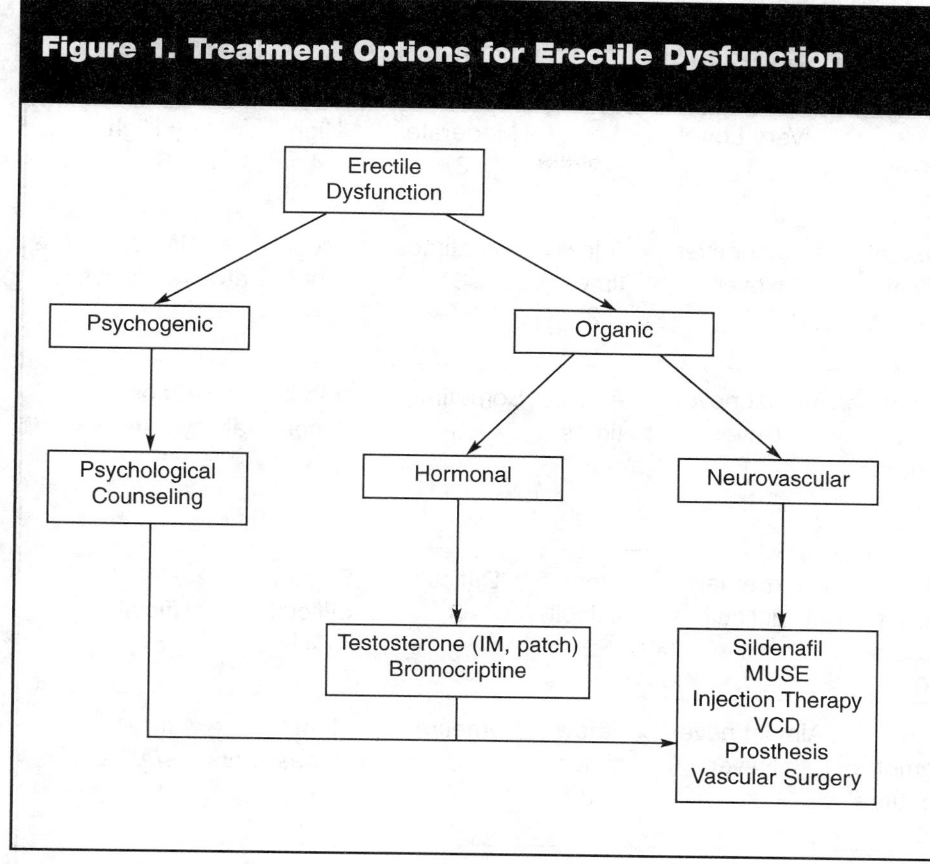

resents the most common therapeutic modality used by the primary care physician.

As primary care practitioners are well aware, this condition can be a difficult and embarrassing topic for many of these individuals to discuss. Moreover, most patients and health care professionals do not have an adequate understanding of the effectiveness, benefit-to-risk ratio, and safety profiles of available treatment options. Hence, it has been estimated that only 5-10% of men with erectile dysfunction will seek medical intervention.[4] Since this is one of the most undertreated conditions in the United States, the evaluation and management of impotence has become a clinical imperative for primary care physicians, as well as specialists who have fueled expansion of numerous men's impotence clinics.[5]

Given the results of evidence-based trials confirming the effectiveness, safety, tolerance, and patient satisfaction improvements seen with sildenafil therapy, primary care physicians have a mandate to screen for and treat all eligible patients who meet diagnostic criteria for ED. What may be under-appreciated by the clinician is that improving sexual "functional" capacity in a man who meets diagnostic criteria for ED is as relevant and medically—and certainly, psychologically—essential as improving functional capacity in the patient with COPD, heart disease, or osteoarthritis.

Up until 10-15 years ago, erectile dysfunction was, for the most part, attributed to psychogenic factors such as life stressors, performance anxiety, and related factors. However, current studies show that up to 90% of men with ED have underlying organic pathology as the principal cause or contributing factor to their condition.[11] The common denominator in all organic impotence is either humoral, vascular, neurogenic, or anatomic derangements; frequently, a combination of these factors may be at work. One group of investigators rated the organic causes of impotence in decreasing order of frequency: arterial, venous, neurological, and endocrine.[12]

Importantly, the overall benefit-to-risk ratio for sildenafil-based treatment of ED may be higher than it is for most common outpatient conditions. This is because successfully treated ED patients report high rates of satisfaction with medical care, which reflects effectiveness of treatment, an acceptable side effect profile, improved well being, and the desire to comply with therapy over the long term. In contrast to ED, many common conditions—among them, allergies, COPD, CHF, and coronary heart disease—require extensive, and sometimes costly, laboratory or radiographic assessment to confirm the diagnosis and risk-stratify patients into appropriate treatment groups. Moreover, compliance with medications to treat chronic conditions may be less than satisfactory and because side effects frequently are troublesome, the benefit-to-risk ratio can be less than ideal.

In these respects, outpatient management of ED with sildenafil offers unique advantages as compared to other conditions. First, because the diagnosis of ED usually can be made expeditiously from the history in the office setting. *(Please see Table 2)*, and because pharmacotherapy is effective, from a time management perspective, confirmation of the diagnosis of ED may be more efficient, cost-effective, and accurate than the diagnosis of such conditions as heart failure, asthma, or arthritis.

Consequently, from a clinical relevance perspective, this condition demands the attention of primary care physicians, as well as urological specialists, in all men who are or wish to be sexually active. Failure to adequately diagnose and treat ED may have a profound impact on a man's sexual, emotional, physical, and psychiatric health. From a necessity-to-treat perspective, failure to identify and treat individuals with ED can result in compromised quality of life, low self-esteem, chronic anxiety, impaired family relations, and perhaps even clinical depression. In summary, despite availability of highly effective and safe treatment for this condition with sildenafil, men are underdiagnosed, undertreated, and in general, underserved when it comes to management of disorders related to their sexual health.

Table 2. Sexual Health Inventory for Men (SHIM) During Previous Six Months

1. How do you rate your confidence that you could get an erection?		Very Low 1	Low 2	Moderate 3	High 4	Very High 5
2. When you had erections with sexual stimulation, how often were your erections hard enough for penetration?	No sexual activity 0	Almost never/ Never 1	A few times 2	Sometimes 3	Most times 4	Almost always/Always 5
3. During sexual intercourse, how often were you able to maintain your erection after you had penetrated (entered) your partner?	Did not attempt intercourse 0	Almost never/ Never 1	A few times 2	Sometimes 3	Most times 4	Almost always/Always 5
4. During sexual intercourse, how difficult was it to maintain your erection to completion of intercourse?	Did not attempt intercourse 0	Extremely difficult 1	Very difficult 2	Difficult 3	Slightly difficult 4	Not difficult 5
5. When you attempted sexual intercourse, how often was it satisfactory to you?	Did not attempt intercourse 0	Almost never/ Never 1	A few times 2	Sometimes 3	Most times 4	Almost always/Always 5

To administer the Sexual Health Inventory for Men (SHIM), patients answer each of the questions in the SHIM on a scale from 0 to 5, where "0" indicates no activity, "1" is the most negative response, and "5" is the most positive response. Overall scores on the SHIM range from 1 to 25. Higher scores indicate better erectile function, with a score of 20 or higher indicating a normal degree of erectile functioning. Low scores (10 or less) indicate moderate to severe erectile dysfunction. The scale can be given at the initial or follow-up visits as a means to facilitate patient-physician communication about erectile function or sexual satisfaction.

Recent Safety Data in Hypertension, Diabetes, and Heart Disease: Confirmation of Excellent Tolerance and Lack of Adverse Cardiovascular Effects

Newly published clinical trial data provide additional confirmation of the safety of sildenafil in eligible patient populations.[13] Recent reviews in the *American Journal of Cardiology* provide compelling placebo-controlled safety data for sildenafil treatment in ED. A number of conclusions supported the safety and acceptable toleration profile of sildenafil in several patient subgroups frequently encountered by the primary care practitioner. Although specific trials will be discussed below, from a practical, primary care perspective the following conclusions about sildenafil safety were reported in a recent review and should be entered into the benefit-to-risk equation for ED treatment:

• The clinical effects of sildenafil on blood pressure are modest and independent of dosage or plasma level.

• The effects of sildenafil on blood pressure are modest, even in those patients taking multiple antihypertensive medications. Specifically, in a separate controlled interaction study of sildenafil and amlodipine (Norvasc®), the mean additional reduction in supine blood pressure was 8mm Hg systolic and 7 mm Hg diastolic.

• No statistically significant difference in the rate of serious cardiovascular adverse events was noted between patients treated with sildenafil and placebo.

• Sildenafil is associated with a low incidence of adverse effects.

• With respect to drug interactions, sildenafil combined with a CYP3A4 inhibitor can increase plasma levels of sildenafil; however, increased systemic exposure did not appear to decrease patient tolerability.[13]

Growing confirmation of sildenafil's acceptable safety profile in diverse patient subgroups—i.e., disease-free individuals as well as those with heart disease, diabetes, hypertension, and other associated conditions—has emerged from a number of recent studies and clinical trials.[13-17] In one important study, 32 male cardiac patients (ages 38-74, mean 49.3 years) completed

Table 3. Medical History for ED

- Chronic medical illness (e.g., diabetes, anemia, renal failure, heart disease)
- Medications/Recreational drug use (e.g., antihypertensives, antidepressants, alcohol, cocaine)
- Artheresclerotic vascular risk factors (e.g., hypercholesterolemia, hypertension, diabetes, family history)
- Pelvic/perineal/penile trauma (e.g., bicycling injury)
- Past surgery (e.g., radical prostatectomy, laminectomy, vascular bypass surgery)
- Neurological illness (e.g., spinal cord injury, multiple sclerosis, lumosacral disc disease)
- Endocrinologic illness (e.g., hypogonadism, hyperprolactinemia, thyroid disorders)
- Psychiatric illness (e.g., depression, anxiety)
- Sexually transmitted diseases (e.g., gonorrhea)
- Obesity

a conventional stress test, using standard ergometric equipment. Every subject underwent an initial, control stress test, and then received 100 mg sildenafil. One hour later, during maximal sildenafil plasma concentration, subjects underwent a second stress test, with echocardiographic examination. The investigators reported that no ischemic changes were detected after sildenafil intake, and no significant differences in systolic or diastolic blood pressure, heart rate, or cardiac output could be attributed to sildenafil.[14]

In another study, the efficacy and safety of sildenafil therapy were evaluated for a 12-week period in 224 men (n=136, sildenafil; n=88, placebo) with cardiovascular disease (CVD) and erectile dysfunction. The subjects had been taking a number of CVD medications—calcium channel blockers, beta-blockers, and/or ACE inhibitors—for six months, but not nitrate therapy. The 50 mg sildenafil starting dose could be adjusted to 100 mg or 25 mg based on therapeutic response and tolerability. Efficacy measures included a global efficacy question (GEQ): "Has the treatment improved your erections?" and data on sexual intercourse recorded in a patient event log. Adverse events over the 12-week period were monitored.[15] The rates of discontinuation were comparable for the two groups.

The 224 men had a number of CVDs including hypertension (83%), previous MI (19%), coronary artery disease (17%), angina (17%), and previous coronary artery bypass (14%). Flushing (17%), headache (15%), and dyspepsia (4%) were the most frequent adverse events. The GEQ assessment showed that 24% of patients with CVD and ED on placebo reported improved erections as compared to 71% on sildenafil (P=0.0001 versus placebo). The percentage of all attempts at sexual intercourse that were successful were 26+/-6% on placebo as compared to 75 +/- 5% on sildenafil (P=0.0001 versus placebo). Moreover, the mean number of successful attempts at sexual intercourse/week was 0.26 +/- 0.13 for placebo subjects as compared to 1.2 +/- 0.10 for those on sildenafil (P=0.0001 versus placebo). The investigators concluded that sildenafil significantly improved erectile function and the number of successful attempts at sexual intercourse, and that it was well-tolerated in men with ED and CVD who were not on nitrate therapy.[15]

Another group led by a Harvard Medical School investigator pooled the results of 53 studies (30 of them double-blinded, [DB] placebo-controlled; 23 open-label [OL] trials of sildenafil) in which treatment was undertaken for a period of 6 weeks to 2 years.[16] Exclusionary criteria included hypotension (BP < 90/50 mm Hg); uncontrolled hypertension (BP > 170/110 mm Hg); a recent (< 6 months) history of unstable cardiovascular disease, MI, or stroke; and regular nitrate therapy.

The results strongly support the safety of sildenafil in this patient population. As of March 31, 1999, report the authors, total exposure in the 53 clinical trials was 6884 patient years for sildenafil (964 DB trials, 5920 OL trials) and 543 patient-years for placebo. There were 44 nonfatal and 11 fatal MIs among sildenafil users versus 5 nonfatal and 1 fatal Mis for the placebo group. There were 29 deaths from any cause among those receiving sildenafil and 4 among those receiving placebo. Overall, the incidence rates of MI and death were comparable and not significantly different from patients receiving sildenafil and and those receiving placebo; in addition, the incidence rates for the combined endpoint of MI or death were not significantly different. The authors conclude that these data are reassuring and suggest that treatment of ED with sildenafil and resumption of sexual activity are not associated with even a moderate increase in cardiac risk.[16]

In another small study,[18] sildenafil was studied in 14 men with severe heart disease. In all the patients, at least one major coronary artery demonstrated > 70% occlusion. They also had other risk factors including smoking, diabetes, and hypertension. Patients were given sildenafil—they did not engage in sexual activity while on the drug—and then had cardiovascular and pulmonary parameters measured while lying down before and 45 minutes after taking a dose of sildenafil. On most measures of blood pressure and blood flow, sildenafil did not appear to have any significant effects, and none of the subjects experience serious side effects, i.e., hypotension, chest, or similar symptoms that could be attributed to sildenafil. The researchers concluded that that oral sildenafil has no direct adverse cardiovascular affects in men with severe coronary artery disease, and point out that the drug is safe for this subgroup of patients, provided their condition is stable and they are not on nitrates.[18]

From a primary care perspective, these are reassuring studies, and suggest that, given certain exclusionary criteria, men with CVD can be considered eligible candidates for ED therapy. A few caveats, however, should be kept in mind. First, the physical and/or psychological stress of sexual activity per se can be excessive in some individuals, especially those who have not engaged in this activity for extended periods or who have severely compromised left ventricular function. Accordingly, the American College of Cardiology and the American Heart Association both recommend that patients with stable coronary heart disease (who are not on nitrates) should be evaluated for the risks and benefits of sexual activity according to their physiological state and planned program of sexual activity. On occasion, especially in patients with a complicated CVD history and/or those who are taking multiple cardiac medications, a definitive assessment may require referral to a cardiologist for stress testing, pulmonary function testing, or other evaluations of physiological capacity commensurate with strenuous (i.e., sexual) exercise. These decisions will be made on the basis of clinical judgment, with the understanding that common sense is always advised when transitioning patients from a sedentary lifestyle devoid of sexual activity to one in which sildenafil-facilitated sexual activity becomes a normal part of life.[18]

Diabetic patients are at high risk for acquiring ED and therefore it is not surprising that the safety and efficacy of sildenafil has been extensively studied in this patient population.[19-21] Recent reports confirm clinical usefulness of this medication in both Type I and Type II diabetics. In one study of about 220 men with Type II diabetes, the estimated percentage of successful attempts at sexual intercourse increased from 13.2% at baseline to 58.8% at the end of a 12-week treatment course.[19] In comparison, the success rates among patients in the placebo group did not change.

Two additional analyses have presented an analysis of combined data from 11 randomized, double-blind, placebo-controlled trials evaluating both safety and efficacy of sildenafil in more than 800 diabetic and 1600 non-diabetic men.[20,21] The first of these studies, conducted at the Oschner Medical Institution in New Orleans, showed that 59% of men with Type I and 63% with Type II diabetes experienced overall improvements in their erections with sildenafil (compared with 18% and 17%, respectively, in the placebo groups). An accompanying safety, discontinuation rate, and adverse event (AE) analysis of the same study population revealed that sildenafil was equally well tolerated among patients with Type I and Type II diabetes, and that fewer than 2% discontinued due to AEs.[21] The most common AEs were headache, flushing, dyspepsia, and dizziness. There were no incidents of syncope or postural hypotension in this study group.[21]

Based on these studies and other recent reports, sildenafil has been shown safe and effective in a number of patient subgroups, including those with CVD and diabetes. Accordingly, patients satisfying the following three criteria appear to constitute excellent candidates for sildenafil therapy: 1) those with diabetes and heart disease who are suitable candidates for the drug because they demonstrate a clinical indication (i.e., ED) for its use; 2) those who have been appropriately screened to ensure they are not at risk for incurring potential harmful drug-drug interaction (i.e., nitrates and sildenafil are contraindicated in combination); and 3) those with demonstrated physical capacity to participate in sex-related activity without adverse consequences.

A Streamlined and Time-Efficient Approach for Identifying ED Patients

Assessment of ED requires a focused history and open communication. Moreover, primary care practitioners can optimize patient outcomes in ED by identifying patient populations most suitable for pharmacotherapy. Studies demonstrate that use of sildenafil for treatment of ED is safe and effective when this medication is used appropriately in eligible patient populations.[13-21] Eligible patients are determined on the basis of clinical judgement, based on history, physical, and when appropriate, additional laboratory testing. It should be stressed that eligible populations can be young or old, with or without comorbid conditions, as long as they meet clinical criteria of ED and their history suggests that sexual activity is well tolerated from a physiological, exercise-based perspective.

A directed, focused, and understanding approach to the patient with possible ED will optimize identification of these individuals in the office setting. From a clinical, quality-of-life, and patient satisfaction perspective, when it comes to sexual function, "It is better to ask than not to ask." Physicians have a mandate to inquire about sexual function and approach this condition as they would any other medical illness or compromise in functional capacity. The physician should ask gently, ask with compassion, and ask about specifics; but unless there are clear reasons not to investigate, a history-based inquiry into the functional status of a man's sexual health should be a routine part of every clinical evaluation.

This is a sound approach because, to a great degree, physicians must rely on their patients' subjective perceptions and sexual histories in order to determine whether drug therapy for ED is indicated. A systematic inquiry regarding sexual health is especially important in individuals known to have risk factors for ED. These include diabetes, hypertension, hyperlipidemia, smoking, renal disease and depression. In addition, men who are obese, who have waistlines greater than 36 inches, limited physical activity, and excessive alcohol consumption also are at higher risk for acquiring ED.[22] *(Please See Table 1.)* Considering the large number of risk factors, from a practical, screening standpoint in the primary care setting, evaluation for ED should be routine in every male 30 years of age or older.

In particular, patients with renal disease on hemodialysis (HD) are especially prone to ED, with one study showing that more than 80% of male patients on HD meet the diagnostic criteria of ED, which was severe in more than 50% of those evaluated.[23] Strategies for decreasing the impact of ED in such high-risk populations should be a priority for primary care physicians as well as specialists. However, it should be stressed that such SHIM-based, ED evaluations also should be conducted in otherwise healthy men who are in their 30s and 40s—as well as in individuals 50 years and older, since a portion of the decline in ED over time is age-dependent.[24]

Identification of men who are likely to have ED has been refined by recent surveys looking at men free of major chronic diseases.[22] One group selected 1981 U.S. male health professionals age 51-88 years, as age-matched healthy controls for a study of quality of life related to prostate cancer. The men

Table 4. Drugs Commonly Associated with Erectile Dysfunction

ANTIHYPERTENSIVES
Thiazide, diuretics, beta blockers, calcium channel blockers, angiotensin converting enzyme inhibitors
ANTIDEPRESSANTS
Tricyclic antidepressants, selective serotonin reuptake inhibitors
ANTIARRHYTHMICS
Digoxin
ANTI-ANDROGENS
GnRH agonists, ketoconazole, spironolactone
H2 BLOCKERS
Cimetidine
RECREATIONAL DRUGS
Alcohol, marijuana, cocaine, heroin

included in this study were free of chronic disease, including heart disease and diabetes. Data about ED were gathered via mailed questionnaires in 1988. Erectile function was measured using the following question from the UCLA Prostate Cancer Index: "How would you rate your ability to have an erection during the last four weeks?" Men who reported very poor or poor ability were classified as having dysfunction.

Results from the study indicate that the 671 (34%) with ED were more likely to be older, hypertensive, and weigh more. After simultaneously controlling for age, smoking, and hypertension, men with a larger waist were significantly more likely to report ED. For example, men with a 42-inch waist had an odds ratio of 1.96 (95% Cl 1.48, 2.59) for ED compared to men with a 32-inch waist. Compared to men with the lowest level of physical activity, men who exercised about 30 minutes/day had an odds ratio of 0.59 (95% Cl 0.42, 0.83) for ED. The practical clinical lesson is that primary care practitioners should have an increased index of suspicion for ED in mild-to-moderately obese men and those who do not engage in regular exercise.[22]

Not infrequently, the first and earliest manifestations of ED can present prior to the onset of such conditions as diabetes, heart disease, and prostate disease. This emphasizes the importance of fostering physician-patient communication regarding sexual health issues in men who otherwise appear to be in good health. In the course of a physician-generated history, these "healthy-appearing" patients may report they are experiencing a gradual and subtle—yet significant—deterioration in erectile function. It is important to identify this target group since, from the standpoint of patient selection and satisfaction, these men are highly motivated to optimize life quality parameters, of which sexual function is given high priority.

With respect to patient-identification, one can think about age-associated deterioration in erectile function in terms of the Erectile Dysfunction Morbidity Continuum (or Erectile Dysfunction Manifestation Continuum, EDMC). In this model, ED is viewed as a spectrum disease that begins with minimal abnormalities in erectile function and terminates in complete impotence as the most severe manifestation of ED. According to this model, the chronological Erectile Dysfunction Morbidity Continuum (EDMC) begins with relative erectile competence at age 18 and incremental deterioration to near complete erectile dysfunction in a significant percentage of individuals by age 90. Although the etiology of declining erectile function has not been precisely delineated, it may be the result of evolving co-morbid conditions and/or age-related factors.

Each of the symptoms suggestive of ED can be evaluated—and to some degree quantitated based on patient impressions—by using the SHIM tool. *(Please see Table 2.)* In fact, the diagnosis of ED usually can be made in less than 3 minutes. These manifestations may include, but are not limited to, ability to achieve an erection, hardness of erection, ability to achieve an erection rapidly, maintaining an erection, maintaining an erection for sufficiently long periods to complete intercourse, and general level of satisfaction with sexual activity.

In summary, a systematic inquiry regarding sexual health is especially important in individuals known to have risk factors for ED. These include diabetes, hypertension, hyperlipidemia, smoking, and depression. In addition a thorough inquiry regarding sexual health is especially important in all individuals taking antihypertensive and psychotropic medications.

Younger Patients with ED: High Prevalence and Priority, High Satisfaction Rate, and Optimal Outcomes and Safety Profile

Because ED has been linked to comorbid conditions such as diabetes, heart disease, and prostate disease—conditions that are more likely to involve older patients—many physicians have failed to appreciate the importance and clinical benefits of diagnosing and treating ED in men who are in their 30s, and 40s, as well as those individuals 50 years and older. Ironically, men who indicate that they are participating in sexual activity frequently are excellent candidates for screening with a SHIM and, when indicated, treatment with sildenafil therapy; for reasons outlined below, these individuals require a quick and efficient history to identify the possibility of ED.

Although the rationale for screening sexually active men may not be immediately obvious, the fact is, sexually active individuals can still suffer from mild, perceptible, but clinically and functionally significant impairments of erectile function. In other words, simply because a patient indicates he is participating in sexual activity does not mean that erectile function is unimpaired. Consequently, even when the history indicates a man is participating in sexual activity, a SHIM is still absolutely necessary, because a significant percentage (up to 35%) of these individuals will still meet clinical/diagnostic criteria for ED.[3,5,24,25]

The precise prevalence of ED among younger patients has been clarified in an epidemiological, population-based survey conducted in Northeastern Brazil.[24] Although this population may have charcteristics different from those seen in U.S. males, the findings in this study reveal important ED prevalence data that is applicable to male populations in general, including those in the United States. The investigators conducted a population-based survey in a cluster sample of men 40 to 70 years of age, using a 25-30 minute interviewer administered questionnaire. Of the 602 men eventually studied, some degree of ED characterized as between "minimal and complete" was found in 40% of the overall subjects questioned. Not unexpectedly, the prevalence of ED was associated with age ($p < 0.000$), but the rates of ED among younger men was much higher than primary care physicians might anticipate. The rate of ED increased from 28.5% in men between the ages 40-44, to 32% (ages 45-49), 47.5% (ages 50-54), 40.4% (ages 55-59), 57.5% (ages 60-64) and 5.4% (ages 65-70).(26) From a patient detection perspective, it is interesting to note that such lifestyle characteristics as caffeine consumption ($p = 0.050$ and alcohol use ($p = 0.001$) were significantly associated with ED. The authors concluded that ED is a common health problem in men aged 40-70, and that younger populations are also at significant risk for this condition.

Patient satisfaction tends to be high in the younger patient with ED. Because younger men generally are more sexually active than older men, those individuals between the ages of 30 and 55 with documented ED, even in its milder forms, are likely to derive greater benefits-from overall patient satisfaction to improved mood-over the long term than a cohort of elderly men with multiple comorbid conditions, in whom sexual activity may play a less important role in day-to-day life. Thus, the clinical importance of screening and aggressive treatment of younger individuals with ED cannot be overemphasized.

A recent study conducted in the Netherlands demonstrated that both in the eyes of patients and in the eyes of the general public the enhanced quality of life effects afforded by sildenafil is perceived as substantial.

Communicate, Evaluate, and Medicate

Multiple studies have shown that, when it comes to a sexual history, primary care physicians are not engaging their patients often enough in discussions related to their state of sexual health, and, specifically, about matters related to erectile function. A recent investigation has confirmed that patients may be reluctant to communicate important information about their sexual health, unless they perceive their physicians are receptive to such discussions. One study confirms that 7 out of 10 people who ultimately are diagnosed with sexual dysfunction do not bring up their concerns during the course of a physical exam or history. In another survey, 40-50% of patients coming in to urology clinic for non-ED related problems had ED as a primary or co-diagnosis.

Once the diagnosis of ED is established, a detailed medical history may suggest one or more underlying etiologies. These include endocrinologic disease, psychiatric conditions, diabetes, vascular disease, and other etiologies. A detailed drug history is an essential part of an ED evaluation, since many commonly used drug classes have been associated with ED, among them, antihypertensives, antidepressants, and recreational drugs

Evaluation of Erectile Dysfunction in The Primary Care Setting. As with any medical condition, the initial evaluation relies on a detailed history and physical examination. An important aspect of the preliminary assessment is to determine if psychogenic factors are the principal causes of erectile dysfunction.[1,2] A thorough medical and sexual history should be performed. (*Please see Table 3.*) The physician should try to elicit social or psychological factors that could be potential causes of the problem. Particular attention should be given to medical conditions, medications, and history of prior pelvic surgical procedures. (*Please see Table 4.*) Physical examination should focus on abnormalities of sexual characteristics and inspection of the genitalia for evidence of trauma, plaques, or testicular abnormalities. A careful neurologic examination must be performed as well.

With respect to laboratory testing, there are differing views as to the recommended extent of testing. Some authors have advocated a complete laboratory work-up, including complete blood count, chemistries, and hormonal tests (testosterone, prolactin, etc.). Most clinicians, however, only obtain basic labs and pursue hormonal testing based on clinical suspicion.[25] In a recent study, one group recommended serum testosterone measurement in all impotent patients over age 50.[26] However, in patients younger than 50 years, these investigators advocated serum testosterone determination only in cases of low sexual desire and abnormal physical findings They also advocated serum prolactin measurement only in patients with low sexual desire, gynecomastia, and/or testosterone less than 4 ng/mL.[8]

Nocturnal penile tumescence (NPT) studies have been advocated as a method to differentiate between psychogenic and organic impotence. Although traditionally this has been a difficult test to perform (requiring the patient to stay in a sleep lab), machines like the Rigiscan allow for ambulatory monitoring of erections and rigidity. There is no consensus to the utility and validity of NPT studies, and numerous studies have deemed it unreliable.[27,28] Currently, this study is not as widely used as in previous years.

Emerging Pharmacotherapeutic Options: Questions to Ask and Issues to Consider When Comparing Newly Introduced Agents for ED with Currently Available Medications

New therapies are being developed for treatment of ED, and each agent considered for this condition requires careful scrutiny to evaluate efficacy, safety, and potentially serious adverse consequences. It is important to note that introduction to market

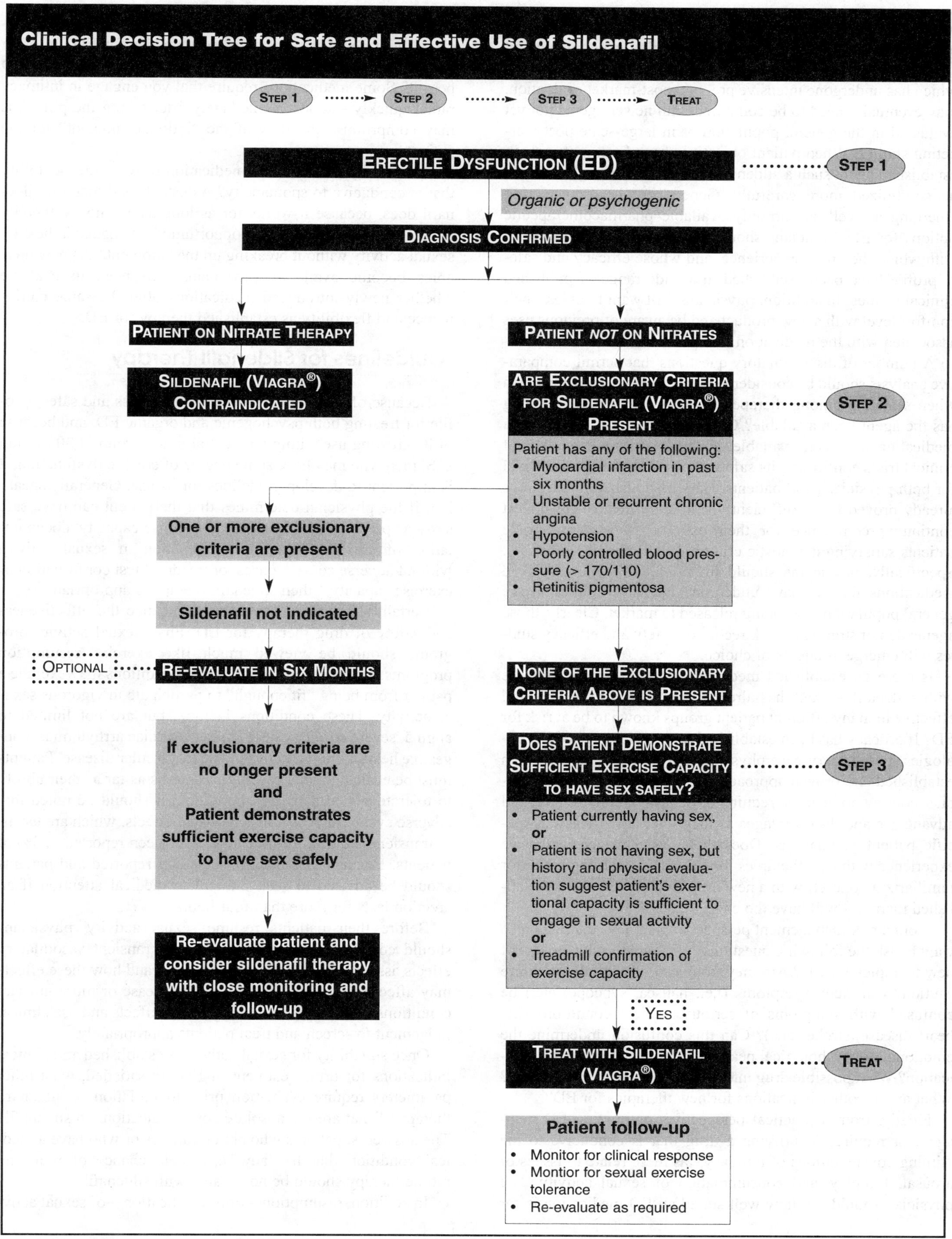
Clinical Decision Tree for Safe and Effective Use of Sildenafil
STEP 1
STEP 2
STEP 3
TREAT
ERECTILE DYSFUNCTION (ED)
STEP 1
Organic or psychogenic
DIAGNOSIS CONFIRMED
PATIENT ON NITRATE THERAPY
SILDENAFIL (VIAGRA®) CONTRAINDICATED
PATIENT NOT ON NITRATES
ARE EXCLUSIONARY CRITERIA FOR SILDENAFIL (VIAGRA®) PRESENT
STEP 2
Patient has any of the following:
• Myocardial infarction in past six months
• Unstable or recurrent chronic angina
• Hypotension
• Poorly controlled blood pressure (> 170/110)
• Retinitis pigmentosa
One or more exclusionary criteria are present
Sildenafil not indicated
OPTIONAL
RE-EVALUATE IN SIX MONTHS
If exclusionary criteria are no longer present and Patient demonstrates sufficient exercise capacity to have sex safely
Re-evaluate patient and consider sildenafil therapy with close monitoring and follow-up
NONE OF THE EXCLUSIONARY CRITERIA ABOVE IS PRESENT
DOES PATIENT DEMONSTRATE SUFFICIENT EXERCISE CAPACITY TO HAVE SEX SAFELY?
STEP 3
• Patient currently having sex, or
• Patient is not having sex, but history and physical evaluation suggest patient's exertional capacity is sufficient to engage in sexual activity or
• Treadmill confirmation of exercise capacity
YES
TREAT WITH SILDENAFIL (VIAGRA®)
TREAT
Patient follow-up
• Monitor for clinical response
• Montior for sexual exercise tolerance
• Re-evaluate as required

of a new medication for ED treatment was delayed because more data were required to establish its safety in certain patient subgroups. As such, the established safety profile of sildenafil, which has undergone intensive pre- and post-market evaluation, may eventually need to be compared with newer agents not yet evaluated in the general population or in large-scale post-marketing studies. When patient objectives have been met with an established agent such a sildenafil, use of a newer agent should be scrutinized more carefully. Generally, when considering emerging as well as currently available pharmacotherapeutic options for ED, clinicians should give priority to medications with which they have experience, and whose efficacy and safety profile have been established in a wide range of published clinical studies. In addition, physicians will want to assess their comfort level with a new product and be aware of previous uses associated with the medication.

A number of discriminatory questions that permit comparative analysis should be considered by the primary care physician when selecting among therapeutic options for ED. How long has the agent been available? Generally speaking, the longer a medication has been available, and the larger the number of clinical trials confirming its safety, the greater the comfort level for both physicians and patients. Have established medications already proved to be sufficiently safe and effective to support continuing confidence for their use? If so, all appropriate patients satisfying diagnostic criteria for ED should be treated. Specifically, physicians should investigate whether approved medications for ED have undergone intensive studies in the general population after being released to market. Clearly, those agents demonstrating a track record of safety and efficacy studies will emerge as agents of choice.

Is there an established medication for ED—as is the case with sildenafil—which has already been shown to be safe and effective in many different patient groups known to be at risk for ED? If efficacy has been established for a wide range of ED etiologies, the primary care physician may want to stay with an established and proven approach and recognize that new therapies coming to market require close evaluation of potential advantages and disadvantages as they relate to efficacy in specific patient populations. Does the physician have extensive experience with new therapies for ED? If the learning curve for familiarizing oneself with a new drug is likely to be slow, established therapies will have the edge.

From a risk management perspective, the physician will also want to ask the following questions: What are the side effects of new therapies for ED? Are they troublesome enough to require caution? Can such symptoms (i.e., nausea, syncope, etc.) be confused with symptoms of serious medical conditions (i.e. heart disease, stroke, etc.)? Can this confusion undermine the emotional or psychological peace of mind when using the medication? What possible drug interactions do new therapies have? What are the other indications for new therapies for ED?

Finally, from a practical perspective, optimizing ED management requires identifying a drug that is conducive to the "timing considerations of intimacy," as these relate to issues of arousal, foreplay, and consummation of sexual activity. The physician should ask how well suited an ED medication is for the patient's intimate needs. What are the time constraints associated with new versus established therapies for ED? In other words, how much time for intimacy does a medication for ED permit? Some medications require that you engage in intimacy rather quickly—almost immediately after taking the pill. This may compromise the flow of the "intimate moment" for the patient.

Specifically, does an ED medication provide the flexibility that is conducive to spontaneity? As established therapy, sildenafil does, because it works for as long as 3-4 hours, thereby opening a longer "window of opportunity" to engage in healthy sexual activity without breaking up the "moment." As new therapies become available, physicians will need to evaluate whether newly introduced medications offer the same convenience and flexibility as established therapy for ED.

Guidelines for Sildenafil Therapy

Because of sildenafil's proven effectiveness and safety profile for treating both psychogenic and organic ED, and because of its growing use within a potential target group of 30 million U.S. men who may have some degree of erectile dysfunction, it is important to develop guidelines for its use. Generally speaking, if the physician determines that the patient can have safe sex—as predicted by the patient's exercise capacity, documentation of current or recent participation in sexual activity without adverse consequences, or treadmill test confirmation of exercise capacity—then sildenafil therapy is appropriate.

Certain strategies, however, will enhance the effectiveness and safety of drug therapy for ED. First, sexual activity programs should be viewed much like exercise resumption programs. In this regard, a number of conditions may exclude a patient from being "fit enough" to participate in vigorous sexual activity. These conditions include, but are not limited to angina, severe coronary heart disease, cardiac arrhythmias, congestive heart failure, COPD, and neurovascular disease. Patients must be evaluated on a case-by-case basis as far as their ability to tolerate sexual activity. In addition, it should be noted that adverse events such as transient visual effects, which are usually transient and mild-to-moderate, have been reported in 3% of patients. Priapism has been infrequently reported and patients should be advised to seek immediate medical attention if an erection lasts for more than four hours.

Before their patients resume sexual activity, physicians should consider the possible mild and transient vasodilatory effects associated with sildenafil therapy, and how these effects may affect underlying cardiovascular disease or more unusual conditions. Physicians should note these effects and use clinical judgement to screen and treat patients appropriately.

Once suitability for sexual activity is established and clinical indications for drug treatment of ED are satisfied, what other parameters require evaluation prior to initiation of sildenafil therapy? What are the absolute contraindications to sildenafil? The answer is, patients who are on nitrates or who have a medical condition that has any reasonable chance of requiring nitrate therapy should be not treated with sildenafil.

In addition, resumption—or intensification—of sexual activity requires counseling from the physician, as would any exercise resumption program. Physiological safety is a prerequisite to pharmacological safety. The physician should instruct the patient to start low and increase activity gradually. Specifically, patients on a "sexual resumption program" should be counseled to resume activity on a measured basis. Initially, for example, the patient may be encouraged to use sildenafil on day one and then evaluate their toleration to sexual exertion over the next day or two. Additional use of this drug to treat ED should accelerate at a moderate pace—one that is commensurate with the patient's exercise capacity and that avoids overexertion. The key point is that the sexual activity resumption program should be tailored to the patient's specific needs and exercise tolerance.

In conclusion, sildenafil (Viagra®) is a highly effective and safe medication in individuals who, on the basis of a sexual history—and, when necessary, noninvasive confirmation of adequate exercise capacity commensurate with exertional demands of sexual activity—require treatment for ED. From a practical perspective, this condition is underdiagnosed, and therefore, undertreated. This is the case for both older and younger men with ED. Consequently, a routine, systematic, and time-efficient screening approach in the primary care setting will identify a large number of patient subgroups who meet the diagnostic criteria of ED, and who can benefit from sildenafil therapy. This population includes both younger and older men, patients with and without comorbid conditions, and individuals who report they are "having sexual activity," but who upon more thorough screening (i.e., SHIM) will meet the criteria for ED. High-benefit, low-risk therapy with sildenafil treatment in the primary care setting should be extended to all eligible patients meeting diagnostic criteria for ED.

References

1. O'Keefe M, Hunt DK. Assessment and treatment of impotence. *Med Clin North Am* 1995;79:415-434.
2. Butler RN, Lewis MI, Hoffman E, et al. Love and sex after 60: How to evaluate and treat the impotent older man. A roundtable discussion: Part 2. *Geriatrics* 1994;49:27-32.
3. Feldman HA, Goldstein I, Hatzichristou DG, et al. Impotence and its medical and psychological correlates: Results of the Massachusetts male aging study. *J Urol* 1994;151:54-61.
4. Gillenwater JY. International impotence education month, November 1997. *AUA News* 1997;2:11.
5. Overmyer M. Impotence clinics find what medicine has overlooked. *Urology Times* 1996;24:1.
6. Benson GS, Boileau MA. The penis: Sexual function and dysfunction. In: Gillenwater JY, Grayhack JT, Howards SS, Duckett JW, (eds): *Adult and Pediatric Urology*, Third Ed. St. Louis: Mosby; 1996:1951-1995.
7. Carrier S, Brock G, Kour NW, et al. Pathophysiology of erectile dysfunction. *Urology* 1993:42:468-481.
8. Lue TF. Impotence: A patient's goal-directed approach to treatment. *World J Urol* 1990;8:67-72.
9. Jarow JP, Nana-Sinkam P, Sabbagh M, et al. Outcome analysis of goal directed therapy for impotence. *J Urol* 1996;155: 1609-1612.
10. Lewis RW, Barrett DM. Modern management of male erectile dysfunction. AUA Update Series, 1995, Vol XIV, Lesson 20, pp 162-167.
11. Chaabouni MN, Mhiri MN, Hassan T, et al. Diagnostic and therapeutic approach in organic impotence. *Ann Urol* (Paris) 1994;28:148-156.
12. Chaabouni MN, Mhiri MN, Hassan T, et al. Diagnostic and therapeutic approach in organic impotence. *Ann Urol* (Paris) 1994;28:148-156.
13. Randall Zussman, MD, *American Journal of Cardiology*, March 4, 1999.
14. Vardi Y, Bulus M, et al. Ergometric studies for evaluating sildenafil effect in cardiac patients. May 2, 2000. American Urological Association 95th Annual Meeting. Abstract No. 886. Atlanta, Georgia
15. Olsson AM, Personn CA. Sildenafil Citrate for the treatment or erectile dysfunction in men with cardiovascular disease. Abstract 888. May 2, 2000. Americal Urological Association 95th Annual Meeting. Atlanta, Georgia
16. Mittleman M, Glasser DB, et al. Incidence of Myocardial Infarction and Death in 53 Clinical Trials of Viagra® (Sildenafil Citrate). Oral Presentation, Session 807. March 14, 2000. American College of Cardiology 49th Annual Scientific Session; Anaheim, California.
17. Olsson AM, Persson, CA, for Swedish Sildenafil Investigators Group. Efficacy and Safety of Viagra® in Men With Cardiovascular Disease and Erectile Dysfunction. Poster Presentation-Session 1202, March 15, 2000. American College of Cardiology 49th Annual Scientific Session; Anaheim, California.
18. Herrman HC, et al. Safety of Viagra® in Men With Heart Disease. *N Engl J Med* 2000; 342: 1622-1626.
19. Boulton AJM, et al. Viagra® Efficacy Patients with Type II Diabetes. American Diabetes Association 60th Scientific Session. San Antonio, Texas.
20. Blonde L, et al. Oschner Medical Clinic. Efficacy of Viagra® on Erectile Function in Type I and Type II Diabetes. American Diabetes Association 60th Scientific Session. San Antonio, Texas.
21. Guay AT, et al. Viagra®-related Adverse Events in Patients with Type I and II diabetes. American Diabetes Association 60th Scientific Session. San Antonio, Texas.
22. Rimm EB, Bacon CG, et al. Body weight, physical activity, and alcohol consumption in relation to erectile dysfunction among U.S. male health professional free of major chronic diseases. Abstract No. 1073. American Urological Association 95th Annual Meeting, May 1, 2000. Atlanta, Georgia.
23. Rosas SE, Joffe BL, et al. Prevalence of erectile dysfunction in hemodialysis patients. American Urological Association 95th Annual Meeting, May 1, 2000. Atlanta, Georgia.
24. Moreira ED, Glasser DB. A cross-sectional population-based study of erectile dysfunction epidemiology in Northeastern Brazil. Abstract No. 65. American Urological Association 95th Annual Meeting, April 29, 2000. Atlanta, Georgia.
25. Johnson AR 3d, Jarow JP. Is routine endocrine testing of impotent men necessary? *J Urol* 1992;147:1542-1543.
26. Buvat J, Lemaire A. Endocrine screening in 1,022 men with erectile dysfunction: Clinical significance and cost-effective

strategy. *J Urol* 1997;158:1764-1767.

27. Djamilian M, Stief CG, Hartmann U, et al. Predictive value of real-time RigiScan monitoring for the etiology of organogenic impotence. *J Urol* 1993;149:1269-1271.
28. Steers WD. Impotence evaluation (editorial). *J Urol* 1993; 149:1284.
29. Lehmann K, Schopke W, Hauri D. Subclinical trauma to perineum: A possible etiology of erectile dysfunction in young men. *Eur Urol* 1995;27:306-310.
30. Bemelmans BL, Meuleman EJ, Doesburg WH, et al. Erectile dysfunction in diabetic men: The neurological factor revisited. *J Urol* 1994;151:884-889.
31. Borirakchanyavat S, Lue TF. Evaluation of impotence. *Infec Urol* 1997;10:12-23.
32. Kaufman JM, Borges FD, Fitch WP 3d, et al. Evaluation of erectile dysfunction by dynamic infusion cavernosometry and cavernosography (DICC). Multi-institutional study. *Urology* 1993;41:445-451.
33. Yaman LS, Kilic S, Sarica K, et al. The place of acupuncture in the management of psychogenic impotence. *Eur Urol* 1994; 26:52-55.
34. Morales A, Johnston B, Heaton JW, et al. Oral androgens in the treatment of hypogonadal impotent men. *J Urol* 1994;152: 1115-1118.
35. Montague DK, Barada JH, Belker AM, et al. Clinical guidelines panel on erectile dysfunction: Summary report on the treatment of organic erectile dysfunction. *J Urol* 1996;156:2007-2011.
36. Raifer J. Impotence: The quick work-up (editorial). *J Urol* 1996;156:1951.
37. Cookson MS, Nadif PW. Long-term results with vacuum constriction device. *J Urol* 1993;149:290-294.
38. Stolk, E, Jan, JV, et al. The Impact of Erectile Dysfunction on Quality of Life. May 2, 2000. Abstract No 1070; Americal Urological Association 95th Annual Meeting. Atlanta, Georgia.

Acute Scrotal Pain

Robert Schwab, MD

Most emergency physicians will encounter several patients with testicular torsion during their careers, and undoubtedly they will see others with undifferentiated scrotal pain.[1] However, few physicians can rely on experience when making diagnostic and therapeutic decisions. Instead, clinicians mush develop a rational stepwise approach to patients with acute scrotal pain.

Unfortunately, there are no precise guidelines for the management of patients with acute scrotal pain. The history and physical examination are often unreliable, even in the hands of experienced practitioners.[2,3] Diagnostic studies are helpful but 1) are not universally available, 2) often fail to provide definitive information, and 3) are surrounded by disagreement as to which is most reliable. And all agree that none of the available studies is 100% accurate.[4,7]

Furthermore, the delay associated with performing and interpreting these studies may lead to loss of testicular function, prompting some urologists to recommend operative exploration in all cases.[8] Other urologic authorities point out that such a policy results in unnecessary surgery and its attendant risks in an unacceptably large number of patients.[9]

The following discussion provides physicians with information that clarifies decision making in cases of acute scrotal pain. The author begins with a review of the relevant anatomy of the scrotum and scrotal contents and discusses risk factors and pathogenesis related to the development of common scrotal disorders. The chapter continues with a discussion of the utility of available diagnostic studies and indications for their use and concludes by presenting a rational approach to the diagnosis and management of acute scrotal emergencies.

Acute Scrotal Emergencies: Etiology and Pathophysiology

Testicular Torsion. The yearly incidence of testicular torsion is estimated at one case per 4,000 males younger than 25 years old.[10] There are two distinct peaks of incidence: 1) in newborns and 2) in teenagers (between 12 and 16 years of age).[11] However, in one study, 20% of patients between the ages of 20 and 29 with acute scrotal pain were found to have testicular torsion,[8] and cases of testicular torsion have been documented in men older than age 40.[12,13]

Neonatal testicular torsion is not associated with definable anatomic abnormalities but is thought to occur as a result of general laxity of the gubernacular attachment of the testis to the scrotal floor.[14] Conversely, developmental abnormalities are thought to play an essential role in the occurrence of testicular torsion in all other age groups. Abnormal inferior and posterior attachment of the testis to the scrotal floor and posterior wall by an overly long mesorchium can predispose to torsion, as can a tunica vaginalis that invests the entire testicle and a portion of the distal spermatic cord. This anatomical

Figure 1. Anatomic Variations in Testicular Torsion

A B C D

A, Normal anatomy. B, The "bell-clapper" deformity. C, Loose epididymal attachment to the testis. D, Torsed testis with transverse lie.

Used with permission: Edelsberg JS, Surh YS. The acute scrotum. *Emerg Med Clin N Am* 1988;6:521.

Figure 2. Torsion of Appendages

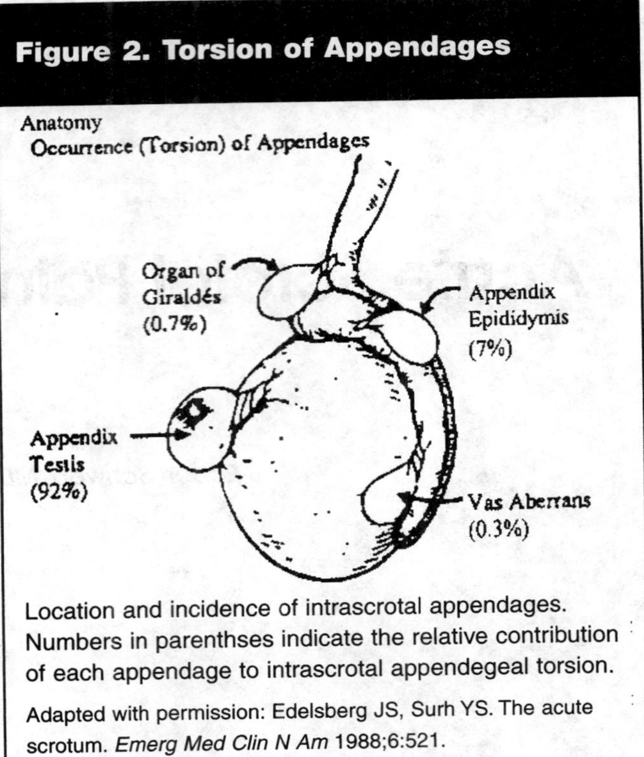

Location and incidence of intrascrotal appendages. Numbers in parenthses indicate the relative contribution of each appendage to intrascrotal appendegeal torsion.

Adapted with permission: Edelsberg JS, Surh YS. The acute scrotum. *Emerg Med Clin N Am* 1988;6:521.

variant is designated as the "bellclapper" deformity. *(Please see Figure 1.)*

The event precipitating torsion may include trauma, certain body movements, or cremasteric muscle contraction.[11] Rotation of the testicle most commonly occurs in a lateral-to-medial direction and may involve 90 to 140 degrees of rotation.[14] Venous congestion and edema precede arterial occlusion, which leads to ischemia and hemorrhagic infarction.[14]

Tissue changes and, ultimately, testicular function are closely related to the duration of torsion. In an animal model, loss of Sertoli cell (sperm-producing) function was demonstrable after four to six hours of ischemia, and Leydig cell (testosterone-producing) function persisted for approximately 10 hours.[15] Several studies suggest a similar pattern in human testicular torsion, with testicular salvage rates of approximately 80% or better in patients operated on within six hours of the onset of pain.[8,11,14-17] Patients operated on after 10 hours of symptoms showed a testicular salvage rate of only 20%, and after 24 hours, salvage was almost nonexistent.[11,15-20]

These studies defined "salvage" as the absence of atrophy on follow-up but did not investigate testicular function. It appears that testicular exocrine function declines rapidly with ischemia and that fertility is adversely affected regardless of duration of torsion." Additionally, some evidence suggests that testes predisposed to torsion have reduced baseline sperm counts,[21] making them even more vulnerable to brief periods of ischemia.

Despite these data, reports of testicular salvage in patients with symptoms for longer than 24 hours exist.[22] The number of twists in the cord influence the rapidity of ischemia and infarction,[23] as does the occurrence of intermittent torsion." Moreover. spontaneous detorsion may occur. Because none of these conditions can be assessed reliably pre-operatively. it is impossible to recommend withholding exploration on the basis of symptom duration alone.[19]

Appendage Torsion. Four testicular appendages have been identified: the appendix testis, the appendix epididymis, the paradidymis (organ of Giraldes), and the vas aberrans. *(Please see Figure 2.)* The appendix testis accounts for over 90% of all cases of appendage torsion, with the appendix epididymis being involved in nearly all the remaining cases.[25,26] The appendix testis is particularly susceptible to torsion because it is attached to the testis by a stalk.[25]

The peak incidence of appendage torsion occurs between ages 10 and 13[25,26] but also has been documented in older patients.[27] The majority of cases are associated with vigorous activity or local trauma.[25] Torsion leads to the progression from venous congestion and edema to arterial occlusion, ischemia, and infarction of the appendage. Edema and inflammation of adjacent structures, including formation of a reactive hydrocele, result in diffuse swelling of the scrotal contents.[25-27]

Epididymitis affects over 500,000 patients per year in the United States.[28] Young adults between the ages of 19 and 35 are affected most commonly, although it is not unusual to encounter infants, adolescents, and older men presenting with this malady.[28,29] Although previously thought to be a disease of primarily idiopathic origin, it is now accepted that a causative organism can be identified in over 80% of patients with acute epididymitis.[30,31]

The pathogenesis and management are influenced by the patient's age. Nearly half of prepubertal patients with epididymitis have associated urogenital anomalies.[28,32] One example involves enterovesicular fistula with resulting coliform infection of the urine and epididymis.[32]

Sexually transmitted pathogens predominate in the 19 to 35 age group. However, because young males are becoming sexually active at an earlier age, teenagers may present with epididymitis caused by sexually transmitted organisms before as well as at puberty. *Chlamydia trachomatis* is the most common organism isolated, found in one-third to over one-half of affected patients in the 19 to 35 age group.[31,33-37] *Neisseria gonorrhoeae* is the next most common.[30] The role of *Ureaplasma urealyticum* in epididymitis is unclear, but it may be a causative agent in sexually active males.[26]

Patients older than age 40 most commonly have coliform epididymitis secondary to a urinary tract infection and may demonstrate an underlying urogenital abnormality.[28] Many of these patients develop epididymitis following a genitourinary procedure.[29]

Regardless of patient age or etiologic agent, the pathogenesis frequently involves direct extension of infected urine through the vas deferens to the epididymis.[28,38] Entry into the ejaculatory duct and vas deferens may be facilitated by conditions that distort the prostatic urethra or ejaculatory duct, including distal urethral obstruction, prostate surgery, detrusor-sphincter dyssynergia, and inflammatory changes secondary to infection.[28] Recent urodynamic research suggests that elevated voiding pressure alone (without evidence of distal obstruction) may be a predisposing factor in the development of epididymitis.[39]

Other infectious agents include *Mycobacterium tuberculosis*, which can occur inpatients with systemic tuberculosis or after topical therapy for bladder cancer;[40] *Haemophilus influenzae*; *Trichomonas vaginalis*; and *Brucella* species.[28,41] Epididymitis also has been reported as a side effect of amiodarone therapy.[42]

Other Conditions. Emergency physicians should be aware of several other important causes of scrotal pain. Tumors, either intra- or extratesticular, may cause pain as a result of necrosis, hemorrhage, or pressure on surrounding structures. Orchitis may result from viral infection; bacterial extension from epididymitis; or, on occasion, syphilis, mycobacteria, or fungal infection. Mumps is the most common viral etiology; orchitis occurs in 15% to 30% of postpubertal males with mumps.

A hydrocele may represent fluid within the tunica vaginalis or within a remnant of the peritoneal diverticulum forming the inguinal canal. Most are painless, so clinicians should consider the possibility of underlying infection or malignancy with a painful scrotal mass. Likewise, a painful varicocele, or dilated spermatic cord veins, suggests the presence of retroperitoneal pathology. Hematoma is usually the result of trauma but also may occur in patients with blood dyscrasias or tumors. Vasculitis of the scrotum and scrotal contents may occur in patients with Henoch-Schonlein purpura.

Cutaneous pathology also may cause acute scrotal pain. infection with herpes simplex virus type 2 may cause pain that typically begins two to four days before the appearance of an erythematous, vesicular rash. A scrotal wall abscess may occur due to minor trauma or poor hygiene. Fournier's gangrene also known as Fournier's necrotizing fasciitis) is one of the most serious of all scrotal pathologies and is a true urologic emergency. A mixed aerobic and anaerobic necrotizing subcutaneous infection produces dermal gangrene and massive scrotal swelling. Usually occurring secondary to perirectal disease or minor trauma, with a predilection for diabetic or uncompromised patients, this syndrome has a mortality ate exceeding 20%.[43]

Important referred sources of scrotal pain include an ilioinguinal hernia. a leaking abdominal aortic aneurysm, renal alculi, and ilioinguinal-iliohypogastric nerve entrapment.

Correlation Between Age and Etiology. Despite numerous studies,[2,8,9,45-48] definitive conclusions regarding the final diagnoses of patients presenting with acute scrotal pain cannot be given. There has been no prospective study of all such patients presenting to the emergency department; most recommendations for management are based on retrospective series involving admitted pediatric patients. However, available data indicate that the relative probabilities of testicular torsion, torsion of a testicular appendage, and epididymitis vary dramatically with the age of the patient.

Acute scrotal pathology is uncommon in children younger than 10 years old,[8] with the exception of extravaginal testicular torsion, which occurs in the neonate. In children 10 to 19 years of age, testicular torsion accounts for 20% to 40% of all cases,[8,9,49] with torsion of an appendage accounting for an equal percentage. Among patients age 20 to 29, torsion accounts for approximately 20% of cases,[8] with epididymitis accounting for 75% of patients presenting with acute scrotal pain in this age group. After age 30, epididymitis accounts for nearly all cases of acute scrotal pain,[8] with hernia and referred pain the next most common etiologies. Torsion has been reported in this age group but is rare.[12,50]

Expediting Accurate Assessment and Prompt Diagnosis

Recognizing Life-threatening Conditions. As with any presenting complaint, the initial ED assessment of the patient with non-traumatic scrotal pain is directed toward detection of life-threatening conditions. After ensuring adequate airway, breathing, and circulation, clinicians immediately should consider three conditions: Foumier's gangrene, ruptured or leaking abdominal aortic aneurysm, and strangulated inguinal hernia.

In its fullest form, Fournier's gangrene presents as scrotal swelling, erythema, and crepitus, usually associated with systemic toxicity, in a diabetic or otherwise immunosuppressed patient. The presence of a pulsatile mass or abdominal bruit or inequality of femoral pulsations in a patient with longstanding hypertension should suggest abdominal aortic aneurysm with referred pain to the scrotum. A strangulated inguinal hernia usually can be differentiated from primary scrotal pathology by its position high in the scrotum and by the presence of a normal testis inferior to the swelling. The presence of fever and peritoneal signs suggests strangulation of an incarcerated hernia.

Obtaining Clues from the History. After ruling out these three life-threatening conditions, the emergency physician must distinguish between testicular torsion, torsion of a scrotal appendage, epididymitis, or other scrotal pathology.

Ask about the onset and character of the pain. Sudden severe pain is more typical of torsion, whereas patients with epididymitis generally report a gradual onset of discomfort, which can progress to severe pain. Inquire about the presence of fever, chills, penile discharge, or dysuria, which suggests an infectious disease. Note any recent history of trauma, viral syndrome (especially mumps), or urologic procedures, and obtain a sexual history.

Past medical history should focus on congenital urologic abnormalities, genitourinary infections, or other urologic problems. A previous episode of similar scrotal pain that resolved spontaneously suggests spontaneous detorsion. If the patient has had testicular torsion previously, with or especially without orchiopexy, then recurrent torsion is extremely likely. Inquire about conditions that predispose to infection, such as diabetes mellitus, human immunodeficiency virus infection, chemotherapy, radiation therapy, or chronic immunosuppressive therapy.

Performing a systematic physical examination. Physical examination of the patient with acute scrotal pain is difficult because of the extreme sensitivity of the scrotal contents, as well as the patient's anxiety. However, a careful examination is mandatory in

Table 1. Clinical Risk Factors for Testicular Torsion[2]

High Risk
1. Palpable knot in spermatic cord
2. Abnormal testicular (epididymal) position or lie (either testicle)
3. Previous torsion without orchiopexy

Moderate Risk
1. Sudden onset, without antecedent symptoms
2. Nausea and/or vomiting
3. Age 10 to 19
4. Previous torsion with orchiopexy
5. Swollen, tender testicle
6. History of spontaneously resolving similar episodes

order to make accurate evaluation and treatment decisions. At times, the urologic consultant may need to perform an anesthetic spermatic cord block to relieve severe pain and allow an adequate examination of the scrotal contents.

Observe the scrotum for evidence of erythema, swelling, ecchymosis, skin lesions, and asymmetry. Erythema, warmth, and induration of the scrotum is consistent with cellulitis but is commonly present with epididymitis or testicular torsion. Look for a small area of bluish discoloration beneath the scrotal skin this may indicate torsion of a scrotal appendage. Transillumination of the scrotal contents also may reveal the "blue dot" sign. In the absence of swelling, observe the lie and relative position of the two testes with the patient standing. Because congenital anomalies predisposing to torsion usually are bilateral, transverse lie of the unaffected testicle is indirect evidence strongly supporting the diagnosis of torsion.

Palpate the scrotal contents gently but thoroughly, beginning on the unaffected side. Note areas of tenderness or crepitus as well as the relative positions of the testes. Epididymitis usually is associated with an obviously enlarged, markedly tender epididymis in conjunction with a nontender or minimally tender and normally positioned testis. In epididymo-orchitis, however, the distinction between epididymal and testicular swelling and tenderness is less obvious.

With testicular torsion, the affected testicle is enlarged, tender. and retracted superiorly relative to the unaffected side. The epididymis usually is tender, and rarely, a knot is palpable in the spermatic cord itself. Additional clues to the presence of torsion include abnormal axis of the testis and abnormal position of the epididymis relative to the contralateral testis. *(Please see Table 1.)* Exacerbation or palliation of the pain with elevation of the affected testicle (Prehn's sign) cannot reliably distinguish epididymitis from torsion.[3,14]

Torsion of a testicular appendage can be difficult to distinguish from testicular torsion. Pain from a twisted appendage is similar to, but usually much less severe than testicular torsion. Patients frequently wait several days before persistence of pain prompts them to seek medical care. The key feature of diagnosis is point tenderness over the superior pole of the involved testis or epididymis with a normal examination of the contralateral scrotal contents.

Testicular tumors are identified by the presence of a firm, irregular contour of the testicle. Significant tenderness in the presence of a tumor suggests hemorrhage into the tumor.

Examine the penis, looking for urethral inflammation or discharge, which suggests the presence of infection. Inspect the groin for skin lesions and evidence of cellulitis. Gently palpate the inguinal canal for evidence of hernia or inguinal adenopathy. Examine the abdomen, seeking areas of localized tenderness, muscle guarding, or rebound tenderness. Rectal examination is mandatory in all patients with scrotal pain to rule out prostatitis, which may be associated with epididymitis.

A normal scrotal examination in a patient with scrotal pain suggests referred pain, most often from the upper urinary tract. Diagnoses to be considered include nephrolithiasis, perinephric abscess, pyelonephritis, or renal mass. Abdominal pathology and inguinal hernias also can cause scrotal pain, as can entrapment or irritation of the ilioinguinal, iliohypogastric, or genitofemoral nerves.

Clinical Assessment Determines Immediate Intervention

Based on the history and physical examination, the emergency physician must estimate the likelihood of the patient having testicular torsion. Any patient with sudden onset of pain; a swollen tender testicle; and abnormal position or lie of either testicle requires emergent urologic consultation and should undergo operative exploration of the scrotum without further diagnostic studies.

Patients older than age 20 with a non-tender testicle and an obviously swollen, tender epididymis likewise do not require additional diagnostic studies except for a urinalysis, urethral Gram's stain and culture for *N. gonorrhoeae*, and immunofluorescence smear or culture for *C. trachomatis*. Clinicians should examine midstream urine for pyuria or bacteriuria and should send the sample for culture and sensitivity.

The presence of pyuria does not reliably indicate infection, but bacteriuria or positive urethral discharge Gram's stain in a patient with scrotal tenderness suggests the diagnosis of epididymitis. Patients between the ages of 10 and 19 and those with an unreliable or uncertain examination require urologic consultation and possibly further diagnostic studies. *(Please see Figure 3.)*

Adjunctive Diagnostic Studies: Indications and Limitations

Proper use of adjunctive diagnostic studies in the patient with acute scrotal pain and swelling requires that the clinician keep in mind one key principle: Testicular torsion is a clinical diagnosis. If the emergency physician is unable to exclude testicular torsion with absolute certainly, immediate urologic consultation is indicated 1) to evaluate the need for urgent scrotal exploration and 2) to determine the appropriateness of obtaining available diagnostic studies in patients not considered candidates for acute exploration (i.e., those in whom a clinical diagnosis other than torsion is considered).

Doppler Ultrasound Stethoscope. The Doppler stethoscope is a rapid, noninvasive bedside procedure that the emergency physician should perform in all patients with acute scrotal pain. The

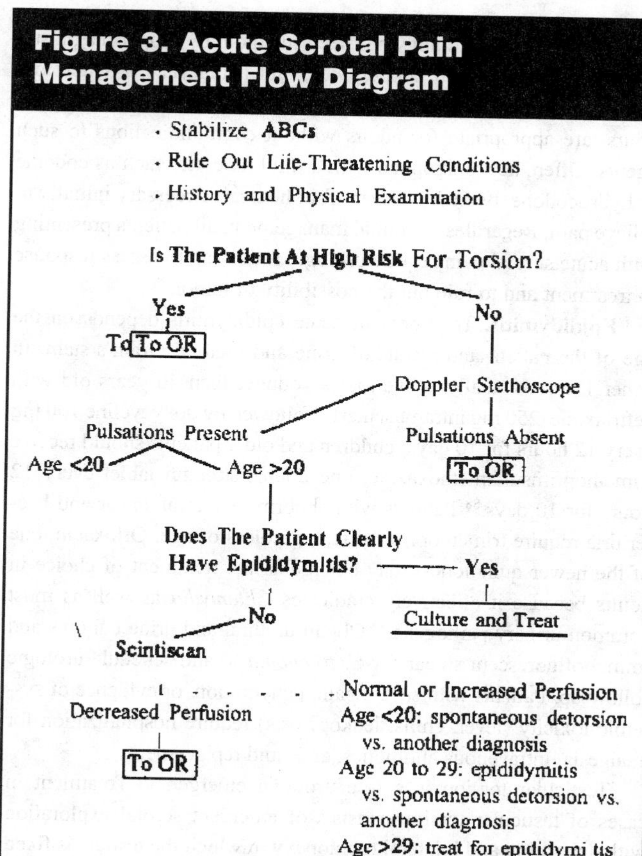

theoretical utility of the Doppler examination is based on its ability to detect pulsatile blood flow. The stethoscope is inexpensive and small, and the technique is simple and reproducible.

To perform the Doppler test, gently grasp the scrotum above the testicle, stretching the scrotal skin tightly over the testicle. Apply the Doppler probe over the inferior testicular pole, and auscultate for blood flow, Absence of pulsatile blood flow suggests testicular torsion and is an indication for surgical exploration. The presence of pulsatile blood flow may indicate an intact blood supply to the testicle or may represent auscultation of scrotal wall blood flow.

To differentiate between the two sources, use the *funicular compression test.*[52] With the Doppler probe in place, compress the spermatic cord. Disappearance of pulsatile blood flow with compression confirms the presence of testicular blood supply. Always examine the unaffected testicle to compare the quality of blood flow to the two testicles.

Early studies of the Doppler examination reported 100% accuracy in differentiating torsion from epididymitis.[52-56] Subsequent large clinical series have identified a significant incidence of false-negative Doppler studies, especially in patients presenting after 24 hours of pain.[4,57,58] Data from these studies suggest that the overall diagnostic accuracy of Doppler examination is approximately 80% but that its sensitivity is an unacceptably low 45% to 60%.[59]

The diagnostic accuracy of the study diminishes with later presentations[4,58,60] largely because of relative hyperemia. However, even early presentations may be undetected because of either partially intact blood supply or detection of blood flow proximal to the site of torsion.[58] *(Please see Figure 4.)* Unfortunately, funicular compression would not have excluded these false-negative examinations.

Figure 4. Misleading Doppler Examination

Diagram shows misleading case owing to reflection of ultrasonic waves by funicular blood flow in vessels proximal to torsion.

Used with permission: Rodriquez DD, Rodriguez WC, Riveria JJ, et al. Doppler ultrasound versus testicular scanning in the evaluation of the acute scrotum. *J Urol* 1981;125343.

Clearly, Doppler examinations that detect pulsatile blood flow are not sufficient to rule out the diagnosis of torsion and should not by themselves determine further evaluation or therapy. Conversely, the unilateral absence of flow in the proper clinical context is a strong indication for surgical exploration.

Radionuclide scintigraphy has been cited as the most useful diagnostic adjunct in the emergency evaluation and management of patients with acute scrotal pain.[6,22,61] In some centers, the test requires less than 30 minutes to complete, and widespread applicability is limited only by equipment and technician availability.

Testicular scanning alone cannot provide anatomic details and precise diagnoses, so clinicians should use it only to assess the perfusion status of the scrotum and scrotal contents.

Diagnostic Accuracy. Numerous studies investigating the utility of testicular scanning in the evaluation of the acute scrotum have demonstrated a sensitivity for detecting testicular torsion of approximately 90% or greater.[24,61-69] False-negative examinations have occurred because of technical errors and, more importantly, incomplete torsion[49] or spontaneous detorsion[68] emphasizing the importance of clinical correlation. Not unexpectedly, the specificity of scanning for testicular torsion is much lower, on the order of 60%.[61] Abscess, hydrocele, hernia, appendage torsion, tumor, and epididymo-orchitis all have been reported to mimic torsion on scintiscan.[63] Because many of these entities can be associated with vascular compromise, the specificity of the test for the detection of perfusion abnormalities is undoubtedly much higher. Furthermore, clinicians should not use radionuclide scanning in the evaluation of the neonate or very young child because it has been shown to be inaccurate, presumably because of inadequate magnification.[61]

Scintigraphy has been shown to be equally accurate in the evaluation of epididymitis, with a reported diagnostic accuracy of 85% to 95%.[22,62-68] Most of the patients in these studies were given a final diagnosis based on clinical course rather than apathologic diagnosis, but the characteristic scan results obtained supported the final diagnosis. Perhaps most notably, the accuracy of scintigraphy for delineating perfusion alone, rather than making a specific diagnosis, exceeds 95%, regardless of the final diagnosis.[61]

Ultrasonography. Ultrasonographic examination provides a rapid, noninvasive method for investigating scrotal pathology.[70] The examination requires less than 30 minutes to complete, and the equipment is somewhat less sophisticated than that for scintigraphy.[71] An experienced technician and radiologist are required to properly perform and interpret the test.

The major advantage of sonography over scintigraphy is sonography's ability to provide precise anatomic detail. The superficial location of the scrotal contents allows the use of high-frequency transducers, which provide excellent resolution.[70] The size, configuration, and appearance of the scrotal contents can be determined and correlated with findings on physical examination. However. ultrasonography provides no information on perfusion status, and the presence of testicular ischemia must be inferred indirectly from the appearance of the testicular tissue.

The use of ultrasonography in investigating acute scrotal pathology has been well-studied. There is little controversy regarding ultrasound's ability to distinguish between intra- and extratesticular pathology and reliably diagnose certain entities, including hydrocele, tumor. varicocele, and hematoma.[7,61,72-78] In cases of epididymitis, testicular torsion, and torsion of an appendage, however, the data suggest an unacceptable degree of uncertainty in relying on ultrasonographic findings alone.

Although some studies have described early, reliable testicular tissue changes secondary to ischemia,[7,79] others have reported difficulty diagnosing early torsion[72] or in distinguishing torsion from severe epididymo-orchitis or hemorrhage.[75,80] One large study reported an overall accuracy of 65% for the diagnosis of non-tumors.[73] Another study directly comparing ultrasound to scintigraphy indicated scintigraphy was more accurate for diagnosing torsion or epididymitis[63] Consequently, most authorities recommend scintigraphy as the initial examination of choice when the diagnosis of testicular torsion is a possibility.[5,6,9,26,49,61,81,82] However, ultrasonography may offer valuable information when the diagnosis is unclear by physical examination or scintigraphy. By delineating anatomic detail, ultrasonography may help to avoid unnecessary surgery due to false-positive scintiscans. Other potential indications for ultrasound include the following: to define locations of nonpalpable testis;

- to define scrotal contents when scintiscan is equivocal;
- to provide additional anatomic information:
- when neoplasm or other mass is suspected;
- post-traumatic scrotal pain.

Other imaging modalities being studied for use in evaluating the acute scrotum include color Doppler sonography and magnetic resonance imaging. Preliminary results suggest that both are highly sensitive and specific in differentiating torsion from epididymitis.[83-88] In fact, in some centers, color Doppler scanning is becoming the preferred study for diagnosing epididymitis and eventually may replace other procedures for confirming this diagnosis. However, firm recommendations for other uses must await larger, definitive studies.

Treatment of Acute Scrotal Emergencies

With the exception of clear-cut epididymitis, most patients with acute scrotal pain are managed in consultation with the urologist. Conservative therapy for patients with epididymitis or those in whom significant scrotal pathology has been ruled out by proper diagnostic studies includes scrotal support, ice, and analgesia. Non-steroidal anti-inflammatory agents, such as ibuprofen 600 mg every eight hours, are appropriate for adults without contraindications to such agents. Often, acetaminophen with a mild narcotic, such as codeine or hydrocodone, two tablets every four hours, is necessary initially to relieve pain, Regardless of initial management, all patients presenting with acute scrotal pain require urologic follow-up to assess response to treatment and to rule out the possibility of tumor.

Epididymitis. Treatment of acute epididymitis depends on the age of the patient and results of urine and urethral Gram's stain. In general, treat sexually active males younger than 40 years old with ceftriaxone, 250 mg intramuscularly, followed by doxycycline 100 mg every 12 hours for 10 days; children and older patients should receive trimethoprimsulfamethoxazole, one double-strength tablet every 12 hours for 10 days.[88] Patients with abnormal urethral smear and bacteriuria require trimethoprim-sulfa, regardless of age. Ofloxacin, one of the newer quinolones, may emerge as the treatment of choice in adults because it effectively eradicates *Chlamydia* as well as most common urinary pathogens.[90] Obtain urethral and urine cultures and immunofluorescent smear for *C. trachomads*, and schedule urologic follow-up. Patients with severe pain, dehydration, or evidence of systemic toxicity (fever, chills, leukocytosis) require hospitalization for analgesia, intravenous antibiotics, and fluid replacement.

Testicular torsion is a true urologic emergency. Treatment in cases of testicular torsion consists of emergent scrotal exploration with derotation and bilateral orchiopexy in which the testicle is fixed to the scrotal wall. The emergency physician's primary responsibility is to ensure that the patient is readied for surgery without delay.

While the patient is being prepared for surgery, the emergency physician may attempt manual detorsion of the torsed testicle. Several studies suggest that detorsion improves salvage rate;[91,92] however, the technique may be painful or difficult, even in experienced hands.

Although some authors recommend focal anesthesia prior to attempting detorsion,[92] most agree that relief of pain is an important indicator of successful detorsion.[1,92] Because torsion most commonly occurs in a medial direction, clinicians should attempt detorsion with counterclockwise rotation of the right testicle and clockwise rotation of the left testicle (viewed from the supine patient's feet). Rotate the testicle in 180 degree increments until pain relief occurs: caudal-to-cranial rotation may be required initially to relieve cremasteric spasm.[92] Increase in pain is an indication to attempt detorsion in the opposite direction. Relief of pain with return of pulsations by Doppler is indicative of successful detorsion but does not obviate the need for surgery.

Torsed Appendage. Definitive therapy for a torsed appendage is operative removal; a number of authors, however, advocate a trial of conservative therapy when the pre-operative diagnosis of torsed appendage is made.[9,19,48,93] Surgery is reserved for patients with an uncertain diagnosis or persistent pain.

References

1. Lindsey D, Stanisic TH. Diagnosis and management of testicular torsion: Pitfalls and perils. *Am J Emerg Mod* 1988; 6:42.

2. Knight PJ, Vassy LE. The diagnosis and treatment of the acute scrotum in children and adolescents. *Ann Surg* 1984; 200:664.
3. Haynes BE, Bessen HA, Haynes VE. The diagnosis of testicular torsion. *JAMA* 1983;249:2522.
4. Haynes BE. Doppler ultrasound failure in testicular torsion. *Ann Emerg Med* 1984;13:1103.
5. Walther TR, Weigand JV. The acute scrotum. *Top Emerg Med* 1991;13:15.
6. Chen DCP, Holder LE, Melloul M. Radionuclide scrotal imagining: Further experience with 210 patients. Part 1: Anatomy, pathophysiology, and methods.*J Nucl Med* 1983; 24:735.
7. Hrivak H, Filley RA. Sonography of the scrotum. *Invest Radiol* 1983;18:112.
8. Cass AS, Cass BP. Veeraraghavan K. Immediate exploration of the unilateral acute scrotum in young male subjects. *J Urol* 1980;124:829.
9. Caldamone AA, Valvok JR, Altebarmakian VK, et al. Acute-scrotal swelling in children. *J Pediatr Surg* 1984;19:581.
10. Williamson RCN. Torsion of the testis and allied conditions. *Br J Surg* 1985;63:465.
11. Skoglund RW. McRoberts JW. Radge 11. Torsion of the spermatic cord: A review of the literature and an analysis of 70 new cases. *J Urol* 1970;104:604.
12. Brewer ME, Glasgow BJ. Adult testicular torsion. *Urology* 1986;27:356.
13. Tolia BM, Mewman HR. Testicular torsion in adults. Plea for its consideration early in clinical evaluation of acute scrotum. *Urology* 1977;10:150.
14. Ransler CW. Allen TD. Torsion of the spermatic cord. *Urol Clin North Am* 1982;9:245.
15. Smith GI. Cellular changes for graded testicular ischemia. *J Urol* 1955; 13:355.
16. Donohue RE. Utley WI. Torsion of spermatic cord. *Urology* 1978;11:33.
17. Bartsch G, Grank S, Marberger H, et al. Testicular torsion: Late results with special regard to fertility and endocrine function. *J Urol* 1980;124:375.
18. Lee LM, Wright JE. McLoughlin MC. Testicular torsion in the adult. *J Urol* 1983;139:1023.
19. Hastie KJ, Charlton CA. Indications for conservative management of acute scrotal pain in children. *Br J Surg* 1990;77:309.
20. Witherington R. Jarrell TS. Torsion of the spermatic cord in adults. *J Urol* 1990;143:62.
21. Anderson JB, Williamson RCN. The fate of the human testes following trilateral torsion of the spermatic cord. *Br J Urol* 1986;58:698.
22. Chen DCP, Holder LE. Melloul M. Radionuclide scrotal imaging: Further experience with 210 patients. Part II: Results and discussion. *J Nucl Med* 1983;24:841.
23. Sonda LP. Lapidis ,I. Experimental torsion of the spermatic cord. *Surg Forum* 1961;12:502.
24. Schulsinger D, Glassberg K, Strashun A. Intermittent torsion: Association with horizontal tie of the testicle. *J Urol* 1991; 145:1053.
25. Skoglund RW, McRoberts JW, Radge H. Torsion of testicular appendages: Presentation of 43 new cases and a collective review. *J Urol* 1970;04:598.
26. Edelsberg JS, Stith YS. The acute scrotum. *Emerg Med Clin North Am* 988;6:521.
27. Altaffer LE, Steele SM. Torsion of testicular appendages in men. *J Urol* 980;124:56.
28. Sufrin G. Acute epididymitis. *Sex Transm Dis* 1981; 8(Suppl):132.
29. Kaver 1, Matzkin H. Braf ZF. Epididymo-orchitis: A retrospective study ,of 122 patients. *J Fam Pract* 1990; 30:548.
30. Berger RE, Alexander E.R. Hanisch JP, et al. Etiology, manifestations, and therapy of acute epididymitis: Prospective study of 50 cases. *J Urol* 1979;21:750.
31. Melekos MD, Asbach HW. Epididymitis: Aspects concerning etiology and treatment. *J Urol* 1987;138:83.
32. Siegel A, Snyder H, Duckett JW. Epididymitis in infants and boys: Underlying urogenital anomalies and efficacy of imaging modalities. *J Urol* 1987;138:1100.
33. Robinson AI, Grant .IB, Spencer KC, et al. Acute epididymitis: Why patient and consort must be investigated. *Br J Urol* 1990;66:642.
34. Dibie A, Taylor-Robinson D, Thomas BJ, et al. Acute epididymitis: A microbiological and ultrasonographic study.*Br J Urol* 1989;63:90.
35. De long Z, Pontonnier F, Plante P, et al. The frequency of Chlamydia trachomatis in acute epididymitis. *Br J Urol* 1988;62:76.
36. Pearson RC, Baumber CD, McGhie D,Thambar IV. The relevance of Chlamydia trachomatis in acute epididymitis in young men. *Br J Urol* 1988:62:72.
37. Grant JB, Costello CB, Sequeira PJ,Blacklock NJ. The role of Chlamydia trachomatis in epididymitis. *Br J Urol* 1987; 60:355.
38. Rinker JR, Hancock CV, Henderson WD. A statistical study of unilateral prophylactic vasectomy in the prevention of epididymitis: 1029 cases. *J Urol* 1970;104:303.
39. Thind P, Gerstenberg TC, Bilde T. Is micturition disorder a pathogenic factor in acute epididymitis? An evaluation of simultaneous bladder pressure and urine flow in men with previous acute epididymitis. *J Urol* 1990;143:323.
40. George VK, Russell CL, Harrison BD. Green NA. Tuberculous epididymo-orchitis following intravesical BCG. *Br J Uro1* 1990;66:101.
41. Khan MS, Humayoon MS, Al Manee MS. lipididymo-orchitis and brucellosis. *Br J Urol* 1989;63:87.
42. Ibsen HH, Frandsen F, Brandup F, Moller M. Epididymitis caused by treatment with amiodarone. *Genitourin Med* 1989; 65:257.
43. Wolach MD, MacDermott JP, Stone AR, deVere White RW. Treatment and complications of Foumier's gangrene. *Br J Urol* 1989;64:3-10.
44. Melville K, Schultz EA, Dougherty JM. Ilioinguinal-ilioltypogastric nerve entrapment. *Ann Emerg Med* 1990;19:925.
45. Flanigan KC, DeKemian JB, Persky L. Acute scrotal pain and swelling in children: A surgical emergency. *Urology* 1981;27:51.

46. Anderson PAM, Giacomantonio JM. The acutely painful scrotum in children. *Can Med Assoc J* 1985;132:1153.
47. Melckos MD, Asbach HW. Markou SA. Etiology of acute scrotum in 100 boys with regard to age distribution. *J Urol* 1988;139:1023.
48. Hastie KJ, Charlton CA. Indications for conservative management of acute scrotal pain in children. *Or J Surg* 1990;77:309.
49. Mendel JB, Taylor GA, Trcves S, et al. Testicular torsion in children: Scintigraphic assessment. *Pediatr Radiol* 1985; 15:110.
50. Perry S, Hoopingarner D, Askins D. Testicular torsion in the older patient. *Ann Emerg Med* 1983;12:319.
51. Rabinowitz R. The importance of the acmasteric reflex in acute scrotal swelling in children. *J Urol* 1984; 132:89.
52. Pedersen JF, Holm HH, Hald T. Torsion of the testis diagnosed by ultrasound. *J Urol* 1975;113:66.
53. Thompson IM, Latourette H, Chadwick S, et al. Diagnosis of testicular torsion using Doppler ultrasonic flowmeter. *Urology* 1975;6:706.
54. Perri AJ, Slachta GA, Feldman AE, et al. The Doppler stethoscope and the diagnosis of the acute scrotum. *J Urol* 1976;116:598.
55. Milleret R. Doppler ultrasound diagnosis of testicular cord torsion. *ICU* 1976;4:425.
56. Iuchtman M, Zoireff L, Assa J. Doppler flowmeter in the differential diagnosis of the acute scrotum in children. *J Urol* 1979;121:221.
57. Nasrallah PF, Manzone D, King IR. Falsely negative Doppler examinations in testicular torsion. *J Urol* 1977:118:194.
58. Rodriguez DD, Rodriguez WC, Rivera JJ, et al. Doppler ultrasound versus testicular scanning in the evaluation of the acute scrotum. *J Urol* 1981:125:343.
59. Bickerstaff KI, Sethia K, Murie JA. Doppler ultrasonography in the diagnosis of acute scrotal pain. *Br J Surg* 1988; 75:238.
60. Brereton RJ. Limitations of the Doppler flow meter in the diagnosis of the "acute scrotum" in boys. *Br J Urol* 1981; 53:380.
61. Lutzker LG, Zuckier LS. Testicular scanning and other applications of radionuclide imaging of the genital tract. *Semin Nucl Med* 1990; 20:159.
62. Vordermark JS, Buck AS, Brown SR, et al. The testicular scan: Usc in diagnosis and management of acute epididymitis. *JAMA* 1981;245:2512.
63. Chen DCP, Holder LE, Kaplan GN. Correlation of radionuclide imaging and diagnostic ultrasound in scrotal diseases. *J Nucl Med* 1986;27:1774.
64. Hahn LC, Nadel NS, Gittcr Mil, et al. Testicular scanning: A new modality for the preoperative diagnosis of testicular torsion. *J Urol* 1975;113:60.
65. Hitch DC, Gilday DL, Shandling B, et al. A new approach to the diagnosis of testicular torsion. *J Ped Surg* 1976;I1:537.
66. Riley TW, Mosbaugh PG, Coles JL, et al. Use of radioisotope scan in evaluation of intrascrotal lesions. *J Urol* 1976;116:472.
67. Abu-SIciman R, Ho JE, Gregory JG. Scrotal scanning: Present value and limits of interpretation. *Urology* 1979: 13:326.
68. Mueller DL, Amundson GM, Rubin SZ, et al. Acute scrotal abnormalities in children: Diagnosis by combined sonography and scintigraphy. *AJR* 1988;150:643.
69. Dunn EK, Maccha RJ, Chauhan PS, et al. Scintiscan for acute intrascrotal conditions. *Clin Nucl Med* I986;11:381.
70. Fournier CR, Laing FC, McAnnich JW. Scrotal ultrasonography and the managemat of testicular trauma. *Urol Clin North Am* 1989;16:377.
71. Martin B, Conte J. Ultrasonography of the acute scrotum. *J Clin Ultrasound* 1987;15:37.
72. Fournier GR, Laing FC, Jeffrey RB, McAnnich JW. High resolution scrotal ultrasonography: A highly sensitive but nonspecific diagnostic technique. *J Urol* 1985;134:490.
73. Hrivak H, Jeffrey RB. Sonography of acute scrotal abnormalities. *Radiol Clin North Am* 1983;21:595.
74. Fowler RC, Chennells PM, Ewing R. Scrotal ultrasonography: A clinical evaluation. *Br J Radiol* 1987; 60:649.
75. Off DP, Skolnick ML. Sonographic examination of the abnormal scrotum. *Clin Radiol* 1990;31:109.
76. Willscher MK, Conway JF, Daly KJ, et al. Scrotal ultrasonography. *J Urol* 1983;130:931.
77. Finkelstein MS, Rosenberg HK, Snyder HM, Duckett JW. Ultrasound evaluation of scrotum in pediatrics. *Urology* 1986;27:1.
78. Howe D, Foster ME, Gateley C, et al. Clinical value of scrotal ultrasound in the investigation of scrotal pathology. *Br J Urol* 1988;62:263.
79. Bird K, Rosenfield AT, Taylor KJW. Ultrasonography in testicular torsion. *Radiology* 1983;147:527.
80. Arger PH, Mulhem CB, Coleman BG, et al. Prospective analysis of the value of scrotal ultrasound. *Radiology* 1981; 141:763.
81. Noe FIN, Jenkins CR. Evaluation of acute scrotal pain and/or swelling. In: McCullough DL. cd. *Difficult Diagnoses in Urology.* New York: Churchill Livingstone: 1988.
82. May DC, Lesh P, Lewis S, Anderson RJ. Evaluation of acute scrotum pain with testicular scanning. *Ann Emerg Med* 1985; 14:696.
83. Middleton WD, Siegel BA, Melson CI, et al. Acute scrotal disorders: Prospective comparison of color Doppler US and testicular scintigraphy. *Radiology* 1990;177:177.
84. Burks DD, Markey BJ, Burkhard TK, et al. Suspected testicular torsion and ischemia: Evaluation with color Doppler sonogaphy. *Radiology* 1990;175:815.
85. Trambent MA, Mattrey RF, Levine D, Berthoty DP. Subacute scrotal pain: Evaluation of torsion versus epiclidymitis with MR imaging. *Radiology* 1990;175:53.
86. Tzika AA, Vigneron DB, Hricak H, et al. P-31 MR spectroscopy in assessing testicular torsion: Rat model. *Radiology* 1989;172:753.
87. Mevorach RA, Lemer RM, Greenspan BS, et al. Color Dopplier ultrasound compared to a radionuclide scanning of spermatic cord torsion in a canine model. *J Urol* 1991; 145:428.
88. Horstman WG, Middleton WD, Melson GL. Scrotal inflammatory disease: Color Doppler US findings. *Radiology*

1991:179:55.
89. Nieh PT. Epididymitis. In: Rakel RE, ed. *Conn's Current Therapy*. Philadelphia: WB Saunders; 1991.
90. Sanford JP. *Guide to Antimicrobial Therapy 1991*. West Bethesda, MD: Antimicrobial Therapy Inc.; 1991:44.
91. Cattolica EV. Preoperative manual detorsion of the toned spermatic cord. *J Urol* 1985;133:903.
92. Kiesling VJ, Schroeder DE, Pauljev P, et al. Spermatic cord block and manual reduction: Primary treatment for spermatic cord torsion. *J Urol* 1984;32:921.
93. McCombe AW, Scobie WG. Torsion of scrotal contents in children. *Br Urol* 1988:61:148.

Obstructive Uropathy

Harrison Alter, MS, MD
Eric Snoey, MD

Urinary tract obstruction is a relatively common but potentially serious clinical phenomenon, and optimal clinical approaches may be elusive to the emergency physician. Because obstructive processes can range from congenital posterior urethral valves, to urolithiasis, to the normal condition of pregnancy, effective management requires accurate diagnosis. Autopsy-based studies estimate incidences of obstruction to be 3% in adults and 2% in children.[1] The most common causes in males occur at the extremes of age—boys with congenital anatomic abnormalities and older men with prostatism. Among females, physiological ureteral obstruction occurs in up to 65% of pregnancies.[1]

This chapter will focus primarily on urolithiasis and its importance in the practice of emergency medicine. It will briefly touch upon the renal pathophysiology of obstructive uropathy, as well as review other causes of urinary obstruction.

Urolithiasis

Epidemiology. Kidney stones occur frequently in the ED population. An annual incidence of 16 per 10,000 population in the United States was cited in an extrapolation of 1974 hospital discharge data, though this figure may be conservative.[2]

Urolithiasis affects males more commonly by a ratio 2:1 to 4:1, peaking in the fourth to sixth decades. Whites are more commonly affected than blacks at a ratio of about 3:1. The risk of developing urolithiasis in middle-aged white men, a high-risk group, is approximately 1% per year.

The incidence of renal calculi exhibits geographic and seasonal variability as well. Australians are more commonly affected than North Americans, while within North America, inhabitants of the Southeast are at highest risk. Seasonal peak incidence appears to lag about two months behind peak local temperature, which may parallel peak intake of high-oxalate content foods. Earlier theories relating geographic patterns of stone formation to dehydration have been largely discredited.[3]

Pathogenesis. *Composition.* It is interesting to note that 80% of all stones contain calcium. The majority of the remaining 20% comprise struvite and uric acid stones, which develop in alkaline and acid urine, respectively. Cystine stones account for fewer than 1%.[4]

Anatomy. Kidney stones arise within the collecting ducts and grow in the renal pelvis, only resulting in symptoms as they obstruct the ureteropelvic junction or proceed down the ureter. Some stones never make it beyond the renal pelvis, being too large to pass the ureteropelvic junction. If a stone is to move on, however, the first likely point of obstruction is at the ureteropelvic junction, the "headwaters" of the drainage. Internal diameter there can be as small as 2-3 mm. Common stones are unlikely to fix in the next segment, the abdominal spindle, which can pass a 10 mm ureterolith. The ureter narrows to about 4 mm as it passes into the pelvis crossing over the iliac vasculature, and it narrows again in the posterior pelvis as it crosses under the hypogastric vessels. The last obstacle for a passing stone is the ureterovesicular junction, where the lumen may be as narrow as 1 mm.

Pathophysiology. The end product of the complex process of glomerular filtration and tubular excretion/reabsorption is supersaturated filtrate urine. Any alterations in the degree of supersaturation of calcium, oxalate, ammonium, uric acid, or citrate, may predispose urine to crystal formation, as will the availability of a ready nidus for crystal growth, known as a nucleus.[6]

A low urine-output state, once thought to account for a significant proportion of stone disease, is now believed to account for fewer than 5-15% of stones but may be a co-factor in up to 50% of calcium-containing stones.[7,8] High dietary calcium, also thought to contribute significantly to stone formation, may actually be inversely related to stone risk.[9] In contrast, a rise in dietary oxalate results in disproportionate increases in urinary oxalate excretion and appears to play a major role in the formation of calcium oxalate stones, the most common calculi in the United States.[10] Oxalate-rich diets are heavy in coffee, tea, cola, and beer, as well as chocolate, nuts, citrus, and spinach. Some authors theorize that the seasonal and geographic variations in incidence are merely reflective of similar variations in diet. For example, a high rate of disease in the South after the summer months correlates with a high rate of iced tea consumption. High urinary oxalate concentrations can also be found in patients with Crohn's disease, short gut syndrome, and other functional disturbances in absorption.

Urinary citrate inhibits stone formation in two important ways: formation of a *soluble* citrate-calcium compound that leaves less free calcium to form crystals; and direct inhibition of calcium crystallization. Therefore, low urinary citrate, occurring idiopathically or in Type 4 renal tubular acidosis and chronic diarrheal syndromes, may be an important etiologic factor implicated in about 30% of stone formers.[7] Primary hyperparathyroidism, an uncommon cause of hypercalciuria and stones, must be considered since it may be amenable to surgical correction. Idiopathic stone formation, the largest category of disease, is thought to arise as a result of abnormalities contributing to increased enteric absorption of calcium.

Uric acid stones are largely a phenomenon associated with hyperuricemia and only rarely occur in the absence of clinical gout. Hyperuricemia unassociated with clinical gout can provide a nidus for calcium crystallization and may occur in up to 25% of calcium oxalate stones.

Cystine stones result from a hereditary defect in the renal tubular reabsorption of cystine, ornithine, lysine, and arginine, generally found in younger patients. Lastly, struvite stones, which can propagate into the "staghorn"-type calculi, are formed in a urinary environment created by the presence of urea-splitting bacteria. These organisms, which include *Proteus*, *Klebsiella*, *Pseudomonas*, *Entercoccus*, and *Morganella* species yet notably exclude *Escherichiae*, create an alkaline environment. Cleaving urea promotes the availability of free ammonium that compounds rapidly with magnesium and phosphate to form the struvite stone. Ureteral obstruction that involves struvite stones suggests a high-risk patient due to the implied associated urinary tract infection, though true staghorn calculi rarely obstruct.

The pathophysiological model of unilateral obstruction primarily addresses stone disease, although ureteral impingement from a pelvic cancer and post-operative ureteral injury also are common mechanisms. There is a widely cited belief that the uninfected kidney can tolerate one week of complete obstruction without serious sequelae. This belief appears to be based upon small dog studies in the 1950s and 1970s that demonstrated complete recovery of GFR after seven days of ureteral ligation. The degree of recovery after this window was found to be proportional to the duration of ligation up to 40 days. After 40 days, recovery of renal function was unlikely in the animals.[11-13] The dog data are supplemented by a handful of case reports describing recovery of renal function in humans following presumed obstruction of 28-150 days' duration.[14]

Despite the suggestion of reversibility, there is evidence suggesting renal injury during the period of obstruction, beginning after the first 24 hours.[15,16] There is significant dropout of functioning nephrons, down to about 40% of normal after the first day of complete obstruction. Florid renal macrophage infiltration progresses, both as a function of cytokine transmission and as a direct result of mechanical obstruction, resulting in renal scarring. What is not currently known is the degree to which such renal insufficiency places the affected kidney at risk for further insult, including insult from IV contrast, NSAIDs, or infection. Therefore, it seems wise not to depend upon the theoretic one-week window and instead to recommend urgent specialty referral in patients with persistently obstructing stones.

Diagnosis. *History and Physical Examination*. There is legitimate controversy among practicing emergency physicians as to whether a firm diagnosis of urolithiasis must be established in the ED or if a presumptive diagnosis is adequate with close referral. Indeed, since the vast majority of patients with stones have an uncomplicated course, the emergency physician may choose to accept a presumptive diagnosis of calculus disease while ruling out infection and eliminating other items on the differential diagnosis, including leaking abdominal aortic aneurysm, appendicitis, renovascular occlusion, and acute tubular necrosis. *(Please see Table 1.)*

As with many common problems facing the emergency physician, an accurate history is critical in the diagnosis of urolithiasis. A presumptive diagnosis will rely heavily upon the presence of a clinical triad: unilateral costovertebral angle pain, abrupt in onset, associated with hematuria. *(Please see Figure 1.)* The patient who presents with this scenario has a 90% probability of having a stone.[17] Radiation of pain to the abdomen and groin may also be a helpful historical feature, present in up to 70% of patients.[17] Ureteropelvic junction stones produce aching back pain related to distention. Pain from a stone in the distal ureter may radiate to the testes or ovaries, as a result of their common embryologic origin and shared autonomic innervation. Stones in the ureterovesicular junction can create urinary tenesmus.

The character of the pain may provide another clue to the diagnosis. The patient with calculus disease seems unable to find a comfortable position, an observation that weighs against intra-abdominal processes that result in peritoneal irritation. The term renal colic may be a misnomer, since the pain is only colicky in nature if the stone lodges, dislodges, and lodges again in the ureter. More typically, the pain rises to a crescendo over 15-30 minutes and persists until the stone lodges or passes to a wider portion of the ureter. Associated symptoms are largely nonspecific. Nausea and vomiting, found in 50-80% of patients, and dysuria, present in 25%, predominate.[17]

Both calcium-containing stones and cystine stones may be associated with a positive family history. A history of prior stone is important, since the recurrence rate is high—50% within five years.[19]

The physical exam is primarily helpful in excluding other potential causes of the patient's presenting complaint. Hypertension and tachycardia may occur in response to the pain. Temperature greater than 100.5°F is important in that it occurs in only 5% of patients with uncomplicated ureteral calculi; fever should alert the clinician to the possibility of proximal infection.[17] Point or rebound abdominal tenderness does not rule out the diagnosis of urolithiasis, but it is not part of the classical presentation. Costovertebral angle tenderness may suggest a proximal stone but is also worrisome for the presence of infection. Symptomatic abdominal aortic aneurysm is of particular concern in older patients; the emergency physician should attempt to palpate the abdominal aorta and both femoral pulses.

Laboratory. Microscopic urinalysis is the linchpin of the laboratory evaluation of urolithiasis. Microscopic hematuria is present in 70-80% of patients, and is part of the classical triad of acute onset costovertebral angle pain with hematuria.[5] Absence of hematuria suggests either a 100% ureteral occlusion, lab error, or a chance event.[17] Low-grade pyuria can exist in uncomplicated urolithiasis, but more than 3 WBC/hpf in the presence of bactiuria indicates a possible infection.

Urine pH is also worth noting. Acid urine suggests uric acid calculi, though they may act only as the nucleus for a calcium-containing stone. Acid urine also rules out renal tubular acidosis as a cause for the stone. Alkaline urine raises the suspicion of urease-producing organisms and the presence of infection.

Other laboratory evaluation rarely affects management decisions. A complete blood count may demonstrate an elevated WBC count, which, in the moderate range, can be attributed to the stress response. Hypokalemia in the presence of low bicarbonate may be useful in diagnosing renal tubular acidosis. A serum creatinine establishes normal renal function prior to the use of intravenous contrast material. Further laboratory evaluation, including uric acid, serum calcium, and analysis of a passed stone is best undertaken during the follow-up phase of care.

Radiographic. The ideal radiographic study in patients with urolithiasis provides diagnostic, anatomic, and functional information.

Historically, physicians have relied upon the "KUB" (kidneys, ureters, bladder) plain film as the study of choice in urolithiasis. This modality, which provides only anatomic data, has been supplanted by more effective imaging techniques. The frequently cited claim that 90% of stones are visible on KUB is based upon data from the early part of the century that has never been reproduced in the modern era.

Several studies from the 1980s demonstrate that the sensitivity and specificity of KUB varies between 50% and 85%, with a negative predictive value—its ability to rule out urolithiasis—as low as 22%. KUB is equally unreliable when interpreted by radiologists or emergency physicians.[17,20-22] While many clinicians continue to use KUBs to influence their decision to proceed to IVP, this strategy has been shown not to be cost-effective and to add little information to the decision-making process.[22] One study reported that a positive KUB in the setting of the classic triad improved sensitivity from 90% to 98%. However, the authors made no comment on the impact of a negative KUB, an important consideration in a test known to have a high false-negative rate.[17] In the contemporary era, the only role for KUB may be as an adjunct to ultrasonography, since it may serve the operator as a roadmap for identifying a stone. KUB actually increases the sensitivity of the ultrasound.[23] Some urologists also may use KUB to follow a stone expectantly.

The intravenous pyelogram (IVP) remains the urologists' study of choice, both out of custom and for the functional data it may convey. Classic IVP findings supporting the presence of a stone include a dense nephrogram with delayed excretion on the affected side and interruption of the dye column. A delayed nephrogram, usually of more than two hours, suggests clinically important obstructive nephropathy. Extravasation of contrast, a rare finding, may be seen in ureteral "blowout" and necessitates prompt urological consultation.

Convention aside, however, the IVP may not be optimal for the ED evaluation of ureteral calculi. Most of the studies demonstrating its efficacy were performed with patients referred for the study who had presumably undergone adequate bowel preparation. Even in ideal conditions, there is a 10-15% false-negative rate, usually due to non-occlusive stones that are also radiolucent (typically uric acid) or stones obscured by the urographic medium.[24] In ED patients, who typically have poor bowel preparation, the study can be even more difficult to interpret. False-positive results may be incurred in the setting of acute tubular necrosis when sloughed cells may obstruct the ureter. Ureteral thrombus and transitional cell carcinoma may create a similar appearance. These conditions mimic an obstructive radiolucent stone.

Although claims of the health risks of IVP may be overstated, it is not an entirely benign procedure. Most recent estimates of the risk of a contrast reaction place the incidence in the 1:75,000 range, with contrast nephropathy occurring in 1.5-15% of patients.[25] Although pre-existing renal insufficiency is the only clearly established risk factor for contrast nephropathy, other conditions, including diabetes, dehydration, multiple myeloma, congestive heart failure, and peripheral vascular disease have all been cited as posing increased risk in contrast administration.[25] In addition, excretory urography can be very time-consuming, occasionally requiring up to 24 hours before definitive results are obtained, thereby extending a patient's stay in the ED.

One of the newer proposed modalities for evaluation of ureteral calculi is ultrasound. In experienced hands, ultrasound is excellent at detecting intracalyceal stones, very proximal stones larger than 5 mm, and, when performed with a full bladder, distal stones stuck at the ureterovesicular junction.[27] Ultrasound can also detect hydronephrosis, which correlates with the degree of obstruction in a manner similar to IVP. When performed in conjunction with KUB, ultrasound demonstrates a favorable receiver operating characteristic (ROC) curve in comparison to IVP.[23] However, in another recent study, this method missed three cases out of 18 diagnosed by CT.[28] Furthermore, the emergency physician who relies upon ultrasound should be aware of a series of reports demonstrating nondilated obstructive uropathy, including cases of obstructive urolithiasis.[26,29,30]

The more recent addition of Doppler to the ultrasound exam can add important functional information. Doppler can assess both intrarenal pressures and distal ureterovesicular jets, a further clue to the degree of obstruction.[31] Although not widely available, non-ionic intravenous sonographic contrast materials promise to greatly enhance the effectiveness of ultrasound in this setting.

In 1995, Smith and Rosenfield et al published a landmark article which established the use of non-contrast helical CT (NCHCT) in imaging urolithiasis. The authors found NCHCT to be more sensitive than IVP, since even radiolucent stones lit up, and equally specific.[32]

Table 1. Differential Diagnoses in Renal Colic

- Pyelonephritis
- Peritonitis, including appendicitis and diverticulitis
- Biliary colic
- Abdominal aortic aneurysm
- Renovascular compromise, including renal artery or vein thrombosis
- Cancer, especially renal
- Endometriosis
- Ovarian torsion

While the urine flow component of kidney function cannot be assessed, the obstructive component (e.g., hydronephrosis or hydroureter) is reliably evident. Furthermore, in an estimated 10% of cases, NCHCT identified an extra-urologic source for a patient's complaint.

Findings on NCHCT characteristic of urolithiasis include: perinephric stranding consistent with hydronephrosis, dilatation of the collecting system, and the presence of a brightly opaque density in the kidney or ureter. Even non-calcium-containing stones will give this rather dramatic presentation. In the initial study, most patients were scanned with 10 mm cuts (although some centers currently use 7 mm sections) with acquisition time averaging about one second per segment. Radiation exposure per unit of tissue is small, as the scanner operates in a corkscrew fashion, and there is no need for IV or PO contrast material.

One of the criticisms of this technique has been its increased cost. This is an imprecise allegation; it is actually an increased *charge*. In fact, in many centers, radiology groups elect to set their charge for the use of NCHCT for evaluation of flank pain with hematuria at a pace with IVP to promote appropriate use of their imaging services.

Urologists have been slow to embrace NCHCT for two reasons: CT cannot provide data about concentrating function within the kidney, and it offers a nontraditional axial perspective on the anatomy rather than the more familiar coronal image of IVP. With the latter obstacle in mind, new CT software permits *curved planar reformatting*, a coronal reconstitution of the kidneys, ureters, and bladder. In one recent study, this system outperformed axial images by defining calculi in three cases in which the axial images were equivocal.[28]

Despite its advantages, helical CT scanning is currently available only at larger institutions, and ultrasound is highly operator-dependent. Therefore, the IVP remains a popular study with many ED physicians, and its flaws do not obviate its usefulness in the radiographic evaluation of renal colic.

Differential Diagnosis. The panoply of imaging options for suspected ureteral calculi begs the question: Why bother? If the clinical presentation is 90% sensitive, and more than half of all stones pass spontaneously, what is the value of ED diagnosis, assuming infected obstruction has been ruled out?[33,34] This debate exists on many levels; for the emergency physician, the matter of differential diagnosis is paramount.

Table 1 depicts the main points of the differential diagnosis. There are a few entities, such as aortic aneurysm or appendicitis, in which missing the diagnosis could lead to significant morbidity or mortality. This suggests one approach to the patient with suspected stone disease: make it a diagnosis of exclusion, and study all the catastrophic alternatives instead. However, in a disease entity so common and so easy to definitively diagnose, this approach seems wasteful.

And why proceed in the setting of "clinical certainty"? While the clinical and laboratory diagnosis is 90% sensitive, its *specificity* is not known. With a high sensitivity and unknown specificity, we are at risk for treating and referring as stones many cases that are not stones. Contemporary medicine demands appropriate use of subspecialty referral; in the case of kidney stones, imaging may be required. Finally, definitive diagnosis is also relevant in the ED because patients in distress look to their physician for some degree of reassurance, and definitive prognosis regarding stone passage or the need for surgery requires an imaging study.

One common management strategy is to defer the ultimate diagnosis to the follow-up clinician. Based upon the patient's response to therapy, the need for imaging or other ancillary testing can be more selectively applied, with substantial cost savings. This approach, however, begs the question of whether an ED imaging study results in an important change in management. A recent study specifically addressing the use of IVP argues for a more liberal use of ED imaging.[35] The author studied emergency physicians caring for patients with suspected ureteral colic over a one-year period and assessed the degree to which obtaining the IVP changed management. In nearly a quarter of the patients, the study forced consideration of an alternative diagnosis, and 40% of the studies yielded an unexpected result. Nearly two-thirds of the studies changed management based on pre- and post-IVP questionnaires. The use of routine imaging resulted in hospitalization of some patients who would otherwise have been sent home and allowed discharge of some who had been marked for admission. The author did not offer data on outcomes, or compare the strategy of emergency department IVP to outpatient referral. However, the results are compelling.

Given the inconclusive state of research on the subject, however, the practicing emergency physician remains well within the standard of care in electing to make a presumptive diagnosis in the setting of the classic presentation of renal colic.

Treatment. The patient's foremost preoccupations are pain and, by extension, pain control. The options available include nonsteroidal anti-inflammatory medications, narcotics, or both.

The proposed mechanism of NSAID efficacy relates to their anti-prostaglandin effects. Even partial obstruction of the urinary tract results in increased pressure in the renal pelvis, stimulating renal prostaglandin release, especially PGE_2. This substance has a vasodilatory effect on the afferent arteriole, leading to further increased pressure. Prostaglandins also mediate the phasic and tonic contractile activity of ureteric smooth muscle.[38] Therefore, the three effects that promote pain—pressure, spasm, and the local inflammatory response—all are potentially remediable by the action of an NSAID. Two studies demonstrate the efficacy of ketorolac for renal colic, one of them head-to-head with meperidine.[36,37] If ketorolac is unavailable, rectal indomethacin also has been demonstrated efficacious in comparison with narcotic analgesia.[38] However, some patients may require the addition of a potent parenteral narcotic, such as IV morphine, when NSAIDs are not enough, and the ED physician is certainly within the standard of care in relying upon narcotics alone.

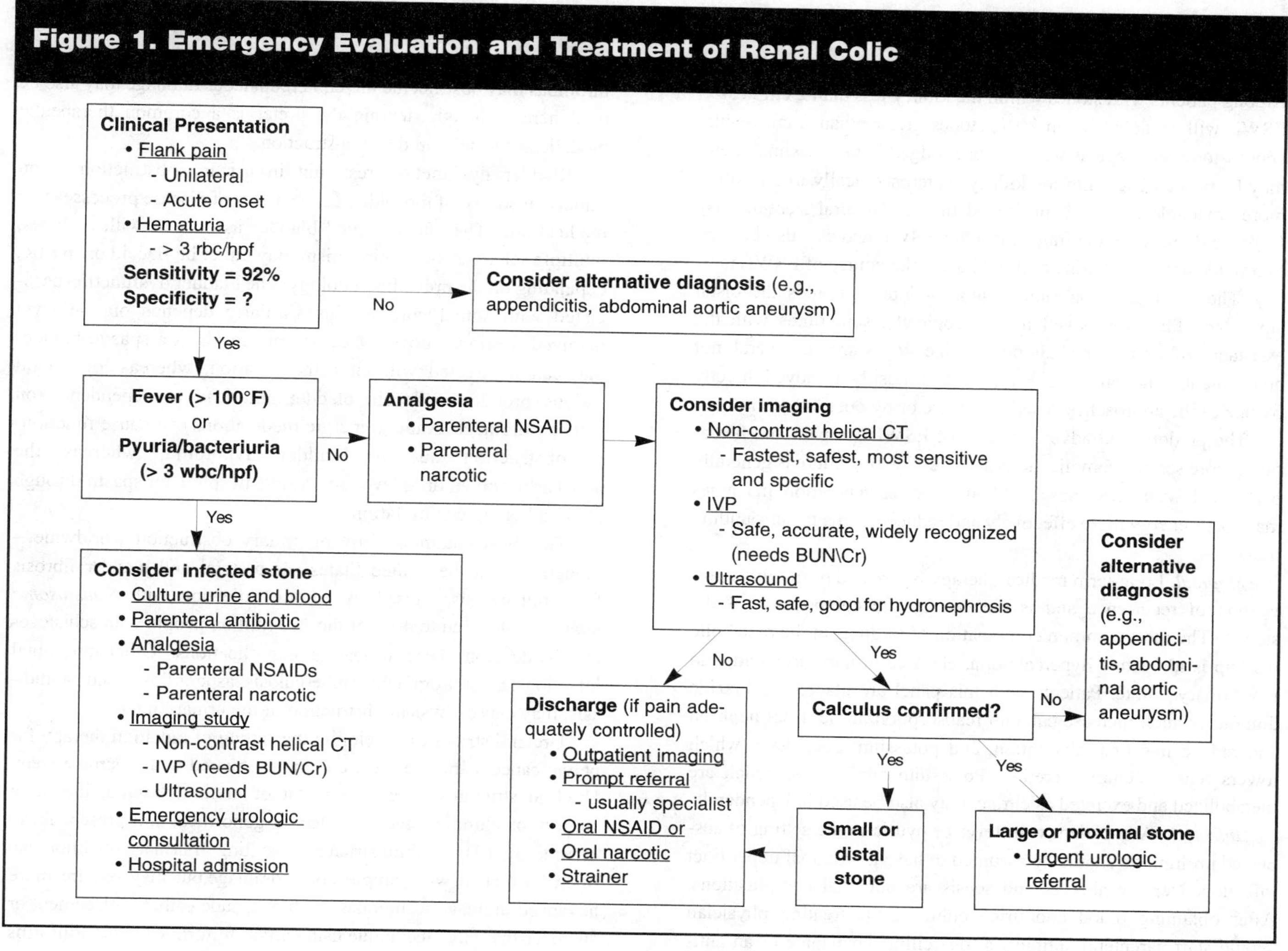

Hydration remains the standard of care despite some controversy. The theory challenging its use centers on the problem of increased flow leading to increased intrarenal back-pressure and worsening compression of nephrons. This question requires more study before reversal of this common practice can be recommended. Glucagon, diuretics, and antispasmodics have all been tried without success, and none is indicated in the acute setting, although the osmotic diuresis from IVP dye has been reported to promote stone passage. One recent study using nifedipine and methylprednisolone in combination showed promise in hastening stone passage.[33]

Hospital admission is occasionally warranted. It should be reserved for those patients with a proximal infection, a solitary kidney, intractable pain, or dehydration. Some authors advocate hospitalizing patients with complete obstruction as well.[5] All patients with ureteral calculi will require follow-up to ensure resolution of symptoms and to initiate stone analysis and consideration for a metabolic work-up, the results of which may dictate long-term therapy. The necessity for subspecialty follow-up may depend on the radiographic findings. Signs of obstruction and large stones unlikely to pass spontaneously suggest prompt referral within 72 hours. Patients with smaller, distal stones can be deferred for up to two weeks, with instructions to return sooner if their pain persists. Those physicians who elect to make the definitive diagnosis outside the department by scheduling an outpatient imaging study with urologic follow-up must ensure that the referral will be prompt.

At discharge, patients are given a set of strainers, with instructions to use them with every void. Oral NSAIDs are typically adequate for outpatient pain control but may be supplemented with oral narcotics and anti-emetics. Patients should make an effort to remain well-hydrated, although some authors question the utility of such a strategy since agents that inhibit crystallization are diluted out at the same rate as those that promote stone formation.[3,39] Common recommendations for hydration include drinking two glasses of liquid every two hours, half of it as water, or drinking until the urine is clear. Alternatively, the patient can be discharged with dipsticks and instructions to keep the urine specific gravity at about 1.010.[40] Obvious caveats apply regarding return to the ED, and include fever, chills, and dysuria (worrisome symptoms of infection), or worsening pain.

Long-Term Treatment. *Surgical. Table 2* demonstrates the relationship between size of stones and likelihood of passage, allowing the surgeon and patient together to balance the risks and benefits of surgical treatment.[34] Asymptomatic stones are rarely treated, regardless of location; the classic exception is an airline pilot, who can little afford a sudden bout of renal colic.

Once it is determined that some intervention is required, the strategy depends upon the location and size of the stone. Calculi trapped within the kidney may be treated with extracorporeal shock-wave lithotripsy (ESWL) alone or with percutaneous nephrolithotomy. Among patients with stones within the kidney less than 2 cm in size, ESWL will be definitive in 80%; stones greater than 2 cm require nephrostomy drainage as well. A stone lodged in the proximal ureter may be pushed back into the kidney ureteroscopically to a position more amenable to ESWL or treated in situ. Ureteral stenting may facilitate drainage of the fragments after ESWL and can also be used to provide temporary urine outflow during the course of ESWL therapy. The most common stone requiring intervention is the distal stone, and this is removed ureteroscopically, sometimes with the assistance of a basket or balloon. Cystine stones are, in general, not amenable to fragmentation by ESWL and must be removed directly by one of the approaches described above or by open lithotomy.

The predominant adverse effects of ESWL are pain and hematuria; more serious complications are rare. The procedure is generally performed with anaesthesia, although newer-generation machines may focus energy more effectively and reduce trauma to surrounding tissue.

Medical. Long-term medical therapy is directed primarily at prevention of recurrence and is dictated by the composition of the stone.[42] The most common combination of findings in the metabolic workup is idiopathic hypercalciuria, elevated urinary uric acid, and low urinary citrate. Patients with this panel are placed on thiazide diuretics, which increase calcium reabsorption at the distal nephron and reduce intestinal absorption, and potassium phosphate, which lowers renal calcium excretion. Potassium alkali salts, which are metabolized and excreted as citrate, may also be used independently.

Infection. Any patient with fever or pyuria in the setting of suspected urolithiasis should be assumed to have a proximal upper tract infection. Nephric abscess and sepsis are potential complications. After obtaining blood and urine cultures, the treating physician should start parenteral antibiotics (ticarcillin/clavulanate or an anti-pseudomonal third-generation cephalosporin is recommended) and obtain urologic consultation for urgent drainage.[43]

Other Causes of Obstructive Uropathy

Intrinsic Processes. Intrinsic causes of urinary obstruction refer to those disease processes, systemic or local, that arise from the urinary system itself. Intrarenal pathologies include nephrocalcinosis, primarily seen in patients receiving alkylating chemotherapy agents. The disease process relates to the high serum uric acid levels associated with necrosis of some tumors, mainly lymphomas and leukemias. Similar phenomena are seen in patients given high-dose sulfadiazine or acyclovir therapy in the primary treatment of HIV-related illnesses. In multiple myeloma, the accumulation of Bence-Jones proteins can lead to precipitation in the renal tubules resulting in complete obstruction and renal failure. Urgent urologic referral for percutaneous nephrostomy drainage offers the best hope of promoting the recovery of renal function. Nevertheless, the incidence of irreversible renal damage is high among patients with multiple myeloma, and renal failure continues to be the leading cause of death in these patients.[1]

Papillary necrosis is an acute process seen in a variety of systemic diseases, including sickle cell disease, anti-inflammatory agent overuse, amyloid, pyelonephritis, and diabetes. Necrotic renal papillae slough into the collecting system, where they may easily be mistaken for a radiolucent obstructing stone on IVP. Similarly, in the setting of severe hematuria (hemophilia, polycystic kidney disease), thrombus may obstruct the ureter. Percutaneous drainage may also be tried here, although stenting the ureter is a common therapeutic modality, especially in distal obstruction.

Bladder dysfunction resulting in urinary obstruction is an important source of morbidity for a variety of disease processes and medications. The "neurogenic" bladder associated with diabetes, multiple sclerosis, or Parkinsonism may either be flaccid or spastic, depending on the prevailing etiology. The bladder dysfunction associated with spinal cord lesions similarly depends on the level involved. Lesions above S4 commonly result in a spastic bladder that can be treated without catheterization, whereas low sacral lesions produce a flaccid bladder and lead to dependency on catheter drainage. Anticholinergic medications can cause functional obstruction due to bladder hypotonia, whereas the anti-Parkinsonian drug levodopa results in sphincter spasm through alpha-adrenergic stimulation.

The most common cause of urinary obstruction worldwide—though rare in the United States—is ureteral and bladder fibrosis from bilharziasis, caused by chronic infection with *Schistosoma haematobium*. Ten to 40% of the 100 million people with schistosomiasis develop these uropathic complications. Other microbial infections, most prominently tuberculosis, aspergillosis, and candidiasis, may cause physical obstruction of the urinary tract.

Ureteral strictures develop in the setting of radiation therapy for pelvic cancers and are most commonly treated with a simple stent. Urethral strictures arise as a result of urethral trauma, including surgery or chronic infection, such as gonorrhea, and present fairly often to the ED. Urethral strictures resulting in urinary retention can often be treated with simple Foley drainage,but may require more advanced drainage techniques, such as Coude catheter placement or an "over-the-wire" technique using a fine filiform catheter. Filiforms are designed to reduce the incidence of false passage in the male urethra, a common complication of attempted drainage in the setting of urethral stricture.[44] If the treating physician is unfamiliar with the use of such devices, and urologic consultation is remote, percutaneous suprapubic drainage is a simple and low-morbidity alternative.[45] In the setting of prior suprapubic procedures, however, the percutaneous approach becomes more dangerous, and surgical consultation is advisable.

Extrinsic Processes. *Urologic Causes.* The most common etiologies of urinary obstruction in the United States relate to compression of the urinary outflow tract by adjacent structures. Of these, benign prostatic hyperplasia (BPH) is the largest single cause. It is estimated that 75% of men over age 70 experience symptoms of outflow obstruction, and, in 1990, over 300,000 men underwent transurethral resection of the prostate (TURP) at an estimated cost of $2.2 billion.[46]

The classic presentation of BPH includes decreased force of the urinary stream, difficulty initiating the stream, and nocturia. The digital rectal examination (DRE) will reveal an enlarged gland with a firm consistency similar to that of the tip of the nose, although the exam can be unreliable. Objective evidence may include an increased post-void residual. Greater than 100 cc is suggestive of outlet obstruction. In fact, an older man who is unable to void and requires catheter drainage is a well-recognized presentation of BPH to the ED. Transrectal ultrasound (TRUS) has also been used to estimate gland

Table 2. Passage Rates Based on Stone Size and Location

SIZE	NUMBER OF STONES PASSED		
	Proximal	Middle	Distal
1 mm	—	1 (100)	12 (85)
2 mm	5 (100)	5 (83)	67 (93)
3 mm	3 (42)	5 (55)	67 (69)
4 mm	4 (20)	5 (62)	29 (55)
5 mm	2 (6)	4 (57)	15 (45)
6 mm	0 (0)	0 (0)	2 (25)
7-9 mm	0 (0)	0 (0)	0 (0)
10-12 mm	0 (0)	—	—

Used with permission: Morse RM, Resnick MI. Ureteral calculi: Natural history and treatment in the era of advanced technology. *J Urol* 1991;145:263.

size and stratify patients for therapy, although the great variability in its positive predictive value limits this modality to an ancillary role at present.[47]

Therapy for BPH ranges from temporizing measures such as transurethral or suprapubic catheterization, to medical management with alpha-1-adrenergic antagonists and 5-alpha-reductase inhibitors, to more definitive surgical procedures like the TURP or open prostatectomy. The indications and timing of intervention are generally dictated by the patient's symptom complex. But when the Agency for Health Care Policy and Research (AHCPR) issued its 1994 clinical practice guidelines for the evaluation and treatment of BPH, the vagaries of this approach were somewhat rectified. Relative indications for operative intervention were based, in part, upon a large longitudinal study demonstrating the four factors that most closely correlated with the eventual need for surgery: age of the patient, change in size or force of the urine stream, sensation of incomplete voiding, and enlarged prostate on DRE.[48] Incontinence was negatively correlated to the need for subsequent surgery, and hesitancy, still a part of the guidelines, did not survive multivariate analysis as a predictor of surgery.

Absolute indications for surgery, based on the AHCPR guidelines, include refractory urinary retention, recurrent UTIs, recurrent or persistent gross hematuria, bladder stones or evidence of renal failure. Relative indications are based on the degree to which the disease impacts upon the patients' daily activities.[46]

The clinical complications of BPH are limited to its effects on renal function, either as a consequence of recurrent infection or direct obstructive nephropathy. The incidence of renal dysfunction in BPH, based on IVP data, is estimated at 5-15%. However, more sensitive nuclear medicine testing demonstrates reduced glomerular filtration rates in as many as 54% of patients.[15] In the ED, evidence of outlet obstruction should be addressed with urgent drainage via transurethral or suprapubic catheter. Assuming no acute renal failure, the patient may be referred with a leg bag to a urologist for outpatient evaluation.

A major concern in the setting of bladder obstruction in a male patient is the possibility of carcinoma of the prostate, second only to lung cancer as a cause of cancer death in American men. This diagnosis should be suspected when DRE reveals a hard nodule or asymmetric prostate. Definitive evaluation involves a needle biopsy. The use of the prostate-specific antigen assay as a screening device is best left to the discretion of the treating physician.[47] Bladder cancer also may cause obstruction and should be suspected in the setting of obstructive uropathy associated with constitutional symptoms.

Gynecologic and Obstetric Causes. The only malignancy more likely than bladder cancer to cause urinary obstruction is cervical cancer.[15] Due to the anatomic proximity to the bladder neck, obstruction will complicate about 30% of cases of cervical cancer. It is a serious complication associated with shortened median survival and reduced five-year survival rates in all pelvic cancers.[49] Patients likely to benefit from urinary diversion are those for whom further treatment options for the malignancy exist. Other groups fare more poorly because the diversion procedures carry significant morbidity and do not themselves prolong life, even in acute renal failure.[50] Clearly, emergent referral is useful in this setting, allowing the specialist the widest window in which to consult with the patient facing a difficult decision.

Uterine fibroid tumors, particularly in the cervical distribution or large posterior fibroids in the retroflexed uterus, may cause bladder neck obstruction. Endometriosis may also cause obstruction and represents a true diagnostic challenge. By contrast, uterine prolapse and subsequent compression of the ureters by the uterine vascular supply is rarely a subtle presentation. Lastly, more than 50% of postoperative cases of inadvertent ureteral injury result from gynecologic surgery.[1]

Hydronephrosis and hydroureter are common during pregnancy and should not be considered pathologic. These usually occur around the 20th week and affect two-thirds of patients.[1] Although the pathophysiology has classically been attributed to direct compression by the uterus, some authors propose that the smooth-muscle-relaxant effect of progesterone better explains the timing of the phenomenon, which is relatively early in the ascent of the fundus. Regardless of the mechanism, the importance of the finding is that it can mask pathological obstruction of another cause. Thus, recurrent urinary tract complaints in the pregnant patient must be viewed with special attentiveness to obstructive nephropathy. Ultrasound indices to account for acceptable degrees of obstruction have been well-described.

The pregnant patient who complains of sudden-onset abdominal pain and oliguria should raise the suspicion for incarcerated uterus. This occurs at about week 12, as the gravid uterus outgrows the pelvis. The anatomically retroflexed uterus may become "wedged" within the pelvis and compress anteriorly on the bladder neck. Generally, bimanual reduction by the obstetrician is effective.

Miscellaneous Causes. There are numerous other causes of obstructive uropathy extrinsic to the urinary tract. Of particular interest to the emergency physician are:

- Pelvic fractures and hematoma, compressing the ureter;[51,52]
- Retroperitoneal fibrosis involving the ureter, associated with a wide variety of conditions, including abdominal aortic aneurysm, scarring from appendiceal or diverticular abscess, gonorrhea, and Henoch-Schönlein purpura;
- Congenital abnormalities, such as congenital ureteropelvic junction obstruction; a hyperplastic condition; ureteral folds, valves, and strictures; and posterior urethral valves in boys.

Bilateral Urinary Obstruction

The degree to which the kidney tolerates obstruction depends first upon whether the insult is unilateral or bilateral and then upon the degree and the duration of obstruction. In no case is the science of obstructive uropathy conclusive, and many mysteries remain.

The pathophysiology of unilateral obstruction is discussed above, and the mechanisms of bilateral disease appear to be similar. Although injury appears to be slower in onset, the consequences of bilateral obstruction (i.e., post-renal azotemia and renal failure) are much more severe.[15] In many cases, the clinician can undertake a temporizing procedure in the ED and relieve the obstruction. Sometimes, however, as with a pelvic mass compressing both ureters, bladder catheterization is not helpful, and emergent consultation is indicated. Timely treatment is paramount, however, because the duration of obstruction—as with urolithiasis—is inversely related to the degree of renal recovery.[53]

If temporizing measures are undertaken in the ED, the clinician must be aware of the risk of post-obstructive diuresis. This phenomenon occurs in the relief of longstanding bilateral obstruction, and probably relates to abnormal salt retention. Onset may be immediate or delayed for several hours; output ranges between 8 and 20 L per day. Treatment involves close monitoring of vital signs, urine output, and electrolytes. Since the output has a sodium concentration of approximately 80 mEq/L, replacement with half-normal saline is recommended until the syndrome subsides, usually within a week.[15]

Summary

Obstructive uropathy is most commonly associated with calculus disease. The chief priorities in approaching the patient with renal colic are pain control, ruling-out infection, and establishing the correct diagnosis. Pain control is best achieved with parenteral NSAIDs, although narcotics are also acceptable. Infection should also be suspected in patients with fever or pyuria, and this constitutes a true emergency in the presence of obstruction. Once infection has been excluded, the ultimate diagnosis can be confirmed either in the ED or as an outpatient. The best diagnostic study is non-contrast CT, although IVP and ultrasound are widely used as well. Patients with suspected obstructive stones should be seen well before one week lapses. Although no human data exist, it is believed that the uninfected kidney can tolerate at least one week of complete obstruction without irreversible damage, requiring that these patients receive expedited follow-up. Other causes of urinary tract obstruction are numerous, but prostatic hypertrophy and cancer should be prominent in the clinician's mind.

References

1. Curhan GC, Zeidel ML. Urinary tract obstruction. In: Brenner BM, ed. *The Kidney.* 5th ed. Philadelphia: WB Saunders; 1996:1936-1958.
2. Sierakowski R, Finlayson B, Landes RR, et al. The frequency of urolithiasis in hospital discharge diagnoses in the United States. *Invest Urol* 1978;16:438-441.
3. Ljunghall S, Fellstrom B, Johansson G. Prevention of renal stones by a high fluid intake? *Eur Urol* 1988;14:381-385.
4. Wilson DM. Clinical and laboratory approaches for evaluation of urolithiasis. *J Urol* 1989;141:770-774.
5. Stewart C. Urolithiasis. *Emerg Med Clin North Am* 1988;6:617-630.
6. Coe FL, Parks JH, Asplin JR. The pathogenesis and treatment of kidney stones. *N Engl J Med* 1992;327:1141-1152.
7. Levy FL, Adams-Huet B, Pak CYC. Ambulatory evaluation of urolithiasis: An update of a 1980 protocol. *Am J Med* 1995;98:50-59.
8. Preminger GM. The metabolic evaluation of patients with recurrent urolithiasis: A review of comprehensive and simplified approaches. *J Urol* 1989;141:760-763.
9. Curhan GC, Willett WC, Rimm EB, et al. A prospective study of dietary calcium and other nutrients and the risk of symptomatic kidney stones. *N Engl J Med* 1993;328:833-838.
10. Yendt ER, Cohanim M. Clinical and laboratory approaches for evaluation of urolithiasis. *J Urol* 1989;141:764-769.
11. Kerr WS. Effects of complete ureteral obstruction in dogs on kidney function. *Am J Physiol* 1956;521-526.
12. Widén T. Restitution of kidney function after induced urinary stasis of varying duration. *Acta Chir Scand* 1957;113:507-510.
13. Vaughan ED, Jr, Gillenwalter JY. Recovery following complete chronic unilateral ureteral occlusion: Functional, radiographic and pathologic alterations. *J Urol* 1971;106:27-34.
14. Shapiro SR, Bennett AH. Recovery of renal function after prolonged unilateral ureteral obstruction. *J Urol* 1976;115:136-140.
15. Yarger WE. Urinary tract obstruction. In: Brenner BM, Rector F, ed. *The Kidney.* 4th ed. Philadelphia: WB Saunders; 1991:1768-1808.
16. Diamond JR. Macrophages and progressive renal disease in experimental hydronephrosis. *Am J Kid Dis* 1995;26:133-140.
17. Elton TJ, Roth CS, Berquist TH, et al. A clinical prediction rule for the diagnosis of ureteral calculi in emergency departments. *J Gen Intern Med* 1993;8:57-62.
18. Jenkins AD. Calculus formation. In: Gillenwalter J, et al, eds. *Adult and Pediatric Urology.* 3rd ed. St. Louis: Mosby-Year Book; 1996:461-486.
19. Coe FL, Keck J, Norton ER. The natural history of calcium urolithiasis. *JAMA* 1977;238:1519-1523.
20. Roth CS, Bowyer BA, Berquist TH. Utility of the plain abdominal radiograph for diagnosing ureteral calculi. *Ann Emerg Med* 1985;14:311-315.
21. Zangerle KF, Iserson KV, Bjelland JC. Usefulness of abdominal flat plate radiographs in patients with suspected ureteral calculi. *Ann Emerg Med* 1985;14:316-319.
22. Mutgi A, Williams JW, Nettleman M. Renal colic: Utility of the plain abdominal Roentgenogram. *Arch Intern Med* 1991;151:1589-1592.
23. Haddad MC, Sharif HS, Shahed MS, et al. Renal colic: Diagnosis and outcome. *Radiology* 1992;184:83-88.
24. LeRoy AJ. Diagnosis and treatment of urolithiasis: Current perspectives. *Am J Roentgenol* 1994;163:1309-1313.
25. Pollack HM, Banner MP. Current status of excretory urography: A premature epitaph. *Urol Clin North Am* 1985;12:585-601.

26. Haddad MC, Sharif HS, Abomelha MS, et al. Management of renal colic: Redefining the role of the urogram. *Radiology* 1992;184:35-36.
27. Vritska TJ, Hattery RR, King BF, et al. Role of ultrasound in medical management of patients with renal stone disease. *Urol Radiol* 1992;14:131-138.
28. Sommer FG, Jeffrey RB, Jr, Rubin GD, et al. Detection of ureteral calculi in patients with suspected renal colic: Value of reformatted noncontrast helical CT. *Am J Roentgenol* 1995;165:509-513.
29. Spital A, Valvo JR, Segal AJ. Nondilated obstructive uropathy. *Urology* 1988;31:478-482.
30. Spital A, Spataro R. Nondilated obstructive uropathy due to a ureteral calculus. *Am J Med* 1995;98:509-511.
31. Burge H, Middleton WD, McClennan BL, et al. Ureteral jets in healthy subjects and in patients with unilateral ureteral calculi: Comparison with color Doppler US. *Radiology* 1991;180:437-442.
32. Smith RC, Rosenfeld AT, Choe KA, et al. Acute flank pain: Comparison of non-contrast-enhanced CT and intravenous urography. Radiology 1995;194:789-794.
33. Borghi L, Meschi T, Amato F, et al. Nifedipine and methylprednisolone in facilitating ureteral stone passage: A randomized, double-blind, placebo-controlled study. *J Urol* 1994;152:1095-1098.
34. Morse RM, Resnick MI. Ureteral calculi: Natural history and treatment in an era of advanced technology. *J Urol* 1991;145:263-265.
35. Wrenn K. Emergency intravenous pyelography in the setting of possible renal colic: Is it indicated? *Ann Emerg Med* 1995;26:304-307.
36. Oosterlinck W, Philips NH, Charig C, et al. A double-blind single-dose comparison of intramuscular ketorolac tromethamine and pethidine in the treatment of renal colic. *J Clin Pharmacol* 1990;30:336-341.
37. Larsen LS, Miller A, Allegra JR. The use of intravenous ketorolac for the treatment of renal colic in the emergency department. *Am J Emerg Med* 1993;11:197-199.
38. Cordell WH, Larson TA, Lingeman JE, et al. Indomethacin suppositories versus intravenously titrated morphine for the treatment of ureteral colic. *Ann Emerg Med* 1994;23:262-269.
39. Pak CYC, Sakhee K, Crowther C, et al. Evidence justifying a high fluid intake in treatment of urolithiasis. *Ann Intern Med* 1980;93:36-39.
40. McCormack M, Dessureault J, Guitard M. The urine specific gravity dipstick: A useful tool to increase fluid intake in stone forming patients. *J Urol* 1991;146:1475-1477.
41. O'Brien WM, Rotolo JE, Pahira JJ. New approaches in the treatment of renal calculi. *Am Fam Physician* 1987:36:181-194.
42. Preminger GM. Renal calculi: Pathogenesis, diagnosis and medical therapy. *Sem Nephrol* 1992;12:200-216.
43. Sanford JP, Gilbert DN, Sande MA. *The Sanford Guide to Antimicrobial Therapy.* 26th ed. Dallas: Antimicrobial Therapy, Inc; 1996:23.
44. Heyman AM, Kogler P, Vogel M, et al. Slipover urethral instrument system. *J Urol* 1982;128:759.
45. Zbaraschuk I, Berger RE, Hedges JR. Genitourinary procedures. In: Roberts JR, Hedges JR, eds. *Clinical Procedures in Emergency Medicine,* 2nd ed. Philadelphia: WB Saunders; 1991:867-889.
46. Jacobsen SJ, Girman CJ, Guess HA, et al. New diagnostic and treatment guidelines for benign prostatic hyperplasia: Potential impact in the United States. *Arch Intern Med* 1995;155:477-481.
47. Hostetler RM, Mandel IG, Marshburn J. Prostate cancer screening. *Med Clin North Am* 1996;80:83-98.
48. Arrighi HM, Guess HA, Metter, EJ, et al. Symptoms and signs of prostatism as risk factors for prostatectomy. *Prostate* 1990;16:253-261.
49. Lau MWM, Temperley DE, Mehta S, et al. Urinary tract obstruction and nephrostomy drainage in pelvic malignant disease. *Br J Urol* 1995;76:565-569.
50. Harrington KJ, Pandha HS, Kelley SA, et al. Palliation of obstructive nephropathy due to malignancy. *Br J Urol* 1995;76:101-107.
51. Flint P, Allen CF. Pelvic fracture complicated by bilateral ureteral obstruction: Case report. *J Trauma* 1994;36:285-287.
52. Kluger Y, Altman GT, Deshmukh R, et al. Acute obstructive uropathy secondary to pelvic hematoma compressing the bladder: Report of two cases. *J Trauma* 1993;35:477-478.
53. Thadhani R, Pascual M, Bonventre JV. Acute renal failure. *N Engl J Med* 1996;334:1448-1460.

End-Stage Renal Disease

Walter G. Belleza, MD

The patient with end-stage renal disease (ESRD) is a diagnostic and therapeutic challenge for the emergency physician. Clinical presentations range from the nearly asymptomatic patient with laboratory evidence of mild hyperkalemia to the patient with fulminate pulmonary edema or cardiac arrest. Within a narrow window of time and with limited data, the emergency physician must initiate potentially treacherous therapeutic maneuvers for a patient functioning within narrow metabolic boundaries.

By definition, ESRD occurs when a patient's kidneys can no longer sustain life without the aid of dialysis therapy or a renal transplant. It is at the end point of chronic renal failure where the majority of clinical complications occur. Chronic renal failure (CRF) implies that an irreversible reduction in renal function exists, and recovery of that function is unlikely.

Nearly every organ system suffers in ESRD. If profound enough and not treated accordingly, ESRD results in the uremic syndrome. The uremic syndrome is a constellation of multisystemic complications that result from the accumulation of nitrogenous wastes and metabolic by-products. Symptoms may range from fluid overload and congestive heart failure to encephalopathy and coma. To prevent this and other systemic derangements, patients are started on either peritoneal dialysis or hemodialysis. Dialysis therapy can be life-saving but also can cause its own complications. In this chapter, the authors review the complex constellation of problems associated with ESRD from the perspective of the emergency physician.

Demographics

An estimation of the number of patients suffering from ESRD is provided by the United States Renal Data Systems (USRDS). Current worldwide estimates indicate a gradual increase in the number of patients entering dialysis therapy, with the United States having the highest rate.[1] As of 1993, statistics from USRDS demonstrate that more than 220,000 patients suffer from ESRD, with an annual growth rate of 8-9%.[2] Some projections indicate that the number of dialysis enrollees will exceed 250,000 by the year 2000.[4] The increase in numbers may also be due to more diabetic and elderly patients being accepted for dialysis therapy. In addition, there is a growing population of patients with predialysis renal insufficiency who may require treatment. As of 1990, this group was estimated to number between 648,000 and 708,000 patients.[5]

In the United States, the most common causes of chronic renal failure, in decreasing incidence, are: diabetes, hypertension, glomerulonephritis, cystic renal disease, and interstitial nephritis.[6] A disproportionate number of patients with ESRD are young, urban-dwelling blacks who suffer from severe, untreated hypertension.[1,4]

Table 1. Differential Diagnosis of Altered Mental Status in Patients with ESRD

Structural Lesions	**Metabolic**
Subdural hematoma	Elemental intoxication (copper, nickel)
Normal pressure hydrocephalus	Drug intoxication
Cerebrovascular accident (hemorrhagic, embolic)	Meningitis/encephalitis
Cerebral abscess	Seizures
Post traumatic	Hypermagnesemia
	Hypernatremia/hyponatremia
Cardiovascular	Hypoxia
Arrhythmia	Hypercalcemia
Myocardial infarction	Hyperglycemia/Hypoglycemia
Hypertension/Hypotension	Hyperparathyroidism
	Nonketotic hyperosmolar coma
Other	Hypophosphatemia
Excessive ultrafiltration	
Wernicke encephalopathy	
Dialysis/Dementia	

Pathophysiology

After receiving a pathogenic insult, the kidney can either recover and continue to function normally, develop chronic renal insufficiency, or progress to ESRD. Factors that influence disease progression include the severity and type of the primary insult, presence of other chronic diseases (hypertension, diabetes, HIV), age, and continuing insult (infection, obstruction). Once chronic renal insufficiency is established, and plasma creatinine exceeds 1.5-2.0 mg/dL, progression to ESRD occurs with an almost linear decline in the glomerular filtration rate (GFR).[7] Although the aforementioned exogenous factors can serve to accelerate functional decline, disease progression still occurs in their absence. This is due to many intrinsic processes that are poorly understood.

If the original insult results in irreversible injury, the remaining functional glomerular units become hyperperfused. This results in increases in glomerular capillary pressure that become injurious by inducing histological changes that cause glomerular hypertrophy, fusion of epithelial foot processes, and mesangial expansion.[7-9] The mesangial expansion causes the eventual collapse of the capillary lumens and the eventual appearance of patchy glomerulosclerosis.

In addition to causing cellular changes, this hyperfunction induces an "injury response" that involves cellular elements, chemical mediators, and biologically active compounds and results in glomerular and tubulointerstitial damage. Implicated cellular elements include macrophages, monocytes, leukocytes, and platelets.[8,9] Once attracted to the damaged area, these elements help initiate an inflammatory cascade involving chemical mediators such as interleukin-1, platelet activating factor, thromboxane A2, and heparinase.[8,9] The chemical mediator interleukin-1 promotes attachment of inflammatory cells such as neutrophils and monocytes and stimulates the release of thromboxane A2. Thromboxane A2 serves as a vasoconstrictor that decreases glomerular perfusion and promotes platelet aggregation. Platelets, in turn, release platelet-derived growth factor that promotes growth of fibroblasts and proliferation of smooth muscle cells and the release of prostaglandins and leukotrienes that perpetuate the inflammatory cascade.

Clinical Effects

Cardiovascular Complications. Cardiovascular and cerebrovascular complications account for 15-30% of deaths in patients suffering from chronic renal failure.[19-22] Although not considered an independent risk factor for heart disease, chronic renal failure may coexist with other proven cardiac risk factors, such as diabetes, hypertension, and hypercholesterolemia. In addition, ESRD makes control of these conditions more difficult. Cardiovascular conditions that are likely to require emergent evaluation and treatment are hypertension, congestive heart failure (CHF) or pulmonary edema, myocardial ischemia, pericardial disease, and dysrhythmias.

Hypertension. Hypertension in the patient with chronic renal failure is a multifactorial problem. Secondary complications of renal failure, such as volume overload, sodium imbalance, elevated catecholamine levels, and derangements in the renin-angiotensin system, can be superimposed on a pre-existing hypertensive condition.[23,24] A hypertensive emergency exists when signs of severe progressive end-organ damage (e.g., encephalopathy, CHF, cardiac ischemia) occur in the presence of elevated blood pressure. Although a hypertensive emergency does not usually occur until the diastolic blood pressure exceeds 130 mmHg, it can occur at levels as low as 110 mmHg.

Congestive Heart Failure/Pulmonary Edema. As with other complications in renal failure, CHF involves multiple pathophysiologic mechanisms. In addition to primary cardiac dysfunction, volume overload, positive sodium balance, high output failure from anemia, and arteriovenous fistulas are major contributing factors. Cardiac dysfunction can result from hypertension, left ventricular hypertrophy, cardiac ischemia, cardiomyopathy, electrolyte abnormalities, dysrhythmias, and hyperparathyroidism.[21,23,24,26-28] Although the most common cause of CHF and pulmonary edema in patients with ESRD is volume overload, all of the previously mentioned factors can cause heart failure and should be considered in the differential diagnosis. Volume overload may range between 5-10 L and can result from a seemingly innocuous ingestion of food or fluid.

Pericardial Disease. Prior to widespread dialysis therapy, pericarditis occurred in more than 50% of ESRD patients and was a harbinger of early demise. However, the current incidence is between 2%-19% and can occur in patients not receiving dialysis as well as those undergoing dialysis.[35] In patients not receiving dialysis, its presence indicates the need to initiate therapy. In patients currently on dialysis, pericarditis indicates the presence of stresses such as trauma and infection or the need for a more aggressive dialysis regimen. The exact pathophysiologic process in under-dialyzed patients is unknown but is thought to be secondary to retained metabolic byproducts.

The most common chief complaint is substernal, nonexertional, sharp pleuritic chest pain. The pain can increase by moving, yawning, and lying supine. It is relieved by sitting upright and can predate diagnostic evidence by 1-2 weeks. Other complaints include shortness of breath, cough, weight loss, fever, and malaise. Clues that indicate significant effusion are new dysrhythmias, frequent episodes of hypotension during dialysis, or a decreasing need to medically control hypertension in a previously hypertensive patient.[23]

Dysrhythmia. Coronary artery disease (CAD), cardiac dysfunction, electrolyte disorders, and the use of potentially proarrhythmic medication are common occurrences in patients with ESRD.[14,39,40] These factors, along with pericardial disease, decreased oxygen delivery from chronic anemia, and dialysis-induced hypotension, can predispose patients to dysrhythmias. Common dysrhythmias include atrial fibrillation and flutter, PVCs, and non-sustained ventricular tachycardia.[41-44] Dysrhythmias may be precipitated by any condition that impairs cardiac oxygen delivery, and electrolyte disorders such as hyperkalemia, hypercalcemia, and hypermagnesemia.

Coronary Artery Disease. CAD and myocardial ischemia commonly occur in patients with ESRD.[19-22,43] The presence of left ventricular hypertrophy, an AV fistula, and fluid overload may increase cardiac oxygen demand, while chronic anemia can decrease oxygen availability. It was previously thought that the incidence of myocardial ischemia was more prevalent among patients with renal failure and ESRD. Recent studies have shown that, when adjustments are made for age and coexisting disease, there is no significant difference between this population and others. The differential diagnosis of chest pain should include pericarditis, pleural effusion, aortic dissection, pneumothorax, infection, and pulmonary embolism.

Acute Neurologic Complications. Neurologic dysfunction is a well-known consequence of ESRD and can involve the central and peripheral nervous systems.[65,66] Complications range from neuropathies and the restless leg syndrome to lethargy and coma. The challenge for the physician is to distinguish between acute, chronic, and potentially life-threatening disorders. Two significant problems that may be seen in the ED are the dialysis disequilibrium syndrome and mental status changes.

Dialysis Disequilibrium Syndrome. This well-known complication usually occurs during or shortly after dialysis. Neurologic symptoms include headache, weakness, restlessness, confusion, seizures, and coma. The syndrome results when the removal of solutes from the blood is too rapid to allow an equilibration between the central nervous system and the rest of the body.[24,48] It occurs more frequently in patients who have more severe metabolic derangements prior to dialysis and in those undergoing a more aggressive dialysis regimen. The syndrome is a diagnosis of exclusion, and other etiologies, such as infection, CVA, uremic encephalopathy, hypoxia, subdural hematoma, and drug intoxication, should be considered.

Altered Mental Status. The list of problems that can cause mental-status change in patients with ESRD is extensive. *(See Table 1.)* In addition to common conditions such as stroke, medication effects, and hypoglycemia, complications from the dialysis process must be considered. These include hypotension, the disequilibrium syndrome, dysrhythmia, and spontaneous CNS hemorrhage.[63] Acute onset may indicate cerebrovascular accidents, dysrhythmias, or trauma. A history of slow onset and dialysis noncompliance may indicate uremic encephalopathy.

Hematological Complications. Bleeding and anemia are common occurrences in patients with ESRD. In addition to an underlying platelet dysfunction, bleeding can occur secondary to concurrent heparin administration during dialysis. Anemia can be a consequence of ESRD but can result from an acute hemorrhagic episode. The challenge for the ED physician is to identify the acuity of these conditions and initiate appropriate therapy.

Common sites of bleeding include vascular access sites and the gastrointestinal tract.[72] Spontaneous hemorrhage into the subdural, retropharyngeal, and retroperitoneal spaces can also occur.[12,61-63] Any area of progressive swelling and pain may harbor occult hemorrhage.

Infectious Complications. Infection is the second most common cause of mortality and morbidity in patients with ESRD and accounts for 15-40% of deaths in this population.[26,46] In addition to compromised humoral and cellular immune responses, patients often have indwelling peritoneal or vascular access devices that serve as ports of entry for infectious agents.[47,48] Conditions that may act as immunosuppressants are chronic uremia, malnutrition, iron overload from transfusion, and electrolyte disorders. Areas such as the urinary tract and lungs have diminished local defenses, making them more susceptible to infection. Other contributing factors to urinary infection include bladder stasis, dysmotility, and underlying structural disease. Complaints of dysuria and frequency may be absent because of decreased urinary flow.

The patient with ESRD should be viewed as an immunocompromised host. Because of this, the presence of fever should prompt an extensive evaluation. Patients may present with fever, chills, hypothermia, joint pain, constitutional complaints, and symptoms referable to the site of infection. Common sites of infection include the lung, urinary tract, vascular access sites, and the peritoneum. Vascular access sites and peritoneal catheters are the most common sources of infection in patients undergoing hemodialysis and peritoneal dialysis, respectively.[50-52]

Electrolyte Complications. Electrolyte abnormalities are the hallmark of chronic renal failure. While many of these complications are not life-threatening and respond to hemodialysis, hyperkalemia, hypercalcemia, and hypermagnesemia can result in clinical decompensation if not treated. These conditions are rare in the compliant and adequately dialyzed patient but can occur due to dietary indiscretion and dialysis noncompliance.

Hyperkalemia. Causes of hyperkalemia include pharmacological agents, dietary and dialysis noncompliance, rhabdomyolysis, metabolic acidosis, and catabolic states. Medications that produce hyperkalemia include: nonselective beta blockers, calcium channel blockers, succinylcholine, and digoxin if taken in toxic doses.[54,55] Tissue breakdown from rhabdomyolysis results in release of intracellular potassium. Extracellular potassium shifts occur with metabolic acidosis.

There are no specific clinical or physical manifestations that can aid in early diagnosis of hyperkalemia. Because clinical presentation can range from cardiac arrest to mild constitutional symptoms, a high index of suspicion for this problem should be maintained in any patient with ESRD who presents to the ED. Although most patients are asymptomatic, the most common complaint is weakness.[34] Because the most important consequence of hyperkalemia is increased cardiac irritability, an ECG should be obtained early.

Hypercalcemia and Hypermagnesemia. Hypercalcemia and hypermagnesemia by themselves, or in conjunction with hyperkalemia, can increase cardiac irritability and potentiate cardiac dysrhythmias. Though not a common consequence of renal failure, hypercalcemia and hypermagnesemia can occur due to the inadvertent use of common medications—phosphate binders, vitamin D analogues, and calcium supplements in hypercalcemia, and magnesium-containing antacids and lithium therapy in hypermagnesemia. As in hyperkalemia, patients often present with a variety of clinical complaints that range from weakness and malaise to cardiopulmonary instability and coma.

Patients with mild hypercalcemia are often asymptomatic but generally have clinical signs once the level exceeds 11.5 mg/dL. Presentation may include nausea, vomiting, fatigue, muscle weakness, and abdominal pain. Mental status changes, such as lack of concentration, confusion, and coma may also occur.[24] Although most physical findings are nonspecific, signs of long-standing hypercalcemia such as band keratopathy may be present.

Hypermagnesemia inhibits the presynaptic release of acetylcholine and norepinephrine. Although most side effects involve neural tissue, magnesium also affects vascular smooth muscle and cardiac tissue. Nausea and vomiting can occur at levels of 4-5 mEq/L (2.0-2.5 mmol/L), loss of deep tendon reflexes and mental status changes occur at levels of 4-7 mEq/L (2.0-3.5 mmol/L), and respiratory paralysis occurs at levels of 10-15 mEq/L (5.0-7.5 mmol/L). Other signs include hypotension, lethargy, and paralysis.

Emergent Complications of Dialysis Therapy

The objective of dialysis therapy is the removal of toxins, metabolic waste products, and excess volume from the vascular space. Through the processes of ultrafiltration and diffusion, solutes and material pass from the vascular space to a dialysate solution by crossing semipermeable membranes located either intraperitoneally (peritoneal dialysis) or externally (hemodialysis). By adjusting the duration of therapy and the nature of the dialysate material, specific changes can be made in the constitution of a patient's plasma. Although many complications can occur from dialysis therapy, those likely to require emergent evaluation involve instability during the dialysis process, mechanical defects, and infection. Because unique problems occur in peritoneal dialysis and hemodialysis, they will be discussed separately.

Peritoneal Dialysis. Peritoneal dialysis involves the sterile introduction of dialysate fluid into the peritoneum through a surgically implanted catheter. The dialysate fluid is then allowed to equilibrate with the patient's plasma for a specific amount of time (dwell time). By adjusting the dialysate material and the length of dwell time, the consistency of a patient's plasma can be adjusted. The fluid is later withdrawn under sterile conditions. Although multiple modalities of peritoneal dialysis are available, the one most commonly used is continuous ambulatory peritoneal dialysis (CAPD). In this modality, the dwell time lasts from 4-6 hours and treatment is performed by the patient four times daily. Because of its ease of use, avoidance of hemodynamic instability from rapid volume shifts, and freedom from use of a dialysis center, CAPD is favored by younger patients, the elderly, and those with severe cardiovascular problems. Because CAPD is relatively stable, conditions such as hypotension, chest pain, and neurological deficits should not be attributed to the dialysis process.

Mechanical Complications. Mechanical complications include obstruction and leakage from the catheter site. Patients will notice either an inability to infuse or properly remove dialysate fluid. This can be due to kinking of the catheter tubing, intraperitoneal migration, or obstruction from overlying omentum or peritoneal debris.[59]

Infection. Infection is the most common complication that afflicts the patient receiving peritoneal dialysis, and it occurs an average of once every nine months.[30] In addition to diffuse abdominal pain and dialysate fluid that becomes cloudy, infected peritoneal dialysis patients may experience nausea, vomiting, fevers, and chills. The most common infectious agents are skin-inhabiting *Staphylococcus epidermidis* and *Staphylococcus aureus*.[46,50,67] Infection is usually due to a break in aseptic technique during dialysis exchange. Other organisms include gram-negative organisms such as *Escherichia coli*, *Pseudomonas*, *Enterobacter*, and fungal species such as *Candida*.[46,50,67]

In addition to microbial infection, peritonitis can occur secondary to allergic reactions to the dialysis catheters (eosinophilic peritonitis) or dialysate fluid (sclerosing peritonitis). While eosinophilic peritonitis is a self-limited condition, sclerosing peritonitis may result in abdominal adhesions that require discontinuation of peritoneal dialysis. If adhesions are severe, surgical lysis may be required.

Hemodialysis. Hemodialysis involves exchanges between a patient's plasma and a dialysate bath through semipermeable membranes. Vascular access is achieved either through a temporary large intravenous double lumen catheter or repeated cannulation of a permanent, surgically constructed, arterio-venous fistula. Fistula construction uses either native or animal vasculature or synthetic material. The fistula usually connects the patient's radial artery to a large vein in the patient's nondominant arm in an end-to-side or side-to-side fashion. Complications involve mechanical obstruction, infection, hemorrhage, and hemodynamic instability during or after dialysis therapy.

Mechanical Complications. The most common mechanical problem with vascular access devices is obstruction from thrombosis, which is usually caused by venous hyperplasia at the venous end of the graft's anastomotic site. Thrombosis can also result from trauma, inadvertent compression while sleeping, or during compression of a graft hemorrhage. Mechanical obstruction may result from inadvertent kinking of the graft site. The likelihood of obstruction is increased following dialysis from a combination of a low-flow state and hypercoaguable condition.[30,68] Obstruction can also occur in temporary double lumen devices.

History may reveal a loss of the bruit or thrill at the fistula site. If obstruction of a double lumen occurs, severe extremity edema can result. Temporary devices may be inadvertently or intentionally removed with resultant hemorrhage.

Infection. The most common source of infection in patients undergoing hemodialysis treatment is the access site. In addition to symptoms of a localized process, infection of access sites can cause metastatic infection involving the vertebrae, joints, and cardiac valves.[34] Joints commonly infected include the wrist, knee, and shoulder. The aortic valve is most frequently infected from metastatic infections. As in peritoneal dialysis, gram-positive skin flora such as *S. aureus* and *S. epidermidis* are the usual causative agents. Infection usually results from frequent handling and cannulation as well as breaks in aseptic technique.

Table 2. Cannulation of Dialysis Vascular Grafts

- Avoid improper placement by documenting function (bruit, thrill) and avoid cannulation of possible aneurysms and pseudoaneurysms
- Adhere to strict sterile technique and firmly, but not occlusively, compress access site for 5-10 min after use
- Avoid use of tourniquets (use finger compression) and multiple punctures
- If IV infusions are to be performed:
  —safely secure all catheters with tape
  —use infusion pump or "pressure bag" apparatus if high-pressure access is cannulated
  —standard intravenous infusion devices may be used if low pressure access is cannulated, or if a precise infusion rate is not required

Adapted from: Wolfson AB, Levy M. The patient with chronic renal insufficiency following renal transplantation. In: *Emergency Care of the Compromised Host*. Philadelphia: J.B. Lippincott Co.; 1994:413-432.

Although localized warmth, tenderness, and erythema may indicate infection, their absence does not exclude the possibility of infection. In fact, as many as one-third of patients will have no localizing signs and may only complain of constitutional symptoms such as malaise, fever, chills, nausea, and vomiting.[23,30]

Hemorrhage. Bleeding is a common problem with vascular access sites. This is due to frequent cannulation, platelet dysfunction, and use of heparin during dialysis. Unlike "natural grafts," the walls of synthetic devices cannot collapse and are more prone to hemorrhage and formation of pseudoaneurysm. A pseudo-aneurysm is a pulsatile hematoma with a pseudocapsule, while an aneurysm is a true expansion of the vessel wall. Both can produce hemorrhagic complications. An additional cause of bleeding is the AV fistula or graft that is used prematurely prior to adequate maturation after implantation.

Hemodynamic Instability. Hypotension commonly occurs during dialysis and is usually due to a combination of underlying autonomic dysfunction and decreased cardiac output from acute depletion in intravascular volume. The decrease in vascular volume occurs from fluid removal in patients who enter dialysis either euvolemic or relatively hypovolemic. Other possibilities include: cardiac dysfunction from ischemia, arrhythmia, or pericardial effusion, infection, sepsis, antihypertensive use, pulmonary embolism, air embolism, and anaphylaxis. Anaphylaxis can occur at the initiation of dialysis treatment and may be a reaction to the dialyzer membrane, the sterilizer used in cleaning the dialysis machine, or bacterial endotoxins.[63] Dialysis personnel should provide records that document the time of occurrence, any coexisting symptoms, and any diagnostic or therapeutic measures.

Air Embolism. Air embolism is a rare but potentially lethal complication of dialysis therapy that results from passage of air from either an external mechanical malfunction in the circuit or from the dialyzer itself. The dialyzer may be a source of air if refrigerated dialysate containing dissolved air is used.

Clinical presentation depends on the amount of air introduced and the position that the patient is in at the time. Although complications can result from as little as 5 mL of air, larger amounts are required to produce cardiovascular collapse. If the patient is upright, a rushing sensation to the head may soon be followed by neurological dysfunction. Patients lying supine may complain of chest pain or shortness of breath. Those in the Trendelenburg position are fortunate because air will pass into the lower extremities, sparing the heart but demonstrating patchy cyanosis on the lower extremities.

Prehospital Care

Initial prehospital support emphasizes the ABCs with initiation of any required resuscitative measures per pre-established ACLS protocols and rapid transport to an appropriate institution. If an airway is required, EMS personnel should be aware that patients with ESRD can have clotting dysfunction and that tracheal intubation may result in inadvertent hemorrhage.[10-12] If the patient can breathe spontaneously, the sitting position may be helpful. Oxygen should be administered via high-flow delivery systems. Efforts to obtain peripheral IV access should be made but should not delay transport. Field attempts at cannulation of vascular grafts should be avoided. Although pharmacologic therapy is limited in the field, early measures include the use of furosemide (Lasix) and nitroglycerin if congestive heart failure is suspected. Nitroglycerin also addresses cardiac ischemia.

Pre-hospital caregivers should attempt to obtain historical information from the patient and family members. Aside from the past medical history, helpful information includes length, frequency, compliance, and duration of any dialysis and medical treatments, previous renal complications, prescription and non-prescription drug use, and any illicit drug use.

ED Care

General Resuscitative Measures. Patient status must be assessed quickly and stabilized prior to initiating any diagnostic evaluation. As with any medical emergency, the ABCs (airway, breathing, circulation) consistently take precedence. In addition to stabilization measures, patients should be placed on a cardiac monitor and continuous pulse oximeter, receive an ECG, and have appropriate laboratory studies obtained shortly after arrival. If hemorrhage is suspected, blood should be sent for type and crossmatch.

Airway. The patient with ESRD can develop respiratory distress from conditions that afflict the general population (pneumonia, myocardial infarction, pulmonary embolism) and those that occur with increasing frequency among dialysis patients (volume overload, cardiac/pleural effusion).

The airway can be secured by a variety of measures, including nasotracheal or oral intubation. If mechanical ventilation is chosen, extreme care should be taken to avoid traumatic intubation. Patients with ESRD may have a severe bleeding diathesis and may bleed spontaneously into the retropharyngeal space.[10-12] Although succinylcholine can cause hyperkalemia, its use is not contraindicated in patients with ESRD unless severe hyperkalemia is suspected as the cause of compromise.[13,14] Vecuronium (Norcuron) may also be used, but pancuronium should be avoided in patients with glomerular filtration rate (GFR) less than 10 mL/min because of possible recurarization after initial recovery.

Breathing. Once the airway has been secured adequate oxygenation should be administered via high-flow oxygen or by mechanical means. A possible option in the ED is the use of continuous positive airway pressure (CPAP) techniques. CPAP's efficacy in avoiding intubation in patients with pulmonary edema secondary to cardiac dysfunction and fluid overload from ESRD has been shown in several studies.[14-18]

Circulation. To avoid any complications with vascular graft cannulation, peripheral access is ideal. If this is not possible, or if intravascular monitoring is required, central venous access should be obtained. If neither of these can be done and IV access is needed quickly, the vascular graft can be cannulated as a last resort. *(Please see Table 2.)*

Diagnostic Evaluation. *History/Physical.* As with any other medical problem, treatment begins with a thorough history and physical examination. Information should be obtained from the patient, family members, other physicians, and dialysis center personnel. The history should ideally seek to establish the patient's baseline functional and medical status; the duration, etiology, and any complications from ESRD; and the level of compliance with dialysis, medical, and dietary therapy.

Evaluation of cardiovascular complications such as myocardial ischemia, dysrhythmias, and hypertensive crisis should be approached in the same manner as in those patients with normal renal function. The physical exam must include a thorough cardiopulmonary, cerebrovascular, and neurological evaluation. Signs of volume overload must be sought in patients with congestive heart failure. Complaints of chest pain should prompt consideration of aortic dissection and pericarditis as well as cardiac ischemia. Signs of aortic dissection may include a new diastolic murmur and pulse/pressure differentials in the extremities.

The evaluation of pericarditis can be difficult because physical findings such as the pericardial friction rub may not be audible until well after the onset of symptoms.[35] The rub is best auscultated along the left sternal border at the third and fourth intercostal spaces using the diaphragm of the stethoscope. It can have a one-, two-, or three-component character, and its presence along with pain is highly suggestive of pericarditis.[36] The presence of pulsus paradoxus, a decrease in systolic blood pressure greater than 10 mmHg during inspiration, should raise suspicion of significant pericardial effusion.

The patient with ESRD should be viewed as an immunocompromised host, and nonspecific complaints as well as fever should prompt consideration of infection. Significant information includes the duration of symptoms, focal complaints, previous infectious complications, HIV status, recent hospitalizations, vaccination status, any recent dental or medical instrumentation, and any illicit drug use. If the patient is sexually active, a social history with an emphasis on high-risk behavior is important. If the patient is receiving dialysis, the time and occurrence of any fever should be sought. Fever that occurs early in dialysis or shortly after cessation is usually secondary to infection. If fever occurs during dialysis, a "pyrogen" reaction may be causative.

The physical exam must include close inspection of the likely infectious sites, such as the lung, urinary tract, peritoneum, and catheter access sites. If the patient is diabetic, the oropharynx, integument, and extremities should be carefully inspected. A cardiopulmonary exam should focus on any new murmurs, signs of pulmonary consolidation, and manifestations of embolic disease. If the patient has fever and abdominal pain signs of other intra-abdominal processes, such as pancreatitis, appendicitis, cholecystitis, or mesenteric ischemia, an abscess must be sought before the diagnosis of CAPD peritonitis is made. Sexually active patients should receive a thorough pelvic and rectal exam. Joints should be checked for metastatic infection if a vascular graft is infected.

If patients are receiving peritoneal dialysis or hemodialysis, catheter and vascular access sites should be closely examined for erythema, fluctuance, discharge, and tenderness. As mentioned previously, an alarming one-third of patients with vascular access infections will manifest no symptoms.[23,30,50] If a vascular shunt is used, its functional integrity should be established. Loss of the bruit or thrill may indicate occlusion. Signs of aneurysm or pseudoaneurysm may include pain, thinning of the overlying skin, exposure of graft material, or impingement of adjacent structures. Aneurysms are a common nidus of infection and may "seed" distant sites, such as the joints, vertebrae, and cardiac valves.

Diagnostic Studies. Because nonspecific complaints may indicate a serious condition, initial diagnostic studies should include at least a 12-lead ECG, electrolytes, and cardiac monitoring. If clinically indicated, a CBC, coagulation studies, ABG, chest x-ray, blood cultures, urinalysis, lumbar puncture, therapeutic drug levels, and toxicology screen should be obtained. It should be noted that patients undergoing hemodialysis can demonstrate low leukocyte counts following dialysis, and, because of impaired cellular response, may not show the expected "left shift" of immature forms in the setting of infection.

The 12-lead ECG is an important tool because it may detect subtle changes secondary to pericardial disease, electrolyte disorders, and ischemia. Early ECG changes in pericarditis include diffuse ST segment elevations with a concave upward contour as well as PR segment depression. Later, the ST segments may return to baseline. The T wave amplitude may decrease and eventually invert in those leads that had ST segment elevation.[73] However, ECG diagnosis can be complicated by the presence of baseline ST-T wave changes often present in this population. ECG evidence of tamponade includes widespread decreases in QRS voltage and electrical alternans. Electrical alternans refers to changing levels of QRS voltage heights in an ECG that occurs when the heart changes position because of its suspension in a fluid-filled pericardium.

Electrolyte disorders such as hyperkalemia, hypercalcemia, and hypermagnesemia may produce characteristic ECG changes. The ECG changes found in hyperkalemia may not correlate with the level of elevation.

In hypercalcemia, a decreased QT interval is the most reliable ECG change and usually occurs at levels greater than 13 mg/dL.[7] Additional changes include prolongation of the PR interval and QRS complex, increased QRS voltage, and T-wave flattening.[7] At higher levels, atrioventricular block can progress to complete heart block. Hypermagnesemia may demonstrate bradycardia, heart block, and asystole. Morphologic changes include prolongation of the PR, QRS, and QT intervals.

Interpretation of chest radiographs may be difficult. Chronic volume overload may make radiographic diagnosis of pneumonia difficult if prior films are not available for comparison.

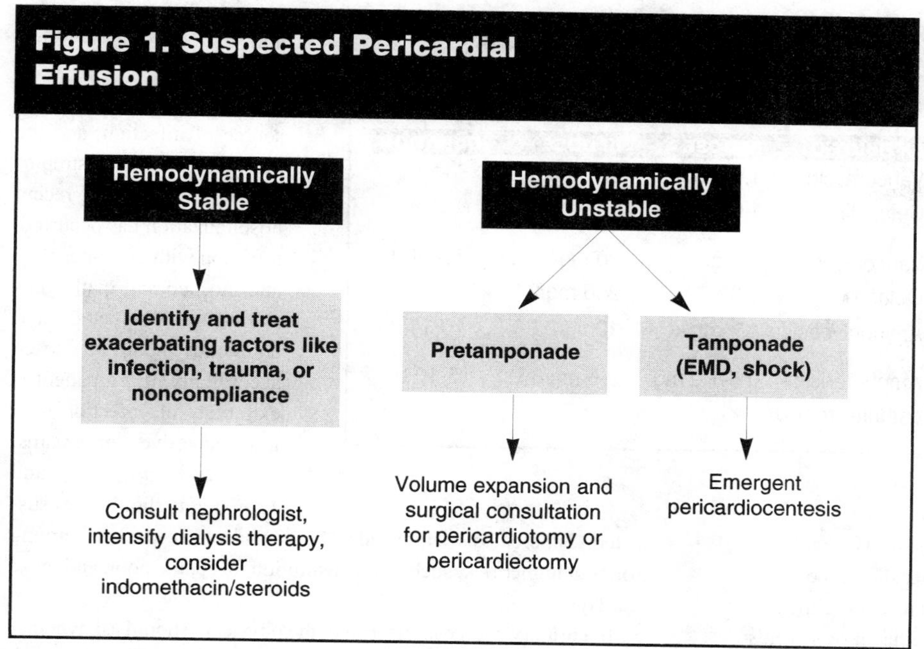

If peritonitis is suspected in patients receiving CAPD, at least 150 cc of peritoneal fluid should be obtained. Peritoneal fluid should be grossly examined for color and character and sent for Gram's stain, cell count, and culture. Peritonitis is diagnosed by the presence of a white cell count greater than 100 cells/mm^3 with a predominance of polymorphonuclear cells.[67] If a predominance of eosinophils or mononuclear cells is found, diagnoses of eosinophilic peritonitis or tubercles peritonitis, respectively, should be considered. Although a Gram's stain exam has a low predictive value, it may help in the early diagnosis of fungal peritonitis. Blood cultures are usually negative in peritonitis.

Additional studies may include a CT scan for suspected intracranial processes or an echocardiogram for suspected pericardial effusion or tamponade.

Specific Treatment Modalities

Hypertensive Complications. Hypertensive complications in patients with ESRD are usually due to volume overload or medical noncompliance. The ideal treatment for hypertensive emergencies caused by volume overload is dialysis. If emergent dialysis is unavailable, parenteral therapy should be started.

The treatment goal in a hypertensive emergency is to reduce the blood pressure in a rapid and controlled fashion. Reasonable goals are to reduce the blood pressure by 20-30% or to a level of 160/100 mmHg in the first 24 hours.[7,23] If a cerebrovascular accident is suspected, drastic reduction should be avoided and a mean arterial pressure (MAP) maintained at a level of 120-160 mmHg to insure adequate cerebral perfusion.[7,25]

If signs of hypertensive crisis exist, parenteral therapy using nitroprusside at an initial dose of 0.3 mcg/kg/min is the drug of choice. It acts as both an alpha- and beta-adrenergic blocker and can reduce both cardiac preload and afterload. Potential thiocynate toxicity can be avoided by limiting infusion to less than 48 hours, initiating early dialysis, and maintaining levels between 5 and 10 mg/dL.

If nitroprusside is unavailable, nitroglycerin may be used and is a safe and effective venodilator. If immediate intravenous access is unavailable, nitroglycerin can be given sublingually every five minutes x 3 with blood pressure checked frequently. Subsequently, nitroglycerin can be infused intravenously at an initial rate of 5 mcg/min.

Other potentially useful agents include combination alpha- and beta-blockers (IV labetalol), diuretics, IV ACE inhibitors, and calcium-channel blockers. 100 mL of 30% sorbitol given orally or rectally may be used if the hypertensive condition exists in the presence of pulmonary edema. It acts by creating an osmotic gradient between the gastrointestinal tract and the vascular space.

Congestive Heart Failure/Pulmonary Edema. The most common exacerbating factor causing congestive heart failure in patients with ESRD is volume overload, but other factors to consider are cardiac ischemia, dysrhythmia, hypertensive emergency, and medication/dialysis noncompliance. The first goal of treatment is to insure hemodynamic stability. Presence of cardiogenic shock may require infusion of vasopressor agents such as dopamine or inotropes such as dobutamine. If anemia is suspected of causing high-output failure or contributing to myocardial ischemia, infusion of packed red cells should be considered. Central venous pressure monitoring may be required with these modalities to avoid volume overload.

Hemodialysis or peritoneal dialysis are the preferred methods of removing excess volume. Because lack of immediate availability may limit their use in some centers, pharmacotherapy should be used as a temporizing measure.

Safe and effective agents immediately available include nitroglycerin, morphine sulfate, and furosemide.[30-33] These agents act by reducing cardiac preload through venodilation. Nitroglycerin 0.4 mg SL q 5 can be given initially and followed by an IV drip started at 5 mcg/min titrated to effect while avoiding hypotension. Morphine 2-5 mg IV decreases preload and decreases patient anxiety. Frequent dosing should be avoided to prevent respiratory depression. Though ineffective in initiating diuresis in an anuric patient, furosemide 80-120 mg IV can cause venodilation with consequent decreases in left ventricular filling pressures and pulmonary capillary wedge pressures.[33]

Additional agents include nitroprusside and sorbitol. Nitroprusside started at 0.3 mcg/kg/min acts as both a preload and afterload reducer, thereby decreasing left ventricular pressure and cardiac oxygen demand; 100 mL of 30% sorbitol given orally or rectally promotes an osmotic shift between the vascular space and the gut.[7,34] Its late onset of action (1-6 hours) and copious diarrhea may make management in the ED difficult. Phlebotomy should be avoided.

Pericardial Disease. The patient's hemodynamic status will dictate the therapeutic approach to pericarditis or pericardial tamponade. *(Please see Figure 1.)* If the patient is hemodynamically stable, exacerbating factors such as trauma, infection, dialysis non-compliance,

Table 3. Antibiotic Treatment for CAPD-Associated Peritonitis

CLINICAL CONDITION	INFECTIOUS AGENT	ANTIBIOTIC	IV DOSE	IP DOSE	DURATION
Mild to moderate	Coagulase-negative *Staphylococcus*	Vancomycin	1.0-1.5 mg	30 mg/kg/2 L	7-10 d
		Cefazolin	1.0 g	250 mg/2 L	
Moderate to severe	*Stapylococcus aureus*	Vancomycin	1.5 g	30 mg/kg/2 L	10-14 d
		Cefazolin	1.0 g	250 mg/2 L	
	Gram negatives	Aminoglycoside	1.7 mg/kg	10mg/2 L	10-14 d
Insidious to severe	Fungi	Amphotericin+ catheter removal	0.5-1.0 mg	2-6 mg/6 L	7-10 d

and medications should be identified and corrected. The patient's nephrologist should be informed, and arrangements should be made to either initiate dialysis or intensify the patient's current regimen. If the patient is complaining of pain or fever, indomethacin or steroids may be used for relief once other sources of fever and chest pain have been ruled out.

If the patient is hemodynamically unstable, the patient should be prepared for pericardiocentesis. Because of potential complications such as myocardial laceration, dysrhythmia, iatrogenic tamponade and hepatic laceration, pericardiocentesis should be deferred for those patients in shock.[38] If the patient is mildly unstable but responds to volume expansion with saline or mannitol, immediate surgical consultation should be made and the patient prepared for either pericardiotomy or pericardiectomy.

Dysrhythmias. Treatment of specific dysrhythmias should follow currently recommended guidelines, with specific dose adjustment. If cardiac arrest exists, hyperkalemia should be suspected and 10-20 mL of 10% calcium chloride or 15-20 mL of 10% calcium gluconate should be given over 10-15 minutes. Calcium should be avoided if digitalis toxicity is suspected, as it may worsen the dysrhythmia. The only ACLS protocol drug to avoid is bretylium. If ischemia is suspected, treatment should include aspirin, nitrates, heparin, and possible thrombolytics.

Cardiac Ischemia. There is no significant alteration in the management of myocardial infarction and ischemia in patients suffering from chronic renal failure and ESRD.

Aspirin, nitrates, heparin, and thrombolytics should be used according to currently established guidelines. Because underlying anemia impairs oxygen delivery, transfusion with packed red blood cells should be considered. Hemodialysis should be avoided during this period.

Infections

General Considerations. Specific treatment regimens are based on likely foci of infection and the patient's underlying renal function. In the unstable septic patient, cultures should be obtained and vancomycin 1g IV and gentamycin 1.7 mg/kg started empirically. This regimen provides coverage for the likely gram-positive and gram-negative organisms that commonly infect this population. Diabetics, patients with HIV, and those suspected of nosocomial pathogens require therapy tailored to likely pathogens, local resistance patterns, and any previous culture results.

Pneumonia is a common source of infection, and the most likely agent is streptococcal pneumonia. If recent hospitalization has occurred, infection with gram-negative and nosocomial pathogens should be suspected, and antibiotics should be chosen accordingly. If the patient is extremely ill, infection with gram-negative organisms, *Staphylococcus,* and *Legionella* should be suspected. Tuberculosis should also be considered, especially among groups at higher risk, such as the institutionalized, the poor, and those with HIV.[53]

If a urinary source is suspected, the physician should ask whether the patient suffers from polycystic kidney disease. These patients require lipid-soluble antibiotics (clindamycin, chloramphenicol, trimethoprim/ sulfamethoxazole) and surgical consultation if intrarenal or perinephric abscesses are suspected.

Peritonitis. ED care of peritoneal dialysis patients with peritonitis should include quick dialysate exchange (which helps alleviate pain and remove peritoneal debris) and intravenous and intraperitoneal antibiotics. The initial antibiotics chosen should have anti-staphylococcal coverage. Additional considerations should be made for gram-negative organisms and methicillin-resistant strains of *Staphylococcus.*

Other therapeutic agents include heparin and rifampin. Heparin given intraperitoneally at a dose of 500 units/lL of dialysate for 3-5 days helps prevent obstruction of the catheter and prevents formation of fibrin that acts as a haven for microbial growth. Rifampin is usually administered for relapsing peritonitis. It acts by penetrating the bacterial protective sanctuaries of peritoneal cellular debris and the biofilm located in and around dialysate catheters. Fortunately, the majority of patients with peritonitis can be treated as outpatients if they are clinically stable, reliable, and able to maintain adequate nutrition. *(Please see Table 3.)*

Hospital admission is mandatory for patients who cannot maintain nutritional balance, who show signs of clinical instability, and are suspected of having either fungal or sclerosing peritonitis. Fungal peritonitis requires removal of the dialysis catheter, systemic antifungal therapy, and nutritional support. Sclerosing peritonitis requires removal of the catheter, discontinuation of peritoneal dialysis, and surgery for complications secondary to abdominal adhesions.

Vascular Access Infection. If access site infection is suspected, the patient's nephrologist should be informed. Concerns of vascular access site aneurysms or thrombosis should lead to vascular surgery consultation as well. Initial treatment should be vancomycin 1g IV × 1, and gentamycin 1.7 mg/kg ×1 if gram-negative infection is suspected. The long half-life (5-7 days) and antimicrobial spectrum of these agents make them ideal agents for outpatient treatment. Patients with hemodynamic instability, graft compromise, or inability to maintain adequate nutrition require admission.

Electrolyte Disorders

Hyperkalemia. Treatment goals in hyperkalemia are to insure cardiac stability, facilitate translocation of extracellular potassium, and enhance excretion. The immediate goal in hyperkalemia is to stabilize the myocardium by administering 10% calcium chloride or 10% calcium gluconate. These agents should be given immediately to patients in cardiac arrest or to patients exhibiting signs of rhythm instability.

Following initial stabilization, agents that help translocate extracellular potassium should be administered. These include beta-agonists, IV insulin, and sodium bicarbonate.

Beta-agonists and insulin act by stimulating the cellular Na^+K^+ ATPase pump to translocate extracellular potassium.[54,55,56] Albuterol, 20 mg in 4 mL NS given by nebulizer can lower potassium by 1.0 mmol/L and has few side effects. Ten to 20 units of regular insulin IV along with 50 cc of D_{50} can lower potassium levels by 0.6-1.0 mmol/L over one hour. Because hypoglycemia is a potential side effect, initial therapy should be followed by IV D_5W.

The role of sodium bicarbonate is controversial. Some studies have not proven its efficacy, but current emergency medicine sources advocate its use. The dose is 50 mEq IV over 5-10 minute.[7,57-60,71]

The ideal means of potassium removal is dialysis, but its rapid availability limits its use. Sodium polystyrene sulfate (Kaexylate) can be given either orally or rectally and exchanges potassium for sodium using the gastrointestinal tract. Kaexylate 25 g/25 cc of 70% sorbitol orally, or 50 g/50 cc of 70% sorbitol rectally, removes 0.5-1.0 mmol of potassium for every gram of kaexylate. Sodium overload can result from Kaexylate treatment, so close monitoring is required.

Disposition. Patients who are symptomatic require admission to a monitored setting. Those having cardiovascular instability need an intensive care unit. Patients with mild elevations (5.5-6.0) who demonstrate no ECG manifestations and who are asymptomatic may receive conservative therapy (albuterol, insulin/glucose, and Kaexylate) and be discharged, if the patient's nephrologist is notified and agrees. Such patients must be reliable, and hemodialysis must be arranged in a timely fashion. If compliance is in question, the patient should be admitted to insure that dialysis takes place.

Hypercalcemia. Unlike patients with normal renal function, fluids and diuretics are ineffective in the treatment of hypercalcemic patients with ESRD. Those with levels between 12 mg/dL and 15 mg/dL can often await timely dialysis. Those with levels greater than 15 mg/dL require emergent treatment regardless of symptoms. This involves IV fluids if the patient's volume is depleted, salmon calcitonin intravenously at 5 MRC U/kg q6hr, and prompt dialysis. Although the effects of steroids are delayed, their use should be considered.

Hypermagnesemia. Treatment goals are to insure respiratory stabilization, cardiac stability, and magnesium elimination. Mechanical ventilation may be required if respiratory depression is significant. Ten mL of 10% calcium chloride or calcium gluconate IV should be given for cardiac instability and may be repeated twice every 5-20 minutes. Elimination is best achieved through hemodialysis.

Hematologic Complications

Spontaneous Hemorrhage. Treatment involves insuring hemodynamic stability, and prevention of further hemorrhage. Resuscitative measures include direct pressure, establishing large-bore IV access, and infusion of crystalloid and/or packed red blood cells as appropriate. If compression is required at the dialysis catheter site, excessive pressure should be avoided to prevent occlusion of the catheter. Persistent bleeding may indicate the presence of an aneurysm or pseudoaneurysm. Tourniquet use above the vascular catheter should be avoided unless fulminate hemorrhage is present

Correction of suspected coagulopathy may require specific pharmacological therapy. If heparin is a suspected factor in major bleeding, protamine 0.5 mg/100 units of heparin used can be given. It is best given within 30 minutes of the last heparin dose. To correct platelet dysfunction, DDAVP, 0.3 mcg/kg in 50 cc of NS IV or 3 mcg/kg nasally can be administered.[64] A subcutaneous dose of 0.4 mcg/kg can also be used, but absorption may be erratic. Ten bags of Cryoprecipitate can also be administered.[11] Dialysis can help correct the bleeding diathesis, but its emergent use may be limited by lack of immediate availability.

Traumatic Hemorrhage. The patient with ESRD who is injured should be approached in the same fashion as other trauma victims. Resuscitation should follow standard ATLS protocols.

Volume resuscitation should use both crystalloid solutions and blood products as indicated. Because lactated ringer's solution contains 4 mEq/L of potassium, it should be avoided because of its potential to cause hyperkalemia. Anemia is a common occurrence among patients with ESRD, and even minor blood loss may impair oxygen delivery; transfusion with packed red blood cells should be considered early. Crossmatching patients may be difficult due to the presence of red cell antibodies from previous transfusion.

Neurologic Complications

Altered Mental Status. In general, the evaluation and management of altered mental status in the patient with ESRD is the same as for other patients. A higher index of suspicion, however, should be maintained for spontaneous subdural hemorrhage. In addition, the dialysis disequilibrium syndrome should be kept as a diagnosis of exclusion. Treatment involves infusion of osmotically active fluid such as mannitol or hypertonic saline. The patient's nephrologist should be consulted prior to initiating therapy.

If a seizure occurs or is suspected, there is no contraindication to using phenytoin, phenobarbital, or diazepam. Because of decreased protein binding, phenytoin should be loaded to achieve a level between 5-10 mcg/mL.

Dialysis-Associated Complications

Peritoneal Catheter Obstruction. Treatment in the ED should be limited to manipulating the patient's position in an attempt to relieve the obstruction. Definitive treatment using a trochar device and thrombolytic agents is limited to the surgical consultant.

Vascular Catheter Obstruction. Since it is difficult to differentiate between a mechanical and thrombotic obstruction, angiography must be performed promptly. Urokinase 2500- 5000 IU can be given if the obstruction is acute, and the vascular surgeon has been consulted. This should be done as soon as possible to preserve function.

If a double-lumen catheter device is obstructed, gentle aspiration may be corrective. Urokinase or streptokinase may also be given. Forceful irrigation must be avoided to prevent distal embolization.

Vascular Access Hemorrhage. Treatment of hemorrhage in the ED is limited to firm, nonocclusive pressure for 5-10 minutes and identification of any correctable bleeding disorder. Observation should continued for 1-2 hours to assure homeostasis. A vascular surgeon should be consulted if functional compromise, rapid expansion, or if imminent rupture is suspected. If rupture occurs, a tourniquet should be applied proximal to the site and resuscitative measures begun.

Air Embolism. If air embolism is suspected, all venous lines should be clamped immediately; the patient should be placed in the left lateral decubitus position and given 100% oxygen. This allows the air to be trapped at the apex of the right ventricle. If the patient develops air embolism while in Trendelenburg, he or she should be left in that position. If the patient is in arrest, percutaneous aspiration of air with an intracardiac needle is required. Additional treatments include IV corticosteroids for cerebral edema and heparin or low molecular weight dextran to improve microcirculation.

Dialysis-Induced Hypotension. Treatment should be tailored to the underlying condition. Most episodes of hypotension respond to volume infusion administered in the dialysis unit. If a patient presents with continuing instability despite early resuscitative measures, etiologies other than modest volume deficits must be investigated. To treat the hypotension, small aliquots of volume in 100-200 mL increments should be given with close monitoring. If a patient is mildly symptomatic and all underlying factors, such as arrhythmia, cardiac dysfunction, and infection, can be ruled out, the hypotension may be treated with food and fluids containing sodium.

Summary

The incidence of ESRD has been progressively increasing over the past two decades. Because of an increasing geriatric population and acceptance of patients with conditions such as severe hypertension, diabetes, and HIV into dialysis therapy, this trend will most likely continue. As a result, the emergency physician is increasingly likely to encounter the many potential complications of ESRD.

ESRD and its complications are difficult entities to manage in both the chronic and acute care settings. The problems that cause rapid decompensation in the ED involve cardiovascular conditions, infections, metabolic disorders, and complications secondary to dialysis therapy. Thorough knowledge is required if the emergency physician is to successfully evaluate and treat this complicated patient population.

References

1. Port FK. Worldwide demographics and international trends in end stage renal disease. *Kidney Int* 1993;43:S4-S7.
2. United States Renal Disease System. *1993 Annual Data Report.* National Institute of Diabetes and Digestion and Kidney Diseases. Bethesda, MD; 1993:1-100.
3. Eggers PW. Projections of the end stage renal disease population to the year 2000. In: *Challenges for Public Health Statistics in the 1990s: Proceedings of the 1989 Public Health Conference on Records and Statistics.* Hyatsville, MD: U.S. Dept of Health and Human Services, Centers for Disease Control, National Center for Health Statistics; 1989:121-126.
4. Moore MA, Blythe WB, and the National High Blood Pressure Education Program. National High Blood Pressure Education Program Working Group report on hypertension and chronic renal failure. *Arch Intern Med* 1991;151: 1280-1287.
5. Strauss MJ, Port FK. An estimate of the size of the U.S. predialysis population with anemia, *Am J Kidney Dis* 1993;21: 264-269.
6. Ismail N, Becker BN. Treatment options and strategies in uremia: Current trends and future directions. *Semin Nephrol* 1994;14:282-299.
7. Wolfson AB. Chronic renal failure and dialysis. In: Rosen P, Barkin RM. *Emergency Medicine Concepts and Clinical Practice.* 3rd ed. St. Louis: Mosby-Year Book; 1992:1928-1943.
8. Klahr S, Schreiner G, Ichikawa I. The progression of renal disease. *N Engl J Med* 1988;318:1657-1666.
9. Jacobson HR. Chronic renal failure: pathophysiology. *Lancet* 1991;338:419-425.
10. Minno GD, Martinez J. Platelet dysfunction in uremia. *Am J Med* 1985;79:552-559.
11. Janson PA, Jubelirer SJ. Treatment of the bleeding tendency in uremia with crypoprecipitate. *N Engl J Med* 1980;303: 1318-1322.
12. Handa SP, Colwell B. Spontaneous retropharyngeal bleeding in a patient on chronic hemodialysis. *Nephron* 1993;64: 485-486.
13. Nancarrow C, Mather LE. Pharmacokinetics in renal failure. *Anaes Intensive Care* 1983;11:350-358.
14. Huff SJ, Whelan TV. CPAP as adjunctive treatment of severe pulmonary edema in patients with ESRD. *Am J Emerg Med* 1994;12:388.
15. Vainasen IT, Rasanen J. Continous positive airway pressure and supplemental oxygen in the treatment of cardiogenic pulmonary edema. *Chest* 1994;92:481-485.
16. Fitzpatrick M, Nelson J. Continous positive airway pressure as an adjunct in treatment of cardiogenic pulmonary edema. *Ann Emerg Med* 1990;21:1045.
17. Bersten AD, Holt AE., et al. Treatment of severe cardiogenic pulmonary edema with continous positive airway pressure delivered by face mask. *N Engl J Med* 1991;325:1825-1836.
18. Ansari A, Kaupke CJ. Cardiac pathology in patients with end stage renal disease maintained on hemodialysis. *Int J Artif Organs* 1993;16:31-36.
19. Ma KW, Greene EL, Raij L. Cardiovascular risk factors in chronic renal failure and hemodialysis populations. *Am J Kidney Dis* 1992;19:505-513.
20. Rostand SG, Brunzell JD, et al. Cardiovascular complications in renal failure. *J Am Soc Nephrol* 1991;2:1053-1061.
21. Greaves SC, Sharpe DN: Cardiovascular disease in patients with end-stage renal failure. *Aust N Z J Med* 1991;22: 152-159.
22. Kreastinos D, Paraskevaidis I, et al. Painless myocardial ischemia in chronic hemodialyzed patients: A real event? *Nephron* 1992;60:164-170.
23. Zarconi J, Phinney, B. Special considerations in the patient with chronic renal failure in the ICU. In: *The High Risk Patient: Management of the Critically Ill.* Baltimore:

Williams & Wilkins; 1995.
24. Kim KE, Swartz C. Cardiovascular complications in end-stage renal disease. In: Schrier RW, Gottschalk CW. *Diseases of the Kidney,* 5th ed. Boston: Little, Brown, and Co; 1993: 2817-2844.
25. Calhou DA, Oparil S. Treatment of hypertensive crisis. *N Engl J Med* 1990;323:1177-1183.
26. Harney JD, Parfrey PS. Cardiac disease in uremia. *Semin Nephrol* 1994;14:245-252.
27. Parferey PS, Harnett JD. Congestive heart failure in dialysis patients. *Arch Intern Med* 1988;148:1519-1526.
28. Gehm L, Propp DA. Pulmonary edema in the renal failure patient. *Am J Emerg Med* 1989;7:336-338.
29. Kohen, JA, Opsahl JA. Deceptive patterns of uremic pulmonary edema. *Am J of Kidney Dis* 1986;8:456-460.
30. Hodde LA, Sandroni S. Emergency department evaluation and management of dialysis patient complications. *J Emerg Med* 1992;10:317-334.
31. Sacchetti A, McCabe H. ED management of acute congestive heart failure in renal dialysis patients. *Am J Emerg Med* 1993;11:644-647.
32. Wolfson AB, Singer I. Hemodialysis-related emergencies—part II. *J Emerg Med* 1987;5:533-543.
33. Kraus PA, Lipman J, Becker PJ. Acute preload effect of furosemide. *Chest* 1990;98:124-128.
34. Cloonan CC, Gatrell CB, Cushner HM. Emergencies in continous dialysis patients: Diagnosis and management. *Am J Emerg Med* 1990;134-148.
35. Rostand SC, Rutsky EA. Pericarditis in end-stage renal disease. *Cardiol Clin* 1990;8:701-707.
36. Shabetai R. Diseases of the pericardium: Pericardial disease. In: Hurst JW, Schlant RC. *The Heart,* 7th ed. New York: Mcgraw Hill; 1992;1348-1374.
37. Kim KE, Swartz C. Cardiovascular complications of end-stage renal disease. In: Schrier RW, Gottschalk CW. *Diseases of the Kidney.* 5th ed. Boston: Little, Brown, and Co.; 1993:2817-2844.
38. Hammerman H, Kloner RA. Pericardial diseases. In: Kloner RA. *The Guide to Cardiology.* 2nd ed. New York: Le Jacq Communications; 1990:383-394.
39. Parfrey PS. Cardiac and cerebrovascular disease in chronic uremia. *Am J Kidney Dis* 1993;21:77-80.
40. Parfrey PS, et al. Congestive heart failure in dialysis patients. *Arch Intern Med* 1988;148:1519-1523.
41. Shapira OM, Bar-Khayim Y. ECG changes and cardiac arrhythmias in chronic renal failure patients on hemodialysis. *J Electrocardiog* 1992;25;273-279.
42. Blumberg A, Hausermann M, et al. Cardiac arrhythmias in patients on maintenance hemodialysis. *Nephron* 1983;33: 91-95.
43. Morrison G, Michelson EL, et al. Mechanisms and prevention of cardiac arrhythmias in chronic hemodialysis patients. *Kidney Int* 1980;17:811-819.
44. Kimura K, Tabei K. Cardiac arrhythmias in hemodialysis patients. *Nephron* 1989;53:201-207.
45. Singhal PC, Barth RH, Ginsberg NS, et al. Determinants of creatinine kinase activity in dialysis patients. *Am J Nephrol* 1988;8:220-224.
46. Goldman M, Vanherwheghen JL. Bacterial infections in chronic hemodialysis patients: Epidemiologic and pathophysiologic aspects. *Adv Nephrol* 1990;19:315-332.
47. Zibaria GB, Rohr MS, et al. Complications from permanent hemodialysis vascular access. *Surgery* 1988; 681-686.
48. Jameson MD, Wiegamann TB. Principles, uses, and complications of hemodialysis. *Med Clin North Am* 1990;74: 945-960.
49. Goldblum SE, Reed WP. Host defenses and immunologic alterations associated with chronic hemodialysis. *Ann Intern Med* 1980;93:597-613.
50. Dobkin JF, Miller MH, et al. Septicemia in patients on chronic hemodialysis. *Ann of Intern Med* 1978;88:28-33.
51. Andrew OT, Shoenfield PY, et al. Tuberculosis in patients with end-stage renal disease. *Am J Med* 1980;68:59-67.
52. Rimmer JM, Horn JF, Gennari J. Hyperkalemia as a complication of drug therapy. *Ann Intern Med* 1987;147:867-869.
53. Papadakis MA, Wexman MP, Fraser C, et al. Hyperkalemia complicating digoxin toxicity in a patient with renal failure. *Am J Kidney Dis* 1985;5:64-66.
54. Allon M. Treatment and prevention of hyperkalemia in end-stage renal disease. *Kidney Int* 1993;43:1197-1209.
55. Liou HH, Chiang SS. Hypokalemic effects of IV infusion on nebulization of salbutamol in patients with chronic renal failure: Comparative study. *Am J Kidney Dis* 1994;23:266-271.
56. Allon M, Copkney C. Albuterol and insulin for treatment of hyperkalemia in hemodialysis patients. *Kidney Int* 1990;38: 869-972.
57. Blumberg A, Weidmann P, Shaw S, et al. Effect of various therapeutic approaches on plasma potassium and major regulating factors in terminal renal failure. *Am J Med* 1988;85: 507-512.
58. Blumber A, Weidmann P, Ferrari P. Effects on prolonged bicarbonate administration on plasma potassium in terminal renal failure. *Kidney Int* 1992;41:369-374.
59. Wolfson AB, Levy M. The patient with chronic renal insufficiency following renal transplantation. In: Herr RD, Cydulka RK. *Emergency Care of the Compromised Patient.* 1st ed. Philadehphia: JP Lippincott Co.; 1994:416-432.
60. Walter FG, Lowe RA. Disorders of potassium metabolism. In: Harwood-Nuss A, Linden C, et al. *The Clinical Practice of Emergency Medicine,* 1st ed. Philadelphia: JP Lippincott Co.; 1991:999-1001.
61. Ellison R, Corroa W, Fox M, et al. Spontaneous mediastinal hemorrhage in patients on chronic hemodialysis. *Ann Intern Med* 1988;95:704-706.
62. Bora S, Kleinfled M. Subcapsular liver hematoma in a patient on chronic hemodialysis. *Ann Intern Med* 1980;93:574.
63. Blagg CR. Acute complications associated with hemodialysis. In: Maher JF. *Replacement of Renal Function by Dialysis.* 3rd ed. Dordecht: Kluwer Academic Publishers; 1989:750-771.
64. Carvalho ACA. Bleeding in uremia: A clinical challenge. *N Engl J Med* 1983;308:38-39.
65. Nielsen VK. The peripheral nerve function in chronic renal failure. *Acta Med Scand* 1971;190:105-111.
66. Fraser CL, Arieff AI. Nervous system complications in uremia. *Ann Intern Med* 1988;109:143-153.
67. Saklayen MG. CAPD peritonitis: Incidence, pathogens, diag-

nosis, and management. *Med Clin North Am* 1990;74: 997-1010.

68. Wolfson AB, Singer I. Hemodialysis-related emergencies—Part 1. *J Emerg Med* 1987;5:533-543.
69. Bernstein JM, Erk SD. Choice of antibiotics, pharmacokinetics, and dose adjustments in acute and chronic renal failure. *Med Clin North Am* 1990;74:1059-1076.
70. Bennett WM, Aronoff GR, et al. Drug prescribing in renal failure: Dosing guidelines for adults. *Am J Kidney Dis* 1993; 3:155-180.
71. Wilson RF. Fluid and electrolyte problems. In: Tintinalli JE, Krome RL, Ruiz E. *Emergency Medicine: A Comprehensive Study Guide.* 3rd ed. New York: McGraw-Hill; 1992:72-74.
72. Nichols, A. Atherosclerosis in chronic renal failure: A historical perspective. *Scott Med J* 1983:28:270.
73. Pratt DF, Bissen HA. Acute pericarditis and cardiac tamponade. In: *The Clinical Practice of Emergency Medicine.* 32nd ed. Philadelphia: Lippincott-Raven; 1996:617-619.

Urinary Incontinence

Neeraj Kohli, MD
Andrew C. Steele, MD

Urinary incontinence, defined as the involuntary loss of urine that is objectively demonstrable and a social or hygienic problem, is a condition that affects approximately 13 million Americans in community and institutional settings. Despite its prevalence and an estimated annual direct cost of more than $15 billion, most affected individuals do not seek help for incontinence primarily because of embarrassment or because they are not aware that help is available.[1] Urinary incontinence has a profound psychosocial effect on individuals, their families, and caregivers. It can result in loss of self esteem, social isolation, sexual dysfunction, and a decrease in ability to maintain an independent lifestyle. When patients do seek help, many clinicians are hesitant or inexperienced to discuss, diagnose, or treat the problem. It is expected that urinary incontinence will continue to be a significant healthcare problem in the elderly and institutionalized populations and will increase as the population continues to age and there is growing awareness and media attention given to this condition. The following paper will review the pathophysiology, diagnosis, and office management of urinary incontinence, with emphasis given on the role of the primary care provider.

Epidemiology

Although demographic surveys report that urinary incontinence affects 10-35% of adults and at least half of the 1.5 million nursing home residents in the United States, this number is most likely underweighted, as many patients who suffer from this condition are reluctant to report the problem to their healthcare provider due to embarrassment and social stigma. Although the prevalence of urinary incontinence increases with age, it should not be considered a normal part of the aging process. Among the population between 15 and 64 years of age, the prevalence of urinary incontinence in men ranges between 1.5-5.0%, and in women from 10-30%.[2] Incontinence is 2-3 times more common among women than men, and is primarily related to gender-specific risk factors, such as childbirth and menopause, that adversely affect pelvic support structures and result in stress urinary incontinence. Although urinary incontinence is commonly regarded as a condition affecting older, multiparous women, it is also common in young, nulliparous women and is particularly associated with strenuous physical exercise.

In the elderly population, urinary incontinence can affect 15-30% of women older than the age of 60 and more than 50% of nursing home residents.[3] It is one of the major causes of institutionalization of the elderly in this country despite the fact that one-third of all cases may be due to transient factors

Table 1. Reversible Causes and Risk Factors for Urinary Incontinence

- Immobility/chronic degenerative disease
- Impaired cognition
- Medications
- Morbid obesity
- Diuretics
- Smoking
- Fecal impaction
- Delirium
- Low fluid intake
- Environmental barriers
- High-impact physical activities
- Diabetes
- Stroke
- Estrogen deprivation
- Pelvic muscle weakness
- Childhood nocturnal enuresis
- Race
- Pregnancy/vaginal delivery/episiotomy

that may be readily treatable or undergo spontaneous remission. Appropriate diagnosis and management of urinary incontinence in the elderly by the primary care provider can have a profound effect on quality of life and may prevent the need for subsequent nursing home admission.

The economic effect of urinary incontinence has been scarcely reported due to the inability to obtain reliable prevalence, risk factor, and cost data, and because of wide diversification of treatment modalities. Recent data, estimated at more than $15 billion annually, does not consider indirect costs, such as loss of productivity due to morbidity/mortality and time costs of unpaid caregivers treating and caring for the incontinent patient. As public awareness of this condition continues to increase, it is expected that the financial costs of treating this disorder will also proportionately rise. Unfortunately, the majority of these expenditures have been directed toward control measures rather than cure options, resulting in minimal improvement. Of the $15 billion spent annually on this disorder, only 1% of this amount was spent on the diagnosis and permanent treatment of this disorder, while 60% was spent on palliative measures.[4]

Due to the increased incidence of incontinence, studies have shown that an effective prevention program would result in a reduction of approximately 50,000 annual cases.[5] Reversible conditions or risk factors associated with incontinence are presented in Table 1. Although no controlled clinical trial data exist to support the fact that risk factor interventions would result in significant reduction of incontinence incidents, severity, or prevalences, these programs are easy to institute and may result in other medically related benefits. These include weight loss and smoking cessation programs, control of hypertension and diabetes, maintenance on estrogen replacement therapy and pelvic muscle exercise programs, and alteration or adjustment of current medications. Patient education and routine follow-up are the cornerstones for an effective risk reduction program with regard to urinary incontinence.

Anatomy and Physiology of the Normal Continence Mechanism

The exact mechanism of continence in the healthy adult is incompletely understood. Current concepts emphasize a complex interaction between the bladder and urethra dependent on intact enervation and anatomic support of the bladder neck, especially in females. The bladder is a muscular organ with two primary functions—bladder storage at rest and bladder emptying during contraction. Both phases are regulated by the autonomic nervous system, with sympathetic enervation from T10 to L2 coming via the hypogastric nerve and parasympathetic enervation coming from S2 to S3 via the pelvic plexus. This system can be modulated by somatic nerves that innervate the pelvic floor and external urethral sphincter.

Disorders that affect bladder storage (filling phase) cause urinary incontinence, while disorders of emptying (voiding phase) cause voiding dysfunction and urinary retention. In some patients, especially women, abnormalities during filling and voiding may coexist. As urinary incontinence is primarily related to the storage phase, a detailed description of the physiology of normal micturition (voiding phase) is beyond the scope of this paper.

The mechanism of continence is complex. At rest, the bladder is a muscular reservoir that holds increasing volumes of urine while maintaining a low, resting pressure (accommodation) due to compliance of the bladder wall. Simultaneous sympathetic stimulation of beta adrenergic receptors within the bladder wall and inhibition of parasympathetic activity causes detrusor relaxation. Continence is maintained by a high resting pressure in the urethra at the urethrovesical junction (bladder neck) due to the musculature of the internal and external urethral sphincter, mucosal coaptation of the urethral lumen, and sympathetic stimulation of alpha adrenergic receptors in the urethra. (*Please see Figure 1.*)

During increases in intra-abdominal pressure, the pressure gradient between the bladder and urethra is maintained by equal transmission of pressure to the bladder and proximal urethra to ensure continence. In the female, the external urethral sphincter and levator ani muscle complex serve as a secondary continence mechanism by a reflex contraction, with resulting bladder neck closure during increased abdominal pressure. In addition, the vagina, slung like a hammock below the urethra by its lateral fascial attachments, functions as a backboard against which the bladder neck is compressed during valsalva maneuvers. During micturition, a coordinated change in the pressure relationship between the bladder (detrusor muscle) and urethra occurs. Voiding is initiated by voluntary relaxation of the pelvic musculature and urethral sphincter, followed by a detrusor contraction mediated by parasympathetic cholinergic receptors in the bladder. With an increase in bladder pressure and a decrease in urethral pressure, the pressure gradient favors micturition and bladder emptying occurs.

Urinary incontinence may occur due to abnormal increases in bladder pressure or decreases in urethral pressure that alter the low bladder pressure-high urethral pressure relationship that maintains continence at rest. Abnormal increases in bladder pressure are primarily due to spontaneous detrusor contractions (detrusor instability) with a reflex relaxation of the urethral sphincter that results in urinary leakage. Increased bladder pressure may also be due to overfilling of the bladder beyond its capacity and compliance resulting in overflow incontinence. Abnormal decreases in urethral pressure may be static or dynamic. A decrease in resting urethral tone can be caused by injury to the sphincter enervation or musculature (intrinsic sphincter deficiency). Abnormal bladder neck function in dynamic states of increased abdominal pressure or valsalva is seen in female patients with genuine stress incontinence. With relaxation of the pelvic floor muculature and fascial supports, the proximal urethra exhibits rotational descent outside the zone of abdominal pressure transmission and no longer has a fixed backboard for mechanical compression. As a result, increases in intra-abdominal pressure cause only elevated intravesical pressure, which overcomes the resting intraurethral pressure, resulting in loss of urine.

An adequate understanding of the normal continence mechanism as well as specific abnormalities resulting in urinary incontinence is critical in determining the underlying etiology and formulating an effective treatment plan. Diagnostic evaluation is based on understanding normal bladder function at rest and assessing the lower urinary tract within these parameters.

Classification of Urinary Incontinence

Urinary incontinence is a symptom, a sign, and a condition. The International Continence Society has created a classification of urinary incontinence.[6] Accurate diagnosis of the type of incontinence will determine the appropriate treatment plan.

Genuine stress incontinence is the involuntary loss of urine that occurs when, in the absence of a detrusor contraction, the intravesical pressure exceeds the maximum urethral pressure. It is most common in women who typically complain of urinary leakage with cough, exercise, laughing, valsalva maneuver, and other activities that increase intra-abdominal pressure. Patients with severe stress incontinence may report constant leakage with minimal exertion. Genuine stress incontinence is due to urethral hypermobility or intrinsic sphincter deficiency. Urethral hypermobility, the most common cause of genuine stress incontinence, occurs when there is loss of the anatomic support of the bladder neck, allowing the proximal urethra to be displaced outside the abdominal pressure zone during straining. McGuire and colleagues have classified subtypes I, IIA, and IIB, depending on the amount of descent of the bladder base at rest and with straining.[7] This damage to the bladder neck supports may be the result of pregnancy and vaginal delivery, tissue atrophy that results from advancing age and estrogen withdrawal, or continuous stressors, such as obesity and chronic coughing. With intrinsic sphincter deficiency, the urethra exhibits decreased resting tone and no longer functions as a sphincter. Even at rest, it loses the ability to maintain a normal continence mechanism. More common in women, it is often associated with a history of pelvic radiation, previous anti-incontinence surgery, advancing age, and deenervation injuries, resulting in overt disruption of the sphincteric musculature. These patients most commonly demonstrate a fixed, rigid urethral tube, with a nonfunctioning sphincter (lead pipe

Figure 1. Physiologic Basis of Storage and Voiding

FILLING/STORAGE

Inhibition of parasympathetics

Stimulation of sympathetics: alpha-contraction beta-relaxation

Stimulation of somatic nerves to striated urogenital sphincter

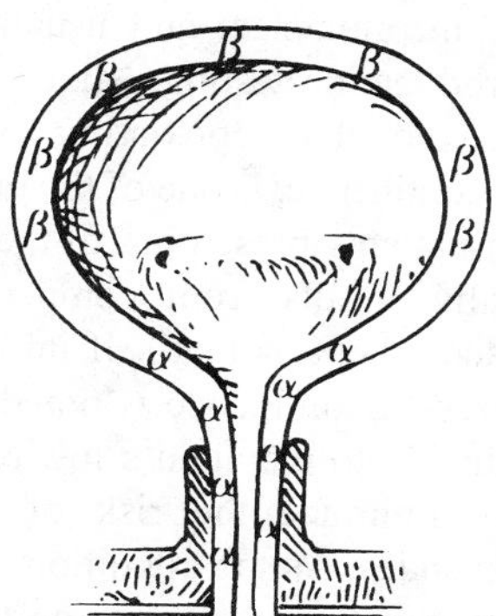

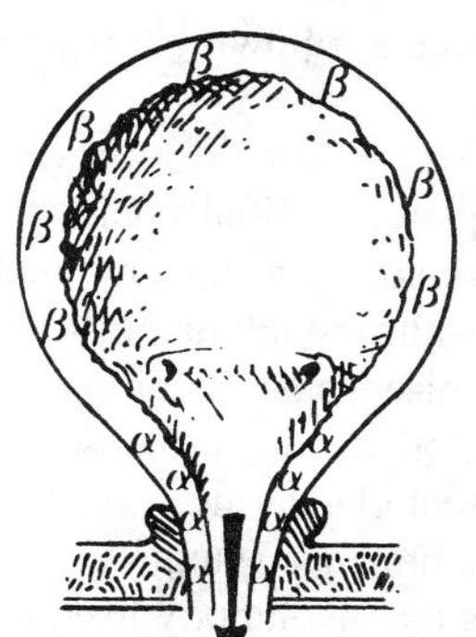

VOIDING

Stimulation of parasympathetics

Inhibition of sympathetics

Inhibition of somatic nerves to striated urogenital sphincter

Physiologic basis of storage and voiding based on characteristic distribution of sympathetic and parasympathetic receptors. Reprinted with permission from Mosby Year-Book Inc. from Walters MD and Karram MM. *Clinical Urogynecology* 1993;1-19.

Figure 2. Diagnosis/Treatment Algorithm for Urinary Incontinence

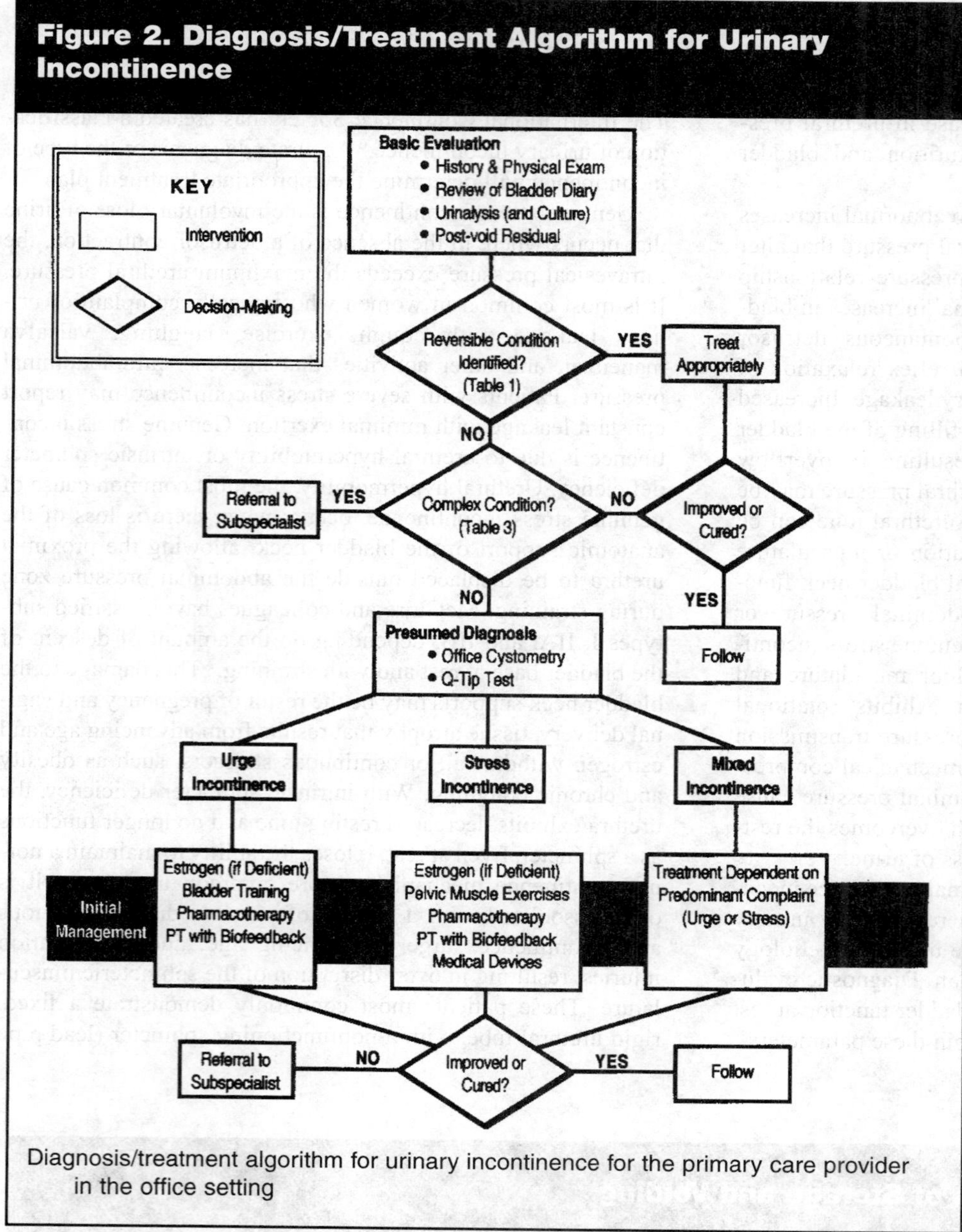

Diagnosis/treatment algorithm for urinary incontinence for the primary care provider in the office setting

urethra or Type III incontinence). In men, it is most often associated with urethral damage that occurs following transurethral resection of the prostate.

Potential stress incontinence can occur in women with advanced pelvic prolapse. These patients initially have loss of bladder neck support and resulting incontinence. Continued prolapse of the anterior vaginal wall results in kinking of the urethra with improvement of incontinent episodes but incomplete bladder emptying. Subsequent reduction of the prolapse with a pessary or surgery without concurrent bladder neck support will result in reestablishment of the incontinence symptoms.

Urge incontinence is defined as the involuntary loss of urine associated with a sudden and strong desire to void (urgency). Normal micturition is under voluntary control. Spontaneous uninhibited detrusor overactivity can result in detrusor contractions with reflex urethral relaxation and urinary incontinence. Overactive detrusor function in the absence of a known neurologic abnormality is called detrusor instability; overactivity due to its disturbance of the nervous control mechanisms is termed detrusor hyperreflexia. Patients with this condition complain of an inability to control voiding and experience sudden urgency to void, which is sometimes unsuppressible. These patients commonly report coexisting urinary frequency (> 7 times/day), nocturia (> 1 time/night), enuresis, and, occasionally, pelvic pain. Although detrusor instability is most often iatrogenic, secondary causes include urinary tract infection, anti-incontinence surgery, bladder stones or foreign bodies, and bladder cancer. Suburethral diverticulum, an outpouching of the urethral mucosa, can also occasionally present with irritative bladder symptoms, such as urgency and frequency.

Detrusor hyperreflexia with impaired contractility (DHIC) is a rare disorder that may occur in some patients—especially the elderly or patients with neurologic lesions. This paradoxical condition is characterized by detrusor overactivity in combination with decreased detrusor contractility. These patients present with urge incontinence in combination with urinary retention. Diagnosis is difficult, as it can mimic other types of incontinence, and usually requires complex multichannel urodynamic testing. Mixed incontinence, a condition characterized by coexisting stress incontinence and urge incontinence, is one of the most common types of incontinence in patients presenting to their primary care physician. It typically results from compensatory responses that the stress incontinent patient self initiates. Once the initial symptom of stress incontinence is noted, the patient begins to urinate frequently to maintain a low residual of urine in the bladder and to minimize the risk of further stress-related incontinent episodes. As the condition worsens, the degree of urinary frequency increases and the bladder accommodates to a lower capacity. When the bladder distends beyond its now reduced capacity, the patient experiences sensory urgency or detrusor instability with or without associated urinary leakage and irri-

Table 2. Medications Causing Incontinence

ACE Inhibitors	**Anticholinergics**
Enalapril	Hyoscyamine
Anti-Parkinsonism Agents	Oxybutinin
Benzotropine	**Antihypertensives**
Trihexyphenidyl	Prazosin
Benzodiazepines	Terazosin
Valium	Alpha-methyl dopa
Bethanocol	Reserpine
Cisapride	**Beta-blockers**
Diuretics	Pindolol
Furosemide	**Neuroleptics**
Hydrochlorothiazide	Thioridazine
Diospyramide	Chloropromazine
Alcohol	Haloperidol
Calcium-Channel Blockers	Clozapine
Verapamil	
	Over-the-counter Cough Preparations

tative symptoms, such as frequency, urgency, and nocturia. Often, however, one symptom, stress, or urge is more bothersome to the patient than the other, and therapeutic intervention is based on the predominant symptomatology.

Overflow incontinence is the uncontrollable loss of urine associated with overdistention of the bladder. This is usually caused by an underactive or acontractile detrusor or bladder outlet/urethral obstruction leading to overdistention and overflow. Failure of the bladder to empty adequately with large post-void residuals may by idiopathic, but it is usually found in conjunction with drugs, diabetic neuropathy, spinal cord injury, or radical pelvic surgery, which causes de-enervation of the detrusor muscle. In men, overflow incontinence is associated with obstruction due to prostatic hypertrophy or urethral stricture. In women, it can be associated with advance pelvic prolapse, which causes bladder outlet obstruction due to kinking of the bladder neck. Increased bladder capacities with a large post-void residual urine volume will clarify the diagnosis.

Other types of incontinence are less common but should be considered in the appropriate clinical context. Functional incontinence refers to urine loss that occurs due to factors outside the urinary tract, such as chronic impairment of physical or cognitive functioning. This type of incontinence is typically found in the elderly immobile nursing home resident. Reflex incontinence is the loss of urine due to detrusor hyperreflexia, involuntary urethral relaxation, or both in the absence of the sensation usually associated with the desire to void. This condition is most commonly seen in patients with neuropathic bladder or urethral dysfunction due to neurologic injury. Transient and reversible causes for incontinence are often identified, particularly in elderly patients. A useful mnemonic for common reversible causes of incontinence is DIAPPERS—Delirium, Infection, Atrophic urethritis, Pharmaceuticals, Psychological factors, Endocrine disorders, Restricted mobility, and Stool impaction. Often, treatment of the inciting factor will result in immediate cure of urinary leakage. Extraurethral causes of incontinence should be included in the differential diagnosis. This is particularly relevant for women with a history of pelvic surgery, radiation, or obstetric delivery. Etiologic entities include urinary fistulas (ureterovaginal, vesicovaginal, or urethrovaginal), ectopic ureter, and urethral diverticulum. A detailed pelvic exam is required for diagnosis.

Evaluation of Urinary Incontinence

The evaluation of patients with urinary incontinence is directed toward: 1) clarifying a patient's symptoms; 2) objectively documenting loss of urine; 3) determining the etiology of the incontinence; and 4) identifying patients who require further consultation and complex testing. The large majority of patients can be appropriately diagnosed and managed in the primary care setting, and few will require outside referrals unless they have a complex condition or desire surgical correction. A step-by-step diagnostic algorithm that includes a history, physical examination, and appropriate office testing is useful in the evaluation of the incontinent patient. (*Please see Figure 2.*)

Accurate diagnosis of urinary incontinence begins with a careful review of the patient's history. The history should focus on the duration, characteristics, and severity of the incontinence, with particular attention to precipitating factors and reversible causes. Cystitis, foreign body, or tumor should be suspected in patients with acute onset of symptoms while chronic etiologies, such as urethral hypermobility, intrinsic sphicter deficiency, and idiopathic detrusor instability, should be considered for long-standing complaints. Concurrent lower urinary tract symptoms (i.e., dysuria, urgency, pelvic pain, dyspareunia) as well as symptoms related to the gastrointestinal tract (i.e., constipation, fecal incontinence) and genital tract (i.e., pelvic prolapse, abnormal vaginal discharge) should also be discussed. Objective assessment of the patient's incontinence using a bladder diary is recommended. We routinely ask patients to keep a two-day record of fluid intake, voids, and incontinent episodes with precipitating events prior to their first visit. This is subsequently reviewed with the patient in order to assess if the patient will benefit from behavioral or dietary modification, such as increased fluid intake, change in voiding pattern, or dietary restriction. A detailed medical and surgical history should be obtained to rule out diabetes, thyroid disease, spinal cord injury, cerebral vascular accidents, urethral sphincter damage, or fistula conditions. As incontinence increases with advanced age, a detailed drug history is particularly important as many of these elderly patients are on multiple medications. A variety of medications can induce urinary incontinence directly by acting on the bladder and/or urethra or indirectly by inducing cough or pelvic muscle relaxation mechanisms. Pharmacotherapy may induce any of the subtypes of urinary incontinence previously discussed. (*Please see Table 2.*) In women, estrogen status should be determined as hypoestrogenism can contribute to recurrent cystitis, detrusor instability, and stress incontinence. Patients should also be questioned about a history of recurrent urinary tract infection, kidney stones, bladder pain, or hematuria.[8]

Following a general physical exam and mental status assessment, clinical evaluation of the lower urinary tract should begin with a detailed neurologic exam of the perineum and lower extremities. Normal sensation in the perineal dermatomes and the back of the leg confirms intact sensory enervation of the lower urinary tract. Sacral reflex activity is tested via two reflexes. In the anal reflex, stroking the skin adjacent to the anus causes reflex contraction of the external anal sphincter while the sacral (bulbocavernosus) reflex involves contraction of the bulbocavernosus and ischiocavernosus muscles in response to tapping or squeezing of the clitoris. Pelvic floor muscle tone can be assessed by voluntary contraction of the anal sphincter and vagina during a bimanual exam.

In women, a pelvic exam should be performed to assess the external genitalia, perineal sensation, presence of pelvic organ prolapse (cystocele, enterocele, rectocele, uterine prolapse), estrogen status, and pelvic muscle strength. During inspection, particular attention should be given to the assessement and grading of pelvic organ prolapse to rule out urethral hypermobility and potential stress incontinence. A bimanual exam with rectovaginal exam should be done to rule out pelvic masses compressing the bladder. In men, a rectal exam should be performed to test for perineal sensation or rectal mass and to evaluate the consistency and size of the prostate.

The patient should be examined with a full bladder so that observation of urine loss can be performed by having the individual cough vigorously, either in the standing or supine position. If instantaneous leakage occurs with cough, stress urinary incontinence is likely while urge incontinence (detrusor instability) should be considered with delayed or sustained leakage. In women, urethral hypermobility due to loss of bladder neck support can most easily be assessed using a simple cotton swab test. A sterile, lubricated cotton swab is inserted transurethrally into the bladder and then withdrawn slowly until definite resistance is felt, indicating that the cotton swab is at the bladder neck. The resting angle of the cotton swab in relation to the horizontal is measured, and the patient is then asked to cough or perform a valsalva maneuver; the maximum straining angle from the horizontal is then measured. Although no standardized data is available to differentiate abnormal from

Figure 3. Complex Multichannel Urodynamics with Pressure Catheters

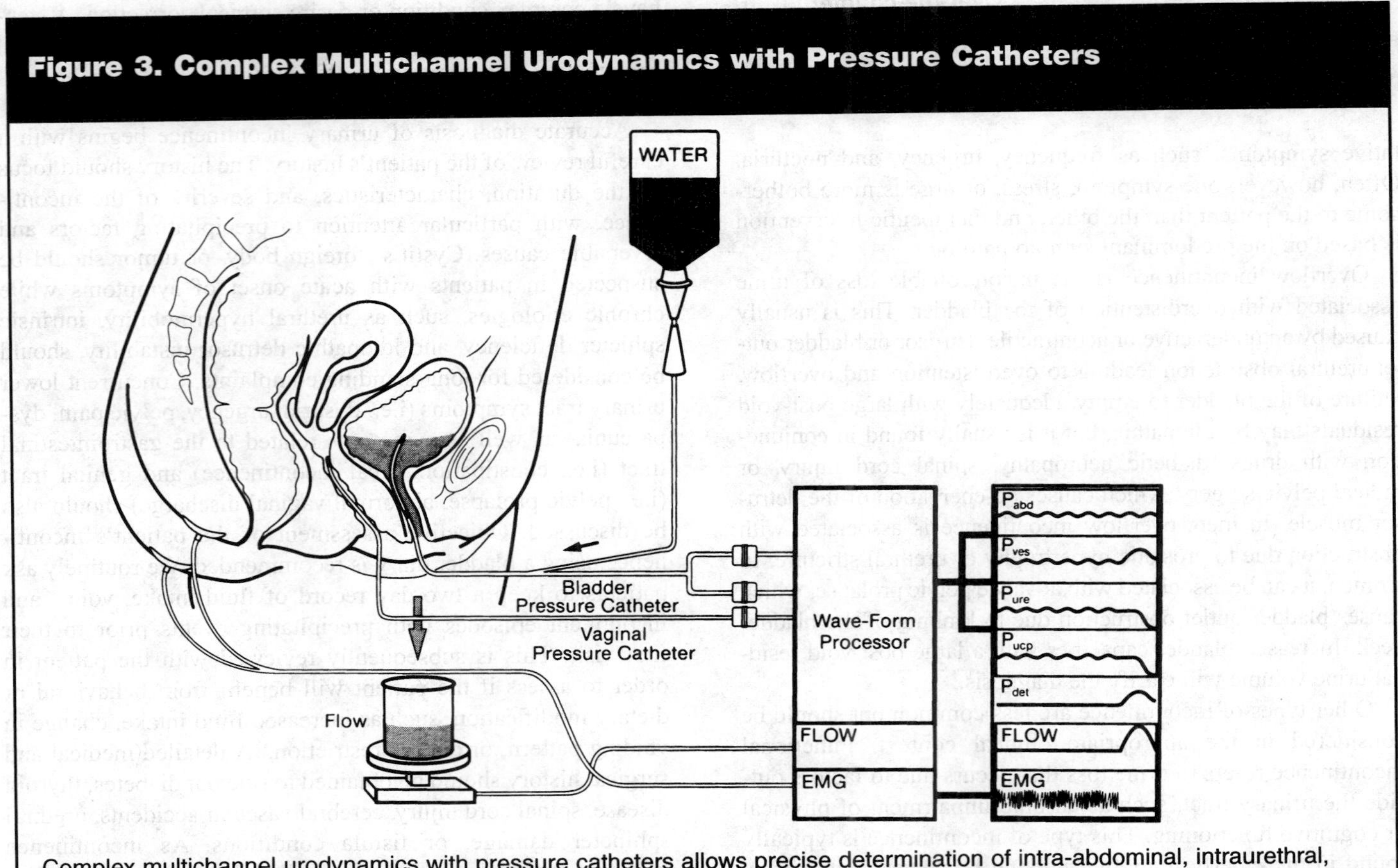

Complex multichannel urodynamics with pressure catheters allows precise determination of intra-abdominal, intraurethral, and detrusor/urethral pressures. Reprinted with permission from Mosby Year-Book Inc. Walters MD, Karram MM. *Clinical Urogynecology* 1993;1:65.

Figure 4. Simple Office Cystometry

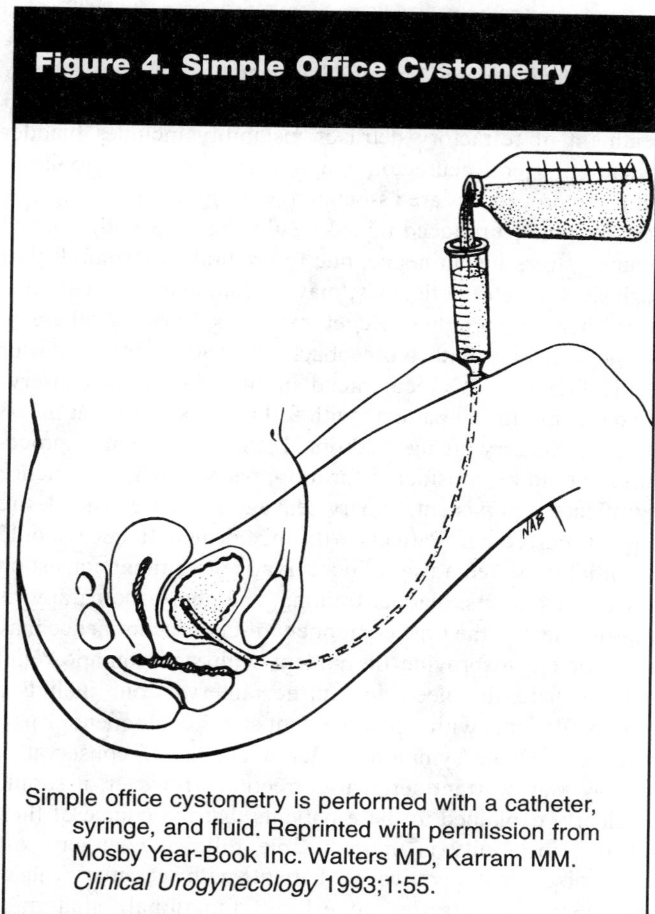

Simple office cystometry is performed with a catheter, syringe, and fluid. Reprinted with permission from Mosby Year-Book Inc. Walters MD, Karram MM. *Clinical Urogynecology* 1993;1:55.

normal measurements, most clinicians have adopted a 30° deflection as a cutoff for urethral hypermobility.

Initial diagnostic testing should include a post-void residual to rule out overflow incontinence and incomplete bladder emptying, and a urinalysis and/or urine culture to rule out urinary tract infection. After a normal void, a post-void residual urine volume is determined using a catheterization or bladder scan. Although values for normal bladder emptying may vary with age, a post-void residual should be less than 25% of the total bladder volume and below 100 cc. Patients with high post-void residual measurement may experience overflow incontinence. A catheterized sample of urine should be obtained for urinalysis or urine culture. We have found that clean catch urine specimens are routinely contaminated and do not provide accurate data with regard to urinary tract infection. Cystitis is the leading cause of acute urinary incontinence in younger women. Based on initial evaluation and testing, a preliminary diagnosis can be made. Further office testing, such as simple cystometry, can be performed at the time of the initial exam or be reserved for subsequent visits. We find that it is an inexpensive test that is easy to perform and provides important initial data; we recommend it be done at the initial evaluation. In addition, it allows simultaneous measurement of a post-void residual and collection of a catheterized urine specimen.

Cystometry is used to measure the pressure volume relationship of the bladder as it distends and contracts and determine abnormalities of the bladder with respect to detrusor activity, sensation, capacity, and compliance. Complex cystometry (multichannel urodynamics) uses specialized equipment with pressure catheters to record abdominal, bladder, and urethral pressures and determines specific detrusor activity through subtracted calculations. (*Please see Figure 3.*) In contrast, simple office cystometry can readily be performed in the office and requires a stopwatch, red rubber catheter, 50 mL syringe, and sterile water or saline. The patient should be initially evaluated with a full bladder. The patient is allowed to void normally in a private setting, and the time to void and amount of urine void are recorded. (This process is called uroflow.) The patient then returns to the examination room where a transurethral catheter is inserted into the bladder lumen to check a post-void residual and to obtain a sterile urine specimen for urinalysis or culture. With the transurethral catheter in place, a 50 mL catheter tip syringe with its bulb removed is attached to the catheter and held approximately 15 cm above the pubic symphysis. With the patient in the sitting or standing position, the bladder is filled by pouring sterile water or saline into the syringe at a medium fill rate, attempting to keep the water level in the syringe constant. (*Please see Figure 4.*) During bladder filling, the patient is asked to report first bladder sensation, initial urge to void, and maximum bladder capacity. Normal values are 100-200 cc, 200-400 cc, and 400-600 cc, respectively. Decreased bladder capacity is suggestive of urgency-frequency syndromes and urge incontinence.

The water level is closely monitored during filling, as a rise with or without associated urgency or urinary leakage may be indicative of an uninhibited bladder contraction, suggesting detrusor instability. Unfortunately, rises in intravesical pressure may result from a detrusor contraction or valsalva maneuver and, therefore, are not diagnostic of detrusor overactivity. It may be helpful to ask the patient to inspire during a noted rise in intravesical pressure, as women can rarely increase their intra-abdominal pressure during inspiration. Once the bladder is filled to maximum capacity, the transurethral catheter is removed and the patient is examined in the supine or lithotomy position and standing position. The patient is asked to perform provocative maneuvers, such as coughing, heel jumping, and valsalva. Urethral hypermobility and urinary leakage are evaluated. Loss of small amounts of urine simultaneous with cough suggests a diagnosis of stress incontinence. Prolonged loss of urine leaking 5-10 seconds after cough or no urine loss with provocation indicates that other causes of incontinence, especially detrusor instability, may be present.[9] Patients with reduced bladder capacity with co-existing urge-related complaints most likely have underlying detrusor instability and should be treated accordingly.

Additional evaluation, including blood testing, multichannel urodynamic testing, and radiographic studies, should be considered on an individualized basis. Blood testing, including BUN, creatinine, glucose, and calcium, is recommended if compromised renal function is suspected or if polyuria is present. Urine cytology and cystoscopy are not necessary in the routine initial evaluation of the incontinent patient but may be

Table 3. Complex Conditions Requiring Further Consultation or Testing

- Complicated history
- Office cystometry inconclusive
- Frequency, urgency, and pain syndromes unresponsive to conservative therapy
- Stress incontinence before surgical correction
- Recurrent urinary loss after previous surgery for stress incontinence
- Urge-related symptoms with gross or microscopic hematuria
- Nocturnal enuresis unresponsive to previous therapy
- Complaints of stress incontinence with absence of urethral hypermobility
- Advanced pelvic prolapse before surgical correction
- Co-existing neurologic disorders or diabetes mellitus
- Urge incontinence unresponsive to previous therapy
- Age older than 65
- Continuous urinary leakage
- Lower urinary tract dysfunction after pelvic radiation or radical pelvic surgery

helpful for patients with persistent symptoms or coexisting hematuria.

After a presumptive diagnosis has been made, the patient should be treated appropriately and re-evaluated in 6-8 weeks. Referral to a subspecialist will depend on various factors, such as the clinician's experience and comfort level with the diagnosis and management of urinary incontinence, access to urodynamic testing equipment, and healthcare referral patterns. However, patients with significant pelvic prolapse and concurrent urinary tract symptoms, recurrent incontinence, anatomic abnormalities, voiding dysfunction, and co-existing neurologic disorders may benefit from a urogynecologic or urologic consultation. (*Please see Table 3.*) The role of the subspecialist should include comprehensive urodynamic testing, interpretation of these findings, and further management including surgery as appropriate.

Treatment of Urinary Incontinence

The appropriate treatment of urinary incontinence primarily depends on accurate diagnosis of the underlying etiology. Patients with isolated urge incontinence (detrusor instability) are best treated with conservative treatment options, including bladder retraining and pharmacologic therapy, with the primary goal being to expand bladder capacity to a functional level with resulting inhibition of spontaneous bladder spasms. Patients with detrusor instability refractory to first-line therapy may be candidates for polypharmacotherapy, biofeedback, psychotherapy, or functional electrical stimulation. Surgical treatment of refractory detrusor instability includes bladder distention, sacral neurectomy, and augmentation cystoplasty, but these procedures are associated with significant complications and have produced mixed results. Patients with isolated genuine stress incontinence, due to urethral hypermobility or intrinsic sphincter deficiency, may be candidates for conservative therapy including Kegel exercises, pharmacotherapy, physical therapy with biofeedback, electrical stimulation, or medical devices. We recommend an initial course of conservative therapy for all patients with follow-up assessment in 2-3 months. Surgery using traditional anti-incontinence procedures should be considered for those patients who experience significantly persistent urinary leakage or those who desire surgical correction. Patients with mixed incontinence should be initially offered a trial of conservative treatment consisting of Kegel exercises, bladder training, and pharmacotherapy, as improvement in the urge component of their incontinence may be sufficient to provide the patient with symptomatic relief and alleviate the need for further intervention, including surgery. Patients with a predominant stress component or persistence of their symptoms after a course of conservative therapy may warrant surgical correction. However, it should be clearly explained to these patients that the course of their detrusor instability is unpredictable following surgery and may worsen postoperatively.[10] Patients with secondary causes of incontinence (reflex, overflow, functional, anatomic) should be treated on an individual basis. Patients with significant voiding dysfunction, anatomic abnormalities, and recurrent incontinence pose a challenging problem to the primary care provider. These patients will often require additional testing or complex procedures and urogynecologic or urologic consultation is recommended.

Behavioral Modification

Behavioral modification is useful in the treatment of many types of urinary incontinence and may include dietary restriction, toileting assistance, bladder retraining, and pelvic muscle rehabilitation. Patients with urge incontinence may benefit from dietary restriction of caffeine, alcohol, chocolate, and spicy food, as these can all cause bladder irritation. Routine or scheduled toileting should be offered to incontinent patients on a consistent schedule and is recommended in the treatment of functional incontinence. The mainstay of treatment for urge and mixed incontinence is bladder training with pharmacotherapy. However, several reports demonstrate that bladder training is effective in reducing episodes of stress incontinence, although the exact etiology of this effect is unclear.[11] Bladder training (timed voiding) helps to progressively distend the bladder and allows the patient to regain critical control over voiding patterns. The patient is instructed to void at pre-assigned times during the waking hours. The initial voiding interval is set at less than the patient's current voiding interval, and this is gradually increased on a weekly basis over an eight-week period. Patients are encouraged to try to suppress the sudden urge to void in between these designated intervals. Regular monitoring and positive reinforcement by review of the bladder diary provides continued feedback to the patient.

Pelvic muscle rehabilitation, or Kegel's exercise, can reduce the severity of incontinent episodes by strengthening the pelvic muscles and re-establishing support to the bladder neck continence mechanism.[12] Although pelvic muscle exercises are used predominantly in the treatment of stress urinary incontinence in women with poor pelvic supports and in men post-prostatectomy, there is evidence that it is also useful in patients with urge or mixed incontinence. Unfortunately, only 30% of women can perform pelvic floor exercises correctly following verbal instruction. We recommend simple biofeedback or referral to a physical therapist.[13] Simple biofeedback can be performed in the office at the time of the bimanual exam with the clinician asking the patient to squeeze her levator muscles while two fingers are placed in the vagina. Care must be given to discourage the patient from performing a Valsalva maneuver or tightening her gluteus muscles. Pelvic floor exercises can be enhanced using biofeedback with intravaginally pressure probes or mechanical devices, such as graduated vaginal cone weights. A typical regimen of pelvic floor exercises is based on sets of short and long contractions performed 2-4 times daily. Under this regimen, patients with mild-to-moderate incontinence can expect 60-70% improvement in their symptoms.[14]

Electrical stimulation has been shown to be effective in the treatment of stress, urge, and mixed incontinence. This treatment modality involves the use of non-implantable vaginal or anal sensors or surface electrodes to stimulate a reflex arc in the sacral micturition center and produce a contraction of the pelvic musculature and urethral sphincter with an accompanying reflex inhibition of the detrusor muscle. This treatment modality is especially useful in the patient who is unable to properly perform pelvic muscle exercises or in patients with an acontractile levator muscle. Electrical stimulation is usually given twice daily for 15 minutes and can be performed in the office or at home using a portable generator. Treatment should be continued 8-12 weeks depending on the underlying etiology and on symptomatic improvement. Several studies addressing long-term follow-up after pelvic floor electrical stimulation have reported cure rates ranging from 54-77%.[15]

Pharmacotherapy

Pharmacotherapy is the mainstay for the treatment of urge incontinence but can also be used for stress urinary incontinence as an adjunct to other nonsurgical modalities or in patients who do not desire surgical correction. Medications used in the treatment of urinary incontinence function by either relaxing the overactive detrusor muscle in women with urge incontinence or increasing urethral sphincter tone in patients with stress incontinence. Anticholinergic and antispasmodic agents are

Table 4. Pharmacologic Agents for the Treatment of Urinary Incontinence

Medication (brand name)	Dosage	Mechanism of Action	Indication
Oxybutynin (Ditropan)	2.5 mg bid - 5mg tid	Anticholinergic/ Spasmolytic	Urge incontinence
Hyoscyamine (Levsin, Cystospaz)	0.15 mg tid to qid 0.375 mg bid to tid (extended release)	Anticholinergic	Urge incontinence
Flavoxilate (Urispas)	100 -200 mg tid to qid	Anticholinergic/ Spasmolytic	Urge incontinence
Tolterodine (Detrol)	2 mg bid	Anticholinergic	Urge incontinence
Propantheline bromide (Pro-Banthine)	7.5 mg tid	Anticholinergic	Urge incontinence
Phenylpropanolamine (Entex)	5 mg bid	Alpha-adrenergic stimulation	Stress incontinence
Psuedoephedrine (Sudafed)	60 mg qid	Alpha-adrenergic stimulation	Stress incontinence
Imipramine (Tofranil)	25-75 mg daily	Anticholinergic and alpha - adrenergic stimulation	Urge incontinence Stress incontinence
Estrogen (Premarin)	0.625 mg po or vaginally, daily	Beneficial effects on urethral mucosa and sphincter	Urge incontinence Stress incontinence

recommended as the first-line pharmacologic therapy for patients with detrusor instability. These medications mediate the parasympathetic control of the bladder and treat detrusor instability by producing bladder relaxation. Commonly used medications are listed in Table 4. Oxybutynin has long been considered the primary anticholinergic agent of choice. It also has a smooth muscle relaxant and local anesthetic properties. The recommended dose is 2.5-5 mg orally tid-qid, but we find that many elderly patients experience significant side effects at this dosage. We routinely start patients on 2.5 mg/po/bid and then titrate up based on improvement of symptoms and occurrence of side effects. The primary side effects of anticholinergic medications include dry mouth, constipation, blurred vision, change in mental status, and nausea. These medications are contraindicated in patients with narrow angle glaucoma. Other anticholinergic agents, including propantheline, dicyclomine hydrochloride, and flavoxate, may be used as second-line agents in patients with a poor response to oxybutinin. Recently, tolterodine has been introduced as a bladder selective anticholinergic agent that is associated with improved symptoms and reduced side effects. Initial results with its use are encouraging as it is well tolerated in most patients.

Imipramine, a tricyclic antidepressant, has been shown to be effective in the treatment of both stress and urge incontinence. Although the exact mechanism of action is incompletely understood, it seems to work by increasing urethral contractility and suppressing involuntary bladder contractions via its anticholinergic properties. The recommended dosage is 25-100 mg daily. Side effects include orthostatic hypertension, dry mouth, nausea, and hepatic dysfunction. It is contraindicated in patients taking MAO inhibitors.

Calcium channel blockers, such as nifedipine, verapamil, and terodiline, work by blocking the influx of extra-cellular calcium, which is important for detrusor muscle contraction. They have been used extensively in the treatment of detrusor instability in Europe but are still currently under investigation for use in the United States. Side effects include dry mouth, blurred vision, headache, and cardiac arrhythmia. At the present time, these agents are not recommended for general use in the treatment of urinary incontinence.

Alpha-adrenergic agonists, phenylpropanolamine (PPA) and pseudoephedrine, have little effect on the detrusor muscle but can significantly increase urethral pressure by inducing contraction of the urethral sphincter. These agents are useful in the treatment of genuine stress incontinence particularly due to intrinsic sphincter deficiency. Recommended dosage for PPA is 25-100 mg orally in a sustained release form (bid) and for pseudoephedrine, 15-30 mg orally tid. Patients often report improvement in their symptoms within one week. Side effects include drowsiness, dry mouth, and hypertension.

Estrogen replacement, either oral or vaginal, should be used as an adjuctive pharmacologic agent for postmenopausal women with stress urinary incontinence or mixed incontinence. Although the exact mechanisms by which estrogen therapy improves incontinence symptoms is unknown, various theories have been proposed. Estrogen has been shown to alter the vaginal pH and decrease the frequency of urinary tract infections. In addition, estrogen-induced cytologic changes in the urethral mucosa may lead to improve coaptation and re-creation of the mucosal seal. Estrogen may also augment periurethral vascularity with improved function of the smooth and striated periurethral muscles.[16] Finally, the combination of alpha-agonists and estrogen may have synergistic effects. Conjugated estrogen can be administered either orally or vaginally and progestin should be added in patients who have an intact uterus. Side effects include irregular vaginal bleeding, breast tenderness, weight gain, and nausea. Estrogen is contraindicated in patients with a history of breast or gynecologic malignancy.[17]

Medical Devices

Medical devices for the management of urinary incontinence include absorbent products, vaginal support devices, and urethral products.[18] The widespread use of absorbant pads for the symptomatic control of urinary incontinence has prolonged research and technological advances in the treatment of this socially debilitating condition. Often marketed as "adult diapers" or "absorbant undergarments," these products provide palliative control and often dissuade the patient from seeking medical attention for incontinence that is usually readily treatable. Given the variety of surgical and nonsurgical management options today, current use of absorbant products should be reserved for long-term care of patients with chronic, intractable urinary incontinence.

Medical devices, classified as obstructive or supportive, are designed primarily for the treatment of stress urinary incontinence or mild mixed incontinence due to urethral hypermobility or intrinsic sphincter deficiency. (*Please see Figure 5.*) Urethral plugs and patches are placed in or over the urethra to occlude the lumen and prevent urinary leakage with increases in abdominal pressure. Complications include urinary tract infection, hematuria, migration of the device into the bladder, and persistent incontinence. Vaginal devices include diaphragms, pessaries, and tampons. These devices function by providing intravaginal support to the bladder neck during episodes of increased abdominal pressure. Complications related to intravaginal devices are less common and include vaginal discharge and pelvic discomfort. Success rates from medical devices have been found to vary depending on the severity of incontinence. Vierhout and Lose have reported subjective success rates ranging from 40-60% depending on the type of device.[19]

Surgical Correction

Although a comprehensive discussion of the various surgical procedures used in the treatment of incontinence is beyond the scope of this paper, it may be helpful to briefly review the major classes of surgery to assist the primary care clinician in providing preliminary information to the patient regarding his/her surgical options. Surgery is used primarily in the treatment of genuine stress urinary incontinence due to urethral hypermobility or intrinsic sphincter deficiency.

In female patients with urethral hypermobility, the goal of the surgical procedure is to restore normal anatomic bladder

Figure 5. Medical Devices for Incontinence

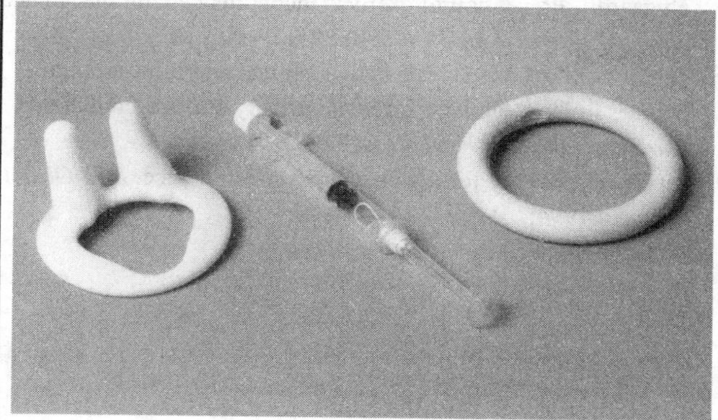

Medical Devices for Incontinence include pessary devices with and without support (left and right) and urethral plugs (center)

neck support and prevent descent during increased abdominal pressure. This can be done by a retropubic urethropexy, a transvaginal needle suspension procedure, or a suburethral sling. The retropubic urethropexy is performed through a small suprapubic laparotomy incision, which provides access to the retropubic space. Vaginal tissue underneath the urethra is then suspended to the pubic symphysis (Marshall-Marchetti-Krantz urethropexy) or Cooper's ligament (Burch colposuspension). Recently, the retropubic procedures have been performed laparoscopically with equivalent cure rates on short-term follow-up. The transvaginal needle suspension procedure is mainly performed via the vaginal route with a small abdominal incision. The retropubic space is entered vaginally and support tissue on either side of the urethra is grasped and sutured in a helical stitch. These sutures are then transferred above the anterior rectus fascia to the suprapubic incision via a long needle carrier. Tie down over the rectus fascia results in elevation and stabilization of the bladder neck. The suburethral sling is performed in a similar manner but uses a synthetic or natural graft underneath the urethra rather than incorporating the periurethral tissue in a helical stitch. Risks of these procedures include bleeding, infection, damage to the lower urinary tract, recurrent incontinence, and postoperative urinary retention. In a meta-analysis performed by Jarvis, the long-term success rates for the retropubic urethropexy, transvaginal needle suspension, and suburethral sling have been reported to be 80%, 70%, and 85%, respectively.[20]

In patients with intrinsic sphincter deficiency, the goal of the surgical procedure is to restore the normal continence mechanism by compressing the urethra at the bladder neck. This can be done by a suburethral sling, an artificial urinary sphincter, or periurethral collagen injections. The suburethral sling has been previously described. The artificial urinary sphincter involves placement of a mechanical prosthesis around the bladder neck which can inflate and deflate depending on the need for continence or voiding. Periurethral collagen injections involve injection of bulk enhancing agents, most commonly cross-linked bovine dermal collagen, around the urethra until closure of the internal urethral meatus occurs. This procedure is commonly performed under local anesthesia in the office setting. Risks of these procedures include infection, recurrent incontinence, and postoperative urinary retention.

Newer Techniques

Recently, a number of medical and surgical advances have been made in the treatment of urinary incontinence. A variety of new medications for the treatment of stress and urge incontinence are expected to be released over the next several years. These include new, long-acting delivery systems as well as new pharmacologic agents that should improve treatment outcomes and reduce the incidence of side effects.

Although pharmacotherapy and behavioral modification are still the mainstay of treatment for detrusor instability, patients with persistent urge incontinence may be candidates for newly introduced implantable nerve root stimulators. The implantable electrode is designed to stimulate the dorsal nerve root of S2, S3, and S4, re-establishing a neurologic equilibrium with relief of persistent urge incontinence. Patients initially undergo placement of a subcutaneous test stimulator on an outpatient basis. Those patients who experience at least a 50% reduction in symptoms are candidates for subsequent placement of a permanent implantable device. Initial results have been encouraging, especially since surgical alternatives for refractory urge incontinence are associated with poor outcomes.

For patients with stress incontinence, new laparoscopic procedures are providing good surgical outcomes with fewer complications and reduced hospital stay. New substances for periurethral injection in the treatment of intrinsic sphincter deficiency are being developed to provide long-lasting results with minimal risk. With increased understanding of this condition and greater media attention, it is expected that more treatment options will be available in the future.

Conclusion

Urinary incontinence is a condition that affects more than 13 million Americans in this country. It is expected that this number will continue to grow as our country continues to age. The diagnosis and treatment of this disorder will begin with the primary care provider. A basic understanding of the pathophysiology of the lower urinary tract is vital in diagnosing and treating this condition. Initial diagnosis can usually be made on the first visit after history and physical exam. Many patients may require basic additional testing, which can easily be performed in the office setting. Preliminary treatment modalities will either treat or significantly improve the majority of patients. The small subset of patients who have a complex presentation or require surgery will need further consultation and complex urodynamic testing.

The primary care provider serves as the gatekeeper for this common problem. A step-by-step algorithm with an understanding of the available treatment options will allow the clinician to provide care for this condition and identify those patients who require subspecialist referral. In either case, this care will probably make a long-lasting effect in the medical, social, and psychological well-being of patients suffering from this debilitating condition.

References

1. Fantl JA, et al. *Urinary Incontinence in Adults: Acute and Chronic Management. Clinical Practice Guideline, No. 2, 1996 Update*. Rockville, MD. U.S. Department of Health and Human Services. Public Health Service, Agency for Health Care Policy and Research 1996;2:5-7.
2. Burgio KL, et al. Prevalence, incidence, and correlates of urinary incontinence in healthy, middle-aged women. *J Urol* 1991; 146:1255-1259.
3. Ouslander J, et al. Urinary incontinence in elderly nursing home patients. *JAMA* 1982;248:1194-1198.
4. Baker KR, Bice TW. The influence of urinary incontinence on publicly financed home care services to low income elderly people. *Gerontologist* 1995;35:360-369.
5. Siu AL, et al. The geriatric medical and public health imperative revisited. *J AM Geriat Soc* 1995;43:286-294.
6. International Continence Society Committee on Standardization of Terminology. The standardization of terminology of lower urinary tract function. *Scan J Urol Nephrol* 1988;114(suppl):5-19.
7. McGuire EJ, et al. Clinical assessment of urethral sphincter function. *J Urol* 1993;50:1452-1454.
8. Jenson JK, et al. The role of patient history in the diagnosis of urinary incontinence. *Obstet Gynecol* 1994;83:904-910.
9. Scotti R, Myers D. A simplified urogynecologic workup. *AUGS Quarterly Report* 1990;8(4):1-3.
10. Cardozo LD, Stanton SL. Genuine stress incontinence and detrusor instabiligy—A review of 200 patients. *Br J Obstet Gynaecol* 1980;87:184-190.
11. Fantl JA, et al. Efficacy of bladder training in older women with urinary incontinence. *JAMA* 1991;265:609-613.
12. Tchou DCH, et al. Pelvic floor musculature exercises in treatment of anatomical urinary stress incontinence. *Phys Ther* 1988;68:652-655.
13. Bump RC, et al. Assessment of Kegel pelvic muscle exercise performance after brief verbal instruction. *Am J Obstet Gynecol* 1991;165:322-329.
14. Dougherty M, et al. Graded pelvic muscle exercise. Effect on stress urinary incontinence. *J Reprod Med* 1993;39:684-691.
15. Fantl JA, et al. *Urinary incontinence in Adults: Acute and Chronic Management. Clinical Practice Guideline, No. 2, 1996 Update*. Rockville, MD. U.S. Department of Health and Human Services. Public Health Service, Agency for Health Care Policy and Research 1996;2:42-43.
16. Bhatia NN, et al. Effects of estrogen on urethral function in women with urinary incontinence. *Am J Obstet Gynecol* 1989; 160:176-181.
17. Griebling TL, et al. Female urinary incontinence: New management techniques and technologies. *Mediguide to Urology* 1998;11:1-6.
18. Nygaard I. Prevention of exercise incontinence with mechanical devices. *J Reprod Med* 1995;40:89-94.
19. Vierhout ME, Lose G. Preventive vaginal and intra-urethral devices in the treatment of female urinary stress incontinence. *Curr Opin Obstet Gynecol* 1997;9:325-328.
20. Jarvis GJ. Surgery for genuine stress incontinence. *Br J Obstet Gynecol* 1994;101:371-374.

Part XVII

Psychiatric Disorders

Depression

Alan J. Gelenberg, MD

Major depression is a common disorder, experienced by up to 19% of people at least once during their lives.[1,2] Women are afflicted twice as often as men.[3] The World Health Organization ranked depression fourth among worldwide illnesses in terms of disease burden in 1990, based on quality-adjusted life years, and projects that by the year 2020, it will rise to second place.[4]

Depression levies a heavy burden in terms of work and productivity. It impairs marriages and disrupts families. People with depression are more likely to become involved with alcohol and drugs. They have a much higher morbidity and mortality when they suffer concomitant medical disorders, including heart disease and diabetes.[5,6] Without effective treatment, suicide is an eventual possibility and, among the most severely depressed, lifetime suicide rates may be as high as 15%.[7]

All of the above notwithstanding, depression tends to be underdiagnosed and, even when recognized, insufficiently treated.[8-11] This is unfortunate, not only because of the burdens of the disease as noted above, but because depression usually is an eminently treatable disorder. This chapter will give a brief overview of depression and its manifestations, discuss why it frequently goes unrecognized and undertreated, examine the role of the primary care physician in managing depression, and describe principles of intervention.

Diagnosis and Differential Diagnosis

Almost everybody gets the blues—sometime. When someone experiences a disappointment or a loss, we expect them to be sad or to grieve. Whether experiencing the death of a loved one or facing an unpleasant medical diagnosis, people react with dysphoric emotions.

But grief and natural reactions to stress and loss are time-limited and "dynamic." In other words, the emotions change and evolve. The typical sufferer reaches out adaptively to others—for comfort and alternative ways to get his or her needs met. Even after a profound loss, such as the death of a spouse, the bereaved typically adjusts to the new circumstances and returns to some level of function, although experiencing a deep sense of inner loss and void. If the symptoms of depression still exist after two months, it is likely that bereavement has triggered major depression, which requires clinical attention. If the depressive symptoms associated with bereavement are particularly severe or disabling (including suicidality and psychosis), the diagnosis can be made without delay. In such circumstances, if depression is appropriately treated, the sufferer can return to the active process of grieving and moving on with his or her life.

The criteria for major depression are listed in Table 1. Clinical science has taught us that there is no magical threshold for clinically relevant depression. Any symptoms of depression that last for

Table 1. Diagnostic Criteria—Major Depressive Episode[40]

At least five of the following symptoms have been present during the same two-week period and represent a change from previous functioning (at least 1 must be depressed mood or loss of interest or pleasure):

- Depressed mood most of the day, nearly every day
- Diminished interest or pleasure in activities most of the day, nearly every day
- Poor appetite or weight loss or increased appetite or weight gain
- Insomnia or hypersomnia
- Loss of energy or fatigue
- Psychomotor agitation or retardation
- Feelings of worthlessness or excessive or inappropriate guilt
- Diminished ability to think or concentrate, or indecisiveness
- Recurrent thoughts of death or suicide

The symptoms do not meet criteria for a mixed episode.

The symptoms cause clinically significant distress or impairment in social, occupational, or other important areas of functioning.

The symptoms are not due to the direct physiological effects of a substance or a general medical condition.

The symptoms are not better accounted for by bereavement, and they persist for longer than two months or are characterized by marked functional impairment, morbid preoccupation with worthlessness, suicidal ideation, psychotic symptoms, or psychomotor retardation.

two weeks or longer (or even a shorter period if they are severe, dysfunctional, and/or life-threatening) are problematic and warrant clinical attention. Lower levels of depression, when ongoing, can increase mortality in the elderly[6] and presumably cause loss of function and work productivity and impair family relations. In addition, patients with subthreshold depressive symptoms have a greater risk of developing a major depressive episode. Therefore, even low-grade depression should be monitored carefully.

Evaluation of depression, like the common syndromes of hypertension or arthritis, includes differential diagnostic considerations. It is unnecessary to list all possible medical, neurologic, and toxic causes of depression. Such a list would be unwieldy and doubtlessly incomplete. A clinician should consider any medical clue that might present in the course of a medical history and review of systems. If a medication was introduced (or deleted) within weeks of new-onset depressive symptoms, consider that drug a possible culprit. If there have been weight changes or altered bowel habits, consider that depression may be a symptom of cancer. If there are symptoms and signs of peripheral neuropathy, perhaps a vitamin deficiency could be a cause. Changes in skin and hair texture and temperature tolerance might indicate thyroid dysfunction. Headaches and visual changes could signal a space-occupying brain lesion. These are just examples but indicate the importance of taking a history and review of systems.

Ask about drug and alcohol abuse. Virtually all patients who abuse substances develop mood symptoms. But people with primary depression also are more likely to abuse drugs and alcohol. When in doubt which is the primary disorder, try to get a good longitudinal history from a family member. Modern antidepressant drugs are safe and will not complicate the recovery from substance abuse—even if the "chicken-and-egg dilemma" remains murky. But antidepressants alone usually will not help the substance abuser become abstinent; that requires ongoing rehabilitative treatment aimed toward achieving and maintaining abstinence.

When to Seek a Consultation or Referral

A primary care physician (PCP) should be able to diagnose and treat uncomplicated depression—major or subsyndromal ("minor"). However, consider a consultation with a psychiatrist if the diagnosis or treatment is unclear, if a patient's comorbid conditions may be affected by antidepressant medications, or if the patient does not respond to or comply with treatment. It might be advisable to refer a patient to a psychiatrist if hallucinations or delusions accompany depression or if the patient shows signs of distorted reasoning. Similarly, when taking a psychiatric history in a patient with depression, ask about episodes of elation and overactivity in a patient's past. These may signal the presence of a bipolar disorder that, again, is best referred to a specialist. A patient with a history of poor response to prior antidepressant treatments or serious suicidal potential or someone with severe functional impairment also might be considered for specialty referral.

Reasons for Depression Being Underdiagnosed and Undertreated

Although it is impossible to determine accurately the percentage of individuals with major depression who are undertreated, results from studies of depressed patients in the community, in primary care settings, and in the mental health care arena give an idea of the extent of the problem. Data from these studies suggest that 50-90% of individuals with major depression either do not seek help or receive inadequate treatment.[12-21] The reasons for this phenomenon can be seen as originating from three sources: the patient, the physician, and the health care system.[22]

The Patient

There are many misconceptions about depression that may prevent a person from seeking appropriate treatment. For instance, many people believe that if there is a cause for depression (e.g., the death of a loved one), it does not need to be treated. They also may feel that depression will go away on its own eventually, so they should just get through it. There is a stigma attached to depression that anyone who cannot overcome it on their own is weak, so many people may not want to admit they need help. In addition, the symptoms of depression often leave a person lacking initiative, drive, and hope. They may not seek help because they feel nothing could help. A recent survey found that among individuals with current major depression, having health insurance and having a PCP each increased the odds of receiving antidepressant therapy fourfold.[10] The next important step was the patient trusting the primary provider enough to tell him or her about depressive symptoms; this predicted a tenfold increase in treatment.

The Physician

The PCP is often the first and, in many cases, the only point of contact for a person suffering from depression. In one study, 12% of patients in a primary care setting met criteria for major depression.[23] Unfortunately, physicians are frequently inadequately trained to diagnose and manage this disorder. Depression can hide behind a variety of symptoms, including pain. Physicians need to have both the medical knowledge to "unmask" and treat depression and the interpersonal skills to manage a patient with disturbances in emotional, cognitive, behavioral, and somatic regulation. A physician's lack of knowledge about antidepressant drugs could lead to a patient not receiving adequate doses or treatment for a long enough period. Physicians need to educate patients and their families about the disorder and its treatments. Too often, there is insufficient time for a PCP to attend to psychiatric conditions in a busy practice.

The Health Care System

While health care systems vary in different places around the world, many of them view depression as an acute disorder rather than the chronic, recurring disease that it is. In the United States, patients often are unreimbursed by managed care and insurance companies for their use of mental health services. Physicians are encouraged not to monitor patients frequently early in treatment, try more than one treatment approach, or refer patients to specialists. Health maintenance organizations might also limit the length of therapy.

The Costs of Undertreating Depression

The costs and consequences of inadequately treating depression are significant, both to the individual sufferer and to society. The total annual cost of depression in the United States was estimated to be $43.7 billion in 1990.[24] This includes $12.4 billion in direct costs of treatment and $31.3 billion in indirect costs, such as premature death, absenteeism from work, and reduced productivity. It is estimated that adequate treatment of depression would result in indirect cost savings that would exceed direct costs of depression by $4 billion.

Untreated episodes of major depression can last six months or longer.[25] During an untreated episode, depression can significantly interfere with recovery from comorbid conditions like cancer, diabetes, stroke, and myocardial infarction. Depression similarly can complicate pregnancy, childbirth, and the postpartum. In general, patients with unrecognized or undertreated depression tend to be higher users of medical services than patients without depression; major depression not only causes unexplained physical symptoms but also amplifies the symptoms of other medical illnesses.[26] Untreated depression may get worse (and lead to suicide) or become chronic. The longer the first episode lasts, the greater likelihood of recurrence. In addition, rates of relapse and recurrence increase with each subsequent episode.[27]

Treatment

In the treatment of major depression, the goals are to eliminate all signs and symptoms of depression, restore the patient's ability to function in work and social settings, and, finally, to reduce the likelihood of a relapse or recurrence. When a patient has uncomplicated depression of mild to moderate severity, the first step in the treatment algorithm is to decide between psychotherapy or antidepressant medications. Often, the choice can be made by the patient: some would rather talk, others prefer to take medication. Even though both methods take a number of weeks to achieve full benefit, antidepressant drugs tend to work faster than psychotherapy. Some symptoms, such as insomnia, may respond to medicine even more quickly.

Psychotherapy

Several forms of psychotherapy, such as cognitive behavioral therapy and interpersonal psychotherapy, have been shown in scientific controlled studies to be equal in efficacy to antidepressant medications in mild to moderate depression.[28-30] In some locales, there may not be psychotherapists trained in these techniques. In the absence of professionals with such qualifications, try to find therapists with good professional reputations. If the patient is taking an antidepressant, choose a therapist with a positive attitude about medication. Encourage patients to use their own judgment and not feel obligated to stay with a psychotherapist if the "chemistry" is not right. Moreover, a depressed patient should not stay with the same treatment approach if there has not been at least a moderate degree of benefit after 2-3 months. In such cases, the possibility of adding a medication trial should be seriously considered. Some studies show combined psychotherapy and antidepressant medication to be more effective than either treatment alone.[28]

Medications

For patients with moderate to severe depression, antidepressant medications are considered first-line treatment.[31] Pharmacologic treatment also is recommended for depression with psychotic, melancholic, or atypical symptoms and for patients who:

- do not have access to adequate psychotherapy;
- have responded to medication in the past;
- will need maintenance treatment;
- have had symptoms for more than two years that have not responded to psychosocial intervention; or
- are experiencing significant impairment of work or social functioning.

There are currently available a wide range of antidepressant medicines from different classes *(please see Table 2)*. The majority of U.S. physicians now turns first to selective serotonin reuptake

Table 2. Commonly Used Antidepressant Drugs

GENERIC NAME (TRADE NAME)	STARTING DOSE (MG/D)*	USUAL DOSE (MG/D)
TRICYCLICS AND TETRACYCLICS		
Tertiary amine tricyclics		
Amitriptyline (Elavil)	25-50	100-300
Clomipramine (Anafranil)	25	100-250
Doxepin (Sinequan)	25-50	100-300
Imipramine (Tofranil)	25-50	100-300
Trimipramine (Surmontil)	25-50	100-300
Secondary amine tricyclics		
Desipramine (Norpramin)	25-50	100-300
Nortriptyline (Pamelor)	25	50-200
Protriptyline (Vivactil)	10	15-60
Tetracyclics		
Amoxapine (Ascendin)	50	100-400
Maprotiline (Ludiomil)	50	100-225
SELECTIVE SEROTONIN REUPTAKE INHIBITORS (SSRIS)		
Citalopram (Celexa)	20	20-60†
Fluoxetine (Prozac)	20	20-60†
Fluvoxamine (Luvox)	50	50-300†
Paroxetine (Paxil)	20	20-60†
Sertraline (Zoloft)	50	50-200†
DOPAMINE-NOREPINEPHRINE REUPTAKE INHIBITORS		
Bupropion (Wellbutrin)	150	300
SEROTONIN-NOREPINEPHRINE REUPTAKE INHIBITORS		
Venlafaxine (Effexor)	37.5	75-225
SEROTONIN MODULATORS		
Nefazodone (Serzone)	50	150-300
Trazodone (Desyrel)	50	75-300
NOREPINEPHRINE-SEROTONIN MODULATOR		
Mirtazapine (Remeron)	15	15-45
MONOAMINE OXIDASE INHIBITORS (MAOIS)		
Irreversible, nonselective		
Isocarboxazid (Marplan)	10	20-30
Phenelzine (Nardil)	15	15-90
Tranylcypromine (Parnate)	10	30-60
Reversible MAOI-A (RIMA)		
Moclobemide (Manerix)‡	150	300-600

Adapted from: The American Psychiatric Association Practice Guideline for the Treatment of Patients with Major Depressive Disorder. *Am J Psychiatry* 2000;157:1-45.

* Lower starting dosages are recommended for elderly patients and for those with panic disorder, significant anxiety or hepatic disease, and general comorbidity.

† Dosage varies with diagnosis.

‡ Not available in the United States.

Table 3. Potential Treatments for Side Effects from Antidepressant Drugs[31]

SIDE EFFECT	ANTIDEPRESSANT(S) ASSOCIATED WITH	TREATMENT
Cardiovascular		
Orthostatic hypotension	TCAs, trazodone, nefazodone, MAOIs	Lower dose, discontinue medication, fludrocortisone, add salt to diet
Reduced cardiac output	TCAs	Discontinue medication
Arrhythmias	TCAs	Discontinue medication
Hypertension	Venlafaxine	Lower dose, discontinue medication
Hypertensive crisis	MAOIs	Discontinue medication, intravenous phentolamine
Increase in cholesterol	Mirtazapine	Lower dose, discontinue medication
Anticholinergic		
Dry mouth	TCAs	Pilocarpine oral rinse, gum, candy
Constipation	TCAs	Hydration, bulk laxatives
Urinary hesitancy	TCAs	Bethanechol
Visual changes	TCAs	Pilocarpine eye drops
Delirium	TCAs	Discontinue medication, antipsychotic medication
Sedation	TCAs, trazodone, nefazodone, mirtazapine	Bedtime dosing
Weight gain	TCAs, mirtazapine, MAOIs	Lower dose, change to secondary amine (if TCA required), discontinue medication
Nausea, vomiting	SSRIs, bupropion (SR), venlafaxine (R)	Lower dose, discontinue medication
Insomnia	SSRIs, bupropion	Lower dose, discontinue medication, morning dosing, trazodone at bedtime
Activation	SSRIs, venlafaxine	Lower dose, discontinue medication
Neurologic		
Myoclonus	TCAs, MAOIs	Lower dose, discontinue medication, clonazepam
Extrapyramidal symptoms	Amoxapine, SSRIs	Lower dose, discontinue medication, tardive dyskinesia
Seizures	Bupropion, amoxapine	Lower dose, discontinue medication, antiepileptic medication
Headaches	SSRIs, bupropion	Lower dose, discontinue medication
Sexual side effects		
Arousal, erectile dysfunction	Paroxetine, venlafaxine	Lower dose, discontinue medication, sildenafil, yohimbine, ginkgo, methylphenidate, dextroamphetamine, pemoline
	TCAs, SSRIs	Lower dose, discontinue medication, sildenafil, yohimbine, ginkgo, bethanechol, neostigmine
Orgasm dysfunction	SSRIs, venlafaxine	Lower dose, discontinue medication, granisetron, amantadine, cyproheptadine, sildenafil
	MAOIs, TCAs	Lower dose, discontinue medication, cyproheptadine, amantadine
Priapism	Trazodone	Discontinue medication, surgical correction
Serotonin syndrome	SSRIs, MAOIs, venlafaxine	Discontinue medication
Agranulocytosis	Mirtazapine	Discontinue medication, monitor white blood cell count and granulocyte colony-stimulating factor

TCA = tricyclic antidepressant; SSRI = selective serotonin reuptake inhibitor; MAOI = monoamine oxidase inhibitor inhibitors (SSRIs) for most depressed patients.[31] These are fluoxetine, sertraline, paroxetine, and citalopram. Other antidepressants sometimes considered for first-line use are nefazodone and venlafaxine. Bupropion is usually reserved for a second- or third-line treatment, and although mirtazapine has been available in the United States for more than three years, it still is not widely used by PCPs. The most sedating of the newer antidepressants, mirtazapine shares with bupropion and nefazodone a low incidence of sexual dysfunction. Tricyclic antidepressants, such as amitriptyline and clomipramine, are generally second- or third-line options. The monoamine oxidase inhibitor (MAOI) antidepressants, such as phenelzine, tranylcypromine, and isocarboxazid, are invaluable but usually far down the list of choices due to their side effects and need for dietary and medication restrictions. MAOIs are most commonly prescribed by psychiatrists. St. John's wort is now widely used as an over-the-counter remedy for depression, but its efficacy has yet to be established by rigorous, controlled trials.

There are few differences in comparisons of grouped data. There are dramatic differences in the effectiveness of antidepressants for particular patients.[31] The choice of agent usually is based on the following seven factors:[32]

- side effects (*please see Table 3*);
- safety in overdose;
- the ease with which a therapeutic dose can be achieved;
- the patient's (or family's) history of response;
- cost;
- half-life; and
- the effect of the medication (or its side effects) on underlying medical conditions.

When a patient taking an antidepressant takes other medications concomitantly, potential interactions also must be considered. Pharmacodynamic interactions involve additive effects, such as cardiac conduction effects or sedation. We now know more about pharmacokinetic interactions, as pharmacology studies have

Table 4. P450 Isoenzymes—Potential Antidepressant Drug Interactions

Isoenzyme	Metabolizes	Inhibited by
2D6	SSRIs: Fluoxetine N-desmethylcitalopram Norfluoxetine Paroxetine Tricyclic antidepressants Amitriptyline Clomipramine Desipramine Imipramine N-desmethylclomipramine Nortriptyline Trimipramine Other: Venlafaxine	Fluoxetine Paroxetine Sertraline Clomipramine
1A2	Amitriptyline Clomipramine Imipramine	Fluvoxamine
3A4	Nefazodone Sertraline Venlafaxine Some tricyclics Trazodone	Fluoxetine Fluvoxamine Nefazodone Sertraline
2C19	Amitriptyline Clomipramine Imipramine	Fluoxetine Fluvoxamine Sertraline

demonstrated which among the drug-metabolizing enzymes of the cytochrome P450 system are influenced by different medications *(please see Table 4)*.

Treatment Failure

Approximately 50% of patients fail to respond adequately to initial treatment with an antidepressant medication.[31] Some improvement should be observable (by family members if not by the patient) within about two weeks. If benefit is not apparent within 2-3 weeks, the dose should be raised. If a patient is beginning to achieve benefits, on the other hand, it is best to let the dose stay where it is. Full accrual of benefits from an antidepressant may take 8-12 weeks.[33] If the patient does not respond within this time frame, it may be due to an inappropriate diagnosis; coexisting general medical conditions; psychiatric disorders or complicating psychosocial factors that are impeding recovery; or noncompliance with treatment. These factors should be reviewed and addressed. If the patient's lack of response is not due to any of these factors, another (preferably non-MAOI) antidepressant should be tried. The primary care doctor should become familiar with the dosing and side effects of a few antidepressants and know them well. If a patient fails to improve after two or three trials of different antidepressants, it may be worthwhile to refer the patient to a psychiatrist.

Continuation and Maintenance Treatment

If a patient has responded favorably to an antidepressant, continue that drug at the therapeutic dose for at least six months. If the patient then has been entirely free of symptoms for at least two months, gradually taper and discontinue the medication. Educate the patient and family members to be on the alert for a future episode and to bring it immediately to clinical attention. Stay in contact with the patient to assess potential recurrences.

Tricyclic antidepressants are associated with a group of common symptoms upon discontinuation, including gastrointestinal or general medical symptoms such as vomiting, nausea, diarrhea, headache, fatigue, and malaise; sleep abnormalities; akathisia and parkinsonism; and paradoxical behavioral activation resulting in hypomanic or manic symptoms.[34] These symptoms usually begin 24-48 hours after the last dose and may last as long as one month. A withdrawal syndrome has also been reported in association with some of the serotonin reuptake inhibitor antidepressants.[35] It generally begins 2-3 days after the last dose, although sometimes it starts during the taper (indicating that the taper is too rapid). The symptoms—which are often described as "flu-like" and include dizziness, lethargy, paresthesia, nausea, vivid dreams, irritability, and lowered mood—generally abate within three weeks.

There is a role for maintenance therapy in depression. It is rarely appropriate after a single episode of depression but might be considered in very severe cases or when there is a heavy family history, particularly for patients who have attempted suicide.[36] After two closely spaced or severe episodes of depression, maintenance therapy should be considered. Patients with three or more lifetime episodes of depression should take antidepressant medication (or be in some form of effective psychotherapy) indefinitely. Prophylactic treatment should also be considered for patients who are older than 50 years when they have their first episode. Maintenance treatment should use the same dosage of the same drug that was used in the acute and continuation phases.[37]

Table 5. Obstacles and Solutions to Adherence Problems

Obstacle	Solution
Attitudes/misconceptions	Patient/family education
Side effects	Side effect monitoring, dose adjustment, adjunctive agents, medication switch
Euthymia leading to treatment discontinuation	Patient/family education
Symptom worsening	Symptom monitoring, psychotherapy, medication changes
Suboptimal functioning or psychosocial problems	Support, formal therapy, rehabilitative efforts
Discouragement	Patient/family groups (e.g., Depressive and Manic Depressive Association, National Alliance for the Mentally Ill, Mental Health Association)

Adapted from: Rush AJ. *J Clin Psychiatry* 1999;60: 21-26.

Relapse and Recurrence

Symptom breakthroughs occur in 10-20% of patients during continuation or maintenance treatment.[32] When symptoms return before full recovery, they are considered to be part of the previous episode of depression (i.e., a relapse). If symptoms occur following recovery, they are considered the start of a new episode (i.e., a recurrence). Symptoms must be absent for six months or longer for the patient to be considered completely recovered.[38] Symptom breakthroughs may result from intermittent adherence to treatment, the addition of alcohol, a concurrent illness, increased stress, or possibly the beginning of a bipolar disorder. Support, close observation, and possibly an increase in dose are necessary.

Compliance

Many individuals who make the effort to get treatment for depression do not stick with it. Reasons for noncompliance include the delay in the onset of effects from antidepressant medications or psychotherapy, the need to continue taking medication after symptoms have remitted, and the adverse effects of medications *(please see Table 5)*. The following six messages, delivered to the patient by the primary care provider, can help patients adhere to antidepressant therapy:[39]

- Take medication daily.
- Antidepressants must be taken for at least 2-4 weeks for a noticeable effect.
- Continue medication even when feeling better.
- Do not stop medication without checking with physician.
- Call with any questions.
- Mild side effects are common and often improve after 7-10 days.

These messages take less than one minute to be delivered slowly and clearly to the patient. Patients should be given this advice at the start of treatment and at every follow-up visit.

Summary and Conclusions

Major depression is a serious medical illness that often goes unrecognized and, even when diagnosed, inadequately treated. This article has reviewed the burden of depression on individuals and on the community, the diagnosis and treatment of this disorder, and reasons why many patients do not get the help they need. To ensure that depressed patients receive optimal therapy and adhere to their treatment regimen, PCPs must learn about antidepressant medications and take the time to educate patients and their families about the illness and its treatments.

Psychiatric neuroscience is pushing knowledge and treatment potential forward in the field of depression. New pharmacotherapies, as well as new magnetic, electrical, and neurosurgical interventions, are being studied. In the meantime, the treatment of depression can be gratifying to clinicians, patients, and family members alike. It is extremely rewarding to see a smile reemerge on a face that has been furrowed with worry lines and pessimism.

References

1. Weissman MM, et al. Cross-national epidemiology of major depression and bipolar disorder. *JAMA* 1996;276:293-299.
2. Blazer DG, et al. The prevalence and distribution of major depression in a national community sample: The National Comorbidity Survey. *Am J Psychiatry* 1994;151:979-986.
3. Gelenberg AJ, Delgado PL. Depression. In: Gelenberg AJ and Bassuk EL, eds. *The Practitioner's Guide to Psychoactive Drugs*. 4th ed. New York: Plenum; 1997:19-97.
4. Murray CJL, Lopez AD (eds.) *The Global Burden of Disease: A Comprehensive Assessment of Mortality and Disability from Diseases, Injuries, and Risk Factors in 1990 and Projected to 2020: Summary*. Cambridge, MA: The Harvard School of Public Health on behalf of The World Health Organization and The World Bank; Distributed by Harvard University Press; 1996.
5. Gelenberg AJ. Morbidity, mortality, and mood. *Biol Ther Psychiatry Newsletter* 1994;17:9-11.
6. Whooley MA, et al. Association between depressive symptoms and mortality in older women. *Arch Intern Med* 1998;158:2129-2135.
7. Keller MB. The difficult depressed patient in perspective. *J Clin Psychiatry* 1993;54(Suppl 2):4-8.
8. Gelenberg A. Depression is still underrecognized and undertreated. *Arch Int Med* 1999;159:1657-1658.
9. Davidson JRT, Meltzer-Brody SE. The underrecognition and undertreatment of depression: What is the breadth and depth of the problem? *J Clin Psychiatry* 1999;60(Suppl 7):4-11.
10. Druss BG, et al. Underuse of antidepressants in major depression: Prevalence and correlates in a national sample of young adults. *J Clin Psychiatry* 2000;61:234-237.
11. Dunner DL, et al. Depression and the introduction of SSRIs. *J Clin Psychiatry* 1999;17(Monograph 3):4-15.
12. Robins LN, et al. An overview of psychiatric disorders in America. In: Robins LN and Regier DA (eds.) *Psychiatric Disorders in America: The Epidemiologic Catchment Area Study*. New York: Free Press;1991:328-366.
13. Keller MB, et al. Treatment received by depressed patients. *JAMA* 1982;248:1848-1855.
14. Kessler RC, et al. Prevalence, correlates, and course of minor depression and major depression in the National Comorbidity Survey. *J Affect Disord* 1997;45:19-30.
15. Keller MB, et al. Treatment for chronic depression with sertraline and imipramine: Preliminary blinded response rate and high rates of undertreatment in the community. *Psychopharmacol Bull* 1995;31:205-212.
16. Shelton RC, et al. The undertreatment of dysthymia. *J Clin Psychiatry* 1997;58:59-65.
17. Katon W, et al. Adequacy and duration of antidepressant treatment in primary care. *Med Care* 1992;30:67-76.
18. Simon GE, von Korff M. Recognition, management, and outcomes of depression in primary care. *Arch Fam Med* 1995;4:99-105.
19. Wells KB, et al. Use of minor tranquilizers and antidepressant medications by depressed outpatients: Results from the Medical Outcomes Study. *Am J Psychiatry* 1994;151:694-700.
20. Goethe JW, et al. A comparison of adequately vs inadequately treated depressed inpatients. *J Nerv Ment Dis* 1988;24:75-80.
21. Keller MB, et al. Long-term outcome of episodes of major depression: Clinical and public health significance. *JAMA* 1984;252:788-792.
22. Hirschfeld RM, et al. The National Depressive and Manic-Depressive Association consensus statement on the undertreatment of depression. *JAMA* 1997;277:333-340.
23. Spitzer RL, et al. Utility of a new procedure for diagnosing mental disorders in primary care. The PRIME-MD 1000 study. *JAMA* 1994;272:1749-1756.
24. Greenberg PE, et al. The economic burden of depression in 1990. *J Clin Psychiatry* 1993;54:405-418.
25. Judd LL. The clinical course of unipolar major depressive disorders. *Arch Gen Psychiatry* 1997;54:989-991.
26. Von Korff M, et al. Disability and depression among high utilizers of health care. A longitudinal analysis. *Arch Gen Psychiatry* 1992;49:91-100.
27. Keller MB, Boland RJ. Implications of failing to achieve successful long-term maintenance treatment of recurrent unipolar major depression. *Biol Psychiatry* 1998;44: 348-360.
28. Weissman MM, Markowitz JC. Interpersonal psychotherapy: Current status. *Arch Gen Psychiatry* 1994;51:599-606.

29. Gloaguen V, et al. A meta-analysis of the effects of cognitive therapy in depressed patients. *J Affect Disorder* 1998;49:59-72.
30. Scott J. Cognitive therapy of affective disorders: A review. *J Affect Disord* 1996;37:1-11.
31. American Psychiatric Association. Practice guideline for the treatment of patients with major depressive disorder (revision). *Am J Psychiatry* 2000;157(Suppl 4):1-45.
32. Depression Guideline Panel. Clinical Practice Guideline: Depression in Primary Care: Treatment of Major Depression. Rockville, MD: US Dept of Health and Human Services, Agency for Health Care Policy and Research. 1993;2. AHCPR publication 93-0551.
33. Thase ME. Long-term nature of depression. *J Clin Psychiatry* 1999;60(Suppl 14):3-9.
34. Zajecka J, et al. Discontinuation symptoms after treatment with serotonin reuptake inhibitors: A literature review. *J Clin Psychiatry* 1997;58:291-297.
35. Coupland NJ, et al. Serotonin reuptake inhibitor withdrawal. *J Clin Psychopharmacol* 1996;16:356-362.
36. Greden JF. Antidepressant maintenance medications: When to discontinue and how to stop. *J Clin Psychiatry* 1993; 54(Suppl 8):39-45.
37. Rush AJ. Strategies and tactics in the management of maintenance treatment for depressed patients. *J Clin Psychiatry* 1999;60(Suppl 14):21-26.
38. Frank E, et al. Conceptualization and rationale for consensus definitions of terms in major depressive disorder: Remission, recovery, relapse, and recurrence. *Arch Gen Psychiatry* 1991;48:51-855.
39. Lin EH, et al. The role of the primary care physician in patients' adherence to antidepressant therapy. *Med Care* 1995;33:67-74.
40. American Psychiatric Association. *Diagnostic and Statistical Manual of Mental Disorders*. 4th ed. Washington DC: American Psychiatric Association; 1994.

Suicide

Barbara Dwyer, RN, MA

Suicidal patients are among the most frequent visitors to emergency departments.[1-6] Although emergency physicians always have been on the front lines of suicide prevention, evaluating suicidal patients who request assistance or arrive after a suicide attempt is a delicate process and requires genuine interest. Covertly suicidal persons may present with baffling somatic complaints, making their underlying suicidal ideation easy to overlook.

Patients frequently seek medical care shortly before suicide attempts.[8,9] According to a classic review, 82% of suicide victims saw a physician within six months (and 53% within one month) of death. Although more than two-thirds of these patients had previous suicide attempts or clinical signs of depression, physicians made correct diagnoses in only 38%.[10] In addition, more than half of patients who die by intentional overdose use a single prescription drug.[11]

Suicidal patients provoke anxiety among the emergency department staff.[12,13] Some emergency physicians may feel ill-equipped to evaluate them, because more than 30% of physicians receive no training in psychiatric emergency management. Yet, expecting suicidal patients to volunteer their plans risks missing key symptoms and underlying depression.[14]

This chapter reviews the risk factors and epidemiology of suicide and presents a practical approach for evaluation of suicidal patients. The article presents a step-by-step management plan, including admission and discharge criteria, recommendations for proper protection, and guidelines for avoiding medicolegal pitfalls.

Recognizing Suicidal Patients: Looking Beyond Stereotypes

Suicide attempts occur during times of acute crisis, such as a major loss, trauma, or depression. Regardless of the precipitating factors, all suicidal persons have three common features.

First, the suicide crisis is time-limited. Second, suicidal patients are always ambivalent about dying, whether consciously or unconsciously. And, third, the suicide event is dyadic, frequently involving attempted revenge at a loved one.[2,3]

In addition to signaling an underlying psychiatric illness, suicidal behavior represents a maladaptive attempt at problem-solving. These patients are in crisis and require protection until they can find less destructive solutions.

Suicide demographics have shifted in the last decade. *(Please see Table 1.)* Elderly white men still account for the highest number of suicides.[15] However, teenage suicides have quadrupled in the last 40 years,[1,7,16-21] and suicide attempts are now recognized more frequently in young children.

The AIDS epidemic also has left its mark. It is estimated that the relative suicide rate for men with AIDS is 36 times that of men who do not have the syndrome.[22]

Table 1. Suicide Demographics

General Considerations
- More than 30,400 suicides were reported to the United States Public Health Service in 1988
- Suicide is the eighth leading cause of death overall
- Suicide is the third leading cause of death among people ages 15-24

Elderly patients
- Elderly white men have the highest suicide rate in the United States[15]
- People ages 75-84 have a suicide rate twice that of people ages 16-24
- Suicide completion ratio in elderly is 1:1, compared with 10:1 in the general population[1,28]
- Risk factors for suicide:[49-55]
  - — Depression
  - — Other psychiatric illnesses
  - — Medical disorders that cause pain and disability
  - — Living alone
  - — Unrecognized dementia

Adolescents
- Adolescent suicide attempts have quadrupled from 2.7 per 100,000 in 1950 to 11.3 in 1988.[1,7,17]
- Hopelessness and depression are strong predictors.[56-58]
- Suicide risk factors:
  - — Family trauma
  - — Turmoil that does not stabilize[59,60]
  - — Domestic violence
  - — Unemployment
  - — Alcoholic parent
  - — Physical or sexual abuse[61-64]
  - — Loss of a family member[24]
  - — Perception of being "expendable" or a family burden [65]
  - — Dissatisfied with level of social support[66]
- Associated contributing factors:
  - — Isolated and withdrawn individuals[63]
  - — Use of alcohol, marijuana, or cocaine
  - — Conduct disorder
  - — Poor school performance
  - — Disputes with peers
  - — Romantic disappointment[68]
  - — Concerns about pregnancy, sexual orientation, and risk of AIDS[16,21,69,70]
  - — Depression/pathological grief in peers of adolescent suicide victims[1]

Minority and ethnic groups
- Suicide rates among black men are lower than among white men
- Suicides among blacks predominately affect young men
- In inner-city Hispanics, suicide rates are disproportionately higher among teenage girls[73]

Medical disorders
- Men with AIDS are at 36 times the risk for suicide than men without the disorder
- Patients with temporal lobe epilepsy have a 25-fold greater risk of suicide than the general population
- Other disorders with increased risk for suicide[1,4]
  - — Cancer
  - — Head injuries
  - — Huntington's disease
  - — Multiple sclerosis
  - — Spinal cord injuries
  - — Anorexia nervosa

In practice, physicians must be alert for suicidal ideation in any patient who appears depressed, abuses alcohol or other drugs, lives in a dysfunctional setting, or who has experienced physical or psychological trauma or some other stressful life event.[2,23]

Predicting Suicide Potential

Although physicians must consider all stated or behavioral threats of suicide to be serious, it is important to be aware of risk factors and predictors.

A previous suicide attempt is probably the most powerful predictor of suicide potential.[20,26] Ten to twenty percent of persons with this history successfully complete suicide.[1,27]

Although women make 60-70% of suicide attempts, men account for 80% of successful suicides.[1,18,27] Suicide attempts are far more common in young patients,[27] whereas the elderly complete their suicides more often.

Pre-existing Psychiatric Illness. Depression, alone or in combination with other psychiatric disorders, is the most common precipitant of suicide.[1,4,28] The affective intensity of depression does not correlate with the degree of lethality, but the degree of hopelessness is a strong predictor.[2] Patients who are "tired of living" or who believe that "things will never get better" are at very high risk.

At the time of death, 90% of suicide victims have a diagnosable psychiatric illness, that in more than half of patients, is an affective illness such as major depression or uni- or bipolar disorder.[1,4] Of note, 60% of psychiatric inpatients who kill themselves do so within six months of leaving the hospital.[1,12,29,30]

Patients with schizophrenia have a high incidence of suicide attempts. Approximately 10% of schizophrenics die by suicide, usually during a depressed episode.[20,31] Agitation, the presence of psychosis (characterized by delusions and hallucinations), and delirium decrease self-control and substantially increase the immediate danger.[20]

Pre-existing anxiety or personality disorder also confers a substantial suicide risk, especially when depression coexists. Twenty percent of deaths among patients with anxiety disorders (including panic attacks) occur by suicide.[12,33] Among people with borderline or antisocial personality disorders, suicide rates range from 4-9.5%.[1,31]

Alcohol figures prominently in suicide.[2,30,34-36] Nearly 25% of suicide victims are alcoholic, and 20% are legally intoxicated at the time of death. Although many people may drink to medicate anxiety, depression, and low self-esteem, alcohol frequently serves to intensify these symptoms and increases disinhibition and impulsiveness.[35]

Alcohol intoxication often plays a central role in "accidental" overdoses, which usually conceal bona fide suicide attempts. In fact, more than half of all suicidal ED patients are intoxicated, yet many are released once they are sober.[36] Unless appropriate intervention is made, patients who are suicidal "only when intoxicated" will be free to make another attempt.

Substance Abuse. Almost any drug can exacerbate pre-existing psychiatric symptoms. Some of the most dangerous agents include depressants and sedatives, cocaine and other stimulants, and hallucinogens (including marijuana and phencyclidine). Drug withdrawal also can produce symptoms that mimic depression, psychosis, or anxiety.

Differing sharply with recent "bad press," current research indicates that selective serotonin reuptake inhibitor antidepressants do not increase suicidal ideation.[37-39] This class of drugs includes fluoxetine (Prozac), sertaline (Zoloft), and the just released paroxetine (Paxil). Several studies show these drugs are equally or more effective than cyclic antidepressants in the treatment of depression and much less lethal when used in overdose.[38,39]

History of Previous Violence. Suicide and other forms of violence, particularly homicide, are closely linked. What is often labeled as homicide may be disguised suicide because 20-40% of murder victims may provoke their assailant to kill them.[3] People who threaten homicide actually are more likely to kill themselves, and physicians must not overlook the potential for assaultive urges in suicidal patients and suicidal urges in homicidal patients.

Victims and witnesses of violence may become suicidal relatively easily. Divorce, incest, and domestic violence are common precipitants.[3] The suicide rate among battered women is eight times greater than that of the general populations.[40] Victims of rape and other violent crimes sometimes attempt to kill themselves, often many weeks or months following the assault.[41] Post-traumatic stress disorder sustained by military combat personnel and disaster survivors confers considerable suicide risk.[42] The patient with a history of cruelty to animals, violent, impulsive, or criminal behavior, family violence, or unexplained "accidents" requires careful scrutiny for suicidal and homicidal ideation. Patients with a family history of suicide are at especially high risk.

Loss, Ambivalence, and Hopelessness. Inability to deal successfully with loss is a common thread among suicidal people. Childhood experiences of parental divorce or death, neglect or abuse, or an alcoholic family predispose a child to vulnerability from future deprivations. These children learn early that they cannot rely on their parents and develop a brittle "pseudo"-maturity.[3] They grow up unable to tolerate life's normal losses without severe disappointment and may avoid intimate relationships in an effort to escape further abandonment. However, any significant loss-such as a job, pet, loved one, health, status, self-image, or independence-awakens feelings of depression and hopelessness.[43]

Recognize the Need to Ask About Suicidal Ideation

Overtly suicidal patients pose few diagnostic problems. Emergency physicians usually can recognize them by the history provided by patients or family. Conversely, covertly suicidal patients often are unrecognized by the ED staff and may present with a wide array of somatic complaints.

In general, physicians should become suspicious of a psychiatric problem and the possibility of underlying suicidal ideation whenever the patient's reason for the ED visit just "doesn't seem to fit."

Subtle indicators often take the form of a midnight visit for seemingly minor complaints, dissatisfaction with the prescribed treatment, unusual requests, or hints of difficulties at home. With children and adolescents, the parent's clinging behavior may provide the only clue that something is awry. People who may feel humiliated, such as those brought to the ED from prisons, also should be questioned carefully.[45] Above all, if the clinical encounter feels wrong, physicians should trust their instincts and ask appropriate questions to explore the possibility of suicidal thoughts.

Table 2. Signs and Symptoms of Major Depression[74]

Depressed mood (irritability in children or adolescents)
Diminished interest or pleasure in usual activities
Significant weight loss or gain
Insomnia or hypersomnia
Psychomotor agitation or retardation
Fatigue or loss of energy
Feelings of worthlessness or excessive guilt (which may be delusional)
Diminished ability to think or concentrate
Recurrent thoughts of death or suicidal ideation

Adapted from *DSM-III-R*

Gauging Suicide Potential

Interviewing a potentially suicidal patient involves being aware of risk factors and focusing on verbal and behavioral cues. Deciding whether patients are genuinely suicidal or simply making a suicidal gesture is of critical importance. Unfortunately, this distinction may be difficult to make and often blurs or changes rapidly. What is most important, however, is that the physician determines the problem that the suicidal behavior is intended to solve and gauges whether the patient has met this objective.[1-3]

Silently Suicidal Patients. Not all suicidal people appear overtly depressed. Many present with "depressive equivalents," which commonly are somatic complaints such as headaches, gastrointestinal problems, back pain, insomnia, malaise, and other nonspecific symptoms. Patients frequently are unable to correlate physical distress with underlying psychic pain. Unless physicians ask specifically, covertly suicidal patients are susceptible to slipping through the diagnostic cracks.

Directed Questions. The physician first should address the presenting complaint by asking general questions about the patient's situation. The evaluation should include a thorough mental status examination along with careful observation for evidence of delirium, psychosis, or hallucinations.

The clinician should inquire specifically about signs and symptoms of depression *(Please see Table 2)* and gradually lead into more directed questions concerning suicide, including:[2,3]

- "Have you ever felt so badly that you thought about killing yourself?"
- "Do you have thoughts of hurting yourself now?"
- "What plans have you made to do this?"

Most suicidal patients will be honest if the interviewer asks these questions in a straightforward, non judgmental manner. Patients who have not considered suicide usually say so emphatically. It is

Table 3. Patients at High Risk for Suicide

History of suicide attempt, particularly if it was serious, violent, or carefully planned
Presence of hopelessness
Family history of suicide
Social isolation and loneliness
Recent loss of a loved one, especially if no other emotional supports are available
Psychosis, particularly if "command hallucinations" are present
Presence of manic-depressive illness
History of impulsive behavior
Presence of other forms of violence or hostility
Chronic or terminal illness
Organic brain syndrome
Alcoholism or drug abuse
Family turmoil (incest, child abuse, spousal violence)
Withdrawal of family members from the patient
Covert or overt "death wish" by family member
Older, single man
Severe insomnia
Physician feels anxiety or fear about patient, even in the absence of definite evidence

impossible to put the idea of suicide into someone's mind. Clearly, most depressed patients are relieved by an opportunity to discuss their concerns openly.

How Effective Was the Attempt? Patients who have failed to accomplish their intent—whether it was their death or mobilizing a response from others—are at high risk for subsequent suicide attempts. Consider the intent, the methods used, and efforts to be stopped as predictors of future attempts.

Some helpful questions are:

- "Were you trying to kill yourself?"
- "Are you surprised that you survived?
- "Are you glad that you're alive now?"

If the answers indicate a wish to die at the time of the attempt, continued ambivalence, or an ongoing desire to die, the patient will probably make another suicide attempt.

The more violent the method used—firearms, jumping from a high building, hanging—generally correlates with the seriousness of the suicide attempt. However, less deadly methods only may reflect naivete. Patients intent upon suicide may believe that 10 20-mg fluoxetine tablets will be fatal, but survive only because they chose a relatively innocuous substance. Other patients who wish only to call attention to their plight may survive because they misjudged the lethality of their method.

People who want to die usually try to avoid discovery. For example, patients who carefully plan an attempt, procure the means, and then rent a hotel room represent a highly significant attempt, even if they call for help at the last moment. A theatrical suicide attempt generally is a suicidal gesture, although this behavior can progress to a highly lethal situation if patients do not accomplish what they intended.

How Imminent is the Danger? Helping patients through the crisis almost invariably changes their minds. However, physicians must determine the patient's immediate plans.

Ask directly about the presence of suicidal thoughts. If the patient does not volunteer a specific suicide plan, ask, "Do you have a plan to kill yourself?"

If the answer is yes, ask about the details. The presence of a specific plan increases the danger, particularly if the patient has made preparations. Does the plan involve a highly lethal method, and is the patient able to carry it out? (Someone who has vague thoughts of "ending it all" is at significantly less risk than a patient who owns a gun and plans to shoot himself "unless things get better.") The more specific the plan, the greater the risk.

Has the patient rehearsed the plan? People who carefully plan the attempt (hoarding pills, loading a gun, fashioning a noose) are preparing to die.

Ask, "What do you expect to happen if you try to kill yourself?" People who don't really expect to die have significantly less risk than those who envision others missing them or attending their funeral.

The response to these questions should indicate whether a suicide attempt is imminent. Also, ask the patient specifically about the presence of auditory hallucinations and look for evidence of psychosis (inappropriate affect, loose associations, bizarre talk or behavior). Re-evaluate the risk factors *(See Table 3)* and talk to the family and significant others.

The Patient's Potential to Hurt Others always requires evaluation. Inquire about homicidal tendencies by asking the following:

- "Did you ever want to hurt anyone beside yourself?"
- "Do you want to hurt anyone right now?"
- "Whom do you want to hurt?"
- "How do you plan to do this?"

By asking these questions directly, patients perceive that the physician is taking them seriously. Weigh the answers carefully and consider the circumstances and risk factors. Patients with a history of psychosis, violent behavior, previous suicide attempts, or family history of suicide should be considered for hospitalization.

Protecting Suicidal Patients

Protecting patients until their crisis has passed is the central goal of emergency management. Suicidal episodes usually last only a few hours or days. Immediate treatment includes determining whether patients require hospitalization, obtaining psychiatric consultation, and laying the groundwork for long-term intervention. Except for rare cases, it is unwise to discharge any patient who threatens or attempts suicide. On occasion, some patients may be managed as outpatients provided they are not imminently suicidal, have verifiable family support systems available, and have specific arrangements for early psychiatric follow-up.

Suicide Precautions. Protecting the patient from self-harm is the first priority. ED staff members never should leave suicidal patients unobserved. Someone must accompany these patients at all times, even if they need to use the rest room. All potentially harmful objects (e.g., glass bottles, mirrors, surgical sutures and instruments, medication) must be removed from the vicinity.

Patients must relinquish all possessions that could be used to inflict injury, especially belts, neckties, bras, long shoelaces, sharp buckles, and pins. Patients who refuse to empty their pockets, handbags, or other belongings must be searched in a safe environment by security personnel. Requiring patients to turn over harmful objects not only helps to protect the patient, but also protects the staff in the event that the patient becomes assaultive.

Indications for Restraints. Restraints are indicated immediately for patients who attempt to harm themselves or anyone else. Offer patients one chance to accept voluntary restraints (or medication). However, once the decision to restrain is made, the physician and the ED staff should not bargain with the patient, should not waiver, and should not cease efforts until the patient is restrained safely.[3,45]

The most experienced team member should direct the effort, and only that person should give instructions. Restraint team members must develop a specific plan because a disorganized effort may exacerbate the situation. Clear the room of all but five of the strongest people, who should remove their neckties, eyeglasses, and weapons. Inform the patient that their behavior is unacceptable and that they need restraints for self-protection.[45] First, attempt voluntary restraint by asking the patient to lie face down on the stretcher.

If the patient does not respond, the team should approach the patient calmly and with authority. Each person should immobilize one extremity (by the knee in the legs; by the elbow in the arms) while another team member applies leather restraints. Adults should be restrained in the prone position and elderly people are restrained on their side. After applications of the restraints, the patient should be searched for concealed weapons or other dangerous objects and should be examined for evidence of fractures or other injuries sustained during the restraint.

Physicians must document the reason for using restraints, how the patient was restrained, and the presence or absence of injuries. Restrained patients require continuous observation, protection from aspiration of gastric contents, hourly position changes, and frequent vital signs.

Chemical Restraints. Patients who remain agitated or violent may require sedation. Haloperidol (5.0 mg IM) alone or in combination with lorazepam (2.0-4.0 mg IM) will be sufficient to calm most acute symptoms.[46] Offer patients the option of taking the oral concentrated form of haloperidol (10 mg), which is absorbed almost as rapidly as the intramuscular preparation.

Psychiatric Consultation and Hospital Admission

Physicians should obtain psychiatric consultation to confirm the degree of suicidal risk and to help plan subsequent management. Immediate consultation is mandatory for high-risk patients, especially those who are hallucinating or who have impaired impulse control, or if there is any doubt regarding disposition. These patients generally require psychiatric hospitalization, antidepressant and neuroleptic drugs, and are best managed by a psychiatrist during the acute crisis.

Admission Criteria. Suicidal patients require protection, ideally in a psychiatric unit, until they can envision less destructive solutions to their problems. Do not hesitate to offer voluntary hospitalization. Most genuinely suicidal patients will be relieved. If a patient who requires hospitalization refuses, physicians in all states are authorized to involuntarily admit patients who pose a danger to themselves or others.

Table 4. Indications for Hospitalizing Suicidal Patients

Refusal to follow the treatment plan
Inability to control suicidal impulses
Refusal to answer questions about suicidal intentions or plans
Family and friends remain concerned that the suicide risk is high
The clinician is still concerned that the patient may be suicidal, even though objective evidence is lacking
The patient lives alone or in a chaotic situation
The crisis has not passed
The patient falls into any of the high-risk categories

In general, hospitalize patients who:

- acknowledge that they are suicidal
- appear highly suicidal to ED staff and family, even if specific evidence is lacking
- have made a suicide attempt and have any of the high-risk factors
- have attempted suicide with the intent to die, particularly if they have not regained hope
- live alone or in a dysfunctional or chaotic setting
- refuse to answer questions about suicidal thoughts or plans
- are psychotic or have underlying psychiatric illness
- refuse to follow a treatment plan
- cause doubt as to whether they may make another suicide attempt. (This includes inability to define what problem the person was attempting to solve via suicidal behavior and whether that problem was solved)

The consulting psychiatrist can help determine whether an open or locked psychiatric unit is appropriate. Patients who first require medical treatment in the intensive care setting or on a medical/surgical floor pose special problems. These patients may make subsequent suicide attempts in the hospital, and non-psychiatric staff may feel uneasy about monitoring them. These patients should have close supervision (e.g., ideally one-to-one staffing) and continued suicide precautions. Patients who are psychotic or highly impulsive require a locked psychiatric unit where they can undergo close observation and be restrained as necessary.

Discharge Criteria. Even patients who do not require hospitalization should undergo psychiatric consultation, both for their own protection and for medicolegal reasons. It is usually safe to discharge patients who meet all of the following criteria:[2] 1) have regained hope; 2) are not psychotic; 3) have a stable, supportive living situation; 4) will follow the treatment plan; and 5) the suicide crisis has passed.

However, in all cases, the emergency physician should contact the psychiatrist before discharge. Ideally, the psychiatrist should evaluate the patient in the ED before discharge. If the psychiatrist is unavailable, arrange a telephone consultation. For all discharged patients, make an appointment with a psychiatrist for the following day. Avoid prescribing antidepressants or anxiolytics because these agents may obscure further diagnosis or may be used in a suicide attempt.

Patients who are discharged must agree to follow a treatment

Table 5. Do's and Don'ts in Managing Suicidal Patients

Do
- Ask about the possibility of suicide
- Take threats seriously
- Be cautious when alcohol is involved
- Ask about family history of depression or alcoholism
- Use family and friends as treatment allies when appropriate
- Be alert to subtle communications, such as "I may not make my next appointment," or "why should I care how I feel?"
- Be suspicious of accidents that may be covert suicide attempts (e.g., one-person car accidents, accidental overdoses)

Don't
- Do not assume that patients who make gestures by overdose are not serious about suicide
- Do not assume that patients who have made multiple suicide attempts are not serious about killing themselves
- Do not prescribe any medication in lethal quantities
- Do not be hostile or judgmental
- Do not suggest "how to do it right next time"

plan, which is best kept simple and put in writing. First, they must be able to make a "suicide contract," which is an agreement to contact or come to the ED if further suicidal impulses arise. Second, patients and families must agree to remove all pills, poisons, and weapons from the home. A family member or other reliable person must stay with the patient until follow-up is obtained.

Physicians must make specific follow-up arrangements, (i.e., a specific appointment time the following day) and should be certain that the patient is able to get to the appointment. Also, the physician should verify the patient's and family's correct names, addresses and telephone numbers. All involved parties must understand and agree on the treatment plan.

Most important, physicians must have no doubts about the patient's reliability for upholding the agreement. If any doubt exists, the patient should be admitted for observation.

Medical-legal Considerations

Most non-psychiatrists are uncertain about the potential medicolegal implications of treating suicidal patients. In general, legal standards expect physicians to be able to predict the degree of suicide risk or potential but do not hold them legally responsible for a subjective error unless they fail to initiate reasonable treatment.[47,48]

For the emergency physician, it is always safer to err on the side of inpatient observation and conservative care, at least until psychiatric consultation can be obtained.

Explaining that all states allow physicians to hospitalize patients who present a threat to themselves or others may encourage suicidal persons to opt for voluntary hospitalization. If necessary, the emergency physician can involuntarily admit a suicidal patient without fear of legal retribution.

In all cases, detailed documentation is necessary regarding the emergency intervention and treatment, and the rationale for selecting that particular intervention.

Effective Intervention For Suicidal Patients

Suicidal crises are episodic and will pass when patients receive definitive treatment. During the crisis period, physicians can help best by not reacting to the patient's often provocative and disagreeable behavior, but rather by focusing on their distress and pointing the way to assistance. By recognizing the risk factors for suicide, protecting suicidal patients from self-harm, and providing appropriate psychiatric intervention, emergency physicians can intervene effectively to help prevent death and limit psychiatric morbidity in patients with suicidal ideation.

References

1. Buzan RD, Weissberg MP. Sulfide: Risk factors and therapeutic considerations in the emergency department. *J Emerg Med* 1992;10:335.
2 Weissberg MP, Dwyer BJ, Suskauer SH: The suicide crisis: Preventing the final act. *Emerg Med Reports* 1985; 6:105.
3. Weissberg MP. *Dangerous Secrets: Maladaptive Responses to Stress.* New York, WW Norton, 1983.
4. Buzan RD, Weissberg MP. Suicide: Risk factors and prevention in medical practice. *Ann Rev Med* 1992;43:37.
5. Hansagi H, Edhag 0, Allbeck P. High consumers of health care in emergency units: How to improve their quality of care. *QA Health Care* 1991;3:51.
6. Hansagi H, Allbeck P, Edhag 0, Magnusson G. Frequency of emergency department attendances as a predictor of mortality: Nine year follow up of a population-based cohort. *J Pub Health Med* 1990;12:39.
7. Aschkenasy JR, Clark DC, Zinn LD, Richtsmeier A7. The nonpsychiatric physician's responsibility for the suicidal adolescent. *NY State J Med* 1992;92:97.
8 Isacsson G, Boethius G, Bergman U. Low level of antidepressant prescription for people who later commit suicide: 15 years of experience from a population-based drug database in Sweden. *Acta Psychiatr Scand* 1992;85:444.
9. Beaumont G, Hetsel W. Patients at risk of suicide and overdose. *Psychopharmacol* 1992;106(suppl):S123.
10. Murphy GE. The physicians responsibility for suicide. 2. Errors of omission. *Ann Intern Med* 1975;82:305.
11. Murphy GE. The physicians responsibility for suicide 1. Errors of commission. *Ann Intern Med* 1975;82:301.
12. Motto JA, Bostram A. Empirical indicators of near-term suicide risk. *Crisis* 1990; 1152.
13. Suokas J, Lonnquivist J. Work stress has negative effects on the attitudes of emergency department personnel toward patients who attempt suicide. *Actn Psychiatr Scand*

1989;79:474.

14. Meehan PJ, Lamb JA, Saltzman LE, O'Carrpll PW. Attempted suicide among young adults: Progress toward a meaningful estimate of prevalence. *Am J Psychiatry* 1992;149:41.
15. Mellick E, Buckwater KC, Stolley JM. Suicide among elderly white men. Development of a profile. *J Psychosoc Nursing Mental Health Serv* 1992;30:29.
16. Bushong C, Cloverdale J, Battaglia J. Adolescent mental health: A review of preventive interventions. *Texas Med* 1992;88:62.
17, Centers for Disease Control. Attempted suicide among young high school students-United States, 1990. *MMWR Morbid Mortal Wkly Rep* 1991;40:633.
18. National Center for Health Statistics. Advance report of final mortality statistics, 1988. Monthly vital statistics report 39(suppl). Hyatsville, MD: Public Health Service, 1990.
19. Earls F, Escobar JI,Manson SM. Suicide in minority groups: epidemiologic and cultural perspectives. In: Blumenthal SJ, Kupfer DJ (eds). *Suicide Over the Life Cycle: Risk Factors, Assessment, and Treatment of Suicidal patients.* Washington, American Psychiatric Press, 1990.
20. Hoffmann DP, Dubovsky SL. Depression and suicide assessment. *Emerg Med Clin North Am* 1991;9:107.
21. Lamb J. Pusker KR. School-based adolescent mental health project survey of depression, suicidal ideation, and anger.) *Child Adolesc Psychiatr Ment Health Nurs* 1991:4:101.
22. Perry S, Jacobsberg L, Fishman B. Suicidal ideation and HIV testing. *JAMA* 1990;262:679.
23. Keitner GI, Ryan CE, Miller IW, et al. Family functioning, social adjustment, and recurrence of suicidality. *Psychiatry* 1990;53:17.
24. DeVanna M, Patemiti S, Milievich C, et al. Recent life events and attempted suicide. *J Affective Disorders* 1990;18:51.
2.5. Petronis KR, Samuels JF, Moscicki EK, Anthony JC. An epidemiologic investigation of potential risk factors for suicide attempts. *Soc Psychiatry Psychiatr Epidemiol* 1990;25:193.
26. Ojehagen A, Regnell G, Traskman- Bendz L. Deliberate selfpoisoning: Repeaters and non- repeaters admitted to an intensive care unit. *Acta Psychiatrica Scanda* 1991;84:266.
27. Robins LN, Kulbock PA. Epidemiologic studies in suicide. In: Frances AJ, Hales RE (eds). *Am Psychiatric Press Rev Psychiatry* 1988;289.
28. Nordentoft M, Rubin PJ. Suicide among psychiatric patients. *Ugeskrift For Laeger* 1992;154:1481.
29. Weissberg MP. The meagerness of physicians' training in emergency psychiatric intervention. *Acad Med* 1990;65:747.
30. Neilsen B, Wang AG, Brille-Brahe U. Attempted suicide in Denmark. A five-year follow-up. *Acta Psychiatrica Scand* 1990;81:250.
31. Peterson LG, Bongar B. Repetitive suicidal crises: Characteristics of repealing versus non-repeating suicidal visitors to a psychiatric emergency service. *Psychopathology* 1990;23:136.
32. Noyes R Jr. Suicide and panic disorder: A review. *J Affective Disord* 1991;22:1.
33. Lepine JP, Chignon JM, Teherani M. Suicide attempts in patients with panic disorder. *Arch Gen Psychiatry* 1993;50:144.
34. Seidel JS. Emergency medical services and the adolescent patient. *J Adolesc Health* 1991;12:95.
35. Biro M, Selakovic-Bursic S, Kapamadzija B. The role of depressive disorders in the suicidal behavior of alcoholics. *Crisis* 1992;12:64.
36. Jayaram G, Janofsky JS, Fischer PJ. The emergency petition process in Maryland. *Bull Am Acad Psychiatry Law* 1990; 18:373.
37. Montgomery SA. Suicide and antidepressants. *Drugs* 1992; 43(suppl 2):24.
38. Molcho A, Stanley M. Antidepressants and suicide risk: Issues of chemical and behavioral toxicity. *J Clin Psychopharmacol* 1992;12(2 suppl):13S.
39. Montgomery SA, Montgomery DB, Green M, et al. Pharmacotherapy in the prevention of suicidal behavior. *J Clin Psychopharmacol* 1992;12(2 suppl):27S.
40. Bergman B, Brismar B. Suicide attempts by battered wives. *Acta Psychiatr Scand* 83:380.
41. Dwyer BJ, Hicks DJ, Weissberg MP. Sensitive emergency management of rape victims. *Emerg Med Reports* 1988; 9:21.
42. Hendin H, Haas AP. Suicide and guilt of 17 SD in Vietnam combat veterans. *Am J Psychiatry* 1991;148:57;6.
43. Bron B, Strack M, Rudolph G. Childhood experiences of loss and suicide attempts. Significance in major depressive states of major depressed and dysthymic or adjustment disordered patients. *J Affective Disord* 1991;23:165.
44. Winkler GE. Assessing and responding to suicidal jail inmates. *Comm Mental Health J* 1992;28:317.
45. Dwyer BJ, Weissberg MP. Safe strategies for recognizing and managing violent patients. *Emerg Med Reports* 1987;8:256.
46. Dubin WR. Overcoming danger with violent patients: Guidelines for safe and effective managment. *Emerg Med Reports* 1992;13:105-112
47. Feinsilver DL. The suicidal patient: Clinical and legal issues. *Hosp Pract* 1983;18:14E.
48. Berman AL, Cohen-Sandler R. Suicide and the standard of care: Optimum vs. acceptable. *Suicide Life Threat Behav* 1982;12:114.
49. Tobias CR, Pary R, Lippman S. Preventing suicide in older people. *Am Fam Physician* 1992;45:1707.
50. Merril J, Owens J. Age and attempted suicide. *Acta Psychiatr Scand* 1990;82:385.
51. Lyness JM, Conwell Y, Nelson JC. Suicide attempts in elderly psychiatric inpatients. *J Am Geriatr Soc* 1992;40:3.
52. Frierson RL. Suicide attempts by the old and the very old. *Arch Intern Med* 1991;151:141.
53. Butler RN, Finkel SI, Lewis Ml, et al. Aging and mental health: diagnosis of dementia and depression. *Geriatrics* 1992;47:49.
54. Margo GM, Finkel JA. Early dementia as a risk factor for suicide. *Hosp Commun Psychiatry* 1990;41:676.
55. Canetto S. Gender and suicide in the elderly. *Suicide Life Threat Behav* 1992;22:80.
56. Bhatara VS. Early detection of adolescent mood disorders. *So Dakota J Med* 1992;45:75.

57. Swedo SE, Rettew DC, Kuppenheimer M, et al. Can adolescent attempters be distinguished from at-risk adolescents? *Pediatrics* 1991;88:6.
58. Simonds JF, McMahon T, Armstrong D. Young suicide attempters compared with a control group: Psychological, affective, and attitudinal variables. *Suicide Life Threat Behav* 1991;21:134.
59. Miller KE, King CA, Shain BN, Naylor MW. Suicidal adolescents' perceptions of their family environment. *Suicide Life Threat Behav* 1992;22:226.
60. de Wilde EJ, Kienhorst JC, Diekstra RF, Wolters WH. The relationship between adolescent suicidal behavior and life events in childhood and adolescence. *Am J Psychiatry* 1992;149:45.
61. Marttunen MJ, Aro HM, Lonnqvist JK. Adolescent suicide: Endpoint of long-term difficulties. *J Am Acad Child Adolesc Psychiatry* 1992;31:649.
62. Krarup G, Neilsen B, Rask P, Petersen P. Childhood experiences and repeated suicidal behavior. *Acta Psychiatr* Scand 1991;83:16.
63. Kienhorst CW, deWilde EJ, Diekstra RF, Wolters RH. Differences between adolescent suicide attempters and depressed adolescents. *Acta Psychiatr Scand* 1992;85:222.
64. Riggs S, Alario AJ, McHorney C. Health risk behaviors and attempted suicide in adolescents who report prior maltreatment. *J Pediatr* 1990;116:815.
65. Woznica JG, Shapiro JR. An analysis of adolescent suicide attempts: The expendable child. *J Pediatr Psychol* 1990;15:789.
66. D'Atillo JP, Campbell BM, Lubold P, et al. Social support and suicide potential: Preliminary findings for adolescent populations. *Psycholog Rep* 1992;70:76.
67. Myers K, McCauley E, Calderon R, et al. Risks for suicidality in major depressive disorder. *J Am Acad Child Adolesc Psychiatry* 1991;30:64.
68. Kalogerakis MG. Emergency evaluation of adolescents. *Hosp Common Psychiatry* 1992;43:617.
69. Slap GB, Vorters DF, Chaudhuri GB, Centor RM. Risk factors for attempted suicide during adolescence. *Pediatrics* 1989;84:762.
70. Remafedi G, Farrow JA, Deisher RW. Risk factors for attempted suicide in gay and bisexual youth. *Pediatrics* 1991;87:869.
71. Brent DA, Perper J, Moritz G, et al. Psychiatric effects of exposure to suicide among the friends and acquaintances of adolescent suicide victims. *J Am Acad Child Adolesc Psychiatry* 1992; 31:629.
72. Griffith EEH, Bell CC. Recent trends in suicide and homicide among blacks. *JAMA* 1989;262:2265.
73. Razin AM, O'Dowd MA, Nathan A, et al. Suicidal behavior among inner-city Hispanic adolescent females. *Gen Hosp Psychiatry* 1991;13:45.
74. American Psychiatric Association. Reference to the Diagnostic Criteria from *DSM-III-R*. Washington DC, 1987:128-129.

Panic Disorder

Randy A. Sansone, MD
Lori A. Sansone, MD

Panic disorder is a common psychiatric diagnosis in the primary care setting. Symptoms are intense and disabling. Misdiagnosis can result in the unwarranted and excessive use of resources. The following chapter that reviews panic disorder includes a discussion of description, epidemiology, etiology, diagnosis, treatment, and outcome. In many cases, effective treatment of panic disorder can be undertaken in the primary care setting.

Description

According to DSM-IV,[1] panic disorder is defined by recurrent panic attacks as well as a one-month history of concern, worry, or behavioral change as a consequence of these attacks. The classic or typical panic attack is highlighted by cardiac symptoms and characterized by at least four of the following: palpitations or accelerated heart rate, sweating, tremulousness, shortness of breath, choking sensation, chest pain or discomfort, nausea or abdominal distress, light-headedness or dizziness, derealization (i.e., the perception that things outside oneself don't appear normal or real), fears of dying, fears of losing control or going crazy, paresthesias (particularly around the mouth or fingertips), and chills or hot flushes. These symptoms are intense, well circumscribed, last approximately 15 minutes, and can be difficult to discern from a genuine heart attack. As an example, 38% of patients who were referred to cardiology clinics for the evaluation of chest pain met criteria for panic disorder.[2]

There appear to be other versions or subtypes of panic disorder[3] in addition to those highlighted by cardiac symptoms. These include a respiratory version in which respiratory symptoms predominate (e.g., hyperventilation), a gastrointestinal version highlighted by intense, discrete episodes of queasiness and nausea, and a vestibular version characterized by light-headedness.[4,5] The comparative prevalence of these subtypes is unknown, although the cardiac version of panic disorder appears to be the most common. All versions are characterized by well-circumscribed symptoms with no long-term medical sequelae. Whether treatment differences exist among the subtypes of panic remains unknown.

Epidemiology

Prevalence. Community surveys indicate that the lifetime prevalence of panic disorder is about 3% internationally[6] and 3.6% among the U.S. general population.[7,8] The prevalence of panic disorder in the primary care setting is estimated around 7%. According to the National Comorbidity Study,[9] the lifetime prevalence of panic disorder among men is 2% and among women 5%. Women may have a greater likelihood of comorbid social phobia or post-traumatic stress disorder.[10]

Onset. The onset of panic has a bimodal distribution with one peak in the teens to early 20s and a second in the mid-30s to early 40s.[11] However, there are case reports of late-onset panic disorder[12];

the clinical and demographic profiles of these patients have been found to be similar to those of early-onset patients.[12]

Timing of Attacks. The symptoms of panic disorder may have seasonal overtones, with exacerbation during the winter months.[13] Panic attacks may also occur during sleep,[14-16] which may indicate greater psychiatric comorbidity, including mood and anxiety disorders as well as a history of trauma.[17]

With regard to times of hormonal change in women, up to 40% of patients experience premenstrual exacerbation of panic.[18] During pregnancy, up to 20% of women with panic disorder experience worsening of symptoms,[19] whereas during the postpartum, 35% experience symptom exacerbation.[20,21] Finally, triphasic oral contraceptives[22] and progesterone[23] have been linked with exacerbations of panic symptoms in predisposed individuals.

Healthcare Use. Of those diagnosed with panic disorder, twice as many seek care in medical settings such as a primary care physician's office or an emergency department compared to mental health settings.[24] Not surprisingly, panic disorder patients demonstrate high rates of use of both psychiatric[25] and nonpsychiatric services.[26-28] Even compared with other anxiety disorders, panic disorder patients have higher levels of healthcare use.[29] As expected, quality of life among these patients is meaningfully diminished.[30]

Etiology

The explicit cause of panic disorder remains unknown, although a variety of factors have been implicated. Because of this, we conceptualize panic disorder as a final common pathway disorder with multiple contributory factors *(please see Figure)*.

Figure. Contributory Substrates for Panic Disorder

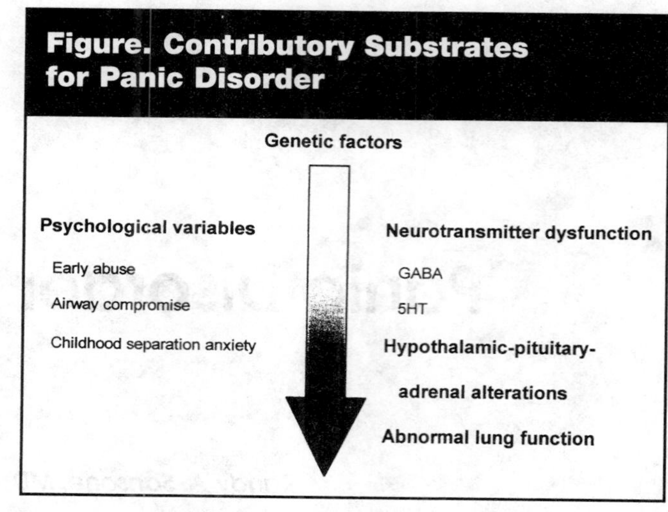

Psychological Variables. A number of psychological variables have been reported as causative factors. For example, sexual abuse,[31,32] a nonspecific contributory factor for many types of psychopathology, as well as physical abuse[33] and chaotic families-of-origin[34] have been associated with panic disorder. Airway compromise (e.g., near-drowning, choking, airway obstruction) has been found among some patients with panic disorder.[35] Finally, there has been an association between separation anxiety in childhood (e.g., fears of leaving home, separating from parents, staying overnight with friends, going to school) and panic disorder in adulthood.[36-38]

Nonpsychological Variables. A number of neurotransmitters have been implicated, including GABA,[39] serotonin,[40,41] and neuropeptide Y.[42] Alterations in the hypothalamic-pituitary-adrenal axis[43] and abnormal lung function[44] have also been identified as potential causative factors. Genetic factors appear to be relevant among some patients and families[45-47] and hypersensitivity to CO_2 challenge may identify those with a greater likelihood of genetic predisposition.[48,49] The intersection of these various risk factors is likely to enhance the probable expression of panic disorder in a given individual.

Exacerbating Factors. Psychosocial stressors appear to exacerbate panic episodes, as well as illness, certain types of drugs (e.g., stimulants, marijuana), antidepressants initially prescribed at routine doses, and weight loss.

Diagnosis

Pattern of Symptom Expression. The diagnosis of panic disorder is based on: 1) the epidemiological context (e.g., age, gender); 2) type and pattern of symptoms; and 3) the exclusion of medical causes. With regard to epidemiology, most convincing is the initial emergence of symptoms during one of the bimodal peaks of onset regardless of the current age of the patient as well as female gender.

Symptoms that reflect the classic panic attack (i.e., cardiac subtype) are highly suggestive of the diagnosis. The symptom pattern is distinctive and characterized by intense, recurrent, and dramatic symptoms during a discrete but brief period (e.g., 15 minutes), with no medical deterioration over time (i.e., months to years). The symptoms of panic disorder usually worsen with stress but, paradoxically, many patients focus on their physiological symptoms and initially appear to dismiss stress factors. With continued exploration, the clinician can usually elicit a relationship between emerging panic attacks and psychosocial stressors.

Medical Evaluation/Differential Diagnosis. Medical evaluation focuses on the predominant symptom complex (i.e., cardiac, respiratory, gastrointestinal, vestibular). The extent of the evaluation is dependent upon the context of the presentation; the more atypical the history, the more necessary a detailed medical work-up. With the cardiac subtype, medical evaluation in suspicious cases might include an echocardiogram, electrocardiogram, or event monitor to exclude certain cardiac conditions such as severe mitral valve prolapse or paroxysmal supraventricular tachycardia,[50] both of which may mimic panic symptoms.

Regardless of panic-disorder subtype, we advise obtaining a thyroid-stimulating hormone (TSH) on all patients presenting with possible panic disorder to exclude the rare possibility of thyroid storm. Also, a drug and caffeine history (including cocaine, marijuana, amphetamines, and caffeine) should be obtained, as exposure may mimic or exacerbate panic attacks.[51]

A rare diagnosis that may be confused with panic disorder is severe paroxysmal hypertension, or pseudopheochromocytoma. This condition is characterized by abrupt elevations in blood pressure and acute physical symptoms that may be confused with panic attacks (e.g., headache, chest pain, dizziness, nausea, palpitations, flushing, diaphoresis).[52] These episodes last from 30 minutes to several hours and are apparently not provoked by psychosocial stressors or accompanied by feelings of panic. Afflicted patients tend to fail treatment with anti-hypertensives and may respond to psychotherapy, alpha or beta blockers, tricyclic antidepressants, or selective serotonin reuptake inhibitors.[52]

Psychometric Scales. To date, there is not a formally recognized panic disorder scale that is generally accepted for use. The MINI Patient Health Survey[53] is a brief self-report survey that explores major depression, alcohol dependence, social phobia, and panic disorder. The panic disorder subscale consists of four primary questions and may be of value in the primary care setting as a screening measure. Shear et al[54] have developed the Panic Disorder Severity Scale, a seven-item interview that assesses the severity of panic.

Comorbid Psychiatric Conditions. Up to 70% of patients with panic disorder have a comorbid psychiatric disorder.[27] The relationship between and among these comorbid disorders is unknown. Comorbid psychiatric conditions include agoraphobia (50%), alcoholism,[55] major depression,[56,57] other anxiety disorders,[58] and personality disorders.[58] Weissman et al[59] found that, compared with other psychiatric disorders, there was a substantial risk of suicidal ideation and attempts among panic disorder patients. However, several investigators attribute this finding to psychiatric comorbidity, not to panic disorder itself.[60,61]

Treatment

Overview. For most patients, the treatment of panic disorder entails several components including psychotropic medication, cognitive-behavioral intervention, and exercise. The preceding interventions can be initiated in the primary care setting. Patients with trauma histories, significant psychosocial stressors, and/or separation difficulties may benefit from psychotherapy. Finally, among those with agoraphobia, systematic desensitization is recommended.

Psychotropic Medication. Several classes of psychotropic medication appear to be efficacious in the treatment of panic disorder. These include the selective serotonin reuptake inhibitors (SSRIs), tricyclic antidepressants (TCAs), benzodiazepines, and monoamine oxidase inhibitors (MAOIs).[1] In the primary care setting, SSRIs and TCAs have the best risk/benefit ratio, with SSRIs emerging as first-line therapy.[62] Whether prescribing an SSRI or a TCA, these drugs need to be started in very low doses and gradually titrated to a therapeutic dose to prevent an overly activating response in the patient (i.e., jitteriness, worsening of panic symptoms). For panic disorder, the duration of the drug-evaluation trial for an antidepressant is approximately six weeks with beneficial effects accruing up to 12 weeks.[1]

The SSRIs, currently the starting point of pharmacologic treatment, include five members: fluoxetine, sertraline, citalopram, paroxetine, and fluvoxamine. SSRIs have the advantages of mild side effect profiles, no addiction, and safety in overdose.[63] Limitations include sexual dysfunction among some patients (e.g., decreased libido, delayed orgasm), discontinuation syndromes (i.e., the emergence in some patients of acute symptoms in response to the abrupt cessation of the SSRI), and the possibility of drug interactions via the P-450 isoenzyme system.

Both sertraline and paroxetine have been approved by the FDA for use in panic disorder,[64] although the remainder of the SSRIs have been found effective as well.[65-67] In comparing sertraline and paroxetine in terms of possible side effects, sertraline is more likely to cause loose stools. Paroxetine is more likely to cause mild sedation, dry mouth, constipation, and sexual dysfunction.

Sertraline can be initiated at 12.5 mg per day and gradually titrated (i.e., increased by 12.5 mg every 4-7 days or as tolerated) to the usual effective dose, which is 50 mg per day. Paroxetine can be initiated at 10 mg per day and gradually titrated (increased by 10 mg every 4-7 days or as tolerated) to the usual effective dose, which is 20 mg per day. On occasion, some patients may be sensitive to these recommended initial starting doses. In these cases, starting doses of both drugs can be reduced to 6.25 mg of sertraline or 5 mg of paroxetine (i.e., ¼ of sertraline 25 mg or ½ of paroxetine 10 mg). When cutting apart pills, patients report no significant pill fragmentation or unpleasant taste.

TCAs also are effective in the treatment of panic disorder. They are a reasonable consideration when either cost is a barrier to SSRI treatment or there are failed drug trials with SSRIs. As with SSRIs, the initial dose should be very small, for example 10 mg of imipramine. Unlike SSRIs, TCAs have both anticholinergic and cardiovascular effects and are lethal in overdose. However, some patients may respond to TCAs and not to SSRIs.

Among the benzodiazepines, alprazolam and clonazepam are well-recognized interventions for panic disorder. Both are high-potency benzodiazepines and both carry the risk of physiological addiction and withdrawal.[68,69] Benzodiazepines can also precipitate disinhibited behavior[70] and depression[70,71] as well as impair recent memory[72,73] and psychomotor performance.[74] They may be helpful among some patients for rapid symptom control while awaiting the effects of an antidepressant medication. However, their combined use with an antidepressant may sabotage the antidepressant trial due to the patient's recognition of the immediate efficacy of the benzodiazepine. In addition, we believe that benzodiazepines should not be prescribed in patients with prior drug or alcohol abuse histories.

The fourth and final group of antipanic medications are the MAOIs. While effective, these medications require strict adherence to low-tyramine diets as well as the avoidance of many medications; admixtures may precipitate hypertensive crises. Therefore, while an academic possibility, few patients in clinical practice are willing to undergo these restrictions or risk a hypertensive crisis.

At times, monotherapy may be insufficient for symptom control, and the addition of a second drug (i.e., augmentation strategy) may be helpful. In the primary care setting, one uncomplicated option includes gabapentin (an anticonvulsant). While not approved by the FDA for use in psychiatric disorders, gabapentin appears to have an augmenting effect among some patients. Unlike other anticonvulsants, gabapentin does not require initial laboratory studies or ongoing serum levels. It is renally excreted, has few drug interactions, and is safe in overdose. We usually begin with 100 mg at bedtime and titrate to 300 or 400 mg per day. Augmenting effects with these drugs are usually apparent in 2-3 weeks or longer.

The duration of pharmacological treatment for panic disorder remains unknown. The minimum duration is probably one year. However, patients with long histories of the disorder and significant functional impairment may continue on lifelong treatment.

Cognitive-Behavioral Intervention. Cognitive-behavioral intervention has been found efficacious in the treatment of panic disorder,[75] whether in group[76] or abbreviated[77] format. The combination of cognitive-behavioral therapy with psychotropic

Table. Treatment of Panic Disorder in the Primary Care Setting

(1) **Initiate antidepressant trial** (SSRI: sertraline or paroxetine; low-dose to start)

(2) **Provide patient with cognitive-behavioral resources**

(3) **Recommend exercise**

(4) **Weigh risks/benefits of benzodiazepine** (rapid, time-limited control of symptoms)

↓

Titrate antidepressant to recommended dose

(sertraline: 50 mg per day; paroxetine: 40 mg per day)

↓

Continue drug-evaluation trial for 6 weeks

↓

Response	**Partial Response**	**No response**
Continue at least 1 year to lifelong	Consider dose increase or augmentation strategy (buspirone or gabapentin)	Undertake 2nd SSRI trial

No response to 2nd SSRI trial → Partial Response (consider dose increase or augmentation strategy) or:

No Response

Consider 3rd SSRI or TCA

Consider psychiatric referral

medication is reported as more effective than either treatment alone.[78] Most clinicians, particularly primary care physicians, do not have the time to undertake this type of treatment in the office setting. In response to this dilemma, we have provided a list of several books and manuals for patients who teach cognitive-behavioral techniques.

Exercise. Few studies in the psychiatric literature have examined the effects of exercise on any disorder, but one in panic patients found significant clinical improvement compared with the placebo group.[79]

Psychotherapy. Psychotherapy can be helpful in resolving acute stressors[80] as well as sorting out trauma-related issues. There is currently an available treatment manual for mental health professionals on this type of therapy.[81]

Systematic Desensitization. Nearly half of the patients with panic disorder also have agoraphobia. The academic intervention is to recommend systematic desensitization, which is reasonable in those locales that have a therapist trained in this procedure. For communities that do not have this resource, clinicians may rely on the sections in the cognitive-behavioral manuals that deal with this procedure.

Management in the Primary Care Setting. In the Table, we have outlined the general management strategy for treating panic disorder patients in the primary care setting. We believe that partial responses or treatment failures are most often due to comorbidity. In these cases, referral to a psychiatrist for further evaluation and treatment is suggested. For cases involving psychosocial stressors and/or trauma, referral to a mental health professional for psychotherapy is advised.

Clinical Pitfalls. In our experience, the most common clinical errors in the treatment of panic disorder include the following: 1) initial doses of antidepressant that exceed those recommended, resulting in an overly activating effect; 2) use of a benzodiazepine among those patients with alcohol and substance abuse histories, resulting in addiction; 3) benzodiazepine coprescription with an antidepressant that unintentionally sabotages a successful antidepressant trial; 4) inadequate drug-evaluation trial (i.e., < 6 weeks); 5) patient resistance to taking medication[82]; and 6) partial responses due to psychiatric or medical comorbidity.

Outcome

The long-term outcome of panic appears to be variable. Approximately one-third of patients attain a stable remission, a third experience exacerbations and relapses, and a third appear to have a chronic course.[83-86] These data indicate that a subgroup of panic disorder patients have a chronic course with rare remissions.[87]

Coexisting psychiatric disorders such as major depression[88,89] and personality disorders[90,91] have empirically been associated with poorer outcomes. The role of comorbid anxiety disorders such as social phobia or generalized anxiety requires further study, although agoraphobia may predict an unfavorable course.[86] A higher risk of suicide has been reported among panic patients,[59] but this risk appears attributable to comorbid psychiatric conditions.[92] Finally, women may have less favorable outcomes compared with men.[93]

On a final note, Battaglia and colleagues found that from generation to generation, the onset of panic disorder was earlier in each succeeding generation.[94] This finding, called "anticipation," requires additional study to determine if illness-affected parents are more sensitive to earlier signs of the disorder in their children.

Conclusion

Panic disorder patients are relatively common in clinical practice. There appear to be multiple contributory factors for this disorder and diagnosis is based upon the epidemiology, pattern and type of symptoms, and the exclusion of medical causes among those with atypical presentations. Treatment in the primary care setting consists of antidepressants (SSRIs being first-line), use of cognitive-behavioral techniques (patient handouts), and recommendation of exercise. Psychiatric comorbidity often accounts for partial or nonresponsiveness, and psychiatric referral is advised. Psychotherapy can be useful for patients with stressors and trauma histories, and agoraphobia may be addressed through systematic desensitization. Future studies of this perplexing disorder need to explore the efficacy of other newer antidepressants and drug combinations, panic disorder subtypes and differences in treatment, outcome factors among special populations (especially women), and prevention strategies. All of these empirical endeavors need to consider effective use of assessment and treatment resources.

References

1. American Psychiatric Association. Practice guidelines for the treatment of patients with panic disorder. *Am J Psychiatry* 1998;155:1S-34S.
2. Dammen T, Arnesen H, Ekeberg O, et al. Panic disorder in chest pain patients referred for cardiological outpatient investigation. *J Intern Med* 1999;245:497-507.
3. Bouwer C, Stein DJ. Association of panic disorder with a history of traumatic suffocation. *Am J Psychiatry* 1997;154: 1566-1570.
4. Stein MB, Asmundson GJG, Ireland D, et al. Panic disorder in patients attending a clinic for vestibular disorders. *Am J Psychiatry* 1994;151:1697-1700.
5. Ball S, Shekhar A. Basilar artery response to hyperventilation in panic disorder. *Am J Psychiatry* 1997;154:1603-1604.
6. Rouillon F. Epidemiology of panic disorder. *Hum Psychopharmacol* 1997;12:S7-S12.
7. Klerman GL, Weissman MM, Ouellette R, et al. Panic attacks in the community. Social morbidity and health care utilization. *JAMA* 1991;265:742-746.
8. Rosenbaum JF, Moroz G, Bowden CL. Clonazepam in the treatment of panic disorder with or without agoraphobia: A dose-response study of efficacy, safety, and discontinuance. *J Clin Psychopharmacol* 1997;17:390-400.
9. Kessler RC, McGonagle KA, Zhao S, et al. Lifetime and 12-month prevalence of DSM-III-R psychiatric disorders in theUnited States. Results from the National Comorbidity Survey. *Arch Gen Psychiatry* 1994;51:8-19.
10. Turgeon L, Marchand A, Dupuis G. Clinical features in panic disorder with agoraphobia: A comparison of men and women.*J Anxiety Disord* 1998;12:539-553.
11. Eaton WW, Kessler RC, Wittchen HU, et al. Panic and panic disorder in the United States. *Am J Psychiatry* 1994;151:413.
12. Hassan R, Pollard A. Late-life-onset panic disorder: Clinical and demographic characteristics of a patient sample. *J Geriatr Psychiatry Neurol* 1994;7:84-88.
13. Marriott PF, Greenwood KM, Armstrong SM. Seasonality in panic disorder. *J Affect Disord* 1994;31:75-80.
14. Lepola U, Koponen H, Lienonen E. Sleep in panic disorders. *J Psychosom Res* 1994;38:105-111.
15. Labbate LA, Pollack MH, Otto MW, et al. Sleep panic attacks: An association with childhood anxiety and adult psychopathology. *Biol Psychiatry* 1994;36:57-60.
16. Rosenfield DS, Furman Y. Pure sleep panic: Two case reports and a review of the literature. *Sleep* 1994;17: 462-465.
17. Freed S, Craske MG, Greher MR. Nocturnal panic and

trauma. *Depress Anxiety* 1999;9:141-145.

18. Kaspi SP, Otto MW, Pollack MH, et al. Premenstrual exacerbation of symptoms in women with panic disorder. *J Anxiety Disord* 1994;8:131-138.
19. Cohen LS, Sichel DA, Dimmock JA, et al. Impact of pregnancy on panic disorder: A case series. *J Clin Psychiatry* 1994;55:284-288.
20. Cohen LS, Sichel DA, Dimmock JA, et al. Postpartum course in women with preexisting panic disorder. *J Clin Psychiatry* 1994;55:289-292.
21. Hertzberg T, Wahlbeck K. The impact of pregnancy and puerperium on panic disorder: A review. *J Psychosom Obstet Gynaecol* 1999;20:59-64.
22. Deci PA, Lydiard RB, Santos AB, et al. Oral contraceptives and panic disorder. *J Clin Psychiatry* 1992;53:163-165.
23. Wagner KD, Berensen AB. Norplant-associated major depression and panic disorder. *J Clin Psychiatry* 1994;55: 478-480.
24. Katerndahl DA, Realini JP. Where do panic attack sufferers seek care? *J Fam Pract* 1995;40:237-243.
25. Kessler RC, Zhao S, Katz, et al. Past-year use of outpatient services for psychiatric problems in the National Comorbidity Survey. *Am J Psychiatry* 1999;156:115-123.
26. Salvador-Carulla L, Segui J, Fernandez-Cano P, et al. Costs and offset effect in panic disorders. *Br J Psychiatry* 1995; 166:23-28.
27. Roy-Byrne PP, Stein MB, Russo J, et al. Panic disorder in the primary care setting: Comorbidity, disability, service utilization, and treatment. *J Clin Psychiatry* 1999;60: 492-499.
28. Barsky AJ, Delamater BA, Orav JE. Panic disorder patients and their medical care. *Psychosomatics* 1999;40:50-56.
29. Greenberg PE, Sisitsky T, Kessler RC, et al. The economic burden of anxiety disorders in the 1990s. *J Clin Psychiatry* 1999;60:427-435.
30. Candilis PJ, McLean RY, Otto MW, et al. Quality of life in patients with panic disorder. *J Nerv Ment Dis* 1999;187: 429-434.
31. Moisan D, Engels ML. Childhood trauma and personality disorder in 43 women with panic disorder. *Psychol Rep* 1995;76:1133-1134.
32. Stein MB, Walker JR, Anderson G, et al. Childhood physical and sexual abuse in patients with anxiety disorders and in a community sample. *Am J Psychiatry* 1996;153: 275-277.
33. David D, Giron A, Mellman TA. Panic-phobic patients and developmental trauma. *J Clin Psychiatry* 1995;56:113-117.
34. Warner V, Mufson L, Weissman MM. Offspring at high and low risk for depression and anxiety: Mechanisms of psychiatric disorder. *J Am Acad Child Adolesc Psychiatry* 1995;34:786-797.
35. Alkin T. Near-drowning experiences and panic disorder. *Am J Psychiatry* 1999;156:667.
36. Lipsitz JD, Martin LY, Mannuzza S, et al. Childhood separation anxiety disorder in patients with adult anxiety disorders. *Am J Psychiatry* 1994;151:927-929.
37. Battaglia M, Bertella S, Politi E, et al. Age at onset of panic disorder: Influence of familial liability to the disease and of childhood separation anxiety disorder. *Am J Psychiatry* 1995; 152:1362-1364.
38. Shear MK. Factors in the etiology and pathogenesis of panic disorder: Revisiting the attachment-separation paradigm. *Am JPsychiatry* 1996;153:S125-S136.
39. Paul SM. Anxiety and depression: A common neurobiological substrate? *J Clin Psychiatry* 1988;49:S13-S16.
40. Sheehan DV, Raj BA, Trehan RR, et al. Serotonin in panic disorder and social phobia. *Int Clin Psychopharmacol* 1993; 8:63-77.
41. Paniccia GS, Rapaport MH. Serotonin receptors, social phobia and panic disorder. *Int Rev Psychiatry* 1995;7: 131-140.
42. Boulenger JP, Jerabek I, Jolicoeur FB, et al. Elevated plasma levels of neuropeptide Y in patients with panic disorder. *Am J Psychiatry* 1996;153:114-116.
43. Abelson JL, Curtis GC. Hypothalamic-pituitary-adrenal axis activity in panic disorder: 24-hour secretion of corticotropin and cortisol. *Arch Gen Psychiatry* 1996;53:323-331.
44. Perna G, Marxconi C, Battaglia M, et al. Subclinical impairment of lung airways in patients with panic disorder. *BiolPsychiatry* 1994;36:601-605.
45. Weissman MM. Family genetic studies of panic disorder. *J Psychiatr Res* 1993;27:69-78.
46. Goldstein RB, Weissman MM, Adams PB, et al. Psychiatric disorders in relatives of probands with panic disorder and/or major depression. *Arch Gen Psychiatry* 1994;51:383-394.
47. Kendler KS, Walters EE, Truett KR, et al. A twin-family study of self-report symptoms of panic-phobia and somatization. *Behav Genet* 1995;25:499-515.
48. Perna G, Bertani A, Caldirola D, et al. Family history of panic disorder and hypersensitivity to CO_2 in patients with panic disorder. *Am J Psychiatry* 1996;153:1060-1064.
49. Bellodi L, Perna G, Caldirola D, et al. CO_2-induced panic attacks: A twin study. *Am J Psychiatry* 1998;155:1184-1188.
50. Lessmeier TJ, Gamperling D, Johnson-Liddon V, et al. Unrecognized paroxysmal supraventricular tachycardia. Potential for misdiagnosis as panic disorder. *Arch Int Med* 1997;157:537-543.
51. Charney DS, Heninger GR, Jatlow PI. Increased anxiogenic effects of caffeine in panic disorders. *Arch Gen Psychiatry* 1985;42:233-243.
52. Mann SJ. Severe paroxysmal hypertension (pseudopheochromocytoma). Understanding the cause and treatment. *Arch Intern Med* 1999;159:670-674.
53. Sheehan DV, Lecrubier Y, Harnett Sheehan K, et al. The validity of the Mini International Neuropsychiatric Interview (MINI) according to the SCID-P and its reliability. *Eur Psychiatry* 1997;12:232-241.
54. Shear MK, Brown TA, Barlow DH, et al. Multicenter collaborative panic disorder severity scale. *Am J Psychiatry* 1997; 154:1571-1575.
55. Lepola U. Alcohol and depression in panic disorder. *Acta Psychiatr Scand* 1994;89:33-35.
56. Starcevic V, Uhlenhuth EH, Kellner R, et al. Comorbidity in panic disorder. *Psychiatry Res* 1993;46:285-293.
57. Servant D, Parquet PJ. Early life events and panic disorder: Course of illness and comorbidity. *Prog Neuro-*

Psychopharmacol Biol Psychiatry 1994;18:373-379.
58. Pollack MH, Otto MW. Long-term pharmacologic treatment of panic disorder. *Psychiatr Ann* 1994;24:291.
59. Weissman MM, Klerman GL, Markowitz JS, et al. Suicidal ideation and suicide attempts in panic disorder and attacks. *N Engl J Med* 1989;321:1209-1214.
60. Borden JW. Panic disorder and suicidality: Prevalence and risk factors. *J Anxiety Disord* 1994;8:217-225.
61. Cox BJ, Direnfeld DM, Swinson RP, et al. Suicidal ideation and suicide attempts in panic disorder and social phobia. *Am J Psychiatry* 1994;151:882-887.
62. Wade AG. Antidepressants in panic disorder. *Int Clin Psychopharmacol* 1999;14:S13-S17.
63. Renaud J, Birmaher B, Wassick SC, et al. Use of selective serotonin reuptake inhibitors for the treatment of childhood panic disorder: A pilot study. *J Child Adolesc Psychopharmacol* 1999;9:73-83.
64. Sheehan DV. Current concepts in the treatment of panic disorder. *J Clin Psychiatry* 1999;60:16-21.
65. Pecknold JC, Luthe L, Iny L, et al. Fluoxetine in panic disorder: Pharmacologic and tritiated platelet imipramine and paroxetine binding study. *J Psychiatry Neurosci* 1995;20:193-198.
66. de Beurs E, van Balkom AJ, Van Dyck R, et al. Long-term outcome of pharmacological and psychological treatment for panic disorder with agoraphobia: A 2-year naturalistic follow-up. *Acta Psychiatr Scand* 1999;99:59-67.
67. Michelson D, Pollack M, Lydiard RB, et al. Continuing treatment of panic disorder after acute response: Randomised, placebo-controlled trial with fluoxetine. The fluoxetine panic disorder study group. *Br J Psychiatry* 1999;174:213-218.
68. Pecknold JC. Discontinuation reactions to alprazolam in panic disorder. *J Psychiatr Res* 1993;27:155-170.
69. Kan CC, Breteler MH, Zitman FG. High prevalence of benzodiazepine dependence in out-patient users, based on the DSM-III-R and ICD-10 criteria. *Acta Psychiatr Scand* 1997;96:85-93.
70. O'Sullivan GH, Noshirvani H, Basoglu M, et al. Safety and side-effects of alprazolam: Controlled study in agoraphobia with panic disorder. *Br J Psychiatry* 1994;165:79-86.
71. Rosenbaum JF, Pollock RA, Otto MW, et al. Integrated treatment of panic disorder. *Bull Menninger Clin* 1995; 59:A4-A26.
72. Cassano GB, Toni C, Petracca A, et al. Adverse effects associated with the short-term treatment of panic disorder with imipramine, alprazolam or placebo. *Eur Neuropsychopharmacol* 1994;4:47-53.
73. Curran HV, Bond A, O'Sullivan G, et al. Memory functions, alprazolam and exposure therapy: A controlled longitudinal study of agoraphobia with panic disorder. *Psychol Med* 1994;24:969-970.
74. Rickels K, Lucki I, Schweizer E, et al. Psychomotor performance of long-term benzodiazepine users before, during, and after benzodiazepine discontinuation. *J Clin Psychopharmacol* 1999;19:107-113.
75. Rangaswami K, Kaliappan KV. Cognitive-behavioural management of panic disorder: An update. *Indian J Clin Psychol* 1995;22:45-51.
76. Otto MW, Pollack MH, Penava SJ, et al. Group cognitive-behavior therapy for patients failing to respond to pharmacotherapy for panic disorder: A clinical case series. *Behav Res Ther* 1999;37:763-770.
77. Clark DM, Salkovskis PM, Hackmann A, et al. Brief cognitive therapy for panic disorder: A randomized controlled trial. *J Consult Clin Psychol* 1999;67:583-589.
78. Ballenger JC. Panic disorder: Efficacy of current treatments. *Psychopharmacol Bull* 1993;29:477-486.
79. Broocks A, Bandelow B, Pekrun G, et al. Comparison of aerobic exercise, clomipramine, and placebo in the treatment of panic disorder. *Am J Psychiatry* 1998;155:603-609.
80. Busch F, Milrod B, Cooper A, et al. Psychodynamic approaches to panic disorder. *J Psychother Pract Res* 1995; 5:73-83.
81. Milrod B, Busch F, Cooper A, et al. *Manual of Panic-Focused Psychodynamic Psychotherapy*. Washington DC: AmericanPsychiatric Association; 1997.
82. Hofmann SG, Barlow DH, Laszlo AP, et al. Pretreatment attrition in a comparative treatment outcome study on panic disorder. *Am J Psychiatry* 1998;155:43-47.
83. Rosenberg NK, Rosenberg R. Three years follow-up of panic disorder patients: A naturalistic study. *Scand J Psychol* 1994; 35:254-262.
84. Faravelli C, Paterniti S, Scarpato A. 5-year prospective, naturalistic follow-up study of panic disorder. *Compr Psychiatry* 1995;36:271-277.
85. Brown TA, Barlow DH. Long-term outcome in cognitive-behavioral treatment of panic disorder: Clinical predictors and alternative strategies for assessment. *J Cons Clin Psychol* 1995;63:754-765.
86. Katschnig H, Amering M. The long-term course of panic disorder and its predictors. *J Clin Psychopharmacol* 1998; 18:6S-11S.
87. Wittchen HU, Essau CA. Epidemiology of panic disorder: Progress and unresolved issues. *J Psychiatr Res* 1993;27:47-68.
88. Scheibe G, Albus M. Prospective follow-up study lasting 2 years in patients with panic disorder with and without depressive disorders. *Eur Arch Psychiatry Clin Neurosci* 1994;244:39-44.
89. Hollifield M, Katon W, Skipper B, et al. Panic disorder and quality of life: Variables predictive of functional impairment. *Am J Psychiatry* 1997;154:766-772.
90. Noyes R, Reich J, Christiansen J, et al. Outcome of panic disorder. Relationship to diagnostic subtypes and comorbidity. *Arch Gen Psychiatry* 1990;47:809-818.
91. Fava G, Zielezny M, Savron G, et al. Long-term effects of behavioural treatment for panic disorder with agoraphobia. *Br J Psychiatry* 1995;166:87-92.
92. Hornig CD, McNally RJ. Panic disorder and suicide attempt: A reanalysis of data from the Epidemiologic Catchment Area study. *Br J Psychiatry* 1995;167:76-79.
93. Yonkers KA, Zlotnick C, Allsworth J, et al. Is the course of panic disorder the same in women and men? *Am J Psychiatry* 1998;155:596-602.
94. Battaglia M, Bertella S, Bajo S, et al. Anticipation of age at onset in panic disorder. *Am J Psychiatry* 1998;155:590-595.

Suggested Reading

1. Wilson RR. *Don't Panic: Taking Control of Anxiety Attacks*. New York, NY: HarperCollins; 1996.
2. Rachman S. *Panic Disorder: The Facts*. New York, NY: Oxford University Press; 1996.
3. *Getting Treatment for Panic Disorder: Information for Patients, Families, and Friends.* Bethesda, MD: National Institutes of Health, National Institute of Mental Health; 1995.
4. Swede S, Jaffe S. *The Panic Attack Recovery Book*. New York, NY: New American Library; 1987.
5. Kleinknecht RA. *Mastering Anxiety: The Nature and Treatment of Anxious Conditions*. New York, NY: Plenum Press; 1991.
6. Puerifoy RZ. *Anxiety, Phobias, and Panic: Taking Charge and Conquering Fear*. Lifeskills; 1988.

Other Resources

1. National Institute of Mental Health, Panic Campaign, 5600 Fishers Lane, Room 7C-02, Rockville, MD 20857; 1-800-64-PANIC (brochures on panic disorder).
2. Anxiety Disorders Association of America, 6000 Executive Boulevard, Suite 513, Rockville, MD 20852; 301-231-8368.

Borderline Personality Disorder

Randy A. Sansone, MD
Lori A. Sansone, MD

The term "borderline," originally coined by Stern in 1938,[1] was an effort to describe a group of patients who appeared neurotic, yet were prone to brief psychotic experiences. Stern conceptualized these individuals as literally existing between the borders of neurosis and psychosis, or on the "borderline." At the present time, borderline personality is conceptualized as a unique personality disorder highlighted by chronic self-regulatory disturbances and self-destructive behavior. This disorder is commonly encountered in the primary care setting and can be challenging both to diagnose and treat.

Description

Borderline personality is a personality disorder characterized by longstanding self-regulatory disturbances and self-destructive behavior. Examples of self-regulatory disturbances include difficulties with modulating eating behavior (anorexia nervosa, bulimia nervosa, obesity), substance use (prescription and illicit substance abuse), mood (chronic anxiety and/or depression), spending (over-extension on credit cards, gambling, bankruptcies), sexual behavior (promiscuity), and interpersonal relationships (boundary difficulties). Examples of self-destructive behavior include self-mutilation (e.g., cutting, burning, hitting oneself), suicide attempts, and physically abusive relationships. Despite pervasive deficits with self-regulation and repetitive self-destructive behavior, these individuals may appear extremely intact during brief superficial encounters. Hence, this particular personality disorder is characterized by the complex enigma of an intact social façade coupled with internal behavioral chaos.

Epidemiology

Prevalence. According to the *Diagnostic and Statistical Manual of Mental Disorders, Fourth Edition* (DSM-IV), 2% of the general population suffers from borderline personality disorder (BPD).[2] However, Stone suggests that up to 10% of the general population may harbor symptoms of this disorder.[3]

Gender Distribution. According to DSM-IV, more women than men suffer from BPD.[2] However, our experience suggests fairly equal gender distribution—although females often display histrionic overtones whereas males display antisocial overtones. This impression is supported by other investigators, who indicate that gender appears to play an important role in the personality stylings, or axis II comorbidity, of individuals with BPD.[4] Zanarini et al found that males were more likely to demonstrate passive-aggressive, narcissistic, sadistic, and antisocial personality characteristics while both sexes demonstrated equal rates of dependent personality features.[4]

Socioeconomic and Educational Factors. We are not aware of any controlled studies specifically examining the socioeconomic and educational attainment of individuals with BPD. However, BPD appears to exist along a continuum of functionality, from lower functioning individuals who populate state hospitals and community mental health centers to those at the opposite end of the continuum, with considerable educational and professional attainment.

Cultural Influences. Little research has been undertaken in the area of BPD and cross-cultural phenomena. Paris suggests that BPD is more prevalent in North America and Europe.[5] Comparing Western vs. Japanese cultures, Moriya et al found a lower prevalence of substance abuse among Japanese subjects with BPD, as well as greater enmeshment in masochistic relationships with parents.[6] In contrast, Ikuta et al concluded that borderline psychopathology is nearly identical among Japanese and American patients.[7] BPD may truly vary in prevalence from culture to culture, or it may be that the expression of BPD is modified through the influences of culture, resulting in different manifestations of the disorder in different cultures.

Etiology

Environmental and Genetic Factors. The explicit etiology of BPD remains unknown. However, in numerous studies, repetitive trauma (e.g., sexual, emotional, and physical abuse; witnessing of violence) by a caretaker during the early developmental years has been associated with BPD in adulthood.[8-14] Zanarini found early developmental trauma present in 85% of those with BPD.[8] Indeed, in examining four different approaches to BPD diagnosis, we found that those subjects with histories of abuse had a significantly greater number of BPD confirmations on study measures (core borderline disorder) compared with nonabused participants.[14] Not all studies support the childhood-abuse hypothesis.[15] It may be that other forms of abuse not examined in these studies play a significant contributory role and/or the unexpectedly high frequency of abuse in the general population may be washing out genuine relationships with BPD on a statistical level.

In addition to childhood maltreatment, there may be other contributory variables to the development of BPD among some individuals including a predisposing or vulnerable temperament,[16] traumatic triggering events,[16] inconsistent treatment by the caretaker,[17] and the patient's perception of a negative family environment.[18] While there may be a genetic contribution to BPD, this variable remains controversial.[19,20]

Biological Findings. Only a small number of studies have examined biological abnormalities among patients with BPD. Because of small sample sizes, their clinical significance remains unknown, but these studies may eventually confirm consistent contributory biological factors.

De la Fuente et al found hypometabolism in the premotor and prefrontal cortex of 10 patients with BPD.[21] Chotai et al reported higher cerebrospinal fluid levels of 5-HIAA and HVA among borderline patients with lower impulsivity scores, suggesting a protective function of serotonin against suicide and impulsivity in a subgroup of patients.[22] Among 20 borderline patients, De la Fuente et al found a 40% incidence of abnormal EEG studies characterized by diffuse, slow activity.[23] In a controlled study, New et al found that borderline patients (n = 14) had significantly lower serum cholesterol levels compared with 28 patients with other types of personality disorders.[24] Coccaro et al found, among personality-disordered subjects, biological abnormalities relating to impulsivity and aggression, including an inverse relationship with central serotonin and a direct relationship with cerebrospinal fluid arginine vasopressin.[25,26]

These biological studies are limited by small sample sizes and the lack of homogeneity among BPD samples. In addition, the reported correlations don't necessarily imply causality. However, these intriguing relationships may eventually lead to the identification of consistent biological abnormalities among those with BPD, some of which may, indeed, be causally related to symptoms.

Comorbidity

Psychiatric Comorbidity. Investigators have determined that, compared with others, individuals with BPD are significantly more likely to have multiple psychiatric (i.e., Axis I) diagnoses.[27,28] Not only is the number of Axis I diagnoses predictive for BPD, but a combination of mood disorder and impulse disorder diagnoses is particularly suggestive.[4] While the prevalence of most Axis I disorders appears similar for both males and females, males are more likely to have a lifetime diagnosis of substance abuse compared with eating disorders among females.[4]

In a population of 379 participants with BPD, Zanarini et al determined the lifetime prevalences of several Axis I disorders.[4] For anxiety disorders, the lifetime prevalence was 88%, major depression 83%, substance use disorders 64%, post-traumatic stress disorder 56%, eating disorders 53%, panic disorder 48%, dysthymia 39%, and somatoform disorders 10%. In contrast to non-BPD patients, those with BPD were more likely to be diagnosed with major depression, bipolar disorder, panic disorder, social or specific phobia, post-traumatic stress disorder, obsessive-compulsive disorder, eating disorder NOS, and any somatoform disorder.[4]

Medical Comorbidity. Few studies have explored specific medical conditions and their comorbidity with BPD. However, BPD has been associated with somatization disorder,[29] somatic preoccupation,[30] rheumatoid arthritis,[31] plastic surgery requests on multiple body areas,[32] and HIV infection.[33] Among male veterans, Streeter et al found traumatic head injury in 42% of those with BPD compared with only 4% among controls.[34] We are in the midst of a chronic pain study in a family practice setting and, to date, have found that nearly two-thirds of participants have BPD according to a highly structured interview (i.e., is chronic pain a self-regulation difficulty among some individuals?).

In the primary care setting, borderline patients may manifest self-destructive behavior in relation to their medical care. We found that a significant minority of family practice patients

(7%) acknowledged the active sabotage of their medical care.[35] Reported behaviors included exposing oneself to an infected person on purpose, damaging oneself on purpose, misusing prescription medication to worsen a medical condition, not following directions given by medical personnel to purposefully prolong illness, and coming into contact with a known allergen to harm self. Medically self-harming behavior among patients in primary care settings has been empirically associated with borderline personality.[36]

Although the relationship of BPD to specific medical conditions and illness behavior is not well studied, patients with either trauma histories or borderline personality symptomatology appear to demonstrate greater health care use[37,38] (e.g., greater number of telephone contacts to the facility, physician visits, and prescriptions).[38] This observation may have a significant effect on the clinician's practice perspective, especially regarding the issue of capitation.

Diagnosis

The diagnosis of BPD in the primary care setting can be readily missed due to the brevity of office encounters and the intact social facade of these patients. Indeed, studies indicate that mental health clinicians under-diagnose BPD compared with researchers using structured interviews.[39] This observation underscores the importance of developing an effective diagnostic assessment strategy.

DSM-IV Criteria. The DSM-IV2 criteria for the diagnosis of BPD are shown in Table 1. These nine features provide the cornerstone for diagnosing borderline personality; confirmation of diagnosis requires that five or more features be present.

Gunderson Criteria. In conjunction with other investigators, Gunderson developed the Diagnostic Interview for Borderlines, which is a semi-structured research interview.[40] This interview contains five descriptive features for BPD that can be organized around the acronym P-I-S-I-A and adapted to the clinical setting (*please see Table 2*). While not a substitute for the DSM-IV criteria, these five features describe the borderline syndrome quite well.

Because of their specificity, the features listed under "Impulsivity" and "Affect" are particularly useful as screening questions. In exploring impulsivity, the line of questioning might progress as follows: "Have you ever had anorexia, bulimia, or been obese? Have you ever had any drug or alcohol difficulties? Have you ever had problems managing money—credit card difficulties, gambling, or bankruptcies? Have you ever physically damaged yourself on purpose? For example, have you ever cut, burned, or hit yourself? Banged your head? Pulled out hair or eyelashes? Have you had any suicide attempts? Have you been in any abusive relationships? Have you engaged in any high-risk hobbies or behaviors?" With regard to affect, the question might be phrased: "Back to the age of 15, what percent of the time have you been in a normal mood—no depression, no anxiety, no emptiness, no anger?" Impulsivity is usually longstanding and may be characterized by symptom substitution over time. Characteristic responses to "normal mood since the age of 15" are typically 20% or less (*see Table 2*).

Table 1. DSM-IV Criteria for Borderline Personality Disorder

- Frantic efforts to avoid real or imagined abandonment
- A pattern of unstable and intense interpersonal relationships characterized by alternating between extremes of idealization and devaluation
- Identity disturbance: markedly and persistently unstable self-image or sense of self
- Impulsivity in at least two areas that are potentially self-damaging (e.g., spending, sex, substance abuse, reckless driving, binge eating)
- Recurrent suicidal behavior, gestures, or threats, or self-mutilating behavior
- Affective instability due to a marked reactivity of mood (e.g., intense episodic dysphoria, irritability, or anxiety usually lasting a few hours and only rarely more than a few days)
- Chronic feelings of emptiness
- Inappropriate, intense anger or difficulty controlling anger (e.g., frequent displays of temper, constant anger, recurrent physical fights)
- Transient, stress-related paranoid ideation or severe dissociative symptoms

* *At least five criteria are required for diagnosis.*

Self-Harm Inventory. The Self-Harm Inventory (SHI)[41] is a self-report measure that can be used in the primary care setting to screen for BPD. It is based upon the concept that longstanding and multiple self-destructive behaviors are characteristic of BPD. In this regard, Gunderson and Singer noted that impulsivity and self-harm behavior were the two characteristics most commonly and consistently associated with BPD.[42] Indeed, Mack identified self-harm behavior as the behavioral specialty of individuals with BPD (i.e., the defining characteristic of the disorder).[43]

Developed among both psychiatric and primary-care populations, the SHI contains 22 yes/no items. Each item is preceded by the statement, "Have you ever intentionally, or on purpose…" Each "yes" response is scored (i.e., pathological). Using a cut-off score of 5, this measure was able to correctly identify 84% of subjects compared with the Diagnostic Interview for Borderlines.[40] We recommend using the SHI as a screening measure among those primary care patients with suspicious symptoms, noting that the cut-off score of 5 is suggestive of BPD (*see Appendix 1*).

Interestingly, there may be different behavioral manifestations of BPD in different medical-specialty settings. For example, using the SHI, we examined for differences among women with BPD in psychiatric vs. primary care samples.

Table 2. Gunderson Features for Borderline Personality Disorder

P	***Psychotic/quasi-psychotic episodes***: transient, fleeting, and brief in nature; may include depersonalization, derealization, dissociation, rage reactions, paranoia in which the patient subsequently recognizes the illogical nature of their suspiciousness, fleeting or isolated hallucinations or delusions, and unusual reactions to drugs; episodes tend to be persistent over the patient's lifetime.
I	***Impulsivity***: longstanding and ongoing; specific behaviors may be stable over time, co-exist with other behaviors, or replace each other over time (i.e., symptom substitution); impulsivity includes both: ***Self-regulation difficulties:*** (e.g., eating disorders including anorexia and bulimia nervosa, and obesity; drug/alcohol problems; money management difficulties including credit-card difficulties, bankruptcies, and gambling; promiscuity; mood regulation difficulties). ***Self-destructive behaviors:*** (e.g., self-mutilation such as hitting, cutting, burning, or biting oneself; suicide attempts; sadomasochistic relationships with others; high-risk hobbies such as parachuting or racing cars; high-risk behaviors such as frequenting dangerous bars or jogging in parks at night; recurrent accidents).
S	***Social adaptation***: superficially intact social facade; if the individual demonstrates high academic or professional achievement, performance is usually inconsistent and erratic.
I	***Interpersonal relationships***: chronically chaotic and unsatisfying relationships with others; the relationship style is characterized by "dichotomous relatedness," wherein social relationships tend to be very superficial and transient, and personal relationships tend to be extremely intense, manipulative and dependent; there may be intense fears of being alone as well as rage with the primary caretaker.
A	***Affect***: chronically dysphoric or labile since adolescence with the predominant affects being anxiety, anger, depression, and/or emptiness.

While most self-destructive behaviors were similar in prevalence among both samples, "overdosed" and "hit self" were more common in the psychiatric sample whereas "abused laxatives" was more common in the primary care sample.[44] These data suggest the possibility of behavioral differences among different populations of patients with BPD.

Presentations in the Primary Care Setting

Although the clinical manifestations of BPD in the primary care setting are varied,[45-47] in comparison with the psychiatric setting, the psychodynamics and diagnostic features remain constant. We have summarized some of the many possible presentations in Table 3. These presentations should be regarded as suspicious for, rather than diagnostic of, BPD and might function as an impetus to undertake a screening for BPD using P-I-S-I-A or the SHI.

Table 3. Possible Clinical Manifestations of BPD in the Primary Care Setting

- Chronic mood disorders (e.g., depression,[71] anxiety, mood lability)
- Impulse problems (e.g., eating disorders including obesity,[72] substance abuse, promiscuity, money-management difficulties)
- Self-destructive behavior (e.g., self-mutilation, multiple suicide attempts, abusive relationships, high-risk hobbies or behaviors, recurrent accidents)
- Multiple Axis I psychiatric diagnoses[27]
- Multiple sensitivities or self-reported allergies to medications[73]
- Extensive and chronic somatic preoccupation[30]
- Sabotage of medical care[35]
- Chronic pain syndromes[61,62]
- Exotic or "fashionable" medical syndromes (e.g., food allergies, chronic fatigue syndrome, fibromyalgia, multiple chemical sensitivities, hypoglycemia)[74]

In addition to the clinical manifestations of BPD, there may be a number of interpersonal dynamics that suggest BPD (*please see Table 4*). Most of these dynamics reflect a very strong or over-active attachment drive to others,[48,49] which is characteristic of BPD. How these attachment dynamics relate to the etiology of BPD remains to be determined.

Management Suggestions

Conservative Medical Management. Investigators have noted among BPD patients greater frequencies of violence and maltreatment in adulthood,[50] which may relate to an underlying masochistic dynamic that develops as an outgrowth of childhood abuse. Through this dynamic, borderline patients may unintentionally lure physicians into inappropriate treatment (i.e., maltreatment). Examples of this include seducing the physician into the overprescription of medications (particularly analgesics, benzodiazepines, and weight-loss medications), multiple referrals for unnecessary surgeries including abdominal or plastic surgery, unusual treatment strategies (e.g., colonic irrigation, self-administration of analgesics via catheter, intra-rectal administration of estrogen), and unnecessary and high-risk referrals (e.g., cardiac catheterization).

Table 4. Interpersonal Dynamics That Suggest Borderline Personality Disorder

- Splitting (intrapsychic splitting: perceiving in absolutes or extremes; interpersonal splitting: polarizing others into conflict)
- Use of transitional objects[75] (i.e., the use of tangible objects), which are related or associated with another person, for soothing; (e.g., adults with teddy bears)
- Rapid transference (unexpected, rapid emotional enmeshment with the clinician/staff)
- Tests of caring (e.g., unusual or impractical requests, such as unnecessary housecalls, designed to consolidate the patient as a favorite of the clinician; seduction into unethical behavior)
- First-name address (i.e., immediately addressing the clinician by the first name)
- Boundary violations (repeated attempts to enter into the clinician's professional or personal life; with the former, examples include repeated calls and appointments; with the latter, examples include obtaining the clinician's beeper or home telephone number, stopping by the clinician's house, performing special service activities for the physician to foster attachment)
- Intermittant childlike demeanor (evidence of periodic regression such as a childlike voice and/or regressed appearance)
- Crisis-oriented professional relationship (i.e., frequent personal crises and tragedies requiring calls to and appointments with the clinician)

Defined Treatment Plan. At the outset of a new-patient encounter, define your practice standards and established treatment approach to the patient's primary problems. This may precipitate the negotiation of medication weans, new drug trials, and different types of interventions. Avoid accommodating borderline patients at the expense of your own medical comfortability. Always carefully document your proposed treatment plan in the medical record to avoid any misinterpretation by the patient, staff, or cross-covering physicians.

Firm Boundaries. Maintain clear and consistent professional boundaries with the patient. Retain a neutral emotional tone during encounters, particularly during conflict situations. Avoid informality, when possible, such as hallway chats. Be prepared for and avoid the accommodation of unusual requests (e.g., stopping by the patient's home to drop off a prescription).

Structured Office Environment. Maintain a stable and consistent office environment for the patient. This may entail having the same nursing staff, the same employee in the business office, and the same physician work with the patient whenever possible. It may even be helpful to use the same examination room.

Accomodation of Attachment Needs. Anticipate the attachment demands of these patients. They may require multiple brief office visits to sustain their own stability. Keep appointments brief, if possible, but be sensitive to their needs to secure an attachment with you.

Limit Setting. Be prepared to establish limits, and to do so in a supportive fashion. Because of the self-regulatory disturbances of these individuals, they will ultimately require various types of limits in their relationships with others. Anticipate this process, establish limits quickly when difficulties emerge, and frame those limits as "an effort to protect our professional relationship and keep it functioning smoothly." Framing a limit in the context of attachment is usually an effective method for supporting the borderline patient.

Avoidance of Sensitive Psychological Issues. Be hesitant to explore psychological issues in an in-depth manner. Psychological exploration in any individual, borderline or not, results in some degree of regression, and borderline individuals may regress precipitously. When complex psychological concerns arise (e.g., abuse dynamics, suicidal thoughts), clarify your professional limits and suggest a referral to a mental health professional.

Use of Psychotropic Medication. Should the patient express concerns about depression and anxiety, consider limited psychotropic intervention. There is no known drug or drug combination specifically for BPD. In the field of psychiatry, many clinicians advocate a symptom-specific approach (i.e., antidepressants for depression, anticonvulsants for impulsivity, antipsychotics for pronounced quasi-psychotic phenomena).[51,52]

In the primary care setting, the use of SSRI-type antidepressants appears to be a conservative intervention as these medications have mild side effects; are safe in overdose with the possible exception of citalopram;[53,54] and have positive effects on mood, impulsivity,[55-57] and post-traumatic stress symptoms.[58] (Among psychiatric prescribers, SSRIs may be recommended in high doses.)

An additional conservative medication strategy might include the prescription of gabapentin.[59] Gabapentin may be prescribed either as an augmenting agent (i.e., enhancing the effects of the primary medication), or for the intervention of specific symptoms such as panic, anxiety, or impulsivity.

Medication trials in borderline patients are typified by medication sensitivity, idiosyncratic responses to medications, and partial responses. Begin psychotropic medications at low dosages and advance slowly. Anticipate potential problems with side effects. Should the patient not experience meaningful benefit, suggest a referral to a psychiatrist, framing the referral as "the need to consult a specialist in psychotropic medication."

In the primary care setting, we would advise caution with benzodiazepines (self-regulatory difficulties may lead to addiction; alprazolam has been associated with behavioral dyscontrol in BPD patients[60]), tricyclic antidepressants or lithium (impulsivity may result in a lethal overdose), combinations of psychotropic medications with not-yet studied effects (e.g., SSRI and a tricyclic-risk of drug interactions via the P-450 isoenzyme system), and multiple psychotropic drugs (e.g., antidepressant, anxiolytic, hypnotic, mood stabilizer, and antipsychotic).

Acceptance of Limited Symptom Resolution. Be alert to the complex medical complaints of many of these patients. Consider that full resolution of symptoms may not occur as medical complaints may function to secure an ongoing attachment to the clinician. On the contrary, antidepressant treatment, including SSRIs and venlafaxine,[61,62] may diminish somatic symptoms among some patients.

Acceptance of Personal Limits. Recognize your own limits. These challenging patients can be highly stressful. A personal consultation (formal or informal case review of difficult patients) with a mental health professional may assist the clinician in the management of these difficult patients.

Psychiatric Referral. Psychiatric referral can be helpful in a number of ways including the confirmation of a BPD diagnosis, pharmacological management of the patient, and assessment for psychological treatment options. In general, lower functioning patients are limited to supportive-maintenance treatment, which consists of assisting individuals with daily life tasks and here/now problem-solving. Higher functioning patients may be candidates for psychodynamic psychotherapy.

Outcome

There is little available outcome research in the area of BPD. In examining the issue of suicide, Gunderson found that 75% of patients acknowledged attempts.[63] Concurrent mood disorder and/or substance abuse appear to heighten the risk of attempts.[64] As for completed suicide, studies indicate that the rate increases with the length of follow-up, with up to 10% of patients suiciding over a 20-year period.[65-67] Better prognostic outcomes are associated with comorbid obsessive-compulsive features and those with eating disorders.[68] A history of sexual abuse[69] and high levels of impulsivity and poor premorbid functioning[70] are associated with poor outcomes. In our experience, those individuals with antisocial features also have poor outcomes. We are aware of no studies examining medical outcomes (e.g., diabetes, hypertension) among primary care patients with BPD.

Conclusion

The diagnosis and management of BPD patients in the primary care setting is a genuine challenge. Strategies include being alert to the associated clinical features (i.e., self-regulation difficulties, self-destructive behavior), consolidating a diagnostic approach, and maintaining a conservative and structured clinical interface. These individuals can be difficult patients, but can be managed in the primary care setting with patience and perserverance. Regardless, they remain true enigmas, with their intact facades concealing the genuine turmoil that lies beneath the social surface.

References

1. Stern A. Psychoanalytic investigation of therapy in the borderline group of neuroses. *Psychoanal Q* 1938;7:467-489.
2. American Psychiatric Association. *Diagnostic and Statistical Manual of Mental Disorders*. 4th ed. Washington, DC: American Psychiatric Assocation; 1994.
3. Stone MH. Borderline personality disorder. In: Michels R, Cavenar JO, Jr., eds. *Psychiatry*. 2nd ed. Philadelphia, Pa: Lippincott; 1986:1-15.
4. Zanarini MC, Frankenburg FR, Dubo ED, et al. Axis II comorbidity of borderline personality disorder. *Compr Psychiatry* 1998;39:296-302.
5. Paris J. Cultural factors in the emergence of borderline pathology. *Psychiatry* 1996;59:185-192.
6. Moriya N, et al. Diagnosis and clinical features of borderline personality disorder in the east and west: A preliminary report. *Compr Psychiatry* 1993;34:418-423.
7. Ikuta N, et al. Comparison of American and Japanese outpatients with borderline personality disorder. *Compr Psychiatry* 1994;35:382-385.
8. Zanarini MC, Williams AA, Lewis RE, et al. Reported pathological childhood experiences associated with the development of borderline personality disorder. *Am J Psychiatry* 1997;154: 1101-1106.
9. Sansone RA, Sansone LA, Wiederman MW. The prevalence of trauma and its relationship to borderline personality symptoms and self-destructive behaviors in a primary care setting. *Arch Fam Med* 1995;4:439-442.
10. Zanarini MC, Gunderson JG, Marino MF, et al. Childhood experiences of borderline patients. *Compr Psychiatry* 1989;30: 18-25.
11. Herman JL, Perry JC, van der Kolk BA. Childhood trauma in borderline personality disorder. *Am J Psychiatry* 1989;146: 490-495.
12. Ogata SN, Silk KR, Goodrich S, et al. Childhood sexual and physical abuse in adult patients with borderline personality disorder. *Am J Psychiatry* 1990;147:1008-1013.
13. Brown GR, Anderson B. Psychiatric morbidity in adult inpatients with childhood histories of sexual and physical abuse. *Am J Psychiatry* 1991;148:55-61.
14. Sansone RA, Gaither GA, Songer DA. The relationships among childhood abuse, borderline personality, and self-harm behavior in psychiatric inpatients. Submitted.
15. Fossati A, Madeddu F, Maffei C. Borderline personality disorder and childhood sexual abuse: a meta-analytic study. *J Pers Disord* 1999;13:268-280.
16. Zanarini MC, Frankenburg FR. Pathways to the development of borderline personality disorder. *J Pers Disord* 1997;11:93-104.
17. Zanarini MC, et al. Risk factors associated with the dissociative experiences of borderline patients. *J Nerv Ment Dis* 2000;188: 26-30.
18. Gunderson JG, Lyoo IK. Family problems and relationships for adults with borderline personality disorder. *Harv Rev Psychiatry* 1997;4:272-278.
19. Torgersen S. Genetics in borderline conditions. *Acta Psychiatr Scand Suppl* 1994;379:19-25.

20. Torgersen S. Genetics of patients with borderline personality disorder. *Psychiatr Clin N Am* 2000;23:1-9.
21. De la Fuente JM, Goldman S, Stanus E, et al. Brain glucose metabolism in borderline personality disorder. *J Psychiatr Res* 1997;31:531-541.
22. Chotai J, Kullgren G, Asberg M. CSF monoamine metabolites in relation to the diagnostic interview for borderline patients (DIB). *Neuropsychobiology* 1998;38:207-212.
23. De la Fuente JM, Tugendhaft P, Mavroudakis N. Electroencephalographic abnormalities in borderline personality disorder. *Psychiatry Res* 1998;77:131-138.
24. New AS, Sevin EM, Mitropoulou V, et al. Serum cholesterol and impulsivity in personality disorders. *Psychiatry Res* 1999; 85:145-150.
25. Coccaro EF, Berman ME, Kavoussi RJ, Hauger RL. Relationship of prolactin response to d-fenfluramine to behavioral and questionnaire assessments of aggression in personality-disordered men. *Biol Psychiatry* 1996;40:157-164.
26. Coccaro EF, et al. Cerebrospinal fluid vasopressin levels: correlates with aggression and seotonin function in personality-disordered subjects. *Arch Gen Psychiatry* 1998;55:708-714.
27. Zanarini MC, Frankenburg FR, Dubo ED, et al. Axis I comorbidity of borderline personality disorder. *Am J Psychiatry* 1998;155:1733-1739.
28. Zimmerman M, Mattia JI. Axis I diagnostic comorbidity and borderline personality disorder. *Compr Psychiatry* 1999;40: 245-252.
29. Hudziak JJ, et al. Clinical study of the relation of borderline personality disorder to Briquet's Syndrome (Hysteria), somatization disorder, antisocial personality disorder, and substance abuse disorders. *Am J Psychiatry* 1996;153:1598-1606.
30. Sansone RA, Wiederman MW, Sansone LA. Adult somatic preoccupation and its relationship to childhood trauma. Violence Vict (in press).
31. Marcenaro M, et al. Rheumatoid arthritis, personality, stress response style, and coping with illness. A preliminary survey. *Ann N Y Acad Sci* 1999;876:419-425.
32. Napoleon A. Personality and plastic surgery. *Ann Plast Surg* 1993;31:193-208.
33. Ellis D, Collis I, King M. A controlled comparison of HIV and general medical referrals to a liaison psychiatry service. *AIDS Care* 1994;6:69-76.
34. Streeter CC, Van Reekum R, Shorr RI, Bachman DL. Prior head injury in male veterans with borderline personality disorder. *J Nerv Ment Dis* 1995;183:577-581.
35. Sansone RA, Wiederman MW, Sansone LA, Mehnert-Kay S. Sabotaging one's own medical care. *Arch Fam Med* 1997;6: 583-586.
36. Sansone RA, Wiederman MW, Sansone LA. Medically self-harming behavior and its relationship to borderline personality symptoms and somatic preoccupation among internal medicine patients. *J Nerv Ment Dis* 2000;188:45-47.
37. Sansone RA, Wiederman MW, Sansone LA. Borderline personality symptomatology, experience of multiple types of trauma, and health care utilization among women in a primary care setting. *J Clin Psychiatry* 1998;59:108-111.
38. Sansone RA, Sansone LA, Wiederman MW. Borderline personality disorder and health care utilization in a primary care setting. *South Med J* 1996;89:1162-1165.
39. Zimmerman M, Mattia JI. Differences between clinical and research practices in diagnosing borderline personality disorder. *Am J Psychiatry* 1999;156:1570-1574.
40. Kolb JE, Gunderson JG. Diagnosing borderline patients with a semistructured interview. *Arch Gen Psychiatry* 1980;37:37-41.
41. Sansone RA, Wiederman MW, Sansone LA. The Self-Harm Inventory (SHI): Development of a scale for identifying self-destructive behaviors and borderline personality disorder. *J Clin Psychol* 1998;54:973-983.
42. Gunderson JG, Singer MT. Defining borderline patients: an overview. *Am J Psychiatry* 1975;132:1-10.
43. Mack J. *Borderline States: An Historical Perspective*. New York, NY: Grune & Stratton; 1975.
44. Sansone RA, et al. Patterns of self-harm behavior among women with borderline personality symptomatology: psychiatric versus primary care samples. *Gen Hosp Psychiatry* 2000;22:174-178.
45. Sansone RA, Sansone LA. Borderline personality disorder: office diagnosis and management. *Am Fam Physician* 1991;44:194-198.
46. Sansone RA, Sansone LA. Borderline personality disorder: interpersonal and behavioral problems that sabotage treatment success. *Postgrad Med* 1995;97:169-179.
47. Sansone RA, Sansone LA. Borderline personality disorder: chaos behind the facade. *Women's Psychiatr Health* 1996;5:1-3, 7, 11.
48. West M, et al. Borderline disorder and attachment pathology. *Can J Psychiatry* 1993;38:S16-S22.
49. Arkema PH. The borderline personality and transitional relatedness. *Am J Psychiatry* 1981;138:172-177.
50. Zanarini MC, et al. Violence in the lives of adult borderline patients. *J Nerv Ment Dis* 1999;187:65-71.
51. Soloff PH. Psychopharmacology of borderline personality disorder. *Psychiatr Clin North Am* 2000;23:169-192.
52. Hirschfeld RM. Pharmacotherapy of borderline personality disorder. *J Clin Psychiatry* 1997;58:48-52.
53. Personne M, Sjoberg G, Persson H. Citalopram overdose-review of cases treated in Swedish hospitals. *J Toxicol Clin Toxicol* 1997;35:237-240.
54. Ostrom M, et al. Fatal overdose with citalopram. *Lancet* 1996;348:339-340.
55. Soloff P. Special feature: Psychobiologic perspectives on treatment of personality disorders. *J Personal Disord* 1997; 11:336-344.
56. Kavoussi RJ, Liu J, Coccaro EF. Open trial of sertaline in personality disordered patients with impulsive aggression. *J Clin Psychiatry* 1994;55:137-141.
57. McElroy S, et al. Placebo-controlled trial of sertraline in the treatment of binge eating disorder. *Am J Psychiatry* 2000; 157:1004-1006.
58. Brady K, et al. Efficacy and safety of sertraline treatment of posttraumatic stress disorder. *JAMA* 2000;283:1837-1844.
59. Letterman L, Markowitz JS. Gabapentin: A review of published experience in the treatment of bipolar disorder and other psychiatric conditions. *Pharmacotherapy* 1999;19:565-572.
60. Gardner DL, Cowdry RW. Alprazolam-induced dyscontrol

in borderline personality disorder. *Am J Psychiatry* 1985;142: 98-100.

61. Markovitz PJ, Wagner SC. Venlafaxine in the treatment of borderline personality disorder. *Psychopharmacol Bull* 1995; 31:773-777.
62. Markovitz PJ. Pharmacotherapy of impulsivity, aggression, and related disorders. In: Stein D, Hollander E, eds. *Aggression and Disorders of Impulse Control*. Sussex, UK: J Wiley and Sons; 1995:263-287.
63. Gunderson JG. *Borderline Personality Disorders*. Washington DC: American Psychiatric Press; 1984.
64. Fine MA, Sansone RA. Dilemmas in the management of suicidal behavior in individuals with borderline personality disorder. *Am J Psychother* 1990;44:160-171.
65. Pope HG Jr, Jonas JM, Hudson JI, et al. The validity of DSM-III borderline personality disorder: A phenomenologic, family history, treatment response, and long-term follow-up study. *Arch Gen Psychiatry* 1983;40:23-30.
66. Paris J, Brown R, Nowlis D. Long-term follow-up of borderline patients in a general hospital. *Compr Psychiatry* 1987;28: 530-535.
67. Stone MH, Stone DK, Hurt SW. The natural history of borderline patients treated by intensive hospitalization. *Psychiatr Clin North Am* 1987;10:185-206.
68. Stone MH. *The Fate of Borderline Patients*. New York, NY: Guilford Press; 1990.
69. Paris J, Zweig-Frank H, Guzder H. The role of psychological risk factors in recovery from borderline personality disorder. *Compr Psychiatry* 1993;34:410-413.
70. Links PS, Mitton JE, Steiner M. Predicting outcome for borderline personality disorder. *Compr Psychiatry* 1990;31:490-498.
71. Markowitz JC, et al. Prevalence and comorbidity of dysthymic disorder among psychiatric outpatients. *J Affect Disord* 1992; 24:63-71.
72. Sansone RA, Sansone LA, Wiederman MW. The comorbidity, relationship and treatment implications of borderline personality and obesity. *J Psychosom Res* 1997;43:541-543.
73. Sansone RA, Gentile J, Markert RJ. Drug allergies among patients with borderline personality symptomatology. *Gen Hosp Psychiatry* 2000;22:289-293.
74. Righter EL, Sansone RA. Managing somatic preoccupation. *Am Fam Physician* 1999;59:3113-3120.
75. Morris H, Gunderson JG, Zanarini MC. Transitional object use and borderline psychopathology. *Am J Psychiatry* 1986;143: 1534-1538.

Obsessive Compulsive Disorder

Jerald Kay, MD
Deborah Y. Liggan, MD

Obsessive-compulsive disorder (OCD) is characterized by recurrent, persistent, intrusive, often repugnant obsessions and/or compulsions performed by the patient to allay overwhelming anxiety. Obsessions are unwanted, repetitive, irresistible thoughts or urges. In spite of their senseless and repugnant qualities, attempts to banish them are to no avail. Compulsions are stereotyped repetitive behaviors designed to produce or prevent some feeling magically connected to the behavior. There is a subjective sense of being compelled—often associated with a simultaneous desire to resist. Insight into the perverse and senseless nature of these frequently bizarre rituals is usually preserved. Evidence exists that early detection and assertive treatment are important for minimizing the impairment experienced. However, OCD is often called a silent epidemic in that patients underreport symptoms or complain of depression or nonspecific anxiety instead of obsessions and compulsions. The primary care physician might be the only health professional who has regular contact with a patient who has this debilitating disorder. Diagnosis is not difficult if the clinician is aware of its prevalence and the different ways it is expressed.

Definition

As many as 5 million Americans may be suffering from serious functional impairment due to this chronic anxiety disorder. Many of these patients initially present to primary care physicians where they go undiagnosed. Often, patients are hesitant to reveal what they consider to be "crazy" or "odd" symptoms to physicians. Their obsessions are intense, intrusive, unwanted thoughts, such as concerns about bodily wastes and secretions, unfounded fears, need for exactness, symmetry, neatness, excessive religious concerns, perverse sexual thoughts, and intrusions of words, phrases, or music. Usually, the person attempts to ignore or suppress such thoughts or to neutralize them with some other thought or action. Compulsions consist of the subjective urge to repeat meaningless and irrational rituals, such as checking, counting, cleaning, washing, touching, smelling, hoarding, and rearranging. *(Please see Figures 1 and 2.)* The person feels driven to perform compulsions in response to an obsession or according to rules that must be rigidly applied. Compulsions are excessively time consuming—taking more than an hour a day—or cause marked distress or significant impairment. The patient is aware of the irrationality of his or her behavior but feels compelled to continue nevertheless. The reluctance of patients to divulge their obsessive-compulsive symptoms is compounded by the fact that many physicians were trained in an era when OCD was thought to be a rare con-

Figure 1. Obsessive Symptoms at Admission

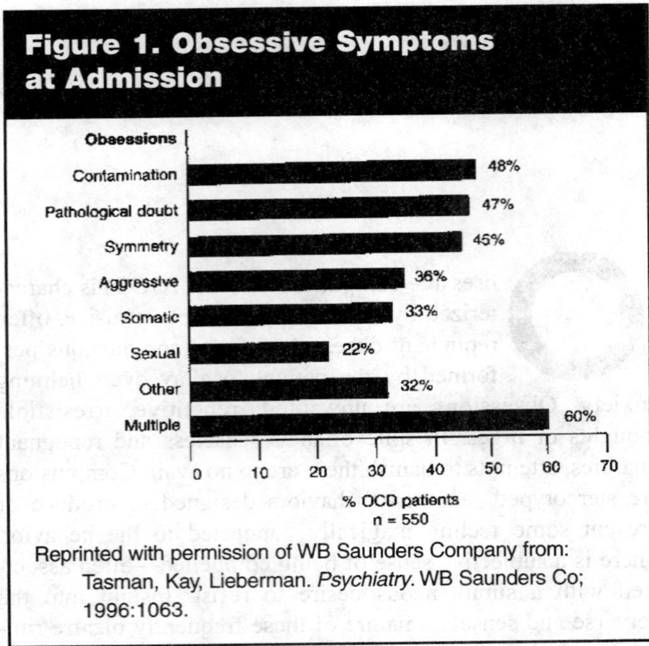

Reprinted with permission of WB Saunders Company from: Tasman, Kay, Lieberman. *Psychiatry.* WB Saunders Co; 1996:1063.

dition and fail to ask routine screening questions for obsessions and compulsions.

Epidemiology

Until the mid 1980s, OCD was considered extremely rare. However, the results of the Epidemiological Catchment Area Study (ECA) conducted in 1984 revealed that OCD is the fourth most common psychiatric disorder (after the phobias, substance use disorders, and major depressive disorder). OCD has a six-month prevalence of 1.6% and a life-time prevalence of 2.5%. Age of onset has a bimodal distribution, with one peak in childhood and another peak in adulthood. The disorder begins most often in adolescence and early adulthood. The disabling condition afflicts more than 1% of children and adolescents.[1,2] Thirty-one percent of first episodes occur between ages 10 and 15, with 75% developing by age 30.[3] Early onset tends to be associated more frequently with tics and male gender, whereas those whose symptoms emerge later in life are more likely to be female and associated with eating disorders or depression. The overall gender ratio is approximately 1:1. However, higher frequency of cleaning rituals, fear of contamination, and avoidant behavior has been found in women, whereas primary obsessive slowness, sexual obsessions, and fear of social situations are prevalent in men.[4,5]

Etiology

At least some predisposition to obsessional behavior is inherited. However, most cases have no single precipitating event or stressor. A model based on the psychological concept of conditioning has been used to understand the development of obsessions and compulsions.[6] If a person is preoccupied with fears of contamination from germs, repetitive hand washing usually decreases the anxiety caused by these fears. The compulsion becomes a conditioned response to anxiety. Because of the tension-reducing aspect of the compulsion, this learned behavior becomes reinforced and eventually fixed.[7] By performing a compulsion, contact with the fear-evoking stimulus (i.e., dirt) is not maintained, and the cycle linking obsessions and compulsions is maintained. *(Please see Figure 3.)*

Environmental causes may also play a role in the cause of OCD or may affect symptom severity. Environmental factors, such as postinfectious antineuronal cross-reactivity in a small number of patients recovering from a course of streptococcal infection with Group A beta-hemolytic streptococci (GABHS) may play a role in OCD etiology. Some children may develop a predisposition to OCD after experiencing a streptococcal infection. A biological marker for a variant of rheumatic fever may identify children at risk of developing OCD after an untreated streptococcal infection. Researchers from Rockefeller University and the National Institutes of Mental Health suggest that OCD may be triggered by an abnormal reaction to streptococcal bacteria by the immune system.[8,9] Antibodies may go to the healthy brain and attack the caudate and subthalamic nuclei, causing a variant of rheumatic fever. In this process, the antibodies alert white blood cells to attack the healthy brain tissue, mistaking it for bacteria.

In contrast to childhood-onset OCD, an adult-onset neurobiologic subtype of OCD has also been proposed for some cases of OCD. Pregnancy and childbirth are particularly strong risk factors for new onset OCD. Recent reports suggest that women may have an increased risk for the onset of OCD during pregnancy and the puerperium.[10-12] Oxytocin, a nonapeptide produced in the hypothalamus, mediates several systemic functions (e.g., uterine contractions and the milk letdown reflex) and several CNS-related functions, such as attachment. In this subgroup of patients, CSF oxytocin has been correlated with OCD severity.

Pathophysiology

Serotonin dysfunction and certain neurocircuits are thought to be involved in OCD behavior.

Although OCD is hypothesized to be a manifestation of primary serotonin dysregulation, multiple neurotransmitters with serotonergic and dopaminergic activity are most likely involved in the cause of OCD. Serotonin has been implicated in mediating impulsivity, suicidality, aggression, and anxiety. Dysregulation of this behaviorally inhibitory neurotransmitter could possibly contribute to the repetitive obsessions and ritualistic behaviors seen in OCD patients. *(Please see Figure 4.)*

Functional neuroimaging studies of patients with OCD are consistent with right frontal lobe dysfunction. The neurobiological basis for OCD is suggested by: 1) OCD symptoms are found in conjunction with selected neurologic disorders; 2) Neuropsychological abnormalities are found in patients with OCD; 3) There are beneficial effects of psychosurgical procedures for some patients; and 4) There are consistent abnormalities found with structural and functional brain imaging in patients with OCD.[13]

Figure 2. Compulsive Symptoms at Admission

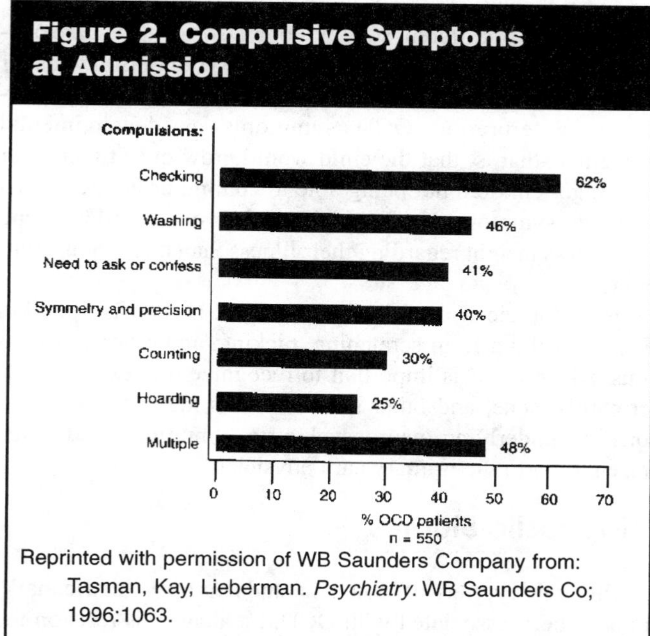

Reprinted with permission of WB Saunders Company from: Tasman, Kay, Lieberman. *Psychiatry.* WB Saunders Co; 1996:1063.

Clinical Features

OCD encompasses a broad range of symptoms that clinically can be grouped into four symptom categories:[14] 1) Cleanliness and washing—consistently paired washing and cleaning compulsions with contamination obsessions; 2) Aggression and checking—aggressive, sexual, and religious obsessions and checking compulsions; 3) Symmetry and ordering—combined compulsions of ordering and arranging, counting compulsions, and repeating rituals with obsessions of symmetry; and 4) Hoarding—hoarding obsessions correlated with hoarding behaviors and other collecting compulsions. *The Diagnostic and Statistical Manual of Mental Disorders*' criteria for OCD is depicted in Table 1.[15]

The most common obsession is concerned with contamination by dirt or germs; the accompanying compulsion is washing. Patients may spend several hours daily washing their hands, showering, or cleaning. They typically try to avoid sources of contamination, such as doorknobs, electrical switches, and newspapers. While they recognize that nothing will happen if they resist washing, they refuse to touch even their own bodies, knowing that if they do, they will not be at ease unless they perform extensive washing rituals.

Checkers are obsessed with doubt, usually tinged with guilt, and are frequently concerned that if they do not check carefully enough they will harm others. However, their checking often contributes to even greater doubt, which leads to further checking. Often, these patients will enlist the help of family and friends to ensure that they have checked enough or correctly. The checker ultimately resolves a particular doubt, only to have it replaced by a new one. Resistance, which, in this case, is the attempt to refrain from checking, leads to difficulty in concentrating and to exhaustion from the endless intrusion of nagging uncertainties. Common examples of such doubts are a fear of causing a fire, leading to checking the stove, to the extent that the patient cannot leave home; or a fear of hurting someone while driving, leading to repetitive driving back over the same spot after hitting a bump in the road. Hoarding behaviors can be seen as a corollary to checking behavior. Patients may refuse to throw out junk mail, old newspapers, or used tissues, for example, because they fear throwing away something important in the process.

Figure 3. Learning Theory of OCD

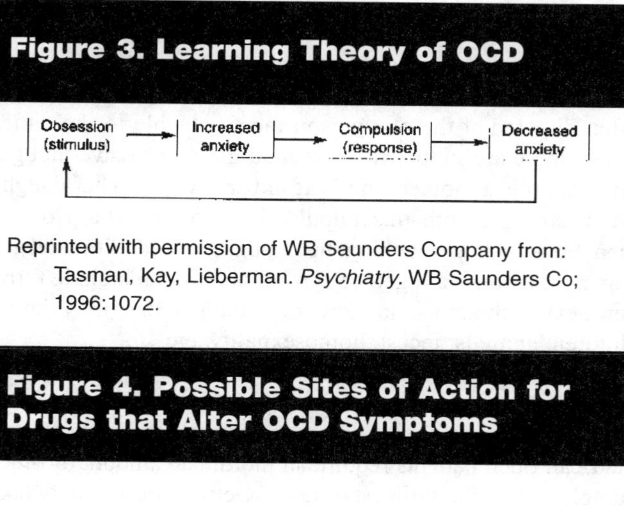

Reprinted with permission of WB Saunders Company from: Tasman, Kay, Lieberman. *Psychiatry.* WB Saunders Co; 1996:1072.

Figure 4. Possible Sites of Action for Drugs that Alter OCD Symptoms

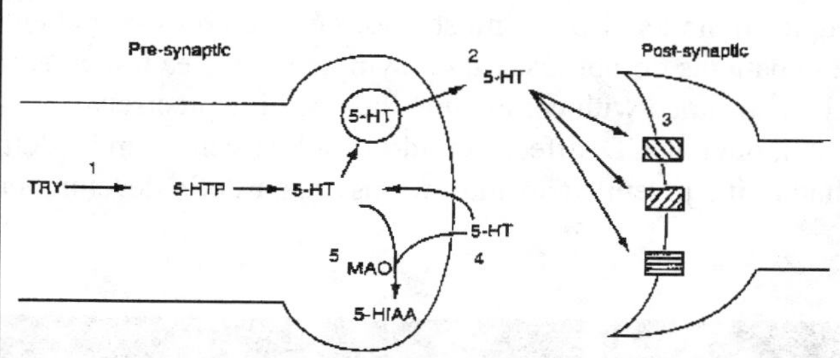

Diagram of a serotonin (5-HT) synapse describes several of the possible sites of action for drugs that alter OCD symptoms. At 1, the rate-limiting step in serotonin synthesis, L-tryptophan (TRY) is hydroxylated to 5-hydroxytryptophan (5-HTP). After serotonin is formed, it is sequestered into vesicles that are released at the presynaptic cell membrane (2). Fenfluramine increases this release. Once released, serotonin can interact with a number of different postsynaptic receptors (3). Several selective agonists (buspirone, m-chlorophenylpiperazine) have been developed to activate each of these serotonin receptor subtypes. Metergoline is a nonselective antagonist, blocking serotonin effects at each of these sites. The inactivation of serotonin is mediated by reuptake (4), the step inhibited by clomipramine, fluvoxamine, and fluoxetine. Finally (5), serotonin is either metabolized to its metabolite, 5-hydroxyindeleacetic acid (5-HIAA), by the enzyme monoamine oxidase (MAO), or recycled back into vesicles for release.

Reprinted with permission of WB Saunders Company from Tasman, Kay, Lieberman. *Psychiatry.* WB Saunders Co; 1996:1070.

Obsessional impulses may be aggressive or sexual, such as intrusive impulses of stabbing one's spouse or raping one's child. When the obsession is an aggressive impulse, it is most often directed at the one person most valuable to the patient. Often, there are subtle rituals around these obsessive thoughts. For example, a mother who is afraid she will stab her daughter might struggle with this impulse by avoiding sharp objects, then by avoiding touching her daughter, and ultimately, by leaving the house altogether. Sexual obsessions include forbidden sexual thoughts, images, or impulses that may involve children, animals, incest, homosexuality, etc.

Obsessional slowness involves the need to have objects or events in a certain order or position, to do and undo certain motor actions in an exact way, or to have things perfectly symmetrical. Such patients require an inordinate amount of time to complete even the simplest of tasks. Getting dressed may take a couple of hours. Unlike most obsessive-compulsive patients, these patients do not resist their symptoms. Instead, they seem to be consumed with completing their routine precisely.

Although OCD affects children, adolescents, and adults, whether it's juvenile and adult forms are part of a developmental continuum or different subtypes of a disorder that share phenotypic features remains unknown. OCD symptoms in younger children may not be identified readily. This may be due to parents misinterpreting OCD symptoms as developmental problems—that is, that the child would grow out of them—or to younger children not being able to communicate the severity of their symptoms as effectively as older ones. Children tend to have less insight regarding their illness than their adult counterparts.[16]

Dermatological manifestations of OCD consist of skin lesions resulting from scratching, picking, and other self-injurious behaviors. It is important to recognize that excoriations, dermatitis, acne, and other skin disorders may be manifestations of underlying neuropsychiatric conditions and often present only to the primary care physician.

Diagnostic Studies

Although a variety of biological and neuropsychiatric markers have been associated with OCD, the diagnosis rests on the psychiatric examination and history. Routine inquiry during the

Table 1. DSM-IV Diagnostic Criteria for Obsessive-Compulsive Disorder

A. Either obsessions or compulsions:

Obsessions as defined by (1), (2), (3), and (4):

1. Recurrent and persistent thoughts, impulses, or images that are experienced, at some time during the disturbance, as intrusive and inappropriate and that cause marked anxiety or distress.
2. The thoughts, impulses, or images are not simply excessive worries about real-life problems.
3. The person attempts to ignore or suppress such thoughts, impulses, or images or to neutralize them with some other thought or action.
4. The person recognizes that the obsessional thoughts, impulses, or images are a product of his or her own mind (not imposed from without as in thought insertion).

Compulsions as defined by (1) and (2):

1. Repetitive behaviors (e.g., handwashing, ordering, checking) or mental acts (e.g., praying, counting, repeating words silently) that the person feels driven to perform in response to an obsession or according to rules that must be applied rigidly.
2. The behaviors or mental acts are aimed at preventing or reducing distress or preventing some dreaded event or situation; however, these behaviors or mental acts are either not connected in a realistic way with what they are designed to neutralize or prevent or are clearly excessive.

B. At some point during the course of the disorder, the person has recognized that the obsessions or compulsions are excessive or unreasonable. Note: This does not apply to children.

C. The obsessions or compulsions cause marked distress, are time consuming (take more than 1 hour a day), or significantly interfere with the person's normal routing, occupational (or academic) functioning, or usual social activities or relationships.

D. If another Axis I disorder is present, the content of the obsessions or compulsions is not restricted to it (e.g., preoccupation with food in the presence of an eating disorder; hair pulling in the presence of trichotillomania; concern with appearance in the presence of body dysmorphic disorder; preoccupation with drugs in the presence of a substance use disorder; preoccupation with having a serious illness in the presence of hypochondriasis; preoccupation with sexual urges or fantasies in the presence of a paraphilia; or guilty ruminations in the presence of major depressive disorder).

E. The disturbance is not due to the direct physiological effects of a substance (e.g., a drug of abuse, a medication) or a general medical condition.

Specify if:

With poor insight: if, for most of the time during the current episode, the person does not recognize that the obsessions and compulsions are excessive or unreasonable.

review of systems regarding recurrent, intrusive thoughts or repetitive rituals can increase detection. Likewise, any complaint of anxiety or panic should be carefully investigated using a similar inquiry to rule out OCD. *(Please see Table 2.)* The four screening questions in Table 2 have an 85% sensitivity for OCD patients. If the answer to one of these questions is positive, the patient should be screened more fully with the symptom checklist and 10-item severity rating scale of the Yale-Brown Obsessive Compulsive Scale (Y-BOCS).

Differential Diagnosis

The differential diagnosis of OCD can be challenging. *(Please see Figure 5.)* Many patients prefer to keep their symptoms private from others and seek help for conditions caused by the OCD symptoms without identifying OCD as the problem. For example, studies have reported high frequency of medical patients in dermatology clinics who exhibited contamination obsessions and washing compulsions that produced

Table 2. Screening Questions for OCD

- Do you have to wash your hands over and over?
- Do you have to check things repeatedly?
- Do you have thoughts that come into your mind that cause distress and that you can't stop thinking about?
- Do you need to complete actions over and over until they are just right or in a certain way before you can move on to the next thing?

Table 3. Yale-Brown Obsessive-Compulsive Scale Symptom Checklist

Aggressive Obsessions
- Fear might harm others
- Fear might harm self
- Violent or horrific images
- Fear of blurting out obsessions or insults
- Fear of doing something embarrassing
- Fear of acting on other impulses (e.g., robbing a bank, stealing groceries, overeating)
- Fear of being responsible for things going wrong (e.g., others will lose their job because of patient)
- Fear something terrible might happen (e.g., fire, burglary)
- Other

Contamination Obsessions
- Concerns or disgust with bodily waste (e.g., urine, feces, saliva)
- Concern with dirt or germs
- Excessive concern with environmental contaminants (e.g., asbestos, radiation, toxic wastes)
- Excessive concern with household items (e.g., cleansers, solvents, pets)
- Concerned will become ill
- Concerned will become ill (aggressive)
- Other

Sexual Obsessions
- Forbidden or perverse sexual thoughts, images, or impulses
- Content involves children
- Content involves animals
- Content involves incest
- Content involves homosexuality
- Sexual behavior toward others (aggressive)
- Other

Hoarding or Collecting Obsessions

Religious Obsessions

Obsession with Need for Symmetry or Exactness

Miscellaneous Obsessions
- Need to know or remember
- Fear of saying certain things
- Fear of not saying things just right
- Intrusive (neutral) images
- Intrusive nonsense sounds, words, or music
- Other

Somatic Obsession-Compulsion

Cleaning or Washing Compulsions
- Excessive or ritualized hand washing
- Excessive or ritualized showering, bathing, brushing the teeth, or grooming
- Involves cleaning of household items or inanimate objects
- Other measures to prevent contact with contaminants

Counting Compulsions

Checking Compulsions
- Checking that did not or will not harm others
- Checking that did not or will not harm self
- Checking that nothing terrible did or will happen
- Checking for contaminants
- Other

Repeating Rituals

Ordering or Arranging Compulsions

Miscellaneous Compulsions
- Mental rituals (other than checking or counting)
- Need to tell, ask, or confess
- Need to touch
- Measures to prevent
  - Harm to self
  - Harm to others
  - Terrible consequences
- Other

Reprinted with permission of WB Saunders Company from: Tasman, Kay, Lieberman. *Psychiatry.* WB Saunders Co;. 1996:1062.

Figure 5. Differential Diagnosis of OCD

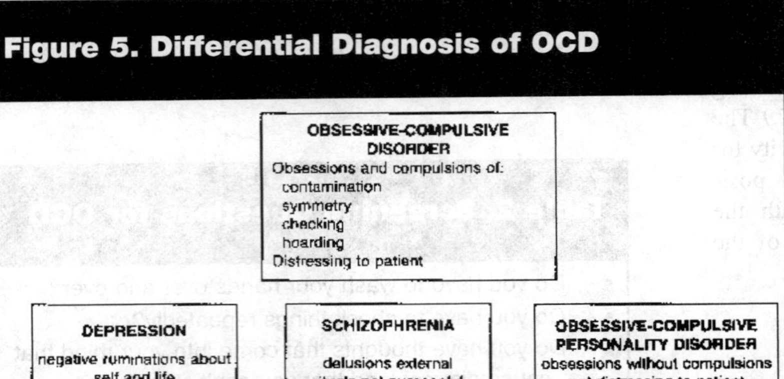

Reprinted with permission of WB Saunders Company from: Tasman, Kay, Lieberman. *Psychiatry*. WB Saunders Co; 1996:1073.

Figure 6. Flow Chart of Treatment Options for OCD

Treatment of OCD
Pharmacotherapy
Also consider
Behavioral therapy
1st-line SRIs:
sertraline—200 mg
fluvoxamine 300 mg
2nd-line SRIs:
clomipramine—250 mg
fluoxetine—80 mg
paroxetine—60 mg
Exposures with response prevention
Augmentors:
buspirone, lithium,
clonazepam,
trazodone,
alprazolam,
liothyronine
Also consider
Because of poor response.
1. Poor compliance
2. Comorbid depression
3. Use/Abuse of CNS depressants
4. Delusions
Try a 2nd SRI
Still unresponsive
For personality disorder
1. Psychotherapy
2. Day program
3. Halfway houses
For severely disabled patients
Consider psychosurgery:
1. After a minimum of two adequate medications
2. After behavioral treatment
3. Without severe personality disorder

Reprinted with permission of WB Saunders Company from: Tasman, Kay, Lieberman. *Psychiatry*. WB Saunders Co; 1996:1073.

dermatitis. In children, careful evaluation is needed to rule out normal developmental variations, depression, and autistic disorders.

A number of issues may be raised regarding the differential diagnosis of OCD. First, there may be some similarities in the diagnosis of OCD and obsessive-compulsive personality disorder. Both disorders reveal a preoccupation with aggression and control; however, OCD symptoms cause great distress to the patient, whereas the patient with personality disorder rarely resists his or her compulsive character and seldom has a sense of compulsion. Second, it may be difficult to distinguish between an obsession, such as contamination, and a delusion, such as being poisoned. The difference here is that an obsession is resisted and recognized as having an internal origin. A delusion is not resisted and is believed to be external. The schizophrenic is also distinguished by disorganized thinking and poor social functioning. If a schizophrenic patient has rituals, they are usually not purposeful and are in response to a threatening external force perceived by the patient.

Another important diagnostic issue concerns depression, the most common complication of OCD. At the clinical level, these illnesses often seem inseparable—one worsening or improving in synchronicity with the other. However, in other clinical cases, OCD symptoms may remain in remission while depression recurs. Depression can express itself through ruminations, but these are generally negative appraisals of the patient's self or life situation rather than the typical OCD patient's obsessions regarding contamination, symmetry, blasphemy, etc. It is important to note that in a study of 100 patients with OCD, 67% had a lifetime history of major depression. Some patients with OCD view their depressive symptoms as occurring secondary to the demoralization and hopelessness accompanying their symptoms of OCD, and report that they would not be depressed if they did not have OCD. Other patients view their major depressive symptoms as occurring independently of the symptoms of OCD. Symptoms of OCD in some patients intensify during depressive episodes, while other patients report that their OCD symptoms are less intense during depression because they feel too apathetic to be as concerned with their obsessions and too fatigued to perform compulsions.

Management

The goals of treatment are to reduce both the frequency and intensity of symptoms, although few patients experience a cure. Treatment response is generally considered to constitute at least a 25% reduction in OCD symptoms as measured by the Y-BOS score. It is misleading to assume that the drastic changes in the management of OCD in the last 10 years have simplified the management of this disorder. With the development of new selective serotonin reuptake inhibitors (SSRIs), attention has now focused on the need for long-term maintenance, on safety and efficacy in the pediatric ages, and on applicability in compulsive-like spectrum disorders. To optimally treat patients suffering from OCD, the clinician needs to integrate various approaches. A combination of pharmacotherapy and behavior therapy is the treatment of choice for OCD.[17] It is unusual for OCD patients to respond fully to either psychotherapeutic or pharmacologic interventions alone. A flow chart that outlines treatment options for OCD is shown in Figure 6.

The SSRIs differ among themselves, just as they do when compared with clomipramine, on specific pharmacokinetic

Table 4. Considerations in Patients with Obsessive-Compulsive Disorder in Whom Initial Treatment Fails

- Was the diagnosis correct?
- Is there an Axis II disorder, especially schizotypal or obsessive-compulsive personality disorder?
- Are there comorbid diagnoses that could interfere with treatment response?
- Is there a major depressive disorder?
- Are there obsessive thoughts, overvalued ideas, or delusions?
- Was the pharmacotherapy trial adequate?
- Was a known effective agent used?
- Was the dose adequate?
- Was the duration of treatment long enough?
- Was behavioral therapy performed?
- Were an adequate number of sessions attended?
- Did the patient comply with homework assignments?
- Was there cognitive impairment inhibiting the ability to implement treatment?
- Was there concurrent use of central nervous system depressants that affected ability to attend to evoked anxiety?

properties, which affect dosage issues, therapeutic monitoring, side effect profile, and drug-drug interaction. The prescribing physician is left with choosing from the SRI/SSRI family, which includes clomipramine, fluoxetine, sertraline, paroxetine, and fluvoxamine. Although clomipramine has been the most extensively studied, it has the greatest anticholinergic side effect profile of the agents. This may be desirable for patients who require a more sedating medication at bedtime or during the day. In patients with a high risk of suicide, clomipramine would not be the first choice of agents since it can be toxic in overdoses. In contrast, the SSRIs offer a less anticholinergic side effect profile but may be associated with more complaints of headaches, nausea, insomnia, and agitation. Generally, if an individual has had no response to the SSRI at 10-12 weeks, another SSRI may be attempted. Failure to respond to one SSRI does not necessarily predict failure to respond to another SSRI. With aggressive treatment, 80-90% of patients experience some improvement in their symptoms, although few patients become symptom free.

Behavior techniques most consistently effective in reducing compulsive rituals and obsessive thoughts are exposure to the feared situation or object, and response prevention in which the patient resists the urge to perform the compulsion after exposure. Exposure consists of asking the patient to interact with stimuli that result in the obsession or ritualistic behavior. Response prevention consists of delaying, diminishing, or discontinuing anxiety-reducing rituals. Behavior therapy produces the largest changes in rituals, such as compulsive cleaning or checking, whereas changes in obsessive thoughts are less predictable. However, 15-25% of patients refuse to engage in behavioral treatment or drop out early in treatment because it is so anxiety provoking. Family members need to help patients by not participating in the compulsive behavior and by supporting treatment compliance.

If a patient does not respond to a full dose of SSRI for at least 12 weeks and systematic behavior therapy has already been tried, consider other selective serotonin reuptake inhibitors. If the patient still does not respond after an adequate trial, consider augmenting the SSRI with buspirone (15-60 mg/d), trazodone (100-200 mg/d), lithium (300-600 mg/d), or L-tryptophan (2-4 mg/d), each for approximately one month. It is advisable to refer the patient for pharmacological consultation. *(Please see Table 4.)* Severe refractory obsessive-compulsive patients may benefit from neurosurgery, which disconnects the outflow pathways from the orbitofrontal cortex.[18]

Disposition

In most cases, no particular stress or event precipitates the onset of OCD symptoms, and following an insidious onset there is a chronic and often progressive course. The natural history of OCD may be characterized by waxing and waning symptoms, but more than half of patients have chronic courses. Without treatment, symptoms usually remain constant or worsen. The disorder has a major impact on daily functioning, with some patients spending all their waking hours consumed with their obsessions and rituals. Patients are often socially isolated, marry at an older age, and have high celibacy rates (particularly in males) and a low fertility rate. Early age of onset is predictive of poor prognosis and multiple obsessions and compulsions.[17] OCD symptoms are often exacerbated by depression. Moreover, persons with OCD and comorbid psychiatric illness have a significantly higher rate of suicide attempts.

Summary

OCD is a common but underrecognized disorder, characterized by repetitive thoughts and behaviors that cause significant functional impairment. Diagnosis is not difficult if one is aware of its prevalence and the different ways it is expressed. Because OCD patients often attempt to conceal their symptoms, it is incumbent on clinicians to screen for OCD, since appropriate treatment can often result in improved quality of life. There have been many new developments in the management of obsessive-compulsive disorder during the past decade. Only the selective serotonin reuptake inhibitors (SSRIs) and clomipramine are consistent in controlling obsessive-compulsive symptoms. To maximize recovery, patients must undergo behavioral therapy along with drug therapy. In many communities, self-help groups exist for OCD. As in other self-help groups, OCD group members share their experiences, educate one another, provide mutual support, and reduce the individual's sense of being alone with this disorder.

References

1. Flament M, et al. Obsessive-compulsive disorder in adolescence: An epidemiologic study. *J Am Acad Child Adolesc Psychiatry* 1988;27:764-771.
2. Valleni-Basile LA, et al. Frequency of obsessive-compulsive disorder in a community sample of adolescents. *J Am Acad Child Adolesc Psychiatry* 1994;33:782-791.
3. Black JL. Obsessive-compulsive disorder: A clinical update. *Mayo Clin Proc* 1992;67:266-275.
4. Marks IM. *Fears, Phobias and Rituals*. Oxford: Oxford University Press; 1987.
5. Roy A. Obsessive-compulsive phenomenology. Outcome and comparison with hysterical neurosis. *Compr Psychiatry* 1979; 20:528-531.
6. Minichiello WE, et al. Age of onset of major subtypes of obsessive-compulsive disorder. *J Anxiety Disord* 1990;4:147-150.
7. Rachman SL, Hodgson RJ. *Obsessions and Compulsions*. Englewood Cliffs, NJ: Prentice Hall; 1980.
8. Swedo S. Sydenham's chorea: A model for childhood autoimmune neuropsychiatric disorders. *JAMA* 1994;272:1788-1791.
9. Swedo S, et al. Identification of children with pediatric autoimmune neuropsychiatric disorders associated with streptococcal infections by a marker associated with rheumatic fever. *Am J Psychiatry* 1997;154:110-112.
10. Buttolph ML, Holland A. Obsessive-compulsive disorders in pregnancy and childbirth. In: Jenike M, Baer L, Minichiello WE, eds. *Obsessive Compulsive Disorders, Theory and Management*. Chicago, IL: Yearbook Medical Publishers; 1990.
11. Neziroglu F, et al. Onset of obsessive-compulsive disorder in pregnancy. *Am J Psychiatry* 1992;149:947-950.
12. Sichel DA, et al. Postpartum obsessive compulsive disorder: A case series. *J Clin Psychiatry* 1993;54:156-159.
13. Trivedi M. Functional neuroanatomy of obsessive-compulsive disorder. *J Clin Psychiatry* 1996;57(suppl):26-35.
14. Leckman JF, et al. Symptoms of obsessive-compulsive disorder. *Am J Psychiatry* 1997;154:911-917.
15. *Diagnostic and Statistical Manual of Mental Disorders*. DSM-IV. 4th ed. Washington, DC: American Psychiatric Press; 1994.
16. Foa EB, Kozak MJ. The DSM-IV field trial: Obsessive-compulsive disorder. *Am J Psychiatry* 1995;152:90-96.
17. Griest JH, et al. Efficacy and tolerability of serotonin transport inhibitors in obsessive-compulsive disorder: A meta-analysis. *Arch Gen Psychiatry* 1995;52:53-60.
18. Mindus P, Jenike M. Neurosurgical treatment of malignant obsessive-compulsive disorder. *Psychiatr Clin North Am* 1992;15:921-938.
19. Ackerman DL, et al. Predictors of treatment response in obsessive-compulsive disorder: Multivariate analyses from a multicenter trial of clomipramine. *J Clin Psychopharmacol* 1994;14:247-254.

Eating Disorders

Randy A. Sansone, MD
Lori A. Sansone, MD
Michael W. Widerman, PhD

The eating disorders anorexia and bulimia nervosa continue to be clinical concerns for all primary care physicians. These disorders show no sign of abating in prevalence, perhaps because both are perpetuated by dieting behavior, body preoccupation, and a drive for thinness—all crucial elements for "success" in a culture plagued with overweight individuals. In the United States, one-third of all adults[1] as well as one-half of black and Hispanic women are overweight.[2] The diet industry is flourishing, including avid interest in pharmaceutical agents that will control eating behavior. These are the sociocultural times that perpetuate body scrutiny and fears of fatness. These are the times of eating disorders.

Eating Disorder Diagnoses

In the *Diagnostic and Statistical Manual of Mental Disorders,* Fourth Edition (DSM-IV), there are three general categories of eating disorder diagnoses.[3] Two represent relatively homogeneous disorders (i.e., anorexia nervosa, bulimia nervosa), and a third category (i.e., eating disorder, not otherwise specified) encompasses a variety of other eating disordered behaviors.

Anorexia Nervosa. According to the criteria in DSM-IV, anorexia nervosa is characterized by: 1) a body weight that is below normal (i.e., < 85% of expected body weight); 2) intense fears of weight gain despite being underweight; 3) body image disturbance resulting in the misperception of one's weight or shape, undue self-evaluation based upon weight, or denial of the seriousness of the current low weight; and 4) in postmenarchal females, the absence of at least three consecutive menstrual cycles.[3] For a DSM-IV diagnosis of anorexia nervosa, individuals must meet all four criteria.

There are two subtypes of anorexia nervosa. The first, *restricting type,* is characterized by restrictive eating patterns that do not entail binge-eating or purging behavior. The second, *binge-eating/purging type,* includes binge-eating episodes followed by purging behavior. Although the definition of a clinical binge is yet to be defined in terms of calories or food volume, a practical guide in the clinical setting is 2500 calories, or 2.5 times the normal amount of food. Binges are characterized by a lack of control over food intake during a discrete period of time (usually < 2 hours). Purging behaviors entail acute and active efforts to eradicate ingested calories and may include self-induced vomiting and/or the use of laxatives, diuretics, or enemas. In the primary care setting, a substantial number of patients may present with sub-syndromal eating disorders (i.e., eating disorder behaviors that are either very time-limited or do not meet full criteria for diagnosis).

Bulimia Nervosa. According to DSM-IV, bulimia nervosa is characterized by: 1) episodes of binge eating; 2) recurrent inappropriate behaviors that are intended to compensate for the ingested calories or prevent weight gain (e.g., self-induced vomiting; the use of laxatives, diuretics, or enemas; fasting; excessive exercise); 3) a frequency of bulimic episodes, on average, of at least twice per week for a period of three months; and 4) undue self-evaluation based on body weight or shape.[3] For a DSM-IV diagnosis of bulimia nervosa, all criteria must be met.

Bulimia nervosa is further sub-divided into two groups: 1) purging type and 2) non-purging type. In the clinical setting, bulimia nervosa, purging type, is the most frequent eating disorder diagnosis. Purging type is characterized by compensatory purging behaviors such as self-induced vomiting or the use of laxatives, diuretics, or enemas. An unusual example is the avoidance of insulin use in diabetes, resulting in glycosuria, to control weight following binges.[4] Non-purging type is characterized by compensatory behaviors that are non-invasive yet counter-regulatory; examples include fasting or excessive exercise. As in anorexia nervosa, individuals in the primary care setting may present with sub-syndromal bulimia nervosa (e.g., experimentation with purging behaviors following episodes of overeating).

Eating Disorder, Not Otherwise Specified. This DSM-IV diagnosis is reserved for those eating disorder patterns that fall outside the descriptions of anorexia or bulimia nervosa.[3] Examples include low-weight patients who routinely purge small amounts of food (i.e., restricter purgers) or bulimic individuals in whom criteria are not met regarding frequency of episodes.

Binge-Eating Disorder. Within the appendix, DSM-IV also includes criteria for diagnostic proposals, primarily constructed by researchers, which are provided for further study.[3] Included in this appendix is one final eating disorder diagnosis, binge-eating disorder. Like bulimia nervosa, binge-eating disorder is characterized by episodes of binge eating. The binge-eating episodes must meet at least three of the following criteria: 1) eating more rapidly than normal; 2) eating until uncomfortably full; 3) eating despite not feeling physically hungry; 4) eating alone due to embarrassment about the quantities of food being consumed; and 5) experiencing a negative effect after eating (e.g., disgust with oneself, depressed feelings, guilt). In addition, there must be marked distress with binge eating and a binge-eating frequency of at least two days a week for six months. Individuals with binge-eating disorder do not use any inappropriate compensatory methods such as purging behaviors, fasting, or excessive exercise. Many, if not most, of these individuals are overweight, and among a significant minority, there may be a comorbid diagnosis of borderline personality disorder.[5] Because this eating disorder remains a diagnostic proposal, the remainder of this article will focus primarily on anorexia and bulimia nervosas.

Epidemiology

Precise data regarding the epidemiology of eating disorders in the United States are scant, but it is clear that eating disorders are most prevalent among adolescent and young adult women. Within this group, the prevalence of anorexia nervosa appears to be 0.5-1% compared to the 1-3% prevalence for bulimia nervosa.[6,7] The prevalence among males in the same age range is about one-tenth that of females.[3] The onset of anorexia nervosa typically occurs during adolescence, whereas the onset of bulimia nervosa usually occurs later, during adolescence or early adulthood.

There has been much speculation about the apparent increased incidence of eating disorders, but research suggests that the incidence has not increased as much as the public and medical recognition of these disorders.[6,8] More importantly, from a clinical perspective, disordered eating exists along a continuum of severity, with subclinical or sub-syndromal cases being at least twice as prevalent as those meeting full diagnostic criteria.[9]

Etiology of Eating Disorders

Eating disorders are conceptualized as multi-factorial disorders (i.e., disorders due to a variety of causes) that culminate in a final common pathway. One etiological factor is cultural influences. As the affluent North American culture struggles with overweight and obesity, the body ideal becomes that which is most difficult to achieve—the physique of thinness. Both anorexia and bulimia nervosa are eating disorders that are preceded by dieting behavior.

In examining genetic factors, studies suggest that, compared with controls, family members of individuals with eating disorders, especially bulimia nervosa, appear to have significantly higher rates of mood disorders,[10] substance abuse,[11] and other psychiatric disorders.[12] In addition, serotonin appears intimately involved with satiety. These findings broach the possibility of a non-specific but contributory factor at a genetic (e.g., neurotransmitter) level.

Many individuals with eating disorders, particularly those with anorexia nervosa, have a personality style highlighted by perfectionism, strong needs to achieve, and obsessive-compulsive behaviors.[13] This psychological style readily compliments the rigors inherent in dieting behavior (i.e., counting calories or fat grams, scheduling and timing exercise, categorizing foods as acceptable or not), and in turn, successful dieting and weight loss reinforce the illusion of self-control and mastery.

Some individuals exist in family environments that are excessively health- or weight-conscious. These families tend to overly emphasize body weight, eating behavior, food selection, and exercise. A more ominous family factor is sexual abuse, in which the eating disorder symptoms function as a means to avoid further abuse through the loss of sexual characteristics that are attractive to others.[14] A variety of interpersonal factors may contribute to the development of an eating disorder.[14] For example, the normal developmental demands of separation-individuation from the family can be suspended through the development of a debilitating eating disorder. The eating disorder may function as a form of non-verbal protest to parents, particularly in families where open protest is not normally tolerated. Achieving the fantasized ideal body may fulfill the limitless expectations of adolescence as well as result in a unique arena of competition with peers. Finally, in a world that appears devoid of caring, eating disorder symptoms may function to elicit validating emotional responses, such as concern, from family and peers.

In addition to the preceding contributory factors, among many cases, there is an acute situational event that precipitates the onset of eating disorder symptoms. Examples of these include parental divorce, loss of a significant relationship, or a family relocation. These situational stressors appear to mobilize the various underlying risk factors of an individual, resulting in the need for enhanced control or emotional homeostasis, which is actualized through the emergence of eating disorder symptoms.

Office Demeanor of the Patient

Anorexia Nervosa. When the individual suffering from anorexia nervosa presents to the primary care physician for evaluation of weight loss or a condition related to weight loss (e.g., amenorrhea), there is often an indifference to the eating disorder symptoms. Emaciated individuals with anorexia nervosa are often aloof, irritable, dysphoric, withdrawn, and hostile. These features are due to the biological stress of malnutrition and starvation as well as the patient's fear that treatment will entail weight gain. On occasion, some patients deny obvious signs and symptoms (e.g., hair loss, cold insensitivity, fatigue), dieting efforts, body preoccupation, or concern about weight loss. Others focus on specific symptoms such as amenorrhea or sleep disturbance, while avoiding disclosure of the underlying eating disorder.

Bulimia Nervosa. Individuals with bulimia nervosa are typically engaging, expressive, and interactive. Although many suffer from mood disorders or mood lability, the professional encounter is far more social than those with individuals suffering from anorexia nervosa. Although some individuals with bulimia nervosa attempt to hide symptoms, many, if not most, respond candidly to compassionate inquiries about related signs and symptoms.

Assessment

Anorexia Nervosa. In the assessment of anorexia nervosa, the history is of utmost importance in confirming DSM-IV criteria, particularly the verification of dieting behavior. Indications of dieting behavior include preoccupation with body weight or specific body areas, attempts to restrict calories and fatty foods, frequent weighings, mirror gazing, conversation that is riddled with food and weight content, meal avoidance, preoccupation with clothes size, and attempts to hide weight loss with bulky clothing. An accurate history may need to be elicited from a parent or significant other.

During the initial appointment, the physical examination should include blood pressure, height, and weight in underwear and gown. General physical findings include emaciation as well as evidence of slowed metabolic and physiological functions. *(Please see Figure.)* The patient may have lanugo, a fine, downy body hair that is particularly prominent on the arms, torso, and face, and may be an adaptive attempt to maintain body heat in the presence of depleted body fat.

Physical examination may disclose cardiovascular complications, which are fairly common and the most likely cause of death in anorexia nervosa.[15] In addition to bradycardia and orthostatic hypotension, findings may include abnormalities in mitral valve motion, decreased left ventricular chamber dimension and mass, reduction in cardiac index due to low stroke index and heart rate, higher peripheral resistance, and systolic dysfunction.[16] Across studies, the crude mortality rate in anorexia nervosa is approximately 6%, which is, in part, contributed to by sudden death.[17]

During psychological assessment, the patient may appear indifferent to the weight loss (denial). On mental status examination, affect is typically flat, and eye contact is poor. The patient's eyes may have a lackluster appearance due to the effects of starvation. Other observations may include impairment in concentration, lack of cooperation, limited verbalization, and dysphoric mood.

Affective disorders are difficult to assess in patients with poor nutritional intake or starvation. Many of the effects of the starvation state itself mimic depression (e.g., fatigue, dysphoria, irritability, poor concentration, sleep disturbance). Therefore, in low-weight patients, a diagnosis of underlying affective disorder should be tempered with an awareness of the contributory effects of starvation.

In addition to affective disorders, eating disorder patients may suffer from personality disorder.[13] Personality disorders are grouped into three clusters (i.e., A, B, C) according to descriptive similarities. Among restricting individuals with anorexia nervosa, the most common personality disturbances are those in Cluster C (e.g., fearful or anxious personality styles such as avoidant, obsessive-compulsive, dependent personality disorders).[13] Among those with binge-purge behaviors, Cluster B personality disturbances are most common (e.g., dramatic, erratic, or emotional personality styles such as borderline, histrionic, narcissistic personality disorders).[13]

A general laboratory screen is usually sufficient in the assessment of anorexia nervosa. Among individuals who purge, the determination of electrolyte status is the most imminent concern, particularly serum potassium status. Although individuals with anorexia nervosa may demonstrate a variety of laboratory abnormalities *(please see Table)*,[18,19] these usually manifest only in extreme cases of starvation. An electrocardiogram is indicated in those individuals with cardiac symptoms, extremely low body weight (loss of > 25% of the original body weight), or histories of exposure to Syrup of Ipecac.

In general, starvation effects are most pronounced among individuals with acute and extreme weight loss and older individuals. Those individuals with previous histories of medical complications at specific low body weights (e.g., cardiac arrhythmias including conduction blocks) need to be carefully monitored during relapses to the same threshold weight.

Bulimia Nervosa. As in anorexia nervosa, the history is paramount to the DSM-IV diagnosis of bulimia nervosa. Binge eating patterns appear to develop in the aftermath of restrictive dieting efforts, and, therefore, a history of dieting behavior is usually present. It is important to screen for the presence of clearly defined binge-eating episodes as well as all possible compensatory behaviors (e.g., self-induced vomiting; the use of laxatives, diuretics, enemas, Syrup of Ipecac; food restriction; exercise).

On physical examination, findings are closely related to the method of purging or compensatory behavior.[20,21] Self-induced vomiting, the most common form of purging in a clinical population, has varying frequencies from occasional to multiple times per day. Whereas some patients are able to spontaneously vomit, most induce a gag reflex. Food types seem to vary in their ease of purgation, and binge foods may be selected, in part, for this characteristic. In addition, self-induced vomiting may be facilitated by volume loading, fluid loading, or manual abdominal pressure.

Self-induced vomiting tends to precipitate upper gastrointestinal complications. Dental erosion, or perimylolysis, may result in discoloration of tooth enamel, temperature sensitivity of the teeth, spaces or gaps between teeth, loose fillings or amalgams due to the erosion of the supporting tooth, and a receding distal surface of the upper front teeth (note that the tongue protects the lower front teeth during vomiting). In extreme cases, the deterioration in dentition may result in extensive crown work (particularly the six upper front teeth) or dentures.

Salivary gland enlargement (parotid and/or submandibular) occurs in some individuals who induce vomiting. The enlargement is nearly always bilateral, and the glands may be tender to palpation. Among

Table. Possible Laboratory Abnormalitiesin Anorexia Nervosa[18,19]

HEMATOLOGIC
Anemia
Leukopenia
Thrombocytopenia
Reduced erythocyte sedimentation rate
Impaired cell-mediated immunity
METABOLIC
Hypercholesterolemia
Hypocalcemia
Hypomagnesemia
Hypophosphatemia
Hypokalemia (vomiting, laxatives, diuretics)
ENDOCRINOLOGIC
Hypercortisolemia
Hypoglycemia
Elevated growth hormone levels
Reduced estrogen levels
Reduced basal levels of luteinizing and follicle-stimulating hormones
GASTROINTESTINAL
Elevated liver function tests
Elevated amylase (vomiting)

those individuals who are susceptible to this complication, enlargement recedes in 4-6 weeks with the cessation of vomiting. We are aware of no long-term medical complications related to salivary gland enlargement.

When vomiting is induced by a gag reflex using the hand or fingers, there may be small cuts, excoriations, or calluses on the hand, particularly in the area of the knuckles. These findings are usually unilateral and involve the dominant hand.

The exposure of the upper gastrointestinal tract to gastric acid may result in frequent sore throats as well as esophageal irritation (i.e., heartburn). Vomiting due to any cause may result in aspiration and a resulting chemical pneumonitis. In addition, the internal forces generated with the act of vomiting may precipitate small mucosal tears along the gastroesophageal juncture (Mallory-Weiss tears), resulting in hematemesis. On very rare occasion, the muscular layer of the esophagus or stomach may rupture during self-induced vomiting (Borhaave's syndrome, which has a reported mortality rate of 25%[22]).

Finally, some individuals with eating disorders use Syrup of Ipecac to induce vomiting. The active emetic agent, emetine, has a long half-life, accumulates with frequent dosing, and induces cardiac arrhythmias.[23] Emetine is also known to cause myopathies resulting in muscle weakness of the neck and proximal muscles of the extremities.[23]

Like self-induced vomiting, laxative abuse varies in frequency and amount. While some individuals use laxatives only episodically, others ingest 10-20 or more per day. In our practice, we have had three individuals who ingested 150 laxative units per day and one patient who sporadically ingested 500 units per day. Laxative abuse can cause acute as well as chronic lower gastrointestinal complications.

The acute effects of laxative loads may include abdominal distention, discomfort, pain, and bloating; nausea; vomiting; and constipation. Chronic laxative abuse may lead to laxative dependence (i.e., reliance on laxatives, no significant physiological damage) or cathartic colon (i.e., physiological damage to the colon characterized by thinning of the muscular and mucosal layers, loss of propulsion, areas of spasm called pseudostrictures, and low-grade inflammation).

The abuse of senna or cascara-containing laxatives may produce a discoloration of the lower colon and rectum (melanosis coli), which causes no physiological impairment and disappears 4-12 months after discontinuing laxatives. In addition, laxatives that contain phenolphthalein can result in fixed drug eruptions in sensitive individuals. Fixed drug eruptions are inflammatory reactions on the skin surface that resolve leaving residual pigmentation. Re-exposure to the offending agent results in an inflammatory response in the same location (i.e., "fixed"), and the subsequent resolution is characterized by a deepening of the pigmentation.

In our experience, diuretic abuse is the least frequent form of purgation among eating disorder patients, particularly those in younger age groups. Some individuals who abuse diuretics appear to have unusual forms of body image disturbance (i.e., dysmorphophobic features) that impede treatment efforts to discontinue these drugs. Diuretic abuse, like self-induced vomiting and laxative abuse, can lower serum potassium levels. When potassium levels are chronically low, it is possible to develop hypokalemic nephropathy. Therefore, in addition to acute potassium depletion and its medical complications (e.g., paresthesias, fatigue, cardiac arrhythmias, tetany, seizures), chronic potassium depletion takes its toll. Diuretic abuse should always be suspected in patients with unexpectedly low serum potassium levels without other co-existing medical problems or associated prescribed medications.

The focus of psychological assessment is the determination of possible comorbid psychiatric conditions. In bulimia nervosa, acute mood disturbances may be 1) intermittent (e.g., episodic lability and irritability) and directly related to eating disorder behaviors or 2) sustained (i.e., a bonafide affective disorder). Therefore, the clinical task is to determine if acute affective symptoms among patients with bulimia nervosa are sustained to a degree that they meet criteria for major depression (e.g., at least 2 weeks in duration). Bulimic symptoms, themselves, may have a seasonal pattern[24] or undergo premenstrual exacerbation,[25] both observations suggesting a mood component among some individuals.

Borderline personality disorder may be a comorbid psychiatric condition, especially in the presence of impulsive behaviors such as binge eating and purging. Borderline personality is a longstanding disorder characterized by chronic impulsivity (i.e., self-regulation difficulties, self-destructive behavior), unstable interpersonal relationships, and dysphoric affect which is coupled with an intact social facade. It is highlighted by chronic self-destructive behavior. Among individuals with eating disorder symptoms and self-destructive behaviors that are unrelated to food and weight issues (e.g., suicide attempts, promiscuity, substance abuse), this personality disorder is likely. Studies indicate that the co-existence of eating disorder symptoms and substance abuse is highly associated with a diagnosis of borderline personality disorder.[26] The presence of comorbid borderline personality disorder in an eating disorder patient indicates that treatment will be more complicated and long-term, and behavioral improvement will evolve slowly, as illustrated in those with substance abuse.[27] For further information about borderline personality disorder in the primary care setting, the reader is referred to other sources.[28,29]

Other psychiatric comorbidity may include dysthymia (chronic depression) or panic disorder (the latter sometimes associated with the weight loss, itself). Patients with trauma histories may have symptoms of post-traumatic stress disorder including dissociative symptoms.

Laboratory examination among individuals with bulimia nervosa is usually unremarkable, with the exception of an occasionally low serum potassium level. Therefore, in most instances, a general laboratory screen is sufficient. In the absence of a low serum potassium level, cardiac symptoms, or a pre-existing cardiac history, an electrocardiogram is not routinely indicated. Electrocardiograms are indicated in those individuals using Syrup of Ipecac.

Less frequent findings may include hyperamylasemia (which may correlate to the frequency of binging and purging);[30] and hypocalcemia, hyperchloremia, and steatorrhea (which may be associated with laxative abuse).

Management in the Primary Care Setting

Anorexia Nervosa. An ongoing task in the management of anorexia nervosa is to weigh the patient with each visit. Weighings should be standardized. For individuals not previously overweight, weight loss of more than 25% of the previous body weight will require referral to a structured refeeding program in a specialized inpatient or day treatment program for eating disorder patients. In patients with lesser degrees of weight loss, outpatient psychological management by a mental health professional with experience in eating disorders is indicated.

The primary care physician should review and address laboratory abnormalities, including hypokalemia and abnormal cardiac findings. Avoid the treatment of starvation-induced hypothyroidism, as thyroid replacement may accelerate weight loss. A DEXA scan should be considered for patients with low body weight of more than six months duration.[31] To protect the patient's bone mass, preventive hormonal replacement therapy may be initiated,[31] although low-weight patients may not evidence significant benefit.[32]

Triage comorbid psychiatric conditions, when present. For example, quickly address imminent problems (e.g., suicidal ideation will require psychiatric hospitalization) and assess pre-existing depression, which will require antidepressant treatment. In low-weight patients, avoid antidepressants with marked cardiovascular effects (e.g., tricyclic antidepressants), and elect antidepressants with anti-obsessional features (i.e., selective serotonin reuptake inhibitors). Note, however, that responses to antidepressant medications are tempered by the starvation state, which may be the cause of, or a contributory factor to, the current psychiatric symptoms. To date, no psychotropic medication has been shown to consistently induce weight gain or change the core features of anorexia nervosa.[33] Consider psychiatric consultation for patients with extensive psychiatric comorbidity, with atypical presentations, or who are unresponsive to routine intervention.

The primary care physician should engage a mental health professional who is experienced in the treatment of eating disorders to begin psychological treatment with the patient. Anorexia nervosa is a psychiatric disorder, and the earlier the psychological intervention, the better the prognosis. Psychological intervention may include a structured outpatient refeeding program, cognitive-behavioral therapy, individual psychotherapy, and/or group or family therapy. Support groups may also be helpful. For a given individual, the various contributory etiologies generally dictate which treatments are selected.

During the ongoing psychological treatment, continue to provide medical support, including periodic assessment of electrolytes for patients who purge, monitoring of body weight, and education and support to family members and the patient with regard to the disorder and the treatment. Among some patients, acute medical intervention will be indicated for emergent medical complications such as cardiac arrhythmias. Among others, education will be important (e.g., a body weight within approximately 90% of standard body weight for height is usually necessary for a return of menses).[34]

When treating the patient with an eating disorder, address purging behaviors with the following recommendations. For patients who induce vomiting, encourage the use of fluoride-containing toothpastes, fluoride treatments through the dentist, and sodium bicarbonate rinses after vomiting. For patients who are laxative-dependent, encourage gradual weaning of laxatives, gradual increase in dietary fiber, adequate hydration, and the use of non-stimulant laxatives should constipation develop in the future. Patients who undergo laxative weaning will also need reassurance and support regarding the fluid retention that may develop shortly after the cessation of laxatives. Barium studies may be indicated in the rare patient who has symptoms or a history suggestive of cathartic colon. For patients who abuse diuretics, discontinue prescribed diuretics, actively discourage over-the-counter diuretic use, monitor serum potassium levels, and observe the patient for rebound edema. An electrocardiogram should be obtained in those patients who are abusing Syrup of Ipecac.

Bulimia Nervosa. The recommendations for bulimia nervosa are similar to those for anorexia nervosa, with the following modifications. First, because most individuals with bulimia nervosa are within a normal weight range, an initial weighing is probably sufficient unless the patient begins to lose weight. Second, electrolyte status is most important in the assessment of the majority of patients with bulimia nervosa, particularly serum potassium levels. Third, psychiatric comorbidity may include personality disorder (particularly borderline personality), substance abuse, and/or mood disorder. Comorbidity may indicate the need for psychiatric consultation. Fourth, it is essential to consult a mental health professional with experience in the treatment of eating disorders. Psychological treatment may entail cognitive-behavioral therapy, individual psychotherapy, group therapy with other bulimic individuals, and nutritional counseling. Most individuals can be treated in an outpatient setting. Fifth, continuing medical support most frequently entails: 1) periodic evaluation and treatment of electrolyte status; 2) review of interventions for specific purging behaviors, as noted previously; 3) encouraging routine contact with a dentist; and 4) prescription of antidepressants.

In our experience, the use of antidepressants is a low-risk, potentially high-yield intervention. We recommend beginning with fluoxetine, sertraline, or paroxetine (i.e., selective serotonin reuptake inhibitors). Antidepressants appear to reduce binge/purge behavior, even in the absence of a mood disorder.[33] In addition, selective serotonin reuptake inhibitors alleviate the ruminative, obsessive psychological style that characterizes many of these patients.

The collaborative efforts of the primary care physician and the mental health professional are of paramount importance in treating patients with eating disorders. In many cases, there may be a team of professionals including a primary care physician, psychiatrist, nonphysician mental health professional, dietitian, and support group leader. Eating disorders exist along a behavioral continuum, and those patients with more severe and frequent eating disordered behaviors will require more professional support.

Outcome of Eating Disorders

Anorexia Nervosa. Outcome studies in the field of eating disorders are fraught with methodological concerns (e.g., inpatient vs outpatient populations, prevalence of comorbid personality disorders, determination of outcome measures). In one recent study, one-fourth of patients fully recovered, while two-thirds subsequently developed bulimic behavior.[35] A general clinical maxim is that one-third of patients fully recover, one-third improve, and one-third remain meaningfully impaired. This latter third is characterized by psychiatric comorbidity, particularly personality disorder. In addition, lower weight at treatment entry appears to be a predictor for lower weight at long-term follow-up.[36] Other long-term concerns in individuals with anorexia nervosa include osteoporosis secondary to reduced bone mass,[32,37] decreased fertility[38] as well as a higher risk of prematurity and perinatal mortality,[39] persistent gray matter volume deficits after weight recovery,[40] and mortality (around 6%).[17,35] Abnormally low serum albumin levels (< 36 g/L) and low body weight (< 60% of average), at initial examination, may be predictors of a lethal course.[41]

Bulimia Nervosa. The long-term outcome for women with bulimia nervosa remains unclear.[42] Greater impulsivity may be a predictor variable for poor outcome.[43] In our clinical experience, relapse rates are fairly high and parallel increases in psychosocial stressors. In one study, one-third of patients relapsed within two years of treatment; relapse was associated with younger age and higher frequency of self-induced vomiting before treatment.[44]

Other long-term concerns in bulimia nervosa include dental erosion and hypokalemic nephropathy. In addition, up to 50% of normal-weight women with bulimia nervosa have disturbed menstrual function that may be associated with an abnormal 24-hour luteinizing hormone secretion, particularly if current weight is less than 85% of past high weight.[45]

Summary

The treatment and outcome of patients with eating disorders is clearly a concern for all professionals in primary care settings. Studies indicate that patients who endorse eating disorder symptoms on questionnaire, as well as obese individuals (a significant number who probably have binge-eating disorder), have greater healthcare utilization in the primary care setting.[46,47] The primary care physician is in a unique role—one that may facilitate early diagnosis of these patients. Early diagnosis is a fundamental element in the successful treatment of individuals with eating disorders.[48]

References

1. Kuczmarski RJ, Flegal KM, Campbell SM, et al. Increasing prevalence of overweight among US adults: The national health and nutrition examination surveys, 1960-1991. *JAMA* 1994; 272:205-211.
2. Rand CS, Kuldau JM. The epidemiology of obesity and self-defined weight problem in the general population: Gender, race, age, and social class. *Int J Eat Disord* 1990;9:329-343.
3. American Psychiatric Association. *Diagnostic and Statistical Manual of Mental Disorders,* Fourth Edition. Washington, DC: American Psychiatric Association; 1994.
4. Hudson JI, Hudson MS, Wentworth SM. Self-induced glycosuria. A novel method of purging in bulimia. *JAMA* 1983;249:2501.
5. Specker S, de Zwaan M, Raymond N, et al. Psychopathology in subgroups of obese women with and without binge eating disorder. *Compr Psychiatry* 1994;35:185-190.
6. Fombonne E. Anorexia nervosa: no evidence of an increase. *Br J Psychiatry* 1995;166:462- 471.
7. Hsu LKG. Epidemiology of the eating disorders. *Psychiatr Clin North Am* 1996;19:681-700.
8. Fombonne E. Is bulimia nervosa increasing in frequency? *Int J Eat Disord* 1996;19:287-296.
9. Shisslak CM, Crago M, Estes LS. The spectrum of eating disturbances. *Int J Eat Disord* 1995;18:209-219.
10. Kuntz B, Groze V, Yates WR. Bulimia: A systemic family history perspective. *Fam Soc J Contemp H* 1992;73:604-612.
11. Kasset JA, Gershon ES, Maxwell ME, et al. Psychiatric disorders in the first-degree relatives of probands with bulimia nervosa. *Am J Psychiatry* 1989;146:1468-1471.
12. Boumann CE, Yates WR. Risk factors for bulimia nervosa: A controlled study of parental psychiatric illness and divorce. *Addict Beh* 1994;19:667-675.
13. Dennis AB, Sansone RA. Treatment of patients with personality disorders. In: Garner DM, Garfinkel PE, eds. *Handbook of Treatment for Eating Disorders.* New York: Guilford; 1997: 437-449.
14. Johnson CL, Sansone RA, Chewning M. Good reasons why young women would develop anorexia nervosa: The adaptive context. *Pediatr Ann* 1992;21:731-737.
15. Sharp CW, Freeman CP. The medical complications of anorexia nervosa. *Br J Psychiatry* 1993;162:452-462.
16. de Simone G, Scalfi L, Galderisi M, et al. Cardiac abnormalities in young women with anorexia nervosa. *Br Heart J* 1994; 71: 287-292.
17. Neumarker KJ. Mortality and sudden death in anorexia nervosa. *Int J Eat Disord* 1997;21:205-212.
18. Mehler PS. Eating disorder 1. Anorexia nervosa. *Hosp Pract* 1996;31:109-113.
19. Haller E. Eating disorders: A review and update. *West J Med* 1992;157:658-662.
20. Sansone RA. Complications of hazardous weight-loss methods. *Am Fam Physician* 1984;30:141-146.

21. Sansone RA, Sansone LA. Medical complications in bulimia nervosa. In: Alexander Mott L, Lumsden DB, eds. *Understanding Eating Disorders: Anorexia Nervosa, Bulimia Nervosa and Obesity.* New York: Taylor & Francis; 1994:181-201.
22. Larsen K, Skov Jensen B, Axelsen F. Perforation and rupture of the esophagus. *Scand J Thorac Cardiovasc Surg* 1983;17:311-316.
23. Board of Directors of the American Society of Hospital Pharmacists. *AHFS Drug Information.* Bethesda, MD: Author; 1997.
24. Blouin A, Blouin J, Aubin P, et al. Seasonal patterns of bulimia nervosa. *Am J Psychiatry* 1992;149:73-81.
25. Gladis MM, Walsh BT. Premenstrual exacerbation of binge eating in bulimia. *Am J Psychiatry* 1987;144:1592-1595.
26. Sansone RA, Fine MA, Nunn JL. A comparison of borderline personality symptomatology and self-destructive behavior in women with eating, substance abuse, and both eating and substance abuse disorders. *J Pers Disord* 1994;8:219-228.
27. Sansone RA, Dennis AB. The treatment of eating disorder patients with substance abuse and borderline personality disorder. *Eat Disord* 1996;4:180-186.
28. Sansone RA, Sansone L. Borderline personality disorder: Office diagnosis and management. *Am Fam Physician* 1991; 44:194-198.
29. Sansone RA, Sansone LA. Borderline personality disorder: Interpersonal and behavioral problems that sabotage treatment success. *Postgrad Med* 1995;97:169-179.
30. Gwirtsman HE, Kaye WH, George DT, et al. Hyperamylasemia and its relationship to binge-purge episodes: Development of a clinical relevant laboratory test. *J Clin Psychiatry* 1989;50:196-204.
31. Hergenroeder AC. Bone mineralization, hypothalamic amenorrhea, and sex steroid therapy in female adolescents and young adults. *J Pediatr* 1995;126:683-689.
32. Klibanski A, Biller BM, Schoenfeld DA, et al. The effects of estrogen administration on trabecular bone loss in young women with anorexia nervosa. *J Clin Endocrinol Metab* 1995;80:898-904.
33. Johnson WG, Tsoh JY, Varnado PJ. Eating disorders: Efficacy of pharmacological and psychological interventions. *Clin Psychol Rev* 1996;16:457-478.
34. Golden NH, Jacobson MS, Schebendach J, et al. Resumption of menses in anorexia nervosa. *Arch Pediatr Adolesc Med* 1997; 151:16-21.
35. Eckert ED, Halmi KA, Marchi P, et al. Ten-year follow-up of anorexia nervosa: Clinical course and outcome. *Psychol Med* 1995;25:143-156.
36. Hebebrand J, Himmelmann GW, Herzog W, et al. Prediction of low body weight at long-term follow-up in acute anorexia nervosa by low body weight at referral. *Am J Psychiatry* 1997;154:566-569.
37. Rigotti NA, Neer RM, Skates SJ, et al. The clinical course of osteoporosis in anorexia nervosa. A longitudinal study of cortical bone mass. *JAMA* 1991;265:1133-1138.
38. Andersen AE. Sexuality and fertility: Women with anorexia nervosa and bulimia. *Med Aspects Hum Sex* 1986;20:138-143.
39. Brinch M, Isager T, Tolstrup K. Anorexia nervosa and motherhood: Reproduction pattern and mothering behavior of 50 women. *Acta Psychiatr Scand* 1988;77:611-617.
40. Lambe EK, Katzman DK, Mikulis DJ, et al. Cerebral gray matter volume deficits after weight recovery from anorexia nervosa. *Arch Gen Psychiatry* 1997;54:537-542.
41. Herzog W, Deter HC, Fiehn W, Petzold E. Medical findings and predictors of long-term physical outcome in anorexia nervosa: A prospective, 12-year follow-up study. *Psychol Med* 1997; 27:269-279.
42. Keel PK, Mitchell JE. Outcome in bulimia nervosa. *Am J Psychiatry* 1997;154:313-321.
43. Sohlberg S, Norring C, Holmgren S, Rosmark B. Impulsivity and long-term prognosis of psychiatric patients with anorexia nervosa/bulimia nervosa. *J Nerv Ment Dis* 1989;177:249-258.
44. Olmsted MP, Kaplan AS, Rockert W. Rate and prediction of relapse in bulimia nervosa. *Am J Psychiatry* 1994;151:738-743.
45. Weltzin TE, Cameron J, Berga S, Kaye WH. Prediction of reproductive status in women with bulimia nervosa by past high weight. *Am J Psychiatry* 1994;151:136-138.
46. Sansone RA, Wiederman MW, Sansone LA. Healthcare utilization among women with eating disordered behavior. *Am J Man Care* 1997;3:1721-1723.
47. Sansone RA, Sansone LA, Wiederman MW. The relationship between obesity and medical utilization among women in a primary care setting. *Int J Eat Disord* (in press).
48. Woodside DB. A review of anorexia nervosa and bulimia nervosa. *Curr Probl Pediatr* 1995;25:67-89.

Violent Patients

William R. Dubin, MD

The threat of violence is an increasing concern in modem society and health care delivery settings. Within the hospital setting, the emergency department (ED) appears to be the clinical site at highest risk for violence. Because EDs are open 24 hours a day and provide unrestricted access to the public, the staff constantly is exposed to an unscreened, and potentially high-risk population for violent behavior.[1]

Two recent studies documented the level of violence encountered in the ED. A one-year retrospective study revealed that police were called in approximately twice a day to help prevent a violent episode.[2] More than 25% of these incidents required physical restraint or removal of the offender from the premises. Approximately 4% represented serious threats to the ED staff, and frequently involved weapons, physical abuse, or an oral threat.

In a survey of ED medical directors of residency programs in emergency medicine and members of the Council of Teaching Hospitals with an annual ED census of 40,000 or more patient visits, 32% of the 127 respondents reported at least one oral threat a day, and 18% noted weapons were displayed as a threat at least once a month. Nearly 60% noted at least one threat of violence with a weapon against a staff member during the preceding five years, 43% reported physical attacks on medical staff at least once a month, and 80.3% reported that at least one staff member had been injured by a violent patient. Perhaps most alarming, nine respondents described an act of violence that resulted in death.

The threat of an armed patient also is a major concern. Four percent to 8% of patients seen in psychiatric emergency services have weapons.[4-6] In a recent study, the first six months of screening ED patients for weapons with a metal detector yielded 33 handguns; 1,324 knives: 97 mace-type sprays: and many other hazardous items. Variables such as age, ethnicity, marital status, or diagnosis did not differentiate weapon-carrying patients from those who did not carry weapons.[6]

Even though the risk of violence is inherent in clinical emergency practice, several key steps can be taken to minimize the risk. Establishing and maintaining a safe working environment is predicated on the development of a comprehensive aggression management protocol. Although many clinicians may believe that aggression management involves finding the fastest acting medication that can be given intramuscularly, comprehensive and effective aggression management encompasses more than medication and involves a philosophy and protocol that must be embraced by the entire treatment staff.

This chapter provides a detailed approach to the ED evaluation and management of violent patients. Such an approach includes understanding the dynamics of violence, establishing a secure environment for patient evaluation, recognizing the prodromal syndrome of violence, knowing the differential diagnosis for violence, developing an understanding of psychological and psychopharmacological treatments, and having knowledge of appropriate restraint techniques.

It is difficult to prioritize treatment into a hierarchical protocol. Frequently, multiple interventions occur simultaneously. Therefore, the order of discussion does not necessarily suggest that one intervention is more important or takes precedence over another. Treatments should be implemented based on the clinical situation.

The Dynamics of Violence

The successful management of aggression is predicated on an understanding of the dynamics of violence. Violence is a reaction against overwhelming feelings of passivity and helplessness. A patient's hypermasculine behavior is commonly an overreaction to a strong sense of impotence, helplessness, and inability to control the environment.[9] These feelings usually are exacerbated before an episode of physical violence.

Medical personnel may inadvertently provoke a violent episode by responding to a threatening patient in an authoritarian and aggressive manner. Such a response intensifies the patient's feelings of helplessness. To avoid an intervention perceived as provocation by the patient, ED personnel must understand their own reactions to a threatening or violent patient.

Staff Attitudes as a Precipitant of Violence. Members of the ED staff may respond to aggressive behavior with fear, anxiety, or frustration. A common reaction is that violent patients belong in jail or are untreatable psychopaths or drug abusers.[10] ED personnel may feel vulnerable in the presence of a violent patient, fearing that the patient may become aggressive if expectations are not fulfilled. Other emergency providers may feel angry and helpless because the patient's behavior could reflect poorly on the professional abilities of emergency care providers, or because the violent patient may do something for which the ED professional will be held liable.

Staff members who feel terrorized may project their fears onto the patient and perceive the patient as being more hostile and threatening than he or she actually is. This expectation of violence may actually cause it. In fact, victims of assault often convey at least a partly rejecting attitude or are provocative towards patients before being assaulted.

Multiple factors, including socioeconomic, racial, ethnic, religious, and educational differences impose barriers between staff and patients. Often these forces lie dormant and manifest only when staff members deal with more difficult or threatening patients.

The ED staff may develop attitudes and feelings about patients based on a single piece of history or behavior. Subsequent responses to the patient may be punitive and repressive, often provoking violence from the patient. For example, staff members often have very little tolerance for substance abusers; patients who induce their own illnesses (e.g., suicide attempts); or psychiatric patients, including those diagnosed with "borderline" personality disorder. In fact, just the mention of the diagnosis borderline may conjure up fantasies of patients who am belligerent, dramatic, suicidal, attention seeking, and disruptive. Once these images are evoked, staff react to patients as though they are disruptive even when such behavior is not present. Three types of distorted thinking may develop towards such patients:[12]

• *Arbitrary references*—forming conclusions based on inadequate or incorrect data; for example, "Nothing will help this patient; he has always been like this."

• *All or nothing thinking*—viewing situations in extreme black and white categories: for instance, "I won't take any grief from a patient like this."

• *Personalization*—taking too much blame or too much credit for the patient's condition; "I'm the only one who truly understands this patient."

Denial as an Impediment to Recognizing the Risk of Violence. A major stumbling block in the management of aggression is the psychological defense of denial. Denial occurs by unconsciously allaying anxiety by disavowing thoughts, feelings, or external reality factors that are consciously intolerable. The threat of violence is extremely anxiety provoking. The most effective way to combat anxiety and fear is to deny that the risk of violence exists. Therefore, clinicians often ignore clinical data or behavior that suggest a patient may become violent. For example, rather than acknowledging anxiety and fear of intimidating patients, the physician may attempt to project an image of false machismo, fearlessness, and confidence. Other manifestations of denial are failure to obtain pertinent data regarding the patient's previous history of violence or arrests, or failure to question the patient about current aggressive behavior.

Differential Diagnosis of Violence

When dealing with violent patients, the first and most critical task in an ED setting is to differentiate organic mental syndromes from functional psychiatric illness. Major diagnostic considerations include delirium, alcohol and drug intoxications or withdrawal, schizophrenia or mania. and personality disorders.[13] *(Please see Table 1.)* Failure to diagnose delirium or substance intoxication or withdrawal can result in increased morbidity and mortality. For rapid screening of organic mental syndromes, the presence of any one of the following indicators should prompt a search for an organic etiology:[13]

• patient older than 40 years of age with no previous psychiatric history;
• disorientation;
• lethargy or stupor;
• abnormal vital signs;
• visual hallucinations;
• illusions.

A laboratory evaluation that quickly rules out life threatening medical illness includes a complete blood count, electrolytes, glucose, blood urinary nitrogen, and an electrocardiogram. Toxicology and alcohol blood screens can also be helpful if the results can be obtained quickly. If these tests are negative and the patient presents with an acute mental status change (hours to days), computerized axial tomography followed by lumbar puncture should be considered.

Aggression secondary to medical illness usually results from relatively common syndromes, such as hypoglycemia, hypoxia, a post-ictal state, or delirium tremens.[13] *(Please see Table 2.)* When violence is secondary to a medical problem, treatment focuses on correcting the underlying medical problem. If patients are not cooperative and their combativeness hinders or prevents an appropriate medical evaluation, physicians should implement the psychological and psychopharmacologic treatment strategies discussed below.

Predicting Violence

The successful management of aggression is predicated on the ability to predict which patients are most likely to become violent.[14] Once such a prediction is made, rapid intervention can defuse the risk of violence. Violence usually does not occur without warning. There is a prodromal syndrome that is characterized by three behaviors: increasing anxiety and tension; verbal abuse and profanity; and increasing hyperactivity. These escalating behaviors usually do not occur in discrete stages but often overlap and sometimes occur simultaneously.

The earliest phase of escalation is the patient's increasing anxiety and tension. Patients often manifest this behavior in their body movements: rigid postures. literally "having their back up in the air," clenching fists and jaws, visibly pulsating temporal arteries. They may have a fixed, mean looking faces. Physicians may observe this tension, but often do not consider it in the context of the potential for violence.

In the second stage of escalation, as tension and anxiety increase, patients become verbally abusive and profane. Mistakes in clinical management in this phase could increase the risk of violence. If the ED staff personalize the abuse, their emotional reaction will cloud clinical judgment as thoughts focus more on retaliation than evaluation. Staff members may react with verbal aggressiveness and counter-threats, thereby increasing the patient's feelings of helplessness and the probability of violence.

Verbal abuse, like violent behavior, is a defense against feelings of helplessness and passivity and must be viewed in the context of the patient's overall predicament—being evaluated and treated by a staff of strangers, while (sometimes) being handcuffed or restrained against his or her will. Proceeding with the clinical evaluation in an effort to understand the etiology of the patient's symptoms, rather than reacting to abusive behavior and speech generally, will facilitate treatment and lead to the appropriate clinical intervention.

The most important predictor of imminent violence is the patient's motor behavior. Most assaults are preceded by a period of increasing hyperactivity. Hyperactive patients should be evaluated immediately and at no time should such a patient be ignored. Patients who cannot sit in an examination room and keep pacing the halls should be considered emergencies and require immediate intervention.

Table 1. Differential Diagnosis of Violent Patients

Delirium
Sudden onset
Disorientation
Waxing and waning of symptoms
Visual hallucinations
Illusions
Known medical illness
Patient on medication for medical illness
No previous psychiatric history

Alcohol or drug intoxication or withdrawal
Tremor
Pupillary changes
Hyperreflexia
Nystagmus
Slurred speech
Ataxia
Autonomic hyperactivity (tachycardia, mild hypertension)
History of drug or alcohol use
Physical signs of drug use (needle tracks, nasal septum erosion)
Requests for controlled substances

Personality disorder
Absence of hallucinations, delusions, disorganized thought
Orientation intact
History of impulsive behaviors including self-mutilation, suicide gestures or attempts, sexual promiscuity, drug abuse, shoplifting, excessive spending
History of antisocial behavior, including stealing, drug use, destroying property, frequent physical fights, engaging in an illegal occupation

Schizophrenia or mania
Gradual onset
Hallucinations
Delusions, especially persecutory
Disorganized thought
Orientation intact
History of psychiatric illness

Used with permission: Dubin. WR, Weiss KJ. *Handbook of Psychiatric Emergencies*. Springhouse, PA: Springhouse Corporation; 1991.

Psychological Approaches to the Management of Violence

Verbal Intervention. The dilemma with using verbal intervention effectively is that it takes time—the one commodity that most emergency physicians do not have. The initial intervention of developing rapport with the patient, therefore, may be delegated to a nurse. It is critical that the patient does not feel overwhelmed or pressured by the physician's own sense of urgency. When patients detect this haste and urgency, their own anxiety, sense of isolation, and withdrawal intensify. This is the one issue that makes treatment of violent patients in the ED so difficult. The physician must be able to convey to patients the sense that unlimited time is available to hear them out even though, in reality, only five or 10 minutes are available. This sudden shift in the physician's pace is difficult but essential to the successful management of these patients.

Most violent patients are terrified of losing control and welcome efforts to prevent them from acting out. The physician can reduce the patient's anxiety and fear by maintaining a humane, respectful manner. Empathic verbal intervention is the most effective method of calming an agitated, fearful, panicky patient. A patient who is treated with honesty, dignity, and respect is more likely to believe that help is at hand.

The physician should address the patient formally, using Mr., Mrs., or Miss to convey respect. Begin the interview with benign topics such as the patient's age, schooling, or occupation, and

Table 2. Common Organic Causes of Violent Behavior

Drugs
Alcohol (intoxication, withdrawal, espeically delirium tremens)
Amphetamines
Cocaine
Sedative-hypnotic intoxication or withdrawal
Phencyclidine
LSD

Diseases
Hypoglycemia
Hypoxia
Meningitis
Head trauma
Electrolyte imbalance
Anemia
Dementia
Vitamin deficiencies
Endocrinopathies
Post-ictal states

avoid a hasty discussion of the patient's reasons for aggressiveness. If the patient does not respond to this initial intervention, do not feel rejected or rebuffed, even when the patient is hostile. With gentle persistence, most patients eventually will talk to the physician because they welcome the interview as an outlet for their tension.

An important element in the psychological treatment of the violent patient is to address the patient's affect (the visible manifestation of their feelings). The importance of allowing patients to talk about their feelings cannot be over-emphasized because it enables the physician to establish a therapeutic rapport. Some clinicians mistakenly believe an angry patient will explode if he talks about what is bothering him. The most effective way to calm patients is to encourage them to talk about their angry feelings. Ask the patient to explain what is upsetting him, what's making him angry, and acknowledge his feelings by comments such as "I can see you are angry," "I understand how you feel," or "I might feel the same way." Efforts to help relieve such intense feelings with logic and rationalization will only exacerbate the angry feelings rather than attenuate them. It is important to let patients ventilate their feelings and get what is bothering them "off their chest." Allowing patients to talk about their feelings will open the door for catharsis and may eliminate their need for further aggression.

Talking allows the patient an outlet for the tension that is being generated. Carefully phrased comments such as "I can understand how you feel" or "this must be terribly upsetting to be brought to an emergency department and not know what is happening or going to happen" may advance the interview. The physician also can empathize with the patient by trying to view the situation from his or her perspective.

One of the most effective ways to facilitate rapport is to offer food or drink, which usually calms a hostile patient and confirms the sense of concern. A patient is unlikely to become assaultive toward someone who has fed him. Offer only cold drinks to potentially violent patients. because hot drinks can be used as a weapon.

Observing the Patient's Behavior. Many patients make verbal threats. To avoid overreacting, note the patient's behavior during the threatening behavior. Although the patient is hostile and angry, his or her behavior may indicate that an assault is not imminent. For example, patients who put their hands in their pockets, cross their ams, or assume some other nonthreatening posture usually pose no danger, even if they are making loud verbal threats. In contrast, the patient who refuses to cooperate with any requests poses a higher risk of violence.

Setting Limits. Most patients will respond to the expectation of self-control. However, an aggressive patient's behavior may worsen if certain limits are not set during the interview. Thus, clearly inform the patient that violence is unacceptable and describe the consequences if violence occurs. A clinician can set limits directly or indirectly.[15] Using the direct approach, the physician can clearly specify the required behavior in positive terms "do this" rather than negative terms "don't do that." The direct approach, which is the most effective for confused or disorganized patients with a psychotic or organic disorder. may require frequent refocusing and reorienting of the patient by repeating the directives.

Using an indirect approach decreases the patient's will to resist by forcing him or her to choose from several acceptable alternatives (e.g., "You have a choice: You can stop yelling profanity and cursing at the staff, or if you feel that you cannot control yourself, you can sit in the seclusion room with the security guard until I have time to interview you"). Because opposing a single directive is easier than deciding between two alternatives, the patient's resistance is reduced. In addition, a single directive often is provocative and viewed as a challenge. With two choices, a patient feels a sense of control and may choose the desired alternative. The indirect approach is most effective for a patient who is not confused or severely disorganized.

Rapid Tranquilization for Controlling Violent Patients

Rapid tranquilization (RT) is a safe and effective method for controlling agitated, potentially assaultive or violent patients.[18] RT is effective across all diagnostic categories regardless of the etiology of the aggression; is effective in psychosis secondary to schizophrenia or mania; and curbs aggression related to dementia, delirium, or alcohol and substance abuse or withdrawal. *(Please see Table 3.)* RT is accomplished by administering a standard dose of antipsychotic medication over 30 to 60 minutes to treat severe agitation, anxiety, tension, hyperactivity, or excitement. Most patients respond to RT within 30 to 60 minutes. Core psychotic symptoms, such as delusions and hallucinations, do not remit with a few doses of medication and require weeks of drug therapy for remission.

Agents for Rapid Tranquilization. Recent research indicates that the combination of antipsychotic medication with lorazepam is more effective than antipsychotic medication alone.[19-21] Haloperidol (5 mg IM) or thiothixene (10 mg) in combination with lorazepam (2 mg IM) in the same syringe usually will be sufficient to control most acute symptoms. Some clinicians use haloperidol (5 mg IM) with

Table 3. Rapid Tranquilization of the Violent Patient

Cause of Violent Behavior	Drug Intervention*
Schizophrenia, mania, or other psychosis	Lorazepam (Ativan) 2-4 mg IM combined with haloperidol (Haldol) 5 mg IM or thiothixene (Navane) 10 mg IM
	or RT with an antipsychotic alone
	Thiothixene (Navane) 10 mg IM or 20 mg concentrate
	Haloperidol (Haldol) 5 mg IM or 10 mg concentrate
	Noxapine (Loxitane) 10 mg IM or 25 mg concentrate PO
Personality disorder	Lorazepam (Ativan) l-2 mg PO every one to two hours or 24 mg IM (0.05 mg/kg) every one to two hours
Alcohol withdrawal states**	For agitation, tremors, or change in vital signs: Chlordiazepoxide (Librium) 25-50 mg PO every four to six hours
	For elderly patients or patients with liver disease: Lorazepam 2 mg PO every 2 hours
	For extreme agitation: Lorazepam 2-4 mg IM every hour or rapid tranquilization of patient not controlled with benzodiazepines
Cocaine and amphetamine intoxication	For mild to moderate agitation: Diazepam (Valium) 10 mg PO every eight hours
	For severe agitation: Thiothixene 20 mg concentrate or 10 mg IM; haloperidol 10 mg concentrate or 5 mg IM
Phencylidine intoxication	For hyperactivity, mild agitation, tension, anxiety, excitement: Diazepam 10-30 mg PO or lorazepam 2-4 mg IM (0.05 mg/kg)
	For severe agitation and excitement with hallucinations, delusions, bizarre behavior: Haloperidol 5-10 mg IM every 30 to 60 minutes

* All doses given at 30- to 60-minute intervals; one-half dose for medically ill or older patients

** Rapid tranquilization in alcohol withdrawal states is for severe agitation and behavioral control. The actual treatment of withdrawal is with a cross-tolerant medication.

Used with permission: Dubin, WR, Weiss KJ. *Handbook of Psychiatric Emergencies*. Springhouse, PA: Springhousc Corporation; 1991.

lorazepam (4 mg IM). If only antipsychotic medications are used, the use of oral concentrate provides an alternative to the IM route *(please see dosing guidelines in Table 3)*. The use of concentrate has been found to be effective and consistent with the dynamics of violence, i.e. the patient has a choice and is able to participate in treatment. The use of IV antipsychotic medication in treating psychiatric emergencies has not been well-studied in the ED.

Administer medication at hourly intervals. Most patients will respond to one to three doses. Although ceiling doses for RT have not been established, high doses of antipsychotic medication alone or in combination with lorazepam generally are safe and well tolerated.[22-24] In medically compromised or older patients (> 65 years of age) dosing should be reduced to half of that recommended for younger patients.

Prior to administration, clearly explain to the patient why the medication is needed. For example, say, "You seem to be restless and nervous. This medication will make you feel calm and help stop the voices that you are hearing." Using terms such as "violent," "out of control," "crazy thoughts," "agitated," or "strange behavior" as reasons for the medication will further agitate a patient.

Adverse effects. Side effects during RT generally are few, mild, and reversible. By far the most common side effect is extrapyramidal symptoms (EPS).[16,17,19] Most studies have found that less than 10% of patients develop EPS within the first 24 hours of RT. EPS is not dose-related and can occur after one dose. The most common EPS is a dystonic reaction, which is sudden in onset, can be bizarre in presentation, and often leads to a misdiagnosis of hysterical conversion reaction.

Dystonic reactions, which consist of involuntary turning or twisting movements produced by massive and sustained muscle contractions, usually involve muscles of the back, neck, and oral area. Extension of the back (opisthotonos) or severe backward arching (retrocollis) or sideways twisting (torticollis) of the neck may occur. The eyes may be pulled upward in a painful manner (oculogyric crisis). At times, patients may complain of thickness of the tongue or difficulty swallowing.

The most serious form of dystonia is laryngospasm, during which contraction of the Laryngeal muscles can compromise the airway and lead to severe respiratory distress. Although extremely rare, clinicians should be alert to its possible occurrence.

A side effect that frequently can be misdiagnosed as psychotic decompensation is akathisia, literally, "inability to sit still." Patients feel uncomfortably restless and pacing is their only relief. They often describe feeling "unable to relax," "tense," "wound up like a spring," "irritable," or "like jumping out of my skin." Severe akathisia can lead to a rapid psychotic decompensation, and in its severest manifestation, patients have committed suicide and homicide.

The treatment for dystonia and akathisia is the same.[16,17] Administer benztropine (Cogentin). 2 mg, or diphenhydramine (Benadryl), 50 mg IM or IV. These doses can be repeated at five-minute intervals up to three doses. Generally, relief occurs within one to three minutes after injection. Relief is dramatic in most patients, but a small minority of patients may not respond. In these cases, diazepam (Valium), 10 mg IV or lorazepam (Ativan), 2 to 4 mg IV or IM may be helpful. The combination of lorazepam with an antipsychotic during RT may further reduce the incidence of EPS.

Alternative Agents for RT. Several other medications have been used successfully in RT, although they have not been evaluated extensively. Midazolam, a benzodiazepine that recently was reported as safe and extremely rapid in onset, was found to produce dramatic response three to six minutes after IM administration of 2.5 to 3.0 mg.[25] However, IV midazolam has been associated with respiratory depression and respiratory arrest. IV midazolam should be given slowly, with the initial dose of 1 mg IV; the total IV dose should not exceed 2.5 mg.

Another agent, droperidol 5 to 10 mg IM is reported to be rapidly effective in assaultive or severely agitated patients.[26] An analog of haloperidol, droperidol has no antipsychotic action but does have sedating properties. The main side effect of droperidol is EPS.

Although barbiturates, especially sodium amytal, have been used to sedate agitated patients, no published data currently support their use in RT.[27] Such risks as tolerance, lethal overdosage, withdrawal symptoms, and interaction with other medication make barbiturates a poor choice for RT.

Occasionally, clinicians voice concern that RT will obscure the patient's mental status and, therefore, medication should be withheld until a diagnosis is made. This can lead to withholding effective treatment and prolonging the risks to both patient and staff. Psychiatric diagnosis is not made on a single mental status evaluation. In fact, definitive psychiatric treatment does not begin in the ED. Occasionally, clinicians choose to withhold antipsychotic medication because of their concern that it will obscure or worsen underlying medical conditions, and therefore prefer to forcibly restrain patients while attempting a physical clinical evaluation and laboratory work-up. Besides the questionable accuracy of a physical clinical examination performed on a restrained, agitated patient, restraints are not without significant risks.

Table 4. Guidelines for Using Restraints

At least four persons should assist with restraining the patient while a fifth staff member controls the patient's head and prevents biting. At no time should only one or two persons try to restrain a patient. Leather restraints are the safest and surest type of restraint.

Explain to the patient why he or she is being restrained. Give the patient a few seconds to comply, but do not negotiate. At a prearranged signal, the team grabs the patient and brings him to the floor in a backward motion without injuring him. The team applies restraints, then moves the patient to the seclusion room.

A staff member should always be visible to reassure the patient who is being restrained.

Restrain the patient with legs spread-eagle and one arm restrained to the side and the other arm restrained over the patient's head.

Remove all dangerous objects from the patient, including rings, shoes, matches, pens, and pencils.

Place restraints so that intravenous fluids can be given if necessary.

Raise the patient's head slightly to decrease his feelings of vulnerability and to reduce the possibility of aspiration.

After the patient is in restraints, begin treatment using verbal intervention or rapid tranquilization.

Remove one restraint at a time at 5-minute intervals until the patient has only two restraints on. Remove both of these restraints at the same time. Never leave only one limb in restraints.

Adapted with permission: Dubin WR. Weiss KJ. Emergency psychiatry. In Michels R, et al, eds. *Psychiatry.* Vol 2. Philadelphia: JB Lippincott Co; 1985.

Using a Show of Force

When verbal and pharmacologic interventions fail to control an aggressive patient, a judicious show of force frequently will avert violence. The key to a successful show of force is to recognize the potential for violence and to alert security personnel and other staff members before the behavior escalates to violence. Controlling the patient is more difficult if violence occurs before summoning help. Security personnel should always be called in a non-threatening manner. The use of a code phrase is a non-provocative way to call for help (e.g., "Would you see if Dr. Armstrong is available?"). The arrival of security personnel conveys to the patient that violent impulses will be controlled. A patient should not be made to feel that security personnel are there to challenge or threaten. Ideally, security guards should be visible but non-threatening, and in most cases, should not be brought into the interview room.

The Portland Veterans Administration Medical Center initiated a violence control program that resulted in a 91.6% decrease in violent incidents.[28] This was done by identifying patients at risk for violence and entering a flag in the patient's computerized and automated data base within the medical center. The flag alerted staff to the patient's potential for violence, and security personnel were in attendence with the patient throughout the visit.

Too often, security staff members are viewed as a physical force whose only goal is to intimidate and dominate, which they often do quite successfully, thus provoking more aggression. Security officers should be in-serviced routinely about mental illness and the principles of effective intervention for violence and should be seen as part of a treatment team and not merely as a physical force to subdue patients.

Physical Restraints

When all interventions fail to reduce a patient's threatening behavior, a physical restraint protocol is indicated. A minimum of four staff members (one controlling each extremity), preferably five (to control the head) should be used to restrain a patient. When staff arrive, the emergency physician should tell the staff why they were called and direct procedures.[29] *(Please see Table 4.)* Relinquish control only if another staff member is more skilled and experienced in managing such situations. Restraining a patient is an integral part of treatment. Once the decision is made to restrain a patient, restraints should be used immediately and without discussion or negotiation with the patient.

Restraints should be used in the following situations?

• to prevent imminent harm to the patient or staff members when other means of control are ineffective or inappropriate;

• to prevent serious disruption of treatment or significant damage to property;

• to decrease patient stimulation;

• to respond to the patient's request for them.

Restraints am contraindicated in a patient with an unstable medical condition, including infection, cardiac illness, disorders of body temperature regulation, metabolic illness, or orthopedic problems. A patient with delirium or dementia may experience a worsening of symptoms secondary to the sensory deprivation induced by restraints.

Managing the Armed Patient

The greatest threat to ED personnel comes from a patient who has a weapon. In addition to guns and knives, weapons also may include a chair, an ashtray, a telephone, or a crutch. If the patient admits to carrying a weapon, recognize it as a symbol of defense against feelings of helplessness and passivity.

Immediately requesting that the patient relinquish the weapon may heighten these feelings and further exacerbate agitation. Notify hospital security so they can be available if the patient tries to use the weapon. If the patient volunteers to surrender the weapon, do not accept it directly. Instead ask the patient to put it on the floor or table, and take it at the end of the interview. Abruptly taking a weapon may trigger a reflex response in which the patient will attack. If the patient threatens to use the weapon, try not to exacerbate feelings of helplessness, impotence, or shame. The most effective approach is to speak to the patient in a calm manner and admit fear and anxiety saying "I would like to help you, but I feel threatened and frightened by the weapon. I have difficulty listening to you under these circumstances.[31] This may be sufficient to disarm the patient. Verbal or physical aggressiveness will provoke an assault.[31,33] All EDs should develop weapon screening protocols. Metal detectors are a successful way to disarm patients in a non-confrontational manner and almost all patients accept this as part of the ED visit.

Securing The Environment

The issues of environmental safety rarely are considered in the management of aggressive patients. Such concerns usually do not occur until a violent event occurs. However, all EDs should establish a secure environment for the patient, staff, and clinicians so that assessment and treatment can be completed without danger. The evaluation is particularly risky in terms of safety because, in most cases, ED staff members have little or no knowledge of the patient's history of violence or of other risk factors that increase the likelihood of violence. Therefore, a wide range of options should be considered when interviewing unscreened, unknown patients. Determine whether to interview the patient alone in a room with the door open and the staff outside the door or in a room with additional staff members present. At times, it is prudent to interview the patient in the hallway with security personnel present. The most extreme option is to interview the patient while he or she is in physical restraints.

If the interview takes place in a room with the door closed, a system to indicate danger should exist. This may be in the form of a panic button or a prearranged message to someone in the ED. Some institutions use portable warning devices such as the "man down" system (Motorola) which utilizes a mercury switch that is activated when the wearer is in a prone position. An alarm pen works on a similar principal.

Carefully note the furniture and decorations that are used in rooms chosen to interview violent or potentially violent patients. Chairs, pictures, ashtrays, and other small objects can make dangerous weapons. Large bulky chairs with rounded comers may be preferable to light metal or wood chairs.

Limiting Violent Episodes

The violent patient presents one of the most difficult challenges for the emergency clinician. However, when these patients are approached in a manner that uses a treatment approach based on an understanding of the dynamics of violence, a dramatic and significant change in most patients' behavior can occur. Verbal intervention coupled with judicious use of rapid tranquilization will resolve most violent episodes. The techniques of aggression management should be taught to all staff and periodically reviewed. Violent patients can be managed successfully and the risk to staff significantly decreased when a preplanned, comprehensive team approach to aggression management is implemented.

References

1. *Guidelines for Protecting the Safety and Health of Health Care Workers*. Washington, DC: U.S. Department of Health and Human Services, Superintendent of Documents, U.S. Government Printing Office; 1988.
2. Pane GA, Winiarski AM, Salness KA. Aggression directed toward emergency department staff at a university teaching hospital. *Ann Emerg Med* 1991;20:283-286.
3. Lavoie FW. Carter GL, Danzi DF, et al. Emergency department violence in United States teaching hospitals. *Ann Emerg Med* 1988;17:1127-1233.
4. Anderson AA, Ghali AY. Bansil RK. Weapon carrying among patients in a psychiatric emergency room. *Hosp Community Psychiatry* 1989;40:845-847.
5. Privitera MR. Springer MO, Perlmutter RA. To search or not to search: Is there a clinical profile of a patient harboring a weapon? *Gen Hosp Psychiatry* 1986;8:442-447.
6. McNeil DE, Binder RL. Patients who bring weapons to the psychiatric emergency room. *J Clin Psychiatry* 1987;48: 230-233.
7. Thompson BM, Nunn 1, Kramer I, et al. Disarming the department: Weapon screening and improved security to create a safer emergency department environment. *Ann Emerg Med* 1988:17:419.
8. Lion JR. *Evaluation and Management of the Violent Patient.* Springfield. IL: Charles C. Thomas; 1972.
9. Bach-y-Rita G, Lion JR, Climent CE, et al. Episodic dyscontrol: A study of 130 violent patients. *Am J Psychiatry* 1971; 127:14731478.
10. Lion JR, Pasternak SA. Counter transference reaction to violent patients. *Am J Psychiatry* 1973;13D:207-210.
11. Maier, GJ, Stava LJ. Morrow BR. A Model for understanding and managing Cycles of aggression among psychiatric inpatients. *Hosp Community Psychiatry* 1987;38:520-524.
12. Hanke H. *Handbook of Emergency Psychiatry*. Lexington, MA: The Collamore Press; 1984.
13. Dubin WR. Weiss KJ. *Handbook of Psychiatric Emergencies.* Springhouse, PA: Springhouse Corporation; 1991.
14. Dubin WR. Evaluating and managing the violent patient. *Ann Emerg Med* 1981;10:481-481.
15. Thackrey M. *Therapeutics for Aggression: Psychological and Physical Crisis Intervention*. New York: Human Sciences Press; 1987.
16. Dubin WR, Weiss KJ, Dom JM. Pharmacotherapy of psychiatric emergencies. *J Clin Psychopharmacol* 1986:6:210-222.
17. Dubin WR, Feld JA. Rapid tranquilization of the violent patient. *Am J Emerg Med* 1989;7:313-320.
18. Dubin WR, Waxman HM; Weiss KJ et al. Rapid tranquilization: The efficacy of oral concentrate. *J Clin Psychiatry* 1985;46:475-478.
19. Dubin WR. Rapid tranquilization: Antipsychotics or benzodiazepines? *J Clin Psychiatry* 1988;49 (suppl): 5-11.
20. Garta-Trevino ES, Hollister LE. Overall JE, et al. Efficacy of combinations of intramuscular antipsychotics and sedative-hypnotics for control of psychotic agitation. *Am J Psychiatry* 1989;146:1598-1601.
21. Battaglia J, Dubin WR, Kang J, et al. Rapid tranquilization of agitated psychotic patients in the emergency room. Presented at the annual meeting of the American College of Emergency Physicians; Boston, Oct. 8, 1991.
22. Tesar GE, Murray GB, Cassem NH. Use of high-dose intravenous haloperidol in the treatment of agitated cardiac patients. *J Clin Psychopharmacol* 1985;5:344-347.
23. Adams F. Neuropsychiatric evaluation and treatment of delirium in the critically ill cancer patient. *Cancer Bull* 1984; 36:156-160.
24. Dudley DL., Rowlett DB, Loebel PJ. Emergency use of intravenous haloperidol. *Gen Hosp Psychiatry* 1979; 1:240-246.
25. Mendoza R, Djenderedjian AH, Adams J, et al. Midazolam in acute psychotic patients with hyperarousal. *J Clin Psychiatry* 1987;48:291-292.
26. Resnick M, Burton BT. Droperidol vs. haloperidol in the initial management of acutely agitated patients. *J Clin Psychiatry* 1984;45:298-299.
27. Fish DN. Treatment of delirium in the critically ill patient. *Clin Pharm* 1991:10:456-466
28. Drummond DJ, Span LF, Gordon GIL Hospital violence reduction among high-risk patients. *JAMA* 1989;261: 2531-2534.
29. Dubin WR, Weiss KJ. Emergency psychiatry. In: Michels R, et al, ed. *Psychiatry*. Philadelphia: JB Lippincott Company; 1985.
30. Task Force Report A22. *Seclusion and Restraint: The Psychiatric Uses.* Washington, DC: American Psychiatric Association; 1985.
31. Dubin WR, Wilson SJ, Mercer, C. Assaults against psychiatrists in outpatient settings. *J Clin Psychiatry* 1988;49: 338-345.
32. Ruben I, Wolkon G, Yamamoto J. Physical attacks on psychiatric residents by patients. *J New Ment Dis* 1980;168: 243-245.
33. Tardiff K. *Assessment and Management of Violent Patients.* Washington, DC: American Psychiatric Press; 1989.

Somatization Disorders

Richard J. Schuster, MD, FACP

Somatization disorders are the bane of a primary care physician's office. These patients often create frustration on the part of the caregivers and bewilderment and disbelief on the part of third-party payors. This chapter provides helpful guidelines for the practitioner in identifying these patients in a practice and offers constructive management techniques with attention to cost-containment. In an increasing managed care market, care for these patients will certainly become more and more challenging.

Introduction

The clinician is all too often confronted by patients who are convinced that there is something wrong with them in the face of normal findings. The physician frequently suspects that there is a hidden agenda but is unable to understand the dynamics. The encounter often ends with mutual dissatisfaction by the patient and the physician.

A patient scenario may help develop the concepts and management of somatization disorder.

Case Study. A 31-year-old male presents to the office with chest pain. He has had it intermittently for four weeks. It occurs at rest and with activity. It is a retrosternal pressure sensation that does not radiate. The patient becomes diaphoretic but not short of breath. He has no palpitations. He plays basketball in a league at work and has had pain sometimes while playing but has never stopped playing because of the pain. He is a manager at a local corporation and is doing well in his high pressured job.

His father had a "heart attack," two years ago. Upon further questioning, you find his father was discharged from the hospital two days after admission and takes no medicines.

His past medical history is notable for "mono" at age 14, resulting in a loss of one year of school for the patient. He had an arthroscopy of the knee at age 18 for chronic knee pain, an appendectomy at age 23, and an upper endoscopy and colonoscopy for long-standing abdominal pain at age 26. At age 28, he had a cystoscopy for an ill-defined urinary problem. Two years ago, the patient had a work-up for headache and visual loss that included a "normal" CT Scan, MRI, and EEG. A neurologist told him "there's nothing wrong with you," and was "nasty" to the patient.

His resting ECG is normal. An exercise tolerance test is done, with normal results after 15 minutes of exercise.

After informing the patient that all of the tests are normal, he states that he has very good insurance and asks, "aren't there any other tests to do?" The next question he asks is, "Maybe you should send me to a specialist; don't they know more than you do?" You explain that no further consultations are required for now.

One month later, the patient presents to you with a history of intense mid-epigastric pain, present "most" of the time for the past two weeks. He has had two episodes of emesis this week, which he says look like "coffee grounds." He tells you that he came back to you because he trusts you. You are the first doctor who took him seriously.

This case highlights many of the issues faced in somatization disorder. At the end of the discussion, the management plan for this patient will be reviewed.

Definition

Details of the medical history are critical in the diagnosis of somatization disorder. These patients will typically report a history of multiple "medical problems" beginning at a relatively early age.[1] Reviewing old medical records is essential to confirm previous evaluations and treatments and to clearly identify if diagnoses were actually made. All too often "colitis" turns out to be irritable bowel, "asthma," an extended upper respiratory infection, and "chronic mono" an unexplained, prolonged episode of fatigue with normal complete blood count and negative mono spot. A history of gastrointestinal illness is particularly common.[2] Multiple surgeries are often an important clue.[3] Patients with somatization disorder frequently have surgeries for pain-related problems. A hallmark in the definition of somatization disorder is the absence of objective findings.[4] Many medical conditions are associated with poorly defined diagnoses. The clinician is required to make a "clinical diagnosis." These patients have an extraordinary record of normal or near-normal tests and procedures. Even surgeries are often associated with normal findings. The appendectomy demonstrated "minimal inflammation;" the gallbladder had a "thickened wall with no acute inflammation;" and the arthroscopy of the knee failed to find the cartilage damage expected pre-operatively.

Patients with somatization disorder often deny any psychological component.[4] They have complex and often purely subconscious mechanisms driving their medical care seeking behavior. When asked directly if there is or may be an emotional component, they declare most emphatically that there is no active psychological issue. When pushed on this, they become defensive and angry at the physician. The doctor-patient relationship may begin to unravel. Patients with somatization disorder are not malingerers and do not generally have conscious factors driving their behavior.

The physician's ego is often fed into the relationship with a somatization disorder patient.[3] The patient reports that the last doctor was no good, but the current doctor is "the best." The patient will have very high expectations about the care they expect delivered. They will often speak of the physician's reputation as a great diagnostician. Unfortunately, just when the diagnosis of somatization disorder should be entertained, the physician's ego is being reinforced that a "bright and sophisticated" patient has finally discovered the physician's qualities. *(Please see Table 1.)*

Table 1. Definition of Somatization Disorder

- History of multiple medical problems
- History of multiple surgeries
- Health problems begin at early age
- Absence of objective findings
- Denial of psychological component
- High expectation of physician performance

Epidemiology

Many patients present to their primary care physician with problems that never result in a well-defined diagnosis. Of primary care visits, 25-50% result from primarily psychosocial factors that manifest themselves as somatic symptoms.[5] Patients who fulfill all of the formal criteria for somatization disorder are much smaller in number, representing about 0.1% of the population.[1,6] A primary care physician with 2000 patients, therefore, will have two patients in his or her practice that have a true somatization disorder. They will stand out in that physician's practice once they are diagnosed because of their heavy use of services and emotional demands on the primary care physician. Many patients who present to a primary care provider with unexplained or inordinately intense symptoms will have an undifferentiated somatiform disorder, a much more loosely defined disorder.

Somatization disorder is more common in rural settings and in a less educated population.[7] The incidence of somatization disorder will vary in different cultures. Irish Americans are less likely to present with somatic symptoms than are Italian Americans. There is a higher incidence of somatization in the Latino culture, although that varies among the Latino cultures, with a greater incidence in the Puerto Rican community than the Mexican. The Asian cultures also vary, but there are some subcultures with somatization greater than the American average. These disorders may have a variable incidence in different cultures because of increased life stresses in some groups, especially recent immigrant cultures. It is also theorized that some cultures interdict individuals from consciously expressing stress or anxiety, driving them to present with somatic symptoms instead.[8]

These patients receive expensive and often dangerous care. In the era of managed care, patients with somatization disorder consume significant resources and often raise anxiety in physicians who are trying to limit "unnecessary" tests, consultations, and therapies.[9] They use three times more ambulatory medical services than patients without somatization disorder.[10] Their total health care use is 10 times greater than the population average.[11] It is important to note that somatization may occur in a family. Children of somatizers present to emergency rooms 12 times more often and miss nine times more school than children of unaffected parents.[12]

One of the most unfortunate clinical, professional, and economic features of somatization disorder is the high incidence of iatrogenic-induced problems.[13] What often begins purely as a psychosomatic disorder becomes a mixture of psychiatric and organic problems as the patient collects multiple complications from multiple procedures and treatments. Because organic diagnoses are often illusive, ever more complex, dangerous, and

Table 2. DSM-IV Diagnostic Criteria—Somatization Disorder[1]

A. A history of many physical complaints beginning before age 30 years that occur over a period of several years and result in treatment being sought of significant impairment in social, occupational, or other important areas of functioning.

B. Each of the following criteria must have been met, with individual symptoms occurring at any time during the course of the disturbance:

Four pain symptoms: A history of pain related to at least four different sites or functions (e.g., head, abdomen, back, joints, extremities, chest, rectum, during menstration, during sexual intercourse, or during urination).

Two gastrointestinal symptoms: A history of at least two gastrointestinal symptoms other than pain (e.g., nausea, bloating, vomiting other than during pregnancy, diarrhea, or intolerance of several different foods).

One sexual symptom: A history of at least one sexual or reproductive symptom other than pain (e.g., sexual indifference, erectile or ejaculatory dysfunction, irregular menses, excessive menstrual bleeding, vomiting throughout pregnancy).

One psuedoneurological symptom: A history of at least one symptom or deficit suggesting a neurological condition not limited to pain (conversion symptoms such as impaired coordination or balance, paralysis or localized weakness, difficulty swallowing or lump in throat, aphonia, urinary retention, hallucinations, loss of touch or pain sensation, double vision, blindness, deafness, seizures; dissociative symptoms such as amnesia; or loss of consciousness other than fainting).

C. Either (1) or (2):

1. After appropriate investigation, each of the symptoms in Criterion B cannot be fully explained by a known general medical condition or the direct effects of a substance (e.g., a drug of abuse, a medication).

2. When there is a related general medical condition, the physical complaints or resulting social or occupational impairment are in excess of what would be expected from the history, physical examination, or laboratory findings.

D. The symptoms are not intentionally produced or feigned (as in factitious disorder or malingering).

expensive tests are done in quest of the diagnosis that will never be made.

Etiology

There are a variety of psychological explanations for the cause of somatization disorder. Many, but not all, patients will have a history of sexual abuse.[14,15] This will be frequently either denied by the patient or not be part of their conscious memories. It is critical for the physician to appreciate that this psychological process is subsconscious.[14] One theory proposes that the patient is subconsciously unable to express his or her psychic stress and finds socially acceptable ways to show that he or she is "sick."[14] Kaplan describes a number of more complex theories.[4] The psychodynamic theory proposes that the expression of somatic symptoms demonstrates an underlying psychological conflict. Furthermore, the secondary gain the patient receives from the health care system supplies much needed nurturing and support.[4] The neurobiologic theory proposes a problem of central nervous system regulation, possibly related to the corpora callosa connections between the two hemispheres. The sociocultural theory is supported by the different incidences of somatization disorder seen in different cultures. When emotional expression is culturally unacceptable, an individual may express their emotions through a somatic presentation of symptoms. This theory contends that these patients are not psychodynamically disturbed but are simply communicating from one culture (theirs) to another culture (the physician's). In the behavioral theory, it is proposed that physicians can drive patients to somatizing behavior by obligating patients to present and express somatic symptoms as the only way they will get attention from providers.[16] Managed care, particularly discounted fee-for-service, produces time pressures on practitioners that result in much more "testing" than "talking."[9]

Diagnosis

Engel has stressed that in psychosomatic disorders it is critical to make an active diagnosis, rather than ruling out all other diseases and making the diagnosis by exclusion.[17] Making the prospective diagnosis of somatization disorder will help avoid that pitfall.[4] The chief somatic symptom must be addressed. It is key to validate the diagnosis with carefully selected tests. The modern diagnostician must be disciplined to avoid the fruitless quest for the rare disease or unusual presentation of a common disease.

The formal diagnostic criteria are listed in Table 2. Many patients who present to a primary care provider have an undifferentiated somatiform disorder that is less well defined. *(Please see Table 3.)* This is by far the more common, although less dramatic problem. Many patients with the cultural and behavioral origins to their problems often will have an undifferentiated somatiform disorder. It is the physician's responsibility to determine where along the continuum of somatization the patient is and, therefore, how strenuously the diagnostic criteria must be met. Two key features in somatization disorder to emphasize are the presentation of multiple unexplained medical problems

Table 3. DSM-IV Diagnostic Criteria—Undifferentiated Somatoform Disorder[1]

A. One or more physical complaints (e.g., fatigue, loss of apetite, gastrointestinal or urinary complaints).

B. Either (1) or (2):
1. After appropriate investigation, the symptoms cannot be fully explained by a known general medical condition or the direct effects of a substance (e.g., a drug of abuse, a medication)
2. When there is a related general medical condition, the physical complaints or resulting social or occupational impairment is in excess of what would be expected from the history, physical examination, or laboratory findings

C. The symptoms cause clinically significant distress or impairment in social, occupational, or other important areas of functioning.

D. The duration of the disturbance is a least six months.

E. The disturbance is not better accounted for by another mental disorder (e.g., another somatoform disorder, sexual dysfunction, mood disorder, anxiety disorder, sleep disorder, or psychotic disorder).

F. The symptom is not intentionally produced or feigned (as in factitious disorder or malingering).

Table 4. DSM-IV Diagnostic Criteria—Hypocondriasis[1]

A. Preoccupation with fears of having, or the idea that one has, a serious disease based on the person's misinterpretation of bodily symptoms.

B. The preoccupation persists despite appropriate medical evaluation and reassurance.

C. The belief in criterion A is not delusional intensity (as in delusional disorder, somatic type) and is not restricted to a circumscribed concern about appearance (as in body dysmorphic disorder).

D. The preoccupation causes clinically significant distress or impairment in social, occupational, or other important areas of functioning.

E. The duration of the disturbance is at least six months.

F. The preoccupation is not better accounted for by generalized anxiety disorder, obsessive-compulsive disorder, panic disorder, a major depressive episode, separation anxiety, or another somatoform disorder.

before age 30 and the persistent nature of their symptoms over a period of time.

The differential diagnosis requires an understanding of some of the similar psychosomatic disorders as well as classic psychiatric diagnoses.[4,3,18] Anxiety disorders, including panic attacks, are extremely common presenting problems to the primary care provider.[19] Patients with anxiety disorders have predominantly autonomic system symptoms, often involving multiple organ systems. Usually, these symptoms have occurred over too short a period of time and involve too many organ systems to be consistent with a somatization disorder. Depression is very frequently seen by the primary care physician and may well present with primarily somatic symptoms.[20,21] Usually, depressed patients have the biological symptoms and signs of depression, but some have "masked depression," which causes them to focus on more somatic symptoms. The diagnosis of depression may be best confirmed by a therapeutic trial of antidepressants.[4] It appears that there are a significant number of patients who simultaneously have somatization, depression, and anxiety. These people had childhood experiences, often deprivation, that resulted in the development of all three psychiatric disorders.[22]

Somatization disorder is one of the overlapping somatoform disorders. A common confusion exists between somatization disorder and hypochondriasis. *(Please see Table 3.)* Hypochondriasis is an enhanced or magnified response to a normal sensation.[1] Patients often worry they have a very specific disease, often focusing on a particular organ system or diagnosis.[3] Somatization disorder patients have multiple symptoms involving multiple organ systems. A conversion disorder is also one of the somatoform disorders. *(Please see Table 4.)* Like somatization disorder, this is an unconscious process. The symptoms often have symbolic meaning to the patient and are non-physiologic in character.[3] The challenge to the physician is to uncover the symbolic significance of the symptom to the patient. They often occur during times of major emotional stress. Like somatization disorder, these patients often have significant secondary gain, receiving special attention from friends, relatives, colleagues, or employers.[4] Finally, pain disorder, formerly known as psychogenic pain, is also included in the somatoform disorders. *(Please see Table 5.)* First described by Engel, it is a disorder identified by pain that is inappropriate in character and intensity in light of the physical problem identified.[23] Pain is a purely subjective phenomena experienced only by the patient, with no objective criteria the physician can use to validate the symptoms. Like somatization disorder, these patients often have a psychic "need" to suffer. The pain often occurs as a response to a loss, either real or perceived. The pain may result from guilt associated with feelings of aggressiveness or forbidden sexual desire. These patients may well respond to antidepressants, raising the question of whether this may actually be a variant of depression.[24]

Somatization disorder is a difficult diagnosis to make. There is no laboratory test that is diagnostic. Organic diseases must be carefully and appropriately considered. Overlapping psychiatric diagnoses must be reviewed. The diagnosis then becomes a clinical one. In common clinical practice, the strictest diagnostic

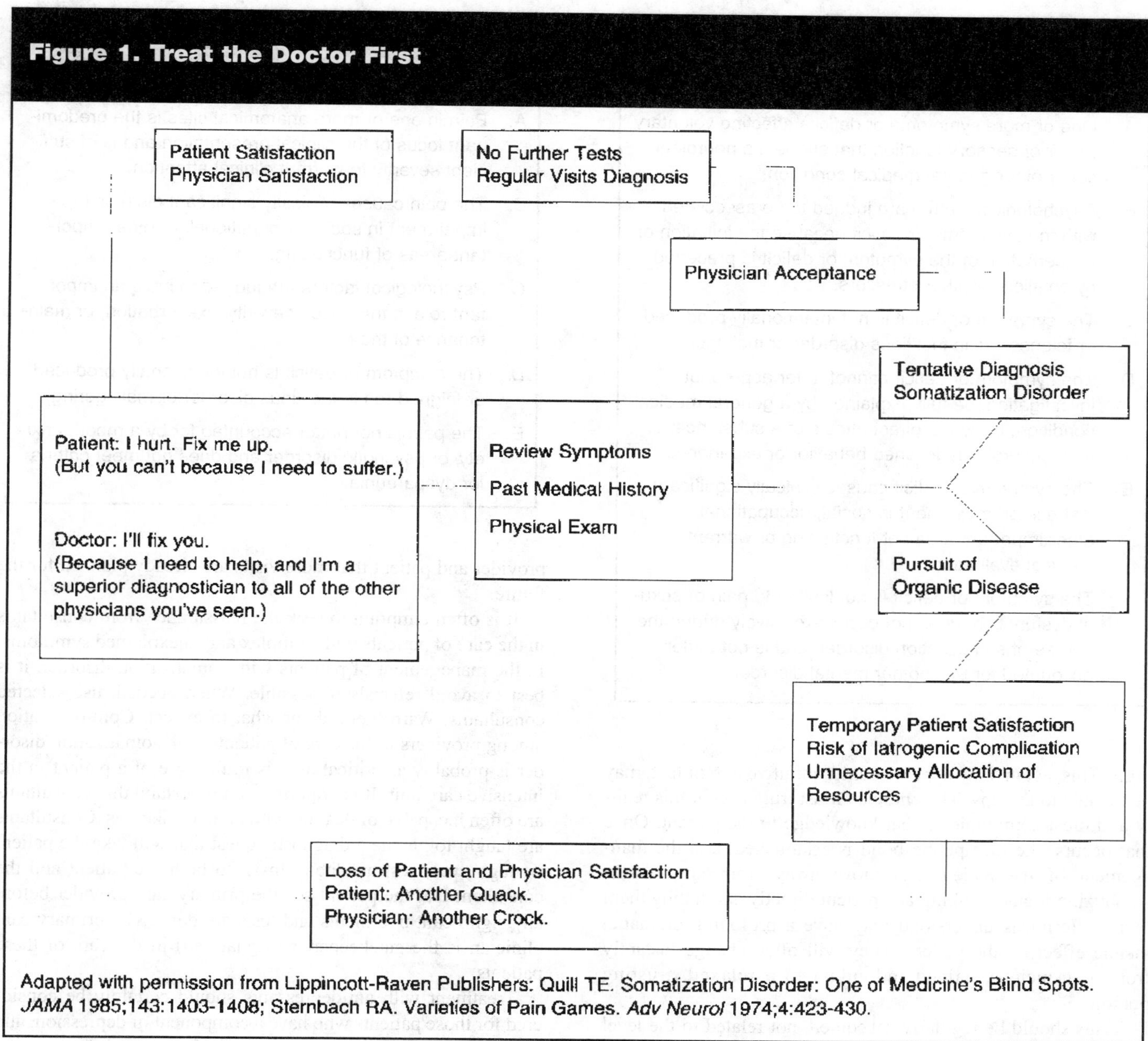

Adapted with permission from Lippincott-Raven Publishers: Quill TE. Somatization Disorder: One of Medicine's Blind Spots. *JAMA* 1985;143:1403-1408; Sternbach RA. Varieties of Pain Games. *Adv Neurol* 1974;4:423-430.

criteria cannot always be met, and the primary care provider must rely on a summation of the data available to make the diagnosis. It may be helpful to review the situation with a skilled mental health professional (psychiatrist, psychologist, or trained counselor) or refer the patient for a formal consultative opinion. This type of collaborative effort may secure the diagnosis and allow a more sophisticated approach to therapy.

Treatment

"Treat the doctor first, the patient second," may be the sentinel message for practitioners. Quill eloquently describes this particular "doctor's dilemma."[3] *(Please see Figure 1.)* The solution is so challenging for clinicians because much of it is counter-intuitive to our routine practice of medicine. The physician must be able to tolerate the inherent risk in a lack of certainty of the diagnosis. Just as is done with pharmacotherapy, a therapeutic trial of a primarily behavioral approach to a patient will often help to secure the diagnosis of somatization disorder. If the provider views this limited diagnostic approach as a therapeutic trial, which can be interrupted any time by more aggressive testing if symptoms change, it may be easier to proceed with the tentative therapy of somatization disorder.

The next essential element of therapy is to understand the psychodynamics of the patient's need to be sick and the clinician's need not to perform unnecessary and dangerous tests and treatments. Remember that this is often a subconscious process. If the provider denies that the patient has a problem, the patient will simply increase or change the symptoms to "prove" they really are ill. It is key to acknowledge that the patient is suffer-

Table 5. DSM-IV Diagnostic Criteria—Conversion Disorder[1]

A. One or more symptoms or deficits affecting voluntary motor or sensory function that suggest a neurological or other general medical condition.

B. Psychological factors are judged to be associated with the symptoms or deficit because the initiation or exacerbation of the symptom or deficit is preceded by conflicts or other stressors.

C. The symptom or deficit is not intentionally produced or feigned (as in factitious disorder or malingering).

D. The symptom or deficit cannot, after appropriate investigation, be fully explained by a general medical condition, or by the direct effects of a substance, or as a culturally sanctioned behavior or experience.

E. The symptom or deficit causes clinically significant distress or impairment in social, occupational, or other important areas of functioning or warrants medical evaluation.

F. The symptom or deficit is not limited to pain or sexual dysfunction, does not occur exclusively during the course of somatization disorder, and is not better accounted for by another mental disorder.

Table 6. DSM-IV Diagnostic Criteria—Pain Disorder[1]

A. Pain in one or more anatomical sites is the predominant focus of the clinical presentation and is of sufficient severity to warrant clinical attention.

B. The pain causes clinically significant distress or impairment in social, occupational, or other important areas of functioning.

C. Psychological factors are judged to have an important role in the onset, severity, exacerbation, or maintenance of the pain.

D. The symptom or deficit is not intentionally produced or feigned (as in factitious disorder or malingering).

E. The pain is not better accounted for by a mood, anxiety, or psychotic disorder and does not meet criteria for dyspareunia.

ing.[25] This, again, may appear counter-intuitive but, in fact, may be the key to therapy. The clinician must truly accept this reality and must communicate that knowledge to the patient. Once that occurs, the therapeutic bond is established, and the management of the patient can move away from an organic, somatizing focus. Looking at a patient directly and telling them their suffering is understood may have a profound, dramatic, visible effect on the patient. They will often change instantly from a suspicious, pained individual to a relaxed, trusting person.

Visits should be regularly scheduled, not related to the level of "sickness." Encounters with patients must not focus on symptoms. This again is not how physicians are typically taught to practice medicine. Why see them if they're not "sick?" Why not ask them what's wrong? If patients can be freed from having to report symptoms, then clinicians free themselves from having to pursue those symptoms. The practitioner must understand that the patient is coming in to share their suffering with the doctor, not to receive a diagnostic test or even a medication. Review symptoms that the patient raises, examine what is appropriate, but focus time and energy on more general issues. A very brief regional exam may give a powerful sense of security to many patients with somatization disorder. The patient wants time and attention, not tests and treatments. A long, insight-oriented psychotherapy session is not the goal or skill of the primary care practitioner. A visit that is too brief will make the patient suspicious that the provider doesn't really care. The traditional 15-minute visit may be just right, with the understanding by both provider and patient that more visits are already planned for the future.

It is often tempting to seek the reassurance from consultants in the care of patients with complex and unexplained symptoms. In the management of patients with somatization disorder, it is best to avoid referrals if possible. When needed, use selected consultants. Warn them about what to expect. Communication among providers in the care of patients with somatization disorder is probably as critical as it is in the care of a patient in the intensive care unit. It is important to understand that consultants are often incapable of dealing with patients like this. Consultants are taught to pursue a diagnostic quest that will take the patient through every test available. Insist to both the patient and the consultant that the patient see the primary care provider before any significant treatments and tests are done. The primary care clinician is the gatekeeper (and guardian) in the care of these patients.

Treatment with antidepressants should certainly be considered for those patients who have a component of depression, and they may provide some improvement, but there is no specific pharmacotherapy for somatization disorder.[4]

Psychiatric consultation is inevitably done once the diagnosis of somatization disorder is established or seriously entertained by the primary care provider. Occasionally insight-oriented psychotherapy is effective, but typically the patient returns to the primary care physician much more quickly than the physician would hope, with no evident "improvement." Recently, short-term group therapy has been used with some success. Patients have fewer somatic symptoms and used fewer health care resources, which results in net economic savings in spite of the added costs of psychiatric services.[26] On a long-term basis, the psychiatrist may serve as a background advisor to the primary care physician on the ongoing behavioral management of the patient. The primary clinician may feel more secure with long-term support, but the patient will often refuse to return to the psychiatrist on a routine basis.[3,25,27]

Table 7. Treatment of Somatization Disorder

- Physician acceptance
- Acknowledge suffering
- Regularly scheduled visits
- Time and attention
- Avoid focus on symptoms
- Avoid tests, referrals, and medications
- Evaluate new symptoms appropriately

The primary provider must always be ready for the next set of symptoms. Even in the ideal therapeutic relationship between the physician and the patient with somatization disorder, the patient will present with new, unexpected symptoms. It is critical to diagnose carefully, as it is possible that this time the symptoms will represent a true organic illness. The sophisticated practitioner learns to rely on clinical judgment, performing the key tests to demonstrate the relatively low likelihood of a new organic problem, avoiding referral to a consultant for extensive evaluation of the new problem. Patients with somatization disorder often have significant organic problems in addition to their psychiatric problem.[3] Both sets of problems must be managed simultaneously and obviously quite differently.

Case Management

The patient scenario can now be reviewed and appropriate management understood. The relatively young age for the presentation of chest pain in this patient reduces the probability that this represents coronary artery disease. It does not eliminate that possibility, however. His prior medical history is impressive, with surgeries and significant health problems before age 30. The prolonged histories of abdominal pain and knee pain should be noted. The patient's criticism of the previous physician should not be ignored. Subconsciously, he is now raising the expectations and obligations of his new doctor. Although the probability of significant coronary artery disease is low, an electrocardiogram and exercise tolerance test are appropriate. The normal results should provide enough re-assurance to the primary care physician that a thallium treadmill or cardiology referral is not indicated, even in the face of pressure from the patient. A near-term follow-up visit should be requested by the physician. That visit should not focus on the chest pain, but generally on the patient's life, lifestyle, and work. The provider should propose, maybe insist, on regular monthly visits, indefinitely.

The presentation of new symptoms of nausea and hematemesis, are not clearly related to the chest pain. This patient could easily have peptic ulcer disease or gastritis. An investigation of his new symptoms will require either endoscopic or radiological studies.

The patient will be back again, whether his abdominal pain is a separate diagnosis or part of his somatization disorder. Anticipate new symptoms, make regularly scheduled visits, accept his "suffering," and retain the bond that has been formed with him.

Summary

Lidz has summarized the tremendous management challenge of the patient with somatization disorder.[28]

Good physicians have always known that the majority of their patients come to them because of emotional difficulties. People turn to physicians, the clergy, and attorneys for help with problems with which they cannot cope alone, but physicians are in a particularly difficult position. Patients come to them with physicial complaints derived from emotional difficulties and problems in living of which patients are unaware because they seek to banish them from consciousness in order to retain their equanimity, but for which substitute physical symptoms occur.[28]

There are few problems in primary care that demonstrate more clearly that patience and compassion are the hallmarks of the excellent physician.

References

1. American Psychiatric Association. *Diagnosis and Statistical Manual of Mental Disorders,* Fourth Edition. Washington: American Psychiatric Association; 1994.
2. Drossman DA, et al. Sexual and physical abuse and gastrointestinal illness. Review and recommendations. *Ann Intern Med* 1995;123: 782-94.
3. Quill TE. Somatization disorder: One of medicine's blind spots. *JAMA* 1985;143:1403-1408.
4. Kaplan C, Mack L, Gordon GH. Somatization in primary care: Patients with unexplained and vexing medical complaints. *J Gen Int Med* 1988;3:177-190.
5. Katon W. The prevalence of somatization in primary care. *Comp Psychiatry* 1984;25:208-215.
6. Myren J, et al. Psychopharmacologic drugs in the treatment of the irritable bowel syndrome. *Ann Gastroenterol Hepatol Paris* 1984;20:117-123.
7. Swartz M, et al. Somatization disorder in a community population. *Am J Psychiatry* 1986;143:1403-1408.
8. Castillo R, Waitzkin H, et al. Somatization in primary care, with a focus on immigrants and refugees. *Arch Fam Med* 1995;4:637-646.
9. Barsky AJ, Borus JF. Somatization and medicalization in the era of managed care. *JAMA* 1995;274:1931-1934.
10. Swartz M. Somatization Disorder. In: Robins, LN (ed). *Psychiatric Disorder in America.* New York: Free Press; 1990:220-257.
11. Smith GR, et al. Patients with multiple unexplained symptoms; their characteristics, functional health, and health care utilization. *Arch Intern Med* 1986;146:69-72.
12. Livingston R, et al. Families who somatize. *J Dev Behav Pediatr* 1995;16:42-46.
13. Fink P. Surgery and medical treatment in persistent somatizing patients. *J Psychosom Res* 1992;36:439-447.
14. Margo KL, Margo GM. The problem of somatization in family practice. *Am Fam Phy* 1994;49:1873-1879.
15. Walker EA, et al. Dissociation in women with chronic pelvic pain. *Am J Psych* 1992;149:534-537.
16. Balint M. *The Doctor, the Patient, and the Illness.* New York: International Universities Press; 1957.
17. Engel GL. The clinical application of the biopsychosocial model.

Am J Psych 1980;137:535-544.

18. Noyes R, et al. Somatization: Diagnosis and management. *Arch Fam Med* 1995;4:790-795.
19. Shear MK, Schulberg HC. Anxiety disorders in primary care. *Bull Menninger Clin* 1995;59(Suppl A);A73-85.
20. Betrus PA, et al. Women and somatization: Unrecognized depression. *Health Care Women Int* 1995;16:287-297.
21. Williams JW, et al. Depressive disorders in primary care: Prevalence, functional disability, and identification. *J Gen Intern Med* 1995;10:7-12.
22. Portegijs PJ, et al. A troubled youth: Relations with somatization, depression and anxiety. *Fam Pract* 1996;13:1-11.
23. Engel GL. 'Psychogenic' pain and the pain-prone patient. *Am J Med* 1959;26:899-918.
24. Blumer D, et al. The pain-prone disorder. *Psychosomatics* 1981;22: 395-402.
25. Lipsitt D. Primary care of the somatizing patient: A collaborative model. *Hospital Practice* 1996;31:77-88.
26. Kashner TM, et al. Enhancing the health of somatization disorder patients. Effectiveness of short-term group therapy. *Psychosomatics* 1995;36:462-470.
27. Craig TKJ, et al. The South London Somatization Study, I: Longitudinal Course and the Influence of Early Life Experience. *Br J Psychiatry* 1993;163:579-588.
28. Lidz T. *The Person: His and Her Development Throughout the Life Cycle.* New York: Basic Books; 1983.
29. Sternbach RA. Varieties of pain games. *Adv Neurol* 1974;4: 423-430.

The Alcoholic Patient: Neurological, Cardiac, Pulmonary, and Renal Complications

Rita K. Cydulka, MD, FACEP
George Eversman, MD

Alcohol. Few drugs wreak so much havoc so often and with such predictability. And to complicate matters, alcoholic patients are frequently uncooperative, have more than one underlying disease, and a compliance profile that is usually less than optimal. Critical diagnostic findings may be obscured by ethanol intoxication, and disposition decisions are complicated by the patient's compromised capacity for vigilant self-care and appropriate follow-up. Add to these pitfalls that chronic alcoholics tend to be poor historians and that the range of medical and surgical disorders afflicting them can fill a textbook of medicine, and it is clear why these patients are prone to falling between the diagnostic cracks.

Although alcoholic patients are frequent users of emergency care, physician recognition of various alcohol-related diseases is poor.[1] Some alcohol-related conditions require immediate lifesaving interventions, whereas others require hospital admission or outpatient referral for resolution. Whatever the diagnosis and ultimate disposition, recognition of chronic alcohol abuse as a cause for these problems is imperative so that early care can be instituted.

This chapter focuses on neurological, cardiac, pulmonary, and renal complications associated with chronic alcoholism. Prompt recognition of alcohol-associated complications, cost-effective strategies for patient assessment, and targeted management techniques are emphasized in order to guide emergency physicians through the complicated conditions related to ethanol-induced pathology.

Background

Ethanol is one of the most commonly abused drugs in the world. Of the estimated 90 million Americans who drink alcoholic beverages, 10 million drink sufficient quantities of ethanol to be considered "problem drinkers," whereas 6 million individuals have developed physical or emotional dependence.[1] In this country alone, the annual cost of lost productivity and health expenses related to alcoholism is estimated to be $117 billion, and as many as 40% of all admissions to the hospital are associated with alcohol-related disorders.[1]

Approach to the Patient

General Principles. First, it should be stressed that however uncooperative, violent, or abusive alcoholic patients may be, this high-risk subgroup requires the same diagnostic scrutiny and therapeutic vigilance that is customarily applied in other emergency encounters. In fact, because signs, symptoms, and clinical presentations in general may be altered by acute intoxication, alcoholic patients require an even higher index of suspicion in order to detect potentially life-threatening disorders—among them, myocardial infarction (MI), subdural hematoma, pneumonia, gastrointestinal hemorrhage—than do individuals who are not known to be chronic

Table 1. Nervous System Complications Associated with Alcohol Abuse

Seizures
Wernicke-Korsakoff's syndrome
Dementia
Cerebellar degeneration
Central pontine myelinolysis
Polyneuropathy
Mononeuropathy
Fetal alcohol syndrome
Marchiafava

abusers of ethanol. Consequently, a targeted, cost-effective approach to emergency assessment of alcoholic patients requires a working knowledge of common ethanol-induced medical disorders.

Second, it is well-known that alcoholic patients represent a medically and medico-legally treacherous subgroup of emergency encounters. For example, determining whether a patient's altered mental status or abnormal vital signs are due to alcohol alone or whether they are manifestations of coexistent infectious, metabolic, or traumatic (e.g., intracranial hemorrhage, ruptured spleen) disorders remains a daily challenge in most EDs. With this in mind, several prudent caveats are in order. In the unstable patient, as well as in those intoxicated individuals with atypical or worrisome findings, it is clearly preferable to aggressively search non-alcohol-related causes of altered mental status, even if definitive assessment requires such costly noninvasive imaging studies as CT or MRI scanning.

Finally, research has confirmed the axiom that the long duration and unpredictable actions of alcohol and its effects on multiple target organs underscore the necessity of careful initial and continuing clinical reevaluation of clinically intoxicated patients.[2] In other words, the emergency physician should search both early and late for reasons other than, or in addition to, alcohol that might explain altered mental status, hypotension, seizures, or metabolic derangements.

Clinical Syndromes. Expeditious management of the alcoholic is facilitated if the extensive differential diagnosis of ethanol-induced disease is both fully appreciated by the emergency practitioner and is considered early in the clinical decision-making process. This approach will generate targeted evaluations and guide the clinician toward the most likely diagnosis. In this vein, it should be stressed that ethanol abuse has been shown to produce toxic effects in almost every organ system in the body. Many of these medical conditions can be attributed to the direct toxic effects of ethanol, whereas others are indirect sequelae that may result from nutritional deficiency or predisposition to trauma.

Medical and surgical syndromes associated with alcohol abuse can be divided into five major categories: 1) acute alcohol intoxication; 2) alcohol dependence or "alcoholism"; 3) acute alcohol withdrawal syndrome; 4) alcohol-related trauma; and 5) medical complications and syndromes. Acute alcohol withdrawal syndromes and medical complications related to alcohol abuse are the focus of this series of articles.

Differential Diagnosis. Neurological complications of alcohol abuse are extremely common and range from trauma-induced, intracranial catastrophes and stroke to chronic myopathies and nutrition-related dementia. Cardiac complications include congestive cardiomyopathy, hypertension, and cardiac arrhythmias. The effects of ethanol on hematopoiesis extend to all cell lines and nearly all blood components involved in hemostasis, producing clinical syndromes that include thrombocytopenia and impaired coagulation. Ethanol also affects all arms of the body's immune system, resulting in an increase in the incidence and severity of infections, especially pneumonia. Moreover, alcohol is the second-leading identified cause of cancer, exceeded in its carcinogenic potential only by tobacco.[2] Cancers associated with heavy use of alcohol include squamous cell carcinoma of the head and neck, esophageal carcinoma, and liver carcinoma.

From a metabolic perspective, alcohol can alter metabolism of carbohydrates, proteins, and lipids, leading to symptomatic hypoglycemia, hypoalbuminemia, and elevated serum triglycerides. Abnormalities of sodium, potassium, phosphorus, and magnesium are common in alcoholics, and severe binge drinkers may manifest alcoholic ketoacidosis, especially when sudden cessation is accompanied by protracted nausea and vomiting. Endocrine problems include hypogonadism and infertility, and a Cushing-like syndrome. Both acute and chronic myopathy have been linked to ethanol misuse, whereas dermatologic conditions associated with alcohol abuse include psoriasis, discoid eczema, and superficial infections.

Alcohol-Related Disorders of the Nervous System

Current research suggests that ethanol-related neurologic disorders may be caused by a combination of neurotoxic effects produced by ethanol or its metabolites, nutritional factors, and genetic predisposition.[1,3-5] In addition, ethanol and its oxidative metabolite acetaldehyde may directly damage both the developing and mature nervous systems.[1] Given the wide-spread prevalence of these conditions, emergency evaluation and triage decisions are made easier when peripheral and central nervous system (CNS) disorders associated with alcohol abuse are considered early in the evaluation process. *(See Table 1.)* Finally, because alcohol intoxication can alter find-ings on the physical exam—especially mental status and neurological testing—an ethanol level should be obtained as a baseline in all patients.

Wernicke-Korsakoff's Syndrome. Wernicke's encephalopathy is a common and preventable disorder caused by a deficiency of thiamine that, in alcoholics, can result from a combination of inadequate dietary intake, reduced gastrointestinal absorption, decreased hepatic storage, and impaired use of the vitamin.[3] Only a subset of thiamine-deficient alcoholics develop full-blown Wernicke's encephalopathy, but exactly how thiamine deficiency leads to brain lesions remains unclear.

Because the diagnosis can be problematic, the emergency physician should maintain a high index of suspicion for this disorder. In fact, one large study reported that acute Wernicke's encephalopathy was correctly diagnosed before death in only 1 of 22 patients, suggesting that the classical clinical triad of encephalopathy, ophthalmoplegia, and ataxia is either rare, not properly elicited, or poorly recognized.[3] In fact, only one-third of patients with acute Wernicke's encephalopathy present with this classic clinical triad, whereas most patients are profoundly disoriented, indifferent, inattentive, and may have an agitated delirium.[3] If untreated, patients with Wernicke's encephalopathy may progress from a decreased level of consciousness, to stupor and coma, to death.[3]

The physical exam should focus on examination of the extraocular muscle groups. Oculomotor abnormalities, including nystagmus, lateral rectus palsy, and conjugate-gaze palsies occur in 96% of patients, and reflect lesions of the oculomotor, abducens, and vestibular nuclei, respectively.[1] Gait ataxia occurs in 87% of patients and probably reflects a combination of polyneuropathy, cerebellar involvement, and vestibular paresis.[6] The hallmark of the encephalopathic stage is characterized by global confusion, in which patients are frequently disoriented to place and time, cannot recognize familiar people, and are so inattentive that they are unable to maintain a coherent conversation.[4] Although CT scanning occasionally reveals low-density diencephalic abnormalities in acute Wernicke's encephalopathy,[7] it should be stressed that the diagnosis must be made promptly on clinical grounds in order to avoid delays in treatment. When the diagnosis cannot be confirmed but the index of suspicion is high, the low risk and potential benefits of administering thiamine far outweigh the consequences of delaying therapy.

With prompt administration of thiamine (100 mg IV stat, followed by 100 mg/d IV for at least 5 days), ocular signs improve within hours to days, whereas ataxia and confusion will improve within days to weeks.[4] Because IV administration of glucose can precipitate Wernicke's encephalopathy in thiamine-deficient patients, if glucose is administered in conjunction with thiamine, it should follow thiamine infusion.[3] For the most part, gastrointestinal malabsorption of thiamine in alcoholics renders oral treatment unreliable.

A majority of patients, including those who are treated, may be left with sequelae, including horizontal nystagmus, ataxia, and a potentially disabling memory disorder known as Korsakoff syndrome, which can be diagnosed by the emergency physician. Unfortunately, memory changes and personality changes are only reversed in 25% of patients who are adequately treated. The clinical hallmark of Korsakoff syndrome is anterograde amnesia.[4] These patients also suffer from confabulation and retrograde amnesia, especially with respect to events occurring just prior to the onset of illness. Confabulation seems to be more marked acutely and is less noticeable as the patient adjusts to his illness. Unfortunately, there is no proven treatment for Korsakoff syndrome, although some reports tout the efficacy of the alpha-2-adrenergic agonist clonidine.[4]

Dementia. Although cognitive deficits are usually mild, many alcoholics have stable and severe cognitive dysfunction ranging from selective anterograde and retrograde amnesia to dementia. In fact, performance on neuropsychological tests is impaired in 50-70% of sober alcoholic patients, most of whom do not have readily treatable disorders.[1] Premorbid intellectual deficits, direct ethanol neurotoxicity and various neurologic complications of alcoholism, including a deficiency of thiamine or nicotinic acid, recurrent head trauma, hepatocerebral degeneration, and Marchiafava Bignami disease may contribute to these problems.

Marchiafava Bignami disease is a rare disorder characterized by necrosis of the corpus callosum and adjacent subcortical white matter that occurs predominantly in malnourished alcoholics. The course may be acute, subacute, or chronic, and it is marked by dementia, spasticity, dysarthria, and inability to walk. Patients may lapse into coma and die, survive for many years in a demented condition, or occasionally recover. Lesions can be identified with use of CT or MRI.[5]

Cerebellar Degeneration. The precise cause(s) of alcoholic cerebellar degeneration is not known, but its similarity to cerebellar lesions seen in Wernicke's encephalopathy suggests that thiamine deficiency may be an important factor.[1] It has also been suggested that alcoholic cerebellar degeneration may be directly related to electrolyte abnormalities. Evidence for direct toxic effect of ethanol as the cause is poor.

Clinical signs and symptoms of alcoholic cerebellar degeneration generally occur after 10 or more years of excessive ethanol use. Typically, it is a gradual, progressive disorder that develops over weeks to months but may also evolve over years or, in some cases, may commence abruptly.[1] Mild or stable cases may suddenly become worse. Ataxia, which primarily affects the gait, is the most common manifestation of cerebellar degeneration. Limb ataxia and dysarthria occur more frequently than in Wernicke's encephalopathy, whereas nystagmus is rare.

The diagnosis of alcoholic cerebellar ataxia is based on the clinical history and neurological examination. CT scan or MRI may show cerebellar cortical atrophy, but half the alcoholic patients with this finding on CT scan are not ataxic on examination.[8] Because of the possible role of thiamine deficiency in this disorder, patients should be given 100 mg of thiamine IV for 5 days. Abstinence from alcohol and resumption of adequate nutritional intake may lead to stabilization or improvement of the neurologic deficit.[9]

Central Pontine Myelinolysis. Central pontine myelinolysis is a rare disorder of the cerebral white matter.[6] Involvement of the corticospinal tract causes paraparesis or quadriparesis, and demyelination of the corticobulbar tracts leads to dysarthria, dysphagia, and an inability to protrude the tongue. Deep tendon reflexes may be increased, decreased, or normal, and Babinski's sign may be present. Disorders of conjugate eye movement may be noted and reflect extension of the lesion in the pons or associated Wernicke's lesions. Disproportionate involvement of motor function may produce the "locked-in" syndrome, in which the patient is conscious but has no motor function to indicate mental alertness.

Cerebral spinal fluid examination in this condition is usually normal. Occasionally, nonspecific increases in protein level or myelin basic protein are detected. MRI is more sensitive than CT scanning for detecting pontine lesions, but even the results of MRI may be unremarkable early in the disease.[10] Radiographic lesions may resolve as the patient recovers. There is no specific treatment for central pontine myelinolysis.

Neuropathy. Alcoholic patients have a high incidence of peripheral nerve disorders, including polyneuropathies and mononeuropathies. Alcoholic polyneuropathy is thought to result from inadequate nutrition, specifically thiamine deficiency and other B-vitamin deficiencies.[3] It is a gradually progressive disorder associated with symptoms and signs that reflect involvement of sensory, motor, and autonomic nerves. Manifestation are usually symmetric and predominantly distal. Symptoms include numbness, paresthesia, and gait ataxia. The most common neurologic signs are loss of deep tendon reflexes, defective perception of touch and vibration sensation,

Table 2. Cardiovascular Manifestations and Syndromes Associated With Alcoholism

Alcoholic heart muscle disease (cardiomyopathy)
Cardiac dysrhythmias—sinus tachycardia, ventricular extrasystoles, atrial fibrillation
"Holiday heart" syndrome
Congestive heart failure
Hypertension
Possible sudden death

and weakness. Autonomic disturbances are less common but, when present, are associated with increased mortality.[2]

Patients with alcoholic polyneuropathy should receive parenteral thiamine supplementation. Improved nutrition, along with abstinence of alcohol intake, is associated with a good prognosis.[1] Alcohol-related mononeuropathy is usually a pressure-related palsy that is treated with splinting, physical and occupational therapy, and abstinence.

Neuromuscular Disease. Both acute and chronic myopathy have been linked to ethanol misuse. Clinically, the two are very distinct entities. Acute alcoholic myopathy is characterized by muscle pain, swelling, and weakness that evolve rapidly and is associated with an elevation of creatine kinase (CK). This condition is much more common in men and frequently follows binge drinking. Conversely, chronic alcoholism myopathy is almost as common among women and is more frequently associated with chronic ethanol misuse. While weakness may be prominent, the condition is slower to evolve and is neither associated with the severe muscle pain nor is there a markedly elevated CK level.[11]

Patients with acute alcoholic myopathy can exhibit a wide range of symptoms and functional impairment, from relatively mild symptoms with transient elevation of the MM-CK fraction to frank rhabdomyolysis with myoglobinuria. Although muscle aches usually are generalized, focal symptoms may occur, especially in the upper legs and calves, in which case the presentation may have to be differentiated from thrombophlebitis. Most episodes of acute alcoholic myopathy are self-limited and resolve over days to weeks. Chronic alcoholic myopathy is characterized by gradual, progressive, and predominantly proximal muscle weakness evolving over weeks to months. Recovery can occur with abstinence but may take months.[12]

Finally, it should be emphasized that alcoholics are at risk for acute myopathy secondary to trauma, seizures, delirium tremens (DTs), and electrolyte depletion. In this regard, low levels of potassium, phosphate, and magnesium have all been associated with myopathic symptoms. Although alcoholics are predisposed to skeletal trauma while intoxicated, they may be more susceptible to fracture because of a higher incidence of osteoporosis, for which alcoholism is a known risk factor.[13]

Seizures. The issue of whether alcohol-related seizures are caused by alcohol itself or are secondary to alcohol withdrawal has not been settled. What is clear, however, is that alcohol abuse as an etiology for seizures carries a poor prognosis.[8-10] CT scans of the head obtained in 259 patients with a first time, alcohol-related generalized seizure ("related" was defined as a seizure clinically associated with recent abstinence from alcohol and with no other obvious etiology for the convulsion) revealed 16 patients with unsuspected intracranial lesions.[9] Accordingly, any patient in whom the etiology of a seizure, especially if it is the first episode, is unclear should be thoroughly evaluated with a careful physical examination, serum electrolytes, and head CT scan prior to discharge from the ED.

Fetal Alcohol Syndrome. Fetal alcohol syndrome is characterized by prenatal and postnatal growth retardation, microcephaly, neurologic abnormalities, facial dysmorphology, and other congenital anomalies. The full syndrome occurs in 6% of the offspring of alcoholic mothers.[14] More often, heavy intrauterine exposure to ethanol is associated with a constellation of less severe abnormalities. For example, prenatal exposure to more than three drinks per day triples the risk of a subnormal IQ at the age of 4. The risk of cranial facial abnormalities also correlates with the amount of ethanol intake early in the first trimester, a time when pregnancy is frequently unrecognized.[14,15] Women seen in the ED who are pregnant and exhibit signs of alcohol misuse should be counseled regarding fetal alcohol syndrome and should be referred for alcohol treatment.

Cardiovascular Manifestations and Syndromes

The association between excessive alcohol consumption and a variety of cardiovascular conditions, many of which present with acute, life-compromising manifestations, is well-established. *(Please see Table 2.)* Therapy will almost always require abstinence in combination with pharmacologic agents, as outlined in the following sections.

Alcoholic Heart Muscle Disease. Because of the known association between alcohol and heart disease, all patients with signs or symptoms suggestive of cardiovascular pathology should be screened for alcohol misuse, preferably with the CAGE questionnaire; a lifetime drinking history must always be obtained. Unfortunately, no blood marker is available for diagnosing alcoholic heart muscle disease, although underlying cardiac abnormalities may be detected by stress-testing or two-dimensional echocardiography.

Alcoholic heart muscle disease must be strongly considered in ethanol-abusing individuals who present to the ED with symptoms suggestive of congestive heart failure (CHF). Interestingly, although beneficial effects of mild ethanol consumption have been shown with respect to coronary artery disease, excessive ethanol consumption can result in alcoholic heart muscle disease, also known as alcoholic cardiomyopathy. Alcoholic heart muscle disease is characterized by clinical features consistent with dilated cardiomyopathy. The metabolic basis of alcoholic heart muscle disease is probably multifactorial, and there is evidence that left ventricular dysfunction may be reversible with abstention from alcohol.[16] Of historical importance is the fact that alcoholic heart muscle disease occurs in patients with a history of excessive daily ethanol consumption (i.e., alcohol intake of > 80 g of ethanol per day) for 10 years or more.[16]

Although alcoholic cardiomyopathy was once thought to be more common in alcoholic men than in alcoholic women, recent studies reveal that alcoholic cardiotoxicity does not spare the female population.[17] Finally, alcoholic heart muscular disease is more common than previously suspected, with one study showing that

Table 3. Treatment Protocol for Alcohol Withdrawal Syndrome

MILD ALCOHOL WITHDRAWAL SYNDROMES

For Adrenergic Hyperactivity:

Benzodiazepines:*

- Diazepam 5-20 mg po/dose q2-6h
- Lorazepam 2 mg po/dose q2-6h **or**
- Chlordiazepoxide 25-100 mg po q2-6h
- Clonidine 0.2 mg po **or**
- Propranolol 40 mg po

* Reduce dose in elderly and in those with hepatic disease. Reevaluate every few hours to determine proper repeat dosage. These drugs are contraindicated in patients with asthma, bradycardia, or CHF.

For Nutritional Deficiency:

- Multivitamins
- Magnesium sulfate 20% 2 cc in each buttock
- 1 mg/d folate po
- 100 mg thiamine po

For Seizures:

- (if there is magnesium deficiency) 6 g IV 10% solution over 3-4 hours

Watch for respiratory depression and impaired renal function

IF HOSPITAL ADMISSION REQUIRED FOR MODERATE-TO-SEVERE ALCOHOL WITHDRAWAL SYNDROME

For Adrenergic Hyperactivity:

Benzodiazepines:*

- Diazepam 5-10 mg IV aliquots until calm q1-4h **or**
- Lorazepam 2-5 mg IV aliquots until calm q2-4h **or**
- Chlordiazepoxide 25 mg IV aliquots until calm q2-4h

*Reduce dose in the elderly and in those with hepatic disease. Reevaluate every few hours to determine proper repeat dosage. These drugs are contraindicated in patients with asthma, bradycardia, or CHF.

For Dehydration:

- 200-1000 mL/h D_5RL or D_5NS

For Nutritional Deficiency:

- Thiamine 100 mg IV
- Multivitamins—1 ampule with first liter of fluids
- Magnesium—6 g IV 10% solution over 3-4 hours

Seizure Precautions:

- None indicated

For Seizures:

- Same as for mild withdrawl

For Hyperthermia:

- Cooling blankets may be required

asymptomatic patients with cirrhosis exhibited a significantly lower left ventricular ejection fraction and significant decreases in left ventricular compliance as compared to non-alcoholics.[17,18]

Congestive Heart Failure. CHF is the most common and dreaded complication of alcoholic cardiomyopathy. As might be expected, clinical signs and symptoms of alcohol-induced CHF are identical to those observed in CHF caused by other precipitants, including coronary heart disease. Pharmacotherapy of symptoms associated with CHF caused by alcoholic cardiomyopathy also is similar and includes vasodilators, digitalis, diuretics, and ACE inhibitors.[18] Recent studies reported in abstract form at the 1995 American Heart Association meetings suggest that oral administration of the calcium blocker amlodipine—when added to a regimen already consisting of ACE inhibitors, digoxin, and diuretics—may significantly reduce mortality rates in patients with Stage III-IV CHF caused by non-ischemic (i.e., alcoholic) etiologies.[19]

The most important factor influencing outcomes in these patients, however, is abstinence, which has been shown to produce improvement in about 60% of patients.[17,18] In contrast, without abstinence, only 10% of patients will demonstrate improvement.[18] All patients with alcohol-associated cardiovascular disease should be referred to their primary care physician or to a cardiologist for follow-up care.

Cardiac Dysrhythmias. In the alcoholic patient, cardiac dysrhythmias, including sinus tachycardia, ventricular extrasystoles, or atrial fibrillation, may be the first manifestation of CHF, MI, concurrent drug toxicity (e.g., cocaine), or electrolyte abnormalities (e.g., hypokalemia, hypomagnesemia). However, atrial or ventricular arrhythmias, especially paroxysmal tachycardia or atrial fibrillation, can also occur after episodes of binge drinking in susceptible individuals, a syndrome known as the "holiday heart." One landmark study on ethanol-induced arrhythmias revealed that alcohol was the primary cause or contributor to new-onset atrial fibrillation in 63% of patients younger than age 65 seen in that ED.[20] Of these individuals, 33% who presented with new onset of atrial fibrillation required digitalis to facilitate conversion to normal sinus rhythm. Overall, 89% of patients eventually converted to sinus rhythm within 24 hours.20 Another study confirms the recurrent nature of this condition; 40% of patients presenting with new-onset atrial fibrillation due to alcohol had a recurrence within several years.[21]

Management of "holiday heart" supraventricular tachyarrhythmias is relatively straightforward. If the patient with atrial fibrillation is symptomatic (angina, cerebral hypoperfusion, or shortness of breath) or has other evidence of cardiac disease, rate control may be achieved with diltiazem administered as 0.25 mg/kg by IV bolus, at a usual starting dose of approximately 20 mg. This can be followed

Table 4. Pulmonary Complications of Ethanol Abuse

Aspiration
Pneumonia
Hyposemia and respiratory failure (multiple etiologies)
Rib fractures (trauma)
Tuberculosis (debilitated host)

by 0.35 mg/kg (approximately 25 mg) in 15 minutes if rate control is not achieved. Simultaneously, a drip consisting of 10 mg in 250 cc of normal saline to be infused over an hour should be started. Alternatively, digoxin 0.5 mg IV in a bolus fashion may be administered, followed by 0.25 mg IV in one hour, followed by 0.25 mg to be repeated again in another hour if rate control has not yet been achieved.

Patients with new-onset atrial fibrillation should also have other non-alcohol-related causes, such as thyrotoxicosis, pulmonary embolism, MI, and pulmonary disease, ruled out. All patients with new-onset atrial fibrillation who demonstrate a persistent, rapid ventricular response that is unresponsive to therapy should be admitted to the hospital for observation and treatment.

A final cautionary note is required. Although many alcohol-induced cardiac conditions are self-limited, respond to abstinence, and are not life-threatening, some studies suggest a higher incidence of sudden cardiac death in heavy drinkers. In this regard, one important investigation found that patients who imbibe more than six alcoholic beverages per day have a much higher incidence of sudden cardiac death than those who drink less.[22]

Hypertension. Although acute ethanol administration or ingestion appears to lower blood pressure, consumption of three or more drinks per day results in a dose-dependent increase in blood pressure, which returns to normal within weeks of abstinence.[23-25] Accordingly, ED patients who have newly diagnosed hypertension or who have hypertension that has been poorly controlled on medication should be questioned about their alcohol intake. In alcohol misusers, the proportion of patients who are hypertensive may be as high as 50%.[25] In patients with essential hypertension who drank up to 80 g of ethanol per day, one study demonstrated that abstinence significantly reduced blood pressure, whereas resumption of alcohol intake increased both systolic and diastolic pressure 48 hours after ethanol consumption.[26]

Although several studies have shown a reduction in the incidence of coronary artery disease and MI in response to mild-to-moderate ethanol consumption (up to 50 g of alcohol per day), it is unclear whether there is a beneficial effect of ethanol in patients with established coronary artery disease.[16] These protective effects, which presumably are mediated by elevated levels of high-density lipoprotein (HDL) cholesterol, are associated with consistent intake rather than binge drinking. Plasma fibrinolytic activity also increases with ethanol consumption. Finally, it is important to note that although moderate alcohol intake reduces the incidence of coronary artery disease, it increases mortality due to hemorrhagic stroke, hypertension, and accidents.

Alcohol Withdrawal Syndrome

Confirmed alcoholics presenting with symptoms, signs, or clinical findings related to the heart or CNS should always be considered candidates for alcohol withdrawal syndrome. Generally speaking, symptoms reflecting CNS and cardiac hyperactivity usually begin within 6-12 hours of decreasing alcohol intake, peak in intensity on day 2 or 3, and improve by day 4 or 5. Many alcoholics wake up in the morning with some signs of withdrawal. Predominant features of alcohol withdrawal include hand tremors (the "shakes"); autonomic nervous system hyperactivity (i.e., agitation and elevated temperature, heart rate, blood pressure, and respiratory rate); and sweats, insomnia, and bad dreams. Psychiatric symptoms include anxiety or depression, whereas common gastrointestinal manifestations consist of nausea, vomiting, and diarrhea. About 5% of alcoholics experience severe withdrawal symptoms that are accompanied by a state of confusion and hallucinations.[1,27]

A small percentage of alcoholics demonstrate one or two generalized seizures, usually commencing within 48 hours of stopping drinking or decreasing alcohol intake. These seizures, known as "rum fits," are rarely focal in nature, occur in short bursts, and do not indicate the presence of an underlying seizure disorder. They require no treatment and are usually self-limited.[3] Although in many cases the seizures of mild withdrawal are benign and require no treatment, other causes of seizures should be sought. In addition, many of the patients who have withdrawal seizures may progress to DTs. Such patients require observation and may benefit from treatment with benzodiazepines if they have continued tremors and other symptoms of withdrawal.

Carrying a 1-5% mortality rate, DTs are characterized by symptoms of withdrawal that have progressed to include confusion; delusion; hallucinations; severe agitation; and persistent, generalized seizures. Initial therapy of seizures should include IV benzodiazepines. For seizures associated with hypomagnesemia, administer 4 g 10% magnesium sulfate solution IV over 10 minutes. All patients with DTs should be monitored carefully in the intensive care unit. Associated illnesses, especially pneumonia, pancreatitis, and hepatitis, occur frequently and contribute to poor outcomes.[1,27]

Treatment goals in alcohol withdrawal include hydration, mild tranquilization, vitamin repletion, prevention of progression, and recognition of underlying coexistent disorders. *(Please see Table 3.)* Accordingly, all patients should be administered multivitamins with 1 mg folate and 50-100 mg thiamine daily for at least a week. Dehydrated patients should be given IV fluids as needed, using either D5 Ringer's lactate or D5 normal saline. Potassium depletion, if present, should be addressed promptly, especially in the face of severe vomiting. Magnesium must also be replaced, with either an IM injection (2 cc of a 20% solution once daily) or 6 g in a 10% solution given IV over several hours.[3] The CNS symptoms of withdrawal can be alleviated by administering another CNS depressant (usually a benzodiazepine) and gradually decreasing the levels given over a three- to five-day period. The goal is to use a drug with a high margin of safety, to alleviate the symptoms on day 1, and then to decrease the dose by about 20% per day over a several-day tapering course. The average patient requires 25-50 mg of chlordiazepoxide, lorazepam 1-2 mg, or 10 mg diazepam po every 4-6 hours on the first day. Patients with severe withdrawal will require IV benzodiazepine administration.[4,6,7] An adrenergic blocking

Table 5. Management of Selected Life-Threatening Neurologic and Cardiac Complications

SEIZURES

Treatment for alcohol-withdrawal seizures not indicated unless:

1. Secondary to magnesium deficiency; 6 g 10% $MgSO_4$ over 3-4 hours
2. Status epilepticus
   - IV diazepam 5-10 mg aliquots until controlled
   - IV lorazepam 2 mg aliquots until controlled
   - IV phenytoin 18-20 mg/kg (rate < 50 mg/min)
   - IV phenobarbital 15-20 mg/kg (rate < 50 mg/min)

WERNICKE-KORSAKOFF'S SYNDROME

Thiamine 100 mg/d IV x 5 days
Abstinence

ATRIAL FIBRILLATION

For rate control:

- Digoxin 0.5 mg IV, then 0.25 mg q1-2h up to 1 mg or
- Diltiazem 0.25 mg/kg IV bolus followed by 0.35 mg/kg in 15 minutes

If no response:

- 10 mg drip over 1 hour
- Admit to hospital if inadequate response

agent may be a useful adjunct to control adrenergic hyperactivity. Propranolol 40 mg po or 0.5-1.0 mg IV is usually effective. Clonidine 0.2 mg has also been used with some success in this setting.[4,5,7,27]

Adjunctive supportive therapy in the patient with symptoms suggestive of alcohol withdrawal or alcohol withdrawal seizures consists of empiric administration of an "alcohol cocktail." One such regimen uses D5 normal saline at a rate of 200 cc per hour (the rate should be decreased in patients with ascites, CHF, or evidence of fluid overload). To this liter bag are added two amps MVI-12 (multivitamins), 1-5 mg folate, 40 meq potassium, 5 g magnesium, and 100 mg thiamine. The two amps of MVI-12 will provide, among other things, niacin (100 mg) to avoid pellagra.

Patients with mild abstinence symptoms who are in good physical condition, have no history of DTs or seizures, and who have solid social support systems at home may be detoxified as outpatients. Such individuals require meticulous evaluation in the ED, as well as treatment with oral vitamins. A trustworthy spouse or significant other may be given a one- to two-day supply of benzodiazepines for administration to the patient, who must return for daily evaluation of vital signs. If signs or symptoms of withdrawal worsen, the patient should be advised to return to the ED immediately.[1,27]

Pulmonary Complications

Alcohol consumption predisposes to pulmonary infection via a number of independent mechanisms. In addition to ethanol-mediated immunosuppression, glottic reflexes are suppressed in alcoholics, predisposing them to aspiration;[28] the cough reflex also may be impaired.[29] Although aspiration most often leads to infection with anaerobic oropharyngeal flora (*Bacteroides fragilis*) or gram-negative bacilli (*Klebsiella*), chemical pneumonitis from gastric contents regurgitated during an alcoholic stupor must also be considered in the differential diagnosis.[30] Even in the absence of aspiration, the general debilitation, poor nutrition, and high prevalence of chronic obstructive pulmonary disease (COPD) and cigarette smoking in this patient population predispose to development of lower respiratory tract infection with such community-acquired pathogens as *Streptococcus pneumoniae* and *Haemophilus influenzae*. The possibility of tuberculosis should always be considered. *(Please see Table 4.)*

In addition, binge drinking may contribute to, or directly precipitate, compromises in respiratory function that predispose to pulmonary infection. For example, the alcoholic patient is at risk for sustaining chest wall trauma secondary to falls, which may produce rib fractures associated with incomplete respiratory excursion secondary to splinting. Muscle weakness secondary to the electrolyte deficiencies also may develop. Adult respiratory distress syndrome (ARDS) or noncardiogenic pulmonary edema complicates 9-13% of patients with acute alcoholic pancreatitis.[31]

The high risk of developing infectious pulmonary complications in this patient population mandates extreme vigilance when evaluating alcoholic patients with respiratory complaints, even when fever is absent. Almost without exception, a chest x-ray, pulse oximetry, and complete blood count should be obtained to rule out pneumonia. Although a small percentage of non-intoxicated patients may be managed as outpatients, in general, the overwhelming majority of debilitated alcoholic patients with radiographic evidence of pneumonia should be hospitalized. The reasons for this disposition strategy are numerous: These individuals are likely to be poorly compliant with oral antibiotic intake, have compromised host defense mechanisms, are more likely to have underlying pulmonary disease, and may be infected with virulent organisms (e.g., *Bacteroides, Klebsiella*) that fall out of the usual spectrum of community-acquired offending agents. Consequently, 2-3 days of parenteral antibiotic therapy, combined with supportive care, represents the most prudent approach in this patient population.

Finally, hypoxemia in the patient with cirrhosis can have multiple etiologies. In addition to pneumonia and COPD, ascites may compromise arterial oxygen by restricting respiratory excursion or even leaking across the diaphragm and creating a hydrothorax.[32] Development of new vascular precapillary shunts in the lung parenchyma, the cause of which is unknown, is a unique cause of hypoxemia in patients with cirrhosis of the liver. Another contributing factor to arterial desaturation in the patient with cirrhosis is the rightward shift of the oxyhemoglobin dissociation curve, which, in part, is caused by hyperventilation and respiratory alkalosis. The exact pathophysiology of increased respiratory drive is not known.[33]

Renal Complications

A potent diuretic and inhibitor of antidiuretic hormone (AD), ethanol produces both direct and indirect effects on renal regulation of fluid, solute, and electrolyte homeostasis. Ethanol-abusing patients who present with muscle weakness, cardiac arrhythmias, fatigue, altered mental status, or muscle cramps should be evaluated for the possibility of electrolyte disturbances, including hypokalemia, hyponatremia, hypomagnesemia, and hypophosphatemia. Obtaining a serum BUN and creatinine level may help determine the patient's state of intravascular hydration, although it should be emphasized that BUN levels in patients with severe liver disease may be extremely low due to poor hepatic function. In these cases, a low urinary sodium level (< 10 meq) may provide confirmatory evidence of severe intravascular volume depletion or, alternatively, suggest the presence of hepatorenal syndrome.

In the setting of severe hepatic failure, ethanol abuse has also been associated with varying degrees of renal insufficiency, including kidney failure. A life-threatening complication, hepatorenal syndrome is characterized by diminished renal function in the presence of severe liver disease. An ominous complication that frequently follows gastrointestinal bleeding, sepsis, or severe hepatic failure, the syndrome is characterized by oliguria with low urine sodium (< 10 meq/L), and high urine osmolality with no evidence of hypovolemia or prerenal azotemia. Hepatorenal syndrome may reverse if there is resolution of hepatic pathology. The precise pathogenesis of this condition is unknown, but it appears to be associated with intrarenal vasoconstriction and redistribution of renal blood flow. The patient with alcoholic cirrhosis is also at risk for developing prerenal azotemia secondary to diuretics or dehydration; ATN secondary to hypotension, hemorrhage or sepsis; renal insufficiency secondary to nephrotoxic medications (e.g., aminoglycosides, NSAIDs); and pyelonephritis.[34]

Ethanol is one of the most commonly recognized causes of rhabdomyolysis and has been estimated to be the etiologic factor in over 20% of all cases.[35] Although alcoholics are at risk for traumatic crush syndromes, they may also suffer from non-traumatic rhabdomyolysis. ATN from rhabdomyolysis should be suspected when an alcoholic presents with evidence of acute renal insufficiency in the setting of oliguria, muscle tenderness, or swelling and characteristic biochemical findings.

To support the diagnosis, the supernatent of freshly voided and centrifuged urine can be tested for reactivity with orthotolidin (Hematest). If positive, a urine sample should be sent for a specific myoglobin assay. Other biochemical findings in rhabdomyolysis include an elevated CK level (usually > 24,000 IU), a disproportionate elevation of creatinine in relation to urea nitrogen, and biochemical evidence of a hypercatabolic state (exaggerated hyperphosphatemia, severe hyperkalemia, acidosis, and profound hyperuricemia).[36] Treatment requires maintenance of adequate urine volume with hydration and diuretics, as well as alkalinization of the urine with sodium bicarbonate.

Finally, the possibility of ethylene glycol ingestion (as an alcohol substitute) should always be considered in the alcoholic who presents with sudden, unexplained renal insufficiency. If ethylene glycol ingestion is suspected, a search should be conducted for calcium oxalate crystals in the urine. This finding, in conjunction with an unexplained anion gap acidosis, is strongly suggestive of the diagnosis.

Summary

From both a diagnostic and therapeutic perspective, experienced emergency physicians have come to appreciate that alcoholic patients pose a substantial risk for stumbling into a number of pitfalls. Because of the life-threatening nature of cardiac, pulmonary, and neurological conditions associated with ethanol abuse, special vigilance is mandatory for individuals presenting with complaints referable to these organ systems. For example, determining whether a patient's altered mental status or abnormal vital signs are due to the direct effects of alcohol alone, or whether they are manifestations of coexistent disorders requires a systematic approach to patient assessment. When indicated, therapy must be initiated promptly and according to established protocols *(Please see Table 5.)*

Clearly, alcohol-related causes should always be considered first. But in the unstable patient, as well as in those intoxicated individuals with atypical or worrisome findings, it is imperative to search out non-alcohol-related causes as well, even if definitive assessment requires such costly noninvasive imaging studies as CT or MRI scanning. The patient's final disposition is a matter of clinical judgment, although erring on the conservative side is well-advised. Finally, attempts by the emergency physician—in conjunction with supportive counseling from social service resources, if available—to initiate alcohol recovery programs remain a critical component of patient management.

References

1. Charness ME, Simon RP, Greenberg DA. Ethanol and the nervous system. *N Engl J Med* 1989;321:442-454.
2. Johnson RH, Robinson BJ. Mortality in alcoholics with autonomic neuropathy. *J Neurol Surg Psych* 1988;51: 476-480.
3. Victor M, Adams RD, Collins GH. The Wernicke-Korsakoff syndrome and related neurologic disorders due to alcoholism and malnutrition. In: Adams RD, Victor M, eds. *Contemporary Neurology Series*. Vol 3. Philadelphia: FA Davis; 1989:1-28.
4. Butters E. Alcoholic Korsakoff syndrome: An update. *Semin Neurol* 1984;4:226-244.
5. Kawamura M, Shiota J, Yagishita T. Marchiafava-Bignami disease: Computed tomographic scan in magnetic resonance imaging. *Ann Neurol* 1985;18:103-104.
6. Victor M, Adams RD, Mancall EL. A restrictive form of cerebellar cortical degeneration occurring in alcoholic patients. *Arch Neurol* 1979;71:579-688.
7. McDowell JR, Leblanc HJ. Computer tomographic findings in Wernicke-Korsakoff syndrome. *Arch Neurol* 1984;41: 453-454.
8. Hillbom M, Muuronen A, Holm L, et al. The clinical versus radiological diagnosis of alcoholic cerebellar degeneration. *J Neurol Sci* 1986;73:45-53.
9. Diener HC, Dichgans J, Bacher M, et al. Improvement of ataxia in alcoholic cerebellar atrophy through alcohol abstinence. *J Neurol* 1984;231:258-262.
10. Miller GM, Baker HL, Okazaki H. Central pontine myelinolysis and its imitators: MR findings. *Radiology* 1988; 168:795-802.
11. Martin FC, Slavin G, Levi AJ. Alcoholic muscle disease. *Br Med Bull* 1982;38:53-56.
12. Haller RG, Knochel JE. Skeletal muscle disease in alcoholism. *Med Clin North Am* 1984;68:91-103.
13. Moniz C. Alcohol and bone. Br Med Bull 1994;50:67-75.

14. Streissguth AP, Barr HM, Sampson PD, et al. IQ at age 4 in relation to maternal alcohol use and smoking during pregnancy. *Devel Psychol* 1989;25:3-11.
15. Ernhart CB, Sokol RJ, Martier S, et al. Alcohol teratogenicity in the human: A detailed assessment of specificity, critical period, and threshold. *Am J Obstet Gynecol* 1987;156: 33-39.
16. Preedy VR, Richardson PJ. Ethanol-induced cardiovascular disease. *Brit Med Bull* 1994;50:152-163.
17. Kupari M, Koskinen P. Comparison of the cardiotoxicity of ethanol in women versus men. *Am J Cardiol* 1992;70: 645-649.
18. Davidson DM. Cardiovascular effects of alcohol. *West J Med* 1989;151:430-439.
19. Packer MC, et al. Prospective Amlodipine Survival Evaluation (PRAISE) trial. AHA Meeting Abstract. March 1995.
20. Lowenstein SR. The role of alcohol in new-onset atrial fibrillation. *Arch Intern Med* 1983;143:1882-1891.
21. Koskinen P. A four-year prospective follow-up study of the role of alcohol in recurrences of atrial fibrillation. *J Intern Med* 1991;230:423-426.
22. Warramethee G, Shaper AG. Alcohol and sudden death. *Br Heart J* 1992;68:443-448.
23. Schuckit MA. Alcohol and alcoholism. In: Isselbacher KJ, Adams RD, eds. *Harrison's Principles of Internal Medicine.* 13th ed. New York: McGraw-Hill; 1994:2420-2428.
24. Yamada Y, Ishizaki M, Kido T, et al. Alcohol, high blood pressure, and serum gamma-glutamyl transpeptidase level. *Hypertension* 1991;18:819-826.
25. Saunder JB, Beevers DG, Paton A. Alcohol-induced hypertension. *Lancet* 1981;ii:653-656.
26. Potter JF, Beevers DG. Pressor effect of alcohol in hypertension. *Lancet* 1984;i:119-122.
27. Doll R, Peto R. The causes of cancer; quantitative estimates of avoidable risks of cancer in the United States today. *J Natl Cancer Inst* 1981;66:1191-1265.
28. Naugesten WJ, Klepsen RG. A probable mechanism for laryngeal resistance to pneumonia. *J Infect Dis* 198s;63:94.
29. Berkowitz A, et al. The effect of ethanol on the cough reflex. *Clin Sci Molec Med* 1973;45:527-531.
30. Fuxench-Lopez Z, Ramirez-Ronda CH. Pharyngeal flora in ambulatory alcoholic patients: Prevalence of gram-negative bacilli. *Arch Intern Med* 1978;138:1815-1816.
31. Hayes MF, et al. Adult respiratory distress syndrome in association with acute pancreatitis. *Am J Surg* 1974;127:314.
32. Johnston RF, Loo RV. Hepatic hydrothorax: Studies to determine the source of fluid and report of thirteen cases. *Ann Intern Med* 1964;61:385.
33. Krumpe PE, et al. Alcohol and the respiratory tract. *Med Clin North Am* 1984;68:201-219.
34. Boyer TD. Major sequelae of cirrhosis. In: Wyngaarden JB, Smith LH, eds. *Cecil Textbook of Medicine.* 18th ed. Philadelphia: WB Saunders; 1988:852.
35. Gabow PA, et al. The spectrum of rhabdomyolysis. *Medicine* 1982;61:141-152.
36. Koffler A, et al. Acute renal failure due to nontraumatic rhabdomyolysis. *Ann Intern Med* 1976;85:23-28.

The Alcoholic Patient: Gastrointestinal, Infectious, Metabolic, and Hematologic Complications

Rita K. Cydulka, MD, FACE
George Eversman, MD

When diagnosing and treating complications associated with chronic ethanol misuse, several cautionary strategies should be employed, among them, searching aggressively for non-alcohol-related causes of symptoms. In clinically intoxicated patients with gastrointestinal, infectious, metabolic, hematologic, endocrine, and dermatologic sequelae of chronic alcoholism,[1] careful initial, comparative, and continuing clinical reevaluation is called for.

Some complications of alcoholism produce conditions that can be stabilized in the emergency department (ED), while other conditions require more comprehensive evaluation, especially those involving the gastrointestinal system. Dreaded because of their propensity to produce life-threatening hemorrhagic and infectious complications, gastrointestinal problems associated with chronic alcohol misuse include not only alcoholic hepatitis and cirrhosis, but also esophageal reflux, esophageal cancer, gastritis, gastrointestinal hemorrhage, diarrhea, and pancreatitis. Drug-drug interactions, alcohol-induced hematologic disorders, and serious metabolic derangements round out the constellation of conditions that the emergency practitioner must be prepared to recognize promptly and manage expeditiously.

This chapter outlines cost-effective assessment strategies and diagnostic clues that suggest the presence of gastrointestinal, metabolic, infectious, or hematologic complications of acute and chronic ethanol misuse.

Pharmacologic Considerations

Because alcohol can affect the metabolism of many different drugs, initial evaluation of the acutely intoxicated patient or the individual known to be a chronic misuser of ethanol should always include consideration of possible drug-drug interactions. For example, depression of the central nervous system (CNS) is enhanced by the additive effects of alcohol when combined with a number of different drugs, including antihistamines, barbiturates, phenothiazines, tricyclic antidepressants, and chloral hydrate. Prolongation in bleeding time induced by salicylates may be further elevated by concurrent alcohol consumption. In addition, ethanol can precipitate lactic acidosis when given with phenformin and, through an unknown mechanism, increases the chance of acquiring hepatitis in patients on isoniazid. Finally, a small but clinically significant percentage of chronic alcoholics taking "therapeutic" doses of acetaminophen can develop severe hepatotoxicity as a result of induction of hepatotoxic intermediate metabolites generated by P450 cytochrome oxidase system.[2-4]

Ethanol can also have antagonistic or additive effects on drugs with which it shares metabolic pathways. Ethanol stimulates increased microsomal oxidation. With acute ingestion of ethanol, there may be competition for these metabolic pathways, which may slow metabolism of the drug and, in turn, produce transient elevations

Table 1. Gastrointestinal Complications of Alcohol Abuse

- Gastroesophageal reflux
- Esophageal carcinoma
- Gastritis
- Mallory-Weiss tear
- Esophageal varices
- Peptic ulcer disease (possibly)
- Diarrhea
- Liver disease
  - Fatty liver
  - Alcoholic hepatitis
  - Cirrhosis/ascites
  - Hepatic encephalopathy
  - Spontaneous bacterial peritonitis
  - Acute liver failure
  - Hepatic carcinoma
- Pancreatitis—chronic and acute
  - Pancreatic pseudocyst
  - Hemorrhagic pseudocyst
  - Infected pseudocyst

in drug level (e.g., phenytoin). Conversely, in alcoholics who are abstaining, metabolism may be accelerated, producing increases in drug clearance and lower serum drug levels. In this regard, the half-lives of phenytoin, tolbutamide, and warfarin have been shown to be significantly shorter in abstaining alcoholics than in nondrinkers.[5]

Perhaps the best-known ethanol-drug interaction is the "Antabuse" reaction. In this syndrome, alcohol consumption that occurs after premedication with disulfiram (Antabuse) produces such symptoms as flushing, nausea, vomiting, chest pain, abdominal cramps, diaphoresis, palpitations, vertigo, blurred vision, dyspnea, hyperventilation, tachypnea, hypotension, confusion, and psychotic episodes within 5-15 minutes after ingestion. A number of other drugs also can induce similar Antabuse-like symptoms, among them metronidazole, chloramphenicol, chlorpropamide, griseofulvin, nitrofurantoin, sulfonamides, and some cephalosporins. Treatment for this reaction is symptomatic and includes monitoring for seizures and arrhythmias.

Gastrointestinal Complaints, Complications, and Syndromes

Gastrointestinal complications in alcoholics are common and, not infrequently, present as life-threatening emergencies. *(Please see Table 1.)* Initial evaluation in the ED will usually guide the physician toward a reasonable working diagnosis and appropriate disposition, although definitive diagnosis most often requires a more comprehensive—and invasive—in-hospital evaluation.

Common Gastrointestinal Syndromes. Not surprisingly, gastrointestinal disorders are extremely common in patients with a history of chronic ethanol misuse.[6] For example, alcohol impairs lower esophageal sphincter function and decreases frequency of peristaltic contractions in the distal esophagus, a combination that sets the stage for reflux esophagitis. Patients usually present with burning, dyspepsia, and abdominal discomfort commencing shortly after consumption of alcohol or a heavy meal. Complications of gastroesophageal reflux disease include severe erosive esophagitis, bleeding, stricture formation, and the development of Barrett's esophagus. Treatment of esophagitis in the alcoholic requires abstention from alcohol as well as the standard antireflux drug regimen, which includes H2-blockers (ranitidine or famotidine), proton pump blockers (prilohsec), and/or antacids.[6] *(Please see Table 2.)*

In addition to its effects on the gastroesophageal sphincter (GES), alcohol also interferes with the integrity of the gastromucosal barrier, permitting back diffusion of ions along their electrochemical gradients. The clinical consequence is acute gastritis, which produces anorexia, dyspepsia, and abdominal pain. Patients with acute gastritis will have endoscopic evidence of gastritis, including patchy mucosal erythema, erosions, petechiae, and exudate.[6] From a historical perspective, other mucosal irritants, such as aspirin and nonsteroidal anti-inflammatory drugs (NSAIDs), can potentiate alcohol-mediated gastric damage and increase the likelihood of bleeding.

A significant percentage of patients with a history suggestive of alcoholic gastritis will have minor, self-limited hemorrhagic episodes that do not require hospitalization. Distinguishing these patients from those with more serious hemorrhage can be difficult, but it is not impossible. In general, patients with alcoholic gastritis who can be considered for discharge and careful follow-up include individuals with normal initial vital signs who have no evidence of guaiac-positive stools or active bleeding based on nasogastric tube evaluation, are at low risk for esophageal varices, and who remain stable after 1-2 hours of observation in the ED. If gastric ulceration is strongly suspected, a course of H2 blockers is reasonable, whereas if the condition is thought to be alcohol-mediated, cessation of drinking must be a part of the treatment plan.

Although most cases of alcoholic gastritis are self-limited, gastritis is the most frequent cause of non-life-threatening gastrointestinal bleeding in heavy drinkers. Alcohol-induced gastritis is reversible within hours to days of abstinence.[6] In contrast to the studies linking ethanol and gastritis, there is no evidence implicating alcohol as a cause of peptic ulcer disease; however, the incidence of duodenal ulcers is higher in alcoholics than in non-alcoholics.[7]

Chronic heavy drinking that is associated with violent vomiting can produce longitudinal tears in the mucosa at the gastroesophageal junction, a disruption that can cause severe upper gastrointestinal hemorrhage. Fortunately, in most patients, the bleeding ceases spontaneously. Continued bleeding may require vasopressin infusion therapy or angiographic embolization. Surgery is rarely needed.[8] On rare occasions, retching may be so violent as to cause a spontaneous rupture of the esophagus, or Boerhaave's syndrome.

Diarrhea is another common complaint in binge-drinking alcoholics and may contribute significantly to dehydration and electrolyte deficiencies of potassium, magnesium, and phosphate.

There is no single etiology and no specific treatment for binge drinker's diarrhea. Intestinal malabsorption with significant weight loss is found in one-third to one-half of binge drinkers. Steatorrhea has been attributed to reversible pancreatic insufficiency, which may be correctable with abstinence and nutritious diet. Recent studies also suggest that protein-losing enteropathy may be an important cause of protein malnutrition in chronic alcoholics.[9,10]

Fatty Liver. Although fatty liver is present in 90% of chronic alcohol abusers, this condition is usually asymptomatic.[11] Although only 8-30% of long-term alcohol abusers will develop alcoholic cirrhosis,[12] a minority of individuals will not progress beyond the stage of fatty liver despite persistent drinking. Some of this variation in individual susceptibility is accounted for by differences in cumulative amounts, duration, and pattern of drinking. Additional environmental factors, such as infection with hepatitis viruses, may contribute to the development of alcoholic liver disease. In this regard, an increased prevalence of hepatitis B markers has been reported in both alcoholics and patients with alcoholic liver disease.[13]

Most patients with fatty liver are asymptomatic and are detected coincidentally when nontender hepatomegaly is discovered during the course of a physical examination. If symptomatic, however, patients with fatty liver may complain of malaise, anorexia, nausea, abdominal discomfort, mild jaundice, and tender hepatomegaly. Rarely, patients have massive steatosis or severe clinical cholestasis. The diagnosis is confirmed with liver biopsy. With abstinence, fatty liver resolves histologically in 4-6 weeks and usually is a benign disease. It does not predispose to cirrhosis. Treatment consists of abstinence from alcohol and consumption of a nutritionally balanced diet.[14]

Alcoholic Hepatitis. Difficult to diagnose because of its protean manifestations, alcoholic hepatitis is characterized by a variable presentation that ranges from the asymptomatic patient to individuals in extremis suffering from florid acute liver failure. As a rule, the illness develops gradually over weeks and is accompanied by anorexia, vomiting, jaundice, weight loss, low-grade fever, and abdominal pain.[14] It should be stressed, however, that only 60% of patients presenting with alcoholic hepatitis have jaundice, whereas 28% have weight loss, 18% have abdominal pain, and 23% are febrile.[15]

Diagnosis. Elevation in bilirubin and serum liver enzymes are the most common laboratory findings in patients with acute alcoholic hepatitis. Hyperbilirubinemia is usually mild and liver enzymes are elevated. Alkaline phosphatase is rarely greater than five times normal. The white blood cell (WBC) count and mean corpuscular volume (MCV) are usually mildly to moderately elevated, and anemia is common.[16] The presence of a total bilirubin level greater than 20 mg/dL, hepatic encephalopathy, a prothrombin time prolonged more than eight seconds beyond control, a serum albumin less than 2 g/dL, and renal failure are poor prognostic indicators.

Treatment. Treatment of alcoholic hepatitis is primarily supportive and should include correction of volume deficits, electrolyte imbalances, and glucose abnormalities, and repletion of deficiencies in phosphorus, potassium, and magnesium. Withdrawal symptoms are common and should be managed with appropriate doses of sedatives. Because hepatic clearance of most sedatives is reduced, benzodiazepines should be administered cautiously. A high-calorie diet is recommended and protein restriction is necessary only for those patients who have hepatic encephalopathy. Correction of folic acid, thiamine, and iron deficiencies is usually necessary. Corticosteroids have several potential therapeutic actions likely to be of benefit in alcoholic hepatitis, although their role in this condition is not established.

As a rule, patients with alcoholic hepatitis should be hospitalized, inasmuch as these individuals are at significant risk for developing secondary life-threatening complications including sepsis, gastrointestinal bleeding, coma, cardiac failure, and renal insufficiency. However, a small percentage of patients (those will mild liver abnormalities, normal coagulation studies, and no evidence of infection) can be managed at home if a supportive environment is available. Liver biopsy should be performed as soon as possible to confirm the diagnosis and to exclude other hepatic pathology that may be amenable to specific therapeutic interventions.[14]

Table 2. Treatment Strategies for Alcohol-Related Gastrointestinal Emergencies

GASTROESOPHAGEAL REFLUX
H2 blockers: ranitidine 150 mg bid po or
Antacids: Maalox 2-4 tsp 20 minutes to 1 hour after meals and at bedtime
GASTRITIS
Abstinence
GASTROINTESTINAL BLEED
IV x 2 L D5 LR or D5 NS—fluid resuscitation
Nasogastric tube
Type and cross for blood
GI or surgery consultation
Admit to hospital
HEPATIC ENCEPHALOPATHY
Correct fluid and electrolyte abnormalities
Discontinue diuretics, opioids, benzodiazepines
Lactulose syrup po or ng 30-50 mL qh until diarrhea occurs
Neomycin 0.5-1.0 g q6h po or ng
Admit to hospital
SPONTANEOUS BACTERIAL PERITONITIS
Antibiotics covering gram-negative coliform bacteria, for example: ampicillin/sulbactam 3 g IV
Admit to hospital
PANCREATITIS
Pain control, hydration

Cirrhosis. Cirrhosis develops in only 8-20% of chronic alcoholics, with most studies suggesting that consumption of more than 120-180 g of alcohol per day for more than 15 years is the critical dose-duration factor.[11] Autopsy evidence indicates that cirrhosis may remain unrecognized in more than 40% of patients, whereas in 20% it is discovered fortuitously on routine examination or during the evaluation of unrelated disease.[17]

Diagnosis. The diagnosis can usually be made with reasonable clinical accuracy in the emergency setting. In most cases, the onset of cirrhosis can be insidious, or it may follow an episode of acute alcoholic hepatitis. The patient may be asymptomatic or may complain of such nonspecific symptoms as fatigue, anorexia, weight loss, nausea, and abdominal discomfort. In contrast, cirrhotic patients also may present to the ED with an urgent or life-threatening syndrome related to

Table 3. Hematologic and Oncologic Complications of Ethanol Abuse

HEMATOLOGIC
Anemia (multiple etiologies)
Coagulation factor deficiencies (K-dependent plus others)
Thrombocytopenia
Thrombocytosis
Antithrombin III deficiency
Thromboembolism
ONCOLOGIC
Squamous cell carcinoma of head and neck
Esophageal carcinoma
Hepatocellular carcinoma

liver failure or portal hypertension, including hepatic encephalopathy, ascites, splenomegaly, or bleeding esophageal varices. Other frequent findings include jaundice, palmar erythema, spider angiomas, parotid and lacrimal gland enlargement, clubbing of the fingers, muscle wasting, and peripheral edema. Men may have decreased body hair, gynecomastia, and/or testicular atrophy.

Over a period of several years, the cirrhotic patient typically becomes emaciated, weak, and chronically jaundiced. Ascites and other signs of portal hypertension become increasingly prominent. Most patients with advanced cirrhosis die in hepatic coma, most often precipitated by hemorrhage from esophageal varices or intercurrent infection. Progressive renal dysfunction often complicates the terminal phase of the illness.[18]

Treatment. Although definitive therapy of cirrhosis is beyond the scope of emergency care, physicians should be familiar with the options so that patients may be counseled regarding currently available therapies. Many agents have been studied in the treatment of cirrhosis. The use of colchicine has proven disappointing.[11] Other agents, such as cyanidanol-3 and polyunsaturated phosphatidylcholine, S-adenosyl-L-methionine, ursodeoxycholic acid, are currently being studied.[11,19,20]

Over the last 10 years, the medical community has generally accepted that patients with end-stage alcoholic liver disease should be eligible for consideration for orthotopic liver transplantation. Both patient and graft survival rates are comparable with results observed in non-alcoholic liver diseases.[11] The most common indications for transplantation are ascites and edema resistant to conventional therapy, repeated episodes of variceal bleeding, recurrent encephalopathy, poor quality of life due to liver failure, or small asymptomatic hepatocellular carcinomas less than 4 cm in diameter detected on routine ultrasound screening.[11]

Acute Liver Failure. Sudden decompensation of liver function can occur with little warning. It may manifest as a rapidly rising bilirubin concentration or prothrombin time or both, worsening ascites, or global mental status change. Although the differential diagnosis of acute liver failure is long and the etiology is often multifactorial, initial evaluation should focus on determining whether there are reversible problems that are amenable to acute therapeutic interventions.

Initial management of cerebral edema associated with acute liver failure should focus on correction of hypoxemia, hypercapnia, and systemic hypertension, which can exacerbate the edema. Elective intubation and hyperventilation may be indicated. After administration of IV thiamine (100 mg), hypoglycemia should be treated with IV infusion of D50 W followed by continuous infusion of either D5 W or D10 W. Coagulopathy with bleeding requires prompt administration of vitamin K, clotting factors using fresh frozen plasma, and, occasionally, cryoprecipitate.[21] Patients with sudden decompensation of liver function should be admitted to the intensive care unit.

Hepatic Encephalopathy. Usually a late manifestation of cirrhosis or a complication of florid liver failure, hepatic encephalopathy typically presents with a variety of neuropsychiatric disturbances, ranging from sleep-wake cycle inversions and subtle decreases in awareness, to personality changes, confusion, and coma. Early evaluation in the ED must focus on recognition of new mental status changes, which may be subtle. On physical examination, fetor hepaticas and asterixis of the hands or tongue may be noted. The patient must be evaluated for head trauma, sepsis, hypoglycemia, dehydration, and electrolyte abnormalities.

Screening of the urine and serum for surreptitious ingestion can be helpful in revealing factors contributing to encephalopathy. Elevation of serum ammonia level helps confirm the diagnosis. Gastrointestinal hemorrhage should be excluded and all sites should be cultured to exclude infection as a cause of encephalopathy. Initial management of hepatic encephalopathy consists of correction of fluid depletion and electrolyte abnormalities. Discontinuation of diuretics, opioids, and benzodiazepines is imperative. Patients with florid manifestations require hospitalization and consultation with a gastroenterologist.[21]

Carcinoma. Alcohol abuse is associated with a higher than normal rate of hepatitis B viral infection.[14] The increased prevalence of hepatic carcinoma in patients with alcoholic liver disease has been ascribed to alcoholic injury with ongoing necrosis and regeneration. Recent reports, however, indicate that the oncogenic effects of the hepatitis B virus may be subtle and may be of even greater significance in liver cancer than is currently thought.[22] Although heavy whiskey drinkers are at greatest risk, wine and beer drinkers are also at greater risk than nondrinkers for developing cancer of the esophagus.[6]

Pancreatitis. After years of heavy ethanol intake, a minority of alcoholics develop acute pancreatic inflammation of variable intensity that ranges from mild edema to hemorrhagic necrosis. In fact, alcohol abuse is responsible for a wide spectrum of pancreatic disorders, among them, acute necrotizing, acute edematous, acute relapsing, chronic relapsing, and painless pancreatitis. Differentiation among these types may be difficult in the emergency environment.

Acute pancreatitis has a low mortality and a high recurrence rate, with frequent progression to chronic pancreatitis. Complications of chronic alcoholic pancreatitis are multiple and include diabetes, frank steatorrhea, pseudocysts, common bile duct obstruction, subcutaneous fat necrosis, bone infarcts, ascites, pleural effusions, and, rarely, pericardial effusion.[23] Gastrointestinal bleeding, which usually manifests as hematemesis or melena, is a known complication of chronic pancreatitis and is usually the result of peptic ulceration, gastritis, or splenic vein thrombosis.

Life-threatening complications of severe, acute alcoholic pancreatitis must be recognized in the ED and include hypovolemic shock, hypocalcemia, hypomagnesemia, hypoalbuminemia, hypoxemia, renal failure, pulmonary complications, coagulopathy, cardiovascular abnormalities, hyperglycemia, psychotic disturbances, pseudocysts, abscess, and bacteremia. With complications that include infection, hemorrhage, or rupture, pseudocysts develop in 5-10% of patients with acute pancreatitis, of which 22-44% will resolve spontaneously.[21] In contrast, pseudocysts associated with chronic pancreatitis are the result of ductal obstruction and resolve spontaneously in only 9% of cases.[21]

Diagnosis. Most patients give a history of 5-10 years of heavy drinking before the onset of the first attack of pancreatitis.[23] After the first attack, patients become susceptible to repeated episodes—usually following a bout of binge drinking— that are characterized by severe upper abdominal, mid-epigastric pain radiating to the back or to both flanks; these symptoms usually are accompanied by nausea and vomiting. In many patients, pain may be relieved partially by sitting up or by lying in bed curled to the right or to the left. Abdominal findings are variable and range from mild tenderness to board-like rigidity.

Serum amylase is elevated in one-third of chronic alcoholics (usually, it is less than three times normal) and, therefore, is an unreliable indicator of acute pancreatitis in this subgroup.[24] An elevated serum lipase test is strongly suggestive of acute pancreatic inflammation. Elevations of serum amylase greater than three times the normal value are highly suggestive of acute pancreatic inflammation.[24] Fever, leukocytosis, and electrolyte disturbances may be present.

A plain radiograph of the abdomen may reveal a duodenal ileus, sentinel loop, and, rarely, pancreatic calcification. An excellent and cost-effective assessment modality for detecting possible complications, ultrasonography has also been used for detecting pseudocysts, evaluating the size of the pancreas, and to diagnose biliary tract abnormalities. Computed tomography (CT) is useful in problematic cases and when complications such as abscess, hemorrhage, or pseudocyst formation are suspected. An ultrasound of the abdomen may reveal an edematous pancreas.

Treatment. Treatment includes relief of pain (meperidine 1 mg/kg IM with an antiemetic agent), aggressive IV hydration, nasogastric suction, placing the patient npo, and, usually, hospitalization. Abstinence from alcohol is essential. Many patients with chronic, recurrent pancreatitis at low risk for complications can be managed as outpatients. If the patient continues to drink, the painful attacks will become more frequent and diabetes and malabsorption will ensue. However, cessation of drinking does not necessarily prevent progressive pancreatic dysfunction. Surgical consultation and intervention is required for patients with chronic pancreatitis who exhibit signs of abscess, hemorrhage into a pseudocyst, cyst erosion into viscera, and rupture of a pancreatic pseudocyst.

Patients with fever and an apparent pseudocyst seen on abdominal ultrasound or CT scan should have a needle aspiration of the fluid performed by an experienced radiologist, gastroenterologist, or surgeon; a Gram's stain and a culture of the fluid must be evaluated. If infection is strongly suspected, treatment with ampicillin-sulbactam 3 g IV plus gentamycin 1.5-2.0 mg/kg IV and metronidazole 750 mg IV should be started immediately. Either open surgical drainage or drainage with percutaneous catheters may also be necessary.[21]

Table 4. Infectious Disease Complications

Suppression of granulocyte function
Inhibition of cellular and humoral immunity
Increased susceptibility to infections, including:

- aspiration pneumonia
- *Klebsiella* pneumonia
- anaerobic abscess
- tuberculosis
- spontaneous bacterial peritonitis
- furunculosis

Hematologic Complications

The toxic effects of ethanol on hematopoiesis extend to all cell lines and include nearly all cellular and humoral components required for hemostasis. In fact, the vast spectrum of anemias associated with chronic alcoholism reads like a table of contents to a hematology textbook: bone marrow suppression, megaloblastosis, iron deficiency, sideroblastic anemia, thrombocytopenia, disorders of platelet aggregation, and hemolysis are just some of the consequences of ethanol abuse. Because of the wide range of hematologic complications—and because multiple causes for anemia often exist within the same patient—the alcoholic with anemia presents a formidable diagnostic challenge. *(Please see Table 3.)*

In general, anemias associated with ethanol abuse can be classified into three categories: 1) direct toxic effects; 2) nutritional deficiency; and 3) anemias due to hepatic disease.[25]

Folate Deficiency. Ethanol not only interferes with folate metabolism, but also predisposes to dietary deficiency of this important vitamin. As a result, chronic alcoholism is the leading cause of folate deficiency in the United States.[26,27] On peripheral blood smear, macroovalocytes and hypersegmented neutrophils are strongly suggestive of megaloblastic anemia caused by folate deficiency. Hypersegmentation of neutrophils is observed in 98% of these patients, is the first peripheral blood abnormality to occur, and can take as long as two weeks to resolve after initiation of therapy.[27] Interestingly, alcoholics who indulge primarily in beer seldom develop this deficiency, as beer is rich in folic acid. Most victims of folate-deficiency anemia are wine and whiskey drinkers.[28]

Iron Deficiency. Iron deficiency anemia in the alcoholic is usually the result of gastrointestinal blood loss. Not only can other anemias, such as those associated with folate deficiency, mask the microcytic changes usually associated with iron deficiency, but other entities, such as infection and hepatic cirrhosis, may alter the laboratory values of several markers that are useful in its detection, including serum ferritin and total iron binding.[27]

Hemolysis can also play a role in the alcoholic with anemia. Although hemolysis occurs in alcoholics with very low levels of serum phosphate,[29] more often, splenomegaly associated with cirrhosis and portal hypertension are accompanied by sequestration of erythrocytes. Cirrhosis also leads to changes in the production of serum lipoproteins, which ultimately affect the composition of cell membranes. Early changes in red blood cells appear as target cells, which actually have some advantage in terms of survival.[25] As hepat-

Table 5. Metabolic and Electrolyte complications in the Alcoholic Patient

METABOLIC
Altered metabolism of carbohydrates
• Alcohol-induced hypoglycemia
• Alcoholic ketoacidosis
Altered metabolism of proteins
• Inhibited synthesis of albumin, transferrin, etc.
Altered metabolism of lipids
• Hyperlipidemia
ELECTROLYTE DERANGEMENTS AND RENAL SYNDROMES
Hypo- or hypernatremia
Hypotonicity
Hypokalemia
Hypophosphatemia
Hypomagnesemia
Hypocalcemia, often secondary to hypomagnesemia
Altered solute and electrolyte regulation
Renal insufficiency (multiple etiologies) including myoglobinuria

ic diseas progresses, red cell membrane changes become more pronounced and the patient can develop spur cells or acanathocytes. Spur cells can lead to severe hemolytic anemia and may produce hematocrits less than 30%. Prognosis, in general, is poor.[27]

Thrombocytopenia. Thrombocytopenia is a well-recognized complication of ethanol misuse, with platelet counts of less than 150,000/mL occurring in more than 80% of patients hospitalized for withdrawal.[30] Reduced platelet production as well as reduced survival time contribute to thrombocytopenia. Acute ethanol ingestion is directly toxic to platelet production. Within 2-3 days of stopping alcohol, platelet counts rise, reaching a peak in 10-14 days.[61] This peak platelet count can be significantly higher than normal and may require an additional 2-3 weeks to return to baseline. During this period of thrombocytosis, the alcoholic patient is at risk for thromboembolism.[25]

Coagulopathy. As in anemia, nutritional deficiencies can affect hemostasis. Folic acid deficiency contributes to thrombocytopenia. Alcoholics whose diets are deficient in vitamin K can manifest deficiencies of the vitamin K-dependent coagulation factors (II, IV, IX, X). Hepatic cirrhosis further complicates hemostasis in the alcoholic. Portal hypertension, gastrointestinal varices, and splenomegaly, combined with deficient production of fibrinogen, vitamin K-dependent factors, and thrombocytopenia, place the alcoholic patient at risk for massive and refractory hemorrhage. In the event of refractory hemorrhage, platelet transfusion, replacement of fibrinogen with cryoprecipitate, and replacement of coagulation factors with fresh frozen plasma will be required.[25]

Finally, antithrombin III levels are consistently depressed in hepatic cirrhosis. Antithrombin III, which is synthesized in the liver, inhibits activated coagulation factors, in particular factor X. Deficiency can lead to the seemingly paradoxical condition of spontaneous thrombosis in the patient with severe hepatic cirrhosis.[25]

The Immune System and Infectious Disease

Because ethanol is a potent inhibitor of the immune defense system, emergency physicians must maintain a high index of suspicion for underlying infections, especially in the lungs, abdomen, and soft tissues. In this regard, alcohol-induced neutropenia has been demonstrated in patients suffering from an acute infection.[31] In addition, chronic ethanol ingestion causes lymphopenia,[32] suppresses lymphocyte blast transformation,[35] natural killer cell activity,[33,34] and antibody-directed cellular cytotoxicity.[33]

Pneumonia. Pneumonia in the alcoholic patient may be severe and, in most cases, requires hospitalization. *(See Table 4.)* This patient population is at risk for developing complications such as pulmonary necrosis, cavitation, and empyema. Usual pathogens include *Streptococcus pneumoniae*, *Klebsiella*, anaerobes, *Haemophilus influenzae*, and *Mycobacterium tuberculosis*. Pneumococcal pneumonia may be accompanied by severe headache and delirium, which suggest the need for lumbar puncture to rule out associated meningitis.

Anaerobic pneumonia is thought to result from aspiration of oropharyngeal secretions. The location of the pneumonia is dependent on the body position at the time of aspiration. If aspiration occurs when the patient is supine, the apical segment of the lower lobe is most often involved. When the patient is on his or her side, the lateral and posterior segments of the upper lobe are affected. Symptoms of anaerobic pneumonia, with or without abscess formation, are usually more gradual and insidious in onset than with other commonly implicated pathogens. *Klebsiella* pneumonia can evolve into abscess, pulmonary fibrosis, and bronchiectasis. Haemophilus pneumonia tends to be more severe and is often associated with extrapulmonary complications.

Ethanol suppression of cell-mediated immunity plays a major role in contributing to the higher incidence of tuberculosis in the alcoholic. One study performed in New York City indicated that tuberculosis rates in alcoholics far exceeded those in drug addicts.[36,37] The rate of relapse for tuberculosis has been shown to be 2-3 times higher in alcoholics due in no small part to poor compliance with anti-tuberculosis therapy.[38]

Spontaneous Bacterial Peritonitis (SBP). Spontaneous bacterial peritonitis is characterized by bacterial infection in ascitic fluid without associated gut perforation. This serious condition has been reported to occur in 10-27% of cirrhotic patients with ascites on hospital admission.[21] The most frequently implicated pathogens include *Escherichia coli, Klebsiella,* and streptococcal species. Pathogenesis may involve hematogenous seeding from the intestine, lungs, or other sources. If multiple organisms are present on Gram's stain of the fluid, a secondary peritonitis, such as that which might be caused by gastrointestinal perforation, should be suspected.

Diagnosis. Despite its high mortality rate, spontaneous bacterial peritonitis may produce subtle clinical findings. The diagnosis must be suspected by the emergency physician in any patient with new-onset or worsening ascites, as well as in any patient with ascites and fever, new leukocytosis, diffuse abdominal pain, or new or worsening hepatic encephalopathy. The diagnosis is confirmed with a small-volume paracentesis (20-35 mL), which can be performed safely by introducing a 20-gauge needle into an area that is dull to percussion in the left lower quadrant. This procedure should only be attempted, however, if the prothrombin time is prolonged by no more than five seconds and if the platelet count approaches 100,000. Fluid should be Gram's stained and assayed for total WBC count and leukocyte differential. In addition, a 10 mL sample should be inoculated directly into blood culture bottles in order to maximize yield of bacterial cultures.

Treatment. The presence of either bacteria on Gram's stain or a polymorphonuclear count greater than 250/mm^3 confirms a diagnosis of SBP and warrants immediate administration of antibiotics with activity against gram-negative coliform bacteria and anaerobes. A reasonable regimen would be ampicillin/sulbactam 3 g IV q4-6h. Aminoglycosides are relatively contraindicated in the cirrhotic patient.[21] The initial findings of a negative Gram's stain or polymorphonuclear count of fewer than 250 cells/mm^3 does not entirely exclude subacute bacterial peritonitis. Patients with confirmed or suspected subacute bacterial peritonitis warrant hospitalization.

Miscellaneous Infections. Cirrhosis also predisposes the alcoholic to spontaneous bacteremia. Most causes of spontaneous bacteremia are caused by *E. coli*, but other pathogens have been implicated, including pneumococcus, group A strep, *Clostridium perfringens*, and the marine vibrios. Non-typhoidal salmonella septicemia and cutaneous *Corynebacterium* diphtheria infections are more common in alcoholics. Patients with peritovenous shunts placed for intractable ascites have an infection rate as high as 25%.[39] Alcohol may play a role in the development of listeriosis, sporotrichosis, and aeromonas, as well as AIDS, but definitive studies are lacking.[40,41]

Malignancy

Alcohol is the second leading identified cause of cancer, exceeded only by tobacco.[42] While its role in carcinogenesis is not always clear, there can be no mistaking its association with a number of malignancies. The association of squamous cell carcinoma of the head and neck with chronic ethanol ingestion is well-recognized. Studies consistently demonstrate a significant increased risk of squamous cell carcinoma of the oral cavity (including tongue), pharynx, and larynx.[42,43] Tobacco and alcohol carry significant individual risks for head and neck cancer, and when used in combination, they appear to act synergistically. In western countries, about 80% of esophageal cancer can be attributed to alcohol and tobacco use.[43] Interestingly, there is no association with pancreatic cancer, despite the documented toxicity associated with ethanol consumption.[44]

Metabolic and Electrolyte Derangements

Alcohol can alter the metabolism of carbohydrates, proteins, and lipids. Ethanol has been shown to inhibit gluconeogenesis. Many alcoholics whose primary source of nutrition consists of the empty calories of ethanol can significantly deplete their hepatic glycogen reserves. The combination of inhibited gluco-neogenesis and a starvation state can lead to the uncommon, but well-known, syndrome of alcohol-induced hypoglycemia. Symptoms of hypoglycemia may be delayed several hours after the last dose of alcohol, and the response to IV glucose can likewise be delayed several hours. This delay may be an ominous sign indicative of severe underlying cerebral damage. After initial glucose repletion, patients with alcohol-induced hypoglycemia should be continued on IV D10 W until they are able to take adequate oral carbohydrates.[45]

Table 6. Miscellaneous Complications of Acute Alcoholic Intoxication and Chronic Ethanol Misuse

ENDOCRINE DISORDERS

Hypogonadism and feminization (in the male)
Pseudo-Cushing syndrome

MUSCULOSKELETAL COMPLICATIONS

Myopathy, acute and chronic
Osteoporosis
Osteonecrosis
Gout with hyperuricemia

DERMATOLOGIC COMPLICATIONS

Increased incidence of:

- Psoriasis
- Discoid eczema
- Superficial infections (fungal)

May aggravate:

- Porphyria cutanea tarda

DRUG REACTIONS AND INTERACTIONS

Antabuse reaction
Slowed drug metabolism
Accelerated drug metabolism
Additive sedative effects
Idiosyncratic reactions

Alcoholic Ketoacidosis. Although relatively uncommon, alcoholic ketoacidosis (AKA) is a relatively underdiagnosed complication of ethanol abuse that, if suspected, should be diag nosed in the emergency setting. Pathophysiology of alcoholic ketoacidosis begins with the starvation state. Cortisol, growth hormone, and catecholamine levels increase while insulin falls. Peripheral adipose tissue undergoes lipolysis to release free fatty acids. Ethanol normally suppresses ketogenesis, but when the alcoholic stops drinking, this inhibition is suspended and, as a result, fatty acids are converted by the liver to ketones to serve as metabolic fuel for the nutritionally deprived body. Some patients may even be alkalemic.[45-47]

Chronic alcoholics who have recently been on a binge and stopped drinking are at highest risk for developing this condition, which typically presents with abdominal pain, nausea, vomiting, and signs of intravascular volume depletion. These symptoms are frequently related to such alcohol-associated diseases as pancreatitis, gastroenteritis, or alcoholic hepatitis. The overwhelming majority of patients present within 1-3 days after their last drink. Laboratory exam usually reveals an elevated anion gap metabolic acidosis. Initial serum ketone assessment is frequently weakly reactive or even negative due to the preponderance of betahydroxybutyrate, which is not detected by the nitroprusside reaction (Acetest). This can lead to a seemingly paradoxical condition as serum ketones appear to increase with hydration and treatment of AKA. In fact, much of the betahydroxybutyrate has merely been converted to acetoacetate upon improvement in the

Table 7. Treatment of Common Alcohol-Related Disorders

ALCOHOL-INDUCED HYPOGLYCEMIA

Initial D50 IV, then D10 W IV until adequate po

ALCOHOLIC KETOACIDOSIS

Dehydration with glucose containing IVF, e.g., D5 NS

COAGULOPATHY

Vitamin K-dependent factor deficiency:
Vitamin K
Other faction deficiency:
Fresh frozen plasma
Fibrinogen:
Cryoprecipitate

FOLATE DEFICIENCY

Folate 1 mg po or IV qd

MYOGLOBINURIA

High-volume alkaline diuresis (IVF, mannitol, bicarbonate)

PNEUMONIA

IV antibiotics and admission depending on clinical setting and Gram's stain. Usual pathogens include: *Pneumococcus, Klebsiella, Haemophilus,* anaerobes, and tuberculosis

ELECTROLYTE IMBALANCES

Hypernatremia: IVF rehydration if volume depleted
Hyponatremia:
Depends on etiology and volume status (fluid restriction for beer drinker's syndrome or SIADH)
Volume repletion, if dehydrated, with D5 NS
Hypokalemia: po K + (i.e., 20 meq per tbsp in 10% solution; 1 tbsp po q8h with food) for mild hypokalemia (3.0-3.5 meq/L)
- 10-20 meq/h IV if moderate or severe
- should be on ECG monitor
- concentration not to exceed 40 meq/L
- not through central line
- may supplement with po

Hypophosphatemia: Usually safest to replete po (1-2 tbsp of phosphosoda q8h)
If symptomatic and level less than 1 mg/dL, then 2.5 mg/kg PO_4 IV as Na + or K + salt over 6 hours
Hypomagnesemia:
Asymptomatic—Milk of magnesium 30 cc po q6h
Symptomatic or level—1.0 meq/L
- $MgSO_4$ 2 g IM q4h to total 10 g on 1st day
- $MgSO_4$ 5 g IV over five hours

Refractory seizures or ventricular dysrhythmias thought secondary to hypomagnesemia: 2 g $MgSO_4$ IV over 5 minutes. May repeat once in 5 min up to 6 g over 3-4 hours for seizures

redox state. Treatment consists of volume repletion with D5 NS and potassium replacement as required.[45,47]

Electrolyte Disturbances. Electrolyte abnormalities are common in alcoholics. *(Please see Table 5.)* Hyponatremia can result from water intoxication, from increased antidiuretic hormone secondary to liver disease, and hypotonic replacement of isotonic gastrointestinal fluid losses. Hypotonicity and hyponatremia place the patient at risk for changes in sensorium, seizures, and even central pontine myelinosis.[48,49]

Potassium deficits in alcoholics can be severe and can result from a number of causes. Inadequate dietary intake, magnesium deficiency, diuresis, gastrointestinal tract losses, and increased renal excretion due to hyperaldosteronism have been implicated. Clinical manifestations of hypokalemia include cardiac arrhythmias, QT-segment prolongation resulting in torsades de pointes,[50] adynamic ileus, muscle weakness, myalgias, frank paralysis, and respiratory arrest.[51,52]

Hypophosphatemia is common in alcoholics. Phosphate plays important roles in bone and cell membrane composition, energy generation and storage, nucleic acid synthesis, and hydrogen ion buffering. Resorption of phosphate occurs in the proximal tubules and is inhibited by parathyroid hormone. Hypokalemia and hypomagnesemia also can cause a phosphate diuresis. Clinically, hypophosphatemia manifests with paresthesias and muscle weakness, which is typically proximal initially and can progress to cause respiratory arrest. Hypophosphatemia can interfere with hematopoiesis, impair tissue oxygenation secondary to a decrease in 2,3 DPG, cause a nonanion gap metabolic acidosis through bicarbonate wasting, and, when severe, may even result in rhabdomyolysis.

Oral repletion of phosphate is the preferred route in the stable patient with serum levels less than 2.5 mg/dL and can be achieved with phosphosoda 1-2 tablespoons q8h[53] or with milk, which is also high in phosphate. IV replacement is indicated if the serum level is less than 1.0 and the patient is symptomatic. Relative contraindications include renal failure secondary to rhabdomyolysis and hypercalcemia. One regimen consists of IV phosphate 2.5 mg/kg as the sodium or potassium salt over six hours.[54]

Alcoholism is the most common cause of hypomagnesemia. Magnesium deficiency, which has already been mentioned as contributing to hypokalemia and hypophosphatemia, can also lead to hypocalcemia. Hypomagnesemia results in a peripheral unresponsiveness to parathyroid hormone and can ultimately blunt its secretion. Symptomatic hypocalcemia can be refractory to any treatment other than magnesium repletion.[55]

Magnesium contributes to bone structure, acts as a cofactor for enzymes, and is necessary for energy metabolism. Like potassium, it exists primarily in the intracellular state in soft tissue. Only 1% of magnesium stores are extracellular, and measured serum levels do not adequately reflect total body magnesium. A major means of loss occurs when there is failure to reabsorb magnesium in the proximal tubules of the kidney.[56]

Clinically and neurologically, hypomagnesemia can manifest symptoms very similar to those seen in alcohol withdrawal, and some have proposed that this is more than coincidence.[48,54] Likewise, there is some evidence that suggests that alcohol withdrawal seizures may in some cases be due to magnesium deficiency.[54] It may be efficacious to empirically treat patients with alcohol withdrawal and alcohol withdraw seizures with magnesium.

In the case of seizures or refractory ventricular arrhythmias thought to be secondary to hypomagnesemia, 2 g of IV magnesium sulfate can be given over five minutes and can be repeated again in five minutes. Lesser symptoms can be treated more cautiously.[54] Magnesium sulfate given IV should be administered slowly with close attention to blood pressure. Replacement can be accomplished by giving 2 g of magnesium sulfate IV over 20-60 minutes and followed by 5 gm IV q8h. Upon discharge, the patient can be sent home on oral therapy consisting of 7.08.5% magnesium hydroxide (milk of magnesium) 30 cc q6h.[48,49,54]

Endocrine Dysfunction

Historical concern regarding deleterious effects of alcohol ingestion on reproductive function is reflected in biblical writings as well as in the ancient Greeks' proscription of alcohol consumption on the day of matrimony.[57] Both hypogonadism and feminization is commonly recognized in the male alcoholic.[58,59] Manifestations include testicular atrophy, impotence, loss of libido, decreased hair growth, reduced prostatic size, and oligospermia. Signs of hyperestrogenism include gynecomastia, vascular spiders, and female fat distribution. In women, menstrual irregularities are frequent: amenorrhea is commonly seen but menorrhagia is also observed. As a consequence, fertility is decreased.[57] Although optimal treatment of the hypogonadal alcoholic is abstinence, there are no data regarding the recovery of gonadal function with alcohol cessation.[57]

Some chronic alcoholics manifest clinical and laboratory features resembling Cushing's syndrome, which differs from true Cushing's disease in being transient. Features of the clinical syndrome include weakness, fatigue, low back pain, plethora, moon face, truncal obesity, easy bruisability, thin skin, purple abdominal striae, increased pigmentation, hirsutism, buffalo hump, peripheral muscle wasting, decreased bone maturation, hypertension, glucose intolerance, and osteoporosis. Finally, parotid gland inflammation can be a manifestation of chronic alcohol abuse.

Dermatologic Disorders

Among the wide range of miscellaneous disorders associated with alcohol toxicity, dermatologic conditions are some of the most common. *(Please see Table 6.)* Well-known are the cutaneous stigmata of alcoholic liver disease, including pubic and axillary hair loss, palmar erythema, and spider nevi. The latter have been shown to closely correlate with the presence of esophageal varices, as the nevi typically occur in those areas drained by the superior vena cava.[60] Skin conditions such as psoriasis, discoid eczema and superficial infections such as tinea pedis and pityriasis versicolor are more common in those who misuse alcohol and, therefore, serve as markers for ethanol abuse long before terminal alcohol-related conditions emerge.

Summary

Although many alcohol-related disorders associated with the gastrointestinal system and infection require hospitalization for definitive evaluation, the majority of life-threatening conditions must nevertheless be recognized and stabilized within the province of the ED. In particular, the physician must maintain a high index of suspicion for hepatic encephalopathy, acute and chronic gastrointestinal hemorrhage, spontaneous bacterial peritonitis, anaerobic pneumonia, and AKA. A comprehensive laboratory-based database—which should include a CBC, chest x-ray, amylase, ETOH level, liver function tests, electrolytes, and urinary sodium and ketones, when indicated—will help guide patient assessment and disposition. Therapy should follow established treatment protocols. *(Please see Table 7.)*

Patients should be counseled to pursue alcohol treatment programs, especially when serious alcohol-related complications compromise longevity.

References

1. Johnson RH, Robinson BJ. Mortality in alcoholics with autonomic neuropathy. *J Neurol Surg Psych* 1988;51: 476-480.
2. McClain CJ. Potentiation of acetaminophen hepatotoxicity by alcohol. *JAMA* 1980;244:251.
3. Interactions of drugs with alcohol. Med Lett 1981;23:33-34.
4. Osborn H. Alcohol toxicodynamics and clinical correlations. In: Schwartz GR, et al, eds. *Principles and Practice of Emergency Medicine*. 3rd ed. Philadelphia: Lea Febiger; 1992:3023-3038.
5. Kater RMH. Accelerated metabolism of drugs in alcoholics. *Gastroenterology* 1969;56:412.
6. Burbige EJ, Lewis DR, Halsted CH. Alcohol and the gastrointestinal tract. *Med Clin North Am* 1984;68:77-89.
7. McGuigan JE. Peptic ulcer and gastritis. In: Isselbacher KJ, ed. *Harrison's Principles of Internal Medicine.* 13th ed. New York: McGraw Hill; 1994:1363-1382.
8. Goyal RK. Diseases of the esophagus. In: Isselbacher KJ, ed. *Harrison's Principles of Internal Medicine.* 13th ed. New York: McGraw Hill; 1994:1361.
9. Persson J. Alcohol and the small intestine. *Scand J Gastroenterol* 1991;26:3-15.
10. Bouchouch AM, Nalpas B, Berger M, et al. Recovery from disturbed colonic transient transport time after alcohol withdrawal. *Dis Col Rect* 1991;34:111-114.
11. Sherman DIN, Williams R. Liver damage: Mechanisms and management. *Br Med Bull* 1994;50:124-138.
12. Grant BF, Dufour MC, Harford TC. Epidemiology of alcoholic liver disease. *Sem Liver Dis* 1988;8:12-25.
13. Saunders JB, Wodak AD, Morgan-Capner P, et al. Importance of markers of hepatitis B virus in alcoholic liver disease. *BMJ* 1983;286:1851-1854.

14. Pimstone NR, French SW. Alcoholic liver disease. *Med Clin North Am* 1984;68:39-56.
15. Woods FE, Hitchcoff M, Meyer A. Alcoholic hepatitis. *Am Fam Physician* 1993;47:1171-1178.
16. Rockey DC. Utility of liver function tests in alcoholic patients. *West J Med* 1992;156:319-321.
17. Salaspura MP, Lieber CS. Alcoholic liver disease. In: *Wright R, ed. Liver and Biliary Diseases*. Philadelphia: WB Saunders Co; 1979:103-145.
18. Podolsky DK, Isselbacher K. Alcohol related liver disease and cirrhosis. In: Isselbacher KJ, ed. *Harrison's Principles of Internal Medicine.* 13th ed. New York: McGraw Hill; 1994:1483-1486.
19. Ferenci P, Dragosics B, Dittrich H, et al. Randomized control trial of silymarin treatment in patients with cirrhosis of the liver. *J Hepatol* 1989;9:105-113.
20. Leiber CS, Casini A, Decarli G, et al. Adenosyl-L methilnine attenuates alcohol induced liver injury in the baboon. *Hepatology* 1990;11:165-172.
21. Horth KS, Quinn P. The patient with chronic intestinal disease. In: Herr RD, Cydulka RK, eds. *Emergency Care of the Compromised Patient.* 1st ed. Philadelphia: JB Lippincott; 1994:475-490.
22. Bechrot C, Napas B, Courouce AM, et al. Evidence that hepatitis B virus has a role in liver cell carcinoma and alcoholic liver disease. *N Engl J Med* 1982;306:1384-1387.
23. Geokas MC. Ethanol and the pancreas. *Med Clin North Am* 1984;68:57-75.
24. Gumate V. Serum lipase: A better test to diagnose acute alcoholic pancreatitis. *Am J Med* 1992;92:239-244.
25. Larkin EC, Watson-Williams EJ. Alcohol and the blood. *Med Clin North Am* 1984;68:105-120.
26. Weston CFM. Pancytopenia and folate deficiency in alcoholics. *Postgrad Med J* 1987;63:117-120.
27. Girard DE, Kumar KL, McAfee JH. Hematologic effects of acute and chronic alcohol abuse. *Hematol Oncol Clin North* Am 1987;1:321-334.
28. Lindenbaum J. Folate and vitamin B12 deficiencies in alcoholism. *Semin Hematol* 1980;17:119.
29. Jacob HS, Amsden T. Acute hemolytic anemia with rigid red cells in hypophosphatemia. *N Engl J Med* 1971;285:1446.
30. Cowan DH. Effect of alcoholism on hemostatis. *Semin Hematol* 1980;17:137.
31. McFarland W, Libre EP. Abnormal leukocyte response in alcoholism. *Ann Intern Med* 1963;59:865-877.
32. Liu YK. Effects of alcohol on granulocytes and lymphocytes. *Semin Hematol* 1980;17:130-136.
33. MacGregor RR. Alcohol and immune defense. JAMA 1986;256:1474-1479.
34. Wrenn K. The febrile alcoholic in the emergency department. *Am J Emerg Med* 1991;9:57-60.
35. Tisman G, Herbert V. In vitro myelosuppression and immunosuppression by ethanol. *J Clin Invest* 1973;52: 1410-1414.
36. Waxman SP, Goldfrank LR. The homeless patient. In: Herr RD, Cydulka RK, eds. *Emergency Care of the Compromised Patient.* 1st ed. Philadelphia: JB Lipincott; 1994:731-746.
37. Friedman LN, et al. Tuberculosis screening in alcoholics and drug addicts. *Am Rev Respir Dis* 1987;136:1188.
38. Segarra F, Sherman DS. Relapses in pulmonary tuberculosis. *Dis Chest* 1967;51:59.
39. Epstein M. Peritoneovenous shunt in the management of ascites and the hepatorenal syndrome. *Gastroenterology* 1982;82:790.
40. Sternbach GL. Infections in alcoholic patients. Emerg Med *Clin North Am* 1990;8:793-803.
41. Adams HG, Jordan C. Infections in the alcoholic. *Med Clin North Am* 1984;68:179-199.
42. Doll R, Peto R. The causes of cancer; quantitative estimates of avoidable risks of cancer in the United States today. *J Natl Cancer Inst* 1981;66:1191-1265.
43. Wynder EL, Bross IJ. A study of etiological factors in cancer of the esophagus. Cancer 1961;14:389-413.
44. Breeden JH. Alcohol, alcoholism, and cancer. *Med Clin North Am* 1984;68:163-177.
45. Williams HE. Alcoholic hypoglycemia and ketoacidosis. Med Clin North Am 1984;68:33-38. 46. Isselbacher KJ. Metabolic and hepatic effects of alcohol. *N Engl J Med* 1977;296:612-616.
47. Adams SL. Alcoholic ketoacidosis. *Emerg Med Clin North Am* 1990;8:749-759.
48. Ragland G. Electrolyte abnormalities in the alcoholic patient. *Emerg Med Clin North Am* 1990;8:761-773.
49. Kaysen G, Noth RH. The effects of alcohol on blood pressure and electrolytes. *Med Clin North Am* 1984;68: 221-246.
50. Schweitzer P, Mark H. Torsades de pointes caused by disopyramide and hypokalemia. *Mt Sinai J Med* 1982;49: 110-114.
51. Martin ML, Hamilton R, West MF. *Potassium. Emerg Med Clin North Am* 1986;4:131-144.
52. Duffens KR. Disorders of potassium balance. In: Silverstein SR, Frommer B, eds. *Emergency Management of Metabolic and Endocrine Disorders*. Rockville: Aspen; 1988:93-124.
53. Lentz RD, et al. The treatment of severe hypophosphatemia. *Ann Intern Med* 1978;89:941.
54. Degnen CJ. Emergencies of calcium, phosphate, and magnesium balance. In: Silverstein SR, Frommer B, eds. *Emergency Management of Metabolic and Endocrine Disorders.* Rockville: Aspen; 1988:125-146.
55. Estep H, et al. Hypokalemia due to hypomagnesemia and reversible parathyroid hormone unresponsiveness. *J Clin Endocrinol* 1969;29:842-848.
56. Sullivan JF, et al. Serum magnesium in chronic alcoholism. *Ann NY Acad Sci* 1969;162:947.
57. Noth RH, Walter RM. The effects of alcohol on the endocrine system. *Med Clin North Am* 1984;68:133-146.
58. Bergonzi, M. Gynakomastie und lebercirrhose. *Virchows Arch Pathol* 1969;293:697-723.
59. Morgan MY, Pratt EO. Sex, alcohol and the developing fetus. *Br Med Bull* 1982;38:43-52.
60. Foutch PG, et al. Cutaneous vascular spiders in cirrhotics patients: Correlation with haemorrhage from oesophageal varices. *Am J Gastroenterology* 1988;83:723-726.

Continuing Medical Education Questions

3. Pediatric Meningitis, p. 19

1. The most common form of bacterial meningitis in the immunocompetent child older than 3 months of age is:
   A. *Haemophilus influenzae*
   B. Group B *Streptococcus*
   C. *Neisseria meningitidis*
   D. *S. pneumoniae*
   E. *Listeria monocytogenes*

2. In children with indwelling CSF shunts, which of the following organisms is/are common causes of acute bacterial meningitis?
   A. *Haemophilus influenzae*
   B. *Staphylococcus aureus*
   C. *Neisseria meningitidis*
   D. *S. pneumoniae*
   E. All of the above

3. Normal CSF findings in the neonate (up to 1 month of age) include:
   A. Protein of 100 mg/dL
   B. WBC count of 50 cells/hpf
   C. Protein of 200 mg/dL
   D. None of the above; all are abnormal

4. If a child younger than age 1 presents with fever and altered mental status, with no evidence of trauma after history and physical examination:
   A. A CT scan should always be done prior to the LP
   B. An LP is indicated if there are no indications of bleeding diatheses, increased intracranial pressure (other than a bulging fontanelle), or a hemodynamic instability
   C. An LP should never be done in a child with a bulging fontanelle
   D. A CBC and toxicology screen should be done first

5. Empiric antibiotic therapy for the child with acute bacterial meningitis and an indwelling CSF shunt (i.e., VP shunt) would be:
   A. Gentamicin and ampicillin
   B. Ceftriaxone and ampicillin
   C. Ceftriaxone or cefotaxime plus vancomycin
   D. Ceftazidime

6. Viral meningitis:
   A. Can be consistently differentiated from bacterial meningitis on the basis of typical CSF characteristics
   B. Is common in late summer due to various enteroviruses
   C. Can usually be clinically distinguished from bacterial meningitis
   D. Always is benign with a good prognosis

6. Pediatric Code and Resuscitation Organization, p. 53

1. Which of the following phases does not occur in the team organizational view?
   A. Prehospital phase
   B. Maintenance phase
   C. Transfer phase
   D. Entry phase
   E. Family notification phase

2. Which of the following is a component activity of a resuscitation process?
   A. A patient with life or limb at risk or at least a perceived risk
   B. Defined leadership (physician and nursing)
   C. Procedures and interventions potentially performed on a patient
   D. A diversity of personnel experience, skills, and expertise potentially required
   E. All of the above

3. The anatomic survey of the patient occurs during which one of the following components of the patient organizational view?
   A. Prehospital
   B. Primary survey
   C. Resuscitation
   D. Secondary survey
   E. Definitive care

4. Which of the following is not a resuscitation team member role?
   A. Critical incident stress debriefing
   B. Equipment preparation
   C. Vital sign procurement or intravenous access
   D. Procedures performance
   E. Documentation

5. In regard to code organization training, all of the following are correct except:
   A. There are many established systems for teaching code team organization
   B. Mock codes are most effective as training tools when they are realistic while protecting the self-confidence of those in training
   C. One important area of training is the megacode format, in which ATLS and ACLS tenets are practiced and reviewed

D. Teaching the process of code organization is a second important training emphasis
E. Other important training areas include emergency alternatives to intravenous and airway access

6. Which of the following statements about job aids in code organization is/are true?
A. The most commonly recognized job aids are checklists containing all the specific task elements for which accuracy and oversight prevention are mandatory
B. Specially designed forms such as well-organized trauma resuscitation records can greatly increase the efficiency of documentation
C. The Broselow resuscitation tape is becoming a standard piece of equipment in most EDs
D. Wall information charts or posters containing valuable reference information can be strategically placed on resuscitation room walls
E. All of the above

7. All of the following statements are true about pediatric code organization except:
A. A distinct fund of knowledge and additional assessment and procedural skills are necessary for the effective management of pediatric resuscitations
B. The demanding pediatric problems of intravenous and airway access must be efficiently managed during pediatric resuscitations
C. Because pediatric resuscitations are quite common, team member expertise, training, and skill maintenance is less problematic
D. Drug calculations are complicated by the need to remember weight-related dosages, have an accurate estimate of the child's weight, and to flawlessly calculate and administrate the medication to the child
E. The small size of the patient frequently makes team member access for procedures a distinct problem with children

7. Cervical Spine Injury, p. 61

1. Normal soft tissue widths and bony measurement widths viewing a lateral cervical spine radiograph in a 6-year-old include:
A. A predental (atlantodental) space of 6 mm
B. A retropharyngeal space at C2 of 8 mm
C. A retropharyngeal space at C6 of 12 mm
D. A 3 mm subluxation of the anterior aspect of the spinous process anterior to the posterior cervical line

2. Cervical spine pseudosubluxation refers to:
A. Excess laxity of the transverse ligament in children so that the predental space is widened compared to adults
B. A normal cervical spine variant in children whereby the anterior aspect of the spinous process of C2 is subluxed > 2 mm anterior to the posterior cervical line
C. Anterior displacement of the vertebral body of C2 on C3 or C3 on C4 due to normal inherent ligamentous laxity of the cervical spine in children
D. Ligamentous injury following whiplash injury when no radiographic abnormality is seen

3. Comparison of adult and pediatric cervical spine anatomy reveals that:
A. Adults typically have a wider atlantodental interval compared to children.
B Placement of young children on standard spine boards allows for neutral positioning of the cervical spine during transportation
C. Children more frequently manifest SCIWORA
D. By age 5, children generally manifest adult patterns of cervical spine injuries

4. Dens fractures in children typically:
A. Are standard type I-III fractures involving either the tip of the odontoid, the entire odontoid, or the odontoid and some of the body of C2
B. Cause immediate spinal cord injuries due to the proximity of the odontoid C1 to the spinal cord
C. Cause occipital pain due to injury of the greater occipital nerve
D. Occur because the atlantotransverse portion of the cruciate ligament is extremely weak in children

5. Risk factors for atlantoaxial subluxation include:
A. Juvenile rheumatoid arthritis
B. Down syndrome
C. Congenital hypoplasia of the dens
D. All of the above

6. Which of the following is true of children with SCIWORA?
A. Subtle bony injuries are usually present on plain films
B. Neurologic deficits are maximal at the time of injury
C. MRI imaging is the radiographic procedure of choice beyond the acute injury phase
D. The injury typically occurs in children 8-12 years old

7. At what level do most cervical spine injuries occur in children younger than 8 years old?
A. C1-C2
B. C3-C4
C. C5-C6
D. C7-T1

8. In which of the following cases is cervical spine radiography required?
A. A child with a severe distracting injury
B. A child with midline tenderness
C. A child injured in a diving accident who has altered mental status
D All of the above

9. Cardiac Emergencies, p. 85

1. Signs, symptoms, and laboratory findings that are consistent with acute graft rejection include:
A. Poor feeding and/or lethargy

B. Tachycardia
C. Decreased QRS voltage
D. Increasing heart size on chest x-ray
E. All of the above

2. Which of the following is true regarding CHF?
A. Diuretic therapy is appropriate initial therapy except in cases of dehydration
B. The pathophysiology is similar in all cases
C. Cyanotic infants never have CHF
D. CHF is present in all children with a diagnosis of VSD

3. Hypercyanotic spells can be induced by all of the following except:
A. Fever
B. Exercise
C. Erythromycin
D. Chlorpromazine

4. The precipitating factors that decompensate a child with CHF include:
A. Infection
B. Fever
C. Tachy- or bradyarrhythmia
D. Infective endocarditis
E. All of the above

10. Sedation for the Pediatric Patient, p. 93

1. All of the following are complications encountered when administering sedation except:
A. Crossover titration
B. Stacking
C. Shifting baseline
D. Cumulation
E. Recovery

2. Which one of the following medications provides analgesia, amnesia, and sedation?
A. Fentanyl
B. Alfentanil
C. Propofol
D. Ketamine
E. Midazolam

3. Deep sedation is easiest to achieve with which of the following routes of administration?
A. Intranasal
B. Oral
C. Intravenous
D. Rectal

4. Emergence reactions with use of ketamine can be prevented or eliminated by:
A. Lowering the dose
B. IM administration
C. Giving atropine first
D. Giving fentanyl first
E. Giving midazolam

5. Benzodiazepines affect the CO_2 response curve by:
A. Shifting the curve to the right
B. Shifting the curve to the right and increasing the slope
C. Shifting the curve to the right and decreasing the slope
D. Shifting the curve to the left
E. Shifting the curve to the left and increasing the slope

12. Pediatric Seizures, p. 117

1. Epilepsy is defined as:
A. Convulsions in a child younger than 17 years of age
B. Generalized tonic-clonic seizures with fever
C. Two or more seizures not provoked by specific events
D. A psychological convulsion triggered by stress
E. An illness which can only be diagnosed by EEG

2. A CT or MRI study may be helpful in the evaluation of a child with:
A. A generalized tonic-clonic seizure
B. An absence seizure
C. A partial complex seizure
D. Rolandic epilepsy
E. Diagnosis of infantile spasm

3. Absence seizures can be distinguished from partial complex seizures by:
A. The difference in loss of consciousness
B. The occurrence of a staring episode
C. The length of the seizure
D. The age of occurrence
E. An EEG that shows typical three-per-second spikes

4. The majority of children who present to the ED with a seizure experience:
A. A febrile seizure
B. A partial complex seizure
C. A non-febrile seizure
D. An absence seizure
E. An infantile spasm

5. Status epilepticus is best treated by:
A. Restraining patients with soft restraints and placing an oropharyngeal bite block between the teeth to prevent injuries to the tongue
B. Protecting the airway and then giving a bolus of phenytoin of 18 mg/kg
C. Intramuscular injection of paraldehyde as a first drug of choice
D. Administration of benzodiazepines after the airway is secured
E. Cooling measures and per rectum administration of acetaminophen

6. The occurrence of a simple febrile seizure is determined by all of the following except:

A. The age of the patient
B. The level of fever
C. Hereditary factors
D. Underlying illness
E. The race of the patient

7. The treatment sequence following a simple febrile seizure is:
A. Antipyretics, assurance of the caretaker, prophylactic phenobarbital, follow-up with primary care physician
B. Antipyretics, benzodiazepines in the ED, assurance of caretaker, follow-up with primary care physician
C. Bedside glucose level, antipyretics, assurance of caretaker, outpatient EEG, follow-up with pediatric neurologist
D. Bedside glucose level, antipyretics, assurance of caretaker, follow-up with primary care physician
E. Bedside glucose level, assurance of caretaker, follow-up with primary care physician

8. The drug of choice to control a seizure disorder in the neonatal period is:
A. Phenobarbital
B. Phenytoin
C. Valproate
D. Benzodiazepines
E. Carbamazepine

14. Shock, p. 137

1. Symptoms and signs of SVT in newborns and infants include all of the following except:
A. Increased feeding
B. Tachypnea
C. Lethargy
D. Vasoconstriction

2. The initial management of a 6-month-old infant with clinically stable SVT should be:
A. Administration of digitalis
B. Administration of verapamil
C. Application of ice water to the face
D. Application of ocular pressure

3. Which of the following is not a determinant of oxygen delivery?
A. Cardiac output
B. Heart rate
C. Hemoglobin
D. Blood pressure

4. The most common type of shock seen in the pediatric population is:
A. Distributive shock
B. Cardiogenic shock
C. Hypovolemic shock
D. Spinal shock

5. Which of the following is not the proper treatment for obstructive sleep apnea in young children?
A. Weight loss
B. Nasal CPAP
C. Surgery
D. Racemic epinephrine

6 Proper treatment of a hypotensive patient with pericardial effusion consists of all of the following except:
A. Vigorous fluid administration
B. Dobutamine
C. Pericardiocentesis
D. Neo-synephrine

7. Which of the following agents is most appropriate for treating a 2-week-old infant presenting with cardiogenic shock?
A. Verapamil
B. Digitalis
C. Nifedipine
D. Prostaglandin E1

8. Which of the following is not appropriate for patients with possible ventricular tachycardia?
A. Magnesium
B. Verapamil
C. Adenosine
D. Phenytoin

15. Tachyarrhythmias, p. 149

1. Children younger than 1 year of age who have SVT should not be given either intravenous propranolol or:
A. Intravenous procainamide
B. Intravenous verapamil
C. Intravenous adenosine
D. Oral propranolol
E. Oral procainamide

2. A left bundle-branch block pattern seen during tachycardia in infants is almost always compatible with a diagnosis of:
A. Atrial flutter
B. Ventricular tachycardia
C. Wolff-Parkinson-White syndrome
D. Congenital heart disease
E. Supraventricular tachycardia

3. All of the following may indicate an underlying diagnosis of long QT syndrome except:
A. Seizures
B. Left bundle-branch block
C. T wave alternans
D. Torsades de pointes
E. Congenital deafness

4. Adenosine may be effective in terminating most tachyarrhythmias due to:
A. AV node reentry
B. Atrial flutter
C. Ventricular fibrillation

D. Torsades de pointes
E. Atrial fibrillation

5. Common presentations of SVT in infants include all of the following except:
A. Sweating
B. Poor feeding
C. Irritability
D. Tachypnea
E. Syncope

6. One of the most common arrhythmias seen in patients late after repair of congenital cardiac defects is:
A. Atrial fibrillation
B. Ventricular tachycardia
C. AV node reentry SVT
D. Torsades de pointes
E. Atrial flutter

16. Infants and Children with HIV, p. 157

1. Which of the following is the most appropriate treatment for an infant with PCP pneumonia?
A. Discharge on oral Septra for the next week with a recheck physician visit in the next 2-3 days
B. Outpatient treatment with oral Septra and oral prednisone
C. Obtain an arterial blood gas and discharge if the oxygen saturation is > 95%
D. Admit to the hospital and treat with Septra and steroids

2. Which of the following confirms the diagnosis of HIV in a 12-month-old infant?
A. Two consecutive positive IgG tests (ELISA or Western blot)
B. A positive IgM antibody assay
C. A positive IgG test in the mother
D. Two positive tests consisting of either polymerase chain reaction, HIV culture, or p24 antigen assay

3. Which of the following is true concerning bacteremia in infants with HIV?
A. Encapsulated organisms (e.g., *S. pneumoniae* and *H. influenzae* type b) are common pathogens
B. Fever (noted on ED arrival) is an unreliable sign of bacteremia.
C. Salmonella gastroenteritis frequently leads to bacteremia
D. All of the above

4. Side effects of zidovudine (AZT) therapy include:
A. Anemia, leukopenia, and thrombocytopenia
B. Hepatitis
C. Cardiomyopathy
D. All of the above

5. Chest radiographs in *Pneumocystis carinii* pneumonia typically reveal:
A. Lobar infiltrates
B. Hilar lymphadenopathy
C. Bilateral interstitial infiltrates
D. Pleural effusions

17. Sickle Cell Disease, p. 169

1. The most common cause of death in adult patients with sickle cell disease is:
A. Acute cerebrovascular accident
B. Acute chest syndrome
C. Acute splenic sequestration crisis
D. High-output cardiac failure
E. Sickle cell intrahepatic cholestasis

2. In adult patients, all of the following are associated with increased risk of early death in sickle cell anemia except:
A. Acute chest syndrome
B. Baseline WBC above 15,000 cell/m^3
C. High level of fetal hemoglobin
D. Renal failure
E. Seizures

3. Which of the following concerning acute splenic sequestration crisis is incorrect?
A. It is uncommon in adults with HbSS disease
B. It is classically defined as an increase in hemoglobin concentration of at least 2g/dL.
C. Laboratory studies usually reveal a marked reticulocytosis
D. Clinical findings may include sudden weakness, pallor of lips and mucous membranes, tachycardia, tachypnea, and abdominal fullness

4. Which of the following statements concerning Acute CVA in sickle cell disease is correct?
A. Recurrent stroke in children is most common one year after the initial stroke
B. Ischemic stroke is most common in children
C. Simple transfusions is indicated in children with ischemic stroke
D. Stroke in adults with SCD is usually due to large vessel occlusion
E. In children, stroke is most common in the 6-month to 1-year age group

5. Which of the following statements about acute chest syndrome is correct?
A. Acute chest syndrome only occurs in adults
B. Adult patients are usually febrile
C. Rib and sternal infections, and fat and/or pulmonary emboli have all been identified as causes
D. Hydroxyurea has no affect on the incidence of acute chest syndrome

6. Which of the following is correct concerning the use of meperidine in the treatment of acute vaso-occlusive crisis?
A. Meperidine is the least commonly used analgesic in the emergency department management of acute vaso-occlusive crisis

B. Nor-meperidine has a half-life that is one-half that of meperidine
C. Nor-meperidine is a toxic metabolite of meperidine which can cause seizures
D. Meperidine does not accumulate in patients with normal renal function
E. Meperidine is the drug of choice for the treatment of acute vaso-occlusive crisis

7. All of the following concerning acute vaso-occlusive crisis are true except:
A. Most patients with SCD are able to treat most of their painful episodes at home
B. No specific laboratory test is pathognomonic of painful crisis
C. Oxygen therapy is indicated in all patients with painful crisis
D. Acute painful crisis is responsible for 90% of hospital admissions in patients with SCD
E. Factors known to precipitate acute painful episodes include dehydration, infection, and psychological stress

8. Which of the following is true of transfusions in SCD?
A. Patients with SCD should be transfused to a HCT of 40-45% for optimal oxygen carrying capacity
B. Exchange transfusion are indicated in adults with hemorrhagic strokes
C. Aplastic crisis is initially treated with exchange transfusion
D. Patients with SCD with severe, symptomatic anemia usually require simple blood transfusion.
E. It is recommended that priapism be treated with red cell transfusion

18. Envenomations in Children, p. 179

1. What is the best treatment for children who suffer coagulopathy from crotalid envenomation?
A. Vitamin K
B. Antivenom
C. Transfusion
D. Fresh frozen plasma

2. Which prehospital therapy/first aid is safe and may be beneficial in the treatment of pediatric envenomations?
A. Electric shock
B. Tourniquet
C. Venom extraction
D. Incision and suction

3. Children may present with which of the following after widow spider envenomation?
A. Unexplained crying
B. Diaphoresis
C. Muscle cramping
D. All of the above

4. What is the best treatment for children with brown spider envenomation?
A. Local wound care
B. Hyperbaric oxygen
C. Dapsone
D. Steroids

5. Children are at increased risk for which complication following bark scorpion envenomation?
A. Necrosis
B. Infection
C. Rhabdomyolysis
D. Respiratory paralysis

21. Medical Hardware, p. 211

1. The most common problem related to a CSF shunt is:
A. Infection
B. Obstruction
C. Fracture of the tubing
D. Valve dysfunction

2. The most common organism causing CSF shunt infection is/are:
A. *Staphylococcus epidermis*
B. *Staphylococcus aureus*
C. Gram-negative organisms
D. *H. influenzae*

3. The most common presenting complaint of a child with a CSF shunt obstruction is:
A. Headache
B. Vomiting
C. Lethargy
D. Irritability

4. After a shunt is placed or revised, most infection will occur within:
A. Less than six months
B. 6-12 months
C. 12-18 months
D. More than 18 months

5. Maneuvers to open an occluded line that is due to a blood clot include all of the following except:
A. Urokinase bolus
B. Attempt to aspirate the clot
C. Continuous infusion of urokinase
D. Forcefully flushing the catheter to dislodge the clot

6. Removal of an indwelling line is almost always necessary for:
A. Exit-site infection
B. Tunnel infections
C. Bacteremia due to a line infection
D. Fever without a source on initial presentation

7. Blood drawn from an indwelling line can be used for all of the following tests except:
A. CBC
B. Electrolytes

C. Coagulation tests
D. Type and screen

8. Which of the following is true for gastrostomy button replacement?
A. A radiographic imaging study should be ordered whenever a replacement gastrostomy tube is inserted
B. A radiographic imaging study should be ordered only if a new gastrostomy tube is inserted into an immature tract
C. Dislodged gastrostomy buttons do not need to be emergently replaced; instead they should be referred to a surgeon the following day
D. A smaller gastrostomy button should never be inserted

22. Urinary Tract Infections, p. 223

1. Significant risk factors for development of UTI include all of the following except:
A. Family history of UTI
B. Premature birth
C. Bladder outlet obstruction
D. Circumcision
E. Constipation

2. UTI occurs in 1% of full-term infants. In premature infants, UTI occurs in:
A. 0.5%
B. 1.0%
C. 3.0%
D. 5.0%
E. 10.0%

3. An indication for admission in pediatric patients with UTI includes:
A. Fever
B. Elevated white count
C. Age younger than three months
D. First time UTI
E. Family history of UTI

4. Symptoms of upper UTI include:
A. Dysuria
B. Fever
C. Vomiting
D. Fever and vomiting
E. All of above

5. Vesicoureteral reflux occurs in approximately what percentage of children with UTI?
A. 10%
B. 20%
C. 40%
D. 75%
E. 90%

6. According to the article, which of the following may parenthetically present with symptoms identical to lower bacterial UTI?
A. Chlamydia
B. Urethritis
C. Viral hemorrhagic cystitis
D. None of the above

7. On standard UA, which of the following findings is most specific and sensitive for establishing a diagnosis of UTI?
A. Presence of hematuria on chemical strip test
B. Presence of pyuria on chemical strip test
C. Combined presence of pyuria and bacteriuria on urine microanalysis
D. None of the above

26. Occult Bacteremia, p. 263

1. Which of the following is true concerning OB?
A. All children with OB have temperatures ≥ 38°C
B. Febrile children with otitis media and upper respiratory infections have the same rate of OB as febrile children with no source of infection
C. Observation variables (e.g., YOS) are an accurate method for determining a child's risk for harboring OB
D. Children who attend day care centers have a decreased risk of developing OB

2. Which of the following techniques will increase the speed and rate of the detection of positive blood cultures?
A. Using at least 3 mL of blood per bottle
B. Obtaining two or more different sets of cultures
C. Use of a specialized atmospheric pressure monitors that measure any increase or decrease in internal atmospheric pressure due to gas production or use (e.g., DIFCO ESP technique)
D. All of the above

3. All of the following may be used for identifying the presence of OB except:
A. Temperature elevation
B. Blood cultures
C. Immune status
D. Use of antipyretics
E. Appearance of patient

4. Untreated OB due to *Streptococcus pneumoniae:*
A. Progresses to a serious bacterial infection in about 25% of cases
B. Progresses to meningitis in about 10% of cases
C. Causes a WBC count ≥ 20,000 cells/mm^3 in most cases
D. Clears spontaneously in most cases

5. ACEP's clinical policy for managing febrile children 1-24 months old with fever and no source includes which of the following?
A. Mandatory blood culture on all children with fever ≥ 39°C
B. Urinalysis on all febrile female children with fever ≥ 39°C
C. Consideration of a CBC, lumbar puncture, blood culture, and empiric treatment with antibiotics for well-appearing children with fever ≥ 40°C

D. Lumbar puncture on all children less than 6 months old with temperatures ≥ 40°C

6. Untreated OB due to *Haemophilus influenzae:*
   A. Progresses to a serious bacterial infection in about 25% of cases.
   B. Progresses to meningitis in about 25% of cases
   C. Is less likely to lead to a serious bacterial infection compared to untreated *S. pneumoniae* OB
   D. Causes a WBC count ≥ 20,000 cells/mm³ in most cases

7. At what age cut-off can the absence of meningeal signs be relied upon to exclude meningitis in a febrile child who is alert and awake?
   A. 6 months
   B. 12 months
   C. 24 months
   D. 5 years

27. Pneumonia, p. 271

1. Pneumonia in an adolescent is most commonly due to:
   A. *Streptococcus pneumoniae*
   B. *Mycoplasma*
   C. *Chlamydia*
   D. *Hemophilus influenzae*
   E. Adenovirus

2. The drug of choice for the patient in question #1 is:
   A. A macrolide
   B. Amoxicillin-clavulanate
   C. Penicillin
   D. Ciprofloxin
   E. None of the above

3. A 10-year-old has the sudden onset of a fever (T = 40°C) and a cough, WBC count of 20,000 with a lobar consolidation on the chest radiograph. The most likely etiology (or pneumonia syndrome) is:
   A. Bacterial
   B. Viral
   C. Tuberculosis
   D. Atypical (mycoplasma)
   E. Atypical (chlamydia)

4. A 3 year old has the gradual onset of upper-respiratory infection symptoms, with a low grade fever (T = 100.7°F), a cough, and an interstitial pattern on the chest radiograph. The most likely pathogen is:
   A. *Streptococcus pneumoniae*
   B. *Hemophilus influenzae*
   C. *Mycoplasma*
   D. *Chlamydia*
   E. Respiratory synctival virus

5. The antibiotic of choice for the patient in question # 4 is:
   A. Tetracycline
   B. Erythromycin
   C. Sulfonamide
   D. Amoxicillin-clavulanate
   E. None of the above

6. The antibiotic of choice for "afebrile pneumonia of infancy" is:
   A. Tetracycline
   B. Erythromycin
   C. Sulfonamide
   D. Amoxicillin-clavulanate
   E. None of the above

7. An 8 year old has the sudden onset of fever (T = 40.2°C) with a cough, rales on the lung examination, and lobar consolidation on the chest radiograph. The most likely organism causing the pneumonia is:
   A. *Mycoplasma*
   B. *Chlamydia*
   C. *Streptococcus pneumoniae*
   D. *Hemophilus influenza*
   E. Adenovirus

8. Assuming there is no antibiotic resistance (beta-lactamase negative), which of the following antibiotic should be used in this patient?
   A. Erythromycin
   B. Sulfisoxazole
   C. Penicillin
   D. Tetracycline
   E. Ribavirin

28. Stridor in Children, p. 287

1. Which of the following statements is correct about the glottic and subglottic airway?
   A. This part of the airway is soft and easily distensible resulting in a greater risk of obstruction
   B. Myriad congenital conditions can cause obstruction at the glottic and subglottic level, but vocal cord paralysis is by far the most common cause
   C. Drooling is almost never associated with partial obstruction at this level, and its presence would indicate that a lesion is not at the level of the glottis or trachea
   D. Stridor is heard with both inspiration and expiration
   E. A hoarse sounding or muffled voice is heard with diseases of the glottic and subglottic area.

2. All of the following are important clues to be used in identifying the cause of a child's upper airway obstruction or stridor except:
   A. Aperture (nares)
   B. Acoustics
   C. Acuity of onset
   D. Air-shadow interface (radiographs)
   E. Airway examination

3. Which of the following features is not suggestive of impending airway obstruction for children with croup?
   A. Age greater than 6 months

B. Rest stridor
C. Cyanosis
D. Decreased level of consciousness
E. Hypoxia

4. Which one of the following statements about radiographic presentations of airway disease is incorrect?
A. As many as 30% of all patients with epiglottitis have radiographs that are initially read as normal by radiologists
B. Never send an unaccompanied child in whom a life-threatening disorder is suspected to a separate radiology suite
C. It is sometimes appropriate for stable children suspected of having epiglottitis to have a portable radiograph of the lateral neck
D. A retropharyngeal space wider than 7 mm anterior to the inferior border of the second cervical vertebral body may suggest abnormal widening of this space
E. In children with croup, plain radiographs of the chest are probably more useful than soft-tissue radiographs of the neck

5. Which of the following statements about retropharyngeal abscesses is accurate?
A. Retropharyngeal abscesses are a rare but serious cause of subglottic airway obstruction
B. The microbial agent most likely to cause an abscess is *Haemophilus influenzae* type b
C. Because of the location of the retropharyngeal abscess, the head is often flexed to help open the child's airway
D. Computed tomography is more accurate than plain radiography at detecting retropharyngeal abscesses
E. A retropharyngeal abscess is a type of peritonsillar abscess which occurs specifically in school-age children

6. All of the following statements concerning diseases of the supraglottic airway are correct except:
A. Drooling can be a prominent feature if an obstruction is present
B. When stridor is present with supraglottic obstruction, it most frequently occurs with expiration
C. Disease processes of the supraglottic area may be associated with a muffled or "hot-potato" voice
D. The lack of surrounding cartilage makes this part of the airway easily distensible and collapsible
E. Disorders that cause supraglottic obstruction have the potential to rapidly obstruct this part of the airway

7. All of the following statements about laryngotracheobronchitis are correct except:
A. Viral croup is the most common infectious cause of acute upper airway obstruction in children, accounting for more than 90% of all cases of stridor and 20,000 hospital admissions per year
B. The stridor associated with croup occurs from mucosal and submucosal edema of the subglottic portion of the airway
C. Stridor is usually biphasic, although it is often louder on inspiration
D. Prodromal upper respiratory symptoms, such as nasal congestion, mild cough, and fever, often precede the development of stridor
E. The typical age of laryngotracheobronchitis is about 12 months

29. Treatment of Acute Otitis Media, p. 299

1. Otitis media with effusion is characterized by:
A. Fever
B. Ear pain or tugging
C. Non-specific signs and symptoms of infection
D. A middle ear effusion without symptoms
E. Gross hearing deficits

2. Which of the following is one of the most common complications of otitis media?
A. Perforation of the tympanic membrane
B. Brain abscess
C. Cholesteatoma
D. Meningitis
E. Facial nerve injury

3. Examination of the ear in children with acute otitis media commonly reveals each of the following except:
A. A bulging tympanic membrane
B. An absent light reflex
C. Clear bony landmarks
D. An air-fluid level behind the tympanic membrane
E. A hyperemic tympanic membrane

4. Regarding the microbiology of acute otitis media:
A. Bacterial beta-lactamase production is uncommon
B. *S. aureus* infection is common in older children
C. *M. catarrhalis* is a common pathogen
D. Viral organisms are the sole cause of most infections
E. Penicillin-resistant *S. pneumoniae* is rare

5. Acute otitis media that does not respond to initial antibiotic therapy:
A. Is an indication for corticosteroid therapy
B. Is an indication for myringotomy with tube placement
C. Renders other first-line antibiotics inappropriate
D. Is seen in at about 10% of cases
E. Frequently results in permanent hearing loss

6. Indications for patient reevaluation after 48 hours of antibiotic therapy for otitis media include:
A. Rising temperature
B. Increasing irritability
C. Development of lethargy
D. Development of anorexia and vomiting
E. All of the above

7. Which antibiotics has been approved for five days of therapy for acute otitis media in children?
A. Amoxicillin
B. Clarithromycin

C. Azithromycin
D. Amoxicillin-clavulanate
E. None of the above

8. Which of the following is not a common organism isolated in acute otitis media?
A. *Streptococcus pneumoniae*
B. *Haemophilus influenzae*
C. *Moraxella catarrhalis*
D. *Escherichia coli*

31. The Battered Child, p. 319

1. Which of the following statements is true about the bones of a child?
A. Periosteal reaction on x-ray indicates that a fracture has occurred
B. Perfect realignment is needed to ensure adequate growth in all fractures of childhood
C. Children are more likely to sustain a fracture than a sprain
D. Salter-Harris type I fractures have the worst prognosis for subsequent growth

2. Which of the following statements is true about radiographic evolution of child abuse?
A. Skeletal survey is rarely indicated in a child older than 5 years
B. A normal skeletal survey will rule out child abuse
C. Bone scan should be performed on all children with suspected abuse
D. It is very unusual to find additional fractures in a skeletal survey when abuse is strongly suspected

3. Which of the following histories is most consistent with a non-accidental injury?
A. A 3-year-old child sustains an oblique fracture to the tibia after running and tripping
B. A 6-month-old child fell out of his father's arms and sustained a linear parietal skull fracture. A CT scan of the head was otherwise normal
C. A 2-year-old child fell off a slide and has a supracondylar fracture of the elbow
D. A 2-month-old infant rolled out of bed and has a midshaft femur fracture

4. Which of these fractures is diagnostic of child abuse?
A. Oblique fractures of the distal tibia in a 2 year old
B. A bucket handle fracture of the distal humerus
C. Salter-Harris II fracture of the radius
D. Torus fracture of the distal radius

5. A 1-year-old girl has history of not moving her arm for one day. The family denies any history of trauma. An x-ray reveals a midshaft humeral fracture. The next step in the work up of this child wold be:
A. Order a CT scan of the head to rule out a chronic subdural hematoma
B. Order liver enzymes to help rule out intra-abdominal injury
C. Obtain a skeletal survey to rule out other fractures
D. Apply a sling and swath and have the patient follow up with orthopedics

6. Which of the following fractures is likely to be unintentional?
A. Posterior rib fracture
B. Metaphyseal lucency
C. Avulsion fracture of the lateral tip of the clavicle
D. Supracondylar fracture of the humerus

7. In children younger than 1 year, what percentage of femur fractures have been estimated to be intentional?
A. 20%
B. 30%
C. 80%
D. 60%

32. Meningitis, p. 329

1. The annual incidence of bacterial meningitis in the United States is:
A. Between 4-10 cases per 100,000
B. 10-15 cases per 100,000
C. 4-10 cases per 10,000
D. None of the above

2. In what percentage of patients with ABM do generalized seizures occur?
A. 40%
B. 50%
C. 70%
D. None of the above

3. Which common clinical symptom of ABM is absent in up to 40% of elderly patients?
A. Fever
B. Hypothermia
C. Confusion
D. Seizures

4. Which group of patients should have a CT evaluation before undergoing lumbar puncture?
A. Immunosuppressed patients
B. Alcoholics
C. Elderly patients
D. All of the above

5. Preadministration of oral antibiotics decreases the:
A. Total CSF white blood cell count
B. Glucose
C. Glucose serum ratio
D. None of the above

6. Which of the following is the antibiotic of choice when gram-positive cocci is discovered?
A. Penicillin G
B. Vancomycin

C. Ampicillin
D. Gentamycin

7. A presentation with papilledema may suggest which alternate diagnosis?
A. Venous sinus thrombosis
B. Brain abscess
C. Subdural hematoma
D. All of the above

33. Evaluation of Fever, p. 341

1. In most cases, a temperature higher than 41.5°C reflects which of the following?
A. Hyperthermia
B. True fever
C. Sepsis
D. None of the above

2. For each degree Celsius rise in temperature, a patient's basal metabolic rate may increase as much as:
A. 5%
B. 25%
C. 15%
D. 30%
E. 35%

3. The diagnosis of what percent of febrile illnesses can be made on the basis of a history and physical examination?
A. 50%
B. 70-85%
C. 10-20%
D. 100%
E. 25%

4. In a febrile patient with frank bradycardia, a physician should consider:
A. Viral myocarditis and bacterial endocarditis
B. Rheumatic fever and Lyme disease
C. Concurrent use of medications such as beta-blockers
D. The presence of underlying cardiac conduction disease
E. All of the above

5 Purpuric lesions are characteristic of:
A. Vasculitis
B. Meningococcemia
C. Thrombocytopenia
D. Cellulitis
E. None of the above

6. In the literature, the presence of urine infection has been characterized according to which criteria?
A. 10,000-100,000 CFUs/mL of a single urinary pathogen
B. 100 CFUs/mL of a single urinary pathogen in a "symptomatic" female patient
C. 1000 CFUs/mL of a single urinary pathogen from a catheterized specimen
D. All of the above

7. The false-negative incidence of a fecal leukocyte test is approximately:
A. 15%
B. 5%
C. 50%
D. 75%
E. 22%

8. Cardinal signs and symptoms of adult meningitis include:
A. Kernig's sign
B. Fever
C. Brudzinski's sign
D. Headache
E. All of the above

34. Causes of Fever, p. 349

1. Many drugs can produce fever through several different mechanisms. These mechanisms include:
A. Febrile responses caused by impurities in the drug
B. Induction of pyrogen release
C. Disorders in thermo-regulation
D. Hypersensitivity reactions
E. All of the above

2. What percent of patients with angiographically proven pulmonary thromboemboli will exhibit fever?
A. One-half
B. Two-thirds
C. 90%
D. 10%
E. 15%

3. The most common malignancies associated with fever are:
A. Hodgkin's and non-Hodgkin's lymphomas
B. Hepatoma and atrial myxoma
C. Leukemia and hypernephroma
D. All of the above

4. Post partum fever occurs in what percent of vaginal deliveries?
A. 2-4%
B. 15-18%
C. About 30%
D. 12%
E. 50%

5. The most common cause of emphysematous pyelonephritis is:
A. *K. pneumoniae*
B. *P. mirables*
C. *P. aeruginosa*
D. *E. coli*
E. *E. aerogenes*

6. What is the most common offending agent in infective endocarditis?
A. *E. coli*
B. *Klebsiella pneumoniae*
C. *Staphylococcus aureus*

D. *Mycobacterium tuberculosis*
E. *H. influenza*

7. Disseminated cytomegalovirus (CMV) infection typically occurs in patients with CD4 counts of:
A. 100/mm³
B. 200/mm³ or greater
C. 150/mm³
D. less than 25/mm³
E. 500/mm³

35. Fever in the Returning Traveler, p. 357

1. Which vaccine is the least efficacious?
A. Japanese encephalitis
B. Hepatitis A
C. Yellow fever
D. Cholera

2. Which traveler is at higher risk for contracting cholera and/or typhoid fever?
A. History of renal insufficiency
B. Taking H2-blocker for a history of gastritis
C. Taking oral hypoglycemic for adult onset diabetes
D. Recent viral upper respiratory tract infection

3. Which pathogen has the shortest incubation time?
A. Dengue fever
B. Malaria
C. Leishmaniasis
D. Rabies
E. Typhoid fever

4. Which describes the rash of typhoid?
A. Petechiae on arms and legs
B. Pruritic papules on back
C. Transient pink macules on chest and abdomen
D. Icteric patches

5. Which disease produces thrombocytopenia and leukopenia?
A. Pyogenic abscess
B. Leishmaniasis
C. Japanese encephalitis
D. Dengue fever

6 Which species of malaria is the most prevalent worldwide?
A. *Plasmodium falciparum*
B. *Plasmodium vivax*
C. *Plasmodium malariae*
D. *Plasmodium ovale*

36. Community-Acquired Pneumonia, p. 365

1. Even with appropriate follow-up treatment, patients with CAP may have which of the following symptoms that last for several months?
A. Sputum production
B. Dyspnea
C. Fatigue
D. Cough and chest pain
E. All of the above

2. The most common etiologic agent identified in patients with CAP is:
A. *Legionella*
B. *Streptococcus pneumoniae*
C. *Staphylococcus aureus*
D. *Klebsiella pneumoniae*
E. *H. influenzae*

3. *Klebsiella pneumoniae* occurs in all of the following except:
A. Patients younger than 1 year of age
B. Alcholoics
C. Nursing home patients
D. Patients older than 40 years

4. *Moraxella catarrhalis* can cause infection in patients with:
A. Lung cancer
B. Diabetes mellitus
C. Cerebral vascular disease
D. COPD
E. All of the above

5. Acinetobacter can be found colonizing on what percent of the skin of normal patients?
A. 50%
B. 12%
C. 25%
D. 5%
E. 95%

6. Which of the following organisms causes Q fever?
A. *Eikenella corrodens*
B. *Bacillus cerius*
C. *Moraxella catarrhalis*
D. *Coxiella burnetii*
E. *Chlamydia*

7. What pathogens are commonly found in patients with COPD?
A. *H. influenzae* and *Mycoplasma*
B. *H. influenzae* and *M. catarrhalis*
C. *Legionella*
D. *Staphylococcus aureus*
E. *S. pneumoniae*

8. Prospective studies determining the causes of CAP in adults have failed to identify the cause in what percent of cases?
A. 40-60%
B. 70%
C. 20%
D. 89-90%
E. 10%

37. Outpatient Management of Bacterial Infections in the Lower Respiratory Tract, p. 395

1. Antimicrobial coverage in patients with ABE/COPD typically requires using an antibiotic that covers which of the following organism(s)?
   A. *S. pneumoniae*
   B. *M. catarrhalis*
   C. *H. influenzae*
   D. All of the above
   E. None of the above

2. Antimicrobial coverage in patients with CAP typically requires using an antibiotic that covers the following organism(s):
   A. *S. pneumoniae* and *C. pneumoniae.*
   B. *M. catarrhalis* and *Legionella.*
   C. *H. influenzae* and *Mycoplasma pneumoniae.*
   D. All of the above
   E. None of the above

3. As a rule, antimicrobial therapy is indicated in patients who have at least two of the following three symptoms:
   A. increased wheezing, fever, or rhinorrhea.
   B. increased purulence, malaise, and rhinorrhea.
   C. increasing purulence of sputum, increasing sputum volume, or increasing cough/dyspnea.
   D. All of the above
   E. None of the above

4. Use of antibiotics for "chronic prophylaxis" against ABE/COPD should be:
   A. encouraged in older patients with emphysema.
   B. encouraged in younger patients with recurrent acute bronchitis.
   C. encouraged in patients on oxygen therapy.
   D. discouraged.

5. Which of the following antibiotics are approved as a five-day course for the treatment of ABE/COPD?
   A. TMP/SMX and clarithromycin
   B. Clarithromycin and levofloxacin
   C. Clarithromycin and azithromycin

38. Urinary Tract Infections: Diagnosis and Evaluation, p. 417

1. In children younger than 2 years of age with a urinary tract infection (UTI), one of the most common presenting complaints at evaluation is:
   A. vomiting.
   B. dysuria.
   C. abdominal pain.
   D. fever.

2. Which of the following populations has a 10-15% risk of developing renal scarring, subsequent hypertension, and end-stage renal disease from pyelonephritis?
   A. Pediatric
   B. Adult
   C. Pregnant
   D. Elderly

3. The most common (> 50%) anatomic abnormality associated with UTIs in infants is:
   A. renal calculus.
   B. urethral stricture.
   C. vesico-ureteral reflux.
   D. bladder spasm.

4. The most common uropathogen in adult patients with UTIs is:
   A. *Proteus mirabilis.*
   B. *Escherichia coli.*
   C. *Klebsiella.*
   D. Enterococci.

5. Significant adverse effects and drug interactions associated with fluoroquinolones include all of the following except:
   A. cardiotoxity in patients taking medications that prolong the QT interval.
   B. tendonitis, arthritis, and tendon rupture.
   C. acute renal failure.
   D. increased risk of theophylline and digoxin toxicity.

6. In acute cystitis, which of the following antibiotics is now recommended as a first-line agent in most adult populations?
   A. TMP/SMX
   B. Amoxicillin/clavulinic acid
   C. Nitrofurantoin
   D. Fluoroquinolone

7. Patients receiving digoxin and quinolones have increased risk of digoxin toxicity and should be monitored for which of the following?
   A. Nausea
   B. Vomiting
   C. Cardiac arrhythmias
   D. All of the above

39. Antibiotic Therapy for Urinary Tract Infections, p. 433

1. Analysis of 1991-1996 Medicare claims showed that UTI was the most common diagnosis in women older than age 65.
   A. True
   B. False

2. Choice and intensity of antimicrobial treatment with UTI should be determined by which of the following?
   A. Severity of the illness
   B. Patient tolerance
   C. Cost
   D. Susceptibility of the infecting organism
   E. All of the above

3. Fluoroquinolones are a better choice for treating uncomplicated UTI under which of the following condition or conditions?

A. In areas where *E. coli* resistance to TMP/SMX is greater than 10%-20%
B. For patients with allergies to sulfa or other drugs
C. In patients returning for failed antibiotic treatment after having used non-fluoroquinolone antibiotics for UTI
D. All of the above
E. None of the above

4. In certain regions of the United States, resistance among *E. coli* to TMP/SMX has risen to as high as:
A. 4%.
B. 14%.
C. 24%.
D. 64%.
E. None of the above

5. Superior bacteriologic and clinical cure rates seen with a seven-day course of ciprofloxacin, compared to a 14-day course of TMP/SMX, and reduced overall treatment costs, suggest ciprofloxacin should be considered an agent of choice in female patients with acute pyelonephritis.
A. True
B. False

6. In young women with uncomplicated UTI, the preferred duration of treatment with ciprofloxacin or TMP-SMX is:
A. three days.
B. five days.
C. seven days.
D. 10 days.
E. 14 days.

7. Patients with which of the following should be admitted to the hospital for parenteral antibiotics?
A. Vomiting
B. Severe pain and nausea
C. Dehydration
D. Inability to take oral fluids or medications
E. All of the above

40. Tuberculosis, p. 443

1. Each of the following has been implicated in the resurgence of tuberculosis except:
A. The AIDS epidemic
B. Drug-resistant strains of bacteria
C. Less effective generic drug preparations
D. Cutbacks in tuberculosis treatment programs

2. The most common clinical manifestation of tuberculosis infection is:
A. Primary pulmonary disease
B. Reactivation pulmonary disease
C. Extrapulmonary disease
D. Disseminated disease

3. Each of the following is considered a risk factor for tuberculosis except:
A. Prolonged cough
B. Tuberculosis exposure
C. Unexplained fever
D. History of bacterial pneumonia

4. Tuberculosis associated with HIV infection requires special considerations because:
A. Extrapulmonary disease is more common
B. Drug therapy is different
C. PPD skin testing is likely to cause tissue necrosis
D. AFB smears of the sputum are likely to be falsely positive

5. ED patients suspected of having undiagnosed tuberculosis should have all of the following initiated except:
A. Placement in an isolation room
B. Initiation of antituberculosis medication
C. PPD skin testing
D. Chest radiograph

6. The most common cause of death in children with TB is:
A. Osteomyelitis
B. Tuberculosis meningitis
C. Miliary TB
D. Sepsis
E. None of the above

7. Extrapulmonary disease is seen in approximately what percentage of children?
A. 10%
B. 20%
C. 30%
D. 40%
E. 50%

41. Lyme Disease, p. 453

1. The most common tick vector of Lyme disease in the eastern United States, *Ixodes scapularis:*
A. Is only found in the New England states
B. Has a bite that is noticed by nearly all patients diagnosed with Lyme disease
C. Can transmit babesiosis and ehrlichiosis as well
D. Requires 72 hours of attachment to the host to transmit disease

2. Ehrlichiosis is another tick-borne disease that:
A. Can present with non-specific findings such as fevers, chills, myalgias, and arthralgias
B. Is generally associated with a high WBC count and hyperamylasemia
C. Is an intra-erythrocytic parasite similar to malaria
D. Should be treated only after serologic confirmation or a positive PCR test of blood

3. Regarding the pathophysiology of Lyme disease, all the following statements are true except:

A. Following the bite of a tick infected with *B. burgdorferi*, substances in tick saliva help the organism establish infection in the skin
B. The spirochete immediately invades host blood vessels and travels to the CNS within the first two days of infection
C. *B. burgdorferi* has a tropism for skin, CNS, cardiac, and articular tissues
D. Some tick bites are responsible for transmitting multiple infecting organisms

4. The diagnosis of Lyme disease:
A. Always requires a positive serology for confirmation
B. Is most reliably made by seeing EM in an epidemiologically appropriate setting
C. Always requires Western blot confirmation of a positive ELISA test
D. Requires the patient to have traveled to one of the eight endemic states

5. Possible treatment of a patient with EM and 7th nerve palsy might include all the following regimens except:
A. one month of doxycycline
B. one month of amoxicillin
C. IV ceftriaxone if the patient had pleocytosis in the CSF
D. IV clindamycin and ciprofloxcacin

6. All of the following are true of erythema migrans (EM) except:
A. Classic EM is a flat red rash with central clearing found 7-10 days after the bite of an infected Ixodes tick
B. Only about a third of early Lyme disease patients have EM
C. A typical EM rash may appear uniform in color, centrally darkened, vesicular, or necrotic
D. Untreated, EM will disappear on its own in several weeks

7. Regarding serologic testing for Lyme disease, which of the following statements is false?
A. ELISA tests may be falsely positive in patients with certain viral infections, other spirochetal infections, and patients with malignancies and immunologic disorders
B. In early Lyme disease, serologic testing may be falsely negative because it can take several weeks for the host to mount an antibody response to *B. burgdorferi*
C. Western blot testing should be done to confirm positive ELISA tests
D. All patients with a positive ELISA test should be treated for Lyme disease

42. Influenza, p. 463

1. Package inserts to zanamivir contain a relative caution to:
A. patients with liver disease.
B. children younger than age 12.
C. patients with congestive heart failure (CHF).
D. patients with a history of bronchospasm.
E. elderly patients in nursing homes.

2. Primary control of influenza epidemics is dependent on:
A. chemoprophylaxis of all susceptible persons with amantadine/rimantadine.
B. chemoprophylaxis of high-risk patients with zanamivir/oseltamivir.
C. an effective, timely vaccination program.
D. quarantine of suspected cases.

3. From a diagnostic perspective, the most important factor(s) in a patient history is (are) the typically abrupt onset of which of the following systemic symptom(s)?
A. Headache
B. Fever
C. Myalgias and malaise
D. Chills accompanied by cough and sore throat
E. All of the above

4. Early onset of respiratory distress in a previously healthy adult influenza patient indicates:
A. presence of secondary lobar pneumonia.
B. myocarditis and congestive heart failure.
C. need for specific antibiotic therapy.
D. onset of status asthmaticus triggered by viral infection.
E. presence of progressive viral pneumonia.

5. Clinically useful confirmation of influenza infection may be obtained most efficiently by:
A. viral culture.
B. serum antibody titers.
C. rapid immunoassay (or assay) kits.
D. WBC and chest x-ray.
E. gram stain of sputum.

6. Clinically significant side effects of oseltamivir include:
A. CNS disturbance (confusion, vertigo, lassitude).
B. exacerbation of COPD or asthma.
C. GI upset, with nausea and vomiting.
D. significant drug interactions.
E. known teratologic effects.

7. The elderly often present with which of the following symptom complex, which is uncommon in other age groups?
A. Respiratory distress
B. Generalized malaise with myalgias
C. Depressed CNS function with lassitude, confusion, and memory loss
D. Reye's syndrome
E. Acute laryngotracheobronchitis

8. Infants with influenza may present to the emergency room with symptoms of:
A. acute laryngotracheobronchitis/croup.
B. classic bronchiolitis.
C. sepsis.
D. febrile seizures.
E. All of the above

51. Neuromuscular Transmission Failure, p. 547

1. Which of the following statements is correct?
   A. Myasthenia gravis most frequently presents with extremity weakness
   B. Almost 75% of the time, patients with myasthenia gravis have bulbar palsy at the time of initial presentation
   C. Myasthenic weakness worsens with rest
   D. It is not known whether D-penicillamine is an iatrogenic cause of myasthenia gravis

2. Which of the following is correct regarding diagnosis of myasthenia gravis?
   A. ACh-R antibodies are present in 90-95% of patients with myasthenia
   B. Up to 19% of the patients with MG do not have ACh-R antibody detectable by radioimmunoasssay
   C. The clinical presentation and disease spectrum of the seronegative patients is similar to those of seropositive patients
   D. All are correct

3. Which of the following statements is correct?
   A. Myasthenic crisis refers to rapid deterioration with involvement of respiratory muscles in the myasthenic patient
   B. Up to 20% of the patients will experience one episode of crisis
   C. Patients with an associated thymoma have higher risk for crisis
   D. Anticholinesterase medications should be stopped in suspected crisis
   E. All are correct

4. Which of the following statements regarding botulinum toxin is correct?
   A. Its action is on the postsynaptic membrane
   B. Ingestion of the toxin leads to muscular weakness without autonomic symptoms
   C. Up to 40% of the patients with clinical botulism may not have *C. botulinum* in the stool
   D. Antibiotics are indicated in infant botulism

5. Which of the following medications compromises neuromuscular transmission?
   A. Magnesium
   B. Aminoglycosides
   C. Flurorquinolones
   D. All of the above

6. In milder forms of transmission failure, subtle bulbar manifestations will predominate. They include which of the following?
   A. Difficulty chewing
   B. Blurry vision
   C. Changes in speech
   D. Drooping eyelids
   E. All of the above

7. Which group of disorders is characterized by persistent ACh in the synapse?
   A. Synaptic transmission disorders
   B. Postsynaptic disorders
   C. Presynaptic disorders
   D. None of the above

8. Limb weakness is the initial symptom in what percentage of patients with myasthenia gravis?
   A. 50%
   B. 80%
   C. Fewer than 10%
   D. 35%
   E. 90%

52. Subarachnoid Hemorrhage, p. 559

1. Subarachnoid hemorrhage is found in approximately how many Americans each year?
   A. 5000
   B. 10,000
   C. 30,000
   D. 75,000
   E. 1,000,000

2. Other than trauma, the most common cause of subarachnoid hemorrhage is:
   A. Arteriovenous malformations
   B. Saccular aneurysms
   C. Mycotic aneurysms
   D. Stimulant abuse
   E. Osler-Weber-Rendu disease

3. Intracranial aneurysms are more common in the posterior circulation of the brain.
   A. True
   B. False

4. Common causes of not considering the diagnosis of subarachnoid hemorrhage include all but which of the following?
   A. Lack of a "classic" presentation
   B. Failure to recognize that some patients present atypically
   C. Focus on the blood pressure or ECG abnormalities
   D. Failure to recognize that a head injury may have been the result of a spontaneous SAH
   E. Confusion with acute arbovirus encephalitis

5. CT scanning is most sensitive in diagnosing subarachnoid hemorrhage:
   A. In the first 12 hours
   B. In the first three days
   C. After the first week
   D. When the patient's hematocrit is less than 30%
   E. When the spinal fluid is positive for xanthochromia by spectrophotometry

6. Which of the following finding on an LP most strongly suggests a subarachnoid hemorrhage?

A. WBCs count greater than 5/mm^3
B. RBCs count 400 in the first tube diminishing to 10 in the third tube
C. Xanthochromia of the supernatant
D. Protein count of higher than 100 mg/dL
E. CSF pressure of less than 15 cm of water

7. Once a diagnosis of subarachnoid hemorrhage is established in the ED, assuming that the airway is not a problem at the time, the priority is:
A. Administering 40 mg of nimodipine PO
B. Starting a nitroprusside drip to bring the BP to less than 120 systolic
C. Consultation with a neurosurgeon and arranging cerebral angiography
D. Administering phenobarbital to prophylax against seizures
E. Putting in a urinary catheter to measure the urine output

8. Definitive therapy of a ruptured aneurysm of the anterior cerebral artery in an awake patient is currently:
A. Inserting an endovascularly placed coil
B. Intrathecal tPA to prevent bleeding
C. Nimodipine to prevent vasospasm
D. Surgical clipping of the aneurysm
E. Vitrectomy

53. Stroke: Clinical Presentations, p. 569

1. Lacunar infarctions present with:
A. Aphasia
B. Pure motor hemiparesis
C. Cranial nerve palsies
D. Hemineglect

2. Neglect syndromes are common in:
A. MCA infarctions
B. Lateral medullary syndrome
C. PICA infarction
D. Posterior cerebral artery infarction

3. The World Health Organization definition of stroke is:
A. A neurological deficit accompanied by focal dysfuncion
B. A neurological deficit of sudden onset accompanied by focal dysfunction and symptoms lasting more than 24 hours
C. Neurological events that have a duration shorter than 24 hours
D. Neurological deficit of sudden onset that is unaccompanied by or accompanied by focal dysfunction

4. In patients younger than 60, the predominance of stroke is:
A. Male to female, 3:2
B. Female to male, 2:4
C. Female to male, 3:2
D. Male to female, 2:4

5. The most common cause of focal neurologic deficits are:
A. Embolic infarctions
B. Intracranial hemorrhage
C. Thrombotic cerebral infarctions
D. None of the above

6. Patients with Wernicke's aphasia:
A. Show no deficit in the ability to vocalize, but, in the acute phase, use speech containing few understandable words
B. Demonstrate an abnormality in the execution of a task
C. Demonstrate deficits of attention
D. None of the above

7. The most common transient symtom of a TIA is:
A. Paresis
B. Dizziness or vertigo
C. Headache
D. Diminished pulse

54. Stroke: Evaluation and Management, p. 581

1. The correct dose of corticosteroid in acute stroke is:
A. Dexamethasone, 10 mg IV
B. Methylprednisone, 120 mg IV
C. Prednisone, 60 mg PO
D. Should not be used

2. An early finding of large infarct on noncontrast CT of the brain is:
A. Sulcal effacement
B. Normal CT of the brain
C. Midline shift
D. Well-defined hypodensity

3. The appropriate dose of t-PA is:
A. 1.0 mg/kg, max dose of 100 mg
B. 0.7 mg/kg, max dose of 90 mg
C. 0.9 mg/kg, max dose of 90 mg
D. 0.8 mg/kg, max dose of 100 mg

4. Risk factors for cardioembolism include:
A. Second-degree heart block
B. Mitral regurgitation
C. Right bundle-branch block
D. Mitral stenosis

5. The percentage of acute ischemic stroke patients who qualify for thrombolytic treatment is estimated to be:
A. 25%
B. Less than 10%
C. 50%
D. 90%

55. Spinal Cord Injuries, p. 591

1. Central cord syndrome will classically present with which of the following clinical findings?
A. Paralysis below the injury with preservation of position sense and vibratory sensation
B. Distal upper extremity weakness greater than proximal upper extremity weakness greater than lower extremity weakness

C. Paralysis below the injury with preservation of pain and temperature sensation
D. Complete motor and sensory loss below the injury

2. A C8 cervical cord injury will present with which of the following motor findings?
A. Decreased elbow flexion
B. Decreased wrist extension
C. Decreased finger flexion
D. Decreased elbow extension

3. An elderly patient with underlying cervical spine arthritis suffers a spinal cord injury as a result of excessive hyperextension of the cervical spine. Which of the following incomplete spinal cord injury syndromes would be most likely to occur?
A. Anterior cord syndrome
B. Posterior cord syndrome
C. Central cord syndrome
D. Brown-Sequard syndrome

4. Spinal shock often presents with which of the following vital sign patterns?
A. Hypertension and bradycardia
B. Hypotension and bradycardia
C. Hypertension and tachycardia
D. Hypotension and tachycardia

5. What percentage of head injured patients have an associated spinal injury?
A. 0-5%
B. 5-10%
C. 10-15%
D. 15-20%

6. How sensitive is a single lateral view of the cervical spine in identifying a cervical spine fracture?
A. 90-100%
B. 80-90%
C. 70-80%
D. 60-70%

7. Hypercapnic respiratory failure may ensue because of impaired phrenic nerve interruption to the diaphram with high cervical cord injury at or above which of the following levels?
A. C4
B. C5
C. C6
D. C7

8. When should steroids be administered to a patient with an acute spinal cord injury?
A. After neurosurgical consultation
B. As soon as the neurologic deficit is recognized
C. Just prior to transfer to a regional spinal cord center
D. After definitive open reduction of a vertebral fracture is performed

61. Migraine, p. 645

1. Up to what percent of headaches evaluated in emergency departments and by primary care physicians are thought to be due to muscle contraction?
A. 10%
B. 30%
C. 90%
D. 50%

2. Frequent findings in the patient with common migraine include:
A. photophobia.
B. sonophobia.
C. vomiting.
D. anorexia.
E. all of the above.

3. Headache pain in ophthalmoplegic migraine is associated with:
A. ocular muscle weakness.
B. ptosis.
C. extraocular paralysis.
D. pupillary changes.
E. All of the above.

4. Migraine equivalent refers to a condition in which a migraine sufferer experiences autonomic nervous system effects resulting in:
A. edema.
B. chest pain.
C. visual changes.
D. intense headache pain.
E. Both A and B are correct.

5. Cluster headaches are characterized by:
A. unilateral, excruciating facial pain often lasting for days.
B. lacrimation.
C. ipsilateral nasal congestion.
D. Both B and C are correct.

6. A history in the headache patient should include:
A. location.
B. mitigating factors.
C. prodromal symptoms.
D. quality.
E. All of the above.

7. Sumatriptan's mechanism of action is vasoconstriction, which is mediated through which of the following receptor sites?
A. Serotonin
B. Dopamine
C. Adrenergic
D. All of the above.

8. What percent of cluster headaches will resolve with 4% lidocaine (or cocaine hydrochloride)?
A. 5%
B. 80%
C. 20%
D. 40%

62. Status Epilepticus, p. 657

1. Neuronal damage from status epilepticus is thought to result primarily from:
   A. Hypoxia
   B Hypotension
   C. Abnormal CNS electrical activity
   D. Acidosis

2. Population studies reveal that the most common cause of status epilepticus in the adult population is:
   A. Alcohol-related
   B. Anticonvulsant discontinuation
   C. Meningitis
   D. Acute or remote stroke

3. Studies show that the most effective anticonvulsant in terminating status epilepticus that is refractory to optimal doses of lorazepam and phenytoin is:
   A. Phenobarbital
   B. Midazolam
   C. Propofol
   D. No clear data exist for next choice

4. Indications for request for stat EEG in treating a patient with seizures include:
   A. Suspicion of subtle generalized convulsive status epilepticus in an unresponsive patient with small twitching movements
   B. Failure of a patient to improve level of consciousness 20 minutes following clinical termination of seizures
   C. A patient with generalized convulsive status epilepticus when treatment included airway management, intubation, mechanical ventilation, and maintenance of neuromuscular blockade for adequate ventilation
   D. All of the above

5. Subtle generalized status epilepticus may be used to best describe which of the following?
   A. A comatose patient who recently had convulsive seizures and now has only intermittent arm twitching, but generalized seizure activity continues on EEG
   B. Partial complex status epilepticus or absence status epilepticus
   C. The quiet period between seizures
   D. Psychogenic seizures

6. Nonconvulsive status epilepticus is a term best employed for?
   A. A comatose patient who recently had convulsive seizures and now has only intermittent arm twitching, but generalized seizure activity continues on EEG
   B. Partial complex status epilepticus or absence status epilepticus
   C. The quiet period between seizures
   D. Psychogenic seizures

7. The following drugs may be useful in treating refractory generalized convulsive status epilepticus:
   A. Propofol
   B. Midazolam
   C. Pentobarbital
   D. All of the above

8. A clinical definition for GCSE includes continuous generalized convulsions lasting for:
   A. Two hours
   B. One hour
   C. 30 minutes
   D. Five minutes

67. Pulmonary Embolism: Etiology and Clinical Features, p. 717

1. Patients at high risk of death from PE include all of the following except:
   A. Patients with comorbid disease (cancer, CHF, COPD)
   B. Elderly patients
   C. Patients with right ventricular failure secondary to PE
   D. Young infants

2. All of the following are true of diagnostic studies except:
   A. D-dimer is sensitive but not specific for PE
   B. Alveolar dead space analysis can detect small changes in pulmonary artery flow
   C. Echocardiogram is useful in identifying PE in the unstable patient
   D. Computed tomography is very sensitive for peripheral pulmonary emboli

3. All of the following statements are correct about patients with PE except:
   A. Dyspnea, tachypnea, or pleuritic chest pain occur in 97% of patients with PE
   B. The triad of hemoptysis, dyspnea, and pleuritic chest pain is rare
   C. Almost all young people with PE have known risk factors and abnormal vital signs
   D. PE may present in unusual ways in the elderly and in paraplegics

4. All of the following regarding V/Q scans are correct except:
   A. There's an overall interobserver disagreement rate of 20%
   B. An "OK" scan rules out PE
   C. Twelve percent of patients with low-probability scans may have PE
   D. Combining clinical assessment with V/Q scanning provides greatest accuracy

5. All of the following occur in PE except:
   A. Kussmaul's sign
   B. Friction rub
   C. Venous cords in the lower extremity
   D. Fever greater than 103°F

6. All of the following regarding diagnostic studies are true except:
   A. Chest x-rays may be abnormal in 84% of patients with PE

B. Hampton's hump, Westermark and Fleishner's signs are common and accurate chest x-ray findings
C. ECG changes may include signs of right ventricular overload
D. Nearly 25% of patients with PE will have room air PO_2 > 80 mmHg

7. The most common precipitant(s) of thromboembolic disease are:
A. Trauma and surgery
B. Antithrombin III deficiency
C. Neoplasms
D. Nephrotic syndrome

8. All of the following are correct except:
A. MRI can distinguish pneumonia from PE
B. Angiography has minimal morbidity and mortality
C. A normal Doppler ultrasound of the lower extremities rules out the diagnosis of PE
D. Lung scanning substantiates or excludes PE in only half of all patients with PE

68. Pulmonary Embolism: Diagnosis and Management, p. 729

1. Patients who present in extremis:
A. Benefit from large volumes of crystalloid
B. May require thrombolysis in the presence of strong clinical suspicion
C. Should be immediately sent to angiography
D. Comprise about 25% of all ED patients with PE

2. Which of the following statements about heparin therapy is true?
A. Bleeding occurs in less than 1% of patients
B. Loading dose is 100-150 U/kg
C. Drip is 1000 U/h
D. It is mandatory to measure PTT prior to beginning heparin

3. LMWH:
A. Has its primary effect on platelet aggregation
B. Has a greater incidence of bleeding than unfractionated heparin
C. Dosing is based upon PTT
D. Is safe and effective in pregnancy

4. Adequate anticoagulation:
A. Rules out PE as a diagnostic consideration
B. Is defined as an INR between 2 and 3 for patients on coumadin
C. Results in a recurrent embolism rate of 1-2%
D. Obviates the need for vena caval filter, even in the presence of recurrent emboli

5. PE in pregnancy:
A. Is responsible for 15% of all deaths in pregnant women
B. Does not represent a risk to the fetus
C. Should never be diagnosed using V/Q scan
D. Is treated with coumadin

6. Thrombolysis in the treatment of PE:
A. Decreases mortality
B. Must be given via intrapulmonary route
C. May be given empirically to patients undergoing CPR if PE is strongly suspected
D. Has no significant role due to extensive bleeding complications

7. Which of the following statements is true?
A. Liberal use of V/Q scanning may be necessary to distinguish pleurisy from PE
B. Response to nonsteroidal anti-inflammatory drugs rules out PE
C. Acute pneumonia rarely mimics PE
D. Chest pain associated with crack cocaine is crushing in nature and is not pleuritic, as in PE

69. Allergic Diseases Update, p. 741

1. Allergic rhinitis is most common during:
A. Infancy
B. Childhood and adolescence
C. Middle age
D. Elderly

2. Which one of the following statements is correct?
A. First-generation antihistamines are more effective than second-generation in treatment of allergic rhinitis
B. Side-effect profiles of first- and second-generation antihistamines are essentially the same
C. First-generation antihistamines are associated with torsades des pointes when combined with antimicrobial medicines
D. First-generation antihistamines should be prescribed with caution in the elderly and in children

3. Which of the following antihistamines is associated with torsades des pointes?
A. Fexofenadine (Allegra)
B. Cetirizine (Zyrtec)
C. Loratadine (Claritan)
D. Terfenadine (Seldane)

4. Which of the following statements is correct?
A. There are significant differences in onset of action among second-generation antihistamines
B. Second-generation antihistamines are not differentiated based on half-lives
C. All second-generation antihistamines are associated with significant sedation
D. Second-generation antihistamines generally are less expensive than first-generation ones

5. Nasal steroids:
A. Are not useful in allergic rhinitis

B. Are associated with significant side effects that limit their use
C. Are fundamental in the treatment of perennial allergic rhinitis
D. Are effective within hours

6. Which statement is true regarding urticaria and angioedema?
A. Autoimmune disorders are the most common cause
B. Laboratory workup is fundamental in establishing an etiology
C. Treatment includes epinephrine in patients with airway compromise
D. Oral steroids should not be given

7. Which of the following is true regarding anaphylaxis?
A. Anaphylactic and anaphylactoid reactions have significantly different therapeutic implications
B. Snake bites and oral penicillin are the most common causes of fatal anaphylactic reactions
C. Patients most commonly die from overwhelming sepsis or direct neurotoxic effects of the inciting substance.
D. Most patients have immediate symptoms that resolve with proper therapy, but some have a second episode after initial recovery

8. Regarding epinephrine in the treatment of anaphylaxis:
A. IV epinephrine should be initial therapy in all patients
B. Racemic epinephrine is contraindicated in adults
C. Slow, low-dose IV infusions are preferred over fast, high-dose ones
D. All forms of epinephrine are contraindicated in pregnant patients and those with underlying cardiovascular disease

73. Electrocardiographic Diagnosis: Evaluating Patients With Chest Pain, p. 779

1. According to the article, what range of percentage of patients with proven infarction have been found to have an ECG that is diagnostic?
A. 10-15%
B. 30-40%
C. 25-50%
D. 30-50%

2. AMI is the most common diagnosis in adult chest-pain patients with STE.
A. True
B. False

3. In the case of AMI, the hyperacute T wave can be detected as early as:
A. Two hours after the onset of coronary occlusion and transmural infarction
B. 30 minutes after the onset of coronary occlusion and transmural infarction
C. 10 minutes after the onset of occlusion and infarction
D. None of the above

4. The absence of reciprocal change, or reciprocal ST segment depression, can reliably rule out the presence of AMI.
A. True
B. False

5. Which of the following signs commonly appears in continuing myocardial infarction after the hyperacute T wave but before the development of STE?
A. Q wave
B. Giant R wave
C. T wave inversion
D. None of the above

6. Posterior AMI:
A. Refers to infarction of the dorsal area of the heart, and, in most cases, involves occlusion of either the left circumflex or right coronary artery and its posterior descending branch
B. Most often occurs in conjunction with acute inferior or lateral myocardial infarction
C. Is rarely isolated
D. All of the above

7. In right ventricular AMI:
A. The 12-lead ECG reveals typical STE in the inferior leads as well as STE in the right precordial leads
B. Decreasing magnitude of STE in the V1 to V4 distribution is noted
C. Additional lead applications can be used to define injury
D. All of the above

8. Patients with inferior wall AMI manifest reciprocal changes in what percentage of cases?
A. 20%
B. 40%
C. 75%
D. 10%

74. Electrocardiographic Diagnosis: Specific Clinical Syndromes, p. 793

1. All of the following statements regarding electrocardiographic LVH and associated ST/T wave changes are true except:
A. The rule of appropriate discordance applies
B. They are frequently not recognized and therefore misdiagnosed as ischemic change in chest pain patients
C. ST segment elevation is always seen in all leads with prominent QRS complexes due to LVH
D. LVH-related ST segment changes are relatively permanent

2. Electrocardiographic features of LVH include all of the following except:
A. Poor R wave progression in the right- to mid-precordial leads
B. Prominent ST segment depression in the right precordial leads
C. QS complexes are usually seen in leads V1 and V2
D. Associated STE frequently has a concave morphology

3. In acute pericarditis, all of the following electrocardiographic findings are correctly matched with the ECG stage except:
   A. Resolution - stage 4
   B. STE - stage 1
   C. T wave inversion - stage 3
   D. Q wave formation – stage 2

4. Electrocardiographic features of acute pericarditis include all of the following except:
   A. ST segment elevation
   B. T wave inversion
   C. QRS complex widening
   D. PR segment depression

5. Benign early repolarization is characterized electrocardiographically by all of the following except:
   A. Prominent T waves
   B. Poor R wave progression
   C. ST segment elevation with J point elevation
   D. Peaked T waves similar to the hyperacute T wave of hyperkalemia

6. Features useful in distinguishing between acute pericarditis and benign early repolarization include all of the following except:
   A. The presence of q waves in BER
   B. The PR/ST discordant ratio
   C. PR segment depression in acute pericarditis
   D. None of the above

7. WPW syndrome is characterized on the ECG by all of the following except:
   A. PR segment depression
   B. QRS widening
   C. Delta wave
   D. PR interval shortening

77. Pericardial Disease, p. 825

1. Constrictive pericarditis:
   A. Is commonly seen soon after radiation therapy is given
   B. Can often be definitively treated in the ED
   C. Is often first suspected by calcifications seen on chest radiograph
   D. Is not often confused with the clinical presentation of hepatic cirrhosis

2. Cardiac tamponade in the trauma patient:
   A. Often develops prior to the patient's presentation to the ED
   B. Can often be managed by observation while waiting for arrival of consultants
   C. Requires urgent pericardiocentesis or thoracotomy
   D. Is commonly seen in blunt trauma patients

3. Which of the following is a characteristic symptom of pericarditis that aids in distinguishing it from acute myocardial ischemia?
   A. Intense diaphoresis unrelated to fever
   B. Dyspnea at rest and exertion
   C. Exacerbation of pain during inspiration and with rotation of the thorax
   D. Tachycardia out of proportion to the degree of discomfort exhibited by the patient

4. Bacterial pericarditis:
   A. Occurs more frequently than viral pericarditis
   B. Carries a higher mortality rate than viral pericarditis
   C. Results in tamponade less often than viral pericarditis
   D. Can be distinguished from viral pericarditis by ECG changes

5. Typical ECG findings of viral pericarditis include:
   A. an anatomic distribution of ST-T wave changes with reciprocal changes in opposing leads
   B. Evolutionary changes over time characterized by the development of deep Q-wave climbs in the limb and precordial leads
   C. Early T-wave depression progressing to diffuse ST-T elevations over a period of weeks
   D. Diffuse PR depression reflecting subepicardial injury to the atria

6. When performing a therapeutic pericardiocentesis:
   A. Parasternal approach is considered the first choice approach
   B. There is no risk of inducing cardiac tamponade
   C. ED thoracotomy is not indicated for cardiac arrest during this procedure
   D. If no fluid is aspirated during the procedure, this is not proof that tamponade is absent

7. Concerning traumatic cardiac tamponade:
   A. A one-to-three component friction rub is commonly present
   B. It most commonly results from blunt chest trauma
   C. It is caused by stab wounds to the chest more often than gunshot wounds to the chest
   D. Hemodynamic compromise may be severe with accumulation of as little as 100 cc of fluid if the time course of accumulation is rapid

8. The best diagnostic test for pericardial effusion or tamponade is:
   A. Chest radiograph
   B. 2D echocardiography
   C. CT scan
   D. ECG

79. Acute Myocardial Infarction: Thrombolysis and Procedural Revascularization, p. 847

1. In the GUSTO-I Trial the 30-day mortality rates for accelerate t-PA with heparin versus streptokinase with heparin, respectively, were:
   A. 10.2% and 12.3%
   B. 9.3% and 9.9%
   C. 8.3% and 9.3%
   D. 6.3% and 7.3%
   E. None of the above

2. Based on a review of patients entered into the NRMI-2 (National Registry of Myocardial Infarction-2) Study, there is a suggestion that:
   A. Lower body weight patients may benefit from weight-adjusted dosing of thrombolytic agents, in terms of lower fewer bleeding complications
   B. There is no need to consider body weight when dosing thrombolytics
   C. Bleeding complications cannot be prevented
   D. All of the above
   E. None of the above

3. For PTCA to be considered an alternative to thrombolytic therapy, the procedure should be:
   A. Performed in timely fashion, preferably within 60-90 minutes of arrival
   B. Performed by people skilled in the procedure, preferably performing more than 75 PTCA procedures per year
   C. Performed in institutions with high volume of procedures with experienced support staff
   D. All of the above
   E. None of the above

4. PTCA is recommended preferentially especially in the following patients:
   A. Those at high risk for intracranial bleeding
   B. Individuals who fail to qualify for thrombolytic therapy
   C. Patients in cardiogenic shock
   D. All of the above
   E. None of the above

5. Most bleeding complications of thrombolytic therapy:
   A. Occur in the brain
   B. Occur in the GI tract
   C. Occur in the GU tract
   D. Occur at vascular access sites
   E. None of the above

6. The most serious complication of thrombolytic therapy with t-PA is:
   A. Transient hypotension
   B. Allergic reactions
   C. Intracranial hemorrhage
   D. Immune complex disease
   E. None of the above

7. Thrombolytics should not be used in patients older than age:
   A. 60
   B. 65
   C. 70
   D. 75
   E. None of the above

8. Lidocaine should be avoided in accelerated idioventricular rhythms associated with thrombolysis
   A. True
   B. False

81. Reperfusion and Revascularization Therapies, p. 865

1. The theoretical and practical advantages of PCI over primary fibrinolysis include:
   A. larger patient eligibility pool.
   B. lower risk of intracranial bleeding.
   C. significantly higher initial reperfusion rate.
   D. All of the above

2. The GUSTO-III trial revealed that, because of its greater fibrin specificity, accelerated tPA may be superior to rPA in what group of patients?
   A. Those who present more than four hours after onset of symptoms
   B. Those who present within one hour of symptom onset
   C. Those who present within 30 minutes of symptom onset
   D. Those who present within two hours of symptom onset

3. Which of the following factors is included in the TIMI risk-stratification scheme?
   A. Age 65 or older
   B. Known coronary artery disease (CAD)
   C. Two or more episodes of resting angina during the 24 hours prior to presentation
   D. Prior chronic aspirin intake for CAD prevention
   E. All of the above

4. The generally accepted therapeutic window for administration of a fibrinolytic agent after the onset of ST-segment elevation AMI is:
   A. 2 hours.
   B. 4 hours.
   C. 18 hours.
   D. 12 hours.
   E. 24 hours.

5. No evidence of benefit from fibrinolytic therapy is found in patients who:
   A. have ST-elevation.
   B. have ST-elevation and present fewer than four hours after chest pain onset.
   C. lack either appropriate ST-segment elevation or the development of a new LBBB.
   D. None of the above

6. In the ASSENT-3 trial, the combination of full-dose TNK-tPA plus enoxaparin produced 30-day mortality rates of about:
   A. 1.2%.
   B. 5.2%.
   C. 10%.
   D. 22.2%.
   E. None of the above

7. In the STOPAMI Trial, comparing coronary stenting plus abciximab vs. primary fibrinolysis with tPA, the investigators concluded that a greater degree of myocardial salvage was seen in:

A. the coronary stenting group.
B. the tPA group.

8. Fibrinolysis is not effective in patients with AMI who present with cardiogenic shock. This is most likely due to:
A. a significantly lower coronary perfusion pressure.
B. a significantly higher coronary perfusion pressure.
C. the occlusive thrombus being overexposed to the fibrinolytic agent.
D. None of the above

86. Congestive Heart Failure: Initial Assessment and Stabilization, p. 935

1. Data from large clinical trials indicate that patients with CHF have a five-year mortality rate of:
A. Approximately 50%
B. 25%
C. 10%
D. 75%

2. It is estimated that approximately 75% of patients with heart failure are:
A. 80 years of age or older
B. Older than ages 65-70
C. In the 55-60 year age group
D. None of the above

3. The most common causes of of CHF encountered by the emergency physician include:
A. Hypertension
B. Alcoholic cardiomyopathy
C. Coronary artery disease
D. All of the above

4. Specific disease states that induce diastolic heart failure include:
A. Infiltrative myocardial disease
B. Pericardial disease
C. Hypertrophic cardiomyopathy
D. Coronary ischemia
E. All of the above

5. What diagnosis should be considered in a patient who presents with tachycardia, is hypertensive, and has no previous history of heart failure?
A. Hypothyroidism
B. Upper respiratory tract infection
C. Thyrotoxicosis
D. None of the above

6. Which of the following is not a sensitive indicator for heart failure?
A. Cardiac monitor
B. Physical findings
C. 12-lead EKG
D. Chest x-ray

7. A study indicated that what percent of eligible patients currently enrolled in managed care plans were receiving beta-blockers following their MI?
A. 35-65%
B. 15%
C. 80-90%
D. 5%

8. In the PRECISE study, carvedilol produced what percent reduction in combined risk of death or all-cause hospitalization?
A. 12%
B. 58%
C. 76%
D. 39%

87. Congestive Heart Failure: Targeted Therapy and Invasive Interventions, p. 945

1. It should be stressed that hyperkalemia can occur with spironolactone, and this adverse consequence of drug therapy is more likely to occur in patients already taking which of the following drug(s)?
A. Diuretics
B. Digoxin
C. ACEIs
D. Isordil
E. None of the above

2. In the PRAISE-1 study, amlodipine decreased all-cause mortality and was found to lower the risk of death by what percentage in patients with nonischemic cardiomyopathy?
A. 25%
B. 33%
C. 40%
D. 45%
E. None of the above

3. According to the article, digoxin levels should be measured in all patients presenting to the ED with which of the following?
A. Cardiac symptoms
B. Rhythm abnormalities
C. Deterioration in CHF
D. Unexplained clinical findings suggestive of possible drug toxicity
E. All of the above

4. Diuretics have been proven to be useful for symptomatic improvement in patients with heart failure, especially in those individuals with evidence of congestion, including:
A. Dyspnea on exertion
B. Edema
C. Orthopnea
D. B and C
E. A, B, and C

5. Potential side effects of administration of diuretics may include which of the following?
A. Electrolyte abnormalities, especially potassium depletion,

which may be a more pronounced loss if more than one diuretic is necessary for control (follow electrolytes vigilantly in patients on digoxin therapy).
B. Activation of the neurohormonal cascade, which is known to be deleterious in patients with heart failure.
C. Pre-renal azotemia and hypotension, which are usually secondary to overdiuresis or progression of heart failure associated with decreased renal perfusion
D. All of the above

6. Beta-adrenergic agonsists and phosphodiesterase inhibitors work by:
A. Decreasing myocardial contractility
B Increasing myocardial contractility
C. Neither decreasing nor increasing myocardial contractility
D. Maintaining myocardial contractility
E. None of the above

7. At what dose is it recommended to start dobutamine?
A. 1 mcg/kg/min
B. 2-5 mcg/kg/min
C. 6-8 mcg/kg/min
D. 9-11 mcg/kg/min
E. None of the above

8. Conditions that most commonly lead to the development of pulmonary edema include which of the following?
A. Myocardial ischemia
B. Fluid excess and volume overload
C. Medication noncompliance
D. Arrhythmias
E. All of the above

91. Deep Venous Thrombosis: Risk Factor Assessment and Diagnosis, p. 993

1. Surgery and trauma are responsible for what percent of all thromboembolic disease resulting from hypercoagulable state and immobility?
A. 10%
B. 40%
C. 90%
D. 75%
E. 80%

2. Increased estrogen occurs in a patient:
A. During all stages of pregnancy
B. After elective abortion
C. During treatment with oral contraceptive pills
D. During the first three months post-partum
E. All of the above

3. Clinical examination alone is able to confirm what percent of DVT cases?
A. 20-30%
B. 50%
C. 5%
D. 60-70%

4. Radiologists disagree on the interpretation of what percent of venography cases?
A. 50%
B. Less than 5%
C. At least 10%
D. 75%

5. A sonographer can distinguish a fresh clot from an old clot based on:
A. Collateral flow
B. Echogenicity
C. Homogeneity
D. All of the above

6. Duplex scanning:
A. Is most sensitive for clots below the knee
B. Is less sensitive for clots below the knee
C. Detects 30% of distal thrombi
D. Is more likely to detect non-occluding thrombi

7. What percent of patients with suspected thrombosis and a negative ultrasound later prove to have DVT?
A. 10%
B. 25%
C. 2-3%
D. 40-45%

8. Bilateral leg swelling can be caused by:
A. Liver disease
B. Nephrotic syndrome
C. Capillary leak syndrome
D. Pregnancy
E. All of the above

92. Deep Venous Thrombosis: Patient Management and Anticoagulation, p. 1005

1. Heparin:
A. Causes significant bleeding in about 7-30% of patients
B. Causes complications in patients at a rate of 1-2% per day
C. Has a narrow therapeutic window
D. All of the above

2. Which of the following is not an absolute contraindication to heparin?
A. Active internal bleeding
B. Iliofemoral thrombosis
C. Malignant hypertension
D. CNS neoplasm
E. Recent and significant trauma

3. LMWH:
A. Is valued for its anticoagulant effect
B. Primarily effects thrombin and platelet aggregation
C. Usually does not elevate PTT
D. Does not inhibit factor X-a

4. Compared to heparin, streptokinase poses:
   A. A three-fold risk of significant bleeding
   B. 5% less risk of significant bleeding
   C. Twice as much risk of significant bleeding
   D. 25% less risk of significant bleeding

5. What percent of calf thrombi will propagate?
   A. 2-5%
   B. 32%
   C. 10%
   D. 59%

6. Duplex scanning in pregnant wome is safe and accurate:
   A. Only after 24 weeks of gestation
   B. Only after 32 weeks of gestation
   C. Prior ot 20 weeks ao gestation
   D. Prior to 30 weeks of gestation

7. What might differentiate between old and new DVT?
   A. A combination of clinical suspicion and D-dimer testing
   B. A combination of serial venous ultrasonography and lung scanning
   C. A combination of nuclear magnetic imaging and fibrinogen leg scanning
   D. All of the above

93. Anticoagulation and Antiplatelet Therapy: Aspirin, Glycoprotein IIb/IIIa Inhibitors, and ADP Platelet Receptor Antagonists, p. 1015

1. Which of the following statements is true?
   A. Arterial thrombi mostly consist of fibrin
   B. Venous thrombi mostly consist of fibrin
   C. Arterial thrombi mostly consist of platelets
   D. Venous thrombi mostly consist of platelets

2. Which patient is most likely to benefit from daily aspirin?
   A. Patient with history of deep vein thrombosis
   B. Healthy male, age 40, non-smoker
   C. A 60-year-old male with recent myocardial infarction
   D. 85-year-old normotensive, non-smoking woman with no history of neurologic or cardiovascular ischemia

3. Which of the following statement is true regarding clopidogrel?
   A. It is commonly associated with thrombocytopenia
   B. It is commonly associated with neutropenia
   C. It is not related structurally to ticlopidine
   D. Blood counts must be checked on a regular basis
   E. Its most common side effects are rash, diarrhea, and abdominal pain.

4. How is abciximab different from eptifibatide and tirofiban?
   A. It may be used in unstable angina whether cardiac catheterization is planned
   B. It may be used only when cardiac catheterization is planned within 24 hours
   C. It is available in both oral and intravenous forms
   D. It should not be used concomitantly with aspirin
   E. It may be used in acute non-Q-wave myocardial infarction

5. The ADP Plate receptor antagonists have an onset of action that:
   A. Is similar to aspirin
   B. Is faster than aspirin
   C. Is slower than aspirin
   D. Is faster or slower than aspirin depending on the patient's liver function

6. The preferred initial treatment of choice in patients with high-risk atrial fibrillation is:
   A. Warfarin
   B. Aspirin
   C. Ticlopidine
   D. None of the above

7. GP IIa/IIIb inhibitors can be combined with thrombolytic agents in treatment protocols for acute MI.
   A. True
   B. False

8. Aspirin is the drug of choice for prevention of DVT and PE.
   A. True
   B. False

97. Atrial Fibrillation, p. 1059

1. Which of the following statements concerning the epidemiology of atrial fibrillation is correct?
   A. Atrial fibrillation is an uncommon arrhythmia
   B. The prevalence of atrial fibrillation increases with age
   C. Atrial fibrillation is usually not associated with coexistant heart or systemic disease
   D. Atrial fibrillation and stroke are unrelated

2. Which of the following is not a cause of atrial fibrillation?
   A. Thyrotoxicosis
   B. Valvular heart disease
   C. Parasitosis
   D. Hypertensive heart disease

3. Which of the following drugs is contraindicated for rate control in heart failure?
   A. Digoxin
   B. Amiodarone
   C. Propranolol
   D. Diltiazem

4. What is the ideal drug for rate control in thyrotoxicosis?
   A. Digoxin
   B. Beta-blocker
   C. Flecainide
   D. Propafenone

5. What is the ideal drug for rapid atrial fibrillation due to an accessory pathway such as Wolff-Parkinson-White?
   A. Digoxin

B. Diltiazem
C. Propranolol
D. Procainamide

6. Which of the following is a contraindication to the use of ibutilide?
A. Hypomagnesemia
B. Fasting state
C. History of SVT
D. An INR in the range of 2-3

7. What is the most common proarrhythic effect of ibutilide?
A. Mutifocal atrial tachycardia
B. Ventricular fibrillation
C. Asystole
D. Polymorphic ventricular tachycardia

8. Which of the following statements concerning hospitalization of patients with new onset atrial fibrillation is correct?
A. All patients must be admitted to rule out myocardial infarction
B. Only patients with decompensated heart failure require admission
C. Patients may beadmitted for cardiovascular instability or for attempts at cardioversion
D. Hospitalization is never indicated

98. Syncope, p. 1069

1. Patients undergoing evaluation of syncope require all of the following except:
A. History of event
B. Family history
C. CT scan
D. ECG
E. Physical examination

2. Which of the following syncopal patients is not at risk for increased mortality or sudden death?
A. A 75-year-old with dilated cardiomyopathy
B. A 10-year-old male with onset of symptoms while running
C. A previously healthy 14-year-old female with benign family history
D. A 30-year-old with sudden onset syncope, headache, nausea, and ataxic gait
E. A 20-year-old man with increased Q-T interval on EKG

3. CT scan or MRI is indicated in which of the following?
A. All syncope patients older than 60 years
B. A 25-year-old patient with visual symptoms preceding loss of consciousness
C. A 35-year-old syncopal patient with family history of seizure disorder
D. A 40-year-old patient with pronator-drift on neurologic examination

4. Which of the following types of agents has been recently shown to be a particular cause of drug syncope in the elderly?
A. Selective serotonin reuptake inhibitors
B. Antihistamines
C. Benzodiazepines
D. Thyroid hormone replacement agents
E. Antiemetics

5. Carotid sinus massage may be helpful in the examination of which of the following patients?
A. Syncopal patient with carotid bruits
B. Syncopal patient with history of cerebrovascular infarction one year previously
C. Young adult patient with frequent unexplained falls and occasional syncope
D. Patient with pacemaker and automated defibrillator due to history of ventricular tachycardia

6. A history of syncope that accompanies exercise in a pediatric patient should increase suspicion of all of the following except:
A. Long Q-T syndrome
B. Congenital aortic stenosis
C. Hypertrophic cardiomyopathy
D. Sick sinus syndrome
E. Anomalous origin of the left coronary artery from the sinus of Valsalva

101. Acute Appendicitis, p. 1101

1. What percentage of the cases of appendicitis are seen in the 10-30 year age group?
A. 10%
B. 69%
C. 25%
D. 91%

2. "Classical" presentations of appendicitis are reported in what percentage of patients?
A. 5-10%
B. 29%
C. 50-60%
D. 85%

3. Which presenting sign or symptom is most likely to be seen in appendicitis?
A. Anorexia with nausea and vomiting
B. Migration of pain to the RLQ as time progresses
C. Rebound abdominal tenderness
D. RLQ tenderness on physical exam
E. Low-grade temperature

4. Ultrasound findings consistent with acute appendicitis include all but which of the following?
A. Dilated appendix lumen
B. Presence of periappendiceal fluid
C. A compressible appendix
D. Greater than 6 mm outer wall to outer wall diameter

5. Which of the following is true concerning the WBC in appendicitis?

A. The WBC may be normal in up to 20-45% of elderly patients with appendicitis
B. A WBC over 15,000 cells/mm^3 means the patient has a perforation
C. During observation of a patient with suspected appendicitis, a rising WBC is diagnostic of appendicitis
D. If the patient has both a normal WBC and differential, then they do not have appendicitis

6. Which of the following is commonly found in litigation for failure to diagnose appendicitis?
A. Documentation of a rectal exam or pelvic exam
B. Documentation of adequate follow-up instructions
C. Documentation of serial abdominal exams
D. Discharge diagnosis of gastroenteritis

102. Infectious Diarrhea, p. 1117

1. Which of the following statements is true regarding the treatment of infectious diarrhea?
A. Most clear liquids provide adequate sodium and potassium for the rehydration of infants
B. Fluoroquinolones are recommended for the empiric antibiotic treatment of acute infectious enteritis
C. Empiric antibiotic use does not increase the risk of prolonged *Salmonella* carriage
D. There is no risk of salicylate toxicity in patients who use bismuth salicylate
E. Clonidine has been demonstrated to be efficacious in the treatment of acute infectious enteritis

2. Which pathogen is associated with toxin-mediated food poisoning?
A. *Bacillus cereus*
B. *Yersinia enterocolitica*
C. *Campylobacter jejuni*
D. *Salmonella typhi*
E. *Giardia lamblia*

3. Which pathogen is sought on routine stool culture?
A. *Vibrio cholerae*
B. *Campylobacter jejuni*
C. Enteroinvasive *E. coli*
D. Enterohemorrhagic *E. coli*
E. *Clostridium difficile*

4. Which of the following is an invasive organism that causes inflammatory diarrhea?
A. *Vibrio cholerae*
B. Enterotoxigenic *Escherichia coli*
C. Calcivirus
D. *Campylobacter jejuni*
E. *Vibrio vulnificus*

5. All of the following are risk factors for acquiring acute infectious diarrhea except:
A. Day care center participation
B. Rustic travel
C. Ingestion of undercooked poultry or beef
D. Exposure to individuals with acute infectious gastroenteritis
E. Urban dwelling

6. Which of the following does not suggest an enteroinvasive pathogen?
A. Fever
B. Fecal leukocytes
C. Vomiting
D. Rice-water stools
E. Abdominal pain

7. Risk factors that increase the likelihood of yielding bacteria by stool culture include:
A. Fecal leukocytes
B. Vomiting preceding diarrhea
C. Fewer than four stools per day
D. A peripheral WBC count of greater than 15,000 cells/mm^3
E. A sour-fruity odor to the stool

8. Which pet is not associated with Salmonella carriage?
A. Snakes
B. Turtles
C. Ducklings
D. African pygmy hedgehogs
E. Tropical fish

103. Ischemic Bowel Syndromes, p. 1127

1. The most extensive bowel injury pattern seen intraoperatively is in patients with:
A. Mesenteric venous thrombosis
B. Nonocclusive mesenteric ischemia
C. Mesenteric arterial thrombosis
D. Mesenteric arterial emboli

2. All of the following physical exam findings are expected in a late presentation of AMI except:
A. Abdominal percussion tenderness
B. Abdominal pain out of proportion to physical findings
C. Rigid abdomen
D. involuntary guarding with shock

3. The first radiological evaluation that should be done on a patient suspected of having acute mesenteric ischemia is:
A. Abdominal ultrasound
B. Visceral angiography
C. Abdominal and chest x-rays
D. Computed tomography
E. Magnetic resonance imaging

4. The most common finding in early mesenteric ischemia on plain films is:
A. Air fluid levels
B. Free intra-abdominal air
C. Ileus
D. Normal
E. Splenic flexure cut off sign

5. Findings highly suggestive of AMI on plain radiography include all of the following except:
   A. Pneumatosis
   B. Portal venous gas
   C. Free intra-abdominal air
   D. Thumbprinting of abdominal wall

6. What is the appropriate initial management of patients diagnosed as angiography with nonocclusive mesenteric ischmeia without peritoneal findings?
   A. Urokinase infusion
   B. Exploratory laparotomy
   C. Intra-arterial papaverine infusion
   D. Systemic heparinization

7. Visceral pain:
   A. Is derived from receptors located in the parietal peritoneum
   B. Is triggered by such stimuli as touch, cutting, ischemia, pressure, heat, or inflammation
   C. Produces guarding
   D. Is triggered by such stimuli as smooth-muscle contraction or spasm, distention or stretching, and ischemia, but not by physical palpation or temperature

8. The majority of mesenteric arterial emboli lodge in the:
   A. Superior mesenteric artery (SMA)
   B. The celiac trunk
   C. The inferior mesenteric artery (IMA)
   D. None of the above

105. Foodborne Illness, p. 1145

1. The most common fish borne illness in the United States is:
   A. Ciguatera
   B. Scombroid
   C. Paralytic shellfish poisoning
   D. Tetrodotoxin

2. With which toxin does food not taste normal?
   A. *Ciguatera*
   B. *Scombroid*
   C. Staphylococcal toxin
   D. *B. cereus* emetic toxin

3. Ciguatera does not usually affect which system?
   A. Gastrointestinal
   B. Neurologic
   C. Cardiovascular
   D. Dermatologic

4. Primary treatments of suspected ciguatera poisoning include which of the following?
   A. Steroids
   B. Opiates
   C. Mannitol
   D. Phenobarbital

5. Primary treatment of suspected scombroid poisoning include which of the following?
   A. Steroids
   B. Diphenhydramine
   C. Mannitol
   D. Naloxone

6. Staphylococcal enterotoxin is most common in which foods?
   A. Potato and macaroni salads
   B. Milk and milk products
   C. Fish and shellfish
   D. Ham and chicken

7. One study found that in about 83% of cases, bloody and watery diarrhea with leukocytes resulted from:
   A. *Salmonella*
   B. *Shigella*
   C. *Campylobacter*
   D. All of the above

8. The leading cause of bacterial food poisoning is:
   A. *Salmonella*
   B. *Campylobacter*
   C. *E. coli* O157:47
   D. *C. botulinum*

116. Abnormal Vaginal Bleeding, p. 1265

1. Menorrhagia is defined as blood loss greater than:
   A. 20 mL per period
   B. 40 mL per period
   C. 60 mL per period
   D. 80 mL per period

2. Polymenorrhea is:
   A. Bleeding at intervals 35 days to 6 months
   B. Bleeding at intervals less than 21 days
   C. Bleeding at intervals 21 days to 35 days
   D. No bleeding for 6 months
   E. Bleeding between regular cycles

3. Breakthrough or intermenstrual bleeding while on OCPs is usually due to:
   A. Pregnancy
   B. Missed OCPs or variable ingestion time
   C. Antibiotics
   D. Anticonvulsants

4. The secretory surge occurs:
   A. Just prior to ovulation
   B. Just prior to menses
   C. Just after menses
   D. After implantation of the fertilized egg

5. In evaluating the amount of blood loss in the ED, the best objective parameter is:
   A. A woman's own perception of increased loss
   B. The number of pads used

C. The presence of iron-deficiency anemia
D. Having to switch from tampons to pads

6. Common systemic causes of menorrhagia include all of the following except:
A. Hypothyroidism
B. Liver failure
C. Coagulopathies
D. COPD

7. Uterine leiomyomas:
A. Are usually symptomatic
B. When discovered, can be assumed to be the cause of abnormal vaginal bleeding
C. May cause cyclic, profuse bleeding
D. Are found in only 10% of women overall

8. For the unstable patient with abnormal uterine bleeding, the agent with quickest onset of action is:
A. Intravenous premarin
B. NSAIDs
C. OCPs
D. Danazol

117. Preeclampsia/Eclampsia, p. 1275

1. The risk of developing preeclampsia is decreased in:
A. Nulliparous women
B. Women who smoke
C. Women conceiving by a new partner
D. Sisters and daughters of women with a history of preeclampsia

2. In women who develop preeclampsia, microscopic examination of uterine spiral arteries reveals:
A. Trophoblastic invasion of arterial walls, converting these vessels to low-resistance, high-flow vessels
B. No specific abnormalities
C. A failure of trophoblastic invasion, resulting in vessels that retain their responsiveness to pressors
D. No abnormalities, except in severe disease

3. Which finding is consistent with mild preeclampsia?
A. Blood pressure of 190/120 mmHg at 35 weeks' gestation
B. Diminished fibrinogen level, elevated fibrin split products, prolonged PT, PTT, and bleeding from multiple sites
C. A generalized, tonic-clonic seizure lasting one minute
D. Blood pressure of 120/80 mmHg, 2+ proteinuria, and generalized edema in an otherwise asymptomatic woman at 25 weeks' gestation

4. Patients who are ultimately diagnosed with the HELLP syndrome:
A. Often present with subtle, nonspecific symptoms
B. Have a better prognosis than those with preeclampsia
C. Can be managed at home if compliance with instructions seems likely
D. Often present with jaundice and fulminant hepatic failure

5. Initial imaging studies for patients with severe preeclampsia and neurologic symptoms should include:
A. Cranial CT scanning
B. Cranial MRI
C. EEG
D. Skull x-rays

6. Which of the following laboratory abnormalities may be useful as an early indication of developing preeclampsia?
A. Elevated serum bilirubin
B. Elevated serum uric acid
C. Decreased serum fibrinogen
D. Prolonged prothrombin time

7. Which of the following is true regarding cardiopulmonary resuscitation of patients with preeclampsia/eclampsia?
A. CPR is contraindicated in patients with a gravid uterus
B. The risk of neurologic sequelae to the fetus is independent of time from cardiac arrest to delivery
C. Perimortem caesarean section should be delayed until perfusing rhythm is restored
D. Early perimortem caesarean section improves fetal and maternal outcome

8. The definition of severe preeclampsia includes:
A. Polyuria
B. Hematuria
C. 1+ to 2+ proteinuria
D. Evidence of hemolysis

118. Pelvic Inflammatory Disease, p. 1283

1. Long-term sequelae such as ectopic pregnancy and infertility occur in about what percentage of cases of PID?
A. 5%
B. 15%
C. 25%
D. 35%
E. 45%

2. The triad of lower abdominal tenderness, adnexal tenderness, and pain on manipulation of the cervix are reported in up to:
A. 30% of cases of PID
B. 60% of cases of PID
C. 90% of cases of PID
D. None of the above

3. PID is thought to result from:
A. Descending infection from tuobo-ovarian structures to cervix
B. Ascending infection from anal structures to cervix
C. Descending infection from renal structures to salpinx
D. Ascending infection from cervix and vagina to upper portion of the genital tract
E. None of the above

4. Generally speaking, antibiotic treatment of PID requires multiple drug regimens active against:

A. Gram-positive cocci, *Neisseria gonorrhoeae*, and anaerobes
B. *Chlamydia pneumoniae*, *Neisseria gonorrhoeae*, and anaerobes
C. *Chlamydia trachomatis*, gram-positive cocci, and *Neisseria gonorrhoeae*
D. *Chlamydia trachomatic*, *Neisseria gonorrhoeae*, anaerobes and gram-negative organisms
E. None of the above

5. All FDA-approved antimicrobial regimens for treatment of PID are included in the current CDC Guidelines for treatment of PID.
A. True
B. False

6. Pelvic ultrasound is:
A. Not the "gold standard" for diagnosis of PID
B. Has a sensitivity rate of up to 93% for identifying tubal and ovarian pathology
C. Useful for making the diagnosis of tubo-ovarian abscess
D. Should be performed if a pelvic mass is suspected
E. All of the above

7. The following is an FDA-approved treatment course for PID:
A. Azithromycin IV (500 mg qD for 1-2 days) followed by oral azithromycin 250 mg orally one daily to complete a course of therapy of 7 days plus metronidazole 500 mg orally twice daily for 14 days (when required for anaerobic infection)
B. Azithromycin 500 mg PO for 1-2 days, followed by azithromycin 250 mg orally once daily to complete a course of therapy of 7 days plus metronidazole 500 mg orally twice daily for 14 days (when required for anaerobic infection)
C. Azithromycin 500 mg PO once daily to complete a course of therapy of 7 days plus metronidazole 500 mg orally twice daily for 14 days (when required for anaerobic infection)
D. None of the above
E. All of the above

119. Sexually Transmissable Diseases, p. 1293

1. Male to female transmission of gonorrhea is the most efficient transmission vector.
A. True
B. False

2. The incubation period for gonorrhea ranges from three to seven days, and the disease usually manifests symptoms within:
A. 7-9 days after exposure
B. 10-14 days after exposure
C. 15-21 days after exposure
D. More than 21 days after exposure
E. None of the above

3. What percentage of people harboring gonorrhea are thought to be asymptomatic?
A. 20%
B. 30%
C. 40%
D. 50%
E. None of the above

4. The sensitivity rate for a gram stain evaluation of a cervical specimen site is about:
A. 5%
B. 10%
C. 15%
D. 20%
E. None of the above

5. The two forms of gonococcus-mediated resistance are:
A. Plasmid-mediated and chromosome-mediated resistance
B. Plasminogen-mediated and chromosome-mediated resistance
C. Plasminogen-mediated and lysosome-mediated resistance
D. None of the above

6. Increasing resistance to what CDC-approved antibiotic for treatment of gonococcus has been reported in Asia?
A. Cephalosporins
B. Azithromycin
C. Quinolones
D. Macrolides
E. None of the above

7. A one-dose treatment for uncomplicated chlamydial infection is:
A. Tetracycline
B. Cefixime
C. Ciprofloxacin
D. Azithromycin
E. None of the above

8. Chlamydia infection increases the risk of HIV infection.
A. True
B. False

127. Inflammatory Conditions, Head and Neck, p. 1363

1. Intracranial complication should be suspected in which of these patients with otitis media?
A. A patient with a 35 dB conductive hearing loss and an air fluid level in the middle ear
B. A patient with mild otalgia and purulent material draining from the EAC
C. A patient with a red, bulging tympanic membrane
D. A patient with sensorineural hearing loss and purulent material draining from the EAC

2. Necrotizing otitis externa:
A. Can lead to cavernous sinus thrombosis
B. Is usually caused by *Staphylococcus aureus*
C. Is less common in diabetics
D. Usually begins in the middle ear

3. Group A beta-hemolytic streptococcal pharyngitis:
A. Is more common in the summer and fall
B. Can be detected 99% of the time by rapid antigen test

C. Can be treated with erythromycin
D. Can lead to rheumatic fever in up to 10% of patients

4. The diagnosis of epiglottitis in a child is suggested by:
A. The presence of a steeple sign on AP radiograph of the neck
B. Drooling and dysphagia
C. A barky cough
D. A gradual onset of symptoms

5. Sinusitis:
A. Most commonly occurs in the maxillary sinus
B. Is best diagnosed by plain sinus radiographs
C. Can result in exacerbation of asthma
D. Is less common in patients with Kartagener's syndrome

6. Which of the following statements is false?
A. Deep neck abscesses are commonly polymicrobial
B. Deep neck abscesses are more common in diabetics and immunocompromised patients
C. Deep neck abscesses occur most commonly in the peritonsillar area
D. Deep neck abscesses are easily differentiated clinically from deep space cellulitis

7. Which of the following statements is correct?
A. Mumps parotitis can be unilateral or bilateral
B. Parotitis can be easily distinguished from cat scratch disease
C. HIV commonly causes microabscesses of the parotid gland
D. Adenovirus is the most common viral etiology of parotitis

129. Ophthalmologic Emergencies, p. 1383

1. Which of the following is not true about hyphemas?
A. Rebleeding occurs most frequently in the first five days
B. Aminocaproic acid decreases the risk of rebleed
C. Patients must be hospitalized
D. Rebleed with increased IOP can cause corneal bloodstaining

2. With regard to ocular and adnexal lacerations, which of the following are true?
A. Marginal lid lacerations medial to the perimeter could possibly involve the canaliculus
B. Most conjunctival lacerations do not require surgical repair
C. Scleral lacerations due to blunt trauma occur most often at the limbus or in the area posterior to the insertion of the rectus muscles
D. All of the above

3. Orbital fractures need to be repaired if there is:
A. Diplopia in central 20° of the eye.
B. Ptosis of the globe
C. Significant enophthalmos
D. All of the above

4. Traumatic retinal detachments are most often:
A. Seen with retinal flap tears due to vitreous separation
B. Diagnosed at the time of injury
C. In the inferotemporal and superonasal quadrant
D. In the superotemporal and inferonasal quadrant

5. Pre-auricular adenopathy is found in conjunction with many viral eye infections and with which of the following bacterial infections?
A. *Staphylococcus*
B. *Streptococcus*
C. *Gonococcus*
D. *Pseudomonas*
E. None of the above

6. Which of the following conditions require emergent treatment?
A. Central retinal artery occlusion
B. Ocular chemical burn
C. Angle closure glaucoma
D. Endophthalmitis
E. All of the above

7. Which of the following retinal causes of visual loss most commonly presents with no afferent pupillary defect?
A. Central retinal artery occlusion
B. Retinal detachment
C. Central retinal vein occlusion
D. Age-related macular degeneration
E. None of the above

140. Altered Mental Status, p. 1505

1. Which of the following signs or symptoms characterize(s) dementia?
A. Loss of intellectual function
B. Memory disturbances
C. Impairment in thinking and judgment
D. Personality changes
E. All of the above

2. All of the following are characteristic of delirium except:
A. Symptoms are global in nature
B. It is usually chronic with onset over several months
C. It is common in the elderly
D. It is a commonly associated with chronic dementia

3. After Alzheimer's disease, the most common cause of dementia is:
A. Delirium
B. Chronic hypoglycemia
C. Multi-infarct dementia associated with cerebrovascular disease
D. Infection

4. The following medication(s) can produce anticholinergic side effects:
A. Diphenhydramine
B. Antipsychotics
C. Tricyclic antidepressants
D. Anti-Parkinsonian drugs
E. All of the above

5. The sensitivity and specificity of the Confusion Assessment Method for detecting delirium is about:
   A. 30%
   B. 50%
   C. 70%
   D. 90%

6. CT scanning in patients with delirium may be especially helpful if:
   A. The diagnosis of hypoglycemia is confirmed
   B. The patient is septic
   C. The patient has a focal neurologic finding or history of head trauma
   D. the patient has loss of memory

7. With respect to use of restraints for hyperactive patients in the ED, which of the following is true?
   A. Physical restraints are preferable to chemical restraints
   B. Leather restraints are almost always needed
   C. Chemical restraints are usually preferrable to physical restraints
   D. Most sedating drugs used as chemical restraints do not have anticholinergic or extrapyramidal properties

8. Which of the following patient subgroup(s) generally require admission to the hospital:
   A. Hemodynamic instability
   B. Sepsis
   C. CNS structural lesions
   D. Serious electrolyte abnormalities
   E. All of the above

152. Winter Sports-Related Injuries, p. 1637

1. The most common ski injury seen today is:
   A. spiral fracture of the tibia
   B. Anterior dislocation of the shoulder
   C. Knee ligament strains
   D. Patellar dislocation
   E. Peroneal tendon dislocation

2. When do most ski injuries occur?
   A. Early in the morning—dawn patrol
   B. Night skiing
   C. About suppertime
   D. Just after breakfast
   E. Last run of the day

3. Beginners are more likely to be hurt on a snowboard than on skis?
   A. True
   B. False

4. Cold injuries are about what percentage of reported cross-country ski injuries?
   A. 10%
   B. 20%
   C. 30%
   D. 40%
   E. 75%

159. Hand Injuries, p. 1709

1. When examining the patient with a hand injury, radiographs should be obtained:
   A. For penetrating injuries of the hand
   B. For simple dislocations of the finger
   C. When examining a hand infection
   D. In all but the most minor of hand lacerations or contusions

2. A metacarpal neck fracture of the fifth metacarpal is often called:
   A. A Bennet's fracture
   B. A Boxer's fracture
   C. A Tuft's fracture
   D. A Brewerton's fracture

3. A devascularized digit should be:
   A. Immersed in ice water
   B. Immersed in milk
   C. Carefully cleaned of all debris and nonviable tissue
   D. Placed in saline soaked gauze and put on ice

4. Dislocation of the MCP joint can cause:
   A. An unstable joint
   B. A joint that requires surgical reduction
   C. Rupture of the volar plate
   D. All of the above

5. Froment's sign is useful in testing:
   A. Damage to the flexor carpi ulnaris
   B Damage to the median nerve
   C. Damage to ulnar nerve
   D. Damage to the radial nerve

6. Major clues to the loss of senation in the hand include:
   A. FLinch reaction to sharp/dull testing
   B. Loss of capillary refill in the digit
   C. Loss of sweating
   D. Increased pain on flexion of the digit

7. The median nerve supplies the:
   A. Web space between thumb and first finger
   B. The fifth finger
   C. Dorsal surface of the proximal first and second fingers
   D. All of above

160. COX-2 Specific Inhibitors, p. 1721

1. To completely inhibit the COX-2 without affecting the COX-1, the COX-2 specific NSAID would need to be at least:
   A. 20 times more potent against COX-2 than COX-1.
   B. 50 times more potent against COX-2 than COX-1.
   C. 80 times more potent against COX-2 than COX-1.

D. 100 times more potent against COX-2 than COX-1.
E. 150 times more potent against COX-2 than COX-1.

2. COX-2 selective drugs may have the following advantages over traditional NSAIDs, except:
A. They inhibit mainly inducible COX-2 enzymes found at inflammatory sites and spare the constitutive COX-1 enzymes.
B. They can be given in patients taking warfarin.
C. They do not interfere with platelet activity, since platelets express only COX-1 enzymes and, thus, can be given during surgery.
D. They can theoretically be given in patients with asthma, since bronchial inflammatory cells produce cytokine-induced COX-2.
E. Both celecoxib and rofecoxib can be given to patients with sulfa allergy.

3. Side effects of COX-2 selective NSAIDs are reported to be few but include which one of the following?
A. peripheral edema
B. increased risk of gastritis
C. increased risk of renal insufficiency
D. prolonged bleeding time
E. exacerbation of asthma

4. Approximately what percentage of NSAID prescriptions are written for patients 60 years of age or older?
A. 20%
B. 30%
C. 40%
D. 50%

5. Production of the COX-2 isoform is induced by:
A. elevated PGE2 levels.
B. proinflammatory substances.
C. hyperkalemia.
D. hypertension.

6. Of 5285 patients studied who received celecoxib over a 1-6 month period, how many experienced significant upper GI bleeding?
A. 0.04%
B. 0.08%
C. 0.10%
D. 5%

165. Bioterrorism, p. 1783

1. The mortality rate of untreated anthrax is:
A. about 10%
B. about 20%
C. about 50%
D. about 80%
E. about 100%

2. The mortality rate of anthrax in patients who are treated more than 48 hours after the onset of symptoms is:
A. about 10%
B. about 20%
C. about 50%
D. about 80%
E. None of the above

3. The FDA has recently approved which antibiotic for people exposed to inhaled anthrax?
A. Norfloxacin
B. Levofloxacin
C. Ciprofloxacin
D. Grepafloxacin
E. None of the above

4. The most likely infection to be encountered from a bioterrorist threat from *Bacillus anthracis* spores would be:
A. mucocutaneous anthrax.
B. gastrointestinal anthrax.
C. neuromuscular anthrax.
D. inhalational anthrax.
E. None of the above

5. The recommended oral treatment course for post-exposure treatment of individuals exposed to inhaled anthrax is:
A. ciprofloxacin 500 mg PO BID for 14 days.
B. ciprofloxacin 500 mg PO BID for 21 days.
C. ciprofloxacin 500 mg PO BID for 30 days.
D. ciprofloxacin 500 mg PO BID for 60 days.
E. None of the above

6. Inhalation anthrax has an incubation period of how long?
A. 24 hours
B. 1-6 days
C. 2 weeks
D. 30 days
E. None of the above

7. The treatment for severe brucellosis (bone, joint, heart, CNS infection) includes a combination of doxycycline (100 mg bid) plus an aminoglycoside for four weeks.
A. True
B. False

166. Volatile Substance Abuse, p. 1795

1. Distal renal tubular acidosis is most commonly associated with which of the following substances?
A. Gasoline
B. Methylene chloride
C. Nitrites
D. Toluene

2. The practice of inhaling solvent vapors after pouring them over a piece of cloth is called:
A. bagging
B. gasping
C. huffing
D. sniffing

3. Which of the following statements regarding methylene chloride is true?
   A. Delayed production of carbon monoxide may contribute to toxicity
   B. It is a common ingredient of typewriter correction fluid
   C. Its use is epidemiologically linked to Kaposi's sarcoma
   D. Its use is more common among Native Americans

4. Which of the following may be indicated in the treatment of amyl nitrite toxicity?
   A. Cimetidine (Tagamet)
   B. Dimercaprol (BAL)
   C. Methylene blue
   D. N-acetylcysteine (Mucomyst)
   E. Prussian blue

5. Which of the following may be seen with long-term solvent abuse?
   A. Cerebral infarction
   B. Paranoid psychosis
   C. Parkinsonism
   D. Peripheral neuropathy
   E. All of the above

6. Which of the following statements is true?
   A. Although VSA has been linked to marijuana use, there is no association between VSA and IV drug abuse
   B. Inhalant use begins in grades 10-12 and increases steadily until graduation from high school
   C. The majority of VSA deaths occur from abuse of "whippets."
   D. VSA is most commonly practiced in groups of adolescents
   E. Warning labels are effective deterrents in the elimination of VSA

7. Which of the following solvents is matched correctly with its source?
   A. Cigarette lighter—toluene
   B. Fire extinguisher—methylene chloride
   C. Paint stripper—bromochromodifluoromethane
   D. Typewriter correction fluid—trichloroethane
   E. Whipped cream canisters—amyl nitrite

168. Alcohol Withdrawal Syndromes, p. 1811

1. Which statement regarding the CAGE screening tool is incorrect?
   A. Have you ever felt the need to cut down on your drinking?
   B. Have you ever associated with drinkers?
   C. Have you ever felt guilty about something you've done when you've been drinking?
   D. Have you ever had an eye-opener in the morning to get going?

2. Alcohol withdrawal syndromes include:
   A. Delirium tremens
   B. Seizures
   C. Hallucinosis
   D. All of the above

3. Which is true regarding the treatment of alcohol withdrawal?
   A. Treatment should begin only when symptoms occur
   B. When alcohol dependency is established, appropriate action must be taken to prevent or treat withdrawal symptoms
   C. All patients should receive a standard dose of benzodiazepines
   D. Only a few patients with alcohol dependency will eventually need to be treated for withdrawal on admission to the hospital

4. All of the following diagnoses of patients with alcohol dependency require hospital admission except:
   A. Boxer's fracture of non-dominant hand
   B. Nausea and vomiting with evidence of dehydration
   C. Severe withdrawal
   D. Pneumonia

5. Which of the following management strategies is most accurate regarding the ED treatment of alcohol-related seizures?
   A. Load with phenytoin; observe and discharge when no longer post-ictal
   B. Observe and discharge when alert and oriented
   C. Administer 2 mg of lorazepam, observe for six hours.
   D. Administer 2 mg of lorazepam and admit for 24 hours

6. Which of the following statements is false?
   A. Alcohol abuse and the risk of alcohol withdrawal are underrecognized by physicians
   B. The use and abuse of alcohol has declined in the United States during the last decade
   C. It is preferable to predict and prevent AWS rather than wait for the onset of symptoms
   D. The major impediment to referral is the scarcity of resources

7. Assessment of alcohol withdrawal severity includes all of the following except:
   A. Vital signs
   B. Tremor
   C. Visual and tactile disturbances
   D. Long-term memory

176. Foreign Body Removal, p. 1887

1. Which of the following is an advantage of xeroradiograms in the detection of foreign bodies?
   A. Muted contrast
   B. Lower resolution
   C. Edge enhancement
   D. Decreased patient radiation dose
   E. Ready availability at all hours

2. Which of the following techniques is/are suitable for removal of cactus spines?
   A. Pounding the spines to break them up
   B. Use rubber cement to pull them out

C. Leave them in place, as they will eventually fall out
D. Soak the area in very hot (110°F) water to soften the spines before removal
E. All of the above

3. Which of the following techniques would be helpful in the removal of a hardened steel ring in a patient whose finger is very swollen?
A. Cutting it with a standard ring cutter
B. Lowering the finger below the level of the heart
C. Making a single cut and then bending the ring with a pair of hemostats
D. Making two cuts and removing the ring in two pieces
E. Scoring the ring with a diamond cutting wheel

4. What is the most common presenting symptom of a nasal foreign body?
A. Unilateral nasal discharge
B. Bilateral nasal discharge
C. Sinusitis
D. Irritation of the nasal septum
E. Swelling and edema of the nose

5. What is the safest technique to remove a rounded foreign body that is impacted in the external ear canal of a combative 3-year-old child?
A. Slide a Fogarty catheter past the object, inflate it, and pull it out
B. Use a blunt hook to engage the object and pull it out
C. Attempt to irrigate the foreign body out with normal saline
D. Consult an ENT specialist to arrange for anesthesia and operative removal
E. Attempt to grasp the object with a hemostat

6. Complications of retained foreign body include:
A. Pain
B. Infection
C. Nerve damage
D. Vascular damage
E. All of the above

7. Wood foreign bodies:
A. Do not cause inflammation
B. Are very reactive and require removal
C. Are benign except for cedar
D. Never require removal
E. Do not require complete removal if fragmentation occurs

8. Potential complications of removal of ear foreign bodies include:
A. Tympanic membrane perforation
B. Laceration of the auditory canal
C. Damage to the ossicles
D. Hearing loss
E. All of the above

181. Bedside Ultrasonography, p. 1931

1. Which of the following statements is true regarding image quality?
A. A tissue velocity of 331 meters per second is optimal
B. A conducting gel does not affect image quality
C. A higher frequency probe improves resolution
D. Acoustic windows do not affect image quality
E. Probes emitting longer wavelengths improve resolution

2. Which statement is true regarding the US examination of the trauma patient:
A. US can differentiate between ascites, urine, and free fluid
B. Free fluid flows to one specific area within the abdominal cavity
C. US is comparable to contrast CT for identifying specific organ injury
D. The multiple view trauma examination for the ED is completed in approximately 10 minutes
E. Free fluid is typically anechoic

3. Which of the statements regarding a possible pseudosac is true?
A. The presence of a yolk sac rules out an ectopic pregnancy
B. Cardiac activity can sometimes be seen within the pseudosac
C. Pseudosacs occur in 25% of ectopic pregnancies
D. A fetal pole can sometimes be seen within the pseudo sac

4. Which of the following is a cause of pseudohydronephrosis?
A. Obstructive uropathy
B. Pregnancy
C. Dehydration
D. Staghorn calculi with shadowing
E. Retroperitoneal fibrosis

5. Sonographic criteria for acute cholecystitis include:
A. The presence of gallstones
B. Sludge
C. S sonographic Murphy's sign
D. Wall thickening
E. All of the above

6. The following statement is true regarding echogenicity:
A. The renal pyramids are echogenic
B. Lung tissue is anechoic
C. The renal capsule is slightly more hypoechoic than the cortex
D. Metal foreign bodies are typically hypoechoic
E. Fat and fluid can appear similar within the pericardial sac

7. The sonographic hallmark of a large pulmonary embolus includes:
A. Diastolic collapse of right-sided chambers
B. A large, thin-walled hypokinetic right ventricle
C. Globally decreased contractility
D. Hyperdynamic right-sided chambers
E. Small right-sided chambers with a hyperdynamic left ventricle

8. Which statement is true regarding the accurate measurement of the aorta?
   A. Measure the AP diameter in longitudinal section, from inner wall to outer wall
   B. Measure the AP width in longitudinal section, from outer wall to outer wall
   C. Measure the lateral width in transverse section, from inner wall to outer wall
   D Measure perpendicular to the aorta, from outer to inner wall
   E. Measure the AP width in transverse section, from outer wall to outer wall

182. Magnetic Resonance Imaging, p. 1941

1. In a patient with profound neurologic deficits after neck injury and a normal five-view c-spine series, the best sequence of further studies to obtain the most accurate prognostic and treatment related information would be:
   A. Only MRI needed.
   B. Flexion-extension views, then CT, then MRI
   C. CT; if positive, then nothing further
   D. CT; then MRI regardless of CT result

2. MRI is considered inferior to CT in the diagnosis of:
   A. Osteomyelitis
   B. Fracture
   C. Herniated nucleus pulposa
   D. Multiple sclerosis

3. The spin echo sequence of an MRI study can be adjusted to:
   A. Control the temperature gradient in a tissue specimen
   B. Bring out certain magnetic resonance characteristics of a given type of tissue
   C. Differentiate between long and cancellous bone
   D. Decrease the side effects of magnetism

4. Nuclear magnetic resonance relies upon all of the following properties, except:
   A. The magnetic behavior of spinning dipolar atoms
   B. The proportionality of an atom's precession frequency to the strength of an external magnetic field
   C. The response of certain atoms in a magnetic field when subject to radiofrequency energy
   D. The energy levels of electrons

5. MRI angiography:
   A. Involves the injection of a safe, non-ionic contrast material into the peripheral circulation
   B. Can only be used for venous studies
   C. Can be used to evaluate both venous and arterial flow
   D. Is commonly performed in the ED

6. In an elderly patient with a strong suspicion of having an anterior cruciate ligament tear, MRI:
   A. Should be performed as soon as possible
   B. May have therapeutic as well as diagnostic value
   C. Is probably not needed
   D. Is not sensitive enough to detect the tear

7. An MRI image weighted for T1 effects will show tissue with a high lipid content:
   A. As a bright area
   B. In shades of red
   C. Will not be able to distinguish from bone
   D. Will be opaque

8. Regarding head injuries, MRI is primarily of value in the:
   A. First two hours post injury
   B. Pediatric population
   C. Evaluation of patients with persistent post-concussion symptoms who have had negative CT studies
   D. Evaluation of acute hematomas

188. Obstructive Uropathy, p. 1999

1. A high urinary pH in a patient with renal colic should alert the physician to:
   A. The presence of renal tubular acidosis
   B. A higher risk of infection
   C. Laboratory error necessitating repeat lab tests
   D. A high risk of gout

2. The smallest caliber of the urinary outflow tract can be found at:
   A. The ureteropelvic junction
   B. The ureterovesicular junction
   C. The abdominal spindle
   D. The urethral meatus

3. All of the following are correct regarding imaging in renal colic except:
   A. Non-contrast helical CT of the abdomen is more sensitive than IVP in calculus disease and is equally specific
   B. KUB can reliably and cost-effectively be used to screen for patients who may require IVP
   C. No role has yet been established for MRI in renal colic
   D. Imaging in the ED may be indicated if the clinical diagnosis is in doubt, if prognostic information is desired, or to avoid inappropriate referral

4. The factor most predictive of renal injury in unilateral obstruction is:
   A. Duration of obstruction greater than one week
   B. Location of the obstruction at the ureteropelvic junction
   C. Presence of a "staghorn" calculus
   D. Presence of a lymphocytic infiltration in the renal parenchyma

5. All of the following are true regarding the diagnosis of ureteral calculi except:
   A. Radiations of the pain to the groin is seen in 70% of patients
   B. Hematuria is not part of the classic triad
   C. Calcium-containing stones and cystine stones may be associated with a positive family history
   D. Leukocytosis may be present in the absence of infection

6. Regarding the use of KUB in patients with urolithiasis:
   A. KUB increases the sensitivity of ultrasound
   B. KUB has no role in following a stone expectantly
   C. The negative predictive value is very high
   D. A negative KUB obviates the need for IVP

7. All of the following factors may contribute to kidney stone formation except:
   A. A family history of stone disease
   B. A diet high in calcium
   C. A diet high in oxalate
   D. Low urinary citrate

8. Non-steroidal anti-inflammatory agents:
   A. Have no role in treating the pain of renal colic
   B. Are effective pain relievers due to their prostaglandin effects
   C. Should never be used in conjunction with narcotics
   D. May relieve urinary tract spasm in patients with renal colic

189. End-Stage Renal Disease, p. 2009

1. Therapeutic approach to a patient with pericardial effusion or tamponade is based on:
   A. The patient's ECG changes such as electrical alternans
   B. The presence of pulsus paradoxus
   C. The patient's hemodynamic status
   D. The results of the patient's echocardiogram

2. The only drug used in ACLS resuscitation that should be avoided in ESRD patients is:
   A. Procainamide
   B. Beta-blocker agents
   C. Lidocaine
   D. Bretylium

3. Treatment of choice in severe hypermagnesemia is:
   A. Sodium bicarbonate
   B. Kaexylate
   C. calcium chloride/calcium gluconate
   D. insulin with glucose

4. Emergency therapy of vascular access thrombosis may include:
   A. Irrigation and infusion of the site with normal saline
   B. Heparin
   C. Thrombolytic agents and immediate vascular surgery consult
   D. "Outpatient" consultation and discharge

5. Therapy for hemorrhage at the vascular access site includes:
   A. Thorough "packing" of the hemorrhagic site
   B. Tourniquet use
   C. Firm, nonocclusive compression for 30 minutes
   D. Firm, nonocclusive compression followed by timely vascular surgical consultation

6. Cardiovascular and cerebrovascular complications account for what percentage of deaths in patients suffering from chronic renal failure?
   A. 95%
   B. 15-30%
   C. 75%
   D. less than 5%

7. Which acute neurological complication usually occurs during or shortly after dialysis?
   A. Altered mental status
   B. Dialysis disequilibrium syndrome
   C. Restless leg syndrome
   D. Lethargy

8. What is the second most common cause of mortality and morbidity in patients with ESRD?
   A. Hematological complications
   B. Hyperkalemia
   C. Infection
   D. Pericardial disease

Index

B

C

D

G

H

I

N

O

P

T

Y

Z

Appendix A

QUICK CONSULT® GUIDE TO CLINICAL TRIALS IN THROMBOSIS MANAGEMENT

YEAR 2001-2002 UPDATE

Acute Coronary Syndromes • Venous Thromboembolic Disease • Thrombosis Prophylaxis in the Medically Ill • Thrombosis Treatment • Patient Recognition

Authors: **Kurt Kleinschmidt, MD, FACEP**, Associate Professor, University of Texas Southwestern Medical Center, Dallas, TX; Associate Medical Director, Emergency Services Department, Parkland Memorial Hospital, Dallas, TX; **Adam Miller, MD, FACEP,** Associate Professor, University of Texas Southwestern Medical Center, Dallas, TX; Associate Medical Director, Emergency Services Department, Parkland Memorial Hospital, Dallas, TX

Project Editor-in-Chief: **Gideon Bosker, MD, FACEP,** Assistant Clinical Professor, Section of Emergency Services, Yale University School of Medicine, Associate Clinical Professor, Oregon Health Sciences University, Editor-in-Chief, *Clinical Consensus Reports*®

ASSENT-II — ASESSMENT OF THE SAFETY AND EFFICACY OF A NEW THROMBOLYTIC

TRIAL FULL NAME
Single-bolus tenecteplase compared with front-loaded tPA in acute myocardial infarction: the ASSENT-2 double-blind randomized trial

PUBLICATION DATA
Lancet 1999; 354:716-722

STUDY DATES
1997-1998

AUTHOR(S)

CLINICAL TRIAL SUMMARY

This was a multicenter, randomized, double-blind comparison of tPA (up to 100 mg over 1 hour) vs. tenecteplase (30-50 mg depending on weight in a single 10 second bolus) in 16,949 patients with STEMI presenting within 6 hours of the onset of chest pain. All patients received aspirin and heparin. The primary endpoint, 30-day mortality, occurred in 6.18% of the tenecteplase group and in 6.15% of the tPA group (p = NS). Intracranial hemorrhage occurred equally, in 0.93% vs. 0.94% of the respective groups. Tenecteplase was associated with fewer non-cerebral bleeding complications (26.4% vs. 29.0%; p = 0.0003) and with less need for blood transfusion (4.3% vs. 5.5%; p = 0.0002).

BOTTOM LINE

Tenecteplase and tPA resulted in equal 30-day mortality; tenecteplase was associated with fewer non-cerebral bleeding complications.

ACUTE CORONARY SYNDROMES

CLINICAL TRIAL FEATURES, THERAPEUTICS AND ENDPOINTS

DISEASE STATES
- [x] ACS
- [x] STEMI/QMI
- [ ] NSTEMI/NQMI
- [ ] UA
- [ ] VTE
- [ ] DVT
- [ ] PE
- [ ] CVA

MEDICATIONS
- [ ] **Platelet Antagonist**
  - [ ] Aspirin
  - [ ] Clopidogrel
  - [ ] IIb/IIIa Receptor Antagonist
    - [ ] Abciximab
    - [ ] Eptifibatide
    - [ ] Lamifiban
    - [ ] Tirofiban
- [ ] **Heparin**
- [ ] **LMWH**
  - [ ] Enoxaparin
  - [ ] Dalteparin
  - [ ] Nadroparin
  - [ ] Tinzaparin
  - [ ] Reviparin
- [ ] **Direct Thrombin Inhibitor**
  - [ ] Hirudin
  - [ ] Hirulog
- [x] **Fibrinolytic / Thrombolytic**
  - [x] **Alteplase**
  - [ ] Reteplase
  - [x] **Tenecteplase**
  - [ ] Anistreplase
  - [ ] Streptokinase
- [ ] **Other cardiac medications (captopril, magnesium, nitrates)**

PROCEDURES
- [ ] Angioplasty
- [ ] Stent
- [ ] CABG
- [ ] PCI

THERAPEUTIC ENDPOINT
- [x] **Treatment**
- [ ] Prophylaxis

CLINICAL ENVIRONMENT
- [x] **Inpatient**
- [ ] Outpatient

FIBRINOLYTICS

GISSI — GRUPPO ITALIANO PER LO STUDIO DELLA STREPTOCHINASI NELL'INFARTO MIOCARDICO

TRIAL FULL NAME
Effectiveness of IV thrombolytic treatment in acute myocardial infarction

PUBLICATION DATA
Lancet 1986; 1:397-401

STUDY DATES
1984 to 1985

AUTHOR(S)
GA Feruglio, C DeVita, A Selvini, E Ambrosioni, G Mezzanotte, M Bruno, M Anselmi, et al

CLINICAL TRIAL SUMMARY

This was a randomized, multicenter, unblinded comparison of streptokinase (1.5 MU over 1 hour) vs. nothing in 11,806 patients with STEMI who presented within 12 hours of onset of symptoms. Use of anticoagulants and antiplatelet agents were low but comparable between groups. The primary endpoint, in-hospital mortality (90% of patients were in-house 14-21 days), occurred in 10.7% of the streptokinase group and in 13.0% of the controls (p = 0.0002). Benefit was best if treatment occurred early; there was a trend towards superiority from 6-12 hours and statistical significance if < 6 hours.

BOTTOM LINE

Streptokinase reduced mortality in patients with STEMI and it worked best if initiated within 6 hours of onset of symptoms.

ACUTE CORONARY SYNDROMES

CLINICAL TRIAL FEATURES, THERAPEUTICS AND ENDPOINTS

DISEASE STATES
- [x] ACS
- [x] STEMI/QMI
- [ ] NSTEMI/NQMI
- [ ] UA
- [ ] VTE
- [ ] DVT
- [ ] PE
- [ ] CVA

MEDICATIONS
- [x] **Platelet Antagonist**
  - [ ] Aspirin
  - [ ] Clopidogrel
  - [ ] IIb/IIIa Receptor Antagonist
    - [ ] Abciximab
    - [ ] Eptifibatide
    - [ ] Lamifiban
    - [ ] Tirofiban
- [ ] **Heparin**
- [ ] **LMWH**
  - [ ] Enoxaparin
  - [ ] Dalteparin
  - [ ] Nadroparin
  - [ ] Tinzaparin
  - [ ] Reviparin
- [ ] **Direct Thrombin Inhibitor**
  - [ ] Hirudin
  - [ ] Hirulog
- [x] **Fibrinolytic / Thrombolytic**
  - [ ] Alteplase
  - [ ] Reteplase
  - [ ] Tenecteplase
  - [ ] Anistreplase
  - [x] **Streptokinase**
- [ ] **Other cardiac medications (captopril, magnesium, nitrates)**

PROCEDURES
- [ ] Angioplasty
- [ ] Stent
- [ ] CABG
- [ ] PCI

THERAPEUTIC ENDPOINT
- [x] **Treatment**
- [ ] Prophylaxis

CLINICAL ENVIRONMENT
- [x] **Inpatient**
- [ ] Outpatient

FIBRINOLYTICS

GISSI-2 | GRUPPO ITALIANO PER LO STUDIO DELLA SOPRAVVIVENZA NELL'INFARTO MIOCARDICO

TRIAL FULL NAME

GISSI-2: A factorial randomized trial of tPA versus streptokinase and heparin versus no heparin among 12,490 patients with acute myocardial infarction

PUBLICATION DATA

Lancet 1990; 336: 65-71

STUDY DATES

1988 to 1989

AUTHOR(S)

GA Feruglio, C DeVita, A Selvini, E Ambrosioni, G Mezzanotte, M Bruno, M Anselmi, et al

CLINICAL TRIAL SUMMARY

This was a randomized, multicenter, open label comparison of (1) streptokinase 1.5 MU over 1 hour vs. tPA 100 mg over 3 hours; and (2) SQ heparin BID vs. nothing. The 12490 patients had CP within 6 hours and STEMI. Endpoints were death or severe change in LVEF as per Echocardiogram. Endpoints occurred in 23.1% of the tPA group vs. 22.5% of the STK group (p= NS) and in 22.7% of the heparin group vs. 22.9% in the no heparin group (p = NS). While major bleeding occurred significantly more in the STK plus heparin group, the overall incidence of stroke was similar in all groups.

BOTTOM LINE

Streptokinase and tPA were similarly safe and associated with equal death or change in LVEF in patients with STEMI who received subcutaneous heparin

ACUTE CORONARY SYNDROMES

CLINICAL TRIAL FEATURES, THERAPEUTICS AND ENDPOINTS

DISEASE STATES

☑ ACS ☑ STEMI/QMI ☐ NSTEMI/NQMI ☐ UA
☐ VTE ☐ DVT ☐ PE ☐ CVA

MEDICATIONS

- ☐ **Platelet Antagonist**
  - ☐ Aspirin
  - ☐ Clopidogrel
  - ☐ IIb/IIIa Receptor Antagonist
    - ☐ Abciximab
    - ☐ Eptifibatide
    - ☐ Lamifiban
    - ☐ Tirofiban
- ☑ **Heparin**
- ☐ **LMWH**
  - ☐ Enoxaparin
  - ☐ Dalteparin
  - ☐ Nadroparin
  - ☐ Tinzaparin
  - ☐ Reviparin
- ☐ **Direct Thrombin Inhibitor**
  - ☐ Hirudin
  - ☐ Hirulog
- ☑ **Fibrinolytic / Thrombolytic**
  - ☑ **Alteplase**
  - ☐ Reteplase
  - ☐ Tenecteplase
  - ☐ Anistreplase
  - ☑ **Streptokinase**
- ☐ **Other cardiac medications (captopril, magnesium, nitrates)**

PROCEDURES

☐ Angioplasty ☐ Stent
☐ CABG ☐ PCI

THERAPEUTIC ENDPOINT

☑ Treatment ☐ Prophylaxis

CLINICAL ENVIRONMENT

☑ Inpatient ☐ Outpatient

FIBRINOLYTICS

GUSTO | GLOBAL UTILIZATION OF STREPTOKINASE AND TISSUE PLASMINOGEN ACTIVATOR FOR OCCLUDED CORONARY ARTERIES

TRIAL FULL NAME

An International Randomized Trial Comparing Four Thrombolytic Strategies for Acute Myocardial Infarction

PUBLICATION DATA

NEJM 1993; 329:673-82

STUDY DATES

1990 to 1993

AUTHOR(S)

E Topol, R Califf, F Nan de Werf, PW Armstrong, P Alward, G Barbash, E Bates, A Betriu, JP Boissel, J Chesebro, J Col, D de Bono, J Gore, A Guerci, et al

CLINICAL TRIAL SUMMARY

This randomized, multi-national, trial compared four thrombolytic regimens: STK plus SQ heparin vs. STK plus IV heparin vs. accelerated tPA (given over 1½ hours) plus IV heparin vs. accelerated tPA plus STK plus IV heparin. The 41,021 patients had STEMI and CP $\leq$ 6 hours. The primary endpoint, 30 day mortality rates, for the four groups, respectively, were: 7.2%, 7.4%, 6.3%, and 7.0%. This represented a 14% (p = 0.001) reduction in mortality with tPA compared to the two STK-only strategies. Hemorrhagic stroke occurred in 0.49%, 0.54%, 0.72%, and 0.94%, respectively. This represented an increase of hemorrhagic strokes for tPA (p = 0.03) and for the combination strategy (p < 0.001). A combined end-point of death or disabling stroke was significantly lower in the accelerated tPA group than in the STK-only groups (6.9% vs. 7.8%; p = 0.006).

BOTTOM LINE

Alteplase given over 1½ hours with IV heparin resulted in a significant survival benefit over STK that was somewhat offset by a significant increase in hemorrhagic strokes.

ACUTE CORONARY SYNDROMES

CLINICAL TRIAL FEATURES, THERAPEUTICS AND ENDPOINTS

DISEASE STATES

☑ ACS ☑ STEMI/QMI ☐ NSTEMI/NQMI ☐ UA
☐ VTE ☐ DVT ☐ PE ☐ CVA

MEDICATIONS

- ☐ **Platelet Antagonist**
  - ☐ Aspirin
  - ☐ Clopidogrel
  - ☐ IIb/IIIa Receptor Antagonist
    - ☐ Abciximab
    - ☐ Eptifibatide
    - ☐ Lamifiban
    - ☐ Tirofiban
- ☑ **Heparin**
- ☐ **LMWH**
  - ☐ Enoxaparin
  - ☐ Dalteparin
  - ☐ Nadroparin
  - ☐ Tinzaparin
  - ☐ Reviparin
- ☐ **Direct Thrombin Inhibitor**
  - ☐ Hirudin
  - ☐ Hirulog
- ☑ **Fibrinolytic / Thrombolytic**
  - ☑ **Alteplase**
  - ☐ Reteplase
  - ☐ Tenecteplase
  - ☐ Anistreplase
  - ☑ **Streptokinase**
- ☐ **Other cardiac medications (captopril, magnesium, nitrates)**

PROCEDURES

☐ Angioplasty ☐ Stent
☐ CABG ☐ PCI

THERAPEUTIC ENDPOINT

☑ Treatment ☐ Prophylaxis

CLINICAL ENVIRONMENT

☑ Inpatient ☐ Outpatient

FIBRINOLYTICS

GUSTO III — GLOBAL USE OF STRATEGIES TO OPEN OCCLUDED CORONARY ARTERIES

TRIAL FULL NAME
A comparison of Reteplase with Alteplase for Acute Myocardial Infarction

PUBLICATION DATA
NEJM 1997; 337:1118-23

STUDY DATES
1995 to 1997

AUTHOR(S)
E Topol, R Califf, F Nan de Werf, PW Armstrong, P Alward, G Barbash, E Bates, A Betriu, JP Boissel, J Chesebro, J Col, D de Bono, J Gore, A Guerci, et al.

CLINICAL TRIAL SUMMARY

This randomized, multi-national trial compared reteplase (10 MU twice, 30 minutes apart) vs. tPA (bolus plus infusion, up to 100 mg over 90 minutes). The 15,059 patients had CP within six hours of presentation and had a ST-elevation or a BBB on ECG. The primary endpoint, 30 day mortality, occurred in 7.5% of the reteplase group and in 7.2% of the tPA group; p = 0.54. Stroke occurred in 1.64% and 1.79%, respectively. The two regimens were equal in efficacy and safety.

BOTTOM LINE

Reteplase and alteplase resulted in equal efficacy and safety for the treatment of AMI.

ACUTE CORONARY SYNDROMES

CLINICAL TRIAL FEATURES, THERAPEUTICS AND ENDPOINTS

DISEASE STATES
- ☑ **ACS** ☑ **STEMI/QMI** ❑ NSTEMI/NQMI ☑ **UA**
- ❑ VTE ❑ DVT ❑ PE ❑ CVA

MEDICATIONS
- ❑ **Platelet Antagonist**
  - ❑ Aspirin
  - ❑ Clopidogrel
  - ❑ IIb/IIIa Receptor Antagonist
    - ❑ Abciximab
    - ❑ Eptifibatide
    - ❑ Lamifiban
    - ❑ Tirofiban
- ❑ **Heparin**
- ❑ **LMWH**
  - ❑ Enoxaparin
  - ❑ Dalteparin
  - ❑ Nadroparin
  - ❑ Tinzaparin
  - ❑ Reviparin
- ❑ **Direct Thrombin Inhibitor**
  - ❑ Hirudin
  - ❑ Hirulog
- ☑ **Fibrinolytic / Thrombolytic**
  - ☑ **Alteplase**
  - ☑ **Reteplase**
  - ❑ Tenecteplase
  - ❑ Anistreplase
  - ❑ Streptokinase
- ❑ **Other cardiac medications (captopril, magnesium, nitrates)**

PROCEDURES
- ❑ Angioplasty ❑ Stent
- ❑ CABG ❑ PCI

THERAPEUTIC ENDPOINT
- ☑ **Treatment** ❑ Prophylaxis

CLINICAL ENVIRONMENT
- ☑ **Inpatient** ❑ Outpatient

FIBRINOLYTICS

ISIS — INTERNATIONAL STUDIES OF INFARCT SURVIVAL

TRIAL FULL NAME
Randomized factorial trial of high-dose IV streptokinase, of oral aspirin and of IV heparin in acute myocardial infarction

PUBLICATION DATA
European Heart Journal (1987) 8, 634-642

STUDY DATES
1983 to 1985

AUTHOR(S)
R Collins, M Conway, D Alexopoulos, S Yusuf, P Sleight, N Brooks, R Bowes, A Marshall, S Harding, G Maskell, J Sanderson, B Mittra, D Hunt, D Tibbutt, H Sterry, D Jackson, A Scrimgeour, L Lim, P Appleby, S Parish, R Peto

CLINICAL TRIAL SUMMARY

This was a randomized, placebo-controlled, 2 X 2 X 2 factorial designed comparison of (1) streptokinase 1.5 MU over one hour vs. placebo, (2) aspirin 325 mg q 48 hours vs. placebo, and (3) IV heparin (infusion but not bolus) starting 12 hours after STK vs. placebo. The 619 patients had CP within 24 hours of admission with suspected MI (ECG changes not required!). Endpoints were reinfarction during hospitalization or death up to one year. Streptokinase was associated with more reinfarction (3.9% vs. 2.9% placebo; p = NS) but decreased mortality (7.5% vs. 9.7% in-hospital; 6.1% vs. 8.7% after discharge; p = NS for both). While aspirin was associated with similar reinfarction frequency (3.2% vs. 3.9% placebo; p = NS) and deaths after discharge (7.0% vs. 6.9% with placebo; p = NS), in-hospital deaths were decreased (6.1% vs. 10.5%; $p < 0.05$). Heparin was associated with a similar frequency of reinfarction or deaths (p = NS). Streptokinase was associated with more allergic reactions, hypotension/bradycardia, vomiting, and minor bleeding than placebo but less total stroke. This trial was the pilot for ISIS-2.

BOTTOM LINE

Streptokinase caused a non-significant decrease in mortality in patients with suspected MI who had CP $\leq$ 24 hours while ASA significantly decreased in-hospital deaths.

ACUTE CORONARY SYNDROMES

CLINICAL TRIAL FEATURES, THERAPEUTICS AND ENDPOINTS

DISEASE STATES
- ☑ **ACS** ☑ **STEMI/QMI** ☑ **NSTEMI/NQMI** ☑ **UA**
- ❑ VTE ❑ DVT ❑ PE ❑ CVA

MEDICATIONS
- ☑ **Platelet Antagonist**
  - ☑ **Aspirin**
  - ❑ Clopidogrel
  - ❑ IIb/IIIa Receptor Antagonist
    - ❑ Abciximab
    - ❑ Eptifibatide
    - ❑ Lamifiban
    - ❑ Tirofiban
- ☑ **Heparin**
- ❑ **LMWH**
  - ❑ Enoxaparin
  - ❑ Dalteparin
  - ❑ Nadroparin
  - ❑ Tinzaparin
  - ❑ Reviparin
- ❑ **Direct Thrombin Inhibitor**
  - ❑ Hirudin
  - ❑ Hirulog
- ☑ **Fibrinolytic / Thrombolytic**
  - ❑ Alteplase
  - ❑ Reteplase
  - ❑ Tenecteplase
  - ❑ Anistreplase
  - ☑ **Streptokinase**
- ❑ **Other cardiac medications (captopril, magnesium, nitrates)**

PROCEDURES
- ❑ Angioplasty ❑ Stent
- ❑ CABG ❑ PCI

THERAPEUTIC ENDPOINT
- ☑ **Treatment** ❑ Prophylaxis

CLINICAL ENVIRONMENT
- ☑ **Inpatient** ❑ Outpatient

FIBRINOLYTICS

ISIS-2 | SECOND INTERNATIONAL STUDY OF INFARCT SURVIVAL

TRIAL FULL NAME

Randomized trial of IV streptokinase, oral aspirin, both or neither among 17,187 cases of suspected acute myocardial infarction

PUBLICATION DATA

Lancet August 13 1988

STUDY DATES

1986 to 1988

AUTHOR(S)

R Collins, M Conway, D Alexopoulos, S Yusuf, P Sleight, N Brooks, R Bowes, A Marshall, S Harding, G Maskell, J Sanderson, B Mittra, D Hunt, D Tibbutt, H Sterry, D Jackson, A Scrimgeour, L Lim, P Appleby, S Parish, R Peto

CLINICAL TRIAL SUMMARY

This was a randomized, multi-national comparison of four regimes: STK 1.5 MU over 1 hour vs. 160 mg aspirin qd for one month vs. both active treatments vs. neither treatment. The 17187 patients had CP within 24 hours of presentation and were suspected to have MI; ECG changes were not required. Endpoints were vascular death at 5 weeks and up to a median of 10 months from discharge. Five-week vascular mortality was 9.2% with STK versus 12.0% without ($p < 0.00001$) and 9.4% with aspirin versus 11.8% without ($p < 0.0001$). The combination of STK and aspirin was significantly better than either agent used alone; resulting in a five-week mortality of 8.0 % versus 13.2% in those receiving neither agent ($p < 0.001$). Cerebral hemorrhage occurred in 0.1% of those receiving STK versus in none those not ($p < 0.02$) while overall strokes were similar between groups.

BOTTOM LINE

Streptokinase and ASA, individually and particularly in combination, result in significantly decreased mortality in patients with suspected MI who present with ≤ 24 hours of CP.

ACUTE CORONARY SYNDROMES

CLINICAL TRIAL FEATURES, THERAPEUTICS AND ENDPOINTS

DISEASE STATES

☑ ACS ☑ STEMI/QMI ☑ NSTEMI/NQMI ☑ UA
❑ VTE ❑ DVT ❑ PE ❑ CVA

MEDICATIONS

☑ **Platelet Antagonist**
- ☑ **Aspirin**
- ❑ Clopidogrel
- ❑ IIb/IIIa Receptor Antagonist
  - ❑ Abciximab
  - ❑ Eptifibatide
  - ❑ Lamifiban
  - ❑ Tirofiban

❑ **Heparin**

❑ **LMWH**
- ❑ Enoxaparin
- ❑ Dalteparin
- ❑ Nadroparin
- ❑ Tinzaparin
- ❑ Reviparin

❑ **Direct Thrombin Inhibitor**
- ❑ Hirudin
- ❑ Hirulog

☑ **Fibrinolytic / Thrombolytic**
- ❑ Alteplase
- ❑ Reteplase
- ❑ Tenecteplase
- ❑ Anistreplase
- ☑ **Streptokinase**

❑ **Other cardiac medications (captopril, magnesium, nitrates)**

PROCEDURES

❑ Angioplasty ❑ Stent
❑ CABG ❑ PCI

THERAPEUTIC ENDPOINT

☑ **Treatment** ❑ Prophylaxis

CLINICAL ENVIRONMENT

☑ **Inpatient** ☑ **Outpatient**

FIBRINOLYTICS

ISIS-3 | THIRD INTERNATIONAL STUDY OF INFARCT SURVIVAL COLLABORATIVE GROUP

TRIAL FULL NAME

ISIS-3: A randomized comparison of streptokinase vs. tissue plasminogen activator vs. anistreplase and of aspirin plus heparin vs. aspirin alone among 41,299 cases of suspected acute MI

PUBLICATION DATA

Lancet 1992; 339: 753-766

STUDY DATES

1989 to 1991

AUTHOR(S)

R Collins, M Conway, D Alexopoulos, S Yusuf, P Sleight, N Brooks, R Bowes, A Marshall, S Harding, G Maskell, J Sanderson, B Mittra, et al

CLINICAL TRIAL SUMMARY

This was a multicenter, randomized, 3X2 factorial design (1) blinded comparison of STK 1.5 MU over one hour vs. tPA 100 mg over 3 hours vs. anisoylated plasminogen-streptokinase (APSAC) over 3 minutes; and (2) unblinded comparison of SQ heparin 12,500 IU BID X 1week vs. nothing. The 41299 patients had CP within 24 hrs. of admission and had suspected MI; ECG changes were not required. All received aspirin. Endpoints were in-hospital reinfarction or 35 day mortality. The STK and APSAC groups had similar reinfarction and mortality rates. Streptokinase was associated with more allergic problems and non-cerebral bleeds but APSAC was associated with more cerebral hemorrhage. Compared to STK, tPA was associated with significantly more strokes (1.39% vs. 1.04%; $p < 0.01$) and cerebral hemorrhage (0.66% vs. 0.24%; $p < 0.00001$); but with fewer reinfarctions (2.93% vs. 3.47%; $p < 0.02$). Steptokinase and tPA had similar 35 day and 6 month mortality. In comparison with aspirin alone, the addition of heparin was associated with increased non-cerebral bleeding or need for transfusion (1.9% vs. 0.8%; $p < 0.01$) and cerebral hemorrhage (0.56% vs. 0.40%; $p < 0.05$); however, total strokes were comparable. At one week, heparin was associated with decreased mortality (7.4% vs. 7.9%; $p = 0.06$). However, by day 35, there was no difference between groups. Both the heparin results and the tPA vs. STK results mirrored those of GISSI 2.

BOTTOM LINE

Compared to STK, tPA was associated with reduced reinfarction rates but increased cerebral hemorrhage and strokes. They had similar mortality. Heparin, in addition to aspirin, was associated with increased cerebral and non-cerebral bleeding with reduced mortality at one week that was no longer evident by day 35.

ACUTE CORONARY SYNDROMES

CLINICAL TRIAL FEATURES, THERAPEUTICS AND ENDPOINTS

DISEASE STATES

☑ ACS ☑ STEMI/QMI ☑ NSTEMI/NQMI ☑ UA
❑ VTE ❑ DVT ❑ PE ❑ CVA

MEDICATIONS

☑ **Platelet Antagonist**
- ☑ **Aspirin**
- ❑ Clopidogrel
- ❑ IIb/IIIa Receptor Antagonist
  - ❑ Abciximab
  - ❑ Eptifibatide
  - ❑ Lamifiban
  - ❑ Tirofiban

☑ **Heparin**

❑ **LMWH**
- ❑ Enoxaparin
- ❑ Dalteparin
- ❑ Nadroparin
- ❑ Tinzaparin
- ❑ Reviparin

❑ **Direct Thrombin Inhibitor**
- ❑ Hirudin
- ❑ Hirulog

☑ **Fibrinolytic / Thrombolytic**
- ❑ Alteplase
- ❑ Reteplase
- ❑ Tenecteplase
- ☑ **Anistreplase**
- ☑ **Streptokinase**

❑ **Other cardiac medications (captopril, magnesium, nitrates)**

PROCEDURES

❑ Angioplasty ❑ Stent
❑ CABG ❑ PCI

THERAPEUTIC ENDPOINT

☑ **Treatment** ❑ Prophylaxis

CLINICAL ENVIRONMENT

☑ **Inpatient** ☑ **Outpatient**

FIBRINOLYTICS

LATE | LATE ASSESSMENT OF THROMBOLYTIC EFFICACY

TRIAL FULL NAME
Late assessment of thrombolytic efficacy study with tPA 6-24 hours after onset of acute myocardial infarction

PUBLICATION DATA
Lancet 1993; 342:759-766

STUDY DATES
1989 to 1992

AUTHOR(S)
Not available

CLINICAL TRIAL SUMMARY

This was a multicenter, randomized, double-blind comparison of tPA (100 mg over 3 hours) vs. placebo in 5711 patients with STEMI who presented 6-24 hours after the onset of chest pain. All patients received aspirin and heparin during the second half of the study. Mortality at 35 days was 8.9% for the tPA group and 10.3% for the placebo group (p = 0.07). For those treated within 12 hours, mortality was 8.9% vs 12.0% (p = 0.023), respectively. For those treated at 12-24 hours, mortality was 8.7% vs. 9.2% (p = 0.65), respectively. The tPA group had an increase in hemorrhagic strokes, but by 6 months, the number of disabled in each group due to all strokes was the same. It was concluded that the time window for thrombolysis should be extended to at least 12 hours from symptom onset.

BOTTOM LINE

Patients receiving tPA within 12 hours of symptom onset, not just within 6 hours, retained a benefit in mortality.

ACUTE CORONARY SYNDROMES

CLINICAL TRIAL FEATURES, THERAPEUTICS AND ENDPOINTS

DISEASE STATES
- ☑ **ACS** ☑ **STEMI/QMI** ❑ NSTEMI/NQMI ❑ UA
- ❑ VTE ❑ DVT ❑ PE ❑ CVA

MEDICATIONS
- ☑ **Platelet Antagonist**
  - ☑ **Aspirin**
  - ❑ Clopidogrel
  - ❑ IIb/IIIa Receptor Antagonist
    - ❑ Abciximab
    - ❑ Eptifibatide
    - ❑ Lamifiban
    - ❑ Tirofiban
- ❑ **Heparin**
- ❑ **LMWH**
  - ❑ Enoxaparin
  - ❑ Dalteparin
  - ❑ Nadroparin
  - ❑ Tinzaparin
  - ❑ Reviparin
- ❑ **Direct Thrombin Inhibitor**
  - ❑ Hirudin
  - ❑ Hirulog
- ☑ **Fibrinolytic / Thrombolytic**
  - ☑ **Alteplase**
  - ❑ Reteplase
  - ❑ Tenecteplase
  - ❑ Anistreplase
  - ❑ Streptokinase
- ❑ **Other cardiac medications (captopril, magnesium, nitrates)**

PROCEDURES
- ❑ Angioplasty ❑ Stent
- ❑ CABG ❑ PCI

THERAPEUTIC ENDPOINT
- ☑ **Treatment** ❑ Prophylaxis

CLINICAL ENVIRONMENT
- ☑ **Inpatient** ❑ Outpatient

FIBRINOLYTICS

MITI | MYOCARDIAL INFARCTION TRIAGE AND INTERVENTION

TRIAL FULL NAME
Prehospital-Initiated vs. Hospital-Initiated Thrombolytic Therapy: The Myocardial Infarction Triage and Intervention Trial

PUBLICATION DATA
JAMA 1993; 270:1211-1216

STUDY DATES
1991

AUTHOR(S)
Weaver WD, Cerqueira M, Hallsstrom AP, et al

CLINICAL TRIAL SUMMARY

This was a multicenter, randomized, open-label comparison of both aspirin and tPA being started prehospitally vs. after arrival. The 360 patients had CP for < 6 hours and had STEMIs with the ECGs having been transmitted to a physician in a base station. The primary endpoint was the composite of death, stroke, serious bleeding, and infarct size. Time to initial treatment was decreased by prehospital administration from 110 min to 77 min (p < 0.001). However, there was no significant difference between prehospital or hospital administration in the composite score (p = 0.64), mortality (5.7% vs. 8.1%; p = NS), ejection fraction, or infarct size. Treatment within 70 minutes of CP onset, whether in the hospital or in the field, did result in significant improvements in all the outcome parameters. Complications were comparable between groups.

BOTTOM LINE

Efficacy and safety were not affected by the pre-hospital, versus in-hospital, administration of tPA. Treatment within 70 minutes of symptom onset minimized complications.

ACUTE CORONARY SYNDROMES

CLINICAL TRIAL FEATURES, THERAPEUTICS AND ENDPOINTS

DISEASE STATES
- ☑ **ACS** ☑ **STEMI/QMI** ❑ NSTEMI/NQMI ❑ UA
- ❑ VTE ❑ DVT ❑ PE ❑ CVA

MEDICATIONS
- ☑ **Platelet Antagonist**
  - ☑ **Aspirin**
  - ❑ Clopidogrel
  - ❑ IIb/IIIa Receptor Antagonist
    - ❑ Abciximab
    - ❑ Eptifibatide
    - ❑ Lamifiban
    - ❑ Tirofiban
- ❑ **Heparin**
- ❑ **LMWH**
  - ❑ Enoxaparin
  - ❑ Dalteparin
  - ❑ Nadroparin
  - ❑ Tinzaparin
  - ❑ Reviparin
- ❑ **Direct Thrombin Inhibitor**
  - ❑ Hirudin
  - ❑ Hirulog
- ☑ **Fibrinolytic / Thrombolytic**
  - ☑ **Alteplase-tPA**
  - ❑ Reteplase
  - ❑ Tenecteplase
  - ❑ Anistreplase
  - ❑ Streptokinase
- ❑ **Other cardiac medications (captopril, magnesium, nitrates)**

PROCEDURES
- ❑ Angioplasty ❑ Stent
- ❑ CABG ❑ PCI

THERAPEUTIC ENDPOINT
- ☑ **Treatment** ❑ Prophylaxis

CLINICAL ENVIRONMENT
- ☑ **Inpatient** ❑ Outpatient

FIBRINOLYTICS

TIMI | **THROMBOLYSIS IN MYOCARDIAL INFARCTION**

TRIAL FULL NAME
The Thrombolysis in Myocardial Infarction Trials: Phase 1 Findings

PUBLICATION DATA
NEJM 1985; 312(14) 932-936

STUDY DATES
1984 to 1985

AUTHOR(S)
Not available

CLINICAL TRIAL SUMMARY

This was a multicenter, randomized, double-blinded comparison of streptokinase (STK; 1.5 MU over 1 hour) vs. tissue type plasminogen activator (tPA; 80 mg over 3 hours) in 290 patients with STEMI. All patients received heparin. The primary endpoint was TIMI grade 2 or 3 flow at 90 minutes. The trial was stopped early because of the significant findings. Ninety-minute Grade 2 or 3 flow occurred in 60% of the tPA group and in 35% of the streptokinase group. Major bleeding was comparable between groups.

BOTTOM LINE

Tissue plasminogen activator produced significantly better TIMI grade2 or 3 flow than STK at 90 minutes.

ACUTE CORONARY SYNDROMES

CLINICAL TRIAL FEATURES, THERAPEUTICS AND ENDPOINTS

DISEASE STATES

- ☑ **ACS** ☑ **STEMI/QMI** ❑ NSTEMI/NQMI ❑ UA
- ❑ VTE ❑ DVT ❑ PE ❑ CVA

MEDICATIONS

- ❑ **Platelet Antagonist**
  - ❑ Aspirin
  - ❑ Clopidogrel
  - ❑ IIb/IIIa Receptor Antagonist
    - ❑ Abciximab
    - ❑ Eptifibatide
    - ❑ Lamifiban
    - ❑ Tirofiban
- ☑ **Heparin**
- ❑ **LMWH**
  - ❑ Enoxaparin
  - ❑ Dalteparin
  - ❑ Nadroparin
  - ❑ Tinzaparin
  - ❑ Reviparin
- ❑ **Direct Thrombin Inhibitor**
  - ❑ Hirudin
  - ❑ Hirulog
- ☑ **Fibrinolytic / Thrombolytic**
  - ☑ **Alteplase**
  - ❑ Reteplase
  - ❑ Tenecteplase
  - ❑ Anistreplase
  - ☑ **Streptokinase**
- ❑ **Other cardiac medications (captopril, magnesium, nitrates)**

PROCEDURES

- ❑ Angioplasty ❑ Stent
- ❑ CABG ☑ **PCI**

THERAPEUTIC ENDPOINT

- ☑ **Treatment** ❑ Prophylaxis

CLINICAL ENVIRONMENT

- ☑ **Inpatient** ❑ Outpatient

FIBRINOLYTICS

ESSENCE — Efficacy and Safety of Subcutaneous Enoxaparin in Non-Q Wave Coronary Events

Trial Full Name
A comparison of low molecular weight heparin with unfractionated heparin for unstable coronary artery disease

Publication Data
NEJM 1997; 337:447-52

Study Dates
1994 to 1996

Author(s)
Cohen M, Demers C, Gurfinkel EP, et al

Clinical Trial Summary

This was a randomized, double-blind, placebo-controlled, parallel-group, multicenter trial comparing enoxaparin 1 mg/kg q 12 hours vs. IV heparin. The 3,171 patients had CP within 24 hours and either ECG changes or documented CAD. The risk of death, MI, or recurrent angina was significantly lower in the patients receiving enoxaparin than in those getting UFH at 14 days (16.6% vs. 19.8%; p = 0.019) and at 30 days (19.8% vs. 23.3%; p = 0.016). The difference was primarily due to the need for less revascularization in the enoxaparin group. Major bleeding was comparable between groups. Follow-up on these patients have revealed that the benefit is maintained out to one year.

Bottom Line

Compared to heparin, enoxaparin significantly reduced the 30 day incidence of death, MI, or need for urgent revascularization in patients with ischemic CP.

ACUTE CORONARY SYNDROMES

Clinical Trial Features, Therapeutics and Endpoints

Disease States
- ☑ **ACS** ❑ STEMI/QMI ☑ **NSTEMI/NQMI** ☑ **UA**
- ❑ VTE ❑ DVT ❑ PE ❑ CVA

Medications
- ☑ **Platelet Antagonist**
  - ❑ Aspirin
  - ❑ Clopidogrel
  - ☑ **IIb/IIIa Receptor Antagonist**
    - ☑ **Abciximab**
    - ❑ Eptifibatide
    - ❑ Lamifiban
    - ❑ Tirofiban
- ☑ **Heparin**
- ☑ **LMWH**
  - ☑ **Enoxaparin**
  - ❑ Dalteparin
  - ❑ Nadroparin
  - ❑ Tinzaparin
  - ❑ Reviparin
- ❑ **Direct Thrombin Inhibitor**
  - ❑ Hirudin
  - ❑ Hirulog
- ❑ **Fibrinolytic / Thrombolytic**
  - ❑ Alteplase
  - ❑ Reteplase
  - ❑ Tenecteplase
  - ❑ Anistreplase
  - ❑ Streptokinase
- ❑ **Other cardiac medications (captopril, magnesium, nitrates)**

Procedures
- ❑ Angioplasty ❑ Stent
- ❑ CABG ❑ PCI

Therapeutic Endpoint
- ☑ **Treatment** ❑ Prophylaxis

Clinical Environment
- ☑ **Inpatient** ❑ Outpatient

LOW MOLECULAR WEIGHT HEPARIN

FRAX.I.S — FRAxiparine in Ischaemic Syndromes

Trial Full Name
Comparison of two treatment durations (6 days and 14 days) of a low molecular weight heparin with a 6-day treatment of unfractionated heparin in the initial management of unstable angina or non-Q wave myocardial infarction: FRAX.I.S.

Publication Data
European Heart Journal (1999) 20, 1553-1562

Study Dates
1995 to 1997

Author(s)
Alain Leizorovicz

Clinical Trial Summary

This was a multicenter, prospective, randomized, double-blind, comparison of IV heparin for 6 days vs. the LMWH nadroparin for 6 days vs. nadroparin for 14 days. The 3,468 patients had CP within 48 hours of presentation and ECG changes. The endpoint was the composite cardiac death, MI, refractory angina, or recurrence of UA on day 14 (primary), or day 6 or at 3 months (secondary). At 14 days the composite outcome occurred in 18% of the heparin group, 18% of the 6-day nadroparin group, and in 20% of the 14 days nadroparin group (p = NS). No differences existed between groups at 6 days or 3 months. While major bleeding was comparable between groups at day 6, it occurred in 3.5% of the 14 day nadroparin group vs. 1.6% in the IV heparin group (p = 0.0035).

Bottom Line

Nadroparin and IV heparin provide similar efficacy and safety during the first 6 days of management of UA or NQMI; however, 14 days of nadroparin resulted in significantly increased bleeding.

ACUTE CORONARY SYNDROMES

Clinical Trial Features, Therapeutics and Endpoints

Disease States
- ☑ **ACS** ❑ STEMI/QMI ☑ **NSTEMI/NQMI** ☑ **UA**
- ❑ VTE ❑ DVT ❑ PE ❑ CVA

Medications
- ❑ **Platelet Antagonist**
  - ❑ Aspirin
  - ❑ Clopidogrel
  - ❑ IIb/IIIa Receptor Antagonist
    - ❑ Abciximab
    - ❑ Eptifibatide
    - ❑ Lamifiban
    - ❑ Tirofiban
- ☑ **Heparin**
- ☑ **LMWH**
  - ❑ Enoxaparin
  - ❑ Dalteparin
  - ☑ **Nadroparin**
  - ❑ Tinzaparin
  - ❑ Reviparin
- ❑ **Direct Thrombin Inhibitor**
  - ❑ Hirudin
  - ❑ Hirulog
- ❑ **Fibrinolytic / Thrombolytic**
  - ❑ Alteplase
  - ❑ Reteplase
  - ❑ Tenecteplase
  - ❑ Anistreplase
  - ❑ Streptokinase
- ❑ **Other cardiac medications (captopril, magnesium, nitrates)**

Procedures
- ❑ Angioplasty ❑ Stent
- ❑ CABG ❑ PCI

Therapeutic Endpoint
- ☑ **Treatment** ❑ Prophylaxis

Clinical Environment
- ☑ **Inpatient** ☑ **Outpatient**

LOW MOLECULAR WEIGHT HEPARIN

FRIC | FRAGMIN IN UNSTABLE CORONARY ARTERY DISEASE STUDY

TRIAL FULL NAME
Comparison of low molecular weight heparin with unfractionated heparin acutely and with placebo for 6 weeks in the management of unstable coronary artery disease

PUBLICATION DATA
Circulation 1997; 96:61-68

STUDY DATES
1993 to 1996

AUTHOR(S)
Klein W, Buchwald A, Hillis SE, et al

CLINICAL TRIAL SUMMARY

This was a prospective, randomized, multinational, comparison of (Phase 1) dalteparin 120 IU/kg q 12 hours SQ vs. IV heparin for up to six days (unblinded); and (Phase 2) dalteparin 7500 IU q day vs. placebo from days 6-45 in the outpatient setting (double-blinded). The 1,482 patients had CP within 72 hours of presentation and ECG changes. The primary endpoint was death, MI, or recurrent angina up to 45 days. In phase one, the composite endpoint occurred in 7.6% of the heparin group and in 9.3% in the dalteparin group (p = NS). Interestingly, dalteparin was associated with significantly more death than heparin (1.5% vs. 0.4%; p = 0.05). In the 45 day phase 2, the composite end point occurred in 12.3% of both groups; reflecting no additional benefit with the long term administration.

BOTTOM LINE

Six days of dalteparin and heparin provided equal outcomes in patients with CAD and prolonged treatment with dalteparin yielded no additional benefit over ASA alone.

ACUTE CORONARY SYNDROMES

CLINICAL TRIAL FEATURES, THERAPEUTICS AND ENDPOINTS

DISEASE STATES
☑ **ACS** ❑ STEMI/QMI ☑ **NSTEMI/NQMI** ☑ **UA**
❑ VTE ❑ DVT ❑ PE ❑ CVA

MEDICATIONS
❑ **Platelet Antagonist**
- ❑ Aspirin
- ❑ Clopidogrel
- ❑ IIb/IIIa Receptor Antagonist
  - ❑ Abciximab
  - ❑ Eptifibatide
  - ❑ Lamifiban
  - ❑ Tirofiban

☑ **Heparin**
☑ **LMWH**
- ❑ Enoxaparin
- ☑ **Dalteparin**
- ❑ Nadroparin
- ❑ Tinzaparin
- ❑ Reviparin

❑ **Direct Thrombin Inhibitor**
- ❑ Hirudin
- ❑ Hirulog

❑ **Fibrinolytic / Thrombolytic**
- ❑ Alteplase
- ❑ Reteplase
- ❑ Tenecteplase
- ❑ Anistreplase
- ❑ Streptokinase

❑ **Other cardiac medications (captopril, magnesium, nitrates)**

PROCEDURES
❑ Angioplasty ❑ Stent
❑ CABG ❑ PCI

THERAPEUTIC ENDPOINT
☑ **Treatment** ❑ Prophylaxis

CLINICAL ENVIRONMENT
☑ **Inpatient** ☑ **Outpatient**

LOW MOLECULAR WEIGHT HEPARIN

FRISC | FRAGMIN DURING INSTABILITY IN CORONARY ARTERY DISEASE

TRIAL FULL NAME
Low-molecular-weight heparin during instability in coronary artery disease

PUBLICATION DATA
Lancet 1996:347: 561-68

STUDY DATES
1992

AUTHOR(S)
Lars Wallentin

CLINICAL TRIAL SUMMARY

This was a prospective, multicenter, double-blind, randomized, placebo-controlled, comparison of dalteparin 120 IU/kg q 12 hours vs. placebo. The 1,506 patients had CP within 72 hours of presentation and ECG changes. The primary endpoints of death or new MI were lower in the dalteparin group at 6 days (1.8% vs. 4.8%;p = 0.001) and at 40 days (8.0% vs. 10.7%; p = 0.042), but not at 150 days (15.5% vs. 14.0%; p = 0.41). Major bleeding was comparable between groups.

BOTTOM LINE

Compared to placebo, inpatient SQ dalteparin reduced the incidence of death or new MI up to 40 days but not up to 150 days, in patients with ischemic CP and ECG changes.

ACUTE CORONARY SYNDROMES

CLINICAL TRIAL FEATURES, THERAPEUTICS AND ENDPOINTS

DISEASE STATES
☑ **ACS** ❑ STEMI/QMI ☑ **NSTEMI/NQMI** ☑ **UA**
❑ VTE ❑ DVT ❑ PE ❑ CVA

MEDICATIONS
☑ **Platelet Antagonist**
- ❑ Aspirin
- ❑ Clopidogrel
- ❑ IIb/IIIa Receptor Antagonist
  - ❑ Abciximab
  - ❑ Eptifibatide
  - ❑ Lamifiban
  - ❑ Tirofiban

❑ **Heparin**
☑ **LMWH**
- ❑ Enoxaparin
- ☑ **Dalteparin**
- ❑ Nadroparin
- ❑ Tinzaparin
- ❑ Reviparin

❑ **Direct Thrombin Inhibitor**
- ❑ Hirudin
- ❑ Hirulog

❑ **Fibrinolytic / Thrombolytic**
- ❑ Alteplase
- ❑ Reteplase
- ❑ Tenecteplase
- ❑ Anistreplase
- ❑ Streptokinase

❑ **Other cardiac medications (captopril, magnesium, nitrates)**

PROCEDURES
❑ Angioplasty ❑ Stent
❑ CABG ❑ PCI

THERAPEUTIC ENDPOINT
☑ **Treatment** ❑ Prophylaxis

CLINICAL ENVIRONMENT
☑ **Inpatient** ❑ Outpatient

LOW MOLECULAR WEIGHT HEPARIN

FRISC II — FRAGMIN AND FAST REVASCULARIZATION DURING IN STABILITY IN CORONARY ARTERY DISEASE

TRIAL FULL NAME
Invasive compared with non-invasive treatment in unstable coronary artery disease: FRISC II prospective randomized multicentre study

PUBLICATION DATA
Lancet 1999; 354: 701-707 and 708-15 (two articles)

STUDY DATES
1996 to 1998

AUTHOR(S)
Wallentin, E Swahn, G Kontny, S Husted, B Lagerqvist, E Stahle, et al

CLINICAL TRIAL SUMMARY

This was a prospective, randomized, multicenter comparison with parallel arms. It included (1) a comparison of an early invasive (within 7 days) strategy versus early medical therapy (with PCI only used if problems occurred) and (2) a double-blind comparison of long term (3 months) twice-daily SQ dalteparin versus placebo. During the early in-hospital phase, all patients received either IV heparin or dalteparin in an unblinded fashion; this trial was NOT a comparison of in-hospital dalteparin with any other product. Primary endpoints were death or MI. The 2,457 patients had ischemic symptoms, consistent with either unstable angina or MI, within 48 hours of presentation plus either ECG changes or serum marker elevation. The primary endpoint, relative to the invasive versus medical management strategy, was the composite of death and MI after 6 months. Relative to the comparison of dalteparin with placebo, the primary endpoint was the composite at 3 months. At 6 months, the composite endpoint occurred in 9.4% of the invasive group and in 12.1% of the non-invasive group (p = 0.031). Anginal symptoms and readmissions were halved by the invasive strategy. Benefits were best in high-risk patients. Results were independent of dalteparin use. There was no difference in strokes between groups. In the dalteparin vs. placebo comparison, the composite endpoint occurred in 6.7% and 8.0%, respectively (p = 0.17).

BOTTOM LINE

Early (within 7 days) invasive therapy compared to medical management of patients with ACS (with ECG changes or marker elevation) resulted in fewer deaths or MIs. Dalteparin therapy for 3 months in the same population had similar outcomes as did the placebo arm.

ACUTE CORONARY SYNDROMES

CLINICAL TRIAL FEATURES, THERAPEUTICS AND ENDPOINTS

DISEASE STATES
☑ **ACS** ☑ **STEMI/QMI** ☑ **NSTEMI/NQMI** ☑ **UA**
☐ VTE ☐ DVT ☐ PE ☐ CVA

MEDICATIONS
- ☐ **Platelet Antagonist**
  - ☐ Aspirin
  - ☐ Clopidogrel
  - ☐ IIb/IIIa Receptor Antagonist
    - ☐ Abciximab
    - ☐ Eptifibatide
    - ☐ Lamifiban
    - ☐ Tirofiban
- ☐ **Heparin**
- ☑ **LMWH**
  - ☐ Enoxaparin
  - ☑ **Dalteparin**
  - ☐ Nadroparin
  - ☐ Tinzaparin
  - ☐ Reviparin
- ☐ **Direct Thrombin Inhibitor**
  - ☐ Hirudin
  - ☐ Hirulog
- ☐ **Fibrinolytic / Thrombolytic**
  - ☐ Alteplase
  - ☐ Reteplase
  - ☐ Tenecteplase
  - ☐ Anistreplase
  - ☐ Streptokinase
- ☐ **Other cardiac medications (captopril, magnesium, nitrates)**

PROCEDURES
☑ **Angioplasty** ☑ **Stent**
☑ **CABG** ☑ **PCI**

THERAPEUTIC ENDPOINT
☑ **Treatment** ☐ Prophylaxis

CLINICAL ENVIRONMENT
☑ **Inpatient** ☑ **Outpatient**

LOW MOLECULAR WEIGHT HEPARIN

NADROPARIN IN UNSTABLE ANGINA

TRIAL FULL NAME
Low Molecular Weight Heparin (LMWH) versus Regular Heparin or Aspirin in the treatment of Unstable Angina and Silent Ischemia

PUBLICATION DATA
JACC 1995; 26:313-8

STUDY DATES
1993 to 1994

AUTHOR(S)
Gurfinkel E., Eustaquio J., M Ricardo, et al

CLINICAL TRIAL SUMMARY

This prospective, randomized, single-blind trial enrolled 219 patients who had CP within 24 hours of presentation and either ECG changes or prior documentation of CAD. Patients received either (A) aspirin alone, (B) aspirin plus IV heparin, or (C) aspirin plus the LMWH nadroparin SQ. The primary endpoints were recurrent angina, MI, or need for urgent intervention. Recurrent angina occurred less frequently in the aspirin plus nadroparin group (21%) compared to the aspirin alone group (37%; p = 0.03) or the aspirin plus IV heparin group (44%; p = 0.002). Myocardial infarction occurred in 7 patients in group A, 4 in group B, and none in group C (C vs. A; p = 0.01). Urgent revascularization was performed in 9 patients in group A, 7 in group B, and one in group C (C vs. A; p = 0.01). Major bleeding was comparable among groups. This was the first trial comparing a LMWH with UFH in ACS.

BOTTOM LINE

Aspirin plus nadroparin (compared to aspirin plus IV heparin) reduced the incidence of recurrent angina, MI, or need for urgent intervention in patients with acute ischemia.

ACUTE CORONARY SYNDROMES

CLINICAL TRIAL FEATURES, THERAPEUTICS AND ENDPOINTS

DISEASE STATES
☑ **ACS** ☐ STEMI/QMI ☑ **NSTEMI/NQMI** ☑ **UA**
☐ VTE ☐ DVT ☐ PE ☐ CVA

MEDICATIONS
- ☑ **Platelet Antagonist**
  - ☑ **Aspirin**
  - ☐ Clopidogrel
  - ☐ IIb/IIIa Receptor Antagonist
    - ☐ Abciximab
    - ☐ Eptifibatide
    - ☐ Lamifiban
    - ☐ Tirofiban
- ☑ **Heparin**
- ☑ **LMWH**
  - ☐ Enoxaparin
  - ☐ Dalteparin
  - ☑ **Nadroparin**
  - ☐ Tinzaparin
  - ☐ Reviparin
- ☐ **Direct Thrombin Inhibitor**
  - ☐ Hirudin
  - ☐ Hirulog
- ☐ **Fibrinolytic / Thrombolytic**
  - ☐ Alteplase-tPA
  - ☐ Reteplase
  - ☐ Tenecteplase
  - ☐ Anistreplase
  - ☐ Streptokinase
- ☐ **Other cardiac medications (captopril, magnesium, nitrates)**

PROCEDURES
☐ Angioplasty ☐ Stent
☐ CABG ☐ PCI

THERAPEUTIC ENDPOINT
☑ **Treatment** ☐ Prophylaxis

CLINICAL ENVIRONMENT
☑ **Inpatient** ☐ Outpatient

LOW MOLECULAR WEIGHT HEPARIN

NICE 3 | NATIONAL INVESTIGATORS COLLABORATING ON ENOXAPARIN

TRIAL FULL NAME
The Use of Enoxaparin and IIb/IIIa Antagonists in Acute Coronary Syndromes, including PCI

PUBLICATION DATA
Abstract presented at the European Congress of Clinical Cardiology in August, 2000

STUDY DATES
Not available

AUTHOR(S)
JJ Ferguson, E Antman, E Bates, et al

CLINICAL TRIAL SUMMARY

This was a prospective, open label, non-randomized observational safety study on the combination of enoxaparin with IIb/IIIa antagonists in patients undergoing catheterization. The 661 patients were admitted with an acute coronary syndrome, received a glycoprotein IIb/IIIa antagonist and enoxaparin 1 mg/kg, and were to undergo angiography and potential PCI or CABG. If it had been more than 8 hours since the last enoxaparin administration, then the patient received an additional 0.3 mg/kg IV in the lab. Tirofiban, eptifibatide, and abciximab were given to 217, 252, and 147 patients, respectively. The primary endpoint, non-CABG bleeding during the initial hospitalization, occurred in 1.9%. This is comparable to the average of 2.0% seen in prior trials of patients undergoing PCI.

BOTTOM LINE

The combination of enoxaparin and a IIb/IIIa antagonist does not result in an excess of non-CABG bleeding.

ACUTE CORONARY SYNDROMES

CLINICAL TRIAL FEATURES, THERAPEUTICS AND ENDPOINTS

DISEASE STATES
☑ ACS ☑ STEMI/QMI ❑ NSTEMI/NQMI ☑ UA
❑ VTE ❑ DVT ❑ PE ❑ CVA

MEDICATIONS
- ☑ Platelet Antagonist
  - ❑ Aspirin
  - ❑ Clopidogrel
  - ☑ IIb/IIIa Receptor Antagonist
    - ☑ Abciximab
    - ☑ Eptifibatide
    - ❑ Lamifiban
    - ☑ Tirofiban
- ❑ Heparin
- ☑ LMWH
  - ☑ Enoxaparin
  - ❑ Dalteparin
  - ❑ Nadroparin
  - ❑ Tinzaparin
  - ❑ Reviparin
- ❑ Direct Thrombin Inhibitor
  - ❑ Hirudin
  - ❑ Hirulog
- ❑ Fibrinolytic / Thrombolytic
  - ❑ Alteplase-tPA
  - ❑ Reteplase
  - ❑ Tenecteplase
  - ❑ Anistreplase
  - ❑ Streptokinase
- ❑ Other cardiac medications (captopril, magnesium, nitrates)

PROCEDURES
☑ Angioplasty ❑ Stent
☑ CABG ☑ PCI

THERAPEUTIC ENDPOINT
☑ Treatment ❑ Prophylaxis

CLINICAL ENVIRONMENT
☑ Inpatient ❑ Outpatient

LOW MOLECULAR WEIGHT HEPARIN

TIMI 11B | THROMBOLYSIS IN MYOCARDIAL INFARCTION TRIAL

TRIAL FULL NAME
Enoxaparin prevents death and cardiac ischemic events in unstable angina/non-Q wave myocardial infarction

PUBLICATION DATA
Circulation 1999; 100:1593-1601

STUDY DATES
1996 to 1998

AUTHOR(S)
Antman E, McCabe C, Gurfinkel E, et al

CLINICAL TRIAL SUMMARY

This was a double-blind, randomized trial comparing (Acute phase) enoxaparin 30 mg IV bolus followed by 1 mg/kg q 12 hours SQ vs. IV heparin for up to 8 days; and (outpatient phase) enoxaparin 40-60 mg SQ q 12 hours with placebo for up to 43 days. The 3,910 patients had CP and either CAD history, ECG changes, or marker elevation. The primary end points were death, MI, or urgent revascularization up to 43 days. At 8 days, the composite occurred in 14.5% in the UFH group and 12.4% in the enoxaparin group ($p = 0.048$). At 43 days, it occurred in 19.7% and 17.3% of the respective groups ($p = 0.048$). While major hemorrhage was comparable during the acute phase, it occurred in 1.5% of the heparin group and 2.9% of the enoxaparin group at 43 days ($p = 0.021$). Thus, while enoxaparin was superior to heparin during the acute phase; outpatient treatment was associated with more major hemorrhage but no further relative decrease in events.

BOTTOM LINE

Compared to heparin, enoxaparin significantly reduced the incidence of death, MI, or need for revascularization in patients with UA/NQMI; however, extended therapy yielded no further benefit but did result in increased bleeding complications.

ACUTE CORONARY SYNDROMES

CLINICAL TRIAL FEATURES, THERAPEUTICS AND ENDPOINTS

DISEASE STATES
☑ ACS ❑ STEMI/QMI ☑ NSTEMI/NQMI ☑ UA
❑ VTE ❑ DVT ❑ PE ❑ CVA

MEDICATIONS
- ❑ Platelet Antagonist
  - ❑ Aspirin
  - ❑ Clopidogrel
  - ❑ IIb/IIIa Receptor Antagonist
    - ❑ Abciximab
    - ❑ Eptifibatide
    - ❑ Lamifiban
    - ❑ Tirofiban
- ☑ Heparin
- ☑ LMWH
  - ☑ Enoxaparin
  - ❑ Dalteparin
  - ❑ Nadroparin
  - ❑ Tinzaparin
  - ❑ Reviparin
- ❑ Direct Thrombin Inhibitor
  - ❑ Hirudin
  - ❑ Hirulog
- ❑ Fibrinolytic / Thrombolytic
  - ❑ Alteplase
  - ❑ Reteplase
  - ❑ Tenecteplase
  - ❑ Anistreplase
  - ❑ Streptokinase
- ❑ Other cardiac medications (captopril, magnesium, nitrates)

PROCEDURES
❑ Angioplasty ❑ Stent
❑ CABG ☑ PCI

THERAPEUTIC ENDPOINT
☑ Treatment ❑ Prophylaxis

CLINICAL ENVIRONMENT
☑ Inpatient ☑ Outpatient

LOW MOLECULAR WEIGHT HEPARIN

ANTIPLATELET TRIALISTS' COLLABORATION

TRIAL FULL NAME
Collaborative overview of randomized trials of antiplatelet therapy-I: Prevention of myocardial infarction, and stroke by prolonged antiplatelet therapy in various categories of patients

PUBLICATION DATA
BMJ 1994; 308:81-105

STUDY DATES
Articles by 1990

AUTHOR(S)
R Collins, R Peto, C Baigent, P Sandercock, D Dunbabin, C Warlow, et al

CLINICAL TRIAL SUMMARY

This paper is an overview of 145 randomized trials of "prolonged" antiplatelet therapy (various agents) available by March 1990. Trials included 70,000 high-risk patients (acute MI, history of MI, stroke or TIA, history of angina, peripheral vascular disease, or history of vascular surgery) and 30,000 low-risk patients who were followed for 1-3 years. Among high risk patients, anti-platelet agents reduced progression to MI or to stroke by ~ 33% and to vascular death by ~ 16% (each with a $p < 0.00001$). Among low risk patients (primary prevention), the one-third reduction in progression to MI was offset by a non-significant increase in stroke. Various antiplatelet regimens were tested. There was no evidence that either high dose aspirin or any other antiplatelet regimen was more effective than once daily aspirin at 75-325 mg.

BOTTOM LINE

Antiplatelet therapy in patients with known vascular disease significantly reduces progression to MI, stroke, or vascular death. Aspirin at 75-325 mg qd was as effective as any therapy.

ACUTE CORONARY SYNDROMES

CLINICAL TRIAL FEATURES, THERAPEUTICS AND ENDPOINTS

DISEASE STATES
- [x] **ACS**
- [ ] STEMI/QMI
- [ ] NSTEMI/NQMI
- [ ] UA
- [ ] VTE
- [ ] DVT
- [ ] PE
- [x] **CVA**

MEDICATIONS
- [x] **Platelet Antagonist**
  - [x] **Aspirin**
  - [ ] Clopidogrel
  - [ ] IIb/IIIa Receptor Antagonist
    - [ ] Abciximab
    - [ ] Eptifibatide
    - [ ] Lamifiban
    - [ ] Tirofiban
- [ ] **Heparin**
- [ ] **LMWH**
  - [ ] Enoxaparin
  - [ ] Dalteparin
  - [ ] Nadroparin
  - [ ] Tinzaparin
  - [ ] Reviparin
- [ ] **Direct Thrombin Inhibitor**
  - [ ] Hirudin
  - [ ] Hirulog
- [ ] **Fibrinolytic / Thrombolytic**
  - [ ] Alteplase
  - [ ] Reteplase
  - [ ] Tenecteplase
  - [ ] Anistreplase
  - [ ] Streptokinase
- [ ] **Other cardiac medications (captopril, magnesium, nitrates)**

PROCEDURES
- [ ] Angioplasty
- [ ] Stent
- [ ] CABG
- [ ] PCI

THERAPEUTIC ENDPOINT
- [ ] Treatment
- [x] **Prophylaxis**

CLINICAL ENVIRONMENT
- [ ] Inpatient
- [x] **Outpatient**

ASPIRIN

CANADIAN MULTICENTER TRIAL

TRIAL FULL NAME
Aspirin, Sulfinpyrazone, or Both in unstable angina

PUBLICATION DATA
NEJM 1985; 313: 1369-75

STUDY DATES
1979 to 1983

AUTHOR(S)
Cairns J, Gent M, Singer J, et al

CLINICAL TRIAL SUMMARY

This was a randomized, double-blind, placebo-controlled comparison of aspirin 325 mg QID, sulfinpyrazone, both, or neither. The 555 patients had UA, were enrolled within 8 days of hospitalization, and took the medications during the 2 year treatment and follow-up period. Endpoints, cardiac death or MI, occurred in 8.6% of the aspirin groups and in 17.0% of the non-aspirin groups ($p = 0.008$). Gastrointestinal side effects were 29% more common in the aspirin group than the other (p 0.014, including more bleeding. There was no change in outcome with sulfinpyrazone.

BOTTOM LINE

Aspirin reduced death or MI in patients who were hospitalized with UA; however, the high dose in this trial was associated with increased gastrointestinal and bleeding complications.

ACUTE CORONARY SYNDROMES

CLINICAL TRIAL FEATURES, THERAPEUTICS AND ENDPOINTS

DISEASE STATES
- [x] **ACS**
- [ ] STEMI/QMI
- [ ] NSTEMI/NQMI
- [x] **UA**
- [ ] VTE
- [ ] DVT
- [ ] PE
- [ ] CVA

MEDICATIONS
- [x] **Platelet Antagonist**
  - [x] **Aspirin**
  - [ ] Clopidogrel
  - [ ] IIb/IIIa Receptor Antagonist
    - [ ] Abciximab
    - [ ] Eptifibatide
    - [ ] Lamifiban
    - [ ] Tirofiban
- [ ] **Heparin**
- [ ] **LMWH**
  - [ ] Enoxaparin
  - [ ] Dalteparin
  - [ ] Nadroparin
  - [ ] Tinzaparin
  - [ ] Reviparin
- [ ] **Direct Thrombin Inhibitor**
  - [ ] Hirudin
  - [ ] Hirulog
- [ ] **Fibrinolytic / Thrombolytic**
  - [ ] Alteplase
  - [ ] Reteplase
  - [ ] Tenecteplase
  - [ ] Anistreplase
  - [ ] Streptokinase
- [ ] **Other cardiac medications (captopril, magnesium, nitrates)**

PROCEDURES
- [ ] Angioplasty
- [ ] Stent
- [ ] CABG
- [ ] PCI

THERAPEUTIC ENDPOINT
- [x] **Treatment**
- [ ] Prophylaxis

CLINICAL ENVIRONMENT
- [x] **Inpatient**
- [x] **Outpatient**

ASPIRIN

ISIS-2 | SECOND INTERNATIONAL STUDY OF INFARCT SURVIVAL

TRIAL FULL NAME

Randomized trial of IV streptokinase, oral aspirin, both or neither among 17,187 cases of suspected acute myocardial infarction

PUBLICATION DATA

Lancet August 13 1988

STUDY DATES

1986 to 1988

AUTHOR(S)

R Collins, M Conway, D Alexopoulos, S Yusuf, P Sleight, N Brooks, R Bowes, A Marshall, S Harding, G Maskell, J Sanderson, B Mittra, D Hunt, D Tibbutt, H Sterry, D Jackson, A Scrimgeour, L Lim, P Appleby, S Parish, R Peto

CLINICAL TRIAL SUMMARY

This was a randomized, multi-national comparison of four regimes: STK 1.5 MU over 1 hour vs. 160 mg aspirin qd for one month vs. both active treatments vs. neither treatment. The 17187 patients had CP within 24 hours of presentation and were suspected to have MI; ECG changes were not required. Endpoints were vascular death at 5 weeks and up to a median of 10 months from discharge. Five-week vascular mortality was 9.2% with STK versus 12.0% without ($p < 0.00001$) and 9.4% with aspirin versus 11.8% without ($p < 0.0001$). The combination of STK and aspirin was significantly better than either agent used alone; resulting in a five-week mortality of 8.0 % versus 13.2% in those receiving neither agent ($p < 0.001$). Cerebral hemorrhage occurred in 0.1% of those receiving STK versus in none those not ($p < 0.02$) while overall strokes were similar between groups.

BOTTOM LINE

Streptokinase and ASA, individually and particularly in combination, result in significantly decreased mortality in patients with suspected MI who present with ≤ 24 hours of CP.

ACUTE CORONARY SYNDROMES

CLINICAL TRIAL FEATURES, THERAPEUTICS AND ENDPOINTS

DISEASE STATES

☑ ACS ☑ STEMI/QMI ☑ NSTEMI/NQMI ☑ UA
❑ VTE ❑ DVT ❑ PE ❑ CVA

MEDICATIONS

- ☑ **Platelet Antagonist**
  - ☑ **Aspirin**
  - ❑ Clopidogrel
  - ❑ IIb/IIIa Receptor Antagonist
    - ❑ Abciximab
    - ❑ Eptifibatide
    - ❑ Lamifiban
    - ❑ Tirofiban
- ❑ **Heparin**
- ❑ **LMWH**
  - ❑ Enoxaparin
  - ❑ Dalteparin
  - ❑ Nadroparin
  - ❑ Tinzaparin
  - ❑ Reviparin
- ❑ **Direct Thrombin Inhibitor**
  - ❑ Hirudin
  - ❑ Hirulog
- ☑ **Fibrinolytic / Thrombolytic**
  - ❑ Alteplase
  - ❑ Reteplase
  - ❑ Tenecteplase
  - ❑ Anistreplase
  - ☑ **Streptokinase**
- ❑ **Other cardiac medications (captopril, magnesium, nitrates)**

PROCEDURES

❑ Angioplasty ❑ Stent
❑ CABG ❑ PCI

THERAPEUTIC ENDPOINT

☑ **Treatment** ❑ Prophylaxis

CLINICAL ENVIRONMENT

☑ **Inpatient** ☑ **Outpatient**

ASPIRIN

ISIS-3 | THIRD INTERNATIONAL STUDY OF INFARCT SURVIVAL COLLABORATIVE GROUP

TRIAL FULL NAME

ISIS-3: A randomized comparison of streptokinase vs. tissue plasminogen activator vs. anistreplase and of aspirin plus heparin vs. aspirin alone among 41,299 cases of suspected acute MI

PUBLICATION DATA

Lancet 1992; 339: 753-766

STUDY DATES

1989 to 1991

AUTHOR(S)

R Collins, M Conway, D Alexopoulos, S Yusuf, P Sleight, N Brooks, R Bowes, A Marshall, S Harding, G Maskell, J Sanderson, B Mittra, et al

CLINICAL TRIAL SUMMARY

This was a multicenter, randomized, 3X2 factorial design (1) blinded comparison of STK 1.5 MU over one hour vs. tPA 100 mg over 3 hours vs. anisoylated plasminogen-streptokinase (APSAC) over 3 minutes; and (2) unblinded comparison of SQ heparin 12,500 IU BID X 1week vs. nothing. The 41,299 patients had CP within 24 hrs. of admission and had suspected MI; ECG changes were not required. All received aspirin. Endpoints were in-hospital reinfarction or 35 day mortality. The STK and APSAC groups had similar reinfarction and mortality rates. Streptokinase was associated with more allergic problems and non-cerebral bleeds but APSAC was associated with more cerebral hemorrhage. Compared to STK, tPA was associated with significantly more strokes (1.39% vs. 1.04%; $p < 0.01$) and cerebral hemorrhage (0.66% vs. 0.24%; $p < 0.00001$); but with fewer reinfarctions (2.93% vs. 3.47%; $p < 0.02$). Steptokinase and tPA had similar 35 day and 6 month mortality. In comparison with aspirin alone, the addition of heparin was associated with increased non-cerebral bleeding or need for transfusion (1.9% vs. 0.8%; $p < 0.01$) and cerebral hemorrhage (0.56% vs. 0.40%; $p < 0.05$); however, total strokes were comparable. At one week, heparin was associated with decreased mortality (7.4% vs. 7.9%; $p = 0.06$). However, by day 35, there was no difference between groups. Both the heparin results and the tPA vs. STK results mirrored those of GISSI 2.

BOTTOM LINE

Compared to STK, tPA was associated with reduced reinfarction rates but with increased cerebral hemorrhage and strokes. They had similar mortality rates. Heparin, in addition to aspirin, was associated with increased cerebral and non-cerebral bleeding with a reduced mortality at one week that was no longer evident by day 35.

ACUTE CORONARY SYNDROMES

CLINICAL TRIAL FEATURES, THERAPEUTICS AND ENDPOINTS

DISEASE STATES

☑ ACS ☑ STEMI/QMI ☑ NSTEMI/NQMI ☑ UA
❑ VTE ❑ DVT ❑ PE ❑ CVA

MEDICATIONS

- ☑ **Platelet Antagonist**
  - ☑ **Aspirin**
  - ❑ Clopidogrel
  - ❑ IIb/IIIa Receptor Antagonist
    - ❑ Abciximab
    - ❑ Eptifibatide
    - ❑ Lamifiban
    - ❑ Tirofiban
- ☑ **Heparin**
- ❑ **LMWH**
  - ❑ Enoxaparin
  - ❑ Dalteparin
  - ❑ Nadroparin
  - ❑ Tinzaparin
  - ❑ Reviparin
- ❑ **Direct Thrombin Inhibitor**
  - ❑ Hirudin
  - ❑ Hirulog
- ☑ **Fibrinolytic / Thrombolytic**
  - ❑ Alteplase
  - ❑ Reteplase
  - ❑ Tenecteplase
  - ☑ **Anistreplase**
  - ☑ **Streptokinase**
- ❑ **Other cardiac medications (captopril, magnesium, nitrates)**

PROCEDURES

❑ Angioplasty ❑ Stent
❑ CABG ❑ PCI

THERAPEUTIC ENDPOINT

☑ **Treatment** ❑ Prophylaxis

CLINICAL ENVIRONMENT

☑ **Inpatient** ☑ **Outpatient**

ASPIRIN

RISC | RESEARCH GROUP ON INSTABILITY IN CORONARY ARTERY DISEASE

TRIAL FULL NAME
Risk of myocardial infarction and death during treatment with low dose aspirin and IV heparin in men with unstable coronary artery disease

PUBLICATION DATA
Lancet 1990; 336: 827-30

STUDY DATES
1985 to 1988

AUTHOR(S)
L. Wallentin, U Berglund, O Svensson, F Landgren, J Fridn, PO Andersson, JO Magnusson, BO Ryden, B Hedback, B Sinnnerstad, et al

CLINICAL TRIAL SUMMARY

This was a prospective, randomized, double-blind, multicenter, 2 X 2 factorial designed comparison of (1) aspirin 75 mg qd vs. placebo vs. (2) IV heparin 5000 U boli q 6 hour for five days vs. placebo. The 796 men had UA or NQMI. The combined endpoint of death or MI was reduced by aspirin (vs. placebo) at 5 days (2.5% vs. 5.8%; p = 0.03) and at 90 days (6.5% vs. 17.0%; p < 0.0001). Heparin had no significant effect on outcome, although the group treated with aspirin and heparin had the lowest number of events during the initial 5 days.

BOTTOM LINE

Aspirin significantly reduced death or MI in patients with UA or NQMI while bolus heparin therapy, when combined with aspirin, reduced events compared to other groups during the five day administration period.

ACUTE CORONARY SYNDROMES

CLINICAL TRIAL FEATURES, THERAPEUTICS AND ENDPOINTS

DISEASE STATES
- ☑ **ACS** ☑ **STEMI/QMI** ☑ **NSTEMI/NQMI** ☑ **UA**
- ❑ VTE ❑ DVT ❑ PE ❑ CVA

MEDICATIONS
- ☑ **Platelet Antagonist**
  - ☑ **Aspirin**
  - ❑ Clopidogrel
  - ☑ **IIb/IIIa Receptor Antagonist**
    - ❑ Abciximab
    - ❑ Eptifibatide
    - ❑ Lamifiban
    - ☑ **Tirofiban**
- ❑ **Heparin**
- ❑ **LMWH**
  - ❑ Enoxaparin
  - ❑ Dalteparin
  - ❑ Nadroparin
  - ❑ Tinzaparin
  - ❑ Reviparin
- ❑ **Direct Thrombin Inhibitor**
  - ❑ Hirudin
  - ❑ Hirulog
- ❑ **Fibrinolytic / Thrombolytic**
  - ❑ Alteplase
  - ❑ Reteplase
  - ❑ Tenecteplase
  - ❑ Anistreplase
  - ❑ Streptokinase
- ❑ **Other cardiac medications (captopril, magnesium, nitrates)**

PROCEDURES
- ☑ **Angioplasty** ❑ Stent
- ❑ CABG ☑ **PCI**

THERAPEUTIC ENDPOINT
- ☑ **Treatment** ❑ Prophylaxis

CLINICAL ENVIRONMENT
- ☑ **Inpatient** ❑ Outpatient

ASPIRIN

HEPARIN THERAPY IN UNSTABLE ANGINA

TRIAL FULL NAME
Adding Heparin to Aspirin reduces the incidence of myocardial infarction and death in patients with unstable angina

PUBLICATION DATA
JAMA 1996; 276:811-815

STUDY DATES
Not applicable

AUTHOR(S)
Oler A, Whooley M, J Oler, D Grady

CLINICAL TRIAL SUMMARY

This was a meta-analysis of 6 randomized, controlled trials that compared aspirin plus heparin with aspirin alone in patients with UA or NQMI. The trials had varied degrees of blinding. Endpoints, death or MI during the heparin infusion, occurred in 7.9% of the aspirin plus heparin group and in 10.4% of the aspirin alone group (p = 0.06).

BOTTOM LINE

Heparin, in addition to aspirin, reduced the occurrence of death or MI during the infusion in patients with UA or NQMI. and effective as IV heparin as medication adjuncts.

ACUTE CORONARY SYNDROMES

CLINICAL TRIAL FEATURES, THERAPEUTICS AND ENDPOINTS

DISEASE STATES
- ☑ **ACS** ❑ STEMI/QMI ☑ **NSTEMI/NQMI** ☑ **UA**
- ❑ VTE ❑ DVT ❑ PE ❑ CVA

MEDICATIONS
- ☑ **Platelet Antagonist**
  - ☑ **Aspirin**
  - ❑ Clopidogrel
  - ❑ IIb/IIIa Receptor Antagonist
    - ❑ Abciximab
    - ❑ Eptifibatide
    - ❑ Lamifiban
    - ❑ Tirofiban
- ☑ **Heparin**
- ❑ **LMWH**
  - ❑ Enoxaparin
  - ❑ Dalteparin
  - ❑ Nadroparin
  - ❑ Tinzaparin
  - ❑ Reviparin
- ❑ **Direct Thrombin Inhibitor**
  - ❑ Hirudin
  - ❑ Hirulog
- ❑ **Fibrinolytic / Thrombolytic**
  - ❑ Alteplase
  - ❑ Reteplase
  - ❑ Tenecteplase
  - ❑ Anistreplase
  - ❑ Streptokinase
- ❑ **Other cardiac medications (captopril, magnesium, nitrates)**

PROCEDURES
- ❑ Angioplasty ❑ Stent
- ❑ CABG ❑ PCI

THERAPEUTIC ENDPOINT
- ☑ **Treatment** ❑ Prophylaxis

CLINICAL ENVIRONMENT
- ☑ **Inpatient** ❑ Outpatient

UNFRACTIONATED HEPARIN

RISC | RESEARCH GROUP ON INSTABILITY IN CORONARY ARTERY DISEASE

TRIAL FULL NAME
Risk of myocardial infarction and death during treatment with low dose aspirin and IV heparin in men with unstable coronary artery disease

PUBLICATION DATA
Lancet 1990; 336: 827-30

STUDY DATES
1985 to 1988

AUTHOR(S)
L. Wallentin, U Berglund, O Svensson, F Landgren, J Fridn, PO Andersson, JO Mangnusson, BO Ryden, B Hedback, B Sinnnerstad, et al

CLINICAL TRIAL SUMMARY

This was a prospective, randomized, double-blind, multicenter, 2 X 2 factorial designed comparison of (1) aspirin 75 mg qd vs. placebo vs. (2) IV heparin 5000 U boli q 6 hour for five days vs. placebo. The 796 men had UA or NQMI. The combined endpoint of death or MI was reduced by aspirin (vs. placebo) at 5 days (2.5% vs. 5.8%; p = 0.03) and at 90 days (6.5% vs. 17.0%; p < 0.0001). Heparin had no significant effect on outcome, although the group treated with aspirin and heparin had the lowest number of events during the initial 5 days.

BOTTOM LINE

Aspirin significantly reduced death or MI in patients with UA or NQMI while bolus heparin therapy, when combined with aspirin, reduced events compared to other groups during the five day administration period.

ACUTE CORONARY SYNDROMES

CLINICAL TRIAL FEATURES, THERAPEUTICS AND ENDPOINTS

DISEASE STATES
☑ **ACS** ☑ **STEMI/QMI** ☑ **NSTEMI/NQMI** ☑ **UA**
☐ VTE ☐ DVT ☐ PE ☐ CVA

MEDICATIONS
- ☑ **Platelet Antagonist**
  - ☑ **Aspirin**
  - ☐ Clopidogrel
  - ☑ **IIb/IIIa Receptor Antagonist**
    - ☐ Abciximab
    - ☐ Eptifibatide
    - ☐ Lamifiban
    - ☑ **Tirofiban**
- ☐ **Heparin**
- ☐ **LMWH**
  - ☐ Enoxaparin
  - ☐ Dalteparin
  - ☐ Nadroparin
  - ☐ Tinzaparin
  - ☐ Reviparin
- ☐ **Direct Thrombin Inhibitor**
  - ☐ Hirudin
  - ☐ Hirulog
- ☐ **Fibrinolytic / Thrombolytic**
  - ☐ Alteplase
  - ☐ Reteplase
  - ☐ Tenecteplase
  - ☐ Anistreplase
  - ☐ Streptokinase
- ☐ **Other cardiac medications (captopril, magnesium, nitrates)**

PROCEDURES
☑ **Angioplasty** ☐ Stent
☐ CABG ☑ **PCI**

THERAPEUTIC ENDPOINT
☑ **Treatment** ☐ Prophylaxis

CLINICAL ENVIRONMENT
☑ **Inpatient** ☐ Outpatient

UNFRACTIONATED HEPARIN

GISSI-3 | GRUPPO ITALIANO PER LO STUDIO DELLA SOPRAVVIVENZA NELL'INFARTO MIOCARDICO

TRIAL FULL NAME
Effects of lisinopril and transdermal glyceryl trinitrate singly and together on 6-week mortality and ventricular function after acute myocardial infarction

PUBLICATION DATA
Lancet 1994; 343: 1115-22

STUDY DATES
1991 to 1993

AUTHOR(S)
GA Feruglio, C DeVita, A Selvini, E Ambrosioni,G Mezzanotte, M Bruno, M Anselmi, et al

CLINICAL TRIAL SUMMARY

This was a multicenter, randomized, open label, 6 week, 2 X 2 factorial comparison of (1) lisinopril 10 mg qd for 6 weeks vs. nothing, and (2) transdermal glyceryl trinitrate X 14 hours per day vs. nothing. The 18,895 patients had CP within 24 hours of randomization with ST deviation in ^{3} 1 lead(s). Endpoints were death and the combination of death plus CHF (clinically or per ECHO) at 6 weeks. Lisinopril was associated with both decreased mortality (6.3% vs. 7.1%; p = 0.03) and combined endpoint (15.6% vs. 17.0%; p = 0.009). Nitrates had no affect on mortality (6.5% with vs. 6.9% without) nor on the combined endpoint (15.9% with vs. 16.7% without). The combination of agents yielded no further benefit beyond that of lisinopril alone.

BOTTOM LINE

In patients with < 24 hours of CP and STEMI (ECG change in ≥ 1 lead), lisinopril resulted in decreased mortality at 6 weeks when compared to nothing. Nitrates had no effect on mortality.

ACUTE CORONARY SYNDROMES

CLINICAL TRIAL FEATURES, THERAPEUTICS AND ENDPOINTS

DISEASE STATES
☑ **ACS** ☑ **STEMI/QMI** ☐ NSTEMI/NQMI ☑ **UA**
☐ VTE ☐ DVT ☐ PE ☐ CVA

MEDICATIONS
- ☐ **Platelet Antagonist**
  - ☐ Aspirin
  - ☐ Clopidogrel
  - ☐ IIb/IIIa Receptor Antagonist
    - ☐ Abciximab
    - ☐ Eptifibatide
    - ☐ Lamifiban
    - ☐ Tirofiban
- ☐ **Heparin**
- ☐ **LMWH**
  - ☐ Enoxaparin
  - ☐ Dalteparin
  - ☐ Nadroparin
  - ☐ Tinzaparin
  - ☐ Reviparin
- ☐ **Direct Thrombin Inhibitor**
  - ☐ Hirudin
  - ☐ Hirulog
- ☑ **Fibrinolytic / Thrombolytic**
  - ☐ Alteplase
  - ☐ Reteplase
  - ☐ Tenecteplase
  - ☐ Anistreplase
  - ☐ Streptokinase
- ☑ **Other cardiac medications (captopril, magnesium, nitrates)**

PROCEDURES
☐ Angioplasty ☐ Stent
☐ CABG ☐ PCI

THERAPEUTIC ENDPOINT
☑ **Treatment** ☐ Prophylaxis

CLINICAL ENVIRONMENT
☑ **Inpatient** ☐ Outpatient

OTHER CARDIAC MEDICATIONS

HART-II

TRIAL FULL NAME
A randomized comparison of low molecular weight heparin and unfractonated heparin adjunctive to tPA thrombolysis and aspirin

PUBLICATION DATA
Presented at the American College of Cardiology Meeting, March 2000

STUDY DATES
Not available

AUTHOR(S)
Ross A

CLINICAL TRIAL SUMMARY

This was a randomized comparison of IV heparin (4000-5000 U bolus plus infusion at 15 U/kg/hour for 72 hours) vs. enoxaparin (30 mg IV followed by 1 mg/kg SQ q 12 hours for 72 hours) as an adjunct with tPA in 400 patients with STEMI. The endpoints were safety and TIMI grade 2 or 3 flow at 90 minutes after tPA and again at 5-7 days. Angiograms were read blinded as to treatment groups. Intracranial hemorrhage and fatality were comparable between groups. At 90 minutes, TIMI grade 2 or 3 flow occurred in 80.1% of the enoxaparin group and in 75.1% of the heparin group (p = NS). At one-week follow-up, target vessel occlusion had occurred in 5.9% of the enoxaparin group and in 9.8% of the heparin group (p = NS).

BOTTOM LINE

In patients with STEMI receiving alteplase, enoxaparin was as safe and effective as IV heparin as medication adjuncts.

ACUTE CORONARY SYNDROMES

CLINICAL TRIAL FEATURES, THERAPEUTICS AND ENDPOINTS

DISEASE STATES
☑ ACS ☑ STEMI/QMI ❑ NSTEMI/NQMI ❑ UA
❑ VTE ❑ DVT ❑ PE ❑ CVA

MEDICATIONS
- ❑ **Platelet Antagonist**
  - ❑ Aspirin
  - ❑ Clopidogrel
  - ❑ IIb/IIIa Receptor Antagonist
    - ❑ Abciximab
    - ❑ Eptifibatide
    - ❑ Lamifiban
    - ❑ Tirofiban
- ☑ **Heparin**
- ☑ **LMWH**
  - ☑ **Enoxaparin**
  - ❑ Dalteparin
  - ❑ Nadroparin
  - ❑ Tinzaparin
  - ❑ Reviparin
- ❑ **Direct Thrombin Inhibitor**
  - ❑ Hirudin
  - ❑ Hirulog
- ❑ **Fibrinolytic / Thrombolytic**
  - ❑ Alteplase
  - ❑ Reteplase
  - ❑ Tenecteplase
  - ❑ Anistreplase
  - ❑ Streptokinase
- ❑ **Other cardiac medications (captopril, magnesium, nitrates)**

PROCEDURES
❑ Angioplasty ❑ Stent
❑ CABG ❑ PCI

THERAPEUTIC ENDPOINT
☑ **Treatment** ❑ Prophylaxis

CLINICAL ENVIRONMENT
☑ **Inpatient** ❑ Outpatient

OTHER CARDIAC MEDICATIONS

ISIS-4 INTERNATIONAL STUDIES OF INFARCT SURVIVAL

TRIAL FULL NAME
A randomized factorial trial assessing early oral captopril , oral mononitrate, and IV magnesium sulfate in 58,050 patients with suspected acute myocardial infarction

PUBLICATION DATA
Lancet 1995; 345:669-85

STUDY DATES
1991 to 1993

AUTHOR(S)
R Collins, M Conway, D Alexopoulos, S Yusuf, P Sleight, N Brooks R Bowes, A Marshall, S Harding,G Maskell, J Sanderson, B Mittra, D Hunt, D Tibbutt, H Sterry, D Jackson, A Scrimgeour, L Lim, P Appleby, S Parish, R Peto

CLINICAL TRIAL SUMMARY

This was a multicenter, randomized, 2 X 2 X 2 factorial design trial in the management of 58,050 patients with suspected (ECG changes not required) MI who presented within 24 hours of symptom onset. The three arms were (1) captopril 50 mg BID vs. placebo for 1 month, (2) mononitrate 60 mg qd vs. placebo for 1 month, and (3) open label IV magnesium 80 mmoles over 24 hours without placebo. Treatments were started immediately after the first hour of thrombolytic therapy or sooner if no thrombolytic. Seventy-percent of the patients received a thrombolytic and 94% received antiplatelet therapy. Captopril reduced 5-week mortality from 7.7% to 7.2% (p = 0.02) and benefit was maximal in higher risk patients including those with hypotension or CHF. Mortality was not reduced by mononitrate (7.3% vs. 7.5% with placebo) nor by magnesium (7.6% vs. 7.2% with nothing).

BOTTOM LINE

Captopril resulted in a significantly reduced 5-week mortality in patients with suspected (ECG changes not required) MI. Neither oral mononitrate nor IV magnesium affected mortality.

ACUTE CORONARY SYNDROMES

CLINICAL TRIAL FEATURES, THERAPEUTICS AND ENDPOINTS

DISEASE STATES
☑ ACS ☑ STEMI/QMI ☑ NSTEMI/NQMI ❑ UA
❑ VTE ❑ DVT ❑ PE ❑ CVA

MEDICATIONS
- ❑ **Platelet Antagonist**
  - ❑ Aspirin
  - ❑ Clopidogrel
  - ❑ IIb/IIIa Receptor Antagonist
    - ❑ Abciximab
    - ❑ Eptifibatide
    - ❑ Lamifiban
    - ❑ Tirofiban
- ❑ **Heparin**
- ❑ **LMWH**
  - ❑ Enoxaparin
  - ❑ Dalteparin
  - ❑ Nadroparin
  - ❑ Tinzaparin
  - ❑ Reviparin
- ❑ **Direct Thrombin Inhibitor**
  - ❑ Hirudin
  - ❑ Hirulog
- ❑ **Fibrinolytic / Thrombolytic**
  - ❑ Alteplase
  - ❑ Reteplase
  - ❑ Tenecteplase
  - ❑ Anistreplase
  - ❑ Streptokinase
- ☑ **Other cardiac medications (captopril, magnesium, nitrates)**

PROCEDURES
❑ Angioplasty ❑ Stent
❑ CABG ❑ PCI

THERAPEUTIC ENDPOINT
☑ **Treatment** ❑ Prophylaxis

CLINICAL ENVIRONMENT
☑ **Inpatient** ❑ Outpatient

OTHER CARDIAC MEDICATIONS

SHOCK | SHOULD WE EMERGENTLY REVASCULARIZE OCCLUDED CORONARIES FOR CARDIOGENIC SHOCK

TRIAL FULL NAME
Early Revascularization in Acute Myocardial Infarction Complicated by Cardiogenic Shock

PUBLICATION DATA
NEJM 1999; 341: 625-34

STUDY DATES
1993 to 1998

AUTHOR(S)
Hochman J, Sleeper L, Webb JG, et al

CLINICAL TRIAL SUMMARY

This was a multicenter, randomized comparison of emergency revascularization (PTCA or CABG within 6 hours) vs. initial medical stabilization in patients with acute MI and cardiogenic shock. The 302 patients had ST elevation, Q-waves, or new LBBB and had both clinical (SBP < 90 mm Hg) and hemodynamic (cardiac index < 2.2) criteria for shock. Mortality was the primary (30 days) and secondary (6 and 12 months) outcome. Over 80% of both groups had balloon pump counterpulsation. Mortality for the revascularization and medical groups were comparable at 30 days (47% vs. 56%; p = 0.11). Revascularization reduced mortality at 6 months (50% vs. 63%; p = 0.027). Twelve-month mortality was not reported despite being a defined secondary endpoint. The authors recommended that emergency revascularization be strongly considered for patients with acute MI complicated by cardiogenic shock.

BOTTOM LINE

In patients with cardiogenic shock, revascularization within 6 hours did not significantly reduce overall mortality at 30 days; however, it did result in a significant survival benefit at 6 months.

ACUTE CORONARY SYNDROMES

CLINICAL TRIAL FEATURES, THERAPEUTICS AND ENDPOINTS

DISEASE STATES
- ☑ ACS ☑ STEMI/QMI ❏ NSTEMI/NQMI ❏ UA
- ❏ VTE ❏ DVT ❏ PE ❏ CVA

MEDICATIONS
- ❏ **Platelet Antagonist**
  - ❏ Aspirin
  - ❏ Clopidogrel
  - ❏ IIb/IIIa Receptor Antagonist
    - ❏ Abciximab
    - ❏ Eptifibatide
    - ❏ Lamifiban
    - ❏ Tirofiban
- ❏ **Heparin**
- ❏ **LMWH**
  - ❏ Enoxaparin
  - ❏ Dalteparin
  - ❏ Nadroparin
  - ❏ Tinzaparin
  - ❏ Reviparin
- ❏ **Direct Thrombin Inhibitor**
  - ❏ Hirudin
  - ❏ Hirulog
- ❏ **Fibrinolytic / Thrombolytic**
  - ❏ Alteplase
  - ❏ Reteplase
  - ❏ Tenecteplase
  - ❏ Anistreplase
  - ❏ Streptokinase
- ❏ **Other cardiac medications (captopril, magnesium, nitrates)**

PROCEDURES
- ☑ **Angioplasty** ❏ Stent
- ☑ **CABG** ☑ **PCI**

THERAPEUTIC ENDPOINT
- ☑ **Treatment** ❏ Prophylaxis

CLINICAL ENVIRONMENT
- ☑ **Inpatient** ❏ Outpatient

OTHER CARDIAC MEDICATIONS

SPAMI | STENT PRIMARY ANGIOPLASTY IN MYOCARDIAL INFARCTION

TRIAL FULL NAME
Coronary Angioplasty with or without Stent Implantation for Acute Myocardial Infarction

PUBLICATION DATA
NEJM 1999; 341:1949-56

STUDY DATES
No data

AUTHOR(S)
Grines C., Cox D., et al

CLINICAL TRIAL SUMMARY

This was a multicenter, randomized comparison of primary PTCA with PTCA accompanied by implantation of a heparin-coated stent. The 900 patients presented within 12 hours of the onset of CP and had ST elevation in ³ 2 leads. The primary endpoint was the composite of death, reinfarction, disabling stroke, or target vessel revascularization at 6 months. Ninety-percent of all patients received ticlopidine, 99% aspirin, and 5% abciximab. Stent placement was associated with improved outcomes for angina (11.3% vs. 16.9%; p = 0.02), target vessel revascularization (7.7% vs. 17.0%; p < 0.001), and the combined end point (12.6% vs. 20.1%; p < 0.01). The improved combined outcome was entirely due to the need for less revascularization. Mortality was comparable between groups. Restenosis at 6.5 months occurred less often in the stent group (20.3% vs. 33.5%; p < 0.001). In patients with acute myocardial infarction, routine implantation of a stent has clinical benefits beyond those of primary coronary angioplasty.

BOTTOM LINE

Compared to PTCA alone, stent placement in patients with STEMI significantly reduced the composite of death, reinfarction, disabling stroke, or target vessel revascularization at 6 months. The difference was primarily due to the need for less revascularization.

ACUTE CORONARY SYNDROMES

CLINICAL TRIAL FEATURES, THERAPEUTICS AND ENDPOINTS

DISEASE STATES
- ☑ ACS ☑ STEMI/QMI ❏ NSTEMI/NQMI ❏ UA
- ❏ VTE ❏ DVT ❏ PE ❏ CVA

MEDICATIONS
- ❏ **Platelet Antagonist**
  - ❏ Aspirin
  - ❏ Clopidogrel
  - ❏ IIb/IIIa Receptor Antagonist
    - ❏ Abciximab
    - ❏ Eptifibatide
    - ❏ Lamifiban
    - ❏ Tirofiban
- ❏ **Heparin**
- ❏ **LMWH**
  - ❏ Enoxaparin
  - ❏ Dalteparin
  - ❏ Nadroparin
  - ❏ Tinzaparin
  - ❏ Reviparin
- ❏ **Direct Thrombin Inhibitor**
  - ❏ Hirudin
  - ❏ Hirulog
- ❏ **Fibrinolytic / Thrombolytic**
  - ❏ Alteplase
  - ❏ Reteplase
  - ❏ Tenecteplase
  - ❏ Anistreplase
  - ❏ Streptokinase
- ❏ **Other cardiac medications (captopril, magnesium, nitrates)**

PROCEDURES
- ☑ **Angioplasty** ☑ **Stent**
- ☑ **CABG** ☑ **PCI**

THERAPEUTIC ENDPOINT
- ☑ **Treatment** ❏ Prophylaxis

CLINICAL ENVIRONMENT
- ☑ **Inpatient** ❏ Outpatient

OTHER CARDIAC MEDICATIONS

STOP AMI | STENT VERSUS THROMBOLYSIS FOR OCCLUDED CORONARY ARTERIES IN PATIENTS WITH ACUTE MYOCARDIAL INFARCTION

TRIAL FULL NAME

Coronary Stenting plus Platelet Glycoprotein IIb/IIIa Blockage compared with Tissue Plasminogen activator in Acute Myocardial Infarction

PUBLICATION DATA

NEJM 2000; 343:385-91

STUDY DATES

1997 to 1999

AUTHOR(S)

Schomig A., Kastrati A., Dirschinger J et al

CLINICAL TRIAL SUMMARY

This was a multicenter, randomized comparison of thrombolysis (tPA 100 mg over 90 minutes) vs. PTCA with a stent plus abciximab. The 140 patients presented within 12 hours of the onset of symptoms and had ST elevation in ³ 2 leads. Both groups received aspirin and heparin. The stent group also received ticlopidine 250 mg BID for one-month. The primary endpoint was left ventricular (LV) infarct size as measured by serial scintigraphic studies with Tc 99m sestamibi. The secondary endpoint was a composite of death, reinfarction, and stroke within 6 months. The median infarct size in the stent + abciximab group was 14.3% vs. 19.4% in the tPA group (p = 0.02). The composite endpoint occurred less often in the stent + abciximab group (8.5% vs. 23.2%; p = 0.02).

BOTTOM LINE

Compared to alteplase alone, patients with STEMI receiving coronary stenting plus abciximab had significantly better myocardial salvage and 6 month incidence of death, reinfarction, and stroke.

ACUTE CORONARY SYNDROMES

CLINICAL TRIAL FEATURES, THERAPEUTICS AND ENDPOINTS

DISEASE STATES

- ☑ **ACS** ☑ **STEMI/QMI** ❑ NSTEMI/NQMI ❑ UA
- ❑ VTE ❑ DVT ❑ PE ❑ CVA

MEDICATIONS

- ☑ **Platelet Antagonist**
  - ☑ **Aspirin**
  - ❑ Clopidogrel
  - ☑ **IIb/IIIa Receptor Antagonist**
    - ☑ **Abciximab**
    - ❑ Eptifibatide
    - ❑ Lamifiban
    - ❑ Tirofiban
- ❑ **Heparin**
- ❑ **LMWH**
  - ❑ Enoxaparin
  - ❑ Dalteparin
  - ❑ Nadroparin
  - ❑ Tinzaparin
  - ❑ Reviparin
- ❑ **Direct Thrombin Inhibitor**
  - ❑ Hirudin
  - ❑ Hirulog
- ☑ **Fibrinolytic / Thrombolytic**
  - ☑ **Alteplase**
  - ❑ Reteplase
  - ❑ Tenecteplase
  - ❑ Anistreplase
  - ❑ Streptokinase
- ❑ **Other cardiac medications (captopril, magnesium, nitrates)**

PROCEDURES

- ☑ **Angioplasty** ☑ **Stent**
- ❑ CABG ☑ **PCI**

THERAPEUTIC ENDPOINT

- ☑ **Treatment** ❑ Prophylaxis

CLINICAL ENVIRONMENT

- ☑ **Inpatient** ❑ Outpatient

OTHER CARDIAC MEDICATIONS

TIMI 14 | THROMBOLYSIS IN MYOCARDIAL INFARCTION 14 TRIAL

TRIAL FULL NAME

Abciximab Facilitates the Rate and Extent of Thrombolysis

PUBLICATION DATA

Circulation 1999; 99:2720-2732

STUDY DATES

1997 to 1998

AUTHOR(S)

Antman E, Giugliano R., Gibson CM, et al

CLINICAL TRIAL SUMMARY

This was a multicenter, randomized, open-label comparison of various combinations of abciximab, thrombolytics, and IV heparin in the management of 888 patients with STEMI presenting within 12 hours of onset of CP. Arms included (1) tPA 100mg over 90 minutes alone, (2) abciximab bolus and 12 hour infusion alone, and (3) abciximab plus varied does of tPA (20 mg to 65 mg) or streptokinase (500,000 U to 1.5 MU). The heparin bolus was 60 U/kg in patients who received abciximab and 70 U/kg in those who did not receive abciximab. The primary endpoint, TIMI grade 3 flow, occurred more in the tPA plus abciximab group than in the tPA alone group at 60 minutes (72% vs. 43%; p = 0.0009) and at 90 minutes (77% vs. 62%; p = 0.02). The rates of major hemorrhage were 6% in patients receiving tPA alone, 3% with abciximab alone, 10% with streptokinase plus abciximab, and 1% with tPA plus abciximab with low-dose heparin. Efficacy and safety were most optimal for a tPA dose that was one-half the standard dose. Abciximab facilitates the rate and extent of thrombolysis, producing early, marked increases in TIMI 3 flow when combined with half the usual dose of tPA.

BOTTOM LINE

Compared to full dose tPA alone, abciximab combined with tPA 50 mg in patients with STEMI resulted in significantly improved TIMI grade 3 flow at 60 and 90 minutes.

ACUTE CORONARY SYNDROMES

CLINICAL TRIAL FEATURES, THERAPEUTICS AND ENDPOINTS

DISEASE STATES

- ☑ **ACS** ☑ **STEMI/QMI** ❑ NSTEMI/NQMI ☑ **UA**
- ❑ VTE ❑ DVT ❑ PE ❑ CVA

MEDICATIONS

- ☑ **Platelet Antagonist**
  - ❑ Aspirin
  - ❑ Clopidogrel
  - ☑ **IIb/IIIa Receptor Antagonist**
    - ☑ **Abciximab**
    - ❑ Eptifibatide
    - ❑ Lamifiban
    - ❑ Tirofiban
- ☑ **Heparin**
- ❑ **LMWH**
  - ❑ Enoxaparin
  - ❑ Dalteparin
  - ❑ Nadroparin
  - ❑ Tinzaparin
  - ❑ Reviparin
- ❑ **Direct Thrombin Inhibitor**
  - ❑ Hirudin
  - ❑ Hirulog
- ☑ **Fibrinolytic / Thrombolytic**
  - ☑ **Alteplase**
  - ❑ Reteplase
  - ❑ Tenecteplase
  - ❑ Anistreplase
  - ☑ **Streptokinase**
- ❑ **Other cardiac medications (captopril, magnesium, nitrates)**

PROCEDURES

- ❑ Angioplasty ❑ Stent
- ❑ CABG ❑ PCI

THERAPEUTIC ENDPOINT

- ☑ **Treatment** ❑ Prophylaxis

CLINICAL ENVIRONMENT

- ☑ **Inpatient** ❑ Outpatient

OTHER CARDIAC MEDICATIONS

GUSTO 11B — GLOBAL USE OF STRATEGIES TO OPEN OCCLUDED CORONARY ARTERIES

TRIAL FULL NAME
A comparison of recombinant hirudin with heparin for the treatment of acute coronary syndromes

PUBLICATION DATA
NEJM 1996; 335: 775-82

STUDY DATES
1994 to 1995

AUTHOR(S)
Topol E

CLINICAL TRIAL SUMMARY

This was a multicenter, double-blind comparison of IV heparin vs. IV hirudin (0.1 mg/kg bolus then 0.1 mg/kg/hour infusion). The 12,142 patients had CP within 12 hours of presentation and ECG changes consistent with either MI or UA. The primary end point of death or nonfatal MI was reached in 9.8% of the heparin group and in 8.9% (p = 0.06) of the hirudin group at 30 days. Major or moderate bleeding occurred more often in the hirudin group, 8.8%, than in the heparin group, 7.7%; (p = 0.03).

BOTTOM LINE

Compared with heparin, hirudin resulted in a nearly significant improvement in death or MI in patients with CP and ECG changes; however, it also resulted in significantly more bleeding.

ACUTE CORONARY SYNDROMES

CLINICAL TRIAL FEATURES, THERAPEUTICS AND ENDPOINTS

DISEASE STATES
- ☑ **ACS** ☑ **STEMI/QMI** ☑ **NSTEMI/NQMI** ☑ **UA**
- ☐ VTE ☐ DVT ☐ PE ☐ CVA

MEDICATIONS
- ☐ **Platelet Antagonist**
  - ☐ Aspirin
  - ☐ Clopidogrel
  - ☐ IIb/IIIa Receptor Antagonist
    - ☐ Abciximab
    - ☐ Eptifibatide
    - ☐ Lamifiban
    - ☐ Tirofiban
- ☑ **Heparin**
- ☐ **LMWH**
  - ☐ Enoxaparin
  - ☐ Dalteparin
  - ☐ Nadroparin
  - ☐ Tinzaparin
  - ☐ Reviparin
- ☑ **Direct Thrombin Inhibitor**
  - ☑ **Hirudin**
  - ☐ Hirulog
- ☐ **Fibrinolytic / Thrombolytic**
  - ☐ Alteplase
  - ☐ Reteplase
  - ☐ Tenecteplase
  - ☐ Anistreplase
  - ☐ Streptokinase
- ☐ **Other cardiac medications (captopril, magnesium, nitrates)**

PROCEDURES
- ☐ Angioplasty ☐ Stent
- ☐ CABG ☐ PCI

THERAPEUTIC ENDPOINT
- ☑ **Treatment** ☐ Prophylaxis

CLINICAL ENVIRONMENT
- ☑ **Inpatient** ☐ Outpatient

DIRECT THROMBIN INHIBITORS

HIRULOG ANGIOPLASTY STUDY INVESTIGATORS

TRIAL FULL NAME
Treatment with bivalirudin (hirulog) as compared with heparin during coronary angioplasty for unstable or post infarction angina

PUBLICATION DATA
NEJM 1995; 333:764-9

STUDY DATES
1993 to 1994

AUTHOR(S)
Bittl J, Strony J, Brinker J, et al

CLINICAL TRIAL SUMMARY

This was a double-blind, randomized comparison of IV hirulog (1 mg/kg bolus then 4 hour infusion at 2.5 mg/kg/hour then a 14-20 hour infusion at 0.2 mg/kg/hour) vs. IV heparin (125 IU/kg bolus with 15 IU/kg/hour infusion) administered just before angioplasty. The 4098 patients had CP due to unstable or postinfarction angina and were scheduled to undergo angioplasty. The primary end points were death in the hospital, MI, abrupt vessel closure, or rapid clinical deterioration of cardiac origin. Hirulog and heparin resulted in similar study end-point frequency (11.4% vs. 12.2%; p = NS) but hirulog was associated with less major bleeding (3.8% vs. 9.8%; p > 0.001).

BOTTOM LINE

Bivalirudin was as effective as high-dose heparin in preventing ischemic complications in patients who underwent angioplasty for UA and it carried a lower risk of bleeding.

ACUTE CORONARY SYNDROMES

CLINICAL TRIAL FEATURES, THERAPEUTICS AND ENDPOINTS

DISEASE STATES
- ☑ **ACS** ☐ STEMI/QMI ☐ NSTEMI/NQMI ☑ **UA**
- ☐ VTE ☐ DVT ☐ PE ☐ CVA

MEDICATIONS
- ☐ **Platelet Antagonist**
  - ☐ Aspirin
  - ☐ Clopidogrel
  - ☐ IIb/IIIa Receptor Antagonist
    - ☐ Abciximab
    - ☐ Eptifibatide
    - ☐ Lamifiban
    - ☐ Tirofiban
- ☑ **Heparin**
- ☐ **LMWH**
  - ☐ Enoxaparin
  - ☐ Dalteparin
  - ☐ Nadroparin
  - ☐ Tinzaparin
  - ☐ Reviparin
- ☑ **Direct Thrombin Inhibitor**
  - ☐ Hirudin
  - ☑ **Hirulog**
- ☐ **Fibrinolytic / Thrombolytic**
  - ☐ Alteplase
  - ☐ Reteplase
  - ☐ Tenecteplase
  - ☐ Anistreplase
  - ☐ Streptokinase
- ☐ **Other cardiac medications (captopril, magnesium, nitrates)**

PROCEDURES
- ☑ **Angioplasty** ☐ Stent
- ☐ CABG ☐ PCI

THERAPEUTIC ENDPOINT
- ☑ **Treatment** ☐ Prophylaxis

CLINICAL ENVIRONMENT
- ☑ **Inpatient** ☐ Outpatient

DIRECT THROMBIN INHIBITORS

OASIS-2 — ORGANIZATION TO ASSESS STRATEGIES FOR ISCHEMIC SYNDROMES

TRIAL FULL NAME
Effects of recombinant hirudin (lepirudin) compared with heparin on death, myocardial infarction, refractory angina, and revascularization procedures in patients with acute myocardial ischaemia without ST elevation: a randomized trial

PUBLICATION DATA
Lancet 1999; 353:429-38

STUDY DATES
1996 to 1998

AUTHOR(S)
S Yusuf, J Pogue, S Anan, M Flather, K Fox, G Tognoni, et al

CLINICAL TRIAL SUMMARY

This was a double-blind, randomized comparison of the direct thrombin inhibitor IV recombinant hirudin (0.4 mg/kg bolus then 0.15 mg/kg/hour infusion) vs. IV heparin. The 10,141 patients had CP within 12 hours of presentation and either a history of CAD or ECG changes. The primary outcome of death or new MI at 7 days occurred in 4.2% of the heparin group vs. 3.6% of the hirudin group (p = 0.077). If recurrent angina were also assessed, this composite outcome occurred in 6.7% and 5.6% of the groups, respectively (p = 0.019). Major bleeding occurred more often in the hirudin group (1.2%) than in the heparin group (0.7%; p = 0.01); however, there was no difference in life threatening events.

BOTTOM LINE

Compared to heparin, recombinant hirudin resulted in a nearly significant improvement in the incidence of CV death, MI, and refractory angina in patients with UA or NSTEMI; however, it was also associated with an increase in major bleeding.

ACUTE CORONARY SYNDROMES

CLINICAL TRIAL FEATURES, THERAPEUTICS AND ENDPOINTS

DISEASE STATES
- ☑ **ACS** ☐ STEMI/QMI ☑ **NSTEMI/NQMI** ☑ **UA**
- ☐ VTE ☐ DVT ☐ PE ☐ CVA

MEDICATIONS
- ☐ **Platelet Antagonist**
  - ☐ Aspirin
  - ☐ Clopidogrel
  - ☐ IIb/IIIa Receptor Antagonist
    - ☐ Abciximab
    - ☐ Eptifibatide
    - ☐ Lamifiban
    - ☐ Tirofiban
- ☐ **Heparin**
- ☐ **LMWH**
  - ☐ Enoxaparin
  - ☐ Dalteparin
  - ☐ Nadroparin
  - ☐ Tinzaparin
  - ☐ Reviparin
- ☑ **Direct Thrombin Inhibitor**
  - ☑ **Hirudin**
  - ☐ Hirulog
- ☐ **Fibrinolytic / Thrombolytic**
  - ☐ Alteplase
  - ☐ Reteplase
  - ☐ Tenecteplase
  - ☐ Anistreplase
  - ☐ Streptokinase
- ☐ **Other cardiac medications (captopril, magnesium, nitrates)**

PROCEDURES
- ☐ Angioplasty ☐ Stent
- ☐ CABG ☐ PCI

THERAPEUTIC ENDPOINT
- ☑ **Treatment** ☐ Prophylaxis

CLINICAL ENVIRONMENT
- ☑ **Inpatient** ☐ Outpatient

DIRECT THROMBIN INHIBITORS

TIMI 9B — THROMBOLYSIS AND THROMBIN INHIBITION IN MYOCARDIAL INFARCTION

TRIAL FULL NAME
Hirudin in Acute Myocardial Infarction

PUBLICATION DATA
Circulation 1996; 94: 911-921

STUDY DATES
1994 to 1995

AUTHOR(S)
E Antman

CLINICAL TRIAL SUMMARY

This was a multinational, randomized comparison of IV hirudin (0.1 mg/kg bolus then 0.1 mg/kg/hour infusion) vs. IV heparin. The 3,002 patients had CP within 12 hours of presentation and STEMI or new BBB; all received a thrombolytic (tPA or STK). The primary end point was death, recurrent nonfatal MI, or development of CHF or Cardiogenic Shock by 30 days. The endpoint occurred in 11.9% of the heparin group and 12.9% of the hirudin group (p = NS). Major bleeding complications were comparable between groups.

BOTTOM LINE

Heparin and Hirudin, in combination with a thrombolytic, resulted in equal ischemic complications and safety.

ACUTE CORONARY SYNDROMES

CLINICAL TRIAL FEATURES, THERAPEUTICS AND ENDPOINTS

DISEASE STATES
- ☑ **ACS** ☑ **STEMI/QMI** ☐ NSTEMI/NQMI ☑ **UA**
- ☐ VTE ☐ DVT ☐ PE ☐ CVA

MEDICATIONS
- ☐ **Platelet Antagonist**
  - ☐ Aspirin
  - ☐ Clopidogrel
  - ☐ IIb/IIIa Receptor Antagonist
    - ☐ Abciximab
    - ☐ Eptifibatide
    - ☐ Lamifiban
    - ☐ Tirofiban
- ☑ **Heparin**
- ☐ **LMWH**
  - ☐ Enoxaparin
  - ☐ Dalteparin
  - ☐ Nadroparin
  - ☐ Tinzaparin
  - ☐ Reviparin
- ☑ **Direct Thrombin Inhibitor**
  - ☑ **Hirudin**
  - ☐ Hirulog
- ☑ **Fibrinolytic / Thrombolytic**
  - ☑ **Alteplase**
  - ☐ Reteplase
  - ☐ Tenecteplase
  - ☐ Anistreplase
  - ☑ **Streptokinase**
- ☐ **Other cardiac medications (captopril, magnesium, nitrates)**

PROCEDURES
- ☐ Angioplasty ☐ Stent
- ☐ CABG ☐ PCI

THERAPEUTIC ENDPOINT
- ☑ **Treatment** ☐ Prophylaxis

CLINICAL ENVIRONMENT
- ☑ **Inpatient** ☐ Outpatient

DIRECT THROMBIN INHIBITORS

CAPRIE

TRIAL FULL NAME
A randomized, blinded, trial of clopidogrel versus aspirin in patients at risk of ischaemic events

PUBLICATION DATA
Lancet 1996; 348: 1329-39

STUDY DATES
1992-1995

AUTHOR(S)
M Gent, D Beaumont, J Blanchard, et al

CLINICAL TRIAL SUMMARY

This was a randomized, double-blind comparison of clopidogrel 75 mg qd vs. aspirin 325 mg qd. The 19,185 patients had previous atherosclerotic vascular disease. Endpoints were stroke, MI, or vascular death during the 1-3 year follow-up. Endpoints occurred in 5.3% of the clopidogrel group and in 5.83% of the aspirin group (p = 0.043). Safety profiles were comparable.

BOTTOM LINE

Compared with aspirin, long-term use of clopidogrel significantly reduces the incidence of ischemic stroke, MI, or vascular death in patients with atherosclerotic vascular disease.

ACUTE CORONARY SYNDROMES

CLINICAL TRIAL FEATURES, THERAPEUTICS AND ENDPOINTS

DISEASE STATES
☑ ACS ☑ STEMI/QMI ☑ NSTEMI/NQMI ☑ UA
❑ VTE ❑ DVT ❑ PE ☑ CVA

MEDICATIONS
☑ **Platelet Antagonist**
- ☑ **Aspirin**
- ☑ **Clopidogrel**
- ❑ IIb/IIIa Receptor Antagonist
  - ❑ Abciximab
  - ❑ Eptifibatide
  - ❑ Lamifiban
  - ❑ Tirofiban

❑ **Heparin**
❑ **LMWH**
- ❑ Enoxaparin
- ❑ Dalteparin
- ❑ Nadroparin
- ❑ Tinzaparin
- ❑ Reviparin

❑ **Direct Thrombin Inhibitor**
- ❑ Hirudin
- ❑ Hirulog

❑ **Fibrinolytic / Thrombolytic**
- ❑ Alteplase
- ❑ Reteplase
- ❑ Tenecteplase
- ❑ Anistreplase
- ❑ Streptokinase

❑ **Other cardiac medications (captopril, magnesium, nitrates)**

PROCEDURES
❑ Angioplasty ❑ Stent
❑ CABG ❑ PCI

THERAPEUTIC ENDPOINT
❑ Treatment ☑ **Prophylaxis**

CLINICAL ENVIRONMENT
❑ Inpatient ☑ **Outpatient**

ANTI ADP

CURE — CLOPIDOGREL IN UNSTABLE ANGINA TO PREVENT RECURRENT EVENTS

TRIAL FULL NAME
The clopidogrel in Unstable angina to prevent Recurrent Events trial program

PUBLICATION DATA
Eur Heart J 2000: 2033-2041

STUDY DATES

AUTHOR(S)
SR Mehta, S Yusuf, S Anan, et al

CLINICAL TRIAL SUMMARY

This was a randomized, double-blind, multicenter, comparison of clopidogrel (300 mg load followed by 75 mg daily) with aspirin vs. aspirin alone in a secondary prevention trial. The 12,563 patients had UA or NQMI, received standard medical care, and were followed up for a mean of 9 months. The primary endpoints of cardiovascular death, MI, stroke, or refractory ischemia, were decreased by 20% in the clopidogrel group. Benefit achieved by 30 days was maintained though the follow up period.

BOTTOM LINE

For secondary prevention, compared to aspirin alone, clopidogrel plus with aspirin significantly reduced the incidence of new atherosclerotic disease events.

ACUTE CORONARY SYNDROMES

CLINICAL TRIAL FEATURES, THERAPEUTICS AND ENDPOINTS

DISEASE STATES
☑ ACS ☑ STEMI/QMI ☑ NSTEMI/NQMI ☑ UA
❑ VTE ❑ DVT ❑ PE ❑ CVA

MEDICATIONS
☑ **Platelet Antagonist**
- ☑ **Aspirin**
- ☑ **Clopidogrel**
- ❑ IIb/IIIa Receptor Antagonist
  - ❑ Abciximab
  - ❑ Eptifibatide
  - ❑ Lamifiban
  - ❑ Tirofiban

❑ **Heparin**
❑ **LMWH**
- ❑ Enoxaparin
- ❑ Dalteparin
- ❑ Nadroparin
- ❑ Tinzaparin
- ❑ Reviparin

❑ **Direct Thrombin Inhibitor**
- ❑ Hirudin
- ❑ Hirulog

❑ **Fibrinolytic / Thrombolytic**
- ❑ Alteplase
- ❑ Reteplase
- ❑ Tenecteplase
- ❑ Anistreplase
- ❑ Streptokinase

❑ **Other cardiac medications (captopril, magnesium, nitrates)**

PROCEDURES
❑ Angioplasty ❑ Stent
❑ CABG ❑ PCI

THERAPEUTIC ENDPOINT
❑ Treatment ☑ **Prophylaxis**

CLINICAL ENVIRONMENT
❑ Inpatient ☑ **Outpatient**

ANTI ADP

CAPTURE

TRIAL FULL NAME

Randomized placebo-controlled trial of abciximab before and during coronary intervention in refractory unstable angina

PUBLICATION DATA

Lancet 1997; 349: 1429-35

STUDY DATES

1993-1995

AUTHOR(S)

ML Simoons, W Rutsch, A Vahanian, J Adgey, A Maseri, C Vassanelli, et al

CLINICAL TRIAL SUMMARY

This was a multicenter, randomized comparison of abciximab (0.25 mg/kg bolus then 0.125 mcg/kg/hour for 12 hours) vs. placebo. The 1,265 patients had refractory UA despite medical therapy and had undergone angiography revealing culprit lesions. Patients then received abciximab or placebo and then underwent PCI. The primary endpoint was the occurrence of death, MI, or urgent intervention for recurrent ischemia at 30 days. The end point occurred in 11.3% of the abciximab patients and 15.9% of the placebo group (p = 0.012). The rate of MI was lower in the abciximab group than in the placebo group before PCI (0.6% vs. 2.1%) and during PCI (2.6% vs. 5.5%). However, major bleeding occurred more often in the abciximab group (3.8% vs 1.9%; p = 0.043). Meticulous wound care was not done in this trial. Outcomes were comparable at 6 months.

BOTTOM LINE

Abciximab significantly reduced the incidence of death, MI, or need for repeat intervention at 30 days in patients with refractory UA who underwent a PCI; however, major bleeding was increased.

ACUTE CORONARY SYNDROMES

CLINICAL TRIAL FEATURES, THERAPEUTICS AND ENDPOINTS

DISEASE STATES

☑ **ACS** ❑ STEMI/QMI ❑ NSTEMI/NQMI ☑ **UA**
❑ VTE ❑ DVT ❑ PE ❑ **CVA**

MEDICATIONS

☑ **Platelet Antagonist**
- ❑ Aspirin
- ❑ Clopidogrel
- ☑ **IIb/IIIa Receptor Antagonist**
  - ☑ **Abciximab**
  - ❑ Eptifibatide
  - ❑ Lamifiban
  - ❑ Tirofiban

❑ **Heparin**
❑ **LMWH**
- ❑ Enoxaparin
- ❑ Dalteparin
- ❑ Nadroparin
- ❑ Tinzaparin
- ❑ Reviparin

❑ **Direct Thrombin Inhibitor**
- ❑ Hirudin
- ❑ Hirulog

❑ **Fibrinolytic / Thrombolytic**
- ❑ Alteplase
- ❑ Reteplase
- ❑ Tenecteplase
- ❑ Anistreplase
- ❑ Streptokinase

❑ **Other cardiac medications (captopril, magnesium, nitrates)**

PROCEDURES

☑ **Angioplasty** ❑ Stent
☑ **CABG** ☑ **PCI**

THERAPEUTIC ENDPOINT

☑ **Treatment** ❑ Prophylaxis

CLINICAL ENVIRONMENT

☑ **Inpatient** ❑ Outpatient

IIB/IIIA WITH PROCEDURAL CORONARY INTERVENTION

EPIC — EVALUATION OF 7E3 FOR THE PREVENTION OF ISCHEMIC COMPLICATIONS

TRIAL FULL NAME

Use of Monoclonal Antibody Directed Against the platelet glycoprotein IIb/IIIa receptor in high-risk coronary angioplasty

PUBLICATION DATA

NEJM 1994; 330: 956-61

STUDY DATES

1991-1992

AUTHOR(S)

R M. Califf, N Shadoff, E Bates, W Knopf, T Aversano, P Gurbe, et al

CLINICAL TRIAL SUMMARY

This was a multicenter, prospective, randomized, double-blind comparison of abciximab (0.25 mg/kg bolus then 10 mcg/min infusion) vs. abciximab (0.25 mg/kg bolus without infusion) vs. placebo. The 2099 patients were to undergo elective, urgent, or emergent PCI. The primary end points were death, MI, or unplanned PCI at 30 days. The endpoint occurred in 12.8% of the placebo group and in 8.3% of the abciximab bolus + infusion group (p = 0.008). The abciximab bolus only groups did not result in a significant reduction of the outcome parameters. Major bleeding occurred twice as often in the abciximab group (14%) as the placebo group (7%; p = 0.001). Attention to vascular hemostasis was poor in this first major abciximab trial.

BOTTOM LINE

Abciximab bolus plus infusion significantly reduced the incidence of death, MI, or unplanned PCI in patients who were undergoing PCI. Abciximab was also associated with a significant increase in bleeding, albeit attempts at vascular hemostasis were poor.

ACUTE CORONARY SYNDROMES

CLINICAL TRIAL FEATURES, THERAPEUTICS AND ENDPOINTS

DISEASE STATES

☑ **ACS** ☑ **STEMI/QMI** ☑ **NSTEMI/NQMI** ☑ **UA**
❑ VTE ❑ DVT ❑ PE ❑ CVA

MEDICATIONS

☑ **Platelet Antagonist**
- ❑ Aspirin
- ❑ Clopidogrel
- ☑ **IIb/IIIa Receptor Antagonist**
  - ☑ **Abciximab**
  - ❑ Eptifibatide
  - ❑ Lamifiban
  - ❑ Tirofiban

❑ **Heparin**
❑ **LMWH**
- ❑ Enoxaparin
- ❑ Dalteparin
- ❑ Nadroparin
- ❑ Tinzaparin
- ❑ Reviparin

❑ **Direct Thrombin Inhibitor**
- ❑ Hirudin
- ❑ Hirulog

❑ **Fibrinolytic / Thrombolytic**
- ❑ Alteplase
- ❑ Reteplase
- ❑ Tenecteplase
- ❑ Anistreplase
- ❑ Streptokinase

❑ **Other cardiac medications (captopril, magnesium, nitrates)**

PROCEDURES

☑ **Angioplasty** ☑ **Stent**
☑ **CABG** ☑ **PCI**

THERAPEUTIC ENDPOINT

☑ **Treatment** ❑ Prophylaxis

CLINICAL ENVIRONMENT

☑ **Inpatient** ❑ Outpatient

IIB/IIIA WITH PROCEDURAL CORONARY INTERVENTION

EPILOG | EVALUATION OF PTCA TO IMPROVE LONG-TERM OUTCOME WITH ABCIXIMAB GPIIB/IIIA BLOCKADE

TRIAL FULL NAME
Platelet Glycoprotein IIb/IIIa receptor blockade and low-dose heparin during percutaneous coronary revascularization

PUBLICATION DATA
NEJM 1997; 336: 1689-96

STUDY DATES
1995

AUTHOR(S)
EJ Topol, RM Cliff, AM Lincoff, JE Tcheng, CF Cabot, HF Weisman, et al

CLINICAL TRIAL SUMMARY

This was a multicenter, randomized, double-blind, placebo-controlled, three-armed, comparison of abciximab (0.25 mg/kg bolus then 0.125 mcg/kg/hour for 12 hours) with low-dose or standard-dose heparin (70 IU/kg or 100 IU/kg bolus, respectively; each followed by further weight- and algorithm-based boli) vs. placebo with standard heparin. The 2,792 patients were undergoing elective or urgent PCI. The primary end points were death, MI, or urgent revascularization within 30 days. The end point occurred in 11.7% of the placebo group and in 5.3% of the abciximab (with low or standard dosed heparin) group ($p < 0.001$). Major bleeding was comparable among the 3 groups. Wound care was more meticulous than in the previous CAPRIE or EPIC trials.

BOTTOM LINE

Abciximab plus heparin significantly reduced death, MI, or urgent revascularization at 30 days in patients who were undergoing a PCI.

ACUTE CORONARY SYNDROMES

CLINICAL TRIAL FEATURES, THERAPEUTICS AND ENDPOINTS

DISEASE STATES
- ☑ ACS ❑ STEMI/QMI ❑ NSTEMI/NQMI ☑ UA
- ❑ VTE ❑ DVT ❑ PE ❑ CVA

MEDICATIONS
- ☑ **Platelet Antagonist**
  - ☑ **Aspirin**
  - ❑ Clopidogrel
  - ☑ **IIb/IIIa Receptor Antagonist**
    - ☑ **Abciximab**
    - ❑ Eptifibatide
    - ❑ Lamifiban
    - ❑ Tirofiban
- ☑ **Heparin**
- ❑ **LMWH**
  - ❑ Enoxaparin
  - ❑ Dalteparin
  - ❑ Nadroparin
  - ❑ Tinzaparin
  - ❑ Reviparin
- ❑ **Direct Thrombin Inhibitor**
  - ❑ Hirudin
  - ❑ Hirulog
- ❑ **Fibrinolytic / Thrombolytic**
  - ❑ Alteplase
  - ❑ Reteplase
  - ❑ Tenecteplase
  - ❑ Anistreplase
  - ❑ Streptokinase
- ❑ **Other cardiac medications (captopril, magnesium, nitrates)**

PROCEDURES
- ☑ **Angioplasty** ☑ **Stent**
- ❑ CABG ☑ **PCI**

THERAPEUTIC ENDPOINT
- ☑ **Treatment** ❑ Prophylaxis

CLINICAL ENVIRONMENT
- ☑ **Inpatient** ❑ Outpatient

IIB/IIIA WITH PROCEDURAL CORONARY INTERVENTION

EPISTENT | EVALUATION OF PLATELET IIB/IIIA INHIBITOR FOR STENTING

TRIAL FULL NAME
Randomized placebo-controlled and balloon-angioplasty-controlled trial to assess safety of coronary stenting with use of platelet glycoprotein-IIb/IIIa blockade

PUBLICATION DATA
Lancet 1998; 352:87-92

STUDY DATES
1996 to 1997

AUTHOR(S)
E J Topol, AM Lincof, RM Califf, JE Tcheng, et al

CLINICAL TRIAL SUMMARY

This was a multicenter, randomized, double-blind comparison of stent placement plus abciximab (0.25 mg/kg bolus then 0.125 mcg/kg/hour for 12 hours) vs. PTCA plus abciximab vs. stent placement plus placebo. The 2,399 patients were undergoing elective or urgent PCI. The primary end points were death, MI, or need for urgent revascularization at 30 days. The endpoint occurred in 10.8% of the stent plus placebo group, 5.3% ($p < 0.001$) of the stent plus abciximab group, and 6.9% ($p = 0.007$) of the PTCA plus abciximab group. Death and large MI occurred less with abciximab: 7.8% with placebo, 3.0% ($p < 0.001$) with stent plus abciximab, and 4.7% ($p = 0.01$) with angioplasty plus abciximab. Major bleeding complications were comparable among groups. Meticulous wound care was used in this trial.

BOTTOM LINE

Abciximab significantly reduced the incidence of death, MI, or need for urgent revascularization at 30 days in patients undergoing either stent placement or PTCA

ACUTE CORONARY SYNDROMES

CLINICAL TRIAL FEATURES, THERAPEUTICS AND ENDPOINTS

DISEASE STATES
- ☑ ACS ☑ STEMI/QMI ☑ NSTEMI/NQMI ☑ UA
- ❑ VTE ❑ DVT ❑ PE ❑ CVA

MEDICATIONS
- ☑ **Platelet Antagonist**
  - ❑ Aspirin
  - ❑ Clopidogrel
  - ☑ **IIb/IIIa Receptor Antagonist**
    - ☑ **Abciximab**
    - ❑ Eptifibatide
    - ❑ Lamifiban
    - ❑ Tirofiban
- ❑ **Heparin**
- ❑ **LMWH**
  - ❑ Enoxaparin
  - ❑ Dalteparin
  - ❑ Nadroparin
  - ❑ Tinzaparin
  - ❑ Reviparin
- ❑ **Direct Thrombin Inhibitor**
  - ❑ Hirudin
  - ❑ Hirulog
- ❑ **Fibrinolytic / Thrombolytic**
  - ❑ Alteplase
  - ❑ Reteplase
  - ❑ Tenecteplase
  - ❑ Anistreplase
  - ❑ Streptokinase
- ❑ **Other cardiac medications (captopril, magnesium, nitrates)**

PROCEDURES
- ☑ **Angioplasty** ☑ **Stent**
- ❑ CABG ☑ **PCI**

THERAPEUTIC ENDPOINT
- ☑ **Treatment** ❑ Prophylaxis

CLINICAL ENVIRONMENT
- ☑ **Inpatient** ❑ Outpatient

IIB/IIIA WITH PROCEDURAL CORONARY INTERVENTION

IMPACT-II — INTEGRILIN TO MINIMIZE PLATELET AGGREGATION AND CORONARY THROMBOSIS II

TRIAL FULL NAME
Randomized placebo-controlled trial of effect of eptifibatide on complications of percutaneous coronary intervention: IMPACT-II

PUBLICATION DATA
Lancet 1997; 349:1422-28

STUDY DATES
1993 to 1994

AUTHOR(S)
JE Tcheng, AM Lincoff, KN Sigmon, KL Lee, MM Kitt, RM Califf, EJ Topol, et al

CLINICAL TRIAL SUMMARY

This was a multicenter, randomized, double-blind, comparison of (1) eptifibatide 135 mcg/kg bolus with 0.5 mcg/kg/min infusion, (2) eptifibatide 135 mcg/kg bolus with 0.75 mcg/kg/min infusion, and (3) placebo in 4010 patients receiving elective, urgent, or emergency PCI. The PCI was started within 1 hour of drug administration. All patients received aspirin. The primary endpoint was the 30 day composite of death, MI, or need for repeat PCI or CABG. The composite endpoint occurred in 11.4% of placebo group, 9.9% of the high-dose eptifibatide group ($p = 0.22$), and in 9.2% of the low dose eptifibatide group ($p = 0.063$). Major bleeding was comparable among groups.

BOTTOM LINE

Low-dose eptifibatide during PCI resulted in a trend towards a reduced rate of death, MI, or need for repeat revascularization at 30 days.

ACUTE CORONARY SYNDROMES

CLINICAL TRIAL FEATURES, THERAPEUTICS AND ENDPOINTS

DISEASE STATES
- ☑ **ACS** ☑ **STEMI/QMI** ☑ **NSTEMI/NQMI** ☑ **UA**
- ❑ VTE ❑ DVT ❑ PE ❑ CVA

MEDICATIONS
- ☑ **Platelet Antagonist**
  - ❑ Aspirin
  - ❑ Clopidogrel
  - ☑ **IIb/IIIa Receptor Antagonist**
    - ❑ Abciximab
    - ☑ **Eptifibatide**
    - ❑ Lamifiban
    - ❑ Tirofiban
- ❑ **Heparin**
- ❑ **LMWH**
  - ❑ Enoxaparin
  - ❑ Dalteparin
  - ❑ Nadroparin
  - ❑ Tinzaparin
  - ❑ Reviparin
- ❑ **Direct Thrombin Inhibitor**
  - ❑ Hirudin
  - ❑ Hirulog
- ❑ **Fibrinolytic / Thrombolytic**
  - ❑ Alteplase
  - ❑ Reteplase
  - ❑ Tenecteplase
  - ❑ Anistreplase
  - ❑ Streptokinase
- ❑ **Other cardiac medications (captopril, magnesium, nitrates)**

PROCEDURES
- ☑ **Angioplasty** ❑ Stent
- ❑ CABG ☑ **PCI**

THERAPEUTIC ENDPOINT
- ☑ **Treatment** ❑ Prophylaxis

CLINICAL ENVIRONMENT
- ☑ **Inpatient** ❑ Outpatient

IIB/IIIA WITH PROCEDURAL CORONARY INTERVENTION

RESTORE — RANDOMIZED EFFICACY STUDY OF TIROFIBAN FOR OUTCOMES AND RESTENOSIS

TRIAL FULL NAME
Effects of Platelet Glycoprotein IIb/IIIa Blockade with Tirofiban on Adverse Cardiac Events in patients with Unstable Angina or Acute Myocardial Infarction undergoing Coronary Angioplasty

PUBLICATION DATA
Circulation 1997; 96:1445-1453

STUDY DATES
1995

AUTHOR(S)
SB King III, P Hanrath, W Paulus, JA Sosa, D Muller, JR Resar, W Herzog, et al

CLINICAL TRIAL SUMMARY

This was a randomized, double-blind, comparison of tirofiban (10 mcg/kg bolus with 0.15 mcg/kg/min infusion for 36 hours) vs. placebo in 2141 patients receiving PCI within 72 hours of presentation with UA or MI. All patients received aspirin and heparin. The primary endpoint was the composite of death, MI, or need for repeat PCI or CABG. At 2 days, the endpoint had occurred in 8.7% of the placebo group and in 5.4% of the tirofiban group ($p < 0.005$). However, by 30 days, the respective occurrences were 12.2% and 10.3% ($p = 0.160$). Major bleeding was comparable among groups.

BOTTOM LINE

Tirofiban reduced the incidence of death, MI, or need for revascularization at 2 days but not by 30 days when used in patients with UA or MI who received a PCI.

ACUTE CORONARY SYNDROMES

CLINICAL TRIAL FEATURES, THERAPEUTICS AND ENDPOINTS

DISEASE STATES
- ☑ **ACS** ❑ STEMI/QMI ☑ **NSTEMI/NQMI** ☑ **UA**
- ❑ VTE ❑ DVT ❑ PE ❑ CVA

MEDICATIONS
- ☑ **Platelet Antagonist**
  - ☑ **Aspirin**
  - ❑ Clopidogrel
  - ❑ **IIb/IIIa Receptor Antagonist**
    - ❑ Abciximab
    - ❑ Eptifibatide
    - ❑ Lamifiban
    - ❑ Tirofiban
- ☑ **Heparin**
- ❑ **LMWH**
  - ❑ Enoxaparin
  - ❑ Dalteparin
  - ❑ Nadroparin
  - ❑ Tinzaparin
  - ❑ Reviparin
- ❑ **Direct Thrombin Inhibitor**
  - ❑ Hirudin
  - ❑ Hirulog
- ❑ **Fibrinolytic / Thrombolytic**
  - ❑ Alteplase
  - ❑ Reteplase
  - ❑ Tenecteplase
  - ❑ Anistreplase
  - ❑ Streptokinase
- ❑ **Other cardiac medications (captopril, magnesium, nitrates)**

PROCEDURES
- ❑ Angioplasty ❑ Stent
- ❑ CABG ❑ PCI

THERAPEUTIC ENDPOINT
- ☑ **Treatment** ❑ Prophylaxis

CLINICAL ENVIRONMENT
- ☑ **Inpatient** ☑ **Outpatient**

IIB/IIIA WITH PROCEDURAL CORONARY INTERVENTION

TARGET

TRIAL FULL NAME
A direct comparison of tirofiban and abciximab during percutaneous coronary revascularization and stent placement

PUBLICATION DATA
Presented at the American Heart Association Meeting; Scientific Sessions 2000

STUDY DATES
No data

AUTHOR(S)
Moliterno DJ, Topol EJ

CLINICAL TRIAL SUMMARY

This was a multicenter, randomized double-blind, double-dummy, comparison of abciximab (0.25 mg/kg bolus with 0.125 mcg/kg/min infusion X 12 hours) vs. tirofiban (10 mcg/kg bolus with 0.15 mcg/kg/min infusion for 36 hours) in 4812 patients undergoing non-emergency PCI with stent placement. All patients received aspirin, heparin, and clopidogrel. The primary endpoint was the composite of death, MI, or urgent target vessel revascularization at 30 days. This composite occurred in 6.01% of the abciximab group and in 7.55% of the tirofiban group (p = 0.037). This difference was primarily due to the difference in MI. This was the first head-to-head trial of two GP IIb/IIIa inhibitors.

BOTTOM LINE

Compared to tirofiban, abciximab significantly reduced the incidence of death, MI, or urgent target vessel revascularization at 30 days in patients undergoing non-emergency PCI.

ACUTE CORONARY SYNDROMES

CLINICAL TRIAL FEATURES, THERAPEUTICS AND ENDPOINTS

DISEASE STATES
- ☑ **ACS** ☐ STEMI/QMI ☐ NSTEMI/NQMI ☑ **UA**
- ☐ VTE ☐ DVT ☐ PE ☐ CVA

MEDICATIONS
- ☑ **Platelet Antagonist**
  - ☐ Aspirin
  - ☐ Clopidogrel
  - ☑ **IIb/IIIa Receptor Antagonist**
    - ☑ **Abciximab**
    - ☐ Eptifibatide
    - ☐ Lamifiban
    - ☑ **Tirofiban**
- ☐ **Heparin**
- ☐ **LMWH**
  - ☐ Enoxaparin
  - ☐ Dalteparin
  - ☐ Nadroparin
  - ☐ Tinzaparin
  - ☐ Reviparin
- ☐ **Direct Thrombin Inhibitor**
  - ☐ Hirudin
  - ☐ Hirulog
- ☐ **Fibrinolytic / Thrombolytic**
  - ☐ Alteplase
  - ☐ Reteplase
  - ☐ Tenecteplase
  - ☐ Anistreplase
  - ☐ Streptokinase
- ☐ **Other cardiac medications (captopril, magnesium, nitrates)**

PROCEDURES
- ☐ Angioplasty ☑ **Stent**
- ☐ CABG ☑ **PCI**

THERAPEUTIC ENDPOINT
- ☑ **Treatment** ☐ Prophylaxis

CLINICAL ENVIRONMENT
- ☑ **Inpatient** ☐ Outpatient

IIB/IIIA WITH PROCEDURAL CORONARY INTERVENTION

GUSTO-4 — GLOBAL UTILIZATION OF STEPTOKINASE AND TPA FOR OCCLUDED CORONARY ARTERIES

TRIAL FULL NAME
GUSTO 4 Acute Coronary Syndromes

PUBLICATION DATA
Abstract at the European Society of Cardiology Congress; August 2000

STUDY DATES
1990 to 1993

AUTHOR(S)
Simoons M

CLINICAL TRIAL SUMMARY

This was a multicenter, randomized comparison of placebo vs. abciximab infusions (0.25 mg/kg bolus then either a 24 vs. 48 hour infusion at 0.125 mcg/kg/hour) in 7800 patients with CP and either ST depression on ECG or marker elevation. Percutaneous coronary intervention was not planned. The primary endpoint was the composite of death or MI at 30 days. The endpoint occurred in 8.0% of the placebo group, 8.2% of the 24 hour abciximab group, and 9.1% of the 48 hour abciximab group (p = NS). Major bleeding occurred in 0.3%, 0.6%, and 1.0% of the groups, respectively. A substudy compared dalteparin (974 patients) with IV heparin. There was no difference in the primary endpoint between the groups.

BOTTOM LINE

Neither 24 nor 48 hour infusions of abciximab significantly reduced the 30 day incidence of death or MI in patients with UA or NSTEMI. In addition, dalteparin also did not affect outcome in comparison to IV heparin.

ACUTE CORONARY SYNDROMES

CLINICAL TRIAL FEATURES, THERAPEUTICS AND ENDPOINTS

DISEASE STATES
- ☑ **ACS** ☐ STEMI/QMI ☑ **NSTEMI/NQMI** ☑ **UA**
- ☐ VTE ☐ DVT ☐ PE ☐ CVA

MEDICATIONS
- ☑ **Platelet Antagonist**
  - ☐ Aspirin
  - ☐ Clopidogrel
  - ☑ **IIb/IIIa Receptor Antagonist**
    - ☑ **Abciximab**
    - ☐ Eptifibatide
    - ☐ Lamifiban
    - ☐ Tirofiban
- ☑ **Heparin**
- ☑ **LMWH**
  - ☐ Enoxaparin
  - ☑ **Dalteparin**
  - ☐ Nadroparin
  - ☐ Tinzaparin
  - ☐ Reviparin
- ☐ **Direct Thrombin Inhibitor**
  - ☐ Hirudin
  - ☐ Hirulog
- ☐ **Fibrinolytic / Thrombolytic**
  - ☐ Alteplase
  - ☐ Reteplase
  - ☐ Tenecteplase
  - ☐ Anistreplase
  - ☐ Streptokinase
- ☐ **Other cardiac medications (captopril, magnesium, nitrates)**

PROCEDURES
- ☐ Angioplasty ☐ Stent
- ☐ CABG ☐ PCI

THERAPEUTIC ENDPOINT
- ☑ **Treatment** ☐ Prophylaxis

CLINICAL ENVIRONMENT
- ☑ **Inpatient** ☐ Outpatient

IIB/IIIA ± PROCEDURAL CORONARY INTERVENTION

PARAGON — Platelet IIb/IIIa Antagonism for the Reduction of Acute coronary syndrome events in a Global Organization Network trial

Trial Full Name
International, Randomized, controlled trial of Lamifiban, Heparin, or both in Unstable Angina

Publication Data
Circulation 1998; 97:2386-2395

Study Dates
1995 to 1996

Author(s)
E Topol, R Califf, F Van de Werf, E Paolasso, DJ Moliterno, et al

Clinical Trial Summary

This was a randomized, double-blind, five arm comparison of placebo vs. high dose lamifiban (with or without heparin) vs. low dose lamifiban (with or without heparin). Drugs were administered for 3-5 days. The 2282 patients had CP within 12 hours plus ECG changes. End points included the composite of all-cause mortality or MI within 30 days (primary) or 6 months (secondary). Percutaneous coronary intervention was discouraged. No difference was found at 30 days. At 6 months, the composite rate was 13.7% in the low-dose lamifiban (with or without heparin) group and 17.9% in the placebo group ($p < 0.05$). However, major bleeding complications occurred in 10.5% of the lamifiban plus heparin group compared to 5.9% with heparin alone ($p < 0.05$). Differentiating the outcomes of those who received PCI from those who id not is difficult. These results are curious in that no difference existed at 30 days and also that the high-dose lamifiban group did not result in improvement (not considering bleeding issues).

Bottom Line

Lamifiban significantly reduced the incidence of death or MI at 6 months but not at 30 days in patients with UA and ECG changes; however, there was a significant increase in major bleeding.

ACUTE CORONARY SYNDROMES

Clinical Trial Features, Therapeutics and Endpoints

Disease States
- ☑ **ACS** ☐ STEMI/QMI ☑ **NSTEMI/NQMI** ☑ **UA**
- ☐ VTE ☐ DVT ☐ PE ☐ CVA

Medications
- ☑ **Platelet Antagonist**
  - ☐ Aspirin
  - ☐ Clopidogrel
  - ☑ **IIb/IIIa Receptor Antagonist**
    - ☐ Abciximab
    - ☐ Eptifibatide
    - ☑ **Lamifiban**
    - ☐ Tirofiban
- ☐ **Heparin**
- ☐ **LMWH**
  - ☐ Enoxaparin
  - ☐ Dalteparin
  - ☐ Nadroparin
  - ☐ Tinzaparin
  - ☐ Reviparin
- ☐ **Direct Thrombin Inhibitor**
  - ☐ Hirudin
  - ☐ Hirulog
- ☐ **Fibrinolytic / Thrombolytic**
  - ☐ Alteplase
  - ☐ Reteplase
  - ☐ Tenecteplase
  - ☐ Anistreplase
  - ☐ Streptokinase
- ☐ **Other cardiac medications (captopril, magnesium, nitrates)**

Procedures
- ☐ Angioplasty ☐ Stent
- ☐ CABG ☐ PCI

Therapeutic Endpoint
- ☑ **Treatment** ☐ Prophylaxis

Clinical Environment
- ☑ **Inpatient** ☐ Outpatient

IIB/IIIA ± PROCEDURAL CORONARY INTERVENTION

PRISM — Platelet Receptor Inhibition in Ischemic Syndrome Management

Trial Full Name
A comparison of Aspirin plus Tirofiban with Aspirin plus Heparin for Unstable Angina

Publication Data
NEJM 1998; 338:1498-505

Study Dates
1994 to 1996

Author(s)
H White, M Espeland, G FitzGerald, M Verstraete, M Cohen, LS Dreifus, et al

Clinical Trial Summary

This was a randomized, double-blind comparison of a 48-hour infusion of IV tirofiban (0.6 mcg/kg/min X 30 min then 0.15 mcg/kg/min) vs. IV heparin (5000 IU bolus then 1000 IU/hour). The 3,232 patients had CP within 24 hours plus either ECG changes, marker elevation, or evidence of prior coronary artery disease. Percutaneous coronary intervention was discouraged during the infusion. The primary endpoint; a composite of death, MI, or refractory ischemia at 48 hours; occurred in 3.8% of the tirofiban group and in 5.6% of the heparin group ($p < 0.05$). At 30 days, the rate of composite end point was similar in the two groups (15.9% vs. 17.1% in heparin group). Mortality was reduced at 30 days by tirofiban, 3.6% to 2.3% ($p < 0.05$). Major bleeding was equal between the two groups, 0.4% in each.

Bottom Line

Tirofiban significantly reduced the incidence of death, MI, or refractory ischemia at 2 days, but not at 30 days in patients with ACS. Differentiating the outcome of those treated with vs. without PCI is difficult.

ACUTE CORONARY SYNDROMES

Clinical Trial Features, Therapeutics and Endpoints

Disease States
- ☑ **ACS** ☐ STEMI/QMI ☑ **NSTEMI/NQMI** ☑ **UA**
- ☐ VTE ☐ DVT ☐ PE ☐ CVA

Medications
- ☑ **Platelet Antagonist**
  - ☐ Aspirin
  - ☐ Clopidogrel
  - ☑ **IIb/IIIa Receptor Antagonist**
    - ☐ Abciximab
    - ☐ Eptifibatide
    - ☐ Lamifiban
    - ☑ **Tirofiban**
- ☐ **Heparin**
- ☐ **LMWH**
  - ☐ Enoxaparin
  - ☐ Dalteparin
  - ☐ Nadroparin
  - ☐ Tinzaparin
  - ☐ Reviparin
- ☐ **Direct Thrombin Inhibitor**
  - ☐ Hirudin
  - ☐ Hirulog
- ☐ **Fibrinolytic / Thrombolytic**
  - ☐ Alteplase
  - ☐ Reteplase
  - ☐ Tenecteplase
  - ☐ Anistreplase
  - ☐ Streptokinase
- ☑ **Other cardiac medications (captopril, magnesium, nitrates)**

Procedures
- ☐ Angioplasty ☐ Stent
- ☐ CABG ☐ PCI

Therapeutic Endpoint
- ☑ **Treatment** ☐ Prophylaxis

Clinical Environment
- ☑ **Inpatient** ☐ Outpatient

IIB/IIIA ± PROCEDURAL CORONARY INTERVENTION

PRISM-PLUS — PLATELET RECEPTOR INHIBITION IN ISCHEMIC SYNDROME MANAGEMENT IN PATIENTS LIMITED BY UNSTABLE SIGNS AND SYMPTOMS

TRIAL FULL NAME
Inhibition of the Platelet Glycoprotein IIb/IIIa receptor with Tirofiban in Unstable Angina and Non-Q wave infarction

PUBLICATION DATA
NEJM 1998; 338:1488-97

STUDY DATES
1994 to 1996

AUTHOR(S)
Theroux, Pierre

CLINICAL TRIAL SUMMARY

This was a randomized, double-blind comparison of 48-hour infusions of either tirofiban alone, heparin alone, or both tirofiban and heparin. The 1,915 patients had CP within 12 hours of presentation and either EKG changes or CK-MB elevation. The primary and secondary end points were the composite of death, new MI, or refractory ischemia at 7 days, 30 days, or 6 months. The tirofiban alone group was stopped prematurely because of excess mortality at seven days (4.6% vs. 1.1% in the heparin alone group). The composite-endpoints at 7 days (12.9% vs. 17.9%), 30 days (18.5% vs. 22.3%), and 6 months (27.7% vs. 32.1%) were lower among the patients receiving tirofiban plus heparin vs. heparin alone (all with $p < 0.05$). Percutaneous coronary intervention was discouraged during the 48 hour infusion and encouraged thereafter; 54% were revascularized. Bleeding complications were similar among groups. The authors concluded that when administered with heparin and aspirin, tirofiban was associated with a lower incidence of ischemic events in patients with ACS than in those receiving only heparin and aspirin.

BOTTOM LINE

Tirofiban, in combination with heparin and aspirin, reduced deaths, MI, or refractory ischemia in patients with ECG changes or marker elevation; outcomes of those who received a PCI could not be differentiated from those who did not.

ACUTE CORONARY SYNDROMES

CLINICAL TRIAL FEATURES, THERAPEUTICS AND ENDPOINTS

DISEASE STATES
- ☑ **ACS** ☐ STEMI/QMI ☑ **NSTEMI/NQMI** ☑ **UA**
- ☐ VTE ☐ DVT ☐ PE ☐ CVA

MEDICATIONS
- ☑ **Platelet Antagonist**
  - ☑ **Aspirin**
  - ☐ Clopidogrel
  - ☑ **IIb/IIIa Receptor Antagonist**
    - ☐ Abciximab
    - ☐ Eptifibatide
    - ☐ Lamifiban
    - ☑ **Tirofiban**
- ☑ **Heparin**
- ☐ **LMWH**
  - ☐ Enoxaparin
  - ☐ Dalteparin
  - ☐ Nadroparin
  - ☐ Tinzaparin
  - ☐ Reviparin
- ☐ **Direct Thrombin Inhibitor**
  - ☐ Hirudin
  - ☐ Hirulog
- ☐ **Fibrinolytic / Thrombolytic**
  - ☐ Alteplase
  - ☐ Reteplase
  - ☐ Tenecteplase
  - ☐ Anistreplase
  - ☐ Streptokinase
- ☐ **Other cardiac medications (captopril, magnesium, nitrates)**

PROCEDURES
- ☐ Angioplasty ☐ Stent
- ☐ CABG ☑ **PCI**

THERAPEUTIC ENDPOINT
- ☑ **Treatment** ☐ Prophylaxis

CLINICAL ENVIRONMENT
- ☑ **Inpatient** ☐ Outpatient

IIB/IIIA ± PROCEDURAL CORONARY INTERVENTION

PURSUIT — PLATELET GLYCOPROTEIN IIB/IIIA UNSTABLE ANGINA: RECEPTOR SUPPRESSION USING INTEGRILIN THERAPY TRIAL

TRIAL FULL NAME
Inhibition of Platelet Glycoprotein IIb/IIIa with Eptifibatide in patients with ACS

PUBLICATION DATA
NEJM, 1998; 339:436-43

STUDY DATES
1995 to 1997

AUTHOR(S)
E Topol, R Califf, M Simoons, R Diaz, E Paolasso, R A. Harrington, et al

CLINICAL TRIAL SUMMARY

This was a randomized, double-blind, worldwide comparison of ≤ 72 hour infusions of placebo vs. one of two eptifibatide doses. The 10,948 patients had CP within 24 hours plus either an ECG change or an elevation of the CKMB. The low dose eptifibatide arm was dropped early in the trial after the safety of the higher dose was evident. Heparin use was optional; PCI was done at physician discretion. The primary end point, a composite of death or non-fatal MI at 30 days, occurred in 14.2% of the eptifibatide group and in 15.7% of the placebo group ($p < 0.05$). The benefit was apparent by 96 hours. Thirty-eight percent received revascularization; no difference in outcome was found in patients treated without a revascularization procedure. Outcomes within four regions of the world correlated with the frequency of revascularization within the regions. Major bleeding occurred in 10.6% of the eptifibatide group vs. 9.1% of the placebo group ($p < 0.05$).

BOTTOM LINE

Eptifibatide significantly reduced the incidence of death or MI at 30 days in patients with ECG changes or CKMB elevations; however, this benefit was not clear in patients who did not received PCI and the rate of major bleeding was increased.

ACUTE CORONARY SYNDROMES

CLINICAL TRIAL FEATURES, THERAPEUTICS AND ENDPOINTS

DISEASE STATES
- ☑ **ACS** ☐ STEMI/QMI ☑ **NSTEMI/NQMI** ☑ **UA**
- ☐ VTE ☐ DVT ☐ PE ☐ CVA

MEDICATIONS
- ☑ **Platelet Antagonist**
  - ☑ **Aspirin**
  - ☐ Clopidogrel
  - ☑ **IIb/IIIa Receptor Antagonist**
    - ☐ Abciximab
    - ☑ **Eptifibatide**
    - ☐ Lamifiban
    - ☐ Tirofiban
- ☐ **Heparin**
- ☐ **LMWH**
  - ☐ Enoxaparin
  - ☐ Dalteparin
  - ☐ Nadroparin
  - ☐ Tinzaparin
  - ☐ Reviparin
- ☐ **Direct Thrombin Inhibitor**
  - ☐ Hirudin
  - ☐ Hirulog
- ☐ **Fibrinolytic / Thrombolytic**
  - ☐ Alteplase
  - ☐ Reteplase
  - ☐ Tenecteplase
  - ☐ Anistreplase
  - ☐ Streptokinase
- ☐ **Other cardiac medications (captopril, magnesium, nitrates)**

PROCEDURES
- ☐ Angioplasty ☐ Stent
- ☐ CABG ☐ PCI

THERAPEUTIC ENDPOINT
- ☑ **Treatment** ☐ Prophylaxis

CLINICAL ENVIRONMENT
- ☑ **Inpatient** ☐ Outpatient

IIB/IIIA ± PROCEDURAL CORONARY INTERVENTION

IMPACT-AMI | INTEGRILIN TO MINIMIZED PLATELET AGGREGATION AND CORONARY THROMBOSIS-AMI

TRIAL FULL NAME
Combined Accelerated Tissue-Plasminogen Activator and Platelet Glycoprotein IIb/IIIa Integrin Receptor Blockade with Integrilin in Acute Myocardial Infarction

PUBLICATION DATA
Circulation 1997; 95: 847-854

STUDY DATES
1993 to 1995

AUTHOR(S)
E Mohman, NS Kleiman, G Gacioch et al

CLINICAL TRIAL SUMMARY

This was a multicenter, randomized, dose-ranging comparison of eptifibatide (Integrilin) with placebo in patients presenting within 6 hours of onset of acute MI. All received tPA 100 mg over one hour, aspirin, and heparin. In phase 1 (132 patients), 6 eptifibatide doses were compared with placebo. In phase 2 (48 patients), the highest eptifibatide dose was compared in a double-blind fashion with placebo. The primary outcome was TIMI 3 flow at 90 minutes. TIMI grade 3 flow occurred in 66% of the high-dose eptifibatide group and in 39% of the placebo group- (p =0.006). Complications were similar for the two groups.

BOTTOM LINE

In this dose-ranging trial, eptifibatide, compared to placebo, significantly improved the frequency of TIMI grade 3 perfusion at 90 minutes in patients with STEMI who concomitantly received tPA, ASA, and IV heparin.

ACUTE CORONARY SYNDROMES

CLINICAL TRIAL FEATURES, THERAPEUTICS AND ENDPOINTS

DISEASE STATES
☑ **ACS** ☑ **STEMI/QMI** ☐ NSTEMI/NQMI ☐ UA
☐ VTE ☐ DVT ☐ PE ☐ CVA

MEDICATIONS
- ☑ **Platelet Antagonist**
  - ☐ Aspirin
  - ☐ Clopidogrel
  - ☑ **IIb/IIIa Receptor Antagonist**
    - ☐ Abciximab
    - ☑ **Eptifibatide**
    - ☐ Lamifiban
    - ☐ Tirofiban
- ☐ **Heparin**
- ☐ **LMWH**
  - ☐ Enoxaparin
  - ☐ Dalteparin
  - ☐ Nadroparin
  - ☐ Tinzaparin
  - ☐ Reviparin
- ☐ **Direct Thrombin Inhibitor**
  - ☐ Hirudin
  - ☐ Hirulog
- ☐ **Fibrinolytic / Thrombolytic**
  - ☐ Alteplase
  - ☐ Reteplase
  - ☐ Tenecteplase
  - ☐ Anistreplase
  - ☐ Streptokinase
- ☐ **Other cardiac medications (captopril, magnesium, nitrates)**

PROCEDURES
☐ Angioplasty ☐ Stent
☐ CABG ☐ PCI

THERAPEUTIC ENDPOINT
☑ **Treatment** ☐ Prophylaxis

CLINICAL ENVIRONMENT
☑ **Inpatient** ☐ Outpatient

IIB/IIIA IN ACUTE MYOCARDIAL INFARCTION

SPEED | STRATEGIES FOR PATENCY ENHANCEMENT IN THE EMERGENCY DEPARTMENT

TRIAL FULL NAME
Trial of abciximab with and without low-dose reteplase for acute myocardial infarction

PUBLICATION DATA
Circulation 2000; 101:2788-2794

STUDY DATES
1997 to 1998

AUTHOR(S)
EJ Topol, EM Ohman, E Barnathan, RM Califf, KL Lee, et al

CLINICAL TRIAL SUMMARY

This was a randomized, multicenter, two-phased, dose-finding comparison of abciximab plus reteplase in patients with acute MI presenting within 12 hours of symptom onset. In phase A (n = 241), patients received abciximab plus one of six reteplase dosing strategies (none, 5 U, 7.5 U, 10 U, 5 U + 2.5 U, or 5 U + 5 U). In phase B (n = 224), the best combination from phase A (abciximab plus reteplase 5 U + 5 U) was compared with reteplase alone (10 U + 10 U). All patients received aspirin and heparin. Primary endpoint was TIMI grade 3 flow at 60-90 minutes. In phase A, TIMI grade 3 flow occurred in 62% of the abciximab-reteplase (5+5) group and in 27% of the abciximab only group (p = 0.001). In phase B, TIMI grade 3 flow occurred in 54% of the abciximab-reteplase (5+5) group and in 47% of the reteplase (10U + 10 U) only patients (p = 0.32). Major bleeding in phase B occurred in 9.8% of the abciximab-reteplase (5+5) group and in 3.7% of the reteplase alone group (p = NS). This was the pilot trial for the GUSTO IV AMI trial.

BOTTOM LINE

In this dose-ranging trial, adding abciximab to half-dose reteplase improved the TIMI grade 3 flow non-significantly in patients with STEMI.

ACUTE CORONARY SYNDROMES

CLINICAL TRIAL FEATURES, THERAPEUTICS AND ENDPOINTS

DISEASE STATES
☑ **ACS** ☑ **STEMI/QMI** ☐ NSTEMI/NQMI ☐ UA
☐ VTE ☐ DVT ☐ PE ☐ CVA

MEDICATIONS
- ☑ **Platelet Antagonist**
  - ☑ **Aspirin**
  - ☐ Clopidogrel
  - ☑ **IIb/IIIa Receptor Antagonist**
    - ☑ **Abciximab**
    - ☐ Eptifibatide
    - ☐ Lamifiban
    - ☐ Tirofiban
- ☐ **Heparin**
- ☐ **LMWH**
  - ☐ Enoxaparin
  - ☐ Dalteparin
  - ☐ Nadroparin
  - ☐ Tinzaparin
  - ☐ Reviparin
- ☐ **Direct Thrombin Inhibitor**
  - ☐ Hirudin
  - ☐ Hirulog
- ☐ **Fibrinolytic / Thrombolytic**
  - ☐ Alteplase
  - ☐ Reteplase
  - ☐ Tenecteplase
  - ☐ Anistreplase
  - ☐ Streptokinase
- ☐ **Other cardiac medications (captopril, magnesium, nitrates)**

PROCEDURES
☐ Angioplasty ☐ Stent
☐ CABG ☐ PCI

THERAPEUTIC ENDPOINT
☑ **Treatment** ☐ Prophylaxis

CLINICAL ENVIRONMENT
☑ **Inpatient** ☐ Outpatient

IIB/IIIA IN ACUTE MYOCARDIAL INFARCTION

FRISC II — Fragmin and Fast Revascularization during Instability in Coronary artery disease

Trial Full Name
Invasive compared with non-invasive treatment in unstable coronary artery disease: FRISC II prospective randomized multicentre study

Publication Data
Lancet 1999; 354: 701-707 and 708-15 (two articles)

Study Dates
1996 to 1998

Author(s)
L Wallenti E Swahn, G Kontny, S Husted, B Lagerqvist, E Stahle, et al

Clinical Trial Summary

This was a prospective, randomized, multicenter comparison with parallel arms. It included (1) a comparison of an early invasive (within 7 days) strategy versus early medical therapy (with PCI only used if problems occurred) and (2) a double-blind comparison of long term (3 months) twice-daily SQ dalteparin versus placebo. During the early in-hospital phase, all patients received either IV heparin or dalteparin in an unblinded fashion; this trial was NOT a comparison of in-hospital dalteparin with any other product. Primary endpoints were death or MI. The 2,457 patients had ischemic symptoms, consistent with either unstable angina or MI, within 48 hours of presentation plus either ECG changes or serum marker elevation. The primary endpoint, relative to the invasive versus medical management strategy, was the composite of death and MI after 6 months. Relative to the comparison of dalteparin with placebo, the primary endpoint was the composite at 3 months. At 6 months, the composite endpoint occurred in 9.4% of the invasive group and in 12.1% of the non-invasive group ($p = 0.031$). Anginal symptoms and readmissions were halved by the invasive strategy. Benefits were best in high-risk patients. Results were independent of dalteparin use. There was no difference in strokes between groups. In the dalteparin vs. placebo comparison, the composite endpoint occurred in 6.7% and 8.0%, respectively ($p = 0.17$).

Bottom Line

Early (within 7 days) invasive therapy compared to medical management of patients with ACS (with ECG changes or marker elevation) resulted in fewer deaths or MIs. Dalteparin therapy for 3 months in the same population had similar outcomes as did the placebo arm.

Acute Coronary Syndromes

Clinical Trial Features, Therapeutics and Endpoints

Disease States
- ☑ ACS ☑ STEMI/QMI ☑ NSTEMI/NQMI ☑ UA
- ☐ VTE ☐ DVT ☐ PE ☐ CVA

Medications
- ☐ Platelet Antagonist
  - ☐ Aspirin
  - ☐ Clopidogrel
  - ☐ IIb/IIIa Receptor Antagonist
    - ☐ Abciximab
    - ☐ Eptifibatide
    - ☐ Lamifiban
    - ☐ Tirofiban
- ☐ Heparin
- ☑ LMWH
  - ☐ Enoxaparin
  - ☑ Dalteparin
  - ☐ Nadroparin
  - ☐ Tinzaparin
  - ☐ Reviparin
- ☐ Direct Thrombin Inhibitor
  - ☐ Hirudin
  - ☐ Hirulog
- ☐ Fibrinolytic / Thrombolytic
  - ☐ Alteplase
  - ☐ Reteplase
  - ☐ Tenecteplase
  - ☐ Anistreplase
  - ☐ Streptokinase
- ☐ Other cardiac medications (captopril, magnesium, nitrates)

Procedures
- ☑ Angioplasty ☑ Stent
- ☑ CABG ☑ PCI

Therapeutic Endpoint
- ☑ Treatment ☐ Prophylaxis

Clinical Environment
- ☑ Inpatient ☑ Outpatient

Invasive or Not in NSTEMI or Unstable Angina

TACTICS / TIMI 18

Trial Full Name
Treat angina with Aggrastat plus determine Cost of Therapy with an Invasive or Conservative Strategy

Publication Data
Presented at the American Heart Association, Scientific Sessions 2000

Study Dates
No data

Author(s)
Cannon

Clinical Trial Summary

This was a randomized, multicenter, comparison of an early invasive (INV) versus early conservative (CONS) strategy in 2220 patients with UA or NSTEMI. All patients received tirofiban, aspirin, and heparin. The INV group had angiography done within 48 hours of presentation with revascularization if appropriate. The primary endpoint was the composite of death, MI, or need for rehospitalization for ACS. The endpoint occurred in 7.4% of the INV group and in 10.5% of the CONS group ($p = 0.009$) at 30 days and in 15.9% vs. 19.4% of the respective groups at six months. Per the six-month data, patient populations that benefited from the INV strategy were those with ECG changes (16.4% vs. 26.3% of CONS group; $p = 0.006$) or troponin elevations (14.3% vs. 24.2% of CONS group; $p < 0.001$). Low risk patients had comparable outcomes with the two strategies.

Bottom Line

Among patients with UA or NSTEMI, those with ECG changes or troponin elevations had a significantly reduced incidence of death, MI, or need for rehospitalization at one and 6 months if angiography with revascularization as needed was routinely done within 48 hours of admission.

Acute Coronary Syndromes

Clinical Trial Features, Therapeutics and Endpoints

Disease States
- ☑ ACS ☐ STEMI/QMI ☑ NSTEMI/NQMI ☑ UA
- ☐ VTE ☐ DVT ☐ PE ☐ CVA

Medications
- ☑ Platelet Antagonist
  - ☑ Aspirin
  - ☐ Clopidogrel
  - ☑ IIb/IIIa Receptor Antagonist
    - ☐ Abciximab
    - ☐ Eptifibatide
    - ☐ Lamifiban
    - ☑ Tirofiban
- ☐ Heparin
- ☐ LMWH
  - ☐ Enoxaparin
  - ☐ Dalteparin
  - ☐ Nadroparin
  - ☐ Tinzaparin
  - ☐ Reviparin
- ☐ Direct Thrombin Inhibitor
  - ☐ Hirudin
  - ☐ Hirulog
- ☑ Fibrinolytic / Thrombolytic
  - ☐ Alteplase
  - ☐ Reteplase
  - ☐ Tenecteplase
  - ☐ Anistreplase
  - ☐ Streptokinase
- ☐ Other cardiac medications (captopril, magnesium, nitrates)

Procedures
- ☐ Angioplasty ☐ Stent
- ☑ CABG ☑ PCI

Therapeutic Endpoint
- ☑ Treatment ☐ Prophylaxis

Clinical Environment
- ☑ Inpatient ☐ Outpatient

Invasive or Not in NSTEMI or Unstable Angina

TAMI | THROMBOLYSIS AND ANGIOPLASTY IN MYOCARDIAL INFARCTION

TRIAL FULL NAME
A randomized trial of immediate versus delayed elective angioplasty after IV tissue plasminogen activator in acute myocardial infarction

PUBLICATION DATA
NEJM 1987; 317:581-8

STUDY DATES
1985 to 1986

AUTHOR(S)
Topol E, Califf R, George BS, et al

CLINICAL TRIAL SUMMARY

This was a randomized comparison of immediate vs. delayed (at 7-10 days) PTCA in 386 patients with MI treated initially with tPA 150 mg over 5 hours. Patients had CP for ≤ 4 hours before presentation and STEMI. All had angiography done after thrombolysis was begun and those with PTCA-suitable lesions were randomized. Endpoints included reocclusion and LVEF on angiography done 7-10 days after interventions. All films were read blinded. Post thrombolytic angiography was associated with an average drop in hematocrit of 12 points and 18% of the patients required transfusions. Improvement in global LVEF and reocclusion (11% in the immediate PTCA group and 13% in the delayed PTCA group) were similar in the two groups.

BOTTOM LINE

Immediate angiography with PCI after full-dose thrombolytics in patients with STEMI resulted in no better LVEF or reocclusion rates, but did result in significantly more bleeding.

CLINICAL TRIAL FEATURES, THERAPEUTICS AND ENDPOINTS

DISEASE STATES
- ☑ **ACS** ☑ **STEMI/QMI** ☐ NSTEMI/NQMI ☐ UA
- ☐ VTE ☐ DVT ☐ PE ☐ CVA

MEDICATIONS
- ☐ **Platelet Antagonist**
  - ☐ Aspirin
  - ☐ Clopidogrel
  - ☐ IIb/IIIa Receptor Antagonist
    - ☐ Abciximab
    - ☐ Eptifibatide
    - ☐ Lamifiban
    - ☐ Tirofiban
- ☐ **Heparin**
- ☐ **LMWH**
  - ☐ Enoxaparin
  - ☐ Dalteparin
  - ☐ Nadroparin
  - ☐ Tinzaparin
  - ☐ Reviparin
- ☐ **Direct Thrombin Inhibitor**
  - ☐ Hirudin
  - ☐ Hirulog
- ☑ **Fibrinolytic / Thrombolytic**
  - ☑ **Alteplase**
  - ☐ Reteplase
  - ☐ Tenecteplase
  - ☐ Anistreplase
  - ☐ Streptokinase
- ☐ **Other cardiac medications (captopril, magnesium, nitrates)**

PROCEDURES
- ☑ **Angioplasty** ☐ Stent
- ☐ CABG ☑ **PCI**

THERAPEUTIC ENDPOINT
- ☑ **Treatment** ☐ Prophylaxis

CLINICAL ENVIRONMENT
- ☑ **Inpatient** ☐ Outpatient

INVASIVE OR NOT IN NSTEMI OR UNSTABLE ANGINA

TIMI IIIB

TRIAL FULL NAME
Effects of Tissue Plasminogen Activator and a Comparison of Early Invasive and Conservative Strategies in Unstable Angina and Non-Q-wave Myocardial Infarction

PUBLICATION DATA
Circulation 1994; 89:1545-1556

STUDY DATES
1989 to 1992

AUTHOR(S)
E Braunwald, C McCabe, CP Cannon, J E Muller, et al

CLINICAL TRIAL SUMMARY

This was a randomized, 2 X 2 factorial design comparison of (1) tPA (up to 80 mg over 90 min and started within 25 hours of any pain.) vs. placebo and (2) an early invasive strategy (catheterization within 48 hours followed by appropriate management) vs. early conservative strategy (catheterization only if initial medical therapy failed). All received aspirin and heparin. The 1,473 patients had CP within 24 hours of enrollment, either ECG changes or documented CAD, and a diagnosis of UA or NQMI. The primary end point for the tPA vs. placebo comparison (death, MI, or failure of initial therapy at 6 weeks) occurred in 54.2% of the tPA group and in 55% of the placebo group (p = NS). Death or MI occurred in 7.4% of the tPA group and in 4.9% of the placebo group (p = 0.04). Four intracranial hemorrhages occurred in the tPA group vs. none in the placebo group (p = 0.06). The endpoint for the comparison of the two strategies (death, MI, or an unsatisfactory symptom-limited exercise stress test at 6 weeks) occurred in 18.1% of the early conservative group and in 16.2% of the early invasive group (p = NS). Patients in the early invasive group also had increased days of hospitalization and of rehospitalization and more use of antianginal drugs.

BOTTOM LINE

The use of alteplase in patients with NQMI or UA was associated with increased death or later MI and with a near statistically significant increase in intracranial hemorrhage. Early catheterization, after thrombolytic therapy, was associated with no difference in death, MI, or poor stress tests at 6 weeks, but it did result in the need for significantly more hospitalization days.

CLINICAL TRIAL FEATURES, THERAPEUTICS AND ENDPOINTS

DISEASE STATES
- ☑ **ACS** ☐ STEMI/QMI ☑ **NSTEMI/NQMI** ☑ **UA**
- ☐ VTE ☐ DVT ☐ PE ☐ CVA

MEDICATIONS
- ☐ **Platelet Antagonist**
  - ☐ Aspirin
  - ☐ Clopidogrel
  - ☐ IIb/IIIa Receptor Antagonist
    - ☐ Abciximab
    - ☐ Eptifibatide
    - ☐ Lamifiban
    - ☐ Tirofiban
- ☐ **Heparin**
- ☐ **LMWH**
  - ☐ Enoxaparin
  - ☐ Dalteparin
  - ☐ Nadroparin
  - ☐ Tinzaparin
  - ☐ Reviparin
- ☐ **Direct Thrombin Inhibitor**
  - ☐ Hirudin
  - ☐ Hirulog
- ☑ **Fibrinolytic / Thrombolytic**
  - ☑ **Alteplase**
  - ☐ Reteplase
  - ☐ Tenecteplase
  - ☐ Anistreplase
  - ☐ Streptokinase
- ☐ **Other cardiac medications (captopril, magnesium, nitrates)**

PROCEDURES
- ☑ **Angioplasty** ☐ Stent
- ☑ **CABG** ☑ **PCI**

THERAPEUTIC ENDPOINT
- ☑ **Treatment** ☐ Prophylaxis

CLINICAL ENVIRONMENT
- ☑ **Inpatient** ☐ Outpatient

INVASIVE OR NOT IN NSTEMI OR UNSTABLE ANGINA

VANQWISH | VETERANS AFFAIRS NON-Q-WAVE INFARCTION STRATEGIES IN HOSPITAL

TRIAL FULL NAME
Outcomes in Patients with Acute Non-Q-wave Myocardial Infarction randomly assigned to an invasive as compared with a conservative management strategy

PUBLICATION DATA
NEJM 1998; 338:1785-92

STUDY DATES
1993 to 1996

AUTHOR(S)
Boden W, O'Rourke RA, Crawford MH, et al

CLINICAL TRIAL SUMMARY

This was a randomized, multicenter comparison of early coronary angiography with revascularization as needed vs. medical management in 920 patients with NQMI. The medical management group could also go onto PTCA or CABG if their course became complicated. Follow-up of an average 23 months occurred with a combined primary end point of death or MI. The number of patients reaching end point was 152 in the invasive group and 139 in the conservative group (p = 0.35).

BOTTOM LINE

The incidence of death or MI at 23 months in patients who had NQMI was comparable between groups treated with routine early angiography with revascularization as needed vs. those receiving medical management with angiography being done only if patient course deteriorated.

CLINICAL TRIAL FEATURES, THERAPEUTICS AND ENDPOINTS

DISEASE STATES
- ☑ **ACS** ☐ STEMI/QMI ☑ **NSTEMI/NQMI** ☐ UA
- ☐ VTE ☐ DVT ☐ PE ☐ CVA

MEDICATIONS
- ☐ **Platelet Antagonist**
  - ☐ Aspirin
  - ☐ Clopidogrel
  - ☐ IIb/IIIa Receptor Antagonist
    - ☐ Abciximab
    - ☐ Eptifibatide
    - ☐ Lamifiban
    - ☐ Tirofiban
- ☐ **Heparin**
- ☐ **LMWH**
  - ☐ Enoxaparin
  - ☐ Dalteparin
  - ☐ Nadroparin
  - ☐ Tinzaparin
  - ☐ Reviparin
- ☐ **Direct Thrombin Inhibitor**
  - ☐ Hirudin
  - ☐ Hirulog
- ☐ **Fibrinolytic / Thrombolytic**
  - ☐ Alteplase
  - ☐ Reteplase
  - ☐ Tenecteplase
  - ☐ Anistreplase
  - ☐ Streptokinase
- ☐ **Other cardiac medications (captopril, magnesium, nitrates)**

PROCEDURES
- ☑ **Angioplasty** ☐ Stent
- ☑ **CABG** ☑ **PCI**

THERAPEUTIC ENDPOINT
- ☑ **Treatment** ☐ Prophylaxis

CLINICAL ENVIRONMENT
- ☑ **Inpatient** ☐ Outpatient

INVASIVE OR NOT IN NSTEMI OR UNSTABLE ANGINA

CAST | CHINESE ACUTE STROKE TRIAL

TRIAL FULL NAME
Randomized placebo-controlled trial of early aspirin use in 20000 patients with acute ischemic stroke

PUBLICATION DATA
Lancet 1997; 349: 1641-49

STUDY DATES
1993-1997

AUTHOR(S)
ZM Chen, R Collins, LS Liu, HC Pan, et al

CLINICAL TRIAL SUMMARY

This was a multicenter, randomized, double-blind comparison of 4-week use of aspirin 160 mg qd vs. placebo in 21,106 patients with suspected ischemic stroke. A CT scan before entry was not required. Primary endpoints were death from any cause, physical dependence, or complications at 4 weeks. Death occurred in 3.3% of the aspirin group and in 3.9% of the placebo group (p = 0.04). Recurrent ischemic strokes occurred in 1.6% of the aspirin group and in 2.1% of the placebo group (p= 0.01) while there was a nonsignificant increase in hemorrhagic strokes in the aspirin group (1.1% vs. 0.9%; p > 0.1). Death or dependence at discharge occurred in 30.5% of the aspirin group and in 31.6% of the placebo group (p 0.08). Combined with the International Stroke Trial, aspirin produces a small but real reduction of about 10 deaths or recurrent strokes per 1000 during the first few weeks.

BOTTOM LINE

In patients with ischemic stroke, aspirin use for 4 weeks resulted in a small but significant reduction in 4 week mortality or stroke recurrence without significantly increasing intracranial hemorrhage.

STROKE

CLINICAL TRIAL FEATURES, THERAPEUTICS AND ENDPOINTS

DISEASE STATES
- ☐ ACS ☐ STEMI/QMI ☐ NSTEMI/NQMI ☐ UA
- ☐ VTE ☐ DVT ☐ PE ☑ **CVA**

MEDICATIONS
- ☐ **Platelet Antagonist**
  - ☑ **Aspirin**
  - ☐ Clopidogrel
  - ☐ IIb/IIIa Receptor Antagonist
    - ☐ Abciximab
    - ☐ Eptifibatide
    - ☐ Lamifiban
    - ☐ Tirofiban
- ☐ **Heparin**
- ☐ **LMWH**
  - ☐ Enoxaparin
  - ☐ Dalteparin
  - ☐ Nadroparin
  - ☐ Tinzaparin
  - ☐ Reviparin
- ☐ **Direct Thrombin Inhibitor**
  - ☐ Hirudin
  - ☐ Hirulog
- ☐ **Fibrinolytic / Thrombolytic**
  - ☐ Alteplase
  - ☐ Reteplase
  - ☐ Tenecteplase
  - ☐ Anistreplase
  - ☐ Streptokinase
- ☐ **Other cardiac medications (captopril, magnesium, nitrates)**

PROCEDURES
- ☐ Angioplasty ☐ Stent
- ☐ CABG ☐ PCI

THERAPEUTIC ENDPOINT
- ☑ **Treatment** ☑ **Prophylaxis**

CLINICAL ENVIRONMENT
- ☑ **Inpatient** ☑ **Outpatient**

ASPIRIN

IST | INTERNATIONAL STROKE TRIAL

TRIAL FULL NAME
The International Stroke Trial (IST): a randomized trial of aspirin, subcutaneous heparin, both, or neither among 19435 patients with acute ischaemic stroke

PUBLICATION DATA
Lancet 1997; 349: 1569-81

STUDY DATES
1991 to 1996

AUTHOR(S)
PAG Sandercock

CLINICAL TRIAL SUMMARY

This was a multicenter, randomized, unblinded, 2 X 2 factorial designed comparison of 14 days of (1) SQ heparin (two doses: 5000 U or 12500 U BID) vs. nothing, and (2) aspirin 300 mg qd vs. nothing for the prophylaxis against untoward events. The 19435 patients had suspected ischemic strokes within 48 hours of presentation. A head CT was done before randomization in most patients. The primary endpoints were death at 14 days and death or dependency at 6 months. Deaths at 14 days occurred in 9.0% of the aspirin group and 9.4% of the placebo group (p = NS; 4 fewer deaths per 1000). At 6 months, less death or dependence occurred in the aspirin group (62.2% vs. 63.5%; p = 0.07; 13 fewer per 1000); however, once adjusted for baseline prognosis, the difference was significant (p = 0.03). At 14 days, recurrent stokes occurred in 2.8% of the aspirin group and in 3.9% of the placebo group (p < 0.01) while hemorrhagic strokes were comparable between groups (0.9% vs. 0.8%, respectively). Neither heparin regimen offered clinical advantage. Combined with the Chinese Acute Stroke Trial, aspirin produced a small but real reduction of about 10 deaths or recurrent strokes per 1000 during the first few weeks.

BOTTOM LINE

Compared to placebo, aspirin use for 14 days by patients with ischemic strokes resulted in non-significant reductions in 14 day mortality and 6 month mortality plus physical dependence. Aspirin did significantly reduce the 14 day recurrence of stroke. Neither heparin regimen offered clinical advantage.

STROKE

CLINICAL TRIAL FEATURES, THERAPEUTICS AND ENDPOINTS

DISEASE STATES
- ❑ ACS ❑ STEMI/QMI ❑ NSTEMI/NQMI ❑ UA
- ❑ VTE ❑ DVT ❑ PE ☑ **CVA**

MEDICATIONS
- ☑ **Platelet Antagonist**
  - ☑ **Aspirin**
  - ❑ Clopidogrel
  - ❑ IIb/IIIa Receptor Antagonist
    - ❑ Abciximab
    - ❑ Eptifibatide
    - ❑ Lamifiban
    - ❑ Tirofiban
- ☑ **Heparin**
- ❑ **LMWH**
  - ❑ Enoxaparin
  - ❑ Dalteparin
  - ❑ Nadroparin
  - ❑ Tinzaparin
  - ❑ Reviparin
- ❑ **Direct Thrombin Inhibitor**
  - ❑ Hirudin
  - ❑ Hirulog
- ❑ **Fibrinolytic / Thrombolytic**
  - ❑ Alteplase
  - ❑ Reteplase
  - ❑ Tenecteplase
  - ❑ Anistreplase
  - ❑ Streptokinase
- ❑ **Other cardiac medications (captopril, magnesium, nitrates)**

PROCEDURES
- ❑ Angioplasty ❑ Stent
- ❑ CABG ❑ PCI

THERAPEUTIC ENDPOINT
- ☑ **Treatment** ☑ **Prophylaxis**

CLINICAL ENVIRONMENT
- ☑ **Inpatient** ☑ **Outpatient**

ASPIRIN

ATLANTIS | ALTEPLASE THROMBOLYSIS FOR ACUTE NON-INTERVENTIONAL THERAPY IN ISCHEMIC STROKE

TRIAL FULL NAME
Recombinant Tissue-Type Plasminogen Activator (Alteplase) for Ischemic Stroke 3 to 5 Hours After Symptom Onset

PUBLICATION DATA
JAMA 1999; 282: 2019-2026

STUDY DATES
1993-1998

AUTHOR(S)
Clark W, Wissman S, Albers G, et al

CLINICAL TRIAL SUMMARY

This was a randomized, double-blind, multicenter, comparison of tPA (0.9 mg/kg over 1 hour) vs. placebo in 613 patients with acute ischemic stroke who were treated between 3-5 hours after symptoms began. A CT was required to rule out ICH. Two CT scans were repeated at up to 37 days. Patients with signs of cerebral ischemia in > one-third of the territory of the middle cerebral artery were excluded because of the poor outcomes in this group in ECASS-I. The primary outcome, excellent neurologic recovery at 90 days according to an NIHSS score of ≤ 1, occurred in 32% of the placebo group and in 34% of the tPA group (p = 0.65). Functional outcome measures were comparable between groups. At 10 days, all types of ICH were significantly increased in the tPA group; symptomatic ICH in 1.1% vs. 7.0%, p < 0.001; asymptomatic ICH in 4.7% vs. 11.4%, p = 0.004; and fatal ICH in 0.3% vs. 3.0%, p < 0.001. Mortality at 90 days was 6.9% with placebo and 11.0% with tPA (p = 0.09).

BOTTOM LINE

In comparison to placebo, neurologic outcomes of patients treated with tPA between 3-5 hours after symptom onset are similar. All types of intracranial bleeding occurred significantly more with tPA.

STROKE

CLINICAL TRIAL FEATURES, THERAPEUTICS AND ENDPOINTS

DISEASE STATES
- ❑ ACS ❑ STEMI/QMI ❑ NSTEMI/NQMI ❑ UA
- ❑ VTE ❑ DVT ❑ PE ☑ **CVA**

MEDICATIONS
- ❑ **Platelet Antagonist**
  - ❑ Aspirin
  - ❑ Clopidogrel
  - ❑ IIb/IIIa Receptor Antagonist
    - ❑ Abciximab
    - ❑ Eptifibatide
    - ❑ Lamifiban
    - ❑ Tirofiban
- ❑ **Heparin**
- ❑ **LMWH**
  - ❑ Enoxaparin
  - ❑ Dalteparin
  - ❑ Nadroparin
  - ❑ Tinzaparin
  - ❑ Reviparin
- ❑ **Direct Thrombin Inhibitor**
  - ❑ Hirudin
  - ❑ Hirulog
- ☑ **Fibrinolytic / Thrombolytic**
  - ☑ **Alteplase**
  - ❑ Reteplase
  - ❑ Tenecteplase
  - ❑ Anistreplase
  - ❑ Streptokinase
- ❑ **Other cardiac medications (captopril, magnesium, nitrates)**

PROCEDURES
- ❑ Angioplasty ❑ Stent
- ❑ CABG ❑ PCI

THERAPEUTIC ENDPOINT
- ☑ **Treatment** ❑ Prophylaxis

CLINICAL ENVIRONMENT
- ☑ **Inpatient** ❑ Outpatient

FIBRINOLYTICS

ECASS II | EUROPEAN-AUSTRALASIAN ACUTE STROKE STUDY

TRIAL FULL NAME
Randomized placebo-controlled trial of early aspirin use in 20000 patients with acute ischemic stroke

PUBLICATION DATA
Lancet 1998; 352:1245-1251

STUDY DATES
1996-1998

AUTHOR(S)

CLINICAL TRIAL SUMMARY

This was a multicenter, randomized, double-blind comparison of tPA (0.9 mg/kg up to 90 mg over 1 hour; same regimen as NINDS) vs. placebo in 800 patients with acute moderate-severe stroke. Groups were stratified as to whether presentation was < 3 hours or 3-6 hours. Patients were excluded if brain swelling exceeded 33% of the middle-cerebral artery territory. CT scans were mandatory and readings were done by providers with special training. The primary endpoint, a determination of favorable outcome according to a modified Rankin scale, occurred in 40.3% of the tPA group and in 36.6% of the placebo group (p = 0.27). For patients treated within 3 hours, a favorable outcome occurred in 42% of the tPA group and in 38% of the placebo group (p = 0.63). Mortality was comparable between groups as 30 and 90 days. Various neurologic outcome scales were used as secondary endpoints; some showed trends towards improvement with tPA. Symptomatic intracranial hemorrhage occurred in 8.8% of the tPA group and in 3.4% of the placebo group.

BOTTOM LINE

In patients with acute ischemic stroke who were treated within 3 hours or 6 hours, tPA, in comparison with placebo, resulted in similar mortality and clinical outcomes according to a modified Rankin scale. More intracranial hemorrhage occurred with tPA.

STROKE

CLINICAL TRIAL FEATURES, THERAPEUTICS AND ENDPOINTS

DISEASE STATES
- ☐ ACS ☐ STEMI/QMI ☐ NSTEMI/NQMI ☐ UA
- ☐ VTE ☐ DVT ☐ PE ☑ **CVA**

MEDICATIONS
- ☐ **Platelet Antagonist**
  - ☐ Aspirin
  - ☐ Clopidogrel
  - ☐ IIb/IIIa Receptor Antagonist
    - ☐ Abciximab
    - ☐ Eptifibatide
    - ☐ Lamifiban
    - ☐ Tirofiban
- ☐ **Heparin**
- ☐ **LMWH**
  - ☐ Enoxaparin
  - ☐ Dalteparin
  - ☐ Nadroparin
  - ☐ Tinzaparin
  - ☐ Reviparin
- ☐ **Direct Thrombin Inhibitor**
  - ☐ Hirudin
  - ☐ Hirulog
- ☑ **Fibrinolytic / Thrombolytic**
  - ☑ **Alteplase**
  - ☐ Reteplase
  - ☐ Tenecteplase
  - ☐ Anistreplase
  - ☐ Streptokinase
- ☐ **Other cardiac medications (captopril, magnesium, nitrates)**

PROCEDURES
- ☐ Angioplasty ☐ Stent
- ☐ CABG ☐ PCI

THERAPEUTIC ENDPOINT
- ☑ **Treatment** ☐ Prophylaxis

CLINICAL ENVIRONMENT
- ☑ **Inpatient** ☐ Outpatient

FIBRINOLYTICS

MAST-E | MULTICENTER ACUTE STROKE TRIAL-EUROPE

TRIAL FULL NAME
Thrombolytic Therapy with Streptokinase in Acute Ischemic Stroke

PUBLICATION DATA
NEJM 1996; 335: 145-50

STUDY DATES
1992 to 1994

AUTHOR(S)
Marc Hommel

CLINICAL TRIAL SUMMARY

This was a multicenter, randomized, double-blind, comparison of STK 1.5 MU over one hour vs. placebo in the treatment of acute stroke within 6 hours of onset. The 310 patients had focal neurologic deficits due to ischemia in the territory of the middle cerebral artery and had moderate-to-severe injury. The primary outcome, the combination of death or severe disability (Rankin score ³ 3) at 6 months, occurred equally in the groups (156 in STK group and 154 in placebo group). Mortality was significantly higher in the STK group at 10 days (34% vs. 18%; p = 0.002) and at 6 months (47% vs. 38%; p = 0.06), Symptomatic intracranial hemorrhage occurred more with STK than with placebo (21.2% vs. 2.6%; p < 0.001).

BOTTOM LINE

In patients with acute ischemic stroke being treated within 6 hours, streptokinase is associated with a significant increase in both mortality and symptomatic intracranial hemorrhage.

STROKE

CLINICAL TRIAL FEATURES, THERAPEUTICS AND ENDPOINTS

DISEASE STATES
- ☐ ACS ☐ STEMI/QMI ☐ NSTEMI/NQMI ☐ UA
- ☐ VTE ☐ DVT ☐ PE ☑ **CVA**

MEDICATIONS
- ☐ **Platelet Antagonist**
  - ☐ Aspirin
  - ☐ Clopidogrel
  - ☐ IIb/IIIa Receptor Antagonist
    - ☐ Abciximab
    - ☐ Eptifibatide
    - ☐ Lamifiban
    - ☐ Tirofiban
- ☐ **Heparin**
- ☐ **LMWH**
  - ☐ Enoxaparin
  - ☐ Dalteparin
  - ☐ Nadroparin
  - ☐ Tinzaparin
  - ☐ Reviparin
- ☐ **Direct Thrombin Inhibitor**
  - ☐ Hirudin
  - ☐ Hirulog
- ☑ **Fibrinolytic / Thrombolytic**
  - ☐ Alteplase
  - ☐ Reteplase
  - ☐ Tenecteplase
  - ☐ Anistreplase
  - ☑ **Streptokinase**
- ☐ **Other cardiac medications (captopril, magnesium, nitrates)**

PROCEDURES
- ☐ Angioplasty ☐ Stent
- ☐ CABG ☐ PCI

THERAPEUTIC ENDPOINT
- ☑ **Treatment** ☐ Prophylaxis

CLINICAL ENVIRONMENT
- ☑ **Inpatient** ☐ Outpatient

FIBRINOLYTICS

MAST-I | MULTICENTRE ACUTE STROKE TRIAL-ITALY

TRIAL FULL NAME
Randomized controlled trial of streptokinase, aspirin, and combination of both in treatment of acute ischaemic stroke

PUBLICATION DATA
Lancet 1995; 346: 1509-14

STUDY DATES
1991 to 1995

AUTHOR(S)
Not available

CLINICAL TRIAL SUMMARY

This was a randomized, multicenter, 2 X 2 factorial designed, open trial comparing (1) STK with aspirin, (2) aspirin alone, (3) STK alone, and (4) neither agent in 622 patients with acute ischemic stroke presenting within 6 hours of symptom onset. Streptokinase was dosed at 1.5 MU over one hour and aspirin was at 300 mg/day for 10 days. A CT scan was required before randomization. Streptokinase increased mortality at 10 days (26.5% vs. 11.6%; p < 0.00001) and at 6 months (36% vs. 24%); however, it was associated with improved disability at 6 months (27% vs. 40%). No significant differences existed for the aspirin vs. no aspirin group. Ten day mortality in the STK alone group was 34% compared to 13% in the group with neither (p < 0.00001) 19% in the STK only group, and 10% in the aspirin alone group.

BOTTOM LINE

Streptokinase within 6 hours of the onset of ischemic stroke resulted in a significant increase in 10 day and a near significant increase in 6 month mortality. Six month death or disability was comparable between STK and non-STK groups and also between aspirin vs. no aspirin groups.

STROKE

CLINICAL TRIAL FEATURES, THERAPEUTICS AND ENDPOINTS

DISEASE STATES
☐ ACS ☐ STEMI/QMI ☐ NSTEMI/NQMI ☐ UA
☐ VTE ☐ DVT ☐ PE ☑ **CVA**

MEDICATIONS
- ☑ **Platelet Antagonist**
  - ☑ **Aspirin**
  - ☐ Clopidogrel
  - ☐ IIb/IIIa Receptor Antagonist
    - ☐ Abciximab
    - ☐ Eptifibatide
    - ☐ Lamifiban
    - ☐ Tirofiban
- ☐ **Heparin**
- ☐ **LMWH**
  - ☐ Enoxaparin
  - ☐ Dalteparin
  - ☐ Nadroparin
  - ☐ Tinzaparin
  - ☐ Reviparin
- ☐ **Direct Thrombin Inhibitor**
  - ☐ Hirudin
  - ☐ Hirulog
- ☑ **Fibrinolytic / Thrombolytic**
  - ☐ Alteplase
  - ☐ Reteplase
  - ☐ Tenecteplase
  - ☐ Anistreplase
  - ☑ **Streptokinase**
- ☐ **Other cardiac medications (captopril, magnesium, nitrates)**

PROCEDURES
☐ Angioplasty ☐ Stent
☐ CABG ☐ PCI

THERAPEUTIC ENDPOINT
☑ **Treatment** ☑ **Prophylaxis**

CLINICAL ENVIRONMENT
☑ **Inpatient** ☑ **Outpatient**

FIBRINOLYTICS

NINDS | NATIONAL INSTITUTE OF NEUROLOGICAL DISORDERS AND STROKE

TRIAL FULL NAME
Tissue Plasminogen Activator for Acute Ischemic Stroke

PUBLICATION DATA
NEJM 1995; 333: 1581-7

STUDY DATES
1991 to 1994

AUTHOR(S)
KM Welch, BC Tilley, J Marler

CLINICAL TRIAL SUMMARY

This was a randomized, double-blind, comparison of tPA (0.9 mg/kg over 1 hour) vs. placebo in the treatment of acute stroke with treatment started within 3 hours of the onset of symptoms in 624 patients. Exclusion criteria included prior stroke or head injury within 3 months, major surgery within 14 days, previous intracranial hemorrhage, a SBP > 185 or DBP > 110 mmHg, rapidly improving or minor symptoms, symptoms consistent with a subarachnoid hemorrhage, GI or urinary hemorrhage within 3 weeks, an arterial puncture at a noncompressible site within 7 days, or a seizure at the onset of stroke. Patients were also excluded if aggressive treatment was required in order to lower their blood pressure. The primary outcomes, at 3 months, were four measures of neurologic status (Barthel index, modified Rankin scale, Glasgow outcome scale, and the NIHSS 42-point scale). At 24 hours, neurologic outcomes were comparable between groups. At 3 months, the tPA group had significantly better outcomes according to all four scales. The clinical significance of these outcomes has been debated. At 36 hours, symptomatic ICH occurred significantly more in the tPA group (4.2% vs. 0.3%; p < 0.001). Mortality at three months was 17% in the tPA group and 21% in the placebo group.

BOTTOM LINE

Patients with ischemic strokes treated within 3 hours with tPA had significant improvement in their clinical outcomes according to 4 stroke scales; however, there was a significant increase in symptomatic intracranial hemorrhage.

STROKE

CLINICAL TRIAL FEATURES, THERAPEUTICS AND ENDPOINTS

DISEASE STATES
☐ ACS ☐ STEMI/QMI ☐ NSTEMI/NQMI ☐ UA
☐ VTE ☐ DVT ☐ PE ☑ **CVA**

MEDICATIONS
- ☐ **Platelet Antagonist**
  - ☐ Aspirin
  - ☐ Clopidogrel
  - ☐ IIb/IIIa Receptor Antagonist
    - ☐ Abciximab
    - ☐ Eptifibatide
    - ☐ Lamifiban
    - ☐ Tirofiban
- ☐ **Heparin**
- ☐ **LMWH**
  - ☐ Enoxaparin
  - ☐ Dalteparin
  - ☐ Nadroparin
  - ☐ Tinzaparin
  - ☐ Reviparin
- ☐ **Direct Thrombin Inhibitor**
  - ☐ Hirudin
  - ☐ Hirulog
- ☑ **Fibrinolytic / Thrombolytic**
  - ☑ **Alteplase**
  - ☐ Reteplase
  - ☐ Tenecteplase
  - ☐ Anistreplase
  - ☐ Streptokinase
- ☐ **Other cardiac medications (captopril, magnesium, nitrates)**

PROCEDURES
☐ Angioplasty ☐ Stent
☐ CABG ☐ PCI

THERAPEUTIC ENDPOINT
☑ **Treatment** ☐ Prophylaxis

CLINICAL ENVIRONMENT
☑ **Inpatient** ☐ Outpatient

FIBRINOLYTICS

ENOXAPARIN FOR HOME-BASED TREATMENT OF DVT

TRIAL FULL NAME
A comparison of low-molecular-weight heparin administered primarily at home with unfractionated heparin administered in the hospital for proximal deep-vein thrombosis

PUBLICATION DATA
NEJM 1996; 334: 677-81

STUDY DATES
1992 to 1995

AUTHOR(S)
Levine M, Gent M, J Hirsh, et al

CLINICAL TRIAL SUMMARY

This was a randomized comparison of inpatient IV heparin vs. outpatient (primarily) SQ enoxaparin 1 mg/kg q 12 hours in 500 patients with proximal DVTs. Primary endpoints were symptomatic recurrence of thromboembolic (TE) disease at 90 days or bleeding during study drug administration. Exclusion criteria were extensive including, PE, bleeding, coexisting medical conditions, and likely noncompliance; only 33% of patients were eligible. Recurrent TE disease occurred in 5.3% of the enoxaparin group and in 6.7% of the heparin group (p = NS). Bleeding complications were comparable.

BOTTOM LINE

In patients with proximal-vein thrombosis, treatment with enoxaparin at home was effective and safe.

VENOUS THROMBOEMBOLISM

CLINICAL TRIAL FEATURES, THERAPEUTICS AND ENDPOINTS

DISEASE STATES
- ☐ ACS ☐ STEMI/QMI ☐ NSTEMI/NQMI ☐ UA
- ☑ VTE ☑ DVT ☐ PE ☐ CVA

MEDICATIONS
- ☐ **Platelet Antagonist**
  - ☐ Aspirin
  - ☐ Clopidogrel
  - ☐ IIb/IIIa Receptor Antagonist
    - ☐ Abciximab
    - ☐ Eptifibatide
    - ☐ Lamifiban
    - ☐ Tirofiban
- ☑ **Heparin**
- ☑ **LMWH**
  - ☑ **Enoxaparin**
  - ☐ Dalteparin
  - ☐ Nadroparin
  - ☐ Tinzaparin
  - ☐ Reviparin
- ☐ **Direct Thrombin Inhibitor**
  - ☐ Hirudin
  - ☐ Hirulog
- ☐ **Fibrinolytic / Thrombolytic**
  - ☐ Alteplase
  - ☐ Reteplase
  - ☐ Tenecteplase
  - ☐ Anistreplase
  - ☐ Streptokinase
- ☐ **Other cardiac medications (captopril, magnesium, nitrates)**

PROCEDURES
- ☐ Angioplasty ☐ Stent
- ☐ CABG ☐ PCI

THERAPEUTIC ENDPOINT
- ☑ **Treatment** ☐ Prophylaxis

CLINICAL ENVIRONMENT
- ☑ **Inpatient** ☑ **Outpatient**

HOME TREATMENT FOR DEEP VENOUS THROMBOSIS

TASMAN STUDY GROUP

TRIAL FULL NAME
Treatment of venous thrombosis with IV unfractionated heparin administered in the hospital as compared with subcutaneous low-molecular-weight heparin administered at home

PUBLICATION DATA
NEJM 1996; 334: 682-7

STUDY DATES
No data

AUTHOR(S)
Koopman M, Prandoni P, F Piovella, et al

CLINICAL TRIAL SUMMARY

This was a randomized comparison of inpatient IV heparin vs. outpatient (primarily) SQ nadroparin q 12 hours in 400 patients with proximal DVTs. Primary endpoints were symptomatic recurrence of thromboembolic (TE) disease at 6 months or major bleeding by 3 months. Exclusion criteria included suspected PE, DVT/PE within 2 years, shortened life expectancy, and likely noncompliance; 69% of patients were eligible. Recurrent TE disease occurred in 6.9% of the nadroparin group and in 8.6% of the heparin group (p = NS). Bleeding complications were comparable.

BOTTOM LINE

In patients with proximal-vein thrombosis, treatment with nadroparin at home was effective and safe.

VENOUS THROMBOEMBOLISM

CLINICAL TRIAL FEATURES, THERAPEUTICS AND ENDPOINTS

DISEASE STATES
- ☐ ACS ☐ STEMI/QMI ☐ NSTEMI/NQMI ☐ UA
- ☑ VTE ☑ DVT ☐ PE ☐ CVA

MEDICATIONS
- ☐ **Platelet Antagonist**
  - ☐ Aspirin
  - ☐ Clopidogrel
  - ☐ IIb/IIIa Receptor Antagonist
    - ☐ Abciximab
    - ☐ Eptifibatide
    - ☐ Lamifiban
    - ☐ Tirofiban
- ☑ **Heparin**
- ☑ **LMWH**
  - ☐ Enoxaparin
  - ☐ Dalteparin
  - ☑ **Nadroparin**
  - ☐ Tinzaparin
  - ☐ Reviparin
- ☐ **Direct Thrombin Inhibitor**
  - ☐ Hirudin
  - ☐ Hirulog
- ☐ **Fibrinolytic / Thrombolytic**
  - ☐ Alteplase
  - ☐ Reteplase
  - ☐ Tenecteplase
  - ☐ Anistreplase
  - ☐ Streptokinase
- ☐ **Other cardiac medications (captopril, magnesium, nitrates)**

PROCEDURES
- ☐ Angioplasty ☐ Stent
- ☐ CABG ☐ PCI

THERAPEUTIC ENDPOINT
- ☑ **Treatment** ☐ Prophylaxis

CLINICAL ENVIRONMENT
- ☑ **Inpatient** ☑ **Outpatient**

HOME TREATMENT FOR DEEP VENOUS THROMBOSIS

THE COLUMBUS INVESTIGATORS

TRIAL FULL NAME
Low-molecular weight heparin in the treatment of patients with venous thromboembolism

PUBLICATION DATA
NEJM 1997; 337: 657-62

STUDY DATES
1994-1995

AUTHOR(S)
HR Buller, M Gent, et al

CLINICAL TRIAL SUMMARY
This was a multicenter, randomized, unblinded comparison of SQ reviparin (at three different doses based on weight) BID vs. IV heparin for the management of 1021 patients with confirmed DVT/PE. Patients receiving the reviparin could be treated a home. The primary endpoints were recurrence of VTE disease, major bleeding, or death at 12 weeks. Twenty-seven percent had a PE. Among those treated with reviparin, 27% were never admitted to the hospital and 15% were discharged home in less than 3 days. Recurrent VTE disease occurred in 5.3% of the reviparin group and in 4.9% of the heparin group (p = NS). Major bleeding and mortality rates were comparable between groups.

BOTTOM LINE
Reviparin was as safe and effective as IV heparin in the inpatient or outpatient treatment of DVT or PE.

VENOUS THROMBOEMBOLISM

CLINICAL TRIAL FEATURES, THERAPEUTICS AND ENDPOINTS

DISEASE STATES
❑ ACS ❑ STEMI/QMI ❑ NSTEMI/NQMI ❑ UA
☑ **VTE** ☑ **DVT** ☑ **PE** ❑ CVA

MEDICATIONS
❑ **Platelet Antagonist**
- ❑ Aspirin
- ❑ Clopidogrel
- ❑ IIb/IIIa Receptor Antagonist
  - ❑ Abciximab
  - ❑ Eptifibatide
  - ❑ Lamifiban
  - ❑ Tirofiban

☑ **Heparin**
☑ **LMWH**
- ❑ Enoxaparin
- ❑ Dalteparin
- ❑ Nadroparin
- ❑ Tinzaparin
- ☑ **Reviparin**

❑ **Direct Thrombin Inhibitor**
- ❑ Hirudin
- ❑ Hirulog

❑ **Fibrinolytic / Thrombolytic**
- ❑ Alteplase
- ❑ Reteplase
- ❑ Tenecteplase
- ❑ Anistreplase
- ❑ Streptokinase

❑ **Other cardiac medications (captopril, magnesium, nitrates)**

PROCEDURES
❑ Angioplasty ❑ Stent
❑ CABG ❑ PCI

THERAPEUTIC ENDPOINT
☑ **Treatment** ❑ Prophylaxis

CLINICAL ENVIRONMENT
☑ **Inpatient** ☑ **Outpatient**

LOW MOLECULAR WEIGHT HEPARINS IN PULMONARY EMBOLISM

ENOXAPARIN CLINICAL TRIAL GROUP

TRIAL FULL NAME
Subcutaneous Enoxaparin Once or Twice Daily Compared with Intravenous Unfractionated Heparin Treatment of Venous Thromboembolic Disease

PUBLICATION DATA
Ann Intern Med 2001; 134: 191-202

STUDY DATES

AUTHOR(S)
G Merli, TI Spiro, Carl-Gustav Olsson, et al

CLINICAL TRIAL SUMMARY
This was a randomized, multicenter, inpatient comparison of SQ enoxaparin 1 mg/kg BID vs. SQ enoxaparin 1.5 mg/kg q 12 hours vs. IV heparin in the management of 900 patients with acute DVT and/or PE. Administration of the two-enoxaparin regimes was blinded while IV heparin use was unblinded. Primary endpoints were recurrence of VTE disease, hemorrhage, or other adverse events at 3 months. Thirty-two percent had a PE. Symptomatic VTE disease recurred in 4.1% of the heparin group, 4.4% of the enoxaparin qd group, and in 2.9% of the enoxaparin q 12 hours group (p = NS). Major bleeding and other adverse events were comparable between groups.

BOTTOM LINE
Enoxaparin once- or twice-a-day is as effective and safe as IV heparin in the management of DVT and/or PE.

VENOUS THROMBOEMBOLISM

CLINICAL TRIAL FEATURES, THERAPEUTICS AND ENDPOINTS

DISEASE STATES
❑ ACS ❑ STEMI/QMI ❑ NSTEMI/NQMI ❑ UA
☑ **VTE** ☑ **DVT** ☑ **PE** ❑ CVA

MEDICATIONS
❑ **Platelet Antagonist**
- ❑ Aspirin
- ❑ Clopidogrel
- ❑ IIb/IIIa Receptor Antagonist
  - ❑ Abciximab
  - ❑ Eptifibatide
  - ❑ Lamifiban
  - ❑ Tirofiban

☑ **Heparin**
☑ **LMWH**
- ☑ **Enoxaparin**
- ❑ Dalteparin
- ❑ Nadroparin
- ❑ Tinzaparin
- ❑ Reviparin

❑ **Direct Thrombin Inhibitor**
- ❑ Hirudin
- ❑ Hirulog

❑ **Fibrinolytic / Thrombolytic**
- ❑ Alteplase
- ❑ Reteplase
- ❑ Tenecteplase
- ❑ Anistreplase
- ❑ Streptokinase

❑ **Other cardiac medications (captopril, magnesium, nitrates)**

PROCEDURES
❑ Angioplasty ❑ Stent
❑ CABG ❑ PCI

THERAPEUTIC ENDPOINT
☑ **Treatment** ❑ Prophylaxis

CLINICAL ENVIRONMENT
☑ **Inpatient** ❑ Outpatient

LOW MOLECULAR WEIGHT HEPARINS IN PULMONARY EMBOLISM

THESEE — TINZAPARINE OU HEPARINE STANDARD: EVALUATIONS DANS L'EMBOLIE PULMONAIRE STUDY REPORT

TRIAL FULL NAME
A comparison of Low-molecular weight heparin with unfractionated heparin for acute pulmonary Embolism

PUBLICATION DATA
NEJM 1997; 337:663-9

STUDY DATES
1995 to 1996

AUTHOR(S)
Simonneau G, Sors H, Charbonnier B, et al

CLINICAL TRIAL SUMMARY

This was a multicenter, randomized, unblinded comparison of IV heparin vs. tinzaparin SQ qd. The 612 patients had acute, symptomatic pulmonary embolism not requiring thrombolytic therapy. The primary endpoint was recurrent thromboembolism, major bleeding, or death at 8 days and 3 months. The endpoint occurred in 2.9% of the heparin group and 3% of the tinzaparin group (p = NS) at day 8 and in 7.1% and 5.9% of the respective groups (p = NS) by 3 months. Bleeding complications were comparable between groups.

BOTTOM LINE

Immediate angiography with PCI after full-dose thrombolytics in patients with STEMI resulted in no better LVEF or reocclusion rates, but did result in significantly more bleeding.

VENOUS THROMBOEMBOLISM

CLINICAL TRIAL FEATURES, THERAPEUTICS AND ENDPOINTS

DISEASE STATES
- ❑ ACS ❑ STEMI/QMI ❑ NSTEMI/NQMI ❑ UA
- ☑ **VTE** ❑ DVT ☑ **PE** ❑ CVA

MEDICATIONS
- ❑ **Platelet Antagonist**
  - ❑ Aspirin
  - ❑ Clopidogrel
  - ❑ IIb/IIIa Receptor Antagonist
    - ❑ Abciximab
    - ❑ Eptifibatide
    - ❑ Lamifiban
    - ❑ Tirofiban
- ☑ **Heparin**
- ☑ **LMWH**
  - ❑ Enoxaparin
  - ❑ Dalteparin
  - ❑ Nadroparin
  - ☑ **Tinzaparin**
  - ❑ Reviparin
- ❑ **Direct Thrombin Inhibitor**
  - ❑ Hirudin
  - ❑ Hirulog
- ❑ **Fibrinolytic / Thrombolytic**
  - ❑ Alteplase
  - ❑ Reteplase
  - ❑ Tenecteplase
  - ❑ Anistreplase
  - ❑ Streptokinase
- ❑ **Other cardiac medications (captopril, magnesium, nitrates)**

PROCEDURES
- ❑ Angioplasty ❑ Stent
- ❑ CABG ❑ PCI

THERAPEUTIC ENDPOINT
- ☑ **Treatment** ❑ Prophylaxis

CLINICAL ENVIRONMENT
- ☑ **Inpatient** ❑ Outpatient

LOW MOLECULAR WEIGHT HEPARINS IN PULMONARY EMBOLISM

ENOXAPARIN IN MEDICINE STUDY GROUP

TRIAL FULL NAME
A Multicenter Randomized Double-blind Study of Enoxaparin Compared with Unfractionated Heparin in the Prevention of Venous Thromboembolic Disease in Elderly In-patients Bedridden for an Acute Medical Illness

PUBLICATION DATA
Thromb Haemost 1996; 76:529-34

STUDY DATES
1990 to 1991

AUTHOR(S)
Bergmann J, Neuhart E

CLINICAL TRIAL SUMMARY

This was a multicenter, randomized, double-blind comparison of SQ enoxaparin 20 mg qd vs. SQ heparin 5000U q 12 hours for the prophylaxis against VTE disease. The 442 patients had an acute medical illness, were 65 years old or more, and had a recent reduction of mobility. The primary endpoint was the occurrence of VTE disease as seen on fibrinogen uptake test. VTE disease was found in 4.8% of the enoxaparin group and 4.6% of the heparin group (for equivalency p = 0.0005). Bleeding complications were comparable between groups.

BOTTOM LINE

Enoxaparin 20mg SQ qd for 10 days is as effective and safe as heparin 5000IU SQ q 12 hours in the prevention of VTE disease in bedridden, elderly, in-patients with an acute medical illness.

VENOUS THROMBOEMBOLISM

CLINICAL TRIAL FEATURES, THERAPEUTICS AND ENDPOINTS

DISEASE STATES
- ❑ ACS ❑ STEMI/QMI ❑ NSTEMI/NQMI ❑ UA
- ☑ **VTE** ❑ DVT ❑ PE ❑ CVA

MEDICATIONS
- ❑ **Platelet Antagonist**
  - ❑ Aspirin
  - ❑ Clopidogrel
  - ❑ IIb/IIIa Receptor Antagonist
    - ❑ Abciximab
    - ❑ Eptifibatide
    - ❑ Lamifiban
    - ❑ Tirofiban
- ☑ **Heparin**
- ☑ **LMWH**
  - ☑ **Enoxaparin**
  - ❑ Dalteparin
  - ❑ Nadroparin
  - ❑ Tinzaparin
  - ❑ Reviparin
- ❑ **Direct Thrombin Inhibitor**
  - ❑ Hirudin
  - ❑ Hirulog
- ❑ **Fibrinolytic / Thrombolytic**
  - ❑ Alteplase
  - ❑ Reteplase
  - ❑ Tenecteplase
  - ❑ Anistreplase
  - ❑ Streptokinase
- ❑ **Other cardiac medications (captopril, magnesium, nitrates)**

PROCEDURES
- ❑ Angioplasty ❑ Stent
- ❑ CABG ❑ PCI

THERAPEUTIC ENDPOINT
- ❑ Treatment ☑ **Prophylaxis**

CLINICAL ENVIRONMENT
- ☑ **Inpatient** ❑ Outpatient

VENOUS THROMBOEMBOLISM PROPHYLAXIS IN MEDICAL PATIENTS

NADROPARIN FOR PREVENTION OF VTE IN MEDICAL PATIENTS

TRIAL FULL NAME
Subcutaneous Low-Molecular-Weight Heparin versus Standard Heparin and the Prevention of Thromboembolism in Medical Inpatients

PUBLICATION DATA
Haemostasis 1996; 26:127-139

STUDY DATES
No data

AUTHOR(S)
Harenberg J., Schmitz-Huebner U, Roebruck P., et al

CLINICAL TRIAL SUMMARY

This was a multicenter, randomized, double-blind comparison of SQ fraxiparine 36 mg qD vs. SQ heparin 5000 U TID for the prophylaxis against VTE disease in medical in-patients. The 1590 patients had to be in-house for at least 10 days and have at least one risk factor for VTE disease (excess weight, varicosis, or history of previous VTE or arterial disease or estrogen use). Primary endpoints were occurrence of DVT/PE at day 10 or change in clot size based upon compression sonography done at admission and at discharge. Endpoints occurred in 4 of the heparin group and in 6 of the fraxiparine group (for equivalency p = 0.012). Major bleeding complications were comparable between groups.

BOTTOM LINE

SQ Fraxiparine 36 mg qd and SQ heparin 5000 U TID provide comparable safety and efficacy in the prophylaxis for VTE disease in medical patients who are hospitalized and who have ^{3} 1 risk factor.

VENOUS THROMBOEMBOLISM

CLINICAL TRIAL FEATURES, THERAPEUTICS AND ENDPOINTS

DISEASE STATES
❑ ACS ❑ STEMI/QMI ❑ NSTEMI/NQMI ❑ UA
☑ **VTE** ❑ DVT ❑ PE ❑ CVA

MEDICATIONS
❑ **Platelet Antagonist**
- ❑ Aspirin
- ❑ Clopidogrel
- ❑ IIb/IIIa Receptor Antagonist
  - ❑ Abciximab
  - ❑ Eptifibatide
  - ❑ Lamifiban
  - ❑ Tirofiban

☑ **Heparin**
☑ **LMWH**
- ❑ Enoxaparin
- ❑ Dalteparin
- ☑ **Nadroparin**
- ❑ Tinzaparin
- ❑ Reviparin

❑ **Direct Thrombin Inhibitor**
- ❑ Hirudin
- ❑ Hirulog

❑ **Fibrinolytic / Thrombolytic**
- ❑ Alteplase
- ❑ Reteplase
- ❑ Tenecteplase
- ❑ Anistreplase
- ❑ Streptokinase

❑ **Other cardiac medications (captopril, magnesium, nitrates)**

PROCEDURES
❑ Angioplasty ❑ Stent
❑ CABG ❑ PCI

THERAPEUTIC ENDPOINT
❑ Treatment ☑ **Prophylaxis**

CLINICAL ENVIRONMENT
☑ **Inpatient** ❑ Outpatient

VENOUS THROMBOEMBOLISM PROPHYLAXIS IN MEDICAL PATIENTS

MEDENOX | PROPHYLAXIS IN MEDICAL PATIENTS WITH ENOXAPARIN TRIAL

TRIAL FULL NAME
A comparison of enoxaparin with placebo for the prevention of venous thromboembolism in acutely ill medical patients

PUBLICATION DATA
NEJM 1999; 341: 793-800

STUDY DATES
1996 to 1998

AUTHOR(S)
Samama M, Cohen A, Darmon J-Y, et al

CLINICAL TRIAL SUMMARY

This was a multicenter, double-blind, randomized comparison of SQ enoxaparin qd (20 mg vs. 40 mg) vs. placebo for prophylaxis against VTE disease. The 866 patients were medical patients who were going to be hospitalized at least 6 days and have either Class III or IV CHF, acute respiratory failure, or one of various medical conditions associated with one additional risk factor for VTE. Primary endpoints were occurrence of venographically demonstrated DVT at 14 days and occurrence of VTE disease at up to 110 days. VTE disease developed in 14.9% of the placebo group, 5.5% of the 40 mg enoxaparin group ($p < 0.001$), and 15% of the 20 mg enoxaparin group (p = NS). Benefit was maintained at three months. Bleeding complications were comparable between groups.

BOTTOM LINE

Venous thromboembolic disease occurs in 15% of general medical patients. Enoxaparin 40 mg SQ qd safely reduces the risk of VTE disease in patients with acute medical illnesses.

VENOUS THROMBOEMBOLISM

CLINICAL TRIAL FEATURES, THERAPEUTICS AND ENDPOINTS

DISEASE STATES
❑ ACS ❑ STEMI/QMI ❑ NSTEMI/NQMI ❑ UA
☑ **VTE** ❑ DVT ❑ PE ❑ CVA

MEDICATIONS
❑ **Platelet Antagonist**
- ❑ Aspirin
- ❑ Clopidogrel
- ❑ IIb/IIIa Receptor Antagonist
  - ❑ Abciximab
  - ❑ Eptifibatide
  - ❑ Lamifiban
  - ❑ Tirofiban

❑ **Heparin**
☑ **LMWH**
- ☑ **Enoxaparin**
- ❑ Dalteparin
- ❑ Nadroparin
- ❑ Tinzaparin
- ❑ Reviparin

❑ **Direct Thrombin Inhibitor**
- ❑ Hirudin
- ❑ Hirulog

❑ **Fibrinolytic / Thrombolytic**
- ❑ Alteplase
- ❑ Reteplase
- ❑ Tenecteplase
- ❑ Anistreplase
- ❑ Streptokinase

❑ **Other cardiac medications (captopril, magnesium, nitrates)**

PROCEDURES
❑ Angioplasty ❑ Stent
❑ CABG ❑ PCI

THERAPEUTIC ENDPOINT
❑ Treatment ☑ **Prophylaxis**

CLINICAL ENVIRONMENT
☑ **Inpatient** ❑ Outpatient

VENOUS THROMBOEMBOLISM PROPHYLAXIS IN MEDICAL PATIENTS